BRUNNER & SUDDARTH'S

CANADIAN TEXTBOOK OF MEDICAL-SURGICAL NURSING

4th edition

Mohamed Toufic El Hussein, PhD, RN, NP
Associate Professor, School of Nursing and Midwifery
Faculty of Health, Community, and Education
Mount Royal University
Adjunct Associate Professor
Faculty of Nursing
University of Calgary
Acute Care Nurse Practitioner, Medical Cardiology
Coronary Care Unit
Rockyview General Hospital
Calgary, Alberta

Joseph Osuji, PhD, RN
Associate Professor, School of Nursing and Midwifery
Faculty of Health, Community, and Education
Mount Royal University
Calgary, Alberta
Visiting Associate Professor
Department of Nursing Sciences
University of Nigeria, Nsukka
Enugu Campus
Nigeria

Authors of *Brunner & Suddarth's Textbook of Medical-Surgical Nursing,* 14th Edition

Janice L. Hinkle, PhD, RN, CNRN
Fellow
Villanova University College of Nursing
Villanova, Pennsylvania

Kerry H. Cheever, PhD, RN
Professor and Chairperson
Helen S. Breidegam School of Nursing
Moravian College
Bethlehem, Pennsylvania

Wolters Kluwer

Philadelphia • Baltimore • New York • London
Buenos Aires • Hong Kong • Sydney • Tokyo

Vice President and Publisher: Julie K. Stegman
Director, Nursing Education Content Publishing: Renee A. Gagliardi
Director of Product Development: Jennifer K. Forestieri
Senior Product Development Editor: Meredith L. Brittain
Freelance Development Editor: Rose G. Foltz
Editorial Coordinator: Tim Rinehart
Marketing Manager: Sarah Schuessler
Editorial Assistant: Molly Kennedy
Production Project Manager: David Saltzberg
Design Coordinator: Steve Druding
Art Coordinator: Jennifer Clements
Manufacturing Coordinator: Karin Duffield
Prepress Vendor: Aptara, Inc.

Fourth Canadian edition.

9 8 7 6 5 4 3 2 1

Printed in China

Library of Congress Cataloging-in-Publication Data available upon request.
Library of Congress Control Number: 2019945805
978-1-9751-0803-8

---

shop.lww.com

CCS0919

Contributors

Contributors to the Fourth Canadian Edition*

Lisa Acorn, RN, BN, CIC
Infection Control Practitioner, Central Zone
Alberta Health Services
Red Deer, Alberta

Joanne Bouma, RN, MN
Associate Professor
Faculty of Health and Community Studies
Department of Nursing and Midwifery
Mount Royal University
Calgary, Alberta

Lindsay Burnett, RN, BScN, MN
Clinical Nurse Educator
Unit 30/31 Burns, Plastic & ENT Surgery
Foothills Medical Centre
Calgary, Alberta

Pamela Cawley, PhD, RN
Dean of Health Sciences
Douglas College
New Westminster, British Columbia

Jennifer Densmore, BN, MN, RN
Nurse Educator
Centre for Nursing Studies
St. John's, Newfoundland

Mohamed Toufic El Hussein, PhD, RN, NP
Associate Professor, School of Nursing and Midwifery
Faculty of Health, Community, and Education
Mount Royal University
Adjunct Associate Professor
Faculty of Nursing
University of Calgary
Acute Care Nurse Practitioner, Medical Cardiology
Coronary Care Unit
Rockyview General Hospital
Calgary, Alberta

Holly A. Feist, BN, MN, RN, ACCN
Assistant Professor
Course Coordinator–Emergency Stream
Advanced Studies in Critical Care Nursing (ACCN)
Mount Royal University
Calgary, Alberta

Joan Harris, RN, BSc, MHSc
Assistant Professor
Advanced Studies in Critical Care Nursing (ACCN)–ICU Stream
Calgary, Alberta

Bernice Heinrichs, BN, RN, CIC
Infection Prevention and Control Professional
Alberta Health Services
Red Deer, Alberta

Tanya Heuver, BScN, MN, RN
Assistant Professor, Bachelor of Science in Nursing
Mac Ewan University
Edmonton, Alberta

Sandra P. Hirst, RN, PhD, GNC(C)
Associate Professor
University of Calgary
Calgary, Alberta

Lance Hoddinott, RN
Emergency Management Officer
Emergency/Disaster Management–Calgary Zone
Calgary, Alberta

Kelly Power-Kean, MHS, NP, RN
BN & MNNP Program Faculty
Center for Nursing Studies/Memorial University
St. John's, Newfoundland

Alice S.W. Khin, MBBS, MSc (Int. Med)
Faculty Lecturer, Nursing
University of Alberta
Edmonton, Alberta

Annette M. Lane
Associate Professor
Faculty of Health Disciplines
Centre for Nursing and Health Studies
Athabasca University
Athabasca, Alberta

Eric Lavoie, NP, MN, FAA
Specialist in Musculoskeletal Injuries and Pain
Adjunct Clinical Associate Professor, Faculty of Nursing
University of Calgary
Calgary, Alberta

Lisa McKendrick-Calder, RN, BScN, MN
Assistant Professor
MacEwan University
Edmonton, Alberta

Lucia New, RN, BScN, MBA
Program Head
Saskatchewan Collaborative Bachelor of Science in Nursing (SCBScN)
Undergraduate Adjunct Professor
University of Regina
Regina, Saskatchewan

*For a list of the contributors to the online ancillaries for this title, go to thepoint.lww.com/Hussein4e.

Colleen Norris, PhD, RN
Associate Professor, Faculty of Nursing
University of Alberta
Edmonton, Alberta

Kärin Olson, PhD, RN
Associate Professor, Faculty of Nursing
University of Alberta
Edmonton, Alberta

Joseph Osuji, PhD, RN
Associate Professor
School of Nursing and Midwifery
Faculty of Health, Community, and Education
Mount Royal University
Calgary, Alberta

Charlotte Pooler, PhD, RN
Clinician Scientist
Alberta Health Services
Edmonton, Alberta

Ron Prince, RN, MN, NP
Nurse Practitioner
Division of Neurosurgery
Department of Clinical Neuroscience
Foothills Medical Center
Alberta Health Services
Calgary, Alberta

Ruhina Rana, RN, BSN, BA, MN(c)
Faculty, Bachelor of Science in Nursing
Douglas College
New Westminster, British Columbia

James A. Rankin, PhD, ACNP
Professor and Acute Care
Nurse Practitioner
University of Calgary/Alberta Health Services
Calgary, Alberta

Marlette B. Reed, BEd, MA
Community Chaplain
Calgary, Alberta

Rhonda Roedler, BSc. Pharm, ACPR, Pharm D, CDE
Pharmacy Clinical Practice Leader
Pharmacy Services
South Health Campus
Alberta Health Services
Calgary, Alberta

Rebecca Stares, RCSW, MSW
Spirited Connections Counselling
Calgary, Alberta

Nicole Tegg
Research Assistant
Faculty of Nursing
University of Alberta
Edmonton, Alberta

Karen Lynn Then, PhD, NP
Professor and Acute Care Nurse Practitioner
University of Calgary/Alberta Health Services
Calgary, Alberta

Carla Wells, RN, PhD, GNC(C)
Retired from Western Regional School of Nursing
Adjunct Professor
Grenfell Campus
School of Arts and Social Science
Memorial University of Newfoundland
St. John's, Newfoundland

Stephanie Zettel, MN, BN, BSc (Honours)
Associate Professor
School of Nursing and Midwifery
Mount Royal University
Calgary, Alberta

Contributors to the Third Canadian Edition

Vera Caine, PhD, RN
Associate Professor
Faculty of Nursing
University of Alberta
Edmonton, Alberta

Sandra J. Carless, MN, BScN, RN
Faculty Lecturer
Faculty of Nursing
University of Alberta—Augustana Campus
Camrose, Alberta

Pamela Cawley, PhD, RN
Dean of Health Sciences
Douglas College
New Westminster, British Columbia

Shelley Cobbett, EdD, RN
Assistant Professor, BScN Program
Dalhousie University
Halifax, Nova Scotia

Alison M. Gooley, MSc(HP), BScN, RN
Faculty Lecturer
Faculty of Nursing
University of Alberta
Edmonton, Alberta

Melanie J. Hamilton, MN, BN, RN
Theory Courses Coordinator
NESA BN Faculty
Lethbridge College
Lethbridge, Alberta

Bernice Heinrichs, BN, RN, CIC
Infection Prevention and Control Professional
Alberta Health Services
Red Deer, Alberta

Shauna Houk, MN, RN
Assistant Director, Undergraduate Studies
Assistant Professor, School of Nursing
Dalhousie University
Halifax, Nova Scotia

Jim Hunter, MSN, RN
Clinical Placement Coordinator, Nursing
British Columbia Institute of Technology
Burnaby, British Columbia

Mohamed Toufic El Hussein, PhD, RN, NP
Associate Professor, School of Nursing and Midwifery
Faculty of Health, Community, and Education
Mount Royal University
Adjunct Associate Professor
Faculty of Nursing
University of Calgary
Acute Care Nurse Practitioner, Medical Cardiology
Coronary Care Unit
Rockyview General Hospital
Calgary, Alberta

Joan Jacobson, MN, BScN, RN
Nursing Instructor
Grande Prairie Regional College
Grande Prairie, Alberta

Paul Jeffrey, MN, RN(EC), NP-Adult
Professor, Nursing
Humber Institute of Technology and Advanced Learning
Toronto, Ontario

Willy Kabotoff, MN, RN
Faculty Lecturer
Faculty of Nursing
University of Alberta
Edmonton, Alberta

Hossein Khalili, PhD, MScN, BScN, RN
Professor, The Western-Fanshawe Collaborative BScN Program
School of Nursing, Fanshawe College
Adjunct Faculty, Western University
Associate Editor, The Clinical Teacher
London, Ontario

Alice S.W. Khin, MBBS, MSc (Int. Med)
Faculty Lecturer, Nursing
University of Alberta
Edmonton, Alberta

Kari Krell, MN, BScN, RN
Instructor
Faculty of Health and Community Studies
MacEwan University
Edmonton, Alberta

Kathryn Martin, BScN, RN, MHSA
Faculty Lecturer
Faculty of Nursing
University of Alberta
Edmonton, Alberta

Lisa McKendrick-Calder, RN, BScN, MN
Assistant Professor
MacEwan University
Edmonton, Alberta

Donna McLean, PhD, RN, NP
Nurse Practitioner, Cardiac Sciences
Mazankowski Alberta Heart Institute
Nurse Practitioner, Internal Medicine/Family Medicine
Misericordia Communiy Hospital—Covenant Health
Edmonton, Alberta

Sean McMurtry, MD, PhD, FRCPC
Associate Professor of Medicine
University of Alberta
Edmonton, Alberta

Nadine Moniz, MN, BScN, RN
Faculty Lecturer
Faculty of Nursing
University of Alberta
Edmonton, Alberta

Joseph Osuji, PhD, RN
Associate Professor
School of Nursing and Midwifery
Faculty of Health, Community, and Education
Mount Royal University
Calgary, Alberta

Raj Padwal, MD, MSc
Associate Professor
Division of General Internal Medicine
University of Alberta
Edmonton, Alberta

Charlotte Pooler, PhD, RN
Clinician Scientist
Alberta Health Services
Edmonton, Alberta

Ann Ranson Ratusz, PhD, MSc, BScN, RN
Faculty Lecturer of Nursing
University of Alberta
Edmonton, Alberta

David Reid, MN, RN
Lecturer
Arthur Labatt Family School of Nursing
Western University
London, Ontario

Lisa Rock, MN, BN, RN
Quality Improvement Nurse Educator
Prince Albert Parkland Health Region
Prince Albert, Saskatchewan

Carolyn J.M. Ross, PhD, RN
Associate Professor
Assistant Dean, Undergraduate Programs
Faculty of Nursing
University of Alberta
Edmonton, Alberta

D. Lynn Skillen, PhD, RN
Professor Emerita
University of Alberta
Edmonton, Alberta

Glenna V. Swiniarski
Undergraduate Nursing Student
Faculty of Nursing
University of Alberta
Edmonton, Alberta

Saman Maleki Vareki, PhD
Postdoctoral Fellow
LAWSON Health Research Institute
London, Ontario

Jim Wohlgemuth, MN, RN, CTN-B
Nursing Instructor
Grande Prairie Regional College
Grande Prairie, Alberta

Jason Woytas, MN, RN
Faculty Lecturer
University of Alberta
Edmonton, Alberta

Contributors to the 14th U.S. Edition

Marianne Adam, PhD, RN, CRNP
Assistant Professor of Nursing
RN to BSN Program Coordinator
Pennsylvania State University
Schuylkill Haven, Pennsylvania

Chapter 43: Assessment of Digestive and Gastrointestinal Function

Julie Adkins, DNP, APN, FNP-BC, FAANP
Family Nurse Practitioner
West Frankfort, Illinois

Chapter 63: Assessment and Management of Patients With Eye and Vision Disorders

Jennifer L. Bartlett, PhD, RN-BC, CNE, CHSE
Assistant Professor
Georgia Baptist College of Nursing of Mercer University
Atlanta, Georgia

Chapter 45: Management of Patients With Oral and Esophageal Disorders

Tara Bilofsky, ACNP-BC, MS
Acute Care Nurse Practitioner
St. Luke's University Health Network-Allentown
Allentown, Pennsylvania

Chapter 21: Respiratory Care Modalities

Susan Bonini, MSN, RN
Senior Instructor
Integrated Nursing Pathway Program Coordinator
University of Colorado College of Nursing
Anschutz Medical Campus
Aurora, Colorado

Chapter 31: Assessment and Management of Patients With Hypertension

Lisa Bowman, RN, MSN, CRNP, CNRN
Nurse Practitioner
Jefferson Hospital for Neuroscience
Thomas Jefferson University Hospital
Philadelphia, Pennsylvania

Chapter 67: Management of Patients With Cerebrovascular Disorders

Jo Ann Brooks, PhD, RN, FAAN, FCCP
System Vice President, Quality and Safety
Indiana University Health
Indianapolis, Indiana

Chapter 23: Management of Patients With Chest and Lower Respiratory Tract Disorders

Chapter 24: Management of Patients With Chronic Pulmonary Disease

Sherry Burrell, PhD, RN, CNE
Assistant Professor
Villanova University College of Nursing
Villanova, Pennsylvania

Chapter 46: Management of Patients With Gastric and Duodenal Disorders

Wendy Cantrell, DNP, CRNP
Assistant Professor
Manager of Clinical Research
University of Alabama at Birmingham Department of Dermatology
Birmingham, Alabama

Chapter 61: Management of Patients With Dermatologic Disorders

Lauren Cantwell, RN, MS, ACNP-BC, ACNPC, CNS, CCNS, CCRN, CHFN
Advanced Heart Failure/Transplant Nurse Practitioner
Inova Heart and Vascular Institute
Falls Church, Virginia

Chapter 28: Management of Patients With Structural, Infectious, and Inflammatory Cardiac Disorders

Kim Cantwell-Gab, MN, ACNP-BC, ANP-BC, CVN, RVT, RDMS
Nurse Practitioner, Cardiology
Providence Medical Group-Cardiology
Medford, Oregon

Chapter 30: Assessment and Management of Patients With Vascular Disorders and Problems of Peripheral Circulation

Patricia E. Casey, MSN, RN, CPHQ, AACC
Associate Director, NCDR Training and Orientation
American College of Cardiology
Washington, DC

Chapter 26: Management of Patients With Dysrhythmias and Conduction Problems

Jill Cash, RN, MSN, APRN-BC
Family Nurse Practitioner
Vanderbilt University Medical Center
Westhaven Family Practice
Franklin, Tennessee

Chapter 38: Assessment and Management of Patients With Rheumatic Disorders

Chapter 64: Assessment and Management of Patients With Hearing and Balance Disorders

Kerry H. Cheever, PhD, RN
Professor and Chairperson
Helen S. Breidegam School of Nursing
Moravian College
Bethlehem, Pennsylvania

Chapter 1: Health Care Delivery and Evidence-Based Nursing Practice

Chapter 47: Management of Patients With Intestinal and Rectal Disorders

Chapter 48: Assessment and Management of Patients With Obesity

Elise Colancecco, MSN, RN
Instructor
Helen S. Breidegam School of Nursing
Moravian College
Bethlehem, Pennsylvania

Chapter 42: Management of Patients With Musculokeletal Trauma

Moya Cook, RN, MSN, APN
Family Nurse Practitioner
Marion, Illinois

Chapter 13: Fluid and Electrolytes: Balance and Disturbance

Linda Carman Copel, PhD, RN, PMHCNS, BC, CNE, ANEF, NCC, FAPA
Professor
Villanova University College of Nursing
Villanova, Pennsylvania
Chapter 4: Health Education and Health Promotion
Chapter 6: Individual and Family Homeostasis, Stress, and Adaptation
Chapter 59: Assessment and Management of Problems Related to Male Reproductive Processes

Elizabeth Petit de Mange, PhD, RN
Assistant Professor
Villanova University College of Nursing
Villanova, Pennsylvania
Chapter 52: Assessment and Management of Patients With Endocrine Disorders

Nancy Donegan, MPH, RN
Independent Consultant
Washington, DC
Chapter 71: Management of Patients With Infectious Diseases

Paulette Dorney, PhD, RN, CCRN
Assistant Professor
Helen S. Breidegam School of Nursing
Moravian College
Bethlehem, Pennsylvania
Chapter 21: Respiratory Care Modalities

Diane Dressler, MSN, RN, CCRN-R
Clinical Assistant Professor Emerita
Marquette University College of Nursing
Milwaukee, Wisconsin
Chapter 27: Management of Patients With Coronary Vascular Disorders
Chapter 29: Management of Patients With Complications From Heart Disease

Debra Drew, MS, RN-BC (retired), ACNS-BC (retired), AP-PMN
Clinical Nurse Specialist, Pain Management
Minneapolis, Minnesota
Chapter 12: Pain Management

Phyllis Dubendorf, MSN, RN, CCNS, CNRN, CRNP-BC
Clinical Nurse Specialist
Hospital of the University of Pennsylvania
Philadelphia, Pennsylvania
Chapter 66: Management of Patients With Neurologic Dysfunction

Susan M. Fallone, MS, RN, CNN
Retired Clinical Nurse Specialist, Adult and Pediatric Dialysis
Albany Medical Center Hospital
Albany, New York
Chapter 53: Assessment of Kidney and Urinary Function

Janice Farber, PhD, RN, CNOR
Assistant Professor
Helen S. Breidegam School of Nursing
Moravian College
Bethlehem, Pennsylvania
Chapter 7: Overview of Transcultural Nursing

Eleanor Fitzpatrick, RN, MSN, CCRN, AGCNS-BC, ACNP-BC
Clinical Nurse Specialist
Thomas Jefferson University Hospital
Philadelphia, Pennsylvania
Chapter 49: Assessment and Management of Patients With Hepatic Disorders
Chapter 50: Assessment and Management of Patients With Biliary Disorders

Trudy Gaillard, PhD, RN, CDE
Assistant Professor
University of Cincinnati College of Nursing
Cincinnati, Ohio
Chapter 51: Assessment and Management of Patients With Diabetes

Dawn Goodolf, PhD, RN
Assistant Professor
Director of RN to BSN and Accelerated Postbaccalaureate Programs
Helen S. Breidegam School of Nursing
Moravian College
Bethlehem, Pennsylvania
Chapter 39: Assessment of Musculoskeletal Function

Beth Gotwals, PhD, RN
Associate Professor
Helen S. Breidegam School of Nursing
Moravian College
Bethlehem, Pennsylvania
Chapter 2: Community-Based Nursing Practice
Home Care Checklists

Theresa Lynn Green, PhD, MSc(HRM), BScN, RN
Professor
School of Nursing, Queensland University of Technology
Queensland, Australia
Chapter 10: Principles and Practices of Rehabilitation

Debbie Gunter, MSN, APRN, ACHPN
Palliative Care and Family Nurse Practitioner
Emory Healthcare
Atlanta, Georgia
Chapter 22: Management of Patients With Upper Respiratory Tract Disorders

Jamie Heffernan, MSN, RN, CCRN-K, NE-BC
Patient Care Director
New York-Presbyterian/Weill Cornell
New York, New York
Chapter 62: Management of Patients With Burn Injury

Janice L. Hinkle, PhD, RN, CNRN
Fellow
Villanova University College of Nursing
Villanova, Pennsylvania
Chapter 55: Management of Patients With Urinary Disorders

Lisa J. Jesaitis, RN, MS, CHFN, ACNP
Acute Care Nurse Practitioner
MedStar Georgetown University Hospital Arrhythmia Service
Washington, DC
Chapter 28: Management of Patients With Structural, Infectious, and Inflammatory Cardiac Disorders

Tamara Kear, PhD, RN, CNS, CNN
Assistant Professor
Villanova University College of Nursing
Villanova, Pennsylvania
Chapter 54: Management of Patients With Kidney Disorders

Elizabeth Keech, PhD, RN
Adjunct Clinical Assistant Professor
Villanova University College of Nursing
Villanova, Pennsylvania
Chapter 11: Health Care of the Older Adult

Kathleen Kelleher, DMH, WHNP-BC, CBCN, DVS
Coordinator, Women's Health Nurse Practitioner
Breast Surgery Atlantic Health System
Pompton Plains, New Jersey
Chapter 58: Assessment and Management of Patients With Breast Disorders

Lynne Kennedy, PhD, MSN, RN, RNFA, CHPN, CNOR, CLNC, CHTP, Alumnus CCRN
Program Coordinator
Women's Services, Minimally Invasive Gynecology and Palliative Care
Inova Fair Oaks Hospital
Fairfax, Virginia
Chapter 17: Preoperative Nursing Management
Chapter 18: Intraoperative Nursing
Chapter 19: Postoperative Nursing Management

Mary Beth Flynn Makic, PhD, CNS, CCNS, CCRN-K, FAAN, FNAP
Professor
University of Colorado College of Nursing
Denver, Colorado
Chapter 14: Shock and Multiple Organ Dysfunction Syndrome

Katrina Nice Masterson, RN, DNP, FNP-BC, DCNP
Educational Coordinator
Randall Dermatology
West Lafayette, Indiana
Chapter 60: Assessment of Integumentary Function

Jennifer McCaughey, MSN, BS, RNC-MNN, CCE
Clinical Educator
Women and Children's Services
Inova Fair Oaks Hospital
Fairfax, Virginia
Chapter 57: Management of Patients With Female Reproductive Disorders

Melissa V. Moreda, BSN, RN, CCRN, CNRN, SCRN
Clinical Nurse IV
Duke Raleigh Hospital
Raleigh, North Carolina
Chapter 70: Management of Patients With Oncologic or Degenerative Neurologic Disorders

Donna Nayduch, MSN, RN, ACNP, TCRN
Assistant Vice President of Trauma
HCA North Florida Division
Ocala, Florida
Chapter 72: Emergency Nursing
Chapter 73: Terrorism, Mass Casualty, and Disaster Nursing

Kathleen Nokes, PhD, RN, FAAN
Professor Emerita
Hunter College and Graduate Center, CUNY
New York, New York
Chapter 36: Management of Patients With Immunodeficiency Disorders

Kristen Overbaugh, PhD, RN, ACNS-BC, CHPN
Clinical Assistant Professor
School of Nursing
University of Texas Health Science Center San Antonio
San Antonio, Texas
Chapter 20: Assessment of Respiratory Function

Janet Parkosewich, DNSc, RN, FAHA
Nurse Researcher
Yale New Haven Hospital
New Haven, Connecticut
Chapter 25: Assessment of Cardiovascular Function

Mae Ann Pasquale, PhD, RN
Assistant Professor of Nursing
Cedar Crest College
Allentown, Pennsylvania
Chapter 40: Musculoskeletal Care Modalities

Beth A. Bednarz Pruski, RN, MSN, CCRN
Program Manager, National Cardiovascular Data Registries (NCDR)
American College of Cardiology
Washington, DC
Chapter 26: Management of Patients With Dysrhythmias and Conduction Problems

Sue Pugh, MSN, RN, CNRN, CRRN, CNS-BC, FAHA
Patient Care Manager
Neuroscience Unit (NSU) and Neuroscience Critical Care Unit (NSCCU)
Johns Hopkins Bayview Medical Center
Baltimore, Maryland
Chapter 69: Management of Patients With Neurologic Infections, Autoimmune Disorders, and Neuropathies

JoAnne Reifsnyder, PhD, RN, FAAN
Executive Vice President and Chief Nursing Officer
Genesis HealthCare
Kennett Square, Pennsylvania
Chapter 16: End-of-Life Care

Rebecca Wildman Repetti, RN, ANP-BC
Nurse Practitioner, Thoracic Oncology Service
Memorial Sloan Kettering Cancer Center
New York, New York
Chapter 35: Assessment of Immune Function

Marylou V. Robinson, PhD, FNP
Associate Professor of Nursing
Pacific Lutheran University
Tacoma, Washington
Chapter 41: Management of Patients With Musculoskeletal Disorders

Erin Sarsfield, MSN, RN, CCRN-K
Clinical Nurse Specialist, Medical and Heart and Vascular Critical Care
Penn State Health Milton S. Hershey Medical Center
Hershey, Pennsylvania
Chapter 44: Digestive and Gastrointestinal Treatment Modalities

Susan Scholtz, PhD, RN
Associate Professor
Helen S. Breidegam School of Nursing
Moravian College
Bethlehem, Pennsylvania

Chapter 3: Critical Thinking, Ethical Decision Making, and the Nursing Process

Ethical Dilemma charts

Lindsey R. Siewert, RN, MSN, APRN, CCNS, CCRN-K
Clinical Nurse Specialist, Neuroscience/Stroke Coordinator
Norton Healthcare
Louisville, Kentucky

Chapter 65: Assessment of Neurologic Function

Suzanne C. Smeltzer, RN, EdD, ANEF, FAAN
Professor and Director, Center for Nursing Research
Villanova University College of Nursing
Villanova, Pennsylvania

Chapter 9: Chronic Illness and Disability

Jennifer Specht, PhD, RN
Assistant Professor
Widener University
Chester, Pennsylvania

Chapter 5: Adult Health and Nutritional Assessment

Chapter 48: Assessment and Management of Patients With Obesity

Cindy Stern, RN, MSN, CCRP
Senior Administrator, Penn Cancer Network
Abramson Cancer Center of the University of Pennsylvania
Philadelphia, Pennsylvania

Chapter 15: Management of Patients With Oncologic Disorders

Julie G. Stover, RN, MSN, CRNP
Women's Health Nurse Practitioner
Lancaster, Pennsylvania

Chapter 56: Assessment and Management of Female Physiologic Processes

Kimberly A. Subasic, PhD, MS, RN
Associate Professor
University of Scranton
Scranton, Pennsylvania

Chapter 8: Overview of Genetics and Genomics in Nursing
Genetics in Nursing Practice charts

Carole Sullivan, DNP, RN
Director
Deaconess VNA Home Care and Hospice
Eldorado, Illinois

Chapter 37: Assessment and Management of Patients With Allergic Disorders

Unit-opening case studies, Units 1–9

Mary Laudon Thomas, MS, CNS, AOCN
Hematology Clinical Nurse Specialist
VA Palo Alto Health Care System
Palo Alto, California

Chapter 32: Assessment of Hematologic Function and Treatment Modalities

Chapter 33: Management of Patients With Nonmalignant Hematologic Disorders

Chapter 34: Management of Patients With Hematologic Neoplasms

Kristin Weitmann, RN, MSN, ACNP
Acute Care Nurse Practitioner
Optum
Wauwatosa, Wisconsin

Chapter 27: Management of Patients With Coronary Vascular Disorders

Chapter 29: Management of Patients With Complications From Heart Disease

Marie Wilson, RN, MSN, CCRN, CNRN, CRNP
Nurse Manager
Neuroscience Intensive Care Unit
Thomas Jefferson University Hospital
Philadelphia, Pennsylvania

Chapter 68: Management of Patients With Neurologic Trauma

Reviewers

Monique Bacher, RN, BScN, MSN/Ed
Year 2 Coordinator and Professor, Practical Nursing Program
Sally Horsfall Eaton School of Nursing
George Brown College
Toronto, Ontario

Kelly Kidd, RN, BScN, MN
Coordinator, Practical Nursing Program
School of Health & Community Studies
Algonquin College
Pembroke, Ontario

Kari Krell, MN, RN, PhD(c)
Assistant Professor
Faculty of Nursing
MacEwan University
Edmonton, Alberta

Kathleen Mawhinney, RN, MN
Senior Instructor
Department of Nursing and Health Sciences
University of New Brunswick Saint John
Saint John, New Brunswick

Jane Moore, RN, APN, PhD
Associate Professor
Department of Nursing
Brock University
St. Catharines, Ontario

Marg Olfert, RN, MN, EdD
Assistant Professor
School of Nursing and Midwifery
Mount Royal University
Calgary, Alberta

Margot Rykhoff, RN, BScN, MA(Ed)
Professor, Collaborative Nursing Degree Program
Humber Institute of Technology and Advanced Learning
Oakville, Ontario

Bonny Taylor, MSN, RN
Instructor
School of Nursing
University of British Columbia—Okanagan
Kelowna, British Columbia

Barbara Thompson, RN, BScN, MScN
Professor, Collaborative Bachelor of Science in Nursing Program
Sault College
Sault Ste. Marie, Ontario

Preface

As we complete the second decade of the 21st century, nursing continues to be influenced by the expansion of science and technology and by social, cultural, economic, and environmental changes throughout the world. At the same time, today's nurses are faced with the many challenges that result from the acute shortage of nurses throughout health care settings. This worldwide nursing shortage has resulted in the need for nurses to have increasingly high levels of nursing knowledge and skills in meeting the acute care, long-term care, and health promotion needs of individuals and groups. Nurses must be particularly skilled in critical thinking and clinical decision making as well as in consulting and collaborating with other members of the interprofessional health care team.

Along with the challenges that today's nurses confront, there are many opportunities for them to provide skilled, compassionate nursing care in a variety of health care settings, for patients in various stages of illness, and for patients across the age continuum. At the same time, there are significant opportunities for fostering health promotion activities for individuals and groups; this is an integral part of providing nursing care.

About the Fourth Canadian Edition

This fourth Canadian edition builds on the 14th U.S. edition of *Brunner & Suddarth's Textbook of Medical-Surgical Nursing* and is designed to assist nursing students in preparing for their roles and responsibilities within the complex health care system. A goal of the textbook is to provide balanced attention to both the art and science of adult medical-surgical nursing. The focus of the textbook is on physiologic, pathophysiologic, psychosocial, and spiritual concepts as they relate to nursing care. Emphasis is placed on integrating a variety of concepts from other disciplines such as nutrition, pharmacology, and gerontology. Throughout the textbook, particular attention has been placed on addressing the nursing care and health care needs of older adults and people with disabilities, both of which are important priorities in the education of tomorrow's health care professionals. In addition, content relative to nursing research findings and evidence-based practice has been expanded to provide opportunities for the nurse to refine clinical decision-making skills.

Canadian contributors have reviewed each chapter and have changed the following as needed: drug names, names of tests and procedures, spelling, laboratory values to the international system of units, and all measurements to their metric equivalents. Whenever possible, the contributors have added Canadian citations, references, and research studies, and have provided Canadian statistics related to disease entities.

This fourth Canadian edition includes new and updated material that reflects the differences in Canadian nursing practice in terms of the health care system, community health, ethics, culture, epidemiology, pain management, gerontology, infection control, nursing and medical management, pharmacology, diagnostic tests and investigations, as well as support groups and Web resources specific to Canada. Chapters have been significantly updated to reflect the latest evidence.

Considering the significance of interprofessional practice (IPP) and collaborative practice, a new chapter on the topic of delegation has been added to this edition. In addition, a chapter on spirituality in nursing practice has been added to highlight concepts and interventions necessary for competent practice and to ensure that all aspects of individual care—physiologic, psychological, cultural, and spiritual—have been addressed.

In an attempt to mitigate the confusion that stems from using the term "diagnosis" due to its medical connotations, and to move away from treating patients as diagnoses rather than as individuals, we have used nursing priorities instead of NANDA nursing diagnoses in this edition. We would appreciate receiving any feedback on this approach via email at mesurg2020@gmail.com.

Organization

Brunner & Suddarth's Canadian Textbook of Medical-Surgical Nursing, 4th edition, is organized into 16 units. Units 1 through 4 cover core concepts related to medical-surgical nursing practice. Units 5 through 16 discuss adult health conditions that are treated medically or surgically. Each unit covering adult health conditions is structured in the following way to facilitate understanding:

- The first chapter in the unit covers assessment and includes a review of normal anatomy and physiology of the body system being discussed.
- The subsequent chapters in the unit cover management of specific disorders. Pathophysiology, clinical manifestations, assessment and diagnostic findings, medical management, and nursing management are presented. Special Nursing Process sections, provided for selected conditions, clarify and expand on the nurse's role in caring for patients with these conditions.

Features

Brunner & Suddarth's Canadian Textbook of Medical-Surgical Nursing, 4th edition, has been revised and updated to reflect the complex nature of nursing practice today. This textbook includes many features to help you gain and apply the knowledge that you need to pass NCLEX and successfully meet the challenges and opportunities of clinical practice. In addition, features have been developed specifically to help you fulfill the varied roles that nurses assume in practice.

Opening Features That Start With the End in Mind

Unit-opening features put the patient first and highlight competent nursing as well as application of the nursing process.

- **A Case Study with QSEN Competency Focus** opens each unit and provides discussion points focusing on one competency from the QSEN Institute: patient-centered care, interdisciplinary teamwork and collaboration, evidence- based practice, quality improvement, safety, or informatics. This feature helps you consider the knowledge, skills, and abilities required for the delivery of safe, quality patient care. For your convenience, a list of these case studies, along with their location in the book, appears in the "Case Studies in This Book" section later in this front matter.
- **Learning Objectives** give an overview of each chapter and identify learning goals to help focus reading and studying.
- A **Glossary** provides a list of key terms and definitions at the beginning of each chapter, providing a review of vocabulary words before reading the material and a useful reference and study tool.

Features to Develop the Nurse as Practitioner

One of the central roles of the nurse is to provide holistic care to patients and their families, both independently and through collaboration with other health care professionals. Special features throughout chapters are designed to assist readers with clinical practice.

- **Nursing Process sections** are organized according to the nursing process framework—the basis for all nursing practice—and help clarify the nurse's responsibilities in caring for patients with selected disorders.
- **Plans of Nursing Care**, provided for selected disorders, illustrate how the nursing process is applied to meet the patient's health care and nursing needs.
- **Assessment charts** focus on data that should be collected as part of the assessment step of the nursing process.
- **Risk Factors charts** outline factors that can impair health.
- **Pharmacology charts and tables** display important considerations related to administering medications and monitoring drug therapy.
- **Quality and Safety Nursing Alerts** offer tips for best clinical practice and red-flag safety warnings to help avoid common mistakes.
- **Critical Care icons** identify nursing considerations for the critically ill patient.
- **Genetics in Nursing Practice charts** summarize and highlight nursing assessments and management issues related to the role of genetics in selected disorders.
- In addition to a new chapter on obesity, **Obesity Considerations icons** identify content related to obesity or to the nursing care of patients with obesity.
- **Gerontologic Considerations**, identified with an icon applied to headings, charts, and tables, highlight information that pertains specifically to the care of the older adult patient.
- **Physiology/Pathophysiology figures** include illustrations and algorithms describing normal physiologic and pathophysiologic processes.

Features to Develop the Nurse as Educator

Health education is a primary responsibility of the nursing profession. Nursing care is directed toward promoting, maintaining, and restoring health; preventing illness; and helping patients and families adapt to the residual effects of illness. Patient education and health promotion are central to all of these nursing activities.

- **Patient Education charts and icons** help the nurse prepare the patient and family for procedures, assist them in understanding the patient's condition, and explain to them how to provide self-care.
- **Health Promotion charts** review important points that the nurse should discuss with the patient to prevent common health problems from developing.
- **Home Care Checklists** review points that should be covered as part of home care education prior to discharge from the health care facility.

Features to Develop the Nurse as Patient Advocate

Nurses advocate for patients by protecting their rights (including the right to health care) and assisting patients and their families in making informed decisions about health care.

- **Ethical Dilemma charts** provide a clinical scenario, discussion points, and questions to help analyze fundamental ethical principles related to the dilemma.

Features to Develop the Nurse as Researcher

Nurses identify potential research problems and questions to increase nursing knowledge and improve patient care. The use and evaluation of research findings in nursing practice are essential to further the science of nursing.

- **Nursing Research Profiles** identify the implications and applications of nursing research findings for evidence-based nursing practice.

Features to Facilitate Learning

In addition to practice-oriented features, special features have been developed to help readers learn key information.

- **New! Unfolding Patient Stories**, written by the National League for Nursing, are an engaging way to begin meaningful conversations in the classroom. These vignettes, which appear throughout the text near related content, feature patients from Wolters Kluwer's *vSim for Nursing | Medical-Surgical* and DocuCare products; however, each Unfolding Patient Story in the book stands alone, not requiring purchase of these products. For your convenience, a list of these case studies, along with their location in the book, appears in the "Case Studies in This Book" section later in this front matter.
- **Critical Thinking Exercises** foster critical thinking and challenge you to apply textbook knowledge to clinical scenarios. Evidence-based practice (EBP) questions encourage you to apply best evidence from research findings to nursing interventions. Prioritization (PQ) questions ask you to consider the priorities for nursing care for specific patients and conditions.
- **References and Suggested Readings** lists at the end of each chapter include updated, current sources of

additional information; Web sites; agencies; and patient education materials.

A Comprehensive Package for Teaching and Learning

To further facilitate teaching and learning, a carefully designed ancillary package has been developed to assist faculty and students.

Instructor Resources

Tools to assist you with teaching your course are available upon adoption of this text on thePoint at http://thepoint.lww.com/Hussein4e.

- A thoroughly revised and augmented **Test Generator** contains NCLEX-style questions mapped to chapter learning objectives.
- **PowerPoint Presentations** provide an easy way to integrate the textbook with your students' classroom experience; multiple choice and true/false questions are included to promote class participation.
- An **Image Bank** lets you use the photographs and illustrations from this textbook in your course materials.
- **Strategies for Effective Teaching** provides general tips for instructors related to preparing course materials and meeting student needs.
- Access to all **Student Resources** is provided so that you can understand the student experience and use these resources in your course as well.

Student Resources

An exciting set of free learning resources is available on thePoint to help students review and apply vital concepts in medical-surgical nursing. Multimedia engines have been optimized so that students can access many of these resources on mobile devices. Students can access all these resources at http://thepoint.lww.com/Hussein4e using the codes printed in the front of their textbooks.

- **NCLEX-Style Review Questions** from the U.S. edition, totalling more than 1,800 questions, help students review important concepts and practice for NCLEX.
- Interactive learning resources appeal to a variety of learning styles. Icons in the text direct readers to relevant resources:
  - **Concepts in Action Animations** bring physiologic and pathophysiologic concepts to life.
  - **Interactive Tutorials** review key information for common or complex medical-surgical conditions. Tutorials include graphics and animations and provide interactive review exercises as well as case-based questions.
  - **Practice & Learn Case Studies** present case scenarios and offer interactive exercises and questions to help students apply what they have learned.
  - **Watch & Learn Video Clips** reinforce skills from the textbook and appeal to visual and auditory learners.
- **Learning Objectives** give an overview of each chapter and identify learning goals to help focus reading and studying.
- **Interactive Activities** review key concepts in medical-surgical nursing from the textbook, providing tutorials, case studies, and CRNE-style quiz questions.
- **Journal Articles** offer access to current articles relevant to each chapter and available in Wolters Kluwer journals to familiarize students with nursing literature.

vSim for Nursing

vSim for Nursing, jointly developed by Laerdal Medical and Wolters Kluwer Health, offers innovative scenario-based learning modules consisting of Web-based virtual simulations, course learning materials, and curriculum tools designed to develop critical thinking skills and promote clinical confidence and competence. vSim for Nursing | Medical-Surgical includes 10 virtual simulations based on the National League for Nursing Volume I Complex patient scenarios. Students can progress through suggested readings, pre- and postsimulation assessments, documentation assignments, and guided reflection questions, and will receive an individualized feedback log immediately upon completion of the simulation. Throughout the student learning experience, the product offers remediation back to trusted Lippincott resources, including *Brunner & Suddarth's Textbook of Medical-Surgical Nursing* (the U.S. edition) as well as Lippincott Nursing Advisor and Lippincott Nursing Procedures—two online, evidence-based, clinical information solutions used in health care facilities throughout the United States. This innovative product provides a comprehensive patient-focused solution for learning and integrating simulation into the classroom.

Contact your Wolters Kluwer sales representative or visit http://thepoint.lww.com/vsim for options to enhance your medical-surgical nursing course with vSim for Nursing.

Lippincott DocuCare

Lippincott DocuCare combines Web-based academic EHR simulation software with clinical case scenarios, allowing students to learn how to use an EHR in a safe, true-to-life setting, while enabling instructors to measure their progress. Lippincott DocuCare's nonlinear solution works well in the classroom, simulation lab, and clinical practice.

Contact your Wolters Kluwer sales representative or visit http://thepoint.lww.com/DocuCare for options to enhance your medical-surgical nursing course with DocuCare.

Acknowledgements

We gratefully acknowledge our Canadian contributors who took on the challenge of continuing to "Canadianize" and update this edition of *Brunner & Suddarth's Canadian Textbook of Medical-Surgical Nursing*.

At Mount Royal University, we thank:

- Our students who are using the textbook and who have provided us with helpful suggestions

- Our colleagues who have supported us through the process of bringing 74 chapters to production

At Wolters Kluwer, we thank Meredith Brittain, Senior Product Development Editor, for her patience and commitment to this project, and Rose Foltz, Freelance Developmental Editor, for her timely and thorough feedback during the editing process. Thanks also to Tim Rinehart, Editorial Coordinator, and to Corey Wolfe, Instructional Services Consultant, for their support.

Mohamed Toufic El Hussein, PhD, RN, NP
Joseph Osuji, PhD, RN

Contents

UNIT 1 Basic Concepts in Nursing 2

1 Health Care Delivery and Nursing Practice 4

2 Community-Based Nursing Practice 13

3 Critical Thinking, Ethical Decision Making, and the Nursing Process 21

4 Health Education and Health Promotion 37

5 Adult Health and Nutritional Assessment 52

6 Delegation 73

7 Spirituality in Nursing Practice 80

UNIT 2 Biophysical and Psychosocial Concepts in Nursing Practice 88

8 Perspectives in Transcultural Nursing 90

9 Homeostasis, Stress, and Adaptation 101

10 Individual and Family Considerations Related to Illness 120

11 Genetics and Genomics Perspectives in Nursing 130

12 Chronic Illness and Disabilities 155

13 Principles and Practices of Rehabilitation 174

14 Health Care of the Older Adult 210

15 Hospice, Palliative, and End-of-Life Care 238

UNIT 3 Concepts and Challenges in Patient Management 264

16 Pain Management 266

17 Fluid and Electrolytes: Balance and Disturbance 296

18 Shock and Multiple Organ Dysfunction Syndrome 341

UNIT 4 Perioperative Concepts and Nursing Management 370

19 Preoperative Nursing Management 372

20 Intraoperative Nursing Management 392

21 Postoperative Nursing Management 412

UNIT 5 Gas Exchange and Respiratory Function 436

22 Assessment of Respiratory Function 438

23 Management of Patients With Upper Respiratory Tract Disorders 470

24 Management of Patients With Chest and Lower Respiratory Tract Disorders 504

25 Management of Patients With Chronic Pulmonary Disease 563

26 Respiratory Care Modalities 601

UNIT 6 Cardiovascular and Circulatory Function 650

27 Assessment of Cardiovascular Function 652

28 Management of Patient With Dysrhythmias and Conduction Problems 691

29 Management of Patients With Coronary Vascular Disorders 729

30 Management of Patients With Structural, Infections, and Inflammatory Cardiac Disorders 777

31 Management of Patients With Complications From Heart Disease 803

32 Assessment and Management of Patients With Vascular Disorders and Peripheral Circulation Concerns 834

33 Assessment and Management of Patients With Hypertension 877

UNIT 7 Digestive and Gastrointestinal Function 896

34 Assessment of Digestive and Gastrointestinal Function 898

35 Management of Patients With Oral and Esophageal Disorders 918

36 Gastrointestinal Intubation and Special Nutritional Modalities 947

37 Management of Patients With Gastric and Duodenal Disorders 976

38 Management of Patients With Intestinal and Rectal Disorders 997

39 Assessment and Management of Patients With Hepatic Disorders 1051

40 Assessment and Management of Patients With Biliary Disorders 1106

UNIT 8 Metabolic and Endocrine Function 1134

41 Assessment and Management of Patients With Diabetes Mellitus 1136

42 Assessment and Management of Patients With Obesity 1191

43 Assessment and Management of Patients With Endocrine Disorders 1213

UNIT 9 Urinary Tract Function 1260

44 Assessment of Renal and Urinary Tract Function 1262

45 Management of Patients With Kidney Disorders 1282

46 Management of Patients With Urinary Disorders 1331

UNIT 10 Reproductive Function 1370

47 Assessment and Management of Female Physiologic Processes 1372

48 Management of Patients With Female Reproductive Disorders 1411

49 Management of Patients With Breast Disorders 1445

50 Assessment and Management of Problems Related to Male Reproductive Disorders 1479

UNIT 11 Immunologic and Hematologic Function 1514

51 Assessment of Immune Function 1516

52 Management of Patients With Immune Deficiency Disorders 1533

53 Assessment and Management of Patients With Allergic Disorders 1571

54 Assessment and Management of Patients With Hematologic Disorders 1598

55 Management of Patients With Infectious Diseases 1697

56 Assessment and Management of Patients With Rheumatic Disorders 1731

UNIT 12 Integumentary Function 1762

57 Assessment of Integumentary Function 1764

58 Management of Patients With Dermatologic Conditions 1782

59 Management of Patients With Burn Injury 1835

UNIT 13 Sensorineural Function 1878

60 Assessment and Management of Patients With Eye and Vision Disorders 1880

61 Assessment and Management of Patients With Hearing and Balance Disorders 1925

UNIT 14 Neurologic Function 1956

62 Assessment of Neurologic Function 1958

63 Management of Patients With Neurologic Dysfunction 1987

64 Management of Patients With Cerebrovascular Disorders 2028

65 Management of Patients With Neurologic Trauma 2056

66 Management of Patients With Neurologic Infections, Autoimmune Disorders, and Neuropathies 2088

67 Management of Patients With Oncologic or Degenerative Disorders 2116

68 Oncology: Nursing Management in Cancer Care 2149

UNIT 15 Musculoskeletal Function 2212

69 Assessment of Musculoskeletal Function 2214

70 Musculoskeletal Care Modalities 2232

71 Management of Patients With Musculoskeletal Disorders 2265

72 Management of Patients With Musculoskeletal Trauma 2298

UNIT 16 Other Acute Problems 2336

73 Emergency Nursing 2338

74 Terrorism, Mass Casualty, and Disaster Nursing 2380

Index 2403

Case Studies in This Book

QSEN Cases That Open Each Unit

Unit 1 **Basic Concepts in Nursing**
The Community With an Identified Health Problem 2

Unit 2 **Biophysical and Psychosocial Concepts in Nursing Practice**
Providing Care for a Patient With a Communication Barrier 88

Unit 3 **Concepts and Challenges in Patient Management**
A Patient With Debilitating Pain 264

Unit 4 **Perioperative Concepts and Nursing Management**
A Patient Recovering From Abdominal Surgery 370

Unit 5 **Gas Exchange and Respiratory Function**
A Patient With Impaired Cough Reflex 436

Unit 6 **Cardiovascular and Circulatory Function**
Avoiding a Near Miss With Anticoagulation Therapy 650

Unit 7 **Digestive and Gastrointestinal Function**
Promoting Self-Care in the Patient With a New Ostomy 896

Unit 8 **Metabolic and Endocrine Function**
Ensuring Open Communication and Appropriate Delegation 1134

Unit 9 **Urinary Tract Function**
Decreasing Central Line–Associated Bloodstream Infections 1260

Unit 10 **Reproductive Function**
Incorporating Technology in Managing a Patient With Newly Diagnosed Prostate Cancer 1370

Unit 11 **Immunologic and Hematologic Function**
Supporting the Patient With Systemic Lupus Erythematosus 1514

Unit 12 **Integumentary Function**
Managing a Patient With a Pressure Ulcer 1762

Unit 13 **Sensorineural Function**
Supporting a Patient Who Values Independence 1878

Unit 14 **Neurologic Function**
Evaluating Increased Hypertension in a Neurology Clinic 1956

Unit 15 **Musculoskeletal Function**
Developing a Team Approach to Care in the Home Setting 2212

Unit 16 **Other Acute Problems**
Ensuring Equitable Patient Assignments in an Emergency Department 2336

Unfolding Cases That Appear Within Chapters

Chapter 4 Health Education and Health Promotion
Unfolding Patient Stories: Vincent Brody, Part 1 47

Chapter 9 Homeostasis, Stress, and Adaptation
Unfolding Patient Stories: Skyler Hansen, Part 1 116

Chapter 19 Preoperative Nursing Management
Unfolding Patient Stories: Vernon Watkins, Part 1 384

Chapter 24 Management of Patients With Chest and Lower Respiratory Tract Disorders
Unfolding Patient Stories: Kenneth Bronson, Part 1 513

Chapter 25 Management of Patients With Chronic Pulmonary Disease
Unfolding Patient Stories: Jennifer Hoffman, Part 1 594

Chapter 28 Management of Patient With Dysrhythmias and Conduction Problems
Unfolding Patient Stories: Kenneth Bronson, Part 2 708

Chapter 29 Management of Patients With Coronary Vascular Disorders
Unfolding Patient Stories: Carl Shapiro, Part 1 737

Chapter 41 Assessment and Management of Patients With Diabetes Mellitus
Unfolding Patient Stories: Skyler Hansen, Part 2 1160

Chapter 44 Assessment of Renal and Urinary Tract Function
Unfolding Patient Story: Lloyd Bennett, Part 1 1274

Chapter 48 Management of Patients With Female Reproductive Disorders
Unfolding Patient Stories: Doris Bowman, Part 1 1442

Chapter 53 Assessment and Management of Patients With Allergic Disorders
Unfolding Patient Stories: Jennifer Hoffman, Part 2 1579

Chapter 54 Assessment and Management of Patients With Hematologic Disorders
Unfolding Patient Stories: Lloyd Bennett, Part 2 1607

Chapter 57 Assessment of Integumentary Function
Unfolding Patient Stories: Vincent Brody, Part 2 1771

Chapter 60 Assessment and Management of Patients With Eye and Vision Disorders
Unfolding Patient Stories: Vernon Watkins, Part 2 1892

Chapter 62 Assessment of Neurologic Function
Unfolding Patient Stories: Marilyn Hughes, Part 1 1973

Chapter 68 Oncology: Nursing Management in Cancer Care
Unfolding Patient Stories: Doris Bowman, Part 2 2157

Chapter 72 Management of Patients With Musculoskeletal Trauma
Unfolding Patient Stories: Marilyn Hughes, Part 2 2306

Chapter 73 Emergency Nursing
Unfolding Patient Stories: Carl Shapiro, Part 2 2376

BRUNNER & SUDDARTH'S

CANADIAN TEXTBOOK OF MEDICAL-SURGICAL NURSING

4th edition

UNIT 1

Basic Concepts in Nursing

Case Study

THE COMMUNITY WITH AN IDENTIFIED HEALTH PROBLEM

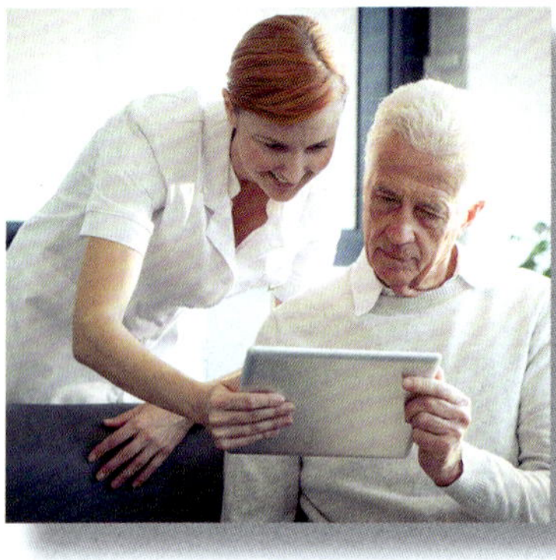

A nurse working in an urgent care clinic that serves an economically depressed urban area notes a high incidence of older patients with dehydration and heatstroke in the summer months. The nurse verifies the observations by accessing data about hospital admissions for dehydration and heatstroke. The nurse determines that many of the admitted patients live in the area served by the clinic and that many of the patients live alone and have chronic illnesses. The nurse sees the need for a plan that includes a community response to this situation. The plan includes arranging an education program about the prevention of dehydration; a community telehealth program with potential to increase adherence to prescribed therapy for older adults who are chronically ill, and a support buddy system in which neighbours or volunteers call or visit older adults in their own homes during critical periods in the summer.

QSEN Competency Focus: Informatics

The complexities inherent in today's health care system challenge nurses to demonstrate integration of specific interdisciplinary core competencies that are aimed at ensuring the delivery of safe and quality patient care (Institute of Medicine, 2003). The Quality and Safety Education for Nurses project (QSEN, 2017; Cronenwett, Sherwood, Barnsteiner, et al., 2007) provides a framework for the knowledge, skills, and attitudes (KSAs) required for nurses to demonstrate competency in these key areas, which include ***patient-centred care***, ***interdisciplinary teamwork and collaboration***, ***evidence-based practice***, ***quality improvement***, ***safety***, and ***informatics.*** *According to the* Canadian Association of Schools of Nursing (CASN, 2014), the Registered Nurse "Uses information and communication technologies to support information synthesis in accordance with professional and regulatory standards in the delivery of patient/client care."

Informatics Definition: Use information and technology to communicate, manage knowledge, mitigate error, and support decision making.

SELECTED PRE-LICENSURE KSAs	APPLICATION AND REFLECTION
Knowledge	
Identify essential information that must be available in a common database to support patient care in the community.	Describe what type of information the nurse will need to include in reporting results to the project manager for additional funding or resources. Describe ways in which the use of telehealth can potentially decrease hospitalization rates for patients monitored in the home for chronic conditions.
Skills	
Seek education about how information is managed in care settings and in the community before providing care.	Describe the type of training the nurse would need in order to use telehealth competently. Identify how the nurse can ensure quality outcomes for these older adult patients.
Attitudes	
Value nurse's involvement in design, selection, implementation, and evaluation of information technologies to support patient care.	The role of the nurse is vital in choosing which patients to monitor. How might the nurse determine which patients should be selected for the telehealth program? What barriers can the nurse anticipate with using technology at home?

Canadian Association of Schools of Nursing (CASN). (2014). *Nursing informatics entry to practice competencies for Registered Nurses*. Retrieved June 12, 2019, from https://www.casn.ca/2014/12/nursing-informatics-entry-practice-competencies-registered-nurses-2; Cronenwett, L., Sherwood, G., Barnsteiner, J., et al. (2007). Quality and safety education for nurses. Nursing Outlook, *55*(3), 122–131; Institute of Medicine. (2003). *Health professions education: A bridge to quality*. Washington, DC: National Academies Press; and QSEN Institute. (2017). *QSEN competencies: Definitions and pre-licensure KSAs*. Retrieved June 12, 2019, from www.qsen.org/competencies/pre-licensure-ksas

1 Health Care Delivery and Nursing Practice

Adapted by Joseph Osuji and Mohamed Toufic El Hussein

Learning Objectives

On completion of this chapter, the learner will be able to:

1. Define nursing, health, wellness, and health promotion.
2. Recognize and define the principles of the Canada Health Act.
3. Identify common nursing care delivery models.
4. Define primary health care (PHC).
5. List the principles of PHC.
6. Describe factors contributing to changes in the health care system and their impact on health care and the nursing profession.
7. Describe the caregiver, leadership, and research roles of nurses.
8. Discuss advanced nursing practice roles.
9. Describe models that foster interdisciplinary collaborative practice and promote safety and quality outcomes in the practice of health care.

Organized nursing in Canada began in the 17th century with the settlement by France of the parts of North America that were then known as Acadia and New France. The provision of nursing care was one of the first services offered to settlers and Aboriginal people alike. For example, only 27 years after the foundation of Quebec City, the Augustinian Sisters founded the Hôtel-Dieu de Québec, the first hospital of New France. After the **British North America Act of 1867**, Roman Catholic nursing sisters continued to play an instrumental role in the development of nursing and health care in every region of the country. For example, during the late 1800s and early 1900s, the Grey Nuns of Montreal spearheaded the creation of an impressive network of hospitals across the Canadian Prairies. Although religious orders no longer play a predominant role in health care delivery in the 21st century, their legacy is alive and well through new generations of nurses and through the institutions they created and once managed. The nurses of today continue to be essential to the delivery and organization of health care services (Paul & Ross-Kerr, 2011).

The Health Care System and the Nursing Profession

Although the delivery of nursing care has been affected by changes occurring in the health care system, the definition of nursing has continued to distinguish nursing care and identify the major aspects of nursing care.

Nursing Defined

Since the time of Florence Nightingale, who wrote in 1859 that the goal of nursing was "to put the patient in the best condition for nature to act upon him," nursing leaders have described nursing as both an art and a science. However, the definition of nursing has evolved over time. The International Council of Nurses (ICN) states:

> Nursing encompasses autonomous and collaborative care of individuals of all ages, families, groups, and communities, sick or well and in all settings. Nursing includes the promotion of health, prevention of illness, and the care of the ill, disabled, and dying people. Advocacy, promotion of safe environment, research, participation in shaping health policy and in patient and health systems management, and education are also key nursing roles. (ICN, 2018)

In Canada, there are three regulated nursing professions: registered nurses ([RNs], includes also nurse practitioners [NP]); practical nurses, who use the designation "licensed practical nurse" in some provinces and the designation "registered practical nurse" in other provinces; and registered psychiatric nurses, who are unique to western Canada. The supply of RNs grew by 8.9% from 2007 to 2016 (from 274,274 in 2007 to 298,743 in 2016). Since 2013, there has been a decline (3.2%) in the number of RN graduates obtaining a licence to practise in Canada (Canadian Institute for Health Information [CIHI], 2018).

Because the regulation of health care professionals is under provincial jurisdiction in Canada, the provincial nursing associations—or colleges, as they are most often called—regulate individual nurses (See appropriate provincial **Regulated Health Professions** Act). In some provinces, registration of all nurses is under one college, while in other provinces each group of nurses has its own regulating college. The cases of Ontario and Alberta are used to provide examples of these two types of systems. In Ontario, RNs and registered practical nurses are both regulated by the College of Nurses of Ontario. In Alberta, RNs, licensed practical nurses, and registered psychiatric nurses each have their own regulating college—the College and Association of Registered Nurses of Alberta, College of Licensed Practical Nurses of Alberta, and College of Registered Psychiatric Nurses of Alberta, respectively. Provincial regulatory bodies set standards of practice and expect ethical practice from their members. An example of a code of ethics is the Canadian Nurses Association (CNA)'s *Code of Ethics for Registered Nurses* (CNA, 2017), which is used by most RN regulatory bodies in Canada.

The Patient/Client: Consumer of Nursing and Health Care

The central figure in health care services is, of course, the patient. The term *patient*, which is derived from a Latin verb meaning "to suffer," has traditionally been used to describe a person who is a recipient of care. For some, this term has a connotation of dependence. For this reason, many nurses prefer to use the term *client*, which is derived from a Latin verb meaning "to lean," connoting alliance and interdependence. However, for many, the term *client* has a mercantile connotation, which makes its use even more negative than the term *patient*. The term *patient* is used throughout this book, with the understanding that either term is acceptable.

The patient who seeks care for a health concern or concerns (increasing numbers of people have multiple health concerns) is also an individual person, a member of a family, and a member of the community. Patients' needs vary depending on their health issues, associated circumstances, and past experiences. Many patients seeking care have become more knowledgeable about health care options and expect a collaborative approach with the nurse and other health team members in the quest for optimal health (van den Hooff & Goossensen, 2015). Among the nurse's important functions in health care delivery are identifying and prioritizing the patient's immediate, ongoing, and long-term needs and working in concert with the patient to address them.

The Patient's Basic Needs

Certain needs are basic to all people. Some of these needs are more important than others. Once an essential need is met, people often experience a need on a higher level of priority.

Maslow's Hierarchy

Maslow (1954) ranked human needs as follows: physiologic needs; safety and security; sense of belonging and affection; esteem and self-respect; and self-actualization, which includes self-fulfillment, desire to know and understand, and aesthetic needs. Lower-level needs always remain, but a person's ability to pursue higher-level needs indicates movement toward psychological health and well-being. Such a hierarchy of needs is a useful framework that can be applied to the various nursing models for assessment of a patient's strengths, limitations, and need for nursing interventions (Fig. 1-1).

Health Care in Transition

Changes occurring in health care delivery and nursing are the result of societal, economic, technologic, scientific, and political forces that have evolved throughout the 20th and 21st centuries. Among the most significant changes are shifts in population demographics, particularly the increase in the aging population and the cultural diversity of the population; changing patterns of diseases; increased technology; increased consumer expectations; higher costs of health care and changes in health care financing; and other health care reform efforts. These changes have led to institutional restructuring, staff reduction and cross-training, increased outpatient care services, decreased lengths of hospital stay, and increased health care in community and home settings. Such changes have dramatically influenced where nurses practice. These

Glossary

British North America Act of 1867: legislation that led to the creation of the Canadian Confederation, and made health care a matter of provincial jurisdiction

Canada Health Act: a federal health legislation enacted in 1984 that includes five principles that must be respected across the country

continuous quality improvement (CQI): the ongoing examination of processes used to provide care, with the aim of improving quality by assessing and improving those processes that might improve patient care outcomes and patient satisfaction

evidence-based practice (EBP): a best practice derived from valid and reliable research studies that also considers the health care setting, patient preferences and values, and clinical judgment

interprofessional collaborative practice: employing multiple health professionals to work together with patients, families, and communities to deliver best practices, thus ensuring best patient outcomes

regulated health profession: a health profession whose members are regulated by a professional college which has the legislated mandate to protect the public

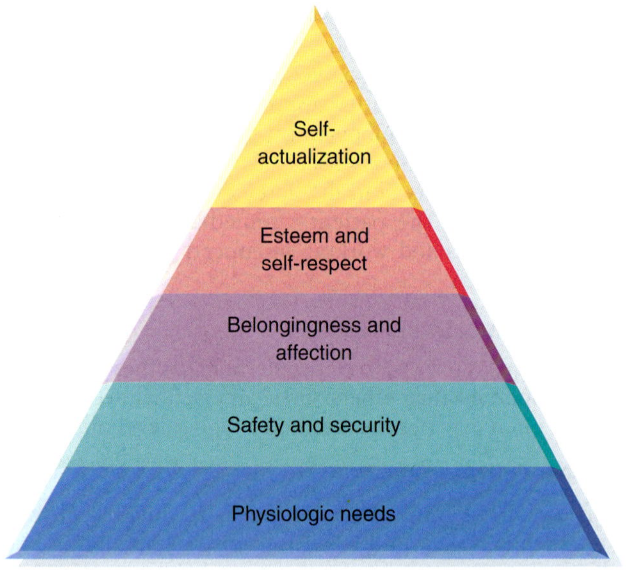

FIGURE 1-1. This scheme of Maslow's hierarchy of needs shows how a person moves from fulfillment of basic needs to higher levels of needs, with the ultimate goal being integrated human functioning and health.

changes have influenced society's view of health and illness and affected the focus of nursing and health care.

As the proportion of the population reaching age 65 years has increased, and with the shift from acute illnesses to chronic illnesses, the traditional disease management and care focus of the health care professions has expanded. There is increasing concern about emerging infectious diseases, chronic disease conditions, trauma, obesity, and bioterrorism. Thus, health care must focus more on disease prevention, health promotion, and management of chronic conditions and disability than in previous times. This shift in focus coincides with a nationwide emphasis on cost control and resource management directed toward providing safe, cost-efficient, and cost-effective health care services to the population as a whole.

Organization and Financing of Health Care Services in Canada

The passage of the British North America Act of 1867 made health care in Canada a matter of provincial jurisdiction, and the Constitutional Act of 1982 reconfirmed this division of power. In practice, it means that because provincial governments have this constitutional authority, it takes considerable efforts and compromise/negotiation to obtain the provincial and federal consensus necessary to establish policies that have a national scope. However, because Canadians see health care and the provision of health care services as a key priority, the federal government has played an increasing role in fostering the development of national policies through cost-sharing initiatives. In 1955, the provincial and federal governments agreed to establish hospital insurance, which led to the Hospital Insurance and Diagnostic Act of 1957. In 1964, the Royal Commission on Health Services recommended that it would be important to also add the provision of medical services to the national program. This recommendation led to the passage of the Medical Care Act of 1968. Although all provincial governments entered into these partnerships, the development in the following decades of provincial variations, such as the introduction of extra-billing and user fees, concerned federal authorities and brought about the **Canada Health Act** of 1984 (Ross-Kerr, 2011).

The Canada Health Act

The Canada Health Act stipulates that health care insurance plans must be publicly administered, universal, comprehensive, accessible, and portable. Providing an exhaustive definition of these principles is beyond the scope of this chapter, but in brief, the plan must be operated and administered on a nonprofit basis by a public authority responsible to the provincial government; 100% of the insured individuals in a province are entitled to the services that are provided under this plan; the plan must insure all services offered by hospitals and physicians and, where permitted, by other health care professionals; these services must be reasonably accessible; and when moving from one province to another, or when temporarily absent from their province (but within Canada), residents must continue to be covered (Health Canada, 2017). Current issues related to the financing of health care services are further addressed in the section of this chapter on economic pressures.

Models of Nursing Care Delivery

Several organizational methods or models that vary greatly from one facility to another and from one set of patient circumstances to another may be used to carry out nursing care. These methods and models have changed over the years and have included functional nursing, team nursing, primary nursing, and patient-focused or patient-centred care. A review of these models is beyond the scope of this chapter. Of note, health care agencies may use elements of a variety of models in the actual delivery of care, and there is much variation across Canada.

Health, Wellness, and Health Promotion

Health

How health is perceived depends on how health is defined. The World Health Organization (WHO) defines *health* in the preamble to its constitution as a "state of complete physical, mental, and social well-being and not merely the absence of disease and infirmity" (WHO, 2014, p. 1). Although commonly cited worldwide, this definition has been criticized for being too utopian—after all, it is not possible for anyone to achieve *complete* physical, mental, and social well-being (Pender, Murdaugh, & Parsons, 2015). The WHO definition of health does not allow for any variation in degrees of wellness or illness; the concept of a health–illness continuum allows for a greater range in describing a person's health status. By viewing health and illness on a continuum, it is possible to consider a person as being neither completely healthy nor completely ill. Instead, a person's state of health is ever-changing and has the potential to range from high-level wellness to extremely poor health and imminent death. Use of the health–illness continuum makes it possible to regard a person as simultaneously possessing degrees of both health and illness. On the health–illness continuum, even people with a chronic illness or disability may attain a high level of wellness if they are successful in meeting their health potential within the limits of their chronic illness or disability.

Wellness

Wellness and *health* are related terms that nurses often use interchangeably. However, for some, wellness is a broader concept that is like a journey taken by people in their quest for well-being.

Wellness involves being proactive and being involved in self-care activities aimed toward a state of physical, psychological, and spiritual well-being. Wellness is conceptualized as having four components: (1) the capacity to perform to the best of one's ability, (2) the ability to adjust and adapt to varying situations, (3) a reported feeling of well-being, and (4) a feeling that "everything is together" and harmonious (Hood, 2018). With this in mind, nurses must aim to promote positive changes that are directed toward health and well-being. The sense of wellness has a subjective aspect that addresses the importance of recognizing and responding to patient's individuality and diversity in health care and nursing.

Health Promotion

In Canada, the 1974 report *A New Perspective on the Health of Canadians, a Working Document*, also known as the Lalonde report, brought to the forefront the concept of health promotion. The Lalonde report suggested that medical care was not the most important determinant of health and changes in lifestyle and environment played the greatest role in improving the health of populations.

The WHO and Canada played a central role in creating a new vision of health promotion that recognizes that social factors are paramount to the health of populations. In 1986, Canada hosted the first international conference on health promotion, at which was promulgated the Ottawa Charter for Health Promotion. In this charter, health promotion is defined, as follows:

> [T]he process of enabling people to increase control over, and to improve, their health. To reach a state of complete physical, mental, and social well-being, an individual or group must be able to identify and to realize aspirations, to satisfy needs, and to change or cope with the environment. (WHO, 1986, p. 1)

People are increasingly knowledgeable about health and take more interest in and responsibility for their health and well-being. Organized self-care education programs emphasize health promotion, disease prevention, management of illness, self-care, and collaborative use of the professional health care system. Web sites, chat groups, and social media applications promote sharing of experiences and information about self-care with others who have similar conditions, chronic diseases, or disabling conditions. The advent of mobile wireless computer technologies (e.g., Fitbit) and novel informatics tools (e.g., Step counts) have had the effect of tailoring health promotion activities to meet individual preferences (Pender et al., 2015). Researchers have begun to take advantage of these popular technologic advancements by developing population-based registries.

According to the Public Health Agency of Canada (PHAC), the "new" health promotion recognizes that a series of factors, known as determinants of health, have a profound impact on the health of individuals and populations. These factors are income and social status, social support networks, employment and working conditions, education, physical environment, social environment, biology and genetic endowment, personal health practices and coping skills, healthy child development, health services, gender, and culture (PHAC, 2018a). The *Population Health Approach* endorsed by the PHAC is concerned with addressing the determinants of health for the population as a whole (PHAC, 2018b).

Primary Health Care

The primary health care (PHC) model, first introduced by the Alma-Ata Declaration of 1978, is important in the Canadian context, especially because there is a renewed interest by governments, who see it as a way to sustain our publicly funded health care system (Reutter & Ogilvie, 2011). It is also congruent with the principles of the Canada Health Act. PHC is defined as follows:

> Essential health care made universally accessible to individuals and families in the community by means acceptable to them, through their full participation and at a cost that the community and country can afford. It forms an integral part both of the country's health system of which it is the nucleus and of the overall social and economic development of the community. (WHO, 1978)

PHC is based on five principles that are seen as essential if a nation wishes to improve the health of its population: services must be accessible to the population; this population must be involved in the planning and operation of services; intersectoral and interdisciplinary collaboration are essential because determinants of health cannot be addressed by one type of provider alone and by only the health care sector; technologies must be adapted to the given context; and a focus on health promotion and prevention of illness and injury must be present (Reutter & Ogilvie, 2011).

Influences on Health Care Delivery

The health care delivery system is constantly adapting as the population shifts its health care needs and expectations change. The shifting demographics of the population, the increase in chronic illnesses and disability, the greater emphasis on health care costs, and technologic advances have resulted in changing emphases in health care delivery and in nursing.

Population Demographics

Changes in the population in general are affecting the need for and the delivery of health care. The 2016 Canadian census indicated that there were 35,151,728 people in the country (Statistics Canada, 2018a). Population growth is attributed in part to improved public health services and improved nutrition.

Not only is the population increasing, but also its composition is changing. The decline in birth rate and the increase in life span due to improved health care have resulted in fewer school-age children and more senior citizens, many of whom are women. Much of the population resides in highly congested urban areas, with a steady migration of members of ethnic minorities to the inner cities and a migration of members of the middle class to suburban areas. The number of people who are homeless, including entire families, has increased significantly. The population has become more culturally diverse as increasing numbers of people from different national backgrounds enter the country.

Because of population changes, the health care needs of people of specific ages, of women, and of diverse groups of people in specific geographic locations are altering the effectiveness of traditional means of providing health care. As a result, far-reaching changes in the overall health care delivery system are necessary.

Aging Population

The older population in Canada has increased significantly and will continue to grow in future. According to the 2016 census, 5.9 million people, representing 16.9% of the Canadian population, were aged 65 years or older. Among these, there were 8,230 centenarians (Statistics Canada, 2018b). The health care needs of older adults are complex and demand significant investments, both in human resources and financially. Many older Canadians live with multiple chronic conditions. As the Canadian population continues to age, it will become increasingly imperative to provide services that make it easier for older people to remain in their homes and continue to have fulfilling lives. See Chapter 14 for more details about the health care of the older adult.

Cultural Diversity

An appreciation for the diverse characteristics and needs of people from varied ethnic and cultural backgrounds is important in health care and nursing.

The term "Aboriginal Peoples" includes First Nations, Inuit, and Métis populations in Canada (Royal Commission on Aboriginal Peoples, 1996), and is usually written as Aboriginal Peoples (First Nations, Inuit, and Métis). There are over 605 Aboriginal communities in Canada and each one is unique in terms of history, language, cultural beliefs, and ceremonies. About 6% (2.1 million) of the Canadian population have identified themselves as Aboriginal and of these, 1.5 million are First Nations; others include the Inuit and the Métis (Statistics Canada, 2018c).

The Truth and Reconciliation Commission of Canada held meetings (2010 to 2014) across Canada to hear first-hand from some of the 150,000 Aboriginal men and women who as children were taken from their families and forced to attend Indian residential schools. Many of the children were physically, emotionally, and sexually abused (Woods, 2013). Bombay, Matheson, and Anisman (2014) have written about the intergenerational impact of the residential schools and the implications for health policy and the concept of historical trauma. In 2013, new information was released about federal research projects conducted on Aboriginal children in residential schools, which included severely limited diets for children between 1942 and 1952 (Woods, 2013), and giving antibiotics inappropriately, which resulted in deafness.

More than 250 ethnic origins were identified in the 2016 National Household Survey, and visible minorities now constitute 22.3% of the Canadian population (Statistics Canada, 2018d). As the cultural composition of the population changes, it is increasingly important to address cultural considerations in the delivery of health care. Patients from diverse sociocultural groups not only bring various health care beliefs, values, and practices to the health care setting, but also have a variety of risk factors for some disease conditions and unique reactions to treatment. These factors significantly affect a person's responses to health care issues or illnesses, to caregivers, and to the care itself. Unless these factors are assessed for, understood, and respected by health care providers, the care delivered may be ineffective, and health care outcomes may be negatively affected.

Culture is defined as learned patterns of behaviour, beliefs, and values that are shared by a particular group of people. Included among the many characteristics that distinguish cultural groups are the manner of dress, language spoken, values, rules or norms of behaviour, gender-specific practices, economics, politics, law and social control, artifacts, technology, dietary practices, and health beliefs and practices. Health promotion, illness prevention, causes of sickness, treatment, coping, caring, dying, and death are part of every culture. Every person has a unique belief and value system that has been shaped at least in part by his or her cultural environment. This belief and value system guide the person's thinking, decisions, and actions. It provides direction for interpreting and responding to illness and disability and to health care.

To promote an effective nurse–patient relationship and positive outcomes of care, nursing care must be culturally safe and competent, appropriate, and sensitive to cultural differences. All attempts should be made to help patients retain their unique cultural characteristics/identities. Providing special foods that have significance and arranging for religious observances may enable patients to maintain a feeling of wholeness at a time when they may feel isolated from family and community.

Knowing the cultural and social significance that particular situations have for each patient helps the nurse avoid imposing a personal value system when the patient has a different point of view. In most cases, cooperation with the plan of care occurs when communication among the nurse, the patient, and the patient's family is directed toward understanding the situation or the concern and respecting each other's goals.

Changing Patterns of Disease

During the past 50 years, the health issues of Canadians have changed significantly. Although many infectious diseases have been controlled or eradicated, others, such as tuberculosis, acquired immunodeficiency syndrome (AIDS), and sexually transmitted infections, are on the rise. An increasing number of infectious agents are becoming resistant to antibiotic therapy as a result of widespread and inappropriate use of antibiotics. Obesity has become a major health concern, and the multiple comorbidities that accompany it, such as hypertension, heart disease, diabetes, and cancer, add significantly to its associated mortality (see Chapter 42).

The prevalence of chronic illnesses and disability is increasing because of the lengthening of life span of Canadians and the advances in care and treatment options for conditions, such as cancer, human immunodeficiency virus (HIV) infection, and cystic fibrosis. In addition, improvements in care for trauma and other serious acute health problems have meant that many people with these conditions live decades longer than in the past. Because the majority of health issues seen today are chronic in nature, many people are learning to maximize their health within the constraints of chronic illness and disability.

As chronic conditions increase, health care broadens from a focus on cure and eradication of disease to include the prevention or rapid treatment of exacerbations of chronic conditions. Nursing, which has always encouraged patients to take control of their health and wellness, has a prominent role in the current focus on management of chronic illness and disability.

Advances in Technology and Genetics

Advances in technology and genetics have occurred rapidly during the past several decades. Sophisticated techniques and devices, such as robot-assisted technology, have revolutionized treatments making it possible to perform many procedures and tests on an outpatient basis. Increased knowledge and understanding of genetics and genomics have resulted in expanded screening, diagnostic testing, and treatments for a variety of conditions (see Chapter 11).

The sophisticated communication systems that connect most parts of the world, with the capability of rapid storage, retrieval, and dissemination of information, have stimulated brisk change as well as swift obsolescence in health care delivery strategies. Using health information technology (HIT) to improve the quality, efficacy, or delivery of health care is an interdisciplinary field of study called health informatics. Advances in genetics and HIT have also resulted in many ethical issues for the health care system, health care providers, patients, families, and society. Nurses must not only be cognizant of advances in HIT, but also become adept in its use as their practice settings and population requires.

Demand for Quality Health Care

Nurses in acute care settings work with other health care team members to maintain quality care while facing pressures to discharge patients and decrease staffing costs. Nurses in hospitals now care for patients who are hospitalized for relatively few days. Nurses in the community care for patients who need high-technology acute care services as well as long-term care at home. The importance of effective discharge planning and quality improvement cannot be overstated. Acute care nurses must also work with community-based nurses and others in community settings to ensure continuity of care.

Quality Improvement and Evidence-Based Practice

The general public has become increasingly interested in and knowledgeable about health care and health promotion. This awareness has been stimulated by television, newspapers, magazines, and other communications media as well as by political debate. The public has also become very health conscious and subscribes to the belief that health and quality health care constitute a basic right, rather than a privilege for a chosen few, and desires care that is both personalized and delivered in a timely manner. Over the last three decades, new systems of quality assurance (QA) and delivery have gradually emerged. Three of them—**continuous quality improvement (CQI)** and **evidence-based practice (EBP)**, clinical pathways and care mapping, and case management—are discussed in more detail.

Continuous Quality Improvement and Evidence-Based Practice

Seeking to ensure the quality of patient care, Canadian hospitals have adopted, over time, various methods aimed at improving quality. The adoption of these methods has also been linked with the aim of meeting accreditation standards. Since 1958, the Canadian Council on Health Services Accreditation, formerly known as the Canadian Council on Hospital Accreditation, has the mandate to provide accreditation programs. In the 1970s and the 1980s, the presence of a QA program was one of its standards of accreditation. Although well-intentioned, QA programs were found to have limitations including, for example, their cost-effectiveness and department-specific focus, which limited opportunities for interdisciplinary involvement to solve problems needing the involvement of more than a single discipline. In light of this, in the early 1990s, attention shifted from achieving predetermined standards to using processes of CQI (Cummings & Wong, 2011).

CQI emphasizes the importance of improving the care processes used by organizations, that improvement must be continuous, customers must be the focus, leaders must be committed, staff education is essential to ensure a motivated workforce, and that cultural transformation is a long-term proposition. In contrast with QA, which was department and disciplinary focused, CQI is system wide and interdisciplinary. The principles of quality improvement are recognized in the current accreditation standards of the Canadian Council on Hospital Services Accreditation (Cummings & Wong, 2011).

If care is to be of the best possible quality and continuously improve, it follows that practice must be based on evidence. In other words, health professionals must incorporate the latest research findings in their practice. However, it is increasingly recognized that health professionals face challenges in locating and using research findings. This is why research on knowledge utilization and knowledge transfer is such a growing field of research.

Clinical Pathways and Care Mapping

First developed in the United States, the use of clinical pathways, or care mapping, is increasingly common in Canada. Clinical pathways are tools for tracking a patient's progress toward achieving positive outcomes within specified time frames. Clinical pathways based on current literature and clinical expertise have been developed for patients with certain diagnosis-related groups (DRGs) (e.g., heart failure, ischemic stroke, fractured hip), for high-risk patients (e.g., those receiving chemotherapy), and for patients with certain common health problems (e.g., diabetes, chronic pain). The pathways indicate key events, such as diagnostic tests, treatments, activities, medications, consultation, and education, that must occur within specified times for patients to achieve the desired and timely outcomes.

A case manager often facilitates and coordinates interventions to ensure that the patient progresses through the key events and achieves the desired outcomes. Nurses who provide direct care have an important role in the development and use of clinical pathways through their participation in researching the literature and then developing, piloting, implementing, and revising clinical pathways. In addition, nurses monitor outcome achievement and document and analyze variances.

Other EBP tools used for planning patient care are care mapping, clinical guidelines, algorithms, multidisciplinary action plans (MAPs), and clinical pathways. These tools are used to move patients toward predetermined outcome markers. Algorithms are used more often in acute situations to determine a particular treatment based on patient information or response. Care maps, clinical guidelines, and MAPs help facilitate coordination of care and education throughout hospitalization and after discharge.

Because care mapping and guidelines are used for conditions in which a patient's progress often defies prediction, specific time frames for achieving outcomes are excluded. A patient with a highly complex condition or multiple underlying illnesses may benefit more from care mapping or guidelines than from clinical pathways, because the use of outcome milestones (rather than specific time frames) is more realistic.

Through case management and the use of clinical pathways or care mapping, patients and the care they receive are continually assessed from preadmission to discharge—and in many cases after discharge to home care and community settings. Continuity of care, effective utilization of services, and cost containment are the major benefits for society and for the health care system. Nurses who provide direct care have an important role in the development and use of these tools through participation in researching the literature and then developing, piloting, implementing, and revising the tools as needed.

Case Management

Case management is a system of coordinating health care services to ensure cost-effectiveness, accountability, and quality care. The premise of case management is that the responsibility for meeting patient needs rests with one person or team whose goals are to provide the patient and family with access to required services, to ensure coordination of these services, and to evaluate how effectively these services are delivered.

Since the 1980s, case management has become prominent in American hospitals. In Canada, case management is primarily used for care delivered in the community, such as home care services. Nurses or other members of the health care team (e.g., occupational therapists and social workers) serve as case managers. Case managers may carry out a variety of roles, depending on the way in which services are organized in a health region. They may be responsible for the care of individual clients or groups of clients and may also have responsibility at the level of program, organizations, or service delivery systems. A case manager may serve as clinical expert, communicator, collaborator, navigator, manager, advocate, and professional (National Case Management Network, 2012).

Roles of the Nurse

The professional nurse in hospital/institutional, community-based or public health, and home care settings has three major roles: the caregiver role, which includes teaching and collaborating; the leadership role; and the research role. Although each role carries specific responsibilities, these roles relate to one another and are found in all nursing positions. These roles are designed to meet the immediate and future health care and nursing needs of the population.

Caregiver Role

The caregiver role involves the actions taken by nurses to meet the health care and nursing needs of individual patients, their families, significant others, and the community. This role is a dominant one for nurses in primary, secondary, and tertiary health care settings and in-home care and community nursing. It is achieved through use of critical thinking, clinical judgment, and the nursing process, all of which are key tools for nursing practice. Nurses help patients meet their needs by using direct intervention, by teaching patients and family members to perform care, and by coordinating and collaborating with other disciplines to provide needed services.

Leadership Role

The leadership role is often viewed as a role assumed by nurses who have titles that suggest leadership and who are the leaders of large groups of nurses or related health care professionals. However, demonstrating leadership skills is required within all nursing positions. For example, when advocating for patients, staff nurses must be able to convince others and to do this they must possess attributes of leadership (Grossman & Valiga, 2016).

Nursing leadership involves four components: decision making, relating, influencing, and facilitating. Each of these components promotes change and the ultimate outcome of goal achievement. Basic to the entire process is effective communication, which determines the success of the process and achievement of goals. The components of the leadership process are appropriate during all phases of the nursing process and in all settings.

Research Role

The primary task of nursing research is to contribute to the scientific base of nursing knowledge and practice. Studies are needed to determine the effectiveness of nursing interventions and nursing care. The science of nursing grows through research, leading to the generation of scientifically based rationale for nursing practice and patient care. This process is the basis of EBP, with a resultant increase in the quality of patient care, and improved outcomes.

The research role is considered to be a responsibility of all nurses. Nurses are constantly alert for nursing problems and important issues related to patient care that can serve as a basis for the identification of researchable questions. Nurses with a background in research methods can use their research knowledge and skills to initiate and implement timely, relevant studies.

Nurses directly involved in patient care are often in the best position to identify potential research questions, and their clinical insights are invaluable. Nurses also have a responsibility to become actively involved in ongoing research studies. This may involve facilitating the data collection process, or it may include actual collection of data. Explaining the study to patients and their families and to other health care professionals is often of invaluable assistance to the researcher who is conducting the study.

Above all, nurses must use research findings in their nursing practice; the use, validation, replication, dissemination, and evaluation of research findings further the science of nursing. As stated previously, EBP requires the critique of the best evidence available in research-based studies and validating their saliency to nursing practice. Nurses need to continually be aware of studies that are directly related to their own area of clinical practice and critically analyze those studies to determine the applicability of their implications for specific patient populations. Relevant conclusions and implications can be used to improve patient care.

Advanced Nursing Practice Roles

Professional nursing is adapting to meet changing health needs and expectations. One such adaptation is through advanced nursing practice, which has developed to better respond to the needs of the population (Schober, 2016). As stated by the CNA (2008, p. ii):

> "Advanced nursing practice is an umbrella term describing an advanced level of clinical nursing practice that maximizes the use of graduate educational preparation, in-depth nursing knowledge and expertise in meeting the health needs of individuals, families, groups, communities and populations"

Advanced practice nurses usually have a graduate degree in nursing. Two advanced nursing practice roles exist in Canada: the clinical nurse specialist (CNS) and the NP.

The CNS has been present in Canada since the 1960s (CNA, 2016). A *CNS* is "a registered nurse who holds a master's or doctoral degree in nursing with expertise in a clinical nursing specialty: uses in-depth knowledge and skills, advanced judgment and clinical experience in a nursing specialty to assist in providing solutions for complex health care issues" (CNA, 2008, p. 40). The primary role of CNSs is to integrate care across the health care continuum through three spheres of influence—the patient, the nurse, and the health care system. In each of these spheres of influence, the goal of CNS practice is to monitor and improve aggregate patient outcomes and nursing care.

An *NP* is "a registered nurse with additional educational preparation and experience who possesses and demonstrates the competencies to autonomously diagnose, order and interpret diagnostic tests, prescribe pharmaceuticals, and perform specific procedures within the legislated scope of practice" (CNA, 2008, p. 41). NPs are not as common in Canada as they are in the United States. The role initially emerged in the late 1960s, but had almost disappeared by the 1980s. After renewed interest from employers and governments in the 1990s, legislation regulating NP practice was enacted. The numbers of NPs are on the rise in Canada, and has increased steadily since 2007 (CIHI, 2018).

In general, initial care, ambulatory health care, and anticipatory guidance are all becoming increasingly important in nursing practice. Advanced practice roles enable nurses to function interdependently with other health care professionals and to establish a more collegial relationship with physicians. As changes in health care continue, the role of advanced practice nurses, especially in primary care settings, is expected to increase in terms of scope, responsibility, and recognition.

Interprofessional Collaboration

This chapter has explored the changing roles of nursing. Many references have been made to the significance of nurses as members of the health care team. As team members, nurses develop and maintain solid working relationships with other health care professionals in order to obtain the best possible outcomes for patients. As interprofessional collaboration is becoming increasingly critical, the Canadian Interprofessional Health Collaborative (CIHC) has developed a competency framework to assist educators in fostering the development of new practitioners who will be well-prepared for this type of collaboration (CIHC, 2010). **Interprofessional collaborative practice** involves employing multiple health professionals to work together with patients, families, and communities to deliver best practices, thus assuring best patient outcomes. Interprofessional teamwork is viewed as central to this model, which incorporates the interdisciplinary core competencies.

Critical Thinking Exercises

1. Your clinical assignment is in a long-term care facility. Identify a patient care issue (e.g., nutritional status) that could be improved. Describe the mechanism that is available within a clinical facility to address such quality improvement issues.
2. You are planning the discharge of an older patient who has several chronic medical conditions. A case manager has been assigned to this patient. How would you explain the role of the case manager to the patient and her husband?
3. **ebp** You are assigned to care for a hospitalized patient with obesity, with a history of diabetes, and a new diagnosis of stable angina. There is a clinical nurse specialist

(CNS) assigned to provide consistent, quality care for this patient from hospital admission to discharge. Identify the evidence that supports the effectiveness of CNSs in supervising care of patients and promoting positive patient outcomes. What is the strength of the evidence? How might this specific patient's care be affected?

REFERENCES AND SELECTED READINGS

Books

Canadian Nurses Association (CNA). (2017). *Code of ethics for registered nurses*. Ottawa, ON: Author.

Cummings, G. G., & Wong, C. A. (2011). Quality of care: Quality assurance and improvement to culture of patient safety. In J. C. Ross-Kerr, & M. J. Wood (Eds.). *Canadian nursing issues and perspectives* (5th ed., pp. 210–227). Toronto, ON: Elsevier Mosby.

Grossman, S. C., & Valiga, T. M. (2016). *The new leadership challenge creating the future of nursing* (5th ed.). Philadelphia, PA: F. A. Davis Company.

Hood, L. (2018). *Leddy & Pepper's conceptual bases of professional nursing* (9th ed.). Philadelphia, PA: Lippincott Williams & Wilkins.

Lalonde, M. (1974). *A new perspective on the health of Canadians, a working document*. Ottawa, ON: Department of National Health and Welfare.

Maslow, A. (1954). *Motivation and personality*. New York: Harper.

Paul, P., & Ross-Kerr, J. C. (2011). Nursing in Canada, 1600 to the present: A brief account. In J. C. Ross-Kerr, & M. J. Wood (Eds.). *Canadian nursing issues and perspectives* (5th ed., pp. 17–41). Toronto, ON: Elsevier Mosby.

Pender, N. J., Murdaugh, C. L., & Parsons, M. A. (2015). *Health promotion in nursing practice* (7th ed.). Upper Saddle River, NJ: Pearson Education.

Reutter, L., & Ogilvie, L. (2011). Primary health care: Challenges and opportunities for the nursing profession. In J. C. Ross-Kerr, & M. J. Wood (Eds.). *Canadian nursing issues and perspectives* (5th ed., pp. 185–207). Toronto, ON: Elsevier Mosby.

Ross-Kerr, J. C. (2011). The Canadian health care system. In J. C. Ross-Kerr, & M. J. Wood (Eds.). *Canadian nursing issues and perspectives* (5th ed., pp. 3–17). Toronto, ON: Elsevier Mosby.

Schober, M. (2016). *Introduction to advanced nursing practice: An international focus*. Cham, Switzerland: Springer International Publishing.

World Health Organization (WHO). (1978). *Primary health care: Report of the international conference on primary health care, Alma-Ata. USSR*. Geneva, Switzerland: Author.

World Health Organization (WHO). (1986). *Ottawa charter for health promotion*. Geneva, Switzerland: Author.

World Health Organization (WHO). (2014). *Constitution of the World Health Organization* (45th ed.). New York: Author.

Journals and Electronic Documents

Bombay, H., Matheson, K., & Anisman, H. (2014). The intergenerational effects of Indian residential schools: Implications for the concept of historical trauma. *Transcultural Psychiatry*, *51*(3), 320–338.

Canadian Interprofessional Health Collaborative (CIHC). (2010). *A national interprofessional competency framework*. Ottawa, ON: Queens' Printer. Retrieved from http://www.cihc.ca/files/CIHC_IPCompetencies_Feb1210r.pdf

Canadian Institute for Health Information (CIHI). (2018). Regulated Nurses 2016. Retrieved from: https://secure.cihi.ca/free_products/regulated-nurses-2016-report-en-web.pdf

Canadian Nurses Association (CNA). (2008). *Advanced nursing practice: A national framework*. Ottawa, ON: Author. Retrieved from https://www.cna-aiic.ca/~/media/cna/page-content/pdf-en/anp_national_framework_e.pdf

Canadian Nurses Association (CNA). (2016). *Position statement: Clinical nurse specialist*. Ottawa, ON: Author. Retrieved from https://www.cna-aiic.ca/-/media/cna/page-content/pdf-en/clinical-nurse-specialist-position-statement_2016.pdf

Canadian Nurses Association (CNA). (2018). *Nursing statistics*. Retrieved August 23, 2018, from https://www.cna-aiic.ca/en/nursing-practice/the-practice-of-nursing/health-human-resources/nursing-statistics

Dahrouge, S., Muldoon, L., Ward, N., et al. (2014). Roles of nurse practitioners and family physicians in community health centres. *Canadian Family Physician*, *60*(11), 1020–1027.

Health Canada. (2017). *Canada Health Act overview*. Ottawa, ON: Author. Retrieved from https://www.canada.ca/en/health-canada/services/health-care-system/canada-health-care-system-medicare/canada-health-act.html

International Council of Nurses (ICN). (2018). *The ICN definition of nursing*. Retrieved August 25, 2018, from https://www.icn.ch/nursing-policy/nursing-definitions

National Case Management Network (NCMN). (2012). *Canadian core competency profile for case management providers*. Retrieved August 25, 2018, from http://www.ncmn.ca/Resources/Documents/core_competency_english-2014.pdf

Public Health Agency of Canada (PHAC). (2018a). *What determines health?*. Ottawa, ON: Author. Retrieved from http://www.phac-aspc.gc.ca/ph-sp/determinants/index-eng.php

Public Health Agency of Canada (PHAC). (2018b). *What is the Population Health Approach?* Ottawa, ON: Author. Retrieved from https://www.canada.ca/en/public-health/services/health-promotion/population-health/population-health-approach.html

Royal Commission on Aboriginal Peoples. (1996). *Royal commission report on Aboriginal peoples*. Retrieved from https://www.aadnc-aandc.gc.ca/eng/1100100014597/1100100014637

Statistics Canada. (2018a). *A portrait of the population aged 85 and older in 2016 in Canada*. Ottawa, ON: Author. Retrieved January 5, 2018, from http://www12.statcan.gc.ca/census-recensement/2016/as-sa/98-200-x/2016004/98-200-x2016004-eng.cfm

Statistics Canada (2018b). *2016 census topic: Population and dwelling counts*. Retrieved from: https://www12.statcan.gc.ca/census-recensement/2016/rt-td/population-eng.cfm

Statistics Canada. (2018c). *Ethnic and cultural origins of Canadians: Portrait of a rich heritage*. Ottawa, ON: Author. Retrieved January 5, 2018, from http://www12.statcan.gc.ca/census-recensement/2016/as-sa/98-200-x/2016016/98-200-x2016016-eng.cfm

Statistics Canada (2018d). *Immigration and ethnocultural diversity highlight tables, 2016 census*. Retrieved from: https://www12.statcan.gc.ca/census-recensement/2016/dp-pd/hlt-fst/imm/index-eng.cfm

van den Hooff, S. L., & Goossensen, A. (2015). Ethical considerations on the value of patient knowledge in long-term care: A qualitative study of patients suffering from Korsakoff's syndrome. *Nursing Ethics*, *22*(3), 377–388.

Woods, M. (2013, June 11). We can't lose another generation. *Edmonton Journal*, p. A12. Retrieved from http://www.pressreader.com/canada/edmonton-journal/20130611/281719792138997

2 Community-Based Nursing Practice

Adapted by Joseph Osuji and Mohamed Toufic El Hussein

Learning Objectives

On completion of this chapter, the learner will be able to:

1. Discuss recent changes in the health care system that have increased the need for medical-surgical nurses to practice in community-based settings.
2. Compare the differences and similarities between community-based and hospital nursing.
3. Describe the discharge planning process in relation to home care preparation.
4. Explain methods for identifying community resources and making referrals.
5. Discuss how to prepare for a home visit and how to conduct the visit.
6. Identify personal safety precautions a home care nurse takes when making home visits.
7. Describe the various types of nursing functions provided in ambulatory care facilities, in occupational health and school nursing programs, to people who are homeless, and to those with alcohol or drug addictions.

The changes that have occurred in the health care system and society in the past two decades have increased the need for care in ambulatory settings and in the home. These changes have created a demand for highly skilled and well-prepared nurses to provide community-based care.

The delivery of community health care occurs within the Canadian health care system, also known as *Medicare*. This system reflects the values that define Canadian culture: social justice, equity, and community. Guided by the Canada Health Act, passed in 1984, the system is based on the fundamental principle that all members of Canadian society, including the most vulnerable, are entitled to health care. Within the Canadian health care system, there has been a trend toward more health care being delivered within communities. This shift is partly due to ongoing implementation of a long-held Canadian belief that health promotion services are a critical component of the country's health care system. The more recent factors contributing to this trend include advancements in scientific knowledge and technology leading to improved diagnostics and treatment, and thus earlier hospital discharge (Kozier, Erb, Berman, et al., 2018).

As more health care delivery shifts into the community, more nurses are working in a variety of public health and community-based settings. These settings include public health departments, ambulatory health clinics, long-term care facilities, prenatal and well-baby clinics, hospice agencies, industrial settings (as occupational health nurses), shelters for people who are homeless, and clinics, nursing centres, home care agencies, urgent care centres, same-day surgical centres, short-stay correctional facilities, and patients' homes.

Nurses in these settings often deliver care without direct on-site supervision or the support of other health care personnel. They must be self-directed, flexible, adaptable, and tolerant of various lifestyles and living conditions.

Community-based nursing occurs in a variety of settings and is directed toward people and families with needs related to illness, injury, or disability. A community is an interacting population of individuals living together within a larger social structure. While community-based nurses may care for patients recovering from an acute illness, many times the interventions needed result from chronic illness (Stanhope, Lancaster, Jakubec, et al., 2017). Home health care is a major aspect of community-based care.

Community-Based Care

Community-based nursing is a philosophy of care of individuals and families. The care is provided in a community as the individual or family move among various kinds of service providers outside of hospitals (Stanhope et al., 2017). Although the phrase "community-based nursing" is often interchanged with "community health nursing," a distinction should be made. The phrase "community health nursing" has generally been equated to "**public health nursing**." Public health nursing is a specialty focused on total populations, although care may be given to individuals. Community-based nursing is broader and may incorporate community health–public health nursing; it is focused on individuals and families rather than total populations. Community-based nursing also includes home care nursing, school health nursing, and a host of other nursing services provided to individuals and groups in the community (Fig. 2-1).

Nurses in community-based practice provide preventive care at three levels: primary, secondary, and tertiary. **Primary prevention** focuses on health promotion and prevention of illness or disease, including interventions such as teaching about healthy lifestyles. **Secondary prevention** centres on health maintenance and is aimed at early detection and prompt intervention to prevent or minimize loss of function and independence, including interventions such as health screening and health risk appraisal. **Tertiary prevention** focuses on minimizing deterioration and improving quality of life, including rehabilitation to assist patients in achieving their maximum potential by working through their physical or psychological challenges. Home care nurses often focus on tertiary preventive nursing care, although primary and secondary prevention are also addressed. Nurses practicing in the community need to be self-directed, flexible, adaptable, and accepting of various lifestyles and living conditions. To function effectively, nurses in these settings must have expertise in independent decision making, critical thinking, assessment, health education, community resources, and competence in basic nursing care (Allender, Rector, & Warner, 2014).

In addition, nurses in community settings must be culturally competent, as culture plays a role in the delivery of care and there are many opportunities for culturally diverse interactions (Canadian Association of Schools of Nursing, 2018). Cross-cultural health encounters are especially common in Canada because of the diverse ethnic and Aboriginal peoples' (First Nations, Inuit, and Métis) populations in the country (Kozier et al., 2018). Increasingly, health care providers in Canada are from diverse cultural backgrounds as well (Babenko-Mould & Elliott, 2015). Developing cultural competence involves awareness and self-reflection, willingness to explore cultural expressions in health and illness, and delivery of interventions that are congruent with the patient's culture (see Chapter 8) (Dreachslin, Gilbert, & Malone, 2013).

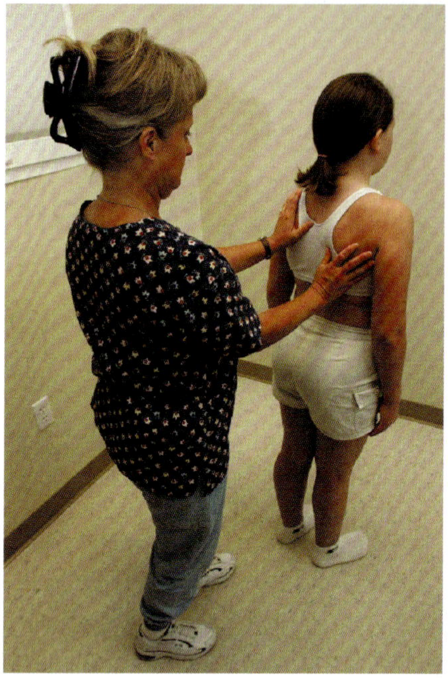

FIGURE 2-1. Community-based nursing takes many forms and focuses. Here, the school nurse performs screening for scoliosis.

Community-based nursing practice focuses on promoting and maintaining the health of individuals and groups, preventing and minimizing the progression of disease, and improving quality of life (Stanhope et al., 2017). Although nursing interventions used by public health nurses may involve individuals, families, or small groups, the central focus remains promotion of health and prevention of disease in the entire community. The actions of community health nurses may include provision of direct care to patients and families as well as political advocacy to secure resources for aggregate populations (e.g., the aging population or individuals experiencing homelessness). The community health nurse may function as an epidemiologist, a case manager for a group of patients, a coordinator of services provided to an aggregate of patients, an occupational health nurse, a school nurse, a visiting nurse, or a parish nurse (in parish nursing, the members of the

Glossary

community-based nursing: nursing care of individuals and families that is designed to (1) promote and maintain health and (2) prevent disease. It is provided as patients transition through the health care system to health-related services outside of the hospital setting, to manage acute and chronic conditions

primary prevention: health care delivery focused on health promotion and prevention of illness or disease

public health nursing: a specialty practice of nursing that combines the discipline of public health with nursing; it is considered a specialty practice within community-oriented nursing that focuses on population health

secondary prevention: health care delivery centred on health maintenance and aimed at early detection of disease, with prompt intervention to prevent or minimize loss of function and independence

tertiary prevention: health care delivery focused on minimizing deterioration associated with disease and improving quality of life through rehabilitation measures religious community—the parish—are the recipients of care). The commonality of these various roles is that the nurse maintains a focus on community needs as well as on the needs of the patient. The primary concepts of community-based nursing care are self-care and preventive care within the context of culture and community. Two other important concepts are continuity of care and collaboration. Some community-based nursing fields have become specialties in their own right, such as school health nursing and home care nursing.

Home Care

Home care nursing is a unique aspect of community-based nursing and a major player in posthospital care for patients who return home to complete recuperation following an acute illness episode or exacerbation of chronic illness. Home health agencies can also provide advanced technologies in the home setting. All together, these services provided in the home setting, work to maximize the patient's ability to function at his or her highest level of wellness (Allender et al., 2014).

Home care visits are made by nurses who work for home care agencies, public health agencies, and visiting nurse associations; by nurses who are employed by hospitals; and by parish nurses who voluntarily work with the members of their religious communities to promote health. Such visits may also be part of the responsibilities of school nurses, clinic nurses, or occupational health nurses. Home health care agencies are continuing to employ more nurses. Because of the high acuity levels of patients, nurses with acute care and critical care experience are in demand in this field.

The type of nursing services provided to patients in their homes varies from agency to agency. Nurses from home care or hospice agencies make home visits to provide skilled nursing care, follow-up care, and teaching to promote health and prevent complications. Hospice nursing has become a specialty area of nursing practice in which nurses provide palliative care in patients' homes and within hospice centres, thus promoting comfort, peace, and dignity to patients who are dying. Clinic nurses may conduct home visits as part of patient follow-up. Public health, parish, and school nurses may make visits to provide anticipatory guidance to high-risk families and follow-up care to patients with communicable diseases. Many home care patients are acutely ill, and many have chronic health problems and disabilities, requiring nurses to provide more education and monitoring to the patients and families. Holistic care is provided in the home through the collaboration of an interdisciplinary team that includes professional nurses; home care aides; social workers; physical, speech, and occupational therapists; pharmacists; and physicians. An interdisciplinary approach is used to provide health and social services with oversight of the total health care plan by a case manager, clinical nurse specialist, or nurse practitioner.

Basic home care services are provided to Canadians through programs operated by territorial or provincial governments. The basic services covered may vary from province to province or territory. Private payment or insurance coverage is therefore sometimes required to cover costs not publicly funded.

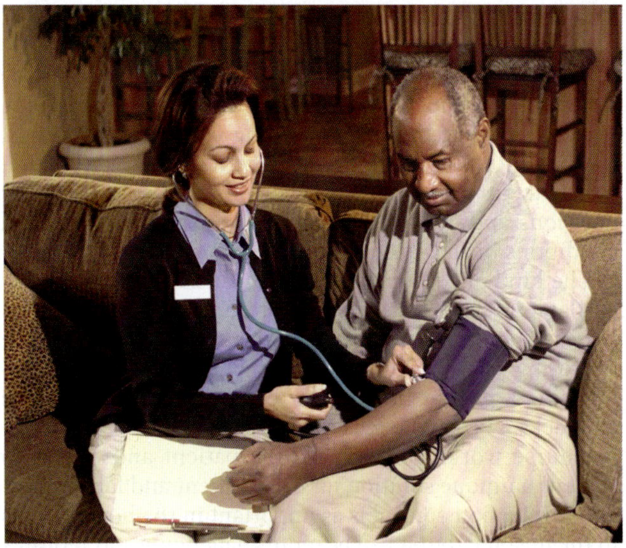

FIGURE 2-2. Assessment is an important part of any home health visit.

Older adults are the most frequent users of home care services. To be eligible for service, the patient must be ill, homebound, and in need of skilled nursing services.

Health care visits may be intermittent or periodic, and case management via telephone or via Internet may be used to promote communication with home care consumers. The nurse instructs the patient and family about skills and self-care strategies and about health maintenance and promotion activities (e.g., nutritional counselling, exercise programs, stress management). Nursing care includes skilled assessment of the patient's physical, psychological, social, and environmental status (Fig. 2-2). Nursing interventions may include intravenous (IV) therapy and injections, parenteral nutrition, venipuncture, catheter insertion, pressure ulcer treatment, wound care, ostomy care, and patient and family teaching. Complex technical equipment, such as dialysis machines and ventilators, is often part of home health care (Allender et al., 2014; Stanhope et al., 2017). Nurses have a role in evaluating the safety and effectiveness of technology in the home setting. In addition, "telehealth" is an emerging trend in home health care; this facilitates exchange of information via telephone lines between patients and nurses regarding health information such as blood glucose readings, vital signs, and cardiac parameters (Stanhope et al., 2017). Use of a broad spectrum of computer and Internet resources, such as webcams, also facilitates exchange of information.

Nursing in the Home Setting

The home care nurse is a guest in the patient's home and must have permission to visit and give care. The nurse has minimal control over the lifestyle, living situation, and health practices of the patients he or she visits. This lack of full decision-making authority can create a conflict for the nurse and may lead to issues in the nurse–patient relationship. To work successfully with patients in any setting, the nurse must be nonjudgmental and convey respect for patients' beliefs, even if they differ sharply from the nurse's. This can be difficult when a patient's lifestyle involves activities that a nurse considers harmful or unacceptable, such as smoking, use of alcohol, drug abuse, or overeating.

The cleanliness of a patient's home may not meet the standards of a hospital. Although the nurse can provide teaching points about maintaining clean surroundings, the patient and family decide whether they will implement the nurse's suggestions. The nurse must accept their decisions and deliver the care required regardless of the conditions of the setting (Lundy & Janes, 2016).

The kind of equipment, supplies, and resources usually available in acute care settings are often unavailable in a patient's home. The nurse has to learn to improvise when providing care, such as when changing a dressing or catheterizing a patient in a regular bed that is not adjustable and lacks a bedside table (Allender et al., 2014). At times, the nurse works closely with the patient and others to achieve a unique solution for each patient and family situation. Infection control is as important in the home as it is in the hospital, but it can be more challenging and requires creative approaches. As in any situation, it is important to cleanse one's hands before and after giving direct patient care, even in a home that does not have running water. A waterless, alcohol-based hand cleanser is a useful product for hand decontamination. If aseptic technique is required, the nurse needs to have a plan for implementing this technique before going to the home. This applies also to Routine Practices and Additional Precautions (Health Canada, 2018) and disposal of bodily secretions and excretions. If injections are given, the nurse uses a closed container to dispose of syringes. Injectable and other medications must be kept out of the reach of children during visits and must be stored in a safe place if they are to remain in the house.

Friends, neighbours, or family members may ask the nurse about the patient's condition. A patient has a right to confidentiality, and information should be shared only with the patient's permission. If the nurse carries the patient's health record into the house, it must be put in a secure place to prevent it from being picked up by others or misplaced.

Discharge Planning for Home Care

Discharge planning is an important part of making the transition from the acute care setting to the home care setting. Discharge planning begins with the patient's admission to the hospital and must consider the possible need for follow-up home care. Several different personnel (e.g., social workers, home care nurses, and case managers) or agencies may be involved in the planning process.

The development of a comprehensive discharge plan requires collaboration with other professionals at both the referring agency and the home care agency, as well as the community agencies that provide specific resources upon discharge. The process involves identifying the patient's needs and developing a thorough plan to meet them. It is essential to have open lines of communication with family members to ensure their understanding and cooperation.

Community Resources and Referrals

As case managers, community-based nurses may make referrals to other team members, such as home health aides and social workers. These nurses work collaboratively with the health team and the referring agency or person. Continuous coordinated care among all health care providers involved in a patient's care is essential to avoid duplication of effort by the various personnel caring for the patient.

A community health nurse is knowledgeable about community resources available to patients as well as services provided by local agencies, eligibility requirements, and any possible charges for the services. Most communities have directories of health and social service agencies that the nurse can consult. These directories are continually updated as resources change. If a community does not have a resource booklet, an agency may develop one for its staff. It should include the commonly used community resources that patients need as well as the costs of the services and eligibility requirements. The telephone book and Internet are often useful in helping patients identify the location and accessibility of grocery and drug stores, banks, health care facilities, ambulances, physicians, dentists, pharmacists, social service agencies, and senior citizens' programs. In addition, a patient's place of worship or parish may be an important resource for services.

The community health nurse is responsible for informing the patient and family about the community resources available to meet their needs. During initial and subsequent home visits, the nurse helps the patient and family identify these community services and encourages them to contact the appropriate agencies. When appropriate, nurses may make the initial contact.

Home Visits

Most agencies have a policy manual that states their philosophy and procedures and defines the services they provide. Becoming familiar with these policies is an essential step before initiating a home visit. It is also important to know the agency's policies and the provincial/territorial law regarding what actions to take if the nurse finds a patient who has died, encounters an abusive situation in the family, determines that a patient cannot safely remain at home, or observes a situation that possibly indicates malicious harm to the community at large.

Before making a home visit, the nurse reviews the patient's referral form and other pertinent data concerning the patient. It may be necessary to contact the referring agency if the purpose for the referral is unclear or if important information is missing. The first step is to call the patient to obtain permission to visit, schedule a time for the visit, and verify the address. This initial phone conversation provides an opportunity to introduce oneself, identify the agency, and explain the reason for the visit. If a patient does not have a telephone, the nurse should see if the people who made the referral have a number where a phone message can be left for the patient. If an unannounced visit to a patient's home must be made, the nurse should ask permission to come in before entering the house. Explaining the purpose of the referral at the outset and setting up the times for future visits before leaving are also recommended.

Most agencies provide nurses with bags that contain standard supplies and equipment needed during home visits. It is important to keep the bag properly stocked and to bring any additional items that might be needed for the visit.

Personal Safety Precautions

Community nurses pay particular attention to personal safety, because their practice settings are often in unknown environments. Based on the principle of due diligence, agencies are required to inform employees of at-risk working environments. Agencies have policies and procedures concerning the promotion of safety for clinical staff, and training is provided to facilitate personal safety. Environments are proactively assessed for safety by the individual nurse and agency.

Whenever a nurse makes a home visit, the agency should know the nurse's schedule and the locations of the visits. The nurse needs to learn about the neighbourhood and obtain directions to the destination. A plan of action should always be established in case of emergencies. If a dangerous situation is encountered during the visit, the nurse should return to the agency and contact his or her supervisor or law enforcement officials, or both. Suggested precautions to take when making a home visit are presented in Chart 2-1.

CHART 2-1

Safety Precautions in Home Care

- Learn, or preprogram a cellular phone with the telephone numbers of the agency, police, and emergency services.
- Let the agency know your daily schedule and the telephone numbers of your patients so that you can be located if you do not return when expected.
- Know where the patient lives before leaving to make the visit and carry a map or GPS for quick referral.
- Keep your car in good working order and have sufficient gas in the tank.
- Park the car near the patient's home and lock it during the visit.
- Do not drive an expensive car or wear expensive jewelry when making visits.
- Know the regular bus schedule and know the routes when using public transportation or walking to the patient's house.
- Carry agency identification and have enough change to make telephone calls in case you get lost or have problems. Most agencies provide cellular phones for their nurses so that the agency can contact the nurse, and so that the nurse can contact the agency in case of an emergency or unexpected situation.
- When making visits in high-crime areas, visit with another person rather than alone.
- Schedule visits only during daylight hours.
- Never enter a patient's home uninvited.
- If you do not feel safe entering a patient's home, leave the area.
- Become familiar with the layout of the house, including exits from the house.
- If a patient or family member is intoxicated, hostile, or obnoxious, reschedule the visit and leave.
- If a family member is having a serious argument or abusing the patient or anyone else in the household, reschedule the visit, contact your supervisor, and report the abuse to the appropriate authorities.

Initial Home Visit

The first visit sets the tone for subsequent visits and is a crucial step in establishing the nurse–patient relationship. The situations encountered can vary depending on numerous factors. Patients may be in pain and unable to care for themselves. Families may be overwhelmed and doubt their ability to care for their loved one. They may not understand why the patient was sent home from the hospital before being totally rehabilitated. They may not comprehend what home care is or why they cannot have 24-hour nursing services. It is critical that the nurse try to convey an understanding of what the patient and family are experiencing and how the illness is affecting their lives.

During the initial home visit, which usually lasts up to an hour, the patient is evaluated and a plan of care is established to be followed or modified on subsequent visits. The nurse informs the patient of the agency's practices, policies, and hours of operation.

The initial assessment includes evaluating the individual patient, the home environment, the patient's self-care abilities or the family's ability to provide care, and the patient's need for additional resources. Identification of possible hazards, such as cluttered walk areas, potential fire risks, air or water pollution, or inadequate sanitation facilities, is also part of the initial assessment.

One important aspect of the transition from hospital to home is self-management of the medication regimen. Older adults may have multiple prescribers or may use alternative therapies such as herbal remedies as well as vitamins and other over-the-counter medications. The home health nurse may promote medication management by assisting with discrepancies such as wrong dosages, duplicate medications, omissions, or use of a medication for something other than the prescribed reason (Lancaster, Marek, Bub, et al., 2014). Some home health agencies mandate medication reconciliation at each visit, and the nurse as case manager works to develop a plan for future discharge from home health services.

Documentation considerations for home visits follow fairly specific regulations. The patient's needs and the nursing care given are documented accurately. The medical diagnosis and specific detailed information on the functional limitations of the patient are usually part of the documentation. The goals and the actions appropriate for attaining them need to be identified. Expected outcomes of the nursing interventions are stated in terms of patient behaviours and are to be realistic and measurable. They reflect the nursing diagnosis or the patient's conditions and specify those actions that address the patient's issues. Many digital and electronic innovations have been developed for use in home and community care, and some agencies provide home care nurses with handheld computers for documenting the condition of the patient, and results of the visit (Jones, 2016).

Determining the Need for Future Visits

While conducting an assessment of the patient's situation, the nurse evaluates the need for future visits and the frequency with which those visits may need to be made. To make these judgments, the nurse may find it helpful to consider the questions listed in Chart 2-2. With each subsequent visit, these same factors are evaluated to determine

CHART 2-2

Assessing the Need for Home Visits

Current Health Status
- How well is the patient progressing?
- How serious are the present signs and symptoms?
- Has the patient shown signs of progressing as expected? Or does it seem that recovery will be delayed?

Home Environment
- Are worrisome safety factors apparent?
- Are family or friends available to provide care? Or is the patient alone?

Level of Self-Care Ability
- Is the patient capable of self-care?
- What is the patient's level of independence?
- Is the patient ambulatory? Or bedridden?
- Does the patient have sufficient energy? Or is he or she frail and easily fatigued?
- Does the patient need and use assistive devices?

Level of Nursing Care Needed
- What level of nursing care does the patient require?
- Does the care require basic skills or more complex interventions?

Prognosis
- What is the expectation for recovery in this particular instance?
- What are the chances that complications may develop if nursing care is not provided?

Educational Needs
- How well has the patient or family grasped the teaching points made?
- Is there a need for further follow-up and retraining?
- What level of proficiency does the patient or family show in carrying out the necessary care?

Mental Status
- How alert is the patient?
- Are there signs of confusion or thinking difficulties?
- Does the patient tend to be forgetful or have a limited attention span?

Level of Adherence
- Is the patient following the instructions provided?
- Does the patient seem capable of following the instructions?
- Are the family members helpful, or are they unwilling or unable to assist in caring for the patient as expected?

the continuing health needs of the patient. As progress is made and the patient, with or without the help of significant others, becomes more capable of self-care and more independent, the need for home visits may decline.

Ending the Visit

As the visit comes to a close, it is important to summarize the main points of the visit for the patient and family and to identify expectations for future visits or patient achievements. The following points should be considered:

- What are the main points the patient or family should remember from the visit?
- What positive attributes have been noted about the patient and the family that will give them a sense of accomplishment?
- What were the main points of the teaching plan or the treatments needed to ensure that the patient and family understand what they must do? A written set of instructions should be left with the patient or family; provided they can read and see (alternative formats include video or audio recordings). Printed material should be in the patient's primary language and in large print when indicated.
- Whom should the patient or family call in case someone needs to be contacted immediately? Are current emergency telephone numbers readily available? Is telephone service available, or can an emergency cell phone service be provided?
- What signs of complications should be reported immediately?
- What is the date and time of the next visit? Will a different nurse make the visit? How frequently and for how long will visits be made (if determinable at this time)?

Other Community-Based Health Care Settings

Ambulatory Settings

Ambulatory health care is provided for patients in community- or hospital-based settings. The types of agencies that provide ambulatory health care are medical clinics, ambulatory care units, urgent care centres, cardiac rehabilitation programs, mental health centres, student health centres, community outreach programs, and nursing centres. Neighbourhood health centres provide services to patients who live in a geographically defined area. The centres may operate in freestanding buildings, storefronts, or mobile units. Agencies may provide ambulatory health care in addition to other services, such as offering an adult day care or health program. The kinds of services offered and the patients served depend on the agency's mission.

Nursing responsibilities in ambulatory health care settings include providing direct patient care, conducting patient intake screenings, treating patients with acute or chronic illnesses or emergency conditions, referring patients to other agencies for additional services, teaching patients self-care activities, and offering health education programs that promote health maintenance.

Nurses also work as clinic managers, direct the operation of clinics, and supervise other health team members. Nurse practitioners, educated in primary care, often practice in ambulatory care settings with a focus on gerontology, pediatrics, family or adult health, or women's health.

Nurses can play an important part in facilitating the function of the ambulatory care facility.

Occupational Health Programs

In Canada, health and safety standards in the workplace are legislated by provincial and territorial governments. The legislated standards are directed at creating safer and healthier work conditions. It is in an employer's interest to provide as safe a working environment as possible, because the result is reduced costs associated with employee absenteeism, hospitalization, and disability.

Occupational health nurses may work in solo units in industrial settings, or they may serve as consultants on a limited or part-time basis. They may be members of an interdisciplinary team composed of a variety of personnel such as nurses, physicians, exercise physiologists, health educators, counsellors, dietitians, safety engineers, and industrial hygienists. Occupational health nurses may:

- Provide direct care to employees who become ill or injured
- Conduct health education programs for company staff members
- Set up health programs aimed at establishing specific health behaviours, such as eating properly and getting enough exercise
- Monitor employees' hearing, vision, blood pressure, or blood glucose
- Track exposure to radiation, infectious diseases, and toxic substances, reporting results to government agencies as necessary

Occupational health nurses must be knowledgeable about government regulations pertaining to occupational health and safety and be familiar with other pertinent legislations.

School Health Programs

School health programs provide services to students and may also serve the school's community. School-age children and adolescents with health conditions are at major risk for underachieving or failing in school. The leading health conditions of elementary school children are injuries, infections (including influenza and pneumonia), malnutrition, dental disease, and cancer. The leading health concerns of high school students are alcohol and drug abuse, injuries, homicide, pregnancy, eating disorders, sexually transmitted infections (STIs), sports injuries, dental disease, and mental and emotional issues. Contemporary school health issues that are being examined include school violence, which may affect students' and teachers' physical and emotional health, and the increasing numbers of children and adolescents who are overweight or have obesity.

Ideally, school health programs have an interdisciplinary health team consisting of physicians, nurses, dentists, social workers, counsellors, school administrators, parents, and students. The school may serve as the site for a family health clinic that offers primary health and mental health services to children and adolescents as well as to all family members in the community. Nurse practitioners perform physical examinations and diagnose and treat students and families for acute and chronic illnesses within the scope of their practice. These clinics are cost effective and benefit students from low-income families who lack access to traditional health care.

School nurses play a number of roles, including care provider, health educator, consultant, and counsellor. They collaborate with students, parents, administrators, and other health and social service professionals regarding student health issues. School nurses perform health screenings, provide basic care for minor injuries and concerns, administer medications, monitor the immunization status of students and families, identify children with health concerns, provide teaching related to health maintenance and safety, and monitor the weight of children in order to facilitate prevention and treatment of obesity. They need to be knowledgeable about provincial/territorial and local regulations affecting school-age children, such as ordinances for excluding students from school because of communicable diseases or parasites such as lice or scabies.

School nurses are also health education consultants for teachers. In addition to providing information on health practices, teaching health classes, and participating in the development of the health education curriculum, school nurses educate teachers and classes when a student has a special issue, a disability, or a disease such as hemophilia, asthma, or human immunodeficiency virus (HIV) infection.

Care for People Who Are Experiencing Homelessness

While exact figures are unknown, it is estimated that 350,000 people are homeless each night in Canada (Gaetz, Dej, Richter, et al., 2016). The homeless population includes increasing numbers of women with children (often victims of abuse) and older adults. People who are homeless are a heterogeneous group, including members of dysfunctional families, the unemployed, and those who cannot find affordable housing. A significant number of persons who are homeless are chronically mentally ill and/or abuse alcohol or other drugs.

People who are homeless often have difficulty gaining access to health care. Because of numerous obstacles, they seek health care late in the course of a disease and deteriorate more quickly than other patients. Many of the health problems they experience are related in large part to their living situations. Street life exposes people who are homeless to the extremes of hot and cold environments and a culture of drugs, alcohol, and violence, all of which compound their health risks.

Persons who are homeless have high rates of trauma, tuberculosis, upper respiratory tract infections, poor nutrition and anemia, lice, scabies, peripheral vascular problems, STIs, dental issues, arthritis, hypothermia, skin disorders, and foot problems. Common chronic health conditions of people who are homeless include diabetes, hypertension, heart disease, AIDS, and mental illness. These health conditions are made more difficult by living on the street and by being discharged to a transitory, homeless shelter where follow-up is unlikely. Shelters are frequently overcrowded and unventilated, promoting the spread of communicable diseases such as tuberculosis.

Community health nurses who work with people who are homeless need to be nonjudgmental, patient, and understanding. They must be skilled in dealing with people who have a wide variety of health problems and needs and recognize that individualized treatment strategies are required in highly unpredictable contexts. Nursing interventions are aimed at assessing health care needs of people who live on the streets and in shelters, providing nursing care, and attempting to obtain other appropriate health care services for all people. Governments of many Canadian cities as well as officials of smaller communities are committed to locating/building appropriate housing and are making significant progress in reducing the number of people who are homeless. In 2007, Cathy Crowe (a street nurse in Toronto for 15 years) and a group of 10 activists who were homeless co-wrote a book—*Dying for a Home: Homeless Activists Speak Out*. The message is a call for nurses to advocate for the right to housing as a necessary prerequisite to health.

Critical Thinking Exercises

1 Recall a difficult discharge planning situation in which you have been involved. Evaluate the effectiveness of the processes used to accomplish the goals. What changes could have been made that would have improved the processes and the outcomes?

2 ebp An older adult man with diabetes is being referred for home care after discharge from the hospital, and he will need glucose monitoring and teaching. He has no family at home; his wife died 3 years ago, and his only daughter lives several hundred kilometres away. During the nurse's initial visit to the man's home, the nurse learns that he has difficulty seeing and therefore cannot read. What is the evidence for conducting a safety assessment of the home environment for older adult patients and for patients with visual limitations? Evaluate the strength of the evidence. What assessment criteria would you use to determine the needs of the patient's home care situation?

3 A 58-year-old woman who is an accountant and ready for discharge from the hospital has just experienced a mild stroke due to undiagnosed hypertension. Assessment reveals complete return of function and ability to perform ADLs. The woman impatiently states that "it's over and done, thank goodness, it's tax season and they need me back at work." Further discussion reveals she has not seen a health care practitioner since the birth of her children 30 years ago. Develop a teaching plan for this patient with rationale for including specific content and plans to use specific teaching approaches.

REFERENCES AND SELECTED READINGS

Books

Allender, J. A., Rector, C., & Warner, K. D. (2014). *Community & public health nursing: Promoting the public's health* (8th ed.). Philadelphia, PA: Lippincott Williams & Wilkins.

Crowe, C. (2007). *Dying for a home: Homeless activists speak out*. Toronto, ON: Between the Lines.

Dreachslin, J. L., Gilbert, M. J., & Malone, B. (2013). *Diversity and cultural competence in health care: A systems approach*. San Francisco, CA: Jossey-Bass.

Homeward Trust Edmonton. (2012). *Homeward Trust Edmonton 2012 Annual report*. Retrieved from http://www.homewardtrust.ca/images/files/2013-06-19-17-15HT%20Annual%20Report%202012%20WEB.pdf

Kozier, B., Erb, G., Berman, A., et al. (2018). *Fundamentals of Canadian nursing: Concepts, process, and practice* (4th ed.). Toronto, ON: Prentice Hall.

Lundy, K. S., & Janes, S. (2016). *Community health nursing: Caring for the public's health* (3rd ed.). Burlington, MA: Jones & Bartlett.

Stanhope, M., Lancaster, J., Jakubec, S. L., et al. (2017). *Community health nursing in Canada* (3rd ed.). Toronto, ON: Elsevier Canada.

Journals and Electronic Documents

Babenko-Mould, Y., & Elliott, J. (2015). Internationally educated nursing students' experiences of integration in the hospital setting. *Journal of Nursing Education and Practice*, *5*(9), 100–109.

Canadian Association of Schools of Nursing. (2018). *Educating nurses to address socio-cultural, historical, and contextual determinants of health among Aboriginal peoples*. Retrieved from https://www.casn.ca/2014/12/educating-nurses-address-socio-cultural-historical-contextual-determinants-health-among-aboriginal-peoples/

Canadian Nursing Students' Association. (2015). *Cultural safety in the context of Aboriginal health in nursing education*. Retrieved August 27, 2018, from http://cnsa.ca/wp-content/uploads/2016/01/NA-Position-Statement-Cultural-Safety-in-the-Context-of-Aboriginal-Health-in-Nursing-Education.pdf

Covel, C., Primeau, M., Kilpatrick, K., et al. (2017). Internationally educated nurses in Canada: Predictors of workforce integration. *Human Resources for Health*, *15*(1), 26.

Gaetz, S., Dej, E., Richter, T., et al. (2016). *The state of homelessness in Canada 2016*. Retrieved January 4, 2018, from http://homelesshub.ca/sites/default/files/SOHC16_final_20Oct2016.pdf

Health Canada. (2018). *Routine practices and additional precautions for preventing the transmission of infection in healthcare settings*. Retrieved September 11, 2018, from https://www.canada.ca/en/public-health/services/infectious-diseases/nosocomial-occupational-infections/routine-practices-additional-precautions-preventing-transmission-infection-healthcare-settings.html

Jones, K. (2016). *New technology: Empowering better health and home care*. Retrieved August 25, 2018, from http://www.homeandlong-termcare.ca/ew-technology-empowering-better-health-and-homecare/

Lancaster, R., Marek, K. D., Bub, L. D., et al. (2014). Medication regimens of frail older adults after discharge from home health care. *Home Healthcare Nurse*, *32*(9), 536–542.

Romanow, R. J. (2002). *Building on values: The future of health care in Canada—Final Report*. Retrieved from: http://publications.gc.ca/collections/Collection/CP32-85-2002E.pdf

Royal Commission on Aboriginal Peoples. (1996). *Royal commission report on Aboriginal peoples*. Retrieved from http://www.aadnc-aandc.gc.ca/eng/1307458586498/1307458751962

Resources

Aboriginal Nurses Association of Canada (ANAC): http://indigenousnurses.ca/

The Canadian Association for Occupational Health Nurses (COHNA): http://www.cohna-aciist.ca

The Canadian Association for Parish Nursing Ministry (CAPNM): http://www.capnm.ca

Canadian Nurses Association: https://www.cna-aiic.ca/en

Canadian Public Health Association: http://www.cpha.ca

Community Health Nurses of Canada (CHNC): https://www.chnc.ca/en/?lang=switch1

Health Canada: http://www.hc-sc.gc.ca

National Aboriginal Health Organization (NAHO): https://casw-acts.ca/en/national-aboriginal-health-organization

National Advisory Committee on Immunization: http://www.phac-aspc.gc.ca/naci-ccni/index-eng.php

Public Health Agency of Canada: http://www.phac-aspc.gc.ca

Victorian Order of Nurses: http://www.von.ca/

3 Critical Thinking, Ethical Decision Making, and the Nursing Process

Adapted by Joseph Osuji and Mohamed Toufic El Hussein

Learning Objectives

On completion of this chapter, the learner will be able to:

1. Define the characteristics of critical thinking and critical thinkers.
2. Describe the critical thinking process.
3. Define ethics and nursing ethics.
4. Identify several ethical dilemmas common to the medical-surgical area of nursing practice.
5. Specify strategies that can be helpful to nurses in ethical decision making.
6. Describe the components of the nursing process.
7. Develop a plan of nursing care for a patient using strategies of critical thinking.

In today's health care arena, nurses face increasingly complex issues and situations resulting from advanced technology, greater acuity of patients in both hospital and community settings, an aging population, and complex disease processes, as well as ethical issues and cultural factors. The decision-making part of the problem-solving activities of nurses has become increasingly multifaceted and requires **critical thinking**, based on sound ethical principles.

Critical Thinking

Critical thinking is a multidimensional skill, a cognitive or mental process or set of procedures. It involves reasoning and purposeful, systematic, reflective, rational, outcome-directed thinking based on a body of knowledge, as well as examination and analysis of all available information and ideas. Thoughts must not be taken at "face value"; rather, they must be analyzed and assessed for clarity, accuracy, relevance, depth, breadth, and logicalness (The Critical Thinking Community, 2013). Although many definitions of critical thinking have been offered in various disciplines, some consistent themes within those definitions are (1) a strong formal and informal foundation of knowledge; (2) willingness to pursue or ask questions; and (3) ability to develop solutions that are new, even those that do not fit the standard or current state of knowledge or attitudes. Willingness and openness to various viewpoints are inherent in critical thinking, and it is also important to reflect on the current situation (Chan, 2013). Critical thinking includes metacognition, the examination of one's own reasoning or thought processes, to help refine thinking skills. Independent judgments and decisions evolve from a sound knowledge base and the ability to synthesize information within the context in which it is presented. Nursing practice in today's society requires the use of high-level critical thinking skills. Critical thinking enhances clinical decision making, helping to identify patient needs and the best nursing actions that will assist patients in meeting those needs. This cognitive process is critical to effective use of the **nursing process** (Perez-Rivas, Martin-Iglesias, Pacheco del Cerro, et al., 2015).

As previously stated, critical thinking is a conscious, outcome-oriented activity. It is not erratic but rather is systematic and organized. Alfaro-LeFevre (2015) identified critical thinkers as people who ideally are active thinkers, fair minded, open minded, persistent, empathic, independent in thought, good communicators, honest, organized and systematic, proactive, flexible, realistic, humble, cognizant of the rules of logic, curious and insightful, and creative and committed to excellence. Critical thinkers are inquisitive truth seekers who are open to alternative solutions that might surface. The skills involved in critical thinking are developed over time through effort, practice, and experience.

Critical Thinking in Nursing Practice

Critical thinking enhances clinical decision making, helping to identify patient's needs and to determine the best nursing actions that will assist the patient in meeting those needs. Nurses must use critical thinking skills in all practice settings—acute care, ambulatory care, extended care, and the home and community. Regardless of the setting, each patient situation is viewed as unique and dynamic. The unique factors that patients and nurses bring to the health care situation are considered, studied, analyzed, and interpreted. Interpretation of the information then allows nurses to focus on those factors that are most relevant and most significant to the clinical situation. Decisions about what to do and how to do it are then developed into a plan of action.

In addition, much emphasis is placed on nurses basing their clinical actions on research, using evidence-based practice. Skills needed in critical thinking include interpretation, analysis, inference, explanation, **evaluation**, self-reflection, and self-regulation. Critical thinking requires strong background knowledge and knowledge of key concepts as well as logical thinking. Nurses use this disciplined process to validate the accuracy of data and the reliability of any assumptions they have made, and they then carefully evaluate the effectiveness of what they have identified as the necessary actions to take. Critical thinking is also reflective, involving metacognition, active evaluation, and refinement of the thinking process. Metacognition involves reflective thinking as well as awareness of the nursing skills needed for patient-centred care (Alfaro-LeFevre, 2015). Nurses engaged in critical thinking consider the possibility of cultural differences and personal bias when interpreting data and determining appropriate actions (see Chapter 8). Critical thinkers must be insightful and have a sense of fairness and integrity; the courage to question personal ethics; and the perseverance to strive continuously to minimize the effects of egocentricity, ethnocentricity, and other biases on the decision-making process (Alfaro-LeFevre, 2015).

Certain cognitive or mental activities are key components of critical thinking as it relates to nurses. Critical thinkers:

- Identify the priorities that will determine the nurse's plan of patient-centred care.
- Gather pertinent data from the patient's chart and **assessments** to determine why certain developments have occurred and to determine if additional data are needed to address the situation accurately.
- Validate the information presented to make sure that it is accurate and compare it with any pre-existing data. Information should be evidence based.

Glossary

assessment: the systematic collection of data to determine the patient's health status and any actual or potential health problems

collaborative problems: specific pathophysiologic manifestations that nurses monitor to detect onset or changes in status

critical thinking: a process of insightful thinking that utilizes multiple dimensions of one's cognition to develop conclusions, solutions, and alternatives that are appropriate for the given situation

deontologic or formalist theory: an ethical theory that states rational beings are ethically bound to act from a "sense of duty" independent of the ends or consequences

ethics: the formal, systematic approach used to understand, analyze, and evaluate matters of right and wrong as they relate to well-being

evaluation: determination of the patient's responses to the nursing interventions and the extent to which the outcomes have been achieved

implementation: actualization or carrying out of the plan of care through nursing interventions

moral dilemma: situation in which a clear conflict exists between two or more moral principles or competing moral claims that may be incompatible

moral distress: conflict that arises within oneself when a person is aware of the correct course of action but institutional constraints stand in the way of pursuing the correct action

moral problem: competing moral claim or principle; one claim or principle is clearly dominant

moral uncertainty: conflict that arises within a person when he or she cannot accurately define what the moral situation is or what moral principles apply but has a strong feeling that something is not right

morality: the adherence to informal personal values

nursing diagnoses: a clinical judgment concerning an individual's, family's, group's, or community's actual or potential health problems, state of health promotion, or potential risk that can be managed by independent nursing interventions

nursing process: a deliberate and systematic problem-solving approach for meeting people's health care and nursing needs; common components are assessment, diagnosis, planning, implementation, and evaluation

planning: development of goals and outcomes, as well as a plan of care designed to assist the patient in resolving the diagnosed problems and achieving the identified goals and desired outcomes

teleologic theory or consequentialism: the theoretical basis of ethics, which focuses on the ends or consequences of actions, such as utilitarianism

utilitarianism: a teleologic theory of ethics based on the concept of achieving "the greatest good for the greatest number" of people who may be affected by the action

- Analyze the information to determine its significance and to identify the formation of clusters or patterns that point to certain conclusions.
- Utilize logical thinking, past clinical experiences, theoretical knowledge, and intuitive thinking to assess the status of the patient's condition. Anticipate the patient's needs and outcomes while acknowledging personal bias and cultural influences.
- Maintain a flexible attitude that facilitates thinking and inquiry and consider all possibilities.
- Utilize inductive and deductive reasoning to identify available options and analyze each in terms of its advantages and disadvantages.
- Formulate decisions that reflect creativity and independent decision making.
- Demonstrate personal humility in terms of one's knowledge deficits and willingly seek additional information to assist with decision making.
- Exhibit the courage to seek new, innovative approaches to patient-centred care. Detach their personal viewpoints from situations and look at things objectively, a process called *bracketing*.

Critical thinking requires going beyond basic problem solving into a realm of inquisitive exploration, looking for all relevant factors that affect the issue, and being an "out-of-the-box" thinker. Nurses' ongoing quest for "best practice" clearly demonstrates intellectual integrity, a component of critical thinking.

Critical thinking and decision making are thought to be associated with improved clinical expertise. Critical thinking is the foundation of the process of clinical reasoning and clinical judgment (Alfaro-LeFevre, 2015). Using critical thinking to develop a plan of nursing care requires considering the human factors that might influence the plan. Nurses interact with patients, families, and other health care providers in the process of providing appropriate, individualized nursing care.

Nurses must use critical thinking skills in all practice settings—acute care, ambulatory care, extended care, and the home and community—and must view each patient situation as unique and dynamic. The unique factors that patients and nurses bring to the health care situation are considered, studied, analyzed, and interpreted. Interpretation of the information then allows nurses to focus on those factors that are most relevant and most significant to the clinical situation. Decisions about a nursing plan, priority of actions, and measurable outcomes are developed into an action plan.

In decision making related to the nursing process, nurses use cognitive and metacognitive skills as well as logical reasoning to set priorities. These skills include systematic and comprehensive assessment, recognition of assumptions and inconsistencies, verification of reliability and accuracy, identification of missing information, distinguishing relevant from irrelevant information, support of the evidence with facts and conclusions, priority setting with timely decision making, determination of patient-specific outcomes, and reassessment of responses and outcomes (Alfaro-LeFevre, 2015). All of these data are examined within the context of a solid knowledge base. For example, nurses use critical thinking, clinical reasoning, and decision-making skills in providing genetics-related nursing care when they:

- Assess and analyze family history data for genetic risk factors.
- Identify those individuals and families in need of referral for genetic testing or counselling.
- Ensure the privacy and confidentiality of genetic information.
- Maintain a knowledge base that is current and based on evidence-based research.

Because developing the skill of critical thinking involves experiential learning and practice, critical thinking exercises are offered at the end of each chapter as a means of honing the reader's ability to think critically. Some exercises include questions that stimulate the reader to seek information about evidence-based practice relative to the clinical situation described, whereas others challenge the reader to identify priority assessments and interventions. Additional exercises may be found in the study guide that accompanies the text. The questions listed in Chart 3-1 can serve as a guide in working through the exercises. It is important to remember that each clinical situation is unique and calls for an individualized approach that fits its unique set of circumstances. As critical thinking may require consideration of ethical principles and cultural contexts, these concepts are discussed in this chapter and in Chapter 8.

Ethical Nursing Care

There has been a heightened interest in the field of ethics in an attempt to gain a better understanding of how these issues influence us. Specifically, the focus on ethics in health care has intensified in response to controversial developments, including advances in technology and genetics, as well as diminished health care and financial resources.

Today, sophisticated technology can prolong life well beyond the time when death would have occurred in the past. Expensive experimental procedures, medications, equipment, and devices are available for attempting to preserve life, even when such attempts are likely to fail. The development of technologic support has influenced the quality and delivery of nursing care at all stages of life and also has contributed to an increase in average life expectancy. For example, the prenatal period has been influenced by genetic screening, in vitro fertilization, the harvesting and freezing of embryos, and prenatal surgery. Premature neonates who once would have died early in life now may survive because of advances in technology. Patients who would have died of organ failure are living longer because of organ or stem cell transplantation.

These advances in technology have been a mixed blessing. Questions have been raised about whether it is appropriate to use such technology, and if so, under what circumstances. Although many patients do achieve a better quality of life, others face extended suffering as a result of efforts to prolong life, usually at great expense. Ethical issues also surround those practices or policies that seem

CHART 3-1

The Inquiring Mind: Critical Thinking in Action

Throughout the critical thinking process, a continuous flow of questions evolves in the thinker's mind. It is not sufficient to rely solely on the acquisition of knowledge or a set of problem-solving skills; rather, it is the combination of one's application of knowledge, analysis of the situation, synthesis, and evaluation that promotes effective critical thinking inquiry. Although posing questions will vary according to the particular clinical situation, certain general inquiries can serve as a basis for reaching conclusions and determining a course of action.

When faced with a patient situation, seeking answers to some or all of the following questions may help to determine those actions that are most appropriate:

- What relevant assessment information do I need, and how do I interpret this information? What is the most effective way to gather this information? What does this information tell me? What contextual factors must be considered when gathering this information? What are the priority assessments?
- Have I identified the most important assessments and findings? Does the information I have gathered point to any other problems that I should consider?
- Have I gathered all of the necessary information (signs and symptoms, laboratory values, medication history, emotional factors, mental status)? Is anything missing?
- Is there anything that needs to be reported immediately? Do I need to seek additional assistance?
- What risks factors are specific to this patient? Which risk factors are of the highest priority? What must I do to minimize these risks?
- What possible complications must I anticipate?
- What are the most important problems in this situation? Do the patient and the patient's family recognize the same problems?
- What are the desired outcomes for this patient? Which have the highest priority? Do the patient and I agree on these points?
- What is going to be my first action in this situation? Why is this action a priority?
- How can I construct a plan of care to achieve the goals?
- Are there any age-related factors involved, and will they require some special approach? Will I need to make some change in the plan of care to take these factors into account?
- How do the family dynamics affect this situation, and will they affect my actions or the plan of care?
- Are there cultural factors that I must address and consider?
- Am I dealing with an ethical issue here? If so, how am I going to resolve it?
- Has any nursing research been conducted on this subject? What are the nursing implications of this research for care of this patient? What is the strength of the evidence found from research?

Adapted from Brudvig, T. J., Dirkes, A., Dutta, P., et al. (2013). Critical thinking in health care professional students: A systematic review. *Journal of Physical Therapy Education*, *27*(3), 12–25.

to allocate health care resources unjustly on the basis of age, race, gender, disability, or social mores. Older adults may be at risk for being denied health care because of their advanced age and the bias known as ageism. See Chapter 14 for a further discussion of ageism.

The ethical dilemmas nurses may encounter in the medical-surgical nursing arena are numerous and diverse and occur in all settings. An awareness of underlying philosophical concepts helps nurses use reason to work through these dilemmas. Basic concepts related to moral philosophy, such as ethics and its terminology, theories, and approaches, are included in this chapter. Understanding the role of the professional nurse in ethical decision making, not only helps nurses articulate their ethical positions and develop the skills needed to make ethical decisions, but also assists them use the nursing process to develop plans of care from an ethical perspective.

Ethics versus Morality

The terms **ethics** and **morality** are used to describe beliefs about right and wrong and to suggest appropriate guidelines for action. In essence, ethics is the formal, systematic study of moral beliefs, whereas morality is the adherence to informal personal values. Because the distinction between *ethics* and *morality* is slight, the two terms are often used interchangeably.

Ethics Theories

One classic theory in ethics is **teleologic theory or consequentialism**, which focuses on the ends or consequences of actions. The best-known form of this theory, **utilitarianism**, is based on the concept of "the greatest good for the greatest number." The choice of action is clear under this theory, because the action that maximizes good over bad is the correct one. The theory poses difficulty when one must judge intrinsic values and determine whose good is the greatest. In addition, it is important to ask whether good consequences can justify any amoral actions that might be used to achieve them.

Another theory in ethics is the **deontologic or formalist theory**, which argues that ethical standards or principles exist independently of the ends or consequences. In a given situation, one or more ethical principles may apply. Nurses have a duty to act based on the one relevant principle, or the most relevant of several ethical principles. Problems arise with this theory when personal and cultural biases influence the choice of the most primary ethical principle.

Approaches to Ethics

There are three approaches to ethics: meta-ethics, applied ethics, and relational ethics. An example of meta-ethics (understanding the concepts and linguistic terminology used in ethics) in the health care environment is analysis of the concept of informed consent. Nurses are aware that patients must give consent before surgery, but sometimes a question arises as to whether a patient is truly informed. Delving more deeply into the concept of informed consent would be a meta-ethical inquiry.

CHART 3-2

Common Ethical Principles

The following common ethical principles may be used to validate moral claims.

Autonomy

This word is derived from the Greek words *autos* ("self") and *nomos* ("rule" or "law"), and therefore refers to self-rule. In contemporary discourse it has broad meanings, including individual rights, privacy, and choice. Autonomy entails the ability to make a choice free from external constraints.

Beneficence

Beneficence is the duty to do good and the active promotion of benevolent acts (e.g., goodness, kindness, charity). It may also include the injunction not to inflict harm (see nonmaleficence).

Confidentiality

Confidentiality relates to the concept of privacy. Information obtained from an individual will not be disclosed to another unless it will benefit the person or there is a direct threat to the social good.

Double Effect

This is a principle that may morally justify some actions that produce both good and evil effects.

All four of the following criteria must be fulfilled:

1. The action itself is good or morally neutral.
2. The agent sincerely intends the good and not the evil effect (the evil effect may be foreseen but is not intended).
3. The good effect is not achieved by means of the evil effect.
4. There is proportionate or favourable balance of good over evil.

Fidelity

Fidelity is promise keeping; the duty to be faithful to one's commitments. It includes both explicit and implicit promises to another person.

Justice

From a broad perspective, justice states that like cases should be treated alike. A more restricted version of justice is *distributive justice*, which refers to the distribution of social benefits and burdens based on various criteria that may include the following:

- Equality
- Individual need
- Individual effort
- Societal contribution
- Individual merit
- Legal entitlement

Retributive justice is concerned with the distribution of punishment.

Nonmaleficence

This is the duty not to inflict harm as well as to prevent and remove harm. Nonmaleficence may be included within the principle of beneficence, in which case nonmaleficence would be more binding.

Paternalism

Paternalism is the intentional limitation of another's autonomy, justified by an appeal to beneficence or the welfare or needs of another. Under this principle, the prevention of evil or harm takes precedence over any potential evil caused by interference with the individual's autonomy or liberty.

Respect for Persons

Respect for persons is frequently used synonymously with *autonomy*. However, it goes beyond accepting the notion or attitude that people have autonomous choices, to treating others in such a way that enables them to make choices.

Sanctity of Life

This is the perspective that life is the highest good. Therefore, all forms of life, including mere biologic existence, should take precedence over external criteria for judging quality of life.

Veracity

Veracity is the obligation to tell the truth and not to lie or deceive others.

An example of applied ethics is when a specific discipline identifies ethical problems within that discipline's practice. Various disciplines use the frameworks of general ethical theories and principles and apply them to specific problems within their domain. Common ethical principles that apply in nursing include autonomy, beneficence, confidentiality, double effect, fidelity, justice, nonmaleficence, paternalism, respect for people, sanctity of life, and veracity. Brief definitions of these important principles can be found in Chart 3-2.

Nursing ethics may be considered a form of applied ethics because it addresses moral situations that are specific to the nursing profession and patient care. Some ethical problems that affect nursing may also apply to the broader area of bioethics and health care ethics. Nursing has its own professional code of ethics.

Relational ethics is a third approach to discussing ethics. According to Pollard (2015), "the central tenets of Relational Ethics are mutual respect, engagement, embodied knowledge, environment, and uncertainty. The most important of these is mutual respect, followed closely by engagement. Responsibility for the other is inherent in the relational ethic concept of mutual respect." The focus becomes asking the ethical question rather than trying to solve the ethical problem, like answering the question "what is the right thing to do?"

Moral Situations

Many situations exist in which ethical analysis is needed. Some are **moral dilemmas**, situations in which a clear conflict exists between two or more moral principles or competing moral claims, and nurses must choose the lesser of two evils. Other situations represent **moral problems**, in which there may be competing moral claims or principles, but one claim or principle is clearly dominant. Some situations result in **moral uncertainty**, when one cannot accurately define what the moral situation is or what moral principles apply but has a strong feeling that something is not right. Still other situations may result in **moral distress**, in which one is aware of the correct course of action but constraints stand in the way of pursuing the correct action.

For example, a patient tells a nurse that if he is dying he wants all possible measures taken to save his life. However, the surgeon and family have made the decision not to tell the patient that he is terminally ill and not to resuscitate him if he stops breathing. From an ethical perspective, the patient should be told the truth about his diagnosis and should have the opportunity to make decisions about treatment. Ideally, this information should come from the physician, with the nurse present to assist the patient in understanding the terminology and to provide further support, if necessary. In this situation, a moral problem exists because of the competing moral claims of the family and physician, who wish to spare the patient distress, and the nurse, who wishes to be truthful with the patient. If the patient's competency were questionable, a moral dilemma would exist because no dominant principle would be evident. The nurse could experience moral distress if the hospital threatened disciplinary action or job termination because the information is disclosed to the patient without the agreement of the physician or the family, or both.

It is essential that nurses freely engage in dialogue concerning moral situations, even though such dialogue is difficult for everyone involved. Improved interdisciplinary communication is supported when all members of the health care team can voice their concerns and come to an understanding of the moral situation. The use of an ethics consultant or consultation team could be helpful to assist the health care team, patient, and family to identify the moral dilemma and possible approaches to the dilemma. Nurses should be familiar with agency policy supporting patient self-determination and resolution of ethical issues.

Types of Ethical Problems in Nursing

As a profession, nursing is accountable to the society. Collectively, Canadian nursing has formally defined its standards of accountability through the *Code of Ethics for Registered Nurses* (Canadian Nurses Association [CNA], 2017). This code is structured around values and responsibilities that are providing safe, compassionate, competent, and ethical care; promoting health and well-being; promoting and respecting informed decision making; preserving dignity; promoting justice; and being accountable (CNA, 2017). The code offers an ideal framework for nurses to use in ethical decision making. Ethical issues have always affected the role of the professional nurse.

The accepted definition of professional nursing has inspired a new advocacy role for nurses. The International Council of Nurses (ICN, 2018, p. 1) states:

> Nursing encompasses autonomous and collaborative care of individuals of all ages, families, groups and communities, sick or well and in all settings. Nursing includes the promotion of health, prevention of illness, and the care of ill, disabled and dying people. Advocacy, promotion of a safe environment, research, participation in shaping health policy and in patient and health systems management, and education are also key nursing roles.

This definition supports the claim that nurses must be actively involved in the decision-making process regarding ethical concerns surrounding health care and human responses. Efforts to enact this standard may cause conflict in health care settings in which the traditional roles of the nurse are delineated within a bureaucratic structure. If, however, nurses learn to present ethical conflicts within a logical, systematic framework, struggles over jurisdictional boundaries may decrease. Health care settings in which nurses are valued members of the team promote interdisciplinary communication and may enhance patient care. To practice effectively in these settings, nurses must be aware of ethical issues and assist patients in voicing their moral concerns.

Nursing theories that incorporate the biopsychosocial–spiritual dimensions emphasize a holistic viewpoint, with humanism or caring at the core. As the nursing profession strives to delineate its own theory of ethics, caring and compassion are often cited as moral foundations. For nurses to embrace this professional ethos, they must be aware not only of major ethical dilemmas, but also of those daily interactions with health care consumers that frequently give rise to less easily identifiable ethical challenges. Although technologic advances and diminished resources have been instrumental in raising numerous ethical questions and controversies, including life-and-death issues, nurses should not ignore the many routine situations that involve ethical considerations. Some of the most common issues faced by nurses today include confidentiality, use of restraints, truth-telling, trust, refusing care, end-of-life concerns, and palliative care.

Confidentiality

All nurses should be aware of the confidential nature of information obtained in daily practice. If information is not pertinent, they should question whether it is prudent to document it in a patient's record. In the practice setting, discussion of patients with other members of the health care team is often necessary. However, these discussions should occur in a private area where it is unlikely that the conversation will be overheard. Nurses should also be aware that the use of family members or hospital ancillary personnel as interpreters for patients who are not fluent in English language or who are deaf violates patients' rights of confidentiality. The hospital or institution should provide translation services for non–English-speaking patients and interpreters for those who use sign language.

Another threat to confidentiality is the widespread use of computer-based technologies and people's easy access to them. The growing demand for telehealth innovations and the increasing use of this new method can result in unchecked access to health information. In addition, personal and health information is often made available to numerous individuals and corporate stakeholders, which may increase the potential for misuse of health care information. Because of the possibility of maleficence (see Chart 3-2), sensitivity to the principle of confidentiality is essential.

Restraints

The use of restraints (including physical and pharmacologic measures) and patient seclusions are additional issues with ethical overtones. It is important to weigh carefully the risks of limiting a person's autonomy and increasing the risk of injury by using restraints against the risks of not using restraints; they have been documented as resulting in physical harm and death. Before restraints are used, other strategies, such as asking family members to sit with the patient, should be tried. The Patient Safety Institute of Canada considers physical restraint never a part of treatment, under any circumstances. Further, any restraint should be considered an intervention of last resort and should, at most, only be used temporarily in a behavioural emergency (The Patient Safety Education Program Canada [PSEP], 2018).

Trust Issues

Truth-telling or veracity is one of the basic principles in the nurse–patient relationship. Truth-telling is based upon the principle of autonomy and the patient's "rational capacity for self-determination" (Vaughn, 2016).

Three ethical dilemmas in clinical practice that can directly conflict with this principle are the use of placebos (nonactive substances used for treatment), not revealing a diagnosis to a patient, and revealing a diagnosis to people other than the patient with the diagnosis. All involve the issue of trust, which is an essential element in the nurse–patient relationship.

Placebos may be used in experimental research, in which a patient is involved in the decision-making process and is aware that placebos are being used in the treatment regimen. However, the use of a placebo as a substitute for an active drug to show that a patient does not have actual symptoms of a disease is deceptive, and this practice may severely undermine the nurse–patient relationship.

Informing a patient of his or her diagnosis when the family and physician have chosen to withhold information is a common ethical situation in nursing practice. The nursing staff may often use evasive comments with the patient as a means of maintaining professional relationships with other health practitioners. This area is indeed complex, because it challenges a nurse's integrity. Strategies nurses could consider include the following:

- Not lying to the patient
- Providing all information related to nursing procedures and diagnoses
- Communicating the patient's requests for information to the family and physician—the family is often unaware of the patient's repeated questions to the nurse; with a better understanding of the situation, the family members may change their perspective
- Make referral to institutional ethics committee when not sure of line of action

Although providing the information may be the morally appropriate behaviour, the manner in which the patient is told is important. Nurses must be compassionate and caring while informing patients; disclosure of information merely for the sake of patient autonomy does not convey respect for others. Family support or the support of a spiritual advisor (e.g., chaplain) may be needed to reduce the impact of distressing information or a poor prognosis.

Refusing to Provide Care

Any nurse who feels compelled to refuse to provide care for a particular type of patient faces an ethical dilemma. The reasons given for refusal range from a conflict of personal values to fear of injury to self or the patient. However, there is an ethical obligation to care for all patients, and nurses must be accountable. In the section on "Being Accountable," the *Code of Ethics for Registered Nurses* includes the following statement:

> If nursing care is requested that is in conflict with the nurse's moral beliefs and values but in keeping with professional practice, the nurse provides safe, compassionate, competent and ethical care until alternative care arrangements are in place to meet the person's needs or desires. If nurses can anticipate a conflict with their conscience, they have an obligation to notify their employers. (CNA, 2017)

To avoid facing these ethical situations, a nurse can follow certain strategies. For example, when applying for a job, one should ask questions regarding the patient population. If the applicant is uncomfortable with a particular situation, then not accepting the position would be an option. Denial of care, or providing substandard nursing care to some members of our society, is not an acceptable nursing practice.

End-of-Life Issues

Dilemmas that centre on death and dying are prevalent in medical-surgical nursing practice and frequently initiate ethical discussion (CNA, 2017). The dilemmas are compounded by the fact that the idea of curing is paramount in health care. With advanced technology, it may be difficult to accept the fact that nothing more can be done or that technology may prolong life but at the expense of comfort and quality of life. Focusing on the caring as well as the curing role may assist nurses in dealing with these difficult ethical situations. End-of-life issues are discussed in detail in Chapter 15. Many people who are terminally ill seek legal options for a peaceful and dignified death. Nurses who deliver palliative care must understand that their actions are targeted at relieving pain and suffering and not hastening death. End-of-life issues shift the focus from curative care to palliative and end-of-life care. Needs of patients and families require holistic a nd interdisciplinary approaches. End-of-life issues that often involve ethical dilemmas include pain control, "do not resuscitate" orders, life support measures, and administration of food and fluids. These issues are discussed in detail in Chapter 15.

Preventive Ethics

When a nurse is faced with two conflicting alternatives, it is his or her moral decision to choose the lesser of the two evils. Various preventive strategies are available to help nurses anticipate or avoid certain kinds of ethical dilemmas. Frequently, dilemmas occur when health care practitioners are unsure of the patient's wishes because the patient is unconscious or too cognitively impaired to communicate directly. Encouraging patients to prepare advance directives serves in the prevention of these dilemmas.

Advance Directives

An advance directive is a legal document that specifies a person's wishes prior to illness (and before hospitalization) and provides valuable information that may assist health care providers in decision making (Health Canada, 2018). This directive is used only if the person is unable to speak for him or herself, and it is revoked if the person regains the ability to make decisions. Whereas one tends to think that the advance directive contains information about treatments that are not to be initiated or maintained, it can also provide the direction that active, potentially lifesaving treatment is to occur. An advance directive usually includes the name of a substitute decision maker who has agreed to make decisions that respect the instructions contained within the document.

Each province and two of the three territories have advance directive legislation with information on what to include and how to ensure that the directive is legally binding. All advance directives in Canada are about future health care decisions. There are fines or other penalties in place if an advance directive is not followed. The provinces and territories have laws that regulate how individuals can arrange for another person to manage their financial affairs if they become physically unable to do so themselves (power of attorney). This type of power of attorney ends if the signer becomes mentally incompetent. Of more importance is the durable power of attorney, in which an individual identifies another person to make health care decisions on his or her behalf. In this type of directive, the person may have clarified his or her wishes concerning a variety of medical situations. The benefit of a durable power of attorney is that it continues even if the signer becomes mentally incompetent.

The heightened interest in ethical decision making has resulted in many continuing education programs, ranging from seminars or workshops to full-semester courses offered by local colleges or professional organizations. In addition, nursing and medical journals contain articles on ethical issues, and numerous textbooks on clinical ethics or nursing ethics are available. These are valuable resources because they cover the ethical theory and dilemmas of practice in greater depth. The CNA also has publications available to assist nurses with ethical decision making.

Ethics Committees

Institutional ethics committees exist in many hospitals to assist clinicians with ethical dilemmas. The purpose of these interdisciplinary committees varies among institutions. In some hospitals, the committees exist solely for the purpose of developing policies, whereas in others, they may have a strong educational or consultation focus. These committees usually are composed of people with some advanced training in ethics and are important resources for the health care team, patient, and family. Nurses with a particular interest or expertise in the area of ethics can serve as members of these committees, which are valuable resources for staff nurses.

Ethical Decision Making

Ethical dilemmas are common and diverse in nursing practice. Situations vary, and experience indicates that there are no clear solutions to these dilemmas, which may be referred to as a slippery slope (Pozgar, 2016). However, the fundamental philosophical principles are the same, and the process of moral reflection helps nurses justify their actions. The systematic approach to ethical decision making can follow the steps of the nursing process. Ethics charts contained in all units within this text present case scenarios that challenge the reader to identify the ethical principles involved that may or may not be in conflict (see Chart 3-2). Chart 3-3 outlines the steps of an ethical analysis that may be used to resolve the moral dilemmas presented in these charts.

The Nursing Process

Definition

The nursing process is a deliberate problem-solving approach for meeting people's health care and nursing needs. Although the steps of the nursing process have been stated in various ways by different writers, the common components cited are assessment, diagnosis, **planning**, **implementation**, and evaluation (Carpenito, 2017). The traditional steps are defined as follows:

1. *Assessment:* The systematic collection of data to determine the patient's health status and any actual or potential health problems. (Analysis of data is included as part of the assessment. Analysis may also be identified as a separate step of the nursing process.)
2. *Diagnosis:* Identification of the following two types of patient problems:
   - *Nursing diagnoses:* Clinical judgment on actual or potential health problems that can be managed by independent nursing interventions.
   - *Collaborative problems:* "Certain physiologic complications that nurses monitor to detect onset or changes in status. Nurses manage **collaborative problems** using physician-prescribed and nurse-prescribed interventions to minimize the complications of the events" (Carpenito, 2017, p. 9).
3. *Planning:* Development of goals and outcomes, as well as a plan of care designed to assist the patient in resolving the diagnosed problems and achieving the identified goals and desired outcomes
4. *Implementation:* Actualization of the plan of care through nursing interventions
5. *Evaluation:* Determination of the patient's responses to the nursing interventions and the extent to which the outcomes have been achieved

Dividing the nursing process into distinct steps serves to emphasize the essential nursing actions that must be taken to address the patient's **nursing diagnoses** and manage any collaborative problems or complications. However, dividing the process into separate steps is artificial—the process

CHART 3-3

Steps of an Ethical Analysis

The following are guidelines to assist nurses in ethical decision making. These guidelines reflect an active process in decision making, similar to the nursing process detailed in this chapter.

Assessment

1. Assess the ethical/moral situations of the problem. This step entails recognition of the ethical, legal, and professional dimensions involved.
   a. Does the situation entail substantive moral problems (conflicts among ethical principles or professional obligations)?
   b. Are there procedural conflicts? (e.g., Who should make the decisions? Any conflicts among the patient, health care providers, family, and guardians?)
   c. Identify the significant people involved and those affected by the decision.

Planning

1. Collect information.
   a. Include the following information: the medical facts, treatment options, nursing diagnoses, legal data, and the values, beliefs, and religious components.
   b. Make a distinction between the factual information and the values/beliefs.
   c. Validate the patient's capacity, or lack of capacity, to make decisions.
   d. Identify any other relevant information that should be elicited.
   e. Identify the ethical/moral issues and the competing claims.

Implementation

1. List the alternatives. Compare alternatives with applicable ethical principles and professional code of ethics. Choose either of the frameworks below, or other frameworks, and compare outcomes.
   a. *Utilitarian approach:* Predict the consequences of the alternatives; assign a positive or negative value to each consequence; choose the consequence that predicts the highest positive value or "the greatest good for the greatest number."
   b. *Deontologic approach:* Identify the relevant moral principles; compare alternatives with moral principles; appeal to the "higher-level" moral principle if there is a conflict.

Evaluation

1. Decide and evaluate the decision.
   a. What is the best or morally correct action?
   b. Give the ethical reasons for your decision.
   c. What are the ethical reasons against your decision?
   d. How do you respond to the reasons against your decision?

functions as an integrated whole, with the steps being interrelated, interdependent, and recurrent (Fig. 3-1). Chart 3-4 presents an overview of the nursing activities involved in applying the nursing process. Note that the use of the nursing process requires critical thinking and consideration of common ethical principles to ensure that a truly comprehensive plan is developed.

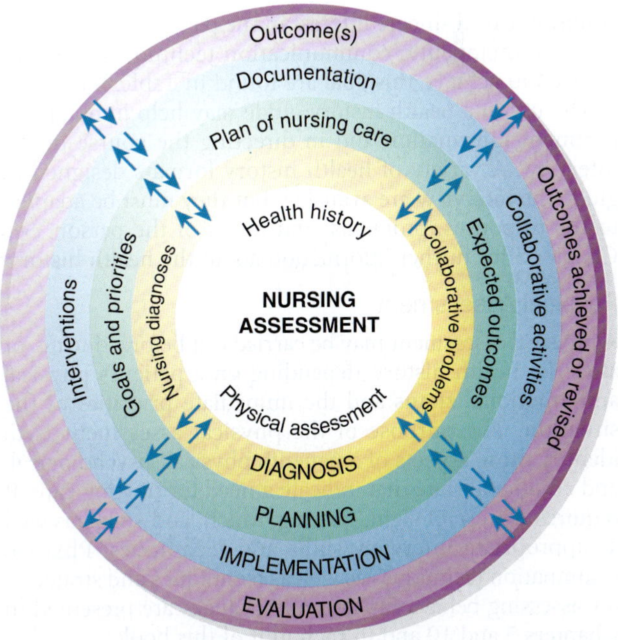

FIGURE 3-1. The nursing process is depicted schematically in this circle. Starting from the innermost circle, nursing assessment, the process moves outward through the formulation of nursing diagnoses and collaborative problems; planning, with setting of goals and priorities in the nursing plan of care; implementation and documentation; and, finally, the ongoing process of evaluation and outcomes.

Using the Nursing Process

Assessment

According to Carpenito (2017), the initial or baseline assessment is a systematic process of collecting predetermined data during the first contact with the patient. Data are gathered through the health history and the physical assessment. In addition, ongoing assessment and monitoring are crucial to remain aware of changing patient needs and the effectiveness of nursing care.

Health History

The health history is conducted to determine a person's state of wellness or illness and is best accomplished as part of a planned interview. The interview is a personal dialogue between a patient and a nurse that is conducted to obtain information. The nurse's approach to the patient largely determines the amount and quality of the information that is received. To achieve a relationship of mutual trust and respect, the nurse must have the ability to

CHART 3-4

Steps of the Nursing Process

Assessment

1. Conduct the health history.
2. Perform the physical assessment.
3. Interview the patient's family or significant others.
4. Study the health record.
5. Organize, analyze, synthesize, and summarize the collected data.

Diagnosis

NURSING DIAGNOSIS

1. Identify the patient's nursing problems.
2. Identify the defining characteristics of the nursing problems.
3. Identify the etiology of the nursing problems.
4. State nursing diagnoses concisely and precisely.

COLLABORATIVE PROBLEMS

1. Identify potential problems or complications that require collaborative interventions.
2. Identify health team members with whom collaboration is essential.

Planning

1. Assign priority to the nursing diagnoses.
2. Specify the goals.
   a. Develop immediate, intermediate, and long-term goals.
   b. State the goals in realistic and measurable terms.
3. Identify nursing interventions appropriate for goal attainment.
4. Establish expected outcomes.
   a. Make sure that the outcomes are realistic and measurable.
   b. Identify critical times for the attainment of outcomes.
5. Develop the written plan of nursing care.
   a. Include nursing diagnoses, goals, nursing interventions, expected outcomes, and critical times.
   b. Write all entries precisely, concisely, and systematically.
   c. Keep the plan current and flexible to meet the patient's changing problems and needs.
6. Involve the patient, family or significant others, nursing team members, and other health team members in all aspects of planning.

Implementation

1. Put the plan of nursing care into action.
2. Coordinate the activities of the patient, family or significant others, nursing team members, and other health team members.
3. Record the patient's responses to the nursing actions.

Evaluation

1. Collect data.
2. Compare the patient's actual outcomes with the expected outcomes. Determine the extent to which the expected outcomes were achieved.
3. Include the patient, family or significant others, nursing team members, and other health care team members in the evaluation.
4. Identify alterations that need to be made in the nursing diagnoses, collaborative problems, goals, nursing interventions, and expected outcomes.
5. Continue all steps of the nursing process: assessment, diagnosis, planning, implementation, and evaluation.

communicate a sincere interest in the patient. Examples of effective therapeutic communication techniques that can be used to achieve this goal are found in Table 3-1.

The use of a health history guide may help in obtaining pertinent information and in directing the course of the interview. A variety of health history formats designed to guide the interview are available, but they must be adapted to the responses, problems, and needs of the person. See Chapter 5 for further information about the health history.

Physical Assessment

A physical assessment may be carried out before, during, or after the health history, depending on a patient's physical and emotional status and the immediate priorities of the situation. The purpose of the physical assessment is to identify those aspects of a patient's physical, psychological, and emotional state that indicate a need for nursing care. It requires the use of sight, hearing, touch, and smell, as well as appropriate interview skills and techniques. Physical examination techniques as well as techniques and strategies for assessing behaviours and role changes are presented in Chapters 5 and 10 and in each unit of this book.

Other Components of the Assessment

Additional relevant information should be obtained from the patient's family or significant others, from other members of the health team, and from the patient's health record or chart. Depending on the patient's immediate needs, this information may have been completed before the health history and the physical assessment were obtained. A review of past medical history or records from previous admissions may provide important and relevant information to be considered. Whatever the sequence of events, it is important to use all available sources of pertinent data to complete the nursing assessment.

Recording the Data

After the health history and physical assessment are completed, the information obtained is recorded in the patient's permanent record. These records, which are more commonly becoming electronic (i.e., electronic health records [EHRs]), provide a means of communication among members of the health care team and facilitate coordinated planning and continuity of care (Perez-Rivas et al., 2015). The record fulfills other functions as well:

- It serves as the legal and business record for a health care agency and for the professional staff members who are responsible for the patient's care. A variety of systems are used for documenting patient care, and each health care agency selects the system that best meets its needs.
- It serves as a basis for evaluating the quality and appropriateness of care and for reviewing the effective use of patient care services.
- It provides data that are useful in research, education, and short- and long-range planning.

TABLE 3-1 Therapeutic Communication Techniques

Technique	Definition	Therapeutic Value
Listening	Active process of receiving information and examining one's reactions to the messages received	Nonverbally communicates nurse's interest in patient
Silence	Periods of no verbal communication among participants for therapeutic reasons	Gives patient time to think and gain insights, slows the pace of the interaction, and encourages the patient to initiate conversation, while conveying the nurse's support, understanding, and acceptance
Restating	Repeating to the patient what the nurse believes is the main thought or idea expressed	Demonstrates that the nurse is listening and validates, reinforces, or calls attention to something important that has been said
Reflection	Directing back to the patient his or her feelings, ideas, questions, or content	Validates the nurse's understanding of what the patient is saying and signifies empathy, interest, and respect for the patient
Clarification	Asking the patient to explain what he or she means or attempting to verbalize vague ideas or unclear thoughts of the patient to enhance the nurse's understanding	Helps to clarify the patient's feelings, ideas, and perceptions and to provide an explicit correlation between them and the patient's actions
Focusing	Questions or statements to help the patient develop or expand an idea	Allows the patient to discuss central issues and keeps communication goal directed
Broad openings	Encouraging the patient to select topics for discussion	Indicates acceptance by the nurse and the value of the patient's initiative
Humour	Discharge of energy through the comic enjoyment of the imperfect	Promotes insight by bringing repressed material to consciousness, resolving paradoxes, tempering aggression, and revealing new options; a socially acceptable form of sublimation
Informing	Providing information	Helpful in health teaching or patient education about relevant aspects of patient's well-being and self-care
Sharing perceptions	Asking the patient to verify the nurse's understanding of what the patient is thinking or feeling	Conveys the nurse's understanding to the patient and has the potential to clarify confusing communication
Theme identification	Underlying issues or problems experienced by the patient that emerge repeatedly during the course of the nurse–patient relationship	Allows the nurse to best promote the patient's exploration and understanding of important problems
Suggesting	Presentation of alternative ideas for the patient's consideration relative to problem solving	Increases the patient's perceived options or choices

Adapted from Stuart, G. W. (2012). *Principles and practice of psychiatric nursing* (10th ed.). St Louis, MO: Mosby.

Diagnosis

The assessment component of the nursing process serves as the basis for identifying nursing diagnoses and collaborative problems. Soon after the completion of the health history and the physical assessment, nurses organize, analyze, synthesize, and summarize the data collected and determine the patient's need for nursing care.

Nursing Diagnosis

Nursing diagnoses, the first taxonomy created in nursing, have fostered autonomy and accountability in nursing and have helped delineate the scope of practice.

North American Nursing Diagnosis Association (NANDA) International is the official organization responsible for developing the taxonomy of nursing diagnoses and formulating nursing diagnoses acceptable for study. Approved nursing diagnoses are compiled and categorized by NANDA International in a taxonomy that is updated to maintain currency. The revised diagnostic labels (and associated definitions and defining characteristics, as well as risk factors for potential problems) identified by NANDA International (Herdman & Kamitsuru, 2018) have been generally accepted, but ongoing validation, refinement, and expansion based on clinical use and research are encouraged.

Choosing a Nursing Diagnosis

When identifying the nursing diagnoses for a particular patient, nurses must first identify the commonalities among the assessment data collected. These common features lead to the categorization of related data that reveal the existence of a problem and the need for nursing intervention. The identified problems are then defined as specific nursing diagnoses. Nursing diagnoses represent actual or potential health problems, state of health promotion, or potential risks that can be managed by independent nursing actions.

It is important to remember that nursing diagnoses are not medical diagnoses; they are not medical treatments prescribed by the physician, and they are not diagnostic studies. Rather, they are succinct statements in terms of specific patient problems that guide nurses in the development of the nursing plan of care.

To give additional meaning to the nursing diagnosis, the characteristics and etiology of the problem are identified and included as part of the diagnosis. For example, the nursing diagnoses and their defining characteristics and etiology for a patient who has anemia may include the following:

- Activity intolerance related to weakness and fatigue
- Ineffective tissue perfusion related to decreased hemoglobin
- Imbalanced nutrition—less than body requirements related to fatigue and inadequate intake of essential nutrients

Collaborative Problems

In addition to nursing diagnoses and their related nursing interventions, nursing practice involves certain situations and interventions that do not fall within the definition of nursing diagnoses. These activities pertain to potential problems or complications that are medical in origin and require collaborative interventions with the physician and other members of the health care team. The term *collaborative problem* is used to identify these situations.

Collaborative problems are certain physiologic complications that nurses monitor to detect changes in status or onset of complications. Nurses manage collaborative problems using physician- and nurse-prescribed interventions to minimize complications (Carpenito, 2017). When treating collaborative problems, a primary nursing focus is monitoring patients for the onset of complications or changes in the status of existing complications. The complications are usually related to the disease process, treatments, medications, or diagnostic studies. The nurse recommends nursing interventions that are appropriate for managing the complications and implements the treatments prescribed by the physician. According to Carpenito (2017), collaborative problems do not have patient goals; therefore, the approach to evaluation is different from a nursing diagnosis. The algorithm in Figure 3-2 depicts the differences between nursing diagnoses and collaborative problems. After the nursing diagnoses and collaborative problems have been identified, they are recorded on the plan of nursing care.

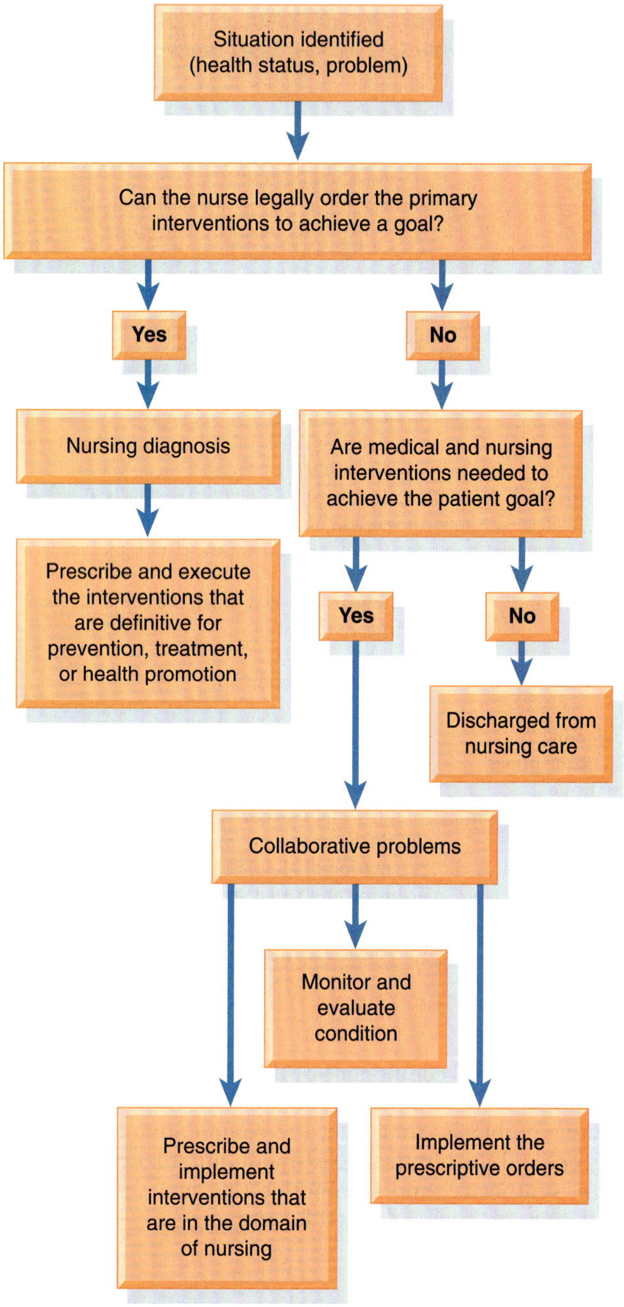

FIGURE 3-2. Differentiating nursing diagnoses and collaborative problems. (Redrawn from Carpenito, L. J. [2017]. *Nursing diagnosis: Application to clinical practice* [15th ed.]. Philadelphia, PA: Lippincott Williams & Wilkins.)

Planning

Once the nursing diagnoses have been identified, the planning component of the nursing process begins. This phase involves the following steps:

1. Assigning priorities to the nursing diagnoses and collaborative problems
2. Specifying expected outcomes
3. Specifying the immediate, intermediate, and long-term goals of nursing action
4. Identifying specific nursing interventions appropriate for attaining the outcomes
5. Identifying interdependent interventions
6. Documenting the nursing diagnoses, collaborative problems, expected outcomes, nursing goals, and nursing interventions on the plan of nursing care
7. Communicating to appropriate personnel any assessment data that point to health care needs that can best be met by other members of the health care team

Setting Priorities

Assigning priorities to the nursing diagnoses and collaborative problems is a joint effort by the nurse and the patient or family members. Any disagreement about priorities is resolved in a way that is mutually acceptable. Consideration must be given to the urgency of the problems, with the most critical problems receiving the highest priority. The Maslow's hierarchy of needs provides one framework for prioritizing problems, with importance being given first to physical needs; once those basic needs are met, higher-level needs can be addressed. See Chapter 1 for a further discussion of the Maslow's hierarchy.

Establishing Expected Outcomes

Expected outcomes of the nursing interventions, identified either as long term or short term, are written in terms of the patient's behaviours and the time period in which the outcomes are to be met. The outcomes must be attainable and quantifiable (Carpenito, 2017). Resources for identifying appropriate expected outcomes include the Nursing Outcomes Classification (NOC) (Moorhead, Swanson, Johnson, et al., 2018) and standard outcome criteria established by health care agencies for people with specific health problems. These outcomes can be associated with nursing diagnoses and interventions and can be used when appropriate. However, the NOC may need to be adapted to establish realistic criteria for the specific patient involved.

The expected outcomes that define the desired behaviour of the patient are used to measure the progress made toward resolving the problem. The expected outcomes also serve as the basis for evaluating the effectiveness of the nursing interventions and for deciding whether additional nursing care is needed or whether the plan of care needs to be revised.

Establishing Goals

After the priorities of the nursing diagnoses and expected outcomes have been established, goals (immediate, intermediate, and long term) and the nursing actions appropriate for attaining the goals are identified. The patient and family are included in establishing goals for the nursing actions. Immediate goals are those that can be attained within a short period. Intermediate and long-term goals require a longer time to be achieved and usually involve preventing complications and other health problems and promoting self-care and rehabilitation. For example, goals for a patient with a nursing diagnosis of impaired physical mobility related to pain and edema following total knee replacement may be stated as follows:

- Immediate goal: Stands at bedside for 5 minutes 6 to 12 hours after surgery
- Intermediate goal: Ambulates 15 to 20 minutes with walker or crutches in hospital and home
- Long-term goal: Ambulates independently 1 to 2 km each day

Determining Nursing Actions

In planning appropriate nursing actions to achieve the desired goals and outcomes, the nurse, with input from the patient and significant others, identifies individualized interventions based on the patient's circumstances and preferences that address each outcome. Interventions should identify the activities needed and who will implement them, as well as the frequency. Determination of interdisciplinary activities is made in collaboration with other health care providers as needed. The patient's medications and other prescribed treatments should be integrated into the plan of care to assist the nurse in determining how all interventions contribute to resolution of the identified problems.

The nurse identifies and plans patient teaching and demonstration as needed to assist the patient in learning certain self-care activities. Planned interventions should be ethical and appropriate to the patient's culture, age, and gender. Standardized interventions, such as those found on institutional care plans or in the Nursing Interventions Classification (NIC) (Butcher, Bulechek, Dochterman, et al., 2018), can be used. It is important to individualize prewritten interventions to promote optimal effectiveness for each patient. Actions of nurses should be based on established standards.

Implementation

The implementation phase of the nursing process involves carrying out the proposed plan of nursing care. The nurse assumes responsibility for the implementation and coordinates the activities of all those involved in implementation, including the patient and family, other members of the nursing team, and other members of the health care team, so that the schedule of activities facilitates the patient's recovery. The plan of nursing care serves as the basis for implementation, as described below:

- The immediate, intermediate, and long-term goals are used as a focus for the implementation of the designated nursing interventions.
- While implementing nursing care, the nurse continually assesses the patient and his or her response to the nursing care.
- Revisions are made in the plan of care as the patient's condition, problems, and responses change and when reordering of priorities is required.

Implementation includes direct or indirect execution of the planned interventions. It is focused on resolving the patient's nursing diagnoses and collaborative problems and achieving expected outcomes, thus meeting the patient's health needs.

The following are examples of nursing interventions:

- Reposition the patient every 2 hours around the clock
- Teach and reinforce the use of guided imagery to reduce pain prior to invasive procedures
- Monitor oral and intravenous fluid intake to ensure that 2,000 mL of fluids has been received
- Position the patient in an upright position in a chair for 15 minutes before meals
- Apply lanolin to the patient's lips every 2 hours and as needed (i.e., pro re nata [prn])
- Teach the patient and family the correct way to apply a wedge splint prior to sleep
- Promote a therapeutic relationship

Judgment, critical thinking, and good decision-making skills are essential in the selection of appropriate evidence-based and ethical nursing interventions. All nursing interventions are patient focused and outcome directed and are implemented with compassion, confidence, and a willingness to accept and understand the patient's responses. Note that implementation is nursing action. Therefore, statements involving implementation always start with a verb.

Although many nursing actions are independent, others are interdependent, such as carrying out prescribed treatments, administering medications and therapies, and collaborating with other health care team members to accomplish specific expected outcomes and to monitor and manage potential complications. Such interdependent functioning is just that—interdependent. Requests or orders from other health care team members should not be followed blindly but should be assessed critically and questioned when necessary. The implementation phase of the nursing process ends when the nursing interventions have been completed.

Evaluation

Evaluation, the final step of the nursing process, allows the nurse to determine the patient's response to the nursing interventions and the extent to which the objectives have been achieved. The plan of nursing care is the basis for evaluation. The nursing diagnoses, collaborative problems, priorities, nursing interventions, and expected outcomes provide the specific guidelines that dictate the focus of the evaluation. Through evaluation, the nurse can answer the following questions:

- Were the nursing diagnoses and collaborative problems accurate?
- Did the patient achieve the expected outcomes within the critical time periods?
- Have the patient's nursing diagnoses been resolved?
- Have the collaborative problems been resolved?

- Do priorities need to be reordered?
- Have the patient's nursing needs been met?
- Should the nursing interventions be continued, revised, or discontinued?
- Have new problems evolved for which nursing interventions have not been planned or implemented?
- What factors influenced the achievement or lack of achievement of the objectives?
- Should changes be made in the expected outcomes and outcome criteria?

Objective data that provide answers to these questions are collected from all available sources (e.g., patients, families, significant others, health care team members). These data are included in patients' records and must be substantiated by direct patient observation before the outcomes are documented.

Documentation of Outcomes and Revision of Plan

Outcomes are documented concisely and objectively. Documentation should relate outcomes to the nursing diagnoses and collaborative problems, describe the patient's responses to the interventions, indicate whether the outcomes were met, and include any additional pertinent data. As noted previously, the nurse individualizes a plan of care for each patient's particular circumstances. An example of an individualized plan of nursing care is given in Chart 3-5.

The plan of care is subject to change as a patient's needs change, as the priorities of needs shift, as needs are resolved, and as additional information about a patient's state of health

Plan of Nursing Care

Chart 3-5. Example of an Individualized Plan of Nursing Care

Mrs. T.C., a 52-year-old elementary school teacher, was admitted to the nursing unit from the emergency department. She had had a gnawing pain on her right side radiating to her back for 3 days. She now describes her pain as "excruciating after eating or drinking." In the past 48 hours she has been vomiting about 2 to 3 hours after she eats. She has not had anything to eat or drink for the past 12 hours.

Mrs. T.C. stated that she had not been successful in adhering to the weight reduction diet that had been prescribed by her physician and that she had rapidly lost, then regained, weight several times in the past year and a half. She stated, "My life is just too busy—I work late hours planning lessons and have to buy my meals out a lot." She indicated that in addition to her work, she and her husband share the responsibility for raising their three young children.

Admission physical examination revealed BP 132/84, P 104, R 22, T 37.8°C, height 1.7 m, weight 92 kg, skin warm, no jaundice. She stated that her urine has been "a strange gold colour" and her stools were "greyish." She was admitted with the diagnosis of acute cholecystitis. The physician's orders on admission included monitor vital signs every 4 hours; IV of Lactated Ringers in D5% Dextrose 125 mL per hour; 1,500-calorie, low-fat liquid diet and progress to low-fat soft diet if no pain in 16 hours; morphine sulphate 2 mg IV every 2 hours as needed; notify physician for sudden increase in frequency or intensity of pain; promethazine 12.5 mg IV every 4 hours as needed for nausea or vomiting.

Nursing Diagnoses

- Acute pain related to distended cystic duct and inflamed or infected gallbladder
- Risk for deficient fluid volume related to vomiting and decreased intake
- Ineffective coping related to role and responsibilities at work and home
- Imbalanced nutrition—more than body requirements, related to knowledge deficit about sedentary lifestyle, poor food choices and eating pattern

Collaborative Problems

- Risk for cystic duct necrosis or perforation
- Obesity

Goals

Immediate

- Relief of pain
- Prevent fluid volume deficit and electrolyte imbalance
- Promote rest
- Early detection of any complications

Intermediate

- Initiation of lifestyle alterations to decrease stress and facilitate rest

Long Term

- Alteration of lifestyle to reduce emotional and environmental stressors
- Compliance with dietary regimen
- Weight reduction

NURSING INTERVENTIONS	EXPECTED OUTCOMES	OUTCOMES
1. Monitor BP, pulse, temperature, and respirations every 4 hours.	1. Vital signs within normal limits	1. BP range 110/62–128/78 with pain relief measures; temperature 36.6°–37.1°C; pulse range 74–88; respirations 18–22
2. Monitor pain status with accompanying abdominal assessment every 2 hours, or more frequently, as needed. a. Assess pain characteristics every 2 hours or as needed.	2. Experiences pain relief; abdominal assessment within normal limits	2. Verbalized decrease in pain from severe (8) to low (2) intensity within 10 minutes after morphine administered; no pain radiation to back Abdomen soft and nontender

Plan of Nursing Care

Chart 3-5. Example of an Individualized Plan of Nursing Care, *Continued*

NURSING INTERVENTIONS	EXPECTED OUTCOMES	OUTCOMES
b. Assess abdomen every 2 hours or with pain assessment. c. Use nonpharmacologic measures (pillows, repositioning, etc.) as desired and tolerated by patient for pain relief. d. Administer analgesic at regular intervals as needed, and assess response.		
3. Monitor and support fluid and electrolyte status: a. Monitor weight. b. I&O c. Monitor skin turgor and temperature. d. Monitor serum electrolytes. e. Monitor colour and consistency of urine and stool output. f. Encourage low-fat liquid intake if pain free. g. Administer promethazine as prescribed to control or relieve vomiting.	3. Fluid balance maintained; electrolytes within normal limits	3. Weight 92.9 kg on admission and 90.2 kg after 2-day period Urinary output adequate in relation to oral and IV intake Skin warm and supple, good recoil Electrolytes in normal range Urine dark amber in colour, no sediment; stools soft, formed, light brown No vomiting reported
4. Promote atmosphere conducive to physical and mental rest: a. Encourage alternation of rest and activity. b. Encourage limitation of visitors and interactions that are stress producing.	4. Alternates periods of rest and activity Limits visitors to family in the evenings Avoids stress-producing interactions	4. Rested in bed 2 hours in morning and 2 hours in afternoon; disconnected phone during rest periods 8 hours uninterrupted sleep at night; husband and children visit 2 hours in evening; patient calm and relaxed after visits Accurately described relationship between stress, sedentary lifestyle, and obesity
5. Assist patient to alter lifestyle to decrease stress: a. Discuss relationship between emotional stress and physiologic function. b. Encourage patient to identify stress-producing stimuli. c. Encourage patient to identify adjustments necessary to reduce stress relative to the home and work setting.	5. Describes stress, sedentary lifestyle, and obesity as precursors to alteration in physiologic functioning Identifies lifestyle factors that produce stress	5. Identified the following stressors: Demands of job Excessive involvement in children's school and recreational activities
6. Encourage patient to identify sedentary lifestyle, obesity, and repetitive weight loss and gain as physiologic and emotional stressors; request consultation with dietitian and reinforce instructions given.	6. Identifies lifestyle adjustments necessary to reduce stress Discusses lifestyle adjustments with family	6. Identified need to stop taking work home with her Consulted with husband and children; will alternate with husband in attending children's activities; all family members supportive
7. Teach importance of maintaining low-fat liquid diet and progression toward long-term low-fat diet. Teach food and menu choices low in fat.	7. Identifies harmful effects of obesity and high-fat foods Makes plans for losing weight Makes plans for preplanned meals Identifies foods/menu choices low in fat	7. Accurately described effects of obesity and intake of high-fat foods on overall physical health and well-being Plans to attend Weight Watchers; has had success with this program in the past Identified that preparing low-fat lunches at home the night before work is a good preplanning option

is collected. As the nursing interventions are implemented, the patient's responses are evaluated and documented, and the plan of care is revised accordingly. A well-developed, continuously updated plan of care is the greatest assurance that the patient's nursing diagnoses and collaborative problems are addressed and his or her basic needs are met.

Framework for a Common Nursing Language: Combining NANDA, NIC, and NOC

Various frameworks or taxonomies can be used for determining nursing diagnoses (e.g., NANDA-I), establishing outcomes (e.g., NOC), and designing interventions (e.g., NIC). Ultimately, a framework that uses a language common to all aspects of nursing, regardless of the classification system, is desirable. Although still controversial and in its infancy, significant efforts have been made toward accomplishing this goal of unifying the language of nursing. In 2001, a taxonomy of nursing practice was developed for the harmonization of NANDA-I, NIC, and NOC. This three-part combination links nursing diagnoses, accompanying interventions, and outcomes, organizing them in the same way. Such organization of concepts in a common language may facilitate the process of critical thinking because interventions and outcomes are more accurately matched with appropriately developed nursing diagnoses (Carpenito, 2017).

Critical Thinking Exercises

1. **pq** A 50-year-old man with morbid obesity is admitted to your unit with a severe asthma attack. He reports extreme shortness of breath and chest pain. What are the priorities for data collection for this patient's current condition? How would these priorities change if the client is in no acute distress and not having chest pain?
2. You are assigned to care for a 40-year-old man with terminal metastatic cancer. Three days ago, he became unresponsive and was admitted to the intensive care unit (ICU). The palliative care physician shares with you that he is going to strongly recommend using terminal sedation for this patient and asks you for your support with the family. The patient's girlfriend, the designated health care representative, is in favour of the palliative care plan; however, the patient's mother vehemently opposes this option and protests that this is "murder." The patient's 16-year-old daughter wants "everything done" for him. You realize the difficulty the family is experiencing and request an ethics committee consult. What ethical principles should be examined when exploring this dilemma? What legal issues should be taken into consideration? Who has the decision-making authority in this case?
3. **ebp** You are caring for a patient with another nursing student, and the student shares that he administered a wrong medication to the patient but is afraid to share this with the faculty and nurses. The patient was given an antihypertensive agent that was not due for another 12 hours. The patient appears to be "OK" at this time, and it is 2 hours after the medication was given. What actions should be taken? Should this information be communicated to your faculty supervisor? What is the care priority for the patient? What evidence supports or does not support disclosure of medication administration errors to patients? What steps would you take and in what order?

REFERENCES AND SELECTED READINGS

Books

Alfaro-LeFevre, R. (2015). *Critical thinking and clinical judgment: A practical approach to outcome focused thinking* (6th ed.). Toronto, ON: Elsevier Canada.

Butcher, H. K., Bulechek, G. M., Dochterman, J. M., et al. (Eds.). (2018). *Nursing interventions classification (NIC)* (7th ed.). St. Louis, MO: Mosby-Elsevier.

Carpenito, L. J. (2017). *Nursing diagnosis: Application to clinical practice* (15th ed.). Philadelphia, PA: Lippincott Williams & Wilkins.

Herdman, T. H., & Kamitsuru, S. (Eds.). (2018). *Nursing diagnoses: Definitions & classification 2018–2020* (11th ed.). Stuttgart, Germany: Thieme.

Moorhead, S., Swanson, E., Johnson, M., et al. (Eds.). (2018). *Nursing outcomes classification (NOC). Measurement of health outcomes* (6th ed.). St. Louis, MO: Mosby-Elsevier.

Pozgar, G. D. (2016). *Legal and ethical issues for healthcare professionals*. Burlington, MA: Jones and Bartlett.

Stuart, G. W. (2012). *Principles and practice of psychiatric nursing* (10th ed.). St. Louis, MO: Mosby.

Vaughn, L. (2016). *Bioethics: Principles, issues, and cases* (3rd ed.). New York: Oxford University Press.

Journals and Electronic Documents

Brudvig, T. J., Dirkes, A., Dutta, P., et al. (2013). Critical thinking in health care professional students: A systematic review. *Journal of Physical Therapy Education*, 27(3), 12–25.

Canadian Nurses Association (CNA). (2017). *Code of ethics for registered nurses*. Ottawa, ON: Author. Retrieved from https://cna-aiic.ca/on-the-issues/best-nursing/nursing-ethics

Canadian Nurses Association (CNA). (2015). *Respecting choices in end-of-life care: Challenges and opportunities for RNs*. Ottawa, ON: Author. Retrieved from https://canadian-nurse.com/~/media/canadian-nurse/files/pdf%20en/respecting-choices-in-end-of-life-care.pdf

Chan, Z. C. (2013). A systematic review of critical thinking in nursing education. *Nurse Education Today*, 33, 236–240.

The Critical Thinking Community. (2013). *Critical thinkers*. Retrieved January 5, 2018, from www.criticalthinking.org

Health Canada. (2018). *Options and decision-making at end of life*. Retrieved from https://www.canada.ca/en/health-canada/services/options-decision-making-end-life.html

Hofman, H., Schorro, E., Haastert, B., et al. (2015). Use of physical restraints in nursing homes: A multicenter cross-sectional study. *BMC Geriatrics*, 15, 129.

International Council of Nurses (ICN). (2018). *The ICN definition of nursing*. Retrieved from http://www.icn.ch/who-we-are/icn-definition-of-nursing/icn-definition-of-nursing-618.html

The Patient Safety Education Program Canada (PSEP). (2017). *Module 13d: Mental health care: Seclusion and restraint: When all else fails*. Retrieved August 25, 2018, from http://www.patientsafetyinstitute.ca/en/education/PatientSafetyEducationProgram/PatientSafetyEducationCurriculum/Documents/Module%2013d%20Seclusion%20and%20Restraint.pdf

Perez-Rivas, F. J., Martin-Iglesias, S., Pacheco del Cerro, J. L., et al. (2015). Effectiveness of nursing process use in primary care. *International Journal of Nursing Knowledge*, 27(1), 43–48.

Pollard, C. (2015). What is the right thing to do: Use of a relational ethic framework to guide clinical decision-making. *International Journal of Caring Sciences*, 8(2), 362–368.

Resources

Canadian Nurses Association (CNA): http://www.cna-aiic.ca
Dying With Dignity Canada: http://www.dyingwithdignity.ca/
International Council of Nurses (ICN): http://www.icn.ch
NANDA International: http://www.nanda.org/

4 Health Education and Health Promotion

Adapted by Joseph Osuji and Mohamed Toufic El Hussein

Learning Objectives

On completion of this chapter, the learner will be able to:

1. Describe the purposes and significance of health education.
2. Describe the concept of adherence to a therapeutic regimen.
3. Identify variables that affect learning readiness and adult learning abilities.
4. Describe the relationship of the teaching–learning process to the nursing process.
5. Develop an individualized teaching plan for a patient.
6. Identify modifications indicated when teaching patients with disabilities.
7. Define the concepts of health, wellness, and health promotion.
8. Discuss major health promotion theories.
9. Describe the components of health promotion: self-responsibility, nutritional awareness, stress reduction and management, and physical fitness.
10. Specify the variables that affect health promotion activities for adolescents, young and middle-aged adults, and older adults.
11. Describe the role of the nurse in health promotion.

Effective **health education** lays a solid foundation for individual and **community** wellness. **Teaching** is an integral tool that all nurses use to assist patients and families in developing effective health behaviours and altering lifestyle patterns that predispose people to health risks. Health education is an influential factor directly related to positive patient care outcomes.

Purpose of Health Education

Today's health care environment mandates the use of an organized approach to health education so that patients can meet their specific health care needs. Significant factors for nurses to consider when planning patient education include the availability of health care outside the hospital setting, the use of diverse health care providers to accomplish care management goals, and the increased use of complementary and alternative strategies rather than traditional approaches to care. Careful consideration of these factors can provide patients with the comprehensive information that is essential for making informed decisions about health care. Demands from consumers for comprehensive information about their health issues throughout the life span accentuate the need for holistic health education to occur in every patient–nurse encounter.

Teaching, as a function of nursing, is included in provincial standards of practice. For example, see the College and Association of Registered Nurses of Alberta (CARNA, 2013) and the Code of Ethics of the Canadian Nurses Association (CNA, 2017). Health education is an independent function of nursing practice and is a primary nursing responsibility. All nursing care is directed toward promoting, maintaining, and restoring health; preventing illness; and helping people adapt to the residual effects of illness. Many of these nursing activities are accomplished through health education or patient teaching. Nurses who serve as teachers are challenged to focus on the educational needs of communities and to provide specific patient and family education. Health education is important to nursing care because it affects the abilities of people and families to perform important self-care activities.

Every contact an individual nurse has with a patient, whether or not that person is ill or has a disability, should be considered an opportunity for health teaching. Although people have a right to decide whether or not to learn, nurses have the responsibility to present information that motivates people to recognize the need to learn. Therefore, nurses use opportunities in all health care settings to promote **wellness**. Educational environments may include homes, hospitals, community health centres, schools, places of business, service agencies, shelters, correctional facilities, and consumer action or support groups (de Chesnay & Anderson, 2016).

Supporting Informed Decision Making and Self-Care

This emphasis on health education stems in part from the public's right to comprehensive health care, which includes up-to-date health information. It also reflects the emergence of an informed public that is asking more significant questions about health and health care. Because of the importance Canadian society places on health and the responsibility each person has to maintain and promote his or her own health, members of the health care team, specifically nurses, are obligated to make health education available. Without adequate knowledge and education in self-care skills, consumers cannot make informed decisions about their health. Guidance from nurses may assist consumers to obtain health information from trustworthy, credible, and timely Internet resources (Blanch-Hartigan, Blake, & Viswanath, 2014). People with chronic illnesses and disabilities are among those most in need of health education.

As the life span of the population increases, the number of people with chronic illnesses and disabilities also increases. People with chronic illness may need health care information to participate actively in and assume responsibility for self-care. Health education can help those with chronic illness adapt to their illness, identify and manage exacerbations, prevent complications, carry out prescribed therapy, and solve issues when confronted with new situations. It can also help prevent crisis situations and reduce the potential for rehospitalisation resulting from inadequate information about self-care. The goal of health education is to teach people to live life to their healthiest—that is, to strive toward achieving their maximum health potential.

In addition to the public's right to and desire for health education, patient education is also a strategy for promoting self-care at home and in the community, reducing health care costs by preventing illness, effectively managing necessary therapies, avoiding expensive medical interventions, decreasing hospital lengths of stay, and facilitating earlier discharge. For health care agencies, offering community wellness programs is a public relations tool for increasing patient knowledge and satisfaction and for developing a positive image of the institution.

Promoting Adherence to the Therapeutic Regimen

One of the goals of patient education is to encourage people to adhere to their **therapeutic regimen**. **Adherence** to treatment usually requires that a person make one or more lifestyle changes to carry out specific activities that promote and maintain health. Common examples of behaviours facilitating health include taking prescribed medications, maintaining a healthy diet, increasing daily activities and exercise, self-monitoring for signs and symptoms of illness, practicing specific hygiene measures, seeking recommended health evaluations and screening, and performing other therapeutic and preventive measures. When using nursing diagnosis language, the term compliance is used to discuss patient adherence.

Many people do not adhere to their prescribed regimens; rates of adherence are generally low, especially when the regimens are complex or of long duration (e.g., therapy for tuberculosis, multiple sclerosis, and human immunodeficiency virus [HIV] disease, and hemodialysis).

Glossary

adherence: the process of faithfully following guidelines or directions

community: an interacting population of individuals living together within a larger society

feedback: the return of information about the results of input given to a person or a system

health education: a variety of learning experiences designed to promote behaviours that facilitate health

health literacy: the capability of a person to obtain, communicate, process, and understand essential health information for the purpose of securing health care services and for making health care decisions

health promotion: the art and science of assisting people to change their lifestyle toward a higher state of wellness

learning: the act of gaining knowledge, skills, and attitudes

learning readiness: the optimum time for learning to occur; usually corresponds to the learner's perceived need and desire to obtain specific knowledge

nutrition: the science that deals with food and nourishment in humans

physical fitness: the condition of being physically healthy as a result of appropriate exercise and nutrition

reinforcement: the process of strengthening a given response or behaviour to increase the likelihood that the behaviour will continue

self-responsibility: personal accountability for one's actions or behaviours

stress management: behaviours and techniques used to strengthen a person's resources against stress

teaching: assisting another individual to learn

therapeutic regimen: a routine that promotes health and healing

wellness: a condition of good physical and emotional health sustained by a healthy lifestyle

Nonadherence to prescribed therapy has been the subject of many studies (Bender, Gentry, Brufsky, et al., 2014; Claborn, Meier, Miller, et al., 2015; Hooper & Huffman, 2014; Martins, de Souza, & da Silva, 2015; Mitchell, Khoukaz, McNeal, et al., 2014). For the most part, findings have been inconclusive, and no one predominant causative factor has been identified. Instead, a wide range of variables influences the degree of adherence, including the following:

- Demographic variables, such as age, gender, race, socioeconomic status, level of education, and health literacy
- Illness variables, such as the severity of the illness and the relief of symptoms afforded by the therapy
- Therapeutic regimen variables, such as the complexity of the regimen and uncomfortable side effects
- Psychosocial variables, such as intelligence, motivation, availability of significant and supportive people (especially family members), attitudes toward health professionals, acceptance or denial of illness, substance abuse, and religious or cultural beliefs
- Financial variables, especially the direct and indirect costs associated with a prescribed regimen

Nurses' success with health education is determined by ongoing assessment of the variables that affect patients' ability to adopt specific behaviours, to obtain resources, and to maintain a healthy social environment (Edelman, Kudzma, & Mandle, 2014).

Another factor to consider when the nurse is developing strategies to promote patient adherence is the concept of health literacy. A challenge for all health care providers is to improve the health literacy of patients. In establishing suitable health education materials, technologic innovations, and services, providers must communicate health information in plain language and work with patients to promote accurate processing and understanding of the health information. Nurses must consider their knowledge of the myriad factors that affect health literacy in any given population. The primary factors influencing health literacy are the effective use of communication and cultural skills, along with the presentation of health care information, and a basic background of mathematical skills. Without such skills, patients are at risk for being unable to share personal health information, perform self-care management for both acute and chronic health conditions, navigate through health systems and complete health forms, and calculate information such as nutritional information on food labels (Harris, Thomas, & Fox, 2015).

Health literacy skills are basic to understanding the body and how it functions, assessing lifestyle choices along with the variables that cause and perpetuate disease, as well as making health care decisions. If people have low health literacy, the consequence is poor overall health. Deconstructing this cycle of low health literacy leading to poor health status and higher risk of health problems is essential. To increase health literacy, providers must design and distribute accurate health information and must ensure that these health materials are culturally appropriate for various populations. It is imperative to build community partnerships to support education and public health activities. Nurses can be instrumental in performing evaluation research on the educational undertakings that support individuals, groups, or communities. Furthermore, nurses must be directly involved in facilitating change through the development of health care policies that address the promotion of a health literate society (Parnell, 2015).

Nurses' success with health education is determined by both the development of strong **health literacy** and the ongoing assessment of the variables that affect patients' ability to adopt specific behaviours to obtain resources, and maintain a healthy social environment (Edelman et al., 2014). Teaching programs are more likely to succeed if patients have improved health literacy and providers pay careful attention to the variables affecting patient adherence. Both health literacy and the concept of adherence must be considered in the patient's teaching plan. Teaching strategies are discussed later in the chapter.

The problem of nonadherence to therapeutic regimens is substantial and must be addressed before patients can achieve their maximum health potential. Patients' need for knowledge has not been found to be a sufficient stimulus for acquiring knowledge and thereby enabling complete adherence to a health regimen. Teaching directed toward stimulating patient motivation results in varying degrees of adherence. Research suggests that factors such as medication costs, perceived control, and type of health problem must also be considered (Adam & Folds, 2014; Ryan, Fedders, Jennings, et al., 2014; Theofilou, 2013; Wu & Moser, 2014). The variables of choice, establishment of mutual goals, and quality of the patient–provider relationship also influence the behavioural changes that can result from patient education. Many factors are linked to motivation for **learning**.

Using a learning contract or agreement can also be a motivator for learning. Such a contract is based on assessment of patient needs; health care data; and specific, measurable goals (Miller & Stoeckel, 2016). The learning contract is recorded in writing and contains methods for ongoing evaluation. A well-designed learning contract is realistic and positive. In a typical learning contract, a series of measurable goals is established, beginning with small, easily attainable objectives and progressing to more advanced goals. Frequent, positive **reinforcement** is provided as the person moves from one goal to the next. For example, incremental goals such as weight loss of 0.5 to 1 kg per week are more appropriate in a weight reduction program than a general goal such as a 14-kg weight loss.

Gerontologic Considerations

Nonadherence to therapeutic regimens is a significant problem for older adults, leading to increased morbidity, mortality, and cost of treatment (Fang, Robinson, Lauffenburger, et al., 2014; Harold, Briesacher, Peterson, et al., 2013). Many admissions to nursing homes and hospitals are associated with nonadherence.

Older adults frequently have one or more chronic illnesses that are managed with numerous medications, and their disease course may be complicated by periodic acute episodes (Miller, 2015). Older adults may have additional problems that affect adherence to therapeutic regimens, such as increased sensitivity to medications and their side effects, difficulty in adjusting to change and stress, financial constraints, forgetfulness, inadequate support systems, lifetime habits of self-treatment with over-the-counter

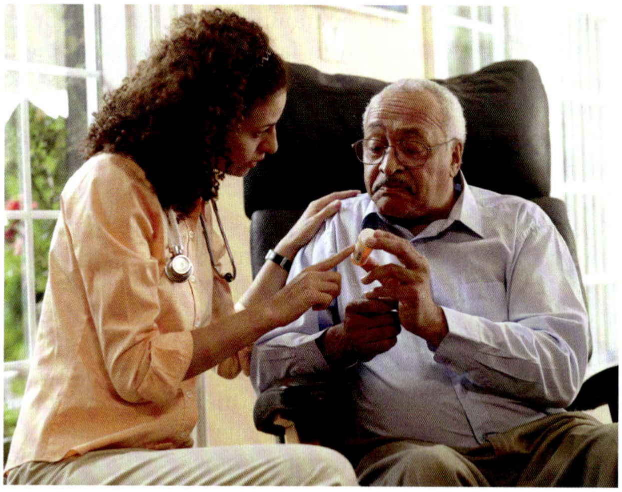

FIGURE 4-1. Taking time to teach patients about their medication and treatment program promotes interest and cooperation. Older adults who are actively involved in learning about their medication and treatment program and the expected effects may be more likely to adhere to the therapeutic regimen.

medications, visual and hearing impairments, and mobility limitations. To promote adherence among older adults, all variables that may affect health behaviour should be assessed (Fig. 4-1). Nurses must also consider that cognitive impairment may be manifested by the older adult's inability to draw inferences, apply information, or understand the major teaching points (Mauk, 2017). The person's strengths and limitations must be assessed to encourage the use of existing strengths to compensate for limitations. Above all, health care professionals must work together to provide continuous, coordinated care; otherwise, the efforts of one health care professional may be negated by those of another.

The Nature of Teaching and Learning

Learning can be defined as acquiring knowledge, attitudes, or skills. Teaching is defined as helping another person learn. These definitions indicate that the teaching–learning process is an active one, requiring the involvement of both teacher and learner in the effort to reach the desired outcome, a change in behaviour. The teacher does not simply give knowledge to the learner but instead serves as a facilitator of learning. Although learning can take place without teachers, most people who are attempting to learn new or altered health behaviours benefit from contact with a nurse. The interpersonal interaction between the person and the nurse who is attempting to meet the person's learning needs may be formal or informal, depending on the method and techniques of teaching.

In general, there is no definitive theory about how learning occurs and how it is affected by teaching. However, learning can be affected by factors such as readiness to learn, the learning environment, and the teaching techniques used (Miller & Stoeckel, 2016).

Learning Readiness

One of the most significant factors influencing learning is a person's **learning readiness**. For adults, readiness is based on culture, personal values, physical and emotional status, and past experiences in learning (Tam, 2014). The "teachable moment" occurs when the content and skills being taught are congruent with the task to be accomplished (Miller & Stoeckel, 2016).

Culture encompasses values, ideals, and behaviours, and the traditions within each culture provide the framework for solving the issues and concerns of daily living. Because people with different cultural backgrounds have different values and lifestyles, choices about health care vary. Culture is a major variable influencing readiness to learn because it affects how people learn and what information can be learned. Sometimes people do not accept health teaching because it conflicts with culturally mediated values. Before beginning health teaching, nurses conduct an individual cultural assessment instead of relying only on generalized assumptions about a particular culture. A patient's social and cultural patterns are appropriately incorporated into the teaching–learning interaction. See Chapter 8.

A person's values include beliefs about behaviours that are desirable and undesirable. The nurse needs to know what value the patient places on health and health care. In clinical situations, patients express their values through their actions and the level of knowledge pursued (de Chesney & Anderson, 2016). When the nurse is unaware of the patient's cultural values, misunderstanding, lack of cooperation, and negative health outcomes may occur (McFarland & Wehbe-Alamah, 2015). A person's values and behaviours can be either an asset or a deterrent to readiness to learn. Therefore, patients are unlikely to accept health education unless their values and beliefs about health and illness are respected (Giger, 2016).

Physical readiness is of vital importance, because until the person is physically capable of learning, attempts at teaching and learning may be both futile and frustrating. For example, a person in acute pain is unable to focus attention away from the pain long enough to concentrate on learning. Likewise, a person who is short of breath concentrates on breathing rather than on learning.

Emotional readiness also affects the motivation to learn. A person who has not accepted an existing illness or the threat of illness is not motivated to learn. A person who does not accept a therapeutic regimen, or who views it as conflicting with his or her present lifestyle, may consciously avoid learning about it. Until the person recognizes the need to learn and demonstrates an ability to learn, teaching efforts may be thwarted. However, it is not always wise to wait for the person to become emotionally ready to learn, because that time may never come unless the nurse makes an effort to stimulate the person's motivation. For example, a person with colon cancer who has a fasting blood sugar twice the expected normal value may focus only on the cancer diagnosis and exclude or deny the health consequences of an abnormal blood sugar.

Illness and the threat of illness are usually accompanied by anxiety and stress. Nurses who recognize such reactions can use simple explanations and instructions to alleviate these anxieties and provide further motivation to learn. Because learning involves behaviour change, it often produces mild anxiety, which can be a useful motivating factor.

Emotional readiness can be promoted by creating a warm, accepting, positive atmosphere and by establishing realistic learning goals. When learners achieve success and a feeling of accomplishment, they are often motivated to participate in additional learning opportunities. One example of a strategy that facilitates learner success is the teach-back technique. This technique is used to evaluate the recall and understanding of the learner after health teaching has occurred. It is a useful, in-the-moment **feedback** and evaluation method because it allows the educator to discover if the learner can effectively verbalize information or demonstrate a particular health behaviour (Miller & Stoeckel, 2016). In addition, the teach-back strategy can be used with family members and caregivers to ascertain if they have retained and understood the health content. Having a strategy to actively involve the adult learner in making health care decisions and performing self-management skills promotes learner receptivity and motivation to integrate health principles into one's daily life. Furthermore, feedback about progress also motivates learning. Such feedback should be presented in the form of positive reinforcement when the learner is successful, and in the form of constructive suggestions for improvement when the learner is unsuccessful.

Experiential readiness refers to past experiences that influence a person's ability to learn. Previous educational experiences and life experiences in general are significant determinants of a person's approach to learning. People with little or no formal education may not be able to understand the instructional materials presented. People who have had difficulty learning in the past may be hesitant to try again. Many behaviours required for reaching maximum health potential require knowledge, physical skills, and positive attitudes. In their absence, learning may be very difficult and very slow. For example, a person who does not understand the basics of adequate **nutrition** may not be able to understand the restrictions of a specific diet. A person who does not view the desired learning as personally meaningful may reject teaching efforts. A person who is not future oriented may be unable to appreciate many aspects of preventive health teaching. Experiential readiness is closely related to emotional readiness, because motivation tends to be stimulated by an appreciation for the need to learn and by those learning tasks that are familiar, interesting, and meaningful.

The Learning Environment

Learning may be optimized by minimizing factors that interfere with the learning process. For example, the room temperature, lighting, noise levels, and other environmental conditions should be appropriate to the learning situation. In addition, the time selected for teaching should be suited to the needs of the individual person. Scheduling a teaching session at a time of day when a patient is fatigued, uncomfortable, or anxious about a pending diagnostic or therapeutic procedure, or when visitors are present, is not conducive to learning. However, if the family is to participate in providing care, the sessions should be scheduled when family members are present so that they can learn any necessary skills or techniques.

Teaching Techniques and Resources

Teaching techniques and methods enhance learning if they are appropriate to the patient's needs. Numerous techniques are available, including the following:

- *Lectures:* Lectures are explanation methods of teaching and should be accompanied by discussion, because discussion affords learners opportunities to express their feelings and concerns, ask questions, and receive clarification.
- *Group teaching:* Group teaching allows people not only to receive needed information but also to feel secure as members of a group (promoting moral support). Assessment and follow-up are imperative to ensure that each person has gained sufficient knowledge and skills. Not all patients relate or learn well in groups.
- *Demonstration and practice:* Demonstration and practice are especially important when teaching skills. The nurse should demonstrate the skill and then give the learner ample opportunity for practice. When special equipment is involved, such as syringes or colostomy bags, it is important to teach with the same equipment that will be used in the home setting to avoid confusion, frustration, and mistakes.
- *Reinforcement and follow-up:* Nurses must allow ample time for patients to learn and provide reinforcement. Follow-up sessions are imperative to promote the learner's confidence in their abilities and to plan for additional teaching sessions.
- *Motivational interviewing:* Pilot research suggests that using motivational interviewing as an enhanced educational method in an acute inpatient setting can increase both patient and caregiver knowledge as well as patient satisfaction following discharge from the acute care setting (Mehta, Cameron, & Battistella, 2014).
- *Electronic, online, or Internet information:* Electronic technologies are used to provide health information. Examples are interactive or noninteractive Internet learning, an online self-paced program, or a structured online course. There are also DVD, CD-ROM, podcasts, and recorded programs available over a television channel.
- *Teaching aids:* Teaching aids include books, pamphlets, pictures, films, slides, audiotapes, models, programmed instruction, other visual aids (e.g., charts), and computer-assisted learning modules. They are invaluable when used appropriately and can save a significant amount of personnel time and related cost. However, all such aids should be reviewed before use to ensure that they meet the patient's learning needs and are free of advertisements that may confuse the patient (see Resources section at the end of the chapter for additional information).

There are specific considerations for teaching special populations. Table 4-1 outlines some of the teaching strategies to use when teaching people with disabilities (see Chapters 13 and 14 for additional teaching strategies for people with disabilities and older adults).

TABLE 4-1 Educating People With Disabilities

Type of Disability	Educational Strategy
Physical, Emotional, or Cognitive Disability	Adapt information to accommodate the person's cognitive, perceptual, and behavioural disabilities. Give clear written and oral information. Highlight significant information for easy reference. Avoid medical terminology or "jargon."
Hearing Impairment	Use slow, directed, deliberate speech. Use sign language or interpreter services if appropriate. Position yourself so that the person can see your mouth if speechreading. Use telecommunication devices (TTY or TDD) for the person with hearing impairment. Use written materials and visual aids, such as models and diagrams. Use captioned videos, films, and computer-generated materials. Teach on the side of the "good ear" if unilateral deafness is present.
Visual Impairment	Use optical devices such as magnifying lens. Use proper lighting and proper contrast of colours on materials and equipment. Use large-print materials. Use Braille materials if appropriate. Convert information to auditory and tactile formats. Obtain audiotapes and talking books. Explain noises associated with procedures, equipment, and treatments. Arrange materials in clockwise pattern.
Learning Disabilities	
Input disability	If visual perceptual disorder: • Explain information verbally, repeat, and reinforce frequently. • Use audiotapes. • Encourage learner to verbalize information received. If auditory perceptual disorder: • Speak slowly with as few words as possible, repeat, and reinforce frequently. • Use direct eye contact to focus person on task. • Use demonstration and return demonstration such as modelling, role playing, and hands-on experiences. • Use visual tools, written materials, and computers.
Output disability	Use all senses as appropriate. Use written, audiotape, and computer information. Review information and give time to interact and ask questions. Use hand gestures and motions.
Developmental disability	Base information and teaching on developmental stage, not chronologic age. Use nonverbal cues, gestures, signing, and symbols as needed. Use simple explanations and concrete examples with repetition. Encourage active participation. Demonstrate information and have the person perform return demonstrations.

Teaching Special Populations

People With Disabilities

When providing health information to people with disabilities, the individual needs of each person must be assessed and incorporated into the teaching plan. Teaching techniques and the imparting of information may need to be altered. The nurse needs to be aware of the **health promotion** needs when teaching specific groups of people with physical disabilities; emotional, psychiatric, or mental health disabilities; hearing, visual, or sensory impairments; learning disabilities; and developmental disabilities. It may be necessary to institute new or modified approaches to teach people with disabilities about their health. See Table 4-1.

Older Adults

Nurses caring for older adults need to be aware of how the usual changes that occur with aging may affect learning abilities and how they can help older people age well. Above all, it is important to recognize that just because a person is older does not mean that he or she cannot learn. Older adults *can* learn and remember if information is paced appropriately, is relevant, and is followed by the appropriate feedback strategies that apply to all learners (Miller, 2015). Because changes associated with aging vary significantly among older people, the nurse conducts a thorough assessment of each person's level of physiologic and psychological functioning before beginning teaching. More information on the physiologic effects of aging can be found in Chapter 14.

Changes in cognition with age may include slowed mental functioning; decreased short-term memory, abstract thinking, and concentration; and slowed reaction time. These changes are often accentuated by the health concerns that cause the older person to seek health care in the first place. Effective teaching strategies include slow-paced presentation of small amounts of material at a time; frequent repetition of information; and the use of reinforcement techniques, such as audiovisual and written materials, and repeated practice sessions. Distracting stimuli should be minimized as much as possible in the teaching environment.

Sensory changes associated with aging also affect teaching and learning. Teaching strategies to accommodate decreased visual acuity include large-print and easy-to-read materials printed on nonglare paper. Because colour discrimination is often impaired, the use of colour-coded or highlighted materials may not be effective. To maximize hearing, teachers speak distinctly with a normal or lowered pitch, facing the person so that speechreading can occur as needed. Visual cues often help reinforce verbal teaching.

Family members should be involved in teaching sessions when possible and appropriate. They provide another source for reinforcement of material and can help the older person recall instructions later. Family members can also provide valuable assessment information about the person's living situation and related learning needs.

The chance of success is maximized when nurses, families, and other health care professionals work collaboratively to facilitate the older person's learning. Successful learning should result in improved self-care management skills, enhanced self-esteem, confidence, and a willingness to learn in the future.

The Nursing Process in Patient Education

The nurse relies on the steps of the nursing process when constructing an individualized teaching plan to meet the patient's teaching and learning needs (Chart 4-1).

Assessment

Assessment in the teaching–learning process is directed toward the systematic collection of data about the person and family's learning needs and readiness to learn. All internal and external variables that affect the patient's readiness to learn are identified. A learning assessment guide may be used for this purpose. Some of the available guides are directed toward the collection of general health information (e.g., smoking cessation), whereas others are specific to medication regimens or disease processes (e.g., stroke risk assessments). Such guides facilitate assessment but must be adapted to the responses, issues, and needs of each person. The nurse organizes, analyzes, synthesizes,

CHART 4-1

Summary of the Nursing Process for Individualized Patient Education

Assessment

1. Assess the person's readiness for health education.
   a. What are the person's health beliefs and behaviours?
   b. What physical and psychosocial adaptations does the person need to make?
   c. Is the learner ready to learn?
   d. Is the person able to learn these behaviours?
   e. What additional information about the person is needed?
   f. Are there any variables (e.g., hearing or visual impairment, cognitive issues, literacy issues) that will affect the choice of teaching strategy or approach?
   g. What are the person's expectations?
   h. What does the person want to learn?
2. Organize, analyze, synthesize, and summarize the collected data.

Nursing Diagnosis

1. Formulate the nursing diagnoses that relate to the person's learning needs.
2. Identify the learning needs, their characteristics, and their etiology.
3. State nursing diagnoses concisely and precisely.

Planning and Goals

1. Assign priority to the nursing diagnoses that relate to the individual's learning needs.
2. Specify the immediate, intermediate, and long-term learning goals established by teacher and learner together.
3. Identify teaching strategies appropriate for goal attainment.
4. Establish expected outcomes.
5. Develop the written teaching plan.
   a. Include diagnoses, goals, teaching strategies, and expected outcomes.
   b. Put the information to be taught in logical sequence.
   c. Write down the key points.
   d. Select appropriate teaching aids.
   e. Keep the plan current and flexible to meet the person's changing learning needs.
6. Involve the learner, family or significant others, nursing team members, and other health care team members in all aspects of planning.

Implementation

1. Put the teaching plan into action.
2. Use language the person can understand.
3. Use appropriate teaching aids and provide Internet resources if appropriate.
4. Use the same equipment that the person will use after discharge.
5. Encourage the person to participate actively in learning.
6. Record the learner's responses to the teaching actions.
7. Provide feedback.

Evaluation

1. Collect objective data.
   a. Observe the person.
   b. Ask questions to determine whether the person understands.
   c. Use rating scales, checklists, anecdotal notes, and written tests when appropriate.
2. Compare the person's behavioural responses with the expected outcomes. Determine the extent to which the goals were achieved.
3. Include the person, family or significant others, nursing team members, and other health care team members in the evaluation.
4. Identify alterations that need to be made in the teaching plan.
5. Make referrals to appropriate sources or agencies for reinforcement of learning after discharge.
6. Continue all steps of the teaching process: assessment, diagnosis, planning, implementation, and evaluation.

and summarizes the assessment data collected and determines the patient's need for teaching.

Nursing Diagnosis

The process of formulating nursing diagnoses makes educational goals and evaluations of progress more specific and meaningful. Teaching is an integral intervention implied by all nursing diagnoses, and for some diagnoses, education is the primary intervention. Examples of nursing diagnoses that help in planning for educational needs are ineffective health maintenance, ineffective self-health management, and decisional conflict. The diagnosis "Deficient knowledge" should be used cautiously, because knowledge deficit is not a human response but a factor relating to or causing the diagnosis. For example, "Ineffective health maintenance related to a lack of information about wound care" is a more appropriate nursing diagnosis than "Deficient knowledge" (Carpenito-Moyet, 2017). A nursing diagnosis that relates specifically to a patient's and family's learning needs serves as a guide in the development of the teaching plan.

Planning

Once the nursing diagnoses have been identified, the planning component of the teaching–learning process is established in accordance with the steps of the nursing process:

1. Assigning priorities to the diagnoses
2. Specifying the immediate, intermediate, and long-term goals of learning
3. Identifying specific teaching strategies appropriate for attaining goals
4. Specifying the expected outcomes
5. Documenting the diagnoses, goals, teaching strategies, and expected outcomes of the teaching plan

The assignment of priorities to the diagnoses should be a collaborative effort by the nurse, the patient, and the family members. Consideration is given to the urgency of the patient's learning needs; the most critical needs should receive the highest priority. The nurse needs to keep in mind that before the teaching strategy can be determined, the goals of learning must be developed.

After the diagnostic priorities have been mutually established, it is important to identify the immediate and long-term goals and the teaching strategies appropriate for attaining the goals. Teaching is most effective when the objectives of both the patient and nurse are in agreement (Bastable, 2014). Learning begins with the establishment of goals that are appropriate to the situation and realistic in terms of the patient's ability and desire to achieve them. Involving the patient and family in establishing goals and in planning teaching strategies promotes their cooperation in the implementation of the teaching plan.

Outcomes of teaching strategies can be stated in terms of expected behaviours of patients, families, or both. Outcomes are to be realistic and measurable, and the critical time periods for attaining them are also identified. The desired outcomes and the critical time periods serve as a basis for evaluating the effectiveness of the teaching strategies.

During the planning phase, the nurse considers the sequence in which the subject matter is presented. Critical information (e.g., survival skills for a patient with diabetes) and material that the person or family identifies to be of particular importance receives high priority. An outline is often helpful for arranging the subject matter and for ensuring that all necessary information is included. In addition, appropriate teaching aids to be used in implementing teaching strategies are prepared or selected at this time.

The entire planning phase concludes with the formulation of the teaching plan. This teaching plan communicates the following information to all members of the nursing team:

- The nursing diagnoses that specifically relate to the patient's learning needs and the priorities of these diagnoses
- The goals of the teaching strategies
- The teaching strategies that are appropriate for goal attainment
- The expected outcomes, which identify the desired behavioural responses of the learner
- The critical time period within which each outcome is expected to be met
- The patient's behavioural responses (which are documented on the teaching plan)

The same rules that apply to writing and revising the plan of nursing care apply to the teaching plan.

Implementation

In the implementation phase of the teaching–learning process, the patient, the family, and other members of the nursing and health care team carry out the activities outlined in the teaching plan. The nurse coordinates these activities.

Flexibility during the implementation phase of the teaching–learning process and ongoing assessment of patient responses to the teaching strategies support modification of the teaching plan as necessary. Creativity in promoting and sustaining the patient's motivation to learn is essential. New learning needs that may arise after discharge from the hospital or after home care visits have ended should also be taken into account.

The implementation phase ends when the teaching strategies have been completed and when the patient's responses to the actions have been recorded. This serves as the basis for evaluating how well the defined goals and expected outcomes have been achieved.

Evaluation

Evaluation of the teaching–learning process determines how effectively the patient has responded to teaching and to what extent the goals have been achieved. An evaluation is made to determine what was effective and what needs to be changed or reinforced. It cannot be assumed that patients have learned just because teaching has occurred; learning does not automatically follow teaching. An important part of the evaluation phase addresses the question, "What can be done to improve teaching and enhance learning?" Answers to this question direct the changes to be made in the teaching plan.

A variety of measurement techniques can be used to identify changes in patient behaviour as evidence that learning has taken place. These techniques include directly observing the behaviour; using rating scales, checklists, or anecdotal notes to document the behaviour; and indirectly measuring results using oral questioning and written tests. All direct measurements are supplemented with indirect measurements whenever possible. Using more than one measuring technique enhances the reliability of the resulting data and decreases the potential for error from a measurement strategy.

In many situations, measurement of actual behaviour is the most accurate and appropriate evaluation technique. Nurses often perform comparative analyses using patient admission data as the baseline. Selected data points observed when nursing care is given and self-care is initiated are compared with the patient's baseline data. In other cases, indirect measurement may be used. Some examples of indirect measurement are patient satisfaction surveys, attitude surveys, and instruments that evaluate specific health status variables.

Measurement is only the beginning of evaluation, which must be followed by data interpretation and value judgments about learning and teaching. These aspects of evaluation are conducted periodically throughout the teaching–learning program, at its conclusion, and at varying periods after the teaching has ended.

Evaluation of learning after teaching that occurs in any setting (e.g., clinics, offices, and hospitals) is essential, because the analysis of teaching outcomes must extend into aftercare. With shortened hospital lengths of stay and with short-stay and same-day surgical procedures, follow-up evaluation is especially important. Coordination of efforts and sharing of information between hospital-based and community-based nursing personnel facilitate post-discharge teaching and home care evaluation.

Evaluation is not the final step in the teaching–learning process but is the beginning of a new patient assessment. The information gathered during evaluation is used to redirect teaching actions, with the goal of improving the patient's responses and outcomes.

Health Promotion

Health teaching and health promotion are linked by a common goal—to encourage people to achieve as high a level of wellness as possible so that they can live maximally healthy lives and avoid preventable illnesses. The call for health promotion has become a cornerstone in health policy because of the need to control costs and reduce unnecessary sickness and death.

Health goals for the nation were originally established in the *Ottawa Charter for Health Promotion* in 1986 with the intent of achieving Health for All by the year 2000 and beyond (World Health Organization [WHO], 2018). The priorities from this initiative were identified as building healthy public policy, creating supportive environments, strengthening community action, developing personal skills, and reorienting health services. The original goals continue to be relevant today. Every few years countries meet to reaffirm the original goals.

Definition

Health promotion may be defined as those activities that assist people in developing resources that maintain or enhance well-being and improve their quality of life. These activities involve people's efforts to remain healthy in the absence of symptoms and do not require the assistance of a health care team member, and occur within or outside of the health system (Haber, 2016; O'Donnell, 2014).

The purpose of health promotion is to focus on the person's potential for wellness and to encourage appropriate alterations in personal habits, lifestyle, and environment in ways that reduce risks and enhance health and well-being. Health promotion is an active process; that is, it is not something that can be prescribed or dictated. It is up to each person to decide whether to make changes to promote a higher level of wellness. Only the individual can make these choices.

Following the catastrophic public event of SARS, the Public Health Agency of Canada (PHAC) was created in 2003, with Dr. Butler-Jones as the first Chief Public Health Officer of Canada. The mission of the PHAC is "promoting and protecting the health of Canadians through leadership, partnership, innovation and action in public health" (PHAC, 2018).

Health and Wellness

The concept of health promotion has evolved because of a changing definition of health and an awareness that wellness exists at many levels of functioning. Health is viewed as a dynamic, ever-changing condition that enables people to function at an optimal potential at any given time. The ideal health status is one in which people are successful in achieving their full potential, regardless of any limitations they might have.

Wellness, a reflection of health, involves a conscious and deliberate attempt to maximize one's health. Wellness does not just happen; it requires planning and conscious commitment and is the result of adopting lifestyle behaviours for the purpose of attaining one's highest potential for well-being. Wellness is not the same for every person. The person with a chronic illness or disability may still be able to achieve a desirable level of wellness. The key to wellness is to function at the highest potential within the limitations over which there is no control, such as a lifelong disability or genetic disorders (Chart 4-2).

A significant amount of research has shown that people, by virtue of what they do or fail to do, influence their own health. Today, many of the major causes of illness are chronic diseases that have been closely related to lifestyle behaviours (e.g., type 2 diabetes mellitus, heart disease, lung and colon cancer, chronic obstructive pulmonary diseases (COPDs), hypertension, cirrhosis, traumatic injury, and HIV disease). To a large extent, a person's health status may be reflective of his or her lifestyle.

Health Promotion Models

Several health promotion models identify health-protecting behaviours and seek to explain what makes people engage in preventive behaviours. A health-protecting behaviour is defined as any behaviour performed by people, regardless

GENETICS IN NURSING PRACTICE

Chart 4-2. Genetic Aspects of Health Education and Promotion

Nurses in all settings should be prepared to incorporate genetics into health education and promotion by:

- Inquiring about patients' and families' desired health outcomes with regard to genetics-related conditions or risk factors
- Referring patients for genetics services when indicated
- Identifying barriers to accessing genetics-related health services
- Offering appropriate genetics information and resources

of their actual or perceived health condition, for the purpose of promoting or maintaining their health, whether or not the behaviour produces the desired outcome (Murdaugh, Parsons, & Pender, 2018). One model, the Health Belief Model, was designed to foster understanding of why some healthy people choose actions to prevent illness while others do not. Another model, the resource model of preventive health behaviour, addresses the ways in which people use resources to promote health (Murdaugh et al., 2018). Nurse educators can use this model to assess how demographic variables, health behaviours, and social and health resources influence health promotion.

The Canadian health promotion initiative, Achieving Health for All, builds on the work of Lalonde (1977), in which four determinants of health—human biology, environment, lifestyle, and the health care delivery system—were identified. Determinants of health were defined as factors and conditions that have an influence on the health of individuals and communities. Since the 1970s, a total of 12 health determinants have been identified, and this number will continue to increase as population health research progresses. Determinants of health provide a framework for assessing and evaluating the population's health.

A model crafted to address organizational and individual health behaviour change is the Awareness, Motivation, Skills, and Opportunity (AMSO) Model. The four components of this model focus on empowering people, understanding their individual priorities, and assisting them to change in personal ways that promote and maintain their optimal level of health. The dimensions of optimal health are physical, emotional, social, intellectual, and spiritual. This model promotes the process of creating and maintaining a balance among these five dimensions (O'Donnell, 2014). Optimal health is a dynamic condition kept in balance by a combination of efforts to sustain awareness, maintain motivation, build skills, and have opportunities to practice positive health behaviours.

The Health Belief Model developed by Becker (1974) is based on the premise that four variables influence the selection and use of health promotion behaviours. **Demographic and disease factors**, the first variable, include patient characteristics such as age, gender, education, employment, severity of illness or disability, and length of illness. **Barriers**, the second variable, are defined as factors leading to unavailability or difficulty in gaining access to a specific health promotion alternative. **Resources**, the third variable, encompass such factors as financial and social support. **Perceptual factors**, the fourth variable, consist of how the person views his or her health status, self-efficacy, and the perceived demands of the illness. Becker demonstrated that these four variables have a positive correlation with a person's quality of life.

The Transtheoretical Model of Change, also known as the Stages of Change Model, is a framework that focuses on the motivation of a person to make decisions that promote healthy behaviour change (DiClemente, 2007; Miller, 2015). Table 4-2 shows the six stages of the model. Research indicates that people seeking assistance from professionals or self-help groups progress through these stages of change (Chaufan, Yeh, & Sigal, 2015; Seebohm, Chaudhary, Boyce, et al., 2013).

Any of the models can serve as an organizing framework for clinical work and research that support the enhancement of health. Research suggests that the application of health promotion models, concepts, and frameworks increases the nurse's understanding of the health promotion behaviours of families and communities (Cha, 2013; Meraviglia, Stuifbergen, Morgan, et al., 2015; Yeun, Baek, & Kim, 2013).

Components of Health Promotion

There are several components of health promotion as an active process: **self-responsibility**, nutritional awareness, stress reduction and management, and **physical fitness**.

TABLE 4-2 Stages in the Transtheoretical Model of Change

Stage	Description
1. Precontemplative	The person is not thinking about making a change.
2. Contemplative	The person is only thinking about change in the near future.
3. Decision making	The person constructs a plan to change behaviour.
4. Action	The person takes steps to operationalize the plan of action.
5. Maintenance	The person works to prevent relapse and to sustain the gains made from the actions taken.
6. Termination	The person has the ability to resist relapse back to unhealthy behaviour(s).

Adapted from DiClemente, C. (2007). The transtheoretical model of intentional behavior change. *Drugs & Alcohol Today*, *7*(1), 29–33; Miller, C. A. (2019). *Nursing for wellness in older adults* (8th ed.). Philadelphia, PA: Lippincott Williams & Wilkins.

Self-Responsibility

Taking responsibility for oneself is the key to successful health promotion. The concept of self-responsibility is based on the understanding that the individual controls his or her life. Each person alone must make the choices that determine how healthy his or her lifestyle is. As more people recognize that lifestyle and behaviour significantly affect health, they may assume responsibility for avoiding high-risk behaviours such as smoking, alcohol and drug abuse, overeating, driving while intoxicated, risky sexual practices, and other unhealthy habits. They may also assume responsibility for adopting routines that have been found to have a positive influence on health, such as engaging in regular exercise, wearing seat belts, and eating a healthy diet.

A variety of techniques have been used to encourage people to accept responsibility for their health, ranging from extensive educational programs to reward systems. No one technique has been found to be superior to any other. Instead, self-responsibility for health promotion is individualized and depends on a person's desires and inner motivations. Health promotion programs are important tools for encouraging people to assume responsibility for their health and to develop behaviours that improve health.

Nutritional Awareness

Nutrition, as a component of health promotion, has become the focus of considerable attention and publicity with the growing epidemic of obesity in Canada. A vast array of books and magazine articles address the topics of special diets; natural foods; and the hazards associated with certain substances, such as sugar, salt, cholesterol, trans fats, carbohydrates, artificial colours, and food additives. It has been suggested that good nutrition is the single most significant factor in determining health status, longevity, and weight control.

Nutritional awareness involves an understanding of the importance of a healthy diet that supplies all of the essential nutrients. Understanding the relationship between diet and disease is an important facet of a person's self-care. Many clinicians believe that a healthy diet is one that substitutes "natural" foods for processed and refined ones and reduces the intake of sugar, salt, fat, cholesterol, caffeine, alcohol, food additives, and preservatives.

Chapter 5 contains further information about the assessment of a person's nutritional status. It describes the physical signs indicating nutritional status, assessment of food intake (food record, 24-hour recall), the dietary guidelines presented in the Canada Food Guide, and calculation of ideal body weight.

Stress Management and Stress Reduction

Stress management and stress reduction are important aspects of health promotion. Studies suggest the negative effects of stress on health and a cause-and-effect relationship between stress and infectious diseases, traumatic injuries (e.g., motor vehicle crashes), and some chronic illnesses. Stress has become inevitable in contemporary societies in which demands for productivity have become excessive. More and more emphasis is placed on encouraging people to manage stress appropriately and to reduce the pressures that are counterproductive. Research suggests that including techniques such as relaxation training, exercise, yoga, and modification of stressful situations in health promotion programs assists patients in dealing with stress (Hartley, Flowers, Lee, et al., 2014; Rao, Raghuram, Nagendra, et al., 2015; Smith, 2014). Further information on **stress management**, including health risk appraisal and stress reduction methods such as the Benson Relaxation Response, can be found in Chapter 9.

Physical Fitness

Physical fitness and exercise are important components of health promotion. Clinicians and researchers (Bruning & Sturek, 2015; Halvarsson, Franzen, & Stahle, 2015; Murimi, Chrisman, McAllister, et al., 2015; Resnick, Nahm, Zhu, et al., 2014; Yoo, Park, Yang, et al., 2014) who have examined the relationship between health and physical fitness have found that a regular exercise program can promote health in the following ways:

- Improve the function of the circulatory system and the lungs
- Decrease cholesterol and low-density lipoprotein levels
- Decrease body weight by increasing calorie expenditure
- Delay degenerative changes such as osteoporosis
- Improve flexibility and overall muscle strength and endurance

An appropriate exercise program can have a positive effect on a person's performance capacity, appearance, and level of stress and fatigue, as well as their general state of physical, mental, and emotional health (Gerber, Jonsdottir, Arvidson, et al., 2015; Groh & Urbancic, 2015; Khazaee-Pool, Sadeghi, Majlessi, et al., 2014). An exercise program should be designed specifically for a given person, with consideration to age, physical condition, and any known cardiovascular or other risk factors. Exercise can be harmful if it is not started gradually and increased slowly in accordance with a person's response.

Unfolding Patient Stories: Vincent Brody • Part 1

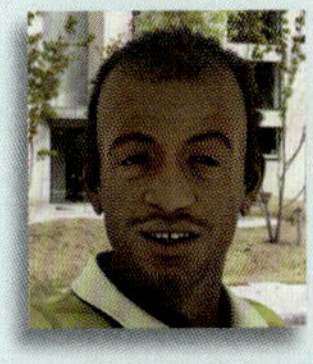

Vincent Brody, a 67-year-old male with chronic obstructive pulmonary disease (COPD), is experiencing increased fatigue. He spends most of the day in a recliner chair watching television and smoking one to two packs per day. His nutritional intake is poor due to shortness of breath. What patient education can the nurse provide to promote self-care behaviours for symptom improvement and a healthier lifestyle? (Vincent Brody's story continues in Chapter 57.)

Care for Vincent and other patients in a realistic virtual environment: ***vSim** for Nursing* (**thepoint.lww.com/vSimMedicalSurgical**). Practice documenting these patients' care in DocuCare (**thepoint.lww.com/DocuCareEHR**).

Health Promotion Strategies Throughout the Life Span

Health promotion is a concept and a process that extends throughout the life span. The health of a child can be

TABLE 4-3 Selected Health Promotion Screening for Adults

Type of Screening	Suggested Time Frame
Routine health examination	Yearly
Blood chemistry profile	Baseline at age 20, then as mutually determined by patient and clinician
Complete blood count	Baseline at age 20, then as mutually determined by patient and clinician
Lipid profile	Baseline at age 20, then as mutually determined by patient and clinician
Hemoccult screening (fecal occult blood)	Yearly after age 50. If positive, follow-up with colonoscopy
Electrocardiogram	Baseline at age 40, then as mutually determined by patient and clinician
Blood pressure	Yearly, then as mutually determined by patient and clinician
Chest x-ray film	Baseline and as needed
Breast self-examination	Optional. However, it is important for both women and men to "be breast aware"—to know how their breasts look and feel, and what changes to look for
Mammogram	Every 2 years for women 50–69 years and then as determined by patient and clinician. For women at increased risk due to family history of breast cancer, begin mammograms 10 years before date of onset in woman's relative
Clinical breast examination (CBE)	Yearly examination by a physician or nurse practitioner is questioned. "There is no direct scientific evidence that CBE reduces breast cancer death rates." (Canadian Breast Cancer Foundation, 2013, p. 1). CBE and mammogram together slightly reduces breast cancer deaths but results in many false positives (Canadian Breast Cancer Foundation)
Gynecologic examination	Yearly
Pap smear	Every 1–3 years for sexually active women to age 70 years
Bone density screening	Based on identification of primary and secondary risk factors (prior to onset of menopause, if indicated)
Nutritional screening	As mutually determined by patient and clinician. (Includes weight, waist measurement, body mass index [BMI], if meeting the requirements of Canada's Food Guide, and amount of sodium, fats, fibre, calcium, vitamin D taken daily)
Digital rectal examination	Yearly for men after age 50
Colonoscopy	Every 5 years after age 50 or as mutually determined by patient and clinician
Prostate examination	Yearly
Prostate-specific antigen	Every 1–2 years after age 50
Testicular examination	Monthly self-examination
Skin examination	Yearly or as mutually determined by patient and clinician
Vision screening glaucoma	Every 2–3 years Baseline at age 40, then every 2–3 years until age 70, then yearly
Dental screening	Every 6 months
Hearing screening	As needed
Health risk appraisal	As needed
Adult Immunizations	
Hepatitis A and B (if not received as a child)	Series of three doses (now, 1 month later, then 5 months after the second date)—for lifetime
Influenza vaccine	Yearly
Pneumococcus	Once at age 60 years (earlier if have respiratory conditions)
Diphtheria, pertussis, tetanus	Every 10 years

Note: Any of these screenings may be performed more frequently if deemed necessary by the patient or recommended by the health care provider.

affected either positively or negatively by the health practices of the mother during the prenatal period. Therefore, health promotion starts before birth and extends through childhood, adolescence, adulthood, and old age (Haber, 2016).

Health promotion includes health screening. The College of Family Physicians of Canada has developed recommendations for periodic health examinations for both adults and children that identify when specific screening interventions are appropriate. Table 4-3 presents general population guidelines.

Adolescents

Health screening has traditionally been an important aspect of adolescent health care. The goal has been to detect health problems at an early age so that they can be treated at this time. Today, health promotion goes beyond the mere screening for disabilities and includes extensive efforts to promote positive health practices at an early age. Because health habits and practices are formed early in life, adolescents should be encouraged to develop positive health attitudes. For this reason, more and more programs are being offered to adolescents to help them develop good health habits. Although the negative results of practices such as smoking, risky sexual activities, alcohol and drug abuse, and poor nutrition are explained in these educational programs, emphasis is also placed on values training, self-esteem, and healthy lifestyle practices. The projects are designed to appeal to a particular age group, with emphasis on learning experiences that are fun, interesting, and relevant.

Young and Middle-Aged Adults

Young and middle-aged adults represent an age group that not only expresses an interest in health and health promotion, but also responds enthusiastically to suggestions that show how lifestyle practices can improve health. Adults are frequently motivated to change their lifestyles in ways that are believed to enhance their health and wellness. Many adults who wish to improve their health turn to health promotion programs to help them make the desired changes in their lifestyles. Many have responded to programs that focus on topics such as general wellness, smoking cessation, exercise, physical conditioning, weight control, conflict resolution, and stress management. Because of the nationwide emphasis on health during the reproductive years, young adults actively seek programs that address prenatal health, parenting, family planning, and women's health issues.

Programs that provide health screening, such as those that screen for cancer, high cholesterol, hypertension, diabetes, abdominal aneurysm, and visual and hearing impairments, are quite popular with young and middle-aged adults. Programs that involve health promotion for people with specific chronic illnesses such as cancer, diabetes, heart disease, and pulmonary disease are also popular. Chronic disease and disability do not preclude health and wellness; rather, positive health attitudes and practices can promote optimal health for people who must live with the limitations imposed by their chronic illnesses and disabilities.

Health promotion programs can be offered almost anywhere in the community. Common sites include local clinics, schools, colleges, recreation centres, churches, and even private homes. Health fairs are frequently held in civic centres and shopping malls. The outreach idea for health promotion programs has served to meet the needs of many adults who otherwise would not avail themselves of opportunities to strive toward a healthier lifestyle.

The workplace has become a centre for health promotion activity for several reasons. Employers have become increasingly concerned about the rising costs of health care insurance to treat illnesses related to lifestyle behaviours, and they are also concerned about increased absenteeism and lost productivity. Some employers use health promotion specialists to develop and implement these programs, and others purchase packaged programs that have already been developed by health care agencies or private health promotion corporations.

Programs offered at the workplace usually include employee health screening and counselling, physical fitness, nutritional awareness, work safety, and stress management and stress reduction. In addition, efforts are made to promote a safe and healthy work environment. Many large businesses provide exercise facilities for their employees and offer their health promotion programs to retirees.

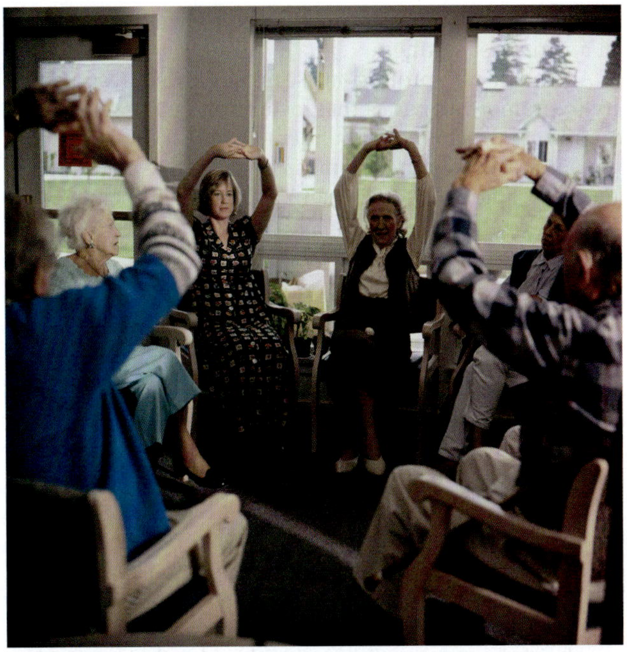

FIGURE 4-2. Health promotion for the older adults includes physical fitness. Here, a nurse teaches exercises at a seniors' centre.

Gerontologic Considerations

Health promotion is as important for older people as it is for others. Although 80% of people older than 65 years have one or more chronic illnesses and many are limited in their activity, older adults as a group experience significant gains from health promotion. Older adults are very health conscious, and most view their health positively and are willing to adopt practices that will improve their health and well-being. Although their chronic illnesses and disabilities cannot be eliminated, these adults can benefit from activities that help them maintain independence and achieve an optimal level of health.

Various health promotion programs have been developed to meet the needs of older Canadians. Both public and private organizations continue to be responsive to health promotion, and more programs that serve older adults are emerging. Many of these programs are offered by health care agencies, churches, community centres, senior citizen residences, and a variety of other organizations. The activities directed toward health promotion for older adults are the same as those for other age groups: physical fitness and exercise, nutrition, safety, and stress management (Fig. 4-2).

Nursing Implications of Health Promotion

By virtue of their expertise in health and health care and their long-established credibility with consumers, nurses play a vital role in health promotion. In many instances, they have initiated health promotion and health screening programs or have participated with other health care personnel in developing and providing wellness services in a variety of settings.

As health care professionals, nurses have a responsibility to promote activities that foster well-being, self-actualization, and personal fulfillment. Every interaction with consumers of health care must be viewed as an opportunity to promote positive health attitudes and behaviours.

Critical Thinking Exercises

1 A female college student with a 2-year history of irritable bowel syndrome makes an appointment to speak with the nurse practitioner at the college health centre to discuss her increased use of antidiarrheal medication. The student states, "I've been very busy with my studies and several activities this semester, and I haven't been eating right." What health promotion components guide the nurse in assessing the student's situation? What is the evidence base for offering information and health programs to help this young adult make appropriate health decisions and establish positive health behaviours? Identify the criteria used to evaluate the strength of the evidence for this practice.

2 After falling from a piece of machinery at a construction site, a 40-year-old man is recuperating at home after being in the hospital. A home care nurse visits three times a week to perform abdominal wound care. During a visit, the man reports that he misses his daily exercise routine and asks when he will be able to resume exercising. Determine the factors that influence his ability to engage in exercise. What factors support the overall relationship between fitness and health? Develop a collaborative plan to assist the man to maintain muscle tone and promote well-being.

3 A 74-year-old woman is volunteering at a local health fair being held at her granddaughter's high school. When the nurse coordinator asks the woman if she would like to participate in the screening events and other informational activities, she replies, "No, thank you. I'm too old to think about health promotion. I just need to take care of the health problems that I already have." What evidence supports the importance of health promotion strategies for the older adult? What information should you include in a discussion with this woman about promoting health in older adults? What type of information, available at various booths at the health fair, would be appropriate for this woman to obtain?

REFERENCES AND SELECTED READINGS

Books

Andrews, M. M., & Boyle, J. S. (2016). *Transcultural concepts in nursing care* (7th ed.). Philadelphia, PA: Wolters Kluwer Health/Lippincott Williams & Wilkins.

Bastable, S. B. (2014). *Nurse as educator: Principles of teaching and learning*. Sudbury, MA: Jones & Bartlett.

Becker, M. H. (Ed.). (1974). *The health belief model and personal health behavior*. Thorofare, NJ: Charles B. Slack.

Canadian Nurses Association (CNA). (2017). *Code of ethics for registered nurses*. Ottawa, ON: Author.

Carpenito-Moyet, L. J. (2017). *Handbook of nursing diagnosis* (15th ed.). Philadelphia, PA: Lippincott Williams & Wilkins.

College and Association of Registered Nurses of Alberta (CARNA). (2013). *Nursing practice standards*. Edmonton, AB: Author.

de Chesnay, M., & Anderson, B. A. (2016). *Caring for the vulnerable: Perspectives in nursing theory, practice, and research* (2nd ed.). Sudbury, MA: Jones & Bartlett.

Edelman, C. L., Kudzma, E. C., & Mandle, C. L. (2014). *Health promotion throughout the life span* (8th ed.). Philadelphia, PA: Elsevier Health Sciences.

Giger, J. N. (2016). *Transcultural nursing: Assessment and intervention* (7th ed.). St. Louis, MO: Elsevier/Mosby.

Haber, D. (2016). *Health promotion and aging: Practical application for health professionals* (7th ed.). New York: Springer.

Lalonde, M. (1977). *New perspectives on the health of Canadians: A working document*. Ottawa, Canada: Minister of Supply and Services.

Mauk, K. L. (2017). *Gerontological nursing: Competencies for care* (4th ed.). Sudbury, MA: Jones & Bartlett.

McFarland, M. R., & Wehbe-Alamah, H. B. (2015). *Leininger's culture care diversity and universality: A worldwide nursing theory* (3rd ed.). Burlington, MA: Jones & Bartlett.

Miller, C. A. (2015). *Nursing for wellness in older adults* (8th ed.). Philadelphia, PA: Lippincott Williams & Wilkins.

Miller, M. A., & Stoeckel, P. R. (2016). *Client education: Theory and practice* (2nd ed.). Sudbury, MA: Jones & Bartlett.

Murdaugh, C. L., Parsons, M. A., & Pender, N. J. (2018). *Health promotion in nursing practice* (8th ed.). Upper Saddle River, NJ: Pearson.

O'Donnell, M. P. (Ed.). (2014). *Health promotion in the workplace*. Troy, MI: American Journal of Health Promotion.

Parnell, T. A. (2015). *Health literacy in nursing: Providing person-centered care*. New York: Springer Publication.

Rootman, I., Pederson, A., Frohlich, K., et al. (Eds.). (2017). *Health promotion in Canada: New perspectives on theory, practice, policy and research* (4th ed.). Toronto, ON: Canadian Scholars.

Tabloski, P. (2013). *Gerontological nursing: The essential guide to clinical practice* (3rd ed.). New York: Pearson.

Touhy, T., Jett, K., Boscart, V., et al. (2018). *Ebersole and Hess' gerontological nursing and healthy aging in Canada* (2nd ed.). Toronto, ON: Elsevier/Mosby.

Journals and Electronic Documents

Adam, J., & Folds, L. (2014). Depression, self-efficacy, and adherence in patients with type 2 diabetes. *The Journal for Nurse Practitioners*, *10*(9), 646–652.

Becker, H., Stuifbergen, A., Oh, H. S., et al. (1993). Self-rated abilities for health practices: A health self-efficacy measure. *Health Values*, *17*, 42–50.

Bender, C. M., Gentry, A. L., Brufsky, A. M., et al. (2014). Influence of patient and treatment factors on adherence to adjuvant endocrine therapy in breast cancer. *Oncology Nursing Forum*, *41*(3), 274–285.

Blanch-Hartigan, D., Blake, K. D., & Viswanath, K. (2014). Cancer survivors' use of numerous information sources for cancer-related information: Does more matter? *Journal of Cancer Education*, *29*, 488–496.

Bruning, R. S., & Sturek, M. (2015). Benefits of exercise training on coronary blood flow in coronary artery disease patients. *Progress in Cardiovascular Diseases*, *57*, 443–453.

Centers for Disease Control and Prevention (CDC). (2016). *Recommended adult immunization schedule—United States, 2016*. Retrieved January 05, 2018, from www.cdc.gov/vaccines/schedules/hcp/adult.html

Cha, C. (2013). Health concept and health promotion process among Korean migrant women. *Health Care for Women International*, *34*, 628–650.

Chaufan, C., Yeh, J., & Sigal, B. (2015). Advancing family health through the garden of eatin': On-site food gardens in early childhood. *American Journal of Public Health*, *105*(4), 625–628.

Claborn, K. R., Meier, E., Miller, M. B., et al. (2015). A systematic review of treatment fatigue among HIV-infected patients prescribed antiretroviral therapy. *Psychology, Health and Medicine*, *20*(3), 255–265.

DiClemente, C. (2007). The transtheoretical model of intentional behavior change. *Drugs & Alcohol Today*, *7*(1), 29–33.

Fang, G., Robinson, J., Lauffenburger, J., et al. (2014). Prevalent but moderate variation across small geographic regions in patient nonadherence to evidence-based preventive therapies in older adults post myocardial infarction. *Medical Care*, *52*(3), 185–193.

Gerber, M., Jonsdottir, I. H., Arvidson, E., et al. (2015). Promoting grade exercise as a part of multimodal treatment in patients diagnosed with stress-related exhaustion. *Journal of Clinical Nursing, 24*, 1904–1915.
Groh, C. J., & Urbancic, J. C. (2015). The impact of a lifestyle change program on the mental health of obese under-served African American women. *Archives of Psychiatric Nursing, 29*, 76–82.
Halvarsson, A., Franzen, E., & Stahle, A. (2015). Balance training with multi-task exercises improves fall-related self-efficacy, gait, balance performance and physical function in older adults with osteoporosis: A randomized controlled study. *Clinical Rehabilitation, 29*(4), 365–375.
Harold, L. R., Briesacher, B. A., Peterson, D., et al. (2013). Cost-related medication nonadherence in older patients with rheumatoid arthritis. *Journal of Rheumatology, 40*(2), 137–143.
Harris, L., Thomas, V., & Fox, M. (2015). The influence of health care literacy on the use of PHRs among older adults. *Medsurg Nursing, 24*(4), 383–385.
Hartley, L., Flowers, N., Lee, M. S., et al. (2014). Tai chi for primary prevention of cardiovascular disease. *The Cochrane Database of Systematic Reviews*, (4), CD010366.
Hooper, L. M., & Huffman, L. E. (2014). Associations among depressive symptoms, well-being, patient involvement, provider cultural competency, and treatment nonadherence: An exploratory study among university student-patients. *Counselling Psychology Quarterly, 27*(3), 241–263.
Khazaee-Pool, M., Sadeghi, R., Majlessi, F., et al. (2014). Effects of physical exercise programme on happiness among older people. *Journal of Psychiatric and Mental Health Nursing, 22*, 47–57.
Martins, M. M., de Souza, J., & da Silva, A. A. (2015). Children and adolescents who are substance users in the psychiatric emergency service. *Acta Paulista de Enfermagem, 28*(1), 13–18.
Mehta, S., Cameron, K., & Battistella, M. (2014). Motivational interviewing: Application to end stage disease patients. *Canadian Association of Nephrology Nurses and Technologists Journal, 24*(4), 19–24.
Meraviglia, M., Stuifbergen, A., Morgan, S., et al. (2015). Low-income cancer survivors' use of health-promoting behaviors. *Medsurg Nursing, 24*(2), 101–106.
Mitchell, J., Khoukaz, T., McNeal, D., et al. (2014). Adverse event management strategies: Optimizing treatment with regorafenib in patients with metastatic colorectal cancer. *Clinical Journal of Oncology Nursing, 18*(2), E19–E25.
Murimi, M., Chrisman, M. S., McAllister, T., et al. (2015). Fostering healthy lifestyles in the African American population. *Health Education & Behavior, 42*(1), 109–116.
Public Health Agency of Canada (PHAC). (2018). *Mission, vision and values*. Retrieved August 25, 2018, from https://www.canada.ca/en/public-health/corporate/mandate.html
Rao, R. M., Raghuram, N., Nagendra, H. R., et al. (2015). Effects of an integrated yoga program on self-reported depression scores in breast cancer patients undergoing conventional treatment: A randomized controlled trial. *Indian Journal of Palliative Care, 21*(2), 174–181.
Resnick, B., Nahm, E. S., Zhu, S., et al. (2014). The impact of osteoporosis, falls, fear of falling, and efficacy expectations on exercise among community-dwelling older adults. *Orthopaedic Nursing, 35*(5), 277–286.
Ryan, J. G., Fedders, M., Jennings, T., et al. (2014). Clinical outcomes and incremental costs from a medication adherence pilot intervention targeting low-income patients with diabetes at risk of cost-related medication nonadherence. *Clinical Therapeutics, 36*(12), 1991–2002.
Seebohm, P., Chaudhary, S., Boyce, M., et al. (2013). The contribution of self-help/mutual aid groups to mental well-being. *Health & social care in the community, 21*(4), 391–401.
Smith, S. A. (2014). Mindfulness-based stress reduction: An intervention to enhance the effectiveness of nurses' coping with work-related stress. *International Journal of Nursing Knowledge, 25*(2), 119–130.
Stirratt, M. J., Curtis, J. R., Danila, M. I., et al. (2018). Advancing the science and practice of medication adherence. *Journal of General Internal Medicine, 33*(2), 216–222.
Tam, M. (2014). Understanding and theorizing the role of culture in the conceptualizations of successful aging and lifelong learning. *Educational Gerontology, 40*(12), 881–893.
Theofilou, P. (2013). Medication adherence in Greek hemodialysis patients: The contribution of depression and health cognitions. *International Journal of Behavioural Medicine, 20*, 311–318.
World Health Organization (WHO). (2018). *The Ottawa Charter for Health Promotion*. Retrieved September 10, 2018, from http://www.who.int/healthpromotion/conferences/previous/ottawa/en/
Wu, J. R., & Moser, D. K. (2014). Type D personality predicts poor medication adherence in patients with heart failure in the USA. *International Journal of Behavioral Medicine, 21*, 833–842.
Yeun, E. J., Baek, S., & Kim, H. (2013). Health promotion behavior in middle-aged Koreans: A cross-sectional survey. *Nursing & Health Sciences, 15*, 461–467.
Yoo, C., Park, S., Yang, D., et al. (2014). Study of the physical condition of middle-aged office and field workers aged 50 and older. *Journal of Physical Therapy Science, 26*, 1575–1577.

Resources

Canadian Nurses Association: https://www.cna-aiic.ca
Canadian Task Force on Preventative Health Care: https://canadiantaskforce.ca/
Centers for Disease Control and Prevention: http://www.cdc.gov
The College of Family Physicians of Canada: http://cfpc.ca
Health Canada: http://www.hc-sc.gc.ca
Public Health Agency of Canada: http://www.phac-aspc.gc.ca/World Health Organization: http://www.who.int/en/

5 Adult Health and Nutritional Assessment

Adapted by Joseph Osuji and Mohamed Toufic El Hussein

Learning Objectives

On completion of this chapter, the learner will be able to:

1. Identify ethical considerations necessary for protecting a person's rights related to data collected in the health history and physical assessment.
2. Describe the components of the holistic health history.
3. Apply culturally competent and culturally safe interviewing skills and techniques to conduct a successful health history, physical examination, and nutritional assessment.
4. Identify genetic aspects nurses incorporate into the health history and physical assessment.
5. Identify modifications needed to obtain a health history and conduct a physical assessment for a person with a disability.
6. Describe the techniques of inspection, palpation, percussion, and auscultation to perform a basic physical assessment.
7. Discuss the techniques of measurement of body mass index, biochemical assessment, clinical examination, and assessment of food intake to assess a person's nutritional status.
8. Describe factors that may contribute to altered nutritional status in high-risk groups such as adolescents and older adults.
9. Conduct a health history and physical and nutritional assessment of a person at home.

The ability to assess patients is a skill integral to nursing, regardless of the practice setting. In all settings in which nurses interact with patients and provide care, eliciting a complete **health history** and using appropriate assessment skills are critical to identifying physical and psychological issues and concerns experienced by the patient. As the first step in the nursing process, patient assessment is necessary to obtain data that enable the nurse to make an accurate nursing diagnosis, identify and implement appropriate interventions, and assess their effectiveness. This chapter includes the complete health history and basic assessment techniques. Because a patient's nutritional status is an important factor in overall health and well-being, nutritional assessment is also addressed in this chapter.

Considerations for Conducting a Health History and Physical Assessment

The Role of the Nurse

All members of the health care team collaborate and use their unique skills and knowledge to contribute to the resolution of patient problems by first obtaining some level of history and assessment (Weber & Kelley, 2018). Various formats for obtaining the health history (the collection of subjective data about the patient's health status) and performing the **physical examination** (the collection of objective data about the patient's health status) have been developed because the focus of each member of the health care team is unique. Regardless of the format, the information obtained by the nurse complements the data obtained by other members of the health care team and focuses on nursing's unique concerns for the patient. The nurse completes a health assessment by obtaining the patient's health history and performing a physical assessment, which can be carried out in a variety of settings. These settings may include an acute care facility, a clinic or outpatient office, a long-term care facility, a school, or the patient's home. Nursing diagnoses are used to determine the appropriate plan of care for the patient and drive nursing interventions and patient outcomes. Nursing diagnoses also provide a standard nomenclature for use in the electronic health record (EHR), enabling clear communication among care team members and the collection of data for continuous improvement in patient care (Herdman & Kamitsuru, 2018).

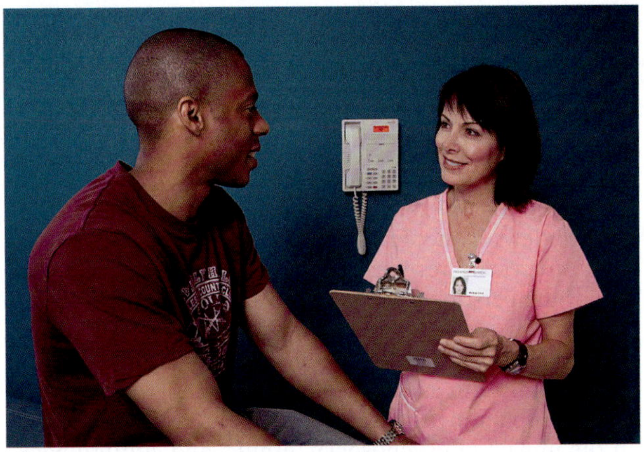

FIGURE 5-1. A comfortable, relaxed atmosphere and an attentive interviewer are essential for a successful clinical interview.

Communicating Effectively

People who seek health care for a specific concern are often anxious. Their anxiety may be increased by fear of potential diagnoses, possible disruption of lifestyle, and other concerns. With this in mind, the nurse attempts to establish rapport, put the patient at ease, encourage honest communication, make eye contact, and listen carefully to the patient's responses to questions about health issues (Fig. 5-1).

When obtaining a health history or performing a physical examination, the nurse is aware of his or her own nonverbal communication as well as that of the patient. The nurse takes into consideration the patient's educational and cultural background as well as language proficiency. Questions and instructions to the patient are phrased in a way that is easily understandable. Technical terms and medical jargon are avoided. In addition, the nurse considers the patient's disabilities or impairments such as hearing, vision, cognitive, and physical limitations. At the end of the assessment, the nurse may summarize and clarify the information obtained and ask the patient if he or she has any questions; this gives the nurse and the patient the opportunity to correct misinformation and add facts that may have been omitted.

Ethical Use of History or Physical Examination Data

Whenever information is elicited from a person through a health history or physical examination, the person has the right to know why the information is sought and how it will be used. For this reason, it is important to explain the purpose of the health history and physical examination, how the information will be obtained, how it will be used, and with whom it will be shared (Bickley, 2017; Stephen, 2012a; Weber & Kelley, 2018). It is also important that the person knows that the decision to participate is voluntary. A private setting for the history interview and physical examination should promote trust and encourage open, honest communication. After the history and examination are completed, the nurse selectively records the data pertinent to the patient's health status. This written record of the patient's history and physical examination findings is then securely maintained and made available only to those health professionals directly involved in the care of the patient.

Increasing Use of Technology

The use of technology to augment the information gathering process has become an increasingly important aspect of obtaining a health history and physical examination. Computerization of health records is becoming more common. **Electronic health records** are thought to enhance continuity of care, improve the quality of care, reduce medical errors, and help reduce health care costs; therefore, their implementation is moving forward on a global scale (Stephen, 2012a). Nurses may need to allow extra time and provide detailed instructions or explanations, depending on age, status, and experience of patient.

Glossary

auscultation: listening to sounds produced within different body structures created by the movement of air or fluid

body mass index (BMI): a calculation done to estimate the amount of body fat of a person

electronic health record (EHR): computerization of health records; also referred to as electronic medical record (EMR)

health history: a series of questions that provides an overview of the patient's current health status

inspection: visual assessment of different aspects of the patient

palpation: examination of different organs of the body using the sense of touch

percussion: the use of sound to examine different organs of the body

physical examination: collection of objective data about the patient's health status

It is important to establish eye contact with the patient during the health history and not focus solely on the computer screen for data entry.

Health History

The health history is a series of questions used to provide an overview of the current health status of the patient. Many nurses are responsible for obtaining a detailed history of the person's current health problems, past medical history, and family history and a review of the person's functional status. This results in a total health profile that focuses on health as well as illness.

When obtaining the health history, attention is focused on the impact of psychosocial, ethnic, and cultural background on a person's health, illness, and health promotion behaviours. The interpersonal and physical environments, as well as the person's lifestyle and activities of daily living, are explored in depth. The format of the health history traditionally combines the medical history and the nursing assessment, although formats based on nursing frameworks, such as functional health patterns, have also become standard. Both the review of systems and the patient profile are expanded to include individual and family relationships, lifestyle patterns, health practices, nutritional assessment, and coping strategies. These components of the health history are the basis of nursing assessment and can be easily adapted to address the needs of any patient population in any setting, institution, or agency (Stephen, 2012a; Weber & Kelley, 2018). Combining the information obtained by the physician and the nurse into one health history prevents duplication of information and minimizes efforts on the part of the patient to provide this information repeatedly. This also encourages collaboration among members of the health care team who share in the collection and interpretation of the data. The health history format discussed in this chapter is only one approach that is useful in obtaining and organizing information about a patient's health status. Some experts consider this traditional format to be inappropriate for nurses, because it does not focus exclusively on the assessment of human responses to actual or potential health problems. Several attempts have been made to develop an assessment format and database with this focus in mind. One example is a nursing database developed by North American Nursing Diagnosis Association (NANDA) International with its 13 domains (Herdman & Kamitsuru, 2018). Although there is support in nursing for using this approach, no consensus for its use has been reached.

The Informant

The informant, or the person providing the health history, may not always be the patient, as in the case of a developmentally delayed, mentally impaired, disoriented, confused, unconscious, or comatose patient. The interviewer assesses the reliability of the informant and the usefulness of the information provided. For example, a patient who is disoriented is often unable to provide reliable information; people who use alcohol and illicit drugs often deny using these substances. The interviewer must make a clinical judgment about the reliability of the information (based on the context of the entire interview) and include this assessment in the record. Chart 5-1 provides special considerations for obtaining a health history from an older adult.

CHART 5-1

Health Assessment in the Older Adult

- Obtain the health history from older adult patients in a calm, unrushed manner.
- Consider possible vision or hearing impairments. Ensure that lighting is adequate but not glaring, and keep distracting noises to a minimum.
- Assume a position that enables the older adult patient to read lips and facial expressions. Sometimes sitting at a 90-degree angle to the patient is helpful because some visual impairments, such as macular degeneration, can limit the patient's vision to only peripheral vision. It is best to ask the patient where the interviewer should sit in relation to the patient to optimize the patient's view of the interviewer.
- Determine if the patient uses a hearing aid and ask the patient to use it during the interview. Check if the patient usually wears glasses and ensure that they are worn as well.
- Be aware that older adults often assume that new physical problems are a result of age rather than a treatable illness. Some of these problems may limit their activities of daily living and lifestyle patterns.
- Ask questions related to changes in the level of functioning. The signs and symptoms of illness in older adults are often more subtle than those in younger adults and may go unreported. A question such as "What interferes most in your daily activities?" may be useful in focusing the clinical evaluation.
- Obtain a complete history of medications used, because many older adult patients take many different kinds of prescription and over-the-counter (OTC) medications.
- Consider including a member of the family in the interview process. Although older adults may experience a decline in mental function, it should not be assumed that they are unable to provide an adequate history. Including a spouse, adult child, sibling, or caretaker may validate information and provide missing details. However, this should be done after obtaining the patient's permission. (Further details about assessment of the older adult are provided in Chapter 14.)

Adapted from Eliopoulos, C. (2018). *Gerontological nursing* (9th ed.). Philadelphia, PA: Lippincott Williams & Wilkins; Weber, J. R., & Kelley, J. H. (2018). *Health assessment in nursing* (5th ed.). Philadelphia, PA: Lippincott Williams & Wilkins.

Components of the Health History

When a patient is seen for the first time by a member of the health care team, the first requirement is that baseline information be obtained (except in emergency situations). The sequence and format of obtaining data about a patient may vary, but the content, regardless of format, usually addresses the same general topics. A traditional approach includes the following: biographical data, chief complaint, present health concern (or history of present illness), past health history, family history, review of systems, and patient profile.

Biographical Data

Biographical information puts the patient's health history into context. This information includes the person's name, address, age, gender, marital status, occupation, and ethnic origins. Most interviewers prefer to wait to ask more personal questions later in the interview, when more trust and confidence have been established or until a patient's immediate or urgent needs have been addressed. A patient who is in severe pain or has another urgent condition is unlikely to have a great deal of patience for an interviewer who is more concerned about marital or occupational status than with quickly addressing the problem at hand.

Chief Complaint

The chief complaint is the issue that brings a person to the attention of the health care professional. Questions such as "Why have you come to the health centre today?" or "Why were you admitted to the hospital?" usually elicit the chief complaint. In the home setting, the initial question might be, "What is bothering you most today?" When an issue is identified, the person's exact words are usually recorded in quotation marks. However, a statement such as "My doctor sent me," should be followed up with a question that identifies the probable reason why the person is seeking health care; this reason is then identified as the chief complaint (Stephen, 2012a; Weber & Kelley, 2018).

Present Health Concern or Illness

The history of the present health concern or illness is the single most important factor in helping the health care team arrive at a diagnosis or determine the person's needs. The physical examination is helpful but often only validates the information obtained from the history. A careful history assists in correct selection of appropriate diagnostic tests. Although diagnostic test results can be helpful, they often support rather than establish the diagnosis.

If the present illness is only one episode in a series of episodes, the entire sequence of events is recorded. For example, a history from a patient whose chief concern is an episode of insulin shock describes the entire course of the diabetes to put the current episode in context. The details of the health concern or present illness are described from onset until the time of contact with the health care team. These facts are recorded in chronologic order, beginning with, for example, "The patient was in good health until..." or "The patient first experienced abdominal pain 2 months prior to seeking help."

The history of the present illness or health concern includes such information as the date and manner (sudden or gradual) in which the problem occurred, the setting in which the concern occurred (at home, at work, after an argument, after exercise), manifestations of the problem, and the course of the illness or concern. This includes self-treatment (including complementary and alternative therapies), medical interventions, progress and effects of treatment, and the patient's perceptions of the cause or meaning of the problem.

Specific symptoms, such as (pain, headache, fever, change in bowel habits) are described in detail, along with the location and radiation (if pain), quality, severity, and duration. The interviewer also asks whether the concern is persistent or intermittent, what factors aggravate or alleviate it, and whether any associated manifestations exist.

Associated manifestations are symptoms that occur simultaneously with the chief complaint. The presence or absence of such symptoms may shed light on the origin or extent of the concern, as well as on the diagnosis. These symptoms are referred to as significant positive or negative findings and are obtained from a review of systems directly related to the chief complaint. For example, if a patient reports a vague symptom, such as fatigue or weight loss, all body systems are reviewed and included in this section of the history. If, on the other hand, a patient's chief complaint is chest pain, only the cardiopulmonary and gastrointestinal systems may be included in the history of the present illness. In either situation, both positive and negative findings are recorded to define the concern further.

Past Health History

A detailed summary of a person's past health is an important part of the health history (Stephen, 2012a). After determining the general health status, the nurse inquires about the immunization status according to the recommendations of the adult immunization schedule and records the dates of immunization (if known) (Public Health Agency of Canada [PHAC], 2018a, 2018b). The nurse also inquires about any known allergies to medications or other substances, along with the type of allergy and adverse reactions. Other relevant material includes information, if known, about the patient's last physical examination, chest x-ray, electrocardiogram, eye examination, hearing test, dental checkup, Papanicolaou (Pap) smear and mammogram (if female), digital rectal examination of the prostate gland (if male), bone density testing, colon cancer screening, and any other pertinent tests. The nurse then discusses previous illnesses and records negative as well as positive responses to a list of specific diseases. Dates of illness or the age of the patient at the time, as well as the names of the primary health care professional and hospital, the diagnosis, and the treatment are noted. The nurse elicits a history of the following areas:

- Childhood illnesses—rubeola, rubella, polio, whooping cough, mumps, measles, chickenpox, scarlet fever, rheumatic fever, strep throat, meningitis
- Adult illnesses
- Psychiatric illnesses
- Injuries—burns, fractures, head injuries
- Hospitalizations
- Surgical and diagnostic procedures
- Current medications—prescription, over-the-counter (OTC), home remedies, complementary, and alternative therapies
- Use of alcohol and other drugs
- Smoking

If a particular hospitalization or major medical intervention is related to the present illness, the account of it is not repeated; rather, the report refers to the appropriate part of the record, such as "See history of present illness" on the patient's health record.

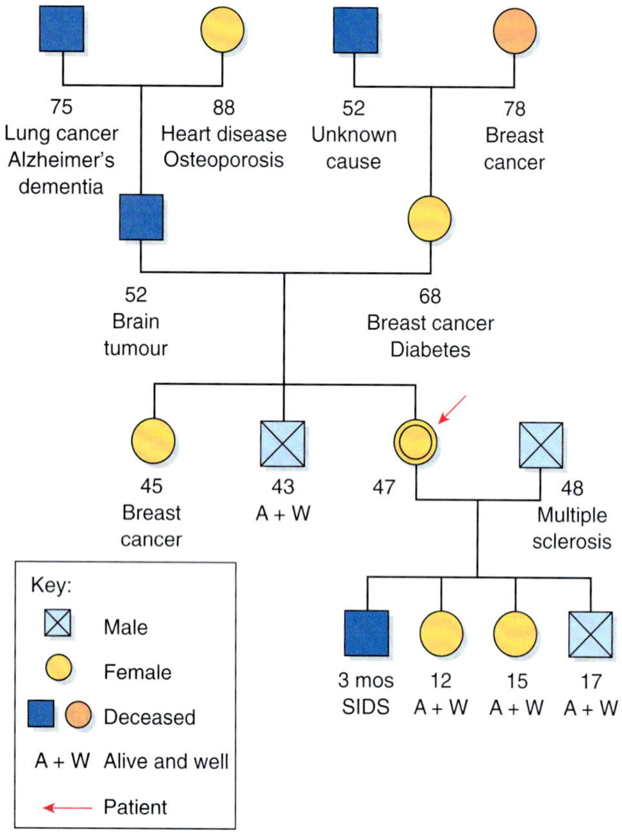

FIGURE 5-2. Diagram (called a genogram) used to record history of family members, including their age and cause of death or, if living, their current health status.

Family History

To identify diseases that may be genetic, communicable, or possibly environmental in origin, the nurse asks about the age and health status, or the age and cause of death of first-order relatives (parents, siblings, spouse, children) and second-order relatives (grandparents, cousins). In general, the following conditions are included: cancer, hypertension, heart disease, diabetes, epilepsy, mental illness, tuberculosis, kidney disease, arthritis, allergies, asthma, alcoholism, and obesity. One of the easiest methods of recording such data is by using the family tree, or genogram (Fig. 5-2). The results of genetic testing or screening, if known, are recorded. Chart 5-2 provides genetic considerations related to health assessment; see also Chapter 11 for a detailed discussion of genetics.

Review of Systems

The review of systems includes an overview of general health as well as symptoms related to each body system. Questions are asked about each of the major body systems for information about past and present symptoms. Reviewing each body system helps reveal relevant data. Negative as well as positive answers are recorded. If a patient responds positively to questions about a particular system, further questioning is used and the information is analyzed carefully. If any illnesses were previously mentioned or recorded, it is not necessary to repeat them in this part of the history. Instead, reference is made to the appropriate place in the health history where the information can be found.

A review of systems can be organized in a formal checklist, which becomes a part of the health history. One advantage of a checklist is that it can be easily audited and is less subject to error than a system that relies heavily on the interviewer's memory.

Patient Profile

In the patient profile, more biographical information is gathered. A complete composite or profile of the patient is critical to analysis of the chief concern and of the person's ability to deal with the concern. A complete patient profile is summarized in Chart 5-3.

At this point in the interview, the information elicited is highly personal and subjective. People are encouraged to express feelings honestly and to discuss personal experiences. It is best to begin with general, open-ended questions and to move to direct questioning when specific facts are needed. Interviews that progress from information that is less personal (birthplace, occupation, education) to information that is more personal (sexuality, body image, coping abilities) often reduce anxiety.

A general patient profile consists of the following content areas: past life events related to health, current medications, education and occupation, environment (physical, spiritual, cultural), lifestyle (patterns and habits), presence of a physical or mental disability, self-concept, sexuality, risk for abuse, and stress and coping response.

Past Life Events Related to Health

The patient profile begins with a brief life history. Questions about place of birth and past places of residence help focus attention on the earlier years of life. Personal experiences during childhood or adolescence that have special significance may be elicited by asking a question such as "Was there anything that you experienced as a child or adolescent that would be helpful for me to know about?" The interviewer's intent is to encourage the patient to make a quick review of his or her earlier life, highlighting information of particular significance. Although many patients may not recall anything significant, others may share information such as a personal achievement, a failure, a developmental crisis, or an instance of physical, emotional, or sexual abuse. The life history includes a brief medication history as appropriate for the patient.

Current Medications

A review of the patient's current medications is necessary to complete a comprehensive health history. Particular attention is given to allergies or adverse reactions to medications. The interviewer should inquire about the use of OTC medications and herbal supplements; patients often include only prescription medications when they list their current medications.

Education and Occupation

Inquiring about current occupation can reveal much about a person's economic status and educational preparation. A statement such as "Tell me about your job," often elicits information about role, job tasks, and satisfaction with the position. Direct questions about past employment and career goals may be asked if the person does not provide this information.

GENETICS IN NURSING PRACTICE

Chart 5-2. Genetic Aspects of Health Assessment

Nursing Assessments

FAMILY HISTORY ASSESSMENT

Obtain information about maternal and paternal sides of family for three generations.

Obtain history of known diseases or disorders for three generations for:

- Clustering of diseases or disorders.
- Early onset of disease or illness (e.g., blood clots in an active, otherwise apparently healthy 30 year old, or colon cancer in a 40 year old).
- Similar disorder or disease in two or more close relatives.
- History of multiple miscarriages, birth defects, or developmental delays.
- Close biologic relationship between parents.

Assess for individual and family perceptions and beliefs around genetics topics through a cultural, social, and spiritual assessment.

Acknowledge ethnic risk for particular genetic disorders.

Determine whether the patient or a direct family member has had an unexpected response to medications or anesthesia.

Recognize and evaluate for patterns of inheritance.

Ascertain family relationships (family structure, roles, communication patterns, support system).

PATIENT ASSESSMENT

Assess physical findings that may suggest a genetic condition (e.g., unusually tall stature—Marfan syndrome; low set ears and epicanthal folds—Down's syndrome).

Is there a presence of two or more dysmorphic features?

Is there a presence of disability (physical or intellectual) or a history of developmental delay?

Assess for conditions that occur in a less-often affected sex (e.g., stuttering in females, breast cancer in males, inguinal hernia in females).

Presence of disease without known risk factors (e.g., hyperlipidemia).

Acknowledge genetic-related risk related to ethnic background.

Identify religious health, spiritual health, beliefs, and practices.

Management Issues Specific to Genetics

Assess patient's understanding of genetic information and factors related to their health risks.

Refer for risk assessment when a hereditary disease or disorder is suspected.

Determine if genetic testing has been performed and if other family members are affected.

Educate patient and family about the Genetic Information Nondiscrimination Act (GINA), passed in 2008.

Offer appropriate genetic information and resources.

Refer to a genetic counselor.

Ensure that consent obtained for genetic testing is voluntary and informed.

Provide support to patients and families with known genetic test results for hereditary disease or disorders, and refer to support groups as indicated.

Participate in the management and coordination of risk reduction measures for those with known gene mutations.

Genetics Resources

Genetic Information Nondiscrimination Act. Retrieved from www.ginahelp.org

It is important to learn about a person's educational background. Asking a person what kind of educational requirements were necessary to attain his or her present job is a more sensitive approach than asking whether he or she graduated from high school. Information about the patient's general financial status may be obtained by questions such as "Do you have any financial concerns at this time?" or "Sometimes there just doesn't seem to be enough money to make ends meet. Are you finding this to be true?"

Environment

The concept of environment includes a person's physical environment and its potential hazards, spiritual awareness, cultural background, interpersonal relationships, and support system.

PHYSICAL ENVIRONMENT. Information is elicited about the type of housing (apartment, duplex, single family) in which the person lives, its location, the level of safety and comfort within the home and neighbourhood, and the presence of environmental hazards (e.g., isolation, potential fire risks, inadequate sanitation). If the patient has a disability, or is homeless or living in a shelter, the nurse asks questions about the patient's home environment.

SPIRITUAL ENVIRONMENT. Spirituality is defined as connectedness with self, others, a life force, or God that allows people to experience self-transcendence and find meaning in life. Spirituality helps many people discover a purpose in life, understand the ever-changing qualities of life, and develop their relationship with God or a higher power. Within the framework of spirituality, people may discover truths about themselves, about the world, and their morality (O'Brien, 2018).

Spiritual behaviour can be expressed through devotion, sacrifice, self-discipline, and spending time in activities that focus on the inner self or the soul. Although religion and nature are two vehicles that people use to connect themselves with God or a higher power, bonds to religious institutions, beliefs, or dogma are not required to experience the spiritual sense of self. Faith, considered the foundation of spirituality, is trust in God and belief in a higher power or something that a person cannot see. The spiritual part of a person views life as a mystery that unfolds over one's lifetime, encompassing questions about meaning, hope, relatedness to a higher power, acceptance or forgiveness, and transcendence (see Chapter 7).

A person's spiritual environment refers to the degree to which he or she thinks about or contemplates their existence, accepts challenges in life, and seeks and finds answers to personal questions. Spirituality may be expressed through identification with a particular religion. Spiritual values and beliefs often direct a person's behaviour and approach to health problems and can influence

CHART 5-3

Patient Profile

Past Events Related to Health
Place of birth
Places lived
Significant childhood/adolescent experiences

Current Medications
Prescription, over-the-counter (OTC), home remedies, complementary and alternative therapies

Education and Occupation
Jobs held in past
Current position/job
Length of time at position
Educational preparation
Work satisfaction and career goals

Financial Resources
Income
Coverage for prescription medications, dental care, treatments (massage, physical therapy, acupuncture, etc.)

Environment
Physical—living arrangements (type of housing, neighbourhood, presence of hazards)
Spiritual—extent to which religion is a part of individual's life; religious beliefs related to perception of health and illness; religious practices
Interpersonal—ethnic background (language spoken, customs and values held, practices used to maintain health or to cure illness); family relationships (family structure, roles, communication patterns, support system); friendships (quality of relationship)

Lifestyle Patterns
Sleep (time person retires, hours per night, comfort measures, awakens rested)
Exercise (type, frequency, time spent)
Nutrition (24-hour diet recall, idiosyncrasies, restrictions)
Recreation (type of activity, time spent)
Caffeine (coffee, tea, cola, chocolate—kind), amount
Smoking (cigarette, pipe, cigar, marijuana—kind), amount per day, number of years, desire to quit
Alcohol—kind, amount, pattern over past year
Drugs—kind, amount, route of administration

Physical or Mental Disability
Presence of a disability (physical or mental)
Effect of disability on function and health access
Accommodations needed to support functioning

Self-Concept
View of self in present
View of self in future
Body image (level of satisfaction, concerns)

Sexuality
Perception of self as a man or woman
Quality of sexual relationships
Concerns related to sexuality or sexual functioning

Risk for Abuse
Physical injury in past
Afraid of partner, caregiver, or family member
Refusal of caregiver to provide necessary equipment or assistance

Stress and Coping Response
Major concerns or problems at present
Daily "hassles"
Past experiences with similar problems
Past coping patterns and outcomes
Present coping strategies and anticipated outcomes
Individual's expectations of family/friends and health care team in problem resolution

responses to sickness. A strong sense of spirituality or religious faith can have a positive impact on health. Spirituality is also a component of hope, and, especially during chronic, serious, or terminal illness, patients and their families often find comfort and emotional strength in their religious traditions or spiritual beliefs. At other times, illness and loss can cause a loss of faith or meaning in life and a spiritual crisis, which can place considerable stress on a person's internal resources and beliefs. It is important that the spiritual beliefs of people and families be acknowledged, valued, and respected for the comfort and guidance they provide. Inquiring about spirituality can identify possible support systems as well as beliefs and customs that need to be considered in planning care. Information is gathered about the extent to which religion is a part of the person's life as well as religious beliefs and practices related to health and illness.

A spiritual assessment may involve asking the following questions:

- Is religion or spirituality important to you?
- If no, what is the most important thing in your life?
- If yes, in what way? For instance:
  - Are there any religious or spiritual practices that are important to you?
  - Do you belong to a faith community or have a place of worship?
  - Do you have any religious or spiritual concerns because of your present health problem?

The nurse should assess spiritual strength further by inquiring about the patient's sense of spiritual well-being, hope, and peacefulness. It is also necessary to assess whether spiritual beliefs and values have changed in response to illness or loss. The nurse assesses current and past participation in religious or spiritual practices and notes the patient's responses to questions regarding spiritual needs to help determine the patient's need for spiritual care. Another simple assessment technique is to inquire about the patient's and the family's desire for spiritual support (O'Brien, 2018).

CULTURAL ENVIRONMENT. When obtaining the health history, the person's cultural and religious backgrounds are taken into account. Cultural attitudes and beliefs about health, illness, health care, hospitalization, the use of medications, and use of complementary and alternative therapies, which are derived from personal experiences, vary according to ethnic, cultural, and religious background. A person from another culture may have different views of personal health practices from those of the health care professional (Skillen, 2012c; Weber & Kelley, 2018). See Chapter 8 for more cultural considerations.

The beliefs and practices that have been shared from generation to generation are known as cultural or ethnic patterns. They are expressed through language, dress, dietary choices, and role behaviours; in perceptions of health and illness; and in health-related behaviours. The influence of these beliefs and customs on how a person reacts to health issues and interacts with health care providers cannot be underestimated. The following questions may assist in obtaining relevant information:

- Where did your parents or ancestors come from? When?
- What language do you speak at home?
- Are there certain customs or values that are important to you?
- Is there anything special you do to keep in good health?
- Do you have any specific practices for treating illness?

FAMILY RELATIONSHIPS AND SUPPORT SYSTEM. An assessment of family structure (members, ages, and roles), patterns of communication, and the presence or absence of a support system is an integral part of the patient profile. Although the traditional family is recognized as a mother, a father, and children, many different types of living arrangements exist within our society. "Family" may mean two or more people bound by emotional ties or commitments. Live-in companions, roommates, and close friends can all play a significant role in a person's support system.

Lifestyle

The lifestyle section of the patient profile provides information about health-related behaviours. These behaviours include patterns of sleep, exercise, nutrition, and recreation, as well as personal habits such as smoking, use of alcohol, caffeine, and the use of illicit drugs. Adequate sleep and nutrition are important to maintain optimal health; therefore, it is important to inquire about usual sleep habits and bedtime routines, as well as perform a nutritional assessment. Although most people readily describe their exercise patterns or recreational activities, many are unwilling to report their smoking, alcohol use, and illicit drug use, and many deny or understate the degree to which they use such substances. Questions such as "What kind of alcohol do you enjoy drinking at a party?" may elicit more accurate information than, "Do you drink?" The specific type of alcohol (e.g., wine, liquor, beer) and the amount ingested per day or per week (e.g., 500 mL of whiskey daily for 2 years) should be described (Bickley, 2017; Stephen, 2012a). The lifestyle of some people includes the use of mood-altering substances. People who engage in substance abuse use illegally obtained drugs, prescribed or OTC medications, and alcohol alone or in combination with other drugs in ineffective attempts to cope with the pressures, strains, and burdens of life. Over time, physiologic, emotional, cognitive, and behavioural problems develop as a result of continuous substance abuse.

If alcohol abuse is suspected, additional information may be obtained by using common alcohol screening questionnaires, such as the CAGE (*C*utting down, *A*nnoyance by criticism, *G*uilty feelings, and *E*ye-openers) (Ewing, 1984), AUDIT (*A*lcohol *U*se *D*isorders *I*dentification *T*est), TWEAK (*T*olerance, *W*orry, *E*ye-opener, *A*mnesia, *K*ut down on drinking) (Chan, Pristach, Welte, et al., 1993), or SMAST (*S*hort *M*ichigan *A*lcohol *S*creening *T*est). The CAGE tool has also been adapted as the CAGE Questions Adapted to Include Drugs (CAGEAID). The MAST (Michigan Alcohol Screening Test) has been updated to include drug use and has a geriatric version (The New York State Office of Alcoholism and Substance Abuse Services [OASAS], 2015).

Similar questions can be used to elicit information about smoking and caffeine consumption. Questions about illicit drug use follow naturally after questions about smoking, caffeine consumption, and alcohol use. A nonjudgmental approach makes it easier for a person to respond truthfully and factually. If street names or unfamiliar terms are used to describe drugs, the person is asked to define the terms used.

Investigation of lifestyle also includes questions about complementary and alternative therapies. According to the Public Health Agency of Canada (PHAC), 70% of Canadians use complementary or alternative therapies (PHAC, 2018c). Other types of therapies include: special diets, prayer, visualization or guided imagery, massage, acupuncture, meditation, herbal products, and many others. Marijuana is used for the management of symptoms, especially pain and anorexia, in several chronic conditions. Since the marijuana plant contains chemicals, called cannabinoids, that may help treat a range of illnesses or symptoms, many people argue that it should be legal for medical purposes. This has led to the legalization of marijuana for medical and recreational use in Canada with effect from 2018.

The assessment of a patient's lifestyle patterns also includes questions about continuing health promotion and health screening practices. The health history assessment should include the type, frequency, and duration of exercise and recreational activities. Inquiry should also include the types of health screenings the patient has completed. If the person has not been involved in these practices in the past, he or she should be educated about their importance and referred to the appropriate health care providers. Nurses should recognize the importance of encouraging culturally competent and health promotion activities (Jongen, McCalman, & Bainbridge, 2017).

Disability

The general patient profile contains questions about any hearing, vision, or other type of physical disability. Mental, sensory, or cognitive disabilities are inquired about as well. The presence of an obvious physical limitation (e.g., using crutches to walk or using a wheelchair to get around) necessitates further investigation. The etiology of the disability should be elicited, and the length of time the patient has had the disability, the impact on function, and health access are important to assess. Chart 5-4 presents specific issues that the nurse considers when obtaining health histories and conducting physical assessments of patients with disabilities. See Chapter 12.

CHART 5-4

Assessing the Health of People With Disabilities

Overview

People with disabilities are entitled to the same level of health assessment and physical examination as people without disabilities. Physical and mental disabilities should be explained in the health history. Patients with mental disabilities are often marginalized from mainstream health care services because of the complexities of their disability. It is appropriate to ask the patient, or caregiver when necessary, what assistance he or she needs rather than assuming that help is needed for all activities or that, if assistance is needed, the patient will ask for it.

Health History

Communication between the nurse and the patient is essential. To ensure that the patient is able to respond to assessment questions and provide needed information, interpreters, assistive listening devices, or other alternative formats (e.g., Braille, large-print forms) may be required.

When interpreters are needed, interpretation services should be arranged. Health care facilities have a responsibility to provide these services without charge to the patient. Family members (especially children) should not be used as interpreters, because doing so violates the patient's right to privacy and confidentiality.

The nurse should speak directly to the patient and not to family members or others who have accompanied the patient. If patients have impaired hearing, they should be encouraged to use their hearing aids or hearing assistance technology during the assessment. The patient should be able to see the nurse's face clearly during the health history so that speechreading and nonverbal clues can be used to aid communication.

The health history should address general health issues that are important to all patients, including sexual history and risk for abuse. It should also address the impact of the patient's disability on health issues and access to care, as well as the effect of the patient's current health problem on their disability. An assessment of whether the patient's quality of life meets their expectations should be included in the health history.

The nurse should verify what the patient has said; if the patient has difficulty communicating verbally, the nurse should ask for clarification rather than assume that it is too difficult for the patient to do so. Most people would rather be asked to explain again than run the risk of being misunderstood.

Physical Examination

Inaccessible facilities remain a major barrier to health care for people with disabilities. Barriers include lack of ramps and grab bars, inaccessible restrooms, small examination rooms, and examination tables that cannot be lowered to allow the patient to move himself or herself onto, or be transferred easily and safely to, the examination table. The patient may need help getting undressed for the physical examination (and dressed again), moving on and off the examination table, and maintaining positions usually required during physical examination manoeuvres. It is important to ask the patient what assistance is needed.

If the patient has impaired sensory function (e.g., lack of sensation, hearing or vision loss), it is important to inform the patient that you will be touching him or her. Furthermore, it is important to explain all procedures and manoeuvres.

Gynecologic examinations should not be deferred because a patient has a disability or is assumed to be sexually inactive. Explanations of the examination are important for all women, and even more so for women with disabilities, because they may have had previous negative experiences. Slow, gentle moving and positioning of the patient for the gynecologic examination and warming the speculum before attempting insertion often minimize spasticity in women with neurologically related disabilities.

Health Screenings and Testing

Many people with disabilities report that they have not been weighed for years or even decades because they are unable to stand for this measurement. Alternative methods (e.g., use of wheelchair scales) are needed to monitor weight and body mass index. This is particularly important because of the increased incidence of obesity and its effects on health status and transfer of persons with disabilities.

Patients with disabilities may require special assistance if urine specimens are to be obtained as part of the visit. They are often able to suggest strategies to obtain urine specimens based on previous experience.

If it is necessary for the nurse to wear a mask during a procedure or if the patient is unable to see the face of the nurse during a procedure, it is important to explain the procedure and the expected role of the patient ahead of time. If the patient is unable to hear or communicate with the nurse or other health care provider verbally during an examination or diagnostic test, a method of communication (e.g., signalling the patient by tapping the arm, signalling the nurse by using a bell) should be established beforehand.

People with disabilities experience difficulties related to obtaining care, challenges accessing health care facilities, perceptions that health professionals are insensitive to their needs, and concerns about the quality of care they receive. Therefore, it is important to ask about health screening and recommendations for screening. In addition, people with disabilities should be asked about their participation in health promotion activities, because inaccessible environments and other barriers may limit their participation in exercise, health programs, and other health promotion efforts such as health screenings.

Adapted from Dunkley, S., & Sales, R. (2014). The challenges of providing palliative care for people with intellectual disabilities: A literature review. *International Journal of Palliative Nursing*, *20*(6), 279–284; Kelly-Campbell, R. J., & Lessoway, K. (2015). Hearing aid and hearing assistance technology use in Aotearoa/New Zealand. *International Journal of Audiology*, *54*(5), 308–315; Sharts-Hopko, N. (2009). Low vision and blindness among midlife and older adults. *Holistic Nursing Practice*, *23*(2), 94–100; Sharts-Hopko, N. C., Smeltzer, S. C., Ott, B. B., et al. (2010). Healthcare experiences of women with visual impairment. *Clinical Nurse Specialist*, *24*(3), 149–153; Smeltzer, S. C., Sharts-Hopko, N. C., Ott, B. B., et al. (2007). Perspectives of women with disabilities on reaching those who are hard to reach. *Journal of Neuroscience Nursing*, *29*(3), 163–171.

Self-Concept

Self-concept refers to a person's view of himself or herself, an image that has developed over many years. To assess self-concept, the interviewer might ask how a person views life, using a question such as "How do you feel about your life in general?" A person's self-concept can be threatened very easily by changes in physical function or appearance or other threats to health. The impact of certain medical conditions or surgical interventions, such as a colostomy or a mastectomy, can threaten body image. The question, "Do you have any particular concerns about your body?" may elicit useful information about self-image.

Sexuality

No area of assessment is more personal than the sexual history. Health care professionals are frequently uncomfortable with such questions and ignore this area of the patient profile or conduct a very cursory interview about this subject. Lack of knowledge about sexuality, preconceived notions (e.g., assuming all people are heterosexual), and anxiety about one's own sexuality may hamper the interviewer's effectiveness in dealing with this subject (Stephen, 2012a).

Sexual assessment can be approached at the end of the interview, at the time interpersonal or lifestyle factors are assessed, or it may be easier to discuss sexuality as a part of the genitourinary history within the Review of Systems. In female patients, a discussion of sexuality would follow questions about menstruation. In male patients, a similar discussion would follow questions about the urinary system.

Effective health care for older adults requires assessment of sexual health. Sexual function may be affected negatively by disease (or treatment), surgery, or aging. In order for the patient to maintain sexual function and optimize quality of life, sexual issues must be addressed. During the sexual history, nurses need to recognize how their practices are influenced by assumptions about sexuality in relation to age, gender, and culture, and not make assumptions based on their own personal beliefs (Ayaz, 2013). In addition, the interviewer should project a nonjudgmental attitude related to sexual preference or toward those who are transgender.

Obtaining the sexual history provides an opportunity to discuss sexual matters openly and gives the person permission to express sexual concerns to an informed professional. The interviewer is nonjudgmental and uses language appropriate to the patient's age and background (Stephen, 2012a). Determining whether a person is sexually active should precede any attempts to explore issues related to sexuality and sexual function. The assessment begins with an orienting sentence such as "Next, I would like to ask about your sexual health and practices." Such an opening may lead to a discussion of concerns related to sexual expression or the quality of a relationship, or to questions about contraception, risky sexual behaviours, and safer sex practices. Examples of other questions are, "How many sexual partners have you had?" and "Are you satisfied with your sexual relationships?"

Care should be taken to initiate conversations about sexuality with older patients and patients with disabilities and not to treat them as asexual people. Questions are worded in such a way that the person feels free to discuss his or her sexuality regardless of marital status or sexual preference. Direct questions are usually less threatening when prefaced with such statements as, "Most people feel that..." or "Many people worry about...." This suggests the normalcy of such feelings or behaviour and encourages the person to share information that might otherwise be omitted because of fear of seeming "different."

If a person answers abruptly or does not wish to carry the discussion any further, then the nurse moves to the next topic. However, introducing the subject of sexuality indicates to the person that a discussion of sexual concerns is acceptable and can be approached again in the future if so desired. Further discussion of the sexual history is presented in Chapters 47 and 50.

Risk for Abuse

Physical, sexual, and psychological abuse is a topic of growing importance in today's society (Stephen, 2012c). Such abuse occurs to people of both genders, of all ages, and from all socioeconomic, ethnic, and cultural groups. Patients rarely discuss this topic unless specifically asked about it. In fact, research shows that the majority of women currently in an abusive relationship have never told a health care professional. Therefore, it is important to ask direct questions, such as:

- Is anyone physically hurting you? Or forcing you to have sexual activities?
- Has anyone ever hurt you physically? Or threatened to do so?
- Are you ever afraid of anyone close to you (your partner, caregiver, or other family members)?

Patients who are older or have disabilities are at increased risk for abuse and should be asked about it as a routine part of assessment. However, when older patients are questioned directly, they rarely admit to abuse. Health care professionals should assess for risk factors, such as high levels of stress or alcoholism in caregivers, evidence of violence, and emotional outbursts, as well as financial, emotional, or physical dependency.

Two additional questions have been found to be effective in uncovering specific types of abuse that may occur only in people with disabilities:

- Does anyone prevent you from using a wheelchair? Cane? Respirator? Other assistive device?
- Does anyone you depend on refuse to help you with an important personal need, such as taking your medicine? Getting to the bathroom? Getting in or out of bed? Bathing? Dressing? Getting food or drink?

If a person's response indicates that abuse is a risk, further assessment is warranted, and efforts are made to ensure the patient's safety and provide access to appropriate community and professional resources and support systems. Further discussion of domestic violence and abuse is presented in Chapter 47.

Stress and Coping Responses

Each person handles stress differently. How well people adapt depends on their ability to cope. During a health history, past coping patterns and perceptions of current stresses and anticipated outcomes are explored to identify the person's overall ability to handle stress. It is especially important to identify expectations that a person may have from family, friends, and caregivers in providing emotional, physical, or financial support. Further discussion of stress and coping is presented in Chapter 9.

Other Health History Formats

The health history format discussed in this chapter is only one possible approach that is useful in obtaining and organizing information about a person's health status. Some experts consider this traditional format to be inappropriate for nurses, because it does not focus exclusively on the assessment of human responses to actual or potential health problems. Several attempts have been made to develop an assessment format and database with this focus in mind. One example is a nursing database based on the NANDA International and its 13 domains: health promotion, nutrition, elimination/exchange, activity/rest, perception/cognition, self-perception, role relationship, sexuality, coping/stress tolerance, life principles, safety/protection, comfort, and growth/development (Herdman & Kamitsuru, 2018). Although there is support in nursing for using this approach, no consensus for its use has been reached. Other examples include electronic systems specific to home care and perioperative nursing.

Groups from the public and private sectors have focused on assessing not only biologic health, but also other dimensions of health. These dimensions include physical, functional, emotional, mental, and social health. Efforts to assess health status have focused on the manner in which disease or disability affects a patient's functional status—that is, the ability of the person to function and perform his or her usual physical, mental, and social activities. An emphasis on functional assessment is viewed as more holistic than the traditional health or medical history. Instruments to assess health status in these ways may be used by nurses along with their own clinical assessment skills to determine the impact of illness, disease, disability, and health concerns on functional status.

Health concerns that are not complex (e.g., earache, sinusitis) and can be resolved in a short period usually do not require the depth or detail that is necessary when a person is experiencing a major illness or health concern. Additional assessments that go beyond the general patient profile may be used if the patient's health concerns are acute and complex or if the illness is chronic.

The person is asked about continuing health promotion and screening practices. If the person has not been involved in these practices in the past, information can be given about their importance and referred to appropriate health care professionals. Research has shown that health promotion is beneficial even for frail older home care clients. One study found that proactively providing older people with health promotion offers a systematic framework to improve the well-being of residents in nursing homes (Helfer, Sommerhalder, Schols, et al., 2015).

Regardless of the assessment format used, the focus of nurses during data collection is different from that of physicians and other health team members. However, the nursing focus complements these other approaches and encourages collaboration among the health care professionals, with each member bringing his or her own expertise and focus to the situation.

Physical Assessment

Physical assessment, or the physical examination, is an integral part of nursing assessment. The basic techniques and tools used in performing a physical examination are described in general in this chapter. The examinations of specific systems, including special manoeuvres, are described in the appropriate chapters throughout the book.

Examination Considerations

The physical examination is usually performed after the health history is obtained. It is carried out in a well-lighted, warm area. The patient is asked to (or helped to) undress and is draped appropriately so that only the area to be examined is exposed. The person's physical and psychological comfort is considered at all times. It is necessary to describe procedures to the patient and explain what sensations to expect before each part of the examination. The examiner's hands are washed before and immediately after the examination. Fingernails are kept short to avoid injuring the patient. If there is a possibility of coming into contact with blood or other body secretions during the physical examination, gloves should be worn.

An organized and systematic examination is the key to obtaining appropriate data in the shortest time. Such an approach encourages cooperation and trust on the part of the patient. The person's health history provides the examiner with a health profile that guides all aspects of the physical examination.

A "complete" physical examination is not routine. Many of the body systems are selectively assessed on the basis of the presenting concern. For example, if a healthy 20-year-old college student requires a physical examination to study abroad and reports no history of neurologic abnormality, the neurologic assessment is brief. Conversely, a history of transient numbness and diplopia (double vision) usually necessitates a complete neurologic investigation. Similarly, a patient with chest pain receives a much more intensive examination of the chest and heart than one with an earache. In general, the health history guides the examiner in obtaining additional data for a complete picture of the patient's health.

The process of learning to perform a physical examination requires repetition and reinforcement in a simulated or clinical setting. Only after basic physical assessment techniques are mastered can the examiner tailor the routine examination to include thorough assessments of particular systems, including special manoeuvres (Bickley, 2017; Skillen, 2012d; Weber & Kelley, 2018).

Components of the Physical Examination

The components of a physical examination include general observations and then a more focused assessment of the pertinent body systems. The tools of the physical examination are the human senses of vision, hearing, touch, and smell. These may be augmented by special tools (e.g., stethoscope, ophthalmoscope, reflex hammer) that are extensions of the human senses; they are tools that anyone can learn to use well. Expertise comes with practice, and sophistication comes with the interpretation of what is seen and heard.

Initial Observations

General inspection begins with the first contact with the patient. Introducing oneself and shaking hands provide opportunities for making initial observations: Is the person old? Or young? How old? How young? Does the person appear to be his or her stated age? Is the person thin? Or has obesity? Does the person appear anxious? Or depressed? Is the person's body structure as expected? Or not? In what way, and how different from the expected? It is essential to pay attention to the details in observation. Vague, general statements are not a substitute for specific descriptions based on careful observation. Consider the following examples:

- "The person appears sick." In what way does he or she appear sick? Is the skin pale, jaundiced, or cyanotic? Is the person grimacing in pain? Or having difficulty breathing? Does he or she have edema? What specific physical features or behavioural manifestations indicate that the person is "sick"?
- "The person appears chronically ill." In what way does he or she appear chronically ill? Does the person appear to have lost weight? People who lose weight secondary to muscle-wasting diseases (e.g., acquired immunodeficiency syndrome [AIDS], malignancy) have a different appearance than those who are merely thin, and weight loss may be accompanied by loss of muscle mass or atrophy. Does the skin have the appearance of chronic illness (i.e., Is it pale? Or does it give the appearance of dehydration? Or loss of subcutaneous tissue)?

These important specific observations are documented in the patient's chart or health record. Among general observations that are noted in the initial examination of the patient are posture and stature, body movements, gait, nutritional status, speech pattern, and vital signs.

Posture

The posture that a person assumes often provides valuable information. Patients who have breathing difficulties (dyspnea) secondary to cardiac disease prefer to sit and may report feeling short of breath when lying flat for even a brief time. Patients with abdominal pain due to peritonitis prefer to lie perfectly still; even slight jarring of the bed causes agonizing pain. In contrast, patients with abdominal pain due to renal or biliary colic are often restless and may pace the room.

Body Movements

Abnormalities of body movement are of two kinds: generalized disruption of voluntary or involuntary movement and asymmetry of movement. The first category includes tremors of a wide variety; some tremors may occur at rest (Parkinson's disease), whereas others occur only on voluntary movement (cerebellar ataxia). Other tremors may exist during both rest and activity (alcohol withdrawal syndrome, thyrotoxicosis). Some voluntary or involuntary movements are described as "fine," and others are "quite coarse." At the extreme are the convulsive movements of epilepsy or tetanus and the choreiform (involuntary and irregular) movements of patients with rheumatic fever or Huntington's disease.

Asymmetry of movement, in which only one side of the body is affected, may occur with disorders of the central nervous system (CNS), primarily in those patients who have had a cerebrovascular accident (stroke). Patients may have drooping of one side of the face, weakness or paralysis of the extremities on one side of the body, and a foot-dragging gait. Spasticity (increased muscle tone) may also be present, particularly in patients with multiple sclerosis.

Nutritional Status

Nutritional status is important to note. Obesity may be generalized as a result of excessive intake of calories, or it may be specifically localized to the trunk in patients who have an endocrine disorder (Cushing's disease) or who have been taking corticosteroids for long periods. Loss of weight may be generalized as a result of inadequate caloric intake, or it may be seen in loss of muscle mass with disorders that affect protein synthesis. Nutritional assessment is discussed in more detail later in this chapter.

Speech Pattern

Speech may be slurred because of CNS disease or because of damage to cranial nerves. Recurrent damage to the laryngeal nerve results in hoarseness, as do disorders that produce edema or swelling of the vocal cords. Speech may be halting, slurred, or interrupted in flow in patients with some CNS disorders (e.g., multiple sclerosis, stroke).

Vital Signs and Pain Assessment

The recording of vital signs is a part of every physical examination (Bickley, 2017; Skillen, 2012d). Blood pressure, pulse rate, respiratory rate, and body temperature measurements are obtained and recorded. Acute changes and trends over time are documented and unexpected changes and values that deviate significantly from a patient's usual values are brought to the attention of the patient's primary health care professional. The "fifth vital sign," pain, is also assessed and documented, if indicated.

Usual oral temperature for most people is 37°C; however, some variation is expected. Some people's usual temperatures can be at 36.6° or 37.3°C. There is an expected diurnal variation of a degree or two in body temperature throughout the day; temperature is usually lowest in the morning and increases during the day to between 37.3° and 37.5°C (99° to 99.5°F), and it then decreases during the night (Skillen, 2012d).

Focused Assessment

Following the general **inspection**, a more focused assessment is conducted. Although the sequence of physical examination depends on the circumstances and on the patient's reason for seeking health care, the complete examination usually proceeds in a head to toe format as follows (Skillen, 2012d):

- Skin, hair, nails
- Head and neck
- Eyes, ears, nose, mouth, and throat
- Spine, thorax, and lungs
- Cardiovascular system (heart and great vessels)
- Breasts and axillae
- Abdomen
- Musculoskeletal system
- Neurologic system
- Arms and legs
- Rectum
- Genitalia

In clinical practice, all relevant body systems are tested throughout the physical examination, not necessarily in the sequence described (Weber & Kelley, 2018). For example, when the face is examined, it is appropriate to check for facial asymmetry and, thus, for the integrity of the fifth and seventh cranial nerves; the examiner does not need to repeat this as part of a neurologic examination. When systems are combined in this manner the patient does not need to change positions repeatedly, which can be exhausting and time consuming.

The traditional sequence in the focused portion of the examination is inspection, **palpation**, percussion, and then **auscultation**, except in the case of an abdominal examination (in which auscultation precedes palpation and percussion).

Inspection

The first fundamental technique is inspection or observation of each relevant body system in more detail as indicated from the health history or the general inspection. Characteristics such as skin colour, presence and size of lesions, edema, erythema, symmetry, and pulsations are noted. Specific body movements that are noted on inspection include spasticity, muscle spasms, and an abnormal gait (Grossman & Porth, 2014).

Palpation

Palpation is a vital part of the physical examination. Many structures of the body, although not visible, may be assessed through the techniques of light and deep palpation (Fig. 5-3). Examples include the superficial blood vessels, lymph nodes, thyroid gland, organs of the abdomen and pelvis, and rectum. When the abdomen is examined, auscultation is performed before palpation and percussion to avoid altering bowel sounds (Roach, 2012; Weber & Kelly, 2018).

Sounds generated within the body, if within specified frequency ranges, also may be detected through touch. For example, certain murmurs generated in the heart or within blood vessels (thrills) may be detected. Thrills cause a sensation to the hand much like the purring of a cat. Voice sounds are transmitted along the bronchi to the periphery of the lung. These may be perceived by touch and may be altered by disorders affecting the lungs. The phenomenon is called *tactile fremitus* and is useful in assessing diseases of the chest. The significance of these findings is discussed in Chapters 22 and 27.

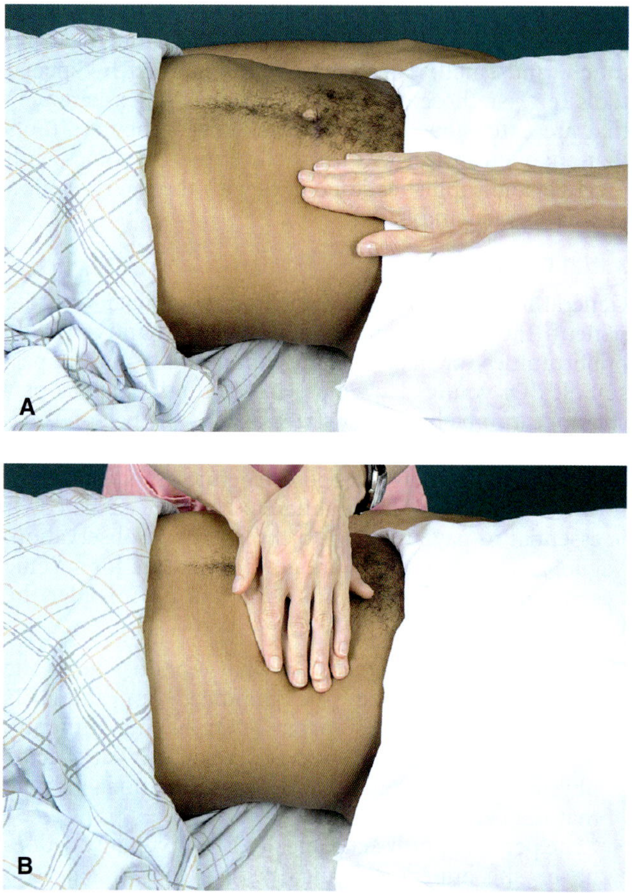

FIGURE 5-3. **A.** Light palpation. **B.** Deep palpation.

Percussion

The technique of percussion translates the application of physical force into sound (Fig. 5-4). It is a skill requiring practice that yields much information about disease processes in the chest and abdomen (Bickley, 2017; Roach, 2012). The principle is to set the chest wall or abdominal

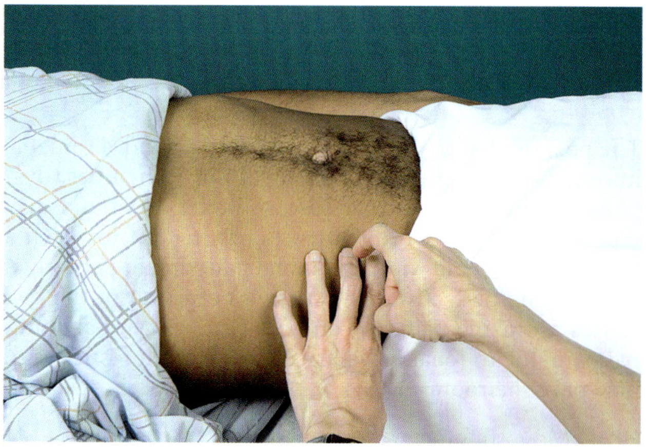

FIGURE 5-4. Percussion technique. The middle finger of one hand strikes the terminal phalanx of the middle finger of the other hand, which is placed firmly against the body. If the action is performed sharply, a brief, resonant tone will be produced. The clarity of the tone depends on the brevity of the action. The intensity of the tone varies with the force used.

wall into vibration by striking it with a firm object. The sound produced reflects the density of the underlying structure. Certain densities produce sounds as **percussion** notes. These sounds, listed in a sequence that proceeds from the least to the most dense, are tympany, hyperresonance, resonance, dullness, and flatness. Tympany is the drum-like sound produced by percussing the air-filled stomach. Hyperresonance is audible when one percusses over inflated lung tissue in a person with emphysema. Resonance is the sound elicited over air-filled lungs. Percussion of the liver produces a dull sound, whereas percussion of the thigh produces a flat sound.

Percussion allows the examiner to assess such usual anatomic details as the borders of the liver and the movement of the diaphragm during inspiration. It is also possible to determine the level of a pleural effusion (fluid in the pleural cavity) and the location of a consolidated area caused by pneumonia or atelectasis (collapse of alveoli). The use of percussion is described further with disorders of the thorax and abdomen (see Chapters 22 and 34).

Auscultation

Auscultation is the skill of listening with a stethoscope to sounds produced within the body created by the movement of air or fluid. Examples include breath sounds, the spoken voice, bowel sounds, heart sounds, and cardiac murmurs. Physiologic sounds may be expected (e.g., first and second heart sounds) or pathologic (e.g., heart murmurs in diastole, crackles in the lung). Some expected sounds may be distorted by abnormalities of structures through which the sound must travel (e.g., changes in the character of breath sounds as they travel through the consolidated lung of a patient with lobar pneumonia).

Sound produced within the body, if of sufficient amplitude, may be detected with the stethoscope, which functions as an extension of the human ear and channels sound. The nurse must avoid touching the tubing or rubbing other surfaces (hair, clothing) during auscultation to minimize extraneous noises. Sounds detected by auscultation are classified according to their intensity (loud or soft), pitch (high or low), duration (length), and quality (musical, raspy, crackling) (Bickley, 2017; Weber & Kelley, 2018).

Sound produced by the body, like any other sound, is characterized by intensity, frequency, and quality. The *intensity*, or loudness, associated with physiologic sound is low; therefore, the use of the stethoscope is needed. The *frequency*, or pitch, of physiologic sound is in reality "noise," in that most sounds consist of a frequency spectrum, as opposed to the single-frequency sounds that we associate with music or a tuning fork. The frequency spectrum may be quite low, yielding a rumbling noise, or comparatively high, producing a harsh or blowing sound. *Quality* of sound relates to overtones that allow one to distinguish among various sounds. Sound quality enables the examiner to distinguish between the musical quality of high-pitched wheezing and the low-pitched rumbling of a diastolic murmur (Skillen, 2012d).

Nutritional Assessment

Nutrition is important to maintain health and to prevent disease and death. When illness or injury occurs, optimal nutrition is essential for healing and resisting infection and other complications. An in-depth nutritional assessment is often integrated into the health history and physical examination. Assessment of nutritional status provides information about obesity, weight loss, undernutrition, malnutrition, deficiencies in specific nutrients, metabolic abnormalities, effects of medications on nutrition, and special issues affecting patients both in hospitals and in the home and other community settings (Day, 2012).

Disorders caused by nutritional deficiency, overeating, or eating unhealthy meals are among the leading causes of illness and death in Canada today. The three leading causes of death—heart disease, cancer, and stroke—are related, in part, to consequences of unhealthy nutrition (Day, 2012). Other examples of health issues associated with poor nutrition include obesity, osteoporosis, cirrhosis, diverticulitis, and eating disorders.

Certain signs and symptoms that suggest possible nutritional deficiency, such as muscle wasting, poor skin integrity, loss of subcutaneous tissue, and obesity, are easy to note because they are specific; these are pursued further. Other physical signs may be subtle and need to be carefully assessed. For example, certain signs that appear to indicate nutritional deficiency may actually reflect other systemic conditions (e.g., endocrine disorders, infectious disease). Others may result from impaired digestion, absorption, excretion, or storage of nutrients in the body (Grossman & Porth, 2014; Weber & Kelly, 2014).

Obesity is a major concern for children, adolescents, and adults in the North America and globally. The World Health Organization (WHO) defines obesity as abnormal or excessive fat accumulation that may impair health. Obesity and being overweight are leading risk factors for global deaths; most of the world's population lives in countries where overweight and obesity kill more people than underweight. In addition, coronary artery disease, diabetes, musculoskeletal disorders, and certain cancers can be attributable to obesity (WHO, 2018). See Chapter 42 for a detailed discussion of obesity.

Life Span Considerations

Adolescents

Adolescence is a time of critical growth and acquisition of lifelong eating habits, and therefore nutritional assessment, analysis, and intervention are critical (Day, 2012). In the past two decades rates of obesity in adolescents have increased at an alarming rate.

Adolescent girls are at particular nutritional risk, because iron, folate, and calcium intakes are below recommended levels and they are a less physically active group compared to adolescent males. Adolescents with other nutritional disorders, such as anorexia and bulimia, have a better chance of recovery if these disorders are identified and treated in the adolescent years rather than in adulthood.

Older Adults

Older adults are also at risk for altered nutrition. Nutritional assessment in the older adult should include inquiry about the patient's current dietary practices as well as a nutritional screening to assess for adequate nutrition. Many older adults adhere to specific diets, such as those low in saturated fat or sodium, for improving or maintaining health. Proper nutrition for an older adult meets daily requirements, maintains ideal body weight, and addresses specific health concerns such as cardiovascular or renal disease (Eliopoulos, 2018).

Inadequate dietary intake in older adults, which may lead to malnutrition and resultant illness and frailty, may result from physiologic changes in the gastrointestinal tract, socioeconomic factors, drug interactions, disease, excessive use of alcohol, and poor dentition or missing teeth. Malnourished patients have an increased risk of morbidity and mortality; malnutrition is also linked to a poorer quality of life in older adults (Rasheed & Woods, 2014). Disorders affecting any part of the gastrointestinal tract can alter nutritional requirements and health status in people of any age; however, they are likely to occur more quickly and more frequently in older persons. Acute and chronic diseases may affect the metabolism and utilization of nutrients, which already are altered by the aging process. Even well older adults may be nutritionally at risk because of decreased odour perception, poor dental health, limited ability to shop and cook, financial hardship, and the fact that they often eat alone (Eliopoulos, 2018).

Moreover, many older adults take multiple prescribed and OTC medications; this is referred to as polypharmacy. The number of adverse reactions increases proportionately with the number of medications taken. Age-related physiologic and pathophysiologic changes may alter the metabolism and elimination of many medications (Eliopoulos, 2018). Medications can influence food intake by producing side effects such as nausea, vomiting, decreased appetite, and changes in cognition. They may also interfere with the distribution, utilization, and storage of nutrients.

Components of Nutritional Assessment

The sequence of assessment of parameters may vary, but evaluation of nutritional status includes one or more of the following methods: measurement of **body mass index** (BMI) and waist circumference, biochemical measurements, clinical examination findings, and dietary data. Measurement of BMI and waist circumference is recommended to determine whether a patient is having obesity (Centers for Disease Control and Prevention [CDC], 2015).

Body Mass Index

BMI is a ratio based on body weight and height. The obtained value is compared to the established standards; however, trends or changes in values over time are considered more useful than isolated or one-time measurements. BMI is highly correlated with body fat, but increased lean body mass, large muscles, edema, or a large body frame can also increase the BMI. People who have a BMI lower than 24 (or who are 80% or less of their desirable body weight for height) are at increased risk for health issues associated with poor nutritional status. In addition, a low BMI is associated with a higher mortality rate among hospitalized patients and community-dwelling older adults. Those who have a BMI of 25 to 29 are considered overweight; those with a BMI of 30 to 39, as having obesity; and those with a BMI greater than 40, as having extreme obesity (Dudek, 2018; WHO, 2018). In analyzing BMI, the nurse is aware that cutoff scores for "normal," "overweight," and "obese" may differ for different ethnic groups. For example, in an Asian population, a BMI of 23 is considered overweight, while a BMI of 27 would be classified as having obesity (World Health Organization, 2004). These scores may also differ by age. For adults 65 years and older, a BMI of 18.5 to 20 increases the risk of morbidity (Brunet, Day, & Mager, 2010; Day, 2012; Weber & Kelley, 2018).

It is important to assess for usual body weight and height and to compare these values with ideal weight. Current weight does not provide information about recent changes in weight; therefore, patients are asked about their usual body weight. Loss of height may be due to osteoporosis, an important problem related to nutrition, especially in postmenopausal women. A loss of 2 or 3 in of height may indicate osteoporosis (Brunet et al., 2010; Day, 2012).

In addition to the calculation of BMI, waist circumference measurement is particularly useful for adult patients who are categorized as being of normal weight or overweight (Dudek, 2018). To measure waist circumference, have patient stand with feet 25 to 30 cm apart. A tape measure is placed in a horizontal plane around the abdomen halfway between the costal margin and the iliac crest (Fig. 5-5). The measurement is taken after the patient exhales. A waist circumference greater than 102 cm for men or 88 cm for women indicates excess abdominal fat. Those with a high waist circumference are at increased risk for diabetes, dyslipidemias, hypertension, stroke, cardiovascular disease, and atrial fibrillation (Tigbe, Granat, Sattar, et al., 2017).

Biochemical Assessment

Biochemical assessment reflects both the tissue level of a given nutrient and any abnormality of metabolism in the utilization of nutrients. These determinations are made from studies of serum (albumin, transferrin, retinol-binding protein, electrolytes, hemoglobin, vitamin A, carotene, vitamin C, and total lymphocyte count) and

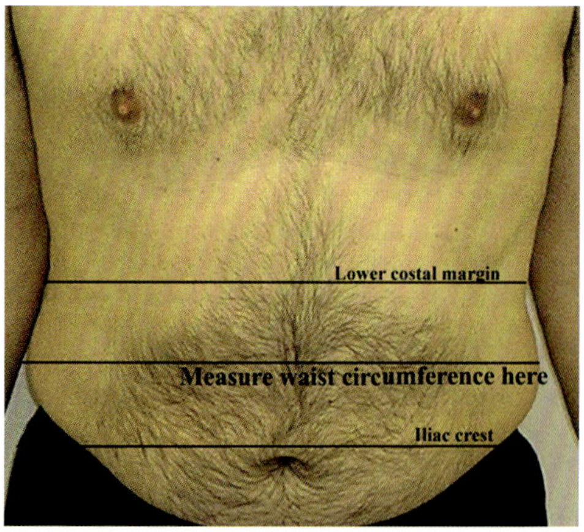

FIGURE 5-5. Measuring waist circumference.

studies of urine (creatinine, thiamine, riboflavin, niacin, and iodine). Some of these tests, while reflecting recent intake of the elements detected, can also identify below-normal levels when there are no clinical symptoms of deficiency.

Low serum albumin and prealbumin levels are most often used as measures of protein deficit in adults. Albumin synthesis depends on normal liver function and an adequate supply of amino acids. Because the body stores a large amount of albumin, the serum albumin level may not decrease until malnutrition is severe; therefore, its usefulness in detecting recent protein depletion is limited. Decreased albumin levels may be caused by overhydration, liver or renal disease, or excessive protein loss due to burns, major surgery, infection, or cancer. Serial measurements of prealbumin levels are also used to assess the results of nutritional therapy. Prealbumin, also called thyroxin-binding protein, is a more sensitive indicator of protein status than albumin, but the test is more expensive and therefore less frequently ordered (Dudek, 2018).

Additional laboratory data, such as levels of transferrin and retinol-binding protein, anergy panels, and lymphocyte and electrolyte counts, are used in many institutions. Transferrin is a protein that binds and carries iron from the intestine through the serum. Because of its short half-life, transferrin levels decrease more quickly than albumin levels in response to protein depletion. Although measurement of retinol-binding protein is not available from many laboratories, it may be a useful means of monitoring acute, short-term changes in protein status. The total lymphocyte count may be reduced in people who are acutely malnourished as a result of stress and low-calorie feeding and in those with impaired cellular immunity. Anergy, the absence of an immune response to injection of small concentrations of recall antigen under the skin, may also indicate malnutrition because of delayed antibody synthesis and response. Serum electrolyte levels provide information about fluid and electrolyte balance and kidney function. The creatinine/height index calculated over a 24-hour period assesses the metabolically active tissue and indicates the degree of protein depletion, comparing expected body mass for height with actual body cell mass. A 24-hour urine sample is obtained, and the amount of creatinine is measured and compared to expected ranges based on the patient's height and gender. Values lower than expected may indicate loss of lean body mass and protein malnutrition (Fischbach & Dunning, 2015).

Clinical Examination

The state of nutrition is often reflected in a person's appearance. Although the most obvious physical sign of good nutrition is an appropriate body weight with respect to height, body frame, and age, other tissues can serve as indicators of general nutritional status and adequate intake of specific nutrients; these include the hair, skin, teeth, gums, mucous membranes, mouth and tongue, skeletal muscles, abdomen, lower extremities, and thyroid gland (Table 5-1). Specific aspects of clinical examination that are useful in identifying nutritional deficits include an examination and assessment of skin for turgor, edema, elasticity, dryness, subcutaneous tone, poorly healing wounds and ulcers, purpura, and bruises. The musculoskeletal examination also provides information about muscle wasting and weakness.

TABLE 5-1 Physical Indicators of Nutritional Status

Indicator	Signs of Adequate Nutrition	Signs of Inadequate Nutrition
General appearance	Alert, responsive, energetic	Listless, appears acutely or chronically ill
Hair	Shiny, lustrous; minimal loss, healthy scalp	Dull and dry, brittle, depigmented, easily plucked; thin and sparse, flaking scalp
Face	Skin colour uniform; smooth, moist	Skin dark over cheeks and under eyes, skin flaky, face swollen or hollow/sunken cheeks
Eyes	Bright, clear, moist	Eye membranes pale, dry (xerophthalmia); increased vascularity, cornea soft (keratomalacia)
Lips	Pink colour, smooth	Swollen and puffy; angular lesion at corners of mouth (cheilosis)
Tongue	Deep red in appearance; surface papillae present	Smooth appearance, swollen, beefy-red, sores, atrophic papillae
Teeth	Straight, no crowding, no dental caries, uniform bright colour	Dental caries, missing teeth, mottled appearance (fluorosis), malpositioned, dentures no longer fit
Gums	Firm, pink colour, margins tight around teeth	Spongy, bleed easily, marginal redness, recession
Thyroid	No enlargement of the thyroid	Thyroid enlargement (simple goitre)
Skin	Smooth, uniform colour, moist, warm	Rough, dry, flaky, swollen, pale, pigmented; lack of or excess fat under skin
Nails	Firm, pink	Spoon shaped, ridged, brittle
Skeleton	Erect posture, no malformation	Poor posture, bending of ribs, bowed legs, or knock knees
Muscles	Well developed, firm	Flaccid, poor tone, wasted, underdeveloped
Extremities	No tenderness or edema	Weak and tender; edematous
Abdomen	Flat	Scaphoid (concave or hollow), protruding
Nervous system	Reflexes present	Decreased or absent ankle and knee reflexes
Weight	Appropriate for height, age, and body build	Overweight or underweight

Dietary Data

Commonly used methods of determining individual eating patterns include the food record, the 24-hour food recall, and a dietary interview. Each of these methods helps estimate whether food intake is adequate and appropriate. If these methods are used to obtain the dietary history, instructions should be given to the patient about measuring and recording food intake.

Methods of Collecting Data

FOOD RECORD. The food record is used most often in nutritional status studies. A person is instructed to keep a record of food actually consumed over a period of time, varying from 3 to 7 days, and to accurately estimate and describe the specific foods consumed. Food records are fairly accurate if the person is willing to provide factual information and is able to estimate food quantities. Another option is to photograph all foods consumed.

24-HOUR RECALL. As the name implies, the 24-hour recall method is a recall of food intake over a 24-hour period. A person is asked to recall all foods eaten during the previous day and to estimate the quantities of each food consumed. Because information does not always represent usual intake, at the end of the interview the patient is asked whether the previous day's food intake was typical. To obtain supplementary information about the typical diet, it is also necessary to ask how frequently the person eats foods from the major food groups.

DIETARY INTERVIEW. The success of the interviewer in obtaining information for dietary assessment depends on effective communication, which requires that good rapport be established to promote respect and trust. The interviewer explains the purpose of the interview. The interview is conducted in a nondirective and exploratory way, allowing the respondent to express feelings and thoughts while encouraging him or her to answer specific questions. The manner in which questions are asked influences the respondent's cooperation. The interviewer must be nonjudgmental and avoid expressing disapproval, either by verbal comments or by facial expression.

Character of General Intake. Several questions may be necessary to elicit the information needed. Assumptions are not made about the size of servings; instead, questions are phrased so that quantities are more clearly determined. For example, to help determine the size of one hamburger, the patient may be asked, "How many servings were prepared with the kilogram of meat you bought?" Another approach to determining quantities is to use food models of known sizes in estimating portions of meat, cake, or pie, or to record quantities in common measurements, such as cups or spoonfuls (or the size of containers, when discussing intake of bottled beverages).

In recording a particular combination dish, such as a casserole, it is useful to ask about the ingredients, recording the largest quantities first. When recording quantities of ingredients, the interviewer notes whether the food item was raw or cooked and the number of servings provided by the recipe. When a patient lists the foods for the recall questionnaire, it may help to read back the list of foods and ask whether anything was forgotten, such as fruit, cake, candy, between-meal snacks, or alcoholic beverages.

Additional information obtained during the interview includes methods of preparing food, sources available for food (including donated foods and food bank use), food-buying practices, use of vitamin and mineral supplements, and amount of income available for food purchases.

Cultural and Religious Considerations. An individual's culture determines to a large extent which foods are eaten and how they are prepared and served. Culture and religious practices together often determine whether certain foods are prohibited and whether certain foods and spices are eaten on certain holidays or at specific family gatherings. Because of the importance of culture and religious beliefs to many individuals, it is important to be sensitive to these factors when obtaining a dietary history. It is, however, equally important not to stereotype individuals and assume that because they are from a certain culture or religious group, they adhere to specific dietary customs. One particular area of consideration is the presence of fish and shellfish in the diet, where they come from (farmed vs. wild), and the method of preparation. These methods may put certain populations at risk for toxicity due to contaminants. Culturally sensitive versions of Canada's Food Guide are available in a variety of languages and for First Nations, Inuit, and Metis (Government of Canada, 2018).

Evaluating Dietary Information

After obtaining basic dietary information, the nurse evaluates the patient's dietary intake and communicates the information to the dietitian and the rest of the health care team for more detailed assessment and for clinical nutrition intervention. If the goal is to determine whether the patient generally eats a healthful diet, his or her food intake may be compared with the dietary guidelines outlined in "*Eating well with Canada's Food Guide.*" The Food Guide divides foods into five major groups (grains, vegetables, fruits, milk products, and meat and beans), plus fats and oils. Recommendations are provided for variety in the diet, proportion of food from each food group, and moderation in eating fats, oils, and sweets. A person's food intake is compared with recommendations based on various food groups for different age groups and activity levels (Government of Canada, 2018).

If nurses or dietitians are interested in knowing about the intake of specific nutrients, such as vitamin A, iron, or calcium, the patient's food intake is analyzed by consulting a list of foods and their composition and nutrient content. The diet is analyzed in terms of grams and milligrams of specific nutrients. The total nutritive value is then compared with the recommended dietary allowances specific for the patient's age category, gender, and special circumstances such as pregnancy or lactation.

Fat intake and cholesterol levels are additional aspects of the nutritional assessment. Trans fats are produced when hydrogen atoms are added to mono- or polyunsaturated fats to produce a semisolid product such as margarine. Trans fats, which are contained in many baked goods and restaurant foods, are a concern, because increased amounts of trans fats have been associated with increased risk for heart disease and stroke. Canada was the first country to require the inclusion of trans fats information on food labels.

Factors Influencing Nutritional Status in Various Situations

One sensitive indicator of the body's gain or loss of protein is its nitrogen balance. An adult is said to be in nitrogen equilibrium when the nitrogen intake (from food) equals the nitrogen output (in urine, feces, and perspiration); it is a sign of health. A positive nitrogen balance exists when nitrogen intake exceeds nitrogen output and indicates tissue growth, such as occurs during pregnancy, childhood, recovery from surgery, and rebuilding of wasted tissue. A negative nitrogen balance indicates that tissue is breaking down faster than it is being replaced. In the absence of an adequate intake of protein, the body converts protein to glucose for energy. This can occur with fever, starvation, surgery, burns, and debilitating diseases. Each gram of nitrogen loss in excess of intake represents the depletion of 6.25 g of protein or 25 g of muscle tissue. Therefore, a negative nitrogen balance of 10 g/day for 10 days could mean the wasting of 2.5 kg (5.5 lb) of muscle tissue as it is converted to glucose for energy.

When conditions that result in negative nitrogen balance are combined with anorexia (loss of appetite), they can lead to malnutrition. Malnutrition interferes with wound healing, increases susceptibility to infection, and contributes to an increased incidence of complications, longer hospital stays, and prolonged confinement of patients to bed.

Patients who are hospitalized may have an inadequate dietary intake because of the illness or disorder that necessitated the hospital stay or because the hospital's food is unfamiliar or unappealing. Patients who are cared for at home may feel too sick or fatigued to shop and prepare food, or they may be unable to eat because of other physical problems or limitations. Limited or fixed incomes or the high costs of medications may result in insufficient money to buy nutritious foods. Patients with inadequate housing or inadequate cooking facilities are unlikely to have an adequate nutritional intake (Day, 2012). Because complex treatments (e.g., mechanical ventilation, intravenous infusions, chemotherapy), once used only in the hospital setting, are now being provided in the home and outpatient settings, nutritional assessment of patients in these settings is an important aspect of home and community-based care.

Many medications influence nutritional status by suppressing the appetite, irritating the oral or gastric mucosa, or causing nausea and vomiting. Others may influence bacterial flora in the intestine or directly affect nutrient absorption so that secondary malnutrition results. People who must take many medications in a single day often report feeling too full to eat. A patient's use of prescription and OTC medications and their effects on appetite and dietary intake are assessed. Many of the factors that contribute to poor nutritional status are identified in Table 5-2.

Analysis of Nutritional Status

Physical measurements (BMI, waist circumference) and biochemical, clinical, and dietary data are used in combination to determine a patient's nutritional status. Often, these data provide more information about the patient's nutritional status than the clinical examination, which may not detect subclinical deficiencies unless they become so advanced that overt signs develop. A low intake of nutrients over a long period may lead to low biochemical levels and, without nutritional intervention, may result in characteristic and observable signs and symptoms (see Table 5-2). A plan of action for nutritional intervention is

TABLE 5-2 Factors Associated With Potential Nutritional Deficits

Factor	Possible Consequences
Dental and oral issues (missing teeth, ill-fitting dentures, impaired chewing, or swallowing)	Inadequate intake of high-fibre foods
NPO for diagnostic testing	Inadequate caloric and protein intake; dehydration
Prolonged use of glucose and saline IV fluids	Inadequate caloric and protein intake
Nausea and vomiting	Inadequate caloric and protein intake; loss of fluid, electrolytes, and minerals
Stress of illness, surgery, and/or hospitalization	Increased protein and caloric requirement; increased catabolism
Wound drainage	Loss of protein, fluid, electrolytes, and minerals
Pain	Loss of appetite; inability to shop, cook, eat
Fever	Increased caloric and fluid requirement; increased catabolism
Gastrointestinal intubation	Loss of protein, fluid, and minerals
Tube feedings	Inadequate amounts; various nutrients in each formula
Gastrointestinal disease	Inadequate intake and malabsorption of nutrients
Alcoholism	Inadequate intake of nutrients; increased consumption of calories without other nutrients; vitamin deficiencies
Depression	Loss of appetite; inability to shop, cook, eat
Eating disorders (anorexia, bulimia)	Inadequate caloric and protein intake; loss of fluid, electrolytes, and minerals
Medications	Inadequate intake due to medication side effects, such as dry mouth, loss of appetite, decreased taste perception, difficulty swallowing, nausea and vomiting, physical problems that limit shopping, cooking, eating; malabsorption of nutrients
Restricted ambulation or disability	Inability to help self to food, liquids, other nutrients

CHART 5-5

Assessing the Home Environment

Physical Facilities (check all that apply)

EXTERIOR

- steps ______
- unsafe steps ______
- porch ______
- litter ______
- noise ______
- inadequate lighting ______
- other ______

______

INTERIOR

- accessible bathroom ______
- level, safe floor surface ______
- number of rooms ______
- privacy ______
- sleeping arrangements ______
- refrigeration ______
- garbage management ______
- animals ______
- adequate lighting ______
- steps/stairs ______
- other ______

______

Safety Hazards found in the patient's current residence (check all that apply)

- none ______
- inadequate floor, roof, or windows ______
- inadequate lighting ______
- unsafe gas/electric appliances ______
- inadequate heating ______
- inadequate cooling ______
- lack of fire safety devices ______
- unsafe floor coverings ______
- inadequate stair rails ______
- lead-based paint ______
- improperly stored hazardous material ______
- improper wiring/electrical cords ______
- other ______

______

Safety Factors (check all that apply)

- fire/smoke detectors ______
- fire extinguisher ______
- carbon monoxide detector ______
- telephone ______
- placement of electrical cords ______
- emergency plan ______
- emergency phone numbers displayed ______
- safe portable heaters ______
- obstacle-free paths ______
- other ______

______

based on the results of the dietary assessment and the patient's clinical profile. To be effective, the plan must meet the patient's need for a healthy diet, maintain (or control) weight, and compensate for increased nutritional needs.

Assessment in the Home and Community

Assessment of people in community settings, including the home, consists of collecting information specific to existing health conditions, including data on the patient's physiologic and emotional status, the community and home environment, the adequacy of support systems or care given by family and other care providers, and the availability of needed resources. In addition, it is important to evaluate the ability of the individual and family to cope with and address their respective needs. The physical assessment in the community and home consists of the same techniques used in the hospital, outpatient clinic, or office setting. Privacy is provided, and the person is made as comfortable as possible. See Chapter 2.

Before the first home visit, the nurse calls the patient's home to determine a convenient time to expect the home care nurse; this also gives the patient's primary caregiver the opportunity to be available. During the home visit, assessment is not limited to physical assessment of the patient. Other aspects of assessment are related to the home environment and support systems (Chart 5-5). The patient may not have family members available to assist him or her and may live alone in substandard housing or in a shelter for the homeless. Therefore, the nurse needs to be aware of resources available in the community and methods of obtaining those resources for the patient.

Critical Thinking Exercises

1 Your health history and physical examination of a young adult male patient alerts you to the possibility of substance abuse. Explain how you would pursue this. What is the evidence base for available assessments to assist in a more comprehensive evaluation? Identify the criteria used to evaluate the strength of the evidence for this practice.

2 **ebp** Your health assessment of a new female college student reveals that she has a high fat intake, has a minimal calcium intake, and gets little exercise. What recommendations would you make for this patient? If the patient is a vegetarian, what dietary instructions would you develop for her? What is the evidence base for the type of instructional method to use with a college student? Identify the criteria used to evaluate the strength of the evidence for this practice.

3 pq A 38-year-old woman is brought by ambulance to the emergency department after a suicide attempt, following the death of her spouse 6 months ago. What types of assessments are necessary to complete a comprehensive admission assessment? What are the priorities in this patient's care? How might your approach to this patient differ if the patient's culture viewed suicidal ideation as a sign of weakness and disrespect for the culture?

REFERENCES AND SELECTED READINGS

Books

Anderson, M. C., Hunter, K., & Bickley, L. S. (2010). The older adult. In T. C. Stephen, D. L. Skillen, R. A. Day, et al. (Eds.). *Canadian Bates' guide to health assessment for nurses* (1st ed., pp. 887–932). Philadelphia, PA: Wolters Kluwer Health/Lippincott Williams & Wilkins.

Bickley, L. S. (2017). *Bates' guide to physical examination and history taking* (12th ed.). Philadelphia, PA: Lippincott Williams & Wilkins.

Brunet, K., Day, R. A., & Mager, D. (2010). Nutritional assessment. In T. C. Stephen, D. L. Skillen, R. A. Day, et al. (Eds.). *Canadian Bates' guide to health assessment for nurses* (1st ed., pp. 167–201). Philadelphia, PA: Wolters Kluwer Health/Lippincott Williams & Wilkins.

Day, R. A. (2012). Nutrition assessment. In T. C. Stephen, D. L. Skillen, R. A. Day, et al. (Eds.). *Canadian Jensen's nursing health assessment: A best practice approach* (1st ed., pp. 152–184). Philadelphia, PA: Wolters Kluwer Health/Lippincott Williams & Wilkins.

Dudek, S. G. (2018). *Nutrition essentials for nursing practice* (8th ed.). Philadelphia, PA: Lippincott Williams & Wilkins.

Eliopoulos, C. (2018). *Gerontological nursing* (9th ed.). Philadelphia, PA: Lippincott Williams & Wilkins.

Fischbach, F., & Dunning, M. B. (2015). *A manual of laboratory and diagnostic tests* (9th ed.). Philadelphia, PA: Lippincott Williams & Wilkins.

Grossman, S. C., & Porth, C. M. (2014). *Porth's pathophysiology: Concepts of altered health states* (9th ed.). Philadelphia, PA: Lippincott Williams & Wilkins.

Harder, N., Skillen, D. L., & Bickley, L. S. (2010). The abdomen. In T. Stephen, D. L. Skillen, R. A. Day, et al. (Eds.). *Canadian Bates' guide to health assessment for nurses* (1st ed., pp. 509–561). Philadelphia, PA: Wolters Kluwer Health/Lippincott Williams & Wilkins.

Herdman, T. H., & Kamitsuru, S. (2018). *Nursing diagnoses: Definitions & classification 2018–2020* (11th ed.). Stuttgart, Germany: Thieme.

Karch, A. M. (2017). *Lippincott's Nursing Drug Guide* (6th ed.). Philadelphia, PA: Wolters Kluwer Health/Lippincott Williams & Wilkins.

O'Brien, M. E. (2018). *Spirituality in nursing* (6th ed.). Sudbury, MA: Jones & Bartlett.

Roach, S. (2012). Abdominal assessment. In T. C. Stephen, D. L. Skillen, R. A. Day, et al. (Eds.). *Canadian Jensen's nursing health assessment: A best practice approach* (1st ed., pp. 602–644). Philadelphia, PA: Wolters Kluwer Health/Lippincott Williams & Wilkins.

Skillen, D. L. (2012a). Older adults. In T. C. Stephen, D. L. Skillen, R. A. Day, et al. (Eds.). *Canadian Jensen's nursing health assessment: A best practice approach* (1st ed., pp. 925–956). Philadelphia, PA: Wolters Kluwer Health/Lippincott Williams & Wilkins.

Skillen, D. L. (2012b). Assessment of social, cultural, and spiritual health. In T. C. Stephen, D. L. Skillen, R. A. Day, et al. (Eds.). *Canadian Jensen's health assessment for nurses: A best practice approach* (1st ed., pp. 231–247). Philadelphia, PA: Wolters Kluwer Health/Lippincott Williams & Wilkins.

Skillen, D. L. (2012c). Techniques of physical examination and equipment. In T. C. Stephen, D. L. Skillen, R. A. Day, et al. (Eds.). *Canadian Jensen's nursing health assessment: A best practice approach* (1st. ed., pp. 231–247). Philadelphia, PA: Wolters Kluwer Health/Lippincott Williams & Wilkins.

Skillen, D. L. (2012d). General survey and vital signs assessment. In T. C. Stephen, D. L. Skillen, R. A. Day, et al. (Eds.). *Canadian Jensen's nursing health assessment: A best practice approach* (1st ed., pp. 91–124). Philadelphia, PA: Wolters Kluwer Health/Lippincott Williams & Wilkins.

Stephen, T. C. (2012a). The interview and therapeutic dialogue. In T. C. Stephen, D. L. Skillen, R. A. Day, et al. (Eds.). *Canadian Jensen's nursing health assessment: A best practice approach* (1st ed., pp. 20–36). Philadelphia, PA: Wolters Kluwer Health/Lippincott Williams & Wilkins.

Stephen, T. C. (2012b). The health history. In T. C. Stephen, D. L. Skillen, R. A. Day, et al. (Eds.). *Canadian Jensen's nursing health assessment: A best practice approach* (1st ed., pp. 37–51). Philadelphia, PA: Wolters Kluwer Health/Lippincott Williams & Wilkins.

Stephen, T. C. (2012c). Documentation and interprofessional communication. In T. C. Stephen, D. L. Skillen, R. A. Day, et al. (Eds.). *Canadian Jensen's nursing health assessment: A best practice approach* (1st ed., pp. 69–88). Philadelphia, PA: Wolters Kluwer Health/Lippincott Williams & Wilkins.

Stephen, T. C. (2012d). Assessment of human violence. In T. C. Stephen, D. L. Skillen, R. A. Day, et al. (Eds.). *Canadian Jensen's nursing health assessment: A best practice approach* (1st ed., pp. 248–264). Philadelphia, PA: Wolters Kluwer Health/Lippincott Williams & Wilkins.

Weber, J. R., & Kelley, J. H. (2018). *Health assessment in nursing* (6th ed.). Philadelphia, PA: Wolters Kluwer Health.

Journals and Electronic Documents

General Assessment

Ayaz, S. (2014). Sexuality and nursing process: A literature review. *Sexuality and Disability*, *31*(1), 3–12.

Centers for Disease Control and Prevention (CDC). (2015). *Assessing your weight*. Retrieved January 05, 2018, from www.cdc.gov/healthyweight/assessing/index.html

Chan, A. W., Pristach, E. A., Welte, J. W., et al. (1993). Use of the TWEAK test in screening for alcoholism/heavy drinking in three populations. *Alcoholism, Clinical and Experimental Research*, *17*(6), 1188–1192.

Dhingra, I., De Sousa, A., & Sonavane, S. (2016). Sexuality in older adults: Clinical and psychosocial dilemmas. *Journal of Geriatric Mental Health*, *3*(2), 131–139.

Duclos-Miller, P. (2016). *Improving nursing documentation and reducing risk*. Retrieved August 27, 2018, from https://hcmarketplace.com/ait-downloadablefiles/download/aitfile/aitfile_id/1806.pdf

Ewing, J. A. (1984). Detecting alcoholism. The CAGE questionnaire. *Journal of the American Medical Association*, *252*(14), 1906.

Government of Canada. (2018). *Canada's food guides*. Retrieved January 05, 2018, from https://www.canada.ca/en/health-canada/services/canada-food-guides.html

Helfer, T., Sommerhalder, K., Schols, J., et al. (2015). A scoping study of health promotion in the nursing home setting: Tannys Helfer. *European Journal of Public Health*, *25*(Suppl 3). doi: https://doi.org/10.1093/eurpub/ckv171.099

Institute for Safe Medication Practices Canada. (2018). *Safer medication use in older persons*. Retrieved from https://www.ismp-canada.org/beers_list/

Jongen, C. S., McCalman, J., & Bainbridge, R. G. (2017). The implementation and evaluation of health promotion services and programs to improve cultural competency: A systematic scoping review. *Frontiers in Public Health*, *5*, 24.

The New York State Office of Alcoholism and Substance Abuse Services (OASAS). (2015). *Elderly alcohol and substance abuse*. Retrieved January 08, 2018, from www.oasas.ny.gov/AdMed/FYI/FYIInDepth-Elderly.cfm

Public Health Agency of Canada (PHAC). (2018a). *Canadian immunization guide: Part 2–Vaccine safety*. Retrieved from https://www.canada.ca/en/public-health/services/publications/healthy-living/canadian-immunization-guide-part-2-vaccine-safety.html

Public Health Agency of Canada (PHAC). (2018b). *Canadian immunization guide: Part 4–Active vaccines*. Retrieved from https://www.canada.ca/en/public-health/services/publications/healthy-living/canadian-immunization-guide-part-4-active-vaccines.html

Public Health Agency of Canada (PHAC). (2018c). *Complementary and alternative health*. Ottawa, ON: Author. Retrieved from http://www.phac-aspc.gc.ca/chn-rcs/cah-acps-eng.php

Rasheed, S., & Woods, R. T. (2014). An investigation into the association between nutritional status and quality of life in older people admitted to hospital. *Journal of Human Nutrition and Dietetics*, *27*(2), 142–151.

Sakellariou, D., & Rotarou, E. S. (2017). Access to healthcare for men and women with disabilities in the UK: Secondary analysis of cross-sectional data. *BMJ Open*, *7*, e016614.

Tigbe, W. W., Granat, M. H., Sattar, N., et al. (2017). Time spent in sedentary posture is associated with waist circumference and cardiovascular risk. *International Journal of Obesity*, *41*(5), 689–696.

Villarosa, A. C., Villarosa, A. R., Salamonson, Y., et al. (2018). The role of indigenous health workers in promoting oral health during pregnancy: A scoping review. *BMC Public Health, 18(1)*, 381.

World Health Organization (WHO). (2018). *Obesity and overweight*. Retrieved January 05, 2018, from www.who.int/mediacentre/factsheets/fs311/en/

WHO. (2004). Obesity: preventing and managing the global epidemic. Report of WHO Consultation (WHO Technical report series 894). Retrieved from https://www.who.int/nutrition/publications/obesity/WHO_TRS_894/en/

Zeran, V. (2016). Cultural competency and safety in nursing education: A case study. *Nursing Education in the Circumpolar North*. Retrieved from http://journals.sfu.ca/nr/index.php/nr/article/view/591

Resources

Alliance of Cannabis Therapeutics: http://marijuana-as-medicine.org/alliance.htm

Canadian Cancer Society, Cancer Information Service: http://www.cancer.ca

Canadian Diabetes Association: http://www.diabetes.ca

Heart and Stroke Foundation of Canada: http://www.heartandstroke.com

Genetics Resources for Nurses and Patients on the Web

Genetic Alliance: http://www.geneticalliance.org

National Organization for Rare Disorders: http://www.rarediseases.org

6 Delegation

Adapted by Sandra P. Hirst and Rebecca Stares

Learning Objectives

On completion of this chapter, the learner will be able to:

1. Define the terms delegation, accountability, and supervision.
2. Identify the five rights of delegation.
3. Describe the principles and process of delegation.
4. Discuss delegation within the context of a diverse ethnic team.
5. Identify the responsibilities of a nurse related to delegation.
6. Describe the significance of delegation within professional nursing practice.
7. Identify strategies that will help nurses learn how to delegate effectively.

What Does Delegation Mean?

Nursing is complex and multifaceted; it is difficult for one person to complete every task. Due to an increasing global shortage of nurses, professional regulated nurses are increasingly dependent on unregulated health care workers to assist in the provision of safe client care. There are numerous definitions of the term **delegation** in the Canadian nursing literature. The College of Nurses of Ontario defines delegation as "a formal process through which a regulated health professional (**delegator**) who has the authority and competence to perform a procedure under one of the controlled acts delegates the performance of that procedure to another individual (**delegatee**)" (p. 6). The Canadian Nurses Protective Society (2000) describes delegation as occurring when either the employer or the nurse transfers authority to a health care worker in a selected situation to do work traditionally performed by a nurse. Through successful delegation, regulated nurses can concentrate on more complex nursing activities (Stonehouse, 2015). It does not involve transferring **accountability** for the outcome of the function or intervention although the delegatee is responsible to successfully perform the task. It is important to remember that when a nurse delegates care, he or she is aware of the scope of practice (or job description) of the person to whom the care is delegated. Nurses cannot delegate tasks that compromise the essential elements of the nursing process and require the specialized knowledge, judgment, and/or skill of a regulated nurse. Effective nurse delegators are advocates for quality client care.

Delegation of Nursing Care

Health care in Canada involves the participation of clients, significant others, and a diverse team of health care professionals. The involvement of all team members in a cooperative, coordinated, and interprofessional approach is essential to provide quality client care. With this understanding, it is the responsibility of the nurse to understand how and when to appropriately delegate. The role of the nurse has evolved to that of delegating, directing, guiding, and oversight of client care. The nurse needs delegation skills to protect the health, safety, and welfare of clients. Delegation is client specific, meaning that the delegatee can do the delegated task only for that client. The College of Registered Nurses of Nova Scotia (2015) recommends delegation of activities only when it is in the client's best interest, and only "for those clients who are stable with predictable outcomes, there is minimal potential risk, and the task does not require application of the nursing process. As client outcomes become less predictable, the nurse is less likely to delegate to other healthcare workers because of the risk to client safety."

An example of such delegation is as follows: A regulated nurse and an **unregulated health worker** are working an evening shift on an acute surgical unit. They are assigned 18 patients. The nurse, who is entering the room of patient who has been stable for 18 hours to do a routine postoperative assessment, is approached by the unregulated worker. The worker informs the nurse that a fresh postop patient has just come onto the unit. The nurse is required to take the report from the recovery room transfer staff.

The nurse requests the unregulated worker to complete the postop assessment and report back the results. The worker has the competencies to complete the assessment.

In this example, it is important to recognize who is accountable and who is responsible within the delegation of the task. The nurse delegating the fleet enema remains accountable for the appropriateness of the delegation and for the quality of the task performed by the unregulated health care worker. In addition, the health care worker, who accepts the delegated task, must agree that he or she is the correct person to undertake it. In other words, the worker has taken responsibility to complete the task.

To meet the needs of clients, regulated nurses must delegate aspects of care to other members of the health care team, including unregulated health care workers. The role of unregulated workers is defined by the organization that employs them. It is often a challenge for a nurse to delegate to an unskilled worker. Such workers may have some knowledge and training but this will vary depending on the experience and training that they bring to the position. They may never have had the opportunity or training to perform some tasks. There is a lack of evidence on the effectiveness of delegation interventions and strategies by nurses to unregulated health care workers.

A regulated nurse can only succeed if he or she is an effective delegator. It is an important skill in nursing and a skill deficit can have serious consequences for clients. However, recent studies have suggested that this is an underdeveloped skill in new nurses (Jones, Hamilton, & Murry, 2015). Magnusson, Allan, Horton, et al.'s (2017) study investigated how newly qualified nurses learn to organize, delegate, and supervise patient care on acute care units when working with and supervising health care assistants. Ethnographic case studies were conducted in three hospitals and the researchers used thematic analysis to examine the data collected. Five styles of how newly qualified nurses delegated care to health care assistants were identified: the do-it-all nurse, who finished most of the work themselves; the justifier, who overly explained the reasons for decisions and was sometimes defensive; the buddy, who wanted to be everybody's friend and avoided assuming authority; the role model, who hoped that others would copy their best practice but had no strategy of ensuring how; and the inspector, who was very much aware of personal accountability and constantly checked the work of others. Most nurses need to learn the skills of delegation through education and work experience.

Through success delegation, nurses concentrate on complicated nursing tasks (Stonehouse, 2015). The literature shows that regulated nurses are often confused about delegation, their roles, and their responsibilities (Gransjön Craftman, Grape, Ringnell, et al., 2016; Mueller & Vogelsmeier, 2013). Often nurses struggle with which tasks they can delegate because of the different levels of unregulated health care workers including; student nurses, nursing assistants, care aides, and support workers (Hasson, McKenna, & Keeney, 2013; Johnson, Magnusson, Allan, et al., 2015). Other contributing factors to delegation difficulties between nurses and health care worker include role uncertainty, lack of trust, concern about who is accountable, fears of reciprocity, lack of clear communication, staffing mixes, and attitudes (Johnson et al., 2015).

One important thing to remember is that the regulated nurse maintains accountability for the decisions regarding what tasks to delegate. Safe care depends on safe delegation and that requires regulated nurses to appropriately plan and communicate delegated tasks. Failure to safely and appropriately delegate care activities could result in poor client outcomes. Research has identified the increase in the occurrence of "missing" care may be due to ineffective delegation by the nurse as a substantial issue (Griffiths, Ball, Drennan, et al., 2014; McMullen, Kozik, Myers, et al., 2017). Cipriano (2010) reported that delegation is an underdeveloped skill among nurses and one that is difficult to measure. The success or failure of delegation depends on a positive two-way relationship of mutual respect and trust between the nurse and the health care worker who assumes responsibility for a specific task. This dynamic exchange between the regulated nurse and the health care worker requires effective communication, constant evaluation, feedback, and modification to achieve the results needed to meet client care goals.

Delegation is sometimes confused with accountability. Each nurse is accountable for his or her actions and the consequences of them. This means that each nurse is responsible to ensure that legislative requirements and practice standards of one's professional jurisdiction are

Glossary

accountability: being answerable to oneself and others for one's own choices, decisions, and actions as measured against a standard

competency: competencies describe the attitudes, knowledge, skills, and reasoning a nurse must have to practise safely and ethically in a specific role and setting

critical thinkers: critical thinkers in nursing demonstrate the metacognition skills of information seeking, analyzing, discriminating, applying practice standards, clinical reasoning, and decision making

delegatee: one who is delegated a nursing responsibility

delegation: reassigning a task or intervention to a nonregulated health worker (delegatee) who otherwise would not be authorized to perform it

delegator: one who delegates a nursing responsibility

supervision: a practice activity of directing, guiding, and influencing the outcome of an individual's performance of an undertaking

unregulated health worker: individuals who are not regulated by the province/territory and are trained to assist nurses by performing client care tasks as allowed by the employer organization. There are numerous job titles for such employees, including: nursing assistant, nursing auxiliary, health care aide, unregulated assistive personnel, and personal support worker followed regardless of the setting in which one is employed. The nurse delegating the task remains accountable for the appropriateness of the delegation.

Delegation and work assignment are different. Assignment to an unregulated health care worker occurs when the required task falls within the unregulated worker's job description and training, as defined by the employer. Delegation to unregulated health care workers occurs when the required task is performed primarily by nurses and is outside the job description and training of the unregulated worker. In the earlier example, the nurse delegated the administration of the enema to the unregulated worker. **Supervision** involves providing guidance or direction, support, evaluation, and follow-up by the nurse for the purpose of achieving appropriate outcomes for the care which was delegated. Supervision may be either direct or indirect. The term "direct supervision" means being immediately present to guide or direct while indirect supervision means supervising from a distance but being available within a specified time frame. Nurses supervise activities by having the unregulated health care worker report regularly to the nurse and by periodically observing the unregulated health care worker's activities.

Benefits of Delegation

Delegation is beneficial as it may promote the most efficient use of another individual's knowledge and skill and give regulated nurses the opportunity to extend their services to a greater number of clients. These benefits apply to the regulated nurse, delegatee, and the employer organization.

For the Regulated Nurse

Effective delegation allows the nurse to use more advanced nursing skills in care and facilitates more frequent observations of clients. It can result in increased productivity because several team members are involved in a specific task or activity at a given point in time. In addition, the development of effective delegation skills can contribute to the personal and professional growth of the regulated nurse. This contributes to job satisfaction (Yoon, Kim, & Shin, 2016). One other reason to develop good delegation skills is to protect yourself, as a regulated nurse. If you are aware of what you can and cannot do as a nurse and you assign tasks accordingly, then you are less likely to breach your professional practice standards. You reduce your risk of legal liability for your actions.

For the Delegatee

Participation in decision making can contribute to an increase in personal self-esteem and feeling of empowerment in the delegatee. It can also contribute to their enhanced understanding of organizational policy and work. The development of these skills can improve career opportunities.

For the Organization

Health care workers can leave an organization if they believe that their abilities are not being appropriately utilized. Through effective delegation, tasks are matched against knowledge and skills, thereby producing higher quality of work. This contributes to the success of an organization. Effective delegation can result in faster and more effective decision making. It also permits numerous team members to perform the same tasks so that if one worker becomes ill or an emergency arises, which requires them to perform tasks that are not part of their usual work responsibilities, they are familiar with the task components.

Guiding Principles of Delegation

Delegation is the transfer of authority to perform a specific nursing task in a specific situation to a competent individual. It is one of the most challenging activities for the nurse. There is often more nursing care required than there are nurses to provide that care. In addition, not all care needed for a client requires a professional nurse. Nurses must work within an interprofessional team and work with individuals of varying knowledge, skills, and experience. The delegation process requires critical thinking and self-reflection by the nurse (Chart 6-1).

Remembering Accountability

It is important to remember what that the nurse is responsible for in the delegation process. This includes:

- Assessing the client's needs
- Making the decision to delegate
- Planning for the identified outcome
- Assessing the ability and skills of the delegatee
- Giving clear directions and obtaining agreement from the delegatee
- Evaluating the outcomes of the delegatee and for the client
- Documenting as per organizational policy

Setting Priorities

Proper delegation also requires priority setting, which is defined as the ordering of nursing problems using concepts of urgency and importance in order to have a preferential sequence for nursing actions.

A number of factors have been identified as potentially influencing priority setting, including unit organization, models of care, nurse–client relationship, and the critical thinking skills of the regulated nurse to establish priorities.

Evaluating Delegation

Many regulated nurses do not take the time to evaluate the outcomes of their delegation. This may perhaps be due to high workloads or difficulty in confronting the delegatee when concerns arise. Evaluating can help to prevent mistakes and help to improve communication between the regulated nurse and the delegatee. Some delegators avoid giving delegatees negative feedback but this is not fair to the delegatees and is avoidance of responsibilities. If mistakes are not discussed, then they are likely to be repeated. Delegators should also provide commendations when tasks have been successfully completed.

CHART 6-1

Delegator's Self-Reflection

Should I Delegate?

- What is the context of the situation, and what is the environment?
- Who is available to be the delegatee?
- Does this task provide an opportunity to help develop the potential delegatee's skills?
- Is this a one-time task? If it needs to be repeated, if so, how often?
- Are there ethical considerations?
- What is the potential for an adverse outcome if I delegate the task and it is not done well?
- What are the knowledge, clinical reasoning, and psychomotor skills needed to perform the task? Does the potential delegatee have these skills?
- What level of communication with team members is needed to perform the task?
- Who is responsible for documentation upon completion of the task?

What Information Is Needed to Complete the Task?

- How is the task to be accomplished?
- What resources are needed for the task?
- What is the time frame for its completion?
- When and what information should be reported? And to whom?
- What is the process for seeking clarification about what is to be delegated?

What Is My Follow-Up Responsibility?

- What level of supervision do I need to provide?
- What frequency of monitoring do I need to do to make sure the task gets done?
- How will the completion of the task be verified and documented (if needed)?
- How will unexpected problems in completing the task be resolved? Who will address them?

How Do I Evaluate the Delegation?

- Was the delegation successful?
- Did the task get accomplished in a timely manner?
- How much support did I need to provide? Was it adequate?
- Did I provide appropriate feedback and follow-up?
- Did I give positive feedback if deserved?
- Did I document as needed?
- Did I report to the health care team if needed?

Promoting Collaboration and Teamwork

Effective delegation requires collaboration and positive interpersonal relationships between nurses and all members of the health care team. Each brings different knowledge and skills to the care of the client. The nurse's communication and leadership style influences the success of delegation. Effective leadership includes successful delegation (Drescher, 2017). Transformational leadership was identified by Yoon et al. (2016) as influencing the nurse's confidence in delegating, perhaps because they can develop a collaborative culture.

Immigration patterns are changing the composition of the Canadian health care workforce. The employers are aware of the need to recruit and retain a culturally diverse workforce that reflects this country's change in demographics. This means that regulated nurses work with team members from diverse ethnic and religious backgrounds. Such diversity when reflected in language, cultural beliefs, and practices may influence the effectiveness of communication between the delegator and delegate.

Regulated nurses can use the decision tree in Figure 6-1 to determine if it is appropriate to delegate a specific nursing task in a particular setting to another team member, such as an unregulated worker.

The Five Rights of Delegation

Right task: the function falls within the delegatee's role description or is included as part of the written policies and procedures of the nursing practice setting. It is important for the nurse to know the nursing practice legislation and standards of the jurisdiction in which one is practising. In addition, most employers have policies and procedures that describe what tasks can be delegated. This is important because different employers may have differing standards of delegation. For example, many continuing care facilities assign practical nurses (registered nursing assistants) as charge nurses. They may also give medications depending on the policies of the employer.

Right circumstance: the health condition of the client must be stable and the outcomes of the delegated task predictable. If the client's condition changes, the delegatee must communicate this to the nurse, and the nurse must reassess the situation and the appropriateness of the delegation.

Right person: the nurse along with the employer and the delegatee is responsible for ensuring that the delegatee possesses the appropriate knowledge and skills to perform the activity. This means that the regulated nurse must know the **competency** level, job description, individual level of skill, and education level of the potential delegatee. Job descriptions will provide a broad overview of what an individual is expected to do, but the nurse must know the individual's capabilities, experience, and skills.

Right directions and communication: the right direction and communication is required of the nurse when tasks are delegated. Each situation where delegation occurs should be specific to the client, the nurse, and the delegatee. The regulated nurse is expected to communicate specific instructions for the delegated task to the delegatee; the delegatee, as part of two-way communication, should ask any clarifying questions. This communication includes any client information that needs to be collected, the method for collecting the information, the time frame for reporting the results to the regulated nurse, and additional information pertinent to the situation. The nurse should ensure that the delegatee understands that he or she cannot make any decisions or modifications in carrying out the activity without first consulting the regulated nurse. It is important to create an atmosphere where the delegatee feels comfortable to say that he or she is not competent or able to complete the task. For a guideline,

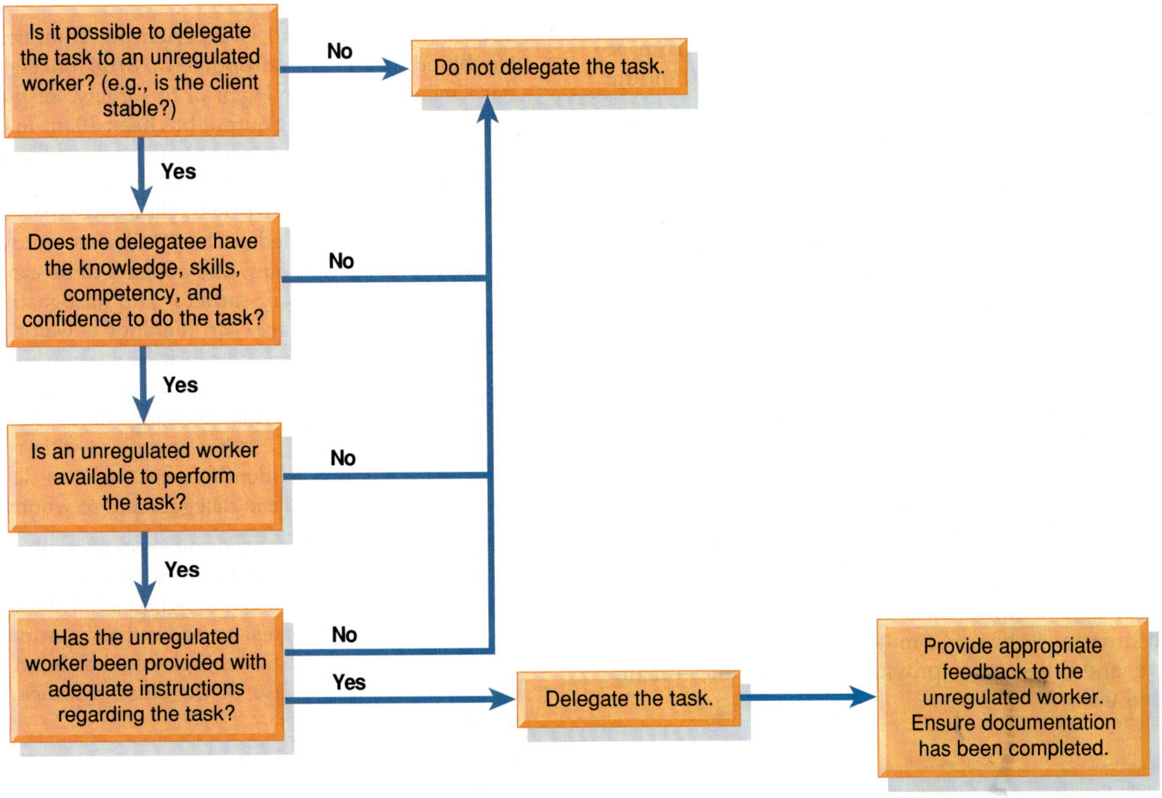

FIGURE 6-1. Delegation decision tree for assessment of delegation.

follow the four Cs—be clear, concise, correct, and complete. The delegatee must understand the terms of the delegation, agree to accept the delegated task, and report back to the delegator.

Right supervision and evaluation: the nurse remains accountable for the total care delivery. Consequently, the regulated nurse is responsible for monitoring the delegated activity, following up with the delegatee at its completion, and evaluating client outcomes. The delegatee is responsible for communicating client information to the nurse during the delegation situation. The nurse should be ready and available to intervene as necessary. The nurse should ensure appropriate documentation of the task is completed.

Delegation skills are developed by the nurse over time. Delegation involves an awareness of the total client care needs for the clients assigned, as well as a thorough knowledge of the capabilities and competencies of staff members. When used appropriately, it is a vital tool for the nurse that results in safe, competent, and efficient client care. Because nurses' time is often limited, effective delegation is essential for quality client care. Nurses can use the strategies in Chart 6-2 to effectively delegate.

CHART 6-2

Strategies for Effective Delegation

- Plan ahead
- Identify necessary knowledge and skills
- Identify who is available to perform the task
- Select the most capable person
- Communicate task clearly
- Empower the delegatee
- Set a timeline and monitor progress
- Evaluate performance
- Reward accomplishment
- Complete required documentation

Common Factors That May Hinder Delegation

There are a number of factors that might hinder effective delegation. Some of these factors are discussed as follows.

Inadequate Staffing

In health care organizations, inadequate means that there are too few staff working, or those that are available do not possess the requisite knowledge and skills for the task that might be delegated to them.

Underdelegating

Underdelegating can occur when the nurse believes that delegation can be interpreted as a lack of ability on their part to accomplish identified tasks. They might fear the loss of control. It might also be caused by a fear that delegatees will resent having work delegated to them. Nurses lacking professional experience are less likely to delegate owing to a lack of supervisory experience.

Overdelegating

Nurses may overdelegate if their time management skills are not well developed or they waste their time trying to get organized. Some nurses do it because they are unsure of their ability to designate a specific task (Ekström & Idvall, 2015). Other delegators may lack an understanding of the appropriateness of delegation.

Resistance to Delegation

When delegatees resist delegation, the nurse might decide to do the task themselves. This should be discouraged. Instead, talking to the delegatee might identify why tasks are not being accomplished and acted on immediately to reduce or eliminate obstructing factors. A common reason for resistance to delegation is the nurse's failure to appreciate the perspective of the delegatee. Delegatees may have heavy workloads and feel that they cannot accomplish additional tasks. Other delegatees may feel that they lack the necessary knowledge and skills required or perhaps lack the self-confidence. If the nurse feels that the delegatee does have the requisite knowledge and abilities, then promoting the delegatee's self-confidence might be necessary. Resistance to authority is also a reason for resistance. In such situations, the nurse must remain calm but also be assertive, and if necessary, provide clear guidelines for the delegated task.

Strategies to Help Nurses Learn How to Delegate Effectively

There are a number of strategies that nurse leaders may initiate to help their colleagues effectively delegate. Provincial and territorial nursing jurisdictional authorities need to work with the Canadian Nurses Association and other national nursing organizations to define what nursing tasks can be delegated to unregulated health care workers. "Nationally standardized delegation requirements for nursing tasks would maintain patient safety" (Yoon et al., 2016, p. 682).

Unregulated workers require education on the importance of reporting and documentation (Johnson et al., 2015). This responsibility will often fall on orientation facilitators and on-site health care educators. These educators may also provide continuing education opportunities for regulated nurses, including a focus on leadership skills to promote effective delegation, since few undergraduate programs offer such content (Saccomano & Pinto-Zipp, 2014).

Mentoring can also promote the learning of effective delegation skills by the nurse. A regulated and unregulated worker may be partnered together on several shifts. This provides each with the opportunity to learn about the knowledge and skills that the other possesses, and to develop healthy interpersonal relationships. Allan, Magnusson, Evans, et al. (2016) called this invisible learning.

Critical Thinking Exercises

1 As the team leader on a 12-hour shift, you have three regulated nurses working with you and two unregulated health care workers to care for 56 patients. One client, Mrs. Chang, is 6-hour postoperative after extensive abdominal surgery and is experiencing complications. Her blood pressure has dropped to 78/64 mm Hg from a baseline of 132/84 mm Hg prior to surgery. Respirations are shallow. Her urinary output has been 30 mL in the last 3 hours. It is extremely concentrated and reddish tinged. Another patient, Mrs. Lladro, 6 hours postsurgery, from a hiatus hernia repair is trying to climb over the side rails of her bed, and has pulled out her IV. She has removed her nasal prongs several times. She appears to be experiencing delirium. Her urinary catheter and nasogastric tube currently remain in place. Mr. Jennings is waiting for a continuing care bed but is currently wandering in and out of other patients' rooms looking for his pet dog. What are the factors to consider when deciding what tasks to delegate to team members? What specifics within the case study will help you to identify what tasks to delegate? Identify what tasks you can delegate and to whom.

2 Brian Swan is an experienced nurse on an acute 38-bed medical unit. He returned to work this week following knee surgery. Brian has been assigned all of the patients in the three rooms closest to the nurses' station. How would you respond to staff complaints that Brian has an easy assignment because of his close distance to the nurses' station?

REFERENCES AND SELECTED READINGS

Books

Marquis, B. L., & Huston, C. J. (2017). *Leadership roles and management functions in nursing: Theory and application* (9th ed.). Philadelphia, PA: Wolters Kluwer.

Motacki, K., & Burke, K. (2016). *Nursing delegation and management of patient care—e-book*. St. Louis, MO: Elsevier Health Sciences.

Journals and Electronic Documents

Allan, H. T., Magnusson, C., Evans, K., et al. (2016). Delegation and supervision of healthcare assistants' work in the daily management of uncertainty and the unexpected in clinical practice: Invisible learning among newly qualified nurses. *Nursing Inquiry*, 23(4), 377–385, 1–29. Retrieved from http://discovery.ucl.ac.uk/1523729/1/Evans_Invisible%20Learning15072016accepted2.pdf

Canadian Nurses Association. (2018). *Evidence-informed decision-making and nursing practice [Position statement]*. Ottawa, Canada: Author. Retrieved from https://www.cna-aiic.ca/-/media/cna/page-content/pdf-en/evidence-informed-decision-making-and-nursing-practice-position-statement_dec-2018.pdf?la=en&hash=F67B89BDF7AADF342AC928B5A3FB0F98C3E190D3

Canadian Nurses Protective Society. (2000). *Delegation to other health care workers*. Retrieved from https://www.cnps.ca/index.php?page=90

Cipriano, P. (2010). Overview and summary: Delegation dilemmas: Standards and skills for practice. *OJIN: The Online Journal of Issues in Nursing*, 15(2).

College of Nurses of Ontario. (2018). *Practice guidelines: Authorizing mechanisms*. Retrieved February 21, from https://www.cno.org/globalassets/docs/prac/41075_authorizingmech.pdf

College of Registered Nurses of Nova Scotia. (2015). *Assignment and delegation guidelines for registered nurses and licensed practical nurses*. Retrieved February 20, from https://crnns.ca/wp-content/uploads/2015/02/AssignmentandDelegationGuidelines.pdf

College of Registered Nurses of Nova Scotia. (2017). *Assignment and delegation guidelines for registered nurses and licensed practical nurses*. Retrieved from https://crnns.ca/wp-content/uploads/2015/02/AssignmentandDelegationGuidelines.pdf

Drescher, G. (2017). Delegation outcomes: Perceptions of leaders and follower's satisfaction. *Journal of Managerial Psychology*, 32(1), 2–15. Retrieved from https://doi.org/10.1108/JMP-05-2015-0174

Ekström, L., & Idvall, E. (2015). Being a team leader: Newly registered nurses relate their experiences. *Journal of Nursing Management*, *23*(1), 75–86.

Gransjön Craftman, Å., Grape, C., Ringnell, K., et al. (2016). Registered nurses' experience of delegating the administration of medicine to unregulated personnel in residential care homes. *Journal of Clinical Nursing*, *25*(21–22), 3189–3198.

Griffiths, P., Ball, J., Drennan, J., et al. (2014). *The association between client safety outcomes and regulated nurse/healthcare assistant skill mix and staffing levels and factors that may influence staffing requirements*. Retrieved from https://eprints.soton.ac.uk/id/eprint/367526

Hasson, F., McKenna, H. P., & Keeney, S. (2013). Delegating and supervising unregistered professionals: The student nurse experience. *Nurse Education Today*, *33*(3), 229–235.

Johnson, M., Magnusson, C., Allan, H., et al. (2015). 'Doing the writing' and 'working in parallel': How 'distal nursing' affects delegation and supervision in the emerging role of the newly qualified regulated nurse. *Nurse Education Today*, *35*(2), e29–e33.

Jones, T. L., Hamilton, P., & Murry, N. (2015). Unfinished nursing care, missed care, and implicitly rationed care: State of the science review. *International Journal of Nursing Studies*, *52*(6), 1121–1137.

Magnusson, C., Allan, H., Horton, K., et al. (2017). An analysis of delegation styles among newly qualified nurses. *Nursing Standard*, *31*(25), 46–53.

Manitoba College of Registered Nurses. (2018). *Practice direction: Assignment and delegation to unregulated workers*. Retrieved February 20, from https://www.crnm.mb.ca/uploads/document/document_file_40.pdf?t=1527775148

McMullen, S. L., Kozik, C. A., Myers, G., et al. (2017). Improving nursing care: Examining errors of omission. *MedSurg Nursing*, *26*(1), 9–16.

Mueller, C., & Vogelsmeier, A. (2013). Effective delegation: Understanding responsibility, authority, and accountability. *Journal of Nursing Regulation*, *4*, 20–24. Retrieved from https://doi.org/10.1016/S2155-8256(15)30126-5

National Council of State Boards of Nursing. (2016). *National guidelines for nursing delegation*. Retrieved from https://www.ncsbn.org/NCSBN_Delegation_Guidelines.pdf

Saccomano, S. J., & Pinto-Zipp, G. (2014). Integrating delegation into the undergraduate curriculum. *Creative Nursing*, *20*(2), 106–115.

Stonehouse, D. (2015). The art and science of delegation. *British Journal of Healthcare Assistants*, *9*(3), 150–153.

Tourangeau, A., Saari, M. E., Rowe, A., et al. (2015). *The role of nurses in assigning, delegating, teaching and supervising patient care activities to unregulated care providers in home care a jurisdictional scan of legislation, regulation and policy in Canada*. Retrieved from https://www.researchgate.net/publication/283291142_The_Role_of_Nurses_in_Assigning_Delegating_Teaching_and_Supervising_Patient_Care_Activities_to_Unregulated_Care_Providers_in_Home_Care_A_Jurisdictional_Scan_of_Legislation_Regulation_and_Policy_in_Can

Yoon, J., Kim, M., & Shin, J. (2016). Confidence in delegation and leadership of registered nurses in long-term care hospitals. *Journal of Nursing Management*, *24*(5), 676–685.

Resources and Web Sites

American Nurses Association: https://www.nursingworld.org/ana
Canadian Nurses Association: https://www.cna-aiic.ca
Canadian Nurses Protective Society: https://www.cnps.ca
College of Nurses of Ontario: https://www.cno.org
College of Registered Nurses of Nova Scotia: https://crnns.ca
Nursing and Midwifery Board of Australia: https://www.nursingmidwiferyboard.gov.au
Royal College of Nursing: https://www.rcn.org.uk

7 Spirituality in Nursing Practice

Adapted by Marlette B. Reed and Annette M. Lane

Learning Objectives

On completion of this chapter, the learner will be able to:

1. Define the concept of spirituality and list a number of expressions of spirituality.
2. Describe the relationship between spirituality and health.
3. Describe the various ways that patients express their spirituality and how they may reveal spiritual needs.
4. Discuss how nurses can help patients with their spiritual needs.
5. Understand why it is important for nurses to recognize the paradigm through which they process the illnesses/deaths of their patients.
6. Identify ways in which nurses can tend to their own spirituality, in order to support their nursing practice and provide a spiritual presence for patients.
7. Understand when a referral to a professional spiritual caregiver is necessary.

Many years ago, psychiatrist and World War 2 Concentration Camp survivor, Viktor Frankl, made the following statement (1986, xv–xvi): "Man lives in three dimensions: the somatic, the mental, and the spiritual. The spiritual dimension cannot be ignored, for it is what makes us human." Today, depending on the source, there are a number of dimensions, or domains, identified in which we as humans live: the physical, psychological, emotional, social, and spiritual, as well as others such as the environment. Health involves the successful balance and integration of each of these dimensions in a person's life. As such, a person's spirit has a profound effect upon the physical, psychological, emotional, and social self. Conversely, the other facets of an individual's being affect him/her spiritually. Body, mind, and spirit are independent, yet inextricably intertwined.

Science has powerfully aided our understanding of the body and mind (soul); however, the objectivity of this discipline has, in the last several centuries, resulted in a separation between what is considered "medical" treatment and what is not. This sharp delineation is weakening as society is becoming more attuned to the spiritual again. Within the health care system there is an increased acceptance of the need for a comprehensive care plan that addresses the needs of the whole patient. Nurses are expected to give spiritual care (Karadag Arli, Bakan, & Erisik, 2017).

This chapter covers **spirituality** and its common expressions. The relationship between spirituality and health, and how patients may reveal their spiritual needs, will also be examined, along with ways in which nurses can respond to their patients' spiritual needs. Finally, this chapter will discuss the importance of nurses being aware of their own life beliefs/spirituality, so that they can help patients and families who are suffering.

Definition of Spirituality

While there is no universally accepted definition for spirituality (Canfield, Taylor, Nagy, et al., 2016), there are a number of generally agreed upon concepts in this subjective construct. Deconstructing the noun *spirituality* begins with the concept of spirit. One's spirit is his or her energy and life force (Lloyd, 2019), the passion and yearning that motivates his or her life. The life of the human spirit is expressed through one's spirituality. Not to be considered synonymous to **religion** (Lane & Reed, 2019), spirituality is understood to be much broader in scope. It can involve appreciation for (as well as a sense of responsibility toward) nature (Cooper, Brady, Steen, et al., 2016) and beauty.

A key component of spirituality is *meaning,* which can relate to activities that are significant to the individual and others impacted by it; it may also relate to "ultimate meanings"—those larger-than-life questions that occur in crisis. *What happens when we die?* is an example. In this context, social worker Evan Senreich (2013) defines spirituality as "each person's unique relationship to what is unknowable about existence" (p. 553). One's spirituality reflects his or her world view regarding human experience. The practice of religion can be a valuable way of conceptualizing and expressing one's spirituality; however, it is not a requirement, as many people express the life force within them through broad guiding principles. For example, the "Golden Rule" is expressed by many world religions, as well as by many people's spiritual codes: "Do to others as you would have them do to you" is sometimes expressed as "Do good and good will come back to you." Profound transcendent experiences of joy and awe happen to those who practice religious faith and to those who do not (Hodge, 2013).

Expressions of Spirituality

The number and variety of expressions of the individual life force—the spirits of human beings—are as diverse as people themselves. The way in which individuals express spirituality is tied into the values and activities that guide their lives and that give them meaning in life (including "ultimate meanings"). These values and activities can include the following:

- a love of nature/environment
- the practice of a religious faith
- art
- music
- caring for others
- beauty
- social justice
- physical fitness/mastery
- a love of animals
- making the world a better place.

Spirituality is all about connection (Brown, 2018; Smith-Trudeau, 2019)—connection to self, to others, and perhaps to the Divine. All of the above can be experienced in a superficial way, but if people are deeply connected to one of the above, they will be passionate about it, their life's meaning will be entwined with it, their extra hours (or perhaps their working hours too), will be filled with it. For the individual for whom one of the above is a life motivator, the loss of it, through illness, death, job lay off, etc., becomes very significant. If all of one's meaning is found in only one area, and that area is compromised, broken or destroyed, then the very core of this individual will be disrupted (Lane & Reed, 2017).

The Relationship Between Spirituality and Health

Within the last couple of decades, a number of studies have examined the relationship between spirituality (or religion as part of spirituality) and health. While some studies question the linkage of spirituality and health, others reveal that spirituality positively impacts the health of individuals.

Spirituality, and related activities, may impact psychological health (Chung, Wong, Chen, et al., 2016). For instance, Chung et al. (2016) examined the impact of praise dance (dance that praises and thanks God) upon quality of life and the psychological health of 256 Chinese adult women. The women practiced praise dance with other women and a coach three times per week for 4 weeks and then weekly by themselves or with others for 8 weeks. The researchers found a significant improvement in the psychological health of women, irrespective of their religious backgrounds (Chung et al., 2016).

Spirituality has been shown to benefit aging adults. For example, in one research study, meaning in life was found to have a direct relationship with emotional and functional well-being among residents of nursing homes (Haugan, 2013). In another study, residents of nursing homes who were cognitively intact and who experienced **self-transcendence** and meaning in life, both of which are components of spirituality, had significantly improved quality of life (Haugan, Moksnes, & Lohre, 2016).

Glossary

posttraumatic growth: posttraumatic growth refers to positive changes in relationships with others, self-perception, and an appreciation of life and openness to spirituality in response to a trauma or stressful event.

religion: a codified system of beliefs, faith and worship, usually involving community gatherings, standard of conduct and rituals. The practice of religion is a subset of one's spirituality.

sacred objects: in the context of religion, objects that are dedicated to God, such as a copy of religious writings, and are treated specially. In a broadly spiritual sense, an item that is so important to an individual, that it is treated specially.

sacred space: a place that is set apart to honour something, someone or a belief. This can be a physical space (a chapel, for instance) or the term can be used metaphorically: "Her weekly time with her mother was a sacred space in her life."

self-transcendence: the overcoming of the limits of the individual self and its desires in spiritual contemplation and realization. This term is often used in relation to facing into and overcoming challenging situations in the natural world through inner resources of the mind and the spirit.

spirituality: the expression of the essence of a person (spirit); values, passions, expressions of meaning and purpose.

spiritual teddy bears: a term coined by Vance, Moore, Farr, et al. (2008) meaning an object of comfort that can give someone spiritual (existential) comfort in a time of stress.

Self-transcendence is related to lower rates of depression in aging individuals (Kim, Hayward, & Reed, 2014). Purpose in life, as part of spirituality, is strongly related to improved mental and physical health outcomes in aging adults.

If older adults do not possess significant self-transcendence—the ability to overcome challenging situations in the natural world through the inner resources of the mind and the spirit—can this be increased?

To answer the question about increasing self-transcendence in older adults, McCarthy, Ling, Bowland, et al. (2015) examined the impact of a psychoeducational program with 19 older adults living in the community. The conceptual model of self-transcendence upon which the psychoeducational model was based included relationships with others, introspection, creativity, contemplation of the world, and spirituality. The 8-week program involved activities such as music, journaling, meditation, and seeking the sacred to increase self-transcendence. The researchers found that self-transcendence improved among the intervention group, as compared to the control group (McCarthy et al., 2015).

In serious illness, spirituality may be an effective coping mechanism for individuals. Meaning in life, as part of spirituality, may strengthen individuals' will to live with life-threatening illness. For instance, in one study, researchers interviewed 14 individuals living with amyotrophic lateral sclerosis (ALS) to examine how they create meaning despite their illness (Ozanne, Graneheim, & Strang, 2013). Despite experiencing anxiety regarding life and death, these individuals found meaning through connections with family and friends, giving help to others and receiving help, and accepting their circumstances (Ozanne et al., 2013). In individuals with HIV/AIDS, spirituality/faith helped individuals accept their diagnosis, gave them hope, and kept them moving forward in life (da Cruz, dos Santos Cordeiro, Marques, et al., 2017). Spirituality has also been linked to higher quality of life in women with breast cancer (Al-Natour, Al Momani, & Qandil, 2017). For those receiving palliative care, the practices of faith and spirituality gave hope and strength and enhanced individuals' sense of well-being (Asgeirsdottir, Sigurbjornsson, Traustadottir, et al., 2013).

Although these studies link spirituality with well-being in individuals experiencing illness, research also suggests that *caregivers* of those with illness may be helped by the spirituality of their ailing loved ones. For instance, Tan, Lim, Kuek, et al. (2015) found that caregivers of loved ones with cancer experienced enhanced well-being when their ill relatives made meaning of their cancer experience.

Spirituality may also enhance **posttraumatic growth** (Rzeszutek, Oniszczenko, & Kwiatkowska, 2017). Posttraumatic growth refers to positive changes in relationships with others, self-perception, and an appreciation of life and openness to spirituality in response to a trauma or a stressful event (Wang, Lee, & Yates, 2019). Rzeszutek et al. (2017) found that meaning-focused strategies, such as a return to religion and acceptance, were linked to posttraumatic growth in 250 individuals with rheumatoid arthritis. Similarly, in a study examining attachment to God and religious coping in individuals with cancer or renal disease, researchers found that a secure attachment to God led to a willingness to fight the illness (as opposed to feeling hopeless), and hence, resulted in better adjustment to disease (Cassibba, Papagna, Calabrese, et al., 2014).

How Patients Reveal Spiritual Needs

Patients express their spirituality or reveal their spiritual needs in different ways, according to how they view spirituality. Some modes of expression may clearly indicate spiritual beliefs, while other behaviours may be less obvious.

Overt Expressions of Spirituality

For some patients who are open about their spirituality, their expressions may involve having religious objects in their hospital room. These objects, such as a picture of a holy leader or a copy of sacred writings, are a concrete presence of religious and/or spiritual beliefs, helping to tie the physical world to the transcendent (Gabel, 2017), and this connection is especially important in times of stress, such as illness or hospitalization (Reed, Lane, & Hirst, 2016). The physicality of the object is important to some, and an individual may experience that object as unconditional love and comfort from God (Gabel, 2017).

Other patients may ask for a spiritual advisor, such as a minister, priest, rabbi, or imam. The critically ill person may well have some spiritual matters to address. Sometimes, patients may not present with spiritual issues at the beginning of their hospitalization, but may suddenly have some spiritual care needs when their health deteriorates. For instance, an individual who has not practiced formalized religion in his adult life may have entered hospital thinking that he would be quickly discharged, and hence, had initially not indicated any spiritual distress. But now, with a diagnosis of a terminal illness and imminent death, religious practices that had been important in his upbringing may take on renewed value. If this patient is expressing anxiety and remarks that he would like to see a clergyperson, the course of action is easily discerned.

In other situations, spiritual needs may not be visible during the daytime, but become overt at night. For example, some patients may ask to speak with nurses, especially during the night, when patients are alone with their thoughts, and fears and spiritual concerns come to the forefront. If patients move into a discussion of their fear of dying, unfinished business with family members, or fear for the future, for example, the nurse should recognize that they are voicing spiritual concerns.

Less Obvious Expressions of Spirituality or Spiritual Distress

In a study of patients receiving hemodialysis, Mulder and Sikken-Kersten (2016) examined the diaries kept by six participants during their hemodialysis sessions. Patients were to include in their diaries thoughts and feelings during treatment, and the researchers focused on writings related to spirituality and quality of life. The diary entries revealed that the spiritual presence of the nurses, who truly saw and heard patients' concerns, helped participants to endure the isolation of illness; telling their stories to nurses was important and a necessary part of their spiritual expressions (Mulder & Sikken-Kersten, 2016). Telling their stories is more than idle conversation for patients; it is vital for them to express spirituality and find meaning out of illness.

Sometimes patients will express spiritual needs through trying to gain control of their surroundings (Lane & Reed, 2017). A common example is a patient who continually pushes the call bell; when the nurse enters the room, the need for help is minor—and perhaps something the patient could have handled without assistance. A patient who continually pushes the call bell may be displaying evidence of anxiety. The patient may be fearful or experiencing existential issues. *Am I going to die? Who am I now that I have this disease, or cannot do what I once could do? If I don't die, how do I go on with life?* Some patients have expressed their distress by stating, "I can't live and I can't die!" These are all important existential questions and statements that are inherently spiritual.

Saunders, a leader in the hospice movement, used the term *total pain* (Scrignaro, Marini, Magrin, et al., 2018). This occurs when the spiritual/existential issues are not addressed, and a person's *physical* pain levels cannot be managed by what would normally take care of them. At times like this, a referral to a chaplain or a faith leader (if there is one) may be helpful.

How Nurses Can Address Patients' Spiritual Needs

Nurses have a number of ways to address the spiritual needs of their patients. Aiding patients with their spiritual needs may occur in a formalized manner, or it may occur informally, almost intuitively.

Gerontologic Considerations

Part of the spiritual work with older patients is to facilitate patients' telling of their life stories. This involves gentle questioning and patience (Reed et al., 2016). Understanding Erikson's developmental stages (1982), older adults review their lives in order to find a sense of meaning. The end-of-life developmental task for the older adult is to achieve *integrity*—meaning wholeness. This process involves an older adult reviewing his or her life and deriving a sense of meaning and achievement (Wren, 2016); to not do this, in Erikson's model, is *despair.* The older adult patient who has a serious diagnosis is inclined to review his or her life—expressing joys and regrets. The insightful nurse can look for themes in the patient's life and help the patient identify them. "Wow, Bill, you've helped a lot of people in your life; you must feel so good about that!" (Interestingly, many older adults will push aside the compliment: "I just did what needed to be done…"). However, the spiritual work of the nurse is to identify themes and highlight their importance; this aids the older adult patient to achieve *integrity*. Using a different model—McGee and Myers—this activity helps to strengthen the patient's sacred relationship with the self (2014); interestingly, these researchers speak of the value of this type of activity for those with early to moderate stage Alzheimer's: the sense of self, of personhood, can feel tenuous to the one with dementia; discussion about the past (which the individual can be helped to recall) can strengthen that sacred relationship.

Respecting Patients' Spiritual/Faith Beliefs

The Canadian Nurses Association (CNA) proposed a position statement about nurses' role in responding to patients' spiritual needs (2010). Within this position statement, the CNA affirms the importance of patients' spirituality and that being attentive to patients' spiritual needs is part of nursing practice. Within this statement, however, the CNA advises that nurses need to demonstrate sensitivity toward and respect for the diversity of beliefs their patients hold (CNA, 2010). In other words, the spiritual needs of the patients take preference over the personal beliefs of the nurse (Lane & Reed, 2019).

Formalized Ways to Address Spirituality

On some acute care units, staff may conduct a spiritual/religious assessment: What religion (if any) does the patient hold? Is there a spiritual leader to be contacted? Would the patient like to have a visit from a hospital chaplain? This type of formal assessment is particularly necessary in end-of-life circumstances. A Roman Catholic may wish to have the Sacrament of the Sick in his dying. If staff have no knowledge of this, a sudden passing may result in him missing out on receiving a rite that which was important to him.

A more in-depth spiritual assessment may also be conducted. Rather than focusing solely upon a faith or a spiritual advisor, such assessments ask patients about meaning in their lives, their passions, where they place their hope, what they regret in their lives, their experiences with forgiveness, and what nourishes their souls. Well-known spiritual assessments include the FICA Spiritual History Tool, the HOPE Questions for Spiritual Assessment and the Open Invite Mnemonic (see Saguil & Phelps, 2012).

Nonformalized Ways to Address Spirituality

Beyond formalized assessments, another way nurses can recognize and honour the spiritual needs of patients is to create **sacred space** (Roseman, 2016). Creating sacred space involves "creat(ing) space for a healing presence greater than ourselves" (Roseman, 2016, p. 11). That space allows patients to share their fears and to do so feeling safe and valued. If the nurse, or the patient, does not believe in a Greater Presence, another way to look at this is to *hold space* (Plett, 2016). Holding space means to be fully present with another in need: to provide the time and space for that person to grieve or to be angry, for example, without trying to fix the situation. It is to journey with them without judgment. Being heard deeply is so profound for people in need that sometimes they feel as if that space is sacred; it certainly is connection (Brown, 2018; Smith-Trudeau, 2019).

Nurses also can honour their patients' spirituality by recognizing objects that are clearly sacred to them. Pargament and colleagues spoke about the work of making sacred ("sanctifying" is the religious term, which means to set apart for holy purposes, by both religious and nonreligious people of objects and activities in their lives). Though the object may be ordinary, the significance placed upon it by the patient makes it sacred to them (Pargament, 2007, 2008). It is important for the nurse to recognize that these objects—religious, such as a siddur (Jewish prayer book) or a mala (Buddhist prayer beads), or not specifically religious, such as a blanket—are important to their patients and to show respect for their patients' belief systems.

To illustrate, a patient in an end-of-life situation had been newly admitted, and the chaplain went to visit and conduct the spiritual assessment. This gentleman was Mormon, and he wore undergarments in keeping with his faith. As he was no longer mobile, he counted on staff support in changing his bedclothes, washing, etc. It was very important to him that the practice of wearing these undergarments be respected; they were, by his church, made sacred ("sanctified"). By respecting this practice and his faith, the staff would be respecting him. The chaplain assured him that this would be communicated to staff, and care would be taken in the washing of these garments. Coming to the end of his life, he needed spiritual care; had his belief system not been respected, he may not have been willing to receive spiritual care from the chaplain or his nurses.

Spiritual "teddy bears" are another less formalized way nurses can tend to the spiritual needs of their patients. Since childhood we have sought ways to self-soothe. The child who sucks her thumb when going to a sitter's house will later wrap herself in a special blanket to bring comfort. When patients are experiencing disruption to their lives—through serious medical/surgical issues—they may greatly benefit from what Vance et al. (2008) call "**spiritual teddy bears**." Patients who have had heart surgery often receive a heart-shaped red pillow to hug; this provides pain relief (the action of squeezing the pillow on top of one's chest), but also something cute to squeeze (emotional pain relief). Sometimes, ministers may give out *prayer blankets* knitted by people who then prayed a blessing upon them. Patients of a variety of faiths have found these objects significant—as the blanket itself provided warmth and because, for the patient, the knowledge that others care and worked to produce a beautiful blanket, and asked God to bless the one receiving it, provided comfort for the spirit of the one who received it.

Unofficial spiritual assessments are done regularly by nursing staff, whether they recognize this or not. By getting to know a patient, staff become familiar with what is important and meaningful to that individual. That which is important will be brought up directly by the patient, or hinted at through oblique references in conversation, through decorations in their room, and through those who come to visit. By being alert to this, and through effective charting, the staff on the floor can get to know what interests and motivates their patients.

At times, astute nurses will recognize restlessness in the patient that is existential in nature. As previously noted, a patient may try to exercise control in ways that are not appropriate. It is a perceptive nurse who evaluates spirituality informally, is in touch with his/her own existential needs, and who recognizes this and sees the behaviour as more than simply "bad." He or she will recognize that a person who has lost control in a key area of life (health) may try to seize control in other ways (Lane & Reed, 2019). While inappropriate behaviour is not to be ignored, understanding some of the motivations behind it can ameliorate a staff's approach.

A significant aspect of providing effective spiritual care is to attend to the dignity of the patient. As an example, patients who are incontinent can feel utter humiliation. Providing dignified care involves treating patients with worth and value, facilitating their independence as much as possible, being sensitive to their needs, protecting their privacy, and communicating with them when providing care (Lin, Watson, & Tsai, 2013). Chart 7-1 examines how nurses can uphold the dignity of their patients. This type of connection cares for the patient, upholds personhood, and builds the spirit; it makes the difference between having tasks done *for/with* them, rather than *to* them (Hirst, Lane, & Reed, 2013).

There are situations when providing spiritual care is taxed by the patient's challenges, such as cognitive impairment or the patient being comatose. In these situations, what does spiritual care entail? First, the nurse who is

NURSING RESEARCH PROFILE

Chart 7-1. Characteristics of Dignified Care by Staff in Iranian Acute Care Facilities

Manookian, A., Cheraghi, M. A., & Nasrabadi, A. N. (2014). Factors influencing patients' dignity: A qualitative study. *Nursing Ethics*, *21*(3), 323–334.

Purpose
The purpose of this study was to examine the factors that promote or compromise patient dignity.

Design
This study was a qualitative study utilizing semi-structured interviews with 14 participants who had been hospitalized. Inductive content analysis was used to identify themes.

Findings
Research participants (as former patients) felt that dignity involved being treated with respect, having health care providers who were humble, calm, and polite, who smiled at them and provided compassionate care, and who maintained patients' confidences and privacy.

Nursing Implications
The researchers noted that how nurses treat patients, through their words and behaviours, preserves or threatens patients' dignity. They also determined the importance of nurses communicating with their patients and having enough time with them in interactions.

astute in spiritual care for those with cognitive impairment, or for those who are comatose, will honour spiritual practices that were important to these patients in the past (Reed et al., 2016). This may necessitate checking with family members about former spiritual practices that were meaningful to these patients. If reading from holy writings was important to the patient, the nurse can encourage family members to continue this practice, or, if family members are not available, read a brief portion to the patient when able. The tone and cadence of the reader's voice may be of comfort to the patient. (Even if the spiritual practices were once important to the patient, the nurse or family member should still ask permission to read from the holy writings to the patient [Reed et al., 2016]). If the patient is comatose, one should explain to the patient that they are going to read to them from the holy writings sitting on the patient's night table, so that the patient—at whatever level of awareness—has a sense that something is being done with/for them, rather than to them. Or, the nurse can play music for the patient that was once meaningful to him or her (with the consent of the roommate). According to Pargament's theory (2007), the holy writings or music are **sacred objects** that comfort the individual.

The nurse may, if time permits, just sit quietly, attentively, with the patient; the nurse also may speak gentle words of reassurance. While there may not be a response, it is generally recognized that unresponsive patients are more aware than they look (Tapson, Sierotowicz, Marks-Maran, et al., 2015); as they say in palliative care when encouraging a loved one to speak to their beloved in the bed, "Hearing is the last sense to go."

The Spirituality of the Nurse

Being in touch—connected—with who one is, is essential for every nurse. The acuity of patients' illnesses, and hence their needs, will test the nurse's belief system repeatedly. Throughout a nursing career, individuals will need to process difficult situations on the job through their own spiritual lenses, allowing them to cope with the stresses of the work. Consciously processing the losses and challenges through the nurse's own belief system will lead to spiritual growth, a healthier nursing practice, and will guard against burn out.

What are spiritual lenses? They are the "glasses" through which a nurse looks at the world; it includes a nurse's belief system and world view. On units where patients regularly die, nurses must be able to find enduring connections with the patients who die, while emotionally moving on (Task 4 of Mourning, Worden, 2018). This means the nurse needs to be able to process the loss of a patient by metaphorically relocating that person: "He's in my heart." "I'll always remember her." "He is in heaven." This enables the nurse to move on, knowing that this person continues to matter and that he or she won't be "lost" to the nurse. (It is a common issue in unresolved grief that mourners fear moving on, because they think that in doing so, they may forget their loved one.)

It is also critical that nurses understand their own spiritual lenses and beliefs, because situations will occur that will challenge personal beliefs or ethics and nurses must avoid bias toward or against a patient. A patient's belief system or expression of spirituality may produce strong emotions—positively or negatively—in the nurse who is providing care. A negative response can be due to a nurse's beliefs, experiences in the past, or because of things he or she has been taught. A nurse's professional code (as per the 2010 Canadian Nurses' Association position statement on Nurses and Spirituality) requires respect of each person's beliefs; deeper than the written code, the honouring of others is an essential part of the nurse's spiritual practice. Many health care institutions provide training for their staff in developing awareness of diverse religious and spiritual practices; embedded in that goal of awareness is the understanding (and hope) that this will lead to self-awareness and respect for others.

It is not uncommon to have personal belief system challenged when working as nurses. What do sensitive, conscientious nurses do about this? First, nurses must recognize their own spiritual lenses, using one of the tools mentioned earlier in the chapter, such as the FICA Spiritual History Tool or the HOPE Questions for Spiritual Assessment (see Saguil & Phelps, 2012). This type of evaluation can help nurses connect more deeply with themselves, perhaps allowing them an appreciation of what has been built into their own lives through parents, interactions with others, and the institutions of personal formation (schools, faith communities, community groups).

Nurses can reflect on the following question: Are there areas in my work that grate against my world view? If so, this will cause some cognitive dissonance and emotional turmoil for the nurse. It may cause moral distress (van Wijlen, 2017). Nurses must work through those conflicts, to bring congruity between their belief systems and the working environment. This may mean getting some help from a professional—a counsellor or a minister—to work with the nurse's belief system in order to bring that peace. Gently stretching one's beliefs to incorporate what he or she is experiencing can be growth producing. If it is impossible (a stark collision of personal values and the work environment), it may be necessary to find work in a different specialty. For instance, a nurse who does not ethically agree with Medical Assistance in Dying (MAID) might decline to work on a unit where this is carried out.

As nurses develop professionally through practice, courses and reading, they also need to attend to their own spiritual lives. For different people this will mean different things. For example, for the nurse who loves nature and challenging herself physically, recreation (literally, re-*creation*) on the weekend might mean a trip to the mountains to ski. For another, it will be a phone call to a valued friend. For another, it might be spending some quiet time in the sacred writings of their faith or journaling (van Wijlen, 2017). Ideally, the individual will find meaning in through various activities, so that *renew*-al will be achieved through a variety of means.

When to Refer a Patient to a Spiritual Care Professional

When patients' spiritual needs exceed the expertise of nurses, referral to a spiritual care professional is necessary. Often, nurses do not have the time to extensively address the spiritual concerns of patients. In these situations, it is helpful to have people trained in dealing with spiritual needs—clergy members from different faiths who are employed as hospital chaplains—to offer as a resource for those in need. Many people do not have their own clergy—as only about 13% of Canadians regularly attend a worship service (and hence have connection with a spiritual caregiver of their faith) (Hiemstra & Stiller, 2016). When a referral needs to be made, the nurse can request a chaplain who can assist the patient through a mutual faith perspective. If the institution's policies and procedures allow, the chaplain could contact (with the patient's expressed desire) a minister/imam/priest/rabbi from the community to come in. A hospital with a limited Spiritual Care department can put together a list of community religious visitors to provide spiritual care. These individuals are vetted by the hospital and have gone through training regarding institutional spiritual care; requisite screening through police checks and references helps to ensure safety (physical, emotional, and spiritual) for the patient.

A nurse who makes a referral to the hospital chaplain or another religious caregiver is not abdicating responsibility; such a referral is an effective way to meet the patient's religious and spiritual needs. It also can help prevent burn out. Part of the nurse's care of his or her own spiritual self is to guard against over-extending into areas in which expertise is lacking. It is also dignifying for the patient, who is the focus of the spiritual care, to receive religious care that is appropriate. The nurse, by providing presence and dignity, still provides spiritual care.

It also should be noted that a patient's religious/spiritual needs should not be a forum for the health care professional to proselytize. The need of the *patient*, not the nurse, is what determines the type of spiritual care that a patient receives (Lane & Reed, 2019).

REFERENCES AND SELECTED READINGS

Books

Erikson, E. H. (1982). *The life cycle completed: A review*. New York: Norton.

Frankl, V. E. (1986). *The doctor and the soul* (2nd ed.). New York: Vintage.

Hiemstra, R., & Stiller, K. (2016). Religious attendance and affiliation in Canada. In *Trust Centre for Theological Schools (New Year)*. Retrieved January 30, 2018, from http://www.intrust.org/Magazine/Issues/New-Year-2016/Religious-affiliation-and- attendance-in-Canada

Lane, A. M., & Reed, M. B. (2017). *Making meaning in older age: Bringing together the pieces of your life*. Winnipeg, MB: Word Alive Press.

Lane, A. M., & Reed, M. B. (2019). *Older adults: Understanding and facilitating transitions* (3rd ed.). Dubuque, IA: Kendall Hunt.

Pargament, K. (2007). *Spiritually integrated psychotherapy: Understanding and addressing the sacred*. New York: The Guilford Press.

Worden, J. W. (2018). *Grief counseling and grief therapy: A handbook for the mental health practitioner* (5th ed.). New York: Springer Publishing.

Journals and Electronic Documents

Al-Natour, A., Al Momani, S. M., Qandil, A. M. A. (2017). The relationship between spirituality and quality of life of Jordanian women diagnosed with breast cancer. *Journal of Religion and Health*, *56*, 2096–2108.

Asgeirsdottir, G. H., Sigurbjornsson, E., Traustadottir, R., et al. (2013). "To cherish each day as it comes": A qualitative study of spirituality among persons receiving palliative care. *Supportive Care in Cancer*, *21*, 1445–1451.

Brown, B. (2018). *Defining spirituality. Brene Brown blog*. Retrieved April 8, 2019, from https://brenebrown.com/blog/2018/03/27/defining-spirituality/

Canadian Nurses Association (CNA). (2010). *Position statement: Spirituality, health and nursing practice*. Retrieved February 21, 2018, from http://www.cna-aiic.ca/~/media/cna/page-content/pdf-en/ps111_spirituality_2010_e.pdf?la = en

Canfield, C., Taylor, D., Nagy, K., et al. (2016). Critical care nurses' perceived need for guidance in addressing spirituality in critically ill patients. *American Journal of Critical Care*, *25*(3), 206–211.

Cassibba, R., Papagna, S., Calabrese, M., et al. (2014). The role of attachment to God in secular and religious/spiritual ways of coping with serious disease. *Mental Health, Religion, & Culture*, *17*(3), 252–261.

Chung, J. W., Wong, B. Y., Chen, J. H., et al. (2016). Effects of praise dance on the quality of life of Chinese women. *The Journal of Alternative and Complementary Medicine*, *22*(12), 1013–1019.

Cooper, N., Brady, E., Steen, H., et al. (2016). Aesthetic and spiritual values of ecosystems: Recognising the ontological and axiological plurality of cultural ecosystem 'services'. *Ecosystem Services*, *21*, 218–222.

da Cruz, D. S., dos Santos Cordeiro, R., Marques, D. K., et al. (2017). Experience of patients with HIV/AIDS and the influence of religiosity/spirituality when coping with the disease. *Journal of Nursing—UFPE On line*, *11*, 4089–4895.

Gabel, S. (2017). D. W. Winnicott, transitional objects and the creation of the divine. *Mental Health, Religion & Culture*, *20*(8), 741–755.

Haugan, G. (2013). Meaning-in-life in nursing home patients: A valuable approach for enhancing psychological and physical well-being? *Journal of Clinical Nursing*, *23*, 1830–1844.

Haugan, G., Moksnes, U. K., & Lohre, A. (2016). Intra-personal transcendence, meaning-in-life and nurse-patient interaction: Powerful assets for quality of life in cognitively intact nursing home patients. *Scandinavian Journal of Caring Sciences*, *30*, 790–801.

Hirst, S. P., Lane, A. M., & Reed, M. B. (2013). Personhood in nursing homes: An ethnographic study. *Indian Journal of Gerontology*, *27*(1), 69–87.

Hodge, D. R. (2013). Implicit spiritual assessment: An alternative approach for assessing client spirituality. *Social Work*, *58*(3), 223–230.

Karadag Arli, S, Bakan, A. B., & Erisik, E. (2017). An investigation of the relationship between nurses' views on spirituality and spiritual care and their level of burnout. *Journal of Holistic Nursing*, *35*(3), 214–220.

Kim, S. S., Hayward, R. D., & Reed, P. (2014). Self-transcendence, spiritual perspective, and sense of purpose in family caregiving relationships: A mediated model of depression symptoms in Korean older adults. *Aging & Mental Health*, *18*(7), 905–913.

Lin, Y. P., Watson, R., & Tsai, Y. F. (2013). Dignity in care in the clinical setting: A narrative review. *Nursing Ethics*, *20*(2), 168–177.

Lloyd, J. (2019). A hospital is the place to heal a ravaged body, but what about a wounded spirit?. *Australian Nursing & Midwifery Journal*, *26*(6), 23.

McCarthy, V. L., Ling, J., Bowland, S., et al. (2015). Promoting self-transcendence and well-being in community-dwelling older adults. A pilot study of a psycho-educational intervention. *Geriatric Nursing*, *36*, 431–437.

McGee, J., & Myers, D. (2014). Sacred relationships, strengthened by community, can help people with mild or early-stage Alzheimer's. *Generations*, *38*(1), 61–67.

Mulder, A., & Sikken-Kersten, L. (2016). Spirituality during hemodialysis: A pilot study. *Nephrology Nursing Journal*, *43*(4), 323–329.

Musich, S., Wang, S. S., Kraemer, S., et al. (2018). Purpose in life and positive health outcomes among older adults. *Population Health Management*, *21*(2), 139–147.

Ozanne, A. O., Graneheim, U. H., & Strang, S. (2013). Finding meaning despite anxiety over life and death in amyotrophic lateral sclerosis. *Journal of Clinical Nursing*, *22*, 2141–2149.

Pargament, K. (2008). The sacred character of community life. *American Journal of Community Psychology*, *41*(1/2), 22–34.

Plett, H. (2016). What it really means to hold space for someone. *Uplift*. Retrieved February 23, 2018, from https://upliftconnect.com/hold-space/

Reed, M. B., Lane, A. M., & Hirst, S. P. (2016). Spiritual care for those with dementia: A case study. *Journal of Religion, Spirituality, & Aging*, *28*(4), 338–348.

Roseman, J. L. (2016). Creating sacred space. *Alternative and Complementary Therapies*, *22*(1), 9–13.

Rzeszutek, M., Oniszczenko, W., & Kwiatkowska, B. (2017). Stress coping strategies, spirituality, social support, and posttraumatic growth in a Polish sample of rheumatoid arthritis patients. *Psychology, Health & Medicine*, *22*(9), 1082–1088.

Saguil, A., & Phelps, K. (2012). The spiritual assessment. *American Family Physician*, *86*(6), 546–550.

Scrignaro, M., Marini, E., Magrin, M. E., et al. (2018). Emotive and cognitive processes in cancer patients: Linguistic profiles of post-traumatic growth. *European Journal of Cancer Care*, *27*, 1–8.

Senreich, E. (2013). An inclusive definition for spirituality for social work education and practice. *Journal of Social Work Education*, *49*(4), 548–563.

Smith-Trudeau, P. (2019). Spirituality: A very misunderstood word. *Vermont Nurse Connection*, *22*(2), 1–3.

Tan, J. Y., Lim, H., Kuek, N. M., et al. (2015). Caring for the caregiver while caring for the patient: Exploring the dyadic relationship between patient spirituality and caregiver quality of life. *Supportive Care in Cancer*, *23*, 3403–3406.

Tapson, K., Sierotowicz, W., Marks-Maran, D., et al. (2015). 'It's the hearing that is last to go': A case of traumatic head injury. *British Journal of Nursing*, *24*(5), 277–281.

Vance, D. E., Moore, B. S., Farr KF, et al. (2008). Procedural memory and emotional attachment in Alzheimer disease: Implications for meaningful and engaging activities. *The Journal of Neuroscience Nursing*, *40*, 96–102.

van Wijlen, J. (2017). Healing the healer: A caring science approach to moral distress in new graduate nurses. *International Journal for Human Caring*, *21*(1), 15–19.

Wang, X., Lee, M. Y., & Yates, N. (2019). From past trauma to post-traumatic growth: The role of self in participants with serious mental illnesses. *Social Work in Mental Health*, *17*(2), 149–172.

Wren, R. (2016). Effect of life review on quality of life for older adults living in nursing homes. *Physical & Occupational Therapy in Geriatrics*, *34*(4), 186–204.

Resources

Canadian Association for Spiritual Care: http://www.spiritualcare.ca/profession/

Canadian Hospice Palliative Care Foundation: http://www.chpca.net/

Canadian Nurses Association Position Statement on Spirituality, Health, and Nursing Practice: http://www.cna-aiic.ca/~/media/cna/page-content/pdf-en/ps111_spirituality_2010_e.pdf?la=en

Canadian Virtual Hospice: http://www.virtualhospice.ca

UNIT 2

Biophysical and Psychosocial Concepts in Nursing Practice

Case Study

PROVIDING CARE FOR A PATIENT WITH A COMMUNICATION BARRIER

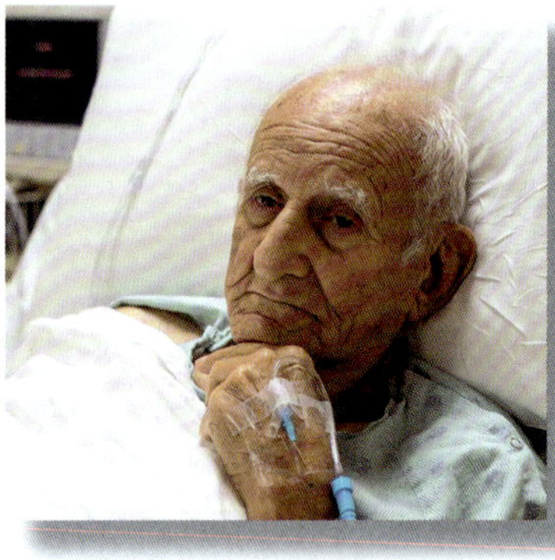

An 80-year-old man whose primary language is Spanish is brought into the emergency department (ED) by his grandson after slipping and falling in the garage. The grandson tells the triage nurse that his grandfather can understand a little bit of English but mainly speaks Spanish. He tells the nurse that his grandfather is allergic to morphine and to make sure that he is not given any. After his grandfather is triaged, the grandson leaves for work. A couple of hours later, the patient is in pain, and the physician orders morphine 5 mg IM. The patient becomes agitated and subsequently goes into respiratory arrest as a result of receiving the medication. He is resuscitated but suffers long-term effects of the hypoxia. A root cause analysis or incident report is requested, and the nurse who cared for the patient in the ED is part of the team.

QSEN Competency Focus: Safety

The complexities inherent in today's health care system challenge nurses to demonstrate integration of specific interdisciplinary core competencies that are aimed at ensuring the delivery of safe and quality patient care (Institute of Medicine, 2003). The Quality and Safety Education for Nurses project (QSEN, 2017; Cronenwett, Sherwood, Barnsteiner, et al., 2007) provides a framework for the knowledge, skills, and attitudes (KSAs) required for nurses to demonstrate competency in these key areas, which include ***patient-centred care***, ***interdisciplinary teamwork and collaboration***, ***evidence-based practice***, ***quality improvement***, ***safety***, and ***informatics.***

Health organizations must create a trusting work environment where nurses are able to report safety issues and adverse events without fear of retribution, and thus reduce the likelihood of future adverse events.

Safety Definition: Minimize risk of harm to patients and providers through both system effectiveness and individual performance.

SELECTED PRE-LICENSURE KSAs	APPLICATION AND REFLECTION
Knowledge	
Describe processes used in understanding causes of error and allocation of responsibility and accountability (such as root cause analysis or incident reports, or failure mode effect analysis).	What is a root cause analysis (RCA) or incident report? What role does the nurse have as part of this process? What is the intended outcome of an effective RCA?
Skills	
Participate appropriately in analyzing errors and designing system improvements. Engage in root cause analysis rather than blaming when errors or near misses occur.	Upon review of the case, it is discovered that the information from the grandson about the medication allergy was not documented in the EMR upon admission. What role could the communication barrier between the patient and staff have played in the error occurring? What processes could be put into place to ensure this documentation is not missed? What should happen to the nurse who had the knowledge and did not document it? How can this become a learning process, without placing blame, in order to improve patient outcomes in future situations?
Attitudes	
Value relationship between national safety campaign (Canadian Patient Safety Institute, 2018) and implementation in local practices and practice settings.	Discuss national safety goals that are established to reduce medication errors and adverse drug effects. Think about the level at which these goals are identified and developed. How might a nurse in the ED be part of implementing national safety goals into local practice?

EMR, electronic medical record.

Canadian Patient Safety Institute. (2018). *Medication Without Harm—Canada's contribution to a global effort to reduce medication errors*. Retrieved June 14, 2019, from https://www.patientsafetyinstitute.ca/en/NewsAlerts/News/Pages/Medication-Without-Harm-2018-09-14.aspx; Cronenwett, L., Sherwood, G., Barnsteiner, J., et al. (2007). Quality and safety education for nurses. Nursing Outlook, *55*(3), 122–131; Institute of Medicine. (2003). *Health professions education: A bridge to quality*. Washington, DC: National Academies Press; and QSEN Institute. (2017). *QSEN competencies: Definitions and pre-licensure KSAs*. Retrieved June 12, 2019, from www.qsen.org/competencies/pre-licensure-ksas

8 Perspectives in Transcultural Nursing

Adapted by Alice S.W. Khin

Learning Objectives

On completion of this chapter, the learner will be able to:

1. Identify key components of cultural assessment.
2. Apply transcultural nursing principles, concepts, and theories when providing nursing care to individuals, families, groups, and communities.
3. Develop strategies for planning, providing, and evaluating culturally competent and culturally safe nursing care for patients from diverse backgrounds.
4. Critically analyze the influence of culture on nursing care decisions and actions for patients.
5. Discuss the impact of diversity and health care disparities on health care delivery.

In the health care delivery system, as in society, nurses interact with people of similar as well as diverse cultural backgrounds. People may have different frames of reference about health and varied health care needs. Nurses often practice transcultural nursing, in providing care to clients and families across cultural variations. Acknowledging, respecting, and adapting to the cultural needs of patients and significant others are important components of nursing care. In addition, facilitating access to culturally appropriate health care is critical to ensure holistic nursing care. To be able to best serve culturally diverse populations, nurses must understand a number of concepts related to **culture** including cultural competence and cultural safety.

Cultural Concepts

The concept of culture and its relationship to the health care beliefs and practices of the patient and his or her family or significant others provide the foundation for transcultural nursing. This awareness of culture in the delivery of nursing care has been described in different terms and phrases, including respect for cultural diversity; culturally sensitive or comprehensive care; and culturally congruent nursing care (Holland, 2015; Leininger, 2002; Mixer, McFarland, Andrews, et al., 2013). Three important concepts are cultural diversity, cultural competence, and cultural safety.

Culture is commonly defined as the knowledge, belief, art, morals, laws, customs, and any other capabilities and habits acquired by humans as members of a society. During the past century, and especially during recent decades, hundreds of definitions of culture have been offered that integrate these themes and the themes of ethnic variations of a population based on race, nationality, religion, language, physical characteristics, and geography. To fully appreciate the broad impact of culture, factors such as disabilities, gender, social class, physical appearance (e.g., weight, height), ideologies (political views), or sexual orientation must be integrated into the definition of culture as well (Marzilli, 2014).

Madeleine Leininger (2002), founder of the specialty called transcultural nursing, writes that culture involves learned and transmitted knowledge about values, beliefs, rules of behaviour, and lifestyle practices that guide designated groups in their thinking and actions in patterned ways. Giger (2013) defines transcultural nursing as a research-focused, client-based practice field of culturally competent nursing. Transcultural nursing addresses the differences and similarities among cultures in relation to health, health care, and illness, with consideration of patient values, beliefs, and practices. Culture develops over time as a result of exposure to social and religious structures and intellectual and artistic manifestations, and each individual person, including each nurse, is culturally unique (Giger, 2013).

Ethnic culture has four basic characteristics:

- It is learned from birth through language and socialization.
- It is shared by members of the same cultural group, and it includes an internal sense and external perception of distinctiveness.

- It is influenced by specific conditions related to environmental and technical factors and to the availability of resources.
- It is dynamic and ever changing.

With the exception of the first characteristic, cultures related to aging, physical appearance, lifestyle, and other less frequently acknowledged aspects also share the above characteristics.

Cultural diversity has also been defined in a number of ways. Often, differences in skin colour, religion, and geographic area are the only elements used to identify diversity, with ethnic minorities being considered the primary sources of cultural diversity. However, there are many other possible sources of cultural diversity. To truly acknowledge an increasingly culturally diverse population, the nurse must be prepared for and able to work with patients in a way that recognizes and respects their diversity (McClimens, Brewster, & Lewis, 2014).

Culturally competent nursing care is defined as effective, individualized care that demonstrates respect for the dignity, personal rights, preferences, beliefs, and practices of the person receiving care, while acknowledging the biases of the caregiver and preventing these biases from interfering with the care provided. Culturally competent nursing care is a dynamic process that requires comprehensive knowledge of culture-specific information and an awareness of, and sensitivity to, the effect that culture has on the care situation. It requires that the nurse integrate cultural knowledge, awareness of his or her own cultural perspective, client access to culturally appropriate care, and the patient's cultural perspectives when preparing and implementing a plan of care (Giger, 2013). Understanding the diversity within cultures, such as **subcultures**, is also important.

Culturally safe nursing care is more than being aware of cultural difference and more than acknowledging these differences. Therefore it is more than culturally competent nursing care. Cultural humility—addressing one's cultural knowledge deficit(s) by exploring the patient's needs from the patient's cultural perspective and exploring one's own cultural beliefs and how they might conflict with the patient's beliefs—is a critical step toward becoming culturally competent. Cultural humility requires a commitment to learning that considers each individual's unique viewpoint (Isaacson, 2014). It implies that while we cannot be competent in another's culture, we may learn our own biases through self-reflection, thereby, becoming open to others' cultures. Cultural humility requires active listening and encourages self-reflection and self-awareness (Isaacson, 2014).

This type of care recognizes that systematic marginalization has occurred in society over time and that this has had an impact and continues to have an impact on populations. For example, residential schools are a tragic example of practices that marginalized children from First Nations and that continues to negatively impact the health of First Nations' people. In 2014, the Truth and Reconciliation Commission completed its travels across Canada to record Aboriginal people's experiences in residential schools, particularly loss of language, violence, and sexual abuse.

Bilingualism, Multiculturalism, Subcultures, and Minorities

Canada is a bilingual and multicultural nation. The Official Languages Act of 1969 established that French and English are Canada's two official languages. In 1971, Prime Minister Trudeau introduced Canada's first official policy on multiculturalism, "Multiculturalism Within a Bilingual Framework." In 1988, the *Canadian Multiculturalism Act* was proclaimed, thus making multiculturalism a defining characteristic of Canadian society. In this Act, multiculturalism is conceptualized through three themes: "Recognizing diversity; promoting understanding; and promoting equality and eliminating barriers" (Government of Canada, Justice Laws Website, 2018).

- Aboriginal Canadians (status Indians, nonstatus Indians, Métis, and Inuit) and Canadians of French and British origins are considered the founding nations of Canada. The Aboriginal peoples of Canada have a younger population than the non-Aboriginal population. New data

Glossary

culture: the knowledge, belief, art, morals, laws, customs, and any other capabilities and habits acquired by humans as members of society

culturally competent nursing care: effective, individualized care that demonstrates respect for the dignity, personal rights, preferences, beliefs, and practices of the person receiving care, while acknowledging the biases of the caregiver and preventing these biases from interfering with the care provided

culturally safe nursing care: goes beyond cultural competence in that it brings nurses to also recognize systemic discrimination that has, or has had, a negative impact on a particular group. Cultural competence includes recognizing the power imbalance between a health professional and a nurse. In Canada, the Aboriginal Nurses Association of Canada has been a champion of cultural safety

cultural nursing assessment: a systematic appraisal or examination of individuals, families, groups, and communities in terms of their cultural beliefs, values, and practices

ethnocentrism: making a value judgment on another culture from the vantage point of one's own culture

minority: group of people whose physical or cultural characteristics differ from the majority of people in a society

subculture: relatively large groups of people who share characteristics that identify them as a distinct entity

transcultural nursing: nursing care to patients and families across cultural variations from the National Household Survey (NHS) show that 1,400,685 people had an Aboriginal identity in 2011, representing 4.3% of the total Canadian population. Aboriginal people accounted for 3.8% of the population enumerated in the 2006 Census, 3.3% in the 2001 Census, and 2.8% in the 1996 Census (Statistics Canada, 2017). Through immigration, Canada has welcomed people of other origins who have also contributed to making this country one of the most culturally and ethnically diverse nations in the world. According to Statistics Canada, more than 17 million people from all over the world have made Canada their home since Confederation in 1867. In 2011, 20.6% of Canadians were foreign born which is the largest proportion among the G8 countries:

- 6,264,800—The number of people who identified themselves as a member of a visible **minority** group in 2011. Combined, the three largest visible minority groups—South Asians, Chinese, and Blacks—accounted for 61.3% of the visible minority population in 2011. They were followed by Filipinos, Latin Americans, Arabs, Southeast Asians, West Asians, Koreans, and Japanese.
- Over 200—The number of ethnic origins reported in 2011 (Statistics Canada, 2017).

Although culture is a universal phenomenon, it takes on specific and distinctive features for a particular group because it encompasses all of the knowledge, beliefs, customs, and skills acquired by the members of that group. When such groups function within a larger cultural group, they are referred to as subcultures.

The term subculture is used for relatively large groups of people who share characteristics that identify them as a distinct entity (McFarland & Wehbe-Alamah, 2015). Examples of Canadian subcultures based on ethnicity (i.e., subcultures with common traits such as physical characteristics, language, or ancestry) include First Nations, French Canadians, and Eastern European Canadians. Each of these subcultures can be further divided. For example, First Nations include diverse groups such as Mohawk, Cree, and Blackfoot, to name a few.

Subcultures may also be based on religion (e.g., Anglican, Greek Orthodox, Judaism), occupation (e.g., registered nurses, physicians, other members of the health care team), disability (e.g., the deaf community), or illness. In addition, subcultures may be based on age (e.g., infants, children, adolescents, adults, older adults), gender (e.g., male, female), sexual orientation (e.g., homosexual, bisexual, heterosexual), or geographic location (e.g., Newfoundlanders, Québécois, Westerners).

Nurses should also be sensitive to cultural tensions that may arise.

Differences between individuals in subcultures in a designated group add to the challenge to plan and provide culturally competent care. Cultural competence begins with cultural awareness and understanding how it influences thinking about those from other cultures. Such examination facilitates comparison of the nurse's own culture with others, so that the nurse can ultimately become sensitive to and accepting of those with different cultural backgrounds (Rew, Becker, Chontichachalalauk, et al., 2014). Nurses must refrain from culturally stereotyping patients. Instead, nurses should consult patients or significant others regarding personal values, beliefs, preferences, and cultural identification. This strategy is also applicable for members of nonethnic subcultures.

Minorities

The term minority refers to a group of people whose physical or cultural characteristics differ from the majority of people in a society. At times, minorities may be singled out or isolated from others in society or treated in different or unequal ways. The concept of "minority" varies widely and must be understood within a specific context. For example, men may be considered a minority within the nursing profession, but they constitute a majority within the field of engineering. Similarly, while Francophones are the minority in Canada, they are the majority in Québec. Who constitutes a minority or a majority may also change over time; therefore, the minority of today could be the majority of tomorrow. Finally, because the term *minority* may connote inferiority, attention needs to be paid to ensure that it is used appropriately and in the right context.

Health Disparities

Health disparities—higher rates of morbidity, mortality, and burden of disease in a population or community than found in the overall population—are significant in ethnic, aboriginal, and racial minorities. Ethnic, aboriginal, and racial minorities are disproportionately burdened with cancer, heart disease, diabetes, human immunodeficiency virus infection/acquired immunodeficiency syndrome, and other conditions. They receive a lower quality of health care than nonminorities and are at greater risk for declining health. Health disparities also occur with women, gay, lesbian, and transgender people, as well as with people who have disabilities. Many reasons are cited for these disparities, including low socioeconomic status, health behaviours, limited access to health care because of poverty or disability, systemic environmental factors, and direct and indirect manifestations of discrimination.

Transcultural Nursing

Transcultural nursing, a term sometimes used interchangeably with cross-cultural, intercultural, or multicultural nursing, refers to research-focused practice that focuses on patient-centred, culturally competent nursing (Giger, 2013). Transcultural nursing incorporates the care (caring) values, beliefs, and practices of people and groups from a particular culture without imposing the nurse's cultural perspective on the patient. The underlying focus of transcultural nursing is to provide culture-specific and culture-universal care that promotes the well-being or health of individuals, families, groups, communities, and institutions (Giger, 2013; Leininger, 2002). All people as well as the community or institution at large benefit when culturally competent care is provided. When the care is delivered beyond a nurse's national boundaries, the term *international* or *transnational nursing* is often used.

Although many nurses, anthropologists, and others have written about the cultural aspects of nursing and health care, Leininger (2002) developed a comprehensive research-based theory called Culture Care Diversity and

Universality to promote culturally congruent nursing for people of different or similar cultures. This means promoting recovery from illness, preventing conditions that would limit the patient's health or well-being, or facilitating a peaceful death in ways that are culturally meaningful and appropriate. Nursing care needs to be tailored to fit the patient's cultural values, beliefs, and lifestyles.

Leininger's theory stresses the importance of providing culturally congruent nursing care (meaningful and beneficial health care tailored to fit the patient's cultural values) through culture care accommodation and culture care restructuring. *Culture care accommodation* refers to professional actions and decisions that nurses make on behalf of those in their care to help people of a designated culture achieve a beneficial or satisfying health outcome. *Culture care restructuring* or repatterning refers to professional actions and decisions that help patients reorder, change, or modify their lifestyles toward new, different, or more beneficial health care patterns. At the same time, the patient's cultural values and beliefs are respected, and a better or healthier lifestyle results. Other terms and definitions that provide further insight into culture and health care include the following:

- *Acculturation:* the process by which members of a cultural group adapt to or take on the behaviours of another group
- *Cultural blindness:* the inability of people to recognize their own values, beliefs, and practices and those of others because of strong ethnocentric tendencies (the tendency to view one's own culture as superior to others)
- *Cultural imposition:* the tendency to impose one's cultural beliefs, values, and patterns of behaviour on a person or people from a different culture
- *Cultural taboos:* activities or behaviours that are avoided, forbidden, or prohibited by a particular cultural group

Culturally Competent and Culturally Safe Nursing Care

"Cultural competence is defined as the gradually developed capacity of nurses to provide safe and quality healthcare to clients with different cultural backgrounds" (Cai, 2016). According to the Canadian Nurses Association (CNA) "[c]ultural competence includes valuing diversity, knowing about cultural mores and traditions of the populations being served and being sensitive to these... while caring for the individual."

For the CNA (2010), the responsibility for the provision of culturally competent care is shared between nurses, professional and regulatory nursing organizations, accreditation organizations, educational institutions, health service delivery organizations, and governments.

Agency policies are important to achieve culturally competent and culturally safe care. Policies that promote culturally competent care establish flexible regulations pertaining to visitors (number, frequency, and length of visits), provide translation services for non–English or non–French-speaking patients, and prepare staff to provide care for patients with different cultural values (The Joint Commission, 2014). Culturally competent and culturally safe policies are developed to promote an environment in which the traditional healing, spiritual, and religious practices of patients are respected and encouraged, and where systemic discrimination is also acknowledged and where efforts are made to address the impact of that discrimination on the health of people, and improve practice. Relational ethics can be useful in helping nurses to move from cultural competence to cultural safety.

Giger and Davidhizar (Giger, 2013) created an assessment model to guide nurses in exploring cultural phenomena that might affect nursing care. They identified communication, space, time orientation, social organization, environmental control, and biologic variations as relevant phenomena. This model has been used in various patient care settings to provide data essential to the provision of culturally competent care.

Cross-Cultural Communication

Establishment of an environment of cultural safety and respect begins with effective communication, which occurs not only through words, but also through body language and other cues, such as voice, tone, and loudness. Nurse–patient interactions, as well as communication among members of a multicultural health care team, are dependent on the ability to understand and be understood. Communication barriers frequently exist between nurses and patients, especially when they are from different cultural backgrounds (Giger, 2013).

Besides the two official languages (English and French), there are approximately 150 different languages spoken in Canada. Obviously, nurses cannot become fluent in all languages, but certain strategies for fostering effective cross-cultural communication are necessary when providing care for patients who are not fluent in English or French. Cultural needs should be considered when choosing an interpreter. The interpreter's voice quality, pronunciation, use of silence, use of touch, and use of nonverbal communication should also be considered (Giger, 2013). Ideally, the interpreter should not be a member of the patient's family because it may violate privacy or interfere with the communication of the patient's wishes as opposed to the wishes of the family member. During illness, patients of all ages may regress, and the regression often involves language skills. Chart 8-1 summarizes suggested strategies for overcoming language barriers. Nurses should also assess how well patients and families have understood what has been said. The following cues may signify a lack of effective communication:

- *Efforts to change the subject:* This could indicate that the listener does not understand what was said and is attempting to talk about something more familiar.
- *Absence of questions:* Paradoxically, this often means that the listener is not grasping the message and therefore has difficulty formulating questions to ask.
- *Inappropriate laughter:* A self-conscious giggle may signal poor comprehension and may be an attempt to disguise embarrassment.
- *Nonverbal cues:* A blank expression may signal poor understanding. However, among some Asian Canadians, it may reflect a desire to avoid overt expression of emotion. Avoidance of eye contact may be a cultural expression of respect for the speaker in some Aboriginal and Asian cultures.

CHART 8-1

Overcoming Language Barriers

- Greet the patient using the last or complete name. Avoid being too casual or familiar. Point to yourself and say your name. Smile.
- Proceed in an unhurried manner. Pay attention to any effort by the patient or the family to communicate.
- Speak in a low, moderate voice. Avoid talking loudly. Remember that there is a tendency to raise the volume and pitch of your voice when the listener appears not to understand. The listener may perceive that you are shouting or angry.
- Organize your thoughts. Repeat and summarize frequently. Use audiovisual aids when feasible.
- Use short, simple sentence structure, and speak in the active voice.
- Use simple words, such as "pain" rather than "discomfort." Avoid medical jargon, idioms, and slang. Avoid using contractions, such as don't, can't, won't.
- Use nouns repeatedly instead of pronouns. *Example:* Do not say: "He has been taking his medicine, hasn't he?" Do say: "Does Juan take his medicine?"
- Pantomime words (use gestures) and simple actions while verbalizing them.
- Give instructions in the proper sequence. *Example:* Do not say: "Before you rinse the bottle, sterilize it." Do say: "First, wash the bottle. Second, rinse the bottle."
- Discuss one topic at a time and avoid giving too much information in a single conversation. Avoid using conjunctions. *Example:* Do not say: "Are you cold and in pain?" Do say (while pantomiming/gesturing): "Are you cold?" "Are you in pain?"
- Talk directly to the patient rather than to the person who accompanied him or her.
- Validate whether the person understands by having him or her repeat instructions, demonstrate the procedure, or act out the meaning.
- Use any words that you know in the person's language. This indicates that you are aware of and respect the patient's primary means of communicating.
- Be aware of culturally based gender and age differences and diverse socioeconomic, educational, and tribal or regional differences when choosing an interpreter.
- Contact hospitals for a list of language interpreters such as trained bilingual staff or interpreting services via person, telephone, or video. The use of untrained individuals and minors should be avoided.

Adapted from Jarvis, C. (2016). *Physical examination & health assessment* (7th ed.). St. Louis, MO: Elsevier Saunders.

Culturally Mediated Characteristics

Nurses should be aware that patients act and behave in a variety of ways, in part because of the influence of culture on behaviours and attitudes. However, although certain attributes and attitudes are frequently associated with particular cultural groups, as described in the rest of this chapter, it is important to remember that not all people from the same cultural background share the same behaviours and views. Although nurses who fail to consider patients' cultural preferences and beliefs are considered insensitive and possibly indifferent, nurses who assume that all members of any one culture act and behave in the same way run the risk of stereotyping people. As previously stated, the best way to avoid stereotyping is to view each patient as an individual and to assess the patient's cultural preferences. A thorough culture assessment using a culture assessment tool or questionnaire (see later discussion) is very beneficial.

Many aspects of care may be influenced by the diverse cultural perspectives held by health care providers, patients, families, or significant others. One example is the issue of informed consent and full disclosure. In general, nurses may argue that patients have the right to full disclosure concerning their disease and prognosis and may believe that advocacy means working to provide that disclosure. However, family members in some cultural backgrounds may believe it is their responsibility to protect and spare the patient (their loved one) knowledge about a terminal illness. Similarly, patients may in fact not want to know about their condition and may expect their family members to "take the burden" of that knowledge and related decision making. Nurses should not decide that a family or patient is simply wrong or that a patient must know all of the details of his or her illness regardless of the patient's preference. Similar concerns may be noted when patients refuse pain medication or treatment because of cultural beliefs regarding pain or beliefs in divine intervention or faith healing.

Determining the most appropriate and ethical approach to patient care requires an exploration of the cultural aspects of these situations. Self-examination and recognition of one's own cultural bias and worldview, as discussed earlier, play a major part in helping the nurse resolve cultural and ethical conflicts. Nurses must promote open dialogue and work with patients, families, physicians, and other health care providers to reach the culturally appropriate solution for the individual patient.

Space and Distance

People tend to regard the space in their immediate vicinity as an extension of themselves. The amount of space they need between themselves and others to feel comfortable is a culturally determined phenomenon.

Because nurses and patients usually are not consciously aware of their personal space requirements, they frequently have difficulty understanding different behaviours in this regard. For example, one patient may perceive the nurse sitting close to him or her as an expression of warmth and care; another patient may perceive the nurse's act as a threatening invasion of personal space.

If the patient appears to position himself or herself too close or too far away, the nurse should consider cultural preferences for space and distance. Ideally, the patient should be permitted to assume a position that is comfortable to him or her in terms of personal space and distance. The nurse should be aware that the wheelchair of a person with a disability is considered an extension of the person; therefore, the nurse should ask the person's permission before moving or touching the wheelchair. Because a significant amount of communication during nursing care requires close physical contact, the nurse should be aware that having personal space promotes self-identity by allowing opportunities for patient self-expression (Giger, 2013).

Eye Contact

Eye contact is also a culturally determined behaviour. Although most nurses have been taught to maintain eye contact when speaking with patients, some people from certain cultural backgrounds may interpret this behaviour differently. The nurse who is aware that eye contact may be culturally determined can better understand the patient's behaviour and provide an atmosphere in which the patient can feel comfortable.

Time

Attitudes about time vary widely among cultures and can be a barrier to effective communication between nurses and patients. Views about punctuality and the use of time are culturally determined, as is the concept of waiting. Symbols of time, such as watches, sunrises, and sunsets, represent methods for measuring the duration and passage of time (Giger, 2013).

For most health care providers, time and promptness are extremely important. For example, nurses frequently expect patients to arrive at an exact time for an appointment, although patients are often kept waiting by health care providers who are running late. Health care providers are likely to function according to an appointment system in which there are short intervals of perhaps only a few minutes. However, for patients from some cultures, time is a relative phenomenon, with little attention paid to the exact hour or minute. Time may also be determined according to traditional times for meals, sleep, and other activities or events. For people from some cultures, the present is of the greatest importance, and time is viewed in broad ranges rather than in terms of a fixed hour. Being flexible in regard to schedules is the best way to accommodate these differences.

Value differences also may influence a person's sense of priority when it comes to time. For example, responding to a family matter may be more important to a patient than meeting a scheduled health care appointment. Allowing for these different views is essential in maintaining an effective nurse–patient relationship. Scolding or acting annoyed at patients for being late undermines their confidence and may result in further missed appointments or indifference to health care suggestions.

Touch

The meaning people associate with touching is culturally determined to a great degree. In some cultures, male health care providers may be prohibited from touching or examining certain parts of the female body. Similarly, it may be inappropriate for females to care for males. Sometimes it is impolite to touch a person's head if the person believes the spirit is residing there. Therefore, assessment of the head or evaluation of a head injury requires permission of the patient or a family member, if the patient is not able to give permission.

Observance of Holidays

People from all cultures observe certain civil and religious holidays. Nurses should familiarize themselves with major observances for members of the cultural groups they serve. Information about these observances is available from various sources, including religious organizations, hospital chaplains, and patients themselves. Routine health appointments, diagnostic tests, surgery, and other major procedures should be scheduled to avoid observances patients identify as significant. If not contraindicated, efforts should also be made to accommodate patients and families or significant others who wish to perform cultural and religious rituals in the health care setting.

Diet

The cultural meanings associated with food vary widely but usually include one or more of the following: relief of hunger; promotion of health and healing; prevention of disease or illness; expression of caring for another; promotion of interpersonal closeness among individual people, families, groups, communities, or nations; and promotion of kinship and family alliances. Food may also be associated with strengthening of social ties; celebration of life events (e.g., birthdays, marriages, funerals); expression of gratitude or appreciation; recognition of achievement or accomplishment; validation of social, cultural, or religious ceremonial functions; facilitation of business negotiations; and expression of affluence, wealth, or social status.

Culture determines which foods are served and when they are served, the number and frequency of meals, who eats with whom, and who receives the choicest portions. Culture also determines how foods are prepared and served, how they are eaten (with chopsticks, hands, or fork, knife, and spoon), and where people shop (e.g., ethnic grocery stores, specialty food markets). Culture also determines the impact of excess weight and obesity on self-esteem and social standing. In some cultures, physical bulk is viewed as a sign of affluence and health (e.g., a healthy baby is a chubby baby).

Religious practices may include fasting (e.g., Mormons, Roman Catholics, Buddhists, Jews, Muslims) and abstaining from selected foods at particular times (e.g., Roman Catholics abstain from meat on Ash Wednesday and on Fridays during Lent). Practices may also include the ritualistic use of food and beverages (e.g., Passover dinner, consumption of bread and wine during religious ceremonies). Chart 8-2 summarizes some dietary practices of selected religious groups.

Many groups tend to feast, often in the company of family and friends, on selected holidays. These culturally based dietary practices are especially significant in the care of patients with diabetes, hypertension, gastrointestinal disorders, obesity, and other conditions in which diet plays a key role in the treatment and health maintenance regimen.

Biologic Variations

Along with psychosocial adaptations, nurses must also consider the physiologic impact of culture on patients' response to treatment, particularly medications. Data have been collected for many years regarding differences in the effect some medications have on people of diverse ethnic or cultural origins. Genetic predispositions to different

CHART 8-2

Prohibited Foods and Beverages of Selected Religious Groups

Hinduism

All meats
Animal shortenings

Islam

Pork
Alcoholic products and beverages (including extracts, such as vanilla and lemon)
Animal shortenings
Gelatin made with pork, marshmallow, and other confections made with gelatin
Note: Halal food is lawful food that may be consumed according to tenets of the Koran whereas *Haram* is food that is unlawful to consume.

Judaism

Pork
Predatory fowl
Shellfish and scavenger fish (e.g., shrimp, crab, lobster, escargot, catfish). Fish with fins and scales is permissible
Mixing milk and meat dishes at same meal
Blood by ingestion (e.g., blood sausage, raw meat)
Note: Packaged foods will contain labels identifying kosher ("properly preserved" or "fitting") and pareve (made without meat or milk) items.

Mormonism (Church of Jesus Christ of Latter-Day Saints)

Alcohol
Beverages containing caffeine stimulants (coffee, tea, colas, and selected carbonated soft drinks)

Seventh-Day Adventism

Alcohol
Beverages containing caffeine stimulants (coffee, tea, colas, and selected carbonated soft drinks)
Pork
Certain seafood, including shellfish
Fermented beverages
Note: Optional vegetarianism is encouraged.

rates of metabolism cause some patients to be prone to adverse reactions to the standard dose of a medication, whereas other patients are likely to experience a greatly reduced benefit from the standard dose of the medication. General polymorphism—biologic variation in response to medications resulting from patient age, gender, size, and body composition—has long been acknowledged by the health care community. Nurses must be aware that ethnicity and related factors such as values and beliefs regarding the use of herbal supplements, dietary intake, and genetic factors can affect the effectiveness of treatment and compliance with the treatment regimen (Giger, 2013).

Complementary and Alternative Therapies

Complementary therapies, also referred to as alternative therapies when they replace Western medicine, can be defined as any therapies that are outside of conventional Western medicine. The Fraser Institute Canada (2017) reported that more than three quarters of Canadians (79%) had used at least one complementary or alternative therapy sometime in their lives in 2016. This compares to 74% in 2006 and 73% in 1997. Complementary and alternative interventions are classified into two main categories: natural products or mind and body practices (National Institutes of Health [NIH], National Center for Complementary and Integrative Health [NCCIH], 2015).

- *Natural products* include herbs (also known as botanicals), vitamins and minerals, and probiotics. These are widely marketed to consumers and often sold and used as dietary supplements.
- *Mind and body practices* include large and diverse procedures and techniques given or taught by trained practitioners or teachers and include practices such as yoga, meditation, chiropractic and osteopathic manipulation, massage therapy, acupuncture, relaxation techniques, and tai chi.

Patients may choose to seek a complementary or alternative approach to conventional medical or surgical therapies. Nurses should work with patients to develop effective, personalized health strategies that might include the use of natural products and mind and body practices to promote individual health and well-being. Nurses must assess all patients for the use of complementary therapies, be alert to the danger of natural product–drug interactions or conflicting treatments, and be prepared to provide information to patients about treatments that may be harmful or helpful, based upon best evidence from research findings. However, nurses must be accepting of patients' beliefs and right to autonomy—that is, to control their own care. As patient advocates, nurses facilitate the integration of conventional medical, complementary, and alternative therapies.

Causes of Illness

People may view illness differently. Three major views, or paradigms, attempt to explain the causes of disease and illness: the biomedical or scientific view, the naturalistic or holistic perspective, and the magico-religious view.

Biomedical or Scientific View

The biomedical or scientific worldview prevails in most health care settings and is embraced by most nurses and other health care providers. The basic assumptions underlying the biomedical perspective are that all events in life have a cause and effect, that the human body functions much like a machine, and that all of reality can be observed and measured (e.g., blood pressures, partial pressure of arterial oxygen [PaO_2] levels, intelligence tests). One example of the biomedical or scientific view is the bacterial or viral explanation of communicable diseases.

Naturalistic or Holistic

The naturalistic or holistic perspective is another viewpoint that explains the cause of illness. According to this view, the forces of nature must be kept in natural balance or harmony.

One example of a naturalistic belief is the yin/yang theory, in which health is believed to exist when all aspects of a person are in perfect balance or harmony. Rooted in the ancient Chinese philosophy of Taoism (which translates as "The Way"), the yin/yang theory proposes that all organisms and objects in the universe consist of yin and yang energy. The seat of the energy forces is within the autonomic nervous system, where balance between the opposing forces is maintained during health. Yin energy represents the female and negative forces, such as emptiness, darkness, and cold, whereas the yang forces are male and positive, emitting warmth and fullness. Foods are classified as cold (yin) or hot (yang) in this theory and are transformed into yin and yang energy when metabolized by the body. Cold foods are eaten when a person has a hot illness (e.g., fever, rash, sore throat, ulcer, infection), and hot foods are eaten when a person has a cold illness (e.g., cancer, headache, stomach cramps, "cold"). The yin/yang theory is the basis for Eastern or Chinese medicine and is embraced by some Asian Canadians.

Some Hispanic and Arab groups also embrace the hot/cold theory of health and illness. The four humours of the body—blood, phlegm, black bile, and yellow bile—regulate basic bodily functions and are described in terms of temperature and moisture. The treatment of disease consists of adding or subtracting cold, heat, dryness, or wetness to restore the balance of these humours. Beverages, foods, herbs, medicines, and diseases are classified as hot or cold according to their perceived effects on the body, not their physical characteristics. According to the hot/cold theory, the person as a whole, not just a particular ailment, is significant. People who embrace the hot/cold theory maintain that health consists of a positive state of total well-being, including physical, psychological, spiritual, and social aspects of the person.

According to the naturalistic worldview, breaking the laws of nature creates imbalances, chaos, and disease. People who embrace the naturalistic paradigm use metaphors such as "the healing power of nature" and view illness as an intruding agent but as a part of life's rhythmic course and an outward sign of disharmony within.

Magico-Religious

The third major way in which people view the world and explain the causes of illness is the magico-religious worldview. This view's basic premise is that the world is an arena in which supernatural forces dominate, and that the fate of the world and those in it depends on the action of supernatural forces for good or evil. People who adhere to this view believe in voodoo or witchcraft. Faith healing is based on religious beliefs, whereas various healing rituals may be found in many religions.

Of course, it is possible to hold a combination of worldviews, and many patients offer more than one explanation for the cause of their illness. As a profession, nursing largely embraces the scientific or biomedical worldview, but some aspects of holism have begun to gain popularity, including a wide variety of techniques for managing chronic pain, such as hypnosis, therapeutic touch, and biofeedback. Belief in spiritual power is also held by many nurses who credit supernatural forces with various unexplained phenomena related to patients' health and illness states. Regardless of the view held and whether the nurse agrees with the patient's beliefs in this regard, it is important to be aware of how the person views illness and health and to work within this framework to promote patient care and well-being.

Folk Healers

People of some cultures believe in folk or indigenous healers. For example, nurses may find that some Hispanic Canadian patients may seek help from a *curandero* or *curandera, espiritualista* (spiritualist), *yerbo* (herbalist), or *sabador* (healer who manipulates bones and muscles). Some Haitian Canadian patients may seek assistance from voodoo priest. Aboriginal Canadian patients may seek assistance from a shaman or medicine man or woman. Asian Canadian patients may mention that they have visited herbalists, acupuncturists, or bone setters. Several cultures have their own healers, most of whom speak the native tongue of that culture, make house calls, and charge significantly less than healers practicing in the conventional medical health care system.

People seeking complementary and alternative therapies have expanded the practices of folk healers beyond their traditional populations, so the nurse should ask the patient about use of folk healers regardless of the patient's cultural background. It is best not to disregard the patient's belief in folk healers or try to undermine trust in the healers. To do so may alienate the patient and drive him or her away from receiving the prescribed care. Nurses should make an effort to accommodate the patient's beliefs while also advocating the treatment proposed by health science (Chart 8-3).

Cultural Nursing Assessment

Cultural nursing assessment refers to a systematic appraisal or examination of individuals, families, groups, and communities in terms of their cultural beliefs, values, and practices. The purpose of such an assessment is to provide culturally competent care (Giger, 2013). In an effort to establish a database for determining a patient's cultural background, nurses have developed cultural assessment tools, scales, and questionnaires to measure cultural needs of patients (Shen, 2015), and to ensure that transcultural considerations are included in the plan of care. Giger and Davidhizar's model has been used to design nursing care from health promotion to nursing skills activities (Giger, 2013). The information presented in this chapter and the general guidelines presented in Chart 8-4 can be used to direct nursing assessment of culture and its influence on a patient's health beliefs and practices. Yet, despite the availability of tools designed to facilitate performing cultural assessments, recent research findings suggest that many nurses feel unprepared to perform cultural assessments and provide culturally competent care for ethnic minority patients (Chart 8-5) (Alpers & Hanssen, 2014).

Additional Cultural Considerations: Know Thyself

Because the nurse–patient interaction is the focal point of nursing, nurses should consider their own cultural

CHART 8-3

Ethical Dilemma: When May Folk Remedies Be Considered Harmful or Complementary?

Case Scenario

You are working in an urban neighbourhood health clinic. A 78-year-old woman who is a Chinese immigrant presents with a 5-day history of chills, low-grade fever, pallor, dry, nonproductive cough, and fatigue. The woman's adult daughter has brought her to the clinic, and they both insist on the daughter being present during assessment. When you begin to listen to the woman's lung sounds, you incidentally note that she has round, bruised areas in regions of her back in a symmetric pattern. A few of the marks appear to be infected at the sites where small amounts of blood were suctioned. You ask her how this happened, and her daughter interjects, "That is from cupping, but it didn't seem to work right this time, because she is still very sick. That is the reason we are here now." You have heard that in Chinese communities, wet cupping is practiced as a folk remedy and that the intent of this treatment is to remove inflammation.

Discussion

There are many folk remedies that immigrants to the United States may continue to use to treat various ailments. Some of these may be complementary to traditional Western medicine, whereas others may be considered harmful therapies in that they may result in delays to seek traditional routes to treatment or may otherwise result in harm to the patient. It is important to determine if this procedure is complementary and if the patient regularly sees a licensed primary provider to provide her with comprehensive health care. The way of thinking about culture is evolving from an essentialist, ethnocentric perspective to a more open, and inclusive way of understanding the people we care for (Vandenberg, 2010). Therefore nurses must be cognizant when their own ethnocentrism is present during interactions with patients of a different culture—that is, a belief that the nurse's culturally accepted way of practicing health care is inherently superior to another culturally acceptable health care practice.

Analysis

Describe the ethical principles that are in conflict in this case (see Chart 3-3). Which principle should have pre-eminence as you proceed with your assessment of this patient?

Describe any concerns that you may have regarding preservation of the patient's autonomy. What steps might you take to assure that her autonomy is preserved?

Cupping is a relatively common folk remedy among many people from southeastern Asian cultures. How can you determine whether the marks you find on this patient signify that she may be a victim of elder abuse rather than a willing recipient of a folk remedy? How do you ensure that the patient is not harmed (i.e., ensure nonmaleficence)? How do you ascertain if she is receiving health care to treat any existing health problems?

Assume that you find that the patient has full capacity to make competent decisions and that she does indeed value the traditional practice of cupping. How do you professionally reconcile that she has sought to treat her illness with a folk remedy before seeking traditional care? Does her right to make an autonomous decision over her health care trump your desire that she seek traditional health care sooner (or, in this case, does the principle of autonomy outweigh the dual principles of beneficence and nonmaleficence)?

Ludwick, R., & Silva, M. C. (2000). Ethics: Nursing around the world: Cultural values and ethical conflicts. *Online Journal of Issues in Nursing, 5*(3). Retrieved August 27, 2016, from www.nursingworld.org/MainMenuCategories/ANAMarketplace/ANAPeriodicals/OJIN/Columns/Ethics/CulturalValuesandEthicalConflicts.aspx

orientation when conducting assessments of patients and their families and friends. The following guidelines may prove useful to nurses who want to provide culturally appropriate care:

- Know your own cultural attitudes, values, beliefs, and practices.
- Regardless of "good intentions," recognize that everyone has cultural "baggage" that ultimately results in **ethnocentrism**.
- In general, it is easier to understand those whose cultural heritage is similar to your own, while viewing those who are unlike you as strange and different.
- Maintain a broad, open attitude. Expect the unexpected. Enjoy surprises.
- Avoid seeing all people as alike; that is, avoid cultural stereotypes, such as "all Chinese like rice" or "all Italians eat spaghetti."
- Try to understand the reasons for any behaviour by discussing commonalities and differences with representative of ethnic groups different from your own.
- If a patient has said or done something that you do not understand, ask for clarification. Be a good listener. Most patients will respond positively to questions that arise from a genuine concern for and interest in them.
- If at all possible, speak the patient's language (even simple greetings and social courtesies are appreciated). Avoid feigning an accent or using words that are ordinarily not part of your vocabulary.
- Be yourself. There are no right or wrong ways to learn about cultural diversity.

The Future of Transcultural Nursing Care

Until the late 1970s, the majority of Canadian immigrants were of European origin. Since the 1980s, Asian and Middle Eastern immigration has been greater than European immigration. This had led to an increasing proportion of visible minorities. Therefore, institutions must develop culturally sensitive policies and provide a climate that fosters the provision of culturally competent care by nurses.

As the population becomes more culturally diverse, efforts need to be made to facilitate the recruitment and successful program completion of nursing students from varied origins. Nurses, who reflect the multicultural complexion of our society, must learn to acknowledge and adapt to diversity among their colleagues in the workplace. Nurses will be expected to provide culturally competent and culturally safe nursing care for patients. Nurses must work effectively with patients, one another, and other health care team members whose ancestry reflects the multicultural complexion of contemporary society.

CHART 8-4

Assessing for Patients' Cultural Beliefs

Communication

Do you like communicating with friends, family, and acquaintances?

- When asked a question, do you usually respond?
- If you have something important to discuss with your family, how would you approach them?

Space

- When you talk with family members, how close do you stand?
- When you talk with acquaintances, how close do you stand?
- If a stranger touches you, how do you react or feel?
- If a loved one touches you, how do you react or feel?
- Are you comfortable with the distance between us now?

Social Organization

- What are some activities that you enjoy?
- What are your hobbies, or what do you do when you have free time?
- Do you believe in a Supreme Being?
- How do you worship that Supreme Being?
- What is your role in your family/unit system?

Time

- What kind of timepiece do you wear daily?
- If a nurse tells you that you will receive a medication "in about a half hour," how much time will you allow before calling the nurse station?

Environmental Control

- Is it acceptable for you to have visitors drop in unexpectedly?
- Do you use home remedies? Which home remedies worked? Will you use them in the future?
- What is your definition of "good health"?
- What is your definition of illness or "poor health"?

Biologic Variations

- What diseases or illnesses are common in your family?
- Who usually helps you to cope during a difficult time?
- What foods do you and your family like to eat? What foods are family favourites or are considered traditional?

Nursing Process Utilization

- Note whether the patient has become culturally assimilated or observes own cultural practices.
- Incorporate data into the plan of nursing care.

Adapted from Giger, J. (2013). *Transcultural nursing: Assessment and intervention* (6th ed.). St. Louis, MO: Elsevier.

NURSING RESEARCH PROFILE

Chart 8-5. Self-Assessed Cultural Competency of Nurses

Alpers, L., & Hanssen, I. (2014). Caring for ethnic minority patients: A mixed-method study of nurses' self-assessment of cultural competency. *Nursing Education Today*, *34*(6), 999–1004.

Purpose

Research shows that nurses lack cultural competence, which may negatively affect treatment and care for ethnic minority patients. The purpose of this study was to investigate how medical unit (MU) nurses and psychiatric unit (PU) nurses assess their own cultural competency in caring for patients with minority backgrounds. The topics assessed included the following: intercultural knowledge, knowledge of medical traditions and differences in illness etiology, symptom assessment, and in-service education and availability of advice.

Design

This study used a mixed-methods study research design of nurses' self-assessment of cultural competency. Three focus group interviews were conducted with both MU and PU nurse participants to develop a Likert scale survey to learn about the participants' experiences working with ethnic minority patients. Survey items were designed to operationalize cultural competency, with an emphasis on gauging nurse participants' experience and knowledge. SPSS was used to analyze the quantitative data; hermeneutic thematic analysis was used for the qualitative data.

Findings

A total of 145 MU nurse participants and 100 PU nurse participants completed the survey. Participants lacked knowledge about a wide range of subjects, such as how to communicate well through an interpreter, how to handle nursing care with family and small children present, and how to appropriately care for a female patient who has been circumcised. They also expressed a lack of knowledge about various cultural expressions that may be important to hospitalized ethnic minority patients. Survey responses highlighted that 20% of the MU nurse participants and 28% of the PU nurse participants indicated that they had adequate intercultural knowledge, while 44% of both groups of nurse participants indicated that they had inadequate knowledge to give ethnic minority patients good treatment and care. There was no effect of years of practice experience on participants' self-rated intercultural knowledge.

Nursing Implications

Study findings suggest that experience alone is not adequate to develop cultural competency. Years of practice experience does not equip nurses with adequate knowledge to perform intercultural symptom assessment and render culturally competent treatment and care. Formal education, in-service classes, feedback, and access to relevant information are needed in order to facilitate the delivery of culturally competent nursing care.

Critical Thinking Exercises

1 You are assigned to care for a hospitalized patient whose cultural background is Hispanic. You know little about this culture. What is the evidence base for use of a cultural assessment tool to ensure that cultural considerations are included in the nursing plan of care? What is the strength of that evidence? What resources are available to you to promote culturally competent care? Explain why it is important to examine your own feelings about each patient's cultural beliefs and practices.

2 An 84-year-old man who is originally from Vietnam is hospitalized in the neurosurgical intensive care unit with a cerebrovascular accident (CVA, stroke). His immediate family members insist on staying with him around the clock, and many extended family members visit each day, staying late into the night. His prognosis is poor, and when his attending physician discusses discontinuing his life support therapy with his family members who are his legal next of kin, they acquiesce but request that all family members be allowed to remain present to witness his death. Policies in the intensive care unit do not permit more than three family members to be with a patient at any given time. The staff members complain that they have difficulty completing their tasks with other critically ill patients because of the distractions they face from the multiple family members visiting this man. How can you help the nursing staff explore the meaning of the family's behaviour and understand their own negative feelings about this behaviour? Devise a strategy that will help resolve this situation.

3 As a diabetes educator, you are consulted about providing initial teaching services for a young Arab woman who is admitted to the hospital with a new diagnosis of diabetes. Her husband insists that he must be present for any teaching you perform. During your initial meeting with the patient and her husband, you note that the patient does not make eye contact and defers all questions you pose to her husband. You wish to initiate her diabetes teaching and begin a teaching plan for her. What aspects of the patient's and family's background would you want to further assess to determine the need for continuing assessment and care? Identify culturally sensitive methods you might use to ensure that the patient receives the diabetes teaching she requires. What resources might you use to assist you in providing the teaching?

REFERENCES AND SELECTED READINGS

Books

Giger, J. N. (2013). *Transcultural nursing: Assessment and intervention* (6th ed.). St. Louis, MO: Elsevier.

Jarvis, C. (2016). *Physical examination & health assessment* (7th ed.). St. Louis, MO: Elsevier Saunders.

Leininger, M. M. (Ed.). (2001). *Culture care diversity and universality: A theory of nursing*. New York: National League for Nursing Press.

McFarland, M. R., & Wehbe-Alamah, H. B. (2015). *Leininger's cultural care diversity and universality: A worldwide nursing theory* (3rd ed.). Burlington, MA: Jones & Bartlett.

Journals and Electronic Documents

Alpers, L. M., & Hanssen, I. (2014). Caring for ethnic minority patients: A mixed-method study of nurses' self-assessment of cultural competency. *Nurse Education Today*, *34*(6), 999–1004.

Cai, D. (2016). A concept analysis of cultural competence. *International Journal of Nursing Sciences*, *3*(3), 268–273.

Canadian Nurses Association. (2018). *Promoting cultural competence in nursing: Position statement*. Ottawa, ON: Author. Retrieved from https://www.cna-aiic.ca/-/media/cna/page-content/pdf-en/position_statement_promoting_cultural_competence_in_nursing.pdf?la=en&hash=4B394DAE5C2138E7F6134D59E505DCB059754BA9

CNA. (2010). *Promoting cultural competence in nursing*. Retrieved from: https://www.cna-aiic.ca/~/media/cna/page-content/pdf-en/ps114_cultural_competence_2010_e.pdf?la=en

The Fraser Institute. (2017). *Complementary and alternative medicine: Use and public attitudes 1997, 2006, and 2016*. Retrieved from https://www.fraserinstitute.org/studies/complementary-and-alternative-medicine-use-and-public-attitudes-1997-2006-and-2016

Government of Canada, Justice Laws Website. (2018). *Canadian Multiculturalism Act (R.S.C., 1985, c. 24 (4th Supp))*. Retrieved from https://laws-lois.justice.gc.ca/eng/acts/c-18.7/page-1.html?wbdisable=true

Health Canada. (2018). *Diseases that affect First Nations and Inuit communities*. Ottawa, ON: Author. Retrieved from https://www.canada.ca/en/indigenous-services-canada/services/first-nations-inuit-health/diseases-health-conditions.html

Holland, A. (2015). The lived experience of teaching about race in cultural nursing education. *Journal of Transcultural Nursing Education*, *26*(1), 92–100.

Isaacson, M. (2014). Clarifying concepts: Cultural humility or competency. *Journal of Professional Nursing*, *30*(3), 251–258.

The Joint Commission. (2014). *Crosswalk of joint commission hospital program and the national CLAS standards*. Retrieved October 6, 2015, from www.jointcommission.org/topics/health_equity.aspx

Leininger, M. (2002). Culture care theory: A major contribution to advance transcultural nursing knowledge and practices. *Journal of Transcultural Nursing*, *13*(3), 189–192.

Mareno, N., & Hart, P. (2014). Cultural competency among nurses with undergraduate and graduate degrees: Implications for nursing education. *Nursing Education Perspectives*, *35*(2), 83–88.

Marzilli, C. (2014). Concept analysis of culture applied to nursing. *Creative Nursing*, *20*(4), 227–233.

McClimens, A., Brewster, J., & Lewis, R. (2014). Recognising and respecting patients' cultural diversity. *Nursing Standard*, *28*(28), 45–52.

Mixer, S. J., McFarland, M. R., Andrews, M. M., et al. (2013). Exploring faculty health and wellbeing: Creating a caring scholarly community. *Nurse Education Today*, *33*(12), 1471–1476.

National Institutes of Health (NIH), National Center for Complementary and Integrative Health (NCCIH). (2015). *Complementary, alternative, or integrative health: What's in a name?* Retrieved October 10, 2015, from nccih.nih.gov/health/integrative-health

Rew, L., Becker, H., Chontichachalalauk, J., et al. (2014). Cultural diversity among nursing students: Reanalysis of the cultural awareness scale. *Journal of Nursing Education*, *53*(2), 71–76.

Shen, Z. (2015). Cultural competence models and cultural competence assessment instruments in nursing: A literature review. *Journal of Transcultural Nursing*, *26*(3), 308–321.

Statistics Canada. (2017). *2017 Canada Day…by the numbers*. Retrieved from https://www.statcan.gc.ca/eng/dai/smr08/2017/smr08_219_2017

Vandenberg, H. (2010). Culture theorizing past and present: trends and challenges. *Nursing philosophy*, *11*, 238–249.

Resources

Organizations

Council on Nursing and Anthropology: http://conaa.org/

Language Line Solutions (provides written and oral translation in 140 languages): http://www.languageline.com

National Black Nurses Association: https://www.nbna.org

National Center for Complementary and Integrative Health: https://nccih.nih.gov/

Office of Minority Health: http://www.omhrc.gov

Transcultural Nursing Society: https://tcns.org

9 Homeostasis, Stress, and Adaptation

Adapted by Joseph Osuji and Mohamed Toufic El Hussein

Learning Objectives

On completion of this chapter, the learner will be able to:

1. Relate the principles of internal constancy, homeostasis, stress, and adaptation to the concept of steady state.
2. Identify the significance of the body's compensatory mechanisms in promoting adaptation and maintaining the steady state.
3. Identify and compare physiologic and psychosocial stressors.
4. Compare the sympathetic–adrenal–medullary and hypothalamic–pituitary responses to stress.
5. Describe the general adaptation syndrome (GAS) as a theory of adaptation to biologic stress.
6. Describe the relationship of the process of negative feedback to the maintenance of the steady state.
7. Compare the adaptive processes of hypertrophy, atrophy, hyperplasia, dysplasia, and metaplasia.
8. Describe the inflammatory and reparative processes.
9. Assess the health patterns of a person and determine their effects on maintenance of the steady state.
10. Identify ways in which maladaptive responses to stress can increase the risk of illness and cause disease.
11. Identify individual and group measures that are useful in reducing stress.

When the body is threatened or suffers an injury, its response may involve functional and structural changes; these changes may be adaptive (having a positive effect) or maladaptive (having a negative effect). The defense mechanisms that the body uses determine the difference between **adaptation** and maladaptation—health and **disease**. This chapter discusses homeostasis, **stress**, adaptation, health problems associated with maladaptation, and the ways nurses can intervene to reduce stress and its health-related effects.

Fundamental Concepts

Each body system performs specific functions to sustain optimal life for an organism. Compensatory mechanisms for adjusting internal conditions promote the usual steady state of the organism and its survival. These mechanisms are compensatory in nature and work to restore balance in the body. An example of this restorative effort is the development of rapid breathing (hyperpnea) after intense exercise in an attempt to compensate for an oxygen deficit and excess lactic acid accumulated in the muscle tissue.

Pathophysiologic processes result when cellular injury occurs at such a rapid rate that the body's compensatory mechanisms can no longer make the adaptive changes necessary to remain healthy. An example of a pathophysiologic change is the development of heart failure; the body reacts by retaining sodium and water and increasing venous pressure, which worsens the condition. These pathophysiologic responses give rise to symptoms that are reported by patients or signs that are observed by patients, nurses, or other health care providers. These observations, plus a sound knowledge of physiologic and pathophysiologic processes, can assist in determining the existence of a problem and can guide nurses in planning the appropriate course of action.

Steady State

Physiologic mechanisms must be understood in the context of the body as a whole. Each person, as a living system, has both an internal and an external environment, between which information and matter are continuously exchanged. Within the internal environment, each organ, tissue, and cell is also a system or subsystem of the whole, each with its own internal and external environment, each exchanging information and matter (Fig. 9-1). The goal of the interaction of the body's subsystems is to produce a dynamic balance or steady state (even in the presence of change), so that all subsystems are in harmony with each other. Four concepts—constancy, homeostasis, stress, and adaptation—are key to the understanding of steady state.

Claude Bernard, a 19th-century French physiologist, developed the biologic principle that for life there must be a constancy or "fixity of the internal milieu" despite changes in the external environment. The internal milieu was the fluid that bathed the cells, and the constancy was the balanced internal state maintained by physiologic and biochemical processes. His principle of "constancy" implied a static process (homeostasis).

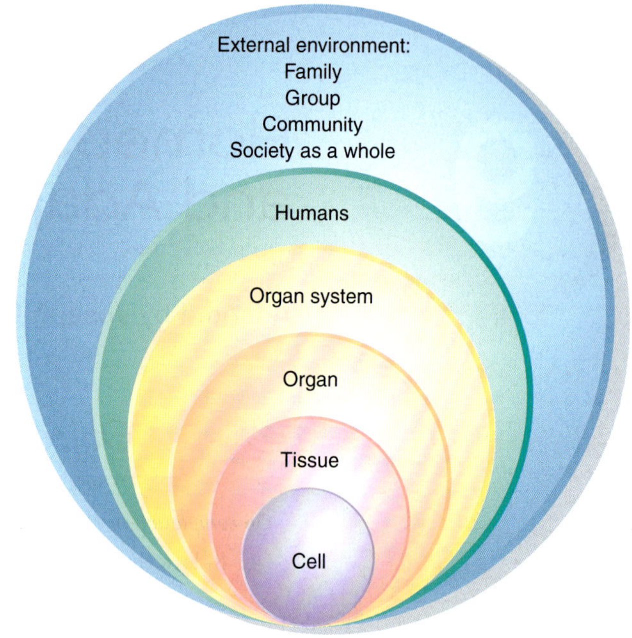

FIGURE 9-1. Constellation of systems. Each system is a subsystem of the larger system (suprasystem) of which it is a part. In this figure, the cells represent the smallest system and are a subsystem of all other systems.

Homeostasis refers to a **steady state** within the body. When a change or stress occurs that causes a body function to deviate from its stable range, processes are initiated to restore and maintain dynamic balance. When these adjustment processes or compensatory mechanisms are

Glossary

adaptation: a change or alteration designed to assist in adjusting to a new situation or environment

adrenocorticotropic hormone (ACTH): a hormone produced by the anterior lobe of the pituitary gland that stimulates the secretion of cortisol and other hormones by the adrenal cortex

antidiuretic hormone (ADH): a hormone secreted by the posterior lobe of the pituitary gland that constricts blood vessels, elevates blood pressure, and reduces the excretion of urine

catecholamines: any of the group of amines (such as epinephrine, norepinephrine, or dopamine) that serves as neurotransmitters

coping: the cognitive and behavioural strategies used to manage the stressors that tax a person's resources

disease: an abnormal variation in the structure or function of any part of the body

dysplasia: bizarre cell growth resulting in cells that differ in size, shape, or arrangement from other cells of the same tissue type

glucocorticoids: the group of steroid hormones, such as cortisol, that are produced by the adrenal cortex; they are involved in carbohydrate, protein, and fat metabolism and have anti-inflammatory properties

gluconeogenesis: the formation of glucose by the liver from noncarbohydrate sources, such as amino acids and the glycerol portion of fats

guided imagery: the mindful use of a word, phrase, or visual image to achieve relaxation or direct attention away from uncomfortable sensations or situations

homeostasis: a steady state within the body; the stability of the internal environment

hyperplasia: an increase in the number of new cells of a tissue

hypoxia: inadequate supply of oxygen to the cell

inflammation: a localized, protective reaction of tissue to injury, irritation, or infection, manifested by pain, redness, heat, swelling, and sometimes loss of function

metaplasia: a cell transformation in which there is conversion of one type of mature cell into another type of cell

negative feedback: feedback that decreases the output of a system

positive feedback: feedback that increases the output of a system

steady state: a stable condition that does not change over time, or when change in one direction is balanced by change in an opposite direction

stress: a disruptive condition that occurs in response to adverse influences from the internal or external environments

stressor: an internal or external event or situation that creates the potential for physiologic, emotional, cognitive, or behavioural changes not adequate, steady state is threatened, function becomes disordered, and dysfunctional responses occur. This can lead to disease, which is a threat to steady state. Disease is an unexpected variation in the structure or function of any part of the body. It disrupts function and therefore can limit freedom of action.

Stress and Adaptation

Stress is a state produced by a change in the environment that is perceived as challenging, threatening, or damaging to a person's dynamic balance or equilibrium. The person may feel unable to meet the demands of the new situation. The change or stimulus that evokes this state is the stressor. The nature of the stressor is variable; an event or change that is stressful for one person may not be stressful for another, and an event that produces stress at one time and place may not do so at another time and place. A person appraises and copes with changing situations. The desired goal is adaptation or adjustment to the change so that the person is again in equilibrium and has the energy and ability to meet new demands. This is the process of coping with stress, a compensatory process that has physiologic and psychological components.

Adaptation is a constant, ongoing process that requires a change in structure, function, or behaviour so that a person is better suited to the environment; it involves an interaction between the person and the environment. The outcome depends on the degree of "fit" between the skills and capacities of the person, the type of social support available, and the various challenges or stressors encountered. As such, adaptation is an individual process: Each person has varying abilities to cope or respond. As new challenges are met, this ability to cope and adapt can change, thereby providing the person with a wide range of adaptive ability. Adaptation occurs throughout the life span as the person encounters many developmental and situational challenges, especially related to health and illness. The goal of adaptation is optimal wellness.

Because both stress and adaptation may exist at different levels of a system, it is possible to study these reactions at the cellular, tissue, and organ levels. Biologists are concerned mainly with subcellular components or with subsystems of the total body. Behavioural scientists, including many nurse researchers, study stress and adaptation in individuals, families, groups, and societies; they focus on how a group's organizational features are modified to meet the requirements of the social and physical environment in which the group exists. In any system, the desired goals of adaptation are survival, growth, and reproduction.

Overview of Stress

Types of Stressors

Each person operates at a certain level of adaptation and regularly encounters a certain amount of change. Such change is expected; it contributes to growth and enhances life. A stressor can upset this equilibrium. A stressor may be defined as an internal or external event or situation that creates the potential for physiologic, emotional, cognitive, or behavioural changes in an individual.

Stressors exist in many forms and categories. They may be described as physical, physiologic, or psychosocial. Physical stressors include cold, heat, and chemical agents; physiologic stressors include pain and fatigue. An example of a psychosocial stressor is fear (e.g., fear of failing an examination, losing a job, and waiting for a diagnostic test result). Stressors can also occur as expected life transitions that require some adjustment, such as going from childhood into puberty, getting married, or giving birth.

Stressors have also been classified as (1) day-to-day frustrations or hassles; (2) major complex occurrences involving large groups; and (3) stressors that occur less frequently and involve fewer people. The first group, the day-to-day stressors, includes such common occurrences as getting caught in a traffic jam, experiencing computer downtime, and having an argument with a spouse or roommate. These experiences vary in effect. For example, encountering a rainstorm while you are vacationing at the beach will most likely evoke a more negative response than it might at another time. These daily hassles have been shown to have a greater health impact than major life events because of the cumulative effect they have over time. They can lead to high blood pressure, palpitations, or other physiologic changes (Schonfels, Brailovskaia, Bieda, et al., 2015).

The second group of stressors influences larger groups of people, sometimes even entire nations. These include events of history, such as terrorism and war, experienced either directly in the war zone or indirectly through live news coverage. The demographic, economic, and technologic changes occurring in society also serve as stressors. The tension produced by any stressor is sometimes a result not only of the change itself, but also of the speed with which the change occurs.

The third group of stressors has been studied most extensively and concerns relatively infrequent situations that directly affect people. This category includes the influence of life events such as death, birth, marriage, divorce, and retirement. It also includes the psychosocial crises that occur in the life cycle stages of the human experience. More enduring chronic stressors may include having a permanent disability or **coping** with the need to provide long-term care to a frail older parent.

Duration may also be used to categorize stressors, as in the following:

- An acute, time-limited stressor, such as studying for final examinations
- A stressor sequence—a series of stressful events that result from an initial event such as job loss or divorce
- A chronic intermittent stressor, such as daily hassles
- A chronic enduring stressor that persists over time, such as chronic illness, a disability, or poverty

Stress as a Stimulus for Disease

Relating life events to illness (the theoretical approach that defines stress as a stimulus) has been a major focus of psychosocial studies. Research has revealed that people under constant stress have a high incidence of psychosomatic disease.

Holmes and Rahe (1967) developed life event scales that assign numerical values, called life-change units, to typical life events. Because the items in the scales reflect events that require a change in a person's life pattern, and stress is defined as an accumulation of changes in one's life that require psychological adaptation, one can theoretically predict the likelihood of illness by checking off the number of recent events and deriving a total score. The Recent Life Changes Questionnaire (Tausig, 1982) contains 118 items such as death, birth, marriage, divorce, promotions, serious arguments, and vacations. The items include both desirable and undesirable events.

Sources of stress for people have been well researched (Lavoie, 2013; Prince, Chappelle, McDonald, et al., 2015; Shudifat & Al-Husban, 2015). People typically experience distress related to alterations in their physical and emotional health status, changes in their level of daily functioning, and decreased social support or the loss of significant others (Boland, Lee, & Bleck, 2015; Parker, Sricharoenchai, Raparla, et al., 2015; Su, Lau, Mak, et al., 2013; Taylor, 2013). Fears of immobilization, isolation, loneliness, sensory changes, financial problems, and death or disability increase a person's anxiety level. Loss of one's role or perceived purpose in life can cause intense discomfort. Any of these identified variables, plus myriad other conditions or demands are likely to cause ineffective coping, and a lack of effective coping skills is often a source of additional distress for the person. When a person endures prolonged or unrelenting suffering, the outcome is frequently the development of a stress-related illness. Nurses have the skills to assist people to alter their distressing circumstances and manage their responses to stress, as discussed later in the chapter.

Psychological Responses to Stress

After recognizing a stressor, a person consciously or unconsciously reacts to manage the situation. This is termed the mediating process. A theory developed by Lazarus (1991a) emphasizes cognitive appraisal and coping as important mediators of stress. Appraisal and coping are influenced by antecedent variables, including the internal and external resources of the individual person.

Appraisal of the Stressful Event

Cognitive appraisal (Lazarus, 1991a; Lazarus & Folkman, 1984) is a process by which an event is evaluated with respect to what is at stake (primary appraisal) and what might and can be done (secondary appraisal). What a person sees as being at stake is influenced by his or her personal goals, commitments, or motivations. Important factors include how important or relevant the event is to the person, whether the event conflicts with what the person wants or desires, and whether the situation threatens the person's own sense of strength and ego identity.

Primary appraisal results in the situation being identified as either nonstressful or stressful. Secondary appraisal is an evaluation of what might and can be done about the situation. Reappraisal, a change of opinion based on new information, may occur. The appraisal process is not necessarily sequential; primary and secondary appraisal and reappraisal may occur simultaneously.

The appraisal process contributes to the development of an emotion. Negative emotions such as fear and anger accompany harm/loss appraisals, and positive emotions accompany challenge. In addition to the subjective component or feeling that accompanies a particular emotion, each emotion also includes a tendency to act in a certain way. For example, unprepared students may view an unexpected quiz as threatening. They might feel fear, anger, and resentment and might express these emotions through hostile behaviour or comments.

Lazarus (1991a) expanded his initial ideas about stress, appraisal, and coping into a more complex model relating emotion to adaptation. He called this model a "cognitive–motivational–relational theory," with the term *relational* "standing for a focus on negotiation with a physical and social world" (p. 13). A theory of emotion was proposed as the bridge to connect psychology, physiology, and sociology: "More than any other arena of psychological thought, emotion is an integrative, organismic concept that subsumes psychological stress and coping within itself and unites motivation, cognition, and adaptation in a complex configuration" (p. 40).

Coping With the Stressful Event

Coping consists of the cognitive and behavioural efforts made to manage the specific external or internal demands that tax a person's resources and may be emotion focused or problem focused. Coping that is emotion focused seeks to make the person feel better by lessening the emotional distress. Problem-focused coping aims to make direct changes in the environment so that the situation can be managed more effectively. Both types of coping usually occur in a stressful situation. Even if the situation is viewed as challenging or beneficial, coping efforts may be required to develop and sustain the challenge—that is, to maintain the positive benefits of the challenge and to ward off any threats. In harmful or threatening situations, successful coping reduces or eliminates the source of stress and relieves the emotion generated.

Appraisal and coping are affected by internal characteristics such as health, energy, personal belief systems, commitments, or life goals, self-esteem, control, mastery, knowledge, problem-solving skills, and social skills. The characteristics that have been studied in nursing research are health-promoting lifestyles and resilience (Harper, Bruce, Hosek, et al., 2014; Herrick, Egan, Coulter, et al., 2014; McDonald, Jackson, Wilkes, et al., 2013). Resilience is considered both a personal trait and a process. Researchers have defined resilience as the ability of a person to function well in stressful situations such as traumatic events and other types of adverse situations (Theron, Theron, & Malindi, 2013). A resilient individual maintains flexibility even in difficult circumstances and controls strong emotional reactions using appropriate communication and problem-solving skills. Factors that play a role in building a person's resilience are having strong, supportive relationships with family members and other individuals and being exposed to positive role models. A resilient individual knows when to take action, when to step back and rely on others, and when to stop to reenergize and nurture the self. Researchers have found positive support for resilience as a significant variable that positively influences rehabilitation and overall improvement after a challenging or traumatic experience (Bertisch, Rath, Long, et al., 2014; Guccione, 2014; Monden, Trost, Catalano, et al., 2014;

Muir & Strnadova, 2014; Trief, Sandberg, Dimmock, et al., 2013; Zoellner & Feeny, 2014).

A health-promoting lifestyle buffers the effect of stressors. From a nursing practice standpoint, this outcome—buffering the effect of stressors—supports nursing's goal of promoting health. In many circumstances, promoting a healthy lifestyle is more achievable than altering the stressors.

Physiologic Response to Stress

The physiologic response to a stressor, whether it is physical or psychological, is a protective and adaptive mechanism to maintain the homeostatic balance of the body. When a stress response occurs, it activates a series of neurologic and hormonal processes within the brain and body systems. The duration and intensity of the stress can cause both short- and long-term effects. A stressor can disrupt homeostasis to the point where adaptation to the stressor fails, and a disease process results.

Selye's Theory of Adaptation

Hans Selye developed a theory of adaptation that profoundly influenced the scientific study of stress (1976). Selye first described a syndrome consisting of enlargement of the adrenal cortex; shrinkage of the thymus, spleen, lymph nodes, and other lymphatic structures; and the appearance of deep, bleeding ulcers in the stomach and duodenum. He identified this as a nonspecific response to diverse, noxious stimuli.

General Adaptation Syndrome

Selye then developed a theory of adaptation to biologic stress that he named the general adaptation syndrome (GAS), which has three phases: alarm, resistance, and exhaustion. During the alarm phase, the sympathetic "fight-or-flight" response is activated with release of **catecholamines** and the onset of the **adrenocorticotropic hormone** (ACTH)–adrenal cortical response. The alarm reaction is defensive and anti-inflammatory but self-limited. Because living in a continuous state of alarm would result in death, people move into the second stage, resistance. During the resistance stage, adaptation to the noxious stressor occurs, and cortisol activity is still increased. If exposure to the stressor is prolonged, the third stage, exhaustion, occurs. During the exhaustion stage, endocrine activity increases, and this has negative effects on the body systems (especially the circulatory, digestive, and immune systems) that can lead to death. Stages one and two of this syndrome are repeated, in different degrees, throughout life as the person encounters stressors.

Selye compared the GAS with the life process. During childhood, too few encounters with stress occur to promote the development of adaptive functioning, and children are vulnerable. During adulthood, a number of stressful events occur, and people develop resistance or adaptation. During the later years, the accumulation of life's stressors and wear and tear on the organism again decrease people's ability to adapt, resistance falls, and eventually death occurs.

Local Adaptation Syndrome

According to Selye, a local adaptation syndrome also occurs. This syndrome includes the inflammatory response and repair processes that occur at the local site of tissue injury. The local adaptation syndrome occurs in small, topical injuries, such as contact dermatitis. If the local injury is severe enough, the GAS is activated as well.

Selye emphasized that stress is the nonspecific response common to all stressors, regardless of whether they are physiologic, psychological, or social. The many conditioning factors in each person's environment account for why different demands are experienced by different people as stressors. Conditioning factors also account for differences in the tolerance of different people for stress. Some people may develop diseases of adaptation, such as hypertension and migraine headaches, whereas others are unaffected.

Interpretation of Stressful Stimuli by the Brain

Physiologic responses to stress are mediated by the brain through a complex network of chemical and electrical messages. The neural and hormonal actions that maintain homeostatic balance are integrated by the hypothalamus, which is located in the centre of the brain surrounded by the limbic system and the cerebral hemispheres. The hypothalamus is made up of a number of nuclei and integrates autonomic nervous system mechanisms that maintain the chemical constancy of the internal environment of the body. Together with the limbic system, which contains the amygdala, hippocampus, and septal nuclei, along with other structures, the hypothalamus regulates emotions and many visceral behaviours necessary for survival (e.g., eating, drinking, temperature control, reproduction, defense, aggression).

Each of the brain structures responds differently to stimuli. The cerebral hemispheres are concerned with cognitive functions: thought processes, learning, and memory. The limbic system has connections with both the cerebral hemispheres and the brain stem. In addition, the reticular activating system (RAS), a network of cells that forms a two-way communication system, extends from the brain stem into the midbrain and limbic system. This network controls the alert or waking state of the body.

In the stress response, afferent impulses are carried from sensory organs (eye, ear, nose, skin) and internal sensors (baroreceptors, chemoreceptors) to nerve centres in the brain. The response to the perception of stress is integrated in the hypothalamus, which coordinates the adjustments necessary to return to homeostatic balance. The degree and duration of the response vary; major stress evokes both sympathetic and pituitary adrenal responses.

Neural and neuroendocrine pathways under the control of the hypothalamus are also activated in the stress response. Initially, there is a sympathetic nervous system discharge, followed by a sympathetic–adrenal–medullary discharge. If the stress persists, the hypothalamic–pituitary system is activated (Fig. 9-2).

Sympathetic Nervous System Response

The sympathetic nervous system response is rapid and short lived. Norepinephrine is released at nerve endings that are in direct contact with their respective end organs to cause an increase in function of the vital organs and a state of general body arousal. The heart rate is increased and peripheral vasoconstriction occurs, raising the blood pressure. Blood is also shunted away from abdominal

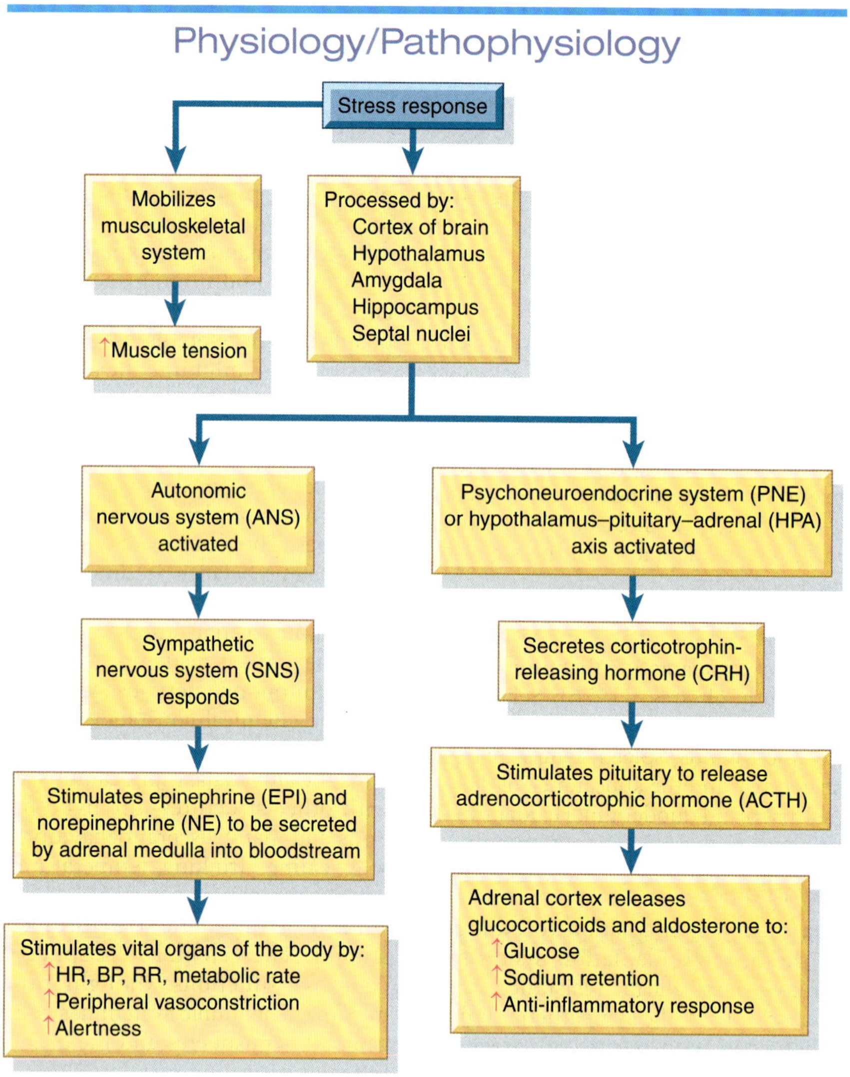

FIGURE 9-2. The physiologic response to stress. The body is prepared through brain activation of the autonomic nervous system and psychoneuroendocrine system commonly referred to as the hypothalamus–pituitary–adrenal axis to cope with stress.

organs. The purpose of these responses is to provide better perfusion of vital organs (brain, heart, skeletal muscles). Blood glucose is increased, supplying more readily available energy. The pupils are dilated, and mental activity is increased; a greater sense of awareness exists. Constriction of the blood vessels of the skin limits bleeding in the event of trauma. The person is likely to experience cold feet, clammy skin and hands, chills, palpitations, and "knots" in the stomach. Typically, the person appears tense, with the muscles of the neck, upper back, and shoulders tightened; respirations may be rapid and shallow, with the diaphragm tense.

Sympathetic–Adrenal–Medullary Response

In addition to its direct effect on major end organs, the sympathetic nervous system stimulates the medulla of the adrenal gland to release the hormones epinephrine and norepinephrine into the bloodstream. The action of these hormones is similar to that of the sympathetic nervous system and has the effect of sustaining and prolonging its actions. Epinephrine and norepinephrine are catecholamines that stimulate the nervous system and produce metabolic effects that increase the blood glucose level and increase the metabolic rate. The effect of the sympathetic–adrenal–medullary responses is summarized in Table 9-1. This effect is called the "fight-or-flight" reaction (Grossman & Porth, 2014).

Hypothalamic–Pituitary Response

The longest-acting phase of the physiologic response, which is more likely to occur in persistent stress, involves the hypothalamic–pituitary pathway. The hypothalamus secretes corticotropin-releasing factor, which stimulates the anterior pituitary to produce ACTH, which in turn stimulates the adrenal cortex to produce **glucocorticoids**, primarily cortisol (Grossman & Porth, 2014). Cortisol stimulates protein catabolism releasing amino acids, stimulates liver uptake of amino acids and their conversion to glucose (**gluconeogenesis**), and inhibits glucose uptake (anti-insulin action) by many body cells but not those of the brain and heart. These cortisol-induced metabolic effects provide the body with a ready source of energy during a stressful

TABLE 9-1 Sympathetic–Adrenal–Medullary Response to Stress

Effect	Purpose	Mechanism
Increased heart rate and blood pressure	Better perfusion of vital organs	Increased cardiac output due to increased myocardial contractility and heart rate; increased venous return (peripheral vasoconstriction)
Increased blood glucose level	Increased available energy	Increased liver and muscle glycogen breakdown; increased breakdown of adipose tissue triglycerides
Mental acuity	Alert state	Increase in amount of blood shunted to the brain from the abdominal viscera and skin
Dilated pupils	Increased awareness	Contraction of radial muscle of iris
Increased tension of skeletal muscles	Preparedness for activity, decreased fatigue	Excitation of muscles; increase in amount of blood shunted to the muscles from the abdominal viscera and skin
Increased ventilation (may be rapid and shallow)	Provision of oxygen for energy	Stimulation of respiratory centre in medulla; bronchodilation
Increased coagulability of blood	Prevention of hemorrhage in event of trauma	Vasoconstriction of surface vessels

situation. This effect has some important implications. For example, a person with diabetes who is under stress, such as that caused by an infection, needs more insulin than usual. Any patient who is under stress (e.g., illness, surgery, trauma, or prolonged psychological stress) catabolizes body protein and needs supplements.

The actions of the catecholamines (epinephrine and norepinephrine) and cortisol are the most important in the general response to stress. Other hormones that play a role are **antidiuretic hormone** (ADH) released from the posterior pituitary and aldosterone released from the adrenal cortex. ADH and aldosterone promote sodium and water retention, which is an adaptive mechanism in the event of hemorrhage or loss of fluids through excessive perspiration. ADH has also been shown to influence learning and may thus facilitate coping in new and threatening situations. Secretion of growth hormone and glucagon stimulates the uptake of amino acids by cells, helping to mobilize energy resources. Endorphins, which are endogenous opioids, increase during stress and enhance the threshold for tolerance of painful stimuli. They may also affect mood and have been implicated in the so-called high that long-distance runners experience. The secretion of other hormones is also affected, but their adaptive function is less clear.

Immunologic Response

Research findings show that the immune system is connected to the neuroendocrine and autonomic systems. Lymphoid tissue is richly supplied by autonomic nerves capable of releasing a number of different neuropeptides that can have a direct effect on leukocyte regulation and the inflammatory response. Neuroendocrine hormones released by the central nervous system and endocrine tissues can inhibit or stimulate leukocyte function. The wide variety of stressors a person experiences may result in different alterations in autonomic activity and subtle variations in neurohormone and neuropeptide synthesis. All of these possible autonomic and neuroendocrine responses can interact to initiate, weaken, enhance, or terminate an immune response.

The study of the relationships among the neuroendocrine system, the central and autonomic nervous systems, and the immune system and the effects of these relationships on overall health outcomes, is called *psychoneuroimmunology.* Because one's perception of events and one's coping styles determine whether, and to what extent, an event activates the stress response system, and because the stress response affects immune activity, one's perceptions, ideas, and thoughts can have profound neurochemical and immunologic consequences. Studies have demonstrated altered immune function in people who are under stress (Jain & Chandel, 2013; Polloni, Ferruzza, Ronconi, et al., 2015; Schwitalla, 2014). Other studies have identified certain personality traits, such as decisiveness, assertiveness, compassion, helpfulness, and conscientiousness, as having positive effects on health (Hankonen, Konttinen, & Absetz, 2014; Jokela, Pulkki-Raback, Elovaino, et al., 2014; Skodova & Lajciakova, 2013). As research continues, this field of study will likely uncover to what extent and by what mechanisms people can consciously influence their immunity.

Maladaptive Responses to Stress

The stress response, as indicated earlier, facilitates adaptation to threatening situations, and is retained from humans' evolutionary past. The "fight-or-flight" response, for example, is an anticipatory response that mobilized the bodily resources of our ancestors to deal with predators and other harsh factors in their environment. This same mobilization comes into play in response to emotional stimuli unrelated to danger. For example, a person may get an "adrenaline rush" when competing over a decisive point in a ball game, or when excited about attending a party.

When responses to stress are ineffective, they are referred to as *maladaptive*. Maladaptive responses are chronic, recurrent responses or patterns of response that do not promote the goals of adaptation. The goals of adaptation are somatic or physical health (optimal wellness); psychological health or having a sense of well-being (happiness, satisfaction with life, morale); and enhanced social functioning, which includes work, social life, and family (positive relationships). Maladaptive responses that threaten these goals include faulty appraisals and inappropriate coping (Lazarus, 1991a).

The frequency, intensity, and duration of stressful situations contribute to the development of emotions and subsequent patterns of neurochemical discharge. By appraising situations adequately and coping appropriately, it is possible to anticipate and defuse some of these situations. For example, frequent stressful encounters (e.g., marital discord) might be avoided with better communication and problem solving, or a pattern of procrastination (e.g., delaying work on tasks) could be corrected to reduce stress when deadlines approach.

Coping processes that include the use of alcohol or drugs to reduce stress increase the risk of illness. Other inappropriate coping patterns may increase the risk of illness less directly. For example, people who demonstrate "type A" behaviours, including impatience, competitiveness, and achievement orientation, have an underlying aggressive approach to life and are more prone than others to develop stress-related illnesses. Type A behaviours increase the output of catecholamines, the adrenal–medullary hormones, with their attendant effects on the body. Additional forms of inappropriate coping include denial, avoidance, and distancing. Denial may be illustrated by the woman who feels a lump in her breast but downplays its seriousness and delays seeking medical attention. The intent of denial is to control the threat, but it may also endanger life.

Models of illness frequently include stress and maladaptation as precursors to disease. A general model of illness, based on Selye's theory, suggests that any stressor elicits a state of disturbed physiologic equilibrium. If this state is prolonged or the response is excessive, it increases the susceptibility of the person to illness. This susceptibility, coupled with a predisposition in the person (from genetic traits, health, or age), leads to illness. If the sympathetic adrenal–medullary response is prolonged or excessive, a state of chronic arousal develops that may lead to high blood pressure, arteriosclerotic changes, and cardiovascular disease. If the production of ACTH is prolonged or excessive, behaviour patterns of withdrawal and depression are seen. In addition, the immune response is decreased, and infections and tumours may develop.

Selye (1976) proposed a list of disorders known as diseases of maladaptation: high blood pressure (including hypertension of pregnancy), diseases of the heart and blood vessels, diseases of the kidney, rheumatic diseases and inflammatory diseases of the skin and eyes, infections, allergic and hypersensitivity diseases, nervous and mental diseases, sexual dysfunction, digestive diseases, metabolic diseases, and cancer. Research continues on the complex interconnections between stress, coping (adaptive and maladaptive), and disease (Akyil & Erguney, 2013; Barre, Padmaja, Saxena, et al., 2015; Cevik & Erguney, 2013; Epel & Lithgow, 2014; McVicar, Ravalier, & Greenwood, 2014; Smith, Fortune, Phillips, et al., 2014).

CHART 9-1

Assessing for Stress

Be alert for the following:

- Bruxism (grinding of teeth)
- Changes in menstrual cycle
- Change in appetite
- Concentration difficulties
- Diarrhea
- Difficulty sleeping
- Dry mouth
- Emotional lability
- Excessive perspiration
- Fatigue
- Feeling weak or dizzy
- Gastrointestinal distress
- Headaches
- Hyperactivity
- Increased substance use or abuse
- Increased use of tobacco
- Increased body tension
- Intense or increased anxiety
- Impulsive behaviours
- Loss of interest in life activities
- Nausea or vomiting
- Nervous habits
- Nervous laughter
- Overpowering urge to act out
- Pain in back, neck, or other parts of the body
- Palpitations
- Prone to injury
- Restlessness
- Strong startle response
- Tremors
- Unintentional weight loss or gain
- Urinary frequency

Adapted from Rice, V. H. (Ed.). (2012). *Handbook of stress, coping, and health: Implications for theory, research, and practice* (2nd ed.). Thousand Oaks, CA: Sage; Selye, H. (1976). *The stress of life* (Rev. ed.). New York: McGraw-Hill.

Indicators of Stress

Indicators of stress and the stress response include both subjective and objective measures. Chart 9-1 lists signs and symptoms that may be observed directly or reported by a person. They are psychological, physiologic, or behavioural and reflect social behaviours and thought processes. Some of these reactions may be coping behaviours. Over time, each person tends to develop a characteristic pattern of behaviour during stress to warn that the system is out of balance.

Laboratory measurements of indicators of stress have helped in understanding this complex process. Blood and urine analyses can be used to demonstrate changes in hormonal levels and hormonal breakdown products. Blood levels of catecholamines, glucocorticoids, ACTH, and eosinophils are reliable measures of stress. Serum cholesterol and free fatty acid levels can be used to measure stress. When the body experiences distress, there are changes in adrenal hormones such as cortisol and aldosterone. As the levels of these chemicals increase, there is a simultaneous release of additional cholesterol into the general circulation. Both physical and psychological distress can trigger an elevated cholesterol level. In addition, the results of immunoglobulin assays are increased when a person is exposed to a variety of stressors, especially infections and immunodeficiency conditions. With greater attention to the field of neuroimmunology, improved laboratory measures are likely to follow.

In addition to using laboratory tests, researchers have developed questionnaires to identify and assess stressors, stress, and coping strategies. The work of Rice (2012), a compilation of information gained from research on stress, coping, and health, includes some of these questionnaires.

Nursing Implications

It is important for nurses to realize that the optimal point of intervention to promote health is during the stage when a person's own compensatory processes are still functioning effectively. A major role of nurses is the early identification of both physiologic and psychological stressors. Nurses should be able to relate the presenting signs and symptoms of distress to the physiology they represent and identify a person's position on the continuum of function, from health and compensation to pathophysiology and disease.

For example, if an anxious, middle-aged woman presented for a checkup and was found to be overweight with a blood pressure of 150/85 mm Hg, the nurse would counsel her with respect to diet, stress management, and activity. The nurse would also encourage weight loss and discuss the woman's intake of salt (which affects fluid balance) and caffeine (which provides a stimulant effect). The patient and the nurse would identify both individual and environmental stressors and discuss strategies to decrease her lifestyle stress, with the ultimate goal being to create a healthy lifestyle and prevent hypertension and its sequelae.

Stress at the Cellular Level

Pathologic processes may occur at all levels of the biologic organism. If the cell is considered the smallest unit or subsystem (tissues being aggregates of cells, organs aggregates of tissues, and so on), the processes of health and disease or adaptation and maladaptation can all occur at the cellular level. Indeed, pathologic processes are often described by scientists at the subcellular or molecular level.

The cell exists on a continuum of function and structure, ranging from the usual cell, to the adapted cell, to the injured or diseased cell, to the dead cell (Fig. 9-3). Changes from one state to another may occur rapidly and may not be readily detectable, because each state does not have discrete boundaries, and disease represents disruption of usual processes. The earliest changes occur at the molecular or subcellular level and are not perceptible until steady-state functions or structures are altered. With cell injury, some changes may be reversible; in other instances, the injuries are lethal. For example, tanning of the skin is an adaptive, morphologic response to exposure to the rays of the sun. However, if the exposure is continued, sunburn and injury occur, and some cells may die, as evidenced by desquamation ("peeling").

Different cells and tissues respond to stimuli with different patterns and rates of response, and some cells are more vulnerable to one type of stimulus or stressor than others. The cell involved, its ability to adapt, and its physiologic state are determinants of the response. For example, cardiac muscle cells respond to **hypoxia** (inadequate oxygenation) more quickly than do smooth muscle cells.

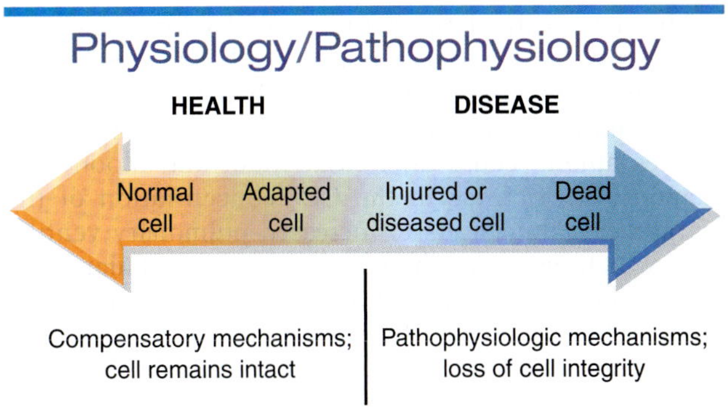

FIGURE 9-3. The cell on a continuum of function and structure. Changes in the cell are not as easily discerned as the diagram depicts, and the point at which compensation subsides and pathophysiology begins is not clearly defined.

Other determinants of cellular response are the type or nature of the stimulus, its duration, and its severity. For example, neurons that control respiration can develop a tolerance to regular, small amounts of a barbiturate, but one large dose may result in respiratory depression and death.

Control of the Steady State

The concept of the cell as existing on a continuum of function and structure includes the relationship of the cell to compensatory mechanisms, which occur continuously in the body to maintain the steady state. Compensatory processes are regulated primarily by the autonomic nervous system and the endocrine system, with control achieved through **negative feedback**.

Negative Feedback

Negative feedback mechanisms throughout the body monitor the internal environment and restore homeostasis when conditions shift out of the usual range. These mechanisms work by sensing deviations from a predetermined set point or range of adaptability and triggering a response aimed at offsetting the deviation. Blood pressure, acid–base balance, blood glucose level, body temperature, and fluid and electrolyte balance are examples of functions regulated through such compensatory mechanisms.

Most of the human body's control systems are integrated by the brain with feedback from the nervous and endocrine systems. Control activities involve detecting deviations from the predetermined reference point and stimulating compensatory responses in the muscles and glands of the body. The major organs affected are the heart, lungs, kidneys, liver, gastrointestinal tract, and skin. When stimulated, these organs alter their rate of activity or the amount of secretions they produce. Because of this, they have been called the "organs of homeostasis or adjustment."

In addition to the responses influenced by the nervous and endocrine systems, local responses consisting of small feedback loops in a group of cells or tissues are possible. The cells detect a change in their immediate environment and initiate an action to counteract its effect. For example, the accumulation of lactic acid in an exercised muscle stimulates dilation of blood vessels in the area to increase blood flow and improve the delivery of oxygen and removal of waste products.

The net result of the activities of feedback loops is homeostasis. A steady state is achieved by the continuous, variable action of the organs involved in making the adjustments and by the continuous exchange of chemical substances among cells, interstitial fluid, and blood. For example, an increase in the CO_2 concentration of the extracellular fluid leads to increased pulmonary ventilation, which decreases the CO_2 level. On a cellular level, increased CO_2 raises the hydrogen ion concentration of the blood. This is detected by chemosensitive receptors in the respiratory control centre of the medulla of the brain. The chemoreceptors stimulate an increase in the rate of discharge of the neurons that innervate the diaphragm and intercostal muscles, which increases the rate of respiration. Excess CO_2 is exhaled, the hydrogen ion concentration returns to a steady state, and the chemically sensitive neurons are no longer stimulated (Grossman & Porth, 2014).

Positive Feedback

Another type of feedback, **positive feedback**, perpetuates the chain of events set in motion by the original disturbance instead of compensating for it. As the system becomes more unbalanced, disorder and disintegration occur. There are some exceptions to this; blood clotting in humans, for example, is an important positive feedback mechanism.

Cellular Adaptation

Cells are complex units that dynamically respond to the changing demands and stresses of daily life. They possess a maintenance function and a specialized function. The maintenance function refers to the activities that the cell must perform with respect to itself; specialized functions are those that the cell performs in relation to the tissues and organs of which it is a part. Individual cells may cease to function without posing a threat to the organism. However, as the number of dead cells increases, the specialized functions of the tissues are altered, and health is threatened.

Cells can adapt to environmental stress through structural and functional changes. Some of these adaptations include cellular hypertrophy, atrophy, **hyperplasia**, **dysplasia**, and **metaplasia** (Table 9-2). These adaptations reflect changes in the usual cell in response to stress. If the stress is unrelenting, cellular injury and death may occur.

Hypertrophy and atrophy lead to changes in the size of cells and hence the size of the organs they form. Compensatory hypertrophy is the result of an enlarged muscle mass and commonly occurs in skeletal and cardiac muscles that experience a prolonged, increased workload. One example is the bulging muscles of the athlete who engages in body building.

Atrophy can be the consequence of disease, decreased use, decreased blood supply, loss of nerve supply, or inadequate nutrition. Disuse of a body part is often associated with the aging process and immobilization. Cell size and organ size decrease, and the structures principally affected are the skeletal muscles, the secondary sex organs, the heart, and the brain.

Hyperplasia is an increase in the number of new cells in an organ or tissue. As cells multiply and are subjected to increased stimulation, the tissue mass enlarges. This mitotic response (a change occurring with mitosis) is reversible when the stimulus is removed. This distinguishes hyperplasia from neoplasia or malignant growth, which continues after the stimulus is removed. Hyperplasia may be hormonally induced. An example is the increased size of the thyroid gland caused by thyroid-stimulating hormone (secreted from the pituitary gland) when a deficit in thyroid hormone occurs.

Dysplasia is bizarre cell growth resulting in cells that differ in size, shape, or arrangement from other cells of the same tissue type. Dysplastic cells have a tendency to become malignant; dysplasia is seen commonly in epithelial cells in the bronchi of people who smoke.

Metaplasia is a cell transformation in which there is a conversion of one type of mature cell into another type of cell. This serves a protective function, because less-transformed

TABLE 9-2 Cellular Adaptation to Stressors

Adaptation	Stimulus	Example
Hypertrophy—increase in cell size leading to increase in organ size	Increased workload	Leg muscles of runner Arm muscles in tennis player Cardiac muscle in person with hypertension
Atrophy—shrinkage in size of cell, leading to decrease in organ size	Decrease in: Use Blood supply Nutrition Hormonal stimulation Innervation	Secondary sex organs in aging person Extremity immobilized in cast
Hyperplasia—increase in number of new cells (increase in mitosis)	Hormonal influence	Breast changes of girl in puberty or of pregnant woman Regeneration of liver cells New red blood cells in blood loss
Dysplasia—bizarre changes in the appearance of cells	Reproduction of cells with resulting alteration of their size and shape	Alterations in epithelial cells of the skin or the cervix, producing irregular tissue changes that could be the precursors of a malignancy
Metaplasia—transformation of one adult cell type to another (reversible)	Stress applied to highly specialized cell	Changes in epithelial cells lining bronchi in response to smoke irritation (cells become less specialized)

cells are more resistant to the stress that stimulated the change. For example, the ciliated columnar epithelium lining the bronchi of people who smoke is replaced by squamous epithelium. The squamous cells can survive; loss of the cilia and protective mucus, however, can have damaging consequences.

Cellular Injury

Injury is defined as a disorder in steady-state regulation. Any stressor that alters the ability of the cell or system to maintain optimal balance of its adjustment processes leads to injury. Structural and functional damage then occurs, which may be reversible (permitting recovery) or irreversible (leading to disability or death). Homeostatic adjustments are concerned with the small changes within the body's systems. With adaptive changes, compensation occurs and a new steady state may be achieved. With injury, steady-state regulation is lost, and changes in functioning ensue.

Causes of disorder and injury in the system (cell, tissue, organ, body) may arise from the external or internal environment (Fig. 9-4) and include hypoxia, nutritional imbalance, physical agents, chemical agents, infectious agents, immune mechanisms, genetic defects, and psychogenic factors. The most common causes are hypoxia (oxygen deficiency), chemical injury, and infectious agents. In addition, the presence of one injury makes the system more susceptible to another injury. For example, inadequate oxygenation and nutritional deficiencies make the system vulnerable to infection. These agents act at the cellular level by damaging or destroying:

- The integrity of the cell membrane, necessary for ionic balance
- The ability of the cell to transform energy (aerobic respiration, production of adenosine triphosphate)
- The ability of the cell to synthesize enzymes and other necessary proteins
- The ability of the cell to grow and reproduce (genetic integrity)

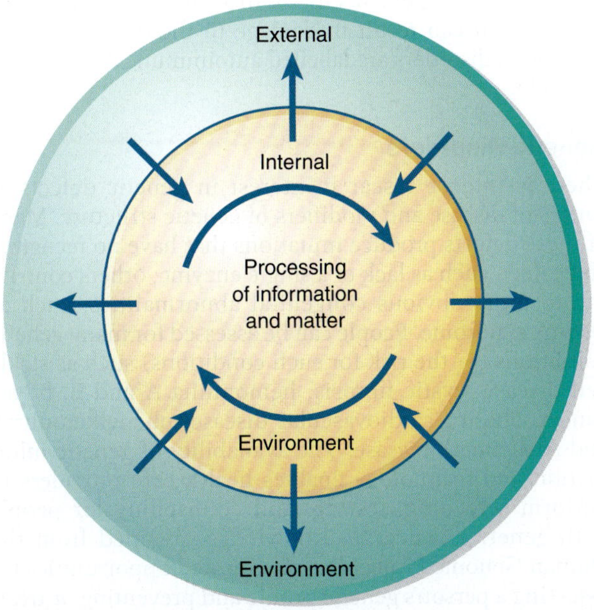

FIGURE 9-4. Influences leading to disorder may arise from the internal environment and the external environment of the system. Excesses or deficits of information and matter may occur, or there may be faulty regulation of processing.

Hypoxia

Inadequate cellular oxygenation (hypoxia) interferes with the cell's ability to transform energy. Hypoxia may be caused by a decrease in blood supply to an area, a decrease in the oxygen-carrying capacity of the blood (decreased hemoglobin), a ventilation/perfusion or respiratory problem that reduces the amount of arterial oxygen available, or a problem in the cell's enzyme system that makes it unable to use oxygen.

The usual cause of hypoxia is ischemia, or deficient blood supply. Ischemia is commonly seen in myocardial cell injury in which arterial blood flow is decreased because of atherosclerotic narrowing of blood vessels. Ischemia also results from intravascular clots (thrombi or emboli) that may form and interfere with blood supply. Thrombi and emboli are common causes of cerebrovascular accidents (strokes, brain attacks). The length of time different tissues can survive without oxygen varies. For example, brain cells most often succumb in 3 to 6 minutes. If the condition leading to hypoxia is slow and progressive, collateral circulation may develop, whereby blood is supplied by other blood vessels in the area. However, this mechanism is not highly reliable.

Nutritional Imbalance

Nutritional imbalance refers to a relative or absolute deficiency or excess of one or more essential nutrients. This may be manifested as undernutrition (inadequate consumption of food or calories) or overnutrition (caloric excess). Caloric excess to the point of obesity overloads cells in the body with lipids. By requiring more energy to maintain the extra tissue, obesity places a strain on the body and has been associated with the development of disease, especially pulmonary and cardiovascular disease.

Specific deficiencies arise when an essential nutrient is deficient or when there is an imbalance of nutrients. Protein deficiencies and avitaminosis (deficiency of vitamins) are typical examples. An energy deficit leading to cell injury can occur if there is insufficient glucose, or insufficient oxygen to transform the glucose into energy. A lack of insulin, or the inability to use insulin, may also prevent glucose from entering the cell from the blood. This occurs in diabetes mellitus, a metabolic disorder that can lead to nutritional deficiency, as well as in a host of short- and long-term life-threatening complications.

Physical Agents

Physical agents, including temperature extremes, radiation, electrical shock, and mechanical trauma, can cause injury to the cells or to the entire body. The duration of exposure and the intensity of the stressor determine the severity of damage.

Temperature

When a person's temperature is elevated, hypermetabolism occurs and the respiratory rate, heart rate, and basal metabolic rate all increase. With fever induced by infections, the hypothalamic thermostat may be reset at a higher temperature and then return to normal when the fever abates. The increase in body temperature is achieved through physiologic mechanisms. Body temperatures greater than 41°C (106°F) indicate hyperthermia, because the physiologic function of the thermoregulatory centre breaks down and the temperature soars. This physiologic condition occurs in people who have heat stroke. Eventually, the high temperature causes coagulation of cell proteins, and cells die. The body must be cooled rapidly to prevent brain damage.

The local response to burn injury is similar. There is an increase in metabolic activity and, as heat increases, proteins coagulate and enzyme systems are destroyed. In extreme situations, charring or carbonization occurs. For more information about burn injuries, see Chapter 59.

Extremes of low temperature, or cold, cause vasoconstriction. Blood flow becomes sluggish and clots form, leading to ischemic damage in the involved tissues. With still lower temperatures, ice crystals may form, and cells may burst.

Radiation and Electrical Shock

Radiation is used for diagnosis and treatment of diseases. Ionizing forms of radiation may cause injury by their destructive action. Radiation decreases the protective inflammatory response of the cell, creating a favourable environment for opportunistic infections. Electrical shock produces burns as a result of the heat generated when electrical current travels through the body. It may also unexpectedly stimulate nerves, leading, for example, to fibrillation of the heart.

Mechanical Trauma

Mechanical trauma can result in wounds that disrupt the cells and tissues of the body. The severity of the wound, the amount of blood loss, and the extent of nerve damage are significant factors in the outcome.

Chemical Agents

Chemical injuries are caused by poisons, such as lye, which have a corrosive action on epithelial tissue, or by heavy metals, such as mercury, arsenic, and lead, each of which has its own specific destructive action. Many other chemicals are toxic in certain amounts, in certain people, and in specific tissues. For example, excessive secretion of hydrochloric acid can damage the stomach lining; large amounts of glucose can cause osmotic shifts, affecting the fluid and electrolyte balance; and too much insulin can cause unusual levels of glucose in the blood (hypoglycemia) and can lead to coma.

Drugs, including prescribed medications, can also cause chemical poisoning. Some people are less tolerant of medications than others and manifest toxic reactions at the usual or customary dosages. Aging tends to decrease tolerance to medications. Polypharmacy (taking many medications at one time) also occurs frequently in the aging population and is a problem because of the unpredictable effects of the resulting medication interactions.

Alcohol (ethanol) is also a chemical irritant. In the body, alcohol is broken down into acetaldehyde, which has a direct toxic effect on liver cells that leads to a variety of liver abnormalities, including cirrhosis in susceptible people. Disordered liver cell function leads to complications in other organs of the body.

Infectious Agents

Biologic agents known to cause disease in humans are viruses, bacteria, rickettsiae, mycoplasmas, fungi, protozoa, and nematodes. The severity of the infectious disease depends on the number of microorganisms entering the body, their virulence, and the host's defenses (e.g., health, age, immune responses).

Some bacteria, such as those that cause tetanus and diphtheria, produce exotoxins that circulate and create cell damage. Others, such as gram-negative bacteria, produce endotoxins when they die. Tubercle bacilli induce an immune reaction.

Viruses, the smallest living organisms known, survive as parasites of the living cells they invade. Viruses infect specific cells. Through a complex mechanism, viruses replicate within cells and then invade other cells, where they continue to replicate. An immune response is mounted by the body to eliminate the viruses, and the cells harbouring the viruses can be injured in the process. Typically, an inflammatory response and immune reaction are the physiologic responses of the body to viral infection.

Disordered Immune Responses

The immune system is an exceedingly complex system, the purpose of which is to defend the body from invasion by any foreign object or foreign cell type, such as cancerous cells. This is a steady-state mechanism, but like other adjustment processes it can become disordered, and cellular injury results. The immune response detects foreign bodies by distinguishing non-self substances from self substances and destroying the non-self entities. The entrance of an antigen (foreign substance) into the body evokes the production of antibodies that attack and destroy the antigen (antigen–antibody reaction).

The immune system may function as expected or it may be hypo- or hyperactive. When it is hypoactive, immunodeficiency diseases occur; when it is hyperactive, hypersensitivity disorders occur. A disorder of the immune system itself can result in damage to the body's own tissues. Such disorders are labelled autoimmune diseases (see Unit 11).

Genetic Disorders

There is intense research interest in genetic defects as causes of disease and modifiers of genetic structure. Many of these defects produce mutations that have no recognizable effect, such as lack of a single enzyme; others contribute to more obvious congenital abnormalities, such as Down's syndrome. People can be assessed for many genetic conditions (or the risk for such conditions) such as sickle cell disease, cystic fibrosis, hemophilia A and B, breast cancer, obesity, cardiovascular disease, phenylketonuria, and Alzheimer's disease. The availability of genetic information and technology enables health care providers to perform screening, testing, and counselling for people with genetics concerns. Knowledge obtained from the Human Genome Project has also created opportunities for assessing a person's genetic profile and preventing or treating diseases. Diagnostic genetics and gene therapy have the potential to identify and modify genes before they begin to express traits that would lead to disease or disability. (For further information, see Chapter 11.)

Cellular Response to Injury: Inflammation

Cells or tissues of the body may be injured or killed by any of the agents (physical, chemical, infectious) described earlier. When this happens, an inflammatory response (or inflammation) naturally occurs in the healthy tissues adjacent to the site of injury. Inflammation is a defensive reaction intended to neutralize, control, or eliminate the offending agent and to prepare the site for repair. It is a nonspecific response (not dependent on a particular cause) that is meant to serve a protective function. For example, inflammation may be observed at the site of a bee sting, in a sore throat, in a surgical incision, and at the site of a burn. Inflammation also occurs in cell injury events, such as strokes and myocardial infarctions.

Inflammation is not the same as infection. An infectious agent is only one of several agents that may trigger an inflammatory response. An infection exists when the infectious agent is living, growing, and multiplying in the tissues and is able to overcome the body's usual defenses.

Regardless of the cause, a general sequence of events occurs in the local inflammatory response. This sequence involves changes in the microcirculation, including vasodilation, increased vascular permeability, and leukocytic cellular infiltration (Fig. 9-5). As these changes take place, five cardinal signs of inflammation are produced: redness, heat, swelling, pain, and loss of function.

The transient vasoconstriction that occurs immediately after injury is followed by vasodilation and an increased rate of blood flow through the microcirculation to the area of tissue damage. Local heat and redness result. Next, the structure of the microvascular system changes to accommodate the movement of plasma protein from the blood into the tissues. Following this increase in vascular permeability, plasma fluids (including proteins and solutes) leak into the inflamed tissues producing swelling. Leukocytes migrate through the endothelium and accumulate in the tissue at the site of the injury. The pain that occurs is attributed to the pressure of fluids or swelling on nerve endings and to the irritation of nerve endings by chemical mediators released at the site. Bradykinin is one of the chemical mediators suspected of causing pain. Loss of function is most likely related to the pain and swelling, but the exact mechanism is not completely known.

As blood flow increases and fluid leaks into the surrounding tissues, the formed elements (red blood cells, white blood cells, and platelets) remain in the blood, causing it to become more viscous. Leukocytes (white blood cells) collect in the vessels, exit, and migrate to the site of injury to engulf offending organisms and to remove cellular debris in a process called phagocytosis. Fibrinogen in the leaked plasma fluid coagulates, forming fibrin for clot formation, which serves to wall off the injured area and prevent the spread of infection.

Chemical Mediators of Inflammation

Injury initiates the inflammatory response, but chemical substances released at the site induce vascular changes. Foremost among these chemicals are histamine and kinins. Histamine is present in many tissues of the body but is concentrated in the mast cells. It is released when injury occurs and is responsible for the early changes in

Physiology/Pathophysiology

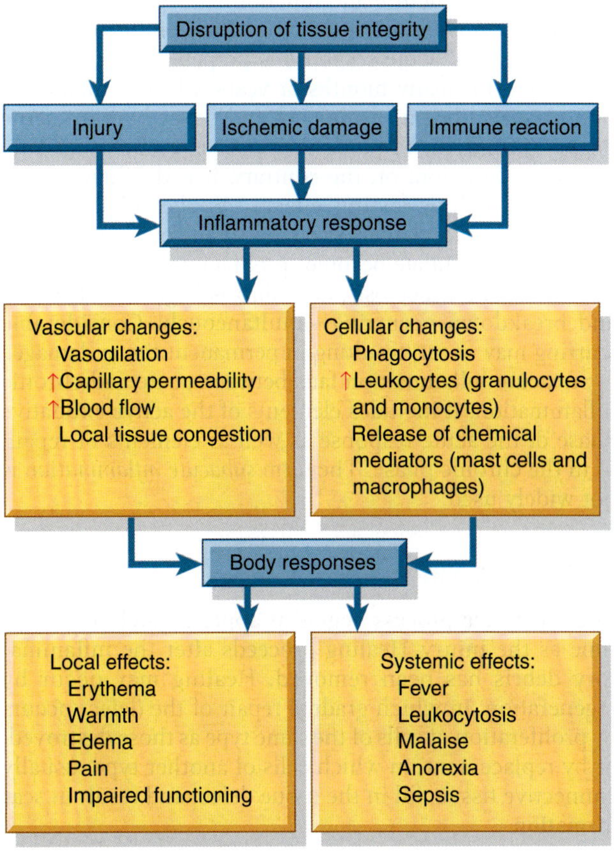

FIGURE 9-5. Inflammatory response.

vasodilation and vascular permeability. Kinins increase vascular dilations and permeability and attract neutrophils to the area. Prostaglandins, another group of chemical substances, are also suspected of causing increased vascular permeability (Grossman & Porth, 2014).

Systemic Response to Inflammation

The inflammatory response is often confined to the site, causing only local signs and symptoms. However, systemic responses can also occur. Fever is the most common sign of a systemic response to injury, and it is most likely caused by endogenous pyrogens (internal substances that cause fever) released from neutrophils and macrophages (specialized forms of leukocytes). These substances reset the hypothalamic thermostat, which controls body temperature, and produce fever. Leukocytosis, an increase in the synthesis and release of neutrophils from bone marrow, may occur to provide the body with greater ability to fight infection. During this process, general, nonspecific symptoms develop, including malaise, loss of appetite, aching, and weakness.

Types of Inflammation

Inflammation is categorized primarily by its duration and the type of exudate produced. It may be acute, subacute, or chronic. Acute inflammation is characterized by the local vascular and exudative changes described previously and usually lasts less than 2 weeks. An acute inflammatory response is immediate and serves a protective function.

After the causative agent is removed, the inflammation subsides and healing takes place with the return of usual or near-usual structure and function.

Chronic inflammation develops if the injurious agent persists and the acute response is perpetuated. Symptoms are present for many months or years. Chronic inflammation may also begin insidiously and never have an acute phase. The chronic response does not serve a beneficial and protective function; on the contrary, it is debilitating and can produce long-lasting effects. As the inflammation becomes chronic, changes occur at the site of injury and the nature of the exudate becomes proliferative. A cycle of cellular infiltration, necrosis, and fibrosis begins, with repair and breakdown occurring simultaneously. Considerable scarring may occur, resulting in permanent tissue damage.

Subacute inflammation falls between acute and chronic inflammation. It includes elements of the active exudative phase of the acute response as well as elements of repair, as in the chronic phase. The term *subacute inflammation* is not widely used.

Cellular Healing

The reparative process begins at approximately the same time as the injury. Healing proceeds after the inflammatory debris has been removed. Healing may occur by regeneration, in which gradual repair of the defect occurs by proliferation of cells of the same type as those destroyed, or by replacement, in which cells of another type, usually connective tissue, fill in the tissue defect and result in scar formation.

Regeneration

The ability of cells to regenerate depends on whether they are labile, permanent, or stable. Labile cells multiply constantly to replace cells worn out by usual physiologic processes; these include epithelial cells of the skin and those lining the gastrointestinal tract. Permanent cells include neurons—the nerve cell bodies, not their axons. Destruction of neurons is permanent, but axons may regenerate. If usual activity is to return, tissue regeneration must occur in a functional pattern, especially in the growth of several axons. Stable cells in some organ systems have a latent ability to regenerate. Under usual physiologic processes, they are not shed and do not need replacement, but if they are damaged or destroyed, they are able to regenerate. Examples include functional cells of the kidney, liver, and pancreas. Cells in other organs, such as the brain, for example, do not regenerate.

Replacement

The condition of the host, the environment, and the nature and severity of the injury affect the processes of inflammation, repair, and replacement. Depending on the extent of damage, repair and replacement may occur by first-, second-, or third-intention healing. In first-intention healing, the wound edges are approximated, as in a surgical wound. Little scar formation occurs, and the wound healing occurs without granulation. In second-intention healing, the edges are not approximated and the wound fills with granulation tissue. The process of repair takes longer and may result in scar formation, with loss of specialized function. For example, people who have recovered from myocardial infarction have abnormal electrocardiographic tracings because the electrical signal cannot be conducted through the connective tissue that has replaced the infarcted area. In third-intention healing, the wound edges are not approximated and healing is delayed. For more information about wound healing see Chapter 21.

Nursing Implications

In the assessment of people who seek health care, both objective signs and subjective symptoms are the primary indicators of existing physiologic processes. The following questions are addressed:

- Are the heart rate, respiratory rate, and temperature normal?
- What emotional distress may be contributing to the patient's health issues?
- Are there other indicators of steady-state deviation?
- What are the patient's blood pressure, height, and weight?
- Are there any problems in movement or sensation?
- Are there any problems with affect, behaviour, speech, cognitive ability, orientation, or memory?
- Are there obvious impairments, lesions, or deformities?

Objective evidence can be obtained from laboratory data, such as electrolytes, blood urea nitrogen, blood glucose, and urinalysis results. Further signs of change are seen in diagnostic studies such as computed tomography (CT), magnetic resonance imaging (MRI), and positron emission tomography (PET). Further information on diagnostic studies can be found in assessment chapters of each unit of the book.

In making a nursing diagnosis, the nurse must relate the symptoms or problems reported by the patient to the existing physical signs. Management of specific biologic disorders is discussed in subsequent chapters; however, nurses can assist any patient to respond to stress-inducing biologic or psychological disorders with stress management interventions.

Stress Management: Nursing Interventions

Stress or the potential for stress is ubiquitous—that is, it is both everywhere and anywhere. Indeed, nursing students experience stressors that can negatively affect their academic and clinical performance (Chart 9-2) (Shudifat & Al-Husban, 2015). Anxiety, frustration, anger, and feelings of inadequacy, helplessness, or powerlessness are emotions often associated with stress. In the presence of these emotions, the customary activities of daily living may be disrupted—for example, a sleep disturbance may occur, eating and activity patterns may be altered, and family processes or role performance may be disrupted.

Many nursing diagnoses are possible for patients suffering from stress. Stress may be manifested as ineffective coping patterns, impaired thought processes, or disrupted relationships. Because human responses to stress are varied, as are the sources of stress, arriving at an accurate diagnosis allows interventions and goals to be more specific and leads to improved outcomes.

CHART 9-2

Information Addressed in Health Risk Questionnaires

Demographic data: age, gender, race, ethnic background
Personal and family history of diseases and health problems
Lifestyle choices:

- Eating, sleeping, exercise, smoking, drinking, sexual activity, and driving habits
- Stressors at home and on the job
- Role relationships and associated stressors

Physical measurements:

- Blood pressure
- Height, weight, body mass index (BMI)
- Laboratory analyses of blood and urine

Participation in high-risk behaviours

Stress management is directed toward reducing and controlling stress and improving coping. The need to prevent illness, improve the quality of life, and decrease the cost of health care makes efforts to promote health essential, and stress control is a significant health promotion goal. Stress reduction methods and coping enhancements can derive from either internal or external sources. For example, healthy eating habits and relaxation techniques are internal resources that help reduce stress, and a broad social network is an external resource that helps reduce stress. Goods and services that can be purchased are also external resources for stress management. It may be easier for people with adequate financial resources to cope with constraints in the environment, because their sense of vulnerability to threat is decreased compared to those without adequate financial resources.

Promoting a Healthy Lifestyle

A health-promoting lifestyle provides internal resources that aid in coping, and it buffers or cushions the impact of stressors. Lifestyles or habits that contribute to the risk of illness can be identified through a health risk appraisal, an assessment method designed to promote health by examining a person's habits, and recommending changes when a health risk is identified.

Health risk appraisals involve the use of health risk questionnaires to estimate the likelihood that people with a given set of characteristics will become ill. It is hoped that if people are provided with this information, they will adopt healthy behaviours (e.g., stop smoking, have periodic screening examinations) to improve their health. Questionnaires typically address the information presented in Chart 9-2.

The personal information is compared with average population risk data, and the risk factors are identified and weighed. From this analysis, a person's risks and major health hazards are identified. Further comparisons with population data can estimate how many years will be added to a person's life span if the suggested changes are made. However, research has not yet demonstrated that providing people with such information ensures that they will change their behaviours. The single most important factor for determining health status is social class, and within a social class the research suggests that the major factor influencing health is level of education (Bastable, Gramet, Jacobs, et al., 2014).

Enhancing Coping Strategies

Butcher, Bulechek, Dochterman, et al. (2018) identifies "coping enhancement" as a nursing intervention and defines it as "assisting a patient to adapt to perceived stressors, changes, or threats that interfere with meeting life demands and roles" (Chart 9-3). The nurse can build on the patient's existing coping strategies, as identified in the health appraisal, or teach new strategies for coping if necessary.

The five predominant ways of coping with illness identified in a review of 57 nursing research studies were as follows (Jalowiec, 1993):

- Trying to be optimistic about the outcome
- Using social support
- Using spiritual resources (Skillen, 2012)
- Trying to maintain control either over the situation or over feelings
- Trying to accept the situation

Other ways of coping included seeking information, reprioritizing needs and roles, lowering expectations,

CHART 9-3

Coping Enhancement: Nursing Interventions

Definition

Assisting a patient to adapt to perceived stressors, changes, or threats that interfere with meeting life demands and roles.

Selected Activities

Use a calm, reassuring approach and provide an atmosphere of acceptance for patients and families.
Assist the patient and family in developing an objective appraisal of the event.
Provide factual information concerning diagnosis, treatment, and prognosis as needed.
Encourage an attitude of realistic hope as a way of dealing with feelings of helplessness.
Acknowledge the patient's spiritual/cultural background and encourage the use of spiritual resources if desired.
Foster constructive methods of dealing with life problems for patients and families.
Assist the patient and family to identify appropriate short- and long-term goals.
Appraise the needs and desires for social support and assist the patient and family to identify available support systems.
Assist the patient to identify positive strategies to deal with limitations, manage needed lifestyle or role changes, and work through the losses of chronic illness and/or disability if appropriate.

Adapted from Butcher, H. K., Bulechek, G. M., Dochterman, J. M. M., et al. (2018). *Nursing Interventions classification (NIC)-e-book* (7th Ed). Elsevier Health Science.

making compromises, comparing oneself to others, planning activities to conserve energy, taking things one step at a time, listening to one's body, and using self-talk for encouragement.

Unfolding Patient Stories: Skyler Hansen • Part 1

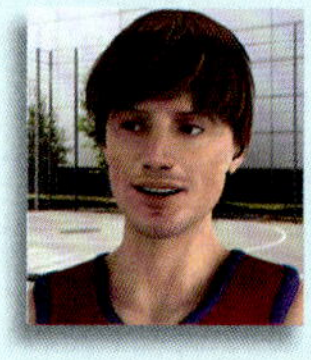

Skyler Hansen is an 18-year-old male recently diagnosed with type 1 diabetes. He lives with his parents and two younger siblings and is active in high school sports. He now requires insulin injections, glucose monitoring, and a diabetic diet. Examine how the psychological, physical, and teaching needs for managing a new diagnosis can be a great source of stress to the patient and the family. How can the nurse enhance his ability to cope with and adapt to diabetes management? (Skyler Hansen's story continues in Chapter 41.)

Care for Skyler and other patients in a realistic virtual environment: ***vSim** for Nursing* (**thepoint.lww.com/vSimMedicalSurgical**). Practice documenting these patients' care in DocuCare (**thepoint.lww.com/DocuCareEHR**).

Teaching Relaxation Techniques

Relaxation techniques are a major method used to relieve stress. The goal of relaxation training is to produce a response that counters the stress response. When this goal is achieved, the action of the hypothalamus adjusts, decreasing sympathetic and parasympathetic nervous system activity. The sequence of physiologic effects and their signs and symptoms are then interrupted, thus reducing psychological stress. This is a learned response and requires practice to achieve. Commonly used techniques include progressive muscle relaxation, the Benson relaxation response, and relaxation with **guided imagery** (all discussed later). Other relaxation techniques include meditation, breathing techniques, massage, Reiki, music therapy, biofeedback, and the use of humour.

The different relaxation techniques share four similar elements: (1) a quiet environment; (2) a comfortable position; (3) a passive attitude; and (4) a mental device (something on which to focus one's attention, such as a word, phrase, or sound).

Progressive Muscle Relaxation

Progressive muscle relaxation involves tensing and releasing the muscles of the body in sequence and sensing the difference in feeling. It is best if the person lies on a soft cushion, in a quiet room, breathing easily. Someone usually reads the instructions in a low tone in a slow and relaxed manner, or a recording of the instructions may be played. The person tenses the muscles in the entire body (one muscle group at a time), holds, senses the tension, and then relaxes. As each muscle group is tensed, the person keeps the rest of the body relaxed. Each time the focus is on feeling the tension and relaxation. When the exercise is completed, the entire body should be relaxed (Benson, 1993; Benson & Stark, 1996).

CHART 9-4

The Benson Relaxation Response

1. Pick a brief phrase or word that reflects your basic belief system.
2. Choose a comfortable position.
3. Close your eyes.
4. Relax your muscles.
5. Become aware of your breathing and start using your selected focus word.
6. Maintain a passive demeanour.
7. Continue for a set period of time.
8. Practice the technique twice daily.

Adapted from Benson, H. (1993). The relaxation response. In D. Goleman, & J. Gurin (Eds.). *Mind-body medicine: How to use your mind for better health*. Yonkers, NY: Consumer Reports Books.

Benson's Relaxation Response

The Benson relaxation response (Chart 9-4) combines meditation with relaxation. Along with the repeated word or phrase, a passive demeanour is essential. If other thoughts or distractions (noises, pain) occur, Benson recommends not fighting the distraction but simply continuing to repeat the focus phrase. Time of day is not important; however, the exercise works best on an empty stomach (Benson, 1993; Benson & Proctor, 1984; Benson & Stark, 1996).

Relaxation With Guided Imagery

Simple guided imagery is the mindful use of a word, phrase, or visual image for the purpose of distracting oneself from distressing situations or consciously taking time to relax or reenergize. A nurse can help a person select a pleasant scene or experience, such as watching the ocean or dabbling the feet in a cool stream. This image serves as the mental device in this technique. As the person sits comfortably and quietly, the nurse guides the person to review the scene, trying to feel and relive the imagery with all of the senses. A recording may be made of the description of the image, or commercial recordings for guided imagery and relaxation can be used. Other relaxation techniques include meditation, breathing techniques, massage, Reiki, music therapy, biofeedback, and the use of humour.

Educating About Stress Management

Two commonly prescribed nursing educational interventions—providing sensory information and providing procedural information (e.g., preoperative education)—aim to reduce stress and improve the patient's coping ability. This preparatory education includes giving structured content, such as a lesson in childbirth preparation to expectant parents, a review of how an implantable cardioverter defibrillator works to a patient with heart disease, or a description of sensations a patient will experience during cardiac catheterization. These techniques may alter the person–environment relationship such that something that might have been viewed as harmful or a threat will now be perceived more positively. Giving patients information also reduces the emotional response so that they can concentrate and solve problems more effectively (Christaki, Kokkinos, Costarelli, et al., 2013; Kells, Rogers, Oppenheimer, et al., 2013; Miller & Stoeckel, 2016).

Enhancing Social Support

The nature of social support and its influence on coping have been studied extensively. Social support has been demonstrated to be an effective moderator of life stress. Such support has been found to provide people with several different types of emotional information (Carpenter, Carpenter, Kimbel, et al., 2015; Cho, Jae, Choo, et al., 2014; Duax, Bohnert, Rausch, et al., 2014). The first type of information leads people to believe that they are cared for and loved. This emotional support appears most often in a relationship between two people in which mutual trust and attachment are expressed by helping one another meet their emotional needs. The second type of information leads people to believe that they are esteemed and valued. This is most effective when others in a group recognize a person's favourable position within that group, demonstrating the individual's value. Known as esteem support, this elevates the person's sense of self-worth. The third type of information leads people to feel that they belong to a network of communication and mutual obligation. Members of this network share information and make goods and services available to the members as needed.

Social support also facilitates a person's coping behaviours; however, this depends on the nature of the social support. People can have extensive relationships and interact frequently; however, the necessary support comes only when people feel a deep level of involvement and concern, not when they merely touch the surface of each other's lives. The critical qualities within a social network are the exchange of intimate communications and the presence of solidarity and trust.

Emotional support from family and significant others provides love and a sense of sharing the burden. The emotions that accompany stress are unpleasant and often increase in a spiralling fashion if relief is not provided. Being able to talk with someone and express feelings openly may help a person gain mastery of the situation. Nurses can provide this support; however, it is important to identify the person's social support system and encourage its use. People who are "loners," who are isolated, or who withdraw in times of stress have a high risk of coping failure.

Because anxiety can also distort a person's ability to process information, it helps to seek information and advice from others who can assist with analyzing the threat and developing a strategy to manage it. Again, this use of others helps people maintain mastery of a situation and self-esteem.

Thus, social networks assist with management of stress by providing people with:

- A positive social identity
- Emotional support
- Material aid and tangible services
- Access to information
- Access to new social contacts and new social roles

Recommending Support and Therapy Groups

Support groups exist especially for people in similar stressful situations. Groups have been formed by people with ostomies; women who have had mastectomies; and people with cancer or other serious diseases, chronic illnesses, and disabilities. There are groups for single parents, substance abusers and their family members, homicide bereavement, and victims of child abuse. Professional, civic, and religious support groups are active in many communities (Hundt, Robinson, Arney, et al., 2015; Wittenberg-Lyles, Goldsmith, & Reno, 2014; Wnuk, 2015). Encounter groups, assertiveness training programs, and consciousness-raising groups help people modify their usual behaviours in their transactions with their environment. Many find that being a member of a group with similar problems or goals has a releasing effect that promotes freedom of expression and exchange of ideas.

The Role of Stress in Health Patterns

As previously noted, a person's psychological and biologic health, internal and external sources of stress management, and relationships with the environment are predictors of health outcomes. These factors are directly related to the person's health patterns. The nurse has a significant role and responsibility in identifying the health patterns of the patient receiving care. If those patterns are not achieving physiologic, psychological, and social balance, the nurse is obligated, with the assistance and agreement of the patient, to seek ways to promote balance.

Although this chapter has presented some physiologic mechanisms and perspectives on health and disease, the way that one copes with stress, the way one relates to others, and the values and goals held are also interwoven into those physiologic patterns. To evaluate a patient's health patterns and to intervene if a disorder exists require a total assessment of the person. Specific disorders and their nursing management are addressed in greater depth in other chapters.

Critical Thinking Exercises

1 **pq** A 74-year-old man recently became a widower, stopped driving a car, and has moved from his home to a retirement community. He depends on his extended family members to provide for his transportation and shopping needs. He has hypertension and thyroid and coronary artery diseases. This patient has become increasingly sad since moving to his new home. Identify the priorities, approach, and techniques that you would use to assess this patient's health promotion needs.

2 **ebp** A patient experiences burns to the upper extremities after being involved in a kitchen fire. Describe the manner in which homeostasis has been disrupted and the compensatory mechanisms that are evident. How does the patient's medical treatment support the body's compensatory mechanisms? Determine the evidence-based nursing interventions that are appropriate for promoting the healing process.

3 A 70-year-old woman recently moved to a retirement community where she lives independently. A nurse practitioner assesses this patient's health promotion needs. The family's health history reveals that her mother had type 2 diabetes and thyroid disease, and that her father had hypertension and coronary artery disease. This patient has limited resources and support networks for making necessary lifestyle changes. What evidence exists to support the nurse practitioner's initiating strategies to promote a healthy lifestyle? What is the evidence that supports intervention to limit or prevent maladaptive responses from occurring with this woman? Describe the strength of the evidence regarding the effectiveness of lifestyle changes in promoting health in older adults.

REFERENCES AND SELECTED READINGS

Books

Bastable, S., Gramet, P., Jacobs, K., et al. (2014). *Health professional as educator: Principles of teaching and learning*. Sudbury, MA: Jones & Bartlett.

Benson, H. (1993). The relaxation response. In D. Goleman, & J. Gurin (Eds.). *Mind-body medicine: How to use your mind for better health*. Yonkers, NY: Consumer Reports Books.

Benson, H., & Proctor, W. (1984). *Beyond the relaxation response*. New York: Berkley Books.

Benson, H., & Stark, M. (1996). *Timeless healing*. New York: Scribner.

Butcher, H. K., Bulechek, G. M., Dochterman, J. M., et al. (2018). *Nursing interventions classification (NIC)-E-Book*. Oxford, UK: Elsevier Health Science.

El-Hussein, M. T., Power-Kean, K., Zettel, S., et al. (2018). *Understanding pathophysiology* (1st Canadian ed.). Ontario, Canada: Elsevier.

Fauci, A. (Ed.). (2006). *Harrison's principles of internal medicine* (16th ed.). New York: McGraw-Hill.

Grossman, S. C., & Porth, C. M. (2014). *Porth's Pathophysiology: Concepts of altered health status* (9th ed.). Philadelphia, PA: Lippincott Williams & Wilkins.

Herdman, T. H., & Kamitsuru, S. (Eds.). (2018). *Nursing diagnoses: Definitions & classification 2018–2020* (11th ed.). Stuttgart, Germany: Thieme.

Jalowiec, A. (1993). Coping with illness: Synthesis and critique of the nursing literature from 1980–1990. In J. D. Barnfather, & B. L. Lyon (Eds.). *Stress and coping: State of the science and implications for nursing theory, research, and practice*. Indianapolis, IN: Sigma Theta Tau International.

Lazarus, R. S. (1991a). *Emotion and adaptation*. New York: Oxford University Press.

Lazarus, R. S. (1993). Why we should think of stress as a subset of emotion. In L. Goldberger, & S. Breznitz (Eds.). *Handbook of stress: Theoretical and clinical aspects* (2nd ed.). New York: The Free Press.

Lazarus, R. S., & Folkman, S. (1984). *Stress, appraisal, and coping*. New York: Springer Publishing Co.

Miller, M. A., & Stoeckel, P. R. (2016). *Client education: Theory and practice* (2nd ed.). Sudbury, MA: Jones & Bartlett.

Rice, V. H. (Ed.). (2012). *Handbook of stress, coping, and health: Implications for theory, research, and practice* (2nd ed.). Thousand Oaks, CA: Sage.

Selye, H. (1976). *The stress of life* (Rev. ed.). New York: McGraw-Hill.

Skillen, D. L. (2012). Assessment of social, cultural, & spiritual health. In T. C. Stephen, D. L. Skillen, R. A. Day, et al. (Eds.). *Jensen's Canadian health assessment for nurses: A best practice approach* (1st Canadian ed.). Philadelphia, PA: Wolters Kluwer Health/Lippincott Williams & Wilkins.

Zoellner, L. A., & Feeny, N. C. (Eds.). (2014). *Facilitating resilience and recovery following trauma*. New York: Guilford Press.

Journals

Akyil, R. C., & Erguney, S. (2013). Roy's adaptation model-guided education for adaptation to chronic obstructive pulmonary disease. *Journal of Advanced Nursing*, *69*(5), 1063–1075.

Alasad, J. A., Abu Tabar, N., & Ahmad, M. M. (2015). Patients' experience of being in intensive care units. *Journal of Critical care*, *30*(4), 859.e7–e11.

Alhurani, A. S., Dekker, R., Ahmad, M., et al. (2018). Stress, cognitive appraisal, coping, and event free survival in patients with heart failure. *Heart & Lung*, *47*(3), 205–210.

Austin, W., Gable, E., Leier, B., et al. (2009). Compassion fatigue: The experience of nurses. *Ethics and Social Welfare*, *3*(2), 195–214.

Baczewska, B., Kropornicka, B., Sepiolo, J., et al. (2015). Acceptance of illness and satisfaction with life among patients with arterial hypertension. *Health Problems of Civilization*, *9*(3), 31–38.

Barre, V. P., Padmaja, G., Saxena, R. K., et al. (2015). Impact of medical interventions on stress and quality of life in patients with cancer. *Indian Journal of Palliative Care*, *21*(2), 203–208.

Baumann, S. (2007). Recovering from abuse: A comparison of three paths. *Nursing Science Quarterly*, *20*(4), 342–348.

Bekyarova, G., Tzaneva, M., Hristova, M., et al. (2014). Melatonin protection against burn-induced liver injury. A review. *Central European Journal of Medicine*, *9*(1), 148–158.

Bertisch, H., Rath, L., Long, C., et al. (2014). Positive psychology in rehabilitation medicine: A brief report. *NeuroRehabilitation*, *34*(3), 573–585.

Boland, T. A., Lee, V. H., & Bleck, T. P. (2015). Stress-induced cardiomyopathy. *Critical Care Medicine*, *43*(3), 686–693.

Caldeira, S., & Timmins, F. (2016). Resilience: Synthesis of concept analyses and contribution to nursing classifications. *International Nursing Review*, *63*(2), 191–199.

Carpenter, G. S., Carpenter, T. P., Kimbel, N. A., et al. (2015). Social support, stress, and suicidal ideation in professional firefighters. *American Journal of Health Behavior*, *39*(2), 191–196.

Cevik, R. C., & Erguney, S. (2013). Roy's adaptation model-guided education for adaptation to chronic obstructive pulmonary disease. *Journal of Advanced Nursing*, *69*(5), 1063–1075.

Chien, W. T., & Yick, S. Y. (2016). An investigation of nurses' job satisfaction in a private hospital and its correlates. *The Open Nursing Journal*, *10*, 99.

Christaki, E., Kokkinos, A., Costarelli, V., et al. (2013). Stress management can facilitate weight loss in Greek overweight and obese women: A pilot study. *Journal of Human Nutrition and Dietetics*, *26*(1), 132–139.

Cho, J. H., Jae, S. Y., Choo, I. H., et al. (2014). Health-promoting behavior among women with abdominal obesity: A conceptual link to social support and perceived stress. *Journal of Advanced Nursing*, *70*(6), 1381–1390.

Chung, M. C., Jones, R. C., Harding, S. A., et al. (2016). Posttraumatic stress disorder among older patients with chronic obstructive pulmonary disease. *The Psychiatric Quarterly*, *87*(4), 605–618.

DeForge, R., Ward-Griffin, C., St-Amant, O., et al. (2017). Evaluating dementia home care practices: The reification of care norms. *Journal of Aging Studies*, *43*, 23–31.

Dorsett, P., Geraghty, T., Sinnott, A., et al. (2017). Hope, coping and psychosocial adjustment after spinal cord injury. *Spinal Cord Series and Cases*, *3*, 17046.

Duax, J. M., Bohnert, K. M., Rauch, S. A., et al. (2014). Posttraumatic stress disorder symptoms, levels of social support, and emotional hiding in returning veterans. *Journal of Rehabilitation Research and Development*, *51*(4), 571–578.

Duncan, G. J., Magnuson, K., & Votruba-Drzal, E. (2017). Moving beyond correlations in assessing the consequences of poverty. *Annual Review of Psychology*, *68*, 413–434.

Epel, E. S., & Lithgow, G. J. (2014). Stress biology and aging mechanisms: Toward understanding the deep connection between adaptation to stress and longevity. *The Journals of Gerontology. Series A, Biological Sciences and Medical Sciences*, *69*(1), S10–S16.

Fisher, A. B., & Forman, H. J. (2014). Antioxidants in the intensive care unit. *American Journal of Respiratory and Critical Care Medicine*, *189*(8), 1007–1008.

Fox, S., Lydon, S., Byrne, D., et al. (2018). A systematic review of interventions to foster physician resilience. *Postgraduate Medical Journal*, *94*, 162–170.

Geiker, N. R. W., Astrup, A., Hjorth, M. F., et al. (2018). Does stress influence sleep patterns, food intake, weight gain, abdominal obesity and weight loss interventions and vice versa? *Obesity Reviews*, *19*(1), 81–97.

Grant, L., & Kinman, G. (2014). Emotional resilience in the helping professions and how it can be enhanced. *Health and Social Care Education*, *3*(1), 23–34.

Guccione, A. A. (2014). Resilience and self-efficacy as mediators of quality of life in geriatric rehabilitation. *Topics in Geriatric Rehabilitation*, *30*(3), 164–169.

Hankonen, N., Konttinen, H., & Absetz, P. (2014). Gender-related personality traits, self-efficacy, and social support: How do they relate to women's waist circumference change? *Journal of Health Psychology, 19*(10), 1291–1301.

Harper, G. W., Bruce, D., Hosek, S. G., et al. (2014). Resilience processes demonstrated by gay and bisexual men living with HIV: Implications for intervention. *AIDS Patient Care and STDs, 28*(12), 666–676.

Herrick, A. L., Egan, J. E., Coulter, R. W., et al. (2014). Raising sexual minority youths' health levels by incorporating resiliencies into health promotion efforts. *American Journal of Public Health, 104*(2), 206–210.

Holmes, T. H., & Rahe, R. H. (1967). The social readjustment rating scale. *Journal of Psychosomatic Research, 11*, 213–218.

Holton, M. K., Barry, A. E., & Chaney, J. D. (2016). Employee stress management: An examination of adaptive and maladaptive coping strategies on employee health. *Work, 53*(2), 299–305.

Huang, L. B., Tsai, Y. F., Liu, C. Y., et al. (2017). Influencing and protective factors of suicidal ideation among older adults. *International Journal of Mental Health Nursing, 26*(2), 191–199.

Hundt, N. E., Robinson, A., Arney, J., et al. (2015). Veterans' perspectives on benefits and drawbacks of peer support for posttraumatic stress disorder. *Military Medicine, 180*(8), 851–856.

Izaguirre, A., & Calvete, E. (2015). Children who are exposed to intimate partner violence: Interviewing mothers to understand its impact on children. *Child Abuse & Neglect, 48*, 58–67.

Jain, M., & Chandel, N. S. (2013). Rethinking antioxidants in the intensive care unit. *American Journal of Respiratory Care Medicine, 188*(11), 1283–1285.

Jokela, M., Pulkki-Raback, L., Elovaino, M., et al. (2014). Personality traits as risk factors for stroke and coronary heart disease mortality: Pooled analysis of three cohort studies. *Journal of Behavioral Medicine, 37*, 881–889.

Kells, M., Rogers, J., Oppenheimer, S. C., et al. (2013). The teachable moment captured: A framework for nurse-led smoking cessation interventions for parents of hospitalized children. *Public Health Nursing, 30*(5), 468–473.

Lazarus, R. S. (1991b). Cognition and motivation in emotion. *American Psychologist, 46*(4), 352–367.

Lazarus, R. S. (1991c). Progress on a cognitive-motivational-relational theory of emotion. *American Psychologist, 46*(8), 819–834.

Lavoie, J. A. (2013). Eye of the beholder: Perceived stress, coping style, and coping effectiveness among discharged psychiatric patients. *Archives of Psychiatric Nursing, 27*, 185–190.

Makam, A. N., Nguyen, O. K., Xuan, L., et al. (2018). Factors associated with variation in long-term acute care hospital vs skilled nursing facility use among hospitalized older adults. *JAMA Internal Medicine, 178*(3), 399–405.

McDonald, G., Jackson, D., Wilkes, L., et al. (2013). Personal resilience in nurses and midwives: Effects of a work-based educational intervention. *Contemporary Nurse, 45*(1), 134–143.

McVicar, A., Ravalier, J. M., & Greenwood, C. (2014). Biology of stress revisited: Intracellular mechanisms and the conceptualization of stress. *Stress and Health, 30*(4), 272–279.

Modecki, K. L., Zimmer Gembeck, M. J., & Guerra, N. (2017). Emotion regulation, coping, and decision making: three linked skills for preventing externalizing problems in adolescence. *Child Development, 88*(2), 417–426.

Monden, K. R., Trost, Z., Catalano, D., et al. (2014). Resilience following spinal cord injury: A phenomenological view. *Spinal Cord, 52*, 197–201.

Muir, K., & Strnadova, I. (2014). Whose responsibility? Resilience in families of children with developmental disabilities. *Disability & Society, 29*(6), 922–937.

O'Shea, E., Timmons, S., O'Shea, E., et al. (2017). Key stakeholders' experiences of respite services for people with dementia and their perspectives on respite service development: A qualitative systematic review. *BMC Geriatrics, 17*(1), 282.

Otaghi, M., Nazarpour, B., Taghinegad, H., et al. (2018). The effect of care plan based on Roy Adaptation Model on the spiritual well-being of women with breast cancer. *Analysis*, 22, 92.

Parker, A. M., Sricharoenchai, T., Raparla, S., et al. (2015). Posttraumatic stress disorder in critical illness survivors: A metaanalysis. *Critical Care Medicine, 43*(5), 1121–1129.

Pimenta, F., Maroco, J., Ramos, C., et al. (2014). Predictors of weight variation and weight gain in peri-and post-menopausal women. *Journal of Health Psychology, 19*(8), 993–1002.

Polloni, L., Ferruzza, E., Ronconi, L., et al. (2015). Perinatal stress and food allergy: A preliminary study on maternal reports. *Psychology, Health & Medicine, 20*(6), 732–741.

Prince, L., Chappelle, W. L., McDonald, K. D., et al. (2015). Reassessment of psychological distress and post-traumatic stress disorder in United States Air Force distributed common ground system operators. *Military Medicine, 180*(3), 171–178.

Princip, M., Gattlen, C., Meister-Langraf, R. E., et al. (2018). The role of illness perception and its association with posttraumatic stress at three months following acute myocardial infarction. *Frontiers in Psychology, 9*, 941.

Sampaio, C. V. S., Lima, M. G., & Ladeia, A. M. (2017). Meditation, health and scientific investigations: review of the literature. *Journal of Religion and Health, 56*(2), 411–427.

Schonfels, P., Brailovskaia, J., Bieda, A., et al. (2015). The effects of daily stress on positive and negative mental health: Mediation through self-efficacy. *International Journal of Clinical and Health Psychology, 28*(3), 256–266.

Schwitalla, S. (2014). Tumor cell plasticity: The challenge to catch a moving target. *Journal of Gastroenterology, 49*, 618–627.

Shields, G. S., & Slavich, G. M. (2017). Lifetime stress exposure and health: A review of contemporary assessment methods and biological mechanisms. *Social and Personality Psychology Compass, 11*(8), e12335.

Shudifat, R. M., & Al-Husban, R. Y. (2015). Perceived sources of stress among first-year nursing students in Jordan. *Journal of Psychosocial Nursing and Mental Health Services, 53*(6), 37–43.

Skodova, Z., & Lajciakova, P. (2013). The effect of personality traits and psychosocial training on burnout syndrome among healthcare students. *Nurse Education Today, 33*, 1311–1315.

Smith, A., Fortune, Z., Phillips, R., et al. (2014). UPBEAT study patients' perceptions of the effect of coronary heart disease on their lives: A cross-sectional sub-study. *International Journal of Nursing Studies, 51*, 1500–1506.

Su, X., Lau, J. T., Mak, W. W., et al. (2013). Perceived discrimination, social support, and perceived stress among people living with HIV/AIDS in China. *AIDS Care, 25*(2), 239–248.

Tam-Tham, H., Nettel-Aguirre, A., Silvius, J., et al. (2016). Provision of dementia-related services in Canada: a comparative study. *BMC Health Services Research, 16*(1), 184.

Tausig, M. (1982). Measuring life events. *Journal of Health and Social Behavior, 23*(1), 52–64.

Taylor, C. J. (2013). Physiological stress response to loss of social influence and threats to masculinity. *Social Science & Medicine, 103*, 51–59.

Theron, L. C., Theron, A. M., & Malindi, M. J. (2013). Toward an African definition of resilience: A rural South African community's view of resilient Basotho youth. *Journal of Black Psychology, 39*(1), 63–87.

Thomson, A. K., Heyworth, J. S., Girschik, J., et al. (2014). Beliefs and perceptions about the causes of breast cancer: a case-control study. *BMC Research Notes, 7*(1), 558.

Trief, P. M., Sandberg, J. G., Dimmock, J. A., et al. (2013). Personal and relationship challenges of adults with type 1 diabetes: A qualitative focus group study. *Diabetes Care, 36*, 2483–2488.

Wittenberg-Lyles, E., Goldsmith, J., & Reno, J. (2014). Perceived benefits and challenges of an oncology nurse support group. *Clinical Journal of Oncology Nursing, 18*(4), E71–E76.

Wnuk, M. (2015). Religious-spiritual sources of hope and the meaning of life in alcohol co-dependent subjects receiving support in self-help groups. *Journal of Substance Use, 20*(3), 194–199.

Yi-Frazier, J. P., Fladeboe, K., Klein, V., et al. (2017). Promoting Resilience in Stress Management for Parents (PRISM-P): An intervention for caregivers of youth with serious illness. *Families, Systems, & Health, 35*(3), 341.

Resources

Centre for Stress Management: http://www.managingstress.com/articles/definition.htm

Inflammation—The Key to Chronic Disease: http://www.womentowomen.com/inflammation/default.aspx

Institute of HeartMath: Empowering Heart-Based Living: http://www.heartmath.org/

Stress: The Silent Killer: http://holisticonline.com/stress/stress_GAS.htm

The Psychology of "Stress": http://www.guidetopsychology.com/stress.htm

10 Individual and Family Considerations Related to Illness

Adapted by Annette M. Lane and Marlette B. Reed

Learning Objectives

On completion of this chapter, the learner will be able to:

1. Describe a psychosocial typology of illness.
2. Discuss human responses to illness, such as anxiety, depression, and grief.
3. Discuss the challenges of extenuating circumstances, such as posttraumatic stress disorder (PTSD) and dying and death.
4. Discuss the concepts of healthy and unhealthy coping.
5. Understand the reasons for substance abuse and consider how the nurse can identify substance abuse problems.
6. Assess the impact of illness on the patient's family and on family functioning.
7. Identify nursing actions that promote effective coping for both patients and their families.

When individuals encounter threats to their health, they often experience an assault to their personhood, or sense of self. Their previous view of themselves, perhaps as strong and in control, may be replaced by feelings of powerlessness, fear, and uncertainty. In response to physical symptoms and altered self-concept, individuals seek ways to manage not only the physical aspect of their illness, but also the psychological responses to their illness and to their new and unanticipated life. Similarly, **family** members may experience worry about a loved one's symptoms, or express shock when a diagnosis is determined, or even display fear for the loved one's future. In addition, family members often wonder how the illness will impact the individual as well as themselves. How will they support their family member, and what will that support entail? This chapter examines the individual and family response to illness according to Rolland's (2018) psychosocial typology of illness. Common responses to illness, including **anxiety**, **depression**, and loss and **grief**, are discussed. Extenuating circumstances, such as **posttraumatic stress disorder (PTSD)** and dying and death, are also addressed, along with coping methods of individuals and family considerations in illness. Finally, this chapter considers how nurses can assess and intervene in situations where individuals are experiencing challenging illnesses.

Psychosocial Typology of Illness

Rolland's psychosocial typology (2018) of illness provides a useful framework for nurses to understand how individuals and families respond to illness, depending in part upon the illness trajectory. Rolland (2018) classified illness according to the following categories: onset, course, outcome, and incapacitation. The onset of illness may be acute or gradual. The skills needed by individuals to respond effectively to each type of onset are different (Rolland, 2018). For example, individuals and family members will likely respond differently to the shock of an acute illness, such as a myocardial infarction (MI), as compared to an illness with a gradual onset, such as multiple sclerosis (MS).

Individuals who experience an MI, for instance, may feel shock, anger, and intense fear (Heart and Stroke Foundation Canada, 2018). Fear may be related not only to the fear of death, but also to the apparent suddenness of the MI. As a result, individuals commonly experience anxiety (Abu-Ruz & Masa'Deh, 2017) and depression (Page, Davidson, Edward, et al., 2010) following a cardiac event. Family members need to mobilize crisis management skills in a short period of time.

In contrast, individuals with MS may experience fear and grief prior to diagnosis and may undergo multiple tests over an extended period of time before this diagnosis is reached (Multiple Sclerosis Foundation, 2016), and then experience some relief for the fact that a diagnosis is finally made. As the onset of symptoms has been more gradual, family members have had time to adjust to changes in the health of their loved one (Rolland, 2018).

The course of illness also impacts how patients and families experience an illness. Rolland (2018) considered the course of illness to include three types: progressive, constant, and relapsing/episodic. An example of a progressive illness course is Alzheimer's disease (AD). The symptoms of AD are generally continuous but become more severe over time (Alzheimer Society of Canada, 2018). Family members of an individual with AD experience extreme fatigue caregiving for their loved one over the course of years. In contrast, an example of a constant course of illness is when an individual experiences a spinal cord injury resulting in paraplegia. While there is a sudden and dramatic change in functioning, the individual's health status stabilizes after the event (Lane & Reed, 2015). The relapsing/episodic course of illness involves periods of stability that are interspersed with acute flare-ups. An example of such an illness is asthma. Although family members have periods of stability where they can gather strength, they live with a sense of impending danger of a possible acute emergency.

The outcome refers to the likelihood that the illness will result in death or will shorten an individual's life span (Rolland, 2018). For example, individuals who have advanced cancer are faced with great uncertainty about how long they have to live and may experience resignation and challenges coping (Brown & de Graaf, 2013). Family members share in that uncertainty and experience the range of emotions that come with it. Family members may struggle with wanting intimacy with their dying loved one as well as wanting to distance themselves from the individual (Rolland, 2018). Some family members may detach emotionally before their loved one has passed away, presenting a challenging situation for staff when other family members are hurt by this.

Incapacitation refers to the amount of disability caused by the illness (Rolland, 2018). The incapacitation may impact cognition (e.g., AD), the senses (such as blindness), or functionality (e.g., rheumatoid arthritis). The onset of incapacitation, such as a spinal cord injury (as noted above) is sudden and severe and requires the family to mobilize resources from the time of the injury. When the onset of incapacitation is slower, such as in MS, the family has more time to adjust to the illness and mobilize supports (Rolland, 2018).

Rolland (2018) included one more important aspect of coping with disability: stigma. Nurses must be aware of the fact that when an illness is stigmatized, coping may be more difficult. Conditions that may carry a stigma include HIV/AIDS (Costelloe, Kemppainen, Brion, et al., 2015), severe mental illness such as schizophrenia (Abiri, Oakley, Hitchcock, et al., 2016), or facial and other deformities. In addition, family members of patients with such conditions may also experience stigma, either through the responses of others toward their loved one or toward themselves (Liegghio, 2017). One man, whose sister was dying of Creutzfeldt–Jakob disease, said, sitting on the floor outside his sister's hospital room, "How do you tell people that she is dying of the human form of Mad Cow disease?" Only those closest to the patient were permitted to visit; her brother felt that people had pulled away from *him*, with this unusual diagnosis his sister had received.

Responses to Illnesses

As noted previously, individuals may experience anxiety, depression, and grief in relation to their illnesses. Understanding this is important, as individuals who are anxious or depressed will visit emergency departments more often than those who are not (Abar, Holub, Lee, et al., 2017). Such individuals may also experience higher levels of pain related to their illness (Brandt, Zvolensky, Daumas, et al., 2016) and may have poorer health outcomes (Amoozegar, Patten, Becker, et al., 2017). Some individuals may seek to quell feelings of anxiety and depression through substances such as alcohol. The following section addresses anxiety, depression, and grief related to illness.

Anxiety

All people experience some degree of anxiety (a tense emotional state) as they face new, challenging, or threatening life situations. In clinical settings, fear of the unknown, unexpected news about one's health, and impairment of bodily functions engender anxiety (Legg, Andrews, Huynh, et al., 2015). Although a mild level of anxiety can mobilize a person to take a position, act on the task that needs to be done, or learn to alter lifestyle habits, more severe anxiety can be paralyzing (Legg et al., 2015). When patients receive unwelcome news about results of diagnostic studies, they are certain to experience anxiety. Different patients manifest the physiologic, emotional, and behavioural signs and symptoms of anxiety in different ways.

Nursing Implications

Early clinical observations of anxiety are essential components of nursing care (Chart 10-1). A high level of anxiety is very uncomfortable for the patient and may exacerbate

Glossary

anxiety: an emotional state characterized by feelings of apprehension, discomfort, restlessness, or worry

depression: state in which a person feels sad, distressed, and hopeless, with little to no energy for usual activities

family: a group whose members are related by reciprocal caring, mutual responsibilities, and loyalties

grief: a universal response to any loss

posttraumatic stress disorder (PTSD): the development of severe anxiety-type symptoms after the experience of a traumatic life event

substance abuse: a maladaptive pattern of drug use that causes physical and emotional harm with the potential for disruption of daily life

CHART 10-1

Assessing for Anxiety

Be alert for the following:

Physiologic Indicators

- Appetite change
- Headaches
- Muscle tension
- Fatigue or lethargy
- Weight change
- Digestive upsets
- Palpitations
- Restlessness
- Difficulty sleeping

Emotional/Cognitive Indicators

- Forgetfulness
- Low productivity
- Feeling dull
- Poor concentration
- Negative attitude
- Confusion
- Whirling mind
- Boredom
- Negative self-talk
- Anxiety
- Frustration
- Depression
- Crying periods
- Irritability
- Worrying

Relational Indicators

- Isolation
- Loneliness

Adapted from Jenkins, E., & Musto, L. (2019). Anxiety, obsessive-compulsive and related disorders. In W. Austin, D. Kunyk, C. A. Peternelj-Taylor, & M. A. Boyd (Eds.). *Psychiatric & mental health nursing for Canadian practice* (4th ed., pp. 512–539). Philadelphia, PA: Wolters Kluwer.

CHART 10-2

Managing Anxiety

- Listen actively and allow patient to discuss personal feelings.
- Use positive remarks and dwell on the positive aspects of life in the "here and now."
- Discuss the importance of safety and the patient's overall sense of well-being.
- Explain all procedures, policies, medications, or protocols for care.
- Explore coping strategies and work with the patient to practice them effectively (e.g., breathing, progressive relaxation, visualization, imagery).
- Use distraction as necessary to relax and prevent self from being overwhelmed.

Adapted from Hegadoren, K., & Lasiuk, G. (2015). Anxiety and obsessive-compulsive disorders. In W. Austin, & M. A. Boyd (Eds.). *Psychiatric & mental health nursing for Canadian practice* (3rd ed., pp. 480–504). Philadelphia, PA: Wolters Kluwer.

physiologic distress. For example, a postoperative patient who is in pain may discover that anxiety intensifies the sensation of pain (Sherman, Winch, Koukoulis, et al., 2015). A patient newly diagnosed with type 1 diabetes mellitus may be worried and fearful and therefore unable to focus on or complete essential self-care activities. Many medical conditions (e.g., a breast lump or heart condition) cause anxiety. Many assessment findings alert the nurse to patients with moderate to severe anxiety.

Nurses must be vigilant about patients who worry excessively and deteriorate in emotional, social, or occupational functioning. If participation in the therapeutic regimen (e.g., administration of insulin) becomes a problem because of extreme anxiety, nursing interventions must be immediately initiated. Caring strategies emphasize ways for the patient to verbalize feelings and fears and to identify sources of anxiety. The need to teach and promote effective coping abilities and the use of relaxation techniques are the priorities of care. In some cases, antianxiety medication may be prescribed. Chart 10-2 provides a list of basic nursing principles that are useful to assist patients in managing severe anxiety. Chapter 9 presents additional information about stress and the relaxation response.

Depression

Depression is a common response to health issues and is an underdiagnosed condition, particularly in hospitalized patients (Dennis, Kadri, & Coffey, 2012). People may become depressed as a result of injury (Ahl, Lindgren, Cao, et al., 2017) or illness, may be suffering from an earlier loss that is compounded by a new health issue, or may seek health care for somatic manifestations of depression. The cause of depression is multifaceted and includes an interaction of genetic, biologic, social, and psychological factors (Canadian Mental Health Association, 2014a).

Clinical depression is distinguished from everyday feelings of sadness by its duration and severity (Canadian Mental Health Association, 2014a). Most people occasionally feel down or depressed, but these feelings are short lived and do not result in impaired functioning. The American Psychiatric Association (2013) describes the diagnostic criteria for depression. Unfortunately, only one out of three persons who are depressed receives an appropriate diagnosis and treatment (American Psychiatric Association, 2013).

Not all individuals with depression present in a sad manner. Many function appropriately in their interactions with the outside world by exerting great effort and forcing themselves to mask their distress. Sometimes they are successful at hiding their depression for months or years and astonish family members and others when they finally admit that they are seriously depressed. Some people, particularly older adults, experience depression but may seek treatment for somatic concerns (Dennis et al., 2012). Individuals with depression may present with chest or abdominal pain (Abar et al., 2017), or aggression, irritability, violence, **substance abuse**, risky behaviour, or somatic complaints such as headaches and chronic pain.

CHART 10-3

Risk Factors for Depression

- Family history
- Stressful situations
- Prior episodes of depression
- Onset before age 40 years
- Medical comorbidity
- Past suicide attempts
- Lack of support systems
- History of physical or sexual abuse
- Current substance abuse

Adapted from Rupcich, C. (2019). Depressive, bipolar, and related disorders. In W. Austin, D. Kunyk, C. A. Peternelj-Taylor, & M. A. Boyd (Eds.). *Psychiatric & mental health nursing for Canadian practice* (4th ed., pp. 474–511). Philadelphia, PA: Wolters Kluwer.

Nursing Implications

Because any loss in function, change in role, or alteration in body image is a possible antecedent to depression, nurses in all settings encounter patients who are depressed or who have thought about suicide. Depression is suspected if changes in the patient's thoughts or feelings and a loss of self-esteem are noted. Chart 10-3 lists risk factors for depression. Depression can occur at any age, and it is diagnosed more frequently in women than in men. When caring for older patients, nurses should be aware that decreased mental alertness, withdrawal-type responses, or emphasis on physical symptoms may be indicative of depression.

Talking with the patient about his or her fears, sharing relevant personal information, showing interest and acceptance, and communicating clearly have been found to help alleviate a sense of helplessness and worthlessness expressed by patients who are depressed (Parcival, Donovan, Kessler, et al., 2017). Helping the patient to talk about actual or potential losses, as well as his/her grief, may lessen the depressive response to illness. It may also be possible to help the patient identify and decrease negative self-talk and unrealistic expectations and show how these contribute to depression. The nurse monitors the patient for the onset of new concerns because depression adversely affects physical health and self-care activities. All patients with depression should be evaluated by psychiatry to determine if they would benefit from antidepressant therapy or mental health support following discharge from hospital.

In addition to the measures previously listed, psychoeducational programs, the establishment of support systems, and counselling can reduce depression-related distress. Psychoeducational programs can help patients and their families understand depression, treatment options, and coping strategies.

NURSING ALERT

In crisis situations, it is imperative that patients be referred to psychiatrists, psychiatric nurse specialists, advanced practice psychiatric mental health nurses, or crisis centres.

Nurses need to explain to patients that depression is a medical illness and not a sign of personal weakness and that effective treatment will allow them to feel better and stay emotionally healthy (Canadian Mental Health Association, 2014a).

Suicide

Suicide is the ninth leading cause of death in Canada. Approximately 10 Canadians die by suicide each day and approximately 90% of these individuals were living with a mental health issue (Public Health Agency of Canada, 2016). While women attempt suicide more often than men, men die more often of suicide because of the lethality of the methods chosen (Public Health Agency of Canada, 2016).

Risk factors for suicide include a prior suicide attempt, family history of suicide, a serious physical or mental health problem, substance abuse, a significant loss through death or divorce, and social isolation (Canadian Mental Health Association, 2014b). High-risk populations include some First Nations and Metis communities, Inuit peoples, youth (those between 15 and 24 years of age), and older men (Government of Canada, 2016). See Chart 10-4 for risk factors for suicide.

Loss and Grief

Grief is a normal response to illness, as illness experiences often include loss. This is particularly the case when the illness changes the expected life span of an individual (e.g., metastatic cancer), or when illness impacts what a person can do (e.g., activities of daily living, paid employment, ability to play sports), how the person appears to others (e.g., changes in appearance due to scleroderma), or how the individual perceives him/herself (a person who was athletic and is now in a wheelchair due to a spinal injury). Illness may impact self-esteem, as well as how one perceives him/herself, resulting in chronic sorrow (Weingarten, 2012).

People grieve in different ways, and there is no timeline for completing the bereavement process. The time of

CHART 10-4

Risk Factors for Suicide

- Age younger than 20 or older than 65 years
- Gender—women make more attempts, men are more successful
- Childhood trauma (abuse)
- Family history of suicide
- Severe depression
- Severe, intractable pain
- Chronic, debilitating medical problems
- Substance abuse
- Lethal suicide plan
- Previous suicide attempt

Adapted from Santa Mina, E. (2019). Self-harm behaviour and suicide. In W. Austin, D. Kunyk, C. A. Peternelj-Taylor, & M. A. Boyd (Eds.). *Psychiatric & mental health nursing for Canadian practice* (4th ed., pp. 374–400). Philadelphia, PA: Wolters Kluwer.

grieving often depends on the significance of the loss, the anticipation of or preparation for the loss, the person's emotional stability and maturity, and the person's coping abilities.

Regardless of the duration of the grieving process, there are two basic goals: (1) healing the self and (2) incorporating that loss into one's life and moving forward. Other factors that influence grieving are the type of loss, previous life experiences with various changes and transitions, religious beliefs (Klass, 2014), cultural background (Rosenblatt, 2017), and personality characteristics. Some individuals may resort to abusing prescription medications, illegal drugs, or alcohol if they find it difficult to cope with the loss; the grief process is then complicated by the use of addictive substances (Masferrer, Garre-Olmo, & Caparros, 2017).

Nursing Implications

Nurses identify patients and family members who are grieving and work with them to accomplish the four major tasks of the grief process: (1) acceptance of the loss, (2) acknowledgement of the intensity of the pain of the loss, (3) adaptation to life after the loss, and (4) cultivation of new relationships and activities (Worden, 1991). Nurses assess for levels of depression in grief. Grief is a universal experience in significant loss; and depression is not uncommon in grief. However, the skilled nurse can differentiate between the depression that will run its course as the loss is grieved, and that which will need professional help.

The physical response to grief includes crying, headaches, chest pain, loss of appetite, weakness, fatigue, aches and pains, as well as difficulties with sleep (Granek, Ben-David, Shapira, et al., 2017). Symptoms such as chest pain should be assessed medically to rule out cardiac problems. Further, a patient whose grief is compromising the ability to care for the self and manage illness should be provided psychological support. Because grief also impacts the family, the patient's loved ones should be offered support as well (Mendes, 2017).

Extenuating Circumstances

Posttraumatic Stress Disorder

In medical-surgical settings, especially in emergency departments, burn units, and rehabilitation centres, nurses care for extremely anxious patients who have experienced overwhelming events that may be outside the range of usual human experience. In response to these extenuating circumstances, individuals may suffer from PTSD. The American Psychiatric Association (2013) describes the symptoms and characteristic presentations of PTSD. Events that place people at risk for PTSD include rape, violence (Bender, Eynan, O'Grady, et al., 2016) (including family violence), torture, terrorist attacks, fire, earthquakes (Gokcen, Sahingöz, & Annagur, 2013), and military combat (Fry, 2016). Patients who have experienced a traumatic event are often frequent users of the health care system, seeking treatment for the overall emotional and physical trauma that they experienced.

Symptoms of PTSD can occur hours to years after the trauma is experienced. Acute PTSD is defined as the experience of symptoms for less than a 3-month period. Chronic

CHART 10-5

Assessing for Posttraumatic Stress Disorder (PTSD)

Be alert for the following:

Psychological/Behavioural Indicators

- Anxiety/fear
- Anger
- Depression
- Hypervigilance
- Nightmares or flashbacks
- Intrusive thoughts related to trauma
- Memory impairments
- Restlessness and irritability
- Strong startle response
- Substance abuse
- Feelings of estrangement
- Feelings of helplessness, worthlessness, hopelessness, or powerlessness
- Inability to concentrate

Adapted from McCay, E. A. (2019). Care of persons with a history of abuse. In W. Austin, D. Kunyk, C. A. Peternelj-Taylor, & M. A. Boyd (Eds.). *Psychiatric & mental health nursing for Canadian practice* (4th ed., pp. 877–918). Philadelphia, PA: Wolters Kluwer.

PTSD is defined as the experience of symptoms lasting longer than 3 months. In the case of delayed PTSD, up to 6 months may elapse between the trauma and the manifestation of symptoms (American Psychiatric Association, 2013). Please see Chart 10-5 for assessment of PTSD.

Nurses must be aware that PTSD or posttraumatic stress syndrome (PTSS) (manifesting many of the symptoms of PTSD but not meeting the full criteria for PTSD) may come from hospitalization. Studies show that individuals treated for acute coronary syndrome may experience symptoms of PTSD (Sundquist, Chang, Parsons, et al., 2016), as well as those treated in the ICU (Warlan, Howland, & Connelly, 2016). Also, family members of individuals in critical care units (Petrinic, 2017; Trevick & Lord, 2017) or parents of children in a neonatal intensive care unit (Aftyka, Rybojad, Rosa, et al., 2017) may experience PTSD symptoms.

Nurses may also experience PTSD or trauma symptoms due to their work. Although studies usually report on PTSD symptoms among nurses who work in critical care areas, PTSD has also been documented among nurses who work in other high-stress work environments such as operating rooms and emergency departments (McMeekin, Hickman, Douglas, et al., 2017; Mealer, Jones, & Meek, 2017). Resilience, however, decreases the risks of developing PTSD (Mealer et al., 2017). See Chart 10-6 for a study examining PTSD and resilience in intensive care nurses.

Nursing Implications

The incidence of PTSD is thought to be very low in the overall population; however, Statistics Canada reported a lifetime prevalence of 8% (2015). In high-risk groups, such as those in the military, or individuals who have been traumatized through assaults or natural disasters, the risk is much higher. Nurses must consider which of their

NURSING RESEARCH PROFILE

Chart 10-6. Factors Affecting Resilience and Development of Posttraumatic Stress Disorder in Critical Care Nurses

Mealer, M., Jones, J., & Meek, P. (2017). Factors affecting resilience and development of posttraumatic stress disorder in critical care nurses. *American Journal of Critical Care*, *26*(3), 184–192. doi: https://doi.org/10.4037/ajcc2017798

Purpose

The purpose of this study was to identify individual and group characteristics that impact resilience and to determine if the individual or group characteristics have a direct or indirect impact upon posttraumatic stress disorder (PTSD). Further, the researchers examined personal characteristics of resilience.

Design

The researchers conducted a secondary analysis of data using a statistical modeling program Mplus to examine surveys sent to 3,500 American critical care nurses. Surveys examined the prevalence of PTSD, burnout, anxiety, depression, and resilience. Researchers examined 744 completed surveys.

Findings

Nurses who worked in intensive care units (other than medical) and scored high for resilience were 18% to 50% less likely to experience PTSD than nurses with lower resilience scores. Nurses who possessed graduate degrees were 18% more likely to experience PTSD than those with baccalaureate degrees.

Nursing Implications

The researchers raised concerns about the findings that working in a medical intensive care unit and having a graduate degree can impact the development of PTSD. They suggested the importance of a resilience training program for nurses that includes exposure therapy, exercise, cognitive-behavioural therapy, and mindfulness-based stress reduction to lower the risks of PTSD.

patients are at risk for PTSD and recognize common symptoms associated with it.

The sensitivity and caring of the nurse create the interpersonal relationship necessary to work with patients who have PTSD. These patients are physically compromised and are struggling emotionally with situations that are not considered part of normal human experience, situations that violate the commonly held perceptions of human social justice.

While nurses on medical/surgical units are not directly involved in the treatment of patients' symptoms of PTSD, knowledge about what treatment entails is useful. Treatment of patients with PTSD includes several essential components: establishing a trusting relationship, addressing and working through the trauma experience, and teaching the coping skills needed for recovery and self-care. The patient's progress can be influenced by the ability to cope with the various aspects of both the physical and the emotional distress.

Dying and Death

Coping with the death of a loved one or with anticipation of one's own death is considered the ultimate challenge. The idea of death is threatening and anxiety provoking to many people. Kübler-Ross (1975, p. 1) stated: "The key to the question of death unlocks the door of life.... For those who seek to understand it, death is a highly creative force." Common fears of those who are dying are fear of the unknown, pain, suffering, loneliness, loss of the body, and loss of personal control.

Dying and death also raise existential questions in those who are dying, as well as their family members (Lane & Reed, 2015). Individuals ask questions such as "Has my life counted?" They may also ask spiritual questions, such as "What will happen to me after I die?" See Chapter 7 for more information.

Healthy and Unhealthy Coping Strategies

Coping refers to an individual's ability to face, deal with, overcome, or adapt to adverse situations. Individuals who cope well with adverse circumstances have strong internal resources (e.g., resilience, problem-solving skills, spirituality, humour, hope) (Frederick, Purrington, & Dunbar, 2016; Jones, Simpson, Briggs, et al., 2016), strong support systems (e.g., family, friends) (Stutts, Bills, Erwin, et al., 2015), and have learned effective coping strategies in childhood through family modelling.

If individuals have not developed healthy coping methods throughout their lives, they may resort to unhealthy behaviours to cope when under stress. These behaviours may include substance abuse (Rodriquez, Gregorich, Livaudais-Toman, et al., 2017), overeating, and isolating themselves. While these unhealthy coping behaviours are problematic in everyday life, they can be dangerous when individuals are experiencing acute onset illnesses such as MIs, or chronic illnesses such as diabetes. Abusing alcohol, for example, is a problem for a healthy individual; but for the person with type 1 diabetes, a drinking binge triggered by stress can lead to ketoacidosis (Hillson, 2015) and even death.

Substance Abuse

Substance abuse is an issue for some people. For instance, The Chief Public Health Officer's Report on the State of Public Health Agency of Canada (2015) stated that in 2013, 3.1 million Canadians consumed enough alcohol to be at risk for immediate harm or injury and that 4.4 million were at risk for chronic health problems, such as cirrhosis of the liver (Public Health Agency of Canada, 2015). Cigarette smoking has declined in Canada since the beginning of the 21st century, with 16% of individuals 15 years of age and older smoking, as compared to 25% in 2001 (Government of Canada, 2013). While this is a noteworthy decrease in the percentage of smokers, there is still a considerable number of smokers in Canada, particularly when the health impact of smoking is considered. Drugs like fentanyl have become part of Canada's illicit drug market and resulted in hundreds of deaths since 2015 (Jaimet, 2017).

As noted earlier, some people use mood-altering substances as a coping mechanism. People who engage in substance abuse use illegally obtained drugs, prescribed or over-the-counter medications, and alcohol alone or in combination with other drugs in ineffective attempts to cope with the pressures, strains, and burdens of life (Centre for Addiction and Mental Health, 2012). They are unable to make healthy decisions and to solve problems effectively. Typically, they are also unable to identify and implement adaptive behaviours. Some people may respond to personal illness or the illness of a loved one by using those substances to decrease emotional pain. It is not uncommon for nurses to encounter a relative of a dying patient, come to visit near the end of the patient's life, drunk; the imminent passing and the visit are numbed with alcohol. Over time, physiologic, emotional, cognitive, and behavioural problems develop as a result of continuous substance abuse. These problems cause distress for people, their families, and their communities.

Nursing Implications

Substance abuse is encountered in all clinical settings. Intoxication and withdrawal are two common substance abuse issues. Nurses may treat patients who have experienced trauma as a result of intoxication. Other patients who are active substance abusers enter the primary care setting with a diagnosis other than that of substance abuse. Many do not disclose the extent of their substance use. The nurse who performs a substance use assessment can detect the patient's utilization of denial or lack of knowledge about the harmful effects of psychoactive substances.

A number of tools are available to nurses to assess drug and alcohol abuse. Examples of such instruments are the CAGE Questionnaire (Ewing, 1984) and the Michigan Alcohol Screening Test (MAST) (Selzer, 1971). The CAGE questionnaire has been revised to include drug abuse (Basu et al., 2016). The MAST has been revised (Oklahoma University, n.d.), and a geriatric version (MAST-G) has been evaluated (Kano et al., 2014). Information that is commonly addressed in substance abuse questionnaires is summarized in Chart 10-7.

Family Considerations in Illness

The family (a group related by reciprocal caring, mutual responsibilities, and loyalties) plays a central role in the life of the patient and is a major part of the context of the patient's life. It is within families that people grow, are nurtured, acquire a sense of self, develop beliefs and values about life, and progress through life's developmental stages (Fig. 10-1). Families are also the first source for socialization and teaching about health and illness. Families prepare their own members with strategies for balancing closeness with separateness and togetherness with individuality. A major role of families is to provide physical and emotional resources to maintain health and a system of support in times of crises, such as in illness and disability.

CHART 10-7

Assessing for Substance Abuse

Be alert for the following:

- Past and recurrent use of a particular substance
- Patient's understanding of substance use as a problem
- Age or circumstances when substance was first used and last used
- Length and duration of substance use
- Preferred method of substance use
- Amount of substance used
- How substance is procured
- Effect of or reaction to substance after use
- Previous attempts to cease or decrease substance use

Health problems often affect the family's ability to function (Wright & Leahey, 2013). Five family functions are viewed as essential to the growth of individuals and families. The first function, *management*, involves the use of power, decision making about resources, establishment of rules, provision of finances, and future planning—responsibilities assumed by the adults of the family. The second function, *boundary setting*, makes clear distinctions between the generations and the roles of adults and children within the family structure. The third function, *communication*, is important to individual and family growth; healthy families have a full range of clear, direct, and meaningful communication among their members. The fourth function is *education and support*. Education involves modelling skills for living a physically, emotionally, and socially healthy life. Support is manifested by actions that tell family members they are cared about and loved; it promotes health and is seen as a critical factor in coping with crises and illness situations. The fifth function, *socialization*, involves families' transmission of culture and the acceptable behaviours needed to perform adequately in the home and in the world (Wright & Leahey, 2013).

Nursing Implications

When a family member becomes ill, injured, or disabled, all members of the family are affected. Depending on the

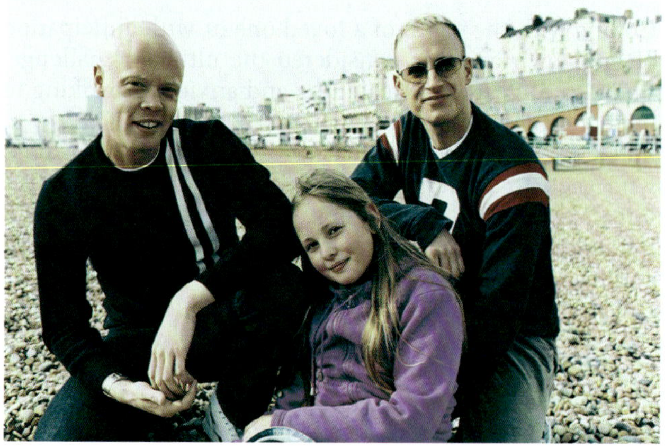

FIGURE 10-1. There are many types of families.

nature of the health problem, family members may need to modify their existing lifestyles or even restructure their lives.

There are many degrees of family functioning. Nurses assess family functioning to determine how a particular family copes with the impact of the health condition. If the family is chaotic or disorganized, promoting coping skills becomes a priority in the plan of care. The family with pre-existing problems may require additional assistance throughout the current health situation (Lane & Reed, 2015). In performing a family assessment, the nurse evaluates the present family structure and function. Areas of appraisal include demographic data, developmental information (keeping in mind that different family members can be in different developmental stages simultaneously), family structure, family functioning, and coping abilities. The role the environment plays in family health is also assessed (Wright & Leahey, 2013).

Interventions with family members are based on strengthening coping skills through direct care, fostering communication skills, and providing education. Healthy family communication has a strong influence on the quality of family life and can help the family make appropriate choices, consider alternative strategies, or persevere through complex circumstances (Wright & Leahey, 2013). Within a family system, for example, a particular patient may be undergoing extensive surgery for cancer while the partner has cardiac disease, an adult child has type 1 diabetes, and a grandchild has been in a car accident and is injured. In this situation, there are multiple health concerns along with competing developmental tasks and needs. Despite the obvious concerns of the family members, both individually and collectively, a crisis may or may not be present. The family may be coping effectively, or it may be in crisis or unable to handle the situation. Ideally, the health care team conducts a careful and comprehensive family assessment, develops interventions tailored to handle the stressors, implements the specified treatment protocols, and facilitates the construction of social support systems. The health care team may also take into consideration Rolland's psychosocial typology of illness (2018) in recognizing the types of illness and their subsequent demands upon the family.

The use of existing family strengths, resources, and education is augmented by therapeutic family interventions. The nurse's primary goals are to maintain and improve the patient's present level of health and to prevent physical and emotional deterioration. Next, the nurse intervenes in the cycle that the illness creates: patient illness, stress for other family members, new illness in other family members, and additional patient stress. Negative patterns can be derailed if the nurse helps family members identify thinking processes that are defeating how they respond to the illness and resultant stresses (Wright & Leahey, 2013). Understanding that individuals under stress often forget to employ healthy coping methods, the nurse can help family members identify coping methods that have worked in the past, and consider how they can use these same strategies when dealing with the current issues (Lane & Reed, 2015). Referrals to community supports may help family members over a period of months, even when the patient has been discharged home.

Critical Thinking Exercises

1. A 60-year-old woman who survived an earthquake is in a hospital emergency department for treatment of severe lacerations. She tells the nurse she is fearful that her spouse, who was already admitted to the hospital with a fractured hip, is alone and suffering. She states, "I am nervous about his condition and that he will go to surgery before I see him. I know that he will feel better if he knows that I am all right, too. Please, let me see him!" What assessment data should be collected to determine measures that will most likely allay this patient's anxiety? What evidenced-based nursing interventions are appropriate for assisting the woman through the trauma that she experienced? What complementary or alternative interventions might be helpful to this woman? Discuss the strength of the evidence. Identify the criteria used to evaluate the strength of the evidence for the strategies.
2. The night before a patient's major cardiac surgery, the nurse learns her patient has lost both his wife and his adult son in the past 6 months. What physiologic, emotional, and behavioural indicators should the nurse be alert for in assessing grieving? Generate a list of possible nursing diagnoses for this patient. Identify the nursing interventions that would be most appropriate for each of the possible nursing diagnoses and evaluation criteria for these interventions.

REFERENCES AND SELECTED READINGS

Books

American Psychiatric Association. (2013). *Diagnostic and statistical manual of mental disorders (DSM—5)*. Arlington, VA: Author.

Kübler-Ross, E. (1975). *Death: The final stage of growth*. Englewood Cliffs, NJ: Prentice-Hall.

Lane, A. M., & Reed, M. B. (2015). *Older adults: Understanding and facilitating transitions* (2nd ed.). Dubuque, IA: Kendall Hunt.

Rolland, J. (2018). *Helping couples and families navigate illness and disability: An integrated approach*. New York: The Guilford Press.

Worden, J. W. (1991). *Grief counseling and grief therapy: A handbook for the mental health practitioner*. New York: Springer.

Wright, L. M., & Leahey, M. (2013). *Nurses and families: A guide to family assessment and intervention* (6th ed.). Philadelphia, PA: F.A. Davis.

Journals and Electronic Documents

Abar, B., Holub, A., Lee, J., et al. (2017). Depression and anxiety among emergency department patients: Utilization and barriers to care. *Academic Emergency Medicine*, *24*, 1286–1289.

Abiri, S., Oakley, L. D., Hitchcock, M. E., et al. (2016). Stigma related avoidance in people living with severe mental illness (SMI): Findings of an integrative review. *Community Mental Health Journal*, *52*, 251–261.

AbuRuz, M. E., & Masa'Deh, R. (2017). Gender differences in anxiety and complications early after acute myocardial infarction. *The Journal of Cardiovascular Nursing*, *32*(6), 538–543.

Aftyka, A., Rybojad, B., Rosa, W., et al. (2017). Risk factors for the development of post-traumatic stress disorder and coping strategies in mothers and fathers following infant hospitalisation in the neonatal intensive care unit. *Journal of Clinical Nursing*, *26*, 4436–4445. https://doi.org/10.1111/jocn.13773

Ahl, R., Lindgren, R., Cao, Y., et al. (2017). Risk factors for depression following traumatic injury: An epidemiological study from a Scandinavian trauma center. *Injury—International Journal of the Care of the Injured*, *48*(5), 1082–1087. doi: http://doi.org/10.1016/j.injury.2017.03.019

Alzheimer Society of Canada. (2018). Stages of Alzheimer's disease. Retrieved January 14, 2018, from http://www.alzheimer.ca/en/Home/About-dementia/Alzheimer-s-disease/Stages-of-Alzheimer-s-disease

Amoozegar, F., Patten, S. B., Becker, W. J., et al. (2017). The prevalence of depression and the accuracy of depression screening tools in migraine patients. *General Hospital Psychiatry*, *48*, 27–31. doi: http://dx.doi.org/10.1016/j.genhosppsych.2017.06.006

Basu, D., Ghosh, A., Hazari, N., et al. (2016). Use of family CAGE_AID questionnaire to screen the family members for diagnosis of substance dependence. *Indian Journal of Medical Research, 143*(6), 722–730. doi 10.4103/0971-5916.191931

Bender, A., Eynan, R., O'Grady, J., et al. (2016). Best practice intervention for post-traumatic stress disorder among transit workers. *Work*, *54*, 59–71.

Bonanno, A., & Esmaeli, B. (2012). Cancer and facial disfigurement: Reducing survivors' stigma in social interaction. *Clinical Journal of Oncology Nursing*, *16*(2), 153–159.

Brandt, C., Zvolensky, M., Daumas, S., et al. (2016). Pain-related anxiety in relation to anxiety and depression among persons living with HIV/AIDS. *AIDS Care*, *28*(4), 432–435.

Brown, P., & de Graaf, S. (2013). Considering a future which may not exist: The construction of time and expectations amidst advanced-stage cancer. *Health, Risk & Society*, *15*(6-7), 543–560. http://dx.doi.org/10.1080/13698575.2013.830081

Call, J. B., & Shafer, K. (2018). Gendered manifestations of depression and help seeking among men. *American Journal of Men's Health*, *12*(1), 41–51.

Canadian Mental Health Association. (2014a). *Depression and bipolar disorder*. Retrieved January 22, 2018, from https://cmha.ca/wp-content/uploads/2015/12/Depression-and- Bipolar-NTNL-brochure-2014-web.pdf

Canadian Mental Health Association. (2014b). *Preventing suicide*. Retrieved February 18, 2018, from https://cmha.ca/wp-content/uploads/2016/02/Preventing-Suicide-NTNL-brochure- 2014-web.pdf

Centre for Addiction and Mental Health. (2012). Addiction. Retrieved February 18, 2018, from http://www.camh.ca/en/hospital/health_information/a_z_mental_health_and_addiction_information/drug-use-addiction/Pages/addiction.aspx

Costelloe, S., Kemppainen, J., Brion, J., et al. (2015). Impact of anxiety and depressive symptoms on perceptions of stigma in persons living with HIV disease in rural versus urban North Carolina. *AIDS Care*, *27*(12), 1425–1428. http://dx.doi.org/10.1080/09540121.2015.1114993

da Costa, B. R. C., & Pinto, I. C. J. F. (2017). Stress, burnout and coping in health professionals: A literature review. *Journal of Psychology and Brain Studies*, *1*, 1–8.

Dennis, M., Kadri, A., & Coffey, J. (2012). Depression in older people in the general hospital. A systematic review of screening instruments. *Age and Ageing*, *41*, 148–154.

Ewing, J. (1984). Detecting alcoholism: The CAGE questionnaire. *JAMA*, *252*, 1907–1907.

Frederick, T., Purrington, S., & Dunbar, S. (2016). Differentiation of self, religious coping, and subjective well-being. *Mental Health, Religion, & Culture*, *19*(6), 553–564. http://dx.doi.org/10.1080/13674676.2016.1216530

Fry, M. (2016). Post traumatic stress disorder. *Practice Nurse*, *46*(2), 30–34.

Gokcen, C., Sahingöz, M., & Annagur, B. (2013). Does a non-destructive earthquake cause posttraumatic stress disorder? A cross sectional study. *European Child & Adolescent Psychiatry*, *22*(5), 295–299.

Government of Canada. (2013). Canadian tobacco use monitoring survey (CTUMS): 2012 summary. Retrieved February 06, 2018, from https://www.canada.ca/en/health-canada/services/publications/healthy-living/canadian-tobacco-use-monitoring-survey-summary-2012.html

Government of Canada. (2016). Suicide in Canada. Retrieved February 19, 2018, from https://www.canada.ca/en/public-health/services/suicide-prevention/suicide-canada.html

Granek, L., Ben-David, M., Shapira, S., et al. (2017). Grief symptoms and difficult patient loss for oncologists in response to patient death. *Psycho-Oncology*, *26*, 960–966.

Heart and Stroke Foundation Canada. (2018). Reacting to a diagnosis. Retrieved February 20, 2018, from http://www.heartandstroke.ca/heart/recovery-and-support/emotions-and-feelings/reacting-to-a-diagnosis

Hillson, R. (2015). Diabetes and alcohol. *Practical Diabetes*, *32*(6), 195–196.

Jaimet, K. (2017). The fentanyl crisis. *The Canadian Nurse*. Retrieved February 06, 2018, from https://www.canadian-nurse.com/en/articles/issues/2017/january-february-2017/the-fentanyl-crisis

Johns Hopkins Medicine. *CAGE-AID*. Retrieved February 18, 2018, from https://www.hopkinsmedicine.org/johns_hopkins_healthcare/downloads/cage%20substan ce%20screening%20tool.pdf

Jones, K., Simpson, G. K., Briggs, L., et al. (2016). Does spirituality facilitate adjustment and resilience among individuals and families after SCI? *Disability & Rehabilitation*, *38*(10), 921–935.

Kano, M. Y., Santos, M. A., & Pillon, S. C. (2014). Use of alcohol in the elderly: transcultural validation of the Michigan Alcoholism Screening Test—Geriatric Version (MAST-G). *Revista da Escola de Enfermagem da USP [Internet]*, *48*(4), 649–656. Retrieved from http://www.scielo.br/pdf/reeusp/v48n4/0080-6234-reeusp-48-04-648.pdfhttp://www.scielo.br/pdf/reeusp/v48n4/0080-6234-reeusp-48-04-648.pdf

Klass, D. (2014). Grief, consolation, and religions: A conceptual framework. *Omega (Westport)*, *69*(1), 1–18. doi: http://dx.doi.org/10.2190/OM.69.1.a

Legg, A., Andrews, S., Huynh, H., et al. (2015). Patients' anxiety and hope: Predictors and adherence intentions in an acute care context. *Health Expectations*, *18*, 3034–3043.

Liegghio, M. (2017). 'Not a good person': Family stigma of mental illness from the perspective of younger siblings. *Child & Family Social Work*, *22*, 1237–1245.

Masferrer, L., Garre-Olmo, J., & Caparros, B. (2017). Is complicated grief a risk factor for substance abuse? A comparison of substance-users and normative grievers. *Addiction Research & Theory*, *25*(5), 361–367.

McMeekin, D. E., Hickman, R. L., Douglas, S., et al. (2017). Stress and coping of critical care nurses after unsuccessful cardiopulmonary resuscitation. *American Journal of Critical Care*, *26*(2), 128–135. doi: https://doi.org/10.4037/ajcc2017916

Mealer, M., Jones, J., & Meek, P. (2017). Factors affecting resilience and development of posttraumatic stress disorder in critical care nurses. *American Journal of Critical Care*, *26*(3), 184–192. doi: https://doi.org/10.4037/ajcc201798

Mendes, A. (2017). A community nurse's role in supporting a 'good' experience of grief. *British Journal of Community Nursing*, *22*(11), 566–567.

Multiple Sclerosis Foundation. (2016). Common questions: If my tests are inconclusive, is it all in my head? Retrieved January 12, 2018, from https://msfocus.org/multiple-sclerosis- faqs.aspx

Oklahoma University. (n.d.). MAST revised. Retrieved February 18, 2018, from http://www.ou.edu/cwtraining/assets/pdf/handouts/1009/MAST.pdf

Page, K., Davidson, P., Edward, K. L., et al. (2010). Recovering from an acute cardiac event—the relationship between depression and life satisfaction. *Journal of Clinical Nursing*, *19*, 736–743.

Parcival, J., Donovan, J., Kessler, D., et al. (2017). 'She believed in me'. What patients with depression value in their relationship with practitioners. A secondary analysis of multiple qualitative data sets. *Health Expectations*, *20*(1), 85–97.

Petrinic, A. (2017). Post-intensive care syndrome in family decision makers of long-term acute care hospital patients. *American Journal of Critical Care*, *26*(5), 416–422. doi: http://doi.org/10.4037/ajcc2017414

Public Health Agency of Canada. (2015). The Chief Public Health Officer's report on the state of public health in Canada 2015—Alcohol consumption in Canada. Retrieved February 06, 2018, from http://healthycanadians.gc.ca/publications/department-ministere/state-public-health-alcohol-2015-etat-sante-publique-alcool/alt/state-phac-alcohol-2015-etat-aspc-alcool-eng.pdf

Public Health Agency of Canada. (2016). Suicide in Canada: Infographic. Retrieved February 18, 2018, from https://www.canada.ca/en/public-health/services/publications/healthy-living/suicide-canada-infographic.html

Rodriquez, E. J., Gregorich, S., Livaudais-Toman, J., et al. (2017). Coping with stress by unhealthy behaviors: A re-evaluation among older adults by race/ethnicity. *Journal of Aging and Health*, *29*(5), 805–825.

Rosenblatt, P. (2017). Researching grief: Cultural, relational, and individual possibilities. *Journal of Loss and Trauma*, *22*(8), 617–630.

Selzer, M. L. (1971). The Michigan alcohol screening test (MAST): The quest for a new diagnostic instrument. *American Journal of Psychiatry*, *127*(12), 1653–1658.

Sherman, K. A., Winch, C. J., Koukoulis, A., et al. (2015). The effect of monitoring on 'processing style' on post-surgical neuropathic pain in women with breast cancer. *European Journal of Pain*, *19*(4), 585–592.

Statistics Canada. (2015). Section B—Anxiety disorders—Post-traumatic stress disorder. Retrieved February 12, 2018, from http://statcan.gc.ca/pub/82-619-m/2012004/sections/sectionb-eng.htm#a6

Stutts, L. A., Bills, S. E., Erwin, S. R., et al. (2015). Coping and posttraumatic growth in women with limb amputations. *Psychology, Health &*

Medicine, *20*(6), 742–752. http://dx.doi.org/10.1080/13548506.2015.1009379

Sundquist, K., Chang, B., Parsons, F., et al. (2016). Treatment rates for PTSD and depression in recently hospitalized cardiac patients. *Journal of Psychosomatic Research*, *86*, 60–62. doi:http://dx.doi.org/10.1016/j.jpsychores.2016.05.007

Trevick, S. A., & Lord, A. (2017). Post-traumatic stress disorder and complicated grief are common in caregivers of neuro-ICU patients. *Neurocritical Care*, *26*, 436–443.

Warlan, H., Howland, L., & Connelly, C. (2016). Detection of post-traumatic stress symptoms in patients after discharge from intensive care. *American Journal of Critical Care*, *25*(6), 509–515. doi: http://dx.doi.org/10.4037/ajcc2016573

Weingarten, K. (2012). Sorrow: A therapist's reflection on the inevitable and the unknowable. *Family Process*, *51*, 440–455.

Resources

Alcoholics Anonymous: http://www.aa.org
Anxiety Disorders Association of Canada: http://www.anxietycanada.ca
Canadian Association on Gerontology: http://cagacg.ca/
Canadian Mental Health Association: http://cmha.ca/bins/index.asp
Canadian Psychiatric Association: http://www.cpa-apc.org
Canadian Psychological Association: http://www.cpa.ca
Centre for Addiction and Mental Health: http://camh.net
Compassionate Friends of Canada, Inc.: http://www.tcfcanada.net
Mood Disorders Society of Canada: https://mdsc.ca/
Schizophrenia Society of Canada: http://www.schizophrenia.ca
Veterans Affairs Canada: http://www.vac-agg.gc.ca

11 Genetics and Genomics Perspectives in Nursing

Adapted by Mohamed Toufic El Hussein and Joseph Osuji

Learning Objectives

On completion of this chapter, the learner will be able to:

1. Describe the role of the nurse in integrating genetics and genomics in nursing care.
2. Conduct a comprehensive genetics- and genomics-based assessment.
3. Identify the common patterns of inheritance of genetic disorders.
4. Identify ethical, legal, and social issues in nursing related to genetics and genomics.
5. Apply the principles, concepts, and theories of genetics and genomics to individuals, families, groups, and communities.

The completion of the **Human Genome Project** has had a monumental impact on the application of **genetics** and **genomics** in all sectors of health care. Some evidence of this genetic revolution is noted with the development of tests that screen and diagnose genetic alterations, so that diseases may be identified and treated earlier (e.g., certain types of breast and ovarian cancers). These advancements also have been useful in generating translational research, which has spurred advances in **pharmacogenetics**, which aims to identify the best medications that can be used to treat an individual patient with a given disease. These advancements have also spurred the development of electronic health records, which give health care providers quick access to each individual patient's comprehensive family health history and personal health risk factors (Cramer, Adjei, & Labhasetwar, 2015). Precision Medicine is a major national initiative that supports both short- and long-term research initiatives aimed at facilitating genetic and genomic advances in health care (Ashley, 2015; The White House, 2015). Goals of the Precision Medicine Initiative are expected to further advance personalized medicine, which tailors health care at the individual level by using a patient's genomic information, often called *genetic makeup* or *genomic profile*.

Identification of the genetic and genomic factors associated with disease, including gene–gene function and gene–environment interactions, contributes to the development of more effective therapies customized to that particular patient's genetic makeup and the genomic profile of his or her disease. The term genetics applies to single genes and their impact on relatively rare single gene disorders, whereas genomics is the study of the interaction of all genes in the human **genome**, environmental factors, and their interactions with each other (Consensus Panel, 2009; National Institute of Health (NIH), 2015). The study of **epigenetics** focuses on changes in the expression of a given gene (Conley, Biesecker, Gonsalves, et al., 2013). Genetic and genomic profiles allow health care providers to prescribe individualized and effective treatment for each patient, to identify and follow individuals at high risk for disease, and to avoid adverse drug reactions (Ashley, 2015). New genomic-based strategies for disease detection, management, and treatment are being utilized, making personalized medicine a reality (Table 11-1).

To meet the challenges of personalized medicine, nurses must understand the role of genetics as it relates to inheritance patterns, and stay abreast of new technologies and treatments of genetic- and genomic-based health care. Nurses are a vital link between the patient and health care services; patients often turn to nurses first with questions about a family history of risk factors, information regarding genetics, and genetic tests and interpretations. The incorporation of genetics and genomics is relevant to all aspects of the nursing process. For instance, genetics and genomics should be included in health assessments, in devising nursing diagnoses, as appropriate, in planning nursing interventions that are specific to the patient and based upon the patient's diagnosis and genetic makeup, in implementing interventions that support the identification of and response to genetic-related health needs, and

TABLE 11-1 Transition From the Medical Era to the Genomic Era of Personalized Medicine

	Medical Era	Genomic Era of Personalized Medicine
Defining characteristics	• Considers single genes • Waits for disease symptoms to appear • Treats symptoms of presenting disease • Uses trial-and-error approach to treatment • Tailors medication administration according to clinical trials	• Considers interaction of genes with one another and the environment • Identifies genetic predisposition and optimizes risk reduction to prevent disease • Treats underlying genetic cause of disease • Uses personalized approach tailored to the genetic/genomic profile of the individual and the disease • Adapts medication administration per clinical trials *and* personalized genetic response to medication

in evaluating responses to medications based upon pharmacogenetics (Consensus Panel, 2009). This chapter offers a foundation for the clinical application of genetic and genomic principles in medical-surgical nursing; outlines the nurse's role in genetic counselling and evaluation; addresses important legal, ethical, and social issues; and provides related information and resources for nurses and patients.

Genomic Framework for Nursing Practice

The unique contribution of nursing to genomic medicine is its holistic perspective that takes into account each person's intellectual, physical, spiritual, social, cultural, biopsychologic, ethical, and aesthetic experiences. Because genomics addresses all of the genes of a given individual's human genome working together as a whole, genomics expands nursing's holistic view. Genetics and genomics are the basis of physiologic and pathophysiologic development, human health and disease, and health outcomes. Knowledge and interpretation of genetic and genomic information, gene-based testing, diagnosis, and treatment broaden the holistic view of nursing. Such expertise in genetics and genomics is basic to nursing practice and its holistic approach to patient care.

The *Essentials of Genetics and Genomic Nursing* (Consensus Panel, 2009) provides a framework for integrating

Glossary

carrier: person who is heterozygous; possessing two different alleles of a gene pair

chromosome: microscopic structures in the cell nucleus that contain genetic information and are constant in number in a species (e.g., humans have 46 chromosomes)

deoxyribonucleic acid (DNA): the primary genetic material in humans consisting of nitrogenous bases, a sugar group, and phosphate combined into a double helix

dominant: a genetic trait that is usually expressed when a person has a gene mutation on one of a pair of chromosomes and the "normal" form of the gene is on the other chromosome

epigenetics: the study of the regulation of gene expression

genetics: the scientific study of heredity; how specific traits or predispositions are transmitted from parents to offspring

genome: the total genetic complement of an individual genotype

genomics: the study of the human genome, including gene sequencing, mapping, and function

genotype: the genes and the variations therein that a person inherits from his or her parents

Human Genome Project: an international research effort aimed at identifying and characterizing the order of every base in the human genome

mutation: a heritable alteration in the genetic material

nondisjunction: the failure of a chromosome pair to separate appropriately during meiosis, resulting in abnormal chromosome numbers in reproductive cells (gametes)

pedigree: a diagrammatic representation of a family history

pharmacogenetics: the study of the safety and efficacy of medication administration based on a person's genotype

phenotype: a person's entire physical, biochemical, and physiologic makeup, as determined by the person's genotype and environmental factors predisposition testing: testing that is used to determine the likelihood that a healthy person with or without a family history of a condition will develop a disorder

prenatal screening: testing that is used to identify whether a fetus is at risk for a birth defect such as Down's syndrome or spina bifida (e.g., multiple marker maternal serum screening in pregnancy)

presymptomatic testing: genetic testing that is used to determine whether persons with a family history of a disorder, but no current symptoms, have the gene mutation (e.g., testing for Huntington's disease)

recessive: a genetic trait that is expressed only when a person has two copies of a mutant autosomal gene or a single copy of a mutant X-linked gene in the absence of another X chromosome

variable expression: variation in the degree to which a trait is manifested; clinical severity

X-linked: located on the X chromosome

CHART 11-1

Essential Nursing Competencies for Genetics and Genomics

Professional Responsibilities

1. Recognition of attitudes and beliefs related to genetic and genomic science
2. Advocacy for genetic and genomic services
3. Incorporation of genetic and genomic technologies and information into practice
4. Demonstration of personalizing genetic and genomic information and services
5. Provide autonomous, informed genetic- and genomic-related decision making

Professional Practice

1. Integrate and apply genetic and genomic knowledge to nursing assessment
2. Identify clients who may benefit from specific genetic and genomic resources, services, or technologies
3. Facilitate referrals for genetic and genomic services
4. Provide education, care, and support related to the interpretation of genetic or genomic tests, services, interventions, or treatments

Adapted from Consensus Panel on Genetic/Genomic Nursing Competencies. (2009). *Essentials of genetic and genomic nursing: Competencies, curricular guidelines, and outcome indicators* (2nd ed.). Silver Spring, MD: American Nurses Association.

genetics and genomics into nursing practice (Chart 11-1). This document includes a philosophy of care that recognizes when genetic and genomic factors play a role or could play a role in a person's health. This means assessing predictive genetic and genomic factors using family history and the results of genetic tests effectively, informing patients about genetics and genomic concepts, understanding the personal and societal impact of genetics and genomic information, and valuing the privacy and confidentiality of genetics and genomic information (Consensus Panel, 2009). In addition, there is formal consensus regarding higher-level competencies in the application of genetics and genomics for nurses with graduate degrees (Greco, Tinley, & Seibert, 2012).

A person's response to genetics and genomics information, genetic testing, or genetics-related conditions may be either empowering or disabling. Genetic and genomic information may stigmatize people if it affects how they view themselves or how others view them. Nurses help individuals and families learn how genetic traits and conditions are passed on within families as well as how genetic and environmental factors influence health and disease (Consensus Panel, 2009). Nurses facilitate communication among family members, the health care system, and community resources, and they offer valuable support to patients and families. All nurses should be able to recognize when a patient is asking a question related to genetic or genomic information and should know how to obtain genetics information by gathering family and health histories and conducting physical and developmental assessments. This allows nurses to provide appropriate genetics resources and support to patients and families (Consensus Panel, 2009).

For example, when nurses assess patients' cardiovascular risk, they can expand their assessment to include information about family history of hypertension, hypercholesterolemia, and clotting disorders. Knowledge that genes are involved in the control of lipid metabolism, insulin resistance, blood pressure regulation, clotting factors, and vascular lining function helps individualize care based on the patient's genetic and genomic risk profile.

Essential to a genetic and genomic framework in nursing is the awareness of one's attitudes, experience, and assumptions about genetics and genomics concepts and how these are manifested in one's own practice (Consensus Panel, 2009). To develop awareness of these attitudes, experiences, and assumptions, the nurse examines his or her own:

- Beliefs or values about health as well as family, religious, or cultural beliefs about the cause of illness; and how one's values or biases affect understanding of genetic conditions
- Philosophical, theologic, cultural, and ethical perspectives related to health and how these perspectives influence one's use of genetics information or services
- Level of expertise about genetics and genomics
- Experiences with birth defects, chronic illnesses, and genetic conditions along with one's view of such conditions as disabling or empowering
- Attitudes about the right to access and other rights of individuals with genetic disorders
- View and assumptions about DNA and beliefs about the value of information about one's risk for genetic disorders
- Beliefs about reproductive options
- View of genetic testing and engineering
- Approach to patients with disabilities

Integrating Genetic and Genomic Knowledge

Scientific developments and advances in technology have increased the understanding of genetics, resulting in better understanding of relatively rare diseases such as phenylketonuria (PKU) or hemophilia that are related to **mutations** of a single gene inherited in families. Scientists are able to characterize inherited metabolic variations that interact over time and lead to common diseases such as cancer, diabetes, heart disease, and dementia (Carroll, 2017). The transition from genetics to genomics has increased understanding of how multiple genes act and control biologic processes. Most health conditions are now believed to be the result of a combination of genetic and environmental influences (Roadmap Epigenomics Consortium, 2015).

Genes and Their Role in Human Variation

Genes are central components of human health and disease. The Human Genome Project has shown how basic human genetics is to human development, health, and disease (National Institutes of Health [NIH], 2014a). Knowledge that specific genes are associated with specific genetic conditions makes diagnosis possible, even in the unborn. Many common conditions have genetic causes and many more associations between genetics, health, and disease are likely to be identified. Genomics is the study of the interaction of genes with other genes and environmental factors.

Genes and Chromosomes

A person's unique genetic constitution, called a **genotype**, is made up of approximately 25,000 genes (Romanoski & Glass, 2015). A person's **phenotype**, the observable characteristics of his or her genotype, includes physical appearance and other biologic, physiologic, and molecular traits. Environmental influences modify every person's phenotype, even phenotypes with a major genetic component. This concept of genotype and phenotype applies to a person's total genome and the respective traits of his or her genetic makeup.

The concept of genotype and phenotype also applies to specific diseases. For example, in hypercholesterolemia, the genotype refers to the genes that control lipid metabolism, and the phenotype may be manifested in various corresponding ways. The genotype involves mutations in low-density lipoprotein (LDL) receptors and in one of the apolipoprotein genes. The phenotype is characterized by early onset of cardiovascular disease, high levels of LDL, skin xanthomas, and a family history of heart disease. An individual's genotype, consisting of normal functioning genes as well as some mutations, is characterized by physical and biologic traits that may predispose to disease.

Human growth, development, and disease occur as a result of both genetic and environmental influences and interactions. The contribution of genetic factors may be large or small. For example, in a person with cystic fibrosis or PKU, the genetic contribution is significant. In contrast, the genetic contribution underlying a person's response to infection may be less applicable.

A single gene is conceptualized as a unit of heredity. A gene is composed of a segment of **deoxyribonucleic acid (DNA)** that contains a specific set of instructions for making the protein or proteins needed by body cells for proper functioning. Genes regulate both the types of proteins made and the rate at which proteins are produced. The structure of the DNA molecule is referred to as a double helix. The essential components of the DNA molecule are sugar–phosphate molecules and pairs of nitrogenous bases. Each nucleotide contains a sugar (deoxyribose), a phosphate group, and one of four nitrogenous bases: adenine (A), cytosine (C), guanine (G), and thymine (T). DNA is composed of two paired strands, each made up of a number of nucleotides. The strands are held together by hydrogen bonds between pairs of bases (Fig. 11-1).

Genes are arranged in a linear order within **chromosomes**, which are located in the cell nucleus. In humans, 46 chromosomes occur in pairs in all body cells except oocytes (eggs) and sperm, in which each contain only 23 chromosomes. Twenty-two pairs of chromosomes, called autosomes, are the same in females and males. The 23rd pair is referred to as the gender chromosome. A female has two X chromosomes, whereas a male has one X and one Y chromosome. At conception, each parent normally gives one chromosome of each pair to his or her child. As a result, children receive half of their chromosomes from their fathers and half from their mothers (Fig. 11-2).

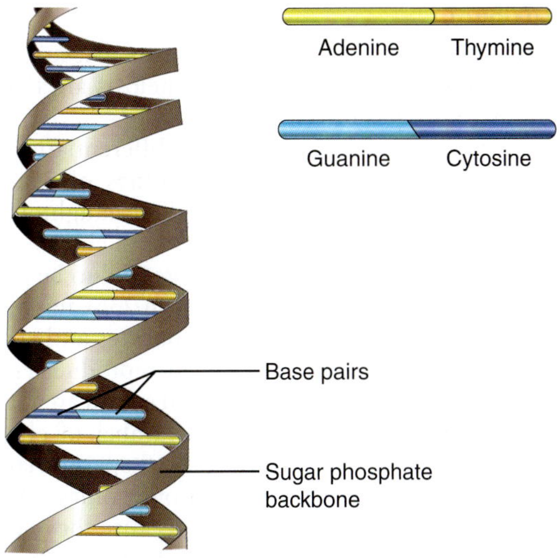

FIGURE 11-1. DNA is a double helix formed by base pairs attached to a sugar–phosphate backbone. DNA carries the instructions that allow cells to make proteins. DNA is made up of four chemical bases. (Redrawn from Genetics Home Reference. http://ghr.nlm.nih.gov/handbook/illustrations/dnastructure)

Careful examination of DNA sequences from many people shows that these sequences have multiple versions in a population. The different versions of these sequences are called alleles. Sequences found in many forms are said to be polymorphic, meaning that there are at least two common forms of a particular gene.

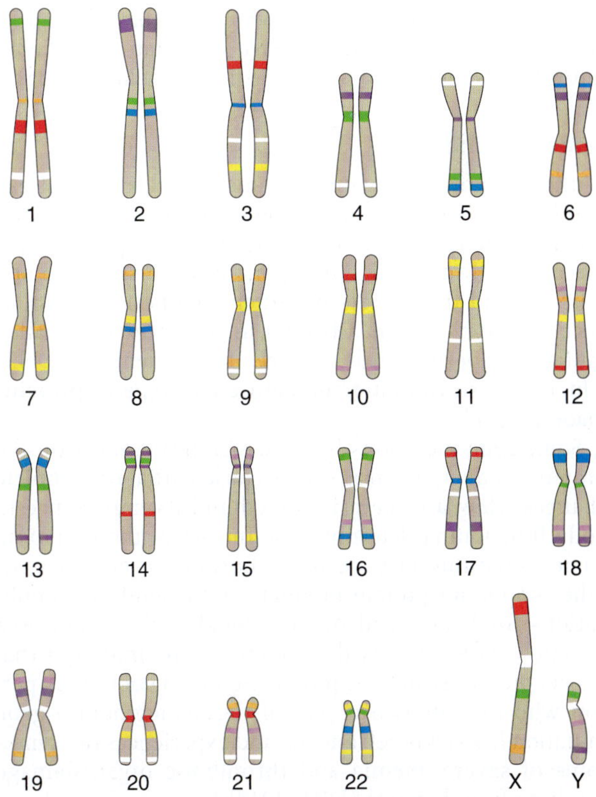

FIGURE 11-2. Each human cell contains 23 pairs of chromosomes, which can be distinguished by their size and unique banding patterns. This set is from a male, because it contains a Y chromosome. Females have two X chromosomes. (Redrawn from Genetics Home Reference. http://ghr.nlm.nih.gov/handbook/basics/howmanychromosomes)

Cell Division

The human body grows and develops as a result of the process of cell division. Mitosis and meiosis are two distinctly different types of cell division.

Mitosis is involved in cell growth, differentiation, and repair. During mitosis, the chromosomes of each cell duplicate. The result is two cells, called daughter cells, each of which contains the same number of chromosomes as the parent cell. The daughter cells are said to be diploid because they contain 46 chromosomes in 23 pairs. Mitosis occurs in all cells of the body except oocytes and sperm.

Meiosis, in contrast, occurs only in reproductive cells and is the process by which oocytes and sperm are formed. During meiosis, a reduction in the number of chromosomes takes place, resulting in oocytes or sperm that contain half the usual number, or 23 chromosomes. Oocytes and sperm are referred to as haploid because they contain a single copy of each chromosome, compared to the usual two copies in all other body cells. During meiosis, as the paired chromosomes come together in preparation for cell division, portions cross over, and an exchange of genetic material occurs before the chromosomes separate. This event, called recombination, creates greater diversity in the makeup of oocytes and sperm.

During the process of meiosis, a pair of chromosomes may fail to separate completely, creating a sperm or oocyte that contains either two copies or no copy of a particular chromosome. This sporadic event, called **nondisjunction**, can lead to either a trisomy or a monosomy. Down's syndrome is an example of trisomy, in which people have three copies of chromosome number 21. Turner's syndrome is an example of monosomy, in which girls have a single X chromosome, causing them to have short stature and infertility (U.S. National Library of Medicine [NLM], 2015a).

Gene Mutations

Within each cell, many intricate and complex interactions regulate and express human genes. Gene structure and function, transcription and translation, and protein synthesis are all involved. Alterations in gene structure and function and the process of protein synthesis may influence a person's health. Changes in gene structure, called mutations, permanently change the sequence of DNA, which in turn can alter the nature and type of proteins made (Fig. 11-3).

Some gene mutations have no significant effect on the protein product, whereas others cause partial or complete changes. How a protein is altered and its importance to body functioning determine the impact of the mutation. Gene mutations may occur in hormones, enzymes, or other important protein products, with significant implications for health and disease. Sickle cell anemia is a genetic condition caused by a small gene mutation that affects protein structure, producing hemoglobin S. A person who inherits two copies of the hemoglobin S gene mutation has sickle cell anemia and experiences the symptoms of severe anemia and thrombotic organ damage resulting from hypoxia (NIH, 2014b).

Other gene mutations include deletion (loss), insertion (addition), duplication (multiplication), or rearrangement (translocation) of a longer DNA segment. Duchenne muscular dystrophy, myotonic dystrophy, Huntington's disease,

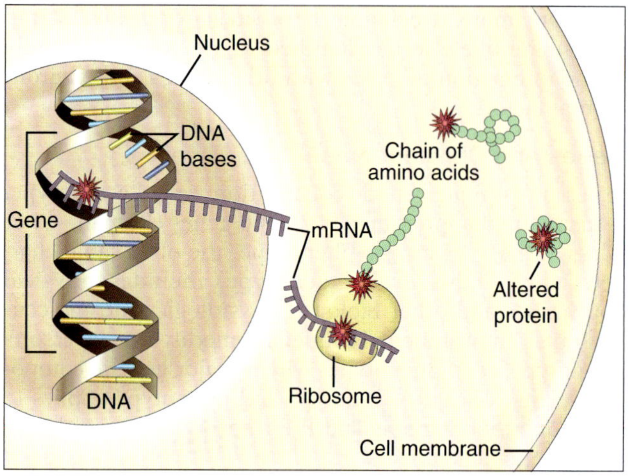

FIGURE 11-3. When a gene contains a mutation, the protein encoded by that gene is likely to be abnormal. Sometimes the protein is able to function, although it does so imperfectly. In other cases, it is totally disabled. The outcome depends not only on how the mutation alters the protein's function but also on how vital that particular protein is to survival.

and fragile X syndrome are examples of conditions caused by gene mutations.

Gene mutations may be inherited or acquired. Inherited or germline gene mutations are present in the DNA of all body cells and are passed on in reproductive cells from parent to child. Germline or hereditary mutations are passed on to all daughter cells when body cells replicate (Fig. 11-4). The gene that causes Huntington's disease is one example of a germline mutation.

Spontaneous mutations take place in individual oocytes or sperm at the time of conception. A person who carries the new "spontaneous" mutation may pass on the mutation to his or her children. Achondroplasia, Marfan's syndrome, and neurofibromatosis type 1 are examples of

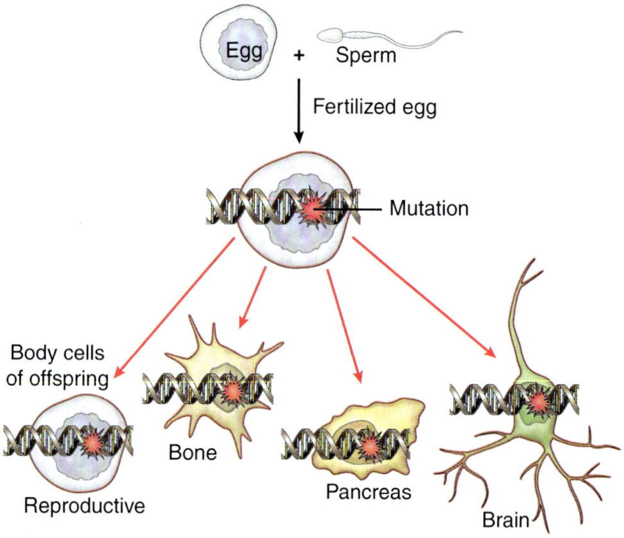

FIGURE 11-4. Hereditary mutations are carried in the DNA of the reproductive cells. When reproductive cells containing mutations combine to produce offspring, the mutation is present in all of the offspring's body cells. (Redrawn from the National Cancer Institute. http://www.cancer.gov/cancertopics/understandingcancer/genetesting/Slide11)

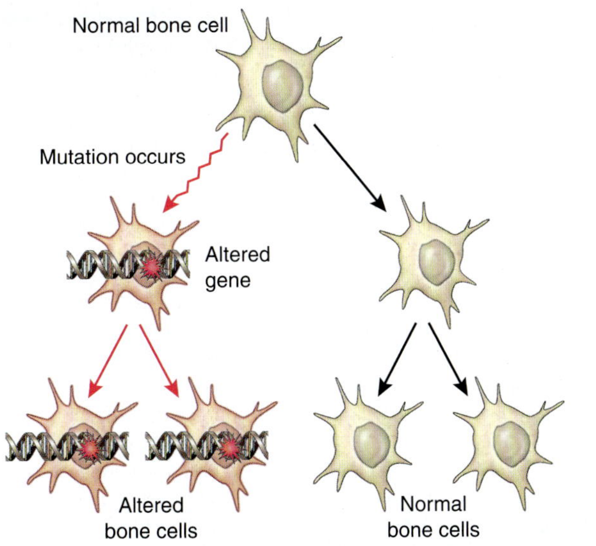

FIGURE 11-5. Acquired mutations develop in DNA during a person's lifetime. If the mutation arises in a body cell, copies of the mutation will exist only in the descendants of that particular cell. (Redrawn from the National Cancer Institute. http://www.cancer.gov/cancertopics/understandingcancer/genetesting/Slide12)

genetic conditions that may occur in a single family member as a result of spontaneous mutation.

Acquired mutations take place in somatic cells and involve changes in DNA that occur after conception, during a person's lifetime. Acquired mutations develop as a result of cumulative changes in body cells other than reproductive cells (Fig. 11-5). Somatic gene mutations are passed on to the daughter cells derived from that particular cell line.

Gene mutations occur in the human body all the time. Cells have built-in mechanisms by which they can recognize mutations in DNA, and in most situations, they correct the changes before they are passed on by cell division. However, over time, body cells may lose their ability to repair damage from gene mutations, causing an accumulation of genetic changes that may ultimately result in diseases such as cancer and possibly other conditions of aging, such as Alzheimer's disease (Roadmap Epigenomics Consortium, 2015).

Genetic Variation

Genetic variations occur among all people. Single nucleotide polymorphisms (SNPs, referred to as "snips") is the term used to identify common genetic variations that occur most frequently throughout the human genome. SNPs are changes in a single nucleotide (an A, T, C, or G) of the DNA sequence. For example, a normal DNA sequence of AAGGT could change to ATGG; in this case, there is one single nucleotide change from A to T. Most SNPs do not alter normal cell function. Some SNPs do alter gene function and may influence disease development. Knowledge about SNPs that affect biologic function will help pinpoint individuals who may be more prone to common diseases such as cancer, diabetes, and heart disease. Information on SNPs has helped to clarify why some individuals metabolize drugs differently (Korf & Rehm, 2013). For example, a polymorphism or SNP can alter protein or enzyme activity of medications. If the SNP causes a variation in drug transport or drug metabolism, the drug's action, half-life, or excretion could lead to lack of drug response or drug toxicity.

Inheritance Patterns

Nursing assessment of the patient's health includes obtaining and recording family history information in the form of a genogram (**pedigree**). This is a first step in establishing the pattern of inheritance. Nurses need to be familiar with mendelian patterns of inheritance and genogram construction and analysis to help identify patients and families who may benefit from further genetic counselling, testing, and treatment (Consensus Panel, 2009).

Mendelian conditions are genetic conditions that are inherited in fixed proportions among generations. They result from gene mutations that are present on one or both chromosomes of a pair. A single gene inherited from one or both parents can cause a mendelian condition. Mendelian conditions are classified according to their pattern of inheritance: autosomal dominant, autosomal recessive, and X linked. The terms **dominant** and **recessive** refer to the trait, genetic condition, or phenotype but not to the genes or alleles that cause the observable characteristics (NLM, 2015a).

Autosomal Dominant Inheritance

Autosomal dominant inherited conditions affect female and male family members equally and follow a vertical pattern of inheritance in families (Fig. 11-6). A person who has an autosomal dominant inherited condition carries a gene mutation for that condition on one chromosome of a pair. Each of that person's offspring has a 50% chance of inheriting the gene mutation for the condition and a 50% chance of inheriting the normal version of the gene (Fig. 11-7). Offspring who do not inherit the gene mutation do not develop the condition and do not have an increased chance for having children with the same condition. Table 11-2 presents characteristics and examples of different patterns of inherited conditions.

Autosomal dominant conditions often manifest with varying degrees of severity. Some affected people may have

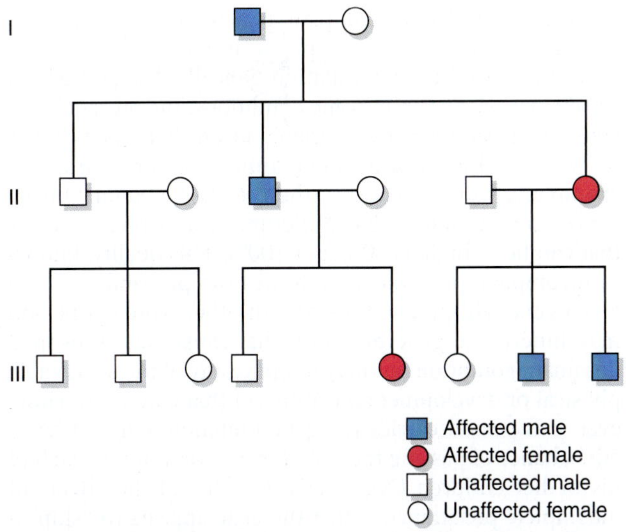

FIGURE 11-6. Three-generation genogram (pedigree) illustrating autosomal dominant inheritance.

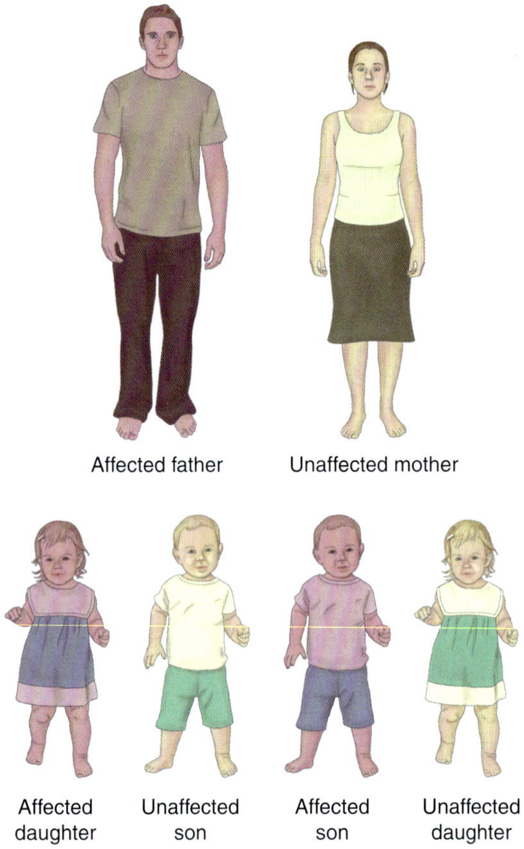

FIGURE 11-7. In dominant genetic disorders, if one affected parent has a disease-causing allele that dominates its normal counterpart, each child in the family has a 50% chance of inheriting the disease allele and the disorder. (Redrawn from Genetics Home Reference. http://ghr.nlm.nih.gov/handbook/illustrations/autodominant)

TABLE 11-2 Patterns of Mendelian Inheritance

Characteristics	Examples
Autosomal Dominant Inherited Conditions	
Vertical transmission in families Males and females equally affected Variable expression among family members and others with condition Reduced penetrance (in some conditions) Advanced paternal age associated with sporadic cases	Hereditary breast/ovarian cancer syndrome Familial hypercholesterolemia Hereditary nonpolyposis colorectal cancer Huntington's disease Marfan's syndrome Neurofibromatosis
Autosomal Recessive Inherited Conditions	
Horizontal pattern of transmission seen in families Males and females equally affected Associated with consanguinity (genetic relatedness) Associated with particular ethnic groups	Cystic fibrosis Galactosemia Phenylketonuria Sickle cell anemia Tay-Sachs disease Canavan disease
X-Linked Recessive Inherited Conditions	
Vertical transmission in families Males predominantly affected	Duchenne muscular dystrophy Hemophilia A and B Wiskott-Aldrich syndrome Protan and deutan forms of colour blindness
Multifactorial Inherited Conditions	
Occur as a result of combination of genetic and environmental factors May recur in families Inheritance pattern does not demonstrate characteristic pattern of inheritance seen with other mendelian conditions	Congenital heart defects Cleft lip and/or palate Neural tube defects (anencephaly and spina bifida) Diabetes mellitus Osteoarthritis High blood pressure

Adapted from Dwyer, T. M., Glaser, R. L., & Mason, T. M. (2016). Inheritance patterns in human phenotypes and types of genetic disorders. In C. E. Kasper, T. A. Schneidereith, & F. R. Lashley (Eds.). *Lashley's essentials of clinical genetics in nursing practice* (pp. 65–114). New York: Springer Publishing Company; U.S. National Library of Medicine. Genetic Home Reference (NLM). (2015a). *What are the different ways in which a genetic condition can be inherited?* Retrieved June 30, 2015, from ghr.nlm.nih.gov/handbook/inheritance/inheritancepatterns

significant symptoms, whereas others may have only mild ones. This characteristic is referred to as **variable expression**; it results from the influences of genetic and environmental factors on clinical presentation.

Another phenomenon observed in autosomal dominant inheritance is penetrance, or the percentage of persons known to have a particular gene mutation who actually show the trait. Almost complete penetrance is observed in conditions such as achondroplasia, in which nearly 100% of people with the gene mutation typically display traits of the disease. However, in some conditions, the presence of a gene mutation does not invariably mean that a person has or will develop an autosomal inherited condition. For example, a woman who has the *BRCA1* hereditary breast cancer gene mutation has a lifetime risk of breast cancer that can be as high as 80%, not 100%. This quality, known as incomplete penetrance, indicates the probability that a given gene will produce disease. In other words, a person may inherit the gene mutation that causes an autosomal dominant condition but may not have any of the observable physical or developmental features of that condition. However, this person carries the gene mutation and still has a 50% chance of passing the gene for the condition to each of his or her children (NLM, 2015b). One of the effects of incomplete penetrance is that the gene appears to "skip" a generation, thus leading to errors in interpreting family history and in genetic counselling. Examples of other genetic conditions with incomplete penetrance include otosclerosis (40%) and retinoblastoma (80%) (Porth, 2017).

Autosomal Recessive Inheritance

In contrast to autosomal dominant conditions, autosomal recessive conditions have a pattern that is more horizontal than vertical; relatives of a single generation tend to have the condition (Fig. 11-8). Autosomal recessive conditions are frequently seen among particular ethnic groups and usually occur more often in children of parents who are related by blood, such as first cousins (see Table 11-2).

In autosomal recessive inheritance, each parent carries a gene mutation on one chromosome of the pair and a normal gene on the other chromosome. The parents are said to be **carriers** of the gene mutation. Unlike people with an autosomal dominant condition, carriers of a gene mutation for a recessive condition do not have symptoms of the genetic condition. When carriers have children together, there is a 25% chance that each child may inherit

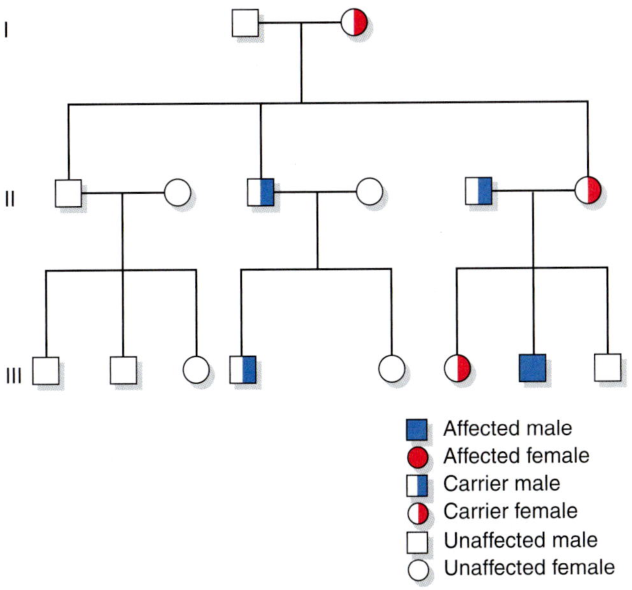

FIGURE 11-8. Three-generation genogram (pedigree) illustrating autosomal recessive inheritance.

the gene mutation from both parents and have the condition (Fig. 11-9). Gaucher's disease, cystic fibrosis, sickle cell anemia, and PKU are examples of autosomal recessive conditions (NLM, 2015a).

X-Linked Inheritance

X-linked conditions may be inherited in recessive or dominant patterns (see Table 11-2). In both, the gene mutation is located on the X chromosome. All males inherit an X chromosome from their mothers and a Y chromosome from their fathers for a normal sex constitution of 46,XY. Because males have only one X chromosome, they do not have a counterpart for its genes, as do females. This means that a gene mutation on the X chromosome of a male is expressed even though it is present in only one copy. Females, on the other hand, inherit one X chromosome from each parent for a normal sex constitution of 46,XX. A female may be an unaffected carrier of a gene mutation, or she may be affected if the condition results from a gene mutation causing an X-linked dominant condition. Either the X chromosome that she received from her mother or the X chromosome she received from her father may be passed on to each of her offspring, and this is a random occurrence.

The most common pattern of X-linked inheritance is that in which a female is a carrier for a gene mutation on one of her X chromosomes. This is referred to as X-linked recessive inheritance in which a female carrier has a 50% chance of passing on the gene mutation to a son, who would be affected, or to a daughter, who would be a carrier like her mother (Fig. 11-10). Examples of X-linked recessive conditions include factor VIII and factor IX hemophilia, severe combined immunodeficiency, and Duchenne muscular dystrophy.

Multifactorial Inheritance and Complex Genetic Conditions

Many birth defects and common health conditions such as heart disease, high blood pressure, cancer, osteoarthritis, and diabetes occur as a result of interactions of multiple gene

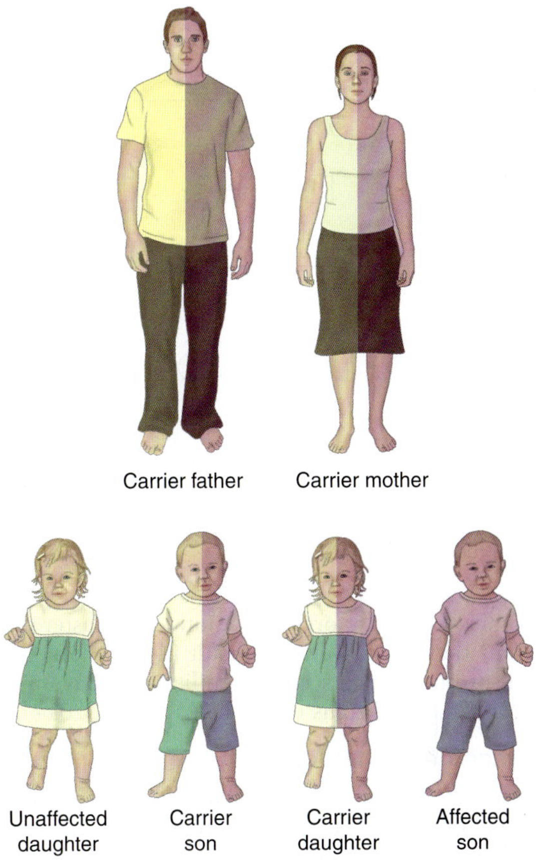

FIGURE 11-9. In diseases associated with altered recessive genes, both parents—although disease free themselves—carry one normal allele and one altered allele. Each child has one chance in four of inheriting two abnormal alleles and developing the disorder; one chance in four of inheriting two normal alleles; and two chances in four of inheriting one normal and one altered allele, and therefore being a carrier like both parents. (Redrawn from Genetics Home Reference. http://ghr.nlm.nih.gov/handbook/illustrations/autorecessive)

mutations and environmental influences. Thus, they are called multifactorial or complex conditions (see Table 11-2). Other examples of multifactorial genetic conditions include neural tube defects such as spina bifida and

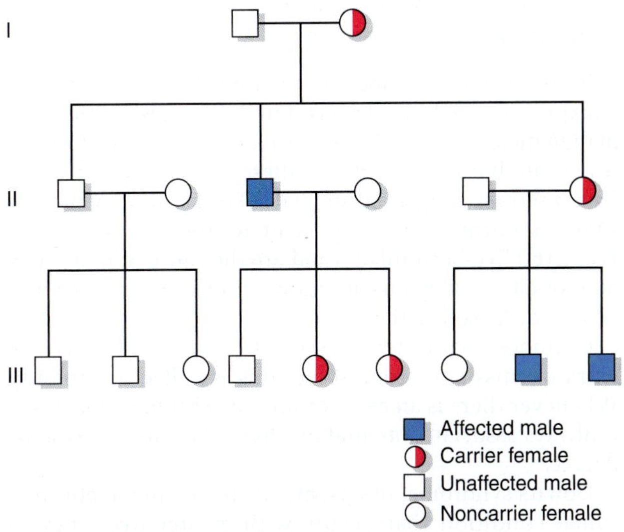

FIGURE 11-10. Three-generation genogram (pedigree) illustrating X-linked recessive inheritance.

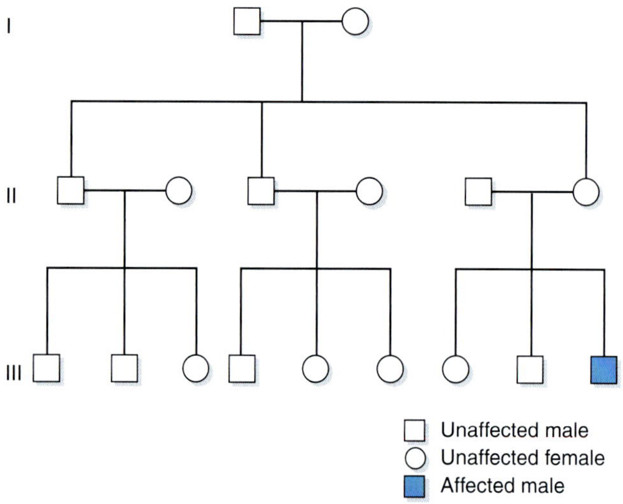

FIGURE 11-11. Three-generation genogram (pedigree) illustrating multifactorial conditions.

anencephaly. Multifactorial conditions may cluster in families, but they do not always result in the characteristic pattern of inheritance seen in families who have mendelian inherited conditions (Fig. 11-11) (Porth, 2017).

Nontraditional Inheritance

Although mendelian conditions manifest with a specific pattern of inheritance in some families, many diseases and traits do not follow these simple patterns. A variety of factors influence how a gene performs and is expressed. Different mutations in the same gene can produce variable symptoms in different people, as in cystic fibrosis. Different mutations in several genes can lead to identical outcomes, as in Alzheimer's disease. Some traits involve simultaneous mutation in two or more genes. A recently observed phenomenon, imprinting, can determine which of a pair of genes (the mother's or the father's) is silenced or activated. This form of inheritance has been observed in Angelman syndrome, a severe form of mental retardation and ataxia (NIH, 2015a).

Chromosomal Differences and Genetic Conditions

Differences in the number or structure of chromosomes are a major cause of birth defects, intellectual disabilities, and malignancies (NLM, 2015c). In Canada, about 350,000 babies are born each year. Of these babies 2% to 3% will have a serious congenital anomaly (Porth, 2017). Chromosomal abnormalities are present in approximately 1 of every 160 live-born infants and are the cause of more than 50% of all spontaneous abortions or miscarriages (Dwyer, Glaser, & Mason, 2016).

Chromosomal differences most commonly involve an extra or missing chromosome; this is called aneuploidy. Whenever there is an extra or missing chromosome, there is always associated mental or physical disability to some degree.

Down's syndrome, or trisomy 21, is a common chromosomal condition that occurs with greater frequency in pregnancies of women who are 35 years of age or older. A person with trisomy 21 has a complete extra chromosome 21, which causes a particular facial appearance and increased risk of congenital heart defects, thyroid and vision problems, and mental retardation. Other examples of chromosomal differences include trisomy 13 and trisomy 18, both more severe than Down's syndrome, and conditions involving extra or missing sex chromosomes, such as Turner's syndrome (NIH, 2013a).

Chromosomal differences may also involve a structural rearrangement within or between chromosomes. These are less common than chromosomal conditions in which there is an extra or missing chromosome (NIH, 2015b; NLM, 2015c). People who carry "balanced" chromosome rearrangements have all of their chromosomal material, but it is rearranged. Women with a "balanced" chromosomal rearrangement have an increased risk of spontaneous pregnancy loss and of having children with an unbalanced chromosomal arrangement that may result in physical or mental disabilities. Known carriers of these chromosomal differences are offered prenatal counselling and testing.

Chromosome studies may be needed at any age, depending on the indication. Two common indications are a suspected diagnosis such as Down's syndrome and a history of two or more unexplained pregnancy losses. Chromosome studies are accomplished by obtaining a tissue sample (e.g., blood, skin, amniotic fluid), preparing and staining the chromosomes, and analyzing them under a microscope. The microscopic study of chromosomes, called cytogenetics, is used with new molecular techniques such as fluorescent in situ hybridization (FISH), which permits more detailed examination of chromosomes (Korf & Rehm, 2013). FISH is useful to detect small abnormalities and to characterize chromosomal rearrangements.

Genetic and Genomic Technologies in Practice

One of the most immediate applications of new genetic and genomic discoveries is the development of genetic tests that can be used to detect a trait, diagnose a genetic condition, and identify people who have a genetic predisposition to a disease such as cancer or heart disease. Another emerging application is pharmacogenetics, which involves the use of genetic testing to identify genetic variations that relate to the safety and efficacy of medications and gene-based treatments, so that individualized treatment can be developed. Future applications may include the use of gene chips to map a person's individual genome for genetic variations that may lead to disease. Some nurses are involved in caring for patients who are undergoing genetic testing and gene-based treatments. Knowledge of the clinical applications of modern genetic and genomic technologies enables nurses to inform and support patients and to provide high-quality genetics-related health care (Consensus Panel, 2009).

Genetic Testing

Genetic testing is the primary tool used to identify individuals predisposed to specific genetic diseases. Genetic tests provide information that can lead to the diagnosis of inherited conditions or other conditions with a known genetic contribution.

CHART 11-2

Ethical Dilemma: Can Predictive Genetic Testing Threaten Patient Autonomy?

Case Scenario

Ashley is a 34-year-old woman who is a patient in the family care clinic. Her sister just gave birth to a child who was born with fragile X syndrome (a genetic mutation associated with intellectual disabilities and impaired social development). Although her first child, a daughter, has not demonstrated any signs of this disorder, Ashley is requesting to have predictive genetic testing (PGT) on her 5-year-old daughter to determine if she is a carrier of fragile X syndrome.

Discussion

The Human Genome Project initiative has spearheaded the development of technology that can identify conditions with genetic origins in patients who have no demonstrable symptoms but may carry a mutated gene. Although not evidencing the disorder, future offspring of a patient who carries the mutation may have the disorder. PGT may be done to identify patients who may be carriers for inherited genetic disorders such as fragile X syndrome.

One of the legal and ethical concerns raised by health care providers regarding pediatric genetic screening addresses the value of testing for disorders that cannot be cured or ameliorated. In this particular case, the data obtained from this screening will not be used to medically benefit the health of Ashley's daughter. The American College of Medical Genetics contends that ultimately, the best interest of the person tested must be the focus of PGT. Arguably, Ashley's daughter will have the right to give informed consent to this procedure as an adult, should she choose to do so.

Analysis

Describe the ethical principles that are in conflict in this case (see Chapter 3). Which principle do you believe should have pre-eminence in deciding whether or not parents have the right to have PGT in a child who will not medically benefit from the findings?

- Do the benefits outweigh the risks of PGT in the child? Identify the stakeholders who could benefit from the findings of PGT.
- Are there any professional guidelines that you can turn to for help in determining the ethical issues that still remain around PGT? If so, what are they, and how can they help?

Clayton, E. W., McCullough, L. B., Biesecker, L. G., et al. (2014). Addressing the ethical challenges in genetic testing and sequencing of children. *The American Journal of Bioethics, 14*(3), 3–9; Porry, P., Shabani, M., & Howard, H. C. (2014). Is there a right time to know? The right not to know and genetic testing in children. *Journal of Law, Medicine, & Ethics, 42*(1), 19–27.

In genetic testing, approaches may be genotypic or phenotypic. Genotypic methods involve analysis of the chromosomes and genes directly, using specific laboratory techniques to learn whether a genetic alteration related to a specific disease or condition is present. This testing may be DNA based, chromosomal, or biochemical. Phenotypic methods examine the familial or biologic presentation of disease and include assessment of the patient's personal or family history and medical factors influencing his or her disease as well as testing for gene products such as protein markers in body fluids or diseased tissues. The family history, which is considered the first genetic test, is discussed later in this chapter (see Family History Assessment). It is expected that all nurses will know how to use this genetic tool.

Another phenotypic approach involves searching for gene products, such as proteins and enzymes that can clinically indicate a genetic abnormality. For example, germline mutations in the repair genes *MLH1*, *MSH2*, *MSH6*, and *PMS2* are responsible for hereditary early-onset colorectal cancer. Colorectal tumours are now tested to measure the presence or absence of these proteins using immunohistochemistry, a routine type of pathology test. Tumours that stain negative for one of those proteins signify malfunction of the gene whose protein is missing. Patients with absent or negative protein expression in their tumours (e.g., MLH1 protein–negative) can proceed with genetic testing for a germline *MLH1* mutation (Harkness, Barrow, Newton, et al., 2015).

Genetic testing can be used for a variety of purposes in prenatal, pediatric, and adult populations. Prenatal testing is widely used for **prenatal screening** and diagnosis of such conditions as Down's syndrome. Carrier testing is used to determine if a person carries a recessive allele for an inherited condition (e.g., cystic fibrosis, sickle cell anemia, Tay–Sachs disease) and therefore risks passing it on to his or her children. Genetic testing is also used widely in newborn screening. In Canada, it is available for an increasing number of genetic conditions (e.g., PKU, galactosemia).

Diagnostic testing is used to detect the presence or absence of a particular genetic alteration or allele to identify or confirm a diagnosis of a disease or condition (e.g., myotonic dystrophy, fragile X syndrome) (Chart 11-2). Increasingly, genetic tests are being used to predict drug response and to design specific and individualized treatment plans or personalized medicine. For example, genetic testing is used to identify specific gene variants that can predict the effectiveness of treatments of human immunodeficiency virus infection, atherothrombosis, thrombophilia, hyperlipidemia, breast cancer, pain management, hepatitis C, rheumatoid arthritis, leukemia, depression, and bipolar disorder (Johnson, 2013; Korf & Rehm, 2013). Selected examples of current uses of genetic tests are shown in Table 11-3.

Nurses are increasingly participating in patient's genetic testing, especially in the area of taking family histories and patient education. They contribute by ensuring informed health choices and consent, advocating for privacy and confidentiality with regard to genetic test results, and helping patients understand the complex issues involved (Porth, 2017).

Genetic Screening

Genetic screening, in contrast to genetic testing, applies to testing of populations or groups independent of a

TABLE 11-3 Selected Genetic Tests: Examples of Current Uses

Purpose of Genetic Test	Type of Genetic Test
Carrier Testing	
Cystic fibrosis	DNA analysis
Tay–Sachs disease	Hexosaminidase A activity testing and DNA analysis
Canavan disease	DNA analysis
Sickle cell anemia	Hemoglobin electrophoresis
Thalassemia	Complete blood count and hemoglobin electrophoresis
Diagnosis	
Down's syndrome	Chromosomal analysis
Fragile X syndrome	DNA analysis
Myotonic dystrophy	DNA analysis
Presymptomatic Testing	
Huntington's disease	DNA analysis
Myotonic dystrophy	DNA analysis
Susceptibility Testing	
Hereditary breast/ovarian cancer	DNA analysis
Hereditary nonpolyposis colorectal cancer	DNA analysis

Adapted from U.S. National Library of Medicine. Genetics Home Reference (NLM). (2015e). *What are the types of genetic tests?* Retrieved November 24, 2015, from ghr.nlm.nih.gov/handbook/testing/uses

positive family history or symptom manifestation. Genetic screening, as defined in 1975 by the Committee for the Study of Inborn Errors of Metabolism of the National Academy of Sciences (Simopoulos, 2009), has several major aims. The first aim is to improve management; that is, to identify people with treatable genetic conditions that could prove dangerous to their health if left untreated. For example, newborns are screened for an increasing number of conditions, including PKU, congenital hypothyroidism, and galactosemia. The second aim is to provide reproductive options to people with a high probability of having children with severe, untreatable diseases and for whom genetic counselling, prenatal diagnosis, and other reproductive options could be helpful and of interest. For example, people of Ashkenazi Jewish descent (Jews of Eastern European origin) are screened for conditions such as Tay–Sachs disease and Canavan disease. The third aim is to screen pregnant women to detect birth defects such as neural tube defects and Down's syndrome. Genetic screening may also be used for public health purposes to determine the incidence and prevalence of a birth defect or to investigate the feasibility and value of new genetic testing methods. Most commonly, genetic screening occurs in prenatal and newborn programs. Table 11-4 gives examples of types of genetic screening.

Testing and Screening for Adult-Onset Conditions

Adult-onset conditions with a genetic or genomic basis are manifested in later life. Often clinical signs or symptoms occur only in late adolescence or adulthood, and disease is clearly observed to run in families. Some of these conditions are attributed to specific genetic mutations and follow either an autosomal dominant or an autosomal recessive inheritance pattern. However, the majority of adult-onset conditions are considered to be genomic or multifactorial. Examples of multifactorial conditions include heart disease, diabetes, and arthritis. Genomic or multifactorial influences involve interactions among several genes (gene–gene interactions) and between genes and the environment (gene–environment interactions), as well as the individual's lifestyle (Waters, Muff, & Hamilton, 2014).

Nursing assessment for adult-onset conditions is based on family history, personal and medical risk factors, and identification of associated diseases or clinical manifestations (the phenotype). Knowledge of adult-onset conditions and their genetic bases (i.e., mendelian vs. multifactorial conditions) influences the nursing considerations for genetic testing and health promotion. Table 11-5 describes selected adult-onset conditions, their age of onset, pattern of inheritance, and risk factors, both genetic and environmental.

If a single gene accounts for an adult-onset condition in a symptomatic person, diagnostic testing is used to

TABLE 11-4 Applications for Genetic Screening

Timing of Screening	Purpose	Examples
Preconception screening	For autosomal recessive inherited genetic conditions that occur with greater frequency among individuals of certain ethnic groups	Cystic fibrosis—all couples, but especially Northern European Caucasian, and Ashkenazi Jewish Tay-Sachs disease—Ashkenazi Jewish Sickle cell anemia—African American, Puerto Rican, Mediterranean, Middle Eastern Alpha-thalassemia—Southeast Asian, African American
Prenatal screening	For genetic conditions that are common and for which prenatal diagnosis is available when a pregnancy is identified at increased risk	Neural tube defects—spina bifida, anencephaly Down's syndrome Other chromosomal abnormalities—trisomy 18
Newborn screening	For genetic conditions for which there is specific treatment	Phenylketonuria (PKU) Galactosemia Homocystinuria Biotinidase deficiency

Adapted from U.S. National Library of Medicine. Genetics Home Reference (NLM). (2015e). *What are the types of genetic tests?* Retrieved November 24, 2015, from ghr.nlm.nih.gov/handbook/testing/uses

TABLE 11-5 Selected Adult-Onset Disorders

Clinical Description	Age of Onset	Genetic Inheritance	Molecular Genetics	Test Availability
Neurologic Conditions				
Early-onset familial Alzheimer's disease (EOFAD) Progressive dementia, memory failure, personality disturbance, loss of intellectual functioning associated with cerebral cortical atrophy, beta-amyloid plaque formation, and intraneuronal neurofibrillary tangles	<60–65 years; often <55 years	A.D.	PSEN1 (14q24) mutations in *presenilin 1* gene; (30–70% of pathogenic variants) APP (21q21.3); (10–15% of pathogenic variants) PSEN2 (14q24.2); (<5% of pathogenic variants)	Presymptomatic
Late-onset familial Alzheimer's disease Progressive dementia, cognitive decline	60–65 years		Apolipoprotein E (19q13) *APOE* gene product	Presymptomatic
Frontotemporal dementia with parkinsonism-17 Dementia and/or parkinsonism: Slowly progressive behavioural changes, language disturbances and/or extrapyramidal signs, rigidity, bradykinesia, and saccadic eye movements	40–60 years	A.D.	*MAPT* gene (linked to 17q21.1)	Diagnostic and presymptomatic
Huntington's disease Widespread degenerative brain change with progressive motor loss; both voluntary disability and involuntary disability, cognitive decline, chorea (involuntary movements) at later stage, psychiatric disturbances	Mean age, 35–44 years	A.D.	*HTT HD* gene (4p16)	Diagnostic and presymptomatic
Neuromuscular Disorders				
Spinocerebellar ataxia type 6 Slowly progressive cerebellar ataxia, dysarthria, and nystagmus	Mean age, 43–52 years	A.D.	*CACNA1A* gene (19p13)	Diagnostic and presymptomatic
Spinocerebellar ataxia type 1 Ataxia, dysarthria, and bulbar dysfunction	Mean age, 30–40 years	A.D.	*ATXN1* gene (6p22–p23)	Diagnostic and presymptomatic
Spinocerebellar ataxia type 2 Slow saccadic eye movement, peripheral neuropathy, decreased deep tendon reflexes, dementia	Mean age, 30–40 years	A.D.	*ATXN2* gene (12q24.1)	Diagnostic and presymptomatic
Spinocerebellar ataxia type 3 Progressive cerebellar ataxia and various other neurologic symptoms including dystonic-rigid syndrome, parkinsonian syndrome or combined dystonia, and peripheral neuropathy	Mean age onset in 30s	A.D.	*ATXN3* gene (14q21)	Diagnostic and presymptomatic
Myotonic muscular dystrophy type 1 Cataracts and myotonia or muscle wasting and weakness, frontal balding and electrocardiographic changes (heart block or dysrhythmia), diabetes in 5% of all cases	20–70 years	A.D. with variable penetrance	DMPK CTG trinucleotide repeat expansion	Diagnostic
Familial amyotrophic lateral sclerosis Progressive loss of motor function with predominantly lower motor neuron manifestations	50–70 years	Both A.D. and A.R.	ALS1 (*SOD1*) test for gene product superoxide/dismutase	Diagnostic
Hematologic Conditions				
Hereditary hemochromatosis High absorption of iron by gastrointestinal mucosa resulting in excessive iron storage in liver, skin, pancreas, heart, joints, and testes. Abdominal pain, weakness, lethargy, and weight loss are early symptoms. Untreated individuals can present with skin pigmentation, diabetes, hepatic fibrosis or cirrhosis, congestive heart failure, dysrhythmias, or arthritis.	40–60 years in males; after menopause in females	A.R.	*HFE* gene (6p21) C282Y mutation	Diagnostic and presymptomatic

continued >

TABLE 11-5 Selected Adult-Onset Disorders (Continued)

Clinical Description	Age of Onset	Genetic Inheritance	Molecular Genetics	Test Availability
Factor V Leiden thrombophilia				
Poor anticoagulant response to activated protein C with increased risk for venous thromboembolism and increased risk for fetal loss during pregnancy	30s; during pregnancy in females	A.D.	F5 (1q23) 1691G>A mutation; abnormal coagulation factor V	Diagnostic and presymptomatic
Polycystic kidney disease dominant				
Most common genetic disease in humans. Manifests with renal cysts, liver cysts, and occasionally intracranial/aortic aneurysm and hypertension. Loss of glomerular filtration can lead to kidney failure.	Variable onset; all carriers have detectable disease by ultrasonography at age 30 years	A.D.	PKD1 (16p13) polycystin; (approx. 85% of pathogenic variants) PKD2 (4q21–q23) polysystin 2; (approx. 15% of pathogenic variants)	Diagnostic and presymptomatic
Diabetes type 2				
Insulin resistance and impaired glucose tolerance	Variable onset most often >30 years	M.F.	Insulin promoter factor 1 (IPF-1); *CAPN10* gene polymorphism (single nucleotide polymorphism)	Research
			Interaction of $NIDDM_1$ chromosome 2 and several candidate genes on chromosomes 1, 2, 3, and 15 (CYP19)	Research
Cardiovascular disease				
Familial hypercholesterolemia; elevated low-density lipoprotein levels leading to coronary artery disease, xanthoma, and corneal arcus.	40–50 years	A.D.	LDLR (19p13.2) (60–80% of pathogenic variants) PCSK9 (1p323) (3% of pathogenic variants) APOB (2p24.1) (1–5% of pathogenic variants)	Diagnostic
Hyperlipidemia				
Elevated cholesterol and triglycerides associated with premature coronary disease and peripheral vascular disease	30–40 years	A.R.	*APOE* gene (19q13)	Clinical testing related to Alzheimer's/research
Alpha-1 antitrypsin deficiency				
60–70% small airway and alveolar wall destruction; emphysema, especially at base; chronic obstructive pulmonary disease	35-year-old smoker; 45-year-old nonsmoker	M.F. in A.R fashion	*SERPINA1* (14q32.12)	Diagnostic and presymptomatic
Oncology Conditions				
Multiple endocrine neoplasia				
Familial medullary thyroid cancer: Medullary thyroid cancer, pheochromocytoma, and parathyroid abnormalities	Early adulthood 40–50 years	A.D.	*RET* gene (10q11) MEN1 (11q13.1); (80–90% of pathogenic variants)	Presymptomatic
Breast cancer				
BRCA1/2 hereditary breast/ovarian cancer: Breast, ovarian, prostate, and colon (*BRCA1*); breast, ovarian, and other cancers (*BRCA2*)	30–70 years; often <50 years	A.D.	*BRCA1* gene (17q21) BRCA2 (13q12 DNA analysis)	Presymptomatic Presymptomatic
Lynch syndrome				
Colorectal, endometrial, bladder, gastric, biliary, and renal cell cancers as well as atypical endometrial hyperplasia and uterine leiomyosarcoma	<50 years	A.D.	MLH1 (3p21); (50% of pathogenic variants) MSH2 (2p22–p21); (40% of pathogenic variants) MSH6 (2p16); (7–10% of pathogenic variants) PMS2 (7p22); (<5% of pathogenic variants)	Presymptomatic and diagnostic

TABLE 11-5 Selected Adult-Onset Disorders (Continued)

Clinical Description	Age of Onset	Genetic Inheritance	Molecular Genetics	Test Availability
Li–Fraumeni syndrome				
Soft tissue sarcoma, breast cancer, leukemia, osteosarcoma, melanoma, and other cancers often including colon, pancreas, adrenal cortex, and brain	Often <40 years	A.D.	*TP53* gene (17q13); test for protein product	Presymptomatic and diagnostic
Cowden's syndrome				
Breast, nonmedullary (papillary or follicular) thyroid cancer; breast fibroadenomas and noncancerous thyroid modules or goitre; multiple buccal mucosa papillomas (cobblestone-line papules), facial trichilemmomas, gastrointestinal polyps; high-arched palate, thickened furrowed tongue, megalencephaly, and pectus excavatum.	40–50 years for cancer; teens—20 years for mucocutaneous lesions	A.D.	*PTEN* gene (10q23); gene product test	Presymptomatic and research

Adapted from Genetests. (2015a). GeneReviews. Retrieved July 12, 2015, from www.genetests.org; Online Mendelian Inheritance of Man. (2013a). *Alpha-1-antitrypsin deficiency (number 613490)*. Retrieved November 24, 2015, from www.omim.org/entry/613490?search=alpha1-antitrypsin%20deficiency&highlight=deficiency%20 alpha1%20alpha1antitrypsin%20antitrypsin; Online Mendelian Inheritance of Man. (2013b). *Beta-2-adrenergic receptor; ADRB2 (number 109690)*. Retrieved July 2, 2015, from www.omim.org/entry/109690?search=number%3A%28109690%20OR%20600807%20OR%20605238%29&highlight=605238%20600807%20109690

confirm a diagnosis to assist in the plan of care and management. Diagnostic testing for adult-onset conditions is most frequently used with autosomal dominant conditions, such as Huntington's disease or factor V Leiden thrombophilia, and with autosomal recessive conditions such as hemochromatosis. In families with known adult-onset conditions or with a confirmed genetic mutation in an affected family member, **presymptomatic testing** provides asymptomatic people with information about the presence of a genetic mutation and about the likelihood of developing the disease. Presymptomatic testing is considered for people in families with a known adult-onset condition in which either a positive or a negative test result indicates an increased or reduced risk of developing the disease, affects medical management, or allows earlier treatment of a condition.

Huntington's disease has served as the model for presymptomatic testing because the presence of the genetic mutation predicts disease onset and progression. Although preventive measures are not yet available for Huntington's disease, the genetics information enables health care professionals to develop a clinical, supportive, and psychological plan of care. Indeed, the presence of a single gene mutation has implications for the risk of developing many types of cancer; therefore, presymptomatic testing has become the standard of care so that early planning and implementation of select medical measures may reduce that risk (Leoz, Carballal, Moreira, et al., 2015).

Genomic Conditions

The foremost factor that may influence the development and severity of disease is a person's genomic makeup. In the absence of a single disease-causing gene, it is thought that multiple genes and other environmental factors are related to the onset of most adult diseases. For some diseases, the interactions among several genes and other environmental or metabolic events affect disease onset and progression. Specific gene–gene interactions or SNPs can confer susceptibility to disease. Most susceptibility testing is conducted in the research setting to identify candidate genes for diseases such as Alzheimer's disease, psychiatric conditions, heart disease, hypertension, and hypercholesterolemia (Conley et al., 2013; Korf & Rehm, 2013). Susceptibility testing helps distinguish variations within the same disease or response to treatment. For example, no single gene is associated with osteoporosis. Several polymorphisms on candidate genes related to the vitamin D receptor, estrogen and androgen receptors, and regulation of bone mineral density (BMD) have been shown to contribute to osteoporosis and fracture risk. Moreover, diet and exercise have a strong interaction with the polymorphisms regulating BMD (Cosman, de Beur, LeBoff, et al., 2014).

Some genomic tests may predict treatment response. For example, people may present with similar clinical signs and symptoms of asthma but have different responses to glucocorticoid (GC) treatment. Mutations in genes that regulate GC (i.e., corticosteroid) receptors are helpful to classify people with asthma as sensitive or resistant to treatment with corticosteroids (Online Mendelian Inheritance in Man, 2013b).

Population Screening

Population screening, the use of genetic testing for large groups or entire populations, to identify late-onset conditions is under development. For a test to be considered for population screening, there must be (1) sufficient information about gene distribution within populations, (2) accurate prediction about the development and progression of disease, and (3) appropriate medical management for asymptomatic people with a mutation. Currently, population screening is offered in some ethnic groups to identify cancer-predisposing genes. For example, the Ashkenazi Jewish have a greater chance of having a specific genetic mutation in the *BRCA1* or *BRCA2* gene. People with one of these *BRCA* mutations have approximately an 80% risk of breast cancer, a 40% to 65% risk of ovarian cancer (*BRCA1* carriers), a 20% risk of ovarian cancer (*BRCA2* carriers), and a 16% risk of prostate cancer (Genetests, 2015b). The identification of one of these mutations gives patients options for cancer screening as well as chemoprevention or prophylactic mastectomy or oophorectomy. Population screening is also being explored for other adult-onset conditions such as type 2 diabetes, heart disease, and hereditary hemochromatosis (iron overload disorder).

The Nursing Role in Testing and Screening for Adult-Onset Conditions

Nurses will be expected to participate in explaining risk and genetic predisposition, supporting informed health decisions and opportunities for prevention and early intervention, clarifying legal protections and risks related to genetic testing or health concerns, and protecting patients' privacy. Nurses must be alert for family histories that indicate multiple generations (autosomal dominant inheritance) or multiple siblings (autosomal recessive inheritance) are affected with the same condition or that the onset of disease is earlier than expected (e.g., multiple generations with early-onset hyperlipidemia). Possible adult-onset conditions are discussed with other members of the health care team for appropriate resources and referral. When a family history of disease is identified, a patient is made aware that this is a risk factor for disease; resources and referral are then provided. It is the patient's decision whether or not to pursue a genetic testing workup. For example, if a 45-year-old woman presents for her annual gynecology visit and reports a family history of colon cancer in multiple paternal relatives, including her father, the nurse should discuss the family history with the gynecologist. In addition, the woman should be alerted to the risk of colon cancer based on the family history and given information about possible genetic testing and referral for a colonoscopy.

If the existence of a mutation for an adult-onset condition in a family is identified, at-risk family members can be referred for predisposition testing. If the patient is found to carry the mutation, the nurse provides him or her with information and referral for risk-reduction measures and information about the risk to other family members. In that discussion, the nurse assures the patient that the test results are private and confidential and will not be shared with others, including family members, without the patient's permission. If the patient is an unaffected family member, the nurse discusses inheritance and the risk of developing the disease, provides support for the decision-making process, and offers referral for genetics services.

Predisposition testing is used for at-risk family members if the existence of a mutation for an adult-onset condition in a family is identified. Presymptomatic testing provides asymptomatic people with information about the presence of a genetic mutation and about the likelihood of developing the disease.

Personalized Genomic Treatments

Information about genes and their variations is helping researchers identify genetic differences that predispose certain people to more aggressive diseases and affect their responses to treatment. Genetics and genomics have revolutionized the field of oncology because genetic mutations are the basis for the development and progression of all cancers. In the medical era, individuals with cancer faced treatment based on the stage of the cancer, lymph node involvement, and spread to distant organs. Treatments for a particular type of cancer, stage for stage, were similar. Now, in the genomic era of personalized medicine, cancer is treated on the basis of genetic makeup. For example, women with early-stage breast cancer (i.e., tumour diameter less than 2 cm, estrogen receptor–positive tumours, no lymph node involvement) have often received chemotherapy. In the past, deciding which of these women would benefit the most from chemotherapy was unclear. Currently, a gene tumour profile of these women's tumours can be used to predict which women are more likely to have an aggressive cancer. Genetic testing helps clinicians to provide personalized care and the most effective treatment based on the genetic signature of the tumour treatment, called *targeted therapy,* tries to match the treatment to the specific malfunctioning genes expressed in the tumour, or to selectively inhibit genetic factors that promote cancer growth (Genetests, 2015b).

The use of individualized genetic and genomic data is rapidly resulting in personalized treatment for some common diseases.

Pharmacogenomics

The difference between genetics and genomics, described earlier in this chapter, aptly corresponds to the terms pharmacogenetics and pharmacogenomics, which combine pharmacology and genetics/genomics. Pharmacogenetics refers to the study of the effect of variations in a single gene on drug response and toxicity. The field of pharmacogenetics has evolved so that it has become a broader genomic-based approach that recognizes the interaction of multiple genes and the environment on drug response. Pharmacogenomics refers to the study of the combined effect of variations in many genes on drug response and toxicity and involves methods that rapidly identify which genetic variations influence a drug's effect. Pharmacogenomics involves the search for genetic variations associated with medication metabolism and efficacy, with the goal of tailoring treatment to each individual's genomic makeup (NLM, 2015d).

It has long been known that patients differ in their response to medications. The genetic and genomic variations in drug metabolism account largely for the differences in drug response and drug-related toxicities. Drug metabolism involves genetically controlled protein/enzyme activity for absorption, distribution, drug–cell interaction, inactivation, and excretion, metabolic processes that are known as pharmacokinetics. The cytochrome P450 (CYP) family genes play a key role in the pharmacokinetic process of drug metabolism (Johnson, 2013). Once a drug reaches its target cell, other genes such as those regulating cell receptors and cell signalling control the drug's effect, known as pharmacodynamics. Single genes may affect drug response. More commonly, drug response involves the interaction of multiple genes, the host, and the effects of other drugs. Figure 11-12 is a

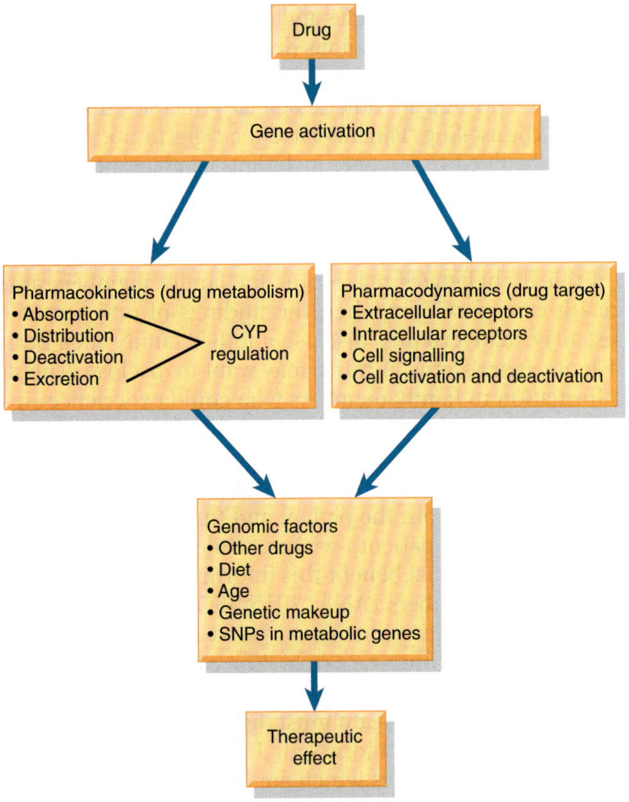

FIGURE 11-12. Simplified schematic representation of the multiple, complex, genetic-regulated mechanisms involved in pharmacokinetics (cytochrome [CYP]-dependent) and pharmacodynamics, along with other genomic and environmental factors affecting drug metabolism and treatment effect. SNP, single nucleotide polymorphism.

schematic display of the genetic and genomic influences on drug metabolism and treatment effect.

SNPs, described earlier, are common genetic variations that occur most frequently throughout the human genome and often contribute to variations in enzymatic activity that affect drug metabolism. The CYPs, a family of enzymes, play a key role in the pharmacokinetic process of drug metabolism. More than 300 variations (SNPs) of genes that control CYP activation and deactivation have been identified. Researchers have created a catalogue of CYP variations because of their role in drug metabolism (HUGO Gene Nomenclature Committee [HGNC], 2015).

Four classes of CYP metabolic activity levels have been identified based on a person's CYP genotype and the corresponding drug response: (1) poor metabolizers, (2) intermediate metabolizers, (3) extensive metabolizers, and (4) ultrarapid metabolizers (Ingelman-Sundberg, 2004). Poor metabolizers have a specific SNP variation in a CYP gene that causes little or no enzyme function, resulting in very little or no drug metabolism and higher blood levels of active drug because the drug cannot be absorbed or excreted. Conversely, ultrarapid metabolizers have SNP variations that cause increased enzyme activity, resulting in rapid absorption, distribution, and excretion of a drug. Ultrarapid metabolizers have lower drug blood levels, usually with inadequate therapeutic response or longer treatment time to achieve therapeutic results. Both poor metabolizers and ultrarapid metabolizers are predisposed to adverse drug reactions. Poor metabolizers may have adverse effects or toxicities from high blood levels of drugs and need a lower dose, whereas ultrarapid metabolizers have inadequate treatment response because of lower drug blood levels and may need a higher dose or more frequent dosing. Table 11-6 shows examples of differences in drug response in poor versus ultrarapid metabolizers. Intermediate metabolizers have reduced enzyme activity levels and metabolize drugs at a slower than normal rate. Because intermediate metabolizers have some enzyme activity, they may have differences in treatment response. Extensive metabolizers have normal enzyme activity levels and normal drug metabolism. Differences in metabolism of other medications occur with other genetic variations.

Nurses have traditionally monitored and reported drug response and drug adverse effects. Clinical guidelines for pharmacogenomic testing for several drugs, such as warfarin (Coumadin), abacavir (Ziagen), trastuzumab (Herceptin), mercaptopurine (Purinethol), and irinotecan (Camptosar), are currently being tested (NIH, 2014c). Pharmacogenomic testing offers patients and health care providers more information about drug dosage, time to achieve response, and risk of adverse effects. Nurses will provide education about a particular patient's genomic profile for drug metabolism and explain the rationale for the recommended dosage and likelihood of adverse effects.

TABLE 11-6 Examples of Clinical Effects of Cytochrome P450 Enzyme Variations

		Effects	
Enzyme	**Drug**	***Poor Metabolizer***	***Ultrarapid Metabolizer***
CYP2C9	Warfarin	Bleeding	Longer treatment time to achieve stable dosing
	Phenytoin	Ataxia	Not established
CYP2C19	Diazepam	Sedation	Poor response
CYP2D6	Tricyclic antidepressants	Cardiotoxicity	No response to recommended dose; need 10-fold increase in dose
	Selective serotonin reuptake inhibitors	Nausea	Not established
	Antipsychotics	Parkinson-like effects	Longer treatment time and higher drug costs

Adapted from Genetests. (2015a). GeneReviews. Retrieved July 12, 2015, from www.genetests.org/; HUGO Gene Nomenclature Committee (HGNC). (2015). *Cytochrome P450*. Retrieved July 9, 2015, from www.genenames.org/cgi-bin/search?search_type=all&search=cytochrome+P450&submit=Submit; Johnson, J. A. (2013). Pharmacogenetics in clinical practice: How far have we come and where are we going? *Pharmacogenomics*, *14*(7), 835–843.

Nurses will continue to incorporate information about gender differences, food interactions, and drug compliance into patient education (Consensus Panel, 2009).

Ethical, Legal, and Social Issues Surrounding Genetics

The rapid application of genetics and genomics across all sectors of health care has had implications for gathering, recording, and sharing personal health information. An ethical foundation provides nurses with a holistic framework for handling these issues with integrity and provides a basis for communicating genetic and genomic information to a patient, a family, other care providers, community agencies and organizations, and society. Nurses must consider their responsibilities in handling genetic and genomic information and strive to ensure that informed decision making occurs, that patient and family health information is kept private and confidential, and that access to and justice in health care is available to everyone (Badzek, Henaghan, Turner, et al., 2013).

Ethical Concerns

Ethical principles of beneficence (i.e., to do good) and nonmaleficence (i.e., to do no harm), as well as autonomy, justice, fidelity, and veracity, are used to resolve ethical dilemmas that may arise in clinical care. Respect for people is the ethical principle underlying all nursing care. Using these principles and the values of caring, nurses can promote thoughtful discussions that are useful when patients and families are facing genetics- and genomics-related health and reproductive decisions and consequences (Consensus Panel, 2009; International Society of Nurses in Genetics [ISONG], 2014). The ethical principles of autonomy, fidelity, and veracity are also important (American Nurses Association [ANA], 2015). (Further information about ethics is included in Chapter 3.)

Ethical questions relating to genetics and genomics occur in all settings and at all levels of nursing practice. At the level of direct patient care, nurses participate in providing genetic information, testing, and gene-based therapeutics. They offer patient care based on the values of self-determination and personal autonomy. To be as fully informed as possible, patients need appropriate, accurate, and complete information given at a level and in a form so that they and their families can make well-informed personal, medical, and reproductive health decisions. Nurses can help patients clarify values and goals, assess understanding of information, protect their rights, and support their decisions. Nurses can advocate for patient autonomy in health decisions. Several resources and position statements have been developed to guide genetic-related nursing practice (Consensus Panel, 2009; ISONG, 2014).

Respecting the patient's right to self-determination—that is, supporting decisions that reflect the patient's personal beliefs, values, and interests—is a central principle in directing how nurses provide genetic and genomic information and counselling. Nurses and others participating in genetic counselling make every attempt to respect the patient's ability to make autonomous decisions. Recognizing one's own attitudes and beliefs (see Chart 11-1) and how communication of genetic and genomic information may be influenced by those attitudes and beliefs is a first step toward assuring patients' autonomous decision making.

Confidentiality of genetic and genomic information and respect for privacy are other essential principles underlying genetic counselling. Patients have the right to not have test results divulged to anyone, including insurers, physicians, employers, or family members. Some patients pay for testing themselves so that insurers will not learn of the test, and others use a different name for testing to protect their privacy.

Ethical challenges may occur for family members and health care providers when the findings of one person's test may inadvertently disclose another family member's risk or carrier status. A nurse may want to disclose genetic information to family members who could experience significant harm if they do not know such information. However, the patient may have other views and may wish to keep this information from the family, resulting in an ethical dilemma for both the patient and the nurse. The nurse must honour the patient's wishes, while explaining to the patient the potential benefit this information may have for other family members (ANA, 2015; ISONG, 2014).

Ethical considerations must be reviewed as part of genetic and genomic research. For example, before an individual participates in genetic and genomic clinical research, the research team must discuss how any incidental findings will be addressed. Incidental findings are genetic-related illnesses which are found secondary to the intended goals of the research project or intended testing (Christenhusz, Devriendt, & Dierickx, 2013).

Canadian College of Medical Geneticists (https://www.ccmg-ccgm.org/) is responsible about issuing policy statements that list conditions known to be treatable and should be reported to the patient if found incidentally during clinical research.

Legal Aspects of Personalized Health Care

The Canadian College of Medical Geneticists continuously issues policies and guidelines to protect Canadians from genetic discrimination. This organization's purpose is to protect Canadians against improper use of genetic and genomic information in insurance and employment decisions. The Canadian College of Medical Geneticists is particularly helpful for people who carry a gene mutation but are asymptomatic for the illness. The act prohibits health insurers from denying coverage to a healthy person or charging higher insurance rates based on a person's genetic predisposition to a disease. The Canadian College of Medical Geneticists offers legal protection with regard to health insurance and employment. The act also prevents employers from using a person's genetic and genomic information to make decisions about hiring, job placement, promotion, or firing.

Ancestry, Cultural, Social, and Spiritual Concerns Related to Genetic and Genomic Practice

Genetics assessment addresses the ancestry of patients and families, as well as their ethnicity. This information helps identify individual patients and groups who could benefit from genetic testing for carrier identification, prenatal diagnosis, and susceptibility testing. For example,

NURSING RESEARCH PROFILE

Chart 11-3. Family Health History, Genetic Testing, and Feasibility of Pedigree Development

Pettey, C. M., McSweeney, J. C., Stewart, K. E., et al. (2015). Perceptions of family history and genetic testing and feasibility of pedigree development among African Americans with hypertension. *European Journal of Cardiovascular Nursing, 14*(1), 8–15.

Purpose

African Americans are the largest ethnic group at risk for hypertension (HTN) and cardiovascular disease. Due to the multifactorial inheritance of these illnesses, it is challenging for health care providers to identify a person at risk for HTN prior to clinical presentation. The purpose of this research was to determine the feasibility of creating pedigrees using the *U.S. Surgeon General's My Family Health Portrait.*

Design

Twenty-nine African American adults with HTN were recruited from a faith-based urban clinic. The mixed methods research design consisted of demographic data, ethnographic interviews, and the completion of the *My Family Health Portrait* for each participant. The *My Family Health Portrait* was collected but required a moderate amount of assistance by the researchers due to the high reading level needed to complete the forms. Upon completion of the *My Family Health Portrait,* a pedigree was created based upon the information that was obtained. The pedigrees and demographic data were completed using descriptive analysis. The pedigree was then used to guide the personal interviews (ranging from 30 to 60 minutes). Interviews were audiotaped and transcribed verbatim. Qualitative analysis was used to identify themes and code the interviews.

Findings

The use of medical terminology and overall design of the Web site was at a 12th-grade reading level and determined to be too high for the participants to comprehend. Themes from the interviews indicated that the participants were aware that family members had HTN but were not aware of specific details or did not understand the inheritance pattern. Some believed that having a family history of HTN influenced their behaviours while others believed that HTN was a matter of fate. The majority of the participants stated that they would participate in genetic testing for HTN.

Nursing Implications

It is important for nurses to be aware of genetic health literacy and offer means to assist patients in recognizing genetic health risks. The visual representation of a family pedigree, which may be developed using the *My Family Health Portrait* online tool, can aid the nurse in assessing patients' patterns of inheritance and health risks. In addition, viewing a family pedigree may motivate patients to be more engaged in health-related behaviours that will decrease their risk for familial diseases, such as HTN.

carrier testing for sickle cell anemia is routinely offered to people of African American descent, and carrier testing for Tay–Sachs disease and Canavan disease is offered to people of Ashkenazi Jewish descent. The American College of Obstetricians and Gynecologists (ACOG) recommends that members of at-risk racial and ethnic populations be offered carrier testing (ACOG Committee on Genetics, 2014a). ACOG and the American College of Medical Genetics (ACMG) recommend that all couples, particularly those of Northern European and Ashkenazi Jewish ancestry, be offered carrier screening for cystic fibrosis (ACOG Committee on Genetics, 2014b). Ideally, carrier testing is offered before conception to allow people who are carriers to make decisions about reproduction. Prenatal diagnosis is offered and discussed when both partners of a couple are found to be carriers.

It is also important to inquire about the patient's ethnic backgrounds when assessing for susceptibilities to adult-onset conditions such as hereditary breast or ovarian cancer. For example, a *BRCA1* cancer-predisposing gene mutation seems to occur more frequently in women of Ashkenazi Jewish descent. Therefore, asking about ethnicity can help identify people with an increased risk of cancer gene mutations (Iqbal, Ginsburg, Rochon, et al., 2015).

Nurses also should consider their patients' views about the significance of a genetic condition and its effect on self-concept, as well as patients' perception of the role of genetics in health and illness, reproduction, and disability. Patients' social and cultural backgrounds determine their interpretations and values about information obtained from genetic testing and evaluation and thus influence their perceptions of health, illness, and risk (Chart 11-3). Family structure, decision making, and educational background contribute in the same way (Consensus Panel, 2009).

Assessment of the patients' beliefs, values, and expectations regarding genetic testing and genetic and genomic information helps nurses provide appropriate information about the specific genetics or genomics topic. For example, in some cultures, people believe that health means the absence of symptoms and that the cause of illness is supernatural. Patients with these beliefs may initially reject suggestions for presymptomatic or carrier testing. However, by including resources such as family, cultural, and religious community leaders when providing genetics- or genomics-related health care, nurses can help ensure that patients receive information in a way that transcends social, cultural, and economic barriers (Boucher, Habin, & Underhill, 2014).

Applications of Genetics and Genomics in Nursing Practice

Nurses who provide genetics- and genomics-related health care blend the principles of human genetics with nursing care in collaboration with other professionals, including genetic specialists, to foster improvement, maintenance, and restoration of patients' health. Genetics-related nursing practice involves the care of people who have genetic conditions, those who may be predisposed to develop or pass on genetic

GENETICS IN NURSING PRACTICE

Chart 11-4. Genetics Family History: An Essential Tool for All Nurses

A well-documented family history can be used to:

- Assess risk of certain diseases
- Decide on testing strategies, such as what genetic and other diagnostic tests to order
- Establish a pattern of inheritance
- Identify other family members who are at increased risk
- Identify shared environmental risk factors
- Calculate risks
- Assess risk of passing on conditions to children
- Determine and recommend treatments that modify disease risk
- Making decisions about management or surveillance
- Develop patient rapport
- Educate patients

Key questions to ask about each family member include:

- What is the current age or what was the age at death?
- What is the ethnic background (some genetic conditions are more common in certain ethnic groups)?
- Is there a history of:
  - Multiple pregnancy losses/stillbirths?
  - Unexplained infertility?
  - Birth defects?
  - Mental retardation or developmental delay?
  - Learning disabilities?
  - Medical problems in children whose parents are closely related (second cousins or closer)?
  - Congenital or juvenile blindness, cataracts, hearing loss, or deafness?
  - Very short or very tall stature?
  - Several close relatives with the same or related conditions (e.g., breast or colon cancer, diabetes, heart disease, asthma, stroke, high blood pressure, kidney disease)?
  - Occurrence of a common condition with earlier age of onset than is usual (e.g., breast or colon cancer, hearing loss, dementia, heart disease)?

Adapted from Welch, B. M., Dere, W., & Schiffman, J. D. (2015). Family health history: The case for better tools. *JAMA, 313*(7), 1711–1712; Mayo Clinic. (2014). *Medical history: Compiling your medical family tree.* Retrieved July 12, 2015, from www.mayoclinic.org/healthy-lifestyle/adult-health/in-depth/medical-history/art-20044961; U.S. National Library of Medicine (NLM). (2015g). *Medline Plus. Family history*. Retrieved on July 12, 2015, from www.nlm.nih.gov/medlineplus/familyhistory.html#cat59.

conditions, and those who are seeking genetic information and referral for additional genetics services. The application of genomic information has been integrated into clinical practice areas of preconception, preimplantation, and prenatal testing, newborn screening, disease susceptibility, screening and diagnosis, prognosis and therapeutic decisions, and in monitoring disease recurrence (Calzone, Jenkins, Bakos, et al., 2013). The Genomic Nursing State of the Science Advisory Panel acknowledges that genomics is a fundamental, yet critical component, to nursing practice across the health care continuum and has mapped 67 genomic nursing research topics to the National Institute of Nursing Research Strategic Plan (Calzone et al., 2013).

Nurses are positioned to support patients and families with genetics- and genomics-related health concerns by ensuring that their health choices are informed ones and by advocating for the privacy and confidentiality of genetic and genomic information and for equal access to genetic testing and treatments (Badzek et al., 2013). Nurses are expected to attend to the genetic and genomic health care needs of the patient (Kirk & Marshallay, 2013).

Genetics and Genomics in Health Assessment

Assessment of a person's genetic and genomic health status is an ongoing process. Nurses collect information that can help identify individuals and families who have actual or potential genetics- or genomics-related health concerns or who may benefit from further genetics information, counselling, testing, and treatment. This process can begin before conception and continue throughout the life span. Nurses evaluate family and past medical histories, including prenatal history, childhood illnesses, developmental history, adult-onset conditions (in adults), past surgeries, treatments, and medications; this information may relate to the genetic or genomic condition at hand or to a condition being considered. (See Chapter 5 for more information on assessing past medical history.) Nurses also identify the patient's ethnic background and conduct a physical assessment to gather pertinent genetics information. The assessment also includes information about culture, spiritual beliefs, and ancestry. Health assessment includes determining a patient's or family's understanding of actual or potential genetics- or genomics-related health concerns and awareness of how these issues are communicated within a family (Boucher et al., 2014).

Family History Assessment

Nurses in any practice setting can assess families' genetics histories to identify the presence of a genetic trait, inherited condition, or predisposition. Targeted questions are used to identify genetic and genomic conditions for which further information, education, testing, or treatment can be offered (Chart 11-4). After consultation and collaboration with other health care providers and specialists, further genetic testing and evaluation is offered for the trait or condition in question. The genetics family history is used to make a diagnosis, identify testing strategies, and establish a pattern of inheritance. It includes at least three generations, as well as information about the current and past health status of all family members, including the age at onset of any illnesses, cause of death, and age at death. Nurses also can inquire about medical conditions that are known to have a heritable component and for which genetic testing may be available. Nurses obtain information about the presence of birth defects, mental retardation, familial traits, or similarly affected family members (Stephen, 2012).

CHART 11-5

Indications for Making a Genetics Referral

Prepregnancy and Prenatal

- Maternal age of 35 years or greater at expected time of delivery
- Previous child with a chromosome problem
- Positive alpha-fetoprotein profile screening test
- Previous child with a birth defect or family history of birth defects
- Pregnancy history of two or more unexplained miscarriages
- Maternal conditions such as diabetes, epilepsy, or alcoholism
- Exposures to certain medications or drugs during pregnancy
- Family history of mental retardation
- Either member of the couple has a birth defect such as cleft lip or palate, spina bifida, or congenital heart defect
- Either member of the couple has a chromosome abnormality

Pediatric

- Positive newborn screening test
- One or more major birth defects
- Unusual (dysmorphic) facial features
- Developmental delay/mental retardation
- Suspicion of a metabolic disorder
- Unusually tall or short stature, or growth delays
- Known chromosomal abnormality

Adult

- Intellectual disability without a known cause
- Unexplained infertility or multiple pregnancy losses
- A personal or family history of thrombotic events
- Adult-onset conditions such as hemochromatosis, hearing loss, visual impairment
- Family history of an adult-onset neurodegenerative disorder (e.g., Huntington's disease)
- Features of a genetic condition such as neurofibromatosis (*café au lait* spots, neurofibromas on the skin), Marfan's syndrome (unusually tall stature, dilation of the aortic root), others
- Personal or family history of cardiovascular disorders known to be associated with genetic factors such as cardiomyopathy or long QT syndrome
- Family history of cancers known to be associated with specific genes such as hereditary breast/ovarian cancer or hereditary nonpolyposis colorectal cancer (HNPCC)
- Family history of early-onset cancers and familial clustering of related tumours

Adapted from Pletcher, B. A., Toriello, H. V., Noblin, S. J., et al. (2007). Indications for genetic referral: A guide for healthcare providers. *Genetics in Medicine*, *9*(6), 385–389.

Nurses also consider the closeness of the relationship (genetic relatedness or consanguinity) among family members when assessing the risk of genetic conditions in couples or families. For example, when obtaining a preconception or prenatal family history, it is important for the nurse to ask if the prospective parents have common ancestors (i.e., are they first cousins?). This is important because people who are related have more genes in common than those who are unrelated, thus increasing their chance of having children with an autosomal recessive inherited condition such as cystic fibrosis. Ascertaining genetic relatedness provides direction for genetic counselling and evaluation. It may also serve as an explanation for parents who have a child with a rare autosomal recessive inherited condition or for a person who is similarly affected.

When the assessment of family history reveals that a patient has been adopted, genetics- and genomics-based health assessment becomes more challenging. Every effort is made to help the patient obtain as much information as possible about his or her biologic parents, including their ethnic backgrounds.

Questions about previous miscarriage or stillbirth are included in genetics health assessments to identify possible chromosomal conditions. Nurses inquire about any history of family members with inherited conditions or birth defects; maternal health conditions such as type 1 diabetes, seizure disorders, or PKU, which may increase the risk for birth defects in children; and about exposure to alcohol or other drugs during pregnancy. Maternal age is also noted; women who are 35 years of age or older who are considering pregnancy and childbearing or who are already pregnant should be offered prenatal diagnosis (e.g., testing through amniocentesis) because of the association between advanced maternal age and chromosomal abnormalities such as Down's syndrome.

Physical Assessment

Physical assessment may provide clues that a particular genetic or genomic condition is present in a person and family. Family history assessment may serve as a guide to focus the physical assessment. For example, a history of familial hypercholesterolemia would alert the nurse to assess for symptoms of hyperlipidemias (xanthomas, corneal arcus, abdominal pain of unexplained origin). As another example, a family history of neurofibromatosis type 1, an inherited condition involving tumours of the central nervous system, would prompt the nurse to carry out a detailed assessment of closely related family members. Skin findings such as *café au lait* spots, axillary freckling, or tumours of the skin (neurofibromas) would warrant referral for further evaluation, including genetic evaluation and counselling (NLM, 2015f).

If a genetic or genomic condition is suspected as a result of a family history or physical assessment, the nurse, as a part of his or her role, and in collaboration with the health care team, may initiate further discussion of genetics and genomic information, offering and discussing genetic tests and suggesting a referral for further genetic evaluation (Chart 11-5).

Psychosocial Assessment

Psychosocial assessment is an essential nursing component of the genetics health assessment to understand the potential impact of new genetic and genomic information

CHART 11-6

Assessing Psychosocial Genetic Health

The assessment of a client's psychosocial genetic health is based on the nurse's professional responsibility to "demonstrate in practice the importance of tailoring genetic and genomic information and services to clients based on their culture, religion, knowledge level, literacy and preferred language."

The nurse assesses:

- Educational level and understanding of the genetic condition or concern in the family
- Desired goals and health outcomes in relation to the genetic condition or concern
- Family rules regarding disclosure of medical information (e.g., some families may not reveal a history of a disease such as cancer or mental illness during the family history assessment)
- Family rules, boundaries, and cultural practices as well as personal preference about knowing genetic information
- Past coping mechanisms and social support
- Ability to make an informed decision (e.g., is the patient under stress from family situations, acute or chronic illness, or medications that may impair the patient's ability to make an informed decision?)

Adapted from Consensus Panel on Genetic/Genomic Nursing Competencies. (2009). *Essentials of genetic and genomic nursing: Competencies, curricular guidelines, and outcome indicators* (2nd ed.). Silver Spring, MD: Author.

on the patient and family and how they may cope with this information (Chart 11-6).

Genetic Counselling and Evaluation Services

People seek genetic counselling for a variety of reasons and at different stages of life. Some are seeking preconception or prenatal information, others are referred after the birth of a child who has a birth defect or suspected genetic condition, and still others are seeking information for themselves or their families because of the presence of, or a family history of, a genetic condition. Regardless of the timing or setting, genetic counselling is offered to all people who have questions about genetics or genomics and their health.

As the contribution of genetics and genomics to the health–illness continuum is recognized, genetic counselling will become a responsibility of all health care professionals in clinical practice. Nurses are in an ideal position to assess the patient's health and genetics family history and to make referrals for specialized diagnosis and treatment. They offer anticipatory guidance by explaining the purpose and goals of a referral. They collaborate with other health care providers in giving supportive and follow-up counselling and coordinating follow-up and case management.

Genetics Services

Genetics services provide genetics information, education, and support to patients and families. Medical geneticists, genetics counsellors, and advanced practice nurses in genetics provide specific genetics services to patients and families who are referred by their primary or specialty health care providers. A team approach is often used to obtain and interpret complex family history information, evaluate and diagnose genetic conditions, interpret and discuss complicated genetic test results, support patients throughout the evaluation process, and offer professional and family support. Patients participate as team members and decision makers throughout the process. Genetics services enable patients and their families to learn and understand relevant aspects of genetics and genomics, to make informed health decisions, and to receive support as they integrate personal and family genetic and genomic information into daily living.

Genetic counselling may take place over an extended period and may entail more than one counselling session, which may include other family members. The components of genetic counselling are outlined in Chart 11-7. Although genetic counselling may be offered at any point during a patient's life span, counselling issues are often relevant to the life stage in which counselling is sought (NIH, 2013b). Some examples are presented in Chart 11-8.

CHART 11-7

Components of Genetic Counselling

Information and Assessment Sources

- Reason for referral
- Family history
- Medical history/records
- Relevant test results and other medical evaluations
- Social and emotional concerns
- Relevant cultural, educational, and financial factors

Analysis of Data

- Family history
- Physical examination as needed
- Additional laboratory testing and procedures (e.g., echocardiogram, ophthalmology, or neurologic examination)

Communication of Genetic Finding

- Natural history of disorder
- Pattern of inheritance
- Reproductive and family health issues and options
- Testing options
- Management and treatment issues

Counselling and Support

- Identify individual and family questions and concerns
- Identify existing support systems
- Provide emotional and social support
- Refer for additional support and counselling as indicated

Follow-Up

- Written summary to referring primary care providers and family
- Coordination of care with primary care providers and specialists
- Additional discussions of test results or diagnosis

Adapted from Genetics Home Reference. *Genetic consultation*. Retrieved August 16, 2015, from www.ghr.nlm.nih.gov/handbook/consult?show=all#consultation

CHART 11-8

Genetic Counselling Across the Life Span

Prenatal Issues

- Understanding prenatal screening and diagnosis testing
- Implications of reproductive choices
- Potential for anxiety and emotional distress
- Effects on partnership, family, and parental–fetal bonding

Newborn Issues

- Understanding newborn screening results
- Potential for disrupted parent–newborn relationship on diagnosis of a genetic condition
- Parental guilt
- Implications for siblings and other family members
- Coordination and continuity of care

Pediatric Issues

- Caring for children with complex medical needs
- Coordination of care
- Potential for impaired parent–child relationship
- Potential for social stigmatization

Adolescent Issues

- Potential for impaired self-image and decreased self-esteem
- Potential for altered perception of family
- Implications for lifestyle and family planning

Adult Issues

- Potential for ambiguous test results
- Identification of a genetic susceptibility or diagnosis without an existing cure
- Effect on marriage, reproduction, parenting, and lifestyle
- Potential impact on insurability and employability

Adapted from Dwyer, T. M., Glaser, R. L., & Mason, T. M. (2016). Inheritance patterns in human phenotypes and types of genetic disorders. In C. E. Kasper, T. A. Schneidereith, & F. R. Lashley (Eds.). *Lashley's essentials of clinical genetics in nursing practice* (pp. 65–114). New York: Springer Publishing Company.

Providing Precounselling Information

All genetics specialists, including nurses who participate in the genetic counselling process and those with access to a person's genetics information, must honour a patient's desire for confidentiality. Genetics information should not be revealed to family members, insurance companies, employers, and schools if the patient so desires, even if keeping the information confidential is difficult.

Preparing the patient and family, promoting informed decision making, and obtaining informed consent are essential in genetic counselling. Nurses assess the patient's capacity and ability to give voluntary consent. This includes assessment of factors that may interfere with informed consent, such as hearing loss, language differences, cognitive impairment, and the effects of medication. Nurses make sure that a person's decision to undergo testing is not affected by coercion, persuasion, or manipulation. Because information may need to be repeated over time, nurses offer follow-up discussion as needed (Consensus Panel, 2009).

The genetics service to which a patient or family is referred for genetic counselling will ask the nurse for background information for evaluation. Genetics specialists need to know the reason for referral, the patient's or family's reason for seeking genetic counselling, and potential genetics-related health concerns. For example, a nurse may refer a family with a new diagnosis of hereditary breast or ovarian cancer for counselling or to discuss the likelihood of developing the disease and the implications for other family members. The family may have concerns about confidentiality and privacy. The nurse and the genetics specialist tailor the genetic counselling to respond to these concerns.

With the patient's permission, genetics specialists will request the relevant test results and medical evaluations. Nurses obtain permission from the patient and, if applicable, from other family members to provide medical records that document the genetic condition of concern. In some situations, evaluation of more than one family member may be necessary to establish a diagnosis of a genetic disorder. Nurses explain that the medical information is needed to ensure that appropriate information and counselling (including risk interpretation) are provided.

The genetics service asks nurses about the emotional and social status of the patient and family. Genetics specialists want to know the coping skills of patients and families who have recently learned of the diagnosis of a genetic disorder as well as what type of genetics information is being sought. Nurses help identify cultural and other issues that may influence how information is provided and by whom. For example, for patients with hearing loss, a sign interpreter's services may have to be arranged. For those with vision loss, alternative forms of communication may be necessary. Genetics professionals prepare for the genetic counselling and evaluation with these relevant issues in mind (NIH, 2013b).

Preparing Patients for Genetics Evaluation

Before a genetic counselling appointment, the nurse discusses with the patient and family the type of family history information that will be collected during the consultation. Family history collection and analysis are comprehensive and focus on information that may be relevant to the genetics- or genomics-related concern in question. The genetic analysis always includes assessment for any other potentially inherited conditions for which testing, prevention, and treatment may be possible.

A physical examination may be performed by the medical geneticist to identify specific clinical features that are diagnostic of a genetic condition. The examination also helps determine if further testing is needed to diagnose a genetic disorder. This examination generally involves assessment of all body systems, with a focus on specific physical characteristics considered for diagnosis. Nurses describe the diagnostic evaluations that are part of a genetics consultation and explain their purposes.

Communicating Genetic and Genomic Information to Patients

After the family history and physical examination are completed, the genetics team reviews the information gathered before beginning genetic counselling with the patient and family. The genetics specialists meet with the patient and family to discuss their findings. If the information gathered confirms the presence of a genetic condition in a family, genetics specialists discuss with the patient the natural history of the condition, the pattern of inheritance, and the implications of the condition for reproductive and general health. When appropriate, specialists also discuss relevant testing and management options.

Providing Support

The genetics team provides support throughout the counselling session and identifies personal and family concerns. Genetics specialists use active listening to interpret patient concerns and emotions, seek and provide feedback, and demonstrate understanding of those concerns. Genetics specialists suggest referral for additional social and emotional support. Genetics specialists discuss pertinent patient and family concerns and needs with nurses and primary health care teams so that they can provide additional support and guidance (Kirk & Marshallay, 2013; NIH, 2013b). Nurses assess the patient's understanding of the information given during the counselling session, clarify information, answer questions, assess patient reactions, and identify support systems.

Follow-Up After Genetic Evaluation

As follow-up to genetic evaluation and counselling, genetics specialists prepare a written summary of the evaluation and counselling session for the patient and, with the patient's consent, send this summary to the primary health care provider as well as other providers identified by the patient as participants in care. The consultation summary outlines the results of the family history and physical and laboratory assessments, provides a discussion of the specific diagnosis (if made), reviews the inheritance and associated risk of recurrence for the patient and his or her family, presents reproductive and general health options, and makes recommendations for further testing and management. The nurse reviews the summary with the patient and identifies information, education, and counselling for which follow-up genetic counselling may be useful (Kirk & Marshallay, 2013).

Follow-up genetic counselling is always offered because some patients and families need more time to understand and discuss the specifics of a genetic test or diagnosis, or they may wish to review reproductive options again later, when pregnancy is being considered. Follow-up counselling is also offered to patients when further evaluation and counselling of extended family members is recommended (Kirk & Marshallay, 2013).

As part of follow-up, nurses can educate patients about sources of information about genetic and genomic issues. Some resources that provide the most up-to-date and reliable genetic and genomic information are available on the Internet (see Resources at the end of this chapter).

Genetics and Genomics Tomorrow

The pace of genetic and genomic research is transforming our understanding of the role of genetics and genomics in health and disease. In addition, it is increasing clinical opportunities for presymptomatic prediction of illness based on a patient's genetic makeup. Genetic research is now focused on identifying the genetic and environmental causes of common diseases such as diabetes, heart disease, and asthma. The studies are opening the doors for many advances in the prevention and treatment of both rare and common diseases (NIH, 2014d).

As applications of genetics and genomics to health and disease develop, genetic testing may be used to scan all of a patient's genetic material so that disease risk variants can be identified and early interventions and treatments can be determined. Personalized medicine will continue to expand, and many treatments and interventions for medical conditions will be chosen on the basis of what genetic testing indicates about a patient's genetic makeup. Nurses will be on the front line in communicating genetic and genomic information to patients, families, and communities. Patients, families, and communities will also expect that health care providers, including nurses, will use new genetic and genomic information and technologies in the provision of care. It is, therefore, imperative that all nurses become fluent in the language of genetics and genomics so that they can provide effective nursing care (Consensus Panel, 2009).

Critical Thinking Exercises

1 A 16-year-old African American male is trying out for the football team. He has been complaining of joint pain for the past 3 days. During his last football practice, he was rushed to the hospital due to severe respiratory compromise. What immediate assessment questions should the nurse include? His parents deny any prior history of respiratory difficulty. Upon further investigation, it is learned that the patient has sickle cell disease. How does this relate to his joint pain? What is the inheritance pattern of sickle cell disease? What is unique with this type of inheritance pattern? Should the parents be treated for sickle cell disease? To help during this sickle cell crisis, how might pharmacogenetics be applied to best manage pain? What questions should the patient and his parents be asked regarding pain control? What evidence related to pain medications supports the discussion?

2 A 51-year-old man is admitted to the hospital with complaint of lower extremity pain. Upon assessment, the right calf is warm to touch and edematous. The pedal pulse is not palpable but able to be attained by Doppler. What critical questions should the nurse include in the admission assessment? The patient becomes diaphoretic and short of breath. Oxygen is applied and an x-ray is obtained. The findings from the x-ray indicate that the patient has three small blood clots in his lung. Based on these new findings, what additional questions should be asked? Hematology reports confirm that the patient has factor V Leiden thrombophilia. What concerns should the nurse discuss with the patient? Warfarin (Coumadin) will be started according to hospital protocol for a diagnosis of deep vein thrombosis. How might principles of pharmacogenetics be applied while monitoring the effectiveness of the warfarin? Knowing that factor V Leiden thrombosis is an autosomal dominant condition, what genetic information needs to be shared with the patient? What recommendations will be made for the patient's family?

3 A 34-year-old man is diagnosed with hypertrophic cardiomyopathy after experiencing chest pain and shortness of breath while exercising. The physician explains that this is a hereditary condition known to have an autosomal dominant pattern of inheritance. The patient has two young sons, 2 and 5 years of age. His mother is living but his father died from cardiac problems at the age of 60 years. During your assessment, you take a family history and complete a three-generation pedigree including the information that is known. Draw the pedigree illustrating autosomal dominant inheritance. What advice should be given to this patient regarding genetic testing?

REFERENCES AND SELECTED READINGS

Book

Carroll, E. W. (2017). Genetic control of cell function and inheritance. In R. A. Hannon, & C. M. Porth (Eds.). *Porth pathophysiology: Concepts of altered health states* (2nd Canadian ed.). Philadelphia, PA: Wolters Kluwer Health/Lippincott Williams & Wilkins.

Consensus Panel on Genetic/Genomic Nursing Competencies. (2009). *Essentials of genetic and genomic nursing: Competencies, curricular guidelines, and outcome indicators* (2nd ed.). Silver Spring, MD: American Nurses Association.

Dwyer, T. M., Glaser, R. L., & Mason, T. M. (2016). Inheritance patterns in human phenotypes and types of genetic disorders. In C. E. Kasper, T. A. Schneidereith, & F. R. Lashley (Eds.). *Lashley's essentials of clinical genetics in nursing practice* (pp. 65–114). New York: Springer Publishing Company.

Porth, C. M. (2017). Genetic and congenital disorders. In R. A. Hannon, & C. M. Porth (Eds.). *Porth pathophysiology: Concepts of altered health states* (2nd Canadian ed., pp. 128–149). Philadelphia, PA: Wolters Kluwer Health/Lippincott Williams & Wilkins.

Stephen, T. C. (2012). The health history. In T. C. Stephen, D. L. Skillen, R. A. Day, S. Jensen (Eds.). *Canadian Jensen's nursing health assessment: A best practice approach* (pp. 37–51). Philadelphia, PA: Wolters Kluwer Health/Lippincott Williams and Wilkins.

Journals and Electronic Documents

American College of Obstetricians and Gynecologists (ACOG) Committee on Genetics. (2014a). *Committee opinion. Committee on Genetics. Number 442 (replaces 298). Preconception and prenatal carrier screening for genetic diseases in individuals of eastern European Jewish descent.* Retrieved July 10, 2015, from www.acog.org/-/media/Committee-Opinions/Committee-on-Genetics/co442.pdf?dmc=1&ts=20150710T1049586049

American College of Obstetricians and Gynecologists (ACOG) Committee on Genetics. (2014b). *Committee opinion. Committee on Genetics. Number 486. Update on carrier screening for cystic fibrosis* (pp. 1–4). Retrieved July 10, 2015, from www.acog.org/-/media/Committee-Opinions/Committee-on-Genetics/co486.pdf?dmc=1&ts=20150710T1033593218p

American Nurses Association (ANA). (2015). The code of ethics for nurses with interpretive statements. Retrieved from http://www.nursingworld.org/MainMenuCategories/EthicsStandards/CodeofEthicsforNurses

Ashley, E. A. (2015). The precision medicine initiative: A new national effort. *JAMA, 313*(21), 2119–2120.

Badzek, L., Henaghan, M., Turner, M., et al. (2013). Ethical, legal, and social issues in the translation of genomics into health care. *Journal of Nursing Scholarship, 45*(1), 15–24.

Boucher, J., Habin, K., & Underhill, M. (2014). Cancer genetics and genomics: Essentials for oncology nurses. *Clinical Journal of Oncology Nursing, 18*(3), 355–359.

Calzone, K. A., Jenkins, J., Bakos, A. D., et al. (2013). A blueprint for genomic nursing science. *Journal of Nursing Scholarship, 45*(1), 96–104.

Christenhusz, G. M., Devriendt, K., & Dietrickx, K. (2013). To tell or not tell? A systematic review of ethical reflections on incidental findings arising in genetics contexts. *European Journal of Human Genetics, 21*(3), 248–255.

Conley, Y. P., Biesecker, L. G., Gonsalves, S., et al. (2013). Current and emerging technology approaches in genetics. *Journal of Nursing Scholarship, 45*(1), 5–14.

Cosman, F., de Beur, S. J., LeBoff, M. S., et al. (2014). Clinician's guide to prevention and treatment of osteoporosis. *Osteoporosis International, 25*(10), 2359–2381.

Cramer, S. A., Adjei, I. M., & Labhasetwar, V. (2015). Advancements in the delivery of epigenetic drugs. *Expert Opinion Drug Delivery, 12*(9), 1501–1512.

Genetests. (2015b). *Breast cancer*. Retrieved June 30, 2015, from https://www.breastcancer.org/symptoms/testing/genetic

Greco, K. E., Tinley, S., & Seibert, D. (2012). *Essential genetic and genomic competencies for nurses with graduate degrees.* Retrieved July 11, 2015, from www.nursingworld.org/MainMenuCategories/EthicsStandards/Genetics-1/Essential-Genetic-and-Genomic-Competencies-for-Nurses-With-Graduate-Degrees.pdf

Harkness, E. F., Barrow, E., Newton, K., et al. (2015). Lynch syndrome caused by MLH1 mutations is associated with an increased risk of breast cancer: A cohort study. *Journal of Medical Genetics, 52*(8), 553–556.

HUGO Gene Nomenclature Committee (HGNC). (2015). *Cytochrome P450*. Retrieved July 9, 2015, from www.genenames.org/cgi-bin/search?search_type=all&search=cytochrome+P450&submit=Submit

Ingelman-Sundberg, M. (2004). Pharmacogenetics of cytochrome P450 and its applications in drug therapy: The past, present and future. *Trends in Pharmacological Sciences, 25*(4), 193–200.

International Society of Nurses in Genetics (ISONG). (2014). Retrieved from https://www.isong.org/resources/Documents/ISONG%20White%20paper%20on%20GINA%20approved%20May%202018.pdf

Iqbal, J., Ginsburg, O., Rochon, P., et al. (2015). Differences in breast cancer stage at diagnosis and cancer-specific survival by race and ethnicity in the United States. *JAMA, 313*(2), 165–173.

Johnson, J. A. (2013). Pharmacogenetics in clinical practice: How far have we come and where are we going? *Pharmacogenomics, 14*(7), 835–843.

Kirk, M., & Marshallay, M. (2013). Providing nursing care and support to individuals and families with genetic/genomic healthcare needs. *Nursing Standard, 28*(16), 39–46.

Korf, B. R., & Rehm, H. L. (2013). New approaches to molecular diagnosis. *JAMA, 309*(14), 1511–1521.

Leoz, M. L., Carballal, S., Moreira, L., et al. (2015). The genetic basis of familial adenomatous polyposis and its implications for clinical practice and risk management. *The Application of Clinical Genetics, 8*, 95–107.

National Institutes of Health. National Human Genome Research Institute (NIH). (2013a). *Learning about Turner syndrome*. Retrieved from: www.genome.gov/19519119

National Institutes of Health (NIH). National Human Genome Research Institute. (2013b). *Frequently asked questions about genetic counseling*. Retrieved July 9, 2015, from www.genome.gov/19016905

National Institutes of Health (NIH). National Human Genome Research Institute. (2014a). *All about the Human Genome Project*. Retrieved July 5, 2015, from www.genome.gov/10001772

National Institutes of Health (NIH). National Human Genome Research Institute. (2014b). *Learning about sickle cell disease*. Retrieved July 8, 2015, from www.genome.gov/10001219

National Institutes of Health. National Human Genome Research Institute (NIH). (2014c). *Frequently asked questions about pharmacogenomics*. Retrieved from: www.genome.gov/27530645#al-3

National Institutes of Health. National Human Genome Research Institute (NIH). (2014d). *New horizons and research activities*. Retrieved from: www.genome.gov/27527636

National Institutes of Health (NIH). National Human Genome Research Institute. (2015a). *Talking glossary of genetic terms*. Retrieved July 7, 2015, from www.genome.gov/Glossary/index.cfm?id=92

National Institutes of Health (NIH). National Human Genome Research Institute. (2015b). *Chromosome abnormalities*. Retrieved June 30, 2015, from www.genome.gov/11508982

National Institutes of Health (NIH). National Human Genome Research Institute. (2015c). *Policy and program analysis branch*. Retrieved July 9, 2015, from www.genome.gov/10001087

Online Mendelian Inheritance in Man. (2013b). *Beta-2-adrenergic receptor; ADRB2 (number 109690)*. Retrieved July 2, 2015, from www.omim.org/entry/109690?search=number%3A%28109690%20OR%20600807%20OR%20605238%29&highlight=605238%20600807%20109690

Roadmap Epigenomics Consortium. (2015). Integrative analysis of 111 reference human epigenomes. *Nature*, *518*(7539), 317–330.

Romanoski, C. E., & Glass, C. K. (2015). Roadmap for regulation: Differentiation enhanced. *Nature*, *518*(7539), 314–315.

Simopoulos, A. P. (2009). Genetic screening: Programs. Principles, and research—thirty years later. *Public Health Genomics*, *12*, 105–111.

U.S. National Library of Medicine (NLM). Genetics Home Reference. (2015a). *What are the different ways in which a genetic condition can be inherited?* Retrieved June 30, 2015, from ghr.nlm.nih.gov/handbook/inheritance/inheritancepatterns

U.S. National Library of Medicine. Genetics Home Reference (NLM). (2015b). *What are reduced penetrance and variable expressivity?* Retrieved from: ghr.nlm.nih.gov/handbook/inheritance/penetranceexpressivity

U.S. National Library of Medicine (NLM). Genetics Home Reference. (2015c). *Can changes in the structure of chromosomes affect health and development?* Retrieved June 30, 2015, from ghr.nlm.nih.gov/handbook/mutationsanddisorders/structuralchanges

U.S. National Library of Medicine (NLM). Genetics Home Reference. (2015d). *What is pharmacogenomics?* Retrieved July 9, 2015, from ghr.nlm.nih.gov/handbook/genomicresearch/pharmacogenomics

U.S. National Library of Medicine (NLM). Genetics Home Reference. (2015f). *Neurofibromatosis type 1*. Retrieved July 9, 2015, from ghr.nlm.nih.gov/condition/neurofibromatosis-type-1

Waters, E. A., Muff, J., & Hamilton, J. G. (2014). Multifactorial beliefs about the role of genetics and behavior in common health conditions: Prevalence and associations with participant characteristics and engagement in health behaviors. *Genetics in Medicine*, *16*, 913–921.

The White House. (2015). *Fact sheet: President Obama's precision medicine initiative*. Retrieved June 2, 2015, from www.whitehouse.gov/the-press-office/2015/01/30/fact-sheet-president-obama-s-precision-medicine-initiative

Resources

Biologics and Genetic Therapies Directorate (BGTD) of Health Canada, Director's General Office: http://www.hc-sc.gc.ca/dhp-mps/brgtherap/activit/index-eng.php

Canadian Association of Genetic Counsellors (CAGC): http://www.cagc-accg.ca

Canadian Cancer Society/Société canadienne du cancer, National Office: http://www.cancer.ca

Canadian Directory of Genetic Support Groups, Support Group Directory, Regional Medical Genetics Centre: http://www.lhsc.on.ca/programs/medgenet

Canadian Genetic Disease Network: https://www.cifar.ca/research/programs/genetic-networks

Canadian Organization for Rare Disorders (CORD): https://www.raredisorders.ca/

Canadian Paediatric Surveillance Program (CPSP): http://www.cps.ca/English/Surveillance/CPSP/index.htm

Canadian Society for molecular biosciences: https://csmb-scbm.ca/

Genetic Resources Ontario: http://www.geneticresourcesontario.ca/Genome British Columbia: http://www.genomebc.ca/ethics/newsletter.htm

Genome Program: http://www.genomecanada.ca

Inherited Metabolic Disorders: http://www.ihsc.on.ca/programs/rmgc/met/metabolic.htm

Public Health Agency of Canada: http://www.hc-sc.gc.ca/hpb/lcdc

12 Chronic Illness and Disabilities

Adapted by Joseph Osuji and Mohamed Toufic El Hussein

Learning Objectives

On completion of this chapter, the learner will be able to:

1. Compare and contrast the concepts of chronic illness, chronic disease, and disability.
2. Identify factors related to the increasing incidence of chronic conditions.
3. Describe characteristics of chronic conditions and their implications for people with chronic conditions and for their families.
4. Describe the phases of chronic conditions.
5. Specify the advantages and disadvantages of various models of disability.
6. Apply the nursing process to the care of the patient with chronic conditions.

Chronic health problems affect people of all ages—they occur in the very young, the middle aged, and the very old. Chronic conditions do, however, increase in frequency with age, and older people often have multiple chronic disorders (Public Health Agency of Canada, 2013). Chronic illnesses are found in all socioeconomic, ethnic, cultural, and racial groups; certain diseases, however, occur more frequently in some groups than in others. **Chronic diseases** may refer to **noncommunicable diseases**, chronic conditions, or chronic disorders. In contrast, **chronic illness** refers to the human experience of living with a chronic disease or condition. Chronic illness includes the individual's perception of the experience of having a chronic disease or condition and the individual's and others' responses to it, including health care professionals (Kramer-Kile, Osuji, Larsen, et al., 2014). Individuals' and their families' values and previous experiences determine their perception and beliefs about the condition, which in turn affect their illness and wellness behaviours. Their values are influenced by a number of demographic, socioeconomic, technologic, cultural, and environmental variables. Only the individual and the family really know what it is like to live with chronic illness.

Poverty, cultural or language barriers, and social or geographic isolation often act as barriers to receiving preventive screening measures such as mammography, cervical screening, and routine checkups.

The Phenomenon of Chronicity

Chronic diseases are long-term health conditions that affect one's well-being and function in an episodic, continuous, or progressive way over many years of life. Although each chronic disease or condition has its own specific physiologic characteristics, chronic conditions share common features. Many chronic conditions, for example, have pain and fatigue as associated symptoms. Other common symptoms are sleep disturbances and difficulty adjusting to the onset and uncertainty of a chronic condition (Lorig, Holman, Sobel, et al., 2012). Many people with chronic health conditions and **disability** function independently with only minor inconvenience to their everyday lives; others, however, require frequent and close monitoring or placement in long-term care facilities. Certain conditions require advanced technology for survival, as in the late stages of chronic obstructive lung disease or end-stage renal disease, or intensive care or mechanical ventilation for periods of weeks, months, or years. People with disorders such as these have been described as being chronically critically ill, although there is no consensus on a definition of chronic critical illness.

Many chronic conditions require complicated therapeutic regimens to successfully manage them. Unlike the term *acute*, which implies a curable and relatively short disease course, *chronic* describes a prolonged trajectory and conditions are generally incurable. It is this characteristic of duration that often makes managing chronic conditions so difficult for those who must live with them on a day-to-day basis throughout their life span.

Some chronic conditions have little effect on quality of life, whereas others have a major effect because they result in disability. However, it is important to note that not all disabilities are a result of chronic illness, and not all chronic illnesses cause disability (Drum, 2014). Unlike the term *acute*, which implies a curable and relatively short disease course, the term *chronic* describes a long disease course that may be incurable. This often makes managing chronic conditions difficult for those who live with them. Although chronic conditions often cannot be cured, nurses can and do make a difference in the illness experience with quality nursing care in the absence of a cure (Kramer-Kile et al., 2014).

Psychological and emotional reactions of people to acute and chronic conditions and changes in their health status are described in detail in this chapter. People who develop chronic conditions may react with shock, disbelief, depression, anger, resentment, or a number of other emotions when they are initially diagnosed. How people react and cope with chronic conditions over time is usually similar to how they react to other events in their lives, depending, in part, on their understanding of the condition and their perception about its disruption of their own and their family's lives. Adjustment to chronic illness is affected by various factors:

- Personality before the illness
- Unresolved anger or grief from the past
- Suddenness, extent, and duration of lifestyle changes necessitated by the illness
- Family and individual resources for dealing with stress
- Stages of the individual/family life cycle
- Previous experience with illness and crises

Psychological, emotional, and cognitive reactions to chronic conditions are likely to occur at the initial onset, but they may also recur if symptoms worsen or recur after a period of remission. Symptoms associated with chronic illnesses are often unpredictable, and some are perceived as crisis events by people and their families, who must contend with both the uncertainty of chronic illness and the changes it brings to their lives. This chapter describes some of the problems and challenges faced by people living with chronic conditions and offers a guide to nursing assessment and intervention when providing care to people with chronic illness.

Definition of Chronic Conditions

Chronic conditions are health problems with associated symptoms or disabilities that require long-term management over 3 months or longer. Chronic diseases or conditions are often defined as medical conditions or health problems with associated symptoms or disabilities that require long-term management. No single definition for chronic disease exists, but it is generally accepted that chronic diseases are those that persist for months or years rather than days or weeks (Goodman, Posner, Huang, et al., 2013). Considered from this perspective, "chronic conditions" cover a broad array of what could appear on the surface as disparate health problems. A specific condition may be a result of illness, persistent communicable infectious disease (e.g., human immunodeficiency virus [HIV]/acquired immunodeficiency syndrome [AIDS]), genetic factors, or injury. It may also be a consequence of life circumstances or health-limiting behaviours that began earlier in life.

Chronic diseases or disorders are one of the major health and development challenges of the 21st century because of their global human, social, and financial consequences. Although chronic diseases affect all countries, their impact is more severe in low- and middle-income countries (i.e., South American, African, and Asian countries), where the majority of premature deaths due to chronic diseases occur. Their impact is particularly devastating to poor and vulnerable populations. Chronic diseases also referred to as noncommunicable diseases, cause

Glossary

chronic disease: medical or health problem with associated symptoms or disabilities that require long-term management; has also been referred to as noncommunicable disease, chronic condition, or chronic disorder

chronic illness: the experience of living with a chronic disease or condition; the individual's perception of the experience and the individual's and others' responses to the chronic disease or condition

disability: restriction or lack of ability to perform an activity in a normal manner; the consequences of impairment in terms of an individual's functional performance and activity. Disabilities represent disturbances at the level of the person (e.g., bathing, dressing, communication, walking, grooming)

impairment: loss or abnormality of psychological, physiologic, or anatomic structure or function at the organ level (e.g., dysphagia, hemiparesis); an abnormality of body structure, appearance, and organ or system function resulting from any cause

multiple chronic conditions (MCC): presence of more than one chronic disease or condition, which increases the complexity of care as well as morbidity and mortality rates

noncommunicable diseases: a group of conditions that are not caused by an acute infection; many are considered chronic diseases and are often due to unhealthy behaviours

secondary health conditions: any physical, mental, or social disorder resulting directly or indirectly from an initial disabling condition; a condition to which a person with a disability is more susceptible because of having a primary disabling condition more deaths than all other causes combined. Deaths due to chronic disease are expected to increase globally from 38 million in 2012 to 52 million per year by 2030 (World Health Organization [WHO], 2014a).

Management of chronic conditions includes learning to live with symptoms or disabilities and coming to terms with identity changes resulting from having a chronic condition. It also consists of carrying out the lifestyle changes and regimens designed to control symptoms and prevent complications. Although some people assume what might be called a "sick role" identity, most people with chronic conditions do not consider themselves to be sick or ill and try to live as normal a life as possible. Only when complications develop or symptoms interfere with activities of daily living (ADLs) do most people with chronic health conditions think of themselves as being sick or disabled.

Prevalence and Causes of Chronic Conditions

The most frequently occurring chronic diseases account for 7 of the 10 leading causes of death and are responsible for more than two thirds of the deaths that occur globally. They include cardiovascular disease, cancers, diabetes, and chronic lung diseases (WHO, 2014a, 2014b). Chronic conditions occur in people of every age group, socioeconomic level, and culture. It is estimated that more than 16 million Canadians live with at least one chronic disease (Chronic Disease Prevention Alliance of Canada, 2018). Three out of five people over the age of 25 live with a chronic condition and four out of five are at risk (Public Health Agency of Canada [PHAC], 2013). Five chronic diseases—cancers, cardiovascular disease, stroke, chronic lower respiratory disease, and diabetes—kill more than 165,000 Canadians yearly and are the major causes of premature death and hospitalization (Statistics Canada, 2018a). Cancer is the leading cause of death in Canada at 29.8%, followed by cardiovascular disease at 19.7%.

The cost of treating chronic conditions in Canada runs into billions of dollars annually and has remained on the increase due to a number of factors, including our aging population, longer life with chronic disease, rising drug and treatment costs, economic inflation, and new technology (Kramer-Kile et al., 2014).

Chronic diseases are a global issue that affects both rich and poor nations. Chronic conditions have become the major cause of health-related problems in developed countries as well as in the developing countries, which are also trying to cope with new and emerging infectious diseases. In almost all countries, chronic diseases are the major cause of death among adults. Four of every five deaths occur in countries characterized as low or middle income, where people tend to develop chronic diseases at younger ages, suffer longer, and die sooner than people in high-income countries. In contrast to common belief, the total number of people dying from chronic disease is twice that of patients dying from infectious (including HIV infection), maternal, and perinatal conditions, and nutritional deficiencies combined (WHO, 2014a, 2014b). The number of people worldwide who die because of chronic disease is higher than all other diseases combined. Most of these chronic diseases and complications of chronic illness are preventable, emphasizing the importance of health promotion across the globe. Although chronic diseases or illnesses are common, people have many myths or misunderstandings about them (Table 12-1).

Some of the reasons that chronic diseases are becoming more prevalent globally include the following:

- A decrease in mortality from infectious diseases (e.g., smallpox, diphtheria, AIDS-related infections) and from acute conditions because of prompt and aggressive management of acute conditions (e.g., myocardial infarction, trauma)
- Lower infant mortality and increases in life expectancy due to successful public health measures, medical advances, and technology
- Improved screening and diagnostic procedures and aggressive management of acute conditions
- Tendency for the development of single or multiple chronic diseases with advancing age
- Lifestyle factors and consumption patterns such as poor nutrition, obesity, tobacco use, physical inactivity, unmanaged psychosocial stress, and unsafe sexual practices (Kramer-Kile et al., 2014)

Physiologic changes in the body often occur before the appearance of symptoms of chronic disease. Therefore, the goal of emphasizing healthy lifestyles early in life is to improve overall health status and slow the development of such disorders. Major risk factors for chronic disease, which represent a growing challenge to public health, include unhealthy eating habits, decreased energy expenditure associated with a sedentary lifestyle, increasing age, and tobacco use and alcohol consumption (WHO, 2014a). In addition, serious psychiatric or mental illness puts people at greater risk for chronic illness than the general population and leads to higher morbidity and mortality rates of chronic diseases.

Recently, much greater emphasis has been placed on the adoption of healthy lifestyles, beginning in childhood. This is not a new idea in Canada; in fact, Lalonde's *A New Perspective on the Health of Canadians*, an influential Canadian health policy document (Lalonde, 1974), framed health or disease as the result of lifestyle choices and self-imposed risks. Although the "new perspective" emphasized that a variety of factors constitute the "health field" (social and physical environments, health care services, biology, and lifestyle), lifestyle choices and risks have received the most attention in relation to chronic disease. Epp's Framework for Health Promotion (Epp, 1986) and the 1986 Ottawa Charter for Health Promotion also emphasized the importance of enhancing personal skills and knowledge in relation to health and the development of community and individual capacities in maintaining good health and preventing chronic disease. Although many chronic diseases can be prevented or postponed, factors that place people at significantly higher risk for developing any number of chronic diseases remain prevalent.

According to the World Health Report 2010, the major risk factors include:

- tobacco use
- the harmful use of alcohol
- raised blood pressure (or hypertension)

TABLE 12-1 Myths and Truths About Chronic Disease

Common Misconceptions About Chronic Disease	The Reality About Chronic Disease
1. Everyone dies of something.	Chronic illnesses typically do not result in sudden death but often result in progressive illness and disability. People with chronic disease often die slowly, painfully, and prematurely.
2. People can live to old age even if they lead unhealthy lives (smoke, have obesity).	While there are exceptions (some people who live unhealthy lives live to old age, and some people who live healthy lives develop chronic illnesses), most chronic illnesses can be traced to modifiable risk factors and can be prevented by eliminating these risks.
3. Solutions for chronic disease prevention and control are expensive and not feasible for low- and middle-income countries.	A full range of chronic disease interventions are very cost effective for all regions of the world, including the poorest. Many of these interventions are inexpensive to implement. Chronic disease is increasing rapidly around the world, including in low- and middle-income countries.
4. There is nothing that can be done and chronic diseases cannot be prevented.	The major causes of chronic diseases are known, and if these risk factors were eliminated, at least more than 80% of heart disease, stroke, and type 2 diabetes and more than 40% of cancers would be prevented.
5. If individuals develop chronic disease as a result of unhealthy "lifestyles," they have only themselves to blame.	Individual responsibility can have its full effect only if individuals have equal access to a healthy life and are supported to make healthy choices. Poor people often have limited choices about the food they eat, their living conditions, and access to education and health care.
6. Certain chronic diseases primarily affect men.	Chronic diseases, including heart disease, affect women and men almost equally. Almost half of all deaths attributed to chronic illness occur in women.
7. Chronic diseases primarily affect old people.	Almost half of chronic disease deaths occur prematurely in people younger than 70 years.
8. Chronic diseases mainly affect rich (affluent) people.	Poor people are much more likely than the wealthy to develop chronic diseases and as a result are more likely to die. Chronic diseases cause substantial financial burden and result in extreme poverty.
9. The priority of low- and middle-income countries should be on control of infectious diseases.	Although infectious diseases are an issue, low- and middle-income countries are experiencing a dramatic increase in chronic disease risk factors and deaths, especially in urban settings.
10. Chronic diseases affect mostly high-income countries.	Eighty percent of deaths attributed to chronic disease are in low- and middle-income countries. The prevalence of chronic diseases in low- and middle-income countries is rapidly growing.

Adapted from World Health Organization (WHO). (2005). *Widespread misunderstandings about chronic disease—and the reality. Facing the Facts #2*. Retrieved January 23, 2016, from www.who.int/chp/chronic_disease_report/media/Factsheet2.pdf

- physical inactivity
- raised cholesterol
- overweight/obesity
- unhealthy diet
- raised blood glucose

The WHO (2013) has identified high-impact, cost-effective interventions to prevent premature death due to chronic disease or chronic conditions that can be implemented even in settings with limited resources. These interventions are summarized in Chart 12-1.

Patient education to prevent chronic disease or reduce its severity or effects is another important component of the nurse's role in working with patients to identify risks for chronic disease and to identify strategies to reduce those risks. Health promotion and patient education are discussed in detail in Chapter 4 of this book.

Characteristics of Chronic Conditions

Sometimes it is difficult for people who are disease free to understand the profound effect that chronic illness often has on the lives of patients and their families. It is easy for health professionals to focus on the illness or disability itself while overlooking the person who has the disorder. In all illnesses, but even more so with chronic conditions, the illness cannot be separated from the person. People with chronic illness must contend with it daily (Lorig et al., 2012). To properly manage their chronic condition, individuals often have to find the time, and the social and financial resources, to participate in physically and psychologically beneficial activities, work with health care professionals to follow treatment guidelines, monitor their health and make decisions about their health and lifestyle and that of their family, and manage the effects of the illness on their physical, psychological, and social well-being. To relate to what people must cope with or to plan effective interventions, nurses must understand the multiple characteristics of a chronic illness.

- Psychological and social issues: Managing chronic illness involves more than treating medical problems. Associated psychological and social issues must also be addressed, because living for long periods with illness

CHART 12-1

Interventions According to Risk Factors

Tobacco

- Reduce affordability of tobacco by increasing its costs
- Legally mandate smoke-free environments in all indoor workplaces, public places, and public transport
- Disseminate warnings about dangers of tobacco and tobacco smoke through mass media campaigns and ban all forms of tobacco advertising, promotion, and sponsorship

Harmful Use of Alcohol

- Reduce affordability of alcohol by increasing its costs
- Limit availability of alcohol
- Ban all forms of alcohol advertising and promotions

Diet and Physical Activity

- Promote reduction of dietary salt intake and replacement of trans fats with unsaturated fats
- Implement public awareness programs on diet and physical activity
- Promote and protect breastfeeding (reduces risk of obesity later in life)

Cardiovascular Disease and Diabetes

- Promote glycemic control for diabetes mellitus and control of hypertension using medication therapy
- Counsel individuals who have had a heart attack or stroke and those persons at high risk of a fatal or nonfatal cardiovascular event in the next 10 years
- Initiate acetylsalicylic acid (aspirin) use for acute myocardial infarction

Cancer

- Promote hepatitis B immunization to prevent liver cancer
- Promote screening and early treatment of precancerous lesions to prevent cervical cancer

Adapted from World Health Organization (WHO). (2013). *Global action plan for the prevention and control of noncommunicable diseases, 2013–2020*. Geneva, Switzerland: World Health Organization.

symptoms and disability can threaten identity, bring about role changes, alter body image, and disrupt lifestyles. These changes require continuous adaptation and accommodation, depending on age and situation in life. Each decline in functional ability requires physical, emotional, and social adaptation for patients and their families.

- Phases of illness: Chronic conditions usually involve many different phases over the course of a person's lifetime. There can be acute periods, stable and unstable periods, flare-ups, and remissions. Each phase brings its own set of physical, psychological, and social problems, and each requires its own regimens and types of management.
- Therapeutic regimens: Keeping chronic conditions under control requires persistent adherence to therapeutic regimens. Failing to adhere to a treatment plan or to do so consistently increases the risks of developing complications and accelerating the disease process. However, the realities of daily life, including the impact of culture, values, and socioeconomic factors, affect the degree to which people adhere to a treatment regimen. Managing a chronic illness takes time, requires knowledge and planning, and can be uncomfortable and inconvenient. It is not unusual for patients to stop taking medications or alter dosages because of side effects that are more disturbing or disruptive than symptoms of the illness, or to cut back on regimens they consider overly time consuming, fatiguing, or costly.
- Development of other chronic conditions: One chronic disease can lead to the development of other chronic conditions. Diabetes, for example, can lead to neurologic and vascular changes that may result in visual, cardiac, and kidney diseases and erectile dysfunction. The presence of a chronic illness also contributes to a higher risk of morbidity and mortality in patients admitted to the intensive care unit with acute health conditions as well as greater utilization of clinical services during hospitalization.
- Family life: Chronic illness affects the entire family. Family life can be dramatically altered as a result of role reversals, unfilled roles, loss of income, time required to manage the illness, decreases in family socialization activities, and the costs of treatment. Family members often become caregivers for the person with chronic illness while trying to continue to work and keep the family intact. Stress and caretaker fatigue are common with severe chronic conditions, and the entire family may need care (Golics, Basra, Salek, et al., 2013). However, some families are able to master the treatment regimen and changes that accompany chronic illness as well as make the treatment regimen a routine part of life. Furthermore, they are able to keep the chronic illness from becoming the focal point of family life.
- Home life: The day-to-day management of illness is largely the responsibility of people with chronic disorders and their families (Lorig et al., 2012). As a result, the home, rather than the hospital, is the centre of care in chronic conditions. Hospitals, clinics, physicians' offices, nursing homes, nursing centres, and community agencies (home care services, social services, and disease-specific associations and societies) are considered adjuncts or backup services to daily home management.
- Self-management: The management of chronic conditions is a process of discovery. People can be taught how to manage their conditions. However, each patient must discover how their own body reacts under varying circumstances—for example, what it is like to be hypoglycemic, what activities are likely to bring on angina, and how these or other conditions can best be prevented and managed.
- Collaborative process: Managing chronic conditions must be a collaborative process that involves many different health care professionals working together with patients and their families to provide the full range of services that are often needed for management at home. The medical, social, and psychological aspects of chronic health problems are often complex, especially in severe conditions.
- Health care costs: The medical management of chronic conditions is expensive. Billions of dollars in direct and indirect costs are spent every year on health care for

people with chronic conditions. The costs are incurred from hospitalizations, medications, and productivity losses related to premature short- and long-term disability or death. Overall health care costs are not likely to decrease until there is a substantial downward trend in the incidence of chronic conditions and the costs of chronic health care. Living with a chronic condition is also costly for individuals and families, as there are many out-of-pocket costs involved in the medical management of illness (e.g., travel to treatment centres, costs for uninsured services, costs of medications) as well as the additional burdens introduced when there is a loss of income or job security due to prolonged absence from work.

- Lost income: Direct out-of-pocket expenses represent a significant percent of income, especially in low- and middle-income families. These expenses include high copays and deductibles that must be paid out of pocket. Those with serious chronic disorders may have difficulty paying for care, resulting in bankruptcy or having to rely on family or friends to pay for health insurance or health care. People from low-income groups who do not receive adequate health care get sicker and die sooner from chronic diseases than those from groups with higher levels of education, greater financial resources, and access to care (WHO, 2014a). If a family's primary income earner becomes ill, chronic diseases can result in drastic loss in income with inadequate funds for food, education, and health care. Furthermore, affected families may become unstable and impoverished (WHO, 2014a).
- Ethical issues: Chronic conditions raise difficult ethical issues for patients, families, health care professionals, and society. Problematic questions include how to establish cost controls, how to allocate scarce resources (e.g., organs for transplantation), and what constitutes quality of life and when life support should be withdrawn.
- Living with uncertainty: Having a chronic illness means living with uncertainty. Although health care providers may be aware of the usual progression of a chronic disease such as Parkinson's disease or multiple sclerosis, no one can predict with certainty a person's illness course because of individual variation. Even when a patient is in remission or symptom free, he or she often fears that the illness will reappear.

Chronic illness is something that people must live with and manage on a daily basis. The focus of nursing is on human responses to disruption in health and understanding how self-management makes sense from within the life as lived (Chart 12-2).

NURSING RESEARCH PROFILE

Chart 12-2. Older Adults and Disability

Hassani, P., Izadi-Avanji, F. S., Rakhshan, et al. (2017). A phenomenological study on resilience of the elderly suffering from chronic disease: A qualitative study. *Psychology Research and Behavior Management*, *10*, 59.

Purpose

The ability to adapt positively to significant pressures or changes in health is referred to as resilience and is often recognized as an important factor in an individual's ability to cope to the fullest of his/her abilities. Resilience is a key factor in improving health and attenuating problems caused by chronic diseases in older adults. Resilience is seen as being increasingly important as an individual ages, has been shown to influence health-related behaviours, and is linked to psychological well-being and better outcomes for patients suffering from chronic conditions. Having a clear understanding of the meaning of resilience in a specific population can be of great help in taking efficient steps toward better health services. This study aimed at understanding the meaning of resilience for hospitalized older adults who experience chronic conditions.

Design

This study utilized the descriptive phenomenologic approach/method to understand the concept of resilience among older adults suffering from chronic diseases. A total of 22 older adults study participants were selected purposefully and were interviewed in 24 sessions. The collected data were recorded and analyzed through Colaizzi's method.

Findings

Through the research, the authors identified the following four themes, with associated subthemes, that characterize resilience in this population:

1. Meaning of resilience in the participants' experiences
   a. The art of overcoming pain and suffering
   b. Adapt to health problem of senescence
   c. Accepting life with the chronic disease
   d. Patience and trust in God
2. Growth context as a prologue of resilience
   a. Growth background
3. External factors contributing to resilience
   a. Welfare
   b. Received support
   c. Deprivation and shortage
   d. Attitudes toward an older adult with health problem
4. Personal factors to overcome illness
   a. Enthusiasm for following up the treatment program
   b. Aversion to physical dependence
   c. Hope for improvement
   d. Motivation and purpose
   e. Being content with one's belongings and blessings

The researchers concluded that improvement in resilience is associated with a patient-oriented approach.

Nursing Implications

In an effort to improve patient outcomes, a focus on increasing his/her resilience is important. Providers of health services might make proper interventions based on unique needs of patients to improve their resilience and ability to overcome health problems. These can be performed by family members, health team, and related organizations and bodies.

The Challenges of Managing Chronic Conditions

Chronic conditions have implications for everyday living and management issues for individuals and their families as well as for society at large. Most importantly, efforts can fruitfully be directed at preventing chronic conditions since many can be traced, at least in part, to behaviours such as smoking and overeating. Thus, changes in lifestyle can result in the prevention of some chronic conditions, or at least a delay in their onset until a later age. Nurses can play an important role in facilitating healthy lifestyles.

Once a chronic condition has occurred, the focus shifts from disease prevention to managing symptoms and staying well by avoiding complications (e.g., eye problems in the person with diabetes) and the development of other acute illnesses (e.g., pneumonia in a person with chronic obstructive lung disease). Quality of life, often overlooked by health professionals in their approach to care of people with chronic conditions, is also important. Health-promoting behaviours, such as exercise, are essential to quality of life in people who have chronic illnesses and disabilities, as they help to maintain functional status.

Although coworkers, extended family, and health care professionals are affected by the problems of people with chronic illnesses, the problems of living with chronic conditions are most acutely experienced by people living with these conditions as well as their immediate families. It is they who feel the greatest impact with lifestyle changes that directly affect quality of life. Nurses provide direct care, especially during acute episodes, but they also provide the education and assist in mobilizing resources and other supports that enable people to integrate their illness into their lives and maintain quality of life despite their illness. To understand what nursing care is needed, it is important to appreciate the complexity of the issues that people with chronic illness and their families contend with and manage on a daily basis. Some of the challenges of living with chronic conditions include the following:

- Alleviating and managing symptoms
- Psychologically adjusting to and physically accommodating disabilities
- Preventing and managing crises and complications
- Carrying out regimens as prescribed
- Validating individual self-worth and family functioning
- Managing threats to identity and fulfill social roles
- Normalizing individual and family life as much as possible
- Finding meaning in the illness experience
- Living with altered time, social isolation, and loneliness
- Establishing the networks of support and resources that can enhance quality of life
- Returning to a satisfactory way of life after an acute debilitating episode (another myocardial infarction or stroke) or reactivation of a chronic condition
- Dying with dignity and comfort

Many people with chronic disease or chronic illness must face an additional challenge—the need to deal with **multiple chronic conditions (MCC)** (Ward, Schiller, & Goodman, 2014). The symptoms or treatment of a second chronic condition may aggravate the first chronic condition. Patients need to be able to deal with their various chronic conditions separately as well as in combination and to coordinate the health care and directions they receive, often from more than one health care professional. The challenges of living with and managing a chronic illness are well known, and people with chronic illnesses often report receiving inadequate care, information, services, and counselling. This provides an opportunity for nurses to assume a more active role in addressing many of the issues experienced, coordinating care, and serving as an advocate for patients who need additional assistance to manage their illness while maintaining a quality of life that is acceptable to them.

Understanding Chronic Illness

There are a number of theoretical frameworks that are useful in understanding the human experience of chronic illness. Paterson's Shifting Perspectives Model (Paterson, 2001, 2003) facilitates an understanding of chronic illness as lived according to people's needs and situations rather than according to predictable stages or phases. Miller (2000) framed chronic illness as an experience that challenges one's perceptions of power—with power defined as the ability to provide and care for self, to direct others regarding self-care, and to retain the status of ultimate decision maker regarding care. Chronic illness should be understood in terms of its disruption of the life story of individuals.

The Trajectory Model of Chronic Illness, a nursing model based on many years of interdisciplinary research on chronic illness, will be used to describe the phases and the role of nurses in the trajectory of chronic illness. Table 12-2 describes the different phases of chronic illness and the focus of nursing care during different phases. In this model, the term *trajectory* refers to the path or course that the chronic illness follows. The course of an illness can be thought of as a trajectory that can be managed or shaped over time, to some extent, through proper illness management strategies (Corbin, 1998). It is important to keep in mind that the course of a patient's chronic illness may be too uncertain to predict with any degree of accuracy. Furthermore, not all phases occur in all patients; some phases do not occur at all, and some phases may recur. Each phase is characterized by different medical and psychosocial issues. For example, the needs of a patient with a stroke who is a good candidate for rehabilitation are very different from the needs of a patient with terminal cancer. By thinking in terms of phases and individual patients within a phase, nurses can target their care more specifically to each person. Not every chronic condition is necessarily life threatening, and not every patient passes through each possible phase of a chronic condition in the same order.

Using the trajectory model enables the nurse to put the present situation into the context of what might have happened to the patient in the past—that is, the life factors and understandings that might have contributed to the present state of the illness. In this way, the nurse can more readily address the underlying issues and problems.

TABLE 12-2 Phases in the Trajectory Model of Chronic Illness

Phase	Description	Focus of Nursing Care
Pretrajectory	Genetic factors or lifestyle behaviours that place a person or community at risk for a chronic condition.	Refer for genetic testing and counselling if indicated; provide education about prevention of modifiable risk factors and behaviours.
Trajectory onset	Appearance or onset of noticeable symptoms associated with a chronic disorder; includes period of diagnostic workup and announcement of diagnosis; may be accompanied by uncertainty as patient awaits a diagnosis and begins to discover and cope with implications of diagnosis.	Provide explanations of diagnostic tests and procedures and reinforce information and explanations given by primary provider; provide emotional support to patient and family.
Stable	Illness course and symptoms are under control as symptoms, resulting disability, and everyday life activities are being managed within limitations of illness; illness management centred in the home.	Reinforce positive behaviours and offer ongoing monitoring; provide education about health promotion; and encourage participation in health-promoting activities and health screening.
Unstable	Characterized by an exacerbation of illness symptoms, development of complications, or reactivation of an illness in remission. Period of inability to keep symptoms under control or reactivation of illness; difficulty in carrying out everyday life activities. May require more diagnostic testing and trial of new treatment regimens or adjustment of current regimen, with care usually taking place at home.	Provide guidance and support; reinforce previous patient education.
Acute	Severe and unrelieved symptoms or the development of illness complications necessitating hospitalization, bed rest, or interruption of the person's usual activities to bring illness course under control.	Provide direct care and emotional support to the patient and the family members.
Crisis	Critical or life-threatening situation requiring emergency treatment or care and suspension of everyday life activities until the crisis has passed.	Provide direct care; collaborate with other health care team members to stabilize patient's condition.
Comeback	Gradual recovery after an acute period and learning to live with or overcome disabilities and return to an acceptable way of life within the limitations imposed by the chronic condition or disability; involves physical healing, limitations stretching through rehabilitative procedures, psychosocial coming-to-terms, and biographical reengagement with adjustments in everyday life activities.	Assist in coordination of care; rehabilitative focus may require care from other health care providers; provide positive reinforcement for goals identified and accomplished.
Downward	Illness course characterized by rapid or gradual worsening of a condition; physical decline accompanied by increasing disability or difficulty in controlling symptoms; requires biographical adjustment and alterations in everyday life activities with each major downward step.	Provide home care and other community-based care to help patient and family adjust to changes and come to terms with these changes; assist patient and family to integrate new treatment and management strategies; encourage identification of end-of-life preferences and planning.
Dying	Final days or weeks before death; characterized by gradual or rapid shutting down of body processes, biographical disengagement and closure, and relinquishment of everyday life interests and activities.	Provide direct and supportive care to patients and their families through palliative care or hospice programs.

Adapted from Corbin, J. M. (1998). The Corbin and Strauss chronic illness trajectory model: An update. *Scholarly Inquiry for Nursing Practice*, *12*(1), 33–41.

Implications for Nursing

Working with people living with one or more chronic conditions certainly requires dealing with the medical aspects of the condition(s), but the essential contribution of nurses to chronic illness care lies in seeking to base that care on a holistic understanding of what living with the illness means to the person physically, emotionally, and socially. This holistic approach to care requires nurses to draw upon their entire repertoire of knowledge and skills, including knowledge from the social and psychological sciences. People often respond to illness, health teaching, and regimens in ways that are different from the expectations of health care providers.

Nursing Care of People Living With Chronic Conditions

Nursing care of people living with chronic conditions is varied and occurs in an assortment of settings. It can include provision of direct care or supportive care. Such care is often provided in the clinic or physician's office, the hospital, or the home, depending on the status of the illness.

Examples of direct care may include assessing the patient's physical status, providing wound care, managing and overseeing medication regimens, and performing other technical tasks. The availability of this type of nursing care is one of the main reasons patients can remain at home and return to a somewhat normal life after an acute episode of illness.

Because much of the day-to-day responsibility for managing chronic conditions rests with the individual and family, nurses often provide supportive care unless the person is hospitalized. Supportive care may include ongoing monitoring, teaching, counselling, serving as an advocate, making referrals, coordinating services, mobilizing resources, and case managing. Providing supportive care is just as important as the performance of technical care. For example, through ongoing monitoring that might take place either in the home or a nursing clinic, such as a heart failure clinic, a nurse might detect impending complications, such as signs of heart failure. The nurse might detect these signs before they are noticeable to the person and could make a referral (call the physician or consult the medical protocol in a clinic) for medical evaluation, thereby preventing a lengthy hospitalization.

Working with people with chronic illness requires not only dealing with the medical aspects of their disorder but also working with the whole person—physically, emotionally, and socially. This holistic approach to care requires nurses to draw on their knowledge and skills, including knowledge from the social sciences and psychology in particular. People often respond to illness, health education, and regimens in ways that differ from the expectations of health care providers. Although quality of life is usually affected by chronic illness, especially if the illness is severe, patients' perceptions of what constitutes quality of life often drive their management behaviours or affect how they view advice about health care. Nurses and other health care professionals need to recognize this, even though it may be difficult to see patients make unwise choices and decisions about lifestyles and disease management. People have the right to receive care without fearing ridicule or refusal of treatment, even if their behaviours (e.g., smoking, substance abuse, overeating, and failure to follow health care providers' recommendations) may have contributed to their chronic disorder.

Each phase of chronic illness brings with it different concerns, both medical and psychosocial. The needs of a person who has had a stroke and is a good candidate for rehabilitation, for example, are very different from those of a person with terminal cancer. By thinking in terms of phases, and where the person may be in relation to these phases, nurses can target their care more specifically to each person.

Care by Phase: Applying the Nursing Process

The focus of care for people with chronic conditions is determined by the unique needs of the person and family and the particular phase of illness. Care is organized by the nursing process, incorporating assessment, diagnosis, planning, implementation, and evaluation.

Step 1: Identifying the Trajectory Phase

The first step is assessment of the person to determine the specific phase (see Table 12-2). Assessment enables the nurse to identify the medical or psychosocial problems likely to be encountered in a phase. For instance, the problems associated with having an acute myocardial infarction are very different from those likely to be encountered with the same person, 10 years later, dying at home of heart failure. The kinds of direct care, referrals, teaching, and emotional support needed in each situation are different as well. Complementary and alternative therapies are often used by people living with chronic conditions, so it becomes important for the nurse to also assess for the use of such regimens.

Step 2: Establishing and Prioritizing Goals

Once the phase of illness has been identified and the related medical and psychosocial issues have been explored, the next step involves establishing the goals of care. The establishment of goals must be a collaborative effort and starts with the person, family, and nurse working together. The attainment of a goal is unlikely if it is primarily the nurse's goal, and goals must be consistent with the abilities, desires, motivations, and resources of the person and family in their context. In the following example, goals are determined collaboratively and then written in the language of the nursing process.

An older adult male with severe progressive COPD reports increasing difficulty breathing, with the oxygen level set at 2 L/min. This interferes with his ability to carry out ADLs, limits the activities he and his wife can do together, and has decreased his enjoyment of life. He worries for his frail wife's health and feels he cannot ask for her assistance with his care. He asks the nurse for help. The nursing diagnosis for this problem might be "activity intolerance related to less than adequate intake of oxygen secondary to lung disease," and the mutually agreed upon goal of care might be to increase his ability to care for himself and engage in some social activities with his wife. Nursing interventions related to this goal might include exploring with him and his wife strategies such as pacing his activities, eating small nutritious meals frequently throughout the day to maintain energy, and avoid limiting diaphragmatic movement with a full stomach, as well as exploring how he might obtain assistance with the most demanding ADLs.

Step 3: Establishing a Plan to Achieve Desired Outcomes

Once goals have been established, the next step consists of establishing a realistic and mutually agreed upon plan for achieving them and identifying specific criteria that can be used to assess progress. A plan of care for the man with COPD who reports a decreased ability to engage in valued activities and self-care, for example, might include assisting him to prioritize his activities so he can carry out those that are most important to him before he becomes too short of breath and tired. It might also include exploring how he feels about having someone assist him at home on a regular basis and, if he agrees to have help, assisting him and his wife to check on the availability and any costs associated with such services. The plan must be broken down into manageable and achievable steps, and the identification of the person responsible for each task of this plan is also essential.

In addition, identification of the environmental, social, and psychological factors that might interfere with or facilitate achieving the desired outcome is an important part of planning. Again, in the case of the man with COPD, for example, not having sufficient resources could prevent him and his wife from seeking additional support services. The nurse may want to explore carefully the issue of resources with them and, if there are financial constraints, enlist the services of a social worker, with their consent, to explore possible community resources.

Step 4: Implementing the Plan and Interventions

The next step is the intervention phase. Possible interventions include providing direct care, serving as an advocate, teaching, counselling, making referrals, and case managing (arranging for resources). For example, if the man with COPD reports after prioritizing his ADLs that showering each morning is the most important self-care activity for him, then perhaps having a home health aide come early in the morning to help with the shower may be the best arrangement. The home health aide could also help with breakfast, make the bed, and straighten up the house. In this way, the man would use less energy doing these daily tasks. After showering and dressing, he might also want to plan a daily rest period, such as sitting down with a crossword puzzle or reading which may help him overcome some of his sense of breathlessness. Pacing activity this way may help him feel more rested and able to go for a short outing with his wife or visit friends.

Physicians prescribe therapies, such as medications and diet, and give directions for how much, when, and how they are to be used. Nurses, however, by virtue of their broad knowledge base, are equipped to help people develop the strategies needed to live with both the symptoms and therapies associated with chronic conditions. It is important to work individually with each person and family to identify the best ways to integrate treatment regimens into their daily living activities. In chronic illness management, two tasks are of key importance: (a) incorporating disease management regimens into life in a way that controls symptoms, keeps the disease stable, and is manageable within one's life context; and (b) addressing the psychological, social, and emotional issues that often accompany chronic disease and that can potentially hinder one's ability to self-care and live well.

Diagnosis and medical treatment by physicians are important aspects of chronic illness care, but they are only part of the disease management picture. Other essential components include teaching, counselling, supporting, problem solving, arranging, and case management in collaboration with people living with chronic disease, with the goal of enabling people to live well with their disease, and preserve autonomy and independence. Saving the life of a person with an acute myocardial infarction in the intensive care unit, for example, is a positive outcome, but he or she will likely relapse if not supported in making the lifestyle changes necessary to reduce the probability of another heart attack. Seeking to understand the person's perspective on illness management, and supporting his or her efforts to make sense of treatment regimens and to live life well within the limits of his or her disabilities, is one of the most important aspects of health care delivery and nursing care for people living with chronic illness.

Step 5: Following Up and Evaluating the Effectiveness of Interventions

The final step involves following up to determine if the problem is resolving or being managed and if the patient and the family are able to adhere to the treatment plan. Follow-up may uncover new problems resulting from the intervention, problems that interfere with the ability of the patient and the family to carry out the plan, or previously unexpected problems. A primary goal is to maintain the stability of the chronic condition while preserving the patient's sense of control, identity, independence, and accomplishment. Alternative strategies or revisions to the initial plan may be warranted based on evaluation and follow-up.

Helping the patient and the family to integrate changes into their lifestyle is an important part of the process. Change takes time, patience, and creativity and often requires encouragement from the nurse. Validation of the patient's progress is important for enhancing self-esteem and reinforcing behaviours. If no progress is made, or if progress toward goals seems too slow, it may be necessary to redefine the goals, the intervention, or the time frame. The nurse must realize and accept that some people will not change. Patients share responsibility for management of their conditions, and outcomes are as much related to their ability to accommodate the illness and carry out regimens as they are to nursing intervention (Lorig et al., 2012).

As the collaborative treatment and management plan progresses, it is important to continually assess the effectiveness of interventions. In chronic illness, maintaining the stability of the condition while at the same time preserving the person's control over his or her life and a sense of identity and accomplishment are the primary goals. Success may be defined, however, as merely making progress toward a goal when an individual finds it difficult to implement rapid and drastic changes in the way that they do things. Nurses cannot expect that the sedentary person with high blood pressure, for example, is going to develop a sudden passion for exercise. Nor can they expect that working people can easily rearrange their day to accommodate time-consuming regimens such as special diets or complex medication schedules. Bringing about change takes time, patience, creativity, encouragement, respect, and trust from the nurse. Validation by the nurse for each small increment toward goal accomplishment is important for enhancing self-esteem and reinforcing behaviours. If no progress is made or if progress toward goals seems slow, it may be necessary to redefine the goals or the time frame. Nurses must also realize that some people will be unable to follow their management plan; it may be a choice, or it may be a reflection of life circumstances that limit their ability to engage in what the nurse views as positive self-care. Some people, for example, are unable to give up smoking despite advanced COPD. As well, it is not unusual to find people with the diagnosis of diabetes unable to follow their diabetic diets. When people are having difficulty carrying out regimens or are unable or reluctant to change their lifestyles, the most helpful response is not a judgmental one; helpful self-care strategies emerge when nurses maintain respectful, collaborative, trusting partnerships with patients and families.

Promoting Home and Community-Based Care

Teaching Self-Care

Because chronic conditions are so costly to people, families, and society, two of the major goals of nursing today are the prevention of chronic conditions and the care of people with them. This requires promoting healthy lifestyles and encouraging the use of safety and disease prevention measures, such as wearing seat belts and obtaining immunizations. Prevention should also begin early in life and continue throughout life. Education on self-care may need to address interactions among the patient's chronic conditions as well as skills necessary to care for the individual diseases and their interactive effects.

Patient and family education is an important nursing role that may make the difference in the ability of the patient and the family to adapt to chronic conditions. Well-informed, educated patients are more likely than uninformed patients to be concerned about their health and do what is necessary to maintain it. They are also more likely to manage symptoms, recognize the onset of complications, and seek health care early. Knowledge is the key to making informed choices and decisions during all phases of the chronic illness trajectory.

Despite the importance of educating the patient and the family, the nurse must recognize that patients recently diagnosed with serious chronic conditions and their families may need time to understand the significance of their condition and its effect on their lives. Education must be planned carefully so that it is not acute. Furthermore, it is important to assess the impact of a new diagnosis of chronic illness on a patient's life and the meaning of self-management to the patient.

The nurse who cares for patients with chronic conditions in the hospital, clinic, home, or any other setting should assess each patient's knowledge about their illness and its management; the nurse cannot assume that patients with a long-standing chronic condition have the knowledge necessary to manage the condition. Patients' learning needs change as the chronic condition changes and their personal situations change. The nurse must also recognize that patients may know how their body responds under certain conditions and how best to manage their symptoms. Contact with patients in any setting offers nurses the ideal opportunity to reassess patients' learning needs and provide additional education about a chronic condition and its management.

Educational strategies and materials should be adapted to the individual patient so that the patient and the family can understand and follow recommendations from health care providers. For instance, educational materials should be tailored for people with low literacy levels and available in several languages and in various alternative formats (e.g., Braille, large print, audiotapes). It may be necessary to provide sign language interpreters.

Continuing Care

Chronic illness management is a collaborative process between the person with the illness, the family, nurse, and other health care professionals. Collaboration is not limited to hospital settings; rather, it is important in all settings and throughout the illness trajectory. Keeping an illness stable over time requires careful and continued monitoring of symptoms and attention to management regimens. Detecting problems early and assisting people to develop appropriate management strategies can make a significant difference in outcomes.

Most chronic conditions are managed in the home. Therefore, care and teaching during hospitalization should focus on what the person needs to know about the condition in order to manage once discharged to home. Nurses in all settings should be aware of the resources and services available in a community and should make the arrangements (before hospital discharge if the person is hospitalized) necessary to secure those resources and services. When appropriate, home care services are contacted directly. The home care nurse will reassess how the person and family are adapting to the chronic condition and its treatment and will continue or revise the plan of care accordingly.

Because chronic conditions occur worldwide and the world is increasingly interconnected, nurses need to think beyond the individual level to the community and global levels. In terms of illness prevention and health promotion, this entails wide-ranging efforts to assess people for risk factors for chronic illness (e.g., blood pressure and diabetes screening, stroke risk assessments) and group teaching related to illness prevention and management.

Also, in terms of factors operating in the larger context, there are many considerations at the level of the health care system, health policy, and society in general that require the attention of health care professionals. The Chronic Care Model (Wagner, Davis, Schaefer, et al., 1999) is an internationally endorsed model that proposes paying attention to six interrelated elements in improving chronic illness care. These elements are community resources and policies, the organization of the health system, self-management support, delivery system design and structure (team-based care), decision support and evidence-based care, and integrated clinical information systems. Paying attention to these elements and a process of evidence-based change have been found to foster productive interactions between informed patients who take an active part in their care and providers with resources and expertise. Barr, Robinson, Marin-Link, et al. (2003) have created an expansion of this model in which health promotion and population health concepts, such as healthy public policy, supportive environments, and activated communities, are included. Nurses have a professional mandate to improve population health and reduce the incidence and impact of chronic illness. The Canadian Nurses Association (CNA) code of ethics states that nurses should recognize and work "to address organizational, social, economic and political factors that influence health and well-being within the context of nurses' role in the delivery of care" (CNA, 2017, p. 24). Good public health policy requires an understanding of the broad determinants of health and not only includes policies that support healthy behaviours such as nonsmoking, exercise, and good nutrition but also extends to address socioenvironmental risk factors such as poverty, poor working conditions, and educational disadvantage.

While it is not realistic to expect all registered nurses to become policy experts or activists, it is realistic to expect nurses to be able to assess, identify, and articulate the impact of some of these broader factors and capitalize on opportunities to effect policy change through professional or advocacy organizations.

Telehealth (use of electronic data and telecommunications technologies to support long-distance clinical health care, patient and professional health-related education, public health, and health administration) has been used effectively to provide care for patients with chronic illness. It is particularly useful in monitoring patients with chronic conditions living in remote and rural areas. It has also been used to deliver selected medical and nursing interventions (e.g., counselling) and provide ongoing education and support.

Nursing Care for Special Populations With Chronic Illness

When providing care and teaching, the nurse considers a variety of factors (e.g., age, gender, culture, and ethnicity) that influence susceptibility to chronic illness and the ways people respond to chronic disorders. Certain populations, for example, tend to be more susceptible to certain chronic conditions. Populations at high risk for specific conditions can be targeted for special teaching and monitoring programs. People of different cultures and genders tend to respond to illness differently; being aware of these differences is extremely important. For cultures in which the ill person relies heavily on family support, families must be involved and made part of the nursing care plan. As Canada becomes more multicultural and ethnically diverse, and as the general population ages, nurses need to be aware of how an individual's culture and age facilitate or hinder chronic illness management. As such, nurses should be prepared to adapt the care they give accordingly.

Overview of Disability

Definitions of Disability

A person is considered to have a disability (limitation in performance or function in everyday activities) if he or she has difficulty talking, hearing, seeing, walking, climbing stairs, lifting or carrying objects, performing ADLs, doing school work, or working at a job. A severe disability is present if a person is unable to perform one or more activities, uses an assistive device for mobility, or needs help from another person to accomplish basic activities. People are also considered severely disabled if they receive federal benefits because of an inability to work.

According to the WHO (2001), *disability* is an umbrella term for impairments, activity limitations, participation restrictions, and environmental factors, and **impairment** is a loss or abnormality in body structure or physiologic function, including mental function. A person's functioning or disability is viewed as a dynamic interaction between health conditions (i.e., diseases, disorders, injuries, trauma) and contextual factors (i.e., personal and environmental factors) (WHO, 2001). The term *societal participation* is used in the WHO classification system in place of *handicap* to acknowledge the fact that the environment is always interacting with people to either assist or hinder participation in life activities and that the environment may have a greater impact on an individual's ability to participate in life activities than does the physical, mental, or emotional condition.

According to the WHO (2014c), over 1 billion people, or about 15% of the global population, have some type of disability. Between 110 and 190 million adults worldwide have significant difficulties in function due to disability. The number of people with disabilities is increasing and is expected to continue to climb as people with early-onset disabilities, chronic disorders, and severe trauma survive (Gostin, 2015).

Approximately one in seven Canadians aged 15 years or older has some form of disability. Statistics Canada reports that in 2012, almost 14% of the Canadian population aged 15 years or older reported having a disability that limited their daily activities (Statistics Canada, 2018b), and this number is expected to increase in the coming decades due to the aging of the population. More than half of persons with disabilities are women, irrespective of age. On average, women also live longer, making them more likely to develop age-related chronic conditions that lead to disability. Canada's Aboriginal (First Nations, Inuit, and Métis) population has higher rates of disabilities than the rest of Canada.

For years, people with disabilities have been discriminated against in employment, public accommodations, and public and private services including health care. The needs of people with disabilities in health care settings produce many challenges to health care providers—how to communicate effectively if there are communication deficits, the additional physical demands for mobility, and time required to provide assistance with self-care routines during hospitalization. Physicians and nurses may not know the specific needs of individuals with disability and may fail to provide services for them.

Characteristics of Disability

Categories and Types of Disability

Disabilities can be categorized as developmental disabilities, acquired disabilities, and age-associated disabilities. Developmental disabilities are those that occur any time from birth to 22 years of age and result in impairment of physical or mental health, cognition, speech, language, or self-care. Examples of developmental disabilities are spina bifida, cerebral palsy, Down's syndrome, and muscular dystrophy. Some developmental disabilities occur as a result of birth trauma or severe illness or injury at a very young age, whereas many developmental disabilities are genetic in origin (see Chapter 13). Acquired disabilities may occur as a result of an acute and sudden injury (e.g., traumatic brain injury; spinal cord injury; and traumatic amputation due to traffic crashes, falls, burns, or acts of violence such as intimate partner violence and war and military conflicts), acute nontraumatic disorders (e.g., stroke, myocardial infarction), or progression of a chronic disorder (e.g., arthritis, multiple sclerosis, Parkinson's disease, chronic obstructive pulmonary disease, heart disease, blindness due to diabetic retinopathy) (WHO, 2014c).

Many people with disabilities are at risk for **secondary health conditions** (e.g., pressure ulcers, urinary tract infections, low bone density, depression) because of a narrow margin of health. Therefore, attention needs to be given to assessment, prevention when possible, and management of secondary health conditions or disorders that occur (Newland, Jenson, Budhathoki, et al., 2015).

Types of disability include sensory disabilities that affect hearing or vision; learning disabilities that affect the ability to learn, remember, or concentrate; disabilities that affect the ability to speak or communicate; and disabilities that affect the ability to work, shop, and care for oneself, or access health care. Many disabilities are visible; however, invisible disabilities are often as disabling as those that can be seen. Some disabilities affect only instrumental activities of daily living (IADLs), whereas others affect ADLs. People can be temporarily disabled because of an injury or acute exacerbation of a chronic disorder but later return to full functioning.

Although different impairments may result from different types of disabilities, there are some similarities across disabilities. People with disabilities are often considered by society to be dependent and needing to be cared for by others; however, many people with disabilities are highly functioning, independent, productive people who are capable of caring for themselves and others, having children and raising families, holding a full-time job, and making significant and major contributions to society. Like other people, those with disabilities often prefer to live in their own homes with family members. Most people with disabilities are able to live at home independently. Some patients live alone in their own homes and use home care services. However, alternative living arrangements may be necessary; these include assisted living facilities, long-term care facilities, and group homes.

Models of Disability

Several models of disability have been used to address or explain the issues encountered by people with disabilities (Drum, 2014). Chart 12-3 briefly describes these models of disability. The interface model, developed by a nurse, promotes care designed to be empowering rather than care that promotes dependency. It takes into account the disabling condition and its disabling effects. Furthermore, it promotes the view that people with disabilities are capable, responsible people who are able to function effectively despite having a disability. The interface model can serve as a basis for the role of nurses as advocates for the removal of barriers to health care and for the examination of how society and health care professionals contribute to discrimination by viewing disability as an abnormal state.

Disability versus Disabling Disorders

Regardless of which definition or model of disability is adopted, one can understand the pathophysiology and physical changes related to a disabling condition or injury without understanding the concept of disability. The nurse caring for patients with pre-existing disabilities or

CHART 12-3

Models of Disability

Medical Model

The medical model equates people who are disabled with their disabilities and views disability as a problem of the person, directly caused by disease, trauma, or other health condition, that requires medical care provided in the form of individual treatment by professionals. Health care providers, rather than people with disabilities, are viewed as the experts or authorities. Management of the disability is aimed at cure or the person's adjustment and behaviour change. The model is viewed as promoting passivity and dependency. People with disabilities are viewed as tragic.

Rehabilitation Model

The rehabilitation model emerged from the medical model. It regards disability as a deficiency that requires a rehabilitation specialist or other helping professional to fix the problem. People with disabilities are often perceived as having failed if they do not overcome the disability.

Social Model

The social model, which is also referred to as the barriers or disability model, views disability as socially constructed and as a political issue that is a result of social and physical barriers in the environment. Its perspective is that disability can be overcome by removal of these barriers.

Biopsychosocial Model

The biopsychosocial model integrates the medical and social models to address perspectives of health from a biologic, individual, and social perspective. Critiques of this model have suggested that the disabling condition, rather than the person and the experience of the person with a disability, remains the defining construct of the biopsychosocial model.

Functional Model

The functional model is driven by the World Health Organization's *International Classification of Functioning, Disability and Health* (*ICF*). Disability is considered an umbrella term for impairments, activity limitations, participation restrictions, and their interaction with environmental factors. The ICF addresses components of health rather than consequence of disease.

Interface Model

The interface model is based on the life experience of the person with a disability and views disability at the intersection (i.e., interface) of the medical diagnosis of a disability and environmental barriers. It considers rather than ignores the diagnosis. The person with a disability, rather than others, defines the problems and seeks or directs solutions.

Adapted from Drum, C. E. (2014). The dynamics of disability and chronic conditions. *Disability and Health Journal*, *7*(1), 2–5.

new disabilities must recognize the impact of a disability on current and future health and well-being, the ability to participate in self-care or self-management, and the ability to obtain required health care and health screening. Nursing management—from assessment through evaluation of the effectiveness of nursing interventions—must be examined to ensure that appropriate modifications have been made so that people with disabilities can receive health care equal to that of people without disabilities. Furthermore, nurses as well as other health care providers need to examine their facilities and procedures to ensure that the needs of people with various disabilities can be adequately addressed. Although the health care needs of people with disabilities generally do not differ from those of the general population, some disabilities create special needs and necessitate the use of special accommodations.

Significance of "People-First" Language

It is important to all people, both those with and without disabilities, that they not be equated with their illness or physical condition. Therefore it is important to refer to all people using "people-first" language. This means referring to the person first: "the patient with diabetes" rather than "the diabetic" or the "diabetic patient"; the "person with a disability" rather than the "disabled woman"; "women with disabilities" rather than the "disabled"; and "people who are wheelchair users" rather than "wheelchair bound." This simple use of language conveys the message that the person, rather than the illness or disability, is of greater importance to the nurse. Often the person with disability must educate the health care professionals.

The Role of the Nurse

Because of unfavourable interactions with health care providers, including negative attitudes, insensitivity, and lack of knowledge, people with disability may avoid seeking medical intervention or health promotion programs and activities. For this reason, and because the number of individuals with disability is increasing, nurses must acquire knowledge and skills and be accessible to assist these individuals in maintaining a high level of wellness.

Nurses are in key positions to influence the architectural design of health care settings and the selection of equipment that promotes ease of access and health. Padded examination tables that can be raised or lowered make transfers easier for people with a disability. Birthing chairs benefit women with disability during yearly pelvic examinations and Pap smears and for urologic evaluations. Ramps, grab bars, and raised and padded toilet seats benefit many persons who have orthopedic disabilities and need routine physical examination and monitoring (e.g., bone density measurements).

Nurses can provide expert health promotion education classes that are targeted to those with a disability. Classes on nutrition and weight management are extremely important to individuals who are wheelchair dependent and need assistance with transfers. Safe sex classes are needed by adolescents and young adults who have spinal cord or traumatic brain injury, because the threats of AIDS and unplanned pregnancy exist for these populations just as they do for the population in general. Other healthy behaviours about which persons with neurologic disabilities need education include avoiding alcohol and nonprescription medications while taking antispasmodic and anticonvulsant medications. Nurses should teach all survivors of strokes and patients with diabetes how to monitor their own blood pressure or glucose levels. The warning signs and symptoms of stroke, heart attack, and cancer, as well as how to access help, should also be taught to all persons with a disability.

As active members of society, people with disabilities are no longer an invisible minority. An increased awareness of the needs of people with disabilities will bring about changes to improve their access and accommodate their needs.

Patient Responses to Disability

Disability can occur at any age and may result from an acute incident, such as stroke or trauma, or from the progression of a chronic condition, such as arthritis or multiple sclerosis. A person with a disability may experience many losses, including loss of function, independence, social role, status, and income. A patient and his or her family members experience a range of emotional reactions to these losses. The reactions may progress from disorganization and confusion to denial of the disability, grief over the lost function or body part, depression, anger, and, finally, acceptance of the disability. The reactions may subside over time and may recur at a later time, especially if chronic illness is progressive and results in increasing losses. Not all patients experience all of the stages, although most do exhibit grief. Patients who exhibit grief should not be blithely encouraged to "cheer up." The nurse should show a willingness to listen to the patient talk about the disability and should understand that grief, anger, regret, and resentment are all part of the healing process.

The patient's pre-existing coping abilities play an important role in the adaptation process—one patient may be particularly independent and determined, while another may be dependent and seem to lack personal power. One goal of rehabilitation is to help the patient gain a positive self-image through effective coping. The nurse must recognize different coping abilities and identify when the patient is not coping well or not adjusting to the disability (Chart 12-4), or when older adults facing disability have concerns (Chart 12-5). The patient and family may benefit from participating in a support group or talking with a mental health professional to achieve this goal. Refer to Chapter 9 for a detailed discussion of adaptive and maladaptive responses to illness.

Disability and Sexuality Issues

An important issue confronting the patient with a disability, and a vital component of self-concept, is sexuality. Sexuality involves not only biologic sexual activity but also one's concept of masculinity or femininity. It affects the way a person reacts to others and is perceived by them, and it is expressed not only by physical intimacy but also by caring and emotional intimacy.

CHART 12-4

Patient Education: Learning to Cope With Disabilities

The following points may be useful in teaching patients how to reduce their energy output and conserve their strength to achieve a meaningful lifestyle.

Take Control of Your Life

- Face the reality of your disability.
- Emphasize areas of strength.
- Remain outward looking.
- Seek inventive ways to tackle problems.
- Share concerns and frustrations.
- Maintain and improve general health.
- Plan for recreation.

Have Well-Defined Goals and Priorities

- Keep priorities in order; eliminate nonessential activities.
- Plan and pace your activities.

Organize Your Life

- Plan each day.
- Organize work.
- Perform tasks in steps.
- Distribute heavy work throughout the day or week.

Conserve Energy

- Rest before undertaking difficult tasks.
- Stop the activity before fatigue occurs.
- Continue with an exercise conditioning program to strengthen muscles.

Control Your Environment

- Try to be well organized.
- Keep possessions in the same place so that they can be found with a minimum of effort.
- Store equipment (personal care, crafts, work) in a box or basket.
- Use energy-conservation and work-simplification techniques.
- Keep work within easy reach and in front of you.
- Use adaptive equipment, self-help aids, and labour-saving devices.
- Recruit assistance from others; delegate when necessary.
- Take safety precautions.

Sexuality problems faced by patients with disabilities include limited access to information about sexuality, lack of opportunity to form friendships and loving relationships, impaired self-image, and low self-esteem. The person with a disability may have physical and emotional difficulties that interfere with sexual activities. For example, diabetes and spinal cord injury may affect the ability to have an erection. The patient who has suffered a heart attack or stroke may fear having a life-threatening event (e.g., another heart attack or stroke) during sexual activity. He or she may fear the loss of bowel or bladder control during intimate moments. Changes in desire for sex and in the quality of sexual activities can occur for the patient and the partner, who may be too involved as the caregiver to have desire and energy for sexual activities.

Unfortunately, society and some health care providers contribute to these problems by ignoring patients' sexuality and by viewing persons with disabilities as asexual. Health care providers' own discomfort and lack of knowledge related to sexuality issues prevent them from providing the patient with disability and his or her partner interventions that promote healthy intimacy. Nurses caring for persons with disability must recognize and address sexual issues in order to promote feelings of self-worth, which are essential to total rehabilitation. The nurse should give the patient "permission" to discuss sexuality concerns and show a willingness to listen and help the patient overcome these concerns. The "PLISSIT" model, initially described by Annon (1976), is a framework frequently used in planning and setting priorities related to the sexual health of a patient. There are four stages of the model: "P" or permission giving, the nurse and/or patient bring up the topic of sexuality as a way of allowing more specific concerns to be raised; "LI" (limited information) is where limited information about sexuality and sexual functioning is provided; "SS" (specific suggestions) allows more specific suggestions to be provided to deal with issues—if the nurse is unable to give specific suggestions, a referral should be made; "IT" (intensive therapy) is where a qualified practitioner provides individualized therapy. The level of intervention by the nurse depends on that clinician's level of experience and knowledge working with patients with specific sexual health issues.

The nurse also has the key role to provide appropriate patient education about how specific disabilities affect sexual function. For example, arthritis produces fatigue and morning stiffness, making planned afternoon sex a

CHART 12-5

Concerns of Older Adults Facing Disability

- Loss of independence, which is a source of self-respect and dignity
- Increased potential for discrimination or abuse
- Increased social isolation
- Added burden on spouse, who may also have impaired health
- Less access to community services and health care
- Less access to religious institutions
- Increased vulnerability to declining health secondary to other disorders, reduced physiologic reserve, or pre-existing impairments of mobility and balance
- Fears and doubts about the ability to learn or relearn self-care activities, exercises, and transfer and independent mobility techniques
- Inadequate support system for successful rehabilitation

better alternative; spinal cord injury may impair erections and ejaculations; and traumatic brain injury may produce an increased or decreased interest in sexual behaviour. Women with spinal cord injuries may have questions regarding contraception, pregnancy, and labour and delivery. Classes, books, movies, and support groups are useful tools to help patients learn about sexuality and disability. When open discussion and education about disability and sexuality do not result in a patient's achievement of his or her sexuality goals, the nurse should refer the patient for ongoing counselling with a sex counsellor or therapist. The patient may need training in communication and in social and assertiveness skills to develop desired relationships.

Fatigue

People with disabilities frequently experience fatigue and fatigue is a specific, common effect of brain injury. Physical and emotional weariness may be caused by discomfort and pain associated with a chronic health problem, deconditioning associated with prolonged periods of bed rest and immobility, impaired motor function requiring excessive expenditure of energy to ambulate, and the frustrations of performing ADLs. Ineffective coping with the disability, unresolved grief, and depression can also contribute to fatigue. The patient can use coping strategies to manage the psychological impact of the disability and pain management techniques to control the associated discomforts. (Refer to Chapter 16 for a discussion of pain management.) In addition, the nurse can teach the patient to manage fatigue through priority setting and energy-conserving techniques.

Nursing Care of Patients With Disabilities

As active members of society, people with disabilities are no longer an invisible minority. An increased awareness of their needs will bring about changes to improve access and accommodations. Modification of the physical environment permits access to public and private facilities and services, including health care, and nurses can serve as advocates for people with disabilities to eliminate discriminatory practices.

Nursing Considerations During Hospitalization

During hospitalization, as well as during periods of acute illness or injury or while recovering from surgery, patients with pre-existing disabilities may require assistance with carrying out ADLs that they could otherwise manage at home independently and easily. Patients should be asked preferences about approaches to carrying out their ADLs, and assistive devices they require should be readily available. Careful planning with patients to ensure that the hospital room is arranged with their input enables them to manage as independently as possible. For example, patients who have paraplegia may be able to transfer independently from bed to wheelchair; however, if the bed is left in an elevated position, they may be unable to do so. If patients usually use service animals to assist them with ADLs, it is necessary to make arrangements for the accommodation of these animals. If patients with hearing loss or vision impairment are hospitalized, it is essential to establish effective communication strategies. Alternative methods for these patients to communicate with the health care team must be put in place and used, and all staff members must be aware that some patients are not able to respond to the intercom or telephone. If patients have vision impairment, it is necessary to orient them to the environment and talk to them in a normal tone of voice. It may be necessary to obtain a referral with a speech–language therapist or communication specialist to assist in identifying alternative methods (use of sounds, gestures, eye movements) between the nurse and the patient when the patient has a severe cognitive disability that affects speech.

Health Promotion and Prevention

Health care providers often neglect health promotion concerns of people with disabilities, who may be unaware of these concerns. For example, people who have had hearing loss since childhood may lack exposure to information about AIDS through radio and television. People with lifelong disabilities may not have received information about general health issues as children, and people with new onset as well as lifelong disabilities may not receive encouragement to participate in health promotion activities. Therefore, nurses should take every opportunity to emphasize the importance of participation in health promotion activities (e.g., healthy diet, exercise, social interactions) and preventive health screening.

The management of some disabilities increases the risk of illness, and in some people, health screening (e.g., bone density testing, gynecologic examinations, mammography) may be required earlier in life or more frequently. Referrals by nurses to accessible sites for screening may be needed because many imaging centres are inaccessible. In addition, nursing consultation with physical therapists may be needed to identify creative ways of enabling people with disabilities to exercise safely, because exercise facilities are also often inaccessible for people with disabilities.

General health promotion strategies and health-screening recommendations for all men and women also apply to those with disabilities. Although physical limitations, cognitive impairments, and structural and attitudinal barriers existing in clinical facilities may make it difficult for some men and women to obtain health care and preventive health screening, the presence of a disability should not be used as a reason or excuse to defer recommended screening. Rather, the presence of a disability may *increase* the risk of secondary health conditions or disorders that require screening and follow-up. Just as people without disabilities should have regular screening tests, such as mammography or testicular and prostate examinations, so should people with disabilities. Nurses are often in a position to influence decisions about how equipment and procedures can be adapted to meet the special needs of their patients, whether these needs are cognitive, motor, or communicative.

The effect of the disabling condition on health risks should be considered. For example, the risk of osteoporosis may be increased in women and men whose disabilities limit their ability to participate in weight-bearing exercise or who use medications that contribute to bone loss. Although people with disabilities have an increased risk of osteoporosis at a younger age than people without disabilities, little attention is given to prevention, detection, and treatment of osteoporosis, despite the increased risk for falls associated with many disabling disorders.

Nurses can provide expert health promotion education classes that are targeted to people with disabilities and refer them to accessible online resources. Classes on nutrition and weight management are extremely important to people who are wheelchair users and need assistance with transfers. Safer sex classes are needed by adolescents and young adults who have spinal cord injury, traumatic brain injury, or developmental disabilities, because the threats of sexually transmitted infections and unplanned pregnancy exist for these populations just as they do for the population in general.

The need for health promotion in the areas of establishing relationships, sex, pregnancy, and childbearing is as great in people with disabilities, including those with intellectual and cognitive disabilities, as people without disabilities. However, societal attitudes and bias against sexual relationships and childbearing in people with disabilities often result in their exclusion from discussions about these issues as well as failure to take their interest and questions seriously. Approaching these topics at the point of interest and knowledge level of a patient with a disability is important for sexual health. Furthermore, addressing sexual issues is important to prepare people with disabilities, who are at risk of sexual and other forms of abuse, to distinguish between healthy and abusive or exploitative sexual interactions and relationships.

Other healthy behaviours about which people with neurologic disabilities need education include avoiding alcohol and nonprescription medications while taking antispasmodic and anticonvulsant medications.

Critical Thinking Exercises

1 A 25-year-old graduate student is diagnosed with fibromyalgia after several years of visiting physicians and being told that her symptoms were "all in your mind." Due to chronic fatigue and pain, she often missed days from school and eventually withdrew from school. Her husband is not very supportive, as he too thinks the disease is "in her head." How would you help this woman learn to cope with her condition and the damages to her self-esteem? How would you involve her husband in the process?

2 A 43-year-old Aboriginal woman tells you that she is always thirsty and has frequent yeast infections. She also tells you that she has not had a Pap smear or any kind of physical examination since her last child was born 8 years ago because she lives a full day's travel from the health clinic, has no reliable means of transportation, and has no one to care for her four children while she is away. What would you tell this woman? How would y[illegible] her to obtain health care?

3 **ebp** A 43-year-old woman experienced a spi[illegible]cord injury 4 years ago as a result of a diving mishap. She has been admitted to the hospital for treatment of a stage IV pressure ulcer. The health history reveals that the patient has not been following recommendations for skin care and other health practices, including health screening. However, she indicates that she is ready to begin to take a more active role in self-care to avoid development of further pressure ulcers. What recommendations would you make to her for self-care to prevent secondary conditions and disabilities and for health screening? What is the evidence base for your recommendations? What criteria would you use to evaluate the strength of the evidence? Develop an evidence-based plan of care for her.

4 A 30-year-old woman with spina bifida uses crutches and occasionally a motorized scooter for long distance ambulation. She is being seen in an obstetrician/nurse midwifery practice because she and her partner want to explore the possibility of pregnancy and childbearing. She is a successful attorney who has had occasional hospitalizations for acute urinary tract infections with high fevers. What are the risks and benefits of pregnancy and childbearing for this woman and her partner? What nursing assessments are indicated at the time of her first visit? What are the nursing implications for her if she decides to become pregnant? What nursing care and teaching would be warranted as she progresses through a pregnancy?

REFERENCES AND SELECTED READINGS

Books

Bodenheimer, T., & Willard-Grace, R. (2016). The chronic care model and the transformation of primary care. In J. Mechanick, & R. Kushner (Eds.). *Lifestyle medicine* (pp. 89–96). Cham, Switzerland: Springer.

Epp, J. (1986). Achieving health for all: A framework for health promotion. Ottawa, ON: Health and Welfare Canada. Retrieved from http://www.frcentre.net/library/AchievingHealthForAll.pdf

Falvo, D., & Holland, B. E. (2017). *Medical and psychosocial aspects of chronic illness and disability*. Burlington, MA: Jones & Bartlett Learning.

Kramer-Kile, M., Osuji, J., Larsen, P., et al. (2014). *Chronic illness in Canada: Impact and intervention*. Burlington, MA: Jones & Bartlett Publishing.

Lalonde, M. (1974). *A new perspective on the health of Canadians, a working document*. Ottawa, ON: Government of Canada.

Lorig, K., Holman, H., Sobel, D., et al. (2012). Living a healthy life with chronic conditions. Boulder CO: Bull Publishing Company.

Miller, J. F. (2000). Coping with chronic illness: Overcoming powerlessness (3rd ed.). Philadelphia, PA: FA Davis.

World Health Organization (WHO). (2001). *International classification of functioning, disability and health—ICF*. Geneva, Switzerland: Author.

World Health Organization (WHO). (2013). *Global action plan for the prevention and control of noncommunicable diseases, 2013–2020*. Geneva, Switzerland: Author.

World Health Organization (WHO). (2014a). *Global status report on noncommunicable diseases 2014*. Geneva, Switzerland: Author.

World Health Organization (WHO). (2014b). *Noncommunicable diseases country profiles, 2014*. Geneva, Switzerland: Author.

Journals and Electronic Documents

Allegranzi, B., Kilpatrick, C., Storr, J., et al. (2017). Global infection prevention and control priorities 2018–22: A call for action. *The Lancet Global Health*, 5(12), e1178–e1180.

Andermann, A. (2016). Taking action on the social determinants of health in clinical practice: A framework for health professionals. *Canadian Medical Association Journal*, *188*(17–18), E474–E483.

Anton, S. D., Woods, A. J., Ashizawa, T., et al. (2015). Successful aging: Advancing the science of physical independence in older adults. *Ageing Research Reviews*, *24*, 304–327.

Annon, J. S. (1976). The PLISSIT Model: A proposed conceptual scheme for the behavioral treatment of sexual problems. *Journal of Sex Education and Therapy*, 2:1, 1–15, DOI: 10.1080/01614576.1976.11074483

Baptista, D. R., Wiens, A., Pontarolo, R., et al. (2016). The chronic care model for type 2 diabetes: A systematic review. *Diabetology & Metabolic Syndrome*, *8*(1), 7.

Barr, V. J., Robinson, S., Marin-Link, B., et al. (2003). The expanded chronic care model: An integration of concepts and strategies from population health promotion and the chronic care model. *Hospital Quarterly*, *7*(1), 73–82.

Belanger, M., Poirier, M., Jbilou, J., et al. (2014). Modelling the impact of compliance with dietary recommendations on cancer and cardiovascular disease mortality in Canada. *Public Health*, *128*(3), 222–230.

Blyth, F. M., & Noguchi, N. (2017). Chronic musculoskeletal pain and its impact on older people. *Best Practice & Research Clinical Rheumatology*, *31*, 160–168.

Boxell, E. M., Amoaku, W. M., & Bradley, C. (2017). Healthcare experiences of patients with age-related macular degeneration: Have things improved? Cross-sectional survey responses of Macular Society members in 2013 compared with 1999. *BMJ Open*, *7*(2), e012790.

Brathwaite, A. C., & Lemonde, M. (2017). Exploring health beliefs and practices of Caribbean immigrants in Ontario to prevent type 2 Diabetes. *Journal of Transcultural Nursing*, *28*(1), 15–23.

Canadian Nurses Association (CNA). (2017). *Code of ethics for registered nurses*. Ottawa, ON: Author. Retrieved from https://www.cna-aiic.ca/html/en/Code-of-Ethics-2017-Edition/files/assets/basic-html/page-1.html#

Chronic Disease Prevention Alliance of Canada. (2018). *CDPAC Reducing chronic disease in Canada*. Retrieved January 13, 2018, from http://www.cdpac.ca/content.php?doc=330

Corbin, J. M., & Strauss, A. (1991). A nursing model for chronic illness management based upon the trajectory framework. *Scholarly Inquiry for Nursing Practice*, *5*(3), 155–174.

Corbin, J. M. (1998). The Corbin and Strauss chronic illness trajectory model: An update. *Scholarly Inquiry for Nursing Practice*, *12*(1), 33–41.

Dixon-Ibarra, A., Nery-Hurwit, M., Driver, S., et al. (2017). Using health promotion guidelines for persons with disabilities to develop and evaluate a physical activity program for individuals with multiple sclerosis: A feasibility study. *Evaluation and Program Planning*, *61*, 150–159.

Drum, C. E. (2014). The dynamics of disability and chronic conditions. *Disability and Health Journal*, *7*(1), 2–5.

Ellenbecker, C. H., Fawcett, J., Jones, E. J., et al. (2017). A staged approach to educating nurses in health policy. *Policy, Politics, & Nursing Practice*, *18*(1), 44–56.

Eriksson, E., Wejåker, M., Danhard, A., et al. (2017). Living with a spouse with chronic illness–The challenge of balancing demands and resources. *BMC Public Health, 19*: 422. https://doi.org/10.1186/s12889-019-6800-7

Gee, P. M., Greenwood, D. A., Paterniti, D. A., et al. (2015). The eHealth enhanced chronic care model: A theory derivation approach. *Journal of Medical Internet Research*, *17*(4), e86.

Goldstein, I., Kim, N. N., Clayton, A. H., et al. (2017). Hypoactive sexual desire disorder: International Society for the Study of Women's Sexual Health (ISSWSH) expert consensus panel review. *Mayo Clinic Proceedings*, *92*(1), 114–128.

Golics, C. J., Basra, M. K., Salek, M. S., et al. (2013). The impact of patients' chronic disease on family quality of life: An experience from 26 specialties. *International Journal of General Medicine*, *6*, 787–798.

Goodman, R. A., Posner, S. F., Huang, E. S., et al. (2013). Defining and measuring chronic conditions: Imperatives for research, policy, program, and practice. *Preventing Chronic Disease*, *10*, E66.

Gostin, L. O. (2015). The Americans with Disabilities Act at 25: The highest expression of American values. *Journal of the American Medical Association*, *313*(22), 2231–2235.

Gunn, H., Cameron, M., Hoang, P., et al. (2018). The relationship between physiological and perceived fall risk in people with multiple sclerosis: Implications for assessment and management. *Archives of Physical Medicine and Rehabilitation*, *99*, 2022–2029.

Henderson, R., Montesanti, S., Crowshoe, L., et al. (2018). Advancing indigenous primary health care policy in Alberta, Canada. *Health Policy, 122(6), 638–644*.

Hodge, J. G., Jr., Wetter, S. A., Chronister, D., et al. (2017). Redefining public health emergencies: The opioid epidemic. *Jurimetrics*, *58*(1), 1–15.

Hovey, R. B., Delormier, T., McComber, A. M., et al. (2017). Enhancing indigenous health promotion research through two-eyed seeing: A hermeneutic relational process. *Qualitative Health Research*, *27*(9), 1278–1287.

Hucker, A., & McCabe, M. P. (2015). Incorporating mindfulness and chat groups into an online cognitive behavioral therapy for mixed female sexual problems. *The Journal of Sex Research*, *52*(6), 627–639.

Hummel, S. B., van Lankveld, J. J., Oldenburg, H. S., et al. (2015). Internet-based cognitive behavioral therapy for sexual dysfunctions in women treated for breast cancer: Design of a multicenter, randomized controlled trial. *BMC Cancer*, *15*(1), 321.

Jackson, B., & Huston, P. (2016). Social determinants of health: Advancing health equity to improve health: The time is now. *Canada Communicable Disease Report*, *42*(Suppl 1), S1-1.

Jaeger, P. T. (2018). Designing for diversity and designing for disability: New opportunities for libraries to expand their support and advocacy for people with disabilities. *The International Journal of Information, Diversity, & Inclusion*, *2*(1/2).

Johansson, H., Kanis, J. A., Odén, A., et al. (2014). A meta analysis of the association of fracture risk and body mass index in women. *Journal of Bone and Mineral Research*, *29*(1), 223–233.

Karvonen, S., Kestilä, L. M., & Mäki-Opas, T. E. (2018). Who needs the sociology of health and illness? A new agenda for responsive and interdisciplinary sociology of health and medicine. *Frontiers in Sociology*, *3*, 4.

Kehler, D. S., Ferguson, T., Stammers, A. N., et al. (2017). Prevalence of frailty in Canadians 18–79 years old in the Canadian Health Measures Survey. *BMC Geriatrics*, *17*(1), 28.

Kingsberg, S. A., & Woodard, T. (2015). Female sexual dysfunction: Focus on low desire. *Obstetrics & Gynecology*, *125*(2), 477–486.

Krahn, G. L., Walker, D. K., & Correa-De-Araujo, R. (2015). Persons with disabilities as an unrecognized health disparity population. *American Journal of Public Health*, *105*(S2), S198–S206.

Krueger, H., Krueger, J., & Koot, J. (2015). Variation across Canada in the economic burden attributable to excess weight, tobacco smoking and physical inactivity. *Canadian Journal of Public Health*, *106*(4), e171–e177.

Krueger, H., Williams, D., Ready, A. E., et al. (2013). Improved estimation of the health and economic burden of chronic disease risk factors in Manitoba. *Chronic Diseases and Injuries in Canada*, *33*(4), 236–246.

Leggio, M., Lombardi, M., Caldarone, E., et al. (2017). The relationship between obesity and hypertension: An updated comprehensive overview on vicious twins. *Hypertension Research*, *40*(12), 947–963.

Lenzen, S. A., Daniëls, R., van Bokhoven, M. A., et al. (2017). Disentangling self-management goal setting and action planning: A scoping review. *PLoS One*, *12*(11), e0188822.

Lewis, B. A., Napolitano, M. A., Buman, M. P., et al. (2017). Future directions in physical activity intervention research: Expanding our focus to sedentary behaviors, technology, and dissemination. *Journal of Behavioral Medicine*, *40*(1), 112–126.

Lontchi-Yimagou, E., Mapa-Tassou, C., Dehayem, M. Y., et al. (2017). The effect of free diabetes care on metabolic control and on health-related quality of life among youths with type 1 diabetes in Cameroon. *BMJ Open Diabetes Research and Care*, *5*(1), e000397.

Marzolini, S., Brooks, D., Oh, P., et al. (2018). Aerobic with resistance training or aerobic training alone post stroke: A secondary analysis from a randomized clinical trial. *Neurorehabilitation and Neural Repair*, *32*(3), 209–222.

McColl, M. A., Jaiswal, A., & Roberts, L. (2017). *A review of federal disability policy in Canada*. Retrieved from http://www.disabilitypolicyalliance.ca/wp-content/uploads/2016/02/dispol-3rded-federal-final-240417.pdf

McGlynn, N., Kirsh, V. A., Cotterchio, M., et al. (2015). Shift work and obesity among Canadian women: A cross-sectional study using a novel exposure assessment tool. *PLoS One*, *10*(9), e0137561.

Murnaghan, D., Morrison, W., Griffith, E. J., et al. (2013). Knowledge exchange systems for youth health and chronic disease prevention: A tri provincial case study. *Chronic Diseases and Injuries in Canada*, *33*(4), 257–266.

Newland, P., Jenson, M. P., Budhathoki, C., et al. (2015). Secondary health conditions in individuals with multiple sclerosis: A cross-sectional web-based survey analysis. *Journal of Neuroscience Nursing*, *47*(3), 124–130.

Northwood, M., Ploeg, J., Markle Reid, M., et al. (2018). Integrative review of the social determinants of health in older adults with multimorbidity. *Journal of Advanced Nursing*, *74*(1), 45–60.

O'Brien, M. W., Robinson, S. A., Frayne, R., et al. (2018). Achieving Canadian physical activity guidelines is associated with better vascular function independent of aerobic fitness and sedentary time in older adults. *Applied Physiology, Nutrition, and Metabolism*, *43*, 1003–1009.

Paterson, B. L. (2001). The shifting perspectives model of chronic illness. *Journal of Nursing Scholarship, 33*, 21–26.

Paterson, B. L. (2003). The koala has claws: Applications of the shifting perspectives model in research of chronic illness. *Qualitative Health Research, 13*, 981–984.

Phelan, S. K. (2011). Constructions of disability: A call for critical reflexivity in occupational therapy. *Canadian Journal of Occupational Therapy*, *78*, 164–172.

Plamondon, K., Walters, D., Campbell, S., et al. (2017). Promoting equitable global health research: A policy analysis of the Canadian funding landscape. *Health Research Policy and Systems*, *15*(1), 72.

Prince, M. J., Wu, F., Guo, Y., et al. (2015). The burden of disease in older people and implications for health policy and practice. *Lancet*, *385*(9967), 549–562.

Public Health Agency of Canada (PHAC). (2013). *Preventing chronic diseases strategic plan 2013–2016*. Retrieved from http://publications.gc.ca/collections/collection_2014/aspc-phac/HP35-39-2013-eng.pdf

Ramjan, L., Cotton, A., Algoso, M., et al. (2016). Barriers to breast and cervical cancer screening for women with physical disability: A review. *Women & Health*, *56*(2), 141–156.

Robinson, C. A. (2017). Families living well with chronic illness: The healing process of moving on. *Qualitative Health Research*, *27*(4), 447–461.

Sinu, E., Parthasarathy, B. N., Reddy, K., et al. (2018). Needs of persons with neurological disorders. *Indian Journal of Psychiatric Social Work*, *9*(1), 29–37.

Staebler, S., Campbell, J., Cornelius, P., et al. (2017). Policy and political advocacy: Comparison study of nursing faculty to determine current practices, perceptions, and barriers to teaching health policy. *Journal of Professional Nursing*, *33*(5), 350–355.

Statistics Canada. (2018a). *Leading causes of death, by total population, by age group*.Retrieved January 14, 2018, from http://www.statcan.gc.ca/tables-tableaux/sum-som/l01/cst01/hlth36a-eng.htm

Statistics Canada. (2018b). *A profile of persons with disabilities among Canadians aged 15 years or older, 2012*. Retrieved January 18, 2018 from http://www.statcan.gc.ca/pub/89-654-x/89-654-x2015001-eng.htm#a1

Stienstra, D. (2018). Canadian disability policies in a world of inequalities. *Societies*, *8*(2), 1–13.

Stretton, C. M., Mudge, S., Kayes, N. M., et al. (2017). Interventions to improve real-world walking after stroke: A systematic review and meta-analysis. *Clinical Rehabilitation*, *31*(3), 310–318.

Tao, Z., Shi, A., & Zhao, J. (2015). Epidemiological perspectives of diabetes. *Cell Biochemistry and Biophysics*, *73*(1), 181–185.

Waddell, A., Audette, K., DeLong, A., et al. (2016). A hospital-based interdisciplinary model for increasing nurses' engagement in legislative advocacy. *Policy, Politics, & Nursing Practice*, *17*(1), 15–23.

Wagner, E. H., Davis, J., Schaefer, M., et al. (1999). A survey of leading chronic disease management programs: Are they consistent with the literature? *Managed Care Quarterly*, *7*(3), 56–66.

Ward, B. W., Schiller, J. S., & Goodman, R. A. (2014). Multiple chronic conditions among US adults: A 2012 update. *Preventing Chronic Disease*, *11*, E62. http://dx.doi.org/10.5888/pcd11.130389

Woodward, B., Smart, D., & Benavides-Vaello, S. (2016). Modifiable factors that support political participation by nurses. *Journal of Professional Nursing*, *32*(1), 54–61.

World Health Organization (WHO). (2014c). *Disability and health. Fact sheet No 352*. Retrieved July 18, 2015, from www.who.int/mediacentre/factsheets/fs352/en/

World Health Organization (WHO). (2017). *Noncommunicable diseases: Progress monitor 2017*. Retrieved from https://www.who.int/nmh/publications/ncd-progress-monitor-2017/en/

Resources

Canadian Fitness and Lifestyle Research Institute: https://www.cflri.ca/

Chronic Disease Prevention Alliance of Canada: http://www.cdpac.ca/

Council of Canadians with Disabilities: http://www.ccdonline.ca/en/

Health Canada, Commission on the Future of Health Care in Canada (Romanow Commission Web site): http://www.hc-sc.gc.ca/english/care/romanow/index1.html

Health in Action, Alberta Healthy Living Program: https://www.albertahealthservices.ca/info/Page8930.aspx

Public Health Agency of Canada, Health Promotion and Chronic Disease Prevention in Canada: Research, Policy and Practice: http://www.phac-aspc.gc.ca/publicat/cdic-mcc/index.html

Rights of People with Disabilities: https://www.canada.ca/en/canadian-heritage/services/rights-people-disabilities.html

World Health Organization, Chronic Diseases and Health Promotion: http://www.who.int/chp/en/

13 Principles and Practices of Rehabilitation

Adapted by Joseph Osuji and Mohamed Toufic El Hussein

Learning Objectives

On completion of this chapter, the learner will be able to:

1. Describe the goals of rehabilitation.
2. Discuss the interprofessional approach to rehabilitation.
3. Identify physical and emotional reactions exhibited by patients with disabilities.
4. Use the nursing process as a framework for care of patients with self-care deficits, impaired physical mobility, impaired skin integrity, and altered patterns of elimination.
5. Describe nursing strategies appropriate for promoting self-care through activities of daily living (ADLs).
6. Describe nursing strategies appropriate for promoting mobility and ambulation and the use of assistive devices.
7. Describe risk factors and related nursing measures to prevent development of pressure injuries.
8. Incorporate bladder training and bowel training into the plan of care for patients with bladder and bowel problems.
9. Describe the significance of continuity of care from the health care facility to the home or extended care facility for patients who need rehabilitative assistance and services.

Rehabilitation is a goal-oriented process that enables people with acute or chronic disorders, including those with physical, mental, or emotional disabilities or **impairments**; activity limitations; and participation restrictions to (1) identify, reach, and maintain optimal physical, sensory, intellectual, psychological, and/or social functional levels and (2) focus on existing abilities to facilitate independence, self-determination, and social integration (Camicia, Black, Farrell, et al., 2014; Kearney & Cronin, 2014; Miller, 2014). During rehabilitation, patients adjust to disabilities by learning how to use available resources with a focus on overall health promotion (Hyde & Kautz, 2014).

Rehabilitation is a dynamic, health-oriented process that assists an ill person or a person with disability (restriction in performance or function in everyday activities) to achieve the greatest possible level of physical, mental, spiritual, social, and economic functioning. The rehabilitation process helps the patient achieve an acceptable quality of life with dignity, self-respect, and independence and is designed for people with physical, mental, or emotional disabilities. During rehabilitation—sometimes called **habilitation**—the patient adjusts to the disability by learning how to use resources and to focus on existing abilities. In habilitation, abilities—not disabilities—are emphasized. **Prehabilitation** focuses on strength training preoperatively to promote functional recovery and prevention of complications post surgery.

Rehabilitation is an integral part of nursing because every major illness or injury carries the threat of disability or impairment, which involves decreased function. The principles of rehabilitation are basic to the care of all patients, and rehabilitation efforts should begin during the initial contact with a patient. Ultimately, the goal of rehabilitation nursing is to assist the patient to attain and maintain optimum health as defined by the patient (Bamm, Rosenbaum, Wilkins, et al., 2015; Chang & Johnson, 2013;

Dean, Siegert, & Taylor, 2012). If restoring the debilitated patient's ability to function independently or at a pre-illness or pre-injury level of functioning is not possible, the aims of rehabilitation are to maximize independence and prevent secondary disability as well as to promote a quality of life acceptable to the patient. This includes assessing and treating physical as well as psychological disorders and comorbidities after illness or injury (Craig, Perry, Guest, et al., 2015).

Rehabilitation services are required by more people than ever before because of advances in technology that save or prolong the lives of patients who are seriously ill, injured, and disabled. Increasing numbers of patients who are recovering from serious illnesses or injuries are returning to their homes and communities with ongoing needs. Every patient, regardless of age, gender, ethnic group, socioeconomic status, or diagnosis, has a right to rehabilitation services (Chart 13-1).

The Rehabilitation Team

Rehabilitation is a creative, dynamic process that requires a team of professionals working together with patients and families. The interdisciplinary team members include health professionals who make unique contributions to the rehabilitation process. Communication, collaboration, understanding of roles, and educational levels of team members are all important considerations in building an effective interdisciplinary team (Papadimitriou & Cott, 2015; Strasser, Burridge, Falconer, et al., 2014; White, Gutierrez, Mclaughlin, et al., 2013). In addition to nurses, members of the rehabilitation team may include physicians, nurse practitioners, physiatrists, physical therapists, occupational therapists, recreational therapists, speech–language therapists, psychologists, psychiatric liaison nurses, spiritual advisors, social workers, vocational counselors, orthotists or prosthetists, and sex counselors.

CHART 13-1

Ethics and Related Issues

Access to Rehabilitation Services

SITUATION

Most communities have citizens who are poor and homeless and who are more at risk for community violence. In turn, violence often creates life-threatening and disabling conditions. After a victim of violence has been treated and stabilized, the health care team identifies rehabilitation needs. You are concerned about your patient's inability to perform self-care and demonstrate safe mobility skills and wonder how your patient will manage after discharge.

DILEMMA

Although your patient needs a secure living environment to recover and manage a disability, you recognize the patient's right to autonomy in making decisions about health and living conditions. As a health care provider, you recognize there are costs associated with an individual's personal decisions, and affordable follow-up care may or may not be available.

DISCUSSION

Who determines the length of stay and level of care? Who will take care of patients who need longer-term rehabilitation but services are not readily available? Should the level of rehabilitation services being offered depend on the patient's past history of complying with therapy and self-care?

Nurses assume an equal or, depending on the circumstances of the patient, a more critical role than other members of the health care team in the rehabilitation process. The evidence-based plan of care that nurses develop must be approved by the patient and family and is an integral part of the rehabilitation process (Clark & Bassett, 2014; Clark-Wilson, Giles, & Baxter, 2014). See Chart 13-2 for

Glossary

activities of daily living (ADLs): self-care activities including bathing, grooming, dressing, eating, toileting, and bowel and bladder care

adaptive device: a type of assistive technology that is used to change the environment or help a person to modify the environment (e.g., a ramp that can be used in place of steps for someone in a wheelchair)

assistive device: a type of assistive technology that helps people with disabilities perform a given task (e.g., a lap board with pictures to assist a person who cannot talk to communicate)

assistive technology: any item, piece of equipment, or product system that is used to improve the functional capabilities of individuals with disabilities; this term encompasses both assistive devices and adaptive devices

habilitation: making able; learning new skills and abilities to meet maximum potential

impairment: loss or abnormality of psychological, physiologic, or anatomic structure or function at the organ level (e.g., dysphagia, hemiparesis); an abnormality of body structure, appearance, and organ or system function resulting from any cause

instrumental activities of daily living (IADLs): complex aspects of independence including meal preparation, grocery shopping, household management, finances, and transportation

prehabilitation: preoperative rehabilitation to help patients build reserve capacity in order to promote positive outcomes. The musculoskeletal, cardiovascular, and pulmonary systems are often the focus of prehabilitation (Shoemaker, Gibson, & Saagman, 2013)

pressure injuries: breakdown of the skin due to prolonged pressure and insufficient blood supply, usually at bony prominences

rehabilitation: making able again; relearning skills or abilities or adjusting existing functions

NURSING RESEARCH PROFILE

Chart 13-2. Understanding Interdisciplinary Teams in Rehabilitation Practice

White, M. J., Gutierrez, A., Mclaughlin, C., et al. (2013). A pilot study to examine interdisciplinary teams from the perspective of the rehabilitation nurse, the occupational therapist and the physiotherapist. *Rehabilitation Nursing*, *38*(3), 142–152.

Purpose

The Institute of Medicine identifies interdisciplinary teams (IDTs) being able to work well together as one of five core competencies of health care workers. A literature review on teams identified communication, collaboration, understanding of roles, and educational levels of team members as key themes. Based on these themes, the study team developed a survey to assess perceptions of teams by rehabilitation nurses, physical therapists, and occupational therapists.

Design

A prospective pilot study of a convenience sample ($N = 106$) of 79 rehabilitation nurses, 14 physical therapists, and 13 occupational therapists was conducted to assess perceptions of IDTs and facilitators and barriers for teamwork. A survey was developed that asked about demographic characteristics of team members and open-ended questions about barriers and facilitators for effective teams.

Findings

Four major themes emerged from the pilot study: communication and collaboration, experience, education, and knowledge of roles. Education and experience levels of IDT members are facilitators in IDTs. Communication is both a barrier and a facilitator for IDT effectiveness. Understanding the roles and responsibilities of other IDT members is important to enable the team to function effectively.

Nursing Implications

Learning how to be effective team members, understanding concepts of team development, and participating in teams need to be emphasized in nursing education. Mentorship and team building support should be provided in work settings. All disciplines should come to the team understanding how to participate effectively, with good communication skills essential to develop effective IDTs.

a Nursing Research Profile on multiprofessional and interdisciplinary teamwork in the rehabilitation setting. Principles that undergird the process of patient-centred, rehabilitation-focused care include the following:

- Rehabilitation encompasses all domains of personhood: physical, psychosocial, emotional, cultural, spiritual, and cognitive (Chang & Johnson, 2013).
- Rehabilitation is a continuous process.
- Rehabilitation requires active patient participation.
- Rehabilitation is goal directed.
- Rehabilitation requires multiprofessional and interdisciplinary teamwork (Camicia et al., 2014; Dean et al., 2012; Kolar, 2014; O'Sullivan, Schmitz, & Fulk, 2013).

In working toward maximizing independence, nurses affirm the patient as an active participant and essential part of the health care delivery process (Bamm et al., 2015). Indeed, the patient is a key member of the rehabilitation team, the focus of the team's effort, and the one who determines the final outcomes of the rehabilitation process. The patient participates in goal setting, in learning to function using their remaining abilities, and in adjusting to living with disabilities. Nurses also recognize the importance of informal caregivers as support team members in the rehabilitation process circle of care (Hanson, Armstrong, Green, et al., 2012; Knudson-Martin, Huenergardt, Lafontant, et al., 2015; Price & Lau, 2013). The patient's family is also incorporated into the team. Families are dynamic systems; therefore, the disability of one member affects other family members. Only by incorporating the family into the rehabilitation process can the family system adapt to the change in one of its members. The family provides ongoing support, participates in problem solving, and learns to participate in providing ongoing care.

The nurse develops a therapeutic and supportive relationship with the patient and family. The nurse emphasizes the patient's assets and strengths, positively reinforcing the patient's efforts to improve self-concept and self-care abilities. During nurse–patient interactions, the nurse actively listens, encourages, and shares patient and family successes. Using the nursing process, the nurse develops a plan of care designed to facilitate rehabilitation, restore and maintain optimal health, and prevent complications (Clarke, 2014).

Coping with the disability, fostering self-care, identifying mobility limitations, and managing skin care and bowel and bladder training are areas that frequently require nursing care. The nurse acts as a caregiver, educator, counselor, patient advocate, case manager, and consultant. The nurse is often responsible for coordinating the total rehabilitative plan and collaborating with and coordinating the services provided by all members of the health care team, including home care nurses, who are responsible for directing patient care after the patient returns home.

Areas of Specialty Rehabilitation

Although rehabilitation is a component of every patient's care, there are specialty rehabilitation programs established in general hospitals, free-standing rehabilitation hospitals, and outpatient facilities. The Accreditation Canada and the Commission for the Accreditation of Rehabilitation Facilities (CARF) have set standards for these programs and monitor compliance with them.

Specialty rehabilitation programs meet the needs of patients with various disabilities:

- Stroke recovery programs and traumatic brain injury rehabilitation emphasize cognitive remediation, assisting patients to compensate for memory, perceptual, judgment, and safety deficits as well as teaching self-care and mobility skills. Other goals include assisting patients to swallow food safely and communicate effectively. In addition to stroke and brain injury, other neurologic disorders treated include multiple sclerosis, Parkinson's disease, amyotrophic lateral sclerosis, and nervous system tumours.

- Spinal cord injury rehabilitation programs have increased since World War II. Integral components of the programs include understanding the effects and complications of spinal cord injury; neurogenic bowel and bladder management; sexuality and male fertility enhancement; self-care, including prevention of skin breakdown; bed mobility and transfers; and driving with adaptive equipment. The programs also focus on vocational assessment, training, and reentry into employment and the community.
- Orthopedic rehabilitation programs provide comprehensive services to patients with traumatic or nontraumatic amputations, patients undergoing joint replacements, and patients with arthritis. Learning to be independent with a prosthesis or a new joint is a major goal of the program. Pain management, energy conservation, and joint protection are other goals.
- Cardiac rehabilitation, for patients who have had myocardial infarction, begins during the acute hospitalization and continues on an outpatient basis. Emphasis is placed on monitored, progressive exercise; nutritional counselling; stress management; sexuality; management of hypertension; and smoking cessation.
- Pulmonary rehabilitation programs may be appropriate for patients with restrictive or chronic obstructive pulmonary disease or ventilator dependency. Respiratory therapists help the patient achieve more effective breathing patterns. The programs also teach energy-conservation techniques, self-medication, and home airway management.
- Comprehensive pain management programs are available for sufferers of chronic pain, especially low back pain. These programs focus on alternative pain treatment modalities, exercise, supportive counselling, and vocational evaluation.
- Comprehensive burn rehabilitation programs may serve as step-down units from intensive care burn units. Although rehabilitation strategies are implemented immediately in acute care, a program focused on progressive joint mobility, self-care, and ongoing counselling is imperative for the patient with burns. (See the Rehabilitation Phase of Burn Care section in Chapter 59.)
- Pediatric rehabilitation programs meet the needs of children with developmental and acquired disabilities, including cerebral palsy, spina bifida, traumatic brain injuries, and spinal cord injuries.
- Cancer rehabilitation helps a person with cancer obtain the best physical, social, psychological, and work-related functioning during and after cancer treatment (http://www.cancer.net).
- Psychiatric (mental health) rehabilitation is the process of restoration of community functioning and well-being of an individual diagnosed with a mental disorder and who may be considered to have a psychiatric disability. A team of rehabilitation professionals seeks to effect change in a person's environment and in a person's ability to deal with his/her environment, so as to facilitate improvement in symptoms or personal distress.

As in all areas of nursing practice, nurses who work in the area of rehabilitation must be skilled and knowledgeable about care of patients with substance abuse. For all individuals with disability, including adolescents, the nurse must assess actual or potential substance abuse. In Canada, 13.6% of all Canadians are considered high-risk drinkers (8.9% of women drinkers, 25.1% of men drinkers). The use of illicit drugs is generally limited to cannabis only. About 28.7% of Canadians report using only cannabis during their lifetime, and 11% used only cannabis during the past year. In Canada, medicinal marijuana has been available for symptom relief for a variety of conditions, including cancer, multiple sclerosis, spinal cord injury, HIV/AIDS, arthritis, and epilepsy. It has been used to treat such symptoms as severe pain and/or persistent muscle spasms, seizures, nausea, weight loss, cachexia, and anorexia (http://www.medicalmarijuana.ca).

Parental alcoholism is one of the strongest predictors of substance abuse. Alcohol abuse rates for people with disability may be twice as high as the general population.

Fifty percent of spinal cord injuries are related to substance abuse, and approximately 50% of all patients with traumatic brain injury were intoxicated at the time of injury (Substance Abuse and Mental Health Services Administration [SAMHSA], 2014).

Substance abuse is a critical issue in rehabilitation, especially for individuals with a disability who are attempting to gain employment via vocational rehabilitation. The rates of substance abuse, including alcohol abuse, in people with disabilities are two to four times as high (Glazier & Kling, 2013) as in the general population, and this increased abuse is associated with numerous risks that may have an adverse impact. These risks include medication and health problems, societal enabling (i.e., acceptance and tolerance of substance abuse by key social and cultural groups), a lack of identification of potential problems, and a lack of accessible and appropriate prevention and treatment services. Treatment for alcoholism and drug dependencies includes a thorough physical and psychosocial evaluation; detoxification; counselling; medical treatment; psychological assistance for the patient and family; treatment of any coexisting psychiatric illness; and referral to community resources for social, legal, spiritual, or vocational assistance. Length of treatment and the rehabilitation process depends on the individual's needs. Self-help groups are also encouraged, although attendance in such groups (e.g., Alcoholics Anonymous, Narcotics Anonymous) poses various challenges for the person who has neurologic deficits, is confined to a wheelchair, or must adapt to encounters with able-bodied attendees who may not understand disability. All specialty areas of rehabilitation require implementation of the nursing process as described in this chapter.

Assessment of Functional Ability

Comprehensive assessment of functional capacity is the basis for developing a rehabilitation program. Functional capacity measures a person's ability to perform ADLs as well as **instrumental activities of daily living (IADLs)**. ADLs include activities performed to meet basic needs, such as personal hygiene, dressing, toileting, eating, and moving. IADLs include activities that are necessary for independent living, such as the ability to shop for and prepare meals, use the telephone, clean, manage finances, and travel.

The nurse observes the patient performing specific activities (e.g., eating, dressing) and notes the degree of independence; the time taken; the patient's mobility, coordination, and endurance; and the amount of assistance required. Good joint motion, muscle strength, cardiovascular reserve, and an intact neurologic system are also carefully assessed, because functional ability depends on these factors as well. Observations are recorded on a functional assessment tool. These tools provide a way to standardize assessment parameters and supply a scale or score against which improvements may be measured. They also clearly communicate the patient's level of functioning to all members of the rehabilitation team. Rehabilitation staff uses these tools to provide an initial assessment of the patient's abilities and to monitor the patient's progress in independence.

Worldwide, one of the most frequently used tools to assess the patient's level of independence is the Functional Independence Measure (FIM) (Keith, Granger, Hamilton, et al., 1987). The FIM is a minimum data set, measuring 18 items. It provides a common or standard language that is not discipline specific. The self-care items measured are eating, bathing, grooming, dressing the upper body, dressing the lower body, and toileting. The FIM also assesses sphincter control; locomotion, including stairs; and communication, social interaction, and cognition. A WeeFIM instrument is used for children. Each of the 18 items is rated with a 7-level scale, where 1 represents complete dependence and 7 represents complete independence. (The 18-item FIM instrument is the property of Uniform Data System for Medical Rehabilitation, a division of UB Foundation Activities, Inc.) The Alpha FIM, a short version of the FIM, is used frequently within 72 hours of admission in acute care settings to measure functional independence and the amount of assistance the patient needs to perform ADLs.

Occupational therapists in Canada use the Canadian Occupational Performance Measure as an individualized, client-centred measure to detect change in a client's self-perception of occupational performance over time (Yang et al., 2017). There are many other assessment tools designed to evaluate function in persons with specific disabling conditions, such as the PULSES profile (Granger, Albrecht, & Hamilton, 1979), Barthel Index (Mahoney & Barthel, 1965), Patient Evaluation Conference System (PECS) (Harvey & Jellinek, 1981), and Disability Rating Scale (DRS) (Wright, 2011).

In addition to the detailed functional assessment, the nurse assesses the patient's physical, mental, emotional, spiritual, social, and economic status. Secondary problems related to the disability, such as muscle atrophy and deconditioning, are assessed, as are residual strengths unaffected by disease or disability. Other areas that require nursing assessment include potential for altered skin integrity, altered bowel and bladder control, and sexual dysfunction.

Nursing Process

The Patient With Self-Care Deficits in Activities of Daily Living

Activities of daily living (ADLs) are those self-care activities that the patient must accomplish each day to meet personal needs. ADLs include personal hygiene/bathing, dressing/grooming, feeding, and toileting. Many patients are unable to perform such activities easily. An ADL program is started as soon as the rehabilitation process begins, because the ability to perform ADLs is frequently the key to independence, return to the home, and reentry into the community.

Assessment

The nurse must observe and assess the patient's ability to perform ADLs to determine the level of independence in self-care and the need for nursing intervention. The activity of bathing requires obtaining bath water and utensils, washing, and drying the body after bathing. Dressing requires getting clothes from the closet, putting on and taking off clothing, and fastening the clothing. Self-feeding requires using utensils to bring food to the mouth and chewing and swallowing the food. The activity of toileting includes removing clothing to use the toilet, cleansing oneself, and readjusting clothing. Grooming activities include combing hair, brushing teeth, shaving or applying makeup, and washing the hands. Patients who can sit up and raise their hands to their head can begin self-care activities.

In addition, the nurse needs to be aware of the patient's medical conditions, the effect that they have on the ability to perform ADLs, and the family's involvement in the patient's ADLs. This information is valuable in setting goals and developing the plan of care to maximize self-care.

Nursing Diagnosis

Based on the assessment data, major nursing diagnoses for the patient may include the following:

- Self-care deficit: bathing/hygiene, dressing/grooming, feeding, toileting

Planning and Goals

The major goals of the patient include the following using an **adaptive device** or devices as appropriate: bathing/hygiene independently or with assistance, dressing/grooming independently or with assistance, feeding independently or with assistance, and toileting independently or with assistance. Another goal is that the patient with a self-care deficit expresses satisfaction with the extent of independence in self-care activities.

Nursing Interventions

Repetition, practice, and demonstrations help patients achieve maximum independence in personal care activities. The nurse's role is to provide an optimal learning environment that minimizes distractions. The nurse can identify the patient's optimal time to work on activities, encourage concentration, identify endurance issues that may affect safety, and provide cues and reminders to patients with specific disabilities (e.g., hemiparesis or hemineglect) (Hyde & Kautz, 2014). Patients with impaired mobility, sensation, strength, or dexterity may need to use **assistive devices** to accomplish self-care.

Fostering Self-Care Abilities

To learn methods of self-care effectively, the patient must be motivated. An "I'd rather do it myself" attitude is encouraged. The nurse must also help the patient identify the safe limits of independent activity; knowing when to ask for assistance is particularly important.

The nurse teaches, guides, and supports the patient who is learning or relearning how to perform self-care activities. Consistency in instructions and assistance given by health care providers facilitates the learning process. Recording the patient's performance provides data for evaluating progress and may be used as a source for motivation and morale building (Chart 13-3).

Often, a simple manoeuvre requires concentration and the exertion of considerable effort on the part of the patient with a disability; therefore, self-care techniques need to be adapted to accommodate the individual patient's lifestyle. There is usually more than one way to accomplish a self-care activity, so common sense and a little ingenuity may promote increased independence. For example, a person who cannot quite reach his or her head may be able to do so by leaning forward. Encouraging the patient to participate in a support group may also help the patient to discover inventive or creative solutions to self-care problems. Pre-existing cultural norms may influence the degree of self-care the patient is willing to consider. Cultural and ethnic beliefs about hygiene can vary among individuals and families. The nurse must recognize these beliefs, work through any issues with the patient and family, and communicate pertinent findings to the rehabilitation team.

Recommending Adaptive and Assistive Devices

If the patient has difficulty in performing an ADL, an adaptive or assistive device (self-help device) may be useful. The term assistive technology is a term used to describe either assistive or adaptive devices that could be used to improve the functioning of individuals living with disabilities. A large variety of assistive devices are available commercially or can be fabricated by the nurse, the occupational therapist, the patient, or the family. The devices may include built-up handles on toothbrushes or razors; long, curved handles on mirrors or shoe horns; suction cups to hold items in place; shower chairs; raised toilet seats; and universal cuffs to grip self-care items. The nurse should be alert to "gadgets" coming on the market and evaluate their potential for usefulness. Of course, the nurse must exercise professional judgment and caution in recommending devices, because unscrupulous vendors have marketed unnecessary, overly expensive, or useless items to patients in the past.

NURSING ALERT

To avoid injury or bleeding, people who take anticoagulant medication should be encouraged to use an electric razor. Women may wish to consider depilatory creams or electrolysis.

A wide selection of computerized assistive devices is available, or devices can be designed to help individual patients with severe disabilities to function more independently. The booklet entitled *Access to Assistive Technology in Canada: A Jurisdictional Scan of Programs* (Agewell, 2017) can be a useful resource for these patients.

Helping the Patient Accept Limitations

If the patient has a severe disability, independent self-care may be an unrealistic goal; in this situation, the rehabilitation nurse teaches the patient how to direct his or her own care. The patient may require a personal attendant to perform ADLs. Family members may not be appropriate for providing bathing/hygiene, dressing/grooming, feeding, and toileting assistance, and a spouse may have difficulty providing bowel and bladder care for the patient and maintaining the role of sexual partner. If a personal caregiver is needed, the person with a disability or family members must

CHART 13-3

Educating Patients About Activities of Daily Living

1. Define the goal of the activity with the patient. Be realistic. Set short-term goals that can be accomplished in the near future.
2. Identify several approaches to accomplish the task (e.g., there are several ways to put on a given garment).
3. Select the approach most likely to succeed.
4. Specify the approach on the patient's care plan and the patient's level of accomplishment on the progress notes.
5. Identify the motions necessary to accomplish the activity (e.g., to pick up a glass, extend arm with hand open; place open hand next to glass; flex fingers around glass; move arm and hand holding glass vertically; flex arm toward body).
6. Focus on gross functional movements initially, and gradually include activities that use finer motions (e.g., buttoning clothes, eating with a fork).
7. Encourage the patient to perform the activity up to maximal capacity within the limitations of the disability.
8. Monitor the patient's tolerance.
9. Minimize frustration and fatigue.
10. Support the patient by giving appropriate praise for effort put forth and for acts accomplished.
11. Assist the patient to perform and practice the activity in real-life situations.

learn how to manage an employee effectively. The nurse assists the patient in accepting self-care dependency. Independence in other areas, such as social interaction, should be emphasized to promote a positive self-concept.

Evaluation

Expected Patient Outcomes

Expected patient outcomes may include the following:

1. Demonstrates independent self-care in bathing/hygiene or with assistance, using adaptive devices as appropriate
   a. Bathes self at maximal level of independence
   b. Uses adaptive devices effectively
   c. Reports satisfaction with level of independence in bathing/hygiene
2. Demonstrates independent self-care in dressing/grooming or with assistance, using adaptive devices as appropriate
   a. Dresses/grooms self at maximal level of independence
   b. Uses adaptive devices effectively
   c. Reports satisfaction with level of independence in dressing/grooming
   d. Demonstrates increased interest in appearance
3. Demonstrates independent self-care in feeding or with assistance, using adaptive and assistive devices as appropriate
   a. Feeds self at maximal level of independence
   b. Uses adaptive and assistive devices effectively
   c. Demonstrates increased interest in eating
   d. Maintains adequate nutritional intake
4. Demonstrates independent self-care in toileting or with assistance, using adaptive and assistive devices as appropriate
   a. Toilets self at maximal level of independence
   b. Uses adaptive and assistive devices effectively
   c. Indicates positive feelings regarding level of toileting independence
   d. Experiences adequate frequency of bowel and bladder elimination
   e. Does not experience incontinence, constipation, urinary tract infection, or other complications

Nursing Process

The Patient With Impaired Physical Mobility

Patients who are ill or injured are frequently placed on bed rest or have their activities limited. Problems commonly associated with immobility include weakened muscles, joint contracture, and deformity. Each joint of the body has a normal range of motion; if the range is limited, the functions of the joint and of the muscles that move the joint are impaired, and painful deformities may develop. Nurses must identify patients at risk for such complications.

Another problem frequently seen in rehabilitation nursing is an altered ambulatory/mobility pattern. The patient with a disability may be either temporarily or permanently unable to walk independently. The nurse assesses the mobility of the patient and designs care that promotes independent mobility within the prescribed therapeutic limits.

If a person is not able to exercise and move the joints through their full range of motion, contractures may develop. A contracture is a shortening of the muscle and tendon that leads to deformity and limits joint mobility. When the contracted joint is moved, the patient experiences pain; in addition, more energy is required to move when joints are contracted and deformed.

Assessment

At times, a patient's mobility is restricted because of pain, paralysis, loss of muscle strength, systemic disease, an immobilizing device (e.g., cast, brace), or prescribed limits to promote healing. Assessment of the patient's mobility includes positioning, ability to move, muscle strength and tone, joint function, and the prescribed mobility limits. The nurse may need to collaborate with the physical therapist or other team members to assess mobility.

During position change, transfer, and ambulation activities, the nurse assesses the patient's abilities, the extent of disability, and residual capacity for physiologic adaptation. The nurse observes for orthostatic hypotension, pallor, diaphoresis, nausea, tachycardia, and fatigue.

If a patient is not able to ambulate without assistance, the nurse assesses the ability to balance, transfer, and use assistive devices (e.g., crutches, walker). Crutch walking requires high energy expenditure and produces considerable cardiovascular stress; so older people with reduced exercise capacity, decreased arm strength, and problems with balance because of old age and multiple diseases may be unable to use them. A walker is more stable and may be a better choice for such patients. The nurse assesses the patient's ability to use various devices that promote mobility. If a patient uses an orthosis—an external appliance that provides support, prevents or corrects deformities, and improves function—the nurse monitors the patient for effective use and potential problems associated with its use (e.g., reddened or pressure areas).

Nursing Diagnosis

Based on the assessment data, major nursing diagnoses for the patient may include the following:

- Impaired physical mobility
- Activity intolerance/poor endurance
- Risk for injury
- Risk for contractures or footdrop
- Impaired walking
- Impaired wheelchair mobility
- Impaired bed mobility
- Deconditioning

Planning and Goals

The major goals of the patient may include absence of contracture and deformity, maintenance of muscle strength and joint mobility, independent mobility, and increased activity tolerance.

Nursing Interventions

Positioning to Prevent Musculoskeletal Complications

Deformities and contractures can often be prevented by proper positioning. Maintaining correct body alignment when the patient is in bed is essential regardless of the position selected. During each contact with the patient, the nurse evaluates the patient's position and assists the patient to achieve proper positioning and alignment. The most common positions that a patient assumes in bed are supine (dorsal) and side-lying (lateral). The nurse helps the patient assume these positions and supports the body in correct alignment with pillows (Chart 13-4). At times, a splint (e.g., for the wrist or hand) may be fabricated by the occupational therapist to support a joint and prevent deformity. The nurse must ensure proper use of the splint and provide skin care.

CHART 13-4

Positioning a Patient in Bed

Supine (Dorsal) Position

1. Align the head with the spine, both laterally and anteroposteriorly.
2. Position the trunk to minimize hip flexion.
3. Flex the arms at the elbow, and rest the hands against the lateral abdomen.
4. Extend the legs with a small, firm support under the popliteal area.
5. Support the heels off the mattress with a small pillow or towel roll at the ankles.
6. Point the toes straight up using protective boots to prevent footdrop.
7. Place trochanter rolls under the greater trochanters to prevent external rotation of the hip.

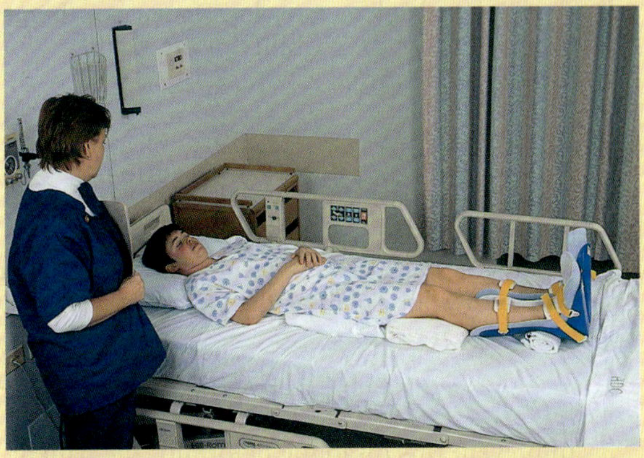

Side-Lying (Lateral Position)

1. Align the head with the spine, and support it with a pillow.
2. Properly align the body; avoid twisting at the shoulders, waist, or hips.
3. Flex shoulders and elbows, and support the upper arm with a pillow.
4. Position the uppermost hip joint slightly forward, and support the leg in a position of slight abduction by a pillow.
5. Place and support the feet in neutral dorsiflexion.
6. Support the back with a pillow.

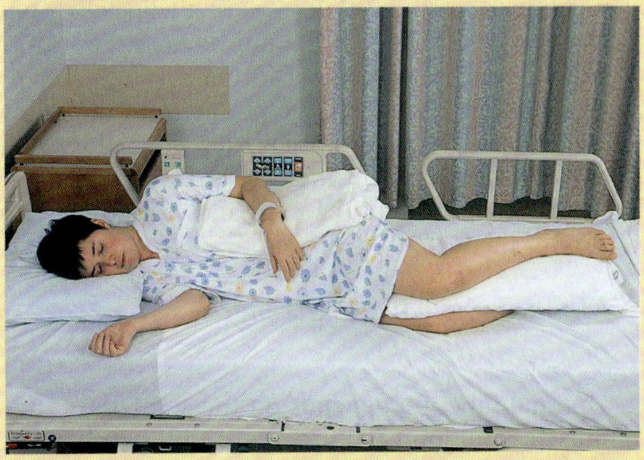

Prone (on Abdomen) Position

1. Turn the head laterally, and align it with the rest of the body.
2. Abduct and externally rotate the arms at the shoulder joint; flex the elbows.
3. Place a small, flat support under the pelvis, extending from the level of the umbilicus to the upper third of the thigh.
4. Maintain the lower extremities in a neutral position.
5. Suspend the toes over the edge of the mattress.

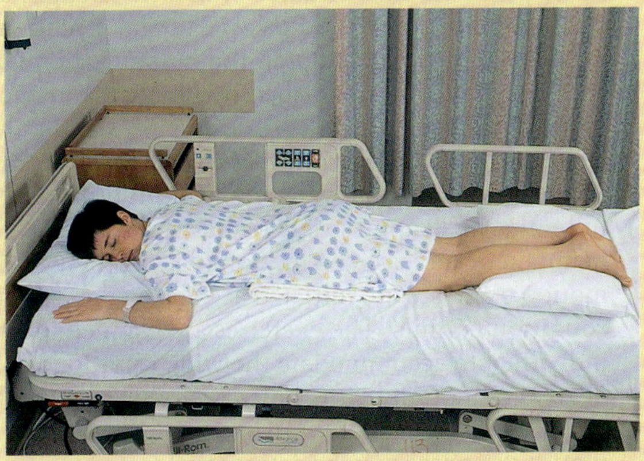

Note: Side rails of bed are down for photographic purposes; they should remain raised if the patient is at risk for falling.

PREVENTING EXTERNAL ROTATION OF THE HIP. Patients who are in bed for any period of time may develop external rotation deformity of the hip because the ball-and-socket joint of the hip has a tendency to rotate outward when the patient lies on his or her back. A trochanter roll (i.e., a flannel sheet or bath towel folded in thirds lengthwise and rolled toward the patient or a commercially manufactured roll) extending from the crest of the ilium to the midthigh prevents this deformity; with correct placement, it serves as a mechanical wedge under the projection of the greater trochanter.

PREVENTING FOOTDROP. Footdrop is a deformity in which the foot is plantar flexed (the ankle bends in the direction of the sole of the foot). If the condition continues without correction, the patient will not be able to hold the foot in a normal position and will be able to walk only on his or her toes, without touching the ground with the heel of the foot. The deformity is caused by contracture of both the gastrocnemius and soleus muscles. Damage to the peroneal nerve or loss of flexibility of the Achilles tendon may result in footdrop.

NURSING ALERT

Prolonged bed rest, lack of exercise, incorrect positioning in bed, and the weight of bedding that forces the toes into plantar flexion are factors that contribute to footdrop.

To prevent this disabling deformity, the patient is positioned to sit at 90 degrees in a wheelchair with feet on the footrests or flat on the floor. Footdrop splints may be applied at bedtime.

The patient is encouraged to perform the following ankle exercises several times each hour: dorsiflexion and plantar flexion of the feet, flexion and extension (curl and stretch) of the toes, and eversion and inversion of the feet at the ankles.

Maintaining Muscle Strength and Joint Mobility

Optimal function depends on the strength of the muscles and joint motion, and active participation in ADLs promotes maintenance of muscle strength and joint mobility. Active and passive range-of-motion exercises may be included in the nursing care plan or are prescribed and performed by physical and occupational therapists.

PERFORMING RANGE-OF-MOTION EXERCISES. Range of motion is movement of a joint through its full range in all appropriate planes (Chart 13-5). To maintain or increase the motion of a joint, range-of-motion exercises are initiated as soon as the patient's condition permits. The exercises are planned for the individual to accommodate the wide variation in the degrees of motion that people of varying body builds and age groups can attain (Chart 13-6). Range-of-motion exercises may be active (performed by the patient under the supervision of the nurse), assisted (with the nurse helping if the patient cannot do the exercise independently), or passive (performed by the nurse).

The joint to be exercised is supported, the bones above the joint are stabilized, and the body part distal to the joint is moved through the range of motion of the joint. For example, the humerus must be stabilized while the radius and ulna are moved through their range of motion at the elbow joint.

The joint should not be moved beyond its free range of motion; the joint is moved to the point of resistance and stopped at the point of pain. If muscle spasms are present, the joint is moved slowly to the point of resistance. Gentle, steady pressure is then applied until the muscle relaxes, and the motion is continued to the joint's final point of resistance.

To perform assisted or passive range-of-motion exercises, the patient must be in a comfortable supine position with arms at the sides and knees extended. Good body posture is maintained during the exercises. The nurse also uses good body mechanics during the exercise session.

PERFORMING THERAPEUTIC EXERCISES. Therapeutic exercises are prescribed by the physical therapist and performed with their assistance and the guidance of a nurse. Technology is used to assist the use of therapeutic exercises. These include continuous passive motion (CPM) and joint active system (JAS) splints (http://www.jointactivesystems.com). Research is also underway to evaluate the use of computerized robots with gentle, compliant behaviour that could be used with stroke (Colombo, Sterpi, Mazzone, et al.,

CHART 13-5

Range-of-Motion Terminology

Abduction: movement away from the midline of the body
Adduction: movement toward the midline of the body
Flexion: bending of a joint so that the angle of the joint diminishes
Extension: the return movement from flexion; the joint angle is increased
Rotation: turning or movement of a part around its axis
Internal: turning inward, toward the centre
External: turning outward, away from the centre
Dorsiflexion: movement that flexes or bends the hand back toward the body or the foot toward the leg
Palmar flexion: movement that flexes or bends the hand in the direction of the palm
Plantar flexion: movement that flexes or bends the foot in the direction of the sole
Pronation: rotation of the forearm so that the palm of the hand is down
Supination: rotation of the forearm so that the palm of the hand is up
Opposition: touching the thumb to each fingertip on same hand
Inversion: movement that turns the sole of the foot inward
Eversion: movement that turns the sole of the foot outward

CHART 13-6

Performing Range-of-Motion Exercises

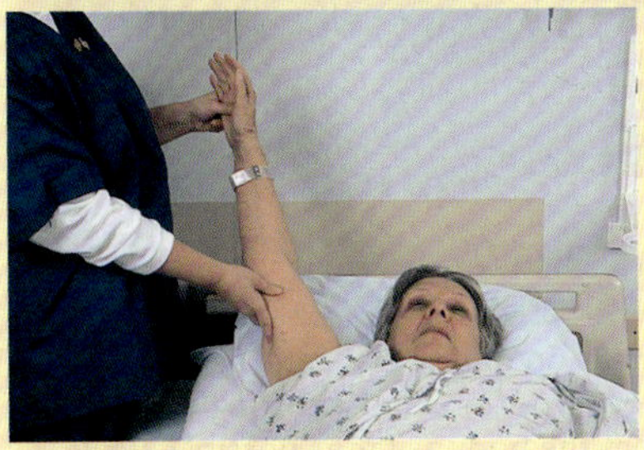

Abduction of shoulder. Move arm from side of body to above the head, then return arm to side of body or neutral position (adduction).

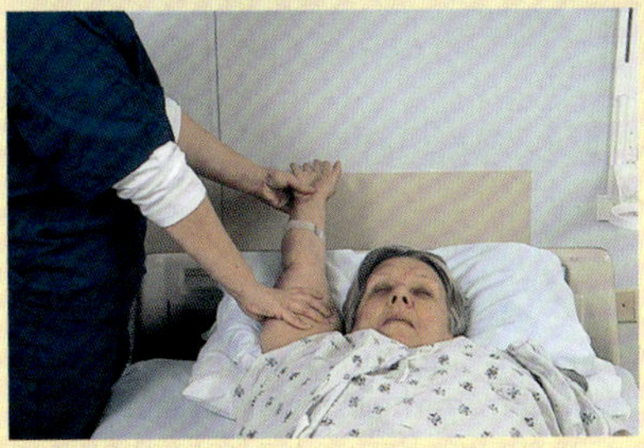

Forward flexion of shoulder. Move arm forward and upward until it is alongside of head.

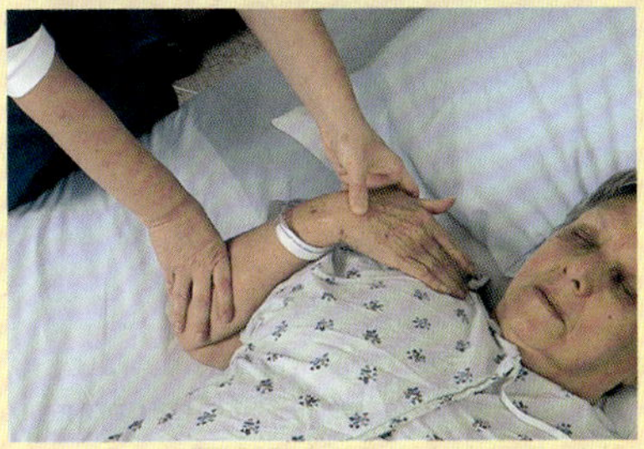

Flexion of elbow. Bend elbow, bringing forearm and hand toward shoulder, then return forearm and hand to neutral position (arm straight).

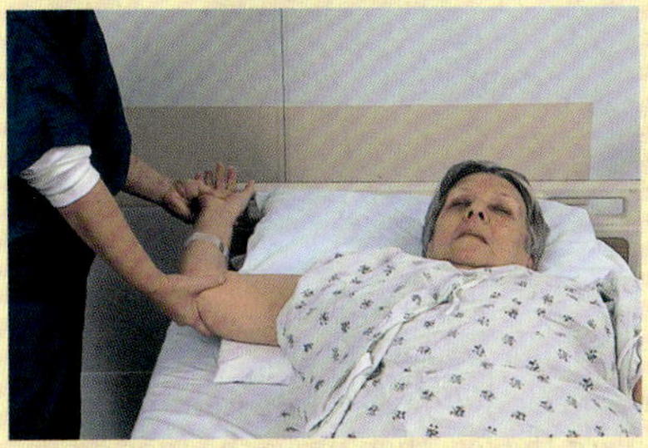

External rotation of shoulder. With arm at shoulder height, elbow bent at a 90-degree angle, and palm toward feet, turn upper arm until palm and forearm point backward.

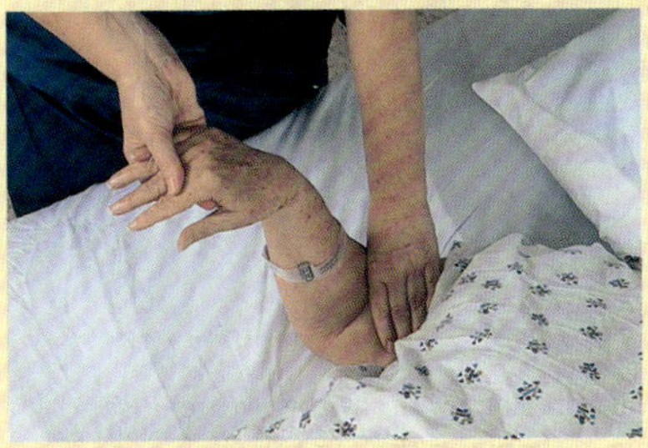

Pronation of forearm. With elbow at waist and bent at a 90-degree angle, turn hand so that palm is facing down.

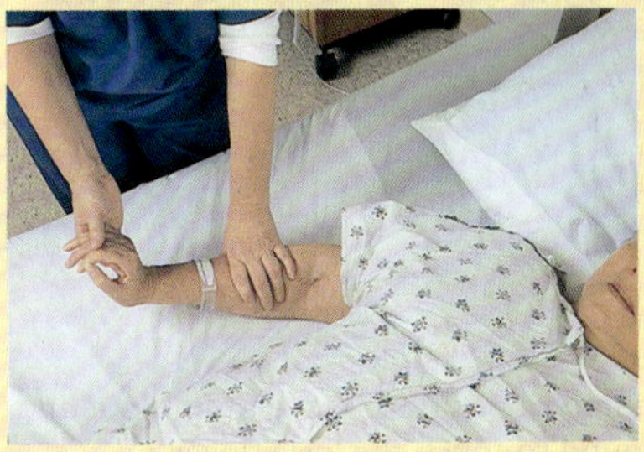

Wrist extension.

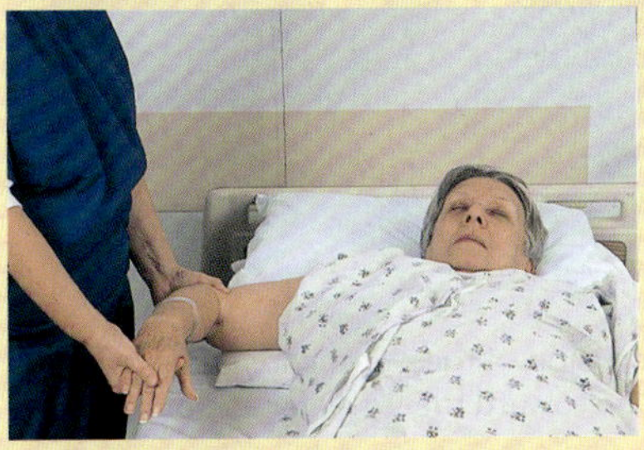

Internal rotation of shoulder. With arm at shoulder height, elbow bent at a 90-degree angle, and palm toward feet, turn upper arm until the palm and forearm point forward.

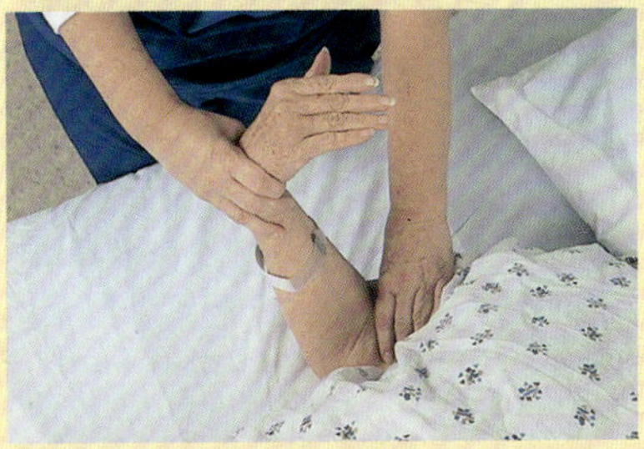

Supination of forearm. With elbow at waist and arm bent at a 90-degree angle, turn hand so that palm is facing up.

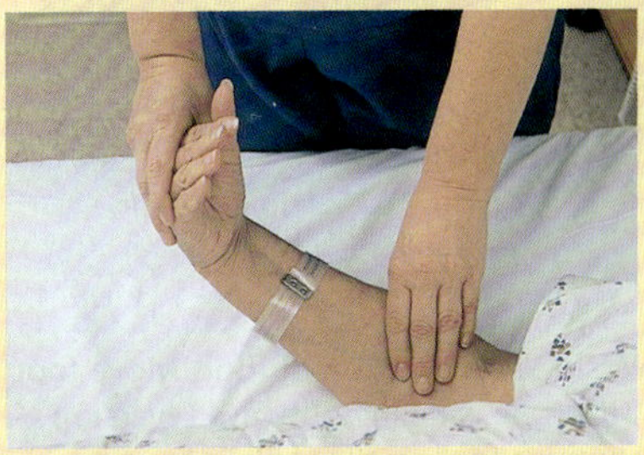

Flexion of wrist. Bend wrist so that palm is toward forearm. Straighten to a neutral position.

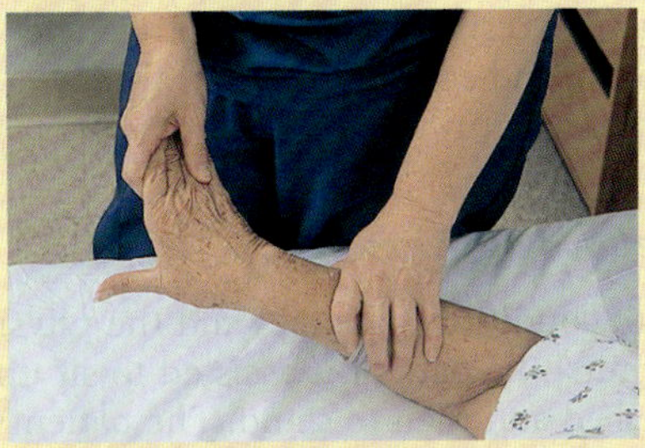

Ulnar deviation. Move hand sideways so that the side of hand on which the little finger is located moves toward forearm.

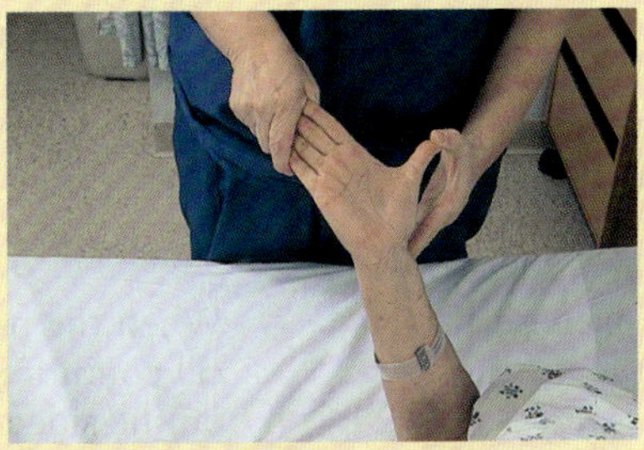

Extension of fingers.

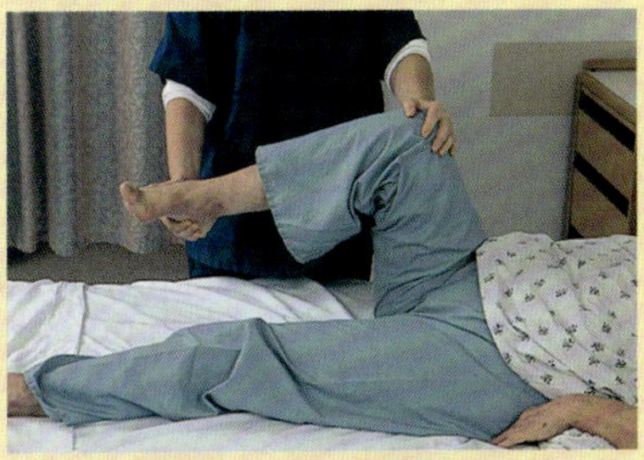

Hip and knee at 90 degrees. Cradle knee and cup heel. Move foot toward midline and then away from patient.

continued >

CHART 13-6 Performing Range-of-Motion Exercises (Continued)

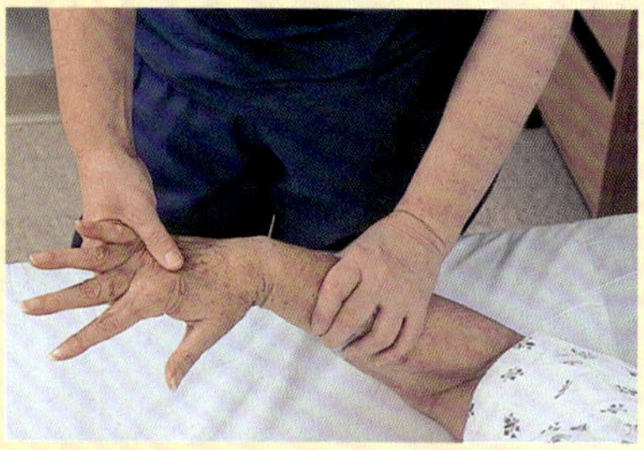
Radial deviation. Move hand sideways so that side of hand on which thumb is located moves toward forearm.

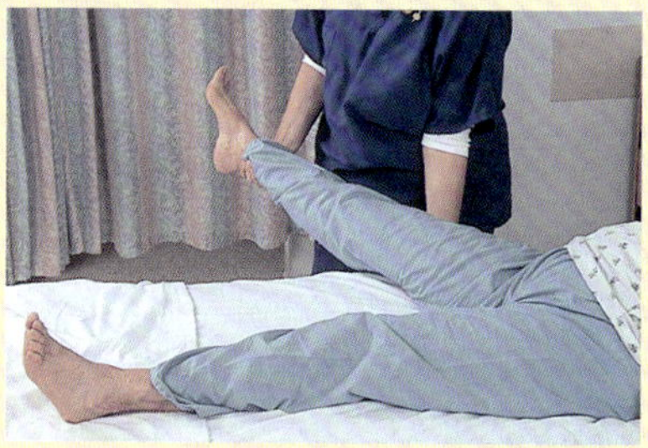
Abduction–adduction of hip. Move leg outward from the body as far as possible, as shown. Return leg from abducted position to neutral position and across the other leg as far as possible.

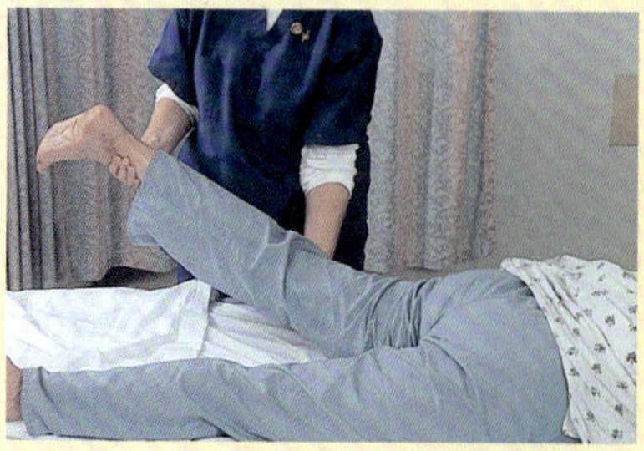
Extension of hip. Place the patient in a prone position, and move leg backward from the body as far as possible, while stabilizing the pelvis. It can also be done in side-lying position.

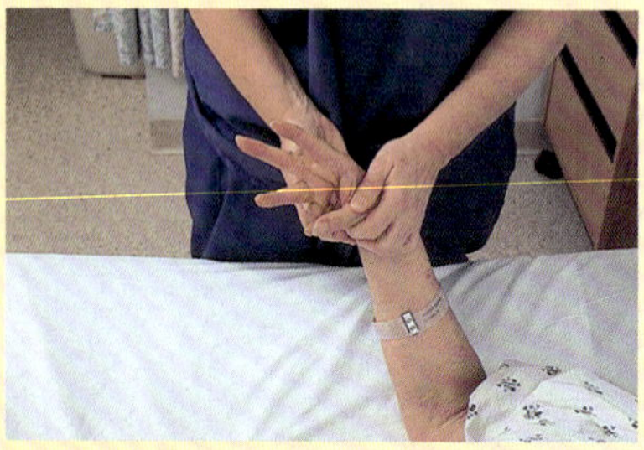
Thumb opposition. Move thumb out and around to touch the little finger.

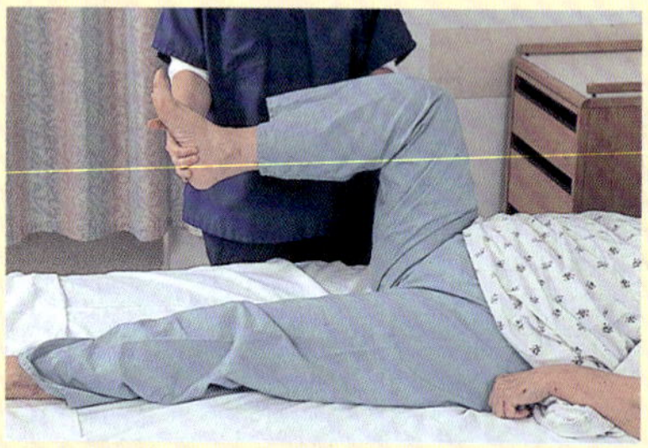
Flexion of the hip and the knee. Bend hip by moving the leg forward as far as possible. Return leg from the flexed position to the neutral position.

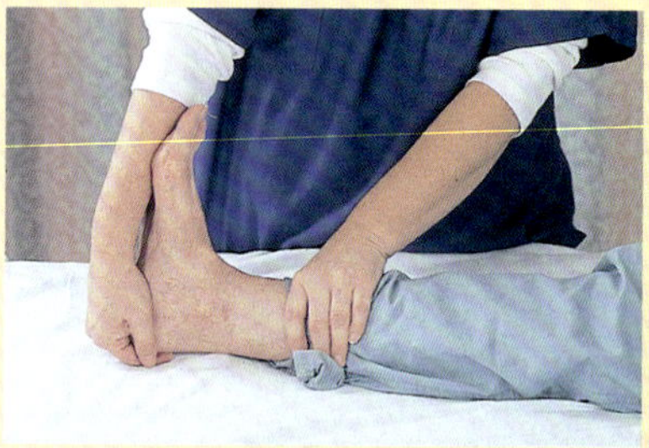
Dorsiflexion of foot. Move foot up and toward the leg, then move the foot down and away from the leg (plantar flexion).

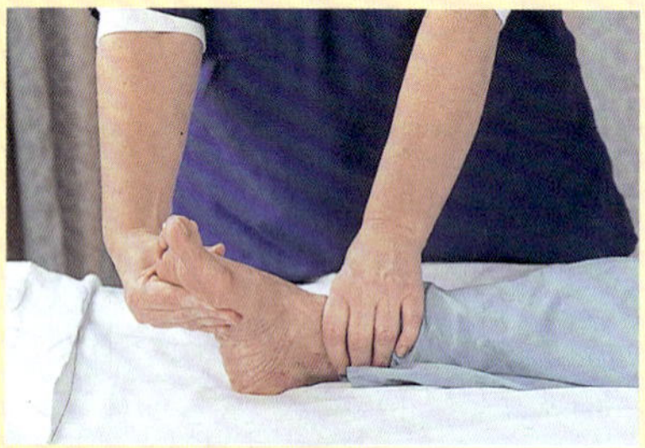
Inversion and eversion of foot. Move foot so that sole is facing outward (eversion), then move foot so that sole is facing inward (inversion).

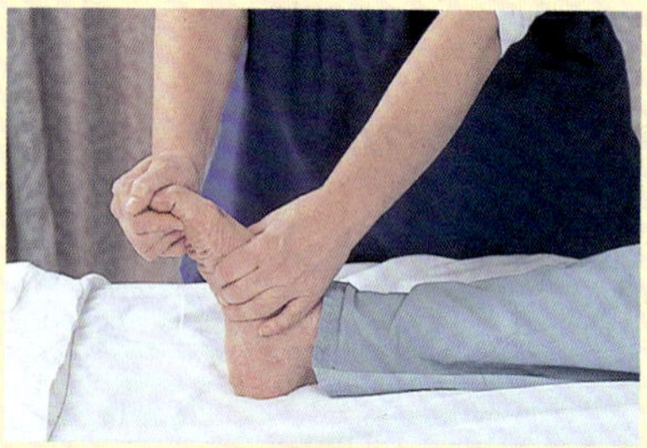
Flexion of toes. Bend the toes toward the ball of foot.

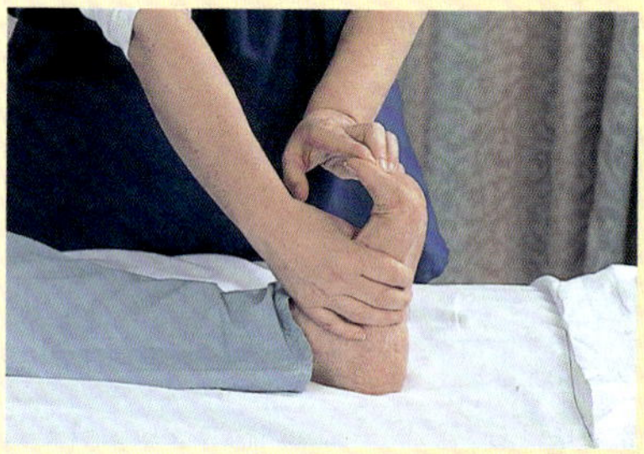
Extension of toes. Straighten toes, and pull them toward the leg as far as possible.

2013) and spinal cord–injured patients (Gizzi et al., 2012).

The patient should have a clear understanding of the goal of the prescribed exercise. Written instructions about the frequency, duration, and number of repetitions, as well as simple line drawings of the exercise, help to ensure adherence to the exercise program. Return demonstration of the exercise also helps the patient and family to follow the instructions correctly.

When performed correctly, exercise assists in maintaining and building muscle strength, maintaining joint function, preventing deformity, stimulating circulation, developing endurance, and promoting relaxation. Exercise is also valuable in helping to restore motivation and the well-being of the patient. (Weight-bearing exercises may increase bone density.) There are five types of exercise: passive, active-assistive, active, resistive, and isometric. The description, purpose, and action of each of these exercises are summarized in Table 13-1.

Promoting Independent Mobility

When the patient's condition stabilizes and the physical condition permits, the patient is assisted to sit up on the side of the bed and then to stand. The patient's tolerance of this activity is assessed. Orthostatic (postural) hypotension may develop when the patient assumes a vertical position. Because of inadequate vasomotor reflexes, blood pools in the splanchnic (visceral) area and in the legs, resulting in inadequate cerebral circulation. If indicators of orthostatic hypotension (e.g., drop in blood pressure,

TABLE 13-1 Therapeutic Exercises

	Description	Purposes	Action
Passive	An exercise carried out by the therapist or the nurse without assistance from the patient	To retain as much joint range of motion as possible; to maintain circulation	Stabilize the proximal joint and support the distal part; move the joint smoothly, slowly, and gently through its full range of motion; avoid producing pain
Active-assistive	An exercise carried out by the patient with the assistance of the therapist or the nurse, or with the assistance of equipment	To encourage normal muscle function	Support the distal part, and encourage the patient to take the joint actively through its range of motion; give no more assistance than is necessary to accomplish the action; short periods of activity should be followed by adequate rest periods
Active	An exercise accomplished by the patient without assistance	To increase muscle strength	When possible, active exercise should be performed against gravity; the joint is moved through full range of motion without assistance; make sure that the patient does not substitute another joint movement for the one intended
Resistive	An active exercise carried out by the patient working against resistance produced by either manual or mechanical means	To provide resistance to increase muscle power	The patient moves the joint through its range of motion while the therapist resists slightly at first and then with progressively increasing resistance; sandbags and weights can be used and are applied at the distal point of the involved joint; the movements should be performed smoothly
Isometric or muscle setting	Alternately contracting and relaxing a muscle while keeping the part in a fixed position; this exercise	To maintain strength when a joint is immobilized	Contract or tighten the muscle as much as possible without moving the joint, hold for several seconds, then let go and relax; breathe deeply

pallor, diaphoresis, nausea, tachycardia, dizziness) are present, the activity is stopped, and the patient is assisted to a supine position in bed.

Some disabling conditions, such as spinal cord injury, acute brain injury, and other conditions that require extended periods in the recumbent position, prevent patients from assuming an upright position at the bedside. Several strategies can be used to assist a patient to assume a 90-degree sitting position. First, a reclining wheelchair with elevating leg rests allows a slow and controlled progression from a supine position to a 90-degree sitting position. A tilt table—a board that can be tilted in 5- to 10-degree increments from a horizontal to a vertical position—may also be used. The tilt table promotes vasomotor adjustment to positional changes and helps the patient with limited standing balance and limited weight-bearing activities to avoid the decalcification of bones and low bone mass associated with disuse syndrome and lack of weight-bearing exercise.

Edema of the limbs is a common problem for patients with disability. Various assessment techniques are used to determine the type of compression therapy that may be needed. Assessment tests include serum albumin (to detect signs of chronic insufficiency), ankle brachial index (ABI), and a positive pressure gradient (PPG) test. In an acute care setting, patients on bed rest may be managed with light compression, such as antiembolism (AE) stockings. In a rehabilitation setting, Tubergrip may be used for light compression, or a wrap product such as a Profore bandage. Once edema is reduced the patient may be fitted for pressure gradient stockings (PGS) to help manage long-term edema. A vasopressor medication may also be administered to manage orthostatic hypotension, by enhancing the blood return from the extremities to the heart. Elastic compression stockings are used to prevent venous stasis. For some patients, a compression garment (leotard) or snug-fitting abdominal binder and elastic compression bandaging of the legs are needed to prevent venous stasis and ensuing orthostatic hypotension. When the patient is standing, the feet are protected with a pair of properly fitted shoes. Extended periods of standing are avoided because of venous pooling and pressure on the soles of the feet. The nurse monitors the patient's blood pressure and pulse and observes for signs of orthostatic hypotension and cerebral insufficiency (e.g., the patient reports feeling faint and weak), which suggest intolerance of the upright position. If the patient does not tolerate the upright position, the nurse should recline the patient and elevate the patient's legs.

New strategies are being developed to safely lift or position patients who have morbid obesity. These include specialized equipment, new procedures, and extensive training (Liko North America, 2008).

ASSISTING THE PATIENT WITH TRANSFER. A transfer is the movement of a patient from one place to another (e.g., bed to chair, chair to commode, wheelchair to tub). As soon as the patient is permitted out of bed, transfer activities are started. The nurse assesses the patient's ability to participate actively in the transfer and determines in conjunction with an occupational therapist or physical therapist the required adaptive equipment to promote independence and safety. A wheelchair with brake extensions, removable and detachable armrests, and leg rests minimizes structural obstacles during the transfer. Tub seats or benches make transfers in and out of tubs easier and safer. Raised, padded commode seats may also be warranted for patients who must avoid flexing the hips greater than 90 degrees when transferring to a toilet. If warranted (e.g., post–total hip replacement), the nurse will also teach the patient hip precautions (i.e., no adduction past the midline, no flexion greater than 90 degrees, and no internal rotation). Pillows can be used to keep the hip in correct alignment.

It is important that the patient maintain muscle strength and, if possible, perform push-up exercises to strengthen the arm and shoulder extensor muscles. The push-up exercise requires the patient to sit upright in bed; a book is placed under each of the patient's hands to provide a hard surface, and the patient is instructed to push down on the book, raising the body. The nurse encourages the patient to raise and move the body in different directions by means of these push-up exercises. Pulley exercises may be used once the patient is more mobile.

The nurse, or physical or occupational therapist, teaches the patient how to transfer. There are several methods of transferring from the bed to the wheelchair when the patient is unable to stand, and the technique chosen should be appropriate for the patient, considering his or her abilities and disabilities. It is helpful for the nurse to demonstrate the technique. If the therapist is involved in teaching the patient to transfer, the nurse and the therapist must collaborate so that consistent instructions are given to the patient. During transfer, the nurse assists and coaches the patient. Figure 13-1 shows weight-bearing and non–weight-bearing transfer.

Mechanical lifts/ceiling lifts and sit-to-stand lifts are being used in health care facilities to decrease the risk of injury to both patients and health care workers, until the patient has made progress to transfer with appropriate aids.

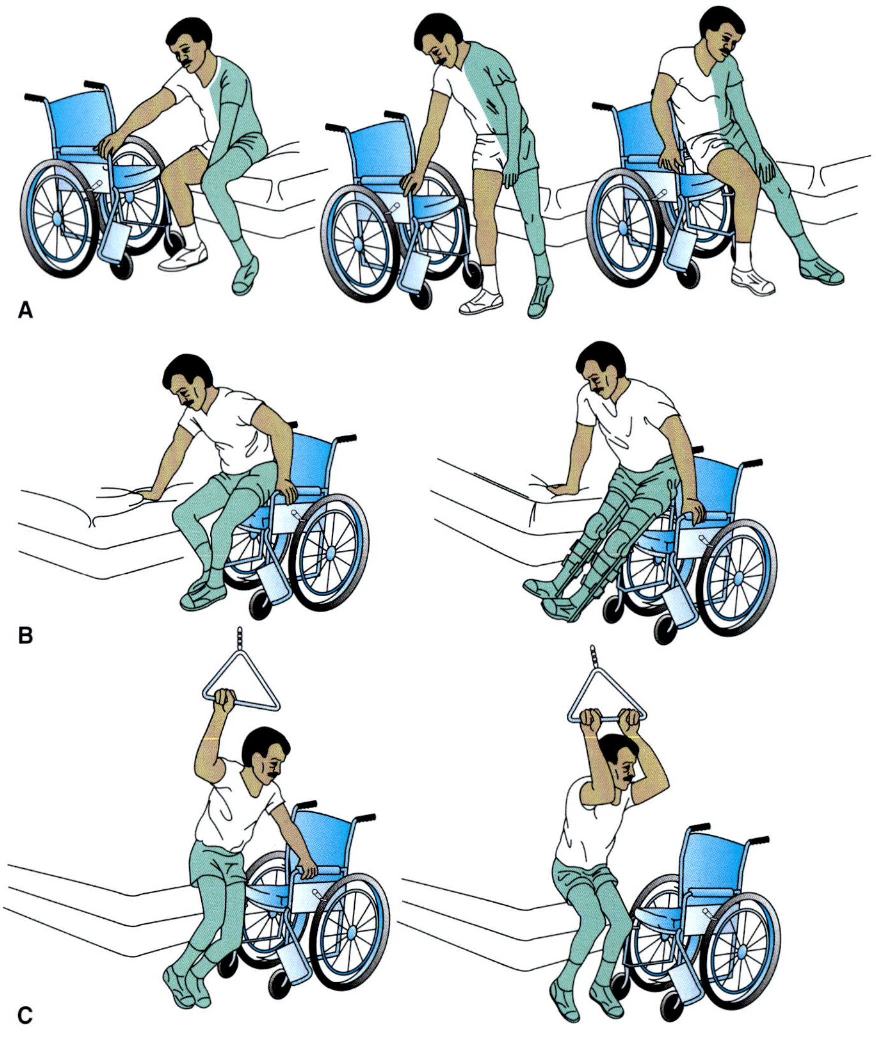

FIGURE 13-1. Methods of patient transfer from the bed to a wheelchair. The wheelchair is in a locked position. *Coloured areas* indicate non–weight-bearing body parts. **A.** Weight-bearing transfer from bed to chair. The patient stands up, pivots until his back is opposite the new seat, and sits down. **B.** (**left**) Non–weight-bearing transfer from chair to bed. (**right**) With legs braced. **C.** (**left**) Non–weight-bearing transfer, combined method. (**right**) Non–weight-bearing transfer, pull-up method.

If the patient's muscles are not strong enough to overcome the resistance of body weight, a polished lightweight board (transfer board) may be used to bridge the gap between the bed and the chair. The patient slides across on the board with or without assistance from a caregiver. This board may also be used to transfer the patient from the chair to the toilet or bathtub bench. It is important to avoid the effects of shear on the patient's skin while sliding across the board. The nurse should make sure that the patient's fingers do not curl around the edge of the board during the transfer, because the weight of the patient's body can crush them as the patient moves across the board. Safety is a primary concern during a transfer:

- Wheelchairs and beds must be locked before the patient transfers.
- Detachable arm- and footrests are removed to make getting in and out of the chair easier and to decrease the risk of skin tears from exposed metal.
- One end of the transfer board is placed under the patient's buttocks and the other end on the surface to which the transfer is being made (e.g., the chair).
- The patient is instructed to lean forward, push up with his or her hands, and then slide across the board to the other surface.

The nurse frequently assists weak and incapacitated patients out of bed. The nurse supports and guides the patient during position changes, protecting the patient from injury. Transfer belts are often helpful to provide a safe and secure place for the nurse or therapist to hold on to the patient. The nurse uses a stroke sling or transfer belt to avoid pulling on the weak or paralyzed upper extremity to prevent dislocation of the shoulder. The patient is assisted to move toward the stronger side (Chart 13-7).

Note: Hospitals and health regions are beginning to adopt safe patient handling educational programs for nursing staff. Such programs focus on assessment of the patient in order to safely move, lift, or transfer a patient (Alberta Health Services, 2012). In the home setting, getting in and out of bed and performing chair, toilet, and tub transfers are difficult for patients with weak musculature and loss of hip, knee, and ankle motion. A bed ladder may help the patient get in and out of bed. The height of a chair can be raised with cushions on the seat or with hollowed-out blocks placed under the chair legs. Grab bars can be attached to the wall near the toilet and tub to provide leverage and stability.

PREPARING FOR AMBULATION. Regaining the ability to walk is a prime morale builder. However, to be prepared for ambulation—whether with a brace, walker, cane, or crutches—the patient must strengthen the muscles required. Exercise, therefore, is the foundation of preparation. The nurse and therapist instruct and supervise the patient in these exercises.

For ambulation, the quadriceps muscles, which stabilize the knee joint, and the gluteal muscles, are strengthened. To perform quadriceps-setting exercises, the patient contracts the quadriceps muscle by attempting to push the popliteal area against the mattress and at the same time raising the heel. The patient maintains the muscle contraction until a count of five and relaxes for a count of five. The exercise is repeated 10 to 15 times hourly. Exercising the quadriceps muscles prevents flexion contractures of the knee.

In gluteal setting, the patient contracts or "pinches" the buttocks together to the count of five, relaxes for the count of five, and repeats 10 to 15 times hourly. If ambulatory aids (i.e., walker, cane, crutches) are to be used, the muscles of the upper extremities are exercised and strengthened. Weight

CHART 13-7

Assisting the Patient Out of Bed

Technique for Moving the Patient to the Edge of the Bed

1. Move head and shoulders of patient toward the edge of the bed.
2. Move feet and legs to the edge of the bed. (The patient is now in a crescent position, which gives good range of motion to the lateral trunk muscles.)
3. Place both arms well under the patient's hips. Next, tighten (set) your upper leg muscles and abdomen.
4. Straighten your back while moving the patient toward you.

Technique for Sitting the Patient on the Edge of the Bed

1. Place arm and hand under the patient's shoulders.
2. Instruct the patient to push into the bed with the elbow while you lift the patient's shoulders with one arm and swing the legs over the edge of the bed with the other. (Gravity pulls the legs downward, which aids in raising the patient's trunk.)
3. If patient is able to side-lie, this technique is easier than from a supine position.

Technique for Assisting the Patient to Stand

1. Position the patient's feet so that they will be well grounded.
2. Face the patient while firmly grasping each side of the patient's rib cage with your hands, or use a transfer belt.
3. Push your knee against one knee of the patient.
4. Rock the patient forward to a standing position. (Your knee is pushed against the patient's knee as he or she comes to the standing position.)
5. Ensure that the patient's knees are "locked" (in full extension) while standing. (Locking the patient's knees is a safety measure for those who are weak or have been in bed for some time.)
6. Give the patient enough time to establish balance.
7. Pivot the patient into a sitting position in the chair.

shifts are useful. While in a sitting position, the patient raises the body by pushing the hands against the chair seat or mattress. The patient should be encouraged to do push-up exercises while in a prone position as well. Pull-up exercises using an exercise/resistance band while lifting the body are also effective for conditioning. The patient is taught to raise the arms above the head and then lower them in a slow, rhythmic manner while holding weights. Gradually, the weight is increased. The hands are strengthened by squeezing a rubber ball.

Typically, the physical therapist designs exercises to help the patient develop the sitting and standing balance, stability, and coordination needed for ambulation. After sitting and standing balance are achieved, the patient uses parallel bars. Under the supervision of the physical therapist, the patient practices shifting weight from side to side, lifting one leg while supporting weight on the other, and then walking between the parallel bars.

A patient who is ready to begin ambulation must be fitted with the appropriate ambulatory aid, instructed about the prescribed weight-bearing limits (e.g., non–weight-bearing, partial weight–bearing ambulation), and taught how to use the aid safely. The nurse continually assesses the patient for stability and adherence to weight-bearing precautions and protects the patient from falling. The nurse provides contact guarding by holding on to a transfer belt that the patient wears around the waist. The patient should wear sturdy, well-fitting shoes and be advised of the dangers of wet or highly polished floors and throw rugs. The patient should also learn how to ambulate on inclines, uneven surfaces, and stairs.

Ambulating With an Assistive Device: Crutches, a Walker, or a Cane

Crutches are for partial weight–bearing or non–weight-bearing ambulation. Good balance, adequate cardiovascular reserve, strong upper extremities, and erect posture are essential for crutch walking. Ambulating a functional distance (at least the length of a room or house) or manoeuvring stairs on crutches requires significant arm strength, because the arms must bear the patient's weight (Fig. 13-2). The nurse or physical therapist determines which gait is best.

A walker provides more support and stability than a cane or crutches do. A pick-up walker is best for patients with poor balance and poor cardiovascular reserve, and a rolling walker, which allows automatic walking, is best for patients who cannot lift. A cane helps the patient walk with balance and support and relieves the pressure on weight-bearing joints by redistributing weight.

Before patients can be considered to be independent in walking with crutches, a walker, or a cane, they should learn to sit, stand from sitting, and go up and down stairs using the device. Table 13-2 describes how patients can ambulate and manoeuvre using each of the three devices and nursing actions to support using assistive devices.

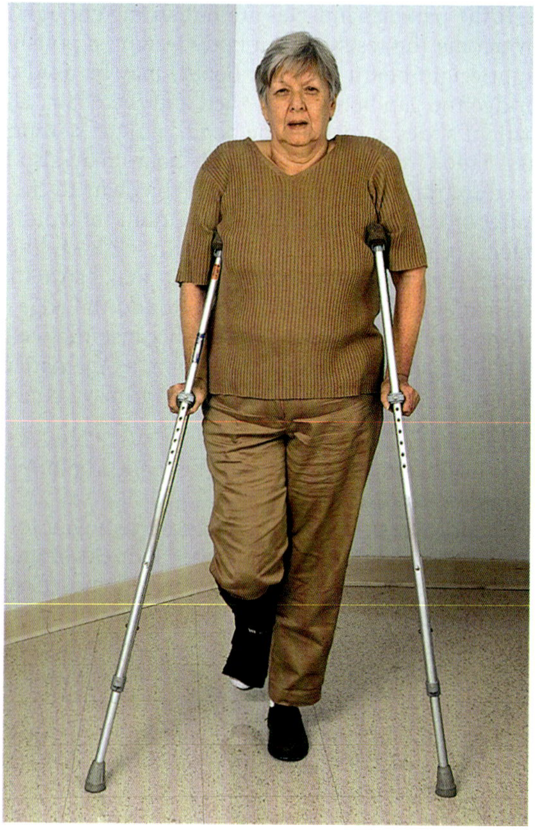

FIGURE 13-2. Crutch walking. The tripod position for basic crutch stance.

AMBULATING WITH CRUTCHES. Patients who are prescribed partial weight–bearing or non–weight-bearing ambulation may use crutches. The nurse or physical therapist should determine whether crutches are appropriate for the patient, because good balance, adequate cardiovascular reserve, strong upper extremities, and erect posture are essential for crutch walking. Muscle groups important for crutch walking include the following:

- Shoulder depressors—to stabilize the upper extremity and prevent shoulder hiking
- Shoulder adductors—to hold the crutch top against the chest wall
- Arm flexors, extensors, and abductors (at the shoulder)—to move crutches forward, backward, and sideways
- Forearm extensors—to prevent flexion or buckling; important in raising the body for swinging gait
- Wrist extensors—to enable weight bearing on hand pieces
- Finger and thumb flexors—to grasp the hand piece

TEACHING CRUTCH WALKING. The nurse or physical therapist explains and demonstrates to the patient how to use the crutches. The patient learns standing balance by standing on the unaffected leg by a chair. To help the patient maintain balance, the

TABLE 13-2 Nursing Actions Involved in Using Assistive Devices

	Crutches	Walker	Cane
Patient Preparation			
Adjusting device to fit patient	Measure patient standing or lying down: If standing, set crutch length approximately 5 cm (2 in) below axilla. If lying down, measure from anterior fold of axilla to sole of the foot and add 5 cm. If using patient's height, subtract 40 cm (16 in) to obtain crutch height. Adjust hand grip to allow 20–30 degrees of flexion at elbow. Use foam rubber pad on underarm piece to relieve pressure of crutch.	Adjust height to individual patient. Patient's arms should be in 20–30 degrees of flexion at elbows when hands are resting on hand grips.	With patient flexing elbow at 30-degree angle, hold handle of cane level with greater trochanter and place tip of cane 15 cm (6 in) lateral to base of fifth toe. Fit cane with gently flaring tip that has flexible, concentric rings to provide stability, absorb shock, and enable greater speed and less fatigue with walking.
Assessment	Assess safety. Crutches should have large rubber tips, and patients should wear firm-soled, well-fitting shoes. Assess balance by asking patient to stand on unaffected leg by a chair. Assess stability and stamina (tolerance). Sweating and shortness of breath indicate that rest is necessary.	Assess safety. Patients should wear firm-soled, well-fitting shoes. Assess stability and stamina (tolerance). Sweating and shortness of breath indicate that rest is necessary.	Assess safety. Patients should wear firm-soled, well-fitting shoes. Assess stability and stamina (tolerance). Sweating and shortness of breath indicate that rest is necessary.
Interventions and patient education	Assist with balance by using a transfer belt or holding patient near waist. Have patient practice shifting weight and maintaining balance. Protect patient from falls. To maximize stability, encourage patient to use tripod stance, with crutches to the front and sides of toes. Have patient perform prescribed preparatory exercises to strengthen shoulder girdle and upper extremity muscles.[a]	Walk with patient, holding at waist if needed for balance. Instruct patient to never pull self up using walker and to look up when walking. Discuss full, partial, or non weight bearing as prescribed. Protect patient from falls.	Walk with patient, holding at waist if needed for balance. Have patient hold cane in hand opposite to affected extremity, if possible, to widen the base of support and reduce stress on involved extremity. Instruct patient to move opposite arm and leg together. Protect patient from falls.
Ambulation			
Gait/action used	Determine which gait is best (see Chart 10-5, Tripod Gait)[b] Four-point Three-point Two-point Swing-to Swing-through	Instruct patient to: Pick up walker: lift device and move it forward with each step. Rolling walker: roll device forward and walk automatically.	Instruct patient to: Advance cane at the same time that the affected leg is moved forward. Keep cane fairly close to body to prevent leaning. Bear down on cane when unaffected extremity begins swing phase.
Sitting	Instruct patient to: Grasp hand piece for control. Bend forward slightly while assuming sitting position. Place affected leg forward to prevent weight bearing and flexion while sitting.	Instruct patient to hold walker on hand grips for stability.	
Standing	Instruct patient to: Move forward to edge of chair, and keep unaffected leg slightly under seat. Place both crutches on side of affected extremity. Push down on hand piece while rising to standing position.	Instruct patient to: Push off chair or bed to come to a standing position. Rolling walker: if walker has a brake, apply it before standing. Lift walker, placing it in front of self while leaning slightly forward. Walk into walker, supporting weight on hands when advancing. Balance on feet. Lift walker and place it in front of self again.	Instruct patient to: Push off chair or bed to come to a standing position. Hold cane for stability. Step forward on unaffected extremity. Swing cane and affected extremity forward in a normal walking gait.

continued >

TABLE 13-2 Nursing Actions Involved in Using Assistive Devices (Continued)

	Crutches	Walker	Cane
Going down stairs	Instruct patient to: Walk forward as far as possible. Advance crutches to lower step; advance affected leg, then unaffected leg.	Continue pattern.	Instruct patient to: Step down on affected extremity. Place the cane and then unaffected extremity on down step.
Going up stairs	Instruct patient to: Advance unaffected leg first up next step. Advance crutches and affected extremity. Unaffected leg goes up first.	n/a	Instruct patient to: Step up on unaffected extremity. Place cane and affected extremity up on step.

[a]For patients who cannot support their weight through the wrist and hand because of arthritis or fracture, platform crutches that support the forearm and allow the weight to be borne through the elbow are available. If weight is borne on the axilla, the pressure of the crutch can damage the brachial plexus nerves, producing "crutch paralysis."

[b]Teach patients two gaits so that they can change from one to another to avoid fatigue. In addition, a faster gait can be used when walking an uninterrupted distance, and a slower gait can be used for shorter distances or in crowded places.

n/a, not applicable.

nurse holds the patient near the waist or uses a transfer belt.

The patient is taught to support his or her weight on the hand pieces. (For patients who are unable to support their weight through the wrist and hand because of arthritis or fracture, platform/gutter crutches that support the forearm and allow the weight to be borne through the elbow are available.) If weight is borne on the axilla, the pressure of the crutch can damage the brachial plexus nerves, producing "crutch paralysis."

For maximum stability, the patient first assumes the tripod position by placing the crutches about 20 to 25 cm (8 to 10 in) in front and to the side of his or her toes (see Fig. 13-2). (This base of support is adjusted according to the height of the patient; a tall person requires a broader base of support than does a short person.) In this position, the patient learns how to shift weight and maintain balance.

Before teaching crutch walking, the nurse or therapist determines which gait will be best for the patient. The selection of the crutch gait depends on the type and severity of the disability and on the patient's physical condition, arm and trunk strength, and body balance. The patient should be taught two gaits so that he or she can change from one to another. Shifting crutch gaits relieves fatigue because each gait requires the use of a different combination of muscles (if a muscle is forced to contract steadily without relaxing, the circulation of the blood to that part is decreased). A faster gait can be used when walking an uninterrupted distance and a slower gait can be used for short distances or in crowded places. The more common gaits are the 4-point, the 2-point, the 3-point, and the swing-to and swing-through gaits. The sequence of movements for each of these gaits is depicted in Chart 13-8.

The nurse walks with the patient who is just learning how to ambulate with crutches, holding on to the transfer belt as needed for balance. During this time, the nurse continually assesses the patient's stability and stamina, as prolonged periods of bed rest and inactivity affect a patient's strength and endurance. Sweating and shortness of breath are indications that crutch-walking practice should be stopped and the patient permitted to rest.

TEACHING MANOEUVRING TECHNIQUES. Before a patient is considered to be independent in crutch walking, he or she needs to learn to sit in a chair, stand from sitting, and go up and down the stairs.

To sit down

1. Grasp the crutches at the hand pieces for control.
2. Bend forward slightly while assuming a sitting position.
3. Place the affected leg forward to prevent weight bearing and flexion.

To stand up

1. Move forward to the edge of the chair with the strong leg slightly under the seat.
2. Place both crutches in the hand on the side of the affected extremity.
3. Push down on the hand piece while raising the body to a standing position.

To go downstairs

1. Walk forward as far as possible on the step.
2. Advance crutches to the lower step. The weaker leg is advanced first and then the stronger one. In this way, the stronger extremity shares with the arms the work of raising and lowering the body weight.

To go upstairs

1. Advance the stronger leg first up to the next step.
2. Advance the crutches and the weaker extremity. Note that the strong leg goes up first and comes down last. A memory device for the patients is, "Up with the good, down with the bad."

AMBULATING WITH A WALKER. A walker provides more support and stability than a cane or crutches. There are several types of walkers: standard walkers, two-wheeled walkers, four-wheeled walkers, and plat-

CHART 13-8

Crutch Gaits

Shaded areas are weight bearing. *Arrow* indicates advance of foot or crutch. (Read chart from bottom, starting with beginning stance.)

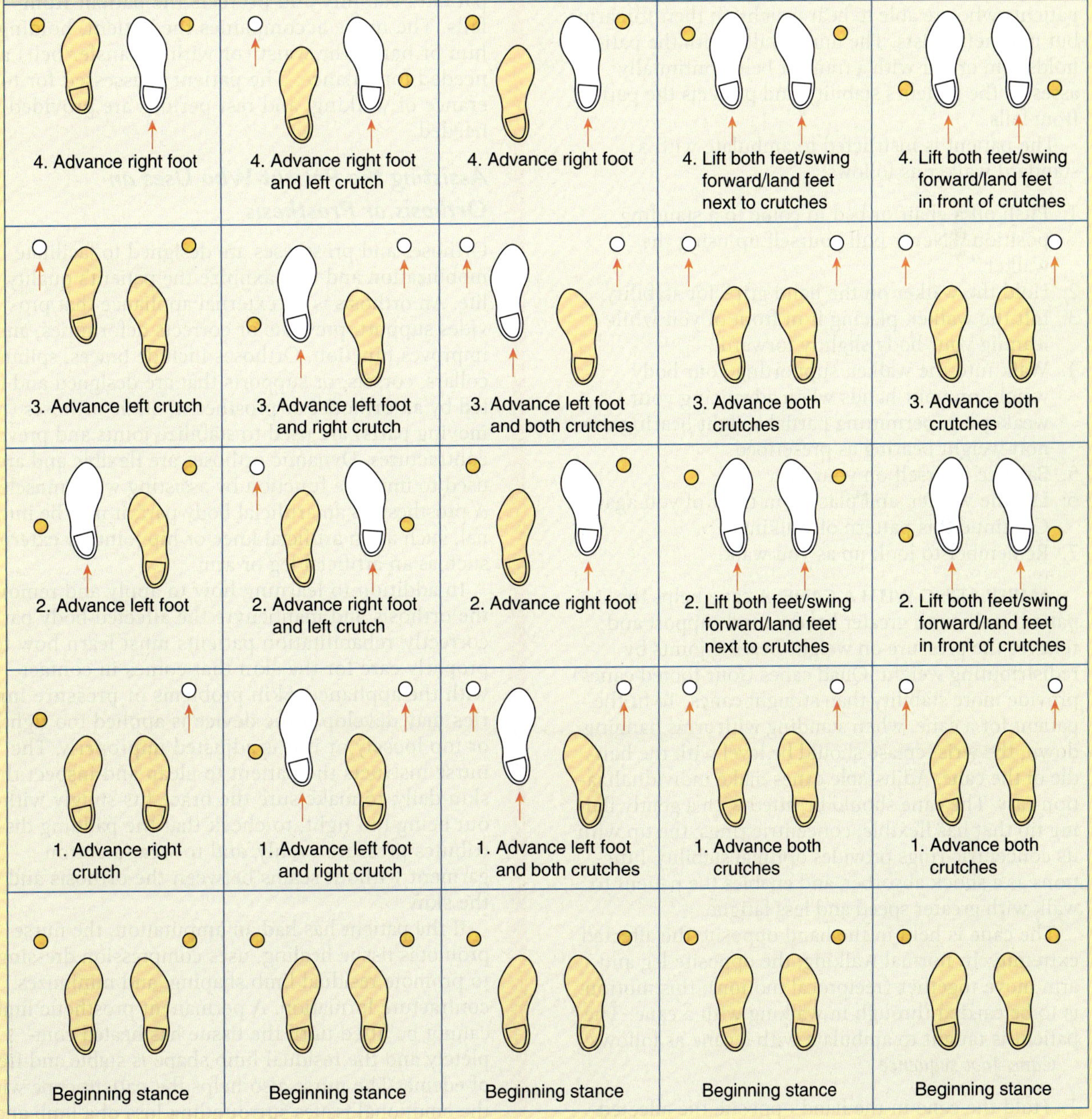

4-POINT GAIT	2-POINT GAIT	3-POINT GAIT	SWING TO	SWING THROUGH
• Partial weight bearing both feet • Maximal support provided • Requires constant shift of weight	• Partial weight bearing both feet • Provides less support • Faster than a 4-point gait	• Non–weight bearing • Requires good balance • Requires arm strength • Faster gait • Can use with walker	• Weight bearing both feet • Provides stability • Requires arm strength • Can use with walker	• Weight bearing • Requires arm strength • Requires coordination/balance • Most advanced gait
4. Advance right foot	4. Advance right foot and left crutch	4. Advance right foot	4. Lift both feet/swing forward/land feet next to crutches	4. Lift both feet/swing forward/land feet in front of crutches
3. Advance left crutch	3. Advance left foot and right crutch	3. Advance left foot and both crutches	3. Advance both crutches	3. Advance both crutches
2. Advance left foot	2. Advance right foot and left crutch	2. Advance right foot	2. Lift both feet/swing forward/land feet next to crutches	2. Lift both feet/swing forward/land feet in front of crutches
1. Advance right crutch	1. Advance left foot and right crutch	1. Advance left foot and both crutches	1. Advance both crutches	1. Advance both crutches
Beginning stance	Beginning stance	Beginning stance	Beginning stance	Beginning stance

form (gutter) walkers. A standard walker, which has no wheels (i.e., one that has to be picked up and moved with each step forward), does not permit a natural walking pattern and is useful for patients who have poor balance or limited cardiovascular reserve or who cannot use crutches. A two-wheeled walker allows automatic walking and is used by patients who cannot lift or who inappropriately carry a pick-up walker. The height of the walker is adjusted to the patient. When the patient's arms are hanging down, the wrist creases should be at the same height as the handgrips. The patient should wear sturdy, well-fitting shoes. A four-wheeled walker is used, usually in the community, when balance and ambulation are stable and the patient is able to use hand brakes appropriately. A platform (gutter) walker is used for patients who are able to bear weight on their forearms but not their wrists. The nurse walks with the patient, holds him or her with a transfer belt, continually assesses the patient's stability, and protects the patient from falls.

The patient is instructed to ambulate with a standard walker as follows:

1. Push off a chair or bed to come to a standing position. "Never pull yourself up using the walker."
2. Hold the walker on the hand grips for stability.
3. Lift the walker, placing it in front of you while leaning your body slightly forward.
4. Walk into the walker, supporting your body weight on your hands when advancing your weaker leg, permitting partial weight bearing or non-weight bearing as prescribed.
5. Balance yourself on your feet.
6. Lift the walker, and place it in front of you again. Continue this pattern of walking.
7. Remember to look up as you walk.

AMBULATING WITH A CANE. A cane helps the patient walk with greater balance and support and relieves the pressure on weight-bearing joints by redistributing weight. Quad canes (four-footed canes) provide more stability than straight canes. To fit the patient for a cane, when standing with arms hanging down, the wrist crease should be level with the handle of the cane. Adjustable canes make individualization easy. The cane should be fitted with a gently flaring tip that has flexible, concentric rings; the tip with its concentric rings provides optimal stability, functions as a shock absorber, and enables the patient to walk with greater speed and less fatigue.

The cane is held in the hand opposite the affected extremity. In normal walking, the opposite leg and arm move together (reciprocal motion); this motion is to be carried through in walking with a cane. The patient is taught to ambulate with a cane as follows:

Cane–foot sequence

1. Hold the cane in the hand opposite the affected extremity to widen the base of support and to reduce the stress on the involved extremity. If the patient is unable to use the cane in the opposite hand, the cane may be used on the same side.
2. Advance the cane at the same time the affected leg is moved forward.
3. Keep the cane fairly close to the body to prevent leaning.
4. Bear down on the cane when the unaffected extremity begins the swing phase.

To go up and down the stairs using the cane

1. Step up on the unaffected extremity.
2. Place the cane and affected extremity up on the step.
3. Reverse this procedure for descending steps ("up with the good, down with the bad").

As for all patients beginning ambulation with an ambulatory aid, the nurse continually assesses the patient's stability and protects the patient from falls. The nurse accompanies the patient, holding him or her at the waist (or with a transfer belt) as needed for balance. The patient is assessed for tolerance of walking, and rest periods are provided as needed.

Assisting the Patient Who Uses an Orthosis or Prosthesis

Orthoses and prostheses are designed to facilitate mobilization and to maximize the patient's quality of life. An orthosis is an external appliance that provides support, prevents or corrects deformities, and improves function. Orthoses include braces, splints, collars, corsets, or supports that are designed and fitted by an orthotist or prosthetist. Static orthoses (no moving parts) are used to stabilize joints and prevent contractures. Dynamic orthoses are flexible and are used to improve function by assisting weak muscles. A prosthesis is an artificial body part; it may be internal, such as an artificial knee or hip joint, or external, such as an artificial leg or arm.

In addition to learning how to apply and remove the orthosis and manoeuvre the affected body part correctly, rehabilitation patients must learn how to properly care for the skin that comes in contact with the appliance. Skin problems or **pressure injuries** may develop if the device is applied too tightly or too loosely or if it is adjusted improperly. The nurse instructs the patient to clean and inspect the skin daily, to make sure the brace fits snugly without being too tight, to check that the padding distributes pressure evenly, and to wear a cotton garment without seams between the orthosis and the skin.

If the patient has had an amputation, the nurse promotes tissue healing, uses compression dressings to promote residual limb shaping, and minimizes contracture formation. A permanent prosthetic limb cannot be fitted until the tissue has healed completely and the residual limb shape is stable and free of edema. The nurse also helps the patient cope with the emotional issues surrounding loss of a limb and encourages acceptance of the prosthesis. The prosthetist, the nurse, and the physician collaborate to provide instructions related to skin care and care of the prosthesis.

Evaluation

Expected Patient Outcomes

Expected patient outcomes may include the following:

1. Demonstrates improved physical mobility
   a. Maintains muscle strength and joint mobility
   b. Does not develop contractures
   c. Participates in an exercise program
2. Transfers safely
   a. Demonstrates assisted transfers
   b. Performs independent transfers
3. Ambulates with maximum independence
   a. Uses the ambulatory aid safely
   b. Adheres to the weight-bearing prescription
   c. Requests assistance as needed
4. Demonstrates increased activity tolerance
   a. Does not experience episodes of orthostatic hypotension
   b. Reports absence of fatigue with ambulatory efforts
   c. Gradually increases the distance and speed of ambulation

Nursing Process

The Patient With Impaired Skin Integrity

Both prevention and treatment of pressure injuries are costly in terms of health care dollars, hospital length of stay, and quality of life for patients at risk. All possible efforts should be made to prevent skin breakdown.

Patients confined to bed for long periods, patients with motor or sensory dysfunction, and patients who experience muscular atrophy and reduction of padding between the overlying skin and the underlying bone are prone to pressure injuries. Pressure injuries are localized areas of infarcted soft tissue that occur when pressure applied to the skin over time is greater than normal capillary closure pressure, which is about 25 to 32 mm Hg. Critically ill patients have a lower capillary closure pressure and are at greater risk for pressure injuries. The initial sign of pressure is erythema (redness of the skin) caused by reactive hyperemia, which normally resolves in less than 1 hour. Unrelieved pressure results in further skin breakdown. The cutaneous tissues become broken or destroyed, leading to progressive destruction and necrosis of underlying soft tissue, and the resulting pressure injury is painful and slow to heal. In addition to significant pain and suffering, the consequences of developing a pressure injury include increased morbidity and mortality and higher medical costs and resource use, and lower odds of discharge to the community.

Assessment

NURSING ALERT

Pressure injuries are associated with increased costs of treatment and length of hospital stay as well as diminished quality of life for patients. It is imperative that nurses perform a skin assessment on every patient admitted to a hospital, inpatient rehabilitation facility, or skilled nursing facility. Scales such as the Braden scale may be used to facilitate systematic assessment and quantification of a patient's risk for pressure injury, although the nurse should recognize that the reliability of these scales is not well established for all patient populations.

Immobility

When a person is immobile and inactive, pressure is exerted on the skin and subcutaneous tissue by objects on which the person rests, such as a mattress, chair seat, or cast. The development of pressure injuries is directly related to the duration of immobility—If pressure continues long enough, small vessel thrombosis and tissue necrosis occur and a pressure injury results. Weight-bearing bony prominences are most susceptible to pressure injury development because they are covered only by skin and small amounts of subcutaneous tissue. Susceptible areas include the sacrum and coccygeal areas, ischial tuberosities (especially in people who sit for prolonged periods), greater trochanter, heel, knee, malleolus, medial condyle of the tibia, fibular head, scapula, and elbow (Fig. 13-3).

Specific nursing actions related to assessing risk include:

- Evaluate level of mobility.
- Note safety and assistive devices (e.g., restraints, splints).
- Assess neurovascular status.
- Evaluate circulatory status (e.g., peripheral pulses, edema).
- Note present health problems.
- Evaluate nutritional and hydration status.
- Review the results of the patient's laboratory studies, including hematocrit, hemoglobin, electrolytes, albumin, prealbumin, transferrin, and creatinine.
- Determine presence of incontinence.
- Review current medications.

Impaired Sensory Perception or Cognition

Patients with sensory loss, impaired level of consciousness, or paralysis may not be aware of the discomfort associated with prolonged pressure on the skin and therefore may not change their position themselves to relieve the pressure. This prolonged pressure impedes blood flow, reducing nourishment

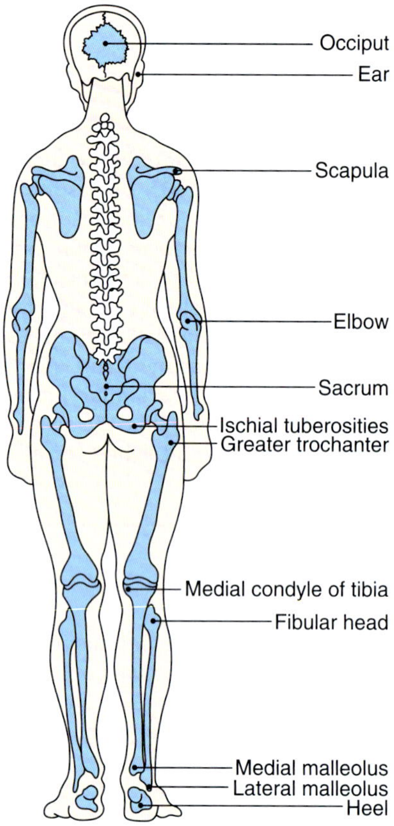

FIGURE 13-3. Areas susceptible to pressure ulcers.

of the skin and underlying tissues. A pressure injury may develop in a short period.

Decreased Tissue Perfusion

Any condition that reduces the circulation and nourishment of the skin and subcutaneous tissue (altered peripheral tissue perfusion) increases the risk of pressure injury development. Patients with diabetes mellitus experience an alteration in microcirculation. Similarly, patients with edema have impaired circulation and poor nourishment of the skin tissue. Patients who have obesity have large amounts of poorly vascularized adipose tissue, which is susceptible to breakdown.

Altered Nutritional Status

Nutritional deficiencies, anemias, and metabolic disorders also contribute to pressure injury development. Anemia, regardless of its cause, decreases the blood's oxygen-carrying ability and predisposes a patient to pressure injury formation. Patients who have low protein levels or who are in a negative nitrogen balance experience tissue wasting and inhibited tissue repair. Serum albumin is a sensitive indicator of protein deficiency; lowered serum albumin levels are associated with hypoalbuminemic tissue edema and increased risk of pressure injuries. Specific nutrients, such as vitamin C and trace minerals, are needed for tissue maintenance and repair.

Friction and Shear

Mechanical forces also contribute to the development of pressure injuries. Friction is the resistance to movement that occurs when two surfaces are moved across each other. Shear is created by the interplay of gravitational forces (forces that push the body down) and friction. When shear occurs, tissue layers slide over one another, blood vessels stretch and twist, and the microcirculation of the skin and subcutaneous tissue is disrupted. Evidence of deep tissue damage may be slow to develop and may present through the development of a draining tract. The sacrum and heels are most susceptible to the effects of shear. Pressure injuries from friction and shear occur when the patient slides down in bed (Fig. 13-4) or when the patient is moved or positioned improperly (e.g., dragged up in bed). Spastic muscles and paralysis increase the patient's vulnerability to pressure injuries related to friction and shear.

Increased Moisture

Prolonged contact with moisture from perspiration, urine, feces, or drainage produces maceration (softening) of the skin. The skin reacts to the caustic substances in the excreta or drainage and becomes irritated. Moist, irritated skin is more vulnerable to pressure breakdown. Once the skin breaks, the area may be invaded by microorganisms (e.g., streptococci, staphylococci, *Pseudomonas aeruginosa, Escherichia coli*), and infection may occur. That is, foul-smelling infectious drainage is present, and the lesion may enlarge and allow a continuous loss of serum, which may further deplete the body of essential protein needed for tissue repair and maintenance. The lesion may continue to enlarge and extend deep into the fascia, muscle, and bone, with multiple sinus tracts radiating from the pressure injury. With extensive local infection, systemic infection may follow, frequently caused by gram-negative organisms and may result in sepsis.

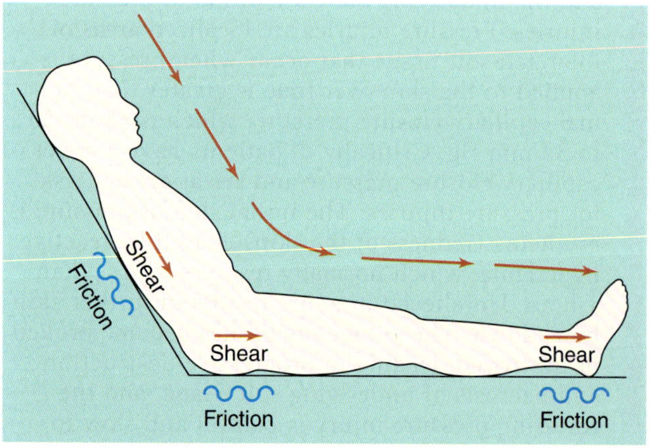

FIGURE 13-4. Mechanical forces contribute to pressure injury development. As the person slides down or is improperly pulled up in bed, ***friction*** resists this movement. ***Shear*** occurs when one layer of tissue slides over another, disrupting microcirculation of skin and subcutaneous tissue.

Gerontologic Considerations

Older adults have a number of age-related changes which increase the risk of skin breakdown, including reduced skin elasticity, decreased collagen, and muscle/tissue atrophy. Polypharmacy and concomitant medical conditions may affect wound healing. Decreased inflammatory response, little subcutaneous padding over bony prominences, and decreased nutritional intake are commonly seen in the older adult and increase the risk of pressure injuries and delay wound healing (Kohr, 2014).

Bariatric Considerations

In 2014, an international collaborative comprising members from the U.S. National Pressure Ulcer Advisory Panel (NPUAP), European Pressure Ulcer Advisory Panel (EPUAP), and the Pan Pacific Pressure Injury Advisory Panel (PPPIAP) released the *Prevention and Treatment of Pressure Ulcers; Clinical Practice Guideline* (Dunk & Carville, 2016; National Pressure Ulcer Advisory Panel, 2014). These updated guidelines include recommendations for adults who have obesity with specific organization-level considerations, recommendations for the bariatric individual, as well as recommendations for bed and equipment selection and repositioning. Please see the NPUAP Web site link at the end of this chapter to review the quick reference guideline.

CHART 13-9

Risk Factors for Pressure Ulcers

- Prolonged pressure on tissue
- Immobility, compromised mobility
- Loss of protective reflexes, sensory deficit/loss
- Poor skin perfusion, edema
- Malnutrition, hypoproteinemia, anemia, vitamin deficiency
- Friction, shearing forces, trauma
- Incontinence of urine or feces
- Altered skin moisture: excessively dry, excessively moist
- Advanced age, debilitation
- Equipment: casts, traction, restraints
- Skin problems on admission

Adapted from DiVita, M. A., Granger, C. V., Goldstein, R., et al. (2015). Risk factors for development of new or worsened pressure ulcers among patients in inpatient rehabilitation facilities in the United States: Data from the Uniform Data System for Medical Rehabilitation. *Physical Medicine & Rehabilitation, 7*(6), 599–612.; Dunk, A. M., & Carville, K. (2016). The international clinical practice guideline for prevention and treatment of pressure ulcers/injuries. *Journal of Advanced Nursing, 72*(2), 243–244.; García-Fernández, F. P., Agreda, J. J., Verdú, J., et al. (2014). A new theoretical model for the development of pressure ulcers and other dependence-related lesions. *Journal of Nursing Scholarship, 46*(1), 28–38.; Stifter, J., Yao, Y., Lodhi, M. K., et al. (2015). Nurse continuity and hospital-acquired pressure ulcers: A Comparative Analysis Using an Electronic Health Record "Big Data" Set. *Nursing Research, 64*(5), 361–371.

Assessment of Risk

In assessing the patient for the potential risk for pressure injury development, the nurse assesses the patient's mobility, sensory perception, cognitive abilities, tissue perfusion, nutritional status, friction and shear forces, sources of moisture on the skin, and age. The nurse performs the following:

- Assesses the total skin condition at least twice a day
- Inspects each pressure site for erythema
- Assesses areas of erythema for a blanching response
- Inspects for dry skin, moist skin, and breaks in skin
- Determines the presence of incontinence
- Notes any drainage and odour
- Evaluates the level of mobility
- Notes restrictive devices (e.g., restraints, splints)
- Evaluates circulatory status (e.g., peripheral pulses, edema)
- Assesses the neurovascular status
- Evaluates the nutritional and hydration status
- Reviews the patient's record for laboratory studies, including hematocrit, hemoglobin, electrolytes, albumin, transferrin, and creatinine
- Notes any present health problems
- Reviews current medications

Validated scales such as the Braden or Norton scale may be used to facilitate systematic assessment and quantification of a patient's risk for pressure injury. The Spinal Cord Injury Pressure Ulcer Scale (SCIPUS) is used to measure the risk for pressure injury development for individuals with a spinal cord injury who are in a rehabilitation centre (Salzberg et al., 1996). Chart 13-9 presents a list of risk factors for the development of pressure injuries. For stages and categories of pressure injuries, see http://www.npuap.org.

If a pressure area is noted, the nurse documents its size and location and may use a grading system to describe its severity. For any pressure injury, it can be upgraded from one stage to another (i.e., from stage 1 to stage 3); however pressure injuries are not downgraded (i.e., from stage 3 to stage 2). Instead it would be described as either a healing or a healed stage 3 pressure injury.

The appearance of purulent drainage or foul odour suggests an infection. With an extensive pressure injury, deep pockets of infection are often present. Drying and crusting of exudate may be present. Infection of a pressure injury may advance to osteomyelitis, pyarthrosis (pus formation within a joint cavity), sepsis, and septic shock.

Nursing Diagnosis

Based on the assessment data, the nursing diagnoses may include the following:

- Risk for impaired skin integrity
- Impaired skin integrity (related to immobility, decreased sensory perception, decreased tissue perfusion, decreased nutritional status, friction and shear forces, increased moisture, or advanced age)

Planning and Goals

The major goals for the patient include relief of pressure and may include any or all of the following: improved mobility, improved sensory perception, improved tissue perfusion, improved nutritional status, minimized friction and shear forces, dry surfaces in contact with skin, and healing of the pressure injury, if present.

Nursing Interventions

Relieving Pressure

Frequent changes of position are needed to relieve and redistribute the pressure on the patient's skin and to promote blood flow to the skin and subcutaneous tissues. This can be accomplished by instructing the patient to change position or by turning and repositioning the patient. The patient's family members should be educated about how to position and turn the patient at home to prevent pressure injuries. Shifting weight allows the blood to flow into the ischemic areas and helps tissues recover from the effects of pressure. Attention should be paid to patient migration (moving down in the bed) in those on bed rest, particularly when the head of the bed is elevated (Wiggermann, Kotowski, Davis, et al., 2015).

For patients who spend long periods in a wheelchair, pressure can be relieved by:

- *Push-ups:* The patient pushes down on armrests and raises buttocks off the seat of the chair.
- *One half push-up:* The patient repeats the push-up on the right side and then the left, pushing up on one side by pushing down on the armrest.
- *Moving side to side:* The patient moves from one side to the other while sitting in the chair.
- *Shifting:* The patient bends forward with the head down between the knees (if able) and constantly shifts in the chair.

Positioning the Patient

The degree of ability to move independently—the comfort, fatigue, loss of sensation, overall physical and mental status, and specific disorder—influences plans for changing position. Patients should be positioned laterally, prone, and dorsally in sequence unless a position is not tolerated or is contraindicated. Generally, those who experience discomfort after 30 to 60 minutes of lying prone need to be repositioned. The recumbent position is preferred to the semi-Fowler's position because of increased supporting body surface area in this position.

Patients able to shift their weight every 15 to 20 minutes and move independently may change total position every 2 to 4 hours. Indications for routine repositioning every 2 hours or more frequently include loss of sensation, paralysis, coma, and edema.

In addition to regular turning, small shifts of body weight, such as repositioning of an ankle, elbow, or shoulder, are necessary. The skin is inspected at each position change and assessed for temperature elevation. If redness or heat is noted or if the patient complains of discomfort, pressure on the area must be relieved.

Another way to relieve pressure over bony prominences is the bridging technique, accomplished through the correct positioning of pillows. Just as a bridge is supported on pillars to allow traffic to move underneath, so can the body be supported by pillows to allow for space between bony prominences and the mattress. Runway Slider Sets are a combination of special friction-reducing bedspreads and draw sheets which are available to aid in repositioning patients while reducing friction and shear during the transferring process (i.e., repositioning in bed) (Alberta Health Services, 2012). A pillow or commercial heel protector may be used to support the heels off the bed when the patient is supine. Offloading using pillows involves turning the patient in increments and placing pillows to support the patient in that position. The patient can be supported using pillows in a side-lying position off the trochanter. Frequent small shifts of body weight may be the most effective strategy. Placing a small rolled towel or sheepskin padding under a shoulder or hip will allow a return of blood flow to the skin in the area on which the patient is sitting or lying. The towel or sheepskin is moved around the patient's pressure points in a clockwise fashion. A turning schedule can help the family keep track of the patient's turns, especially patients who are high risk and cannot get out of bed (Stifter, Yao, Lodhi, et al., 2015).

Using Pressure-Relieving Devices

At times, special equipment and beds may be needed to help relieve the pressure on the skin. These devices are designed to provide support for specific body areas or to distribute pressure evenly.

A patient who sits in a wheelchair for prolonged periods should have wheelchair cushions fitted and adjusted on an individualized basis, using pressure measurement techniques as a guide to selection and fitting. The aim is to redistribute pressure away from areas at risk for pressure injuries; but no cushion is able to eliminate excessive pressure completely. The patient should be reminded to shift weight frequently and to rise for a few seconds every 15 minutes while sitting in a chair (Fig. 13-5).

Static support devices (such as high-density foam, air, or liquid mattress overlays) distribute pressure evenly by bringing more of the patient's body surface into contact with the supporting surface. Gel-type flotation pads and air-fluidized beds reduce pressure. The weight of a body floating on a fluid system is evenly distributed over the entire supporting surface (according to Pascal's law). Therefore, as the patient's body sinks into the fluid, additional surface becomes available for weight bearing, body weight per unit area is decreased, and there is less pressure on the body parts.

Specialized beds have been designed to prevent pressure on the skin. Dynamic support surfaces, such as low air-loss pockets, alternately inflate and deflate

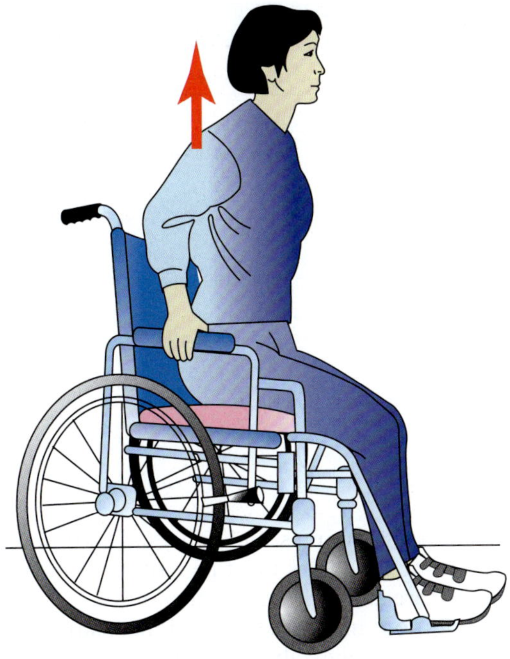

FIGURE 13-5. Wheelchair push-up to prevent ischial pressure ulcers. These push-ups should become an automatic routine (every 15 minutes) for the person with paraplegia. The person should stay up, out of contact with the seat for several seconds. The wheels are kept in the locked position during the exercise.

sections to change support pressure for very high-risk patients who are critically ill and debilitated and cannot be repositioned to relieve pressure. Kinetic beds change pressure by means of rocking movements of the bed that redistribute the patient's weight and stimulate circulation. These beds are frequently used with patients who have injuries due to multiple trauma.

Improving Mobility

The patient is encouraged to remain active and is ambulated whenever possible. When sitting, the patient is reminded to change positions frequently to redistribute weight. Active and passive exercises increase muscular, skin, and vascular tone. Activity stimulates circulation, which relieves tissue ischemia—the forerunner of pressure injuries. For the patient at risk for pressure injuries, turning and exercise schedules are essential—repositioning must occur around the clock.

Improving Sensory Perception

The nurse helps the patient recognize and compensate for altered sensory perception. Depending on the origin of the alteration (e.g., decreased level of consciousness, spinal cord lesion), specific interventions are selected. Strategies to improve cognition and sensory perception may include stimulating the patient to increase awareness of self in the environment, encouraging the patient to participate in self-care, or supporting the patient's efforts toward active compensation for loss of sensation (e.g., a patient with paraplegia lifting up from the sitting position every 15 minutes). When decreased sensory perception exists, the patient and caregiver are taught to inspect potential pressure areas visually every morning and evening, using a mirror if necessary, for evidence of pressure injury development.

Improving Tissue Perfusion

Exercise and repositioning improve tissue perfusion. Massage of erythematous areas is avoided because damage to the capillaries and deep tissue may occur. New research is underway to develop an undergarment that would help increase tissue perfusion for those patients at risk of developing pressure injuries. The Smart-e-Pants delivers an electrical stimulation to susceptible areas to stimulate muscle contraction to help increase blood flow and simulate "fidgeting" in patients who are unable to do so themselves (such as those with SCI or advanced MS) (SMART Team, 2014).

NURSING ALERT

The nurse should avoid massaging reddened areas, as this may increase the damage to already traumatized skin and tissue.

In patients who have evidence of compromised peripheral circulation (e.g., edema), positioning and elevation of the edematous body part to promote venous return and diminish congestion improve tissue perfusion. In addition, the nurse or family must be alert to environmental factors (e.g., wrinkles in sheets, pressure of tubes) that may contribute to pressure on the skin and diminished circulation, and remove the source of pressure.

Improving Nutritional Status

The patient's nutritional status must be adequate, and a positive nitrogen balance must be maintained, because pressure injuries develop more quickly and are more resistant to treatment in patients with nutritional disorders. A high-protein diet with protein supplements may be helpful. Iron preparations may be necessary to raise the hemoglobin concentration so that tissue oxygen levels can be maintained within acceptable limits. Ascorbic acid (vitamin C) is necessary for tissue healing. Other nutrients associated with healthy skin include vitamin A, B vitamins, zinc, and sulphur. With balanced nutrition and hydration, the skin is able to remain healthy, and damaged tissues can be repaired (Table 13-3).

To assess the nutritional status response to therapeutic strategies, the nurse monitors the patient's hemoglobin, albumin, and body weight weekly. Nutritional assessment is described in further detail in Chapter 5.

Reducing Friction and Shear

Shear occurs when the patient is pulled, is allowed to slump, or moves by digging heels or elbows into the

TABLE 13-3 Nutritional Requirements to Promote Healing of Pressure Ulcers

Nutrient	Rationale	Recommended Amount
Protein	Tissue repair	1.25–1.50 g/kg/day
Calories	Spare protein Restore normal weight	30–35 calories/kg/day
Water	Maintain homeostasis	1 mL/calorie fed or 30 mL/kg/day
Multivitamin	Promote collagen formation	1 daily
Vitamin C	Promote collagen synthesis Support integrity of capillary wall	500–1,000 mg daily
Zinc sulphate	Cofactor for collagen formation and protein synthesis Normal lymphocyte and phagocyte response	220 mg daily
Vitamin A	*Caution:* An excess can cause an excessive inflammatory response that could impair healing	–

mattress. Raising the head of the bed by even a few centimetres increases the shearing force over the sacral area; therefore, it is important to keep the head of the bed at less than 30 degrees whenever possible. Proper positioning with adequate support is also important when a patient is sitting in a chair. Polyester sheepskin pads and friction-reducing sheets are thought to reduce shear and friction and may be used with at-risk patients.

NURSING ALERT

To avoid shearing forces when repositioning the patient, the nurse lifts and avoids dragging the patient across a surface.

Minimizing Irritating Moisture

Continuous moisture on the skin must be prevented by meticulous hygienic measures. Perspiration, urine, stool, and drainage must be removed from the skin promptly. The soiled skin should be washed immediately with mild soap and water and blotted dry with a soft towel. The skin may be lubricated with a bland lotion to keep it soft and pliable. Drying agents and powders are avoided. Topical barrier ointments (e.g., zinc oxide) may be helpful in protecting the skin of patients who are incontinent.

Absorbent pads that wick moisture away from the body should be used to absorb drainage. Patients who are incontinent need to be checked *regularly, toileted regularly*, and have their wet incontinence pads and bed sheets changed promptly. Skin must be cleansed and dried promptly. (A no-rinse cleanser is preferable for cleansing due to the pH-balanced formula.) Skin should be patted dry, since rough drying will damage fragile tissue.

Promoting Pressure Injury Healing

Regardless of the stage of the pressure injury, the pressure on the area must be eliminated because the injury will not heal until all pressure is removed. The patient must not lie or sit on the pressure injury, even for a few minutes. Individualized positioning and turning schedules must be written in the plan of nursing care and followed meticulously.

In addition, inadequate nutritional status and fluid and electrolyte abnormalities must be corrected to promote healing. Wounds that drain body fluids and protein place the patient in a catabolic state and predispose to hypoproteinemia and serious secondary infections. Protein deficiency must be corrected to heal the pressure injury. Carbohydrates are necessary to "spare" the protein and to provide an energy source. Vitamin C and trace elements, especially zinc, are necessary for collagen formation and wound healing.

STAGE I PRESSURE INJURIES. To permit healing of stage I pressure injuries, the pressure is removed to allow increased tissue perfusion, nutritional and fluid and electrolyte balance are maintained, friction and shear are reduced, and moisture to the skin is avoided.

STAGE II PRESSURE INJURIES. Stage II pressure injuries have broken skin. In addition to measures listed for stage I pressure injuries, a moist environment, in which migration of epidermal cells over the injury surface occurs more rapidly, should be provided to aid wound healing. The injury is gently cleansed with sterile saline solution. Use dressings that maintain a moist (but not wet) environment for healing and minimizing the loss of fluids and proteins from the body.

STAGE III AND IV PRESSURE INJURIES. Stage III and IV pressure injuries are characterized by extensive tissue damage. In addition to measures listed for stage I, these advanced draining, necrotic pressure injuries must be cleaned (débrided) to create an area that will heal. Necrotic, devitalized tissue favours bacterial growth, delays granulation, and inhibits healing. Wound cleaning and dressing may be uncomfortable; therefore, the nurse must prepare the patient for the procedure by explaining what will occur and administering prescribed analgesia.

Débridement may be accomplished by mechanical flushing of necrotic and infective exudate, application of prescribed enzyme preparations that dissolve necrotic tissue, or surgical dissection. Wet-to-damp dressings are no longer used due to increased pain with removal of gauze, prolongation of wound healing, and the possibility of wound infection.

If an eschar covers the injury, it is removed surgically to ensure a clean, vitalized wound. Exudate may be absorbed by dressings or special hydrophilic powders, beads, or gels. Wound cultures of infected pressure injuries may be used to guide selection of antibiotic therapy.

After the pressure injury is clean, a topical treatment is prescribed to promote healing. New granulation tissue must be protected from reinfection, drying, and damage, and care should be taken to prevent pressure and further trauma to the area. Multiple agents and protocols are used to treat pressure injuries, but consistency is an important key to success. Negative pressure wound therapy can be used to assist granulation and improve vascular blood flow (Webster et al., 2019). For chronic, noninfected injuries that are healing by secondary intention (healing of an open wound from the base upward by laying down new tissue), vacuum-assisted closure (VAC) may be used. VAC involves the use of a negative-pressure sponge dressing in the wound to increase blood flow, increasing formation of granulation tissue and nutrient uptake and decreasing bacterial load.

Hyperbaric oxygen therapy involves either the application of topical oxygen at increased pressure directly to the wound or placing the patient into a hyperbaric oxygen chamber. Both methods of hyperbaric oxygen therapy promote wound healing by stimulating new vascular growth and aiding in the preservation of damaged tissue (Dauwe, Pulikkottil, Lavery, et al., 2014). In a recent systematic review, Stoekenbroek, Santema, Legemate, et al. (2014) reported that hyperbaric oxygen therapy improves healing in patients with diabetic leg injuries; however, more studies are needed prior to routinely introducing this therapy into clinical practice.

Objective evaluation of the pressure injury (e.g., measurement of the pressure injury, inspection for granulation tissue) for response to the treatment protocol must be made every 4 to 6 days. Taking photographs at weekly intervals is a reliable strategy for monitoring the healing process, which may take weeks to months to complete.

Surgical intervention is necessary when the injury is extensive, when potential complications (e.g., fistula) exist, and when the injury does not respond to treatment. Surgical procedures include débridement, incision and drainage, bone resection, and skin grafting. Osteomyelitis is a possible complication of extensive wounds. More information on osteomyelitis is presented in Chapter 71.

Preventing Recurrence

Recurrence of pressure injuries should be anticipated; therefore, active, preventive intervention and frequent continuing assessments are essential. The patient's tolerance for sitting or lying on the healed pressure area is increased gradually by increasing the time that pressure is allowed on the area in 5- to 15-minute increments. The patient is taught to increase mobility and to follow a regimen of turning, weight shifting, and repositioning. The patient teaching plan includes instruction on strategies to reduce the risk for development of pressure injuries and methods to detect, inspect, and minimize pressure areas. Early recognition and intervention are keys to long-term management of potential impaired skin integrity. Gould, Olney, Nichols, et al. (2014) suggest immobility and incontinence are among modifiable risk factors that contribute to recurrent pressure injury development, particularly in patients with SCI; they suggest the development of structured guidelines to prevent pressure injuries rests on the identification of factors that differ in patients with SCI who have none, one, or more pressure injuries. Identifying potentially modifiable risk factors or protective factors may then lead to evidence-based risk assessment tools and interventions customized to patient-specific risks.

Evaluation

Expected Patient Outcomes

Expected outcomes (facilitated by patient education) may include the following:

1. Maintains intact skin
   a. Exhibits no areas of nonblanchable erythema at bony prominences
   b. Avoids massage of bony prominences
   c. Exhibits no breaks in the skin
2. Limits pressure on bony prominences
   a. Changes position every 1 to 2 hours
   b. Uses techniques to reduce pressure
   c. Uses special equipment as appropriate
   d. Repositions self in wheelchair every 15 minutes
3. Increases mobility
   a. Performs range-of-motion exercises
   b. Adheres to the turning schedule
   c. Advances sitting time as tolerated
4. Sensory and cognitive ability improved
   a. Demonstrates an improved level of consciousness
   b. Remembers to inspect potential pressure injury areas every morning and evening
5. Demonstrates improved tissue perfusion
   a. Exercises to increase circulation
   b. Elevates body parts susceptible to edema
6. Attains and maintains adequate nutritional status
   a. Verbalizes the importance of protein and vitamin C in the diet
   b. Eats a diet high in protein and vitamin C
   c. Maintains hemoglobin, electrolyte, albumin, transferrin, and creatinine levels at acceptable levels
7. Avoids friction and shear
   a. Avoids positioning with head of bed greater than 30 degrees for extended periods
   b. Uses sheepskin padding and heel protectors when appropriate

   c. Lifts the body instead of sliding it across surfaces
8. Maintains clean, dry skin
   a. Avoids prolonged contact with wet or soiled surfaces
   b. Keeps the skin clean and dry
   c. Uses lotion to keep dry skin lubricated
9. Experiences healing of the pressure injury
   a. Avoids pressure on the area
   b. Improves nutritional status
   c. Participates in a therapeutic regimen
   d. Demonstrates behaviours to prevent new pressure injuries
   e. States early indicators of pressure injury development

Nursing Process

The Patient With Altered Elimination Patterns

Urinary incontinence and bowel incontinence or constipation and impaction are problems that often occur in patients with disabilities. Incontinence curtails the person's independence, causing embarrassment and isolation. Based on structured oral interviews conducted to collect data on bothersome urinary or fecal incontinence in adults aged 50 and older, 20% of women and 6.4% of men reported urinary incontinence (less than once/month, a few times/month, a few times/week, or every day/night) (Gorina, Schappert, Bercovitz, et al., 2014; Roe, Flanagan, & Maden, 2015). Fecal incontinence (leakage of gas, mucus, liquid or solid stool at least monthly) was reported by 8.2% of women and 8.4% of men (Wu, Matthews, Vaughan, et al., 2015). Internationally, nearly 55% of nursing home residents will experience bowel and/or bladder incontinence at some point (Mandl, Halfens, & Lohrmann, 2015). For patients with disabilities who experience constipation, complete and predictable evacuation of the bowel is the goal. If a bowel routine is not established, the patient may experience abdominal distention; small, frequent oozing of stool; or impaction.

Urinary distention and bowel constipation and impaction are particularly dangerous for a spinal cord patient with an injury above T6. Autonomic hyperreflexia (dysreflexia) is a potentially life-threatening condition involving the autonomic nervous system and is caused by a variety of stimuli, including bladder or bowel fullness.

Assessment

Urinary incontinence may result from multiple causes, including urinary tract infection, detrusor instability, bladder outlet obstruction or incompetence, neurologic impairment, bladder spasm or contracture, and inability to reach the toilet in time.

The health history is used to assess bladder and bowel function, symptoms associated with dysfunction, physiologic risk factors for elimination problems, perception of micturition and defecation cues, and functional toileting abilities. Previous and current fluid intake and voiding patterns may be helpful in designing the plan of nursing care. A record of times of voiding and amounts voided is kept for at least 48 hours. In addition, episodes of incontinence and associated activity (e.g., coughing, sneezing, lifting), fluid intake time and amount, and medications are recorded. This record is analyzed and used to determine patterns and relationships of incontinence to other activities and factors.

The ability to get to the bathroom, to manipulate clothing, and to use the toilet are important functional factors that may be related to incontinence. Related cognitive functioning (perception of the need to void, verbalization of the need to void, and ability to learn to control urination) must also be assessed. In addition, the nurse reviews the results of the diagnostic studies (e.g., urinalysis, urodynamic tests, postvoid residual [PVR] volumes). Refer to the accompanying Gerontologic Considerations section for factors that affect urinary elimination patterns in the older adult.

Bowel incontinence and constipation may result from multiple causes, such as diminished or absent sphincter control, cognitive or perceptual impairment, neurogenic factors, diet, and immobility. The origin of the bowel problem must be determined.

The nurse assesses the patient's usual bowel patterns, nutritional patterns, use of laxatives, gastrointestinal problems (e.g., colitis), bowel sounds, anal reflex and tone, and functional abilities. The character and frequency of bowel movements are recorded and analyzed.

Gerontologic Considerations

Factors That Alter Urinary Elimination Patterns in the Older Adult

Decreased bladder capacity
Decreased muscle tone
Increased residual volumes
Delayed perception of elimination cues
Use of medications that alter elimination patterns, such as diuretics (increase volume of urine produced), sedatives (alter bladder sensitivity to cues), and adrenergics or anticholinergics (cause urinary retention)
Functional immobility
Sedentary lifestyle

Nursing Diagnosis

Based on the assessment data, major nursing diagnoses may include the following:

- Functional urinary incontinence
- Urge urinary incontinence
- Reflex urinary incontinence
- Stress urinary incontinence
- Impaired urinary elimination

- Overflow urinary incontinence
- Urinary retention
- Constipation
- Bowel incontinence

Planning and Goals

The major goals of the patient may include control of urinary incontinence or urinary retention, control of bowel incontinence, and regular elimination patterns.

Nursing Interventions

Promoting Urinary Continence

After the nature of the urinary incontinence has been identified, a nursing plan of care is developed based on analysis of the assessment data. Various approaches to promotion of urinary continence have been designed. Most approaches attempt to condition the body to control urination or to minimize the occurrence of unscheduled urination. Selection of the approach depends on the cause and type of the patient's incontinence. For the program to be successful, the patient's participation and desire to avoid incontinence episodes are crucial, and an optimistic attitude with positive feedback for even slight gains is essential for success.

Accurate recording of intake and output and of the response to selected strategies is essential for evaluation. For some patients, urinary retention may be an issue, particularly with some medical conditions and/or recent removal of an indwelling urinary catheter. After voiding, obtaining a PVR using a specialized ultrasound device ("bladder scanner") provides useful information as to how much urine remains in the bladder. In the absence of a PVR measuring device, the nurse relies on other assessments (such as palpation of the bladder) to determine the presence of residual urine. If residual urine is present, the patient may attempt to void a second time; this is commonly referred to as double voiding. If there is still a significant amount of urine present, an In and Out catheterization may be performed as ordered by the physician.

At no time should the fluid intake be restricted to decrease the frequency of urination. Sufficient fluid intake (2,000 to 3,000 mL/day according to patient needs) must be ensured (concentrated urine is a bladder irritant; caffeine is also a bladder irritant and intake should be minimized). Most of the fluids should be consumed before evening to minimize the need to void frequently during the night.

NURSING ALERT

Carbonated soft drinks, milk shakes, alcohol, tomato juice, and citrus fruit juices are alkaline-producing drinks that promote bacterial growth in the urine. Patients should be encouraged to drink more acid-producing fluids (e.g., cranberry and Cranapple juice) to reduce the chance of urinary tract infection. Water is a preferred fluid because it flushes the kidneys and bladder.

The goal of bladder training is to restore the bladder to normal function. Bladder training can be used with cognitively intact patients who are experiencing urge incontinence. A voiding and toileting schedule is formulated based on analysis of the assessment data. The schedule specifies times for the patient to try to empty the bladder using a bedpan, toilet, or commode. Privacy should be provided during voiding efforts. The interval between voiding times in the early phase of the bladder training period is short (90 to 120 minutes). The patient is encouraged not to void until the specified voiding time. Voiding success and episodes of incontinence are recorded. As the patient's bladder capacity and control increase, the interval is lengthened. Usually, there is a temporal relationship between drinking, eating, exercising, and voiding. The alert patient can participate in recording intake, activity, and voiding and can plan the schedule to achieve maximum continence. Barrier-free access to the toilet and modification of clothing can help the patient with functional incontinence to achieve self-care in toileting and continence.

Habit training is used to try to keep the patient dry by strict adherence to a toileting schedule and may be successful with stress, urge, or functional incontinence. In the case of a person who is confused, the caregiver takes the person to the toilet according to the schedule before involuntary voiding occurs. Simple cuing and consistency promote success. Periods of continence and successful voidings are positively reinforced.

Biofeedback is a system through which the patient learns consciously to contract excretory sphincters and control voiding cues. Cognitively intact patients who have stress or urge incontinence may gain bladder control through biofeedback.

Pelvic floor exercises (Kegel exercises) strengthen the pubococcygeus muscle. The patient is instructed to tighten pelvic floor muscles for 4 seconds 10 times, and this is repeated 4 to 6 times a day. Daily practice is essential. These exercises are helpful for women who are cognitively intact. **Stopping and starting the stream during urination is not recommended to increase control**. Suprapubic tapping or stroking of the inner thigh may produce voiding by stimulating the voiding reflex arc in patients with reflex incontinence. However, this method is not always effective, owing to a lack of detrusor sphincter muscle coordination. As the bladder reflexively contracts to expel urine, the bladder sphincter reflexively closes, producing a high residual urine volume and an increased incidence of urinary tract infection.

Intermittent self-catheterization is an appropriate alternative for managing reflex incontinence, urinary retention, and overflow incontinence due to an overdistended bladder. Technique is extremely important. The emphasis of patient teaching is on regular emptying of the bladder using a clean technique. Patients on an intermittent catheterization program reuse and clean catheters with a nonresidue dish soap and water and lay them flat until completely dry inside and out. Aseptic intermittent catheterization technique is required in health care institutions because of the potential for bladder infection from resistant organisms. Intermittent self-catheterization may be difficult for patients with limited mobility, dexterity, or vision; however, family members can be taught the procedure. Self-catheterization is also particularly pertinent for patients with SCI, because most of these patients do not have voluntary control of urination. Even those patients with spinal cord injuries who can voluntarily void should measure their residual urine (the amount of urine that remains in the bladder after voluntary or involuntary voiding) by self-catheterization.

Indwelling catheters are avoided if at all possible because of the high incidence of urinary tract infections with their use. Short-term use may be needed during treatment of severe skin breakdown due to continued incontinence. Patients with disability who are unable to perform intermittent self-catheterization may require an indwelling or suprapubic catheter for long-term bladder management. A fluid intake of 2,000 to 3,000 mL/day should be encouraged.

External catheters (condom catheters) and leg bags to collect spontaneous voidings may be used for male patients with reflex incontinence. The appropriate design and size must be chosen for maximal success, and the patient or caregiver must be taught how to apply the condom catheter and how to provide daily hygiene, including skin inspection. Instruction on emptying the leg bag must also be provided, and modifications can be made for patients with limited hand dexterity. External collection devices for women do exist, but difficulties with fit have precluded widespread use.

Due to the risk of falls when accessing the washroom or other devices used with toileting a patient, a variety of strategies should be in place to reduce the risk. These include utilizing a night light; ensuring commodes, bedpans, and urinals are in easy reach and close proximity to the bed; and maintaining a clear path to the bathroom/commode. Patients who get out of bed quickly and without waiting for a nurse may benefit from wearing antislip socks to bed, and bed alarms may be necessary to monitor patient activity.

Incontinence pads (or briefs) are used only as a last resort, because they only manage rather than solve the incontinence problem. Also, they have a negative psychological effect on the patient because many people think of them as diapers. Every effort should be made to reduce the incidence of incontinence episodes through the other methods that have been described. Incontinence pads may be useful at times for patients with stress or total incontinence to protect clothing, but they should be avoided whenever possible. When incontinence pads are used, they should wick moisture away from the body to minimize contact of moisture and excreta with the skin. Wet incontinence pads must be changed promptly, the skin cleansed, and a moisture barrier applied to protect the skin.

Patients may be referred for further studies to assess kidney function and promote long-term bladder health. Renal function tests assess kidney function; urodynamic studies assess bladder and urethral function.

Promoting Bowel Continence

The goals of a bowel training program are to develop regular bowel habits and to prevent uninhibited bowel elimination. Regular, complete emptying of the lower bowel results in bowel continence. A bowel-training program takes advantage of the patient's natural reflexes. Regularity, timing, nutrition and fluids, exercise, and correct positioning promote predictable defecation.

The nurse records defecation time, character of stool, nutritional intake, cognitive abilities, and functional self-care toileting abilities for 5 to 7 days. Analysis of this record is helpful when designing a bowel program for the patient with fecal incontinence. (The Bristol Stool Chart is a useful resource and can be found online through a key word search or at this url: http://www.sthk.nhs.uk/library/documents/stoolchart.pdf.)

Consistency in implementing the plan is essential. A regular time for defecation is established, and attempts at evacuation should be made within 15 minutes of the designated time daily. Natural gastrocolic and duodenocolic reflexes occur about 30 minutes after a meal; therefore, after breakfast is one of the best times to plan for bowel evacuation. However, if the patient had a previously established habit pattern at a different time of day, it should be followed.

The anorectal reflex may be stimulated by rectal suppository (e.g., glycerin) or by mechanical stimulation (e.g., digital stimulation and/or disimpaction with a lubricated gloved finger or anal dilator). Mechanical stimulation should be used only in patients with disability who have no voluntary motor function and no sensation as a result of injuries above the sacral segments of the spinal cord, such as quadriplegic, high paraplegic, or severely brain–injured patients. The technique is not effective in patients who do not have an intact sacral reflex arc (e.g., those with flaccid paralysis). Mechanical stimulation, suppository insertion, or both should be initiated about 30 minutes before the scheduled bowel elimination time, and the interval between stimulation and defecation is noted for subsequent modification of the bowel program. Once the bowel routine is well established, stimulation with a suppository may not be necessary.

The patient should assume the normal squatting position (knees higher than the hips) and be in a private bathroom for defecation if at all possible, although a padded commode chair or bedside toilet is an acceptable alternative. Seating time is limited in patients who are at risk for skin breakdown. Bedpans should be avoided. A patient with disability who is unable to sit on a toilet should be positioned on the left side with legs flexed and the head of the bed elevated 30 to 45 degrees to increase intra-abdominal pressure. Protective padding is placed behind the buttocks. When possible, the patient is instructed to bear down and to contract the abdominal muscles. Massaging the abdomen from right to left facilitates movement of feces in the lower tract.

Preventing Constipation

The record of bowel elimination, character of stool, food and fluid intake, level of activity, bowel sounds, medications, and other assessment data are reviewed to develop the plan of care. Multiple approaches may be used to prevent constipation. The diet should be well balanced and should include adequate intake of high-fibre foods (vegetables, fruits, bran) to prevent hard stools and to stimulate peristalsis. Fluid intake should be between 2 and 3 L/day unless contraindicated. Prune juice or fig juice (120 mL) taken 30 minutes before a meal once daily is helpful in some cases when constipation is a problem. Physical activity and exercise are encouraged, as is self-care in toileting. The patient is encouraged to respond to the natural urge to defecate. Privacy during toileting is provided. Stool softeners, bulk-forming agents, mild stimulants, and suppositories may be prescribed to stimulate defecation and to prevent constipation.

Evaluation

Expected Patient Outcomes

Expected patient outcomes may include the following:

1. Demonstrates control of bowel and bladder function
   a. Experiences no episodes of incontinence
   b. Avoids constipation
   c. Achieves independence in toileting
   d. Expresses satisfaction in the level of bowel and bladder control
2. Achieves urinary continence
   a. Uses a therapeutic approach appropriate to the type of incontinence
   b. Maintains adequate fluid intake
   c. Washes and dries the skin after episodes of incontinence
3. Achieves bowel continence
   a. Participates in a bowel program
   b. Verbalizes the need for a regular time for bowel evacuation
   c. Modifies the diet to promote continence
   d. Uses bowel stimulants as prescribed and needed
4. Experiences relief of constipation
   a. Uses a high-fibre diet, fluids, and exercise to promote defecation
   b. Responds to the urge to defecate

Promoting Home, Community-Based, and Transitional Care

An important goal of rehabilitation is to assist the patient to return to the home environment after learning to manage the disability. A referral system maintains continuity of care when the patient is transferred to the home or to a long-term care facility. The plan for discharge is formulated when the patient is first admitted to the hospital, and discharge plans are made with the patient's functional potential in mind.

Educating Patients About Self-Care

Significant expenditures of time and resources are necessary to ensure that patients gain the skills and confidence to self-manage their health effectively after discharge from the hospital (Schmidt, 2013). Formal programs provide patients with effective strategies for interpreting and managing disease-specific issues and skills needed for problem solving, as well as building and maintaining self-awareness and self-efficacy. Self-care programs often use multifaceted approaches, including didactic teaching, group sessions, individual learning plans, and Web-based resources. When planning the approach to self-care, the nurse must consider the individual patient's knowledge, experience, social and cultural background, level of formal education, and psychological status. The preparation for self-care must also be spread out over the course of the recovery period, and it must be monitored and updated regularly as the patient masters aspects of self-care. Preparation for self-care is also highly relevant for informal caregivers of patients in rehabilitation.

When a patient is discharged from acute care or a rehabilitation facility, informal caregivers, typically family members, often assume the care and support of the patient. Although the most obvious care tasks involve physical care (e.g., personal hygiene, dressing, meal preparation), other elements of the caregiving role include psychosocial support and a commitment to this supportive role. Thus, the nurse must assess the patient's support system (family, friends) well in advance of discharge. The positive attitudes of family and friends toward the patient, their disability, and the return home are important in making a successful transition to home. Not all families can carry out the arduous programs of exercise, physical therapy, and personal care that the patient may need. They may not have the resources or stability to care for family members with a severe disability. The physical, emotional, economic, and energy strains of a disabling condition may overwhelm even a stable family. Members of the rehabilitation team must not judge the family but rather should provide supportive interventions that help the family to attain its highest level of function.

The family members need to know as much as possible about the patient's condition and care so that they do not fear the patient's return home. The nurse develops methods to help the patient and family cope with problems that may arise. For example, the nurse may develop an ADL checklist individualized for the patient and family to ensure that the family is proficient in assisting the patient with certain tasks (Chart 13-10).

Continuing and Transitional Care

A home care or transitional care nurse may visit the patient prior to discharge, interview the patient and the family,

CHART 13-10

HOME CARE CHECKLIST • Managing the Therapeutic Regimen at Home

At the completion of education, the patient and/or caregiver will be able to:

- State the impact of disability on physiologic and psychological functioning.
- State changes in lifestyle (e.g., diet, activity) necessary to maintain health.
- State the name, dose, side effects, frequency, and schedule for all medications.
- State how to obtain medical supplies after discharge.
- Identify durable medical equipment needs, proper usage, and maintenance necessary for safe utilization:
  - [ ] Wheelchair—manual/power
  - [ ] Cushion
  - [ ] Grab bars
  - [ ] Sliding board
  - [ ] Mechanical lift
  - [ ] Raised padded commode seat
  - [ ] Padded commode wheelchair
  - [ ] Bedside commode
  - [ ] Crutches
  - [ ] Walker
  - [ ] Cane
  - [ ] Prosthesis
  - [ ] Orthosis
  - [ ] Shower chair
  - [ ] Specialty bed
- Demonstrate usage of adaptive equipment for activities of daily living (ADLs):
  - [ ] Long-handled sponge
  - [ ] Reacher
  - [ ] Universal cuff
  - [ ] Plate mat and guard
  - [ ] Rocker-knife, spork, weighted utensils
  - [ ] Special closures for clothing
  - [ ] Other
- Demonstrate mobility skills:
  - [ ] Transfers: bed to chair; in and out of toilet and tub; in and out of car
  - [ ] Negotiate ramps, curbs, stairs
  - [ ] Assume sitting from supine position
  - [ ] Turn side to side in bed
  - [ ] Manoeuvre wheelchair; manage arm and leg rests; lock brakes
  - [ ] Ambulate safely using assistive devices
  - [ ] Perform range-of-motion exercises
  - [ ] Perform muscle-strengthening exercises
- Demonstrate skin care:
  - [ ] Inspect bony prominences every morning and evening
  - [ ] Identify stage I pressure injury and actions to take if present
  - [ ] Change dressings for stage II to IV pressure ulcers
  - [ ] State dietary requirements to promote healing of pressure ulcers
  - [ ] Demonstrate pressure relief at prescribed intervals
  - [ ] State sitting schedule and demonstrate weight lifts in wheelchair
  - [ ] Demonstrate adherence to bed turning schedule, bed positioning, and use of bridging techniques
  - [ ] Apply and wear protective boots at prescribed times
  - [ ] Demonstrate correct wheelchair sitting posture
  - [ ] Demonstrate techniques to avoid friction and shear in bed
  - [ ] Demonstrate proper hygiene to maintain skin integrity
- Demonstrate bladder care:
  - [ ] State schedule for voiding, toileting, and catheterization
  - [ ] Identify relationship of fluid intake to voiding and catheterization schedule
  - [ ] State how to perform pelvic floor exercises
  - [ ] Demonstrate clean self-intermittent catheterization and care of catheterization equipment
  - [ ] Demonstrate indwelling catheter care
  - [ ] Demonstrate application of external condom catheter
  - [ ] Demonstrate application, emptying, and cleaning of urinary drainage bag
  - [ ] Demonstrate application of incontinence pads and performing perineal hygiene
  - [ ] State signs and symptoms of urinary tract infection
  - [ ] State signs and symptoms of urinary catheter blockage

HOME CARE CHECKLIST • Managing the Therapeutic Regimen at Home (Continued)

- Demonstrate bowel care:
  - [ ] State optimum dietary intake to promote evacuation
  - [ ] Identify schedule for optimum bowel evacuation and know how to alter schedule as needed
  - [ ] Demonstrate techniques to increase intra-abdominal pressure; Valsalva manoeuvre; abdominal massage; leaning forward
  - [ ] Demonstrate techniques to stimulate bowel movements: ingesting warm liquids; digital stimulation; insertion of suppositories
  - [ ] Demonstrate optimum position for bowel evacuation: on toilet with knees higher than hips; left side in bed with knees flexed and head of bed elevated 30 to 45 degrees
  - [ ] Identify complications and corrective strategies for bowel retraining: constipation, impaction, diarrhea, hemorrhoids, rectal bleeding, anal tears
- Identify community resources for peer and caregiver/family support:
  - [ ] Identify sources of support (e.g., friends, relatives, faith community)
  - [ ] Identify phone numbers of support groups for people with disabilities and their caregivers/families
  - [ ] State meeting locations and times
- Demonstrate how to access transportation:
  - [ ] Identify locations of wheelchair accessibility for public buses or trains
  - [ ] Identify phone numbers for private wheelchair van
  - [ ] Contact Division of Motor Vehicles for handicapped parking permit
  - [ ] Contact Division of Motor Vehicles for driving test when appropriate
  - [ ] Identify resources for adapting private vehicle with hand controls or wheelchair lift
- Identify vocational rehabilitation resources:
  - [ ] State name and phone number of vocational rehabilitation counselor
  - [ ] Identify educational opportunities that may lead to future employment
- Identify community resources for recreation:
  - [ ] State local recreation centres that offer programs for people with disabilities
  - [ ] Identify leisure activities that can be pursued in the community
- Identify the need for health promotion and screening activities
  - [ ] State how to reach primary provider with questions if complications arise
  - [ ] State time and date of follow-up appointments

and review the ADL sheet to learn which activities the patient can perform. This helps to ensure that continuity of care is provided and that the patient does not regress yet maintains the independence gained while in the hospital or rehabilitation setting. The family may need to purchase, borrow, or improvise needed equipment, such as safety rails, a raised toilet seat or commode, or a tub bench. Ramps may need to be built or doorways widened to allow full access.

Family members are taught how to use equipment and are given a copy of the equipment manufacturer's instruction booklet, the names of resource people, lists of equipment-related supplies, and locations where they may be obtained. A written summary of the care plan is included in family education. The patient and family members are reminded about the importance of routine health screening and other health promotion strategies.

A network of support services and communication systems may be required to enhance opportunities for independent living. The nurse uses collaborative, administrative skills to coordinate these activities and pull together the network of care (Chart 13-11). The nurse also provides skilled care, initiates additional referrals when indicated, and serves as a patient advocate and counselor when obstacles are encountered. The nurse continues to reinforce prior patient education and helps the patient to set and achieve attainable goals. The degree to which the patient adapts to the home and community environment depends on the confidence and self-esteem developed during the rehabilitation process and on the acceptance, support, and reactions of family members, employers, and community members.

There is a growing trend toward independent living by people with severe disabilities, either alone or in groups that share resources. Preparation for independent living should include training in managing a household and working with personal care attendants as well as training in mobility. The goal is integration into the community—living and working in the community with accessible housing, employment, public buildings, transportation, and recreation.

State rehabilitation administration agencies provide services to assist people with disabilities in obtaining the help they need to engage in gainful employment. These services include diagnostic, medical, and mental

NURSING RESEARCH PROFILE

Chart 13-11. Caregivers

Allen, J., Hutchinson, A. M., Brown, R., et al. (2018). User experience and care for older people transitioning from hospital to home: Patients' and carers' perspectives. *Health Expectations*, *21*(2), 518–527.

Purpose

Transitioning from hospital or rehabilitation services to home is complex and challenging for many older people living with chronic health conditions, and the burden on caregivers can be great. As mentioned by the authors of this study, "Transitional care facilitates safe and timely transfer of patients between levels of care and across care settings and includes communication between practitioners, assessment and planning, preparation, medication reconciliation, follow-up care and self-management education." The objective of this study was to describe the experience of caregivers and patients in the process of transitioning.

Design

The research study design was qualitative descriptive utilizing participant interviews as primary method of data collection. Nineteen patients and seven caregivers were interviewed regarding their experience in transitioning from hospital to home in an Australian health care setting. The interview data were analysed using thematic analysis.

Results

Research participants emphasized their need for independence during the transition process and perceived a range of social processes that supported their independence at home. The themes identified and explored by the researchers were supportive relationships with carers, caring relationships with health-care practitioners, seeking information, discussing and negotiating the transitional care plan, and learning to self-care.

Nursing Implications

These findings and themes contribute to our understanding that quality transitional care should focus on patients' need to work collaboratively with caregivers to regain independence. Social processes supporting the capacities of patients and carers should be at the forefront in implementing transitional care for patients.

According to the authors, "future transitional care interventions should emphasize strategies to enable negotiation for suitable supports and assist care recipients to overcome barriers identified in this study."

health services. Counselling, training, placement, and follow-up services are available to help people with disabilities select and obtain jobs.

If the patient is transferred to a long-term care facility, the transition is planned to promote continued progress. Independence gained continues to be supported, and progress is fostered. Adjustment to the facility is promoted through communication. Family members are encouraged to visit, to be involved, and to take the patient home on weekends and holidays if possible.

Complementary and Alternative Therapies

Individuals with disabilities may seek a variety of different therapies. For some, therapeutic horseback riding influences the whole body and has a profound effect on all body systems. Pet therapy and canine companion programs have reduced stress and promoted coping for many disabled persons. Some animals, including simian monkeys, can pick up the phone, retrieve small assistive devices, assist with drinking beverages, or assist with activating emergency calls. The "working" animals provide companionship as well as physical assistance for older adults and persons with disability who may live alone.

Nurses can also encourage persons with disability to take advantage of community programs. T'ai chi classes improve muscle strength, balance, and coordination and can help to prevent falls in the older adults. Persons with disabilities, including wheelchair users, can participate in T'ai chi classes for improved balance, coordination, muscle strength and control, and a sense of well-being.

Daily journal writing has helped depressed individuals and their families overcome many emotionally draining reactions to adverse circumstances. Nurses are instrumental in teaching patients and family members this cost-effective technique. Relaxation exercises can also be taught by the nurse and encouraged in all settings, including the hospital, rehabilitation setting, outpatient areas, and the home.

Follow-Up Care

A home care nurse may visit the patient in the hospital, interview the patient and family, and review the ADL sheet to learn which activities the patient can perform. This helps ensure continuity of care and that the patient does not regress but instead maintains the independence gained while in the hospital or rehabilitation setting. The family may need to purchase, borrow, or improvise needed equipment, such as safety rails, a raised toilet seat or commode, or a tub bench. Ramps may need to be built or doorways widened to achieve full access.

Agencies are available to provide services to assist people with disability in obtaining the help they need to engage in gainful employment. These services include diagnostic, medical, and mental health services. Counselling, training, placement, and follow-up services are available to help people with disabilities select and attain jobs.

If the patient is transferred to an extended care facility, the transition is planned to promote continued progress.

Independence gained continues to be supported, and progress is fostered. Adjustment to the extended care facility is facilitated through communication. The family is encouraged to visit, to be involved, and to take the patient home on weekends and holidays if possible.

Critical Thinking Exercises

1 The patient who has just been admitted to your unit in the rehabilitation hospital is a 58-year-old woman who is recovering from a stroke. She has paralysis on one side, but speech is intact. In discussing the patient's level of functioning with the physical rehabilitation team, describe the kinds of self-care activities that you would assess in developing a rehabilitation plan for the patient.

2 **ebp** A 22-year-old man who sustained a spinal cord injury with resulting paraplegia (Level L1–L2) is being discharged to his home. He will be cared for by family and will continue physical and occupational therapy as an outpatient. Family members are particularly concerned about what they can do to prevent pressure injuries. Describe the instructions you would give the patient and the family about prevention of pressure injuries. What is the evidence base that supports the appropriateness of these instructions, and how strong is this evidence? What criteria did you use to determine the strength of the evidence for interventions that assist in the prevention of pressure injuries?

3 You are caring for a 48-year-old male patient post lower limb amputation who is experiencing difficulty adjusting to his physical deficits, thus limiting his participation in rehabilitation sessions. You wish to create the necessary "space" for this patient so that he may practice the tasks and activities requisite to successful rehabilitation, without becoming unduly frustrated, but are unsure what approach to take. Identify a specific evidence-based question related to this patient in order to conduct a relevant and focused literature search. What key words would you use in this search, and what sources would be appropriate to search?

REFERENCES AND SELECTED READINGS

Books

Alberta Health Services. (2012). *It's your move*. Edmonton, AB: Author.

Bryant, R., & Nix, D. (2015). *Acute and chronic wounds-E-book*. Elsevier Health Sciences.

Chang, E., & Johnson, A. (Eds.). (2013). *Chronic illness and disability: Principles for nursing practice* (2nd ed.). St. Louis, MO: Elsevier Health Sciences.

Csiernik, R., & Rowe, W. S. (Eds.). (2017). *Responding to the oppression of addiction: Canadian social work perspectives*. Toronto, ON: Canadian Scholars' Press.

Dean, S. G., Siegert, R. J., & Taylor, W. J. (2012). *Interprofessional rehabilitation: A person-centred approach. Chichester: Wiley-Blackwell.*

Falvo, D., & Holland, B. E. (2017). *Medical and psychosocial aspects of chronic illness and disability*. Burlington, MA: Jones & Bartlett Learning.

Johansson, C., & Chinworth, S. A. (2018). *Mobility in context: Principles of patient care skills*. FA Davis Philadelphia.

Kohr, R. (2014). Skin integrity and wound care. In P. A. Potter, & A. G. Perry (Eds.). *Fundamentals of nursing* (5th ed.). Toronto, ON: Elsevier Canada.

Kolar, P. (Ed.). (2014). *Clinical rehabilitation*. Prague: Alena Kobesová.

National Pressure Ulcer Advisory Panel. (2014). Prevention and treatment of pressure ulcers: Clinical practice guideline. Osborne Park, Western Australia: Cambridge Media.

O'Sullivan, S. B., Schmitz, T. J., & Fulk, G. (Eds.) (2013). *Physical rehabilitation*. Philadelphia, PA: FA Davis Company.

Substance Abuse and Mental Health Services Administration (SAMHSA). (2014). *Results from the 2013 National Survey on Drug Use and Health: Summary of National Findings, NSDUH Series H-48, HHS Publication No. (SMA) 14–4863*. Rockville, MD: Author.

Wright, J. (2011). Disability rating scale. In Kreutzer, J., DeLuca, J., & Caplan, B., eds. *Encyclopedia of clinical neuropsychology*. New York, NY: Springer, 862–863.

Journals and Electronic Documents

Agewell. (2017). *Project 8.2: Aging, disability and technology—Understanding and advancing Canadian policies for technology access.* Retrieved September 21, 2018, from http://agewell-nce.ca/wp-content/uploads/2015/09/age-well_jurisdictional-scan_2017_June-30_FINAL.pdf

Amin, K., & Lucioni, A. (2018). Stress urinary incontinence management in the patient with overactive bladder. *Current Bladder Dysfunction Reports, 13*(3), 111–117.

Arora, M., Harvey, L. A., Chhabra, H. S., et al. (2017). The reliability of measuring wound undermining in people with spinal cord injury. *Spinal Cord, 55*(3), 304–306.

Bamm, E. L., Rosenbaum, P., Wilkins, S., et al. (2015). Performance of the measures of processes of care for adults and service providers in rehabilitation settings. *Patient Related Outcome Measures, 6*, 157–165.

Boyko, T. V., Longaker, M. T., & Yang, G. P. (2018). Review of the current management of pressure ulcers. *Advances in Wound Care, 7*(2), 57–67.

Brubaker, L., & Wolfe, A. J. (2017). Microbiota in 2016: Associating infection and incontinence with the female urinary microbiota. *Nature Reviews Urology, 14*(2), 72.

Camicia, M., Black, T., Farrell, J., et al. (2014). The essential role of the rehabilitation nurse in facilitating care transitions: A White Paper by the Association of Rehabilitation Nurses. *Rehabilitation Nursing, 39*(1), 3–15.

Clarke, D. J. (2014). Nursing practice in stroke rehabilitation: Systematic review and meta-ethnography. *Journal of Clinical Nursing, 23*(9–10), 1201–1226.

Clark, H., & Bassett, S. (2014). An application of the health action process approach to physiotherapy rehabilitation adherence. *Physiotherapy Theory and Practice, 30*(8), 527–533.

Clark-Wilson, J., Giles, G. M., & Baxter, D. M. (2014). Revisiting the neurofunctional approach: Conceptualizing the core components for the rehabilitation of everyday living skills. *Brain Injury, 28*(13–14), 1646–1656.

Colombo, R., Sterpi, I., Mazzone, A., et al. (2013). Robot aided neurorehabilitation in sub-acute and chronic stroke: Does spontaneous recovery have a limited impact on outcome? *NeuroRehabilitation, 33*(4), 621–629.

Cosco, T. D., Howse, K., & Brayne, C. (2017). Healthy ageing, resilience and wellbeing. *Epidemiology and Psychiatric Sciences, 26*(6), 579–583.

Craig, A., Perry, K. N., Guest, R., et al. (2015). Prospective study of the occurrence of psychological disorders and comorbidities after spinal cord injury. *Archives of Physical Medicine and Rehabilitation, 96*(8), 1426–1434.

Dauwe, P. B., Pulikkottil, B. J., Lavery, L., et al. (2014). Does hyperbaric oxygen therapy work in facilitating acute wound healing: A systematic review. *Plastic and Reconstructive Surgery, 133*(2), 208e–215e.

Deepika, A., Devi, B. I., & Shukla, D. (2017). Predictive validity of disability rating scale in determining functional outcome in patients with severe traumatic brain injury. *Neurology India, 65*(1), 83–86.

Dennerlein, J. T., O'day, E. T., Mulloy, D. F., et al. (2017). Lifting and exertion injuries decrease after implementation of an integrated hospital-wide safe patient handling and mobilisation programme. *Occupational and Environmental Medicine, 74*, 336–343.

Dossa, A., Bokhour, B., & Hoenig, H. (2012). Care transitions from the hospital to home for patients with mobility impairments: Patient and family caregiver experiences. *Rehabilitation Nursing, 37*(6), 277–285.

Dunk, A. M., & Carville, K. (2016). The international clinical practice guideline for prevention and treatment of pressure ulcers/injuries. *Journal of Advanced Nursing*, n/a-n/a. doi: 10.1111/jan.12614

El-Guebaly, N. (2014). A Canadian perspective on addiction treatment. *Substance Abuse, 35*(3), 298–303.

Gallacher, J., Mitchell, C., Heslop, L., et al. (2012). Resilience to health related adversity in older people. *Quality in Ageing and Older Adults, 13*(3), 197–204.

Gizzi, L., Nielson, J. F., Felici, F., et al. (2012). Motor modules in robot aided walking. *Journal of NeuroEngineering and Rehabilitation, 9*(76). Retrieved from http://www.jneuroengrehab.com/content/9/1/76

Glazier, R. E., & Kling, R. N. (2013). Recent trends in substance abuse among persons with disabilities compared to that of persons without disabilities. *Disability and Health Journal, 6*(2), 107–115.

Gorina, Y., Schappert, S., Bercovitz, A., et al. (2014). Prevalence of incontinence among older Americans. *Vital & Health Statistics*, (36), 1–33.

Gould, L. J., Olney, C. M., Nichols, J. S., et al. (2014). Spinal cord injury survey to determine pressure ulcer vulnerability in the outpatient population. *Medical Hypotheses, 83*(5), 552–558.

Granger, C. V., Albrecht, G. L., & Hamilton, B. B. (1979). Outcomes of comprehensive medical rehabilitation: Measurement by PULSES profile and the Barthel Index. *Archives of Physical Medicine and Rehabilitation, 60*(4), 145–154.

Han, G., & Ceilley, R. (2017). Chronic wound healing: A review of current management and treatments. *Advances in Therapy, 34*(3), 599–610.

Hanga, K., DiNitto, D. M., Wilken, J. P., et al. (2017). A person-centered approach in initial rehabilitation needs assessment: Experiences of persons with disabilities. *ALTER-European Journal of Disability Research/ Revue Européenne de Recherche sur le Handicap, 11*(4), 251–266.

Hanson. L. C., Armstrong, T. D., Green, M. A., et al. (2012). Circles of care: Development and initial evaluation of a peer support model for African Americans with advanced cancer. *Health Education & Behavior, 40*(5), 536–543.

Harvey, D., Foster, M., Quigley, R., et al. (2018). Care transition types across acute, sub-acute and primary care: Case studies of older people with complex conditions and their carers. *Journal of Integrated Care, 26(3), 189–198.*

Harvey, R. F., & Jellinek, H. M. (1981). Functional performance assessment: A program approach. *Archives of Physical Medicine and Rehabilitation, 62*(9), 456–460.

Hyde, Y. M., & Kautz, D. D. (2014). Enhancing health promotion during rehabilitation through information-giving, partnership-building, and teach-back. *Rehabilitation Nursing, 39*(4), 178–182.

Jha, S., Walters, S. J., Bortolami, O., et al. (2018). Impact of pelvic floor muscle training on sexual function of women with urinary incontinence and a comparison of electrical stimulation versus standard treatment (IPSU trial): A randomised controlled trial. *Physiotherapy, 104*(1), 91–97.

Kearney, P. M., & Cronin, N. (2014). Guest editorial: Rehabilitation and disability nursing: Let the cousins marry. *Journal of the Australasian Rehabilitation Nurses Association, 17*(2), 7–9.

Keith, R. A., Granger, C. V., Hamilton, B. B., et al. (1987). The functional independence measure: A new tool for rehabilitation. *Advances in Clinical Rehabilitation, 1*, 6–18.

Knight, E. (2017). A summary of addiction services in a Canadian city: Preliminary results from an internet-based scoping study. *Drug & Alcohol Dependence, 171*, e107.

Knudson-Martin, C., Huenergardt, D., Lafontant, K., et al. (2015). Competencies for addressing gender and power in couple therapy: A socioemotional approach. *Journal of Marital and Family Therapy, 41*(2), 205–220.

Konkolÿ Thege, B., Colman, I., El-Guebaly, N., et al. (2015). Substance-related and behavioural addiction problems: Two surveys of Canadian adults. *Addiction Research & Theory, 23*(1), 34–42.

Liko North America. (2008). *Lift systems for bariatric patients*. Retrieved September 21, 2018, from http://www.liko.com/Documents/en/LiftingNeeds/Bariatric/BariatricLiftsystems_ProdLeafl_EN.pdf

López-Medina, I. M., Gil-García, E., Sánchez-Criado, V., et al. (2016). Patients' experiences of sexual activity following myocardial ischemia. *Clinical Nursing Research, 25*(1), 45–66.

Mahoney, F. I., & Barthel, D. W. (1965). Functional evaluation: The Barthel Index. *Maryland State Medical Journal, 14*, 61–65.

Mandl, M., Halfens, R. J., & Lohrmann, C. (2015). Incontinence care in nursing homes: A cross-sectional study. *Journal of Advanced Nursing, 71*(9), 2142–2152.

McEachern, J., Ahamad, K., Nolan, S., et al. (2016). A needs assessment of the number of comprehensive addiction care physicians required in a Canadian setting. *Journal of Addiction Medicine, 10*(4), 255.

Miller, E. T. (2014). Ripple effect. *Rehabilitation Nursing, 39*(4), 167–168.

Mona, L. R., Cameron, R. P., & Clemency Cordes, C. (2017). Disability culturally competent sexual healthcare. *American Psychologist, 72*(9), 1000–1010.

Mortenson, W. B., Thompson, S. C., Wright, A. L., et al. (2018). A Survey of Canadian occupational therapy practices to prevent pressure injuries among wheelchair users via weight shifting. *Journal of Wound, Ostomy and Continence Nursing, 45*(3), 213–220.

Moyer, R., Ikert, K., Long, K., et al. (2017). The value of preoperative exercise and education for patients undergoing total hip and knee arthroplasty: A systematic review and meta-analysis. *JBJS Reviews, 5*(12), e2.

Newton, K., Wordsworth, M., Allan, A. Y., et al. (2017). Negative pressure wound therapy for traumatic wounds (Protocol). *Cochrane Database of Systematic Reviews*, (1).

Nieuwenhuizen, M. G., de Groot, S., Janssen, T. W., et al. (2014). Canadian Occupational Performance Measure performance scale: Validity and responsiveness in chronic pain. *Journal of Rehabilitation Research and Development, 51*(5), 727–746.

Overmars-Marx, T., Thomése, F., & Meininger, H. (2017). Social inclusion in the neighbourhood and the professional role identity of group home staff members: Views and experiences of staff regarding neighbourhood social inclusion of people with intellectual disabilities. *Society, Health & Vulnerability, 8*(1).

Papadimitriou, C., & Cott, C. (2015). Client-centred practices and work in inpatient rehabilitation teams: Results from four case studies. *Disability and Rehabilitation, 37*(13), 1135–1143.

Price, M., & Lau, F. Y. (2013). Provider connectedness and communication patterns: Extending continuity of care in the context of the circle of care. *BMC Health Services Research, 13*(1), 309.

Roe, B., Flanagan, L., & Maden, M. (2015). Systematic review of systematic reviews for the management of urinary incontinence and promotion of continence using conservative behavioural approaches in older people in care homes. *Journal of Advanced Nursing, 71*(7), 1464–1483.

Salzberg, C. A., Byrne, D. W., Cayten, C. G., et al. (1996). A new pressure ulcer risk assessment scale for individuals with spinal cord injury. *American Journal of Physical Medicine Rehabilitation, 75*:96–104.

Schmidt, A. S. (2013). Outcome trends post discharge from inpatient rehabilitation to the community. *Rehabilitation Nursing, 38*(6), 284–296.

Shahram, S. Z., Bottorff, J. L., Kurtz, D. L., et al. (2017). Understanding the life histories of pregnant-involved young aboriginal women with substance use experiences in three Canadian cities. *Qualitative Health Research, 27*(2), 249–259.

Shoemaker, M. J., Gibson, C., & Saagman, S. (2013). Preoperative exercises in individuals undergoing total knee arthropasty: State of the evidence. *Topics in Geriatric Rehabilitation, 29*(1), 2–16.

Sidani, S., Reeves, S., Hurlock-Chorostecki, C., et al. (2018). Exploring differences in patient-centered practices among healthcare professionals in acute care settings. *Health Communication, 33*(6), 716–723.

SMART Team. (2014). *Smart-e-Pants – A new tool to prevent pressure ulcers*. http://www.smartneuralprostheses.med.ualberta.ca/team-news/smart-e-pants-a-new-tool-to-prevent-pressure-ulcers

Stifter, J., Yao, Y., Lodhi, M. K., et al. (2015). Nurse continuity and hospital-acquired pressure ulcers. *Nursing Research, 64*(5), 361–371.

Stinear, C. M., Byblow, W. D., Ackerley, S. J., et al. (2017). Predicting recovery potential for individual stroke patients increases rehabilitation efficiency. *Stroke, 48*(4), 1011–1019.

Stoekenbroek, R. M., Santema, T. B., Legemate, D. A., et al. (2014). Hyperbaric oxygen for the treatment of diabetic foot ulcers: A systematic review. *European Journal of Vascular and Endovascular Surgery, 47*(6), 647–655.

Strasser, D. C., Burridge, A. B., Falconer, J. A., et al. (2014). Toward spanning the quality chasm: An examination of team functioning measures. *Archives of Physical Medicine and Rehabilitation, 95*(11), 2220–2223.

Supervía, M., Medina-Inojosa, J. R., Yeung, C., et al. (2017). Cardiac rehabilitation for women: A systematic review of barriers and solutions. *Mayo Clinic Proceedings, 92*(4), 565–577.

Thylén, I., & Brännström, M. (2015). Intimate relationships and sexual function in partnered patients in the year before and one year after a myocardial infarction: A longitudinal study. *European Journal of Cardiovascular Nursing, 14*(6), 468–477.

Vowden, K., & Vowden, P. (2017). Wound dressings: Principles and practice. *Surgery (Oxford), 35*(9), 489–494.

Webster, J., Liu, Z., Norman, G., et al. Negative pressure wound therapy for surgical wounds healing by primary closure. *Cochrane Database of*

Systematic Reviews 2019, Issue 3. Art. No.: CD009261. DOI: 10.1002/14651858.CD009261.pub4

White, M. J., Gutierrez, A., Mclaughlin, C., et al. (2013). A pilot for understanding interdisciplinary teams in rehabilitation practice. *Rehabilitation Nursing, 38*(3), 142–152.

Wiggermann, N., Kotowski, S., Davis, K., et al. (2015). The effect of patient migration in bed on torso elevation. *Nursing Research, 64*(3), 221–225.

Wu, J. M., Matthews, C. A., Vaughan, C. P., et al. (2015). Urinary, fecal, and dual incontinence in older US adults. *Journal of the American Geriatrics Society, 63*(5), 947–953.

Yang, S., Lin, C., Lee, Y., et al. (2017). The Canadian occupational performance measure for patients with stroke: A systematic review. *Journal of Physical Therapy Science, 29*(3), 548–555. doi: 10.1589/jpts.29.548.

Resources

American Society of Clinical Oncology: http://www.cancer.net

Assistive Technology Industry Association: http://www.atia.org

Association of Rehabilitation Nurses: http://www.rehabnurse.org

Canadian Association of Rehabilitation Nurses: http://www.oarn.ca/join.php

Canadian Association of Rehabilitation Professionals Inc.: http://www.carpnational.org/

Commission on Accreditation of Rehabilitation Facilities Canada: http://www.carfcanada.org

Functional Independence Measure (FIM) instrument license, Canadian Institute for Health Information: http://www.cihi.ca/nrs

Joint Active System Splints: http://www.jointactivesystems.com

MedicalMarijuana.ca. (2014). *Who is eligible:* http://www.medicalmarijuana.ca/for-patients/who-is-eligible

National Rehabilitation Information Center (NARIC): http://www.naric.com

Ontario Association of Rehabilitation Nurses: http://www.oarn.ca

Rick Hansen Foundation. (2014). *What we do:* https://www.rickhansen.com/

Safe Lifting Portal: https://ohsonline.com/articles/2007/04/safe-lifting-portal-designed-to-back-nurses.aspx

Stroke Engine. (2014): http://www.strokengine.ca

Substance Abuse Resources and Disability Issues: https://medicine.wright.edu/sardi

14 Health Care of the Older Adult

Adapted by Sandra P. Hirst and Rebecca Stares

Learning Objectives

On completion of this chapter, the learner will be able to:

1. Describe the aging Canadian population based on demographic trends.
2. Describe the significance of preventive health care and health promotion for older persons.
3. Compare and contrast the physiologic aspects of aging in older persons with those of middle-aged adults.
4. Identify the common physical and mental health conditions of aging and their effects on the functioning of older persons and their families.
5. Identify the role of the nurse in meeting the health care needs of the older patient.
6. Specify nursing implications related to medication therapy in older people.
7. Examine the concerns of older persons and their families in the home and community, in the acute care setting, and in the long-term care facility.
8. Discuss the potential economic effect on health care of the large aging population in Canada.

Aging, the expected process of time-related change, begins with birth and continues throughout life. Canadians are living longer, and thus the number of older Canadians is the most rapidly expanding segment of the population. Therefore, whenever nurses work with an adult population, they are likely to encounter a majority of older patients. This chapter presents theories of aging, expected age-related changes, health concerns associated with aging, and ways nurses can address the health issues of older persons.

Overview of Aging

Demographics of Aging

Life expectancy, the average number of years that a person can be expected to live, has risen dramatically in the past 100 years. In 2016, there were over three quarters of a million (770,780) people aged 85 and older living in Canada, representing 2.2% of the Canadian population overall (Statistics Canada, 2017b). It is estimated that by the end of 2080, 25% of Canadians will be 65 years of age or older (see https://www.canada.ca/en/employment-social-development/programs/seniors-action-report.html).

As the older population increases, the number of people who live to a very old age is dramatically increasing. The centenarian population (i.e., those aged 100 and older) was the fastest growing age group between 2011 and 2016, by 41.35%, to reach 8,230 people (Statistics Canada, 2017b).

By region, the Atlantic provinces are aging more quickly than other parts of Canada. The 2016 Census reported that Nova Scotia, New Brunswick, Prince Edward Island, and Newfoundland have an average of 19% of their population over 65 years of age compared to 12% in Alberta (Statistics Canada, 2017a). In part, this is a result of having a number of younger people moving out of these provinces to find employment.

Although the majority of older persons enjoy good health, available Statistics Canada (2012a) data identifies that 35.2% of adults 65 years of age and older report a disability. Women are more likely to report disabilities than men. Chronic disease is the major cause of disability; cardiovascular disease, cancer, and respiratory diseases continued to be the three leading causes of death in people 65 years of age and older in Canada (http://www.statcan.gc.ca/pub/82-625-x/2017001/article/14776-eng.htm). See Chapter 12 for a further discussion of chronic illness and disabilities.

Health Status of the Older Adult

The majority of deaths in Canada occur in people 65 years of age and older, and half of these are caused by cancer, heart disease, and stroke. However, due to improvements in the prevention and early detection and treatment of diseases, there has been a noticeable impact on the health of people 65 years of age and older. In the past 50 years, there has been a decline in overall deaths and, specifically, deaths from heart disease and more recently cancer. Between 2009 and 2013, there was a significant decline in all of the top 10 leading causes of death; deaths from heart disease and stroke declined 5.5% and 1.8%, respectively but those from cancer increased 1.1% (Statistics Canada, 2017d).

The majority of older Canadians report their health to be very good or excellent; however, positive health reports declined with advancing age (Public Health Agency of Canada, 2014). In 2014, the proportion of females reporting very good or excellent health decreased with age starting at 35 years. For males, it decreased with age between 35 and 64 years, and then again after age 74. Females had a higher rate of very good or excellent heath compared to men only in the 55 to 64 age groups. For all other ages, there was no significant difference between the sexes (Statistics Canada, 2016). For institutionalized older adults, perceived health is related to mortality. Those older adults reporting a negative self-perceived health were more likely to die than those reporting a positive health status. The trends in health promotion and disease prevention activities, such as improved nutrition, decreased smoking, increased exercise, and early detection and treatment of risk factors such as hypertension and elevated serum cholesterol levels have had a positive impact on health status.

Many chronic conditions commonly found among older people can be managed, limited, and even prevented. In a recent Canadian study, researchers found that physically active older persons reported significantly fewer "general health visits" than their inactive counterparts (Fisher, Harrison, Reeder, et al., 2015). Older people are more likely to maintain good health and functional independence if encouraged to do so and if appropriate community-based support services are available (Levasseur, Généreux, Bruneau, et al., 2015). Nurses are challenged to

Glossary

activities of daily living (ADLs): basic personal care activities; bathing, dressing, grooming, eating, toileting, and transferring

advance directive: a formal, legally endorsed document that provides instructions for care ("living will")

ageism: a bias that discriminates, stigmatizes, and disadvantages older people based solely on their chronologic age

comorbidity: having more than one illness at the same time (e.g., diabetes mellitus and congestive heart failure)

delirium: an acute, confused state that begins with disorientation that if not immediately evaluated and treated, can progress to changes in level of consciousness, irreversible brain damage, and sometimes death

dementia: broad term for a syndrome characterized by a general decline in higher brain functioning, such as reasoning, with a pattern of eventual decline in ability to perform even basic activities of daily living, such as toileting and eating

depression: the most common affective (mood) disorder of old age; results from changes in reuptake of the neurochemical serotonin in response to chronic illness and emotional stresses related to the physical and social changes associated with the aging process

elder abuse: the physical, emotional, or financial harm to an older person by one or more of the individual's children, caregivers, or others; includes neglect

enduring power of attorney: a formal, legally endorsed document that identifies a proxy decision maker who can make decisions if the signer becomes incapacitated

geriatrics: the study of old age that includes the physiology, pathology, diagnosis, and management of the disorders and diseases of older adults

gerontologic/geriatric nursing: that specializes in the nursing process as it relates to the assessment, nursing diagnosis, planning, implementation, and evaluation of older persons in all environments, including acute, intermediate, and skilled care as well as in the community

gerontology: the combined biologic, psychological, and sociologic study of older persons within their environments

instrumental activities of daily living (IADLs): activities that are essential for independent living, such as shopping, cooking, housework, using the telephone, managing medications and finances, and being able to travel by car or public transportation

orientation: a person's ability to recognize who and where he or she is in a time continuum; used to evaluate one's basic cognitive status

polypharmacy: the administration of multiple medications at the same time; common in older persons with several chronic illnesses

presbycusis: the decreased ability to hear high-pitched tones that naturally begins in midlife as a result of irreversible inner ear changes

presbyopia: the decrease in visual accommodation that occurs with advancing age

sundowning: increased confusion at night

promote positive lifelong health behaviours among all populations because the impact of unhealthy behaviours and choices can result in chronic disease.

Nursing Care of the Older Adult

Gerontology, the scientific study of the aging process, is an interprofessional field that draws from the biologic, psychological, and sociologic sciences. **Geriatrics** is the practice (medical or nursing) that focuses on the physiology, pathology, diagnosis, and management of the disorders and diseases of older adults. Because aging is an expected process, care for older adults cannot be limited to one discipline but is best provided through a cooperative effort. An interprofessional approach to providing care combines expertise and resources to provide comprehensive geriatric assessment and intervention. Nurses collaborate with the team to obtain appropriate services for patients and provide a holistic approach to care.

Gerontologic/geriatric nursing is the field of nursing that specializes in the care of older adults. The Gerontological Nursing Competencies and Standards of Practice was originally developed in 1996 by the Canadian Gerontological Nursing Association and revised in 2010. The nurse gerontologist can be either a specialist or a generalist providing comprehensive nursing care to older people by combining the basic nursing process of assessment, diagnosis, planning, implementation, and evaluation with a specialized knowledge of aging. Gerontologic nursing is provided in acute care, skilled and assisted-living facilities, the community, and home settings. The goals of care include promoting and maintaining functional status and helping older adults identify and use their strengths to achieve optimal independence.

Nurses who have obtained the Canadian Nurses Association (CNA's) certification in gerontology have specialized knowledge of the acute and chronic changes specific to older people. The use of gerontologic advanced practice nurses in long-term care has proved to be very effective; when they use current scientific knowledge about clinical issues to collaborate with nursing home staff, significantly less deterioration in the overall health issues of patients occurs (Dellefield, Castle, McGilton, et al., 2015; Kaasalainen, Ploeg, Donald, et al., 2015).

In a 1-year pilot study in Calgary, Alberta, two nurse practitioners (NPs) were assigned to six supportive living sites (Lazar, Bent, Shapkin, et al., 2013). The results included a decrease in the number of patient transfers to emergency departments, an increase in the number of patients who could remain in the facility for a longer period of time, and an increase in the number of palliative patients who could remain in the facility until the end of their lives. As well, the NPs assisted agency staff in increasing their clinical assessment skills. The positive study results has led to eight full-time NP positions providing care for 1,080 patients in 20 sites in Calgary.

Nurses who work in all areas of adult medical–surgical nursing encounter older patients and must be knowledgeable and skilled in meeting their needs. It is important that nurses and caregivers who work with patients who are older understand that aging is not synonymous with disease and that the effects of the aging process alone are not the primary contributors to disability and disease. As research and scientific knowledge increase, it is becoming apparent that aging is a highly complex process.

Functional assessment is a common framework for assessing older people. Age-related changes, as well as additional risk factors such as disease and the effects of medications, can result in a negative impact on function. Assessing the functional consequences of aging and proposing practical interventions help maintain and improve the health of older adults. The goal is to help older people maintain maximum functional level and dignity despite physical, social, and psychological losses. Early intervention can prevent complications of many health conditions and help maximize the quality of life.

Theories of Aging

Aging has been defined chronologically by the passing of time—subjectively, as in how a person feels, and functionally, as in changes in physical or mental capabilities. The many theories of aging attempt to provide a framework in which to understand aging from different perspectives. Each theory is useful to the clinician because it provides a framework and insight into the differences among older patients. In addition to the biologic, developmental, and sociologic theories of aging, Hirst, Lane, and Miller (2015) examined the functional consequences theory, which challenges nurses to consider the effects of expected age-related changes as well as the damage incurred through disease or environmental and behavioural risk factors when planning care. Hirst et al. suggest that nurses can alter the outcome for patients through nursing interventions that address the consequences of these changes. Age-related changes and risk factors may negatively interfere with patient outcomes and actually impair patient activity and quality of life. For example, usual age-related changes in vision may increase sensitivity to glare. Alterations in the environment that reduce glare may enhance patient comfort and safety. In contrast, the development of cataracts, which is not an expected age-related change, also may increase sensitivity to glare. The nurse differentiates between expected age-related changes that cannot be reversed and risk factors that can be modified. Doing so is useful in designing appropriate nursing interventions that have a positive impact on patient outcomes for older adults—most importantly, for quality of life.

Age-Related Changes

The well-being of older people depends on physical, psychosocial, mental, social, economic, and environmental factors. A total assessment includes an evaluation of all major body systems, social and mental status, and the ability of a person to function independently despite having a chronic illness or disability.

Physical Aspects of Aging

As previously mentioned, intrinsic aging (from within the person) refers to those changes caused by the aging process that are genetically programmed and essentially universal within a species. Universality is the major criterion used to distinguish usual aging from pathologic changes

GENETICS IN NURSING PRACTICE

Chart 14-1. Genetics Concepts and the Older Adult

Genetic conditions in the older adult may occur from a specific gene mutation or arise as a result of a genetic predisposition combined with other factors (multifactorial). The following are examples of some adult-onset genetic conditions:

- Colon cancer
- Hemochromatosis
- Huntington's disease
- Polycystic kidney disease
- Alzheimer's disease

The following are some examples of diseases with multifactorial components, which may include a genetic predisposition, in the older adult:

- Diabetes
- Emphysema
- Heart disease

FAMILY HISTORY ASSESSMENT SPECIFIC TO THE OLDER ADULT

- Collect and assess family history on both maternal and paternal sides of the family for three generations.
- Determine whether genetic testing has occurred with other family members.
- Assess for individual and family perceptions and beliefs around topics related to genetics.

PATIENT ASSESSMENT SPECIFIC TO THE OLDER ADULT AND GENETIC ILLNESS

- Assess the older adult patient's knowledge and understanding of genetics, genetic testing, and gene-based therapies.
- Assess the patient's understanding of genetic information and decipher health literacy needs.
- Perform cultural, social, and spiritual assessment.
- Assess patient's communication capacities so that communication strategies about genetics are tailored to their needs and abilities.
- Identify patient's support system.

Management Issues Specific to Genetics and the Older Adult

- Refer for further genetic counselling and evaluation as warranted so that family members can discuss inheritance, risk to other family members, and availability of genetic testing and gene-based interventions.
- Offer appropriate genetic information and resources that take into consideration the older patient's literacy needs.
- Evaluate the older patient's understanding before, during, and after the introduction of genetic information and services.
- Take the time to clearly explain the concepts of genetic testing to older patients and provide written information that reinforces the topic of discussion.
- Participate in the management and coordination of care of older patients with genetic conditions and individuals predisposed to develop or pass on a genetic condition.

Genetics Resources

U.S. Department of Health and Human Services: provides information about health literacy and older adults, www.health.gov/communication/literacy/olderadults/literacy.htm

associated with illness. However, people age quite differently and at different rates, so chronologic age is often less predictive of obvious aging characteristics than other factors, such as one's genetics (see Chart 14-1) and lifestyle. For example, extrinsic aging results from influences outside the person. Air pollution and excessive exposure to sunlight are examples of extrinsic factors that may hasten the aging process and that can be eliminated or reduced.

Cellular and extracellular changes of aging cause a change in physical appearance and a decline in function. Measurable changes in shape and body makeup occur. The body's ability to maintain homeostasis becomes increasingly diminished with cellular aging, and organ systems cannot function at full efficiency because of cellular and tissue deficits. Cells become less able to replace themselves, and they accumulate a pigment known as lipofuscin. A degradation of elastin and collagen causes connective tissue to become stiffer and less elastic. These changes result in diminished capacity for organ function and increased vulnerability to disease and stress.

Table 14-1 summarizes the signs and symptoms of age-related changes in the functioning of body systems. More in-depth information about age-related changes can be found in the chapters pertaining to each organ system. Specifics of diseases, medical and surgical management, as well as nursing interventions are also presented in the related chapters.

Cardiovascular System

Heart disease is the second cause of death in older adults after cancer. Ischemic heart disease is the leading cause of hospitalization, and it is also a major cause of morbidity and mortality among the senior population in Canada. Age-related changes reduce the efficiency of the heart and contribute to decreased compliance of the heart muscle. These changes include myocardial hypertrophy, which changes left ventricular strength and function; fibrosis and stenosis of the valves; and decreased pacemaker cells (Huether & McCance, 2016). As a result, the heart valves become thicker and stiffer, and the heart muscle and arteries lose their elasticity, resulting in a reduced stroke volume. Calcium and fat deposits accumulate within arterial walls, and veins become increasingly tortuous, increasing arterial resistance; this increases the workload of the heart.

It is difficult to differentiate between age- and disease-related changes in cardiovascular function because of the significant influence of behavioural factors on cardiovascular health. When cross-cultural studies are conducted, cardiovascular changes that in the past were thought to be age related do not consistently appear. For example, the higher blood pressure found in older adults in Western societies does not occur in less-developed societies and may be a result of different lifestyle behaviours rather than expected age-related changes (Hirst et al., 2015). Under

TABLE 14-1 Age-Related Changes in Body Systems and Health Promotion Strategies

Changes	Subjective and Objective Findings	Health Promotion Strategies
Cardiovascular System		
Decreased cardiac output; diminished ability to respond to stress; heart rate and stroke volume do not increase with maximum demand; slower heart recovery rate; increased blood pressure	Complaints of fatigue with increased activity Increased heart rate recovery time *Optimal blood pressure:* ≤120/80 mm Hg *Prehypertension:* >120–139/80–89 mm Hg *Hypertension:* ≥140/90 mm Hg	Exercise regularly; pace activities; avoid smoking; eat a low-fat, low-salt diet; participate in stress-reduction activities; check blood pressure regularly; adherence to medications; weight control (body mass index <25 kg/m^2).
Respiratory System		
Increase in residual lung volume; decrease in muscle strength, endurance, and vital capacity; decreased gas exchange and diffusing capacity; decreased cough efficiency	Fatigue and breathlessness with sustained activity; decreased respiratory excursion and chest/lung expansion with less effective exhalation; difficulty coughing up secretions	Exercise regularly; avoid smoking; take adequate fluids to liquefy secretions; receive yearly influenza immunization and pneumonia vaccine at 65 years of age; avoid exposure to upper respiratory tract infections.
Integumentary System		
Decreased subcutaneous fat, interstitial fluid, muscle tone, glandular activity, and sensory receptors, resulting in atrophy and decreased protection against trauma, sun exposure, and temperature extremes; diminished secretion of natural oils and perspiration; capillary fragility	Thin, wrinkled, and dry skin; increased fragility, more easily bruised, and sunburned; complaints of intolerance to heat; prominent bone structure	Limit sun exposure to 10–15 minutes daily for vitamin D (use protective clothing and sunscreen); dress appropriately for temperature; stay hydrated; maintain a safe indoor temperature; take shower rather than hot tub bath if possible; lubricate skin with lotions that contain petroleum or mineral oil.
Reproductive System		
Female: Vaginal narrowing and decreased elasticity; decreased vaginal secretions *Male:* Gradual decline in fertility, less firm testes, and decreased sperm production *Male and female:* Slower sexual response	*Female:* Painful intercourse; vaginal bleeding following intercourse; vaginal itching and irritation; delayed orgasm *Male:* Less firm erection and delayed erection and achievement of orgasm	*Female:* May require vaginal estrogen replacement; gynecology/urology follow-up; use a lubricant with sexual intercourse.
Musculoskeletal System		
Loss of bone density; loss of muscle strength and size; degenerated joint cartilage	Height loss; prone to fractures; kyphosis; back pain; loss of strength, flexibility, and endurance; joint pain	Weight-bearing exercise regularly (three times a week); recommend bone density screening; take calcium and vitamin D supplements as prescribed.
Genitourinary System		
Decrease in detrusor muscle contractility, bladder capacity, flow rate, ability to withhold voiding; increase in residual urine *Male:* Benign prostatic hyperplasia *Female:* Relaxed perineal muscles; detrusor instability leads to urge incontinence; urethral dysfunction (stress urinary incontinence)	Urinary retention; irritative voiding symptoms including frequency, feeling of incomplete bladder emptying, multiple nighttime voiding Urgency/frequency syndrome; decreased "warning time"; drops of urine lost with cough, laugh, position change	Drink adequate fluids but limit drinking in evenings; avoid bladder irritants (e.g., caffeinated beverages, alcohol, artificial sweeteners); do not wait long periods between voiding; empty bladder completely when voiding; wear easily manipulated clothing; consider urologic workup. Women: perform pelvic floor muscle exercises, preferably learned via biofeedback.
Gastrointestinal System		
Decreased sense of thirst, smell, and taste; decreased salivation; difficulty swallowing food; delayed esophageal and gastric emptying; reduced gastrointestinal motility	Risk of dehydration, electrolyte imbalances, and poor nutritional intake; complaints of dry mouth; complaints of fullness, heartburn, and indigestion; constipation, flatulence, and abdominal discomfort; risk for aspiration	Use ice chips, mouthwash; brush, floss, and massage gums daily; receive regular dental care; eat small, frequent meals; sit up while and after eating and avoid heavy activity after eating; limit antacids; eat a high-fibre, low-fat diet; limit laxatives; toilet regularly; drink adequate fluids.
Nervous System		
Decrease in brain volume and cerebral blood flow. Reduced speed in nerve conduction	Slower to respond and react; learning may take longer; increased vulnerability to delirium with illness, anesthesia, even changes in environmental cues such as a room change; increased risk of fainting and falls	Pace teaching; with hospitalization, encourage visitors; enhance sensory stimulation; with sudden confusion, look for cause; encourage slow rising from a resting position and practice fall prevention measures.

TABLE 14-1 Age-Related Changes in Body Systems and Health Promotion Strategies (Continued)

Changes	Subjective and Objective Findings	Health Promotion Strategies
Special Senses		
Vision: Presbyopia; diminished ability to focus on close objects; decreased ability to tolerate glare; pupils become more rigid and lenses more opaque; decreased contrast sensitivity; decrease in aqueous humor	Holds objects far away from face; complains of glare; poor night vision and "dry" eye; difficulty adjusting to changes in light intensity; decreased ability to distinguish colours	Wear eyeglasses and use sunglasses outdoors; avoid abrupt changes from dark to light; use adequate indoor lighting with area lights and nightlights; use large-print books; use magnifier for reading; avoid night driving; use contrasting colours for colour coding; avoid glare of shiny surfaces and direct sunlight.
Hearing: Presbycusis; decreased ability to hear high-frequency sounds; tympanic membrane thinning and loss of resiliency; difficulty with sound discrimination especially in noisy environment	Gives inappropriate responses; asks people to repeat words; strains forward to hear; can result in social isolation and increases vulnerability for delirium during hospitalization	Recommend a hearing examination; reduce background noise; face person; enunciate clearly; speak with a low-pitched voice; use nonverbal cues; rephrase questions.
Taste and smell: Decreased ability to taste and smell	Decreased recognition of familiar smells including recognizing spoiled food or a gas stove left on; decreased enjoyment of food; uses excessive sugar and salt	Encourage use of lemon, spices, herbs; recommend smoking cessation.

Adapted from Carpenter, H. (2015). Summer sun safety. *American Nurse Today, 10*(7), 46 and Oster, K. A., & Oster, C. A. (2015). Special needs population: Care of the geriatric patient population in the perioperative setting. *AORN Journal, 101*(4), 444–456.

usual circumstances, the cardiovascular system can adapt to age-related changes, and an older person is unaware of any significant decline in cardiovascular performance. However, when challenged, the cardiovascular system of an older person is less efficient under conditions of stress and exercise and when life-sustaining activities are needed.

Careful assessment of older people is necessary because they often present with different symptoms than those seen in younger patients. Older people are more likely to have dyspnea or neurologic symptoms associated with heart disease, and they may experience mental status changes or report vague symptoms such as fatigue, nausea, and syncope. Rather than the typical substernal chest pain associated with myocardial ischemia, older patients may report burning or sharp pain or discomfort in an area of the upper body. Complicating the assessment is the fact that many older patients have more than one underlying disease. When a patient reports symptoms related to digestion and breathing and upper extremity pain, cardiac disease must be considered. The absence of chest pain in an older patient is not a reliable indicator of the absence of heart disease.

Hypotension may be a concern. The risk of orthostatic and postprandial hypotension increases significantly after 75 years of age (Hirst et al., 2015). A patient experiencing hypotension should be counselled to rise slowly (from a lying, to a sitting, to a standing position), to avoid straining when having a bowel movement, and to consider having five or six small meals each day, rather than three, to minimize the hypotension that can occur after a large meal. Extremes in temperature, including hot showers and whirlpool baths, should be avoided.

Respiratory System

The respiratory system is the one system that seems to be the most able to compensate for the functional changes of aging. In general, healthy, nonsmoking, older adults show very little decline in respiratory function; however, there are substantial individual variations. The age-related changes that do occur are subtle and gradual, and healthy older adults are able to compensate for these changes. Diminished respiratory efficiency as well as reduced maximal inspiratory and expiratory force may occur as a result of calcification and weakening of the muscles of the chest wall. Lung mass decreases, and residual volume increases (Huether & McCance, 2016).

Conditions of stress, such as illness, may increase the demand for oxygen and affect the overall function of other systems. Like cardiovascular diseases, respiratory diseases manifest more subtly in older adults than in younger adults and do not necessarily follow the typical pattern of cough, chills, and fever. Older adults may exhibit headache, weakness, lethargy, anorexia, dehydration, and mental status changes (Hirst et al., 2015).

Smoking is the most significant risk factor for respiratory and other diseases. Therefore, a major focus of health promotion activities should be on smoking cessation and avoidance of environmental smoke. Pneumonia and influenza together are the eighth leading cause of death in people older than 65 years of age (Statistics Canada, 2017d). Education to promote the use of recommended vaccines is an essential nursing intervention. A pneumococcal vaccine that prevents 85% to 90% of all cases of pneumonia is available, and it is effective in preventing 75% of cases in people older than 65 years of age. Influenza vaccination is less effective in preventing influenza in the older adult than in the younger population, but it reduces influenza-related deaths, hospitalizations, and other complications (Hirst et al., 2015; National Advisory Committee on Immunization [NACI], 2016).

Activities that help older people maintain adequate respiratory function include regular exercise, appropriate fluid intake, pneumococcal vaccination, yearly influenza immunizations, and avoidance of people who are ill. Hospitalized older persons should be frequently reminded to cough and take deep breaths, particularly postoperatively, because their decreased lung capacity and decreased cough efficiency predispose them to atelectasis and respiratory infections.

Integumentary System

The functions of the skin include protection, temperature regulation, sensation, and excretion. With aging, changes occur that affect the function and appearance of the skin. There is a decrease of epidermal proliferation, and the dermis becomes thinner. Elastic fibres are reduced in number, and collagen becomes stiffer. Subcutaneous fat diminishes, particularly in the extremities, but gradually increases in other areas, such as the abdomen (men) and thighs (women), leading to an overall increase in body fat in older people (Hirst et al., 2015). Decreased numbers of capillaries in the skin result in diminished blood supply. These changes cause a loss of resiliency and wrinkling and sagging of the skin. The skin becomes drier and more susceptible to burns, injury, and infection. Hair pigmentation may change and balding may occur; genetic factors strongly influence these changes. These changes in the integument reduce tolerance to temperature extremes and sun exposure.

Lifestyle practices are likely to have a large impact on skin changes. Therefore, strategies to promote healthy skin function include not smoking, avoiding exposure to the sun, using a sun protection factor (SPF) of 30 or higher, using emollient skin cream containing petrolatum or mineral oil, avoiding hot soaks in the bathtub, and maintaining optimal nutrition and hydration. Older adults should be encouraged to have any changes in the skin examined, because early detection and treatment of precancerous or cancerous lesions are essential for the best outcome.

Reproductive System

Sexuality is no longer considered pertinent only to the young. However, research about sexuality among older adults, especially in women, has not been extensive. Ovarian production of estrogen and progesterone ceases with menopause. Changes occurring in the female reproductive system include thinning of the vaginal wall, along with a shortening of the vagina and a loss of elasticity; decreased vaginal secretions, resulting in vaginal dryness, itching, and decreased acidity; involution (atrophy) of the uterus and ovaries; and decreased pubococcygeal muscle tone, resulting in a relaxed vagina and perineum. Without the use of water-soluble lubricants, these changes may contribute to vaginal bleeding and painful intercourse.

In older men, the testes become less firm but men up to 90 years of age continue to produce viable sperm. In about the sixth decade of life, production of testosterone begins to diminish (Handelsman, Sikaris, & Ly, 2016). Decreased libido and erectile dysfunction may develop but are more likely to be associated with factors other than age-related changes. These risk factors include cardiovascular disease; neurologic disorders; diabetes; respiratory disease; pain; and medications such as vasodilators, antihypertensive agents, and tricyclic antidepressants.

In both older men and women, it may take longer to become sexually aroused, longer to complete intercourse, and longer before sexual arousal can occur again. Although a less intense response to sexual stimulation and a decline in sexual activity occurs with increasing age, sexual desire does not disappear. Men may experience a decline in sexual function related to health conditions or interference from medications. Women may lose their partner; the absence of a partner is often the primary factor causing lack of sexual activity. Many couples are unaware of the causes of decreased libido or erectile dysfunction and are often reluctant to discuss decreased sexual function. There are many methods of improving the quality of sexual interactions such as through medication, but the assessment and communication require sensitivity and expert knowledge in the field of sexual dysfunction. If sexual dysfunction is present, referral to a gynecologist, urologist, or sex therapist may be warranted.

Genitourinary System

The genitourinary system continues to function adequately in older people, although there is a decrease in kidney mass, primarily because of a loss of nephrons. However, there is a decline in the glomerular filtration rate with age (Cohen, Nardi, Krause, et al., 2014). Changes in renal function may be due to a combination of aging and pathologic conditions such as hypertension. The changes most commonly seen include a decreased filtration rate, diminished tubular function with less efficiency in resorbing and concentrating the urine, and a slower restoration of acid–base balance in response to stress. In addition, older adults who take medications may experience serious consequences due to decline in renal function because of impaired absorption, decreased ability to maintain fluid and electrolyte balance, and decreased ability to concentrate urine.

Certain genitourinary disorders are more common in older adults than in the general population. At least one in four middle-aged or older women in Canada suffers from urinary incontinence, while fewer men have this disorder. Unfortunately, this condition is often mistakenly viewed as an expected consequence of aging. Costly and embarrassing, it should be evaluated, because in many cases it is reversible or can be treated (Canadian Continence Foundation, 2014). Urinary incontinence is discussed in more detail in Chapter 45. Benign prostatic hyperplasia (enlarged prostate gland), a common finding in older men, causes a gradual increase in urine retention and overflow incontinence.

Changes in the urinary tract increase the susceptibility to urinary tract infections. Adequate consumption of fluids and more frequent voiding are important nursing interventions that reduce the risk of bladder infections and also help decrease urinary incontinence.

Gastrointestinal System

Digestion of food is less influenced by age-related changes than by the risk of poor nutrition. Older people can adjust to the age-related changes but may have difficulty purchasing, preparing, and enjoying their meals. The sense of smell diminishes as a result of neurologic changes and environmental factors such as due to smoking, medications, and vitamin B_{12} deficiency. The ability to recognize sweet, sour, bitter, or salty foods diminishes over time, altering satisfaction with food. Salivary flow does not decrease in healthy adults, but about 30% of older people may experience a dry mouth as a result of medications and diseases (Hirst et al., 2015). Difficulties with chewing and swallowing are generally associated with disease.

Experts disagree on the extent of gastric changes that occur as a result of normal aging. However, there does appear to be a modest slowing of gastric motility, which results in delayed emptying of stomach contents and early satiety (feeling of fullness). Diminished secretion of gastric acid and pepsin, seemingly the result of pathologic conditions rather than normal aging, reduces the absorption of iron, calcium, and vitamin B_{12}. Absorption of nutrients in the small intestine, particularly calcium and vitamin D, appears to diminish with age. Functions of the liver, gallbladder, and pancreas are generally maintained, although absorption and tolerance to fat may decrease. The incidence of gallstones and common bile duct stones increases progressively with advancing years.

Difficulty in swallowing, or dysphagia, increases with age and is a major health care concern in older patients. Aging alters some aspects of the swallowing function, and it is a frequent complication of stroke and a significant risk factor for development of pneumonia. This serious condition can be life threatening. It is caused by interruption or dysfunction of neural pathways, such as can occur with a stroke. Dysphagia may also result from dysfunction of the striated and smooth muscles of the gastrointestinal tract in patients with Parkinson's disease and in patients with disorders such as multiple sclerosis (MS), poliomyelitis, and amyotrophic lateral sclerosis (ALS) (i.e., Lou Gehrig's disease). Aspiration of food or fluid is the most serious complication and can occur in the absence of coughing or choking.

Constipation is a common pathologic condition that affects as many as 80% of institutionalized and 45% of community-dwelling older people (Hirst et al., 2015). Symptoms of mild constipation are abdominal discomfort and flatulence, while more serious constipation leads to fecal impaction that contributes to diarrhea around the impaction, fecal incontinence, and obstruction. Predisposing factors for constipation include lack of dietary bulk, prolonged use of laxatives, and use of some medications, inactivity, insufficient fluid intake, and excessive dietary fat. Ignoring the urge to defecate may also be a contributing factor.

Practices that promote gastrointestinal health include regular toothbrushing and flossing; receiving regular dental care; eating small, frequent meals; avoiding heavy activity after eating; eating a high-fibre, low-fat diet; drinking enough fluids; and avoiding the use of laxatives and antacids. Understanding that there is a direct correlation between loss of smell and taste perception and food intake helps caregivers intervene to maintain older patients' nutritional health.

Nutritional Health

The social, psychological, and physiologic functions of eating influence the dietary habits of older people. Increasing age alters nutrient requirements; the older adult requires fewer calories and a more nutrient-rich, healthy diet in response to alterations in body mass and a more sedentary lifestyle. Recommendations include reducing fat intake while consuming sufficient protein, vitamins, minerals, and dietary fibre for health and disease prevention. Decreased physical activity and a slower metabolic rate reduce the number of calories needed by older adults to maintain an ideal weight. As previously stated, age-related changes that alter pleasure in eating include a decrease in taste and smell. Older people are likely to maintain a taste for sweetness but require more sugar to achieve a sweet flavour. They also may lose the ability to differentiate sour, salty, and bitter tastes. Apathy, immobility, **depression**, loneliness, poverty, inadequate knowledge, and poor oral health also contribute to suboptimal nutrient intake. Budgetary constraints and physical limitations may interfere with food shopping and meal preparation.

Health promotion includes encouraging a varied diet that is low in sodium and saturated fats and high in vegetables, fruits, and fish. Education regarding healthy foods versus foods with inadequate nutrients is helpful. The incidence of obesity in Canadians as old as 80 years of age has reached epidemic proportions, and this greatly increases the incidence of chronic illnesses such as diabetes and cardiovascular diseases.

No more than 30% of dietary calories should be consumed as fat. Protein intake may need to be increased in later adulthood to maintain adequate nitrogen equilibrium (Munro, Gersovitz, & Young, 2018). Carbohydrates, a major source of energy, should supply 55% to 60% of the daily calories. Simple sugars should be avoided, while complex carbohydrates should be encouraged. Potatoes, whole grains, brown rice, and fruit are sources of minerals, vitamins, and fibre and should be encouraged. Drinking 8 to 10 eight-ounce glasses of water per day is recommended unless contraindicated by a medical condition. A multivitamin each day helps meet daily nutritional needs. Adults older than 70 years of age should have a daily calcium intake to 1,200 mg, and 800 IU of vitamin D to maintain bone heath (Health Canada, 2012).

Undernutrition may also be an issue for older adults; as many as 40% to 60% of hospitalized and 40% to 85% of nursing home patients are malnourished. A recent unintentional weight loss may be a result of an illness or other factors, such as depression, that may have serious consequences and affect a person's ability to maintain health and fight illness. Many people are unaware of dietary deficits. Nurses are in an ideal position to identify nutritional issues among their patients and to work within the patient's own framework of knowledge of his or her health status to improve health behaviours. The Canadian Guidelines for Body Weight Classification in Adults is an update of the weight classification system that has been in use in Canada since 1988 (Health Canada, 2015). The system uses two measures to indicate health risks: the body mass index (BMI) and the waist circumference (WC). Chapter 5 provides more information on nutritional assessment.

Sleep

Sleep disturbances affect more than 50% of adults 65 years of age or older. Older people tend to take longer to fall asleep, awaken more easily and frequently, and spend less time in deep sleep. Consequently, they may feel that their sleep is less satisfactory (Hirst et al., 2015). Although older adults require as much sleep as younger people, they may experience variations in their usual sleep–wake

NURSING RESEARCH PROFILE

Chart 14-2. Structured Exercise

Ng, T. K., Kwan, R. L. C., Lo, S. K., et al. (2017). A tailor-made exercise program for improving balance and mobility in older adults with type 2 diabetes. *Journal of Gerontological Nursing, 44*(2), 41–48.

Purpose

The researchers examined the effectiveness of an exercise program designed for improving postural control and mobility in older adults with type 2 diabetes.

Design

Ninety-three older adults aged 65 years plus, who were diagnosed with type 2 diabetes and who could walk unaided, were recruited. They were divided into two groups. The intervention group received exercise training focused on ankle strengthening and mobility twice a week for 10 weeks. The control group did not participate in an exercise program.

Findings

Exercise training focusing on the ankle is effective in enhancing the postural stability of older adults with type 2 diabetes and can also be effective in improving single-leg standing balance and mobility.

Nursing Implications

Nurses should consider this intervention to reduce the risk of falls among older adults with diabetes.

cycles, and the lack of quality sleep at night often creates the need for napping during the day. Older people are more likely to awaken because of factors such as noise, pain, or nocturia.

The incidence of sleep apnea (a sleep disorder characterized by brief periods in which respirations are absent) increases with age. Having insomnia symptoms and a sleep-related disorder (snoring, choking, or pauses in breathing) is associated with significantly impaired daytime functioning and longer psychomotor reaction times compared with having either condition (Canadian Thoracic Association, 2014). Sleep apnea is discussed in more detail in Chapter 42.

The nurse often observes patients while they are sleeping and can identify problems. The nurse also can recommend sleep hygiene behaviours such as avoiding use of the bed for activities other than sleeping (or sex), maintaining a consistent bedtime routine, avoiding or limiting daytime napping, limiting alcohol intake to one or two drinks a day, and avoiding caffeine and nicotine after noon.

Musculoskeletal System

Intact musculoskeletal and neurologic systems are essential for the maintenance of safe mobility, performance of **activities of daily living (ADLs)** (basic personal care activities), and **instrumental activities of daily living (IADLs)** (activities that are essential for independent living), thus allowing older adults to remain safe and live independently in the community. Age-related changes that affect mobility include alterations in bone remodeling, leading to decreased bone density, loss of muscle mass, deterioration of muscle fibres and cell membranes, and degeneration in the function and efficiency of joints. These factors are discussed in detail in Unit 15.

Without exercise, a gradual, progressive decrease in bone mass begins before 40 years of age. The cartilage of joints also progressively deteriorates in middle age. Degenerative joint disease is found in most adults older than 70 years of age, and weight-bearing joint and back pain is a common concern. Excessive loss of bone density results in osteoporosis, which leads to potentially life-altering hip and vertebral fractures. Osteoporosis is preventable.

The axiom "use it or lose it" is very relevant to the physical capacity of older adults. Nurses play an important role by encouraging older adults to participate in a regular exercise program (Chart 14-2). The benefits of regular exercise cannot be overstated. Aerobic exercises are the foundation of programs of cardiovascular conditioning, but resistance and strength training as well as flexibility exercises are essential components of an exercise program. Even late in life, in adults who are very old and frail, it is generally believed that exercise has the benefits of increasing strength, aerobic capacity, flexibility, and balance.

Nervous System

Homeostasis is difficult to maintain with aging, but most older people function adequately and retain their cognitive and intellectual abilities in the absence of pathologic changes. However, usual aging changes in the nervous system can affect all parts of the body.

The structure and function of the nervous system change with advanced age, and a reduction in cerebral blood flow accompanies nervous system changes. Reports of the loss of nerve cells are highly varied with variations in neuron loss in different parts of the brain (Huether & McCance, 2016). The loss of nerve cells contributes to a progressive loss of brain mass.

In addition, the synthesis and metabolism of the major neurotransmitters are also reduced. Because nerve impulses are conducted more slowly, older people take longer to respond and react. The autonomic nervous system performs less efficiently, and postural hypotension, which causes people to lose consciousness or feel lightheaded when standing up quickly, may occur. Neurologic changes can affect gait and balance, which may interfere with mobility and safety. Nurses advise older people to allow a longer time to respond to a stimulus and to move more deliberately.

This slowed reaction time puts older people at risk for falls and injuries, as well as driving errors. Even though older adults spend less time driving compared with younger people, older people are just as likely to be involved in motor vehicle crashes that result in serious injury or death. Older people who are driving unsafely should receive a driving fitness evaluation (Hirst et al.,

2015). This is often administered by an occupational therapist in conjunction with a neuropsychologist, who conducts more detailed cognitive testing.

Mental function is threatened by physical or emotional stresses. A sudden onset of confusion may be the first symptom of an infection or change in physical condition (e.g., pneumonia, urinary tract infection, medication interactions, and dehydration).

Sensory System

People interact with the world through their senses. Sensory losses associated with old age affect all sensory organs, and it can be devastating not to be able to see to read or watch television, hear conversation well enough to communicate, or discriminate taste well enough to enjoy food. Audiometry results from the 2012–2015 Canadian Health Measures Survey (Statistics Canada, 2016) indicated that for adults from 20 to 79 years, 40% experienced at last a slight hearing loss in one or both ears. For those between 60 and 79 years, 78% reported a hearing loss. Men (47%) were significantly more likely to have hearing loss compared with females (32%). An uncompensated alteration in a sensory loss negatively affects the functional ability and quality of life of the older person.

Sensory Loss Versus Sensory Deprivation

Sensory loss can often be compensated for by assistive devices such as glasses and hearing aids. In contrast, sensory deprivation is the absence of stimuli in the environment or the inability to interpret existing stimuli (perhaps as a result of a sensory loss). Sensory deprivation can lead to boredom, confusion, irritability, disorientation, and anxiety. A decline in sensory input can mimic a decline in cognition that is in fact not present. Meaningful sensory stimulation provided to the older person is often helpful in correcting this problem. In some situations, one sense can substitute for another in observing and interpreting stimuli. Nurses can enhance sensory stimulation in the environment with colours, pictures, textures, tastes, smells, and sounds. The stimuli are most meaningful if they are interpreted to older people and if the stimuli are changed often. People who are cognitively impaired tend to respond well to touch and to familiar music.

Vision

As new cells form on the outside surface of the lens of the eye, the older central cells accumulate and become yellow, rigid, dense, and cloudy, leaving only the outer portion of the lens elastic enough to change shape (accommodate) and focus at near and far distances. As the lens becomes less flexible, the near point of focus gets farther away. This condition, **presbyopia**, usually begins in the fifth decade of life and requires the person to wear reading glasses to magnify objects. In addition, the yellowing, cloudy lens causes light to scatter and make the older person sensitive to glare. The ability to differentiate the colour blue from green decreases. The pupil dilates slowly and less completely because of increased stiffness of the muscles of the iris, so the older person takes more time to adjust when going to and from light and dark settings and needs brighter light for close vision. Pathologic visual conditions are not an expected part of aging, but the incidence of eye diseases (most commonly cataracts, glaucoma, diabetic retinopathy, and age-related macular degeneration) increases in older people.

Age-related macular degeneration is the primary cause of vision loss in older adults. More than 25% of people older than 75 years of age have some signs of this disease, and 6% to 8% have advanced disease associated with severe vision loss. Macular degeneration does not affect peripheral vision, which means that it does not cause blindness. However, it affects central vision, colour perception, and fine detail, greatly affecting common visual skills such as reading, driving, and seeing faces. Risk factors include sunlight exposure, cigarette smoking, and heredity, and people with fair skin and blue eyes may be at increased risk. Sunglasses and hats with visors provide some protection, and stopping smoking is paramount in preventing the disease. Although there is no definitive treatment and no cure that restores vision, several treatment options are available, depending on factors such as the location of the abnormal blood vessels. Anti-VEGF treatments are a group of medicines which reduce new blood vessel growth or edema (swelling) and have been found to be beneficial for the wet type of acute macular degeneration (Tolentino, Dennrick, John, et al., 2015). The earlier this condition is diagnosed, the greater the chances of preserving sight. More information on altered vision can be found in Chapter 60.

Hearing

Auditory changes begin to be noticed at about 40 years of age. Environmental factors, such as exposure to noise, medications, and infections, as well as genetics, may contribute to hearing loss as much as age-related changes. **Presbycusis** is a gradual, sensorineural loss that progresses from the loss of the ability to hear high-frequency tones to a generalized loss of hearing. It is attributed to irreversible inner ear changes. Older people often cannot follow conversation because tones of high-frequency consonants (the sounds *f, s, th, ch, sh, b, t, p*) all sound alike. Hearing loss may cause older people to respond inappropriately, misunderstand conversation, and avoid social interaction. This behaviour may be erroneously interpreted as confusion. Wax buildup or other correctable problems may also be responsible for hearing difficulties. A properly prescribed and fitted hearing aid may be useful in reducing some types of hearing deficits. Chapter 61 discusses alterations in hearing.

Taste and Smell

Of the four basic tastes (sweet, sour, salty, and bitter), sweet tastes are particularly dulled in older people. Blunted taste may contribute to the preference for salty, highly seasoned foods, but herbs, onions, garlic, and lemon can be used as substitutes for salt to flavour food.

Changes in the sense of smell are related to cell loss in the nasal passages and in the olfactory bulb in the brain. Environmental factors such as long-term exposure to toxins (e.g., dust, pollen, smoke) contribute to cellular damage.

Psychosocial Aspects of Aging

Successful psychological aging is reflected in the ability of older people to adapt to physical, social, and emotional losses and to achieve life satisfaction. Because changes in life patterns are inevitable over a lifetime, older people need resiliency and coping skills when confronting stresses and change. A positive self-image enhances risk taking and participation in new, untested roles.

Although attitudes toward older people differ in ethnic subcultures, a subtle theme of **ageism**—prejudice or discrimination against older people—predominates in our society, and many myths surround aging. Ageism is based on stereotypes, simplified and often untrue beliefs that reinforce society's negative image of older people. Although older people make up an extremely heterogeneous and increasingly a racially and ethnically diverse group, negative stereotypes are attributed to all older people.

Fear of aging and the inability of many to confront their own aging process may trigger ageist beliefs. Retirement and perceived nonproductivity are also responsible for negative feelings, because a younger working person may falsely see older people as not contributing to society, as draining economic resources, and may actually feel that they are in competition with children for resources. Concern about the large numbers of older people leaving the workforce (baby boomers began to turn age 65 in 2011) is fuelling this debate.

Many negative images are so common in society that older people themselves often believe and perpetuate them. An understanding of the aging process and respect for each person as an individual can dispel the myths of aging. If older adults are treated with dignity and encouraged to maintain autonomy, the quality of their lives will improve.

Stress and Coping in the Older Adult

Coping patterns and the ability to adapt to stress develop over the course of a lifetime and remain consistent later in life. Experiencing success in younger adulthood helps a person develop a positive self-image that remains solid through old age. A person's abilities to adapt to change, make decisions, and respond predictably are also determined by past experiences. A flexible, well-functioning person will probably continue as such. However, losses may accumulate within a short period of time and may become overwhelming. The older person often has fewer choices and diminished resources to deal with stressful events. Common stressors of old age include usual aging changes that impair physical function, activities, and appearance; disabilities from injury or chronic illness; social and environmental losses related to loss of income and decreased ability to perform previous roles and activities; and the deaths of significant others. Many older adults rely strongly on their spiritual beliefs for comfort during stressful times.

Living Arrangements

Most older people want to remain in their own homes; in fact, they function best in their own environment. The family home and familiar community may have strong emotional significance for them, and this should not be ignored. However, with advanced age and increasing disability, adjustments to the environment may be required to allow older adults to remain in their own homes or apartments. Additional family support or more formal support such as Meals on Wheels or transportation services may be necessary to compensate for declining function and mobility.

Many older people have adequate financial resources and good health even until very late in life; therefore, they have many housing options. About one third (33.0%) of older women were living alone in 2016, compared with 17.5% of men. The proportion of older women living alone decreased compared to 2001 (38.3%), whereas, the percentage of older women living in a couple relationship (married or common-law) increased from 44.4% in 2001 to 51.4% in 2016. This trend was especially evident among women aged 80 and older as the proportion of those living in as a couple increased from 19.9% in 2001 to 27.6% in 2016. Older women are more likely to live alone than older men. They have a higher life expectancy and they also tend to marry men older than themselves. As a result, they are more often widowed than men. However, since the 1970s, men have seen larger gains in their life expectancy and this has led to couples living together longer (Statistics Canada, 2017).

Older people tend to relocate in response to changes in their lives such as retirement or widowhood, a significant deterioration in health, or disability. According to the 2016 Census, 6.8% of Canadians aged 65 years and older were living in a nursing home or residence for senior citizens; this proportion increases to 30.0% among those 85 years and older (Garner, Tanuseputro, Manuel, et al., 2018). The type of housing they choose depends on their reason for moving (Canadian Mortgage and Housing Corporation, 2015). With increasing disability and illness, older people may move to retirement facilities or assisted-living communities that provide some support such as meals, transportation, and housekeeping but allow them to live somewhat independently. If they develop a serious illness or disability and can no longer live independently or semi-independently, they may need to move to a setting where additional support is available. Older people may move in with a relative or to a nursing home or an assisted-living facility near a child's home. However, the likelihood of living in a nursing home or seniors' residence is lower for individuals who were not born in Canada.

Sometimes, older adults or couples move in with adult children. This can be a rewarding experience as the children, their parents, and the grandchildren interact and share household responsibilities (Fig. 14-1). It can also be stressful, depending on family dynamics. Adult children and their older parents may choose to pool their financial resources by moving into a house that has an attached "in-law suite." This arrangement provides security for the older adult and privacy for both families.

Unfortunately, many older people and their adult children make housing decisions in times of crisis, such as during a serious illness or after the death of a spouse. Older people and their families often are unaware of all of the ramifications of shared housing and assuming care for an increasingly dependent person. Families can be helped by anticipatory guidance and long-term planning before a crisis occurs. Older adults should participate in decisions that affect them as much as possible.

Continuing Care Retirement Communities

Continuing care retirement communities (CCRCs) provide three levels of living arrangements and care and are becoming more popular. CCRCs consist of independent single–dwelling houses or apartments for people who can manage all of their day-to-day needs; assisted-living

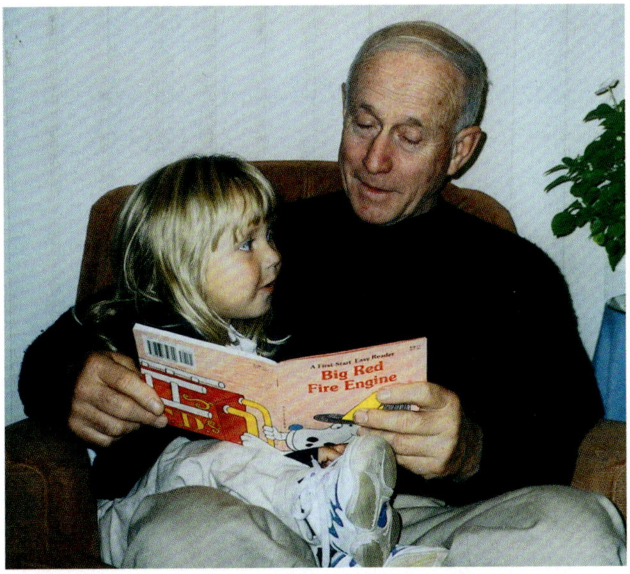

FIGURE 14-1. Families are an important source of psychosocial and physical support for older people and youngsters alike. Caring interaction among grandchildren, grandparents, and other family members typically contributes to the health of all.

apartments for those who need limited assistance with their daily living needs; and skilled nursing services when continuous nursing assistance is required. CCRCs usually contract for a large down payment before the resident moves into the community. This payment gives a person or couple the option of residing in the same community from the time of total independence through the need for assisted or skilled nursing care. Decisions about living arrangements and health care can be made before any decline in health status occurs. CCRCs also provide continuity at a time in an older adult's life when many other factors, such as health status, income, and availability of friends and family members, may be changing.

Assisted-Living Facilities

Assisted-living facilities are an option when an older person's physical or cognitive changes necessitate at least minimal supervision or assistance. Assisted living allows for a degree of independence while providing minimal nursing assistance with administration of medication, assistance with ADLs, or other chronic health care needs. Other services, such as laundry, cleaning, and meals, may also be included.

Long-Term Care Facilities

Many types of nursing homes, nursing facilities, or long-term care facilities offer continuous nursing care. Contrary to the myth of family abandonment and the fear of "ending up in a nursing home," the actual admission age has increased to 85 years or more for most residents (Statistics Canada, 2018). However, the actual number of older people who reside in long-term care facilities has risen due to the large increase in the aging population and the use of nursing homes today for short-term rehabilitation.

In Canada, long-term care is not included under the *Canada Health Act* therefore creating no uniformity of access across the country. In most provinces, long-term care is partly subsidized publicly after an income test is completed and personal contribution is determined. Services are provided by a mix of public (government-owned), non-profit, and private for-profit organizations. As governments face rising health costs, many provinces contract care to for-profit facilities (Canadian Foundation for Health Care Improvement, 2014). Some adults choose to have long-term care insurance as a means of paying, at least in part, for the cost of long-term services should they become necessary. For older people who are living in nursing homes and who are medically stable, even though they may have multiple chronic and debilitating health issues, costs are primarily paid out of pocket by the patient. Family members are not responsible for nursing home costs. When a person's financial resources become exhausted as a result of prolonged nursing home care, the patient may apply for public subsidy.

An increasing number of skilled nursing facilities offer subacute care. This area of the facility offers a high level of nursing care that may either avoid the need for a resident to be transferred to a hospital from the nursing home or allow a hospitalized patient to be transferred back to the nursing facility sooner.

The Role of the Family

Planning for care and understanding the psychosocial issues confronting older people must be accomplished within the context of the family. If dependency needs occur, the spouse often assumes the role of primary caregiver. In the absence of a surviving spouse, an adult child usually assumes caregiver responsibilities and may eventually need help in providing or arranging for care and support.

Two common myths in Canadian society are that adult children and their aged parents are socially alienated, and that adult children abandon their parents when health and other dependency problems arise. In reality, the family has been and continues to be an important source of support for older people; similarly, older family members provide a great deal of support to younger family members.

Although adult children are not financially responsible for their older parents, social attitudes and cultural values often dictate that adult children should provide services and assume the burden of care if their aged parents cannot care for themselves. Among older adults who need assistance, more than 80% received some or all of their care from informal caregivers (Canadian Institute for Health Information [CIHI], 2014a).

Caregiving, which may continue for many years, can become a source of family stress. For prolonged periods, it is not uncommon for caregivers to neglect their own emotional and health needs. In addition, because many people tend to have children later in life, they may face the competing demands of caring for their aging parents while caring for their own dependent children. Furthermore, because of smaller family sizes, fewer numbers of siblings are available to help with parental care issues. If community agencies or adult children cannot provide care, elders are at high risk for institutionalization.

Cognitive Aspects of Aging

Cognition can be affected by many variables, including sensory impairment, physiologic health, environment, and psychosocial influences. Older adults may experience temporary changes in cognitive function when hospitalized or admitted to skilled nursing facilities, rehabilitation centres, or long-term care facilities. These changes are related to differences in the environment or in medical therapy or to alteration in role performance. A commonly used assessment tool is the Mini-Mental State Examination (MMSE).

Intelligence

When intelligence test scores from people of all ages are compared, test scores for older adults show a progressive decline beginning in midlife. However, research has shown that environment and health have a considerable influence on scores, and that certain types of intelligence (e.g., spatial perceptions and retention of nonintellectual information) decline, whereas others (e.g., problem-solving ability based on past experiences, verbal comprehension, mathematical ability) do not. Cardiovascular health, a stimulating environment, high levels of education, occupational status, and income all appear to have a positive effect on intelligence scores in later life.

Learning and Memory

Many factors affect the ability of older people to learn and remember and to perform well in testing situations. Older adults who have higher levels of education, good sensory function, good nutrition, and jobs that require complex problem-solving skills continue to demonstrate intelligence, memory, and the capacity for learning. Part of the challenge in testing older adults is determining what is actually being tested (e.g., speed of response) and whether the test results are indicative of an expected age-related change, a sensory deficit, or poor health. However, age differences continue to emerge even with untimed tests and when the tests are controlled for variations in motor and sensory function. In general, there is a decline in fluid intelligence, the biologically determined intelligence used for flexibility in thinking and problem solving. Crystallized intelligence that is gained through education and lifelong experiences (e.g., verbal skills) remains intact. This is termed the *classic aging pattern of intelligence*. Despite these slight declines, many older people continue to learn and participate in varied educational experiences (Boltz, Capezuti, Fulmer, et al., 2016).

Good health and motivation are important influences on learning (see Chart 14-3).

CHART 14-3

Health Promotion: Nursing Strategies for Promoting Cognitive Function

Nurses can support the processes by which older adults learn by using the following strategies:

- Supply mnemonics to enhance recall of related data.
- Encourage ongoing learning.
- Link new information with familiar information.
- Use visual, auditory, and other sensory cues.
- Encourage learners to wear prescription glasses and hearing aids.
- Provide glare-free lighting.
- Provide a quiet, nondistracting environment.
- Set short-term goals with input from the learner.
- Prioritize the most important information and focus on the priority information.
- Keep teaching periods short.
- Pace learning tasks according to the endurance of the learner.
- Encourage verbal participation by learners.
- Reinforce successful learning in a positive manner.

Pharmacologic Aspects of Aging

Because an increasing number of chronic conditions affect older people, older people use more medications than any other age group. Although older persons account for only 15% of the Canadian population, they are estimated to account for 40% of all spending on prescribed drugs and 60% of public drug program spending (CIHI, 2014a), and 49% of all nonprescription medications (Rochon, Schmader, & Sokol, 2012). Although these medications improve health and well-being by relieving pain and discomfort, treating chronic illnesses, and curing infectious processes, adverse drug reactions are common because of medication interactions, multiple medication effects, incorrect dosages, and the use of multiple medications (**polypharmacy**). On average, 54.6% of older persons are using more than five medications each day (CIHI, 2014a). The potential for drug–drug interactions increases with increased medication use and with multiple coexisting diseases (**comorbidity**) that affect the absorption, distribution, metabolism, and elimination of the medications. Such interactions are responsible for numerous emergency department and physician visits, which cost billions of dollars annually.

Medications such as antipsychotics, anticoagulants, diuretics, and antiepileptics carry high risks for older patients and are often inappropriately prescribed (Institute for Safe Medication Practices Canada, 2012). An effective resource for identifying potentially risky drug interactions and adverse effects in older adults is *Beers Criteria for Potentially Inappropriate Medication Use in the Elderly* (Radcliff, Yue, Rocco, et al., 2015).

Any medication is capable of altering nutritional status, and the nutritional health of the older person may already be compromised by a marginal diet or by chronic disease and its treatment. Medications can affect the appetite, cause nausea and vomiting, irritate the stomach, cause constipation or diarrhea, and decrease absorption of nutrients. In addition, these medications may alter electrolyte balance as well as carbohydrate and fat metabolism. For example, antacids cause thiamine deficiency; laxatives diminish absorption; antibiotics and phenytoin (Dilantin) reduce utilization of folic acid; and phenothiazines, estrogens, and corticosteroids increase food intake and cause weight gain.

Combining multiple medications with alcohol, as well as with over-the-counter and herbal medications, complicates the problem. For example, St. John's wort, a common herbal supplement used for mild depression, decreases the anticoagulant effect of warfarin (Coumadin) and interacts with many other medications metabolized in the liver (Cattanach & Sibindi, 2016).

TABLE 14-2 Altered Drug Responses in Older People

Age-Related Changes	Effect of Age-Related Change	Applicable Medications
Absorption		
Reduced gastric acid; increased pH (less acid)	Rate of drug absorption—possibly delayed	Vitamins
Reduced gastrointestinal motility; prolonged gastric emptying	Extent of drug absorption—not affected	Calcium
Distribution		
Decreased circulating plasma proteins and total body water	Serious alterations in drug binding to plasma proteins (the unbound drug gives the pharmacologic response); highly protein-bound medications have fewer binding sites, leading to increased effects and accelerated metabolism and excretion.	*Selected highly protein-binding medications:* Oral anticoagulants (warfarin) Oral hypoglycemic agents (sulfonylureas) Barbiturates Calcium channel blockers Furosemide (Lasix) Nonsteroidal anti-inflammatory drugs (NSAIDs) Sulfonamides Quinidine Phenytoin (Dilantin)
Reduced cardiac output	Decreased perfusion of many bodily organs	
Impaired peripheral blood flow	Decreased perfusion	
Increased or decreased percentage of body fat	Proportion of body fat increases with age, resulting in increased ability to store fat-soluble medications; this causes drug accumulation, prolonged storage, and delayed excretion.	*Selected fat-soluble medications:* Barbiturates Diazepam (Valium) Lidocaine Phenothiazines (antipsychotics) Ethanol Morphine
Decreased lean body mass	Decreased body volume allows higher peak levels of medications.	
Metabolism		
Decreased cardiac output; decreased size of the liver; diminished intestinal and portal vein blood flow	Decreased metabolism and delay of breakdown of medications, resulting in prolonged duration of action, accumulation, and drug toxicity	All medications metabolized by the liver
Excretion		
Decreased renal blood flow; loss of functioning nephrons; decreased renal efficiency	Decreased rates of elimination and increased duration of action; danger of accumulation and drug toxicity	*Selected medications with prolonged action:* Aminoglycoside antibiotics Cimetidine (Tagamet) Chlorpropamide (Diabinese) Digoxin Lithium Procainamide

Adapted from Comerford, K. C. (2015). *Nursing 2015 drug handbook*. Philadelphia, PA: Wolters Kluwer.

Altered Pharmacokinetics

Alterations in absorption, metabolism, distribution, and excretion occur as a result of aging and may also result from drug and food interactions. Absorption may be affected by changes in gastric pH and a decrease in gastrointestinal motility. Drug distribution may be altered as a result of decrease in body water and increase in body fat. Usual age-related changes and diseases that alter blood flow, liver and renal function, or cardiac output may affect distribution and metabolism (Table 14-2).

Nursing Implications

Prescription principles that have been identified as appropriate for older patients include "start low and go slow" and keep the medication regimen as simple as possible (Le Couteur, McLachlan, & Hilmer, 2017). A comprehensive assessment that begins with a thorough medication history, including use of alcohol, recreational drugs, and over-the-counter and herbal medications, is essential. It is best to ask the patient or reliable informants to provide all medications for review. Ascertaining the patient's understanding of when and how to take each medication as well as the purpose of each medication allows the nurse to assess the patient's knowledge about and adherence with the medication regimen. The patient's beliefs and concerns about the medications should be identified. It is helpful to ask patients if they believe that a given medication is helpful.

Nonadherence leads to significant morbidity and mortality among older adults. The many contributing factors include the number of medications prescribed, the complexity of the regimen, difficulty opening containers, inadequate patient education, financial cost, and the disease or medication interfering with the patient's life. Furthermore, visual and hearing issues may make it difficult to read or to hear directions.

Multifaceted interventions tailored to the individual patient are the most effective strategies in improving adherence. The following steps can help patients manage their medications and improve adherence:

- Explain the purpose, adverse effects, and dosage of each medication.
- Provide the medication schedule in writing.
- Encourage the use of standard containers without safety lids (if there are no children in the household).
- Suggest the use of a multiple-day, multiple-dose medication dispenser to help the patient adhere to the medication schedule.
- Remove old, unused medications and take to a pharmacy for disposal.
- Encourage the patient to inform the primary health care professional about the use of over-the-counter medications and herbal agents, alcohol, and recreational drugs.
- Encourage the patient to keep a list of all medications, including over-the-counter and herbal medications, in his or her purse or wallet to share with the primary care professional at each visit and in case of an emergency.
- Review the medication schedule periodically and update it as necessary.
- Recommend using one supplier for prescriptions; pharmacies frequently track patients and are likely to notice a prescription problem such as duplication or contraindications in the medication regimen.
- If the patient's adherence is doubtful, identify a reliable family member or friend who might monitor the patient for adherence.

Mental Health Issues in the Older Adult

Changes in cognitive ability, excessive forgetfulness, and mood swings are not a part of usual aging. These symptoms should not be dismissed as age-related changes; a thorough assessment may reveal a treatable, reversible physical or mental condition. Changes in mental status may be related to many factors, such as alterations in diet and fluid and electrolyte balance, fever, or low oxygen levels associated with many cardiovascular and pulmonary diseases. Cognitive changes may be reversible when the underlying condition is identified and treated. However, the susceptibility to depression, **delirium**, and incidence of **dementia** increases with age. Older adults are less likely than younger people to acknowledge or seek treatment for mental health symptoms. Therefore, health professionals need to recognize, assess, refer, collaborate, treat, and support older adults who exhibit noticeable changes in intellect or affect.

Depression

Mood disorders are among the most common types of psychological disorders in Canada. They can contribute to stress, or problems with social relationships, as well as poor health. Depression is the most common affective or mood disorder of old age. Between 10% and 15% of older Canadians suffer from depression, and of those, 2% are older people residing in the community. The incidence of depression is higher among the institutionalized older adults, ranging from 30% to 40% (Canadian Mental Health Association Ontario, 2012).

Depression among older adults can follow a major precipitating event or loss and is often related to chronic illness or pain. It may also be secondary to a medication interaction or an undiagnosed physical condition. Signs of depression include feelings of sadness, fatigue, diminished memory and concentration, feelings of guilt or worthlessness, sleep disturbances, appetite disturbances with excessive weight loss or gain, restlessness, impaired attention span, and suicidal ideation. Even mild depression with symptoms that do not meet the criteria for a major depression reduces quality of life and function (Centers for Disease Control and Prevention, 2012). The risk of suicide increases in depressed patients, especially older Caucasians and men over 90 years. This supports the need for routine assessment of patients for depression and risk for suicide. Geriatric depression may be confused with dementia. However, the cognitive impairment resulting from depression is a result of apathy rather than decline in brain function. When depression and medical illnesses coexist, as they often do, neglect of the depression can impede physical recovery. Assessing the patient's mental status, including depression, is vital and must not be overlooked. Two commonly used assessment tools are the MMSE and the Geriatric Depression Scale (GDS).

Depression is highly responsive to treatment but is often not recognized and therefore is undertreated. Initial management involves evaluation of the patient's medication regimen and eliminating or changing any medications that contribute to depression. Furthermore, treatment of underlying medical conditions that may produce depressive symptoms may alleviate the depression. For mild depression, nonpharmacologic measures such as exercise, bright lighting, increasing interpersonal interactions, cognitive therapy, and reminiscence therapy are effective (Centre for Addiction and Mental Health, 2012). However for major depression, antidepressants and short-term psychotherapy, particularly in combination, are effective in older adults. Newer atypical antidepressants, such as bupropion (Wellbutrin), venlafaxine (Effexor), mirtazapine (Remeron), and nefazodone (Serzone), as well as selective serotonin reuptake inhibitors, such as paroxetine (Paxil), may be used.

Tricyclic antidepressants can be an effective medication for depression in some patients. However, medications with anticholinergic, cardiac, and orthostatic adverse effects, as well as interactions with other medications, should be used with care to avoid medication toxicity, hypotensive events, and falls. It may take 4 to 6 weeks for symptoms to diminish, and during this period, nurses offer support and encouragement. In life-threatening cases, electroconvulsive therapy has proved effective.

Alcohol and Drug Abuse

While alcohol consumption declines with advancing age (World Health Organization, 2014), evidence has shown that drinking occasions tend to become more frequent among older adults (Britton, Ben-Shlomo, Benzeval, et al., 2015). There is also evidence of a cohort effect, with successive birth cohorts reporting an increase in alcohol consumption across all age groups, including older persons (Meng, Holmes, Hill-McManus, et al., 2014).

Alcohol abuse is especially dangerous in older people because of age-related changes in renal and liver function as well as the high risk of interactions with prescription medications and the resultant adverse effects. Alcohol- and drug-related problems in older people often remain hidden because many older adults deny their habit when questioned. Assessing for drug and alcohol use with direct questions in a nonaccusatory manner should be part of the routine physical assessment. More information and specific assessment tools can be found in Chapter 5.

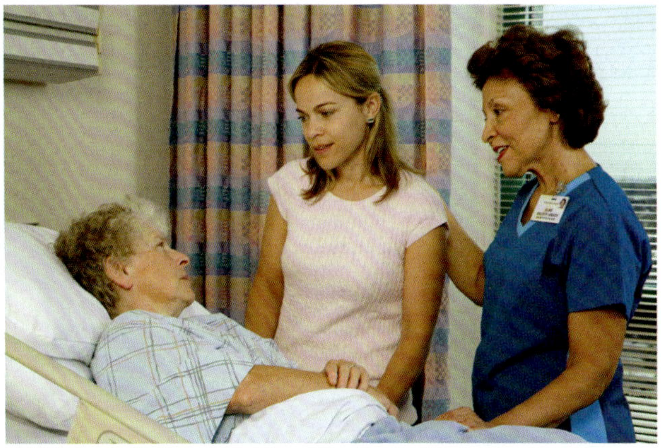

FIGURE 14-2. Talking to family members may increase the comfort of patients with delirium.

Delirium

Delirium, often called acute confusional state, begins with confusion and progresses to disorientation. It is a common and life-threatening complication for the hospitalized older adult and the most frequent complication of hospitalization, occurring in up to 50% of hospitalized older people (O'Regan et al., 2013). Patients may experience an altered level of consciousness, ranging from stupor (hypoalert–hypoactive) to excessive activity (hyperalert–hyperactive); alternatively, they may have a combination of these two types (mixed). Thinking is disorganized, and the attention span is short. Hallucinations, delusions, fear, anxiety, and paranoia may also be evident. Patients who tend to be hyperalert and hyperactive demand more attention from nurses and thus are easier to diagnose, whereas those who are hypoalert or hypoactive tend to be less problematic and pose diagnostic difficulties. Recognition of delirium can also be complicated in patients with the mixed type of disorders. Patients with the hypoalert–hypoactive type of delirium have higher mortality rates and even poorer outcomes of care because the delirium tends not to be recognized and treated (El Hussein & Hirst, 2016).

Attentive clinical assessment is essential because delirium is sometimes mistaken for dementia (Table 14-3 compares dementia and delirium). It helps to know an individual patient's usual mental status and whether the changes noted are long term, which probably represents dementia, or are abrupt in onset, which is more likely delirium.

Delirium occurs secondary to a number of causes, including physical illness, medication or alcohol toxicity, dehydration, fecal impaction, malnutrition, infection, head trauma, lack of environmental cues, and sensory deprivation or overload. Older adults are particularly vulnerable to acute confusion because of their decreased biologic reserve and the large number of medications they may take. Nurses need to recognize the implications of the acute symptoms of delirium (agitation, disorientation, and fearfulness) (Mossello, Tesi, Di Santo, et al., 2018) and report them immediately. Because of the acute and unexpected onset of symptoms and the unknown underlying cause, delirium is a medical emergency. If the delirium goes unrecognized and the underlying cause is not treated, permanent, irreversible brain damage or death can follow.

The most effective strategy is prevention, which includes therapeutic activities for cognitive impairment, early mobilization, controlling pain, minimizing the use of psychoactive drugs, preventing sleep deprivation, enhancing communication methods (particularly eye glasses and hearing aids) for vision and hearing impairment, maintaining oxygen levels and fluid and electrolyte balance, and preventing surgical complications.

Once delirium occurs, treatment of the underlying cause is most important. Therapeutic interventions vary depending on the cause. Delirium increases the risk of falls; therefore, management of patient safety and behavioural issues is essential. Because medication interactions and toxicity are often implicated, nonessential medications are discontinued. Nutritional and fluid intake is supervised and monitored. The environment should be quiet and calm. To increase function and comfort, the nurse provides familiar environmental cues and encourages family members or friends to touch and talk to the patient (Fig. 14-2). Ongoing mental status assessments using prior mental cognitive status as a baseline are helpful in evaluating responses to treatment and upon admission to a hospital or extended-care facility. If the underlying problem is adequately treated, the patient often returns to baseline within several days. Several resources specific to delirium are included in the Resources section at the end of the chapter.

Dementia

The cognitive, functional, and behavioural changes that characterize dementia eventually destroy a person's ability to function. The symptoms are usually subtle in onset and often progress slowly until they are obvious and devastating. The two most common types of dementia are Alzheimer's disease (AD), which accounts for 63% of cases, and vascular or multi-infarct dementia, which accounts for 20% of cases. Other non-Alzheimer dementias include Parkinson's disease, acquired immunodeficiency syndrome (AIDS)-related dementia, and Pick's disease; these types of dementia account for fewer than 20% of cases (Alzheimer Society of Canada, 2018). Approximately 1.5% of the Canadian population presently have dementia; it is estimated that 1.1 million people will have dementia by 2038 (Alzheimer Society of

TABLE 14-3 Summary of Differences Between Dementia and Delirium

	Dementia		
	Alzheimer's Disease (AD)	**Vascular (Multi-Infarct) Dementia**	**Delirium**
Etiology	Early onset (familial, genetic [chromosomes 14, 19, 21]) Late-onset sporadic—etiology unknown	Cardiovascular (CV) disease Cerebrovascular disease Hypertension	Drug toxicity and interactions; acute disease; trauma; chronic disease exacerbation Fluid and electrolyte disorders
Risk factors	Advanced age; genetics	Pre-existing CV disease	Pre-existing cognitive impairment
Occurrence	70% of dementias	10–20% of dementias	7–61% among hospitalized people
Onset	Slow	Often abrupt Follows a stroke or transient ischemic attack	Rapid, acute onset A harbinger of acute medical illness
Age of onset	Early-onset AD: 30–65 years Late-onset AD: 65+ years Most commonly: 85+ years	Most commonly 50–70 years	Any age, although predominantly in older persons
Gender	Males and females equally	Predominantly males	Males and females equally
Course	Chronic, irreversible; progressive, regular, downhill	Chronic, irreversible Fluctuating, stepwise progression	Acute onset Hypoalert–hypoactive Hyperalert–hyperactive Mixed hypo–hyper
Duration	2–20 years	Variable; years	Lasts 1 day to 1 month
Symptom progress	Onset insidious: *Early*—mild and subtle *Middle and late*—intensified Progression to death (infection or malnutrition)	Depends on location of infarct and success of treatment; death attributed to underlying CV disease	Symptoms are fully reversible with adequate treatment; can progress to chronicity or death if underlying condition is ignored.
Mood	Depression common	Labile: mood swings	Variable
Speech/language	Speech remains intact until late in disease: *Early*—mild anomia (cannot name objects); deficits progress until speech lacks meaning; echoes and repeats words and sounds; mutism *Early*—no motor deficits	May have speech deficit/aphasia depending on location of lesion	Fluctuating; often cannot concentrate long enough to speak May be somnolent
Physical signs	*Middle*—apraxia (cannot perform purposeful movement) *Late*—Dysarthria (impaired speech) *End stage*—loss of all voluntary activity; positive neurologic signs	According to location of lesion: focal neurologic signs, seizures Commonly exhibits motor deficits	Signs and symptoms of underlying disease
Orientation	Becomes lost in familiar places (topographic disorientation) Has difficulty drawing three-dimensional objects (visual and spatial disorientation) Disorientation to time, place, and person—with disease progression		May fluctuate between lucidity and complete disorientation to time, place, and person
Memory	Loss is an early sign of dementia; loss of recent memory is soon followed by progressive decline in recent and remote memory		Impaired recent and remote memory; may fluctuate between lucidity and confusion
Personality	Apathy, indifference, irritability: *Early disease*—social behaviour intact; hides cognitive deficits *Advanced disease*—disengages from activity and relationships; suspicious; paranoid delusions caused by memory loss; aggressive; catastrophic reactions		Fluctuating; cannot focus attention to converse; alarmed by symptoms (when lucid); hallucinations; paranoid
Functional status, activities of daily living	Poor judgment in everyday activities; has progressive decline in ability to handle money, use telephone, use computer and other electronic devices, function in home and workplace		Impaired
Attention span	Distractible; short attention span		Highly impaired; cannot maintain or shift attention
Psychomotor activity	Wandering, hyperactivity, pacing, restlessness, agitation		Variable; alternates between high agitation, hyperactivity, restlessness, and lethargy
Sleep–wake cycle	Often impaired; wandering and agitation at nighttime		Takes brief naps throughout day and night

Adapted from Grossman, S. C., & Porth, C. M. (2014). *Pathophysiology: Concepts of altered health states* (9th ed.). Philadelphia, PA: Lippincott Williams & Wilkins.

Canada, 2018). The passing of Bill C-233 by the federal government, in June 2017, identifies a national strategy for AD and other dementias.

Alzheimer's Disease

AD is a progressive, irreversible, degenerative neurologic disease that begins insidiously and is characterized by gradual losses of cognitive function and disturbances in behaviour and affect. Although AD can occur in people as young as 40 years of age, it is uncommon before 65 years of age. Although the prevalence of AD increases dramatically with increasing age, affecting as many as half of those 85 years of age and older, it is important to note that AD is not an expected part of aging. Without a cure or any preventive measures, it is estimated that 770,811 Canadians will have this disease by 2038 (Alzheimer Society of Canada, 2018).

There are numerous theories about the cause of age-related cognitive decline. Although the greatest risk factor for AD is increasing age, many environmental, dietary, and inflammatory factors also may determine whether a person suffers from this cognitive disease. AD is a complex brain disorder caused by a combination of various factors that may include genetics, neurotransmitter changes, vascular abnormalities, stress hormones, circadian changes, head trauma, and the presence of seizure disorders.

AD can be classified into two types: familial or early-onset AD and sporadic or late-onset AD. Familial AD is rare, accounting for less than 5% of all cases, and is frequently associated with genetic mutations (Alzheimer Society of Canada, 2018). It occurs in middle-aged adults. If family members have at least one other relative with AD, then there is a familial component, which nonspecifically includes both environmental triggers and genetic determinants.

Pathophysiology

Specific neuropathologic and biochemical changes are found in patients with AD. These include neurofibrillary tangles (tangled masses of nonfunctioning neurons) and senile or neuritic plaques (deposits of amyloid protein, part of a larger protein called amyloid precursor protein in the brain) (see Fig. 14-3). The neuronal damage occurs primarily in the cerebral cortex and results in decreased brain size. Similar changes are found in the normal brain tissue of older adults, but to a lesser extent. Cells that use the neurotransmitter acetylcholine are principally affected by AD. At the biochemical level, the enzyme active in producing acetylcholine, which is specifically involved in memory processing, is decreased.

Scientists have been studying complex neurodegenerative diseases such as AD and have focused on two key issues: whether a gene might influence a person's overall risk of developing the disease, and whether a gene might influence some particular aspect of a person's risk, such as the age at which the disease begins (age at onset). There are genetic differences in early- and late-onset forms of AD. Researchers are conducting tests to explain what predisposes people to develop the plaques and neurofibrillary tangles that can be seen at autopsy in the brains of patients with AD. Understanding the complex ways in which aging

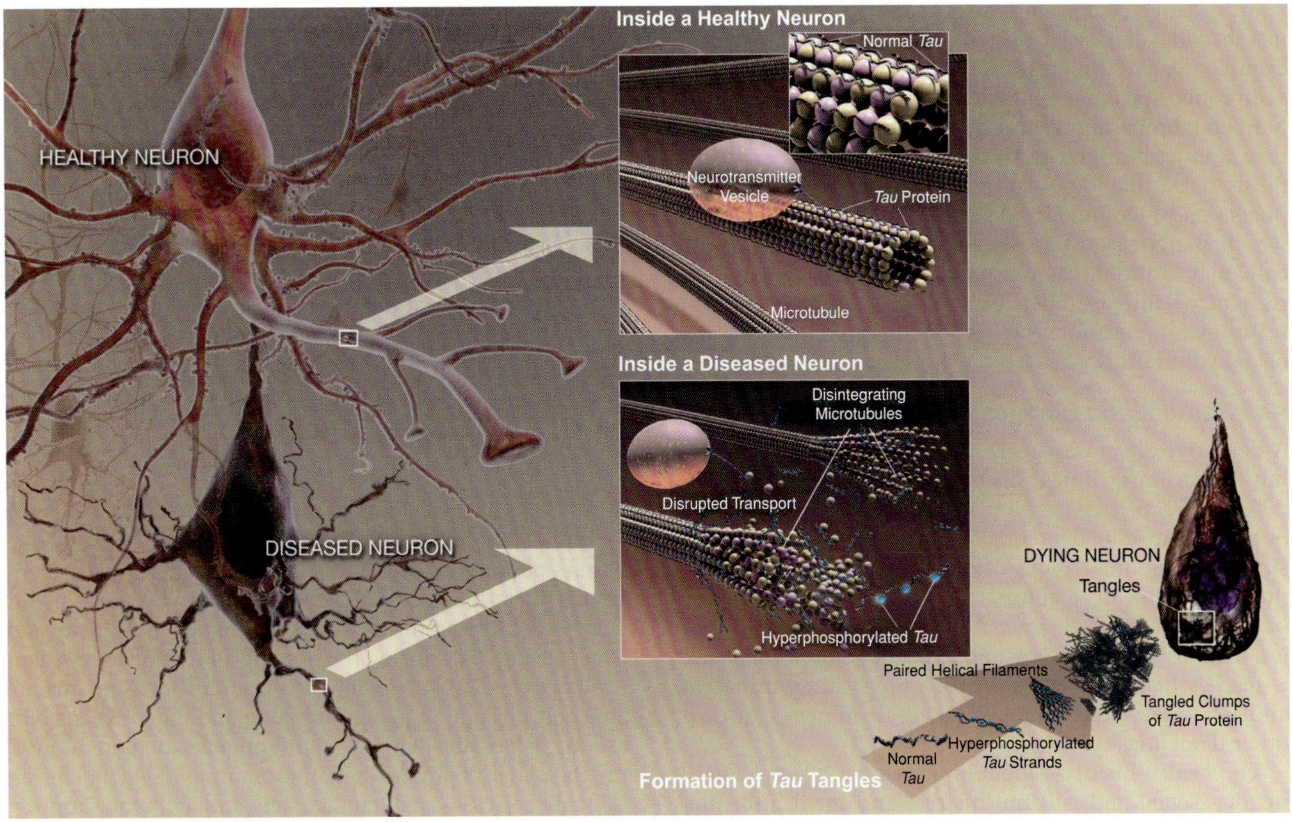

FIGURE 14-3. Healthy and diseased neurons and formation of tau tangles. (From National Institute on Aging, National Institutes of Health, Alzheimer's Disease Education and Referral Center. Retrieved at www.nia.nih.gov/alzheimers/scientific-images.)

and genetic and nongenetic factors affect brain cells over time, eventually leading to AD, continues to increase. Researchers have discovered how amyloid plaques form and cause neuronal death, the possible relationship between various forms of tau protein and impaired function, the roles of inflammation and oxidative stress, and the contribution of brain infarctions to the disease (Alzheimer Society of Canada, 2018).

Clinical Manifestations

In the early stages of AD, forgetfulness and subtle memory loss occur. Patients may experience small difficulties in work or social activities but have adequate cognitive function to compensate for the loss and continue to function independently. With further progression of AD, the deficits can no longer be concealed. Forgetfulness is manifested in many daily actions; patients may lose their ability to recognize familiar faces, places, and objects and they may become lost in a familiar environment. They may repeat the same stories because they forget that they have already told them. Trying to reason with people with AD and using reality **orientation** only increases their anxiety without increasing function. Conversation becomes difficult, and word-finding difficulties occur. The ability to formulate concepts and think abstractly disappears; for example, a patient can interpret a proverb only in concrete terms. Patients are often unable to recognize the consequences of their actions and therefore exhibit impulsive behaviour. For example, on a hot day, a patient may decide to wade in the city fountain fully clothed. Patients have difficulty with everyday activities, such as operating simple appliances and handling money.

Personality changes are also usually evident. Patients may become depressed, suspicious, paranoid, hostile, and even combative. Progression of the disease intensifies the symptoms: speaking skills deteriorate to nonsense syllables, agitation and physical activity increase, and patients may wander at night. Eventually, assistance is needed for most ADLs, including eating and toileting, because dysphagia and incontinence develop. The terminal stage, in which patients are usually immobile and require total care, may last months or years. Occasionally, patients may recognize family members or caregivers. Death occurs as a result of complications such as pneumonia, malnutrition, or dehydration.

Assessment and Diagnostic Findings

A definitive diagnosis of AD can be made only at autopsy, but an accurate clinical diagnosis can be made in about 80% to 90% of cases. The most important goal is to rule out other causes of dementia or reversible causes of confusion, such as other types of dementia, depression, delirium, alcohol or drug abuse, or inappropriate drug dosage or drug toxicity (Alzheimer Society of Canada, 2018). AD is a diagnosis of exclusion, and a diagnosis of probable AD is made when the medical history, physical examination, and laboratory tests have excluded all known causes of other dementias.

The health history—including medical history, family history, social and cultural history, and medication history—and the physical examination, including functional and mental health status, are essential to the diagnosis of probable AD. Diagnostic tests, including complete blood count, chemistry profile, and vitamin B_{12} and thyroid hormone levels, as well as screening with electroencephalography, computed tomography (CT), magnetic resonance imaging (MRI), and examination of the cerebrospinal fluid may all refute or support a diagnosis of probable AD.

Depression can closely mimic early-stage AD and coexists in many patients. Therefore, assessing the patient for underlying depression is important to rule this out. Tests such as the MMSE are useful for screening (Alzheimer Society of Canada, 2018). Both CT and MRI of the brain are useful for excluding hematoma, brain tumour, stroke, normal-pressure hydrocephalus, and atrophy but are not reliable in making a definitive diagnosis of AD. Infections and physiologic disturbances, such as hypothyroidism, Parkinson's disease, and vitamin B_{12} deficiency, can cause cognitive impairment that may be misdiagnosed as AD. Biochemical abnormalities can be excluded through examination of the blood and cerebrospinal fluid.

Medical Management

The primary goal is to manage the cognitive and behavioural symptoms. There is no cure and no way to slow the progression of the disease. Three Health Canada–approved medications are available to treat AD symptoms; however, none of these agents stops the progression of the disease. The cholinesterase inhibitors (CEIs) donepezil hydrochloride (Aricept), rivastigmine tartrate (Exelon), and galantamine hydrobromide (Razadyne [formerly known as Reminyl]), enhance acetylcholine uptake in the brain, thus maintaining memory skills for a period of time; these medications are used for mild to moderate symptoms. A new medication (Ebixa), a receptor agonist, can be used for management of moderate to severe symptoms. Cognitive ability may improve within 6 to 12 months of therapy, but cessation of the medications results in disease progression and cognitive decline. It is recommended that treatment continue at least through the moderate stage of the illness. Combination of a CEI with memantine may be useful for mild to moderate cognitive symptoms (Alzheimer Society of Canada, 2018).

Behavioural issues such as agitation and psychosis can be managed by behavioural and psychosocial therapies. Associated depression and behavioural concerns can also be treated pharmacologically if other interventions fail. Because symptoms change over time, all patients with AD who take medications should be reevaluated routinely, and the nurse should document and report both positive and negative responses to medications (Boltz et al., 2016).

Nursing Management

Nurses play an important role in the recognition of dementia, particularly in hospitalized older adults, by assessing for signs (e.g., repeating or asking the same thing over and over, getting lost) during the nursing admission assessment (Boltz et al., 2016). Nursing interventions for dementia are aimed at promoting patient function and independence for as long as possible. Other important goals include promoting the patient's physical safety, promoting independence in self-care activities, reducing anxiety and agitation, improving communication, providing for socialization and intimacy, promoting adequate nutrition, promoting balanced activity and rest, and supporting and educating family caregivers. These nursing interventions apply to all patients with dementia, regardless of cause.

SUPPORTING COGNITIVE FUNCTION. Because dementia of any type is degenerative and progressive, patients display a decline in cognitive function over time. In the early phase of dementia, minimal cuing and guidance may be all that are needed for the patient to function fairly independently for a number of years. However, as the patient's cognitive ability declines, family members must provide more and more assistance and supervision. A calm, predictable environment helps people with dementia interpret their surroundings and activities. Environmental stimuli are limited, and a regular routine is established. A quiet, pleasant manner of speaking, clear and simple explanations, and use of memory aids and cues help minimize confusion and disorientation and give patients a sense of security. Prominently displayed clocks and calendars may enhance orientation to time. Colour-coding the doorway may help patients who have difficulty locating their room. Active participation may help patients maintain cognitive, functional, and social interaction abilities for a longer period. Physical activity and communication have also been demonstrated to slow some of the cognitive decline of AD.

PROMOTING PHYSICAL SAFETY. A safe home and hospital environment allows the patient to move about as freely as possible and relieves the family of constant worry about safety. To prevent falls and other injuries, all obvious hazards are removed and hand rails are installed in the home. A hazard-free environment allows the patient maximum independence and a sense of autonomy. Adequate lighting, especially in halls, stairs, and bathrooms, is necessary. Nightlights are helpful, particularly if the patient has increased confusion at night (**sundowning**). Driving is prohibited, and smoking is allowed only with supervision. The patient may have a short attention span and be forgetful. Wandering behaviour can often be reduced by gentle persuasion or distraction. Restraints should be avoided because they increase agitation. Doors leading from the house must be secured. Outside the home, all activities must be supervised to protect the patient, and the patient should wear an identification bracelet or neck chain in case of separation from the caregiver.

PROMOTING INDEPENDENCE IN SELF-CARE ACTIVITIES. Pathophysiologic changes in the brain make it difficult for people with AD to maintain physical independence. Patients are assisted to remain functionally independent for as long as possible. One way to do this is to simplify daily activities by organizing them into short, achievable steps so that the patient experiences a sense of accomplishment. Frequently, occupational therapists can suggest ways to simplify tasks or recommend adaptive equipment. Direct patient supervision is sometimes necessary, but maintaining personal dignity and autonomy is important for people with AD, who should be encouraged to make choices when appropriate and to participate in self-care activities as much as possible.

REDUCING ANXIETY AND AGITATION. Despite profound cognitive losses, patients are sometimes aware of their diminishing abilities. Patients need constant emotional support that reinforces a positive self-image. When loss of skills occurs, goals are adjusted to fit the patient's declining ability.

The environment is kept familiar and noise-free. Excitement and confusion can be upsetting and may precipitate a combative, agitated state known as a catastrophic reaction (overreaction to excessive stimulation). The patient may respond by screaming, crying, or becoming abusive (physically or verbally); this may be the patient's only way of expressing an inability to cope with the environment. When this occurs, it is important to remain calm and unhurried. Forcing the patient to proceed with the activity only increases the agitation. It is better to postpone the activity until later, even to another day. Frequently, the patient quickly forgets what triggered the reaction. Measures such as moving to a familiar environment, listening to music, stroking, rocking, or distraction may quiet the patient. Structuring activity is also helpful. Becoming familiar with a particular patient's predicted responses to certain stressors helps caregivers avoid similar situations.

Patients with dementia who have progressed to the late stages of the disease often reside in nursing homes and are predominantly cared for by unregulated personnel. Dementia education for caregivers is essential to minimize patient agitation and can be effectively taught by geriatric NPs.

IMPROVING COMMUNICATION. To promote the patient's interpretation of messages, the nurse should remain unhurried and reduce noises and distractions. Use of clear, easy-to-understand sentences to convey messages is essential because patients frequently forget the meaning of words or have difficulty organizing and expressing thoughts. In the earlier stages of dementia, lists and simple written instructions that serve as reminders may be helpful. In later stages, the patient may be able to point to an object or use nonverbal language to communicate. Tactile stimuli, such as hugs or hand pats, are usually interpreted as signs of affection, concern, and security.

PROVIDING FOR SOCIALIZATION AND INTIMACY NEEDS. Because socialization with friends can be comforting, visits, letters, and phone calls are encouraged. Visits should be brief and nonstressful; limiting visitors to one or two at a time helps reduce overstimulation. Recreation is important, and people with dementia are encouraged to participate in simple activities. Realistic goals for activities that provide satisfaction are appropriate. Hobbies and activities such as walking, exercising, and socializing can improve the quality of life. The nonjudgmental friendliness of a pet may provide stimulation, comfort, and contentment. Care of plants or of a pet can also be satisfying and an outlet for energy.

AD does not eliminate the need for intimacy. Patients and their spouses may continue to enjoy sexual activity. Spouses should be encouraged to talk about any sexual concerns, and sexual counselling may be necessary. Simple expressions of love, such as touching and holding, are often meaningful.

PROMOTING ADEQUATE NUTRITION. Since mealtime can be a pleasant social occasion or a time of upset and distress, it should be kept simple and calm, without confrontations. Patients prefer familiar foods that look appetizing and taste good. To avoid any "playing" with food, one dish is offered at a time. Food is cut into small pieces to prevent choking. Liquids may be easier to swallow if they are converted to gelatin. Hot food and beverages are served warm, and the temperature of the foods should be checked to prevent burns.

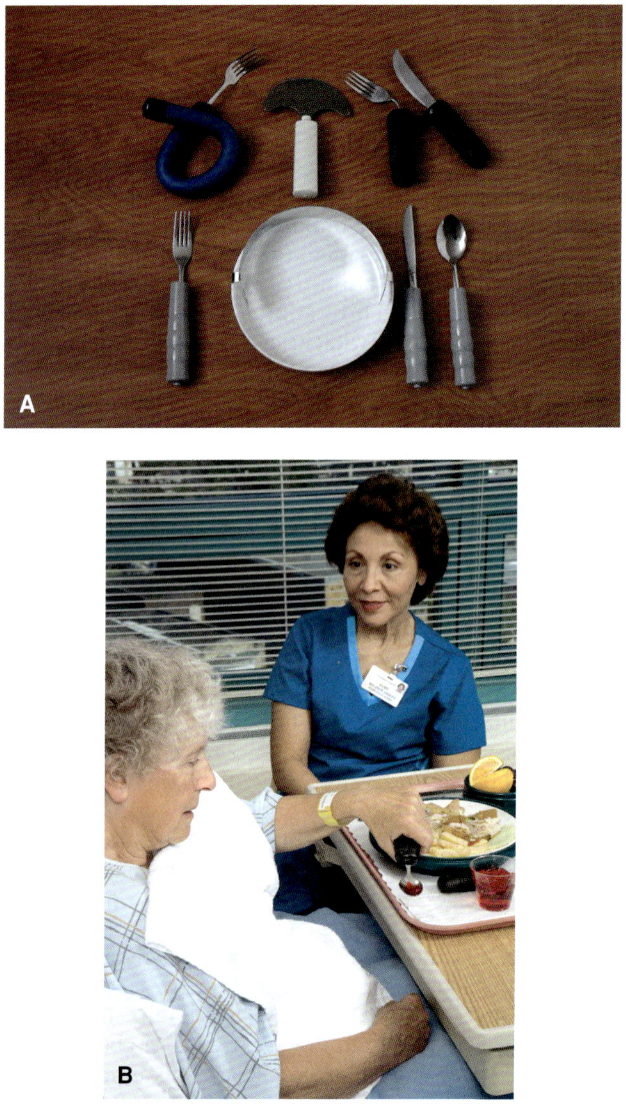

FIGURE 14-4. A. Assistive feeding devices make it easy for patients to grasp and get food on utensils. B. Assistive feeding devices may be required for patients who are weak, fatigued, or paralyzed or have neuromuscular impairment.

When lack of coordination interferes with self-feeding, adaptive equipment is helpful (see Fig. 14-4). Some patients may do well eating with a spoon or with their fingers. If this is the case, an apron or a smock, rather than a bib, is used to protect clothing. As deficits progress, it may become necessary to feed the patient. Forgetfulness, disinterest, dental issues, lack of coordination, overstimulation, and choking all serve as barriers to good nutrition and hydration.

PROMOTING BALANCED ACTIVITY AND REST. Many patients with dementia exhibit sleep disturbances, wandering, and behaviours that may be considered inappropriate. These behaviours are most likely to occur when there are unmet underlying physical or psychological needs. Caregivers identify the needs of patients who are exhibiting these behaviours because further health decline may occur if the source of the problem is not corrected. Adequate sleep and physical exercise are essential. If sleep is interrupted or the patient cannot fall asleep, music, warm milk, or a back rub may help the patient relax. During the day, patients should be encouraged to participate in exercise because a regular pattern of activity and rest enhances nighttime sleep. Long periods of daytime sleeping are discouraged.

SUPPORTING HOME, COMMUNITY-BASED, AND TRANSITIONAL CARE. The emotional burden on the families of patients with all types of dementia is enormous. The physical health of the patient is often very stable, and the mental degeneration is gradual. Family members may cling to the hope that the diagnosis is incorrect and that their relative will improve with greater effort. Family members are faced with numerous difficult decisions (e.g., when the patient should stop driving, when to assume responsibility for the patient's financial affairs). Aggression and hostility exhibited by the patient are often misunderstood by families or caregivers, who feel unappreciated, frustrated, and angry. Feelings of guilt, nervousness, and worry contribute to caregiver fatigue, depression, and family dysfunction.

Neglect or abuse of the patient can occur, and this has been documented in home situations as well as in institutions. If neglect or abuse of any kind—including physical, emotional, sexual, or financial abuse—is suspected, the local adult protective services agency must be notified. The role of the nurse is to report the suspected abuse, not to prove it.

The Alzheimer Society of Canada is a coalition of family members and professionals who share the goals of family support and service, education, research, and advocacy. Family support groups, respite (relief) care, and adult day care may be available through different community resources in which concerned volunteers are trained to provide structure to caregiver support groups. Respite care is a commonly provided service in which caregivers can get away from the home for short periods while someone else tends to the needs of the patient.

Vascular Dementia

Vascular dementia, formerly known as multi-infarct dementia, tends to have a more abrupt onset than AD, and it is characterized by an uneven, stepwise downward decline in mental function associated with a vascular incident such as a subclinical stroke or following cardiac surgery. The clinical course of this type of dementia is unpredictable; as a result, it is sometimes confused with AD, paranoia, or delirium. Diagnosis may be even more difficult if a patient has vascular dementia as well as AD.

Because vascular dementia is associated with hypertension and cardiovascular disease, risk factors (e.g., hypercholesterolemia, history of smoking, diabetes mellitus) are similar (Alzheimer Society of Canada, 2018). Prevention and management are also similar. Therefore, measures to decrease blood pressure and lower cholesterol levels may prevent future mini-infarcts.

Additional Aspects of Health Care of the Older Adult

The nurse needs to consider other health issues of older adults. These include pseudobulbar affect, geriatric syndromes, elder neglect and abuse, as well as ethical and legal issues.

Pseudobulbar Affect

The condition known as pseudobulbar affect involves inappropriate or exaggerated emotional expression, usually episodes of laughing or crying. It is associated with brain injury (e.g., stroke, traumatic brain injury, MS, ALS, AD, and Parkinson's disease). The term "pseudobulbar" refers to damage that occurs in the corticobulbar tracts in the brain (see Chapter 66). The emotional outbursts can cause embarrassment, anxiety, and depression, and often impair quality of life (Yang & Deeks, 2015).

Older adults with pseudobulbar affect can respond appropriately to treatment. Initial management involves evaluation and recognition that this condition can coexist with mood disorders, such as depression, although crying in these patients should not be considered indicative of depression. Pharmacology studies have reported effective management with Nuedexta (dextromethorphan HBr and quinidine sulphate) in patients with ALS, MS, and dementia (Yang & Deeks, 2015).

Geriatric Syndromes

Older people tend to acquire multiple issues and illnesses as they age. The decline of physical function leads to a loss of independence and increasing frailty as well as to susceptibility to both acute and chronic health problems, which generally result from several factors rather than from a single cause. When combined with a decrease in host resistance, these factors can lead to illness or injury. A number of issues commonly experienced by older adults are becoming recognized as geriatric syndromes. These conditions do not fit into discrete disease categories. Examples include frailty, delirium, falls, urinary incontinence, and pressure ulcers (Brown-O'Hara, 2013). Although these conditions may develop slowly, the onset of symptoms is often acute. Furthermore, the presenting symptoms may appear in other body systems before becoming apparent in the affected system. For example, an older patient may present with confusion, and the underlying disease may be a urinary tract infection, dehydration, or a heart attack.

The term *frail* is used to describe older people who are at highest risk for adverse health outcomes. The most widely used criteria include weight loss, weakness, exhaustion or poor endurance, slowness, and low activity. For all geriatric syndromes, older age, functional impairment, cognitive impairment, and impaired mobility are risk factors. Research suggests that frail older adults are at increased risk for falls, hospitalization, disability, and mortality (Lusardi, Fritz, Middleton, et al., 2017).

Impaired Mobility

The causes of decreased mobility are many and varied. Common causes include strokes, Parkinson's disease, diabetic neuropathy, cardiovascular compromise, osteoarthritis, osteoporosis, and sensory deficits. To avoid the downward spiral of immobility, older people should be encouraged to stay as active as possible. During illness, bed rest should be kept to a minimum, even in hospitalized patients, because even brief periods of bed rest quickly lead to deconditioning and, consequently, to a wide range of complications (Covinsky, Pierluissi, Johnston, et al., 2017). When bed rest cannot be avoided, patients should perform active range-of-motion and strengthening exercises with the unaffected extremities, and nurses or family caregivers should perform passive range-of-motion exercises on the affected extremities. Frequent position changes help offset the hazards of immobility. Both the health care staff and the patient's family can assist in maintaining the current level of mobility.

Dizziness

Older people frequently seek help for dizziness, which presents a particular challenge because there are numerous possible causes. For many, the problem is complicated by an inability to differentiate between true dizziness (a sensation of disorientation in relation to position) and vertigo (a spinning sensation). Other similar sensations include near-syncope and disequilibrium. The causes for these sensations range in severity from minor (e.g., buildup of earwax) to severe (e.g., dysfunction of the cerebral cortex, cerebellum, brainstem, proprioceptive receptors, or vestibular system). Even a minor reversible cause, such as earwax impaction, can result in a loss of balance and a subsequent fall and injury. Because dizziness has many predisposing factors, nurses seek to identify any potentially treatable factors related to the condition.

Falls and Falling

Injuries rank eighth as a cause of death for older people, and falls are the leading cause of injury in older adults. Up to 20% to 30% of community-dwelling older people and 45% of nursing home residents fall annually, and about half fall multiple times (Public Health Agency of Canada, 2014). The incidence of falls rises with increasing age. It tends to be highest in people who are 85 years of age and older, and outcomes are worse in these adults. Some causes of falls are treatable.

Although most falls by older adults do not result in injury, a good percentage of falls in this population result in moderate to serious injuries. The most common fracture occurring from falls is hip fracture, which results from both osteoporosis and the situation that provoked the fall. Many older adults who fall and sustain a hip fracture are unable to regain their prefracture ability. Overall, older women who fall sustain a greater degree of injury than do older men.

Causes of falls are multifactorial. Both extrinsic factors such as changes in the environment or poor lighting and intrinsic factors such as physical illness, neurologic changes, or sensory impairment play a role. Mobility difficulties, medication effects, foot problems or unsafe footwear, postural hypotension, visual issues, and tripping hazards are common, treatable causes. Polypharmacy, medication interactions, and use of alcohol precipitate falls by causing drowsiness, decreased coordination, and postural hypotension. Falls have physical dangers as well as serious psychological and social consequences. It is not uncommon for an older person who has experienced a fall to become fearful and lose self-confidence.

Nurses can encourage older adults and their families to make lifestyle and environmental changes to prevent falls. Adequate lighting with minimal glare and shadow can be achieved through the use of small area lamps, indirect lighting, and sheer curtains to diffuse direct sunlight, dull rather than shiny surfaces, and nightlights. Sharply contrasting colours can be used to mark the edges of stairs. Grab bars by the bathtub, shower, and toilet are useful. Loose clothing, improperly fitting shoes, scatter rugs, small objects, and pets create hazards and increase the risk for falls. Older adults function best in familiar settings when the arrangement of furniture and objects remains unchanged.

NURSING ALERT

In institutionalized older people, physical restraints (lap belts; geriatric chairs; vest, waist, and jacket restraints) and chemical restraints (medications) precipitate many of the injuries they were meant to prevent. Documented injuries and deaths resulting from these restraints include strangulation, vascular and neurologic damage, pressure ulcers, skin tears, fractures, increased confusion, and significant emotional trauma. The time required to supervise restrained patients adequately is better used addressing the unmet need that provoked the behaviour that resulted in the use of restraints. Because of the overwhelming negative consequences of restraint use, accrediting agencies of nursing homes and acute care facilities now maintain stringent guidelines concerning their use.

Urinary Incontinence

Urinary incontinence may be acute, occurring during an illness, or may develop chronically over a period of years. Older patients often do not report this very common concern unless specifically asked. Transient causes may be attributed to *d*elirium and *d*ehydration; *r*estricted mobility and restraints; *i*nflammation, *i*nfection, and *i*mpaction; and *p*harmaceuticals and *p*olyuria (the acronym *drip* may be used to remember them). Once identified, the causative factor can be eliminated. Incontinence may also be a result of neurologic or structural abnormalities. Urinary incontinence has been associated with depression and low self-esteem and may reduce the patient's quality of life by causing restriction in social activities.

The pelvic floor serves as the supporting mechanism or "hammock" for the bladder, uterus, and rectum. It may have become weakened as a result of pregnancy, labour and delivery, prior pelvic surgeries, or activities that required prolonged standing or lifting. Dysfunction of the pelvic floor can be greatly improved with Kegel exercises. Other measures that help prevent episodes of incontinence include having quick access to toilet facilities and wearing clothing that can be unfastened easily.

Patients with incontinence should be urged to seek help from appropriate health care professionals because incontinence can be both emotionally devastating and physically debilitating. Nurses who specialize in behavioural approaches to urinary incontinence management can help patients regain full continence or significantly improve the level of continence. Although medications such as anticholinergics may decrease some of the symptoms of urge incontinence (detrusor instability), the adverse effects of these medications (dry mouth, slowed gastrointestinal motility, and confusion) may make them inappropriate choices for older persons. Various surgical procedures are also used to manage urinary incontinence, particularly stress urinary incontinence.

Detrusor hyperactivity with impaired contractility is a type of urge incontinence that is seen predominantly in the older population. In this variation of urge incontinence, patients have no warning that they are about to urinate. They often void only a small volume of urine or none at all and then experience a large volume of incontinence after leaving the bathroom. The nursing staff should be familiar with this form of incontinence and should not show disapproval when it occurs. Many patients with dementia suffer from this type of incontinence, because both incontinence and dementia are a result of dysfunction in similar areas of the brain. Prompted, timed voiding can be of assistance in these patients, although clean intermittent catheterization may be necessary because of post-void residual urine (see Chapter 46).

Increased Susceptibility to Infection

Infectious diseases present a significant threat of morbidity and mortality to older people, in part because of the blunted response of host defenses caused by a reduction in both cell-mediated and humoral immunity (see Chapters 51 and 52). Age-related loss of physiologic reserve and chronic illnesses also contribute to increased susceptibility. Pneumonia, urinary tract infections, tuberculosis (TB), gastrointestinal infections, and skin infections are some of the common infections in older people.

The effects of influenza and pneumococcal infections on older people are also significant. An estimated 10% to 25% of Canadians have influenza each year; more than 12,200 are hospitalized with influenza-related complications, and approximately 3,500 die (Government of Canada, 2017).

The influenza and the pneumococcal vaccinations lower the risks of hospitalization and death in older people. The influenza vaccine, which is prepared yearly to adjust for the specific immunologic characteristics of the influenza viruses at that time, should be administered annually in autumn. Both of these injections can be received at the same time in separate injection sites. Nurses should urge older people to be vaccinated. All health care providers working with older people or high-risk chronically ill people should also be immunized.

TB affects a significant number of older adults. Case rates for TB are highest among those who are 65 or older, with the exception of people with human immunodeficiency virus (HIV) infection. Nursing home residents account for the majority of the cases of TB in older adults. Much of the infection rate is attributed to reactivation of old infection. Pulmonary TB and extrapulmonary TB often have subtle, nonspecific symptoms. This is of particular concern in nursing homes because an active case of TB places patients and staff at risk for infection.

Most provinces' *retirement homes act* suggests that all patients newly admitted to nursing homes have a Mantoux (purified protein derivative [PPD]) test unless there is a history of TB or a previous positive response. All patients whose tests are negative (a positive test is indicated by induration of more than 10 mm at 48 to 72 hours) should have a second test in 1 to 2 weeks. The first PPD serves to boost the suppressed immune response that may occur in older people. Chest x-rays and possibly sputum studies should be used to follow-up on PPD-positive responders and converters. For positive converters, a course of preventive therapy for 6 to 9 months is effective in eliminating active disease. All patients who test negative should be periodically retested (see Chapter 24).

AIDS occurs across the age spectrum. It is increasingly recognized that AIDS does not spare the older segment of society, and many who are living with HIV/AIDS are aging. In the past, male homosexual contact and blood transfusions were the predominant modes of transmission among older patients. Transmission by contaminated blood is now rare and the predominant mode of transmission in older people now is by sexual contact. The most common AIDS-indicator disease in older people is *Pneumocystis* pneumonia (PCP). Wasting syndrome and HIV encephalopathy are also common in older people with HIV infection.

Altered Pain and Febrile Responses

Many altered physical, emotional, and systemic reactions to disease are attributed to age-related changes in older people. Physical indicators of illness that are useful and reliable in young and middle-aged people cannot be relied on for the diagnosis of potential life-threatening problems in older adults. The response to pain in older people may be lessened because of reduced acuity of touch, alterations in neural pathways, and diminished processing of sensory data.

Many older adults who are experiencing a myocardial infarction do not have chest pain. Hiatal hernia or upper gastrointestinal distress is often the cause of chest pain. Acute abdominal conditions may go unrecognized in older people because of atypical signs and absence of pain.

The baseline body temperature for older people is about 0.751°C lower than it is for younger people. In the event of illness, the body temperature of an older person may not be high enough to qualify as a traditionally defined fever. A temperature of 37.8°C, in combination with systemic symptoms, may signal infection. A temperature of 38.3°C almost certainly indicates a serious infection that needs prompt attention. A blunted fever in the face of an infection often indicates a poor prognosis. Temperatures rarely exceed 39.5°C. Nurses are alert to other subtle signs of infection, such as mental confusion, increased respirations, tachycardia, and skin colour.

Altered Emotional Impact

The emotional component of illness in older people may differ from that in younger people. Many older adults equate good health with the absence of old age and believe "you are as old as you feel." An illness that requires hospitalization or a change in lifestyle is an imminent threat to well-being. Admission to the hospital is often feared and actively avoided. Older people admitted to the hospital are at high risk for disorientation, confusion, change in level of consciousness, and other symptoms of delirium, as well as anxiety and fear. In addition, fear of becoming a burden to families often leads to high anxiety in older people. Nurses need to recognize the implications of fear, anxiety, and dependency in older patients. They should encourage autonomy, independent decision making, and early mobilization. A positive and confident demeanour in nurses and family members promotes a positive mental outlook in older patients.

Altered Systemic Response

In an older person, illness has far-reaching repercussions. The decline in organ function that occurs in every system of the aging body eventually depletes the body's ability to respond at full capacity. Illness places new demands on body systems that have little or no reserve to meet the crisis. Homeostasis, the ability of the body to maintain an internal balance of function and chemical composition, is jeopardized. Older people may be unable to respond effectively to an acute illness or, if a chronic health condition is present, they may be unable to sustain appropriate responses over a long period. Furthermore, their ability to respond to definitive treatment is impaired. The altered responses of older adults reinforce the need for nurses to monitor all body system functions closely, being alert to signs of impending systemic complication.

Neglect and Abuse of Older Adults

Older adults who live in communities and institutions can be at risk for abuse and neglect. Because of different definitions and terminology and the pattern of underreporting, a clear picture of the incidence and prevalence of abuse among older adults is lacking. Furthermore, one of the major barriers to fully understanding "**elder abuse**" is that most professionals in all professions, including health care professionals, are not equipped to recognize and report this type of abuse. Both victims and perpetrators are reluctant to report the abuse, and clinicians are unaware of the frequency of the problem.

Neglect is the most common type of abuse. Other forms of abuse include physical, emotional, sexual, and financial abuse. Contributing factors include a family history of violence, mental illness, and drug or alcohol abuse, as well as financial dependency on the older person. In addition, diminished cognitive and physical function or disruptive and abusive behaviour on the part of the older person can lead to caregiver strain and emotional exhaustion. Older people with disabilities of all types are at increased risk for abuse from family members and paid caregivers.

Nurses should be alert to possible senior abuse and neglect. During the health history, in a private portion of the interview, the older person should be asked about abuse. Most provinces require that care providers, including nurses, report suspected abuse. Preventive action should be taken when caregiver strain is evident, before abuse occurs. Early detection and intervention may provide sufficient resources to the family or person at risk to ensure patient safety. Interdisciplinary team members, including the psychologist, social worker, or chaplain, can be enlisted to help the caregiver develop self-awareness, increased insight, and an understanding of the disease or aging process. Community resources such as caregiver support groups or respite services are useful for both the older person and the caregiver.

Health Care Costs of Aging

Many fear that Canada's public health care system will be unsustainable with an aging population. However, three important trends will have an impact. First, older adults have improved health and well-being well into old age. This not only reduces the length of disability and thus dependency but also the possibility of developing acute or chronic health problems. Second is an improved health care service. Despite some concern that health technology advances and new medications are increasing the cost of health care, these developments and advances are having profound effects through reducing the need for and use of health care services. The last trend is the shift of care from more expensive inpatient care settings to outpatient hospital or community care settings (Canadian Medical Association [CMA], 2016).

Home Care

Home care involves the individual patient, the family, and caregivers. Home care nurses are considered skilled generalists who are holistic in their approach to care. In addition to providing skilled nursing care, home care nurses also consider the needs of the family and the impact of the environment and community on the patient situation, and they identify areas for collaboration and referral. Care is episodic (periodic short visits). Home care agencies generally offer several services, including skilled nursing; hospice care; physical, occupational, and speech therapy; and home health aide and homemaker services. Consultation with specialists in nutrition, cardiac, diabetic, and wound care is available. As hospital stays have shortened, the acuity level of home care patients has risen dramatically. "High-tech" therapies such as infusion therapy are frequently available. The primary goal is to promote optimal health and independent function in the home for both patients and their families.

Hospice Services

Hospice is a program of supportive and palliative services for terminally ill patients and their families that includes physical, psychological, social, and spiritual care. In most cases, patients are not expected to live longer than 6 months. The goal of hospice is to improve the quality of life by focusing on symptom management, pain control, and emotional support. Medical and nursing services are provided to keep patients as pain free and comfortable as possible. Hospice services may be incorporated into the care of residents in long-term care facilities and include care for end-stage dementia and other chronic disease such as end-stage congestive heart disease.

Home care and hospice nurses are in a unique position to facilitate discussions about a patient's wishes and goals at the end of life. Too often, discussion regarding end-of-life care is postponed until a crisis occurs, making it difficult or impossible for the patient to be an active participant in the discussion. Home care nurses can assist patients and families by identifying options and initiating conversation about preparing an end-of-life plan. For an in-depth discussion of hospice care, see Chapter 15.

Aging With a Disability

As the life expectancy of people with all types of physical, cognitive, and mental disabilities has increased, individuals must deal with the usual changes associated with aging in addition to their pre-existing disabilities. There are still large gaps in our understanding of the interaction between disabilities and aging, including how this interaction varies depending on the type and degree of disability and other factors such as socioeconomics and gender. For adults without disabilities, the changes associated with aging may be minor inconveniences. For adults with disorders such as polio, MS, and cerebral palsy, aging may lead to greater disability. In addition, many people with disabilities are greatly concerned and fearful about what will happen to them as they age and whether assistance will be available when they need care.

It has been proposed that nurses view people with disabilities as capable, responsible individuals who are able to function effectively despite having a disability. Both the interface and the biopsychosocial models of disability can serve as a basis for the role of nurses as advocates for removal of barriers to health care (Smeltzer, Robinson-Smith, Dolen, et al., 2010). Use of such models would also encourage public policies that support full participation of all citizens through greater availability of personal assistants and affordable and accessible transportation. Other models of disability are discussed in Chapter 12.

Today, children born with intellectual and physical disabilities and those who acquire them early in life are also living into middle and older age. Often, their care has been provided by the family, primarily by the parents. As parents age and can no longer provide the needed care, they seek additional help with the care or long-term care alternatives for their children. However, few services are available at present to support a smooth transition between caregiving by parents and then by others. Research and public policy must focus on supports and interventions that allow people with disabilities who are aging to increase or maintain function within their personal environment as well as in the outside community.

Ethical and Legal Issues Affecting the Older Adult

Nurses play an important role in supporting and informing patients and families when making treatment decisions. This nursing role becomes even more important in the care of aging patients who are facing life-altering and possibly end-of-life decisions. There is the potential for loss of rights, victimization, and other serious problems if a patient has not made plans for personal and property management in the event of disability or death. As advocates, nurses encourage end-of-life discussions and educate older persons to prepare **advance directives** before incapacitation occurs (CNA, 2015).

An advance directive is a document that provides instructions for care or names a proxy decision maker (**enduring power of attorney**). In Canada, not all provinces or territories have legalized advance directives. It is to be implemented if the signer becomes incapacitated. This written document must be signed by the person and by two witnesses, and a copy should be given to the physician and placed in the medical record. The person needs to understand that the advance directive is not meant to be used only when certain (or all) types of medical treatment are withheld; rather, it allows for a detailed description of all health care preferences, including full use of all available medical interventions. The health care proxy may have the authority to interpret the patient's wishes on the basis of medical circumstances and is not restricted to the decisions or situations stated in the advance directives, such as whether life-sustaining treatment can be withdrawn or withheld.

When such serious decisions are made, possibilities exist for significant conflict of values among patients, family members, health care professionals, and the legal representative. Autonomy and self-determination are Western concepts, and people from different cultures may view advance directives as a method for denial of care. Older people from some cultures may be unwilling to consider the future, or they may wish to protect relatives and not want them to be informed about a serious illness. Nurses can facilitate the decision-making process by being sensitive to the complexity of patients' values and respecting their decisions. Directives must be focused on the wishes of the patient, not those of the family or the designated proxy.

If no advance arrangement has been made and the older person appears unable to make decisions, the court may be petitioned for a competency hearing. If the court rules that an older person is incompetent, the judge appoints a guardian—a third party who is given powers by the court to assume responsibility for making financial or personal decisions for that person.

People with communication difficulties or mild dementia may be viewed as incapable of self-determination. Most persons with mild dementia have sufficient cognitive capability to make some, but perhaps not all, decisions. For example, a patient may be able to identify a proxy decision maker yet be unable to select specific treatment options. People with mild dementia may be competent to understand the nature and significance of such decisions.

Critical Thinking Exercises

1 As a new nurse working in a busy medical-surgical unit, you notice that some of the older patients are presenting with a relatively flat affect. What do you suspect may be the cause of this flattened affect? What screening tool(s) would you recommend for these patients? Would you recommend that these tools be used for every older patient? Why? What follow-up would you recommend? What is the strength of the evidence base guiding your assessment, actions, and recommendations?

2 An 82-year-old woman has been admitted to the emergency department three times in the past 6 months for a fall without a major injury. What are some possible causes of these frequent falls? What essential assessments would you perform? What referrals would you make and why?

3 During a posthospitalization home visit for an 81-year-old man with diabetes and an extensive cardiac history, you attempt to do medication reconciliation. The patient admits to some forgetfulness and even confusion about his complex medication schedule. How should you proceed? Identify priorities and strategies that may be helpful to the patient so that he can adhere to the regimen.

REFERENCES AND SELECTED READINGS

Books

Boltz, M., Capezuti, E., Fulmer, T. T., et al. (Eds.). (2016). *Evidence-based geriatric nursing protocols for best practice*. New York: Springer.

Canadian Gerontological Nursing Association. (2010). *Gerontological nursing competencies and standards of practice*. Ottawa, Canada: Author.

Hirst, S. P., Lane, A. M., & Miller, C. A. (2015). *Miller's nursing for wellness in older adults*. Philadelphia, PA: Wolters Kluwer.

Huether, S. E., & McCance, K. L. (2016). *Understanding pathophysiology* (6th ed.). St. Louis, MO: Elsevier.

Le Couteur, D. G., McLachlan, A. J., & Hilmer, S. N. (2017). Principles of medication management. In *Oxford textbook of geriatric medicine* (3rd ed.). Oxford, United Kingdom: Oxford University Press.

Munro, H. N., Gersovitz, M., & Young, V. R. (2018). Human aging: Protein and amino acid metabolism and implications for protein and amino acid requirements. In *Nutritional approaches to aging research* (pp. 58–93). CRC Press.

Tabloski, P. (2009). *Gerontological nursing*. Upper Saddle River, NJ: Pearson Education.

Journals and Electronic Documents

American Geriatrics Society 2015 Beers Criteria Update Expert Panel; Fick, D. M., Semla, T. P., Beizer, J., Brandt, N., Dombrowski, R., . . . & Giovannetti, E. (2015). American Geriatrics Society 2015 updated Beers criteria for potentially inappropriate medication use in older adults. *Journal of the American Geriatrics Society*, *63*(11), 2227–2246.

Alzheimer Society of Canada. (2018). *About dementia*. Retrieved from http://www.alzheimer.ca/en/About-dementia

Britton, A., Ben-Shlomo, Y., Benzeval, M., et al. (2015). Life course trajectories of alcohol consumption in the United Kingdom using longitudinal data from nine cohort studies. *BMC Medicine*, *13*(1), 47.

Brown-O'Hara, T. (2013). Geriatric syndromes and their implications for nursing. *Nursing*, *43*(1), 1–3.

Canadian Continence Foundation. (2014). *Impacts of incontinence in Canada*. Retrieved from http://www.canadiancontinence.ca/pdfs/en-impact-of-incontinence-in-canada-2014.pdf

Canadian Institute for Health Information (CIHI). (2014a). *Commonwealth Fund Survey 2014: Informal caregiving infographic*. Retrieved from https://www.cihi.ca/en/commonwealth-fund-survey-2014-informal-caregiving-infographic

Canadian Institute for Health Information (CIHI). (2014b). *Drug use among seniors on public drug programs in Canada, 2012*. Retrieved from https://secure.cihi.ca/free_products/Drug_Use_in_Seniors_on_Public_Drug_Programs_2012_EN_web.pdf

Canadian Medical Association (CMA). (2016). *The state of seniors health care in Canada*. Retrieved from https://www.cma.ca/En/Lists/Medias/the-state-of-seniors-health-care-in-canada-september-2016.pdf

Canadian Mental Health Association Ontario. (2012). *Seniors and depression*. Retrieved from http://www.ontario.cmha.ca/seniors.asp?cID=5800

Canadian Mortgage and Housing Corporation. (2015). *Housing for older Canadians: The definitive guide to the over-55 market*. Retrieved from https://www.cmhc-schl.gc.ca/odpub/pdf/67514.pdf?fr=1442091635269

Canadian Nurses Association (CNA). (2015). *Joint position statement on the palliative approach to care and the role of the nurse*. Retrieved from https://www.cna-aiic.ca/~/media/cna/page-content/pdf-en/the-palliative-approach-to-care-and-the-role-of-the-nurse_e.pdf

Canadian Thoracic Association. (2014). *Sleep apnea*. Retrieved from https://www.lung.ca/lung-health/lung-disease/sleep-apnea

Cattanach, A., & Sibindi, S. (2016). Warfarin, St John's wort and INR. *Australian Prescriber, 39*(2), 32–33.

Centers for Disease Control and Prevention. (2012). *Program to encourage active, rewarding lives for seniors (PEARLS)—A depression management program for elderly adults*. Retrieved from http://www.cdc.gov/prc/pdf/program-encourage-active-rewarding.pdf

Cohen, E., Nardi, Y., Krause, I., et al. (2014). A longitudinal assessment of the natural rate of decline in renal function with age. *Journal of Nephrology, 27*(6), 635–641.

Covinsky, K., Pierluissi, E., Johnston, C. B., et al. (2017). How can I help older people in hospital get home sooner and prevent deconditioning? *Journal of the American Medical Association, 306*(16), 1782–1793.

Dellefield, M. E., Castle, N. G., McGilton, K. S., et al. (2015). The relationship between registered nurses and nursing home quality: An integrative review (2008-2014). *Nursing Economics, 33*(2), 95–108, 116.

El Hussein, M., & Hirst, S. (2016). Chasing the Mirage: A grounded theory of the clinical reasoning processes that Registered Nurses use to recognize delirium. *Journal of Advanced Nursing, 72*(2), 373–381.

Fisher, K. L., Harrison, E. L., Reeder, B. A., et al. (2015). Is self-reported physical activity participation associated with lower health services utilization among older adults? Cross-sectional evidence from the Canadian Community Health Survey. *Journal of Aging Research, 2015*, 425354.

Folstein, M. F., Folstein, S., & McHugh, P. R. (1975). Mini-mental state. A practical method for grading the cognitive state of patients for the clinician. *Journal of Psychiatric Research, 12*(3), 189–198.

Garner, R., Tanuseputro, P., Manuel, D. G., et al. (2018). *Transitions to long-term and residential care among older Canadians Catalogue no. 82-003-X ISSN 1209–1367*. Retrieved from http://www.statcan.gc.ca/pub/82-003-x/2018005/article/54966-eng.pdf

Government of Canada. (2017). *For health professionals: Flu (influenza)*. Retrieved March 16, 2018, from https://www.canada.ca/en/public-health/services/diseases/flu-influenza/health-professionals-flu-influenza.html#s8

Handelsman, D. J., Sikaris, K., & Ly, L. P. (2016). Estimating age-specific trends in circulating testosterone and sex hormone-binding globulin in males and females across the lifespan. *Annals of Clinical Biochemistry, 53*(3), 377–384.

Health Canada. (2011). *Risk of important drug interactions between St. John's Wort and prescription drugs*. Retrieved from http://www.hc-sc.gc.ca/dhp-mps/medeff/advisories-avis/prof/_2000/hypericum_perforatum_hpc-cps-eng.php

Health Canada. (2012). *Vitamin D and calcium: Updated dietary reference intakes*. Retrieved from http://www.hc-sc.gc.ca/fn-an/nutrition/vitamin/vita-d-eng.php

Health Canada. (2015). *Canadian guidelines for body weight classification in adults*. Retrieved from http://www.hc-sc.gc.ca/fn-an/nutrition/weights-poids/guide-ld-adult/weight_book_tc-livres_des_poids_tm-eng.php

Hypertension Canada. (2013). *Limit salt/sodium intake*. Retrieved from http://www.hypertension.ca/en/hypertension/what-can-i-do/limit-salt-sodium-intake

Hypertension Canada. (2014). *Hypertension diagnosis*. Retrieved from http://www.hypertension.ca/diagnosis

Institute for Safe Medication Practices Canada. (2012). *Safer medication use in older persons*. Retrieved from http://www.ismp-canada.org/beers_list

Kaasalainen, S., Ploeg, J., Donald, F., et al. (2015). Positioning clinical nurse specialists and nurse practitioners as change champions to implement a pain protocol in long-term care. *Pain Management Nursing, 16*(2), 78–88.

Lazar, F., Bent, H., Shapkin, K., et al. (2013). Nurse Practitioners bridge care gap, reduce ER visits for residents in supportive living. *Alberta RN, 69*(2), 32–33.

Leung, A. A., Daskalopoulou, S. S., Dasgupta, K., et al. (2017). Hypertension Canada's 2017 guidelines for diagnosis, risk assessment, prevention, and treatment of hypertension in adults. *Canadian Journal of Cardiology, 33*(5), 557–576.

Levasseur, M., Généreux, M., Bruneau, J. F., et al. (2015). Importance of proximity to resources, social support, transportation and neighborhood security for mobility and social participation in older adults: Results from a scoping study. *BMC Public Health, 15*(1), 503.

Lusardi, M. M., Fritz, S., Middleton, A., et al. (2017). Determining risk of falls in community dwelling older adults: A systematic review and meta-analysis using posttest probability. *Journal of Geriatric Physical Therapy, 40*(1), 1–36.

Meng, Y., Holmes, J., Hill-McManus, D., et al. (2014). Trend analysis and modelling of gender-specific age, period and birth cohort effects on alcohol abstention and consumption level for drinkers in Great Britain using the General Lifestyle Survey 1984–2009. *Addiction, 109*(2), 206–215.

Mossello, E., Tesi, F., Di Santo, S. G., et al. (2018). Recognition of delirium features in clinical practice: Data from the "Delirium Day 2015" National Survey. *Journal of the American Geriatrics Society, 66*, 302–308. Retrieved from https://iris.unito.it/retrieve/handle/2318/1658764/386064/JAGS%20Mossello%20DELIRIUM.pdf

National Advisory Committee on Immunization (NACI). (2016). *A review of the literature of high dose seasonal influenza vaccine for adults 65 years and older*. Retrieved from https://www.canada.ca/content/dam/phac-aspc/migration/phac-aspc/naci-ccni/assets/pdf/influenza-vaccine-65-plus-vaccin-contre-la-grippe-65-plus-eng.pdf

O'Regan, N. A., Fitzgerald, J., Timmons, S., et al. (2013). Delirium: A key challenge for perioperative care. *International Journal of Surgery, 11*(2), 136–144.

Public Health Agency of Canada. (2012). *Elder abuse—It's time to face the reality*. Retrieved from http://www.phac-aspc.gc.ca/ncfv-cnivf/sources/age/age-abuse-broch/index-eng.php

Public Health Agency of Canada. (2014). *Seniors' falls in Canada: Second report*. Retrieved from https://www.canada.ca/content/dam/phac-aspc/migration/phac-aspc/seniors-aines/publications/public/injury-blessure/seniors_falls-chutes_aines/assets/pdf/seniors_falls-chutes_aines-eng.pdf

Public Health Agency of Canada. (2016). *Health status of Canadians 2016: A report of the Chief Public Health Officer*. Ottawa, Canada. Retrieved from http://healthycanadians.gc.ca/publications/department-ministere/state-public-health-status-2016-etat-sante-publique-statut/alt/pdf-eng.pdf

Rochon, P., Schmader, K., & Sokol, H. N. (2012). *Drug prescribing for older adults*. Retrieved from http://www.uptodate.com/contents/drug-prescribing-for-older-adults

Rockwook, K., & Bergman, H. (2012). FRAILTY: A report from the 3rd joint workshop of IAGG/WHO/SFGG. *Canadian Geriatrics Journal, 15*(2), 31–36. Retrieved from http://www.cgjonline.ca/index.php/cgj/article/view/35/77

Schneeberg, A., Bettinger, J. A., McNeil, S., et al. (2014). Knowledge, attitudes, beliefs and behaviours of older adults about pneumococcal immunization, a Public Health Agency of Canada/Canadian Institutes of Health Research Influenza Research Network (PCIRN) investigation. *BMC Public Health, 14*(1), 442.

Smeltzer, S., Robinson-Smith, G., Dolen, M. A., et al. (2010). Disability related content in nursing textbooks. *Nursing Education Perspectives, 31*(3), 148–155.

Statistics Canada. (2012a). *Disability in Canada: Initial findings from the Canadian survey on disability*. Retrieved from http://www.statcan.gc.ca/pub/89-654-x/89-654-x2013002-eng.htm

Statistics Canada. (2012b). *Senior women*. Retrieved from http://www.statcan.gc.ca/pub/89-503-x/2010001/article/11441-eng.htm

Statistics Canada. (2016). *Hearing loss of Canadians, 2012–2015*. Retrieved from https://www.statcan.gc.ca/pub/82-625-x/2016001/article/14658-eng.htm

Statistics Canada. (2017a). *Highlight tables – Age and sex, Census year 2016*. Retrieved from http://www5.statcan.gc.ca/olc-cel/olc.action?objId=98-402-X2016002&objType=46&lang=en&limit=0

Statistics Canada. (2017b). *A portrait of the population aged 85 and older in 2016 in Canada*. Retrieved from http://www12.statcan.gc.ca/census-recensement/2016/as-sa/98-200-x/2016004/98-200-x2016004-eng.pdf

Statistics Canada. (2017c). *Family, households, and marital status: Key results from the 2016 census*. Retrieved from https://www.statcan.gc.ca/daily-quotidien/170802/dq170802a-eng.htm

Statistics Canada. (2017d). *Leading causes of death 2013*. Retrieved from http://www.statcan.gc.ca/pub/82-625-x/2017001/article/14776-eng.htm

Statistics Canada. (2018). *Transitions to long-term and residential care among older Canadians*. Retrieved from https://www150.statcan.gc.ca/n1/pub/82-003-x/2018005/article/54966-eng.htm

Tolentino, M. J., Dennrick, A., John, E., et al. (2015). Drugs in Phase II clinical trials for the treatment of age-related macular degeneration. *Expert Opinion on Investigational Drugs, 24*(2), 183–199.

World Health Organization. (2014). *Global status report on alcohol and health 2014*. Retrieved from http://www.who.int/substance_abuse/publications/global_alcohol_report/msb_gsr_2014_1.pdf

Yang, L. P., & Deeks, E. D. (2015). Dextromethorphan/Quinidine: A review of its use in adults with pseudobulbar affect. *Drugs, 75*(1), 83–90.

Yesavage, J., Brink, T. L., Rose, T. L., et al. (1983). Development and validation of a geriatric screening scale: A preliminary report. *Journal of Psychiatric Research*, *17*(1), 37–49.

Resources and Web Sites

Alzheimer Society of Canada: http://www.alzheimer.ca
Canadian Association on Gerontology: http://www.cagacg.ca
Canadian Association of Schools of Nursing. (2017). Entry-to-practice gerontological care competencies for baccalaureate programs in nursing. Ottawa, Canada: Author.
Canadian Coalition for Seniors' Mental Health: https://ccsmh.ca
Canadian Continence Foundation: http://www.canadiancontinence.ca/EN/
Canadian Foundation for Health Care Improvement: https://www.cfhi-fcass.ca/#
Canadian Gerontological Nursing Association: http://www.cgna.net
Canadian Hospice Palliative Care Association: http://www.chpca.net
Canadian Lung Association: http://www.lung.ca
Canadian National Institute for the Blind (CNIB): http://www.cnib.ca
Canadian Network for the Prevention of Elder Abuse: http://www.cnpea.ca
Centre for Addiction and Mental Health: https://www.camh.ca/
ElderWeb: https://www.seniorliving.org
GeroNurseOnline.*org*: http://www.geronurse-online.org
Hypertension Canada: http://www.hypertension.ca
National Initiative for the Care of the Elderly: http://www.nicenet.ca
Osteoporosis: http://www.osteoporosis.ca
Public Health Agency of Canada: Canadian Best Practices Portal: http://cbpp-pcpe.phac-aspc.gc.ca/public-health-topics/seniors
Veterans Affairs Canada: https://www.veterans.gc.ca/eng

15 Hospice, Palliative, and End-of-Life Care

Adapted by Charlotte Pooler and Kärin Olson

Learning Objectives

On completion of this chapter, the learner will be able to:

1. Discuss historical, legal, and sociocultural context of palliative and end-of-life care.
2. Describe principles and components of palliative and end-of-life care.
3. Discuss general considerations in the care of seriously ill patients and their families.
4. Identify his or her own personal experience with and attitudes toward death and dying.
5. Implement nursing interventions to manage symptoms associated with palliative and end-of-life care.
6. Identify components of advance care planning.
7. Provide culturally and spiritually sensitive care to patients at the end of life and their families.
8. Identify components of uncomplicated grief and mourning, and implement nursing measures to support the patient, family, and professional caregivers.

Nursing and Hospice Palliative Care at the End-of-Life Care

One of the most difficult realities that nurses face is that, despite our very best efforts, patients will die. We cannot change this fact, but we can have a significant and lasting effect on the way in which patients live until they die, the manner in which the death occurs, and the enduring memories of that death for the families. Nursing has a long history of holistic, person- and family-centred care. In this chapter we begin by discussing the key contexts that have shaped palliative and **end-of-life care**. This is followed by a section on key principles of end-of-life care, issues pertaining to the family as the unit of care at the end of life, managing **symptoms** associated with advanced illness, care of the patient and family during the dying process, and professional caregiving issues.

Knowledge about end-of-life decisions and principles of care helps nurses support patients and their families at the end of life in ways that recognize their unique responses to illness and that support their values and goals. Education, clinical practice, and research concerning end-of-life care are evolving, and the need to prepare nurses and other health care professionals to care for the dying has emerged as a priority. At no time in nursing's history has there been a greater opportunity to bring research, education, and practice together to change the culture of dying as well as bring much-needed improvements to care that is relevant across practice settings, age groups, cultural backgrounds, and illnesses.

The Historical, Technologic, Legal, and Sociocultural Contexts of Hospice Palliative Care at the End of Life

Historical Context

In the last century, chronic, degenerative diseases replaced communicable diseases as the major causes of death. With this change, dying generally became a more protracted process, frequently associated with suffering and significant discomfort. Those who are dying now are older than in previous years, and diseases such as cancer and acquired immunodeficiency syndrome (AIDS) have been considered chronic for decades (Jennings, Ryndes, D'Onofrio, et al., 2003). In Canada, cancer remains the leading cause of death followed by heart disease, stroke, and chronic respiratory disease; in 2010, cancer was the fourth cause of hospitalization in all ages and the third cause in adults 45 to 64 years of age (Public Health Agency of Canada, 2016).

Modern **hospice** palliative care began with the work of Dame Cicely Saunders in the 1960s in the United Kingdom. In July 1967, she founded St. Christopher's Hospice, a 60-bed facility for the terminally ill located in England. In Canada, the first facility to provide care for individuals no longer receiving curative treatment was established at St. Boniface General Hospital in Winnipeg in 1974. A second **palliative care** unit was opened in 1974 at the Royal Victoria Hospital in Montreal.

In 2001, Health Canada created the Secretariat on Palliative and End-of-life Care and a year later, the CHPCA published *A Model to Guide Hospice and Palliative Care: Based on the National Principles and Norms of Practice*. The standards included in this document provided the framework for the development of the *Hospice Palliative Care Nursing Standards of Practice*, which were first published in 2002 by the CHPCA in conjunction with the Canadian Nurses Association (CNA). These standards were updated in 2009 and provide the basis for the certification exam in hospice palliative care available through CNA. On December 12, 2017, Royal assent was given to the Framework on Palliative Care in Canada Act, in which the Palliative Care Act of Canada recognizes the importance of ensuring Canadians have access to palliative care (Government of Canada, 2017).

Technologic Context

The technologic advances in health care have extended and improved the quality of life for many, but the ability of technologies to prolong life beyond the point that some would consider meaningful has raised troubling ethical issues. In the latter half of the 20th century, a "technologic imperative" emerged in clinical practice, along with an

Glossary

advance directive: see personal directive; terminology varies across provinces

advance care planning: a broad term to include discussion and documentation of wishes and goals, including medical care, may also include financial decisions and will. Within the health care setting, health professionals and the person may discuss their goals, priorities, wishes for location of care, preferred place of death, and limitations for life-sustaining treatment

assisted suicide: use of pharmacologic agents to hasten the death of a person

autonomy: self-determination; in the health care context, the right of the individual to make choices about the use and discontinuation of medical treatment

bereavement: period during which mourning for a loss takes place

euthanasia: Greek for "good death" or "easy death"; has evolved to mean the intentional killing of an ill or injured human or animal, as an act of mercy for his or her alleged benefit

grief: the personal feelings that accompany an anticipated or actual loss

hospice: a coordinated program of interprofessional care and services for patients at the end of life and their families. Care is provided primarily in the home or specialized settings in the community

interprofessional collaboration: when members of diverse health care disciplines and professions jointly plan, implement, and evaluate care

medical assistance in dying: administration of a substance by a physician or nurse practitioner that causes death to a person at their request, or prescribing or providing of a substance by a physician or nurse practitioner to a person at their request so they may take the substance and cause their own death

mourning: individual, family, group, and cultural expressions of grief and associated behaviours

end-of-life care: comprehensive care for patients and their families in the last days and hours of life, when cure is no longer possible

palliative approach: use of palliative care principles for persons with chronic, life-limiting conditions across the course of their illness, with a focus on quality of life and symptom management

palliative care: services and care to relieve suffering and improve the quality of life for persons who have a life-limiting illness that is usually at an advanced stage

palliative sedation: use of pharmacologic agents, at the request of the terminally ill patient, to induce sedation when symptoms have not responded to other management measures. The purpose of palliative sedation is to relieve intractable symptoms, not to hasten the patient's death

personal directive: a legal document written by the individual that indicates wishes for care, including medical care but excluding financial aspects, with a named agent who will make decisions when the person is not able to communicate their own wishes or does not have the capacity to make decisions

sign: objective indicator that one is not well; assessed by individual or other; may or may not be indicator of disease-related processes

spirituality: the search for meaning and purpose in life, intangible elements that impart meaning and vitality to life, and a connectedness to a higher or transcendent dimension

symptom: subjective indicator that one is not well; perceived by person; may or may not be indicator of disease-related processes

terminal illness: progressive, irreversible illness that is not responding to curative treatment and thus will result in the patient's death expectation among some patients and families, that every available means to extend life must be tried.

In the earlier part of the last century, most deaths occurred at home. Because of this, most families had direct experience "being with" death, providing care to family members at the end of life, and **mourning** for the loss of loved ones. Decisions to apply every available technology to extend life contributed to the shift in the place of death from the home to the hospital or extended care facility. As a result of this shift, families witness death less often. By the early 1970s, when hospice care was just beginning in Canada, technology had become the expected companion of the critically and terminally ill (Waller & Caroline, 2000). The implications of technologic intervention at the end of life continue to be profound, as they affect the societal view of death including how clinicians care for the dying, how family and friends participate in care, how patients and families understand and choose among end-of-life care options, how families prepare for **terminal illness** and death, and the **bereavement** experiences of families.

There is some evidence that the advances in technology have not helped to facilitate a peaceful death. For example, Callahan (1993) found that people viewed death as what happened when medicine fails. A search of the literature indexed in Medline and Cinahl showed a growth in the numbers of studies on technologic issues associated with end-of-life care. For example, McMahan, Knight, Fried, et al. (2013) used a series of focus groups to explore how health care professionals could help families navigate the complex and often technical decisions that need to be made at the end of life. Brummen and Griffiths (2013) found that families were concerned that care in hospital at the end of life could become overly "medicalized" and advocated for provision of care in the home or specialized settings. Attention has been directed to end-of-life care in high technology settings including adult and pediatric critical care, and a **palliative approach** is part of the comprehensive care for critically ill patients in many intensive care units (Aslakson, Curits, & Nelson, 2014; Mauricio & Okhuysen-Cawley, 2010). Stajduhar et al. (2017) reported lower satisfaction by bereaved caregivers of quality in end of life in extended care units, with no difference between intensive care, acute medical care, and palliative care units.

Legal and Ethical Contexts

Legal and ethical issues add to the complexity of decision related to technology use and location of death. In Canada, responsibility for health and justice vary by province. The legislation related to **advance directives** fall within provincial jurisdiction; thus, elements in place in one province may not apply elsewhere. Current information, forms, and legal requirements may be obtained most readily through the local or provincial office of the Public Guardian. However, there are national endeavours designed to facilitate **advance care planning**. In Canada, there are both national and provincial/territorial initiatives and resources, including National Framework led by the CHPCA and National Advanced Care Planning Day (CHPCA, 2012, 2015). Advance care planning is the discussion of wishes and goals for medical treatment and personal care, with family and friends, and may also include health care providers, lawyers, or both. It may include a written plan, referred to as an advanced or **personal directive** which documents the expression of wishes for medical care. A substitute decision maker or named agent may make decisions for a person who is no longer able to do so on their own behalf, guided by relevant advance care planning documents, such as the advance or personal directives (CHPCA, 2012) or medical orders such as Goals of Care Designations (GCD) Order, Do Not Resuscitate (DNR), and Goals of Care (GOC) Orders (Alberta Health Services, 2014; BC Cancer Agency, 2015).

Although the traditional intent of advance directives was to ensure that patients' wishes were honoured, numerous U.S. studies have found that only a minority of adults (20% to 30%) have completed an advance directive and that this tool has limited effects on treatment decisions near end of life (Hickman, Hammes, Moss, et al., 2005). Hickman et al. noted that advance directives are not as successful as initially intended for a number of reasons: the lack of discussion regarding underlying goals and values, lack of discussion regarding preferences for care, the failure to address cultural issues, poor communication between patients and physicians, difficulty accessing resources to develop advance care plans, and the absence of systems to support advance care planning. In a study conducted for Health Canada, Dunbrack (2006) reported similar findings, plus noted that the terminology was confusing and discouraged consumers from participating unless adequate time was provided for discussion. The National Framework noted above builds on work that was supported by Health Canada and conducted by two health authorities, the former Calgary Health Region (now part of Alberta Health Services) and the Fraser Health Authority.

Nurses engage in advance care planning by initiating and documenting conversations with patients about their wishes, by advocating for patient rights and wishes, and by honouring advance directives. Nurses have an ethical and legal obligation to respect advance directives. It is important for the registered nurse to advocate for patient/client wishes, and to know that Canadian law indicates that advance directives be respected.

Sociocultural Context

Separate and apart from the historical, technologic, and legal issues related to end-of-life care, nurses must also consider the unique influences of the patient's own social and cultural context. Each individual experiences terminal illness in a unique way. This experience is shaped substantially by the contexts in which it occurs. Life-threatening illness, life-sustaining treatment decisions, dying, and death all occur in a social environment. Historically, illness was largely considered a foe where battles were either lost or won (Benoliel, 1993). Thus it is not surprising that a care/cure dichotomy emerged in which health care providers viewed cure as the ultimate good and care as second best (Benoliel, 1993). In this dichotomous model, alleviating suffering was not as valued as curing disease, and patients who could not be cured felt distanced from the health care team. Patients and families who internalize this socially constructed meaning of care as second best may fear that any shift from curative goals to goals focused on comfort care will result in no care or poorer-quality care, and that the clinicians on whom they have come to rely will abandon them if they withdraw from the battle for cure.

The view that care as second best results in no care or poorer-quality care is exemplified in the phrase "nothing more can be done for you" sometimes heard by patients with late-stage illness. This statement communicates the belief that there is nothing of value to offer patients who cannot be cured. Nothing could be further from the truth. Even in the "early days" of end-of-life care, authors noted that simply treating the body without attending to the mind and the spirit was unacceptable.

Clinician Attitudes Toward Death

Clinicians' attitudes toward individuals no longer receiving curative treatment influence their abilities to provide care for these individuals. In her seminal work *On Death and Dying*, published in 1969, Kübler-Ross noted that it was common for patients to not be informed about life-threatening diagnoses, particularly cancer, and for physicians and nurses to avoid open discussion of death and dying with their patients (Krisman-Scott, 2000). Kübler-Ross taught the health care community that having open discussion about life and death issues does not harm patients and that the patients in fact welcome such openness. She was openly critical of what she called "a new but depersonalized science in the service of prolonging life rather than diminishing human suffering" (Kübler-Ross, 1969, p. 20).

Clinicians' reluctance to discuss disease and death openly with patients may stem from their own anxieties about death as well as from misconceptions about what and how much patients want to know about their illnesses. In an early study of care of the dying in hospital settings, sociologists Glaser and Strauss (1965) discovered that health care professionals in hospital settings avoided direct communication about dying in the hope that the patient would discover it on his or her own.

Glaser and Strauss (1965) also identified a pattern of clinician behaviour in which those who feared or were uncomfortable discussing death developed and substituted "personal mythologies" for appraisals of what level of disclosure patients actually wanted. For example, clinicians avoided direct communication with patients about the seriousness of their illness based on their beliefs that patients either already knew the truth or would ask if they wanted to know; or that patients would subsequently lose all hope, give up, or be psychologically harmed by disclosure. Glaser and Strauss' findings were published nearly 50 years ago, yet some would argue that their observations remain valid today. Although a growing number of health care providers are becoming comfortable with disclosing information about the seriousness of illness, there is some evidence that the "conspiracy of silence" about dying appears still exists (Marzano, 2009). It is important to remember that information sharing between health professionals, patients, and family is influenced by local cultural practices. For example, in some countries it is customary to not discuss patients' diagnoses with them (Marzano, 2009).

Patient and Family Attitudes Toward Death

Patient and family attitudes toward death play an important part in determining whether end-of-life issues are discussed. Kübler-Ross (1969) was one of the first to discuss the use of a strategy she termed denial to manage distress related to end-of-life concerns. She thought that denial seemed useful because it enabled patients to gain temporary emotional distance from something that was too painful to contemplate fully.

Denial is defined as a defence mechanism in which the person suppresses the existing reality. More recently, researchers have questioned whether patients actually use denial, as it is difficult to distinguish between denial, misconceptions, and strategies that help individuals manage advanced disease and poor prognosis. For example, although denial was described as a theme for family caregivers of persons with terminal illnesses, caregivers described actively being cheerful, avoiding discussion of the illness, and hiding their feelings and being brave so that others were not upset (Riley & Fenton, 2007). Benkel et al. (2010) reported that strategies used by patients and their family members were not the result of denial but new ways to focus, function and cope, having both insight and hope for the future. However, caregivers who perceived they needed to support the patient's denial had conflicted demands and burdens: Four of the 16 interviewed felt they were prevented from participating in advance care planning, including memories, wills, and funerals; nine felt guilty or distressed because they were prevented from reporting symptoms to the physician or nurse; and six used denial to provide relief for themselves (Kogan, Dumas, & Cohen, 2013). Clearly, further research is needed to examine and understand the complex approaches used by patients and families to manage experiences and information related to advanced disease.

It is sometimes a challenge to communicate with patients in a way that acknowledges their preferences for disclosure of information about their illness and that still provides them with unambiguous information. Zerwekh (1994) analyzed stories from 32 hospice nurses and concluded that they were adept at interventions deemed important in care of the dying, namely truth telling and encouraging patient **autonomy**. Zerwekh acknowledged that each individual viewed truth differently, and that hospice nurses participating in the study used communication skills that helped the patient and family discuss end-of-life issues from within this view of the truth. Hospice nurses deliberately spoke about sensitive matters that were usually avoided by others when patients were in transition from curative to end-of-life care. Although individual autonomy and informed consent are valued by health professionals, they must also be considered within cultural and relational perspectives (Rising, 2017). The perspectives on what constitutes truth and on what patients want to know is influenced by local beliefs and values. Thus it is not surprising that issues related to truth-telling raise ethical issues for health care professionals working in multicultural settings (Chater & Tsai, 2008).

Euthanasia, Suicide; Medical Assistance in Dying

As individuals approach the end of their life, symptom management often becomes more difficult and hence quality of life may decline. One consequence of this phenomenon is that debates about **euthanasia**, assisted suicide, and **medical assistance in dying (MAID)** have come to the forefront of public discourse. Euthanasia is the intentional killing of an ill or injured human or animal as an act of mercy. **Assisted suicide** refers to providing another person the means or support to end his or her own life. MAID, also referred to as physician assisted suicide in other countries, involves the prescription and/or administration by a physician or nurse practitioner of a lethal dose of medication for the purpose of ending someone's life in accordance with the wishes of the terminally ill individual (Government of Canada, 2018a). Neither assisted suicide nor MAID is equivalent to withholding or withdrawing treatment, which allows the person to die naturally from the illness or injury. The views of health care providers regarding euthanasia, suicide, and MAID are influenced by many factors including local beliefs and values as well as religious views (Giese, 2009).

Until 2016, euthanasia and MAID were expressly prohibited in Canada under the Criminal Code, and had been opposed by nursing and medical organizations as a violation of their ethical and philosophical traditions. Euthanasia was legalized in other countries such as Belgium, the Netherlands, and Switzerland. At the time of writing, five states in the United States (Oregon, Washington, Montana, Vermont, and California) legally permit MAID. Although the preference to take one's own life over awaiting death has been evident through the ages, the growing discourse regarding assisted suicide adds to the complexity associated with end-of-life care.

In February of 2015, the Supreme Court of Canada ruled that parts of the Criminal Code would need to change to allow MAID to comply with the Charter of Rights and Freedoms. The Government of Canada passed legislation on June 17, 2016 to allow eligible Canadian adults to request MAID, defined as either a physician or nurse practitioner giving or providing a substance resulting in death at the patient's request (Government of Canada, 2018a). Subsequently, under Bill C-14, the Criminal Code and each of the provincial or territorial health and professional-related laws and policies, physicians and nurse practitioners may provide MAID; pharmacists and health care providers may assist; and family members or others may help when asked by the dying person. The legislation does not require any person to provide MAID. The law contains safeguards for implementation, such as free will, informed consent, and eligibility criteria, to which all provinces and territories must adhere (Government of Canada, 2018a). Quebec's legislation on medical aid in dying was enacted prior to the federal law, and aligns with the federal framework. According to federal Canadian reports, between June 2016 and December 2017, approximately half of the medically assisted deaths following the new legislation noted above occurred in hospital settings; and about 2/3 of the persons were diagnosed with cancer (Government of Canada, 2018b).

There is ongoing discussion in Canada on questions regarding the right to end suffering, the need for transparency and clarification of choices, and the commitment to provide funding for comfort and end-of-life care. In Canada, federal legislation recognized the importance of the role of the nurse on the health care team, outlines the roles and ethical obligations, such as providing compassionate care, promoting justice, and respecting patients' wishes, yet addressed the right of each individual's conscientious objection for participation in actions related to MAID (CNA, 2017a).

Whereas proponents of assisted suicide argue that terminally ill individuals should have a legally sanctioned right to make independent decisions about the value of their lives and the timing and circumstances of their deaths, opponents argue for greater access to symptom management and psychosocial support for individuals approaching the end of life. Numerous ethical and legal issues have been raised, including voluntariness, authenticity, mental competence, underlying untreated illness or other suffering, and decision-making capacity of patients who request assisted suicide, and issues of overt or perceived coercion. The Canadian law endeavoured to address these and other considerations. Although MAID has been legalized, additional considerations for assisted suicide are yet to be resolved. Continued dialogue is needed to move forward on this issue.

Principles and Components of Hospice Palliative Care at the End of Life

Historically, hospice referred to a shelter or way station for weary travellers on a pilgrimage. The root of the word *hospice* is *hospes*, meaning "host." In Canada, the term hospice is generally associated with care that is delivered in home-like facilities that provide around the clock for patients who are approaching end of life (CHPCA, 2018). The focus of hospice palliative care is quality of life, including emotional, social, spiritual, and physiologic concerns that often emerge for patients and their families at the end of life.

The work of Kübler-Ross (1969), Saunders and Kastenbaum (1997), and others helped to identify the need for the care provided in hospice, where the impending deaths of patients were accepted, the unit of care was the family, and the focus was on symptom management. This type of care was originally labelled *palliative* care because the focus was on managing symptoms rather than curing disease. In 1990, the World Health Organization (WHO) defined palliative care as the active, total care of patients whose disease is not responsive to treatment. CHPCA broadened the definition of palliative care to incorporate a combination of active and compassionate therapies that provide comfort and support and that involve working with individuals and families who are living with, or dying from, a progressive and advanced life-limiting illness, or those who are bereaved (CHPCA, 2014). WHO acknowledged that a broader definition was needed, and established the following definition in 2002: "Palliative care is an approach that improves the quality of life of patients and their families facing problems associated with life-threatening illness, through prevention and relief of suffering by means of early identification and impeccable assessment and treatment of pain and other problems, physical, psychosocial, and spiritual" (WHO, 2002, p. 84). WHO also defined palliative care for children: "Palliative care for children is the active total care of the child's body, mind and spirit, and also involves giving support to the family. It begins when illness is diagnosed, and continues regardless of whether or not a child receives treatment directed at the disease" (WHO, 2002).

The palliative approach uses principles of palliative care with people and caregivers facing chronic, life-limiting conditions at all stages, not only with a terminal illness or near end of life. These principles are symptom management and relief of suffering, shared decision making, and psychosocial, emotional support with dignity, hope, comfort, and quality of life (CNA, 2015; Kristjanson, Toye, & Dawson, 2003; Kristjanson, 2005; Stajduhar, 2011). Specialized palliative care addresses complex symptoms or issues by a specialized team or professional. The Joint position statement by the CNA, CHPCA, and the Canadian Hospice Palliative Care Nurses Group (CHPC-NG) indicates that registered nurses, nurse practitioners, and clinical nurse specialists all "have a fundamental role in a palliative approach to care" (2015, p. 1).

Of note, in 2007, the WHO published *Cancer Control: Knowledge into Action for Effective Programmes—Palliative Care*. This document is designed to assist governments in assessing palliative care needs and services. In 2015, a Canadian framework was finalized to guide and integrate a palliative approach to care across diverse regions, settings, provinces, diagnoses, and courses of their illness or aging.

Although palliative care is generally understood to be care provided to individuals no longer receiving curative treatment, many aspects of hospice palliative care, such as good symptom management, are easily incorporated into cure-focused treatment plans. Some would argue that in this respect, palliative care is no different from good comprehensive care and that patients should not have to have a terminal illness or be at the end of life in order to receive and benefit from a palliative approach.

Given the multiple dimensions of the illness experience for both patients and their families, palliative care is most effectively delivered by an interprofessional team. The interprofessional team works together to develop and implement a single plan of care. Membership varies depending on the services required to address the identified expectations and needs. Each member of the team contributes his or her knowledge and skill to augment and support the other's contributions. Each member's assessment must take into account others' contributions to allow for holistic management of patients' complex health problems. The provision of palliative care provides an opportunity to examine **interprofessional collaboration** more closely. Interprofessional collaboration may be distinguished from multidisciplinary practice by its focus on communication and cooperation among the various professionals involved, with each member of the team contributing to a single care plan for the patient and family.

Unfortunately, individuals are often referred to palliative care late in the disease trajectory. The reasons for late referral and underuse of services are complex. They may include values and attitudes of health care providers, the inadequate dissemination of existing knowledge about pain and symptom management, lack of information about existing services, health care providers' difficulties in effectively communicating with terminally ill individuals, and insufficient emphasis on palliative care concepts in the education of health care providers. Late referral is also related to the fact that many chronic diseases do not have a predictable "end stage." As a result, patients may experience a long, slow, distressing, and often painful decline in their health status without acknowledgement of their impending death or the benefit of a palliative approach including symptom management and advance care planning.

General Considerations in the Care of Patients With Advanced Illness and Their Families

Many patients suffer unnecessarily when they do not receive adequate attention for the symptoms accompanying serious illness. Careful evaluation of the patient should include not only the physical problems but also the psychosocial and spiritual dimensions of the patient and family's experience of serious illness. This approach contributes to a more comprehensive understanding of how the patient and family's life has been affected by the illness and will lead to nursing care that addresses the needs in every dimension.

Psychosocial Issues

Nurses are responsible for educating patients and families about the possibilities and probabilities inherent in serious illness and for supporting patients as they review their lives, clarify their values, make decisions about treatments, and generally reflect on the end of their lives. The only way to do this effectively is to learn as much as possible about the patient's perspective about his or her illness.

Kübler-Ross (1969) noted that patients in the final stages of life can and will talk openly about their experiences, exposing as a myth the view that patients will be harmed by honest discussion with their caregivers about death. Despite the continued reluctance of health care providers to engage in open discussion about end-of-life issues, many patients want information about their illness and end-of-life choices and are not harmed by open discussion about death (Hoff & Hermeren, 2014). Conversations with patients about their wishes within the context of advance care planning facilitates shared decisions about medical care and promotes important elements of end-of-life care, such as planning for funerals if desired, engaging in meaningful activities, creating memories and legacy projects, and saying final goodbyes.

Communication

As discussed previously, remarkable strides have been made in the ability to prolong life, but attention to care for the dying lags behind. On one level, this comes as no surprise. Each of us will eventually face death, and most would agree that one's own demise is a subject that he or she would prefer not to contemplate. Indeed, Glaser and Strauss (1965) noted that unwillingness in our culture to talk about the process of dying is tied to our discomfort with the notion of particular deaths—those of our patients and our own—rather than talking about death in the abstract, which is more comfortable. Finucane (2002) observed that our struggle to stay alive is a prerequisite to being human. Confronting death in our patients uncovers our own deeply rooted fears.

To develop a level of comfort and expertise in communicating with seriously and terminally ill patients and their families, nurses and other clinicians need to first consider their own experiences with and values concerning illness and death. Reflection, reading, and talking with family members, friends, and colleagues can assist the nurse to examine beliefs about death and dying. Talking with individuals from differing cultural backgrounds can assist the nurse to view personally held beliefs through a different lens and can help to sensitize the nurse to death-related beliefs and practices in other cultures. Discussion with colleagues can also be useful to reveal the values shared by many health care professions and identify diversity in the values of patients in their care. Values clarification and personal death awareness exercises can provide a starting point for self-discovery and discussion.

Skills for Communicating With Individuals Who Have Advanced Illnesses

Nurses need to develop skills and comfort in assessing patient and families' responses to serious illness and in planning interventions that will support their values and choices throughout the continuum of care. Patients and families need ongoing assistance: telling a patient something once is not teaching, and hearing the patient's words is not the same as active listening. Throughout the course of a serious illness, patients and their families will encounter complicated treatment decisions, bad news about disease progression, and recurring emotional responses. In addition to the time of initial diagnosis, lack of response to the treatment course, decisions to continue or withdraw particular interventions, and decisions about hospice care are examples of critical points on the treatment continuum that demand patience, empathy, and honesty from the nurse. Discussing sensitive issues such as serious illness, hopes for survival, and fears associated with death is never easy. However, the art of therapeutic communication can be learned and, like other skills, must be practiced to gain expertise. Similar to other skills, communication should be practiced in a "safe" setting, such as a classroom or clinical skills laboratory with other students or clinicians.

Nurses are with patients in their most vulnerable moments, with a societal and professional recognition that there is a therapeutic relationship to promote well-being. Communication with patients and families within palliative hospice are based on theory, principles, and skills applicable across nursing. Nurses use their therapeutic relationship to provide information, promote understanding, explore options for care, assist in decisions, and facilitate well-being (Arnold & Boggs, 2011). Basic communication skills should be incorporated, including:

- Create an appropriate time and space for the conversation (e.g., a private room, schedule time to be able to be fully present and engaged)
- Be aware of body language (e.g., seated, open forward posture, eye contact)
- Enable the patient/family to lead the conversation (e.g., pick up on cues)
- Explore what they know and their understandings, perceptions
- Be comfortable with silence, listen, acknowledge, and encourage
- Provide information at the depth and rate that the patient and family are able to grasp and understand (e.g., interpret medical or technical information when necessary, evaluate their understanding, check if there are additional questions they might have)

Communication may be ineffective if nurses are uncomfortable or not attending to cues from patients or family members. Examples of ineffective communication include: normalizing statements or experiences; providing false assurance; giving inappropriate advice; using leading or closed questions; or shifting focus away from the concern (Ellershaw & Wilkinson, 2011).

Nursing Interventions When the Patient and Family Receive Bad News

Communicating about a life-threatening diagnosis or about disease progression in any care setting is best accomplished by the interprofessional team—a physician, registered nurse, and social support such as spiritual leader, psychologist, or social worker should collaborate when possible to provide information, facilitate discussion, and address concerns. Most importantly, the presence of the team conveys caring and respect for the patient and family. Creating the right setting is particularly important. If the patient wishes to have family present for the discussion, arrangements should be made to have the discussion at a time that is best for everyone (Griffie, Nelson-Marten, & Muchka, 2004). A quiet area with minimum disturbance should be used. Each clinician who is present should turn off phones, beepers, or other communication devices for the duration of the meeting and should allow sufficient time for the patient and family to absorb and respond to the news. Finally, the space in which the meeting takes place should be conducive to seating all of the participants at eye level. It is difficult enough for patients and families to be the recipients of bad news without having an array of clinicians standing uncomfortably over them at the foot of the patient's bed.

After an initial discussion of a life-threatening illness or progression of a disease, patients and their families will have many questions and may need to be reminded of factual information. Coping with news about a serious diagnosis or poor prognosis is an ongoing process. The nurse needs to be sensitive to these ongoing needs and may need to repeat previously provided information or simply be present while the patient and family react emotionally. The most important intervention the nurse can provide is listening empathetically. Patients and their families need time and support to cope with the changes brought about by serious illness and the prospect of impending death. The nurse who is able to sit comfortably with another's suffering, time and time again, without judgment and without the need to solve the patient and family's problems provides an intervention that is a gift beyond measure. Keys to effective listening include the following:

- Resist the impulse to fill the "empty space" in communication with talk

- Allow the patient and family sufficient time to reflect and respond after asking a question
- Prompt gently: "Do you need more time to think about this?"
- Avoid distractions (noise, interruptions)
- Avoid the impulse to give advice
- Avoid canned responses: "I know just how you feel"
- Ask questions
- Assess understanding—your own and the patient's—by restating, summarizing, and reviewing

Responding With Sensitivity to Difficult Questions

Patients will often direct questions or concerns to nurses before they have been able to fully discuss the details of their diagnosis and prognosis with the physician or the entire health care team. Using open-ended questions allows the nurse to elicit the patient and family's concerns, explore misconceptions and needs for information, and form the basis for collaboration with the physician and other team members. For example, the seriously ill patient may ask the nurse, "Am I dying?" or "I'm not going to make it, am I?" The nurse should avoid making unhelpful responses that dismiss the patient's real concerns or defer the issue to another care provider. This question suggests that the patient sees the nurse as a safe and knowledgeable person with whom to explore their fears and concerns, and is not necessarily asking for a yes or no answer. It is important to avoid making assumptions about why the patient has raised the question, but rather to ask questions to help the nurse learn more about the patient's perceptions and any particular concerns they may have, and follow up with additional questions for clarification. In this example, the nurse might ascertain that the patient's question emanates from a need for specific information—about diagnosis and prognosis from the physician, about the physiology or fears of the dying process from the nurse, or perhaps about financial implications for the family from the social worker. So, the nurse might ask if anything that day started them thinking about that, if they are having some symptoms that are troublesome, if they have any worries at this time, or if they are thinking about plans for the future. The nurse may also express his or her concerns or validate the individual's concerns, (e.g., "I am also worried that you have been in hospital several times this year, so I agree that it's a good time to make a plan).

As a member of the interprofessional team caring for the patient at the end of life, the nurse fills an important role in facilitating the team's understanding of the patient's values and preferences, the family dynamics concerning decision making, and the patient and family's response to treatment and changing health status. Many dilemmas in patient care at the end of life are related to poor communication between team members and the patient and family and failure of team members to communicate effectively with each other. Regardless of the care setting, the nurse can ensure a proactive approach to the psychosocial care of the patient and family. Periodic, structured assessments provide an opportunity for all parties to consider their priorities and plan for an uncertain future. The nurse can assist the patient and family to clarify their values and preferences concerning end-of-life care by using a structured approach. Sufficient time must be devoted to each step so that the patient and family have time to process new information, formulate questions, and consider their options.

Providing Culturally Competent Care at the End of Life

Although death, **grief**, and mourning are universally accepted aspects of living, values, expectations, and practices during serious illness, especially as death approaches and following death, are culturally bound and expressed. Health care providers may find that they are inadequately prepared to assess for and implement care plans that support culturally diverse perspectives, particularly if a language barrier exists.

Many of the elements related to health care decisions in Canada are rooted in the Western notions of autonomy, truth telling, and the acceptability of withdrawing or withholding life-prolonging medical treatment at the end of life (Kwak & Haley, 2005; Rising, 2017). In some families and cultures, interdependence is valued over autonomy, leading to decisions and communication styles that favour shared decision making that involves family members. Personal preferences regarding the use of life-prolonging medical treatments such as cardiopulmonary resuscitation and artificially provided nutrition and hydration at the end of life are examples of values that may vary within cultures.

The nurse's role is to assess the values, preferences, and practices of every patient, regardless of ethnicity, socioeconomic status, or background. The nurse can then share this information with the health care team and facilitate the adaptation of the care plan to accommodate these practices. For example, the nurse may find that a patient prefers to have his or her eldest son make all care decisions, or a patient wants the family to have a discussion before making the decision.

Institutional practices and laws governing informed consent are also rooted in the Western notion of autonomous decision making and informed consent. If a patient wishes to defer decisions to a son, the nurse could work with the team to negotiate informed consent, respecting the patient's right not to participate in decision making and honouring his or her family's cultural practices.

The nurse should assess and document the patient and family's specific beliefs, preferences, and practices regarding end-of-life care, preparation for death, and after-death rituals. Chart 15-1 identifies topics that the nurse should cover and questions that the nurse may use to elicit the information. The nurse must use judgment and discretion about the timing and setting for eliciting this information. Some patients may wish to have a family member speak for them or because of advanced illness may be unable to provide information. The nurse should give the patient and family a context for the discussion, such as "It is very important to us to provide care that addresses your needs and the needs of your family. We want to honour and support your wishes, and want you to feel free to tell us how we are doing, and what we could do to better meet your needs. I'd like to ask you some questions; what you tell me will help me to understand and support what is most

CHART 15-1

Assessing End-of-Life Care Beliefs, Preferences, and Practices

Disclosure/truth telling: "Tell me how you/your family talk about very sensitive or serious matters."

- Content: "Are there any topics that you or your family are uncomfortable discussing?"
- Person responsible for disclosure: "Is there one person in the family who assumes responsibility for obtaining and sharing information?"
- Disclosure practices regarding children: "What kind of information may be shared with children in your family, and who is responsible for communicating with the children?"
- Sharing of information within the family or community group: "What kind/how much information should be shared with your immediate family? Your extended family? Others in the community (e.g., members of a religious community)?"

Decision-making style: "How are decisions made in your family? Who would you like to be involved in decisions about your treatment or care?"

- Individual
- Family centred
- Family elder or patriarch/matriarch
- Deference to authority (such as the physician)

Symptom management: "How would you like us to help you to manage the physical effects of your illness?"

- Acceptability of medications used for symptom relief
- Beliefs regarding expression of pain and other symptoms
- Degree of symptom management desired

Life-sustaining treatment expectations: "Have you thought about what type of medical treatment you or your loved one would want as the end of life is nearing? Do you have an advance directive (living will and/or durable power of attorney)?"

- Nutrition/hydration at the end of life
- Cardiopulmonary resuscitation
- Ventilator
- Dialysis
- Antibiotics
- Medications to treat infection

Desired location of dying: "Do you have a preference about being at home or in some other location when you die?"

- Desired role for family members in providing care: "Who do you want to be involved in caring for you at the end of life?"
- Gender-specific prohibitions: "Are you uncomfortable having either males or females provide your care or your loved one's personal care?"

Spiritual/religious practices and rituals: "Is there anything that we should know about your spiritual or religious beliefs about death? Are there any practices that you would like us to observe as death is nearing?"

Care of the body after the death: "Is there anything that we should know about how a body/your body should be treated after death?"

Expression of grief: "What types of losses have you and your family experienced? How do you and your family express grief?"

Funeral and burial practices: "Are there any rituals or practices associated with funerals or burial that are especially important to you?"

Mourning practices: "How have you and your family carried on after a loss in the past? Are particular behaviours or practices expected or required?"

important to you at this time. You don't need to answer anything that makes you uncomfortable. Is it all right to ask some questions?" The assessment of end-of-life beliefs, preferences, and practices will probably need to be carried out in short segments over a period of time (e.g., across multiple days of an inpatient hospital stay or in conjunction with multiple patient visits to an outpatient setting). The novice nurse's discomfort with asking questions and discussing this type of sensitive content can be reduced by prior practice in a classroom or clinical skills laboratory, observation of interviews conducted by experienced nurses, and partnering with an experienced nurse during the first few assessments.

Goal Setting in Palliative Care at the End of Life

As the treatment goals begin to shift in the direction of comfort care over aggressive disease-focused treatment, symptom relief and patient/family-defined quality of life assume greater prominence in treatment decision making. Patient, family, and clinicians may all be accustomed to an almost automatic tendency to pursue exhaustive diagnostic testing to locate and treat the source of the patient's illness or symptoms. Each decision to shift care from cure to comfort may be an emotional one for the patient and family. They may fear that the support that health care providers gave when the focus was on cure will be withdrawn, and need assurance that comfort and care will be provided.

Throughout the course of the illness, and especially as the patient's functional status and symptoms indicate approaching death, clinicians need to assist the patient and family to determine whether continued diagnostic testing and disease-focused medical treatment are in the patient's best interest. Patients, their families, and their health care providers may be reluctant to forego things like blood tests and x-rays that have become routine throughout earlier phases of illness. The nurse plays an instrumental role in helping the patient, family, and health care team develop a coordinated plan of care that is based on the patient's preferences and that takes their stage of illness into account (Fig. 15-1). The role of the nurse includes initiating and participating in conversations with the patient and family to clarify their goals, expected outcomes, and values as they consider options (Chart 15-2). It is important to continue to support communication among the patient, family and health care team about the wishes, goals and progression of care, with a focus on comfort and alleviation of suffering. Although particulars will vary across settings from acute care to home care, the goal is to support the patient and family before, during, and after death. For example, some patients and families may find it helpful to have a more detailed discussion

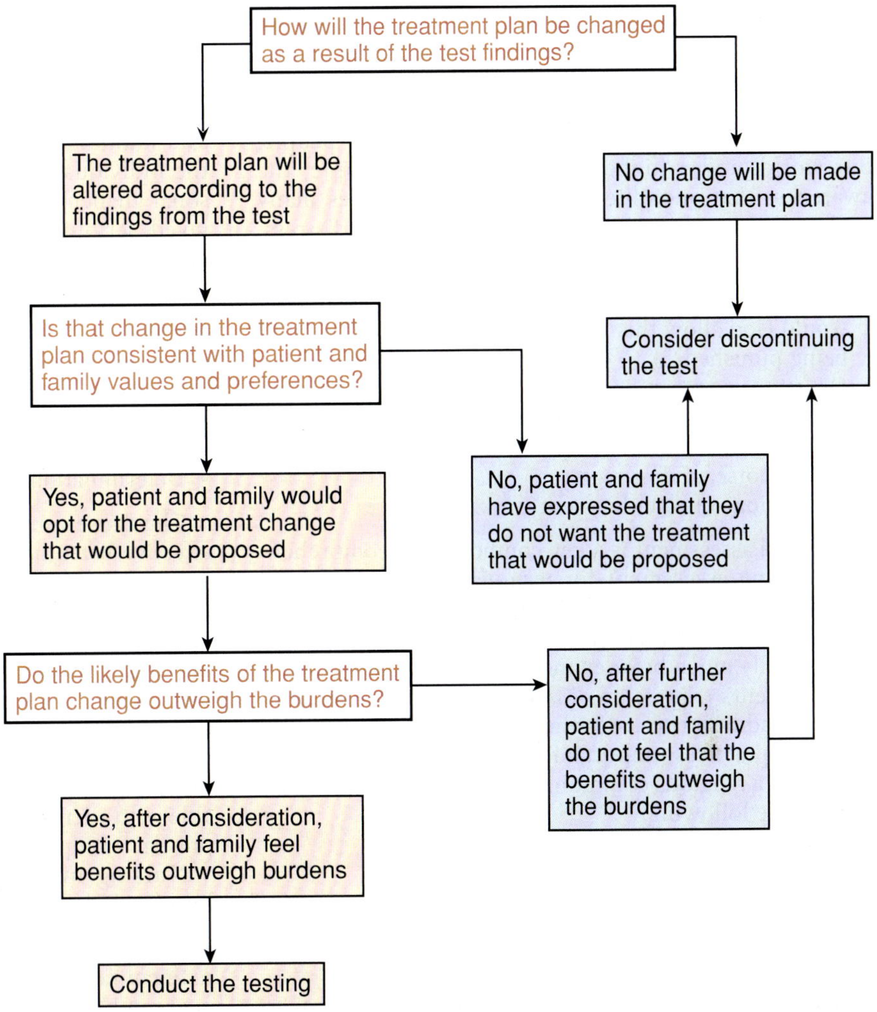

FIGURE 15-1. An algorithm for decision making about diagnostic testing at the end of life.

about treatments that improve comfort and those that may increase the patient's burden or distress. The nurse needs to work with interprofessional colleagues to ensure that the patient and family are referred for continuing psychosocial support, symptom management, and assistance with other care-related challenges (e.g., arranging for home care or hospice support, providing referrals for financial assistance, and sharing information about other programs available from governmental sources, such as compassionate care leave).

Spiritual Care

Attention to the spiritual component of the patient and family's illness experience is not new within the context of nursing care, yet many nurses lack the comfort or skills to assess and intervene in this dimension. **Spirituality** may contain features of religiosity, but the two concepts are not interchangeable (Highfield, 2000). Spirituality includes domains such as how a person derives meaning and purpose from life, one's beliefs and faith, sources of hope, and

CHART 15-2

Assessing the Patient and Family Perspective: Goal Setting in Palliative Care

- **Awareness of diagnosis, illness stage, and prognosis:** "Tell me your understanding of your illness right now."
- **Values:** "Tell me what is most important to you as you are thinking about the treatment options available to you/your loved one."
- **Preferences:** "You've said that being comfortable and pain free is most important to you right now. Where would you like to receive care (home, hospital, long-term care facility, doctor's office), and how can I help?"
- **Expected/desired outcomes:** "What are your hopes and expectations for this (diagnostic test [e.g., computed tomography scan] or treatment)?"
- **Benefits and burdens:** "Is there a point at which you would say that the testing or treatment is outweighed by the burdens it is causing you (e.g., getting from home to the hospital, pain, nausea, fatigue, interference with other important activities)?"

attitudes toward death (Puchalski, Vitillo, Hull, et al., 2014). It is highly personal and refers to our sense of who we are, who we want to be, and what we value. Spirituality encompasses how we seek meaning of life and how we experience ourselves in relationship with other people, our world, and a higher power. For most people, the awareness that one's life may soon be over raises many spiritual issues and may give rise to spiritual distress. **Signs** that may indicate spiritual distress include:

- Questioning of religious faith and beliefs (e.g., "Why would God allow this to happen to me?" or "Why am I being punished?")
- Questions of meaning such as "Why is this happening to me?" or "What does this mean?"
- Expressions of anxiety, hopelessness, guilt, shame, failure, remorse, and/or regret
- Expressions of abandonment

Spiritual assessment is a key component of comprehensive nursing assessment for terminally ill patients and their families. Although the nursing assessment should include religious affiliation if any, spiritual assessment is conceptually much broader and thus is relevant regardless of the patient's expression of religious preference or affiliation. In addition to assessment of the role of religious faith and practices, important religious rituals, and connection to a religious community, the nurse should further explore the following:

- Personal meaning of illness
- Relationship with others and/or higher power
- Sources of meaning and purpose in life
- Significant religious or spiritual practices
- Sources and targets of hope
- Need to give or receive forgiveness or acceptance or to reconcile

Open conversations may enable meaningful interactions and engagement. Family or friends may be given the opportunity to say goodbye or share memories. If able to do so, the patient may find it meaningful to leave a legacy for others, such as cards, letters, photos, or video recordings.

Hope

Kübler-Ross maintained that hope persisted across every stage of terminal illness, noting that "even the most accepting, the most realistic patients left the possibility open for some cure, for the discovery of a new drug, or the "last-minute success in a research project" (1969, p. 139). Frankl (1984), a survivor of the Holocaust, described a human capacity for optimism that could be maintained despite the possibility or even certainty of pain and death. In terminal illness, hope enables people to move forward and engage in life and protects them from being engulfed by suffering and negativity. When hope is viewed this way, it is not limited to cure of the disease and instead focuses on what is achievable in the time remaining. Many patients find hope in working on important relationships and in creating legacies. The terminally ill patient can be extremely resilient, reconceptualizing hope repeatedly as he or she approaches the end of life. Redefining hope is an ongoing progress.

The concept of hope has been delineated and studied by numerous nurse researchers, and its presence has been related to concepts such as spirituality, quality of life, and transcendence. Morse and Doberneck (1995) defined hope as a multidimensional construct that provides comfort to the individual as he or she endures life threats and personal challenges. In their study of patients who had survived serious illness, Morse and Doberneck identified seven universal components of hope:

- Realistic initial assessment of the threat
- Envisioning alternatives and setting goals
- Bracing for negative outcomes
- Realistic assessment of resources
- Solicitation of mutually supportive relationships
- Continuous evaluation for signs reinforcing the goals
- Determination to endure

The nurse can support the patient and family by using effective listening and communication skills and encouraging realistic hope that is specific to the patient and family's needs for information, expectations for the future, and values and preferences concerning the end of life. It is important for the nurse to engage in self-reflection and identify his or her own biases and fears concerning illness, life, and death. As nurses become more skilled in working with seriously ill patients, they can become less determined to "fix" and more willing to listen; more comfortable with silence, grief, anger, and sadness; and more fully present with patients and their families.

Nursing interventions for enabling and supporting hope include the following:

- Listening attentively
- Encouraging sharing of feelings and reflecting on past accomplishments, positive memories, and significant milestones
- Focusing on the individual's strengths and abilities
- Encouraging and supporting patient control over his or her circumstances, choices, and environment whenever possible
- Assisting the patient to explore ways for finding meaning in his or her life
- Encouraging realistic goals
- Maintaining meaningful relationships with family and significant others
- Making referrals for psychosocial and spiritual counselling
- Assisting with the development of support in the home or community when none exist

Managing Symptoms Associated With Advanced Illness

Patients with advanced illnesses experience many of the same symptoms, regardless of their underlying disease processes. These symptoms may be caused by the disease, either directly (e.g., dyspnea due to chronic obstructive lung disease [COPD]) or indirectly (e.g., dyspnea related to pressure due to an abdominal tumour), by the treatment for the disease, or by a coexisting disorder that is unrelated to the disease. Chapter 16 presents assessment principles for pain that include identifying the effect of the pain on the patient's life, the importance of believing the patient's report of the pain and its effect, and the importance of systematic assessment of pain. Similarly, symptoms such as dyspnea, nausea, weakness, and anxiety should be as carefully and systematically assessed and managed. Initial screening for presence and severity should be followed for further description and to guide management, including the patient's goal and understanding, the onset of the symptom, and factors that influence it. Fraser Health Authority has developed an acronym to guide the assessment of symptoms (Fraser Health Authority, 2009). The goal of symptom management is to assess and alleviate each symptom to a level that the patient can tolerate or that has the least amount of burden or distress. Pharmacologic and nonpharmacologic methods for symptom management may be used in combination with medical interventions to modify the physiologic causes of symptoms. For example, some patients who develop pleural effusion secondary to metastatic cancer may experience temporary relief of the associated dyspnea following thoracentesis, an invasive medical procedure in which fluid is drained from the pleural space, while others will experience relief following placement of an indwelling pleural catheter that is drained intermittently. These interventions may be managed in hospital or at home, depending upon community and family resources. Pharmacologic management with low-dose oral morphine is very effective in relieving dyspnea (Kamal, McGuire, Wheeler, et al., 2012), and guided relaxation may reduce the anxiety associated with the sensation of breathlessness when not in an acute state of dyspnea. The principles of pharmacologic symptom management are that one should always give the smallest dose of the medication necessary to achieve the desired effect, avoid polypharmacy, anticipate and manage side effects, and create a therapeutic regimen that is acceptable to the patient based on his or her goals for maximizing quality of life. Patients may elect to endure more severe symptoms in exchange for greater independence, mobility, alertness, or other priorities.

Anticipating and planning interventions for symptoms that have not yet occurred is a cornerstone of palliative and end-of-life care. Patients and family members may manage new and existing symptoms more effectively when they know what to expect. Hospice palliative care services may provide "emergency kits" or ready-to-administer doses of medications that are useful to treat symptoms in advanced illness; they may also provide verbal or written action plans for acute or crisis events. Family members can be instructed to administer a prescribed dose of medication, often avoiding prolonged suffering for the patient as well as rehospitalization for symptom management.

Pain

Pain is a subjective, multidimensional experience. Each person's experience of pain is unique. The perception, expression, and relief of pain are influenced by physical, psychological, social, cultural, and spiritual factors. Therefore, a complete pain assessment and treatment plan must be multidimensional. Recognition of the interrelationships among all of these dimensions of the pain experience is referred to as total pain. Thus, it is important to consider an interprofessional approach to pain assessment and management.

The continued, pervasive undertreatment of pain has been well documented over time in many patient populations, including children as well as adults with cancer, renal disease, heart failure, multiple sclerosis, and amyotrophic lateral sclerosis (ALS) (Jacox, Carr, & Payne, 1994; Reynolds, Drew, & Dunwoody, 2013; Brkovic, Burilovic, & Puljak, 2014; Rivera I, Ajroud-Driss S, Casey P, et al., 2013; De Clercq et al., 2017; Xie et al., 2017). Despite more than two decades of specialized palliative and pain care services in North America and Europe, it is estimated that as many as 70% of patients with advanced cancer experience moderate to severe pain (Wilson et al., 2009; Rayment, Hjermstad, Aass, et al., 2013). The impact of poorly managed pain on patients' psychological, emotional, social, and financial well-being has attracted considerable research interest, but practice has been slow to change.

Nursing Interventions for Pain

A thorough multidimensional pain assessment begins with a physical examination and identifying the pain characteristics through the use of questions. The use of a standardized assessment tool and a systematic approach facilitates communication and consistency in pain assessment. A modification and extension of the PQRST acronym to *OPQRSTUV* may facilitate a thorough and comprehensive assessment of the symptom and the person's experience: Onset, Provoking/Palliating Factors, Quality, Region/Radiation, Severity, Treatment, Understanding/Impact on You and Family, Values/Views and Goals.

The WHO has identified a three-step ladder approach to the management of cancer pain. Types and combinations of analgesics are matched to the patient's level of pain (mild, moderate, and severe). Patients who have an established regimen of analgesics should continue to receive those medications as they approach their end of life. Inability to communicate pain should not be equated with the absence of pain. While most pain can be managed effectively using the oral route, as the end of life nears, patients may be less able to swallow oral medications due to factors such as fatigue, somnolence, or nausea. In these cases, patients who have been receiving opioids should continue to receive equivalent analgesic doses via rectal, subcutaneous, sublingual, or intravenous routes, depending upon their setting of care and stage of illness (Davies, 2016; Kestenbaum et al., 2014). Lipophilic medications such as fentanyl can be effectively delivered by the sublingual or buccal routes for intermittent analgesic, because the small liquid volume is well tolerated even when the patient cannot swallow. As long as the patient continues to receive opioids, a regimen to combat constipation must be implemented. If the patient cannot swallow laxatives or stool softeners, rectal suppositories or enemas may be necessary.

The nurse should teach the family about continuation of comfort measures as the patient approaches the end of life, including how to administer analgesics via alternate routes, and how to assess pain when the patient cannot verbally report pain intensity. Because analgesics administered subcutaneously, orally or rectally may be shorter acting and typically scheduled as frequently as every 4 hours around the clock, there is always a strong possibility that the patient approaching the end of life will die in close proximity to the time of analgesic administration. If the patient is at home, family members administering analgesics need to be prepared for this possibility. They will need reassurance that they did not "cause" the death of the patient by administering a dose of analgesic medication. They also need to be taught about breakthrough cancer pain (pain between doses of analgesic), and when to give an addition "prn" dose to the person in pain who is receiving medications around the clock.

Dyspnea

Dyspnea is a subjective sensation of breathing discomfort, with distinct sensations that vary in intensity, unpleasantness, and significance. As dyspnea is a symptom, it may not necessarily correlate with respiratory rate or oxygen saturation. Although prevalent and one of the most distressing symptoms for the ill individual and his or her family, dyspnea is often underassessed and undertreated.

The causes of dyspnea are often multifactoral, including activation of nociceptors, altered corticolimbic sensations, perceptions of work/effort, sensation of tightness, and intensity of air hunger (Marshall et al., 2012). Patients with primary lung tumours, lung metastases, pleural effusion, COPD, interstitial lung disease such as idiopathic pulmonary fibrosis (IPF), or heart failure may experience significant dyspnea. Although the underlying cause of the dyspnea can be identified and treated in some cases, the burdens of additional diagnostic evaluation and treatment aimed at the physiologic problem may outweigh the benefits. In many circumstances, the focus is on comfort, not cure. The treatment of dyspnea varies depending on the patient's general physical condition and the imminence of death. For example, a blood transfusion may provide temporary symptom relief for the anemic patient earlier in the disease process; however, as the patient approaches the end of life, the benefits of transfusions are typically short lived or absent and the burden of receiving them must also be considered as the person is usually hospitalized.

The meaning of the dyspnea to the patient may increase his or her suffering. For example, the patient may interpret increasing dyspnea as a sign that death is approaching. For others, sensations of breathlessness may invoke frightening images and perceptions of drowning or suffocation, and the resulting cycle of fear and anxiety may create even greater sensations of breathlessness.

Nursing Interventions for Dyspnea

Nursing management of dyspnea for palliative and end-of-life is directed toward pharmacologic management of symptoms for the underlying pathology, monitoring the patient's response to treatment, supporting the patient and family to manage anxiety (which exacerbates dyspnea), altering the perception of the symptom, and conserving energy (Chart 15-3). Pharmacologic intervention is aimed at modifying lung physiology and improving performance as well as altering the perception of the symptom. Bronchodilators and corticosteroids are examples of medications used to treat underlying obstructive pathology, thereby improving overall lung function. Low doses of opioids are very effective in decreasing the perception of dyspnea, presumably by decreasing sensory perception as they do with pain (Marshall et al., 2012). Oxygen may be used to provide comfort, and to target specific oxygen saturation levels for persons with chronic pulmonary disease. A well ventilated room or fan often helps alleviate some sensation of dyspnea, possibly due to the flow of air in the nasal passages.

As discussed, dyspnea may be exacerbated by anxiety, and anxiety may trigger episodes of dyspnea, setting off a respiratory crisis in which patient and family may panic. For patients receiving care at home, the home care nurse and respiratory therapist should collaborate to provide patient and family instruction, including anticipation and management of crisis situations and a clearly communicated emergency or action plan. Patients and families should be instructed about medication administration, condition changes that should be reported to the home care team, and strategies for coping with diminished reserves and increasing symptomatology as the disease progresses. The patient and family need reassurance that the symptom can be effectively managed at home without emergency medical services or hospitalization and that support will be available via telephone or by a home visit. Symptom management, including **palliative sedation**, may be discussed earlier with some patients who indicate in some way that they are afraid of suffocating at the end of life, such as those with COPD or ALS.

CHART 15-3

Palliative Nursing Interventions for Dyspnea

Decrease Anxiety

- Administer prescribed anxiolytic medications as indicated for anxiety or panic associated with dyspnea
- Assist with relaxation techniques, guided imagery
- Provide patient with a means to call for assistance (call bell/light within reach in a hospital or long-term care facility; handheld bell or other device for home)

Treat Underlying Pathology

- Administer prescribed bronchodilators and corticosteroids (obstructive pathology)
- Administer blood products, erythropoietin as prescribed (typically not beneficial in advanced disease)
- Administer prescribed diuretics and monitor fluid balance

Alter Perception of Breathlessness

- Administer prescribed oxygen therapy via nasal cannula, if tolerated; masks may not be well tolerated
- Administer prescribed low-dose opioids via oral route (morphine sulphate is used most commonly)
- Provide air movement in the patient's environment with a portable fan

Reduce Respiratory Demand

- Teach patient and family to implement energy conservation measures
- Place needed equipment, supplies, and nourishment within reach
- For home or hospice care, offer bedside commode, electric bed (with head that elevates)

Fatigue

Fatigue is a common symptom at the end of life. The etiology of fatigue likely varies depending on diagnosis. Most research has focused on cancer-related fatigue. Cancer-related fatigue is associated with feelings of weakness, loss of energy, and tiredness that is out of proportion to the energy expended and that is not relieved by sleep or rest (Olson, 2007). Although its etiology is still uncertain, it likely has roots in both disease processes and treatments. Fatigue is also underrecognized and undertreated, not only in patients with cancer, but in many others, such as persons with chronic pulmonary or cardiac disease.

Nursing Interventions for Fatigue

Several groups have recently published guidelines for the management of fatigue. A group of Canadians with expertise in cancer-related fatigue recently published a clinical practice guideline called, "A Pan-Canadian Practice Guideline: Screening, Assessment and Care of Cancer-Related Fatigue in Adults with Cancer" (Howell, Keller-Olaman, Oliver, et al., 2013). Available in both English and French (http://www.capo.ca/Fatigue_Guideline.pdf), it is considered one of the top guidelines available given its careful assessment of the evidence in this field. The guideline recommends use of tools to screen for fatigue, such as the visual analogue scale for tiredness in the Edmonton Symptom Assessment System, and notes that individuals with a score of 3 or more require further assessment of factors that may be contributing to the fatigue. It also provides information about evidence-based interventions, depending on the results of the assessment, but it is worth noting that most evidence has been obtained by studying individuals currently receiving potentially curative treatment or individuals who are cancer survivors, and there is limited evidence available for fatigue when it occurs at the end of life. Radbruch, Strasser, Elsner, et al., noted that, "in the final stage of life, fatigue may provide protection and shielding from suffering for the patient and thus treatment may be detrimental." As the end of life approaches, it is critically important that the nurse facilitates a plan of care for fatigue that includes patient and family preferences—while some patients may prefer active interventions to manage or perhaps reduce their fatigue, others may experience the fatigue as protective and prefer interventions that support them in their fatigued state.

Anorexia, Dehydration, and Cachexia

Eating and drinking are essential to survival throughout one's lifetime. As patients near the end of life, their bodies' nutritional needs change; their desire for food and fluid may diminish; and they may no longer be able to use, eliminate, or store nutrients and fluids adequately. Eating, feeding, and sharing meals are important social activities in families and communities, and food preparation and enjoyment are linked to happy memories, strong emotions, and hopes for survival. Thus, activities related to food such as food preparation and mealtimes often become battlegrounds where well-meaning family members argue, plead, and cajole to encourage the ill person to eat. It is not unusual for seriously ill patients to become anorexic (lose their appetite) entirely, to develop strong aversions for foods that they have enjoyed in the past, or to crave a particular food to the exclusion of all other foods.

Although causes of anorexia may be controlled for a period of time, progressive anorexia is an expected and natural part of the dying process. Anorexia may be related to or exacerbated by situational variables (e.g., the ability to have meals with the family vs. eating alone in the "sick room"), progression of the disease, treatment for the disease, or psychological distress. The patient and family should be instructed in strategies to manage factors associated with anorexia and to recognize that the person may no longer wish to eat and drink. Table 15-1 summarizes nursing measures and patient and family teaching for managing anorexia.

Cachexia refers to muscle wasting and weight loss associated with end-stage illness, such as cancer, heart failure, and pulmonary disease. Although anorexia may accompany and exacerbate cachexia, it is not the primary cause. Cachexia is associated with changes in metabolism, including hypercatabolism, that lead to depletion of protein stores with weight loss from muscle (Fearon, Strasser, Anker, et al., 2011). The pathophysiology of cachexia in terminal illness is not well understood, and is considered to be multifactoral. The severity of tissue wasting is greater than from reduced food intake alone, and increasing appetite or food intake does not reverse cachexia in the terminally ill.

Anorexia and cachexia differ from starvation (simple food deprivation) in several important ways. First, as noted above, nutritional supplementation alleviates problems associated with starvation but does not replenish lost lean body mass in individuals with anorexia and cachexia. At one time, it was believed that cancer patients with rapidly growing tumours developed cachexia because the tumour created an excessive nutritional demand and diverted nutrients from the rest of the body. Recent research suggests that this is not the case. Rather, cachexia is associated with cytokines, which are produced by the body in response to a tumour. The cytokines are part of a complex inflammatory immune response in patients whose tumours have metastasized. An increase in cytokines occurs not only in cancer but also in heart failure and many other chronic diseases.

Nursing Interventions for Anorexia, Dehydration, and Cachexia

Eating is commonly associated with health and well-being. Consequently, it is often when people are no longer able to eat or drink that the reality of dying is exposed. It is natural for families to be distressed about a loved one's reduced food intake and weight loss (Reid, McKenna, Fitzsimons, et al., 2009). Following a complete assessment, a plan for management of anorexia, dehydration, and cachexia should be developed with the patient, family, and interprofessional team. Both pharmacologic and non-pharmacologic interventions may be considered as part of the plan. Corticosteroids may improve appetite, resulting in increased food intake and quality of life. They have a short-term benefit of approximately 3 weeks. Progestational agents such as megestrol (megestrol acetate) may stimulate the appetite resulting in increased caloric intake and weight gain in a small number of patients, but do not improve survival or quality of life (Arensmeyer, 2012;

TABLE 15-1 Measures for Managing Anorexia

Nursing Interventions	Patient and Family Teaching Tips
Initiate measures to ensure adequate dietary intake without adding stress to the patient at mealtimes	Reduce the focus on "balanced" meals; offer the same food as often as the patient desires it
Assess the impact of medications (e.g., chemotherapy, antiretrovirals) or other therapies (radiation therapy, dialysis) that are being used to treat the underlying illness	Increase the nutritional value of meals. For example, add dry milk powder to milk, and use this fortified milk to prepare cream soups, milkshakes, and gravies
Administer and monitor effects of prescribed treatment for nausea, vomiting, and delayed gastric emptying	
Encourage the patient to eat when effects of medications have subsided	Allow and encourage the patient to eat when hungry, regardless of usual mealtimes
Assess and modify environment to eliminate unpleasant odours and other factors that cause nausea, vomiting, and anorexia	Eliminate or reduce noxious cooking odours, pet odours, or other odours that may precipitate nausea, vomiting, or anorexia
Remove items that may reduce appetite (soiled tissues, bedpans, emesis basins, clutter)	Keep the patient's environment clean, uncluttered, and comfortable
Assess and manage anxiety and depression to the extent possible	Make mealtime a shared experience away from the "sick" room whenever possible Reduce stress at mealtimes Avoid confrontations about the amount of food consumed Reduce or eliminate routine weighing of the patient
Position to enhance gastric emptying.	Encourage the patient to eat in a sitting position; elevate the head of the patient's bed Plan meals (food selection and portion size) that the patient desires Provide small frequent meals if they are easier for patient to eat
Assess for constipation and/or intestinal obstruction	Ensure that the patient and family understand that prevention of constipation is essential, even when the patient's intake is minimal
Prevent and manage constipation on an ongoing basis, even when the patient's intake is minimal	Encourage adequate fluid intake, dietary fibre, and use of bowel program to prevent constipation
Provide frequent mouth care, particularly following nourishment	Assist the patient to rinse after every meal. Avoid mouthwashes that contain alcohol or glycerine, which dry mucous membranes
Ensure that dentures fit properly	Weight loss may cause dentures to loosen and cause irritation. Remove them to inspect the gums and to provide oral care
Administer and monitor effects of topical and systemic treatment for oropharyngeal pain	The patient's comfort may be enhanced if pain medications given on an as-needed basis for breakthrough pain are administered before mealtimes

Bondly & Jatoi, 2015), and have risks, including thromboembolic complications. Promotility agents (metoclopramide or domperidone) may stimulate the gastrointestinal peristalsis and reduce early satiety. Regardless of the approach selected, patient and family education about changes related to eating and drinking at the end of life are important.

Although nutritional supplementation may be an important part of the treatment plan in early or chronic illness, unintended weight loss and dehydration are expected sequelae of progressive illness. As illness progresses, it is important for patients, families, and clinicians to weigh the risks and benefits associated with nutritional supplementation, and based on this information, decide whether it is still warranted. There has been some research in this area, which demonstrated that neither survival nor quality of life increased when terminally ill patients with advanced dementia received enteral feeding (Brooke & Omorogieva, 2015). In patients who are close to death, there are beneficial effects to withholding or withdrawing artificial nutrition and hydration. These benefits include decreased urine output and incontinence, decreased gastric fluids and emesis, decreased pulmonary secretions and respiratory distress, and decreased edema and pressure discomfort.

As the patient approaches the end of life, families and health care providers should offer the patient food that he or she desires and can most easily tolerate. Nurses should instruct the family how to separate feeding from caring by demonstrating love, sharing, and caring by being with the loved one in other ways. Preoccupation with appetite, feeding, and weight loss diverts energy and time that the patient and family could use in other meaningful activities. In addition to treating symptoms that may affect appetite, the following tips promote nutrition for the terminally ill patient:

- Offer small portions of favourite foods
- Do not be overly concerned about a "balanced" diet
- Cool foods may be better tolerated than hot foods
- Offer cheese, eggs, peanut butter, mild fish, chicken, or turkey. Meat (especially beef) may taste bitter and unpleasant
- Add milkshakes, "instant breakfast" drinks, or other liquid supplements
- Add dry milk powder to milkshakes and cream soups to increase protein and calorie content

- Place nutritious foods at the bedside (fruit juices, milkshakes in insulated drink containers with straws)
- Schedule meals when family members can be present to provide company and stimulation
- Avoid arguments at mealtime
- Assist the patient to maintain a schedule of oral care. Rinse the mouth after each meal or snack. Avoid mouthwashes that contain alcohol. Use a soft toothbrush. Treat ulcers or lesions. Make sure that dentures fit well
- Offer ice chips made from frozen fruit juices
- Allow the patient to refuse foods and fluids

Delirium and Depression

Determining the etiology of delirium and of depression is difficult, and sometimes it is difficult to distinguish between them. Screening should be done for depression, whereas delirium may be subtle or evident, but is acute in onset, requiring an assessment tool.

Delirium

Delirium is an acute alteration in cognition that may occur with a severe underlying illness, including those nearing the end of their lives. Many patients may remain alert, arousable, and able to communicate until very close to death. However, others may sleep for long intervals and awaken only intermittently, with eventual somnolence until death. Delirium may be immediately recognizable or be very subtle. Approaches such as the Confusion Assessment Method (CAM) are useful screens for detecting delirium. In some patients, a period of agitated delirium may precede death, while others may experience a state of delirium with reduced arousal. It is important to recognize delirium and to understand its possible coexistence with depression or dementia. Dementia is also associated with cognitive impairment, but its onset is gradual, and the patient's level of consciousness is neither impaired nor fluctuational; persons with depression may also have altered thoughts and concentration. In contrast to dementia, delirium is an acute state of confusion which is of sudden onset over hours or days. It is often reversible and may fluctuate over the course of the day. Risk factors include infections, metabolic/endocrine imbalances, hypoxemia, toxins, tumours, metastases, pain, immobility, medications, CNS alterations, and sleep deprivation. The patient with delirium may become hypoactive, hyperactive, or both. The patient may be listless, restless, irritable, or fearful. Sleep deprivation and hallucinations may occur and worsen the delirium. If treatment of the underlying factors contributing to delirium brings no relief, a combination of hydration with pharmacologic agents may be effective in decreasing delirium. Low doses of haloperidol (Haldol) may reduce hallucinations and agitation, but are not recommended for some clinical populations, including those with Lewy body dementia or Parkinson's disease (Hosker & Bennett, 2016). Benzodiazepines such as lorazepam (Ativan) can reduce anxiety but will not clear the sensorium and may contribute to worsening cognitive impairment or sedation if used alone, but may work well in conjunction with haloperidol for acute agitated delirium (Ferraz Gonçalves et al., 2016).

NURSING INTERVENTIONS FOR DELIRIUM. Interventions are intended to promote the prevention of delirium, or to ensure early recognition of delirium if present. Other symptoms may be mistaken for or contribute to the agitation, and older adults are at particular risk for this problem. If delirium occurs, then nursing interventions focus on reversing it if possible; acknowledging the family's distress over its occurrence; reassuring the family about what is normal; teaching the family how to interact with the patient, ensuring safety for the patient and family; and monitoring the effects of medications used to treat severe agitation.

Confusion may mask the patient's unmet spiritual needs and fears about dying. Spiritual intervention, music therapy, gentle massage, and therapeutic touch may provide some relief. Reducing environmental stimuli, speaking in calm quiet tones, avoiding harsh lighting or very dim lighting (which may produce disturbing shadows), promoting sleep–wake cycles, noting the presence of familiar faces, and providing appropriate gentle reorientation and reassurance are also helpful (Hosker & Bennett, 2016). The nurse communicates clearly, calmly and consistently. If hallucinations are frightening, reassurance is important, but contesting pleasant hallucinations, such as nonpresent butterflies or persons, may only further distress the person.

Depression

Clinical depression should not be accepted as an inevitable consequence of dying, nor should it be confused with sadness and anticipatory grieving, which are usual reactions to the losses associated with impending death. Emotional and spiritual support and control of disturbing physical symptoms are appropriate interventions for situational depression associated with terminal illness. Feeling "low" to having depression is highly prevalent in patient populations with various diseases; for example, Antunes et al. (2015) reported 17.5% depression across a sample from Germany and England of 416 patients with either malignant or nonmalignant diagnoses. Various tools may be used to either screen or assess for depression, such as the Palliative Care Outcome Scale, the Geriatric Depression Scale, and the Hospital Anxiety and Depression Scale–Depression subscale (Antunes et al., 2015).

NURSING INTERVENTIONS FOR DEPRESSION. Patients and their families need to be given space and time to experience sadness and to grieve, but patients should not have to endure untreated depression at the end of their lives. An effective combined approach to clinical depression depends on the individual and the anticipated time until death, with consideration of:

- Management of physical symptoms, including screening for other commonly occurring symptoms, such as loss of appetite, fatigue, nausea, anxiety, constipation
- Attention to emotional and spiritual distress, such as life review/making meaning, music therapy, couples/family therapy
- Dignity therapy, demonstrated to alleviate distress and depression through value of the individual (Martinez et al., 2017)
- Pharmacologic intervention, including psychostimulants, selective serotonin reuptake inhibitors (SSRIs),

and tricyclic antidepressants, although these often require early assessment and intervention than the last days of life

Principles of Palliative Sedation

Effective control of symptoms can be achieved under most conditions, but some patients may experience distressing, intractable symptoms. Although its use remains controversial in some settings and cultures, **continuous palliative sedation therapy** may be offered to patients who are close to death, who have refractory symptoms, and who are experiencing unrelieved suffering (Dean, Cellarius, Henry, et al., 2012). Palliative sedation is distinguished from euthanasia, MAID in that the intent of palliative sedation is to have the person unaware of distressing symptoms, not to hasten the patient's death. Palliative sedation is most commonly used when the patient exhibits dyspnea, agitated delirium, or catastrophic terminal events (e.g., uncontrollable seizures). It is generally considered appropriate in only the most difficult cases. Although there is not yet a consensus document, there is a Canadian framework to guide use (Dean et al., 2012); with implementation varying depending on guidelines and policies of each provincial health authority. Before implementing palliative sedation, the care team must ensure that the following have been addressed:

- The patient and family are aware of the treatment, the reasons for its use, and its outcome; informed consent should be obtained from the patient or the substitute decision maker
- A thorough assessment has been conducted to identify and treat reversible symptom causes
- All pharmacologic and nonpharmacologic approaches to symptom control have been maximized
- The person has a terminal diagnosis and is anticipated to die within 1 to 2 weeks, usually a few hours or days
- A "DNR" order or its equivalent is in place

Palliative sedation is accomplished through a continuous subcutaneous (subcut) or intravenous (IV) infusion, most frequently of a benzodiazepine, in doses adequate to induce a low level of arousal and consciousness (Dean et al., 2012). Analgesics are maintained for effective pain management but are not titrated as sedatives. Essential strategies prior to initiating palliative sedation include the following:

- The option must be discussed with the person, his or her family, and/or the agent or proxy named in an advance directive, the primary physician, and the members of the team providing care.
- The rationale for palliative sedation and the process of consent must be clearly documented.
- The family needs to have time and the opportunity for private conversation before the person enters a deep sleep.
- Providing psychological support to the family is important.

The nurse acts as a collaborating member of the intraprofessional team, providing emotional support to the patient and family, facilitating clarification of values and preferences, initiating and titrating the medication, and providing comfort-focused physical care. Once sedation has been induced, the nurse continues to provide comfort and necessary care, monitor the physiologic effects of the sedation, assess for expected and adverse effects of sedation, monitor the family for distress, support the family during the final hours or days of the patient's life, and ensure communication within the care team and between the team and family.

Providing Support to Patients Who are Actively Dying and Their Families

Providing care to the patient who is close to death and being present at the time of death can be one of the most rewarding experiences a nurse can have. Patients and their families are understandably fearful of the unknown, and the approach of death may prompt new concerns or cause previous fears or issues to resurface. It has often been said that as we age and approach death, we do not become different people—we just become more like ourselves. Families that have always had difficulty communicating old resentments and hurts may experience heightened difficulty as their loved one nears death. In contrast, the time at the end of life can also afford the family the opportunity to resolve old hurts and learn new ways of being a family. Family or friends may take the opportunity to say goodbye; if able to do so, the patient may find it meaningful to leave a legacy, such as a card, letter or recording. Regardless of the setting, dying patients can be made comfortable, space can be made for their loved ones to remain present when they wish, and the opportunity to experience growth and healing can be facilitated by skilled practitioners. Likewise, regardless of setting, patient and families' apprehension surrounding the time of death may be diminished if they know what to expect as death nears and how to respond. See Nursing Research Profile Chart 15-4.

Expected Physiologic Changes When the Patient is Close to Death

Observable, expected changes in the body take place as the patient approaches death and organ systems begin to fail. These changes may occur rapidly, within hours, or they may occur more slowly over a period of days. Nursing care measures aimed at patient comfort should be continued. These measures include pain medications (administered subcutaneously, intravenously, rectally or sublingually), turning, skin care, mouth care, eye care, positioning to facilitate draining of secretions, and protecting the skin from incontinence. The nurse should consult with the physician about discontinuing measures that no longer contribute to patient comfort, such as drawing blood, administering tube feedings, suctioning (in most cases), and invasive or in-depth monitoring, including oxygen saturations. The nurse should prepare the family for the usual, expected changes that accompany the period immediately preceding death. Although the exact time of death cannot be predicted, it is often possible to identify when a patient is very close to death. Hospice programs

NURSING RESEARCH PROFILE

Chart 15-4. Perceptions of Helpful Interventions During End-of-Life Care

Cronin, J., Arnstein, P., & Flanagan, J. (2015). Family members' perceptions of most helpful interventions during end-of-life care. *Journal of Hospice & Palliative Nursing, 17*(3), 223–228.

Purpose

Hospice care and support is directed not just to the patient but to those whom the patient considers family. Numerous studies have provided insight into nurses' perceptions of priorities for, as well as barriers to and facilitators of, end-of-life care. Better understanding of families' needs could improve their experience of hospice care. This study aimed to explore the needs of family members and friends while their loved ones received end-of-life care in a hospital setting.

Design

This was a qualitative study in which the researchers used semi-structured interviews to collect data from a family member or close friend of a patient enrolled in hospice in a hospital setting. Nine potential study participants were identified through convenience sampling on an 18-bed gynecologic oncology unit in a large academic medical centre; seven of the nine agreed to participate. Interview questions focused on perceived helpfulness of nurses' and other staff members' activities, perceptions of communication, and adequacy and helpfulness of referred services (e.g., chaplaincy). Data were compiled as transcripts from handwritten interview notes and analyzed using content analysis techniques.

Findings

Importantly, the principal investigator observed that although she had anticipated that participants might be uncomfortable being interviewed at such a difficult time, she found that participants were not only comfortable, they appreciated the chance to tell their stories and would have been willing to share even more than was requested. Researchers identified four principal themes from the data analysis: (1) family/friend awareness of nursing vigilance provided them with a sense of being cared for; (2) nursing presence enhanced mutual connectedness and appreciation; (3) when death was imminent, family/friends wanted to understand the process, be included in discussions, and be validated after decisions were made; and (4) attention to the environment of care provided peace and relaxation at a difficult time.

frequently provide written information for families so that they know what to expect and what to do as death nears (Chart 15-5).

If they have been prepared for the time of death, families are less likely to panic and will be better able to be with their loved one in a meaningful way. Noisy, gurgling breathing, gasping or moaning may be distressing to the family unless they are informed that the person is usually not aware of these sounds. In most cases, noisy sounds of breathing at the end of life are related to airway secretions and to oropharyngeal relaxation and diminished awareness. Family members may have difficulty believing that the patient is not in distress or that his or her breathing could not be improved by suctioning secretions. Patient positioning and family information and reassurance are the most helpful responses to these sounds. Gasping or intermittent stops in breathing are natural changes in the respiratory centre when death is near.

Respiratory Changes at the End of Life

When death is imminent, the patient may become increasingly unable to clear sputum or oral secretions, which may lead to further impairment of breathing from pooled and/or dried and crusted secretions. As noted above, the sound and appearance of the secretions are often distressing to the family. Family distress over the changes in patient condition may be eased by supportive nursing care. Continuation of comfort-focused interventions and reassurance that the patient is not in any distress can do much to ease family concerns. Gentle mouth care with a moistened swab or very soft toothbrush will help to maintain the integrity of the patient's mucous membranes. In addition, gentle oral suctioning, positioning to enhance drainage of secretions, and sublingual or transdermal administration of anticholinergic drugs (Table 15-2) to reduce the production of secretions will provide comfort to the patient and support to the family. Deeper suctioning may cause significant discomfort to the dying patient and is rarely of any benefit, as secretions will reaccumulate rapidly.

Imminently Dying

Although every death is unique, it is often possible for the experienced clinician to assess that the patient is near death, at times referred to as "actively" or imminently dying. The recognition that death is expected enables opportunities to prepare the family in the final days or hours leading to death. As death nears, the patient may withdraw, sleep for longer intervals, or become somnolent. The family should be encouraged to be with the patient, to speak quietly and reassure him or her of their presence, to stroke or touch him or her, hold hands, or to lie alongside him or her (even in the hospital or long-term care facility) if they are comfortable with this degree of closeness and can do so without causing discomfort to the patient.

Family members may have gone to great lengths to ensure that their loved one will not die alone. However, despite the best intentions and efforts of families and clinicians, the patient's death may occur at a time when no one is present. In any setting, it is unrealistic for family members to be at the patient's bedside 24 hours a day, and it is not unusual for patients to die when the family has

CHART 15-5

Educating the Family: Signs of Approaching Death

The person will show less interest in eating and drinking. For many patients, refusal of food is an indication that they are ready to die. Fluid intake may be limited to that which will keep their mouths from feeling too dry.

- What you can do: Offer, but do not force, fluids and medication. Sometimes, pain or other symptoms that have required medication in the past may no longer be present. For most patients, pain medications will still be needed and can be provided by concentrated oral solutions placed under the tongue or by rectal suppository.

Urinary output may decrease in amount and frequency.

- What you can do: No response is needed unless the patient expresses a desire to urinate and cannot. Call the nurse for advice if you are not sure.

As the body weakens, the patient will sleep more and begin to detach from the environment. He or she may refuse your attempts to provide comfort.

- What you can do: Allow your loved one to sleep. You may wish to sit with him or her, play soft music, or hold hands. Your loved one's withdrawal is normal and is not a rejection of your love.

Mental confusion may become apparent, as less oxygen is available to supply the brain. The patient may report strange dreams or visions.

- What you can do: As he or she awakens from sleep, remind him or her of the day and time, where he or she is, and who is present. This is best done in a casual, conversational way.

Vision and hearing may become somewhat impaired, and speech may be difficult to understand.

- What you can do: Speak clearly but no more loudly than necessary. Keep the room as light as the patient wishes, even at night. Carry on all conversations as if they can be heard, since hearing may be the last of the senses to cease functioning. Many patients are able to talk until minutes before death and are reassured by the exchange of a few words with a loved one.

Secretions may collect in the back of the throat and rattle or gurgle as the patient breathes through the mouth. He or she may try to cough, and his or her mouth may become dry and encrusted with secretions.

- What you can do: If the patient is trying to cough up secretions and is experiencing choking or vomiting, call the nurse for assistance. Secretions may drain from the mouth if you place the patient on his or her side and provide support with pillows.

Cleansing the mouth with moistened mouth swabs will help to relieve the dryness that occurs with mouth breathing. Offer water in small amounts to keep the mouth moist. A straw with one finger placed over the end can be used to transfer sips of water to the patient's mouth.

Breathing may become irregular with periods of no breathing (apnea). The patient may be working very hard to breathe and may make a moaning sound with each breath. As the time of death nears, the breathing remains irregular and may become more shallow and mechanical.

- What you can do: Raising the head of the bed may help the patient breathe more easily. The moaning sound does not mean that the patient is in pain or other distress; it is the sound of air passing over very relaxed vocal cords.

As the oxygen supply to the brain decreases, the patient may become restless. It is not unusual to pull at the bed linens, to have visual hallucinations, or even to try to get out of bed at this point.

- What you can do: Reassure the patient in a calm voice that you are there. Prevent him or her from falling by trying to get out of bed. Soft music or a back rub may be soothing.

The patient may feel hot one moment and cold the next as he or she loses the ability to control body temperature. As circulation slows, the arms and legs may become cool and bluish. The underside of the body may darken. It may be difficult to feel a pulse at the wrist.

- What you can do: Provide and remove blankets as needed. Avoid using electric blankets, which may cause burns because the patient cannot tell you if he or she is too warm. Sponge the patient's head with a cool cloth if this provides comfort.

Loss of bladder and bowel control may occur around the time of death.

- What you can do: Protect the mattress with waterproof padding, and change the padding as needed to keep the patient comfortable.

As people approach death, many times they report seeing gardens, libraries, or family or friends who have died. They may ask you to pack their bags and find tickets or a passport. Sometimes, they may become insistent and attempt to do these chores themselves. They may try getting out of bed (even if they have been confined to bed for a long time) so that they can "leave."

- What you can do: Reassure the patient that it is all right; he or she can "go" without getting out of bed. Stay close, share stories, and be present.

Used with permission from the Hospice of Philadelphia. (2015). *Signs of approaching death*. Philadelphia, PA: Author.

stepped away from the bedside just briefly. Experienced hospice clinicians have observed and reported that some patients appear to "wait" until family members are away from the bedside to die, perhaps to spare their loved ones the pain of being present at the time of death. The nurse can reassure family members by being present intermittently or continuously, modeling behaviours (such as touching and speaking to the patient), providing encouragement in relation to family caregiving, providing reassurance about physiologic changes, and encouraging family rest breaks. Find out if family members want to be present, but also let them know that sometimes patients seem to wait to die until others are absent, even for a few moments. Inform the family that although the person does not seem aware of others around them, we don't know what the patient may or may not hear. It is often helpful to encourage family members to connect by holding the person's hand and, speaking calmly and quietly, tell stories and reminisce together, reminding the person they are cared for and thanking them. Encourage the family to grieve and take breaks, to let others know how they can help, and to express their loss now and afterward.

TABLE 15-2 Pharmacologic Management of Excess Oral/Respiratory Secretions When Death is Imminent

Medication	Suggested Initial Dosing
Atropine 1% ophthalmic (IsoptoAtropine)	1–2 drops PO every 4 hours, scheduled or PRN
Atropine injection	0.4 mg IV/SC/IM every 4 hours, scheduled or PRN
Glycopyrrolate (Robinul)	1 mg PO TID, scheduled or PRN, up to 6 mg/day, or 0.1 mg SC/IM/IV TID PRN
Hyoscyamine (Levsin)	0.125 mg PO/SL every 4 hours PRN, up to 1.5 mg/day
Hyoscyamine extended release (Levbid)	0.375 mg PO every 12 hours, up to 1.5 mg/day
Scopolamine (Transderm Scop)	Apply 1 patch topically behind the ear every 72 hours, up to 3 patches/72 hours

Reprinted with permission from Enclara Pharmacia, Inc. (2015). *Enclara Pharmacia Medication Use Guidelines* (1st ed.). Philadelphia, PA: Author.

When the patient dies while the family is away from the bedside, the family may express feelings of guilt and profound grief and will need emotional support.

The time of death is generally preceded by a period of gradual diminishment of bodily functions in which increasing intervals between respirations, a weakened and irregular pulse, diminishing blood pressure, and skin colour changes or mottling may be observed.

After-Death Care

For the patient who has received adequate management of symptoms and for the family who has received adequate preparation and support, the actual time of death is commonly peaceful and occurs without struggle. The nurse may or may not be present at the time of the patient's death. Inform the family that after the death, they may have some time and space to reflect, say some final goodbyes or be with the deceased. When at all possible, support the religious, spiritual, and cultural rituals during and after death. In some jurisdictions, the certifying physician may authorize the nurse to make the pronouncement of death and sign the death certificate; in others, the nurse may pronounce death and the physician signs the death certificate. The determination of death is made through a physical examination that includes auscultation for the absence of breathing and heart sounds. Immediately on cessation of vital functions, the body will begin to change. The body will become dusky or bluish, waxen appearing, and cool; blood will darken and pool in dependent areas of the body (such as the back and sacrum if the body is in a supine position), and urine and stool may be expelled.

Immediately following the death, the family should be allowed and encouraged to spend time with the deceased. Responses of family members at the time of death vary widely and range from quiet expressions of grief to overt expressions that include wailing and prostration. The family's desires for privacy during their time with the deceased should be honoured. Family members may wish to independently manage or assist with care of the body after death. If the death occurs in a long-term care facility, the nurse follows the facility's procedure for preparation of the body and transportation to the facility's morgue. However, the family's needs to remain with the deceased, to wait until other family members arrive before the body is moved, and to perform after-death rituals should be honoured when at all possible. When an expected death occurs in the home setting, the body is often transported directly to the funeral home by the funeral director. Neither police nor emergency medical services are required; however, home care may go out to support the family.

Grief, Mourning, and Bereavement

A wide range of feelings and behaviours are normal, adaptive, and healthy reactions to the loss of a loved one. Grief refers to the personal feelings that accompany an anticipated or actual loss. Mourning reflects the individual, family, group, and cultural expressions of grief and associated behaviours. Bereavement refers to the period of time during which mourning takes place. Both grief reactions and mourning behaviours change over time as the individual learns to live with the loss. Although the pain of the loss may be tempered by the passage of time, conceptualizations of loss as an ongoing developmental process maintain that time does not heal the bereaved individual completely (Silverman, 2002); that is, the bereaved do not get over a loss entirely, nor do they return to who they were before the loss. Rather, they develop a new sense of who they are and where they now fit in the world.

Anticipatory Grief and Mourning

Denial, sadness, anger, fear, and anxiety are usual grief reactions in the individual with life-threatening illness and those close to him or her. Kübler-Ross (1969) described five common emotional reactions to dying that have been extrapolated to the experience of any loss, although this is questioned today (Table 15-3). Although useful in understanding the overall experience of the dying process, the stages that Kübler-Ross described have been misinterpreted as following a linear, expected trajectory. Not every patient or family member experiences every stage, many patients never reach a stage of acceptance, and patients and families fluctuate on a sometimes day-to-day basis in their emotional responses. Further, while impending loss stresses the patient, those who are close to him or her, and the functioning of the family unit, awareness of dying also provides a unique opportunity for family members to reminisce, resolve relationships, plan for the future, and say goodbye.

TABLE 15-3 Kübler-Ross's Five Stages of Grief

Stage	Nursing Implications
Denial: "This cannot be true." Feelings of isolation. May search for another health care professional who will give a more favourable opinion. May seek unproven therapies	Denial can be an adaptive response, providing a buffer after bad news. It allows time to mobilize defences but can be maladaptive when it prevents the patient or the family from seeking help or when denial behaviours cause more pain or distress than the illness or interfere with everyday functions. Nurses should assess the patient's and family's coping style, information needs, and understanding of the illness and treatment to establish a basis for empathetic listening, education, and emotional support. Rather than confronting the patient with information that he or she is not ready to hear, the nurse can encourage him or her to share fears and concerns. Open-ended questions or statements such as "Tell me more about how you are coping with this new information about your illness" can provide a springboard for expression of concerns
Anger: "Why me?" Feelings of rage, resentment, or envy directed at God, health care professionals, family, others	Anger can be very isolating, and loved ones or clinicians may withdraw. Nurses should allow the patient and family to express anger, treating them with understanding, respect, and knowledge that the root of the anger is grief over impending loss
Bargaining: "I just want to see my grandchild's birth, then I'll be ready...." Patient and/or family plead for more time to reach an important goal. Promises are sometimes made with God	Terminally ill patients are sometimes able to outlive prognoses and achieve some future goal. Nurses should be patient, allow expression of feelings, and support realistic and positive hope
Depression: "I just don't know how my kids are going to get along after I'm gone." Sadness, grief, mourning for impending losses	Normal and adaptive response. Clinical depression should be assessed and treated when present. Nurses should encourage the patient and the family to fully express their sadness. Insincere reassurance or encouragement of unrealistic hopes should be avoided
Acceptance: "I've lived a good life, and I have no regrets." Patient and/or family are neither angry nor depressed	The patient may withdraw as their circle of interest diminishes. The family may feel rejected by the patient. Nurses need to support the family's expression of emotions and encourage them to continue to be present for the patient

Adapted from Kübler-Ross, E. (1969). *On death and dying*. New York: Macmillan.

Individual and family coping with the anticipation of death is complicated by the varied and conflicting trajectories that grief and mourning may assume in the family. For example, while the patient may be experiencing sadness while contemplating role changes that have been brought about by the illness, the patient's spouse or partner may be expressing or holding in feelings of anger about the current changes in role and impending loss of the relationship; others in the family may be engaged in denial or self-protection (e.g., "Dad will get better. He just needs to eat more."), fear (e.g., "Who will take care of us?" or "Will I get sick, too?"), or profound sadness and withdrawal (e.g., going to work and avoiding visiting). Although each of these behaviours is normal, tension may arise when one or more family members perceive that others are less caring, too emotional, or too detached.

The nurse needs to assess the characteristics of the family system and intervene in a manner that supports and enhances the cohesion of the family unit. Parameters for assessing the family facing life-threatening illness are identified in Chart 15-6. The nurse can patiently guide family members to talk about their feelings and understand them in the broader context of anticipatory grief and mourning. Acknowledging and expressing feelings, continuing to interact with the patient in meaningful ways, and planning for the time of death and bereavement are adaptive family behaviours. Professional support provided by grief counsellors in the community, at a local hospital, in the long-term care facility, or associated with a hospice program can help both the patient and family sort out and acknowledge feelings and make the end of life as meaningful as possible.

Grief and Mourning After Death

When a loved one dies, the family members enter a new phase of grief and mourning as they begin to accept the loss, feel the pain of permanent separation, and prepare to live a life without the deceased. Even if the loved one died after a long illness, preparatory grief experienced during the terminal illness will not preclude the grief and mourning that follow the death. Following the patient's death after a long or difficult illness, family members may experience conflicting feelings of relief that the loved one's suffering has ended, compounded by guilt and grief related to unresolved issues or the circumstances of death. Grief work may be especially difficult if the patient's death was painful, prolonged, accompanied by unwanted interventions, or unattended. Families who had no preparation or support during the period of imminence and death may have a more difficult time finding a place for the painful memories.

Although some family members may experience prolonged or complicated mourning, most grief reactions fall within a range of loss, sorrow, and sadness. The feelings are often profound, but the bereaved individual eventually reconciles the loss and finds a way to reengage with his or her life. Grief and mourning are affected by individual characteristics, coping skills, and experiences with illness and death; the nature of the relationship to the deceased; factors surrounding the illness and the death; family dynamics; social support; and cultural expectations and norms. After-death rituals, including preparation of the

CHART 15-6

Assessing for Anticipatory Mourning in the Family Facing Life-Threatening Illness

- **Family constellation**
  - Identify the members who constitute the patient's family.
    - Who is important to the patient?
  - Identify roles and relationships among the family members.
  - Who is the primary caregiver?
  - By what authority is this person the primary caregiver?
- **Cohesion and boundaries**
  - How autonomous/interdependent are family members?
    - Degree of involvement with each other as individuals and as a family
    - Degree of bonding between family members
    - Degree of "teamwork" in the family
    - Degree of reliance on individual family members for specific tasks/roles'
  - How do family members differ in:
    - Personality?
    - Worldview?
    - Priorities?
  - What are the implicit and explicit expectations or "rules" for behaviour within the family?
- **Flexibility and adaptability**
  - What is the family's ability to integrate new information?
  - How does the family manage change?
  - How able are the family members to assume new roles and responsibilities?
- **Communication**
  - What is the style of communication in the family, in terms of:
    - Openness?
    - Directness?
    - Clarity?
  - What are the constraints on communication?
  - What topics are avoided?

body, funeral practices, and burial rituals, are socially and culturally significant ways that members of a family begin to accept the reality and finality of death. Preplanning of funerals is becoming increasingly common, and hospice or palliative home care professionals may assist families to make plans for death, often involving the patient who may wish to take an active planning role. Preplanning the funeral relieves the family of the decision burden in the intensely emotional period following a death. Uncomplicated grief and mourning are characterized by emotional feelings of sadness, anger, guilt, and numbness; physical sensations such as hollowness in the stomach and tightness in the chest, weakness, and lack of energy; cognitions that include preoccupation with the loss and a sense of the deceased as still present; and behaviours such as crying, visiting places that are reminders of the deceased, social withdrawal, and restless overactivity (Worden, 1991).

In general, the period of mourning is an adaptive response to loss during which the mourner comes to accept the loss as real and permanent, acknowledges and experiences the painful emotions that accompany the loss, experiences life without the deceased, overcomes impediments to adjustment, and finds a new way of living in a world without the loved one. Particularly immediately following the death, the mourner begins to recognize the reality and permanence of the loss by talking about the deceased and telling and retelling the story of the illness and death. Societal norms are frequently at odds with the normal grieving processes of individuals, where time excused from work obligations is typically measured in days, and mourners are often expected to get over the loss quickly and get on with life.

In reality, the work of grief and mourning takes time, and avoiding grief work following the death often leads to long-term adjustment difficulties. According to Rando (2000), mourning for a loss involves the "undoing" of psychosocial ties that bind the mourner to the deceased, personal adaptation to the loss, and learning to live in the world without the deceased. Six key processes of mourning allow the individual to accommodate to the loss in a healthy way: recognition of the loss; reaction to the separation, experiencing and expressing the pain of the loss; recollection and reexperiencing the deceased, the relationship, and the associated feelings; relinquishing old attachments to the deceased; readjustment to adapt to the new world without forgetting the old; and reinvestment (Rando, 2000). Similarly, Worden (1991) described four tasks of mourning: acceptance of the reality of the loss, working through the pain of grief, adjusting to the environment in which the deceased is gone, and emotional "relocation" of the deceased in order to move on with life.

Although many individuals complete the work of mourning with the informal support of family and friends, many find that talking with others who have had a similar experience, such as in formal support groups, normalizes the feelings and experiences and provides a framework for learning new skills to cope with the loss and create a new life. Bereavement support groups are often sponsored by hospitals, hospices, and other community organizations. Groups for parents who have lost a child, children who have lost a parent, widows, widowers, and gay men and lesbians who have lost a life partner are some examples of specialized support groups available in many communities. Nursing interventions for those experiencing grief and mourning are identified in Chart 15-7.

Complicated Grief and Mourning

Complicated grief and mourning are characterized by prolonged feelings of sadness and feelings of general worthlessness or hopelessness that persist long after the death, prolonged symptoms that interfere with activities of daily living (anorexia, insomnia, fatigue, panic), or self-destructive behaviours such as alcohol or substance abuse and suicidal ideation or attempts. Complicated grief and mourning require professional assessment and can be treated with pharmacologic and psychological interventions.

CHART 15-7

Nursing Interventions for Grief and Mourning

- **Support the expression of feelings**
  - Encourage the telling of the story using open-ended statements or questions (e.g., "Tell me about your husband")
  - Assist the mourner to find an outlet for his or her feelings: talking, attending a support group, keeping a journal, finding a safe outlet for angry feelings (writing letters that will not be mailed, physical activity)
- **Assess emotional affect, and reinforce the normalcy of feelings**
- **Assess for guilt and regrets**
  - Are you especially troubled by a certain memory or thought?
  - How do you manage those memories?
- **Assess for the presence of social support**
  - Do you have someone to whom you can talk about your husband?
  - Can I help you to find someone you can talk to?
- **Assess coping skills**
- How are you managing day to day?
  - Have you experienced other losses? How did you manage those?
  - Are there things you are having trouble doing?
  - Do you have/need help with specific tasks?
- **Assess for signs of complicated grief and mourning, and offer professional referral**
  - Are you preoccupied with thoughts or the deceased that interfere with your ability to care for yourself?
  - Do you have frequent and prolonged intense emotional pain?

Coping With Death and Dying: Professional Caregiver Issues

Whether practicing in the trauma centre, intensive care unit or other acute care setting, home care, hospice, long-term care, or the many locations where patients and their families receive ambulatory services, nurses are closely involved with complex and emotionally laden issues surrounding loss of life. To be most effective and satisfied with the care they provide, nurses need to attend to their own emotional responses to the losses they witness every day. Well before the nurse exhibits symptoms of stress or burnout, he or she should acknowledge the difficulty of coping with others' pain on a daily basis and put healthy practices in place that will guard against emotional exhaustion. In hospice settings, where death, grief, and loss are expected outcomes of patient care, interprofessional colleagues rely on each other for support, using meeting time to express frustration, sadness, anger, and other emotions; to learn coping skills from each other; and to speak about how they were affected by the lives of those patients who have died since the last meeting. In many settings, staff members organize or attend memorial services to support families and other caregivers, who find comfort in joining each other to remember and celebrate the lives of patients. Finally, healthy personal habits, including diet, exercise, stress reduction activities (such as dance, yoga, T'ai chi, meditation), and sleep, will help to guard against the detrimental effects of stress.

Critical Thinking Exercises

1 Your patient aged 70 years, has metastatic prostate cancer and is receiving home care. In the past, he has received transfusions of packed red blood cells to treat anemia associated with bone marrow involvement. He has received only temporary benefit from the transfusions. The patient's wife has asked that her husband's hemoglobin continue to be checked weekly because she is concerned about his increasing weakness and exertional dyspnea. The interprofessional team is meeting to discuss the patient's treatment plan. The team consensus is that he is unlikely to live more than a few days or weeks. What additional assessment data are needed to determine the wishes and expectations of the patient? Of the wife? What are the team's options for intervention? What are the pros and cons associated with each option?

2 You are conducting your first home care visit to an 88-year-old woman who has been hospitalized three times in the last 4 months with heart failure. She is short of breath, and uses 2-L oxygen continuously. She is confined to bed and is incontinent and has a stage III pressure ulcer on her coccyx. She is not interested in eating and has lost 30 lb in the last 4 months. She is becoming progressively weaker. Her husband, also 88 years, has limited mobility due to arthritis. He has a history of colon cancer and has had a colostomy for the last 10 years. Although he tries to take care of her, it is becoming increasingly difficult for him to do so. They have been married for almost 70 years and are very devoted to each other. What assessments would you carry out and what strategies would you implement to (1) relieve some of the patient's symptoms and discomfort; (2) assist her husband in management of her care; and (3) prepare both of them for her inevitable death?

3 You have been assigned to care for a 34-year-old father of three in the end stages of ALS. He was discharged home from the hospital yesterday and is being admitted to the local visiting nurse association's home palliative care program. During the admission assessment, when you ask him about his religion and beliefs as part of the spiritual assessment that is performed at the time of admission, he says to you, "I don't go to church anymore and I really don't have time for people who want to talk about religion." Should you respond to his comment? If not, why? If so, what will you say? Should you continue with part or all of a spiritual assessment? Explain your rationale. If you continue with the spiritual assessment, what questions would you use in the assessment? Discuss your plan for follow-up.

4 You are a case manager for a 57-year-old woman with pancreatic cancer who is at home and expected to die in the next few weeks. Her husband calls you because her pain has increased over the past 2 days despite increased breakthrough subcutaneous doses of hydromorphone. When you arrive, she is restless, sensitive to touch, and not oriented to place, which is a sudden change. What further assessment and history would you conduct? What would you suspect? What interventions would you initiate with and for the client and family? What would you recommend to the family physician?

REFERENCES AND SELECTED READINGS

Books

Arensmeyer, K. (2012). Nursing management of patients with cancer related anorexia.

Becker, C. A., Wright, G., & Schmit, K. (2017). Perceptions of dying well and distressing death by acute care nurses. *Applied Nursing Research*, *33*, 149–154.

Bellamy, A. (2018). 4 Designing dying well: Toward a new architectural approach of in-patient palliative care environments. *BMJ Supportive and Palliative Care*, *8*(3), 361.

BONDLY, C., & JATOI, A. (2015). Overview of the management of the anorexia/weight loss syndrome. In *Textbook of Palliative Medicine and Supportive Care* (pp. 574–581). CRC Press.

Brkovic, T., Burilovic, E., & Puljak, L. (2016). Prevalence and severity of pain in adult end-stage renal disease patients on chronic intermittent hemodialysis: a systematic review. Patient preference and adherence, 10, 1131.

Brody, B. D., Meltzer, E. C., Feldman, D., et al. (2017). Assessing decision making capacity for Do Not Resuscitate requests in depressed patients: How to apply the "Communication" and "Appreciation" criteria. *HEC Forum*, *29*(4), 303–311.

Callahan, D. (2000). The troubled dream of life: In search of a peaceful death. Georgetown University Press.

Claxton-Oldfield, S. (2018). Volunteering in hospice palliative care in Canada. *The Changing Face of Volunteering in Hospice and Palliative Care*, *96*.

Collins, A., & Leier, B. (2017). Can medical assistance in dying harm rural and remote palliative care in Canada? *Canadian Family Physician*, *63*(3), 186–190.

Connor, S. R. (2017). *Hospice and palliative care: The essential guide*. New York: Routledge.

Dunbrack, J. (2005). The information needs of informal caregivers involved in providing support to a critically ill loved one. Health Canada.

Ellershaw, J., & Wilkinson, S. (Eds.). (2011). Care of the dying: a pathway to excellence. Oxford University Press, USA.

Etkind, S. N., Bone, A. E., Gomes, B., et al. (2017). How many people will need palliative care in 2040? Past trends, future projections and implications for services. *BMC Medicine*, *15*(1), 102.

Fassbender, K. (2018). Consensus Development Conference: Promoting access to quality palliative care in Canada. *Journal of Palliative Medicine*, *21*(S1), S1–S8.

Flannelly, K. J. (2017). Religion and death anxiety. In *Religious beliefs, evolutionary psychiatry, and mental health in America* (pp. 153–164). Cham: Springer.

Frankl, V. E. (1985). Man's search for meaning. Simon and Schuster.

Glaser, B. G., & Strauss, A. L. (1965). Awareness of dying. 1965. London: Weidenfeld and Nicholson.

Greer, J. A., Jackson, V. A., Jacobsen, J. C., et al. (2017). Early palliative care for patients with advanced cancer. In A. M. Vranceanu, J. A. Greer, & S. A. Safren (Eds.). *The Massachusetts general hospital handbook of behavioral medicine* (pp. 277–296). New York: Humana Press.

Hartogh, G. D. (2017). Suffering and dying well: On the proper aim of palliative care. *Medicine, Health Care and Philosophy*, *20*(3), 413–424.

Hui, D., Frisbee-Hume, S., Wilson, A., et al. (2017). Effect of lorazepam with haloperidol vs haloperidol alone on agitated delirium in patients with advanced cancer receiving palliative care: A randomized clinical trial. *JAMA*, *318*(11), 1047–1056.

Iyer, A. S., & Bakitas, M. (2017). Early palliative care in advanced illness: Do right by Mama. *JAMA Internal Medicine*, *177*(6), 761–762.

Jennings, B., Ryndes, T., D'Onofrio, C., & Baily, M. A. (2003). Access to hospice care. Garrison, NY: Hastings Center.

Johnson, T., Cheng, C., Lawand, C., et al. (2018). Access to palliative care in Canada. *International Journal of Population Data Science*, *3*(4).

Kastenbaum, R., & Saunders, D. C. M. (Eds.). (1997). Hospice Care on the International Scene. Springer.

Kristjanson, L. J., Toye, C., & Dawson, S. (2003).

Kübler-Ross, E. (1969). On death and dying. New York: Collier Books.

Leiter, R. (2017). Conversations on dying: A palliative-care pioneer faces his own death. *Journal of Palliative Medicine*, *20*(6), 687.

Martins Pereira, S., Fradique, E., & Hernandez-Marrero, P. (2018). End-of-life decision making in palliative care and recommendations of the Council of Europe: Qualitative secondary analysis of interviews and observation field notes. *Journal of Palliative Medicine*, *21*(5), 604–615.

Oliver, P., Wilson, M., & Malpas, P. (2017). New Zealand doctors' and nurses' views on legalising assisted dying in New Zealand. *The New Zealand Medical Journal*, *130*(1456), 10.

Omilion-Hodges, L. M., Manning, B. L., & Orbe, M. P. (2017). "Context matters:" An exploration of young adult social constructions of meaning about death and dying. *Health Communication*, 1–10.

Osinski, A., Vreugdenhil, G., de Koning, J., et al. (2017). Do-not-resuscitate orders in cancer patients: A review of literature. *Supportive Care in Cancer*, *25*(2), 677–685.

Parker, C. P., Csikai, E. L., & Foster, P. P. (2018). Living and dying well with HIV/AIDS. In R. S. Allen, B. D. Carpenter, M. K. Eichorst (eds.). *Perspectives on Palliative and End-of-Life Care* (pp. 19–43). New York: Routledge.

Peicius, E., Blazeviciene, A., & Kaminskas, R. (2017). Are advance directives helpful for good end of life decision making: A cross sectional survey of health professionals. *BMC Medical Ethics*, *18*(1), 40.

Rando, T. A. (2000). Anticipatory mourning: A review and critique of the literature. *Clinical dimensions of anticipatory mourning: Theory and practice in working with the dying, their loved ones, and their caregivers*, 17–50.

Renz, M., Reichmuth, O., Bueche, D., et al. (2018). Fear, pain, denial, and spiritual experiences in dying processes. *American Journal of Hospice and Palliative Medicine®*, *35*(3), 478–491.

Rosa, W., Estes, T., & Watson, J. (2017). Caring science conscious dying: An emerging metaparadigm. *Nursing Science Quarterly*, *30*(1), 58–64.

Rothman, D. J. (2017). *Strangers at the bedside: A history of how law and bioethics transformed medical decision making*. New York: Routledge.

Seow, H., O'Leary, E., Perez, R., et al. (2018). Access to palliative care by disease trajectory: A population-based cohort of Ontario decedents. *BMJ Open*, *8*(4), e021147.

Sinclair, S., Beamer, K., Hack, T. F., et al. (2017). Sympathy, empathy, and compassion: A grounded theory study of palliative care patients' understandings, experiences, and preferences. *Palliative Medicine*, *31*(5), 437–447.

Swinton, M., Giacomini, M., Toledo, F., et al. (2017). Experiences and expressions of spirituality at the end of life in the intensive care unit. *American Journal of Respiratory and Critical Care Medicine*, *195*(2), 198–204.

Temel, J. S., Greer, J. A., El-Jawahri, A., et al. (2017). Effects of early integrated palliative care in patients with lung and GI cancer: A randomized clinical trial. *Journal of Clinical Oncology: Official Journal of the American Society of Clinical Oncology*, *35*(8), 834–841.

Thomas, K., Lobo, B., & Detering, K. (Eds.). (2017). *Advance care planning in end of life care* (2nd ed.). Oxford, UK: Oxford University Press.

Walkey, A. J., Weinberg, J., Wiener, R. S., et al. (2018). Hospital variation in utilization of life sustaining treatments among patients with do not resuscitate orders. *Health Services Research*, *53*(3), 1644–1661.

Waller, A., & Caroline, N. L. (2000). *Handbook of palliative care in cancer.* Butterworth-Heinemann Medical.

Watchman, K., Hogan, M., Janicki, M., et al. (2017). Dying well with an intellectual disability and dementia? *Journal of Dementia Care*, *25*(4), 28–31.

Wilson, M., Oliver, P., & Malpas, P. (2019). Nurses' views on legalising assisted dying in New Zealand: A cross-sectional study. *International journal of nursing studies*, *89*, 116–124.

Journals and Electronic Documents

Alberta Health Services. (2014). *Goals of care designation (GCD) order*. Retrieved April 10, 2018, from https://www.albertahealthservices.ca/frm-103547.pdf.

Antunes, B., Murtagh, F., Bausewein, C., et al. (2015). Screening for depression in advanced disease: Psychometric properties, sensitivity, and specificity of two items of the Palliative Care Outcome Scale (POS). *Journal of Pain and Symptom Management*, *49*(2), 277–288.

Aslakson, R. A., Curtis, J. R., & Nelson, J. E. (2014). The changing role of palliative care in the ICU. *Critical Care Medicine*, *42*(11), 2418.

BC Cancer Agency. (2015). *Goals of care (GOC) orders*. Retrieved April 10, 2018 from http://www.bccancer.bc.ca/new-patients-site/Documents/ACP-goals-of-care-orders.pdf.

Benkel, I., Wijk, H., & Molander, U. (2010). Using coping strategies is not denial: helping loved ones adjust to living with a patient with a palliative diagnosis. *Journal of Palliative Medicine*, *13*(9), 1119–1123.

Benoliel, J. Q. (1993). The moral context of oncology nursing. In Oncology nursing forum (Vol. 20, No. 10 Suppl, pp. 5–12).

Bindels, L. B., Neyrinck, A. M., Loumaye, A., et al. (2018). Increased gut permeability in cancer cachexia: Mechanisms and clinical relevance. *Oncotarget, 9*(26), 18224.

Brkovic, T., Burilovic, E., & Puljak, L. (2016). "Prevalence and severity of pain in adult end-stage renal disease patients on chronic intermittent hemodialysis: A systematic review." *Patient Preference and Adherence, 10*, 1131.

Brogan, P., Hasson, F., & McIlfatrick, S. (2018). Shared decision-making at the end of life: A focus group study exploring the perceptions and experiences of multi-disciplinary healthcare professionals working in the home setting. *Palliative Medicine, 32*(1), 123–132.

Brooke, J., & Ojo, O. (2015). Enteral nutrition in dementia: A systematic review. *Nutrients, 7*(4), 2456–2468.

Canadian Hospice Palliative Care Association. (2015). *The Way Forward National Framework: A roadmap for an integrated palliative approach to care, The Way Forward initiative*. Retrieved March 29, 2018, from http://www.hpcintegration.ca/media/60044/TWF-framework-doc-Eng-2015-final-April1.pdf.

Canadian Hospice Palliative Care Association (CHPCA) (2018). *FAQs. Where do people receive palliative care?* Retrieved March 28, 2018, from http://www.chpca.net/family-caregivers/faqs.aspx.

Canadian Nurses Association. (2015). *Canadian Nurses Association, Canadian Hospice Palliative Care Association (CHPCA) and the Canadian Hospice Palliative Care Nurses Group (CHPC-NG) Joint Position Statement: The palliative approach to care and the role of the nurse*. Retrieved March 29, 2018, from https://www.cna-aiic.ca/~/media/cna/page-content/pdf-en/the-palliative-approach-to-care-and-the-role-of-the-nurse_e.pdf.

Canadian Nurses Association. (2017a). *Canadian Nurses Association leads the development of a national nursing framework on medical assistance in dying*. Retrieved March 29, 2018, from https://www.cna-aiic.ca/en/news-room/news-releases/2017/cna-leads-the-development-of-a-national-nursing-framework-on-medical-assistance-in-dying#sthash.lJnfyV6z.dpufhttps://www.cna-aiic.ca/en/news-room/news-releases/2017/cna-leads-the-developmnt-of-a-national-nursing-framework-on-medical-assistance-in-dying.

Canadian Nurses Association. (2017b). *Code of ethics for registered nurses*. Retrieved May 5, 2018, from https://www.cna-aiic.ca/~/media/cna/page-content/pdf-en/code-of-ethics-2017-edition-secure-interactive.

Chater, K., & Tsai, C. T. (2008). Palliative care in a multicultural society: a challenge for western ethics. *Australian Journal of Advanced Nursing, 26*(2), 95.

Crawford, J. (2018). Cancer cachexia: Are we ready to take a step forward? *Cancer, 124*(3), 456–458.

Damrauer, J. S., Stadler, M. E., Acharyya, S., et al. (2018). Chemotherapy-induced muscle wasting: Association with NF-κB and cancer cachexia. *European Journal of Translational Myology, 28*(2).

Davies, P. S. (2016). Pharmacologic pain management at the end of life. *The Nurse Practitioner, 41*(5), 26–37.

Dean, M. M., Cellarius, V., Henry, B., Oneschuk, D., & Librach, S. L. (2012). Framework for continuous palliative sedation therapy in Canada. *Journal of palliative medicine, 15*(8), 870–879.

De Clercq, E., Rost, M., Pacurari, N., et al. (2017). Aligning guidelines and medical practice: Literature review on pediatric palliative care guidelines. *Palliative & Supportive Care, 15*(4), 474–489.

Drulovic, J., Basic-Kes, V., Grgic, S., et al. (2015). The prevalence of pain in adults with multiple sclerosis: A multicenter cross-sectional survey. *Pain Medicine, 16*(8), 1597–1602.

Edmonton Zone Palliative Care Program. Including 99 Questions and more about Hospice Palliative Care: A Nurses' handbook. Retrieved March 14, 2014, from http://www.palliative.org/NewPC/_pdfs/education/99QuestionsEbook2013.pdf

Fearon, K., Strasser, F., Anker, S. D., et al. (2011). Definition and classification of cancer cachexia: an international consensus. *The Lancet Oncology, 12*(5), 489–495.

Ferraz Gonçalves, J. A., Almeida, A., Costa, I., et al. (2016). Comparison of haloperidol alone and in combination with midazolam for the treatment of acute agitation in an inpatient palliative care service. *Journal of Pain & Palliative Care Pharmacotherapy, 30*(4), 284–288.

Finucane, T. E. (2002). Care of patients nearing death: Another view. *Journal of the American Geriatrics Society, 50*(3), 551–553.

Giese, C. (2009). German nurses, euthanasia and terminal care: a personal perspective. *Nursing ethics, 16*(2), 231–237.

Government of Canada. (2017). *Justice laws website: Framework on palliative care in Canada Act (S.C. 2017, c. 28)*. Retrieved April 10, 2018, from http://laws-lois.justice.gc.ca/eng/acts/F-31.5/page-1.html.

Government of Canada. (2018a). *Medical assistance in dying*. Retrieved March 27, 2018, from https://www.canada.ca/en/health-canada/services/medical-assistance-dying.html.

Government of Canada. (2018b). *2nd interim report on medical assistance in dying in Canada*. Retrieved March 27, 2018, from https://www.canada.ca/en/health-canada/services/publications/health-system-services/medical-assistance-dying-interim-report-sep-2017.html.

Griffie, J., Nelson-Marten, P., & Muchka, S. (2004). Acknowledging the 'Elephant': Communication in Palliative Care: Speaking the unspeakable when death is imminent. *AJN The American Journal of Nursing, 104*(1), 48–57.

Hickman, S. E., Hammes, B. J., Moss, A. H., & Tolle, S. W. (2005). Hope for the future: achieving the original intent of advance directives. *The Hastings Center Report, 35*(6), S26–S30.

Highfield, M. E. F. (2000). Providing spiritual care to patients with cancer. *Clinical Journal of Oncology Nursing, 4*(3).

Hoff, L., & Hermerén, G. (2014). Identifying challenges to communicating with patients about their imminent death. *The Journal of clinical ethics, 25*(4), 296–306.

Hosker, C. M., & Bennett, M. I. (2016). Delirium and agitation at the end of life. *BMJ*, 353.

Howell, D., Keller–Olaman, S., Oliver, T. K., et al. (2013). A pan-Canadian practice guideline and algorithm: screening, assessment, and supportive care of adults with cancer-related fatigue. *Current oncology, 20*(3), e233.

Jackman, R. W., Floro, J., Yoshimine, R., et al. (2017). Continuous release of tumor-derived factors improves the modeling of cachexia in muscle cell culture. *Frontiers in Physiology, 8*, 738.

Jacox, A., Carr, D. B., & Payne, R. (1994). New clinical-practice guidelines for the management of pain in patients with cancer. *New England Journal of Medicine, 330*(9), 651–655.

Kaasa, S., Laird, B., Balstad, T., et al. (2017). 1611TiPA novel multimodal treatment strategy for cancer cachexia; rationale and motivation for the MENAC (Multimodal–Exercise, Nutrition and Anti-inflammatory medication for Cachexia) trial. *Annals of Oncology, 28*(Suppl 5).

Kamal, A. H., Maguire, J. M., Wheeler, J. L., Currow, D. C., & Abernethy, A. P. (2012). Dyspnea review for the palliative care professional: treatment goals and therapeutic options. *Journal of palliative medicine, 15*(1), 106–114.

Kestenbaum, M. G., Vilches, A. O., Messersmith, S., et al. (2014). Alternative routes to oral opioid administration in palliative care: A review and clinical summary. *Pain Medicine, 15*(7), 1129–1153.

Kogan, N. R., Dumas, M., & Cohen, S. R. (2013). The extra burdens patients in denial impose on their family caregivers. *Palliative & supportive care, 11*(2), 91–99.

Krisman-Scott, M. A. (2000). An historical analysis of disclosure of terminal status. *Journal of Nursing Scholarship, 32*(1), 47–52.

Kristjanson, L. J. (2005). Directions in palliative care nursing research: Impeccable care, timing, and complexity. *CJNR (Canadian Journal of Nursing Research), 37*(2), 13–21.

Kwak, J., & Haley, W. E. (2005). Current research findings on end-of-life decision making among racially or ethnically diverse groups. *The Gerontologist, 45*(5), 634–641.

Leow, M. Q., & Chan, S. W. (2017). The challenges, emotions, coping, and gains of family caregivers caring for patients with advanced cancer in Singapore: A qualitative study. *Cancer Nursing, 40*(1), 22–30.

Litzelman, K., Kent, E. E., & Rowland, J. H. (2018). Interrelationships between health behaviors and coping strategies among informal caregivers of cancer survivors. *Health Education & Behavior, 45*(1), 90–100.

Martínez, M., Arantzamendi, M., Belar, A., et al. (2017). "Dignity therapy", a promising intervention in palliative care: A comprehensive systematic literature review. *Palliative Medicine, 31*(6), 492–509.

Marzano, M. (2009). Lies and pain: Patients and caregivers in the "conspiracy of silence". *Journal of Loss and Trauma, 14*(1), 57–81.

Mauricio, R. V., & Okhuysen-Cawley, R. (2010). The caring continuum: role of the pediatric critical care advanced practice nurse in palliative care program development. *Critical care nursing quarterly, 33*(3), 292–297.

McMahan, R. D., Knight, S. J., Fried, T. R., & Sudore, R. L. (2013). Advance care planning beyond advance directives: perspectives from patients and surrogates. *Journal of pain and symptom management, 46*(3), 355–365.

Morse, J. M., & Doberneck, B. (1995). Delineating the concept of hope. *Image: The Journal of Nursing Scholarship, 27*(4), 277–285.

Mosher, C. E., Ott, M. A., Hanna, N., et al. (2017). Development of a symptom management intervention: Qualitative feedback from advanced lung cancer patients and their family caregivers. *Cancer Nursing, 40*(1), 66.

Moss, K. O., Deutsch, N. L., Hollen, P. J., et al. (2017). Understanding end-of-life decision-making terminology among African American older adults. *Journal of Gerontological Nursing, 44*(2), 33–40.

Ojo, O., & Brooke, J. (2015). Evaluating the association between diabetes, cognitive decline and dementia. *International journal of environmental research and public health, 12*(7), 8281–8294.

Olson, K., Krawchuk, A., & Quddusi, T. (2007). Fatigue in individuals with advanced cancer in active treatment and palliative settings. *Cancer Nursing, 30*(4), E1–E10.

Parliament of Canada. (2016). *Bill C-14. Royal Assent*. Retrieved March 29, 2018 from http://www.parl.ca/DocumentViewer/en/42-1/bill/C-14/royal-assent.

Pötgens, S. A., Sboarina, M., & Bindels, L. B. (2018). Polyunsaturated fatty acids, polyphenols, amino acids, prebiotics: Can they help to tackle cancer cachexia and related inflammation? *Current Opinion in Clinical Nutrition and Metabolic Care, 21*, 458–464.

Public Health Agency of Canada. (2016). *Leading causes of hospitalizations, Canada, 2009/10*. Retrieved April 10, 2018, from https://www.canada.ca/en/public-health/services/reports-publications/leading-causes-death-hospitalization-canada/2009-10-males-females-combined-counts-specific-hospitalization-rate.html.

Puchalski, C. M., Vitillo, R., Hull, S. K., & Reller, N. (2014). Improving the spiritual dimension of whole person care: Reaching national and international consensus. *Journal of Palliative Medicine, 17*(6), 642–656.

Radbruch, L., Strasser, F., Elsner, F., Gonçalves, J. F., Løge, J., Kaasa, S., ... & Research Steering Committee of the European Association for Palliative Care (EAPC). (2008). Fatigue in palliative care patients—an EAPC approach. *Palliative Medicine, 22*(1), 13–32.

Rayment, C., Hjermstad, M. J., Aass, N., Kaasa, S., Caraceni, A., Strasser, F., ... & European Palliative Care Research Collaborative (EPCRC). (2013). Neuropathic cancer pain: prevalence, severity, analgesics and impact from the European Palliative Care Research Collaborative–Computerised Symptom Assessment study. *Palliative medicine, 27*(8), 714–721.

Registered Nurses Association of Ontario. (2011). *Best practice clinical guidelines: End-of-life care during the last days*. Retrieved from http://rnao.ca/bpg/guidelines/endoflife-care-during-last-days-and-hours.

Reid, J., McKenna, H., Fitzsimons, D., & McCance, T. (2009). The experience of cancer cachexia: a qualitative study of advanced cancer patients and their family members. *International journal of nursing studies, 46*(5), 606–616.

Reynolds, J., Drew, D., & Dunwoody, C. (2013). American Society for Pain Management Nursing position statement: pain management at the end of life. *Pain Management Nursing, 14*(3), 172–175.

Riley, J., & Fenton, G. (2007). A terminal diagnosis: The carers' perspective. *Counselling and Psychotherapy Research, 7*(2), 86–91.

Rising, M. L. (2017). Truth telling as an element of culturally competent care at end of life. *Journal of Transcultural Nursing, 28*(1), 48–55.

Rivera, I., Ajroud-Driss, S., Casey, P., et al. (2013). Prevalence and characteristics of pain in early and late stages of ALS. *Amyotrophic Lateral Sclerosis and Frontotemporal Degeneration, 14*(5–6), 369–372.

Sanders, J. J., Chow, V., Enzinger, A. C., et al. (2017). Seeking and accepting: US clergy theological and moral perspectives informing decision making at the end of life. *Journal of Palliative Medicine, 20*(10), 1059–1067.

Silverman, P. R. (2002). Living with grief, rebuilding a world. *Journal of palliative medicine, 5*(3), 449–454.

Solheim, T. S., Laird, B. J., Balstad, T. R., et al. (2017). A randomized phase II feasibility trial of a multimodal intervention for the management of cachexia in lung and pancreatic cancer. *Journal of Cachexia, Sarcopenia and Muscle, 8*(5), 778–788.

Stajduhar, K. I. (2011). Chronic illness, palliative care, and the problematic nature of dying. *CJNR (Canadian Journal of Nursing Research), 43*(3), 7–15.

Stajduhar, K., Sawatzky, R., Cohen, S. R., et al. (2017). Bereaved family members' perceptions of the quality of end-of-life care across four types of inpatient care settings. *BMC Palliative Care, 16*(1), 59.

Statistics Canada. (2018). *Leading causes of death, total population, by age group and sex, Canada, 2011–2015*. Retrieved April 10, 2018, from http://www5.statcan.gc.ca/cansim/a26?lang=eng&id=1020561

Teixeira, R. J., Applebaum, A. J., Bhatia, S., et al. (2018). The impact of coping strategies of cancer caregivers on psychophysiological outcomes: An integrative review. *Psychology Research and Behavior Management, 11*, 207.

Undermann Boggs, K. (2011). Bridges and barriers in the therapeutic relationship. Teoksessa Arnold E & Undermann Boggs K. *Interpersonal Relationships: Professional Communication Skills for Nurses, 4*, 143–165.

Walshe, C., Roberts, D., Appleton, L., et al. (2017). Coping well with advanced cancer: A serial qualitative interview study with patients and family carers. *PLoS One, 12*(1), e0169071.

Wilson, K. G., Chochinov, H. M., Allard, P., et al. (2009). Prevalence and correlates of pain in the Canadian National Palliative Care Survey. *Pain Research and Management, 14*(5), 365–370.

Wooster, M., Stassi, A., Hill, J., et al. (2018). End-of-life decision-making for patients with geriatric trauma cared for in a trauma intensive care unit. *American Journal of Hospice and Palliative Medicine, 35*(8), 1063–1068.

Worden, J. W. (1991). Grieving a loss from AIDS. *The Hospice Journal, 7*(1–2), 143–150.

Xie, K., Gelfman, L., Horton, J. R., et al. (2017). State of research on palliative care in heart failure as evidenced by published literature, conference proceedings, and NIH funding. *Journal of Cardiac Failure, 23*(2), 197–200.

Zerwekh, R. N. (1994). How, Hospice Nurses. *The American journal of nursing, 94*(2), 30–34.

Resources

American Academy of Hospice and Palliative Medicine: http://www.aahpm.org

Canada Hospice and Palliative Care Resources: http://www.cpsonline.info/content/resources/canada.html

Canadian Hospice Palliative Care Association: http://www.chpca.net

Center to Improve Care of the Dying at George Washington University: http://www.gwu.edu/~cicd/

Children's Hospice International: http://www.chionline.org

Fraser Health Authority. Hospice Palliative Care. Retrieved March 14, 2014, from http://www.fraserhealth.ca/your_care/hospice_palliative_care/services/

Health Canada's Secretariat on Palliative and End-of-Life Care: http://www.hc-sc.gc.ca/hcs-sss/palliat/sect/index-eng.php

Hospice Education Institute: http://www.hospiceworld.org/

Hospice Net: https://www.caringcommunity.org/helpful-resources/self-help/death-dying/hospice-net-preparing-for-approaching-death/

Hospice and Palliative Nurses Association (HPNA): http://www.hpna.org

Palliative Care Nursing: http://www.palliativecarenursing.net/index.html

World Health Organization (miscellaneous cancer pages): http://www.who.int/cancer/en/

UNIT 3

Concepts and Challenges in Patient Management

Case Study A PATIENT WITH DEBILITATING PAIN

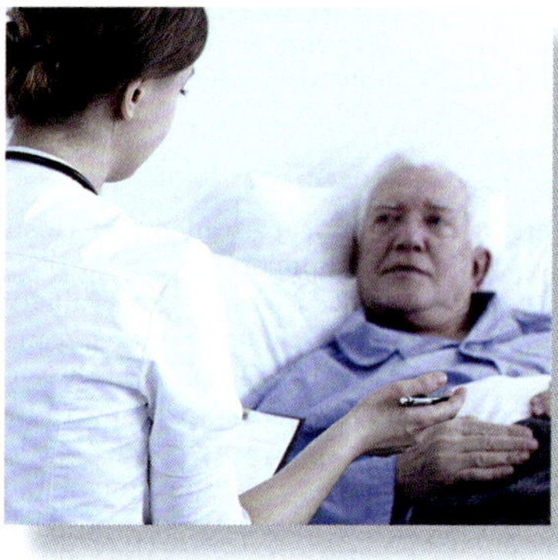

A patient diagnosed with end-stage lung cancer has been admitted to the inpatient hospice unit for pain control. The patient has been in a great deal of pain and discomfort. On admission, the patient asked that he receive the ordered amount of pain medication as scheduled. He has since become nonverbal and difficult to arouse. Upon assessment, the nurse finds that the patient is restless with slow, shallow breathing and is unable to verbalize that he has pain. The family is concerned that the use of pain medication has inhibited the patient's ability to stay alert and affected his breathing. They have requested that pain medication be held until the patient is alert and can ask for it. A family case conference has been booked with the hospice/palliative team.

QSEN Competency Focus: Teamwork and Collaboration

The complexities inherent in today's health care system challenge nurses to demonstrate integration of specific interdisciplinary core competencies that are aimed at ensuring the delivery of safe and quality patient care (Institute of Medicine, 2003). The Quality and Safety Education for Nurses project (QSEN, 2017) provides a framework for the knowledge, skills, and attitudes (KSAs) required for nurses to demonstrate competency in these key areas, which include ***patient-centred care***, ***interdisciplinary teamwork and collaboration***, ***evidence-based practice***, ***quality improvement***, ***safety***, and ***informatics.***

Teamwork and Collaboration Definition: Function effectively within nursing and interprofessional teams, fostering open communication, mutual respect, and shared decision making to achieve quality patient care.

SELECTED PRE-LICENSURE KSAs	APPLICATION AND REFLECTION
Knowledge	
Describe own strengths, limitations, and values in functioning as a member of the team.	Describe the nurse's role in participating in a case conference. How does the role of the nurse differ from other members of the team?
Skills	
Function competently within own scope of practice as a member of the health care team.	Even though the patient is unable to verbalize his pain, what other methods of assessment can the nurse use and rely on to assess pain in this patient? What interventions for pain can a nurse implement as part of a nursing care plan?
Attitudes	
Value different styles of communication used by patients, families, and health care providers. Contribute to resolution of conflict and disagreement.	After the case conference, the hospice team agrees to give the pain medication to the patient as he has requested. The family is displeased with the decision because the patient cannot speak. How can the nurse best diffuse the conflict? Are there other members of the hospice team that may be instrumental in communicating with the family?

Cronenwett, L., Sherwood, G., Barnsteiner, J., et al. (2007). Quality and safety education for nurses. *Nursing Outlook, 55*(3), 122–131; Institute of Medicine. (2003). *Health professions education: A bridge to quality*. Washington, DC: National Academies Press; and QSEN Institute. (2017). *QSEN competencies: Definitions and pre-licensure KSAs*. Retrieved June 12, 2019, from www.qsen.org/competencies/pre-licensure-ksas

16 Pain Management

Adapted by Eric Lavoie

Learning Objectives

On completion of this chapter, the learner will be able to:

1. Compare characteristics of acute pain, procedural pain, chronic pain, and cancer pain.
2. Describe the negative consequences of pain.
3. Describe the pathophysiology of pain.
4. Describe factors that can alter the perception of pain.
5. Demonstrate appropriate use of pain measurement instruments.
6. Explain the physiologic basis of pain relief interventions.
7. Explain the impact of aging on pain.
8. Discuss when opioid tolerance may be a concern.
9. Identify appropriate pain relief interventions for selected groups of patients.
10. Compare the various types of neurosurgical procedures used to treat intractable pain.
11. Develop a plan to prevent and treat the adverse effects of analgesic agents.
12. Use the nursing process as a framework for the care of patients with pain.

Nurses are often the health care providers who have the most contact time with patients. Consequently, nurses are well positioned to assess and treat all types of pain. It is a domain where the nursing profession is a champion, and nurses have a long history of being great advocates. They hold great responsibility in assessing, educating, and treating patients with pain. Given this reality, it behooves all nurses to gain expertise and knowledge in the area of pain nomenclature, pathophysiology, pharmacotherapy, and treatments. Pain is often misunderstood, underreported, and poorly treated. Nonetheless, significant progress has been made with the recent Montreal Declaration by the International Association for the Study of Pain that states access to pain management is a fundamental human right. Nursing's role in pain management has evolved so that the nurse is seen the primary pain manager (Herr, St. Marie, Gordon, et al., 2015). A growing body of evidence is helping providers better understand underlying causes of pain, as well as standard and novel treatments for acute, chronic, non-cancer, and cancer pain.

Definition of Pain

The International Association for the Study of Pain, of which the Canadian Pain Society is a chapter member, is the long-standing authority on pain. The most recent definition agreed upon in 2011 reads as follows: Pain is defined as "**an unpleasant sensory and emotional experience (1) associated with actual or potential tissue damage; or (2) described in terms of such damage**" (Aydede, 2017).

Important nursing considerations:

- The treatment of pain is a basic human right
- Pain is always subjective
- Inability to communicate pain does not mean that the person does not have pain
- The sensation of pain is coupled with an emotional experience (which nurses should explore and validate)

Types and Categories of Pain

The categorization of pain can vary and a rigid distinction between the type(s) of pain a person may be experiencing may not always be possible. It is generally accepted that there are two major categories of pain that reference the duration—acute and chronic (persistent) pain. Chronic pain is further subcategorized as being of cancer or non-cancer origins.

Acute Pain

Acute pain is usually of recent onset and is commonly associated with a specific injury or "noxious" event (i.e., mechanical, thermal, or chemical). Acute pain indicates that damage or injury has occurred. It is time limited and effort should be made to limit the exposure to the "noxious" trigger that is precipitating the pain (Stanos, Tyburki, & Harden, 2016). The current definition of acute pain states: "Acute pain is the physiologic response to and experience of noxious stimuli that can become pathologic, is normally sudden in onset, time limited, and motivates behaviours to avoid potential or actual tissue injury" (Kent, Tighe, Belfer, et al., 2017). **Pain** is significant in that it draws attention to its existence and teaches people to avoid similar potentially painful situations. If no lasting damage occurs and no systemic disease exists, acute pain usually decreases as healing occurs. For definitional purposes, acute pain can last from days to 3 to 6 months (Kent et al., 2017; Stanos et al., 2016). However, the traditional 3 to 6-month time frame is controversial because many acute injuries heal within a few weeks and most heal by 6 weeks (Stanos et al., 2016).

Procedural pain, a form of acute pain, is a brief, intense pain that arises from diagnostic, therapeutic, or preventive procedures. It lasts from seconds to hours. One of the most common sources of procedural pain is needle puncture associated with venipuncture, intravenous cannulation, parenteral drug administration, and lumbar puncture. Wound debridement and wound cleansing also can cause pain, as can many other procedures.

Glossary

addiction: a behavioural pattern of substance use characterized by a compulsion to take the substance (drug or alcohol) primarily to experience its psychic effects

adjuvant analgesic: a drug whose initial use was for another disorder but which later was found to be beneficial for pain. Examples are antidepressants and anticonvulsants

agonist: a substance that when combined with the receptor produces the drug effect or desired effect. Endorphins and morphine are agonists on the opioid receptors

allodynia: pain resulting from a nonpainful stimulus such as a breeze or light touch of clothing

antagonist: a substance that blocks or reverses the effects of the agonist by occupying the receptor site without producing the drug effect

breakthrough pain: a sudden and temporary increase in pain occurring in a patient being managed with opioid analgesia

dependence: occurs when a patient who has been taking opioids experiences a withdrawal syndrome when the opioids are discontinued; often occurs with opioid tolerance and does not indicate an addiction

endorphins and enkephalins: morphine-like substances produced by the body. Primarily found in the central nervous system, they have the potential to reduce pain

multimodal analgesia: using more than one method or modality concurrently for controlling pain to obtain greater benefits and fewer side effects. This may also be referred to as balanced analgesia

nociception: activation of sensory transduction in nerves by thermal, mechanical, or chemical energy impinging on specialized nerve endings; the nerves involved convey information about tissue damage to the central nervous system

nociceptor: a receptor preferentially sensitive to a noxious stimulus

nonnociceptor: nerve fibre that usually does not transmit pain

opioid: a morphine-like compound that produces bodily effects including pain relief, sedation, constipation, and respiratory depression

pain: an unpleasant sensory and emotional experience resulting from actual or potential tissue damage

pain threshold: the point at which a stimulus is perceived as painful

pain tolerance: the maximum intensity or duration of pain that a person is able to endure

patient-controlled analgesia (PCA): self-administration of analgesic agents by a patient instructed about the procedure

phantom limb pain: the sense that an amputated body part is still present. All amputees experience phantom sensations and many people suffer from phantom pain. These sensations arise from damage to peripheral nerves above the site of the amputation

placebo effect (response): analgesia that results from the expectation that a substance will work, not from the actual substance itself

prostaglandins: chemical substances that increase the sensitivity of pain receptors by enhancing the pain-provoking effect of bradykinin

referred pain: pain perceived as coming from an area different from that in which the pathology is occurring

sensitization: a heightened response seen after exposure to a noxious stimulus. Response to the same stimulus is to feel more pain

tolerance: occurs when a person who has been taking opioids becomes less sensitive to their analgesic properties (and usually side effects); characterized by the need for increasing doses to maintain the same level of pain relief

Chronic Pain

Chronic (Non-Cancer) Pain

Chronic pain is constant or intermittent pain that persists beyond the expected healing time; it not necessarily attributed to a specific cause or injury. It is defined as lasting greater than 3 months (McCormick & Law, 2016). It may have a poorly defined onset, and it is often difficult to treat because the cause or origin may be unclear and unrelated to a specific noxious event (Chart 16-1). Despite a patient's efforts to avoid noxious causes of pain, the fight or flight response persists without a known cause. Although acute pain may be a useful signal indicating that something is wrong, chronic pain usually becomes a problem in its own right. In patients presenting with chronic pain, the level of pain reported does not correlate with the degree of tissue damage (Stanos et al., 2016). Unlike acute pain, chronic pain ceases to be protective and becomes central to the dysfunction a patient is experiencing. One in five adult Canadians suffer from chronic pain (Schopflocher, Taenzer, & Jovey, 2011), and an estimated 10% of hospitalized children meet diagnostic criteria that suggests they suffer from chronic pain (Friedrichsdorf, Giordano, Desai Dakoji, et al., 2016). It is also important to note that patients can

CHART 16-1

Pain at the End of Life

Pain is one of the most feared symptoms at the end of life. Many patients experience pain as a terminal illness progresses. The inadequate treatment of cancer pain has been well-documented. In the classic Study to Understand Prognoses and Preferences for Outcomes and Risks of Treatments (SUPPORT) (Murphy et al., 2000), investigators noted that nearly 40% of severely chronically ill and older patients who died in hospitals suffered moderate to severe pain in the last 3 days of life. The suffering caused by unrelieved pain touches all aspects of quality of life (activity, appetite, sleep) and can weaken an already fatigued person. Unrelieved pain can create anxiety and depression, negatively affect relationships, and promote thoughts of suicide.

The Joint Commission's pain standards issued in January 2001 present a unique opportunity to improve care for hospitalized patients. Even though hospices and palliative care agencies are not subject to review by the Joint Commission, many patients with chronic illness who are receiving palliative care may be hospitalized at various times. The standards emphasize pain assessment, patient and family education, continuity of care for symptom management, and evaluation of interventions.

Barriers to Pain Management

Current barriers to pain management include lack of education and fear of addiction.

Lack of Education

Strategies to increase health care professionals' knowledge about pain, pain assessment, and pain management in general and at the end of life are needed to ensure that a patient's pain is effectively addressed. Many studies have increased what is known about pain and pain management. However, the information from these studies must be disseminated to health care professionals to be translated into evidence-based practice. Health care professionals, including nurses, must remain current about the pharmacokinetics and pharmacodynamics of analgesic agents and about new technologies to deliver analgesic medications. Continuing education (CE) can be obtained through conferences, journal articles, and online programs. In a Canadian study, Carlson (2010) reported that "over the past 30 years, postoperative pain relief has been shown to be inadequate." Nurses most likely to adopt evidence-based postoperative care practices are those who are interested in innovation and those who read nursing journals. More studies are needed to evaluate the effect that educational interventions have on health care providers' knowledge about pain and their ability to manage pain effectively (Gunnarsdottir, Donovan, & Ward, 2003).

Addiction Fears

The fear of addiction plays a role even at the end of life. Family members may be hesitant to assist the patient in pain management for fear of the social stigma of addiction. This causes needless pain and suffering. Some health care providers continue to have unfounded fears of contributing to a patient's risk for addiction when administering opioids.

Other Issues Related to Pain Management

Pain management at the end of life requires comprehensive pain assessment and pain management, even though assessment may be hampered by confusion, delirium, or unconsciousness. Caregivers are taught to observe for signs of restlessness or facial expressions as a "proxy" indicator of pain.

Analgesic agents are titrated to find the most effective dose and the best-tolerated route. The nurse and family members assess the effectiveness of the current pain therapy. If the pain is not relieved, a larger dose of medication may be necessary. If the pain continues, another medication may be needed or the patient should be given a different analgesic agent. This process requires frequent assessment to effectively manage pain. The analgesic agent or treatment should be appropriate for the type of pain. For example, neuropathic pain, usually described as burning, tingling, numbness, shooting, stabbing, or electric, requires a different treatment approach than acute pain.

Nonpharmacologic approaches, such as guided imagery and relaxation, can be used to decrease pain and help the patient cope. Careful patient positioning and environmental control are other methods to increase patient comfort.

Respiratory depression is assessed because, over time, the patient's risk for this side effect increases. The rate, depth, and level of consciousness are monitored to determine whether respiratory depression is occurring and requires treatment. A respiratory rate of 6 per minute or greater is usually adequate. If respiratory depression occurs, a decrease in the opioid dose may be indicated. Frequent stimulation to encourage deep breathing may be required until the opioid is metabolized. In the last few days of life, the patient may become restless, which is an indicator of pain. The need to increase the opioid to provide pain relief and the respiratory effects of opioids are considered in decision making. However, comfort should be a priority in the case of a person who clearly is at the end of life.

Side effects from analgesics must be managed. A careful bowel regimen involving diet, bowel stimulants, stool softeners, and/or osmotic agents is instituted to prevent constipation. Vigilance in the assessment, management, and treatment of other side effects is similar to that included in previous discussions.

Careful assessment and management of pain at the end of life can make a "good" death possible by helping patients realize the goal of adequate pain relief throughout the dying process.

have chronic pain with superimposed acute pain, or even an acute exacerbation of their chronic pain. And so, the two main types of pain, acute and chronic, are not mutually exclusive and must be considered and explored to gain a full appreciation of the pain experience.

Cancer-Related Pain

Pain associated with cancer may be acute or chronic; it is poorly understood and complex (Chart 16-1). Cancer pain is present at diagnosis at a frequency of 25% to 50% of patients, whereas 33% of patients develop pain from the cancer treatments (Longo, 2015). Pain in patients with cancer can also be directly associated with the cancer (McCormick, & Law, 2016). Approximately 75% of those with advanced or metastatic disease present with severe pain, which is thought to be from invasion of bony structures, nerves, blood vessels, or mucous membranes (Figura, Smith, & Yu, 2018).

Nociceptive and Neuropathic Pain

Pain can be further categorized by the way it acts on the body, namely, nociceptive (physiologic) pain and neuropathic (pathophysiologic) pain. In a healthy person nociceptive pain is "normal" and an important system to queue the body that noxious stimuli—actual or potential—is present (Hudspith, 2016). In contrast, neuropathic pain is stated to be "initiated or caused by a primary lesion or dysfunction in the nervous system" (Artemiadis & Panagiotis, 2018). Neuropathic pain can be subcategorized as being from a peripheral or a central nervous system (CNS) origin (Chart 16-2).

CHART 16-2

Pain Syndromes and Unusual Severe Pain Problems

Nociceptive Pain Syndromes

Nociceptors (pain receptors) respond to tissue damage, transmitting signals along the peripheral nerves and spinal cord to the brain. Visceral pain is nociceptive pain (see Fig. 16-1) that involves organs.

Arthritis Pain

Various rheumatic diseases, such as osteoarthritis and rheumatoid arthritis, cause pain, which is characterized by joint pain and stiffness. Osteoarthritis is a degenerative joint disease that typically affects the weight-bearing joints and commonly affects older adults. Rheumatoid arthritis is an inflammatory disease affecting weight-bearing and non–weight-bearing joints. It can begin in childhood or in young to middle adulthood. Treatment includes use of nonsteroidal anti-inflammatory drugs (NSAIDs) and thermal therapies.

Fibromyalgia (Fibrositis)

Fibromyalgia, a chronic pain syndrome characterized by generalized musculoskeletal pain, trigger points, stiffness, fatigability, and sleep disturbances, is aggravated by stress and overexertion. The disease primarily affects young women. Treatment consists of NSAIDs, trigger point injections with local anesthetics, tricyclic antidepressants, stress reduction, and regular exercise.

Hemiplegia-Associated Shoulder Pain

Hemiplegia-associated shoulder pain is a pain syndrome that affects as many as 80% of stroke patients. It may result from stretching of the shoulder joint due to the uncompensated pull of gravity on the impaired arm. It may be preventable with functional electrical stimulation of involved shoulder muscles.

Neuropathic Pain Syndromes

Neuropathic pain is caused by a malfunction in the nerves, spinal cord, or brain. It may follow injury or be caused by illness and exposure to chemicals or drugs. The origin of some neuropathic pain may be unknown. The following conditions are associated with neuropathic pain: diabetes, cancer, multiple sclerosis, stroke, human immunodeficiency virus and AIDS, amputation, spinal injury, herpes zoster, and alcoholism. Neuropathic pain syndromes are characterized by tingling or numbness, which evolves to become burning, crushing, or squeezing pain. Those affected by neuropathic pain may be significantly incapacitated. Tricyclic antidepressants and antiepileptic drugs are used as adjuvants for treatment of neuropathic pain.

Complex Regional Pain Syndrome

Complex regional pain syndrome (CRPS) describes a variety of painful conditions that may follow an injury to a limb. It refers to a group of conditions previously described as causalgia, reflex sympathetic dystrophy, and other diagnoses. Although, the main symptom is pain, people also may experience skin changes in the affected limb such as changes in skin colour and temperature, loss of hair and nail growth, and abnormal sweating. Pain is accompanied by weakness and limited range of motion. Treatment includes physical therapy and drugs such as NSAIDs, opioids, and topical anesthetics.

Peripheral Neuropathy

Peripheral neuropathy is caused by damage to peripheral nerves and is an outcome of many diseases. Common causes are endocrine and nutritional disorders (e.g., diabetes and alcoholism), infection (herpes zoster and AIDS), and cancer. In many cases, the etiology of peripheral neuropathy is unknown. The features of peripheral neuropathy include weakness, paresthesia, numbness, and burning pain. Walking and standing become difficult because the patient is unable to identify the position of the joint. Patients risk injury from falls and from inability to feel the development of pressure sores.

Aids-Related Pain

As AIDS progresses, so do problems that produce increasing amounts of pain, such as neuropathy, esophagitis, headaches, postherpetic pain, and abdominal, back, bone, and joint pain. Pain relief interventions are individualized and may consist of NSAIDs, long-lasting opioids such as fentanyl patches, and topical lidocaine. Tricyclic antidepressants may provide comfort in neuropathic and postherpetic pain.

Postherpetic Neuralgia

As immunity for chickenpox (varicella zoster virus) progressively declines over time, the risk of herpes zoster (or shingles) increases. Shingles is an outcome of the reactivation of the dormant virus. Shingles is characterized by pain and a vesicular skin rash located along a sensory nerve pathway (often on the trunk or face). It tends to occur in older adults, and 50% of them will go on to have complications such as postherpetic neuralgia. If antiviral drugs are administered soon after onset of symptoms, the severity and duration of shingles can be reduced. Administration of a zoster vaccine reduces the incidence of shingles by 50% and postherpetic neuralgia by 66% (Shapiro, Kvern, Watson, et al., 2011).

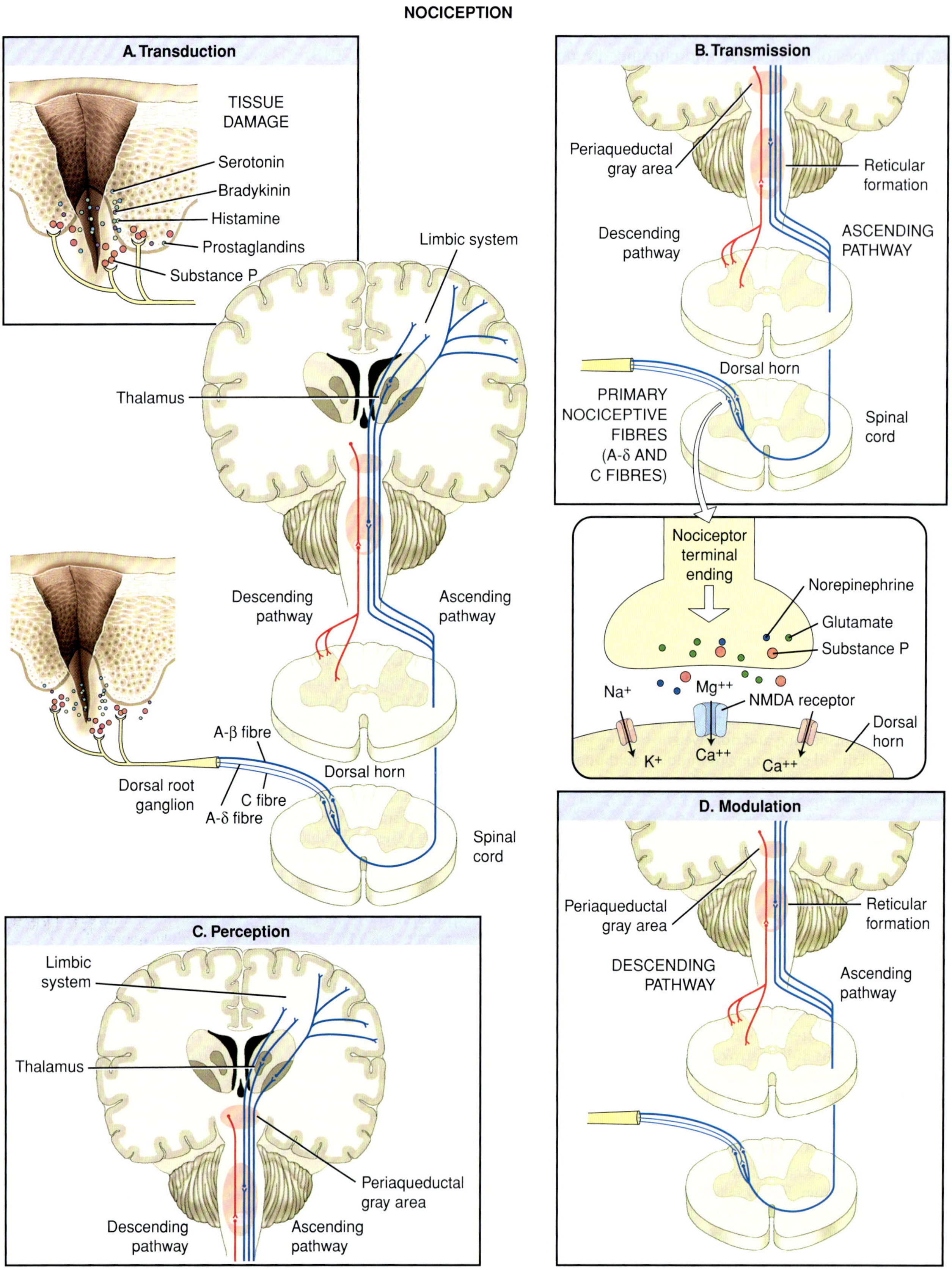

FIGURE 16-1. Nociception. **A.** Transduction. **B.** Transmission. **C.** Perception. **D.** Modulation. (Redrawn from Pasero, C., & McCaffery, M. (2011). *Pain assessment and pharmacologic management* (p. 5). St. Louis, MO: Mosby-Elsevier. Copyright 2011, Pasero C., McCaffery M. Used with permission.)

Nociceptive Pain

After an initial noxious stimulus that actually or potentially damages tissue, the patient's subjective nociceptive pain experience (see Fig. 16-1) can be described by the following processes: transduction, transmission, modulation, and perception (Chart 16-2).

In acute nociceptive pain, the body tends to focus on transduction and transmission and less so, on the modulation or perception (Stanos et al., 2016). Whereas with chronic nociceptive pain, the body shifts its focus on modulation and perception. The following section provides greater foundational knowledge regarding these important concepts in pain to enhance understanding of pharmacologic and nonpharmacologic treatments of pain.

Transduction

Nociception is the act by which the sensation of hot, cold, mechanical, or chemical stimulus is transformed into a signal that can be interpreted by the human body (McEntire, Kirkpatrick, Dueck, et al., 2016). This process involves the activation of **nociceptors** (Fig. 16-1) in the primary afferent neurons which are located in the skin, muscles, and joints (Stanos et al., 2016). The "first pain" sensation is detected by A-delta nociceptor fibres, which is key for quick processing of a pain signal; a "second pain" sensation is felt when the C-fibre nociceptors are activated, producing a dull and more diffuse sensation (Hudspith, 2016). The inflammatory cascade is activated in the body's tissues, becoming a central feature of transduction. Once activated, the inflammatory cascade releases a series of chemical mediators, such as serotonin, bradykinin, histamine, substance P, and **prostaglandins**. These chemical mediators are important to tissue repair but can contribute to increased pain sensation through excess tissue swelling. Not all C-fibres are nociceptors, as there is a subset that is responsible for the sensation of cooling, itch, and some forms of pleasant touch sensations (Hudspith, 2016). The body's normal touch sensation (vibration, pressure, and movement) is mediated by A-beta fibres. (Riquelme, Hatem, & Montoya, 2016).

Transmission

In this phase of the pain process, transmission is the communication of the action potential (electrophysiologic signal) that was first initiated by **nociceptors** (A-delta or C-fibre) from the periphery to the CNS through the spinal cord's dorsal horn (Hudspith, 2016). Sodium, potassium, and calcium channels with varying voltage activation levels play a role in the timing and duration of pain signals. Once these channels are activated by stimuli, chemical messages are transmitted via the neurons to signal an inhibitory or excitatory message. The message travels through the neurons to their respective axon terminals to then release neurotransmitters. The A-delta and C-fibres pass on the nociceptive information of pain through the superficial laminae (I and II) and deep laminae (V and VI) of the dorsal horn of the spine (Stanos et al., 2016). The body, in normal conditions, can modulate the excitatory and inhibitory neurotransmitters to have an appropriate response (i.e., excitatory: brain activity; inhibitory: sleep). An excitatory signal without the appropriate counter inhibition can result in a pain response. Many neurotransmitters are involved in the transmission of pain signals, including excitatory amino acids (e.g., glutamate and aspartate), neurotrophins (e.g., brain-derived neurotrophic factor [BDNF]), and peptides (e.g., substance P, neurokinin A, and calcitonin gene–related peptide [CGRP]); however, the main neurotransmitters are glutamate and substance P (Dissanayake & Dissanayake, 2015; Gatchell et al., 2016). Glutamate acts by transmitting a pain signal by binding to A-delta fibres that transmit the signal to the dorsal horn of the spinal cord. The rapid transmission of acute pain, rising from mechanical or thermal stimuli, usually involves glutamate. In the brain, glutamate's role is highly complex; it can activate pronociceptive (increase pain) receptors in the thalamus and trigeminal nucleus (Gatchell et al., 2016). However, in other areas of the brain, namely the periaqueductal grey and ventrolateral medulla, it can be antinociceptive (decrease pain) (Gatchell et al., 2016). One such pronociceptive receptor that glutamate acts on is *N*-methyl-D-aspartate (NMDA) (Stanos et al., 2016). In normal transmission of healthy neurotransmitter signals, the dorsal horn's sodium channels are only opened by glutamate and do not act on NMDA receptors as they are blocked by magnesium (Stanos et al., 2016). If the sodium channels are depolarized for a prolonged period of time, such as the case in chronic pain, magnesium is then inhibited through a change in the voltage-dependent magnesium receptors. This creates an environment where the dorsal horn is primed to evoke a pain signal with lower threshold. Thus, some pain treatments focus on the blockage of NMDA. Substance P is a more ubiquitous neurotransmitter present on many cytoplasmic and nuclear membranes of many types of cells. It main role is to regulate smooth muscle contractility, epithelial ion transport, vascular permeability, and immune function in the gastrointestinal tract (Gatchell et al., 2016). The secretion of substance P is from nerve and inflammatory cells which subsequently bind to neurokinin-1 (NK-1R) receptors that are located on the C-fibre nociceptor neurons (Xiao et al., 2016). With substance P, the transmission of the pain signal via the dorsal horn of the spinal cord is primarily through its binding with C-fibre nociceptors. It is thought that those who have a high **pain tolerance** appear to be lacking substance P–containing fibres in the dorsal horn area.

Two main pathways carry the pain signal to the brain: the spinothalamic (terminates in thalamus) and spinoreticular (terminates in thalamus and hypothalamus) tracts. The localization of pain is largely controlled by the spinothalamic tract which involves afferent neurons that ascend the spinal cord, utilizing the contralateral spinothalamic tract, to the nuclei within the thalamus. The signals sent through the spinothalamic tract send a signal to the somatosensory cortex and periaqueductal grey matter. This process is involved in the sensory-discriminative, autonomic, and affective aspects of pain. The spinoreticular tract, considered to be an alternate pain pathway to the brain, is important in the emotional aspect of pain. It is considered a more primal response to pain. In the case of pain signals utilizing the spinoreticular tract, it ascends the contralateral cord to reach the brain stem reticular formation and the thalamus and hypothalamus, and terminates at the cortex (Steeds, 2016).

Modulation

The modulation of pain is the body's innate ability to activate inhibitory or excitatory mechanisms and pathways to affect the pain sensation (Dissanayake & Dissanayake, 2015). Fortunately for humans, after the activation of nociceptive pain, the majority of the mechanisms are inhibitory in nature and look to alleviate pain. For example, gamma-aminobutyric acid (GABA) is considered an inhibitory interneuron in the dorsal horn that modulates the transmission of pain. However, if there is injury and/or neuronal damage, the "GABAergic" effect is decreased and counterproductive excitatory amino acids are released, causing a hyperactivation of the NMDA receptors and increasing pain.

Descending pathways come from the cortex to modulate pain transmission at the dorsal horn of the spinal cord. One such descending pathway is called the noradrenergic pathway, of which noradrenaline and serotonin are key neurotransmitters (Stanos et al., 2016). Activation of the noradrenergic pathway results in the decrease of substance P release, hyperpolarizing the sensory afferents (thus preventing more activation) and depolarizing the GABAergic neurons to inhibit pain transmission (Dissanayake & Dissanayake, 2015). In the same pathway, descending serotonergic (5-HT) pathway has both an inhibitory and excitatory effect on pain transmission.

Opioid receptors are an important system in the inhibition of pain with receptors widely distributed in peripheral nerves, spinal cord, and the brain (Benyhe, Zádor, & Ötvös, 2015). There are three main classes of receptors—mu, delta, and kappa—which are activated by endogenous opioid peptides (**enkephalins**, **endorphins**, and dynorphins) and exogenous opioids (Befort, 2015). Morphine is the most commonly used exogenous opioid receptor analgesic drug to modulate pain. Its use reduces the perception of pain by increasing the threshold of noxious stimuli. Generally, mu and delta **agonists** have an analgesic effect and activate reward centres in the brain, whereas kappa receptor activation results in a dysphoric state (Benyhe et al., 2015). Activation of the **opioid** receptors also influences cardiovascular regulation, hormone secretion, immune function, thermoregulation, respiratory function, and gastrointestinal motility, memory, and locomotive activity (Benyhe et al., 2015). From a nursing perspective, the decrease in activity in the respiratory centres, which leads to a hypercapnia, is of particular concern when exogenous opioids are administered.

The cannabinoid system, comprised of lipid neuromodulators called endocannabinoids, has receptors in the CNS and the periphery. Although research around exogenous agonist of cannabinoid receptors is considered to be in its infancy, a growing body of evidence shows that the use of tetrahydrocannabinol (THC)/cannabidiol (CBD) can decrease pain and improve anxiety related to pain (Ibsen, Connor, & Glass, 2017). Cannabinoids (from endogenous or exogenous sources) target CB1 receptors found in the periaqueductal gray, nucleus raphe magnus, dorsal horn, and the periphery (Dissanayake & Dissanayake, 2015).

Perception

Studies involving brain imaging have concluded that the anterior cingulate cortex (ACC) is activated and is an important player in the processing of pain. In the presence of noxious stimuli, the ACC becomes active to process pain but does not seem to alter one's response in terms of behaviours or emotions (Gatchell et al., 2016). The primary somatosensory cortex is thought to be a key player in the sensory aspect of pain, which includes the localization and discrimination of pain intensity (Fig. 16-2) (Steeds, 2016). Beyond the sensation, it also communicates with the motor cortex, which governs the physical and more primitive responses to pain. We are becoming more aware

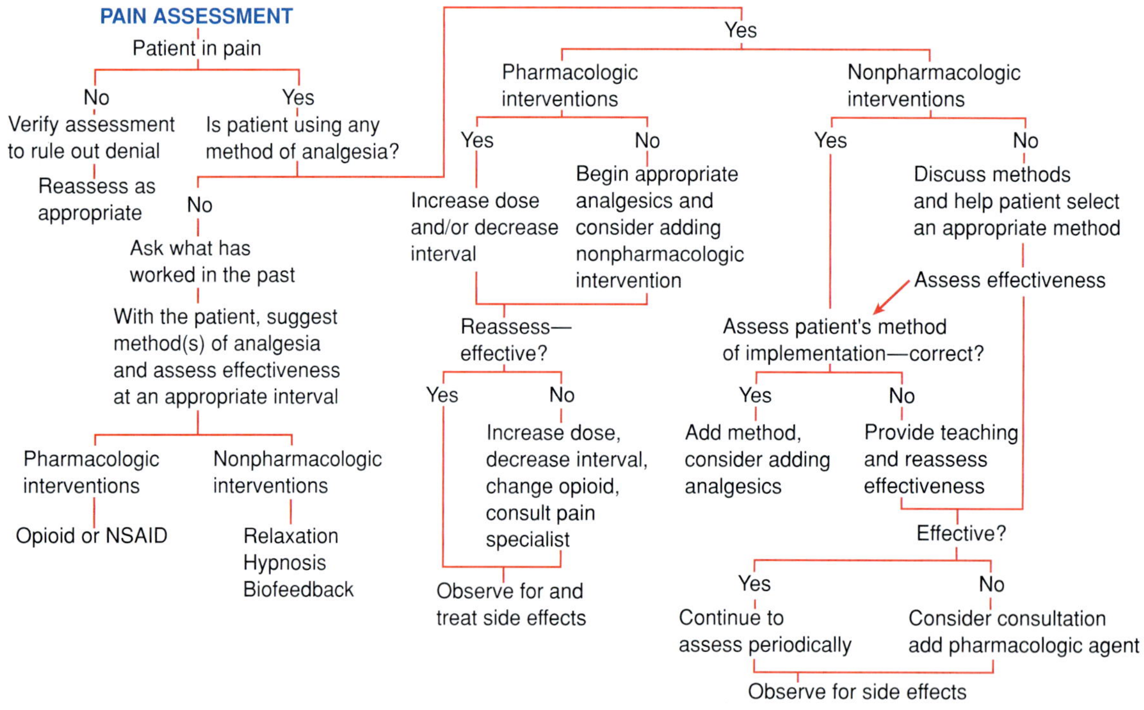

FIGURE 16-2. Examples of pain intensity scales.

that the amygdala, a powerful centre for emotional interpretation and response to input (including pain), is activated by nociceptive pain (Thompson & Neugebauer, 2017). Amygdala activation can drive anxiety and depression type responses to pain. The effects of pain on the brain can cause a "rewiring" of circuits involved in perception of pain and emotional interpretation of pain. Pain scientists agree that this phenomenon in pain is related to pain-activated neuroplasticity of the brain (the concept of rewiring of the brain). Neuroplasticity has a negative connotation when the brain is remodelled to communicate pain. However, neuroplasticity has many positive uses in pain treatments, whereby the brain is rewired positively through cognitive behavioural interventions. This is a bourgeoning field of study in pain neuroscience and psychology.

Neuropathic Pain

Neuropathic pain is pain or abnormal sensations that are caused by a primary lesion or dysfunction of the nervous system (Seth & de Gray, 2016). It affects up to 6% of people, an estimated 2 million Canadians (Kim & Mukovozov, 2017). In essence, neuropathic pain is a significant negative and lasting alteration of the perception of an initial nociceptive signal (Fig. 16-1). The brain and peripheral nervous system reorganize to communicate a disproportionately greater pain sensation whether there is a pain generator or not. Patients with neuropathic pain present with a hyperactive peripheral and/or CNS. To better explain the neurobiologic mechanism of neuropathic pain, it has been theorized that the initial nerve injury can be traumatic or nontraumatic. A traumatic peripheral nerve injury can be the result of a crush, transection, or ligation injury to a nerve, for example, whereas a nontraumatic cause is seen with the application of a neurotoxic substances or metabolic/cellular-mediated nerve damage (West, Bannister, Dickenson, et al., 2015).

Neuropathic pain is a clinical diagnosis that is characterized by dysesthesias (unpleasant sensation), hyperalgesia (disproportionate reaction to pain stimuli), and **allodynia** (pain with an otherwise nonnoxious stimuli). Unlike nociceptive pain, neuropathic pain does not serve a useful purpose (i.e., warning of noxious stimuli) and may be present despite an absence of tissue damage or inflammation.

Central Mechanism of Neuropathic Pain

When a peripheral nerve is stimulated to communicate pain, for reasons that are unclear, it can lead to a negative neuroplastic change in the brain and the spinal cord. There is a downregulation of the pain-relieving descending inhibitory noradrenergic and serotonergic pathways. Repetitive C-fibre activation by noxious stimuli can alter the dorsal horn response with prolonged activation. Local pain inhibition is also reduced within the dorsal horn with evidence of decreased GABA (inhibitory neurotransmitter) secretion. There are neurochemical changes that are mediated by an increase of pain-signalling substances, such as NMDA, neurokinins, and nitric oxide (West et al., 2015). Also, as part of the structural changes that are sometimes spurred on by injury, C-fibre termination in the dorsal horn's substantia gelatinosa (lamina II) is degenerated, and the A-beta fibres involved in normal sensation (and usually only located in laminae III and IV) begin to develop into lamina II, which is central to communicating pain to the brain. This explains why those who have neuropathic pain also have allodynia. Lastly, there is evidence of cortical rewiring and reorganization in the primary somatosensory and motor cortices. For example, some patients with limb amputation may develop phantom pain despite clearly having no afferent input to the somatosensory cortex. In such cases, a rewiring of afferent pathways in the somatosensory cortex results in expanded distribution of the termination of an input signal and recruits uninvolved cortical areas to communicate pain. These cortical changes cause a response in which stimulation of an unrelated area of the body (i.e., touching the face) activates **phantom limb pain** (i.e., in an amputated hand). Some patients with central **sensitization** demonstrate a global pain response to most forms of nonnoxious stimuli (i.e., touch or cold). Extensive rewiring (negative neuroplasticity) may exist in patients with central sensitization.

Peripheral Mechanism of Neuropathic Pain

After an initial traumatic or nontraumatic insult to a peripheral nerve, it will try to repair itself. Some nerves do not heal to their original form, and spontaneous electrical activity can be seen from altered distribution and expression of sodium channels. As a result, ectopic impulses are seen at the dorsal horn in the spine. These nerves are then primed to have a lower threshold for firing, an increased response to noxious stimuli, and can fire with nonnoxious stimuli. Patients can present with a specific area of pain related to a dermatomal or peripheral nerve distribution. For example, peripheral neuropathy is commonly seen in some patients with diabetes who develop peripheral neuropathic pain (usually to their lower limbs) as a result of repeated trauma to nerves from hyperglycemia. A dermatomal presentation of neuropathic pain is seen in those who have postherpetic neuralgia, a condition in which a dormant varicella-zoster virus is awakened in the dorsal ganglion of the spine and causes persistent pain at the specific spinal level of the insult.

Gate Control Theory

The classic gate control theory of pain, described by Melzack and Wall in 1975, was the first to clearly articulate the existence of a pain-modulating system (Melzack, 1996). This theory proposed that stimulation of the skin evokes nervous impulses that are then transmitted by three systems located in the spinal cord. The substantia gelatinosa in the dorsal horn, the dorsal column fibres, and the central transmission cells act to influence nociceptive impulses. The noxious impulses are influenced by a "gating mechanism." Stimulation of the large-diameter fibres inhibits the transmission of pain, thus "closing the gate." Conversely, when smaller fibres are stimulated, the gate is opened. The gating mechanism is influenced by nerve impulses that descend from the brain. This theory proposes a specialized system of large-diameter fibres that activate selective cognitive processes via the modulating properties of the spinal gate. Figure 16-3 shows a schematic representation of a gate control system and nociceptive pathways.

The gate control theory was the first theory to suggest that psychological factors play a role in the perception of pain. The gate control theory guided research toward identifying cognitive behavioural approaches to pain management.

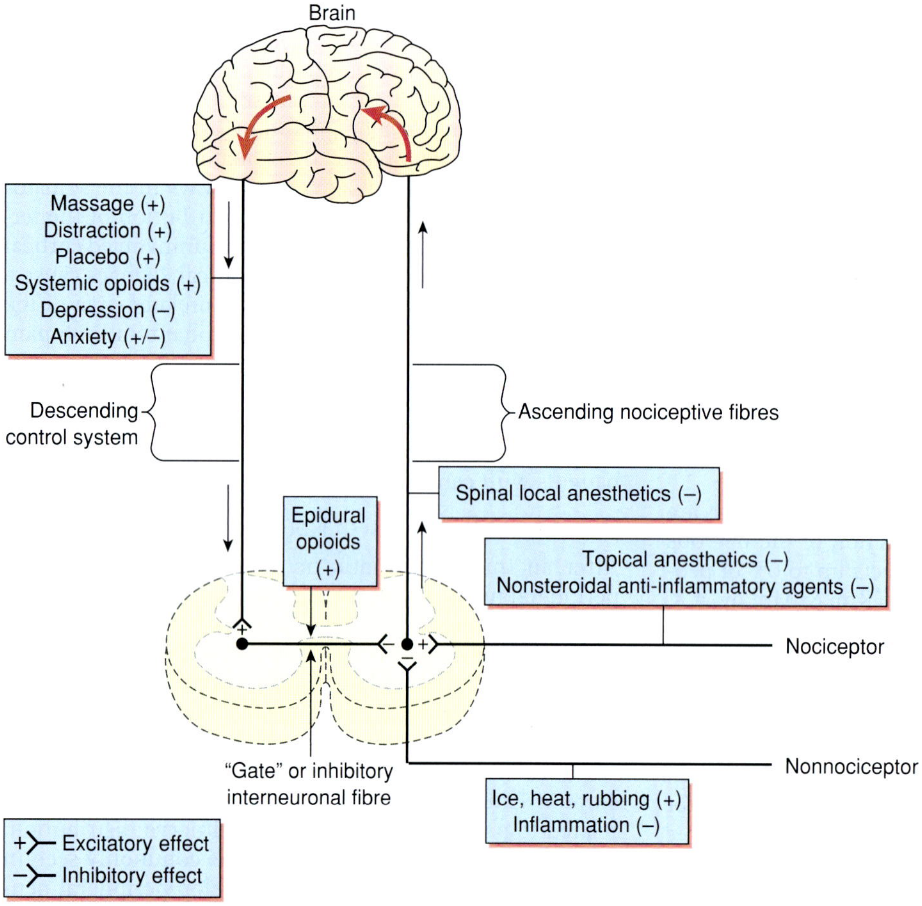

FIGURE 16-3. A schematic representation of the gate control system and aspects of the nociceptive system. The nervous system is made up of stimulatory and inhibitory fibres. For example, stimulation of the nociceptor results in the transmission of an impulse that will be interpreted as pain. When it is stimulated, it will stimulate transmission at the next fibre junction (represented as +>–). The interneuronal fibre is an inhibitory neuron (–>–). When it is stimulated, it, in turn, inhibits or shuts off transmission at the next junction. So a placebo has a (+) stimulatory effect on the descending control system, which has a stimulatory effect (+) on the interneuronal fibre, which has an inhibitory effect (–) on the ascending control system. A topical anesthetic has an inhibitory effect (–) on nerve transmission at the nociceptor level, and a spinal anesthetic has the same impact (–) on the ascending nociceptive fibres (Fig. 16-1).

Therefore, this theory helps explain how interventions such as distraction and music therapy relieve pain (Chart 16-3).

Melzack (1996) extended the gate control theory after studying phantom limb pain. He proposed that a large, widespread network of neurons exists that consists of loops between the thalamus and cortex and between the cortex and the limbic system. Melzack labelled this network the neuromatrix. As information is processed in the neuromatrix, a characteristic pattern emerges. This pattern, referred to as the neurosignature, is a continuous outflow from the neuromatrix. Melzack (1996) theorized that, in the absence of modulating inputs from the missing limb, the active neuromatrix produces a neurosignature pattern that is perceived as pain. The neuromatrix theory highlights the role of the brain in sustaining the experience of pain.

Effects of Pain

Pain has significant economic and social burdens. It is estimated that the cost of pain to the Canadian economy is between $50 and $60 billion dollars (Canadian Pain Society, 2014). Moreover, pain not only affects individual patients (physically and emotionally), but it also affects patients' family and social circles (Dueñas, Ojeda, Salazar, et al., 2016). The prevalence of chronic pain in Canada has reached nearly 20% of the population, and it has been suggested that it is a public health crisis (Schopflocher et al., 2011). The emotional impact of pain in Canada, where there is a perceived negative impact of one's pain on mood, is noted to be 63% of those Canadians suffering from pain (GSK, 2017). Thus it is important that nurses view the assessment and management of pain as critical.

Poorly managed pain (including procedural pain) can have lasting negative effects that can be physical and/or psychological. Inevitably, the stress response is activated, resulting in widespread negative effect on the endocrine, immunologic, and inflammatory systems. For example, nurses caring for already ill patients with superimposed pain may need to pay particular attention to blood pressure, respiration, and cardiac monitoring. From a psychological perspective, poorly managed pain can lead to behaviours of avoidance and catastrophization, and perhaps even a loss of hope. Loss of sleep due to pain is an important consideration when looking at how pain is affecting someone. Lack of sleep leads to poor coping and increased pain. If pain persists, some patients may experience a marked decrease of quality of life. Some may develop depression, decreased ability to work and generate income, or become socially isolated from an inability to participate in social functions. Ultimately, poorly managed acute pain may lead to poor health outcomes.

The Nurse's Role in Assessment and Care of Patients With Pain

The nurse's role in pain management involves performing pain assessment, identifying goals for pain management, providing patient teaching, performing physical care, helping to relieve pain by administering pain-relieving

NURSING RESEARCH PROFILE

Chart 16-3. Effects of Patient-Directed Music

Chlan, L. L., Weinert, C. R., Heiderscheit, A., et al. (2013). Effects of patient-directed music intervention on anxiety and sedative exposure in critically ill patients receiving mechanical ventilator support: A randomized clinical trial. *JAMA*, *309*(22), 2335–2344.

Purpose

Patients who are mechanically ventilated have little control over pharmacologic interventions to decrease anxiety in the intensive care unit (ICU). Sedating medications commonly prescribed to these patients, including analgesic agents, are associated with many adverse effects such as hypotension, bradycardia, gut dysmotility, weakness, and delirium. Interventions are needed that reduce anxiety and minimize the use of sedating medications. This study tested whether listening to self-initiated, patient-directed music (PDM) would reduce anxiety and use of sedating medication in patients who were critically ill and mechanically ventilated.

Design

A sample of 373 patients from 12 ICUs at five hospitals received acute mechanical ventilator support for respiratory failure. Patients who were alert and able to participate were randomized into three groups: (1) PDM; (2) Noise-cancelling headphones (NCHs); and (3) Usual care in the ICU (control).

A research nurse reviewed a starter set of six CDs, a CD player, and headphones with the PDM participants. Patients were prompted to use the music of their choice at least twice daily when feeling anxious or desiring relaxation. The NCH group was encouraged to wear headphones whenever they wanted to block out the noise in the ICU. All patients were assessed daily using a 100-mm visual analogue scale to report anxiety levels. Data about the frequency and doses of sedating medications were also collected.

Findings

The PDM group listened to music for a mean of 79.8 minutes each day, while the NCH group wore NCHs for a mean of 34 minutes each day. At any point in time, the PDM group had lower anxiety scores (19.5 points lower) than patients in the usual care group ($P = 0.003$). Over time, the PDM patients received less frequent and lower doses of sedating medications than the control group or the NCH group.

Nursing Implications

The PDM study was modeled after the concept of patient-controlled analgesia whereby patients report higher satisfaction when they can self-administer their analgesic. This unique approach that involved patients who were mechanically ventilated in self-management of anxiety launches a novel area of clinical research in the ICU. As clinicians seek to minimize the use of sedating medications in patients who are critically ill, PDM may be an appropriate complementary intervention by which patients can self-manage their anxiety and minimize the negative effects of sedating medications.

interventions (including both pharmacologic and nonpharmacologic approaches), assessing the effectiveness of those interventions, monitoring for adverse effects, and advocating for the patient if the prescribed intervention is ineffective in relieving pain. Figure 16-4 depicts a pathway that can be used at the time of assessment to direct clinical decisions for pain management. Specific pain management strategies are discussed later in the chapter.

The highly subjective nature of pain means that pain assessment and management present challenges for all clinicians. Assessment and management of pain requires that the nurse have a good rapport with the person in pain.

The nurse also must be aware of gender, and genetic and cultural considerations in examining the genesis of pain; understanding these factors is important to improved pain outcomes.

Research has found that women and men seem to experience pain differently. A large study on gender differences in pain has shown that, overall, pain is reported more often by women compared to men; however, the statistical difference is arguably small and may not have a clinical impact (Seth & de Gray, 2016). Also, certain conditions seem to be more prevalent in women, namely migraines, fibromyalgia, irritable bowel syndrome, and temporomandibular disorders (Della Volpe, 2016). It is hypothesized that because women secrete higher levels of sex hormones, like estrogen and progesterone, they have a greater pain experience (Della Volpe, 2016). The relationship between sex hormones and pain has been well-documented in the literature. It also appears that men may have greater mu-receptor activation when subjected to pain compared to women (Seth & de Gray, 2016).

Genetic considerations involve individualized perceptions of and responses to pain. An emerging field of study is looking at how "pain genes," of which there are over 200 known subtypes, can improve pain outcomes (Chiorean & Chiorean, 2014).

Regarding cultural considerations in assessing pain syndromes, researchers have found that family-oriented societies have a different perspective as it relates to psychological considerations of pain (Kizilhan, 2016). The experience of pain in these specific populations, as a whole, tends to require the ability to express how disease is impacting their being as whole. Canada has a wonderful diversity of people, so nurses must be able to integrate appropriate cultural considerations into their pain assessments (Chart 16-4). A holistic approach may be most appropriate when working with all populations. This approach highlights the importance of cultural competence when caring for patients and family with pain. An effective model of cross-cultural communication would be to utilize the acronym BELIEF when exploring pain with someone (Epner & Bail, 2012).

*B*elief about health (Why do you think you have pain?)
*E*xplanation (What was/were the precipitating factor(s) to your pain?)
*L*earn (Help me understand your belief around pain?)
*I*mpact (How is your pain impacting you?)
*E*mpathy (I imagine this is very difficult for you?)
*F*eelings (How does this make you feel?)

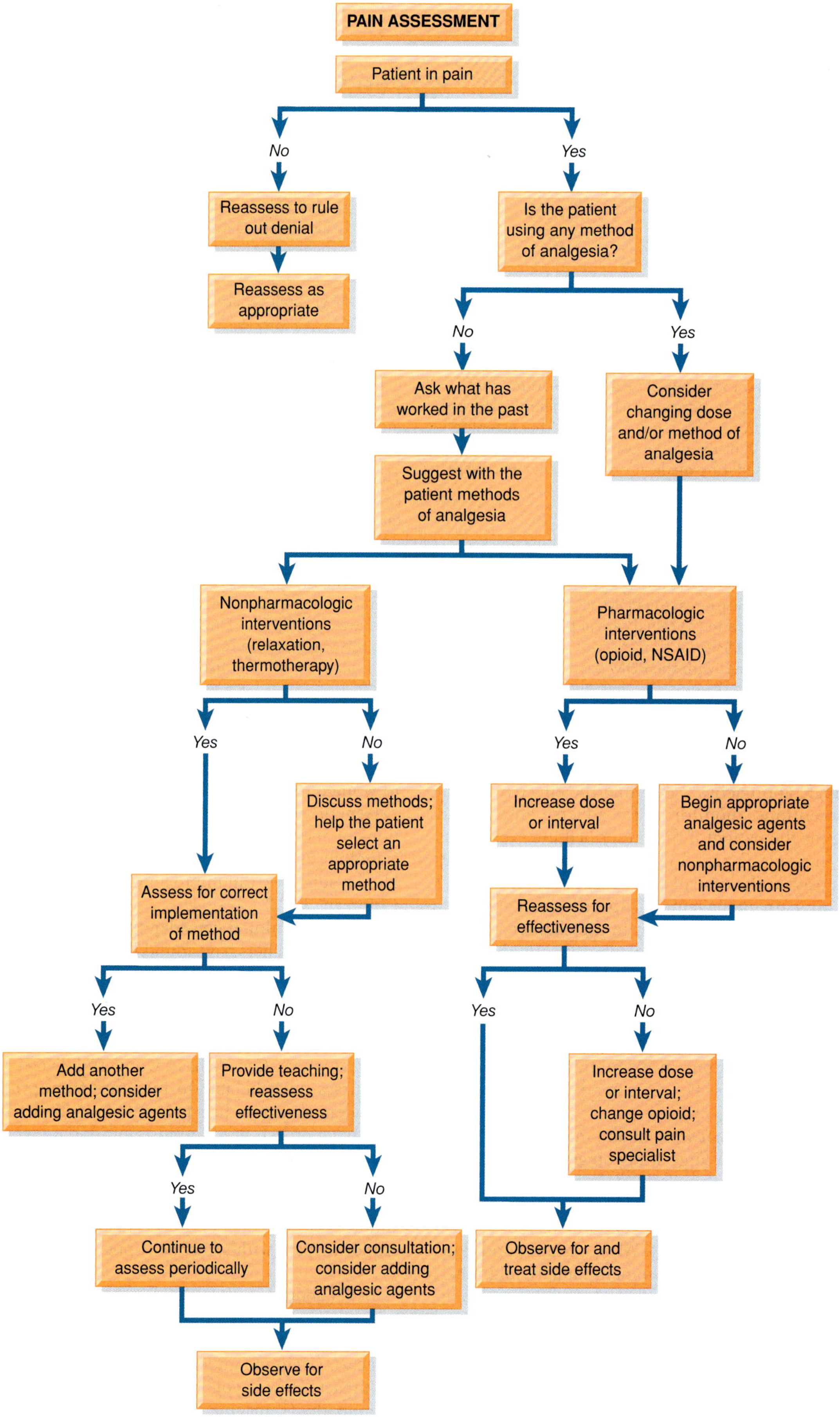

FIGURE 16-4. Pain assessment pathway. NSAID, nonsteroidal anti-inflammatory drug.

CHART 16-4

Ethics and Related Issues

Inadequate Pain Management

SITUATION

When taking over the care of ethnic minority patients at the change of shift from a particular colleague, you usually find these patients to be in a great deal of postoperative pain. Your nonsystematic observations have led you to conclude that these patients receive only a small portion of the analgesia prescribed for them. You have heard a nurse colleague state a belief that people of certain ethnic groups have "no pain tolerance" and are "just looking for drugs."

DILEMMA

Racial biases are difficult to deal with and change. To confront this nurse may not alter the behaviour but will certainly disrupt the working relationships on the unit. It would be easier to look the other way. On the other hand, you believe that the nurse is giving inadequate and unethical care to selected patients and placing them at greater risk for postoperative complications.

DISCUSSION

- What information would you need to collect before acting?
- From whom could you seek counsel?
- Are the two aspects of the dilemma equally important?

Pain Assessment

Given the very subjective nature of pain assessment, it can be challenging to assess and manage pain. The current standard of care in pain assessment involves using a variety of validated self-reported pain scales (Fig. 16-2). Inherently, as these assessments are self-reported, it can lead the health team vulnerable to inaccurate or untruthful reports of pain. That being said, although we are entitled to doubts and opinions, it is not acceptable for it to interfere with appropriate pain management. Nurses conducting pain assessment should first observe the patient as objectively as possible for pain features (grimacing, altered gait, self-soothing by pressure or rubbing, pressured speech, etc.). After careful observation, either through questioning or a chart review, the nurse next obtains a proper history of the presenting illness or concern. Some patients may warrant a complete review of systems with a targeted history related to symptoms:

- Constitutional symptoms: fever, night sweats, unintentional weight loss, fatigue, lymphadenopathy
- Dermatologic: rash, skin lesions, ecchymosis, swelling, redness, deformity
- Head, Eyes, Ears, Nose, Throat (HEENT): eye pain, visual changes, sinus pain, rhinorrhea, epistaxis, globus sensation, change in hearing, tinnitus, vertigo, otalgia, dental decay or infections, oral ulcer
- Endocrine: weight change, heat or cold intolerance, insomnia, soft tissue swelling in the neck, polyuria (i.e., diabetes), polydipsia (i.e., excessive thirst), polyphagia (i.e., excessive hunger).
- Cardiovascular: chest pain, palpitations, syncope, edema, cyanosis, claudication, orthopnea, paroxysmal nocturnal dyspnea
- Pulmonary: shortness of breath, dyspnea with exertion, cough, hemoptysis, wheeze, chest pain
- Gastrointestinal (GI): nausea, vomiting, diarrhea, melena, hematochezia, change in appetite, abdominal pain, change in bowel habits
- Genitourinary (GU): dysuria, frequency, incontinence, hematuria, dysmenorrhea, dyspareunia, pelvic pain
- Musculoskeletal: joint pain, redness or swelling, muscle pain
- Neurologic: headache, muscle weakness, paresthesia, radicular features
- Psychiatric: depression, anxiety, hallucinations, mania, suicidal ideations

NURSING ALERT

Although accepting and responding to the report of pain will undoubtedly result in administering analgesic agents to an occasional patient who does not have pain, doing so ensures that everyone who does have pain receives attentive responses. Health care professionals do not have the right to deprive any patient of appropriate assessment and treatment simply because they believe a patient is not being truthful.

Performing a Comprehensive Pain Assessment: Patient Interview

Nurses must familiarize themselves with pain assessment as it will likely be a central part of their practice. A comprehensive pain assessment should be conducted upon a patient's admission, the start of a shift, a report of new pain, a change in a patient's medical condition (Chart 16-1), or during a procedure. Nurses need to use a disciplined and systematic approach to pain assessment. Factors to consider in a complete pain assessment are the location, quality (description), quantity (intensity), timing, setting, associated symptoms, alleviating factors, aggravating factors, environmental factors, significance to the patient, patient perspective, pain management goal, and functional goal (Rhoads & Petersen, 2018).

Location: Having the patient point to the area of the body involved best determines the location of pain. Some general assessment forms include drawings of human figures, on which the patient is asked to shade in the area involved. This is especially helpful if the pain radiates (**referred pain**). The shaded figures are helpful in determining the effectiveness of treatment or change in the location of pain over time.

Intensity: Have the patient characterize the severity of the pain using a reliable and validated pain scale. Having the various scales available in the patient's native language is best.

- Numeric rating scale: Visual analogue scales (VASs) are useful in assessing the intensity of pain (Fig. 16-2). One version of the scale includes a horizontal 10-cm line with anchors (ends) indicating the extremes of pain. The patient is asked to place a mark indicating where the current pain lies on the line. The left anchor usually represents "none" or "no pain," whereas the right anchor usually represents "severe" or "worst possible pain." To score the results, a ruler is placed along the line, and the distance the patient marked from the left or low end is measured and reported in millimetres or centimetres.

- Wong-Baker FACES pain rating scale: The FACES scale consists of six cartoon faces with word descriptors, ranging from a smiling face on the left for "no pain (or hurt)" to a frowning, tearful face on the right for "worst pain (or hurt)." Patients are asked to choose the face that best reflects their pain. The faces are most commonly numbered using a 0, 2, 4, 6, 8, 10 metric, although 0 to 5 can also be used. Patients are asked to choose the face that best describes their pain. The FACES scale is used in adults and children as young as 3 years (Argoff & Viscusi, 2014). It is important to appreciate that faces scales are self-report tools; clinicians should not attempt to match a face shown on a scale to the patient's facial expression to determine pain intensity. Patients may be able to understand the tool better if it is displayed vertically with no pain as the anchor at the bottom.
- *Faces pain scale-revised (FPS-R):* The FPS-R has six faces to make it consistent with other scales using the 0 to 10 metric. The faces range from a neutral facial expression to one of intense pain and are numbered 0, 2, 4, 6, 8, and 10. As with the Wong-Baker FACES scale, patients are asked to choose the face that best reflects their pain. Faces scales have been shown to be reliable and valid measures in children as young as 4 years of age; however, the ability to optimally quantify pain (identify a number) is not acquired until approximately 8 years of age (Tsze, von Baeyer, Bulloch, et al., 2013). Some research shows that the FPS-R is preferred by both cognitively intact and impaired older and minority populations (Young, et al., 2018).
- Verbal descriptor scale (VDS): A VDS uses different words or phrases to describe the intensity of pain, such as "no pain, mild pain, moderate pain, severe pain, very severe pain, and worst possible pain." The patient is asked to select the phrase that best describes pain intensity.
- Visual analogue scale (VAS): The VAS is a horizontal (sometimes vertical) 10-cm line with word anchors at the extremes, such as "no pain" on one end and "pain as bad as it could be" or "worst possible pain" on the other end. Patients are asked to make a mark on the line to indicate intensity of pain, and the length of the mark from "no pain" is measured and recorded in centimetres or millimetres. Although often used in research, the VAS is impractical for use in daily clinical practice and rarely used in that setting.

Quality (Description): The nurse asks the patient to describe the pain in his or her own words without offering clues. For example, the nurse asks the patient to describe what the pain feels like. The nurse gives the patient sufficient time to describe the pain, and the nurse must record all words in the answer. If the patient cannot describe the quality of the pain, the nurse can suggest words such as burning, aching, throbbing, or stabbing. It is important to document the exact words used by the patient to describe the pain and which words the nurse suggested.

Onset and duration: Sometimes the cause of pain can be determined when time aspects are known. Therefore, the nurse inquires about the onset, duration, relationship between time and intensity (e.g., at what time the pain is the worst), and changes in rhythmic patterns. The nurse asks the patient if the pain began suddenly, or increased gradually. Sudden pain that rapidly reaches maximum intensity is indicative of tissue injury, and immediate intervention is necessary. Pain from ischemia gradually increases and becomes intense over a longer time. The chronic pain of rheumatoid arthritis illustrates the usefulness of determining the relationship between time and intensity because people with rheumatoid arthritis usually report that pain is worse during the night.

Aggravating and alleviating factors: Ask the patient what aggravates and what alleviates the patient's pain.

Effect of pain on function and quality of life: The effect of pain on the ability to perform recovery activities should be regularly evaluated in the patient with acute pain. It is particularly important to ask patients with persistent pain about how pain has affected their lives, what they could do before the pain began that they can no longer do, or what they would like to do but cannot do because of the pain.

Comfort-function goal: For patients with acute pain, identify short-term functional goals and reinforce to the patient that good pain control will more likely lead to successful achievement of the goals. For example, surgical patients are told that they will be expected to ambulate or participate in physical therapy postoperatively. Patients with chronic pain can be asked to identify their unique functional or quality-of-life goals, such as being able to work or walk the dog. Success is measured by progress toward meeting those functional goals (Sullivan, 2017).

Other information: The patient's culture (Chart 16-4), past pain experiences, and pertinent medical history such as comorbidities, laboratory tests, and diagnostic studies are considered when establishing a treatment plan.

For patients who are cognitively impaired, critically ill, comatose, or palliative, special consideration and actions must be taken to properly address this population's unique pain assessment and management needs. To help nurses confidently and competently address pain in the nonverbal patient, evidence-based approaches are available to help. Firstly, the Hierarchy of Pain Assessment can be used to identify and assess pain in patients unable to verbally communicate pain. The following will further examine the Hierarchy of Pain Assessment (Booker & Haedtke, 2016):

Step 1: Determine reliability and verbal ability, and attempt self-report. Some patients who are cognitively impaired may still be able to adequately self-report their pain, thus they should be given an opportunity to do so. If there are concerns about the reliability or mental status of a patient, the nurse can perform a cognitive test (Montreal Cognitive Assessment [MoCA] or Brief Interview for Mental Status [BIMS]). Even a patient who is intubated but not heavily sedated may be able to communicate pain by squeezing a hand or blinking eyes.

Step 2: Identify potential causes or sources of pain (i.e., pathologic, procedural, injury, pharmacologic).

Step 3: Observe for indicators or behaviours suggestive of pain. This is where a validated assessment tool is useful. Specialized assessment tools have been developed to improve clinical decision making with regard to pain; however, these observational assessment tools are not considered equivalent to self-reported validated pain scales (Fig. 16-2). The following are examples of validated tools that are appropriate for different patient populations unable to self-report their pain (Erdek & Gordon, 2014).

- The Faces, Legs, Activity, Cry, and Consolability (FLACC) scale: indicated for use in young children. Scores are assigned after assessing *F*acial expression, *L*eg movement, *A*ctivity, *C*rying, and *C*onsolability, with each of these five categories assigned scores from 0 to 2, yielding a total composite score of 0 to 10. Scores of "0" are interpreted as reflecting that the patient is relaxed and comfortable, scores of "1" to "3" are interpreted as consistent with mild discomfort, scores from "4" to "6" are considered consistent with moderate pain, and scores from "7" to "10" are considered consistent with severe discomfort or pain.
- The Critical-Care Pain Observation Tool (CPOT): indicated for use in patients in critical care units who cannot self-report pain, whether or not they may be intubated. It is also patterned after the FLACC. It has been found that, compared to the FLACC, in the critical care population the CPOT resulted in a more consistent pain assessment (Erdek & Gordon, 2014).
- The *P*ain *A*ssessment *IN* *A*dvanced *D*ementia (PAINAD): indicated for use in adults with advanced dementia who are not able to verbalize their needs. It is comprised of five categories of behaviours to be assessed: breathing, negative vocalization, facial expression, body language, and consolability (Carezzato, Valera, Assis, et al., 2014).

Step 4: Discuss changes in behaviours, mood, and daily functional patterns that may indicate pain with all relevant health care members, family, or friends who may be able to provide further insight into the patient's pain condition. For example, it is important to involve those who know the patient best, whether it is a family member or a nursing aid, and are well placed to provide additional details and corroboration of pain.

Step 5: If pain is suspected, initiate an analgesic trial after comfort and nonpharmacologic measures have been tried. Medication management will be discussed later in this chapter.

Step 6: Develop a multimodal pain treatment plan with measurable comfort-function-mood-behaviour goals. If the analgesic trial did in fact relieve pain, a collaborative approach to a treatment plan should be established, ideally with measurable goals for improved comfort, function, mood, and behaviours.

Reassessing Pain and Setting Goals

Special nursing consideration must be paid to regularly reassessing pain to evaluate the effectiveness of any given treatment, as well as its documentation. The minimum standard suggests that pain should be reassessed with each new report of pain and before and after any pain medication administration. Certainly, the clinical setting and institutional policies will also inform the frequency of a pain assessment, but critical thinking should be used as well. For example, in the postanesthesia care unit (PACU) or emergency room setting, reassessment may be necessary as often as every few minutes, whereas a stable patient in a long-term care setting may only require a pain reassessment every 4 to 8 hours.

In reassessing pain it is important to revisit the patient's goals, in terms of pain reduction and functional outcomes. Motivational interviewing techniques can be used to encourage and empower patients to cocreate a plan with you. To clarify, motivational interviewing techniques are a way of asking questions to cause healthy reflection by a patient, for example, what is something you would like to do but feel like you can't because of your current pain? How do you think we could address your barriers? Some patients may have unrealistic goals for their pain burden reduction; through skilful questioning, nurses can be instrumental in shifting the focus to positive functional outcomes despite a degree of persistent pain in those with chronic symptoms. Goals around sleep, nutrition, pacing, catastrophization, positive social contact, work–life balance, exercise, and play (for children) are also central to having a holistic approach to pain management. The nurse can be a true champion in the area of pain management, having the time and expertise to "quarterback" many core pain management interventions.

Pain Management

Pain can be seen on a continuum where optimal pain relief is multifaceted and relies on providing safe and effective analgesia (Mackey, 2015). Achieving adequate pain control is the responsibility of every member of the health care team. Nursing staff must pay particular attention to assess and address the management of pain interventions whenever patient care is transferred to another nurse or to another unit, or even into the community. Certainly an optimal and safe titration of analgesic agents coupled with adequate reassessments during the course of care is very important, but ultimately the pain management strategy should be to facilitate the patient's functional goals and outcomes, rather than restrict them. For example, narcotics can completely eliminate pain but the patient's function may be largely halted due to the cognitive decline that is seen with high-dose opioid use. This can be where the art of nursing shines. Establishing a trusting nurse–patient relationship can facilitate pain education, and thus ultimately better managed pain. Of course, nurses must believe the patients self-reported pain to begin this trusting relationship. With trust comes the opportunity to educate patients about how pain works, and the pharmacologic and nonpharmacologic strategies currently used to improve pain and functional outcomes. The rest of this chapter will examine pharmacologic and nonpharmacologic strategies to manage pain.

> **NURSING ALERT**
>
> **Pain control is the responsibility of every member of the health care team and begins with systematic assessment and initial analgesic titration, followed by reassessment and analgesic administration throughout the course of care to safely achieve a level of pain that allows patients to meet their functional goals with relative ease.**

Pharmacologic Management of Pain: Multimodal Analgesia

As discussed throughout this chapter, pain is a complex phenomenon involving multiple underlying mechanisms and requires more than one analgesic agent to manage it safely and effectively. The recommended approach for the treatment of all types of pain in all age groups is called ***multimodal analgesia*** (Wick, Grant, & Wu, 2017). A multimodal regimen combines drugs with different underlying mechanisms, which allows lower doses of each of the drugs in the treatment plan, reducing the potential for each to produce adverse effects. Furthermore, multimodal analgesia can result in comparable or greater pain relief than can be achieved with any single analgesic agent (Zhou, Fan, Zhong, et al., 2017).

Timing of Administration

To help patients meet their functional goals and maintain a good quality of life, the nurse uses certain techniques for analgesic administration to ensure that pain is adequately managed. For example, rather than "chasing pain" with pro re nata, or as needed (PRN) administration of analgesic medications, it may be beneficial to schedule around-the-clock (ATC) administration to maintain a stable analgesic blood level. The preventative approach utilized with ATC administration can reduce the "peaks and valleys" of pain relief seen with short-acting analgesics, which can also lead to maladaptive behaviours, such as clock watching (Argoff & Viscusi, 2014). Prevention, with ATC dosing, also reduces a patient's risk of developing undesired side effects (i.e., constipation, pruritus, etc.) and leads to a decreased incidence of substance **dependence** and abuse. When pre-procedure analgesics are needed, or when **breakthrough pain** (pain that surpasses the effectiveness of the ATC dosing) is felt, PRN short-acting medications are deemed most appropriate. A course of short-acting analgesics is necessary at first to reduce the risk of extended adverse reactions.

Routes of Administration

The route selected for administration of an analgesic agent depends on the condition of the individual patient and the desired effect of the medication. Analgesic agents can be administered by parenteral, oral, rectal, transdermal (TD), transmucosal, intraspinal, or epidural routes. Each method of administration has advantages and disadvantages. The route chosen should be based on patient need.

Parenteral Route

Parenteral administration (intramuscular [IM], IV, or subcutaneous) of the analgesic medication produces effects more rapidly than oral administration, but these effects are of shorter duration. Parenteral administration may be indicated if the patient is not permitted oral intake or is vomiting. Medication administered by the IM route enters the bloodstream and is metabolized more slowly than medication given IV. The rate of absorption may be erratic, depending on the site selected and the amount of body fat.

The IV route is the preferred parenteral route in most acute care situations because it is much more comfortable for patients. In addition, peak serum levels and pain relief occur more rapidly and more reliably. Because most analgesic medications peak rapidly (usually within minutes) and are metabolized quickly, an appropriate IV dose is smaller and is prescribed at shorter intervals than an IM dose. Many commonly prescribed analgesics, including opioids, may be administered by IV push or slow push (e.g., over a 5- to 10-minute period) or by continuous infusion with a pump. Continuous infusion provides a steady level of analgesia and is indicated when pain occurs over a 24-hour period, such as after surgery for the first day or two, or in a patient with prolonged pain who cannot tolerate medication by other routes. The dose of analgesic agent is calculated carefully to relieve pain without producing respiratory depression and other side effects.

The subcutaneous route for infusion of opioid analgesic agents is used for patients with severe pain such as cancer pain. In addition, it is particularly useful for patients with limited IV access who cannot take oral medications and for patients who are managing their pain at home. The subcutaneous route is often an effective and convenient way to manage pain, but the dose of opioid that can be infused through this route is limited because of the small volume that can be administered at one time into the subcutaneous tissue.

Oral Route

Oral administration is preferred over parenteral administration if the patient can tolerate medication by mouth, because it is easy and noninvasive. Severe pain can be relieved with oral opioids if the doses are high enough (see Table 16-1). In patients who are terminally ill with prolonged pain, doses may be gradually increased as the disease progresses and causes more pain or as the patient develops a **tolerance** to the medication. If higher doses are increased gradually, they usually provide additional pain relief without producing respiratory depression or sedation. If the route of administration is changed from a parenteral route to the oral route at a dose that is not equivalent in strength (equianalgesic), the smaller oral dose may result in a withdrawal reaction and recurrence of pain.

Rectal Route

The rectal route may be indicated in patients who cannot take medications by any other route. For example, this route may be used for palliative purposes in end-of-life care. The rectum allows passive diffusion of medications and absorption into the systemic circulation. This route of administration can be less expensive and does not involve the skill and expertise required of the parenteral route of administration. Drawbacks are that drug absorption can be unreliable and depends on many factors including rectal tissue health and administrator technique. Some patients may be resistant to or fearful of rectal administration. The rectal route is contraindicated in patients who are neutropenic or thrombocytopenic because of potential rectal bleeding. Diarrhea, perianal abscess or fistula, and abdominoperineal resection are also relative contraindications (MacIntyre & Schug, 2015).

Transdermal Route

The TD route is used to achieve a consistent opioid serum level through absorption of the medication via the skin. It is most often used in the home or hospice care settings for patients with cancer. TD opioids include fentanyl

TABLE 16-1 Selected Opioid Analgesic Agents Commonly Used for Moderate and Severe Pain in Adults

Name	Starting Dose (milligrams)		Comments	Precautions and Contraindications
	Moderate Pain	*Severe Pain*		
Morphine	—	30–60 (oral) 10 (parenteral)	Acts as an agonist at specific opioid receptors in the CNS to produce analgesia, euphoria, and sedation	Use with caution, especially in elderly patients, very ill patients, and those with respiratory impairment. Major risks include respiratory depression, apnea, circulatory depression, respiratory arrest, shock, and cardiac arrest. Obtain history of hypersensitivity to opioids. Monitor patient closely. If prescribed in correct dose, oral preparations (MS Contin) are effective in treating moderate and severe pain
Codeine	15–30 (oral)	60 (oral) up to 360/24 hours	Acts as an agonist at specific opioid receptors in the CNS to produce analgesia, euphoria, and sedation. Is also an antitussive. 10% of people lack the enzyme needed to make codeine active. Codeine may cause more nausea and constipation per unit of analgesia than other mu-agonist opioids	Many preparations of codeine and the other opioids in this table are combinations with nonopioid analgesic agents. Caution must be used in patients with impaired ventilation, bronchial asthma, increased intracranial pressure, or impaired liver function and in elderly and very ill patients
Oxycodone (OxyContin)	5 (oral)	10–20 (oral)	Acts as an agonist at specific opioid receptors in the CNS to produce analgesia, euphoria, and sedation	Caution must be used in patients with impaired ventilation, bronchial asthma, increased intracranial pressure, or impaired liver function and in elderly and very ill patients
Meperidine (Demerol)	50 (oral)	300 (oral) 75 (parenteral)	Acts as an agonist at specific opioid receptors in the CNS to produce analgesia, euphoria, and sedation. Shorter acting than morphine. Meperidine is biotransformed to normeperidine, a toxic metabolite	Normeperidine, a toxic metabolic of meperidine, accumulates with repetitive dosing, causing CNS excitation. High risk for seizures. Should be avoided in patients with impaired renal function who are receiving MAO inhibitors. Is irritating to tissues with repeated intramuscular injections. Chronic use should be avoided. Should not be used for more than 1 or 2 days
Propoxyphene (Darvon)	65–130 (oral)	—	Weak analgesic; acts as an agonist at specific opioid receptors in the CNS to produce analgesia, euphoria, and sedation. Many preparations include nonopioid analgesic agents; biotransformed to potentially toxic metabolite (norpropoxyphene)	Accumulation of propoxyphene and toxic metabolites occurs with repetitive dosing. Overdose is complicated by seizures. Propoxyphene is not recommended for older adults or patients with renal impairment
Hydrocodone (Vicodin)	5–10 (oral)	—	—	Most preparations are combined with nonopioid analgesic agents
Tramadol (Ultram)	50–100 (oral)	—	Unique mechanism; analgesia results from the synergy of two mechanisms. Maximum dose is 400 mg/day	Most common side effects are dizziness, nausea, constipation, and somnolence. Lowers seizure threshold

CNS, central nervous system; MAO, monoamine oxidase.

Adapted from American Pain Society. (2003). *Principles of analgesic use in the treatment of acute pain and cancer pain* (5th ed.). Glenview, IL: American Pain Society; and Karch, A. M. (2012). *Lippincott's nursing drug guide*. Philadelphia, PA: Wolters Kluwer Health/Lippincott Williams & Wilkins.

(Duragesic) and buprenorphine (Suboxone), which are marketed as patches consisting of a reservoir containing the medication and a porous membrane.

Fentanyl was the first commercially available TD opioid. When the fentanyl TD system is first applied to the skin, fentanyl, which is fat soluble, binds to the skin and fat layers. Then it is slowly and systemically absorbed. Therefore, there is a delay in effect while the dermal layer is being saturated. A drug reservoir actually forms in the upper layer of skin. This results in a slowly rising serum level and a slow tapering of the serum level once the patch is removed (see Fig. 16-5).

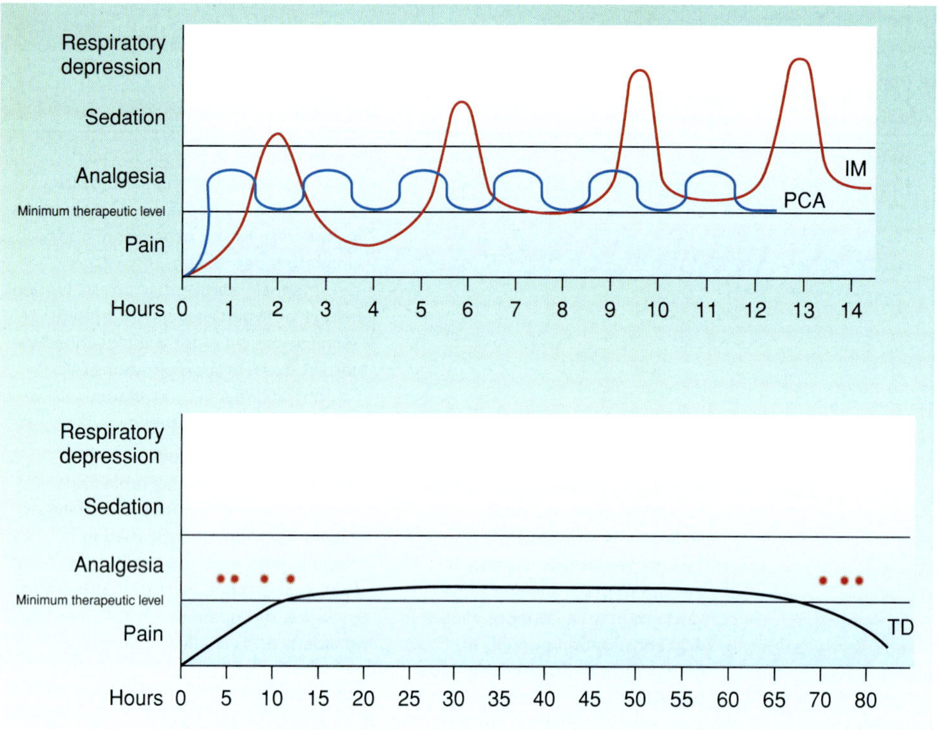

FIGURE 16-5. Relationship of mode of delivery of analgesia to serum analgesic level. **Top**: intramuscular (IM) and intravenous patient-controlled analgesia (PCA). **Bottom**: transdermal (TD) and transmucosal (*) delivery.

Because it takes 12 to 24 hours for the fentanyl levels to gradually increase after application of the first patch, the last dose of sustained-release morphine should be administered at the same time the first patch is applied (Templeman, 2017). TD fentanyl is associated with slightly less constipation than oral opioids. Absorption is increased in febrile patients. A heating pad should never be applied to the area where the patch is applied. TD fentanyl is much more expensive than sustained-release morphine, but it is less costly than methods that deliver parenteral opioids.

Buprenorphine is available in three strengths. It has many of the same advantages as fentanyl and has been shown in limited clinical studies to be associated with a high level of patient adherence and improved quality of life (Bandawar, Kandasamy, Chand, et al., 2015).

Once it is determined that switching from other routes of morphine administration to a TD system is appropriate, the correct dosage or strength for the patch must be calculated. If the patient uses an opioid other than morphine, conversion to milligrams of oral morphine is the first step. After determining how many milligrams of morphine (or morphine equivalents) the patient has been using over 24 hours, an initial dose of TD fentanyl or buprenorphine is calculated (Smith & Pappagallo, 2012). For example, if the patient is using less than 30 mg of morphine or its equivalent, then the lowest dose of buprenorphine TD patch (5µg/hour) should be used; however, a patient requiring 30 to 80 mg of morphine or its equivalent can start at a mid-level dose of buprenorphine (10µg/hour) (Smith & Pappagallo, 2012). Patients switched from morphine to TD patches of either fentanyl or buprenorphine should be assessed not only for pain and potential side effects but also for dependence, reflected by withdrawal symptoms, which may consist of shivering, a feeling of coldness, sweating, headache, and paresthesia (Lalanne, Nicot, Lang, et al., 2016). Patients may require short-acting opioids for breakthrough pain before the systemic opioid delivered through the TD system reaches a therapeutic level.

NURSING ALERT

Conversion tables available for the TD systems should be used only to establish the initial dose of TD fentanyl or buprenorphine when patients switch from oral morphine to the TD route of delivery (and not vice versa). If these tables are inappropriately used to determine the dosages of oral morphine for patients who have been receiving TD fentanyl or buprenorphine, many patients will not achieve satisfactory analgesia and will require an increase in their opioid dose to treat breakthrough pain.

NURSING ALERT

If the conversion table or equation is used incorrectly to calculate a morphine dose, there is a risk of overdose. If a patient requires a change from TD fentanyl or buprenorphine back to oral or IV morphine (as in the case of surgery), the patch should be removed and IV morphine administered on an as-needed basis. Before a new patch is applied, the patient should be carefully checked for any older, forgotten patches, which should be removed and discarded. Patches are replaced every 72 hours.

Transmucosal/Intranasal Route

Patients with cancer pain who are being cared for at home may be receiving continuous opioids using sustained-release morphine, hydromorphone, oxycodone, TD fentanyl or buprenorphine, or other medications. These patients often experience short episodes of severe pain (e.g., after coughing or moving), or they may experience sudden increases in their baseline pain resulting from a change in their condition. These periods, called breakthrough pain, can be well managed with an oral dose of a short-acting transmucosal opioid that has a rapid onset of action. Available transmucosal opioids are fentanyl, buprenorphine, sufentanil, and methadone.

Currently, butorphanol (Apo-Butorphanol), fentanyl (Duragesic), sufentanil (Sufenta), and morphine are the only approved transmucosal opioid analgesic agents commercially available in the form of nasal sprays. Butorphanol is a complex medication that simultaneously acts to induce or promote (agonist) and inhibit or reverse (antagonist) opioid effects. It works like an opioid agonist and an opioid **antagonist** at the same time. Butorphanol in any form cannot be combined with other opioids (e.g., for cancer breakthrough pain), because the antagonist component blocks the action of the opioids the patient is already receiving. The principal use of this agent is for brief, moderate to severe pain, such as migraine headaches.

Intranasal morphine is useful in cancer-related breakthrough pain as it otherwise has a high risk of dependence.

Intraspinal and Epidural Routes

Infusion of opioids or local anesthetic agents into the subarachnoid space (intrathecal space or spinal canal) or epidural space has been used for effective control of pain in postoperative patients and those with chronic pain unrelieved by other methods. A catheter is inserted into the subarachnoid or the epidural space at the thoracic or lumbar level for administration of opioid or anesthetic agents (Fig. 16-6). With intrathecal administration, medication infuses directly into the subarachnoid space and cerebrospinal fluid, which surrounds the spinal cord. With epidural administration, medication is deposited in the dura of the spinal canal and diffuses into the subarachnoid space. It is believed that pain relief from intraspinal administration of opioids is based on the existence of opioid receptors in the spinal cord.

Infusion of opioids and local anesthetic agents through an intrathecal or epidural catheter results in pain relief with fewer side effects, including sedation, than with systemic analgesia. Adverse effects associated with intraspinal administration include spinal headache resulting from loss of spinal fluid when the dura is punctured. This is more likely to occur in younger patients (less than 40 years of age). The dura must be punctured with the intrathecal route, and dural puncture may occur inadvertently with the epidural route. If dural puncture inadvertently occurs, spinal fluid seeps out of the spinal canal. The resultant headache is likely to be more severe with an epidural needle because it is larger than a spinal needle, and therefore more spinal fluid escapes.

Respiratory depression generally peaks 6 to 12 hours after epidural opioids are administered, but it can occur earlier or up to 24 hours after the first injection. Depending on the lipophilicity (affinity for body fat) of the opioid injected, the time frame for respiratory depression can be short or long. Morphine is hydrophilic, and the time for peak effect is longer than that of fentanyl, which is lipophilic. The patient should be monitored closely for at least 24 hours after the first injection and longer if changes in respiratory status or level of consciousness occur. Opioid antagonist agents such as naloxone (Narcan) must be available for IV use if respiratory depression occurs.

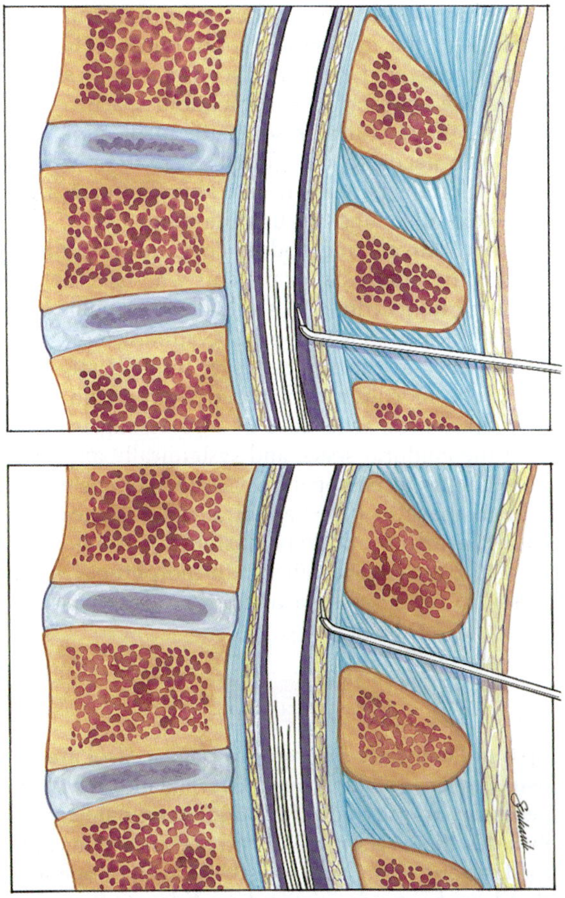

A

B

FIGURE 16-6. Placement of intraspinal catheters for administration of analgesic medications: **A.** Intrathecal route; **B.** Epidural route.

The patient is also observed for urinary retention, pruritus, nausea, vomiting, and dizziness. Precautions must be taken to avoid infection at the catheter site and catheter displacement. Only medications without preservatives are to be administered into the subarachnoid or epidural space because of the potential neurotoxic effects of preservatives.

For patients who have persistent, severe pain that fails to respond to other treatments, or who obtain pain relief only with the risk of serious side effects, medication administered by a long-term intrathecal or epidural catheter may be effective. After the physician tunnels the catheter through the subcutaneous tissue and places the inlet (or port) under the skin, the medication is injected through the skin into the inlet and catheter, which delivers the medication directly into the epidural space. It may be necessary to inject the medication several times a day to maintain an adequate level of pain relief.

For patients who require more frequent doses or continuous infusions of opioid analgesic agents to relieve pain, an implantable infusion device or pump may be used to administer the medication continuously. The medication is administered at a small, constant dose at a preset rate into the epidural or subarachnoid space. The reservoir of the infusion device stores the medication for slow release and needs to be refilled every 1 or 2 months, depending on the patient's needs. This eliminates the need for repeated injections through the skin.

Another delivery method of epidural morphine provides effective analgesia for patients who have undergone major surgical procedures. A single-dose morphine sulphate extended-release liposome may be administered into the epidural space at the lumbar level immediately prior to surgery. The morphine is released slowly from microvesicular liposomes. One dose of 5 to 15 mg is absorbed around the epidural space and systemically and provides up to 48 hours of postoperative analgesia. Side effects are similar to those of other epidural opioids (i.e., nausea, vomiting, pruritus, and hypotension); its use is contraindicated in patients with allergy to morphine, respiratory depression, severe asthma or upper airway obstruction, and circulatory shock.

NURSING ALERT

Epidural catheters inserted for pain control are usually managed by nurses. Baseline information necessary to provide safe and effective pain control includes the level or site of catheter insertion, the medications (e.g., local anesthetic agents, opioids) that have been administered, and the medications anticipated in the future. The infusion rate is increased with caution when anesthetic agents are combined with opioids. Sensory deficits can occur, and patients must be assessed frequently. An infusion with a lower concentration of anesthetic agent allows for administration of a greater concentration of opioid with a lower risk of sensory deficits.

Patient-Controlled Analgesia

Used to manage postoperative pain as well as persistent pain, **patient-controlled analgesia** (PCA) allows patients to control the administration of their own medication within predetermined safety limits. This approach can be used with oral analgesic agents as well as with continuous infusions of opioid analgesic agents by IV, subcutaneous, or epidural routes. PCA can be used in hospitals or in home settings, often in orthopedic cases. The PCA pump permits the patient to receive continuous infusions of medication (basal rates) safely and to administer extra medication (bolus doses) with episodes of increased pain or painful activities. Extra caution and nurse monitoring must be paid to those patients who are opioid naïve, especially when receiving a continuous infusion. A patient experiencing pain can administer small amounts of medication directly into his or her IV, subcutaneous, or epidural catheter by pressing a button. The pump then delivers a preset amount of medication.

A PCA pump is electronically controlled by a timing device. The timer can be programmed to prevent additional doses from being administered until a specified time period has elapsed (lock-out time) and until the first dose has had time to exert its maximal effect. Even if the patient pushes the button multiple times in rapid succession, no additional doses are released. If another dose is required at the end of the delay period, the button must be pushed again to receive the dose. Patients who are controlling their own opioid administration usually become sedated and stop pushing the button before any significant respiratory depression occurs. Nevertheless, assessment of respiratory status remains a major nursing role.

To initiate PCA or any analgesia used at home or in the hospital, it is important to avoid playing "catch-up." Pain should be brought under control before PCA starts, often by the use of an initial, larger bolus dose or loading dose or by administering repeated bolus doses of an IV opioid over short periods until the pain is relieved. Then, after pain control is achieved, the pump is programmed to deliver small doses of medication at preset intervals. The goal is to achieve a minimum therapeutic level of analgesia and to allow the patient to maintain that level by using the PCA pump. The patient is instructed not to wait until the pain is severe before pushing the button to obtain a bolus dose, beyond the basal infusion. A continuous infusion plus bolus doses may be effective with patients who have cancer and require large doses of analgesia and with postsurgical patients. Although this allows more uninterrupted sleep, the risk of sedation increases, especially when the patient has minimal or decreasing pain. It is important to clarify those, if any, who have the ability to use the "PCA-by-proxy" (Anghelescu et al., 2012). If a family member or a caregiver is authorized to do so, special training is necessary to ensure safety and effectiveness of this plan.

NURSING ALERT

Staff, family, and other visitors should be instructed to contact the nurse if they have concerns about pain control rather than pressing the PCA button for the patient.

For some patients who are candidates for PCA but unable to use the PCA equipment, the nurse or a capable family member may be authorized to manage the patient's pain using PCA equipment. This is referred to as authorized agent–controlled analgesia; guidelines are available for the safe administration of this therapy (Cooney, Czarnecki, Dunwoody, et al., 2013).

Pharmacologic Management of Pain

Agents Used to Treat Pain

There are three main groups of analgesics: (1) non-opioid analgesic agents, which include acetaminophen and nonsteroidal anti-inflammatory drugs (NSAIDs); (2) opioid analgesic agents (i.e., morphine, hydromorphone, fentanyl, codeine, etc.); and (3) **adjuvant analgesic** agents (or coanalgesic agents). Adjuvant analgesic agents have a wide variety of mechanisms of action (local anesthetic, anticonvulsants, antidepressants).

Non-opioid Analgesic Agents

Acetaminophen and NSAIDs make up this class of analgesic medications.

Indication, Administration, and Side Effects

NSAIDs are thought to decrease pain and inflammation by inhibiting cyclooxygenase (COX); more specifically, this enzyme catalyzes arachidonic acid to prostaglandin. There are two types of COX, COX-1, and COX-2, and the effects of inhibiting each are different. COX-1 is involved with mediating prostaglandin formation involved in the maintenance of physiologic functions. Two such functions include hemostasis and gut barrier integrity. COX-1 is somewhat ubiquitous in the body. Therefore, inhibiting COX-1 will result in the undesirable effects of gastric ulceration, bleeding, and renal damage. COX-2 mediates prostaglandin formation and is upregulated by exposure to cytokines and mitogens that results in symptoms of pain, inflammation, and fever. Thus, inhibition of COX-2 produces desirable effects.

Three common over-the-counter NSAIDs are aspirin, ibuprofen, and naproxen, and they inhibit both COX-1 and COX-2. Aspirin is infrequently used to treat major acute or chronic pain because it causes frequent and severe side effects, namely increased risk of bleeding due to greater antiplatelet activation. Ibuprofen and naproxen, however, are effective in relieving mild to moderate pain and have a low incidence of adverse effects. Two COX-2 inhibitors are available in Canada, meloxicam and celecoxib. The development of COX-2 inhibitors was driven by a desire to reduce the risk of bleeding that is seen with COX-1 inhibition; however, in decreasing the GI side effects, it unintendedly increased cardiovascular risk of myocardial infarctions, stroke, and heart failure due to a cardioprotective aspect of COX-2 (Bonnie, Ford, & Phillips, 2017).

Ibuprofen (Advil, Motrin), another NSAID that is typically given at doses between 200 mg to 800 mg (or 10 mg/kg/dose for children) every 6 to8 hours, blocks both COX-1 and COX-2 and is effective in relieving mild to moderate pain. It has a low incidence of adverse effects. NSAIDs are very helpful in treating arthritic diseases and may be especially powerful in treating cancer-related bone pain. They have been effectively combined with opioids to treat postoperative and other severe pain. The use of NSAIDs in combination with opioids relieves pain more effectively than opioids alone. In such cases, patients may obtain pain relief with decreased doses of opioid and with fewer side effects.

Acetaminophen, usually taken at doses between 325 mg to 1,000 mg (15 mg/kg/dose for children) every 4 hours, reduces COX-1 and COX-2 by about 50 percent (Bonnie et al., 2017). It is commonly used as an antipyretic. The mechanism of action is not fully understood, but it is thought to inhibit the synthesis of prostaglandins in the CNS, and affects nitric oxide, serotonin, opioid, and cannabinoid signalling pathways. It rarely has the GI side effects typically seen with nonspecific COX inhibition; however, if doses exceed the recommended daily maximum of 4,000 mg/day (3,000 mg/day in older adults) a similar GI risk of bleeding as with NSAIDs is seen. The biggest concern is liver toxicity, and when taken at supertherapeutic doses (above 4,000 mg/dose), acute and possibly fatal liver failure is possible (Smith & Pappagallo, 2012). Acetaminophen combined with NSAIDs or opioids has a synergistic effect and is often used in combination to improve a desired analgesic effect with lower dosing in all medications.

Opioid Analgesic Agents

The goal of administering opioids is to relieve pain and improve functional outcomes and quality of life; therefore, the route, dose, and frequency of administration are determined on an individual basis. Factors that are considered in determining the route, dose, and frequency of medication include the characteristics of the pain (e.g., its expected duration and severity), the overall status of the patient, the patient's response to analgesic medications, and the patient's report of pain. Opioids are administered by oral, IV, subcutaneous, intraspinal, intranasal, rectal, and TD routes. Although the oral route is usually preferred for opioid administration, oral opioids must be given frequently enough and in large enough doses to be effective. Opioid analgesic agents given orally may provide a more consistent serum level than those given intramuscularly.

Opioid Titration

Titration of the opioid dose is usually required at the start, with an opioid naïve patient, and throughout the course of treatment when opioids are given. Whereas patients with cancer pain most often are titrated upward over time for progressive pain, patients with acute pain, particularly postoperative pain, are eventually titrated downward as pain resolves (Busse, Craigie, Juurlink, et al., 2017). The dose and analgesic effect of mu-agonist opioids have no ceiling effect, although the dose may be limited by adverse effects. In light of the opioid epidemic, and an effort to reduce the risk of prescription opioid abuse, the Canadian Opioid Guidelines 2017 state that opioids should be restricted to no greater than 90 mg of morphine equivalents daily (MED), and the maximum prescribed dose should be restricted to 50 mg MED (Busse et al., 2017). The goal of titration is to use the smallest dose that provides satisfactory pain relief with the fewest adverse effects. The time at which the dose can be increased is determined by the onset and peak effects of the opioid and its formulation. For example, the frequency of IV opioid doses during initial titration may be as often as every 5 minutes. In contrast, 48 hours should elapse before the dose of TD fentanyl is increased after the first patch application (Smith & Pappagallo, 2012).

Equianalgesia

Patients who are on long-term opioids inevitably develop a tolerance to the prescribed opioid and thus dose escalation is often required to adequately treat pain. A technique of rotating opioids is often used to mitigate the risk of escalating opioid doses. To do this switch safely, equianalgesic (equal analgesic) charts provide a list of opioids with their respective MED dose to ensure that the proper equivalent dose is given with the new opioid. The Canadian Opioid Guidelines 2017 recommend that an opioid conversion table be used when rotating opioids. A practical recommendation involves reducing the current opioid dose by 10% to

30% while starting the new opioid, then reducing the original opioid dose by 10% to 25% weekly while increasing the new opioid by 10% to 20% weekly (Busse et al., 2017).

Formulation Terminology

The terms *short acting, immediate release,* and *normal release* have been used interchangeably to describe oral opioids that have an onset of action of approximately 30 minutes and a relatively short duration of 3 to 4 hours. The term *immediate release* is misleading because none of the oral analgesic agents have an immediate onset of analgesia; *short acting* is preferred. The terms *modified release, extended release, sustained release, controlled release,* and *long acting* are used to describe opioids that are formulated to release over a prolonged period of time. For the purposes of this chapter, the term *extended release* will be used when discussing these opioid formulations.

Addiction, Physical Dependence, and Tolerance

There is no maximum safe dosage of opioids, nor is there any easily identifiable therapeutic serum level. Both the maximal safe dosage and the therapeutic serum level are relative and individual. Tolerance (the need for increasing doses of opioids to achieve the same therapeutic effect) develops in almost all patients taking opioids for extended periods. Patients requiring opioids over a long term, especially patients with cancer, need increasing doses to relieve pain. After the first few weeks of therapy, their dosing requirements usually level off. Patients who become tolerant to the analgesic effects of large doses of morphine may obtain pain relief by changing to a different opioid. Symptoms of physical dependence may occur when the opioids are discontinued; dependence often occurs with opioid tolerance and does not indicate an addiction.

NURSING ALERT

Although patients may need increasing levels of opioids, they are not addicted. Physical tolerance usually occurs in the absence of addiction. Tolerance to opioids is common and becomes a problem primarily in terms of delivering or administering the medication (e.g., how to administer very large doses of morphine to a patient). On the other hand, addiction is rare and should not be the primary concern of nurses caring for patients in pain.

Addiction is a behavioural pattern of substance use characterized by a compulsion to take the substance (drug or alcohol) primarily to experience its psychic effects. Fear that patients will become addicted or dependent on opioids has contributed to inadequate treatment of pain. This fear, which may be expressed by health care providers as well as patients and their families, results from lack of knowledge about the low risk of addiction.

Addiction after therapeutic opioid administration is so negligible that it should not be a consideration when caring for patients in pain. Therefore, patients and health care providers should be dissuaded from withholding opioid analgesics because of concerns about addiction.

When caring for people with a known history of **addiction**, nurses should consider that each individual person has the right to be treated for pain. The National Academy of Sciences, Engineering, and Medicine (2017) developed a position paper on pain management of patients with addictive disease. It stressed education, communication about methods for pain management, and methods to safely discontinue opioids in this patient population. The opioids should be tapered slowly to prevent withdrawal symptoms.

Opioid Agents

MORPHINE. Morphine is still viewed as the reference drug for equivalence around the world, and in many countries it is used as a first-line opioid in cancer and non-cancer pain. It acts as a mu-receptor agonist on the opioid receptors in the CNS as well in the peripheral nervous system. At the presynaptic level, morphine reduces Ca^{2+} influx in the primary nociceptive afferent neurons, resulting in decreased pronociception neurotransmitter release. At the postsynaptic level, it enhances K^{+} efflux, resulting hyperpolarization of the dorsal horn pain-signalling sensory neurons (leaving no opportunity for pain signals continue) (Smith & Pappagallo, 2012). The net result of the opioid action is a decrease in nociception. Morphine is hydrophilic solubility, and as such, it is a first-line option when intrathecal administration is required for pain management. The onset of action of morphine is patient dependent but as a rule oral (immediate release) takes ~30 minutes for desired effect; and intravenous ~5 to 10 minutes. Morphine has varying durations: immediate release, 3 to 5 hours; extended release, 8 to 24 hours, and epidural or intrathecal in a single dose up to 24 hours; and suppository, 3 to 7 hours (Lexicomp, 2018a). At high doses, caution must be used when administering morphine to a patient with renal impairment as metabolite accumulation can cause neurotoxicity (Lee, Ganta, Horton, et al., 2016).

FENTANYL. Like morphine, fentanyl is a mu-receptor agonist with a similar effect on the CNS and peripheral nervous system. Also, it increases the neurotransmitter dopamine in the pleasure centre of the brain which can cause a slight euphoric feeling (Ramos-Matos & Lopez-Ojeda, 2017). It is known to have a rapid onset as it crosses the blood–brain barrier. This is due to its high lipid solubility (lipophilic). In an acute setting, fentanyl use is ideal as it has little metabolite accumulation, thus no worry of neurotoxicity, and provides rapid analgesia with a short duration of action. In the patient who is hemodynamically unstable, fentanyl can provide pain relief with less hypotension when compared to other opioids. Fentanyl can also be used in a TD form for the treatment of some forms of chronic pain (TD fentanyl is not appropriate for acute pain treatment). It is important to change the TD patch every 48 to 72 hours, depending on the desired effect. In children, it can be used in intranasal form, which has an onset of action of 5 to 10 minutes. In adults, the intramuscular form has an onset of action of 7 to 8 minutes; intravenous has almost immediate effects; TD patch takes 6 hours to take effect; finally, transmucosal fentanyl takes effect in 5 to 15 minutes (Lexicomp, 2018b).

NURSING ALERT

The application of heat (heat packs, heating pads, or hot tubs or showers) directly over the patch can cause increased absorption of transdermal fentanyl, which can lead to life-threatening respiratory depression.

HYDROMORPHONE. Hydromorphone (Dilaudid) is a semi-synthetic opioid that is a mu-receptor agonist and has intermediate hydrophilic and lipophilic properties. It has a similar mechanism of action as morphine with a shorter half-life and a greater impact on sedation (Gulur, 2015). It does not produce metabolite that causes neurotoxicity in those who take high-dose morphine. Otherwise, hydromorphone has a very similar side effect profile as morphine at an equianalgesic dose. It is commonly used for postoperative IV PCA use. It can also be a good option for treatment moderate to severe pain in its oral format.

OXYCODONE. Oxycodone is a semi-synthetic opioid that acts on mu-receptor sites. It is available in oral form only and can be coupled with acetaminophen for a synergistic effect (Percocet). Due to the rise in prescription drug abuse in Canada, the short-acting version is no longer available. Oxycodone controlled release (OxyNeo) is available for those who have daily continuous severe pain (Purdue Pharma, 2018). As the combination oxycodone/acetaminophen uses the immediate action version of oxycodone, it has an onset of action of 10 to 15 minutes, with a peak effect at about 30 to 60 minutes, and a duration of 3 to 6 hours. The extended release form has virtually no peak and has a duration of roughly 12 hours (Lexicomp, 2018c).

METHADONE. Methadone is another synthetic mu-receptor agonist that acts similar to morphine. Unlike morphine, however, it also acts as NMDA antagonist (but not as pronounced as ketamine) (Lexicomp, 2018d). It is primarily used for the treatment of opioid addiction. The reason for its use with this particular patient population is due to its exceptionally long half-life when given in repeated doses. It is usually given orally with an onset of action of 30 to 60 minutes, and a peak effect in continuous dosing of 3 to 5 days. In a one-time single dose format, oral methadone has a duration of 4 to 8 hours. With repeated doses, due to slow release from the liver and other tissues, the duration can increase to 22 to 48 hours (Lexicomp, 2018d). In the patients taking methadone in an effort to reduce opioid withdrawal symptoms there is an increased risk of overdose, particularly with initiation of the treatment. It also generally requires daily witnessed ingestion of methadone by a health team professional. Methadone can cause QT interval prolongation thus giving rise to the likelihood of a lethal cardiac arrhythmia (BC Ministry of Health, 2017). Also, methadone is primarily metabolized by CYP3A4, thus coadministration of medications that inhibit CYP3A4 (such as azole antifungal—ketoconazole and macrolide antibiotic—erythromycin), may cause decreased clearance of methadone and thus increase the risk of toxicity/overdose (Smith & Pappagallo, 2012).

BUPRENORPHINE. Buprenorphine is a partial agonist of mu receptors, antagonist to the kappa-opioid receptors, agonist to the delta-opioid receptors, and partial agonist to the nociception opioid peptide receptors. It is used, in a combination buprenorphine–naloxone form, to treat opioid addiction, all while preventing intravenous abuse. Buprenorphine is also available in an extended release TD form, called Butrans for the treatment of some forms of chronic pain.

TRAMADOL. Tramadol is a dual-action analgesic agent that blocks the reuptake of both serotonin and norepinephrine. This is a newer class of medication used for the treatment of mild to moderate pain. It is considered a synthetic 4-phenyl-piperidine analogue of codeine, which would classify it as an opioid; however, its mode of action differs from other opioids. Tramadol has a low affinity for mu-opioid receptors at about 6,000 times lower than that of morphine (Kizilbash & Ngô-Minh, 2014). Tramadol is used for both acute and chronic pain and is available in oral short-acting and extended-release (Ultram) formulations. A combination tramadol and acetaminophen (Tramacet) is also available. The drug can lower seizure threshold and interact with other drugs that block the reuptake of serotonin, such as the Selective Serotonin Reuptake Inhibitors, putting the patient at risk for serotonin syndrome, characterized by agitation, diarrhea, heart and blood pressure changes, and loss of coordination.

Opioids to Avoid

Codeine is a weak opioid pain reliever and cough suppressant. The precise mechanism of action of codeine is not understood; however, it is known that small amounts of codeine convert to morphine. Metabolic enzyme CYP2D6 is responsible for the conversion of codeine to morphine. Some individuals are considered poor metabolizers, as they do not have the CYP2D6 enzyme. Such patients do not experience the desired analgesic effect. About 5% to 10% of the population, usually from European Caucasian descent, do not have CYP2D6 enzyme. However, about 1% to 2% of the population are ultra-rapid metabolizers. Such patients are at increased risk of initial overdose when taking codeine. North African Ethiopian and Arabs represent 28% of those who are ultra-rapid metabolizers, and up to 10% Caucasian, and 3% Hispanic, Chinese, or Japanese are estimated to have this over active enzyme (Dean, 2017).

Meperidine (Demerol) is an opioid with a similar mechanism of action as morphine; however, the major drawback is the by-production of a metabolite called normeperidine. While meperidine has a half-life of 2 to 5 hours, its neurotoxic metabolite has a much longer half-life of 15 to 30 hours. This creates a clinical dilemma where the dosing frequency necessary for pain control produces an accumulation of normeperidine, which has been associated with delirium and seizures (Friesen, Falk, & Bugden, 2016).

Adverse Effects of Opioid Analgesic Agents

With the administration of opioids by any route, side effects must be considered and anticipated. Clinicians who take steps to minimize the side effects increase the likelihood that the patient will receive adequate pain relief without interrupting therapy to treat the effects.

RESPIRATORY DEPRESSION AND SEDATION. Respiratory depression is the most serious adverse effect of opioid analgesic agents administered by IV, subcutaneous, or epidural routes. However, it is relatively rare because doses administered through these routes are small and tolerance to respiratory depressant effects increases if the dose is increased slowly. The risk of respiratory depression increases with age and with the concomitant use of other opioids or other CNS depressant medications. The risk of respiratory depression also increases when the epidural catheter is placed in the thoracic area and when the intra-abdominal or intrathoracic pressure is increased.

A patient who receives opioids by any route must be assessed frequently for changes in respiratory status. Specific notable changes are shallow respirations and decreasing respiratory rate. Despite the risks associated with their use, IV and epidural opioids are considered safe, with the risks related to epidural administration no greater than those related to IV or other systemic routes of administration. Sedation, which may occur with any method of administering opioids, is likely to occur when opioid doses are increased. However, patients often develop tolerance quickly, so that in a short time they are no longer sedated by the dose that initially caused sedation. Increasing the time between doses or reducing the dose temporarily, as prescribed, usually prevents deep sedation from occurring. Patients at risk for sedation must be monitored closely for changes in respiratory status. Patients are also at risk for problems associated with sedation and immobility. The nurse must initiate strategies to prevent complications such as pressure ulcers.

NURSING ALERT

Opioid-induced respiratory depression is dose related and preceded by increasing sedation. Prevention of clinically significant opioid-induced respiratory depression begins with the administration of the lowest effective opioid dose, careful titration, close nurse monitoring of sedation and respiratory status throughout therapy, and prompt dose reduction when advancing sedation is detected.

NAUSEA AND VOMITING. Nausea and vomiting may occur with opioid use. Usually these effects occur some hours after the initial injection. Patients, especially postoperative patients, may not think to tell the nurse that they are nauseated, particularly if the nausea is mild. However, a patient receiving opioids should be assessed for nausea and vomiting, which may be triggered by a position change and may be prevented by having the patient change positions slowly. Adequate hydration and the administration of antiemetic agents may also decrease the incidence of nausea. Opioid-induced nausea and vomiting often subside within a few days.

CONSTIPATION. Constipation, a common side effect of opioid use, may become so severe that the patient is forced to choose between relief of pain and relief of constipation. This situation can occur in patients after surgery and in patients receiving large doses of opioids to treat cancer-related pain. Preventing constipation must be a high priority in all patients receiving opioids. Whenever a patient receives opioids, a bowel regimen should begin at the same time. Tolerance to this side effect does not occur; rather, constipation persists even with long-term use of opioids.

Several strategies may help prevent and treat opioid-related constipation. Mild laxatives and a high intake of fluid and fibre may be effective in managing mild constipation. Unless contraindicated, a mild laxative and a stool softener should be administered on a regular schedule. However, continued severe constipation often requires the use of a stimulating cathartic agent, such as senna derivatives (Senokot) or bisacodyl (Dulcolax). If oral agents fail, rectal suppositories may be used. Two agents, alvimopan (Entereg) and methylnaltrexone (Relistor) are used for patients with severe opioid-induced constipation because they work as antagonistic agents on the peripheral opioid receptors in the bowel to counteract opioid-induced delays in GI motility. These medications do not reverse the analgesic effects of the opioids (Nelson & Camilleri, 2016).

PRURITUS. When asked about drug allergies, patients with previous hospital experience (especially for surgery) may report that they are "allergic" to morphine. This report should be thoroughly investigated. Commonly, this "allergy" is described as itching only. Pruritus (itching) is a frequent side effect of opioids administered by any route, but it is not an allergic reaction. It can be relieved by administering prescribed antihistamines. Epidurally administered opioids may also cause urinary retention. The patient should be monitored and may require urinary catheterization. Small doses of naloxone (Narcan) may be prescribed to relieve these issues in patients who are receiving epidural opioids for the relief of acute postoperative pain.

Opioid Use With Selected Conditions and Medications

A number of factors may influence the safety and effectiveness of opioid administration. Opioid analgesic agents are primarily metabolized by the liver and excreted by the kidney. Therefore, metabolism and excretion of analgesic medications are impaired in patients with liver or kidney disease, increasing the risk of cumulative or toxic effects. In addition, normeperidine, a metabolite of meperidine (Demerol), may rapidly or unexpectedly accumulate to toxic levels. This is more likely to occur in patients with impaired kidney function and may result in seizures in susceptible patients. Many institutions no longer stock meperidine because of the risks associated with the metabolite normeperidine and because many physicians do not prescribe a high enough dose for it to be effective.

Patients with untreated hypothyroidism are more susceptible to the analgesic effects and side effects of opioids. In contrast, patients with hyperthyroidism may require larger doses for pain relief. Patients with a decreased respiratory reserve from disease or aging may be more susceptible to the depressant effects of opioids and must be carefully monitored for respiratory depression.

Patients who are dehydrated are at increased risk for the hypotensive effects of opioids. Patients, who become hypotensive after the administration of an opioid, should be kept recumbent and rehydrated, unless fluids are contraindicated. Patients who are dehydrated are also more likely to experience nausea and vomiting with opioid use. Rehydration usually relieves these symptoms.

Patients receiving certain other medications, such as monoamine oxidase inhibitors, phenothiazines, or tricyclic antidepressants (TCA), may have an exaggerated response to the depressant effects of opioids. Patients taking these medications should receive small doses of opioids and must be monitored closely. Continued pain in these patients indicates that a therapeutic level of the analgesic has not been achieved. Patients are monitored for sedation even if an analgesic effect has not been obtained.

Adjuvant Analgesic Agents

Local Anesthetic Agents

Local anesthetics work by blocking nerve conduction when applied directly to the nerve fibres. They can be applied directly to the site of injury (e.g., a topical anesthetic spray for sunburn) or infused around nerve fibres. They can also be administered through an epidural catheter.

Local anesthetic agents have been successful in reducing the pain associated with thoracic or upper abdominal surgery when injected by the surgeon intercostally. Local anesthetic agents are rapidly absorbed into the bloodstream, resulting in decreased availability at the surgical or injury site and an increased anesthetic level in the blood, increasing the risk of toxicity. Therefore, a vasoconstrictive agent (e.g., epinephrine or phenylephrine) is added to the anesthetic agent to decrease its systemic absorption and maintain its concentration at the surgical or injury site.

Long-acting local anesthetics (bupivacaine, ropivacaine) may be used perioperatively for postoperative pain relief. The operative wound is infiltrated with the anesthetic during surgery. Postoperative pain and amount of analgesics required after surgery are reduced. When a longer duration of anesthesia is desired, the local anesthetic can be infused continuously using a catheter and pump to deliver the anesthetic to the wound.

Nonopioid Pharmacotherapy for Pain

ANTICONVULSANTS. Although originally developed for the treatment of complex seizures, gabapentinoids (Gabapentin or Pregabalin) are prescribed as standard treatment for neuropathic pain. It is a structural GABA, which binds at the A-delta subunit of voltage-sensitive calcium channels and reduces calcium influx. This medication changes the calcium channel function by decreasing the influx of calcium but does not blunt its secretion. By doing this, it reduces the influx of excitatory neurotransmitters and decreases brain glutamate and glutamine levels. It also increases plasma serotonin levels. It takes about 2 months for this medication to titrate to an effective dose. It is dosed at 300 to 1,800 mg/day in two or three doses, but can be titrated up to the maximum of 3,600 mg/day. Gabapentinoids can cause sedation, dizziness, fatigue, ataxia, weight gain, and dry mouth (Smith & Pappagallo, 2012).

ANTIDEPRESSANTS. Typically, two main classes of antidepressants are used in chronic pain—serotonin and norepinephrine reuptake inhibitors (SNRI) and TCA. They are effective at reducing pain in postherpetic neuralgia, fibromyalgia, central sensitization, knee osteoarthritis, and diabetic peripheral neuropathy (Chart 16-2) (Bonnie et al., 2017). SNRIs, commonly Duloxetine (Cymbalta), block serotonin and noradrenergic reuptake pumps, and while norepinephrine and serotonin have a positive effect on mood and pain, it is thought that the catecholamine blockade is central to pain reduction. The intended pain relieving effect is not noted until days or weeks after treatment initiation. Common side effects include dry mouth, constipation, weight gain, drowsiness, nausea, tremors, and hyperarousal. Some patients may experience episodes of orthostatic hypotension in the 1st week of use. These medications do interact with other medications that increase serotonin levels, which may lead to a dangerous adverse effect called serotonin syndrome (i.e., high body temperature, agitation, tremors, dilated pupils, and diarrhea). Specifically, for TCAs like amitriptyline or nortriptyline, anticholinergics may cause sedative effect, dry mouth, constipation, and blurred vision.

KETAMINE (NMDA ANTAGONIST). Ketamine causes patients to have a dissociative state from their environment, provides analgesia, and has a sedative effect (MacIntyre & Schug, 2015). Ketamine's effect is dose dependent and can be categorized as anesthetic (at high dose), analgesic (at medium dose), and opioid-sparing/antihyperalgesic (at low dose) (Bonnie et al., 2017). It acts by blocking glutamate access to NMDA receptors. It is sometimes used for sedation when children are undergoing a procedure, as it has no respiratory suppression, thus maintaining patent airways with ease. However, it can produce a less desirable side effect of hallucinations, vivid dreams, disorientation, and restlessness. A patient medicated with ketamine will have a nystagmus and hyperclonus. Beyond its use for procedural pain, ketamine compounded into a cream may be used for neuropathic pain for its benefits without the systemic side effects.

CANNABINOIDS. Only recently has modern society begun to use cannabinoids for the treatment of pain in medicine. Some evidence shows that cannabinoids can help with chronic neuropathic pain, cancer-related pain, fibromyalgia, and HIV-associated neuropathy (Bonnie et al., 2017). However, many questions are still to be answered as to the best dose, formulation (THC vs. CBD), administration route, and efficacy. THC has a psychosedative effect, whereas CBD is thought to mainly act on CB1 receptors without negative side effects. Most of the analgesic effect is mediated by CB1 receptors which are broadly located in the brain, spinal cord, peripheral nerves, musculoskeletal muscles, GI tract, and liver.

Gerontologic Considerations

Physiologic changes in older adults require that analgesic agents be administered with caution. Drug interactions are more likely to occur in older adults because of the higher incidence of chronic illness and the increased use of prescription and OTC medications. Although the older adult population is an extremely heterogeneous group, differences in response to pain or medications by patients over this 40-year span (approximately 60 to 100 years) are more likely to be due to chronic illness or other individual factors than to age. Before administering opioid and nonopioid analgesic agents to elderly patients, the nurse obtains a careful medication history to identify potential drug interactions.

Older patients are more sensitive to medications and at an increased risk for drug toxicity (Bettinger, Wegrzyn, & Fudin, 2017). Liver, renal, and GI functions are decreased in older adult patients, resulting in changes in the absorption and metabolism of medications. In addition, changes in body weight, protein stores, and distribution of body fluid alter the distribution of medications in the body. Consequently, medications are not metabolized as quickly, and blood levels of the medications remain higher for a longer period.

Opioid and non-opioid analgesic medications can be administered to older patients but must be used cautiously because of the increased susceptibility to depression of both the nervous and the respiratory systems. Although there is no reason to avoid opioids in patients simply because they are older, meperidine (Demerol) should be avoided because its active and neurotoxic metabolite, normeperidine, is more likely to accumulate and cause CNS excitation and seizures. In addition, because of decreased binding of meperidine by plasma proteins, blood concentrations of the medication twice of those found in younger patients may occur.

In many cases, the initial dose of analgesic medication prescribed for older patients is the same as that for younger patients, or slightly smaller than the usual dose, but because of slowed metabolism and excretion related to aging, the safe interval for subsequent doses may be longer (or prolonged). Older patients may obtain more pain relief for a longer time than do younger patients from the same dose. As a result, smaller and less frequent doses of analgesics may be required.

Nonpharmacologic Methods of Pain Management

Physiotherapy (or Physical Therapy)

Physiotherapists have specialized skills to assess and uniquely address pain that is thought to be from joints, muscles, tendons, or ligaments. Progressive targeted rehabilitation programs are essential to promoting pain self-management and improved overall outcomes in those with pain. Physiotherapists can utilize, but are not limited to, the use of exercise (as medicine), myofascial muscle release techniques, intramuscular stimulation (or medical dry needling), manual therapy, and stretching. In case of chronic refractory pain, a physiotherapist may be used on a semi-regular basis for rescue treatments. This may allow a reduction in medication while still meeting the patient's functional goals.

Exercise

A high level of evidence supports the prescription of exercise in those who are afflicted with osteoarthritic knee or hip pain. Both aerobic and resistance training leads to decreased self-reported levels of pain and increased function. The best outcomes are found with a regular home-based exercise program coupled with a supplemental supervised exercise program (Colledge, 2018). There are also some well-documented positive mental health effects of regular exercises.

Cognitive Behaviour Therapy (CBT)

This is an evidence-based approach that involves therapy with a mental health professional who will help patients change the way they may think about pain and how they manage their pain. Through structured intervention that may include relaxation, distraction, cognitive restructuring, and guided mental exercises, adaptive and healthy coping strategies can be developed to help achieve improved pain and functional outcomes (Wolters Kluwer Health, 2017).

Massage

The gate control theory of pain proposes that stimulation of fibres that transmit nonpainful sensations can block or decrease the transmission of pain impulses. Several nonpharmacologic pain relief strategies, including rubbing the skin and using heat and cold, are based on this theory.

Massage, which is generalized cutaneous stimulation of the body, often concentrates on the back and shoulders. A massage does not specifically stimulate the nonpain receptors in the same receptor field as the pain receptors, but it may have an impact through the descending control system (see previous discussion). Massage also promotes comfort because it produces muscle relaxation (Boyd, Crawford, Paat, et al., 2016).

Thermal Therapies

Ice and heat therapies may be effective pain relief strategies in some circumstances; however, their effectiveness and mechanisms of action need further study (Malanga, Yan, & Stark, 2015). Proponents believe that ice and heat stimulate the nonpain receptors in the same receptor field as the injury.

For greatest effect, ice should be placed on the injury site immediately after injury or surgery. Ice therapy after joint surgery can significantly reduce the amount of analgesic medication required. Ice therapy may also relieve pain if applied later. Care must be taken to assess the skin before treatment and to protect the skin from direct application of the ice. Long applications of ice may result in frostbite or nerve injury.

Application of heat increases blood flow to an area and contributes to pain reduction by speeding healing. Both dry and moist heat may provide some analgesia, but their mechanisms of action are not well understood. Both ice and heat therapy must be applied carefully and monitored closely to avoid injuring the skin. Neither therapy should be applied to areas with impaired circulation or used in patients with impaired sensation.

NURSING ALERT

Heat should not be applied to a painful area that is the site of acute untreated infection (e.g., mastitis, tooth abscess), because it may cause increased pain with increased blood flow to the site.

Transcutaneous Electrical Nerve Stimulation

Transcutaneous electrical nerve stimulation (TENS) uses a battery-operated unit with electrodes applied to the skin to produce a tingling, vibrating, or buzzing sensation in the area of pain. It has been used in both acute and chronic pain relief and is thought to decrease pain by stimulating the nonpain receptors in the same area as the fibres that transmit the pain. This mechanism is consistent with the gate control theory of pain and explains the effectiveness of cutaneous stimulation when applied in the same area as an injury (Johnson, Paley, Howe, et al., 2015).

Relaxation Techniques

Skeletal muscle relaxation is believed to reduce pain by relaxing tense muscles that contribute to the pain. Research findings support the use of relaxation in relieving pain (Blödt, Pach, Roll, et al., 2015).

A simple relaxation technique consists of abdominal breathing at a slow, rhythmic rate. The patient may close both eyes and breathe slowly and comfortably. A constant rhythm can be maintained by counting silently and slowly with each inhalation ("in, two, three") and exhalation ("out, two, three"). When teaching this technique, the nurse may count out loud with the patient at first. Slow, rhythmic breathing may also be used as a distraction technique. Relaxation techniques, as well as other noninvasive pain relief measures, may require practice before the patient becomes skilled in using them. Patients who already know a relaxation technique may need to be reminded to use it to reduce or prevent increased pain.

Almost all people with chronic pain would benefit from some method of relaxation. Regular relaxation periods may help combat the fatigue and muscle tension that occur with and increase chronic pain.

Hypnosis

Hypnosis, which has been effective in relieving pain or decreasing the amount of analgesic agents required in patients with acute and chronic pain, may promote pain relief in particularly difficult situations (e.g., burns). The mechanism by which hypnosis acts is unclear. Its effectiveness depends on the hypnotic susceptibility of the individual (Dillworth, Mendoza, & Jensen, 2012). In some cases, hypnosis may be effective in the first session, with effectiveness increasing in additional sessions. In other cases, hypnosis does not work at all. Usually, hypnosis must be induced by specially skilled people (a psychologist or a nurse with specialized training in hypnosis). Some patients may learn to perform self-hypnosis.

Music Therapy

Music therapy is an inexpensive therapy for the reduction of pain and anxiety. It can be used as part of a multipronged approach to pain management (Holden & Holden, 2013) (Chart 16-3).

Novel Medical Interventions for Pain Management

Stimulation Procedures

Electrical stimulation, or neuromodulation, is a method of suppressing pain by applying controlled low-voltage electrical pulses to the different parts of the nervous system. Electrical stimulation is thought to block painful stimuli (the gate control theory). A surgically implanted device allows the patient to apply pulsed electrical stimulation to the dorsal aspect of the spinal cord to block pain impulses.

Interventional Pain Injections

Some patients with persistent pain may require novel pain injections from an interventional radiologist or physiatrist. Depending on the pathology that is thought to be causing the pain, various injection sites are targeted with various techniques. Usually injections of local anesthetic, corticosteroid, or platelet-rich plasma are focused at damaged joints, nerves, ligaments, or tendons. In another technique, called radiofrequency nerve ablation, the nerve can be temporarily burned to interrupt the pain signal; however, over a period of 12 months, the nerve regrows, causing pain again. A regional pain block, in which a nerve is injected with anesthetic, is commonly used in preoperative settings as it has been found to reduce the incidence of postoperative chronic pain. There is growing interest, research, and evidence that support these novel treatments as important adjuncts in reaching positive function outcomes.

Evaluating Pain Management Strategies

An important aspect of caring for patients in pain is reassessing the pain after the intervention has been implemented. Its effectiveness is based on the patient's assessment of pain, using pain assessment tools. If the intervention was ineffective, the nurse considers other measures. If these are ineffective, pain relief goals need to be reassessed in collaboration with the physician. The nurse serves as the patient's advocate in obtaining additional pain relief.

After interventions have had a chance to work, the nurse asks the patient to rate the intensity of pain. The nurse repeats this assessment at appropriate intervals after the intervention and compares the result with the previous rating. These assessments indicate the effectiveness of the pain relief measures and provide a basis for continuing or modifying the plan of care. A plan of nursing care for a patient with pain is given in Chart 16-5. Expected patient outcomes include the following:

Relief of pain, evidenced when the patient:

- Rates pain at a lower intensity (on a scale of 0 to 10) after intervention
- Rates pain at a lower intensity for longer periods

Correct administration of prescribed analgesic medications, evidenced when the patient or family:

- States correct dose of medication
- Administers correct dose using correct procedure
- Identifies side effects of medication
- Describes actions taken to prevent or correct side effects

Use of nonpharmacologic pain strategies as recommended, evidenced when the patient:

- Reports practice of nonpharmacologic strategies
- Describes expected outcomes of nonpharmacologic strategies

Minimal effects of pain and minimal side effects of interventions, evidenced when the patient:

- Participates in activities important to recovery (e.g., drinking fluids, coughing, ambulating)
- Participates in activities important to self and to family (e.g., family activities, interpersonal relationships, parenting, social interaction, recreation, work)
- Reports adequate sleep and absence of fatigue and constipation

Plan of Nursing Care Chart 16-5. Care of the Patient With Pain

NURSING DIAGNOSIS: Acute Pain
GOAL: Achievement and maintenance of patient's comfort-function goal

NURSING INTERVENTION	RATIONALE	EXPECTED OUTCOMES
1. Perform and document a comprehensive pain assessment.	1. The comprehensive pain assessment is the foundation of the pain treatment plan; documentation ensures communication between team members	• If able, provides information about the pain. • Expresses understanding of the link between function and pain control and establishes a realistic comfort-function goal • Reports a pain intensity that allows participation in important functional activities • If not able to report pain, demonstrates behaviours that indicate pain relief and participation in important functional activities • Expresses satisfaction with the use of nonpharmacologic methods • Tolerates pharmacologic and nonpharmacologic interventions without adverse effects • Demonstrates an understanding of the treatment plan and goals of care
a. Use a reliable and valid tool to determine pain intensity	a. The use of valid and reliable tools helps ensure accuracy and consistency in assessment	
b. Accept the patient's report of pain	b. Accepting the patient's report of pain is the undisputed standard of pain assessment	
c. Assist the patient in establishing a comfort-function goal	c. The comfort-function goal links function to pain control and provides direction for necessary adjustments in the treatment plan to maximize function	
d. Apply the hierarchy of pain measures in patients who are unable to report their pain	d. The use of the hierarchy of pain measures provides a process to ensure pain treatment in the patient who cannot report pain	
2. Administer analgesic agents as prescribed	2. Pharmacologic interventions are the cornerstone of pain management	
3. Offer and educate patient how to use appropriate nonpharmacologic interventions	3. Nonpharmacologic methods are used to supplement pharmacologic interventions	
4. Reassess for degree of pain relief and presence of adverse effects at peak effect time of intervention	4. Reassessment permits evaluation of both the effectiveness and safety of interventions	
5. Obtain additional prescriptions as needed	5. Prescriptions for additional analgesic agents or adjustment in dose are often needed to maximize pain control	
6. Prevent and treat adverse effects	6. Adverse effects are prevented whenever possible and promptly treated to reduce patient discomfort and prevent harm	
7. Educate patient and family about the effects of analgesic agents and the goals of care; explain how adverse effects will be prevented and treated; address fears of addiction	7. An understanding of the treatment plan and goals of care educates patients and their families how to partner with the health care team to optimize pain control	

Critical Thinking Exercises

1 An 82-year-old woman is admitted to the orthopedic unit post hip fracture. She is unable to answer questions about her pain history or her intensity of pain. She is crying and moaning. Her family reports that she has been very forgetful at home and recently diagnosed with dementia. What pain assessment tool would be most helpful in determining whether your pain interventions are helping? What is the strength of the evidence that supports your use of your selected tool?

2 A 47-year-old man who is obese with chronic back pain and chronic opioid use is admitted to the medical unit with acute pancreatitis. His inpatient medications include a long-acting morphine product, intravenous hydromorphone PRN, an anxiolytic medication PRN, an antihistamine for pruritus PRN, and a hypnotic medication for sleep PRN. The patient asks you to give him all his medications at the same time so that he can get some sleep. He asserts that he has done this successfully every night at home for the past year. You are concerned that all these medications are central nervous system depressants and that given together, they could oversedate the patient.

How would you prioritize the medications that he is requesting?

3 A 50-year-old woman with diabetes and bilateral neuropathic leg pain is admitted to the hospital with a leg abscess. She reports excruciating pain during dressing changes. Her only analgesic medication is an oral opioid. Using a multimodal approach, what other interventions (pharmacologic and nonpharmacologic) could be used to better manage her continuous pain as well as the procedural pain of dressing changes?

REFERENCES AND SELECTED READINGS

Books

Apkarian, A. V., Bushnell, M. C., Schweinhardt, P., et al. (2013). Representation of pain in the brain. In S. B. McMahon, M. Koltzenburg, I. Tracey, et al. (Eds.). *Wall and Melzack's textbook of pain* (6th ed.). Philadelphia, PA: Elsevier-Saunders.

Buvanendran, A., Lubenow, T. R., & Droin, J. S. (2013). Postoperative pain and its management. In S. B. McMahon, M. Koltzenburg, I. Tracey, et al. (Eds.). *Wall and Melzack's textbook of pain* (6th ed.). Philadelphia, PA: Elsevier-Saunders.

Centers for Medicare & Medicaid Services (CMS). (2014). *Requirements for hospital medication administration, particularly intravenous (IV) medications and post-operative care of patients receiving IV opioids*. Baltimore, MD: Center for Clinical Standards and Quality/Survey & Certification Group, U.S. Department of Health & Human Services.

Comerford, K. C. (2015). *Nursing 2015 drug handbook*. Philadelphia, PA: Wolters Kluwer.

Dean, L. (2017). Codeine therapy and CYP2D6 genotype. In V. Pratt, H. McLeod, L. Dean, et al., (Eds.). *Medical genetics summaries*. Bethesda, MD: National Center for Biotechnology Information. Retrieved from https://www.ncbi.nlm.nih.gov/books/NBK100662/.

Gagliese, L., & Melzack, R. (2013). Pain in older persons. In S. B. McMahon, M. Koltzenburg, I. Tracey, et al. (Eds.). *Wall and Melzack's textbook of pain* (6th ed.). Philadelphia, PA: Elsevier-Saunders.

Golan, D. E., Tashjian, A. H., & Armstrong, E. J. (2017). *Principles of pharmacology: The pathophysiologic basis of drug therapy* (4th ed.). Baltimore, MD: Wolters Kluwer Health, Lippincott Williams & Wilkins.

Haythornwaite, J. A. (2013). Assessment of pain beliefs, coping, and function. In S. B. McMahon, M. Koltzenburg, I. Tracey, et al. (Eds.). *Wall and Melzack's textbook of pain* (6th ed.). Philadelphia, PA: Elsevier-Saunders.

Heinricher, M. M., & Fields, H. L. (2013). Central nervous system mechanisms of pain modulation. In S. B. McMahon, M. Koltzenburg, I. Tracey, et al. (Eds.). *Wall and Melzack's textbook of pain* (6th ed.). Philadelphia, PA: Elsevier-Saunders.

Hunt, S. P., & Urch, C. E. (2013). Pain, opiates and addiction. In S. B. McMahon, M. Koltzenburg, I. Tracey, et al. (Eds.). *Wall and Melzack's textbook of pain* (6th ed.). Philadelphia, PA: Elsevier-Saunders.

Kim, J., & Mukovozov, I. (Eds.) (2017). *Essential Mednotes—comprehensive medical reference & review for USMLE II and MCCQE I*. Toronto: Thieme.

Kreitzer, M. J., & Koithan, M. (2014). *Integrative nursing*. Oxford, UK: Oxford University Press.

Lehne, R. A. (2013). *Pharmacology for nursing care* (8th ed.). St. Louis, MO: Elsevier Saunders.

Longo, D. L. (2015). Approach to the patient with cancer. In D. Kasper, A. Fauci, S. Hauser, et al. (Eds.). *Harrison's principles of internal medicine* (19th ed.). New York: McGraw-Hill.

MacIntyre, P. E., & Schug, S. A. (2015). *Acute pain management: A practical guide* (4th ed.). Boca Raton, LA: CRC Press; Taylor & Francis Group.

Mantyh, P. W. (2013). Cancer pain: Causes, consequences, and therapeutic opportunities. In S. B. McMahon, M. Koltzenburg, I. Tracey, et al. (Eds.). *Wall and Melzack's textbook of pain* (6th ed.). Philadelphia, PA: Elsevier-Saunders.

Ramos-Matos, C. F., & Lopez-Ojeda, W. (2017). Fentanyl. In: *StatPearls*. Treasure Island, FL: StatPearls Publishing. Retrieved from https://www.ncbi.nlm.nih.gov/books/NBK459275/

Rhoads, J., & Petersen, S. (2018). *Advanced health assessment and diagnostic reasoning* (3rd ed., pp. 2–20). Burlington, MA: Jones & Barlett.

Ringkamp, M., Raja, S. N., Campbell, J. N., et al. (2013). Peripheral mechanisms of cutaneous nociception. In S. B. McMahon, M. Koltzenburg, I. Tracey, et al. (Eds.). *Wall and Melzack's textbook of pain* (6th ed.). Philadelphia, PA: Elsevier-Saunders.

Sandkuhler, J. (2013). Spinal cord plasticity and pain. In S. B. McMahon, M. Koltzenburg, I. Tracey, et al. (Eds.). *Wall and Melzack's textbook of pain* (6th ed.). Philadelphia, PA: Elsevier-Saunders.

Scadding, J. W., & Koltzenburg, M. (2013). Painful peripheral neuropathies. In S. B. McMahon, M. Koltzenburg, I. Tracey, et al. (Eds.). *Wall and Melzack's textbook of pain* (6th ed.). Philadelphia, PA: Elsevier-Saunders.

Schug, S. A. (2013). Opioids: Clinical use. In S. B. McMahon, M. Koltzenburg, I. Tracey, et al. (Eds.). *Wall and Melzack's textbook of pain* (6th ed.). Philadelphia, PA: Elsevier-Saunders.

Smith, H. S. (Ed.). (2013). *Opioid therapy in the 21st century* (2nd ed.). Oxford, UK: Oxford University Press.

Smith, H. S., & Pappagallo, M. (Eds.) (2012). *Essential pain pharmacology: The prescribers Guide* (1st Ed.). Cambridge, UK: Cambridge University Press.

St. Marie, B. (Ed.). (2010). *Core curriculum for pain management nursing. American Society for Pain Management Nursing*. Olathe, KS: Kendall Hunt Professional.

Stanos, P., Tyburki, M., & Harden, N. (2016). Chronic Pain. In *Braddom's Physical Medicine and Rehabilitation* (Ch. 37) pp. 809–833.

Todd, A. J., & Koerber, H. R. (2013) Neuroanatomical substrates of spinal nociception. In S. B. McMahon, M. Koltzenburg, I. Tracey, et al. (Eds.). *Wall and Melzack's textbook of pain* (6th ed.). Philadelphia, PA: Elsevier-Saunders.

Wager, T. D., & Fields, H. L. (2013). Placebo analgesia. In S. B. McMahon, M. Koltzenburg, I. Tracey, et al. (Eds.). *Wall and Melzack's textbook of pain* (6th ed.). Philadelphia, PA: Elsevier-Saunders.

Wickson-Griffiths, A., Kaasalainen, S., & Pokoradi, L. (2018). Nursing roles in managing pain in older adults. In G. Pickering, S. Zwakhalen, & S. Kaasalainen, *Pain management in older adults—A nursing perspective* (pp. 93–108). Cham: Springer.

Journals and Electronic Documents

Anghelescu, D. L., Faughnan, L. G., Oakes, L. L., et al. (2012). Parent-controlled PCA for pain management in pediatric oncology: Is it safe? *Journal of Pediatric Hematology/oncology*, *34*(6), 416–420.

Argoff, C. E, Viscusi, E. R. (2014). The use of opioid analgesics for chronic pain: Minimizing the risk for harm. *The American Journal Of Gastroenterology Supplements*, *2*, 3. Retrieved from http://dx.doi.org/10.1038/ajgsup.2014.3.

Artemiadis A, & Panagiotis, Z. (2018). Neuropathic pain in acute and subacute neuropathies: A systematic review. *Pain Physician*, *21*, 111–120. Retrieved from www.painphysicianjournal.com.

Aydede, M. (2017). Defending the IASP definition of pain. *The Monist*, *100*(4), 439. Retrieved from http://link.galegroup.com.ezproxy.lib.ucalgary.ca/apps/doc/A507658499/AONE?u=ucalgary&sid=AONE&xid=83199974.

Bandawar, M., Kandasamy, A., Chand, P., et al. (2015). Adherence to buprenorphine maintenance treatment in opioid dependence syndrome: A case control study. *Indian Journal of Psychological Medicine*, *37*(3), 330–332.

BC Ministry of Health. (2017). *British Columbia Centre on Substance Use and B.C. Ministry of Health. A guideline for the clinical management of opioid use disorder*. Retrieved from http://www.bccsu.ca/care-guidance-publications/.

Befort, K. (2015). Interactions of the opioid and cannabinoid systems in reward: Insights from knockout studies. *Frontiers in Pharmacology*, *6*, 6.

Benyhe, S., Zádor, F., & Ötvös, F. (2015). Biochemistry of opioid (morphine) receptors: Binding, structure and molecular modelling. *Acta Biologica Szegediensis*, *59*, 17–37.

Bettinger, J., Wegrzyn, E., & Fudin, J. (2017). Pain management in the elderly: Focus on safe prescribing. *Practical Pain Management*, *17*(3). Retrieved from https://www.practicalpainmanagement.com/treatments/pharmacological/opioids/pain-management-elderly-focus-safe-prescribing.

Blödt, S., Pach, D., Roll, S., et al. (2014). Effectiveness of app-based relaxation for patients with chronic low back pain (Relaxback) and chronic neck pain (Relaxneck): Study protocol for two randomized pragmatic trials. *Trials*, *15*, 490.

Bonnie, R., Ford, M., & Phillips, J. (2017). National Academies Of Sciences Engineering and Medicine; Health and Medicine Division; Board on Health Sciences Policy; Committee on Pain Management and Regulatory Strategies to address prescription opioid abuse. *Pain Management and the Opioid epidemic: Balancing societal and individual benefits and risks of prescription opioid use.* Retrieved from https://www.nap.edu/catalog/24781/pain-management-and-the-opioid-epidemic-balancing-societal-and-individual.

Booker, S. Q., & Haedtke, C. (2016). Assessing pain in nonverbal older adults. *Nursing, 46*(5), 66–69.

Boyd, C., Crawford, C. F., Paat, C., et al. (2016). Evidence for massage therapy (EMT) Working Group: The impact of massage therapy on function in pain populations—A systematic review and meta-analysis of randomized controlled trials: Part III, surgical pain populations. *Pain Medicine, 17*(9), 1757–1772.

Busse, J. W., Craigie, S., Juurlink, D. N., et al. (2017). Guideline for opioid therapy and chronic noncancer pain. *Canadian Medical Association Journal, 189*(18), E659–E666. http://doi.org/10.1503/cmaj.170363.

Canadian Pain Society. (2014). *Pain in Canada Fact Sheet.* Retrieved from http://c.ymcdn.com/sites/www.canadianpainsociety.ca/resource/resmgr/docs/pain_fact_sheet_en.pdf

Carezzato, N. L., Valera, G. G., Assis, F., et al. (2014). Instruments for assessing pain in persons with severe dementia. *Dement Neuropsychol, 8*(2), 99–106.

Carlson, C. L. (2010). Prior conditions influencing nurses decisions to adopt evidence-based postoperative pain assessment practices. *Pain Management in Nursing, 11*(4), 245–258.

Chiorean, M. I., & Chiorean, M. A. (2014). Genetics of Pain. *Acta Medica Marisiensis, 59*(4), 231–233.

Colledge, E. (2018). *Prescribing physical activity: Using a vital sign approach.* The Foundation for Medical Practice Education. PBLP. McMaster University. Vol 26 (2).

Cooney, M. F., Czarnecki, M. Dunwoody, C., et al. (2013). American Society for Pain Management Nursing position statement with clinical practice guidelines: Authorized agent controlled analgesia. *Pain Management Nursing, 14*(3), 176–181.

Cornelius, R., Herr, K. A., Gordon, D. B., et al. (2017). Acute pain management in older adults. *Journal of Gerontological Nursing, 43*(2), 18–27.

Cruccu, G., & Truini, A. (2017). A review of neuropathic pain: From guidelines to clinical practice. *Pain and Therapy, 6*(1), 35–42.

Della Volpe, K. (2016). Sex and gender differences in the pain experience. *Practical Pain Management, 16*(2).

Dilworth, T. M., Mendoza, M. E., & Jensen, M. P. (2012). Neurophysiology of pain and hypnosis for chronic pain. *Translational Behavioural Medicine, 2*(1), 65–72.

Dissanayake, D. W., & Dissanayake, D. M. (2015). The physiology of pain: An update and review of clinical relevance. *Journal of the Ceylon College of Physicians, 46*(1–2), 19–23.

Dueñas, M., Ojeda, B., Salazar, A., et al. (2016). A review of chronic pain impact on patients, their social environment and the health care system. *Journal of Pain Research, 9*, 457–467.

Epner, D., & Bail, W. F. (2012). Patient-centered care: The key to cultural competence. *Annals of Oncology, 23* (Suppl 3), 33–42.

Erdek, M., & Gordon, A. H. (2014). Pain management in the critically ill patient. *Practical Management of Pain, 76*, 1015–1022. e2.

Ernstzen, D. V., Louw, Q. A., & Hillier, S. L. (2017). Clinical practice guidelines for the management of chronic musculoskeletal pain in primary healthcare: A systematic review. *Implementation Science, 12*(1), 1.

Figura, N., Smith, J., & Yu, H. M. (2018). Mechanisms of, and adjuvants for, bone pain. *Hematology/oncology Clinics of North America, 32*(3), 447–458.

Friedrichsdorf, S., Giordano, J., Desai Dakoji, K., et al. (2016). Chronic pain in children and adolescents: Diagnosis and treatment of primary pain disorders in head, abdomen, muscles and joints. *Children, 3*(4), 42.

Friesen, K. J., Falk, J., & Bugden, S. (2016). The safety of meperidine prescribing in older adults: A longitudinal population-based study. *BMC Geriatrics, 16*, 100.

Gardner, T., Refshauge, K., McAuley, J., et al. (2018) Goal setting practice in chronic low back pain. What is current practice and is it affected by beliefs and attitudes? *Physiotherapy Theory and Practice.* DOI: 10.1080/09593985.2018.1425785.

Gatchell, R. J., Neblett, R., Kishino, N., et al. (2016). Fear-avoidance beliefs and chronic pain. *Journal of Orthopaedic and Physical Therapy, 46*(2), 38–43.

Grandy, S., Cui, Y., DeClercq, V., et al. (2017). Physical activity levels in Atlantic Canadian arthritis patients.

GSK. (2017). GSK global pain index 2017-Global Research Report. Retrieved from https://www.gsk.com/media/3814/global-pain-index-2017-report.pdf

Guerriero, F., & Reid, M. C. (2017). New opioid prescribing guidelines released in the US: What impact will they have in the care of older patients with persistent pain? *Current Medical Research and Opinion, 33*(2), 275–278.

Gulur, P., Koury, K., Arnstein, P., et al. (2015). Morphine versus hydromorphone: Does choice of opioid influence outcomes? *Pain Research and Treatment*, 2015. http://doi.org/10.1155/2015/482081.

Gunnarsdottir, S., Donovan, H. S., & Ward, S. (2003). Interventions to overcome clinician-and patient-related barriers to pain management. *Nursing Clinics of North America, 38*(3), 419–434.

Häuser, W., Schug, S., & Furlan, A. D. (2017). The opioid epidemic and national guidelines for opioid therapy for chronic noncancer pain: A perspective from different continents. *Pain reports, 2*(3), e599.

Herr K., St. Marie, B., Gordon, D. B., et al. (2015). An interprofessional consensus of core competencies for prelicensure education in pain management: Curriculum application for nursing. *Journal of Nursing Education, 54*(6), 317–327.

Hiragi, S., Yamada, H., Tsukamoto, T., et al. (2018). Acetaminophen administration and the risk of acute kidney injury: A self-controlled case series study. *Clinical epidemiology, 10*, 265.

Holden, R., & Holden, J. (2013). Music: A better alternative than pain? *The British Journal of General Practice, 63*(615), 536.

Horgas, A. L. (2017). Pain assessment in older adults. *Nursing Clinics North America, 52*(3), 375–385.

Horgas, A. L. (2017). Pain management in older adults. *Nursing Clinics of North America, 52*(4), e1–e7.

Hudspith, M. J. (2016). Anatomy, physiology and pharmacology of pain. *Anaesthesia & Intensive Care Medicine, 17*(9), 425–430.

Ibsen, M. S., Connor, M., & Glass, M. (2017). Cannabinoid CB_1 and CB_2 receptor signaling and bias. *Cannabis and Cannabinoid Research.* http://doi.org/10.1089/can.2016.0037.

Johnson, M. I., Paley, C. A., Howe, T. E., et al. (2015). Transcutaneous electrical nerve stimulation for acute pain. *Cochrane Database of Systematic Reviews.* DOI: 10.1002/14651858.CD006142.pub3.

Kellmann, M., Pelka, M., & Beckmann, J. (2018). Psychological relaxation techniques to enhance recovery in sports. *Sport, Recovery and Performance: Interdisciplinary Insights*, 247–259.

Kent, M. L., Tighe, P. J., Belfer, I., et al. (2017). The ACTTION-APS-AAPM Pain Taxonomy (AAAPT) multidimensional approach to classifying acute pain conditions. *Pain Medicine (Malden, Mass.), 18*(5), 947–958.

Kindler, L. L. Bennett, R. M., & Jones, K. D. (2011). Central sensitivity syndromes: Mounting pathophysiologic evidence to link fibromyalgia with other common chronic pain disorders. *Pain Management Nursing, 12*(1), 15–24.

Kizilbash, A., & Ngô-Minh, C. (2014). Review of extended-release formulations of tramadol for the management of chronic non-cancer pain: Focus on marketed formulations. *Journal of Pain Research, 7*, 149–161.

Kizilhan, J. I. (2016). Kulturelle Deutungen des Schmerzes in familienorientierten Gesellschaften. *Der Schmerz.* http://doi.org/10.1007/s00482-016-0127-4.

Lalanne, L., Nicot, C., Lang, J-P., et al. (2016). Experience of the use of ketamine to manage opioid withdrawal in an addicted woman: A case report. *BMC Psychiatry, 16*, 395.

Lee, K., Ganta, N., Horton, J., et al. (2016). Evidence for neurotoxicity due to morphine or hydromorphone use in renal impairment: A systematic review. *Journal of Palliat Medicine, 19*(11), 1179–1187.

Lexicomp. (2018a). *Clinical drug information. Morphine (systemic).* Wolters Kluwer. Retrieved from https://online.lexi.com/lco/action/doc/retrieve/docid/patch_f/1799128#mop.

Lexicomp. (2018b). *Clinical drug information. Fentanyl.* Wolters Kluwer. Retrieved from https://online.lexi.com/lco/action/doc/retrieve/docid/patch_f/6903#f_pharmacology-and-pharmacokinetics.

Lexicomp. (2018c). *Clinical drug information. Oxycodone.* Wolters Kluwer. Retrieved from https://online.lexi.com/lco/action/doc/retrieve/docid/patch_f/7416#f_pharmacology-and-pharmacokinetics.

Lynch, M. E., & Katz, J. (2017). "One Size Fits All" doesn't fit when it comes to long-term opioid use for people with chronic pain.

Makey, S. (2015). The "Continuum of Pain" and the American Academy of Pain Medicine. *Pain Medicine, 16*(3), 413–415.

Malanga, G., Yan, N., & Stark, J. (2014). Mechanisms and efficacy of heat and cold therapies for musculoskeletal injury. *Postgraduate Medicine, 127*(1), 57–65.

McCormick, T., & Law, S. (2016). Assessment of acute and chronic pain. *Anaesthesia & Intensive Care Medicine, 17*(9), 421–424.

McEntire, D. M., Kirkpatrick, D. R., Dueck, N. P., et al. (2016). Pain transduction: A pharmacologic perspective. *Expert Review of Clinical Pharmacology*. http://doi.org/10.1080/17512433.2016.1183481.

Melzack, R. (1996). Gate control theory: On the evolution of pain concepts. *The Journal of Pain, 5*(2), 128–138.

Mu, A., Weinberg, E., Moulin, D. E., et al. (2017). Pharmacologic management of chronic neuropathic pain: Review of the Canadian Pain Society consensus statement. *Canadian Family Physician, 63*(11), 844–852.

Murphy, P., Kreling, B., Kathryn, E., et al. (2000). Description of the SUPPORT intervention. Study to Understand Prognosis and Preferences for Outcomes and Risks of Treatment. *Journal of The American Gerontological Society, 48*(Suppl 5), S154–161.

Nelson, A. D., & Camilleri, M. (2016). Opioid-induced constipation: Advances and clinical guidance. *Therapeutic Advances in Chronic Disease, 7*(2), 121–134.

Panahi, Y., Dehcheshmeh, H. S., Mojtahedzadeh, M., et al. (2018). Analgesic and sedative agents used in the intensive care unit: A review. *Journal of Cellular Biochemistry, 119*(11), 8684–8693.

Pham, P. C., Khaing, K., Sievers, T. M., et al. (2017). 2017 update on pain management in patients with chronic kidney disease. *Clinical Kidney Journal, 10*(5), 688–697.

Purdue Pharma. (2018). *OxyNeo-product monograph*. Retrieved from http://purdue.ca/wp-content/uploads/2018/02/Oxyneo-PM-EN.pdf

Reis, A., Luecke, C., Davis, T. K., et al. (2018). Pain management in pediatric chronic kidney disease. *The Journal of Pediatric Pharmacology and Therapeutics, 23*(3), 192–202.

Reitsma, M. L., Tranmer, J. E., Buchanan, D. M., et al. (2012). The epidemiology of chronic pain in Canadian men and women between 1994 and 2007: Results from the longitudinal component of the National Population Health survey. *Pain Research & Management, 17*(3), 166–172.

Riquelme, I., Hatem, S. M., & Montoya, P. (2016). Abnormal pressure pain, touch sensitivity, proprioception, and manual dexterity in children with autism spectrum disorders. *Neural Plasticity*, 2016. http://doi.org/10.1155/2016/1723401.

Rothaug, J., Weiss, T., & Meissner, W. (2013). How simple can it get? Measuring pain with NRS items or binary items. *Clinical Journal of Pain, 29*(3), 224–232.

Sateia, M. J., Buysse, D. J., Krystal, A. D., et al. (2017). Clinical practice guideline for the pharmacologic treatment of chronic insomnia in adults: An American Academy of Sleep Medicine clinical practice guideline. *Journal of Clinical Sleep Medicine, 13*(02), 307–349.

Savino, F., Vagliano, L., Ceratto, S., et al. (2013). Pain assessment in children undergoing venipuncture: The Wong–Baker faces scale versus skin conductance fluctuations. *PeerJ, 1*, e37.

Schopflocher, D., Taenzer, P., & Jovey, R. (2011). The prevalence of chronic pain in Canada. *Pain Research and Management, 16*(6), 445–450.

Seth, B., & de Gray, L. (2016). Genesis of chronic pain. *Anaesthesia & Intensive Care Medicine, 17*(9), 431–435.

Shapiro, M., Kvern, B., Watson, P., et al. (2011). Update on herpes zoster vaccination: A family practitioners guide. *Canadian Family Physician, 57*(10), 1127–1131.

Steeds, C. E. (2016). The anatomy and physiology of pain. *Surgery (Oxford), 34*(2), 55–59.

Sukcharoen, K., Jeffery, Z., Ratcliffe, L., et al. (2018). Prescribing analgesia for patients with impaired renal function. *British Journal of Hospital Medicine, 79*(5), C74–C77.

Sullivan, M. D.(2017). How chronic pain treatment falls short of patient-centered care. *NEJM Catalyst*. Retrieved from https://catalyst.nejm.org/chronic-pain-care-falls-short/.

Tannenbaum, C., Clow, B., Haworth-Brockman, M., et al. (2017). Sex and gender considerations in Canadian clinical practice guidelines: A systematic review. *CMAJ Open, 5*(1), E66–E73.

Templeman, E. (2017). *How should conversion from oral morphine to fentanyl patches be carried out. UK medicine information. NHS*. Retrieved from https://www.sps.nhs.uk/wp-content/uploads/2017/12/UKMI_QA_Conversion-from-oral-morphine-to-fentanyl-patches_November-2017_Final.docx.

The National Academies of Sciences, Engineering and Medicine. (2017). *Guide to help health clinicians counter the opioid epidemic*. Retrieved from http://www8.nationalacademies.org/onpinews/newsitem.aspx?RecordID=9212017.

Thieme, K., Mathys, M., & Turk, D. C. (2017). Evidenced-based guidelines on the treatment of fibromyalgia patients: Are they consistent and if not, why not? Have effective psychological treatments been overlooked?. *The Journal of Pain, 18*(7), 747–756.

Thompson, J. M., & Neugebauer, V. (2017). Amygdala plasticity and pain. *Pain Research and Management, 2017*. http://doi.org/10.1155/2017/8296501.

Torrance, N., Ferguson, J. A., Afolabi, E., et al. (2013). Neuropathic pain in the community: More undertreated than refractory? *Pain, 154*, 690–699.

Tsze, D. S., von Baeyer, C. L., Bulloch, B., et al. (2013). Validation of self-report pain scales in children. *Pediatrics, 132*(4), e971–e979.

West, S. J., Bannister, K., Dickenson, A. H., et al. (2015). Circuitry and plasticity of the dorsal horn—Toward a better understanding of neuropathic pain. *Neuroscience, 300*, 254–275.

Wick, E. C., Grant, M. C., & Wu, C. L. (2017). Postoperative multimodal analgesia pain management with nonopioid analgesics and techniques: A review. *JAMA Surg, 152*(7), 691–697.

Wolters Kluwer Health. (2017). *Cognitive behavioral therapy for chronic pain: Can CBT help fight the opioid epidemic?* Retrieved May 27, 2018, from www.sciencedaily.com/releases/2017/11/171109131231.htm-www.sciencedaily.com/releases/2017/11/171109131231.htm.

Wong, J. J., Côté, P., Sutton, D. A., et al. (2017). Clinical practice guidelines for the noninvasive management of low back pain: A systematic review by the Ontario Protocol for Traffic Injury Management (OPTIMa) Collaboration. *European journal of pain, 21*(2), 201–216.

Xiao, J., Zeng, S., Wang, X., et al. (2016). Neurokinin 1 and opioid receptors: Relationships and interactions in nervous system. *Translational Perioperative and Pain Medicine, 1*(3), 11–21. http://doi.org/10.1037/neu0000164.Betting.

Young, J. R., Sih, C., Hogg, M. M., et al. (2018). Qualitative assessment of face validity and cross-cultural acceptability of the faces pain scale: "Revised" in Cameroon. *Qualitative Health Research, 28*(5), 832–843.

Zhou, J., Fan, Y., Zhong, J., et al. (2017). Efficacy and safety of multimodal analgesic techniques for preventing chronic postsurgery pain under different surgical categories: A meta-analysis. *Scientific Reports, 7*, 678.

Resources

Canadian Pain Coalition: http://www.rsdcanada.org/parc/english/resources/coalition.htm

Canadian Pain Society: http://www.canadianpainsociety.ca

Chronic Pain Association of Canada: http://www.chronicpaincanada.com

Institute for the Relief of Pain and Disability: http://www.cirpd.org

17 Fluid and Electrolytes: Balance and Disturbance

Adapted by Alice S.W. Khin

Learning Objectives

On completion of this chapter, the learner will be able to:

1. Differentiate between osmosis, diffusion, filtration, and active transport.
2. Describe the role of the kidneys, lungs, and endocrine glands in regulating the body's fluid composition and volume.
3. Identify the effects of aging on fluid and electrolyte regulation.
4. Plan effective care of patients with the following imbalances: fluid volume deficit and fluid volume excess; sodium deficit (hyponatremia) and sodium excess (hypernatremia); potassium deficit (hypokalemia) and potassium excess (hyperkalemia).
5. Describe the cause, clinical manifestations, management, and nursing interventions for the following imbalances: calcium deficit (hypocalcemia) and calcium excess (hypercalcemia); magnesium deficit (hypomagnesemia) and magnesium excess (hypermagnesemia); phosphorus deficit (hypophosphatemia) and phosphorus excess (hyperphosphatemia); chloride deficit (hypochloremia) and chloride excess (hyperchloremia).
6. Explain the roles of the chemical buffers, lungs, and kidneys in maintaining acid–base balance.
7. Compare metabolic acidosis and alkalosis with regard to causes, clinical manifestations, diagnosis, and management.
8. Compare respiratory acidosis and alkalosis with regard to causes, clinical manifestations, diagnosis, and management.
9. Interpret arterial blood gas measurements.

Fluid and electrolyte balance is a dynamic process that is crucial for life and **homeostasis**. Potential and actual disorders of fluid and electrolyte balance occur in every setting, with every disorder, and with a variety of changes that affect healthy people (e.g., increased fluid and sodium loss with strenuous exercise and high environmental temperature, inadequate intake of fluid and electrolytes) as well as those who are ill.

Fundamental Concepts

Nurses need an understanding of the physiology of fluid and electrolyte balance and acid–base balance to anticipate, identify, and respond to possible imbalances (Hannon & Porth, 2017). Nurses also must use effective teaching and communication skills to help prevent and treat various fluid and electrolyte disturbances.

Amount and Composition of Body Fluids

Approximately 60% of the weight of a typical adult consists of fluid (water and electrolytes). Factors that influence the amount of body fluid are age, gender, and body fat. In general, younger people have a higher percentage of body fluid than older adults, and men have proportionately more body fluid than women. People who have obesity have less fluid than those who are thin, because fat cells contain little water. The skeleton also has a low water content. Muscle, skin, and blood have the highest amount of water (Grossman & Porth, 2014).

Body fluid is located in two fluid compartments: the intracellular space (fluid in the cells) and the extracellular space (fluid outside the cells). Approximately two thirds of body fluid is in the intracellular fluid (ICF) compartment and is located primarily in the skeletal muscle mass. Approximately one third is in the extracellular fluid (ECF) compartment (Grossman & Porth, 2014).

The ECF compartment is further divided into the intravascular, interstitial, and transcellular fluid spaces:

- The intravascular space (the fluid within the blood vessels) contains plasma, the effective circulating volume. Approximately 3 L of the average 6 L of blood volume in adults is made up of plasma. The remaining 3 L is made up of erythrocytes, leukocytes, and thrombocytes.
- The interstitial space contains the fluid that surrounds the cell and totals about 11 to 12 L in an adult. Lymph is an interstitial fluid.
- The transcellular space is the smallest division of the ECF compartment and contains approximately 1 L. Examples of transcellular fluids include cerebrospinal, pericardial, synovial, intraocular, and pleural fluids, sweat, and digestive secretions.

As the next section describes, the ECF transports electrolytes; it also carries other substances, such as enzymes and hormones.

Body fluid usually moves between the two major compartments or spaces in an effort to maintain equilibrium between the spaces. Loss of fluid from the body can disrupt this equilibrium. Sometimes fluid is not lost from the body but is unavailable for use by either the ICF or ECF. Loss of ECF into a space that does not contribute to equilibrium between the ICF and the ECF is referred to as a third-space fluid shift, or "third spacing" for short (Papadakis & McPhee, 2016).

Early evidence of a third-space fluid shift is a decrease in urine output despite adequate fluid intake. Urine output decreases because fluid shifts out of the intravascular space; the kidneys then receive less blood and attempt to compensate by decreasing urine output. Other signs and symptoms of third spacing that indicate an intravascular fluid volume deficit (FVD) include increased heart rate, decreased blood pressure, decreased central venous pressure, edema, increased body weight, and imbalances in fluid intake and output (I&O). Examples of causes of third-space fluid losses include intestinal obstruction, pancreatitis, crushing traumatic injuries, bleeding (trauma or dissected aortic aneurysm), peritonitis, and major venous obstruction (Sterns, 2014).

Electrolytes

Electrolytes in body fluids are active chemicals (cations that carry positive charges and anions that carry negative charges). The major cations in body fluid are sodium, potassium, calcium, magnesium, and hydrogen ions. The major anions are chloride, bicarbonate, phosphate, sulphate, and proteinate ions.

These chemicals unite in varying combinations. Therefore, electrolyte concentration in the body is expressed in terms of millimoles (mmol) per litre, a measure of chemical activity, rather than in terms of milligrams (mg), a unit

Glossary

acidosis: an acid-base imbalance characterized by an increase in H^+ concentration (decreased blood pH). A low arterial pH due to reduced bicarbonate concentration is called metabolic acidosis; a low arterial pH due to increased PCO_2 is respiratory acidosis

active transport: physiologic pump that moves fluid from an area of lower concentration to one of higher concentration; active transport requires adenosine triphosphate for energy

ascites: a type of edema in which fluid accumulates in the peritoneal cavity

alkalosis: an acid-base imbalance characterized by a reduction in H^+ concentration (increased blood pH). A high arterial pH with increased bicarbonate concentration is called metabolic alkalosis; a high arterial pH due to reduced PCO_2 is respiratory alkalosis

diffusion: the process by which solutes move from an area of higher concentration to one of lower concentration; does not require expenditure of energy

homeostasis: maintenance of a constant internal equilibrium in a biologic system that involves positive and negative feedback mechanisms

hydrostatic pressure: the pressure created by the weight of fluid against the wall that contains it. In the body, hydrostatic pressure in blood vessels results from the weight of fluid itself and the force resulting from cardiac contraction

hypertonic solution: a solution with an osmolality higher than that of serum

hypotonic solution: a solution with an osmolality lower than that of serum

isotonic solution: a solution with the same osmolality as serum and other body fluids. Osmolality falls within normal range for serum (280 to 300 mOsm/kg)

osmolality: the number of osmoles (the standard unit of osmotic pressure) per kilogram of solution. Expressed as mOsm/kg, osmolality is used more often than the term *osmolarity* to evaluate serum and urine

osmolarity: the number of osmoles (the standard unit of osmotic pressure) per litre of solution. It is expressed as milliosmoles per litre (mOsm/L); describes the concentration of solutes or dissolved particles

osmosis: the process by which fluid moves across a semipermeable membrane from an area of low solute concentration to an area of high solute concentration; the process continues until the solute concentrations are equal on both sides of the membrane

tonicity: fluid tension or the effect that osmotic pressure of a solution with impermeable solutes exerts on cell size because of water movement across the cell membrane of weight. More specifically, a millimole is defined as being equivalent to the electrochemical activity of 1 mg of hydrogen. In a solution, cations and anions are equal in millimoles per litre.

Electrolyte concentrations in the ICF differ from those in the ECF. Because special techniques are required to measure electrolyte concentrations in the ICF, it is customary to measure the electrolytes in the most accessible portion of the ECF, namely, the plasma.

Sodium ions, which are positively charged, far outnumber the other cations in the ECF. Because sodium concentration affects the overall concentration of the ECF, sodium is important in regulating the volume of body fluid. Retention of sodium is associated with fluid retention, and excessive loss of sodium is usually associated with decreased volume of body fluid.

The major electrolytes in the ICF are potassium and phosphate. The ECF has a low concentration of potassium and can tolerate only small changes in potassium concentrations. Therefore, release of large stores of intracellular potassium, typically caused by trauma to the cells and tissues, can be extremely dangerous.

The body expends a great deal of energy maintaining the high extracellular concentration of sodium and the high intracellular concentration of potassium. It does so by means of cell membrane pumps that exchange sodium and potassium ions. Usual movement of fluids through the capillary wall into the tissues depends on **hydrostatic pressure** (the pressure exerted by the fluid on the walls of the blood vessel) at both the arterial and venous ends of the vessel and the osmotic pressure exerted by the protein of plasma. The direction of fluid movement depends on the differences in these two opposing forces (hydrostatic vs. osmotic pressure).

Regulation of Body Fluid Compartments

CONCEPTS IN ACTION

Osmosis and Osmolality

When two different solutions are separated by a membrane that is impermeable to the dissolved substances, fluid shifts through the membrane from the region of low solute concentration to the region of high solute concentration until the solutions are of equal concentration. This **diffusion** of water caused by a fluid concentration gradient is known as **osmosis** (Fig. 17-1A). The magnitude of this force depends on the number of particles dissolved in the solutions, not on their weights. The number of dissolved particles contained in a unit of fluid determines the **osmolality** of a solution, which influences the movement of fluid between the fluid compartments. **Tonicity** is the

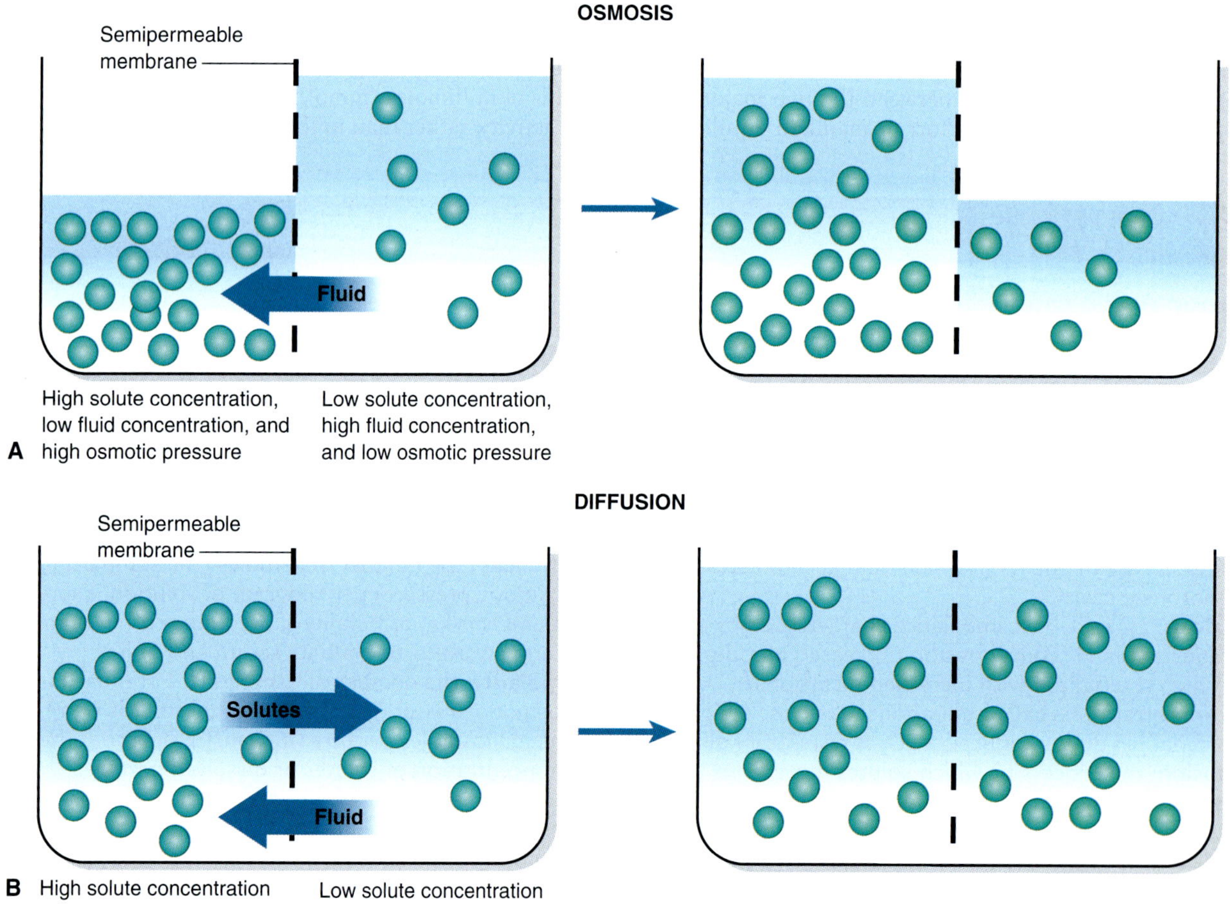

FIGURE 17-1. **A.** Osmosis: movement of fluid from an area of lower solute concentration to an area of higher solute concentration with eventual equalization of the solute concentrations. **B.** Diffusion: movement of solutes from an area of greater concentration to an area of lesser concentration, leading ultimately to equalization of the solute concentrations.

ability of all the solutes to cause an osmotic driving force that promotes water movement from one compartment to another. The control of tonicity determines the normal state of cellular hydration and cell size. Sodium, mannitol, glucose, and sorbitol are effective osmoles (capable of affecting water movement). Three other terms are associated with osmosis: osmotic pressure, oncotic pressure, and osmotic diuresis.

- Osmotic pressure is the amount of hydrostatic pressure needed to stop the flow of water by osmosis. It is primarily determined by the concentration of solutes.
- Oncotic pressure is the osmotic pressure exerted by proteins (e.g., albumin).
- Osmotic diuresis is the increase in urine output caused by the excretion of substances such as glucose, mannitol, or contrast agents in the urine.

Diffusion

Diffusion is the natural tendency of a substance to move from an area of higher concentration to one of lower concentration (see Fig. 17-1B). It occurs through the random movement of ions and molecules (Grossman & Porth, 2014). Examples of diffusion are the exchange of oxygen and carbon dioxide between the pulmonary capillaries and alveoli and the tendency of sodium to move from the ECF compartment, where the sodium concentration is high, to the ICF, where its concentration is low.

Filtration

Hydrostatic pressure in the capillaries tends to filter fluid out of the intravascular compartment into the interstitial fluid. Movement of water and solutes occurs from an area of high hydrostatic pressure to an area of low hydrostatic pressure. The kidneys filter approximately 180 L of plasma per day. Another example of filtration is the passage of water and electrolytes from the arterial capillary bed to the interstitial fluid; in this instance, the hydrostatic pressure results from the pumping action of the heart.

Sodium–Potassium Pump

As previously stated, the sodium concentration is greater in the ECF than in the ICF, and because of this, sodium tends to enter the cell by diffusion. This tendency is offset by the sodium–potassium pump that is maintained by the cell membrane and actively moves sodium from the cell into the ECF. Conversely, the high intracellular potassium concentration is maintained by pumping potassium into the cell. By definition, **active transport** implies that energy must be expended for the movement to occur against a concentration gradient.

Systemic Routes of Gains and Losses

Water and electrolytes are gained in various ways. Healthy people gain fluids by drinking and eating, and their daily average I&O of water is approximately equal (Table 17-1).

Kidneys

The usual daily urine volume in the adult is 1 to 2 L (Grossman & Porth, 2014; Sterns, 2014). A general rule is that the output is approximately 1 mL of urine per kilogram of body weight per hour (1 mL/kg/hr) in all age groups.

TABLE 17-1 Average Daily Intake and Output in an Adult

Intake (mL)		Output (mL)	
Oral intake		Urine	1,500
As water	1,000	Stool	200
In food	1,300	Insensible	
Water of oxidation	200	Lungs	300
		Skin	500
Total gain[a]	2,500	Total loss[a]	2,500

[a]Approximate volumes.

Adapted with permission from Grossman, S. C., & Porth, C. M. (2014). *Porth's pathophysiology: Concepts of altered health states* (9th ed.). Philadelphia, PA: Lippincott Williams & Wilkins.

Skin

Sensible perspiration refers to visible water and electrolyte loss through the skin (sweating). The chief solutes in sweat are sodium, chloride, and potassium. Actual sweat losses can vary from 0 to 1,000 mL or more every hour, depending on factors such as the environmental temperature. Continuous water loss by evaporation (approximately 600 mL/day) occurs through the skin as insensible perspiration, a nonvisible form of water loss (Grossman & Porth, 2014). Fever greatly increases insensible water loss through the lungs and the skin, as does loss of the natural skin barrier (e.g., through major burns; Earhart, Weiss, Rahman, et al., 2015; Sterns, 2014).

Lungs

The lungs usually eliminate water vapour (insensible loss) at a rate of approximately 300 mL every day (Grossman & Porth, 2014). The loss is much greater with increased respiratory rate or depth, or in a dry climate.

Gastrointestinal Tract

The usual loss through the GI tract is 100 to 200 mL daily, even though approximately 8 L of fluid circulates through the GI system every 24 hours. Because the bulk of fluid is usually reabsorbed in the small intestine, diarrhea and fistulas cause large losses.

NURSING ALERT

When fluid balance is critical, all routes of systemic gain and loss must be recorded and all volumes compared. Organs of fluid loss include the kidneys, skin, lungs, and gastrointestinal (GI) tract.

Laboratory Tests for Evaluating Fluid Status

Osmolality is the concentration of fluid that affects the movement of water between fluid compartments by osmosis. Osmolality measures the solute concentration per kilogram in body fluids. It is also a measure of a solution's ability to create osmotic pressure and affect the movement of water. Serum osmolality primarily reflects the concentration of sodium, although blood urea nitrogen (BUN)

TABLE 17-2 Factors Affecting Serum and Urine Osmolality

Fluid	Factors Increasing Osmolality	Factors Decreasing Osmolality
Serum (275–290 mOsm/kg water)	Severe dehydration Free water loss Diabetes insipidus Hypernatremia Hyperglycemia Stroke or head injury Renal tubular necrosis Consumption of methanol or ethylene glycol (antifreeze) High ion gap metabolic acidosis Mannitol therapy Advanced liver disease Alcoholism Burns	Fluid volume excess Syndrome of inappropriate antidiuretic hormone (SIADH) Acute kidney injury Diuretic use Adrenal insufficiency Hyponatremia Overhydration Paraneoplastic syndrome associated with lung cancer
Urine (200–800 mOsm/kg water)	Fluid volume deficit SIADH Congestive heart failure Acidosis Prerenal failure	Fluid volume excess Diabetes insipidus Hyponatremia Aldosteronism Pyelonephritis Acute tubular necrosis

Adapted from Grossman, S. C., & Porth, C. M. (2014). *Porth's pathophysiology: Concepts of altered health states* (9th ed.). Philadelphia, PA: Lippincott Williams & Wilkins.

and glucose also play a major role in determining serum osmolality. Urine osmolality is determined by urea, creatinine, and uric acid. When measured with serum osmolality, urine osmolality is the most reliable indicator of urine concentration. Osmolality is reported as milliosmoles per kilogram of water (mOsm/kg) (Hannon and Porth, 2017).

In healthy adults, serum osmolality is 280 to 300 mmol/kg (Medical Council of Canada, 2019) (https://mcc.ca/objectives/normal-values). Sodium predominates in ECF osmolality and holds water in this compartment. Factors that increase and decrease serum and urine osmolality are identified in Table 17-2. Serum osmolality may be measured directly through laboratory tests or estimated at the bedside by doubling the serum sodium level or by using the following formula:

$$Na^{+} \times 2 = \frac{\text{Glucose}}{18} + \frac{\text{BUN}}{3} = \begin{array}{l}\text{Approximate value}\\ \text{of serum osmolality}\end{array}$$

Osmolarity, another term that describes the concentration of solutions, is measured in millimoles per litre (mmol/L). However, the term osmolality is used more often in clinical practice. The calculated value usually is within 10 mmol of the measured osmolality.

Urine specific gravity measures the kidneys' ability to excrete or conserve water. The specific gravity of urine is compared to the weight of distilled water, which has a specific gravity of 1.000. The usual range of urine specific gravity is 1.010 to 1.025. Urine specific gravity can be measured at the bedside by placing a calibrated hydrometer or urinometer in a cylinder of approximately 20 mL of urine. Specific gravity can also be assessed with a refractometer or dipstick with a reagent for this purpose. Specific gravity varies inversely with urine volume; usually, the larger the volume of urine, the lower the specific gravity is. Specific gravity is a less reliable indicator of concentration than urine osmolality; increased glucose or protein in urine can cause a falsely elevated specific gravity. Factors that increase or decrease urine osmolality are the same as those for urine specific gravity.

BUN is made up of urea, which is an end product of the metabolism of protein (from both muscle and dietary intake), by the liver. Amino acid breakdown produces large amounts of ammonia molecules, which are absorbed into the bloodstream. Ammonia molecules are converted to urea and excreted in the urine. The normal BUN is 3.6 to 7.2 mmol/L. The BUN level varies with urine output. Factors that increase BUN include decreased renal function, GI bleeding, dehydration, increased protein intake, fever, and sepsis. Those that decrease BUN include end-stage liver disease, a low protein diet, starvation, and any condition that results in expanded fluid volume (e.g., pregnancy).

Creatinine is the end product of muscle metabolism. It is a better indicator of renal function than BUN because it does not vary with protein intake and metabolic state. The normal serum creatinine is approximately 62 to 124 mmol/L; however, its concentration depends on lean body mass and varies from person to person. Serum creatinine levels increase when renal function decreases.

Hematocrit measures the volume percentage of red blood cells (erythrocytes) in whole blood and usually ranges from 0.440 to 0.520 for males and 0.397 to 0.470 for females. Conditions that increase the hematocrit value are dehydration and polycythemia, and those that decrease hematocrit are overhydration and anemia.

Urine sodium values change with sodium intake and the status of fluid volume: As sodium intake increases, excretion increases; as the circulating fluid volume decreases, sodium is conserved. Normal urine sodium levels range from 75 to 200 mmol/24 hr. A random specimen usually contains more than 40 mmol/L of sodium. Urine sodium levels are used to assess volume status and are useful in the diagnosis of hyponatremia and acute kidney injury.

Homeostatic Mechanisms

The body is equipped with remarkable homeostatic mechanisms to keep the composition and volume of body fluid within narrow limits of normal. Organs involved in homeostasis include the kidneys, lungs, heart, adrenal glands, parathyroid glands, and pituitary gland (Hannon & Porth, 2017).

Kidney Functions

Vital to the regulation of fluid and electrolyte balance, the kidneys normally filter 180 L of plasma every day in the adult and excrete 1 to 2 L of urine. They act both autonomously and in response to blood-borne messengers, such as aldosterone and antidiuretic hormone (ADH) (Hannon & Porth, 2017). Major functions of the kidneys in maintaining expected fluid balance include the following:

- Regulation of ECF volume and osmolality by selective retention and excretion of body fluids
- Regulation of usual electrolyte levels in the ECF by selective electrolyte retention and excretion
- Regulation of pH of the ECF by retention of hydrogen ions
- Excretion of metabolic wastes and toxic substances

Given these functions, failure of the kidneys results in multiple fluid and electrolyte abnormalities.

Heart and Blood Vessel Functions

The pumping action of the heart circulates blood through the kidneys under sufficient pressure to allow for urine formation. Failure of this pumping action interferes with renal perfusion and thus with water and electrolyte regulation.

Lung Functions

The lungs are also vital in maintaining homeostasis. Through exhalation, the lungs remove approximately 300 mL of water daily in the average adult. Abnormal conditions, such as hyperpnea (abnormally deep respiration) or continuous coughing, increase this loss; mechanical ventilation with excessive moisture decreases it. The lungs also play a major role in maintaining acid–base balance.

Pituitary Functions

The hypothalamus manufactures ADH, which is stored in the posterior pituitary gland and released as needed to conserve water. Functions of ADH include maintaining the osmotic pressure of the cells by controlling the retention or excretion of water by the kidneys and by regulating blood volume (Fig. 17-2).

Adrenal Functions

Aldosterone, a mineralocorticoid secreted by the zona glomerulosa (outer zone) of the adrenal cortex, has a profound effect on fluid balance (see Chart 17-1). Increased secretion of aldosterone causes sodium retention (and thus water retention) and potassium loss. Conversely, decreased secretion of aldosterone causes sodium and water loss and potassium retention.

Cortisol, another adrenocortical hormone, has less mineralocorticoid action. However, when secreted in large quantities (or administered as corticosteroid therapy), it can also produce sodium and fluid retention.

Parathyroid Functions

The parathyroid glands, embedded in the thyroid gland, regulate calcium and phosphate balance by means of parathyroid hormone (PTH). PTH influences bone resorption, calcium absorption from the intestines, and calcium reabsorption from the renal tubules.

Other Mechanisms

Changes in the volume of the interstitial compartment within the ECF can occur without affecting body function. However, the vascular compartment cannot tolerate change as readily and must be carefully maintained to ensure that tissues receive adequate nutrients.

Baroreceptors

The baroreceptors are located in the left atrium and the carotid and aortic arches. These receptors respond to changes in the circulating blood volume and regulate sympathetic and parasympathetic neural activity as well as endocrine activities (Hall, 2015).

As arterial pressure decreases, baroreceptors transmit fewer impulses from the carotid and the aortic arches to the vasomotor centre. A decrease in impulses stimulates the sympathetic nervous system and inhibits the parasympathetic nervous system. The outcome is an increase in cardiac rate, conduction, and contractility and an increase in circulating blood volume. Sympathetic stimulation constricts renal arterioles; this increases the release of aldosterone, decreases glomerular filtration, and increases sodium and water reabsorption.

Renin–Angiotensin–Aldosterone System

Renin is an enzyme that converts angiotensinogen, a substance formed by the liver, into angiotensin I (Hannon & Porth, 2017). Renin is released by the juxtaglomerular cells of the kidneys in response to decreased renal perfusion. Angiotensin-converting enzyme (ACE) converts angiotensin I to angiotensin II. Angiotensin II, with its vasoconstrictor properties, increases arterial perfusion pressure and stimulates thirst. As the sympathetic nervous system is stimulated, aldosterone is released in response to an increased release of renin. Aldosterone is a volume regulator and is also released as serum potassium increases, serum sodium decreases, or adrenocorticotropic hormone (ACTH) increases.

Antidiuretic Hormone and Thirst

ADH and the thirst mechanism have important roles in maintaining sodium concentration and oral intake of fluids. Oral intake is controlled by the thirst centre located in the hypothalamus (Sterns, 2014). As serum concentration or osmolality increases or blood volume decreases, neurons in the hypothalamus are stimulated by intracellular dehydration; thirst then occurs, and the person increases his or her intake of oral fluids. Water excretion is controlled by ADH, aldosterone, and baroreceptors, as mentioned previously. The presence or absence of ADH is the most significant factor in determining whether the urine that is excreted is concentrated or dilute.

Physiology/Pathophysiology

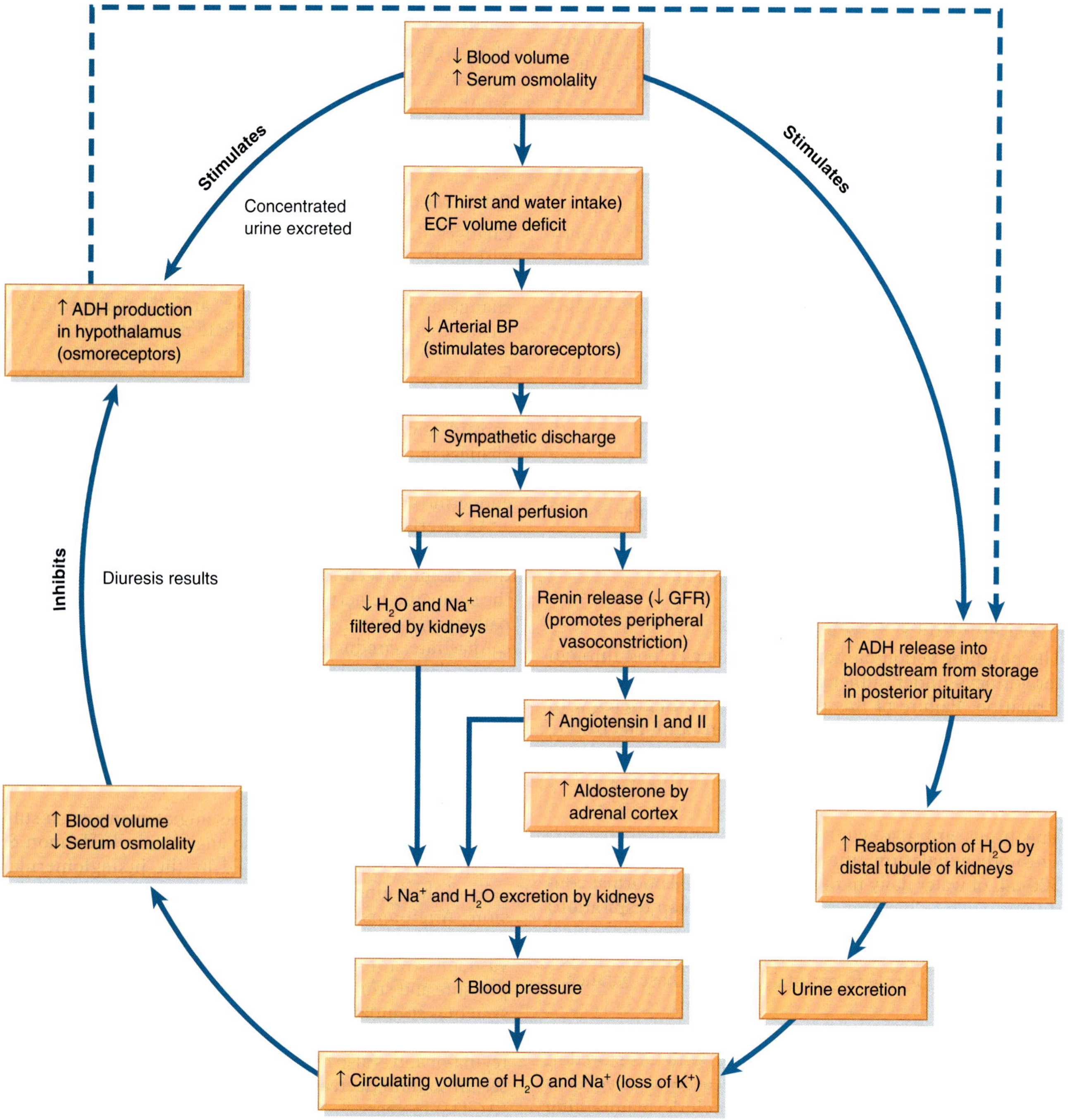

FIGURE 17-2. Fluid regulation cycle. ADH, antidiuretic hormone; BP, blood pressure; ECF, extracellular fluid; GFR, glomerular filtration rate.

Osmoreceptors

Located on the surface of the hypothalamus, osmoreceptors sense changes in sodium concentration. As osmotic pressure increases, the neurons become dehydrated and quickly release impulses to the posterior pituitary, which increases the release of ADH, which then travels in the blood to the kidneys, where it alters permeability to water, causing increased reabsorption of water and decreased urine output. The retained water dilutes the ECF and returns its concentration to normal. Restoration of normal osmotic pressure provides feedback to the osmoreceptors to inhibit further ADH release (see Fig. 17-2).

Release of Atrial Natriuretic Peptide

Natriuretic peptide hormones affect fluid volume and cardiovascular function through the excretion of sodium (natriuresis), direct vasodilation, and the opposition of the rennin–angiotensin–aldosterone system. Four peptides have been identified. The first is atrial natriuretic peptide (ANP) produced by the atrial myocardium with tissue

NURSING RESEARCH PROFILE

Chart 17-1. Monitoring Intake and Output in Patients in the ICU

Diacon, A., & Bell, J. (2014). Investigating the recording and accuracy of fluid balance monitoring in critically ill patients. *South African Journal of Critical Care*, *30*(2), 55–57.

Purpose

Studies suggest that an accurate I&O can have a significant impact on morbidity and mortality in critically ill patients. This study was designed to determine the current practices of fluid balance monitoring of registered nurses in intensive care units (ICUs).

Design

This was a quantitative study using an exploratory, descriptive design. The setting consisted of three ICUs within one hospital group. All three ICUs were similar in terms of patient profiles and size. An audit tool was developed and reviewed by two clinical intensive care nurse experts to determine its face validity. Medical records of patients who were admitted during a certain time frame, within age parameters, and met critical care patient classification were included for sampling purposes. The study used a simple random sampling technique to select records for inclusion. Each patient's recorded fluid balance was calculated for a 24-hour period during the first 48 hours after admission and compared with audited calculations.

Findings

Out of 103 audited ICU patient records, 5 (2%) had a fluid deviation less than 500 mL; 71 (68.9%) had a fluid deviation within 500 mL; 14 (13.5%) were identified as deviating between 500 and 1,000 mL when compared to the audited calculations; 7 (6.8%) showed a deviation between 1,000 and 2,000 mL; and 6 (5.8%) revealed a deviation greater than 2,000 mL when compared to the audited calculations. There was a significant association between the administration of diuretics and inaccurate fluid balance documentation ($p = 0.01$), but no association with any other variables.

Nursing Implications

This study identified that I&O was not being accurately measured in the critically ill patients in the ICUs studied. It is imperative that accurate calculations of fluid balance be an integral part of nursing practice in the ICU setting. Regular outcome-driven audits may help improve practice and thus impact the mortality of patients in the ICU setting.

distribution in the cardiac atria and ventricles. The second is brain natriuretic peptide (BNP) produced by the ventricular myocardium with tissue distribution in the brain and cardiac ventricles (Colucci & Chen, 2014). ANP, also called *atrial natriuretic factor, atrial natriuretic hormone,* or *atriopeptin,* is a peptide that is synthesized, stored, and released by muscle cells of the atria of the heart in response to several factors. These factors include increased atrial pressure, angiotensin II stimulation, endothelin (a powerful vasoconstrictor of vascular smooth muscle that is a peptide released from damaged endothelial cells in the kidneys or other tissues), and sympathetic stimulation. Any condition that results in volume expansion (exercise, pregnancy), calorie restriction, hypoxia, or increased cardiac filling pressures (e.g., high sodium intake, heart failure, chronic kidney disease, atrial tachycardia, or use of vasoconstrictor agents such as epinephrine) increases the release of ANP and BNP. ANP's action decreases water, sodium, and adipose loads on the circulatory system to decrease blood pressure. The action of ANP is therefore directly opposite of the renin–angiotensin–aldosterone system (see Fig. 17-3). The ANP measured in plasma is normally 20 to 77 pg/mL (20 to 77 ng/L). This level increases in acute heart failure, paroxysmal supraventricular tachycardia, hyperthyroidism, subarachnoid hemorrhage, and small cell lung cancer. The level decreases in chronic heart failure and with the use of medications such as enalapril (Vasotec) (Frandsen & Pennington, 2014).

The third peptide is C-type natriuretic peptide (CNP), which has tissue distribution in the brain, ovary, uterus, testis, and epididymis. The fourth peptide is D-type natriuretic peptide (DNP)—the newest peptide with structural similarities to ANP, BNP, and CNP.

Gerontologic Considerations

Usual physiologic changes of aging, including reduced cardiac, renal, and respiratory function and reserve and alterations in the ratio of body fluids to muscle mass, may alter the responses of older adults to fluid and electrolyte changes and acid–base disturbances. Decreased respiratory function can cause impaired pH regulation in older adults with major illness or trauma. Renal function declines with age, as do muscle mass and daily exogenous creatinine production. Therefore, high-normal and minimally elevated serum creatinine values may indicate substantially reduced renal function in older adults.

In addition, the use of multiple medications by older adults can affect renal and cardiac functions, thereby increasing the likelihood of fluid and electrolyte disturbances. Routine procedures, such as the vigorous administration of laxatives or enemas before colon x-ray studies, may produce a serious FVD, necessitating the use of intravenous (IV) fluids to prevent hypotension and other effects of hypovolemia.

Alterations in fluid and electrolyte balance that may produce minor changes in young and middle-aged adults may produce profound changes in older adults. In many older adults, the clinical manifestations of fluid and electrolyte disturbances may be subtle or atypical. For example, fluid deficit may cause delirium in the older adult (see Chapter 14), whereas in the young or middle-aged person, the first sign commonly noticed is increased thirst. Rapid infusion of an excessive volume of IV fluids may produce fluid overload and cardiac failure in older adults. These reactions are likely to occur more quickly and with the administration of smaller volumes of fluid than in healthy

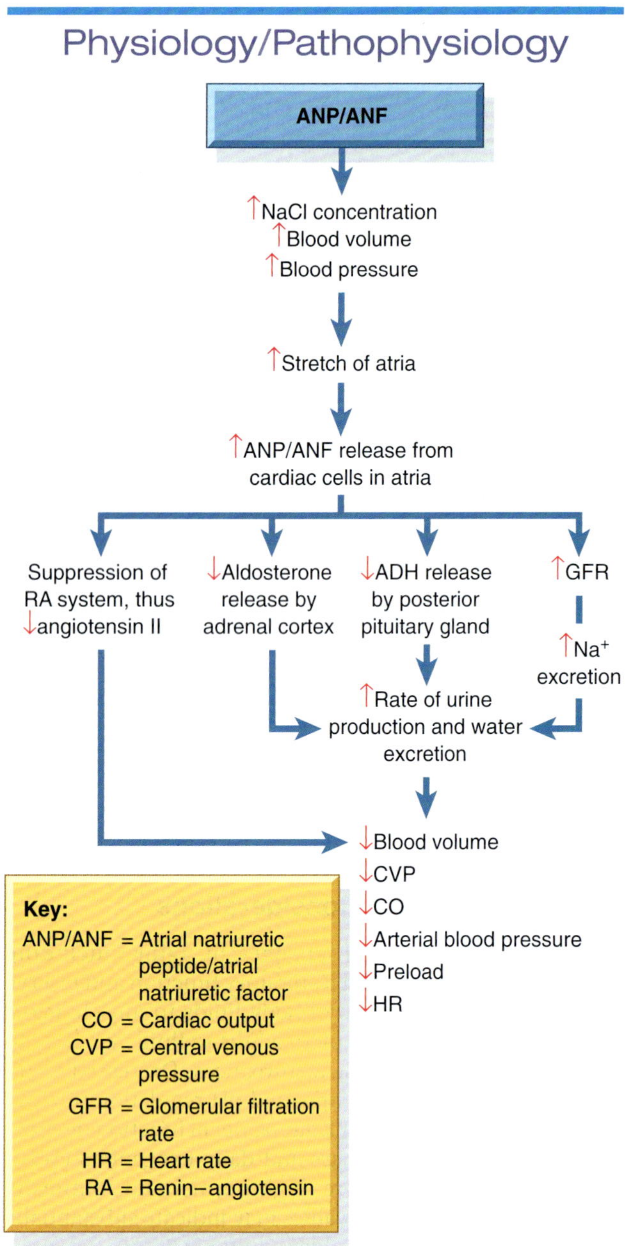

FIGURE 17-3. Role of ANP in maintenance of fluid balance.

young and middle-aged adults because of the decreased cardiac reserve and reduced renal function that accompany aging. Dehydration in older adults is common as a result of decreased kidney mass, decreased glomerular filtration rate, decreased renal blood flow, decreased ability to concentrate urine, inability to conserve sodium, decreased excretion of potassium, and a decrease of total body water.

FLUID VOLUME DISTURBANCES

Hypovolemia

FVD, or hypovolemia, occurs when loss of ECF volume exceeds the intake of fluid. It occurs when water and electrolytes are lost in the same proportion as they exist in normal body fluids, so that the ratio of serum electrolytes to water remains the same. FVD (hypovolemia) should not be confused with dehydration, which refers to loss of water alone, with increased serum sodium levels. FVD may occur alone or in combination with other imbalances. Unless other imbalances are present concurrently, serum electrolyte concentrations remain essentially unchanged.

Pathophysiology

FVD results from loss of body fluids and occurs more rapidly when coupled with decreased fluid intake. FVD can also develop with a prolonged period of inadequate intake. Causes of FVD include abnormal fluid losses, such as those resulting from vomiting, diarrhea, GI suctioning, and sweating; decreased intake, as in nausea or lack of access to fluids (Hall, 2015); and third-space fluid shifts, or the movement of fluid from the vascular system to other body spaces (e.g., with edema formation in burns, **ascites** with liver dysfunction). Additional causes include diabetes insipidus, adrenal insufficiency, osmotic diuresis, hemorrhage, and coma.

Clinical Manifestations

FVD can develop rapidly, and its severity depends on the degree of fluid loss. Clinical signs and symptoms and laboratory findings are presented in Table 17-3.

Assessment and Diagnostic Findings

Laboratory data useful in evaluating fluid volume status include BUN and its relation to serum creatinine concentration. A volume-depleted patient has a BUN elevated out of proportion to the serum creatinine (ratio greater than 20:1). The BUN can be elevated because of dehydration or decreased renal perfusion and function. The cause of hypovolemia may be determined through the health history and physical examination. Also, the hematocrit level is greater than normal because there is a decreased plasma volume (Hall, 2015).

Serum electrolyte changes may also exist. Potassium and sodium levels can be reduced (hypokalemia, hyponatremia) or elevated (hyperkalemia, hypernatremia).

- Hypokalemia occurs with GI and renal losses.
- Hyperkalemia occurs with adrenal insufficiency.
- Hyponatremia occurs with increased thirst and ADH release.
- Hypernatremia results from increased insensible losses and diabetes insipidus.

Urine specific gravity is increased in relation to the kidneys' attempt to conserve water and is decreased with diabetes insipidus. Aldosterone is secreted when fluid volume is low, causing reabsorption of sodium and chloride, resulting in decreased urinary sodium and chloride. Urine osmolality can be greater than 450 mmol/L because the kidneys try to compensate by conserving water.

Gerontologic Considerations

Increased sensitivity to fluid and electrolyte changes in older adults requires careful assessment of

TABLE 17-3 Fluid Volume Disturbances

Imbalance	Contributing Factors	Signs/Symptoms and Laboratory Findings
Fluid volume deficit (hypovolemia)	Loss of water and electrolytes, as in vomiting, diarrhea, fistulas, fever, excess sweating, burns, blood loss, gastrointestinal suction, and third-space fluid shifts; and decreased intake, as in anorexia, nausea, and inability to gain access to fluid. Diabetes insipidus and uncontrolled diabetes mellitus also contribute to a depletion of extracellular fluid volume.	Acute weight loss, ↓ skin turgor, oliguria, concentrated urine, weak rapid pulse, capillary filling time prolonged, low CVP, ↓ blood pressure, flattened neck veins, dizziness, weakness, thirst and confusion, ↑ pulse, muscle cramps, sunken eyes *Labs indicate:* ↑ hemoglobin and hematocrit, ↑ serum and urine osmolality and specific gravity, ↓ urine sodium, ↑ BUN and creatinine, ↑ urine specific gravity and osmolality
Fluid volume excess (hypervolemia)	Compromised regulatory mechanisms, such as renal failure, heart failure, and cirrhosis; overzealous administration of sodium-containing fluids; and fluid shifts (i.e., treatment of burns). Prolonged corticosteroid therapy, severe stress, and hyperaldosteronism augment fluid volume excess.	Acute weight gain, peripheral edema and ascites, distended jugular veins, crackles, elevated CVP, shortness of breath, ↑ blood pressure, bounding pulse and cough, ↑ respiratory rate *Labs indicate:* ↓ hemoglobin and hematocrit, ↓ serum and urine osmolality, ↓ urine sodium and specific gravity

↑ increased; ↓ decreased; BP, blood pressure; BUN, blood urea nitrogen; CVP, central venous pressure.

Adapted from Grossman, S. C., & Porth, C. M. (2014). *Porth's pathophysiology: Concepts of altered health states* (9th ed.). Philadelphia, PA: Lippincott Williams & Wilkins.

I&O of fluids from all sources, assessment of changes in daily weight, careful monitoring of side effects and interactions of medications, and prompt reporting and management of disturbances. It is necessary to monitor skin turgor serially to detect subtle changes. However, assessment of skin turgor is not as valid in older adults because the skin has lost some of its elasticity; therefore, other assessment measures (e.g., slowness in filling of veins of the hands and feet) become more useful in detecting FVD. Skin turgor is best tested over the forehead or the sternum in older adults, because alterations in skin elasticity are less marked in these areas.

The nurse also performs a functional assessment of the ability of the older adult to determine fluid and food needs and to obtain adequate intake in addition to other assessments discussed earlier in this chapter. For example, is the patient cognitively intact, able to ambulate and to use both arms and hands to reach fluids and foods, and able to swallow? Results of this assessment have a direct bearing on how the patient will be able to meet his or her own need for fluids and foods. During an older patient's hospital stay, the nurse provides fluids if the patient is unable to carry out self-care activities.

The nurse should also recognize that some older adults deliberately restrict their fluid intake to avoid embarrassing episodes of incontinence. In this situation, the nurse identifies interventions to deal with the incontinence, such as encouraging the patient to wear protective clothing or devices, to carry a urinal in the car, or to pace fluid intake to allow access to toilet facilities during the day. Older adults without cardiovascular or renal dysfunction should be reminded to drink adequate fluids, particularly in very warm or humid weather.

Medical Management

When planning the correction of fluid loss for the patient with FVD, the primary health care professional considers the maintenance requirements of the patient and other factors (e.g., fever) that can influence fluid needs. If the deficit is not severe, the oral route is preferred, provided the patient can drink. However, if fluid losses are acute or severe, the IV route is required. Isotonic electrolyte solutions (e.g., lactated Ringer's solution, 0.9% sodium chloride) are frequently used to treat the hypotensive patient with FVD because they expand plasma volume. As soon as the patient becomes normotensive, a hypotonic electrolyte solution (e.g., 0.45% sodium chloride) is often used to provide both electrolytes and water for renal excretion of metabolic wastes. These and additional fluids are listed in Table 17-4.

Accurate and frequent assessments of I&O, weight, vital signs, central venous pressure, level of consciousness, breath sounds, and skin colour should be performed to determine when therapy should be slowed to avoid volume overload. The rate of fluid administration is based on the severity of loss and the patient's hemodynamic response to volume replacement (Hall, 2015).

If the patient with severe FVD is not excreting enough urine and is therefore oliguric, the primary health care professional needs to determine whether the depressed renal function is caused by reduced renal blood flow secondary to FVD (prerenal azotemia) or, more seriously, by acute tubular necrosis from prolonged FVD. The test used in this situation is referred to as a fluid challenge test. During a fluid challenge test, volumes of fluid are administered at specific rates and intervals while the patient's hemodynamic response to this treatment is monitored (i.e., vital signs, breath sounds, sensorium, central venous pressure, urine output).

An example of a typical fluid challenge involves administering 100 to 200 mL of normal saline solution over 15 minutes. The goal is to provide fluids rapidly enough to attain adequate tissue perfusion without compromising the cardiovascular system. The response by a patient with FVD but normal renal function is increased urine output and an increase in blood pressure and central venous pressure.

Shock can occur when the volume of fluid lost exceeds 25% of the intravascular volume, or when fluid loss is rapid. Shock and its causes and treatment are discussed in detail in Chapter 18.

TABLE 17-4 Selected Water and Electrolyte Solutions

Solution	Considerations
Isotonic Solutions	
0.9% NaCl (isotonic, also called normal saline [NS]) Na^+ 154 mmol/L Cl^- 154 mmol/L (308 mOsm/L) Also available with varying concentrations of dextrose (the most frequently used is a 5% dextrose concentration)	• An isotonic solution that expands the extracellular fluid (ECF) volume, used in hypovolemic states, resuscitative efforts, shock, diabetic ketoacidosis, metabolic alkalosis, hypercalcemia, mild Na^+ deficit • Supplies an excess of Na^+ and Cl^-; can cause fluid volume excess and hyperchloremic acidosis if used in excessive volumes, particularly in patients with compromised renal function, heart failure, or edema • Not desirable as a routine maintenance solution, as it provides only Na^+ and Cl^- (and these are provided in excessive amounts) • When mixed with 5% dextrose, the resulting solution becomes hypertonic in relation to plasma and, in addition to the above described electrolytes, provides 170 cal/L • Only solution that may be administered with blood products • Tonicity similar to plasma
Lactated Ringer's solution (Hartmann's solution) Na^+ 130 mmol/L K^+ 4 mmol/L Ca^{++} 3 mmol/L Cl^- 109 mmol/L Lactate (metabolized to bicarbonate) 28 mmol/L (274 mOsm/L) Also available with varying concentrations of dextrose (the most common is 5% dextrose)	• An isotonic solution that contains multiple electrolytes in roughly the same concentration as found in plasma (note that solution is lacking in Mg^{++}): provides 9 cal/L • Used in the treatment of hypovolemia, burns, fluid lost as bile or diarrhea, and for acute blood loss replacement • Lactate is rapidly metabolized into HCO_3^- in the body. Lactated Ringer's solution should not be used in lactic acidosis because the ability to convert lactate into HCO_3^- is impaired in this disorder. • Not to be given with a pH >7.5 because bicarbonate is formed as lactate breaks down, causing alkalosis • Should not be used in renal failure because it contains potassium and can cause hyperkalemia • Tonicity similar to plasma
5% dextrose in water (D_5W) No electrolytes 50 g of dextrose	• An isotonic solution that supplies 170 cal/L and free water to aid in renal excretion of solutes • Used in treatment of hypernatremia, fluid loss, and dehydration • Should not be used in excessive volumes in the early postoperative period (when antidiuretic hormone secretion is increased due to stress reaction) • Should not be used solely in treatment of fluid volume deficit, because it dilutes plasma electrolyte concentrations • Contraindicated in head injury because it may cause increased intracranial pressure • Should not be used for fluid resuscitation because it can cause hyperglycemia • Should be used with caution in patients with renal or cardiac disease because of risk of fluid overload • Electrolyte-free solutions may cause peripheral circulatory collapse, anuria in patients with sodium deficiency, and increased body fluid loss • Converts to hypotonic solution as dextrose is metabolized by body. Over time, D_5W without NaCl can cause water intoxication (intracellular fluid volume excess [FVE]) because the solution is hypotonic • Fluid therapy for an extended period of time without electrolytes may result in hypokalemia
Hypotonic Solutions	
0.45% NaCl (half-strength saline) Na^+ 77 mmol/L Cl^- 77 mmol/L (154 mOsm/L) Also available with varying concentrations of dextrose (the most common is a 5% concentration)	• Provides Na^+, Cl^-, and free water • Free water is desirable to aid the kidneys in elimination of solute • Lacking in electrolytes other than Na^+ and Cl^- • When mixed with 5% dextrose, the solution becomes slightly hypertonic to plasma and in addition to the above-described electrolytes, provides 170 cal/L • Used to treat hypertonic dehydration, Na^+ and Cl^- depletion, and gastric fluid loss • Not indicated for third-space fluid shifts or increased intracranial pressure • Administer cautiously, because it can cause fluid shifts from vascular system into cells, resulting in cardiovascular collapse and increased intracranial pressure
Hypertonic Solutions	
3% NaCl (hypertonic saline) Na^+ 513 mmol/L Cl^- 513 mmol/L (1,026 mOsm/L)	• Used to increase ECF volume, decrease cellular swelling • Highly hypertonic solution used only in critical situations to treat hyponatremia • Must be administered slowly and cautiously, because it can cause intravascular volume overload and pulmonary edema • Supplies no calories • Assists in removing intracellular fluid excess
5% NaCl (hypertonic solution) Na^+ 855 mmol/L Cl^- 855 mmol/L (1,710 mOsm/L)	• Highly hypertonic solution used to treat symptomatic hyponatremia • Administer slowly and cautiously, because it can cause intravascular volume overload and pulmonary edema • Supplies no calories
Colloid Solutions	
Dextran in NS or 5% D_5W Available in low-molecular-weight (Dextran 40) and high-molecular-weight (Dextran 70) forms	• Colloid solution used as volume/plasma expander for intravascular part of ECF • Affects clotting by coating platelets and decreasing ability to clot • Remains in circulatory system up to 24 hours • Used to treat hypovolemia in early shock to increase pulse pressure, cardiac output, and arterial blood pressure • Improves microcirculation by decreasing red blood cell aggregation • Contraindicated in hemorrhage, thrombocytopenia, renal disease, and severe dehydration • Not a substitute for blood or blood products

Nursing Management

To assess for FVD, the nurse monitors and measures fluid I&O at least every 8 hours, and sometimes hourly. As FVD develops, body fluid losses exceed fluid intake through excessive urination (polyuria), diarrhea, vomiting, or other mechanisms. Once FVD has developed, the kidneys attempt to conserve body fluids, leading to a urine output of less than 30 mL/hr or 1 ml/kg/hr in an adult. Urine in this instance is concentrated and represents a healthy renal response. Daily body weights are monitored; an acute loss of 0.5 kg represents a fluid loss of approximately 500 mL. (One litre of fluid weighs approximately 1 kg.)

Vital signs are closely monitored. The nurse observes for a weak, rapid pulse and orthostatic hypotension (i.e., a decrease in systolic pressure exceeding 20 mm Hg when the patient moves from a lying to a sitting position). A decrease in body temperature often accompanies FVD, unless there is a concurrent infection.

Skin and tongue turgor are monitored on a regular basis. In a healthy person, pinched skin immediately returns to its usual position when released. This elastic property, referred to as turgor, is partially dependent on interstitial fluid volume. In a person with FVD, the skin flattens more slowly after the pinch is released. In a person with severe FVD, the skin may remain elevated for many seconds. Tissue turgor is best measured by pinching the skin over the sternum, inner aspects of the thighs, or forehead. Tongue turgor is not affected by age (see previous Gerontologic Considerations), and evaluating this may be more valid than evaluating skin turgor. In most people, the tongue has one longitudinal furrow. In the person with FVD, there are additional longitudinal furrows and the tongue is smaller because of fluid loss. The degree of oral mucous membrane moisture is also assessed; a dry mouth may indicate either FVD or mouth breathing.

Urine concentration is monitored by measuring the urine specific gravity. In a volume-depleted patient, the urine specific gravity should be greater than 1.020, indicating healthy renal conservation of fluid.

Mental function is eventually affected in severe FVD as a result of decreasing cerebral perfusion. Decreased peripheral perfusion can result in cold extremities. In patients with relatively normal cardiopulmonary function, a low central venous pressure is indicative of hypovolemia. Patients with acute cardiopulmonary decompensation require more extensive hemodynamic monitoring of pressures in both sides of the heart to determine if hypovolemia exists.

Preventing Hypovolemia

To prevent FVD, the nurse identifies patients at risk and takes measures to minimize fluid losses. For example, if the patient has diarrhea, measures are implemented to control diarrhea and replacement fluids are administered. This includes administering antidiarrheal medications and small volumes of oral fluids at frequent intervals.

Correcting Hypovolemia

When possible, oral fluids are administered to help correct FVD, with consideration given to the patient's likes and dislikes. The type of fluid the patient has lost is also considered and fluids most likely to replace the lost electrolytes are appropriate (Moritz, 2013). If the patient is reluctant to drink because of oral discomfort, the nurse assists with frequent mouth care and provides nonirritating fluids. The patient may be offered small volumes of oral rehydration solutions (e.g., Rehydralyte, Elete, Cytomax). These solutions provide fluid, glucose, and electrolytes in concentrations that are easily absorbed. If nausea is present, antiemetics may be needed before oral fluid replacement can be tolerated.

If the deficit cannot be corrected by oral fluids, therapy may need to be initiated by an alternative route (enteral or parenteral) until adequate circulating blood volume and renal perfusion are achieved. Isotonic fluids are prescribed to increase ECF volume.

Hypervolemia

Fluid volume excess (FVE), or hypervolemia, refers to an isotonic expansion of the ECF caused by the abnormal retention of water and sodium in approximately the same proportions in which they normally exist in the ECF. It is always secondary to an increase in the total body sodium content, which, in turn, leads to an increase in total body water (Hall, 2015). Because there is isotonic retention of body substances, the serum sodium concentration remains essentially normal.

Pathophysiology

FVE may be related to simple fluid overload or diminished function of the homeostatic mechanisms responsible for regulating fluid balance. Contributing factors can include heart failure, kidney injury, and cirrhosis of the liver. Another contributing factor is consumption of excessive amounts of table or other sodium salts. Excessive administration of sodium-containing fluids in a patient with impaired regulatory mechanisms may predispose him or her to a serious FVE as well (Hall, 2015).

Clinical Manifestations

Clinical manifestations of FVE result from expansion of the ECF and include generalized edema, distended neck veins, and pulmonary edema, dyspnea, cough, shortness of breath, and crackles (abnormal lung sounds). Further discussion of clinical signs and symptoms and laboratory findings can be found in Table 17-3.

Assessment and Diagnostic Findings

Laboratory data useful in diagnosing FVE include BUN and hematocrit levels. In FVE, both of these values may be decreased because of plasma dilution. Other causes of abnormalities in these values include low protein intake and anemia. In chronic kidney disease, both serum osmolality and the sodium level are decreased due to excessive retention of water. The urine sodium level is increased if the kidneys are attempting to excrete excess volume. A chest x-ray may reveal pulmonary congestion. Hypervolemia occurs when aldosterone is chronically stimulated (i.e., cirrhosis, heart failure, and nephrotic syndrome). Therefore, the urine sodium level does not increase in these conditions.

Medical Management

Management of FVE is directed at the causes, and if related to excessive administration of sodium-containing fluids, discontinuing the infusion may be all that is needed. Symptomatic treatment consists of administering diuretics and restricting fluids and sodium.

Pharmacologic Therapy

Diuretics are prescribed when dietary restriction of sodium alone is insufficient to reduce edema by inhibiting the reabsorption of sodium and water by the kidneys. The choice of diuretic is based on the severity of the hypervolemic state, the degree of impairment of renal function, and the potency of the diuretic. Thiazide diuretics block sodium reabsorption in the distal tubule, where only 5% to 10% of filtered sodium is reabsorbed. Loop diuretics, such as furosemide (Lasix), bumetanide (Bumex), or torsemide (Demadex), can cause a greater loss of both sodium and water because they block sodium reabsorption in the ascending limb of the loop of Henle, where 20% to 30% of filtered sodium is usually reabsorbed. Generally, thiazide diuretics, such as hydrochlorothiazide (Hydrodiuril) or metolazone (Mykrox, Zaroxolyn), are prescribed for mild to moderate hypervolemia and loop diuretics for severe hypervolemia.

Electrolyte imbalances may result from the effect of the diuretic. Hypokalemia can occur with all diuretics except those that work in the last distal tubule of the nephrons. Potassium supplements can be prescribed to avoid this complication. Hyperkalemia can occur with diuretics that work in the last distal tubule (e.g., spironolactone [Aldactone]), especially in patients with decreased renal function. Hyponatremia occurs with diuresis due to increased release of ADH secondary to reduction in circulating volume. Decreased magnesium levels occur with administration of loop and thiazide diuretics due to decreased reabsorption and increased excretion of magnesium by the kidney.

Azotemia (increased nitrogen levels in the blood) can occur with FVE when urea and creatinine are not excreted due to decreased perfusion by the kidneys and decreased excretion of wastes. High uric acid levels (hyperuricemia) can also occur from increased reabsorption and decreased excretion of uric acid by the kidneys.

Dialysis

If renal function is so severely impaired that pharmacologic agents cannot act efficiently, other modalities are considered to remove sodium and fluid from the body. Hemodialysis or peritoneal dialysis may be used to remove nitrogenous wastes and control potassium and acid–base balance, and to remove sodium and fluid. Continuous renal replacement therapy may also be required. See Chapter 45 for a discussion of these treatment modalities.

Nutritional Therapy

Treatment of FVE usually involves dietary restriction of sodium. According to Health Canada (2017), Canadians consume an average of 2,760 mg of sodium each day, which is almost double the recommended daily amount of sodium. This means that Canadians are still consuming too much sodium, putting them at higher risk of high blood pressure, and therefore heart disease and stroke. It is not surprising that 15,000 to 32,000 Canadians die yearly from this excess sodium intake (Health Canada, 2010). The optimum daily amount of sodium is 2,000 mg daily (Hypertension Canada, 2014). Low sodium diets can range from a mild restriction to as little as 250 mg of sodium per day, depending on the patient's condition. A mild sodium-restricted diet allows only light salting of food (about half the usual amount) in cooking and at the table, and no addition of salt to commercially prepared foods that are already heavily seasoned. All Canadians need to know how to read food labels because 75% of sodium content is from processed foods (Health Canada, 2017). If salt, sodium, or soda is near the top of the ingredient list, the product is probably high in sodium. Of course, foods high in sodium must be avoided. It is the sodium salt, sodium chloride, rather than sodium itself that contributes to edema.

Because about half of ingested sodium is in the form of seasoning, seasoning substitutes can play a major role in decreasing sodium intake. Lemon juice, onions, and garlic are excellent substitute flavourings, although some patients prefer salt substitutes. Most salt substitutes contain potassium and must therefore be used cautiously by patients taking potassium-sparing diuretics (e.g., spironolactone, triamterene [Dyrenium], amiloride [Midamor]). They should not be used at all in conditions associated with potassium retention, such as advanced renal disease. Salt substitutes containing ammonium chloride can be harmful to patients with liver damage.

In some communities, the drinking water may contain too much sodium for a sodium-restricted diet. Depending on its source, water may contain as little as 1 mg or more than 1,500 mg of sodium per quart. Patients may need to use distilled water if the local water supply is very high in sodium. Bottled water can have a sodium content that ranges from 0 to 1,200 mg/L; therefore, if sodium is restricted, the label must be carefully examined for sodium content before purchasing and drinking bottled water. Also, patients on sodium-restricted diets should be cautioned to avoid water softeners that add sodium to water in exchange for other ions, such as calcium. Protein intake may be increased in patients who are malnourished or who have low serum protein levels in an effort to increase capillary oncotic pressure and pull fluid out of the tissues into vessels for excretion by the kidneys.

Nursing Management

To assess for FVE, the nurse measures I&O at regular intervals to identify excessive fluid retention. The patient is weighed daily, and rapid weight gain is noted. An acute weight gain of 1 kg is equivalent to a gain of approximately 1 L of fluid. Breath sounds are assessed at regular intervals in at-risk patients, particularly if parenteral fluids are being administered. The nurse monitors the degree of edema in the most dependent parts of the body, such as the feet and ankles in ambulatory patients and the sacral region in patients confined to bed. Pitting edema is assessed by pressing a thumb into the dorsum of each foot, medial malleolus, and shins for at least 5 seconds, creating a pit or indentation that is evaluated on a scale of 1+ (minimal) to 4+ (severe) (Day, 2012). Peripheral edema of the legs is monitored by measuring the circumference of the extremity with a metric tape measure at four locations: forefoot, smallest circumference above the ankle, largest circumference of the calf, and mid thigh (with knee straight). Both legs are compared. A difference of 1 cm at the ankle, and 2 cm at the calf, usually indicates edema.

Preventing Hypervolemia

Specific interventions vary with the underlying condition and the degree of FVE. However, most patients require sodium-restricted diets in some form, and adherence to the prescribed diet is encouraged. Patients are instructed to avoid over-the-counter (OTC) medications without first checking with a health care professional, because these substances may contain sodium. If fluid retention persists despite adherence to a prescribed diet, hidden sources of sodium, such as the water supply or use of water softeners, should be considered.

Detecting and Controlling Hypervolemia

It is important to detect FVE before the condition becomes severe. Interventions include promoting rest, restricting sodium intake, monitoring parenteral fluid therapy, and administering appropriate medications.

Regular rest periods may be beneficial, because bed rest favours diuresis of edema fluid. The mechanism is probably related to diminished venous pooling and the subsequent increase in effective circulating blood volume and renal perfusion. Sodium and fluid restriction should be instituted as indicated. Because most patients with FVE require diuretics, the patient's response to these agents is monitored. The rate of parenteral fluids and the patient's response to these fluids are also closely monitored. If dyspnea or orthopnea is present, the patient is placed in a semi-Fowler's position to promote lung expansion. The patient is turned and repositioned at regular intervals because edematous tissue is more prone to skin breakdown than normal tissue. Because conditions predisposing to FVE are likely to be chronic, patients are taught to monitor their response to therapy by documenting fluid I&O and body weight changes. The importance of adhering to the treatment regimen is emphasized.

Educating Patients About Edema

Because edema is a common manifestation of FVE, patients need to recognize its symptoms and understand its importance. The nurse gives special attention to edema when teaching the patient with FVE. Edema can occur as a result of increased capillary fluid pressure, decreased capillary oncotic pressure, or increased interstitial oncotic pressure, causing expansion of the interstitial fluid compartment (Hall, 2015). Edema can be localized (e.g., in the ankle, as in rheumatoid arthritis) or generalized (as in cardiac failure and kidney injury). Severe generalized edema is called *anasarca*.

Edema occurs when there is a change in the capillary membrane, increasing the formation of interstitial fluid or decreasing the removal of interstitial fluid. Sodium retention is a frequent cause of the increased ECF volume. Burns and infection are examples of conditions associated with increased interstitial fluid volume. Obstruction to lymphatic outflow, a plasma albumin level less than 15 to 20 g/L, or a decrease in plasma oncotic pressure contributes to increased interstitial fluid volume. The kidneys retain sodium and water when there is decreased ECF volume as a result of decreased cardiac output from heart failure. A thorough medication history is necessary to identify any medications that could cause edema, such as nonsteroidal anti-inflammatory drugs (NSAIDs), estrogens, corticosteroids, and antihypertensive agents.

Ascites is a form of edema in which fluid accumulates in the peritoneal cavity; it results from nephrotic syndrome, cirrhosis, congestive heart failure, and some malignant tumours. The patient commonly reports shortness of breath and a sense of pressure because of pressure on the diaphragm.

The goal of treatment is to preserve or restore the circulating intravascular fluid volume. Thus, in addition to treating the cause of the edema, other treatments may include diuretic therapy, restriction of fluids and sodium, elevation of the extremities, application of antiembolism stockings, paracentesis, dialysis, and continuous renal replacement therapy in cases of kidney injury or life-threatening fluid volume overload (see Chapter 45).

Electrolyte Imbalances

Disturbances in electrolyte balances are common in clinical practice and must be corrected.

Sodium Imbalances

Sodium is the most abundant electrolyte in the ECF; its concentration ranges from 135 to 145 mmol/L and it is the primary determinant of ECF volume and osmolality. Sodium has a major role in controlling water distribution throughout the body, because it does not easily cross the cell wall membrane and because of its abundance and high concentration in the body. Sodium is regulated by ADH, thirst, and the renin–angiotensin–aldosterone system. A loss or gain of sodium is usually accompanied by a loss or gain of water. Sodium also functions in establishing the electrochemical state necessary for muscle contraction and the transmission of nerve impulses (Sahay & Sahay, 2014).

The syndrome of inappropriate secretion of antidiuretic hormone (SIADH) may be associated with sodium imbalance. When there is a decrease in the circulating plasma osmolality, blood volume, or blood pressure, arginine vasopressin (AVP) is released from the posterior pituitary. Oversecretion of AVP can cause SIADH. Patients at risk are older adults, those with acquired immunodeficiency syndrome (AIDS), those on mechanical ventilation, and people taking selective serotonin reuptake inhibitors (SSRIs). Sodium imbalance can develop under simple or complex circumstances. The two most common sodium imbalances are sodium deficit and sodium excess (see Table 17-5).

Sodium Deficit (Hyponatremia)

Hyponatremia refers to a serum sodium level that is less than 135 mmol/L (Sahay & Sahay, 2014). Hyponatremia can present as an acute or chronic form. Acute hyponatremia is commonly the result of a fluid overload in a surgical patient. Chronic hyponatremia is seen more frequently in

TABLE 17-5 Sodium Imbalances

Imbalance	Contributing Factors	Signs/Symptoms and Laboratory Findings
Sodium deficit (hyponatremia) Serum sodium <135 mmol/L	Loss of sodium, as in use of diuretics, loss of GI fluids, renal disease, and adrenal insufficiency. Gain of water, as in excessive administration of D_5W and water supplements for patients receiving hypotonic tube feedings; disease states associated with SIADH, such as head trauma and oat-cell lung tumour; medications associated with water retention (oxytocin and certain tranquilizers); and psychogenic polydipsia. Hyperglycemia and heart failure cause a loss of sodium.	Anorexia, nausea and vomiting, headache, lethargy, dizziness, confusion, muscle cramps and weakness, muscular twitching, seizures, papilledema, dry skin, ↑ pulse, ↓ BP, weight gain, edema *Labs indicate:* ↓ serum and urine sodium, ↓ urine specific gravity and osmolality
Sodium excess (hypernatremia) Serum sodium >145 mmol/L	Fluid deprivation in patients who cannot respond to thirst, hypertonic tube feedings without adequate water supplements, diabetes insipidus, heat stroke, hyperventilation, watery diarrhea, burns, and diaphoresis. Excess corticosteroid, sodium bicarbonate, and sodium chloride administration, and saltwater near-drowning victims.	Thirst, elevated body temperature, swollen dry tongue and sticky mucous membranes, hallucinations, lethargy, restlessness, irritability, simple partial or tonic–clonic seizures, pulmonary edema, hyperreflexia, twitching, nausea, vomiting, anorexia, ↑ pulse, and ↑ BP *Labs indicate:* ↑ serum sodium, ↓ urine sodium, ↑ urine specific gravity and osmolality, ↓ CVP

↑, increased; ↓, decreased; CVP, central venous pressure; BP, blood pressure; GI, gastrointestinal; D_5W, dextrose 5% in water; SIADH, syndrome of inappropriate secretion of antidiuretic hormone.

Adapted from Grossman, S. C., & Porth, C. M. (2014). *Porth's pathophysiology: Concepts of altered health states* (9th ed.). Philadelphia, PA: Lippincott Williams & Wilkins.

patients outside the hospital setting, has a longer duration, and has less serious neurologic sequelae. Another type of hyponatremia is exercise-associated hyponatremia, which is more frequently found in women and those of smaller stature. It can occur during extreme temperatures, because of excessive fluid intake before exercise, or prolonged exercise that results in a decrease in serum sodium (Earhart et al., 2015).

Pathophysiology

Hyponatremia primarily occurs due to an imbalance of water rather than sodium. The urine sodium assists in differentiating renal from nonrenal causes of hyponatremia. Low urine sodium occurs as the kidney retains sodium to compensate for nonrenal fluid loss (i.e., vomiting, diarrhea, sweating). High urine sodium concentration is associated with renal salt wasting (i.e., diuretic use). In dilutional hyponatremia, the ECF volume is increased without any edema.

A deficiency of aldosterone, as occurs in adrenal insufficiency, also predisposes to sodium deficiency. In addition, the use of certain medications, such as anticonvulsants (i.e., carbamazepine [Tegretol], levetiracetam [Keppra]) and SSRIs (fluoxetine [Sarafem], sertraline [Zoloft], paroxetine [Paxil]), increases the risk of hyponatremia (Sahay & Sahay, 2014).

SIADH is seen in hyponatremia as well as hypernatremia. The physiologic disturbances include excessive ADH activity, with water retention and dilutional hyponatremia, and inappropriate urinary excretion of sodium in the presence of hyponatremia. SIADH can be the result of either sustained secretion of ADH by the hypothalamus or production of an ADH-like substance from a tumour (aberrant ADH production). Conditions affecting the central nervous system are associated with SIADH. SIADH is discussed in more detail in Chapters 43 and 65.

Clinical Manifestations

Clinical manifestations of hyponatremia depend on the cause, magnitude, and speed with which the deficit occurs. Poor skin turgor, dry mucosa, headache, decreased saliva production, orthostatic fall in blood pressure, nausea, vomiting, and abdominal cramping occur. Neurologic changes, including altered mental status, status epilepticus, and coma, are probably related to the cellular swelling and cerebral edema associated with hyponatremia. As the extracellular sodium level decreases, the cellular fluid becomes relatively more concentrated and pulls water into the cells (Fig. 17-4). In general, patients with an acute

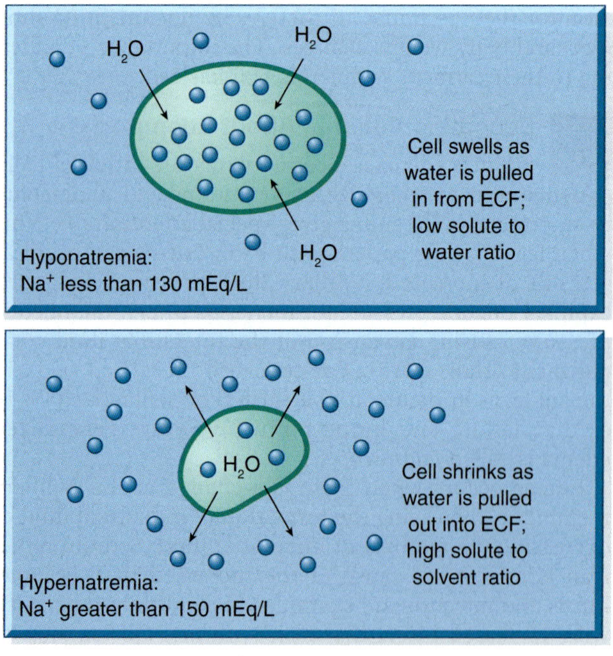

FIGURE 17-4. Effect of extracellular sodium level on cell size.

decrease in serum sodium levels have more cerebral edema and higher mortality rates than do those with more slowly developing hyponatremia. Acute decreases in sodium, developing in less than 48 hours, may be associated with brain herniation and compression of midbrain structures. Chronic decreases in sodium, developing over 48 hours or more, can occur in status epilepticus and cerebral pontine myelinolysis.

Features of hyponatremia associated with sodium loss and water gain include anorexia, muscle cramps, and a feeling of exhaustion. When the serum sodium level decreases to less than 115 mmol/L, edema of brain cells caused by movement of water into brain cells and neuromuscular tissues occurs, with signs of increasing intracranial pressure such as lethargy, confusion, muscle twitching, focal weakness, hemiparesis, papilledema, seizures, and death.

Assessment and Diagnostic Findings

Assessment includes the history and physical examination, including a focused neurologic examination; evaluation of signs and symptoms as well as laboratory test results; identification of current IV fluids, if applicable; and a review of all medications the patient is taking. Regardless of the cause of hyponatremia, the serum sodium level is less than 135 mmol/L; in SIADH, it may be lower than 100 mmol/L. Serum osmolality is also decreased, except in azotemia with the accumulation of toxins. When hyponatremia is due primarily to sodium loss, the urinary sodium content is less than 20 mmol/L, suggesting increased proximal reabsorption of sodium secondary to ECF volume depletion, and the specific gravity is low (1.002 to 1.004). However, when hyponatremia is due to SIADH, the urinary sodium content is greater than 20 mmol/L, and the urine specific gravity is usually greater than 1.012. Although the patient with SIADH retains water abnormally and therefore gains body weight, there is no peripheral edema; instead, fluid accumulates inside the cells. This phenomenon sometimes manifests as pitting edema.

Medical Management

The key to treating hyponatremia is assessment including identifying patients who are at risk and recognizing that the rapidity of the onset of hyponatremia is of primary importance (Morris, Bohm, Nemecek, et al., 2018).

Sodium Replacement

The most common treatment for hyponatremia is careful administration of sodium by mouth, nasogastric tube, or a parenteral route. For patients who can eat and drink, sodium is easily replaced because sodium is consumed abundantly in a regular diet. For those who cannot consume sodium, lactated Ringer's solution or isotonic saline (0.9% sodium chloride) solution may be prescribed. Serum sodium must not be increased by more than 12 mmol/L in 24 hours to avoid neurologic damage due to osmotic demyelination. This condition may occur when the serum sodium concentration is overcorrected (exceeding 140 mmol/L) too rapidly or in the presence of hypoxia or anoxia. It may produce lesions that show symmetric myelin destruction affecting all the fibre tracts that cause paraparesis, dysarthria, dysphagia, and coma. The usual daily sodium requirement in adults is approximately 100 mmol/L provided there are not excessive losses. Selected water and electrolyte solutions are described in Table 17-4.

In SIADH, the administration of hypertonic saline solution alone cannot change the plasma sodium concentration. Excess sodium would be excreted rapidly in highly concentrated urine. With the addition of the diuretic furosemide (Lasix), urine is not concentrated, and isotonic urine is excreted to effect a change in water balance. In patients with SIADH, in whom water restriction is difficult, lithium (Eskalith) or demeclocycline (Declomycin) can antagonize the osmotic effect of ADH on the medullary collecting tubule.

Water Restriction

In a patient with normal or excess fluid volume, hyponatremia is treated by restricting fluid to a total of 800 mL in 24 hours. This is far safer than sodium administration and is usually an effective treatment. However, if neurologic symptoms are severe (e.g., seizures, delirium, coma), as well as in traumatic brain injury, it may be necessary to administer small volumes of a hypertonic sodium solution (Morris et al., 2018) (see Chapter 65). Incorrect use of these fluids is extremely dangerous, because 1 L of 3% sodium chloride solution contains 513 mmol of sodium and 1 L of 5% sodium chloride solution contains 855 mmol of sodium. The prescribed volume of hypertonic saline administered depends on the patient's weight and on current and desired serum sodium levels (Morris et al., 2018). If edema exists alone, sodium is restricted; if edema and hyponatremia occur together, both sodium and water are restricted.

NURSING ALERT

Highly hypertonic sodium solutions (2% to 23% sodium chloride) should be administered only in intensive care settings under close observation, because only small volumes are needed to elevate the serum sodium concentration from a dangerously low level. These fluids are administered slowly and in small volumes, and the patient is monitored closely.

Pharmacologic Therapy

AVP receptor antagonists are new pharmacologic agents that treat hyponatremia by stimulating free water excretion (Morris et al., 2018). IV conivaptan hydrochloride (Vaprisol) use is limited to the treatment of hospitalized patients. It may be a useful therapy for those patients with moderate to severe symptomatic hyponatremia, but is contraindicated in patients with seizures, delirium, or coma, which warrant the use of hypertonic saline.

Nursing Management

The nurse needs to identify and monitor patients at risk of hyponatremia. Early detection and treatment of this disorder are necessary to prevent serious consequences. For patients at risk, the nurse monitors fluid I&O as well as daily body weight. It is also necessary to note abnormal losses of sodium or gains of water, as well as GI manifestations such as anorexia, nausea, vomiting, and abdominal cramping. The nurse must be alert for central nervous system changes, such as lethargy, confusion, muscle twitching, and seizures. Neurologic signs are associated with very low sodium levels that have fallen rapidly because of fluid overloading. Serum sodium is monitored very closely in patients who are at risk for hyponatremia; when indicated, urine sodium and specific gravity are also monitored.

Hyponatremia is a frequently overlooked cause of confusion in older adults, who have an increased risk of hyponatremia because of decreased renal function and thus inability to excrete excess fluids. Administration of prescribed and OTC medications that cause sodium loss or water retention are predisposing factors. A diminished sense of thirst or loss of access to food or fluids may also contribute to the problem.

Detecting and Controlling Hyponatremia

For a patient with abnormal losses of sodium who can consume a general diet, the nurse encourages foods and fluids with high sodium content. For example, broth made with one beef cube contains approximately 900 mg of sodium; 250 mL of tomato juice contains approximately 700 mg of sodium. The nurse also needs to be familiar with the sodium content of parenteral fluids.

If the primary problem is water retention, it is safer to restrict fluid intake than to administer sodium. In normovolemia or hypervolemia, administration of sodium predisposes a patient to fluid volume overload. In severe hyponatremia, the aim of therapy is to elevate the serum sodium level only enough to alleviate neurologic signs and symptoms. It is generally recommended that the serum sodium concentration be increased to no greater than 125 mmol/L with a hypertonic saline solution.

NURSING ALERT

When administering fluids to patients with cardiovascular disease, the nurse assesses for signs of circulatory overload (e.g., cough, dyspnea, puffy eyelids, dependent edema, and weight gain in 24 hours). The lungs are auscultated for crackles.

For the patient taking lithium, the nurse observes for lithium toxicity, particularly when sodium is lost by an abnormal route. In such instances, supplemental salt and fluid are administered. Because diuretics promote sodium loss, the patient taking lithium is instructed not to use diuretics without close medical supervision. For all patients on lithium therapy, adequate salt intake should be ensured.

Excess water supplements are avoided in patients receiving isotonic or hypotonic enteral feedings, particularly if abnormal sodium loss occurs or water is being abnormally retained (as in SIADH). Actual fluid needs are determined by evaluating fluid I&O, urine specific gravity, and serum sodium levels.

Sodium Excess (Hypernatremia)

Hypernatremia is a serum sodium level higher than 145 mmol/L (Sterns, 2014). It can be caused by a gain of sodium in excess of water or by a loss of water in excess of sodium. It can occur in patients with normal fluid volume or in those with FVD or FVE. With a water loss, the patient loses more water than sodium; as a result, the serum sodium concentration increases and the increased concentration pulls fluid out of the cell. This is both an extracellular and an intracellular FVD. In sodium excess, the patient ingests or retains more sodium than water.

Pathophysiology

A common cause of hypernatremia is fluid deprivation in unconscious patients who cannot perceive, respond to, or communicate their thirst. Most often affected are very old, very young, and patients who are cognitively impaired. Administration of hypertonic enteral feedings without adequate water supplements leads to hypernatremia, as does watery diarrhea and greatly increased insensible water loss (e.g., hyperventilation, denuding effects of burns). In addition, both central and nephrogenic diabetes insipidus, which is a decreased ability to concentrate urine due to a defect in the kidney tubules that interferes with water reabsorption, result in hypernatremia if the patient does not experience or cannot respond to thirst, or if fluids are excessively restricted.

Less common causes of hypernatremia are heat stroke, near drowning in sea water (which contains a sodium concentration of approximately 500 mmol/L), and malfunction of hemodialysis or peritoneal dialysis systems. IV administration of hypertonic saline or excessive use of sodium bicarbonate also causes hypernatremia.

Clinical Manifestations

The clinical manifestations of hypernatremia are primarily neurologic and are due to increased plasma osmolality caused by an increase in plasma sodium concentration (Sterns, 2014). Water moves out of the cell into the ECF, resulting in cellular dehydration and a more concentrated ECF (see Fig. 17-4). Clinically, these changes may be manifested by restlessness and weakness in moderate hypernatremia and by disorientation, delusions, and hallucinations in severe hypernatremia. Dehydration (resulting in hypernatremia) is often overlooked as the primary reason for behavioural changes in older adults. If hypernatremia is severe, permanent brain damage can occur (especially in children).

A primary characteristic of hypernatremia is thirst. Thirst is such a strong defender of serum sodium levels in healthy people that hypernatremia never occurs unless the person is unconscious or does not have access to water. However, ill people may have an impaired thirst mechanism. Other signs include a dry, swollen tongue and sticky mucous membranes. Flushed skin; peripheral and pulmonary edema; hypotension; weak and thready pulse; and decreased deep tendon reflexes (DTRs). Body temperature may increase mildly, but it returns to normal after the hypernatremia is corrected.

Assessment and Diagnostic Findings

In hypernatremia, the serum sodium level exceeds 145 mmol/L and the serum osmolality exceeds 300 mmol/L. The urine specific gravity and urine osmolality are increased as the kidneys attempt to conserve water (provided the water loss is from a route other than the kidneys). Patients with nephrogenic or central diabetes insipidus have hypernatremia and produce a dilute urine with a urine osmolality less than 250 mmol/L.

Medical Management

Treatment of hypernatremia consists of a gradual lowering of the serum sodium level by the infusion of a hypotonic electrolyte solution (e.g., 0.3% sodium chloride) or an isotonic nonsaline solution (e.g., dextrose 5% in water [D_5W]). D_5W is indicated when water needs to be replaced without sodium. Clinicians consider a hypotonic sodium solution to be safer than D_5W because it allows a gradual reduction in the serum sodium level, thereby decreasing the risk of cerebral edema. It is the solution of choice in severe hyperglycemia with hypernatremia. A rapid reduction in the serum sodium level temporarily decreases the plasma osmolality below that of the fluid in the brain tissue, causing dangerous cerebral edema. Diuretics also may be prescribed to treat the sodium gain.

There is no consensus about the exact rate at which serum sodium levels should be reduced. As a general rule, the serum sodium level is reduced at a rate no faster than 0.5 to 1 mmol/L to allow sufficient time for readjustment through diffusion across fluid compartments. Desmopressin acetate (DDAVP) may be prescribed to treat diabetes insipidus if it is the cause of hypernatremia (Bichet, 2013).

Nursing Management

As in hyponatremia, fluid losses and gains are carefully monitored in patients who are at risk for hypernatremia. The nurse should assess for abnormal losses of water or low water intake and for large gains of sodium, as might occur with ingestion of OTC medications that have a high sodium content (e.g., Alka-Seltzer). In addition, the nurse obtains a medication history, because some prescription medications have a high sodium content. The nurse also notes the patient's thirst or elevated body temperature and evaluates it in relation to other clinical signs. The nurse monitors for changes in behaviour, such as restlessness, disorientation, and lethargy.

Preventing Hypernatremia

The nurse attempts to prevent hypernatremia by providing fluids at regular intervals, particularly in patients who are debilitated or unconscious and who are unable to perceive or respond to thirst. If fluid intake remains inadequate, the nurse consults with the physician to plan an alternative route for intake, either by enteral feedings or by the parenteral route. If enteral feedings are used, sufficient water should be administered to keep the serum sodium and BUN within expected limits (Moritz, 2013). As a rule, the higher the osmolality of the enteral feeding, the greater is the need for water supplementation.

For patients with diabetes insipidus, adequate water intake must be ensured. If the patient is alert and has an intact thirst mechanism, merely providing access to water may be sufficient. If the patient has a decreased level of consciousness or other disability interfering with adequate fluid intake, parenteral fluid replacement may be prescribed. This therapy can be anticipated in patients with neurologic disorders, particularly in the early postoperative period.

Correcting Hypernatremia

When parenteral fluids are necessary for managing hypernatremia, the nurse monitors the patient's response to the fluids by reviewing serial serum sodium levels and by observing for changes in neurologic signs (Moritz, 2013). With a gradual decrease in the serum sodium level, the neurologic signs should improve. Too-rapid reduction in the serum sodium level renders the plasma temporarily hypo-osmotic to the fluid in the brain tissue, causing movement of fluid into brain cells and dangerous cerebral edema.

Potassium Imbalances

Potassium is the major intracellular electrolyte; in fact, 98% of the body's potassium is inside the cells. The remaining 2% is in the ECF and is important in neuromuscular function. Potassium influences both skeletal and cardiac muscle activity. For example, alterations in its concentration change myocardial irritability and rhythm. Under the influence of the sodium–potassium pump, potassium is constantly moving in and out of cells. The expected serum potassium concentration ranges from 3.5 to 5 mmol/L, and even minor variations are significant. Potassium imbalances are commonly associated with various diseases, injuries, medications (e.g., NSAIDs and ACE inhibitors), and acid–base imbalances (Mount, 2014a). The two most common potassium imbalances are potassium deficit and potassium excess (see Table 17-6).

To maintain potassium balance, the renal system must function, because 80% of the potassium excreted daily leaves the body by way of the kidneys; the other 20% is lost through the bowel and in sweat. The kidneys regulate potassium balance by adjusting the amount of potassium that is excreted in the urine. As serum potassium levels increase, so does the potassium level in the renal tubular cell. A concentration gradient occurs, favouring the movement of potassium into the renal tubule and excretion of potassium in the urine. Aldosterone also increases the excretion of potassium by the kidney. Because the kidneys do not conserve potassium as well as they conserve sodium, potassium may still be lost in urine in the presence of a potassium deficit.

Potassium Deficit (Hypokalemia)

Hypokalemia (serum potassium level below than 3.5 mmol/L) usually indicates a deficit in total potassium stores. However, it may occur in patients with normal potassium stores. When **alkalosis** is present, a temporary shift of serum potassium into the cells occurs (see later discussion).

TABLE 17-6 Potassium Imbalances

Imbalance	Contributing Factors	Signs/Symptoms
Potassium deficit (hypokalemia) Serum potassium <3.5 mmol/L	Diarrhea, vomiting, gastric suction, corticosteroid administration, hyperaldosteronism, carbenicillin, amphotericin B, bulimia, osmotic diuresis, alkalosis, starvation, diuretics, and digoxin toxicity	Fatigue, anorexia, nausea and vomiting, muscle weakness, polyuria, decreased bowel motility, ventricular asystole or fibrillation, paresthesias, leg cramps, ↓ BP, ileus, abdominal distention, hypoactive reflexes. *ECG:* flattened T waves, prominent U waves, ST depression, prolonged PR interval
Potassium excess (hyperkalemia) Serum potassium >5.0 mmol/L	Pseudohyperkalemia, oliguric kidney injury, use of potassium-conserving diuretics in patients with renal insufficiency, metabolic acidosis, Addison's disease, crush injury, burns, stored bank blood transfusions, rapid IV administration of potassium, and certain medications such as ACE inhibitors, NSAIDs, cyclosporine	Muscle weakness, tachycardia → bradycardia, dysrhythmias, flaccid paralysis, paresthesias, intestinal colic, cramps, abdominal distention, irritability, anxiety. *ECG:* tall tented T waves, prolonged PR interval and QRS duration, absent P waves, ST depression

↓, decreased; →, followed by; BP, blood pressure; ECG, electrocardiogram; IV, intravenous; ACE, angiotensin-converting enzyme; NSAIDs, nonsteroidal anti-inflammatory drugs.

Adapted from Grossman, S. C., & Porth, C. M. (2014). *Porth's pathophysiology: Concepts of altered health states* (9th ed.). Philadelphia, PA: Lippincott Williams & Wilkins.

Pathophysiology

Potassium-losing diuretics, such as the thiazides and loop diuretics, can induce hypokalemia (Jensen, Brabrand, Vinholt, et al., 2015). Other medications that can lead to hypokalemia include corticosteroids, sodium penicillin, carbenicillin, and amphotericin B. GI loss of potassium is another common cause of potassium depletion. Vomiting and gastric suction frequently lead to hypokalemia, partly because potassium is actually lost when gastric fluid is lost and because potassium is lost through the kidneys in response to metabolic alkalosis. Because relatively large amounts of potassium are contained in intestinal fluids, potassium deficit occurs frequently with diarrhea, which may contain as much potassium as 30 mmol/L. Potassium deficit also occurs from prolonged intestinal suctioning, recent ileostomy, and villous adenoma (a tumour of the intestinal tract characterized by excretion of potassium-rich mucus).

Alterations in acid–base balance have a significant effect on potassium distribution due to shifts of hydrogen and potassium ions between the cells and the ECF. Respiratory or metabolic alkalosis promotes the transcellular shift of potassium and can have a variable and unpredictable effect on serum potassium. For example, hydrogen ions move out of the cells in alkalotic states to help correct the high pH, and potassium ions move in to maintain an electrically neutral state (see later discussion of acid–base balance).

Hyperaldosteronism increases renal potassium wasting and can lead to severe potassium depletion. Primary hyperaldosteronism is seen in patients with adrenal adenomas. Secondary hyperaldosteronism occurs in patients with cirrhosis, nephrotic syndrome, heart failure, or malignant hypertension.

Because insulin promotes the entry of potassium into skeletal muscle and hepatic cells, patients with persistent insulin hypersecretion may experience hypokalemia, which is often the case in patients receiving high carbohydrate parenteral nutrition.

Patients who are unable or unwilling to eat an adequate diet for a prolonged period are at risk for hypokalemia. This may occur in debilitated older adults, patients with alcoholism, and patients with anorexia nervosa. In addition to poor intake, people with bulimia frequently suffer increased potassium loss through self-induced vomiting, misuse of laxatives, diuretics, and enemas.

Magnesium depletion causes renal potassium loss and must be corrected first; otherwise, urine loss of potassium will continue. Penicillins may produce renal potassium loss by acting as poorly reabsorbable anions and thus increasing distal sodium delivery and sodium–potassium loss.

Clinical Manifestations

Potassium deficiency can result in widespread derangements in physiologic function. Severe hypokalemia can cause death through cardiac or respiratory arrest. Clinical signs rarely develop before the serum potassium level has decreased to less than 3 mmol/L unless the rate of decline has been rapid. Manifestations of hypokalemia include fatigue, anorexia, nausea, vomiting, muscle weakness, leg cramps, decreased bowel motility, paresthesias (numbness and tingling), dysrhythmias, hypotension, and increased sensitivity to digitalis toxicity. If prolonged, hypokalemia can lead to an inability of the kidneys to concentrate urine, causing dilute urine (resulting in polyuria, nocturia) and excessive thirst. Potassium depletion suppresses the release of insulin and results in glucose intolerance. Decreased muscle strength and DTRs can be found on physical assessment.

Assessment and Diagnostic Findings

In hypokalemia, the serum potassium concentration is less than the lower limit of normal. Electrocardiographic (ECG) changes can include flat T waves or inverted T waves or both, suggesting ischemia, and depressed ST segments (Fig. 17-5). An elevated U wave is specific to hypokalemia. Hypokalemia increases sensitivity to digitalis, predisposing the patient to digitalis toxicity at lower digitalis levels. Metabolic alkalosis is commonly associated with hypokalemia (MacLeod-Glover, Mink, Yarema, et al.,

2016). This is discussed further in the section on acid–base disturbances in this chapter.

The source of the potassium loss is usually evident from a careful history. However, if the cause of the loss is unclear, a 24-hour urinary potassium excretion test can be performed to distinguish between renal and extrarenal loss. Urinary potassium excretion exceeding 20 mmol/L/day with hypokalemia suggests that renal potassium loss is the cause.

Medical Management

If hypokalemia cannot be prevented by conventional measures such as increased intake in the daily diet or by oral potassium supplements for deficiencies, then it is treated cautiously with IV replacement therapy (Mount, 2014b). Potassium loss must be corrected daily; administration of 40 to 80 mmol/L/day of potassium is adequate in the adult if there are no abnormal losses of potassium.

For patients who are at risk for hypokalemia, a diet containing sufficient potassium should be provided. Dietary intake of potassium in the average adult is 50 to 100 mmol/L/day. Foods high in potassium include most fruits and vegetables, legumes, whole grains, milk, and meat.

If dietary intake is inadequate for any reason, oral or IV potassium supplements may be prescribed. Many salt substitutes contain 50 to 60 mmol/L of potassium per 5 mL and may be sufficient to prevent hypokalemia.

If oral administration of potassium is not feasible, the IV route is indicated. The IV route is mandatory for patients with severe hypokalemia (e.g., serum level of 2 mmol/L). Although potassium chloride is usually used to correct potassium deficits, potassium acetate or potassium phosphate may be prescribed.

Nursing Management

Because hypokalemia can be life threatening, the nurse needs to monitor for its early presence in patients who are at risk. Fatigue, anorexia, muscle weakness, decreased bowel motility, paresthesias, and dysrhythmias are signals that warrant assessing the serum potassium concentration. When available, the ECG may provide useful information. For example, patients receiving digitalis who are at risk for potassium deficiency should be monitored closely for signs of digitalis toxicity, because hypokalemia potentiates the action of digitalis.

Preventing Hypokalemia

Prevention may involve encouraging the patient at risk to eat foods rich in potassium (when the diet allows). Sources of potassium include fruit juices and bananas, melon, citrus fruits, fresh and frozen vegetables, fresh meats, milk, and processed foods. If the hypokalemia is caused by abuse of laxatives or diuretics, patient education may help alleviate the problem. Part of the health history and assessment should be directed at identifying problems that are amenable to prevention through education. Careful monitoring of fluid I&O is necessary, because 40 mmol/L of potassium is lost for every litre of urine output. The ECG is monitored for changes, and arterial blood gas values are checked for elevated bicarbonate and pH levels.

Correcting Hypokalemia

The oral route is ideal to treat a mild to moderate hypokalemia because oral potassium supplements are absorbed well. Care should be exercised when administering potassium, particularly in older adults, who have lower lean body mass and total body potassium levels and therefore lower potassium requirements. In addition, because of the physiologic loss of renal function with advancing years, potassium may be retained more readily in older than in younger people.

> **NURSING ALERT**
>
> **Oral potassium supplements can produce small bowel lesions; therefore, the patient must be assessed for and cautioned about abdominal distention, pain, or GI bleeding.**

Administering Intravenous Potassium

Potassium should be administered only after adequate urine flow has been established. A decrease in urine volume to less than 20 mL/hr for 2 consecutive hours is an indication to stop the potassium infusion until the situation is evaluated. Potassium is primarily excreted by the kidneys; when oliguria occurs, potassium administration can cause the serum potassium concentration to rise dangerously.

> **NURSING ALERT**
>
> **Potassium is never administered by IV push or intramuscularly to avoid replacing potassium too quickly. IV potassium must be administered using an infusion pump.**

Each health care facility has its own standard of care for the administration of potassium, which should be consulted; however, the maximum concentration of potassium that should be administered on a medical-surgical unit through a peripheral IV line is 20 mmol/100 mL and the rate no faster than 10 to 20 mmol/hr. Concentrations of potassium greater than 20 mmol/100 mL should be administered through a central IV catheter using an infusion pump with the patient monitored by ECG. Caution must be used when selecting the correct premixed solution of IV fluid containing potassium chloride as the concentrations range from 10 to 40 mmol/100 mL. Renal function should be monitored through BUN and creatinine levels and urine output if the patient is receiving potassium replacement. During potassium replacement, smooth muscle hyperactivity can lead to hyperactive bowel sounds, a sign of hyperkalemia.

Potassium Excess (Hyperkalemia)

Hyperkalemia (serum potassium level greater than 5 mmol/L) seldom occurs in patients with normal renal function (Mount, 2014a). Like hypokalemia, hyperkalemia is often caused by iatrogenic (treatment-induced) causes. Although hyperkalemia is less common than hypokalemia, it is usually more dangerous, because cardiac arrest is more frequently associated with high serum potassium levels.

Pathophysiology

The three major causes of hyperkalemia are decreased renal excretion of potassium, rapid administration of potassium, and movement of potassium from the ICF compartment to the ECF compartment. Hyperkalemia is commonly seen in patients with untreated kidney injury, particularly those in whom potassium levels increase as a result of infection or excessive intake of potassium in food or medications. Patients with hypoaldosteronism or Addison's disease are at risk for hyperkalemia, because deficient adrenal hormones lead to sodium loss and potassium retention.

Medications have been identified as a probable contributing factor in more than 60% of hyperkalemic episodes. Medications commonly implicated are potassium chloride, heparin, ACE inhibitors, angiotensin II receptor blockers, captopril, NSAIDs, beta-blockers, and potassium-sparing diuretics (Comerford, 2015). Potassium regulation is compromised in acute and chronic kidney disease, with a glomerular filtration rate less than 10% to 20% of normal.

Improper use of potassium supplements predisposes all patients to hyperkalemia, especially if salt substitutes are used. Not all patients receiving potassium-losing diuretics require potassium supplements, and patients receiving potassium-conserving diuretics should not receive supplements.

> **NURSING ALERT**
>
> **Potassium supplements are extremely dangerous for patients who have impaired renal function and thus decreased ability to excrete potassium. Even more dangerous is the IV administration of potassium to such patients, because serum levels can rise very quickly. Aged (stored) blood should not be administered to patients with impaired renal function, because the serum potassium concentration of stored blood increases due to red blood cell deterioration. It is possible to exceed the renal tolerance of any patient with rapid IV potassium administration, as well as when large amounts of oral potassium supplements are ingested.**

In **acidosis**, potassium moves out of the cells and into the ECF. This occurs as hydrogen ions enter the cells to buffer the pH of the ECF (see later discussion). An elevated ECF potassium level should be anticipated when extensive tissue trauma has occurred, as in burns, crushing injuries, or severe infections. Similarly, it can occur with lysis of malignant cells after chemotherapy (i.e., tumour lysis syndrome).

Pseudohyperkalemia (a variation of hyperkalemia) has a number of causes, the most common being the use of a tight tourniquet around an exercising extremity while drawing a blood sample, producing hemolysis of the sample before analysis. Other causes include marked leukocytosis (white blood cell count exceeding 200,000/mm^3) and thrombocytosis (platelet count exceeding 1 million/mm^3); drawing blood above a site where potassium is infusing; and familial pseudohyperkalemia, in which potassium leaks out of the red blood cells while the blood is awaiting analysis. Lack of awareness of these causes of pseudohyperkalemia can lead to aggressive treatment of a nonexistent hyperkalemia, resulting in serious lowering of serum potassium levels. Therefore, measurements of grossly elevated levels should be verified by retesting.

Clinical Manifestations

The most important consequence of hyperkalemia is its effect on the myocardium. Cardiac effects of elevated serum potassium are usually not significant when the level is less than 7 mmol/L, but they are almost always present when the level is 8 mmol/L or greater. As the plasma potassium level rises, disturbances in cardiac conduction occur. The earliest changes, often occurring at a serum potassium level greater than 6 mmol/L, are peaked, narrow T waves; ST-segment depression; and a shortened QT interval. If the serum potassium level continues to increase, the PR interval becomes prolonged and is followed by disappearance of the P waves. Finally, there is decomposition and widening of the QRS complex (see Fig. 17-5). Ventricular dysrhythmias and cardiac arrest may occur at any point in this progression.

Severe hyperkalemia causes skeletal muscle weakness and even paralysis, related to a depolarization block in muscle. Similarly, ventricular conduction is slowed. Although hyperkalemia has marked effects on the peripheral nervous system, it has little effect on the central nervous system. Rapidly ascending muscular weakness leading to flaccid quadriplegia has been reported in patients with very high serum potassium levels. Paralysis of respiratory and speech muscles can also occur. In addition, GI manifestations, such as nausea, intermittent intestinal colic, and diarrhea, may be evident.

Assessment and Diagnostic Findings

Serum potassium levels and ECG changes are crucial to the diagnosis of hyperkalemia, as discussed previously. Arterial blood gas analysis may reveal both a metabolic and respiratory acidosis. Correcting the acidosis helps correct the hyperkalemia.

Medical Management

An ECG should be obtained immediately to detect changes. Shortened repolarization and peaked T waves are seen initially. To verify results, a repeat serum potassium level should be obtained from a vein without an IV infusing a potassium-containing solution.

In nonacute situations, restriction of dietary potassium and potassium-containing medications may correct the

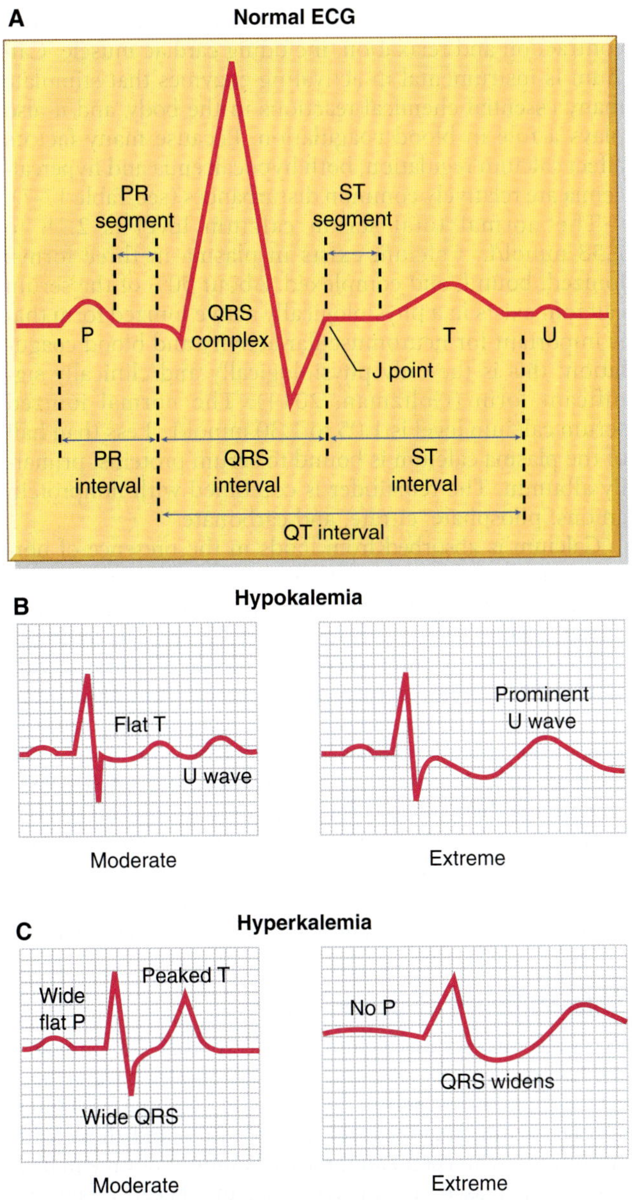

FIGURE 17-5. Effect of potassium on the electrocardiogram (ECG). **A.** Normal tracing. **B.** Hypokalemia: serum potassium level below normal. **Left:** Flattening of the T wave and the appearance of a U wave. **Right:** Further flattening with prominent U wave. **C.** Hyperkalemia: serum potassium level above normal. **Left:** Moderate elevation with wide, flat P wave; wide QRS complex; and peaked T wave. **Right:** ECG changes seen with extreme potassium elevation: widening of QRS complex and absence of P wave.

imbalance. For example, eliminating the use of potassium-containing salt substitutes in a patient who is taking a potassium-conserving diuretic may be all that is needed to deal with mild hyperkalemia.

Prevention of serious hyperkalemia by the administration, either orally or by retention enema, of cation exchange resins (e.g., sodium polystyrene sulfonate [Kayexalate]) may be necessary in patients with renal impairment. Cation exchange resins cannot be used if the patient has a paralytic ileus, because intestinal perforation can occur. Kayexalate binds with other cations in the GI tract and contributes to the development of hypomagnesemia and hypocalcemia; it may also cause sodium retention and fluid overload, and should be used with caution in patients with heart failure.

Emergency Pharmacologic Therapy

If serum potassium levels are dangerously elevated, it may be necessary to administer IV calcium gluconate. Within minutes after administration, calcium antagonizes the action of hyperkalemia on the heart, but it does not reduce the serum potassium concentration. Calcium chloride and calcium gluconate are not interchangeable; calcium gluconate contains 4.5 mmol of calcium and calcium chloride contains 13.6 mmol of calcium. Therefore, caution is required.

Monitoring the blood pressure is essential to detect hypotension, which may result from the rapid IV administration of calcium gluconate. The ECG should be continuously monitored during administration; the appearance of bradycardia is an indication to stop the infusion. The myocardial protective effects of calcium last about 30 minutes. Extra caution is required if the patient has been "digitalized" (i.e., has received accelerated dosages of a digitalis-based cardiac glycoside to reach a desired serum digitalis level rapidly); parenteral administration of calcium sensitizes the heart to digitalis and may precipitate digitalis toxicity.

IV administration of sodium bicarbonate may be necessary to alkalinize the plasma, cause a temporary shift of potassium into the cells, and furnish sodium to antagonize the cardiac effects of potassium. Effects of this therapy begin within 30 to 60 minutes and may persist for hours; however, they are temporary.

IV administration of regular insulin and a hypertonic dextrose solution causes a temporary shift of potassium into the cells. Glucose and insulin therapy has an onset of action within 30 minutes and lasts for several hours. Loop diuretics, such as furosemide (Lasix), increase excretion of water by inhibiting sodium, potassium, and chloride reabsorption in the ascending loop of Henle and distal renal tubule.

Beta-2 agonists, such as albuterol (Proventil, Ventolin), are highly effective in decreasing potassium, but their use remains controversial, because they can cause tachycardia and chest discomfort (Mount, 2014c). Beta-2 agonists move potassium into the cells and may be used in the absence of ischemic cardiac disease. Their use is a stopgap measure that only temporarily protects the patient from hyperkalemia. If the hyperkalemic condition is not transient, actual removal of potassium from the body is required through cation exchange resins, peritoneal dialysis, hemodialysis, or other forms of renal replacement therapy.

Nursing Management

Patients at risk for potassium excess (e.g., those with chronic kidney disease) need to be identified and closely monitored for signs of hyperkalemia. The nurse observes for signs of muscle weakness and dysrhythmias. The presence of paresthesias and GI symptoms such as nausea and intestinal colic is noted. Serum potassium levels, as well as BUN, creatinine, glucose, and arterial blood gas values, are monitored for patients at risk for developing hyperkalemia (Hannon & Porth, 2017).

Preventing Hyperkalemia

Measures are taken to prevent hyperkalemia in patients at risk, when possible, by encouraging the patient to adhere to the prescribed potassium restriction. Potassium-rich foods to be avoided include many fruits and vegetables, legumes, whole-grain breads, meat, milk, eggs, coffee, tea, and cocoa (Dudek, 2013). Conversely, foods with minimal potassium content include butter, margarine, cranberry juice or sauce, ginger ale, gumdrops or jelly beans, hard candy, root beer, sugar, and honey. Labels of cola beverages must be checked carefully because some are high in potassium and some are not.

Correcting Hyperkalemia

It is possible to exceed the tolerance for potassium if administered rapidly by the IV route. Therefore, care is taken to administer and monitor potassium solutions closely. Particular attention is paid to the solution's concentration and rate of administration. Potassium is not added to parenteral solutions on the nursing units but in the pharmacy. IV administration is via a volumetric infusion pump (Mount, 2014c).

It is important to caution patients to use salt substitutes sparingly if they are taking other supplementary forms of potassium or potassium-conserving diuretics. Also, potassium-conserving diuretics, such as spironolactone (Aldactone), triamterene (Dyrenium), and amiloride (Midamor); potassium supplements; and salt substitutes should not be administered to patients with renal dysfunction. Most salt substitutes contain approximately 50 to 60 mmol of potassium per 5 mL (teaspoon).

Calcium Imbalances

More than 99% of the body's calcium is located in the skeletal system; it is a major component of bones and teeth. About 1% of skeletal calcium is rapidly exchangeable with blood calcium, and the rest is more stable and only slowly exchanged. The small amount of calcium located outside the bone circulates in the serum, partly bound to protein and partly ionized. Calcium plays a major role in transmitting nerve impulses and helps regulate muscle contraction and relaxation, including cardiac muscle. Calcium is instrumental in activating enzymes that stimulate many essential chemical reactions in the body, and it also plays a role in blood coagulation. Because many factors affect calcium regulation, both hypocalcemia and hypercalcemia are relatively common disturbances (see Table 17-7).

The normal total serum calcium level is 2.18 to 2.58 mmol/L. Calcium exists in plasma in three forms: ionized, bound, and complexed. About 50% of the serum calcium exists in a physiologically active ionized form that is important for neuromuscular activity and blood coagulation; this is the only physiologically and clinically significant form (Goltzman, 2014). The normal ionized serum calcium level is 1.05 to 1.30 mmol/L. Less than half of the plasma calcium is bound to serum proteins, primarily albumin. The remainder is combined with nonprotein anions: phosphate, citrate, and carbonate.

Calcium is absorbed from foods in the presence of normal gastric acidity and vitamin D. It is excreted primarily in the feces, with the remainder excreted in the urine. The serum calcium level is controlled by PTH and calcitonin. As ionized serum calcium decreases, the parathyroid glands secrete PTH. This, in turn, increases calcium absorption from the GI tract, increases calcium reabsorption from the renal tubule, and releases calcium from the bone. The increase in calcium ion concentration suppresses PTH secretion. When calcium increases excessively, the thyroid gland secretes calcitonin, which briefly inhibits calcium reabsorption from bone and decreases the serum calcium concentration by promoting the entry of calcium into bone tissues and using it for bone synthesis (osteoblast activity).

Calcium Deficit (Hypocalcemia)

Hypocalcemia (serum calcium value lower than 2.18 mmol/L) occurs in a variety of clinical situations. A patient may have a total body calcium deficit (as in osteoporosis) but a normal serum calcium level. Older adults and those with disabilities, who spend an increased amount of time in bed, have an increased risk of hypocalcemia, because bed rest increases bone resorption.

TABLE 17-7 Calcium Imbalances

Imbalance	Contributing Factors	Signs/Symptoms and Laboratory Findings
Calcium deficit (hypocalcemia) Serum calcium <2.18 mmol/L	Hypoparathyroidism (may follow thyroid surgery or radical neck dissection), malabsorption, pancreatitis, alkalosis, vitamin D deficiency, massive subcutaneous infection, generalized peritonitis, massive transfusion of citrated blood, chronic diarrhea, decreased parathyroid hormone, diuretic phase of kidney injury, ↑ PO_4, fistulas, burns, alcoholism	Numbness, tingling of fingers, toes, and circumoral region; positive Trousseau's sign and Chvostek's sign; seizures, carpopedal spasms, hyperactive deep tendon reflexes, irritability, bronchospasm, anxiety, impaired clotting time, ↓ prothrombin, diarrhea, ↓ BP. *ECG:* prolonged QT interval and lengthened ST *Labs indicate:* ↓ Mg^{++}
Calcium excess (hypercalcemia) Serum calcium >2.58 mmol/L	Hyperparathyroidism, malignant neoplastic disease, prolonged immobilization, overuse of calcium supplements, vitamin D excess, oliguric phase of renal failure, acidosis, corticosteroid therapy, thiazide diuretic use, increased parathyroid hormone, and digoxin toxicity	Muscular weakness, constipation, anorexia, nausea and vomiting, polyuria and polydipsia, dehydration, hypoactive deep tendon reflexes, lethargy, deep bone pain, pathologic fractures, flank pain, calcium stones, hypertension. *ECG:* shortened ST segment and QT interval, bradycardia, heart blocks

↑, increased; ↓, decreased; BP, blood pressure; ECG, electrocardiogram.

Adapted from Grossman, S. C., & Porth, C. M. (2014). *Porth's pathophysiology: Concepts of altered health states* (9th ed.). Philadelphia, PA: Lippincott Williams & Wilkins.

Pathophysiology

Several factors can cause hypocalcemia, including primary hypoparathyroidism and surgical hypoparathyroidism. The latter is far more common. Not only is hypocalcemia associated with thyroid and parathyroid surgery, but it can also occur after radical neck dissection and is most likely in the first 24 to 48 hours after surgery. Transient hypocalcemia can occur with massive administration of citrated blood (i.e., massive hemorrhage and shock), because citrate can combine with ionized calcium and temporarily remove it from the circulation.

Inflammation of the pancreas causes the breakdown of proteins and lipids. It is thought that calcium ions combine with the fatty acids released by lipolysis, forming soaps. As a result of this process, hypocalcemia occurs and is common in pancreatitis. Hypocalcemia may be related to excessive secretion of glucagon from the inflamed pancreas, which results in increased secretion of calcitonin.

Hypocalcemia is common in patients with kidney injury, because these patients frequently have elevated serum phosphate levels. Hyperphosphatemia usually causes a reciprocal drop in the serum calcium level. Other causes of hypocalcemia include inadequate vitamin D consumption, magnesium deficiency, medullary thyroid carcinoma, low serum albumin levels, alkalosis, and alcohol abuse. Medications predisposing to hypocalcemia include aluminum-containing antacids, aminoglycosides, caffeine, cisplatin, corticosteroids, mithramycin, phosphates, isoniazid, and loop diuretics.

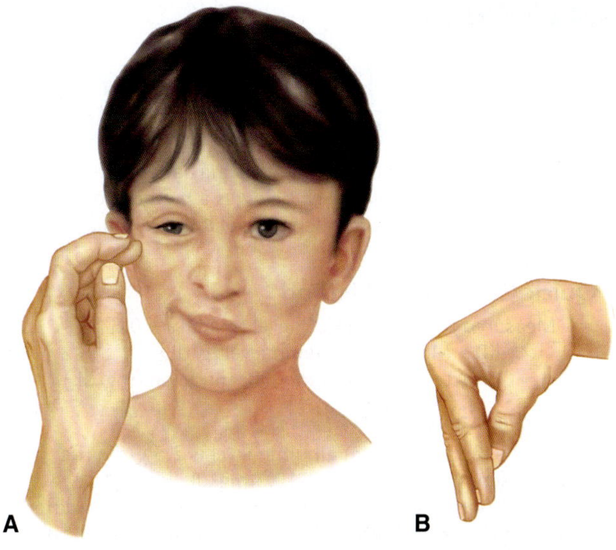

FIGURE 17-6. **A.** Chvostek's sign: a contraction of the facial muscles elicited in response to light tap over the facial nerve in front of the ear. **B.** Trousseau's sign: a carpopedal spasm induced by inflating a blood pressure cuff above systolic blood pressure. (Adapted from Bullock, B. A., & Henze, R. J. [2000]. *Focus on pathophysiology* [p. 173]. Philadelphia, PA: Lippincott Williams & Wilkins.)

Clinical Manifestations

Tetany, the most characteristic manifestation of hypocalcemia and hypomagnesemia, refers to the entire symptom complex induced by increased neural excitability. These symptoms are caused by spontaneous discharges of both sensory and motor fibres in peripheral nerves. Sensations of tingling may occur in the tips of the fingers, around the mouth, and, less commonly, in the feet. Spasms of the muscles of the extremities and face may occur. Pain may develop as a result of these spasms. Hyperactive DTRs are another clinical sign associated with tetany.

Trousseau's sign (Fig. 17-6) can be elicited by inflating a blood pressure cuff on the upper arm to about 20 mm Hg above systolic pressure; within 2 to 5 minutes, carpal spasm (an adducted thumb, flexed wrist and metacarpophalangeal joints, extended interphalangeal joints with fingers together) will occur as ischemia of the ulnar nerve develops. Chvostek's sign consists of twitching of muscles enervated by the facial nerve when the region that is about 2 cm anterior to the earlobe, just below the zygomatic arch, is tapped.

Seizures may occur because hypocalcemia increases irritability of the central nervous system as well as of the peripheral nerves. Other changes associated with hypocalcemia include mental changes such as depression, impaired memory, confusion, delirium, and hallucinations. A prolonged QT interval is seen on the ECG and torsades de pointes, a type of ventricular tachycardia, may occur. Respiratory effects with decreasing calcium include dyspnea and laryngospasm. Signs and symptoms of chronic hypocalcemia include hyperactive bowel sounds, dry and brittle hair and nails, and abnormal clotting.

Osteoporosis is associated with prolonged low intake of calcium and represents a total body calcium deficit, even though serum calcium levels are usually normal. This disorder occurs in many Canadians and is most common in postmenopausal women. It is characterized by loss of bone mass, which causes bones to become porous and brittle and therefore susceptible to fracture. See Chapter 69 for further discussion of osteoporosis.

Assessment and Diagnostic Findings

When evaluating serum calcium levels, the serum albumin level and the arterial pH must also be considered. Because abnormalities in serum albumin levels may affect interpretation of the serum calcium level, it may be necessary to calculate the corrected serum calcium if the serum albumin level is abnormal. For every decrease in serum albumin of 1 g/dL below 4 g/dL, the total serum calcium level is underestimated by approximately 0.8 mg/dL. Chart 17-2 displays a quick method to calculate the corrected serum calcium level.

Clinicians often discount a low serum calcium level in the presence of a similarly low serum albumin level. The ionized calcium level is usually normal in patients with reduced total serum calcium levels and concomitant hypoalbuminemia. When the arterial pH increases (alkalosis), more calcium becomes bound to protein. As a result, the ionized portion decreases. Symptoms of hypocalcemia may occur with alkalosis. Acidosis (low pH) has the opposite effect; that is, less calcium is bound to protein and therefore more exists in the ionized form. However, relatively small changes in serum calcium levels occur in these acid–base abnormalities.

Ideally, the ionized level of calcium should be measured in the laboratory. However, in many laboratories, only the total calcium level is reported; therefore, the concentration of the ionized fraction must be estimated by

CHART 17-2

Calculating Corrected Serum Calcium Level

Abnormalities in serum albumin levels may affect interpretation of the serum calcium level. Below is a method for calculating the corrected serum calcium level if the serum albumin level is abnormal.

Quick Calculation Method

Measured total serum Ca^{++} level (mg/dL) + 0.8
× (4.0 − Measured albumin level [g/dL])
= Corrected total calcium concentration (mg/dL)

Example Calculation

A patient's reported serum albumin level is 2.5 g/dL; the reported serum calcium level is 10.5 mg/dL. First, the decrease in serum albumin level from normal (i.e., the difference from the normal albumin concentration of 4 g/dL) is calculated: 4 g/dL − 2.5 g/dL = 1.5 g/dL. Next, the following ratio is calculated:

0.8 mg/dL: 1 g/dL = X mg/dL: 1.5 mg/dL
X = 0.8 × 1.5 mg/dL
X = 1.2 mg/dL calcium

Finally, 1.2 mg/dL is added to 10.5 mg/dL (the reported serum calcium level) to obtain the corrected total serum calcium level: 1.2 mg/dL + 10.5 mg/dL = 11.7 mg/dL.

simultaneous measurement of the serum albumin level. PTH levels are decreased in hypoparathyroidism. Magnesium and phosphorus levels need to be assessed to identify possible causes of decreased calcium.

Medical Management

Emergency Pharmacologic Therapy

Acute symptomatic hypocalcemia is life threatening and requires prompt treatment with IV administration of a calcium salt. Parenteral calcium salts include calcium gluconate, calcium chloride (Comerford, 2015). Although calcium chloride produces a significantly higher ionized calcium level than calcium gluconate does, it is not used as often because it is more irritating and can cause sloughing of tissue if it infiltrates. Too-rapid IV administration of calcium can cause cardiac arrest, preceded by bradycardia. IV administration of calcium is particularly dangerous in patients receiving digitalis-derived medications, because calcium ions exert an effect similar to that of digitalis and can cause digitalis toxicity, with adverse cardiac effects. Therefore, calcium should be diluted in D_5W and administered as a slow IV bolus or a slow IV infusion using a volumetric infusion pump. The IV site must be observed often for any evidence of infiltration because of the risk of extravasation and resultant cellulitis or necrosis. A 0.9% sodium chloride solution should not be used with calcium because it increases renal calcium loss. Solutions containing phosphates or bicarbonate should not be used with calcium because they cause precipitation when calcium is added. The nurse must clarify with the physician and pharmacist which calcium salt to administer, because calcium gluconate yields 4.5 mmol/L of calcium and calcium chloride provides 13.6 mmol/L of calcium. Calcium replacement can cause postural hypotension; therefore, the patient is kept in bed during IV infusion, and blood pressure is monitored.

Nutritional Therapy

Vitamin D therapy may be instituted to increase calcium absorption from the GI tract; otherwise, the amount of calcium absorbed may not satisfy the body's calcium requirement. In addition, aluminum hydroxide, calcium acetate, or calcium carbonate antacids may be prescribed to decrease elevated phosphorus levels before treating hypocalcemia in the patient with chronic kidney disease. Increasing the dietary intake of calcium to at least 1,000 to 1,500 mg/day in the adult is recommended. Calcium-containing foods include milk products; green, leafy vegetables; canned salmon; sardines; and fresh oysters. Hypomagnesemia can also cause tetany; if the tetany responds to IV calcium, then a low magnesium level is considered as a possible cause in chronic kidney injury.

Nursing Management

It is important to observe for hypocalcemia in at-risk patients. Seizure precautions are initiated if hypocalcemia is severe. The status of the airway is closely monitored, because laryngeal stridor can occur. Safety precautions are taken, as indicated, if confusion is present.

It is important to teach the patient with hypocalcemia what foods are rich in calcium. The nurse also advises the patient to consider calcium supplements if sufficient calcium is not consumed in the diet. Calcium supplements should be taken in divided doses with meals. Alcohol and caffeine in high doses inhibit calcium absorption, and moderate cigarette smoking increases urinary calcium excretion. The patient is also cautioned to avoid the overuse of laxatives and antacids that contain phosphorus, because their use decreases calcium absorption.

The Canadian Cancer Society (2019) recommends 1,000 IU of vitamin D from food sources (e.g., fortified milk) and 1,000 IU as a supplement. Sunlight is not a reliable source of vitamin D in fall and winter months in Canada.

Calcium Excess (Hypercalcemia)

Hypercalcemia (serum calcium value greater than 2.6 mmol/L) is a dangerous imbalance when severe; in fact, hypercalcemic crisis has a mortality rate as high as 50% if not treated promptly.

Pathophysiology

The most common causes of hypercalcemia are malignancies and hyperparathyroidism. Malignant tumours can produce hypercalcemia by a variety of mechanisms. The excessive PTH secretion associated with hyperparathyroidism causes increased release of calcium from the bones and increased intestinal and renal absorption of calcium. Calcifications of soft tissue occur when the calcium–phosphorus product (serum calcium × serum phosphorus) exceeds 70 mmol/L.

Bone mineral is lost during immobilization, and sometimes this causes elevation of total (and especially ionized) calcium in the bloodstream. However, symptomatic hypercalcemia from immobilization is rare; when it does occur, it is virtually limited to people with high calcium turnover rates (e.g., adolescents during a growth spurt). Most cases of hypercalcemia secondary to immobility occur after severe or multiple fractures or spinal cord injury.

Thiazide diuretics can cause a slight elevation in serum calcium levels because they potentiate the action of PTH on the kidneys, reducing urinary calcium excretion. Vitamin A and D intoxication, as well as chronic lithium use and theophylline toxicity, can cause calcium excess. Calcium levels are inversely related to phosphorus levels.

Hypercalcemia reduces neuromuscular excitability because it suppresses activity at the myoneural junction. Decreased tone in smooth and striated muscle may cause symptoms such as muscle weakness, incoordination, anorexia, and constipation. Cardiac standstill can occur when the serum calcium level is about 4.5 mmol/L. Calcium enhances the inotropic effect of digitalis; therefore, hypercalcemia aggravates digitalis toxicity.

Clinical Manifestations

The symptoms of hypercalcemia are proportional to the degree of elevation of the serum calcium level. Anorexia, nausea, vomiting, and constipation are common symptoms of hypercalcemia. Dehydration occurs with nausea, vomiting, anorexia, and calcium reabsorption at the proximal renal tubule. Abdominal and bone pain may also be present. Abdominal distention and paralytic ileus may complicate severe hypercalcemic crisis. Excessive urination due to disturbed renal tubular function produced by hypercalcemia may occur. Severe thirst may occur with polyuria secondary to high solute (calcium) load. Patients with chronic hypercalcemia may develop symptoms similar to peptic ulcer disease because hypercalcemia increases the secretion of acid and pepsin in the stomach.

Confusion, impaired memory, slurred speech, lethargy, acute psychotic behaviour, or coma may occur. The more severe symptoms tend to appear when the serum calcium level is approximately 4 mmol/L or higher. However, some patients become profoundly disturbed with serum calcium levels of only 3 mmol/L. These symptoms resolve as serum calcium levels return to normal after treatment.

Hypercalcemic crisis refers to an acute rise in the serum calcium level to 4.3 mmol/L or higher. Severe thirst and polyuria are often present. Other findings may include muscle weakness, intractable nausea, abdominal cramps, severe constipation, diarrhea, peptic ulcer symptoms, and bone pain. Lethargy, confusion, and coma may also occur. This condition is dangerous and may result in cardiac arrest.

Assessment and Diagnostic Findings

The serum calcium level is greater than 2.6 mmol/L. Cardiovascular changes may include a variety of dysrhythmias (i.e., heart blocks) and shortening of the QT interval and ST segment. The PR interval is sometimes prolonged. The double-antibody PTH test may be used to differentiate between primary hyperparathyroidism and malignancy as a cause of hypercalcemia: PTH levels are increased in primary or secondary hyperparathyroidism and suppressed in malignancy. X-rays may reveal bone changes if the patient has hypercalcemia secondary to a malignancy, bone cavitation, or urinary calculi. The Sulkowitch urine test analyzes the amount of calcium in the urine; in hypercalcemia, dense precipitation is observed due to hypercalciuria.

Medical Management

Therapeutic aims in hypercalcemia include decreasing the serum calcium level and reversing the process causing hypercalcemia. Treating the underlying cause (e.g., chemotherapy for a malignancy, partial parathyroidectomy for hyperparathyroidism) is essential.

Pharmacologic Therapy

Measures include administering fluids to dilute serum calcium and promote its excretion by the kidneys, mobilizing the patient, and restricting dietary calcium intake. IV administration of 0.9% sodium chloride solution temporarily dilutes the serum calcium level and increases urinary calcium excretion by inhibiting tubular reabsorption of calcium. Administering IV phosphate can cause a reciprocal drop in serum calcium. Furosemide (Lasix) is often used in conjunction with administration of a saline solution; in addition to causing diuresis, furosemide increases calcium excretion. Although often overlooked, fluids and medications that contain calcium and dietary sources of calcium should be halted.

Calcitonin can be used to lower the serum calcium level and is particularly useful for patients with heart disease or kidney injury who cannot tolerate large sodium loads. Calcitonin reduces bone resorption, increases the deposition of calcium and phosphorus in the bones, and increases urinary excretion of calcium and phosphorus (Karch, 2012). Although several forms are available, calcitonin derived from salmon is commonly used. Skin testing for allergy to salmon calcitonin is necessary before the hormone is administered. Systemic allergic reactions are possible because this hormone is a protein; resistance to the medication may develop later because of antibody formation. Calcitonin is administered by intramuscular injection rather than subcutaneously, because patients with hypercalcemia have poor perfusion of subcutaneous tissue.

For patients with cancer, treatment is directed at controlling the condition by surgery, chemotherapy, or radiation therapy. Corticosteroids may be used to decrease bone turnover and tubular reabsorption for patients with sarcoidosis, myelomas, lymphomas, and leukemias; patients with solid tumours are less responsive. Some bisphosphonates (e.g., etidronate disodium [Didronel], pamidronate disodium [Aredia], and ibandronate sodium [Boniva]) inhibit osteoclast activity. IV forms can cause fever, transient leukopenia, eye inflammation, nephrotic syndrome, and jaw osteonecrosis (Karch, 2012). Mithramycin, a cytotoxic antibiotic, inhibits bone resorption and thus lowers the serum calcium level. This agent must be used cautiously because it has significant side effects, including thrombocytopenia, nephrotoxicity, rebound hypercalcemia when discontinued, and hepatotoxicity. Inorganic phosphate salts can be administered orally or by nasogastric tube (in the form of Phospho-Soda or Neutra-Phos), rectally (as retention enemas), or intravenously. IV phosphate therapy is used with extreme caution in the treatment of hypercalcemia, because it can cause severe calcification in various tissues, hypotension, tetany, and acute kidney injury.

Nursing Management

It is important to monitor for hypercalcemia in at-risk patients. Interventions such as increasing patient mobility and encouraging fluids can help prevent hypercalcemia, or at least minimize its severity. Hospitalized patients at risk for hypercalcemia should be encouraged to ambulate as soon as possible. Those who are outpatients and receive home care are instructed about the importance of frequent ambulation.

When encouraging oral fluids, the nurse considers the patient's likes and dislikes. Fluids containing sodium should be administered unless contraindicated, because sodium assists with calcium excretion. Patients are encouraged to drink 2.8 to 3.8 L of fluid daily. Adequate fibre in the diet is encouraged to offset the tendency for constipation. Safety precautions are implemented, as necessary, when mental symptoms of hypercalcemia are present. The patient and family are informed that these mental changes are reversible with treatment. Increased calcium increases the effects of digitalis; therefore, the patient is assessed for signs and symptoms of digitalis toxicity. Because ECG changes (premature ventricular contractions, paroxysmal atrial tachycardia, and heart block) can occur, the cardiac rate and rhythm are monitored for any abnormalities.

Magnesium Imbalances

Magnesium is the most abundant intracellular cation after potassium. It acts as an activator for many intracellular enzyme systems and plays a role in both carbohydrate and protein metabolism. The normal serum magnesium level is 0.75 to 0.95 mmol/L. Approximately one third of serum magnesium is bound to protein; the remaining two thirds exists as free cations—the active component (Mg^{++}). Magnesium balance is important in neuromuscular function. Because magnesium acts directly on the myoneural junction, variations in the serum level affect neuromuscular irritability and contractility. For example, an excess of magnesium diminishes the excitability of the muscle cells, whereas a deficit increases neuromuscular irritability and contractility. Magnesium produces its sedative effect at the neuromuscular junction, probably by inhibiting the release of the neurotransmitter acetylcholine. It also increases the stimulus threshold in nerve fibres. Two common magnesium imbalances are magnesium deficit and magnesium excess (see Table 17-8).

Magnesium also affects the cardiovascular system, acting peripherally to produce vasodilation and decreased peripheral resistance. Magnesium is predominantly found in bone and soft tissues and eliminated by the kidneys.

Magnesium Deficit (Hypomagnesemia)

Hypomagnesemia refers to a below-normal serum magnesium concentration (0.75 mmol/L) and is frequently associated with hypokalemia and hypocalcemia. Magnesium is similar to calcium in two aspects: (1) it is the ionized fraction of magnesium that is primarily involved in neuromuscular activity and other physiologic processes, and (2) magnesium levels should be evaluated in combination with albumin levels. About 30% of magnesium is protein bound, principally to albumin. A decreased serum albumin level can therefore reduce the measured total magnesium concentration; however, it does not reduce the ionized plasma magnesium concentration.

Pathophysiology

An important route of magnesium loss is the GI tract. Loss of magnesium from the GI tract may occur with nasogastric suction, diarrhea, or fistulas. Because fluid from the lower

TABLE 17-8 Magnesium Imbalances

Imbalance	Contributing Factors	Signs/Symptoms
Magnesium deficit (hypomagnesemia) Serum magnesium <0.75 mmol/L	Chronic alcoholism, hyperparathyroidism, hyperaldosteronism, diuretic phase of acute kidney injury, malabsorptive disorders, diabetic ketoacidosis, refeeding after starvation, parenteral nutrition, chronic laxative use, diarrhea, acute myocardial infarction, heart failure, decreased serum K^+ and Ca^{++} and certain pharmacologic agents (such as gentamicin, cisplatin, and cyclosporine)	Neuromuscular irritability, positive Trousseau's sign and Chvostek's sign, insomnia, mood changes, anorexia, vomiting, increased tendon reflexes, and ↑ BP. *ECG:* PVCs, flat or inverted T waves, depressed ST segment, prolonged PR interval, and widened QRS
Magnesium excess (hypermagnesemia) Serum magnesium >0.95 mmol/L	Oliguric phase of acute kidney injury (particularly when magnesium-containing medications are given), adrenal insufficiency, excessive IV magnesium administration, diabetic ketoacidosis, and hypothyroidism	Flushing, hypotension, muscle weakness, drowsiness, hypoactive reflexes, depressed respirations, cardiac arrest and coma, diaphoresis. *ECG:* tachycardia → bradycardia, prolonged PR interval and QRS, peaked T waves

↑, increased; →, followed by; BP, blood pressure; ECG, electrocardiogram; IV, intravenous; PVCs, premature ventricular contractions.

Adapted from Grossman, S. C., & Porth, C. M. (2014). *Porth's pathophysiology: Concepts of altered health states* (9th ed.). Philadelphia, PA: Lippincott Williams & Wilkins.

GI tract has a higher concentration of magnesium (10 to 14 mmol/L) than fluid from the upper tract (1 to 2 mmol/L), losses from diarrhea and intestinal fistulas are more likely to induce magnesium deficit than are those from gastric suction. Although magnesium losses are relatively small in nasogastric suction, hypomagnesemia occurs if losses are prolonged and magnesium is not replaced through IV infusion. Because the distal small bowel is the major site of magnesium absorption, any disruption in small bowel function (e.g., intestinal resection or inflammatory bowel disease) can lead to hypomagnesemia. Hypomagnesemia is a common yet often overlooked imbalance in acutely and critically ill patients. It may occur with withdrawal from alcohol and administration of tube feedings or parenteral nutrition.

Alcoholism is currently the most common cause of symptomatic hypomagnesemia in Canada. The serum magnesium level should be measured at least every 2 or 3 days in patients undergoing withdrawal from alcohol. The serum magnesium level may be normal on admission but may decrease as a result of metabolic changes, such as the intracellular shift of magnesium associated with IV glucose administration.

During nutritional replacement, the major cellular electrolytes move from the serum to newly synthesized cells. Therefore, if the enteral or parenteral feeding formula is deficient in magnesium content, serious hypomagnesemia will occur. Because of this, serum magnesium levels should be measured at regular intervals in patients who are receiving parenteral or enteral feedings, especially those who have undergone a period of starvation. Other causes of hypomagnesemia include the administration of aminoglycosides, cyclosporine, cisplatin, diuretics, digitalis, and amphotericin, as well as the rapid administration of citrated blood, especially to patients with renal or hepatic disease. Magnesium deficiency often occurs in diabetic ketoacidosis, secondary to increased renal excretion during osmotic diuresis and shifting of magnesium into the cells with insulin therapy. Other contributing causes are pregnancy, lactation, sepsis, burns, and hypothermia.

Clinical Manifestations

Clinical manifestations of hypomagnesemia are largely confined to the neuromuscular system. Some are due directly to the low serum magnesium level; others are due to secondary changes in potassium and calcium metabolism. Symptoms do not usually occur until the serum magnesium level has dropped to less than 0.75 mmol/L.

Among the neuromuscular changes are hyperexcitability with muscle weakness, tremors, and athetoid movements (slow, involuntary twisting and writhing). Others include tetany, nystagmus, vertigo, generalized tonic–clonic or focal seizures, laryngeal stridor, and positive Chvostek's and Trousseau's signs (see earlier discussion), which occur, in part, because of accompanying hypocalcemia.

Hypomagnesemia may be accompanied by marked alterations in mood. Apathy, depression, apprehension, and extreme agitation have been noted, as well as ataxia, dizziness, insomnia, and confusion. At times, delirium, auditory or visual hallucinations, and frank psychoses may occur.

Magnesium deficiency can disturb the ECG by prolonging the QRS, depressing the ST segment, and predisposing to cardiac dysrhythmias, such as premature ventricular contractions, supraventricular tachycardia, torsades de pointes (a form of ventricular tachycardia), and ventricular fibrillation. Increased susceptibility to digitalis toxicity is associated with low serum magnesium levels. This is important because patients receiving digoxin are also likely to be receiving diuretic therapy, predisposing them to renal loss of magnesium. Hypercalcemia and hypokalemia may be refractory to correction until the magnesium level is corrected.

Assessment and Diagnostic Findings

On laboratory analysis, the serum magnesium level is less than 0.62 mmol/L. Urine magnesium may help identify the cause of magnesium depletion, and levels are measured after a loading dose of magnesium sulphate is administered. Two newer diagnostic techniques (nuclear magnetic resonance spectroscopy and the ion-selective electrode) are sensitive and direct means of measuring ionized serum magnesium levels.

Medical Management

Mild magnesium deficiency can be corrected by diet alone. Principal dietary sources of magnesium include green leafy vegetables, nuts, seeds, legumes, whole grains, seafood, peanut butter, and cocoa.

If necessary, magnesium salts can be administered orally in an oxide or gluconate form to replace continuous losses but can produce diarrhea. Patients receiving parenteral nutrition require magnesium in the IV solution to prevent hypomagnesemia. IV magnesium sulphate must be administered by an infusion pump and at a rate not to exceed 150 mg/min or 67 mEq over 8 hours. Overt symptoms of hypomagnesemia are treated with parenteral administration of magnesium. A bolus dose of magnesium sulphate given too rapidly can produce alterations in cardiac conduction leading to heart block or asystole. Vital signs must be assessed frequently during magnesium administration to detect changes in cardiac rate or rhythm, hypotension, and respiratory distress. Monitoring urine output is essential before, during, and after magnesium administration; the physician is notified if urine volume decreases to less than 100 mL over 4 hours. Calcium gluconate must be readily available to treat hypocalcemic tetany or hypermagnesemia.

Nursing Management

The nurse should be aware of patients at risk for hypomagnesemia and observe them for its signs and symptoms. Patients receiving digitalis are monitored closely, because a deficit of magnesium can predispose them to digitalis toxicity. If hypomagnesemia is severe, seizure precautions are implemented. Other safety precautions are instituted, as indicated, if confusion is observed. Because difficulty in swallowing (dysphagia) may occur in those with magnesium depletion, these patients should be screened for dysphagia.

Teaching plays a major role in treating magnesium deficit, particularly a deficit resulting from abuse of diuretic or laxative medications. In such cases, the nurse instructs the patient about the need to consume magnesium-rich foods. For patients experiencing hypomagnesemia from abuse of alcohol, the nurse provides teaching, counselling, support, and possible referral to alcohol abstinence programs or other professional help.

Magnesium Excess (Hypermagnesemia)

Hypermagnesemia (serum magnesium levels over 0.95 mmol/L) is a rare electrolyte abnormality, because the kidneys efficiently excrete magnesium. A serum magnesium level can appear falsely elevated if blood specimens are allowed to hemolyze or are drawn from an extremity with a tourniquet that was applied too tightly.

Pathophysiology

By far the most common cause of hypermagnesemia is kidney injury (Bansal et al., 2016). In fact, most patients with advanced kidney injury have at least a slight elevation in serum magnesium levels. This condition is aggravated when such patients receive magnesium to control seizures.

Hypermagnesemia can occur in patients with untreated diabetic ketoacidosis when catabolism causes the release of cellular magnesium that cannot be excreted because of profound fluid volume depletion and resulting oliguria. A surplus of magnesium can also result from excessive magnesium administered to treat hypertension of pregnancy or to treat low hypomagnesemia. Increased serum magnesium levels can also occur in adrenocortical insufficiency, Addison's disease, or hypothermia. Excessive use of magnesium-based antacids (e.g., Maalox, Riopan, Mylanta) or laxatives (Milk of Magnesia) and medications that decrease GI motility, including opioids and anticholinergics, can also increase serum magnesium levels. Decreased elimination of magnesium or its increased absorption due to intestinal hypomotility from any cause can contribute to hypermagnesemia. Lithium intoxication can also cause an increase in serum magnesium levels. Extensive soft tissue injury or necrosis as with trauma, shock, sepsis, cardiac arrest, or severe burns can also result in hypermagnesemia.

Clinical Manifestations

Acute elevation of the serum magnesium level depresses the central nervous system as well as the peripheral neuromuscular junction. At mildly increased levels, there is a tendency for lowered blood pressure because of peripheral vasodilation. Nausea, vomiting, weakness, soft tissue calcifications, facial flushing, and sensations of warmth may also occur. At higher magnesium concentrations, lethargy, difficulty speaking (dysarthria), and drowsiness can occur. DTRs are lost, and muscle weakness and paralysis may develop. The respiratory centre is depressed when serum magnesium levels exceed 5 mmol/L. Coma, atrioventricular heart block, and cardiac arrest can occur when the serum magnesium level is greatly elevated and not treated. High levels of magnesium also result in platelet clumping and delayed thrombin formation.

Assessment and Diagnostic Findings

On laboratory analysis, the serum magnesium level is greater than 1.25 mmol/L. Increased potassium and calcium levels are present concurrently. As creatinine clearance decreases to less than 3 mL/min, the serum magnesium levels increase. ECG findings may include a prolonged PR interval, tall T waves, a widened QRS, and a prolonged QT interval, as well as an atrioventricular block.

Medical Management

Hypermagnesemia can be prevented by avoiding the administration of magnesium to patients with kidney injury and by carefully monitoring seriously ill patients who are receiving magnesium salts. In patients with severe hypermagnesemia, all parenteral and oral magnesium salts are discontinued. In emergencies, such as respiratory depression or defective cardiac conduction, ventilatory support and IV calcium gluconate are indicated. In addition, hemodialysis with a magnesium-free dialysate can reduce the serum magnesium to a safe level within hours. Administration of loop diuretics (Lasix) and sodium chloride or lactated Ringer's IV solution enhances magnesium excretion in patients with adequate renal function. IV calcium gluconate antagonizes the cardiovascular and neuromuscular effects of magnesium.

Nursing Management

Patients at risk for hypermagnesemia are identified and assessed. If hypermagnesemia is suspected, the nurse monitors the vital signs, noting hypotension and shallow respirations. The nurse also observes for decreased DTRs and changes in the level of consciousness. Medications that contain magnesium are not administered to patients with kidney injury or compromised renal function, and patients with kidney injury are cautioned to check with their health care providers before taking OTC medications. Caution is essential when preparing and administering magnesium-containing fluids parenterally, because available parenteral magnesium solutions (e.g., 2-mL ampules, 50-mL vials) differ in concentration.

Phosphorus Imbalances

Phosphorus is a critical constituent of all the body's tissues. It is essential to the function of muscle and red blood cells; the formation of adenosine triphosphate (ATP) and of 2,3-diphosphoglycerate, which facilitates release of oxygen from hemoglobin; and the maintenance of acid–base balance, as well as the nervous system and the intermediary metabolism of carbohydrate, protein, and fat. It provides structural support to bones and teeth. Phosphorus is the primary anion of the ICF. About 85% of phosphorus is located in bones and teeth, 14% in soft tissue, and less than 1% in the ECF. The normal serum phosphorus level is 0.8 to 1.5 mmol/L in adults. Phosphorus deficit and phosphorus excess are two common imbalances (see Table 17-9).

Phosphorus Deficit (Hypophosphatemia)

Hypophosphatemia is indicated by a value below 0.8 mmol/L. Although it often indicates phosphorus deficiency,

TABLE 17-9 Phosphorus Imbalances

Imbalance	Contributing Factors	Signs/Symptoms
Phosphorus deficit (hypophosphatemia) Serum phosphorus <0.8 mmol/L	Refeeding after starvation, alcohol withdrawal, diabetic ketoacidosis, respiratory and metabolic alkalosis, ↓ magnesium, ↓ potassium, hyperparathyroidism, vomiting, diarrhea, hyperventilation, vitamin D deficiency associated with malabsorptive disorders, burns, acid–base disorders, parenteral nutrition, and diuretic and antacid use	Paresthesias, muscle weakness, bone pain and tenderness, chest pain, confusion, cardiomyopathy, respiratory failure, seizures, tissue hypoxia, and increased susceptibility to infection, nystagmus
Phosphorus excess (hyperphosphatemia) Serum phosphorus >1.6 mmol/L	Acute kidney injury and chronic kidney disease, excessive intake of phosphorus, vitamin D excess, respiratory and metabolic acidosis, hypoparathyroidism, volume depletion, leukemia/lymphoma treated with cytotoxic agents, increased tissue breakdown, rhabdomyolysis	Tetany, tachycardia, anorexia, nausea and vomiting, muscle weakness, signs and symptoms of hypocalcemia; hyperactive reflexes; soft tissue calcifications in lungs, heart, kidneys, and cornea

↓, decreased.

Adapted from Grossman, S. C., & Porth, C. M. (2014). *Porth's pathophysiology: Concepts of altered health states* (9th ed.). Philadelphia, PA: Lippincott Williams & Wilkins; Medical Council of Canada (MCC). (2019). https://mcc.ca/objectives/normal-values.

hypophosphatemia may occur under a variety of circumstances in which total body phosphorus stores are normal. Conversely, phosphorus deficiency is an abnormally low content of phosphorus in lean tissues that may exist in the absence of hypophosphatemia. It can be caused by an intracellular shift of potassium from serum into cells, by increased urinary excretion of potassium, or by decreased intestinal absorption of potassium.

Pathophysiology

Hypophosphatemia may occur during the administration of calories to patients with severe protein–calorie malnutrition. It is most likely to result from overzealous intake or administration of simple carbohydrates. This syndrome can be induced in any person with severe protein–calorie malnutrition (e.g., patients with anorexia nervosa or alcoholism, debilitated older adults who are unable to eat).

Marked hypophosphatemia may develop in malnourished patients who receive parenteral nutrition if the phosphorus loss is not corrected. Other causes of hypophosphatemia include heat stroke, prolonged intense hyperventilation, alcohol withdrawal, poor dietary intake, diabetic ketoacidosis, respiratory alkalosis, hepatic encephalopathy, and major thermal burns. Low magnesium levels, low potassium levels, and hyperparathyroidism related to increased urinary losses of phosphorus contribute to hypophosphatemia. Loss of phosphorus through the kidneys also occurs with acute volume expansion, osmotic diuresis, use of carbonic anhydrase inhibitors (acetazolamide [Diamox]), and some malignancies. Respiratory alkalosis can cause a decrease in phosphorus because of an intracellular shift of phosphorus.

Excess phosphorus binding by antacids may decrease the phosphorus available from the diet to an amount lower than required to maintain serum phosphorus balance. The degree of hypophosphatemia depends on the amount of phosphorus in the diet compared to the dose of antacid. Phosphate can occur with chronic diarrhea or through severe potassium restriction. Vitamin D regulates intestinal ion absorption; therefore, a deficiency of vitamin D may cause decreased calcium and phosphorus levels, which may lead to osteomalacia (softened, brittle bones).

Clinical Manifestations

Most of the signs and symptoms of phosphorus deficiency appear to result from a deficiency of ATP, 2,3-diphosphoglycerate, or both. ATP deficiency impairs cellular energy resources; diphosphoglycerate deficiency impairs oxygen delivery to tissues, resulting in a wide range of neurologic manifestations, such as irritability, fatigue, apprehension, weakness, numbness, paresthesias, dysarthria, dysphagia, diplopia, confusion, seizures, and coma. Hypoxia leads to an increase in respiratory rate and respiratory alkalosis, causing phosphorus to move into the cells and potentiating hypophosphatemia. Hypophosphatemia may predispose a person to infection. In laboratory animals, hypophosphatemia is associated with depression of the chemotactic, phagocytic, and bacterial activities of granulocytes.

Muscle damage may develop as the ATP level in the muscle tissue declines. Clinical manifestations are muscle weakness, which may be subtle or profound and may affect any muscle group; muscle pain; and at times acute rhabdomyolysis (breakdown of skeletal muscle). Weakness of respiratory muscles may greatly impair ventilation. Hypophosphatemia also may predispose a person to insulin resistance and thus hyperglycemia. Chronic loss of phosphorus can cause bruising and bleeding from platelet dysfunction.

Assessment and Diagnostic Findings

On laboratory analysis, the serum phosphorus level is less than 0.80 mmol/L in adults. When reviewing laboratory results, the nurse should keep in mind that glucose or insulin administration causes a slight decrease in the serum phosphorus level. PTH levels are increased in hyperparathyroidism. Serum magnesium may decrease due to increased urinary excretion of magnesium. Alkaline phosphatase is increased with osteoblastic activity. X-rays may show skeletal changes of osteomalacia or rickets.

Medical Management

Prevention of hypophosphatemia is the goal. In patients at risk for hypophosphatemia, serum phosphate levels should be closely monitored and correction initiated before deficits become severe. Adequate amounts of phosphorus should be added to parenteral solutions, and attention should be paid to the phosphorus levels in enteral feeding solutions.

Severe hypophosphatemia is dangerous and requires prompt attention. Aggressive IV phosphorus correction is usually limited to the patient whose serum phosphorus levels decrease to less than 0.3 mmol/L and whose GI tract is not functioning. Possible dangers of IV administration of phosphorus include tetany from hypocalcemia and calcifications in tissues (blood vessels, heart, lung, kidney, eyes) from hyperphosphatemia. IV preparations of phosphorus are available as sodium or potassium phosphate. The rate of phosphorus administration should not exceed 10 mmol/L/hr, and the site should be carefully monitored because tissue sloughing and necrosis can occur with infiltration. In less acute situations, oral phosphorus replacement is usually adequate.

Nursing Management

The nurse identifies patients who are at risk for hypophosphatemia and monitors them. Because malnourished patients receiving parenteral nutrition are at risk when calories are introduced too aggressively, preventive measures involve gradually introducing the solution to avoid rapid shifts of phosphorus into the cells.

For patients with documented hypophosphatemia, careful attention is given to preventing infection, because hypophosphatemia may alter the granulocytes. In patients requiring correction of phosphorus losses, the nurse frequently monitors serum phosphorus levels and documents and reports early signs of hypophosphatemia (apprehension, confusion, change in level of consciousness). If the patient experiences mild hypophosphatemia, foods such as milk and milk products, organ meats, nuts, fish, poultry, and whole grains should be encouraged. With moderate hypophosphatemia, supplements such as Neutra-Phos capsules (250 mg phosphorus/capsule; 7 mmol/L sodium and potassium), K-Phos (250 mg phosphorus/tablet; 14 mEq potassium), and Fleet's Phospho-Soda (815 mg phosphorus/5 mL) may be prescribed.

Phosphorus Excess (Hyperphosphatemia)

Hyperphosphatemia is a serum phosphorus level that exceeds 1.45 mmol/L in adults.

Pathophysiology

Various conditions can lead to hyperphosphatemia, but the most common is renal failure. Other causes include increased intake, decreased output, or a shift from the intracellular to extracellular space. Conditions such as excessive vitamin D intake, administration of total parenteral nutrition, chemotherapy for neoplastic disease, hypoparathyroidism, metabolic or respiratory acidosis, diabetic ketoacidosis, acute hemolysis, high phosphate intake, profound muscle necrosis, and increased phosphorus absorption may also lead to this phosphorus imbalance. The primary complication of increased phosphorus is metastatic calcification (soft tissue, joints, and arteries), which occurs when the calcium–magnesium product (calcium × magnesium) exceeds 70 mmol/L.

Clinical Manifestations

An increased serum phosphorus level causes few symptoms. Symptoms that do occur usually result from decreased calcium levels and soft tissue calcifications. The most important short-term consequence is tetany. Because of the reciprocal relationship between phosphorus and calcium, a high serum phosphorus level tends to cause a low serum calcium concentration. Tetany can result, causing tingling sensations in the fingertips and around the mouth. Anorexia, nausea, vomiting, bone and joint pain, muscle weakness, hyperreflexia, and tachycardia may occur.

The major long-term consequence is soft tissue calcification, which occurs mainly in patients with a reduced glomerular filtration rate. High serum levels of inorganic phosphorus promote precipitation of calcium phosphate in nonosseous sites, decreasing urine output, impairing vision, and producing palpitations.

Assessment and Diagnostic Findings

On laboratory analysis, the serum phosphorus level exceeds 1.5 mmol/L in adults. The serum calcium level is useful also for diagnosing the primary disorder and assessing the effects of treatments. X-rays may show skeletal changes with abnormal bone development. PTH levels are decreased in hypoparathyroidism. BUN and creatinine levels are used to assess renal function.

Medical Management

When possible, treatment is directed at the underlying disorder. For example, hyperphosphatemia may be related to volume depletion or respiratory or metabolic acidosis. In kidney injury, elevated PTH production contributes to a high phosphorus level and bone disease. Measures to decrease the serum phosphate level and bind phosphorus in the GI tract of these patients include vitamin D preparations such as calcitriol, which is available in both oral (Rocaltrol) and parenteral (Calcijex) forms, and paricalcitol (Zemplar). IV administration of calcitriol does not increase the serum calcium unless its dose is excessive, thus permitting more aggressive treatment of hyperphosphatemia with calcium-binding antacids (calcium carbonate or calcium citrate). Administration of Amphojel with meals is effective but can cause bone and central nervous system toxicity with long-term use. Restriction of dietary phosphate, forced diuresis with a loop diuretic, volume replacement with saline, and dialysis may also lower phosphorus. Surgery may be indicated for removal of large calcium and phosphorus deposits.

Nursing Management

The nurse monitors patients at risk for hyperphosphatemia. If a low phosphorus diet is prescribed, the patient is instructed to avoid phosphorus-rich foods such as hard cheeses, cream, nuts, meats, whole-grain cereals, dried fruits, dried vegetables, kidneys, sardines, sweetbreads, and foods made with milk. When appropriate, the nurse instructs the patient to avoid phosphate-containing substances such as laxatives and enemas. The nurse also teaches the patient to recognize the signs of impending hypocalcemia and to monitor for changes in urine output.

Chloride Imbalances

Chloride, the major anion of the ECF, is found more in interstitial and lymph fluid compartments than in blood. Chloride is also contained in gastric and pancreatic juices, sweat, bile, and saliva. Sodium and chloride make up the largest electrolyte composition of the ECF and assist in determining osmotic pressure. Chloride is produced in the stomach, where it combines with hydrogen to form hydrochloric acid. Chloride control depends on the intake of chloride and the excretion and reabsorption of its ions in the kidneys. A small amount of chloride is lost in the feces.

The normal serum chloride level is 98 to 106 mmol/L. Inside the cell, the chloride level is 4 mmol/L. The serum level of chloride reflects a change in dilution or concentration of the ECF and does so in direct proportion to the sodium concentration. Serum osmolality parallels chloride levels as well. Aldosterone secretion increases sodium reabsorption, thereby increasing chloride reabsorption. The choroid plexus, which secretes cerebrospinal fluid in the brain, depends on sodium and chloride to attract water to form the fluid portion of the cerebrospinal fluid. Bicarbonate has an inverse relationship with chloride. As chloride moves from plasma into the red blood cells (called the chloride shift), bicarbonate moves back into the plasma. Hydrogen ions are formed, which then help release oxygen from hemoglobin. When the level of one of these three electrolytes (sodium, bicarbonate, or chloride) is disturbed, the other two are also affected. Chloride assists in maintaining acid–base balance and works as a buffer in the exchange of oxygen and carbon dioxide in red blood cells. Chloride is primarily obtained from the diet as table salt. The two most common chloride imbalances are chloride deficit and chloride excess (see Table 17-10).

Chloride Deficit (Hypochloremia)

Hypochloremia is a serum chloride level below 98 mmol/L.

Pathophysiology

Hypochloremia can occur with GI tube drainage, gastric suctioning, gastric surgery, and severe vomiting and diarrhea. Administration of chloride-deficient IV solutions, low sodium intake, decreased serum sodium levels, metabolic alkalosis, massive blood transfusions, diuretic therapy, burns, and fever may cause hypochloremia. Administration of aldosterone, ACTH, corticosteroids, bicarbonate, or laxatives decreases serum chloride levels as well. As chloride decreases (usually because of volume depletion), sodium and bicarbonate ions are retained by the kidney to balance the loss. Bicarbonate accumulates in the ECF, which raises the pH and leads to hypochloremic metabolic alkalosis.

Clinical Manifestations

The signs and symptoms of hypochloremia are those of acid–base and electrolyte imbalances (Hannon & Porth, 2017). The signs and symptoms of hyponatremia, hypokalemia, and metabolic alkalosis may also be present. Metabolic alkalosis is a disorder that results in a high pH and a high serum bicarbonate level as a result of excess alkali intake or loss of hydrogen ions. With compensation, the partial pressure of carbon dioxide in arterial blood ($PaCO_2$)

TABLE 17-10 Chloride Imbalances

Imbalance	Contributing Factors	Signs/Symptoms and Laboratory Findings
Chloride deficit (hypochloremia) Serum chloride <98 mmol/L	Addison's disease, reduced chloride intake or absorption, untreated diabetic ketoacidosis, chronic respiratory acidosis, excessive sweating, vomiting, gastric suction, diarrhea, sodium and potassium deficiency, metabolic alkalosis; loop, osmotic, or thiazide diuretic use; overuse of bicarbonate, rapid removal of ascitic fluid with a high sodium content, IV fluids that lack chloride (dextrose and water), draining fistulas and ileostomies, heart failure, cystic fibrosis	Agitation, irritability, tremors, muscle cramps, hyperactive deep tendon reflexes, hypertonicity, tetany, slow shallow respirations, seizures, dysrhythmias, coma *Labs indicate:* ↓ serum chloride, ↓ serum sodium, ↑ pH, ↑ serum bicarbonate, ↑ total carbon dioxide content, ↓ urine chloride level, ↓ serum potassium
Chloride excess (hyperchloremia) Serum chloride >106 mmol/L	Excessive sodium chloride infusions with water loss, head injury (sodium retention), hypernatremia, kidney injury, corticosteroid use, dehydration, severe diarrhea (loss of bicarbonate), respiratory alkalosis, administration of diuretics, overdose of salicylates, Kayexalate, acetazolamide, phenylbutazone and ammonium chloride use, hyperparathyroidism, metabolic acidosis	Tachypnea, lethargy, weakness, deep rapid respirations, decline in cognitive status, ↓ cardiac output, dyspnea, tachycardia, pitting edema, dysrhythmias, coma *Labs indicate:* ↑ serum chloride, ↑ serum potassium and sodium, ↓ serum pH, ↓ serum bicarbonate, normal anion gap, ↑ urinary chloride level

↑, increased; ↓, decreased; IV, intravenous.

Adapted from Grossman, S. C., & Porth, C. M. (2014). *Porth's pathophysiology: Concepts of altered health states* (9th ed.). Philadelphia, PA: Lippincott Williams & Wilkins; Medical Council of Canada (MCC). (2019). https://mcc.ca/objectives/normal-values.

increases to 50 mm Hg. Hyperexcitability of muscles, tetany, hyperactive DTRs, weakness, twitching, and muscle cramps may result. Hypokalemia can cause hypochloremia, resulting in cardiac dysrhythmias. In addition, because low chloride levels parallel low sodium levels, a water excess may occur. Hyponatremia can cause seizures and coma.

Assessment and Diagnostic Findings

In addition to the chloride level, sodium and potassium levels are also evaluated, because these electrolytes are lost along with chloride. Arterial blood gas analysis identifies the acid–base imbalance, which is usually metabolic alkalosis. The urine chloride level, which is also measured, decreases in hypochloremia.

Medical Management

Treatment involves correcting the cause of hypochloremia and the contributing electrolyte and acid–base imbalances. Normal saline (0.9% sodium chloride) or half-strength saline (0.45% sodium chloride) solution is administered by IV to replace the chloride. If the patient is receiving a diuretic (loop, osmotic, or thiazide), it may be discontinued, or another diuretic prescribed.

Ammonium chloride, an acidifying agent, may be prescribed to treat metabolic alkalosis; the dosage depends on the patient's weight and serum chloride level. This agent is metabolized by the liver, and its effects last for about 3 days. Its use should be avoided in patients with impaired liver or renal function.

Nursing Management

The nurse monitors the patient's I&O, arterial blood gas values, and serum electrolyte levels. Changes in the patient's level of consciousness and muscle strength and movement are reported to the physician promptly. Vital signs are monitored, and respiratory assessment is carried out frequently. The nurse provides and teaches the patient about foods with high chloride content. Foods high in chloride include tomato juice, bananas, dates, eggs, cheese, milk, salty broth, canned vegetables, and processed meats. A person who drinks free water (water without electrolytes) or bottled water and excretes large amounts of chloride needs instruction to avoid drinking this kind of water.

Chloride Excess (Hyperchloremia)

Hyperchloremia exists when the serum level of chloride exceeds 106 mmol/L. Hypernatremia, bicarbonate loss, and metabolic acidosis can occur with high chloride levels.

Pathophysiology

High serum chloride levels are almost exclusively a result of iatrogenically induced hyperchloremic metabolic acidosis, stemming from excessive administration of chloride relative to sodium, most commonly as 0.9% normal saline solution, 0.45% normal saline solution, or lactated Ringer's solution. This condition can also be caused by the loss of bicarbonate ions via the kidney or the GI tract with a corresponding increase in chloride ions. Chloride ions in the form of acidifying salts accumulate, and acidosis occurs with a decrease in bicarbonate ions. Head trauma, increased perspiration, excess adrenocortical hormone production, and decreased glomerular filtration can lead to a high serum chloride level.

Clinical Manifestations

The signs and symptoms of hyperchloremia are the same as those of metabolic acidosis: hypervolemia and hypernatremia. Tachypnea; weakness; lethargy; deep, rapid respirations; diminished cognitive ability; and hypertension occur. If untreated, hyperchloremia can lead to a decrease in cardiac output, dysrhythmias, and coma. A high chloride level is accompanied by a high sodium level and fluid retention.

Assessment and Diagnostic Findings

The serum chloride level is 106 mmol/L or greater, the serum sodium level is greater than 145 mmol/L, the serum pH is less than 7.35, and the serum bicarbonate level is less than 22 mmol/L. Urine chloride excretion increases.

Calculation of the serum anion gap is important in analyzing acid–base disorders. The sum of all negatively charged electrolytes (anions) equals the sum of all positively charged electrolytes (cations), with several anions that are not routinely measured leading to an anion gap. It is based primarily on three electrolytes: sodium, chloride, and bicarbonate or serum carbon dioxide (CO_2). A normal anion gap is 8 to 12 mmol/L. A low anion gap may be attributed to hypoproteinemia, whereas an elevated anion gap can be due to metabolic acidosis.

Medical Management

Correcting the underlying cause of hyperchloremia and restoring electrolyte, fluid, and acid–base balance are essential. Hypotonic IV solutions may be administered to restore balance. Lactated Ringer's solution may be prescribed to convert lactate to bicarbonate in the liver, which increases the bicarbonate level and corrects the acidosis. IV sodium bicarbonate may be administered to increase bicarbonate levels, which leads to the renal excretion of chloride ions because bicarbonate and chloride compete for combination with sodium. Diuretics may be administered to eliminate chloride as well. Sodium, chloride, and fluids are restricted.

Nursing Management

Monitoring vital signs, arterial blood gas values, and I&O is important to assess the patient's status and the effectiveness of treatment. Assessment findings related to respiratory, neurologic, and cardiac systems are documented, and changes are discussed with the physician. The nurse teaches the patient about the diet that should be followed to manage hyperchloremia and maintain adequate hydration.

ACID–BASE DISTURBANCES

Acid–base disturbances are commonly encountered in clinical practice. Identification of the specific acid–base imbalance is important in identifying the underlying cause of the disorder and determining appropriate treatment.

Plasma pH is an indicator of hydrogen ion (H^+) concentration. Homeostatic mechanisms keep pH within a normal range (7.35 to 7.45) (Hannon & Porth, 2017). These mechanisms consist of buffer systems, the kidneys, and the lungs. The H^+ concentration is extremely important. The greater the concentration, the more acidic the solution and the lower the pH. The lower the H^+ concentration, the more alkaline the solution and the higher the pH. The pH range compatible with life (6.8 to 7.8) represents a 10-fold difference in H^+ concentration in plasma.

Buffer systems prevent major changes in the pH of body fluids by removing or releasing H^+; they can act quickly to prevent excessive changes in H^+ concentration. Hydrogen ions are buffered by both intracellular and extracellular buffers. The body's major extracellular buffer system is the bicarbonate–carbonic acid buffer system, which is assessed when arterial blood gases are measured. Normally, there are 20 parts of bicarbonate (HCO_3^-) to one part of carbonic acid (H_2CO_3). If this ratio is altered, the pH will change. It is the ratio of HCO_3^- to H_2CO_3 that is important in maintaining pH, not absolute values. CO_2 is a potential acid; when dissolved in water, it becomes carbonic acid ($CO_2 + H_2O = H_2CO_3$). Therefore, when CO_2 is increased, the carbonic acid content is also increased, and vice versa. If either bicarbonate or carbonic acid is increased or decreased so that the 20:1 ratio is no longer maintained, acid–base imbalance results (Moritz, 2013).

Less important buffer systems in the ECF include the inorganic phosphates and the plasma proteins. Intracellular buffers include proteins, organic and inorganic phosphates, and, in red blood cells, hemoglobin.

The kidneys regulate the bicarbonate level in the ECF; they can regenerate bicarbonate ions as well as reabsorb them from the renal tubular cells. In respiratory acidosis and most cases of metabolic acidosis, the kidneys excrete hydrogen ions and conserve bicarbonate ions to help restore balance. In respiratory and metabolic alkalosis, the kidneys retain hydrogen ions and excrete bicarbonate ions to help restore balance. The kidneys obviously cannot compensate for the metabolic acidosis created by kidney injury. Renal compensation for imbalances is relatively slow (a matter of hours or days).

The lungs, under the control of the medulla, control the CO_2 and thus the carbonic acid content of the ECF. They do so by adjusting ventilation in response to the amount of CO_2 in the blood. A rise in the partial pressure of CO_2 in arterial blood ($PaCO_2$) is a powerful stimulant to respiration. Of course, the partial pressure of oxygen in arterial blood (PaO_2) also influences respiration. However, its effect is not as marked as that produced by the $PaCO_2$.

In metabolic acidosis, the respiratory rate increases, causing greater elimination of CO_2 (to reduce the acid load). In metabolic alkalosis, the respiratory rate decreases, causing CO_2 to be retained (to increase the acid load) (Emmett, 2014).

Acute and Chronic Metabolic Acidosis (Base Bicarbonate Deficit)

Metabolic acidosis is a common clinical disturbance characterized by a low pH (increased H^+ concentration) and a low plasma bicarbonate concentration. It can be produced by a gain of hydrogen ion or a loss of bicarbonate. It can be divided clinically into two forms, according to the values of the serum anion gap: high anion gap acidosis and normal anion gap acidosis. The anion gap reflects normally unmeasured anions (phosphates, sulphates, and proteins) in plasma. Measuring the anion gap is essential in analyzing acid–base disorders correctly. The anion gap can be calculated by either one of the following equations:

$$\text{Anion gap} = Na^+ + K^+ - (Cl^- + HCO_3^-)$$
$$\text{Anion gap} = Na^+ - (Cl^- + HCO_3^-)$$

Potassium is often omitted from the equation because of its low level in the plasma; therefore, the second equation is used more often than the first.

The normal value for an anion gap is 8 to 12 mmol/L without potassium in the equation. If potassium is included in the equation, the normal value for the anion gap is 12 to 16 mmol/L. The unmeasured anions in the serum usually account for less than 16 mmol/L of the anion production. An anion gap greater than 16 mmol/L suggests excessive accumulation of unmeasured anions. An anion gap occurs because not all electrolytes are measured. More anions are left unmeasured than cations.

Pathophysiology

Normal anion gap acidosis results from the direct loss of bicarbonate, as in diarrhea, lower intestinal fistulas, ureterostomies, and use of diuretics; early renal insufficiency; excessive administration of chloride; and the administration of parenteral nutrition without bicarbonate or bicarbonate-producing solutes (e.g., lactate). Normal anion gap acidosis is also referred to as hyperchloremic acidosis. A reduced or negative anion gap is primarily caused by hypoproteinemia. Disorders that cause a decreased or negative anion gap are rare compared to those related to an increased or high anion gap.

High anion gap acidosis results from excessive accumulation of fixed acid. If increased to 30 mmol/L or more, then a high anion gap metabolic acidosis is present regardless of the values of pH and HCO_3^-. High ion gap occurs in ketoacidosis, lactic acidosis, the late phase of salicylate poisoning, uremia, methanol or ethylene glycol toxicity, and ketoacidosis with starvation. The hydrogen is buffered by HCO_3^-, causing the bicarbonate concentration to fall. In all of these instances, abnormally high levels of anions flood the system, increasing the anion gap above normal limits (see Table 17-11).

Clinical Manifestations

Signs and symptoms of metabolic acidosis vary with the severity of the acidosis but include headache, confusion, drowsiness, increased respiratory rate and depth, nausea,

TABLE 17-11 Anion Gap in Metabolic Acidosis

	Reduced or Negative Anion Gap	Normal Anion Gap	High Anion Gap
Anion gap without potassium	<8	8–12 mEq/L	>12
Anion gap with potassium	<12	12–16 mEq/L	>16
Clinical significance	Hypoproteinemia	Normal anion gap metabolic acidosis	High anion gap metabolic acidosis

Metabolic acidosis is characterized by a low pH and low plasma bicarbonate concentration. Nurses need to remember that the anion gap is calculated primarily to identify the cause (pathology) of metabolic acidosis (Grossman & Porth, 2014).

and vomiting. Peripheral vasodilation and decreased cardiac output occur when the pH drops to less than 7. Additional physical assessment findings include decreased blood pressure, cold and clammy skin, dysrhythmias, and shock. Chronic metabolic acidosis is usually seen with chronic kidney disease.

Assessment and Diagnostic Findings

Arterial blood gas measurements are valuable in diagnosing metabolic acidosis. Expected blood gas changes include a low bicarbonate level (less than 22 mmol/L) and a low pH (less than 7.35) (Fischbach & Dunning, 2015). The cardinal feature of metabolic acidosis is a decrease in the serum bicarbonate level. Hyperkalemia may accompany metabolic acidosis as a result of the shift of potassium out of the cells. Later, as the acidosis is corrected, potassium moves back into the cells and hypokalemia may occur. Hyperventilation decreases the CO_2 level as a compensatory action. Calculation of the anion gap is helpful in determining the cause of metabolic acidosis. An ECG detects dysrhythmias caused by the increased potassium.

Medical Management

Treatment is directed at correcting the metabolic imbalance (Fischbach & Dunning, 2015). If the problem results from excessive intake of chloride, treatment is aimed at eliminating the source of the chloride. When necessary, bicarbonate is administered. Although hyperkalemia occurs with acidosis, hypokalemia may occur with reversal of the acidosis and subsequent movement of potassium back into the cells. Therefore, the serum potassium level is monitored closely, and hypokalemia is corrected as acidosis is reversed.

In chronic metabolic acidosis, low serum calcium levels are treated before the chronic metabolic acidosis is treated, to avoid tetany resulting from an increase in pH and a decrease in ionized calcium. Alkalizing agents may be administered. Treatment modalities may also include hemodialysis or peritoneal dialysis.

Acute and Chronic Metabolic Alkalosis (Base Bicarbonate Excess)

Metabolic alkalosis is a clinical disturbance characterized by a high pH (decreased H^+ concentration) and a high plasma bicarbonate concentration. It can be produced by a gain of bicarbonate or a loss of H^+ (Hannon & Porth, 2017).

Pathophysiology

Probably the most common cause of metabolic alkalosis is vomiting or gastric suction with loss of hydrogen and chloride ions. The disorder also occurs in pyloric stenosis, in which only gastric fluid is lost. Gastric fluid has an acid pH (usually 1 to 3), and loss of this highly acidic fluid increases the alkalinity of body fluids. Other situations predisposing to metabolic alkalosis include those associated with loss of potassium, such as diuretic therapy that promotes excretion of potassium (e.g., thiazides, furosemide), and excessive adrenocorticoid hormones (as in hyperaldosteronism and Cushing's syndrome).

Hypokalemia produces alkalosis in two ways: (1) the kidneys conserve potassium, and therefore H^+ excretion increases; and (2) cellular potassium moves out of the cells into the ECF in an attempt to maintain near-normal serum levels (as potassium ions leave the cells, hydrogen ions must enter to maintain electroneutrality). Excessive alkali ingestion from antacids containing bicarbonate or from use of sodium bicarbonate during cardiopulmonary resuscitation can also cause metabolic alkalosis.

Chronic metabolic alkalosis can occur with long-term diuretic therapy (thiazides or furosemide), villous adenoma, external drainage of gastric fluids, significant potassium depletion, cystic fibrosis, and the chronic ingestion of milk and calcium carbonate.

Clinical Manifestations

Alkalosis is primarily manifested by symptoms related to decreased calcium ionization, such as tingling of the fingers and toes, dizziness, and hypertonic muscles. The ionized fraction of serum calcium decreases in alkalosis as more calcium combines with serum proteins. Because it is the ionized fraction of calcium that influences neuromuscular activity, symptoms of hypocalcemia are often the predominant symptoms of alkalosis. Respirations are depressed as a compensatory action by the lungs. Atrial tachycardia may occur. As the pH increases and hypokalemia develops, ventricular disturbances may occur. Decreased motility and paralytic ileus may also be evident.

Symptoms of chronic metabolic alkalosis are the same as for acute metabolic alkalosis, and as potassium decreases, frequent premature ventricular contractions or U waves are seen on the ECG.

Assessment and Diagnostic Findings

Evaluation of arterial blood gases reveals a pH greater than 7.45 and a serum bicarbonate concentration greater than

26 mmol/L. The $PaCO_2$ increases as the lungs attempt to compensate for the excess bicarbonate by retaining CO_2. This hypoventilation is more pronounced in semiconscious, unconscious, or debilitated patients than in alert patients. The former may develop marked hypoxemia as a result of hypoventilation. Hypokalemia may accompany metabolic alkalosis.

Urine chloride levels may help identify the cause of metabolic alkalosis if the patient's history provides inadequate information. Metabolic alkalosis is the setting in which urine chloride concentration may be a more accurate estimate of fluid volume than the urine sodium concentration. Urine chloride concentrations help to differentiate between vomiting, diuretic therapy, and excessive adrenocorticosteroid secretion as the causes of the metabolic alkalosis. In patients with vomiting or cystic fibrosis, those receiving nutritional repletion, and those receiving diuretic therapy, hypovolemia and hyperchloremia produce urine chloride concentrations lower than 25 mmol/L. Signs of hypovolemia are not present, and the urine chloride concentration exceeds 40 mEq/L in patients with mineralocorticoid excess or alkali loading; these patients usually have expanded fluid volume. The urine chloride concentration should be less than 15 mmol/L when decreased chloride levels and hypovolemia occur.

Medical Management

Treatment of both acute and chronic metabolic alkalosis is aimed at correcting the underlying acid–base disorder (Fischbach & Dunning, 2015). Because of volume depletion from GI loss, the patient's fluid I&O must be monitored carefully.

Sufficient chloride must be supplied for the kidney to absorb sodium with chloride (allowing the excretion of excess bicarbonate). Treatment also includes restoring normal fluid volume by administering sodium chloride fluids (because continued volume depletion perpetuates the alkalosis). In patients with hypokalemia, potassium is administered as KCl to replace both K^+ and Cl^- losses. H_2 receptor antagonists, such as cimetidine (Tagamet), reduce the production of gastric HCl, thereby decreasing the metabolic alkalosis associated with gastric suction. Carbonic anhydrase inhibitors are useful in treating metabolic alkalosis in patients who cannot tolerate rapid volume expansion (e.g., patients with heart failure).

Acute and Chronic Respiratory Acidosis (Carbonic Acid Excess)

Respiratory acidosis is a clinical disorder in which the pH is less than 7.35 and the $PaCO_2$ is greater than 42 mm Hg. It may be either acute or chronic.

Pathophysiology

Respiratory acidosis is always due to inadequate excretion of CO_2 with inadequate ventilation, resulting in elevated plasma CO_2 concentrations and, consequently, increased levels of carbonic acid. In addition to an elevated $PaCO_2$, hypoventilation usually causes a decrease in PaO_2. Acute respiratory acidosis occurs in emergency situations, such as acute pulmonary edema, aspiration of a foreign object, atelectasis, pneumothorax, overdose of sedatives, sleep apnea, administration of oxygen to a patient with chronic hypercapnia (excessive CO_2 in the blood), severe pneumonia, and acute respiratory distress syndrome. Respiratory acidosis can also occur in diseases that impair respiratory muscles, such as muscular dystrophy, myasthenia gravis, and Guillain–Barré syndrome. Mechanical ventilation may be associated with hypercapnia if the rate of ventilation is inadequate and CO_2 is retained.

Clinical Manifestations

Clinical signs in acute and chronic respiratory acidosis vary. Sudden hypercapnia (elevated $PaCO_2$) can cause increased pulse and respiratory rate, increased blood pressure, mental cloudiness, and a feeling of fullness in the head. An elevated $PaCO_2$, greater than 60 mm Hg, causes cerebrovascular vasodilation and increased cerebral blood flow. Ventricular fibrillation may be the first sign of respiratory acidosis in anaesthetized patients.

If respiratory acidosis is severe, intracranial pressure may increase, resulting in papilledema and dilated conjunctival blood vessels. Hyperkalemia may result as the hydrogen concentration overwhelms the compensatory mechanisms and H^+ moves into cells, causing a shift of potassium out of the cell.

Chronic respiratory acidosis occurs with pulmonary diseases such as chronic emphysema and bronchitis, obstructive sleep apnea, and obesity. As long as the $PaCO_2$ does not exceed the body's ability to compensate, the patient will be asymptomatic. However, if the $PaCO_2$ increases rapidly, cerebral vasodilation will increase the intracranial pressure, and cyanosis and tachypnea will develop. Patients with chronic obstructive pulmonary disease (COPD) who gradually accumulate CO_2 over a prolonged period (days to months) may not develop symptoms of hypercapnia because compensatory renal changes have had time to occur.

NURSING ALERT

If the $PaCO_2$ is chronically higher than 50 mm Hg, the respiratory centre becomes relatively insensitive to CO_2 as a respiratory stimulant, leaving hypoxemia as the major drive for respiration. Oxygen administration may remove the stimulus of hypoxemia, and the patient develops "carbon dioxide narcosis" unless the situation is quickly reversed. Therefore, oxygen is administered only with extreme caution.

Assessment and Diagnostic Findings

Arterial blood gas analysis reveals a pH lower than 7.35, a $PaCO_2$ greater than 42 mm Hg, and a variation in the bicarbonate level, depending on the duration of the acute respiratory acidosis. When compensation (renal retention of bicarbonate) has fully occurred, the arterial pH is within the lower limits of normal. Depending on the cause of respiratory acidosis, other diagnostic measures include monitoring of serum electrolyte levels, chest x-ray for determining any respiratory disease, and a drug screen if an overdose is suspected. An ECG to identify any cardiac involvement as a result of COPD may be indicated as well.

Medical Management

Treatment is directed at improving ventilation; exact measures vary with the cause of inadequate ventilation. Pharmacologic agents are used as indicated. For example, bronchodilators help reduce bronchial spasm, antibiotics are used for respiratory infections, and thrombolytics or anticoagulants are used for pulmonary emboli (see Chapter 26).

Pulmonary hygiene measures are initiated, when necessary, to clear the respiratory tract of mucus and purulent drainage. Adequate hydration (2 to 3 L/day) is indicated to keep the mucous membranes moist and thereby facilitate the removal of secretions. Supplemental oxygen is administered as necessary.

Mechanical ventilation, used appropriately, may improve pulmonary ventilation. Inappropriate mechanical ventilation (e.g., increased dead space, insufficient rate or volume settings, high fraction of inspired oxygen [FiO_2] with excessive CO_2 production) may cause such rapid excretion of CO_2 that the kidneys are unable to eliminate excess bicarbonate quickly enough to prevent alkalosis and seizures. For this reason, the elevated $PaCO_2$ must be decreased slowly. Placing the patient in a semi-Fowler's position facilitates expansion of the chest wall.

Treatment of chronic respiratory acidosis is the same as for acute respiratory acidosis.

Acute and Chronic Respiratory Alkalosis (Carbonic Acid Deficit)

Respiratory alkalosis is a clinical condition in which the arterial pH is greater than 7.45 and the $PaCO_2$ is less than 38 mm Hg. As with respiratory acidosis, acute and chronic conditions can occur.

Pathophysiology

Respiratory alkalosis is always caused by hyperventilation, which causes excessive "blowing off" of CO_2 and, hence, a decrease in the plasma carbonic acid concentration. Causes include extreme anxiety, hypoxemia, early phase of salicylate intoxication, gram-negative bacteremia, and inappropriate ventilator settings that do not match the patient's requirements.

Chronic respiratory alkalosis results from chronic hypocapnia, and decreased serum bicarbonate levels are the consequence. Chronic hepatic insufficiency and cerebral tumours are predisposing factors.

Clinical Manifestations

Clinical signs consist of light-headedness due to vasoconstriction and decreased cerebral blood flow, inability to concentrate, numbness and tingling from decreased calcium ionization, tinnitus, and sometimes loss of consciousness. Cardiac effects of respiratory alkalosis include tachycardia and ventricular and atrial dysrhythmias.

Assessment and Diagnostic Findings

Analysis of arterial blood gases assists in the diagnosis of respiratory alkalosis. In the acute state, the pH is elevated above normal as a result of a low $PaCO_2$ and a normal bicarbonate level. (The kidneys cannot alter the bicarbonate level quickly.) In the compensated state, the kidneys have had sufficient time to lower the bicarbonate level to a near-normal level. Evaluation of serum electrolytes is indicated to identify any decrease in potassium, as hydrogen is pulled out of the cells in exchange for potassium; decreased calcium, as severe alkalosis inhibits calcium ionization, resulting in carpopedal spasms and tetany; or decreased phosphate due to alkalosis, causing an increased uptake of phosphate by the cells. A toxicology screen should be performed to rule out salicylate intoxication.

Patients with chronic respiratory alkalosis are usually asymptomatic, and the diagnostic evaluation and plan of care are the same as for acute respiratory alkalosis.

Medical Management

Treatment depends on the underlying cause of respiratory alkalosis. If the cause is anxiety, the patient is instructed to breathe more slowly to allow CO_2 to accumulate or to breathe into a closed system (such as a paper bag). A sedative may be required to relieve hyperventilation in very anxious patients. Treatment of other causes of respiratory alkalosis is directed at correcting the underlying problem.

Mixed Acid–Base Disorders

Patients can simultaneously experience two or more independent acid–base disorders. A normal pH in the presence of changes in the $PaCO_2$ and plasma HCO_3^- concentration immediately suggests a mixed disorder. An example of a mixed disorder is the simultaneous occurrence of metabolic acidosis and respiratory acidosis during respiratory and cardiac arrest. The only mixed disorder that cannot occur is a mixed respiratory acidosis and alkalosis, because it is impossible to have alveolar hypoventilation and hyperventilation at the same time.

Compensation

Generally, the pulmonary and renal systems compensate for each other to return the pH to normal. In a single acid–base disorder, the system not causing the problem tries to compensate by returning the ratio of bicarbonate to carbonic acid to the normal 20:1. The lungs compensate for metabolic disturbances by changing CO_2 excretion. The kidneys compensate for respiratory disturbances by altering bicarbonate retention and H^+ secretion.

In respiratory acidosis, excess hydrogen is excreted in the urine in exchange for bicarbonate ions. In respiratory alkalosis, the renal excretion of bicarbonate increases, and hydrogen ions are retained. In metabolic acidosis, the compensatory mechanisms increase the ventilation rate and the renal retention of bicarbonate. In metabolic alkalosis, the respiratory system compensates by decreasing ventilation to conserve CO_2 and increase the $PaCO_2$. Because the lungs respond to acid–base disorders within minutes,

TABLE 17-12 Acid–Base Disorders and Compensation

Acid–Base Imbalance	Primary Disturbance	Respiratory Compensation and Predicted Response[a]	Renal Compensation and Predicted Response[a,b]
Metabolic acidosis	↓ pH and HCO_3^- HCO_3^- <22 mEq/L	↑ ventilation and ↓ PCO_2 *1 mEq/L ↓ HCO_3^- → 1 to 1.2 mm Hg ↓ PCO_2*	↑ H^+ excretion and ↑ HCO_3^- reabsorption if no renal disease
Metabolic alkalosis	↑ pH and HCO_3^- HCO_3^- >26 mEq/L	↓ ventilation and ↑ PCO_2 *1 mEq/L ↑ HCO_3^- → 0.7 mm Hg ↑ PCO_2*	↓ H^+ excretion and ↓ HCO_3^- reabsorption if no renal disease
Respiratory acidosis	↓ pH and ↑ PCO_2 PCO_2 >45 mm Hg	None	↑ H^+ excretion and ↑ HCO_3^- reabsorption *Acute: 1 mm Hg ↑ PCO_2 → 0.1 mEq/L ↑ HCO_3^-* *Chronic: 1 mm Hg ↑ PCO_2 →* 0.3 *mEq/L ↑ HCO_3^-*
Respiratory alkalosis	↑ pH and ↓ PCO_2 PCO_2 <35 mm Hg	None	↓ H^+ excretion and ↓ HCO_3^- reabsorption *Acute: 1 mm Hg ↓ PCO_2 → 0.2 mEq/L ↓ HCO_3^-* *Chronic: 1 mm Hg ↓ PCO_2 → 0.4 mEq/L ↓ HCO_3^-*

Note: Predicted compensatory responses are in italics.

[a]If blood values are the same as predicted compensatory values, a single acid–base disorder is present; if values are different, a mixed acid–base disorder is present. (Adrogué, H. J., Gennari F. J., Galla J. H., et al. [2009]. Assessing acid-base disorders. *Kidney International, 76*, 1239–1247.)

[b]Acute renal compensation refers to duration of minutes to several hours; chronic renal compensation refers to a duration of several days.

compensation for metabolic imbalances occurs faster than compensation for respiratory imbalances. Table 17-12 summarizes compensation effects.

Blood Gas Analysis

Blood gas analysis is often used to identify the specific acid–base disturbance and the degree of compensation that has occurred. The analysis is usually based on an arterial blood sample, but if an arterial sample cannot be obtained, a mixed venous sample may be used. Results of arterial blood gas analysis provide information about alveolar ventilation, oxygenation, and acid–base balance. It is necessary to evaluate the concentrations of serum electrolytes (sodium, potassium, and chloride) and carbon dioxide along with arterial blood gas data, because they are often the first sign of an acid–base disorder. The health history, physical examination, previous blood gas results, and serum electrolytes should always be part of the assessment used to determine the cause of the acid–base disorder (Hannon & Porth, 2017). Responding to isolated sets of blood gas results without these data can lead to serious errors in interpretation. Treatment of the underlying condition usually corrects most acid–base disorders. Table 17-13 compares normal ranges of venous and arterial blood gas values. See also Chart 17-3.

TABLE 17-13 Normal Values for Arterial and Mixed Venous Bloods

Parameter	Arterial Blood	Mixed Venous Blood
pH	7.35–7.45	7.32–7.42
PCO_2	35–45 mm Hg	38–52 mm Hg
PO_2[a]	>80 mm Hg	24–48 mm Hg
HCO_3^-	22–26 mEq/L	19–25 mEq/L
Base excess/deficit	±2 mEq/L	±5 mEq/L
Oxygen saturation (SaO_2%)	>94%	65–75%

[a]At altitudes of 3,000 ft and higher, the values for oxygen are decreased.

Adapted from Fischbach, F., & Dunning, M. B. (2015). *A manual of laboratory and diagnostic tests* (9th ed.). Philadelphia, PA: Lippincott Williams & Wilkins.

PARENTERAL FLUID THERAPY

When no other route of administration is available, fluids are administered by IV in hospitals, outpatient diagnostic and surgical settings, clinics, and homes to replace fluids, administer medications, and provide nutrients.

Purpose

The choice of an IV solution depends on the purpose of its administration. Generally, IV fluids are administered to achieve one or more of the following goals:

- To provide water, electrolytes, and nutrients to meet daily requirements
- To replace water and correct electrolyte deficits
- To administer medications and blood products

IV solutions contain dextrose or electrolytes mixed in various proportions with water. Pure, electrolyte-free water can never be administered by IV because it rapidly enters red blood cells and causes them to rupture.

Types of Intravenous Solutions

Solutions are often categorized as **isotonic**, **hypotonic**, or **hypertonic**, according to whether their total osmolality is the same as, less than, or greater than that of blood, respectively (see earlier discussion of osmolality). Electrolyte solutions are considered isotonic if the total electrolyte content (anions + cations) is approximately 310 mmol/L, hypotonic if the total electrolyte content is less than 250 mmol/L, and hypertonic if the total electrolyte content is greater than 375 mmol/L. The nurse must also consider a solution's osmolality, keeping in mind that the osmolality of plasma is approximately 300 mmol/L. For example, a 10% dextrose solution has an osmolality of approximately 505 mmol/L.

Isotonic Fluids

Fluids that are classified as isotonic have a total osmolality close to that of the ECF and do not cause red blood cells

CHART 17-3

Assessing for Arterial Blood Gases

The following steps are recommended to evaluate arterial blood gas values. They are based on the assumption that the average values are:

pH = 7.4
$PaCO_2$ = 40 mm Hg
HCO_3^- = 24 mEq/L

1. *First, note the pH.* It can be high, low, or normal, as follows: A normal pH may indicate perfectly normal blood gases, *or* it may indicate a *compensated* imbalance. A compensated imbalance is one in which the body has been able to correct the pH by either respiratory or metabolic changes (depending on the primary problem). For example, a patient with primary metabolic acidosis starts out with a low bicarbonate level but a normal CO_2 level. Soon afterward, the lungs try to compensate for the imbalance by exhaling large amounts of CO_2 (hyperventilation). As another example, a patient with primary respiratory acidosis starts out with a high CO_2 level; soon afterward, the kidneys attempt to compensate by retaining bicarbonate. If the compensatory mechanism is able to restore the bicarbonate to carbonic acid ratio back to 20:1, full compensation (and thus normal pH) will be achieved.
   pH >7.4 (alkalosis)
   pH <7.4 (acidosis)
   pH = 7.4 (normal)
2. The next step is to determine the primary cause of the disturbance. This is done by evaluating the $PaCO_2$ and HCO_3^- in relation to the pH.
   Example: pH >7.4 (alkalosis)
   a. If the $PaCO_2$ is less than 40 mm Hg, the primary disturbance is respiratory alkalosis. (This situation occurs when a patient hyperventilates and "blows off" too much CO_2. Recall that CO_2 dissolved in water becomes carbonic acid, the acid side of the "carbonic acid-bicarbonate buffer system.")
   b. If the HCO_3^- is greater than 24 mEq/L, the primary disturbance is metabolic alkalosis. (This situation occurs when the body gains too much bicarbonate, an alkaline substance. Bicarbonate is the basic or alkaline side of the "carbonic acid-bicarbonate buffer system.")
   Example: pH <7.4 (acidosis)
   c. If the $PaCO_2$ is greater than 40 mm Hg, the primary disturbance is respiratory acidosis. (This situation occurs when a patient hypoventilates and thus retains too much CO_2, an acidic substance.)
   d. If the HCO_3^- is less than 24 mEq/L, the primary disturbance is metabolic acidosis. (This situation occurs when the body's bicarbonate level drops, either because of direct bicarbonate loss or because of gains of acids such as lactic acid or ketones.)
3. The next step involves determining if compensation has begun. This is done by looking at the value other than the primary disorder. If it is moving in the same direction as the primary value, compensation is underway. Consider the following gases:
   The first set (1) indicates acute respiratory acidosis without compensation (the $PaCO_2$ is high, the HCO_3^- is normal). The second set (2) indicates chronic respiratory acidosis. Note that compensation has taken place—that is, the HCO_3^- has elevated to an appropriate level to balance the high $PaCO_2$ and produce a normal pH.

	pH	$PaCO_2$	HCO_3^-
(1)	7.2	60 mm Hg	24 mEq/L
(2)	7.4	60 mm Hg	37 mEq/L

4. Two distinct acid-base disturbances may occur simultaneously. These can be identified when the pH does not explain one of the changes. When the $PaCO_2$ is ↑ and the HCO_3 is ↓, respiratory acidosis and metabolic acidosis coexist. When the $PaCO_2$ is ↓ and the HCO_3 is ↑, respiratory alkalosis and metabolic alkalosis coexist.
   Example: Metabolic and respiratory acidosis

a. pH	7.2	Decreased acid
b. $PaCO_2$	52	Increased acid
c. HCO_3	13	Decreased acid

5. If metabolic acidosis exists, then calculate the anion gap (AG) to determine the cause of the metabolic acidosis (AG vs. non-AG): AG = Na − (Cl + HCO_3) Normal AG = 10–14 mmol/L
6. Evaluate the patient to determine if the clinical signs and symptoms are compatible with the acid-base analysis.

Adapted from Rogers, K., & McCutcheon, K. (2013). Understanding arterial blood gases. *Journal of Perioperative Practice, 23*(9), 191–197.

to shrink or swell. The composition of these fluids may or may not approximate that of the ECF. Isotonic fluids expand the ECF volume. One litre of isotonic fluid expands the ECF by 1 L; however, it expands the plasma by only 0.25 L because it is a crystalloid fluid and diffuses quickly into the ECF compartment. For the same reason, 3 L of isotonic fluid is needed to replace 1 L of blood loss. Because these fluids expand the intravascular space, patients with hypertension and heart failure should be carefully monitored for signs of fluid overload.

D_5W

A solution of D_5W has a serum osmolality of 252 mmol/L. Once administered, the glucose is rapidly metabolized, and this initially **isotonic solution** then disperses as a hypotonic fluid, one third extracellular and two thirds intracellular. It is essential to consider this action of D_5W, especially if the patient is at risk for increased intracranial pressure. During fluid resuscitation, this solution should not be used, because hyperglycemia can result. Therefore, D_5W is used mainly to supply water and to correct an increased serum osmolality. About 1 L of D_5W provides fewer than 200 kcal and is a minor source of the body's daily caloric requirement.

Normal Saline Solution

Normal saline (0.9% sodium chloride) solution has a total osmolality of 308 mmol/L. Because the osmolality is entirely contributed by electrolytes, the solution remains within the ECF. For this reason, normal saline solution is often used to correct an extracellular volume deficit. Although referred to as "normal," it contains only sodium and chloride and is not identical to ECF. It is used with administration of blood transfusions and to replace large sodium losses, such as in burn injuries. It is not used for heart failure, pulmonary edema, renal impairment, or sodium retention. Normal saline does not supply calories.

Other Isotonic Solutions

Several other solutions contain ions in addition to sodium and chloride and are somewhat similar to the ECF in composition. Lactated Ringer's solution contains potassium and calcium in addition to sodium chloride. It is used to correct dehydration and sodium depletion and replace GI losses. Lactated Ringer's solution contains bicarbonate precursors as well. These solutions are marketed, with slight variations, under various trade names.

Hypotonic Fluids

One purpose of **hypotonic solutions** is to replace cellular fluid, because it is hypotonic compared with plasma. Another is to provide free water for excretion of body wastes. At times, hypotonic sodium solutions are used to treat hypernatremia and other hyperosmolar conditions. Half-strength saline (0.45% sodium chloride) solution, with an osmolality of 154 mmol/L, is frequently used. Multiple electrolyte solutions are also available. Excessive infusions of hypotonic solutions can lead to intravascular fluid depletion, decreased blood pressure, cellular edema, and cell damage. These solutions exert less osmotic pressure than the ECF.

Hypertonic Fluids

When normal saline solution or lactated Ringer's solution contains 5% dextrose, the total osmolality exceeds that of the ECF. However, the dextrose is quickly metabolized, and only the isotonic solution remains. Therefore, any effect on the intracellular compartment is temporary. Similarly, with hypotonic multiple electrolyte solutions containing 5% dextrose, once the dextrose is metabolized, these solutions disperse as hypotonic fluids. Higher concentrations of dextrose, such as 50% dextrose in water, are strongly hypertonic and must be administered into central veins so that they can be diluted by rapid blood flow.

Saline solutions are also available in osmolar concentrations greater than that of the ECF. These solutions draw water from the ICF to the ECF and cause cells to shrink. If administered rapidly or in large quantity, they may cause an extracellular volume excess and precipitate circulatory overload and dehydration. As a result, these solutions must be administered cautiously and usually only when the serum osmolality has decreased to dangerously low levels. **Hypertonic solutions** exert an osmotic pressure greater than that of the ECF.

Other Intravenous Therapies

When the patient is unable to tolerate food, nutritional requirements are often met using the IV route. Solutions may include high concentrations of glucose (such as 50% dextrose in water), protein, or fat to meet nutritional requirements (see Chapter 36). The IV route may also be used to administer colloids, plasma expanders, and blood products. Examples of blood products include whole blood, packed red blood cells, albumin, and cryoprecipitate; these are discussed in more detail in Chapter 54.

Many medications are also delivered by the IV route, either by continuous infusion or intermittent bolus directly into the vein. Because IV medications enter the circulation rapidly, administration by this route is potentially very hazardous. All medications can produce adverse reactions; however, medications administered by the IV route can cause these reactions within seconds to minutes after administration, because the medications are delivered directly into the bloodstream. Administration rates and recommended dilutions for individual medications are available in specialized texts pertaining to IV medications and in manufacturers' package inserts; these should be consulted to ensure safe IV administration of medications.

NURSING ALERT

The nurse must assess the patient for a history of allergic reactions to medications. Although this is important when any medication is to be administered, it is even more important with IV administration, because the medication is delivered directly into the bloodstream.

Nursing Management of the Patient Receiving Intravenous Therapy

The ability to perform venipuncture to gain access to the venous system for administering fluids and medication is an expected nursing skill in many settings. This responsibility includes selecting the appropriate venipuncture site and type of cannula and being proficient in the technique of vein entry. The nurse should demonstrate competency in and knowledge of catheter placement and should follow the rules and regulations, organizational policies and procedures, and practice guidelines of that province's nursing association and the Canadian Nurses Association.

Infusion therapy is initiated by a health care professional who prescribes the type and amount of solution, additives (if any), and rate of flow. When administering parenteral fluids, the nurse monitors the patient's response to the fluids, considering the fluid volume, the fluid content, and the patient's clinical status.

For the procedural guidelines for starting a peripheral IV infusion, go to **thepoint.lww.com/Hussein4e.**

Managing Systemic Complications

IV therapy predisposes the patient to numerous hazards, including both local and systemic complications. Systemic complications occur less frequently but are usually more serious than local complications. They include circulatory overload, air embolism, febrile reaction, and infection.

Fluid Overload

Overloading the circulatory system with excessive IV fluids causes increased blood pressure and central venous pressure. Signs and symptoms of fluid overload include moist crackles on auscultation of the lungs, edema, weight gain, dyspnea, and rapid, shallow respirations. Possible causes include rapid infusion of an IV solution or hepatic, cardiac, or renal disease. The risk of fluid overload and subsequent pulmonary edema is especially increased in older adults with cardiac disease; this is referred to as circulatory overload. Its treatment includes decreasing the IV rate, monitoring vital signs frequently, assessing breath sounds, and placing the patient in a high-Fowler's position. The physician is contacted immediately. This complication can be avoided by using an infusion pump and by carefully monitoring all infusions. Complications of circulatory overload include heart failure and pulmonary edema.

Air Embolism

The risk of air embolism is rare but ever-present. It is most often associated with cannulation of central veins. Manifestations of air embolism include palpitations, dyspnea, and cyanosis; hypotension; weak, rapid pulse; loss of consciousness; and chest, shoulder, and low back pain. Treatment calls for immediately clamping the cannula and replacing a leaking or open infusion system, placing the patient on the left side in the Trendelenburg's position, assessing vital signs and breath sounds, and administering oxygen. Air embolism can be prevented by using locking adapters on all lines, filling all tubing completely with solution, and using an air detection alarm on an IV infusion pump. Complications of air embolism include shock and death. The amount of air necessary to induce death in humans is not known; however, the rate of entry is probably as important as the actual volume of air.

Infection

Pyrogenic substances in either the infusion solution or the IV administration set can cause bloodstream infections. Signs and symptoms include an abrupt temperature elevation shortly after the infusion is started, backache, headache, increased pulse and respiratory rate, nausea and vomiting, diarrhea, chills and shaking, and general malaise. In severe sepsis, vascular collapse and septic shock may occur. See Chapter 18 for a discussion of septic shock.

Infection ranges in severity from local involvement of the insertion site to systemic dissemination of organisms through the bloodstream, as in sepsis. Measures to prevent infection are essential at the time the IV line is inserted and throughout the entire infusion. Prevention includes the following:

- Performing careful hand hygiene before every contact with any part of the infusion system or the patient
- Examining the IV containers for cracks, leaks, or cloudiness, which may indicate a contaminated solution
- Using strict aseptic technique
- Firmly anchoring the IV cannula to prevent to-and-fro motion (e.g., a catheter stabilization device will help)
- Inspecting the IV site daily and replacing a soiled or wet dressing with a dry sterile dressing (antimicrobial agents that should be used for site care include 2% tincture of iodine, 10% povidone–iodine, alcohol, or chlorhexidine gluconate, used alone or in combination)
- Disinfecting injection/access ports with antimicrobial solution before and after each use
- Removing the IV cannula at the first sign of local inflammation, contamination, or complication
- Replacing the peripheral IV cannula every 72 to 96 hours, or as indicated
- Replacing the IV cannula inserted during emergency conditions (with questionable asepsis) as soon as possible
- Using a 0.2-μm air-eliminating and bacteria/particulate retentive filter with non–lipid-containing solutions that require filtration. The filter can be added to the proximal or distal end of the administration set. If added to the proximal end between the fluid container and the tubing spike, the filter ensures sterility and particulate removal from the infusate container and prevents inadvertent infusion of air. If added to the distal end of the administration set, it filters air particles and contaminants introduced from add-on devices, secondary administration sets, or interruptions to the primary system. Filters should be located as close to the catheter insertion site as possible.
- Replacing the solution bag and administration set in accordance with agency policy and procedure
- Infusing or discarding medication or solution within 24 hours of its addition to an administration set
- Changing primary and secondary continuous administration sets every 72 hours, intermittent administration sets every 24 hours, or immediately if contamination is suspected.
- Using administration sets with a twist-lock design

Managing Local Complications

Local complications of IV therapy include infiltration and extravasation, phlebitis, thrombophlebitis, hematoma, and clotting of the needle.

Infiltration and Extravasation

Infiltration is the unintentional administration of a nonvesicant solution or medication into surrounding tissue. This can occur when the IV cannula dislodges or perforates the wall of the vein. Infiltration is characterized by edema around the insertion site, leakage of IV fluid from the insertion site, discomfort and coolness in the area of infiltration, and a significant decrease in the flow rate. When the solution is particularly irritating, sloughing of tissue may result. Close monitoring of the insertion site is necessary to detect infiltration before it becomes severe.

Infiltration is usually easily recognized if the insertion area is larger than the same site of the opposite extremity; however, it is not always so obvious. A common misconception is that a backflow of blood into the tubing proves that the catheter is properly placed within the vein. However, if the catheter tip has pierced the wall of the vessel, IV fluid will seep into tissues as well as flow into the vein. Although blood return occurs, infiltration may have occurred as well. A more reliable means of confirming infiltration is to apply a tourniquet above (or proximal to) the infusion site and tighten it enough to restrict venous flow. If the infusion continues to drip despite the venous obstruction, infiltration is present.

As soon as the nurse detects infiltration, the infusion should be stopped, the IV catheter discontinued, and a

CHART 17-4

Assessing for Infiltration

Grade	Clinical Criteria
0	No clinical symptoms
1	Skin blanched, edema less than 1 in in any direction, cool to touch, with or without pain
2	Skin blanched, edema 1 to 6 in in any direction, cool to touch, with or without pain
3	Skin blanched, translucent, gross edema greater than 6 in in any direction, cool to touch, mild to moderate pain, possible numbness
4	Skin blanched, translucent, skin tight, leaking, skin discoloured bruised, swollen, gross edema greater than 6 in in any direction, deep pitting tissue edema, circulatory impairment, moderate to severe pain, infiltration of any amount of blood products, irritant, or vesicant

Adapted from Infusion Nurses Society. (2011). *Infusion nursing standards of practice*. Norwood, MA: Author.

sterile dressing applied to the site after careful inspection to determine the extent of infiltration. The infiltration of any amount of blood product, irritant, or vesicant is considered the most severe.

The IV infusion should be started in a new site or proximal to the infiltration if the same extremity must be used again. A warm compress may be applied to the site if small volumes of noncaustic solutions have infiltrated over a long period, or if the solution was isotonic with a normal pH; the affected extremity should be elevated to promote the absorption of fluid. If the infiltration is recent and the solution was hypertonic or had an increased pH, a cold compress may be applied to the area. Infiltration can be detected and treated early by inspecting the site every hour for redness, pain, edema, blood return, coolness at the site, and IV fluid leaking from the IV site. Using the appropriate size and type of cannula for the vein prevents this complication. The Infusion Nursing Standards of Practice states that a standardized infiltration scale should be used to document the infiltration (Chart 17-4).

Extravasation is similar to infiltration, with an inadvertent administration of vesicant or irritant solution or medication into the surrounding tissue. Medications such as dopamine, calcium preparations, and chemotherapeutic agents can cause pain, burning, and redness at the site. Blistering, inflammation, and necrosis of tissues can occur. The extent of tissue damage is determined by the concentration of the medication, the quantity that extravasated, the location of the infusion site, the tissue response, and the duration of the process of extravasation.

The infusion must be stopped and the physician notified promptly. The agency's protocol to treat extravasation is initiated; the protocol may specify specific treatments, including antidotes specific to the medication that extravasated, and may indicate whether the IV line should remain in place or be removed before treatment. The protocol often specifies infiltration of the infusion site with an antidote prescribed after assessment by the physician, removal of the cannula, and application of warm compresses to sites of extravasation from vinca alkaloids or cold compresses to sites of extravasation from alkylating and antibiotic vesicants. The affected extremity should not be used for further cannula placement. Thorough neurovascular assessments of the affected extremity must be performed frequently. Reviewing the institution's IV policy and procedures and incompatibility charts and checking with the pharmacist before administering any IV medication, whether peripherally or centrally, are recommended to determine incompatibilities and vesicant potential to prevent extravasation. Careful, frequent monitoring of the IV site, avoiding insertion of IV devices in areas of flexion, securing the IV line, and using the smallest catheter possible that accommodates the vein help minimize the incidence and severity of this complication. In addition, when vesicant medication is administered by IV push, it should be given through a side port of an infusing IV solution to dilute the medication and decrease the severity of tissue damage if extravasation occurs. Extravasation is rated as grade 4 on the infiltration scale.

Phlebitis

Phlebitis is defined as inflammation of a vein, which can be categorized as chemical, mechanical, or bacterial; however, two or more of these types of irritation often occur simultaneously. Chemical phlebitis can be caused by an irritating medication or solution (increased pH or high osmolality of a solution), rapid infusion rates, and medication incompatibilities. Mechanical phlebitis results from long periods of cannulation, catheters in flexed areas, catheter gauges larger than the vein lumen, and poorly secured catheters. Bacterial phlebitis can develop from poor hand hygiene, lack of aseptic technique, failure to check all equipment before use, and failure to recognize early signs and symptoms of phlebitis. Other factors include poor venipuncture technique, catheter in place for a prolonged period, and failure to adequately secure the catheter. Phlebitis is characterized by a reddened, warm area around the insertion site or along the path of the vein, pain or tenderness at the site or along the vein, and swelling. The incidence of phlebitis increases with the length of time the IV line is in place, the composition of the fluid or medication infused (especially its pH and tonicity), the size and site of the cannula inserted, ineffective filtration, inadequate anchoring of the line, and the introduction of microorganisms at the time of insertion. Specific standards for assessing phlebitis appear in Chart 17-5. Phlebitis is graded according to the most severe presenting indication.

Treatment consists of discontinuing the IV line and restarting it in another site, and applying a warm, moist compress to the affected site. Phlebitis can be prevented by using aseptic technique during insertion, using the appropriate-sized cannula or needle for the vein, considering the composition of fluids and medications when selecting a site, observing the site hourly for any complications, anchoring the cannula or needle well, and changing the IV site according to agency policy and procedures.

Thrombophlebitis

Thrombophlebitis refers to the presence of a clot plus inflammation in the vein. It is evidenced by localized pain, redness, warmth, and swelling around the insertion site or

CHART 17-5

Assessing for Phlebitis

Grade	Clinical Criteria
0	No clinical symptoms
1	Erythema at access site with or without pain
2	Pain at access site Erythema, edema, or both
3	Pain at access site Erythema, edema, or both Streak formation Palpable venous cord (2.54 cm [1 in] or shorter)
4	Pain at access site with erythema Streak formation Palpable venous cord (longer than 2.54 cm [1 in]) Purulent drainage

Note: If this scale is not being used in an institution, then the description associated with the number can be used to describe the assessment.

Adapted from Infusion Nurses Society. (2011). *Infusion nursing standards of practice*. Norwood, MA: Author; Norton, L., Ottoboni, L. K., Varady, A., et al. (2013). Phlebitis in amiodarone administration: Incidence, contributing factors, and clinical implications. *American Journal of Critical Care*, *22*(6), 498–505.

along the path of the vein, immobility of the extremity because of discomfort and swelling, sluggish flow rate, fever, malaise, and leukocytosis.

Treatment includes discontinuing the IV infusion; applying a cold compress first, to decrease the flow of blood and increase platelet aggregation, followed by a warm compress; elevating the extremity; and restarting the line in the opposite extremity. If the patient has signs and symptoms of thrombophlebitis, the IV line should not be flushed (although flushing may be indicated in the absence of phlebitis to ensure cannula patency and to prevent mixing of incompatible medications and solutions). The catheter should be cultured after the skin around the catheter is cleaned with alcohol. If purulent drainage exists, the site is cultured before the skin is cleaned.

Thrombophlebitis can be prevented by avoiding trauma to the vein at the time the IV line is inserted, observing the site every hour, and checking medication additives for compatibility.

Hematoma

Hematoma results when blood leaks into tissues surrounding the IV insertion site. Leakage can result if the opposite vein wall is perforated during venipuncture, the needle slips out of the vein, or insufficient pressure is applied to the site after removal of the needle or cannula. The signs of a hematoma include ecchymosis, immediate swelling at the site, and leakage of blood at the insertion site.

Treatment includes removing the needle or cannula and applying light pressure with a sterile, dry dressing; applying ice for 24 hours to the site to avoid extension of the hematoma; elevating the extremity; assessing the extremity for any circulatory, neurologic, or motor dysfunction; and restarting the line in the other extremity if indicated. A hematoma can be prevented by carefully inserting the needle and by using diligent care with patients who have a bleeding disorder, are taking anticoagulant medication, or have advanced liver disease.

Clotting and Obstruction

Blood clots may form in the IV line as a result of kinked IV tubing, a very slow infusion rate, an empty IV bag, or failure to flush the IV line after intermittent medication or solution administrations. The signs are decreased flow rate and blood backflow into the IV tubing.

If blood clots in the IV line, the infusion must be discontinued and restarted in another site with a new cannula and administration set. The tubing should not be irrigated or milked. Neither the infusion rate nor the solution container should be raised, and the clot should not be aspirated from the tubing. Clotting of the needle or cannula may be prevented by not allowing the IV solution bag to run dry, taping the tubing to prevent kinking and maintain patency, maintaining an adequate flow rate, and flushing the line after intermittent medication or other solution administration. In some cases, a specially trained nurse or physician may inject a thrombolytic agent into the catheter to clear an occlusion resulting from fibrin or clotted blood.

Promoting Home, Community-Based, and Transitional Care

Educating Patients About Self-Care

At times, IV therapy is administered in the home setting, in which case much of the daily management rests with the patient and family. Teaching becomes essential to ensure that the patient and family can manage the IV fluid and infusion correctly and avoid complications. Written instructions as well as demonstration and return demonstration help reinforce the key points for all these functions.

Continuing and Transitional Care

Home infusion therapies cover a wide range of treatments, including antibiotic, analgesic, and antineoplastic medications; blood or blood component therapy; and parenteral nutrition. When direct nursing care is necessary, arrangements are made to have a nurse visit the home and administer the IV therapy as prescribed. In addition to implementing and monitoring the IV therapy, the nurse carries out a comprehensive assessment of the patient's condition and continues to teach the patient and family about the skills involved in overseeing the IV therapy setup. Any dietary changes that may be necessary because of fluid or electrolyte imbalances are explained or reinforced during such sessions.

Periodic laboratory testing may be necessary to assess the effects of IV therapy and the patient's progress. Blood specimens may be obtained by a laboratory near the patient's home, or a home visit may be arranged to obtain blood specimens for analysis.

The nurse collaborates with the case manager in assessing the patient, family, and home environment; developing a plan of care in accordance with the patient's treatment plan and level of ability; and arranging for appropriate referral and follow-up if necessary. Any necessary equipment may be provided by the agency or purchased by the patient, depending on the terms of the home care arrangements.

Critical Thinking Exercises

1 You are caring for an 84-year-old patient with chronic kidney disease. You have been given orders to start an IV on the patient after receiving lab results indicating hypocalcemia. What is the best evidence for appropriate treatment in the event of severe hypocalcemia? Which nursing interventions and precautions should you implement for this patient when administering the IV medication? Give your rationale. What will you include in discharge teaching for this patient?

2 A 72-year-old man has been admitted to the hospital. He is confused and unable to give any information. Vital signs: B/P 122/56 sitting and 102/46 standing; HR 84/min, RR 12/min. Serum sodium levels indicate that this patient has hyponatremia. What other electrolyte values will you consider? What are the causes of hyponatremia? What will you include in your assessment of this patient? Give your rationale. What special considerations are needed for this patient because he is an older adult? Give your rationale.

3 A 54-year-old man is sent to the ED by his primary provider. The patient has a history of congestive heart failure and COPD. The physician has requested laboratory tests. Blood gas results are as follows: pH 7.28; HCO_3^- 26; $PaCO_2$ 55 mm Hg. Blood chemistry results are as follows: potassium 4.5 mEq/L; sodium 140 mEq/L; glucose 110 mg/dL. Vital signs: B/P 140/92, HR 90/min, RR 18/min. What is your priority for this patient? Give your rationale. What further diagnostic testing is needed? Give your rationale. What is the rationale for not administering oxygen therapy to this patient immediately?

REFERENCES AND SELECTED READINGS

Books

Buettner, J. R. (2017). *Fast facts for the ER nurse: Emergency department orientation in a nutshell*. New York, NY: Springer Publishing Company.

Comerford, K. C. (2015). *Nursing 2015 drug handbook*. Philadelphia, PA: Wolters Kluwer.

Day, R. A. (2012). Nutrition assessment. In T. C. Stephen, D. L. Skillen, R. A. Day, et al. (Eds.). *Canadian Jensen's guide to health assessment for nurses. A best practice approach* (pp. 167–201). Philadelphia, PA: Wolters Kluwer Health/Lippincott Williams & Wilkins.

Dudek, S. G. (2013). *Nutrition essentials for nursing practice* (7th ed.). Philadelphia, PA: Wolters Kluwer Health/Lippincott Williams & Wilkins.

El-Hussein, M. T., Power-Kean, K., Zettel, S., et al. (2018). *Understanding pathophysiology* (1st Canadian ed.). Milton, ON, Canada: Elsevier.

Fischbach, F., & Dunning, M. B. (2015). *A manual of laboratory and diagnostic tests* (9th ed.). Philadelphia, PA: Lippincott Williams & Wilkins.

Frandsen, G., & Pennington, S. (2014). *Abrams' clinical drug therapy: Rationales for nursing practice* (10th ed.). Philadelphia, PA: Lippincott Williams & Wilkins.

Gorski, L. A. (2018). *Phillips's manual of IV therapeutics: Evidence-based practice for infusion therapy*. Philadelphia, PA: FA Davis.

Grossman, S. C., & Porth, C. M. (2014). *Porth's pathophysiology: Concepts of altered health states* (9th ed.). Philadelphia, PA: Lippincott Williams & Wilkins.

Hall, J. E. (2015). *Guyton and Hall textbook of medical physiology* (13th ed.). Philadelphia, PA: Saunders Elsevier.

Hannon, R. A., & Porth, C. M. (2017). *Porth pathophysiology: Concepts of Altered Health States*. Philadelphia, PA: Wolters Kluwer Health/Lippincott Williams & Wilkins.

Heitz, U., & Horne, M. (2005). *Pocket guide to fluid, electrolyte, and acid-base balance* (5th ed.). St. Louis, MO: Elsevier Mosby.

Karch, A. M. (2012). *2012 Lippincott's nursing drug guide*. Philadelphia, PA: Wolters Kluwer Health/Lippincott Williams & Wilkins.

Matfin, G. (Ed.). (2018). *Endocrine and metabolic medical emergencies: A clinician's guide*. Hoboken, NJ: John Wiley & Sons.

Nair, M., & Peate, I. (2015). *Pathophysiology for nurses at a glance*. Hoboken, NJ: John Wiley & Sons.

Nelms, M., & Sucher, K. (2015). *Nutrition therapy and pathophysiology*. Boston, MA: Nelson Education.

Papadakis M. A., & McPhee. S. J. (2016). *Current medical diagnosis and treatment* (55th ed). New York, NY: McGraw Hill, Education.

Potter, P. A., Perry, A. G., Stockert, P., et al. (2018). *Canadian fundamentals of nursing*. Toronto, ON: Elsevier Health Sciences.

Van Leeuwen, A. M., & Bladh, M. L. (2016). *Textbook of laboratory and diagnostic testing: practical application of nursing process at the bedside*. Philadelphia, PA: FA Davis.

Journals and Electronic Documents

Fluid and Electrolyte Balances and Imbalances

Bansal, A. D., Negoianu, D., & Warburton, K. M. (2016). An Unusual yet "Mg"nificent indication for Hemodialysis. *Seminars in Dialysis, 29*(3), 247–250. https://dx.doi.org/10.1111%2Fsdi.12479

Beatriz, L. V., Gonzalez, C. P., Pascual, B. A., et al. (2018). Secondary hyponatremia to inappropiate secretion of antidiuretic hormone Siadh in diagnosed patient of bladder cancer in treatment with chemotherapy: Exclusion diagnosis? *Journal of Molecular Oncology Research, 2*(2), 36.

Bichet, D. (2013). Treatment of central diabetes insipidus. *UpToDate*. Retrieved February 10, 2016, from www.uptodate.com

Blaine, J., Chonchol, M., & Levi, M. (2015). Renal control of calcium, phosphate, and magnesium homeostasis. *Clinical Journal of the American Society of Nephrology, 10*(7), 1257–1272.

Brindley, J. (2018). Undertaking drug calculations for intravenous medicines and infusions. *Nursing Standard, 32*(20), 55–63.

Canadian Cancer Society. (2019). Should I take Vitmin D supplement. Retrieved from: https://www.cancer.ca/en/prevention-and-screening/reduce-cancer-risk/make-healthy-choices/eat-well/should-i-take-a-vitamin-d-supplement/?region=on

Castillo, M. I., Larsen, E., Cooke, M., et al. (2018). Integrated versus nOn-integrated Peripheral inTravenous catheter. Which Is the most effective systeM for peripheral intravenoUs catheter Management? (The OPTIMUM study): A randomised controlled trial protocol. *BMJ Open, 8*(5), e019916.

Chang, W. P., & Peng, Y. X. (2018). Occurrence of Phlebitis: A systematic review and meta-analysis. *Nursing Research, 67*(3), 252–260.

Colucci, W., & Chen, H. (2014). Natriuretic peptide measurement in heart failure. *UpToDate*. Retrieved February 10, 2016, from www.uptodate.com

Cox, C. L., & Boyd, C. E. (2019). Examination of the cardiovascular system. *Physical Assessment for Nurses and Healthcare Professionals*. Wiley Blackwell: Hoboken New Jersey. Retrieved from https://books.google.ca/books?hl=en&lr=&id=NyiBDwAAQBAJ&oi=fnd&pg=PA67&dq=Cox,+C.+L.,+%26+Boyd,+C.+E.+(2019).&ots=lp2C0UjQTe&sig=djS_21mStHLqsfbXPEmfMpfM9Vw#v=onepage&q&f=false

Daud, A. (2018). Incidence of phlebitis among adult patients with peripheral intravenous catheter in an East Coast Hospital Malaysia. *International Journal of Care Scholars, 1*(2), 5–8.

Decaux, G., Kengne, F. G., Couturier, B., et al. (2018). Mild water restriction with or without urea for the longterm treatment of syndrome of inappropriate antidiuretic hormone secretion (SIADH): Can urine osmolality help the choice? *European Journal of Internal Medicine, 48*, 89–93.

Earhart, E., Weiss, E., Rahman, R., et al. (2015). Effects of oral sodium supplementation on thermoregulation in trained, endurance athletes. *Journal of Sports Science and Medicine, 14*(1), 172–178.

Emmett, M. (2014). Simple and mixed acid–base disorders. *UpToDate*. Retrieved February 9, 2016, from www.uptodate.com

Gavin, N., Lippiatt, R., Northfield, S., et al. (2018). Improving vascular access care for cancer patients. *Infection, Disease & Health, 23*, S6.

Goltzman, D. (2014). Etiology of hypocalcemia in adults. *UpToDate*. Retrieved February 10, 2016, from www.uptodate.com

Health Canada (2010). *Sodium reduction strategy for Canada: Recommendations of the Sodium working group*. Retrieved from: https://www.dietitians.ca/Downloads/Public/sr-position-paper.aspx

Hypertension Canada. (2014). Limit salt/sodium intake. Retrieved from http://www.hypertension.ca/en/hypertension/what-can-i-do/limit-saltsodium-intake

Jensen, H. K., Brabrand, M., Vinholt, P. J., et al. (2015). Hypokalemia in acute medical patients: Risk factors and prognosis." *The American Journal of Medicine, 128*(1), 60–67.

Keogh, S., Marsh, N., Higgins, N., et al. (2014). A time and motion study of peripheral venous catheter flushing practice using manually prepared and prefilled flush syringes. *Journal of Infusion Nursing*, *37*(2), 96–101.

Leggett, T., Williams, J., Daly, C., et al. (2018). Intended hydration strategies and knowledge of exercise-associated hyponatraemia in marathon runners: A questionnaire-based study. *Journal of Athletic Training*, *53*(7), 696–702.

Lin, J., Cheng, Z., Ding, X., et al. (2018). Acid-base and electrolyte managements in chronic kidney disease and end-stage renal disease: Case-based discussion. *Blood Purification*, *45*(1–3), 179–186.

Lo, L. J., & Liu, K. D. (2018). Hyponatremia and hypernatremia. *Critical Care Secrets E-Book*, *150*, 320.

MacLeod-Glover, N., Mink, M., Yarema, M., et al. (2016). Digoxin toxicity: Case for retiring its use in elderly patients? *Canadian Family Physician*, *62*(3), 223–228.

Madiraca, J., & Hoch, C. (2018). Electrolyte series: Calcium and phosphorus. *Nursing2018 Critical Care*, *13*(2), 24–31.

Maly, C., Fan, K. L., Rogers, G. F., et al. (2018). A primer on the acute management of intravenous extravasation injuries for the plastic surgeon. *Plastic and Reconstructive Surgery Global Open*, *6*(4), e1743.

McTavish, A. D., & Sharma, M. P. (2018). Renal physiology: Acid–base balance. *Anaesthesia & Intensive Care Medicine*, *19*(5), 233–238.

Medical Council of Canada (2019). Clinical laboratory tests: Normal Values. Retrieved from https://mcc.ca/objectives/normal-values/

Moritz, M. (2013). Case studies in fluid & electrolyte therapy. *Journal of Infusion Nursing*, *36*(4), 270–277.

Morris, J. H., Bohm, N. M., Nemecek, B. D., et al. (2018). Rapidity of correction of hyponatremia due to syndrome of inappropriate secretion of antidiuretic hormone following Tolvaptan. *American Journal of Kidney Diseases*, *71*(6), 772–782.

Mount, D. B. (2014a). Causes and evaluation of hyperkalemia in adults. *UpToDate*. Retrieved February 10, 2016, from www.uptodate.com

Mount, D. B. (2014b). Clinical manifestations and treatment of hypokalemia in adults. In R. Sterns (Ed.). *UpToDate*. Retrieved February 10, 2016, from www.uptodate.com

Mount, D. B. (2014c). Treatment and prevention of hyperkalemia in adults. In R. Sterns (Ed.). *UpToDate*. Retrieved February 10, 2016, from www.uptodate.com

Palmer, B. F. (2015). Regulation of potassium homeostasis. *Clinical Journal of the American Society of Nephrology*, *10*(6), 1050–1060.

Public Health Agency of Canada. (2018). *Sodium intake of Canadians 2017*. Retrieved from https://www.canada.ca/content/dam/hc-sc/documents/services/publications/food-nutrition/sodium-intake-canadians-2017/2017-sodium-intakes-report-eng.pdf

Robson, J. P., Jr. (2013). A review of hemodialysis vascular access devices: Improving client outcomes through evidence-based practice. *Journal of Infusion Nursing*, *36*(6), 404–410.

Sahay, M., & Sahay, R. (2014). Hyponatremia: A practical approach. *Indian Journal of Endocrinology and Metabolism*, *18*(6), 760–771.

Seliger, S., & Kestenbaum, B. (2018). Commentary on treatment of severe hyponatremia. *Clinical Journal of the American Society of Nephrology*, *13*(4), 650–651.

Sterns, R. H. (2014). Maintenance and replacement fluid therapy in adults. *UpToDate*. Retrieved February 9, 2016, from www.uptodate.com

St-Jules, D. E., Goldfarb, D. S., Pompeii, M. L., et al. (2018). Assessment and misassessment of potassium, phosphorus, and protein in the hemodialysis diet. *Seminars in Dialysis*, *31*(5), 479–486.

Villa, G., Chelazzi, C., Giua, R., et al. (2018). In-line filtration reduces postoperative venous peripheral phlebitis associated with cannulation: A randomized clinical trial. *Anesthesia & Analgesia*, *127*(6), 1367–1374.

Vizcarra, C., Cassutt, C., Corbitt, N., et al. (2014). Recommendations for improving safety practices with short peripheral catheters. *Journal of Infusion Nursing*, *37*(2), 121–124.

Wojnar, D. G., & Bearman, M. (2013). Peripherally inserted central catheter: Compliance with evidence-based indications for insertion in an inpatient setting. *Journal of Infusion Nursing*, *36*(4), 291–296.

Woody, G., & Davis, B. A. (2013). Increasing nurse competence in peripheral intravenous therapy. *Journal of Infusion Nursing*, *36*(6), 413–419.

Resources

Canadian Vascular Access Association: http://www.cvaa.info
Infusion Nurses Society: http://www.ins1.org
Medical council of Canada: https://mcc.ca/objectives/normal-values/
Registered Nurses' Association of Ontario: http://www.rnao.org

18 Shock and Multiple Organ Dysfunction Syndrome

Adapted by Joan Harris and Joanne Bouma

Learning Objectives

On completion of this chapter, the learner will be able to:

1. Describe shock and its underlying pathophysiology.
2. Compare clinical findings of the compensatory, progressive, and irreversible stages of shock.
3. Describe organ dysfunction that may occur with shock.
4. Describe similarities and differences in shock due to hypovolemic, cardiogenic, neurogenic, anaphylactic, and septic shock states.
5. Identify medical and nursing management priorities in treating patients in shock.
6. Identify vasoactive medications used in treating shock, and describe nursing implications associated with their use.
7. Discuss the importance of nutritional support in all forms of shock.
8. Discuss the role of nurses in psychosocial support of patients experiencing shock and their families.
9. Discuss multiple organ dysfunction syndrome.

Shock is a life-threatening condition that results from inadequate tissue perfusion. Many conditions may cause shock; irrespective of the cause, tissue hypoperfusion prevents adequate oxygen delivery to cells, leading to cell dysfunction and death. The progression of shock is neither linear nor predictable, and shock states, especially **septic shock**, comprise an area of aggressive clinical research. Nurses caring for patients with shock and those at risk for shock must understand the underlying mechanisms of the various shock states (i.e., hypovolemic, cardiogenic, neurogenic, anaphylactic, and septic) and recognize the subtle as well as more obvious signs of each of these states. Rapid assessment with early recognition and response to shock states is essential to the patient's recovery.

Overview of Shock

Shock can best be defined as a clinical syndrome that results from inadequate tissue perfusion, creating an imbalance between the delivery of oxygen and nutrients needed to support cellular function (Maier, 2015; Moore, Dyson, Singer, et al., 2015). Adequate blood flow to the tissues and cells requires an effective cardiac pump, adequate vasculature or circulatory system, and sufficient blood volume. If one of these components is impaired, perfusion to the tissues is threatened or compromised. Without treatment, inadequate blood flow to the cells results in poor delivery of oxygen and nutrients, cellular hypoxia, and cell death that progresses to organ dysfunction and eventually death.

Shock affects all body systems. It may develop rapidly or slowly, depending on the underlying cause. During shock, the body struggles to survive, calling on all its homeostatic mechanisms to restore blood flow. Any insult to the body can create a cascade of events resulting in poor tissue perfusion. Therefore, any patient with any disease state may be at risk for developing shock. The primary underlying pathophysiologic process and underlying disorder are used to classify the shock state (e.g., **hypovolemic shock**, **cardiogenic shock**, obstructive shock, **distributive shock** [i.e., neurogenic, anaphylactic, septic]; all discussed later in the chapter).

Regardless of the initial cause of shock, certain physiologic responses are common to all types of shock. These physiologic responses include hypoperfusion of tissues, hypermetabolism, and activation of the inflammatory response. The body responds to shock states by activating the sympathetic nervous system and mounting a hypermetabolic and inflammatory response. Once shock develops, the patient's survival may have more to do with the body's ability to effectively respond to it than with the initial cause of shock. Failure of compensatory mechanisms to effectively restore physiologic balance is the final pathway of all shock states and results in end-organ dysfunction and death (Dellinger, Levy, Rhodes, et al., 2013; Maier, 2015; Wacker & Winters, 2014).

Nursing care of patients with shock requires ongoing systematic assessment. Many of the interventions required in caring for patients with shock call for close collaboration with other members of the health care team and rapid implementation of prescribed therapies. Nurses are in key positions to identify early signs of shock and anticipate rapid therapy.

Normal Cellular Function

Energy metabolism occurs within the cell, where nutrients are chemically broken down and stored in the form of adenosine triphosphate (ATP). Cells use this stored energy to perform necessary functions, such as active transport, muscle contraction, and biochemical synthesis, as well as specialized cellular functions, such as the conduction of electrical impulses. ATP can be synthesized aerobically (in the presence of oxygen) or anaerobically (in the absence of oxygen). Aerobic metabolism yields far greater amounts of ATP per mole of glucose than does anaerobic metabolism; therefore, it is a more efficient and effective means of producing energy. In addition, anaerobic metabolism results in the accumulation of the toxic end product, lactic acid, which must be removed from the cell and transported to the liver for conversion into glucose and glycogen.

Pathophysiology

Cellular Changes

In shock, the cells lack an adequate blood supply and are deprived of oxygen and nutrients; therefore, they must produce energy through anaerobic metabolism. This results in low energy yields from nutrients and an acidotic intracellular environment. Because of these changes, normal cell function ceases (Fig. 18-1). The cell swells and the cell membrane becomes more permeable, allowing electrolytes and fluids to seep out of and into the cell. The sodium–potassium pump becomes impaired; cell structures, primarily the mitochondria, are damaged; and death of the cell results.

Glucose is the primary substrate required for the production of cellular energy in the form of ATP. In stress states, catecholamines, cortisol, glucagon, and inflammatory **biochemical mediators** (i.e., cytokines) are released, causing hyperglycemia and insulin resistance to mobilize glucose for cellular metabolism. Activation of these substances promotes gluconeogenesis, which is the formation of glucose from noncarbohydrate sources such as proteins and fats. Glycogen that has been stored in the liver is converted to glucose through glycogenolysis to meet metabolic needs, increasing the blood glucose concentration (i.e., hyperglycemia).

Continued activation of the stress response by shock states causes a depletion of glycogen stores, resulting in increased proteolysis and eventual organ failure (Moore et al., 2015). The deficit of nutrients and oxygen for normal cellular metabolism causes a buildup of metabolic end products in the cells and interstitial spaces. The clotting cascade, also associated with the inflammatory process, becomes activated, which compounds this pathologic cycle. With significant cell injury or death caused by shock, the clotting cascade is over productive, resulting in small clots lodging in microcirculation, further hampering cellular perfusion (Zarychanski, Abou-Setta, Kanji, et al., 2015). This upregulation of the clotting cascade further

Glossary

anaphylactic shock: circulatory shock state resulting from a severe allergic reaction producing an overwhelming systemic vasodilation and relative hypovolemia

biochemical mediators: messenger substances that may be released by a cell to create an action at that site or be carried by the bloodstream to a distant site before being activated; also called cytokines or *inflammatory mediators*

cardiogenic shock: shock state resulting from impairment or failure of the myocardium

colloids: intravenous solutions that contain molecules that are too large to pass through capillary membranes. Creating an osmotic gradient, pulling fluid into the intravascular space.

crystalloids: intravenous electrolyte solutions that move freely between the intravascular compartment and interstitial spaces

distributive shock: shock state resulting from displacement of blood volume creating a relative hypovolemia and inadequate delivery of oxygen to the cells

hypovolemic shock: shock state resulting from decreased intravascular volume due to fluid loss

multiple organ dysfunction syndrome (MODS): presence of altered function of two or more organs in an acutely ill patient such that interventions are necessary to support continued organ function

neurogenic shock: shock state resulting from loss of sympathetic tone causing relative hypovolemia

sepsis: life-threatening organ dysfunction caused by a dysregulated host response to infection

septic shock: a subset of sepsis in which underlying circulatory and cellular metabolism abnormalities are profound enough to substantially increase mortality

shock: physiologic condition in which there is inadequate blood flow to tissues and cells of the body

systemic inflammatory response syndrome (SIRS): a syndrome resulting from a clinical insult that initiates an inflammatory response that is systemic, rather than localized to the site of the insult

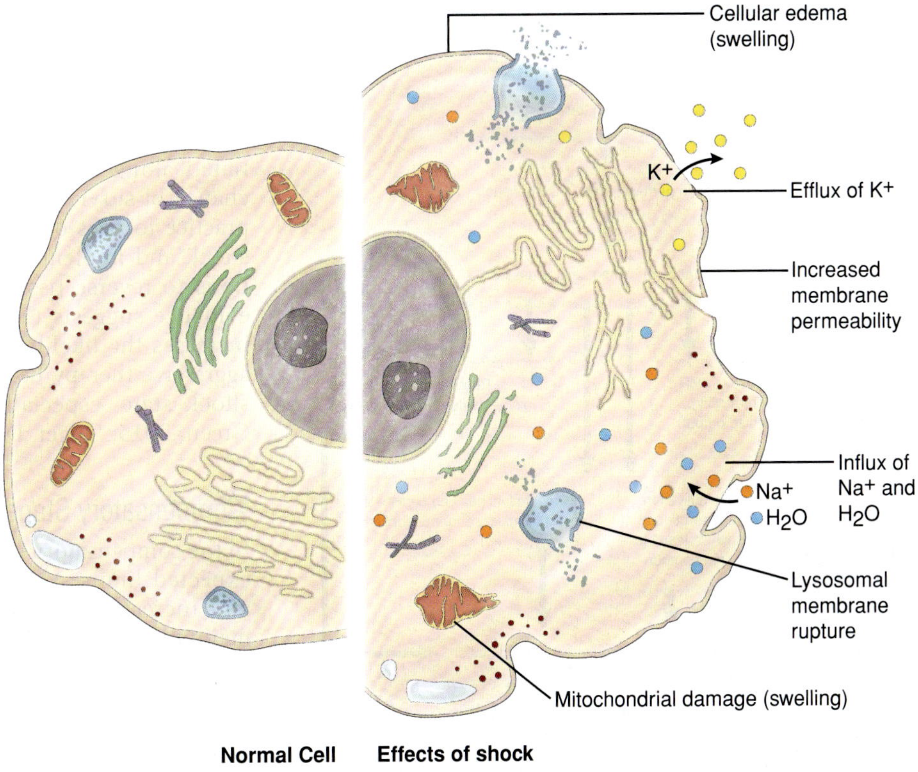

FIGURE 18-1. Cellular effects of shock. The cell swells and the cell membrane becomes more permeable; fluids and electrolytes seep from and into the cell. Mitochondria and lysosomes are damaged, and the cell dies.

compromises microcirculation of tissues, exacerbating cellular hypoperfusion (Moore et al., 2015). Cellular metabolism is impaired, and a self-perpetuating negative situation (i.e., a positive feedback loop) is initiated.

Vascular Responses

Local regulatory mechanisms, referred to as autoregulation, stimulate vasodilation or vasoconstriction in response to biochemical mediators released by the cell, communicating the need for oxygen and nutrients (Moore et al., 2015; Zarychanski et al., 2015). A biochemical mediator is a substance released by a cell or immune cells such as macrophages; the substance triggers an action at a cell site or travels in the bloodstream to a distant site, where it triggers action. Researchers are learning more every day about the physiologic actions of numerous proinflammatory and anti-inflammatory biochemical mediators that are responsible for the complex clinical presentation of shock states (Prucha, Belligan, & Zazula, 2014).

Blood Pressure Regulation

Three major components of the circulatory system—blood volume, the cardiac pump, and the vasculature—must respond effectively to complex neural, chemical, and hormonal feedback systems to maintain an adequate blood pressure (BP) and perfuse body tissues. BP is regulated through a complex interaction of neural, chemical, and hormonal feedback systems affecting both cardiac output and peripheral resistance. This relationship is expressed in the following equation:

Mean arterial BP = Cardiac output × Peripheral resistance

Cardiac output is a product of the stroke volume (the amount of blood ejected from the left ventricle during systole) and heart rate. Peripheral resistance is primarily determined by the diameter of the arterioles.

Tissue perfusion and organ perfusion depend on mean arterial pressure (MAP), or the average pressure at which blood moves through the vasculature. MAP must exceed 65 mm Hg for cells to receive the oxygen and nutrients needed to metabolize energy in amounts sufficient to sustain life (Cestero & Dent, 2015; Dellinger et al., 2013). True MAP can be calculated only by complex methods; however, most digital BP machines provide a MAP reading to guide clinical decisions.

BP is regulated by baroreceptors (pressure receptors) located in the carotid sinus and aortic arch. These pressure receptors are responsible for monitoring the circulatory volume and regulating neural and endocrine activities (see Chapter 17 for further description). When BP drops, catecholamines (epinephrine and norepinephrine) are released from the adrenal medulla. These increase heart rate, contractility, AV node conduction and cause vasoconstriction, restoring BP. Chemoreceptors, also located in the aortic arch and carotid arteries, regulate BP and respiratory rate using much the same mechanism in response to changes in oxygen and carbon dioxide (CO_2) concentrations in the blood. These primary regulatory mechanisms can respond to changes in BP on a moment-to-moment basis.

The kidneys regulate BP by releasing renin, an enzyme needed for the conversion of angiotensin I to angiotensin II, a potent vasoconstrictor. This stimulation of the renin–angiotensin mechanism and the resulting vasoconstriction indirectly lead to the release of aldosterone from the adrenal cortex, which promotes the retention of sodium and water (i.e., hypernatremia). Hypernatremia then stimulates the release of antidiuretic hormone (ADH) by the pituitary gland. ADH causes the kidneys to retain water further in an effort to raise blood volume and BP. These

Physiology/Pathophysiology

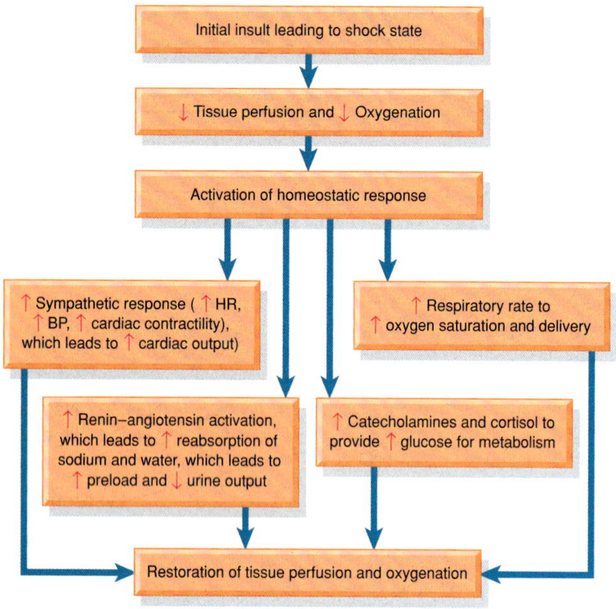

FIGURE 18-2. Compensatory mechanisms in shock.

secondary regulatory mechanisms may take hours or days to respond to changes in BP. The relationship between the initiation of shock and the responsiveness of primary and secondary regulatory mechanisms that compensate for deficits in blood volume, the pumping effectiveness of the heart, or vascular tone, which may result because of the shock state, is noted in Figure 18-2.

Stages of Shock

Shock is believed to progress along a continuum and can be identified as early or late, depending on the signs and symptoms and the overall severity of organ dysfunction. A convenient way to understand the physiologic responses and subsequent clinical signs and symptoms of shock is to divide the continuum into separate stages: compensatory (stage 1), progressive (stage 2), and irreversible (stage 3). The earlier that medical and nursing interventions are initiated along this continuum, the greater the patient's chance of survival. Current research and evidence-based practice focuses on assessing patients at greatest risk for shock and implementing early and aggressive interventions to reverse tissue hypoxia (Green, 2015). Current evidence suggests that the window of opportunity that increases the likelihood of patient survival occurs when aggressive therapy begins within 3 hours of identifying a shock state, especially septic shock (Dellinger, 2015; Green, 2015; Singer, Deutschman, Seymour, et al., 2016).

Compensatory Stage

In the compensatory stage of shock, the BP remains within expected limits. Vasoconstriction, increased heart rate, and increased contractility of the heart contribute to maintaining adequate cardiac output. This results from stimulation of the sympathetic nervous system and subsequent release of catecholamines (epinephrine and norepinephrine). Patients display the often-described "fight or flight" response. The body shunts blood from organs such as the skin, kidneys, and gastrointestinal (GI) tract to the brain, heart, and lungs to ensure adequate blood supply to these vital organs. As a result, the skin is cool and pale, bowel sounds are hypoactive, and urine output decreases in response to the release of aldosterone and ADH.

Clinical Manifestations

Despite a normal BP, the patient shows numerous clinical signs indicating inadequate organ perfusion (Table 18-1). The result of inadequate perfusion is anaerobic metabolism and a buildup of lactic acid, producing metabolic

TABLE 18-1 Clinical Findings in Stages of Shock

Finding	Stage: Compensatory	Progressive	Irreversible
Blood pressure	Normal	Systolic <80–90 mm Hg; MAP <65 mm Hg Requires fluids resuscitation to support blood pressure	Requires mechanical or pharmacologic support
Heart rate	>100 bpm	>150 bpm	Erratic
Respiratory status	>20 breaths/min $PaCO_2$ <32 mm Hg	Rapid, shallow respirations; crackles PaO_2 <80 mm Hg $PaCO_2$ >45 mm Hg	Requires intubation and mechanical ventilation and oxygenation
Skin	Cold, clammy	Mottled, petechiae	Jaundice
Urinary output	Decreased	0.5 mL/kg/hr	Anuric, requires dialysis
Mentation	Confusion	Lethargy	Unconscious
Acid–base balance	Respiratory alkalosis	Metabolic acidosis	Profound acidosis

MAP, mean arterial pressure; $PaCO_2$, partial pressure of arterial carbon dioxide; PaO_2, partial pressure of arterial oxygen.

Adapted from Dellinger, R. P., Levy, M. M., Rhodes, A., et al. (2013). Surviving Sepsis Campaign: International guidelines for management of severe sepsis and septic shock: 2012. *Critical Care Medicine, 41*(2), 580–637; Kleinpell, R., Aitken, L., & Schorr, C. A. (2013). Implications of the new international sepsis guidelines for nursing care. *American Journal of Critical Care, 22*(3), 212–222.

acidosis. The respiratory rate increases in response to the need to increase oxygen to the cells and in compensation for to metabolic acidosis. This rapid respiratory rate facilitates removal of excess CO_2 but raises the blood pH and often causes a compensatory respiratory alkalosis. The alkalotic state causes mental status changes, such as confusion or combativeness. If treatment begins in this stage of shock, the prognosis for the patient is better than in later stages.

Medical Management

Medical treatment is directed toward identifying the cause of the shock, correcting the underlying disorder so that shock does not progress, and supporting those physiologic processes that thus far have responded successfully to the threat. Because compensation cannot be maintained indefinitely, measures such as fluid replacement and medication therapy must be initiated to maintain an adequate BP and MAP to reestablish and maintain adequate tissue perfusion (Dellinger et al., 2013; Green, 2015).

Nursing Management

Early intervention along the continuum of shock is the key to improving the patient's prognosis (Dellinger, 2015; Lee, 2015). The nurse must systematically assess the patient at risk for shock, recognizing subtle clinical signs of the compensatory stage before the patient's BP drops. Early interventions include identifying the cause of shock, administering intravenous (IV) fluids and oxygen, and obtaining necessary laboratory tests to rule out and treat metabolic imbalances or infection. Special considerations related to recognizing early signs of shock in older patients are given in Chart 18-1.

Monitoring Tissue Perfusion

In assessing tissue perfusion, the nurse observes for subtle changes in level of consciousness, vital signs (including pulse pressure), urinary output, skin, respiratory rate, and laboratory values (e.g., base deficit and lactic acid levels). In the compensatory stage of shock, serum sodium and blood glucose levels are elevated in response to the release of aldosterone and catecholamines. If infection is suspected, blood cultures should be obtained prior to administration of prescribed antibiotics; both of these interventions should be given priority in the care of the patient (Dellinger, 2015; Green, 2015).

The nurse monitors the patient's hemodynamic status and promptly reports deviations to the primary provider, assists in identifying and treating the underlying disorder by continuous in-depth assessment of the patient, administers prescribed fluids and medications, and promotes patient safety. Vital signs are key indicators of hemodynamic status and BP is an indirect measure of tissue hypoxia. The nurse should report a systolic BP lower than 90 mm Hg or a drop in systolic BP of 40 mm Hg from baseline or a MAP less than 65 mm Hg (Cestero & Dent, 2015; Dellinger et al., 2013; Green, 2015). If the patient is concurrently diagnosed with an infection or if an infection is suspected, the nurse should promptly notify the primary provider if the patient exhibits any two of the three

CHART 18-1

Recognizing Shock in Older Patients

The physiologic changes associated with aging, coupled with pathologic and chronic disease states, place older adults at increased risk for developing a state of shock and possibly **multiple organ dysfunction syndrome (MODS)**. Older adults can recover from shock if it is detected and treated early with aggressive and supportive therapies. Nurses play an essential role in assessing and interpreting subtle changes in older patients' responses to illness.

- Medications such as beta-blocking agents (metoprolol [Lopressor]) used to treat hypertension may mask tachycardia, a primary compensatory mechanism to increase cardiac output, during hypovolemic states.
- The aging immune system may not mount a truly febrile response (temperature more than 38.3°C [101°F]), however, a lack of a febrile response (temperature less than 37°C [98.6°F]) or an increasing trend in body temperature should be addressed. The patient may also report increased fatigue and malaise in the absence of a febrile response.
- The heart does not function well in hypoxemic states, and the aging heart may respond to decreased myocardial oxygenation with dysrhythmias that may be misinterpreted as a normal part of the aging process.
- There is a progressive decline in respiratory muscle strength, maximal ventilation, and response to hypoxia. Older patients have a decreased respiratory reserve and decompensate more quickly.
- Changes in mentation may be inappropriately misinterpreted as dementia. Older adults with a sudden change in mentation should be aggressively assessed for acute delirium (hypo- and hyperdelirium states) and treated for the presence of infection and organ hypoperfusion.

Adapted from Davis, L. L. (2014). Cardiovascular issues in older adults. *Critical Care Nursing Clinics of North America*, *26*(1), 61–89; Dellinger, R. P., Levy, M. M., Rhodes, A., et al., (2013). Surviving Sepsis Campaign: International guidelines for management of severe sepsis and septic shock: 2012. *Critical Care Medicine*, *41*(2), 580–637; Green, J. M. (2015). Essentials of sepsis management. *Surgical Clinics of North America*, *95*(2), 355–365; Lineberry, C., & Stein, D. E. (2014). Infection, sepsis, and immune function in the older adult receiving critical care. *Critical Care Nursing Clinics of North America*, *26*(1), 47–60; Mayr, F. B., Yende, S., & Angus, D. C. (2014). Epidemiology of severe sepsis. *Virulence*, *5*(1), 4–11.

following signs (Antonelli, DeBacker, Dorman, et al., 2016; Singer et al., 2016) (see later discussion of Septic Shock):

- Respiratory rate ≥22/min
- Altered mentation
- Systolic BP ≤100 mm Hg.

Pulse pressure correlates well with stroke volume. Pulse pressure is calculated by subtracting the diastolic measurement from the systolic measurement. Usually, the pulse pressure is 30 to 40 mm Hg. Widening pulse pressure is indicative of distributive shock. Narrowing or decreased pulse pressure is an **earlier indicator of shock** than a drop in systolic BP and indicates arterial vasoconstriction (deWitt, Joshi, Meislin, et al., 2014; See, Mukhopadhyay, Lau, et al., 2015). This is in contrast to the widening pulse pressure seen with early septic shock.

Decreased or narrowing pulse pressure, an early indication of decreased stroke volume, is illustrated in the following example:

Systolic BP − Diastolic BP = Pulse pressure

Normal pulse pressure:

120 mg Hg − 80 mm Hg = 40 mm Hg

Narrowing of pulse pressure:

90 mm Hg − 70 mm Hg = 20 mm Hg

Elevation of the diastolic BP with release of catecholamines and attempts to increase venous return through vasoconstriction is an early compensatory mechanism in response to decreased stroke volume, BP, and overall cardiac output.

NURSING ALERT

By the time BP drops, damage has already been occurring at the cellular and tissue levels. Therefore, the patient at risk for shock must be assessed and monitored closely before the BP falls.

Continuous central venous oximetry ($Sc\bar{v}O_2$) monitoring may be used to evaluate mixed venous blood oxygen saturation and the severity of tissue hypoperfusion states. A central catheter is introduced into the superior vena cava (SVC), and a sensor on the catheter measures the oxygen saturation of the blood in the SVC as blood returns to the heart and pulmonary system for reoxygenation. A normal $Sc\bar{v}O_2$ value is 70% (Cestero & Dent, 2015; Dellinger et al., 2013). Body tissues use approximately 25% of the oxygen delivered to them during normal metabolism. During states of stress, such as shock, more oxygen is consumed and the $Sc\bar{v}O_2$ saturation is lower, indicating that the tissues are consuming more oxygen.

Interventions focus on decreasing tissue oxygen requirements and increasing perfusion to deliver more oxygen to the tissues. For instance, sedating agents may be administered to lower metabolic demands, the patient's pain may be treated with intravenous (IV) opioid agents, or measures to prevent shivering, all decrease metabolic demands for oxygen. Supplemental oxygen and mechanical ventilation may be required to increase the delivery of oxygen in the blood. Administration of IV fluids and medications supports BP and cardiac output, and the transfusion of packed red blood cells enhances oxygen transport. Monitoring tissue oxygen consumption with $Sc\bar{v}O_2$ is a minimally invasive measure to more accurately assess tissue oxygenation in the compensatory stage of shock before changes in vital signs detect altered tissue perfusion (Dellinger et al., 2013).

In the patient who has an arterial line present, arterial pulse waveform analysis or pulse contour may be used to determine the patient's stroke volume and responsiveness to IV fluid replacement to meet tissue perfusion needs (Cestero & Dent, 2015). This may be used to estimate the patient's stroke volume, thus providing information to guide fluid resuscitation needs. A common limitation in using the arterial pulse waveform device is that cardiac dysrhythmias, severe peripheral vascular disease, and aortic valve regurgitation decrease its accuracy (Cestero & Dent, 2015). Other noninvasive measures that recently have been tried to monitor tissue perfusion include sublingual capnometry and near-infrared spectroscopy (NIRS). Recent research has found that data from these methods are not entirely reliable; therefore, they are no longer in widespread use (Cestero & Dent, 2015).

Although treatments are prescribed and initiated by the primary provider, the nurse usually implements them, operates and troubleshoots equipment used in treatment, monitors the patient's status during treatment, and evaluates the immediate effects of treatment. In addition, the nurse assesses the response of the patient and family to the crisis and its treatment.

Reducing Anxiety

Patients and their families often become anxious and apprehensive when they face a major threat to health and well-being and are the focus of attention of many health care providers. Providing brief explanations about the diagnostic and treatment procedures, supporting the patient during these procedures, and providing information about their outcomes are usually effective in reducing stress and anxiety and thus promoting the patient's physical and mental well-being. Speaking in a calm, reassuring voice and using gentle touch also help ease the patient's concerns. These actions may provide comfort for critically ill, frightened patients (Perrin & Kazanowski, 2015). Research suggests that family members have certain needs during a health-related crisis, including the need for honest, consistent, and thorough communication with health care providers; physical and emotional closeness to the patient; sensing that health care professionals care about their patients; seeing the patient frequently; and knowing exactly what has been done for the patient (Perrin & Kazanowski, 2015).

The nurse should advocate that family members be present during procedures and while patient care is provided. The presence of family provides a necessary connection and support for the patient during a time of crisis. Research suggests that sharing decision making with the patient and the family enhances communication with the health care team, reduces patient anxiety, and improves overall satisfaction with care (Hinkle, Bosslet, & Torke, 2015).

Promoting Safety

The nurse must be vigilant for potential threats to the patient's safety, because a high anxiety level and altered mental status impair judgment. In this stage of shock, patients who were previously cooperative and followed instructions may now disrupt IV lines and catheters and complicate their condition. Close monitoring, frequent reorientation, hourly rounding, and implementing interventions to prevent falls (e.g., bed alarms) are essential.

Progressive Stage

In the second stage of shock, the mechanisms that regulate BP can no longer compensate, and the MAP falls below normal limits. Patients are clinically hypotensive; this is defined as a systolic BP of less than 90 mm Hg or a decrease in systolic BP of 40 mm Hg from baseline. The patient shows signs of declining mental status (Dellinger et al., 2013).

Pathophysiology

Although all organ systems suffer from hypoperfusion at this stage, several events perpetuate the shock syndrome. First, the overworked heart becomes dysfunctional, the body's inability to meet increased oxygen requirements produces ischemia, and biochemical mediators cause myocardial depression (Dellinger et al., 2013; Moore et al., 2015). This leads to failure of the heart even if the underlying cause of the shock is not of cardiac origin. Second, the autoregulatory function of the microcirculation fails in response to the numerous biochemical mediators released by the cells, resulting in increased capillary permeability, with areas of arteriolar and venous constriction further compromising cellular perfusion (Moore et al., 2015). At this stage, the prognosis worsens. The relaxation of precapillary sphincters causes fluid to leak from the capillaries, creating interstitial edema and return of less fluid to the heart. In addition, the inflammatory response to injury is activated, and proinflammatory and anti-inflammatory mediators are released, which activate the coagulation system in an effort to reestablish homeostasis (Levi & van der Poll, 2015). The body mobilizes energy stores and increases oxygen consumption to meet the increased metabolic needs of the underperfused tissues and cells. Anaerobic metabolism ensues, resulting in a buildup of lactic acid and disruption of normal cell function (Green, 2015).

Even if the underlying cause of the shock is reversed, the sequence of compensatory responses to the decrease in tissue perfusion perpetuates the shock state, and a vicious circle ensues. The cellular reactions that occur during the progressive stage of shock are an active area of clinical research. It is believed that the body's response to shock or lack of response in this stage of shock may be the primary factor determining the patient's survival. Early recognition of shock signs and symptoms is essential to improving morbidity and mortality.

Clinical Manifestations

Chances of survival depend on the patient's general health before the shock state as well as the amount of time it takes to restore tissue perfusion. As shock progresses, organ systems decompensate (see Table 18-1).

Respiratory Effects

The lungs, which become compromised early in shock, are affected at this stage. Subsequent decompensation of the lungs increases the likelihood that mechanical ventilation will be needed. Respirations are rapid and shallow. Crackles are heard over the lung fields. Decreased pulmonary blood flow causes arterial oxygen levels to decrease and carbon dioxide levels to increase. Hypoxemia and biochemical mediators cause an intense inflammatory response and pulmonary vasoconstriction, perpetuating pulmonary capillary hypoperfusion and hypoxemia. The hypoperfused alveoli stop producing surfactant and subsequently collapse. Pulmonary capillaries begin to leak, causing pulmonary edema, diffusion abnormalities (shunting), and additional alveolar collapse. This condition is called *acute lung injury* (ALI) as ALI continues, interstitial inflammation and fibrosis are common consequences, leading to acute respiratory distress syndrome (ARDS) (Silva, Pelosi, & Rocco, 2014). Further explanation of ALI and ARDS, as well as their nursing management, can be found in Chapter 24.

Cardiovascular Effects

A lack of adequate blood supply leads to dysrhythmias and ischemia. The heart rate is rapid, sometimes exceeding 150 bpm.

The patient may report chest pain and even suffer a myocardial infarction (MI). Levels of cardiac enzymes (e.g., cardiac troponin I [cTn-I]) increase. In addition, myocardial depression and ventricular dilation may further impair the heart's ability to pump enough blood to the tissues to meet oxygen requirements.

Neurologic Effects

As blood flow to the brain becomes impaired, mental status deteriorates. Changes in mental status occur with decreased cerebral perfusion and hypoxia. Initially, the patient may exhibit subtle changes in behaviour or agitation, confusion, or demonstrate signs of delirium. Subsequently, lethargy increases, and the patient begins to lose consciousness.

Renal Effects

When the MAP falls below 65 mm Hg (Zarbock, Gomez, & Kellum, 2014), the glomerular filtration rate of the kidneys cannot be maintained, and drastic changes in renal function occur. Acute kidney injury (AKI) is characterized by an increase in blood urea nitrogen (BUN) and serum creatinine levels, fluid and electrolyte shifts, acid–base imbalances, and a loss of the renal-hormonal regulation of BP. Urinary output usually decreases to less than 0.5 mL/kg per hour (or less than 30 mL/hr) but may vary depending on the phase of AKI. For further information about AKI, see Chapter 45.

Hepatic Effects

Decreased blood flow to the liver impairs the ability of liver cells to perform metabolic and phagocytic functions. Consequently, the patient is less able to metabolize medications and metabolic waste products, such as ammonia and lactic acid. Metabolic activities of the liver, including gluconeogenesis and glycogenolysis, are impaired. The patient becomes more susceptible to infection as the liver fails to filter bacteria from the blood. Liver enzymes (aspartate aminotransferase [AST], alanine aminotransferase [ALT], lactate dehydrogenase [LDH]) and bilirubin levels are elevated, and the patient develops jaundice.

Gastrointestinal Effects

GI ischemia can cause stress ulcers in the stomach, putting the patient at risk for GI bleeding. In the small intestine, the mucosa can become necrotic and slough off, causing bloody diarrhea. Beyond the local effects of impaired perfusion, GI ischemia leads to bacterial toxin translocation organ dysfunction, in which bacterial toxins enter the bloodstream through the lymphatic system. In addition to causing infection, bacterial toxins can cause cardiac depression, vasodilation, increased capillary permeability, and an intense inflammatory response with activation of additional biochemical mediators. The net result interferes with healthy cellular functioning and their ability to metabolize nutrients (Stapleton, Jones, & Heyland, 2007). Enteral feeding in shock states is recommended, provided motility is not impaired, as it helps protect gut mucosa, prevents bacterial translocation, and reduces the risk of organ dysfunction (Kleinpell, Aitken, & Schorr, 2012).

Hematologic Effects

The combination of hypotension, sluggish blood flow, metabolic acidosis, coagulation system imbalance, and generalized hypoxemia can interfere with usual hemostatic mechanisms. In shock states, the inflammatory cytokines activate the clotting cascade, causing deposition of microthrombi in multiple areas of the body and consumption of clotting factors. The alterations of the hematologic system, including imbalance of the clotting cascade, occur because of overactivation of the inflammatory response (Levi & van der Poll, 2015; Moore et al., 2015). Disseminated intravascular coagulation (DIC) may occur either as a cause or as a complication of shock. In this condition, widespread clotting and bleeding occur simultaneously. Bruises (ecchymoses) and bleeding (petechiae) may appear in the skin. Coagulation times (e.g., prothrombin time [PT], activated partial thromboplastin time [aPTT]) are prolonged. Clotting factors and platelets are consumed and require replacement therapy to achieve hemostasis. Further discussion of DIC appears in Chapter 54.

Medical Management

Specific medical management in the progressive stage of shock depends on the type of shock and its underlying cause. It is also based on the degree of decompensation in the organ systems. Medical management specific to each type of shock is discussed later in this chapter. Although medical management in the progressive stage differs by type of shock, some medical interventions are common to all types. These include the use of appropriate IV fluids and medications to restore tissue perfusion by the following methods:

- Supporting the respiratory system
- Optimizing intravascular volume
- Supporting the pumping action of the heart
- Improving the competence of the vascular system

Other aspects of management may include early enteral nutritional support, targeted hyperglycemic control with IV insulin, use of antacids, histamine-2 (H_2) blockers, or antipeptic agents to reduce the risk of GI ulceration and bleeding.

Tight glycemic control (serum glucose of 4.4 to 5.5 mmol/L) is no longer recommended, as hypoglycemic events associated with regulating tight control in critically ill patients have been found to result in adverse patient outcomes (Marik & Bellomo, 2013). Current evidence suggests that maintaining serum glucose less than 10 mmol/L with insulin therapy and close monitoring is indicated in the management of the critically ill patient (Dellinger et al., 2013).

> **NURSING ALERT**
>
> **Glycemic control is linked to outcomes in the patient in shock. Although tight glycemic control is no longer indicated, evidence shows that maintaining serum glucose less than 10 mmol/L is linked to best outcomes.**

Nursing Management

Nursing care of patients in the progressive stage of shock requires expertise in assessing and understanding shock and the significance of changes in assessment data. Early interventions are essential to the survival of patients; therefore, suspecting that a patient may be in shock and reporting subtle changes in assessment are imperative. Patients in the progressive stage of shock are cared for in the intensive care setting to facilitate close monitoring (hemodynamic monitoring, electrocardiographic [ECG] monitoring, arterial blood gases, serum electrolyte levels, physical and mental status changes); rapid and frequent administration of various prescribed medications and fluids; and possibly interventions with supportive technologies, such as mechanical ventilation, dialysis, and intra-aortic balloon pump.

Working closely with other members of the health care team, the nurse carefully documents treatments, medications, and fluids that are administered, recording the time, dosage or volume, and patient response. In addition, the nurse coordinates both the scheduling of diagnostic procedures that may be carried out at the bedside and the flow of health care personnel involved in the care of patients.

Preventing Complications

The nurse helps reduce the risk of related complications and monitors the patient for early signs of complications. Monitoring includes evaluating blood levels of medications, observing invasive vascular lines for signs of infection, and checking neurovascular status if arterial lines are inserted, especially in the lower extremities. Simultaneously, the nurse promotes the patient's safety and comfort by ensuring that all procedures, including invasive procedures and arterial and venous punctures, are carried out using correct aseptic techniques and that venous and arterial puncture and infusion sites are maintained with the goal of preventing infection. Nursing interventions that reduce the incidence of ventilator-associated pneumonias (VAPs) must also be implemented. These include frequent oral care, aseptic suction technique, turning, and elevating the head of the bed at least 30 degrees to prevent aspiration, and implementing daily interruption of sedation as prescribed to evaluate patient readiness for extubation (Dellinger et al., 2013; Hillier, Wilson, Chamberlain, et al., 2013; Makic, Rauen, Jones, et al., 2015).

Positioning and repositioning of the patient to promote comfort and maintain skin integrity are essential.

The nurse must also be vigilant in assessing for acute delirium, characterized by an acute change in mental status, inattention, disorganized thinking, and altered level of consciousness. Delirium is potentially preventable (Barr, Fraser, Puntillo, et al., 2013). Critically ill patients with delirium have longer mechanical ventilation support needs, experience higher functional decline, and have higher rates of morbidity and mortality than those without delirium. Furthermore, they are at a higher risk of developing post–intensive care syndrome, which manifests as new or worsening impairments in the patient's physical, cognitive, or mental status after a critical illness has resolved and that persists beyond the acute hospitalization (Barr et al., 2013). Delirium should be assessed at a minimum each shift using a standardized delirium assessment tools.

Examples of delirium assessment tools include: The Intensive Care Delirium Screening Checklist (ICDSC) (Bergeron, Dubois, Dumont, et al., 2001) and the Confusion Assessment Method (CAM)-ICU (Vanderbilt University Medical Center, 2013). The ICDSC was developed to assess critically ill patients for delirium based on DSM (Diagnostic and Statistical Manual of Mental Disorders) criteria. Studies to determine the reliability of this tool were done on a variety of ICU patients including patients with neurologic injuries, dementia, and a history of psychiatric disorders.

The ICDSC is broken down into eight categories:

1. Altered level of consciousness (LOC)—RASS
2. Inattention
3. Disorientation
4. Hallucinations or delusions
5. Psychomotor agitation or retardation
6. Inappropriate speech or mood
7. Sleep/wake cycle
8. Symptom fluctuation

One point is given for each category if the symptom is present and a score of 4 or higher is considered positive for delirium (Bergeron et al., 2001).

The CAM-ICU is a modified version of the CAM, specifically designed for use in patients who are critically ill. Nursing interventions that can prevent delirium include engaging the patient in frequent reorientation activities (e.g., to date, time, place), assessing and treating pain, promoting sleep, providing early mobilization activities, and limiting sedation, especially sedation with benzodiazepines (e.g., lorazepam [Ativan]) (Makic, 2013).

Promoting Rest and Comfort

Efforts are made to minimize the cardiac workload by reducing the patient's physical activity and treating pain and anxiety. Because promoting patient rest and comfort is a priority, the nurse performs essential nursing activities in blocks of time, allowing the patient to have periods of uninterrupted rest, which may prevent acute delirium, as noted previously (Barr et al., 2013; Makic, Rauen, Watson, et al., 2014). To conserve the patient's energy, the nurse should protect the patient from temperature extremes (e.g., excessive warmth or cold, shivering), which can increase the metabolic rate and oxygen consumption and thus the cardiac workload.

Supporting Family Members

Because patients in shock receive intense attention by the health care team, families may be overwhelmed and frightened. Family members may be reluctant to ask questions or seek information for fear that they will be in the way or will interfere with the attention given to the patient. The nurse should make sure that the family is comfortably situated and kept informed about the patient's status. Often, families need advice from the health care team to get some rest; family members are more likely to take this advice if they feel that the patient is being well cared for and that they will be notified of any significant changes in the patient's status. A visit from the hospital chaplain may be comforting and provides some attention to the family while the nurse concentrates on the patient. Ensuring patient- and family-centred care is central to the delivery of high-quality care. This helps meet the emotional well-being as well as the physiologic needs of the patient and the family (Giles & Hall, 2013).

Irreversible Stage

The irreversible (or refractory) stage of shock represents the point along the shock continuum at which organ damage is so severe that the patient does not respond to treatment and cannot survive. Despite treatment, BP remains low. Renal and liver failure, compounded by the release of biochemical mediators, creates an acute metabolic acidosis. Anaerobic metabolism contributes to a worsening lactic acidosis. Reserves of ATP are almost totally depleted, and mechanisms for storing new supplies of energy have been destroyed. Respiratory system failure prevents adequate oxygenation and ventilation despite mechanical ventilatory support, and the cardiovascular system is ineffective in maintaining an adequate MAP for tissue perfusion. Multiple organ dysfunction progressing to complete organ failure has occurred, and death is imminent. Multiple organ dysfunction can occur as a progression along the shock continuum or as a syndrome unto itself and is described in more detail later in this chapter.

Medical Management

Medical management during the irreversible stage of shock is similar to interventions and treatments used in the progressive stage. Although the patient may have progressed to the irreversible stage, the judgment that the shock is irreversible can be made only retrospectively on the basis of the patient's failure to respond to treatment. Strategies that may be experimental (e.g., investigational medications, such as immunomodulation therapy) may be tried to reduce or reverse the severity of shock.

Nursing Management

As in the progressive stage of shock, the nurse focuses on carrying out prescribed treatments, monitoring the patient, preventing complications, protecting the patient from injury, and providing comfort. Offering brief explanations to the patient about what is happening is essential even if there is no certainty that the patient hears or understands what is being said. Simple comfort measures, including reassuring touches, should continue to be provided despite the patient's nonresponsiveness to verbal stimuli (Hinkle et al., 2015).

As it becomes obvious that the patient is unlikely to survive, the family must be informed about the prognosis and likely outcome.

Opportunities should be provided throughout the patient's care for the family to see, touch, and talk to the patient. Close family friends or spiritual advisors may be of comfort to the family members in dealing with the inevitable death of their loved one. Whenever possible and appropriate, the patient's family should be approached regarding any living wills, advance directives, or other written or verbal wishes the patient may have shared in the event that he or she became unable to participate in end-of-life decisions. In some cases, ethics committees may assist families and health care teams in making difficult decisions (Hinkle et al., 2015).

During this stage of shock, the family may misinterpret the actions of the health care team. They have been told that nothing has been effective in reversing the shock and that the patient's survival is very unlikely, yet they find physicians and nurses continuing to work feverishly on the patient. Distraught, grieving families may interpret this as a chance for recovery when none exists, and family members may become angry when the patient dies. Conferences with all members of the health care team and the family promote better understanding by the family of the patient's prognosis and the purpose for management measures. Engaging palliative care specialists can be beneficial in developing a plan of care that maximizes comfort and effective symptom management as well as assisting the family with difficult decisions (Perrin & Kazanowski, 2015). During these conferences, it is essential to explain that the equipment and treatments being provided are intended for patient comfort and do not suggest that the patient will recover. Family members should be encouraged to express their wishes concerning the use of life-support measure (Hinkle et al., 2015; Perrin & Kazanowski, 2015).

General Management Strategies in Shock

As described previously and in the discussion of types of shock to follow, management in all types and all phases of shock includes the following:

- Support of the respiratory system with supplemental oxygen and/or mechanical ventilation to provide optimal oxygenation (see Chapter 26)
- Fluid replacement to restore intravascular volume
- Vasoactive medications to restore vasomotor tone and improve cardiac function
- Nutritional support to address the metabolic requirements that are often dramatically increased in shock

Therapies described in this section require collaboration among all members of the health care team.

Fluid Replacement

Fluid replacement, also referred to as fluid resuscitation, is administered in all types of shock. The type of fluids administered and the speed of delivery vary, but fluids are administered to improve cardiac and tissue oxygenation, which in part depends on flow. The fluids administered may include **crystalloids** (electrolyte solutions that move freely between intravascular and interstitial spaces), **colloids** (large-molecule IV solutions), and blood components (packed red blood cells, fresh frozen plasma, and platelets).

Crystalloid and Colloid Solutions

In emergencies, the "best" fluid is often the fluid that is readily available. Fluid resuscitation should be initiated early in shock to maximize intravascular volume. Isotonic crystalloid solutions are often selected because they contain the same concentration of electrolytes as the extracellular fluid and, therefore, can be given without altering the concentrations of electrolytes in the plasma. IV crystalloids commonly used for resuscitation in hypovolemic shock include 0.9% sodium chloride solution (normal saline) and lactated Ringer's solution. Ringer's lactate is an electrolyte solution containing the lactate ion, which should not be confused with lactic acid. The lactate ion is converted to bicarbonate, which helps buffer the overall acidosis that occurs in shock. A disadvantage of using isotonic crystalloid solutions is that some of the volume given is lost to the interstitial compartment and some remains in the intravascular compartment. This occurs as a consequence of capillary permeability that occurs during shock. Diffusion of crystalloids into the interstitial space means that more fluid may need to be given than the amount lost to support tissue perfusion (Perel, Roberts, & Ker, 2013).

Care must be taken when administering isotonic crystalloids to avoid both under- and overresuscitating the patient in shock. Insufficient fluid replacement is associated with a higher incidence of morbidity and mortality from lack of tissue perfusion, whereas excessive fluid administration can cause systemic and pulmonary edema that progresses to ALI, intra-abdominal hypertension (IAH), abdominal compartment syndrome (ACS), and MODS.

ACS is a serious complication that may occur when large volumes of fluid are given. It may also occur after trauma, abdominal surgery, pancreatitis, or **sepsis** (Holodinsky, Roberts, Ball, et al., 2013). In ACS, fluid leaks into the intra-abdominal cavity, increasing pressure that is displaced onto surrounding vessels and organs. Venous return, preload, and cardiac output are compromised. The pressure also elevates the diaphragm, making it difficult to breathe effectively. The renal and GI systems also begin to show signs of dysfunction (e.g., decreased urine output, absent bowel sounds, intolerance of tube feeding). Abdominal compartment pressure can be measured. Normally, it is 0 to 5 mm Hg, and a pressure of 12 mm Hg is considered to be indicative of IAH (Balogh, Lumsdaine, Moore, et al., 2014). If ACS is present, interventions that usually include surgical decompression are necessary to relieve the pressure.

Hypertonic crystalloid solution, often 3% sodium chloride, may be given in patients with shock and traumatic brain injury (Dubick, Shek, & Wade, 2013). These solutions exert a large osmotic force that pulls fluid from the intracellular space to the extracellular space to achieve a fluid balance (Dubick et al., 2013). This osmotic effect results in fewer fluids being administered to restore intravascular volume, which is important in a patient with a head injury and cerebral swelling. Current research suggests that using hypertonic crystalloid solution does not improve patient outcomes and may result in unintended complications (Bulger, May, Kerby, et al., 2011; Dubick et al., 2013). Complications associated with use of hypertonic solutions include excessive serum osmolality, which can cause rapid fluid shifts overwhelming the heart, and hypernatremia.

Generally, IV colloidal solutions are similar to plasma proteins, in that they contain molecules that are too large to pass through capillary membranes. Colloids expand intravascular volume by exerting oncotic pressure, thereby pulling fluid into the intravascular space, increasing intravascular volume. In addition, colloids have a longer duration of action than crystalloids, because the molecules remain within the intravascular compartment longer. Typically, if colloids are used to treat tissue hypoperfusion, albumin is the agent prescribed. Albumin is a plasma protein; an albumin solution is prepared from human plasma and is heated during production to reduce its potential to transmit disease. The disadvantage of albumin is its high cost compared to crystalloid solutions. Resuscitation with colloid solutions has not reduced the risk of morbidity or death compared to resuscitation with crystalloid solutions; moreover, colloids can be considerably more expensive than crystalloid solutions (Annane, Siami, Jaber, et al., 2013; Perel et al., 2013).

NURSING ALERT

With all colloidal solutions, side effects include the rare occurrence of anaphylactic reactions. Nurses must monitor patients closely.

Complications of Fluid Administration

Close monitoring of the patient during fluid replacement is necessary to identify side effects and complications. The most common and serious side effects of fluid replacement are cardiovascular overload and pulmonary edema, and ACS. The patient receiving fluid replacement must be monitored frequently for adequate urinary output, changes in mental status, skin perfusion, and changes in vital signs. Lung sounds are auscultated frequently to detect signs of fluid accumulation. Adventitious lung sounds, such as crackles, may indicate pulmonary edema.

NURSING ALERT

When administering large volumes of crystalloid solutions, monitor the lungs for adventitious sounds and signs and symptoms of interstitial edema, and work of breathing (i.e., increasing effort required for the patient to breathe).

Often, a central venous pressure (CVP) line is inserted (typically into the subclavian or jugular vein) and is advanced until the tip of the catheter rests near the junction of the SVC and the right atrium. The CVP is used to assess preload in the right side of the heart. The CVP value assists in monitoring the patient's response to fluid replacement, especially when it is used in conjunction with additional assessment parameters (e.g., urine output, heart rate, BP response to fluid challenge) (Dellinger et al., 2013; Levy, Rhodes, Phillips, et al., 2015; Yealy, Kellum, Huang, et al., 2014). An expected right atrial pressure value or CVP is 4 to 12 mm Hg or cm H_2O. Several readings are obtained to determine a range, and fluid replacement is continued to achieve a CVP between 8 and 12 mm Hg (Dellinger, 2015; Dellinger et al., 2013). Interpreting blood volume on the basis of CVP readings alone has been recently challenged in the literature; therefore, CVP readings should be used in conjunction with other assessment variables to assess blood volume (Levy et al., 2015; Marik, Baram, & Vahid, 2008; Yealy et al., 2014). Some CVP catheters allow the monitoring of intravascular measures and venous oxygen levels. Assessment of venous oxygenation (venous oxygen saturation [SvO_2], or $Sc\bar{v}O_2$ with a CVP line) may be helpful in evaluating the adequacy of intravascular volume (Dellinger et al., 2013; Rivers, McIntyre, Morro, et al., 2005). Hemodynamic monitoring with arterial lines may be implemented to allow close monitoring of the patient's BP and tissue perfusion. A pulmonary artery catheter may be inserted to assist with closer monitoring of a patient's cardiac status as well as response to therapy. Advances in noninvasive or minimally invasive technology (e.g., esophageal Doppler, arterial pulse contour analysis, cardiac output devices, intrathoracic impedance monitoring) provide additional hemodynamic monitoring options (Cestero & Dent, 2015). (For additional information about hemodynamic monitoring, see Chapter 27.)

Placement of central lines for fluid administration and monitoring requires collaborative practice between the provider and the nurse to ensure that all measures to prevent central line–associated bloodstream infection (CLABSI) are implemented. Several interventions aimed at preventing CLABSI should be implemented collaboratively while the central line is being placed as well as during ongoing nursing management of the central line itself. Chart 18-2 describes the evidence-based ("bundled") interventions that have been found to reduce CLABSI.

Vasoactive Medication Therapy

Vasoactive medications are administered in all forms of shock to improve the patient's hemodynamic stability when fluid therapy alone cannot maintain adequate MAP. Specific medications are selected to correct the particular hemodynamic alteration that is impeding cardiac output. These medications help increase the strength of myocardial contractility, regulate the heart rate, and initiate vasoconstriction.

Vasoactive medications are selected for their action on receptors of the sympathetic nervous system. These receptors are known as alpha-adrenergic and beta-adrenergic receptors. Beta-adrenergic receptors are further classified as beta-1 and beta-2 adrenergic receptors. When alpha-adrenergic receptors

CHART 18-2

Collaborative Practice Interventions to Prevent Central Line–Associated Bloodstream Infections (CLABSIs)

Current best practices can include the implementation of specific evidence-based bundle interventions that when used together (i.e., as a "bundle") improve patient outcomes. This chart outlines specific parameters for the central line bundled collaborative interventions that have been found to reduce central line–associated bloodstream infections (CLABSIs).

What are the five key elements of the central line bundle?

- Hand hygiene
- Maximal sterile barrier precautions during line insertion (see later discussion)
- Chlorhexidine skin antisepsis
- Optimal catheter site selection with avoidance of using the femoral vein for central venous access in adult patients
- Daily review of line necessity, with prompt removal of unnecessary lines

When should hand hygiene be performed in the care of a patient with a central line?

- All clinicians who provide care to the patient should adhere to good hand hygiene practices, particularly:
  - Before and after palpating the catheter insertion site
  - With all dressing changes to the intravascular catheter access site
  - When hands are visibly soiled or contamination of hands is suspected
  - Before donning and after removing gloves

What changes can be made to improve hand hygiene?

- Implement a central line procedure checklist that requires that clinicians perform hand hygiene as an essential step in care.
- Post signage stating the importance of hand hygiene.
- Have soap and alcohol-based hand sanitizers prominently placed to facilitate hand hygiene practices.
- Model hand hygiene practices.
- Provide patient and family education and engage family in hand hygiene practices during visitation.

What are maximal sterile barrier precautions?

- These are implemented during central line insertion:
  - For the primary provider, this means strict compliance with wearing a cap, mask, sterile gown, and sterile gloves. The cap should cover all hair, and the mask should cover the nose and the mouth tightly. The nurse should also wear a cap and a mask.
  - For the patient, this means covering the patient from head to toe with a sterile drape, with a small opening for the site of insertion. If a full-size drape is not available, two drapes may be applied to cover the patient, or the operating room may be consulted to determine how to procure full-size sterile drapes, because these are routinely used in surgical settings.
- Nurses should be empowered to enforce use of a central line checklist to be sure that all processes related to central line placement are properly executed for every line placed.

Which antiseptic should be used to prepare the patient's skin for central line insertion?

- Chlorhexidine skin antisepsis has been proven to provide better skin antisepsis than other antiseptic agents, such as povidone–iodine solutions.
- An alcohol chlorhexidine antiseptic should be applied using a back-and-forth friction scrub for at least 30 seconds; this should not be wiped or blotted dry.
- The antiseptic solution should be allowed time to dry completely before the insertion site is punctured/accessed (approximately 2 minutes).

What nursing interventions are essential to reduce the risk of infection?

- Maintaining sterile technique when changing the central line dressing
- Always performing hand hygiene before manipulating or accessing the line ports
- Wearing clean gloves before accessing the line port
- Performing a 15- to 30-second "hub scrub" using chlorhexidine or alcohol and friction in a twisting motion on the access hub (reduces biofilm on the hub that may contain pathogens)
- Using chlorhexidine-containing dressings in patients older than 2 months
- Consider using antiseptic-containing port protectors to cover connectors

When should central lines be discontinued?

- Assessment for removal of central lines should be included as part of the nurse's daily goal sheets.
- The time and date of central line placement should be recorded and evaluated by staff to aid in decision making.
- The need for the central line access should be reviewed as part of multidisciplinary rounds.
- During these rounds, the "line day" should be stated to remind everyone how long the central line has been in place (e.g., "Today is line day 6").
- An appropriate time frame for regular review of the necessity for a central line should be identified, such as weekly, when central lines are placed for long-term use (e.g., chemotherapy, extended antibiotic administration).

Quality improvement processes that trend CLABSI rates and the compliance with CLABSI bundle prevention strategies have been found to effectively engage the multidisciplinary team in achieving goals to reduce infections related to central lines.

Adapted from Institute for Healthcare Improvement. (2012). How-to guide: Prevent central line-associated bloodstream infection. Retrieved November 28, 2015, from www.ihi.org/knowledge/Pages/Tools/HowtoGuidePreventCentralLineAssociatedBloodstreamInfection.aspx; Marschall, J., Mermel, L. A., Fakih, M., et al. (2014). Strategies to prevent central-line associated blood stream infections in acute care hospitals: 2014 update. *Infection Control and Hospital Epidemiology, 35*(7), 753–771; The Society for Healthcare Epidemiology of America SHEA Guideline Central. (2015). Central line-associated bloodstream infections. Retrieved November 28, 2015, from www.guidelinecentral.com/share/pocketcard/53d67314007df/#i469f5e2f

are stimulated, blood vessels constrict in the cardiorespiratory and GI systems, skin, and kidneys. When beta-1 adrenergic receptors are stimulated, heart rate and myocardial contraction increase. When beta-2 adrenergic receptors are stimulated, vasodilation occurs in the heart and skeletal muscles, and the bronchioles relax. The medications used in treating shock consist of various combinations of vasoactive medications to maximize tissue perfusion by stimulating or blocking the alpha- and beta-adrenergic receptors.

When vasoactive medications are administered, vital signs must be monitored frequently (at least every 15 minutes until stable, or more often if indicated). It is recommended that patients on vasoactive infusions in shock have arterial lines inserted for ongoing and more accurate BP monitoring (Dellinger et al., 2012). Vasoactive medications should be administered through a central venous line, because infiltration and extravasation of some vasoactive medications can cause tissue necrosis and sloughing (Allen, 2014). An IV pump or controller should be used to ensure that the medications are delivered safely and accurately.

Individual medication dosages are usually titrated by the nurse, who adjusts drip rates based on the prescribed dose and the patient's response. Dosages are changed to maintain the MAP at a physiologic level that ensures adequate tissue perfusion (usually greater than 65 mm Hg).

NURSING ALERT

Vasoactive medications should never be stopped abruptly, because this could cause severe hemodynamic instability, perpetuating the shock state.

Dosages of vasoactive medications should be tapered. When vasoactive medications are no longer needed or are necessary to a lesser extent, the infusion should be weaned from medication with frequent monitoring of BP (every 15 minutes). Table 18-2 presents some of the commonly prescribed vasoactive medications used in the treatment of shock. Occasionally, the patient does not respond as expected to vasoactive medications. A current topic of active research is evaluation of patients' adrenal function. Recent studies suggest that critically ill patients should be evaluated for corticosteroid insufficiency (also referred to as relative adrenal insufficiency or critical illness–related corticosteroid insufficiency) and, if this condition is present, corticosteroid replacement (e.g., hydrocortisone) should be considered (Dellinger et al., 2013).

Nutritional Support

Nutritional support is an important aspect of care for patients with shock. Increased metabolic rates during shock increase energy requirements and therefore caloric requirements. Patients in shock may require more than 3,000 calories daily. The release of catecholamines early in the shock continuum causes depletion of glycogen stores in about 8 to 10 hours. Nutritional energy requirements are then met by breaking down lean body mass. In this catabolic process, skeletal muscle mass is broken down even when the patient has large stores of fat or adipose tissue. Loss of skeletal muscle greatly prolongs the patient's recovery time.

Parenteral or enteral nutritional support should be initiated as soon as possible. Enteral nutrition is preferred, promoting GI function through direct exposure to nutrients and limiting infectious complications associated with parenteral feeding (Blaser, Starkopf, Kirsimagi, et al., 2014). Implementation of an evidence-based enteral feeding protocol that is tolerant of increased gastric residual volumes ensures the delivery of adequate nutrition to critically ill patients (Blaser et al., 2014). Gastric residual volume does not predict a patient's risk of aspiration (Blaser et al., 2014). Implementing early enteral nutrition has been found to promote gut-mediated immunity, reduce metabolic response to stress, and improve overall patient morbidity and mortality (Martindale & Warren, 2015).

Stress ulcers occur frequently in acutely ill patients because of the compromised blood supply to the GI tract. Therefore, antacids, H_2 blockers (e.g., famotidine [Pepcid], and proton pump inhibitors (e.g., lansoprazole [Prevacid], esomeprazole magnesium [Nexium]) are prescribed to prevent ulcer formation by inhibiting gastric acid secretion or increasing gastric pH.

Hypovolemic Shock

Hypovolemic shock, the most common type of shock, is characterized by decreased intravascular volume. Body fluid is contained in the intracellular and extracellular

TABLE 18-2 Vasoactive Agents Used in Treating Shock

Medication	Desired Action in Shock	Disadvantages
Inotropic Agents		
Dobutamine (Dobutrex) Dopamine (Intropin) Epinephrine (Adrenaline) Milrinone (Primacor)	Improve contractility, increase stroke volume, increase cardiac output	Increase oxygen demand of the heart
Vasodilators		
Nitroglycerin (Tridil) Nitroprusside (Nipride)	Reduce preload and afterload, reduce oxygen demand of heart	Cause hypotension
Vasopressor Agents		
Norepinephrine (Levophed) Dopamine (Intropin) Phenylephrine (Neo-Synephrine) Vasopressin (Pitressin) Epinephrine (Adrenalin)	Increase blood pressure by vasoconstriction	Increase afterload, thereby increasing cardiac workload; compromise perfusion to skin, kidneys, lungs, gastrointestinal tract

Adapted from Allen, J. M. (2014). Understanding vasoactive medications: Focus on pharmacology and effective titration. *Journal of Infusion Nursing*, *37*(2), 82–86.

CHART 18-3

Risk Factors: Hypovolemic Shock

External: Fluid Losses	Internal: Fluid Shifts
• Trauma	• Hemorrhage
• Surgery	• Burns
• Vomiting	• Ascites
• Diarrhea	• Peritonitis
• Diuresis	• Dehydration
• Diabetes insipidus	• Necrotizing pancreatitis

Adapted from Anderson, M. W., & Watson, G. A. (2013). Traumatic shock: The fifth shock. *Journal of Trauma Nursing, 20*(1), 37–43; Annane, D., Siami, S., Jaber, S., et al. (2013). Effects of fluid resuscitation with colloids vs crystalloids on mortality in critically ill patients presenting with hypovolemic shock: The CRISTAL randomized trial. *JAMA, 310*(17), 1809–1817.

compartments. Intracellular fluid accounts for about two thirds of the total body water. The extracellular body fluid is found in one of two compartments: intravascular (inside blood vessels) or interstitial (surrounding tissues). The volume of interstitial fluid is about three to four times that of intravascular fluid. Hypovolemic shock occurs when there is a reduction in intravascular volume by 15% to 30%, which represents an approximate loss of 750 to 1,500 mL of blood in a 70-kg (154-lb) person (American College of Surgeons, 2012).

Pathophysiology

Hypovolemic shock can be caused by external fluid losses, as in traumatic blood loss, or by internal fluid shifts, as in severe dehydration, severe edema, or ascites (Chart 18-3). Intravascular volume can be reduced both by fluid loss and by fluid shifting between the intravascular and interstitial compartments.

The sequence of events in hypovolemic shock begins with a decrease in the intravascular volume. This results in decreased venous return of blood to the heart and subsequent decreased ventricular filling. Decreased ventricular filling results in decreased stroke volume (amount of blood ejected from the heart) and decreased cardiac output. When cardiac output drops, BP drops and tissues cannot be adequately perfused (Fig. 18-3).

Physiology/Pathophysiology

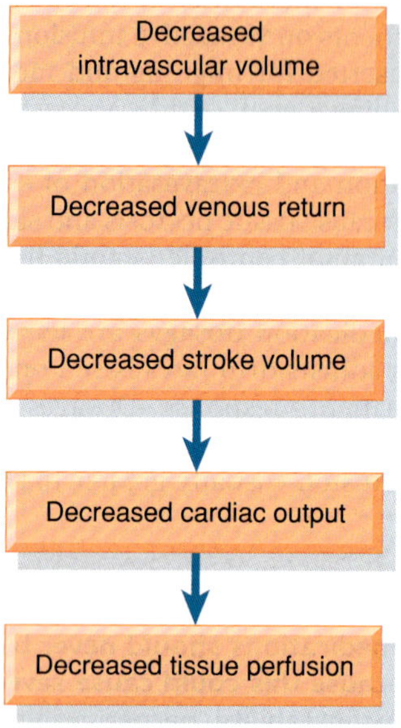

FIGURE 18-3. Pathophysiologic sequence of events in hypovolemic shock.

Medical Management

Major goals in the treatment of hypovolemic shock are to restore intravascular volume to reverse the sequence of events leading to inadequate tissue perfusion, to redistribute fluid volume, and to correct the underlying cause of the fluid loss as quickly as possible. Depending on the severity of shock and the patient's condition, it is likely that efforts will be made to address all three goals simultaneously.

Treatment of the Underlying Cause

If the patient is hemorrhaging, efforts are made to stop the bleeding. This may involve applying pressure to the bleeding site or surgical interventions to stop internal bleeding. If the cause of the hypovolemia is diarrhea or vomiting, medications to treat diarrhea and vomiting are administered while efforts are made to identify and treat the cause. In older patients, dehydration may be the cause of hypovolemic shock.

Fluid and Blood Replacement

Beyond reversing the primary cause of the decreased intravascular volume, fluid replacement is of primary concern. At least two large-gauge IV lines are inserted to establish access for fluid administration. If an IV catheter cannot be quickly inserted, an intraosseous catheter may be used for access in the sternum, legs (tibia), or arms (humerus) to facilitate rapid fluid replacement (Tay, 2015). Multiple IV lines allow simultaneous administration of fluid, medications, and blood component therapy if required. Because the goal of the fluid replacement is to restore intravascular volume, it is necessary to administer fluids that will remain in the intravascular compartment to avoid fluid shifts from the intravascular compartment into the intracellular compartment. Table 18-3 summarizes the fluids commonly used in the treatment of shock.

As discussed earlier, crystalloid solutions such as lactated Ringer's solution or 0.9% sodium chloride solution are commonly used to treat hypovolemic shock as large amounts of fluid must be administered to restore intravascular volume. If hypovolemia is primarily due to blood loss, the American College of Surgeons (2012) recommends administration of 3 mL of crystalloid solution for each millilitre of estimated blood loss. This is referred to as the 3:1 rule. Colloid solutions (e.g., albumin) may also be used. Hetastarch and dextran solutions are not indicated for fluid administration because these agents interfere with platelet aggregation.

Blood products, which are also colloids, may need to be administered, particularly if the cause of the hypovolemic

TABLE 18-3 Fluid Replacement in Shock[a]

Fluids	Advantages	Disadvantages
Crystalloids		
0.9% sodium chloride (normal saline solution)	Widely available, inexpensive	Requires large volume of infusion; can cause hypernatremia, pulmonary edema, abdominal compartment syndrome
Lactated Ringer's	Lactate ion helps buffer metabolic acidosis	Requires large volume of infusion; can cause metabolic acidosis, pulmonary edema, abdominal compartment syndrome
Colloids		
Albumin (5%, 25%)	Rapidly expands plasma volume	Expensive; requires human donors; limited supply; can cause heart failure
Blood Products		
Plasma, packed red blood cells, and platelets	Rapidly replaces volume lost due to hemorrhage	Cross-match type-specific blood is desired for optimal massive transfusion protocols to reduce transfusion-related complications (e.g., transfusion-related acute lung injury, hemolytic reactions, transfusion-associated circulatory overload)

[a]Deliver a minimum of 30 mL/kg of crystalloid.

Adapted from Dellinger, R. P., Levy, M. M., Rhodes, A., et al. (2013). Surviving Sepsis Campaign: International guidelines for management of severe sepsis and septic shock: 2012. *Critical Care Medicine, 41*(2), 580–637; Kleinpell, R., Aitken, L., & Schorr, C. A. (2013). Implications of the new international sepsis guidelines for nursing care. *American Journal of Critical Care, 22*(3), 212–222; McEnvoy, M. T., & Shander A. (2013). Anemia, bleeding, and blood transfusion in the intensive care unit: Causes, risks, costs, and new strategies. *American Journal of Critical Care, 22*(6), eS1–eS13.

shock is hemorrhage. The decision to give blood is based on the patient's lack of response to only crystalloid resuscitation, the volume of blood lost, the need for hemoglobin to assist with oxygen transport, and the necessity to correct the patient's coagulopathy. Patients requiring massive transfusion respond better when blood products are given in a 1:1:1: ratio, meaning units of plasma, platelets, and packed red blood cells (Holcomb, Tiley, Baraniuk, et al., 2015).

Packed red blood cells are administered to replenish the patient's oxygen-carrying capacity in conjunction with other fluids that will expand volume. Plasma and platelets are transfused to assist with coagulation and hemostasis. The need for transfusions is based on the patient's oxygenation needs and coagulation status, which are determined by vital signs, blood gas, chemistry, coagulation laboratory values, and clinical appearance.

Redistribution of Fluid

In addition to administering fluids to restore intravascular volume, positioning the patient properly assists fluid redistribution. A modified Trendelenburg position, also known as passive leg raising (Fig. 18-4) is recommended in hypovolemic shock. Elevation of the legs promotes the return of venous blood and can be used as a dynamic assessment of a patient's fluid responsiveness. Patient's vital signs, specifically a rise in the BP and return of the pulse pressure to normal or near normal is an indication that fluid has been redistributed. Full Trendelenburg position makes breathing difficult and does not increase BP or cardiac output (Dellinger, 2015).

Pharmacologic Therapy

If fluid administration fails to reverse hypovolemic shock, then vasoactive medications that prevent cardiac failure are given. Medications are also administered to reverse the cause of the dehydration. For example, insulin is administered if dehydration is secondary to hyperglycemia, desmopressin (DDAVP) is administered for diabetes insipidus, antidiarrheal agents for diarrhea, and antiemetic medications for vomiting.

Nursing Management

Primary prevention of shock is an essential focus of nursing care. Hypovolemic shock can be prevented in some instances by closely monitoring patients who are at risk for fluid deficits and assisting with fluid replacement before intravascular volume is depleted. In other circumstances, nursing care focuses on assisting with treatment targeted at the cause of the shock and restoring intravascular volume.

General nursing measures include ensuring safe administration of prescribed fluids and medications and documenting their administration and effects. Volumetric IV

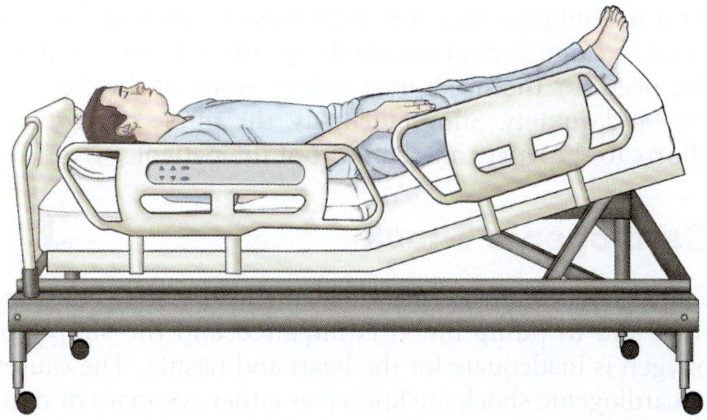

FIGURE 18-4. Proper positioning (modified Trendelenburg) for the patient who shows signs of shock. The lower extremities are elevated to an angle of about 20 degrees; the knees are straight, the trunk is horizontal, and the head is slightly elevated.

pumps should be used to administer vasopressor medications, if prescribed. Another important nursing role is monitoring for complications and side effects of treatment and reporting them promptly.

Administering Blood and Fluids Safely

Administering blood transfusions safely is a vital nursing role. In emergency situations, it is important to acquire blood specimens quickly, to obtain a baseline complete blood count, and to type and cross-match the blood in anticipation of blood transfusions. A patient who receives a transfusion of blood products must be monitored closely for adverse effects (see Chapter 54).

Fluid replacement complications can occur, often when large volumes are administered rapidly. Therefore, the nurse monitors the patient closely for cardiovascular overload, signs of difficulty breathing, a condition known as transfusion-associated circulatory overload. Transfusion-related acute lung injury may occur and is characterized by pulmonary edema, hypoxemia, respiratory distress, and pulmonary infiltrates, usually within hours after massive transfusion (McEnvoy & Shander, 2013). The risk of these complications is increased in older people and in patients with pre-existing cardiac disease, and with increasing number of blood products given. ACS is also a possible complication of excessive fluid resuscitation and may initially present with respiratory symptoms (difficulty breathing) and decreased urine output. Hemodynamic pressures, vital signs, arterial blood gases, serum lactate levels, hemoglobin and hematocrit levels, bladder pressure monitoring, and fluid intake and output (I&O) are among the parameters monitored. Temperature should also be monitored closely to ensure that rapid fluid resuscitation does not cause hypothermia. IV fluids may need to be warmed during the administration of large volumes. Physical assessment focuses on observing the jugular veins for distention and monitoring jugular venous pressure. Jugular venous pressure is low in hypovolemic shock; it increases with effective treatment and is significantly increased with fluid overload and heart failure. The nurse must monitor cardiac and respiratory status closely and report changes in BP, pulse pressure, CVP, heart rate and rhythm, and lung sounds to the primary provider.

Implementing Other Measures

Oxygen is administered to increase the amount of oxygen carried by available hemoglobin in the blood. A patient who is confused may feel apprehensive with an oxygen mask or cannula in place, and frequent explanations about the need for the mask may reduce some of the patient's fear and anxiety. Simultaneously, the nurse must direct efforts to the safety and comfort of the patient.

Cardiogenic Shock

Cardiogenic shock occurs when the heart's ability to contract and to pump blood is impaired and the supply of oxygen is inadequate for the heart and tissues. The causes of cardiogenic shock are known as either coronary or noncoronary. Coronary cardiogenic shock is more common than noncoronary cardiogenic shock and is seen most often in patients with acute MI resulting in damage to a significant portion of the left ventricular myocardium (Tharmaratnam, Nolan, & Jain, 2013). Patients who experience an anterior wall MI are at greatest risk for cardiogenic shock because of the potentially extensive damage to the left ventricle caused by occlusion of the left anterior descending coronary artery. Noncoronary causes of cardiogenic shock are related to conditions that stress the myocardium (e.g., severe hypoxemia, acidosis, hypoglycemia, hypocalcemia, and tension pneumothorax) as well as conditions that result in ineffective myocardial function (e.g., cardiomyopathies, valvular damage, cardiac tamponade, dysrhythmias).

Pathophysiology

In cardiogenic shock, cardiac output, which is a function of both stroke volume and heart rate, is compromised. When stroke volume and heart rate decrease or become erratic, BP falls and tissue perfusion is reduced. Blood supply for tissues and organs and for the heart muscle itself is inadequate, resulting in impaired tissue perfusion. Because impaired tissue perfusion weakens the heart and impairs its ability to pump, the ventricle does not fully eject its volume of blood at systole. As a result, fluid accumulates in the lungs. This sequence of events can occur rapidly or over a period of days (Fig. 18-5).

Clinical Manifestations

Patients in cardiogenic shock may experience the pain of angina, develop dysrhythmias, complain of fatigue, express feelings of doom, and show signs of hemodynamic instability.

Medical Management

The goals of medical management in cardiogenic shock are to limit further myocardial damage and preserve the healthy myocardium and to improve the cardiac function by increasing cardiac contractility and/or decreasing

Physiology/Pathophysiology

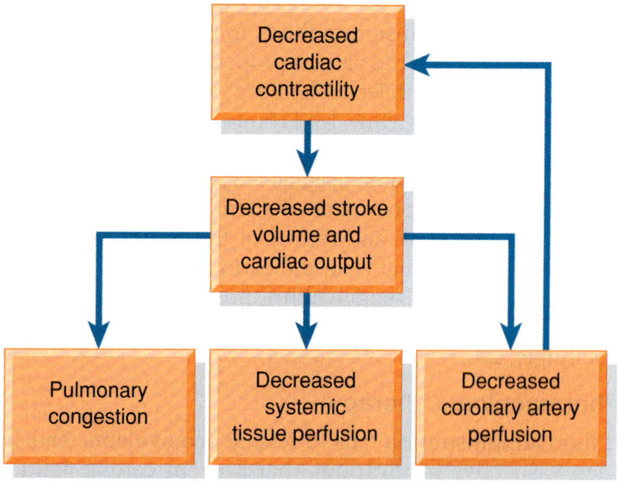

FIGURE 18-5. Pathophysiologic sequence of events in cardiogenic shock.

ventricular afterload by increasing oxygen supply to the heart muscle while reducing oxygen demands (Wacker & Winters, 2014).

Correction of Underlying Causes

As with all forms of shock, the underlying cause of cardiogenic shock must be corrected. It is necessary first to treat the oxygenation needs of the heart muscle to ensure its continued ability to pump blood to other organs. In the case of coronary cardiogenic shock (e.g., acute coronary syndromes, acute MI), the patient may require thrombolytic therapy, a percutaneous coronary intervention (PCI), coronary artery bypass graft (CABG) surgery, intra-aortic balloon pump therapy, or some combination of these treatments (Ng & Yeghiazarians, 2013). In the case of noncoronary cardiogenic shock, interventions focus on correcting the underlying cause, such as replacement of a faulty cardiac valve, correction of a dysrhythmia, correction of acidosis and electrolyte disturbances, or treatment of the tension pneumothorax. If the cause of the cardiogenic shock was related to a cardiac arrest, once the patient is successfully resuscitated, targeted temperature management, also called *therapeutic hypothermia,* may be initiated to actively lower the body temperature to a targeted core temperature (e.g., 32° to 36°C to preserve neurologic function) (American Heart Association, 2015; Subramaniam, Tiruvoipati, & Botha, 2015).

Initiation of First-Line Treatment

Oxygenation

In the early stages of shock, supplemental oxygen is administered by nasal cannula at a rate of 2 to 6 L/min to achieve an oxygen saturation exceeding 95%. Monitoring of arterial blood gas values, pulse oximetry values, and ventilatory effort (i.e., work of breathing) helps determine whether the patient requires a more aggressive method of oxygen delivery (including noninvasive and invasive mechanical ventilation).

Pain Control

If a patient experiences chest pain, IV morphine is administered for pain relief. In addition to relieving pain, morphine dilates the blood vessels. This reduces the workload of the heart by both decreasing the cardiac filling pressure (preload) and reducing the pressure against which the heart muscle has to eject blood (afterload). Morphine also decreases the patient's anxiety.

Hemodynamic Monitoring

Hemodynamic monitoring is initiated to assess the patient's response to treatment. In many institutions, this is performed in the intensive care unit (ICU), where an arterial line can be inserted. The arterial line enables accurate and continuous monitoring of BP and provides a port from which to obtain frequent arterial blood samples without having to perform repeated arterial punctures. A multilumen central venous and pulmonary artery catheter is inserted to allow measurement of myocardial filling pressures, the pulmonary artery pressures, myocardial filling pressures, cardiac output, and pulmonary and systemic resistance.

Laboratory Marker Monitoring

Laboratory biomarkers markers for ventricular dysfunction (e.g., B-type natriuretic peptide) and cardiac enzyme levels and biomarkers (cTn-I), and serum lactate are measured, a transthoracic echocardiography may be performed at the bedside, and serial 12-lead ECGs are obtained to assess the degree of myocardial damage (Tharmaratnam et al., 2013). Continuous ECG and ST-segment monitoring is also used to closely monitor the patient for ischemic changes.

Fluid Therapy

Appropriate fluid administration is also necessary in the treatment of cardiogenic shock. Administration of fluids must be monitored closely to detect signs of fluid overload. Incremental IV fluid boluses are cautiously administered to determine optimal filling pressures for improving cardiac output.

NURSING ALERT

A fluid bolus should never be given rapidly, because rapid fluid administration in patients with cardiac failure may result in acute pulmonary edema.

Pharmacologic Therapy

Vasoactive medication therapy consists of multiple pharmacologic strategies to restore and maintain adequate cardiac output. In coronary cardiogenic shock, the aims of vasoactive medication therapy are improved cardiac contractility, decreased preload and afterload, and stabilized heart rate and rhythm.

Because improving contractility and decreasing cardiac workload are opposing pharmacologic actions, two types of medications may be administered in combination: inotropic agents and vasodilators. Inotropic medications increase cardiac output by mimicking the action of the sympathetic nervous system, activating myocardial receptors to increase myocardial contractility (inotropic action) or increasing the heart rate (chronotropic action). These agents may also enhance vascular tone, increasing preload. Vasodilators are used primarily to decrease afterload, reducing the workload of the heart and the oxygen demand. Vasodilators also decrease preload. Medications commonly combined to treat cardiogenic shock include dobutamine, nitroglycerin, dopamine, and milrinone, which is an inotrope and vasodilator (Brenner & Stevens, 2018) (see Table 18-2).

DOBUTAMINE. Dobutamine produces inotropic effects by stimulating myocardial beta-receptors, increasing the strength of myocardial activity and improving cardiac output. Beta-2-adrenergic receptors are also stimulated, resulting in decreased pulmonary and systemic vascular resistance (decreased afterload).

NITROGLYCERIN. IV nitroglycerin in low doses acts as a venous vasodilator and therefore reduces preload. At higher doses, nitroglycerin causes arterial vasodilation and therefore reduces afterload as well. These actions, in combination with dobutamine, increase cardiac output while minimizing cardiac workload. In addition, vasodilation enhances blood flow to the myocardium, improving oxygen delivery to the weakened heart muscle (Allen, 2014; Ng & Yeghiazarians, 2013).

DOPAMINE. Dopamine is a sympathomimetic agent that has varying vasoactive effects depending on the dosage. It may be used with dobutamine and nitroglycerin to improve tissue perfusion. Doses of 2 to 8 μg/kg/min improve contractility (inotropic action), slightly increase the heart rate (chronotropic action), and may increase cardiac output. Doses that are higher than 8 μg/kg/min predominantly cause vasoconstriction, which increases afterload and thus increases cardiac workload. Because this effect is undesirable in patients with cardiogenic shock, dopamine doses must be carefully titrated.

In severe metabolic acidosis, which occurs in the later stages of shock, metabolic acidosis must first be corrected to ensure maximum effectiveness of vasoactive medications (Allen, 2014; Dellinger et al., 2013).

MILRINONE. Milrinone is a positive inotropic agent used in patients with cardiogenic shock. In addition to its inotropic properties, milrinone causes peripheral vasodilation. Milrinone inhibits the phosphodiesterase-3 intracellular enzyme, preventing the degradation of cyclic adenosine monophosphate (cAMP) within the cell. Increased cAMP levels lead to increased influx of calcium into the cell; in turn, increased intracellular calcium stimulates myocardial contractility. The positive inotropic action of milrinone is independent of β-receptor stimulation in the myocardial cells, making it different from dobutamine and dopamine. Because of this mechanism of action, use of milrinone is preferable in patients who are on β blockers as part of optimal medical therapy (Tariq & Aronow, 2015).

OTHER VASOACTIVE MEDICATIONS. Additional vasoactive agents that may be used in managing cardiogenic shock include norepinephrine, epinephrine, and phenylephrine. Each of these medications stimulates different receptors of the sympathetic nervous system. Vasopressin causes vasoconstriction and increased preload via V1 and V2 receptors while milrinone increases Ca^{++} levels leading to increases contractility and vasodilation (Brenner & Stevens, 2018).

A combination of these medications may be prescribed, depending on the patient's response to treatment. All vasoactive medications have adverse effects, making specific medications more useful than others at different stages of shock. Diuretics such as furosemide may be administered to reduce the workload of the heart by reducing fluid accumulation (see Table 18-2).

ANTIARRHYTHMIC MEDICATIONS. Multiple factors, such as hypoxemia, electrolyte imbalances, and acid–base imbalances, contribute to serious cardiac dysrhythmias in all patients with shock. In addition, as a compensatory response to decreased cardiac output and BP, the heart rate increases beyond normal limits. This impedes cardiac output further by shortening diastole and thereby decreasing the time for ventricular filling. Consequently, antiarrhythmic medications are required to stabilize the heart rate. For a full discussion of cardiac dysrhythmias as well as commonly prescribed medications, see Chapter 28. General principles regarding the administration of vasoactive medications are discussed later in this chapter.

Mechanical Assistive Devices

If cardiac output does not improve despite supplemental oxygen, vasoactive medications, and fluid boluses, mechanical assistive devices are used temporarily to improve the heart's ability to pump. Intra-aortic balloon counterpulsation is one means of providing temporary circulatory assistance (see Chapter 31). Other means of mechanical assistance include left and right ventricular assist devices (VADs) and total temporary artificial hearts (see Chapters 30 and 31). VADs are utilized frequently as bridge therapy to either recovery or heart transplantation. Another short-term means of providing cardiac or pulmonary support to the patient in cardiogenic shock is through an extracorporeal device similar to the cardiopulmonary bypass (CPB) system used in open-heart surgery (see Chapter 29). CPB is used only in emergency situations until definitive treatment, such as heart transplantation, can be initiated.

Nursing Management

Preventing Cardiogenic Shock

Identifying at-risk patients early, promoting adequate oxygenation of the heart muscle, and decreasing cardiac workload can prevent cardiogenic shock. This can be accomplished by conserving the patient's energy, promptly relieving angina, and administering supplemental oxygen. Often, however, cardiogenic shock cannot be prevented. In such instances, nursing management includes working with other members of the health care team to prevent shock from progressing and to restore adequate cardiac function and tissue perfusion.

Monitoring Hemodynamic Status

A major role of the nurse is monitoring the patient's hemodynamic and cardiac status. Arterial lines and ECG monitoring equipment must be well maintained and functioning properly. The nurse anticipates the medications, IV fluids, and equipment that might be used and is ready to assist in implementing these measures. Changes in hemodynamic, cardiac, and pulmonary status and laboratory values are documented and reported promptly. In addition, adventitious breath sounds, changes in cardiac rhythm, and other abnormal physical assessment findings are reported immediately.

Administering Medications and Intravenous Fluids

The nurse plays a critical role in the safe and accurate administration of IV fluids and medications. Fluid overload and pulmonary edema are risks because of ineffective cardiac function and accumulation of blood and fluid in the pulmonary tissues. The nurse documents and records medications and treatments that are administered as well as the patient's response to treatment.

The nurse must be knowledgeable about the desired effects as well as the side effects of medications. For example, it is important to monitor the patient for decreased BP after administering morphine or nitroglycerin. Patients receiving thrombolytic therapy must be monitored for bleeding. Arterial and venous puncture sites must be observed for bleeding, and pressure must be applied at the sites if bleeding occurs. Neurologic assessment is essential after the administration of thrombolytic therapy to assess for the potential complication of cerebral hemorrhage associated with this therapy. IV infusions must be observed closely because tissue necrosis and sloughing may occur if vasopressor medications infiltrate the tissues. When possible, vasoactive medications should be given using central IV lines (Dellinger et al., 2013). Furthermore, the need for the central IV access devices should be reviewed daily to reduce the risk of CLABSIs (Marschall, Mermel, Fakih, et al., 2014). The nurse must also monitor urine output, BUN, and serum creatinine levels to detect decreased renal function secondary to the effects of cardiogenic shock or its treatment.

Maintaining Intra-Aortic Balloon Counterpulsation

The nurse plays a critical role in caring for the patient receiving intra-aortic balloon counterpulsation (see Chapter 31). The nurse makes ongoing timing adjustments of the balloon pump to maximize its effectiveness by synchronizing it with the cardiac cycle. The patient is at risk for circulatory compromise to the leg on the side where the catheter for the balloon has been inserted; therefore, the nurse must check the neurovascular status of the lower extremities frequently.

Enhancing Safety and Comfort

Throughout care, the nurse takes an active role in safeguarding the patient, enhancing comfort, and reducing anxiety. This includes administering medication to relieve chest pain, preventing infection at the multiple arterial and venous line insertion sites, protecting the skin, and monitoring respiratory and renal function. Proper positioning of the patient promotes effective breathing without decreasing BP and may also increase patient comfort while reducing anxiety.

Brief explanations about procedures that are being performed and the use of comforting touch often provide reassurance to the patient and family. The family is usually anxious and benefits from opportunities to see and talk to the patient. Explanations of treatments and the patient's responses are often comforting to family members.

Family presence during emergencies and procedures is becoming a more common practice. Research has explored health care provider and family member perceptions of family presence during procedures and emergent patient treatment, but few studies have explored the patient's perception of family presence. A recent qualitative research study by Twibell, Craig, and Siela (2015) found that most patients do wish to have family present during life-threatening events and procedures. An important finding in this study was that patients wish to decide who will be present; therefore, the health care team should facilitate discussions about family presence with patients before life-threatening events or emergent procedures are necessary (see Chart 18-4).

Distributive Shock

Distributive shock occurs when blood volume pools in peripheral blood vessels. This abnormal displacement of blood volume causes a relative hypovolemia because not enough blood returns to the heart, which leads to inadequate tissue perfusion. The ability of the blood vessels to constrict helps return the blood to the heart. The vascular tone is determined both by central regulatory mechanisms, as in BP regulation, and by local regulatory mechanisms, as in tissue demands for oxygen and nutrients. Therefore, distributive shock can be caused either by a loss of sympathetic tone or by release of biochemical mediators from cells that causes vasodilation.

The varied mechanisms leading to the initial vasodilation in distributive shock provide the basis for the further subclassification of shock into three types: septic shock, **neurogenic shock**, and **anaphylactic shock**. These subtypes of distributive shock cause variations in the pathophysiologic chain of events and are explained here separately. In all types of distributive shock, massive arterial and venous dilation promotes peripheral pooling of blood. Arterial dilation reduces systemic vascular resistance. Initially, cardiac output can be high, both from the reduction in afterload (systemic vascular resistance) and from the heart muscle's increased effort to maintain perfusion despite the incompetent vasculature. Pooling of blood in the periphery results in decreased venous return. Decreased venous return results in decreased stroke volume and decreased cardiac output. Decreased cardiac output, in turn, causes decreased BP and ultimately decreased tissue perfusion. Figure 18-6 presents the pathophysiologic sequence of events in distributive shock.

Physiology/Pathophysiology

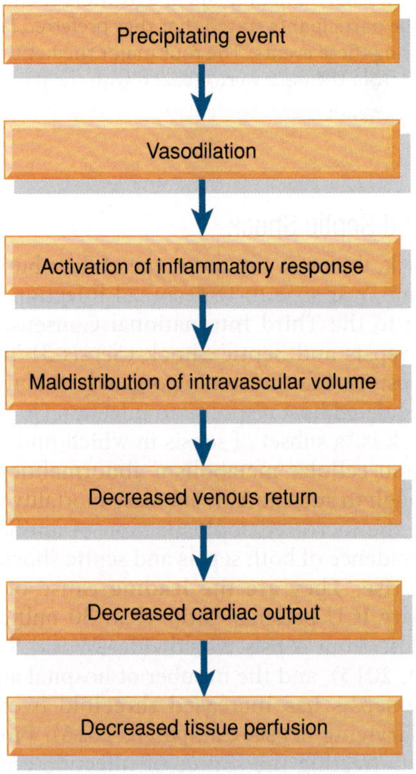

FIGURE 18-6. Pathophysiologic sequence of events in distributive shock.

NURSING RESEARCH PROFILE

Chart 18-4. Family Presence During Life-Threatening Events

Twibell, R. S., Craig, S., Siela, D., et al. (2015). Being there: Inpatients' perceptions of family presence during resuscitation and invasive cardiac procedures. *American Journal of Critical Care*, *24*(6), 108–115.

Purpose

The aim of this study was to explore adult inpatients' perceptions of family presence during resuscitation, near-resuscitation, and unplanned invasive cardiac procedures within hours or days of the life-threatening event.

Design

This was a qualitative, exploratory, descriptive study that enrolled a convenience sample of physiologically stable adult hospitalized patients who had experienced a life-threatening event. Forty-eight participants were interviewed within 13 to 96 hours of the event. Participants were interviewed by one researcher who began each interview session with the same question: "Thinking of your recent life-threatening event here in the hospital, please share your thoughts on having family members present beside you as the care team intervened." All interviews were tape-recorded and transcribed. The research team analyzed the data both independently and collectively until consensus was reached on the major themes that emerged.

Findings

Approximately half of the participants experienced an unplanned cardiac procedure, one fourth experienced resuscitation, and one fourth experienced a near-resuscitation event. There were an equal number of men and women in the study, most were Caucasian (94%), with 33 (69%) participants between 41 and 80 years of age. More than 60% (N = 29) of the participants stated that they preferred family presence during these events. The four major themes that emerged from the data were labelled with the participants' own words. The first theme was "Being there is beneficial." Participants shared the belief that having family present during these events was beneficial to both the family member and the patient. "Being there is hard" was the second theme. Participants expressed that it is hard to decide which family member should be in the room during these events, and also that it is difficult for the chosen family member to watch the events unfold. Most participants felt that the patient or families should decide who should be the family member present during these events, not the health care team. The third theme, "Families in the way" referenced participants' concerns that family members present during these events could interfere in their care because of room space constraints, or because they would likely ask questions of health care providers. The final theme, "Desire for control," referenced participants' desire for control to prevent "out of control" family members being present. None of the participants expressed concern about controlling confidentiality of information.

Nursing Implications

Findings from this study support previous research that suggests that family presence during emergencies and procedures is beneficial to the patient. Important new information that emerged from this study was that patients and their families felt that they should make the decision about family presence, not the health care professionals. Nurses should identify with the patient which family member should be present should a life-threatening event occur. These researchers suggest that this exploratory conversation could occur during the admission process with a review of the patient's advanced directives. Nurses have a key role supporting family members who are present during life-threatening events. Nurses can assist families in understanding the life-threatening events as they unfold, providing support to families during the crisis.

Sepsis and Septic Shock

Septic shock, the most common type of distributive shock, is a systemic response to widespread infection or sepsis. According to the Third International Consensus Definitions for Sepsis and Septic Shock (*Sepsis-3*) Task Force (2016), sepsis is "life-threatening organ dysfunction caused by a dysregulated host response to infection (p. 804)," and septic shock is "a subset of sepsis in which underlying circulatory and cellular metabolism abnormalities are profound enough to substantially increase mortality (p. 806)."

Despite the increased sophistication of antibiotic therapy, the incidence of both sepsis and septic shock has continued to rise. They are the leading cause of death in noncoronary ICU patients. More than 30 million people suffer or die from sepsis worldwide (World Sepsis Day Fact Sheet, 2015), and the number of hospital admissions related to sepsis has increased threefold over the last decade (Surviving Sepsis Campaign, 2016). Finding and aggressively treating the source of infection and quickly restoring tissue perfusion are important interventions that may positively influence the clinical outcome.

According to Statistics Canada (2016), in 2011, 1 in 18 deaths in Canada involved sepsis.

- Deaths involving sepsis increased significantly between 2000 and 2007 and then remained stable between 2007 and 2011.
- Deaths involving sepsis were higher among males than females, although between 2007 and 2011 the difference between the sexes narrowed.
- Sepsis contributed to more than half of all deaths from infectious diseases in Canada during the 2009–2011 time period.

Sepsis can be a community-acquired or a health care–associated problem. Hospital-acquired conditions, which may include hospital-associated infections (i.e., infections not present at the time of admission to the health care setting) in critically ill patients that may progress to septic shock most frequently originate in the bloodstream (bacteremia), lungs (pneumonia), and urinary tract (urosepsis). Other infections include intra-abdominal infections and wound infections. Of increasing concern are bacteremias associated with intravascular catheters and indwelling

CHART 18-5

Risk Factors for Distributive Shock

Septic Shock

- Immunosuppression
- Extremes of age (<1 year and >65 years)
- Malnourishment
- Chronic illness
- Invasive procedures
- Emergent and/or multiple surgeries

Neurogenic Shock

- Spinal cord injury
- Spinal anesthesia
- Depressant action of medications

Anaphylactic Shock

- History of medication sensitivity
- Transfusion reaction
- History of reaction to insect bites/stings
- Food allergies
- Latex sensitivity

Adapted from Anderson, M. W., & Watson, G. A. (2013). Traumatic shock: The fifth shock. *Journal of Trauma Nursing, 20*(1), 37–43; Dellinger, R. P., Levy, M. M., Rhodes, A., et al. (2013). Surviving Sepsis Campaign: International guidelines for management of severe sepsis and septic shock: 2012. *Critical Care Medicine, 41*(2), 580–637; Green, J. M. (2015). Essentials of sepsis management. *Surgical Clinics of North America, 95*(2), 355–365; Kanwar, R., Delasobera, B. E., Hudson, K., et al. (2015). Emergency department evaluation and treatment of cervical spine injuries. *Emergency Medicine Clinics of North America, 33*(2), 241–282; Lineberry, C., & Stein, D. E. (2014). Infection, sepsis, and immune function in the older adult receiving critical care. *Critical Care Nursing Clinics of North America, 26*(1), 47–60; Mayr, F. B., Yende, S., & Angus, D. C. (2014). Epidemiology of severe sepsis. *Virulence, 5*(1), 4–11; Muraro, A., Hoffmann-Sommergruber, K., Holzhauser, T., et al. (2014). EAACI food allergy and anaphylaxis guidelines: Protecting consumers with food allergies, understanding food consumption, meeting regulations and identifying unmet needs. *Allergy, 69*(11), 1464–1472.

urinary catheters (Centers for Medicare & Medicaid Services [CMS], 2014; Institute for Healthcare Improvement [IHI], 2012).

Additional risk factors that contribute to the growing incidence of sepsis are the increased use of invasive procedures and indwelling medical devices, the increased number of antibiotic-resistant microorganisms, and the increasingly older population (Green, 2015). Older adult patients are at particular risk for sepsis because of decreased physiologic reserves, an aging immune system, comorbid conditions and often nonspecific presentation of infection (Davis, 2014; Lineberry & Stein, 2014). Other patients at risk are those undergoing surgical and other invasive procedures, especially patients who have undergone emergency surgery or multiple surgeries (Green, 2015); those with malnutrition or immunosuppression; and those with chronic illness such as diabetes, hepatitis, chronic kidney disease, and immunodeficiency disorders (Lineberry & Stein, 2014) (Chart 18-5).

The incidence of health care–associated infections can be reduced by using strict infection control practices, beginning with thorough hand-hygiene techniques after each encounter with a patient (Dellinger, 2015). Other interventions include implementing programs to prevent central line infection; ensuring early removal of invasive devices that are no longer necessary (e.g., indwelling urinary catheters); implementing prevention programs to prevent ventilator-associated events and pneumonia; promoting early ambulation; timely débriding of wounds to remove necrotic tissue; carrying out standard precautions and adhering to infection prevention/control practices, including the use of meticulous aseptic technique; and properly cleaning equipment and the patient environment.

Pathophysiology

Gram-negative bacteria traditionally have been the most commonly implicated microorganisms in sepsis. However, there is an increased incidence of gram-positive bacterial infections, viral infections, and fungal infections that can also cause sepsis (Wacker & Winters, 2014). Although a site of infection is identified in most cases, up to 30% of patients with sepsis may never have an identifiable site of infection (Surviving Sepsis Campaign, 2016).

When microorganisms invade body tissues, patients exhibit an immune response. This immune response provokes the activation of biochemical cytokines and mediators associated with an inflammatory response, and produces a complex cascade of physiologic events that leads to poor tissue perfusion. Increased capillary permeability, which leads to fluid seeping from the capillaries. Capillary instability and vasodilation interrupt the body's ability to provide adequate perfusion, oxygen, and nutrients to the tissues and cells. The widespread inflammatory response that occurs is called the **systemic inflammatory response syndrome (SIRS)**. SIRS results from a clinical insult that initiates an inflammatory response that is systemic, rather than localized to the site of the insult. The insult may be a significant injury (e.g., multitrauma) or an infection (e.g., sepsis). A patient presenting with manifestations of SIRS may be exhibiting a protective inflammatory response to the initiating insult or may be exhibiting a response to infection, which may lead to sepsis. The clinical criteria used to identify SIRS, which include a temperature >38.3°C (>101°F) or <36°C (<96.8°F), tachycardia, tachypnea, and a white blood cell (WBC) count >12,000 cells/mm^3, less than 4,000 cells/mm^3, or >10% immature WBC (bands), have been found to be not helpful in diagnosing sepsis, however (Singer et al., 2016).

In addition to SIRS, proinflammatory and anti-inflammatory cytokines released during the inflammatory response activate the coagulation system, which begins to form clots whether or not bleeding is present (Moore et al., 2015). This results not only in microvascular occlusions that further disrupt cellular perfusion but also in an inappropriate consumption of clotting factors. The imbalance of the inflammatory response and the clotting and fibrinolysis cascades are considered critical elements of the devastating physiologic progression that occurs in patients with sepsis.

Sepsis is an evolving process that may result in septic shock and life-threatening organ dysfunction if not recognized and treated early. In the early stage of septic shock, BP may remain within normal limits, or the patient may be hypotensive but responsive to fluids. The heart rate increases, progressing to tachycardia. Hyperthermia and fever, with warm, flushed skin and bounding pulses, are present. The respiratory rate is elevated. Urinary output may remain at normal levels or decrease. GI status may be compromised, as evidenced by nausea, vomiting, diarrhea, or decreased gastric motility. Hepatic dysfunction is evidenced by rising bilirubin levels and worsening coagulopathies (e.g., decreasing platelet counts). Signs of hypermetabolism include increased serum glucose and insulin resistance. Subtle changes in mental status, such as confusion or agitation, may be present. The lactate level is elevated because of the maldistribution of blood. Inflammatory markers such as WBC counts, plasma C-reactive protein (CRP), and procalcitonin levels are also elevated (Dellinger et al., 2013; Green, 2015; Moore et al., 2015; Singer et al., 2016).

As sepsis progresses, tissues become less perfused and acidotic, compensation begins to fail, and the patient begins to show signs of organ dysfunction. The cardiovascular system also begins to fail, the BP does not respond to fluid resuscitation and vasoactive agents, and signs of end-organ damage are evident (e.g., AKI, pulmonary dysfunction, hepatic dysfunction, confusion progressing to nonresponsiveness). As sepsis progresses to septic shock, the BP drops, and the skin becomes cool, pale, and mottled. Temperature may be normal or below normal. Heart and respiratory rates remain rapid. Urine production ceases, and multiple organ dysfunction progressing to death occurs.

Medical Management

A significant body of research has been conducted in the past few decades that is aimed at reducing the morbidity and mortality caused by sepsis and septic shock. In 1991, 2003, 2008, 2012, and again in 2016 (i.e., *Sepsis-3*), critical care experts systematically reevaluated the body of research and provided evidence-based recommendations for the acute management of patients with sepsis and septic shock (Dellinger et al., 2013; Singer et al., 2016; Surviving Sepsis Campaign, 2016). Developing and implementing protocols that focus on prevention and early detection and management of patients with sepsis have reduced the mortality of hospitalized patients (Dellinger, 2015; Singer et al., 2016). *Sepsis-3* provides an overview of key concepts and principles germane to sepsis that must be understood in order for physicians and nurses to be able to identify and manage patients with sepsis, including the following (Singer et al., 2016):

- As the leading cause of death from infection, sepsis must be recognized and treated promptly.
- Sepsis is different from infection in that in sepsis there is a dysregulated host response with organ dysfunction, while an infection may cause specific organ dysfunction without a dysregulated host response.
- Sepsis is caused by an interplay between infectious pathogens and a myriad of patient-specific risks, including genetics, age, and the presence of other diseases/disorders.
- The organ dysfunction that occurs with sepsis may not be readily apparent; on the contrary, a new onset of organ dysfunction may be caused by an unrecognized infectious process.

Research efforts are focusing on better identification and early aggressive treatment of patients with sepsis, rapid and effective restoration of tissue perfusion, evaluation and treatment of the patient's immune response, and treatment of dysregulation of the coagulation system that occurs with sepsis (Green, 2015).

Correction of Underlying Causes

Current treatment of sepsis and septic shock involves rapid identification and elimination of the cause of infection. Current goals are to identify and treat patients in early sepsis within 3 hours to optimize patient outcome (Surviving Sepsis Campaign, 2016). Several evidence-based screening tools can be used to help identify patients for sepsis (see later discussion of assessment tools under the section Nursing Management).

In an effort to continue to reduce deaths from sepsis, CMS has launched a *Core Measure* for sepsis, requiring that hospitals demonstrate adherence to 3- and 6-hour timed interventions (see Chart 18-6). The focus on compliance with these evidence-based bundled interventions is to foster early recognition and interventions in patients with sepsis so that patient outcomes improve. These assessments and interventions are collectively referred to as the *Sepsis Bundles* (CMS, 2014).

Rapid identification of the infectious source is a critical element in managing sepsis. Specimens of blood, sputum, urine, wound drainage, and tips of invasive catheters are collected for culture using aseptic technique. IV lines are removed and reinserted at alternate sites. If possible, urinary catheters are removed or changed. Any abscesses are drained, and necrotic areas are debrided. All cultures should be obtained prior to antibiotic administration but should not delay administration of antibiotics as per current guidelines. The guidelines suggest that antibiotics should be initiated within the first hour of treatment of a patient with sepsis (Surviving Sepsis Campaign, 2016).

Fluid Replacement Therapy

Fluid replacement must be instituted to correct tissue hypoperfusion that results from the incompetent vasculature and the inflammatory response. Reestablishing tissue perfusion through aggressive fluid resuscitation is key to the management of sepsis and septic shock (Dellinger et al., 2013; Yealy et al., 2014). An initial fluid challenge, which includes an IV infusion of at least 30 mL/kg of crystalloids over 30 minutes, may be required to aggressively treat sepsis-induced tissue hypoperfusion. In addition to monitoring BP, CVP, fluid responsiveness with passive leg raise, urine output, and serum lactate levels are monitored to assess effectiveness of fluid resuscitation.

Pharmacologic Therapy

If the infecting organism is unknown, the patient is started on broad spectrum until culture and sensitivity reports are received (Dellinger et al., 2013; IHI, 2014a), at which time the antibiotic agents may be changed to agents that are more specific to the infecting organism and less toxic to the patient.

If fluid therapy alone does not effectively improve tissue perfusion, vasopressor agents, specifically norepinephrine, may be initiated to achieve a MAP of 65 mm Hg or higher. Inotropic agents may also be given to provide pharmacologic support to the myocardium. Packed red blood cells may be ordered to support oxygen delivery and transport to the tissues. Neuromuscular blockade agents

CHART 18-6

Surviving Sepsis Campaign Bundle

Complete within 3 hours of patient presentation/symptoms

- Obtain serum lactate level
- Obtain blood culture prior to administration of antibiotics
- Administer prescribed broad-spectrum antibiotics
- Initiate aggressive fluid resuscitation in patients with hypotension or elevated serum lactate (>4 mmol/L):
  - Minimum initial fluid bolus of 30 mL/kg using crystalloid solutions

Complete as soon as possible or within the first 6 hours of patient presentation/symptoms

- Begin vasopressor agents if hypotension is not improved (MAP <65 mm Hg) after initial fluid resuscitation
- If hypotension persists after initial fluid administration (MAP <65 mm Hg) or initial lactate was ≥4 mmol/L, reassess intravascular volume status and tissue perfusion using two of the following assessment parameters:
  - Measure CVP (goal 8–12 mm Hg)

Measure $Sc\bar{v}O_2$ (goal > 70%)

- Bedside cardiovascular ultrasound
- Dynamic assessment of fluid responsiveness with passive leg raise or fluid challenge

Additional interventions and targets for therapy in the early management of sepsis

- Support blood pressure to achieve a urine output >0.5 mL/kg/hr
- Administer vasopressor agents if fluid resuscitation does not restore an effective BP and cardiac output:
  - Norepinephrine centrally given is the initial vasopressor of choice.
  - Epinephrine, phenylephrine, or vasopressin should not be given as the initial vasopressor in septic shock.
- Obtain blood, sputum, urine, and wound cultures and administer broad-spectrum antibiotics:
  - Cultures should be obtained prior to antibiotic administration.
  - Antibiotic administration should occur within 3 hours of admission to the emergency department or within 1 hour of inpatient admission.
- Support the respiratory system with supplemental oxygen and mechanical ventilation.
- Transfuse with packed red blood cells when hemoglobin is <7 g/dL to achieve a target hemoglobin of 7–9 g/dL in adults.
- Provide adequate IV sedation and analgesia; avoid the use of neuromuscular blockade agents when possible.
- Control serum glucose <180 mg/dL with IV insulin therapy.
- Implement interventions and medications to prevent deep vein thrombosis and stress ulcer prophylaxis.
- Discuss advance care planning with patients and families.

Adapted from Centers for Medicare & Medicaid Services. (2014). Improve quality of care during hospital inpatient stays. Retrieved November 28, 2015, from www.cms.gov/Newsroom/MediaReleaseDatabase/Fact-sheets/2014-Fact-sheets-items/2014-08-04-2.html; Dellinger, R. P., Levy, M. M., Rhodes, A., et al. (2013). Surviving Sepsis Campaign: International guidelines for management of severe sepsis and septic shock: 2012. *Critical Care Medicine*, *41*(2), 580–637; Dellinger, R. P. (2015). The future of sepsis performance improvement. *Critical Care Medicine*, *43*(9), 1787–1790; Surviving Sepsis Bundle. (2015). Retrieved 28 November, 2015, from ww.surviving-sepsis.org/SiteCollectionDocuments/SSC_Bundle.pdf

CVP, central venous pressure; MAP, mean arterial pressure; BP, blood pressure; IV, intravenous.

and sedation agents may be required to reduce metabolic demands and provide comfort to the patient. Deep vein thrombosis (DVT) prophylaxis with low-dose unfractionated heparin or low–molecular-weight heparin, in combination with mechanical prophylaxis (e.g., sequential compression devices) should be initiated, as well as medications for stress ulcer prophylaxis (e.g., H_2-blocking agents, proton pump inhibitors).

Nutritional Therapy

Aggressive nutritional supplementation should be initiated within 24 to 48 hours of ICU admission to address the hypermetabolic state present with septic shock (Martindale & Warren, 2015). Malnutrition further impairs the patient's resistance to infection. Enteral feedings are preferred to the parenteral route because of the increased risk of iatrogenic infection associated with IV catheters; however, enteral feedings may not be possible if decreased perfusion to the GI tract reduces peristalsis and impairs absorption.

Nursing Management

Nurses caring for patients in any setting must keep in mind the risks of sepsis and the high mortality rate associated with sepsis and septic shock. All invasive procedures must be carried out with aseptic technique after careful hand hygiene. In addition, IV lines, arterial and venous puncture sites, surgical incisions, traumatic wounds, urinary catheters, and pressure ulcers must be monitored for signs of infection. Nursing interventions to prevent infection need to be implemented in the care of all patients. Nurses should identify patients who are at particular risk for sepsis and septic shock (i.e., older and immunosuppressed patients and those with extensive trauma, burns, or diabetes), keeping in mind that these high-risk patients may not develop typical or classic signs of infection and sepsis. For example, confusion may be the first sign of infection and sepsis older adult patients (Kleinpell, Aitken, & Schorr, 2013).

Sepsis-3 recommends that patients in the ICU setting with infection be monitored for the development of sepsis by using the *Sepsis-Related Organ Failure Assessment Score* (also known as the *Sequential Organ Failure Assessment* [SOFA] score) (Antonelli et al., 2016; Singer et al., 2016; Vincent, Moreno, Takala, et al., 1996). The parameters that are monitored on the SOFA, which include assessment of respiratory rate, platelets, bilirubin, MAP (and use of any vasopressors), serum creatinine, urine output, and Glasgow Coma Scale (GCS) score (see Chapter 66), may all be gathered and assessed by the nurse in the ICU setting. A drop of 2 points or more in a patient's SOFA score from baseline is suggestive of organ dysfunction. In a patient with infection, the presence of organ dysfunction suggests the development of sepsis (Singer et al., 2016).

For a patient not in the ICU setting who has an infection, *Sepsis-3* recommends that the Quick SOFA (qSOFA) scale be used to screen for the development of sepsis. The qSOFA is an easy measurement tool that nurses may readily use; the presence of any two of the three parameters on this scale suggests the development of sepsis. These parameters include a respiratory rate of 22 breaths per minute or higher, a GCS score of less than 15, and a systolic BP of 100 mm Hg or less. The GCS parameter is considered positive for any score less than 15; therefore, any change in the patient's mentation status is considered positive. In order to facilitate ease of use, therefore, *Sepsis-3* recommends that any change in the patient's mentation status be used when computing the qSOFA scale score (Antonelli et al., 2016; Singer et al., 2016). Another assessment tool that is frequently used in hospital-based settings that can identify patients with sepsis is the *Modified Early Warning System* (MEWS) (IHI, 2014b). The nurse assesses the patient for changes in respiratory rate, heart rate, BP, consciousness, temperature, and urine output. Scores ranging from 0 to 3 are assigned to each assessment variable, and MEWS score is greater than 4 are suggestive of the development of sepsis (IHI, 2014b).

When caring for a patient with septic shock, the nurse collaborates with other members of the health care team to identify the site and source of sepsis and the specific organisms involved. The nurse often obtains appropriate specimens for culture and sensitivity. Cultures should be drawn prior to the administration of broad-spectrum antibiotics, but not at the cost of delaying antibiotic administration (Schmidt et al., 2017). The guidelines suggest that antibiotics should be initiated within the first hour of treatment of a patient with sepsis (Surviving Sepsis Campaign, 2016). Early goal-directed therapy (EGDT) protocols have not been shown to improve mortality, however prompt identification of sepsis, attainment of cultures, fluid resuscitation, and antibiotic therapy is essential (Schmidt et al., 2017).

Elevated body temperature (hyperthermia) is common with sepsis and raises the patient's metabolic rate and oxygen consumption. Efforts may be made to reduce the temperature by administering acetaminophen or applying a hypothermia blanket. During these therapies, the nurse monitors the patient closely for shivering, which increases oxygen consumption. Efforts to increase comfort are important if the patient experiences fever, chills, or shivering.

The nurse administers prescribed IV fluids and medications, including antibiotic agents and vasoactive medications, to restore vascular volume. Because of decreased perfusion, serum concentrations of antibiotic agents that are normally cleared by the kidneys and liver may increase and produce toxic effects. Therefore, the nurse monitors blood levels (serum levels of antibiotic agents, procalcitonin, CRP, BUN, creatinine, WBC count, hemoglobin, hematocrit, platelet levels, coagulation studies) and reports changes to the primary provider. As with other types of shock, the nurse monitors the patient's hemodynamic status, fluid intake and output, and nutritional status. Daily weights and close monitoring of serum albumin and prealbumin levels help determine the patient's protein requirements.

Neurogenic Shock

In Neurogenic Shock, vasodilation occurs as a result of a loss of balance between parasympathetic and sympathetic stimulation. Sympathetic stimulation causes vascular smooth muscle to constrict, and parasympathetic stimulation causes vascular smooth muscle to relax or dilate. The patient experiences a predominant parasympathetic stimulation that causes vasodilation lasting for an extended period, leading to a relative hypovolemic state. However, blood volume is adequate, because the vasculature is dilated; the blood volume is displaced, producing a hypotensive (low BP) state. The overriding parasympathetic stimulation that occurs with neurogenic shock causes a drastic decrease in the patient's systemic vascular resistance and bradycardia. Inadequate BP results in the insufficient perfusion of tissues and cells that is common to all shock states.

Neurogenic shock can be caused by spinal cord injury, spinal anesthesia, or other nervous system damage. It may also result from the depressant action of medications or from lack of glucose (e.g., insulin reaction or shock). Neurogenic shock may have a prolonged course (spinal cord injury) or a short one (syncope or fainting). Normally, during states of stress, the sympathetic stimulation causes the BP and heart rate to increase. In neurogenic shock, the sympathetic system is not able to respond to body stressors. Therefore, the clinical characteristics of neurogenic shock are signs of parasympathetic stimulation. It is characterized by dry, warm skin rather than the cool, moist skin seen in hypovolemic shock. Another characteristic is hypotension with bradycardia, rather than the tachycardia that characterizes other forms of shock.

Medical Management

Treatment of neurogenic shock involves restoring sympathetic tone, either through the stabilization of a spinal cord injury or, in the instance of spinal anesthesia, by positioning the patient properly. Specific treatment depends on the cause of the shock. Further discussion of management of patients with a spinal cord injury is presented in Chapter 65. If hypoglycemia (insulin shock) is the cause, glucose is rapidly administered (see Chapter 41).

Nursing Management

It is important to elevate and maintain the head of the bed at least 30 degrees to prevent neurogenic shock when a patient receives spinal or epidural anesthesia. Elevation of the head helps prevent the spread of the anesthetic agent up the spinal cord. In suspected spinal cord injury, neurogenic shock may be prevented by carefully immobilizing the patient to prevent further damage to the spinal cord (Kanwar, Delasobera, Hudson, et al., 2015). Nursing interventions are directed toward supporting cardiovascular and neurologic function until the usually transient episode of neurogenic shock resolves.

Patients with neurogenic shock have a higher risk for venous thromboembolism (VTE) formation because of increased pooling of blood from vascular dilation; this risk is greater in patients with neurogenic shock related to spinal cord injury (Zhang, Wadhwa, Haydel, et al., 2013). The nurse must check the patient daily for any lower extremity pain, redness, tenderness, and warmth. If the patient complains of pain and objective assessment of the calf is suspicious, the patient should be evaluated for DVT. Passive range of motion of the immobile extremities helps promote circulation. Early interventions to prevent VTE include the application of pneumatic compression devices often combined with antithrombotic agents (e.g., low–molecular-weight heparin).

A patient who has experienced a spinal cord injury may not report pain caused by internal injuries. Therefore, in the immediate postinjury period, the nurse must monitor the patient closely for signs of internal bleeding that could lead to hypovolemic shock.

Anaphylactic Shock

Anaphylactic shock is caused by a severe allergic reaction when patients who have already produced antibodies to a foreign substance (antigen) develop a systemic antigen–antibody reaction; specifically, an immunoglobulin E (IgE)–mediated response. This antigen–antibody reaction provokes mast cells to release potent vasoactive substances, such as histamine or bradykinin, and activates inflammatory cytokines, causing widespread vasodilation and capillary permeability. The most common triggers are foods (especially peanuts), medications, and insects (Muraro, Hoffmann-Sommergruber, Holzhauser, et al., 2014). Anaphylaxis has three defining characteristics (Muraro et al., 2014; Triggiani, Montagni, Parente, et al., 2014):

- Acute onset of symptoms
- Presence of two or more symptoms that include respiratory compromise, reduced BP, GI distress, and skin or mucosal tissue irritation
- Cardiovascular compromise from minutes to hours after exposure to the antigen

Signs and symptoms of anaphylaxis may present within 2 to 30 minutes of exposure to the antigen; however, occasionally some reactions may not develop for several hours (Triggiani et al., 2014). The patient may complain of headache, lightheadedness, nausea, vomiting, acute abdominal pain or discomfort, pruritus, and feeling of impending doom. Assessment may reveal diffuse erythema and generalized flushing, difficulty breathing (laryngeal edema), bronchospasm, cardiac dysrhythmias, and hypotension. Characteristics of severe anaphylaxis usually include rapid onset of hypotension, neurologic compromise, respiratory distress, and cardiac arrest (Triggiani et al., 2014). Anaphylactoid reactions present similarly to anaphylaxis but are not mediated by IgE responses. Anaphylaxis and anaphylactoid reactions are often clinically indistinguishable (Muraro et al., 2014).

Medical Management

Treatment of anaphylactic shock requires removing the causative antigen when possible (e.g., discontinuing an antibiotic agent), administering medications that restore vascular tone, and providing emergency support of basic life functions. Fluid management is critical, as massive fluid shifts can occur within minutes due to increased vascular permeability (Muraro et al., 2014). Intramuscular epinephrine is given for its vasoconstrictive action. Diphenhydramine (Benadryl) is administered to reverse the effects of histamine, thereby reducing capillary permeability. These medications are given intravenously. Nebulized medications, such as albuterol (Proventil), may be given to reverse histamine-induced bronchospasm.

If cardiac arrest and respiratory arrest are imminent or have occurred, cardiopulmonary resuscitation is performed. Endotracheal intubation or tracheotomy may be necessary to establish an airway. IV lines are inserted to provide access for administering fluids and medications. Anaphylaxis and specific chemical mediators are discussed further in Chapter 53.

Nursing Management

The nurse has an important role in preventing anaphylactic shock. The nurse must assess all patients for allergies or previous reactions to antigens (e.g., medications, blood products, foods, contrast agents, latex) and communicate the existence of these allergies or reactions to others. In addition, the nurse assesses the patient's understanding of previous reactions and steps taken by the patient and family to prevent further exposure to antigens. When new allergies are identified, the nurse advises the patient to wear or carry identification that names the specific allergen or antigen.

When administering any new medication, the nurse observes all patients for allergic reactions. This is especially important with antibiotics, beta-blockers, angiotensin inhibitors (angiotensin-converting enzyme inhibitors, angiotensin receptor blockers), aspirin, and nonsteroidal anti-inflammatory drugs (Triggiani et al., 2014). Previous adverse drug reactions increase the risk that the patient will develop a reaction to a new medication. If the patient reports an allergy to a medication, the nurse must be aware of the risks involved in the administration of similar medications.

At hospital and outpatient diagnostic testing sites, the nurse must identify patients who are at risk for anaphylactic reactions to contrast agents (radiopaque, dye-like substances that may contain iodine) used for diagnostic tests. The nurse must be knowledgeable about the clinical signs of anaphylaxis, takes immediate action if signs and symptoms occur, and is prepared to begin cardiopulmonary resuscitation if cardiorespiratory arrest occurs.

> **NURSING ALERT**
>
> **Patients with a known allergy to iodine or fish and those who have had previous allergic reactions to contrast agents are at high risk for anaphylactic reactions. This information must be communicated to the staff at the diagnostic testing site, including x-ray personnel.**

Community health and home care nurses who administer medications, including antibiotic agents, in the patient's home or other settings need to be prepared to administer epinephrine subcutaneously or intramuscularly in the event of an anaphylactic reaction.

After recovery from anaphylaxis, the patient and family require an explanation of the event. Furthermore, the nurse provides instruction about avoiding future exposure to antigens and administering emergency medications to treat anaphylaxis (see Chapter 53).

Multiple Organ Dysfunction Syndrome

MODS is altered organ function in acutely ill patients that requires medical intervention to support continued organ function. It is another phase in the progression of shock states. The actual incidence of MODS is difficult to determine, because it develops with acute illnesses that compromise tissue perfusion. Dysfunction of one organ system is associated with 20% mortality, and if more than four organs fail, the mortality may reach 60% (Rossaint & Zarbock, 2015).

Pathophysiology

MODS may be a complication of any form of shock, but it is most commonly seen in patients with sepsis and is a result of inadequate tissue perfusion. The precise mechanism by which MODS occurs remains unknown. However, MODS frequently occurs toward the end of the continuum of septic shock when tissue perfusion cannot be effectively restored. It is not possible to predict which patients who experience shock will develop MODS, partly because much of the organ damage occurs at the cellular level and therefore cannot be directly observed or measured.

The clinical presentation of MODS is insidious; tissues become hypoperfused at both a microcellular and macrocellular level, eventually causing organ dysfunction that requires mechanical and pharmacologic intervention to support organ function. Organ failure usually begins in the lungs, and cardiovascular instability as well as failure of the hepatic, GI, renal, immunologic, and central nervous systems follows (Guirgis, Khadpe, Kuntz, et al., 2014).

Clinical Manifestations

While it is not possible to predict MODS, clinical severity assessment tools may be used to anticipate patient risk of organ dysfunction and mortality. These clinical assessment tools include APACHE (Acute Physiology and Chronic Health Evaluation); SAPS (Simplified Acute Physiology Score); PIRO (Predisposing factors, the Infection, the host Response, and Organ dysfunction); and SOFA score (Gustot, 2011).

In MODS, the sequence of organ dysfunction varies depending on the patient's primary illness and comorbidities prior to experiencing shock. Advanced age, malnutrition, and coexisting disease appear to increase the risk of MODS in acutely ill patients. For simplicity of presentation, the classic pattern is described. Typically, the lungs are the first organs to show signs of dysfunction. The patient experiences progressive dyspnea and respiratory failure that are manifested as ALI or ARDS, requiring intubation and mechanical ventilation (see Chapters 24 and 26). The patient usually remains hemodynamically stable but may require increasing amounts of IV fluids and vasoactive agents to support the BP and cardiac output. Signs of a hypermetabolic state, characterized by hyperglycemia (elevated blood glucose level), hyperlactic acidemia (excess lactic acid in the blood), and increased BUN, are present. The metabolic rate may be 1.5 to 2 times the basal metabolic rate. At this time, there is a severe loss of skeletal muscle mass (autocatabolism) to meet the high-energy demands of the body.

After approximately 7 to 10 days, signs of hepatic dysfunction (e.g., elevated bilirubin and liver function tests) and renal dysfunction (e.g., elevated creatinine and anuria) are evident. As the lack of tissue perfusion continues, the hematologic system becomes dysfunctional, with worsening immunocompromise and increasing risk of bleeding. The cardiovascular system becomes unstable and unresponsive to vasoactive agents, and the patient's neurologic response progresses to a state of unresponsiveness or coma.

The goal of all shock states is to reverse the tissue hypoperfusion and hypoxia. If effective tissue perfusion is restored before organs become dysfunctional, the patient's condition stabilizes. Along the septic shock continuum, the onset of organ dysfunction is an ominous prognostic sign; the more organs that fail, the worse the outcome.

Medical Management

Prevention remains the top priority in managing MODS. Older patients are at increased risk for MODS because of the lack of physiologic reserve and the natural degenerative process, especially immune compromise (Guirgis et al., 2014). Early detection and documentation of initial signs of infection are essential in managing MODS in older adult patients. Subtle changes in mentation and a gradual rise in temperature are early warning signs. Other patients at risk for MODS are those with chronic illness, malnutrition, immunosuppression, or surgical or traumatic wounds.

If preventive measures fail, treatment measures to reverse MODS are aimed at (1) controlling the initiating event, (2) promoting adequate organ perfusion, and (3) providing nutritional support.

Nursing Management

The general plan of nursing care for patients with MODS is the same as that for patients with septic shock. Primary nursing interventions are aimed at supporting the patient and monitoring organ perfusion until primary organ insults are halted. Providing information and support to family members is a critical role of the nurse. It is important that the health care team address end-of-life decisions to ensure that supportive therapies are congruent with the patient's wishes (see Chapter 15).

Promoting Communication

Nurses should encourage frequent and open communication about treatment modalities and options to ensure that the patient's wishes regarding medical management are met. For patients who survive MODS, it is essential that they be informed about the goals of rehabilitation and expectations for progress toward these goals, because massive loss of skeletal muscle mass makes rehabilitation a long, slow process. A strong nurse–patient relationship built on effective communication provides needed encouragement during this phase of recovery.

Promoting Home, Community-Based, and Transitional Care

Educating Patients About Self-Care

Patients who experience and survive shock may have been unable to get out of bed for an extended period of time and are likely to have a slow, prolonged recovery. The patient and family are instructed about strategies to prevent further episodes of shock by identifying the factors implicated in the initial episode (Kleinpell et al., 2013). In addition, the patient and family require education about assessments needed to identify the complications that may occur after the patient is discharged from the hospital. Depending on the type of shock and its management, the patient or family may require education about treatment modalities such as emergency administration of medications, IV therapy, parenteral or enteral nutrition, skin care, exercise, and ambulation. The patient and family are also educated about the need for gradual increases in ambulation and other activity. The need for adequate nutrition is another crucial aspect of teaching.

Continuing and Transitional Care

Because of the physical toll associated with recovery from shock, patients may be cared for in a long-term care facility or rehabilitation setting after hospital discharge. Alternatively, a referral may be made for home, community-based, or transitional care. The nurse assesses the patient's physical status and monitors recovery. The nurse also assesses the adequacy of treatments that are continued at home and the ability of the patient and family to cope with these treatments. The patient is likely to require close medical supervision until complete recovery occurs. The nurse reinforces the importance of continuing medical care and helps the patient and family identify and mobilize community resources.

Critical Thinking Exercises

1 A patient arrives in the preoperative day surgery waiting room. The patient has a sensitivity to peanuts. The waiting room does not have a "no food or drink policy" and several family members are observed eating. The patient's significant other approaches the secretary in the waiting room stating that the patient has a peanut allergy and he is complaining of increasing anxiety, shortness of breath, and chest discomfort. He is flushed, anxious, tachypneic, and visibly uncomfortable. The secretary comments that it is common for preoperative surgery patients to be anxious and encourages the family member to engage in distracting behaviours with the patient. Three minutes later, the patient's significant other approaches the secretary stating that the patient is in extreme distress with worsening shortness of breath and chest discomfort. The secretary calls the preoperative intake nurse to immediately assess the patient. What are the immediate nursing priorities in providing care to this patient? What assessment data are needed to determine whether this patient is experiencing shock? What type of shock do you anticipate the patient may be experiencing and why? What nursing interventions and medical treatments should be anticipated? What additional nursing interventions should be implemented to prevent future adverse medication events for this patient? What follow-up might the nurse provide to the secretary and/or the leadership team related to food and drink in the preoperative waiting areas? Are there quality and safety interventions the nurse can lead to prevent future adverse events associated with food and drink in the preoperative day surgery waiting room?

2 A community-dwelling older woman is admitted to the hospital with a hip fracture after falling at home. Her past medical history includes hypertension and depression; both are well controlled by medications. She is also hard of hearing but does not wear hearing aids. She is now 72 hours post–hip fracture repair. Initial shift assessment reveals the patient to be confused and somewhat combative in behaviour. Should you assess the patient for acute delirium? Why or why not? You know that changes in mental status may be an early sign of sepsis in older adults. How would you assess this patient for the possibility of sepsis? What risk factors place an older patient at higher risk for sepsis? What risk factors does this patient have that placed her at increased risk for sepsis? How would you ensure the accuracy of vital signs and interpretation of vital signs in the older patient experiencing sepsis? What is the evidence base for these risk factors? How would the management of the older adult patient differ from that of a younger patient? What objective assessment data should you convey to the primary provider to support your assessment of possible sepsis? If the patient is thought to have sepsis, what interventions need to be initiated within the next 3- and 6-hour time frames?

3 A 34-year-old patient fell from his roof while doing home repairs. He was found down in his front yard by a passing neighbour. Upon admission to the hospital, he is not responsive to questions. He does not spontaneously move his lower extremities. Vital signs are: BP 92/60, HR 46 bpm, RR 28/min, and temperature 37.0°C (98.6°F). What types of shock do you think that this patient could be experiencing? What risk factors does this patient have for developing a shock state? What therapy and treatments would you anticipate? Describe the rationale for the therapies that you have identified. How would you use the patient's history, assessment, and symptom presentation to help you identify shock states? Describe likely symptoms and the underlying pathophysiology of the shock state.

4 A 47-year-old woman presents to the ED complaining of generalized fatigue, indigestion, uncomfortable chest pain, and shortness of breath. What clinical condition(s)

do you believe the patient may be experiencing? If cardiogenic shock is suspected, what nursing interventions do you anticipate initiating in the care of this patient? What vasopressor and inotropic agents may need to be started? What laboratory analysis will be required in the care of this patient? What risk factors can be identified for this patient related to her presenting condition and subsequent shock state? What educational interventions may be incorporated into the patient's plan of care to optimize her health after hospital discharge? If the primary provider plans to insert a central venous catheter, what essential care is required of the nurse to reduce the risk of CLABSI for the patient?

REFERENCES AND SELECTED READINGS

Books

American College of Surgeons, Committee on Trauma. (2012). *Advanced trauma life support for doctors: Instructors course manual* (9th ed.). Chicago, IL: American College of Surgeons.

Antonelli, M., DeBacker, D., Dorman, T., et al. (2016). Surviving Sepsis campaign responds to Sepsis-3. Mount Prospect, IL: Surviving Sepsis Campaign.

Brenner, G. M., & Stevens, C. (2017). *Brenner and Stevens' Pharmacology E-Book*. Elsevier Health Sciences.

Maier, R. V. (2015). Approach to the patient with shock. In D. Kasper, J. Loscalzo, S. Hauser, et al. (Eds.). *Harrison's principles of internal medicine* (19th ed.). New York: McGraw-Hill Medical.

Journals and Electronic Documents

American Heart Association. (2015). Temperature management after cardiac arrest: An advisory statement by the Advanced Life Support Task Force of the International Liaison Committee on Resuscitation and the American Heart Association Emergency Cardiovascular Care Committee and the Council on Cardiopulmonary, Critical Care, Perioperative and Resuscitation. Retrieved from https://www.ahajournals.org/doi/pdf/10.1161/CIR.0000000000000313

Annane, D., Siami, S., Jaber, S., et al. (2013). Effects of fluid resuscitation with colloids vs crystalloids on mortality in critically ill patients presenting with hypovolemic shock: the CRISTAL randomized trial. *JAMA, 310*(17), 1809–1817.

Balogh, Z., Lumsdaine, W., Moore, E. E., et al. (2014). Post-injury abdominal compartment syndrome: From recognition to prevention. *Lancet, 384*(9952), 1466–1475.

Barr, J., Fraser, G. L., Puntillo, K., et al. (2013). Clinical practice guidelines for the management of pain, agitation, and delirium in adult patients in the intensive care unit. *Critical Care Medicine, 41*(1), 263–306.

Blaser, A. R., Starkopf, J., Kirsimagi, U., et al. (2014). Definition, prevalence, and outcome of feeding intolerance in intensive care: A systematic review and meta-analysis. *Acta Anaesthesiologica Scandinavica, 58*(8), 914–922.

Bergeron, N., Dubois, M. J., Dumont, M., et al. (2001). Intensive Care Delirium Screening Checklist: Evaluation of a new screening tool. *Intensive care medicine, 27*(5), 859–864.

Bulger, E. M., May, S., Kerby, J. D., et al. (2011). Out of hospital hypertonic resuscitation after traumatic hypovolemic shock: A randomized, placebo, controlled trial. *Annals of Surgery, 253*(3), 431–441.

Centers for Medicare & Medicaid Services. (2014). Improve quality of care during hospital inpatient stays. Retrieved November 28, 2015, from www.cms.gov/Newsroom/MediaReleaseDatabase/Fact-sheets/2014-Fact-sheets-items/2014-08-04-2.html

Cestero, R. F., & Dent, D. L. (2015). Endpoints of resuscitation. *Surgical Clinics of North America, 95*(2), 319–336.

Davis, L. L. (2014). Cardiovascular issues in older adults. *Critical Care Nursing Clinics of North America, 26*(1), 61–89.

Dellinger, R. P. (2015). Foreword. The future of sepsis performance improvement. *Critical Care Medicine, 43*(9), 1787–1799.

Dellinger, R. P., Levy, M. M., Rhodes, A., et al. (2013). Surviving Sepsis Campaign: International guidelines for management of severe sepsis and septic shock: 2012. *Critical Care Medicine, 41*(2), 580–637.

deWitt, B., Joshi, R., Meislin, H., et al. (2014). Optimizing oxygen delivery in the critically ill: Assessment of volume responsiveness in the septic patient. *The Journal of Emergency Medicine, 47*(5), 608–615.

Dubick, M. A., Shek, P., & Wade, C. E. (2013). ROC trials update on prehospital hypertonic saline resuscitation in the aftermath of the US-Canadian trials. *Clinics, 68*(6), 883–886.

Giles, T. M., & Hall, K. L. (2013). Qualitative systematic review: The unique experiences of the nurse-family member when a loved one is admitted with a critical illness. *Journal of Advanced Nursing, 70*(7), 1451–1464.

Green, J. M. (2015). Essentials of sepsis management. *Surgical Clinics of North America, 95*(2), 355–365.

Griesdale, D. E., DeSouza, R. J., VanDam, R. M., et al. (2009). Intensive insulin therapy and mortality among critically ill patients: A meta-analysis including NICE-Sugar study data. *Canadian Medical Association Journal, 180*(8), 821–827.

Guirgis, F. W., Khadpe, J. D., Kuntz, G. M., et al. (2014). Persistent organ dysfunction after severe sepsis: A systematic review. *Journal of Critical Care, 29*(3), 320–326.

Gustot, T. (2011). Multiple organ failure in sepsis: Prognosis and role of systemic inflammatory response. *Current Opinion in Critical Care, 17*(2), 153–159.

Hillier, B., Wilson, C., Chamberlain, D., et al. (2013). Preventing ventilator-associated pneumonia through oral care, product selection, and application method: A literature review. *AACN Advanced Critical Care, 24*(1), 38–58.

Hinkle, L. J., Bosslet, G. T., & Torke, A. M. (2015). Factors associated with family satisfaction with end of life care in the ICU: A systematic review. *Chest, 147*(1), 82–93.

Holcomb, J. B., Tiley, B. C., Baraniuk, S., et al. (2015). Transfusion of plasma, platelets, and red blood cells in a 1:1:1 vs a 1:1:2 ration and mortality in patients with severe trauma: The PROPPR randomized clinical trial. *JAMA, 313*(5), 471–482.

Holodinsky J. K., Roberts, D. J., Ball, C. G., et al. (2013). Risk factors for intra-abdominal hypertension and abdominal compartment syndrome among adult intensive care unit patients: A systematic review and meta-analysis. *Critical Care, 17*(5), R249.

Institute for Healthcare Improvement. (2012). How-to guide: Prevent central line–associated bloodstream infection. Retrieved November 28, 2015, from www.ihi.org/knowledge/Pages/Tools/HowtoGuidePreventCentralLineAssociatedBloodstreamInfection.aspx

Institute for Healthcare Improvement. (2014a). Implement the sepsis resuscitation bundle. Retrieved November 29, 2015, from www.ihi.org/resources/Pages/Tools/SevereSepsisBundles.aspx

Institute for Healthcare Improvement (IHI). (2014b). Improving stories: Early warning systems: Scorecards that save lives. Retrieved February 18, 2016, from www.ihi.org/resources/PublishingImages/Image_PatientAssessmentObservationInfusionMonitoring.jpg

Kanwar, R., Delasobera, B. E., Hudson, K., et al. (2015). Emergency department evaluation and treatment of cervical spine injuries. *Emergency Medicine Clinics of North America, 33*(2), 241–282.

Kleinpell, R., Aitken, L., & Schorr, C. A. (2013). Implications of the new international sepsis guidelines for nursing care. *American Journal of Critical Care, 22*(3), 212–222.

Lee, R. (2015). Ask the experts: Time frames for sepsis screening criteria. *Critical Care Nurse, 35*(3), 74–75.

Levi, M., & Poll, T. V. (2015). Coagulation in patients with severe sepsis. *Seminars in Thrombosis and Hemostasis, 41*(1), 9–15.

Levy, M. M., Rhodes, A., Phillips, G. S., et al. (2015). Surviving Sepsis Campaign: Association between performance metrics and outcomes in a 7.5 year study. *Critical Care Medicine, 43*(1), 3–12.

Lineberry, C., & Stein, D. E. (2014). Infection, sepsis, and immune function in the older adult receiving critical care. *Critical Care Nursing Clinics of North America, 26*(1), 47–60.

Makic, M. B. F. (2013). Preventing delirium in postoperative patients. *Journal of PeriAnesthesia Nursing, 28*(6), 404–408.

Makic, M. B. F., Rauen, C. A., Jones, K., et al. (2015). Continuing to challenge practice to be evidence-based. *Critical Care Nurse, 35*(2), 39–50.

Makic, M. B. F., Rauen, C. A., Watson, R., et al. (2014). Examining the evidence to guide practice: Challenging practice habits. *Critical Care Nurse, 34*(2), 28–45; quiz 46.

Marik P. E., & Bellomo, R. (2013). Stress hyperglycemia: An essential survival response. *Critical Care, 17*(2), 305. Retrieved November 29, 2015, from ccforum.com/content/17/2/305

Marik, P. E., Baram, M., & Vahid, B. (2008). Does central venous pressure predict fluid responsiveness? A systematic review of the literature and the tale of seven mares. *Chest, 134*(1), 172–178.

Marschall, J., Mermel, L. A., Fakih, M., et al. (2014). Strategies to prevent central-line associated blood stream infections in acute care hospitals: 2014 update. *Infection Control and Hospital Epidemiology*, *35*(7), 753–771.

Martindale, R. G., & Warren, M. (2015). Should enteral nutrition be started in the first week of critical illness? *Current Opinion in Clinical Nutrition & Metabolic Care*, *18*(2), 202–206.

Mayr, F. B., Yende, S., & Angus, D. C. (2014). Epidemiology of severe sepsis. *Virulence*, *5*(1), 4–11.

McEnvoy, M. T., & Shander, A. (2013). Anemia, bleeding, and blood transfusion in the intensive care unit: Causes, risks, costs, and new strategies. *American Journal of Critical Care*, *22*(6), eS1–eS13; quiz eS14.

Moore, J. P. R., Dyson, A., Singer, M., et al. (2015). Microcirculatory dysfunction and resuscitations: Why when, and how. *British Journal of Anaesthesia*, *115*(3), 366–375.

Muraro, A., Hoffmann-Sommergruber, K., Holzhauser, T., et al. (2014). EAACI food allergy and anaphylaxis guidelines: Protecting consumers with food allergies, understanding food consumption, meeting regulations and identifying unmet needs. *Allergy*, *69*(11), 1464–1472.

Ng, R., & Yeghiazarians, Y. (2013). Post myocardial infarction cardiogenic shock: A review of current therapies. *Journal of Intensive Care Medicine*, *28*(3), 151–165.

Perel, P., Roberts, I., & Ker, K. (2013). Colloids versus crystalloids for fluid resuscitation in critically ill patients (review). *Cochrane Database of Systematic Reviews*, (2), CD000567.

Perrin, K. O., & Kazanowski, M. (2015). Overcoming barriers to palliative care consultation. *Critical Care Nurse*, *35*(5), 44–52.

Prucha, M., Belligan, G., & Zazula, R. (2014). Sepsis biomarkers. *Clinica Chimica Acta*, *440*(2), 97–103.

Rhodes, A., Evans, L. E., Alhazzani, W., et al. (2017). Surviving Sepsis Campaign: International Guidelines for Management of Sepsis and Septic Shock: 2016. *Critical Care Medicine*, *45*(3), 486–552.

Rivers, E. P., McIntyre, L., Morro, D. C., et al. (2005). Early and innovative interventions for severe sepsis and septic shock: Taking advantage of a window of opportunity. *Canadian Medical Association Journal*, *173*(9), 1054–1065.

Rossaint, J., & Zarbock, A. (2015). Pathogenesis of multiple organ failure in sepsis. *Critical Reviews in Immunology*, *35*(4), 277–291.

Schmidt, M., Mandel, J., Sexton, D. J., et al. (2017). Evaluation and management of suspected sepsis and septic shock in adults. UpToDate. Retrieved 29 September, 2017, from https://www. uptodate. com/contents/evaluation-and-management-of-suspected-sepsisand-septic-shock-in-adults

See, K. C., Mukhopadhyay, A., Lau, S. C., et al. (2015). Shock in the first 24 hours of intensive care unit stay: Observational study of protocol-based fluid management. *Shock*, *43*(5), 456–462.

Silva, P. L., Pelosi, P., & Rocco, P. R. M. (2014). Fluids in acute respiratory distress syndrome: Pros and cons. *Current Opinion in Critical Care*, *20*(1), 104–112.

Singer, M., Deutschman, C. S., Seymour, C. W., et al. (2016). The third international consensus definitions for sepsis and septic shock (sepsis-3). *JAMA*, *315*(8), 801–810.

Society for Healthcare Epidemiology of America. (2015). SHEA Guideline Central. Retrieved November 28, 2015, from www.guidelinecentral.com/share/pocketcard/53d67314007df/#i469f5e2f

Stapleton, R. D., Jones, N., & Heyland, D. K. (2007). Feeding critically ill patients: what is the optimal amount of energy?. *Critical care medicine*, *35*(9), S535–S540.

Statistics Canada. (2016). Health at a glance deaths involving sepsis in Canada. Retrieved from https://www150.statcan.gc.ca/n1/pub/82-624-x/2016001/article/14308-eng.htm

Subramaniam, S., Tiruvoipati, R., & Botha, J. (2015). Current advances in the use of therapeutic hypothermia. *Therapeutic Hypothermia and Temperature Management*, *5*(1), 13–16.

Surviving Sepsis Bundle. (2015). Retrieved November 28, 2015, from www.survivingsepsis.org/SiteCollectionDocuments/SSC_Bundle.pdf

Surviving Sepsis Campaign. (2016). International Guidelines for Management of Sepsis and Septic Shock. Retrieved March 15, 2019, from www.survivingsepsis.org

Tariq, S., & Aronow, W. (2015). Use of inotropic agents in treatment of systolic heart failure. *International Journal of Molecular Sciences*, *16*(12), 29060–29068.

Task Force. (2016). The Third International Consensus Definitions for Sepsis and Septic Shock (Sepsis-3). Retrieved from https://www.ncbi.nlm.nih.gov/pmc/articles/PMC4968574/pdf/nihms794087.pdf

Tay, E. T. (2015). Intraosseous access. Medscape. Retrieved November 29, 2015, from reference.medscape.com/article/80431-overview

Tharmaratnam, D., Nolan, J., & Jain, A. (2013). Management of cardiogenic shock complicating acute coronary syndromes. *Heart*, *99*(3), 1614–1623.

Triggiani, M., Montagni, M., Parente, R., et al. (2014). Anaphylaxis and cardiovascular diseases: A dangerous liaison. *Current Opinion in Allergy and Clinical Immunology*, *14*(4), 309–315.

Twibell, R. S., Craig, S., Siela, D., et al. (2015). Being there: Inpatients' perceptions of family presence during resuscitation and invasive cardiac procedures. *American Journal of Critical Care*, *24*(6), 108–115.

Vanderbilt University Medical Center. (2013). ICU delirium and cognitive impairment study group. Retrieved February 15, 2016, from www.icudelirium.org/delirium/monitoring.html

Vincent, J. L., Moreno, R., Takala, J., et al. (1996). The SOFA (Sepsis-related Organ Failure Assessment) score to describe organ dysfunction/failure. On behalf of the Working Group on Sepsis-Related Programs of the European Society of Intensive Care Medicine. *Intensive Care Medicine*, *22*(7), 707–710.

Wacker, D. A., & Winters, M. E. (2014). Shock. *Emergency Medicine Clinics of North America*, *32*(4), 747–758.

World Sepsis Day. Sepsis Fact Sheet. (2015). World Sepsis Day. Retrieved November 29, 2015, from www.world-sepsis-day.org/CONTENTPIC/2015_WSD_FactSheet_long_English.pdf

Yealy, D. M., Kellum J. A., Huang, D. T., et al. (2014). A randomized trial of protocol-based care for early septic shock. *New England Journal of Medicine*, *370*(18), 1683–1693.

Zarbock, A., Gomez, H., & Kellum, J. A. (2014). Sepsis-induced acute kidney injury revisited: Pathophysiology, prevention and future therapies. *Current Opinion in Critical Care*, *20*(6), 588–595.

Zarychanski, R., Abou-Setta, A. M., Kanji S., et al. (2015). The efficacy and safety of heparin in patients with sepsis: A systematic review and meta-analysis. *Critical Care Medicine*, *43*(3), 511–518.

Zhang, S., Wadhwa, R., Haydel, J., et al. (2013). Spine and spinal cord trauma: Diagnosis and management. *Neurologic Clinics*, *31*(1), 183–206.

Resources

Institute for Healthcare Improvement: www.ihi.org
Surviving Sepsis: www.survivingsepsis.org

UNIT 4

Perioperative Concepts and Nursing Management

Case Study: A PATIENT RECOVERING FROM ABDOMINAL SURGERY

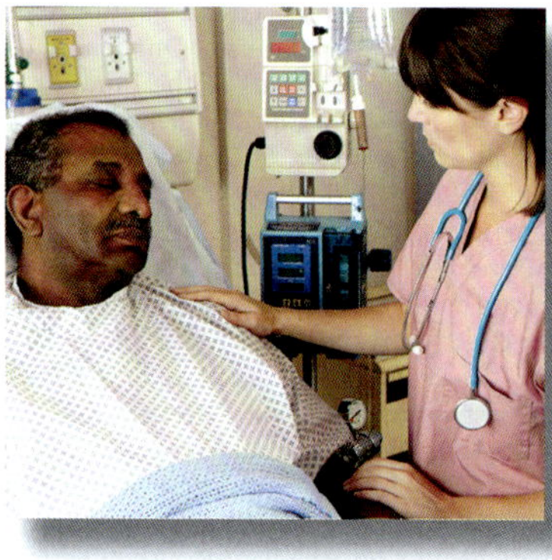

A patient recently diagnosed with lymphoma had a lymph node removed from his right groin area to stage the lymphoma. He is now admitted to the hospital with fever and sepsis from infection of the wound. He is drowsy but easily awakened. The patient is scheduled for surgery tomorrow to debride the wound. The surgeon visits the patient to describe the procedure and the risks and benefits of the surgery. He then asks the nurse to witness the informed consent signed by the patient.

QSEN Competency Focus: Patient-Centred Care

The complexities inherent in today's health care system challenge nurses to demonstrate integration of specific interdisciplinary core competencies that are aimed at ensuring the delivery of safe and quality patient care (Institute of Medicine, 2003). The Quality and Safety Education for Nurses project (QSEN, 2017; Cronenwett, Sherwood, Barnsteiner, et al., 2007) provides a framework for the knowledge, skills, and attitudes (KSAs) required for nurses to demonstrate competency in these key areas, which include ***patient-centred care***, ***interdisciplinary teamwork and collaboration***, ***evidence-based practice***, ***quality improvement***, ***safety***, and ***informatics.***

Patient-Centred Care Definition: Recognize the patient or designee as the source of control and full partner in providing compassionate and coordinated care based on respect for patient's preferences, values, and needs.

SELECTED PRE-LICENSURE KSAs	APPLICATION AND REFLECTION
Knowledge	
Explore ethical and legal implications of patient-centred care.	How would you define ethical patient-centred care? Compare and contrast ethical and legal implications of patient-centred care.
Skills	
Facilitate informed consent.	What is the responsibility of the nurse in obtaining an informed consent? What is within the scope of practice for a nurse in obtaining an informed consent? If the patient has questions about the procedure, how should the nurse respond? Discuss how the nurse would advocate for the patient so that he receives the care that is best for him.
Attitudes	
Acknowledge the tension that may exist between patient rights and the organizational responsibility for professional, ethical care.	Think about your own experience and training with patient rights and informed consent. Why is it important for nurses to demonstrate respect for the principles of informed consent?

Cronenwett, L., Sherwood, G., Barnsteiner, J., et al. (2007). Quality and safety education for nurses. *Nursing Outlook*, *55*(3), 122–131; Institute of Medicine. (2003). *Health professions education: A bridge to quality*. Washington, DC: National Academies Press; and QSEN Institute. (2017). *QSEN competencies: Definitions and pre-licensure KSAs*. Retrieved June 12, 2019, from www.qsen.org/competencies/pre-licensure-ksas

19 Preoperative Nursing Management

Adapted by Ruhina Rana

Learning Objectives

On completion of this chapter, the learner will be able to:

1. Define the three phases of perioperative patient care.
2. Describe a comprehensive preoperative assessment to identify surgical risk factors.
3. Identify considerations related to preoperative nursing care of older adults, patients who are obese, and patients with disabilities.
4. Identify legal and ethical considerations related to obtaining informed consent for surgery.
5. Describe preoperative nursing measures that decrease the risk for infection and other postoperative complications.
6. Describe the immediate preoperative preparation of the patient.
7. Develop a preoperative teaching plan designed to promote the patient's recovery from anesthesia and surgery, thus preventing postoperative complications.

Surgery, whether elective or emergent, is a stressful, complex event. In the past decades, the patient scheduled for elective surgery was admitted to the hospital at least 1 day before surgery for evaluation and preparation; these activities are now often completed before admission to the surgical setting. Today, as a result of advances in technology, surgical techniques and instrumentation, and anesthesia, many surgical procedures take place in outpatient or ambulatory settings in which the patient returns home after recovering from the anesthesia in the postanesthesia care unit (PACU). Often, the surgical patients who require hospital stays are trauma patients, acutely ill patients, patients undergoing major surgery, patients who require emergency surgery, patients who experience complications from surgery, and patients with concurrent medical disorders. As a result, the acuity and complexity of surgical patients and procedures have increased in the inpatient setting. Although each setting (ambulatory, outpatient, or inpatient) offers its own unique advantages for the delivery of patient care, all patients require a comprehensive preoperative nursing assessment and nursing interventions to prepare for surgery.

There is a steady increase in the number of surgeries, both inpatient and day surgeries, across Canada over the years. For example, from 2016 to 2017, Canada recorded over 483,000 in patient surgeries (Canadian Institute for Health Information [CIHI], 2018). Also, wait times for nonemergent surgeries remain a concern for Canadians. Pan-Canadian wait times for hip fracture repair continue to improve, with the percentage of patients receiving surgery within the 48-hour benchmark increasing from 81% in 2012 to 86% in 2016. Pan-Canadian wait times for joint replacement remain unchanged in the last 5 years, with 3 of 4 patients receiving hip or knee replacement surgery within the established benchmark of 182 days; 79% of hip replacement patients and 73% of knee replacement patients received their surgery within the benchmark. There has been a marked increase in procedure volumes since 2012: 22% for hip replacement and 18% for knee replacement (Wait Times for Priority Procedures in Canada, 2017).

Traumatic and emergency surgeries most often result in prolonged hospital stays. Patients who are acutely ill or undergoing major surgery, and patients with concurrent medical disorders, may require supportive supplementary care from other medical disciplines, which can be coordinated more easily within the hospital setting. The high acuity level of surgical inpatients and the greater

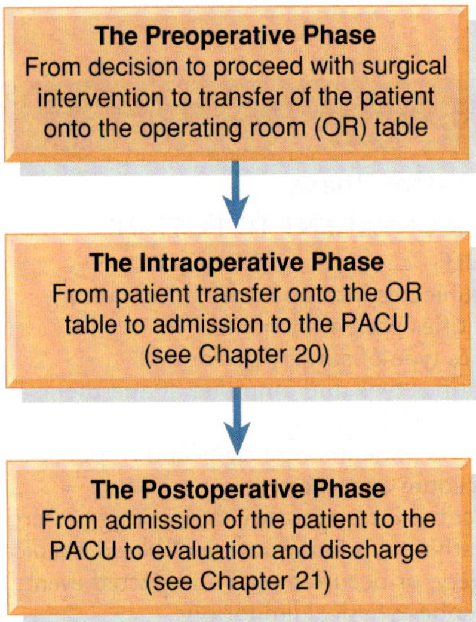

FIGURE 19-1. The perioperative period.

complexity of procedures have placed greater demands on the practice of nursing in this setting.

Although each setting (ambulatory, outpatient, or inpatient) offers its own unique advantages for the delivery of patient care, all patients require a comprehensive preoperative nursing assessment, patient education, and nursing interventions to prepare for surgery.

Perioperative Nursing

Communication, teamwork, and patient assessment are crucial to ensure good patient outcomes in the perioperative setting. Professional perioperative and perianesthesia nursing standards encompass the domains of behavioural response, physiologic response, and patient safety and are used as guides toward development of nursing diagnoses, interventions, and plans. Perioperative nursing, which spans the entire surgical experience, consists of three phases that begin and end at particular points in the sequence of surgical experience events. The field of perioperative and perianesthesia nursing includes a wide variety of nursing functions. The **perioperative period** consists of three phases that begin and end at a particular point in the sequence of events in the surgical experience. See Figure 19-1.

Each **perioperative phase** includes a wide range of activities the nurse performs using the nursing process and based on the standards of practice of the Operating Room Nurses Association of Canada (ORNAC) (2013). Chart 19-1 presents nursing activities characteristic of the three perioperative phases of care. Each phase of the surgical experience is reviewed in more detail in this unit.

Advances in Technology and Anesthesia

Advances in technology have led to more complex procedures, more complicated microsurgical and laser technology, more sophisticated bypass equipment, increased use of laparoscopic and **minimally invasive surgery**, and more sensitive monitoring devices. Surgery today can involve the transplantation of multiple human organs, the implantation of mechanical devices, the reattachment of body parts, and the use of robots and minimally invasive procedures in the OR.

Advances in anesthesia have kept pace with these surgical technologies. More sophisticated monitoring and new pharmacologic agents, such as short-acting anesthetics and more effective antiemetics, have improved postoperative pain management, reduced postoperative nausea and vomiting, and shortened procedure and recovery times.

Surgical Classifications

Surgery may be performed for various reasons. A surgical procedure may be diagnostic (e.g., biopsy, exploratory laparotomy), curative (e.g., excision of a tumour or an inflamed appendix), or reparative (e.g., multiple wound repair). It may be reconstructive or cosmetic (e.g., mammoplasty or a facelift) or palliative (e.g., to relieve pain or alleviate a problem—for instance, a gastrostomy tube may be inserted to compensate for the inability to swallow food). Surgery may also be classified according to the

Glossary

ambulatory surgery: includes outpatient, same-day, or short-stay surgery that does not require an overnight hospital stay

informed consent: the patient's autonomous decision about whether to undergo a surgical procedure, based on the nature of the condition, the treatment options, and the risks and benefits involved

intraoperative phase: period of time that begins with transfer of the patient to the operating room table and continues until the patient is admitted to the postanesthesia care unit

minimally invasive surgery: surgical procedures that use specialized instruments inserted into the body either through natural orifices or through small incisions

perioperative phase: period of time that constitutes the surgical experience; includes the preoperative, intraoperative, and postoperative phases of nursing care

postoperative phase: period of time that begins with the admission of the patient to the postanesthesia care unit and ends after follow-up evaluation in the clinical setting or home

preadmission testing: diagnostic testing performed before admission to the hospital

preoperative phase: period of time from when the decision for surgical intervention is made to when the patient is transferred to the operating room table

CHART 19-1

Examples of Nursing Activities in the Perioperative Phases of Care

Preoperative Phase

PREADMISSION TESTING (PAT)

1. Initiates initial preoperative assessment
2. Initiates teaching appropriate to patient's needs
3. Involves family in interview
4. Verifies completion of preoperative diagnostic testing
5. Verifies understanding of surgeon-specific preoperative orders (e.g., bowel preparation, preoperative shower)
6. Discusses and reviews advanced directive document
7. Begins discharge planning by assessing patient's need for postoperative transportation and care

ADMISSION TO SURGICAL CENTRE

1. Completes preoperative assessment
2. Assesses for risks of postoperative complications
3. Reports unexpected findings or any deviations from normal
4. Verifies that operative consent has been signed
5. Coordinates patient teaching and plan of care with nursing staff and other health team members
6. Reinforces previous teaching
7. Explains phases in perioperative period and expectations
8. Answers patient's and family's questions

In the Holding Area

1. Assesses patient's status, baseline pain, and nutritional status
2. Reviews chart
3. Identifies patient
4. Verifies surgical site and marks site per institutional policy
5. Establishes intravenous line
6. Administers medications if prescribed
7. Takes measures to ensure patient's comfort
8. Provides psychological support
9. Communicates patient's emotional status to other appropriate members of the health care team

Intraoperative Phase

MAINTENANCE OF SAFETY

1. Maintains aseptic, controlled environment
2. Effectively manages human resources, equipment, and supplies for individualized patient care
3. Transfers patient to operating room bed or table
4. Positions patient based on functional alignment and exposure of surgical site
5. Applies grounding device to patient
6. Ensures that the sponge, needle, and instrument counts are correct
7. Completes intraoperative documentation

PHYSIOLOGIC MONITORING

1. Calculates effects on patient of excessive fluid loss or gain
2. Distinguishes normal from abnormal cardiopulmonary data
3. Reports changes in patient's vital signs
4. Institutes measures to promote normothermia

PSYCHOLOGICAL SUPPORT (BEFORE INDUCTION AND WHEN PATIENT IS CONSCIOUS)

1. Provides emotional support to patient
2. Stands near or touches patient during procedures and induction
3. Continues to assess patient's emotional status

Postoperative Phase

TRANSFER OF PATIENT TO POSTANESTHESIA CARE UNIT

1. Communicates intraoperative information
   a. Identifies patient by name
   b. States type of surgery performed
   c. Identifies type and amounts of anesthetic and analgesic agents used
   d. Reports patient's vital signs and response to surgical procedure and anesthesia
   e. Describes intraoperative factors (e.g., insertion of drains or catheters, administration of blood, medications during surgery, or occurrence of unexpected events)
   f. Describes physical limitations
   g. Reports patient's preoperative level of consciousness
   h. Communicates necessary equipment needs
   i. Communicates presence of family or significant others

POSTOPERATIVE ASSESSMENT RECOVERY AREA

1. Determines patient's immediate response to surgical intervention
2. Monitors patient's vital signs and physiologic status
3. Assesses patient's pain level and administers appropriate pain relief measures
4. Maintains patient's safety (airway, circulation, prevention of injury)
5. Administers medications, fluid, and blood component therapy, if prescribed
6. Provides oral fluids if prescribed for ambulatory surgery patient
7. Assesses patient's readiness for transfer to in-hospital unit or for discharge home based on institutional policy (e.g., Aldrete score, see Chapter 20)

SURGICAL NURSING UNIT

1. Continues close monitoring of patient's physical and psychological response to surgical intervention
2. Assesses patient's pain level and administers appropriate pain relief measures
3. Provides teaching to patient during immediate recovery period
4. Assists patient in recovery and preparation for discharge home
5. Determines patient's psychological status
6. Assists with discharge planning

HOME OR CLINIC

1. Provides follow-up care during office or clinic visit or by telephone contact
2. Reinforces previous teaching and answers patient's and family's questions about surgery and follow-up care
3. Assesses patient's response to surgery and anesthesia and their effects on body image and function
4. Determines family's perception of surgery and its outcome

TABLE 19-1 Categories of Surgery Based on Urgency

Classification	Indications for Surgery	Examples
I. Emergent—Patient requires immediate attention; disorder may be life-threatening	Without delay	Severe bleeding Bladder or intestinal obstruction Fractured skull Gunshot or stab wounds Extensive burns
II. Urgent—Patient requires prompt attention	Within 24–30 hours	Acute gallbladder infection Kidney or ureteral stones
III. Required—Patient needs to have surgery	Plan within a few weeks or months	Prostatic hyperplasia without bladder obstruction Thyroid disorders Cataracts
IV. Elective—Patient should have surgery	Failure to have surgery not catastrophic	Repair of scars Simple hernia Vaginal repair
V. Optional—Decision rests with patient	Personal preference	Cosmetic surgery

degree of urgency involved: emergent, urgent, required, elective, and optional (Table 19-1).

Preadmission Testing

Concurrent with the increase in ambulatory surgeries have been changes in the delivery of and payment for health care. The pressure to reduce hospital stays and contain costs has resulted in diagnostic **preadmission testing** (PAT) and preoperative preparation prior to admission. Many facilities have presurgical services department. This department facilitates PAT and initiate the nursing assessment process, which focuses on admission data, such as patients demographics, health history and other information pertinent to the surgical procedure such as appropriate consent forms, patient teaching, assessment by the anesthesiologist and pharmacist as well as the nurse (Rothrock, 2018). The increasing use of ambulatory, same-day, or short-stay surgery means that patients leave the hospital sooner, which increases the need for teaching, discharge planning, preparation for self-care, and referral for home care and rehabilitation services.

Special Considerations During the Perioperative Period

Gerontologic Considerations

The hazards of surgery for older adults are proportional to the number and severity of coexisting health problems and the nature and duration of the operative procedure. The underlying principle that guides the preoperative assessment, surgical care, and postoperative care is that older adult patients have less physiologic reserve (the ability of an organ to return to normal after a disturbance in its equilibrium) than younger patients. According to Watt, Tricco, Talbot-Hamon et al. (2018) pneumonia, wound infection, and venous thromboembolism are the most reported postsurgical complications in older adults in Canada. Cardiac reserves are lower, renal and hepatic functions are depressed, and gastrointestinal activity is likely to be reduced. Dehydration, constipation, and malnutrition may occur. Sensory limitations, such as impaired vision or hearing, and mobility limitations are among common reasons for falls, as well as opioid use (Doaust, Paquet, Moore, et al., 2018). Therefore, the nurse must be alert to maintaining a safe environment. Arthritis is common in older people and may affect mobility, making it difficult for the patient to turn from one side to the other or ambulate without discomfort. Protective measures include adequate padding for tender areas, moving the patient slowly, protecting bony prominences from prolonged pressure, and frequent turning to offload pressure areas at risk to promote circulation.

As the body ages, its ability to perspire decreases. Because decreased perspiration leads to dry, itchy skin that becomes fragile and easily abraded, precautions are taken when moving the older adult. Decreased subcutaneous fat makes older people more susceptible to temperature changes. A lightweight cotton blanket is an appropriate cover when an older adult is moved to and from the OR.

Because the older adult patient may have greater risks during the perioperative period, skilled assessment, careful anesthesia with a geriatric perspective, avoiding certain drugs, and preventing delirium and other complications becomes critical (Sieber & Barnett, 2011).

In addition, the nurse should incorporate pain management information and pain communication skills when teaching the older adult patient how to obtain greater postoperative pain relief (see Providing Patient Teaching).

Patients Who Have Obesity

Like age, obesity increases the risk and severity of complications associated with surgery. In Canada, 60.2% of people are considered overweight or to have obesity (Statistics Canada, 2014). During surgery, fatty tissues are especially susceptible to infection. In addition, obesity increases technical and mechanical problems related to surgery. Therefore, dehiscence (wound separation) and wound infections are more common. Moreover, the patient with obesity may be more difficult to care for because of the excessive weight. It has been estimated that for each [illegible] of excess weight, about 25 additional miles of [illegible]s are needed, and this places increased demands [illegible] heart. The patient tends to have shallow respirations when supine, which increases the risk of hypoventilation and postoperative pulmonary complications. Short thick necks, large tongues, and redundant pharyngeal tissue, along with an increased demand for oxygen and decreased reserves, can make intubation difficult (Magalhaes, Marques, Govêia, et al., 2013). The anesthesiologist or anesthetist also assesses for obstructive sleep apnea (OSA) that is often diagnosed and treated with continuous positive airway pressure (CPAP) preoperatively. The use of CPAP should continue throughout the perioperative period for those diagnosed with or suspected of having (due to obesity) OSA (Chung, Nagappa, Singh, et al., 2016). As the incidence of obesity continues to rise, the care, patient counseling and teaching of such patients will fall on the nurse and allied health care providers to support patients who have obesity (Plourde & Prud'homme, 2012).

Patients With Disabilities

Special considerations for patients with mental or physical disabilities include the need for appropriate assistive devices, modifications in preoperative teaching, and additional assistance with and attention to positioning or transferring. Assistive devices include hearing aids, eyeglasses, braces, prostheses, and other devices. People who are hearing impaired may need a sign interpreter or some alternative communication system perioperatively. If the patient relies on signing or speech (lip) reading and his or her eyeglasses or contact lenses are removed or the health care staff wears surgical masks, an alternative method of communication will be needed. These needs must be identified in the preoperative evaluation and clearly communicated to personnel. Specific strategies for accommodating the patient's needs must be identified in advance. Ensuring the security of assistive devices is important, because these devices are expensive and are likely to be lost.

Most patients are directed to move from the stretcher to the OR table and back again. In addition to being unable to see or hear instructions, the patient with a disability may be unable to move without special devices or a great deal of assistance. The patient with a disability that affects body position (e.g., cerebral palsy, postpolio syndrome, and other neuromuscular disorders) may need special positioning during surgery to prevent pain and injury. Moreover, these patients may be unable to sense whether their extremities are positioned incorrectly.

Patients with respiratory problems related to a disability (e.g., multiple sclerosis, muscular dystrophy) may experience difficulties unless the problems are made known to the anesthesiologist or anesthetist and adjustments are made. These factors need to be clearly identified in the preoperative period and communicated to the appropriate personnel.

Patients Undergoing Ambulatory Surgery

Ambulatory surgery includes outpatient, same-day, or short-stay surgery that does not require an overnight hospital stay but may entail an admission to an inpatient hospital setting for less than 24 hours. During the brief time the patient and family spend in the ambulatory setting, the nurse must quickly and comprehensively assess and anticipate the patient's needs and at the same time begin assessing for complications, and planning for discharge and follow-up home care.

The nurse needs to be sure that the patient and family understand that the patient will first go to the preoperative holding area, then to the OR for the surgical procedure and then to the PACU before being discharged home with the family later that day. Other preoperative teaching content should also be verified and reinforced as needed (see later discussion). The nurse should ensure that any plans for follow-up home care are in place if needed.

Patients Undergoing Emergency Surgery

Emergency surgeries are unplanned and occur with little time for preparation for the patient or the perioperative team. See Chapter 20 for the duties of the members of the perioperative team. The unpredictable nature of trauma and emergency surgery poses unique challenges to the nurse throughout the perioperative period. It is important for the nurse to communicate with the patient and team members as calmly and effectively as possible in these situations.

Factors that affect patients preparing to undergo planned surgery also apply to patients undergoing emergency surgery, but usually in a very condensed time frame. The only opportunity for preoperative assessment may take place at the same time as resuscitation in the emergency department. For the unconscious patient, **informed consent** and essential information, such as pertinent past medical history and allergies, need to be obtained from a family member, if one is available. A quick assessment of the patient is essential to identify all sites of injury if the emergency surgery is due to trauma (see Chapter 73 for more information). The patient, who may have undergone a traumatic experience, may need extra support and explanation of the surgery.

Informed Consent

Informed consent is the patient's autonomous decision about whether to undergo a surgical procedure. Voluntary and written informed consent from the patient is necessary before nonemergent surgery can be performed in order to protect the patient from unsanctioned surgery and protect the surgeon from claims of an unauthorized operation. Although informed consent is a legal mandate, it also helps the patient to prepare psychologically by ensuring that the patient understands the surgery to be performed (Rothrock, 2018).

While the nurse may ask the patient to sign the consent form and witness the signature, it is the surgeon's responsibility to provide a clear and simple explanation of what the surgery will entail, the benefits and possible risks, alternatives, and possible complications as well as what to expect in the early and late postoperative periods. The nurse clarifies the information provided and if the patient requests additional information, the nurse notifies the physician. The nurse ascertains that the consent form has been signed before administering psychoactive premedication, because consent is not valid if it is obtained while the patient is under the influence of medications that can affect judgment and decision-making capacity.

> **NURSING ALERT**
>
> **The signed consent form is placed in a prominent place on the patient's chart and accompanies the patient to the OR.**

Many ethical principles are integral to informed consent (see Chapter 3). Informed consent is necessary in the following circumstances:

- Invasive procedures, such as a surgical incision, a biopsy, a cystoscopy, or paracentesis
- Procedures requiring sedation and/or anesthesia (see Chapter 20)
- A nonsurgical procedure, such as an arteriography, that carries more than a slight risk to the patient
- Procedures involving radiation
- Blood product administration

If of legal age and mentally capable, the patient personally signs the consent form. Otherwise, permission is obtained from a surrogate, who most often is a responsible family member (preferably next of kin) or legal guardian. See Chart 19-2 for criteria for valid informed consent. An emancipated minor (married or independently earning his or her own living) may sign his or her own consent form. Provincial/territorial regulations and agency policy must be followed. In an emergency, it may be necessary for the surgeon to operate as a lifesaving measure without the patient's informed consent. However, every effort must be made to contact the patient's family. In such a situation, contact can be made by telephone, email, fax, or other electronic means.

If the patient has doubts and has not had the opportunity to investigate alternative treatments, he or she may request a second opinion. No patient should be urged or coerced to give informed consent. Refusing to undergo a surgical procedure is a person's legal right and privilege. However, such action must be documented and relayed to the surgeon so that other arrangements can be made. For example, additional explanations may be provided to the patient and family, or the surgery may be rescheduled. Consents for specific procedures such as sterilization, therapeutic abortion, disposal of severed body parts, organ donation, and blood product administration provide additional protection for the patient (Rothrock, 2018).

The consent process can be improved by providing audiovisual materials or multimedia supports to supplement discussion, by ensuring that the wording of the consent form is understandable, and by using other strategies and resources as needed to help the patient understand its content (see Chart 19-2) (Huber, Ihrig, Yass, et al., 2013). It may be necessary to have the consent available in multiple languages or have a trained medical interpreter available. Alternative formats of communication (e.g., Braille, large print, sign interpreter) may be needed if the patient is elderly or has a specific disability that calls for such accommodation.

CHART 19-2

Valid Informed Consent

Voluntary Consent

Valid consent must be freely given, without coercion. Patient must be at least 18 years of age (unless an emancipated minor), consent must be obtained by a physician, and patient's signature must be witnessed by a professional staff member.

Incompetent Patient

Legal definition: individual who is *not* autonomous and cannot give or withhold consent (e.g., individuals who are cognitively impaired, mentally ill, or neurologically incapacitated).

Informed Subject

Informed consent should be in writing. It should contain the following:

- Explanation of procedure and its risks
- Description of benefits and alternatives
- An offer to answer questions about procedure
- Instructions that the patient may withdraw consent
- A statement informing the patient if the protocol differs from customary procedure

Patient Able to Comprehend

If the patient is non-English speaking, it is necessary to provide consent (written and verbal) in a language that is understandable to the client. A trained medical interpreter may be consulted. Alternative formats of communication (e.g., Braille, large print, sign interpreter) may be needed if the patient has a disability that affects vision or hearing. Questions must be answered to facilitate comprehension if material is confusing.

Preoperative Assessment

The goal in the preoperative period is for the patient to be as healthy as possible. Every attempt is made to address risk factors that otherwise may lead to postoperative complications and hinder recovery (Chart 19-3). Before any surgical treatment is initiated, a health history is obtained, a physical examination is performed during which vital signs are noted, and a database is established for future comparisons. The nurse should ask about any allergies and comorbid conditions that may affect anesthesia (Bourdon, 2015). During the physical examination, many factors that have the potential to affect the patient undergoing surgery are considered.

Genetic considerations are also taken into account during assessment to prevent complications with anesthesia (Chart 19-4).

Health care providers should be alert for signs of abuse, which can occur at all ages and to men and women from all socioeconomic, ethnic, and cultural groups (Wang, Brisbin, Loo, et al., 2015). Findings need to be reported

CHART 19-3

Selected Risk Factors for Surgical Complications

- Hypovolemia
- Dehydration or electrolyte imbalance
- Nutritional deficits
- Extremes of age (very young, very old)
- Extremes of weight (emaciation, obesity)
- Infection and sepsis
- Toxic conditions
- Immunologic abnormalities
- Pulmonary disease
  - Obstructive disease
  - Restrictive disorder
  - Respiratory infection
- Renal or urinary tract disease
  - Decreased renal function
  - Urinary tract infection
  - Obstruction
- Pregnancy
  - Diminished maternal physiologic reserve
- Cardiovascular disease
  - Coronary artery disease or previous myocardial infarction
  - Cardiac failure
  - Dysrhythmias
  - Hypertension
  - Prosthetic heart valve
  - Thromboembolism
  - Hemorrhagic disorders
  - Cerebrovascular disease
- Endocrine dysfunction
  - Diabetes mellitus
  - Adrenal disorders
  - Thyroid malfunction
- Hepatic disease
- Cirrhosis
- Hepatitis
- Pre-existing mental or physical disability

accordingly (see Chapter 5 for further discussion of signs of abuse). Blood tests, x-rays, and other diagnostic tests are prescribed when indicated by information obtained from the history and physical examination.

Nutritional and Fluid Status

Optimal nutrition is an essential factor in promoting healing and resisting infection and other surgical complications. Assessment of a patient's nutritional status identifies factors that can affect the patient's surgical course, such as obesity, weight loss, malnutrition, deficiencies in specific nutrients, metabolic abnormalities, and the effects of medications on nutrition. Nutritional needs can be assessed by BMI, waist circumference, and serum albumin (Francon, Chambrier, & Sztark, 2012). See Chapter 5 for further discussion of nutritional assessment.

Any nutritional deficiency, such as malnutrition, should be corrected before surgery to provide adequate protein for tissue repair. The nutrients needed for wound healing are summarized in Table 19-2.

Dehydration, hypovolemia, and electrolyte imbalances can lead to significant problems in patients with comorbid medical conditions or in older adult patients. The severity of fluid and electrolyte imbalances is often difficult to determine. Mild volume deficits may be treated during surgery; however, additional time may be needed to correct pronounced fluid and electrolyte deficits to promote the best possible preoperative condition.

Dentition

The condition of the mouth is an important health factor to assess. Dental caries, dentures, and partial plates are particularly significant to the anesthesiologist or anesthetist, as decayed teeth or dental prostheses may become dislodged during intubation and occlude the airway. This is especially important for the older adult patients, as well as those from underserved communities or who are uninsured or do not have regular dental care.

Drug or Alcohol Use

People who abuse drugs or alcohol frequently deny or attempt to hide it. In such situations, the nurse who is obtaining the patient's health history needs to ask frank questions with patience, care, and a nonjudgmental attitude. See Chapter 5 for an assessment of alcohol and drug use.

Because acutely intoxicated people are susceptible to injury, surgery is postponed if possible. If minor emergency surgery is required, local, spinal, or regional block anesthesia is used. Otherwise, to prevent vomiting and potential aspiration, a nasogastric tube is inserted before general anesthesia is administered.

The person with a history of chronic alcoholism often suffers from malnutrition and other systemic problems that increase surgical risk. Alcohol withdrawal syndrome (i.e., delirium tremens) may be anticipated between 48 and 72 hours after alcohol withdrawal. When it occurs in the **postoperative phase**, a significant mortality rate associated with the cardiac dysrhythmias, cardiomyopathy, and bleeding tendencies often seen in long-term alcohol abuse (Rotevatn, Bøggild, Olesen, et al., 2017).

Respiratory Status

The goal for surgical patients is optimal respiratory function. The patient is taught breathing exercises and the use of an incentive spirometer if indicated. Because ventilation is potentially compromised during all phases of surgical treatment, surgery is usually postponed if the patient has a respiratory infection. Patients with underlying respiratory disease (e.g., asthma, chronic obstructive pulmonary disease) are assessed carefully for current threats to their pulmonary status. Patients also need to be assessed for comorbid conditions such as human immunodeficiency virus (HIV) infection and Parkinson's disease, which may affect respiratory function (Oster & Oster, 2015; West, 2015).

Patients who smoke are urged to stop 4 to 8 weeks before surgery to significantly reduce pulmonary and wound healing complications (Allison & George, 2014). Preoperative smoking cessation interventions can be

GENETICS IN NURSING PRACTICE

Chart 19-4. Genetics Concepts and Perioperative Nursing

Nurses who are caring for patients undergoing surgery need to take various genetic considerations into account when assessing patients throughout the operative experience. Genetic disorders can impact pre-, intra- and postoperative surgical outcomes. In particular, consideration must be given to genetic disorders associated with the delivery of anesthesia as well as other genetic disorders that may increase the risk of postoperative complications. Examples of genetic conditions that may cause complications with anesthesia include the following:

Autosomal Dominant:

- Central core disease
- Hyperkalemic periodic paralysis
- Malignant hyperthermia

Examples of other genetic conditions that must be evaluated and that are associated with perioperative risks include the following:

- Cystic fibrosis (autosomal recessive)
- Duchenne muscular dystrophy (X-linked recessive)
- Ehlers-Danlos syndrome
- Factor V Leiden (autosomal dominant)
- Hemophilia (X-linked)
- Scleroderma

Nursing Assessments

FAMILY HISTORY ASSESSMENT SPECIFIC TO GENETICS AND PERIOPERATIVE NURSING

- Obtain a thorough assessment of personal and family history for three generations, inquiring about prior problems with surgery or anesthesia with specific attention to complications, such as fever, rigidity, dark urine, and unexpected reactions.
- Inquire about any history of musculoskeletal complaints, history of heat intolerance, fevers of unknown origin, or unusual drug reactions.
- Assess for family history of any sudden or unexplained death, especially during participation in athletic events.
- Assess whether any family members have been diagnosed with King-Denborough syndrome, as this is a form of congenital myopathy that places the patient at risk for malignant hyperthermia.

Patient Assessment Specific to Genetics and Perioperative Nursing

- Identify the presence of other inherited genetic disorders that may impact surgical outcomes (e.g., inherited connective tissue, metabolic, bleeding, or neurologic disorders).
- Assess for subclinical muscle weakness.
- Assess for other physical features suggestive of an underlying genetic condition, such as contractures, kyphoscoliosis, and pterygium with progressive weakness.

Management Issues Specific to Genetics

- Inquire whether DNA mutation or other genetic testing has been performed on an affected family member.
- If indicated, refer for further genetic counselling and evaluation so that family members can discuss inheritance, risk to other family members, and availability of diagnostic/genetic testing.
- Offer appropriate genetics information and resources.
- Assess patient's understanding of genetics information.
- Provide support to families with newly diagnosed malignant hyperthermia.
- Participate in management and coordination of care of patients with genetic conditions and individuals predisposed to develop or pass on a genetic condition.

Genetics Resources

Malignant Hyperthermia Association, www.mhaus.org
Genetic Alliance—a directory of support groups for patients and families with genetic conditions, http://www.geneticalliance.org
Gene Clinics—a listing of common genetic disorders with up-to-date clinical summaries, genetic counselling and testing information, http://www.geneclinics.org
International Council of Nurses (ICN)—ICN's statement re: genetics and nursing, http://www.icn.ch/matters_genetics.htm
National Organization of Rare Disorders—a directory of support groups and information for patients and families with rare genetic disorders, http://www.rarediseases.org
OMIM: Online Mendelian Inheritance in Man—a complete listing of inherited genetic conditions: http://www.ncbi.nlm.nih.gov/entrez/query.fcgi?db-OMIM

effective in changing smoking behaviour and reducing the incidence of postoperative complications.

Cardiovascular Status

The goal in preparing any patient for surgery is to ensure a well-functioning cardiovascular system to meet the oxygen, fluid, and nutritional needs of the perioperative period. If the patient has uncontrolled hypertension, surgery may be postponed until the blood pressure is under control. At times, surgical treatment can be modified to meet the cardiac tolerance of the patient. For example, in a patient with obstruction of the descending colon and coronary artery disease, a temporary simple colostomy may be performed rather than a more extensive colon resection that would require a prolonged period of anesthesia.

Hepatic and Renal Function

The presurgical goal is optimal function of the hepatic and renal systems so that medications, anesthetic agents, body wastes, and toxins are adequately metabolized and removed from the body.

The liver plays a significant role in the biotransformation of anesthetic compounds. Therefore, any disorder of the liver has an effect on how anesthetic agents are

TABLE 19-2 Nutrients Important for Wound Healing

Nutrient	Rationale for Increased Need	Possible Deficiency Outcome
Protein	To allow collagen deposition and wound healing to occur	Collagen deposition leading to impaired/delayed wound healing Decreased skin and wound strength Increased wound infection rates
Arginine (amino acid)	To provide necessary substrate for collagen synthesis and nitric oxide (crucial for wound healing) at wound site To increase wound strength and collagen deposition To stimulate T-cell response Associated with various essential reactions of intermediary metabolism	Impaired wound healing
Carbohydrates and fats	Primary source of energy in the body and consequently in the wound-healing process To meet the demand for increased essential fatty acids needed for cellular function after an injury To spare protein To restore normal weight	Signs and symptoms of protein deficiency due to the use of protein to meet energy requirements Extensive weight loss
Water	To replace fluid lost through vomiting, hemorrhage, exudates, fever, drainage, diuresis To maintain homeostasis	Signs, symptoms, and complications of dehydration, such as poor skin turgor, dry mucous membranes, oliguria, anuria, weight loss, increased pulse rate, decreased central venous pressure
Vitamin C	Important for capillary formation, tissue synthesis, and wound healing through collagen formation Needed for antibody formation	Impaired/delayed wound healing related to impaired collagen formation and increased capillary fragility and permeability Increased risk for infection related to decreased antibodies
Vitamin B complex	Indirect role in wound healing through their influence on host resistance	Decreased enzymes available for energy metabolism
Vitamin A	Increases inflammatory response in wounds, reduces anti-inflammatory effects of corticosteroids on wound healing	Impaired/delayed wound healing related to decreased collagen synthesis; impaired immune function Increased risk for infection
Vitamin K	Important for normal blood clotting Impaired intestinal synthesis associated with the use of antibiotics	Prolonged prothrombin time Hematomas contributing to impaired healing and predisposition to wound infections
Magnesium	Essential cofactor for many enzymes that are involved in the process of protein synthesis and wound repair	Impaired/delayed wound healing (impaired collagen production)
Copper	Required cofactor in the development of connective tissue	Impaired wound healing
Zinc	Involved in DNA synthesis, protein synthesis, cellular proliferation needed for wound healing Essential to immune function	Impaired immune response

DNA, deoxyribonucleic acid.

Adapted from Porth, C. M. (2015). *Essentials of pathophysiology: Concepts of altered states* (4th ed.). Philadelphia, PA: Lippincott Williams & Wilkins.

metabolized. Because acute liver disease is associated with high surgical mortality, preoperative improvement in liver function is important. Careful assessment may include various liver function tests (see Chapter 40).

As the kidneys are involved in excreting anesthetic medications and their metabolites, surgery is contraindicated if a patient has acute nephritis, acute renal insufficiency with oliguria or anuria, or other acute renal problems (see Chapter 45). Exceptions include surgeries performed as lifesaving measures or those necessary to improve urinary function (i.e., obstructive uropathy).

Endocrine Function

The patient with diabetes who is undergoing surgery is at risk for hypoglycemia and hyperglycemia. Hypoglycemia may develop during anesthesia or postoperatively from inadequate carbohydrates or excessive administration of insulin. Hyperglycemia, which can increase the risk for surgical wound infection, may result from the stress of surgery, which can trigger increased levels of catecholamine. Other risks are acidosis and glucosuria. Although the surgical risk in the patient with controlled diabetes is no greater than in the patient without diabetes, strict glycemic control (4.4 to 6.1 mmol/L) leads to better outcomes (Khan, Ghali, Cagliero, et al., 2018). Frequent monitoring of blood glucose levels is important before, during, and after surgery (see Chapter 41 for a discussion of the patient with diabetes).

Patients who have received corticosteroids during the year preceding surgery are at risk for adrenal insufficiency. The anesthesiologist or anesthetist and the surgeon must

Ask the patient the following questions. Check "Yes" or "No" in the box.	YES	NO
1. Has a doctor ever told you that you are allergic to latex?		
2. Do you have on-the-job exposure to latex?		
3. Were you born with problems involving your spinal cord?		
4. Have you ever had allergies, asthma, hay fever, eczema, or problems with rashes?		
5. Have you ever had respiratory distress, rapid heart rate, or swelling?		
6. Have you ever had swelling, itching, hives, or other symptoms after contact with a balloon?		
7. Have you ever had swelling, itching, hives, or other symptoms after a dental examination or procedure?		
8. Have you ever had swelling, itching, hives, or other symptoms following a vaginal or rectal examination or after contact with a diaphragm or condom?		
9. Have you ever had swelling, itching, hives, or other symptoms during or within 1 hour after wearing rubber gloves?		
10. Have you ever had a rash on your hands that lasted longer than 1 week?		
11. Have you ever had swelling, itching, hives, runny nose, eye irritation, wheezing, or asthma after contact with any latex or rubber product?		
12. Have you ever had swelling, itching, hives, or other symptoms after being examined by someone wearing rubber or latex gloves?		
13. Are you allergic to bananas, avocados, kiwi, or chestnuts?		
14. Have you ever had an unexplained anaphylactic episode?		

Pre-op RN Signature: ______________________

Patient Name: ______________________

Procedure: ______________________

Scheduled Date / Time: ______________________

Surgeon: ______________________

FIGURE 19-2. Example of a latex allergy assessment form. (Courtesy of Inova Fairfax Hospital, Falls Church, VA.)

be aware of corticosteroid use and the patient will be monitored for signs of adrenal insufficiency.

Patients with uncontrolled thyroid disorders are at risk for thyrotoxicosis (with hyperthyroid disorders) or respiratory failure (with hypothyroid disorders). Therefore, the patient is assessed for a history of these disorders.

Immune Function

During the preoperative assessment, the nurse determines the presence of any allergies and sensitivities (especially related to medications). The patient is asked to identify any substances that precipitated previous allergic reactions, including medications, blood transfusions, contrast agents, latex, and food products, and to describe the signs and symptoms produced by these substances. A sample latex allergy screening questionnaire is shown in Figure 19-2.

Immunosuppression is common with corticosteroid therapy, organ transplantation, radiation therapy, chemotherapy, and disorders affecting the immune system, such as acquired immunodeficiency syndrome (AIDS) and leukemia. The mildest symptoms or slightest temperature elevation must be investigated. Because patients who are immunosuppressed are highly susceptible to infection, great care is taken to ensure strict asepsis.

Previous Medication Use

A medication history is obtained because of the possible effects of medications on the patient's perioperative course, including the possibility of drug interactions. Any medication the patient is using or has used in the past is documented, including over-the-counter (OTC) preparations, herbal agents, and the frequency with which they are used. Many medications have an effect on physiologic functions; interactions of such medications with anesthetic agents can cause serious problems, such as arterial hypotension and circulatory collapse. Medications that cause particular concern are listed in Table 19-3.

The anesthesiologist or anesthetist evaluates the potential effects of prior medication therapy, considering the length of time the patient has used the medication, the physical condition of the patient, and the nature of the proposed surgery (Muluk et al., 2018).

Many patients take self-prescribed or OTC medications. Aspirin is a common OTC medication that inhibits platelet aggregation; therefore, it is prudent to stop aspirin at least 5 to 10 days before surgery if possible, especially for surgeries in which excess bleeding would cause significant complications, such as brain or spinal cord surgeries (Plumer, Seiffert, Punke, et al., 2017). Any use of aspirin or other OTC medications is noted in the patient's chart and conveyed to the anesthesiologist or anesthetist and surgeon.

NURSING ALERT

Because of possible adverse interactions, the nurse must assess and document the patient's use of prescription medications, OTC medications (especially aspirin), herbal agents, and the frequency with which medications are used. The nurse must clearly communicate this information to the anesthesiologist or anesthetist.

The use of natural health products (NHPs), which includes vitamins, minerals, herbal products, homeopathic medicine, traditional Chinese medicines, probiotics, etc., is widespread among patients; 71% of Canadians regularly take these products (Health Canada, 2016). The most commonly used herbal products are echinacea,

TABLE 19-3 Examples of Medications With the Potential to Affect the Surgical Experience

Agent	Effect of Interaction With Anesthetics
Corticosteroids	
Dexamethasone (Dexpak)	Cardiovascular collapse can occur if discontinued suddenly. Therefore, a bolus of corticosteroid may be administered IV immediately before and after surgery
Diuretics	
Hydrochlorothiazide (Microxide)	During anesthesia, may cause excessive respiratory depression resulting from an associated electrolyte imbalance
Phenothiazines	
Chlorpromazine hydrochloride	May increase the hypotensive action of anesthetics
Tranquilizers	
Diazepam (Valium)	May cause anxiety, tension, and even seizures if withdrawn suddenly
Insulins	
Insulin (Humalog)	Interaction between anesthetics and insulin must be considered when a patient with diabetes is undergoing surgery. IV insulin may need to be given to keep the blood glucose within the normal range
Anticoagulants	
Warfarin (Coumadin)	Can increase the risk of bleeding during the intraoperative and postoperative periods; should be discontinued in anticipation of elective surgery. The surgeon will determine how long before the elective surgery the patient should stop taking an anticoagulant, depending on the type of planned procedure and the medical condition of the patient
Anticonvulsant Medications	
Carbamazepine (Tegretol)	IV administration of medication may be needed to keep the patient seizure free in the intraoperative and postoperative periods
Thyroid Hormone	
Levothyroxine sodium (Synthroid)	IV administration may be needed during the postoperative period to maintain thyroid levels
Opioids	
Morphine sulphate (MS Contin)	Long-term use of opioids for chronic pain (≥6 months) in the preoperative period may alter the patient's response to analgesic agents

IV, intravenous.

Adapted from Comerford, K. C. (2015). *Nursing 2015 drug handbook*. Philadelphia, PA: Wolters Kluwer.

ephedra, garlic (*Allium sativum*), ginkgo biloba, ginseng, kava kava (*Piper methysticum*), St. John's wort (*Hypericum perforatum*), licorice (*Glycyrrhiza glabra*), and valerian (*Valeriana officinalis*). However, many patients fail to report the use of NHPs to their health care providers. Because of the potential effects of herbal products on coagulation and potentially lethal interactions with other medications, the nurse must ask surgical patients specifically about the use of these agents, document their use, and inform the surgical team and anesthesiologist. Currently, it is recommended that the use of herbal products be discontinued 2 to 3 weeks before surgery (Rothrock, 2018).

Psychosocial Factors

Most patients have some type of emotional reaction before any surgical procedure, be it obvious or hidden, normal or abnormal. Fears may be related to fear of the unknown or of death, anesthesia, pain, complications, or cancer. Preoperative anxiety may be an anticipatory response to an experience viewed by the patient as a threat to his or her customary role in life, permanent incapacity, body integrity, increased responsibilities or burden on family members, or life itself. Less obvious concerns may occur because of previous experiences with the health care system and people the patient has known with the same condition. Psychological distress directly influences body functioning. Negative physical effects include slow wound healing, increased risk for infection, and complications with anesthesia; therefore, it is imperative to identify any anxiety the patient is experiencing (Bradt, Dileo, & Shim, 2013).

People express fear in different ways. For example, some patients may repeatedly ask many questions, even though answers were given previously. Others may withdraw, deliberately avoiding communication, perhaps by reading, watching television, or talking about trivialities. Consequently, the nurse must be empathetic, listen well, and provide information that helps alleviate concerns.

An important outcome of the psychosocial assessment is determining the extent, role, value and reliability of the patient's support network. Other information, such as usual level of functioning and typical daily activities, may assist in the patient's care and recovery. Assessing the patient's readiness to learn and determining the best approach to maximize comprehension provides the basis for preoperative patient education. This is of particular importance in patients who are developmentally delayed and those who are cognitively impaired, where the approach to patient education and consent will include the legal guardian.

Spiritual and Cultural Safety

Spiritual beliefs play an important role in how people cope with fear and anxiety. Regardless of the patient's religious affiliation, spiritual beliefs can be as therapeutic as medication. Every attempt must be made to help the patient obtain the spiritual support that he or she requests. The nurse respects and supports the beliefs of each patient. Some nurses may avoid the subject of a clergy visit lest the suggestion alarms the patient. Asking whether the patient's spiritual advisor knows about the impending surgery is a caring, nonthreatening approach.

Respecting a patient's cultural values and beliefs facilitates rapport and trust. A thorough assessment includes identifying the ethnic group to which the patient relates and the customs and beliefs the patient holds about illness and health care providers. For example, patients from some cultural groups are unaccustomed to expressing feelings openly. Nurses need to consider this pattern of communication when assessing pain. As a sign of respect, people from some cultural groups may not make direct eye contact with others (Andrews & Boyle, 2016). The nurse should know that this lack of eye contact is not avoidance or a lack of interest.

Perhaps the most valuable nursing skill is listening carefully to the patient, especially when obtaining the history. Invaluable information and insights may be gained through effective communication and interviewing skills. An unhurried, understanding, and caring nurse promotes confidence on the part of the patient.

Preoperative Nursing Interventions

There are a wide range of interventions used to prepare the patient physically and psychologically and to maintain safety.

Providing Patient Education

Nurses have long recognized the value of preoperative instruction (Rothrock, 2018). Each patient is taught as an individual, with consideration for any unique concerns or learning needs. Multiple teaching strategies can be used (e.g., verbal, written, return demonstration), depending on the patient's needs and abilities.

Preoperative education is initiated as soon as possible, beginning in the physician's office, in the clinic, or at the time of PAT when diagnostic tests are performed. During PAT, the nurse or health care provider makes resources available related to patient education, such as written instructions (designed to be copied and given to patients), audiovisual resources, and telephone numbers, to ensure that education continues until the patient arrives for the surgical intervention. When possible, instruction is spaced over a period of time to allow the patient to assimilate information and ask questions as they arise.

Frequently, education sessions are combined with various preparation procedures to allow for an easy and timely flow of information. The nurse should guide the patient through the experience and allow ample time for questions. Education should go beyond descriptions of the procedure and should include explanations of the sensations the patient will experience. Telling the patient that preoperative medication will cause relaxation before the operation is not as effective as also noting that the medication will act quickly and may result in lightheadedness, dizziness, and drowsiness. Knowing what to expect will help the patient anticipate these reactions and attain a superior degree of relaxation. Overly detailed descriptions may increase anxiety in some patients; therefore, the nurse should be sensitive to this, by watching and listening, and provide less detail based on the individual patient's needs.

Unfolding Patient Stories: Vernon Watkins • Part 1

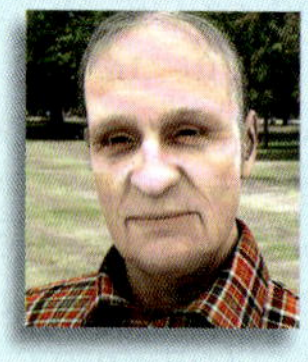

Vernon Watkins, a 69-year-old male, came to the emergency department with severe abdominal pain, and a bowel perforation was diagnosed. He is being prepared for surgery. Significant medical history includes controlled hypertension and smoking for 50 years. What preoperative education should the nurse discuss with Mr. Watkins prior to his emergent surgery? (Vernon Watkins' story continues in Chapter 60.)

Care for Vernon and other patients in a realistic virtual environment: ***vSim** for Nursing* (**thepoint.lww.com/vSimMedicalSurgical**). Practice documenting these patients' care in DocuCare (**thepoint.lww.com/DocuCareEHR**).

Deep Breathing, Coughing, and Incentive Spirometry

One goal of preoperative nursing care is to teach the patient how to promote optimal lung expansion and resulting blood oxygenation after anesthesia. The patient assumes a sitting position to enhance lung expansion. The nurse then demonstrates how to take a deep, slow breath and how to exhale slowly. After practicing deep breathing several times, the patient is instructed to breathe deeply, exhale through the mouth, take a short breath, and cough from deep in the lungs (Chart 19-5). The nurse or respiratory therapist also demonstrates how to use an incentive spirometer, a device that provides measurement and feedback related to breathing effectiveness (see Chapter 26). In addition to enhancing respiration, these exercises may help the patient relax. Research indicates that some patients benefit from intensive inspiratory muscle training in the preoperative period (Tonella, Ratti, Delazari, et al., 2017).

If a thoracic or abdominal incision is anticipated, the nurse demonstrates how to splint the incision to minimize pressure and control pain. The patient places the palms of both hands together, interlacing the fingers snugly. Placing the hands across the incisional site acts as an effective splint when coughing. The patient is also informed that medications to relieve pain are available and are best taken regularly for pain relief so that effective deep-breathing and coughing exercises can be performed. The goal in promoting coughing is to mobilize and remove secretions. Deep breathing before coughing stimulates the cough reflex. If the patient does not cough effectively, atelectasis (collapse of the alveoli), pneumonia, or other lung complications may occur.

Mobility and Active Body Movement

The goals of promoting mobility postoperatively are to improve circulation, prevent venous stasis, and promote optimal respiratory function. The patient is taught that early and frequent ambulation immediately postoperative as tolerated will help to prevent complications.

The nurse explains the rationale for frequent position changes after surgery and then shows the patient how to turn from side to side and how to assume the lateral position without causing pain or disrupting intravenous (IV) lines, drainage tubes, or other equipments. Any special position the patient needs to maintain after surgery (e.g., adduction or elevation of an extremity) is discussed, as is the importance of maintaining as much mobility as possible despite restrictions. Reviewing the process before surgery is helpful, because the patient may be too uncomfortable or drowsy after surgery to absorb new information.

Exercise of the extremities includes extension and flexion of the knee and hip joints (similar to bicycle riding while lying on the side) unless contraindicated by type of surgical procedure (e.g., hip replacement). The foot is rotated as though tracing the largest possible circle with the great toe (see Chart 19-5). The elbow and shoulder are also put through their range of motion. At first, the patient is assisted and reminded to perform these exercises. Later, the patient is encouraged to do them independently. Muscle tone is maintained so that ambulation will be easier. The nurse uses proper body mechanics and encourages the patient to do the same. Whenever the patient is positioned, his or her body needs to be properly aligned. The nurses also teach the safe use of assistive devices (walker, cane, etc.).

Pain Management

A pain assessment includes differentiation between acute and chronic pain so that the patient is prepared to differentiate between acute postoperative pain and chronic conditions such as lower back pain. A pain intensity scale is explained to the patient to promote more effective postoperative pain management. Chapter 16 contains several examples of pain scales. Preoperative pain assessment and teaching for the elderly patient may require additional attention (Chart 19-6).

Postoperatively, medications are administered to relieve pain and maintain comfort without suppressing respiratory function. The patient is encouraged to take the medication as frequently as prescribed during the initial postoperative period for effective pain relief. Anticipated methods of administration of analgesic agents for inpatients include patient-controlled analgesia (PCA), epidural catheter bolus or infusion, patient-controlled perineurial anesthesia (PCPA), or patient-controlled epidural analgesia (PCEA). A patient who is expected to go home will likely receive oral analgesic agents. These methods are discussed with the patient before surgery, and the patient's interest and willingness to use them are assessed.

Cognitive Coping Strategies

Cognitive strategies may be useful for relieving tension, overcoming anxiety, decreasing fear, and achieving relaxation. Examples of such strategies include the following:

- Imagery: Concentrating on a pleasant experience or restful scene.
- Distraction: Thinking of an enjoyable story or recites a favourite poem or song.
- Optimistic self-recitation: Reciting optimistic thoughts ("I know all will go well").
- Music therapy: Listening to soothing music (an easy-to-administer, inexpensive, noninvasive intervention).
- Meditation/mindfulness/prayer (Beiranvand, Noparast, Eslamizade, et al., 2014).

CHART 19-5

Patient Education: Preoperative Instructions to Prevent Postoperative Complications

Diaphragmatic Breathing

Diaphragmatic breathing refers to a flattening of the dome of the diaphragm during inspiration, with resultant enlargement of the upper abdomen as air rushes in. During expiration, the abdominal muscles contract.

1. Practice in the same position you would assume in bed after surgery: a semi-Fowler's position, propped in bed with the back and shoulders well supported with pillows.
2. With your hands resting lightly on the front of the lower ribs, and fingertips against lower chest to feel the movement.

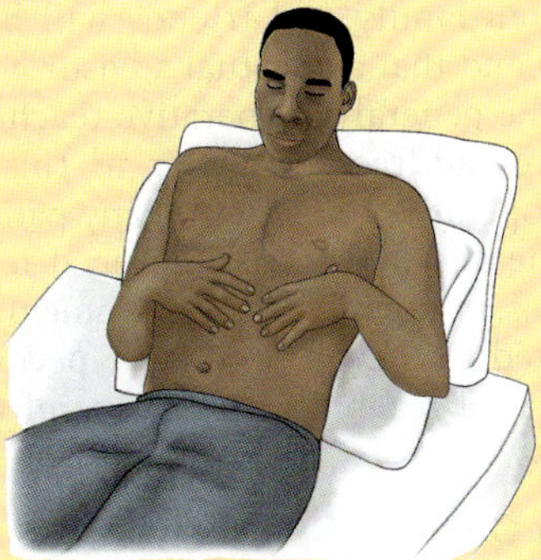

Diaphragmatic breathing

3. Breathe out gently and fully as the ribs sink down and inward toward midline.
4. Then take a deep breath through your nose and mouth, letting the abdomen rise as the lungs fill with air.
5. Hold this breath for a count of five.
6. Exhale and let out all the air through your nose and mouth.
7. Repeat this exercise 15 times with a short rest after each group of five.
8. Practice this twice a day preoperatively.

Coughing

1. Lean forward slightly from a sitting position in bed, interlace your fingers together, and place your hands across the incisional site to act as a splint-like support when coughing.

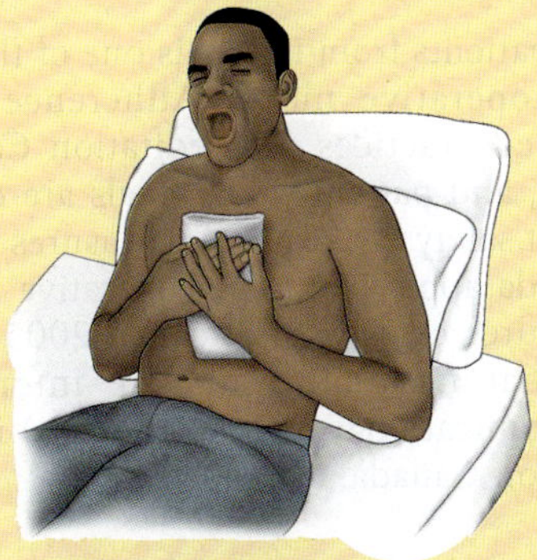

Splinting of chest when coughing

2. Breathe with the diaphragm as described under "Diaphragmatic Breathing."
3. With your mouth slightly open, breathe in fully.
4. "Hack" out sharply for three short breaths.
5. Then, keeping your mouth open, take in a quick deep breath and immediately give a strong cough once or twice. This helps clear secretions from your chest. It may cause some discomfort but will not harm your incision.

Leg Exercises

1. Lie in a semi-Fowler's position and perform the following simple exercises to improve circulation.
2. Bend your knee and raise your foot—hold it a few seconds, then extend the leg and lower it to the bed.

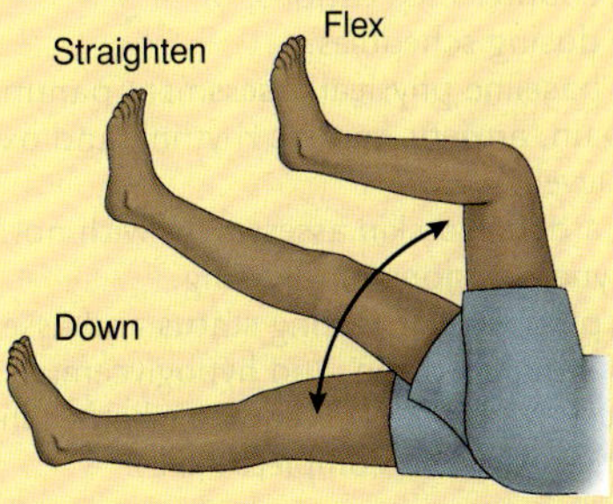

Leg exercises

3. Do this five times with one leg, then repeat with the other leg.
4. Then trace circles with the feet by bending them down, in toward each other, up, and then out.
5. Repeat these movements five times.

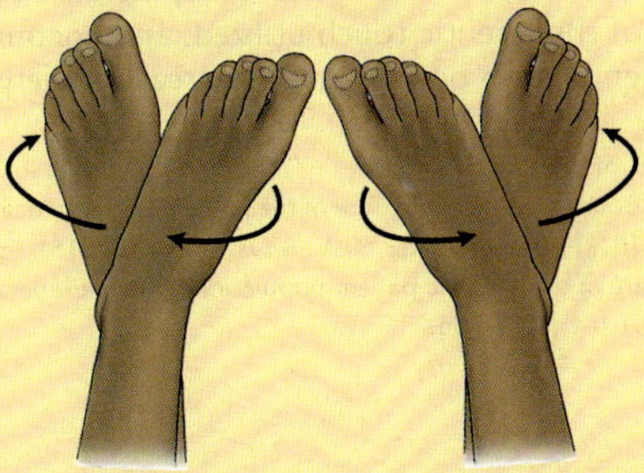

Foot exercises

Turning to the Side

1. Turn on your side with the uppermost leg flexed most and supported on a pillow.
2. Grasp the side rail as an aid to manoeuvre to the side.
3. Practice diaphragmatic breathing and coughing while on your side.

Getting out of Bed

1. Turn on your side.
2. Push yourself up with one hand as you swing your legs out of bed.

CHART 19-6

Preoperative Assessment and Education for Older Adults

Assessment

- Assess for allergies and medical comorbidities.
- Assess the patient's cognitive and sensory function before the surgeon begins the informed consent process.
- Determine the need for a designated support person or power of attorney to complete the informed consent process.
- Review medications to identify potential polypharmaceutical risks to include the following:
  - multiple medications,
  - multiple prescribers,
  - several filling pharmacies,
  - too many forms of medications,
  - over-the-counter medications, or
  - multiple dosing schedules.
- Document baseline physical assessment parameters, including pain, anxiety, cardiac rhythm, and oxygen saturation level.
- Document a detailed skin assessment with notation of areas of dryness, lesions, or bruising.
- Document preoperative fasting status and assess for dehydration, malnutrition, and hypoglycemia.
- Identify social support to determine whether the patient has home assistance to complete ADLs.

Education

- Discuss advanced directives and code status to identify the patient's wishes.
- Educate the patient about the benefits of controlling pain.
- Be prepared to spend additional time, increase the amount of therapeutic touch utilized, and encourage family members to be present to decrease anxiety.

ADLs, activities of daily living.
Adapted from Bourdon, L. (2015). Care of the patient receiving local anesthesia. *AORN Journal, 101*(3), 10–12; Oster, K. A., & Oster, C. A. (2015). Special needs population: Care of the geriatric patient population in the perioperative setting. *AORN Journal, 101*(4), 444–456.

Education for Patients Undergoing Ambulatory Surgery

Preoperative education for the same-day or ambulatory surgical patient comprises all previously discussed patient teaching as well as collaborative planning with the patient and family for discharge and follow-up home care. The major difference in outpatient preoperative education is the teaching environment.

Preoperative teaching content may be presented in a group class, on a videotape, at PAT, or by telephone/teleconference in conjunction with the preoperative interview. In addition to answering questions and describing what to expect, the patient learns when and where to report, what to bring (insurance card, list of medications, and allergies), what to leave at home (jewelry, watch, medications, contact lenses), and what to wear (loose-fitting, comfortable clothes; flat shoes). The nurse in the surgeon's office may initiate teaching before the perioperative telephone contact.

During the final preoperative telephone call, teaching is completed or reinforced as needed and last minute instructions are given. The patient is reminded not to eat or drink as directed and reminded of which medications they can take the morning of surgery.

Providing Psychosocial Interventions

Reducing Anxiety and Decreasing Fear

During the preoperative assessment of psychological factors and spiritual and cultural beliefs, the nurse assists the patient to identify coping strategies that he or she has previously used to decrease fear. Discussions with the patient to help determine the source of fears can help with expression of concerns. The patient benefits from knowing when family and friends will be able to visit after surgery and that a spiritual advisor will be available if desired. The general preoperative teaching and cognitive strategies addressed earlier in this section help decrease preoperative anxiety in many patients. Knowing ahead of time about the possible need for a ventilator, drainage tubes, or other types of equipment helps decrease anxiety related to the postoperative period. Chart 19-7 addresses patient teaching as a means of reducing emotional distress.

Respecting Cultural, Spiritual, and Religious Beliefs

Psychosocial interventions include identifying and respecting cultural, spiritual, and religious beliefs. In some cultures, for example, people are stoic in regard to pain, whereas in others they are more expressive. These responses are recognized as expected for those patients and families and respected by perioperative personnel (Andrews & Boyle, 2016). If patients decline blood transfusions for religious reasons (i.e., Jehovah's Witnesses), this information needs to be clearly identified in the preoperative period, documented, and communicated to the appropriate personnel.

Maintaining Patient Safety

Protecting patients from injury is one of the major roles of the perioperative nurse. Adherence to ORNAC-recommended practices, Accreditation Canada recommendations, and patient safety goals are crucial. Seven main patient safety performance measures from Accreditation Canada apply to the perioperative period. These safety measures came into effect in 2005 and assist in ensuring that national goals are intertwined with required organizational practices (ROPs) in health care (Accreditation Canada, 2018).

Managing Nutrition and Fluids

The major purpose of withholding food and fluid before surgery is to prevent aspiration. Until recently, fluid and food were restricted preoperatively overnight and often longer. However, the Canadian Anesthesiologists' Society (CAS) (2014) reviewed this practice and has made new recommendations for people undergoing elective surgery who are otherwise healthy. Specific recommendations

NURSING RESEARCH PROFILE

Chart 19-7. The Relationship Between Certification of Nurses and Surgical Outcomes

Boyle, D. K., Cramer, E., Potter, C., et al. (2014). The relationship between direct-care RN specialty certification and surgical patient outcomes. *AORN Journal, 100*(11), 511–528.

Purpose

Specialty certification is thought to enhance the safety of patients by validating that standards of practice are met. The purpose of this study was to explore the relationship between specialty-certified nurses in perioperative units and surgical intensive care units (SICUs) and nurse-sensitive patient outcomes. The nurse-sensitive outcomes included central line–associated bloodstream infections (CLABSI), catheter-associated urinary tract infections (CAUTI), hospital-acquired pressure ulcers and unit-acquired pressure ulcers.

Design

This was a retrospective, repeated measures analysis of secondary data from the National Database of Nursing Quality Indicators. Outcomes were examined by unit types and included four specific specialty certifications commonly held by perioperative nurses (certified postanesthesia nurse [CAPA], certified postanesthesia nurse [CPAN], certified nurse operating room [CNOR], certified RN first assistant [CRNFA]). The data were analyzed using an autoregressive generalized linear regression model at the unit level. Patient outcome variables were collected concurrently with the other predictor variables.

Findings

Lower rates of CLABSI in SICUs were significantly associated with higher proportions of CPAN ($\beta = -0.09$, $p = 0.05$) and CNOR/CRNFA ($\beta = -0.17$, $p = 0.00$) certifications in perioperative units. Interestingly, higher proportions of CNOR/CRNFA certification in perioperative units were associated with higher proportions of hospital-acquired pressure ulcers ($\beta = 0.08$, $p = 0.03$) and unit-acquired pressure ulcers ($\beta = 0.13$, $p = 0.00$), possibly because of a higher risk of pressure ulcers in the patient population.

Nursing Implications

Nurses should know that at least in this one study higher rates of nurse certifications were associated with lower rates of CLABSI in SICUs. These findings lend credence to perioperative, SICU, and surgical nurses participating in lifelong learning and continuous professional development, including achievement of specialty certification.

depend on the age of the patient and the type of food eaten. For example, adults may be advised to fast for 8 hours after eating fatty food and 4 hours after ingesting milk products. Many patients are currently allowed clear liquids up to 2 hours before an elective procedure (Gomes, Caporossi, Aguilar-Nascimento, et al., 2017).

Preparing the Bowel

Enemas are not commonly prescribed preoperatively unless the patient is undergoing abdominal or pelvic surgery. In this case, a cleansing enema or laxative may be prescribed the evening before surgery and may be repeated the morning of surgery. This preparation allows satisfactory visualization of the surgical site and prevents trauma to the intestine or contamination of the peritoneum by fecal material. Unless the condition of the patient presents some contraindication, the toilet or bedside commode, rather than the bedpan, is used for evacuating the bowels if the patient is hospitalized during this time. In addition, antibiotics may be prescribed to reduce intestinal flora.

Preparing the Skin

The goal of preoperative skin preparation is to decrease bacteria without injuring the skin. If the surgery is not performed as an emergency, most health care facilities and ambulatory surgical centres have implemented antiseptic skin cleansing protocols. There is an ongoing debate as to the efficacy of skin protocols in preventing SSIs, particularly when the patient is instructed to carry out the preparation independently at home prior to surgery (Chlebicki, Safdar, O'Horo, et al., 2013; Edmiston & Spencer, 2014).

For thoracic surgery, patients may also need to decolonize the throat and nasal cavity with germicidal agents or UV lights.

In general, hair is not removed preoperatively unless the hair at or around the incision site is likely to interfere with the operation. If hair must be removed, electric clippers are used for safe hair removal immediately before the operation. To ensure the correct site, the surgical site is typically marked by the patient and the surgeon in the preoperative waiting area.

Immediate Preoperative Nursing Interventions

WATCH & LEARN

Immediately prior to the procedure the patient changes into a hospital gown that is left untied and open in the back. The patient with long hair may braid it, remove hairpins, and cover the head completely with a disposable paper cap. The mouth is inspected, and dentures or plates are removed. If left in the mouth, these items could easily fall to the back of the throat during induction of anesthesia and cause respiratory obstruction.

Jewelry is not worn to the OR; wedding rings and jewelry or body piercings are removed to prevent injury. If a patient objects to removing a ring, some institutions allow the ring to be securely fastened to the finger with tape. All articles of value, including assistive devices, dentures, glasses, and prosthetic devices, are given to family members or are labeled clearly with the patient's name and stored in a safe and secure place according to the institution's policy.

All patients (except those with urologic disorders) should void immediately before going to the OR. This is particularly important in promoting continence during low abdominal surgery and to make abdominal organs more accessible. Urinary catheterization is performed in the OR as necessary.

Administering Preanesthetic Medication

The use of preanesthetic medication is minimal with ambulatory or outpatient surgery. If prescribed, it is usually administered in the preoperative holding area. If a preanesthetic medication is administered, the patient is kept in bed with the side rails raised, because the medication can cause lightheadedness or drowsiness. During this time, the nurse observes the patient for any untoward reaction to the medications. The immediate surroundings are kept quiet to promote relaxation.

Often, surgery is delayed or OR schedules are changed, and it becomes impossible to request that a medication be given at a specific time. In these situations, the preoperative medication is prescribed "on call to OR." The nurse can have the medication ready to administer as soon as a call is received from the OR staff. It usually takes 15 to 20 minutes to prepare the patient for the OR. If the nurse gives the medication before attending to the other details of preoperative preparation, the patient will have at least partial benefit from the preoperative medication and will have a smoother anesthetic and operative course.

Maintaining the Preoperative Record

Preoperative checklists (Fig. 19-3) contain critical elements that the nurse checks and verifies preoperatively (Rothrock, 2018). The completed chart (with the preoperative checklist, verification form, surgical consent form, all laboratory reports and nurses' record) accompanies the

1. Patient's name: ______ Date: ______ Height: ______ Weight: ______
   Identification band present: ______
2. Informed consent signed: ______ Special permits signed: ______
3. Surgical site: ______ (Ex: Sterilization)
4. History & physical examination report present: ______ Date: ______
5. Laboratory records present: ______
   CBC: ______ Hgb: ______ Urinalysis: ______ Hct: ______

6. Item	Present	Removed
a. Natural teeth		
Dentures; upper, lower, partial	______	______
Bridge, fixed; crown	______	______
b. Contact lenses	______	______
c. Other prostheses—type: ______	______	______
d. Jewelry:		
Wedding band (taped/tied)	______	______
Rings	______	______
Earrings: pierced, clip-on	______	______
Neck chains	______	______
Any other body piercings	______	______
e. Makeup	______	______
Nail polish	______	______

7. Clothing
   a. Clean patient gown ______
   b. Cap ______
   c. Sanitary pad, etc. ______
8. Family instructed where to wait? ______
9. Valuables secured? ______
10. Blood available? ______ Ordered? ______ Where? ______
11. Preanesthetic medication given: ______
    Type ______ Time
12. Voided: ______ Amount: ______ Time: ______ Catheter: ______
    Mouth care given: ______
13. Vital signs: Temperature: ______ Pulse: ______ Resp: ______ Blood Pressure: ______
14. Special problems/precautions: (Allergies, deafness, *etc.*): ______
15. Area of skin preparation: ______
16. ______ Date: ______ Time: ______
    Signature: Nurse releasing patient

FIGURE 19-3. Example of a preoperative checklist.

CHART 19-8

Expected Patient Outcomes in the Preoperative Phase of Care

Relief of anxiety, evidenced when the patient:
- Discusses with the anesthesiologist, anesthetist, or nurse anesthetist concerns related to types of anesthesia and induction
- Verbalizes an understanding of the preanesthetic medication and general anesthesia
- Discusses last minute concerns with the nurse or physician
- Discusses financial concerns with the social worker, when appropriate
- Requests visit with spiritual advisor when appropriate
- Appears relaxed when visited by health care team members

Decreased fear, evidenced when the patient:
- Discusses fears with health care professionals or a spiritual advisor, or both
- Verbalizes an understanding of any expected bodily changes, including expected duration of bodily changes

Understanding of the surgical intervention, evidenced when the patient:
- Participates in preoperative preparation
- Demonstrates and describes exercises he or she is expected to perform postoperatively
- Reviews information about postoperative care
- Accepts preanesthetic medication, if prescribed
- Remains in bed once premedicated
- Relaxes during transportation to the OR or unit
- States rationale for use of side rails
- Discusses postoperative expectations

No evidence of preoperative complications

patient to the OR. Any unusual last-minute observations that may have a bearing on anesthesia or surgery are noted prominently at the front of the chart.

Transporting the Patient to the Presurgical Area

The patient is transferred to the holding area or presurgical suite in a bed or on a stretcher about 30 to 60 minutes before the anesthetic is to be given. The stretcher is made as comfortable as possible, with a sufficient number of blankets to prevent chilling in an air-conditioned room. Evidence supports the use of preoperative warming to increase patient reports of being warm during the perioperative period. The time period and settings (i.e., holding area, surgical suite, or both) for warming are subjects of ongoing investigation (Erdling & Johansson, 2015). A small head pillow is usually provided.

The patient is taken to the preoperative holding area, greeted by name, and positioned comfortably on the stretcher or bed. The surrounding area is kept as quiet as possible to allow the preoperative medication to have maximal effect. Unpleasant sounds or conversation should be avoided, because they may be misinterpreted by a sedated patient.

Patient safety in the preoperative area is a priority. Use of a standard process or procedure to verify patient identification, the surgical procedure, and the surgical site is imperative to maximize patient safety (Canadian Patient Safety Institute, 2016). This allows for prompt intervention if any discrepancies are identified.

Attending to Family Needs

Most hospitals and ambulatory surgery centres have a waiting room where family members and significant others can wait while the patient is undergoing surgery. This room may be equipped with comfortable chairs, televisions, telephones, and light refreshments. Volunteers may remain with the family, offer refreshments, and keep them informed of the patient's progress. After surgery, the surgeon may meet the family in the waiting room and discuss the outcome.

The family and significant others are encouraged not to judge the seriousness of an operation by the length of time the patient is in the OR. A patient may be in the OR much longer than the actual operating time for several reasons:

- Patients are routinely transported well in advance of the actual operating time.
- The anesthesiologist or anesthetist often makes additional preparations that may take 30 to 60 minutes.
- The surgeon may take longer than expected with the preceding case, which delays the start of the next surgical procedure.

After surgery, the patient is taken to the PACU to ensure safe emergence from anesthesia. Family members and significant others waiting to see the patient after surgery are informed that the patient may have certain equipment or devices (e.g., IV lines, indwelling urinary catheter, nasogastric tube, oxygen lines, monitoring equipment, blood transfusion lines) in place when he or she returns from surgery. When the patient returns to the room, the nurse provides explanations regarding the frequent postoperative observations that will be made. It is the responsibility of the surgeon to relay the surgical findings and the prognosis, even when the findings are favourable.

Expected Patient Outcomes

Nurse-sensitive outcomes often include central line–associated bloodstream infections (CLABSI), catheter-associated urinary tract infections (CAUTI), hospital-acquired pressure ulcers, and unit-acquired pressure ulcers. Researchers have reported some patient outcomes are influenced by the level of nurse certification. (See Chart 19-8.)

Critical Thinking Exercises

1 During your preoperative assessment of your patient, a 42-year-old female who is alert and oriented reports that she is having her right breast removed for cancer. The OR

schedule indicates that she is having a left mastectomy. What preoperative assessments are indicated? What nursing interventions are warranted? What should your initial action be?

2 A morbidly obese 55-year-old patient with diabetes and a history of high blood pressure who takes insulin, antihypertensive medication, aspirin, and several herbal supplements daily is scheduled for major abdominal surgery. What preoperative assessments would be appropriate? What instructions would you anticipate for the patient regarding medications and their rationale? What additional preoperative teaching should be undertaken with this patient?

3 A patient is admitted to the same-day surgery unit with a known allergy to latex. What resources would you use to identify evidence-based practices during the perioperative period? Identify the evidence for and the criteria used to evaluate the strength of the evidence for the practices identified for this patient.

REFERENCES AND SELECTED READINGS

Books

Alvarex, A., Brodsky, J. B., Lemmens, H. J., et al. (2014). *Perianesthesia Nursing Core Curriculum: Preprocedure, phase I and phase II PACU nursing* (2nd ed.). St. Louis, MO: Elsevier.

Andrews, M. M., & Boyle, J. S. (2016). *Transcultural concepts in nursing care*. (7th ed.). Philadelphia, PA: Lippincott Williams & Wilkins.

Goodman, T. (2014). *Essentials of perioperative nursing* (5th ed.). Sudbury, MA: Jones & Bartlett.

Hannon, R. A., & Porth, C. M. (2017). *Porth pathophysiology: Concepts of altered health states* (2nd Canadian ed.). Philadelphia, PA: Wolters Kluwer Health/Lippincott Williams & Wilkins.

Herdman, T. H. (Ed.). (2012). *NANDA International Nursing Diagnoses: Definitions & Classification, 2012–2014*. Oxford, UK: Wiley-Blackwell.

Meiner, S. E. (2014). *Gerontologic nursing* (5th ed.). St. Louis, MO: Elsevier Mosby.

Miller, R. D. (2014). *Miller's anesthesia* (8th ed.). New York: Elsevier/Churchill Livingstone.

Porth, C. M. (2015). *Essentials of pathophysiology: Concepts of altered states* (4th ed.). Philadelphia, PA: Lippincott Williams & Wilkins.

Rothrock, J. C. (Ed.). (2018). *Alexander's care of the patient in surgery* (16th ed.). St. Louis, MO: Elsevier.

West, J. B. (2015). *Respiratory physiology: The essentials* (10th ed.). Baltimore, MD: Lippincott Williams & Wilkins.

Journals and Electronic Documents

General

Accreditation Canada. (2018). Required organizational practices 2017. Retrieved from https://store.accreditation.ca/products/required-organizational-practices-handbook-2017-version-2.

Allison, J., & George, M. (2014). Using preoperative assessment and patient instruction to improve patient safety. *AORN Journal, 99*(3), 364–375.

Bourdon, L. (2015). Care of the patient receiving local anesthesia. *AORN Journal, 101*(3), 10–12.

Canadian Anesthesiologists' Society (CAS). (2014). Guidelines to the practice of anesthesia—2018. Retrieved from https://www.ncbi.nlm.nih.gov/pubmed/29243160

Canadian Institute for Health Information (CIHI). (2018). Total number of inpatient surgeries in Canada by type in 2016–2017. Retrieved Sept 10, 2018, from https://www.statista.com/statistics/498422/inpatient-surgery-total-number-canada-by-type/.

Canadian Patient Safety Institute. (2016.) Retrieved from: http://www.patientsafetyinstitute.ca/en/NewsAlerts/News/Pages/Safe-Surgery-Checklist-successes-and-good-catches.aspx

Chlebicki, M. P., Safdar, N., O'Horo, J. C., et al. (2013). Preoperative chlorhexidine shower or bath for prevention of surgical site infection: A meta-analysis. *American Journal of Infection Control, 41*, 167–173.

Edmiston, C. E., & Spencer, M. (2014). Patient care interventions to help reduce the risk of surgical site infections. *AORN Journal, 100*(6), 590–602.

Erdling, A., & Johansson, A. (2015). Core temperature: The intraoperative difference between esophageal versus nasopharyngeal temperatures and the impact of prewarming, age, and weight: A randomized clinical trial. *AANA Journal, 83*(2), 99–105.

Health Canada. (2016). Natural health products. Retrieved from https://www.canada.ca/en/health-canada/services/drugs-health-products/natural-non-prescription/regulation/about-products.html.

Huber, J., Ihrig, A., Yass, M., et al. (2013). Multimedia support for improving preoperative patient education: A randomized controlled trial using the example of radical prostatectomy. *Annals of Surgical Oncology, 20*(1), 15–23.

Khan, N., Ghali A. W., Cagliero, E., et al. (2018). Perioperative management of blood glucose in adults with diabetes mellitus. *UpToDate*. Retrieved from https://www.uptodate.com/contents/perioperative-management-of-blood-glucose-in-adults-with-diabetes-mellitus.

Operating Room Nurses Association of Canada (ORNAC). (2013). Standards, guidelines, and position statements for perioperative registered nursing practice. Retrieved from http://www.ornac.ca/.

Oster, K. A., & Oster, C. A. (2015). Special needs population: Care of the geriatric patient population in the perioperative setting. *AORN Journal, 101*(4), 444–456

Rotevatn, T. A., Bøggild, H., Olesen, C. R., et al. (2017). Alcohol consumption and the risk of postoperative mortality and morbidity after primary hip or knee arthroplasty—A register-based cohort study. *PLoS ONE, 12*(3), e0173083.

Statistics Canada. (2014). Retrieved from https://www.statcan.gc.ca/pub/82-625-x/2015001/article/14185-eng.htm.

The Joint Commission. (2016). 2016 National Patient Safety Goals. Retrieved September 10, 2018, from www.jointcommission.org/standards_information/npsgs.aspx.

Wait Times for Priority Procedures in Canada. (2017). Retrieved from https://www.cihi.ca/sites/default/files/document/wait-times-report-2017_en.pdf.

Preoperative Assessment

Beiranvand, S., Noparast, M., Eslamizade, N., et al. (2014). The effects of religion and spirituality on postoperative pain, hemodynamic functioning and anxiety after cesarean section. *Acta Medica Iranica, 52*(12), 909–915.

Bradt, J., Dileo, C., & Shim, M. (2013). Music interventions for preoperative anxiety. *Cochrane Database of Systematic Reviews, 6*. doi: 10.1002/14651858.CD006908.pub2.

Chung, F., Nagappa, M., Singh, M., et al. (2016). CPAP in the perioperative setting. *Chest, 149*(2), 586–597.

Doaust, R., Paquet, J., Moore, L., et al. (2018). Recent opioid use and fall-related injuries among older patients with trauma. *Canadian Medical Association Journal, 190*(16), E500-506.

Francon, D., Chambrier, C., & Sztark, F. (2012). Nutritional assessment of patients before surgery. *Annales Francaises d'Anesthesie et de Reanimation, 31*(6), 506–511.

Gomes, P. C., Caporossi, C., Aguilar-Nascimento, J. E., et al. (2017). Residual gastric volume evaluation with ultrasonography after ingestion of carbohydrate- or carbohydrate plus glutamine-enriched beverages: A randomized, crossover clinical trial with healthy volunteers. *Arguivos de Gastroenterologia, 54*(1), 33–36.

Magalhaes, E., Marques, F. O., Govêia, C. S., et al. (2013). Use of simple clinical predictors on preoperative diagnosis of difficult endotracheal intubation in obese patients. *Brazilian Journal of Anesthesiology, 63*(3), 262–266.

McGlinch, B. P., Que, F. G., Nelson, J. L., et al. (2006). Perioperative care of patients undergoing bariatric surgery. *Mayo Clinic Proceedings, 81*(10 Suppl), S25–S33.

Milis, E., Eyawo, O., Lockhart, I., et al. (2011). Smoking cessation reduces postoperative complications: A systematic review and meta-analysis. *The American Journal of Medicine, 124*(2), 144–154.

Moller, A., & Villebro, N. (2007). Interventions for preoperative smoking cessation. *Cochrane Database of Systematic Reviews, 3*, CD002294.

Muluk, V., et al. (2018). Perioperative medication management. *UpToDate*. https://www.uptodate.com/contents/perioperative-medication-management.

Plourde, G., & Prud'homme, D. (2012). Managing obesity in adults in primary care. *Canadian Medical Association Journal, 184*(9), 1039–1044.

Plumer, L., Seiffert, M., Punke, M. A., et al. (2017). Aspirin before elective surgery—Stop or continue? A single-center cross-sectional study. *Deutsches Arzteblatt International*, *114*(27/28), 473–480.

Pritchard, M. J. (2012). Pre-operative assessment of elective surgical patients. *Nursing Standard*, 26(30), 51–56.

Renouf, T., Leary, A., & Wiseman, T. (2014). Do psychological interventions reduce preoperative anxiety? *British Journal of Nursing*, *23*(22), 1208–1212.

Sieber, F. E., & Barnett, S. R. (2011). Preventing postoperative complications in the elderly. *Anesthesiology Clinics*, *29*(1), 83–97.

Thanavaro, J. L. (2015). Cardiac risk assessment: Decreasing postoperative complications. *AORN Journal*, *101*(2), 201–212.

Thompson, M., Moe, K., & Lewis, C. P. (2014). The effects of music on diminishing anxiety among preoperative patients. *Journal of Radiology Nursing*, *33*(4), 199–202.

Tonella, R. M., Ratti, L. D. S. R., Delazari, L. E. B., et al. (2017). Inspiratory muscle training in the intensive care unit: A new perspective. *Journal of Clinical Medicine Research*, *9*(11), 929–934.

Wang, X. M., Brisbin, S., Loo, T., et al. (2015). Elder abuse: An approach to identification, assessment and intervention. *Canadian Medical Association Journal*, *187*(8), 575–581.

Watt, J., Tricco, A. C., Talbot-Hamon, C., et al. (2018). Identifying older adults at risk of harm following elective surgery: A systematic review and meta-analysis. *BioMed Central*, *16*, 2.

Webster, J., Osborne, S. R., Gill, R., et al. (2014). Does preoperative oral carbohydrate reduce hospital stay? A randomized trial. *AORN Journal*, *99*(2), 233–242.

Resources

American Society of Metabolic and Bariatric Surgery: http://www.asmbs.org
Association of Perioperative Registered Nurses: http://www.aorn.org
Canadian Anesthesiologists' Society: http://www.cas.ca
Operating Room Nurses Association of Canada (ORNAC): http://www.ornac.ca
The Joint Commission: http://www.jointcommission.org

20 Intraoperative Nursing Management

Adapted by Willy Kabotoff

Learning Objectives

On completion of this chapter, the learner will be able to:

1. Describe the interdisciplinary approach to the care of the patient during surgery.
2. Describe the principles of surgical asepsis.
3. Describe the roles of the surgical team members during the intraoperative phase of care.
4. Identify adverse effects of surgery and anesthesia.
5. Identify the surgical risk factors related to age-specific populations and nursing interventions to reduce those risks.
6. Compare types of anesthesia with regard to uses, advantages, disadvantages, and nursing responsibilities.
7. Use the nursing process to optimize patient outcomes during the intraoperative period.
8. Describe the role of the nurse in ensuring patient safety during the intraoperative period.

The intraoperative experience has undergone many changes and advances that make it safer and less disturbing to patients. Even with these advances, anesthesia and surgery still place the patient at risk for several complications or adverse events. Consciousness or full awareness, mobility, protective biologic functions, and personal control are totally or partially relinquished by the patient when entering the operating room (OR). The staff from the departments of **anesthesia**, nursing, and surgery work collaboratively to implement professional standards of care, to control iatrogenic and individual risks, to prevent complications, and to promote high-quality patient outcomes.

The Surgical Team

The surgical team consists of the patient, the anesthesiologist or certified registered **nurse anesthetist** (CRNA), the surgeon, nurses, and the surgical technologists. The **anesthesiologist** administers the anesthetic agent and monitors the patient's physical status throughout the surgery. The surgeon, nurses, and assistants scrub and perform the surgery. The person in the scrub role, either a nurse or a surgical technologist, provides sterile instruments and supplies to the surgeon during the procedure. The circulating nurse coordinates the care of the patient in the OR and provides any additional needed supplies to the scrub nurse and surgeon. Care provided by the **circulating nurse** includes assisting with patient positioning, preparing the patient's skin for surgery, managing surgical specimens, anticipating the needs of the surgical team, and documenting intraoperative events. Collaboration of the surgical team using evidence-based practice tailored to the specific case results in optimum patient care and improved outcomes.

The Patient

As the patient enters the OR, he or she may feel either relaxed and prepared or fearful and highly stressed. These feelings depend to a large extent on the amount and timing of preoperative sedation and the individual patient's level of fear and anxiety. Fears about loss of control, the unknown, pain, death, changes in body structure or function, previous experiences with surgery or hospitals (personal or of loved ones), and disruption of lifestyle, all contribute to anxiety. These fears can increase the amount of anesthetic medication needed, the level of postoperative pain, and overall recovery time. See Chapter 9 or more information on stress.

The patient is also subject to several risks. Infection, failure of the surgery to relieve symptoms or correct a deformity, temporary or permanent complications related to the procedure or the anesthetic agent, and death are uncommon but potential outcomes of the surgical experience (Chart 20-1). In addition to fears and risks, the patient undergoing sedation and anesthesia temporarily loses both cognitive function and biologic self-protective mechanisms. Loss of pain sense, reflexes, and ability to communicate, subjects the intraoperative patient to possible injury.

Gerontologic Considerations

The older adult patient faces higher risks from anesthesia and surgery compared to the younger adult patient (Gajdos, Kile, Hawn, et al., 2013). There is a progressive loss of skeletal muscle mass in conjunction with an increase in adipose tissue. Statistically, perioperative risk increases with each decade after 60 years of age. Key predictors of perioperative complications in the older adult are the patient's preoperative condition, level of function, and comorbid conditions (Rothrock, 2018). About one third of surgical patients are 65 years of age or older (Oster & Oster, 2015). These numbers will increase with prolongation of the lifespan (Neuman & Bosk, 2013). Even in the healthiest older adult perioperative management is considerably more complex because of comorbidities, more advanced disease, and increased susceptibility to nosocomial illnesses. Age alone confers enough surgical risk that it is a clinical predictor of cardiovascular complications (Meiner, 2014; Smeili & Lotufo, 2015).

Biologic variations of particular importance include age-related cardiovascular and pulmonary changes. The aging heart and blood vessels have decreased ability to respond to stress. Reduced cardiac output and limited cardiac reserve make the older patient vulnerable to changes in circulating volume and blood oxygen levels. Excessive or rapid administration of intravenous (IV) solutions can cause pulmonary edema. A sudden or prolonged decline in blood pressure may lead to cerebral ischemia, thrombosis, embolism, infarction, and anoxia. Reduced gas exchange can result in cerebral hypoxia.

The older adult patient needs lower doses of anesthetic agents due to decreased tissue elasticity (lung and cardiovascular systems) and reduced lean tissue mass. They may often experience an increase in the duration of clinical effects of medications. With decreased plasma proteins,

Glossary

anesthesia: a state of narcosis, analgesia, relaxation, and loss of reflexes

anesthesiologist: physician trained to deliver anesthesia and to monitor the patient's condition during surgery

anesthetic agent: the substance, such as a chemical or gas, used to induce anesthesia

anesthetist: health care professional, such as a nurse anesthetist, who is trained to deliver anesthesia and to monitor the patient's condition during surgery

circulating nurse (or circulator): registered nurse who coordinates and documents patient care in the operating room

epidural anesthesia: state of narcosis, analgesia, relaxation, and loss of reflexes achieved by injecting an anesthetic agent into the epidural space of the spinal cord

general anesthesia: state of narcosis, analgesia, relaxation, and loss of reflexes produced by pharmacologic agents

local anesthesia: injection of a solution containing the anesthetic agent into the tissues at the planned incision site

malignant hyperthermia: a rare life-threatening condition triggered by exposure to most anesthetic agents inducing a drastic and uncontrolled increase in skeletal muscle oxidative metabolism that can overwhelm the body's capacity to supply oxygen, remove carbon dioxide, and regulate body temperature, eventually leading to circulatory collapse and death if untreated. Malignant hyperthermia is often inherited as an autosomal dominant disorder

moderate sedation: previously referred to as conscious sedation, involves use of sedation to depress the level of consciousness without altering the patient's ability to maintain a patent airway and to respond to physical stimuli and verbal commands

monitored anesthesia care: moderate sedation administered by an anesthesiologist

nurse anesthetist: a registered nurse (RN) with advanced educational credentials and significant clinical training. A certified registered nurse anesthetist (CRNA) provides care to patients that require anesthesia or pain management before surgeries or specific types of medical procedures.

regional anesthesia: an anesthetic agent is injected around nerves so that the area supplied by these nerves is anesthetized

restricted zone: area in the operating room where scrub attire and surgical masks are required; includes operating room and sterile core areas

scrub role: registered nurse, licensed practical nurse, or surgical technologist who scrubs and dons sterile surgical attire, prepares instruments and supplies, and hands instruments to the surgeon during the procedure

semirestricted zone: area in the operating room where scrub attire is required; may include areas where surgical instruments are processed

spinal anesthesia: achieved when a local anesthetic agent is introduced into the subarachnoid space of the spinal cord

surgical asepsis: absence of microorganisms in the surgical environment to reduce the risk for infection

unrestricted zone: area in the operating room that interfaces with other departments; includes patient reception area and holding area

CHART 20-1

Potential Adverse Effects of Surgery and Anesthesia

Anesthesia and surgery disrupt all major body systems. Although most patients can compensate for surgical trauma and the effects of anesthesia, all patients are at risk during the operative procedure. These risks include the following:

- Allergic reactions
- Anesthesia awareness
- Cardiac dysrhythmia from electrolyte imbalance or adverse effect of anesthetic agents
- Myocardial depression, bradycardia, and circulatory collapse
- Central nervous system agitation, seizures, and respiratory arrest
- Oversedation or undersedation
- Agitation or disorientation, especially in older adult patients
- Hypoxemia or hypercarbia from hypoventilation and inadequate respiratory support during anesthesia
- Laryngeal trauma, oral trauma, and broken teeth from difficult intubation
- Hypothermia from cool operating room temperatures, exposure of body cavities, and impaired thermoregulation secondary to anesthetic agents
- Hypotension from blood loss or adverse effect of anesthesia
- Infection
- Thrombosis from compression of blood vessels or stasis
- Malignant hyperthermia secondary to adverse effect of anesthesia
- Nerve damage and skin breakdown from prolonged or inappropriate positioning
- Electrical shock or burns
- Laser burns
- Drug toxicity, faulty equipment, and other types of human error

Adapted from Association of PeriOperative Registered Nurses (AORN). (2014). *Association of PeriOperative Registered Nurses (AORN) standards, recommended practice, and guidelines*. Denver, CO: Author; Spruce, L. (2015). Back to basics: Procedural sedation. *AORN Journal*, *101*(3), 345–353.

more of the anesthetic agent remains free or unbound, and the result is more potent action (Misal, Joshi, & Shaikh, 2016).

In addition, body tissues of the older adult are made up predominantly of water while those tissues with a rich blood supply, such as skeletal muscle, liver, and kidneys, shrink as the body ages. Reduced liver size decreases the rate at which the liver can inactivate many anesthetic agents, and decreased kidney function slows the elimination of waste products and anesthetic agents. Other factors that affect the older adult surgical patient in the intraoperative period include the following:

- Impaired ability to increase metabolic rate and impaired thermoregulatory mechanisms increase susceptibility to hypothermia.
- Bone loss (25% in women, 12% in men) necessitates careful manipulation and positioning during surgery.
- Reduced ability to adjust rapidly to emotional and physical stress influences surgical outcomes and requires meticulous observation of vital functions.

All of these factors lead to a higher likelihood of perioperative mortality and morbidity in older adult patients (Oster & Oster, 2015; Penprase & Johnson, 2015). (Further discussion of age-related physiologic changes can be found in Chapter 14.)

Nursing Care

Throughout surgery, nursing responsibilities include providing for the safety and well-being of the patient, coordinating the OR personnel, and performing scrub and circulating activities. Because the patient's emotional state remains a concern, the care initiated by preoperative nurses is continued by the intraoperative nursing staff. The nurse supports coping strategies and reinforces the patient's ability to influence outcomes by encouraging active participation in the plan of care incorporating cultural, ethnic, and religious considerations as appropriate.

As patient advocates, intraoperative nurses monitor factors that can cause injury, such as patient positioning, equipment malfunction, and environmental hazards, and they protect the patient's dignity and interests while the patient is anesthetized. Additional responsibilities include maintaining surgical standards of care and identifying and minimizing risks and complications (The Operating Room Nurses Association of Canada [ORNAC], 2017).

Cultural Diversity

Cultural, ethnic, and religious diversity are important considerations for all health care professionals. Nurses in the perioperative area should be aware of medications that may be prohibited by certain groups (i.e., Muslims and those of the Jewish faith cannot use porcine-based products [heparin {porcine or bovine}], Buddhists may choose not to use bovine products). In certain cultures, the head is a sacred area and staff should allow patients to apply their own surgical cap in this case. When English is the second language of the patient having surgery under **local anesthesia**, personnel with knowledge of anesthesia can be provided who speak the patient's native language (Shapeton, O'Donoghue, VanderWielen, et al., 2017).

The Circulating Nurse

The circulating nurse, a qualified registered nurse, works in collaboration with surgeons, anesthesia providers, and other health care providers to plan the best course of action for each patient (Phillips, 2016; Rothrock, 2018). In this leadership role, the circulating nurse manages the OR and protects the patient's safety and health by monitoring the activities of the surgical team, checking the OR conditions, and continually assessing the patient for signs of injury and implementing appropriate interventions. The main responsibilities of the circulating nurse include verifying consent; coordinating the team; and ensuring cleanliness, proper temperature, humidity, lighting, safe function of equipment, and the availability of supplies and materials. The circulating nurse monitors aseptic practices to avoid breaks in technique while coordinating the movement of related personnel (medical, x-ray, and laboratory), as well as implementing fire safety precautions. The circulating nurse also monitors the patient and documents specific activities throughout the operation to ensure the patient's safety and well-being.

Surgical Safety Checklist

World Health Organization | Patient Safety
A World Alliance for Safer Health Care

Before induction of anaesthesia → **Before skin incision** → **Before patient leaves operating room**

Before induction of anaesthesia

(with at least nurse and anaesthetist)

Has the patient confirmed his/her identity, site, procedure, and consent?
- ☐ Yes

Is the site marked?
- ☐ Yes
- ☐ Not applicable

Is the anaesthesia machine and medication check complete?
- ☐ Yes

Is the pulse oximeter on the patient and functioning?
- ☐ Yes

Does the patient have a:

Known allergy?
- ☐ No
- ☐ Yes

Difficult airway or aspiration risk?
- ☐ No
- ☐ Yes, and equipment/assistance available

Risk of >500ml blood loss (7ml/kg in children)?
- ☐ No
- ☐ Yes, and two IVs/central access and fluids planned

Before skin incision

(with nurse, anaesthetist and surgeon)

- ☐ **Confirm all team members have introduced themselves by name and role.**
- ☐ **Confirm the patient's name, procedure, and where the incision will be made.**

Has antibiotic prophylaxis been given within the last 60 minutes?
- ☐ Yes
- ☐ Not applicable

Anticipated Critical Events

To Surgeon:
- ☐ What are the critical or non-routine steps?
- ☐ How long will the case take?
- ☐ What is the anticipated blood loss?

To Anaesthetist:
- ☐ Are there any patient-specific concerns?

To Nursing Team:
- ☐ Has sterility (including indicator results) been confirmed?
- ☐ Are there equipment issues or any concerns?

Is essential imaging displayed?
- ☐ Yes
- ☐ Not applicable

Before patient leaves operating room

(with nurse, anaesthetist and surgeon)

Nurse Verbally Confirms:
- ☐ The name of the procedure
- ☐ Completion of instrument, sponge and needle counts
- ☐ Specimen labelling (read specimen labels aloud, including patient name)
- ☐ Whether there are any equipment problems to be addressed

To Surgeon, Anaesthetist and Nurse:
- ☐ What are the key concerns for recovery and management of this patient?

This checklist is not intended to be comprehensive. Additions and modifications to fit local practice are encouraged. Revised 1 / 2009 © WHO, 2009

FIGURE 20-1. Surgical safety checklist. (Used with permission from World Health Organization. (2015). New checklist to help make surgery safer. *WHO Bulletin*, *86*(7), 496–576. Retrieved January 24, 2019, from http://apps.who.int/iris/bitstream/10665/44186/2/9789241598590_eng_Checklist.pdf)

In addition, the circulating nurse is responsible for ensuring that the second verification of the surgical procedure and site takes place and is documented (Fig. 20-1). In many institutions, a "time out" takes place prior to induction of anesthesia. Every member of the surgical team verifies the patient's name, procedure, and surgical site using objective documentation and data before beginning the surgery (ORNAC, 2017; World Health Organization [WHO], 2015). Proper patient identification is reviewed in Chapter 19. Research suggests that use of a surgical safety checklist reduces morbidity and mortality (Hayne, Edmondson, Lipsitz, et al., 2017).

NURSING ALERT

It is imperative that the correct patient identity, surgical procedure, and surgical site be verified prior to surgery. The surgical site should be marked by the patient and physician prior to coming to the OR suite during the consent process. The surgical site should be marked by the patient and physician prior to coming to the OR suite during the consent process.

The Scrub Role

The activities of the **scrub role** include performing a surgical hand scrub; donning sterile gloves; setting up the sterile tables; preparing sutures, ligatures, and special equipment (e.g., laparoscope); assisting the surgeon and the surgical assistants during the procedure by anticipating the instruments and supplies that will be required, such as sponges, drains, and other equipment; and performing a surgical count to prevent equipment being retained in the body after surgery. As the surgical incision is closed, the scrub person and the circulator count all needles, sponges, and instruments to be sure they are accounted for and not retained as a foreign body in the patient (ORNAC, 2017; Zejnullahu, Bicaj, Zejnullahu, et al., 2017). Standards call for all sponges to be visible on x-ray and for sponge counts to take place at the beginning of surgery and twice at the end. Tissue specimens obtained during surgery are labelled by the person in the scrub role and sent to the laboratory by the circulator.

The Surgeon

The surgeon performs the surgical procedure, heads the surgical team, and is a licensed physician (MD), osteopath (DO), oral surgeon (DDS or DMD), or podiatrist (DPM) who is specially trained and qualified. Qualifications may include certification by a specialty board; adherence to standards of Accreditation Canada and the Canadian Standards Association; and to hospital standards, admitting practices, and procedures (Phillips, 2016).

The Registered Nurse First Assistant

The registered nurse first assistant (RNFA) is a relative new addition to the Canadian surgical team. The RNFA will practice under the direct supervision of the surgeon. RNFA responsibilities may include handling tissue, providing exposure at the operative field, suturing, and maintaining hemostasis (RNFA Ontario, 2018). The RNFA must be aware of the objectives of the surgery, must have the knowledge and ability to anticipate needs and to work as a skilled member of a team, and must be able to handle any emergency situation in the OR.

The Anesthesiologist and Anesthetist

An anesthesiologist is a physician specifically trained in the art and science of anesthesiology. Anesthesiologist is the term preferred in Canada to represent a medically trained doctor who is educated in anesthesia. An anesthetist is also a qualified and specifically trained health care professional who administers anesthetic medications. In the United States, most anesthetists are nurses who have graduated from an accredited nurse anesthesia program and have passed examinations sponsored by the American Association of Nurse Anesthetists to become a CRNA. In Canada, nurse anesthetists currently work in Ontario and the BC health minister announced in 2012 that this role would be utilized in BC. In BC there are also postdiplomas for RNs and RTs to become anesthesia assistants.

The anesthesiologist assesses the patient before surgery, selects the anesthesia, administers it, intubates the patient if necessary, manages any technical problems related to the administration of the anesthetic agent, and supervises the patient's condition throughout the surgical procedure. Before the patient enters the OR, often at preadmission testing, the anesthesiologist visits the patient to perform an assessment, supplies information, and answers questions. The type of anesthetic agent to be administered, previous reactions to anesthetic medications, and known anatomic abnormalities that would make airway management difficult is also discussed.

Registered nurses working in operating rooms in Canada should be aware that Canadian anesthesiologists use the American Society of Anesthesiologists (ASA) Physical Status Classification System (2008) to determine the patient's status. A patient classified as P2, P3, or P4 has a systemic disease that may or may not be related to the cause of surgery. If a patient with a classification of P1, P2, P3, P4, or P5 requires emergency surgery, an E is added to the physical status designation (e.g., P1E, P2E). P6 refers to a patient who is brain dead and is undergoing surgery as an organ donor (Phillips, 2016).

When the patient arrives in the OR, the anesthesiologist reassesses the patient's physical condition immediately prior to initiating anesthesia. The anesthetic agent is administered, and the patient's airway is maintained through either an intranasal intubation, oral intubation, or a laryngeal mask airway (LMA). During surgery, the anesthesiologist monitors the patient's blood pressure, pulse, and respirations as well as the electrocardiogram (ECG), blood oxygen saturation level, tidal volume, blood gas levels, blood pH, alveolar gas concentrations, and body temperature. A mass spectrometer provides continuous readouts of levels of anesthetic medications in the body and critical concentration levels on display terminals. This information assesses the patient's ability to breathe unassisted or the need for mechanical assistance if ventilation is poor and the patient is not breathing well independently.

The Surgical Environment

The surgical environment is known for its stark appearance and cool temperature. The surgical suite is behind double doors, and access is limited to authorized personnel. External precautions include adherence to principles of **surgical asepsis**; strict control of the OR environment is required, including traffic pattern restrictions. Policies governing this environment address issues such as the health of the staff; the cleanliness of the rooms; the sterility of equipment and surfaces; processes for scrubbing, gowning, and gloving; and OR attire (ORNAC, 2017).

To provide the best possible conditions for surgery, the OR is situated in a location that is central to all supporting services (e.g., pathology, x-ray, and laboratory). The OR has special air filtration devices to screen out contaminating particles, dust, and pollutants.

Accreditation Canada and the CSA work collaboratively to ensure the safe care of individuals in health care. The CSA has developed many standards that relate to the surgical environment and Accreditation Canada has developed accreditation guidelines that apply to the surgical area. The risk of fire in the OR is ever present due to three factors: a source of fuel, an oxygen source, and a mechanism to ignite a fire (ORNAC, 2017). All surgical services personnel must familiarize themselves with the department fire emergency response plan and be competent in the use and safeguards of all combustible materials and equipment in the surgical environment (UpToDate, 2017). Surgical drapes provide an opportunity for oxygen to concentrate; a stray spark could more easily ignite a fire. To further improve safety, electrical hazards, emergency exit clearances, and storage of equipment and anesthetic gases are monitored periodically by official agencies, such as the provincial department of health and Accreditation Canada.

To help decrease microbes, the surgical area is divided into three zones: the **unrestricted zone**, where street clothes are allowed; the **semirestricted zone**, where attire consists of scrub clothes and caps; and the **restricted zone**, where scrub clothes, shoe covers, caps, and masks are worn. The surgeons and other surgical team members wear additional sterile clothing and protective devices during surgery.

ORNAC (2017) recommends specific practices for personnel wearing surgical attire to promote a high level of cleanliness in a particular practice setting. OR attire includes a two piece scrub suit with the top and drawstrings tucked inside the pants. The uniform prevents organisms shed from the perineum, legs, and arms from being released into the immediate surroundings. Wet or soiled garments should be changed.

Masks are worn at all times in the restricted zone of the OR. High-filtration masks decrease the risk of postoperative wound infection by containing and filtering microorganisms from the oropharynx and nasopharynx. Masks should cover the nose and mouth tightly and completely; and adjusted to prevent venting from the sides. Disposable masks have a filtration efficiency exceeding 95%. Masks are changed between patients and should not be worn outside the surgical department. *The mask must be either on or off*; it must not be allowed to hang around the neck.

Headgear completely cover the hair (head and neckline, including beard) so that hair strands, and particles of dandruff or dust do not fall on the sterile field.

It is recommended that shoes be comfortable, supportive and have enclosed toes and heels. Shoe covers are worn when it is anticipated that spills or splashes will occur. If worn, the covers should be changed whenever they become wet, torn, or soiled (Phillips, 2016; Rothrock, 2018).

Barriers such as scrub attire and masks do not entirely protect the patient from microorganisms. Upper respiratory tract infections, sore throats, and skin infections in staff and patients are sources of pathogens and must be reported.

Because artificial fingernails harbour higher numbers of microorganisms than natural fingernails, a ban on artificial nails by OR personnel is supported by the Centers for Disease Control and Prevention (CDC), ORNAC, and the Public Health Agency of Canada.

Principles of Surgical Asepsis

Surgical asepsis prevents the contamination of surgical wounds. The patient's natural skin flora or a previously existing infection may cause postoperative wound infection. Rigorous adherence to the principles of surgical asepsis by OR personnel is basic to preventing surgical site infections.

All surgical supplies, instruments, needles, sutures, dressings, gloves, covers, and solutions that may come in contact with the surgical wound or exposed tissues must be sterilized before use (Li & Ji, 2017). Traditionally, the surgeon, surgical assistants, and nurses prepared themselves by scrubbing their hands and arms with antiseptic soap and water, but this practice is being challenged by research investigating the optimal length of time to scrub and the best preparation to use. In some institutions, an alcohol-based product or scrubless soap is used to prepare for surgery (WHO, n.d.).

In addition to the attire previously discussed, surgical team members wear long-sleeved, sterile gowns and gloves. During surgery, only personnel who have scrubbed, gloved, and gowned may touch sterilized objects. Nonscrubbed personnel refrain from touching or contaminating anything sterile or entering the sterile field.

An area of the patient's skin considerably larger than that requiring exposure during the surgery is meticulously cleansed, and an antiseptic solution is applied (Phillips, 2016). If hair needs to be removed, this is done immediately before the procedure with clippers (not shaved) to minimize the risk of infection (ORNAC, 2017). The remainder of the patient's body is covered with sterile drapes.

Environmental Controls

In addition to the protocols described previously, surgical asepsis requires meticulous cleaning and maintenance of the OR environment. Floors and horizontal surfaces are cleaned between cases with detergent, soap and water or a detergent germicide. Sterilized equipment is inspected regularly to ensure optimal operation and performance.

All equipment that comes into direct contact with the patient must be sterile. Sterilized linens, drapes, and solutions are used. Instruments are cleaned and sterilized in a unit near the OR. Individually wrapped sterile items are used when additional individual items are needed.

To decrease the amount of bacteria in the air, standard OR ventilation provides 15 air exchanges per hour, at least three of which are fresh air (Phillips, 2016). A room temperature of 20° to 23°C (68° to 73°F), humidity between 30% and 60%, and positive pressure relative to adjacent areas are maintained. Staff members shed skin scales, resulting in about 1,000 bacteria-carrying particles (or colony-forming units [CFUs])/cubic foot/min. With the standard air exchanges, air counts of bacteria are reduced from an expected level of 1,000 CFUs/cubic foot/min to 50 to 150 CFUs/cubic foot/min. Systems with high-efficiency particulate air (HEPA) filters are needed to remove particles larger than 0.3 μm (Rothrock, 2018). Unnecessary personnel and physical movement may be restricted to minimize bacteria in the air and to achieve an OR infection rate no greater than 3% to 5% in clean, infection-prone surgery.

Some ORs have laminar airflow units. These units provide 400 to 500 air exchanges per hour (and can result in fewer than 10 CFUs/cubic foot/min during surgery [Phillips, 2016]). The goal for a laminar airflow-equipped OR is an infection rate of less than 1%. An OR equipped with a laminar airflow unit is frequently used for total joint replacement or organ transplant surgery.

Despite using all precautions, wound contamination may inadvertently occur resulting in a nosocomial infection and a prolonged hospitalization. Constant surveillance and conscientious technique in carrying out aseptic practices are necessary to reduce the risk of contamination and infection.

Basic Guidelines for Maintaining Surgical Asepsis

All practitioners involved in the intraoperative phase have a responsibility to provide and maintain a safe environment. Adherence to aseptic practice is part of this responsibility. The basic principles of aseptic technique are as follows:

- All materials in contact with the surgical wound or used within the sterile field must be sterile. Sterile surfaces or articles may touch other sterile surfaces or articles and remain sterile; contact with unsterile objects at any point renders a sterile area contaminated.
- Only the front of surgical gowns is considered sterile from the chest to the level of the sterile field. The sleeves are also considered sterile from 2 in above the elbow to the cuff.
- Sterile drapes are used to create a sterile field (Fig. 20-2). Only the top surface of a draped table is considered sterile. During draping of a table or patient, the sterile drape is held well above the surface to be covered and is

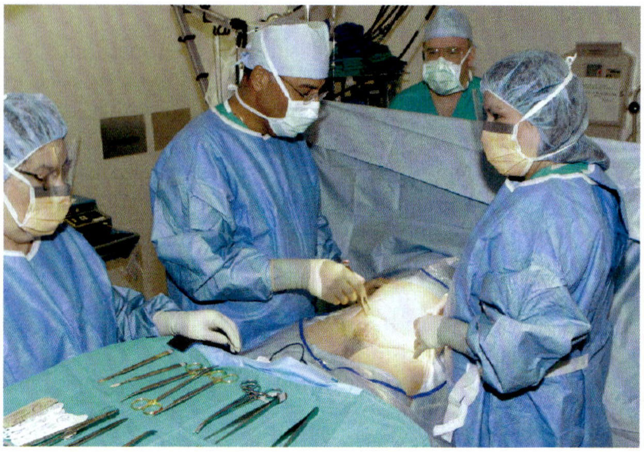

FIGURE 20-2. Proper draping exposes only the surgical site, which decreases the risk for infection.

positioned from front to back. Items are dispensed to a sterile field by methods that preserve the sterility of the items and the integrity of the sterile field. After a sterile package is opened, the edges are considered unsterile. Sterile supplies, including solutions, are delivered to a sterile field or handed to a scrubbed person in such a way that the sterility of the object or fluid remains intact.

- The movements of the surgical team are from sterile to sterile areas and from unsterile to unsterile areas. Scrubbed people and sterile items contact only sterile areas; circulating nurses and unsterile items contact only unsterile areas.
- Movement around a sterile field must not cause contamination of the field. Sterile areas must be kept in view during movement around the area. At least 30 cm distance from the sterile field must be maintained to prevent inadvertent contamination.
- Whenever a sterile barrier is breached, the area is considered contaminated. A tear or puncture of the drape permitting access to an unsterile surface underneath renders the area unsterile. The drape must be replaced.
- Every sterile field is constantly monitored and maintained. Items of doubtful sterility are considered unsterile. Sterile fields are prepared as close as possible to the time of use.
- The administration of hyperoxia (high levels of oxygen) is *not* recommended to reduce surgical site infections.

Robotics

Robot-assisted technology is increasingly part of the intraoperative environment for cardiac, colorectal, general, gynecologic, head and neck, thoracic, and urologic surgeries (Finkelstein, Rabino, Mashiach, et al., 2014). Several types of robotic-driven tools assist in making surgery more precise and less invasive for patients. All practitioners have a responsibility to be knowledgeable about equipment as well as related policies and procedures for its safe use.

Health Hazards Associated With the Surgical Environment

Faulty equipment, improper use of equipment, exposure to toxic substances, as well as infectious waste, cuts, needlestick injuries, radiation, and laser beams are some of the associated hazards in the surgical environment (Phillips, 2016). Internal monitoring of the OR includes the analysis of surface swipe samples and air samples for infectious and toxic agents. In addition, policies and procedures for minimizing exposure to body fluids and reducing the dangers associated with lasers and radiation have been established (ORNAC, 2017).

Unintentional retention of an object (e.g., sponge, instrument) can occur regardless of the size or location of an incision. A retained object can cause wound infection or disruption, abscess formation, and development of fistulas between organs (Zejnullahu et al., 2017).

Laser Risks

ORNAC and the CSA have recommended practices for laser safety (ORNAC, 2017). When lasers are in use, warning signs must be clearly posted. Safety precautions reduce the possibility of exposing the eyes and skin to laser beams, prevent inhalation of the laser plume (smoke and particulate matter), and protect the patient and personnel from fire and electrical hazards. Perioperative personnel should be familiar with the unique features, specific operation, and safety measures for each of the several types of laser used in the practice setting and wear appropriate laser goggles for the type of laser beam in use.

Smoke evacuators are used in some procedures to remove the laser plume from the operative field. This technology protects the surgical team from the potential hazards associated with the generalized smoke plume generated by standard electrocautery units.

Exposure to Blood and Body Fluids

Double gloving is routine in trauma and other types of surgery where sharp bone fragments are present. In addition to the routine scrub suit and double gloves, some surgical personnel wear rubber boots, a waterproof apron, and sleeve protectors. Goggles, or a wrap-around face shield, are worn to protect against splashing when the surgical wound is irrigated or when bone drilling is performed. In hospitals where numerous total joint procedures are performed, a complete bubble mask may be used. This mask provides full-barrier protection from bone fragments and splashes. Ventilation is accomplished through an accompanying hood with a separate air filtration system.

The Surgical Experience

During the surgical procedure, the patient will need sedation, anesthesia, or some combination of these.

Types of Anesthesia and Sedation

Anesthesia today is very safe: It is estimated that the number of anesthesia-related deaths is lower than 1 in 10,000 surgery-related deaths in developed countries (Pignaton, Braz, Kusano, et al., 2016). For the patient, the anesthesia experience consists of having an IV line inserted, if it was not inserted earlier; receiving a sedating agent prior to induction with an anesthetic agent; losing consciousness; being intubated, if indicated; and then receiving a combination of anesthetic agents. Typically the experience is a smooth one, and the patient has no recall of the events.

The main types of anesthesia are general anesthesia, **regional anesthesia**, **moderate sedation**, monitored anesthesia care (MAC), and local anesthesia.

General Anesthesia

Anesthesia is a state of narcosis (severe central nervous system depression produced by pharmacologic agents), analgesia, relaxation, and reflex loss. Patients under general anesthesia are not arousable, not even to painful stimuli. They lose the ability to maintain ventilatory function and require assistance in maintaining a patent airway. Cardiovascular function may be impaired as well.

There is the rare potential for the phenomenon of patients being partially awake while under general anesthesia (referred to as anesthesia awareness). Patients at greatest risk of anesthesia awareness are cardiac, obstetric, and major trauma patients. The entire surgical team must be aware of this phenomenon and help prevent or manage it. General anesthesia consists of four stages, each associated with specific clinical manifestations (Rothrock, 2018):

- *Stage I: beginning anesthesia.* As the patient breathes in the anesthetic mixture, warmth, dizziness, and a feeling of detachment may be experienced. The patient may have a ringing, roaring, or buzzing in the ears and, although still conscious, may sense an inability to move the extremities easily. During this stage, noises are exaggerated; even low voices or minor sounds seem loud and unreal. For this reason, unnecessary noises and motions are avoided when anesthesia begins.
- *Stage II: excitement.* The excitement stage, characterized variously by struggling, shouting, talking, singing, laughing, or crying, is often avoided if the anesthetic agent is administered smoothly and quickly. The pupils dilate, but they contract if exposed to light; the pulse rate is rapid, and respirations may be irregular. Because of the possibility of uncontrolled movements of the patient during this stage, someone must be ready to help the anesthesiologist restrain the patient. Manipulation increases circulation to the operative site and thereby increases the potential for bleeding.
- *Stage III: surgical anesthesia.* Surgical anesthesia is reached by continued administration of the anesthetic vapour or gas. The patient is unconscious and lies quietly on the table. The pupils are small but contract when exposed to light. Respirations are regular, the pulse rate and volume are normal, and the skin is pink or slightly flushed. With proper administration of the anesthetic agent, this stage may be maintained for hours in one of several planes, ranging from light (1) to deep (4), depending on the depth of anesthesia needed.
- *Stage IV: medullary depression.* This stage is reached if too much anesthesia has been administered. Respirations become shallow, the pulse weak and thready, and the pupils widely dilated and will no longer contract when exposed to light. Cyanosis develops and, without prompt intervention, death rapidly follows. If this stage develops, the anesthetic agent is discontinued immediately and respiratory and circulatory support is initiated to prevent death. Stimulants, although rarely used, may be administered; narcotic antagonists can be used if the overdosage is due to opioids.

When opioid agents (narcotics) and neuromuscular blockers (relaxants) are administered, several of the stages are absent. During smooth administration of an anesthetic agent, there is no sharp division between stages I, II, and III, and there is no stage IV. The patient passes gradually from one stage to another, and it is through close observation of the signs exhibited by the patient that an anesthesiologist controls the situation. Pupil response, the blood pressure, and the respiratory and cardiac rates are among the most reliable guides to the patient's condition.

Anesthetic agents used in **general anesthesia** are inhaled and/or administered by IV. Anesthetic medications produce anesthesia because they are delivered to the brain at a high partial pressure that enables them to cross the blood–brain barrier. Relatively large amounts of anesthetic medication must be administered during induction and the early maintenance phases because the anesthetic agent is recirculated and deposited in body tissues. As these sites become saturated, smaller amounts of the anesthetic agent are required to maintain anesthesia because equilibrium or near equilibrium has been achieved between brain, blood, and other tissues. Any condition that diminishes peripheral blood flow, such as vasoconstriction or shock, may reduce the amount of anesthetic medication required. Conversely, when peripheral blood flow is unusually high, as in a muscularly active or apprehensive patient, induction is slower, and greater quantities of anesthetic agents are required because the brain receives a smaller quantity of anesthetic agent.

Inhalation

Inhaled anesthetic agents include volatile liquid agents and gases. Volatile liquid anesthetic agents produce anesthesia when their vapours are inhaled. Some commonly used inhalation agents are included in Table 20-1. All are administered in combination with oxygen and usually with nitrous oxide as well.

Nitrous oxide is the most commonly used gas anesthetic agent. When inhaled, the anesthetic agents enter the blood through the pulmonary capillaries and act on cerebral centres to produce loss of consciousness and sensation. When anesthetic administration is discontinued, the vapour or gas is eliminated through the lungs.

The vapour from an inhalation anesthetic agent may be administered through several methods. An LMA (Fig. 20-3A), a flexible tube with an inflatable silicone ring and cuff, can be inserted into the larynx. An endotracheal tube may be inserted through either the nose (see Fig. 20-3B) or mouth (see Fig. 20-3C) into the trachea, usually by means of a laryngoscope. When in place, the tube seals off the lungs from the esophagus so that, if the patient vomits, stomach contents do not enter the lungs.

Intravenous Administration

General anesthesia can also be produced by the IV administration of various substances, such as barbiturates, benzodiazepines, nonbarbiturate hypnotics, dissociative agents, and opioid agents. Table 20-2 lists commonly used IV anesthetic and analgesic agents, including IV medications used as muscle relaxants in the intraoperative period. These medications may be administered to induce or maintain anesthesia. Although they are often used in combination with inhalation anesthetic agents, they may be

TABLE 20-1 Inhalation Anesthetic Agents

Agent	Administration	Advantages	Disadvantages	Implications/Considerations
Volatile Liquids				
Halothane (Fluothane)	Inhalation; special vaporizer	Not explosive or flammable Induction rapid and smooth Useful in almost every type of surgery Low incidence of postoperative nausea and vomiting	Requires skillful administration to prevent overdose May cause liver damage May produce hypotension Requires special vaporizer for administration	In addition to observation of pulse and respiration postoperatively, blood pressure must be monitored frequently
Enflurane (Ethrane)	Inhalation	Rapid induction and recovery Potent analgesic agent Not explosive or flammable	Respiratory depression may develop rapidly, along with electrocardiogram abnormalities. Not compatible with epinephrine	Observe for possible respiratory depression. Administration with epinephrine may cause ventricular fibrillation
Isoflurane (Forane)	Inhalation	Rapid induction and recovery Muscle relaxants are markedly potentiated	A profound respiratory depressant	Monitor respirations closely, support when necessary, and monitor for malignant hyperthermia
Sevoflurane[a] (Ultane)	Inhalation	Rapid induction and excretion; minimal side effects	Coughing and laryngospasm; trigger for malignant hyperthermia	Monitor for malignant hyperthermia
Desflurane (Suprane)	Inhalation	Rapid induction and emergence; rare organ toxicity	Respiratory irritation; trigger for malignant hyperthermia	Monitor for malignant hyperthermia and dysrhythmias
Gases				
Nitrous oxide (N_2O)	Inhalation (semiclosed method)	Induction and recovery rapid Nonflammable Useful with oxygen for short procedures Useful with other agents for all types of surgery	Poor relaxant Weak anesthetic May produce hypoxia	Most useful in conjunction with other agents with longer action Monitor for chest pain, nausea and vomiting, hypertension, and stroke
Oxygen (O_2)	Inhalation	Can increase O_2 available to tissues	High concentrations are hazardous	Increased fire risk when used with lasers

[a]Currently most popular choice.

Adapted from Association of PeriOperative Registered Nurses (AORN). (2014). *Association of PeriOperative Registered Nurses (AORN) standards, recommended practice, and guidelines*. Denver, CO: Author.

used alone. They may also be used to produce moderate sedation, as discussed later in this chapter.

An advantage of IV anesthesia is that the onset of anesthesia is pleasant; there is no buzzing, roaring, or dizziness associated with the administration of an inhalation anesthetic agent. The duration of action is brief, and the patient awakens with little nausea or vomiting.

The IV anesthetic agents are nonexplosive, require little equipment, and are easy to administer. The low incidence of postoperative nausea and vomiting makes the method

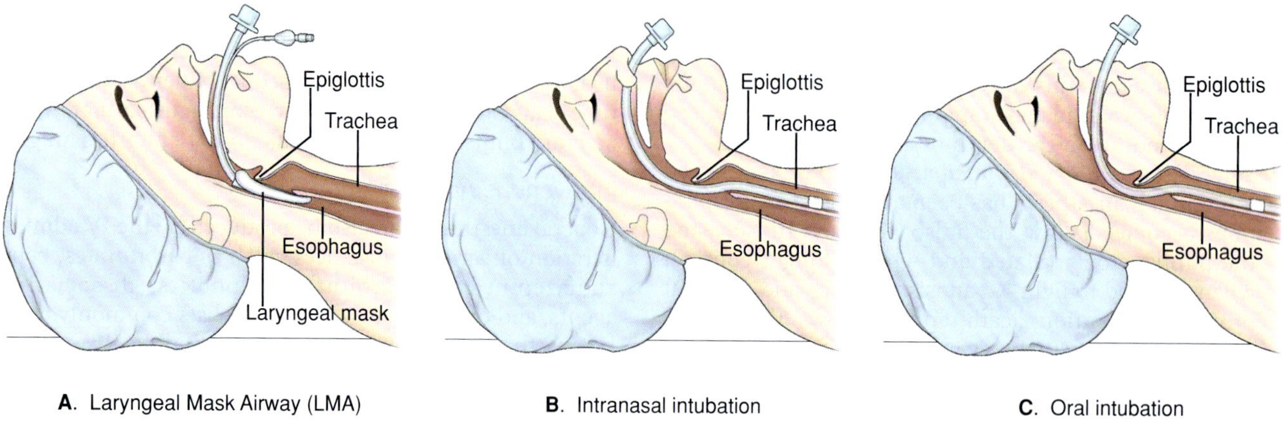

FIGURE 20-3. Anesthetic delivery methods. **A.** laryngeal mask airway (LMA). **B.** Nasal endotracheal catheter (in position with cuff inflated). **C.** Oral endotracheal intubation (in position with cuff inflated).

TABLE 20-2 Commonly Used Intravenous Medications

Medication	Common Usage	Advantages	Disadvantages	Comments
Opioid Analgesic Agents				
Alfentanil (Alfenta)	Surgical analgesia in ambulatory patients	Ultra-short-acting (5–10 minutes) analgesic agent; duration of action 0.5 hours; bolus or infusion		Potency: 750 μg; half-life 1.6 hours
Fentanyl (Sublimaze)	Surgical analgesia: epidural infusion for postoperative analgesia; add to SAB	Good cardiovascular stability; duration of action 0.5 hours	May cause muscle or chest wall rigidity	Most commonly used opioid; potency: 100 μg = 10 mg morphine sulphate; elimination half-life 3.6 hours
Morphine sulphate (MS-Contin)	Preoperative pain; premedication; postoperative pain	Inexpensive; duration of action 4–5 hours; euphoria; good cardiovascular stability	Nausea and vomiting; histamine release; postural ↓ BP and ↓ SVR	Epidural and intrathecal administration for postoperative pain; elimination half-life 3 hours
Remifentanil (Ultiva)	IV infusion for surgical analgesia; small boluses for brief, intense pain	Easily titrated; very short duration; good cardiovascular stability. Ultiva is rapidly metabolized by hydrolysis of the propanoic acid–methyl ester linkage by nonspecific blood and tissue esterases.	Expensive; requires mixing; may cause muscle rigidity	Potency: 25 μg = 10 mg morphine sulphate; 20–30 times potency of alfentanil; elimination half-life 3–10 minutes
Sufentanil (Sufenta)	Surgical analgesia	Duration of action 0.5 hours; prolonged analgesia exceptionally potent (5–10 times more than fentanyl); provides good stability in cardiovascular surgery	Prolonged respiratory depression	Potency: 15 μg = 10 mg morphine sulphate; elimination half-life 2.7 hours
Depolarizing Muscle Relaxants				
Succinylcholine	Relax skeletal muscles for surgery and orthopedic manipulations; short procedures; intubation	Short duration; rapid onset	No known effect on consciousness, pain threshold, or cerebration; fasciculations, postoperative myalgias, dysrhythmias; raises serum K^+ in tissue trauma, muscular disease, paralysis, burns; histamine release is slight; requires refrigeration	Prolonged muscle relaxation with serum cholinesterase deficiency and some antibiotics; may trigger malignant hyperthermia
Nondepolarizing Muscle Relaxants—Intermediate Onset and Duration				
Atracurium besylate (Tracrium)	Intubation; maintenance of skeletal muscle relaxation	No significant cardiovascular or cumulative effects; good with kidney injury	Requires refrigeration; slight histamine release; pregnancy risk category C; do not mix with lactated Ringer's solution or alkaline solutions such as barbiturates	Rapid IV bolus; use cautiously with geriatric and debilitated patients
Cisatracurium besylate (Nimbex)	Intubation; maintenance of skeletal muscle relaxation	Similar to atracurium	No histamine release	Similar to atracurium
Mivacurium (Mivacron)	Intubation; maintenance of skeletal muscle relaxation	Short acting; rapid metabolism by plasma cholinesterase; used as bolus or infusion	Expensive in longer cases	Competes with acetylcholine for receptor sites at the motor end plate, blocking neuromuscular transmission; new; rarely need to reverse; prolonged effect with plasma cholinesterase deficiency

continued >

TABLE 20-2 Commonly Used Intravenous Medications (Continued)

Medication	Common Usage	Advantages	Disadvantages	Comments
Rocuronium (Zemuron)	Intubation; maintenance of relaxation	Rapid onset (dose dependent); elimination via kidney and liver	No known effect on consciousness, pain threshold, or cerebration; vagolytic; may ↑ HR	Duration similar to atracurium and vecuronium
Vecuronium (Norcuron)	Intubation; maintenance of relaxation	No significant cardiovascular or cumulative effects; no histamine release	Requires mixing	Mostly eliminated in bile, some in urine
Nondepolarizing Muscle Relaxants—Longer Onset and Duration				
d-Tubocurarine	Adjunct to anesthesia; maintenance of relaxation		No known effect on consciousness, pain threshold, or cerebration; might cause histamine release and transient ganglionic blockade	Mostly used for pretreatment with succinylcholine
Metocurine (Metubine)	Maintenance of relaxation	Good cardiovascular stability	Slight histamine release	Most commonly used opioid; potency: 100 μg = 10 mg morphine sulphate; elimination half-life 3.6 hours
Pancuronium (Pavulon)	Maintenance of relaxation		May cause ↑ HR and ↑ BP	Used intrathecally and epidurally for postoperative pain; elimination half-life 3 hours
Intravenous Anesthetic Agents				
Diazepam (Valium, Dizac)	Amnesia; hypnotic; relieves anxiety; preoperative	Good sedation	Long acting	Residual effects for 20–90 hours; increased effect with alcohol
Etomidate (Amidate)	Induction of general anesthesia; indicated to supplement low-potency anesthetic agents	Short-acting hypnotic; good cardiovascular stability; fast, smooth induction and recovery	May cause brief period of apnea; pain with injection and myotonic movements	
Ketamine (Ketalar)	Induction; occasional maintenance (IV or IM)	Short acting; profound analgesia; patient maintains airway; good in small children and burn patients	Large doses may cause hallucinations and respiratory depression; chest wall rigidity; laryngeal spasm	Need darkened, quiet room for recovery; often used in trauma cases
Midazolam (Versed)	Hypnotic; anxiolytic; sedation; often used as adjunct to induction	Excellent amnesia; water soluble (no pain with IV injection); short acting	Slower induction than thiopental	Often used for amnesia with insertion of invasive monitors or regional anesthesia; depresses all levels of CNS, including limbic and reticular formation, probably through increased action of GABA, which is major inhibitory neurotransmitter in brain
Propofol (Diprivan)	Induction and maintenance; sedation with regional anesthesia or MAC	Rapid onset; awakening in 4–8 minutes; produces sedation/hypnosis rapidly (within 40 seconds) and smoothly with minimal excitation; decreases intraocular pressure and systemic vascular resistance; rarely is associated with malignant hyperthermia and histamine release	May cause pain when injected; suppresses cardiac output and respiratory drive	Short elimination half-life (34–64 minutes)

TABLE 20-2 Commonly Used Intravenous Medications (Continued)

Medication	Common Usage	Advantages	Disadvantages	Comments
Methohexital sodium (Brevital)	Induction; methohexital slows the activity of brain and nervous system	Ultra-short-acting barbiturate	May cause hiccups	Can be given rectally
Thiopental sodium (Pentothal)	Induction; stops seizures		May cause laryngospasm	Large doses may cause apnea and cardiovascular depression; can be given rectally

BP, blood pressure; CNS, central nervous system; GABA, gamma-aminobutyric acid; HR, heart rate; IM, intramuscular; IV, intravenous; K^+, potassium; MAC, monitored anesthesia care; SAB, subarachnoid block; SVR, stroke volume ratio.

Adapted from Association of PeriOperative Registered Nurses (AORN). (2014). *Association of PeriOperative Registered Nurses (AORN) standards, recommended practice, and guidelines*. Denver, CO: Author; Spruce, L. (2015). Back to basics: Procedural sedation. *AORN Journal, 101*(3), 345–353; Comerford, K. C. (2015). *Nursing 2015 drug handbook*. Philadelphia, PA: Wolters Kluwer.

useful in eye surgery, because in this setting vomiting would increase intraocular pressure and endanger vision in the operated eye. IV anesthesia is useful for short procedures. It is not indicated for children who have small veins or for those who require intubation because of their susceptibility to respiratory obstruction.

IV neuromuscular blockers (muscle relaxants) block the transmission of nerve impulses at the neuromuscular junction of skeletal muscles. Muscle relaxants are used to relax muscles in abdominal and thoracic surgery, relax eye muscles in certain types of eye surgery, facilitate endotracheal intubation, treat laryngospasm, and assist in mechanical ventilation.

Regional Anesthesia

In regional anesthesia, an anesthetic agent is injected around nerves so that the region supplied by these nerves is anesthetized. The effect depends on the type of nerve involved. Motor fibres are the largest fibres and have the thickest myelin sheath. Sympathetic fibres are the smallest and have a minimal covering. Sensory fibres are intermediate. A local anesthetic agent blocks sympathetic nerves more readily than motor nerves. An anesthetic agent cannot be regarded as having worn off until all three systems (motor, sensory, and autonomic) are no longer affected.

The patient receiving regional anesthesia is awake and aware of his or her surroundings unless medications are given to produce mild sedation or to relieve anxiety. The health care team must avoid careless conversation, unnecessary noise, and unpleasant odours; these may be noticed by the patient in the OR and may contribute to a negative response to the surgical experience. The diagnosis must not be stated aloud if the patient is not to know it at this time.

Epidural Anesthesia

Epidural anesthesia is achieved by injecting a local anesthetic agent into the epidural space that surrounds the dura mater of the spinal cord (Fig. 20-4). The administered medication diffuses across the layers of the spinal cord to provide anesthesia and pain relief. In contrast, **spinal anesthesia** involves injection through the dura mater into the subarachnoid space surrounding the spinal cord. Epidural anesthesia blocks sensory, motor, and autonomic functions. Epidural doses are much higher than spinal doses because the epidural anesthetic agent does not make direct contact with the spinal cord or nerve roots.

An advantage of epidural anesthesia is the absence of headache that can result from spinal anesthesia. A disadvantage is the greater technical challenge of introducing the anesthetic agent into the epidural rather than the subarachnoid space. If inadvertent puncture of the dura occurs during epidural anesthesia and the anesthetic agent travels toward the head, high spinal anesthesia can result; this can produce severe hypotension and respiratory depression and arrest. Treatment of these complications includes airway support, IV fluids, and use of vasopressors.

Spinal Anesthesia

Spinal anesthesia is an extensive conduction nerve block that is produced when a local anesthetic agent is introduced into the subarachnoid space at the lumbar level, usually between L4 and L5 (see Fig. 20-4). It produces anesthesia of the lower extremities, perineum, and lower abdomen. For the lumbar puncture procedure, the patient usually lies on the side in a knee–chest position. Sterile technique is used as a spinal puncture is made and the medication is injected through the needle. As soon as the injection has been made, the patient is positioned on his or her back. If a relatively high level of block is sought, the head and shoulders are lowered.

The spread of the anesthetic agent and the level of anesthesia depend on the amount of fluid injected, the speed with which it is injected, the positioning of the patient after the injection, and the specific gravity of the agent. If the specific gravity is greater than that of cerebrospinal fluid (CSF), the agent moves to the dependent position of the subarachnoid space. If the specific gravity is less than that of CSF, the anesthetic agent moves away from the dependent position. The anesthesiologist controls the administration of the agent. Table 20-3 presents types of regional anesthesia agents.

A few minutes after induction of a spinal anesthetic agent, anesthesia and paralysis affect the toes and perineum and then gradually the legs and abdomen. If the anesthetic

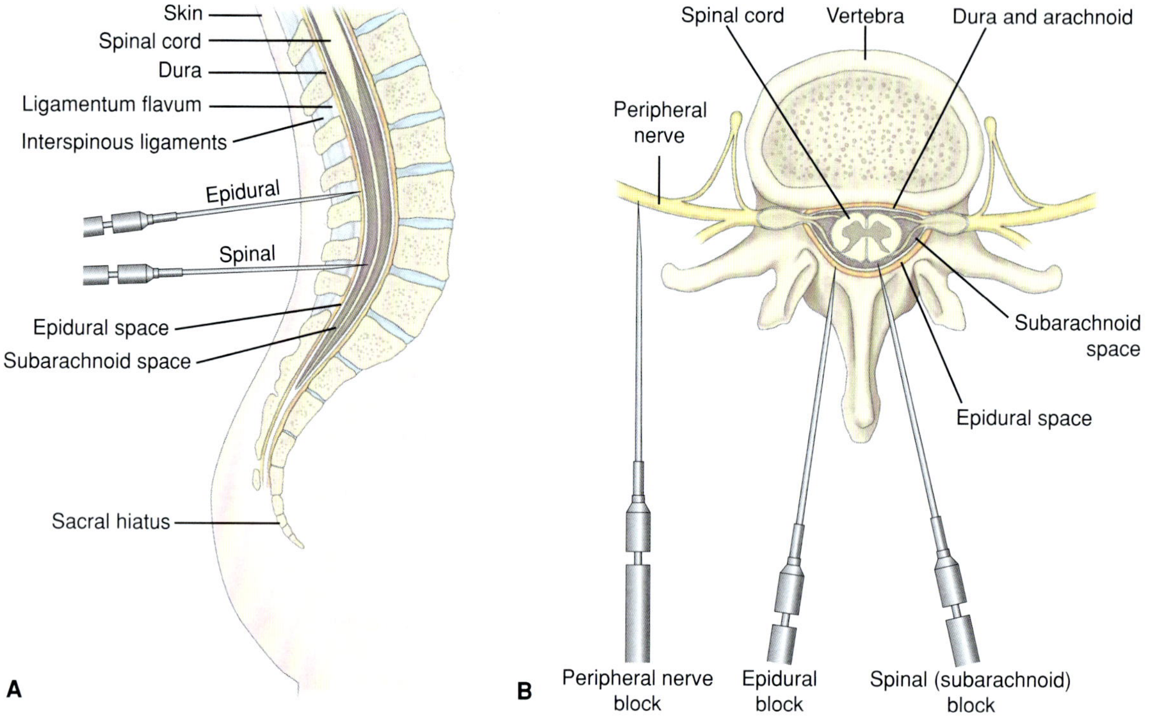

FIGURE 20-4. **A.** Injection sites for spinal and epidural anesthesia. **B.** Cross section of injection sites for peripheral nerve, epidural, and spinal blocks.

agent reaches the upper thoracic and cervical spinal cord in high concentrations, a temporary partial or complete respiratory paralysis results. Paralysis of the respiratory muscles is managed by mechanical ventilation until the effects of the anesthetic agent on the cranial and thoracic nerves have worn off.

Nausea, vomiting, urinary retention, and pain may occur during surgery when spinal anesthesia is used. As a rule, these reactions result from manipulation of various structures, particularly those within the abdominal cavity. Adequate hydration, oxygen, positioning, warming, and the IV administration of appropriate medications may prevent such reactions (O'Neill & Helwig, 2016).

A headache may be an aftereffect of spinal anesthesia. Several factors are related to the incidence of headache: the size of the spinal needle used, the leakage of fluid from the subarachnoid space through the puncture site, and the patient's hydration status. Measures that increase cerebrospinal pressure are helpful in relieving headache. These include maintaining a quiet environment, keeping the patient lying flat, and keeping the patient well hydrated.

TABLE 20-3 Selected Regional and Local Anesthetic Agents

Agent	Administration	Advantages	Disadvantages	Implications/Considerations
Lidocaine (Xylocaine)	Epidural, spinal, peripheral intravenous anesthesia, and local infiltration	Rapid Longer duration of action (compared with procaine) Free from local irritative effect	Occasional idiosyncrasy	Useful topically for cystoscopy Observe for untoward reactions—drowsiness, depressed respiration, seizures
Bupivacaine (Marcaine, Sensoricaine)	Epidural, spinal, peripheral intravenous anesthesia, and local infiltration	Duration is 2–3 times longer than lidocaine	Use cautiously in patients with known drug allergies or sensitivities	A period of analgesia persists after return of sensation; therefore, need for strong analgesic agents is reduced. Greater potency and longer action than lidocaine
Tetracaine (Pontocaine)	Topical, infiltration, and nerve block	Long acting, produces good relaxation	Occasional allergic reaction	More than 10 times as potent as procaine (Novocaine)
Procaine (Novocaine)	Local infiltration		Occasional allergic reaction	Commonly used in oral or dental surgery

In continuous spinal anesthesia, the tip of a plastic catheter remains in the subarachnoid space during the surgical procedure so that more anesthetic medication may be injected as needed. Although this allows for greater control of the dosage, there is greater potential for postanesthetic headache because of the large-gauge needle used.

Local Conduction Blocks

Examples of common local conduction blocks are:

- Brachial plexus block, which produces anesthesia of the arm
- Paravertebral anesthesia, which produces anesthesia of the nerves supplying the chest, abdominal wall, and extremities
- Transsacral (caudal) block, which produces anesthesia of the perineum and, occasionally, the lower abdomen

Moderate Sedation

Moderate sedation, previously referred to as conscious sedation, involves the IV administration of sedatives or analgesic medications to reduce patient anxiety and control pain during diagnostic or therapeutic procedures. It is being used increasingly for specific short-term surgical procedures in hospitals and ambulatory care centres (Leech & Chishti, 2014). The goal is to depress a patient's level of consciousness to a moderate level to enable surgical, diagnostic, or therapeutic procedures to be performed while ensuring the patient's comfort and cooperation with the procedures. With moderate sedation, the patient is able to maintain a patent airway, retain protective airway reflexes, and respond to verbal and physical stimuli.

Moderate sedation can be administered by an anesthesiologist, or other specially trained and credentialed physician or nurse (as applicable to the setting). The patient receiving moderate sedation is never left alone and is closely monitored by a physician or nurse who is knowledgeable and skilled in detecting dysrhythmias, administering oxygen, and performing resuscitation. The continual assessment of the patient's vital signs, level of consciousness, and cardiac and respiratory function is an essential component of moderate sedation. Pulse oximetry, ECG monitor, and frequent measurement of vital signs are used to monitor the patient.

Monitored Anesthesia Care

MAC, also referred to as monitored sedation, is moderate sedation administered by an anesthesiologist who is prepared and qualified to convert to general anesthesia if necessary. The skills of an anesthesiologist may be necessary to manage the effects of a level of deeper sedation to return the patient to the appropriate level of sedation (Barash, Cullen, & Stoelting, 2013). MAC may be used for healthy patients undergoing relatively minor surgical procedures and for some critically ill patients who may be unable to tolerate anesthesia without extensive invasive monitoring and pharmacologic support (Rothrock, 2018).

Local Anesthesia

Local anesthesia is the injection of a solution containing the anesthetic agent into the tissues at the planned incision site. Often it is combined with a local regional block by injecting around the nerves immediately supplying the area. Advantages of local anesthesia are as follows:

- It is simple, economical, and nonexplosive.
- Equipment needed is minimal.
- Postoperative recovery is brief.
- Undesirable effects of general anesthesia are avoided.
- It is ideal for short and minor surgical procedures.

Local anesthesia is often administered in combination with epinephrine. Epinephrine constricts blood vessels, preventing rapid absorption of the anesthetic agent and thus prolonging its local action. Rapid absorption of the anesthetic agent into the bloodstream, which could cause seizures, is also prevented. Agents that can be used as local anesthetic agents are listed in Table 20-3; some of the same agents used in regional anesthesia are used as local anesthetic agents.

Local anesthesia is the preferred method in any surgical procedure in which it can be used. However, contraindications include high preoperative levels of anxiety, because surgery with local anesthesia may increase anxiety. A patient who requests general anesthesia rarely does well under local anesthesia. For some surgical procedures, local anesthesia is impractical because of the number of injections and the amount of anesthetic medication that would be required (e.g., breast reconstruction).

The skin is prepared as for any surgical procedure, and a small-gauge needle is used to inject a modest amount of the anesthetic medication into the skin layers. This produces blanching or a wheal. Additional anesthetic medication is then injected into the skin until an area the length of the proposed incision is anesthetized. A larger, longer needle then is used to infiltrate deeper tissues with the anesthetic agent. The action of the agent is almost immediate, so surgery may begin as soon as the injection is complete. Anesthesia lasts 45 minutes to 3 hours, depending on the anesthetic agent and the simultaneous use of epinephrine.

Potential Intraoperative Complications

The surgical patient is subject to several risks. Potential intraoperative complications include nausea and vomiting, anaphylaxis, hypoxia, hypothermia, and **malignant hyperthermia** (MH).

Anesthesia Awareness

It is important to discuss concerns about intraoperative awareness with patients preoperatively so that they realize that only general anesthesia is meant to create a state of oblivion. All other forms of anesthesia will eliminate pain, but sensation of pushing and pulling tissues may still be recognized, and patients may hear conversations among the operative team. In many cases, patients may be able to respond to questions and involve themselves in the discussion. This is normal and is not what is referred to as anesthesia awareness.

Unintended intraoperative awareness refers to a patient becoming cognizant of surgical interventions while under general anesthesia and then recalling the incident. Neuromuscular blocks, sometimes required for surgical muscle relaxation, intensify the fear of the patient experiencing awareness because they are then unable to communicate during the episode. Indications of the occurrence of anesthesia awareness include an increase in the blood pressure, rapid heart rate, and patient movement. However, hemodynamic changes can be masked by paralytic medication, beta-blockers, and calcium channel blockers; thus, the awareness may remain undetected. Premedication with amnesic agents and avoidance of muscle paralytics except when essential help to preclude its occurrence.

Nausea and Vomiting

Nausea and vomiting, may affect patients during the intraoperative period. If gagging occurs, the patient is turned to the side, the head of the table is lowered, and a basin is provided to collect the vomitus. Suction is used to remove saliva and vomited gastric contents. The advent of new anesthetic agents has reduced the incidence; however, there is no single way to prevent nausea and vomiting. A multimodal approach involving the surgeon, anesthesiologist or anesthetist, and nurse is best (Rother, 2012).

In some cases, the anesthesiologist administers antiemetics preoperatively or intraoperatively to counteract possible aspiration. If the patient aspirates vomitus, an asthma-like attack with severe bronchial spasms and wheezing is triggered. Pneumonitis and pulmonary edema can subsequently develop, leading to extreme hypoxia. Increasing medical attention is being paid to silent regurgitation of gastric contents (not related to preoperative fasting times), which occurs more frequently than previously realized. The volume and acidity of the aspirate determine the extent of damage to the lungs. Patients may be given citric acid and sodium citrate, a clear, nonparticulate antacid to increase gastric fluid pH or a histamine-2 (H_2) receptor antagonist such as cimetidine, ranitidine, or famotidine to decrease gastric acid production (Rothrock, 2018).

Anaphylaxis

Any time a patient comes into contact with a foreign substance, there is the potential for an anaphylactic reaction. Because medications are the most common cause of anaphylaxis, intraoperative nurses must be aware of the type and method of anesthesia used as well as the specific agents (Bourdon, 2015). An anaphylactic reaction can occur in response to many medications, latex, or other substances. The reaction may be immediate or delayed. Anaphylaxis is a life-threatening acute allergic reaction.

Fibrin sealants are used in a variety of surgical procedures, and cyanoacrylate tissue adhesives are used to close wounds without the use of sutures. These sealants have been implicated in allergic reactions and anaphylaxis (Bhat, Banerjee, Barth, et al., 2013). Although these reactions are rare, the nurse must be alert to the possibility and observe the patient for changes in vital signs and symptoms of anaphylaxis when these products are used. See Chapters 18 and 53 for more details about the signs, symptoms, and treatment of anaphylaxis and anaphylactic shock.

Hypoxia and Other Respiratory Complications

Inadequate ventilation, occlusion of the airway, inadvertent intubation of the esophagus, and hypoxia are significant potential complications associated with general anesthesia. Many factors can contribute to inadequate ventilation. Respiratory depression caused by anesthetic agents, aspiration of respiratory tract secretions or vomitus, and the patient's position on the operating table can compromise the exchange of gases. Anatomic variation can make the trachea difficult to visualize and result in insertion of the artificial airway into the esophagus rather than into the trachea. In addition to these dangers, asphyxia caused by foreign bodies in the mouth, spasm of the vocal cords, relaxation of the tongue, or aspiration of vomitus, saliva, or blood can occur. Brain damage from hypoxia occurs within minutes; therefore, vigilant monitoring of the patient's oxygenation status is a primary function of the anesthesiologist and the circulating nurse. Peripheral perfusion is checked frequently, and pulse oximetry values are monitored continuously.

Hypothermia

During anesthesia, the patient's temperature may drop. Glucose metabolism is reduced, and, as a result, metabolic acidosis may develop. This condition is called hypothermia and is indicated by a core body temperature that is 35.0°C or less. Inadvertent hypothermia may occur as a result of a low temperature in the OR, infusion of cold fluids, inhalation of cold gases, open body wounds or cavities, decreased muscle activity, advanced age, or the pharmaceutical agents used (e.g., vasodilators, phenothiazines, general anesthetic medications). Hypothermia can depress neuronal activity and decrease cellular oxygen requirements below the minimum levels normally required for continued cell viability. As a result, it is used to protect function during some surgical procedures (e.g., carotid endarterectomy, cardiopulmonary bypass) and after a cardiac arrest (Wannemacher, Tschannen, Biery, et al., 2017).

If unintentional hypothermia occurs, it must be minimized or reversed. If hypothermia is intentional, the goal is a safe return to normal body temperature. Environmental temperature in the OR can temporarily be set at 25° to 26.6°C. IV and irrigating fluids are warmed to 37°C. Wet gowns and drapes are removed promptly and replaced with dry materials, because wet materials promote heat loss. Whatever methods are used to rewarm the patient, warming must be accomplished gradually, not rapidly. Conscientious monitoring of core temperature, urinary output, ECG, blood pressure, arterial blood gas levels, and serum electrolyte levels is required.

Malignant Hyperthermia

MH is a rare inherited muscle disorder that is chemically induced by anesthetic agents (Sessler, 2016). MH can be triggered by myopathies, emotional stress, heatstroke, neuroleptic malignant syndrome, strenuous exercise exertion, and trauma. It occurs in 1 in 50,000 to 100,000 adults. Mortality from MH had been reported to be as high as 70%; however, with prompt recognition and rapid treatment, it has fallen to less than 10% (Isaak & Steigler, 2015). Susceptible people include those with strong and bulky muscles, a history of muscle cramps or muscle weakness and unexplained temperature elevation, and an unexplained death of a family member during surgery that was accompanied by a febrile response (Riazi, Larach, Hu, et al., 2014).

Pathophysiology

During anesthesia, potent agents such as inhalation anesthetic agents (halothane, enflurane) and muscle relaxants (succinylcholine) may trigger the symptoms of MH (Mahdi, Azadeh, Neshati, et al., 2017). Stress and some medications, such as sympathomimetics (epinephrine), theophylline, aminophylline, anticholinergics (atropine), and cardiac glycosides (digitalis), can induce or intensify such a reaction.

The pathophysiology of MH is related to a hypermetabolic condition that involves altered mechanisms of calcium function in skeletal muscle cells. This disruption of calcium causes clinical symptoms of hypermetabolism, which in turn increases muscle contraction (rigidity) and causes hyperthermia and subsequent damage to the central nervous system.

Clinical Manifestations

The initial symptoms of MH are related to cardiovascular and musculoskeletal activity. Tachycardia is often the earliest sign. Sympathetic nervous stimulation also leads to ventricular dysrhythmia, hypotension, decreased cardiac output, oliguria, and, later, cardiac arrest. With the abnormal transport of calcium, rigidity or tetanus like movements occur, often in the jaw. Generalized muscle rigidity is one of the earliest signs. The rise in temperature is actually a late sign that develops rapidly; body temperature can increase 1° to 2°C every 5 minutes and core body temperature can exceed 42°C in a very short time (Sessler, 2016).

Medical Management

Recognizing symptoms early and discontinuing anesthesia promptly are imperative. Goals of treatment are to decrease metabolism, reverse metabolic and respiratory acidosis, correct dysrhythmias, decrease body temperature, provide oxygen and nutrition to tissues, and correct electrolyte imbalance.

Anesthesia and surgery are postponed. However, if end-tidal CO_2 monitoring and dantrolene sodium (Dantrium) are available and the anesthesiologist is experienced in managing MH, the surgery may continue using a different anesthetic agent (Litman & Joshi, 2014). Although MH usually manifests about 10 to 20 minutes after induction of anesthesia, it can also occur during the first 24 hours after surgery.

Nursing Management

Although MH is uncommon, the nurse must identify patients at risk, recognize the signs and symptoms, have the appropriate medication and equipment available, and be knowledgeable about the protocol to follow. This preparation may be lifesaving for the patient.

Nursing Process

The Patient During Surgery

Intraoperative nurses focus on nursing diagnoses, interventions, and outcomes that surgical patients and their family's experience. Additional priorities include collaborative problems and expected goals.

Assessment

Nursing assessment of the intraoperative patient involves obtaining data from the patient and the patient's medical record to identify factors that can affect care. These serve as guidelines for an individualized plan of patient care. The intraoperative nurse uses the focused preoperative nursing assessment documented on the patient record (Chart 20-2).

Nursing Priorities

Based on the assessment data, some major nursing priorities may include the following:

- Anxiety related to surgical or environmental concerns
- Risk of latex allergy response due to possible exposure to latex in OR environment
- Risk for perioperative positioning injury related to positioning in the OR

CHART 20-2

Ethics and Related Issues

To Resuscitate or Not?

SITUATION

Your ambulatory care centre has developed a policy, authorized through the medical staff that allows for patients to have a do-not-resuscitate order (DNR) in place during a surgical procedure. This policy follows the American Society of Anesthesiologists guidelines for DNR in the OR. You are preparing a patient for surgery, and the anesthesiologist who will be administering the anesthetic agent writes an order for the DNR to be rescinded during surgery. The physician is refusing to talk to the patient concerning the DNR.

PROBLEM

The patient believes his wishes will be followed with regard to resuscitation in the event of a cardiac arrest and the physician does not believe he can administer anesthesia if the DNR is in place.

DISCUSSION

- What are the rights of the patient with regard to advance directives?
- What can you do to advocate for the patient?
- Should you contact the ethics committee of the hospital?
- How do you contact the ethics committee?

- Risk for injury related to anesthesia and surgical procedure
- Disturbed sensory perception (global) related to general anesthesia or sedation

Collaborative Problems/ Potential Complications

Based on the assessment data, potential complications may include the following:

- Nausea and vomiting
- Anaphylaxis
- Hypoxia
- Unintentional hypothermia
- Malignant hyperthermia
- Infection

Planning and Goals

The major goals for care of the patient during surgery include reduced anxiety, absence of latex exposure, absence of positioning injuries, freedom from injury, maintenance of the patient's dignity, and absence of complications.

Nursing Interventions

Reducing Anxiety

The OR environment can seem cold, stark, and frightening to the patient, who may be feeling isolated and apprehensive. When nurses introducing themselves, address the patient by name warmly and frequently, verify details, provide explanations, and encourage and answer questions, they contribute to a sense of professionalism and friendliness that can help the patient feel safe and secure. When discussing what the patient can expect in surgery, the nurse uses basic communication skills, such as touch and eye contact, to reduce anxiety. Attention to physical comfort (warm blankets, padding, and position changes) helps the patient feel more comfortable. Telling the patient who else will be present in the OR, how long the procedure is expected to take, and other details help the patient prepare for the experience and gain a sense of control.

Reducing Latex Exposure

Patients with latex allergies require early identification and communication to all personnel about the presence of the allergy. ORNAC (2017) has recommended standards of care for patients with latex allergy. In most ORs, there are few latex items currently in use, but because there still remain some instances of latex use, maintenance of latex allergy precautions throughout the perioperative period must be observed. For safety, manufacturers and hospital materials managers need to take responsibility for identifying the latex content in items used by patients and health care personnel. (See Chapters 18 and 53 for assessment for latex allergy.)

NURSING ALERT

It is the responsibility of all nurses, and particularly perianesthesia and perioperative nurses, to be aware of latex allergies, necessary precautions, and products that are latex free. Hospital staff is also at risk for development of a latex allergy secondary to repeated exposure to latex products.

Preventing Perioperative Positioning Injury

The patient's position on the operating table depends on the surgical procedure to be performed as well as on the patient's physical condition (Fig. 20-5). The potential for transient discomfort or permanent injury is present, because many positions are awkward. Hyperextending joints, compressing arteries, or pressing on nerves and bony prominences usually results in discomfort simply because the position must be sustained for a long period of time (Rothrock, 2018). Factors to consider include the following:

- The patient should be in as comfortable a position as possible, whether conscious or unconscious.
- The operative field must be adequately exposed.
- An awkward position, undue pressure on a body part, or use of stirrups or traction should not obstruct the vascular supply.
- Respiration should not be impeded by pressure of arms on the chest or by a gown that constricts the neck or chest.
- Nerves must be protected from undue pressure. Improper positioning of the arms, hands, legs, or feet can cause serious injury or paralysis. Shoulder braces must be well padded to prevent irreparable nerve injury, especially when the Trendelenburg position is necessary.
- Precautions for patient safety must be observed, particularly with thin, older patients, or patients with obesity and those with a physical deformity.
- The patient may need light restraint before induction in case of excitement.

The usual position for surgery, called the dorsal recumbent position, is flat on the back. Both arms are positioned at the side of the table, one with the hand placed palm down; the other is carefully positioned on an armboard to facilitate IV infusion of fluids, blood, or medications (see Fig. 20-5A).

The Trendelenburg position usually is used for surgery on the lower abdomen and pelvis to obtain good exposure by displacing the intestines into the upper abdomen. In this position, the head and body are lowered. The patient is held in position by padded shoulder braces (see Fig. 20-5B).

The lithotomy position is used for nearly all perineal, rectal, and vaginal surgical procedures (see Fig. 20-5C). The patient is positioned on the back with the legs and thighs flexed. The position is maintained by placing the feet in stirrups.

A. Patient in position on the operating table for a laparotomy. Note the strap above the knees.

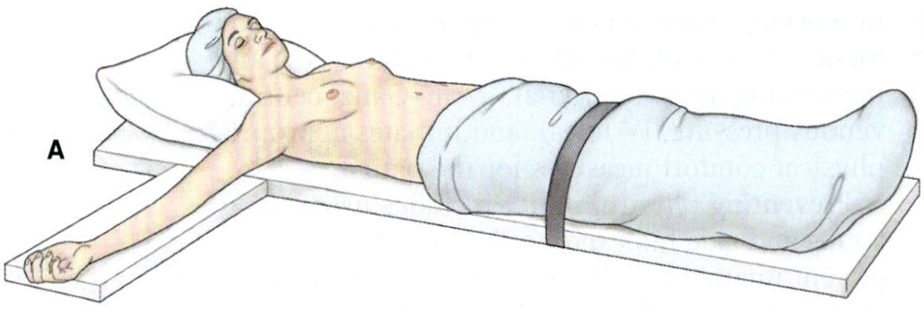

B. Patient in Trendelenburg position on operating table. Note padded shoulder braces in place. Be sure that brace does not press on brachial plexus.

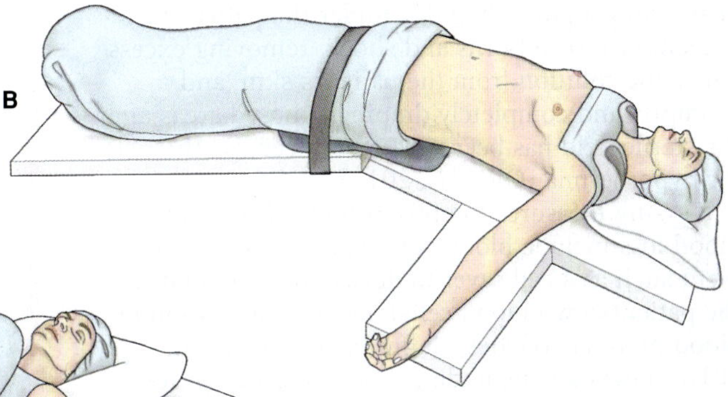

C. Patient in lithotomy position. Note that the hips extend over the edge of the table.

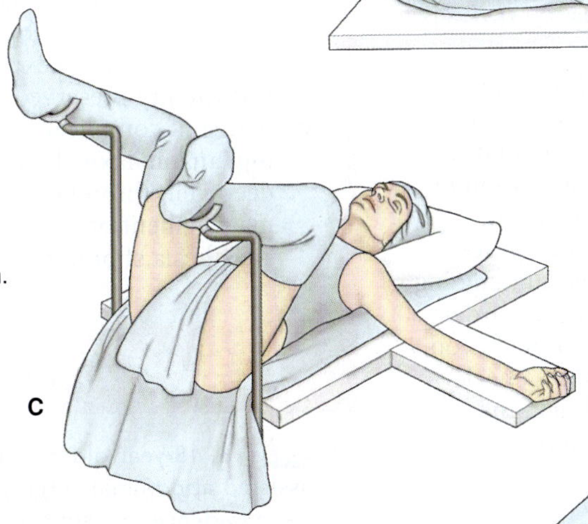

D. Patient lies on unaffected side for kidney surgery. Table is spread apart to provide space between the lower ribs and the pelvis. The upper leg is extended; the lower leg is flexed at the knee and hip joints; a pillow is placed between the legs.

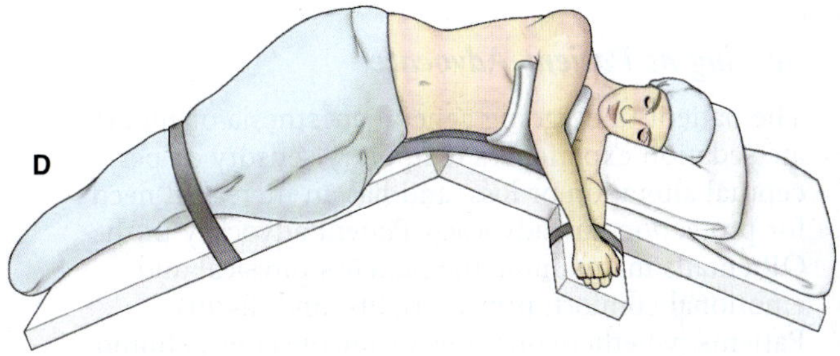

FIGURE 20-5. Positions on the operating table. Captions call attention to safety and comfort features.

The Sims or lateral position is used for renal surgery. The patient is placed on the nonoperative side with an air pillow, 12.5 to 15 cm thick under the loin, or on a table with a kidney or back lift (see Fig. 20-5D).

Protecting the Patient From Injury

A variety of activities are used to address the diverse patient safety issues that arise in the OR. The nurse protects the patient from injury by providing a safe environment. Verifying information, checking the chart for completeness, and maintaining surgical asepsis and an optimal environment are critical nursing responsibilities. Verification that all required documentation is completed is an important function of the intraoperative nurse. A surgical checklist is used prior to induction of anesthesia, before the skin incision is made, and before the patient leaves the OR (see Fig. 20-1). It is important to review the patient's record for the following:

- Correct informed surgical consent, with patient's signature
- Completed records for health history and physical examination
- Results of diagnostic studies
- Allergies (including latex)

In addition to checking that all necessary patient data are complete, the perioperative nurse obtains the necessary equipment specific to the procedure. The need for nonroutine medications, blood components, instruments, and other equipment and supplies is assessed, and the readiness of the room, completeness of physical setup, and completeness of instrument, suture, and dressing setups are determined. Any aspects of the OR environment that may negatively affect the patient are identified. These include physical features, such as room temperature and humidity; electrical hazards; potential contaminants (dust, blood, and discharge on floor or surfaces; uncovered hair; nonsterile attire of personnel; jewelry worn by personnel; chipped or artificial fingernails); and unnecessary traffic. The circulating nurse also sets up and maintains suction equipment in working order, sets up invasive monitoring equipment, assists with insertion of vascular access and monitoring devices (arterial, Swan–Ganz, central venous pressure, IV lines), and initiates appropriate physical comfort measures for the patient.

Preventing physical injury includes using safety straps and side rails and not leaving the sedated patient unattended. Transferring the patient from the stretcher to the OR table requires safe transferring practices. Other safety measures include properly positioning a grounding pad under the patient to prevent electrical burns and shock, removing excess antiseptic solution from the patient's skin, and promptly and completely draping exposed areas after the sterile field has been created to decrease the risk for hypothermia (ORNAC, 2017).

Nursing measures to prevent injury from excessive blood loss include blood conservation using equipment such as a cell saver (a device for recirculating the patient's own blood cells) and administration of blood products (Gabel, Malm, Radulovic, et al., 2016). Few patients undergoing an elective procedure require blood transfusion, but those undergoing high-risk procedures (such as orthopedic or cardiac surgeries) may require an intraoperative transfusion. The circulating nurse anticipates this need, checks that blood has been cross-matched and held in reserve, and is prepared to administer blood.

Serving as Patient Advocate

The patient undergoing general anesthesia or moderate sedation experiences temporary sensory or perceptual alteration or loss, and has an increased need for protection and advocacy. Patient advocacy in the OR entails maintaining the patient's physical and emotional comfort, privacy, rights, and dignity. Patients, whether conscious or unconscious, should not be subjected to excess noise, inappropriate conversation, or, most of all, derogatory comments about the patient's physical appearance, job, personal history, and so forth. Cases have been reported in which seemingly deeply anesthetized patients recalled the entire surgical experience, including disparaging personal remarks made by OR personnel. As an advocate, the nurse never engages in such conversation and discourages others from doing so. Other advocacy activities include minimizing the clinical, dehumanizing aspects of being a surgical patient by making sure the patient is treated as a person, respecting cultural and spiritual values, providing physical privacy, and maintaining confidentiality.

Monitoring and Managing Potential Complications

It is the responsibility of the surgeon and the anesthesiologist to monitor and manage complications. Important functions of the intraoperative nurses include being alert to and reporting changes in vital signs, cardiac dysrhythmias, symptoms of nausea and vomiting, anaphylaxis, hypoxia, hypothermia, and MH and assisting with their management. Maintaining asepsis and preventing infection are responsibilities of all members of the surgical team (Phillips, 2016; Rothrock, 2018). Evidence-based interventions to decrease surgical site infections include appropriate skin preparation and antibiotic administration.

Evaluation

Expected Patient Outcomes

Expected patient outcomes may include the following:

1. Exhibits low level of anxiety while awake during the intraoperative phase of care
2. Has no symptoms of latex allergy
3. Remains free of perioperative positioning injury
4. Experiences no unexpected threats to safety
5. Has dignity preserved throughout OR experience
6. Is free of complications (e.g., nausea and vomiting, anaphylaxis, hypoxia, hypothermia, MH, or deep vein thrombosis) or experiences successful management of adverse effects of surgery and anesthesia should they occur.

Critical Thinking Exercises

1 ebp A 48-year-old man is scheduled to have robotic-assisted abdominal surgery under general anesthesia. Is there evidence that supports that his intraoperative positioning will have any effect on his vital signs? What is the best evidence for how his vital signs should be monitored? What are the best practices that the OR nurse should implement to support the patient and OR team during this minimally invasive surgery?

2 A patient has an identified latex allergy and is undergoing surgery. What resources would you use to identify the current guidelines for avoiding latex exposure for the patient? What is the evidence base for current latex allergy practices? Identify the criteria used to evaluate the strength of the evidence for these practices.

3 A patient has an unintentional temperature of 36°C halfway through surgery. Describe the actions you would take and what parameters you would monitor. How would your actions differ if the patient is at the very end of the surgical procedure?

4 pq Identify the priorities, assessments, and nursing interventions you would implement for a 76-year-old woman who is hard of hearing and is having spinal anesthesia for total knee replacement surgery. How would your priorities, approach, and techniques differ if the patient is having general anesthesia?

REFERENCES AND SELECTED READINGS

Books

Barash, P. G., Cullen, B. F., & Stoelting, R. K. (2013). *Clinical anesthesia* (7th ed.). Philadelphia, PA: Lippincott Williams & Wilkins.
Boltz, M., Capezuti, E., Fulmer, T., et al. (2016). *Evidence-based geriatric nursing protocols for best practice*. New York: Springer Publishing Co.

Bready, L. L., Noorily, S. H., & Hickey, R. (2018). *Decision making in anesthesiology* (5th ed.). St. Louis, MO: Mosby.
Herdman, T. H., & Kamitsura, S. (2018). *Nursing diagnoses: Definitions & classification 2018–2020* (11th ed.). Stuttgart, Germany: Thieme.
Meiner, S. E. (2014). *Gerontologic nursing* (5th ed.). St. Louis, MO: Elsevier Mosby.
Miller, C. A. (2009). *Nursing for wellness in older adults* (5th ed.). Philadelphia, PA: Lippincott Williams & Wilkins.
Phillips, N. (2016). *Berry and Kohn's operating room technique* (13th ed.). St. Louis, MO: Mosby.
Rothrock, J. C. (Ed.). (2018). *Alexander's care of the patient in surgery* (16th ed.). St. Louis, MO: Elsevier.

Journals and Electronic Documents

Bhat, Y. M., Banerjee, S., Barth, B. A., et al. (2013). Tissue adhesives: Cyanoacrylate glue and fibrin sealant. *Gastrointestinal Endoscopy, 78*(2), 209–215. doi: 10.1016/j.gie.2013.04.166
Bourdon, L. (2015). Care of the patient receiving local anesthesia. *AORN Journal, 101*(3), 10–12.
Finkelstein, R., Rabino, G., Mashiach, T., et al. (2014). Effect of preoperative antibiotic prophylaxis on surgical site infections complicating cardiac surgery. *Infection Control & Hospital Epidemiology, 35*(1), 69–74.
Gabel, J., Malm, C. J., Radulovic, V., et al. (2016). Cell saver processing mitigates the negative effects of wound blood on platelet function. *Acta Anaesthesiologica Scandinavia, 60*(7), 901–909. doi: 10.1111/aas.12730
Gajdos, C., Kile, D., Hawn, M. T., et al. (2013). Advancing age and 30-day adverse outcomes after nonemergent general surgeries. *Journal of the American Geriatric Society, 61*(9), 1608–1614. doi: 10.1111/jgs.12401
Hayne, A. B., Edmondson, L., Lipsitz, S. R., et al. (2017). Mortality trends after a voluntary checklist-based surgical safety collaborative. *Annals of Surgery, 266*(6), 923–929. doi: 10.1097/SLA.0000000000002249
Isaak, R. S., & Steigler, M. P. (2015). Review of crisis resource management (CRM) principles in the setting of intraoperative malignant hyperthermia. *Journal of Anesthesiology, 30*(2), 298–306.
Leech, C., & Chishti, A. (2014). Safe sedation for surgeons. *Surgery, 32*(2), 89–92. doi: 10.1016/j.mpsur.2013.12.002
Li, X., & Ji, G. (2017). Evaluation of the direct relationship between bacterial load on contaminated stainless steel surgical instruments and the holding time prior to disinfection and also to analyse the efficacy of different disinfecting solutions. *Biomedical Research, 28*(10), [online].
Litman, R. S., & Joshi, G. P. (2014). Malignant hyperthermia in the ambulatory surgery center: How should we prepare? *Anesthesiology, 120*, 1306–1308. doi: 10.1097/ALN.0000000000000256
Mahdi, N., Azadeh, M., Neshati, P., et al. (2017). Malignant hypothermia: Report of two cases with neglected complication in cardiac surgery. *Journal of Tehran University Heart Center, 12*(4), 175–183.
Misal, U. S., Joshi, S. A., & Shaikh, M. M. (2016). Delayed recovery from anesthesia: A postgraduate educational review. *Anesthesia Essays and Researches, 10*(2), 164–172. doi: 10.4103/0259-1162.165506
Neuman, M. D., & Bosk, C. L. (2013). The redefinition of aging in American surgery. *Milbank Quarterly, 91*(2), 288–315. doi: 10.1111/milq.12014
O'Neill, J., & Helwig, E. (2016). Postoperative management of the physiological effects of spinal anesthesia. *Journal of Perianesthesia Nursing, 31*(4), 330–339. doi: 10.1016/j.jopan.2015.01.018
Operating Room Nurses Association of Canada (ORNAC). (2017). Standards, guidelines, and position statements for perioperative registered nursing practice. Retrieved from http://www.ornac.ca/
Oster, K. A., & Oster, C. A. (2015). Special needs population: Care of the geriatric patient population in the perioperative setting. *AORN Journal, 101*(6), 444–456.
Penprase, B., & Johnson, C. (2015). Optimizing the perioperative nursing role for the older adult surgical patient. *OR Nurse, 8*(4), 26–33.
Pignaton, W., Braz, J. R., Kusano, P. S., et al. (2016). Perioperative and anesthesia-related mortality: An 8 year observational survey from a tertiary teaching hospital. *Medicine, 95*(2), e2208. doi: 10.1097/MD.0000000000002208
Riazi, S., Larach, M., Hu, C., et al. (2014). Malignant Hyperthermia in Canada: Characteristics of Index Anesthetics in 129 Malignant Hyperthermia Susceptible Probands. *International Anesthesia Research Society, 118*(20), 381–387.
RNFA Ontario. (2018). Retrieved from http://www.rnfa-ontario.ca/
Rother, C. (2012). Postoperative nausea and vomiting: Use of antiemetic agents in anesthesia. *Scottish Universities Medical Journal, 1*(1), 89–97.
Sessler, D. (2016). Perioperative thermoregulation and heat balance. *Lancet, 387*(10038), 2655–2664. doi: 1016/S0140-6736(15)00981-2
Shapeton, A., O'Donoghue, M. A., VanderWielen, B., et al. (2017). Anesthesia lost in translation: Perspective and comprehension. *The Journal of Education in Perioperative Medicine, 19*(1), E505.
Smeili, L. A. A., & Lotufo, P. A. (2015). Incidence and predictors of cardiovascular complications and death after vascular surgery. *Arquivos Brasileiros de Cardiologia, 105*(5), 510–518. doi: 10.5935/abc.20150113
UpToDate. (2017). Retrieved from: https://www.uptodate.com/contents/fire-safety-in-the-operating-room
Wannemacher, J., Tschannen, D., Biery, K., et al. (2017). Advanced practice registered nurses on therapeutic hypothermia response teams. *AACN Advanced Critical Care, 28*(4), 332–341. doi: 10.4037/aacnacc2017708
World Health Organization. (n.d.). WHO Surgical Site Infection Prevention Guidelines Web Appendix 10: Summary of a systematic review on surgical hand preparation. Retrieved from: http://www.who.int/gpsc/appendix10.pdf
World Health Organization. (2015). New checklist to help make surgery safer. *WHO Bulletin, 86*(7), 496–576. Retrieved January 24, 2019, from http://apps.who.int/iris/bitstream/10665/44186/2/9789241598590_eng_Checklist.pdf
Zejnullahu, V. A., Bicaj, B. X., Zejnullahu, V. A., et al. (2017). Retained surgical foreign bodies after surgery. *Open Access Macedonian Journal of Medicine, 5*(1), 97–100. doi: 10.3889/oamjms.2017.005

Resources

Canadian Anesthesiologists' Society: http://www.cas.ca
Health Standards Organization: https://healthstandards.org/
The Joint Commission: http://www.jointcommission.org
Operating Room Nurses Association of Canada (ORNAC): http://www.ornac.ca/
Registered Nurse First Assistant (RNFA) Interest Group: Ontario, Canada: http://www.rnfa-ontario.ca

21 Postoperative Nursing Management

Adapted by Ruhina Rana

Learning Objectives

On completion of this chapter, the learner will be able to:

1. Describe the responsibilities of the postanesthesia care unit nurse in the prevention of immediate postoperative complications.
2. Compare postoperative care of the ambulatory surgery patient with that of the hospitalized surgery patient.
3. Identify common postoperative problems and their management.
4. Describe the gerontologic considerations related to postoperative management.
5. Describe variables that affect wound healing.
6. Demonstrate postoperative dressing techniques.
7. Identify assessment parameters appropriate for the early detection of postoperative complications.

The postoperative period extends from the time the patient leaves the operating room (OR) until the last follow-up visit with the surgeon. This may be as short as a day or two or as long as several months. During the postoperative period, nursing care focuses on reestablishing the patient's physiologic equilibrium, alleviating pain, preventing complications, and teaching the patient self-care (Rodriguez, 2015). Careful assessment and immediate intervention assist the patient in returning to optimal function quickly, safely, and as comfortably as possible. Ongoing care in the community through home care, clinic visits, office visits, or telephone follow-up facilitates an uncomplicated recovery.

Care of the Patient in the Postanesthesia Care Unit

The **postanesthesia care unit** (PACU), also called the *recovery room* or *postanesthesia recovery room*, is located adjacent to suite of ORs. Patients still under anesthesia or recovering from anesthesia are placed in this unit for easy access to experienced, highly skilled nurses, anesthesiologists or anesthetists, surgeons, advanced hemodynamic and pulmonary monitoring and support, special equipment, and medications.

Phases of Postanesthesia Care

In some hospitals and ambulatory surgical centres, postanesthesia care is divided into two to three phases (Rothrock, 2014). In the **phase I PACU**, used during the immediate recovery phase, intensive nursing care is provided. In the **phase II PACU**, the patient is prepared for self-care or care in the hospital or an extended care setting. In phase III, which may be on the ward or in surgical daycare, the patient is prepared for discharge. Recliners rather than stretchers or beds are standard in many phase III units, which may also be referred to as step-down, sit-up, or progressive care units. Patients may remain in a PACU unit for as long as 4 to 6 hours, depending on the type of surgery and any pre-existing conditions. In facilities without separate phase I, II, and III units, the patient remains in the PACU and may be discharged home directly from this unit.

Admitting the Patient to the PACU

Transferring the postoperative patient from the OR to the PACU is the responsibility of the anesthesiologist. During transport from the OR to the PACU, the anesthesia provider remains at the head of the stretcher (to maintain the airway), and a surgical team member remains at the opposite end. Transporting the patient involves special consideration of the incision site, potential vascular changes, and exposure. The surgical incision is considered every time the postoperative patient is moved; many wounds are closed under considerable tension, and every effort is made to prevent further strain on the incision. The patient is positioned so that he or she is not lying on and obstructing drains or drainage tubes. Orthostatic hypotension may occur when a patient is moved too quickly from one position to another (e.g., from a lithotomy position to a horizontal position or from a lateral to a supine position), so the patient must be moved slowly and carefully. As soon as the patient is placed on the stretcher or bed, the soiled gown is removed and replaced with a dry gown. The patient is covered with lightweight blankets and warmed. All side rails may be raised to prevent falls.

The nurse who admits the patient to the PACU reviews essential information with the anesthesiologist (Chart 21-1). Monitoring equipment is attached and oxygen applied, and an immediate physiologic assessment is conducted.

CHART 21-1

Anesthesia Provider-to-Nurse Report and Nurse-to-Nurse Report: Information to Convey

Patient name, gender, age
Allergies
Surgical procedure
Length of time in the operating room
Anesthetic agents and reversal agents used
Estimated blood loss/fluid loss
Fluid/blood replacement
Last set of vital signs and any problems during the procedure (e.g., nausea and/or vomiting)
Any complications encountered (anesthetic or surgical)
Medical comorbidities (e.g., diabetes, hypertension)
Considerations for immediate postoperative period (pain management, reversals, ventilator settings)
Language barrier
Location of patient's family
Ideally, the anesthesia provider should not leave the patient until the nurse is satisfied with the patient's airway and immediate condition.

Nursing Management in the PACU

The nursing management objectives for the patient in the PACU are to provide care until the patient has recovered from the effects of anesthesia (e.g., until resumption of motor and sensory functions), is able to protect own airway, oriented, has stable vital signs, and shows no evidence of hemorrhage or other complications (Helvig, Minick, & Patrick, 2014; Noble & Pasero, 2014; Penprase & Johnson, 2015).

Assessing the Patient

Frequent, skilled assessments of the patient's airway, respiratory function, cardiovascular function, skin colour, level of consciousness, and ability to respond to commands are the cornerstones of nursing care in the PACU. The nurse performs and documents a baseline assessment, then checks the surgical site for drainage or hemorrhage and makes sure that all drainage tubes and monitoring lines are connected and functioning. The nurse checks any intravenous (IV) fluids or medications currently infusing and verifies dosage and rate.

After the initial assessment, vital signs are monitored and the patient's general physical status is assessed and documented at least every 15 minutes (CPSBC, 2017). The nurse is usually 1:1 or 1:2, and rarely 1:3, with patients so that they can be closely monitored. The nurse must be aware of any pertinent information from the patient's history that may be significant (e.g., patient is deaf or hard of hearing, has a history of seizures, has diabetes, or is allergic to certain medications or to latex). Administration of the patient's postoperative analgesic requirements is a top priority (Chou, Gordon, de Leon-Casasola, et al., 2016).

Glossary

dehiscence: partial or complete separation of wound edges
evisceration: protrusion of organs through the surgical incision
first-intention healing: method of healing in which wound edges are surgically approximated and integumentary continuity is restored without granulation
phase I PACU: designation of care of surgical patients immediately after surgery and for patients whose condition warrants close monitoring
phase II PACU: designation of care of surgical patients who have been transferred from a phase I PACU because their condition no longer requires the close monitoring provided in a phase I PACU
phase III PACU: setting in which the patient is cared for in the immediate postoperative period. If the patient had ambulatory surgery, then they are prepared for discharge from the facility, otherwise they are transferred to the ward and discharged from there.
postanesthesia care unit (PACU): area where postoperative patients are monitored as they recover from anesthesia; formerly referred to as the recovery room or postanesthesia recovery room
second-intention healing: method of healing in which wound edges are not surgically approximated and integumentary continuity is restored by the process known as granulation
third-intention healing: method of healing in which surgical approximation of wound edges is delayed and integumentary continuity is restored by apposing areas of granulation

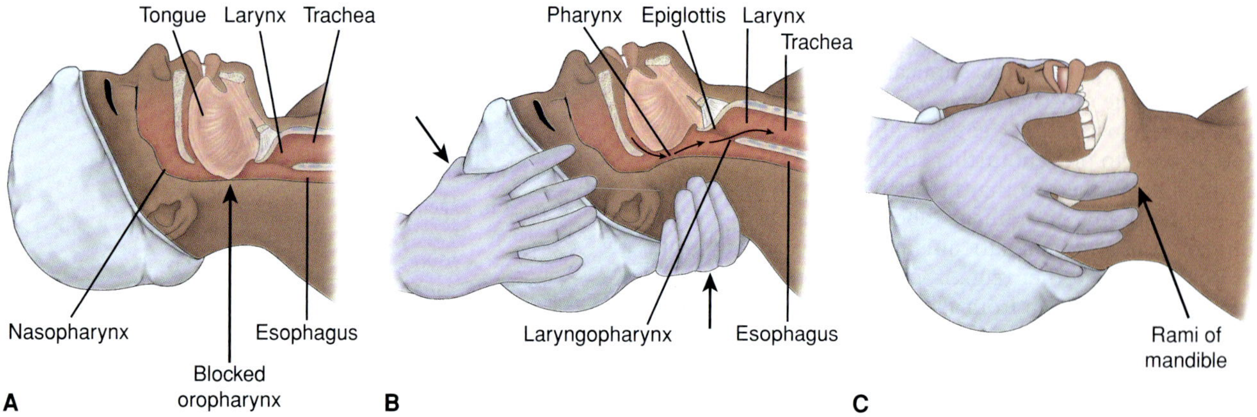

FIGURE 21-1. **A.** A hypopharyngeal obstruction occurs when neck flexion permits the chin to drop toward the chest; obstruction almost always occurs when the head is in the midposition. **B.** Tilting the head back to stretch the anterior neck structure lifts the base of the tongue off the posterior pharyngeal wall. The direction of the *arrows* indicates the pressure of the hands. **C.** Opening the mouth is necessary to correct a valve-like obstruction of the nasal passage during expiration, which occurs in about 30% of unconscious patients. Open the patient's mouth (separate lips and teeth) and move the lower jaw forward so that the lower teeth are in front of the upper teeth. To regain backward tilt of the neck, lift with both hands at the ascending rami of the mandible.

Following surgery, patients who had ketamine as anesthesia must be placed in a quiet, darkened area of the PACU. See Chapter 20, for more information about anesthetic agents.

Maintaining a Patent Airway

The primary objective in the immediate postoperative period is to maintain pulmonary ventilation and thus prevent hypoxemia (reduced oxygen in the blood) and hypercapnia (excess carbon dioxide in the blood). Both can occur if the airway is obstructed and ventilation is reduced. Besides checking the surgeon's orders for and administering supplemental oxygen, the nurse assesses respiratory rate and depth, ease of respirations, oxygen saturation, and breath sounds, including snoring, which can indicate an obstructed airway.

Patients who have experienced prolonged anesthesia usually are unconscious, with all muscles relaxed. This relaxation extends to the muscles of the pharynx. When the patient lies on his or her back, the lower jaw and the tongue fall backward and the air passages become obstructed (Fig. 21-1A). This is called hypopharyngeal obstruction. Signs of occlusion include choking; noisy and irregular respirations; snoring; decreased oxygen saturation scores; and within minutes, a cyanosis of the skin. Because movement of the thorax and the diaphragm does not necessarily indicate that the patient is breathing, the nurse needs to place the palm of the hand at the patient's nose and mouth to feel the exhaled breath.

NURSING ALERT

The treatment of hypopharyngeal obstruction involves tilting the head back and pushing forward on the angle of the lower jaw; as if to push the lower teeth in front of the upper teeth (see Fig. 21-1B,C). This manoeuvre pulls the tongue forward and opens the air passages. This is called a jaw thrust.

The anesthesiologist may leave a hard rubber or plastic airway in the patient's mouth to maintain a patent airway (Fig. 21-2). Such a device should not be removed until signs such as gagging indicate that reflex action is returning. Alternatively, the patient may enter the PACU with an endotracheal tube still in place and may require continued mechanical ventilation. The nurse assists in initiating the use of the ventilator and in the weaning and extubation processes. Some patients, particularly those who have had extensive or lengthy surgical procedures, may be transferred from the OR directly to the intensive care unit (ICU) or from the PACU to the ICU while still intubated and receiving mechanical ventilation. In most facilities the patient is awakened and extubated in the OR (except in cases of trauma or a critically ill patient) and arrives in the PACU breathing without support.

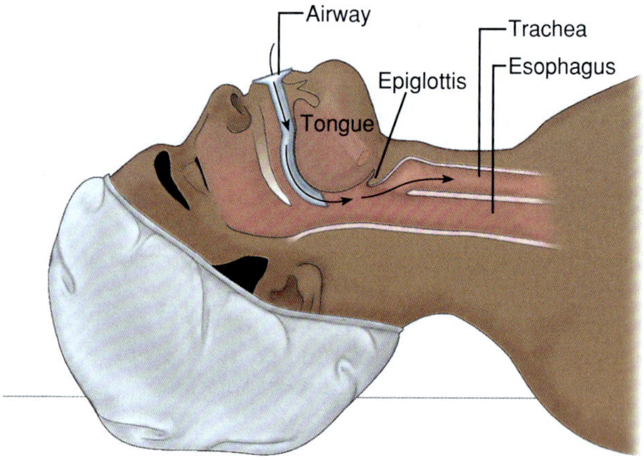

FIGURE 21-2. Use of an airway to maintain a patent airway after anesthesia. The airway passes over the base of the tongue and permits air to pass into the pharynx in the region of the epiglottis. Patients often leave the operating room with an airway in place. The airway should remain in place until the patient recovers sufficiently to breathe normally. As the patient regains consciousness, the airway usually causes irritation and should be removed.

If the teeth are clenched, the mouth may be opened manually but cautiously with a padded tongue depressor. The head of the bed is elevated 15 to 30 degrees unless contraindicated, and the patient is closely monitored to maintain the airway as well as to minimize the risk of aspiration. If vomiting occurs, the patient is turned to the side to prevent aspiration and the vomitus is collected in the emesis basin. Mucus or vomitus obstructing the pharynx or the trachea is suctioned with a pharyngeal suction tip or a nasal catheter introduced into the nasopharynx or oropharynx to a distance of 15 to 20 cm. Caution is necessary in suctioning the throat of a patient who has had a tonsillectomy or other oral or laryngeal surgery because of risk of bleeding and discomfort.

Maintaining Cardiovascular Stability

To monitor cardiovascular stability, the nurse assesses the patient's mental status; vital signs including MAP; cardiac rhythm; heart sounds; pulses; capillary refill; skin temperature, colour, and moisture; and urine output. Central venous pressure, pulmonary artery pressure, and arterial lines are monitored if in place. The nurse also assesses the patency of all IV lines. The primary cardiovascular complications seen in the PACU include hypotension and shock, hemorrhage, hypertension, and dysrhythmias.

Hypotension and Shock

Hypotension can result from blood loss, hypoventilation, position changes, pooling of blood in the extremities, or side effects of medications and anesthetics. The most common cause is loss of circulating volume through blood and plasma loss. If the amount of blood loss exceeds 500 mL (especially if the loss is rapid), replacement is usually indicated.

QUALITY AND SAFETY NURSING ALERT

A systolic blood pressure of less than 90 mm Hg is usually considered immediately reportable. However, the patient's preoperative or baseline blood pressure is used to make informed postoperative comparisons. A previously stable blood pressure that shows a downward trend of 5 mm Hg at each 15-minute reading should also be reported.

Shock, one of the most serious postoperative complications, can result from hypovolemia and decreased intravascular volume (Gallagher & Vacchiano, 2014). The types of shock are classified as hypovolemic, cardiogenic, neurogenic, anaphylactic, and septic shock. The classic signs of hypovolemic shock (the most common type of shock) are pallor; cool, moist skin; rapid breathing; cyanosis of the lips, gums, and tongue; rapid, weak, thready pulse; narrowing pulse pressure; low blood pressure; and concentrated urine. See Chapter 18 for a detailed discussion of shock.

Hypovolemic shock can be avoided largely by the timely administration of IV fluids, blood products, and blood pressure–elevating medications. The primary intervention for hypovolemic shock is volume replacement, with an infusion of lactated Ringer solution, 0.9% sodium chloride solution, colloids, or blood component therapy, depending on the body fluid that was lost (see Chapter 17). Oxygen is administered by nasal cannula, face mask, or mechanical ventilation. If fluid administration fails to reverse hypovolemic shock, then various cardiac, vasodilator, and corticosteroid medications may be prescribed to improve cardiac function and reduce peripheral vascular resistance.

The PACU bed provides easy access to the patient, is easily movable, can readily be positioned to facilitate use of measures to counteract shock. The patient is placed flat with the legs elevated. Respiratory rate, pulse rate, blood pressure, blood oxygen concentration, urinary output, level of consciousness, central venous pressure, pulmonary artery pressure, pulmonary capillary wedge pressure, and cardiac output are monitored to provide continuous information on the patient's respiratory and cardiovascular status until the patient's condition has stabilized.

Other factors can contribute to hemodynamic instability, such as body temperature and pain. The PACU nurse implements measures to manage these factors. The nurse keeps the patient warm (while avoiding overheating to prevent cutaneous vessels from dilating and depriving vital organs of blood), avoids exposure, and maintains normothermia (to prevent vasodilation). Pain control measures are discussed later in this chapter.

Hemorrhage

Hemorrhage is an uncommon yet serious complication of surgery that can result in hypovolemic shock and death. It can present insidiously or emergently at any time in the immediate postoperative period or up to several days after surgery (Table 21-1). The patient presents with hypotension; rapid, thready pulse; disorientation; restlessness; oliguria; and cold, pale skin. The early phase of shock will

TABLE 21-1 Types of Hemorrhage

Classification	Defining Characteristic
Time Frame	
Primary	Hemorrhage occurs at the time of surgery.
Intermediary	Hemorrhage occurs during the first few hours after surgery when the rise of blood pressure to its normal level dislodges insecure clots from untied vessels.
Secondary	Hemorrhage may occur sometime after surgery if a suture slips because a blood vessel was not securely tied, became infected, or was eroded by a drainage tube.
Type of Vessel	
Capillary	Hemorrhage is characterized by a slow, general ooze.
Venous	Darkly coloured blood bubbles out quickly.
Arterial	Blood is bright red and appears in spurts with each heartbeat.
Visibility	
Evident	Hemorrhage is on the surface and can be seen.
Concealed	Hemorrhage is in a body cavity and cannot be seen.

manifest in feelings of apprehension, decreased cardiac output, and vascular resistance. Breathing becomes laboured and "air hunger" will be exhibited; the patient will feel cold and may experience tinnitus. If shock symptoms are left untreated, the patient will continually grow weaker but can remain conscious until near death due to the body's mechanisms to preserve cerebral blood flow (Schiffner, Bischoff, Lehmann, et al., 2017).

Transfusing blood products and determining the cause of hemorrhage are the initial therapeutic measures. The surgical site and incision should always be inspected for bleeding. If bleeding is evident, a sterile gauze pad and a pressure dressing are applied, and the site of the bleeding is elevated to heart level if possible. The patient is placed in the shock position (flat on back; legs elevated at a 20-degree angle; knees kept straight). If hemorrhage is suspected but cannot be visualized, the patient may be taken back to the OR for emergency exploration of the surgical site.

If hemorrhage is suspected, the nurse should be aware of any special considerations related to blood loss replacement. Certain patients may decline blood transfusions for religious or cultural reasons and may identify this request on their advance directives or living will.

Hypertension and Dysrhythmias

Hypertension is common in the immediate postoperative period secondary to sympathetic nervous system stimulation from pain, hypoxia, or bladder distention. Dysrhythmias are associated with electrolyte imbalance, altered respiratory function, pain, hypothermia, stress, and anesthetic agents. Both hypertension and dysrhythmias are managed by treating the underlying causes.

Relieving Pain and Anxiety

The PACU nurse monitors the patient's physiologic status, manages pain, and provides psychological support in an effort to relieve the patient's fears and concerns. The nurse checks the medical record for special needs and concerns of the patient. Opioid and nonopioid analgesics, as well as adjuvants, are administered judiciously and often by IV in the PACU (Luo & Min, 2017). IV opioids provide immediate pain relief and are short-acting, thus minimizing the potential for drug interactions or prolonged respiratory depression while anesthetics are still active in the patient's system. When the patient's condition permits, a close family member may visit in the PACU to decrease the family's anxiety and make the patient feel more secure.

Controlling Nausea and Vomiting

Nausea and vomiting occur in about 10% of patients in the PACU. The nurse should intervene at the patient's first report of nausea to control the problem rather than wait for it to progress to vomiting (Tinsley & Barone, 2013).

NURSING ALERT

At the slightest indication of nausea, the patient is turned completely to one side to promote mouth drainage and prevent aspiration of vomitus, which can cause asphyxiation and death.

Many medications are available to control postoperative nausea and vomiting (PONV) without oversedating the patient; they are commonly administered during surgery as well as in the PACU. Table 21-2 contains examples of medications commonly prescribed to control PONV (Karch, 2016). Ondansetron is an effective antiemetic with few side effects and is frequently the drug of choice. It should be used cautiously in patients with a history of liver impairment or cardiac dysrhythmias. A variety of alternative techniques have been suggested to help control PONV, including deep breathing and aromatherapy (Hodge, McCarthy, & Peirce, 2014; Sites, Johnson, Miller, et al., 2014). (See Chart 21-2.)

TABLE 21-2 Medications Used to Control Postoperative Nausea and Vomiting

Drug Classes	Name	Nursing Implications
GI stimulant	Metoclopramide (Reglan)	Acts by stimulating gastric emptying and increasing GI transit time. Administration recommended at the end of procedure. Available in oral, IM, and IV forms.
Phenothiazine antiemetic	Prochlorperazine (Compazine)	Indicated for control of severe nausea and vomiting. Available in oral, SR, rectal, IM, and IV forms.
Phenothiazine antiemetic antimotion sickness	Promethazine (Phenergan)	Recommended every 4–6 hrs for nausea and vomiting associated with anesthesia and surgery. Available in oral, IM, and IV forms.
Antimotion sickness	Dimenhydrinate (Dramamine)	Indicated for prevention of nausea, vomiting, or vertigo of motion sickness. Available in oral, IM, and IV forms.
Antiemetic	Hydroxyzine (Vistaril, Atarax)	Control of nausea and vomiting and as adjunct to analgesia preoperatively and postoperatively to allow decreased opioid dosage. Available in oral and IM forms.
Antiemetic antimotion sickness	Scopolamine (Transderm Scop)	Used to prevent and control of nausea and vomiting associated with motion sickness and recovery from surgery. Available in oral, transdermal SC, and IM forms.
Antiemetic	Ondansetron (Zofran)	Prevention of postoperative nausea and vomiting. Available in oral, IM, and IV forms. With few side effects, frequently the drug of choice.

GI, gastrointestinal; IM, intramuscular; IV, intravenous; SC, subcutaneous; SR, sustained release.

Adapted from Comerford, K. C. (2015). *Nursing 2015 drug handbook*. Philadelphia, PA: Wolters Kluwer.

NURSING RESEARCH PROFILE

Chart 21-2. The Effectiveness of Aromatherapy for Relief of Postoperative Nausea and Vomiting

Hodge, N. S., McCarthy, M. S., & Peirce, R. M. (2014). A prospective randomized study of the effectiveness of aromatherapy for relief of postoperative nausea and vomiting. *Journal of PeriAnesthesia Nursing, 29*(1), 5–11.

Purpose

Postoperative nausea and vomiting (PONV) is a major concern for patients having surgery under general anesthesia. The purpose of this study was to compare the effectiveness of a placebo unscented inhaler to an aromatherapy inhaler in relieving PONV.

Design

The study used a prospective two-group design. The 121 patients who experienced PONV were randomized into a control group that received a placebo inhaler or another group that received the treatment with aromatics. Patients in both groups evaluated and ranked their nausea before and after therapy using a descriptive scale with 0 equal to "no nausea" and 10 equal to "the worst nausea ever." The patients self-administered the inhalers.

Findings

The initial and follow-up nausea assessment scores in both the placebo and treatment groups decreased significantly ($p < 0.01$), and there was a significant difference between the two groups ($p = 0.03$). Perceived effectiveness of aromatherapy was significantly higher in the treatment group ($p < 0.001$).

Nursing Implications

Nurses working with postoperative patients should be aware that alternatives to pharmacologic intervention are available to control PONV. An aromatherapy inhaler is patient controlled, and it appears to present an effective postoperative nausea treatment.

The risk of PONV ranges from approximately 10% in the PACU to 30% in the first 24 hours of postoperative care (Tinsley & Barone, 2013). These risks include general anesthesia, female gender, nonsmoker, history of PONV, and history of motion sickness (Apfel, Philip, Cakmakkaya, et al., 2012). Surgical risks are increased with PONV due to an increase in intra-abdominal pressure, elevated central venous pressure, the potential for aspiration, increased heart rate and systemic blood pressure, which increase the risk of myocardial ischemia and dysrhythmias. Patients are at increased risk of dehydration, electrolyte disturbances, aspiration, and wound **dehiscence** (Hodge et al., 2014). Postoperative pain is increased as well (McGuire & Bolyanatz, 2014; Rodriguez, 2015). Ongoing research is investigating the most efficacious combination of medications for patients with different risk profiles (Gan, Diemunsch, Habib, et al., 2014).

Gerontologic Considerations

The older adult patient, like all patients, is transferred from the OR table to the bed or stretcher slowly and gently. The effects of this action on blood pressure and ventilation are monitored. Special attention is given to keeping the patient warm as older adult patients are more susceptible to hypothermia. The patient's position is changed frequently to stimulate respirations and to promote circulation and comfort.

The older adult patient may require additional support in the immediate postoperative period if cardiovascular, pulmonary, or renal function is impaired. With careful monitoring, it is possible to detect cardiopulmonary deficits before signs and symptoms are apparent. Changes associated with the aging process, the prevalence of chronic diseases, alteration in fluid and nutrition status, and the increased use of medications result in the need for postoperative vigilance (Oster & Oster, 2015). The older adult patient requires understanding of specific needs such as hypothermia, need for protection of fragile skin, padding and repositioning, depleted energy levels, cardiac and pulmonary issues, postoperative pain, and the sensitivity and metabolic issues related to medication. Having less physiologic reserve, older adult patients require more frequent monitoring. Postoperative confusion and delirium affect as many as 51% of older patients. Acute confusion may be caused by uncontrolled pain and nonjudicious use of opioids; presence of hypoxemia, hypercarbia, metabolic disorders and/or sepsis; use of physical restraints; malnutrition; urinary catheterization; electrolyte and fluid abnormalities; anaemia; increased surgical blood loss and greater intraoperative transfusion; and certain medications (Vijayakumar, Elango, Ganessan, et al., 2014). Providing adequate hydration; reorienting to the environment; and reassessing the doses of sedatives, anesthetics, and analgesics may reduce the risk for confusion. Hypoxia can present as confusion and restlessness, as can blood loss and electrolyte imbalances. Exclusion of all other causes of confusion must precede the assumption that confusion is related to age, circumstances, and medications.

Determining Readiness for Discharge From the PACU

A patient remains in the PACU until fully recovered from the anesthetic agent. Indicators of recovery include stable blood pressure, adequate respiratory function, and adequate oxygen saturation level compared with baseline.

Many hospitals use a scoring system (e.g., Aldrete score) to determine the patient's general condition and readiness for transfer from the PACU (Aldrete & Wright, 1992). Throughout the recovery period, the patient's physical signs are observed and evaluated by means of a scoring system based on a set of objective criteria. This evaluation guide allows an objective assessment of the patient's condition in the PACU (Fig. 21-3). The patient is assessed at regular intervals, and a total score is calculated

Post Anesthesia Care Unit
MODIFIED ALDRETE SCORE

Patient: ______________________ Final score: ______________________

Room: ______________________ Surgeon: ______________________

Date: ______________________ PACU nurse: ______________________

Area of Assessment	Point Score	Upon Admission	After			
			15 min	30 min	45 min	60 min
Activity						
(Able to move spontaneously or on command)						
• Ability to move all extremities	2					
• Ability to move 2 extremities	1					
• Unable to control any extremity	0					
Respiration						
• Ability to breathe deeply and cough	2					
• Limited respiratory effort (dyspnea or splinting)	1					
• No spontaneous effort	0					
Circulation						
• BP 20% of preanesthetic level	2					
• BP 20% –49% of preanesthetic level	1					
• BP 50% of preanesthetic level	0					
Consciousness						
• Fully awake	2					
• Arousable on calling	1					
• Not responding	0					
O_2 Saturation						
• Able to maintain O_2 sat >92% on room air	2					
• Needs O_2 inhalation to maintain O_2 sat >90%	1					
• O_2 sat <90% even with O_2 supplement	0					
Totals:						

Required for discharge from Post Anesthesia Care Unit: 7–8 points

______________________ ______________________

Time of release Signature of nurse

FIGURE 21-3. Postanesthesia care unit record; modified Aldrete score (O_2 sat, oxygen saturation; BP, blood pressure). (Modified from Aldrete, A., & Wright, A. (1992). Revised Aldrete score for discharge. *Anesthesiology News*, *18*(1), 17.)

and recorded on the assessment record. The Aldrete score is usually 7 to 10 before discharge from the PACU. Patients with a score of less than 7 must remain in the PACU until their condition improves or they are transferred to an intensive care area, depending on their preoperative baseline score (Rothrock, 2014).

The patient is discharged from the phase I PACU by the anesthesiologist or to the critical care unit, the medical-surgical unit, the phase II PACU, or home with a responsible family member. In some hospitals and ambulatory care centres, patients are discharged to a **phase III PACU**, where they are prepared for discharge.

Preparing the Postoperative Patient for Direct Discharge

Ambulatory surgical centres frequently only have a step-down PACU similar to a phase II PACU. This type of patient is basically healthy and will be discharged directly to home. Prior to discharge the patient will require verbal and written instructions and information about follow-up care.

Promoting Home, Community-Based, and Transitional Care

To ensure patient safety and recovery, expert patient education and discharge planning are necessary when a patient undergoes same-day or ambulatory surgery. Because anesthetics cloud memory for concurrent events, it is preferred that verbal and written instructions be given to both the patient and the adult who will be accompanying the patient home. Alternative formats (e.g., large print, Braille) of instructions or use of a sign language interpreter may be required to ensure patient and family understanding. A translator may be required if the patient and/or family members do not understand English.

Discharge Preparation

The patient and caregiver (e.g., family member or friend) are informed about expected outcomes and immediate postoperative changes anticipated. Chart 21-3 identifies important teaching points; before discharging the patient, the nurse provides written instructions covering each of those points. Prescriptions are given to the patient. Appropriate telephone numbers are provided, so the patient and caregiver may call with questions and to schedule follow-up appointments.

Although recovery time varies depending on the type and extent of surgery and the patient's overall condition, patients are usually advised to limit activity for 24 to 48 hours. During this time, the patient should not drive a vehicle, drink alcoholic beverages, or perform tasks that require energy or skill. Fluids may be consumed as desired and smaller-than-normal amounts may be eaten at mealtime. Patients are cautioned not to make important decisions at this time because the medications, anesthesia, and surgery may affect their decision-making ability.

Continuing and Transitional Care

Some patients who undergo ambulatory surgery may require referral for home care. These may be elderly or frail patients, those who live alone, and patients with other health care problems or disabilities that might interfere with self-care or resumption of usual activities. The home care nurse assesses the patient's physical status (e.g., respiratory and cardiovascular status, adequacy of pain management, the surgical incision, surgical complications) and the patient's and family's ability to adhere to the recommendations given at the time of discharge. Previous teaching is reinforced as needed. The home care nurse may change surgical dressings, monitor the patency of a drainage system, or administer medications. The patient and family are reminded about the importance of keeping follow-up appointments with the surgeon. Follow-up phone calls from the nurse or surgeon may also be used to assess the patient's progress and to answer any questions.

Care of the Hospitalized Postoperative Patient

Surgical patients who require hospital stays include trauma patients, acutely ill patients, patients undergoing major surgery, patients who require emergency surgery, and patients with a concurrent medical disorder. Seriously

CHART 21-3

HOME CARE CHECKLIST • Discharge After Surgery

At the completion of education, the patient and/or caregiver will be able to:

- Name the procedure that was performed and identify any permanent changes in anatomic structure or function as well as changes in ADLs, IADLs, roles, relationships, and spirituality.
- Identify interventions and strategies (e.g., durable medical equipment, adaptive equipment) used in adapting to any permanent changes in structure or function.
- Describe ongoing postoperative therapeutic regimen, including diet and activities to perform (e.g., walking and breathing exercises) and to limit or avoid (e.g., lifting weights, driving a car, contact sports).
- State the name, dose, side effects, frequency, and schedule for all medications.
- State how to obtain medical supplies and carry out dressing changes, wound care, and other prescribed regimens.
- Describe signs and symptoms of complications.
- State time and date of follow-up appointments.
- Relate how to reach health care provider with questions or complications.
- State understanding of community resources and referrals (if any).
- Identify the need for health promotion (e.g., weight reduction, smoking cessation, stress management), disease prevention, and screening activities.

ill patients and those who have undergone major cardiovascular, pulmonary, or neurologic surgery may be admitted to specialized ICUs for close monitoring and advanced interventions and support. The care required by these patients in the immediate postoperative period is discussed in specific chapters of this book. Patients admitted to the clinical unit for postoperative care have multiple needs and stay for a short period of time. Postoperative care for those surgical patients returning to the general medical-surgical unit is discussed later in this chapter.

Receiving the Patient in the Clinical Unit

The patient's room is readied by assembling the necessary equipment and supplies: IV pole, drainage receptacle holder, suction equipment, oxygen, emesis basin, tissues, disposable pads, blankets, and postoperative documentation forms. When the call comes to the unit about the patient's transfer from the PACU, the need for any additional items is communicated. The PACU nurse reports relevant data about the patient to the receiving nurse (see Chart 21-1).

Usually the surgeon speaks to the family after surgery and relates the general condition of the patient. The receiving nurse reviews the postoperative orders, admits the patient to the unit, performs an initial assessment, and attends to the patient's immediate needs (Chart 21-4).

Nursing Management After Surgery

During the first 24 hours after surgery, nursing care of the hospitalized patient on the medical-surgical unit involves continuing to help the patient recover from the effects of anesthesia (Barash, Cullen, & Stoelting, 2013), frequently assessing the patient's physiologic status, monitoring for complications, managing pain, and implementing measures designed to achieve the long-range goals of independence with self-care, successful management of the therapeutic regimen, discharge to home, and full recovery (Liddle, 2013; Penprase & Johnson, 2015; Rosen, Bergh, Schwartz-Barcott, et al., 2014). In the initial hours after admission to the clinical unit, adequate ventilation, hemodynamic stability, incisional pain, surgical site integrity, nausea and vomiting, neurologic status, and spontaneous voiding are primary concerns. The pulse rate, blood pressure, and respiration rate are recorded at least every 15 minutes for the first hour and every 30 minutes for the next 2 hours. Thereafter, they are measured less frequently if they remain stable. The temperature is monitored every 4 hours for the first 24 hours. Patients usually begin to

CHART 21-4

GUIDELINES for Immediate Postoperative Nursing Interventions

NURSING INTERVENTIONS	RATIONALE
1. Assess breathing and administer supplemental oxygen, if prescribed.	1. Assessment provides a baseline and helps identify signs and symptoms of respiratory distress early.
2. Monitor vital signs and note skin warmth, moisture, and colour.	2. A careful baseline assessment helps identify signs and symptoms of shock early.
3. Assess the surgical site and wound drainage systems. Connect all drainage tubes to gravity or suction as indicated and monitor closed drainage systems.	3. Assessment provides a baseline and helps identify signs and symptoms of hemorrhage early.
4. Assess level of consciousness, orientation, and ability to move extremities.	4. These parameters provide a baseline and help identify signs and symptoms of neurologic complications.
5. Assess pain level; pain characteristics (location, quality); and timing, type, and route of administration of the last dose of analgesic.	5. Assessment provides a baseline of current pain level and assesses effectiveness of pain management strategies.
6. Administer analgesic medications as prescribed and assess their effectiveness in relieving pain.	6. Administration of analgesic agents helps decrease pain.
7. Place the call light, emesis basin, ice chips (if allowed), and bedpan or urinal within reach.	7. Attending to these needs provides for comfort and safety.
8. Position the patient to enhance comfort, safety, and lung expansion.	8. This promotes safety and reduces risk of postoperative complications.
9. Assess IV sites for patency and infusions for correct rate and solution.	9. Assessing IV sites and infusions helps detect phlebitis and prevents errors in rate and solution type.
10. Assess urine output in closed drainage system or use bladder scanner to detect distention.	10. Assessment provides a baseline and helps identify signs of urinary retention.
11. Reinforce the need to begin deep breathing and leg exercises.	11. These activities help prevent complications related to immobility (e.g., atelectasis, VTE).
12. Provide information to the patient and family.	12. Patient education helps decrease the patient's and family's anxiety.

VTE, venous thromboembolism.

Adapted from Association of PeriOperative Registered Nurses (AORN). (2014). *Association of PeriOperative Registered Nurses (AORN) standards, recommended practice, and guidelines*. Denver, CO: Author.

return to their usual state of health several hours after surgery or after awaking the next morning. Although pain may still be intense, many patients feel more alert, less nauseous, and less anxious. They have begun their breathing and leg exercises as appropriate for the type of surgery, and many will have dangled their legs over the edge of the bed, stood, and ambulated a few feet or been assisted out of bed to the chair at least once. Many will have tolerated a light meal and had IV fluids discontinued. The focus of care shifts from intense physiologic management and symptomatic relief of the adverse effects of anesthesia to regaining independence with self-care and preparing for discharge.

Nursing Process

The Hospitalized Patient Recovering From Surgery

WATCH & LEARN

Nursing care of the hospitalized patient recovering from surgery takes place in a compressed time frame, with much of the healing and recovery occurring after the patient is discharged to home or to a rehabilitation centre. The ORNAC Conceptual Model for Perioperative Registered Nursing Practice is a helpful tool used by nurses in the postoperative phase of care (see Chapter 21).

Assessment

Assessment of the hospitalized postoperative patient includes monitoring vital signs and completing a review of systems upon the patient's arrival to the clinical unit (see Chart 21-4) and at regular intervals thereafter.

The nurse monitors for airway patency and any signs of laryngeal edema because pulmonary complications are among the most frequent and serious problems encountered by the surgical patient. The quality of respirations, including depth, rate, and sound, are assessed regularly. Chest auscultation verifies that breath sounds are normal (or abnormal) bilaterally, and the findings are documented as a baseline for later comparisons. Often, because of the effects of analgesic and anesthetic medications, respirations are slow. Shallow and rapid respirations may be caused by pain, constricting dressings, gastric dilation, abdominal distention, or obesity. Noisy breathing may be due to obstruction by secretions or the tongue. Another possible complication is flash pulmonary edema that occurs when protein and fluid accumulate in the alveoli unrelated to elevated pulmonary artery occlusive pressure. Signs and symptoms include agitation; tachypnea; tachycardia; decreased pulse oximetry readings; frothy, pink sputum; and crackles on auscultation.

The nurse assesses the patient's pain level using a verbal or visual analog scale and assesses the characteristics of the pain. The patient's appearance, pulse, capillary refill, respirations, blood pressure, MAP, skin colour, and skin temperature are clues to cardiovascular function. When the patient arrives in the clinical unit, the surgical site is assessed for bleeding, type and integrity of dressings, and presence of drains.

The nurse also assesses the patient's mental status and level of consciousness, speech, and orientation and compares them with the preoperative baseline. Although a change in mental status or postoperative restlessness may be related to anxiety, pain, or medications, it may also be a symptom of oxygen deficit or hemorrhage. These serious causes must be investigated and excluded before other causes are pursued.

General discomfort that results from lying in one position on the operating table, the handling of tissues by the surgical team, the body's reaction to anesthesia, and anxiety are also common causes of restlessness. These discomforts may be relieved by administering the prescribed analgesics, changing the patient's position frequently, and assessing and alleviating the cause of anxiety. If tight, drainage-soaked bandages are causing discomfort, reinforcing or changing the dressing completely as prescribed by the physician may make the patient more comfortable. The bladder is assessed for distention because urinary retention can also cause restlessness.

Nursing Priorities

Based on the assessment data, major nursing priorities may include the following:

- Acute pain
- Anxiety
- Ineffective temperature regulation
- Prevention of shock or hemorrhage
- Immobility
- Airway clearance
- Nutritional management
- Management of constipation
- Prevention of urinary retention
- Proper positioning
- Wound care

Collaborative Problems or Potential Complications

Based on the assessment data, potential complications may include the following:

- Infection
- Pulmonary infection/hypoxia
- Deep vein thrombosis (DVT)
- Hematoma or hemorrhage
- Pulmonary embolism (PE)
- Wound dehiscence or evisceration

Planning and Goals

The major goals for the patient include optimal respiratory function, relief of pain, optimal cardiovascular function, increased activity tolerance, unimpaired wound healing, maintenance of body temperature, and maintenance of nutritional balance. Further goals include resumption of usual pattern of bowel and bladder elimination, identification of any perioperative positioning injury, acquisition of sufficient knowledge to manage self-care after discharge, and absence of complications.

Nursing Interventions

Preventing Respiratory Complications

Respiratory depressive effects of opioid medications, decreased lung expansion secondary to pain, and decreased mobility combine to put the patient at risk for common respiratory complications, particularly atelectasis (alveolar collapse; incomplete expansion of the lung), pneumonia, and hypoxemia (Miskovic & Lumb, 2017; Rothrock, 2014). Atelectasis remains a risk for the patient who is not moving well or ambulating or who is not performing deep-breathing and coughing exercises or using an incentive spirometer. Signs and symptoms include decreased breath sounds over the affected area, crackles, and cough. Pneumonia is characterized by chills and fever, tachycardia, and tachypnea. Cough may or may not be present and may or may not be productive. Hypostatic pulmonary congestion, caused by a weakened cardiovascular system that permits stagnation of secretions at lung bases, may develop; this condition occurs most frequently in older adult patients who are not mobilized effectively. The symptoms are often vague, with perhaps a slight elevation of temperature, pulse, and respiratory rate, as well as a cough. Physical examination reveals dullness and crackles at the base of the lungs. If the condition progresses, the outcome may be fatal.

The types of hypoxemia that can affect postoperative patients are subacute and episodic. Subacute hypoxemia is a constant low level of oxygen saturation when breathing appears normal. Episodic hypoxemia develops suddenly, and the patient may be at risk for cerebral dysfunction, myocardial ischemia, and cardiac arrest. Risk for hypoxemia is increased in patients who have undergone major surgery (particularly abdominal), are obese, or have preexisting pulmonary problems. Hypoxemia is detected by pulse oximetry that measures blood oxygen saturation. Factors that may affect the accuracy of pulse oximetry readings include cold extremities, tremors, atrial fibrillation, acrylic nails, and black or blue nail polish (these colours interfere with the functioning of the pulse oximeter; other colours do not).

Preventive measures and timely recognition of signs and symptoms help avert pulmonary complications. Crackles indicate static pulmonary secretions that need to be mobilized by coughing and deep-breathing exercises. When a mucous plug obstructs one of the bronchi entirely, the pulmonary tissue beyond the plug collapses, resulting in atelectasis.

To clear secretions and prevent pneumonia, the nurse encourages the patient to turn frequently, take deep breaths, cough, and use the incentive spirometer at least every hour. These pulmonary exercises should begin as soon as the patient arrives on the clinical unit and continue until the patient is discharged. Even if he or she is not fully awake from anesthesia, the patient can be asked to take several deep breaths. This helps expel residual anesthetic agents, mobilize secretions, and prevent atelectasis. Careful splinting of abdominal or thoracic incision sites helps the patient overcome the fear that the exertion of coughing might open the incision. Analgesic agents are administered to permit more effective coughing, and oxygen is administered as prescribed to prevent or relieve hypoxia. To encourage lung expansion, the patient is encouraged to yawn or take sustained maximal inspirations to create a negative intrathoracic pressure of −40 mm Hg and expand lung volume to total capacity. Chest physical therapy may be prescribed if indicated. See Chapter 26.

Coughing is contraindicated in patients who have head injuries or who have undergone intracranial surgery (because of the risk for increasing intracranial pressure), as well as in patients who have undergone eye surgery (because of the risk for increasing intraocular pressure) or plastic surgery (because of the risk for increasing tension on delicate tissues).

Early ambulation increases metabolism and pulmonary aeration and, in general, improves all body functions. The patient is encouraged to be out of bed as soon as possible (i.e., on the day of surgery, or no later than the first postoperative day). This practice is especially valuable in preventing pulmonary complications in older patients (Oster & Oster, 2015).

Relieving Pain

Most patients experience some pain after a surgical procedure. Complete absence of pain in the area of the surgical incision may not occur for a few weeks, depending on the site and nature of the surgery, but the intensity of postoperative pain gradually subsides on subsequent days. About one third of patients report severe pain, one third moderate pain, and one third little or no pain (Grossman & Porth, 2014; Rodriguez, 2015). This does not mean that the patients in the last group have no pain; rather, they appear to activate psychodynamic mechanisms that impair the registering of pain ("gate closing" theory and nociceptive transmission). See Chapter 16 for a more detailed discussion of pain.

Many factors (motivational, affective, cognitive, emotional, and cultural) influence the pain experience. The degree and severity of postoperative pain and the patient's tolerance for pain depend on the incision site, the nature of the surgical procedure, the extent of surgical trauma, the type of anesthesia, and route of administration. The preoperative preparation received by the patient (including information about what to expect, reassurance, psychological support, and teaching specific communication techniques related to pain) is a significant factor in decreasing anxiety, apprehension, the amount of postoperative pain, and PONV (Ward, 2014).

Intense pain stimulates the stress response, which adversely affects the cardiac and immune systems.

When pain impulses are transmitted, both muscle tension and local vasoconstriction increase, further stimulating pain receptors. This increases myocardial demand and oxygen consumption. The hypothalamic stress response also results in an increase in blood viscosity and platelet aggregation, increasing the risk of thrombosis and PE.

Often the physician has prescribed different medications or dosages to cover various levels of pain. The nurse discusses these options with the patient to determine the best medication. The nurse assesses the effectiveness of the medication periodically, beginning 30 minutes after administration, or sooner if the medication is being delivered by patient-controlled analgesia (PCA).

OPIOID ANALGESICS. Opioid analgesic agents are commonly prescribed for pain and immediate postoperative restlessness. A preventive approach, rather than an "as needed" (PRN) approach, is more effective in relieving pain. With a preventive approach, the medication is given at prescribed intervals rather than when the pain becomes severe or unbearable. Many patients (and some health care providers) are overly concerned about the risk of drug addiction in the postoperative patient. However, this risk is negligible with the use of opioid medications for short-term pain control (McGuire & Bolyanatz, 2014).

PATIENT-CONTROLLED ANALGESIA. The goal is pain prevention rather than sporadic pain control. Patients recover more quickly when adequate pain relief measures are used, and PCA permits patients to administer their own pain medication when needed. Most patients are candidates for PCA. The two requirements for PCA are an understanding of the need to self-dose and the physical ability to self-dose. The amount of medication delivered by the IV or epidural route and the time span during which the opioid medication is released are controlled by the PCA device. PCA promotes patient participation in care, eliminates delayed administration of analgesics, maintains a therapeutic drug level, and enables the patient to move, turn, cough, and take deep breaths with less pain, thus reducing postoperative pulmonary complications (Rothrock, 2014).

EPIDURAL INFUSIONS AND INTRAPLEURAL ANESTHESIA. Patients undergoing many types of procedures and surgeries benefit from the use of epidural infusion of opioids (Hayes & Gordon, 2015; Rodriguez, 2015). Epidural infusions are used with caution in chest procedures because the analgesic may ascend along the spinal cord and affect respiration. Intrapleural anesthesia involves the administration of a local anesthetic by a catheter between the parietal and visceral pleura. It provides sensory anesthesia without affecting motor function to the intercostal muscles. This anesthesia allows more effective coughing and deep breathing in conditions such as cholecystectomy, renal surgery, and rib fractures, in which pain in the thoracic region would interfere with these exercises.

A local opioid or a combination anesthetic (opioid plus local anesthetic agent) is used in the epidural infusion.

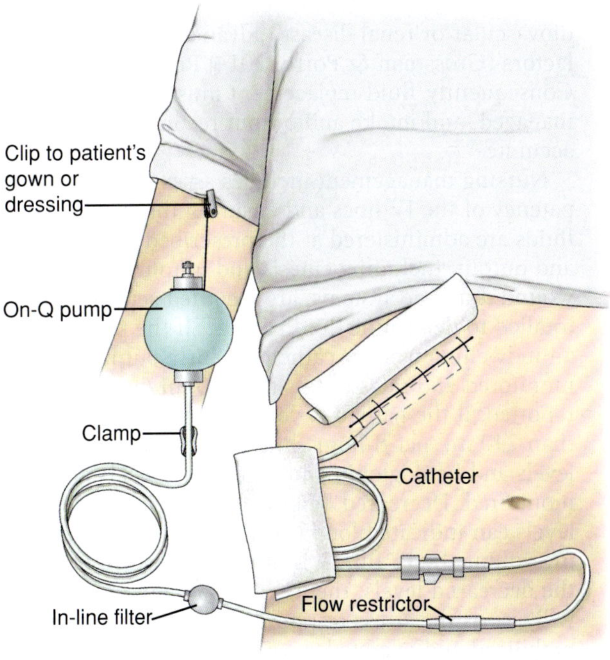

FIGURE 21-4. Subcutaneous pain management system consists of a pump, filter, and catheter that delivers a specific amount of prescribed local anesthetic at the rate determined by the physician. (Redrawn with permission from Kimberly-Clark Corporation, Neenah, WI.)

OTHER PAIN RELIEF MEASURES. For pain that is difficult to control, a subcutaneous pain management system may be used. This is a silicone catheter that is inserted at the site of the affected area. The catheter is attached to a pump that delivers a continuous amount of local anesthetic at a specific amount determined and prescribed by the physician (Fig. 21-4).

Nonpharmacologic measures, such as guided imagery, music, and the implementation of healing touch, have been successful clinical adjuncts used to decrease pain and anxiety (Anderson, Suchicital, Lang, et al., 2015; Kiefer, 2015). Changing the patient's position, using distraction, applying cool washcloths to the face, and providing back massage may be useful in relieving general discomfort temporarily, promoting relaxation, and rendering medication more effective when it is given.

Promoting Cardiac Output

If signs and symptoms of shock or hemorrhage occur, treatment and nursing care are implemented as described in the discussion of care in the PACU.

Although most patients do not hemorrhage or go into shock, changes in circulating volume, the stress of surgery, and the effects of medications and preoperative preparations all affect cardiovascular function. IV fluid replacement is often prescribed for up to 24 hours after surgery or until the patient is stable and tolerating oral fluids. Close monitoring is indicated to detect and correct conditions such as fluid volume deficit, altered tissue perfusion, and decreased cardiac output, all of which can increase the patient's discomfort, place him or her at risk of complications, and prolong the hospital stay. Some patients are at risk of fluid volume excess secondary to existing cardiovascular or renal disease, advanced age, and other factors (Grossman & Porth, 2014; Rothrock, 2014). Consequently, fluid replacement must be carefully managed, and intake and output records must be accurate.

Nursing management includes assessing the patency of the IV lines and ensuring that the correct fluids are administered at the prescribed rate. Intake and output, including emesis and output from wound drainage systems, are recorded separately and totalled to determine fluid balance. If the patient has an indwelling urinary catheter, hourly outputs are monitored and rates of less than 30 mL/hr are reported; if the patient is voiding, an output of less than 240 mL per 8-hour shift is reported. Electrolyte levels and hemoglobin and hematocrit levels are monitored. Decreased hemoglobin and hematocrit levels can indicate blood loss or dilution of circulating volume by IV fluids. If dilution is contributing to the decreased levels, the hemoglobin and hematocrit will rise as the stress response abates and fluids are mobilized and excreted.

Venous stasis from dehydration, immobility, and pressure on leg veins during surgery put the patient at risk for DVT. Leg exercises and frequent position changes are initiated early in the postoperative period to stimulate circulation. Patients should avoid positions that compromise venous return, such as raising the bed's knee gatch, placing a pillow under the knees, sitting for long periods, and dangling the legs with pressure at the back of the knees. Venous return is promoted by antiembolism stockings and early ambulation.

Encouraging Activity

Early ambulation has a significant effect on recovery and the prevention of complications (e.g., atelectasis, hypostatic pneumonia, gastrointestinal [GI] discomfort, circulatory problems) as well as improving anxiety and self-control (Rothrock, 2014). Postoperative activity orders are checked before the patient is assisted to get out of bed, in many instances, on the evening following surgery. Sitting up at the edge of the bed for a few minutes may be all that the patient who has undergone a major surgical procedure can tolerate at first.

Ambulation reduces postoperative abdominal distention by increasing GI tract and abdominal wall tone and stimulating peristalsis. Early ambulation prevents stasis of blood, and thromboembolic events occur less frequently. Pain is often decreased when early ambulation is possible, and the hospital stay is shorter and less costly.

Despite the advantages of early ambulation, patients may be reluctant to get out of bed on the evening of surgery. Reminding them of the importance of early mobility in preventing complications may help patients overcome their fears. When a patient gets out of bed for the first time, orthostatic hypotension, also called postural hypotension, is a concern. Orthostatic hypotension is an abnormal drop in blood pressure that occurs as the patient changes from a supine to a standing position. It is common after surgery because of changes in circulating blood volume and bed rest. Signs and symptoms include a decrease of 20 mm Hg in systolic blood pressure or 10 mm Hg in diastolic blood pressure, weakness, dizziness, and fainting. Older adults are at increased risk for orthostatic hypotension secondary to age-related changes in vascular tone. To detect orthostatic hypotension, the nurse assesses the patient's blood pressure first in the supine position, after the patient sits up, again after the patient stands, and 2 to 3 minutes later. Gradual position change gives the circulatory system time to adjust. If the patient becomes dizzy, he or she is returned to the supine position, and ambulation is delayed for several hours.

To assist the postoperative patient in getting out of bed for the first time after surgery, the nurse:

1. Helps the patient move gradually from the lying position to the sitting position by raising the head of the bed and encourages the patient to splint the incision when applicable.
2. Positions the patient completely upright (sitting) and turned so that both legs are hanging over the edge of the bed.
3. Helps the patient stand beside the bed.

After becoming accustomed to the upright position, the patient may start to walk. The nurse utilizes a transfer belt and remains at the patient's side to give physical support and encouragement. Care must be taken not to tire the patient; the extent of the first few periods of ambulation varies with the type of surgical procedure and the patient's physical condition and age.

Whether or not the patient can ambulate early in the postoperative period, bed exercises are encouraged to improve circulation. Bed exercises consist of the following:

- Arm exercises (full range of motion, with specific attention to abduction and external rotation of the shoulder)
- Hand and finger exercises
- Foot exercises to prevent DVT, foot drop, and toe deformities and to aid in maintaining good circulation
- Leg flexion and leg-lifting exercises to prepare the patient for ambulation
- Abdominal and gluteal contraction exercises

Hampered by pain, dressings, IV lines, or drains, many patients cannot engage in activity without assistance. Helping the patient increase his or her activity level on the first postoperative day is important to prevent complications related to prolonged inactivity. One way to increase the patient's activity is to have the patient perform as much routine personal hygiene care as possible. Setting up the patient to bathe with a bedside wash basin or, if possible, assisting the patient to the bathroom to sit in a chair at the sink not only gets the patient moving but helps restore a sense of self-control and prepares the patient for discharge.

For a safe discharge to home, patients need to be able to ambulate a functional distance (e.g., length of the house or apartment), get in and out of bed unassisted, and be independent with toileting. Patients are encouraged to perform as much as they can and then to call for assistance. The patient and the nurse can collaborate on a schedule for progressive activity that includes ambulating in the room and hallway, sitting out of bed in a chair as well as dressing and/or changing garments/shoes. Assessing the patient's vital signs before, during, and after a scheduled activity helps the nurse and patient determine the rate of progression. By providing physical support, the nurse maintains the patient's safety; by communicating a positive attitude about the patient's ability to perform the activity, the nurse promotes the patient's confidence. The nurse encourages the patient to continue to perform bed exercises, wear pneumatic compression or prescribed antiembolism stockings when in bed, and rest as needed. If the patient has had orthopedic surgery of the lower extremities or will require a mobility aid (i.e., walker, crutches) at home, a physical therapist may be involved the first time the patient gets out of bed to teach him or her to ambulate safely or to use the mobility aid correctly.

Caring for Wounds

WOUND HEALING. Wounds heal by different mechanisms, depending on the condition of the wound. Surgical wound healing occurs in three phases: **first-intention, second-intention,** and **third-intention wound healing** (Chart 21-5) (Rothrock, 2014). With shorter hospital stays, much of the healing takes place at home, and both the hospital and home care nurse should be informed about the principles of wound healing.

Ongoing assessment of the surgical site involves inspection for approximation of wound edges,

CHART 21-5

Wound-Healing Mechanisms

First-Intention Healing

Wounds made aseptically with a minimum of tissue destruction that are properly closed heal with little tissue reaction by first intention (primary union). When wounds heal by **first-intention healing**, granulation tissue is not visible and scar formation is minimal. Postoperatively, many of these wounds are covered with a dry sterile dressing. If a cyanoacrylate tissue adhesive (LiquiBand) has been used to close the incision without sutures, a dressing is contraindicated.

Second-Intention Healing

Second-intention healing (granulation) occurs in infected wounds (abscess) or in wounds in which the edges have not been approximated. When an abscess is incised, it collapses partly, but the dead and dying cells forming its walls are still being released into the cavity. For this reason, a drainage tube or gauze packing is inserted into the abscess pocket to allow drainage to escape easily. Gradually, the necrotic material disintegrates and escapes, and the abscess cavity fills with a red, soft, sensitive tissue that bleeds easily. This tissue is composed of minute, thin-walled capillaries and buds that later form connective tissue. These buds, called *granulations,* enlarge until they fill the area left by the destroyed tissue. The cells surrounding the capillaries change their round shape to become long, thin, and intertwined to form a scar (cicatrix). Healing is complete when skin cells (epithelium) grow over these granulations. This method of repair is referred to as healing by granulation, and it takes place whenever pus is formed or when loss of tissue has occurred for any reason. When the postoperative wound is to be allowed to heal by secondary intention, it is usually packed with saline-moistened sterile dressings and covered with a dry sterile dressing.

Third-Intention Healing

Third-intention healing (secondary suture) is used for deep wounds that either have not been sutured early or break down and are resutured later, thus bringing together two opposing granulation surfaces. This results in a deeper and wider scar. These wounds are also packed postoperatively with moist gauze and covered with a dry sterile dressing.

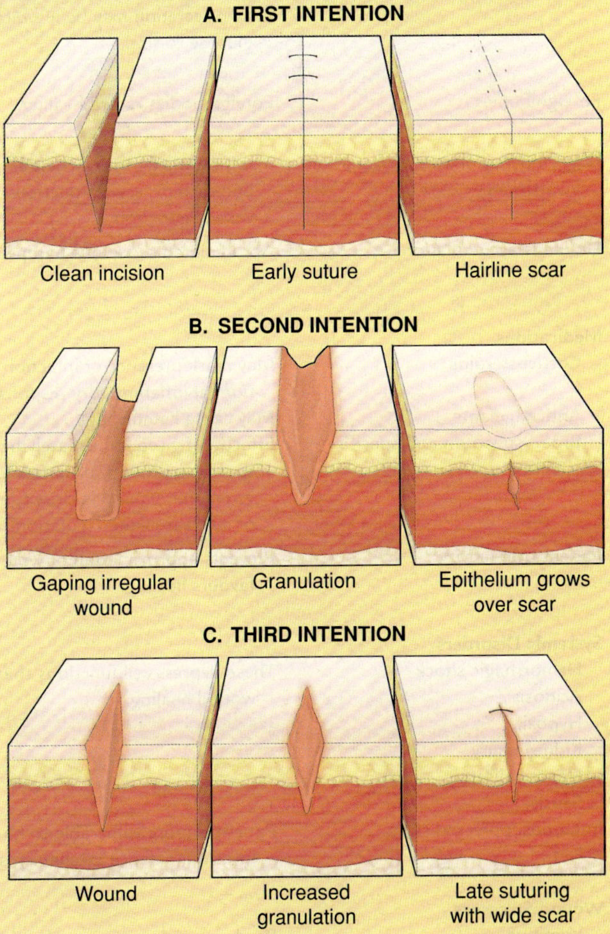

integrity of sutures or staples, redness, discolouration, warmth, swelling, unusual tenderness, or drainage. The area around the wound should also be inspected for a reaction to tape or trauma from tight bandages. As a wound heals, many factors, such as nutrition, cleanliness, rest, and position, determine how quickly healing occurs. These factors can be influenced by nursing interventions. Specific nursing assessments and interventions that address these factors and help promote wound healing are presented in Table 21-3.

TABLE 21-3 Factors Affecting Wound Healing

Factors	Rationale	Nursing Interventions
Age of patient	The older the patient, the less resilient the tissues.	Handle all tissues gently.
Handling of tissues	Rough handling causes injury and delayed healing.	Handle tissues carefully and evenly.
Hemorrhage	Accumulation of blood creates dead spaces as well as dead cells that must be removed. The area becomes a growth medium for organisms.	Monitor vital signs. Observe incision site for evidence of bleeding and infection.
Hypovolemia	Insufficient blood volume leads to vasoconstriction and reduced oxygen and nutrients available for wound healing.	Monitor for volume deficit (circulatory impairment). Correct by fluid replacement as prescribed.
Local Factors		
Edema	Reduces blood supply by exerting increased interstitial pressure on vessels.	Elevate part; apply cool compresses.
Inadequate dressing technique:		
Too small	Permits bacterial invasion and contamination.	Follow guidelines for proper dressing technique.
Too tight	Reduces blood supply carrying nutrients and oxygen.	
Nutritional deficits	Protein–calorie depletion may occur. Insulin secretion may be inhibited, causing blood glucose to rise.	Correct deficits; this may require parenteral nutritional therapy. Monitor blood glucose levels. Administer vitamin supplements as prescribed.
Foreign bodies	Foreign bodies retard healing.	Keep wounds free of dressing threads and talcum powder from gloves.
Oxygen deficit (tissue oxygenation insufficient)	Insufficient oxygen may be due to inadequate lung and cardiovascular function as well as localized vasoconstriction.	Encourage deep breathing, turning, and controlled coughing.
Drainage accumulation	Accumulated secretions hamper healing process.	Monitor closed drainage systems for proper functioning. Institute measures to remove accumulated secretions.
Medications		
Corticosteroids	May mask presence of infection by impairing normal inflammatory response	Be aware of action and effect of medications patient is receiving.
Anticoagulants	May cause hemorrhage	
Broad-spectrum and specific antibiotics	Effective if given immediately before surgery for specific pathology or bacterial contamination. If given after wound is closed, ineffective because of intravascular coagulation.	
Patient overactivity	Prevents approximation of wound edges. Resting favours healing.	Use measures to keep wound edges approximated: taping, bandaging, splints. Encourage rest.
Systemic Disorders		
Hemorrhagic shock Acidosis Hypoxia Kidney injury Hepatic disease Sepsis	These depress cell functions that directly affect wound healing.	Be familiar with the nature of the specific disorder. Administer prescribed treatment. Cultures may be indicated to determine appropriate antibiotic.
Immunosuppressed state	Patient is more vulnerable to bacterial and viral invasion; defence mechanisms are impaired.	Provide maximum protection to prevent infection. Restrict visitors with colds; institute mandatory hand hygiene by all staff.
Wound Stressors		
Vomiting Valsalva maneuver Heavy coughing Straining	Produce tension on wounds, particularly of the torso.	Encourage frequent turning and ambulation, and administer antiemetic medications as prescribed. Assist patient in splinting incision.

Adapted from Edmiston, C. E. Jr, & Spencer, M. (2014). Patient care interventions to help reduce the risk of surgical site infections. *AORN Journal*, *100*(6), 590–602.

CARING FOR SURGICAL DRAINS. Nursing interventions to promote wound healing also include management of surgical drains. Drains are tubes that exit the peri-incisional area, either into a portable wound suction device (closed) or into the dressings (open). Drains allow the escape of fluids that could otherwise serve as a culture medium for bacteria. In portable wound suction, the use of gentle, constant suction enhances drainage of these fluids and collapses the skin flaps against the underlying tissue, thus removing "dead space." Wound drains include the Penrose, Hemovac, and Jackson–Pratt drains (Fig. 21-5). The amount of bloody drainage on the surgical dressing is assessed frequently. Spots of drainage on the dressings are outlined with a pen, and the date and time of the outline are recorded on the dressing so that increased drainage can be easily seen. Output from wound systems is recorded on a regular basis. A certain amount of drainage in a wound drainage system or on the dressing is expected, but excessive amounts should be reported to the surgeon. Increasing amounts of fresh blood on the dressing should be reported immediately. Some wounds are irrigated heavily before closure in the OR, and open drains exiting the wound may be embedded in the dressings. These wounds may drain large amounts of blood-tinged fluid that saturate the dressing. The dressing can be reinforced with sterile gauze bandages; the time at which they were reinforced should be documented. If drainage continues, the surgeon should be notified so that the dressing can be changed. Multiple similar drains are numbered or otherwise labeled (e.g., left lower quadrant, left upper quadrant) so that output measurements can be reliably and consistently recorded.

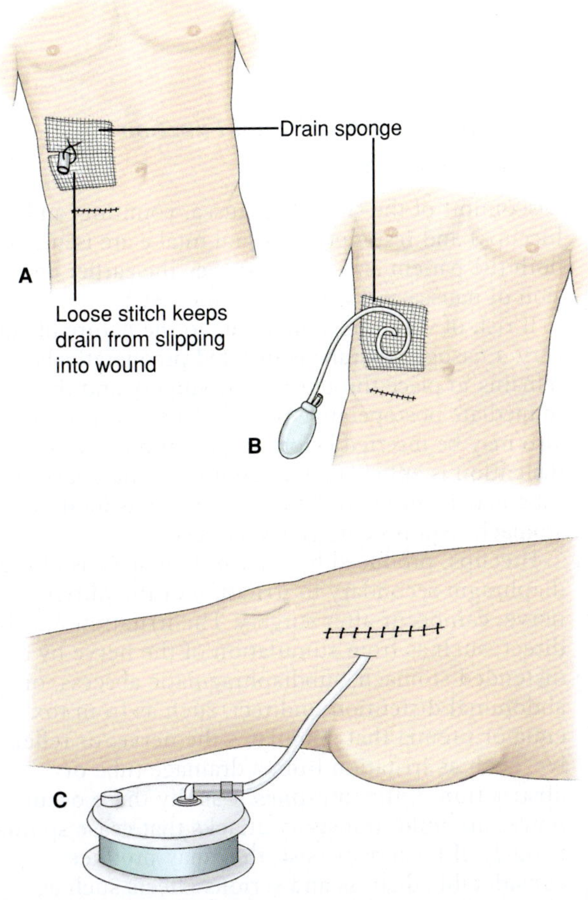

FIGURE 21-5. Types of surgical drains: **A.** Penrose, **B.** Jackson–Pratt, **C.** Hemovac.

CHANGING THE DRESSING. Although the first postoperative dressing is usually changed by a member of the surgical team, subsequent dressing changes in the immediate postoperative period are usually performed by the nurse. A dressing is applied to a wound for one or more of the following reasons: (1) to provide a proper environment for wound healing; (2) to absorb drainage; (3) to splint or immobilize the wound; (4) to protect the wound and new epithelial tissue from mechanical injury; (5) to protect the wound from bacterial contamination and from soiling by feces, vomitus, and urine; (6) to promote hemostasis, as in a pressure dressing; and (7) to provide mental and physical comfort for the patient.

The patient is told that the dressing is to be changed and that changing the dressing is a simple procedure associated with little discomfort. The dressing change is performed at a suitable time (e.g., not at mealtimes or when visitors are present). Privacy is provided, and the patient is not unduly exposed. The nurse should avoid referring to the incision as a *scar* because the term may have negative connotations for the patient. Assurance is given that the incision will shrink as it heals and that the redness will fade.

The nurse performs hand hygiene before and after the dressing change and wears disposable gloves (sterile or clean as needed) for the dressing change itself. Most dressing changes following surgery are sterile. In accordance with standard precautions, dressings are never touched by ungloved hands because of the danger of transmitting pathogenic organisms. The tape or adhesive portion of the dressing is removed by pulling it parallel with the skin surface and in the direction of hair growth. Alcohol wipes or nonirritating solvents aid in removing adhesive painlessly and quickly. The soiled dressing is removed and deposited in a container designated for disposal of biomedical waste.

Gloves are changed and a new dressing applied. If the patient is sensitive to adhesive tape, the dressing may be held in place with hypoallergenic tape. Many tapes are porous to prevent skin maceration. Some wounds become edematous after having been dressed, causing considerable tension on the tape. If the tape is not flexible, the stretching bandage will also cause a shear injury to the skin. This can result in denuded areas or large blisters and should be avoided. An elastic adhesive bandage (Elastoplast, Microfoam-3M) may be used to hold dressings in place over mobile areas, such as the neck or the extremities, or where pressure is required.

CHART 21-6

Patient Education: Wound Care Instructions

Until Sutures Are Removed

1. Keep the wound dry and clean.
   - If there is no dressing, ask your nurse or physician if you can bathe or shower.
   - If a dressing or splint is in place, do not remove it unless it is wet or soiled.
   - If wet or soiled, change dressing yourself if you have been taught to do so; otherwise, call your nurse or physician for guidance.
   - If you have been taught, instruction might be as follows:
     - Cleanse area *gently* with sterile normal saline once or twice daily.
     - Cover with a sterile Telfa pad or gauze square large enough to cover wound.
     - Apply hypoallergenic tape (Dermacel or paper). Adhesive is not recommended because it is difficult to remove without possible injury to the incisional site.
2. Immediately report any of these signs of infection:
   - Redness, marked swelling exceeding ½ in (2.5 cm) from incision site; tenderness; or increased warmth around wound
   - Red streaks in skin near wound
   - Pus or discharge, foul odour
   - Chills or temperature higher than 37.7°C (100°F)
3. If soreness or pain causes discomfort, apply a dry cool pack (containing ice or cold water) or take prescribed acetaminophen tablets (2) every 4–6 hours. Avoid using aspirin without direction or instruction because bleeding can occur with its use.
4. Swelling after surgery is common. To help reduce swelling, elevate the affected part to the level of the heart.
   - Hand or arm
     - Sleep—elevate arm on pillow at side
     - Sitting—place arm on pillow on adjacent table
     - Standing—rest affected hand on opposite shoulder; support elbow with unaffected hand
   - Leg or foot
     - Sitting—place a pillow on a facing chair; provide support underneath the knee
     - Lying—place a pillow under affected leg

After Sutures Are Removed

Although the wound appears to be healed when sutures are removed, it is still tender and will continue to heal and strengthen for several weeks.

1. Follow recommendations of physician or nurse regarding extent of activity.
2. Keep suture line clean; do not rub vigorously; pat dry. Wound edges may look red and may be slightly raised. This is normal.
3. If the site continues to be red, thick, and painful to pressure after 8 weeks, consult the health care provider. (This may be due to excessive collagen formation and should be checked.)

While changing the dressing, the nurse has an opportunity to teach the patient how to care for the incision and change the dressings at home. The nurse observes for indicators of the patient's readiness to learn, such as looking at the incision, expressing interest, or assisting in the dressing change. Information on self-care activities and possible signs of infection is summarized in Chart 21-6.

Maintaining Normal Body Temperature

The patient is still at risk for malignant hyperthermia and hypothermia in the postoperative period. Efforts are made to identify malignant hyperthermia and to treat it early and promptly (Rothrock, 2014; Sessler, 2016).

Patients who have received anesthesia are susceptible to chills and drafts. Hypothermia management extends into the postoperative period to prevent significant nitrogen loss and catabolism. Low body temperature is reported to the physician. The room is maintained at a comfortable temperature, and blankets are provided to prevent chilling. Treatment includes oxygen administration, adequate hydration, and proper nutrition. The patient is also monitored for cardiac dysrhythmias. The risk of hypothermia is greater in the older adult and in patients who were in the cool OR environment for a prolonged period.

Managing Gastrointestinal Function and Resuming Nutrition

Discomfort of the GI tract (nausea, vomiting, and hiccups) and resumption of oral intake are issues for both the patient and the nurse. See the earlier discussion of nausea and vomiting in the PACU.

If risk of vomiting is high due to the nature of surgery, a nasogastric tube is inserted preoperatively and remains in place throughout the surgery and the immediate postoperative period. A nasogastric tube also may be inserted before surgery if postoperative distention is anticipated. In addition, a nasogastric tube may be inserted if a patient who has food in the stomach requires emergency surgery.

Hiccups, produced by intermittent spasms of the diaphragm secondary to irritation of the phrenic nerve, can occur after surgery. The irritation may be direct, such as from stimulation of the nerve by a distended stomach, subdiaphragmatic abscess, or abdominal distention; indirect, such as from toxemia or uremia that stimulates the nerve; or reflexive, such as irritation from a drainage tube or obstruction of the intestines. Usually these occurrences are mild, transitory attacks that cease spontaneously. If hiccups persist, they may produce considerable distress and serious effects such as vomiting, exhaustion, and wound dehiscence. The physician may prescribe phenothiazine medications (e.g., chlorpromazine [Thorazine]) for intractable hiccups.

NURSING ALERT

Any condition that is persistent or considered intractable, such as hiccups, should be reported to the primary provider so that appropriate measures can be implemented.

Once nausea and vomiting have subsided and the patient is fully awake and alert, the sooner he or she can tolerate a usual diet, the more quickly normal GI function will resume. Taking food by mouth stimulates digestive juices and promotes gastric function and intestinal peristalsis. The return to normal dietary intake should proceed at a pace set by the patient. The nature of the surgery and the type of anesthesia directly affect the rate at which normal gastric activity resumes. Liquids are typically the first substances desired and tolerated by the patient after surgery. Water, juice, and tea may be given in increasing amounts. Cool fluids are tolerated more easily than those that are ice cold or hot. Soft foods (gelatin, custard, milk, and creamed soups) are added gradually after clear fluids have been tolerated. As soon as the patient tolerates soft foods well, solid food may be given.

Assessment and management of GI function are important after surgery because the GI tract is subject to uncomfortable or potentially life-threatening complications. Any postoperative patient may suffer from abdominal distention from the accumulation of gas in the intestinal tract. Manipulation of the abdominal organs during surgery may produce a loss of normal peristalsis for 24 to 48 hours, depending on the type and extent of surgery. Even though nothing is given by mouth, swallowed air and GI tract secretions enter the stomach and intestines; if not propelled by peristalsis, they collect in the intestines, producing distention and causing the patient to complain of fullness or pain in the abdomen. Most often, the gas collects in the colon. Abdominal distention is further increased by immobility, anesthetic agents, and the use of opioid medications.

After major abdominal surgery, distention may be avoided by having the patient turn frequently, exercise, and ambulate as early as possible. This also alleviates distention produced by swallowing air, which is common in anxious patients. A nasogastric tube inserted before surgery may remain in place until full peristaltic activity (indicated by the passage of flatus) has resumed. The nurse detects bowel sounds by listening to the abdomen with a stethoscope. Bowel sounds are documented so that diet progression can occur.

Paralytic ileus and intestinal obstruction are potential postoperative complications that occur more frequently in patients undergoing intestinal or abdominal surgery. Refer to Chapter 38 for discussion of treatment.

Promoting Bowel Function

Constipation is common after surgery and can be minor or a serious complication. Decreased mobility, decreased oral intake, and opioid analgesics contribute to difficulty having a bowel movement. In addition, irritation and trauma to the bowel during surgery may inhibit intestinal movement for several days. The combined effect of early ambulation, improved dietary intake, and a stool softener (if prescribed) promotes bowel elimination. Until the patient reports return of bowel function, the nurse should assess the abdomen for distention and the presence and frequency of bowel sounds. If the abdomen is not distended and bowel sounds are present, and if the patient does not have a bowel movement by the second or third postoperative day, the physician should be notified so that a laxative can be administered.

Managing Voiding

Urinary retention after surgery can occur for various reasons. Anesthetics, anticholinergic agents, and opioids interfere with the perception of bladder fullness and the urge to void and inhibit the ability to initiate voiding and completely empty the bladder. Abdominal, pelvic, and hip surgery may increase the likelihood of retention secondary to pain. In addition, some patients find it difficult to use the bedpan or urinal in the recumbent position.

Bladder distention and the urge to void should be assessed at the time of the patient's arrival on the unit and frequently thereafter. The patient is expected to void within 8 hours after surgery (this includes time spent in the PACU). If the patient has an urge to void and cannot, or if the bladder is distended and no urge is felt or the patient cannot void, catheterization is not delayed solely on the basis of the 8-hour time frame. All methods to encourage the patient to void should be tried (e.g., letting water run, applying heat to the perineum). The bedpan should be warm; a cold bedpan causes discomfort and automatic tightening of muscles (including the urethral sphincter). If the patient cannot void on a bedpan, it may be possible to use a commode rather than resorting to catheterization. Male patients are often assisted to sit up or stand beside the bed to use the urinal, but safeguards should be taken to prevent the patient from falling or fainting due to loss of coordination from medications or orthostatic hypotension. If the patient cannot void in the specified time frame, the patient is catheterized and the catheter is removed after the bladder has emptied. Straight intermittent catheterization is preferred over indwelling catheterization because the risk of infection is increased with an indwelling catheter.

Even if the patient voids, the bladder may not necessarily be empty. The nurse notes the amount of urine voided and palpates the suprapubic area for distention or tenderness. A portable ultrasound device may also be used to assess residual volume. Intermittent catheterization may be prescribed every 4 to 6 hours until the patient can void spontaneously and the postvoid residual is less than 50 mL in the middle-aged adult and less than 50 to 100 mL in the older adult (Weber & Kelley, 2013).

Maintaining a Safe Environment

During the immediate postoperative period, the patient recovering from anesthesia should have all side rails up, and the bed should be in the low position. The nurse assesses the patient's level of consciousness and orientation and determines whether the patient can resume wearing his or her eyeglasses or hearing aid, because impaired vision, inability to hear postoperative instructions, or inability to communicate verbally places the patient at risk for injury. All objects the patient may need should be within reach, especially the call bell. Any immediate postoperative orders concerning special positioning, equipment, or interventions should be implemented as soon as possible. The patient is instructed to ask for assistance with any activity. Although restraints are occasionally necessary for the disoriented patient, they should be avoided if at all possible. Agency policy on the use of restraints must be consulted and followed.

Any surgical procedure has the potential for injury due to disrupted neurovascular integrity resulting from prolonged awkward positioning in the OR, manipulation of tissues, inadvertent severing of nerves or blood vessels, or tight bandages. Any orthopedic surgery or surgery involving the extremities carries a risk of peripheral nerve damage. Vascular surgeries, such as replacement of sections of diseased peripheral arteries or inserting an arteriovenous graft, put the patient at risk for thrombus formation at the surgical site and subsequent ischemia of tissues distal to the thrombus. Assessment includes having the patient move the hand or foot distal to the surgical site through a full range of motion, assessing all surfaces for intact sensation, and assessing peripheral pulses, colour, capillary refill, temperature of skin (Rothrock, 2014).

Providing Emotional Support to the Patient and Family

Although patients and families are undoubtedly relieved that surgery is over, anxiety levels may remain high in the immediate postoperative period. Many factors contribute to this anxiety: pain, being in an unfamiliar environment, inability to control one's circumstances or care for oneself, fear of the long-term effects of surgery, fear of complications, fatigue, spiritual distress, altered role responsibilities, ineffective coping, and altered body image are all potential reactions to the surgical experience. The nurse helps the patient and family work through their anxieties by providing reassurance and information and by listening to and addressing their concerns. The nurse describes hospital routines and what to expect in the time until discharge and explains the purpose of nursing assessments and interventions. Informing patients when they will be able to drink fluids or eat, when they will be getting out of bed, and when tubes and drains will be removed helps them gain a sense of control and participation in recovery and engages them in the plan of care. Acknowledging family members' concerns and accepting and encouraging their participation in the patient's care assist them in feeling that they are helping their loved one. The nurse can modify the environment to enhance rest and relaxation by providing privacy, reducing noise, adjusting lighting, providing enough seating for family members, and encouraging a supportive atmosphere.

Managing Potential Complications

The postoperative patient is at risk for complications as outlined below and listed in Table 21-4.

DEEP VEIN THROMBOSIS. Serious potential complications of surgery include DVT and PE (Cionac, Anastase, Munteanu, et al., 2013; Rothrock, 2014).

Prophylactic treatment is common for patients at risk for DVT and PE. Low–molecular-weight or low-dose heparin and low-dose warfarin are anticoagulants that may be used. External pneumatic compression and antiembolism stockings can be used alone or in combination with low-dose heparin. The stress response that is initiated by surgery inhibits the fibrinolytic system, resulting in blood hypercoagulability. Dehydration, low cardiac output, blood pooling in the extremities, and bed rest add to the risk of thrombosis formation. Although all postoperative patients are at some risk, factors such as a history of thrombosis, malignancy, trauma, obesity, indwelling venous catheters, and hormone (e.g., estrogen) use increase the risk. The first symptom of DVT may be a pain or cramp in the calf. Initial pain and tenderness may be followed by a painful swelling of the entire leg, often accompanied by fever, chills, and diaphoresis.

The benefits of early ambulation and leg exercises in preventing DVT cannot be overemphasized, and these activities are recommended for all patients, regardless of their risk. It is important to avoid the use of blanket rolls, pillow rolls, or any form of elevation that can constrict vessels under the knees.

TABLE 21-4 Selected Postoperative Complications

Body System/Type	Complications
Respiratory	Atelectasis, pneumonia, PE aspiration
Cardiovascular	Shock, thrombophlebitis
Neurologic	Delirium, stroke
Skin/wound	Breakdown, infection, dehiscence, evisceration, delayed healing, hemorrhage, hematoma
Gastrointestinal	Constipation, paralytic ileus, bowel obstruction
Urinary	Acute urine retention, urinary tract infection
Functional	Weakness, fatigue, functional decline
Thromboembolic	DVT, PE

Even prolonged "dangling" (having the patient sit on the edge of the bed with legs hanging over the side) can be dangerous and is not recommended in susceptible patients because pressure under the knees can impede circulation. Adequate hydration is also encouraged; the patient can be offered juices and water throughout the day to avoid dehydration. Refer to Chapter 32 for a complete discussion of DVT and to Chapter 24 for discussion of PE.

HEMATOMA. At times, concealed bleeding occurs beneath the skin at the surgical site. This hemorrhage usually stops spontaneously but results in clot (hematoma) formation within the wound. If the clot is small, it will be absorbed and need not be treated. If the clot is large, the wound usually bulges somewhat, and healing will be delayed unless the clot is removed. After the physician removes some of the sutures, the clot can be evacuated and the wound packed lightly with gauze. Healing occurs usually by granulation, or a secondary closure may be performed.

INFECTION (WOUND SEPSIS). The creation of a surgical wound disrupts the integrity of the skin and its protective function. Exposure of deep body tissues to pathogens in the environment places the patient at risk for infection of the surgical site, and a potentially life-threatening complication such as infection increases hospital length of stay, costs of care, and risk of further complications. It is estimated that 14% to 16% of all health care–associated infections are surgical-site infections and 77% of surgical patients who die do so due to sepsis associated with infections (Canadian Patient Safety Institute, 2018).

Multiple factors, including the type of wound, place the patient at potential risk for infection. Surgical wounds are classified according to the degree of contamination. Table 21-5 defines the classification of surgical wounds and SSI rates per category. Patient-related factors include age, nutritional status, diabetes, smoking, obesity, remote infections, endogenous mucosal microorganisms, altered immune response, length of preoperative stay, and severity of illness (Rothrock, 2014). Factors related to the surgical procedure include the method of preoperative skin preparation, surgical attire of the team, method of sterile draping, duration of surgery, antimicrobial prophylaxis, aseptic technique, factors related to surgical technique, drains or foreign material, OR ventilation, length of procedure, and exogenous microorganisms (Edmiston & Spencer, 2014; Pada & Perl, 2015). Other risk factors for wound sepsis include wound contamination, foreign body, faulty suturing technique, devitalized tissue, hematoma, debilitation, dehydration, malnutrition, anemia, obesity, shock, duration of surgical procedure, and associated disorders (e.g., diabetes) (Gadler, Gardiner, & Martinez, 2014). Efforts to prevent wound infection are directed at reducing risks. (Preoperative and intraoperative risks and interventions are discussed in Chapters 19 and 20.) Postoperative care of the wound centres on assessing the wound, preventing contamination and infection before wound edges have sealed, and enhancing healing.

Wound infection may not be evident until at least postoperative day 5. Most patients are discharged before that time, and more than half of wound infections are diagnosed after discharge, highlighting the importance of patient education regarding wound care (Penprase & Johnson, 2015). Signs and symptoms of wound infection include increased pulse rate and temperature; an elevated white blood cell count; wound swelling, warmth, tenderness, or discharge; and incisional pain. Local signs may be absent if the infection is deep. *Staphylococcus aureus* accounts for many postoperative wound infections. Other infections may result from *Escherichia coli, Proteus vulgaris, Aerobacter aerogenes, Pseudomonas aeruginosa*, and

TABLE 21-5 Wound Classification and Associated Surgical Site Infection Risk

Surgical Category	Determinants of Category	Expected Risk of Postsurgical Infection (%)
Clean	Nontraumatic site Uninfected site No inflammation No break in aseptic technique No entry into respiratory, alimentary, genitourinary, or oropharyngeal tracts	1–3
Clean contaminated	Entry into respiratory, alimentary, genitourinary, or oropharyngeal tracts without unusual contamination Appendectomy Minor break in aseptic technique Mechanical drainage	3–7
Contaminated	Open, newly experienced traumatic wounds Gross spillage from gastrointestinal tract Major break in aseptic technique Entry into genitourinary or biliary tract when urine or bile is infected	7–16
Dirty	Traumatic wound with delayed repair, devitalized tissue, foreign bodies, or fecal contamination Acute inflammation and purulent drainage encountered during procedure	16–29

Adapted from Edmiston, C. E. Jr, & Spencer, M. (2014). Patient care interventions to help reduce the risk of surgical site infections. *AORN Journal, 100*(6), 590–602.

other organisms. Although they are rare, beta-hemolytic streptococcal or clostridial infections can be rapid and deadly and need strict infection control practices to prevent the spread of infection to others. Intensive medical and nursing care is essential if the patient is to survive.

When an infection is diagnosed in a surgical incision, the surgeon may remove one or more sutures or staples and, using aseptic precautions, separate the wound edges with a pair of blunt scissors or a hemostat. Once the incision is opened, a drain is inserted. If the infection is deep, an incision and drainage procedure may be necessary. Antimicrobial therapy and a wound care regimen are also initiated.

WOUND DEHISCENCE AND EVISCERATION. Wound dehiscence (disruption of surgical incision or wound) and **evisceration** (protrusion of wound contents) are serious surgical complications (Fig. 21-6). Dehiscence and evisceration are especially serious when they involve abdominal incisions or wounds. These complications result from sutures giving way, from infection, or, more frequently, from marked distention or strenuous cough. They may also occur because of increasing age, anemia, poor nutritional status, obesity, malignancy, jaundice, diabetes, use of steroids, and gender in patients undergoing abdominal surgery (Shanmugam, Fernandez, Evans, et al., 2015).

When the wound edges separate slowly, the intestines may protrude gradually or not at all, and the earliest sign may be a gush of serosanguineous peritoneal fluid from the wound. When a wound ruptures suddenly, coils of intestine may push out of the abdomen. The patient may report that "something gave way." The evisceration causes pain and may be associated with vomiting.

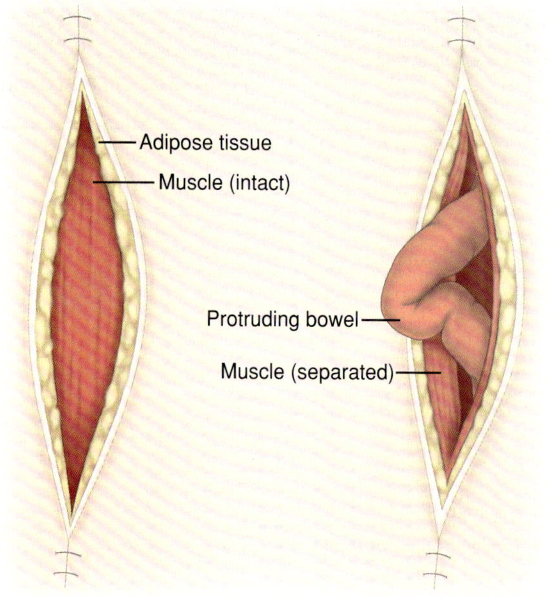

A B

FIGURE 21-6. **A.** Wound dehiscence. **B.** Wound evisceration.

NURSING ALERT

If disruption of a wound occurs, the patient is placed in the low Fowler position and instructed to lie quietly. These actions minimize protrusion of body tissues. The protruding coils of intestine are covered with sterile dressings moistened with sterile saline solution, and the surgeon is notified at once.

An abdominal binder can provide support and guard against dehiscence and often is used along with the primary dressing, especially in patients with weak or pendulous abdominal walls or when rupture of a wound has occurred.

GERONTOLOGIC CONSIDERATIONS. Older adult patients recover more slowly, have longer hospital stays, and are at greater risk for development of postoperative complications. Delirium, pneumonia, decline in functional ability, exacerbation of comorbid conditions, pressure ulcers, decreased oral intake, GI disturbance, and falls are all threats to recovery in the older adult (Ersan, 2013). Expert nursing care can help the older adult avoid these complications or minimize their effects (Phillips, 2016).

Postoperative delirium, characterized by confusion, perceptual and cognitive deficits, altered attention levels, disturbed sleep patterns (Flynn Makic, 2014), and impaired psychomotor skills, is a significant problem for older adults (Meiner, 2014). Causes of delirium are multifactorial (Chart 21-7). Skilled and frequent assessment of mental status and of all physiologic factors influencing mental status helps the nurse plan for care because delirium may be the initial or only indicator of infection, fluid and electrolyte imbalance, or deterioration of respiratory or hemodynamic status in the elderly patient. Factors that determine whether a patient is at risk for delirium include age, history of alcohol abuse, preoperative cognitive function, physical function, serum chemistries, and type of surgery.

Recognizing postoperative delirium and identifying and treating its underlying cause are the goals of care. Postoperative delirium is sometimes mistaken for preexisting dementia or is attributed to age. In addition to monitoring and managing identifiable causes, the nurse implements supportive interventions. Keeping the patient in a well-lit room and close to the nurses' station can reduce sensory deprivation. At the same time, distracting and unfamiliar noises should be minimized. Because pain can contribute to postoperative delirium, adequate pain control without oversedation is essential (Phillips, 2016; Rothrock, 2014).

The patient is reoriented as often as necessary, and staff should introduce themselves each time they come in contact with the patient. Engaging the patient in conversation and care activities and placing a clock and calendar nearby may improve cognitive function. Physical activity should not be neglected while the patient is confused because physical deterioration can worsen delirium and place the patient at increased risk

CHART 21-7

Potential Causes of Postoperative Delirium

- Acid–base disturbances
- Age greater than 80 years
- Fluid and electrolyte imbalance
- Dehydration
- History of dementia-like symptoms
- Hypoxia
- Hypercarbia
- Infection (urinary tract, wound, respiratory)
- Medications (anticholinergics, benzodiazepines, central nervous system depressants)
- Unrelieved pain
- Blood loss
- Decreased cardiac output
- Cerebral hypoxia
- Heart failure
- Acute myocardial infarction
- Hypothermia or hyperthermia
- Unfamiliar surroundings and sensory deprivation
- Emergent surgery
- Alcohol withdrawal
- Urinary retention
- Fecal impaction
- Polypharmacy
- Presence of multiple diseases
- Sensory impairments
- High stress or anxiety levels

for other complications. Physical restraints are to be a last resort. If possible, a family member or staff member is asked to stay with the patient instead. Haloperidol or lorazepam may be administered during episodes of acute confusion, but these medications should be discontinued as soon as possible to avoid side effects.

Other problems confronting the older adult postoperative patient, such as pneumonia, altered bowel function, DVT, weakness, and functional decline, can often be prevented by early and progressive ambulation. Prolonged sitting positions are avoided as they promote venous stasis in the lower extremities. A physical therapy referral may be indicated to promote safe, regular exercise for the older adult.

Urinary incontinence can be prevented by providing easy access to the call bell and the commode and by prompting regular voiding. Early ambulation and familiarity with the room help the patient to become self-sufficient sooner.

Optimal nutritional status is important for wound healing, return of normal bowel function, and fluid and electrolyte balance. The nurse and patient can consult with the dietitian to plan appealing, high-protein meals that provide sufficient fibre, calories, and vitamins. Nutritional supplements, such as Ensure or Boost, may be recommended. Multivitamins, iron, and vitamin C supplements are commonly recommended to aid in tissue healing, formation of new red blood cells, and overall nutritional status.

In addition to monitoring and managing physiologic recovery of the older adult, the nurse identifies and addresses psychosocial needs. The older adult may require much encouragement and support to resume activities, and the pace may be slow. Sensory deficits may require frequent repetition of instructions, and decreased physiologic reserve may necessitate frequent rest periods. The older adult may require extensive discharge planning to coordinate both professional and family care providers, and the nurse, social worker, or nurse case manager may institute the plan for continuing care.

Promoting Home, Community-Based, and Transitional Care

PATIENT SELF-CARE. Patients have always required detailed discharge instructions to become proficient in special self-care needs after surgery; however, shorter hospital stays have increased the amount of information needed while reducing the amount of time in which to provide it. Although needs are specific to individual patients and the procedures they have undergone, general patient education needs for postoperative care have been identified (see Chart 21-3).

CONTINUING AND TRANSITIONAL CARE. Community-based services are frequently necessary after surgery. Older patients, patients who live alone, patients without family support, and patients with pre-existing chronic illness or disabilities are often in greatest need. Planning for discharge involves arranging for necessary services early in the acute care hospitalization for wound care, drain management, catheter care, infusion therapy, and physical or occupational therapy. The home care nurse coordinates these activities and services.

During home care visits, the nurse assesses the patient for postoperative complications by assessment of the surgical incision, respiratory and cardiovascular status, adequacy of pain management, fluid and nutritional status, and the patient's progress in returning to preoperative status. The nurse evaluates the patient's and family's ability to manage dressing changes and drainage systems and other devices and to administer prescribed medications. The nurse may change dressings or catheters if needed. The nurse identifies any additional services that are needed and assists the patient and family to access them. Previous teaching is reinforced, and the patient is reminded to keep follow-up appointments. The patient and family are instructed about signs and symptoms to be reported to the surgeon. In addition, the nurse provides information about how to obtain needed supplies and suggests resources or support groups.

Evaluation

Expected Patient Outcomes

Expected patient outcomes may include the following:

1. Maintains optimal respiratory function
   a. Performs deep-breathing exercises
   b. Displays clear breath sounds
   c. Uses incentive spirometer as prescribed

   d. Splints incisional site when coughing to reduce pain
2. Indicates that pain is decreased in intensity
3. Increases activity as prescribed
   a. Alternates periods of rest and activity
   b. Progressively increases ambulation
   c. Resumes normal activities within prescribed time frame
   d. Performs activities related to self-care
4. Wound heals without complication
5. Maintains body temperature within normal limits
6. Resumes oral intake
   a. Reports absence of nausea and vomiting
   b. Eats at least 75% of usual diet
   c. Is free of abdominal distress and gas pains
   d. Exhibits normal bowel sounds
7. Reports resumption of usual bowel elimination pattern
8. Resumes usual voiding pattern
9. Is free of injury
10. Exhibits decreased anxiety
11. Acquires knowledge and skills necessary to manage therapeutic regimen
12. Experiences no complications

Critical Thinking Exercises

1 A frail 86-year-old woman is admitted to PACU following a hemiarthroplasty of her right hip. She has a history of osteoporosis. She is complaining of pain and difficulty taking a deep breath. How would you prioritize her needs, and what complications would you anticipate? Develop an evidence-based plan of care for her, addressing priorities from admission to the unit until discharge. What resources would you use to identify the current safe practice guidelines? Identify the criteria used to evaluate the strength of the evidence for these practices.

2 A 36-year-old woman who is obese and has had abdominal surgery is admitted to the phase II PACU. Identify what information is essential to obtain during report from the OR, describe the Aldrete scoring system, and explain how you will know when the patient is ready to be discharged from the PACU.

3 A 45-year-old patient who is a smoker is admitted to the postoperative nursing unit after abdominal surgery and is complaining of severe pain. Develop an evidence-based plan of care for this patient, addressing pain relief from admission to the unit until discharge to home. What resources would you use to identify the current pain relief practices? Identify the criteria used to evaluate the strength of the evidence for these practices.

REFERENCES AND SELECTED READINGS

Books

Barash, P. G., Cullen, B. F., & Stoelting, R. K. (2013). *Clinical anesthesia* (7th ed.). Philadelphia, PA: Lippincott Williams & Wilkins.

Comerford, K. C. (2015). *Nursing 2015 drug handbook*. Philadelphia, PA: Wolters Kluwer.

Grossman, S. C., & Porth, C. M. (2014). *Pathophysiology: Concepts of altered health states* (9th ed.). Philadelphia, PA: Lippincott Williams & Wilkins.

Karch, A. M. (2016). *Lippincott's nursing drug guide*. Philadelphia, PA: Lippincott Williams & Wilkins.

Lippincott, Williams, & Wilkins. (2013). *Nursing2013 Drug Handbook*. Philadelphia, PA: Author.

Meiner, S. E. (2014). *Gerontologic nursing* (5th ed.). St. Louis, MO: Elsevier Mosby.

Phillips, N. (2016). *Berry and Kohn's operating room technique* (13th ed.). St. Louis, MO: Mosby.

Rothrock, J. C. (Ed.). (2014). *Alexander's care of the patient in surgery* (15th ed.). St. Louis, MO: Mosby.

Weber, J., & Kelley, J. H. (2013). *Health assessment in nursing* (5th ed.). Philadelphia, PA: Lippincott Williams & Wilkins.

Journals and Electronic Documents

Aldrete, A., & Wright, A. (1992). Revised Aldrete score for discharge. *Anesthesiology News*, *18*(1), 17.

Anderson, J. G., Suchicital, L., Lang, M., et al. (2015). The effects of healing touch on pain, nausea, and anxiety following bariatric surgery: A pilot study. Explore: *The Journal of Science and Healing*, *11*(3), 208–216.

Apfel, C. C., Philip, B. K., Cakmakkaya, O. S., et al. (2012). Who is at risk for postdischarge nausea and vomiting after ambulatory surgery? *Anesthesiology*, *117*(3), 475–86. doi: 10.1097/ALN.0b013e318267ef31

Canadian Patient Safety Institute. (2018). Surgical site infection (SSI). Retrieved from http://www.patientsafetyinstitute.ca/en/Topic/Pages/Surgical-Site-Infection-(SSI).aspx

Chou, R., Gordon, D. B., de Leon-Casasola, O. A., et al. (2016). Management of postoperative pain: A clinical practice guideline from the American pain society, the American society of regional anesthesia and pain medicine, and the American society of anesthesiologists' committee on regional anesthesia, executive committee, and administrative council. *The Journal of Pain*, *17*(2), 131–157. doi: 10.1016/j.jpain.2015.12.008

Cionac Florescu, S., Anastase, D., Munteanu, A., et al. (2013). Venous thromboembolism following major orthopedic surgery. *Maedica: A Journal of Clinical Medicine*, *8*(2), 189–194.

Edmiston, C. E. Jr, & Spencer, M. (2014). Patient care interventions to help reduce the risk of surgical site infections. *AORN Journal*, *100*(6), 590–602.

Ersan, T. (2013). Perioperative management of the geriatric patient, medscape. Retrieved from http://emedicine.medscape.com/article/285433-overview.

Flynn Makic, M. B. (2014). Enhancing sleep in critically ill perianesthesia patients. *Journal of PeriAnesthesia Nursing*, *29*(2), 140–142.

Gadler, T., Gardiner, A., & Martinez, N. (2014). Caring for the postoperative patient with complications presenting to the emergency department. *Advanced Emergency Nursing Journal*, *36*(2), 134–144.

Gallagher, K., & Vacchiano, C. (2014). Reexamining traditional intraoperative fluid administration: Evolving views in the age of goal-directed therapy. *AANA Journal*, *82*(3), 235–242.

Gan, T., Diemunsch, P., Habib, A. S., et al. (2014). Consensus guidelines for the management of postoperative nausea and vomiting. *Anesthesia and Analgesia*, *118*(1), 85–113. doi: 10.1213/ANE.0000000000000002

Guided imagery: Retrieved from https://www.sciencedirect.com/science/article/pii/S1524904217303442

Hayes, K., & Gordon, D. B. (2015). Delivering quality pain management: The challenge for nurses. *AORN Journal*, *101*(3), 328–334; quiz 335–337.

Helvig, A. W., Minick, P., & Patrick, D. (2014). Postoperative management of patients with obstructive sleep apnea: Implications for the medical-surgical nurse. *Medsurg Nursing*, *2*(3), 171–177.

Hodge, N. S., McCarthy, M. S., & Peirce, R. M. (2014). A prospective randomized study of the effectiveness of aromatherapy for relief of postoperative nausea and vomiting. *Journal of PeriAnesthesia Nursing*, *29*(1), 5–11.

Kiefer, D. (2015). Music for postoperative pain. *Integrative Medicine Alert*, *18*(9) [online].

Liddle, C. (2013). How to reduce the risk of deterioration after surgery. *Nursing Times*, *109*(23), 16–17.

Luo, J., & Min, S. (2017). Postoperative pain management in the post-anesthesia care unit: An update. *Journal of Pain Research*, *10*, 2687–2698. doi: 10.2147/JPR.S142889

McGuire, L., & Bolyanatz, P. (2014). Dispelling pain myths. *American Nurse Today*, *9*(7), 8–10.

Miskovic, A., & Lumb, A. B. (2017). Postoperative pulmonary complications. *British Journal of Anesthesia*, *118*(3), 317–334. doi: 10.1093/bja/aex002

Noble, K. A., & Pasero, C. (2014). Opioid-induced ventilatory impairment (OIVI). *Journal of PeriAnesthesia Nursing*, *29*(2), 143–151.

Oster, K. A., & Oster, C. A. (2015). Special needs population: Care of the geriatric patient population in the perioperative setting. *AORN Journal*, *101*(6), 444–456.

Pada, S., & Perl, T. M. (2015). Operating room myths: What is the evidence for common practices? *Current Opinion in Infectious Diseases*, *28*(4), 369–374.

Penprase, B., & Johnson, C. (2015). Optimizing the perioperative nursing role for the older adult surgical patient. *OR Nurse*, *8*(4), 26–33.

Rodriguez, L. (2015). Pathophysiology of pain: Implications for perioperative nursing. *AORN Journal*, *101*(3), 338–344.

Rosen, H. I., Bergh, I. H. E., Schwartz-Barcott, D., et al. (2014). The recovery process after day surgery within the symptom management theory. *Nursing Forum*, *49*(2), 100–110.

Schiffner, R., Bischoff, S. J., Lehmann, T., et al. (2017). Redistribution of cerebral blood flow during severe hypovolemia and reperfusion in a sheep model: Critical role of α1-adrenergic signaling. *International Journal of Molecular Sciences*, *18*(5), 1031. doi: 10.3390/ijms18051031

Sessler, D. (2016). Perioperative thermoregulation and heat balance. *Lancet*, *387*(10038), 2655–2664. doi: 1016/S0140-6736(15)00981-2

Shanmugam, V. K., Fernandez, S., Evans, K. K., et al. (2015). Postoperative wound dehiscence: Predictors and associations. *Wound Repair and Regeneration*, *23*(2), 184–190. doi: 10.1111/wrr.12268

Sites, D. S., Johnson, N. T., Miller, J. A., et al. (2014). Controlled breathing with or without peppermint aromatherapy for postoperative nausea and/or vomiting symptom relief: A randomized controlled trial. *Journal of PeriAnesthesia Nursing*, *29*(1), 12–19.

Tinsley, M. H., & Barone, C. P. (2013). Preventing postoperative nausea and vomiting. *Nursing*, *43*(12), 42–50.

Vijayakumar, B., Elango, P., & Ganessan, R. (2014). Postoperative delirium in elderly patients. *Indian Journal of Anesthesia*, *58*(3), 251–256. doi: 10.4103/0019-5049.135026

Ward, C. W. (2014). Procedure-specific postoperative pain management. *MedSurg Nursing*, *23*(2), 107–110.

Resources

Canadian Anesthesiologists' Society: http://www.cas.ca.
Canadian Pain Society: canadianpainsociety.ca
College of Physicians and Surgeons of BC. (2017). https://www.cpsbc.ca/files/pdf/NHMSFAP-AS-Post-Anesthesia-Care.pdf
Operating Room Nurses of Canada (ORNAC): https://www.ornac.ca/en/standards

UNIT 5

Gas Exchange and Respiratory Function

Case Study

A PATIENT WITH IMPAIRED COUGH REFLEX

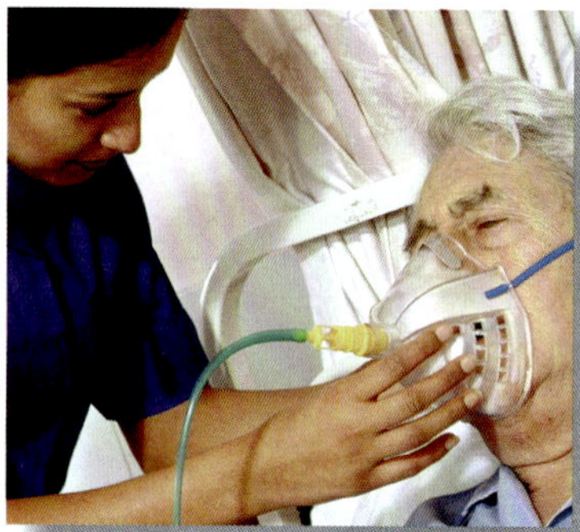

A 57-year-old man with a history of COPD is readmitted for the third time to the hospital within the last year. His vital signs are: Temp 38.11°C; HR 90 and regular; B/P: 142/74; Resp 28. He has a weak cough, diminished breath sounds over the lower left lung field, and a wheeze over the midtracheal area. He can expectorate some sputum, which is thick and greyish-green. He has a history of stroke. Secondary to the stroke, he has impaired gag and cough reflexes and mild weakness of the left side. He is allowed food and fluids because he can swallow safely if he uses the chin-tuck manoeuvre. The nurse manager observes that recently the unit has had an increase in 30-day hospital readmissions of patients with exacerbations of COPD. The manager then asks the nurse to chair a task force to examine how to decrease the rate of 30-day hospital readmissions among patients with COPD.

QSEN Competency Focus: Quality Improvement

The complexities inherent in today's health care system challenge nurses to demonstrate integration of specific interdisciplinary core competencies that are aimed at ensuring the delivery of safe and quality patient care (Institute of Medicine, 2003). The Quality and Safety Education for Nurses project (QSEN, 2017; Cronenwett, Sherwood, Barnsteiner, et al., 2007) provides a framework for the knowledge, skills, and attitudes (KSAs) required for nurses to demonstrate competency in these key areas, which include ***patient-centred care***, ***interdisciplinary teamwork and collaboration***, ***evidence-based practice***, ***quality improvement***, ***safety***, and ***informatics.***

Quality Improvement Definition: Use data to monitor the outcomes of care processes and use improvement methods to design and test changes to continuously improve the quality and safety of health care systems.

SELECTED PRE-LICENSURE KSAs	APPLICATION AND REFLECTION
Knowledge	
Describe strategies for learning about the outcomes of care in the setting in which one is engaged in clinical practice.	Identify why patients with COPD may be at risk for hospital readmissions. Describe how you, as the task force chairperson, could verify whether 30-day hospital readmissions have increased. What data would provide benchmarks for 30-day hospital readmissions?
Skills	
Seek information about outcomes of care for populations served in care setting.	As you analyze the data, you find that there appears to be a higher rate of 30-day hospital readmissions of patients with COPD discharged from the hospital to home compared to those discharged to nursing homes. Describe how you can use this information to develop interventions to decrease 30-day hospital readmissions among patients with COPD.
Attitudes	
Appreciate that continuous quality improvement is an essential part of the daily work of all health professionals.	Reflect on your role in decreasing the rates of 30-day readmission of patients with COPD. How do you feel this will impact your unit, the hospital, local long-term care facilities, home care services, and the quality of life for the patients you provide care for?

Cronenwett, L., Sherwood, G., Barnsteiner, J., et al. (2007). Quality and safety education for nurses. *Nursing Outlook*, *55*(3), 122–131; Institute of Medicine. (2003). *Health professions education: A bridge to quality*. Washington, DC: National Academies Press; and QSEN Institute. (2017). *QSEN competencies: Definitions and pre-licensure KSAs*. Retrieved June 12, 2019, from www.qsen.org/competencies/pre-licensure-ksas

22 Assessment of Respiratory Function

Adapted by Tanya Heuver

Learning Objectives

On completion of this chapter, the learner will be able to:

1. Describe the structures and functions of the upper and lower respiratory tracts.
2. Describe ventilation, diffusion, perfusion, and ventilation–perfusion imbalances.
3. Explain proper techniques utilized to perform a comprehensive respiratory assessment.
4. Discriminate between normal and abnormal assessment findings by inspection, palpation, percussion, and auscultation of the respiratory system.
5. Recognize and evaluate the major symptoms of respiratory dysfunction by applying information from the patient's health history and physical assessment findings.
6. Identify the diagnostic tests used to evaluate respiratory function and related nursing implications.

Disorders of the respiratory system are common and are encountered by nurses in every setting from the community to the intensive care unit. Expert assessment skills must be developed and used to provide the best care for patients with acute and chronic respiratory problems. Alterations in respiratory status have been identified as important predictors of clinical deterioration in hospitalized patients (Helling, Martin, Martin, et al., 2014). In order to differentiate between normal and abnormal assessment findings, an understanding of respiratory function and the significance of abnormal diagnostic test results is essential.

Anatomic and Physiologic Overview

The respiratory system is composed of the upper and lower respiratory tracts. Together, the two tracts are responsible for **ventilation** (movement of air in and out of the airways). The upper respiratory tract, known as the upper airway, warms and filters inspired air so that the lower respiratory tract (the lungs) can accomplish gas exchange. Gas exchange involves delivering oxygen to the tissues through the bloodstream and expelling waste gases, such as carbon dioxide, during expiration. The respiratory system depends on the cardiovascular system for perfusion, or blood flow through the pulmonary system (Porth, 2015).

Anatomy of the Respiratory System

Upper Respiratory Tract

Upper airway structures consist of the nose, sinuses and nasal passages, pharynx, tonsils and adenoids, larynx, and trachea.

Nose

The nose serves as a passageway for air to pass to and from the lungs. It filters impurities and humidifies and warms the air as it is inhaled. The nose is composed of an external and an internal portion. The external portion protrudes from the face and is supported by the nasal bones and cartilage. The anterior nares (nostrils) are the external openings of the nasal cavities.

The internal portion of the nose is a hollow cavity separated into the right and left nasal cavities by a narrow vertical divider, the septum. Each nasal cavity is divided into three passageways by the projection of the turbinates from the lateral walls. The turbinate bones are also called conchae (the name suggested by their shell-like appearance). Because of their curves, these bones increase the mucus membrane surface of the nasal passages and slightly obstruct the air flowing through them (Fig. 22-1).

Air entering the nostrils is deflected upward to the roof of the nose, and it follows a circuitous route before it reaches the nasopharynx. It comes into contact with a large surface of moist, warm, highly vascular, ciliated mucus membrane (called nasal mucosa) that traps practically all the dust and organisms in the inhaled air. The air is moistened, warmed to body temperature, and brought into contact with sensitive nerves. Some of these nerves detect odours; others provoke sneezing to expel irritating dust. Mucus, secreted continuously by goblet cells, covers the surface of the nasal mucosa and is moved back to the nasopharynx by the action of the **cilia** (fine hairs).

Paranasal Sinuses

The paranasal sinuses include four pairs of bony cavities that are lined with nasal mucosa and ciliated pseudostratified columnar epithelium. These airspaces are connected by a series of ducts that drain into the nasal cavity. The sinuses are named by their location: frontal, ethmoidal, sphenoidal, and maxillary (Fig. 22-2). A prominent function of the sinuses is to serve as a resonating chamber in speech. The sinuses are a common site of infection.

Pharynx, Tonsils, and Adenoids

The pharynx, or throat, is a tube-like structure that connects the nasal and oral cavities to the larynx. It is divided

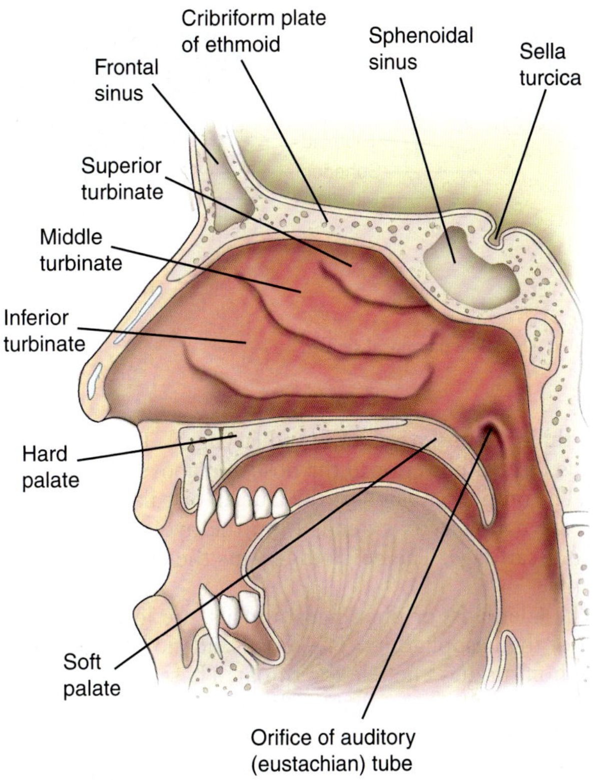

FIGURE 22-1. Cross-section of nasal cavity.

Glossary

apnea: temporary cessation of breathing

bronchophony: abnormal increase in clarity of transmitted voice sounds

bronchoscopy: direct examination of larynx, trachea, and bronchi using an endoscope

cilia: short hairs that provide a constant whipping motion that serves to propel mucus and foreign substances away from the lung toward the larynx

compliance: measure of the force required to expand or inflate the lungs

crackles: soft, high-pitched, discontinuous popping sounds during inspiration caused by delayed reopening of the airways

dyspnea: subjective experience that describes difficulty breathing; shortness of breath

egophony: abnormal change in tone of voice that is heard when auscultating lungs

fremitus: vibrations of speech felt as tremors of chest wall during palpation

hemoptysis: expectoration of blood from the respiratory tract

hypoxemia: decrease in arterial oxygen tension in the blood

hypoxia: decrease in oxygen supply to the tissues and cells

obstructive sleep apnea: temporary absence of breathing during sleep secondary to transient upper airway obstruction

orthopnea: inability to breathe easily except in an upright position

oxygen saturation: percentage of hemoglobin that is bound to oxygen

physiologic dead space: portion of the tracheobronchial tree that does not participate in gas exchange

pulmonary diffusion: exchange of gas molecules (oxygen and carbon dioxide) from areas of high concentration to areas of low concentration

pulmonary perfusion: blood flow through the pulmonary vasculature

respiration: gas exchange between atmospheric air and the blood and between the blood and cells of the body

rhonchi: low-pitched wheezing or snoring sound associated with partial airway obstruction, heard on chest auscultation

stridor: harsh high-pitched sound heard on inspiration, usually without need of stethoscope, secondary to upper airway obstruction

tachypnea: abnormally rapid respirations

tidal volume: volume of air inspired and expired with each breath during normal breathing

ventilation: movement of air in and out of airways

wheezes: continuous musical sounds associated with airway narrowing or partial obstruction

whispered pectoriloquy: whispered sounds heard loudly and clearly upon thoracic auscultation

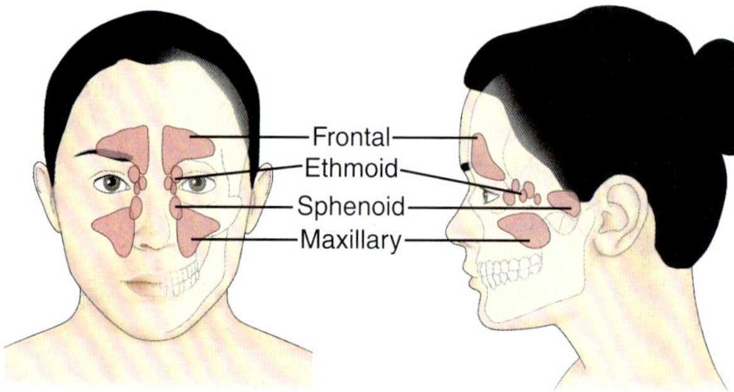

FIGURE 22-2. The paranasal sinuses.

into three regions: nasal, oral, and laryngeal. The nasopharynx is located posterior to the nose and above the soft palate. The oropharynx houses the faucial, or palatine, tonsils. The laryngopharynx extends from the hyoid bone to the cricoid cartilage. The epiglottis forms the entrance to the larynx.

The adenoids, or pharyngeal tonsils, are located in the roof of the nasopharynx. The tonsils, adenoids, and other lymphoid tissues encircle the throat. These structures are important links in the chain of lymph nodes guarding the body from invasion by organisms entering the nose and the throat. The pharynx functions as a passageway for the respiratory and digestive tracts.

Larynx

The larynx, or voice organ, is a cartilaginous epithelium–lined structure that connects the pharynx and the trachea. The major function of the larynx is vocalization. It also protects the lower airway from foreign substances and facilitates coughing. It is frequently referred to as the voice box and consists of the following:

- Epiglottis: A valve flap of cartilage that covers the opening to the larynx during swallowing
- Glottis: The opening between the vocal cords in the larynx
- Thyroid cartilage: The largest of the cartilage structures; part of it forms the Adam's apple
- Cricoid cartilage: The only complete cartilaginous ring in the larynx (located below the thyroid cartilage)
- Arytenoid cartilages: Used in vocal cord movement with the thyroid cartilage
- Vocal cords: Ligaments controlled by muscular movements that produce sounds; located in the lumen of the larynx

Trachea

The trachea, or windpipe, is composed of smooth muscle with C-shaped rings of cartilage at regular intervals. The cartilaginous rings are incomplete on the posterior surface and give firmness to the wall of the trachea, preventing it from collapsing. The trachea serves as the passage between the larynx and the bronchi.

Lower Respiratory Tract

The lower respiratory tract consists of the lungs, which contain the bronchial and alveolar structures needed for gas exchange.

Lungs

The lungs are paired elastic structures enclosed in the thoracic cage, which is an airtight chamber with distensible walls (Fig. 22-3). Ventilation requires movement of the walls of the thoracic cage and of its floor, the diaphragm. The effect of these movements is alternately to increase and decrease the capacity of the chest. When the capacity of the chest is increased, air enters through the trachea (inspiration) because of the lowered pressure within and inflates the lungs. When the chest wall and diaphragm return to their previous positions (expiration), the lungs recoil and force the air out through the bronchi and trachea. Inspiration occurs during the first third of the respiratory cycle, expiration during the later two thirds. The inspiratory phase of **respiration** normally requires energy; the expiratory phase is normally passive, requiring very little energy. In respiratory diseases, such as chronic obstructive pulmonary disease (COPD), expiration requires energy.

PLEURA. The lungs and wall of the thorax are lined with a serous membrane called the pleura. The visceral pleura covers the lungs; the parietal pleura lines the thorax. The visceral and parietal pleura and the small amount of pleural fluid between these two membranes serve to lubricate the thorax and lungs and permit smooth motion of the lungs within the thoracic cavity with each breath.

MEDIASTINUM. The mediastinum is in the middle of the thorax, between the pleural sacs that contain the two lungs. It extends from the sternum to the vertebral column and contains all the thoracic tissue outside the lungs (heart, thymus, certain large blood vessels [i.e., aorta, vena cava], and esophagus).

LOBES. Each lung is divided into lobes. The right lung has upper, middle, and lower lobes, whereas the left lung consists of upper and lower lobes (Fig. 22-4). Each lobe is further subdivided into two to five segments separated by fissures, which are extensions of the pleura.

BRONCHI AND BRONCHIOLES. There are several divisions of the bronchi within each lobe of the lung. First are the lobar bronchi (three in the right lung and two in the left lung). Lobar bronchi divide into segmental bronchi (10 on the right and 8 on the left), which are the structures identified when choosing the most effective postural drainage position for a given patient. Segmental bronchi then divide into subsegmental bronchi. These bronchi are surrounded by connective tissue that contains arteries, lymphatics, and nerves.

The subsegmental bronchi then branch into bronchioles, which have no cartilage in their walls. Their patency depends entirely on the elastic recoil of the surrounding smooth muscle and on the alveolar pressure. The bronchioles contain submucosal glands, which produce mucus that covers the inside lining of the airways. The bronchi and bronchioles are also lined with cells that have surfaces covered with cilia. These cilia create a constant whipping motion that propels mucus and foreign substances away from the lungs toward the larynx.

The bronchioles then branch into terminal bronchioles, which do not have mucus glands or cilia. Terminal bronchioles then become respiratory bronchioles, which are considered to be the transitional passageways between the conducting airways and the gas exchange airways. Up to

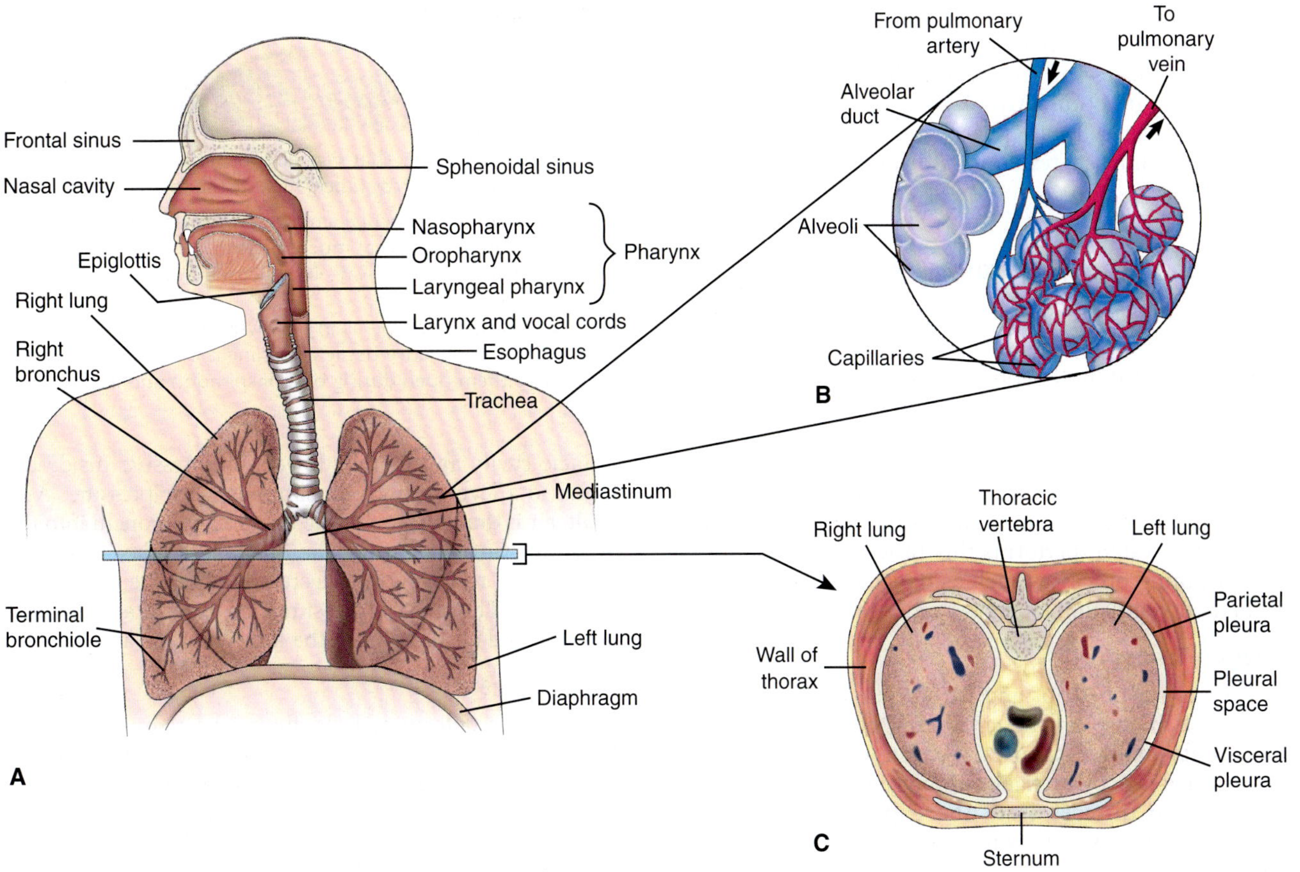

FIGURE 22-3. The respiratory system. **A:** Upper respiratory structures and the structures of the thorax. **B:** Alveoli. **C:** A horizontal cross-section of the lungs.

this point, the conducting airways contain about 150 mL of air in the tracheobronchial tree that does not participate in gas exchange; this is known as **physiologic dead space**. The respiratory bronchioles then lead into alveolar ducts and alveolar sacs and then alveoli. Oxygen and carbon dioxide exchange takes place in the alveoli.

ALVEOLI. The lung is made up of about 300 million alveoli, constituting a total surface area between 50 and 100 m^2 (Porth, 2015). There are three types of alveolar cells. Type I and type II cells make up the alveolar epithelium. Type I cells account for 95% of the alveolar surface area and serve as a barrier between the air and the alveolar

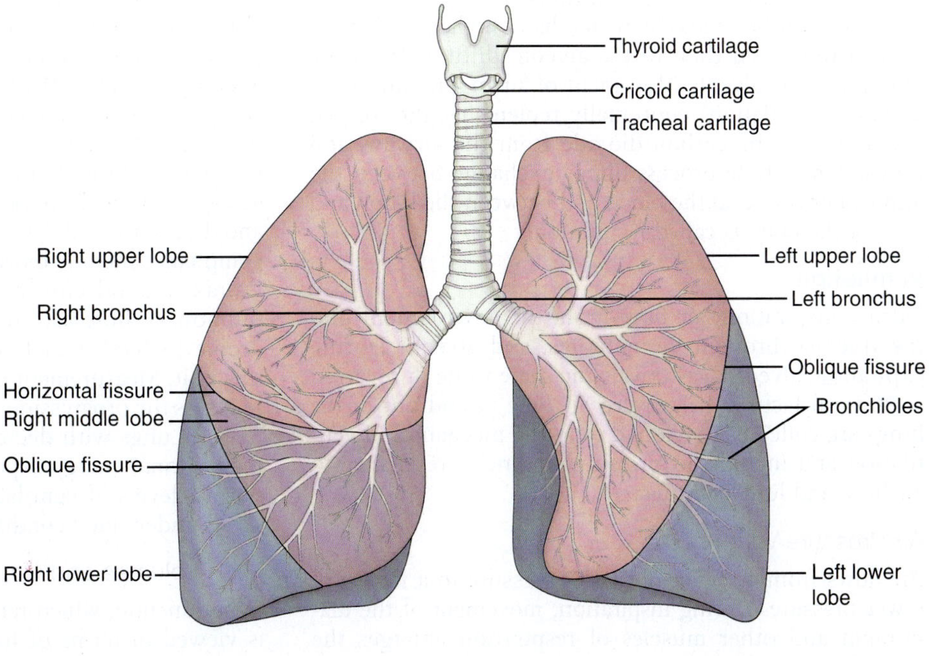

FIGURE 22-4. Anterior view of the lungs. The lungs consist of five lobes. The right lung has three lobes (upper, middle, lower); the left has two (upper and lower). The lobes are further subdivided by fissures. The bronchial tree, another lung structure, inflates with air to fill the lobes.

surface; type II cells account for only 5% of this area but are responsible for producing type I cells and surfactant. Surfactant reduces surface tension, thereby improving the overall lung function. Alveolar macrophages, the third type of alveolar cells, are phagocytic cells that ingest foreign matter and, as a result, provide an important defense mechanism.

Function of the Respiratory System

The cells of the body derive the energy they need from the oxidation of carbohydrates, fats, and proteins. As with any type of combustion, this process requires oxygen. Certain vital tissues, such as those of the brain and the heart, cannot survive for long without a continuous supply of oxygen. However, as a result of oxidation in the body tissues, carbon dioxide is produced and must be removed from the cells to prevent the buildup of acid waste products. The respiratory system performs this function by facilitating life-sustaining processes such as oxygen transport, respiration and ventilation, and gas exchange.

Oxygen Transport

Oxygen is supplied to, and carbon dioxide is removed from, cells by way of the circulating blood. Cells are in close contact with capillaries, the thin walls of which permit easy passage or exchange of oxygen and carbon dioxide. Oxygen diffuses from the capillary through the capillary wall to the interstitial fluid. At this point, it diffuses through the membrane of tissue cells, where it is used by mitochondria for cellular respiration. The movement of carbon dioxide occurs by diffusion in the opposite direction—from cell to blood.

Respiration

After these tissue capillary exchanges, blood enters the systemic veins (where it is called venous blood) and travels to the pulmonary circulation. The oxygen concentration in blood within the capillaries of the lungs is lower than in the lungs' air sacs (alveoli). Because of this concentration gradient, oxygen diffuses from the alveoli to the blood. Carbon dioxide, which has a higher concentration in the blood than in the alveoli, diffuses from the blood into the alveoli. Movement of air in and out of the airways (ventilation) continually replenishes the oxygen and removes the carbon dioxide from the airways and lungs. This whole process of gas exchange between the atmospheric air and the blood and between the blood and cells of the body is called respiration.

Ventilation

During inspiration, air flows from the environment into the trachea, bronchi, bronchioles, and alveoli. During expiration, alveolar gas travels the same route in reverse.

Physical factors that govern air flow in and out of the lungs are collectively referred to as the mechanics of ventilation and include air pressure variances, resistance to air flow, and lung **compliance**.

Air Pressure Variances

Air flows from a region of higher pressure to a region of lower pressure. During inspiration, movement of the diaphragm and other muscles of respiration enlarges the thoracic cavity and thereby lowers the pressure inside the thorax to a level below that of atmospheric pressure. As a result, air is drawn through the trachea and bronchi into the alveoli. During expiration, the diaphragm relaxes and the lungs recoil, resulting in a decrease in the size of the thoracic cavity. The alveolar pressure then exceeds atmospheric pressure, and air flows from the lungs into the atmosphere.

> CHART 22-1
>
> **Causes of Increased Airway Resistance**
>
> Common phenomena that may alter bronchial diameter, which affects airway resistance, include the following:
>
> - Contraction of bronchial smooth muscle—as in asthma
> - Thickening of bronchial mucosa—as in chronic bronchitis
> - Obstruction of the airway—by mucus, a tumour, or a foreign body
> - Loss of lung elasticity—as in emphysema, which is characterized by connective tissue encircling the airways, thereby keeping them open during both inspiration and expiration

Airway Resistance

Resistance is determined chiefly by the radius or size of the airway through which the air is flowing. Any process that changes the bronchial diameter or width affects airway resistance and alters the rate of air flow for a given pressure gradient during respiration (Chart 22-1). With increased resistance, greater-than-normal respiratory effort is required to achieve normal levels of ventilation.

Compliance

Compliance, or distensibility, is the elasticity and expandability of the lungs and thoracic structures. Compliance allows the lung volume to increase when the difference in pressure between the atmosphere and thoracic cavity (pressure gradient) causes air to flow in. Factors that determine lung compliance are the surface tension of the alveoli (normally low with the presence of surfactant) and the connective tissue (i.e., collagen and elastin) of the lungs.

Compliance is determined by examining the volume–pressure relationship in the lungs and the thorax. Compliance is normal (1.0 L/cm H_2O) if the lungs and thorax easily stretch and distend when pressure is applied. High or increased compliance occurs if the lungs have lost their elasticity and the thorax is overdistended (e.g., in emphysema). Low or decreased compliance occurs if the lungs and thorax are "stiff." Conditions associated with decreased compliance include morbid obesity, pneumothorax, hemothorax, pleural effusion, pulmonary edema, atelectasis, pulmonary fibrosis, and acute respiratory distress syndrome (ARDS), which are discussed in later chapters in this unit. Measurement of compliance is one method used to assess the progression and improvement in patients with ARDS. Lungs with decreased compliance require greater-than-normal energy expenditure by the patient to achieve normal levels of ventilation. Compliance is usually measured under static conditions.

Lung Volumes and Capacities

Lung function, which reflects the mechanics of ventilation, is viewed in terms of lung volumes and lung capacities.

TABLE 22-1 Lung Volumes and Lung Capacities

Term	Symbol	Description	Normal Value[a]	Significance
Lung Volumes				
Tidal volume	VT or TV	The volume of air inhaled and exhaled with each breath	500 mL or 5–10 mL/kg	The tidal volume may not vary, even with severe disease.
Inspiratory reserve volume	IRV	The maximum volume of air that can be inhaled after a normal inhalation	3,000 mL	
Expiratory reserve volume	ERV	The maximum volume of air that can be exhaled forcibly after a normal exhalation	1,100 mL	Expiratory reserve volume is decreased with restrictive conditions, such as obesity, ascites, pregnancy.
Residual volume	RV	The volume of air remaining in the lungs after a maximum exhalation	1,200 mL	Residual volume may be increased with obstructive disease.
Lung Capacities				
Vital capacity	VC	The maximum volume of air exhaled from the point of maximum inspiration VC = TV + IRV + ERV	4,600 mL	A decrease in vital capacity may be found in neuromuscular disease, generalized fatigue, atelectasis, pulmonary edema, COPD, and obesity.
Inspiratory capacity	IC	The maximum volume of air inhaled after normal expiration IC = TV + IRV	3,500 mL	A decrease in inspiratory capacity may indicate restrictive disease. May also be decreased in obesity.
Functional residual capacity	FRC	The volume of air remaining in the lungs after a normal expiration FRC = ERV + RV	2,300 mL	Functional residual capacity may be increased with COPD and decreased in ARDS and obesity.
Total lung capacity	TLC	The volume of air in the lungs after a maximum inspiration TLC = TV + IRV + ERV + RV	5,800 mL	Total lung capacity may be decreased with restrictive disease (atelectasis, pneumonia) and increased in COPD.

[a]Values for healthy men; women are 20–25% less.

ARDS, acute respiratory distress syndrome; COPD, chronic obstructed pulmonary disease.

Adapted from West, J. B., & Luks, A. M. (2016). *West's respiratory physiology: The essentials* (10th ed.). Philadelphia, PA: Wolters Kluwer Health/Lippincott Williams & Wilkins.

Lung volumes are categorized as **tidal volume**, inspiratory reserve volume, expiratory reserve volume, and residual volume. Lung capacity is evaluated in terms of vital capacity, inspiratory capacity, functional residual capacity (FRC), and total lung capacity. These terms are described in Table 22-1.

Pulmonary Diffusion and Perfusion

Diffusion is the process by which oxygen and carbon dioxide are exchanged at the air–blood interface. The alveolar–capillary membrane is ideal for diffusion because of its thinness and large surface area. In the normal healthy adult, oxygen and carbon dioxide travel across the alveolar–capillary membrane without difficulty as a result of differences in gas concentrations in the alveoli and capillaries.

Pulmonary perfusion is the actual blood flow through the pulmonary circulation. The blood is pumped into the lungs by the right ventricle through the pulmonary artery. The pulmonary artery divides into the right and left branches to supply both lungs. These two branches divide further to supply all parts of each lung. Normally about 2% of the blood pumped by the right ventricle does not perfuse the alveolar capillaries. This shunted blood drains into the left side of the heart without participating in alveolar gas exchange.

The pulmonary circulation is considered a low-pressure system because the systolic blood pressure in the pulmonary artery is 20 to 30 mm Hg and the diastolic pressure is 5 to 15 mm Hg. Because of these low pressures, the pulmonary vasculature normally can vary its capacity to accommodate the blood flow it receives. However, when a person is in an upright position, the pulmonary artery pressure is not great enough to supply blood to the apex of the lung against the force of gravity. Thus, when a person is upright, the lung may be considered to be divided into three sections: an upper part with poor blood supply, a lower part with maximal blood supply, and a section between the two with an intermediate supply of blood. When a person who is lying down turns to one side, more blood passes to the dependent lung.

Perfusion is also influenced by alveolar pressure. The pulmonary capillaries are sandwiched between adjacent alveoli. If the alveolar pressure is sufficiently high, the capillaries are squeezed. Depending on the pressure, some capillaries completely collapse, whereas others narrow.

Pulmonary artery pressure, gravity, and alveolar pressure determine the patterns of perfusion. In lung disease, these factors vary, and the perfusion of the lung may become very abnormal.

Ventilation and Perfusion Balance and Imbalance

Adequate gas exchange depends on an adequate ventilation–perfusion ($\dot{V}/\dot{Q}$) ratio. In different areas of the lung, the ($\dot{V}/\dot{Q}$) ratio varies. Airway blockages, local changes in compliance, and gravity may alter ventilation. Alterations in perfusion may occur with a change in the pulmonary artery pressure, alveolar pressure, or gravity.

($\dot{V}/\dot{Q}$) imbalance occurs as a result of inadequate ventilation, inadequate perfusion, or both. There are four possible

CHART 22-2

Ventilation–Perfusion Ratios

Normal Ratio (A)

In the healthy lung, a given amount of blood passes an alveolus and is matched with an equal amount of gas **(A)**. The ratio is 1:1 (ventilation matches perfusion).

Low Ventilation–Perfusion Ratio: Shunts (B)

Low ventilation–perfusion states may be called shunt-producing disorders. When perfusion exceeds ventilation, a shunt exists **(B)**. Blood bypasses the alveoli without gas exchange occurring. This is seen with obstruction of the distal airways, such as with pneumonia, atelectasis, tumour, or a mucus plug.

High Ventilation–Perfusion Ratio: Dead Space (C)

When ventilation exceeds perfusion, dead space results **(C)**. The alveoli do not have an adequate blood supply for gas exchange to occur. This is characteristic of a variety of disorders, including pulmonary emboli, pulmonary infarction, and cardiogenic shock.

Silent Unit (D)

In the absence of both ventilation and perfusion or with limited ventilation and perfusion, a condition known as a silent unit occurs **(D)**. This is seen with pneumothorax and severe acute respiratory distress syndrome.

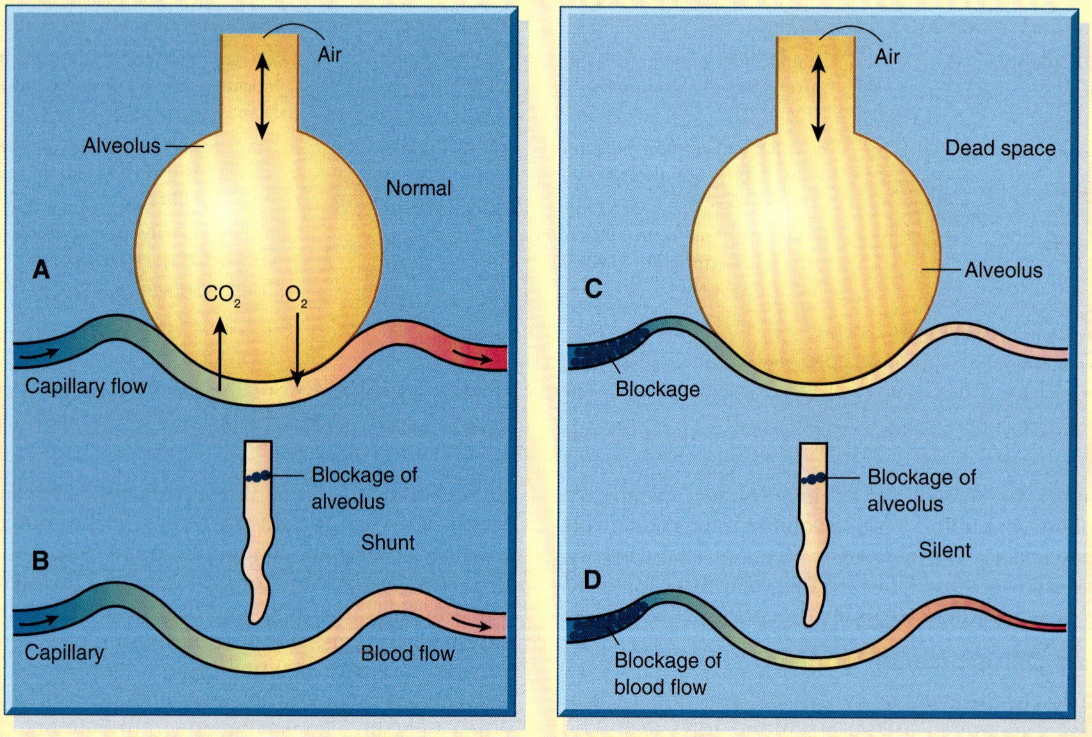

$(\dot{V}/\dot{Q})$ states in the lung: normal $(\dot{V}/\dot{Q})$ ratio, low $(\dot{V}/\dot{Q})$ ratio (shunt), high $(\dot{V}/\dot{Q})$ ratio (dead space), and absence of ventilation and perfusion (silent unit) (see Chart 22-2). $(\dot{V}/\dot{Q})$ imbalance causes shunting of blood, resulting in **hypoxia** (low level of cellular oxygen). Shunting appears to be the main cause of hypoxia after thoracic or abdominal surgery and most types of respiratory failure. Severe hypoxia results when the amount of shunting exceeds 20%. Supplemental oxygen may eliminate hypoxia, depending on the type of $(\dot{V}/\dot{Q})$ imbalance.

Gas Exchange

Partial Pressure of Gases

The air we breathe is a gaseous mixture consisting mainly of nitrogen (78.6%) and oxygen (20.8%), with traces of carbon dioxide (0.04%), water vapor (0.05%), helium, and argon. The atmospheric pressure at sea level is about 760 mm Hg. Partial pressure is the pressure exerted by each type of gas in a mixture of gases. The partial pressure of a gas is proportional to the concentration of that gas in the mixture. The total pressure exerted by the gaseous mixture, whether in the atmosphere or in the lungs, is equal to the sum of the partial pressures.

Based on these facts, the partial pressures of nitrogen and oxygen can be calculated. The partial pressure of nitrogen in the atmosphere at sea level is 78.6% of 760, or 597 mm Hg; that of oxygen is 20.8% of 760, or 158 mm Hg (Grossman & Porth, 2014). Chart 22-3 identifies and defines terms and abbreviations related to partial pressure of gases.

Once the air enters the trachea, it becomes fully saturated with water vapor, which displaces some of the other gases. Water vapor exerts a pressure of 47 mm Hg when it fully saturates a mixture of gases at the body temperature of 37°C (98.6°F). Nitrogen and oxygen are responsible for almost all of the remaining 713 mm Hg pressure. Once this mixture enters the alveoli, it is further diluted by carbon dioxide. In the alveoli, the water vapor continues to exert a pressure of

CHART 22-3

Partial Pressure Abbreviations

P = pressure
PO_2 = partial pressure of oxygen
PCO_2 = partial pressure of carbon dioxide
PAO_2 = partial pressure of alveolar oxygen
$PACO_2$ = partial pressure of alveolar carbon dioxide
PaO_2 = partial pressure of arterial oxygen
$PaCO_2$ = partial pressure of arterial carbon dioxide
PvO_2 = partial pressure of venous oxygen
$PvCO_2$ = partial pressure of venous carbon dioxide
P_{50} = partial pressure of oxygen when the hemoglobin is 50% saturated

47 mm Hg. The remaining 713 mm Hg pressure is now exerted as follows: nitrogen, 569 mm Hg (74.9%); oxygen, 104 mm Hg (13.6%); and carbon dioxide, 40 mm Hg (5.3%).

When a gas is exposed to a liquid, the gas dissolves in the liquid until an equilibrium is reached. The dissolved gas also exerts a partial pressure. At equilibrium, the partial pressure of the gas in the liquid is the same as the partial pressure of the gas in the gaseous mixture. Oxygenation of venous blood in the lung illustrates this point. In the lung, venous blood and alveolar oxygen are separated by a very thin alveolar membrane. Oxygen diffuses across this membrane to dissolve in the blood until the partial pressure of oxygen in the blood is the same as that in the alveoli (104 mm Hg). However, because carbon dioxide is a by-product of oxidation in the cells, venous blood contains carbon dioxide at a higher partial pressure than that in the alveolar gas. In the lung, carbon dioxide diffuses out of venous blood into the alveolar gas. At equilibrium, the partial pressure of carbon dioxide in the blood and in alveolar gas is the same (40 mm Hg). The changes in partial pressure are shown in Figure 22-5.

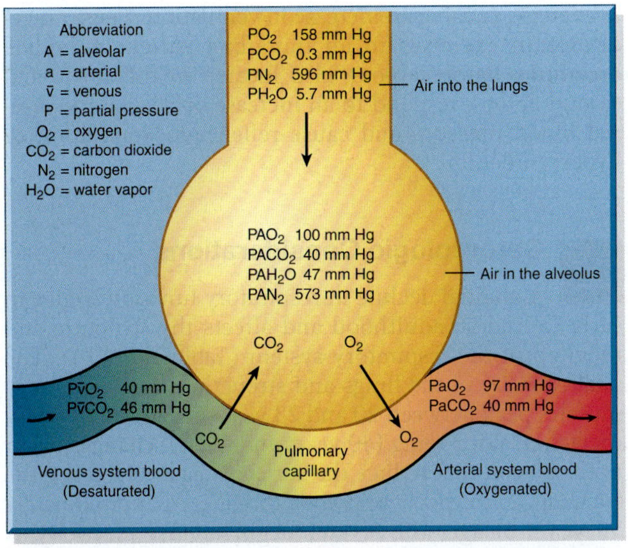

FIGURE 22-5. Changes occur in the partial pressure of gases during respiration. These values vary as a result of the exchange of oxygen and carbon dioxide and the changes that occur in their partial pressures as venous blood flows through the lungs.

Effects of Pressure on Oxygen Transport

Oxygen and carbon dioxide are transported simultaneously either dissolved in blood or combined with hemoglobin in red blood cells. Each 100 mL of normal arterial blood carries 0.3 mL of oxygen physically dissolved in the plasma and 20 mL of oxygen in combination with hemoglobin. Large amounts of oxygen can be transported in the blood because oxygen combines easily with hemoglobin to form oxyhemoglobin:

$$O_2 + Hgb \leftrightarrow HgbO_2$$

The volume of oxygen physically dissolved in the plasma is measured by the partial pressure of oxygen in the arteries (PaO_2). The higher the PaO_2, the greater the amount of oxygen dissolved. For example, at a PaO_2 of 10 mm Hg, 0.03 mL of oxygen is dissolved in 100 mL of plasma. At PaO_2 of 20 mm Hg, twice this amount is dissolved in plasma, and at PaO_2 of 100 mm Hg, 10 times this amount is dissolved.

Therefore, the amount of dissolved oxygen is directly proportional to the partial pressure, regardless of how high the oxygen pressure becomes.

The amount of oxygen that combines with hemoglobin depends on both the amount of hemoglobin in the blood and on PaO_2, but only up to a PaO_2 of about 150 mm Hg. This is measured as O_2 saturation (SaO_2), the percentage of the O_2 that could be carried if all the hemoglobin held the maximum possible amount of O_2. When the PaO_2 is 150 mm Hg, hemoglobin is 100% saturated and does not combine with any additional oxygen. When hemoglobin is 100% saturated, 1 g of hemoglobin combines with 1.34 mL of oxygen. Therefore, in a person with 14 g/dL of hemoglobin, each 100 mL of blood contains about 19 mL of oxygen associated with hemoglobin. If the PaO_2 is less than 150 mm Hg, the percentage of hemoglobin saturated with oxygen decreases. For example, at a PaO_2 of 100 mm Hg (normal value), saturation is 97%; at a PaO_2 of 40 mm Hg, saturation is 70%.

Oxyhemoglobin Dissociation Curve

The oxyhemoglobin dissociation curve (Chart 22-4) shows the relationship between the partial pressure of oxygen (PaO_2) and the percentage of saturation of oxygen (SaO_2). The percentage of saturation can be affected by carbon dioxide, hydrogen ion concentration, temperature, and 2,3-diphosphoglycerate. An increase in these factors shifts the curve to the right, so that less oxygen is picked up in the lungs, but more oxygen is released to the tissues, if PaO_2 is unchanged. A decrease in these factors causes the curve to shift to the left, making the bond between oxygen and hemoglobin stronger. If the PaO_2 is still unchanged, more oxygen is picked up in the lungs, but less oxygen is given up to the tissues. The unusual shape of the oxyhemoglobin dissociation curve is a distinct advantage to the patient for two reasons:

1. If the PaO_2 decreases from 100 to 80 mm Hg as a result of lung disease or heart disease, the hemoglobin of the arterial blood remains almost maximally saturated (94%), and the tissues do not suffer from hypoxia.
2. When the arterial blood passes into tissue capillaries and is exposed to the tissue tension of oxygen (about 40 mm Hg), hemoglobin gives up large quantities of oxygen for use by the tissues.

CHART 22-4

Oxyhemoglobin Dissociation Curve

The oxyhemoglobin dissociation curve is marked to show three oxygen levels:

1. Normal levels—PaO_2 above 70 mm Hg
2. Relatively safe levels—PaO_2 45 to 70 mm Hg
3. Dangerous levels—PaO_2 below 40 mm Hg

The normal (middle) curve (N) shows that 75% saturation occurs at a PaO_2 of 40 mm Hg. If the curve shifts to the right (R), the same saturation (75%) occurs at the higher PaO_2 of 57 mm Hg. If the curve shifts to the left (L), 75% saturation occurs at a PaO_2 of 25 mm Hg.

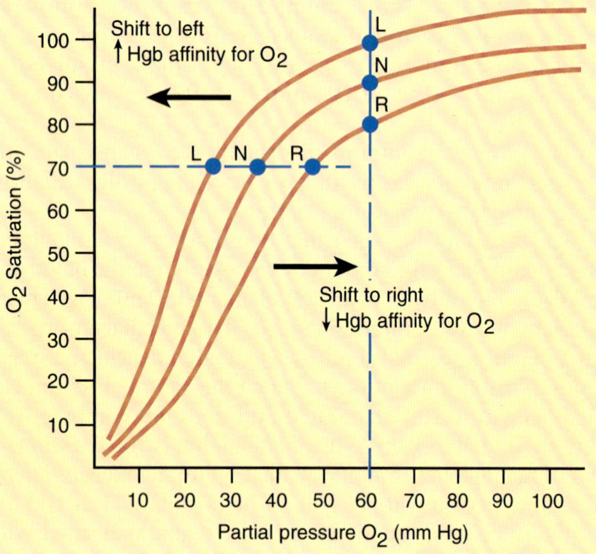

With a normal value for PaO_2 (80 to 100 mm Hg) and SaO_2 (95% to 98%), there is a 15% margin of excess oxygen available to the tissues. With a normal hemoglobin level of 15 mg/dL and a PaO_2 level of 40 mm Hg (SaO_2 75%), there is adequate oxygen available for the tissues but no reserve for physiologic stresses that increase tissue oxygen demand. If a serious incident occurs (e.g., bronchospasm, aspiration, hypotension, or cardiac dysrhythmias) that reduces the intake of oxygen from the lungs, tissue hypoxia results.

An important consideration in the transport of oxygen is cardiac output, which determines the amount of oxygen delivered to the body and affects lung and tissue perfusion. If the cardiac output is normal (5 L/min), the amount of oxygen delivered to the body per minute is normal. Under normal conditions, only 250 mL of oxygen is used per minute, which is approximately 25% of available oxygen. The rest of the oxygen returns to the right side of the heart, and the PaO_2 of venous blood drops from 80 to 100 mm Hg to about 40 mm Hg. If cardiac output falls, however, the amount of oxygen delivered to the tissues also falls and may be inadequate to meet the body's needs.

Carbon Dioxide Transport

At the same time that oxygen diffuses from the blood into the tissues, carbon dioxide diffuses from tissue cells to blood and is transported to the lungs for excretion. The amount of carbon dioxide in transit is one of the major determinants of the acid–base balance of the body. Normally, only 6% of the venous carbon dioxide is removed in the lungs, and enough remains in the arterial blood to exert a pressure of 40 mm Hg. Most of the carbon dioxide (90%) is carried by red blood cells; the small portion (5%) that remains dissolved in the plasma (partial pressure of carbon dioxide [PCO_2]) is the critical factor that determines carbon dioxide movement in or out of the blood.

Although the many processes involved in respiratory gas transport seem to occur in intermittent stages, the changes are rapid, simultaneous, and continuous.

Neurologic Control of Ventilation

Resting respiration is the result of cyclic excitation of the respiratory muscles by the phrenic nerve. The rhythm of breathing is controlled by respiratory centres in the brain. The inspiratory and expiratory centres in the medulla oblongata and pons control the rate and depth of ventilation to meet the body's metabolic demands.

The apneustic centre in the lower pons stimulates the inspiratory medullary centre to promote deep, prolonged inspirations. The pneumotaxic centre in the upper pons is thought to control the pattern of respirations.

Several groups of receptor sites assist in the brain's control of respiratory function. The central chemoreceptors, located in the medulla, respond to chemical changes in the cerebrospinal fluid, which result from chemical changes in the blood. These receptors respond to an increase or decrease in the pH and convey a message to the lungs to change the depth and then the rate of ventilation to correct the imbalance. The peripheral chemoreceptors are located in the aortic arch and the carotid arteries and respond first to changes in PaO_2, then to partial pressure of carbon dioxide ($PaCO_2$) and pH. The Hering–Breuer reflex is activated by stretch receptors in the alveoli. When the lungs are distended, inspiration is inhibited; as a result, the lungs do not become overdistended. In addition, proprioceptors in the muscles and joints respond to body movements, such as exercise, causing an increase in ventilation. Thus, range-of-motion exercises in an immobile patient stimulate breathing. Baroreceptors, also located in the aortic and carotid bodies, respond to an increase or decrease in arterial blood pressure and cause reflex hypoventilation or hyperventilation.

Gerontologic Considerations

A gradual decline in respiratory function begins in early to middle adulthood and affects the structure and function of the respiratory system (Tabloski, 2014). The vital capacity of the lungs and strength of the respiratory muscles peak between 20 and 25 years of age and decrease thereafter. With aging (40 years and older), changes occur in the alveoli that reduce the surface area available for the exchange of oxygen and carbon dioxide. At approximately 50 years of age, the alveoli begin to lose elasticity. A decrease in vital capacity occurs with loss of chest wall mobility, which restricts the tidal flow of air. The amount of respiratory dead space increases with age. These changes result in a decreased diffusion capacity for oxygen

TABLE 22-2 Age-Related Changes in the Respiratory System

	Structural Changes	Functional Changes	History and Physical Findings
Defense mechanisms (respiratory and nonrespiratory)	↓ Number of cilia and ↓ mucus ↓ Cough and gag reflex Loss of surface area of the capillary membrane Lack of a uniform or consistent ventilation and/or blood flow	↓ Protection against foreign particles ↓ Protection against aspiration ↓ Antibody response to antigens ↓ Response to hypoxia and hypercapnia (chemoreceptors)	↓ Cough reflex and mucus ↑ Infection rate History of respiratory infections, COPD, pneumonia. Risk factors: smoking, environmental exposure, TB exposure
Lung	↓ Size of airway ↑ Diameter of alveolar ducts ↑ Collagen of alveolar walls ↑ Thickness of alveolar membranes ↓ Elasticity of alveolar sacs	↑ Airway resistance ↑ Pulmonary compliance ↓ Expiratory flow rate ↓ Oxygen diffusion capacity ↑ Dead space Premature closure of airways ↑ Air trapping ↓ Expiratory flow rates Ventilation–perfusion mismatch ↓ Exercise capacity ↑ Anteroposterior (AP) diameter	Unchanged total lung capacity (TLC) ↑ Residual volume (RV) ↓ Inspiratory reserve volume (IRV) ↓ Expiratory reserve volume (ERV) ↓ Forced vital capacity (FVC) and vital capacity (VC) ↑ Functional residual capacity (FRC) ↓ PaO_2 ↑ CO_2
Chest wall and muscles	Calcification of intercostal cartilages Arthritis of costovertebral joints ↓ Continuity of diaphragm Osteoporotic changes ↓ Muscle mass Muscle atrophy	↑ Rigidity and stiffness of thoracic cage ↓ Respiratory muscle strength ↑ Work of breathing ↓ Capacity for exercise ↓ Peripheral chemosensitivity ↑ Risk for inspiratory muscle fatigue	Kyphosis, barrel chest Skeletal changes ↑ AP diameter Shortness of breath ↑ Abdominal and diaphragmatic breathing ↓ Maximum expiratory flow rates

Adapted from Ramly, E., Kaafarani, H. M. A., & Velmahos, G. C. (2015). The effect of aging on pulmonary function: Implications for monitoring and support of the surgical and trauma patient. *Surgical Clinics of North America, 95*(1), 53–69.

with increasing age, producing lower oxygen levels in the arterial circulation. Older adults have a decreased ability to rapidly move air in and out of the lungs.

Gerontologic changes in the respiratory system are summarized in Table 22-2. Despite these changes, in the absence of chronic pulmonary disease, older adults are able to carry out activities of daily living, but they may have decreased tolerance for, and require additional rest after, prolonged or vigorous activity.

Assessment

Health History

The health history focuses on the physical and functional problems and the effects of these problems on the patient, including the ability to carry out activities of daily living. Several common symptoms related to the respiratory system are discussed in detail below. If the patient is experiencing severe **dyspnea**, the nurse may need to modify or abbreviate the questions asked and the timing of the health history to avoid increasing the patient's breathlessness and anxiety.

In addition to identifying the chief reason why the patient is seeking health care, the nurse tries to determine when the health problem or symptom started, how long it lasted, if it was relieved at any time, and how relief was obtained. The nurse obtains information about precipitating factors, duration, severity, and associated factors or symptoms.

Common Symptoms

The major signs and symptoms of respiratory disease are dyspnea, cough, sputum production, chest pain, wheezing, and **hemoptysis**. The nurse also assesses the impact of signs and symptoms on the patient's ability to perform activities of daily living and to participate in usual work and family activities.

Dyspnea

Dyspnea (subjective feeling of difficult or labored breathing, breathlessness, shortness of breath) is a multidimensional symptom common to many pulmonary and cardiac disorders, particularly when there is decreased lung compliance or increased airway resistance. Dyspnea may also be associated with allergic reactions, anemia, neurologic or neuromuscular disorders, trauma, and advanced disease, and is common at the end of life. Dyspnea predicts adverse clinical outcomes, including increased mortality (Baker, Barsamian, Leone, et al., 2013). Dyspnea can also occur after exercise in people without disease (Porth, 2015).

In general, acute diseases of the lungs produce a more severe grade of dyspnea than do chronic diseases. Sudden dyspnea in a healthy person may indicate pneumothorax (air in the pleural cavity), acute respiratory obstruction, allergic reaction, or myocardial infarction. In immobilized patients, sudden dyspnea may denote pulmonary embolism (PE). Dyspnea and **tachypnea** (abnormally rapid respirations) accompanied by progressive **hypoxemia** (low blood-oxygen level) in a person who has recently experienced lung trauma, shock, cardiopulmonary bypass, or multiple blood transfusions may signal ARDS. **Orthopnea** (shortness of breath when lying flat, relieved by sitting or standing) may be found in patients with heart disease and occasionally in patients with COPD; dyspnea with an expiratory wheeze occurs with COPD. Dyspnea associated with noisy breathing may result from a narrowing of the airway or localized obstruction of a major bronchus by a tumour or foreign body. The high-pitched sound heard (usually on inspiration) when someone is breathing through a partially blocked upper airway is called **stridor**. To help determine the cause of dyspnea, the nurse should ask the following questions:

- Is the shortness of breath related to other symptoms? Is a cough present?
- Was the onset of shortness of breath sudden or gradual?
- At what time of day or night does the shortness of breath occur?
- Is the shortness of breath worse when lying flat?
- How much exertion triggers shortness of breath? Does it occur with exercise? Climbing stairs? At rest?
- How severe is the shortness of breath? On a scale of 1 to 10, if 1 is not at all breathless and 10 is very breathless, how hard is it to breathe?

Because patients use a variety of terms to describe breathlessness, the nurse must explore what these terms mean to each patient. Patients experiencing dyspnea frequently experience fear and anxiety (Dudgeon, 2015; Yorke, 2014). It is especially important to assess the patient's rating of the intensity or distress of breathlessness, what breathing feels like, and its impact on the patient's general health, function, and quality of life. A variety of valid and reliable instruments including various Likert scale types of quality of life tools, the visual analogue scale, and the modified Borg scale are available to assist the nurse in measuring dyspnea. The modified Borg scale is a type of numeric rating scale. The patient is asked to self-rate the difficulty breathing is causing him/her at the present time, with 0 corresponding to no difficulty at all and 10 corresponding to maximal breathing difficulty (Dudgeon, 2015).

Cough

Cough is a reflex that protects the lungs from the accumulation of secretions or the inhalation of foreign bodies. Its presence or absence can be a diagnostic clue because some disorders cause coughing and others suppress it. The cough reflex may be impaired by weakness or paralysis of the respiratory muscles, prolonged inactivity, the presence of a nasogastric tube, or depressed function of the brain's medullary centres (e.g., anesthesia, brain disorders).

Cough results from irritation or inflammation of the mucus membranes anywhere in the respiratory tract and is associated with multiple pulmonary disorders. Mucus, pus, blood, or an airborne irritant, such as smoke or a gas, may stimulate the cough reflex. Common causes of cough include asthma, gastrointestinal reflux disease, infection, and side effects of medications, such as angiotensin-converting enzyme (ACE) inhibitors (Poot, 2014).

To help determine the cause of the cough, the nurse inquires about the onset and time of coughing. Coughing at night may indicate the onset of left-sided heart failure or bronchial asthma (Kaufman, 2012). A cough in the morning with sputum production may indicate bronchitis. A cough that worsens when the patient is supine suggests postnasal drip (rhinosinusitis). Coughing after food intake may indicate aspiration of material into the tracheobronchial tree. A cough of recent onset is usually from an acute infection.

The nurse assesses the character of the cough and associated symptoms. A dry, irritative cough is characteristic of an upper respiratory tract infection of viral origin, or it may be a side effect of ACE inhibitor therapy. An irritative, high-pitched cough can be caused by laryngotracheitis. A brassy cough is the result of a tracheal lesion, and a severe or changing cough may indicate bronchogenic carcinoma. Pleuritic chest pain that accompanies coughing may indicate pleural or chest wall (musculoskeletal) involvement. Violent coughing causes bronchial spasm, obstruction, and further irritation of the bronchi and may result in syncope (fainting).

NURSING ALERT

A nurse interviewing a patient who says he has a dry, irritating cough that is not "bringing anything up" should ask whether he is taking ACE inhibitors.

A persistent cough may affect a patient's quality of life and may produce embarrassment, exhaustion, inability to sleep, and pain. Therefore, the nurse should explore the effect of a chronic cough on the patient and the patient's view about the significance of the cough and its effect on his or her life (Hrisanfow & Hägglund, 2012).

Violent coughing causes bronchial spasm, obstruction, and further irritation of the bronchi and may result in syncope (fainting). A severe, repeated, or uncontrolled cough that is nonproductive is exhausting and potentially harmful.

Sputum Production

A patient who coughs long enough almost invariably produces sputum. Sputum production is the reaction of the lungs to any constantly recurring irritant. It also may be associated with a nasal discharge. The nature of the sputum is often indicative of its cause. A profuse amount of purulent sputum (thick and yellow, green, or rust-coloured) or a change in colour of the sputum is a common sign of a bacterial infection. Thin, mucoid sputum frequently results from viral bronchitis. A gradual increase of sputum over time may occur with chronic bronchitis or bronchiectasis. Pink-tinged mucoid sputum suggests a lung tumour. Profuse, frothy, pink material, often welling up into the throat, may indicate pulmonary edema. Foul-smelling sputum and bad breath point to the presence of a lung abscess, bronchiectasis, or an infection caused by fusospirochetal or other anaerobic organisms.

Chest Pain

Chest pain or discomfort may be associated with pulmonary or cardiac disease. Chest pain associated with pulmonary conditions may be sharp, stabbing, and intermittent, or it may be dull, aching, and persistent. The pain usually is felt on the side where the pathologic process is located, but it may be referred elsewhere—for example, to the neck, back, or abdomen.

Chest pain may occur with pneumonia, PE with lung infarction, pleurisy, or as a late symptom of bronchogenic carcinoma. In carcinoma, the pain may be dull and persistent because the cancer has invaded the chest wall, mediastinum, or spine.

Lung disease does not always cause thoracic pain because the lungs and the visceral pleura lack sensory nerves and are insensitive to pain stimuli. However, the parietal pleura has a rich supply of sensory nerves that are stimulated by inflammation and stretching of the membrane. Pleuritic pain from irritation of the parietal pleura is sharp and seems to "catch" on inspiration; patients often describe it as being "like the stabbing of a knife." Patients are more comfortable when they lay on the affected side because this splints the chest wall, limits expansion and contraction of the lung, and reduces the friction between the injured or diseased pleurae on that side. Pain associated with cough may be reduced manually by splinting the rib cage.

The nurse assesses the quality, intensity, and radiation of pain and identifies and explores precipitating factors and their relationship to the patient's position. In addition, it is important to assess the relationship of pain to the inspiratory and expiratory phases of respiration.

Wheezing

Wheezing is a high-pitched, musical sound heard mainly on expiration (asthma) or inspiration (bronchitis). It is often the major finding in a patient with bronchoconstriction or airway narrowing. **Rhonchi** are low-pitched continuous sounds heard over the lungs in partial airway obstruction. Depending on their location and severity, these sounds may be heard with or without a stethoscope.

Hemoptysis

Hemoptysis (expectoration of blood from the respiratory tract) is a symptom of both pulmonary and cardiac disorders. The onset of hemoptysis is usually sudden, and it may be intermittent or continuous. Signs, which vary from blood-stained sputum to a large, sudden hemorrhage, always merit investigation. The most common causes are:

- Pulmonary infection
- Carcinoma of the lung
- Abnormalities of the heart or blood vessels
- Pulmonary artery or vein abnormalities
- Pulmonary embolus and infarction

Diagnostic evaluation to determine the cause includes chest x-ray, chest angiography, and **bronchoscopy**. A careful history and physical examination are necessary to identify the underlying disorder, irrespective of whether the bleeding involved a small amount of blood in the sputum or a massive hemorrhage. The amount of blood produced is not always proportional to the seriousness of the cause.

First, it is important to determine the source of the bleeding—the gums, nasopharynx, lungs, or stomach. The nurse may be the only witness to the episode. When documenting the bleeding episode, the nurse considers the following points:

- Bloody sputum from the nose or the nasopharynx is usually preceded by considerable sniffing, with blood possibly appearing in the nose.
- Blood from the lung is usually bright red, frothy, and mixed with sputum. Initial symptoms include a tickling sensation in the throat, a salty taste, a burning or bubbling sensation in the chest, and perhaps chest pain, in which case the patient tends to splint the bleeding side. The term hemoptysis is reserved for the coughing up of blood arising from a pulmonary hemorrhage. This blood has an alkaline pH (greater than 7.0).
- If the hemorrhage is in the stomach, the blood is vomited (hematemesis) rather than coughed up. Blood that has been in contact with gastric juice is sometimes so dark that it is referred to as "coffee ground emesis." This blood has an acid pH (less than 7.0).

Past Health, Family, and Social History

After exploring the current problem, the nurse obtains a brief history of events and conditions that could affect the current health status. Specific questions are asked about childhood illnesses, immunizations, chronic medical conditions, injuries, hospitalizations, surgeries, allergies, and current medications (including over-the-counter medications and herbal remedies). Since many lung disorders are related to or exacerbated by tobacco smoke, smoking history (including exposure to second-hand smoke) is also obtained. Smoking history is usually expressed in pack-years, which is the number of packs of cigarettes smoked per day times the number of years the patient smoked. It is important to find out if (and when) the patient quit smoking or is still smoking. The nurse assesses for risk factors and genetic factors that may contribute to the patient's lung condition (Charts 22-5 and 22-6).

In addition, psychosocial factors that may affect the patient are explored (Chart 22-7). These factors include

CHART 22-5

Risk Factors: Respiratory Disease

- Smoking (the single most important contributor to lung disease)
- Exposure to second-hand smoke
- Personal or family history of lung disease
- Genetic makeup
- Exposure to allergens and environmental pollutants
- Exposure to certain recreational and occupational hazards
- Dietary factors, including poor nutrition
- Human immunodeficiency virus infection, overcrowding, and poor immunization rates for certain respiratory infections
- Atypical immune responses in diseases such as asthma

Adapted from Ferkol, T., & Schraufnagel, D. (2014). The global burden of respiratory disease. *Annals of the American Thoracic Society, 11*(3), 404–406.

GENETICS IN NURSING PRACTICE

Chart 22-6. Respiratory Disorders

Various conditions that affect gas exchange and respiratory function are influenced by genetics factors. Some are known to have a direct inherited pathway while others have a strong familial association but the exact inheritance pattern is not entirely clear. The following are examples of respiratory disorders with a known or associated familial component:

- Asthma
- Cystic fibrosis
- Chronic obstructive pulmonary disease
- Alpha-1 antitrypsin deficiency
- Primary ciliary dyskinesia
- Pulmonary fibrosis
- Pulmonary hypertension
- Tuberous sclerosis

Nursing Assessments

FAMILY HISTORY ASSESSMENT

- Assess family history for other family members with histories of respiratory impairment.
- Assess family history for individuals with early-onset chronic pulmonary disease, family history of hepatic disease in infants (clinical symptoms of alpha-1 antitrypsin deficiency).
- Inquire about family history of genetic cystic fibrosis.

PATIENT ASSESSMENT

- Assess for symptoms such as changes in respiratory status associated with asthma (e.g., wheezing, hyperresponsiveness, mucosal edema, and mucus production).
- Assess for multisystem effects characteristic of cystic fibrosis (e.g., productive cough, wheezing, obstructive airways disease, gastrointestinal problems including pancreatic insufficiency, clubbing of the fingers).

Management Issues Specific to Genetics

- Inquire whether DNA mutation or other genetic testing has been performed on affected family members.
- Refer for further genetics counselling and evaluation so that family members can discuss inheritance, risk to other family members, availability of genetic testing, and gene-based interventions.
- Offer appropriate genetics information and resources.
- Assess the patient's understanding of genetics information.
- Provide support to families with newly diagnosed genetic-related respiratory disorders.
- Participate in the management and coordination of care of patients with genetic conditions, individuals predisposed to develop or pass on a genetic condition.

Genetics Resources

American Lung Association—http://www.lungusa.org

Cystic Fibrosis Foundation—http://www.cff.org

Genetic Alliance—a directory of support groups for patients and families with genetic conditions, http://www.geneticalliance.org

Gene Clinics—a listing of common genetic disorders with clinical summaries, genetics counselling, and testing information, http://www.geneclinics.org

National Organization of Rare Disorders—a directory of support groups and information for patients and families with rare genetic disorders, http://www.rarediseases.org

OMIM: Online Mendelian Inheritance in Man—a complete listing of inherited genetic conditions, http://www.ncbi.nlm.nih.gov/entrez/query.fcgi?db=OMIM

anxiety, role changes, family relationships, financial problems, employment status, and the strategies the patient uses to cope with them. Many respiratory diseases are chronic and progressively debilitating and disabling. It is important that the patient with a respiratory disorder understand the condition and be familiar with necessary self-care interventions. The nurse evaluates these factors over time and provides education as needed (Nguyen, Donesky, Reinke, et al., 2013).

Physical Assessment of the Respiratory System

General Appearance

The patient's general appearance may give clues to respiratory status. In particular, the nurse inspects for clubbing of the fingers and notes the skin colour.

Clubbing of the Fingers

Clubbing of the fingers is a change in the normal nail bed. It appears as sponginess of the nail bed and loss of the nail bed angle (see Fig. 22-6). It is a sign of lung disease that is found in patients with chronic hypoxic conditions,

CHART 22-7

Assessing for Psychosocial Factors Related to Pulmonary Disease and Respiratory Function

- What strategies does the patient use to cope with the signs and symptoms and challenges associated with pulmonary disease?
- What effect has the pulmonary disease had on the patient's quality of life, goals, role within the family, and occupation?
- What changes has the pulmonary disease had on the patient's family and relationships with family members?
- Does the patient exhibit depression, anxiety, anger, hostility, dependency, withdrawal, isolation, avoidance, noncompliance, acceptance, or denial?
- What support systems does the patient use to cope with the illness?
- Are resources (relatives, friends, or community groups) available? Do the patient and family use them effectively?

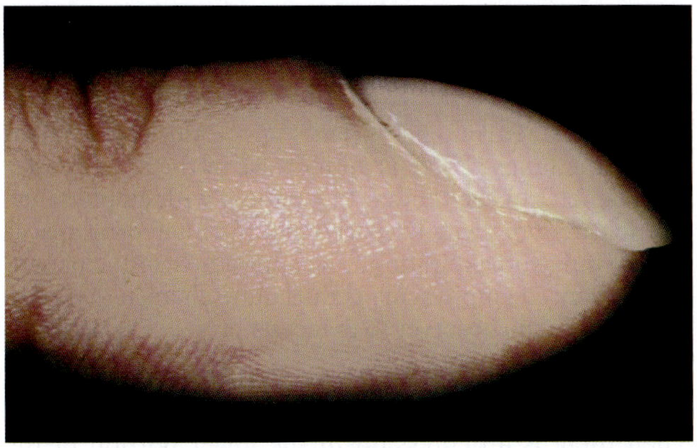

FIGURE 22-6. Clubbed finger. In clubbing, the distal phalanx of each finger is rounded and bulbous. The nail plate is more convex, and the angle between the plate and the proximal nail fold increases to 180 degrees or more. The proximal nail fold, when palpated, feels spongy or floating. Among the many causes are chronic hypoxia and lung cancer.

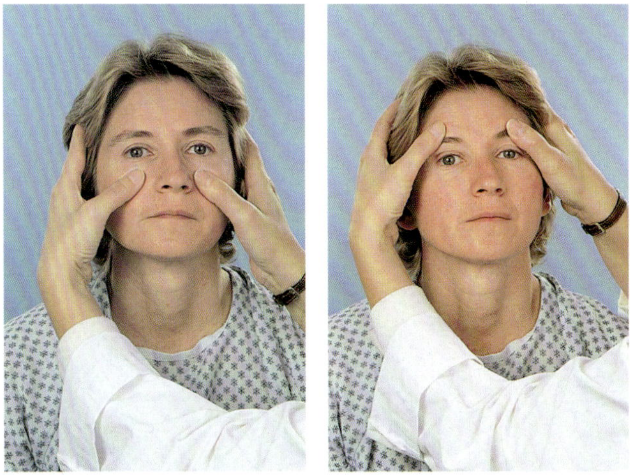

FIGURE 22-7. Technique for palpating the frontal sinuses at left and the maxillary sinuses at right.

chronic lung infections, or malignancies of the lung. Clubbing can also be seen in congenital heart disease and other chronic infections or inflammatory conditions, such as endocarditis or inflammatory bowel disease (Bickley, 2013; Rutherford, 2013).

Cyanosis

Cyanosis, a bluish colouring of the skin, is a very late indicator of hypoxia. The presence or absence of cyanosis is determined by the amount of unoxygenated hemoglobin in the blood. Cyanosis appears when there is at least 5 g/dL of unoxygenated hemoglobin. A patient with a hemoglobin level of 15 g/dL does not demonstrate cyanosis until 5 g/dL of that hemoglobin becomes unoxygenated, reducing the effective circulating hemoglobin to two thirds of the normal level.

A patient with anemia rarely manifests cyanosis, and a patient with polycythemia may appear cyanotic even if adequately oxygenated. Therefore, cyanosis is *not* a reliable sign of hypoxia.

Assessment of cyanosis is affected by room lighting, the patient's skin colour, and the distance of the blood vessels from the surface of the skin. In the presence of a pulmonary condition, central cyanosis is assessed by observing the colour of the tongue and lips. This indicates a decrease in oxygen tension in the blood. Peripheral cyanosis results from decreased blood flow to the body's periphery (fingers, toes, or earlobes), as in vasoconstriction from exposure to cold, and does not necessarily indicate a central systemic problem (Sole, Klein, & Moseley, 2013).

Upper Respiratory Structures

For a routine examination of the upper airway, only a simple light source, such as a penlight, is necessary. A more thorough examination requires the use of a nasal speculum.

Nose and Sinuses

The nurse inspects the external nose for lesions, asymmetry, or inflammation and then asks the patient to tilt the head backward. Gently pushing the tip of the nose upward, the nurse examines the internal structures of the nose, inspecting the mucosa for colour, swelling, exudate, or bleeding. The nasal mucosa is normally redder than the oral mucosa. It may appear swollen and hyperemic if the patient has a common cold, but in allergic rhinitis, the mucosa appears pale and swollen.

Next, the nurse inspects the septum for deviation, perforation, or bleeding. Most people have a slight degree of septal deviation, but actual displacement of the cartilage into either the right or left side of the nose may produce nasal obstruction. Such deviation usually causes no symptoms.

While the head is still tilted back, the nurse inspects the inferior and middle turbinates. In chronic rhinitis, nasal polyps may develop between the inferior and middle turbinates; they are distinguished by their grey appearance. Unlike the turbinates, they are gelatinous and freely movable.

Next, the nurse may palpate the frontal and maxillary sinuses for tenderness (Fig. 22-7). Using the thumbs, the nurse applies gentle pressure in an upward fashion at the supraorbital ridges (frontal sinuses) and in the cheek area adjacent to the nose (maxillary sinuses). Tenderness in either area suggests inflammation. The frontal and maxillary sinuses can be inspected by transillumination (passing a strong light through a bony area, such as the sinuses, to inspect the cavity; Fig. 22-8). If the light fails to penetrate, the cavity likely contains fluid or pus.

Mouth and Pharynx

After the nasal inspection, the nurse assesses the mouth and pharynx, instructing the patient to open the mouth wide and take a deep breath. Usually this flattens the posterior tongue and briefly allows a full view of the anterior and posterior pillars, tonsils, uvula, and posterior pharynx (see Chapter 35, Fig. 35-2). The nurse inspects these structures for colour, symmetry, and evidence of exudate, ulceration, or enlargement. If a tongue blade is needed to depress the tongue to visualize the pharynx, it is pressed firmly beyond the midpoint of the tongue to avoid a gagging response.

Trachea

Next, the position and mobility of the trachea are noted by direct palpation. This is performed by placing the thumb

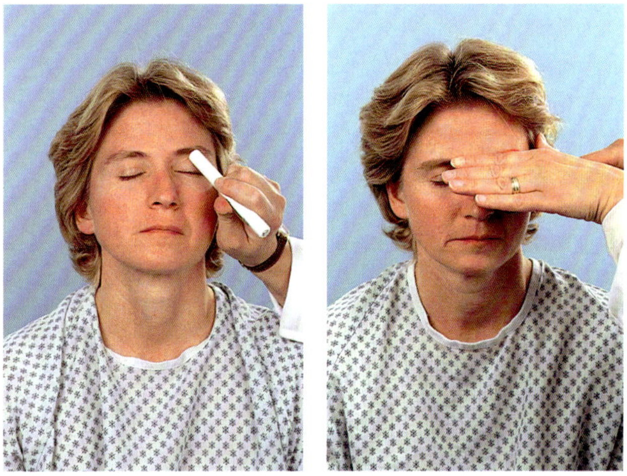

FIGURE 22-8. At left, the nurse positions the light source for transillumination of the frontal sinus. At right, the nurse shields the patient's brow and shines the light. In normal conditions (a darkened room), the light should shine through the tissues and appear as a reddish glow (above the nurse's hand) over the sinus.

and index finger of one hand on either side of the trachea just above the sternal notch. The trachea is highly sensitive, and palpating too firmly may trigger a coughing or gagging response. The trachea is normally in the midline as it enters the thoracic inlet behind the sternum, but it may be deviated by masses in the neck or mediastinum. Pleural or pulmonary disorders, such as a pneumothorax, may also displace the trachea.

Lower Respiratory Structures and Breathing

Assessment of the lower respiratory structures includes inspection, palpation, percussion, and auscultation of the thorax.

Positioning

To assess the posterior thorax and the lungs, the patient should be in a sitting position with arms crossed in front of the chest and hands placed on the opposite shoulders (Bickley, 2013). This position separates the scapulae widely and exposes more lung area for assessment. If the patient is unable to sit, with the patient supine, the nurse should roll the patient from side to side to complete the posterior examination. To assess the anterior thorax and lungs, the patient should be either supine or sitting. The supine position allows easier displacement of the patient's breast tissue, improving the nurse's ability to perform the chest examination.

Thoracic Inspection

Inspection of the thorax provides information about the musculoskeletal structure, the patient's nutritional status, and the respiratory system. The nurse observes the skin over the thorax for colour and turgor and for evidence of loss of subcutaneous tissue. It is important to note asymmetry, if present. In recording or reporting the findings, anatomic landmarks are used as points of reference (Chart 22-8).

CHEST CONFIGURATION. Normally, the ratio of the anteroposterior diameter to the lateral diameter is 1:2. However, there are four main deformities of the chest associated with respiratory disease that alter this relationship: barrel chest, funnel chest (pectus excavatum), pigeon chest (pectus carinatum), and kyphoscoliosis.

Barrel Chest. Barrel chest occurs as a result of overinflation of the lungs. There is an increase in the anteroposterior diameter of the thorax. In a patient with emphysema, the ribs are more widely spaced and the intercostal spaces tend to bulge on expiration. The appearance of the patient with advanced emphysema is thus quite characteristic and often allows the observer to detect its presence easily, even from a distance.

Funnel Chest (Pectus Excavatum). Funnel chest occurs when there is a depression in the lower portion of the sternum. This may compress the heart and great vessels, resulting in murmurs. Funnel chest may occur with rickets or Marfan syndrome.

Pigeon Chest (Pectus Carinatum). A pigeon chest occurs as a result of displacement of the sternum. There is an increase in the anteroposterior diameter. This may occur with rickets, Marfan syndrome, or severe kyphoscoliosis.

Kyphoscoliosis. Kyphoscoliosis is characterized by elevation of the scapula and a corresponding S-shaped spine. This deformity limits lung expansion within the thorax. It may occur with osteoporosis and other skeletal disorders that affect the thorax.

BREATHING PATTERNS AND RESPIRATORY RATES. Observing the rate and depth of respiration is a simple but important aspect of assessment. The normal adult who is resting comfortably takes 14 to 20 breaths per minute (Bickley, 2013). Except for occasional sighs, respirations are quiet and regular in depth and rhythm. This normal pattern is described as eupnea. Certain patterns of respiration are characteristic of specific disease states. Changes in the respiratory rate and rhythm may be the first sign of clinical deterioration in patients who are acutely ill (Philip, Richardson, & Cohen, 2013). The rate and depth of various patterns of respiration are presented in Table 22-3.

NURSING ALERT

There are subtle differences between Cheyne–Stokes and Biot respiration patterns. Between regularly cycled periods of apnea, Cheyne–Stokes respirations demonstrate a regular pattern with the rate and depth of breathing increasing and then decreasing. In Biot respiration, irregularly cycled periods of apnea are interspersed with cycles of normal rate and depth.

Temporary pauses of breathing, or **apnea**, may be noted. When apneas occur repeatedly during sleep, secondary to transient upper airway blockage, the condition is called **obstructive sleep apnea**. In thin people, it is quite normal to note a slight retraction of the intercostal spaces during quiet breathing. Bulging of the intercostal spaces during expiration implies obstruction of expiratory airflow, as in emphysema. Marked retraction on inspiration, particularly if asymmetric, implies blockage of a branch of the respiratory tree. Asymmetric bulging of the intercostal spaces, on

CHART 22-8

Locating Thoracic Landmarks

With respect to the thorax, location is defined both horizontally and vertically. With respect to the lungs, location is defined by lobe.

Horizontal Reference Points

Horizontally, thoracic locations are identified according to their proximity to the rib or the intercostal space under the examiner's fingers. On the anterior surface, identification of a specific rib is facilitated by first locating the angle of Louis. This is where the manubrium joins the body of the sternum in the midline. The second rib joins the sternum at this prominent landmark.

Other ribs may be identified by counting down from the second rib. The intercostal spaces are referred to in terms of the rib immediately above the intercostal space; for example, the fifth intercostal space is directly below the fifth rib.

Locating ribs on the posterior surface of the thorax is more difficult. The first step is to identify the spinous process. This is accomplished by finding the seventh cervical vertebra (*vertebra prominens*), which is the most prominent spinous process. When the neck is slightly flexed, the seventh cervical spinous process stands out. Other vertebrae are then identified by counting downward.

Vertical Reference Points

Several imaginary lines are used as vertical referents or landmarks to identify the location of thoracic findings. The *midsternal line* passes through the centre of the sternum. The *midclavicular line* is an imaginary line that descends from the middle of the clavicle. The *point of maximal impulse* of the heart normally lies along this line on the left thorax.

When the arm is abducted from the body at 90 degrees, imaginary vertical lines may be drawn from the anterior axillary fold, from the middle of the axilla, and from the posterior axillary fold. These lines are called, respectively, the *anterior axillary line*, the *midaxillary line*, and the *posterior axillary line*. A line drawn vertically through the superior and inferior poles of the scapula is called the *scapular line*, and a line drawn down the centre of the vertebral column is called the *vertebral line*. Using these landmarks, for example, the examiner communicates findings by referring to an area of dullness extending from the vertebral to the scapular line between the seventh and tenth ribs on the right.

Lobes of the Lungs

The lobes of the lung may be mapped on the surface of the chest wall in the following manner. The line between the upper and lower lobes on the left begins at the fourth thoracic spinous process posteriorly, proceeds around to cross the fifth rib in the midaxillary line, and meets the sixth rib at the sternum. This line on the right divides the right middle lobe from the right lower lobe. The line dividing the right upper lobe from the middle lobe is an incomplete one that begins at the fifth rib in the midaxillary line, where it intersects the line between the upper and lower lobes and traverses horizontally to the sternum. Thus, the upper lobes are dominant on the anterior surface of the thorax and the lower lobes are dominant on the posterior surface. There is no presentation of the right middle lobe on the posterior surface of the chest.

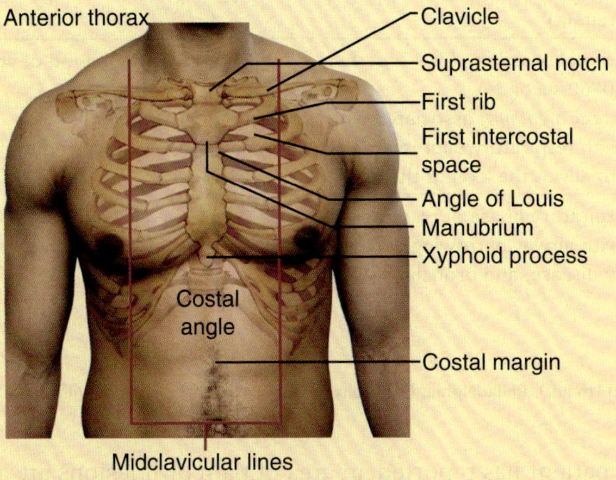

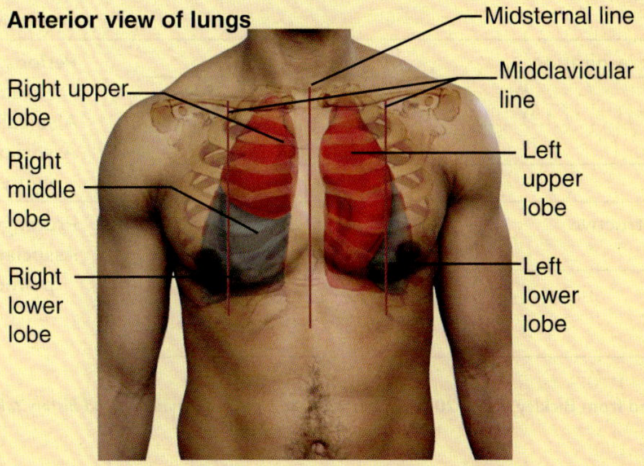

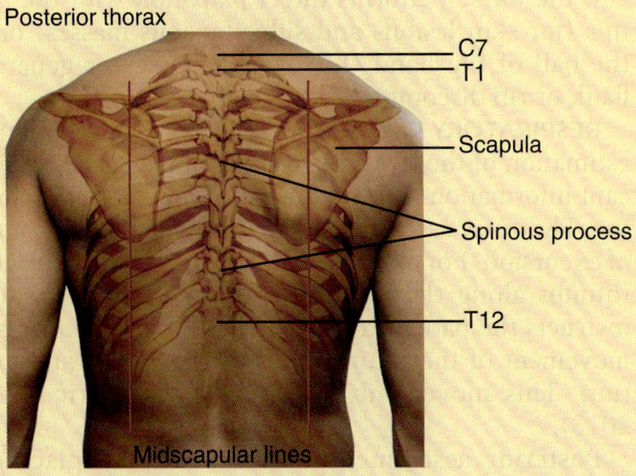

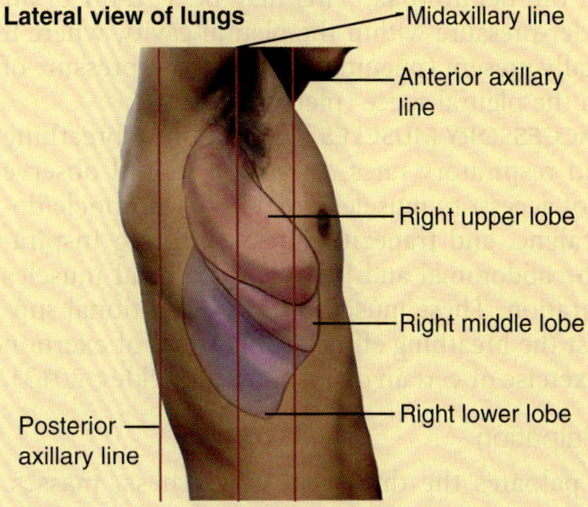

TABLE 22-3 Rates and Depths of Respiration

Type	Description
Eupnea 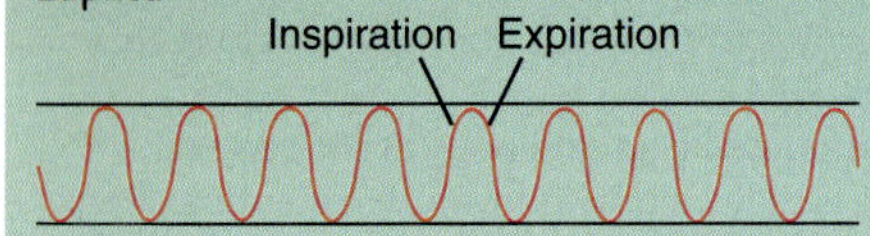	Normal, breathing at 14–20 breaths/min
Bradypnea 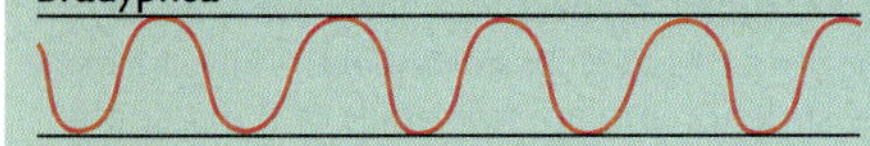	Slower than normal rate (<10 breaths/min), with normal depth and regular rhythm Associated with increased intracranial pressure, brain injury, and drug overdose
Tachypnea 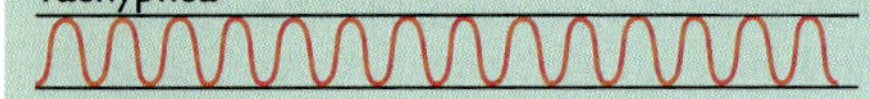	Rapid, shallow breathing >24 breaths/min Associated with pneumonia, pulmonary edema, metabolic acidosis, septicemia, severe pain, or rib fracture
Hypoventilation 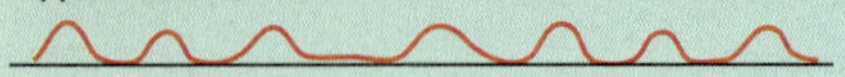	Shallow, irregular breathing
Hyperpnea	Increase depth of respirations
Hyperventilation 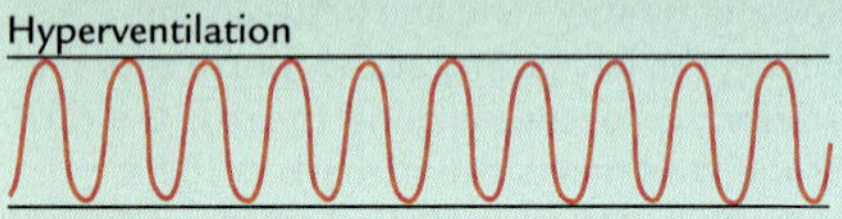	Increased rate and depth of breathing that results in decreased $PaCO_2$ level Inspiration and expiration nearly equal in duration Associated with exertion, anxiety, and metabolic acidosis Called *Kussmaul respiration* if associated with diabetic ketoacidosis or renal origin
Apnea 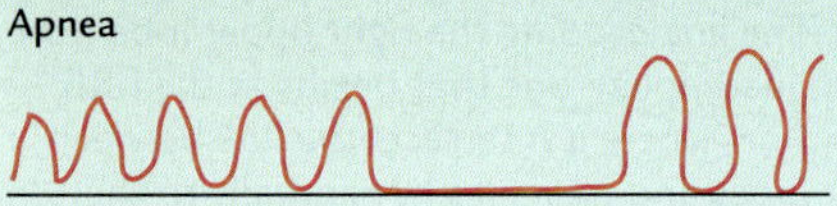	Period of cessation of breathing; time duration varies; apnea may occur briefly during other breathing disorders, such as with sleep apnea; life threatening if sustained
Cheyne–Stokes 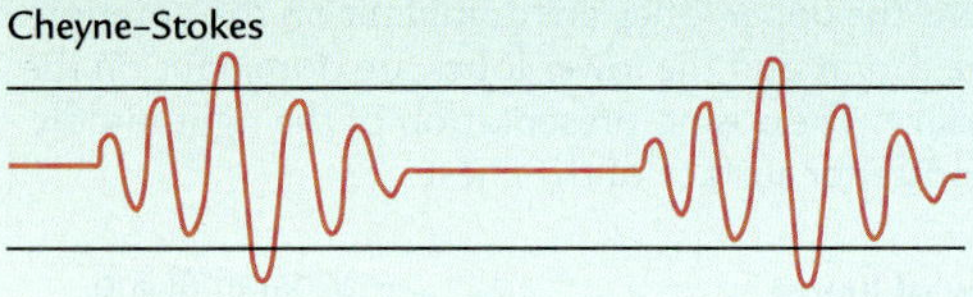	Regular cycle where the rate and depth of breathing increase, then decrease until apnea (usually about 20 seconds) occurs Duration of apnea may vary and progressively lengthen; therefore, it is timed and reported Associated with heart failure and damage to the respiratory centre (drug induced, tumour, trauma)
Biot respiration 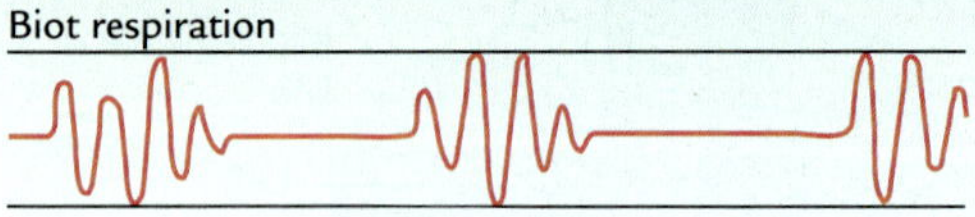	Periods of normal breathing (3–4 breaths), followed by a varying period of apnea (usually 10–60 seconds) Also called *ataxic breathing;* associated with complete irregularity Associated with respiratory depression resulting from drug overdose and brain injury, normally at the level of the medulla
Obstructive 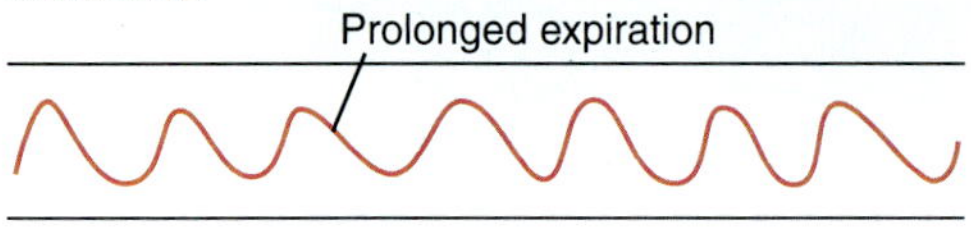	Prolonged expiratory phase of respiration Associated with airway narrowing and seen in asthma, chronic obstructive pulmonary disease, and bronchitis

Adapted from Bickley, L. S. (2013). *Bates' guide to physical examination and history taking* (11th ed.). Philadelphia, PA: Wolters Kluwer Health/Lippincott Williams & Wilkins.

either side of the thorax, is created by an increase in pressure within the hemithorax. This may be a result of air trapped under pressure within the pleural cavity, where it is not normally present (pneumothorax), or the pressure of fluid within the pleural space (pleural effusion).

USE OF ACCESSORY MUSCLES. In addition to breathing patterns and respiratory rates, the nurse should observe for the use of accessory muscles, such as the sternocleidomastoid, scalene, and trapezius muscles during inspiration, and the abdominal and internal intercostal muscles during expiration. These muscles provide additional support to assist the breathing effort during times of exertion as seen in exercise or certain disease states (Bickley, 2013).

Thoracic Palpation

The nurse palpates the thorax for tenderness, masses, lesions, respiratory excursion, and vocal **fremitus**. If the patient has reported an area of pain or if lesions are apparent, the nurse performs direct palpation with the fingertips (for skin lesions and subcutaneous masses) or with the ball of the hand (for deeper masses or generalized flank or rib discomfort).

RESPIRATORY EXCURSION. Respiratory excursion is an estimation of thoracic expansion and may disclose significant information about thoracic movement during breathing. The nurse assesses the patient for range and symmetry of excursion. For anterior assessment, the nurse places the thumbs along the costal margin of the chest wall and instructs the patient to inhale deeply. The nurse observes movement of the thumbs during inspiration and expiration. This movement is normally symmetric (Bickley, 2013).

Posterior assessment is performed by placing the thumbs adjacent to the spinal column at the level of the

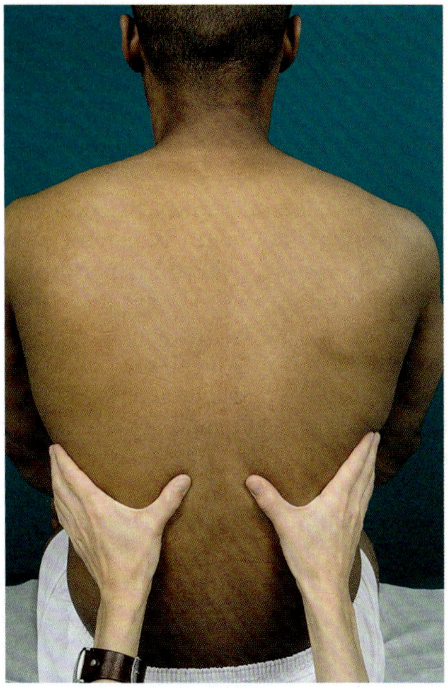

FIGURE 22-9. Method for assessing posterior respiratory excursion. Place both hands posteriorly at the level of T9 or T10. Slide hands medially to pinch a small amount of skin between your thumbs. Observe for symmetry as the patient exhales fully following a deep inspiration.

10th rib (see Fig. 22-9). The hands lightly grasp the lateral rib cage. Sliding the thumbs medially about 2.5 cm (1 in) raises a small skin fold between the thumbs. The patient is instructed to take a full inspiration and to exhale fully. The nurse observes for normal flattening of the skin fold and feels the symmetric movement of the thorax.

Decreased chest excursion may be caused by chronic fibrotic disease. Asymmetric excursion may be due to splinting secondary to pleurisy, fractured ribs, trauma, or unilateral bronchial obstruction.

TACTILE FREMITUS. Tactile fremitus describes vibrations of the chest wall that result from speech detected on palpation. Normally, sounds generated by the larynx travel distally along the bronchial tree to set the chest wall in resonant motion. This is most pronounced with consonant sounds.

Normal fremitus varies on the basis of numerous factors. It is influenced by the thickness of the chest wall, especially muscle, and the subcutaneous tissue associated with obesity. It is also influenced by pitch; lower-pitched sounds travel better through the normal lung and produce greater vibration of the chest wall. Therefore, fremitus is more pronounced in men than in women because of the deeper male voice. Normally, fremitus is most pronounced where the large bronchi are closest to the chest wall, is more prominent on the right side, and is least palpable over the lower lung fields (Bickley, 2013).

The patient is asked to repeat "ninety-nine" or "one, one, one" as the nurse's hands move down the patient's thorax (Bickley, 2013). The vibrations are detected with the palmar surfaces of the hands, or the ulnar aspect of the extended hands, on the thorax. The hand or hands are moved in sequence down the thorax. Corresponding areas of the thorax are compared (see Fig. 22-10). Bony areas are not assessed.

Air does not conduct sound well; however, a solid substance such as tissue does, provided that it has elasticity and is not compressed. Therefore, an increase in solid tissue per unit volume of lung enhances fremitus, and an increase in air per unit volume of lung impedes sound. Patients with emphysema exhibit almost no tactile fremitus. A patient with consolidation of a lobe of the lung from pneumonia has increased tactile fremitus over that lobe.

Thoracic Percussion

Percussion sets the chest wall and underlying structures in motion, producing audible and tactile vibrations. The nurse uses percussion to determine whether underlying

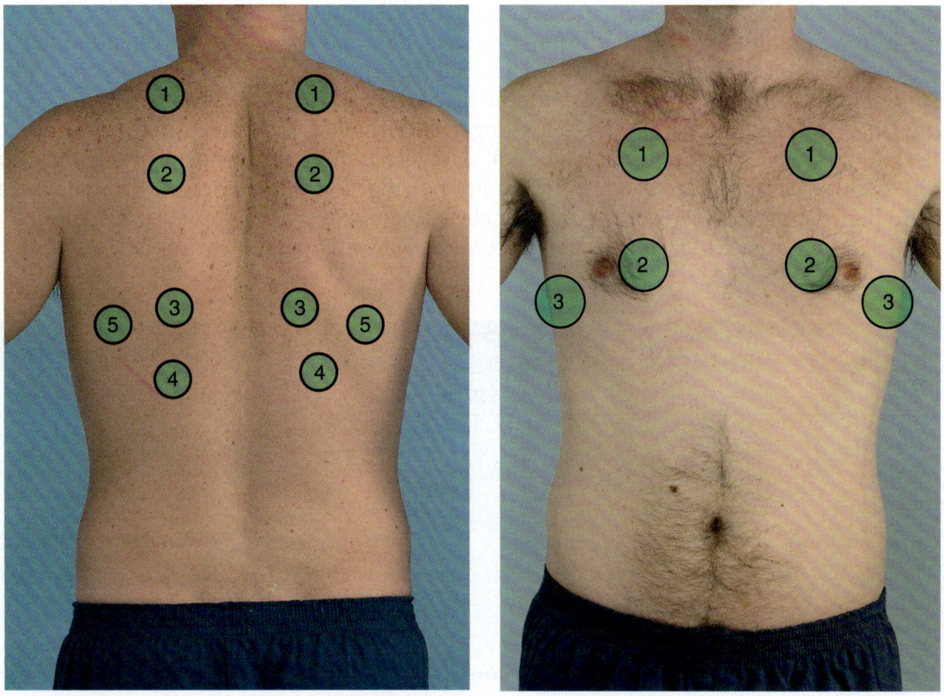

FIGURE 22-10. Palpation sequence for tactile fremitus: posterior thorax (*left*) and anterior thorax (*right*).

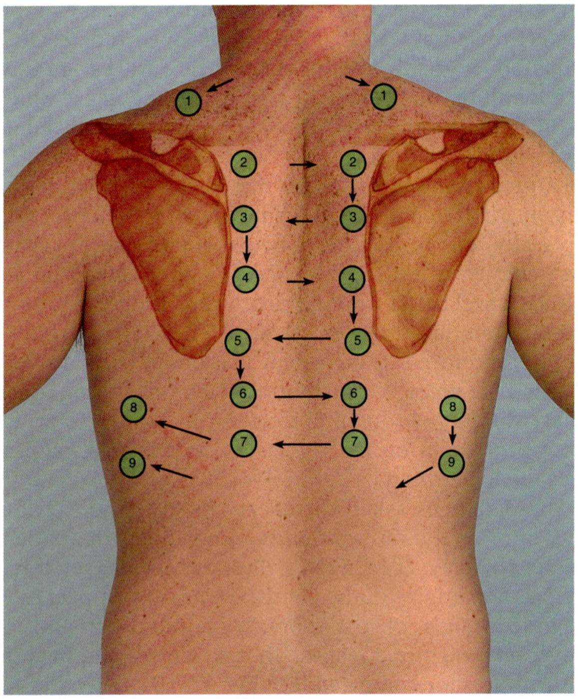

FIGURE 22-11. Percussion of the posterior thorax. With the patient in a sitting position, symmetric areas of the lungs are percussed at 5-cm intervals. This progression starts at the apex of each lung and concludes with percussion of each lateral chest wall.

tissues are filled with air, fluid, or solid material. Percussion also is used to estimate the size and location of certain structures within the thorax (e.g., diaphragm, heart, liver).

Percussion usually begins with the posterior thorax. The nurse percusses across each shoulder top, locating the 5-cm width of resonance overlying the lung apices (see Fig. 22-11). Then the nurse proceeds down the posterior thorax, percussing symmetric areas at intervals of 5 to 6 cm (2 to 2.5 in). To perform percussion, the middle finger of the nondominant hand is firmly placed against the area of the chest wall to be percussed. The distal interphalangeal joint of this finger is struck with the tip of the middle finger of the dominant hand. This finger is partially flexed and percussion occurs in a smooth, dart-like fashion. Bony structures (scapulae or ribs) are not percussed.

To perform percussion over the anterior chest, the nurse begins in the supraclavicular area and proceeds downward, from one intercostal space to the next. Dullness noted to the left of the sternum between the third and fifth intercostal spaces is a normal finding, because that is the location of the heart. Similarly, there is a normal span of liver dullness below the lung at the right costal margin (Bickley, 2013).

The anterior and lateral thorax is examined with the patient in a supine position. If the patient cannot sit up, percussion of the posterior thorax is performed with the patient positioned on the side.

Dullness over the lung occurs when air-filled lung tissue is replaced by fluid or solid tissue. Table 22-4 reviews percussion sounds and their characteristics.

DIAPHRAGMATIC EXCURSION. The normal resonance of the lung stops at the diaphragm. The position of the diaphragm is different during inspiration and expiration.

To assess the position and motion of the diaphragm, the nurse instructs the patient to take a deep breath and hold it while the maximal descent of the diaphragm is percussed. The point at which the percussion note at the midscapular line changes from resonance to dullness is marked with a pen. The patient is then instructed to exhale fully and hold it while the nurse again percusses downward to the dullness of the diaphragm. This point is also marked. The distance between the two markings indicates the range of motion of the diaphragm.

Maximal excursion of the diaphragm may be as much as 8 to 10 cm (3 to 4 in) in healthy, tall young men, but for most people, it is usually 5 to 7 cm (2 to 2.75 in). Normally, the diaphragm is about 2 cm (0.75 in) higher on the right because of the location of the liver. Decreased diaphragmatic excursion may occur with pleural effusion. Atelectasis, diaphragmatic paralysis, or pregnancy may account for a diaphragm that is positioned high in the thorax (Bickley, 2013).

Thoracic Auscultation

Assessment concludes with auscultation of the anterior, posterior, and lateral thorax. Auscultation is useful in assessing the flow of air through the bronchial tree and in evaluating the presence of fluid or solid obstruction in the lung. The nurse auscultates for normal breath sounds, adventitious sounds, and voice sounds.

The nurse places the diaphragm of the stethoscope firmly against the chest wall as the patient breathes slowly and deeply through the mouth. Corresponding areas of the chest are auscultated in a systematic fashion from the apices to the bases and along midaxillary lines. The

TABLE 22-4 Characteristics of Percussion Sounds

Sound	Relative Intensity	Relative Pitch	Relative Duration	Location Example	Examples
Flatness	Soft	High	Short	Thigh	Large pleural effusion
Dullness	Medium	Medium	Medium	Liver	Lobar pneumonia
Resonance	Loud	Low	Long	Normal lung	Simple chronic bronchitis
Hyperresonance	Very loud	Lower	Longer	None normally	Emphysema, pneumothorax
Tympany	Loud	High[a]	Medium	Gastric air bubble or puffed-out cheek	Large pneumothorax

[a]Distinguished mainly by its musical timbre.

Adapted from Bickley, L. S. (2013). *Bates' guide to physical examination and history taking* (11th ed.). Philadelphia, PA: Wolters Kluwer Health/Lippincott Williams & Wilkins.

TABLE 22-5 Breath Sounds

	Duration of Sounds	Intensity of Expiratory Sound	Pitch of Expiratory Sound	Locations Where Heard Normally
Vesicular[a]	Inspiratory sounds last longer than expiratory ones	Soft	Relatively low	Entire lung field except over the upper sternum and between the scapulae
Bronchovesicular	Inspiratory and expiratory sounds are about equal	Intermediate	Intermediate	Often in the first and second interspaces anteriorly and between the scapulae (over the main bronchus)
Bronchial	Expiratory sounds last longer than inspiratory ones	Loud	Relatively high	Over the manubrium, if heard at all
Tracheal	Inspiratory and expiratory sounds are about equal	Very loud	Relatively high	Over the trachea in the neck

[a]The thickness of the bars indicates intensity of breath sounds; the steeper their incline, the higher the pitch of the sounds.

Adapted from Bickley, L. S. (2013). *Bates' guide to physical examination and history taking* (11th ed.). Philadelphia, PA: Wolters Kluwer Health/Lippincott Williams & Wilkins.

sequence of auscultation and the positioning of the patient are similar to those used for percussion. It often is necessary to listen to two full inspirations and expirations at each anatomic location for valid interpretation of the sound heard. Repeated deep breaths may result in symptoms of hyperventilation (e.g., lightheadedness); this is avoided by having the patient rest and breathe normally periodically during the examination.

BREATH SOUNDS. Normal breath sounds are distinguished by their location over a specific area of the lung and are identified as vesicular, bronchovesicular, and bronchial (tubular) breath sounds (Table 22-5).

The location, quality, and intensity of breath sounds are determined during auscultation. When airflow is decreased by bronchial obstruction (atelectasis) or when fluid (pleural effusion) or tissue (obesity) separates the air passages from the stethoscope, breath sounds are diminished or absent. For example, the breath sounds of the patient with emphysema are faint or often completely inaudible. When they are heard, the expiratory phase is prolonged. In the obese or morbidly obese patient, breath sounds may be inaudible. Bronchial and bronchovesicular sounds that are audible anywhere except over the main bronchus in the lungs signify pathology, usually indicating consolidation in the lung (e.g., pneumonia, heart failure). This finding requires further evaluation.

ADVENTITIOUS SOUNDS. An abnormal condition that affects the bronchial tree and alveoli may produce adventitious (additional) sounds. Adventitious sounds are divided into two categories: discrete, noncontinuous sounds (**crackles**), and continuous musical sounds (**wheezes**) (Table 22-6). The duration of the sound is the important distinction to make in identifying the sound as noncontinuous or continuous.

VOICE SOUNDS. The sound heard through the stethoscope as the patient speaks is known as vocal resonance. The nurse should assess voice sounds when abnormal breath sounds are auscultated. The vibrations produced in the larynx are transmitted to the chest wall as they pass through the bronchi and alveolar tissue. Voice sounds are evaluated by having the patient repeat "ninety-nine" or "eee" while the nurse listens with the stethoscope in corresponding areas of the chest from the apices to the bases. With normal physiology, the sounds are faint and indistinct. Pathology that increases lung density, such as pneumonia and pulmonary edema, alters this normal physiologic response and may result in the following sounds:

- **Bronchophony** describes vocal resonance that is more intense and clearer than normal.
- **Egophony** describes voice sounds that are distorted. It is best appreciated by having the patient repeat the letter E. The distortion produced by consolidation transforms the sound into a clearly heard A rather than E.
- **Whispered pectoriloquy** describes the ability to clearly and distinctly hear whispered sounds that should not normally be heard.

Whenever an abnormality is detected on examination, it should be evident using more than one assessment method. A change in tactile fremitus is more subtle and can be missed, but bronchophony can be noted loudly and clearly.

Interpreting Findings

The physical findings for the most common respiratory diseases are summarized in Table 22-7.

Assessment of Respiratory Function in the Acutely or Critically Ill Patient

Assessment of respiratory status is essential for the well-being of the patient who is acutely or critically ill (Sole et al., 2013). Often, such a patient is intubated and receiving mechanical ventilation. This requires that the nurse have expertise in physical assessment, be skilled in monitoring techniques, and be knowledgeable about possible ventilator-induced lung injury (Morris, Whitmer, & Mcintosh, 2013). The nurse reviews the patient's health history, including the history of disorders affecting lung function, signs, and symptoms, and exposure to medications and other agents that can affect the respiratory status. The nurse also observes the patient's respiratory status

TABLE 22-6 Abnormal (Adventitious) Breath Sounds

Breath Sound	Description	Etiology
Crackles		
Crackles in general	Soft, high-pitched, discontinuous popping sounds that occur during inspiration (while usually heard on inspiration, they may also be heard on expiration); may or may not be	Secondary to fluid in the airways or alveoli or to delayed opening of collapsed alveoli Associated with heart failure and pulmonary fibrosis
Coarse crackles	Discontinuous popping sounds heard in early inspiration; harsh, moist sound originating in the large bronchi	Associated with obstructive pulmonary disease
Fine crackles	Discontinuous popping sounds heard in late inspiration; sounds like hair rubbing together; originates in the alveoli	Associated with interstitial pneumonia, restrictive pulmonary disease (e.g., fibrosis); fine crackles in early inspiration are associated with bronchitis or pneumonia
Wheezes		
Wheezes in general	Usually heard on expiration, but may be heard on inspiration depending on the cause	Associated with bronchial wall oscillation and changes in airway diameter Associated with chronic bronchitis or bronchiectasis
Sonorous wheezes (rhonchi)	Deep, low-pitched rumbling sounds heard primarily during expiration; caused by air moving through narrowed tracheobronchial passages	Associated with secretions or tumour
Sibilant wheezes	Continuous, musical, high-pitched, whistle-like sounds heard during inspiration and expiration caused by air passing through narrowed or partially obstructed airways; may clear with coughing	Associated with bronchospasm, asthma, and buildup of secretions
Friction Rubs		
Pleural friction rub	Harsh, crackling sound, like two pieces of leather being rubbed together (sound imitated by rubbing the thumb and finger together near the ear) Heard during inspiration alone or during both inspiration and expiration May subside when the patient holds breath; coughing will not clear sound Best heard over the lower lateral anterior surface of the thorax Sound can be enhanced by applying pressure to the chest wall with the diaphragm of the stethoscope	Secondary to inflammation and loss of lubricating pleural fluid

Adapted from Bickley, L. S. (2013). *Bates' guide to physical examination and history taking* (11th ed.). Philadelphia, PA: Wolters Kluwer Health/Lippincott Williams & Wilkins.

TABLE 22-7 Assessment Findings in Common Respiratory Disorders

Disorder	Tactile Fremitus	Percussion	Auscultation
Consolidation (e.g., pneumonia)	Increased	Dull	Bronchial breath sounds, crackles, bronchophony, egophony, whispered pectoriloquy
Bronchitis	Normal	Resonant	Normal to decreased breath sounds; possible scattered coarse crackles, rhonchi, or wheezes
Emphysema	Decreased	Hyperresonant	Absent or decreased breath sounds; possible crackles, wheezes, or rhonchi
Asthma	Decreased	Resonant to hyperresonant	Wheezes, occasional crackles
Pulmonary edema	Normal	Resonant	Crackles at lung bases, possibly wheezes
Pleural effusion	Decreased to absent but may be increased over large effusion	Dull to flat	Decreased to absent breath sounds, bronchial breath sounds sometimes heard atop of large effusion, possible pleural rub
Pneumothorax	Decreased to absent	Hyperresonant	Absent breath sounds, possible pleural rub
Atelectasis	Absent	Dull	Decreased to absent breath sounds; may be increased in right upper lobe atelectasis

Adapted from Bickley, L. S. (2013). *Bates' guide to physical examination and history taking* (11th ed.). Philadelphia, PA: Wolters Kluwer Health/Lippincott Williams & Wilkins.

to analyze and interpret a variety of clinical findings and laboratory test results. After checking the ventilator settings to make sure that they are set as prescribed and that alarms are always in the "on" position, the nurse must assess for patient–ventilator synchrony and for agitation, restlessness, and other signs of respiratory distress (nasal flaring, excessive use of intercostals and accessory muscles, uncoordinated movement of the chest and abdomen, and a report by the patient of shortness of breath). The nurse must note changes in the patient's vital signs and evidence of hemodynamic instability and report them to the physician, because they may indicate that the mechanical ventilation is ineffective or that the patient's status has deteriorated. It is necessary to assess the position of the patient to be certain that the head of the bed is elevated to prevent aspiration, especially if the patient is receiving enteral feedings. In addition, the patient's mental status should be assessed and compared to previous status. Lethargy and somnolence may be signs of increasing carbon dioxide levels and should not be considered insignificant, even if the patient is receiving sedation or analgesic agents.

Chest auscultation, percussion, and palpation are essential parts of the evaluation of the critically ill patient with or without mechanical ventilation. Assessment of the anterior and posterior lung fields is part of the nurse's routine evaluation. If the patient is recumbent, it is essential to turn the patient to assess all lung fields. Dependent areas must be assessed for normal breath sounds and adventitious sounds. Failure to examine the dependent areas of the lungs can result in missing the findings associated with disorders such as atelectasis or pleural effusion. Percussion is performed to assess for pleural effusion; if pleural effusion is present, the affected lung fields are dull to percussion and breath sounds are absent. A pleural friction rub may also be present.

Tests of the patient's respiratory status are easily performed at the bedside by measuring the respiratory rate (see earlier discussion), tidal volume, minute ventilation, vital capacity, inspiratory force, and compliance. These tests are particularly important for patients who are at risk for pulmonary complications, including those who have undergone chest or abdominal surgery, have had prolonged anesthesia, have pre-existing pulmonary disease, and those who are older adults or obese. These tests are also used routinely for mechanically ventilated patients.

The patient whose chest expansion is limited by external restrictions such as obesity or abdominal distention and who cannot breathe deeply because of postoperative pain or sedation will inhale and exhale a low volume of air (referred to as low tidal volumes). Prolonged hypoventilation at low tidal volumes can produce alveolar collapse (atelectasis). The amount of air remaining in the lungs after a normal expiration (FRC) decreases, the ability of the lungs to expand (compliance) is reduced, and the patient must breathe faster to maintain the same degree of tissue oxygenation. These events can be exaggerated in patients who have pre-existing pulmonary diseases, in older adult patients whose airways are less compliant because the small airways may collapse during expiration, or in patients who have obesity, who have relatively low tidal volumes even when healthy. More details of the assessment of the patient with lung disease, including arterial blood gas (ABG) analysis, are described in subsequent chapters in this unit and in Chapter 16.

NURSING ALERT

The nurse should not rely only on visual inspection of the rate and depth of a patient's respiratory excursions to determine the adequacy of ventilation. Respiratory excursions may appear normal or exaggerated due to an increased work of breathing, but the patient may actually be moving only enough air to ventilate the dead space. If there is any question regarding adequacy of ventilation, auscultation or pulse oximetry (or both) should be used for additional assessment of respiratory status.

Tidal Volume

The volume of each breath is referred to as the tidal volume (see Table 22-1 to review lung capacities and volumes). A spirometer is an instrument that can be used at the bedside to measure volumes. If the patient is breathing through an endotracheal tube or tracheostomy, the spirometer is directly attached to it and the exhaled volume is obtained from the reading on the gauge. In other patients, the spirometer is attached to a face mask or a mouthpiece positioned so that it is airtight, and the exhaled volume is measured.

The tidal volume may vary from breath to breath. To ensure that the measurement is reliable, it is important to measure the volumes of several breaths and to note the range of tidal volumes, together with the average tidal volume.

Minute Ventilation

Respiratory rates and tidal volume alone are unreliable indicators of adequate ventilation, because both can vary widely from breath to breath. However, together the tidal volume and respiratory rate are important because the minute ventilation, which is useful in detecting respiratory failure, can be determined from them. Minute ventilation is the volume of air expired per minute. It is equal to the product of the tidal volume in litres multiplied by the respiratory rate or frequency. In practice, the minute ventilation is not calculated but is measured directly using a spirometer. In a patient receiving mechanical ventilation, minute volume is often monitored by the ventilator and can be viewed on the monitoring screen.

Minute ventilation may be decreased by a variety of conditions that result in hypoventilation. When the minute ventilation falls, alveolar ventilation in the lungs also decreases, and the $PaCO_2$ increases. Risk factors for hypoventilation are listed in Chart 22-9.

Vital Capacity

Vital capacity is measured by having the patient take in a maximal breath and exhale fully through a spirometer. The normal value depends on the patient's age, gender, body build, and weight.

CHART 22-9

Risk Factors for Hypoventilation

- Limited neurologic impulses transmitted from the brain to the respiratory muscles, as in spinal cord trauma, cerebrovascular accidents, tumours, myasthenia gravis, Guillain–Barré syndrome, polio, and drug overdose
- Depressed respiratory centres in the medulla, as with anesthesia, sedation, and drug overdose
- Limited thoracic movement (kyphoscoliosis), limited lung movement (pleural effusion, pneumothorax), or reduced functional lung tissue (chronic pulmonary diseases, severe pulmonary edema)

Adapted from Bulbul, Y., Ayik, S., Ozlu, T., et al. (2014). Frequency and predictors of obesity hypoventilation in hospitalized patients at a tertiary health care institution. *Annals of Thoracic Medicine*, *9*(2), 87–91; Karez, M., & Papadakos, P. J. (2013). Respiratory complications in the postanesthesia care unit: A review of pathophysiological mechanisms. *Canadian Journal of Respiratory Therapy*, *49*(4), 21–29.

NURSING ALERT

Most patients can generate a vital capacity twice the volume they normally breathe in and out (tidal volume). If the vital capacity is less than 10 mL/kg, the patient will be unable to sustain spontaneous ventilation and will require respiratory assistance.

When the vital capacity is exhaled at a maximal flow rate, the forced vital capacity (FVC) is measured. Most patients can exhale at least 80% of their vital capacity in 1 second (forced expiratory volume in 1 second, or FEV_1) and almost all of it in 3 seconds (FEV_3). A reduction in FEV_1 suggests abnormal pulmonary air flow. If the patient's FEV_1 and FVC are proportionately reduced, maximal lung expansion is restricted in some way. If the reduction in FEV_1 greatly exceeds the reduction in FVC (FEV_1/FVC less than 85%), the patient may have some degree of airway obstruction.

Inspiratory Force

Inspiratory force evaluates the effort the patient is making during inspiration. It does not require patient cooperation and therefore is a useful measurement in the unconscious patient. The equipment needed for this measurement includes a manometer that measures negative pressure and adapters that are connected to an anesthesia mask or a cuffed endotracheal tube. The manometer is attached and the airway is completely occluded for 10 to 20 seconds while the inspiratory efforts of the patient are registered on the manometer. The normal inspiratory pressure is about 100 cm H_2O. If the negative pressure registered after 15 seconds of occluding the airway is less than about 25 cm H_2O, mechanical ventilation is usually required because the patient lacks sufficient muscle strength for deep breathing or effective coughing.

Diagnostic Evaluation

A wide range of diagnostic studies may be performed in patients with respiratory conditions. The nurse should educate the patient on the purpose of the studies, what to expect, and any possible side effects related to these examinations prior to testing. The nurse should note trends in results because they provide information about disease progression as well as the patient's response to therapy.

Pulmonary Function Tests

Pulmonary function tests (PFTs) are routinely used in patients with chronic respiratory disorders to aid diagnosis. They are performed to assess respiratory function and to determine the extent of dysfunction, response to therapy, and as screening tests in potentially hazardous industries, such as coal mining and those that involve exposure to asbestos and other noxious irritants. PFTs are also used prior to surgery to screen patients who are scheduled for thoracic and upper abdominal surgical procedures, patients who have obesity, and symptomatic patients with a history suggesting high risk. Such tests include measurements of lung volumes, ventilatory function, and the mechanics of breathing, diffusion, and gas exchange.

PFTs generally are performed by a technician using a spirometer that has a volume-collecting device attached to a recorder that demonstrates volume and time simultaneously. Several tests are carried out because no single measurement provides a complete picture of pulmonary function. The most frequently used PFTs are described in Table 22-8. Technology is available that allows for more complex assessment of pulmonary function. Methods include exercise tidal flow–volume loops, negative expiratory pressure, nitric oxide, forced oscillation, and diffusing capacity for helium or carbon monoxide. These assessment methods allow for detailed evaluation of expiratory flow limitations and airway inflammation.

PFT results are interpreted on the basis of the degree of deviation from normal, taking into consideration the patient's height, weight, age, gender, and ethnicity. Because there is a wide range of normal values, PFTs may not detect early localized changes. The patient with respiratory symptoms usually undergoes a complete diagnostic evaluation, even if the results of PFTs are "normal." Patients with respiratory disorders may be taught how to measure their peak flow rate (which reflects maximal expiratory flow) at home using a spirometer. This allows them to monitor the progress of therapy, to alter medications and other interventions as needed on the basis of caregiver guidelines, and to notify the primary provider if there is inadequate response to their own interventions. (Instructions for home care education are described in Chapter 25, which discusses asthma.)

Arterial Blood Gas Studies

ABG studies aid in assessing the ability of the lungs to provide adequate oxygen and remove carbon dioxide, which reflects ventilation, and the ability of the kidneys to reabsorb or excrete bicarbonate ions to maintain normal body pH, which reflects metabolic states. ABG levels are

TABLE 22-8 Pulmonary Function Tests

Term Used	Symbol	Description	Remarks
Forced vital capacity	FVC	Vital capacity performed with a maximally forced expiratory effort	FVC is often reduced in COPD because of air trapping.
Forced expiratory volume (qualified by subscript indicating the time interval in seconds)	FEV_t (usually FEV_1)	Volume of air exhaled in the specified time during the performance of FVC; FEV_1 is volume exhaled in 1 second	A valuable clue to the severity of the expiratory airway obstruction
Ratio of timed forced expiratory volume to FVC	FEV_t/FVC%, usually FEV_1/FVC%	FEV_t expressed as a percentage of the FVC	Another way of expressing the presence or absence of airway obstruction
Forced expiratory flow	$FEF_{200-1,200}$	Mean forced expiratory flow between 200 and 1,200 mL of the FVC	An indicator of large airway obstruction
Forced midexpiratory flow	$FEF_{25-75\%}$	Mean forced expiratory flow during the middle half of the FVC	Slowed in small airway obstruction
Forced end expiratory flow	$FEF_{75-85\%}$	Mean forced expiratory flow during the terminal portion of the FVC	Slowed in obstruction of smallest airways
Maximal voluntary ventilation	MVV	Volume of air expired in a specified period (12 seconds) during repetitive maximal effort	An important factor in exercise tolerance

COPD, chronic obstructive pulmonary disease.

obtained through an arterial puncture at the radial, brachial, or femoral artery or through an indwelling arterial catheter. Pain (related to nerve injury or noxious stimulation), infection, hematoma, and hemorrhage are potential complications that may be associated with obtaining ABGs (Perry, Potter, & Ostendorf, 2014). ABG levels are discussed in detail in Chapter 16.

Patients whose ABG levels are monitored repeatedly with blood obtained from arterial punctures should receive an explanation of the purpose of the procedure. Because of the nerves in arterial walls, patients often experience pain with repeated ABG level checks but are often unaware of the purpose of the puncture and the fact that the ABG results could make a major difference in their treatment.

Pulse Oximetry

Pulse oximetry, or SpO_2, is a noninvasive method of continuously monitoring the **oxygen saturation** of hemoglobin (SaO_2). Although pulse oximetry does not replace blood gas analysis, it is an effective tool to monitor for subtle or sudden changes in SaO_2 and can easily be used in the home and various health care settings.

A probe or sensor is attached to the fingertip (see Fig. 22-12), forehead, earlobe, or bridge of the nose. The sensor detects changes in oxygen saturation levels by monitoring light signals generated by the oximeter and reflected by blood pulsing through the tissue at the probe. Normal SpO_2 values are more than 95%. Values less than 90% indicate that the tissues are not receiving enough oxygen, in which case further evaluation is needed. SpO_2 values are unreliable in cardiac arrest, shock, and other states of low perfusion (e.g., sepsis, peripheral vascular disease, hypothermia), and when vasoconstrictor medications have been used (Chan, Chan, & Chan, 2013). Additional causes of inaccurate pulse oximetry results include anemia, abnormal hemoglobin, high carbon monoxide level, the use of dyes (e.g., methylene blue), or if the patient has dark skin or is wearing nail polish. Bright light, particularly sunlight, fluorescent and xenon lights, and patient movement (including shivering) also affect accuracy. SpO_2 values cannot reliably detect hypoventilation when supplemental oxygen is in use (Chan et al., 2013).

Cultures

Throat, nasal, and nasopharyngeal cultures can identify pathogens responsible for respiratory infections, such as pharyngitis. Throat cultures are performed in adults with severe or ongoing sore throats accompanied by fever and lymph node enlargement and are most useful in detecting streptococcal infection. Rapid strep tests are now available that can provide results within 15 minutes, often replacing the need for throat cultures. Other sources of infection, such as *Staphylococcus aureus* or *Haemophilus influenzae*, are detected via nasal or nasopharyngeal cultures. Ideally, all cultures should be obtained prior to the initiation of antibiotic therapy. Results usually take between 48 and 72 hours, with preliminary reports available usually within 24 hours. Cultures may be repeated to assess a patient's response to therapy (Pagana & Pagana, 2013).

Sputum Studies

Sputum is obtained for analysis to identify pathogenic organisms and to determine whether malignant cells are present. A sputum specimen also may be obtained to assess for hypersensitivity states (in which there is an increase in eosinophils). Periodic sputum examinations may be necessary for patients receiving antibiotics, corticosteroids, and immunosuppressive medications for prolonged periods because these agents are associated with opportunistic infections.

Expectoration is the usual method for collecting a sputum specimen. The patient is instructed to clear the nose and throat and rinse the mouth to decrease contamination

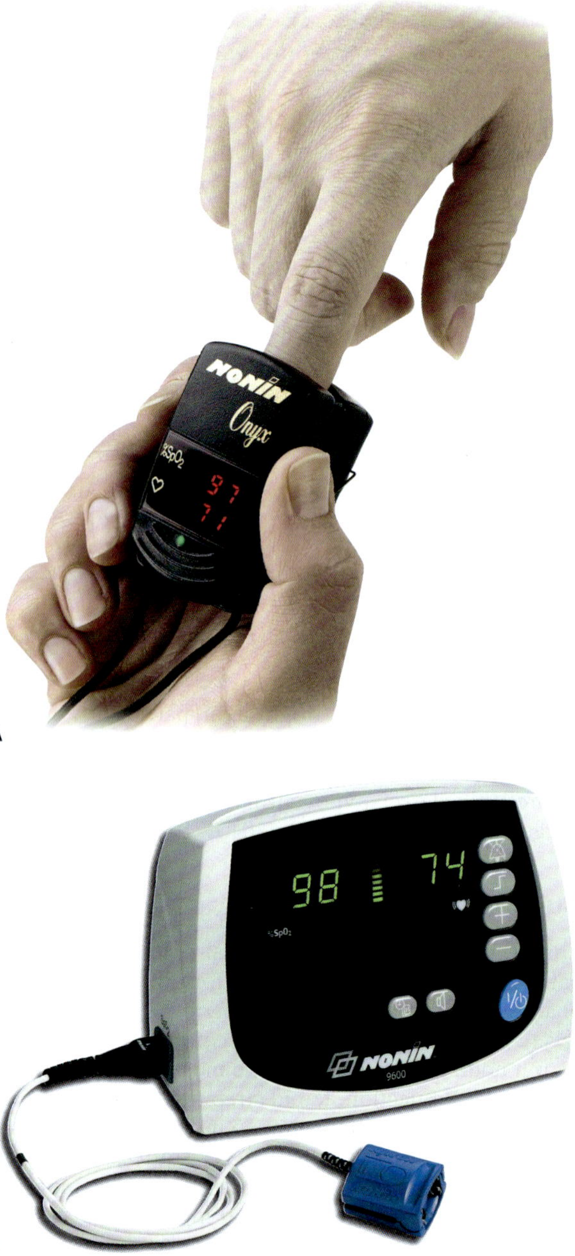

A

B

FIGURE 22-12. Measuring blood oxygenation with pulse oximetry reduces the need for invasive procedures, such as drawing blood for analysis of oxygen levels. **A:** Self-contained digital fingertip pulse oximeter, which incorporates the sensor and the display into one unit. **B:** Table-top model with sensor attached. Memory permits tracking heart rate and oxygen saturation over time.

of the sputum. After taking a few deep breaths, the patient coughs (rather than spits), using the diaphragm, and expectorates into a sterile container.

If the sputum cannot be raised spontaneously, the patient often can be induced to cough deeply by breathing an irritating aerosol of supersaturated saline, propylene glycol, or some other agent delivered with an ultrasonic nebulizer. Other methods of collecting sputum specimens include endotracheal aspiration, bronchoscopic removal, bronchial brushing, transtracheal aspiration, and gastric aspiration (the last is usually done for tuberculosis organisms; see Chapter 24). Generally, the deepest specimens (those from the base of the lungs) are obtained in the early morning after they have accumulated overnight.

The specimen is delivered to the laboratory within 2 hours by the patient or nurse. Allowing the specimen to stand for several hours in a warm room results in the overgrowth of contaminant organisms and may make it difficult to identify the pathogenic organisms (especially *Mycobacterium tuberculosis*). The home care nurse may assist patients who need help obtaining the sample or who cannot deliver the specimen to the laboratory in a timely fashion.

Imaging Studies

Imaging studies, including x-rays, computed tomography (CT), magnetic resonance imaging (MRI), contrast studies, and radioisotope diagnostic scans may be part of any diagnostic workup, ranging from a determination of the extent of infection in sinusitis to tumour growth in cancer.

Chest X-Ray

Normal pulmonary tissue is radiolucent because it consists mostly of air and gases; therefore, densities produced by fluid, tumours, foreign bodies, and other pathologic conditions can be detected by x-ray examination. In the absence of symptoms, a chest x-ray may reveal an extensive pathologic process in the lungs. The routine chest x-ray consists of two views: the posteroanterior projection and the lateral projection. Chest x-rays are usually obtained after full inspiration because the lungs are best visualized when they are well aerated. In addition, the diaphragm is at its lowest level and the largest expanse of lung is visible. Patients, therefore, need to be able to take a deep breath and hold it without discomfort. Chest x-rays are contraindicated in pregnant women.

Nursing Interventions

The nurse should notify the patient that chest x-rays do not require fasting, nor typically cause pain. However, in order to best visualize the lungs, the patient must be able to take a deep breath and hold it without discomfort, while the technician takes the images. The patient will be positioned in a standing, sitting, or recumbent position, in order to obtain the appropriate view of the chest (posterior–anterior, lateral, oblique, or decubitus position). The patient will be asked to wear a gown, remove metal objects from the chest, such as necklaces, and may be given a lead shield to minimize radiation exposure to the thyroid gland, ovaries, or testicles (Pagana & Pagana, 2013).

Computed Tomography

A CT is an imaging method in which the lungs are scanned in successive layers by a narrow-beam x-ray. The images produced provide a cross-sectional view of the chest. Whereas a chest x-ray shows major contrasts between body densities such as bone, soft tissue, and air, a CT scan can distinguish fine tissue density. A CT scan may be used to define pulmonary nodules and small tumours adjacent to pleural surfaces that are not visible on routine chest x-rays and to demonstrate mediastinal abnormalities and hilar adenopathy, which are difficult to visualize with other techniques. Contrast agents are useful when evaluating the mediastinum and its contents, particularly its vasculature. Advancements in CT scanning technology, referred to as multidetection, spiral, or helical CT, enable the chest to be scanned quickly while generating an extensive number of images that can generate a three-dimensional analysis (Pagana & Pagana, 2013). CT pulmonary angiography is now used routinely in place of catheter angiography to diagnose PE (York, Kane, Smith, et al., 2015). Contraindications include allergy to dye, pregnancy, claustrophobia, and morbid obesity, whereas potential complications include acute kidney injury and acidosis secondary to contrast (Pagana & Pagana, 2013).

Nursing Interventions

The nurse should inform patients preparing for CT scans that they will be required to remain supine and still for a short period, typically less than 30 minutes, while a body scanner surrounds them and takes multiple images. Patients typically do not experience claustrophobia during CT scanning but can be given antianxiety medications preprocedure if this is a concern. If a contrast dye is required, patients will need to stay *nil per os* (NPO) for 4 hours prior to the examination. In this case, the nurse should also assess for allergies to iodine or shellfish (Pagana & Pagana, 2013).

Magnetic Resonance Imaging

MRI is similar to a CT scan except that magnetic fields and radiofrequency signals are used instead of radiation. MRI is able to better distinguish between normal and abnormal tissues than CT and, therefore, yields a much more detailed diagnostic image. MRI is used to characterize pulmonary nodules; to help stage bronchogenic carcinoma (assessment of chest wall invasion); and to evaluate inflammatory activity in interstitial lung disease, acute PE, and chronic thrombolytic pulmonary hypertension. Contraindications for MRI include morbid obesity, claustrophobia, confusion and agitation, and having implanted metal or metal support devices that are considered unsafe (Pagana & Pagana, 2013). Various labels and icons are used to indicate whether a medical device is safe or unsafe for use during MRI. Recent improvements in technology have contributed to the design of certain medical devices, such as infusion pumps and ventilators, deemed safe for the MRI room. The nurse should consult with specially trained MRI personnel to clarify the safety of various devices (Wells & Murphy, 2014). Gadolinium-based contrast agents used during MRI may potentially lead to nephrogenic systemic fibrosis in patients with reduced kidney function (Pagana & Pagana, 2013).

Nursing Interventions

Patients scheduled for MRI should be instructed to remove all metal items such as hearing aids, hair clips, and medication patches with metallic foil components (e.g., nicotine patches). Prior to the MRI, the nurse should assess for the presence of implanted metal devices, such as aneurysm clips or a cardiac pacemaker/defibrillator. The nurse should inform patients preparing for MRI that they will need to lie flat and remain still for between 30 to 90 minutes, while the table that they are on moves into a large tubular magnet. Patients should be notified that they will hear a loud humming or thumping noise. Earplugs are typically offered to patients to minimize this noise. Patients will be able to communicate with the MRI staff via a microphone and earphones. The nurse should clarify with the physician or the technologist if the ordered test requires the use of dye or the patient should remain NPO pre-examination. Patients who experience claustrophobia should be offered antianxiety medications preprocedure or be scheduled at a facility that uses an open MRI system (Pagana & Pagana, 2013).

Fluoroscopic Studies

Fluoroscopy is used to assist with invasive procedures, such as a chest needle biopsy or transbronchial biopsy, that are performed to identify lesions. It also may be used to study the movement of the chest wall, mediastinum, heart, and diaphragm; to detect diaphragm paralysis; and to locate lung masses.

Pulmonary Angiography

Pulmonary angiography is used to investigate congenital abnormalities of the pulmonary vascular tree, and less frequently PE, when less invasive tests are inconclusive, but there is a high clinical suspicion for PE (Ma, Yan, Zhou, et al., 2016). To visualize the pulmonary vessels, a radiopaque agent is injected through a catheter, which has been initially inserted into a vein (e.g., jugular, subclavian, brachial, or femoral vein) and then threaded into the pulmonary artery. Contraindications include allergy to the radiopaque dye, pregnancy, and bleeding abnormalities, whereas potential complications include acute kidney injury, acidosis, cardiac dysrhythmias, and bleeding (Pagana & Pagana, 2013).

Nursing Interventions

Prior to the angiography, the nurse should verify that informed consent has been obtained; assess for known allergies that may suggest allergies to radiopaque dye (e.g., iodine and shellfish); assess anticoagulation status and renal function; ensure that the patient has not eaten or had anything to drink preprocedurally as prescribed (normally for 6 to 8 hours); and administer preprocedure medications that may include antianxiety medications, secretion-reducing agents, and antihistamines. The nurse should instruct patients that they may experience a warm flushing sensation or chest pain during the injection of the dye. If an arterial puncture is necessary, the affected extremity will need to be immobilized for a certain amount of time depending on the size of the sheath that was used and the type of arterial closure device employed. Following the procedure, the nurse should closely monitor vital signs, level of consciousness, oxygen saturation, and the vascular access site for bleeding or hematoma, and perform frequent assessment of neurovascular status (Perry et al., 2014).

Radioisotope Diagnostic Procedures (Lung Scans)

Several types of lung scans—($\dot{V}/\dot{Q}$) scan, gallium scan, and positron emission tomography (PET)—are performed to assess normal lung functioning, pulmonary vascular supply, and gas exchange. Pregnancy is a contraindication for these scans.

A ($\dot{V}/\dot{Q}$) lung scan is performed by injecting a radioactive agent into a peripheral vein and then obtaining a scan of the chest to detect radiation. The isotope particles pass through the right side of the heart and are distributed into the lungs in proportion to the regional blood flow, making it possible to trace and measure blood perfusion through the lung. This procedure is used clinically to measure the integrity of the pulmonary vessels relative to blood flow and to evaluate blood flow abnormalities, as seen in PE. The imaging time is 20 to 40 minutes, during which the patient lies under the camera with a mask fitted over the nose and the mouth. This is followed by the ventilation component of the scan. The patient takes a deep breath of a mixture of oxygen and radioactive gas, which diffuses throughout the lungs. A scan is performed to detect ventilation abnormalities in patients who have regional differences in ventilation. It may be helpful in the diagnosis of bronchitis, asthma, inflammatory fibrosis, pneumonia, emphysema, and lung cancer. Ventilation without perfusion is seen with PE.

A gallium scan is a radioisotope lung scan used to detect inflammatory conditions, abscesses, adhesions, and the presence, location, and size of tumours. It is used to stage bronchogenic cancer and to document tumour regression after chemotherapy or radiation. Gallium is injected intravenously, and scans are obtained at intervals (e.g., 6, 24, and 48 hours) to evaluate gallium uptake by the pulmonary tissues.

PET is a radioisotope study with advanced diagnostic capabilities that is used to evaluate lung nodules for malignancy. PET can detect and display metabolic changes in tissue, distinguish normal tissue from diseased tissue (such as in cancer), differentiate viable from dead or dying tissue, show regional blood flow, and determine the distribution and fate of medications in the body. PET is more accurate in detecting malignancies than CT and has equivalent accuracy in detecting malignant nodules when compared with invasive procedures such as thoracoscopy. Images from PET scans are now being superimposed on CT and MRI images to enhance the accuracy of diagnosis (Pagana & Pagana, 2013).

Nursing Interventions

For each of these nuclear scans, the nurse should educate the patient on what to expect. Intravenous access is required. Sometimes, an enema is prescribed prior to a gallium scan to decrease its uptake in the gastrointestinal tract. Chest x-ray should be performed prior to a $(\dot{V}/\dot{Q})$ scanning. Patients should be told that $(\dot{V}/\dot{Q})$ and gallium scans require only a small amount of radioisotopes; therefore, radiation safety measures are not indicated. Normally, the patient may eat or drink prior to $(\dot{V}/\dot{Q})$ or gallium scans. Multiple factors can hinder the uptake of radioactive agents used for a PET scan. The nurse should instruct the patient to avoid caffeine, alcohol, and tobacco for 24 hours prior to the PET scan and abstain from food and fluids for 4 hours prior to the scan. Accurate results depend on an empty bladder; thus, a Foley catheter may be indicated. The nurse should encourage fluid intake postprocedure to facilitate the elimination of radioisotopes in the urine (Pagana & Pagana, 2013).

Endoscopic Procedures

Endoscopic procedures include bronchoscopy, thoracoscopy, and thoracentesis.

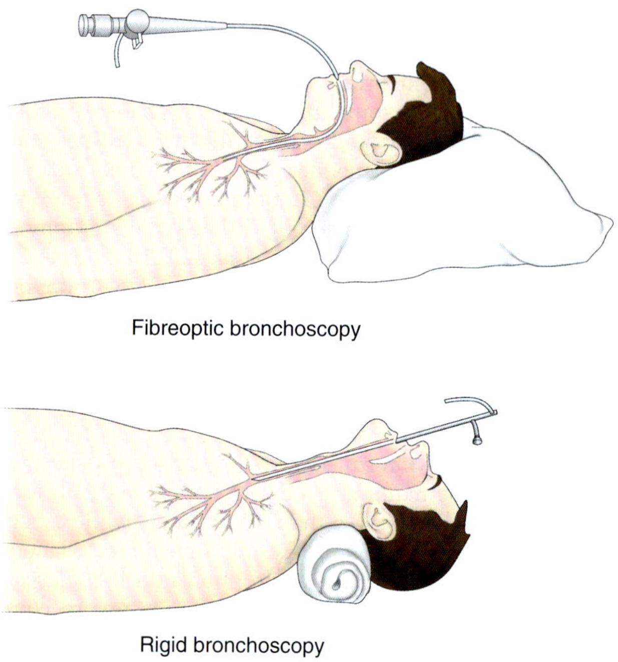

FIGURE 22-13. Endoscopic bronchoscopy permits visualization of bronchial structures. The bronchoscope is advanced into bronchial structures orally. Bronchoscopy permits the clinician not only to diagnose but also to treat various lung problems.

Bronchoscopy

Bronchoscopy is the direct inspection and examination of the larynx, trachea, and bronchi through either a flexible fibreoptic bronchoscope or a rigid bronchoscope (Fig. 22-13). The fibreoptic scope is used more frequently in current practice.

Procedure

The purposes of diagnostic bronchoscopy are: (1) to visualize tissues and determine the nature, location, and extent of the pathologic process; (2) to collect secretions for analysis and to obtain a tissue sample for diagnosis; (3) to determine whether a tumour can be resected surgically; and (4) to diagnose sources of hemoptysis.

Therapeutic bronchoscopy is used to: (1) remove foreign bodies or secretions from the tracheobronchial tree, (2) control bleeding, (3) treat postoperative atelectasis, (4) destroy and excise lesions, and (5) provide brachytherapy (endobronchial radiation therapy). It has also been used to insert stents to relieve airway obstruction that is caused by tumours or miscellaneous benign conditions or that occurs as a complication of lung transplantation.

The fibreoptic bronchoscope is a thin, flexible bronchoscope that can be directed into the segmental bronchi. Because of its small size, its flexibility, and its excellent optical system, it allows increased visualization of the peripheral airways and is ideal for diagnosing pulmonary lesions. Fibreoptic bronchoscopy allows biopsy of previously inaccessible tumours and can be performed at the bedside. It also can be performed through endotracheal or tracheostomy tubes of patients on ventilators. Cytologic examinations can be performed without surgical intervention.

The rigid bronchoscope is a hollow metal tube with a light at its end. It is used mainly for removing foreign substances, investigating the source of massive hemoptysis, or performing endobronchial surgical procedures. Rigid bronchoscopy is performed in the operating room, not at the bedside.

Possible complications of bronchoscopy include a reaction to the local anesthetic, oversedation, prolonged fever, infection, aspiration, vasovagal response, laryngospasm, bronchospasm, hypoxemia, pneumothorax, and bleeding (Pagana & Pagana, 2013; Perry et al., 2014).

Nursing Interventions

Before the procedure, the nurse should verify that informed consent has been obtained. Food and fluids are withheld for 4 to 8 hours before the test to reduce the risk of aspiration when the cough reflex is blocked by anesthesia. The nurse explains the procedure to the patient to reduce fear and decrease anxiety and then administers preoperative medications (usually atropine and a sedative or opioid) as prescribed to inhibit vagal stimulation (thereby guarding against bradycardia, dysrhythmias, and hypotension), suppress the cough reflex, sedate the patient, and relieve anxiety.

NURSING ALERT

Sedation given to patients with respiratory insufficiency may precipitate respiratory arrest.

The patient must remove dentures and other oral prostheses. The examination is usually performed under local anesthesia or moderate sedation; however, general anesthesia may be used for rigid bronchoscopy. A topical anesthetic such as lidocaine (xylocaine) is normally sprayed on the pharynx or dropped on the epiglottis and vocal cords and into the trachea to suppress the cough reflex and minimize discomfort.

After the procedure, the patient must take nothing by mouth until the cough reflex returns, because the preoperative sedation and local anesthesia impair the protective laryngeal reflex and swallowing. Once the patient demonstrates a cough reflex, the nurse may offer ice chips and eventually fluids. In the older adult patient, the nurse assesses for confusion and lethargy, which may be owing to the large doses of lidocaine given during the procedure. The nurse also monitors the patient's respiratory status and observes for hypoxia, hypotension, tachycardia, dysrhythmias, hemoptysis, and dyspnea. Any abnormality is reported promptly. A small amount of blood-tinged sputum and fever may be expected within the first 24 hours (Pagana & Pagana, 2013). The patient is not discharged from the recovery area until adequate cough reflex and respiratory status are present. The nurse instructs the patient and caregivers to report any shortness of breath or bleeding immediately.

Thoracoscopy

Thoracoscopy is a diagnostic procedure in which the pleural cavity is examined with an endoscope (Fig. 22-14).

Procedure

This procedure is performed in the operating room, normally under anesthesia. Small incisions are made into the pleural cavity in an intercostal space at the location

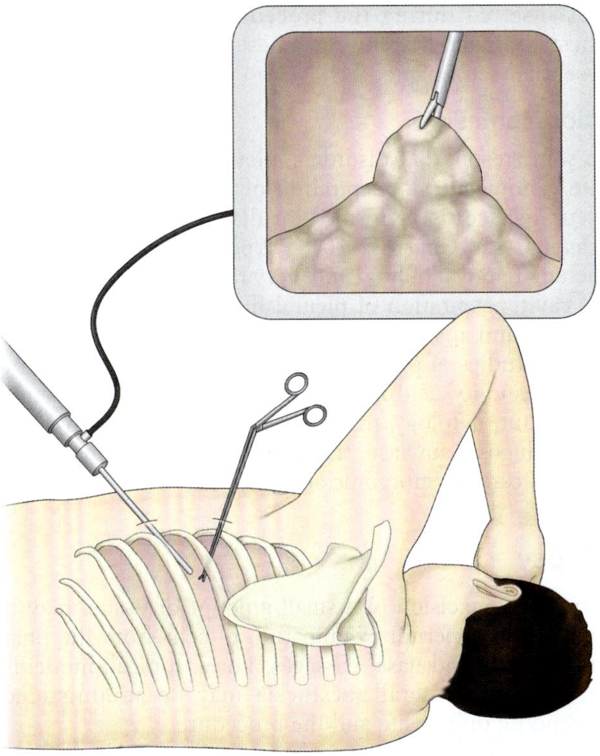

FIGURE 22-14. Endoscopic thoracoscopy. Like bronchoscopy, thoracoscopy uses fibreoptic instruments and video cameras for visualizing thoracic structures. Unlike bronchoscopy, thoracoscopy usually requires the surgeon to make a small incision before inserting the endoscope. A combined diagnostic–treatment procedure, thoracoscopy includes excising tissue for biopsy.

indicated by clinical and diagnostic findings. The fibreoptic mediastinoscope is inserted into the pleural cavity, any fluid present is aspirated, and the pleural cavity is inspected through the instrument. After the procedure, a chest tube may be inserted to facilitate re-expansion of the lung.

Thoracoscopy is primarily indicated in the diagnostic evaluation and treatment of pleural effusions, pleural disease, and tumour staging. Biopsies of the lesions and resection of tissues can be performed under visualization for diagnosis.

Thoracoscopic procedures have expanded with the availability of video monitoring, which permits improved visualization of the lung. Video-assisted thoracoscopy (VATS) may be used in the diagnosis and treatment of empyema, pleural effusion, pulmonary and pleural masses, and pneumothorax. Although VATS does not replace the need for thoracotomy in the treatment of some lung cancers, its use continues to grow, because it is less invasive than open surgical procedures, and hospitalization and recovery are shorter.

Nursing Interventions

The nurse should follow routine preoperative practices, such as ensuring that informed consent is obtained and that the patient remains NPO (has nothing by mouth) prior to the procedure. Postoperatively, the nurse should monitor vital signs, pain level, and respiratory status, and should look for signs of bleeding and infection at the incisional site. Shortness of breath may indicate a pneumothorax and should be reported immediately. If a chest tube was inserted during the procedure, monitoring of the chest drainage system and chest tube insertion site is essential (see Chapter 24).

Thoracentesis

In some respiratory disorders, pleural fluid may accumulate. Thoracentesis (aspiration of fluid and air from the pleural space) is performed for diagnostic or therapeutic reasons (see Chart 22-10). Purposes of the procedure include removal of fluid and, very rarely, air from the pleural cavity; aspiration of pleural fluid for analysis; pleural biopsy; and instillation of medication into the pleural space. Studies of pleural fluid include Gram stain culture and sensitivity, acid-fast staining and culture, differential cell count, cytology, pH, total protein, lactic dehydrogenase, glucose, amylase, triglycerides, and cancer markers such as carcinoembryonic antigen.

Biopsy

Biopsy, the excision of a small amount of tissue, may be performed to permit examination of cells from the pharynx, larynx, and nasal passages. Local, topical, moderate sedation, or general anesthesia may be administered, depending on the site and the procedure.

Pleural Biopsy

Pleural biopsy is accomplished by needle biopsy of the pleura or by pleuroscopy, a visual exploration through a fibreoptic bronchoscope inserted into the pleural space. Pleural biopsy is performed when there is pleural exudate of undetermined origin or when there is a need to culture or stain the tissue to identify tuberculosis or fungi.

Lung Biopsy Procedures

Lung biopsy is performed to obtain tissue for examination when other diagnostic testing indicates potential interstitial lung disease, such as cancer, infection, or sarcoidosis. Several nonsurgical lung biopsy techniques are used because they yield accurate information with low morbidity: transbronchial brushing or needle aspiration, transbronchial lung biopsy, and percutaneous (through-the-skin) needle biopsy. Possible complications for all methods include pneumothorax, pulmonary hemorrhage, and empyema (Pagana & Pagana, 2013).

Procedure

In transbronchial brushing, a fibreoptic bronchoscope is introduced into the bronchus under fluoroscopy. A small brush attached to the end of a flexible wire is inserted through the bronchoscope. Under direct visualization, the area under suspicion is brushed back and forth, causing cells to slough off and adhere to the brush. The catheter port of the bronchoscope may be used to irrigate the lung tissue with saline solution to secure material for additional studies. The brush is removed from the bronchoscope, and a slide is made for examination under the microscope. The brush may be cut off and sent to the pathology laboratory

CHART 22-10

GUIDELINES for Assisting the Patient Undergoing Thoracentesis

Equipment

- Thoracentesis tray (should include standard supplies needed to perform procedure)
- Sterile gloves
- Antiseptic solution
- Local anesthetic
- Sterile collection bottles, laboratory requisition forms, and labels

Implementation

NURSING ACTIONS	RATIONALE
1. Ascertain in advance that a chest x-ray or ultrasound has been ordered and completed and the consent form has been signed.	1. Chest x-ray films are used to localize fluid and air in the pleural cavity and to aid in determining the puncture site. When fluid is loculated (isolated in a pocket of pleural fluid), ultrasound scans are performed to help select the best site for needle aspiration.
2. Take "Time Out" with patient and healthcare providers. Verify patient's identity using at least two identifiers, not including the patient's room number. Verify purpose of procedure and procedure site; assess patient for allergies to latex, antiseptic, or local anesthetic; and review coagulation status (prothrombin time/international normalized ratio [INR] and platelet count).	2. Verification maintains patient safety and prevents potential complications such as allergic reactions and bleeding.
3. Inform the patient about the nature of the procedure as well as: a. The importance of remaining immobile. b. Pressure sensations to be experienced. c. That minimal discomfort is anticipated after the procedure.	3. An explanation helps to orient the patient to the procedure, assists the patient to mobilize resources, and provides an opportunity to ask questions and verbalize anxiety.

GUIDELINES for Assisting the Patient Undergoing Thoracentesis (Continued)

NURSING ACTIONS	RATIONALE
4. Obtain baseline vital signs, oxygen saturation, pain level, and respiratory status. Administer sedation if prescribed.	4. Provides preprocedure assessment data to guide sedation administration and postprocedure assessment. Sedation enables the patient to cooperate with the procedure and promotes relaxation.
5. Position the patient comfortably with adequate supports. If possible, place the patient upright or in one of the following positions: a. Sitting on the edge of the bed with the feet supported and arms on a padded over-the-bed table. b. Straddling a chair with arms and head resting on the back of the chair. c. Lying on the unaffected side with the head of the bed elevated 30 to 45 degrees if unable to assume a sitting position.	5. The upright position facilitates the removal of fluid that usually localizes at the base of the thorax. It expands the ribs and widens the intercostal space to aid needle insertion. A position of comfort helps the patient to relax and prevents patient movement that could contribute to potential complications.
6. Support and reassure the patient during the procedure. a. Prepare the patient for the cold sensation of skin antiseptic solution and for a pressure sensation from infiltration of local anesthetic agent. b. Encourage the patient to refrain from coughing.	6. Sudden and unexpected movement, such as coughing, by the patient can damage the visceral pleura and lung.
7. Expose the entire chest. The site for aspiration is visualized by chest x-ray and percussion. If fluid is in the pleural cavity, the thoracentesis site is determined by the chest x-ray, ultrasound scan, or fluoroscopy and physical findings, with attention to the site of maximal dullness on percussion.	7. If air is in the pleural cavity, the thoracentesis site is usually in the second or third intercostal space in the midclavicular line, because air rises in the thorax.
8. The procedure is performed under aseptic conditions. After the skin is cleansed, the physician uses a small-caliber needle to inject a local anesthetic slowly into the intercostal space.	8. An intradermal wheal is raised slowly; rapid injection causes pain. The parietal pleura is very sensitive and should be well infiltrated with anesthetic before the physician passes the thoracentesis needle through it.
9. The physician advances the thoracentesis needle with the syringe attached. When the pleural space is reached, suction may be applied with the syringe. a. A 20-mL syringe with a three-way stopcock is attached to the needle (one end of the adapter is attached to the needle and the other to the tubing leading to a receptacle that receives the fluid being aspirated). b. If a considerable quantity of fluid is removed, the needle is held in place on the chest wall with a small hemostat.	9. The use of a thoracentesis needle allows proper insertion. a. When a large quantity of fluid is withdrawn, a three-way stopcock serves to keep air from entering the pleural cavity. b. The hemostat steadies the needle on the chest wall. Sudden pleuritic chest pain or shoulder pain may indicate that the needle point is irritating the visceral or the diaphragmatic pleura.
10. After the needle is withdrawn, pressure is applied over the puncture site and a small, airtight, sterile dressing is fixed in place.	10. Pressure helps to stop bleeding, and the airtight dressing protects the site and prevents air from entering the pleural cavity.
11. Advise the patient that a chest x-ray will be obtained after thoracentesis and activity will be limited for the first hour.	11. A chest x-ray verifies that there is no pneumothorax.
12. Record the total amount of fluid withdrawn from the procedure and document the nature of the fluid, its color, and its viscosity. If indicated, prepare samples of fluid for laboratory evaluation. A specimen container with formalin may be needed for a pleural biopsy.	12. The fluid may be clear, serous, bloody, or purulent and provides clues to the pathology. Bloody fluid may indicate malignancy, whereas purulent fluid usually indicates an infection.
13. Monitor the patient at intervals for increasing respiratory rate; asymmetry in respiratory movement; dyspnea; diminished breath sounds; anxiety or restlessness; tightness in chest; uncontrollable cough; blood-tinged, frothy mucus; a rapid pulse; pain; and signs of hypoxemia.	13. Pneumothorax, tension pneumothorax, subcutaneous emphysema, and pyogenic infection are complications of a thoracentesis. Pulmonary edema or cardiac distress can occur after a sudden shift in mediastinal contents when large amounts of fluid are aspirated.

Adapted from Caple, C., & Heering, H. (2016). Thoractentesis: Assisting with. In D. Pravikoff (Ed.). *Nursing practice and skill.* Glendale, CA: CINAHL Information Systems.

for analysis. This procedure is especially useful in the immunologically compromised patient.

In transbronchial needle aspiration, a catheter with a needle is inserted into the tissue through the bronchoscope and aspirated, whereas in transbronchial lung biopsy, biting or cutting forceps are introduced by a fibreoptic bronchoscope to excise the tissue.

In percutaneous needle biopsy, a cutting needle or a spinal-type needle is used to obtain a tissue specimen for histologic study under fluoroscopic or CT guidance. Analgesia may be given before the procedure. The skin over the biopsy site is cleansed and anesthetized and a small incision is made. The biopsy needle is inserted through the incision into the pleura with the patient holding their breath in mid-expiration. The surgeon guides the needle into the periphery of the lesion and obtains a tissue sample from the mass.

Nursing Interventions

After the procedure, recovery and home care are similar to those for bronchoscopy and thoracoscopy. Nursing care involves monitoring the patient for complications such as shortness of breath, bleeding, or infection. In preparation for discharge, the patient and the family are instructed to report pain, shortness of breath, visible bleeding, redness of the biopsy site, or purulent drainage (pus) to the primary provider immediately. Patients who have undergone biopsy are often anxious because of the need for the biopsy and the potential findings; the nurse must consider this in providing postbiopsy care and patient education.

Lymph Node Biopsy

The scalene lymph nodes, which are enmeshed in the deep cervical pad of fat overlying the scalenus anterior muscle, drain the lungs and mediastinum and may show histologic changes from intrathoracic disease. If these nodes are palpable on physical examination, a scalene node biopsy may be performed. A biopsy of these nodes may be performed to detect spread of pulmonary disease to the lymph nodes and to establish a diagnosis or prognosis in such diseases as Hodgkin lymphoma, sarcoidosis, fungal disease, tuberculosis, and carcinoma.

Procedure

Mediastinoscopy is the endoscopic examination of the mediastinum for exploration and biopsy of mediastinal lymph nodes that drain the lungs; this examination does not require a thoracotomy. Biopsy is usually performed through a suprasternal incision. Mediastinoscopy is carried out to detect mediastinal involvement of pulmonary malignancy and to obtain tissue for diagnostic studies of other conditions (e.g., sarcoidosis).

An anterior mediastinotomy is thought to provide better exposure and diagnostic possibilities than a mediastinoscopy. An incision is made in the area of the second or third costal cartilage. The mediastinum is explored, and biopsies are performed on any lymph nodes found. Chest tube drainage is required after the procedure. Mediastinotomy is particularly valuable to determine whether a pulmonary lesion is resectable.

Nursing Interventions

Postprocedure care focuses on providing adequate oxygenation, monitoring for bleeding, and providing pain relief. The patient may be discharged a few hours after the chest drainage system is removed. The nurse should instruct the patient and the family about monitoring for changes in respiratory status, taking into consideration the impact of anxiety about the potential findings of the biopsy on their ability to remember those instructions.

Critical Thinking Exercises

1 A 48-year-old woman with a long history of smoking (40 pack-years) is scheduled for surgery under general anesthesia to remove a lump from her breast. In preparation for surgery, she is scheduled for PFTs, which she refuses to have because she says her breathing is fine and has nothing to do with her breasts. How would you respond to her statement? What impact does her 40 pack-year history of cigarette smoking have on your preoperative, intraoperative, and postoperative assessment?

2 You are obtaining a health history from a 62-year-old patient who is seeking health care because of a persistent cough and extreme fatigue. She mentions that she cannot keep up with her grandchildren and even gets out of breath when reading to them or talking to them on the phone. What specific information about signs and symptoms would you obtain during the health history? How would you modify your physical examination based on your observations? What initial laboratory tests would you anticipate will be ordered for this patient?

3 An 88-year-old man has been recently relocated because his family does not want him to live by himself. He has never been seen at this pulmonary clinic and is here to get acquainted with his new health care providers. He says his lungs are "no good" because he has smoked since he was 18 years old and was exposed to asbestos during the 15 years he worked in shipyards. He brought a folder from his previous health care provider with results of tests that were done during a hospitalization for pneumonia 2 years earlier: PFTs, ABGs, sputum cultures, chest x-ray, and CT scan of the chest. What questions will you ask him about his health history? What tests do you anticipate being repeated at this time and why?

4 A 70-year-old patient who has cancer of the lung has undergone a thoracentesis with removal of 750 mL of pleural fluid to relieve his shortness of breath. Soon after the procedure is completed, the patient reports that his shortness of breath has increased rather than decreased. Based on your knowledge of risks associated with thoracentesis, what assessment data would you obtain from this patient and report to the physician? What additional nursing measures are warranted for the patient at this time? What is the evidence on which your nursing interventions are based? How would you determine the strength of that evidence? How would you respond if the patient had been discharged an hour after the thoracentesis and provided this information to you by telephone from home?

REFERENCES AND SELECTED READINGS

Books

Bickley, L. S. (2013). *Bates' guide to physical examination and history taking* (11th ed.). Philadelphia, PA: Wolters Kluwer Health/Lippincott Williams & Wilkins.

Dudgeon, D. (2015). Dyspnea, terminal secretions, and cough. In B. R. Ferrel, N. Coyle, & J. A. Pace (Eds.). *Oxford textbook of palliative nursing* (4th ed.). Oxford: Oxford University Press.

Grossman, S., & Porth, C. M. (2014). *Porth's pathophysiology: Concepts of altered health states* (9th ed.). Philadelphia, PA: Wolters Kluwer Health/Lippincott Williams & Wilkins.

Pagana, K. S., & Pagana, T. J. (2013). *Mosby's diagnostic and laboratory test reference* (11th ed.). St. Louis, MO: Mosby Elsevier.

Perry, A. G., Potter, P. A., & Ostendorf, W. (2014). *Clinical nursing skills and techniques* (8th ed.). St. Louis, MO: Mosby Elsevier.

Porth, C. M. (2015). *Essentials of pathophysiology* (4th ed.). Philadelphia, PA: Wolters Kluwer Health/Lippincott Williams & Wilkins.

Sole, M. L., Klein, D. G., & Moseley, M. J. (2013). *Introduction to critical care nursing* (6th ed.). St. Louis, MO: Elsevier.

Tabloski, P. A. (2014). *Gerontological nursing* (3rd ed.). Boston: Pearson.

West, J. B., & Luks, A. M. (2016). *West's respiratory physiology: The essentials* (10th ed.). Philadelphia, PA: Wolters Kluwer Health/Lippincott Williams & Wilkins.

Journals

Arber, A., Clackson, C., & Dargan, S. (2013). Malignant pleural effusion in the palliative care setting. *International Journal of Palliative Nursing*, *19*(7), 320–325.

Baker, K., Barsamian, J., Leone, D., et al. (2013). Routine dyspnea assessment on unit admission. *American Journal of Nursing*, *113*(11), 42–49.

Bulbul, Y., Ayik, S., Ozlu, T., et al. (2014). Frequency and predictors of obesity hypoventilation in hospitalized patients at a tertiary health care institution. *Annals of Thoracic Medicine*, *9*(2), 87–91.

Chan, E. D., Chan, M. M., & Chan, M. M. (2013). Pulse oximetry: Understanding its basic principles facilitates appreciation of its limitations. *Respiratory Medicine*, *107*(6), 789–799.

Ferkol, T., & Schraufnagel, D. (2014). The global burden of respiratory disease. *Annals of the American Thoracic Society*, *11*(3), 404–406.

Hayen, A., Herigstad, M., & Pattinson, K. T. (2013). Understanding dyspnea as a complex individual experience. *Maturitas*, *76*(1), 45–50.

Helling, T. S., Martin, L. C., Martin, M., et al. (2014). Failure events in transition of care for surgical patients. *Journal of the American College of Surgeons*, *218*(4), 723–733.

Hrisanfow, E., & Hägglund, D. (2012). Impact of cough and urinary incontinence on quality of life in women and men with chronic obstructive pulmonary disease. *Journal of Clinical Nursing*, *22*(1-2), 97–105.

Kaufman, G. (2012). Asthma update: Recommendations for diagnosis, treatment and management. *Primary Health Care*, *22*(4), 32–39.

Luo, Q., Han, Q., Chen, X., et al. (2013). The diagnosis efficacy and safety of video-assisted thoracoscopy surgery (VATS) in undefined interstitial lung diseases: A retrospective study. *Journal of Thoracic Diseases*, *5*(3), 283–288.

Ma, Y., Yan, S., Zhou, L., et al. (2016). Competitive assessments of pulmonary embolism: Noninvasiveness versus the golden standard. *Vascular*, *24*(2), 217–224.

McLean, B. A. (2012). Acute respiratory failure and intensive measures. *Critical Care Nursing Clinics of North America*, *24*(3), 361–375.

Morris, L. L., Whitmer, A., & Mcintosh, E. (2013). Tracheostomy care and complications in the intensive care unit. *Critical Care Nurse*, *33*(5), 18–22, 24–31.

Nguyen, H. Q., Donesky, D., Reinke, L. F., et al. (2013). Internet-based dyspnea self-management support for patients with chronic obstructive pulmonary disease. *Journal of Pain and Symptom Management*, *46*(1), 43–55.

Philip, K., Richardson, R., & Cohen, M. (2013). Staff perceptions of respiratory rate measurement in a general hospital. *British Journal of Nursing*, *22*(10), 570–574.

Poot, B. (2014). Nurse-led chronic cough clinic: What is the impact on patient waiting times? *Kai Tiaki Nursing Research*, *5*(1), 17–20.

Ramly, E., Kaafarani, H. M. A., & Velmahos, G. C. (2015). The effect of aging on pulmonary function: Implications for monitoring and support of the surgical and trauma patient. *Surgical Clinics of North America*, *95*(1), 53–69.

Rutherford, J. D. (2013). Digital clubbing. *Circulation*, *127*(19), 1997–1999.

Wells, J. L., & Murphy, P. S. (2014). Clearing the runway: An innovative approach to preparing the intensive care unit patient for a magnetic resonance imaging scan. *Journal of Radiology Nursing*, *33*(3), 147–151.

York, N. L., Kane, C. J., Smith, C., et al. (2015). Care of the patient with an acute pulmonary embolism. *Dimensions of Critical Care Nursing*, *34*(1), 3–9.

Yorke, J. (2014). Breathlessness in the community: Part 1—assessment. *Journal of Community Nursing*, *28*(5), 83–90.

Resources

Canadian Lung Association: http://www.lung.ca.

National Heart, Lung, and Blood Institute: http://www.nhlbi.nih.gov/index.htm.

National Lung Health Education Program: http://www.nlhep.org.

Registered Nurses' Association of Ontario: http://www.rnao.org.

23 Management of Patients With Upper Respiratory Tract Disorders

Adapted by Tanya Heuver

Learning Objectives

On completion of this chapter, the learner will be able to:

1. Describe nursing management of patients with upper airway disorders.
2. Compare and contrast the upper respiratory tract infections (URTIs) with regard to cause, incidence, clinical manifestations, management, and the significance of preventive health care.
3. Use the nursing process as a framework for care of patients with upper airway infection.
4. Describe nursing management of the patient with epistaxis.
5. Use the nursing process as a framework for care of patients undergoing laryngectomy.

Upper respiratory tract disorders are those that involve the nose, paranasal sinuses, pharynx, larynx, trachea, or bronchi. Many of these conditions are relatively minor, and their effects are limited to mild and temporary discomfort and inconvenience for the patient. However, others are acute, severe, and life threatening and may require permanent alterations in breathing and speaking. Therefore, the nurse must have expert assessment skills, an understanding of the wide variety of disorders that may affect the upper airway, and an awareness of the impact of these alterations on patients. Because many of these disorders are treated outside the hospital or at home by patients themselves, patient teaching is an important aspect of nursing care. When caring for patients with acute, life-threatening disorders, the nurse needs highly developed assessment and clinical management skills, along with a focus on rehabilitation needs.

UPPER AIRWAY INFECTIONS

Upper airway infections are the most common cause of illness and affect most people on occasion. Some infections are acute, with symptoms that last several days; others are chronic, with symptoms that last for weeks or months or recur. Patients with these conditions seldom require hospitalization. However, nurses working in community settings or long-term care facilities may encounter patients who have these infections. Therefore, it is important for the nurse to recognize the signs and symptoms and to provide appropriate care.

Infections of the upper airway are also known as upper respiratory tract infections (URTIs); the common cold is the most frequently occurring example. URTIs occur when microorganisms such as viruses and bacteria are inhaled. There are many causative organisms, and people are susceptible throughout life. URTIs are the most common reason for seeking health care and for absences from school and work.

URTIs affect the nasal cavity; ethmoidal air cells; and frontal, maxillary, and sphenoid sinuses; as well as the pharynx, larynx, and trachea. About 90% of upper respiratory disorders stem from a viral infection of the upper respiratory passages and subsequent mucous membrane inflammation. On average, adults typically develop two to four URTIs per year because of the wide variety of respiratory viruses that circulate in the community. Although patients are rarely hospitalized for the treatment of URTIs, the nurse can influence patient outcomes in community settings and in long-term facilities through patient teaching. Special considerations with regard to URTIs in older adults are summarized in Chart 23-1.

Rhinitis

Rhinitis is a group of disorders characterized by inflammation and irritation of the mucous membranes of the nose. These conditions can have a significant impact on quality

CHART 23-1

Upper Respiratory Tract Disorders in Older Adults

- Upper respiratory infections in older adults may have more serious consequences if patients have concurrent medical problems that compromise their respiratory or immune status.
- Influenza causes exacerbations of chronic obstructive pulmonary disease and reduced pulmonary function.
- Antihistamines and decongestants used to treat upper respiratory disorders must be used cautiously in older adults because of their side effects and potential interactions with other medications.
- Of Americans 65 years and older, approximately 14.1% have chronic rhinosinusitis (CRS). With anticipated future growth in the older adult population, the need for endoscopic sinus surgery will increase. Older patients with CRS present with symptoms similar to those of younger adults and experience a similar degree of improvement and quality of life after endoscopic sinus surgery.
- The structure of the nose changes with aging; it lengthens and the tip droops from loss of cartilage. This can cause restriction in airflow and predispose older adult patients to geriatric rhinitis, characterized by increased thin, watery sinus drainage. These structural changes may also adversely affect the sense of smell.
- Laryngitis in older adults is common and may be secondary to gastroesophageal reflux disease (GERD). Older adults are more likely to have impaired esophageal peristalsis and a weaker esophageal sphincter. Treatment measures include sleeping with the head of the bed elevated and the use of medications such as histamine-2 receptor blockers (e.g., famotidine [Pepcid], ranitidine [Zantac]) or proton pump inhibitors (omeprazole [Prilosec]).
- Age-related loss of muscle mass and thinning of the mucous membranes can cause structural changes in the larynx that may change characteristics of the voice. In general, the pitch of voice becomes higher in older adult men and lower in older adult women. The voice also "thins" (decreased projection) and may sound tremulous. These changes should be discriminated from signs that could indicate pathologic conditions.

Adapted from American Academy of Otolaryngology. (2015). *Fact sheet: Sinusitis: Special considerations for aging patients*. Retrieved October 8, 2015, from www.entnet.org/content/sinusitis-special-considerations-aging-patients

of life and contribute to sinus, ear, and sleep problems and learning disorders. Rhinitis often coexists with other respiratory disorders, such as asthma. It affects between 10% and 30% of the population worldwide annually. Viral rhinitis, especially the common cold, affects approximately one billion individuals yearly (Krouse & Krouse, 2014).

Rhinitis may be acute or chronic, nonallergic or allergic. It is further classified as seasonal or perennial rhinitis, and is commonly associated with exposure to airborne particles such as dust, dander, or plant pollens in people who are allergic to these substances. Seasonal rhinitis occurs during pollen seasons, and perennial rhinitis occurs throughout the year. Allergic disorders, including allergic rhinitis, are described in detail in Chapter 53.

Pathophysiology

Rhinitis may be caused by a variety of factors, including changes in temperature or humidity; odours; infection; age; systemic disease; use of over-the-counter and prescribed

Glossary

alaryngeal communication: alternative modes of speaking that do not involve the normal larynx; used by patients whose larynx has been surgically removed

aphonia: impaired ability to use one's voice due to disease or injury to the larynx

apnea: cessation of breathing

carcinogen: agent that can cause cancer; carcinogens can be chemicals, viruses, hormones, ionizing radiation, or solid materials

dysphagia: difficulties in swallowing

epistaxis: hemorrhage from the nose due to rupture of tiny, distended vessels in the mucous membrane of any area of the nose

herpes simplex (cold sore): cutaneous viral infection with painful vesicles and erosions on the tongue, palate, gingiva, buccal membranes, or lips

laryngectomy: surgical removal of all or part of the larynx and surrounding structures

laryngitis: inflammation of the larynx; may be caused by voice abuse, exposure to irritants, or infectious organisms

nuchal rigidity: stiffness of the neck or inability to bend the neck

pharyngitis: inflammation of the throat; usually viral or bacterial in origin

rhinitis: inflammation of the mucous membranes of the nose; may be infectious, allergic, or inflammatory in origin

rhinitis medicamentosa: rebound nasal congestion commonly associated with overuse of over-the-counter nasal decongestants

rhinorrhea: drainage of a large amount of fluid from the nose

rhinosinusitis: inflammation of the nares and paranasal sinuses, including frontal, ethmoid, maxillary, and sphenoid sinuses; replaces the term "sinusitis"

tonsillitis: inflammation of the tonsils, usually due to an acute infection

xerostomia: dryness of the mouth from a variety of causes

CHART 23-2

Examples of Common Indoor and Outdoor Allergens

Common Indoor Allergens

- Dust mite feces
- Dog dander
- Cat dander
- Cockroach droppings
- Moulds

Common Outdoor Allergens

- Trees (e.g., oak, elm, western red cedar, ash, birch, sycamore, maple, walnut, cypress)
- Weeds (e.g., ragweed, tumbleweed, sagebrush, pigweed, cockle weed, Russian thistle)
- Grasses (e.g., timothy, orchard, sweet vernal, Bermuda, sour dock, redtop, bluegrass)
- Moulds (*Alternaria, Cladosporium, Aspergillus*)

Adapted from Aljubran, S., & Lockey, R. F. (2014). *Aeroallergens*. Retrieved March 9, 2016, from www.emedicine.medscape.com/article/137911-overview

nasal decongestants; and the presence of a foreign body. Allergic rhinitis may occur with exposure to allergens such as foods (e.g., peanuts, walnuts, Brazil nuts, wheat, shellfish, soy, cow's milk, and eggs), medications (e.g., penicillin, sulfa medications, aspirin, and others with the potential to produce an allergic reaction), and particles in the indoor and outdoor environment (Chart 23-2). The most common cause of nonallergic rhinitis is the common cold (Seidman, Gurgel, Lin, et al., 2015).

Drug-induced rhinitis may occur with antihypertensive agents, such as angiotensin-converting enzyme (ACE) inhibitors and beta blockers; "statins," such as atorvastatin (Lipitor) and simvastatin (Zocor); antidepressants; aspirin; and some antianxiety medications. Other causes of rhinitis are identified in Table 23-1. Figure 23-1 shows the pathologic processes involved in rhinitis and **rhinosinusitis**. Other causes of rhinovirus are identified in Table 23-1.

TABLE 23-1 Causes of Rhinosinusitis

Category	Causes
Vasomotor	Idiopathic Abuse of nasal decongestants (rhinitis medicamentosa) Psychological stimulation (anger, sexual arousal) Irritants (smoke, air pollution, exhaust fumes, cocaine)
Mechanical	Tumour Deviated septum Crusting Hypertrophied turbinates Foreign body Cerebrospinal fluid leak
Chronic inflammatory	Polyps (in cystic fibrosis) Sarcoidosis Wegener's granulomatosis Midline granuloma
Infectious	Acute viral infection Acute or chronic rhinosinusitis Rare nasal infections (syphilis, tuberculosis)
Hormonal	Pregnancy Use of oral contraceptives Hypothyroidism

Adapted from Peters, A. (2015). *Rhinosinusitis: Synopsis*. Retrieved October 8, 2015, from www.worldallergy.org/professional/allergic_diseases_center/rhinosinusitis/sinusitissynopsis.php

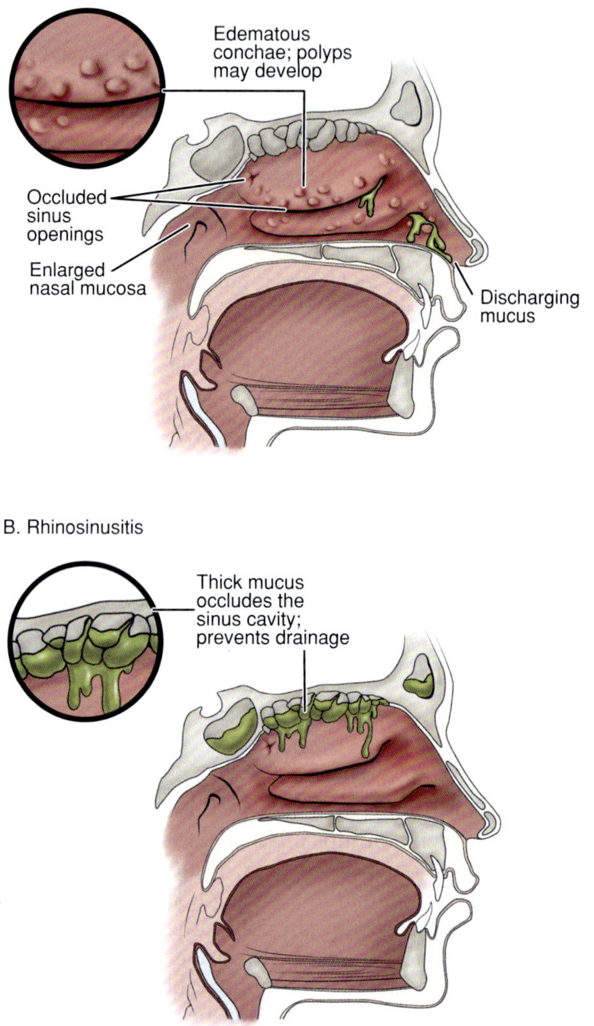

FIGURE 23-1. Pathophysiologic processes in rhinitis and rhinosinusitis. Although pathophysiologic processes are similar in rhinitis and rhinosinusitis, they affect different structures. **A.** In rhinitis, the mucous membranes lining the nasal passages become inflamed, congested, and edematous. The swollen nasal conchae block the sinus openings, and mucus is discharged from the nostrils. **B.** Rhinosinusitis is also marked by inflammation and congestion, with thickened mucous secretions filling the sinus cavities and occluding the openings.

Clinical Manifestations

The signs and symptoms of rhinitis include **rhinorrhea** (excessive nasal drainage, runny nose); nasal congestion; nasal discharge (purulent with bacterial rhinitis); sneezing;

and pruritus of the nose, roof of the mouth, throat, eyes, and ears. Headache may occur, particularly if rhinosinusitis is also present. Nonallergic rhinitis can occur throughout the year.

Medical Management

The management of rhinitis depends on the cause, which may be identified through the history and physical examination. The nurse asks the patient about recent symptoms as well as possible exposure to allergens in the home, environment, or workplace. If viral rhinitis is the cause, medications may be prescribed to relieve the symptoms. In allergic rhinitis, allergy tests may be performed to identify possible allergens. Depending on the severity of the allergy, desensitizing immunizations and corticosteroids may be required (see Chapter 53 for more details). If symptoms suggest a bacterial infection, an antimicrobial agent is used. Patients with nasal septal deformities or nasal polyps may be referred to an ear, nose, and throat specialist.

Pharmacologic Therapy

Medication therapy for allergic and nonallergic rhinitis focuses on symptom relief. Antihistamines and corticosteroid nasal sprays may be useful. Antihistamines remain the most common treatment and are administered for sneezing, pruritus, and rhinorrhea. Examples of commonly prescribed antihistamines are discussed in more detail in Chapter 53. Brompheniramine/pseudoephedrine (Dimetapp) is an example of combination antihistamine/decongestant medications. Cromolyn (NasalCrom), a mast cell stabilizer that inhibits the release of histamine and other chemicals, is also used in the treatment of rhinitis. Oral decongestant agents may be used for nasal obstruction. Use of saline nasal spray can act as a mild decongestant and can liquefy mucus to prevent crusting. Two inhalations of intranasal ipratropium (Atrovent) can be administered in each nostril two to three times per day for symptomatic relief of rhinorrhea. In addition, intranasal corticosteroids may be used for severe congestion, and ophthalmic agents (cromolyn ophthalmic solution 4%) may be used to relieve irritation, itching, and redness of the eyes. Newer allergy treatments include leukotriene modifiers (e.g., montelukast [Singulair], zafirlukast [Accolate]), immunoglobulin E modifiers (e.g., omalizumab [Xolair]), and immunomodulatory medications, which are all part of the revised asthma treatment guidelines and are discussed further in Chapter 25. The choice of medications depends on the symptoms, adverse reactions, adherence factors, risk of drug interactions, and cost to the patient.

Nursing Management

Educating Patients About Self-Care

The nurse instructs the patient with allergic rhinitis to avoid or reduce exposure to allergens and irritants, such as dusts, moulds, animals, fumes, odours, powders, sprays, and tobacco smoke. Patient education is essential when assisting the patient in the use of all medications. To prevent possible drug interactions, the patient is cautioned to read drug labels before taking any over-the-counter medication.

The nurse instructs the patient about the importance of controlling the environment at home and at work. Saline nasal sprays or aerosols may be helpful in soothing mucous membranes, softening crusted secretions, and removing irritants. The nurse instructs the patient in correct administration of nasal medications. To achieve maximal relief, the patient is instructed to blow the nose before applying any medication into the nasal cavity. In addition, the patient is taught to keep the head upright; spray quickly and firmly into each nostril away from the nasal septum; and wait at least 1 minute before administering the second spray. The container should be cleaned after each use and should never be shared with other people to avoid cross-contamination.

In the case of infectious rhinitis, the nurse reviews hand hygiene technique with the patient as a measure to prevent transmission of organisms. This is especially important for those in contact with vulnerable populations such as the very young, older adults, or people who are immunosuppressed (e.g., patients with human immunodeficiency virus [HIV] infection, those taking immunosuppressive medications). In older adults and other high-risk populations, the nurse reviews the value of receiving an influenza vaccination each year to achieve immunity before the beginning of the flu season.

Viral Rhinitis (Common Cold)

Viral rhinitis is the most frequent viral infection in the general population (Krouse & Krouse, 2014). The term common cold often is used when referring to a URTI that is self-limited and caused by a virus. The term cold refers to an infectious, acute inflammation of the mucous membranes of the nasal cavity characterized by nasal congestion, rhinorrhea, sneezing, sore throat, and general malaise. More broadly, the term refers to an acute URTI, whereas terms such as rhinitis, **pharyngitis**, and **laryngitis** distinguish the sites of the symptoms. The term is also used when the causative virus is influenza (the flu). Colds are highly contagious because virus is shed for about 2 days before the symptoms appear and during the first part of the symptomatic phase.

In Canada, colds are more frequent during the late fall and winter seasons. The incidence of viral rhinitis follows a specific pattern during the year, depending on the causative agent. Although viral rhinitis can occur at any time, three periods account for the epidemics in North America: in September, just after the opening of school; in late January; and toward the end of April.

Seasonal changes in relative humidity may affect the prevalence of colds. The most common cold-causing viruses survive better when humidity is low, in the colder months of the year. In Canada, URTIs in children under the age of 18 are the frequent cause of emergency department visits as well as a cause of inpatient hospitalization (CIHI, 2014).

As many as 200 different viruses are responsible for causing colds (National Institute of Allergy and Infectious Diseases, 2015). Rhinoviruses are the most likely causative organisms. Other viruses implicated in the common cold include coronavirus, adenovirus, respiratory syncytial virus, influenza virus, and parainfluenza virus. Because each virus has multiple strains, developing vaccines against

CHART 23-3

Colds and Cold Sores (Herpes Simplex Virus)

Herpes labialis is an infection that is caused by herpes simplex virus type 1 (HSV-1). It is characterized by an eruption of small, painful blisters on the skin of the lips, mouth, gums, tongue, or the skin around the mouth. The blisters are commonly referred to as cold sores or fever blisters. Once the person is infected with this virus, it can lie latent in the cells for a period of time. The incubation period is about 2 to 12 days. Between 50% and 80% of Americans are infected by age 30 years, because HSV-1 is typically transmitted during childhood through nonsexual contact. Herpes labialis is extremely contagious and can be spread through contaminated razors, towels, and dishes. It is activated by overexposure to sunlight or wind, colds, influenza and similar infections, heavy alcohol use, and physical or emotional stress.

Although herpes simplex virus type 2 (HSV-2) typically causes painful vesicular and ulcerative lesions in the genital and anal areas, HSV-1 may also cause genital herpes. Oral–genital contact can spread oral herpes to the genitals (and vice versa). People with active herpetic lesions should avoid oral sex. It is extremely important for patients to understand that the virus can be transmitted by asymptomatic people. Estimates suggest that 80% of people infected are asymptomatic.

Early symptoms of herpes labialis include burning, itching, and increased sensitivity or tingling sensation. These symptoms may occur several days before the appearance of lesions. The lesions appear as macules or papules, progressing to small blisters (vesicles) filled with clear, yellowish fluid. They are raised, red, and painful and can break and ooze. The lesions typically extend through the epidermis and penetrate into the underlying dermis, consistent with a partial-thickness wound. Eventually, yellow crusts slough to reveal pink, healing skin. Typically, the virus is no longer detectable in the lesion or wound 5 days after the vesicle has developed.

Medications used in the management of herpes labialis include acyclovir (Zovirax) and valacyclovir (Valtrex), which help to minimize the symptoms and the duration or length of flare-up. Acetaminophen may be given for analgesia. Topical anesthetics such as lidocaine (Xylocaine) can help in the control of discomfort. Occlusive dressings have been shown to speed the healing process. Not only do such dressings prevent desiccation and scab formation but they also maintain an aqueous wound environment rich in growth factors and matrix materials. However, occlusive dressings are not practical for lip and mucosal lesions. In this case, alternatives include occlusive ointments such as Herpecin-L or docosanol (Abreva).

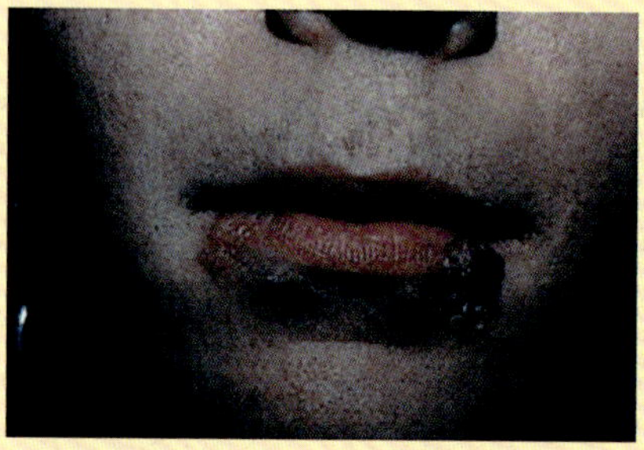

Adapted from Salvaggio, M. R. (2014). *Herpes simplex*. Retrieved October 12, 2015, from www.emedicine.medscape.com/article/218580-overview

each one is almost impossible; therefore, individuals are susceptible to colds throughout life. Immunity after recovery is variable and depends on many factors, including a person's natural host resistance and the specific virus that caused the cold. Despite popular belief, cold temperatures and exposure to cold rainy weather do not increase the incidence or severity of the common cold.

Clinical Manifestations

Signs and symptoms of viral rhinitis are low-grade fever, nasal congestion, rhinorrhea and nasal discharge, halitosis, sneezing, tearing watery eyes, "scratchy" or sore throat, general malaise, chills, and often headache and muscle aches. As the illness progresses, cough usually appears. In some people, the virus exacerbates **herpes simplex**, commonly called a cold sore (Chart 23-3).

The symptoms of viral rhinitis may last from 1 to 2 weeks. If severe systemic respiratory symptoms occur, it is no longer considered viral rhinitis but one of the other acute URTIs. Allergic conditions can affect the nose, mimicking the symptoms of a cold.

Medical Management

Management consists of symptomatic therapy that includes an adequate fluid intake, rest, prevention of chilling, and use of expectorants as needed. Warm salt water gargles soothe the sore throat, and nonsteroidal anti-inflammatory drugs (NSAIDs), such as ibuprofen, relieve aches and pains. Antihistamines are used to relieve sneezing, rhinorrhea, and nasal congestion. Petroleum jelly can soothe irritated, chapped, and raw skin around the nares (National Institute of Allergy and Infectious Diseases, 2015).

Guaifenesin (Mucinex), an expectorant, is available without a prescription and is used to promote removal of secretions. Antimicrobial agents (antibiotics) should not be used, because they do not affect the virus or reduce the incidence of bacterial complications. In addition, their inappropriate use has been implicated in development of organisms resistant to therapy. Topical nasal decongestants, such as oxymetazoline hydrochloride and xylometazoline hydrochloride, may provide temporary relief of sinus congestion and pressure due to colds or allergies (Government of Canada, 2014).

Topical therapy delivers medication directly to the nasal mucosa, and its overuse can produce **rhinitis medicamentosa**, or rebound rhinitis. Most patients treat the common cold with over-the-counter medications that produce moderate clinical benefits, such as relief of symptoms.

In addition, herbal medicines (e.g., echinacea, zinc lozenges, zinc nasal spray) are frequently used to treat the common cold; however, evidence regarding their effectiveness in shortening the symptomatic phase is questionable (Karsch-Volk, Barrett, Keifer, et al., 2015). The inhalation of steam or heated, humidified air has been a mainstay of home remedies for common cold sufferers, but the value of this therapy has not been demonstrated.

Nursing Management

Educating Patients About Self-Care

Most viruses can be transmitted in several ways: direct contact with infected secretions; inhalation of large particles from others' coughing or sneezing; or inhalation of small particles (aerosol) that may be suspended in the air for up to an hour. Implementation of appropriate hand hygiene measures remains the most effective measure to prevent transmission of organisms. The nurse teaches the patient how to break the chain of infection with appropriate handwashing or hand hygiene and the use of tissues to avoid the spread of the virus with coughing and sneezing. The nurse teaches methods to treat symptoms of the common cold and provides both verbal and written information to assist the patient in the prevention and management of URTIs.

Rhinosinusitis

Rhinosinusitis, commonly referred to as sinusitis, means inflammation of the mucosa of the nose and sinus cavities most often due to an infection (Canadian Society of Otolaryngology—Head and Neck Surgery, n.d.). Sinusitis is classified by duration of symptom as acute (less than 4 weeks), subacute (4 to 12 weeks), and chronic (more than 12 weeks). Sinusitis can be a bacterial or viral infection.

Chronic sinusitis, one of the most frequent inflammatory conditions in Canada, affects an estimated 7% of the Canadian population. The economic burden on Canadian health care resources is significant costing approximately $860 million annually (Medical Pharmaceuticals, 2014).

Acute Rhinosinusitis

Acute rhinosinusitis is classified as acute bacterial rhinosinusitis (ABRS) or acute viral rhinosinusitis (AVRS). Recurrent acute rhinosinusitis is characterized by four or more acute episodes of ABRS per year (Rosenfeld, Piccirillo, Chandrasekhar, et al., 2015) and is discussed with chronic rhinosinusitis (CRS).

Pathophysiology

Acute rhinosinusitis usually follows a viral URTI or cold, such as an unresolved viral or bacterial infection, or an exacerbation of allergic rhinitis. Normally, the sinus openings into the nasal passages are clear and infections resolve promptly. However, if their drainage is obstructed by a deviated septum or by hypertrophied turbinates, spurs, or nasal polyps or tumours, sinus infection may persist as a smoldering (persistent) secondary infection or progress to an acute suppurative process (causing purulent discharge).

Nasal congestion, caused by inflammation, edema, and transudation of fluid secondary to URI, leads to obstruction of the sinus cavities (see Fig. 23-1). This provides an excellent medium for bacterial growth. Other conditions that can block the normal flow of sinus secretions include abnormal structures of the nose, enlarged adenoids, diving and swimming, tooth infection, trauma to the nose, tumours, and the pressure of foreign objects. Some people are more prone to rhinosinusitis because exposure to environmental hazards such as paint, sawdust, and chemicals may result in chronic inflammation of the nasal passages.

Bacterial organisms account for more than 60% of the cases of acute sinusitis. Typical pathogens include *Streptococcus pneumoniae, Haemophilus influenzae*, and less commonly *Staphylococcus aureus* and *Moraxella catarrhalis* (Brook, 2015). Biofilms, which consist of organized, heterogeneous communities of bacteria, have been found to be 10 to 1,000 times more resistant to antibiotic treatment and more likely to contribute to host resistance when compared with other bacteria. They serve as bacterial reservoirs that can cause systemic illness when released into the circulation. Although antibiotics kill bacteria in the biofilm margin, cells deep in the biofilm are not affected, allowing for regrowth once antibiotic therapy has been discontinued. Pathogens in the upper respiratory tract that form biofilms include those species listed above as well as *Pseudomonas aeruginosa*. Other organisms that are occasionally isolated include *Chlamydia pneumoniae, Streptococcus pyogenes*, viruses, and fungi (*Aspergillus fumigatus*). Fungal infections occur most often in immunosuppressed patients (Brook, 2015).

Clinical Manifestations

Symptoms of ABRS include purulent nasal drainage (anterior, posterior, or both) accompanied by nasal obstruction or a combination of facial pain, pressure, or a sense of fullness (referred to collectively as facial pain–pressure–fullness), or both (Rosenfeld et al., 2015). The facial pain–pressure–fullness may involve the anterior face or the periorbital region. The patient may also report cloudy or coloured nasal discharge congestion, blockage, or stuffiness as well as a localized or diffuse headache. Patients with ABRS may present with a high fever (39°C or higher). In addition, the occurrence of symptoms for 10 days or more after the initial onset of upper respiratory symptoms indicates ABRS (Brook, 2015).

The symptoms of AVRS are similar to those of ABRS, except the patient does not present with a high fever, nor with the same intensity of symptoms (e.g., there tends to be an absence of facial pain–pressure–fullness), nor with symptoms that persist for as long a period of time. Symptoms of AVRS occur for fewer than 10 days after the onset of upper respiratory symptoms and do not worsen (Tierney, McPhee, & Papadakis, 2015).

Assessment and Diagnostic Findings

A careful history and physical examination are performed. The head and neck, particularly the nose, ears, teeth, sinuses, pharynx, and chest, are examined. There may be tenderness to palpation over the infected sinus area. The sinuses are percussed using the index finger, tapping lightly to determine whether the patient experiences pain. Although less frequently performed, transillumination of the affected area may reveal a decrease in the transmission of light with rhinosinusitis (see Chapter 22). Diagnostic imaging (x-ray, computed tomography [CT], magnetic resonance imaging [MRI]) is not recommended and generally not needed for the diagnosis of acute rhinosinusitis if the patient meets clinical diagnostic criteria (Rosenfeld et al., 2015). When a complication or alternative diagnosis is suspected, CT scans may be indicated because these scans are sensitive to inflammatory changes and bone destruction and identify anatomical variations that can guide sinus surgery if indicated.

To confirm the diagnosis of maxillary and frontal rhinosinusitis and identify the pathogen, sinus aspirates may be obtained. Flexible endoscopic culture techniques and swabbing of the sinuses have been used for this purpose (Seidman, Gurgel, Lin, et al., 2015).

Complications

If untreated, acute rhinosinusitis may lead to severe complications. Local complications include osteomyelitis and mucocele (cyst of the paranasal sinuses). Osteomyelitis requires prolonged antibiotic therapy and at times removal of necrotic bone. Intracranial complications, although rare, include cavernous sinus thrombosis, meningitis, brain abscess, ischemic brain infarction, and severe orbital cellulitis (Tierney et al., 2015). Mucoceles may require surgical treatment to establish intranasal drainage or complete excision with ablation of the sinus cavity. Brain abscesses occur by direct spread and can be life threatening. Frontal epidural abscesses are usually quiescent but can be detected by CT scan.

Medical Management

Treatment of acute rhinosinusitis depends on the cause; oral therapies can include antibiotics for bacterial cases and oral corticosteroids for acute inflammation. The goals of treatment of acute rhinosinusitis are to shrink the nasal mucosa, relieve pain, and treat infection. Because of inappropriate use of antibiotics for nonbacterial illness, including viral rhinosinusitis, and the resulting resistance that has occurred, oral antibiotics should only be prescribed when there is sufficient empiric evidence that the patient has ABRS (e.g., high fever or symptoms that persist for at least 10 days or worsening symptoms following a viral respiratory illness) (Tewfik, 2015). Deep-seated bacterial rhinosinusitis can be a serious infection that requires antibiotic treatment for 2 to 3 weeks.

Treatment of acute rhinosinusitis typically involves nasal saline lavage and decongestants (guaifenesin/pseudoephedrine). Decongestants or nasal saline sprays can increase patency of the ostiomeatal unit and improve drainage of the sinuses. Topical decongestants should not be used for longer than 3 or 4 days. Oral decongestants must be used cautiously in patients with hypertension. Over-the-counter antihistamines, such as diphenhydramine (Benadryl), and prescription antihistamines, such as fexofenadine (Allegra), are used if an allergic component is suspected.

Intranasal corticosteroids have been shown to produce complete or marked improvement in acute symptoms of either bacterial or viral rhinosinusitis; however, they are only recommended for use in patients with a previous history of allergic rhinitis (Krouse & Krouse, 2014; Rosenfeld et al., 2015). Examples of intranasal corticosteroids, side effects, and precautions are presented in Table 23-2.

If the patient continues to have symptoms after 7 to 10 days, the sinuses may need to be irrigated.

Nursing Management

Educating Patients About Self-Care

Patient teaching is an important aspect of nursing care for the patient with acute rhinosinusitis. The nurse instructs the patient about symptoms of complications that require immediate follow-up. Referral to a physician is indicated if periorbital edema and severe pain on palpation occur. The nurse instructs the patient about methods to promote drainage of the sinuses, including humidification of the air in the home and use of warm compresses to relieve pressure. The patient is advised to avoid swimming, diving, and air travel during the acute infection. Patients using tobacco are advised to immediately stop smoking or using any form of tobacco.

Most patients use nasal sprays incorrectly, which can lead to several side effects that include nasal irritation, nasal burning, bad taste, and drainage in the throat or even **epistaxis**. Therefore, if an intranasal corticosteroid is prescribed, it is important to teach the patient the correct

TABLE 23-2 Selected Nasal Corticosteroids and Common Side Effects

Nasal Corticosteroids	Side Effects	Contraindications (for all Nasal Corticosteroids)
Beclomethasone (Beconase)	Nasal irritation, headache, nausea, lightheadedness, epistaxis, rhinorrhea, watering eyes, sneezing, dry nose and throat	Avoid in patients with recurrent epistaxis, glaucoma, and cataracts. Patients who have been exposed to measles/varicella or who have adrenal insufficiency should avoid these medications.
Budesonide (Rhinocort)	Epistaxis, pharyngitis, cough, nasal irritation, bronchospasm	
Mometasone (Nasonex)	Headache, viral infection, pharyngitis, epistaxis, cough, dysmenorrhea, musculoskeletal pain, arthralgia	
Triamcinolone (Nasacort AQ)	Pharyngitis, epistaxis, cough, headache	

Adapted from Peters, A. (2015). *Rhinosinusitis: Synopsis.* Retrieved October 8, 2015, from www.worldallergy.org/professional/allergic_diseases_center/rhinosinusitis/sinusitissynopsis.php use of prescribed nasal sprays through demonstration, explanation, and return demonstration to evaluate the patient's understanding of the correct method of administration. The nurse also teaches the patient about the side effects of prescribed and over-the-counter nasal sprays and about rebound congestion, medicamentosa. Once the decongestant is discontinued, the nasal passages close and congestion results. Appropriate medications to use for pain relief include acetaminophen (Tylenol) and NSAIDs such as ibuprofen (Advil), naproxen sodium (Aleve), and aspirin for adults older than 20 years of age.

The nurse tells patients with recurrent sinusitis to begin decongestants at the first sign of rhinosinusitis. This promotes drainage and decreases the risk of bacterial infection. Patients should also check with their health care provider or pharmacist before using over-the-counter medications because many cold medications can worsen symptoms or other health problems, specifically hypertension.

The nurse stresses the importance of following the recommended antibiotic regimen because a consistent blood level of the medication is critical to treat the infection. The nurse teaches the patient the early signs of a sinus infection and recommends preventive measures such as following healthy practices and avoiding contact with people with URTIs.

The nurse explains to the patient that fever, severe headache, and **nuchal rigidity** (stiffness of the neck or inability to bend the neck) are the signs of potential complications. Patients with chronic symptoms of rhinosinusitis who do not have marked improvement in 4 weeks with continuous medical treatment may be candidates for sinus surgery (Krings, Kallogjeri, Wineland, et al., 2014).

NURSING ALERT

Patients with nasotracheal and nasogastric tubes in place are at risk for development of sinus infections. Thus, accurate assessment of patients with these tubes is critical. Removal of the nasotracheal or nasogastric tube as soon as the patient's condition permits allows the sinuses to drain, possibly avoiding septic complications.

Chronic Rhinosinusitis and Recurrent Acute Rhinosinusitis

The prevalence for CRS in Canada is approximately 2% to 2.5% of the population and occurs more frequently in women than men (Xu, Quan, Faris, et al., 2016). It is diagnosed when the patient has experienced 12 weeks or longer of two or more of the following symptoms: mucopurulent drainage, nasal obstruction, facial pain–pressure–fullness, or decreased sense of smell. It is estimated that in about 40% of patients, CRS is accompanied by nasal polyps (Rosenfeld et al., 2015). Recurrent acute rhinosinusitis is diagnosed when four or more episodes of ABRS occur per year with no signs or symptoms of rhinosinusitis between the episodes. The use of antibiotics in people with recurrent acute rhinosinusitis is even higher than in CRS. Both CRS and recurrent acute rhinosinusitis affect quality of life as well as physical and social function (Rosenfeld et al., 2015).

Pathophysiology

Mechanical obstruction in the ostia of the frontal, maxillary, and anterior ethmoid sinuses (known collectively as the ostiomeatal complex) is the usual cause of CRS and recurrent acute rhinosinusitis. Obstruction prevents adequate drainage of the nasal passages, resulting in accumulation of secretions and an ideal medium for bacterial growth. Persistent blockage in an adult may occur because of infection, allergy, or structural abnormalities. Other associated conditions and factors may include cystic fibrosis, ciliary dyskinesia, neoplastic disorders, gastroesophageal reflux disease, tobacco use, and environmental pollution (Rosenfeld et al., 2015).

Both aerobic and anaerobic bacteria have been implicated in CRS and recurrent rhinosinusitis. Common aerobic bacteria include alpha-hemolytic streptococci, microaerophilic streptococci, and *Staphylococcus aureus*. Common anaerobic bacteria include gram-negative bacilli, *Peptostreptococcus*, and *Fusobacterium*.

In addition, immunodeficiency should be considered in patients with CRS or acute recurrent rhinosinusitis. Acute fulminant/invasive sinusitis is a life-threatening illness and is commonly attributed to *Aspergillus* in immunocompromised patients. Chronic fungal sinusitis also poses a risk. Chronic invasive fungal sinusitis occurs in immunocompromised patients along with fungus ball/mycetoma and allergic fungal sinusitis, the more common forms of chronic fungal sinusitis, which are considered noninvasive conditions in immunocompromised patients. The fungus generally remains contained in the fungus ball, which consists of mucopurulent cheesy or claylike materials within the sinus, but can become invasive when immunosuppression occurs, leading to encephalopathy (Lal, 2015). Symptoms include nasal stuffiness, nasal discharge, and facial pain. Vision loss, headache, and cranial nerve palsies have been identified in patients with a sphenoid sinus fungal ball (Lal, 2015).

Clinical Manifestations

Clinical manifestations of CRS include impaired mucociliary clearance and ventilation, cough (because the thick discharge constantly drips backward into the nasopharynx), chronic hoarseness, chronic headaches in the periorbital area, and facial pain. As a result of chronic nasal congestion, the patient is usually required to breathe through the mouth. Snoring, sore throat, and, in some situations, adenoidal hypertrophy may also occur. Periorbital edema and facial pain are common. These symptoms are generally most pronounced on awakening in the morning. Fatigue and nasal congestion are also common. Many patients experience a decrease in smell and taste and a sense of fullness in the ears.

Assessment and Diagnostic Findings

The health assessment focuses on onset and duration of symptoms. It addresses the quantity and quality of nasal discharge and cough, the presence of pain, factors that relieve or aggravate the pain, and allergies. The Canadian clinical practice guidelines for CRS propose a mnemonic, CPODS (Congestion or fullness; facial Pain, pressure, or fullness; nasal Obstruction or blockage; purulent anterior or posterior nasal Drainage; and Smell disorder) to facilitate recollection of important symptoms seen in patients with CRS. It is essential to obtain any history of comorbid conditions, including asthma, and history of tobacco use. A history of fever, fatigue, previous episodes and treatments, and previous response to therapies is also obtained.

In the physical assessment, the external nose is evaluated for any evidence of anatomical abnormality. A crooked-appearing external nose may imply septal deviation internally. The nasal mucous membranes are assessed for erythema, pallor, atrophy, edema, crusting, discharge, polyps, erosions, and septal perforations or deviations. Appropriate lighting improves visualization of the nasal cavity and should be used in every examination. Pain on examination of the teeth and with tapping with a tongue blade suggests tooth infection (Bickley & Szilagyi, 2013).

Assessment of the posterior oropharynx may reveal purulent or mucoid discharge, which is indicative of an infection caused by CRS. The patients' eyes are examined for conjunctival erythema, tearing, photophobia, and edema of the lids. Additional assessment techniques include transillumination of the sinuses and palpation of the sinuses. The frontal and maxillary sinuses are palpated, and the patient is asked whether this produces tenderness. The pharynx is inspected for erythema and discharge and palpated for cervical node adenopathy (Rosenfeld et al., 2015).

Imaging studies such as x-ray, sinoscopy, ultrasound, CT, and MRI may be used in the diagnosis of CRS. X-ray is an inexpensive and readily available tool to assess disorders of the paranasal sinuses. CT of the paranasal sinuses can identify mucosal abnormalities, sinus ostial obstruction, anatomical variants, sinonasal polyposis, and neoplastic disease. In addition, nasal endoscopy allows for visualization of the posterior nasal cavity, nasopharynx, and sinus drainage pathways and can identify posterior septal deviation and polyps. Osseous destruction, extrasinus extension of the disease process, and local invasion suggest malignancy (Rosenfeld et al., 2015).

Complications

Complications of CRS, although uncommon, include severe orbital cellulitis, subperiosteal abscess, cavernous sinus thrombosis, meningitis, encephalitis, and ischemic infarction. CRS can lead to intracranial infection either by direct spread through bone or via venous channels, resulting in epidural abscess, subdural empyema, meningitis, and brain abscess. Clinical sequelae can include personality changes with frontal lobe abscesses, headache, symptoms of elevated intracranial pressure to include alterations of consciousness, visual changes, focal neurologic deficits, seizures, and, ultimately, coma and death.

Frontal rhinosinusitis can lead to osteomyelitis of the frontal bones. Patients typically present with headache, fever, and a characteristic doughy edema over the involved bone. Ethmoid rhinosinusitis may result in orbital cellulitis, which usually begins with edema of the eyelids and rapidly progresses to ptosis (droopy eyelid), proptosis (bulging eye), chemosis (edema of the bulbar conjunctiva), and diminished extraocular movements. Patients are usually febrile and acutely ill and require immediate attention because pressure on the optic nerve can lead to loss of vision and spread of infection can lead to intracranial infection. Cavernous sinus thrombophlebitis can be a result of extension of infection along venous channels from the orbit, ethmoid, frontal sinuses, or nose. Symptoms may include altered consciousness, lid edema, and proptosis, as well as third, fourth, and sixth cranial nerve palsies.

Medical Management

The goal of treatment is to reduce symptoms and decrease the likelihood of complications by decreasing inflammation and controlling the infectious agents (Kaplan, 2013). Early identification of risk factors guides the selection of treatment and leads to early intervention and ultimately better patient outcomes. Management for CRS includes intranasal corticosteroids and in the presence of symptoms of infection with antibiotics. The course of antibiotic treatment for CRS and recurrent ABRS may be as long as 3 to 4 weeks to effectively eradicate the offending organism (Brook, 2015). The use of intranasal corticosteroids has been shown to reduce the size of nasal polyps and improve nasal symptoms of patients. Steroids administered systemically may also be useful in treating individuals with CRS.

General measures include adequate hydration, steam inhalation 20 to 30 minutes three times per day whenever possible, saline irrigation, and saline nose drops. Patients are instructed to sleep with the head of the bed elevated and to avoid exposure to cigarette smoke and fumes. Patients are cautioned to avoid caffeine and alcohol, which can cause dehydration.

Prescribed medications may be necessary. Although there is no rigorous data to support the use of mucolytics, antihistamines, or decongestants, these medications should help improve symptoms. Medications commonly used for relief of symptoms include loratadine (Claritin), chlorpheniramine (Chlor-Trimeton), and diphenhydramine. For patients with concomitant asthma, leukotriene inhibitors such as montelukast, and zafirlukast may be used (Brook, 2015). Commonly used nasal steroids include mometasone furoate (Nasonex) and fluticasone propionate (Flonase). If allergies are a possible cause of CRS, oral antihistamines or nasal corticosteroids may also be prescribed. Patients with allergic rhinitis may also benefit from the addition of a mast cell stabilizer such as cromolyn.

Surgical Management

If standard medical therapy fails and symptoms persist, endoscopic sinus surgery may be indicated to relieve obstruction, remove diseased mucosa, and restore ventilation (Kaplan, 2013). Minimally invasive surgical procedures are used, reducing postoperative discomfort and producing significant improvement in the patient's quality of life. In particular, endoscopic sinus surgery is associated with either complete or moderate relief of symptoms in more than 85% to 91% of patients (Patel, 2014). Computer-assisted or computer-guided surgery is used to increase the precision of the surgical procedure and to minimize complications (Patel, 2014).

Some of the specific procedures performed include excising and cauterizing nasal polyps, correcting a deviated septum, incising and draining the sinuses, aerating the sinuses, and removing tumours. Antimicrobial agents may be given before and after surgery.

Surgical intervention may be required in acute invasive fungal rhinosinusitis to excise the fungus ball and necrotic tissue and drain the sinuses. Patients require aggressive surgical débridement and drainage as well as systemic antifungal medications.

Nursing Management

Because the patient usually performs care measures for sinusitis at home, nursing management consists mainly of patient teaching.

Educating Patients About Self-Care

Many people with sinus infections tend to blow their nose frequently and with force to clear their nasal passages. However, doing so often increases the symptoms. Therefore, the patient is instructed to blow the nose gently and to use tissue to remove the nasal drainage. Increasing fluid intake, applying local heat (hot wet packs), and elevating the head of the bed promote drainage of the sinuses. The nurse also instructs the patient about the importance of following the prescribed medication regimen. Instructions on the early signs of a sinus infection are provided, and preventive measures are reviewed. The nurse instructs the patient about signs and symptoms that require follow-up and provides these instructions verbally and in writing. Instructions in alternate formats (e.g., large font, patient's language) may be needed to increase the patient's understanding and adherence to the treatment plan. The nurse encourages the patient to follow-up with his or her primary health care provider if symptoms persist.

NURSING ALERT

URTIs, specifically chronic rhinosinusitis and recurrent acute rhinosinusitis, may be linked to primary or secondary immunodeficiency or treatment with immunosuppressive therapy (i.e., for cancer or organ transplantation). Typical symptoms may be blunted or absent due to immunosuppression. Immunocompromised patients are at increased risk for acute or chronic fungal infections; these infections can progress rapidly and become life threatening. Thus, assessment, early reporting of symptoms to the physician, and immediate initiation of treatment are essential.

Pharyngitis

Acute Pharyngitis

Acute pharyngitis is a sudden painful inflammation of the pharynx, the back portion of the throat that includes the posterior third of the tongue, soft palate, and tonsils. It is commonly referred to as a sore throat. In the United States, approximately 15 million health care visits are due to pharyngitis each year (Randel, 2013). Because of environmental exposure to viral agents and poorly ventilated rooms, the incidence of viral pharyngitis peaks during winter and early spring in regions that have warm summers and cold winters. Viral pharyngitis spreads easily in the droplets of coughs and sneezes, as well as from unclean hands that have been exposed to the contaminated fluids.

Pathophysiology

Viral infection causes most cases of acute pharyngitis. Responsible viruses include the adenovirus, influenza virus, Epstein–Barr virus, and herpes simplex virus. Bacterial infection accounts for the remainder of cases. Ten percent of adults with pharyngitis have group A beta-hemolytic streptococcus (GABHS), which is commonly referred to as group A streptococcus (GAS) or streptococcal pharyngitis. Streptococcal pharyngitis warrants the use of antibiotic treatment. When GAS causes acute pharyngitis, the condition is known as strep throat. The body responds by triggering an inflammatory response in the pharynx. This results in pain, fever, vasodilation, edema, and tissue damage, manifested by redness and swelling in the tonsillar pillars, uvula, and soft palate. A creamy exudate may be present in the tonsillar pillars (see Fig. 23-2). Other bacterial

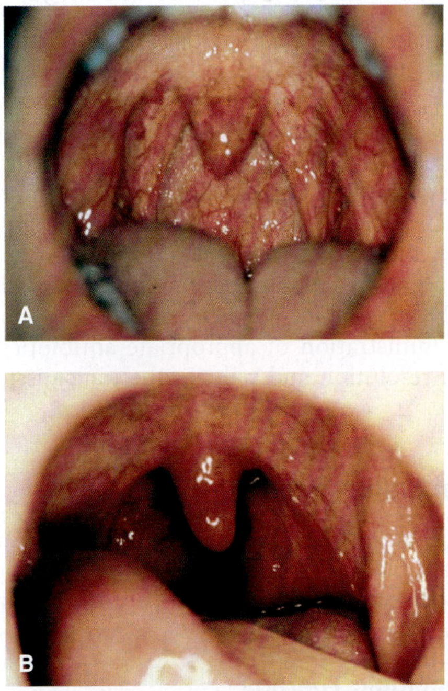

FIGURE 23-2. Pharyngitis—inflammation without exudate. **A.** Redness and vascularity of the pillars and uvula are mild to moderate. **B.** Redness is diffuse and intense. Each patient would probably complain of a sore throat. (From the Wellcome Trust, National Medical Slide Bank, London, UK.)

organisms implicated in acute pharyngitis include groups B and G streptococci, *Neisseria gonorrhoeae, Mycoplasma pneumoniae, C. pneumoniae, Arcanobacterium haemolyticum,* and HIV (Randel, 2013).

Uncomplicated viral infections usually subside promptly, within 3 to 10 days after the onset. However, pharyngitis caused by more virulent bacteria, such as GAS, is a more severe illness. If left untreated, the complications can be severe and life threatening. Complications include sinusitis, otitis media, peritonsillar abscess, mastoiditis, and cervical adenitis. In rare cases, the infection may lead to bacteremia, pneumonia, meningitis, rheumatic fever, and nephritis.

Clinical Manifestations

The signs and symptoms of acute pharyngitis include a fiery-red pharyngeal membrane and tonsils, lymphoid follicles that are swollen and flecked with white-purple exudate, enlarged and tender cervical lymph nodes, and no cough. Fever (higher than 38.3°C), malaise, and sore throat also may be present. Occasionally, patients with GAS pharyngitis exhibit vomiting, anorexia, and a scarlatiniform rash with urticaria known as scarlet fever.

People who have streptococcal pharyngitis suddenly develop a painful sore throat 1 to 5 days after being exposed to the streptococcus bacteria. They usually report malaise, fever (with or without chills), headache, myalgia, painful cervical adenopathy, and nausea. The tonsils appear swollen and erythematous, and they may or may not have an exudate. The roof of the mouth is often erythematous and may demonstrate petechiae. Bad breath is common.

Assessment and Diagnostic Findings

Accurate diagnosis of pharyngitis is essential to determine the cause (viral or bacterial) and to initiate treatment early. Rapid antigen detection testing (RADT) uses swabs that collect specimens from the posterior pharynx and tonsil. RADT is reported to be 90% to 95% sensitive, thus facilitating earlier treatment and earlier symptom improvement and reductions in pathogen transmission. Negative results should be confirmed by a throat culture (Randel, 2013). In most communities, preliminary culture reports are available in 24 hours. Once a definitive diagnosis of GAS is made, administration of appropriate antibiotics hastens symptom resolution and reduces the transmission of the illness.

Medical Management

Viral pharyngitis is treated with supportive measures because antibiotics have no effect on the causal organism. Bacterial pharyngitis is treated with a variety of antimicrobial agents.

Pharmacologic Therapy

If the cause of pharyngitis is bacterial, penicillin is usually the treatment of choice. Penicillin V potassium given for 5 days is the regimen of choice. Penicillin injections are recommended only if there is a concern that the patient will not adhere to therapy (Tierney et al., 2015).

For patients who are allergic to penicillin or have organisms that are resistant to erythromycin (one fifth of GAS and most *Staphylococcus aureus* organisms are resistant to penicillin and erythromycin), cephalosporins, and macrolides (clarithromycin and azithromycin) may be used.

Severe sore throats can also be relieved by analgesic medications. For example, aspirin or acetaminophen can be taken at 4- to 6-hour intervals; if required, acetaminophen with codeine can be taken three or four times daily. Some patients find salt water gargling to be soothing. In severe cases, gargles with benzocaine may relieve symptoms.

Nutritional Therapy

A liquid or soft diet is provided during the acute stage of the disease, depending on the patient's appetite and the degree of discomfort that occurs with swallowing. Cool beverages, warm liquids, and flavoured frozen desserts such as Popsicles are often soothing. Occasionally, the throat is so sore that liquids cannot be taken in adequate amounts by mouth. In severe situations, intravenous (IV) fluids may be needed. Otherwise, the patient is encouraged to drink as much fluid as possible (at least 2 to 3 L per day).

Nursing Management

Nursing care for patients with viral pharyngitis focuses on symptomatic management. For patients who demonstrate signs of strep throat and have a history of rheumatic fever, who appear toxic, who have clinical scarlet fever, or who have symptoms suggesting peritonsillar abscess, nursing care focuses on prompt initiation and correct administration of prescribed antibiotic therapy. The nurse instructs the patient about signs and symptoms that warrant prompt contact with the physician. These include dyspnea, drooling, inability to swallow, and inability to fully open the mouth.

The nurse instructs the patient to stay in bed during the febrile stage of illness and to rest frequently once up and about. Used tissues should be disposed of properly to prevent the spread of infection. The nurse (or the patient or family member, if the patient is not hospitalized) should examine the skin once or twice daily for possible rash, because acute pharyngitis may precede some other communicable diseases (e.g., rubella).

Depending on the severity of the pharyngitis and the degree of pain, warm saline gargles or throat irrigations are used. The benefits of this treatment depend on the degree of heat that is applied. The nurse teaches the patient about these procedures and about the recommended temperature of the solution: high enough to be effective and as warm as the patient can tolerate, usually 40.6° to 43.3°C (105° to 110°F). Irrigating the throat may reduce spasm in the pharyngeal muscles and relieve soreness of the throat.

An ice collar also can relieve severe sore throats. Mouth care may promote the patient's comfort and prevent the development of fissures (cracking) of the lips and oral inflammation when bacterial infection is present. The nurse instructs the patient to resume activity gradually and to delay returning to work or school until after 24 hours of antibiotic therapy. A full course of antibiotic therapy is indicated in patients with strep infection because of the potential complications such as nephritis and rheumatic fever, which may have their onset 2 or 3 weeks after the pharyngitis has subsided. The nurse instructs the patient and family about the importance of taking the full course of therapy and informs them about the symptoms to watch for that may indicate complications.

In addition, the nurse instructs the patient about preventive measures that include not sharing eating utensils, glasses, napkins, food, or towels; cleaning telephones after use; using a tissue to cough or sneeze; disposing of used tissues appropriately; and avoiding exposure to tobacco and secondhand smoke. The nurse also teaches the patient with pharyngitis, especially streptococcal pharyngitis, to replace his or her toothbrush with a new one.

Chronic Pharyngitis

Chronic pharyngitis is a persistent inflammation of the pharynx. It is common in adults who work in dusty surroundings, use their voice to excess, suffer from chronic cough, or habitually use alcohol and tobacco.

There are three types of chronic pharyngitis:

- Hypertrophic: characterized by general thickening and congestion of the pharyngeal mucous membrane
- Atrophic: probably a late stage of the first type (the membrane is thin, whitish, glistening, and at times wrinkled)
- Chronic granular ("clergyman's sore throat"), characterized by numerous swollen lymph follicles on the pharyngeal wall

Clinical Manifestations

Patients with chronic pharyngitis complain of a constant sense of irritation or fullness in the throat, mucus that collects in the throat and can be expelled by coughing, and difficulty swallowing. This is often associated with intermittent postnasal drip that causes minor irritation and inflammation of the pharynx. A sore throat that is worse with swallowing in the absence of pharyngitis suggests the possibility of thyroiditis, and patients with this symptom are referred for evaluation for possible thyroiditis.

Medical Management

Treatment of chronic pharyngitis is based on relieving symptoms, avoiding exposure to irritants, and correcting any upper respiratory, pulmonary, gastrointestinal, or cardiac condition that might be responsible for a chronic cough.

Nasal congestion may be relieved by short-term use of nasal sprays or medications containing ephedrine sulphate (Kondon's Nasal) or phenylephrine hydrochloride (Neo-Synephrine). For a patient with a history of allergy, one of the antihistamine decongestant medications, such as pseudoephedrine (Sudafed) or brompheniramine/pseudoephedrine, is prescribed orally every 4 to 6 hours. Aspirin (for patients older than 20 years of age) or acetaminophen is recommended for its anti-inflammatory and analgesic properties.

For adults with chronic pharyngitis, tonsillectomy is an effective option, if consideration is given to morbidity and complications relating to the surgery. For further information, see the section **Tonsillitis** and Adenoiditis, below.

Nursing Management

Educating Patients About Self-Care

To prevent the infection from spreading, the nurse instructs the patient to avoid contact with others until the fever subsides. The nurse recommends avoidance of alcohol, tobacco, secondhand smoke, and exposure to cold or to environmental or occupational pollutants. The patient may minimize exposure to pollutants by wearing a disposable facemask. The nurse encourages the patient to drink plenty of fluids. Gargling with warm saline solution may relieve throat discomfort. Lozenges keep the throat moistened.

Tonsillitis and Adenoiditis

The tonsils are composed of lymphatic tissue and are situated on each side of the oropharynx. The faucial or palatine tonsils and lingual tonsils are located behind the pillars of fauces and tongue, respectively. They frequently serve as the site of acute infection in children and adults (tonsillitis). Chronic tonsillitis is less common and may be mistaken for other disorders such as allergy, asthma, and sinusitis.

The adenoids or pharyngeal tonsils consist of lymphatic tissue near the centre of the posterior wall of the nasopharynx. Infection of the adenoids frequently accompanies acute tonsillitis. Frequently occurring bacterial pathogens include GABHS, the most common organism. The most common viral pathogen is Epstein–Barr virus, present in 90% of affected adults. Cytomegalovirus may also cause tonsillitis and adenoiditis.

Clinical Manifestations

The symptoms of tonsillitis include sore throat, fever, snoring, and difficulty swallowing. Enlarged adenoids may cause mouth breathing, earache, draining ears, frequent head colds, bronchitis, foul-smelling breath, voice impairment, and noisy respirations. Unusually enlarged adenoids fill the space behind the posterior nares, making it difficult for the air to travel from the nose to the throat and resulting in nasal obstruction. Infection can extend to the middle ears by way of the auditory (eustachian) tubes and may result in acute otitis media, which can lead to spontaneous rupture of the tympanic membranes (eardrums) and further extension of the infection into the mastoid cells, causing acute mastoiditis. The infection also may reside in the middle ear as a chronic, low-grade, smoldering process that eventually may cause permanent deafness.

Assessment and Diagnostic Findings

The diagnosis of acute tonsillitis is primarily clinical, with attention given to whether the illness is viral or bacterial in nature. As in acute pharyngitis, rapid streptococcal antigen test (RSAT) is quick and convenient; however, it is less sensitive than the throat swab culture.

A thorough physical examination is performed, and a careful history is obtained to rule out related or systemic conditions. The tonsillar site is cultured to determine the presence of bacterial infection. In adenoiditis, if recurrent episodes of suppurative otitis media result in hearing loss, comprehensive audiometric assessment is warranted (see Chapter 61).

Medical Management

Tonsillitis is treated through the use of supportive measures that include increased fluid intake, analgesics, salt water gargles, and rest. Bacterial infections are treated with penicillin (first-line therapy) or cephalosporins. Viral tonsillitis is not effectively treated with antibiotic therapy.

Tonsillectomy (with or without adenoidectomy) continues to be a commonly performed surgical procedure and remains the treatment of choice for patients with chronic tonsillitis (Shah, 2018).

A tonsillectomy is indicated if the patient has had repeated episodes of tonsillitis (6 per year) despite antibiotic therapy; hypertrophy of the tonsils and adenoids that could cause obstruction and obstructive sleep apnea (OSA); and/or recurrent peritonsillar abscess (Canadian Society of Otolaryngology—Head and Neck Surgery, 2018). Indications for adenoidectomy include chronic nasal congestion, chronic infection, or as an additional intervention done when ventilating tubes are inserted (Canadian Society of Otolaryngology—Head and Neck Surgery, 2018). An adenoidectomy is a common surgical intervention done almost exclusively on pre-teenage children.

Nursing Management

Providing Postoperative Care

Continuous nursing observation is required in the immediate postoperative and recovery periods because of the significant risk of hemorrhage, which may also compromise the patient's airway (Seshamani, Vogtmann, Gatwood, et al., 2014). In the immediate postoperative period, the most comfortable position is prone, with the patient's head turned to the side to allow drainage from the mouth and pharynx. The nurse must not remove the oral airway until the patient's gag and swallowing reflexes have returned. The nurse applies an ice collar to the neck, and a basin and tissues are provided for the expectoration of blood and mucus.

Symptoms of postoperative complications include fever, throat pain, ear pain, and bleeding. Pain can be effectively controlled with analgesic medications (Paquette, Le May, Lachance Fiola, et al., 2012). Postoperative bleeding, which occurs in only 2% to 4% of tonsillectomy cases, may be classified as primary (occurring within the first 24 hours) or secondary (occurring between 24 hours and 8 days). The blood may be bright red if the patient expectorates it before swallowing it. If the patient swallows the blood, it becomes brown because of the action of the acidic gastric juice. If the patient vomits large amounts of dark blood or bright-red blood at frequent intervals, or if the pulse rate and temperature rise and the patient is restless, the nurse notifies the surgeon immediately. The nurse should have the following items ready for examination of the surgical site for bleeding: a light, a mirror, gauze, curved hemostats, and a waste basin.

Occasionally, suture or ligation of a bleeding vessel is required. In such cases, the patient is taken to the operating room and given general anesthesia. After ligation, continuous nursing observation and postoperative care are required, as in the initial postoperative period. If there is no bleeding, water and ice chips may be given to the patient as soon as desired. The patient is instructed to refrain from too much talking and coughing because these activities can produce throat pain.

Educating Patients About Self-Care

Tonsillectomy and adenoidectomy are usually performed as outpatient surgery and the patient is sent home from the recovery room once awake, oriented, and able to drink liquids and void. The patient and family must understand the signs and symptoms of hemorrhage. As previously stated, bleeding may occur up to 8 days after surgery. The nurse instructs the patient about use of liquid acetaminophen with or without codeine for pain control and explains that the pain will subside during the first 3 to 5 days. The nurse informs the patient about the need to take the full course of any prescribed antibiotic (Drake & Carr, 2017).

Alkaline mouthwashes and warm saline solutions are useful in coping with the thick mucus and halitosis that may be present after surgery. The nurse should explain to the patient that a sore throat, stiff neck, minor ear pain, and vomiting may occur in the first 24 hours. The patient should eat an adequate diet with soft foods, which are more easily swallowed than hard foods. The patient should avoid spicy, hot, acidic, or rough foods. Milk and milk products (ice cream and yogurt) may be restricted because they make removal of mucus more difficult for some patients. The nurse instructs the patient about the need to maintain good hydration. It is important to tell the patient to avoid vigorous tooth brushing or gargling because these activities can cause bleeding. The nurse encourages the use of a cool-mist vaporizer or humidifier in the home postoperatively. The patient should avoid smoking and heavy lifting or exertion for 10 days.

Peritonsillar Abscess

Peritonsillar abscess (also called quinsy) is the most common major suppurative complication of sore throat accounting for roughly 30% of soft tissue head and neck abscesses. It most commonly afflicts adults between the ages of 20 and 40 years, with the incidence roughly the same between men and women (Flores, 2015). This collection of purulent exudate between the tonsillar capsule and the surrounding tissues, including the soft palate, may develop after an acute tonsillar infection that progresses to a local cellulitis and abscess. Several bacteria are typically implicated in the pathogenesis of these abscesses, including *Streptococcus pyogenes*, *Staphylococcus aureus*, *Neisseria* species, and *Corynebacterium* species (Flores, 2015; Shah, 2018). In more severe cases, the infection can spread over the palate and to the neck and chest. Edema can cause airway obstruction, which can be life threatening and is a medical emergency. Peritonsillar abscess can be life threatening with mediastinitis, intracranial abscess, and empyemas resulting from spread of infection. Early detection and aggressive management are essential (Flores, 2015).

Clinical Manifestations

The person with a peritonsillar abscess appears acutely ill with a severe sore throat, fever, trismus (inability to open the mouth), and drooling. Inflammation of the medial pterygoid muscle that lies lateral to the tonsil results in spasm, severe pain, and difficulty in opening the mouth fully. The pain may be so intense that the patient has difficulty swallowing saliva. The patient's breath often smells rancid. Other symptoms include a raspy voice, odynophagia (a severe sensation of burning, squeezing pain while swallowing), **dysphagia** (difficulty swallowing), and otalgia (pain in the ear). Odynophagia is caused by the inflammation of the superior constrictor muscle of the pharynx that forms the lateral wall of the tonsil. This causes pain on lateral movement of the head. The patient may also have tender and enlarged cervical lymph nodes. Examination of the oropharynx reveals erythema of the anterior pillar and soft palate as well as a purulent tonsil on the side of the peritonsillar abscess. The tonsil is pushed inferomedially and the uvula is shifted contralaterally (Flores, 2015).

Assessment and Diagnostic Findings

Emergency department physicians are often required to make the diagnosis of peritonsillar abscess and to decide whether aspiration, an invasive procedure, should be carried out based on the patient's clinical picture. Intraoral ultrasound and transcutaneous cervical ultrasound are used in the diagnosis of peritonsillar cellulitis and abscesses.

Medical Management

Antimicrobial agents and corticosteroid therapy are used for treatment of peritonsillar abscess. Antibiotics (usually penicillin) are extremely effective in controlling the infection and, if they are prescribed early in the course of the disease, the abscess may resolve without needing to be incised. However, if the abscess does not resolve, treatment choices include needle aspiration, incision and drainage under local or general anesthesia, and drainage of the abscess with simultaneous tonsillectomy. Following needle aspiration (discussed below) intramuscular administration of clindamycin (Cleocin) can be used in the outpatient setting, thus reducing both antibiotic and hospital costs. Use of topical anesthetic agents and throat irrigations may be prescribed to promote comfort along with administration of prescribed analgesic agents.

Patients with signs of toxicity or complications require hospitalization for IV antibiotics, imaging studies, observation, and proper airway management.

Surgical Management

Needle aspiration may be preferred over a more extensive procedure due to its high efficacy, low cost, and patient tolerance. The mucous membrane over the swelling is first sprayed with a topical anesthetic and then injected with a local anesthetic. Single or repeated needle aspirations are performed to decompress the abscess. Alternatively, the abscess may be incised and drained. These procedures are performed best with the patient in the sitting position to make it easier to expectorate the pus and blood that accumulate in the pharynx. The patient experiences almost immediate relief. Incision and drainage is also an effective option but is more painful than needle aspiration.

Tonsillectomy is considered for patients who are poor candidates for needle aspiration or incision and drainage. The risk of hemorrhage following tonsillectomy to treat peritonsillar abscess is higher than that of elective tonsillectomy and may be due to the patient's previous use of aspirin for pain relief.

Nursing Management

If the patient requires intubation, cricothyroidotomy, or tracheotomy to treat airway obstruction, the nurse assists with the procedure and provides support to the patient before, during, and after the procedure. The nurse also assists with the needle aspiration when indicated.

The nurse encourages the patient to use prescribed topical anesthetic agents and assists with throat irrigations or the frequent use of mouthwashes or gargles, using saline or alkaline solutions at a temperature of 40.6° to 43.3°C. Gentle gargling after the procedure with a cool normal saline gargle may relieve discomfort. The patient must be upright and clearly expectorate forward. The nurse instructs the patient to gargle *gently* at intervals of 1 or 2 hours for 24 to 36 hours. Liquids that are cool or at room temperature are usually well tolerated. Adequate fluids must be provided to treat dehydration and prevent its recurrence.

The nurse also observes the patient for complications and instructs the patient about signs and symptoms of complications that require prompt attention by the physician. At discharge, the nurse provides verbal and written instructions regarding foods to avoid, when to return to work, and the need to refrain from or cease smoking; it is also important to reinforce the need for continuation of good oral hygiene.

Laryngitis

Laryngitis, an inflammation of the larynx, often occurs as a result of voice abuse or exposure to dust, chemicals, smoke, and other pollutants or as part of a URTI. It also may be caused by isolated infection involving only the vocal cords. Laryngitis is also associated with gastroesophageal reflux (referred to as reflux laryngitis).

Laryngitis is very often caused by the pathogens that cause the common cold and pharyngitis, most commonly viruses. Viral laryngitis is common in the winter and is easily transmitted to others. Laryngitis is often associated with allergic rhinitis or pharyngitis. Bacterial invasion may be secondary. The onset of infection may be associated with exposure to sudden temperature changes, dietary deficiencies, malnutrition, or an immunosuppressed state.

Clinical Manifestations

Signs of acute laryngitis include hoarseness or **aphonia** (complete loss of voice) and severe cough. Chronic laryngitis is marked by persistent hoarseness. Other signs of acute laryngitis include sudden onset made worse by cold dry wind. The throat feels worse in the morning and improves when the patient is indoors in a warmer climate. At times, the patient presents with a dry cough and a dry, sore throat that worsens in the evening hours. If allergies are present, the uvula will be visibly edematous. Many patients also complain of a "tickle" in the throat that is made worse by cold air or cold liquids.

Medical Management

Management of acute laryngitis includes resting the voice, avoiding irritants (including smoking), resting, and inhaling cool steam or an aerosol. If the laryngitis is part of a more extensive respiratory infection caused by a bacterial organism or if it is severe, appropriate antibacterial therapy is instituted. The majority of patients recover with conservative treatment; however, laryngitis tends to be more severe in older adult patients and may be complicated by pneumonia.

For chronic laryngitis, the treatment includes resting the voice, eliminating any primary respiratory tract infection, eliminating smoking, and avoiding secondhand smoke. Topical corticosteroids may be given by inhalation. These preparations have few systemic or long-lasting effects and may reduce local inflammatory reactions. Treatment for reflux laryngitis typically involves use of proton pump inhibitors given once daily.

Nursing Management

The nurse instructs the patient to rest the voice and to maintain a well-humidified environment. If laryngeal secretions are present during acute episodes, expectorant agents are suggested, along with a daily fluid intake of 2 to 3 L to thin secretions. The nurse instructs the patient about the importance of taking prescribed medications, including proton pump inhibitors, and using continuous positive airway therapy at bedtime, if prescribed for OSA. In cases involving infection, the nurse informs the patient that the symptoms of laryngitis often extend a week to 10 days after completion of antibiotic therapy. The nurse instructs the patient about signs and symptoms that require contacting the health care provider. These signs and symptoms include loss of voice with sore throat that makes swallowing saliva difficult, hemoptysis, and noisy respirations. It is important to report continued hoarseness after voice rest or laryngitis that persists for longer than 5 days because of the possibility of malignancy.

Nursing Process

The Patient With Upper Airway Infection

Assessment

A health history may reveal signs and symptoms of headache, sore throat, pain around the eyes and on either side of the nose, difficulty in swallowing, cough, hoarseness, fever, stuffiness, and generalized discomfort and fatigue. Determining when the symptoms began, what precipitated them, what if anything relieves them, and what aggravates them is part of the assessment. The nurse should also determine any history of allergy or the existence of a concomitant illness. Inspection may reveal swelling, lesions, or asymmetry of the nose as well as bleeding or discharge. The nurse inspects the nasal mucosa for abnormal findings such as increased redness, swelling, exudate, and nasal polyps, which may develop in chronic rhinitis. The mucosa of the nasal turbinates may also be swollen (boggy) and pale, bluish-grey. The nurse palpates the frontal and maxillary sinuses for tenderness, which suggests inflammation, and then inspects the throat by having the patient open the mouth wide and take a deep breath. Redness, asymmetry, or evidence of drainage, ulceration, or enlargement of the tonsils and pharynx is abnormal. Palpation of the neck lymph nodes for enlargement and tenderness is necessary.

Nursing Priorities

Based on the assessment data, the patient's major nursing priorities may include the following:

- Airway clearance
- Acute pain
- Communication issues
- Fluid and electrolyte balance
- Patient teaching regarding treatment and prevention or possible surgery

Collaborative Problems/ Potential Complications

Based on assessment data, potential complications include:

- Sepsis
- Meningitis or brain abscess
- Peritonsillar abscess, otitis media, or sinusitis

Planning and Goals

The major goals for the patient may include maintenance of a patent airway, relief of pain, maintenance of effective means of communication, normal hydration, knowledge of how to prevent upper airway infections, and absence of complications.

Nursing Interventions

Maintaining a Patent Airway

An accumulation of secretions can block the airway in patients with an upper airway infection. As a result, changes in the respiratory pattern occur, and the work of breathing increases to compensate for the blockage. The nurse can implement several measures to loosen thick secretions or to keep the secretions moist so that they can be easily expectorated. Increasing fluid intake helps thin the mucus. Use of room vaporizers or steam inhalation also loosens secretions and reduces inflammation of the mucous membranes. To enhance drainage from the sinuses, the nurse instructs the patient about positioning; this depends on the location of the infection or inflammation. For example, drainage for sinusitis or rhinitis is achieved in the upright position. In some conditions, topical or systemic medications, when prescribed, help relieve nasal or throat congestion.

Promoting Comfort

Upper respiratory tract infections (URTIs) usually produce localized discomfort. In sinusitis, pain may occur in the area of the sinuses, or a general headache may be produced. In pharyngitis, laryngitis, or tonsillitis, a sore throat occurs. The nurse encourages the patient to take analgesics, such as acetaminophen with codeine, as prescribed, to relieve this discomfort. A pain intensity rating scale (see Chapter 16) may be used to assess effectiveness of pain relief measures. Other helpful measures include topical anesthetic agents for symptomatic relief of herpes simplex blisters (see Chart 23-3) and sore throats, hot packs to relieve the congestion of sinusitis and promote drainage, and warm water gargles or irrigations to relieve the pain of a sore throat. The nurse encourages rest to relieve the generalized discomfort and fever that accompany many upper airway conditions (especially rhinitis, pharyngitis, and laryngitis). For postoperative care after tonsillectomy and adenoidectomy, an ice collar may reduce swelling and decrease bleeding.

Promoting Communication

Upper airway infections may result in hoarseness or loss of speech. The nurse instructs the patient to refrain from speaking as much as possible and, if possible, to communicate in writing instead. Additional strain on the vocal cords may delay full return of the voice. The nurse encourages the patient and family to use alternative forms of communication, such as a memo pad, sending text messages, or a bell to signal for assistance.

Encouraging Fluid Intake

Upper airway infections lead to fluid loss. Sore throat, malaise, and fever may interfere with a patient's willingness to eat and drink. The nurse provides a list of easily ingested foods to increase caloric intake during the acute phase of illness. These include soups, pudding, yogurt, cottage cheese, high-protein drinks, and Popsicles. The nurse encourages the patient to drink 2 to 3 L of fluid per day during the acute stage of airway infection, unless contraindicated, to thin the secretions and promote drainage. Liquids (hot or cold) may be soothing, depending on the disorder.

Promoting Home, Community-Based, and Transitional Care

EDUCATING PATIENTS ABOUT SELF-CARE. Prevention of most upper airway infections is difficult because of the many potential causes. But because most URTIs are transmitted by hand-to-hand contact, the nurse teaches the patient and family techniques to minimize the spread of infection to others, including frequent handwashing. The nurse advises the patient to avoid exposure to people who are at risk for serious illness if respiratory infection is transmitted (older adults, immunosuppressed people, and those with chronic health problems).

The nurse teaches patients and their families strategies to relieve symptoms of URTIs. It is important to reinforce the need to complete the treatment regimen, particularly when antibiotics are prescribed.

CONTINUING AND TRANSITIONAL CARE. Referral for home care is rare. However, it may be indicated for people whose health status was compromised before the onset of the respiratory infection and for those who cannot manage self-care without assistance. In such circumstances, the home care nurse assesses the patient's respiratory status and progress in recovery. The nurse may advise older adult patients and those at increased risk from a respiratory infection to consider annual influenza and pneumococcal vaccination as recommended by the physician. A follow-up appointment with the primary care provider may be indicated for patients with compromised health status to ensure that the respiratory infection has resolved.

Monitoring and Managing Potential Complications

Although major complications of URTIs are rare, the nurse must be aware of them and assess the patient for them. Because most patients with URTIs are managed at home, patients and their families must be instructed to monitor for signs and symptoms and to seek immediate medical care if the patient's condition does not improve or if the patient's physical status appears to be worsening.

Sepsis or meningitis may occur in patients with compromised immune status or in those with an overwhelming bacterial infection. The patient with a URTI and family members are instructed to seek medical care if the patient's condition fails to improve within several days after the onset of symptoms, if unusual symptoms develop, or if the patient's condition deteriorates. They are instructed about signs and symptoms that require further attention: persistent or high fever, increasing shortness of breath, confusion, and increasing weakness and malaise. The patient with sepsis requires expert care to treat the infection, stabilize vital signs, and prevent or treat septicemia and shock. Deterioration of the patient's condition necessitates intensive care measures (e.g., hemodynamic monitoring and administration of vasoactive medications, IV fluids, nutritional support, corticosteroids) to monitor the patient's status and to support the patient's vital signs. High doses of antibiotics may be administered to treat the causative organism. The nurse's role is to monitor the patient's vital signs, hemodynamic status, and laboratory values, administer needed treatment, alleviate the patient's physical discomfort, and provide explanations, teaching, and emotional support to the patient and family.

Peritonsillar abscess may develop after an acute infection of the tonsils. The patient requires treatment to drain the abscess and receives antibiotics for infection and topical anesthetic agents and throat irrigations to relieve pain and sore throat. Follow-up is necessary to ensure that the abscess resolves; tonsillectomy may be required. The nurse assists the patient in administering throat irrigations and instructs the patient and family about the importance of adhering to the prescribed treatment regimen and recommended follow-up appointments.

In some severe situations, peritonsillar abscess may progress to meningitis or brain abscess. The nurse assesses for changes in mental status ranging from subtle personality changes through drowsiness to coma, nuchal rigidity, and focal neurologic signs that signal increasing cerebral edema around the abscess. Seizures often occur in this situation. Intensive care measures are necessary. High doses of antibiotics may be used to treat the causative organism. The nurse's role is similar to caring for the patient with sepsis in an intensive care setting. The nurse monitors the patient's neurologic status and reports changes immediately to the physician.

Otitis media and rhinosinusitis may develop with URTI. The patient and family are instructed about the signs and symptoms of otitis media and rhinosinusitis and about the importance of follow-up with the primary health care practitioner to ensure adequate evaluation and treatment of these conditions.

Evaluation

Expected patient outcomes may include the following:

1. Maintains a patent airway by managing secretions
   a. Reports decreased congestion
   b. Assumes best position to facilitate drainage of secretions
   c. Uses self-care measures appropriately and consistently to manage secretions during the acute phase of illness
2. Reports relief of pain and discomfort using pain intensity scale
   a. Uses comfort measures: analgesics, hot packs, gargles, rest
   b. Demonstrates adequate oral hygiene
3. Demonstrates ability to communicate needs, wants, level of comfort
4. Maintains adequate fluid and nutrition intake
5. Utilizes strategies to prevent upper airway infections and allergic reactions
   a. Demonstrates hand hygiene techniques
   b. Identifies the value of the influenza vaccine
6. Demonstrates an adequate level of knowledge and performs self-care adequately
7. Becomes free of signs and symptoms of infection
   a. Exhibits normal vital signs (temperature, pulse, respiratory rate)
   b. Absence of purulent drainage
   c. Free of pain in ears, sinuses, and throat
   d. Absence of signs of inflammation
8. Absence of complications
   a. No signs of sepsis: fever, hypotension, deterioration of cognitive status
   b. Vital signs and hemodynamic status normal
   c. No evidence of neurologic involvement
   d. No signs of development of peritonsillar abscess
   e. Resolution of URI without development of otitis media or sinusitis
   f. No signs and symptoms of brain abscess

OBSTRUCTION AND TRAUMA OF THE UPPER RESPIRATORY AIRWAY

Obstructive Sleep Apnea

OSA is a disorder characterized by recurrent episodes of upper airway obstruction and a reduction in ventilation. It is defined as cessation of breathing (**apnea**) during sleep usually caused by repetitive upper airway obstruction. In 2016 and 2017, nearly one third (30%) of Canadian adults were considered to be at intermediate or high risk for OSA, and about 6.4% of Canadians reported being diagnosed with sleep apnea in 2016 and 2017 (Statistics Canada, 2018). OSA interferes with people's ability to obtain adequate rest, thus affecting memory, learning, and decision making.

Risk factors for OSA include obesity, male gender, advanced age, menopause, smoking, and adenotonsillar hypertrophy (Franklin & Lindberg, 2015; Jordan, McSharry, & Malhotra, 2014).

Pathophysiology

The pharynx is a collapsible tube that can be compressed by the soft tissues and structures surrounding it. The tone of the muscles of the upper airway is reduced during sleep. Mechanical factors such as reduced diameter of the upper airway or dynamic changes in the upper airway during sleep may result in obstruction. These sleep-related changes may predispose to upper airway collapse when small amounts of negative pressure are generated during inspiration.

Repetitive apneic events result in hypoxia (decreased oxygen saturation) and hypercapnia (increased concentration of carbon dioxide), which trigger a sympathetic response. As a consequence, patients with OSA have a high prevalence of hypertension. In addition, OSA is associated with an increased risk of myocardial infarction and stroke (cerebrovascular accident), which may be mitigated with appropriate treatment (Downey, 2015).

Clinical Manifestations

OSA, as defined by the International Classification of Sleep Disorders, is characterized by the presence of symptoms or certain comorbidities associated with five or more

CHART 23-4

Assessment: Assessing for Obstructive Sleep Apnea (OSA)

Be alert for the following signs and symptoms of OSA:

- Excessive daytime sleepiness
- Frequent nocturnal awakening
- Insomnia
- Loud snoring
- Morning headaches
- Intellectual deterioration
- Personality changes, irritability
- Impotence
- Systemic hypertension
- Dysrhythmias
- Pulmonary hypertension, cor pulmonale
- Polycythemia
- Enuresis

Adapted from Downey, R. (2015). *Obstructive sleep apnea*. Retrieved October 12, 2015, from www.emedicine.medscape.com/article/295807-overview

predominantly obstructive respiratory events per hour or by 15 or more predominantly obstructive respiratory events per hour in asymptomatic individuals (Kapur et al., 2017). These obstructive respiratory events often include loud snoring with breathing cessation for 10 seconds or longer followed by awakening abruptly with a loud snort as the blood oxygen level drops. Patients with sleep apnea may have anywhere from five apneic episodes per hour to several hundred per night.

Classic signs and symptoms of OSA include the "3S's"—namely, snoring, sleepiness, and significant-other report of sleep apnea episodes. Common signs and symptoms of OSA are presented in Chart 23-4. Symptoms typically progress with increases in weight, aging, and during the transition to menopause (Downey, 2015). Patients are typically unaware of nocturnal upper airway obstruction during sleep. They frequently complain of insomnia including difficulty in going to sleep, nighttime awakenings, and early morning awakenings with an inability to go back to sleep, as well as chronic fatigue and hypersomnolence (daytime sleepiness). When obtaining the health history, the nurse asks the patient about sleeping during normal activities such as eating or talking. Patients with this symptom are considered to have pathologic hypersomnolence (Downey, 2015).

Assessment and Diagnostic Findings

The diagnosis of sleep apnea is based on clinical features plus a polysomnographic finding (sleep study), which is the gold standard for diagnosis of OSA. The test is an overnight study which continuously measures multiple physiologic signals while the patient sleeps. These signals are analyzed as they are related to stages of sleep; measures include those taken by electroencephalogram (EEG), electrooculogram, and chin electromyogram (EMG). In addition, cardiac rhythms and dysrhythmias are monitored with a single-lead electrocardiogram (ECG) and leg movements are recorded by an anterior tibialis EMG. Airflow at the nose and mouth is monitored using both a thermal sensor and a nasal pressure transducer, breathing effort is monitored using inductance plethysmography, and hemoglobin oxygen saturation is monitored by oximetry. The breathing pattern is analyzed for the presence of apneas and hypopneas. Characteristic findings consistent with OSA include apneic episodes occurring in the presence of respiratory muscle effort, clinically significant apneic episodes lasting 10 seconds or longer, and apneic episodes most prevalent during the rapid eye movement (REM) stage of sleep. Sleep disruption from automated patient arousal is usually seen at the termination of an episode of apnea (Downey, 2015).

Medical Management

Patients usually seek medical treatment because their sleeping partners express concern or because they experience excessive sleepiness at inappropriate times or settings (e.g., while driving a car). A variety of treatments are used. Weight loss, avoidance of alcohol, positional therapy (prevents individuals from sleeping on their back), and oral appliances such as mandibular advancement devices (MADs) are the first steps (Downey, 2015).

When applied correctly, a MAD advances the mandible so that it is slightly anterior to the upper front teeth, preventing airway obstruction by the tongue and soft tissue during sleep. A randomized controlled trial that compared the effectiveness of these devices among patients with OSA with the more conventional therapy, continuous positive airway pressure (CPAP), found no difference in short-term outcomes between MAD and CPAP, including daytime sleepiness and quality of life, suggesting that MAD is as effective a treatment as CPAP in patients with mild to moderate OSA (White & Shafazand, 2013). In more severe cases involving hypoxemia and severe hypercapnia, the treatment includes CPAP or bilevel positive airway pressure (BiPAP) therapy with supplemental oxygen via nasal cannula. CPAP is used to prevent airway collapse, whereas BiPAP makes breathing easier and results in a lower average airway pressure. (The use of CPAP and BiPAP is discussed in more detail in Chapter 26.)

CPAP is used to prevent airway collapse, whereas BiPAP makes breathing easier and results in a lower average airway pressure. CPAP has been shown to reduce apnea–hypopnea index and sleepiness (Canadian Agency for Drugs and Technologies in Health [CADTH], 2017). Although these treatments are effective in management of OSA, compliance with treatment continues to be a major concern.

Oral appliances are recommended for patients with mild to moderate OSA who are unable to tolerate CPAP. These oral appliances are either MADs or tongue-retaining devices. Oral appliances have been shown to improve sleepiness and decrease the apnea–hypopnea index, albeit to a lesser extent than seen with treatment with CPAP (CADTH, 2017).

Surgical Management

Surgical procedures also may be performed to correct OSA. Simple tonsillectomy may be effective for patients with larger tonsils when deemed clinically necessary, or when other options have failed or are refused by patients (Morgan, 2015). Uvulopalatopharyngoplasty is the resection of pharyngeal soft tissue and removal of approximately 15 mm of the free edge of the soft palate and uvula. Effective in about 50% of patients, it is more effective in eliminating snoring than apnea. Nasal septoplasty may be performed for gross anatomic nasal septal deformities. Tracheostomy relieves upper airway obstruction but has numerous adverse effects, including speech difficulties and increased risk of infections. These procedures, as well as other maxillofacial surgeries, are reserved for patients with life-threatening dysrhythmias or severe disability who have not responded to conventional therapy (Tierney et al., 2015).

Pharmacologic Therapy

Although medications are not generally recommended for OSA, modafinil (Provigil) has been shown to reduce daytime sleepiness (Downey, 2015). Protriptyline (Triptil) given at bedtime may increase the respiratory drive and improve upper airway muscle tone. Medroxyprogesterone acetate (Provera) and acetazolamide (Diamox) have been used for sleep apnea associated with chronic alveolar hypoventilation, but their benefits have not been well established. The patient must understand that these medications are not a substitute for CPAP, BiPAP, or MAD. Administration of low-flow nasal oxygen at night can help relieve hypoxemia in some patients but has little effect on the frequency or severity of apnea. Further studies on the effectiveness of pharmacologic therapy are needed.

Nursing Management

The patient with OSA may not recognize the potential consequences of the disorder. Therefore, the nurse explains the disorder in terms that are understandable to the patient and relates symptoms (daytime sleepiness) to the underlying disorder. The nurse also instructs the patient and family about treatments, including the correct and safe use of CPAP, BiPAP, and oxygen therapy, if prescribed.

Epistaxis (Nosebleed)

Epistaxis, a hemorrhage from the nose, is caused by the rupture of tiny, distended vessels in the mucous membrane of any area of the nose. Rarely does epistaxis originate in the densely vascular tissue over the turbinates. Most commonly, the site is the anterior septum, where three major blood vessels enter the nasal cavity: (1) the anterior ethmoidal artery on the forward part of the roof (Kiesselbach's plexus), (2) the sphenopalatine artery in the posterosuperior region, and (3) the internal maxillary branches (the plexus of veins located at the back of the lateral wall under the inferior turbinate).

Several risk factors are associated with epistaxis (Chart 23-5).

CHART 23-5

Risk Factors: Epistaxis

- Local infections (vestibulitis, rhinitis, sinusitis)
- Systemic infections (scarlet fever, malaria)
- Drying of nasal mucous membranes
- Nasal inhalation of illicit drugs (e.g., cocaine)
- Trauma (digital trauma as in picking the nose; blunt trauma; fracture; forceful nose blowing)
- Arteriosclerosis
- Hypertension
- Tumour (sinus or nasopharynx)
- Thrombocytopenia
- Use of aspirin
- Liver disease
- Osler–Weber–Rendu syndrome (hereditary hemorrhagic telangiectasia)

Adapted from Nguyen, Q. A. (2015). *Epistaxis.* Retrieved October 12, 2015, from www.emedicine.medscape.com/article/863220-overview

Medical Management

Management of epistaxis depends on its cause and the location of the bleeding site. A nasal speculum, penlight, or headlight may be used to identify the site of bleeding in the nasal cavity. Most nosebleeds originate from the anterior portion of the nose. Initial treatment may include applying direct pressure. The patient sits upright with the head tilted forward to prevent swallowing and aspiration of blood and is directed to pinch the soft outer portion of the nose against the midline septum for 5 or 10 minutes continuously. Application of nasal decongestants (phenylephrine, one or two sprays) to act as vasoconstrictors may be necessary. If these measures are unsuccessful in stopping the bleeding, the nose must be examined using good illumination and suction to determine the site of bleeding. Visible bleeding sites may be cauterized with silver nitrate or electrocautery (high-frequency electrical current). A supplemental patch of Surgicel or Gelfoam may be used (Tierney et al., 2015).

Alternatively, a cotton tampon may be used to try to stop the bleeding. Suction may be used to remove excess blood and clots from the field of inspection. The search for the bleeding site should shift from the anteroinferior quadrant to the anterosuperior, then to the posterosuperior, and finally to the posteroinferior area. The field is kept clear by using suction and by shifting the cotton tampon.

If the origin of the bleeding cannot be identified, the nose may be packed with gauze impregnated with petrolatum jelly or antibiotic ointment; a topical anesthetic spray and decongestant agent may be used before the gauze packing is inserted, or a balloon-inflated catheter may be used (Fig. 23-3). Alternatively, a compressed nasal sponge may be used. Once the sponge becomes saturated with blood or is moistened with a small amount of saline, it will expand and produce tamponade to halt the bleeding. The packing may remain in place for 3 to 4 days if necessary to control bleeding (Nguyen, 2015).

Nursing Management

The nurse monitors the patient's vital signs, assists in the control of bleeding, and provides tissues and an emesis

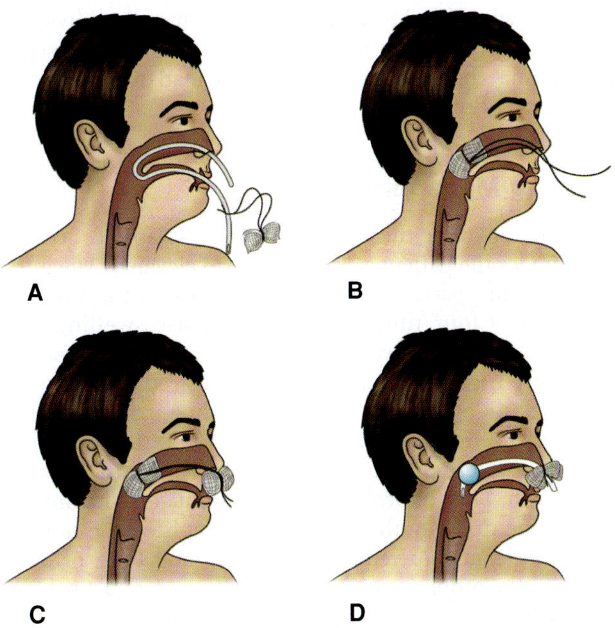

FIGURE 23-3. Packing to control bleeding from the posterior nose. **A.** Catheter is inserted, and packing is attached. **B.** Packing is drawn into position as the catheter is removed. **C.** Strip is tied over a bolster to hold the packing in place with an anterior pack installed "accordion pleat" style. **D.** Alternative method, using a balloon catheter instead of gauze packing.

basin to allow the patient to expectorate any excess blood. It is common for patients to be anxious in response to a nosebleed. Blood loss on clothing and handkerchiefs can be frightening, and the nasal examination and treatment are uncomfortable. Assuring the patient in a calm, efficient manner that bleeding can be controlled can help reduce anxiety. The nurse continuously assesses the patient's airway and breathing as well as vital signs. On rare occasions, a patient with significant hemorrhage requires IV infusions of crystalloid solutions (normal saline) as well as cardiac and pulse oximetry monitoring.

Educating Patients About Self-Care

Once the bleeding is controlled, the nurse instructs the patient to avoid vigorous exercise for several days and to avoid hot or spicy foods and tobacco because this may cause vasodilation and increase the risk of rebleeding. Discharge teaching includes reviewing ways to prevent epistaxis: avoiding forceful nose blowing, straining, high altitudes, and nasal trauma (including nose picking). Adequate humidification may prevent drying of the nasal passages. The nurse explains how to apply direct pressure to the nose with the thumb and the index finger for 15 minutes in the case of a recurrent nosebleed. If recurrent bleeding cannot be stopped, the patient is instructed to seek additional medical attention.

Nasal Obstruction

The passage of air through the nostrils is frequently obstructed by a deviation of the nasal septum, hypertrophy of the turbinate bones, or the pressure of nasal polyps (Moche & Palmer, 2012). Chronic nasal congestion forces the patient to breathe through the mouth, thus producing dryness of the oral mucosa and associated problems including persistent dry, cracked lips. Patients with chronic nasal congestion often suffer from sleep deprivation due to difficulty maintaining an adequate airway while lying flat and during sleep.

Persistent nasal obstruction also may lead to chronic infection of the nose and result in frequent episodes of nasopharyngitis. Frequently, the infection extends to the nasal sinuses. When rhinosinusitis develops and the drainage from these cavities is obstructed by deformity or swelling within the nose, pain is experienced in the region of the affected sinus.

Medical Management

The treatment of nasal obstruction requires the removal of the obstruction, followed by measures to treat whatever chronic infection exists. In many patients, an underlying allergy also requires treatment. Measures to reduce or alleviate nasal obstruction include nonsurgical as well as surgical techniques. Commonly used medications include nasal corticosteroids (see Table 23-2) as well as oral leukotriene inhibitors, such as montelukast. Treatment with nasal corticosteroids for 1 to 3 months is usually successful for treatment of small polyps and may even reduce the need for surgical intervention. A short course of oral corticosteroids (6-day course of prednisone) may be beneficial in the treatment of nasal obstruction due to polyps (Tierney et al., 2015). Additional medications may include antibiotics for the treatment of underlying infection or antihistamines for management of allergies. Hypertrophied turbinates may be treated by applying an astringent agent to shrink them.

A more aggressive approach in treating nasal obstruction caused by turbinate hypertrophy involves surgical reduction of the hypertrophy. Surgical procedures used to treat obstructive nasal conditions are collectively known as functional rhinoplasty. Technical advances with newer techniques provide a number of options for reconstruction and reshaping of the nose (Moche & Palmer, 2012).

Nursing Management

Most of the surgical procedures are performed on an outpatient basis. The nurse explains the procedure after the physician provides the initial description. Postoperatively, the nurse elevates the head of the bed to promote drainage and to alleviate discomfort from edema. Frequent oral hygiene is encouraged to overcome dryness caused by breathing through the mouth. Before discharge from the outpatient or same-day surgical unit, the patient is instructed to avoid blowing the nose with force during the postoperative recovery period. The patient is also instructed about the signs and symptoms of bleeding and infection and when to contact the physician. The patient is provided with written postoperative instructions, including emergency phone numbers.

Fractures of the Nose

The location of the nose makes it susceptible to injury. Nasal fracture is the most common facial fracture and the most common fracture in the body. Fractures of the nose usually result from a direct assault. Nasal fractures may affect the ascending process of the maxilla and the septum. The torn mucous membrane results in a nosebleed. Complications include hematoma, infection, abscess, and avascular or septic necrosis. However, as a rule, serious consequences usually do not occur.

Clinical Manifestations

The signs and symptoms of a nasal fracture are pain, bleeding from the nose externally and internally into the pharynx, swelling of the soft tissues adjacent to the nose, periorbital ecchymosis, nasal obstruction, and deformity. The patient's nose may have an asymmetric appearance that may not be obvious until the edema subsides.

Assessment and Diagnostic Findings

The nose is examined internally to rule out the possibility that the injury may be complicated by a fracture of the nasal septum and a submucosal septal hematoma. Intranasal examination is performed in all cases to rule out septal hematoma (Tierney et al., 2015). Because of the swelling and bleeding that occur with a nasal fracture, an accurate diagnosis can be made only after the swelling subsides.

Clear fluid draining from either nostril suggests a fracture of the cribriform plate with leakage of cerebrospinal fluid. Because cerebrospinal fluid contains glucose, it can readily be differentiated from nasal mucus by means of a dipstick (Dextrostix). Usually, careful inspection or palpation discloses any deviations of the bone or disruptions of the nasal cartilages. An x-ray may reveal displacement of the fractured bones and may help rule out extension of the fracture into the skull.

Medical Management

A nasal fracture very often produces bleeding from the nasal passage. As a rule, bleeding is controlled with the use of packing. Cold compresses are used to prevent or reduce edema. For the patient who has sustained enough trauma to break the nose or any facial bone, the emergency medical team must consider the possibility of a cervical spine fracture. Therefore, it is essential to ensure a patent airway and to rule out a cervical spine fracture. Uncomplicated nasal fractures may be treated initially with antibiotics, analgesic agents, and a decongestant nasal spray.

Treatment of nasal fractures is aimed at restoring nasal function and returning the appearance of the nose to baseline. The patient is referred to a specialist to evaluate the need to realign the bones. Although improved outcomes are obtained when reduction of the fracture is performed during the first 3 hours after the injury, this is often not possible because of the edema. If immediate reduction of the fracture is not possible, it is performed within 3 to 7 days. Timing is important when treating nasal fractures because further delay in treatment may result in significant bone healing, which ultimately may require surgical intervention that includes rhinoplasty to reshape the external appearance of the nose. A septorhinoplasty is performed when the nasal septum needs to be repaired. In patients who develop a septal hematoma, the physician drains the hematoma through a small incision. A septal hematoma that is not drained can lead to permanent deformity of the nose.

Nursing Management

Immediately after the fracture, the nurse applies ice and encourages the patient to keep the head elevated. The nurse instructs the patient to apply ice packs to the nose for 20 minutes four times a day to decrease swelling. The patient who experiences bleeding from the nose (epistaxis) is usually frightened and anxious and needs reassurance. The packing inserted to stop the bleeding may be uncomfortable and unpleasant, and obstruction of the nasal passages by the packing forces the patient to breathe through the mouth. This in turn causes the oral mucous membranes to become dry. Mouth rinses help to moisten the mucous membranes and to reduce the odour and taste of dried blood in the oropharynx and nasopharynx. Use of analgesic agents such as acetaminophen or NSAIDs such as ibuprofen or naproxen is encouraged. When removing the cotton pledgets, the nurse carefully inspects the mucosa for lacerations or a septal hematoma. The nurse instructs the patient to avoid sports activities for 6 weeks.

Laryngeal Obstruction

Obstruction of the larynx because of edema is a serious, often fatal, condition. The larynx is a stiff box that will not stretch. It contains a narrow space between the vocal cords (glottis), through which air must pass. Swelling of the laryngeal mucous membranes may close off the opening tightly, leading to life-threatening hypoxia or suffocation. Edema of the glottis occurs rarely in patients with acute laryngitis, occasionally in patients with urticaria, and more frequently in patients with severe inflammation of the throat, as in scarlet fever. It is an occasional but usually preventable cause of death in severe anaphylaxis (angioedema).

Hereditary angioedema (HAE) is also characterized by episodes of life-threatening laryngeal edema. Laryngeal edema in people with HAE can occur at any age, although young adults are at greatest risk. Risk factors for laryngeal obstruction are given in Table 23-3.

Foreign bodies frequently are aspirated into the pharynx, the larynx, or the trachea and cause a twofold problem. First, they obstruct the air passages and cause difficulty in breathing, which may lead to asphyxia; later, they may be drawn farther down, entering the bronchi or a bronchial branch and causing symptoms of irritation, such as a croupy cough, expectoration of blood or mucus, or laboured breathing. The physical signs and x-ray findings confirm the diagnosis.

Clinical Manifestations

The patient's clinical presentation and x-ray findings confirm the diagnosis of laryngeal obstruction. The patient may demonstrate lowered oxygen saturation; however, normal oxygen saturation should not be interpreted as a sign that the obstruction is not significant. Use of accessory muscles to maximize airflow may occur and is often

TABLE 23-3 Causes of Laryngeal Obstruction

Precipitating Event	Mechanism of Obstruction
History of allergies; exposure to medications, latex, foods (peanuts, tree nuts [e.g., walnuts, pecans]), bee stings	Anaphylaxis
Foreign body	Inhalation/ingestion of meat or other food items, coin, chewing gum, balloon fragments, drug packets (ingested to avoid criminal arrest)
Heavy alcohol consumption; heavy tobacco use	Obstruction from tumour
Family history of airway problems	Suggests angioedema (type I hypersensitivity reaction)
Use of angiotensin-converting enzyme (ACE) inhibitor	Increased risk of angioedema of the mucous membranes
Recent throat pain or recent fever	Infectious process
History of surgery or previous tracheostomy	Possible subglottic stenosis
History of nasogastric tube placement	Nasogastric tube syndrome

Adapted from Reardon, R. F., Mason, P. E., & Clinton, J. E. (2014). Basic airway management and decision-making. In J. D. Roberts (Ed.). *Roberts & Hedges' clinical procedures in emergency medicine* (6th ed.). Philadelphia, PA: Elsevier Saunders.

manifested by retractions in the neck or abdomen during inspirations. Patients who demonstrate these symptoms are at an immediate risk of collapse, and respiratory support (i.e., mechanical ventilation or positive-pressure ventilation) is considered.

Assessment and Diagnostic Findings

A thorough history can be very useful in diagnosing and treating the patient with a laryngeal obstruction. However, emergency measures to secure the patient's airway should not be delayed in order to obtain a history or to perform tests. If possible, the nurse obtains a history from the patient or family about heavy alcohol or tobacco consumption, current medications, history of airway problems, recent infections, pain or fever, dental pain or poor dentition, and any previous surgeries, radiation therapy, or trauma.

Medical Management

Medical management is based on the initial evaluation of the patient and the need to ensure a patent airway. If the airway is obstructed by a foreign body and signs of asphyxia are apparent, immediate treatment is necessary. Emergent manoeuvres to clear an airway obstruction are presented in Chart 23-6. If all efforts are unsuccessful, an immediate tracheotomy is necessary (see Chapter 26 for further discussion). If the obstruction is caused by edema resulting from an allergic reaction, treatment may include immediate administration of subcutaneous epinephrine and a corticosteroid (see Chapter 54). Ice may be applied to the neck in an effort to reduce edema. Continuous pulse oximetry is essential in the patient who has experienced acute upper airway obstruction.

Cancer of the Larynx

Cancer of the larynx is a malignant tumour in and around the larynx (voice box). Squamous cell carcinoma is the most common form of cancer of the larynx (95%). Adenocarcinoma or sarcoma of the larynx is diagnosed less often. In 2017, an estimated 1,150 Canadians were diagnosed with

CHART 23-6

Performing the Abdominal Thrust Manoeuvre

To assist a patient or other person who is choking on a foreign object, the nurse performs the abdominal thrust manoeuvre (sometimes called the Heimlich manoeuvre) according to guidelines set forth by the American Heart Association. (Note: Hands crossed at the neck is the universal sign for choking.)

1. Stand behind the person who is choking.
2. Place both arms around the person's waist.
3. Make a fist with one hand with the thumb outside the fist.
4. Place thumb side of fist against the person's abdomen above the navel and below the xiphoid process.
5. Grasp fist with other hand.
6. Quickly and forcefully exert pressure against the person's diaphragm, pressing upward with quick, firm thrusts.
7. Apply thrusts 6 to 10 times until the obstruction is cleared.
8. The pressure from the thrusts should lift the diaphragm, force air into the lungs, and create an artificial cough powerful enough to expel the aspirated object.

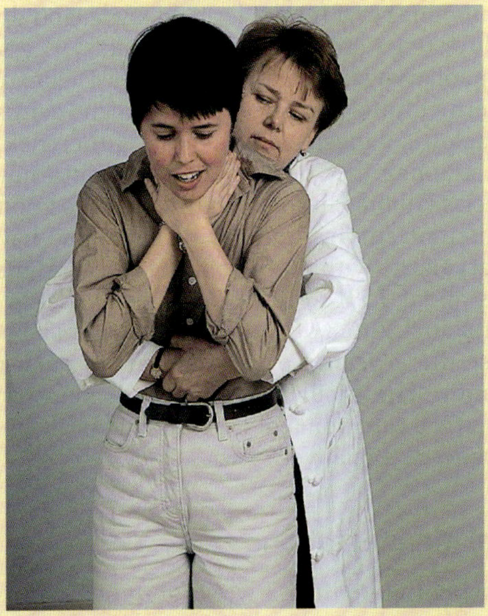

CHART 23-7

Risk Factors: Laryngeal Cancer

Carcinogens

- Tobacco (smoke, smokeless, e-cigarettes, hookahs)
- Combined effects of alcohol and tobacco
- Asbestos
- Secondhand smoke
- Paint fumes
- Wood dust
- Cement dust
- Chemicals
- Tar products
- Mustard gas
- Leather and metals

Other Factors

- Nutritional deficiencies (vitamins)
- History of alcohol abuse
- Genetic predisposition
- Age (higher incidence after 65 years of age)
- Gender (more common in men)
- Race (more prevalent in African Americans and Caucasians)
- Weakened immune system

Adapted from American Cancer Society (ACS). (2015). *What are the risk factors for laryngeal and hypopharyngeal cancers?* Retrieved March 9, 2016, from www.cancer.org/Cancer/LaryngealandHypopharyngealCancer/DetailedGuide/laryngeal-and-hypopharyngeal-cancer-risk-factors

laryngeal cancer, with approximately 440 Canadians dying from laryngeal cancer that same year (Canadian Cancer Society, 2017a).

Carcinogens that have been associated with laryngeal cancer include tobacco (smoke, smokeless) and alcohol and their combined effects (Chart 23-7). Use of chewing tobacco from other countries has increased the risk of laryngeal cancer because of its stronger potency, and the risk of laryngeal cancer may be greater than that associated with cigarette smoking (Canadian Cancer Society, 2017). Occupational exposure to coal dust, steel dust, iron compounds and fumes, formaldehyde, and dust from hard alloys (e.g., still or iron compounds) is associated with hypopharyngeal or laryngeal cancer. Dietary patterns of Western cultures are associated with an increased risk of supraglottic cancer of the larynx. Other risk factors include straining the voice, chronic laryngitis, nutritional deficiencies (riboflavin), and family predisposition.

The lifetime survival rate for patients who have small laryngeal cancers without evidence of spread to the lymph nodes is about 75% to 95%. Recurrence occurs usually within the first 2 to 3 years after diagnosis. The presence of disease after 5 years is often secondary to a new primary malignancy. The incidence of distant metastasis with squamous cell carcinoma of the head and neck (including larynx cancer) is relatively low.

Clinical Manifestations

Hoarseness of more than 2 weeks' duration occurs in the patient with cancer in the glottic area because the tumour impedes the action of the vocal cords during speech. The voice may sound harsh, raspy, and lower in pitch. Affected voice sounds are not early signs of subglottic or supraglottic cancer. The patient may complain of a persistent cough or sore throat and pain and burning in the throat, especially when consuming hot liquids or citrus juices. A lump may be felt in the neck. Later symptoms include dysphagia, dyspnea (difficulty breathing), unilateral nasal obstruction or discharge, persistent hoarseness, persistent ulceration, and foul breath. Cervical lymph adenopathy, unintentional weight loss, a general debilitated state, and pain radiating to the ear may occur with metastasis.

Assessment and Diagnostic Findings

An initial assessment includes a complete history and physical examination of the head and neck. This includes identification of risk factors, family history, and any underlying medical conditions. An indirect laryngoscopy, using a flexible endoscope, is initially performed in the otolaryngologist's office to visually evaluate the pharynx, larynx, and possible tumour. Mobility of the vocal cords is assessed; if normal movement is limited, the growth may affect muscle, other tissue, and even the airway. The neck and the thyroid gland are palpated for enlarged lymph nodes and enlarged thyroid gland. See Nursing Research Profile Chart 23-8 for patterns of symptom severity of patients with cancer of the head and neck.

Diagnostic procedures that may be used include endoscopy, including virtual endoscopy, fine-needle aspiration (FNA) biopsy, CT or MRI scan (American Cancer Society [ACS], 2015). If a tumour of the larynx is suspected on an initial examination, a direct laryngoscopic examination is performed under local or general anesthesia to evaluate all areas of the larynx. In some cases, intraoperative examination obtained by direct microscopic visualization and palpation of the vocal folds may yield a more accurate diagnosis. Samples of the suspicious tissue are obtained for analysis.

The classification, including stage of the tumour (i.e., size and histology of the tumour, presence and extent of cervical lymph node involvement) and location of the tumour serve as a basis for treatment. FNA biopsy may be done as an initial screening procedure to obtain samples of any enlarged lymph nodes in the neck. CT and MRI are used to assess regional adenopathy and soft tissues and to stage and determine the extent of a tumour. MRI is also helpful in posttreatment follow-up to detect a recurrence.

Medical Management

The goals of treatment of laryngeal cancer include cure, preservation of safe, effective swallowing, preservation of useful voice, and avoidance of permanent tracheostoma (Tierney et al., 2015). Treatment options include surgery, radiation therapy, and chemotherapy. The prognosis depends on the tumour stage, the patient's gender and age, and pathologic features of the tumour, including the grade and depth of infiltration. The treatment plan also depends on whether the cancer is an initial diagnosis or a recurrence. In addition, before treatment begins, a complete dental examination is performed to rule out any oral disease.

NURSING RESEARCH PROFILE

Chart 23-8. Patterns of Symptom Severity of Patients With Cancer of the Head and Neck

Haisfield-Wolfe, M. E., Brown, C., Richardson, M. et al. (2015). Variations in symptom severity patterns among oropharyngeal and laryngeal cancer outpatients during radiation treatment: A pilot study. *Cancer Nursing, 38*(4), 279–287.

Purpose

Patients diagnosed with laryngeal and oropharyngeal cancer (head and neck cancer [HNC]) commonly receive radiotherapy (RT) treatment on an outpatient basis. Patients with HNC who receive RT treatment commonly experience disturbing symptoms that include pain, difficulty swallowing, dry mouth, change in taste, lack of appetite, and mouth sores. While it is known that these patients tend to experience these symptoms, the patterns and severity of these symptoms are unknown. This pilot study aimed to identify the individual symptom patterns that patients with HNC experience over the course of 6 weeks of RT treatment.

Design

This was a secondary study derived from a parent study that examined symptoms patients with HNC experience when RT therapy is initiated. The study sites included two university-affiliated outpatient cancer centres located in the eastern United States. There were 21 patients with HNC who consented to participate in this study. Eligible participants were at least 18 years of age, with a new diagnosis of HNC, receiving RT treatment, and able to speak and write English. Sampling yielded 21 participants, 5 with laryngeal cancer, and 16 with oropharyngeal cancer. The Memorial Symptom Assessment Scale, a validated and reliable Likert scale survey that measures 32 symptoms associated with cancer treatment, was used to measure participants' symptoms during RT treatment at the time of midtreatment (week 5), end of treatment (week 9), and 6 weeks posttreatment (week 12). Visual graphical analysis was performed to find patterns of symptoms.

Findings

Participants reported variability in symptoms they experienced over time. The most common symptom experienced was pain; peak pain severity was commonly reported by participants, with no detectable pattern based upon study time points. Difficulty swallowing frequently accompanied pain. The other four symptoms of dry mouth, mouth sores, change in taste, and lack of appetite, along with difficulty swallowing, were commonly experienced during midtreatment and at treatment completion. Three patterns were identified. The first pattern noted increase in symptom severity after RT treatment initiation and declined in severity by midtreatment. The second pattern revealed increase in severity of symptoms posttreatment. The last pattern revealed symptom severity that persisted from RT treatment initiation to the posttreatment period. The small sample size precluded conducting inferential statistical analysis.

Nursing Implications

Findings from this study confirm that patients diagnosed with HNC and who receive RT treatment commonly experience the symptoms of pain, difficulty swallowing, dry mouth, change in taste, lack of appetite, and mouth sores. However, patients' symptoms varied in this pilot both in terms of intensity and patterns over the course of RT treatment. Therefore, nurses should assess patients' symptoms and provide individualized plans of care. In particular, participants in this study reported peak pain intensity at different time points during RT treatment, suggesting that patients with HNC require frequent pain assessment, reassessment, and implementation of proactive preventive pain management strategies.

Any dental problems are resolved, if possible, before surgery and radiotherapy (ACS, 2015).

For patients with early-stage tumours and lesions without lymph node involvement, external beam radiation therapy or conservation surgery (i.e., less invasive surgery, such as vocal cord stripping or cordectomy) may be effective. Other indicated surgical procedures may include transoral endoscopic laser excision or partial **laryngectomy** (NCI, 2015).

Patients should be educated so that they carefully consider the various side effects and complications associated with the different treatment modalities. The presence of lymph node involvement in the neck can affect the outcome. Supraglottic tumours metastasize early and bilaterally even when there appears to be no lymph node involvement at the time of diagnosis. When the neck lymph nodes are involved, the treatment includes surgery, chemoradiation, or both (Tierney et al., 2015).

Surgical Management

The overall goals for the patient undergoing surgical treatment include minimizing the effects of surgery on speech, swallowing, and breathing while maximizing the cure of the cancer (Jenckel & Knecht, 2013). Several different curative procedures are available that can offer voice-sparing results while achieving a positive cure rate for the patient who has an early laryngeal carcinoma. Surgical options include (1) vocal cord stripping, (2) cordectomy, (3) laser surgery, (4) partial laryngectomy, or (5) total laryngectomy.

Vocal Cord Stripping

Stripping of the cord is used to treat dysplasia, hyperkeratosis, and leukoplakia and is often curative for these lesions. The procedure involves removal of the mucosa of the edge of the vocal cord, using an operating microscope. Early vocal cord lesions are initially treated with radiation therapy.

Cordectomy

Cordectomy removes part or all of the vocal cords (Canadian Cancer Society, 2017). This procedure is used for very small tumours or laryngeal cancers on the surface of the glottis (Canadian Cancer Society, 2017). The resulting voice quality is related to the extent of tissue removed.

Laser Surgery

Endoscopic laser surgery, also called transoral laser microsurgery may be used as a treatment option for individuals with early-stage laryngeal tumours (Canadian Cancer Society, 2017). Endoscopic surgery is done through the mouth, where an endoscope with a microscope is passed down the throat. The laser, a narrow, intense beam of light is positioned on the tissue to be treated (Canadian Cancer Society, 2017). Laser surgery also helps preserve laryngeal tissue, so the affected individual can speak, swallow, and breathe as normally as possible (Canadian Cancer Society, 2017). When compared with the results of other treatments for early laryngeal cancer, laser microsurgery is considered to be the method of choice based on patient outcomes (NCI, 2015).

Partial Laryngectomy

A partial laryngectomy is often used for smaller cancers of the larynx and may be performed using endoscopic laser surgery or through a cut in the neck (known as an open partial laryngectomy) (Canadian Cancer Society, 2017) (see Chart 23-8). Individuals with an open partial laryngectomy may need a tracheostomy tube temporarily. The surgery is associated with a very high cure rate. It may also be performed for recurrence when high-dose radiation has failed. A portion of the larynx is removed along with one vocal cord and the tumour; all other structures remain. The airway remains intact, and the patient is expected to have no difficulty swallowing. The voice quality may change, most frequently resulting in a weak or hoarse voice (Canadian Cancer Society, 2017).

Total Laryngectomy

Complete removal of the larynx (total laryngectomy) can provide the desired cure in most advanced laryngeal cancers, when the tumour extends beyond the vocal cords, or for cancer that recurs or persists after radiation therapy. In a total laryngectomy, the laryngeal structures are removed, including the hyoid bone, epiglottis, cricoid cartilage, and two or three rings of the trachea. The tongue, pharyngeal walls, and trachea are preserved. A total laryngectomy results in permanent loss of the voice and a change in the airway, requiring a permanent tracheostomy (Fig. 23-4) (Canadian Cancer Society, 2017). Usually, swallowing is not affected so the individual should be able to eat and drink the same as they did before the surgery.

Surgery is more difficult when the lesion involves the midline structures or both vocal cords. With or without neck dissection, a total laryngectomy requires a permanent tracheal stoma because the larynx that provides the protective sphincter is no longer present. The tracheal stoma prevents the aspiration of food and fluid into the lower respiratory tract. The patient has no voice but has normal swallowing. A total laryngectomy changes the manner in which airflow is used for breathing and speaking, as depicted in Figure 23-4. The patient has significant loss of the natural voice and the need to breathe through an opening (stoma) created in the lower neck. Complications that may occur include a salivary leak, wound infection from the development of a pharyngocutaneous fistula, stomal stenosis, and dysphagia secondary to esophageal stricture. Despite these changes and potential complications, many patients who have undergone a total laryngectomy maintain overall improved quality of life.

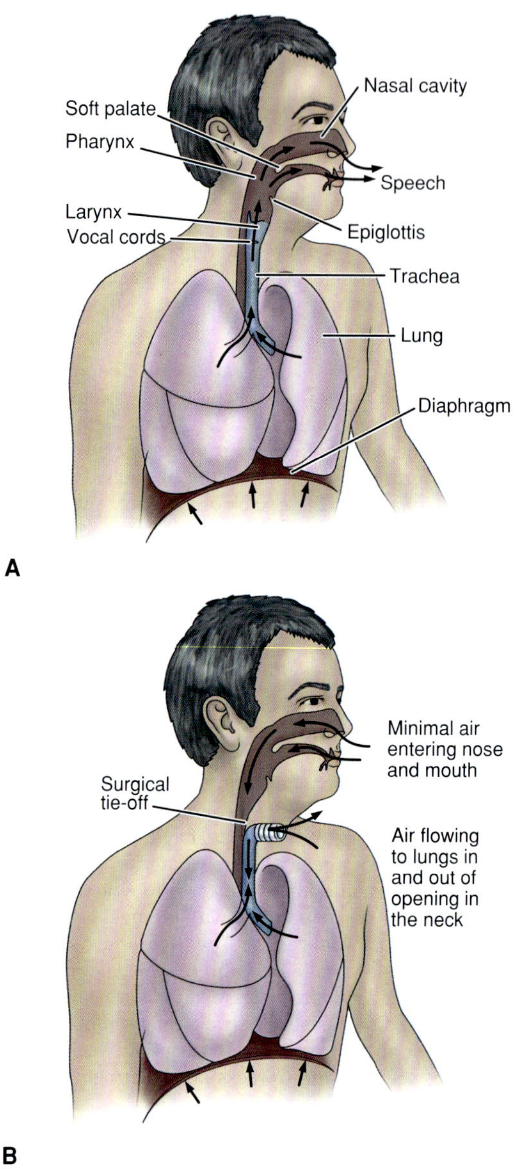

FIGURE 23-4. Total laryngectomy produces a change in airflow for breathing and speaking. **A.** Normal airflow. **B.** Airflow after total laryngectomy.

Radiation Therapy

The goal of radiation therapy is to eradicate the cancer and preserve the function of the larynx. The decision to use radiation therapy is based on several factors, including the staging of the tumour and the patient's overall health status, lifestyle (including occupation), and personal preference. Excellent results have been achieved with radiation therapy in patients with early-stage glottic tumours when only one vocal cord is involved and there is normal mobility of the cord (i.e., with phonation), as well as in small supraglottic lesions. One of the benefits of radiation therapy is that patients retain a near-normal voice. A few may develop chondritis (inflammation of the cartilage) or stenosis; a small number may later require laryngectomy.

Radiation therapy may also be used preoperatively to reduce the tumour size. Radiation therapy is combined with surgery in advanced laryngeal cancer as adjunctive therapy to surgery or chemotherapy and as a palliative measure.

Complications from radiation therapy are a result of external radiation to the head and neck area, which may also include the parotid gland, which is responsible for mucus production. Symptoms may include acute mucositis, ulceration of the mucous membranes, pain, **xerostomia** (dry mouth), loss of taste, dysphasia, fatigue, and skin reactions. Later complications may include laryngeal necrosis, edema, and fibrosis.

Speech Therapy

The patient who undergoes a laryngectomy and the patient's family face potentially complex challenges, including significant changes in the ability to communicate. To minimize anxiety and frustration on the part of the patient and family, it is necessary to discuss the loss or alteration of speech with them. To plan postoperative communication strategies and speech therapy, the speech therapist or pathologist conducts a preoperative evaluation (ACS, 2015). During this time, the nurse discusses with the patient and family methods of communication that will be available in the immediate postoperative period. These include writing, lip speaking and reading, and communication or word boards. A system of communication is established with the patient, family, nurse, and physician and is implemented consistently after surgery.

In addition, a long-term postoperative communication plan for **alaryngeal communication** is developed. The three most common techniques of alaryngeal communication are esophageal speech, artificial larynx (electrolarynx), and tracheoesophageal puncture.

Esophageal Speech

Esophageal speech was the primary method of alaryngeal speech taught to patients until the 1980s. The patient needs the ability to compress air into the esophagus and expel it, setting off a vibration of the pharyngeal esophageal segment. The technique can be taught once the patient begins oral feedings, approximately 1 week after surgery. First, the patient learns to belch and is reminded to do so an hour after eating. Then the technique is practiced repeatedly. Later, this conscious belching action is transformed into simple explosions of air from the esophagus for speech purposes. The speech therapist continues to work with the patient to make speech intelligible and as close to normal as possible. Because it takes a long time to become proficient, the success rate is low (ACS, 2015).

Artificial Larynx

If esophageal speech is not successful, or until the patient masters the technique, an electric larynx may be used for communication. This battery-powered apparatus projects sound into the oral cavity. When the mouth forms words (articulation), the sounds from the electric larynx become audible words. The voice that is produced sounds mechanical, and some words may be difficult to understand. The advantage is that the patient is able to communicate with relative ease while working to become proficient at either esophageal or tracheoesophageal puncture speech.

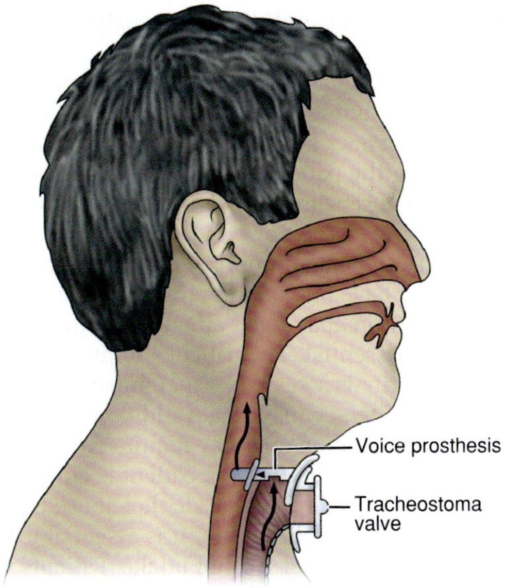

FIGURE 23-5. Schematic representation of tracheoesophageal puncture speech. Air travels from the lung through a puncture in the posterior wall of the trachea into the esophagus and out the mouth. A voice prosthesis is fitted over the puncture site.

Tracheoesophageal Puncture

The third technique of alaryngeal speech is tracheoesophageal puncture (Fig. 23-5). This technique for voice restoration is simple and has few complications. It is associated with high phonation success, good phonation quality, and steady long-term results. This technique is widely used because the speech associated with it most resembles normal speech (the sound produced is a combination of esophageal speech and voice), and it is easily learned. A valve is placed in the tracheal stoma to divert air into the esophagus and out the mouth. Once the puncture is surgically created and has healed, a voice prosthesis (Blom-Singer) is fitted over the puncture site. A speech therapist teaches the patient how to produce sounds. Moving the tongue and lips to form the sound into words produces speech as before. To prevent airway obstruction, the prosthesis is removed and cleaned when mucus builds up.

Nursing Process

The Patient Undergoing Laryngectomy

Assessment

The nurse obtains a health history and assesses the patient's physical, psychosocial, and spiritual domains. The health history addresses the following symptoms: hoarseness, sore throat, dyspnea, dysphagia, and pain or burning in the throat. The physical assessment includes a thorough head and neck examination with an emphasis on the patient's airway. In addition, the neck and thyroid are palpated for swelling, nodularity, or adenopathy.

The nurse also assesses the patient's general state of nutrition, including height and weight and body mass index and reviews laboratory values that assist in determining the patient's nutritional status (albumin, protein, glucose, and electrolyte levels). If treatment includes surgery, the nurse must know the nature of the surgery to plan appropriate care. If the patient is expected to have no voice as a result of the surgical procedure, a preoperative evaluation by the speech therapist is essential. The patient's ability to hear, see, read, and write is assessed. Visual impairment and functional illiteracy may create additional problems with communication and may require creative approaches to ensure that the patient is able to communicate any needs. Because alcohol abuse is a risk factor for cancer of the larynx, it is essential to assess the patient's pattern of alcohol intake. Patients who are accustomed to daily consumption of alcohol are at risk for alcohol withdrawal syndrome (delirium tremens) when alcohol intake is stopped suddenly.

In addition, the nurse assesses the psychological readiness of the patient and family (Chart 23-9). The thought of having cancer is frightening to most people. Fear is compounded by the possibility of permanent voice loss and, in some cases, some degree of disfigurement. The nurse evaluates the patient's and family's knowledge of the planned surgical procedure and expected postoperative course and assesses the patient's and family's coping methods and support systems. The nurse assesses the patient's spirituality needs based on the patient's individual preferences, beliefs, and culture.

Nursing Priorities

Based on all the assessment data, major nursing diagnoses may include the following:

- Patient teaching about the surgical procedure and postoperative course
- Anxiety and depression
- Airway clearance
- Verbal communication
- Nutrition
- Body image and low esteem issues
- Self-care

Collaborative Problems/ Potential Complications

Based on assessment data, potential complications that may develop include the following:

- Respiratory distress (hypoxia, airway obstruction, tracheal edema)
- Hemorrhage, infection, and wound breakdown
- Aspiration
- Tracheostomal stenosis

CHART 23-9

Ethics and Related Issues

Situation

You are the nurse working the morning shift on a medical-surgical unit at your local hospital. You are caring for an 82-year-old man with a new diagnosis of advanced stage IV cancer of the larynx. The surgeon has determined that this patient needs to undergo a total laryngectomy for better control of the disease. Although the patient continues to live at home, he has early signs of senile dementia along with significant weight loss; he is quite debilitated and frail. He has a history of tobacco abuse and continues to smoke one pack of cigarettes per day. He is a widow with two living children: one daughter and one son. Because of his dementia, the patient is not able to sign consent for his total laryngectomy. The patient's daughter has informed the surgeon that she will not agree to sign surgical consent for a total laryngectomy. She is very concerned about the possible outcome of the surgery and has informed you that she knows for certain that her father would not want this surgery and would want to live at home and not in a nursing home facility. The daughter has asked to speak with you regarding her concerns. The patient's son is in agreement with the recommendation for a total laryngectomy and would be willing to sign surgical consent, but he lives out of state and cannot travel at this time. He is estranged from his sister. The patient does not have a designated health care surrogate or power of attorney.

Dilemma

This patient has been diagnosed with a life-threatening illness and needs surgical intervention for control of the disease. He is unable to make medical decisions due to his dementia, and therefore it is now the responsibility of his children in the absence of a spouse to function as his health care surrogate. Based on his physical appearance and condition, he appears to be unable to care for himself. His children are not in agreement regarding the recommended treatment plan. This poses an ethical dilemma that must be resolved so that the patient can receive adequate and timely treatment for his illness and appropriate physical, psychological, and home care should he undergo this procedure.

Discussion

1. Based on the above scenario, what further assessment of the patient's physical and psychosocial condition is needed prior to his surgery and why?
2. What is the relevance for evaluation of the patient's home environment in relation to his need for total laryngectomy?
3. You need to reinforce the education given by the surgeon to the patient's daughter and son regarding the possible complications of a total laryngectomy. Briefly discuss each complication as you would with the patient's daughter and son.
4. What other health care resources should be consulted given the above scenario?
5. Given the patient's dementia, would it be reasonable to communicate to him the plan of care and education about the recommended treatment and possible side effects?

Planning and Goals

The major goals for the patient may include attainment of an adequate level of knowledge, reduction in anxiety, maintenance of a patent airway (patient is able to handle own secretions), effective use of alternative means of communication, attainment of optimal levels of nutrition and hydration, improvement in body image and self-esteem, improved self-care management, and absence of complications.

Nursing Interventions

Providing Preoperative Patient Education

The diagnosis of laryngeal cancer often produces misconceptions and fears. Many people assume that loss of speech and disfigurement are inevitable with this condition. Once the physician explains the diagnosis and discusses treatment options with the patient and family, the nurse clarifies any misconceptions by identifying the location of the larynx, its function, the nature of the planned surgical procedure, and its effect on speech. Further, the patient's ability to sing, laugh, and whistle will be lost. Informational materials (written and audiovisual) about the surgery are given to the patient and family for review and reinforcement. If a complete laryngectomy is planned, the patient must understand that the natural voice will be lost, but that special training can provide a means for communicating. The patient needs to know that until training is started, communication will be possible by using the call light, by writing, or by using a special communication board. The interdisciplinary team conducts an initial assessment of the patient and family. In addition to the nurse in charge of the patient's care and the physician, the team might include an advanced practice nurse or nurse practitioner, speech therapist, respiratory therapist, social worker, dietitian, and home care nurse. The services of a spiritual advisor are made available to the patient and family, as appropriate.

The nurse also reviews equipment and treatments for postoperative care with the patient and family, teaches important coughing and deep breathing exercises, and helps the patient perform return demonstrations. The nurse clarifies the patient's role in the postoperative and rehabilitation periods. The family's needs must also be addressed because family members are often responsible for complex care of the patient in the home.

Reducing Anxiety

Because surgery of the larynx is performed most often for a malignant tumour, the patient may have many questions: Will the surgeon be able to remove all of the tumour? Is it cancer? Will I die? Will I choke? Will I suffocate? Will I ever speak again? What will I look like? Because of these and other questions, the psychological preparation of the patient is as important as the physical preparation.

Any patient undergoing surgery may have many fears. In laryngeal surgery, these fears may relate to the diagnosis of cancer and the possibility of permanent loss of the voice and disfigurement. The nurse provides the patient and family with opportunities to ask questions, verbalize feelings, and discuss perceptions. The nurse should address any questions and misconceptions the patient and family have. During the pre- or postoperative period, a visit from someone who has had a laryngectomy may reassure the patient that people are available to assist, and that rehabilitation is possible.

In the immediate postoperative period, the nurse attempts to spend uninterrupted time with the patient that is focused on building trust and reducing the patient's anxiety. Active listening provides an environment that promotes open communication and allows the patient to verbalize feelings. Clear instructions and explanations are given to the patient and family in a calm, reassuring manner. The nurse listens attentively, encourages the patient, and identifies and reduces environmental stressors. The nurse seeks to learn from the patient what activities promote feelings of comfort and assists the patient in such activities (e.g., listening to music, reading). Relaxation techniques such as guided imagery and meditation are often helpful. The nurse remains with the patient during episodes of severe anxiety and includes the patient in decision making.

Maintaining a Patent Airway

The nurse promotes a patent airway by positioning the patient in the semi-Fowler's or Fowler's position after recovery from anesthesia. This position decreases surgical edema and promotes lung expansion. Observing the patient for restlessness, laboured breathing, apprehension, and increased pulse rate helps identify possible respiratory or circulatory problems. The nurse assesses the patient's lung sounds and reports changes that may indicate impending complications. Medications that depress respiration, particularly opioids, should be used cautiously. However, adequate use of analgesic medications is essential for pain relief because postoperative pain can result in shallow breathing and an ineffective cough. The nurse encourages the patient to turn, cough, and take deep breaths. If necessary, suctioning may be performed to remove secretions, but disruption of suture lines must be avoided. The nurse also encourages and assists the patient with early ambulation to prevent atelectasis, pneumonia, and deep vein thrombosis. Pulse oximetry is used to monitor the patient's oxygen saturation level.

If a total laryngectomy was performed, a laryngectomy tube will most likely be in place. In some instances, a laryngectomy tube is not used; in others it is used temporarily; and in many it is used permanently. The laryngectomy tube, which is shorter than a tracheostomy tube but has a larger diameter, is the patient's only airway. The care of this tube is similar to that for a tracheostomy tube (see Chapter 26). The nurse changes the inner cannula (if present) every 8 hours if it is disposable. If a tracheostomy tube without an inner cannula is used, humidification and suctioning of this tube are essential to prevent formation of mucous plugs. If a T-shaped laryngectomy tube is used, both sides of the T-tube should be suctioned to prevent obstruction due to copious secretions. The nurse should also use secure tracheostomy ties to prevent tube dislodgement. The nurse cleans the stoma daily with soap and water or another prescribed solution and a soft cloth or gauze, taking care to prevent water and soap or solution from entering the stoma. If a non–oil-based antibiotic ointment is prescribed, it is applied around the stoma and suture line. If crusting appears around the stoma, the crusts are removed with sterile tweezers and additional ointment is applied.

Wound drains, inserted during surgery, may be in place to assist in removal of fluid and air from the surgical site. Suction also may be used, but cautiously, to avoid trauma to the surgical site and incision. The nurse observes, measures, and records drainage. When drainage is less than 30 mL/day for 2 consecutive days, the physician usually removes the drains.

Frequently, the patient coughs up large amounts of mucus through this opening. Because air passes directly into the trachea without being warmed and moistened by the upper respiratory mucosa, the tracheobronchial tree compensates by secreting excessive amounts of mucus. Therefore, the patient has frequent coughing episodes and may develop a brassy-sounding, mucus-producing cough. The nurse reassures the patient that these problems will diminish in time, as the tracheobronchial mucosa adapts to the altered physiology.

After the patient coughs, the tracheostomy opening must be wiped clean and clear of mucus. A simple gauze dressing, washcloth, or even paper towel (because of its size and absorbency) worn below the tracheostomy may serve as a barrier to protect the clothing from the copious mucus that the patient may initially expel.

One of the most important factors in decreasing cough, mucus production, and crusting around the stoma is adequate humidification of the environment. Mechanical humidifiers and aerosol generators (nebulizers) increase the humidity and are important for the patient's comfort. The laryngectomy tube may be removed when the stoma is well healed, within 3 to 6 weeks after surgery. The nurse teaches the patient how to clean and change the tube (see Chapter 26) and remove secretions.

Promoting Alternative Communication Methods

Establishing an effective means of communication is usually the ultimate goal in the rehabilitation of the laryngectomy patient. To understand and anticipate the patient's postoperative needs, the nurse works with the patient, speech therapist, and family to encourage use of alternative communication methods. These means of communication are established preoperatively and must be used consistently by all personnel who come in contact with the patient postoperatively. The patient is now unable to use an intercom system. A call bell or hand bell must be placed within easy reach of the patient. A whiteboard is often used for communication, and the nurse documents which hand the patient uses for writing so that the opposite arm can be used for IV infusions.

Writing everything or communicating through gestures can be very time consuming and frustrating. The patient must be given adequate time to communicate his or her needs. The patient may become impatient and angry when not understood.

Promoting Adequate Nutrition and Hydration

Postoperatively, the patient may not be permitted to eat or drink for several days. Alternative sources of nutrition and hydration include IV fluids, enteral feedings through a nasogastric or gastrostomy tube, and parenteral nutrition.

When the patient is ready to start oral feedings, a speech therapist or radiologist may conduct a swallow study (a video fluoroscopy radiology procedure) to evaluate the patient's risk of aspiration. Once the patient is cleared for oral feedings, the nurse explains that thick liquids will be used first because they are easy to swallow. Different swallowing manoeuvres are attempted with various food consistencies. Once the patient is cleared for food intake, the nurse stays with the patient during initial oral feedings and keeps a suction setup at the bedside for needed suctioning. The nurse instructs the patient to avoid sweet foods, which increase salivation and suppress the appetite. Solid foods are introduced as tolerated. The patient is instructed to rinse the mouth with warm water or mouthwash after oral feedings and to brush the teeth frequently.

Because taste and smell are so closely related, taste sensations are altered for a while after surgery because inhaled air passes directly into the trachea, bypassing the nose and the olfactory end organs. In time, however, the patient usually accommodates to this change and olfactory sensation adapts, often with return of interest in eating. The nurse observes the patient for any difficulty in swallowing, particularly when eating resumes, and reports its occurrence to the physician.

The patient's weight and laboratory data are monitored to ensure that nutritional and fluid intake are adequate. In addition, skin turgor and vital signs are assessed for signs of decreased fluid volume.

Promoting Positive Body Image and Self-Esteem

Disfiguring surgery and an altered communication pattern are threats to a patient's body image and self-esteem. The reaction of family members and friends is a major concern for the patient. The nurse encourages the patient to express feelings about the changes brought about by surgery, particularly feelings related to fear, anger, depression, and isolation. Encouraging use of previous effective coping strategies may be helpful. Referral to a support group, such as International Association of Laryngectomees (IAL); WebWhispers;

and an online support group through the Canadian Cancer Society, cancerconnection.ca may help the patient and family deal with the changes in their lives.

Promoting Self-Care Management

A positive approach along with promotion of self-care activities is important when caring for the patient. The patient should begin participating in self-care activities as soon as possible. The nurse assesses the patient's readiness for decision making and encourages the patient to participate actively in performing care. The nurse provides positive reinforcement when the patient makes an effort in self-care. The nurse needs to be a good listener and a support to the family, especially when explaining the tubes, dressings, and drains that are in place postoperatively.

In addition to its work through support groups, the IAL encourages an exchange of ideas and methods for learning and teaching alaryngeal methods of communication. It also works to promote employers' understanding about cancer of the larynx and to enable patients to retain or obtain employment after surgery.

Monitoring and Managing Potential Complications

The potential complications after laryngectomy include respiratory distress and hypoxia, hemorrhage, infection, wound breakdown, aspiration, and tracheostomal stenosis.

RESPIRATORY DISTRESS AND HYPOXIA. The nurse monitors the patient for signs and symptoms of respiratory distress and hypoxia, particularly restlessness, irritation, agitation, confusion, tachypnea, use of accessory muscles, and decreased oxygen saturation on pulse oximetry (SpO_2). Any change in respiratory status requires immediate intervention. Hypoxia may cause restlessness and an initial rise in blood pressure; this is followed by hypotension and somnolence. Cyanosis is a late sign of hypoxia. Obstruction needs to be ruled out immediately by suctioning and by having the patient cough and breathe deeply. Hypoxia and airway obstruction, if not immediately treated, are life threatening.

Other nursing measures include repositioning of the patient to ensure an open airway and administering oxygen as prescribed and used with caution in patients with chronic obstructive pulmonary disease. The nurse should always be prepared for possible intubation and mechanical ventilation. The nurse must be knowledgeable about the hospital's emergency code protocols and skilled in use of emergency equipment. The nurse must remain with the patient at all times during respiratory distress.

HEMORRHAGE. Bleeding from the drains at the surgical site or with tracheal suctioning may signal the occurrence of hemorrhage. The nurse promptly notifies the surgeon of any active bleeding, which can occur at a variety of sites, including the surgical site, drains, and trachea. Rupture of the carotid artery is especially dangerous. Should this occur, the nurse must apply direct pressure over the artery, summon assistance, and provide emotional support to the patient until the vessel is ligated. The nurse monitors vital signs for changes, particularly increased pulse rate, decreased blood pressure, and rapid deep respirations. Cold, clammy, pale skin may indicate active bleeding. IV fluids and blood components may be administered, and other measures implemented to prevent or treat hemorrhagic shock. Management of the patient with shock is discussed in detail in Chapter 16.

INFECTION. The nurse monitors the patient for signs of postoperative infection. These include an increase in temperature and pulse, a change in the type of wound drainage, and increased areas of redness or tenderness at the surgical site. Other signs include purulent drainage, odour, and increased wound drainage. The nurse monitors the patient's white blood cell (WBC) count; a rise in WBCs may indicate the body's effort to combat infection. In older adult patients, infection can be present without an increase in the patient's WBC count; therefore, the nurse must monitor the patient for more subtle signs. WBCs are suppressed in the patient with decreased immune function (e.g., patients with HIV infection, or those receiving chemotherapy or radiation therapy); this predisposes the patient to a severe infection and sepsis. Antimicrobial (antibiotic) medications must be administered as scheduled. All suspicious drainage is cultured, and the patient may be placed in isolation as indicated. Strategies are implemented to minimize the exposure of the patient to microorganisms and their spread to others. The nurse reports any significant change in the patient's status to the surgeon.

WOUND BREAKDOWN. Wound breakdown caused by infection, poor wound healing, development of a fistula, radiation therapy, or tumour growth can create a life-threatening emergency. The carotid artery, which is close to the stoma, may rupture from erosion if the wound does not heal properly. The nurse observes the stoma area for wound breakdown, hematoma, and bleeding and reports their occurrence to the surgeon. If wound breakdown occurs, the patient must be monitored carefully and identified as at high risk for carotid hemorrhage.

ASPIRATION. The patient who has undergone a laryngectomy is at risk for aspiration and aspiration pneumonia due to depressed cough, the sedating effects of anesthetic and analgesic medications, alteration in the airway, impaired swallowing, and the administration of tube feedings. The nurse assesses for the presence of nausea and administers antiemetic medications, as prescribed. The nurse keeps a suction setup available in the hospital and instructs the family to do so at home for use if needed. Patients receiving tube feedings are positioned with the head of the bed at 30 degrees or higher during feedings and for 30 to 45 minutes after tube feedings. Patients receiving oral feedings are positioned with the head of the bed in an upright position for 30 to 45 minutes after feedings. For patients with a nasogastric or gastrostomy tube, the placement of the tube and residual gastric volume must be checked before each feeding. High amounts of residual volume (greater than 50% of previous intake) indicate delayed gastric emptying; this can lead to reflux and aspiration (Tierney et al., 2015). Signs or symptoms of aspiration are reported to the physician immediately.

TRACHEOSTOMAL STENOSIS. Tracheostomal stenosis is an abnormal narrowing of the trachea or the tracheostomy stoma. Infection at the stoma site, excessive traction on the tracheostomy tube by the connecting tubing, and persistent high tracheostomy cuff pressure are risk factors for tracheostomal stenosis. The incidence of this condition varies widely, and it is often preventable. The nurse assesses the patient's stoma for signs and symptoms of infection and reports any evidence of this to the physician immediately. Tracheostomy care is performed routinely. The nurse assesses the connecting tubing (e.g., ventilation tubing) and secures the tubing to avoid excessive traction on the patient's tracheostomy. The nurse ensures that the tracheostomy cuff is deflated (for a patient with a cuffed tube) except for short periods, such as when the patient is eating or taking medications.

Promoting Home, Community-Based, and Transitional Care

EDUCATING PATIENTS ABOUT SELF-CARE. The nurse has an important role in the recovery and rehabilitation of the patient who has had a laryngectomy. In an effort to facilitate the patient's ability to manage self-care, discharge instruction begins as soon as the patient is able to participate. Nursing care and patient teaching in the hospital, outpatient setting, and rehabilitation or long-term care facility must take into consideration the many emotions, physical changes, and lifestyle changes experienced by the patient. In preparing the patient to go home, the nurse assesses the patient's readiness to learn and the level of knowledge about self-care management. The nurse also reassures the patient and family that most self-care management strategies can be mastered. The patient needs to learn a variety of self-care behaviours, including tracheostomy and stoma care, wound care, and oral hygiene. The nurse also instructs the patient about the need for adequate dietary intake, safe hygiene, and recreational activities.

TRACHEOSTOMY AND STOMA CARE. The nurse provides specific instructions to the patient and family about what to expect with a tracheostomy and its management. The nurse teaches the patient and caregiver to perform suctioning and emergency measures and tracheostomy and stoma care. The nurse stresses the importance of humidification at home and instructs the family to obtain and set up a humidification system before the patient returns home. In addition, the nurse cautions the patient and family that air-conditioned air may be too cool or too dry, and therefore irritating for the patient with a new laryngectomy. (See Chapter 26 for details about tracheostomy care.)

HYGIENE AND SAFETY MEASURES. The nurse instructs the patient and family about safety precautions that are needed because of the changes in structure and function resulting from the surgery. Special precautions are needed in the shower to prevent water from entering the stoma. Wearing a loose-fitting plastic bib over the tracheostomy or simply holding a hand over the opening is effective. Swimming is not recommended because a person with a laryngectomy can drown without submerging his or her face. Barbers and beauticians need to be alerted so that hair sprays, loose hair, and powder do not get near the stoma, because they can block or irritate the trachea and possibly cause infection. These self-care points are summarized in Chart 23-10.

The nurse teaches the patient and caregiver the signs and symptoms of infection and identifies indications that require contacting the physician after discharge. A discussion regarding cleanliness and infection control behaviours is essential in the education of the patient. The nurse teaches the patient and family to wash their hands before and after caring for the tracheostomy, to use tissue to remove mucus, and to dispose of soiled dressings and equipment properly. If the patient's surgery included cervical lymph node dissection, the nurse teaches the patient exercises for strengthening the shoulder and neck muscles.

Recreation and exercise are important for the patient's well-being and quality of life, and all but very strenuous exercise can be enjoyed safely. Avoidance of strenuous exercise and fatigue is important because the patient will have more difficulty speaking when tired, which can be discouraging. Additional safety points to address include the need for the patient to wear or carry medical identification, such as a bracelet or card, to alert medical personnel to the special requirements for resuscitation should this need arise. If resuscitation is needed, direct mouth-to-stoma ventilation should be performed. For home emergency situations, prerecorded emergency messages for police, the fire department, or other rescue services can be kept near the phone to be used quickly.

The nurse instructs and encourages the patient to perform oral care on a regular basis to prevent halitosis and infection. If the patient is receiving radiation therapy, synthetic saliva may be required because of decreased saliva production. Patients receiving radiation therapy frequently report dry mouth, change in taste, lack of appetite, and mouth sores (see Chart 23-8) (Haisfield-Wolfe, Brown, Richardson, et al., 2015). The nurse instructs the patient to drink water or sugar-free liquids throughout the day and to use a humidifier at home. Brushing the teeth or dentures and rinsing the mouth several times a day will assist in maintaining proper oral hygiene.

CONTINUING AND TRANSITIONAL CARE. Referral for home, community-based, or transitional care is an important aspect of postoperative care for the patient who has had a laryngectomy and will assist the patient and family in the transition to the home. The home care nurse assesses the patient's general health status and the ability of the patient and family to care for the stoma and tracheostomy. The nurse assesses the surgical incisions, nutritional and respiratory status, and adequacy of pain management. The

CHART 23-10

HOME CARE CHECKLIST • The Patient With a Laryngectomy

At the completion of education, the patient and/or caregiver will be able to:

- Name the procedure that was performed and identify any permanent changes in anatomic structure or function as well as changes in ADLs, IADLs, communication, roles, relationships, and spirituality.
- State the name, dose, side effects, frequency, and schedule for all medications.
- Identify interventions and strategies (e.g., durable medical equipment, oxygen, nebulizer, humidifier) used in adapting to any permanent changes in structure or function.
- Describe ongoing postoperative therapeutic regimen, including stoma care, diet, and activities to perform (e.g., shoulder and neck exercises if a node dissection was performed) and to limit or avoid (e.g., swimming and contact sports).
  - Demonstrate tracheostomy care and tracheal suctioning to clear the airway and handle secretions.
  - Explain the rationale for maintaining adequate humidification with a humidifier or nebulizer.
  - Demonstrate how to clean the skin around the stoma and how to use ointments and tweezers to remove encrustations.
  - State the rationale for wearing a loose-fitting protective cloth at the stoma and covering the stoma when showering or bathing.
  - Discuss the need to avoid sprays, powders, particulates, and cold air from air conditioning and the environment to prevent irritation of the airway.
  - Demonstrate safe technique in changing the laryngectomy/tracheostomy tube.
  - Identify fluid and caloric needs.
  - Describe mouth care and discuss its importance.
  - Identify the signs and symptoms of wound infection and state what to do about them.
  - Describe safety or emergency measures to implement in case of breathing difficulty or bleeding.
  - State the rationale for wearing or carrying special medical identification and ways to obtain help in an emergency.
  - Demonstrate alternative communication methods.
- Relate how to reach primary provider with questions or to report complications.
- State time and date of follow-up appointments.
- Obtain an annual influenza vaccine, and discuss vaccination against pneumonia with the primary provider.
- State understanding of community resources, support groups, and referrals (if any).
- Identify the need for health promotion (e.g., weight reduction, smoking cessation, and stress management), disease prevention, and screening activities.

nurse assesses for signs and symptoms of complications and the patient's and family's knowledge of signs and symptoms to be reported to the physician. During the home visit, the nurse identifies and addresses other learning needs and concerns of the patient and family, such as adaptation to physical, lifestyle, and functional changes, as well as the patient's progress with learning and using new communication strategies. The nurse assesses the patient's psychological status as well. The home care nurse reinforces previous teaching and provides reassurance and support to the patient and family caregivers as needed.

It is important that the person who has had a laryngectomy have regular physical examinations and seek advice concerning any problems related to recovery and rehabilitation. The nurse also reminds the patient to participate in health promotion activities and health screening and about the importance of keeping scheduled appointments with the physician, speech therapist, and other health care providers.

Evaluation

Expected patient outcomes may include the following:

1. Demonstrates an adequate level of knowledge, verbalizing an understanding of the surgical procedure and performing self-care adequately
2. Demonstrates less anxiety and depression
   a. Expresses a sense of hope
   b. Is aware of available community organizations and agencies that provide patient education and support groups
   c. Participates in support group for people with a laryngectomy
3. Maintains a clear airway and handles own secretions; also demonstrates practical, safe, and correct technique for cleaning and changing the tracheostomy or laryngectomy tube
4. Acquires effective communication techniques
   a. Uses assistive devices and strategies for communication (Magic Slate, call bell, picture board, sign language, speechreading, computer aids)

   b. Follows the recommendations of the speech therapist
   c. Demonstrates ability to communicate with new communication strategy
   d. Reports availability of prerecorded messages to summon emergency assistance by telephone
5. Maintains adequate nutrition and fluid intake
6. Exhibits improved body image, self-esteem, and self-concept
   a. Expresses feelings and concerns
   b. Participates in self-care and decision making
   c. Accepts information about support group
7. Adheres to rehabilitation and home care program
   a. Practices recommended speech therapy
   b. Demonstrates proper methods for caring for stoma and laryngectomy or tracheostomy tube (if present)
   c. Verbalizes understanding of symptoms that require medical attention
   d. States safety measures to take in emergencies
   e. Performs oral hygiene as prescribed
8. Absence of complications
   a. Demonstrates a patent airway
   b. No bleeding from surgical site and minimal bleeding from drains; vital signs (blood pressure, temperature, pulse, respiratory rate) are normal
   c. No redness, tenderness, or purulent drainage at surgical site
   d. No wound breakdown
   e. Clear breath sounds; oxygen saturation level within acceptable range; chest x-ray clear
   f. No indications of infection, stenosis, or obstruction of tracheal stoma

Critical Thinking Exercises

1 A 20-year-old male college student comes to the student health clinic with complaints of a sore throat and a fever lasting more than 12 days. Your physical assessment reveals a fiery-red pharyngeal membrane and tonsils with white-purple exudates and a scarlatiniform rash on the chest, abdomen, and axilla. What diagnostic tests and treatment would you anticipate for this patient? What additional nursing measures would be indicated for this patient if he indicates that he is opposed to use of all medications because of his cultural and religious beliefs?

2 A 65-year-old man presents to the family health clinic for a follow-up visit to check his blood pressure (BP), which has been generally high and difficult to control with antihypertensive medications. The patient has obesity, with a body mass index of 38. In addition to his elevated BP, he also reports falling asleep during the day and not feeling like he has slept when he wakes up. You suspect that this patient may have OSA. What risk factors for OSA will your health history focus on? What are the common signs and symptoms of OSA? Describe how a patient with OSA is diagnosed and the treatment(s) that might be prescribed. What is the strength of the evidence that commonly prescribed therapies (such as CPAP) may be effective in alleviating symptoms and improving quality of life for patients with OSA?

3 You are with your family at a company picnic and you see that a coworker is grasping her throat and is unable to speak or cough. You suspect that she is choking. You know that the abdominal thrust is used to remove a foreign object from a conscious adult who is choking. Briefly describe what you would do in this situation. What is the evidence base for your actions? How would you determine the strength of the evidence on which your actions are based?

4 You are the home health nurse for a female patient who has undergone a total laryngectomy for the treatment of cancer of the larynx. You are responsible to provide patient education regarding tracheostomy care and gastric tube feedings. The overall plan is for the patient to begin to assume responsibility for her own care and to consider speech therapy, but the patient and her husband believe she is not yet ready to do so. What are your priorities in terms of assessment of this patient? What is your plan to address the patient's fear, anxiety, communication, and nutritional needs? What is the evidence base for your actions in response to the patient's fear, anxiety, communication, and nutritional needs? How would you assess the strength of the evidence on which your actions are based?

REFERENCES AND SELECTED READINGS

Books

Bickley, L. S., & Szilagyi, P. G. (2013). *Bates' guide to physical examination and history taking* (11th ed.). Philadelphia, PA: Lippincott Williams & Wilkins.

Blondel-Hill, E., & Fryters, S. (2012). *Bugs and drugs 2012* (5th ed.). Edmonton, AB: Alberta Health Services.

De Vita, V., Hellman, S., & Rosenberg, S. (Eds.). (2014). *Cancer: Principles and practice of oncology* (10th ed.). Philadelphia, PA: Lippincott Williams & Wilkins.

Reardon, R. F., Mason, P. E., & Clinton, J. E. (2014). Basic airway management and decision-making. In J. D. Roberts (Ed.). *Roberts & Hedges' clinical procedures in emergency medicine* (6th ed.). Philadelphia, PA: Elsevier Saunders.

Tierney, L., McPhee, S. J., & Papadakis, M. (Eds.). (2015). *Current medical diagnosis and treatment* (54th ed.). New York: McGraw-Hill.

Journals and Electronic Documents

General

Aljubran, S., & Lockey, R. F. (2014). *Aeroallergens*. Retrieved from www.emedicine.medscape.com/article/137911-overview

American Academy of Otolaryngology. (2015). *Fact sheet: Sinusitis: Special considerations for aging patients*. Retrieved from www.entnet.org/content/sinusitis-special-considerations-aging-patients

American Cancer Society (ACS). (2015). *Risk factors for laryngeal and hypopharyngeal cancers*. Retrieved from www.cancer.org/Cancer/LaryngealandHypopharyngealCancer/DetailedGuide/laryngeal-and-hypopharyngeal-cancer-risk-factors

Brook, I. (2015). *Chronic sinusitis*. Retrieved from www.emedicine.medscape.com/article/232791-overview

Canadian Agency for Drugs and Technologies in Health (CADTH). (2017). *Interventions for the treatment of obstructive sleep apnea in adults: A health technology assessment*. Retrieved from https://www.cadth.ca/sites/default/files/pdf/OP0525_OSA_Treatment_HTA_Report.pdf

Canadian Cancer Society (CCS). (2017a). *Laryngeal cancer statistics*. Retrieved from http://www.cancer.ca/en/cancer-information/cancer-type/laryngeal/statistics/?region=ab#ixzz5JYWBiax9
Canadian Cancer Society (CCS). (2017b). *Surgery for laryngeal cancer*. Retrieved from www.cancer.ca/en/cancer-information/cancer-type/laryngeal/treatment/surgery/?region=on#ixzz5JYaqpTCH
Canadian Society of Otolaryngology—Head and Neck Surgery. (n.d.). *Acute sinusitis*. Retrieved from https://www.entcanada.org/education/general-public/public-information-sheets-2/nose/acute-sinusitis/
Canadian Society of Otolaryngology—Head and Neck Surgery. (2018). *Tonsillectomy*. Retrieved from https://www.entcanada.org/education/general-public/public-information-sheets-2/throat/tonsillectomy/
CIHI. (2014). Retrieved from https://secure.cihi.ca/free_products/ED_Report_ForWeb_EN_Final.pdf
Downey, R. (2015). *Obstructive sleep apnea*. Retrieved from www.emedicine.medscape.com/article/295807-overview
Drake, A. F., & Carr, M. M. (2017). *Tonsillectomy*. Retrieved from reference.medscape.com/article/872119-overview#showall
Flores, J. (2015). *Peritonsillar abscess in emergency medicine*. Retrieved from www.emedicine.medscape.com/article/764188-overview
Franklin, K. A., & Lindberg, E. (2015). Obstructive sleep apnea is a common disorder in the population—a review on the epidemiology of sleep apnea. *Journal of Thoracic Disease*, *7*(8), 1311–1322.
Frisch, S., & Guo, A. M. (2013). Diagnostic methods and management strategies of herpes simplex and herpes zoster infections. *Clinics in Geriatric Medicine*, *29*(2), 501–526.
Government of Canada. (2014). *Guidance document—Non-prescription topical nasal decongestants labelling standard*. Retrieved from https://www.canada.ca/en/health-canada/services/drugs-health-products/drug-products/applications-submissions/guidance-documents/non-prescription-drugs-labelling-standards/nonprescription-topical-nasal-decongestants-labelling-standard.html
Haisfield-Wolfe, M. E., Brown, C., Richardson, M., et al. (2015). Variations in symptom severity patterns among oropharyngeal and laryngeal cancer outpatients during radiation treatment: A pilot study. *Cancer Nursing*, *38*(4), 279–287.
Hartl, D. M. (2012). Evidence-based practice: Management of glottis cancer. *Otolaryngology Clinics of North America*, *45*(5), 1143–1161.
Jenckel, F., & Knecht, R. (2013). State of the art in the treatment of laryngeal cancer. *Anticancer Research*, *33*, 4701–4710.
Jordan, A. S., McSharry, D. G., & Malhotra, A. (2014). Adult obstructive sleep apnoea. *The Lancet*, *383*(9918), 736–747. https://doi.org/10.1016/S0140-6736(13)60734-5
Kapur, V. K., Auckley, D. H., Chowdhuri, S., et al. (2017). Clinical practice guideline for diagnostic testing for adult obstructive sleep apnea: An american academy of sleep medicine clinical practice guideline. *Journal of Clinical Sleep Medicine, 13*(03), 479–504.
Karsch-Völk, M., Barrett, B., & Linde, K. (2015). *Echinacea for preventing and treating the common cold. Jama, 313*(6), 618–619.
Krings, J. G., Kallogjeri, D., Wineland, A., et al. (2014). Complications of primary and revision functional endoscopic sinus surgery for chronic rhinosinusitis. *The Laryngoscope*, *124*(4), 838–845.
Krouse, H. J., & Krouse, J. H. (2014). Allergic rhinitis: Diagnosis through management. *The Nurse Practitioner*, *39*(4), 20–28.
Lal, D. (2015). *Fungal sinusitis*. American Rhinologic Society. Retrieved from www.care.american-rhinologic.org/fungal_sinusitis
Luke Rudmik, Medical Pharmaceuticals. (2014). *New evidence suggests Canadians are paying substantial productivity costs associated with refractory chronic rhinosinusitis: Annual price tag $1.3 billion*. Retrieved from https://www.newswire.ca/news-releases/new-evidence-suggests-canadians-are-paying-substantial-productivity-costs-associated-with-refractory-chronic-rhinosinusitis-annual-price-tag-13-billion-513964371.html
Moche, J. A., & Palmer, O. (2012). Surgical management of nasal obstruction. *Oral Maxillofacial Surgery Clinics of North America*, *24*, 229–237.
Morgan, C. (2015). *Surgical approach to snoring and sleep apnea*. Retrieved from www.emedicine.medscape.com/article/868770-overview
National Institute of Allergy and Infectious Diseases. (2015). *Common cold*. Retrieved from www.niaid.nih.gov/topics/commoncold/Pages/default.aspx
Nguyen, Q. A. (2015). *Epistaxis*. Retrieved from www.emedicine.medscape.com/article/863220-overview
Paquette, J., Le May, S., Lachance Fiola, J., et al. (2012). A randomized clinical trial of a nurse telephone follow-up on paediatric tonsillectomy pain management and complications. *Journal of Advanced Nursing*, *69*(9), 2054–2065.
Patel, A. (2014). *Functional endoscopic sinus surgery*. Retrieved from www.emedicine.medscape.com/article/863420-overview
Peters, A. (2015). *Rhinosinusitis: Synopsis*. Retrieved from www.worldallergy.org/professional/allergic_diseases_center/rhinosinusitis/sinusitis-synopsis.php
Randel, A; Infectious Disease Society of America. (2013). IDSA updates: Guideline for managing Group A streptococcal pharyngitis. *American Family Physician*, *88*(5), 338–340.
Rosenfeld, R. M., Piccirillo, J. F., Chandrasekhar, S. S., et al. (2015). Clinical practice guideline (update): Adult sinusitis executive summary. *Otolaryngology—Head and Neck Surgery*, *152*(4), 598–609.
Salvaggio, M. R. (2014). *Herpes simplex*. Retrieved from www.emedicine.medscape.com/article/218580-overview
Seidman, M. D., Gurgel, R. K., Lin, S. Y., et al. (2015). Clinical practice guideline: Allergic rhinitis. *Otolaryngology—Head and Neck Surgery*, *152*(1_suppl), S1–S43.
Seshamani, M., Vogtmann, E., Gatwood, J., et al. (2014). Prevalence of complications from adult tonsillectomy and impact on health care expenditures. *Otolaryngology—Head and Neck Surgery*, *150*(4), 574–581.
Shah, U. K. (2018). *Tonsillitis and peritonsillar abscess: Treatment and management*. Retrieved from emedicine.medscape.com/article/871977-overview#showall
Statistics Canada. (2018). *Health fact sheets: Sleep apnea in Canada, 2016 and 2017*. Retrieved from https://www150.statcan.gc.ca/n1/pub/82-625-x/2018001/article/54979-eng.htm
Tewfik, T. (2015). *Medical treatment for acute sinusitis*. Retrieved from www.emedicine.medscape.com/article/861646-overview
White, D. P., & Shafazand, S. (2013). Mandibular advancement device vs. CPAP in the treatment of obstructive sleep apnea: Are they equally effective in short term health outcomes? *Journal of Clinical Sleep Medicine*, *9*(9), 971–972.
Xu, Y., Quan, H., Faris, P., et al. (2016). Prevalence and incidence of diagnosed chronic rhinosinusitis in Alberta, Canada. *JAMA Otolaryngology—Head and Neck Surgery*, *142*(11), 1063–1069.

Resources

American Cancer Society: http://www.cancer.org
American Lung Association: http://www.lungusa.org
American Sleep Apnea Association: http://www.sleepapnea.org
Canadian Cancer Society—British Columbian and Yukon Division: http://www.bccancer.ca
Canadian Cancer Society—online support group: www.cancerconnection.ca
Canadian Lung Association: http://www.lung.ca
Canadian Medical Association: http://www.cma.ca
Canadian Thoracic Society: http://www.lung.ca/cts
Health Canada: http://www.hc-sc.gc.ca
International Association of Laryngectomees: http://www.larynxlink.com
National Cancer Institute (NCI): http://www.cancernet.nci.nih.gov
National Heart, Lung, and Blood Institute (NHLBI): http://www.nhlbi.nih.gov
National Institute of Allergy and Infectious Diseases: http://www.niaid.nih.gov
National Sleep Foundation: http://www.sleepfoundation.org
Voice Center at Eastern Virginia Medical School, Norfolk: http://www.voice-center.com
WebWhispers: http://www.webwhispers.org
World Allergy Organization: http://www.worldallergy.org

24 Management of Patients With Chest and Lower Respiratory Tract Disorders

Adapted by Tanya Heuver

Learning Objectives

On completion of this chapter, the learner will be able to:

1. Identify patients at risk for atelectasis and nursing interventions related to its prevention and management.
2. Compare the various pulmonary infections with regard to causes, clinical manifestations, nursing management, complications, and prevention.
3. Use the nursing process as a framework for care of the patient with pneumonia.
4. Describe nursing measures to prevent aspiration.
5. Relate pleurisy, pleural effusion, and empyema to pulmonary infection.
6. Relate the therapeutic management techniques of acute respiratory distress syndrome to the underlying pathophysiology of the syndrome.
7. Describe risk factors for and measures appropriate for prevention and management of pulmonary embolism (PE).
8. Describe preventive measures appropriate for controlling and eliminating the problem of occupational lung disease.
9. Discuss the modes of therapy and related nursing management for patients with lung cancer.
10. Describe the complications of chest trauma and their clinical manifestations and nursing management.

Conditions affecting the lower respiratory tract range from acute problems to long-term chronic disorders. Many of these disorders are serious and often life-threatening. The patient with a lower respiratory tract disorder requires care from nurses with astute assessment and clinical management skills as well as an understanding of the impact of the disorder on the patient's quality of life and ability to carry out usual activities of daily living. Patient and family teaching is an important nursing intervention in the management of all lower respiratory tract disorders.

ATELECTASIS

Atelectasis refers to closure or collapse of alveoli and often is described in relation to x-ray findings and clinical signs and symptoms. It is one of the most commonly encountered abnormalities seen on a chest x-ray (Stark, 2015). Atelectasis may be acute or chronic and may cover a broad range of pathophysiologic changes, from microatelectasis (which is not detectable on chest x-ray) to macroatelectasis with loss of segmental, lobar, or overall lung volume. The most commonly described atelectasis is acute atelectasis, which occurs frequently in the postoperative setting or in people who are immobilized and have a shallow, monotonous breathing pattern (Conde & Adams, 2015; Smetana, 2015). Excess secretions or mucous plugs may also cause obstruction of airflow and result in atelectasis in an area of the lung. Atelectasis also is observed in patients with a chronic airway obstruction that impedes or blocks airflow to an area of the lung (e.g., obstructive atelectasis in the patient with lung cancer that is invading or compressing the airways). This type of atelectasis is more insidious and slower in onset (Conde & Adams, 2015; Smetana, 2015).

Pathophysiology

Atelectasis may occur in the adult as a result of reduced alveolar ventilation (nonobstructive atelectasis) or any type of blockage that impedes the passage of air to and from the alveoli (obstructive atelectasis), thus reducing alveolar ventilation (Stark, 2015). Obstructive atelectasis is the most common type and results from reabsorption of gas (trapped alveolar air is absorbed into the blood stream), however outside air cannot replace the absorbed air because of the blockage. As a result, the isolated portion of the lung becomes airless, and the alveoli collapse. This may occur with altered breathing patterns, retained secretions, pain, alterations in small airway function, prolonged supine positioning, increased abdominal pressure, reduced lung volumes due to musculoskeletal or neurologic disorders, restrictive defects, and specific surgical procedures (e.g., upper abdominal, thoracic, or open-heart surgery) (Conde & Adams, 2015).

Patients are at high risk for atelectasis postoperatively due to numerous factors. A monotonous low tidal breathing pattern may cause airway closure and alveolar collapse. This results from the effects of anesthesia or analgesic agents, supine positioning, splinting of the chest wall because of pain, and abdominal distention. Secretion retention, airway obstruction, and an impaired cough reflex or reluctance to cough because of pain may also occur postoperatively (Conde & Adams, 2015). Figure 24-1 shows the pathogenic mechanisms and consequences of acute atelectasis in the postoperative patient.

Atelectasis resulting from bronchial obstruction by secretions may occur in patients with impaired cough mechanisms (e.g., postoperative, musculoskeletal, or neurologic disorders) or in weak, bedridden patients. Atelectasis may also result from excessive pressure on the lung tissue, which restricts normal lung expansion on inspiration (Stark, 2015). Such pressure may be produced by

Glossary

acute lung injury (ALI): an umbrella term for hypoxemic respiratory failure, acute respiratory distress syndrome is a severe form of ALI

acute respiratory distress syndrome (ARDS): nonspecific pulmonary response to a variety of pulmonary and nonpulmonary insults to the lung; characterized by interstitial infiltrates, alveolar hemorrhage, atelectasis, decreased compliance, and refractory hypoxemia

asbestosis: diffuse lung fibrosis resulting from exposure to asbestos fibres

aspiration: inhalation of either oropharyngeal or gastric contents into the lower airways

atelectasis: collapse or airless condition of the alveoli caused by hypoventilation, obstruction to the airways, or compression

central cyanosis: bluish discolouration of the skin or mucous membranes due to hemoglobin carrying reduced amounts of oxygen

consolidation: lung tissue that has become more solid in nature due to collapse of alveoli or infectious process (pneumonia)

cor pulmonale: "heart of the lungs"; enlargement of the right ventricle from hypertrophy or dilation or as a secondary response to disorders that affect the lungs

empyema: accumulation of purulent material in the pleural space

fine-needle aspiration: insertion of a needle through the chest wall to obtain cells of a mass or tumour; usually performed under fluoroscopy or chest computed tomography guidance

hemoptysis: the coughing up of blood from the lower respiratory tract

hemothorax: partial or complete collapse of the lung due to blood accumulating in the pleural space; may occur after surgery or trauma

induration: an abnormally hard lesion or reaction, as in a positive tuberculin skin test

nosocomial: pertaining to or originating from a hospitalization; not present at the time of hospital admission

open lung biopsy: biopsy of lung tissue performed through a limited thoracotomy incision

orthopnea: shortness of breath when reclining or in the supine position

pleural effusion: abnormal accumulation of fluid in the pleural space

pleural friction rub: localized grating or creaking sound caused by the rubbing together of inflamed parietal and visceral pleurae

pleural space: the area between the parietal and visceral pleurae; a potential space

pneumothorax: partial or complete collapse of the lung due to positive pressure in the pleural space

pulmonary edema: increase in the amount of extravascular fluid in the lung

pulmonary embolism: obstruction of the pulmonary vasculature with an embolus; embolus may be due to blood clot, air bubbles, or fat droplets

purulent: consisting of, containing, or discharging pus

restrictive lung disease: disease of the lung that causes a decrease in lung volumes

tension pneumothorax: pneumothorax characterized by increasing positive pressure in the pleural space with each breath; this is an emergency situation, and the positive pressure needs to be decompressed or released immediately

thoracentesis: insertion of a needle into the pleural space to remove fluid that has accumulated and decrease pressure on the lung tissue; may also be used diagnostically to identify potential causes of a pleural effusion

transbronchial: through the bronchial wall, as in a transbronchial lung biopsy

ventilation–perfusion ratio ($\dot{V}/\dot{Q}$): the ratio between ventilation and perfusion in the lung; matching of ventilation to perfusion optimizes gas exchange

Physiology/Pathophysiology

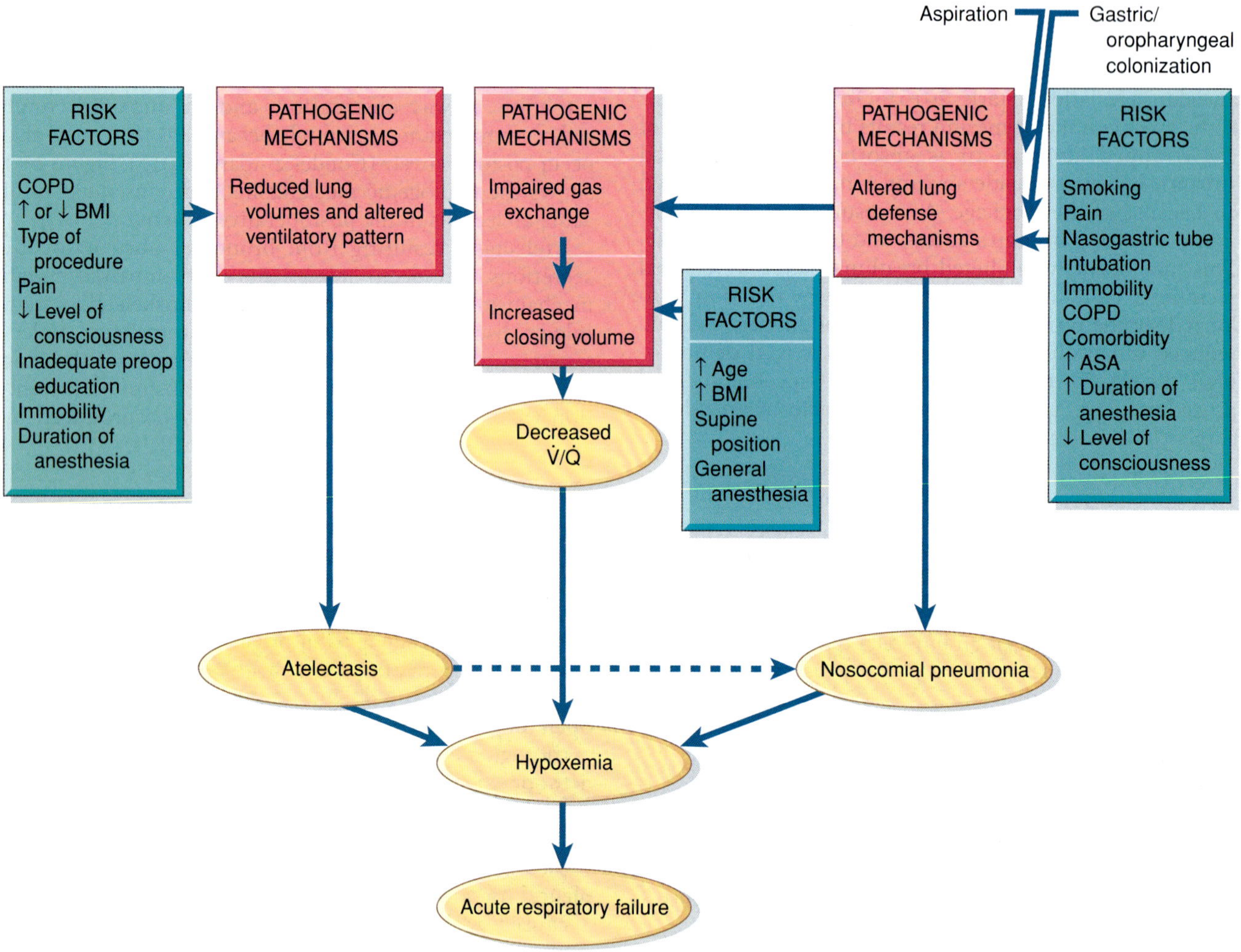

FIGURE 24-1. Relationship of risk factors, pathogenic mechanisms, and consequences of acute atelectasis in the postoperative patient. COPD, chronic obstructive pulmonary disease; BMI, body mass index; ASA, American Society of Anesthesiology physical status; V̇/Q̇, ventilation–perfusion ratio. (Adapted from the work of Jo Ann Brooks-Brunn, DNS, RN, FAAN, FCCP, Indiana University Medical Center, Indianapolis.)

fluid accumulating within the pleural space (**pleural effusion**), air in the pleural space (**pneumothorax**), or blood in the pleural space (**hemothorax**). The **pleural space** is the area between the parietal and the visceral pleurae. Pressure may also be produced by a pericardium distended with fluid (pericardial effusion), tumour growth within the thorax, or an elevated diaphragm.

Clinical Manifestations

The development of atelectasis usually is insidious. Signs and symptoms include cough, sputum production, and increasing dyspnea. In acute atelectasis involving a large amount of lung tissue (lobar atelectasis), marked respiratory distress may be observed. In addition to the above signs and symptoms, dyspnea, tachycardia, tachypnea, pleural pain, and **central cyanosis** (a bluish skin hue that is a late sign of hypoxemia) may be anticipated. The patient characteristically has difficulty breathing in the supine position and is anxious. Signs and symptoms of chronic atelectasis are similar to those of acute atelectasis. Because the alveolar collapse is chronic, infection may occur distal to the obstruction. Thus, the signs and symptoms of a pulmonary infection also may be present.

Assessment and Diagnostic Findings

When clinically significant atelectasis develops, it is generally characterized by increased work of breathing and hypoxemia. The patient may demonstrate an increased respiratory rate and an increased work of breathing. Decreased breath sounds and crackles are heard over the affected area. Atelectasis may be diagnosed by chest x-ray, revealing patchy infiltrates or consolidated areas, before the patient presents with clinical symptoms, or identified by physical assessment in the dependent, posterior, basilar areas of the lungs. Depending on the degree of hypoxemia, pulse oximetry (SpO_2) may demonstrate a low saturation of hemoglobin with oxygen (less than 90%) or a lower than normal partial pressure of arterial oxygen (PaO_2).

NURSING ALERT

Tachypnea, dyspnea, and mild-to-moderate hypoxemia are hallmarks of the severity of atelectasis.

Prevention

Nursing measures to prevent atelectasis include frequent turning, early mobilization, and strategies to expand the lungs and to manage secretions. Deep-breathing manoeuvres (at least every 2 hours) assist in preventing and treating atelectasis. The performance of these manoeuvres requires a patient who is alert and cooperative. Patient education and reinforcement are key to the success of these interventions. The use of incentive spirometry or voluntary deep breathing enhances lung expansion, decreases the potential for airway closure, and may generate a cough. Secretion management techniques may include directed cough, suctioning, aerosol nebulizer treatments followed by chest physical therapy (postural drainage and chest percussion), or bronchoscopy. In some settings, a metered-dose inhaler (MDI) is used to dispense a bronchodilator. Chart 24-1 summarizes measures to prevent atelectasis.

Management

The goal in treating the patient with atelectasis is to improve ventilation and remove secretions. The strategies to prevent atelectasis, which include frequent turning, early ambulation, lung volume expansion manoeuvres (e.g., deep-breathing exercises, incentive spirometry), and coughing also serve as the first-line measures to minimize or treat atelectasis by improving ventilation. Multidisciplinary, evidence-based standardized intervention programs, such as ICOUGH℠ (see Chart 24-2), hold promise in preventing atelectasis (Cassidy, Rosenkranz, McCade, et al., 2013; Smetana, 2015).

CHART 24-1

Preventing Atelectasis

- Change patient's position frequently, especially from supine to upright position, to promote ventilation and prevent secretions from accumulating.
- Encourage early mobilization from bed to chair followed by early ambulation.
- Encourage appropriate deep breathing and coughing to mobilize secretions and prevent them from accumulating.
- Educate/reinforce appropriate technique for incentive spirometry.
- Administer prescribed opioids and sedatives judiciously to prevent respiratory depression.
- Perform postural drainage and chest percussion, if indicated.
- Institute suctioning to remove tracheobronchial secretions, if indicated.

CHART 24-2

ICOUGH℠ Program

- **I**ncentive spirometry
- **C**oughing and deep breathing
- **O**ral care (brushing teeth and using mouthwash twice a day)
- **U**nderstanding (patient and staff education)
- **G**etting out of bed at least three times daily
- **H**ead-of-bed elevation

Adapted from Boston University School of Medicine. *ICOUGH℠*. Retrieved December 1, 2016, from https://www.bumc.bu.edu/surgery/quality-safety/i-cough/

In patients who do not respond to first-line measures or who cannot perform deep-breathing exercises, other treatments such as positive end-expiratory pressure or PEEP therapy (a simple mask and one-way valve system that provides varying amounts of expiratory resistance [usually 10 to 15 cm H_2O]), continuous or intermittent positive pressure breathing (IPPB), or bronchoscopy may be used. Before initiating more complex, costly, and labour-intensive therapies, the nurse should ask several questions:

- Has the patient been given an adequate trial of deep-breathing exercises?
- Has the patient received adequate education, supervision, and coaching to carry out the deep-breathing exercises?
- Have other factors been evaluated that may impair ventilation or prohibit a good patient effort (e.g., lack of turning, mobilization; excessive pain; excessive sedation)?

If the cause of atelectasis is bronchial obstruction from secretions, the secretions must be removed by coughing or suctioning to permit air to reenter that portion of the lung. Chest physical therapy (chest percussion and postural drainage) may also be used to mobilize secretions. Nebulizer treatments with a bronchodilator medication or sodium bicarbonate may be used to assist the patient in the expectoration of secretions. If respiratory care measures fail to remove the obstruction, a bronchoscopy is performed. Although bronchoscopy is an excellent measure to remove secretions and increase ventilation, it is imperative for the nurse to assist the patient with maintaining the patency of the airways after bronchoscopy, using the traditional techniques of deep breathing, coughing, and suctioning. Severe or massive atelectasis may lead to acute respiratory failure, especially in a patient with underlying lung disease. Endotracheal intubation and mechanical ventilation may be necessary.

If atelectasis has resulted from compression of lung tissue, the goal is to decrease the compression. With a large pleural effusion that is compressing lung tissue and causing alveolar collapse, treatment may include **thoracentesis**, removal of the fluid by needle aspiration, or insertion of a chest tube. The measures to increase lung expansion described above also are used.

Management of chronic atelectasis focuses on removing the cause of the obstruction of the airways or the compression of the lung tissue. For example, bronchoscopy may be used to open an airway obstructed by lung cancer or a nonmalignant lesion, and the procedure may involve cryotherapy or laser therapy. If the atelectasis is a result of obstruction caused by lung cancer, an airway stent or radiation therapy to shrink a tumour may be used to open the airways and provide ventilation to the collapsed area. However, in patients who have experienced chronic, long-term collapse, it may not be possible to reopen the airways and reaerate the area of the lung. In some cases, surgical management may be indicated.

RESPIRATORY INFECTIONS

Acute Tracheobronchitis

Acute tracheobronchitis, an acute inflammation of the mucous membranes of the trachea and the bronchial tree, often follows infection of the upper respiratory tract. Patients with a viral infection have decreased resistance and can readily develop a secondary bacterial infection. Adequate treatment of upper respiratory tract infection is one of the major factors in the prevention of acute bronchitis.

Pathophysiology

In acute tracheobronchitis, the inflamed mucosa of the bronchi produces mucopurulent sputum, often in response to infection by *Streptococcus pneumoniae, Haemophilus influenzae,* or *Mycoplasma pneumoniae.* In addition, a fungal infection (e.g., *Aspergillus*) may also cause tracheobronchitis. A sputum culture is essential to identify the specific causative organism. In addition to infection, inhalation of physical and chemical irritants, gases, or other air contaminants can also cause acute bronchial irritation. A subcategory of tracheobronchitis is ventilator-associated tracheobronchitis, which is a common illness in chronically ventilated patients. If managed appropriately, ventilator-associated pneumonia (VAP) may be prevented (Kollef, 2015).

Clinical Manifestations

Initially, the patient has a dry, irritating cough and expectorates a scanty amount of mucoid sputum. The patient may report sternal soreness from coughing and has fever or chills and night sweats, headache, and general malaise. As the infection progresses, the patient may be short of breath, have noisy inspiration and expiration (inspiratory stridor and expiratory wheeze), and produce **purulent** (pus-filled) sputum. In severe tracheobronchitis, blood-streaked secretions may be expectorated as a result of the irritation of the mucosa of the airways.

Medical Management

Antibiotic treatment may be indicated depending on the symptoms, sputum purulence, and results of the sputum culture. Antihistamines are usually not prescribed, because they may cause excessive drying and make secretions more difficult to expectorate. Expectorants may be prescribed, although their efficacy is questionable. Fluid intake is increased to thin the viscous and tenacious secretions. Copious, purulent secretions that cannot be cleared by coughing place the patient at risk for increasing airway obstruction and the development of a more severe lower respiratory tract infection, such as pneumonia. Suctioning and bronchoscopy may be needed to remove secretions. Rarely, endotracheal intubation may be required in cases of acute tracheobronchitis leading to ARF. This may be necessary for patients who are severely debilitated or who have coexisting diseases that also impair the respiratory system.

In most cases, treatment of tracheobronchitis is largely symptomatic. Increasing the vapor pressure (moisture content) in the air will reduce irritation. Cool vapor therapy or steam inhalations may help to relieve laryngeal and tracheal irritation. Moist heat to the chest may relieve the soreness and pain. Mild analgesics or antipyretics may be indicated.

Nursing Management

Acute tracheobronchitis is frequently treated in the home setting. A primary nursing function is to encourage bronchial hygiene, such as increasing fluid intake and directed coughing to remove secretions. The nurse should encourage and assist the patient to sit up frequently to cough effectively and to prevent retention of mucopurulent sputum. If the patient is treated with antibiotics for an underlying infection, it is important to emphasize the need to complete the full course of antibiotics prescribed. Fatigue is a consequence of tracheobronchitis; therefore, the nurse must caution the patient against overexertion, which can induce a relapse or exacerbation of the infection. The patient is advised to rest.

Pneumonia

Pneumonia is an inflammation of the lung parenchyma caused by various microorganisms, including bacteria, mycobacteria, chlamydiae, mycoplasma, fungi, parasites, and viruses (CDC, 2018). *Pneumonitis* is a more general term that describes an inflammatory process in the lung tissue that may predispose a patient to or place a patient at risk for microbial invasion.

Lower respiratory tract infections are a significant issue globally and a leading cause of illness and death in people of all ages. Estimates from 2013 revealed that lower respiratory tract infections were responsible for more than 2.6 million deaths worldwide, making them the fifth leading cause of death overall and the leading infectious cause of death in children under 5 years of age (GBD 2013 Mortality and Causes of Death Collaborators, 2015). In Canada, pneumonia and influenza were the seventh leading causes of death in 2013 accounting for a total of 6,551 deaths (Statistics Canada, 2013).

Classification

Pneumonia can be classified into four types: community-acquired pneumonia (CAP), health care–associated

CHART 24-3

Classifications and Definitions of Pneumonias

- *Community-acquired pneumonia (CAP):* Pneumonia occurring in the community or ≤48 hours after hospital admission or institutionalization of patients who do not meet the criteria for health care–associated pneumonia (HCAP)
- *Health care–associated pneumonia (HCAP):* Pneumonia occurring in a nonhospitalized patient with extensive health care contact with one or more of the following:
  - Hospitalization for ≥2 days in an acute care facility within 90 days of infection
  - Residence in a nursing home or long-term care facility
  - Antibiotic therapy, chemotherapy, or wound care within 30 days of current infection
  - Hemodialysis treatment at a hospital or clinic
  - Home infusion therapy or home wound care
  - Family member with infection due to multidrug-resistant bacteria
- *Hospital-acquired pneumonia (HAP):* Pneumonia occurring ≥48 hours after hospital admission that did not appear to be incubating at the time of admission
- *Ventilator-associated pneumonia (VAP):* A type of HAP that develops ≥48 hours after endotracheal tube intubation

Adapted from File, T. (2016). Risk factors and prevention of hospital-acquired, ventilator-associated and healthcare-associated pneumonia in adults. UpToDate. Last updated January 29, 2016. Retrieved April 23, 2016, from www.uptodate.com/contents/treatment-of-hospital-acquired-ventilator-associated-and-healthcare-associated-pneumonia-in-adults?source=search_result&search=Treatment+of+hospital-acquired%2C+ventilator-associated+and+healthcare-associated+pneumonia+in+adults&selectedTitle=1~150

pneumonia (HCAP), hospital-acquired pneumonia (HAP), and VAP (File, 2016). HCAP was added as a category in 2005 to identify patients at increased risk for multidrug-resistant (MDR) pathogens versus community-acquired pathogens (File, 2016). Chart 24-3 describes the different classifications and definitions of pneumonias. Other subcategories of HCAPs are those in the immunocompromised host and **aspiration** pneumonia. There is overlap in how specific pneumonias are classified, because they may occur in differing settings. Risk factors associated for specific pathogens are shown in Chart 24-4.

Community-Acquired Pneumonia

CAP occurs either in the community setting or within the first 48 hours of hospitalization or institutionalization. CAP is the most common type of pneumonia with most cases occurring during the winter months (National Heart, Lung, and Blood Institute, n.d.). The need for hospitalization for CAP depends on the severity of the pneumonia. The assessment of severity is a critical step in the initial care of individuals diagnosed with CAP. Approximately 50% of patients diagnosed with CAP are at low risk of death and can be safely treated outside of hospital while around 20% are at increased risk (Kolditz, Braeken, Ewig, et al., 2016). The causative pathogens for CAP by site of care are shown in Table 24-1.

The organisms that most frequently cause CAP are *S. pneumoniae, H. influenzae, Moraxella catarrhalis*, rhinovirus, and influenza (Baer, 2017). The specific etiologic agent of CAP is identified in about 50% of the cases. Pneumonia caused by *S. pneumoniae* (pneumococcus) is the most common CAP in people younger than 60 years without comorbidity and in those older than 60 years with comorbidity. It is most prevalent during the winter and spring, when upper respiratory tract infections are most frequent. *S. pneumoniae* is a gram-positive, capsulated, nonmotile coccus that resides naturally in the upper respiratory tract. The organism colonizes the upper respiratory tract and can cause the following types of illnesses: disseminated invasive infections; pneumonia and other lower respiratory tract infections; and upper respiratory tract infections, including otitis media and sinusitis. It may occur as a lobar or bronchopneumonic form in patients of any age and may follow a recent respiratory illness.

H. influenzae is another cause of CAP. It frequently affects older people or those with comorbid illnesses (e.g., chronic obstructive pulmonary disease [COPD], alcoholism, diabetes mellitus). The presentation of this pneumonia is indistinguishable from that of other forms of bacterial CAP. The presentation may be subacute, with

CHART 24-4

Risk Factors: Pneumonia Based Upon Pathogen Type

Risk Factors for Infection With Penicillin-Resistant and Drug-Resistant Pneumococci

- Age >65 years
- Alcoholism
- Beta-lactam therapy (e.g., cephalosporins) in past 3 months
- Immunosuppressive disorders
- Multiple medical comorbidities
- Exposure to a child in a day care facility

Risk Factors for Infection With Enteric Gram-Negative Bacteria

- Residency in a long-term care facility
- Underlying cardiopulmonary disease
- Multiple medical comorbidities
- Recent antibiotic therapy

Risk Factors for Infection With *Pseudomonas aeruginosa*

- Structural lung disease (e.g., bronchiectasis)
- Corticosteroid therapy
- Broad-spectrum antibiotic therapy (>7 days in the past month)
- Malnutrition

TABLE 24-1 Community-Acquired Pneumonia Microbial Causes by Site of Care[a]

	Hospitalized Patients	
Outpatients	Non-ICU	ICU
Streptococcus pneumonia	*S. pneumoniae*	*S. pneumoniae*
Mycoplasma pneumonia	*M. pneumoniae*	*Staphylococcus aureus*
Haemophilus influenza	*Chlamydophila pneumoniae*	*Legionella*
Chlamydia pneumonia	*H. influenzae*	Gram-negative bacilli
Respiratory viruses	*Legionella*	*H. influenzae*

[a]Listed in descending order of frequency at each site.

ICU, intensive care unit.

Adapted from File, T. M. (2016). Treatment of hospital-acquired, ventilator associated and healthcare-associated pneumonia in adults. UpToDate. Last updated January 29, 2016. Retrieved April 23, 2016, from www.uptodate.com/contents/treatment-of-hospital-acquired-ventilator-associated-and-healthcare-associated-pneumonia-in-adults?source=search_result&search=Treatment+of+hospital-acquired%2C+ventilator-associated+and+healthcare-associated+pneumonia+in+adults&selectedTitle=1~150; Marrie, T. J. (2015). Epidemiology, pathogenesis, and microbiology of community-acquired pneumonia in adults. UpToDate. Last updated August 13, 2015. Retrieved April 23, 2016, from www.uptodate.com/contents/epidemiology-pathogenesis-and-microbiology-of-community-acquired-pneumonia-in-adults?source=search_result&search=Epidemiology%2C+pathogenesis%2C+and+microbiology+of+community-acquired+pneumonia+in+adults&selectedTitle=1~145

cough or low-grade fever for weeks before diagnosis. Chest x-rays may reveal multilobed, patchy bronchopneumonia or areas of **consolidation** (tissue that solidifies as a result of collapsed alveoli or pneumonia).

Viruses are the most common cause of pneumonia in infants and children but are relatively uncommon causes of CAP in adults. The chief causes of viral pneumonia in the immunocompetent adult are influenza viruses types A and B, adenovirus, parainfluenza virus, coronavirus, and varicella zoster virus. In immunocompromised adults, cytomegalovirus is the most common viral pathogen, followed by herpes simplex virus, adenovirus, and respiratory syncytial virus. The acute stage of a viral respiratory infection occurs within the ciliated cells of the airways. This is followed by infiltration of the tracheobronchial tree. With pneumonia, the inflammatory process extends into the alveolar area, resulting in edema and exudation. The clinical signs and symptoms of a viral pneumonia are often difficult to distinguish from those of a bacterial pneumonia.

Health Care–Associated Pneumonia

An important distinction of HCAP is that the causative pathogens are often MDR. Consequently, identifying this type of pneumonia in areas such as the emergency department is crucial. Because HCAP is often difficult to treat, initial antibiotic treatment must not be delayed. Initial antibiotic treatment of HCAP is often different from that for CAP due to the possibility of MDR bacteria (File, 2016).

Hospital-Acquired Pneumonia

HAP, also known as **nosocomial** pneumonia, is defined as the onset of pneumonia symptoms more than 48 hours after admission to the hospital. HAP is the second most common and most lethal nosocomial infection, with mortality rates up to 33% (Cunha, 2015). In critical care settings, pneumonia is the most common hospital-acquired infection in patients who are intubated and mechanically ventilated (Public Health Agency of Canada, 2012).

HAP occurs when at least one of three conditions exists: host defenses are impaired, an inoculum of organisms reaches the patient's lower respiratory tract and overwhelms the host's defenses, or a highly virulent organism is present. Certain factors may predispose a patient to HAP because of impaired host defenses. Examples include severe acute or chronic illness, a variety of comorbid conditions, coma, malnutrition, prolonged hospitalization, hypotension, and metabolic disorders. Hospitalized patients are also exposed to potential bacteria from other sources (e.g., respiratory therapy devices and equipment, transmission of pathogens by the hands of health care personnel). Numerous intervention-related factors also may play a role in the development of HAP (e.g., therapeutic agents leading to central nervous system depression with decreased ventilation, impaired removal of secretions, or potential aspiration; prolonged or complicated thoracoabdominal procedures, which may impair mucociliary function and cellular host defenses; endotracheal intubation; prolonged or inappropriate use of antibiotics; use of nasogastric tubes). In addition, immunocompromised patients are at particular risk. HAP is associated with a high mortality rate, in part because of the virulence of the organisms, their resistance to antibiotics, and the patient's underlying disorder.

The common organisms responsible for HAP include the pathogens *Enterobacter* species, *Escherichia coli*, *H. influenzae*, *Klebsiella* species, *Proteus*, *Serratia marcescens*, *P. aeruginosa*, methicillin-sensitive or methicillin-resistant *Staphylococcus aureus* (MRSA), and *S. pneumoniae*. Most patients with HAP are colonized with multiple organisms. Pseudomonal pneumonia, which accounts for 15% of cases of HAP, occurs in patients who are debilitated, those with altered mental status, and those with prolonged intubation or with tracheostomies. Staphylococcal pneumonia, which accounts for more than 30% of cases of HAP but less than 10% of cases of CAP, can occur through inhalation of the organism or spread through the hematogenous route. It is often accompanied by bacteremia and positive blood cultures. Its mortality rate is high. Specific strains of staphylococci are resistant to all available antimicrobials except vancomycin. Overuse and misuse of antimicrobial agents are major risk factors for the emergence of these resistant pathogens. Because MRSA is highly virulent, steps must be taken to prevent its spread (Martel, Bui-Wuan, Carreau, et al., 2013; Nichol, McGeer, Bigelow, et al., 2013). Patients with MRSA are isolated in a private room, and contact precautions (gown, mask, glove, and antibacterial soap) are used to reduce transmission. The number of people in contact with the patient should be minimized, and appropriate precautions must be taken when transporting the patient within or between facilities.

The usual presentation of HAP is a new pulmonary infiltrate on chest x-ray combined with evidence of infection such as fever, respiratory symptoms, purulent sputum, and/or leukocytosis. Development of a cough or increased cough and sputum production are common presentations, along with low-grade fever and general malaise. Pleural effusions, high fevers, and tachycardia are often observed. In the patient who is dehydrated, sputum production may be minimal or absent. Older patients and those with alcoholism, chronic lung disease, or diabetes are at particular risk.

Ventilator-Associated Pneumonia

Hospital-acquired infections are common in the intensive care setting and in individuals with increased severity of illness or injury. Patients who require intubation and mechanical ventilation are at particular risk for developing hospital-acquired infections. Pneumonia that occurs in patients who are intubated and mechanically ventilated is referred to as ventilator-associated pneumonia (VAP) (Safer Healthcare Now, 2012). Mechanical ventilation has been associated with a 3- to 21-fold increased risk of nosocomial pneumonia (Public Health Agency of Canada, 2012).

The incidence of VAP increases with the duration of mechanical ventilation. The estimated rates are 3% per day for the first 5 days, 2% per day for days 6 through 10, and 1% per day thereafter (Amanullah, 2015). VAP is the leading cause of death related to hospital-acquired infections; in individuals diagnosed with VAP, the mortality rate was 46%, as opposed to 32% of ventilated patients who did not develop VAP (Canadian Patient Safety Institute, 2016). Along with increased mortality rates, patients diagnosed with VAP also spend longer periods of time in the intensive care unit, being mechanically ventilated, as well as experience an increase in their total hospital length of stay (Canadian Patient Safety Institute, 2016).

The etiology of VAP typically differs based on the timing of the occurrence of the infection relative to the start of mechanical ventilation. VAP occurring within 96 hours of the onset of mechanical ventilation is usually due to antibiotic-sensitive bacteria that colonize the patient prior to hospital admission, whereas VAP developing after 96 hours of ventilatory support is more often associated with MDR bacteria.

Prevention remains the key to reducing the incidence of VAP (Amanullah, 2015). The Canadian Patient Safety Institute recommends the use of VAP bundles, which are based on evidence-based practices, to reduce the incidence of VAP. The VAP bundle has been most effective when all the elements are included in care of patients. The five key components of the VAP bundle include:

1. Elevate the head of the bed to 45° when possible; otherwise, attempt to maintain the head of the bed at more than 30°
2. Evaluate readiness for extubation daily
3. Use endotracheal tubes with subglottic secretion drainage
4. Conduct oral care and decontamination with chlorhexidine
5. Initiate safe enteral nutrition within 24 to 48 hours of ICU admission (Canadian Patient Safety Institute, 2016).

Pneumonia in the Immunocompromised Host

Pneumonia in the immunocompromised host includes *Pneumocystis carinii* pneumonia (PCP), fungal pneumonias, and *Mycobacterium tuberculosis*. The organism that causes PCP is now known as *Pneumocystis jiroveci* instead of *P. carinii*. The acronym *PCP* still applies because it can be read "*Pneumocystis* pneumonia."

Pneumonia in the immunocompromised host occurs with the use of corticosteroids or other immunosuppressive agents, chemotherapy, nutritional depletion, use of broad-spectrum antimicrobial agents, acquired immunodeficiency syndrome (AIDS), genetic immune disorders, and long-term advanced life-support technology (mechanical ventilation). It is seen with increasing frequency because affected patients represent a growing portion of the patient population. Pneumonia carries a higher morbidity and mortality rate in patients who are immunocompromised than in those who are immunocompetent (Augenbraun, 2014). Patients with compromised immune systems commonly develop pneumonia from organisms of low virulence. In addition, increasing numbers of patients with impaired defenses develop HAP from gram-negative bacilli (*Klebsiella, Pseudomonas, E. coli,* Enterobacteriaceae, *Proteus, Serratia*) (Augenbraun, 2014).

Pneumonia in immunocompromised hosts may be caused by the organisms also observed in CAP or HAP (*S. pneumoniae, S. aureus, H. influenzae, P. aeruginosa, M. tuberculosis*). PCP is rarely observed in the immunocompetent host and is often an initial AIDS-defining complication. Whether the patient is immunocompromised or immunocompetent, the clinical presentation of pneumonia is similar. PCP has a subtle onset with progressive dyspnea, fever, and a nonproductive cough.

Aspiration Pneumonia

Aspiration pneumonia refers to the pulmonary consequences resulting from the entry of endogenous or exogenous substances into the lower airway. This type of pneumonia may occur in the presence of an abnormal gag reflex, swallowing dysfunction, or with the excessive use of alcohol or drugs. The most common form of aspiration pneumonia is bacterial infection from aspiration of bacteria that normally reside in the upper airways. Aspiration pneumonia may occur in the community or hospital setting. Common pathogens are *S. pneumoniae, H. influenzae,* and *S. aureus*. Substances other than bacteria may be aspirated into the lung, such as gastric contents, exogenous chemical contents, or irritating gases. This type of aspiration or ingestion may impair the lung defenses, cause inflammatory changes, and lead to bacterial growth and a resulting pneumonia. (Aspiration is described in more detail at the end of this chapter.)

Pathophysiology

Upper airway characteristics usually prevent potentially infectious particles from reaching the normally sterile lower respiratory tract. Pneumonia arises from normally present flora in a patient whose resistance has been altered, or it results from aspiration of flora present in the oropharynx; patients often have an acute or chronic underlying disease that impairs host defenses. Pneumonia may also result from blood-borne organisms that enter the pulmonary circulation and are trapped in the pulmonary capillary bed.

Pneumonia affects both ventilation and diffusion. An inflammatory reaction can occur in the alveoli, producing an exudate that interferes with the diffusion of oxygen and

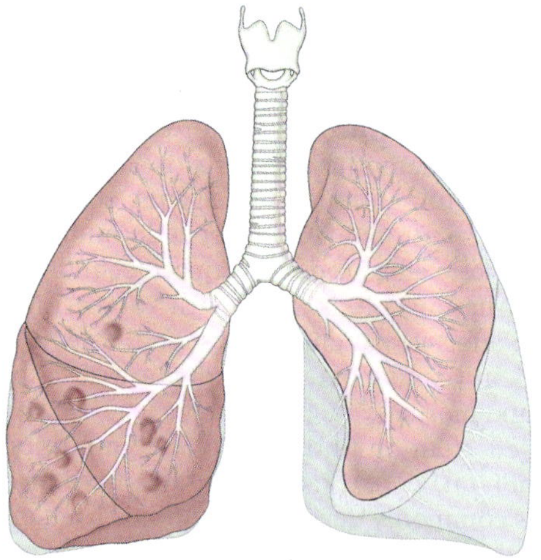

FIGURE 24-2. Distribution of lung involvement in bronchial and lobar pneumonia. (**Left**) In bronchopneumonia, patchy areas of consolidation occur. (**Right**) In lobar pneumonia, an entire lobe is consolidated.

carbon dioxide. White blood cells, mostly neutrophils, also migrate into the alveoli and fill the normally air-containing spaces. Areas of the lung are not adequately ventilated because of secretions and mucosal edema that cause partial occlusion of the bronchi or alveoli, with a resultant decrease in alveolar oxygen tension. Bronchospasm may also occur in patients with reactive airway disease. Because of hypoventilation, a ventilation–perfusion mismatch occurs in the affected area of the lung. Venous blood entering the pulmonary circulation passes through the under-ventilated area and exits to the left side of the heart poorly oxygenated. The mixing of oxygenated and unoxygenated or poorly oxygenated blood eventually results in arterial hypoxemia.

If a substantial portion of one or more lobes is involved, the disease is referred to as lobar pneumonia. The term *bronchopneumonia* is used to describe pneumonia that is distributed in a patchy fashion, having originated in one or more localized areas within the bronchi and extending to the adjacent surrounding lung parenchyma. Bronchopneumonia is more common than lobar pneumonia (see Fig. 24-2).

Risk Factors

Being knowledgeable about the factors and circumstances that commonly predispose people to pneumonia will aid in identifying patients at high risk for the disease (Bartlett, 2015). (Table 24-2 describes risk factors for pneumonia; additional risk factors are travel or exposure to certain environments and residence in a long-term care facility.)

Increasing numbers of patients who have compromised defenses against infections are susceptible to pneumonia. Some types of pneumonia, such as those caused by viral infections, occur in previously healthy people and often follow a viral illness.

Pneumonia is common with certain underlying disorders such as heart failure, diabetes, alcoholism, COPD, and AIDS (Cunha, 2015; File, 2016). Certain diseases also have been associated with specific pathogens. For example, staphylococcal pneumonia has been noted after epidemics of influenza, and patients with COPD are at increased risk for developing pneumonia caused by pneumococci or *H. influenzae*. In addition, cystic fibrosis is associated with respiratory infection caused by pseudomonal and staphylococcal organisms, and PCP has been associated with AIDS. Pneumonias occurring in hospitalized patients often involve organisms not usually found in CAP, including enteric gram-negative bacilli and *S. aureus*.

Clinical Manifestations

Pneumonia varies in its signs and symptoms depending on the type, organism, and the patient's age and underlying disease. It is not possible however to diagnose a specific type of pneumonia by clinical manifestations alone.

Commonly seen clinical manifestations include: pleuritic chest pain, confusion or changes in level of consciousness, cough, fatigue, fever, nausea, vomiting, shortness of breath (Mayo Clinic, 2018). In older adults and immunocompromised patients, a lower than normal body temperature may be present. Purulent sputum or slight changes in respiratory symptoms may be the only sign of pneumonia in patients with COPD. It may be difficult to determine whether an increase in symptoms is an exacerbation of the underlying disease process or an additional infectious process.

Some patients exhibit an upper respiratory tract infection (nasal congestion, sore throat), and the onset of symptoms of pneumonia is gradual and nonspecific. The predominant symptoms may be headache, low-grade fever, pleuritic pain, myalgia, rash, and pharyngitis. After a few days, mucoid or mucopurulent sputum is expectorated. In severe pneumonia, the cheeks are flushed and the lips and nail beds demonstrate central cyanosis.

Signs and symptoms of pneumonia may also depend on underlying conditions. Differing signs occur in patients with other conditions, such as cancer, or in those who are undergoing treatment with immunosuppressants, which lower the resistance to infection. Such patients have fever, crackles, and physical findings that indicate consolidation of lung tissue, including increased tactile fremitus (vocal vibration detected on palpation), percussion dullness, bronchial breath sounds, egophony (when auscultated, the spoken "E" becomes a loud, nasal-sounding "A"), and whispered pectoriloquy (whispered sounds are easily auscultated through the chest wall). These changes occur because sound is transmitted better through solid or dense tissue (consolidation) than through normal air-filled tissue; these sounds are described in Chapter 22.

Assessment and Diagnostic Findings

The diagnosis of pneumonia is made by history, physical examination, chest x-ray, blood culture (bloodstream invasion, called *bacteremia*, occurs frequently), and sputum examination. The sputum sample is obtained by having the patient: (a) rinse the mouth with water to minimize contamination by normal oral flora, (b) breathe deeply several times, (c) cough deeply, and (d) expectorate the raised sputum into a sterile container. More invasive procedures may be used to collect specimens.

Sputum may be obtained by nasotracheal or orotracheal suctioning with a sputum trap or by fibreoptic bronchoscopy (see Chapter 22). Bronchoscopy is often used in

TABLE 24-2 Risk Factors and Preventive Measures for Pneumonia

Risk Factor	Preventive Measure
Conditions that produce mucus or bronchial obstruction and interfere with normal lung drainage (e.g., cancer, cigarette smoking, chronic obstructive pulmonary disease)	Promote coughing and expectoration of secretions. Encourage smoking cessation
Immunosuppressed patients and those with a low neutrophil count (neutropenic)	Initiate special precautions against infection
Smoking (cigarette smoke disrupts both mucociliary and macrophage activity)	Encourage smoking cessation
Prolonged immobility and shallow breathing pattern	Reposition frequently and promote lung expansion exercises and coughing. Initiate suctioning and chest physical therapy if indicated
Depressed cough reflex (due to medications, a debilitated state, or weak respiratory muscles); aspiration of foreign material into the lungs during a period of unconsciousness (head injury, anesthesia, depressed level of consciousness), or abnormal swallowing mechanism	Reposition frequently to prevent aspiration and administer medications judiciously, particularly those that increase risk for aspiration. Perform suctioning and chest physical therapy if indicated
Nothing-by-mouth (NPO) status; placement of nasogastric, orogastric, or endotracheal tube	Promote frequent oral hygiene. Minimize risk for aspiration by checking placement of tube and proper positioning of patient
Supine positioning in patients unable to protect their airway	Elevate head of bed at least 30 degrees
Antibiotic therapy (in very ill people, the oropharynx is likely to be colonized by gram-negative bacteria)	Monitor patients receiving antibiotic therapy for signs and symptoms of pneumonia
Alcohol intoxication (because alcohol suppresses the body's reflexes, may be associated with aspiration, and decreases white cell mobilization and tracheobronchial ciliary motion)	Encourage reduced or moderate alcohol intake (in case of alcohol stupor, position patient to prevent aspiration)
General anesthetic, sedative, or opioid preparations that promote respiratory depression, which causes a shallow breathing pattern and predisposes to the pooling of bronchial secretions and potential development of pneumonia	Observe the respiratory rate and depth during recovery from general anesthesia and before giving medications. If respiratory depression is apparent, withhold the medication and contact the primary provider
Advanced age, because of possible depressed cough and glottic reflexes and nutritional depletion	Promote frequent turning, early ambulation and mobilization, effective coughing, breathing exercises, and nutritious diet
Respiratory therapy with improperly cleaned equipment	Make sure that respiratory equipment is cleaned properly; participate in continuous quality improvement monitoring with the respiratory care department
Transmission of organisms from health care providers	Use strict hand hygiene and gloves. Implement health care provider education

patients with acute severe infection, patients with chronic or refractory infection, or immunocompromised patients when a diagnosis cannot be made from an expectorated or induced specimen and in mechanically ventilated patients. Bronchoscopic techniques may include a protected brush specimen or bronchoalveolar lavage.

Unfolding Patient Stories: Kenneth Bronson • Part 1

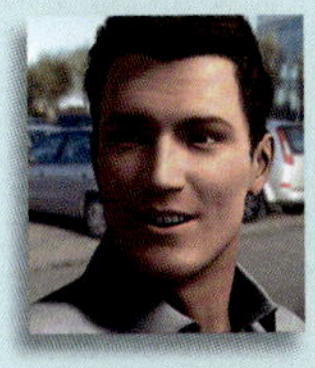

Kenneth Bronson, a 27-year-old man, has a history of fatigue, high fever, and a productive cough for a week and arrives in the emergency department with difficulty breathing. A chest x-ray reveals a right lower lobe pneumonia. What are the clinical manifestations and assessment findings associated with a right lower lobe pneumonia that the nurse should investigate when evaluating the patient? (Kenneth Bronson's story continues in Chapter 28.)

Care for Kenneth and other patients in a realistic virtual environment: ***vSim** for Nursing* (**thepoint.lww.com/vSimMedicalSurgical**). Practice documenting these patients' care in DocuCare (**thepoint.lww.com/**)

Prevention

Pneumococcal vaccination reduces the incidence of pneumonia, hospitalizations for cardiac conditions, and deaths in the older adult population. There are two types of pneumococcal vaccine recommended for adults: a pneumococcal conjugate vaccine (PCV13) and a pneumococcal polysaccharide vaccine (PPSV23).

Medical Management

The treatment of pneumonia includes administration of the appropriate antibiotic as determined by the results of culture and sensitivity if bacteria are identified. However, an etiologic agent is not identified in 50% of CAP cases, and empiric therapy must be initiated (Marrie, 2015). Guidelines exist to guide antibiotic choice; however, the resistance patterns, prevalence of etiologic agents, patient risk factors, and costs and availability of newer antibiotic agents must all be taken into consideration. See Table 24-3. Prompt administration of antibiotics in patients in whom pneumonia is strongly suspected or confirmed is a key treatment measure. Therapy with parenteral agents

(text continued on page 517)

TABLE 24-3 Commonly Encountered Pneumonias

Type (Causal Organism)	Epidemiology	Clinical Features	Treatment	Complications/ Comments
Community-Acquired Pneumonia				
Streptococcal pneumonia (*Streptococcus pneumoniae*)	Most prevalent in winter months More frequent occurrence in African Americans Incidence greatest in older adults and in patients with COPD, heart failure, alcoholism, asplenia, diabetes, and after influenza Leading infectious cause of illness worldwide among young children, people with underlying chronic health conditions, and older adults Mortality rate (in hospitalized adults with invasive disease): 14%	Abrupt onset, toxic appearance, pleuritic chest pain; usually involves ≥1 lobes Lobar infiltrate common on chest x-ray or bronchopneumonia pattern	Severity determines type of antibiotic and route (IV vs. oral) PCN sensitive: PCN, amoxicillin (Amoxil), ceftriaxone (Rocephin), cefotaxime (Claforan), cefprozil (Cefzil), or a macrolide PCN resistant: levofloxacin (Levaquin), moxifloxacin (Avelox), vancomycin (Vancocin), or linezolid (Zyvox)	Shock, pleural effusion, superinfections, pericarditis, and otitis media
Haemophilus influenzae (*Haemophilus influenzae*)	Incidence greatest in alcoholics, older adults, patients in long-term care facilities and nursing homes, patients with diabetes or COPD, and children <5 years of age Accounts for 5–20% of community-acquired pneumonias *Mortality rate:* 30%	Frequently insidious onset associated with upper respiratory tract infection 2–6 weeks before onset of illness; fever, chills, productive cough; usually involves ≥1 lobes Bacteremia is common. Infiltrate, occasional bronchopneumonia pattern on chest x-ray	Severity determines type of antibiotic and route (IV vs. oral) Doxycycline (Vibramycin), second- or third-generation cephalosporin or a fluoroquinolone	Lung abscess, pleural effusion, meningitis, arthritis, pericarditis, epiglottitis
Legionnaires disease (*Legionella pneumophila*)	Highest occurrence in summer and fall May cause disease sporadically or as part of an epidemic Incidence greatest in middle-aged and older men, smokers, patients with chronic diseases, those receiving immunosuppressive therapy, and those in close proximity to excavation sites Accounts for 15% of community-acquired pneumonias *Mortality rate:* 15–50%	Flulike symptoms; high fevers, mental confusion, headache, pleuritic pain, myalgias, dyspnea, productive cough, hemoptysis, leukocytosis Bronchopneumonia, unilateral or bilateral disease, lobar consolidation	Severity determines type of antibiotic and route (IV vs. oral) Azithromycin (Zithromax), moxifloxacin (Avelox), or a fluoroquinolone	Hypotension, shock, and acute renal failure
Mycoplasma pneumoniae (*Mycoplasma pneumoniae*)	Increase in fall and winter Responsible for epidemics of respiratory illness Most common type of atypical pneumonia Accounts for 20% of community-acquired pneumonias; more common in children and young adults Mortality rate: <0.1%	Onset is usually insidious. Patients not usually as ill as in other pneumonias. Sore throat, nasal congestion, ear pain, headache, low-grade fever, pleuritic pain, myalgias, diarrhea, erythematous rash, pharyngitis. Interstitial infiltrates on chest x-ray	Severity determines type of antibiotic and route (IV vs. oral) Macrolides, combination drugs (macrolide plus ampicillin and sulbactam [Unasyn]) or tetracyclines (doxycycline)	Aseptic meningitis, meningoencephalitis, transverse myelitis, cranial nerve palsies, pericarditis, myocarditis

TABLE 24-3 Commonly Encountered Pneumonias (Continued)

Type (Causal Organism)	Epidemiology	Clinical Features	Treatment	Complications/ Comments
Viral pneumonia (influenza viruses types A, B adenovirus, parainfluenza, cytomegalovirus, coronavirus, varicella zoster)	Incidence greatest in winter months Epidemics occur every 2–3 years Most common causative organisms in adults; other organisms in children (e.g., cytomegalovirus and respiratory syncytial virus) Accounts for 20% of community-acquired pneumonias	Patchy infiltrate, small pleural effusion on chest x-ray In most patients, influenza begins as an acute upper respiratory infection; others have bronchitis, pleurisy, and so on, and still others develop gastrointestinal symptoms	Treated symptomatically; treat in high-risk patients; oseltamivir (Tamiflu) or zanamivir (Relenza) (+ other agents depending upon dominant strain [type of virus]) Does not respond to treatment with currently available antimicrobials	Superimposed bacterial infection, bronchopneumonia
Chlamydial pneumonia (*Chlamydophila pneumoniae*)	Reported mainly in college students, military recruits, and older adults May be a common cause of community-acquired pneumonia or observed in combination with other pathogens Mortality rate is low because the majority of cases are relatively mild. Older adults with coexistent infections, comorbidities, and reinfections may require hospitalization	Hoarseness, fever, chills, pharyngitis, rhinitis, nonproductive cough, myalgias, arthralgias Single infiltrate on chest x-ray; pleural effusion possible	Macrolide or doxycycline	Reinfection and acute respiratory failure
Hospital-Acquired and Health Care–Associated Pneumonias				
Pseudomonas pneumonia (*Pseudomonas aeruginosa*)	Incidence greatest in those with pre-existing lung disease, cancer (particularly leukemia); those with homograft transplants, burns; debilitated people; and patients receiving antimicrobial therapy and treatments such as tracheostomy, suctioning, and in postoperative settings. Almost always of nosocomial origin Accounts for 15% of hospital-acquired pneumonias Mortality rate: 40–60%	Diffuse consolidation on chest x-ray; toxic appearance: fever, chills, productive cough, relative bradycardia, leukocytosis	Sensitivity tests guide choice and severity determines type of antibiotic and route (IV vs. oral): ceftazidime (Fortaz), ciprofloxacin (Cipro), cefepime (Maxipime), aztreonam (Azactam), imipenem/cilastatin (Primaxin), meropenem (Merrem), piperacillin (Pipracil), +/− an aminoglycoside	Lung cavitation; has capacity to invade blood vessels, causing hemorrhage and lung infarction; usually requires hospitalization
Staphylococcal pneumonia (*Staphylococcus aureus*)	Incidence greatest in immunocompromised patients, IV drug users, and as a complication of epidemic influenza Commonly nosocomial in origin Accounts for 10–30% of hospital-acquired pneumonias Mortality rate: 25–60% MRSA may also cause community-based infection	Severe hypoxemia, cyanosis, necrotizing infection. Bacteremia is common	Severity determines type of antibiotic and route (IV vs. oral) MSSA: oxacillin or nafcillin MRSA or PCN allergy: vancomycin or linezolid	Pleural effusion/ pneumothorax, lung abscess, empyema, meningitis, endocarditis Frequently requires hospitalization. Treatment must be vigorous and prolonged because disease tends to destroy lung tissue

continued >

TABLE 24-3 Commonly Encountered Pneumonias (Continued)

Type (Causal Organism)	Epidemiology	Clinical Features	Treatment	Complications/ Comments
Klebsiella pneumonia (*Klebsiella pneumoniae* [Friedländer's bacillus-encapsulated gram-negative aerobic bacillus])	Incidence greatest in older adults; alcoholics; patients with chronic disease, such as diabetes, heart failure, COPD; patients in chronic care facilities and nursing homes Accounts for 2–5% of community-acquired and 10–30% of hospital-acquired pneumonias Mortality rate: 40–50%	Tissue necrosis occurs rapidly. Toxic appearance: fever, cough, sputum production, bronchopneumonia, lung abscess. Lobar consolidation, bronchopneumonia pattern on chest x-ray	Severity determines type of antibiotic and route (IV vs. oral) Hospital acquired: cefepime, ceftazidime, imipenem, meropenem, or piperacillin/ tazobactam plus an aminoglycoside or a fluoroquinolone; Community acquired: a levofloxacin plus ciprofloxacin or nitrofurantoin (Macrodantin) or nitrofurantoin macrocrystals	Multiple lung abscesses with cyst formation, empyema, pericarditis, pleural effusion; may be fulminating, progressing to fatal outcome
Pneumonia in the Immunocompromised Host				
Pneumocystis pneumonia (*Pneumocystis jiroveci*)	Incidence greatest in patients with AIDS and patients receiving immunosuppressive therapy for cancer, organ transplantation, and other disorders Frequently seen with cytomegalovirus infection Mortality rate 15–20% in hospitalized patients and fatal if not treated	Pulmonary infiltrates on chest x-ray; nonproductive cough, fever, dyspnea	Severity determines type of antibiotic and route (IV vs. oral) Trimethoprim/ sulfamethoxazole (TMP-SMZ)	Respiratory failure
Fungal pneumonia (*Aspergillus fumigatus*)	Incidence greatest in immunocompromised and neutropenic patients Mortality rate: 15–20%	Cough, hemoptysis, infiltrates, fungus ball on chest x-ray	Severity determines type of antibiotic and route (IV vs. oral) Voriconazole (Vfend); for invasive disease: amphotericin B or liposomal amphotericin B (L-AMB) or caspofungin (Cancidas) Lobectomy for fungus ball	Dissemination to brain, myocardium, and thyroid gland
Tuberculosis (*Mycobacterium tuberculosis*)	Incidence increased in indigent, immigrant, and prison populations; people with AIDS; and the homeless Mortality rate: <1% (depending on comorbidity)	Weight loss, fever, night sweats, cough, sputum production, hemoptysis, nonspecific infiltrate (lower lobe), hilar node enlargement, pleural effusion on chest x-ray	Isoniazid (INH) + rifampin (Rifadin) + ethambutol (Myambutol) + pyrazinamide (PZA) (see section on TB and Table 24.4)	Reinfection and acute respiratory infection
Pneumonia From Aspiration				
Anaerobic bacteria (*S. pneumoniae, H. influenzae, S. aureus*)	Risk: reduced consciousness, dysphagia, disorders of upper GI tract; mechanical disruption of glottic closure (endotracheal tube, tracheostomy, nasogastric feeding)	Abrupt onset of dyspnea, low-grade fever, cough, predisposing condition for aspiration	Severity determines type of antibiotic and route (IV vs. oral) Clindamycin (Cleocin) +/− a fluoroquinolone	Identification of potential aspirate is important for treatment

PCN, penicillin; COPD, chronic obstructive pulmonary disease; IV, intravenous; MSSA, methicillin-sensitive *Staphylococcus aureus;* MRSA, methicillin-resistant *Staphylococcus aureus;* AIDS, acquired immunodeficiency syndrome; TB, tuberculosis; GI, gastrointestinal.

Adapted from Gilbert, D. N., Chambers, H. F., Eliopoulos, G. M., et al. (2015). *The Sanford guide to antimicrobial therapy 2015* (45th ed.). Sperryville, VA: Antimicrobial Therapy, Inc.

usually is changed to oral antimicrobial agents when there is evidence of a clinical response and the patient is able to tolerate oral medications.

Treatment of viral pneumonia is primarily supportive. Hydration is a necessary part of therapy because fever and tachypnea may result in insensible fluid losses. Antipyretics may be used to treat headache and fever; antitussive medications may be used for the associated cough. Warm, moist inhalations are helpful in relieving bronchial irritation. Antihistamines may provide benefit with reduced sneezing and rhinorrhea. Nasal decongestants may also be used to treat symptoms and improve sleep; however, excessive use may cause rebound nasal congestion. Treatment of viral pneumonia (with the exception of antimicrobial therapy) is the same as that for bacterial pneumonia. The patient is placed on bed rest until the infection shows signs of clearing. If hospitalized, the patient is observed carefully until the clinical condition improves.

If hypoxemia develops, oxygen is administered. Pulse oximetry or arterial blood gas analysis is performed to determine the need for oxygen and to evaluate the effectiveness of the therapy. Arterial blood gases may be used to obtain a baseline measure of the patient's oxygenation and acid–base status; however, pulse oximetry is used to continuously monitor the patient's oxygen saturation and response to therapy. More aggressive respiratory support measures include high oxygen concentrations (fraction of inspired oxygen [FiO_2]), endotracheal intubation, and mechanical ventilation. Different modes of mechanical ventilation may be required (see Chapter 26).

Gerontologic Considerations

Pneumonia in older adult patients may occur as a primary diagnosis or as a complication of a chronic disease. Pulmonary infections in older adults frequently are difficult to treat and result in a higher mortality rate than in younger people. Jain et al. (2015) studied approximately 2,500 adults in a population-based surveillance project. They estimated the incidence of hospitalization for pneumonia among adults aged 50 to 64 was four times the incidence as compared to adults 18 to 49 years. For patients between 65 and 79 years, the estimated incidence was nine times the younger population. And, for those at least 80 years of age, the estimated incidence was 25 times higher (Jain, Self, Wunderink, et al., 2015). General deterioration, weakness, abdominal symptoms, anorexia, confusion, tachycardia, and tachypnea may signal the onset of pneumonia. The diagnosis of pneumonia may be missed because the classic symptoms of cough, chest pain, sputum production, and fever may be absent or masked in older adult patients. In addition, the presence of some signs may be misleading. Abnormal breath sounds, for example, may be caused by microatelectasis that occurs as a result of decreased mobility, decreased lung volumes, or other respiratory function changes. Chest x-rays may be needed to differentiate chronic heart failure, which is often seen in older adults, from pneumonia as the cause of clinical signs and symptoms.

Supportive treatment includes hydration (with caution and with frequent assessment because of the risk of fluid overload in older adults); supplemental oxygen therapy; and assistance with deep breathing, coughing, frequent position changes, and early ambulation. All of these are particularly important in the care of older adult patients with pneumonia. To reduce or prevent serious complications of pneumonia in older adults, vaccination against pneumococcal and influenza infections is recommended.

Complications

Shock and Respiratory Failure

Severe complications of pneumonia include hypotension and shock and respiratory failure. These complications are encountered chiefly in patients who have received no specific treatment or inadequate or delayed treatment. These complications are also encountered when the infecting organism is resistant to therapy, when a comorbid disease complicates the pneumonia, or when the patient is immunocompromised.

If the patient is seriously ill, aggressive therapy may include hemodynamic and ventilatory support to combat peripheral collapse, maintain arterial blood pressure, and provide adequate oxygenation. A vasopressor agent may be administered intravenously by continuous infusion and at a rate adjusted in accordance with the pressure response. Corticosteroids may be administered parenterally to combat shock and toxicity in patients who are extremely ill with pneumonia and in apparent danger of dying of the infection. Patients may require endotracheal intubation and mechanical ventilation. Congestive heart failure, cardiac dysrhythmias, pericarditis, and myocarditis also are complications of pneumonia that may lead to shock.

Pleural Effusion

A pleural effusion is an accumulation of pleural fluid in the pleural space (space between the parietal and visceral pleurae of the lung). A parapneumonic effusion is any pleural effusion associated with bacterial pneumonia, lung abscess, or bronchiectasis. After the pleural effusion is detected on a chest x-ray, a thoracentesis may be performed to remove the fluid. There are three stages of para-pneumonic pleural effusions based on pathogenesis: uncomplicated, complicated, and thoracic empyema. An **empyema** occurs when thick, purulent fluid accumulates within the pleural space, often with fibrin development and a loculated (walled-off) area where the infection is located. (Empyema is discussed in greater detail in the Pleural Conditions section.) A chest tube may be inserted to treat pleural infection by establishing proper drainage of the empyema. Sterilization of the empyema cavity requires 4 to 6 weeks of antibiotics, and sometimes surgical management is required.

Nursing Process

The Patient With Pneumonia

Assessment

Nursing assessment is critical in detecting pneumonia. Fever, chills, or night sweats in a patient who also has respiratory symptoms should alert the nurse to the possibility of bacterial pneumonia. A respiratory assessment will further identify the clinical manifestations of pneumonia: pleuritic-type pain, fatigue, tachypnea, use of accessory muscles for breathing, bradycardia or relative bradycardia, coughing, and purulent sputum. It is important to identify the severity, location, and cause of the chest pain, along with any medications or procedures that provide relief. The nurse should monitor the following:

- Changes in temperature and pulse
- Amount, odour, and colour of secretions
- Frequency and severity of cough
- Degree of tachypnea or shortness of breath
- Changes in physical assessment findings (primarily assessed by inspecting and auscultating the chest)
- Changes in the chest x-ray findings

In addition, it is important to assess the older patient for unusual behaviour, altered mental status, dehydration, excessive fatigue, and concomitant heart failure.

Nursing Priorities

Based on the assessment data, the patient's major nursing diagnoses may include the following:

- Airway clearance
- Activity
- Fluid and electrolyte balance
- Nutrition
- Patient teaching

Collaborative Problems/Potential Complications

Based on the assessment data, collaborative problems or potential complications that may occur include the following:

- Continuing symptoms after initiation of therapy
- Sepsis and septic shock
- Respiratory failure
- Atelectasis
- Pleural effusion
- Delirium

Planning and Goals

The major goals for the patient may include improved airway patency, rest to conserve energy, maintenance of proper fluid volume, maintenance of adequate nutrition, an understanding of the treatment protocol and preventive measures, and absence of complications.

Nursing Interventions

Improving Airway Patency

Removing secretions is important because retained secretions interfere with gas exchange and may slow recovery. The nurse encourages hydration (2 to 3 L/day) because adequate hydration thins and loosens pulmonary secretions. Humidification may be used to loosen secretions and improve ventilation. A high-humidity facemask (using either compressed air or oxygen) delivers warm, humidified air to the tracheobronchial tree, helps to liquefy secretions, and relieves tracheobronchial irritation. Coughing can be initiated either voluntarily or by reflex. Lung expansion manoeuvres, such as deep breathing with an incentive spirometer, may induce a cough. To improve airway patency, the nurse encourages the patient to perform an effective, directed cough, which includes correct positioning, a deep inspiratory manoeuvre, glottic closure, contraction of the expiratory muscles against the closed glottis, sudden glottic opening, and an explosive expiration. In some cases, the nurse may assist the patient by placing both hands on the patient's lower rib cage (anteriorly or posteriorly) to focus the patient on a slow deep breath and then manually assisting the patient by applying external pressure during the expiratory phase.

Chest physiotherapy (percussion and postural drainage) is important in loosening and mobilizing secretions (see Chapter 26). Indications for chest physiotherapy include sputum retention not responsive to spontaneous or directed cough, a history of pulmonary problems previously treated with chest physiotherapy, continued evidence of retained secretions (decreased or abnormal breath sounds, change in vital signs), abnormal chest x-ray findings consistent with atelectasis or infiltrates, or deterioration in oxygenation. The patient is placed in the proper position to drain the involved lung segments and then the chest is percussed and vibrated either manually or with a mechanical percussor. The nurse may consult the respiratory therapy department for volume expansion protocols and secretion management protocols that help to direct the respiratory care of the patient and match the patient's needs with appropriate treatment schedules.

After each position change, the nurse encourages the patient to breathe deeply and cough. If the patient is too weak to cough effectively, the nurse may need to remove the mucus by nasotracheal suctioning (see Chapter 26). It may take time for secretions to mobilize and move into the central airways for expectoration. Thus, it is important for the nurse to monitor the patient for cough and sputum production after the completion of chest physiotherapy.

The nurse administers and titrates oxygen therapy as prescribed or via protocols. The effectiveness of oxygen therapy is monitored by improvement in clinical signs and symptoms as well as adequate oxygenation values measured by pulse oximetry or arterial blood gas analysis.

Promoting Rest and Conserving Energy

The nurse encourages the debilitated patient to rest and avoid overexertion and possible exacerbation of symptoms. The patient should assume a comfortable position to promote rest and breathing (e.g., semi-Fowler's) and should change positions frequently to enhance secretion clearance and ventilation/perfusion in the lungs. It is important to instruct outpatients not to overexert themselves and to engage in only moderate activity during the initial phases of treatment.

Promoting Fluid Intake

The respiratory rate of a patient with pneumonia increases because of the increased workload imposed by laboured breathing and fever. An increased respiratory rate leads to an increase in insensible fluid loss during exhalation and can lead to dehydration. Therefore, it is important to encourage increased fluid intake (at least 2 L/day), unless contraindicated.

Maintaining Nutrition

Patients with shortness of breath and fatigue often have a decreased appetite and will take only fluids. Fluids with electrolytes (commercially available drinks, such as Gatorade) may help provide fluid, calories, and electrolytes. Other nutritionally enriched drinks or shakes may be helpful. In addition, fluids and nutrients may be administered intravenously, if necessary.

Promoting Patients' Knowledge

The patient and family are instructed about the cause of pneumonia, management of symptoms of pneumonia, signs and symptoms that should be reported to the physician or nurse, and the need for follow-up. The patient also needs information about factors (both patient risk factors and external factors) that may have contributed to developing pneumonia and strategies to promote recovery and to prevent recurrence. If hospitalized for treatment, the patient is instructed about the purpose and importance of management strategies that have been implemented and about the importance of adhering to them during and after the hospital stay. Explanations should be given simply and in language that the patient can understand. If possible, written instructions and information should be provided, and alternative formats should be provided for patients with hearing or vision loss, if necessary.

Monitoring and Managing Potential Complications

CONTINUING SYMPTOMS AFTER INITIATION OF THERAPY. Patients need to be observed closely for their response to treatment. Patients started on antibiotics usually begin to respond to treatment within 24 to 48 hours after antibiotics are initiated. The patient is monitored for changes in physical status (deterioration of condition or resolution of symptoms) and for persistent recurrent fever, which may be due to medication allergy (signalled possibly by a rash); medication resistance or slow response (greater than 48 hours) of the susceptible organism to therapy; superinfection; pleural effusion; or pneumonia caused by an unusual organism, such as *P. jiroveci* or *Aspergillus fumigatus*. Failure of the pneumonia to resolve or persistence of symptoms despite changes on the chest x-ray raises the suspicion of other underlying disorders, such as lung cancer. As described earlier, lung cancers may invade or compress airways, causing an obstructive atelectasis that may lead to pneumonia.

In addition to monitoring for continuing symptoms of pneumonia, the nurse also monitors for other complications, such as shock and multiple organ dysfunction syndrome (MODS), atelectasis and pleural effusion, and superinfection, which may develop during the first few days of antibiotic treatment.

SHOCK AND RESPIRATORY FAILURE. The nurse assesses for signs and symptoms of shock and respiratory failure by evaluating the patient's vital signs, pulse oximetry values, and hemodynamic monitoring parameters. The nurse reports signs of deteriorating patient status and assists in administering IV fluids and medications prescribed to treat shock. Intubation and mechanical ventilation may be required if respiratory failure occurs. Shock is described in detail in Chapter 18, and care of the patient receiving mechanical ventilation is described in Chapter 26.

PLEURAL EFFUSION. If pleural effusion develops and thoracentesis is performed to remove fluid, the nurse assists in the procedure and explains it to the patient. After thoracentesis, the nurse monitors the patient for pneumothorax or recurrence of pleural effusion. If a chest tube needs to be inserted, the nurse monitors the patient's respiratory status (see Chapter 26 for more information on care of the patient with a chest tube).

DELIRIUM. A patient with pneumonia is assessed for delirium and other more subtle changes in cognitive status; this is especially true in the older adult. The Confusion Assessment Method (CAM) is a commonly used screening tool (see Chapter 14). Confusion, suggestive of delirium, and other changes in cognitive status resulting from pneumonia are poor prognostic signs (File, 2016). Delirium may be related to hypoxemia, fever, dehydration, sleep deprivation, or developing sepsis. The patient's underlying comorbid conditions may also play a part in the development of confusion. Addressing and correcting underlying factors as well as ensuring patient safety are important nursing interventions.

Promoting Home, Community-Based, and Transitional Care

EDUCATING PATIENTS ABOUT SELF-CARE. Depending on the severity of the pneumonia, treatment may occur in the hospital or in the outpatient setting. Patient education is crucial regardless of the setting, and the proper administration of antibiotics is important. In some instances, the patient may be initially treated with IV antibiotics as an inpatient and then be discharged to continue the IV antibiotics in the home setting. It is important that a seamless system of care be maintained for the patient from hospital to home; this includes communication between the nurses caring for this patient in both settings. In addition, if oral antibiotics are prescribed, it is important to teach the patient about their proper administration and potential side effects. The patient should be instructed about symptoms that require contacting the health care provider: difficulty breathing, worsening cough, recurrent/increasing fever, and medication intolerance.

After the fever subsides, the patient may gradually increase activities. Fatigue and weakness may be prolonged after pneumonia, especially in the older. The nurse encourages breathing exercises to promote secretion clearance and volume expansion. A patient who is being treated as an outpatient should be contacted by the health care team or instructed to contact the health care provider 24 to 48 hours after starting therapy. It is important to instruct the patient to return to the clinic or caregiver's office for a follow-up chest x-ray and physical examination. Often, improvement in chest x-ray findings lags behind improvement in clinical signs and symptoms.

The nurse encourages the patient to stop smoking. Smoking inhibits tracheobronchial ciliary action, which is the first line of defense of the lower respiratory tract. Smoking also irritates the mucous cells of the bronchi and inhibits the function of alveolar macrophage cells. The patient is instructed to avoid stress, fatigue, sudden changes in temperature, and excessive alcohol intake, all of which lower resistance to pneumonia. The nurse reviews with the patient the principles of adequate nutrition and rest, because one episode of pneumonia may make the patient susceptible to recurring respiratory tract infections.

CONTINUING AND TRANSITIONAL CARE. Patients who are severely debilitated or who cannot care for themselves may require referral for home, transitional, or community-based care. During home visits, the nurse assesses the patient's physical status, monitors for complications, assesses the home environment, and reinforces previous teaching. The nurse evaluates the patient's adherence to the therapeutic regimen (i.e., taking medications as prescribed; performing breathing exercises; consuming adequate fluid and dietary intake; and avoiding smoking, alcohol, and excessive activity). The nurse stresses to the patient and family the importance of monitoring for complications or exacerbation of the pneumonia. The nurse encourages the patient to obtain an influenza vaccine at the prescribed times, because influenza increases susceptibility to secondary bacterial pneumonia, especially that caused by staphylococci, *H. influenzae*, and *S. pneumoniae* (Aoki, Allen, Stiver, et al., 2012).

Evaluation

Expected patient outcomes may include the following:

1. Demonstrates improved airway patency, as evidenced by adequate oxygenation by pulse oximetry or arterial blood gas analysis, normal temperature, normal breath sounds, and effective coughing
2. Rests and conserves energy by limiting activities and remaining in bed while symptomatic and slowly increasing activities
3. Maintains adequate hydration, as evidenced by an adequate fluid intake and urine output and normal skin turgor
4. Consumes adequate dietary intake, as evidenced by maintenance or increase in body weight without excess fluid gain
5. States an explanation for management strategies
6. Understands management strategies
7. Exhibits no complications
   a. Exhibits acceptable vital signs, pulse oximetry, and arterial blood gas measurements
   b. Reports a productive cough that diminishes over time
   c. Has absence of signs or symptoms of shock, respiratory failure, or pleural effusion
   d. Remains oriented and aware of surroundings
   e. Maintains or increases weight
8. Complies with the treatment protocol and prevention strategies

Aspiration

Aspiration is inhalation of foreign material (e.g., oropharyngeal or stomach contents) into the lungs. Aspiration pneumonia represents 5% to 15% of pneumonias in the hospitalized population.

It is a serious complication that may cause pneumonia and result in the following clinical picture: tachycardia, dyspnea, central cyanosis, hypertension, hypotension, and potentially death. It can occur when the protective airway reflexes are decreased or absent from a variety of factors (Chart 24-5).

NURSING ALERT

When a nonfunctioning nasogastric tube allows the gastric contents to accumulate in the stomach, a condition known as silent aspiration may result. Silent aspiration often occurs unobserved and may be more common than suspected. If untreated, massive inhalation of gastric contents develops in a period of several hours.

CHART 24-5

Risk Factors: Aspiration

- Seizure activity
- Brain injury
- Decreased level of consciousness from trauma, drug or alcohol intoxication, excessive sedation, or general anesthesia
- Flat body positioning
- Stroke
- Swallowing disorders
- Cardiac arrest

Adapted from American Association of Critical-Care Nurses. (2016). AACN practice alert: Prevention of aspiration in adults. *Critical Care Nurse*, *36*(1), e20–e24; Bartlett, J. (2015). Aspiration pneumonia in adults. UpToDate. Last updated June 6, 2015. Retrieved March 19, 2016, from www.uptodate.com/contents/aspiration-pneumonia-in-adults

Pathophysiology

The primary factors responsible for complications after aspiration of gastric contents are the volume and character of the aspirated gastric contents. Aspiration pneumonia develops after inhalation of colonized oral or pharyngeal material. The pathologic process involves an acute inflammatory response to bacteria and bacterial products. Most commonly, the bacteriologic findings include gram-positive cocci, gram-negative rods, and occasionally anaerobic bacteria (Bartlett, 2015).

A full stomach contains solid particles of food. If these are aspirated, the problem then becomes one of mechanical blockage of the airways and secondary infection. Aspiration of gastric contents causes a chemical burn of the tracheobronchial tree and pulmonary parenchyma inflammatory response occurs. This results in the destruction of alveolar–capillary endothelial cells, with a consequent outpouring of protein-rich fluids into the interstitial and intra-alveolar spaces. As a result, surfactant is lost, which in turn causes the airways to close and the alveoli to collapse. Finally, the impaired exchange of oxygen and carbon dioxide causes respiratory failure. During periods of fasting, the stomach contains acidic gastric juice, which, if aspirated, may be very destructive to the alveoli and capillaries. Fecal contamination (more likely seen in intestinal obstruction) increases the likelihood of death because the endotoxins produced by intestinal organisms may be absorbed systemically, or the thick proteinaceous material found in the intestinal contents may obstruct the airway, leading to atelectasis and secondary bacterial invasion.

Prevention

Prevention is the primary goal when caring for patients at risk for aspiration. Examples of risk factors for aspiration include decreased level of consciousness, supine positioning, presence of a nasogastric tube, tracheal intubation and mechanical ventilation, bolus or intermittent feeding delivery methods, and advanced age (Echevarria & Schwoebel, 2012). Aspiration of small amounts of material from the buccal (oral) cavity is not uncommon, particularly during sleep; however, disease as a result of aspiration does not occur in healthy persons because the material is cleared by the mucociliary tree and the macrophages. Witnessed aspiration of large volumes occurs occasionally; however, small-volume clinically silent aspiration is more common.

NURSING ALERT

When a nonfunctioning nasogastric tube allows the gastric contents to accumulate in the stomach, a condition known as silent aspiration may result. Silent aspiration often occurs unobserved and may be more common than suspected. If untreated, massive inhalation of gastric contents develops in a period of several hours.

CHART 24-6

Clinical Practice to Prevent Aspiration

- Maintain head-of-bed elevation at an angle of 30 to 45 degrees, unless contraindicated
- Use sedatives as sparingly as possible
- Before initiating enteral tube feeding, confirm the tip location
- For patients receiving tube feedings, assess placement of the feeding tube at 4-hour intervals, assess for gastrointestinal residuals (<150 mL before next feeding) to the feedings at 4-hour intervals
- For patients receiving tube feedings, avoid bolus feedings in those at high risk for aspiration
- Consult with primary provider about obtaining a swallowing evaluation before oral feedings are started for patients who were recently extubated but were previously intubated for >2 days
- Maintain endotracheal cuff pressures at an appropriate level, and ensure that secretions are cleared from above the cuff before it is deflated.

Adapted from American Association of Critical-Care Nurses. (2016). AACN practice alert: Prevention of aspiration in adults. *Critical Care Nurse, 36*(1), e20–e24; Swaminathan, A. (2015). Aspiration pneumonitis and pneumonia. Medscape, Updated 2015. Retrieved June 8, 2016, from emedicine.medscape.com/article/296198-overview

Compensating for Absent Reflexes

Aspiration is likely to occur if the patient cannot adequately coordinate protective glottic, laryngeal, and cough reflexes. This hazard is increased if the patient has a distended abdomen, is in a supine position, has the upper extremities immobilized by IV infusions or hand restraints, receives local anesthetics to the oropharyngeal or laryngeal area for diagnostic procedures, has been sedated, or has had long-term intubation (see Chart 24-6).

For patients with known swallowing dysfunction or those recently extubated following prolonged endotracheal intubation, a swallowing assessment is necessary. Patients deemed at risk are then assessed by a speech therapist. Besides positioning the patient semirecumbent or upright prior to eating, other helpful techniques may include suggesting a soft diet and encouraging the patient to take small bites. The patient should be instructed to keep the chin tucked and the head turned with repeated swallowing. Straws should not be used.

When vomiting, a person can normally protect the airway by sitting up or turning on the side and coordinating breathing, coughing, gag, and glottic reflexes. If these reflexes are active, an oral airway should not be inserted. If an airway is in place, it should be pulled out the moment the patient gags so as not to stimulate the pharyngeal gag reflex and promote vomiting and aspiration. Suctioning of oral secretions with a catheter should be performed with minimal pharyngeal stimulation.

For patients with an endotracheal tube and feeding tube, the endotracheal cuff pressure should be maintained at greater than 20 cm H_2O (but less than 30 cm H_2O to minimize injury) to prevent leakage of secretions from around the cuff into the lower respiratory tract. In addition, hypopharyngeal suctioning is recommended before the cuff is deflated (AACN, 2016).

Assessing Feeding Tube Placement

When the patient is intubated, aspiration may occur even with a nasogastric tube in place and may result in nosocomial pneumonia. Assessment of tube placement is key to preventing aspiration. The best method for determining tube placement is via an x-ray. Other nonradiologic methods that have been studied; observation of the aspirate and testing of its pH are the most reliable. Gastric fluid may be grassy green, brown, clear, or colourless. An aspirate from the lungs may be off-white or tan mucus. Pleural fluid is watery and usually straw coloured. Gastric pH values are typically lower or more acidic than that of the intestinal or respiratory tract. Gastric pH is usually between 1 and 5, while intestinal or respiratory pH is 7 or higher. There are differences in assessing tube placement with continuous versus intermittent feedings. For intermittent feedings with small-bore tubes, observation of aspirated contents and pH evaluation should be performed. For continuous feedings, the pH method is not clinically useful due to the infused formula.

Patients who receive continuous or timed-interval tube feedings must be positioned properly. The patient receiving a continuous infusion is given small volumes under low pressure in an upright position, which helps to prevent aspiration. Patients receiving tube feedings at timed intervals are maintained in an upright or semirecumbent position (elevation of the head of the bed to a 30- to 45-degree angle) during the feeding and for a minimum of 30 minutes afterward to allow the stomach to partially empty.

Identifying Delayed Stomach Emptying

A full stomach may cause aspiration because of increased intragastric or extragastric pressure. The following clinical situations cause a delayed emptying time of the stomach and may contribute to aspiration: intestinal obstruction; increased gastric secretions in gastroesophageal reflex disease; increased gastric secretions during anxiety, stress, or pain; or abdominal distention because of ileus, ascites, peritonitis, use of opioids and sedatives, severe illness, or vaginal delivery.

Managing the Effects of Prolonged Intubation

Prolonged endotracheal intubation or tracheostomy can depress the laryngeal and glottic reflexes because of disuse. Patients with prolonged tracheostomies are encouraged to phonate and exercise their laryngeal muscles. For patients who have had long-term intubation or tracheostomies, it may be helpful to have a rehabilitation therapist experienced in speech and swallowing disorders work with the patient to assess the swallowing reflex.

Pulmonary Tuberculosis

Tuberculosis (TB) is an infectious disease that primarily affects the lung parenchyma. It also may be transmitted to other parts of the body, including the meninges, kidneys, bones, and lymph nodes. The primary infectious agent, *M. tuberculosis*, is an acid-fast aerobic rod that grows slowly and is sensitive to heat and ultraviolet light.

TB is a worldwide public health problem that is closely associated with poverty, malnutrition, overcrowding, substandard housing, and inadequate health care. Mortality and morbidity rates continue to rise; *M. tuberculosis* infects an estimated one third of the world's population and remains the leading cause of death from infectious disease in the world. In 2014, 9.6 million people were sick with TB throughout the world and there were 1.5 million TB-related deaths (CDC, 2015d).

Throughout the first half of the 20th century, TB was a major cause of morbidity and mortality in Canada. Improvement in general living conditions, public health measures, and the introduction of effective drug treatment have resulted in a significant decline since a peak in the early 1940s. It was thought that by the early part of the 21st century, TB might be eliminated in Canada. The incidence of TB in Canada fell from 7.0 per 100,000 in 1990 to 4.6 per 100,000 in 2016 (Public Health Agency of Canada, 2018). Although the incidence of TB in Canada is low in comparison to the global context, there has been a slight increase in rates over the last 3 years (Public Health Agency of Canada, 2018). Almost 90% of new cases of active TB reported in Canada over the past 3 years have occurred among individuals born in foreign countries or Canadian Indigenous people (Public Health Agency of Canada, 2018).

Transmission and Risk Factors

TB spreads from person to person by airborne transmission. An infected person releases droplet nuclei (generally particles 1 to 5 μm in diameter) through talking, coughing, sneezing, laughing, or singing. Larger droplets settle; smaller droplets remain suspended in the air and are inhaled by the susceptible person. Risk factors for TB are listed in Chart 24-7. The CDC's recommendations for prevention of TB transmission in health care settings are summarized in Chart 24-8.

Pathophysiology

TB begins when a susceptible person inhales mycobacterium bacilli and becomes infected. The bacteria are transmitted through the airways to the alveoli, where they are deposited and begin to multiply. The bacilli also are transported via the lymph system and bloodstream to other parts of the body (kidneys, bones, cerebral cortex) and other areas of the lungs (upper lobes). The body's immune system responds by initiating an inflammatory reaction. Phagocytes (neutrophils and macrophages) engulf many of the bacteria, and TB-specific lymphocytes lyse (destroy) the bacilli and normal tissue. This tissue reaction results in the accumulation of exudate in the alveoli, causing bronchopneumonia. The initial infection usually occurs 2 to 10 weeks after exposure.

Granulomas, new tissue masses of live and dead bacilli, are surrounded by macrophages, which form a protective wall around the granulomas. Granulomas are then transformed to a fibrous tissue mass, the central portion of which is called a *Ghon tubercle*. The material (bacteria and macrophages) becomes necrotic, forming a cheesy mass. This mass may become calcified and form a collagenous scar. At this point, the bacteria become dormant, and there is no further progression of active disease.

After initial exposure and infection, the person may develop active disease because of a compromised or

CHART 24-7

Risk Factors: Tuberculosis

- Close contact with someone who has active TB. Inhalation of airborne nuclei from an infected person is proportional to the amount of time spent in the same air space, the proximity of the person, and the degree of ventilation.
- Immunocompromised status (e.g., those with HIV infection, cancer, transplanted organs, and prolonged high-dose corticosteroid therapy).
- Substance abuse (IV/injection drug users and alcoholics).
- Any person without adequate health care (the homeless; impoverished; minorities, particularly children <15 years and young adults between ages 15 and 44 years).
- Pre-existing medical conditions or special treatment (e.g., diabetes, chronic kidney injury, malnourishment, selected malignancies, hemodialysis, transplanted organ, gastrectomy, and jejunoileal bypass).
- Immigration from or recent travel to countries with a high prevalence of TB (southeastern Asia, Africa, Latin America, Caribbean).
- Institutionalization (e.g., long-term care facilities, psychiatric institutions, prisons).
- Living in overcrowded, substandard housing.
- Being a health care worker performing high-risk activities: administration of aerosolized pentamidine and other medications, sputum induction procedures, bronchoscopy, suctioning, coughing procedures, caring for the immunosuppressed patient, home care with the high-risk population, and administering anesthesia and related procedures (e.g., intubation, suctioning).

TB, tuberculosis.
Adapted from Centers for Disease Control and Prevention. (2012). TB fact sheets-infection control and prevention; TB in specific populations. Last updated September 1, 2012. Retrieved March 26, 2016, from www.cdc.gov/tb/publications/factsheets/specpop.htm

inadequate immune system response. Active disease also may occur with reinfection and activation of dormant bacteria. In this case, the Ghon tubercle ulcerates, releasing the cheesy material into the bronchi. The bacteria then become airborne, resulting in further spread of the disease. Then, the ulcerated tubercle heals and forms scar tissue. This causes the infected lung to become more inflamed, resulting in further development of bronchopneumonia and tubercle formation.

Unless the process is arrested, it spreads slowly downward to the hilum of the lungs and later extends to adjacent lobes. The process may be prolonged and characterized by long remissions when the disease is arrested, only to be followed by periods of renewed activity. Approximately

CHART 24-8

Centers for Disease Control and Prevention Recommendations for Preventing Transmission of Tuberculosis in Health Care Settings

1. Early identification and treatment of persons with active TB
   a. Maintain a high index of suspicion for TB to identify cases rapidly.
   b. Promptly initiate effective multidrug anti-TB therapy based on clinical and drug-resistance surveillance data.
2. Prevention of spread of infectious droplet nuclei by source control methods and by reduction of microbial contamination of indoor air
   a. Initiate AFB isolation precautions immediately for all patients who are suspected or confirmed to have active TB and who may be infectious. AFB isolation precautions include the use of a private room with negative pressure in relation to surrounding areas and a minimum of six air exchanges per hour. Air from the room should be exhausted directly to the outside. The use of ultraviolet lamps and/or high-efficiency particulate air filters to supplement ventilation may be considered.
   b. Persons entering the AFB isolation room should use disposable particulate respirators that fit snugly around the face.
   c. Continue AFB isolation precautions until there is clinical evidence of reduced infectiousness (i.e., cough has substantially decreased and the number of organisms on sequential sputum smears is decreasing). If drug resistance is suspected or confirmed, continue AFB precautions until the sputum smear is negative for AFB.
   d. Use special precautions during cough-inducing procedures.
3. Surveillance for TB transmission
   a. Maintain surveillance for TB infection among health care workers (HCWs) by routine, periodic tuberculin skin testing. Recommend appropriate preventive therapy for HCWs when indicated.
   b. Maintain surveillance for TB cases among patients and HCWs.
   c. Promptly initiate contact investigation procedures among HCWs, patients, and visitors exposed to an untreated, or ineffectively treated, patient with infectious TB for whom appropriate AFB procedures are not in place. Recommend appropriate therapy or preventive therapy for contacts with disease or TB infection without current disease. Therapeutic regimens should be chosen based on the clinical history and local drug-resistance surveillance data.

TB, tuberculosis; AFB, acid-fast bacilli.
Adapted from Centers for Disease Control and Prevention. (2012). TB fact sheet-infection control and prevention. Retrieved March 26, 2016, from www.cdc.gov/tb/publications/factsheets/prevention.htm

10% of people who are initially infected develop active disease (Pozniak, 2016). Some people develop reactivation TB (also called *adult-type TB*). This type of TB results from a breakdown of the host defenses. It most commonly occurs within the lungs, usually in the apical or posterior segments of the upper lobes or the superior segments of the lower lobes.

Clinical Manifestations

The signs and symptoms of pulmonary TB are insidious. Most patients have a low-grade fever, cough, night sweats, fatigue, and weight loss. The cough may be nonproductive, or mucopurulent sputum may be expectorated. **Hemoptysis** also may occur. Both the systemic and pulmonary symptoms are usually chronic and may have been present for weeks to months. The older usually present with less pronounced symptoms than do younger patients. Nonrespiratory disease occurs in about 25% of cases in Canada (CTS & PHAC, 2013). In patients infected with HIV, extrapulmonary disease is more prevalent.

Assessment and Diagnostic Findings

A complete history, physical examination, tuberculin skin test, chest x-ray, acid-fast bacillus smear, and sputum culture are used to diagnose TB. If the person is infected with TB, the chest x-ray usually reveals lesions in the upper lobes, and the acid-fast bacillus smear contains mycobacterium.

Tuberculin Skin Test

The Mantoux test is used to determine if a person has been infected with the TB bacillus. The Mantoux test is a standardized procedure that should be performed only by those trained in its administration and reading. Tubercle bacillus extract (tuberculin), purified protein derivative (PPD), is injected into the intradermal layer of the inner aspect of the forearm, approximately 10 cm below the elbow (Fig. 24-3). Intermediate-strength (5 TU) PPD in a tuberculin syringe with a 1.3 cm 26- or 27-gauge needle is used. The needle, with the bevel facing up, is inserted beneath the skin. Then, 0.1 mL of PPD is injected, creating an elevation in the skin—a wheal or bleb. The site, antigen name, strength, lot number, date, and time of the test are recorded. The test result is read 48 to 72 hours after injection. Tests read after 72 hours tend to underestimate the true size of **induration** (hardening). A delayed localized reaction indicates that the person is sensitive to tuberculin.

A reaction occurs when both induration and erythema (redness) are present. After the area is inspected for induration, it is lightly palpated across the injection site, from the area of normal skin to the margins of the induration. The diameter of the induration (not erythema) is measured in millimetres at its widest part (see Fig. 24-3), and the size of the induration is documented. Erythema without induration is not considered significant.

Interpretation of Results

The size of the induration determines the significance of the reaction. A reaction of 0 to 4 mm is considered not significant; a reaction of 5 mm or greater may be significant in individuals who are considered at risk. An induration of 10 mm or greater is usually considered significant in individuals who have normal or mildly impaired immunity. A significant reaction indicates past exposure to *M. tuberculosis* or vaccination with bacillus Calmette–Guérin (BCG) vaccine. The BCG vaccine is given to produce a greater resistance to developing TB. It is estimated to be effective in 60% to 80% of those who receive it (Roy, Eisenhut, Harris, et al., 2014). However, the United States and Canada no longer routinely use the BCG vaccine (CTS & PHAC, 2013).

A significant (positive) reaction does not necessarily mean that active disease is present in the body. More than 90% of people who are tuberculin-significant reactors do not develop clinical TB. However, all significant reactors are candidates for active TB. In general, the more intense the reaction, the greater the likelihood of an active infection.

A nonsignificant (negative) skin test means the person's immune system did not react to the test and that latent TB infection or TB disease is not likely. It does not exclude TB infection or disease, because patients who are immunosuppressed cannot develop an immune response adequate to produce a positive skin test. This is referred to as anergy.

QuantiFERON-TB Gold In-Tube and T-SPOT

There are two TB blood tests (called interferon–gamma release assays or IGRAs) available in the United States: the QuantiFERON-TB Gold In-Tube (QFT-GIT) test and the T-SPOT. TB blood tests are the preferred diagnostic tests for patients who have received the BCG vaccine and for patients who are not likely to return for a second appointment to look for a reaction to the tuberculin skin test. The results of both of these tests are available within 24 to

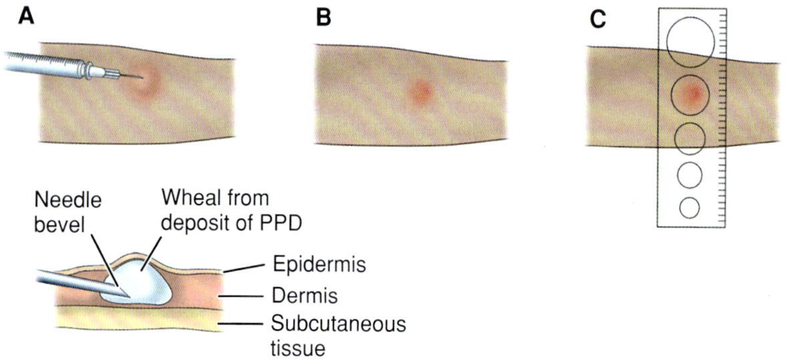

FIGURE 24-3. The Mantoux test for tuberculosis. **A.** Correct technique for inserting the needle involves depositing the PPD subcutaneously with the needle bevel facing upward. **B.** The reaction to the Mantoux test usually consists of a wheal—a hive-like, firm welt. **C.** To determine the extent of the reaction, the wheal is measured using a commercially prepared gauge. A wheal measuring 5 mm or more is considered significant. PPD, purified protein derivative.

36 hours. A positive IGRA signifies that the patient has been infected with TB bacteria and additional tests are needed. A negative IGRA means that the patient's blood did not react to the test and a latent or active TB infection is not likely (CDC, 2015d).

Classification of Tuberculosis

Data from the history, physical examination, skin test, chest x-ray, and microbiologic studies are used to classify TB into one of five classes. A classification scheme provides public health officials with a systematic way to monitor epidemiology and treatment of the disease.

- *Class 0:* No exposure; no infection
- *Class 1:* Exposure; no evidence of infection
- *Class 2:* Latent infection; no disease (e.g., positive PPD reaction but no clinical evidence of active TB)
- *Class 3:* Disease; clinically active
- *Class 4:* Disease; not clinically active
- *Class 5:* Suspected disease; diagnosis pending

Gerontologic Considerations

TB may have atypical manifestations in older patients, whose symptoms may include unusual behaviour and altered mental status, fever, anorexia, and weight loss. Many older patients may have no reaction (loss of immunologic memory) or delayed reactivity for up to a week (recall phenomenon). A second skin test is performed in 1 to 2 weeks. Older adults who live in long-term care facilities are at increased risk for primary and reactivation TB as compared to those in the community (Pagali, Verdoom, Wieland, et al., 2014).

Medical Management

Pulmonary TB is treated primarily with chemotherapeutic agents (anti-TB agents) for 6 to 12 months. A prolonged treatment duration is necessary to ensure eradication of the organisms and to prevent relapse. The continuing and increasing resistance of *M. tuberculosis* to TB medications is a worldwide concern and challenge in TB therapy. Several types of drug resistance must be considered when planning effective therapy:

- *Primary drug resistance:* Resistance to one of the first-line anti-TB agents in a person who has not had previous treatment
- *Secondary or acquired drug resistance:* Resistance to one or more anti-TB agents in a patient undergoing therapy
- *Multidrug resistance:* Resistance to two agents, isoniazid (INH) and rifampin (RMP). The populations at highest risk for multidrug resistance are those who are HIV-positive, institutionalized, or homeless.

The increasing prevalence of drug resistance points out the need to begin TB treatment with four or more medications, to ensure completion of therapy, and to develop and evaluate new anti-TB medications.

Pharmacologic Therapy

In current TB therapy, four first-line medications are used (Table 24-4): INH, RMP, pyrazinamide (PZA), and ethambutol. Combination medications, such as INH/RMP (Rifamate) or INH/RMP/PZA and medications administered twice a week (e.g., rifapentine) are available to help improve patient adherence. Capreomycin, ethionamide, para-aminosalicylate sodium, and cycloserine are second-line medications. Additional potentially effective medications include other aminoglycosides, quinolones, rifabutin, clofazimine, and combinations of medications. Recommended Canadian treatment guidelines for newly diagnosed cases of pulmonary TB have two parts: an initial phase and a continuation phase (CDC, 2015d; PHAC, 2014). People are considered noninfectious after 2 to 3 weeks of continuous medication therapy. The total number of doses taken, not simply the duration of treatment, more accurately determines whether a course of therapy has been completed.

Isoniazid also may be used to treat latent TB infection for those at risk for significant disease, including the following:

- Household family members of patients with active disease
- HIV-infected patients with a PPD test reaction of 5 mm of induration or more
- Patients with fibrotic lesions detected on a chest x-ray, suggestive of old TB, and a PPD reaction of 5 mm of induration or more
- Patients whose current PPD test results show a change from former test results, suggesting recent exposure to TB and possible infection (also called *skin test converters*)
- Users of IV/injectable drugs who have PPD test results of 10 mm of induration or more
- Patients with high-risk comorbid conditions with a PPD result of 10 mm of induration or more

Other candidates for preventive INH therapy are those aged 35 years or younger with PPD test results of 10 mm of induration or more and one of the following criteria:

- Foreign-born individuals from countries with a high prevalence of TB
- High-risk, medically underserved populations
- Institutionalized patients

Prophylactic INH treatment involves taking daily doses for 6 to 12 months. Liver enzyme, blood urea nitrogen, and creatinine levels are monitored monthly. Sputum culture results are monitored for acid-fast bacillus to evaluate the effectiveness of treatment and the patient's compliance with therapy.

Nursing Process

The Patient With Tuberculosis

Assessment

The nurse performs a complete history and physical examination. Clinical manifestations of fever, anorexia, weight loss, night sweats, fatigue, cough,

TABLE 24-4 First-Line Antituberculosis Medications for Active Disease

Commonly Used Agents	Adult Daily Dosage[a]	Most Common Side Effects	Drug Interactions[b]	Nursing Considerations[a]
Isoniazid (INH)	5 mg/kg (300 mg maximum daily)	Peripheral neuritis, hepatic enzyme elevation, hepatitis, hypersensitivity	Phenytoin—synergistic Antabuse Alcohol	Bactericidal Pyridoxine is used as prophylaxis for neuritis. Monitor AST and ALT
Rifampin (Rifadin)	10 mg/kg (600 mg maximum daily)	Hepatitis, febrile reaction, purpura (rare), nausea, vomiting	Rifampin increases metabolism of oral contraceptives, quinidine, corticosteroids, coumarin derivatives and methadone, digoxin, oral hypoglycemics. PAS may interfere with absorption of rifampin	Bactericidal Orange urine and other body secretions Discolouring of contact lenses Monitor AST and ALT
Rifabutin (Mycobutin)	5 mg/kg (300 mg maximum daily)		Avoid protease inhibitors	
Rifapentine (Priftin)	10 mg/kg (600 mg twice weekly)	Hepatotoxicity, thrombocytopenia		Orange-red colouration of body secretions, contact lenses, dentures Use with caution in older adults or in those with renal disease
Pyrazinamide	15–30 mg/kg (2 g maximum daily)[a]	Hyperuricemia, hepatotoxicity, skin rash, arthralgias, GI distress		Bactericidal Monitor uric acid, AST, and ALT
Ethambutol (Myambutol)	15–25 mg/kg (1.6 g maximum daily dose)[a]	Optic neuritis (may lead to blindness; very rare at 15 mg/kg), skin rash		Bacteriostatic Use with caution with renal disease or when eye testing is not feasible. Monitor visual acuity, colour, and discrimination[c]
Combinations: INH + rifampin (e.g., Rifamate)	150-mg and 300-mg caps (2 caps daily)			

[a]Check product labelling for detailed information on dose, contraindications, drug interactions, adverse reactions, and monitoring.

[b]Refer to current literature, particularly on rifampin, because it increases hepatic microenzymes and therefore interacts with many drugs.

[c]Initial examination should be performed at start of treatment.

AST, aspartate transaminase; ALT, alanine transaminase; PAS, para-aminosalicylic acid; GI, gastrointestinal.

Adapted from Gilbert, D. N., Chambers, H. F., Eliopoulos, G. M., et al. (2015). *The Sanford guide to antimicrobial therapy 2015* (45th ed.). Sperryville, VA: Antimicrobial Therapy, Inc.

and sputum production prompt a more thorough assessment of respiratory function—for example, assessing the lungs for consolidation by evaluating breath sounds (diminished, bronchial sounds, crackles), fremitus, egophony, and dullness on percussion. Enlarged, painful lymph nodes may be palpated as well. The nurse also assesses the patient's living arrangements, perceptions and understanding of TB and its treatment, and readiness to learn.

Nursing Priorities

Based on the assessment data, the nursing diagnoses may include the following:

- Airway
- Patient teaching
- Activity

Collaborative Problems/ Potential Complications

Based on the assessment data, collaborative problems or potential complications that may occur include the following:

- Malnutrition
- Adverse side effects of medication therapy: hepatitis, neurologic changes (deafness or neuritis), skin rash, gastrointestinal upset
- Multidrug resistance
- Spread of TB infection (miliary TB)

Planning and Goals

The major goals for the patient include maintenance of a patent airway, increased knowledge about the disease and treatment regimen and adherence to the medication regimen, increased activity tolerance, and absence of complications.

Nursing Interventions

Promoting Airway Clearance

Copious secretions obstruct the airways in many patients with TB and interfere with adequate gas exchange. Increasing fluid intake promotes systemic hydration and serves as an effective expectorant. The nurse instructs the patient about correct positioning to facilitate airway drainage (postural drainage) (see Chapter 26).

Promoting Adherence to the Treatment Regimen

Adherence to the prescribed treatment regimen is key in treating the disease and controlling the spread of infection (Reichman & Lardizabal, 2015). The multiple-medication regimen that a patient must follow can be quite complex. Understanding the medications, schedule, and side effects is important. The patient must understand that TB is a communicable disease and that taking medications is the most effective means of preventing transmission. The major reason treatment fails is that patients do not take their medications regularly and for the prescribed duration. This may be due to side effects or the complexity of the treatment regimen. Risk factors for nonadherence to the drug regimen include patients who have previously failed to complete the course of therapy; patients who are physically, emotionally, or mentally challenged; patients unable to pay for medication; patients actively abusing illicit substances; and patients who do not understand the importance of treatment (Reichman & Lardizabal, 2015).

The nurse educates the patient to take the medication either on an empty stomach or at least 1 hour before meals, because food interferes with medication absorption (although taking medications on an empty stomach frequently results in gastrointestinal upset). Patients taking INH should avoid foods that contain tyramine and histamine (tuna, aged cheese, red wine, soy sauce, yeast extracts), because eating them while taking INH may result in headache, flushing, hypotension, lightheadedness, palpitations, and diaphoresis. Patients should also avoid alcohol because of the high potential for hepatotoxic effects.

In addition, rifampin can alter the metabolism of certain other medications, making them less effective. These medications include beta-blockers, oral anticoagulants such as warfarin (Coumadin), digoxin, quinidine, corticosteroids, oral hypoglycemic agents, oral contraceptives, theophylline, and verapamil (Calan, Isoptin). This issue should be discussed with the primary provider and pharmacist so that medication dosages can be adjusted accordingly. The nurse informs the patient that rifampin may discolour contact lenses and that the patient may want to wear eyeglasses during treatment. The nurse monitors for other side effects of anti-TB medications, including hepatitis, neurologic changes (hearing loss, neuritis), and rash. Liver enzymes, blood urea nitrogen (BUN), and serum creatinine levels are monitored to detect changes in liver and kidney function. Sputum culture results are monitored for AFB to evaluate the effectiveness of the treatment regimen and adherence to therapy.

The nurse instructs the patient about the risk of drug resistance if the medication regimen is not strictly and continuously followed. The nurse carefully monitors vital signs and observes for spikes in temperature or changes in the patient's clinical status. Caregivers of patients who are not hospitalized are taught to monitor the patient's temperature and respiratory status. Changes in the patient's respiratory status are reported to the primary provider.

For patients at risk of nonadherence, programs used in the community setting may include comprehensive case management and directly observed therapy (DOT). In case management, each patient with TB is assigned a case manager who coordinates all aspects of the patient's care. DOT consists of a health care provider or another responsible person who directly observes that the patient ingests the prescribed medications. Although successful, DOT is a resource-intensive program (Reichman & Lardizabal, 2015).

Monitoring and Managing Potential Complications

Promoting Activity and Adequate Nutrition

Patients with TB are often debilitated from a prolonged chronic illness and impaired nutritional status. The nurse plans a progressive activity schedule that focuses on increasing activity tolerance and muscle strength. Anorexia, weight loss, and malnutrition are common in patients with TB. The patient's willingness to eat may be altered by fatigue from excessive coughing, sputum production, chest pain, generalized debilitated state, or cost, if the person has few resources. A nutritional plan that allows for small, frequent meals may be required. Liquid nutritional supplements may assist in meeting basic caloric requirements.

SIDE EFFECTS OF MEDICATION THERAPY. It is important to assess medication side effects, as they are often a reason the patient fails to adhere to the prescribed medication regimen. Efforts are made to reduce the side effects to increase the patient's willingness to take the medications as prescribed.

The nurse instructs the patient to take the medication either on an empty stomach or at least 1 hour before meals, because food interferes with medication absorption (although taking medications on an empty stomach frequently results in gastrointestinal upset). Patients taking INH should avoid foods containing tyramine and histamine (tuna, aged cheese, red wine, soy sauce, yeast extracts). Eating these types of foods while taking INH may result in headache, flushing, hypotension, lightheadedness, palpitations, and diaphoresis.

In addition, RMP can increase the metabolism of other medications, making them less effective. These medications include beta-blockers, oral anticoagulants such as warfarin (Coumadin), digoxin, quinidine, corticosteroids, oral hypoglycemic agents, oral contraceptives, theophylline, and verapamil. This issue should be discussed with the physician and pharmacist so that medication dosages can be adjusted accordingly. The nurse informs the patient that RMP may discolour contact lenses, so the patient may want to wear eyeglasses during treatment. The nurse monitors for other side effects of anti-TB medications, including hepatitis, neurologic changes (hearing loss, neuritis), and rash. Liver enzyme, BUN, and serum creatinine levels are monitored to detect medication-related changes in liver and kidney function. Sputum culture results are monitored for acid-fast bacillus to evaluate the effectiveness of the treatment regimen and adherence to therapy.

MULTIDRUG RESISTANCE. The nurse carefully monitors vital signs and observes for spikes in temperature or changes in the clinical status. The nurse reports any change in the patient's respiratory status to the primary health care provider. The nurse instructs the patient about the risk of drug resistance if the medication regimen is not strictly and continuously followed.

SPREAD OF TUBERCULOSIS INFECTION. The spread of TB infection to nonpulmonary sites of the body is known as miliary TB. It is the result of invasion of the bloodstream by the tubercle bacillus (Ghon tubercle). Usually, it results from late reactivation of a dormant infection in the lung or elsewhere. The origin of the bacilli that enter the bloodstream is either a chronic focus that has ulcerated into a blood vessel or multitudes of miliary tubercles lining the inner surface of the thoracic duct. The organisms migrate from these foci into the bloodstream, are carried throughout the body, and disseminate throughout all tissues, with tiny miliary tubercles developing in the lungs, spleen, liver, kidneys, meninges, and other organs.

The clinical course of miliary TB may vary from an acute, rapidly progressive infection with high fever to a slowly developing process with low-grade fever, anemia, and debilitation. At first, there may be no localizing signs except an enlarged spleen and a reduced number of leukocytes. Within a few weeks, however, the chest x-ray reveals small densities scattered diffusely throughout both lung fields; these are the miliary tubercles, which gradually grow.

The possibility of TB in nonpulmonary sites in the body requires careful monitoring for this very serious form of infection. The nurse monitors vital signs and observes for spikes in temperature as well as changes in renal and cognitive function. Few physical signs may be elicited on physical examination of the chest; however, at this stage, the patient has a severe cough and dyspnea. Treatment of miliary TB is the same as for pulmonary TB.

Promoting Home, Community-Based, and Transitional Care

EDUCATING PATIENTS ABOUT SELF-CARE. The nurse plays a vital role in caring for the patient with TB and the family, which includes assessing the patient's ability to continue therapy at home. The nurse instructs the patient and family about infection control procedures, such as proper disposal of tissues, covering the mouth during coughing, and frequent handwashing. Assessment of the patient's adherence to the medication regimen is imperative because of the risk of developing resistant strains of TB if the regimen is not followed faithfully. In some cases when the patient's ability to comply with the medication regimen is in question, referral to an outpatient clinic for daily medication administration may be required. This is referred to as DOT.

CONTINUING AND TRANSITIONAL CARE. The nurse evaluates the patient's environment, including home or workplace and social setting, to identify other people who may have been in contact with the patient during the infectious stage. It is important to arrange follow-up screening for any contacts of the infected person. Nurses who have contact with the patient in home, shelter, hospital, clinic, or work settings assess the patient's physical and psychological status and ability to adhere to the prescribed treatment. The nurse assesses the patient for adverse effects of medications and adherence to the therapeutic regimen (e.g., taking medications as prescribed, practicing safe hygiene, consuming a nutritious and adequate diet, and participating in an appropriate level of activity). The nurse reinforces previous teaching and emphasizes the importance of keeping scheduled appointments with the primary health care provider. In addition, the patient is reminded of the importance of other health promotion activities and recommended health screening.

Evaluation

Expected patient outcomes may include the following:

1. Maintains a patent airway by managing secretions with hydration, humidification, coughing, and postural drainage
2. Demonstrates an adequate level of knowledge
   a. Lists medications by name and the correct schedule for taking them
   b. Identifies expected side effects of medications
   c. Identifies how and when to contact health care provider
3. Adheres to the treatment regimen by taking medications as prescribed and reporting for follow-up screening
4. Participates in preventive measures
   a. Disposal of used tissues properly
   b. Encourages people who are close contacts to report for testing
   c. Adheres to hand hygiene recommendations
5. Maintains an activity schedule

6. Exhibits no complications
    a. Maintains adequate weight or gains weight, if indicated
    b. Exhibits normal results of tests of liver and kidney function
7. Takes steps to minimize side effects of medications
    a. Takes supplemental vitamins (vitamin B) as prescribed to minimize peripheral neuropathy
    b. Avoids the use of alcohol
    c. Avoids foods containing tyramine and histamine
    d. Has regular physical examinations and blood tests to evaluate liver and kidney function, neuropathy, and hearing and visual acuity

Lung Abscess

A lung abscess is a localized collection of pus caused by microbial infection (Weinberger, Cockrill, & Mandel, et al., 2014). It is generally caused by aspiration of anaerobic bacteria. By definition, the chest x-ray will demonstrate a cavity of at least 2 cm. Patients who have impaired cough reflexes and cannot close the glottis, or those with swallowing difficulties, are at risk for aspirating foreign material and developing a lung abscess. Other at-risk patients include those with central nervous system disorders (seizure, stroke), drug addiction, alcoholism, esophageal disease or compromised immune function, those without teeth and patients receiving nasogastric tube feedings, and those with an altered state of consciousness.

Pathophysiology

Most lung abscesses are a complication of bacterial pneumonia or are caused by aspiration of oral anaerobe into the lung. Abscesses also may occur secondary to mechanical or functional obstruction of the bronchi by a tumour, foreign body, or bronchial stenosis or from necrotizing pneumonias, TB, PE, or chest trauma.

Most abscesses are found in areas of the lung that may be affected by aspiration. The site of the lung abscess is related to gravity and is determined by the patient's position. For patients who are confined to bed, the posterior segment of an upper lobe and the superior segment of the lower lobe are the most common areas. However, atypical presentations may occur, depending on the position of the patient when the aspiration occurred.

Initially, the cavity in the lung may or may not extend directly into a bronchus. Eventually, the abscess becomes surrounded, or encapsulated, by a wall of fibrous tissue. The necrotic process may extend until it reaches the lumen of a bronchus or the pleural space and establishes communication with the respiratory tract, the pleural cavity, or both. If the bronchus is involved, the purulent contents are expectorated continuously in the form of sputum. If the pleura is involved, an empyema results. A communication or connection between the bronchus and pleura is known as a bronchopleural fistula. The organisms frequently associated with lung abscesses are anaerobic; however, aerobic organisms may be involved as well. The organisms vary depending on the underlying predisposing factors (Weinberger et al., 2014).

Clinical Manifestations

The clinical manifestations of a lung abscess may vary from a mild productive cough to acute illness. Most patients have a fever and a productive cough with moderate to copious amounts of foul-smelling, often bloody, sputum. The fever and cough may develop insidiously and may have been present for several weeks before diagnosis. Leukocytosis may be present. Pleurisy or dull chest pain, dyspnea, weakness, anorexia, and weight loss are common.

Assessment and Diagnostic Findings

Physical examination of the chest may reveal dullness on percussion and decreased or absent breath sounds with an intermittent **pleural friction rub** (grating or rubbing sound) on auscultation. Crackles may be present. Confirmation of the diagnosis is made by chest x-ray, sputum culture, and in some cases fibreoptic bronchoscopy. The chest x-ray reveals an infiltrate with an air–fluid level. A computed tomography (CT) scan of the chest may be required to provide more detailed pictures of different cross-sectional areas of the lung.

Prevention

The following measures will reduce the risk of lung abscess:

- Appropriate antibiotic therapy before any dental procedures in patients who must have teeth extracted while their gums and teeth are infected
- Adequate dental and oral hygiene, because anaerobic bacteria play a role in the pathogenesis of lung abscess
- Appropriate antimicrobial therapy for patients with pneumonia

Medical Management

The findings of the history, physical examination, chest x-ray, and sputum culture indicate the type of organism and the treatment required. Adequate drainage of the lung abscess may be achieved through postural drainage and chest physiotherapy. The patient should be assessed for an adequate cough. Some patients need a percutaneous chest catheter placed for long-term drainage of the abscess. Therapeutic use of bronchoscopy to drain an abscess is uncommon. A diet high in protein and calories is necessary because chronic infection is associated with a catabolic state, necessitating increased intake of calories and protein to facilitate healing. Surgical intervention is rare, but pulmonary resection (lobectomy) is performed when there is massive hemoptysis (coughing up of blood) or little or no response to medical management.

Pharmacologic Therapy

IV antimicrobial therapy depends on the results of the sputum culture and sensitivity and is administered for 3 to 6 weeks. Standard treatment of an anaerobic lung infection is clindamycin (Cleocin), ampicillin–sulbactam (Unasyn), or carbapenem (Gilbert et al., 2015). Large IV doses are generally required because the antibiotic must penetrate the necrotic tissue and the fluid in the abscess. The duration of treatment with IV antibiotics is controversial (Bartlett, 2014). Treatment with IV antibiotics may continue for 3 weeks and longer, depending upon the clinical severity and organism involved. Improvement is demonstrated by normal temperature, decreased white blood cell count, and improvement on chest x-ray (resolution of surrounding infiltrate, reduction in cavity size, and absence of fluid). Once improvement is demonstrated, IV antibiotics are discontinued and oral administration of antibiotic therapy is continued for an additional 4 to 12 weeks and sometimes longer. If treatment is stopped too soon, a relapse may occur (Bartlett, 2014).

Nursing Management

The nurse administers antibiotics and IV therapies as prescribed and monitors for adverse effects. Chest physiotherapy is initiated as prescribed to facilitate drainage of the abscess. The nurse teaches the patient to perform deep-breathing and coughing exercises to help expand the lungs. To ensure proper nutritional intake, the nurse encourages a diet high in protein and calories. The nurse also offers emotional support because the abscess may take a long time to resolve.

Promoting Home, Community-Based, and Transitional Care

Educating Patients About Self-Care

The patient who has had surgery may return home before the wound closes entirely or with a drain or tube in place. Thus, the patient or a caregiver needs instruction on how to change the dressings to prevent skin excoriation and odour, how to monitor for signs and symptoms of infection, and how to care for and maintain the drain or tube. The nurse instructs the patient to perform deep-breathing and coughing exercises every 2 hours during the day and shows a caregiver how to perform chest percussion and postural drainage to facilitate expectoration of lung secretions.

CONTINUING AND TRANSITIONAL CARE. Referral for home, transitional, or community-based care may be required by some patients whose condition requires therapy at home. During home visits, the nurse assesses the patient's physical condition, nutritional status, and home environment as well as the patient and family's ability to carry out the therapeutic regimen. Patient teaching is reinforced during home visits, and nutrition counselling is provided with the goal of attaining and maintaining an optimal state of nutrition. To prevent a relapse, the nurse emphasizes the importance of completing the antibiotic regimen and of following the suggestions for rest and appropriate activity. If IV antibiotic therapy is to continue at home, the services of a home care nurse may be arranged to initiate IV therapy and to evaluate its administration by the patient or family. Although most outpatient IV therapy is administered in the home setting, a patient may visit a nearby clinic or physician's office for this treatment. In some cases, patients with lung abscesses may have ignored their health. Therefore, it is important to use this opportunity to address health promotion strategies and health screening with the patient.

PLEURAL CONDITIONS

Pleural conditions are disorders that involve the membranes covering the lungs (visceral pleura) and the surface of the chest wall (parietal pleura) or disorders affecting the pleural space.

Pleurisy

Pathophysiology

Pleurisy (pleuritis) refers to inflammation of both layers of the pleurae (parietal and visceral). Pleurisy may develop in conjunction with pneumonia or an upper respiratory tract infection, TB, or collagen disease; after trauma to the chest, pulmonary infarction, or PE; in patients with primary and metastatic cancer; and after thoracotomy. The parietal pleura has nerve endings; the visceral pleura does not. When the inflamed pleural membranes rub together during respiration (intensified on inspiration), the result is severe, sharp, knifelike pain.

Clinical Manifestations

The key characteristic of pleuritic pain is its relationship to respiratory movement. Taking a deep breath, coughing, or sneezing worsens the pain. Pleuritic pain is restricted in distribution rather than diffuse; it usually occurs only on one side. The pain may become minimal or absent when the breath is held, or it may be localized or radiate to the shoulder or abdomen. Later, as pleural fluid develops, the pain decreases (Weinberger et al., 2014).

Assessment and Diagnostic Findings

In the early period, when little fluid has accumulated, a pleural friction rub can be heard with the stethoscope, only to disappear later as more fluid accumulates and separates the inflamed pleural surfaces. Diagnostic tests may include chest x-rays, sputum examinations, thoracentesis to obtain a specimen of pleural fluid for examination, and less commonly a pleural biopsy.

Medical Management

The objectives of treatment are to discover the underlying condition causing the pleurisy and to relieve the pain. As the underlying disease (pneumonia, infection) is treated, the pleuritic inflammation usually resolves. At the same time, it is necessary to monitor for signs and symptoms of pleural effusion, such as shortness of breath, pain, assumption of a position that decreases pain, and decreased chest wall excursion.

Prescribed analgesics and topical applications of heat or cold provide symptomatic relief. Indomethacin, a nonsteroidal anti-inflammatory drug (NSAID), may provide pain relief while allowing the patient to take deep breaths and cough more effectively. If the pain is severe, an intercostal nerve block may be required (Weinberger et al., 2014).

Nursing Management

Because the patient has considerable pain on inspiration, the nurse can offer suggestions to enhance comfort, such as turning frequently onto the affected side to splint the chest wall and reduce the stretching of the pleurae. The nurse also can teach the patient to use the hands or a pillow to splint the rib cage while coughing.

Pleural Effusion

Pleural effusion, a collection of fluid in the pleural space, is rarely a primary disease process but is usually secondary to other diseases. Normally, the pleural space contains a small amount of fluid (5 to 15 mL), which acts as a lubricant that allows the pleural surfaces to move without friction (Fig. 24-4). Pleural effusion may be a complication of heart failure, TB, pneumonia, pulmonary infections (particularly viral infections), nephrotic syndrome, connective tissue disease, PE, and neoplastic tumours. Bronchogenic carcinoma is the most common malignancy associated with a pleural effusion.

Pathophysiology

In certain disorders, fluid may accumulate in the pleural space to a point where it becomes clinically evident. This almost always has pathologic significance. The effusion can be composed of a relatively clear fluid, or it can be bloody or purulent. An effusion of clear fluid may be a transudate or an exudate. A transudate (filtrates of plasma that move across intact capillary walls) occurs when factors influencing the formation and reabsorption of pleural fluid are altered, usually by imbalances in hydrostatic or oncotic pressures. The finding of a transudative effusion generally implies that the pleural membranes are not diseased. The most common cause of a transudative effusion is heart failure. An exudate (extravasation of fluid into tissues or a cavity) usually results from inflammation by bacterial products or tumours involving the pleural surfaces (Heffner, 2015a).

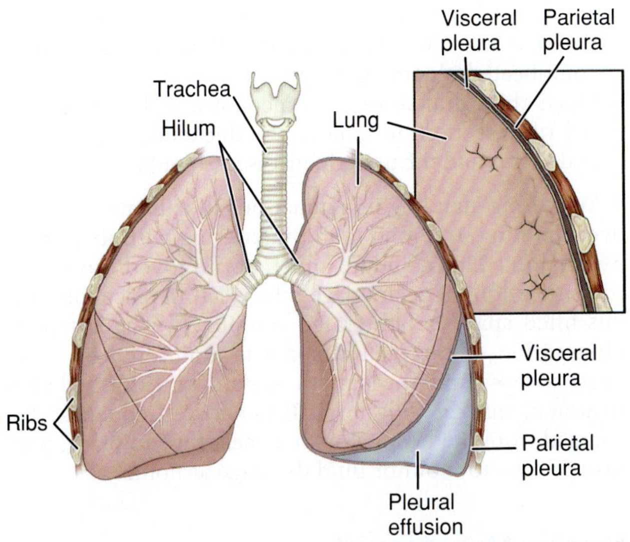

FIGURE 24-4. In pleural effusion, an abnormal volume of fluid collects in the pleural space, causing pain and shortness of breath. Pleural effusion is usually secondary to other disease processes.

Clinical Manifestations

Usually, the clinical manifestations are those caused by the underlying disease. Pneumonia causes fever, chills, and pleuritic chest pain, whereas a malignant effusion may result in dyspnea and coughing. The severity of symptoms is determined by the size of the effusion, the speed of its formation, and the underlying lung disease. A large pleural effusion causes shortness of breath. When a small to moderate pleural effusion is present, dyspnea may be absent or only minimal.

Assessment and Diagnostic Findings

Assessment of the area of the pleural effusion reveals decreased or absent breath sounds, decreased fremitus, and a dull, flat sound when percussed. In an extremely large pleural effusion, the assessment reveals a patient in acute respiratory distress. Tracheal deviation away from the affected side may also be noted.

Physical examination, chest x-ray, chest CT scan, and thoracentesis confirm the presence of fluid. In some instances, a lateral decubitus x-ray is obtained. For this x-ray, the patient lies on the affected side in a side-lying position. A pleural effusion can be diagnosed because this position allows for the "layering out" of the fluid, and an air–fluid line is visible.

Pleural fluid is analyzed by bacterial culture, Gram stain, acid-fast bacillus stain (for TB), red and white blood cell counts, chemistry studies (glucose, amylase, lactic dehydrogenase, protein), cytologic analysis for malignant cells, and pH. A pleural biopsy also may be performed.

Medical Management

The objectives of treatment are to discover the underlying cause, to prevent reaccumulation of fluid, and to relieve discomfort, dyspnea, and respiratory compromise. Specific treatment is directed at the underlying cause (e.g., heart failure, pneumonia, lung cancer, cirrhosis). If the pleural fluid is an exudate, more extensive diagnostic procedures are performed to determine the cause. Treatment for the primary cause is then instituted.

Thoracentesis is performed to remove fluid, to obtain a specimen for analysis, and to relieve dyspnea and respiratory compromise (see Chapter 26). Thoracentesis may be performed under ultrasound guidance. Depending on the size of the pleural effusion, the patient may be treated by removing the fluid during the thoracentesis procedure or by inserting a chest tube connected to a water-seal drainage system or suction to evacuate the pleural space and reexpand the lung.

If the underlying cause is a malignancy, however, the effusion tends to recur within a few days or weeks. Repeated thoracenteses result in pain, depletion of protein and electrolytes, and sometimes pneumothorax. Once the pleural space is adequately drained, a chemical pleurodesis may be performed to obliterate the pleural space and prevent reaccumulation of fluid. Pleurodesis may be performed using a thoracoscopic approach or via a chest tube. Chemically irritating agents (e.g., bleomycin or talc) are instilled in the pleural space. With the chest tube insertion approach, after the agent is instilled, the chest tube is clamped for 60 to 90 minutes, and the patient is assisted to assume various positions to promote uniform distribution of the agent and to maximize its contact with the pleural surfaces (Heffner, 2015b). The tube is unclamped as prescribed, and chest drainage may be continued several days longer to prevent reaccumulation of fluid and to promote the formation of adhesions between the visceral and parietal pleurae.

Other treatments for malignant pleural effusions include surgical pleurectomy, insertion of a small catheter attached to a drainage bottle for outpatient management, or implantation of a pleuroperitoneal shunt. A pleuroperitoneal shunt consists of two catheters connected by a pump chamber containing two one-way valves. Fluid moves from the pleural space to the pump chamber and then to the peritoneal cavity. The patient manually pumps on the reservoir daily to move fluid from the pleural space to the peritoneal space.

Nursing Management

The nurse's role in the care of the patient with a pleural effusion includes implementing the medical regimen. The nurse prepares and positions the patient for thoracentesis and offers support throughout the procedure. The nurse is responsible for making sure the thoracentesis fluid amount is recorded and sent for appropriate laboratory testing. If a chest tube drainage and water-seal system is used, the nurse monitors the system's function and records the amount of drainage at prescribed intervals. Nursing care related to the underlying cause of the pleural effusion is specific to the underlying condition. Care of the patient with a chest tube is discussed in Chapter 26.

If a chest tube is inserted for talc instillation, pain management is a priority and the nurse helps the patient assume positions that are the least painful. However, frequent turning and movement are important to facilitate adequate spreading of the talc over the pleural surface. The nurse evaluates the patient's pain level and administers analgesics as prescribed and as needed.

If the patient is to be managed as an outpatient with a pleural catheter for drainage, the nurse is responsible for educating the patient and family regarding management and care of the catheter and drainage system.

Empyema

An empyema is an accumulation of thick, purulent fluid within the pleural space, often with fibrin development and a loculated (walled-off) area where infection is located (Strange, 2016).

Pathophysiology

Most empyemas occur as complications of bacterial pneumonia or lung abscess. Other causes include penetrating chest trauma, hematogenous infection of the pleural space, nonbacterial infections, or iatrogenic causes (after thoracic surgery or thoracentesis).

At first, the pleural fluid is thin with a low leukocyte count, but it frequently progresses to a fibropurulent stage and, finally, to a stage where it encloses the lung within a thick exudative membrane (loculated empyema).

Clinical Manifestations

The patient is acutely ill and has signs and symptoms similar to those of an acute respiratory infection or pneumonia (fever, night sweats, pleural pain, cough, dyspnea, anorexia, weight loss). If the patient is immunocompromised, the symptoms may be vaguer. If the patient has received antimicrobial therapy, the clinical manifestations may be less obvious.

Assessment and Diagnostic Findings

Chest auscultation demonstrates decreased or absent breath sounds over the affected area, and there is dullness on chest percussion as well as decreased fremitus. The diagnosis is established by a chest x-ray or chest CT scan. Usually, a diagnostic thoracentesis is performed, often under ultrasound guidance.

Medical Management

The objectives of treatment are to drain the pleural cavity and to achieve full expansion of the lung. The fluid is drained and appropriate antibiotics, in large doses, are prescribed based on the causative organism. Sterilization of the empyema cavity requires 4 to 6 weeks of antibiotics (Strange, 2016). Drainage of the pleural fluid depends on the stage of the disease and is accomplished by one of the following methods:

- Needle aspiration (thoracentesis) with a thin percutaneous catheter, if the volume is small and the fluid not too purulent or thick
- Tube thoracostomy (chest drainage using a large-diameter intercostal tube attached to water-seal drainage [see Chapter 26]) with fibrinolytic agents instilled through the chest tube in patients with loculated or complicated pleural effusions
- Open chest drainage via thoracotomy, including potential rib resection, to remove the thickened pleura, pus, and debris and the underlying diseased pulmonary tissue

With long-standing inflammation, an exudate can form over the lung, trapping it and interfering with its normal expansion. This exudate must be removed surgically (decortication). The drainage tube is left in place until the pus-filled space is obliterated completely. The complete obliteration of the pleural space is monitored by serial chest x-rays, and the patient should be informed that treatment may be long term. Patients are frequently discharged from the hospital with a chest tube in place, with instructions to monitor fluid drainage at home.

Nursing Management

Resolution of empyema is a prolonged process. The nurse helps the patient cope with the condition and instructs the patient in lung-expanding breathing exercises to restore normal respiratory function. The nurse also provides care specific to the method of drainage of the pleural fluid (e.g., needle aspiration, closed chest drainage, or rib resection and drainage). When a patient is discharged to home with a drainage tube or system in place, the nurse instructs the patient and family on care of the drainage system and drain site, measurement and observation of drainage, signs and symptoms of infection, and how and when to contact the health care provider. (See The Patient Undergoing Thoracic Surgery in Chapter 26.)

Pulmonary Edema (Noncardiogenic)

Pulmonary edema is defined as abnormal accumulation of fluid in the lung tissue, the alveolar space, or both. It is a severe, life-threatening condition. Pulmonary edema can be classified as cardiogenic or noncardiogenic. (See Chapter 31 for further discussion of cardiogenic pulmonary edema.) Noncardiogenic pulmonary edema occurs due to damage of the pulmonary capillary lining. It may be due to direct injury to the lung (e.g., chest trauma, aspiration, and smoke inhalation), hematogenous injury to the lung (e.g., sepsis, pancreatitis, multiple transfusions, and cardiopulmonary bypass), or injury plus elevated hydrostatic pressures. Management of noncardiogenic pulmonary edema mirrors that of cardiogenic pulmonary edema (see Chapter 31); however, hypoxemia may persist despite high concentrations of supplemental oxygen, due to the intrapulmonary shunting of blood.

Pathophysiology

Pulmonary edema most commonly occurs as a result of increased microvascular pressure from abnormal cardiac function. The backup of blood into the pulmonary vasculature resulting from inadequate left ventricular function causes an increased microvascular pressure, and fluid begins to leak into the interstitial space and the alveoli. Other causes of pulmonary edema are hypervolemia or a sudden increase in the intravascular pressure in the lung. One example of this is in the patient who has undergone pneumonectomy. When one lung has been removed, all cardiac output then goes to the remaining lung. If the patient's fluid status is not monitored closely, pulmonary edema can quickly develop in the postoperative period as the patient's pulmonary vasculature attempts to adapt. This type of pulmonary edema is sometimes termed *flash pulmonary edema*. A second example is called *reexpansion pulmonary edema*. This may be due to a rapid reinflation of the lung after removal of air from a pneumothorax or evacuation of fluid from a large pleural effusion.

Clinical Manifestations

The patient has increasing respiratory distress, characterized by dyspnea, air hunger, and central cyanosis. The patient is usually very anxious and often agitated. As the fluid leaks into the alveoli and mixes with air, a foam or froth is formed. The patient coughs up or the nurse suctions out these foamy, frothy, and often blood-tinged secretions. The patient has acute respiratory distress and may become confused or stuporous.

Assessment and Diagnostic Findings

Auscultation reveals crackles in the lung bases (especially in the posterior bases) that rapidly progress toward the apices of the lungs. These crackles are due to the movement of air through the alveolar fluid. The chest x-ray reveals increased interstitial markings. The patient may be tachycardic, the pulse oximetry values begin to fall, and arterial blood gas analysis demonstrates increasing hypoxemia.

Medical Management

Management focuses on correcting the underlying disorder. If the **pulmonary edema** is cardiac in origin, then improvement in left ventricular function is the goal. Vasodilators, inotropic medications, afterload or preload agents, or contractility medications may be given. Additional cardiac measures (e.g., intra-aortic balloon pump) may be indicated if the patient does not respond. If the problem is fluid overload, diuretics are given, and the patient is placed on fluid restrictions. Oxygen is administered to correct the hypoxemia; in some circumstances, intubation and mechanical ventilation are necessary. The patient is extremely anxious, and morphine is administered to reduce anxiety and control pain.

Nursing Management

Nursing management of the patient with pulmonary edema includes assisting with administration of oxygen and intubation and mechanical ventilation if respiratory failure occurs. The nurse also administers medications (i.e., morphine, vasodilators, inotropic medications, preload and afterload agents) as prescribed and monitors the patient's response. Nursing management in pulmonary edema is described in more detail in Chapter 31.

Acute Respiratory Failure

Respiratory failure is a sudden and life-threatening deterioration of the gas exchange function of the lung. It exists when the exchange of oxygen for carbon dioxide in the lungs cannot keep up with the rate of oxygen consumption and carbon dioxide production by the cells of the body.

ARF is defined as a fall in arterial oxygen tension (PaO_2) to less than 50 mm Hg (hypoxemia) and a rise in arterial carbon dioxide tension ($PaCO_2$) to greater than 50 mm Hg (hypercapnia), with an arterial pH of less than 7.35.

It is important to distinguish between ARF and chronic respiratory failure. Chronic respiratory failure is defined as a deterioration in the gas exchange function of the lung that has developed insidiously or has persisted for a long period after an episode of ARF. The absence of acute symptoms and the presence of a chronic respiratory acidosis suggest the chronicity of the respiratory failure. Two causes of chronic respiratory failure are COPD (discussed in Chapter 25) and neuromuscular diseases (discussed in

Chapter 66). Patients with these disorders develop a tolerance to the gradually worsening hypoxemia and hypercapnia. However, a patient with chronic respiratory failure may develop ARF. This is seen in the COPD patient who develops an exacerbation or infection that causes additional deterioration of the gas exchange mechanism. The principles of management of acute versus chronic respiratory failure are different; the following discussion will be limited to ARF.

Pathophysiology

In ARF, the ventilation or perfusion mechanisms in the lung are impaired. Impaired respiratory system mechanisms leading to ARF include the following:

- Alveolar hypoventilation
- Diffusion abnormalities
- Ventilation–perfusion mismatching
- Shunting

Common causes of ARF can be classified into four categories: decreased respiratory drive, dysfunction of the chest wall, dysfunction of the lung parenchyma, and other causes.

Decreased Respiratory Drive

Decreased respiratory drive may occur with severe brain injury, large lesions of the brain stem (multiple sclerosis), use of sedative medications, and metabolic disorders such as hypothyroidism. These disorders impair the normal response of chemoreceptors in the brain to normal respiratory stimulation.

Dysfunction of the Chest Wall

The impulses arising in the respiratory centre travel through nerves that extend from the brain stem down the spinal cord to receptors in the muscles of respiration. Thus, any disease or disorder of the nerves, spinal cord, muscles, or neuromuscular junction involved in respiration seriously affects ventilation and may ultimately lead to ARF. These include musculoskeletal disorders (muscular dystrophy, polymyositis), neuromuscular junction disorders (myasthenia gravis, poliomyelitis), some peripheral nerve disorders, and spinal cord disorders (amyotrophic lateral sclerosis, Guillain–Barré syndrome, and cervical spinal cord injuries).

Dysfunction of the Lung Parenchyma

Pleural effusion, hemothorax, pneumothorax, and upper airway obstruction are conditions that interfere with ventilation by preventing expansion of the lung. These conditions, which may cause respiratory failure, usually are produced by an underlying lung disease, pleural disease, or trauma and injury. Other diseases and conditions of the lung that lead to ARF include pneumonia, status asthmaticus, lobar atelectasis, PE, and pulmonary edema.

Other Causes

In the postoperative period, especially after major thoracic or abdominal surgery, inadequate ventilation and respiratory failure may occur because of several factors. During this period, for example, ARF may be caused by the effects of anesthetic agents, analgesics, and sedatives, which may depress respiration as described earlier or enhance the effects of opioids and lead to hypoventilation. Pain may interfere with deep breathing and coughing. A mismatch of ventilation to perfusion is the usual cause of respiratory failure after major abdominal, cardiac, or thoracic surgery.

Clinical Manifestations

Early signs are those associated with impaired oxygenation and may include restlessness, fatigue, headache, dyspnea, air hunger, tachycardia, and increased blood pressure. As the hypoxemia progresses, more obvious signs may be present, including confusion, lethargy, tachycardia, tachypnea, central cyanosis, diaphoresis, and finally respiratory arrest. Physical findings are those of acute respiratory distress, including use of accessory muscles, decreased breath sounds if the patient cannot adequately ventilate, and other findings related specifically to the underlying disease process and cause of ARF.

In the early phase of acute respiratory failure, vague signs and symptoms such as restlessness, anxiety, fatigue, and headache make it difficult to determine what the patient is experiencing. However, as oxygenation becomes more impaired, hypoxemia increases and leads to more obvious signs such as tachycardia, tachypnea, circumoral cyanosis, diaphoresis, accessory muscle use, inability to speak in full sentences, and altered mental status. Pain usually is not present. Some patients may progress through these phases over several hours, whereas others may progress within seconds.

Medical Management

The objectives of treatment are to correct the underlying cause and to restore adequate gas exchange in the lung. Intubation and mechanical ventilation may be required to maintain adequate ventilation and oxygenation while the underlying cause is corrected.

Nursing Management

Nursing management of the patient with ARF includes assisting with intubation and maintaining mechanical ventilation (described in Chapter 26). Patients are usually managed in the intensive care unit. The nurse assesses the patient's respiratory status by monitoring the patient's level of response, arterial blood gases, pulse oximetry, and vital signs and assessing the respiratory system. In addition, the nurse assesses the entire respiratory system and implements strategies (e.g., turning schedule, mouth care, skin care, range of motion of extremities) to prevent complications. The nurse also assesses the patient's understanding of the management strategies that are used and initiates some form of communication to enable the patient to express his or her needs to the health care team. Nursing care also addresses the problems that led to ARF. As the patient's status improves, the nurse assesses the patient's knowledge of the underlying disorder and provides teaching as appropriate to address the underlying disorder.

Acute Respiratory Distress Syndrome

Acute respiratory distress syndrome (ARDS) can be thought of as a spectrum of disease, from its milder form (**acute lung injury** [ALI]) to its most severe form of fulminate,

CHART 24-9

Risk Factors: Acute Respiratory Distress Syndrome

- Aspiration (gastric secretions, drowning, hydrocarbons)
- Drug ingestion and overdose
- Hematologic disorders (disseminated intravascular coagulopathy [DIC], massive transfusions, cardiopulmonary bypass)
- Prolonged inhalation of high concentrations of oxygen, smoke, or corrosive substances
- Localized infection (bacterial, fungal, viral pneumonia)
- Metabolic disorders (pancreatitis, uremia)
- Shock (any cause)
- Trauma (pulmonary contusion, multiple fractures, head injury)
- Major surgery
- Fat or air embolism
- Sepsis

life-threatening ARDS. This clinical syndrome is characterized by a severe inflammatory process causing diffuse alveolar damage that results in sudden and progressive pulmonary edema, increasing bilateral infiltrates on chest x-ray, hypoxemia unresponsive to oxygen supplementation regardless of the amount of PEEP, and the absence of an elevated left atrial pressure (Siegel, 2015a). Patients often demonstrate reduced lung compliance. A wide range of factors are associated with the development of ARDS (see Chart 24-9), including direct injury to the lungs (e.g., smoke inhalation) or indirect insult to the lungs (e.g., shock). ARDS has been associated with a mortality rate ranging from 26% to 58% (Siegel, 2015b). The major cause of death in ARDS is nonpulmonary MODS, often with sepsis.

Pathophysiology

ARDS occurs as a result of an inflammatory trigger that initiates the release of cellular and chemical mediators, causing injury to the alveolar capillary membrane. This results in leakage of fluid into the alveolar interstitial spaces and alterations in the capillary bed.

Severe ventilation–perfusion mismatching occurs in ARDS. Alveoli collapse because of the inflammatory infiltrate, blood, fluid, and surfactant dysfunction. Small airways are narrowed because of interstitial fluid and bronchial obstruction. The lung compliance becomes markedly decreased (stiff lungs), and the result is a characteristic decrease in functional residual capacity and severe hypoxemia. The blood returning to the lung for gas exchange is pumped through the nonventilated, nonfunctioning areas of the lung, causing a shunt to develop. This means that blood is interfacing with nonfunctioning alveoli and gas exchange is markedly impaired, resulting in severe, refractory hypoxemia. Figure 24-5 shows the sequence of pathophysiologic events leading to ARDS.

Clinical Manifestations

Clinically, the acute phase of ARDS is marked by a rapid onset of severe dyspnea that usually occurs 12 to 48 hours

Physiology/Pathophysiology

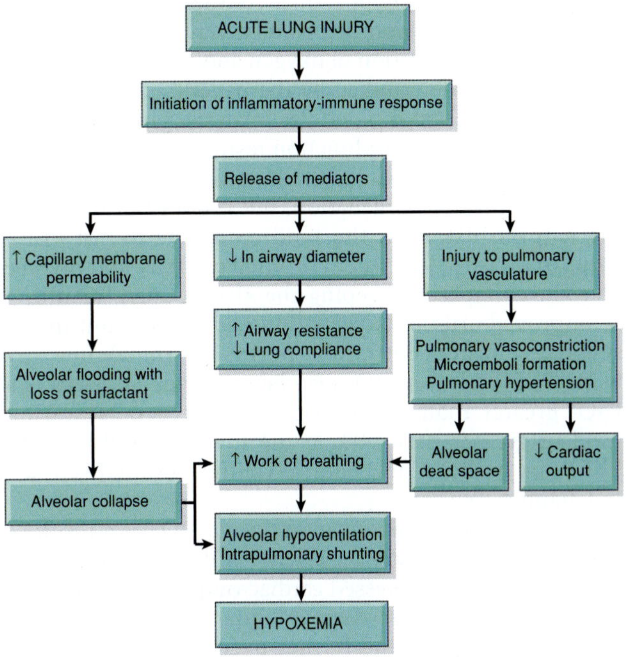

FIGURE 24-5. Pathogenesis and pathophysiology of acute respiratory distress syndrome.

after the initiating event. A characteristic feature is arterial hypoxemia that does not respond to supplemental oxygen. On chest x-ray, bilateral opacities are present. The acute lung injury then progresses to fibrosing alveolitis with persistent, severe hypoxemia. The patient also has increased alveolar dead space (ventilation to alveoli but poor perfusion) and decreased pulmonary compliance ("stiff lungs," which are difficult to ventilate). Clinically, a patient is thought to be in the recovery phase if the hypoxemia gradually resolves, the chest x-ray improves, and the lungs become more compliant.

Assessment and Diagnostic Findings

Intercostal retractions and crackles, as the fluid begins to leak into the alveolar interstitial space, are evident on physical examination. A diagnosis of ARDS is made when the following criteria are met: (1) onset within 1 week of a known clinical insult or new/worsening respiratory symptoms; (2) presence of bilateral opacities on chest x-ray; (3) diagnosis of respiratory failure not fully explained by cardiac failure or fluid overload; (4) presence of hypoxemia and a ratio of partial pressure of oxygen of arterial blood to fraction of inspired oxygen (PaO_2/FiO_2) ≤200 mm Hg (The ARDS Definition Task Force, 2012).

Medical Management

The primary focus in the management of ARDS includes identification and treatment of the underlying condition. Aggressive, supportive care must be provided to compensate for the severe respiratory dysfunction. This supportive therapy almost always includes intubation and mechanical ventilation. In addition, circulatory support, adequate fluid volume, and nutritional support are important. Supplemental oxygen is used as the patient begins the initial spiral of hypoxemia. As the hypoxemia progresses, intubation and mechanical ventilation are instituted. The concentration of oxygen and ventilator settings and modes are determined by the patient's status. This is monitored by arterial blood gas analysis, pulse oximetry, and bedside pulmonary function testing.

PEEP is a critical part of the treatment of ARDS. PEEP usually improves oxygenation, but it does not influence the natural history of the syndrome. The use of PEEP helps to increase functional residual capacity and reverse alveolar collapse by keeping the alveoli open, resulting in improved arterial oxygenation and a reduction in the severity of the ventilation–perfusion imbalance. By using PEEP, a lower FiO_2 may be required. The goal is a PaO_2 greater than 60 mm Hg or an oxygen saturation level of greater than 90% at the lowest possible FiO_2. PEEP and modes of mechanical ventilation are discussed in Chapter 26.

Systemic hypotension may occur in ARDS as a result of hypovolemia secondary to leakage of fluid into the interstitial spaces and depressed cardiac output from high levels of PEEP therapy. Hypovolemia must be carefully treated without causing further overload. IV crystalloid solutions are administered, with careful monitoring of pulmonary status. Inotropic or vasopressor agents may be required. Additional supportive treatments may include prone positioning, sedation, paralysis, and nutritional support (Siegel, 2015b).

Pharmacologic Therapy

There is no specific pharmacologic treatment of ARDS except supportive care. Neuromuscular blocking agents, sedatives, and analgesics may be used to improve patient–ventilator synchronization and help to decrease severe hypoxemia (see later discussion in Ventilator Considerations section). Inhaled nitric oxide (an endogenous vasodilator) may help to reduce $\dot{V}/\dot{Q}$ mismatch and improve oxygenation. Multiple therapies are undergoing clinical evaluation but are not yet approved or supported for widespread clinical use (Siegel, 2015a, 2015b).

Nutritional Therapy

Adequate nutritional support is vital in the treatment of ARDS. Patients with ARDS require 35 to 45 kcal/kg/d to meet caloric requirements. Enteral feeding is the first consideration; however, parenteral nutrition also may be required.

Nursing Management

General Measures

The patient with ARDS is critically ill and requires close monitoring because the condition could quickly change to a life-threatening situation. Most of the respiratory modalities discussed in Chapter 26 are used in this situation (oxygen administration, nebulizer therapy, chest physiotherapy, endotracheal intubation or tracheostomy, mechanical ventilation, suctioning, bronchoscopy). Frequent assessment of the patient's status is necessary to evaluate the effectiveness of treatment.

In addition to implementing the medical plan of care, the nurse considers other needs of the patient. Positioning is important. The nurse should turn the patient frequently to improve ventilation and perfusion in the lungs and enhance secretion drainage. However, the nurse must closely monitor the patient for deterioration in oxygenation with changes in position. Oxygenation in patients with ARDS is sometimes improved in the prone position. This position may be evaluated for improvement in oxygenation and used in special circumstances. Devices and specialty beds are available to assist the nurse in placing the patient in a prone position ("proning") (Hariprashad & Rizzolo, 2013).

The patient is extremely anxious and agitated because of the increasing hypoxemia and dyspnea. The nurse should explain all procedures and provide care in a calm, reassuring manner. It is important to reduce the patient's anxiety because anxiety prevents rest and increases oxygen expenditure. Rest is essential to reduce oxygen consumption, thereby reducing oxygen needs.

Ventilator Considerations

If the patient is intubated and receiving mechanical ventilation with PEEP, several considerations must be addressed. PEEP, which causes increased end-expiratory pressure, is an unnatural pattern of breathing and feels strange to the patient. The patient may be anxious and "fight" the ventilator. Nursing assessment is important to assess for problems with ventilation that may be causing the anxiety reaction: tube blockage by kinking or retained secretions, other acute respiratory problems (e.g., pneumothorax, pain), a sudden drop in the oxygen level, the patient's level of dyspnea, or ventilator malfunction. In some cases, sedation may be required to decrease the patient's oxygen consumption, allow the ventilator to provide full support of ventilation, and decrease the patient's anxiety. Possible sedatives are lorazepam (Ativan), midazolam (Versed), haloperidol (Haldol), propofol (Diprivan), and short-acting barbiturates.

If the PEEP level cannot be maintained despite the use of sedatives, neuromuscular blocking agents, such as pancuronium (Pavulon), vecuronium (Norcuron), atracurium (Tracrium), and rocuronium (Zemuron), may be given to chemically paralyze the patient. This allows the patient to be ventilated more easily. With paralysis, the patient appears unconscious, loses motor function, and cannot breathe, talk, or blink independently. However, the patient retains sensation and is awake and able to hear. The nurse must reassure the patient that the paralysis is a result of the medication and is temporary. Paralysis should be used for the shortest possible time and never without adequate sedation and pain management.

Peripheral nerve stimulators are used to assess nerve impulse transmissions at the neuromuscular junction of select skeletal muscles when neuromuscular blocking agents are used. A "train-of-four" test may be used to measure the level of neuromuscular blockade. With this test, four consecutive stimuli are delivered along the path of a nerve, and the response of the muscle is measured in order to evaluate whether or not stimuli are effectively blocked. Four equal muscle contractions, seen as "twitches," will result if there is no neuromuscular blockade. However, if neuromuscular blockade is present, there will be a loss of

NURSING RESEARCH PROFILE

Chart 24-10. Nurses' Knowledge About Neuromuscular Blocking Agents

Frazee, E. N., Personett, H. A., Bauer, S. R., et al. (2015). Intensive care nurses' knowledge about use of neuromuscular blocking agents in patients with respiratory failure. *American Journal of Critical Care*, *24*(5), 431–439.

Purpose

The purpose of this study was to describe critical care nurses' knowledge of neuromuscular blocking agents (NMBAs). Areas evaluated were the therapeutic properties, adverse effects, and monitoring parameters for patients on NMBAs.

Design

Five academic medical centres were utilized for data collection; medical intensive care nurses' knowledge was evaluated using a web-based survey between May 2012 and May 2013. To be eligible for the study, a nurse must have had more than 25% of his/her clinical practice in an intensive care unit (ICU) with a patient population of more than 50% medical patients. A 16-question survey was designed for this study. The survey had two sections: general knowledge about NMBAs and perceptions of the role of NMBAs in patients with acute respiratory distress syndrome (ARDS).

Findings

Responses were received from 160 nurses, which was 22% of the eligible participants identified by unit leaders at the five academic medical centres. Most of the participants (92%) were able to correctly identify the NMBAs vecuronium and cisatracurium as nonanalgesics. Most of the participants (82%) correctly identified the NMBAs pancuronium and atracurium as nonanxiolytics. Of 6 different NMBAs, nurses identified the elimination properties of these drugs correctly ranging from 28% to 64% of the time. The nurses had variable responses to NMBAs' specific adverse events. Over 75% of nurses identified the relationship between foot drop and NMBAs; however, only 34% identified the independent association of NMBAs and consciousness. The perceived durations of action of NMBAs varied widely.

Nursing Implications

NMBAs are used in patients with ARDS and improve oxygenation, inflammation, and mortality. The ICU nurse is responsible for the safe and effective use of these agents in patients who are critically ill. It is crucial that ICU nurses understand the properties and adverse effects of these drugs. This study demonstrates that focused education and demonstrated competence is necessary for ICU nurses to safely care for this patient population.

twitch height and number, which will indicate the degree of blockade. If all four stimulations result in an absence of twitches, it is estimated that 100% of the receptors are blocked.

The use of neuromuscular blocking agents has many dangers and side effects. The nurse must be sure the patient does not become disconnected from the ventilator, because respiratory muscles are paralyzed and the patient will be apneic. Consequently, the nurse ensures that the patient is closely monitored; all ventilator and patient alarms must be on at all times. Eye care is important as well, because the patient cannot blink, increasing the risk of corneal abrasions. Neuromuscular blockers predispose the patient to venous thromboembolism (VTE), muscle atrophy, foot drop, peptic ulcer disease, and skin breakdown (see Chart 24-10).

NURSING ALERT

Nursing assessment is essential to minimize the complications related to neuromuscular blockade. The patient may have discomfort or pain but cannot communicate these sensations. In addition, frequent oral care and suctioning may be needed.

Analgesia must be given concurrently with neuromuscular blocking agents. The nurse must anticipate the patient's needs regarding pain and comfort. The nurse checks the patient's position to ensure it is comfortable without excessive pressure points and in normal alignment. Talking to and not about the patient while in the patient's presence is important.

In addition, the nurse must describe the purpose and effects of the neuromuscular blocking agents to the patient's family. If family members are unaware that these agents have been given, they may become distressed by the change in the patient's status.

Pulmonary Hypertension

Pulmonary hypertension (PH) is characterized by elevated pulmonary arterial pressure and secondary right heart ventricular failure (Rubin & Hopkins, 2016). It may be suspected in a patient with dyspnea with exertion without other clinical manifestations. Unlike systemic blood pressure, the pulmonary pressures cannot be measured indirectly. In the absence of these measurements, clinical recognition becomes the only indicator of PH. However, PH is a condition that is often not clinically evident until late in its progression. Patients are classified by the World Health Organization (WHO) into five groups based upon the mechanism of PH (Rubin & Hopkins, 2016) (see Chart 24-11).

There are two forms of PH: primary (or idiopathic) pulmonary arterial hypertension and pulmonary arterial hypertension due to a known cause (Kiely et al., 2013). Idiopathic hypertension is an uncommon disease; the incidence is 1 to 3 cases per million persons per year (Kiely et al., 2013). It occurs most often in women 20 to

CHART 24-11

Clinical Classification of Pulmonary Hypertension (PH)

Group 1: Pulmonary Arterial Hypertension (PAH)

- Sporadic idiopathic PAH
- Heritable idiopathic PAH
- Drug- and toxin-induced PAH
- PAH due to diseases such as connective tissues disorders, HIV infection, portal hypertension, congenital heart disease

Group 2: PH due to Left Heart Disease

- Systolic dysfunction
- Diastolic dysfunction
- Valvular heart disease

Group 3: PH due to Chronic Lung Diseases and/or Hypoxemia

- Chronic obstructive pulmonary disease
- Interstitial lung disease
- Mixed restrictive and obstructive lung disease
- Sleep-disordered breathing

Group 4: Chronic Thromboembolic Pulmonary Hypertension (CTEPH)

- Due to thromboembolic occlusion of the proximal or distal pulmonary vasculature

Group 5: PH With Unclear Multifactorial Mechanisms

- Hematologic disorders
- Systemic disorders (e.g., sarcoidosis)
- Metabolic disorders

Adapted from Rubin, L., & Hopkins, W. (2016). Overview of pulmonary hypertension in adults. UpToDate. Last updated February 5, 2016. Retrieved April 23, 2016, from www.uptodate.com/contents/overview-of-pulmonary-hypertension-in-adults?source=search_result&search=Overview+of+pulmonary+hypertension+in+adults&selectedTitle=1~15

40 years of age, either sporadically or in patients with a family history, and is usually fatal within 5 years of diagnosis. There are several possible causes, but the exact cause is unknown (Chart 24-12). The clinical presentation may occur with no evidence of pulmonary or cardiac disease or PE.

In contrast, pulmonary arterial hypertension due to a known cause is more common and results from existing cardiac or pulmonary disease. The prognosis depends on the severity of the underlying disorder and the changes in the pulmonary vascular bed. A common cause of secondary PH is pulmonary artery constriction due to hypoxemia from COPD (**cor pulmonale**).

Pathophysiology

Conditions such as collagen vascular disease, congenital heart disease, portal hypertension, and HIV infection increase the risk for pulmonary arterial hypertension in susceptible patients. Vascular injury occurs with endothelial dysfunction and vascular smooth muscle dysfunction, which leads to disease progression (vascular smooth muscle hypertrophy, adventitial and intimal proliferation [thickening of the wall], and advanced vascular lesion formation). Normally, the pulmonary vascular bed can handle the blood volume delivered by the right ventricle. It has a low resistance to blood flow and compensates for increased blood volume by dilation of the vessels in the pulmonary circulation. However, if the pulmonary vascular bed is destroyed or obstructed, as in PH, the ability to handle whatever flow or volume of blood it receives is impaired, and the increased blood flow then increases the pulmonary artery pressure. As the pulmonary arterial pressure increases, the pulmonary vascular resistance also increases. Both pulmonary artery constriction (as in hypoxemia or hypercapnia) and a reduction of the pulmonary vascular bed (which occurs with pulmonary emboli) result in an increase in pulmonary vascular resistance and pressure. This increased workload affects right ventricular function. The myocardium ultimately cannot meet the increasing demands imposed on it, leading to right ventricular hypertrophy (enlargement and dilation) and failure.

CHART 24-12

Causes of Pulmonary Arterial Hypertension

Idiopathic (Primary) Arterial Hypertension and Pulmonary Arterial Hypertension due to a Known Cause

- Collagen vascular diseases
- Congenital systemic-to-pulmonary shunts
- Portal hypertension
- Altered immune mechanisms (HIV infection)
- Diseases associated with significant venous or capillary involvement
- Chronic thrombotic or embolic disease
- Pulmonary venous hypertension
- Pulmonary vasoconstriction due to hypoxemia
- Chronic obstructive pulmonary disease (COPD), interstitial lung disease, sleep-disordered breathing
- Miscellaneous causes: sarcoidosis, histiocytosis, compression of pulmonary vessels

Clinical Manifestations

Dyspnea is the main symptom of PH, occurring at first with exertion and eventually at rest. Other signs and symptoms include substernal chest pain, weakness, fatigue, syncope, occasional hemoptysis, and signs of right-sided heart failure (peripheral edema, ascites, distended neck veins, liver engorgement, crackles, heart murmur).

Assessment and Diagnostic Findings

Diagnostic testing is used to confirm that PH exists, determine its severity, and identify its causes. Initial diagnostic evaluation includes a history, physical examination, chest x-ray, pulmonary function studies, electrocardiogram (ECG), and echocardiogram. Echocardiography can be used to estimate the pulmonary artery systolic pressure and to assess right ventricular size, thickness, and function. It can also evaluate the right atrial size, left ventricular system, and diastolic function as well as valve function. Right heart catheterization is necessary to confirm the diagnosis of PH and to accurately assess the hemodynamic abnormalities. PH is confirmed with a mean pulmonary artery pressure greater than 25 mm Hg. If left heart disease is identified via echocardiography and correlates with the degree of estimated PH, then exercise testing and both a right and a left heart catheterization may be done to determine the functional severity of the disease and the abnormalities in pressures (left heart filling, pulmonary vascular resistance, transpulmonary gradient) (Rubin & Hopkins, 2016).

Pulmonary function studies may be normal or show a slight decrease in vital capacity (VC) and lung compliance, with a mild decrease in the diffusing capacity. The PaO_2 also is decreased (hypoxemia). An echocardiogram can assess the progression of the disease and rule out other conditions with similar signs and symptoms. A ventilation–perfusion scan or pulmonary angiography detects defects in pulmonary vasculature, such as pulmonary emboli.

Medical Management

The goal of treatment is to manage the underlying cardiac or pulmonary condition. Recommendations regarding therapy are tailored to the patient's individual situation, functional New York Heart Association class, and specific needs (Rubin & Hopkins, 2016). All patients with PH should be considered for the following therapies: diuretics, oxygen, anticoagulation, digoxin, and exercise training. Diuretics and oxygen should be added as needed. Appropriate oxygen therapy reverses the vasoconstriction and reduces the PH in a relatively short time. Most patients with primary PH do not have hypoxemia at rest but require supplemental oxygen with exercise. However, patients with severe right ventricular failure, decreased cardiac output, and progressive disease may have resting hypoxemia and require continuous oxygen supplementation. Anticoagulation should be considered for patients at risk for intrapulmonary thrombosis. Digoxin may improve right ventricular ejection fraction in some patients and may help to control heart rate; however, patients must be monitored closely for potential complications (Rubin & Hopkins, 2016).

Pharmacologic Therapy

Different classes of medications are used to treat PH; these include calcium-channel blockers, prostanoids, endothelin antagonists, and phosphodiesterase-5 inhibitors. The choice of therapeutic agents is based on many facets, including the classification group status of the patient with PH (see Chart 24-11), as well as the cost and the patient's tolerance of the agents (Hopkins & Rubin, 2016). In addition, a vasoreactivity test may be done to identify which medication is best suited for the patient with PH; this is done during cardiac catheterization using vasodilating medications such as nitric oxide. A positive vasoreactivity test occurs when there is a decrease of at least 10 mm Hg in the pulmonary artery pressure with an overall pressure that is less than 40 mm Hg in the presence of both an increased or unchanged cardiac output and a minimally decreased or unchanged systemic blood pressure (Hopkins & Rubin, 2016).

Patients with a positive vasoreactivity test may be prescribed calcium-channel blockers. Calcium-channel blockers have a significant advantage over other medications taken to treat PH in that they may be taken orally and are generally less costly; however, because calcium-channel blockers are indicated in only a small percentage of patients, other treatment options, including prostanoids, are often necessary (Hopkins & Rubin, 2016).

Bosentan, an endothelin receptor antagonist, causes vasodilation and is prescribed for its antihypertensive effects in patients with PH (Hopkins & Rubin, 2016). Other medications, including diuretics, digoxin, anticoagulant therapy, and calcium-channel blockers (nifedipine [Procardia], diltiazem [Cardizem]) may be prescribed. Because calcium-channel blockers are effective in only a small percentage of patients, other treatment options, including prostacyclin, are often necessary (Hopkins & Rubin, 2016).

Prostaglandin (prostacyclin) relaxes vascular smooth muscle by stimulating the production of cyclic adenosine monophosphate (AMP) and inhibiting the growth of smooth muscle cells. Additionally, it inhibits platelet aggregation. Because of its short half-life in the circulation (i.e., 3 minutes), IV prostacyclin (epoprostenol [Flolan]) can be administered only by continuous IV infusion (Hopkins & Rubin, 2016). It helps to decrease PH by reducing pulmonary vascular resistance and pressures and increasing cardiac output. For long-term administration, epoprostenol can be infused with the use of a portable infusion pump connected to a permanent catheter inserted in the subclavian vein. The use of epoprostenol has led to improvement in some patients without lung transplantation, which had previously been the only treatment.

Surgical Management

Lung transplantation remains an option for a select group of patients with PH who are refractory to medical therapy. Bilateral lung or heart–lung transplantation is the procedure of choice. Atrial septostomy may be considered for selected patients with severe disease (Hopkins & Rubin, 2016); this procedure results in shunting of blood from the right side of the heart to the left, decreasing the strain on the right side of the heart and maintaining left ventricular output.

Nursing Management

The major nursing goal is to identify patients at high risk for PH, such as those with COPD, pulmonary emboli, congenital heart disease, and mitral valve disease. The nurse also must be alert for signs and symptoms, administer oxygen therapy appropriately, and instruct patients and their families about the use of home oxygen supplementation. In patients treated with prostacyclin (i.e., epoprostenol or treprostinil), education about the need for central venous access (epoprostenol), subcutaneous infusion (treprostinil), proper administration and dosing of the medication, pain at the injection site, and potential severe side effects is extremely important. Emotional and psychosocial aspects of this disease must be addressed. Formal and informal support groups for patients and families are extremely valuable.

Pulmonary Heart Disease (Cor Pulmonale)

Cor pulmonale is a condition that results from PH, which causes the right side of the heart to enlarge because of the increased work required to pump blood against high resistance through the pulmonary vascular system. This causes right-sided heart failure (Kings, 2014). (See Chapter 31 for further discussion of management of right-sided heart failure.)

In cor pulmonale, the right ventricle of the heart enlarges (with or without right-sided heart failure) as a result of diseases that affect the structure or function of the lung or its vasculature. It is a type of pulmonary arterial hypertension due to a known cause. Any disease affecting the lungs and accompanied by hypoxemia may result in cor pulmonale. The most frequent cause is severe COPD (see Chapter 25), in which changes in the airway and retained secretions reduce alveolar ventilation. Other causes are conditions that restrict or compromise ventilatory function, leading to hypoxemia or acidosis (deformities of the thoracic cage, massive obesity), or conditions that reduce the pulmonary vascular bed (primary idiopathic pulmonary arterial hypertension, pulmonary embolus). Certain disorders of the nervous system, respiratory muscles, chest wall, and pulmonary arterial tree also may be responsible for cor pulmonale.

Pathophysiology

Pulmonary disease can produce physiologic changes that in time affect the heart and cause the right ventricle to enlarge and eventually fail. Any condition that deprives the lungs of oxygen can cause hypoxemia and hypercapnia, resulting in ventilatory insufficiency. Hypoxemia and hypercapnia cause pulmonary arterial vasoconstriction and possibly reduction of the pulmonary vascular bed, as in emphysema or pulmonary emboli. The result is increased resistance in the pulmonary circulatory system, with a subsequent rise in pulmonary blood pressure (PH). A mean pulmonary arterial pressure of 45 mm Hg or more may occur in cor pulmonale. Right ventricular hypertrophy may result, followed by right ventricular failure. In short, cor pulmonale results from PH, which causes the right side of the heart to enlarge because of the increased work required to pump blood against high resistance through the pulmonary vascular system.

Clinical Manifestations

Symptoms of cor pulmonale are usually related to the underlying lung disease, such as COPD. With right ventricular failure, the patient may develop increasing edema of the feet and legs, distended neck veins, an enlarged palpable liver, pleural effusion, ascites, and a heart murmur. Headache, confusion, and somnolence may occur as a result of increased levels of carbon dioxide (hypercapnia). Patients often complain of increasing shortness of breath, wheezing, cough, and fatigue.

Medical Management

The objectives of treatment are to improve the patient's ventilation and to treat both the underlying lung disease and the manifestations of heart disease. Supplemental oxygen is administered to improve gas exchange and to reduce pulmonary arterial pressure and pulmonary vascular resistance. Improved oxygen transport relieves the PH that is causing the cor pulmonale.

Better survival rates and greater reduction in pulmonary vascular resistance have been reported with continuous, 24-hour oxygen therapy for patients with severe hypoxemia. Substantial improvement may require 4 to 6 weeks of oxygen therapy, usually in the home. Periodic assessment of pulse oximetry and arterial blood gases is necessary to determine the adequacy of alveolar ventilation and to monitor the effectiveness of oxygen therapy.

Ventilation is further improved with chest physical therapy and bronchial hygiene manoeuvres, as indicated to remove accumulated secretions, and the administration of bronchodilators. Further measures depend on the patient's condition. If the patient is in respiratory failure, endotracheal intubation and mechanical ventilation may be necessary. If the patient is in heart failure, hypoxemia and hypercapnia must be relieved to improve cardiac function and output. Bed rest, sodium restriction, and diuretic therapy also are instituted judiciously to reduce peripheral edema (to lower pulmonary arterial pressure through a decrease in total blood volume) and the circulatory load on the right side of the heart. Digitalis may be prescribed to relieve PH if the patient also has left ventricular failure, a supraventricular dysrhythmia, or right ventricular failure that does not respond to other therapy.

ECG monitoring may be indicated because of the high incidence of dysrhythmias in patients with cor pulmonale. Any pulmonary infection must be treated promptly to avoid further impaired gas exchange and exacerbations of hypoxemia and pulmonary heart disease. The prognosis depends on whether the PH is reversible. (Management of ARF was presented earlier in this chapter.)

Nursing Management

Nursing care of the patient with cor pulmonale addresses the underlying disorder leading to cor pulmonale as well as the problems related to pulmonary hyperventilation and right-sided cardiac failure. If intubation and mechanical ventilation are required to manage ARF, the nurse assists with the intubation procedure and maintains mechanical ventilation. The nurse assesses the patient's respiratory and cardiac status and administers medications as prescribed.

During the patient's hospital stay, the nurse instructs the patient about the importance of close monitoring (fluid retention, weight gain, edema) and adherence to the therapeutic regimen, especially the 24-hour use of oxygen. Factors that affect the patient's adherence to the treatment regimen are explored and addressed.

Promoting Home, Community-Based, and Transitional Care

Educating Patients About Self-Care

Most of the care and monitoring of the patient with cor pulmonale is performed by the patient and family in the home because it is a chronic disorder. If supplemental oxygen is administered, the nurse instructs the patient and the family in its use. Nutrition counselling is warranted if the patient is on a sodium-restricted diet or is taking diuretics. The nurse teaches the family to monitor for signs and symptoms of right ventricular failure and about emergency interventions and when to call for assistance. Most importantly, the nurse urges the patient to stop smoking.

CONTINUING AND TRANSITIONAL CARE. A referral for home care may be warranted for the patient who cannot manage self-care or for the patient whose physical condition warrants close assessment. During the home visit, the home care nurse evaluates the patient's status and the patient and family members' understanding of the therapeutic regimen and their adherence to it. If oxygen is used in the home, the nurse determines if it is being administered safely and as prescribed. It is important to assess the patient's progress in stopping smoking and to reinforce the importance of smoking cessation with the patient and family. The nurse identifies strategies to assist with smoking cessation and refers the patient and family to community support groups. In addition, the patient is reminded about the importance of other health promotion and screening practices.

CHART 24-13

Risk Factors: Pulmonary Embolism

Venous Stasis (Slowing of Blood Flow in Veins)

Prolonged immobilization (especially postoperative)
Prolonged periods of sitting/travelling
Varicose veins
Spinal cord injury

Hypercoagulability (Due to Release of Tissue Thromboplastin After Injury/Surgery)

Injury
Tumour (pancreatic, gastrointestinal, genitourinary, breast, lung)
Increased platelet count (polycythemia, splenectomy)

Venous Endothelial Disease

Thrombophlebitis
Vascular disease
Foreign bodies (intravenous/central venous catheters)

Certain Disease States (Combination of Stasis, Coagulation Alterations, and Venous Injury)

Heart disease (especially heart failure)
Trauma (especially fracture of hip, pelvis, vertebra, lower extremities)
Postoperative state/postpartum period
Diabetes mellitus
Chronic obstructive pulmonary disease

Other Predisposing Conditions

Advanced age
Obesity
Pregnancy
Oral contraceptive use
History of previous thrombophlebitis, pulmonary embolism
Constrictive clothing

Pulmonary Embolism

Pulmonary embolism refers to the obstruction of the pulmonary artery or one of its branches by a thrombus (or thrombi) that originates somewhere in the venous system or in the right side of the heart. It is associated with significant morbidity and mortality in hospitalized and recently discharged patients (Hull, Merali, Mills, et al., 2013). VTE affects approximately 1–2 in 1,000 Canadian adults per year with about one third of first thromboembolism events being due to a PE (Thrombosis Canada, 2013).

PE is often is associated with trauma, surgery (orthopedic, major abdominal, pelvic, gynecologic), pregnancy, heart failure, age older than 50 years, hypercoagulable states, and prolonged immobility. It also may occur in an apparently healthy person. Risk factors for developing PE are identified in Chart 24-13.

Pathophysiology

Most commonly, PE is due to a blood clot or thrombus. However, there are other types of emboli: air, fat, amniotic fluid, and septic (from bacterial invasion of the thrombus). Although most thrombi originate in the deep veins of the legs, other sites include the pelvic veins and the right atrium of the heart. Venous thrombosis can result from slowing of blood flow (stasis) secondary to damage to the blood vessel wall (particularly the endothelial lining) or changes in the blood coagulation mechanism. Atrial fibrillation also causes PE. An enlarged right atrium in fibrillation causes blood to stagnate and form clots in this area. These clots are prone to travel into the pulmonary circulation.

When a thrombus completely or partially obstructs a pulmonary artery or its branches, the alveolar dead space is increased. The area, although continuing to be ventilated, receives little or no blood flow. Thus, gas exchange is impaired or absent in this area. In addition, various substances are released from the clot and surrounding area, causing regional blood vessels and bronchioles to constrict. This causes an increase in pulmonary vascular resistance. This reaction compounds the ventilation–perfusion imbalance.

The hemodynamic consequences are increased pulmonary vascular resistance from the regional vasoconstriction and reduced size of the pulmonary vascular bed. This results in an increase in pulmonary arterial pressure and, in turn, an increase in right ventricular work to maintain pulmonary blood flow. When the work requirements of the right ventricle exceed its capacity, right ventricular failure occurs, leading to a decrease in cardiac output followed by a decrease in systemic blood pressure and the development of shock.

Clinical Manifestations

The symptoms of PE depend on the size of the thrombus and the area of the pulmonary artery occluded by the thrombus; they may be nonspecific. Signs and symptoms include sudden onset dyspnea, syncope, pleurisy, tachypnea, tachycardia, hypoxemia, and hypotension (Thrombosis Canada, 2013). Chest pain is also common and is usually sudden and pleuritic. It may be substernal and mimic angina pectoris or a myocardial infarction. Other symptoms include anxiety, fever, apprehension, cough, diaphoresis, and hemoptysis. As many as 10% of symptomatic PEs are fatal within the first hour of signs and symptoms (Thrombosis Canada, 2013). It is therefore imperative that nurses recognize the signs and symptoms quickly.

Deep venous thrombosis is closely associated with development of PE. Typically, patients report sudden onset of pain and/or swelling and warmth of the proximal or distal extremity, skin discolouration, and superficial vein distention. The pain is usually relieved with elevation.

A massive embolism is best defined by the degree of hemodynamic instability rather than the percentage of pulmonary vasculature occlusion. It is described as an occlusion of the outflow tract of the main pulmonary artery or the bifurcation of the pulmonary arteries that produces pronounced dyspnea, sudden substernal pain, rapid and weak pulse, shock, syncope, and sudden death. Multiple small emboli can lodge in the terminal pulmonary arterioles, producing multiple small infarctions of the lungs. The clinical picture may mimic that of bronchopneumonia or heart failure. In atypical instances, the disease causes few signs and symptoms, whereas in other instances, it mimics various other cardiopulmonary disorders.

Assessment and Diagnostic Findings

Since death from a PE can occur within the first hour of onset of symptoms, early recognition and diagnosis are priorities. Because the symptoms of PE can vary from few to severe, a diagnostic workup is performed to rule out other diseases. The initial diagnostic workup includes chest x-ray, ECG, peripheral vascular studies, arterial blood gas analysis, and ventilation–perfusion scan.

The chest x-ray is usually normal but may show infiltrates, atelectasis, elevation of the diaphragm on the affected side, or a pleural effusion. The chest x-ray is most helpful in excluding other possible causes. The ECG usually shows sinus tachycardia, PR-interval depression, and nonspecific T-wave changes. Peripheral vascular studies may include impedance plethysmography, Doppler ultrasonography, or venography (see Chapter 32). Test results confirm or exclude the diagnosis of PE. Arterial blood gas analysis may show hypoxemia and hypocapnia (from tachypnea); however, arterial blood gas measurements are normal in up to 20% of patients with PE.

The ventilation–perfusion scan was once the second choice for diagnosis of a PE (with pulmonary angiogram [discussed below] considered the best diagnostic procedure). It is still used, especially in facilities that do not have access to a spiral CT scanner. The ventilation–perfusion scan is minimally invasive, involving the IV administration of a contrast agent. This scan evaluates different regions of the lung (upper, middle, lower) and allows comparisons of the percentage of ventilation and perfusion in each area. This test has a high sensitivity but can be more cumbersome than CT scan and is not as accurate as a pulmonary angiogram.

A high suspicion of PE may warrant a spiral CT scan of the lung, D-dimer assay (blood test for evidence of blood clots), and pulmonary arteriogram. Spiral CT of the chest may also assist in the diagnosis. Spiral CT scan has recently gained popularity for use in the diagnosis of PE; it is more advanced and quicker than routine tomography. The term *spiral* comes from the shape of the path taken by the x-ray beam during scanning. The examination table advances at a constant rate through the scanner while the x-ray tube rotates continuously around the patient, following a spiral path, thus allowing the gathering of continuous data with no gaps between images. Unlike the traditional CT scan, the spiral CT scan evaluates slices as narrow as 1.0 mm, as compared with 5.0 mm slices obtained by traditional CT scan. This allows for a more accurate visualization of a PE. However, spiral CT has limitations. It cannot be performed at the bedside, so unstable patients must be transported to a CT scanner. In addition, IV infusion of contrast agent is necessary for visualization.

The D-dimer assay is becoming a more commonly used method for evaluating patients with possible PE. Because it is a simple test to perform, involving only a venipuncture, it has been studied as a possible method for ruling out PE; it is not used to make the diagnosis of PE. Emergency departments in particular have used this as a rapid, cost-effective test. D-dimer is a product of fibrin degradation and occurs as a result of fibrin lysis. An increased D-dimer value is usually indicative of a clotting abnormality. When a clot is dislodged, similar elevations of clotting factors should be present in the blood, especially in the case of a large embolus.

Pulmonary angiography is considered the best method to diagnose PE; however, it may not be feasible, cost-effective, or easily performed, especially with critically ill patients. The pulmonary angiogram allows for direct visualization under fluoroscopy of the arterial obstruction and accurate assessment of the perfusion deficit. A catheter is threaded through the vena cava to the right side of the heart to inject dye, similar to a cardiac catheterization, and a specially trained team must be available to perform the procedure.

Prevention

For those at risk, the most effective approach to preventing PE is to prevent deep venous thrombosis. Active leg exercises to avoid venous stasis, early ambulation, and use of elastic compression stockings are general preventive measures (Kearon, Aki, Omelas, et al., 2016). Additional

CHART 24-14

HOME CARE CHECKLIST • Prevention of Recurrent Pulmonary Embolism

At the completion of education, the patient and/or caregiver will be able to:

- State the impact of pulmonary embolism on physiologic functioning, ADLs, IADLs, roles, relationships, and spirituality.
- State changes in lifestyle (e.g., diet, activity) necessary to restore health.
- State the name, dose, side effects, frequency, and schedule for all medications.
- Name the anticoagulant prescribed and identify dosage and schedule of administration.
- Describe the need for continued anticoagulant therapy after the initial embolism.
- Describe the importance of follow-up appointments for coagulation tests and appointments with providers.
- Describe potential side effects of coagulation such as bruising and bleeding and identify ways to prevent bleeding.
- Avoid the use of sharps (razors, knives, etc.) to prevent cuts; shave with an electric shaver.
- Use a toothbrush with soft bristles to prevent gum injury.
- Do not take aspirin or antihistamines while taking warfarin sodium (Coumadin).
- Always check with the primary provider before taking any medicine, including over-the-counter medications.
- Avoid laxatives, because they may affect vitamin K absorption.
- Report the occurrence of dark, tarry stools to the primary provider immediately.
- Wear an identification bracelet or carry a medicine card stating that you are taking anticoagulants.
- Describe strategies to prevent recurrent deep venous thrombosis and pulmonary emboli.
- Continue to wear anti-embolism stockings (compression hose) as long as directed.
- Avoid sitting with legs crossed or sitting for prolonged periods of time.
- When travelling, change position regularly, walk occasionally, and do active exercises of moving the legs and ankles while sitting.
- Drink fluids, especially while travelling and in warm weather, to avoid hemoconcentration due to fluid deficit.
- Describe the signs and symptoms of lower extremity circulatory compromise and potential deep venous thrombosis: calf or leg pain, swelling, pedal edema.
- Describe the signs and symptoms of pulmonary compromise related to recurrent pulmonary embolism (e.g., dyspnea, chest pain, anxiety, fever, tachycardia, apprehension, cough, syncope, diaphoresis, hemoptysis).
- Describe how and when to contact the primary provider if symptoms of circulatory compromise or pulmonary compromise are identified.
- Identify the need for health promotion, disease prevention and screening activities

ADL, activities of daily living; IADL, independent activities of daily living.

strategies for prevention are listed in the checklist in Chart 24-14.

Patients who are older than 40 years, whose hemostasis is adequate, and who are undergoing major elective abdominal or thoracic surgery may receive anticoagulant therapy (Kahn, Lim, & Dunn, 2012). Low doses of heparin may be given before surgery to reduce the risk of postoperative deep venous thrombus and PE. Low-dose heparin is thought to enhance the activity of antithrombin III, a major plasma inhibitor of clotting factor X. This regimen is not recommended for patients with an active thrombotic process or for those undergoing major orthopedic surgery, open prostatectomy, or surgery on the eye or brain. Low-molecular-weight heparin (e.g., enoxaparin [Lovenox]) is an alternative therapy. It has a longer half-life, enhanced subcutaneous absorption, a reduced incidence of thrombocytopenia, and reduced interaction with platelets as compared with unfractionated heparin.

Sequential compression devices (SCDs) are often used to prevent venous stasis through compression and relaxation of the calf muscles, similar to the effect of muscle contraction. SCDs have been proven to effectively reduce the risk of deep venous thrombosis when used alone or in combination with anticoagulant therapy (Kearon, Aki, Omelas, et al., 2016). Several types of SCDs, using foot, calf, and thigh-high compression as well as graduated, asymmetric, and circumferential compression, are available. There is little evidence favouring any particular type of compression. Graduated compression involves the sequential movement of air in the sleeve up the leg, followed by relaxation of the sleeve. The advantage of this therapy is the extended duration of compression compared with standard inflation. Asymmetric compression involves inflating only the area on the back of the leg or foot. Circumferential compression involves even compression of the entire leg.

Medical Management

Because PE is often a medical emergency, emergency management is of primary concern. After emergency measures have been taken and the patient's condition stabilizes, the treatment goal is to dissolve (lyse) the existing emboli and prevent new ones from forming. The treatment of PE may include a variety of modalities:

- General measures to improve respiratory and vascular status
- Anticoagulation therapy
- Thrombolytic therapy
- Surgical intervention

Emergency Management

Massive PE is a life-threatening emergency. The immediate objective is to stabilize the cardiopulmonary system. A sudden increase in pulmonary resistance increases the work of the right ventricle, which can cause acute right-sided heart failure with cardiogenic shock. Emergency management consists of the following actions:

- Nasal oxygen is given immediately to relieve hypoxemia, respiratory distress, and central cyanosis; severe hypoxemia may necessitate emergent endotracheal intubation and mechanical ventilatory support.
- IV infusion lines are inserted to establish routes for medications or fluids that will be needed.
- For hypotension that does not resolve with IV fluids, prompt initiation of vasopressor therapy is recommended, with agents that may include dobutamine, dopamine, or norepinephrine.
- Hemodynamic measurements and evaluation for hypoxemia (pulse oximetry or arterial blood gas) are performed. If available, multidetector computed tomographic angiography (MDCTA) will be performed.
- The ECG is monitored continuously for dysrhythmias and right ventricular failure, which may occur suddenly.
- Blood is drawn for serum electrolytes, complete blood count, and coagulation studies.
- If the patient has suffered massive embolism and is hypotensive, an indwelling urinary catheter is inserted to monitor urinary output.
- Small doses of IV morphine or sedatives are given to relieve patient anxiety, to alleviate chest discomfort, to improve tolerance of the endotracheal tube, and to ease adaptation to the mechanical ventilator, if necessary.

General Management

Measures are initiated to improve the patient's respiratory and vascular status. Oxygen therapy is administered to correct the hypoxemia, relieve the pulmonary vascular vasoconstriction, and reduce the PH. Using elastic compression stockings or intermittent pneumatic leg compression devices reduces venous stasis. These measures compress the superficial veins and increase the velocity of blood in the deep veins by redirecting the blood through the deep veins. Elevating the leg (above the level of the heart) also increases venous flow.

Pharmacologic Therapy

Anticoagulation Therapy

Anticoagulant therapy (heparin, warfarin sodium) has traditionally been the primary method for managing acute deep vein thrombosis and PE (Tapson, 2016). Heparin is used to prevent recurrence of emboli but has no effect on emboli that are already present.

Heparin is generally recommended for all patients who have been diagnosed with PE. Generally, a therapeutic heparin dose is administered as a one-time 5,000-U bolus, and a continuous IV infusion is then started to maintain the partial thromboplastin time (PTT) at 1.5 to 2.0 times the normal level.

Heparin administration is associated with several concerns. Because the half-life of heparin is dose dependent, it is difficult, and time consuming to adjust and maintain the IV drip infusion at a therapeutic level; frequent laboratory testing is necessary. With long-term heparin use, there is also the risk of antibody formation and bleeding. Despite the risks, anticoagulation after initial clot formation and dislodgement is necessary because of the high risk for a recurrent thrombus. Therapy may be changed to an oral regimen, such as warfarin (Coumadin) as soon as the patient is able to take oral medications. Heparin must be continued until the international normalized ratio (INR) is within a therapeutic range, typically 2.0 to 2.5. Once the patient starts an oral regimen, it is important that he or she continue to take the same brand of warfarin, because the bioavailability may vary greatly among brands.

High doses of subcutaneous low–molecular-weight heparin or heparinoids may also be used to maintain a therapeutic PTT while oral anticoagulation therapy is being adjusted. Lepirudin (Refludan) and argatroban are alternatives for patients in whom heparin or heparinoids are contraindicated. These agents are direct thrombin inhibitors; therefore, they require less frequent monitoring and dose adjustment. Both medications have contraindications and side effects that the nurse must be aware of before administration. Lepirudin and argatroban are both contraindicated in patients with overt major bleeding and in patients who are hypersensitive to these agents or at high risk for bleeding (e.g., recent cerebrovascular accident [CVA, brain attack], anomaly of vessels or organs, recent major surgery, recent puncture of large vessels, or organ biopsy). Major side effects are bleeding anywhere in the body and anaphylactic reaction resulting in shock or death. Other side effects include fever, abnormal liver function, and allergic skin reaction. All patients must continue to take some form of anticoagulation for at least 3 to 6 months after the embolic event.

Thrombolytic Therapy

Thrombolytic therapy (urokinase, streptokinase, alteplase) also may be used in treating PE, particularly in patients who are severely compromised (e.g., those who are hypotensive and have significant hypoxemia despite oxygen supplementation) (Ouellette, 2015). Thrombolytic therapy resolves the thrombi or emboli more quickly and restores more normal hemodynamic functioning of the pulmonary circulation, thereby reducing PH and improving perfusion, oxygenation, and cardiac output. Bleeding, however, is a significant side effect. Contraindications to thrombolytic therapy include a CVA within the past 2 months, other active intracranial processes, active bleeding, surgery within the past 10 days of the thrombotic event, recent labour and delivery, trauma, or severe hypertension. Consequently, thrombolytic agents are advocated only for PE affecting a significant area of blood flow to the lung and causing hemodynamic instability.

Before thrombolytic therapy is started, prothrombin time, PTT, hematocrit values, and platelet counts are obtained. Heparin is stopped prior to administration of a thrombolytic agent. During therapy, all but essential invasive procedures are avoided because of potential bleeding. If necessary, fresh whole blood, packed red cells, cryoprecipitate, or frozen plasma is administered to replace blood loss and reverse the bleeding tendency. After the thrombolytic infusion is completed (which varies in duration according to the agent used and the condition being treated), the patient is given anticoagulants.

Surgical Management

A surgical embolectomy is rarely performed but may be indicated if the patient has a massive PE or hemodynamic instability or if there are contraindications to thrombolytic therapy. Pulmonary embolectomy requires a thoracotomy with cardiopulmonary bypass technique (Ouellette, 2015).

It may be used for patients who fail to improve with thrombolytic therapy, have contraindications to thrombolytic therapy and have had a massive PE, or must have the clot removed to help reduce right-sided heart failure (Kearon et al., 2016; Tapson, 2016). Although surgical embolectomy ensures removal of the clot, it is not without risk. The procedure has a high intraoperative mortality rate and has typical postoperative complications.

Transvenous catheter embolectomy is a technique in which a vacuum-cupped catheter is introduced transvenously into the affected pulmonary artery. Suction is applied to the end of the embolus, and the embolus is aspirated into the cup. The surgeon maintains suction to hold the embolus within the cup, and the entire catheter is withdrawn through the right side of the heart and out the femoral vein. Catheters are available that pulverize the clot with high-velocity jets of normal saline solution. An inferior caval filter is usually inserted at the time of surgery to protect against a recurrence.

Nursing Management

Minimizing the Risk of Pulmonary Embolism

A key role of the nurse is to identify patients at high risk for PE and to minimize the risk of PE in all patients. The nurse must have a high degree of suspicion for PE in any patient, but particularly in those with conditions predisposing to a slowing of venous return.

Preventing Thrombus Formation

Preventing thrombus formation is a major nursing responsibility. The nurse encourages ambulation and active and passive leg exercises to prevent venous stasis in patients on bed rest. The nurse instructs the patient to move the legs in a "pumping" exercise so that the leg muscles can help increase venous flow. The nurse also advises the patient not to sit or lie in bed for prolonged periods, not to cross the legs, and not to wear constricting clothing. Legs should not be dangled, or feet placed in a dependent position while the patient sits on the edge of the bed; instead, the patient's feet should rest on the floor or on a chair. In addition, IV catheters (for parenteral therapy or measurements of central venous pressure) should not be left in place for prolonged periods.

Assessing the Potential for Pulmonary Embolism

All patients are evaluated for risk factors for thrombus formation and pulmonary embolus. The nurse does a careful assessment of the patient's health history, family history, and medication record. On a daily basis, the patient is asked about pain or discomfort in the extremities. In addition, the extremities are evaluated for warmth, redness, and inflammation.

Monitoring Thrombolytic Therapy

The nurse is responsible for monitoring thrombolytic and anticoagulant therapy. Thrombolytic therapy (streptokinase, urokinase, tissue plasminogen activator) causes lysis of deep vein thrombi and pulmonary emboli, which helps dissolve the clots. During thrombolytic infusion, the patient remains on bed rest, vital signs are assessed every 2 hours, and invasive procedures are limited. Tests to determine prothrombin time or PTT are performed 3 to 4 hours after the thrombolytic infusion is started to confirm that the fibrinolytic systems have been activated. See Chapter 32 for nursing management for the patient receiving anticoagulant or thrombolytic therapy.

NURSING ALERT

Because of the prolonged clotting time, only essential arterial punctures or venipunctures are performed in patients who have received thrombolytics and manual pressure is applied to any puncture site for at least 30 minutes. Pulse oximetry is used to monitor changes in oxygenation. The thrombolytic infusion is discontinued immediately if uncontrolled bleeding occurs.

Managing Pain

Chest pain, if present, is usually pleuritic rather than cardiac in origin. A semi-Fowler's position provides a more comfortable position for breathing. However, it is important to continue to turn the patient frequently and reposition the patient to improve the **ventilation–perfusion ratio** in the lung. The nurse administers opioid analgesics as prescribed for severe pain.

Managing Oxygen Therapy

Careful attention is given to the proper use of oxygen. It is important to ensure that the patient understands the need for continuous oxygen therapy. The nurse assesses the patient frequently for signs of hypoxemia and monitors the pulse oximetry values to evaluate the effectiveness of the oxygen therapy. Deep breathing and incentive spirometry are indicated for all patients to minimize or prevent atelectasis and improve ventilation. Nebulizer therapy or percussion and postural drainage may be used for management of secretions.

Relieving Anxiety

The nurse encourages the stabilized patient to talk about any fears or concerns related to this frightening episode, answers the patient and family's questions concisely and accurately, explains the therapy, and describes how to recognize untoward effects early.

Monitoring for Complications

When caring for a patient who has had PE, the nurse must be alert for the potential complication of cardiogenic shock or right ventricular failure subsequent to the effect of PE on the cardiovascular system. Nursing activities for managing shock are found in Chapter 16.

Providing Postoperative Nursing Care

After surgery, the nurse measures the patient's pulmonary arterial pressure and urinary output. The nurse assesses the insertion site of the arterial catheter for hematoma formation and infection. It is important to maintain the blood pressure at a level that supports perfusion of vital organs. To prevent peripheral venous stasis and edema of the lower extremities, the nurse elevates the foot of the bed and encourages isometric exercises, use of elastic compression stockings, and walking when the patient is permitted out of bed. Sitting is discouraged, because hip flexion compresses the large veins in the legs.

Promoting Home, Community-Based, and Transitional Care

Educating Patients About Self-Care

Before hospital discharge and at follow-up visits to the clinic or during home visits, the nurse instructs the patient about how to prevent recurrence and what signs and symptoms to report immediately. Patient instructions, as presented in Chart 24-14, are intended to help prevent recurrences and side effects of treatment.

Continuing and Transitional Care

During follow-up or home care visits, the nurse monitors the patient's adherence to the prescribed management plan and reinforces previous instructions. The nurse also monitors the patient for residual effects of the PE and recovery. The patient is reminded about the importance of keeping follow-up appointments for coagulation tests and appointments with the primary care provider. The nurse also reminds the patient about the importance of participation in health promotion activities (e.g., immunizations) and health screening.

Sarcoidosis

Sarcoidosis is an inflammatory disease which can affect any of the body's organs or systems (National Sarcoidosis Organization, n.d.). Sarcoidosis affects the normal functioning of the body's immune system, causing it to overreact, forming granulomas or groups of cells that attach to other tissues and organs in the body (National Sarcoidosis Organization, n.d.). It may involve almost any organ or tissue but most commonly involves the lungs, lymph nodes, liver, spleen, central nervous system, skin, eyes, fingers, and parotid glands. The disease is not gender specific, but some manifestations are more common in women. Epidemiologic data are not currently available for Canada specifically; however, the worldwide prevalence is approximately 20 individuals in 100,000) (Canadian Liver Foundation, n.d.).

Pathophysiology

Sarcoidosis is thought to be a hypersensitivity response to one or more agents (bacteria, fungi, virus, chemicals) in people with an inherited or acquired predisposition to the disorder. The hypersensitivity response results in granuloma formation due to the release of cytokines and other substances that promote replication of fibroblasts. In the lung, granuloma infiltration and fibrosis may occur, resulting in low lung compliance, impaired diffusing capacity, and reduced lung volumes (King, 2016).

Clinical Manifestations

A hallmark of this disease is its insidious onset and lack of prominent clinical signs or symptoms. The clinical picture depends on the systems involved. The disease involves the lungs in about 90% of patients but presents with pulmonary symptoms in about 50% of cases. With pulmonary involvement, signs and symptoms may include dyspnea, nonproductive cough, wheezing, and chest pressure (Culver, 2012). Generalized symptoms include anorexia, fatigue, and weight loss. Other signs include uveitis, joint pain, fever, and granulomatous lesions of the skin, liver, spleen, kidney, and central nervous system. The granulomas may disappear or gradually convert to fibrous tissue. With multisystem involvement, the patient has fatigue, fever, anorexia, weight loss, and joint pain.

Assessment and Diagnostic Findings

Chest x-rays and CT scans are used to assess pulmonary adenopathy. The chest x-ray may show hilar adenopathy and disseminated miliary and nodular lesions in the lungs. A mediastinoscopy or **transbronchial** biopsy (in which a tissue specimen is obtained through the bronchial wall) may be used to confirm the diagnosis. In rare cases, an **open lung biopsy** is performed. Diagnosis is confirmed by a biopsy that shows noncaseating granulomas. Pulmonary function test results are abnormal if there is restriction of lung function (reduction in total lung capacity). Arterial blood gas measurements may be normal or may show reduced oxygen levels (hypoxemia) and increased carbon dioxide levels (hypercapnia).

Medical Management

Many patients undergo remission without specific treatment. Corticosteroid therapy may benefit some patients because of its anti-inflammatory effect. Oral corticosteroids have been the most commonly used agents for the relief of symptoms and control of potentially disabling respiratory impairment from pulmonary sarcoidosis. Once begun, corticosteroid therapy is usually continued in tapering doses for 12 months, and longer if the patient has recurrence of symptoms and chest x-ray indications (i.e., continued pulmonary adenopathy) (King, 2014). It is useful for patients with ocular and myocardial involvement, skin involvement, extensive pulmonary disease that compromises pulmonary function, hepatic involvement, and hypercalcemia.

OCCUPATIONAL LUNG DISEASES: PNEUMOCONIOSIS

Pneumoconiosis is a general term given to any lung disease caused by dusts that are breathed in and then deposited deep in the lungs causing damage. Pneumoconiosis is usually considered an occupational lung disease, and includes **asbestosis**, silicosis, and coal workers' pneumoconiosis, also known as "Black Lung Disease" (ALA, 2016). Pneumoconiosis refers to a nonneoplastic alteration of the lung resulting from inhalation of mineral or inorganic dust (e.g., "dusty lung"). Pneumoconiosis is caused by inhalation and deposition of mineral dusts in the lungs, resulting in pulmonary fibrosis and parenchymal changes. Many people with early pneumoconiosis are asymptomatic, but advanced disease often is accompanied by disability and premature death. In 2010, reported mortality rates were 90 per 100,000 population in Canada (PHAC, 2016).

Diseases of the lungs occur in numerous occupations as a result of exposure to organic and inorganic (mineral) dusts and noxious gases (fumes and aerosols). Examples include mineral dusts (asbestos, silica, coal), metal dusts, biologic dusts (spores, mycelia, bird droppings), manufactured fibres (glass or ceramic fibres), and toxic fumes (nitrogen dioxide, sulphur dioxide, chlorine, ammonia). The effects of inhaling these materials depend on the composition of the substance, its concentration, its ability to initiate an immune response, its irritating properties, the duration of exposure, and the individual's response or susceptibility to the irritant. Smoking may compound the problem and may increase the risk of lung cancers in people exposed to the mineral asbestos and other potential carcinogens (ALA, 2016).

Key aspects of any assessment of patients with a potential occupational respiratory history include job and job activities, exposure levels, general hygiene, time frame of exposure, amount of respiratory protection used, and direct versus indirect exposures. Specific information that should be obtained includes the following:

- Exposure to an agent known to cause an occupational disorder
- Length of time from exposure of agent to onset of symptoms
- Congruence of symptoms with those of known exposure-related disorder
- Lack of other more likely explanations of the signs and symptoms

These diseases are not treatable once they develop; however, they are preventable. Therefore, a major role for nurses, especially occupational health nurses, is that of advocate for employees. Occupational health nurses serve as employee advocates, making every effort to promote measures to reduce the exposure of workers to industrial products. Resources for occupational health nurses include provincial and territorial legislation and resources and the Canadian Centre for Occupational Health and Safety (CCOHS). The CCOHS is a federal government agency located in Hamilton, Ontario, that reports to the Parliament of Canada through the federal Minister of Labour. Three stakeholder groups (government [federal, provincial, and territorial], employers, and workers) govern the centre. The mission of CCOHS is to eliminate all Canadian work-related illnesses and injuries by facilitating cooperation among all stakeholder groups, assisting on development and maintenance of policies and programs, and serving as a national source for information about occupational health and safety.

Laws require that the work environment be ventilated properly to remove any noxious agent. Dust control can prevent many of the pneumoconiosis. Dust control includes ventilation, spraying an area with water to control dust, and effective and frequent floor cleaning. Air samples need to be monitored. Toxic substances should be enclosed and placed in restricted areas. Workers must wear or use protective devices (facemasks, hoods, industrial respirators) to provide a safe air supply when a toxic element is present. Employees who are at risk should be carefully screened and monitored. There is a risk of developing serious smoking-related illness (cancer) in industries in which there are unsafe levels of certain gases, dusts, fumes, fluids, and other toxic substances. In addition, there is the potential for second-hand exposure. Asbestos and toxic dusts and substances may be transferred to others through the handling of clothing or shoes that have been exposed. Ongoing educational programs should be designed to teach workers to take responsibility for their own health and to stop smoking and receive an influenza vaccination.

Employees must be informed about all hazardous and toxic substances in the workplace. Specifically, they must be informed about any hazardous or toxic substances they work with, what effects these substances can have on their health, and the measures they can take to protect themselves. The responsibility for implementing these controls inevitably falls on the provincial/territorial governments.

In addition to teaching preventive measures to patients and their families, the nurse assesses patients for a history of exposure to environmental agents (e.g., dusts, fibres, fumes) and makes referrals so that pulmonary function can be evaluated, and the patient can be treated early in the course of the disease. Patients with occupational lung disease often experience increasing chronic dyspnea, cough, and a prolonged illness culminating in respiratory failure. Strategies to prevent superimposed infection are implemented, and the patient and family are assisted in coping with the increasing disability that accompanies occupational lung disease. Home care referrals are often helpful in identifying measures to decrease the patient's dyspnea, ensure appropriate and safe use of oxygen, and make the patient as comfortable as possible. In addition, referral to a pulmonary rehabilitation program may be considered in some patients.

The most common pneumoconiosis are silicosis, asbestosis, and coal worker's pneumoconiosis.

Asbestosis

Asbestosis is a disease characterized by diffuse pulmonary fibrosis from the inhalation of asbestos dust. Current laws restrict the use of asbestos, but many industries used it in the past. Therefore, exposure occurred, and may still occur, in numerous occupations, including asbestos mining and manufacturing, shipbuilding, demolition of structures containing asbestos, and roofing. Materials such as shingles, cement, vinyl asbestos tile, fireproof paint and clothing, brake linings, and filters all contained asbestos at one time, and many of these materials are still in existence. Chronic exposure may also occur by washing clothes that have been in contact with asbestos. Additional diseases related to asbestos exposure include lung cancer, mesothelioma, and asbestos pleural effusion.

Pathophysiology

Inhaled asbestos fibres enter the alveoli, where they are surrounded by fibrous tissue. The fibrous tissue eventually obliterates the alveoli. Fibrous changes also affect the pleura, which thickens and develops plaque. The result of these physiologic changes is a **restrictive lung disease**, with a decrease in lung volume, diminished exchange of oxygen and carbon dioxide, and hypoxemia.

Clinical Manifestations

The onset of the disease is insidious, and the patient has progressive dyspnea, persistent dry cough, mild-to-moderate chest pain, anorexia, weight loss, and malaise. Early physical findings include bibasilar fine, end-inspiratory crackles, and in more advanced cases clubbing of the fingers. Cor pulmonale and respiratory failure occur as the disease progresses. A high proportion of workers who have been exposed to asbestos dust die of lung cancer, especially those who smoke or have a history of smoking. Malignant mesotheliomas may also occur. These are rare cancers of the pleura or peritoneum that are strongly associated with asbestos exposure.

Medical Management

There is no effective treatment for asbestosis, as the lung damage is permanent and often progressive. Management is directed at controlling infection and treating the lung disease. When oxygen–carbon dioxide exchange becomes severely impaired, continuous oxygen therapy may help to improve activity tolerance. The patient must be instructed to avoid additional exposure to asbestos and to stop smoking. A significant contributing cause to mortality in this population is the high incidence of lung carcinoma.

Coal Worker's Pneumoconiosis

Coal worker's pneumoconiosis ("black lung disease") includes a variety of respiratory diseases found in coal workers who have inhaled coal dust over the years. Coal miners are exposed to dusts that are mixtures of coal, kaolin, mica, and silica.

Pathophysiology

When coal dust is deposited in the alveoli and respiratory bronchioles, macrophages engulf the particles (by phagocytosis) and transport them to the terminal bronchioles, where they are removed by mucociliary action. In time, the clearance mechanisms cannot handle the excessive dust load, and the macrophages aggregate in the respiratory bronchioles and alveoli. Fibroblasts appear, and a network of reticulin is laid down surrounding the dust-laden macrophages. The bronchioles and the alveoli become clogged with coal dust, dying macrophages, and fibroblasts. This leads to the formation of the coal macule, which is the primary lesion of the disorder. Macules appear as blackish dots on the lungs. Fibrotic lesions develop, and as the macules enlarge, the weakening bronchioles dilate, with subsequent development of a localized emphysema. The disease begins in the upper lobes of the lungs but may progress to the lower lobes.

Clinical Manifestations

The first signs of coal worker's pneumoconiosis are a chronic cough and sputum production, similar to the signs encountered in chronic bronchitis. As the disease progresses, the patient develops dyspnea and coughs up large amounts of sputum with varying amounts of black fluid (melanoptysis), particularly if the individual is a smoker. Eventually, cor pulmonale and respiratory failure result. The diagnosis may first be made based on chest x-ray findings and a history of exposure.

Medical Management

Preventing this disease is key because there is no effective treatment. Instead, treatment focuses on early diagnosis and management of complications (see Chapter 25 for discussion of emphysema).

Nursing Management

Teaching About Prevention

The occupational health nurse serves as an employee advocate, making every effort to promote measures to reduce the exposure of workers to industrial products. Laws require that the work environment be ventilated properly to remove any noxious agent.

CHEST TUMOURS

Tumours of the lung may be benign or malignant. A malignant chest tumour can be primary, arising within the lung, chest wall, or mediastinum, or it can be a metastasis from a primary tumour site elsewhere in the body. Metastatic lung tumours occur frequently because the bloodstream transports cancer cells from primary cancers elsewhere in the body to the lungs.

Lung Cancer (Bronchogenic Carcinoma)

Lung cancer is the most commonly diagnosed cancer and the leading cause of cancer death in Canada (excluding nonmelanoma skin cancers) (Canadian Cancer Society, 2017). On average, in 2017, 78 Canadians were diagnosed with lung cancer every day, and 58 Canadians died from lung cancer every day (Canadian Cancer Society, 2017). In approximately 57% of patients with lung cancer, the disease has spread to regional lymphatics and other sites by the time of diagnosis (Siegel, Miller, & Jemal, 2015). As a result, the long-term survival rate is low. Overall, the 5-year survival rate is 17% (Siegel et al., 2015).

Pathophysiology

Between 80% and 90% of lung cancers are caused by inhaled carcinogens, most commonly cigarette smoke, other carcinogens include radon gas and occupational and environmental agents (Weinberger et al., 2014). Lung cancers arise from a single transformed epithelial cell in the tracheobronchial airways. A carcinogen binds to a cell's DNA and damages it. This damage results in cellular changes, abnormal cell growth, and eventually a malignant cell. As the damaged DNA is passed on to daughter cells, the DNA undergoes further changes and becomes unstable. With the accumulation of genetic changes, the pulmonary epithelium undergoes malignant transformation from normal epithelium to eventual invasive carcinoma. Evidence indicates that carcinoma tends to arise at sites of previous scarring (TB, fibrosis) in the lung.

Classification and Staging

For purposes of staging and treatment, most lung cancers are classified into one of two major categories: small cell lung cancer (SCLC) and non–small cell lung cancer (NSCLC). Non–small cell lung cancer is further classified with cell types. Squamous cell cancer is usually more centrally located and arises more commonly in the segmental and subsegmental bronchi (Canadian Cancer Society, n.d.). Adenocarcinoma is the most prevalent carcinoma of the lung for both men and women; it presents more peripherally as peripheral masses or nodules and often metastasizes (Canadian Cancer Society, n.d.). Large cell carcinoma (also called *undifferentiated carcinoma*) is a fast-growing tumour that tends to arise peripherally. Bronchioalveolar cell cancer arises from the terminal bronchus and alveoli and is usually slower growing as compared with other bronchogenic carcinomas.

Non–small cell carcinoma represents 70% to 80% of tumours; small cell carcinoma represents 15% to 20% of tumours. In non–small cell carcinoma, the cell types include squamous cell carcinoma (30%), large cell carcinoma (10% to 16%), and adenocarcinoma (31% to 34%), including bronchioalveolar carcinoma (3% to 4%). Most small cell carcinomas arise in the major bronchi and spread by infiltration along the bronchial wall. Small cell cancers account for 20% to 25% of all bronchogenic cancers (Kalemkerian & Gadgeel, 2013).

In addition to cell type, lung cancers also are staged. The stage of the tumour refers to the size of the tumour, its location, whether lymph nodes are involved, and whether the cancer has spread (Kalemkerian & Gadgeel, 2013). Non–small cell lung cancer is staged as 0 to IV. Stage I is the earliest stage with the highest cure rates, while stage IV designates metastatic spread. Estimated 5-year survival rates for the stages of non–small cell lung cancer are as follows: stages IA and IB, 50% to 80%; stage IIA and IIB, 30% to 50%; stage IIIA, 10% to 40%; stage IIIB, 5% to 20%; and stage IV, less than 5% (Walters et al., 2013). Small cell lung cancers are classified as limited or extensive.

Risk Factors

Smoking tobacco, especially cigarettes, is the main cause of lung cancer accounting for more than 85% of lung cancer cases in Canada (Canadian Cancer Society, n.d.). Some of the many chemicals found in tobacco are carcinogenic, meaning they causes alterations to cells in the lungs that can lead to lung cancer. Various other factors have been associated with the development of lung cancer, including second-hand smoke, environmental and occupational exposure, gender, genetics, advanced age, and dietary deficits. Other factors that have been associated with lung cancer include other underlying respiratory diseases, such as COPD and TB.

Tobacco Smoke

The risk of developing lung cancer is about 23 times higher in male smokers and 13 times higher in female smokers compared to lifelong nonsmokers (ACS, 2016). Risk is determined by the pack-year history (number of packs of cigarettes used each day, multiplied by the number of years smoked), the age of initiation of smoking, the depth of inhalation, and the tar and nicotine levels in the cigarettes smoked. The younger a person is when he or she starts smoking, the greater the risk of developing lung cancer. Smokers who use smokeless products as a supplemental source of nicotine will increase their risk of lung cancer (ACS, 2016).

Almost all cases of SCLC are due to cigarette smoking. SCLC is rare in people who have never smoked. It is the most aggressive form of lung cancer, grows quickly, and usually starts in the airways in the centre of the chest (ACS, 2016).

Electronic Cigarettes

Electronic cigarettes are a form of electronic nicotine delivery system. Per the American Cancer Society, there are questions about how safe it is to inhale some substances in the vapor. The amounts of nicotine and other substances a person gets from each cartridge are also unclear and have been found to vary greatly even when comparing same brand cartridges from the same manufacturer (American Cancer Society, 2016).

Second-Hand (Passive) Smoke

Passive smoking has been identified as a possible cause of lung cancer in nonsmokers. In other words, people who are involuntarily exposed to tobacco smoke in a closed environment (home, car, building) are at increased risk for developing lung cancer as compared with unexposed nonsmokers.

Environmental and Occupational Exposure

Various carcinogens have been identified in the atmosphere, including motor vehicle emissions and pollutants from refineries and manufacturing plants. Evidence suggests that the incidence of lung cancer is greater in urban areas as a result of the build-up of pollutants and motor vehicle emissions.

Radon is a colourless, odourless gas found in soil and rocks. For many years it has been associated with uranium mines, but it is now known to seep into homes through ground rock. High levels of radon have been associated with the development of lung cancer, especially when combined with cigarette smoking. Homeowners are advised to have radon levels checked in their houses and to arrange for special venting if the levels are high.

Chronic exposure to industrial carcinogens, such as arsenic, asbestos, mustard gas, chromates, coke oven fumes, nickel, oil, and radiation, has been associated with the development of lung cancer. Laws have been passed to control exposure to such elements in the workplace.

Genetics

Genetic mutations may be one of the risk factors for lung cancer and can cause certain changes in the DNA of lung cells. These changes can lead to abnormal cell growth and, sometimes, cancer. There are inherited gene changes and acquired gene changes. Inherited gene changes probably do not play a large role in lung cancer. Acquired mutations in lung cells often result from exposure to factors in the environment, such as cancer-causing chemicals in tobacco smoke (ACS, 2016). Acquired changes in certain genes, such as the *TP53* or *p16* tumour suppressor genes and the *K-RAS* or *ALK*oncogenes, are thought to be important in the development of NSCLC. Ongoing research will help to both identify additional changes in genes and develop targeted therapies for lung cancer (ACS, 2016) (see Chapter 11).

Dietary Factors

Smokers who eat a diet low in fruits and vegetables have an increased risk of developing lung cancer. The actual active agents in a diet rich in fruits and vegetables have yet to be determined. It has been hypothesized that carotenoids, particularly carotene or vitamin A, may be important. Several ongoing trials may help to determine if carotene supplementation has anticancer properties. Other nutrients, including vitamin E, selenium, vitamin C, fat, and retinoids, are also being evaluated regarding their protective role against lung cancer.

Clinical Manifestations

Often, lung cancer develops insidiously and is asymptomatic until late in its course. The signs and symptoms depend on the location and size of the tumour, the degree of obstruction, and the existence of metastases to regional or distant sites.

The most frequent symptom of lung cancer is cough or change in a chronic cough. People frequently ignore this symptom and attribute it to smoking or a respiratory infection. The cough starts as a dry, persistent cough, without sputum production. When obstruction of airways occurs, the cough may become productive due to infection.

> **NURSING ALERT**
>
> **A cough that changes in character should arouse suspicion of lung cancer.**

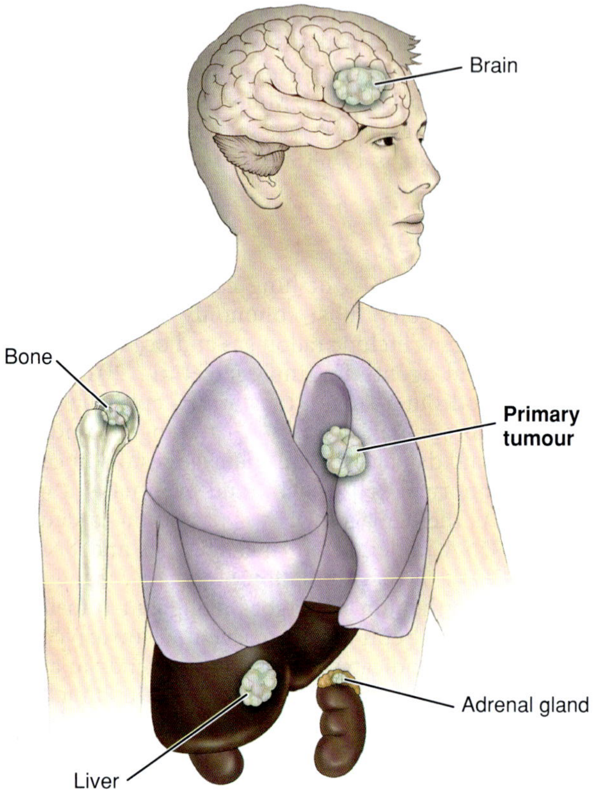

FIGURE 24-6. Frequent sites of lung cancer metastasis.

Dyspnea is prominent in patients early in their disease process, occurring in 35% to 50% of patients (Evans, 2013). Causes of dyspnea may include tumour occlusion of the airway or lung parenchyma, pleural effusion, pneumonia, or complications of treatment. Hemoptysis or blood-tinged sputum may be expectorated. Chest or shoulder pain may indicate chest wall or pleural involvement by a tumour. Pain also is a late manifestation and may be related to metastasis to the bone.

In some patients, a recurring fever occurs as an early symptom in response to a persistent infection in an area of pneumonitis distal to the tumour. In fact, cancer of the lung should be suspected in people with repeated unresolved upper respiratory tract infections. If the tumour spreads to adjacent structures and regional lymph nodes, the patient may present with chest pain and tightness, hoarseness (involving the recurrent laryngeal nerve), dysphagia, head and neck edema, and symptoms of pleural or pericardial effusion. The most common sites of metastases are lymph nodes, bone, brain, contralateral lung, adrenal glands, and liver. See Figure 24-6 for frequent sites of lung cancer metastasis. Nonspecific symptoms of weakness, anorexia, and weight loss also may be present.

Assessment and Diagnostic Findings

If pulmonary symptoms occur in a heavy smoker, cancer of the lung should always be considered. A chest x-ray is performed to search for pulmonary density, a solitary peripheral nodule (coin lesion), atelectasis, and infection. CT scans of the chest are used to identify small nodules not visualized on the chest x-ray and also to serially examine areas for lymphadenopathy.

Fibreoptic bronchoscopy is more commonly used and provides a detailed study of the tracheobronchial tree and allows for brushings, washings, and biopsies of suspicious areas. For peripheral lesions not amenable to bronchoscopic biopsy, a transthoracic **fine-needle aspiration** may be performed under CT or fluoroscopic guidance to aspirate cells from a suspicious area.

A variety of scans may be used to assess for metastasis of the cancer. These may include bone scans, abdominal scans, positron emission tomography (PET) scans, or liver ultrasound or scans. CT of the brain, magnetic resonance imaging (MRI), and other neurologic diagnostic procedures are used to detect central nervous system metastases. Mediastinoscopy or mediastinotomy may be used to obtain biopsy samples from lymph nodes in the mediastinum.

If surgery is a potential treatment, the patient is evaluated to determine whether the tumour is resectable and whether the physiologic impairment resulting from such surgery can be tolerated. Pulmonary function tests, arterial blood gas analysis, ventilation–perfusion scans, and exercise testing may all be used as part of the preoperative assessment.

CHART 24-15

Types of Lung Resection

- Lobectomy: a single lobe of the lung is removed
- Bilobectomy: two lobes of the lung are removed
- Sleeve resection: cancerous lobe(s) is removed and a segment of the main bronchus is resected
- Pneumonectomy: removal of entire lung
- Segmentectomy: a segment of the lung is removed[a]
- Wedge resection: removal of a small, pie-shaped area of the segment
- Chest wall resection with removal of cancerous lung tissue: for cancers that have invaded the chest wall

[a]Not recommended as curative resection for lung cancer.

Medical Management

The objective of management is to provide a cure, if possible. Treatment depends on the cell type, the stage of the disease, and the physiologic status (particularly cardiac and pulmonary status) of the patient. In general, treatment may involve surgery, radiation therapy, or chemotherapy—or a combination of these. Newer and more specific therapies to modulate the immune system (gene therapy, therapy with defined tumour antigens) are under study and show promise in treating lung cancer.

Surgical Management

Surgical resection is the preferred method of treating patients with localized non–small cell tumours, no evidence of metastatic spread, and adequate cardiopulmonary function. If the patient's cardiovascular status, pulmonary function, and functional status are satisfactory, surgery is generally well tolerated. Coronary artery disease, pulmonary insufficiency, and other comorbidities may contraindicate surgical intervention. The cure rate of surgical resection depends on the type and stage of the cancer. Surgery is primarily used for non–small cell carcinomas because small cell cancer of the lung grows rapidly and metastasizes early and extensively. Unfortunately, in many patients with bronchogenic cancer, the lesion is inoperable at the time of diagnosis.

Several different types of lung resections may be performed (Chart 24-15). The most common surgical procedure for a small, apparently curable tumour of the lung is lobectomy (removal of a lobe of the lung). In some cases, an entire lung may be removed (pneumonectomy) (see Chapter 26 for further details).

Radiation Therapy

Radiation therapy may cure a small percentage of patients. It is useful in controlling neoplasms that cannot be surgically resected but are responsive to radiation. Irradiation also may be used to reduce the size of a tumour, to make an inoperable tumour operable, or to relieve the pressure of the tumour on vital structures. It can control symptoms of spinal cord metastasis and superior vena caval compression. Also, prophylactic brain irradiation is used in certain patients to treat microscopic metastases to the brain. Radiation may help to relieve cough, chest pain, dyspnea, hemoptysis, and bone and liver pain. Relief of symptoms may last from a few weeks to many months and is important in improving the quality of the remaining period of life.

Radiation therapy usually is toxic to normal tissue within the radiation field, and this may lead to complications such as esophagitis, pneumonitis, and radiation lung fibrosis. These conditions may impair ventilatory and diffusion capacity and significantly reduce pulmonary reserve. The patient's nutritional status, psychological outlook, fatigue level, and signs of anemia and infection are monitored throughout the treatment. See Chapter 68 for management of the patient receiving radiation therapy.

Chemotherapy

Chemotherapy is used to alter tumour growth patterns, to treat patients with distant metastases or small cell cancer of the lung, and as an adjunct to surgery or radiation therapy. Chemotherapy may provide relief, especially of pain, but it does not usually cure the disease or prolong life to any great degree. Chemotherapy is also accompanied by side effects. It is valuable in reducing pressure symptoms of lung cancer and in treating brain, spinal cord, and pericardial metastasis. See Chapter 68 for a discussion of chemotherapy for the patient with cancer.

The choice of agent depends on the growth of the tumour cell and the specific phase of the cell cycle that the medication affects. In combination with surgery, chemotherapy may be administered before surgery (neoadjuvant therapy) or after surgery (adjuvant therapy). Combinations of two or more medications may be more beneficial than single-dose regimens. A large number of medications are active against lung cancer. A variety of chemotherapeutic agents are used, including alkylating agents (ifosfamide), platinum analogues (cisplatin and carboplatin), taxanes (paclitaxel, docetaxel), vinca alkaloids (vinblastine and vindesine), doxorubicin, gemcitabine, vinorelbine, irinotecan (CPT-11), and etoposide (VP-16). The choice of agent depends on the growth of the tumour cell and the specific phase of the cell cycle that the medication affects. Numerous combinations of chemotherapy are undergoing investigation to identify the optimal regimen to treat differing types of lung cancer.

Palliative Therapy

Palliative therapy may include radiation therapy to shrink the tumour to provide pain relief, a variety of bronchoscopic interventions to open a narrowed bronchus or airway, and pain management and other comfort measures. Location of death (for example, hospital, home, long-term care facility) has been associated with adequacy of symptom management at end of life. Valuation and referral for hospice care are important in planning for comfortable and dignified end-of-life care for the patient and family.

Treatment-Related Complications

A variety of complications may occur as a result of lung cancer treatments. Surgical resection may result in respiratory failure, particularly if the cardiopulmonary system is compromised before surgery. Surgical complications and prolonged mechanical ventilation are potential outcomes. Radiation therapy may result in diminished cardiopulmonary function and other complications, such as pulmonary fibrosis, pericarditis, myelitis, and cor pulmonale. Chemotherapy, particularly in combination with radiation therapy, can cause pneumonitis. Pulmonary toxicity is a potential side effect of chemotherapy.

Nursing Management

Nursing care of the patient with lung cancer is similar to that of other patients with cancer (see Chapter 68) and addresses the physiologic and psychological needs of the patient. The physiologic problems are primarily due to the respiratory manifestations of the disease. Nursing care includes strategies to ensure relief of pain and discomfort and to prevent complications.

Managing Symptoms

The nurse instructs the patient and family about the potential side effects of the specific treatment and strategies to manage them. Strategies for managing such symptoms as dyspnea, fatigue, nausea and vomiting, and anorexia will assist the patient and family to cope with the therapeutic measures.

Relieving Breathing Problems

Airway clearance techniques are key to maintaining airway patency through the removal of excess secretions. This may be accomplished through deep-breathing exercises, chest physiotherapy, directed cough, suctioning, and in some instances bronchoscopy. Bronchodilator medications may be prescribed to promote bronchial dilation. As the tumour enlarges or spreads, it may compress a bronchus or involve a large area of lung tissue, resulting in an impaired breathing pattern and poor gas exchange. At some stage of the disease, supplemental oxygen will probably be necessary.

Nursing measures focus on decreasing dyspnea by encouraging the patient to assume positions that promote lung expansion, breathing exercises for lung expansion and relaxation, and educating the patient on energy conservation and airway clearance techniques. Many of the techniques used in pulmonary rehabilitation can be applied to the lung cancer patient. Depending on the severity of disease and the patient's wishes, a referral to a pulmonary rehabilitation program may be helpful in managing respiratory symptoms.

Reducing Fatigue

Fatigue is a devastating symptom that affects the quality of life in the patient with cancer. It is commonly experienced by the patient with lung cancer and may be related to the disease itself, the cancer treatment and complications (e.g., anemia), sleep disturbances, pain and discomfort, hypoxemia, poor nutrition, or the psychological ramifications of the disease (e.g., anxiety, depression). The nurse is pivotal in thoroughly assessing the patient's level of fatigue, identifying potentially treatable causes, and validating with the patient that fatigue is indeed an important symptom. Educating the patient in energy conservation techniques or referring the patient to a physical therapy, occupational therapy, or pulmonary rehabilitation program may be helpful. In addition, guided exercise has been recently identified as a potential intervention for treating fatigue in cancer patients. This is an important area for research because few studies have been conducted, and only in select populations of patients with cancer.

Providing Psychological Support

Another important part of the nursing care of the patient with lung cancer is psychological support and identification of potential resources for the patient and family (Chart 24-16). Often, the nurse must help the patient and family deal with the following:

- The poor prognosis and relatively rapid progression of this disease
- Informed decision-making regarding the possible treatment options
- Methods to maintain the patient's quality of life during the course of this disease
- End-of-life treatment options

Gerontologic Considerations

At the time of diagnosis of lung cancer, most patients are older than 65 years of age and have stage III or IV disease (Gajra & Jatoi, 2014). Although age is not a significant prognostic factor for overall survival and response to treatment for either non–small cell or small cell lung cancer, older patients have specific needs. Depending on the comorbidities and functional status of older patients, chemotherapy agents, doses, and cycles may need to be adjusted to maintain quality of life. Issues that must be considered in care of older patients with lung cancer include functional status, comorbid conditions, nutritional status, cognition, concomitant medications, and psychological and social support.

CHART 24-16

Ethical Dilemma: Who Makes Difficult Health Care Decisions for Patients Who Lack Capacity?

Case Scenario

As a nurse working on a medical-surgical unit, you are caring for an 84-year-old woman with a history of emphysema and a new diagnosis of adenocarcinoma of the lung. She is a widow with two adult daughters, one of whom she resides with. The surgeon recommends a lobectomy for this patient to better control the disease. The patient has mild-to-moderate Alzheimer's disease and has recently lost 10 lb. She appears debilitated and frail. She has a history of tobacco abuse, and although she no longer smokes, the daughter she resides with smokes two packs of cigarettes per day. Because of her dementia, the patient is not considered to have mental capacity to sign informed consent for the lobectomy. The patient's daughter with whom she resides has informed the surgeon that she will not agree to sign surgical consent for a lobectomy. The daughter has asked to speak with you regarding her concerns. She tells you that she knows for certain that her mother would not want this surgery and would want to continue to live at home and not in a skilled nursing facility. She asks, "Who will take care of Mom after this? I have been told I need to stop smoking if she is going to continue to live with me after the surgery, but I don't see why I need to change my lifestyle. And she always said she would not want to go to a nursing home." The patient's other daughter agrees with the recommendation for a lobectomy and is willing to sign surgical consent. However, this daughter is estranged from her sister and has not had contact with her mother since she moved in with her sister 2 years ago. The patient does not have a designated health care surrogate or a medical power of attorney.

Discussion

This patient has been diagnosed with a life-threatening illness and needs surgical intervention for the control of the disease. She is unable to make medical decisions due to her dementia and lack of mental capacity. The patient's decision-making capacity is determined by the physician on the basis of a clinical assessment. End-of-life decision-making in patients who are terminally ill is complicated because ongoing quality of life must be examined. Although the lobectomy may prolong the patient's life, her loss of the ability to talk and care for herself may compromise her integrity. In the absence of a spouse, her adult daughters are now responsible to function as her health care surrogates since she has no advanced directive and has not appointed a medical power of attorney. She will be unable to care for herself at home postoperatively. Her daughters disagree regarding the recommended treatment plan. Yet, the patient is entitled to receive adequate and timely treatment of her illness and appropriate physical, psychological, and home care should she undergo this procedure.

Analysis

- Describe the ethical principles that are in conflict in this case (see Chart 3-3). Which principle should have preeminence in recommending the best treatment plan for the patient?
- What resources might be available in your hospital/community to help you, your professional colleagues (e.g., the multidisciplinary health care team), and the patient and her family determine what is in the patient's best interests?
- How can you advocate for a patient's autonomy when dementia is present? Is it possible to determine what the patient's wishes would be in this particular situation? Of those involved, who would be best able to make this type of determination?
- Compare and contrast the legal ramifications of an advanced directive and designated power of attorney in a situation where the patient is mentally competent and in a situation where the patient is mentally incompetent.
- For whom do you feel an obligation to advocate for in this situation—the patient, the daughter with whom the patient resides, the other daughter, or perhaps the surgeon? Does any one of these people merit your primary focus of concern, according to the American Nurses Association (2015) Code of Ethics?

References

American Nurses Association. (2015). Code of ethics for nurses with interpretive statements. Washington, DC: American Nurses Publishing, American Nurses Foundation/American Nurses Association.

Kepple, A. L., Azzam, P. N., Gopalan, P., et al. (2015). Decision-making capacity at the end of life. *Progress in Palliative Care*, *23*(3), 133–136.

Tumours of the Mediastinum

Tumours of the mediastinum include neurogenic tumours, tumours of the thymus, lymphomas, germ cell, cysts, and mesenchymal tumours. These tumours may be malignant or benign. These tumours are usually described in relation to location: anterior, middle, or posterior masses or tumours.

Clinical Manifestations

Nearly all symptoms of mediastinal tumours result from the pressure of the mass against important intrathoracic organs. Symptoms may include cough, wheezing, dyspnea, anterior chest or neck pain, bulging of the chest wall, heart palpitations, angina, other circulatory disturbances, central cyanosis, superior vena cava syndrome (i.e., swelling of the face, neck, and upper extremities), marked distention of the veins of the neck and the chest wall (evidence of the obstruction of large veins of the mediastinum by extravascular compression or intravascular invasion), and dysphagia and weight loss from pressure or invasion into the esophagus (Berry, 2015).

Assessment and Diagnostic Findings

Chest x-rays are the major method used initially to diagnose mediastinal tumours and cysts. CT scans are the gold standard for assessment of the mediastinum and surrounding structures. MRI may be used in some circumstances as well as PET scans (Berry, 2015; Thomas & Gould, 2015).

Medical Management

If the tumour is malignant and has infiltrated surrounding tissue, radiation therapy and/or chemotherapy are the therapeutic modalities used when complete surgical removal (discussed below) is not feasible.

Surgical Management

Many mediastinal tumours are benign and operable. The location of the tumour (anterior, middle, or posterior compartments) in the mediastinum dictates the type of incision. The common incision used is a median sternotomy; however, a thoracotomy may be used, depending on the location of the tumour. Additional approaches may include a bilateral anterior thoracotomy (clamshell incision) or video-assisted thoracoscopic surgery (see Chapter 26). The care is the same as for any patient undergoing thoracic surgery. The major complications include hemorrhage, injury to the phrenic or recurrent laryngeal nerve, and infection.

CHEST TRAUMA

Major chest trauma may occur alone or in combination with multiple other injuries. Chest trauma is classified as either blunt or penetrating. Blunt chest trauma results from sudden compression or positive pressure inflicted to the chest wall. Penetrating trauma occurs when a foreign object penetrates the chest wall.

Blunt Trauma

Overall, blunt thoracic injuries are directly responsible for 20% to 25% of all trauma deaths (Mancini, 2014). Although blunt chest trauma is more common than penetrating trauma, it is often difficult to identify the extent of the damage because the symptoms may be generalized and vague. In addition, patients may not seek immediate medical attention, which may complicate the problem.

Pathophysiology

The most common causes of blunt chest trauma are motor vehicle crashes (trauma from steering wheel, seat belt), falls, and bicycle crashes (trauma from handlebars). Mechanisms of blunt chest trauma include acceleration (moving object hitting the chest or patient being thrown into an object), deceleration (sudden decrease in rate of speed or velocity, such as a motor vehicle crash), shearing (stretching forces to areas of the chest causing tears, ruptures, or dissections), and compression (direct blow to the chest, such as a crush injury). Injuries to the chest are often life-threatening and result in one or more of the following pathologic states:

- Hypoxemia from disruption of the airway; injury to the lung parenchyma, rib cage, and respiratory musculature; massive hemorrhage; collapsed lung; and pneumothorax
- Hypovolemia from massive fluid loss from the great vessels, cardiac rupture, or hemothorax
- Cardiac failure from cardiac tamponade, cardiac contusion, or increased intrathoracic pressure

These pathologic states frequently result in impaired ventilation and perfusion leading to ARF, hypovolemic shock, and death.

Assessment and Diagnostic Findings

Since time is critical in treating patients with a traumatic chest injury, it is essential to assess the patient immediately to determine the following: when the injury occurred, mechanism of injury, level of responsiveness, specific injuries, estimated blood loss, recent drug or alcohol use, and prehospital treatment.

The initial assessment of thoracic injuries includes assessment of the patient for airway obstruction, **tension pneumothorax**, open pneumothorax, massive hemothorax, flail chest, and cardiac tamponade (Bernardin & Troquet, 2013). These injuries are life-threatening and need immediate treatment. Secondary assessment would include simple pneumothorax, hemothorax, pulmonary contusion, traumatic aortic rupture, tracheobronchial disruption, esophageal perforation, traumatic diaphragmatic injury, and penetrating wounds to the mediastinum. Although listed as secondary, these injuries may be life-threatening as well, depending on the circumstances.

The physical examination includes inspection of the airway, thorax, neck veins, and breathing difficulty. Specifics include assessing the rate and depth of breathing for abnormalities, such as stridor, cyanosis, nasal flaring, use of accessory muscles, drooling, and overt trauma to the face, mouth, or neck. The chest should be assessed for symmetric movement, symmetry of breath sounds, open chest wounds, entrance or exit wounds, impaled objects, tracheal shift, distended neck veins, subcutaneous emphysema, and paradoxical chest wall motion. In addition, the chest wall should be assessed for bruising, petechiae, lacerations, and burns. The vital signs and skin colour are assessed for signs of shock. The thorax is palpated for tenderness and crepitus; the position of the trachea is also assessed.

The initial diagnostic workup includes a chest x-ray, CT scan, complete blood count, clotting studies, type and cross-match, electrolytes, oxygen saturation, arterial blood gas analysis, and ECG. The patient is completely undressed to avoid missing additional injuries that can complicate care. Many patients with injuries involving the chest have associated head and abdominal injuries that require attention. Ongoing assessment is essential to monitor the patient's response to treatment and to detect early signs of clinical deterioration.

Medical Management

The goals of treatment are to evaluate the patient's condition and to initiate aggressive resuscitation. An airway is immediately established with oxygen support and, in some cases, intubation and ventilatory support. Reestablishing fluid volume and negative intrapleural pressure and draining intrapleural fluid and blood are essential.

The potential for massive blood loss and exsanguination with blunt or penetrating chest injuries is high because of injury to the great blood vessels. Many patients die at the scene or are in shock by the time help arrives. Agitation and irrational and combative behaviour are signs of decreased oxygen delivery to the cerebral cortex. Strategies to restore and maintain cardiopulmonary function include ensuring an adequate airway and ventilation, stabilizing and reestablishing chest wall integrity, occluding any opening into the chest (open pneumothorax), and draining or removing any air or fluid from the thorax to relieve pneumothorax, hemothorax, or cardiac tamponade. Hypovolemia and low cardiac output must be corrected. Many of these treatment efforts, along with the control of hemorrhage, are usually carried out simultaneously at the scene of the injury or in the emergency department. Depending on the success of efforts to control the hemorrhage in the emergency department, the patient may be taken immediately to the operating room. Principles of management are essentially those pertaining to care of the postoperative thoracic patient (see Chapter 26).

Sternal and Rib Fractures

Sternal fractures are most common in motor vehicle crashes with a direct blow to the sternum via the steering wheel. Rib fractures are the most common type of chest trauma and are associated with considerable morbidity and mortality (Mancini, 2014). Most rib fractures are benign and are treated conservatively. Fractures of the first three ribs are rare but can result in a high mortality rate because they are associated with laceration of the subclavian artery or vein. The fifth through ninth ribs are the most common sites of fractures. Fractures of the lower ribs are associated with injury to the spleen and liver, which may be lacerated by fragmented sections of the rib. Older adult patients with three or more rib fractures have been shown to have a fivefold increased mortality rate and a fourfold increased incidence of pneumonia (Mancini, 2014).

Clinical Manifestations

The patient with sternal fractures has anterior chest pain, overlying tenderness, ecchymosis, crepitus, swelling, and the potential of a chest wall deformity. For the patient with rib fractures, clinical manifestations are similar: severe pain, point tenderness, and muscle spasm over the area of the fracture that is aggravated by coughing, deep breathing, and movement. The area around the fracture may be bruised. To reduce the pain, the patient splints the chest by breathing in a shallow manner and avoids sighs, deep breaths, coughing, and movement. This reluctance to move or breathe deeply results in diminished ventilation, collapse of unaerated alveoli (atelectasis), pneumonitis, and hypoxemia. Respiratory insufficiency and failure can be the outcomes of such a cycle.

Assessment and Diagnostic Findings

The patient with a sternal fracture must be closely evaluated for underlying cardiac injuries. A crackling, grating sound in the thorax (subcutaneous crepitus) may be detected with auscultation. The diagnostic workup may include a chest x-ray, rib films of a specific area, ECG, continuous pulse oximetry, and arterial blood gas analysis.

Medical Management

Medical management of the patient with a sternal fracture is directed toward controlling pain, avoiding excessive activity, and treating any associated injuries. Surgical fixation is rarely necessary unless fragments are grossly displaced and pose a potential for further injury.

The goals of treatment for rib fractures are to control pain and to detect and treat the injury. Sedation is used to relieve pain and to allow deep breathing and coughing. Care must be taken to avoid over sedation and suppression of the respiratory drive. Alternative strategies to relieve pain include an intercostal nerve block and ice over the fracture site; a chest binder may decrease pain on movement. The patient is instructed to apply the binder snugly enough to provide support but not enough to impair respiratory excursion. Usually, the pain abates in 5 to 7 days, and discomfort can be controlled with epidural analgesia, patient-controlled analgesia, or nonopioid analgesia. Most rib fractures heal in 3 to 6 weeks. The patient is monitored closely for signs and symptoms of associated injuries.

Flail Chest

Flail chest is frequently a complication of blunt chest trauma from a steering wheel injury. It usually occurs when three or more adjacent ribs (multiple contiguous ribs) are fractured at two or more sites, resulting in free-floating rib segments. It may also result as a combination fracture of ribs and costal cartilages or sternum. As a result, the chest wall loses stability, and there is subsequent respiratory impairment and usually severe respiratory distress.

Pathophysiology

During inspiration, as the chest expands, the detached part of the rib segment (flail segment) moves in a paradoxical manner (pendelluft movement) in that it is pulled inward during inspiration, reducing the amount of air that can be drawn into the lungs. On expiration, because the intrathoracic pressure exceeds atmospheric pressure, the flail segment bulges outward, impairing the patient's ability to exhale. The mediastinum then shifts back to the affected side (Fig. 24-7). This paradoxical action results in increased dead space, a reduction in alveolar ventilation, and decreased compliance. Retained airway secretions and atelectasis frequently accompany flail chest. The patient has hypoxemia, and if gas exchange is greatly compromised, respiratory acidosis develops as a result of carbon dioxide retention. Hypotension, inadequate tissue perfusion, and metabolic acidosis often follow as the paradoxical motion of the mediastinum decreases cardiac output.

Medical Management

As with rib fracture, treatment of flail chest is usually supportive. Management includes providing ventilatory support, clearing secretions from the lungs, and controlling pain. The specific management depends on the degree of respiratory dysfunction. If only a small segment of the

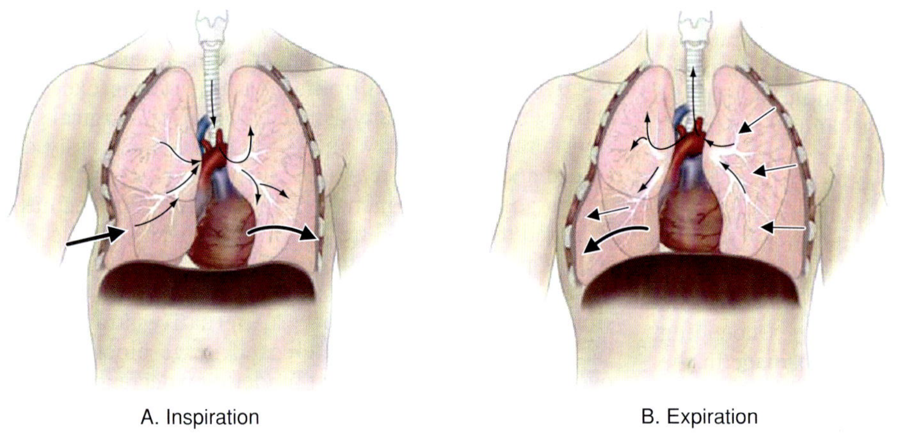

FIGURE 24-7. Flail chest is caused by a free-floating segment of rib cage resulting from multiple rib fractures. **A.** Inspiration. Paradoxical movement on inspiration occurs when the flail rib segment is sucked inward and the mediastinal structures shift to the unaffected side. The amount of air drawn into the affected lung is reduced. **B.** Expiration. On expiration, the flail segment bulges outward, and the mediastinal structures shift back to the affected side.

chest is involved, the objectives are to clear the airway through positioning, coughing, deep breathing, and suctioning to aid in the expansion of the lung and to relieve pain by intercostal nerve blocks, high thoracic epidural blocks, or cautious use of IV opioids.

For mild-to-moderate flail chest injuries, the underlying pulmonary contusion is treated by monitoring fluid intake and appropriate fluid replacement while at the same time relieving chest pain. Pulmonary physiotherapy focusing on lung volume expansion and secretion management techniques is performed. The patient is closely monitored for further respiratory compromise.

For severe flail chest injury, endotracheal intubation and mechanical ventilation are required to provide internal pneumatic stabilization of the flail chest and to correct abnormalities in gas exchange. This helps to treat the underlying pulmonary contusion, serves to stabilize the thoracic cage to allow the fractures to heal, and improves alveolar ventilation and intrathoracic volume by decreasing the work of breathing. This treatment modality requires endotracheal intubation and ventilator support. Differing modes of ventilation are used depending on the patient's underlying disease and specific needs.

In rare circumstances, surgery may be required to more quickly stabilize the flail segment. This may be used in the patient who is difficult to ventilate or the high-risk patient with underlying lung disease who may be difficult to wean from mechanical ventilation.

Regardless of the type of treatment, the patient is carefully monitored by serial chest x-rays, arterial blood gas analysis, pulse oximetry, and bedside pulmonary function monitoring. Pain management is key to successful treatment. Patient-controlled analgesia, intercostal nerve blocks, epidural analgesia, and intrapleural administration of opioids may be used to control thoracic pain.

Pulmonary Contusion

A pulmonary contusion involves injury to the alveolar capillaries, resulting in accumulation of blood and other fluids within the lung tissue (Ganie et al., 2013). Due to the accumulation of excess fluid, gas exchange is impaired thus leading to hypoxia (Ganie et al., 2013).

Pulmonary contusion is associated with chest trauma when there is rapid compression and decompression to the chest wall (i.e., blunt trauma). It represents a spectrum of lung injury characterized by the development of infiltrates and various degrees of respiratory dysfunction and sometimes respiratory failure. A contusion is sustained in 30% to 70% of patients who experience blunt force trauma. Pulmonary contusion may not be evident initially on examination but develops in the posttraumatic period; it may involve a small portion of one lung, a massive section of a lung, one entire lung, or both lungs. Thoracic injury and complications that follow account for up to 25% of blunt trauma mortality (Simon et al., 2012).

Pathophysiology

The primary pathologic defect is an abnormal accumulation of fluid in the interstitial and intra-alveolar spaces. It is thought that injury to the lung parenchyma and its capillary network results in a leakage of serum protein and plasma. The leaking serum protein exerts an osmotic pressure that enhances loss of fluid from the capillaries. Blood, edema, and cellular debris (from cellular response to injury) enter the lung and accumulate in the bronchioles and alveolar surface, where they interfere with gas exchange. An increase in pulmonary vascular resistance and pulmonary artery pressure occurs. The patient has hypoxemia and carbon dioxide retention.

Clinical Manifestations

Pulmonary contusion may be mild, moderate, or severe. The clinical manifestations vary from tachypnea, tachycardia, pleuritic chest pain, hypoxemia, and blood-tinged secretions to more severe tachypnea, tachycardia, crackles, frank bleeding, severe hypoxemia, and respiratory acidosis. Changes in sensorium, including increased agitation or combative irrational behaviour, may be signs of hypoxemia.

In addition, the patient with moderate pulmonary contusion has a large amount of mucus, serum, and frank blood in the tracheobronchial tree; the patient often has a constant cough but cannot clear the secretions. A patient with severe pulmonary contusion has the signs and symptoms of ARDS; these may include central cyanosis, agitation, combativeness, and productive cough with frothy, bloody secretions.

Assessment and Diagnostic Findings

The efficiency of gas exchange is determined by pulse oximetry and arterial blood gas measurements. Pulse oximetry is also used to measure oxygen saturation continuously. The initial chest x-ray may show no changes; changes may not appear for 1 or 2 days after the injury and appear as pulmonary infiltrates on chest x-ray.

Medical Management

Treatment priorities include maintaining the airway, providing adequate oxygenation, and controlling pain. In mild pulmonary contusion, adequate hydration via IV fluids and oral intake is important to mobilize secretions. However, fluid intake must be closely monitored to avoid hypervolemia. Volume expansion techniques, postural drainage, physiotherapy including coughing, and endotracheal suctioning are used to remove the secretions. Pain is managed by intercostal nerve blocks or by opioids via patient-controlled analgesia or other methods. Usually, antimicrobial therapy is administered because the damaged lung is susceptible to infection. Supplemental oxygen is usually given by mask or cannula for 24 to 36 hours.

The patient with moderate pulmonary contusion may require bronchoscopy to remove secretions; intubation and mechanical ventilation with PEEP (see Chapter 26) may also be necessary to maintain the pressure and keep the lungs inflated. Diuretics may be given to reduce edema. A nasogastric tube is inserted to relieve gastrointestinal distention.

The patient with severe contusion may develop respiratory failure and may require aggressive treatment with endotracheal intubation and ventilatory support, diuretics, and fluid restriction. Colloids and crystalloid solutions may be used to treat hypovolemia.

Antimicrobial medications may be prescribed for the treatment of pulmonary infection. This is a common complication of pulmonary contusion (especially pneumonia in the contused segment) because the fluid and blood that extravasate into the alveolar and interstitial spaces serve as an excellent culture medium.

Penetrating Trauma: Stab and Gunshot Wounds

Any organ or structure within the chest is potentially susceptible to traumatic penetration. These organs include the chest wall, lung and pleura, tracheobronchial system, esophagus, diaphragm, and major thoracic blood vessels, as well as heart and other mediastinal structures. The clinical consequence of penetrating trauma to the chest depends on the mechanism of injury, location, associated injuries, and underlying illnesses (Shahani, 2015). Common injuries include pneumothorax and cardiac tamponade.

Stab and gunshot wounds are the most common types of penetrating chest trauma. They are classified according to their velocity. Stab wounds are generally considered of low velocity because the weapon destroys a small area around the wound. Knives and switchblades cause most stab wounds. The appearance of the external wound may be very deceptive, because pneumothorax, hemothorax, lung contusion, and cardiac tamponade, along with severe and continuing hemorrhage, can occur from any small wound, even one caused by a small-diameter instrument such as an ice pick.

Gunshot wounds to the chest may be classified as of low, medium, or high velocity. The factors that determine the velocity and resulting extent of damage include the distance from which the gun was fired, the calibre of the gun, and construction and size of the bullet. A gunshot wound can produce a variety of pathophysiologic changes. A bullet can cause damage at the site of penetration and along its pathway. It also may ricochet off bony structures and damage the chest organs and great vessels. If the diaphragm is involved in either a gunshot wound or a stab wound, injury to the chest cavity must be considered.

Medical Management

The objective of immediate management is to restore and maintain cardiopulmonary function. After an adequate airway is ensured and ventilation is established, the patient is examined for shock and intrathoracic and intra-abdominal injuries. The patient is undressed completely so that additional injuries will not be missed. There is a high risk for associated intra-abdominal injuries with stab wounds below the level of the fifth anterior intercostal space. Death can result from exsanguinating hemorrhage or intra-abdominal sepsis.

The diagnostic workup includes a chest x-ray, chemistry profile, arterial blood gas analysis, pulse oximetry, and ECG. Blood typing and cross-matching are done in case blood transfusion is required. After the status of the peripheral pulses is assessed, a large-bore IV line is inserted. An indwelling catheter is inserted to monitor urinary output. A nasogastric tube is inserted to prevent aspiration, minimize leakage of abdominal contents, and decompress the gastrointestinal tract.

Shock is treated simultaneously with colloid solutions, crystalloids, or blood, as indicated by the patient's condition. Chest x-rays are obtained, and other diagnostic procedures are carried out as dictated by the needs of the patient (e.g., CT scans of chest or abdomen, flat plate x-ray of the abdomen, abdominal tap to check for bleeding).

A chest tube is inserted into the pleural space in most patients with penetrating wounds of the chest to achieve rapid and continuing reexpansion of the lungs. The insertion of the chest tube frequently results in a complete evacuation of the blood and air. The chest tube also allows early recognition of continuing intrathoracic bleeding, which would make surgical exploration necessary. If the patient has a penetrating wound of the heart and great vessels, the esophagus, or the tracheobronchial tree, surgical intervention is required.

Pneumothorax

Pneumothorax occurs when the parietal or visceral pleura is breached, and the pleural space is exposed to positive atmospheric pressure. Normally, the pressure in the pleural space is negative or subatmospheric compared with atmospheric pressure; this negative pressure is required to maintain lung inflation. When either pleura is breached, air enters the pleural space, and the lung or a portion of it collapses. Types of pneumothorax include simple, traumatic, and tension pneumothorax.

Types of Pneumothorax

Types of pneumothorax include simple, traumatic, and tension pneumothorax.

Simple Pneumothorax

A simple, or spontaneous, pneumothorax occurs when air enters the pleural space through a breach of either the parietal or visceral pleura. Most commonly, this occurs as air enters the pleural space through the rupture of a bleb or a bronchopleural fistula. A spontaneous pneumothorax may occur in an apparently healthy person in the absence of trauma due to rupture of an air-filled bleb, or blister, on the surface of the lung, allowing air from the airways to enter the pleural cavity. It may be associated with diffuse interstitial lung disease and severe emphysema.

Traumatic Pneumothorax

Traumatic pneumothorax occurs when air escapes from a laceration in the lung itself and enters the pleural space or enters the pleural space through a wound in the chest wall. It can occur with blunt trauma (e.g., rib fractures) or penetrating chest trauma. It may also occur from abdominal trauma (e.g., stab or gunshot wounds to the abdomen) and from diaphragmatic tears. Traumatic pneumothorax may occur with invasive thoracic procedures (i.e., thoracentesis, transbronchial lung biopsy, insertion of a subclavian line) in which the pleura is inadvertently punctured or with barotrauma from mechanical ventilation.

Traumatic pneumothorax resulting from major injury to the chest is often accompanied by hemothorax (collection of blood in the pleural space resulting from torn intercostal vessels, lacerations of the great vessels, and lacerations of the lungs). Often, both blood and air are found in the chest cavity (hemopneumothorax) after major trauma. Chest surgery can cause what is classified as a traumatic pneumothorax as a result of the entry into the pleural space and the accumulation of air and fluid in the pleural space.

Open pneumothorax is one form of traumatic pneumothorax. It occurs when a wound in the chest wall is large enough to allow air to pass freely in and out of the thoracic cavity with each attempted respiration. Because the rush of air through the hole in the chest wall produces a sucking sound, such injuries are termed *sucking chest wounds*. In such patients, not only does the lung collapse, but the structures of the mediastinum (heart and great vessels) also shift toward the uninjured side with each inspiration and in the opposite direction with expiration. This is termed *mediastinal flutter* or *mediastinal swing*, and it produces serious circulatory problems.

NURSING ALERT

Traumatic open pneumothorax calls for emergency interventions. Stopping the flow of air through the opening in the chest wall is a lifesaving measure.

Tension Pneumothorax

A tension pneumothorax occurs when air is drawn into the pleural space from a lacerated lung or through a small hole in the chest wall. It may be a complication of other types of pneumothorax. In contrast to open pneumothorax, the air that enters the chest cavity with each inspiration is trapped; it cannot be expelled during expiration through the air passages or the hole in the chest wall. In effect, a one-way valve or ball valve mechanism occurs where air enters the pleural space but cannot escape. With each breath, tension (positive pressure) is increased within the affected pleural space. This causes the lung to collapse and the heart, the great vessels, and the trachea to shift toward the unaffected side of the chest (mediastinal shift). Both respiration and circulatory function are compromised because of the increased intrathoracic pressure. The increased intrathoracic pressure decreases venous return to the heart, causing decreased cardiac output and impairment of peripheral circulation.

Clinical Manifestations

The signs and symptoms associated with pneumothorax depend on its size and cause. Pain is usually sudden and may be pleuritic. The patient may have only minimal respiratory distress with slight chest discomfort and tachypnea with a small simple or uncomplicated pneumothorax. If the pneumothorax is large and the lung collapses totally, acute respiratory distress occurs. The patient is anxious, has dyspnea and air hunger, has increased use of the accessory muscles, and may develop central cyanosis from severe hypoxemia.

In assessing the chest for any type of pneumothorax, the nurse assesses tracheal alignment, expansion of the chest, breath sounds, and percussion of the chest. In a simple pneumothorax, the trachea is midline, expansion of the chest is decreased, breath sounds may be diminished, and percussion of the chest may reveal normal sounds or hyperresonance, depending on the size of the pneumothorax.

In a tension pneumothorax, the trachea is shifted away from the affected side, chest expansion may be decreased or fixed in a hyper expansion state, breath sounds are diminished or absent, and percussion to the affected side is hyperresonant. The clinical picture is one of air hunger, agitation, increasing hypoxemia, central cyanosis, hypotension, tachycardia, and profuse diaphoresis. Figure 24-8 compares open and tension pneumothorax.

NURSING ALERT

Relief of tension pneumothorax is considered an emergency measure.

Medical Management

Medical management of pneumothorax depends on its cause and severity. The goal of treatment is to evacuate the air or blood from the pleural space. A small chest tube (28 French) is inserted near the second intercostal space;

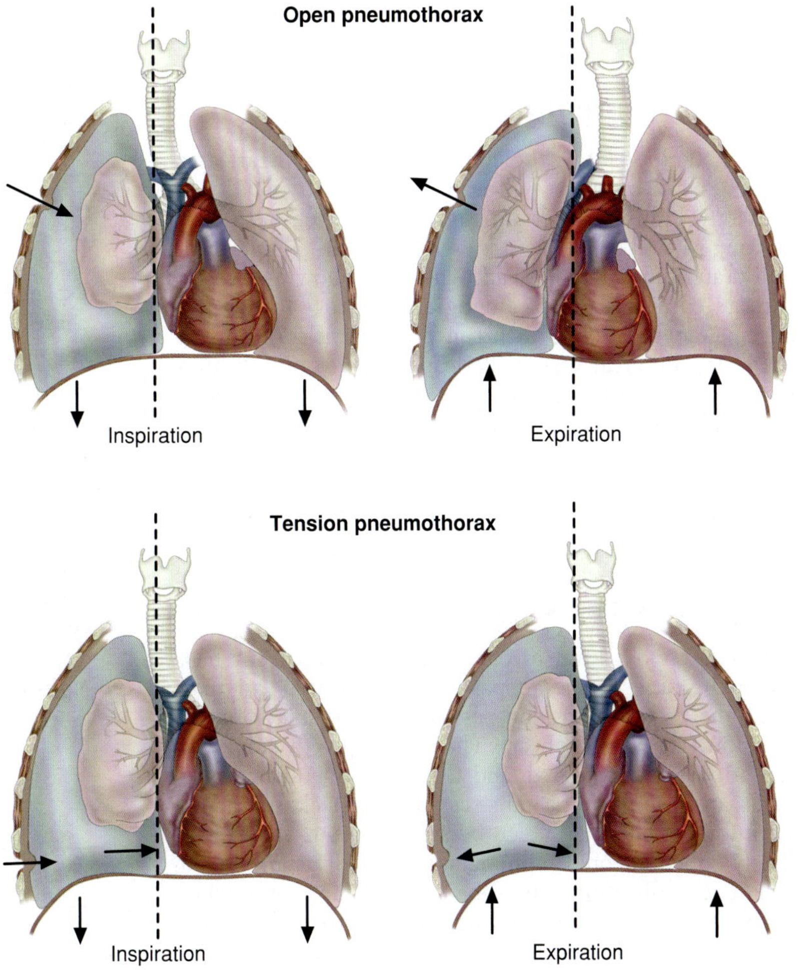

FIGURE 24-8. Open pneumothorax **(top)** and tension pneumothorax **(bottom)**. In open pneumothorax, air enters the chest during inspiration and exits during expiration. A slight shift of the affected lung may occur because of a decrease in pressure as air moves out of the chest. In tension pneumothorax, air enters but cannot leave the chest. As the pressure increases, the heart and great vessels are compressed, and the mediastinal structures are shifted toward the opposite side of the chest. The trachea is pushed from its normal midline position toward the opposite side of the chest, and the unaffected lung is compressed.

this space is used because it is the thinnest part of the chest wall, minimizes the danger of contacting the thoracic nerve, and leaves a less visible scar. If the patient also has a hemothorax, a large-diameter chest tube (32 French or greater) is inserted, usually in the fourth or fifth intercostal space at the midaxillary line. The tube is directed posteriorly to drain the fluid and air. Once the chest tube or tubes are inserted and suction is applied (usually to 20 mm Hg suction), effective decompression of the pleural cavity (drainage of blood or air) occurs.

If an excessive amount of blood enters the chest tube in a relatively short period, an autotransfusion may be needed. This technique involves taking the patient's own blood that has been drained from the chest, filtering it, and then transfusing it back into the patient's vascular system.

In such an emergency, anything may be used that is large enough to fill the chest wound—a towel, a handkerchief, or the heel of the hand. If conscious, the patient is instructed to inhale and strain against a closed glottis. This action assists in reexpanding the lung and ejecting the air from the thorax. In the hospital, the opening is plugged by sealing it with gauze impregnated with petrolatum. A pressure dressing is applied. Usually, a chest tube connected to water-seal drainage is inserted to permit air and fluid to drain. Antibiotics usually are prescribed to combat infection from contamination.

The severity of open pneumothorax depends on the amount and rate of thoracic bleeding and the amount of air in the pleural space. The pleural cavity can be decompressed by needle aspiration (thoracentesis) or chest tube drainage of the blood or air. The lung is then able to reexpand and resume the function of gas exchange. As a rule of thumb, the chest wall is opened surgically (thoracotomy) when more than 1,500 mL of blood is aspirated initially by thoracentesis (or is the initial chest tube output) or when chest tube output continues at greater than 200 mL/hr (Shahani, 2015). The urgency with which the blood must be removed is determined by the respiratory compromise. An emergency thoracotomy may also be performed in the emergency department if there is suggested cardiovascular injury secondary to chest or penetrating trauma. The patient with a possible tension pneumothorax should immediately be given a high concentration of supplemental oxygen to treat the hypoxemia, and pulse oximetry should be used to monitor oxygen saturation. In an emergency situation, a tension pneumothorax can be decompressed or quickly converted to a simple pneumothorax by inserting a large-bore needle (14 gauge) at the second intercostal space, midclavicular line on the affected side. This relieves the pressure and vents the positive pressure to the external environment. A chest tube is then inserted and connected to suction to remove the remaining air and fluid, reestablish the negative pressure, and reexpand the lung. If the lung reexpands and air leakage from the lung parenchyma stops, further drainage may be unnecessary. If a prolonged air leak continues despite chest tube drainage to underwater seal, surgery may be necessary to close the leak.

Cardiac Tamponade

Cardiac tamponade is the compression of the heart as a result of fluid within the pericardial sac. It usually is caused by blunt or penetrating trauma to the chest. A penetrating wound of the heart is associated with a high mortality rate. Cardiac tamponade also may follow diagnostic cardiac catheterization, angiographic procedures, and pacemaker insertion, which can produce perforations of the heart and great vessels. Pericardial effusion with fluid compressing the heart also may develop from metastases to the pericardium from malignant tumours of the breast, lung, and mediastinum and may occur with lymphomas and leukemias, renal failure, TB, and high-dose radiation to the chest. Cardiac tamponade is discussed in detail in Chapter 31.

Subcutaneous Emphysema

No matter what kind of chest trauma the patient has, when the lung or the air passages are injured, air may enter the tissue planes and pass for some distance under the skin (e.g., neck, chest). The tissues give a crackling sensation when palpated, and the subcutaneous air produces an alarming appearance as the face, neck, body, and scrotum become misshapen by subcutaneous air. Fortunately, subcutaneous emphysema is by itself usually not a serious complication. The subcutaneous air is spontaneously absorbed if the underlying air leak is treated or stops spontaneously. In severe cases in which there is widespread subcutaneous emphysema, a tracheostomy is indicated if airway patency is threatened.

Critical Thinking Exercises

1 Your patient, a 44-year-old unemployed man who lives with his 80-year-old mother, has recently been diagnosed with active TB. He has been started on treatment and given specific instructions about his medications. What strategies would you initiate to be sure that he takes his medications correctly? What strategies would you use to ensure that his mother is not infected? How would your care differ if the patient lived alone or were homeless?

2 You are working on a surgical unit. Your patient is a 67-year-old woman who has had surgery to repair a fractured hip that occurred following a fall associated with heavy alcohol use. She has been a heavy smoker for over 35 years and is reluctant to move in bed because of pain. What are the potential postoperative pulmonary complications? What assessment criteria would you use to assess her respiratory status? What interventions would you implement to prevent pulmonary complications in this patient? What changes, if any, would you implement if she had a history of deep vein thrombosis?

3 Your patient has experienced blunt chest trauma following a motor vehicle crash. A chest tube has been inserted to treat a pneumothorax. The chest drainage system has drained 400 mL of light-red fluid during the first 6 hours following the tube's insertion. The patient is unable to recall how he was injured or what has happened to him over the last 24 hours. The patient is experiencing pain requiring opioids and is asking that the chest tube be removed to enable him to walk to the bathroom. What additional information would you obtain through assessment, and what actions would you take? How would you explain to the patient and his family the purpose of the chest tubes? How would you modify your explanation and teaching if he has little understanding of English?

4 You are caring for an 82-year-old woman who was recently transferred to the hospital from a nursing home with the diagnosis of presumed nursing home-acquired pneumonia. She has a nasogastric feeding tube in place and is lethargic, dehydrated, and confused. What strategies would you initiate to prevent aspiration? What nursing care interventions would you use to assess for aspiration? What is the evidence base for the interventions that you consider? How will you evaluate the strength of the evidence? What suggestions might you have regarding appropriate devices for long-term enteral feeding in this patient once she is discharged back to the nursing home?

REFERENCES AND SELECTED READINGS

Books

Gilbert, D. N., Chambers, H. F., Eliopoulos, G. M., et al. (2015). *The Sanford guide to antimicrobial therapy 2015* (45th ed.). Sperryville, VA: Antimicrobial Therapy, Inc.

Weinberger, S. E., Cockrill, B. A., & Mandel, J. (2014). *Principles of pulmonary medicine* (6th ed.). Philadelphia, PA: Elsevier Saunders.

Journals and Electronic Documents

Amanullah, S. (2015). Ventilator-associated pneumonia overview of nosocomial pneumonias. *Medscape*. Last updated December 31, 2015. Retrieved from emedicine.medscape.com/article/304836overview

American Association of Critical Care Nurses (AACN). (2016). AACN practice alert: Prevention of aspiration in adults. *Critical Care Nurse, 36*(1), e20–e24.

American Cancer Society (ACS). (2016). *Learn about cancer: Lung cancer*. Last updated February 8, 2016. Retrieved from www.cancer.org/cancer/lungcancer/index

American College of Surgeons. (2015). *National trauma data bank 2015—annual report*. Retrieved from www.facs.org/quality-programs/trauma/ntdb/docpub

Aoki, F. Y., Allen, U. D., Stiver, H. G., et al. (2013). The use of antiviral drugs for influenza: Guidelines for practitioners 2012/2013. *Canadian Journal of Infectious Diseases & Medical Microbiology, 24*(1), 12.

Augenbraun, M. H. (2014). Pneumonia in immunocompromised patients. *eMedicine/Medscape*. Last updated November 13, 2014. Retrieved from emedicine.medscape.com/article/807846-overview

Baer, S. (2017). *Community-Acquired Pneumonia (CAP)*. Retrieved from https://emedicine.medscape.com/article/234240-overview

Bernardin, B., & Troquet, J. M. (2012). Initial management and resuscitation of severe chest trauma. *Emergency Medicine Clinics, 30*(2), 377–400.

Bartlett, J. G. (2014). *Lung abscess*. Retrieved from www.uptodate.com/contents/lung-abscess

Bartlett, J. (2015). *Aspiration pneumonia in adults*. Retrieved from www.uptodate.com/contents/aspiration-pneumonia-in-adults

Berry, M. F. (2015). *Evaluation of mediastinal masses*. Retrieved from www.uptodate.com/contents/evaluation-of-mediastinal-masses

Canadian Cancer Society. (n.d.). *Risk factors for lung cancer*. Retrieved from http://www.cancer.ca/en/cancer-information/cancer-type/lung/risks/?region=on#ixzz5JjQIqf17

Canadian Cancer Society. (2017). *Lung cancer statistics*. Retrieved from http://www.cancer.ca/en/cancer-information/cancer-type/lung/statistics/?region=on#ixzz5JjM1Ro00 (2017)

Canadian Liver Foundation. (n.d.). *Sarcoidosis*. Retrieved from https://www.liver.ca/patients-caregivers/liver-diseases/sarcoidosis/

Canadian Patient Safety Institute. (2016). *Ventilator-associated pneumonia (VAP)*. Retrieved from http://www.patientsafetyinstitute.ca/en/Topic/Pages/Ventilator-Associated-Pneumonia-(VAP).aspx

Cassidy, M. R., Rosenkranz, P., McCabe, K., Rosen, J. E., & McAneny, D. (2013). I COUGH: reducing postoperative pulmonary complications with a multidisciplinary patient care program. *JAMA surgery, 148*(8), 740–745.

CDC. (2018). Retrieved from https://www.cdc.gov/pneumonia/index.html

Conde, M. V., & Adams, S. G. (2015). Overview of the management of postoperative pulmonary complications. UpToDate. Last updated October 13, 2015. Retrieved from www.uptodate.com/contents/overview-of-the-management-of-postoperative-pulmonary-complications?source=search_result&search=Overview+of+the+management+of+postoperative+pulmonary+complications&selectedTitle=1~150

CTS & PHAC. (2013). Retrieved from http://www.phac-aspc.gc.ca/tbpc-latb/pubs/tb-canada-7/assets/pdf/tb-standards-tb-normes-ch15-eng.pdf

Culver, D. A. (2012). Sarcoidosis. *Immunology and Allergy Clinics of North America, 32*, 487–511.

Cunha, B. A. (2015). Community-acquired pneumonia. *eMedicine/Medscape*. Retrieved from emedicine.medscape.com/article/234240-overview

Echevarria, I. M., & Schwoebel, A. (2012). Development of an intervention model for the prevention of aspiration pneumonia in high-risk patients on a medical-surgical unit. *Medsurg Nursing, 21*(5), 303–308.

Evans, M. (2013). Lung cancer: Needs assessment, treatment and therapies. *British Journal of Nursing, 22*(17), S15–S22.

File, T. M. (2016). *Treatment of hospital-acquired, ventilator-associated and healthcare-associated pneumonia in adults*. Retrieved from www.uptodate.com/contents/treatment-of-hospital-acquired-ventilator-associated-and-healthcare-associated-pneumonia-in-adults?source=search_result&search=Treatment+of+hospital-acquired%2C+ventilator-associated+and+healthcare-associated+pneumonia+in+adults&selectedTitle=1~150

Gajra, A., & Jatoi, A. (2014). Non–small-cell lung cancer in elderly patients: a discussion of treatment options. *Journal of Clinical Oncology, 32*(24), 2562–2569.

Ganie, F., Lone, H., Lone, G., et al. (2013). Lung contusion: A clinico-pathological entity with unpredictable clinical course. *Bulletin of Emergency and Trauma, 1*(1), 7–16.

GBD 2013 Mortality and Causes of Death Collaborators. (2015). Global, regional, and national age-sex specific all-cause and cause-specific mortality for 240 causes of death, 1990–2013: A systematic analysis for the Global Burden of Disease Study 2013. *Lancet, 385*, 117–171.

Hariprashad, A., & Rizzolo, D. (2013). Acute respiratory distress syndrome: An overview for physician assistants. *Journal of the American Academy of Physician Assistants*, 26(9), 23–28.

Heffner, J. E. (2015a). Diagnostic evaluation of pleural effusion in adults: Initial testing. UpToDate. Last updated December 2, 2015. Retrieved from www.uptodate.com/contents/diagnostic-evaluation-of-a-pleural-effusion-in-adults-initial-testing?source=search_result&search=Diagnostic+evaluation+of+pleural+effusion+in+adults%3A+Initial+testing&selectedTitle=1~150

Heffner, J. E. (2015b). Chemical pleurodesis. UpToDate. Last updated April 7, 2015. Retrieved from www.uptodate.com/contents/chemical-pleurodesis?source=search_result&search=Heffner+Chemical+Pleurodesis&selectedTitle=1~56

Hopkins, W., & Rubin, L. (2016). *Treatment of pulmonary hypertension in adults*. Retrieved from www.uptodate.com/contents/treatment-of-pulmonary-hypertension-in-adults?source=search_result&search=Overview+of+pulmonary+hypertension+in+adults&selectedTitle=2~150

Hull, R. D., Merali, T., Mills, A., et al. (2013). Venous thromboembolism in elderly high-risk medical patients: Time course of events and influence of risk factors. *Clinical and Applied Thrombosis/Hemostasis, 19*(4), 357–362.

Jain, S., Self, W. H., Wunderink, R. G., et al. (2015). CDC EPIC Study Team. Community-acquired pneumonia requiring hospitalization among US adults. *New England Journal of Medicine*, 373(5), 415–427.

Kahn, S. R., Lim, W., & Dunn, A. S. (2012). Prevention of VTE in nonsurgical patients: Antithrombotic therapy and prevention of thrombosis 9th ed. American College of Chest Physicians Evidence-Based Clinical Practice Guidelines. *Chest, 141*(Suppl 2), e195S–e226S.

Kalemkerian, G. P., & Gadgeel, S. M. (2013). Modern staging of small cell lung cancer. *Journal of the National Comprehensive Cancer Network, 11*(1), 99–104.

Kearon, C., Aki, E. A., Omelas, J., et al. (2016). Antithrombotic therapy for VTE diseases: Chest guideline and Expert Panel Report. *Chest, 149*, 315–352.

Kiely, D., Elliot, C. A., Sabroe, I., et al. (2013). Pulmonary hypertension: Diagnosis and management. *British Medical Journal, 346*, 1–12.

King, T. (2014). *Treatment of pulmonary sarcoidosis with glucosteroids*. Retrieved from www.uptodate.com/contents/treatment-of-pulmonary-sarcoidosis-with-glucocorticoids?source=search_result&search=Treatment+of+pulmonary+sarcoidosis+with+glucosteroids&selectedTitle=2~98

Kolditz, M., Braeken, D., Ewig, S., et al. (2016). Severity assessment and the immediate and long-term prognosis in community-acquired pneumonia. *Seminars in Respiratory and Critical Care Medicine, 37*, 886–896.

Kollef, M. H. (2015). *Clinical presentation and diagnosis of ventilator-associated pneumonia*. Retrieved from www.uptodate.com/contents/clinical-presentation-and-diagnosis-of-ventilator-associated-pneumonia?source=search_result&search=Clinical+presentation+and+diagnosis+of+VAP&selectedTitle=1~72

Mancini, M. C. (2014). Blunt chest trauma. *eMedicine/Medscape*. Retrieved from emedicine.medscape.com/article/428723-overview

Marrie, T. J. (2015). *Epidemiology, pathogenesis, and microbiology of community-acquired pneumonia in adults*. Retrieved from www.uptodate.com/contents/epidemiology-pathogenesis-and-microbiology-of-community-acquired-pneumonia-in-adults?source=search_result&search=Epidemiology%2C+pathogenesis%2C+and+microbiology+of+community-acquired+pneumonia+in+adults&selectedTitle=1~145

Martel, J., Bui-Wuan, E. F., Carreau, A. M., et al. (2013). Respiratory hygiene in emergency departments: Compliance, beliefs, and perceptions. *American Journal of Infection Control, 41*, 14–18.

Mayo Clinic. (2018). *Pneumonia*. Retrieved from https://www.mayoclinic.org/diseases-conditions/pneumonia/symptoms-causes/syc-20354204

National Heart, Lung, and Blood Institute. (n.d.). Pneumonia. Retrieved from https://www.nhlbi.nih.gov/health-topics/pneumonia

Nichol, K., McGeer, A., Bigelow, P., et al. (2013). Behind the mask: Determinants of nurse's adherence to facial protective equipment. *American Journal of Infection Control, 41*, 8–13.

Ouellette, D. R. (2015). Pulmonary embolism. *eMedicine/Medscape*. Last updated January 30, 2015. Retrieved from www.emedicine.medscape.com/article/300901-overview

Pagali, S. R., Verdoom, B. P., Wieland, M. L., et al. (2014). Infection control and managing tuberculosis at long term care facility: A case report. *The Journal of Post-Acute and Long-Term Care Medicine, 15*(3), B6.

PHAC. (2014). Retrieved from http://www.phac-aspc.gc.ca/tbpc-latb/pubs/tpc-pct/assets/pdf/tpc-pcta-eng.pdf

Pozniak, A. (2016). Clinical manifestations and complications of pulmonary tuberculosis. UpToDate. Last updated January 12, 2016. Retrieved from www.uptodate.com/contents/clinical-manifestations-and-complications-of-pulmonary-tuberculosis?source=search_result&search=Clinical+manifestations+and+complications+of+pulmonary+tuberculosis&selectedTitle=1~150

Public Health Agency of Canada. (2012). *Infection control guidelines for the prevention of healthcare-associated pneumonia*. Retrieved from http://publications.gc.ca/collections/collection_2012/aspc-phac/HP40-54-2010-eng.pdf

Public Health Agency of Canada. (2018). *Tuberculosis 2016*. Retrieved from https://www.canada.ca/en/public-health/services/reports-publications/canada-communicable-disease-report-ccdr/monthly-issue/2018-44/issue-3-4-march-1-2018/article-1-tuberculosis-2016.html

Reichman, L. E., & Lardizabal, A. (2015). *Adherence to tuberculosis treatment*. Retrieved from www.uptodate.com/contents/adherence-to-tuberculosis-treatment/contributors

Roy, A., Eisenhut, M., Harris, R. J., et al. (2014). Effect of BCG vaccination against Mycobacterium tuberculosis infection in children: Systematic review and meta-analysis. *British Medical Journal, 349*, g4643.

Rubin, L., & Hopkins, W. (2016). *Overview of pulmonary hypertension in adults*. Retrieved from www.uptodate.com/contents/overview-of-pulmonary-hypertension-in-adults?source=search_result&search=Overview+of+pulmonary+hypertension+in+adults&selectedTitle=1~150

Safer Healthcare Now. (2012). *Prevent ventilator associated pneumonia: Getting started kit*. Retrieved from http://www.patientsafetyinstitute.ca/en/toolsResources/Documents/Interventions/Ventilator-Associated%20Pneumonia/VAP%20Getting%20Started%20Kit.pdf

Shahani, R. (2015). Penetrating chest trauma. *eMedicine/Medscape*. Updated November 8, 2015. Retrieved from emedicine.medscape.com/article/425698-overview

Siegel, R. L., Miller, K. D., & Jemal, A. (2015). Cancer statistics, 2015. CA: *A cancer journal for clinicians, 65*(1), 5–29.

Siegel, M. D. (2015a). *Acute respiratory distress syndrome: Epidemiology, pathophysiology, pathology and etiology in adults*. Retrieved from www.uptodate.com/contents/acute-respiratory-distress-syndrome-epidemiology-pathophysiology-pathology-and-etiology-in-adults?source=search_result&search=Acute+respiratory+distress+syndrome%3A+epidemiology%2C+pathophysiology%2C+pathology+and+etiology+in+adults&selectedTitle=1~150

Siegel, M. D. (2015b). *Acute respiratory distress syndrome: Prognosis and outcomes in adults*. Retrieved from www.uptodate.com/contents/acute-respiratory-distress-syndrome-prognosis-and-outcomes-in-adults?source=search_result&search=Acute+respiratory+distress+syndrome%3A+Prognosis+and+outcomes+in+adults&selectedTitle=1~150

Simon, B., Ebert, J., Bokhari, F., et al. (2012). Management of pulmonary contusion and flail chest: An Eastern Association for the Surgery of Trauma practice management guideline. *Journal of Trauma and Acute Care Surgery*, *73*(5), S351–S361.

Smetana, G. W. (2015). *Strategies to reduce postoperative pulmonary complications*. Retrieved from www.uptodate.com/contents/strategies-to-reduce-postoperative-pulmonary-complications?source=search_result&search=Strategies+to+reduce+postoperative+pulmonary+complications&selectedTitle=1~150

Stark, P. (2015). *Atelectasis: Types and pathogenesis in adults*. Retrieved from www.uptodate.com/contents/atelectasis-types-and-pathogenesis-in-adults?source=search_result&search=Atelectasis%3A+Types+and+pathogenesis+in+adults&selectedTitle=1~150

Statistics Canada. (2017). *Health Fact: Sheets The 10 leading causes of death, 2013*. Retrieved from https://www150.statcan.gc.ca/n1/pub/82-625-x/2017001/article/14776-eng.htm

Strange, C. (2016). *Parapneumonic effusion and empyema in adults*. Retrieved from www.uptodate.com/contents/parapneumonic-effusion-and-empyema-in-adults?source=search_result&search=Parapneumonic+effusion+and+empyema+in+adults&selectedTitle=1~150

Tapson, V. F. (2016). *Overview of the treatment, prognosis, and follow-up of acute pulmonary embolism in adults*. Retrieved from www.uptodate.com/contents/overview-of-the-treatment-prognosis-and-follow-up-of-acute-pulmonary-embolism-in-adults?source=search_result&search=Tapson+Overview+of+the+treatment%2C+prognosis%2C+and+follow-up+of+acute+pulmonary+embolism+in+adults&selectedTitle=1~150

The ARDS Definition Task Force. (2012). Acute respiratory distress syndrome: The Berlin definition. *Journal of the American Medical Association*, *5*, 1–13.

Thomas, K., & Gould, M. (2015). *Overview of the initial evaluation, diagnosis, and staging of patient with suspected lung cancer*. Retrieved from www.uptodate.com/contents/overview-of-the-initial-evaluation-diagnosis-and-staging-of-patients-with-suspected-lung-cancer?source=search_result&search=Overview+of+the+initial+evaluation%2C+diagnosis%2C+and+staging+of+patient+with+suspected+lung+cancer&selectedTitle=1~150

Thrombosis Canada. (2013). *Pulmonary embolism: Diagnosis and management*. Retrieved from http://thrombosiscanada.ca/wp-content/uploads/2018/04/Pulmonary-Embolism-Diagnosis-2018Apr03.pdf

Walters, S., Maring, C., Coleman, M. P., et al. (2013). Lung cancer survival and stage at diagnosis in Australia, Canada, Denmark, Norway, Sweden and the UK: A population-based study, 2004–2007. *Thorax*, *68*, 551–564.

Resources

Agency for Healthcare Quality and Research: http://www.ahrq.gov
American Lung Association: http://www.lungusa.org
American Thoracic Society: http://www.thoracic.org
Canadian Cancer Society: www.cancer.ca
Canadian Cardiovascular Society: http://www.ccs.ca
Canadian Centre for Occupational Health and Safety: http://www.ccohs.ca
Canadian Council for Tobacco Control: http://www.cctc.ca
Canadian Lung Association: http://www.lung.ca
Canadian Medical Association: http://www.cma.ca
Canadian Thoracic Society: http://www.lung.ca/cts
Centers for Disease Control and Prevention: http://www.cdc.gov
Edmonton Zone Palliative Care Program: http://www.palliative.org
Health Canada: http://www.hc-sc.gc.ca
National Cancer Institute, National Institutes of Health: http://www.cancer.gov
National Heart, Lung and Blood Institute, National Institutes of Health: http://www.nhlbi.nih.gov
Occupational Safety and Health Administration (OSHA), U.S. Department of Labor: http://www.osha.gov
Public Health Agency of Canada: http://www.publichealth.gc.ca
Pulmonary Hypertension Association of Canada: http://www.phacanada.ca/en/
Respiratory Nursing Society: http://www.respiratorynursingsociety.org

25 Management of Patients With Chronic Pulmonary Disease

Adapted by Kelly Power-Kean

Learning Objectives

On completion of this chapter, the learner will be able to:

1. Describe the pathophysiology, clinical manifestations, and treatment of chronic obstructive pulmonary disease (COPD).
2. Discuss the major risk factors for developing COPD and nursing interventions to minimize or prevent these risk factors.
3. Use the nursing process as a framework for care of patients with COPD.
4. Develop an education plan for patients with COPD.
5. Describe the pathophysiology, clinical manifestations, and treatment of bronchiectasis.
6. Identify medical and nursing management of bronchiectasis
7. Describe the pathophysiology, clinical manifestations, and treatment of asthma.
8. Describe asthma self-management strategies.
9. Describe the pathophysiology, clinical manifestations, and treatment of cystic fibrosis.

Chronic obstructive pulmonary disease (COPD) is a leading cause of morbidity and mortality in Canada. Nurses care for patients with COPD across the spectrum of care, from outpatient and home care to emergency department (ED), critical care and hospice settings. To care for these patients, nurses not only need to have astute assessment and clinical management skills, but they also need knowledge of how these disorders can affect patients' quality of life. In addition, the nurse's knowledge of palliative and end-of-life care is important for applicable patients. Patient and family education is an important nursing intervention to enhance self-management in patients with any chronic pulmonary disorder.

Chronic Obstructive Pulmonary Disease

COPD is a preventable and treatable slowly progressive respiratory disease of airflow obstruction involving the airways, pulmonary parenchyma, or both (Vogelmeier, Criner, Martinez, et al., 2017). The parenchyma includes any form of lung tissue, including bronchioles, bronchi, blood vessels, interstitium, and alveoli. The airflow limitation or obstruction in COPD is not fully reversible. Most patients with COPD present with overlapping signs and symptoms of emphysema and chronic bronchitis, which are two distinct disease processes.

COPD may include diseases that cause airflow obstruction (e.g., emphysema, chronic bronchitis) or a combination of these disorders. Other diseases such as cystic fibrosis (CF), bronchiectasis, and asthma are classified as chronic pulmonary disorders. Asthma is considered a distinct, separate disorder and is classified as an abnormal airway condition characterized primarily by reversible inflammation. COPD can coexist with asthma. Both of these diseases have the same major symptoms; however, symptoms are generally more variable in asthma than in COPD. This chapter discusses COPD as a disease and briefly describes chronic bronchitis and emphysema as distinct disease states, providing a foundation for understanding the pathophysiology of COPD. Bronchiectasis, asthma, and CF are discussed separately.

In 2011, COPD caused 4.4% of all deaths in Canada (Statistics Canada, 2015). Over the years COPD has historically caused a higher percentage of deaths among men than among women; however, by 2011 the gap between the sexes had significantly decreased. For men, smoking rates have been steadily declining over the past 55 years corresponding with similar declines in the death rate from COPD observed in since the late 1990s. There has also been a consistent decline in the smoking rate among women since the early 1990s but a decline in the COPD death rate has not yet been observed. The economic burden associated with moderate and severe exacerbations in Canada has been estimated in the range of $646 million to $736 million per annum. It is predicted that COPD will be the third leading cause of death in the world (and for Canadians) by 2020 (GOLD, 2019).

It is estimated that there are over 2 million Canadians living with COPD. The 2015 incidence rate of COPD for persons 35 years of age and older was estimated at 156,500 per 100,000. The Public Health Agency of Canada (PHAC) reports that the likelihood of being affected by COPD increases with age. It is estimated that in 2012–2013, 15% of seniors between the ages of 65 and 69 were living with COPD and for seniors aged 85 years and older, 26% were living with COPD. In younger age groups, women and men are about equally likely to have COPD, while in older age groups, men are more likely to be affected. PHAC (2013) state that this may be due to smoking being more common among men than women. When considering gender comparisons, men are more likely than women to be affected by COPD, however; the gap between men and women has gradually narrowed over the years.

Pathophysiology

People with COPD commonly become symptomatic during the middle adult years, and the incidence of COPD increases with age. Although certain aspects of lung function normally decrease with age—for example, vital capacity and forced expiratory volume in 1 second (FEV_1)—COPD accentuates and accelerates these physiologic changes as described later. In COPD, the airflow limitation is both progressive and associated with an abnormal inflammatory response of the lungs to noxious particles or gases. The inflammatory response occurs throughout the airways, parenchyma, and pulmonary vasculature (GOLD, 2019; British Columbia Medical Association [BCMA], 2017). Because of the chronic inflammation and the body's attempts to repair it, changes and narrowing occurs in airways. In the proximal airways (trachea and bronchi greater than 2 mm in diameter), changes include increased numbers of goblet cells and enlarged submucosal glands, both of which lead to hypersecretion of mucus. In the peripheral airways (bronchioles less than 2-mm diameter), inflammation causes thickening of the airway wall, peribronchial fibrosis, exudate in the airway, and overall airway narrowing (obstructive bronchiolitis). Over time, this injury-and-repair process causes scar tissue formation and narrowing of the airway lumen (GOLD, 2019). Inflammatory and structural changes also occur in the lung parenchyma (respiratory bronchioles and alveoli). Alveolar wall destruction leads to loss of alveolar attachments and a decrease in elastic recoil. Finally, the chronic inflammatory process affects the pulmonary vasculature and causes thickening of the lining of the vessel and hypertrophy of smooth muscle, which may lead to pulmonary hypertension (GOLD, 2019).

Processes related to imbalances of substances (proteinases and antiproteinases) in the lung may be responsible for airflow limitation. When activated by chronic inflammation, proteinases and other substances may be released, damaging the parenchyma of the lung. The parenchymal changes may also be consequences of inflammation, environmental, or genetic factors (e.g., **alpha$_1$-antitrypsin deficiency**).

Early in the course of COPD, the inflammatory response causes pulmonary vasculature changes that are characterized by thickening of the vessel wall. These changes may

Glossary

air trapping: incomplete emptying of alveoli during expiration due to loss of lung tissue elasticity (emphysema), bronchospasm (asthma), or airway obstruction

alpha$_1$-antitrypsin deficiency: genetic disorder resulting from deficiency of alpha$_1$ antitrypsin, a protective agent for the lung; increases patient's risk for developing panacinar emphysema even in the absence of smoking

asthma: a heterogeneous disease, usually characterized by chronic airway inflammation; defined by history of symptoms such as wheeze, shortness of breath, chest tightness, and cough that vary over time and in intensity

bronchiectasis: chronic, irreversible dilation of the bronchi and bronchioles that results from the destruction of muscles and elastic connective tissue; dilated airways become saccular and are a medium for chronic infection

chronic bronchitis: a disease of the airways defined as the presence of cough and sputum production for at least a combined total of 3 months in each of 2 consecutive years

chronic obstructive pulmonary disease: disease state characterized by airflow limitation that is not fully reversible; sometimes referred to as chronic airway obstruction or chronic obstructive lung disease

desaturate: a precipitous drop in the saturation of hemoglobin with oxygen

emphysema: a disease of the airways characterized by destruction of the walls of overdistended alveoli

polycythemia: increase in the red blood cell concentration in the blood; in COPD, the body attempts to improve oxygen-carrying capacity by producing increasing amounts of red blood cells

pressurized metered-dose inhaler: patient-activated medication canister that provides aerosolized medication that the patient inhales into the lungs

spirometry: pulmonary function tests that measure specific lung volumes (e.g., FEV_1, FVC) and rates ($FEF_{25\%-75\%}$); may be measured before and after bronchodilator administration

Physiology/Pathophysiology

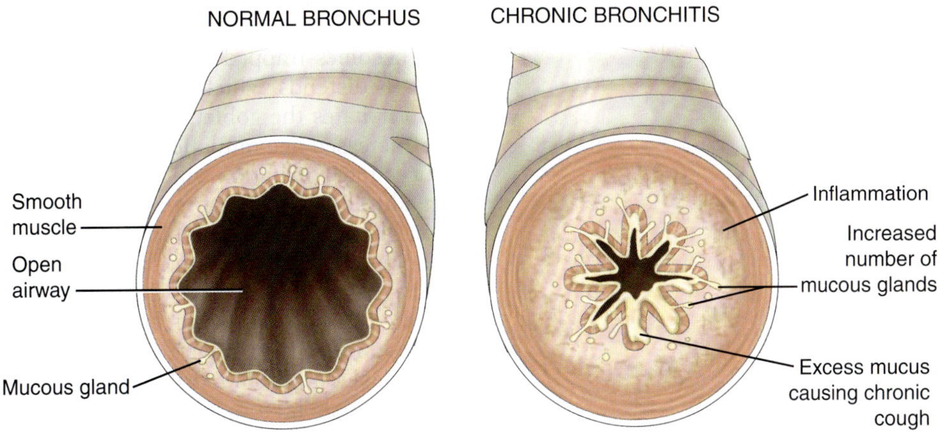

FIGURE 25-1. Pathophysiology of chronic bronchitis as compared with a normal bronchus. The bronchus in chronic bronchitis is narrowed and has impaired airflow due to multiple mechanisms: inflammation, excess mucus production, and potential smooth muscle constriction (bronchospasm).

occur as a result of exposure to cigarette smoke or use of tobacco products or as a result of the release of inflammatory mediators (GOLD, 2019).

Chronic Bronchitis

Chronic bronchitis, a disease of the airways, is defined as the presence of cough and sputum production for at least 3 months in each of 2 consecutive years. Although *chronic bronchitis* is a clinically and epidemiologically useful term, it does not reflect the major impact of airflow limitation on morbidity and mortality in COPD (GOLD, 2019). In many cases, smoke or other environmental pollutants irritate the airways, resulting in hypersecretion of mucus and inflammation. Mucus plugging of the airway reduces ciliary function. Bronchial walls also become thickened, further narrowing the bronchial lumen (see Fig. 25-1). Alveoli adjacent to the bronchioles may become damaged and fibrosed, resulting in altered function of the alveolar macrophages. This is significant because the macrophages play an important role in destroying foreign particles, including bacteria. As a result, the patient becomes more susceptible to respiratory infection. A wide range of viral, bacterial, and mycoplasmal infections can produce acute episodes of bronchitis. Exacerbations of chronic bronchitis are most likely to occur during the winter when viral and bacterial infections are more prevalent.

Emphysema

In emphysema, impaired gas exchange (oxygen, carbon dioxide) results from destruction of the walls of overdistended alveoli. ***Emphysema*** is a pathologic term that describes an abnormal distention of the air spaces beyond the terminal bronchioles, with destruction of the walls of the alveoli (GOLD, 2019). In addition, a chronic inflammatory response may induce disruption of the parenchymal tissues and often progresses slowly for many years. As the walls of the alveoli are destroyed (a process accelerated by recurrent infections), the alveolar surface area in direct contact with the pulmonary capillaries continually decreases. This causes an increase in dead space (lung area where no gas exchange can occur) and impaired oxygen diffusion, which leads to hypoxemia. In the later stages of the disease, carbon dioxide elimination is impaired, resulting in increased carbon dioxide tension in arterial blood (hypercapnia) leading to respiratory acidosis. As the alveolar walls continue to break down, the pulmonary capillary bed is reduced in size. Consequently, resistance to pulmonary blood flow is increased, forcing the right ventricle to maintain a higher blood pressure in the pulmonary artery. Hypoxemia may further increase pulmonary artery pressures (pulmonary hypertension). Cor pulmonale, one of the complications of emphysema, is right-sided heart failure brought on by long-term high blood pressure in the pulmonary arteries. This high pressure in the pulmonary arteries and right ventricle lead to back up of blood in the venous system, resulting in dependent edema, distended neck veins, or pain in the region of the liver (see Chapter 31 for further discussion).

There are two main types of emphysema, based on the changes taking place in the lung (see Fig. 25-2). Both types may occur in the same patient. In the panlobular (panacinar) type of emphysema, there is destruction of the respiratory bronchiole, alveolar duct, and alveolus. All air spaces within the lobule are essentially enlarged, but there is little inflammatory disease. A hyperinflated (hyperexpanded) chest, marked dyspnea on exertion, and weight loss typically occur. To move air into and out of the lungs, negative pressure is required during inspiration, and an adequate level of positive pressure must be attained and maintained during expiration. Instead of being an involuntary passive act, expiration becomes active and requires muscular effort.

In the centrilobular (centroacinar) form, pathologic changes take place mainly in the centre of the secondary lobule, preserving the peripheral portions of the acinus (i.e., the terminal airway unit where gas exchange occurs). Frequently, there is a derangement of ventilation–perfusion ratios, producing chronic hypoxemia, hypercapnia, **polycythemia** (i.e., an increase in red blood cells), and

Physiology/Pathophysiology

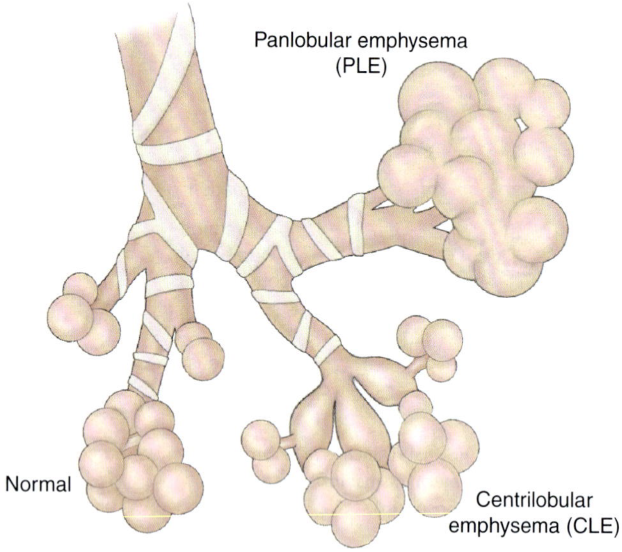

FIGURE 25-2. Changes in alveolar structure in panlobular and centrilobular emphysema. In panlobular emphysema, the bronchioles, alveolar ducts, and alveoli are destroyed, and the air spaces within the lobule are enlarged. In centrilobular emphysema, the pathologic changes occur in the lobule, while the peripheral portions of the acinus are preserved.

episodes of right-sided heart failure. This leads to central cyanosis and respiratory failure. The patient also develops peripheral edema.

Risk Factors

Risk factors for COPD include environmental exposures and host factors (see Chart 25-1). The most important environmental risk factor for COPD worldwide is cigarette smoking. A dose–response relationship exists between the intensity of smoking (pack-year history) and the decline in pulmonary function. Other environmental risk factors include smoking pipes, cigars, and other types of tobacco. Passive smoking (i.e., secondhand smoke) also contributes to respiratory symptoms and COPD (GOLD, 2015). Smoking depresses the activity of scavenger cells and affects the respiratory tract's ciliary cleansing mechanism, which keeps breathing passages free of inhaled irritants, bacteria, and other foreign matter. When smoking damages this cleansing mechanism, airflow is obstructed, and air becomes trapped behind the obstruction. The alveoli greatly distends, which diminishes lung capacity. Smoking also irritates the goblet cells and mucous glands, causing an increased accumulation of mucus, which in turn produces more irritation, infection, and damage to the lung. In addition, carbon monoxide (a by-product of smoking) combines with hemoglobin to form carboxyhemoglobin. Hemoglobin that is bound by carboxyhemoglobin cannot carry oxygen efficiently. Cigarette smoking is the best-studied COPD risk factor; however, it is not the only risk factor and studies have demonstrated nonsmokers may also develop chronic airflow obstruction. Other environmental risk factors for COPD include prolonged and intense exposure to occupational dusts and chemicals, indoor air pollution, and outdoor air pollution (GOLD, 2019).

Host risk factors for COPD include a person's genetic makeup. One well-documented genetic risk factor is a deficiency of alpha$_1$ antitrypsin, an enzyme inhibitor that protects the lung parenchyma from injury (Marciniuk, Hernandez, Balter, et al., 2012). This deficiency may lead to lung and liver disease. Worldwide, alpha$_1$-antitrypsin deficiency impacts between 1/1,700 and 1/5,000 people (American Liver Foundation, 2015). Of patients with COPD, 1% to 2% are found to have severe alpha$_1$-antitrypsin deficiency. This deficiency predisposes young people to rapid development of lobular emphysema, even in the absence of smoking. Among Caucasians, alpha$_1$-antitrypsin deficiency is one of the most common genetically linked lethal diseases. COPD may also result from gene–environment interactions (GOLD, 2019). Genetically susceptible people are sensitive to environmental factors (e.g., smoking, air pollution, infectious agents, and allergens) and eventually develop chronic obstructive symptoms. Carriers of this genetic defect must be identified so that they can modify environmental risk factors to delay or prevent overt symptoms of disease. Genetic counselling should also be offered. Alpha-protease inhibitor replacement therapy, which slows the progression of the disease, is available for patients with this genetic defect and for those with severe disease. However, this intermittent infusion therapy is costly and is required on an ongoing basis.

Other genetic risk factors may predispose a patient to COPD. Work is ongoing to identify specific variants of genes hypothesized to be involved in the development of COPD. These may include specific phenotypes to several chromosomal regions in families with multiple members developing early-onset COPD.

Age is often identified as a risk factor for COPD, but it is unclear whether healthy aging is an independent risk or whether the risk is related to cumulative exposures to risks over time (GOLD, 2019). There is a strong inverse relationship between COPD and lower socioeconomic status. However, perhaps it is not the lower socioeconomic status but how the socioeconomic status places the person at risk of increased patterns of exposure (indoor and outdoor pollutants, crowding, poor nutrition, infections and increased smoking).

CHART 25-1

Risk Factors: Chronic Obstructive Pulmonary Disease

- Exposure to tobacco smoke accounts for an estimated 80% to 90% of chronic obstructive pulmonary disease cases (GOLD, 2019)
- Passive smoking (i.e., second hand smoke)
- Increased age
- Occupational exposure (i.e., dust, chemicals)
- Indoor or outdoor air pollution
- Genetic abnormalities, including a deficiency of alpha$_1$ antitrypsin, an enzyme inhibitor that normally counteracts the destruction of lung tissue by certain other enzymes

Clinical Manifestations

Although the natural history of COPD is variable, it is generally a progressive disease characterized by three primary symptoms: chronic cough, sputum production, and dyspnea (GOLD, 2019). These symptoms often worsen over time. Chronic cough and sputum production often precede the development of airflow limitation by many years. However, not all individuals with cough and sputum production develop COPD. The cough may be intermittent and may be unproductive in some patients (GOLD, 2019). Dyspnea may be severe and interfere with the patient's activities and quality of life. Weight loss is common because dyspnea interferes with eating, and the work of breathing is energy depleting. As the work of breathing increases over time, the accessory muscles are recruited in an effort to breathe. Patients with COPD are at risk for respiratory insufficiency and respiratory infections or COPD exacerbation, which in turn increase the risk for acute and chronic respiratory failure.

In patients with COPD who have a primary emphysematous component, chronic hyperinflation leads to the "barrel chest" thorax configuration. This configuration results from a more fixed position of the ribs in the inspiratory position (due to hyperinflation) and from loss of lung elasticity (see Fig. 25-3). Retraction of the supraclavicular fossae occurs on inspiration, causing the shoulders to heave upward (see Fig. 25-4). In advanced emphysema, the abdominal muscles may also contract on inspiration.

There are systemic or extrapulmonary manifestations of COPD. These include musculoskeletal wasting (see Chapter 5 for discussion of nutrition assessment and Chapter 36 for discussion of nutrition therapy), metabolic syndrome (see Chapter 41), and depression (a frequent comorbidity that accompanies chronic debilitating illnesses). These clinical manifestations beyond the lungs must also be assessed and treated in order to decrease the morbidity and improve the quality of life of the patient with COPD.

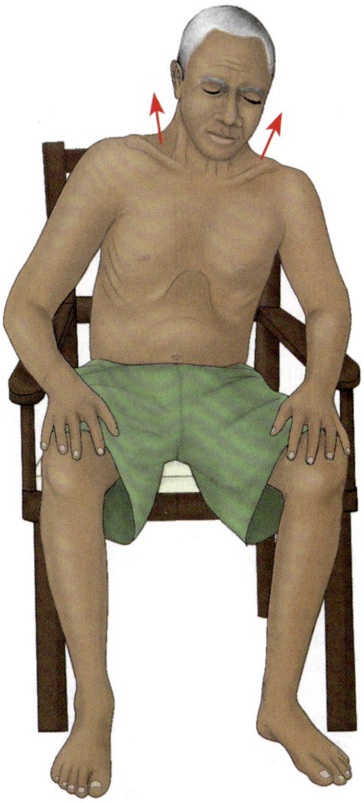

FIGURE 25-4. Typical posture of person with chronic obstructive pulmonary disease—primarily emphysema. The person tends to lean forward and uses the accessory muscles of respiration to breathe, forcing the shoulder girdle upward and causing the supraclavicular fossae to retract on inspiration.

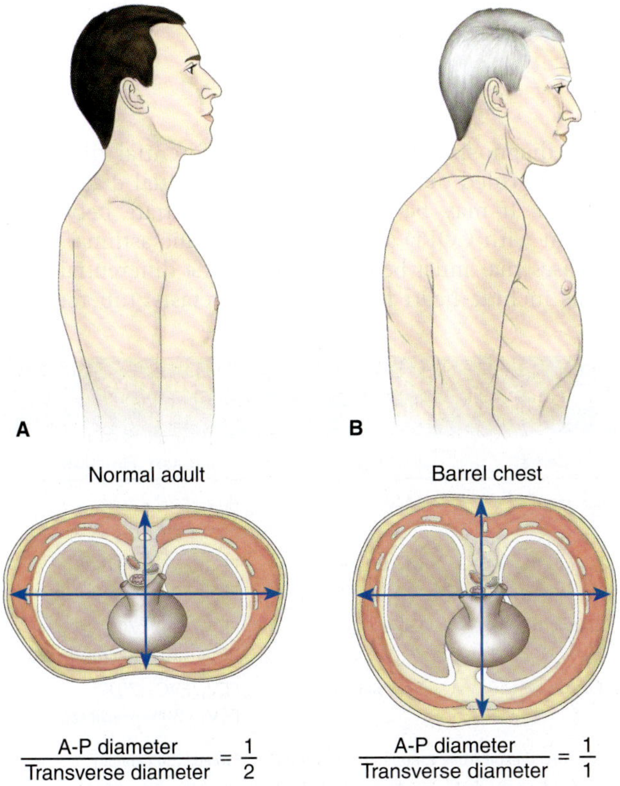

FIGURE 25-3. Characteristics of normal chest wall and chest wall in emphysema. **A.** The normal chest wall and its cross section. **B.** The barrel-shaped chest of emphysema and its cross section.

Assessment and Diagnostic Findings

The nurse obtains a thorough health history for a patient with known or potential COPD. Chart 25-2 lists the key factors to assess for patients with known or suspected COPD. Pulmonary function studies are used to help confirm the diagnosis of COPD, determine disease severity, and follow disease progression. **Spirometry** is used to evaluate airflow obstruction, which is determined by the ratio of FEV_1 to forced vital capacity (FVC). Spirometric results are expressed as an absolute volume and as a percentage of the predicted value using appropriate normal values for gender, age, and height. With obstruction, the patient either has difficulty exhaling or cannot forcibly exhale air from the lungs, reducing the FEV_1. Spirometry is also used to determine reversibility of obstruction after the use of bronchodilators (GOLD, 2015). Spirometry is initially performed, the patient is given an inhaled bronchodilator treatment according to a standard protocol, and then spirometry is repeated. The patient demonstrates a degree of reversibility if the pulmonary function values improve after administration of the bronchodilator.

CHART 25-2

Assessment: Assessing Patients With Chronic Obstructive Pulmonary Disease

Health History

- Has the patient been exposed to risk factors (types, intensity, duration)?
- Does the patient have a past medical history or respiratory diseases/problems, including asthma, allergy, sinusitis, nasal polyps, or respiratory infections?
- Does the patient have a family history of chronic obstructive pulmonary disease or other chronic respiratory diseases?
- How long has the patient had respiratory difficulty?
- What is the pattern of symptom development?
- Does exertion increase the dyspnea? What type of exertion?
- What are the limits of the patient's tolerance for exercise? At what times during the day does the patient complain most of fatigue and shortness of breath?
- Does the patient describe any discomfort or pain in any part of the body? If so, where does it occur, how intense is this pain, when does it occur, and does it interfere with activities of daily living? Is there any intervention that helps to alleviate the pain or discomfort?
- Which eating and sleeping habits have been affected?
- What is the impact of respiratory disease on quality of life?
- What does the patient know about the disease and their condition?
- What is the patient's smoking history (primary and secondary)?
- Is there occupational exposure to smoke or other pollutants?
- What are the triggering events (e.g., exertion, strong odours, dust, exposure to animals)?
- Does the patient have a history of exacerbations or previous hospitalizations for respiratory problems?
- Are comorbidities present?
- How appropriate are current medical treatments?
- Does the patient have available social and family support?
- What is the potential for reducing risk factors (e.g., smoking cessation)?

Physical Assessment

- What position does the patient assume during the interview?
- What are the pulse and the respiratory rates?
- What is the character of respirations? Even and without effort? Other?
- Can the patient complete a sentence without having to take a breath?
- Does the patient contract the abdominal muscles during inspiration?
- Does the patient use accessory muscles of the shoulders and neck when breathing?
- Does the patient take a long time to exhale (prolonged expiration)?
- Is central cyanosis evident?
- Are the patient's neck veins engorged?
- Does the patient have peripheral edema?
- Is the patient coughing?
- What are the colour, amount, and consistency of the sputum?
- Is clubbing of the fingers present?
- What types of breath sounds (i.e., clear, diminished or distant, crackles, and wheezes) are heard? Describe and document findings and locations.
- Are there any sensory deficits?
- Is there short- or long-term memory impairment?
- Is there increasing stupor?
- Is the patient apprehensive?

Arterial blood gas measurements may also be obtained to assess baseline oxygenation and gas exchange and are especially important in advanced COPD. A chest x-ray may be obtained to exclude alternative diagnoses. A computed tomography (CT) chest scan is not routinely obtained in the diagnosis of COPD, but a high-resolution CT scan may help in the differential diagnosis. Finally, screening for alpha$_1$-antitrypsin deficiency may be performed for patients younger than 45 years or for those with a strong family history of COPD, particularly if they have a family history of blood relatives with alpha$_1$-antitrypsin deficiency or COPD that is primarily emphysematous in nature.

COPD is classified into four grades depending on the severity measured by pulmonary function tests, as shown in Table 25-1 (GOLD, 2019). However, pulmonary function is not the only way to assess or classify COPD; pulmonary function is evaluated in conjunction with symptoms, health status impairment with COPD, and the potential for exacerbations (see Table 25-1). Factors that determine the clinical course and survival of patients with COPD include history of cigarette smoking, passive smoking exposure, age, rate of decline of FEV$_1$, hypoxemia, pulmonary artery pressure, resting heart rate, weight loss, reversibility of airflow obstruction and comorbidities.

In diagnosing COPD, several differential diagnoses must be ruled out. The primary differential diagnosis is asthma. It may be difficult to differentiate between a patient with COPD and one with chronic asthma. Other diseases that must be considered in the differential diagnosis include heart failure, bronchiectasis, tuberculosis,

TABLE 25-1 Grades of Chronic Obstructive Pulmonary Disease

Grade	Severity	Pulmonary Function
Grade I	Mild	FEV$_1$/FVC <70% FEV$_1$ ≥80% predicted
Grade II	Moderate	FEV$_1$/FVC <70% FEV$_1$ 50–80% predicted
Grade III	Severe	FEV$_1$/FVC <70% FEV$_1$ <30–50% predicted
Grade IV	Very severe	FEV$_1$/FVC <70% FEV$_1$ <30% predicted

FEV$_1$, forced expiratory volume in 1 second; FVC, forced vital capacity.

Adapted from Global Initiative for Chronic Obstructive Disease. (2015). *Global strategy for the diagnosis, management and prevention of COPD*. Retrieved on April 18, 2016, from www.goldcopd.org/uploads/users/files/GOLD_Report_2015.pdf

obliterative bronchiolitis, and diffuse panbronchiolitis (GOLD, 2019). Key points in determining the diagnosis are the patient history, severity of symptoms, and responsiveness to bronchodilators.

Complications

Respiratory insufficiency and failure are major life-threatening complications of COPD. The acuity of the onset and the severity of respiratory failure depend on baseline pulmonary function, pulse oximetry or arterial blood gas values, comorbid conditions, and the severity of other complications of COPD. Respiratory insufficiency and failure may be chronic (with severe COPD) or acute (with severe bronchospasm or pneumonia in the patient with severe COPD). Acute respiratory insufficiency and failure may necessitate ventilatory support until other acute complications, such as infection, can be treated. (See Chapter 26 for the management of the patient requiring ventilatory support.) Other complications of COPD include pneumonia, chronic atelectasis, pneumothorax, and pulmonary arterial hypertension (cor pulmonale).

Medical Management

Therapeutic strategies for the patient with COPD include promoting smoking cessation as appropriate, prescribing medications that typically include bronchodilators and may include corticosteroids, managing exacerbations, and providing supplemental oxygen therapy as indicated.

Risk Reduction

For patients with stable disease, treatment aims to reduce risk and symptoms. The major risk factor associated with COPD is environmental exposure and it is modifiable. The most important environmental exposure is smoking. Smoking cessation is the single most cost-effective intervention to prevent COPD and to slow its progression (GOLD, 2019). Since smoking is often established in adolescence and early age use is associated with higher levels of dependence primary smoking prevention among adolescence is important (Small, Eastlick Kushner, & Neufeld, 2012). Recent surveys indicate that 16% of all Canadians age 15 years and over smoke cigarettes on a daily or non-daily basis (Health Canada, 2012). Smoking cessation is difficult to achieve and even more difficult to sustain in the long term. Factors associated with continued smoking vary among patients and may include the strength of nicotine addiction, continued exposure to smoking-associated stimuli (at work or in social settings), stress, depression, and habit.

Because multiple factors are associated with continued smoking, successful cessation often requires multiple strategies. Health care providers should promote cessation by explaining the risks of smoking and personalizing the "at-risk" message to the patient. After giving a strong warning about smoking, health care providers should work with the patient to set a definite "quit date." Referral to a smoking cessation program may be helpful. Follow-up within 3 to 5 days after the quit date to review progress and to address any problems is associated with an increased rate of success; this should be repeated as needed. Continued reinforcement with a modality that is individualized to the patient and their lifestyle (e.g., telephone calls, texting, e-mail, or clinic visits) is beneficial. Relapses should be analyzed, and the patient and health care provider should jointly identify possible solutions to prevent future backsliding. It is important to emphasize successes rather than failures. Nicotine replacement—a first-line pharmacotherapy that reliably increases long-term smoking abstinence rates—comes in a variety of forms (gum, inhaler, nasal spray, transdermal patch, sublingual tablet, or lozenge). Bupropion SR (Wellbutrin, Zyban) and nortriptyline (Aventyl), both antidepressants, may also increase long-term quit rates. Other pharmacologic agents include the antihypertensive agent clonidine (Catapres); however, its side effects limit its use. Varenicline (Chantix), a nicotinic acetylcholine receptor partial agonist, may assist in smoking cessation (GOLD, 2019). Patients who are not appropriate candidates for such pharmacotherapy include those with medical contraindications, light smokers (fewer than 10 cigarettes per day), pregnant women, and adolescent smokers.

Smoking cessation can begin in a variety of health care settings—outpatient clinic, nursing centre, pulmonary rehabilitation centre, community, hospital, and in the home. Regardless of the setting, the nurse has the opportunity to teach the patient about the risks of smoking and the benefits of smoking cessation. Various materials, resources, and programs developed by several organizations (e.g., Health Canada Tobacco Control Program, Canadian Lung Association, Canadian Council for Tobacco Control, Canadian Cancer Society; see Resources section) are available to assist with this effort.

Pharmacologic Therapy

Medication regimens used to manage COPD are based on disease severity. For grade I (mild) COPD, a short-acting bronchodilator may be prescribed. For grade II or III COPD, a short-acting bronchodilator and regular treatment with one or more long-acting bronchodilators may be used. For grade III or IV (severe or very severe) COPD, medication therapy includes regular treatment with one or more bronchodilators and/or inhaled corticosteroids for repeated exacerbations.

Bronchodilators

Bronchodilators relieve bronchospasm by improving expiratory flow through widening of the airways and promoting lung emptying with each breath. These medications alter smooth muscle tone and reduce airway obstruction by allowing increased oxygen distribution throughout the lungs and improving alveolar ventilation. Although regular use of bronchodilators that act primarily on the airway smooth muscle does not modify the decline of function or the prognosis of COPD, their use is central in the management of COPD (GOLD, 2019). These agents can be delivered through a **pressurized metered-dose inhaler** (pMDI) or other type of inhaler, by nebulization, or via the oral route in pill or liquid form. Bronchodilators are often given regularly throughout the day as well as on an as-needed basis. They may also be used prophylactically to prevent breathlessness by having the patient use them before an activity, such as eating or walking.

Several devices are available to deliver medication via the inhaled route. These include pMDIs, breath-actuated

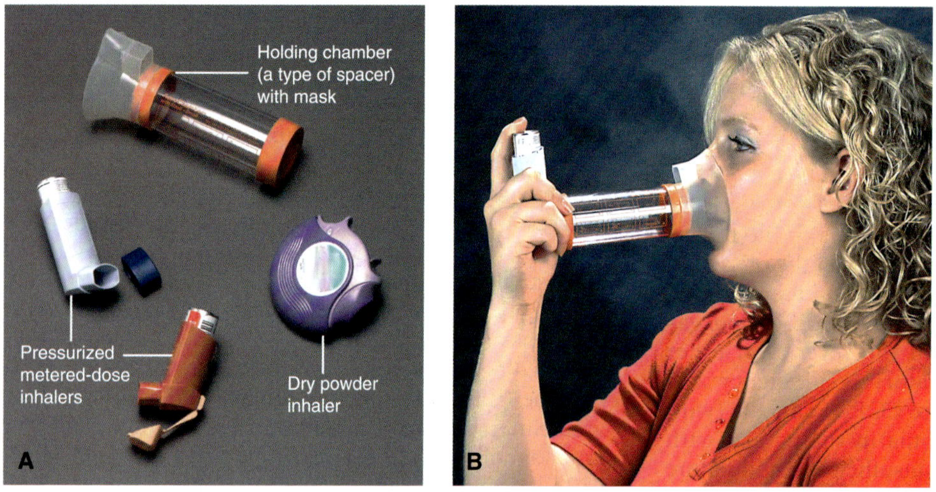

FIGURE 25-5. **A.** Examples of pressurized metered-dose inhalers and spacers. **B.** A pressurized metered-dose inhaler and spacer in use.

pMDIs, dry powder inhalers, spacer or valved-holding chambers, and nebulizers. Attention to effective drug delivery and training in proper inhaler technique is essential. A respiratory therapist is an excellent health care provider to consult on appropriate inhaler technique. The choice of an inhaler device will depend on availability, cost, prescribing physician, insurance coverage, and the skills and ability of the patient (GOLD, 2019).

A **pMDI** is a pressurized device containing an aerosolized powder of medication. A precise amount of medication is released with each activation of the canister. Patients need to be instructed on the correct use of the device. A spacer or valved-holding chamber may also be used to enhance deposition of the medication in the lung and help the patient coordinate activation of the MDI with inspiration. Spacers come in several designs, but all are attached to the pMDI and have a mouthpiece on the opposite end (Fig. 25-5). Other types of inhalers include the diskus inhaler (Serevent) and the Aerolizer inhaler (Foradil). Specific package insert information is available on the use of these inhalers.

A new breath-actuated multidose, dry powder inhaler was approved by Health Canada, albuterol (ProAir Respi-Click). Although this inhaler is prescribed primarily for asthma at this time, it is indicated for treatment or prevention of reversible bronchospasm. COPD may have a component of bronchospasm that can be treated with this drug. In addition, the newly introduced breath-actuated mechanism seems a promising method of delivery. The breath-actuated method minimizes the patient coordination necessary to activate the inhaler on inspiration (Teva Respiratory, 2016).

Several classes of bronchodilators are used that include beta-adrenergic agonists, muscarinic antagonists (anticholinergics), and combination agents. Beta-adrenergic agonists include short-acting beta$_2$-agonists (SABAs) and long-acting beta$_2$-agonists (LABAs). The anticholinergic agents include short-acting muscarinic (anticholinergic) antagonists (SAMAs) and long-acting muscarinic antagonists (LAMAs) (Bellinger & Peters, 2015; GOLD, 2019). Inhaled corticosteroids may also be combined with bronchodilators. These medications may be used in combination to optimize bronchodilation. LABA bronchodilators are more convenient for patient use as compared to short-acting beta$_2$-agonist bronchodilators. Nebulized medications also known as wet nebulizers (nebulization of medication via an air compressor) may also be effective in patients who cannot use a pMDI properly or who prefer this method of administration. However, wet nebulizers are more expensive than other devices and require appropriate cleaning and maintenance (GOLD, 2019) (see Table 25-2).

Corticosteroids

Although inhaled and systemic corticosteroids may improve the symptoms of COPD, they do not slow the decline in lung function. Their effects are less dramatic than in asthma. A short trial course of oral corticosteroids may be prescribed for patients to determine whether pulmonary function improves and symptoms decrease. Long-term treatment with oral corticosteroids is not recommended in COPD and can cause steroid myopathy, leading to muscle weakness, decreased ability to function, and, in advanced disease, respiratory failure (BCMA, 2017; GOLD, 2019). Inhaled corticosteroids are frequently prescribed in COPD.

Combination long-term beta$_2$-agonists plus corticosteroids in one inhaler may be appropriate; examples include formoterol/budesonide (Symbicort), vilanterol/fluticasone furoate (Breo Ellipta) and salmeterol/fluticasone (Advair) (Bellinger & Peters, 2015; GOLD, 2019).

Other Medications

Other pharmacologic treatments that may be used in COPD include alpha$_1$-antitrypsin augmentation therapy, antibiotic agents, mucolytic agents, antitussive agents, vasodilators, and narcotics. Vaccines are also effective in that they prevent exacerbations by preventing respiratory infections. For instance, influenza vaccines can reduce serious morbidity and death in patients with COPD by approximately 50% (GOLD, 2019). It is recommended that people limit their risk through influenza vaccination and smoking cessation. Pneumococcal vaccination also reduces the incidence of pneumonia, hospitalizations for cardiac conditions, and deaths in the general older adult population (GOLD, 2019) (see Chapter 14 for further discussion of pneumococcal vaccination).

Management of Exacerbation

An exacerbation of COPD is defined as an event in the natural course of the disease characterized by acute changes

TABLE 25-2 Aerosol Delivery Devices

Devices/Drugs	Optimal Technique	Therapeutic Issues
Pressurized metered-dose inhaler (pMDI) Beta$_2$-agonists Corticosteroids Cromolyn sodium Anticholinergics	Actuation[a] during a slow (30 L/minute or 3–5 seconds) deep inhalation, followed by 10-second breathhold	Slow inhalation and coordination of actuation may be difficult for some patients. Patients may incorrectly stop inhalation at actuation. Deposition of 50–80% of actuated dose in the oropharynx. Mouth washing and spitting is effective in reducing the amount of drug swallowed and absorbed systemically
Breath-actuated MDI Beta$_2$-agonists	Tight seal around mouthpiece and slightly more rapid inhalation than standard pMDI (see above) followed by 10-second breathhold	May be particularly useful for patients unable to coordinate inhalation and actuation. May also be useful for older patients. Patients may incorrectly stop inhalation at actuation. Cannot be used with currently available spacer/valved-holding chamber (VHC) devices
Dry powder inhaler Beta$_2$-agonists Corticosteroids Anticholinergics	Rapid (1–2 seconds) deep inhalation. Minimally effective inspiratory flow is device dependent	Dose is lost if patient exhales through device after actuating. Delivery may be greater or lesser than pMDIs, depending on device and technique. Delivery is more flow dependent in devices with highest internal resistance. Rapid inhalation promotes greater deposition in larger central airways. Mouth washing and spitting are effective in reducing amount of drug swallowed and absorbed systemically
Spacer or VHC	Slow (30 L/minute or 3–5 seconds) deep inhalation, followed by 10-second breathhold immediately following actuation. Actuate only once into spacer/VHC per inhalation. Rinse plastic VHCs once a month with low concentration of liquid household dishwashing detergent (1:5000 or 1–2 drops per cup of water) and let drip dry	Indicated for patients who have difficulty performing adequate pMDI technique. May be bulky. Simple tubes do not obviate coordinating actuation and inhalation. VHCs are preferred. Spacers or VHCs may increase delivery of inhalational corticosteroids to the lungs
Nebulizer Beta$_2$-agonists Corticosteroids Cromolyn sodium Anticholinergics	Slow tidal breathing with occasional deep breaths. Tightly fitting facemask for those unable to use mouthpiece	Less dependent on patient's coordination and cooperation. May be expensive, time consuming, and bulky; output depends on device and operating parameters (fill volume, driving gas flow); internebulizer and intranebulizer output variances are significant. The use of a facemask reduces delivery to lungs by 50%. Choice of delivery system depends on resources, availability, and clinical judgment of clinician caring for patient There is potential for infections if device is not cleaned properly

[a]Actuation refers to release of dose of medication with inhalation.

Adapted from Gardenhire, D. S., Ari, A., Hess, D., et al. (2013). *A guide to aerosol delivery devices for respiratory therapists* (3rd ed.). Dallas, TX: American Association for Respiratory Care.

(worsening) in the patient's respiratory symptoms beyond the normal day-to-day variations. An exacerbation also leads to change in medication (GOLD, 2019). Primary causes of an acute exacerbation include tracheobronchial infection and air pollution (BCMA, 2017; GOLD, 2019). However, the cause of approximately one third of severe exacerbations cannot be identified (GOLD, 2019). Roflumilast (Daliresp) may be used as a treatment to reduce the risk of exacerbations in patients with severe COPD associated with chronic bronchitis and a history of exacerbations. Roflumilast is a selective phosphodiesterase-4 (PDE4) inhibitor and is taken as a tablet once daily.

Treatment of an exacerbation requires identifying the primary cause (if possible) and administering the specific treatment. Optimization of bronchodilator medications is the first-line therapy and involves identifying the best medication or combinations of medications taken on a regular schedule for a specific patient. Depending on the signs and symptoms, corticosteroids, antibiotic agents, oxygen therapy, and intensive respiratory interventions may also be used. Indications for hospitalization for acute exacerbation of COPD include severe dyspnea that does not respond adequately to initial therapy, confusion or lethargy, respiratory muscle fatigue, paradoxical chest wall movement, peripheral edema, worsening or new onset of central cyanosis, persistent or worsening hypoxemia, and the need for noninvasive or invasive assisted mechanical ventilation (GOLD, 2019). The outcome from an exacerbation of COPD is closely related to the development of respiratory acidosis, the presence of significant comorbidities, and the need for noninvasive or invasive positive-pressure ventilatory support.

The GOLD guidelines (2019) provide indications for assessment, hospital admission, and possible critical care admission for patients with exacerbation of COPD. Indications for hospitalization include marked increase in intensity of symptoms, severe underlying COPD, onset of new physical signs (e.g., the use of accessory muscles, paradoxical chest wall movement, worsening or new onset of central cyanosis, peripheral edema, signs of right heart failure, and reduced alertness), failure to respond to initial medical management, older age, and insufficient home support.

When the patient arrives in an ED, the first line of treatment is supplemental oxygen therapy and rapid assessment to determine if the exacerbation is life-threatening (GOLD, 2019). A short-acting inhaled bronchodilator may be used to assess response to treatment. Oral or intravenous (IV) corticosteroids, in addition to bronchodilators, are recommended in the hospital management of a COPD exacerbation. Antibiotics also benefit patients with COPD because bacterial infections often follow viral infections.

General Principles of Oxygen Therapy

Oxygen therapy can be given as long-term continuous therapy, during exercise, or to prevent acute dyspnea during an exacerbation. The goal of supplemental oxygen therapy is to increase the baseline resting partial pressure of arterial oxygen (PaO_2) to at least 60 mm Hg at sea level and an arterial oxygen saturation (SaO_2) to at least 90% (GOLD, 2019). Long-term oxygen therapy (more than 15 hours per day) has been shown to improve quality of life, reduce pulmonary arterial pressure and dyspnea (GOLD, 2019). Long-term oxygen therapy is usually introduced in very severe COPD, and indications generally include a PaO_2 of 55 mm Hg or less or evidence of tissue hypoxia and organ damage such as cor pulmonale, secondary polycythemia, edema from right-sided heart failure, or impaired mental status (GOLD, 2019). For patients with exercise-induced hypoxemia, oxygen supplementation during exercise may improve performance. No evidence supports the idea that short bursts of oxygen before or after exercise provide any symptomatic relief (GOLD, 2019). Patients who are hypoxemic while awake are likely to be so during sleep. Therefore, nighttime oxygen therapy is recommended as well, and the prescription for oxygen therapy is for continuous, 24-hour use. Intermittent oxygen therapy is indicated for those who **desaturate** (i.e., experience a precipitous drop in hemoglobin molecule saturation with oxygen) only during activities of daily living, exercise, or sleep.

The main objective in treating patients with hypoxemia and hypercapnia is to give sufficient oxygen to improve oxygenation. Patients with COPD who require oxygen may have respiratory failure that is caused primarily by a ventilation–perfusion mismatch. These patients respond to oxygen therapy and should be treated to keep the resting oxygen saturation at or above 90%, which is associated with a PaO_2 of 60 mm Hg or higher (Hooley, 2015). Although the hypoxic drive is often cited as a concern in administering supplemental oxygen to patients with COPD, in actuality it is a very small part of the overall stimulus driving the respiratory system. However, a small subset of patients with COPD and chronic hypercapnia (elevated partial pressure of arterial carbon dioxide [$PaCO_2$] levels) may be more oxygen sensitive; their respiratory failure is caused more by alveolar hypoventilation (hypoxic drive). Administering too much oxygen can result in the retention of carbon dioxide. Patients with alveolar hypoventilation cannot increase ventilation to adjust for this increased CO2 load, leading to worsening of hypercapnia (Spiro, Sivestri, & Agusti, 2012). Monitoring and assessment are essential in the care of patients with COPD on supplemental oxygen. Pulse oximetry is helpful in assessing response to therapy but does not assess $PaCO_2$ levels. In addition, the nurse must evaluate for other factors and medications which could further decrease the respiratory drive—neurologic impairment, fluid and electrolyte issues, and narcotics or sedatives. Optimal oxygenation of patients is important while monitoring for any possible complications of oxygen supplementation (Spiro et al., 2012).

NURSING ALERT

Oxygen therapy is variable in patients with COPD; its aim in COPD is to achieve an acceptable oxygen level without a fall in the pH (increasing hypercapnia).

Surgical Management

Surgical options might be necessary for patients who do not demonstrate symptom improvement with nonsurgical therapies.

Bullectomy

A bullectomy is a surgical option for select patients with bullous emphysema. Bullae are enlarged airspaces that do not contribute to ventilation but occupy space in the thorax; these areas may be surgically excised. These bullae compress areas of the lung and may impair gas exchange. Bullectomy may help reduce dyspnea and improve lung function. It can be performed via video-assisted thoracoscope or a limited thoracotomy incision (see Chapter 26).

Lung Volume Reduction Surgery

Treatment options for patients with advanced or end-stage COPD (grade IV) with a primary emphysematous component are limited, although lung volume reduction surgery is a palliative surgical option that is approved in selected patients. This includes patients with homogeneous disease or disease that is focused in one area and not widespread throughout the lungs. Lung volume reduction surgery involves the removal of a portion of the diseased lung parenchyma. This reduces hyperinflation and allows the functional tissue to expand, resulting in improved elastic recoil of the lung and improved chest wall and diaphragmatic mechanics. This type of surgery does not cure the disease, but it may improve life expectancy, decrease dyspnea, improve lung function and exercise tolerance, and improve the patient's overall quality of life (GOLD, 2019).

Bronchoscopic lung volume reduction therapies are under investigation in clinical research protocols. These bronchoscopic procedures were developed to collapse areas of emphysematous lung and thus improve aeration of the functional lung tissue. Techniques include endobronchial placement of a one-way valve that allows air and mucus to exit the treated area but does not allow air to reenter. Another technique achieves biologic lung volume reduction through bronchoscopic instillation of a sealant or gel, valves or coils into the airway of the hyperinflated lung tissue. Because air can no longer enter the airway, the lung tissue beyond the sealed airway collapses over time. There is insufficient evidence to determine the benefit–risk ratios, cost-effectiveness, and possible roles of these procedures in care of the patient with severe emphysema (GOLD, 2019).

Lung Transplantation

Lung transplantation is a viable option for definitive surgical treatment of severe COPD in selected patients. It has been shown to improve quality of life and functional capacity in a select group of patients with COPD (GOLD, 2019). Limited not only by the shortage of donor organs, it is also a costly procedure with financial implications for months to years because of complications and the need for costly immunosuppressive medication regimens (GOLD, 2019).

Pulmonary Rehabilitation

Pulmonary rehabilitation for patients with COPD is well established and widely accepted as a means to alleviate symptoms and optimize functional status (McCarthy, Casey, Murphy, et al., 2015). The primary goals of rehabilitation are to reduce symptoms, improve quality of life and increase physical and emotional participation in everyday activities (GOLD, 2019). The benefits of this therapy include improvement of exercise capacity, reduction in the perceived intensity of breathlessness, improvement in health-related quality of life, reduction in the number of hospitalizations and days in the hospital, and reduction in the anxiety and depression associated with COPD (GOLD, 2019). Pulmonary rehabilitation services are multidisciplinary and include assessment, education, smoking cessation, physical reconditioning, nutritional counselling, skills training, and psychological support. A successful rehabilitation program is individualized for each patient, is multidisciplinary, and attends to both the physiologic and emotional needs of the patient. Most pulmonary rehabilitation programs include educational, psychosocial, behavioural, and physical components. Patients are taught methods to alleviate symptoms. Breathing exercises, as well as retraining and exercise programs, are used to improve functional status.

Pulmonary rehabilitation is appropriate for patients with grades II through IV COPD (GOLD, 2019). The minimum length of an effective program is 6 weeks; the longer the program, the more effective the results (GOLD, 2019). Programs vary in duration and may be conducted in inpatient, outpatient, or home settings. Program selection depends on the patient's physical, functional, and psychosocial status; insurance coverage; availability of programs; and preference. Pulmonary rehabilitation may also be used therapeutically in other disorders besides COPD, including asthma, CF, lung cancer, interstitial lung disease, thoracic surgery, and lung transplantation.

Nursing Management

Nurses play a key role in identifying potential candidates for pulmonary rehabilitation and in facilitating and reinforcing the material learned in the rehabilitation program. Not all patients have access to a formal rehabilitation program. However, the nurse can be instrumental in educating patients and families as well as facilitating specific services, such as respiratory therapy education, physical therapy for exercise and breathing retraining, occupational therapy for conserving energy during activities of daily living, and nutritional counselling. In addition, numerous educational materials are available to assist the nurse in teaching patients with COPD. Potential resources include the American Thoracic Society, American Association of Cardiovascular and Pulmonary Rehabilitation, Canadian Lung Association, Canadian Thoracic Society, and Health Canada (see Resources section).

Patient Education

Patient education is a major component of pulmonary rehabilitation and includes a broad variety of topics. Depending on the length and setting of the educational program, topics may include normal anatomy and physiology of the lung, pathophysiology and changes with COPD, medications and home oxygen therapy, nutrition, respiratory therapy treatments, symptom alleviation, smoking cessation, sexuality and COPD, coping with chronic disease, communicating with the health care team, and planning for the future (advance directives, living wills, informed decision making about health care alternatives). Education, including that relating to smoking cessation, should be incorporated into all aspects of care for COPD and in many settings (health care provider's offices, clinics, hospitals, home and community health care settings, and comprehensive rehabilitation programs).

Breathing Exercises

The breathing pattern of most people with COPD is shallow, rapid, and inefficient; the more severe the disease, the more inefficient the breathing pattern. With practice, this type of upper chest breathing can be changed to diaphragmatic breathing, which reduces the respiratory rate, increases alveolar ventilation, and sometimes helps to expel as much air as possible during expiration (see Chapter 26 for technique). Pursed-lip breathing helps to slow expiration, prevents collapse of small airways, and helps the patient control the rate and depth of respiration. It also promotes relaxation, enabling the patient to gain control of dyspnea and reduce feelings of panic.

Inspiratory Muscle Training

Once the patient masters diaphragmatic breathing, a program of inspiratory muscle training may be prescribed to help strengthen the muscles used in breathing. This program requires that the patient breathe against resistance for a prescribed amount of time every day. As the resistance is gradually increased, the muscles become better conditioned. Conditioning of the respiratory muscles takes time, and the patient is instructed to continue practicing at home.

Activity Pacing

People with COPD have decreased exercise tolerance during specific periods of the day, especially in the morning on arising, because bronchial secretions have collected in the lungs during the night while the person was lying down. The patient may have difficulty bathing or dressing and may become fatigued. Activities that require the arms to be supported above the level of the thorax may produce fatigue or respiratory distress but may be tolerated better after the patient has been up and moving around for an hour or more. The nurse can help the patient reduce these limitations by planning self-care activities and determining the best time for bathing, dressing, and other daily activities.

Self-Care Activities

As gas exchange, airway clearance, and the breathing pattern improve, the patient is encouraged to assume increasing participation in self-care activities. The patient is taught to coordinate diaphragmatic breathing with activities such as walking, bathing, bending, or climbing stairs. The patient should bathe, dress, and take short walks, resting as needed to avoid fatigue and excessive dyspnea. Fluids should always be readily available, and the patient should begin to drink fluids without having to be reminded. If management of secretions is a problem and some type of postural drainage or airway clearance manoeuver is to be performed at home, the nurse or respiratory therapist instructs and supervises the patient before discharge or in the outpatient setting.

Physical Conditioning

People with COPD of all grades may benefit from exercise training programs. These benefits may include increased exercise tolerance and decreased dyspnea and fatigue (GOLD, 2019). Physical conditioning techniques include breathing exercises and general exercises intended to conserve energy and increase pulmonary ventilation. Graded exercises and physical conditioning programs using treadmills, stationary bicycles, and measured level walks can improve symptoms and increase work capacity and exercise tolerance. Any physical activity that can be performed regularly is helpful. Walking aids may be beneficial (GOLD, 2019). Lightweight portable oxygen systems are available for ambulatory patients who require oxygen therapy during physical activity.

Oxygen Therapy

Oxygen supplied to the home comes in compressed gas, liquid, or concentrator systems. Portable oxygen systems allow the patient to exercise, work, and travel. To help the patient adhere to the oxygen prescription, the nurse explains the proper flow rate and required number of hours for oxygen use as well as the dangers of arbitrary changes in flow rates or duration of therapy. The nurse also reassures the patient that oxygen is not "addictive" and explains the need for regular evaluations of blood oxygenation by pulse oximetry or arterial blood gas analysis.

> **NURSING ALERT**
>
> **The nurse should caution the patient that smoking with or near oxygen is extremely dangerous.**

Nutritional Therapy

Nutritional assessment and counselling are important for patients with COPD. Nutritional status is reflected in severity of symptoms, degree of disability, and prognosis. Significant weight loss is often a major problem; however, excessive weight can also be problematic, although it occurs less often. Most patients with COPD have difficulty gaining and maintaining weight. A thorough assessment of caloric needs and counselling about meal planning and supplementation are part of the rehabilitation process. Continual monitoring of weight and interventions as necessary are important parts of the care of patients with COPD.

Coping Measures

Any factor that interferes with normal breathing quite naturally induces anxiety, depression, and changes in behaviour. Constant shortness of breath and fatigue may make the patient irritable and apprehensive to the point of panic. Restricted activity (and reversal of family roles due to loss of employment), the frustration of having to work to breathe, and the realization that the disease is prolonged and unrelenting may cause the patient to become angry, depressed, and demanding (Simpson & Jones, 2013). Sexual function may be compromised, which also diminishes self-esteem. The nurse should provide education and support to the spouse or significant others and families, because the caregiver role in end-stage COPD can be challenging.

Palliative Care

Palliative care is integral for the patient with advanced COPD. Unfortunately, palliative care is often not considered until the disease is far advanced. The overall goals of palliative care are to manage symptoms and improve the quality of life for patients and families with advanced disease (GOLD, 2019; Rocker, Simpson & Horton, 2015). Areas addressed in palliative care include effective and empathetic communication with patients and families; close attention to pain and other symptoms; psychosocial, spiritual and bereavement support; and coordination of the wide range of medical and social services required with this disease. Palliative care should be considered complementary to hospice and end-of-life care (Rocker et al. 2015) (see Chapter 15).

Nursing Management

Assessing the Patient

Assessment involves obtaining information about current symptoms as well as previous disease manifestations. Chart 25-2 lists sample questions that may be used to obtain a clear history of the disease process. In addition to the history, the nurse also reviews the results of available diagnostic tests.

Achieving Airway Clearance

Bronchospasm, which occurs in many pulmonary diseases, reduces the caliber of the small bronchi and may cause dyspnea, static secretions, and infection. Bronchospasm can sometimes be detected on auscultation with a stethoscope when wheezing or diminished breath sounds are heard. Increased mucus production, along with decreased mucociliary action, contributes to further reduction in the caliber of the bronchi and results in decreased airflow and decreased gas exchange. This is further aggravated by the loss of lung elasticity that occurs with COPD (GOLD, 2019). These changes in the airway require that the nurse monitor the patient for dyspnea and hypoxemia. If bronchodilators or corticosteroids are prescribed, the nurse must administer the medications properly and be alert for potential side effects. The relief of bronchospasm is confirmed by measuring improvement in expiratory flow rates and volumes (the force of expiration, how long it takes to exhale, and the amount of air exhaled) as well as by assessing the dyspnea and making sure that it has lessened.

Diminishing the quantity and viscosity of sputum can clear the airway and improve pulmonary ventilation and gas exchange. All pulmonary irritants should be eliminated or reduced, particularly cigarette smoke, which is the most persistent source of pulmonary irritation. The nurse instructs the patient in directed or controlled coughing, which is more effective and reduces the fatigue associated with undirected forceful coughing. Directed coughing consists of a slow, maximal inspiration followed by breath-holding for several seconds and then two or three coughs. "Huff" coughing may also be effective. The technique consists of one or two forced exhalations (huffs) from low to medium lung volumes with the glottis open.

Chest physiotherapy with postural drainage, intermittent positive-pressure breathing, increased fluid intake, and bland aerosol mists (with normal saline solution or water) may be useful for some patients with COPD. The use of these measures must be based on the response and tolerance of each patient.

Improving Breathing Patterns

Ineffective breathing patterns and shortness of breath are due to the ineffective respiratory mechanics of the chest wall and lung resulting from **air trapping** (i.e., incomplete emptying of alveoli during expiration), ineffective diaphragmatic movement, airway obstruction, the metabolic cost of breathing, and stress. Inspiratory muscle training and breathing retraining may help to improve breathing patterns. Training in diaphragmatic breathing reduces the respiratory rate, increases alveolar ventilation, and sometimes helps to expel as much air as possible during expiration. Pursed-lip breathing helps slow expiration, prevent collapse of small airways, and control the rate and depth of respiration. It also promotes relaxation, which allows the patient to gain control of dyspnea and reduce feelings of panic.

Improving Activity Tolerance

Patients with COPD experience progressive activity and exercise intolerance that may lead to disability. Education is focused on rehabilitative therapies to promote independence in executing activities of daily living. These may include pacing activities throughout the day or using supportive devices to decrease energy expenditure. The nurse evaluates the patient's activity tolerance and limitations and uses education strategies to promote independent activities of daily living. The patient may be a candidate for exercise training to strengthen the muscles of the upper and lower extremities and improve exercise tolerance and endurance. The use of walking aids may be recommended to improve activity levels and ambulation (GOLD, 2019). Other health care professionals (rehabilitation therapist, occupational therapist, physical therapist) may be consulted as additional resources.

Monitoring and Managing Potential Complications

The nurse must assess for various complications of COPD, such as life-threatening respiratory insufficiency and failure as well as respiratory infection and chronic atelectasis, which may increase the risk for respiratory failure. The nurse also monitors for cognitive changes (personality and behavioural changes, memory impairment), increasing dyspnea, tachypnea, and tachycardia, which may indicate increasing hypoxemia and impending respiratory failure.

The nurse monitors pulse oximetry values to assess the patient's need for oxygen and administers supplemental oxygen as prescribed. The nurse also instructs the patient about signs and symptoms of respiratory infection that may worsen hypoxemia and reports changes in the patient's physical and cognitive status to the primary provider.

Bronchopulmonary infections must be controlled to diminish inflammatory edema and to permit recovery of normal ciliary action. Minor respiratory infections that are of no consequence to people with normal lungs can be life-threatening to people with COPD. Infection compromises lung function and is a common cause of respiratory failure in people with COPD. In COPD, infection may be accompanied by subtle changes. The nurse instructs the patient to report any signs of infection, such as a fever or change in sputum colour, character, consistency, or amount. Any worsening of symptoms (increased tightness of the chest, increased dyspnea, fatigue) also suggests infection and must be reported. Viral infections are hazardous to these patients because they are often followed by infections caused by bacterial organisms, such as *Streptococcus pneumoniae* and *Haemophilus influenzae, and Moraxella catarrhalis* (Bartlett & Sethi, 2016).

To prevent infection, the nurse encourages the patient with COPD to be immunized against influenza and pneumococcal pneumonia, because the patient is prone to respiratory infection. In addition, because each patient reacts differently to external exposures (significant air pollution, high or low temperatures, high humidity, strong smells), the nurse must assess the patient's actual and potential triggers that cause bronchospasm so that avoidance or a treatment plan can be established.

Pneumothorax is a potential complication of COPD and can be life-threatening in patients with COPD who have minimal pulmonary reserve. Patients with severe emphysematous changes can develop large bullae, which may rupture and cause a pneumothorax. The development of a pneumothorax may be spontaneous or related to an activity such as severe coughing or large intrathoracic pressure changes. If a rapid onset of shortness of breath occurs, the nurse should quickly evaluate the patient for a potential pneumothorax by assessing the symmetry of chest movement, differences in breath sounds, and pulse oximetry.

Over time, pulmonary hypertension may occur as a result of chronic hypoxemia which causes the pulmonary arteries to constrict and thus leads to this complication. Pulmonary hypertension may be prevented by maintaining adequate oxygenation through an adequate hemoglobin level, improved ventilation–perfusion of the lungs, or continuous administration of supplemental oxygen (if needed).

Promoting Home, Community-Based, and Transitional Care

Educating Patients About Self-Care

When providing education about self-management, the nurse must assess the knowledge of patients and family members about self-care and the therapeutic regimen. The nurse should also consider whether they are comfortable with this knowledge. Familiarity with prescribed medications' potential side effects is essential. In addition patients and family members need to learn the early signs and symptoms of infection and other complications so that they seek appropriate health care promptly. Nurses are key in promoting smoking cessation and educating patients about its importance. Patients diagnosed with COPD who continue to smoke must be encouraged and assisted to quit.

A major area of patient education involves setting and accepting realistic short-term and long-range goals. If the COPD is mild (i.e., grade I), the objectives of treatment are to increase exercise tolerance and prevent further loss of pulmonary function. If the COPD is severe (i.e., grade III), the objectives are to preserve current pulmonary function and relieve symptoms as much as possible. It is important to plan and share the goals and expectations of treatment with the patient. Both the patient and the care provider need patience to achieve these goals.

The nurse instructs the patient to avoid extremes of heat and cold. Heat increases the body temperature, thereby raising oxygen requirements, and cold tends to promote bronchospasm. Air pollutants such as fumes, smoke, dust, and even talcum, lint, and aerosol sprays may initiate bronchospasm. High altitudes aggravate hypoxemia.

A patient with COPD should adopt a lifestyle of moderate activity, ideally in a climate with minimal shifts in temperature and humidity. As much as possible, the patient should avoid emotional disturbances and stressful situations that might trigger a coughing episode. Self-management also includes getting sufficient rest and sleep (see Chart 25-3).

The medication regimen can be quite complex; patients receiving aerosol medications by a pMDI or other type of inhaler may be particularly challenged. The nurse must review educational information and have the patient demonstrate correct pMDI use before discharge, during follow-up visits to a caregiver's office or clinic, and during home visits (see Chart 25-4).

Smoking cessation goes hand in hand with lifestyle changes, and reinforcing the patient's efforts is a key nursing activity. Smoking cessation is the single most important therapeutic intervention for patients with COPD. There are many strategies, including prevention, cessation with or without oral or topical patch medications, and behaviour modification techniques.

Numerous educational materials are available to assist nurses in educating patients with COPD (see Resources at the end of the chapter).

Continuing and Transitional Care

Referral for home, community-based, or transitional care is important to enable assessment of the patient's home environment and physical and psychological status, to evaluate the patient's adherence to the prescribed regimen, and to assess the patient's ability to cope with changes in lifestyle and physical status. Home visits provide an opportunity to reinforce the information and activities learned in the inpatient or outpatient pulmonary rehabilitation program and to have the patient and family

NURSING RESEARCH PROFILE

Chart 25-3. Sleep and Quality of Life in Chronic Obstructive Pulmonary Disease

Geiger-Brown, J., Lindberg, S., Krachman, S., et al. (2015). Self-reported sleep quality and acute exacerbations of chronic obstructive pulmonary disease. *International Journal of COPD, 10*(1), 389–397.

Purpose

The purpose of this secondary analysis study was to characterize sleep quality in patients with clinically stable COPD; describe relationships between sleep quality, concomitant medical conditions and medications; and determine if sleep quality during the clinically stable period was predictive of health-related quality of life or was an independent predictor of exacerbation.

Design

This secondary analysis was from a randomized trial of 1,117 patients with moderate to severe COPD. Measures of quality of life included the Medical Outcomes Study 36-item Short Form Survey and the St. Georges Respiratory Questionnaire. Self-reported sleep quality was measured using the Pittsburgh Sleep Quality Index (PSQI). Higher scores reflect poorer sleep quality (range 0 to 21). Outcomes were measured as time to first exacerbation and exacerbation rate.

Findings

In 53% of participants, sleep quality was rated as low (score >5). This finding was not related to age or severity of airflow obstruction. "Poor" sleepers had worse quality of life measures as compared to "good" sleepers. Comorbidities were more common in the "poor" sleepers. In comparing "poor" and "good" sleepers, unadjusted time to first exacerbation was shorter (190 days vs. 239 days) and exacerbation rate was higher in the "poor" sleepers (1.7 vs. 1.37 per year). Once these data were adjusted for more medications and comorbid conditions, there were no significant differences between the two groups.

Nursing Implications

Sleep quality is an issue in the patient with COPD that has received little attention. Results from this study suggest that sleep quality is related to quality of life. Sleep quality was poor in 53% of the patients at the beginning and end of this clinical trial despite receiving therapy that reduced exacerbations. The nurse should assess sleep quality in the patient with COPD in both the inpatient and outpatient setting. In the outpatient setting, it may be helpful to evaluate patients' self-reported sleep quality, duration of sleep, use of sleep aids and any daytime dysfunction over time to evaluate changes in sleep. In the inpatient setting, the nurse should work closely with the patient to plan care that may improve sleep while in the hospital. At this time it is unknown whether therapy directed at improving sleep can also lead to improved prognosis of COPD.

COPD, chronic obstructive pulmonary disease.

CHART 25-4

Patient Education: Use of Pressurized Metred-Dose Inhaler (pMDI)

The nurse instructs the patient to:

- Remove the cap and hold the inhaler upright
- Shake the inhaler
- Sit upright or stand upright. Breathe out slowly and all the way
- Use one of two techniques: open-mouth technique or closed-mouth technique
  - *Open-mouth technique*
    - Place the pMDI 2 finger widths away from lips
    - With mouth open and tongue flat, tilt outlet of the pMDI so that it is pointed toward the upper back of the mouth
    - Actuate the pMDI and begin to breathe in slowly. Breathe slowly and deeply through the mouth and try to hold breath for 10 seconds
  - *Closed-mouth technique*
    - Place the pMDI between the teeth and make sure the tongue is flat under the mouth-piece and does not block pMDI
    - Seal lips around mouthpiece and actuate the pMDI. Breathe in slowly through the mouth and try to hold breath for 10 seconds
- Repeat puffs as directed, allowing 1 minute between puffs. There is no need to wait for other medications
- Apply the cap to the pMDI for storage
- After inhalation, rinse mouth with water when using a corticosteroid-containing pMDI

The pMDI mouthpiece should be cleaned on a regular basis as should the nozzle of the canister based on the manufacturer's recommendations. As there are many types of inhalers, it is important to follow the manufacturer's instructions for use and care of the inhaler.

Adapted from Gardenhire, D. S., Ari, A., Hess, D., et al. (2013). *A guide to aerosol delivery devices for respiratory therapists* (3rd ed.). Dallas, TX: American Association for Respiratory Care.

demonstrate correct administration of medications and oxygen, if indicated, and performance of exercises. If the patient does not have access to a formal pulmonary rehabilitation program, the nurse provides the education and breathing retraining necessary to optimize the patient's functional status.

The nurse directs patients to community resources, such as pulmonary rehabilitation programs and smoking cessation programs, to help improve patient's ability to cope with their chronic condition and the therapeutic regimen and to provide a sense of worth, hope, and well-being. In addition, the nurse reminds the patient and family about the importance of participating in general health promotion activities and health screening.

Patients with COPD have indicated that information about their end-of-life needs is limited. Areas to discuss regarding end-of-life care may include symptom management quality of life, satisfaction with care, information/communication, use of care professionals, use of differing care facilities, hospital admission, and place of death. It is crucial that patients know what to expect as the disease progresses. In addition, they should have information about their role in decisions regarding aggressiveness of care near the end of life and access to specialists who may help them and their families. As the disease course progresses, a holistic assessment of physical and psychological needs should be undertaken at each hospitalization, clinic visit, or home visit. This helps to gauge the patient's assessment of the progression of the disease and its impact on quality of life and guides planning for future interventions and management (see Chapter 15 for additional information).

Continuing and Transitional Care

Chart 25-5 provides further information on providing nursing care for the patient with COPD.

Bronchiectasis

Bronchiectasis is a chronic, irreversible dilation of the bronchi and bronchioles that results from destruction of muscles and elastic connective tissue. Under the new definition of COPD, it is considered a separate disease process from COPD (GOLD, 2019). Numerous factors can induce or contribute to the development of bronchiectasis. Some of these include recurrent respiratory infections, CF, rheumatic and other systemic diseases, primary ciliary dysfunction, tuberculosis, or immunodeficiency disorders (Barker, 2015a).

Pathophysiology

The inflammatory process associated with pulmonary infections damages the bronchial wall, causing a loss of its supporting structure and resulting in thick sputum that ultimately obstructs the bronchi. The walls become permanently distended and distorted, impairing mucociliary clearance. In saccular bronchiectasis, each dilated peribronchial tube amounts to a lung abscess, the exudate of which drains freely through the bronchus. Bronchiectasis is usually localized, affecting a segment or lobe of a lung, most frequently the lower lobes.

The retention of secretions and subsequent obstruction ultimately cause the alveoli distal to the obstruction to collapse (atelectasis). Inflammatory scarring or fibrosis replaces functioning lung tissue. In time, the patient develops respiratory insufficiency with reduced vital capacity, decreased ventilation, and an increased ratio of residual volume to total lung capacity. There is impairment in the matching of ventilation to perfusion (ventilation–perfusion imbalance) and hypoxemia.

Clinical Manifestations

Characteristic symptoms of bronchiectasis include chronic cough and the production of purulent sputum in copious amounts. Many patients with this disease have hemoptysis. Clubbing of the fingers also is common because of respiratory insufficiency. The patient usually has repeated episodes of pulmonary infection.

Assessment and Diagnostic Findings

Bronchiectasis is not readily diagnosed because the symptoms can be mistaken for those of chronic bronchitis. A

(text continued on page 583)

Plan of Nursing Care — Chart 25-5. Care of the Patient With COPD

NURSING INTERVENTIONS	RATIONALE	EXPECTED OUTCOMES
Nursing Priority: Impaired gas exchange and ineffective airway clearance **Goal:** Improvement in gas exchange		
1. Evaluate current smoking status, educate regarding smoking cessation, and facilitate efforts to quit. a. Evaluate current smoking habits of patient and family b. Educate regarding hazards of smoking and relationship to COPD c. Evaluate previous smoking cessation attempts d. Provide educational materials e. Refer to a smoking cessation program or resource	1. Smoking causes permanent damage to the lung and diminishes the lungs' protective mechanisms. Airflow is obstructed, secretions are increased, and lung capacity is reduced. Continued smoking increases morbidity and mortality in COPD and is also a risk factor for lung cancer	• Identifies the hazards of cigarette smoking • Identifies resources for smoking cessation • Enrolls in a smoking cessation program • Reports success in stopping smoking • Verbalizes types of inhaled toxins • Minimizes or eliminates exposures • Monitors public announcements regarding air quality and minimizes or eliminates exposures during episodes of severe pollution
2. Evaluate current exposure to occupational toxins or pollutants and indoor/outdoor pollution 3. Evaluate current exposures to occupational toxins, indoor and outdoor air pollution (e.g., smog, toxic fumes, and chemicals) 4. Emphasize primary prevention to occupational exposures. This is best achieved by elimination or reduction of exposures in the workplace 5. Educate regarding types of indoor and outdoor air pollution (e.g., biomass fuel burned for cooking and heating in poorly ventilated buildings, outdoor air pollution) 6. Advise patient to monitor public announcements regarding air quality	2. Chronic inhalation of both indoor and outdoor toxins causes damage to the airways and impairs gas exchange	
Nursing Priority: Impaired gas exchange **Goal:** Improvement in gas exchange		
1. Administer bronchodilators as prescribed: a. Inhalation is preferred route b. Observe for side effects: tachycardia, dysrhythmias, central nervous system excitation, nausea, and vomiting c. Assess for correct technique of pressurized metered-dose inhaler (pMDI) or other type of administration	1. Bronchodilators dilate the airways. The medication dosage is carefully adjusted for each patient, in accordance with clinical response	• Verbalizes the need for bronchodilators and for taking as prescribed • Evidences minimal side effects; heart rate near normal, absence of dysrhythmias, normal mentation • Reports a decrease in dyspnea • Shows an improved expiratory flow rate • Uses and cleans respiratory therapy equipment as applicable • Demonstrates diaphragmatic breathing and coughing • Uses oxygen equipment appropriately when indicated • Evidences improved arterial blood gases or pulse oximetry • Demonstrates correct technique for use of pMDI
2. Evaluate effectiveness of nebulizer or pMDI treatments a. Assess for decreased shortness of breath, decreased wheezing or crackles, loosened secretions, and decreased anxiety b. Ensure that treatment is given before meals to avoid nausea and to reduce fatigue that accompanies eating	2. Combining medication with aerosolized bronchodilators is typically used to control bronchoconstriction in an acute exacerbation. In general, however, the pMDI with spacer is the preferred route (less cost and time to treatment)	

Plan of Nursing Care — Chart 25-5. Care of the Patient With COPD, *Continued*

NURSING INTERVENTIONS	RATIONALE	EXPECTED OUTCOMES
3. Instruct and encourage patient in diaphragmatic breathing and effective coughing	3. These techniques improve ventilation by opening airways to facilitate clearing the airways of sputum. Gas exchange is improved, and fatigue is minimized	
4. Administer oxygen by the method prescribed. a. Explain rationale and importance to patient b. Evaluate effectiveness; observe for signs of hypoxemia. Notify physician if restlessness, anxiety, somnolence, cyanosis, or tachycardia is present c. Analyze arterial blood gases, and compare with baseline values When arterial puncture is performed and a blood sample is obtained, hold puncture site for 5 minutes to prevent arterial bleeding and development of ecchymoses d. Initiate pulse oximetry to monitor oxygen saturation e. Explain that no smoking is permitted by the patient or visitors while oxygen is in use	4. Oxygen will correct the hypoxemia. Careful observation of the litre flow or the percentage administered and its effect on the patient is important. These patients generally require low-flow oxygen rates of 1 to 2 L/minute. Periodic arterial blood gases and pulse oximetry help to evaluate adequacy of oxygenation. Smoking may render pulse oximetry inaccurate because the carbon monoxide from cigarette smoke also saturates hemoglobin	

Nursing Priority: Ineffective airway clearance
Goal: Achievement of airway clearance

NURSING INTERVENTIONS	RATIONALE	EXPECTED OUTCOMES
1. Adequately hydrate the patient	1. Systemic hydration keeps secretions moist and easier to expectorate. Fluids must be given with caution if right- or left-sided heart failure is present	• Verbalizes the need to drink fluids • Demonstrates diaphragmatic breathing and coughing • Performs postural drainage correctly • Coughing is minimized • Does not smoke • Verbalizes that pollens, fumes, gases, dusts, and extremes of temperature and humidity are irritants to be avoided • Identifies signs of early infection • Is free of infection (no fever, no change in sputum, lessening of dyspnea) • Verbalizes the need to notify the primary provider at the earliest sign of infection • Verbalizes the need to stay away from crowds or people with colds in flu season • Discusses flu and pneumonia vaccines with the clinician to help prevent infection
2. Instruct in and encourage the use of diaphragmatic breathing and coughing techniques	2. These techniques help to improve ventilation and mobilize secretions without causing breathlessness and fatigue	
3. Assist in administering the nebulizer or pMDI	3. This ensures adequate delivery of medication to the airways	
4. If indicated, perform postural drainage with percussion and vibration in the morning and at night as prescribed	4. This uses gravity to help raise secretions so they can be more easily expectorated or suctioned	
5. Instruct the patient to avoid bronchial irritants such as cigarette smoke, aerosols, extremes of temperature, and fumes	5. Bronchial irritants cause bronchoconstriction and increased mucus production, which then interfere with airway clearance	
6. Educate about early signs of infection that are to be reported to the clinician immediately: a. Increased sputum production b. Change in colour of sputum c. Increased thickness of sputum d. Increased shortness of breath, tightness in chest, or fatigue e. Increased coughing f. Fever or chills	6. Minor respiratory infections that are of no consequence to the person with normal lungs can produce fatal disturbances in the lungs of the person with emphysema. Early recognition is crucial	

continued >

Plan of Nursing Care Chart 25-5. Care of the Patient With COPD, *Continued*

NURSING INTERVENTIONS	RATIONALE	EXPECTED OUTCOMES
7. Administer antibiotics as prescribed.	7. Antibiotics may be prescribed to prevent or treat infection	
8. Encourage patient to be immunized against influenza and *Streptococcus pneumoniae*.	8. People with respiratory conditions are prone to respiratory infections and are encouraged to be immunized	
Nursing Priority: Ineffective breathing pattern **Goal:** Improvement in breathing pattern		
1. Instruct patient in diaphragmatic and pursed-lip breathing 2. Encourage alternating activity with rest periods. Allow the patient to make some decisions (bath, shaving) about care based on the tolerance level 3. Encourage the use of an inspiratory muscle trainer, if prescribed	1. This helps the patient prolong expiration time and decreases air trapping. With these techniques, the patient will breathe more efficiently and effectively 2. Pacing activities permits the patient to perform activities without excessive distress 3. This strengthens and conditions the respiratory muscles	• Practices pursed-lip and diaphragmatic breathing and uses them when short of breath and with activity • Shows signs of decreased respiratory effort and paces activities • Uses inspiratory muscle trainer as prescribed
Nursing Priority: Self-care deficits **Goal:** Independence in self-care activities		
1. Educate patient to coordinate diaphragmatic breathing with activity (e.g., walking, bending) 2. Encourage the patient to begin to bathe self, dress self, walk, and drink fluids. Discuss energy conservation measures 3. Teach postural drainage, if appropriate	1. This will allow the patient to be more active and to avoid excessive fatigue or dyspnea during activity 2. As condition resolves, the patient will be able to do more but needs to be encouraged to avoid increasing dependence 3. This encourages the patient to become involved in self-care. Prepares the patient to manage at home	• Uses controlled breathing while bathing, bending, and walking • Paces activities of daily living to alternate with rest periods to reduce fatigue and dyspnea • Describes energy conservation strategies • Performs same self-care activities as before • Performs postural drainage correctly
Nursing Priority: Activity intolerance **Goal:** Improvement in activity tolerance		
1. Support the patient in establishing a regular regimen of exercise using a treadmill and exercise bicycle, walking, or other appropriate exercises, such as mall walking 2. Assess patient's current level of functioning, and develop exercise plan based on baseline functional status 3. Suggest consultation with physical therapist or pulmonary rehabilitation program to determine an exercise program specific to patient's capability. Have portable oxygen unit available if oxygen is prescribed for exercise	1. Muscles that are deconditioned consume more oxygen and place an additional burden on the lungs. Through regular, graded exercise, these muscle groups become more conditioned, and the patient can do more without getting as short of breath. Graded exercise breaks the cycle of debilitation	• Performs activities with less shortness of breath • Verbalizes the need to exercise daily and demonstrates an exercise plan to be carried out at home • Walks and gradually increases walking time and distance to improve physical condition • Exercises both upper and lower body muscle groups

Plan of Nursing Care

Chart 25-5. Care of the Patient With COPD, *Continued*

NURSING INTERVENTIONS	RATIONALE	EXPECTED OUTCOMES
Nursing Priority: Ineffective coping **Goal:** Attainment of an optimal level of coping		
1. Help the patient develop realistic goals	1. Developing realistic goals will promote a sense of hope and accomplishment rather than defeat and hopelessness	• Expresses interest in the future • Participates in discharge plan • Discusses activities or methods that can be performed to ease shortness of breath • Uses relaxation techniques appropriately • Expresses interest in a pulmonary rehabilitation program
2. Encourage activity to level of symptom tolerance	2. Activity reduces tension and decreases the degree of dyspnea as the patient becomes conditioned	
3. Educate the patient about relaxation techniques or provide a relaxation recording on audiotape, CD, or digital audio available on smart phones or tablets	3. Relaxation reduces stress, anxiety, and dyspnea and helps the patient cope with disability	
4. Enroll patient in a pulmonary rehabilitation program where available	4. Pulmonary rehabilitation programs have been shown to promote a subjective improvement in a patient's status and self-esteem as well as increased exercise tolerance and decreased hospitalizations	
Nursing Priority: Lack of knowledge **Goal:** Adherence to therapeutic program and home care		
1. Help the patient understand short- and long-term goals. a. Educate the patient about disease, medications, procedures, and how and when to seek help b. Refer patient to pulmonary rehabilitation	1. The patient needs to be a partner in developing the plan of care and needs to know what to expect. Education about the condition is one of the most important aspects of care; it will prepare the patient to live and cope with the condition and improve quality of life	• Understands disease and what affects it • Verbalizes the need to preserve existing lung function by adhering to prescribed program • Understands purposes and proper administration of medications • Stops smoking or enrolls in a smoking cessation program • Identifies when and whom to call for assistance
2. Give a strong message to stop smoking. Discuss smoking cessation strategies. Provide information about resource groups (e.g., Canadian Cancer Society, Canadian Lung Association, Government of Canada resources)	2. Smoking causes permanent damage to the lung and diminishes the lungs' protective mechanisms. Airflow is obstructed, and lung capacity is reduced. Smoking increases morbidity and mortality and is also a risk factor for lung cancer	
Collaborative Problem: Atelectasis **Goal:** Absence of atelectasis on x-ray and physical examination		
1. Monitor the respiratory status, including the rate and pattern of respirations, breath sounds, signs and symptoms of respiratory distress, and pulse oximetry	1. A change in respiratory status, including tachypnea, dyspnea, and diminished or absent breath sounds, may indicate atelectasis	• Normal (baseline for patient) respiratory rate and pattern • Normal breath sounds for patient • Demonstrates diaphragmatic breathing and effective coughing • Performs deep-breathing exercises, incentive spirometry as prescribed • Pulse oximetry ≥90%
2. Instruct in and encourage diaphragmatic breathing and effective coughing techniques	2. These techniques improve ventilation and lung expansion and ideally improve gas exchange	
3. Promote the use of lung expansion techniques (e.g., deep-breathing exercises, incentive spirometry) as prescribed	3. Deep-breathing exercises and incentive spirometry promote maximal lung expansion	

continued >

Plan of Nursing Care

Chart 25-5. Care of the Patient With COPD, *Continued*

Collaborative Problem: Pneumothorax
Goal: Absence of signs and symptoms of pneumothorax

NURSING INTERVENTIONS	RATIONALE	EXPECTED OUTCOMES
1. Monitor the respiratory status, including the rate and pattern of respirations, symmetry of chest wall movement, breath sounds, signs and symptoms of respiratory distress, and pulse oximetry	1. Dyspnea, tachypnea, tachycardia, acute pleuritic chest pain, tracheal deviation away from the affected side, absence of breath sounds on the affected side, and decreased tactile fremitus may indicate pneumothorax	• Normal respiratory rate and pattern for patient • Normal breath sounds bilaterally • Normal pulse for patient • Normal tactile fremitus • Absence of pain • Tracheal position is midline • Pulse oximetry ≥90% • Maintains normal oxygen saturation and arterial blood gas measurements for patient • Exhibits no hypoxemia and hypercapnia (or returns to baseline values) • Absence of pain • Symmetric chest wall movement • Lung fully expanded bilaterally on chest x-ray
2. Assess the pulse	2. Tachycardia is associated with pneumothorax and anxiety	
3. Assess for chest pain and precipitating factors	3. Pain may accompany pneumothorax	
4. Palpate for tracheal deviation/shift away from the affected side	4. Early detection of pneumothorax and prompt intervention will prevent other serious complications	
5. Monitor the pulse oximetry and, if indicated, arterial blood gases	5. Recognition of a deterioration in respiratory function will prevent serious complications	
6. Administer supplemental oxygen therapy as indicated	6. Oxygen will correct hypoxemia; administer it with caution	
7. Administer analgesics, as indicated, for chest pain	7. Pain interferes with deep breathing, resulting in a decrease in lung expansion	
8. Assist with chest tube insertion, and use the pleural drainage system as prescribed	8. Removal of air from the pleural space will re-expand the lung	

Collaborative Problem: Respiratory failure
Goal: Absence of signs and symptoms of respiratory failure; no evidence of respiratory failure on laboratory tests

NURSING INTERVENTIONS	RATIONALE	EXPECTED OUTCOMES
1. Monitor the respiratory status, including the rate and pattern of respirations, breath sounds, and signs and symptoms of acute respiratory distress	1. Early recognition of a deterioration in respiratory function will avert further complications, such as respiratory failure, severe hypoxemia, and hypercapnia	• Normal respiratory rate and pattern for patient with no acute distress • Recognizes symptoms of hypoxemia and hypercapnia • Maintains normal arterial blood gases/pulse oximetry or returns to baseline values
2. Monitor the pulse oximetry and arterial blood gases	2. Recognition of changes in oxygenation and acid–base balance will guide in correcting and preventing complications	
3. Administer supplemental oxygen, and initiate mechanisms for mechanical ventilation as prescribed	3. Acute respiratory failure is a medical emergency. Hypoxemia is a hallmark sign. Administration of oxygen therapy and mechanical ventilation, if indicated, are critical to survival	

Collaborative Problem: Pulmonary hypertension
Goal: Absence of evidence of pulmonary hypertension on physical examination or laboratory tests

NURSING INTERVENTIONS	RATIONALE	EXPECTED OUTCOMES
1. Monitor the respiratory status, including the rate and pattern of respirations, breath sounds, pulse oximetry, and signs and symptoms of acute respiratory distress	1. Dyspnea is the primary symptom of pulmonary hypertension. Other symptoms include fatigue, angina, near syncope, edema, and palpitations	• Normal respiratory rate and pattern for patient • Exhibits no signs and symptoms of right-sided failure • Maintains baseline pulse oximetry values and arterial blood gases
2. Assess for signs and symptoms of right-sided heart failure, including peripheral edema, ascites, distended neck veins, crackles, and heart murmur.	2. Right-sided heart failure is a common clinical manifestation of pulmonary arterial hypertension due to increased right ventricular workload	
3. Administer oxygen therapy as prescribed	3. Continuous oxygen therapy is a major component of management of pulmonary arterial hypertension; it prevents hypoxemia thereby reducing pulmonary vascular constriction (resistance) secondary to hypoxemia	

definite sign is prolonged history of productive, chronic cough, with sputum consistently negative for tubercle bacilli. The diagnosis is established by a CT scan, which demonstrates either the presence or absence of bronchial dilation. The advent of high-resolution CT scanning makes it possible to diagnose this disease during its earlier stages.

Medical Management

Treatment objectives are to promote bronchial drainage to clear excessive secretions from the affected portion of the lungs and to prevent or control infection. Postural drainage is part of all treatment plans, because draining the bronchiectatic areas by gravity reduces the amount of secretions and the degree of infection. Sometimes, mucopurulent sputum must be removed by bronchoscopy. Chest physiotherapy, including percussion and postural drainage, is important in the management of secretions. Smoking cessation is important because smoking impairs bronchial drainage by paralyzing ciliary action, increasing bronchial secretions, and causing inflammation of the mucous membranes, resulting in hyperplasia of the mucous glands.

Antibiotics are the cornerstone therapy for management of a bronchiectatic exacerbation. Antimicrobial therapy choice is based on the results of sensitivity studies on organisms cultured from sputum; however, empiric coverage (i.e., broad-spectrum antibiotics that are effective in treating commonly implicated pathogens) is often prescribed initially, pending results of sputum cultures. The most commonly implicated pathogens include *H. influenza,* which may be treated with amoxicillin-clavulanate (Augmentin), *M. catarrhalis,* which can be treated with gemifloxacin (Factive) or levofloxacin (Levaquin), *Staphylococcus aureus,* which responds to clindamycin (Cleocin), and *Pseudomonas aeruginosa,* which may be treated with ciprofloxacin (Cipro) (Barker, 2015b). Because infection with *P. aeruginosa* is associated with a greater rate of lung function deterioration, more aggressive oral or IV antibiotic therapy may be used for a longer duration. For patients with recurrent exacerbations (usually two or more during the past year), a low-dose macrolide antibiotic may be used as preventative, ongoing therapy (Barker, 2015b). In addition, patients should be vaccinated against influenza and pneumococcal pneumonia.

Secretion management is an issue for patients with bronchiectasis. Bronchodilators, which may be prescribed for patients who also have reactive airway disease, may also assist with secretion management. In addition, nebulized mucolytics may help to clear airway secretions. Ensuring adequate hydration and employing chest physiotherapy may also be of help in loosening and thinning secretions (Barker, 2015b).

Surgical intervention, although used infrequently, may be indicated for patients who continues to expectorate large amounts of sputum and have repeated bouts of pneumonia and hemoptysis despite adhering to the treatment regimen. The disease must involve only one or two areas of the lung that can be removed without producing respiratory insufficiency. The goals of surgical treatment are to conserve normal pulmonary tissue and to avoid infectious complications. Diseased tissue is removed, provided that the postoperative lung function will be adequate. It may be necessary to remove a segment of a lobe (segmental resection), a lobe (lobectomy), or rarely an entire lung (pneumonectomy). (See Chart 26-16 for further information.) Segmental resection is the removal of an anatomic subdivision of a pulmonary lobe. In select cases, video-assisted surgery (VATS) segmentectomy or lobectomy may be performed, which is associated with fewer complications and decreased length of stay. The chief advantage is that only diseased tissue is removed and healthy lung tissue is conserved.

The surgery is preceded by a period of careful preparation. The objective is to obtain a dry (free of infection) tracheobronchial tree to prevent complications (atelectasis, pneumonia, bronchopleural fistula, and empyema). This is accomplished by postural drainage or, depending on the location, by direct suction through a bronchoscope. A course of antibacterial therapy may be prescribed. After surgery, care is the same as for any patient who has undergone chest surgery (see Chapter 26).

Nursing Management

Nursing management focuses on alleviating symptoms and helping patients clear pulmonary secretions. Patient education targets eliminating smoking and other factors that increase the production of mucus and hamper its removal. Patient and family are taught to perform postural drainage and to avoid exposure to people with upper respiratory or other infections. If the patient experiences fatigue and dyspnea, he or she is informed about strategies to conserve energy while maintaining as active a lifestyle as possible. The patient is educated about the early signs of respiratory infection and the progression of the disorder so that appropriate treatment can be implemented promptly. The presence of a large amount of mucus may decrease the patient's appetite and result in an inadequate dietary intake, therefore, the patient's nutritional status is assessed, and strategies are implemented to ensure an adequate diet.

Asthma

Asthma is a heterogeneous disease, usually characterized by chronic airway inflammation (GINA [Global Initiative for Asthma], 2015). This chronic inflammatory disease of the airways causes airway hyperresponsiveness, mucosal edema, and mucus production. This inflammation ultimately leads to recurrent episodes of asthma symptoms: cough, chest tightness, wheezing, and dyspnea (Fig. 25-6). It is estimated that the number of Canadians living with diagnosed asthma was 3.8 million, or 10.8% of the population, in 2011/2012 (Public Health Agency of Canada [PHAC], 2018a). The PHAC also state that the 2011/2012 prevalence of asthma increased steadily in childhood, peaking in the 10 to 14 age group for males (22.2%) and the 15 to 19 age group in females (17.0%). Prevalence declined after that until the 30 to 34 age group and remained steady until the 60 to 64 age group, after which there was an increase in prevalence in both males (more pronounced) and females. The majority of individuals with asthma have suboptimal asthma control despite the fact that effective treatments for asthma exist. Subsequent

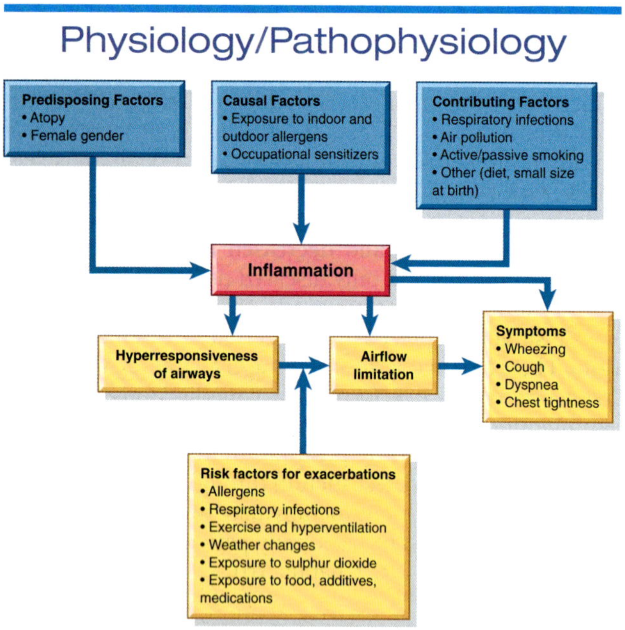

FIGURE 25-6. Pathophysiology of asthma. (Adapted from materials developed for the Global Initiative for Asthma (2015). Global strategy for asthma management and prevention. Available at: www.ginasthma.org.)

costs for hospitalizations, unscheduled health care provider visits, ED visits, drug treatment, and ambulance services for asthma exacerbations resulting from poor asthma control exceed $160 million (Ismaila, Sayani, Marin, et al., 2013). Although asthma is the most common chronic disease of childhood, it can occur at any age. For most patients, asthma is a disruptive disease, affecting school and work attendance, occupational choices, physical activity, and general quality of life. Despite increased knowledge regarding the pathology of asthma and the development of improved medications and management plans, the death rate from the disease continues to rise.

Ethnic and racial disparities affect morbidity and mortality in asthma, which are higher in inner-city African Americans and Latinos (CDC, 2015c). Contributing to these disparities are epidemiology and risk factors, genetics and molecular aspect, inner-city environments, limited community assets, health care access/delivery/and quality, and insufficient health insurance coverage.

Unlike other obstructive lung diseases, asthma is largely reversible, either spontaneously or with treatment. Patients with asthma may experience symptom-free periods alternating with acute exacerbations, which last from minutes to hours or days.

Allergy is the strongest predisposing factor for asthma. Chronic exposure to airway irritants or allergens also increases the risk of asthma. Common allergens can be seasonal (e.g., grass, tree, and weed pollens) or perennial (e.g., mold, dust, roaches, or animal dander). Common triggers for asthma symptoms and exacerbations include airway irritants (e.g., air pollutants, cold, heat, weather changes, strong odours or perfumes, smoke, occupational exposure), foods (e.g., shellfish, nuts), exercise, stress, hormonal factors, viral respiratory tract infections, medications, and gastroesophageal reflux. Most people who have asthma are sensitive to a variety of triggers (Kaufman, 2012).

Pathophysiology

The underlying pathology in asthma is reversible diffuse airway inflammation that leads to long-term airway narrowing. This narrowing, which is exacerbated by various changes in the airway, includes bronchoconstriction, airway edema, airway hyperresponsiveness, and airway remodeling. The interaction of these factors determines the clinical manifestations and severity of asthma (GINA, 2015). Over the course of a lifetime, the impact of increasing pathophysiologic changes and environmental susceptibility leads to an irreversible disease process.

The inflammation leads to obstruction from the following: swelling of the membranes that line the airways (mucosal edema), reducing the airway diameter; contraction of the bronchial smooth muscle that encircles the airways (bronchospasm), causing further narrowing; and increased mucus production, which diminishes airway size and may entirely plug the bronchi.

Asthma is a complex disease process that involves numerous inflammatory and structural cells as well as mediators that lead to the disorder's effects. Mast cells, macrophages, T lymphocytes, neutrophils, and eosinophils all play a key role in the inflammation of asthma. When activated, mast cells release several chemicals called *mediators*. These chemicals, which include histamine, bradykinin, prostanoids, cytokines, leukotrienes, and other mediators perpetuate the inflammatory response, causing increased blood flow, vasoconstriction, fluid leak from the vasculature, attraction of white blood cells to the area, mucous secretion and bronchoconstriction (GINA, 2014). Regulation of these chemicals is the aim of much of the current research regarding pharmacologic therapy for asthma.

During acute exacerbations of asthma, bronchial smooth muscle contraction or bronchoconstriction occurs quickly to narrow the airway in response to an exposure. Acute bronchoconstriction due to allergens results from an immunoglobulin E (IgE)–dependent release of mediators from mast cells; these mediators include histamine, tryptase, leukotrienes, and prostaglandins that directly contract the airway. There are also non–IgE-mediated responses and proinflammatory cytokines (GINA, 2015). In addition, alpha- and beta$_2$-adrenergic receptors of the sympathetic nervous system located in the bronchi play a role. When the alpha-adrenergic receptors are stimulated, bronchoconstriction occurs. The balance between alpha- and beta$_2$-adrenergic receptors is controlled primarily by cyclic 3′,5′-adenosine monophosphate (cAMP). Beta$_2$-receptor stimulation results in increased levels of cAMP, which inhibits the release of chemical mediators and causes bronchodilation.

As asthma becomes more persistent, the inflammation progresses, and other factors may be involved in airflow limitation. These include airway edema, mucus hypersecretion, and the formation of mucus plugs. In addition, airway "remodeling" (i.e., structural changes) may occur in response to chronic inflammation, causing further airway narrowing.

Clinical Manifestations

The three most common symptoms of asthma are cough, dyspnea, and wheezing. In some instances, cough may be the only symptom. Asthma attacks often occur at night or early in the morning, possibly due to circadian variations that influence airway receptor thresholds.

An asthma exacerbation may begin abruptly but most frequently is preceded by increasing symptoms over the previous few days. There is cough, with or without mucus production. At times, the mucus is so tightly wedged in the narrowed airway that the patient cannot cough it up. There may be generalized wheezing (the sound of airflow through narrowed airways), first on expiration and then possibly during inspiration as well. Generalized chest tightness and dyspnea occur. Expiration requires effort and becomes prolonged. As the exacerbation progresses, diaphoresis, tachycardia, and a widened pulse pressure may occur along with hypoxemia and central cyanosis (a late sign of poor oxygenation). Although severe, life-threatening hypoxemia can occur in asthma, it is relatively uncommon. The hypoxemia is secondary to a ventilation–perfusion mismatch and readily responds to supplemental oxygenation.

Symptoms of exercise-induced asthma include maximal symptoms during exercise, absence of nocturnal symptoms, and sometimes only a description of a "choking" sensation during exercise.

Assessment and Diagnostic Findings

To establish the diagnosis, the clinician must determine that periodic symptoms of airflow obstruction are present, airflow is at least partially reversible, and other causes have been excluded. A positive family history and environmental factors, including seasonal changes, high pollen counts, mold, pet dander, climate changes (particularly cold air), and air pollution, are primarily associated with asthma. In addition, asthma is associated with a variety of occupation-related chemicals, foods, and compounds. Comorbid conditions that may accompany asthma include viral infections, gastroesophageal reflux disease, drug-induced asthma, and allergic bronchopulmonary aspergillosis. Other possible allergic reactions that may accompany asthma include eczema, rashes, and temporary edema.

Specific questions in the assessment that may help to evaluate the patient's asthma control include:

- Have your symptoms awakened you at night or in the early morning?
- Have you needed your quick-acting relief medication more than usual?
- Have you needed unscheduled care for your asthma—a call to the primary provider's office, office visit, ED?
- Have your symptoms impacted your normal activities at school/work/sports?

During acute episodes, sputum and blood tests may disclose eosinophilia (elevated levels of eosinophils). Serum levels of IgE may be elevated if allergy is present. Arterial blood gas analysis and pulse oximetry reveal hypoxemia during acute attacks. Initially, hypocapnia and respiratory alkalosis are present. As the patient's condition worsens and he or she becomes more fatigued, the $PaCO_2$ may increase. Because carbon dioxide is 20 times more diffusible than oxygen, it is rare for $PaCO_2$ to be normal or elevated in a person who is breathing very rapidly.

> **NURSING ALERT**
>
> **Normal $PaCO_2$ during an asthma attack may be a signal of impending respiratory failure.**

During an exacerbation, the FEV_1 and FVC are markedly decreased but improve with bronchodilator administration (demonstrating reversibility). Pulmonary function is usually normal between exacerbations. The occurrence of a severe, continuous reaction is referred to as status asthmaticus and is considered life-threatening (see later discussion).

Asthma severity is considered in the selection of the initial type, amount, and schedule of treatments (GINA, 2015); (National Heart Lung and Blood Institute [NHLBI], 2012). Disease severity is classified by current impairment and future risk of adverse events. Impairment is defined by the following factors: nighttime awakenings, the need for short-acting bronchodilators for symptom relief, work/school days missed, ability to engage in normal activities, and quality of life. Lung function is evaluated by spirometry. Assessment of risk of future adverse events is evaluated by numbers of exacerbations, the need for ED care or hospitalizations in the past year, demographic data (gender, ethnicity, nonuse of prescribed inhaled corticosteroid therapy, existing smoking), psychosocial factors and attitudes, and beliefs about taking medication (GINA, 2015; NHLBI, 2012).

Prevention

Patients with recurrent asthma should undergo tests to identify the substances that precipitate the symptoms. Possible causes are dust, dust mites, roaches, certain types of cloth, pets, horses, detergents, soaps, certain foods, molds, and pollens. If the attacks are seasonal, pollens can be strongly suspected. The patient is instructed to avoid the causative agents whenever possible. Knowledge is the key to quality asthma care. Evaluation of impairment and risk are primary methods that help ensure control.

Occupational asthma refers to asthma induced by exposure in the work environment to dusts, vapors, or fumes, with or without a pre-existing diagnosis of asthma. Work-related asthma should be part of the differential diagnosis of every case of adult-onset asthma. A detailed work history evaluation is key to identifying occupational asthma. Immediate treatment is aimed at removing or decreasing the exposure in the patient's environment and following the patient on an ongoing basis. Standard asthma medications may be prescribed to minimize bronchoconstriction and airway inflammation. In certain cases, patients may be impaired or disabled from the disease. Compensation systems are in place to protect a worker; however, these systems are often slow and complex to navigate.

Complications

Complications of asthma may include status asthmaticus, respiratory failure, pneumonia, and atelectasis. Airway obstruction, particularly during acute asthmatic episodes, often results in hypoxemia, requiring the administration

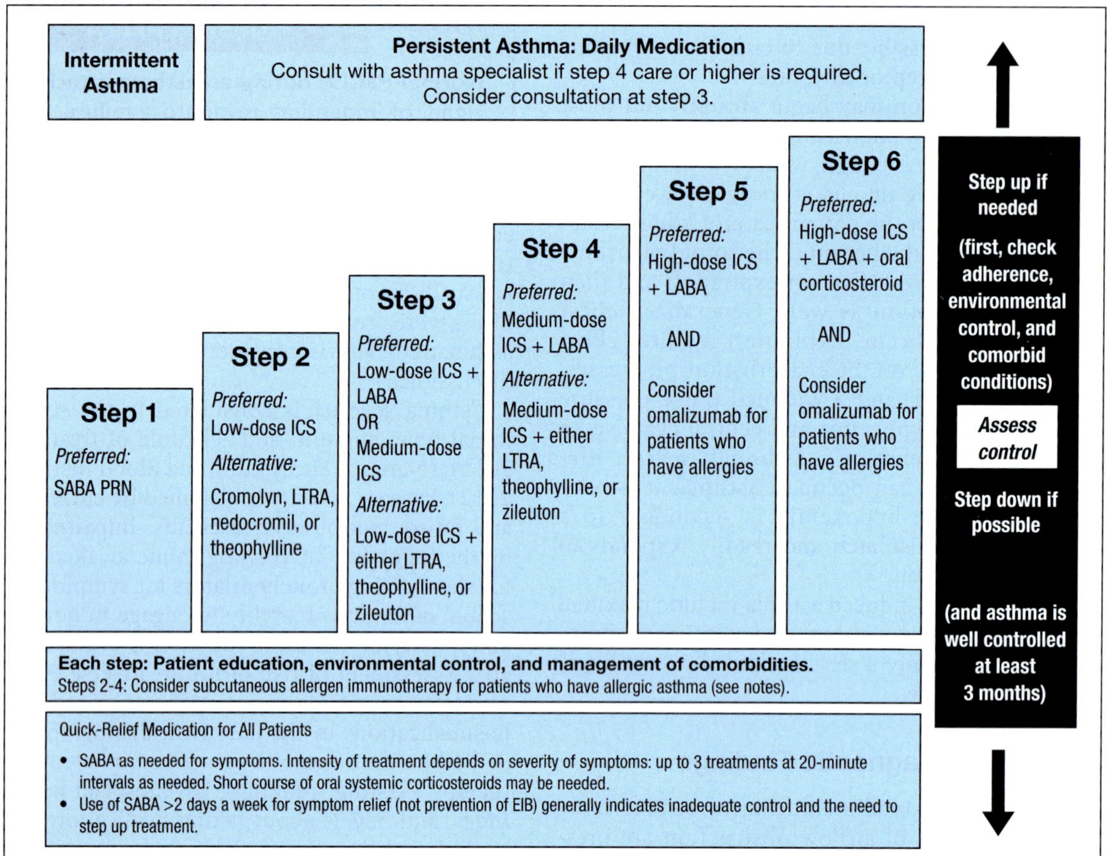

Key: **Alphabetical order is used when more than one treatment option is listed within either preferred or alternative therapy.** EIB, exercise-induced bronchospasm; ICS, inhaled corticosteroid; LABA, inhaled long-acting beta$_2$-agonist; LTRA, leukotriene receptor antagonist; SABA, inhaled short-acting beta$_2$-agonist

Notes:

- The stepwise approach is meant to assist, not replace, the clinical decision making required to meet individual patient needs.
- If alternative treatment is used and response is inadequate, discontinue it and use the preferred treatment before stepping up.
- Zileuton is a less desirable alternative due to limited studies as adjunctive therapy and the need to monitor liver function. Theophylline requires monitoring of serum concentration levels.
- In step 6, before oral systemic corticosteroids are introduced, a trial of high-dose ICS + LABA + either LTRA, theophylline, or zileuton may be considered, although this approach has not been studied in clinical trials.
- Steps 1, 2, and 3 preferred therapies are based on evidence A; step 3 alternative therapy is based on evidence A for LTRA, evidence B for theophylline, and evidence D for zileuton. Step 4 preferred therapy is based on evidence B, and alternative therapy is based on evidence B for LTRA and theophylline and evidence D for zileuton. Step 5 preferred therapy is based on evidence B. Step 6 preferred therapy is based on (EPR—2 1997) and evidence B for omalizumab.
- Immunotherapy for steps 2-4 is based on evidence B for house-dust mites, animal danders, and pollens; evidence is weak or lacking for molds and cockroaches. Evidence is strongest for immunotherapy with single allergens. The role of allergy in asthma is greater in children than in adults.
- Clinicians who administer immunotherapy or omalizumab should be prepared and equipped to identify and treat anaphylaxis that may occur.

FIGURE 25-7. Stepwise approach for managing asthma in youths 12 years and older and adults. (Redrawn and adapted from Expert Panel Report 3. (2007). *Guidelines for the diagnosis and management of asthma.* National Asthma Education and Prevention Program. NIH Publication Number 08-5846. Bethesda, MD: U.S. Department of Health and Human Services, National Heart, Lung and Blood Institute; National Heart, Lung and Blood Institute (NHLBI) (2012). Asthma care quick reference: diagnosing and managing asthma. NIH Publication No. 12-5075. Revised September 2012.)

of oxygen and the monitoring of pulse oximetry and arterial blood gases. Fluids are given because people with asthma are frequently dehydrated from diaphoresis and insensible fluid loss with hyperventilation.

Medical Management

Immediate intervention is necessary because the continuing and progressive dyspnea leads to increased anxiety, aggravating the situation. The NHLBI (2012) and GINA (2015) recommendations are based on the concept of severity and control of asthma along with the domains of reducing impairment and reducing risk as keys to improving care. Primary treatment concerns are impairment of lung function and normal life and risk of exacerbations, decline in lung function, and adverse effects from medications (NHLBI, 2012).

Pharmacologic Therapy

Figure 25-7 shows the pharmacologic treatment of asthma using a stepwise approach. There are two general classes of asthma medications: quick-relief medications for immediate treatment of asthma symptoms and exacerbations and long-acting medications to achieve and maintain control of persistent asthma (see Tables 25-3, 25-4, and 25-5). Because the underlying pathology of asthma is inflammation, control of persistent asthma is accomplished primarily with regular use of anti-inflammatory medications. These medications have systemic side effects when used over the long term. The route of choice for administration of these medications is the pMDI or other type of inhaler, because it allows for topical administration.

Long-Acting Control Medications

Corticosteroids are the most potent and effective anti-inflammatory medications currently available. They are broadly effective in alleviating symptoms, improving airway function, and decreasing peak flow variability. Initially, the inhaled form is used. A spacer should be used with inhaled corticosteroids, and the patient should rinse the mouth after administration to prevent thrush, a common complication of inhaled corticosteroid use. A systemic preparation may be used to gain rapid control of the disease; to manage severe, persistent asthma; to treat moderate to severe exacerbations; to accelerate recovery; and to prevent recurrence.

Cromolyn sodium (Crolom, NasalCrom) and *nedocromil* (Alocril, Tilade) are mild to moderate anti-inflammatory agents and are considered alternative medications for treatment. These medications stabilize mast cells. They also are effective on a prophylactic basis to prevent exercise-induced

(text continued on page 591)

TABLE 25-3 Common Types of Bronchodilator Medications for Chronic Obstructive Pulmonary Disease

Class/Drug (Trade Name)	Method of Administration Inhaler[a]	Nebulizer	Oral	Duration of Action[b]
Beta$_2$-Adrenergic Agonist Agents				
Fenoterol (Berotec N)	X	X	X	SABA
Salbutamol, albuterol (Ventolin)	X	X	X	SABA
Albuterol (ProAir RespiClick)	X	X	X	SABA
Levalbuterol (Xopenex HFA)	X	X		SABA
Terbutaline (Brethine, Brethaire)	X			SABA
Arformoterol (Brovana)	X			LABA
Formoterol (Foradil)	X			LABA
Salmeterol (Serevent Diskus)				LABA
Indacaterol (Arcapta, Onbrez)				LABA
Anticholinergic Agents				
Ipratropium bromide (Atrovent, Ipraxa) tiotropium bromide	X	X		SAMA
(Spiriva) umeclidinium (Incruse Ellipta)	X			LAMA
	X			LAMA
Combination Short-Acting Beta$_2$-Adrenergic Agonist and Anticholinergic Agents				
Fenoterol/ipratropium (Beodual N)	X	X		SABA/SAMA
Salbutamol/ipratropium (Combivent, DuoNeb)	X			SABA/SAMA
Inhaled Corticosteroids (ICS)				
Beclomethasone propionate (Qvar)	X	X		
Budesonide (Pulmicort Flexhaler)	X	X		
Fluticasone propionate (Flovent)	X	X		
Combination Inhaled Corticosteroids and Long Acting Beta$_2$-Adrenergic Agonist				
Budesonide/formoterol (Symbicort)	X			ICS/LABA
Mometasone/formoterol/(Dulera)	X			ICS/LABA
Fluticasone/salmetereol/(Advair Discus)	X			ICS/LABA
Fluticasone furoate/vilanterol (Breo Ellipta)	X			ICS/LABA

[a]Inhaler may include pressurized metered-dose inhaler, dry powdered inhalation with inhaler, or Diskus.

[b]Short acting, 4–6 hours; long acting, 12+ hours.

SABA, short-acting beta$_2$-agonist; LABA, long-acting beta$_2$-agonist; SAMA, short-acting anticholinergic; LAMA, long-acting anticholinergic; ICS, inhaled corticosteroid.

Adapted from Global Initiative for Chronic Obstructive Lung Disease (GOLD). (2015). *Global strategy for the diagnosis, management and prevention of COPD*. Retrieved on April 18, 2016, from www.goldcopd.org/uploads/users/files/GOLD_Report_2015.pdf

TABLE 25-4 Long-Term Medications for Treatment of Asthma (Controller Medications)

Medication	Indications/Mechanisms	Potential Adverse Effects	Nursing Considerations
Inhaled Corticosteroids			
Beclomethasone Propionate (QVAR) Budesonide (Pulmicort Flexhaler) Ciclesonide (Alvesco) Flunisolide (AeroBid) Fluticasone (Flovent) Mometasone furoate (Asmanex) Triamcinolone acetonide (Azmacort)	*Indications* Long-term prevention of symptoms; suppression, control, and reversal of inflammation Reduce need for oral corticosteroid *Mechanisms* Anti-inflammatory; block late reaction to allergen and reduce airway hyperresponsiveness Inhibit cytokine production, adhesion protein activation, and inflammatory cell migration and activation; reverse beta$_2$-receptor down-regulation; inhibit microvascular leakage	Cough, dysphonia, oral thrush (candidiasis), headache In high doses, systemic effects may occur (e.g., adrenal suppression, osteoporosis, skin thinning, and easy bruising)	Instruct patient in correct use of pMDI and use of spacer/holding chamber devices Instruct patient to rinse mouth after inhalation to reduce local side effects
Systemic Corticosteroids			
Methylprednisolone (Medrol) Prednisolone (Prelone) Prednisone (Deltasone, Orasone)	*Indications* For short-term (3–10 days) "burst": to gain prompt control of inadequately controlled persistent asthma For long-term prevention of symptoms in severe persistent asthma: suppression, control, and reversal of inflammation *Mechanisms* Same as inhaled corticosteroids	*Short-term use:* reversible abnormalities in glucose metabolism, increased appetite, fluid retention, weight gain, mood alteration, hypertension, peptic ulcer, and rarely aseptic necrosis *Long-term use:* adrenal axis suppression, growth suppression, dermal thinning, hypertension, diabetes, Cushing syndrome, cataracts, muscle weakness, and, in rare instances, impaired immune function Consideration should be given to comorbidities that could be worsened by systemic corticosteroids	Instruct patient about possible side effects and the importance of taking the medication as prescribed (usually a single dose in the morning daily or on an alternate-day schedule, which may produce less adrenal suppression)
Long-Acting Beta$_2$-Agonists			
Inhaled salmeterol (Serevent Diskus) Formoterol (Foradil Aerolizer)	*Indications* Long-term prevention of symptoms, added to ICS Prevention of exercise-induced bronchospasm *Mechanisms* Bronchodilation; smooth muscle relaxation following adenylate cyclase activation and in crease in cAMP, producing functional antagonism of bronchoconstriction Compared to SABA, salmeterol (but not formoterol) has slower onset of action (15–30 minutes). Both salmeterol and formoterol have longer duration (>12 hours) compared to SABA	Should *not* be used to treat acute symptoms or exacerbations Decreased protection against exercise-induced bronchospasm may occur with regular use Tachycardia, muscle tremor, hypokalemia, ECG changes with overdose. A diminished bronchoprotective effect may occur within 1 week of chronic therapy. Potential risk of uncommon, severe, life-threatening, or fatal exacerbation	Reinforce to patient that these medications should *not* be used to treat acute asthma symptoms or exacerbations Instruct patient about correct use of pMDI or aerolizer inhaler
Oral Albuterol (Proventil) sustained release		Inhaled route is preferred to oral route because LABAs are longer acting and have fewer side effects than oral sustained-release agents	

TABLE 25-4 Long-Term Medications for Treatment of Asthma (Controller Medications) (Continued)

Medication	Indications/Mechanisms	Potential Adverse Effects	Nursing Considerations
Methylxanthines			
Theophylline (Slo-Bid, Theo-Dur) sustained-release tablets and capsules	*Indications* Long-term control and prevention of symptoms in mild persistent asthma or as adjunctive with ICS, in moderate or persistent asthma	Dose-related acute toxicities include tachycardia, nausea and vomiting, tachyarrhythmias (SVT), central nervous system stimulation, headache, seizures, hematemesis, hyperglycemia, and hypokalemia	Maintain steady-state serum concentrations between 5 and 15 mcg/mL
	Mechanisms Bronchodilation; smooth muscle relaxation from phosphodiesterase inhibition and possibly adenosine antagonism May affect eosinophilic infiltration into bronchial mucosa as well as decreased T-lymphocyte numbers in epithelium Increases diaphragm contractility and mucociliary clearance	Adverse effects at usual therapeutic doses include insomnia, gastric upset, aggravation of ulcer or reflux, and difficulty in urination in older males who have prostatism Not generally recommended for exacerbations. There is minimal evidence for added benefit to optimal doses of SABA. Serum concentration monitoring is mandatory Available as sustained-release tablets and capsules	Be aware that absorption and metabolism may be affected by numerous factors that can produce significant changes in steady-state serum theophylline concentrations Instruct patients to discontinue if they experience toxicity Inform patients about the importance of blood tests to monitor serum concentration Instruct patient to check with primary provider before taking any new medication
Combined Medication (corticosteroid/long-acting beta agonist)			
Fluticasone/salmeterol (Advair)	*DPI* 100 mcg/50 mcg 250 mcg/50 mcg 500 mcg/50 mcg *HFA* 45 mcg/21 mcg 115 mcg/21 mcg 230 mcg/21 mcg	Lowest dose of DPI or HFA used for patients whose asthma is not controlled on low- to medium-dose ICS Higher doses of DPI or HFA used for patients whose asthma is not controlled on medium- to high-dose ICS	
budesonide/formoterol (Symbicort) fluticasone furoate/vilanterol (Breo Ellipta)	*HFA pMDI* 80 mcg/4.5 mcg 160 mcg/4.5 mcg 100 mcg/25 mcg	Lower dose used for patients who have asthma not controlled on low- to medium-dose ICS Higher dose used for patients who have asthma not controlled on medium- to high-dose ICS Used if asthma not controlled on long term asthma control medication. Do not use with other long acting beta agonist drugs	
Cromolyn and Nedocromil			
Cromolyn sodium (Crolom, NasalCrom, Intal) Nedocromil (Alocril, Tilade)	*Indications* Long-term prevention of symptoms in mild persistent asthma; may modify inflammation Preventive treatment prior to exposure to exercise or known allergen *Mechanisms* Anti-inflammatory; blocks *early* and late reaction to allergen Stabilizes mast cell membranes and inhibits activation and release of mediators from eosinophils and epithelial cells Inhibits acute response to exercise, cold dry air, and SO_2	Cough and irritation 15–20% of patients complain of an unpleasant taste from nedocromil Dose of cromolyn by pMDI may be inadequate to affect airway hyperresponsiveness Nebulizer delivery may be preferred for some patients Safety is the primary advantage of these agents One dose before exercise or exposure to allergen provides effective prophylaxis for 1–2 hours. Not as effective for exercise-induced bronchospasm as short-acting $beta_2$-agonist	Inform patient that 4–6-week trial may be needed to determine maximum benefit Instruct patient about correct use of inhaler

continued >

TABLE 25-4 Long-Term Medications for Treatment of Asthma (Controller Medications) (Continued)

Medication	Indications/Mechanisms	Potential Adverse Effects	Nursing Considerations
Leukotriene Modifiers			
Leukotriene Receptor Antagonists Montelukast (Singulair)	*Mechanism* Selective competitive inhibitor of CysLT1 receptor *Indications* Long-term control and prevention of symptoms in mild persistent asthma for patients ≥1 y of age May also be used with ICS as combination therapy in moderate persistent asthma	May attenuate EIB in some patients, but less effective than ICS therapy LTRA + LABA should not be used as a substitute for ICS + LABA. No specific adverse effects have been identified Available in tablets and granules	Instruct patient to take at least 1 hour before meals or 2 hours after meals. Inform patient that zafirlukast can inhibit the metabolism of warfarin. INRs should be monitored if patient is taking both medications
Zafirlukast (Accolate)	Long-term control and prevention of symptoms in mild persistent asthma; may also be used with ICS as combination therapy in moderate persistent asthma	Cases of reversible hepatitis have been reported along with rare cases of irreversible hepatic failure resulting in death and liver transplantation Available in tablets	Instruct patients to discontinue use if they experience signs and symptoms of liver dysfunction (right upper quadrant pain, pruritus, lethargy, jaundice, nausea), and to notify their primary provider
5-Lipoxygenase Inhibitor zileuton (Zyflo)	*Mechanism* Inhibits the production of leukotrienes from arachidonic acid, both LTB and the cysteinyl leukotrienes *Indications* Long-term control and prevention of symptoms in mild persistent asthma for patients May be used with ICS as combination therapy in moderate persistent asthma in patients	Elevation of liver enzymes has been reported. Limited case reports of reversible hepatitis and hyperbilirubinemia	Inform patient that zileuton can inhibit the metabolism of warfarin and theophylline. Therefore, the doses of these medications should be monitored accordingly Educate patient about the importance of monitoring medication levels and tests of liver function
Immunomodulators			
Omalizumab (Xolair)	*Indications* Long-term control and prevention of symptoms in adults with moderate or severe persistent allergic asthma inadequately controlled with ICS *Mechanisms* Monoclonal antibody (anti-IgE) that binds to circulating IgE, preventing it from binding to the high-affinity receptors on basophils and mast cells Decreases mast cell mediator release from allergen exposure	Given by subcutaneous injection Anaphylaxis has been reported in 0.2% of treated patients Pain, bruising, and skin reactions (itching, redness, stinging) at injection sites Dose is given either every 2 or 4 weeks and depends on the patient's body weight and IgE level before therapy A maximum of 150 mg can be given in one injection Medication needs to be stored under refrigeration at 2–8°C (35.6–46.4°F) It is unknown if patients will develop significant antibody titers to the drug with long-term administration	Monitor patients for allergic reactions or anaphylaxis following administration Be prepared to initiate emergency treatment if anaphylaxis occurs Instruct patient about signs and symptoms that indicate allergic reaction and immediate action to take Remind patient to continue to take other medications prescribed for treatment of asthma

pMDI, pressurized metered-dose inhaler; ICS, inhaled corticosteroid; cAMP, cyclic 3′,5′-adenosine monophosphate; ECG, electrocardiogram; SABA, inhaled short-acting beta$_2$-agonist; LABA, long-acting beta$_2$-agonist; SVT, supraventricular tachycardia; DPI, dry powder inhaler; HFA, hydrofluoroalkane; SO_2, sulphur dioxide; CysLT1, cysteinyl leukotriene receptor 1; EIB, exercise-induced bronchospasm; LTRA, leukotriene receptor antagonist; INR, international normalized ratio; LTB, leukotriene B; IgE, immunoglobulin E.

Adapted from Global Strategy for Asthma Management and Prevention, Global Initiative for Asthma (GINA). (2015). Retrieved on January 25, 2015, from www.ginasthma.org/local/uploads/files/GINA_Report_2015_Aug11.pdf

TABLE 25-5 Quick-Relief Medications for Treatment of Asthma

Medication	Indications/Mechanisms	Potential Adverse Effects	Nursing Considerations
Inhaled Short-Acting Beta$_2$-Agonists			
Albuterol (AccuNeb, Proventil HFA, Ventolin HFA, ProAir RespiClick) Levalbuterol HFA (Xopenex HFA) Metaproterenol sulphate (Alupent)	*Indications* Relief of acute symptoms; quick-relief medication Preventive treatment for exercise-induced bronchospasm *Mechanisms* Bronchodilation; binds to the beta$_2$-adrenergic receptor, producing smooth muscle relaxation and decreased bronchoconstriction	Tachycardia, muscle tremor, hypokalemia, increased lactic acid, headache, and hyperglycemia. Inhaled route causes few systematic adverse effects. Patients with pre-existing cardiovascular disease, especially older adults, may have adverse cardiovascular reactions with inhaled therapy Lack of effect or need for regular use indicates inadequate asthma control	Instruct patient in correct use of inhaled agents and how to evaluate amount of remaining medication in pressurized metered-dose inhaler. Recommend periodic cleaning of device. Inform patient about possible adverse effects and need to inform primary provider about increased use of medication to control symptoms
Anticholinergics			
Ipratropium (Atrovent)	*Indications* Relief of acute bronchospasm *Mechanisms* Bronchodilation; inhibition of muscarinic cholinergic receptors Reduction in vagal tone of airways May decrease mucous gland secretion	Dryness of mouth and respiratory secretions; may cause increased wheezing in some patients Does not block exercise-induced bronchospasm Is not effective in long-term control of asthma	Instruct patient in correct use of inhaled agents Ensure adequate fluid intake Assess patient for hypersensitivity to atropine, soybeans, peanuts; glaucoma; prostatic hypertrophy
Corticosteroids			
Systemic Methylprednisolone (Medrol) Prednisolone (Prelone) Prednisone (Deltasone, Orasone)	*Indications* For moderate or severe exacerbations to prevent progression of exacerbation, reverse inflammation, speed recovery, and reduce rate of relapse *Mechanisms* Anti-inflammatory; block reaction to allergen and reduce hyperresponsiveness; inhibit cytokine production, adhesion protein activation, and inflammatory cell migration and activation; reverses beta$_2$-receptor down-regulation	Blood glucose abnormalities, increased appetite, fluid retention, weight gain, mood alteration, hypertension, peptic ulcer Consideration must be given to comorbidities that may be worsened by systemic corticosteroids	Explain to patient that action is often rapid in onset, although resolution of symptoms may take 3–10 days Instruct patient about possible side effects and the importance of taking the medication as prescribed

HFA, hydrofluoroalkane.

Adapted from Global Strategy for Asthma Management and Prevention, Global Initiative for Asthma (GINA). (2015). Retrieved on January 25, 2015, from www.ginasthma.org/local/uploads/files/GINA_Report_2015_Aug11.pdf

asthma or in unavoidable exposure to known triggers. These medications are contraindicated in acute asthma exacerbations.

LABAs are used with anti-inflammatory medications to control asthma symptoms, particularly those that occur during the night. These agents are also effective for preventing exercise-induced asthma. LABAs are not indicated for immediate relief of symptoms. Theophylline (Slo-Bid, Theo-Dur) is a mild to moderate bronchodilator that is usually used in addition to inhaled corticosteroids, mainly for relief of nighttime asthma symptoms. Salmeterol (Serevent Diskus) and formoterol (Foradil Aerolizer) have duration of bronchodilation of at least 12 hours. They are used with other medications in long-term control of asthma.

Leukotriene modifiers (inhibitors) or antileukotrienes are a class of medications that include montelukast (Singulair), and zafirlukast (Accolate). Leukotrienes, which synthesized from membrane phospholipids through a cascade of enzymes, are potent bronchoconstrictors that also dilate blood vessels and alter permeability. Leukotriene inhibitors act by either interfering with leukotriene synthesis or blocking the receptors where leukotrienes exert their action. They may provide an alternative to inhaled corticosteroids for mild persistent asthma or may be added to a regimen of inhaled corticosteroids in more severe asthma to attain further control.

Immunomodulators prevent binding of IgE to the high-affinity receptors of basophils and mast cells. Omalizumab

(Xolair) is a monoclonal antibody and may be used for patients with allergies and severe persistent asthma.

Numerous asthma biologic agents are in development. Most of these target a specific cell or mediator and may only be appropriate for a small subset of patients. The future of asthma may be stratification of specific pathway-selective phenotypes in patients; thus, treatment in the future may include individually tailored medications (Choby & Lee, 2015; GINA, 2015).

Quick-Relief Medications

Short-acting beta-adrenergic agonists (SABA) (e.g., albuterol [AccuNeb, Proventil, Ventolin, ProAir RespiClick], levalbuterol [Xopenex HFA], and pirbuterol [Maxair]) are the medications of choice for relieving acute symptoms and preventing exercise-induced asthma. They are used to relax smooth muscle.

Anticholinergics (e.g., ipratropium bromide [Atrovent]) inhibit muscarinic cholinergic receptors and reduce intrinsic vagal tone of the airway. They may be used in patients who do not tolerate short-acting beta$_2$-adrenergic agonists.

Management of Exacerbations

Asthma exacerbations are best managed by early treatment and education, including the use of written action plans as part of any overall effort to educate patients about self-management techniques, especially those with moderate or severe persistent asthma or with a history of severe exacerbations (GINA, 2015; NHLBI, 2012) (see Fig. 25-8). Quick-acting beta$_2$-adrenergic agonist medications are first used for prompt relief of airflow obstruction. Systemic corticosteroids may be necessary to decrease airway inflammation in patients who fail to respond to inhaled beta-adrenergic medications. In some patients, oxygen supplementation may be required to relieve hypoxemia associated with a moderate to severe exacerbation. In addition, response to treatment may be monitored by serial measurements of lung function.

Evidence from clinical trials suggests that antibiotic therapy, whether given routinely or when suspicion of bacterial infection is low, is not beneficial for asthma exacerbations (GINA, 2015). Antibiotics may be appropriate in the treatment of acute asthma exacerbations in patients with comorbid conditions (e.g., fever and

Asthma Action Plan

For: ______ **Doctor:** ______ **Date:** ______

Doctor's Phone Number ______ **Hospital/Emergency Department Phone Number** ______

GREEN ZONE

Doing Well
- No cough, wheeze, chest tightness, or shortness of breath during the day or night
- Can do usual activities

And, if a peak flow meter is used,
Peak flow: more than ______
(80% or more of my best peak flow)
My best peak flow is: ______

Take these long-term-control medicines each day (include an anti-inflammatory).

Medicine	How much to take	When to take it
______	______	______
______	______	______

Identify and avoid and control the things that make your asthma worse, like (list here):
______ ______ ______
______ ______ ______

Before exercise, if prescribed, take: □ 2 or □ 4 puffs ______ 5 to 60 minutes before exercise

YELLOW ZONE

Asthma Is Getting Worse
- Cough, wheeze, chest tightness, or shortness of breath, or
- Waking at night due to asthma, or
- Can do some, but not all, usual activities

-Or-
Peak flow: ______ to ______
(50% to 79% of my best peak flow)

First Add: quick-relief medicine—and keep taking your GREEN ZONE medicine.
______ **(short-acting beta$_2$-agonist)** □ **2 or** □**4 puffs, every 20 minutes for up to 1 hour** □ **Nebulizer, once**

If applicable, remove yourself from the thing that made your asthma worse.

Second **If your symptoms (and peak flow, if used) return to GREEN ZONE after 1 hour of above treatment:**
Continue monitoring to be sure you stay in the green zone.
-Or-
If your symptoms (and peak flow, if used) do not return to GREEN ZONE after 1 hour of above treatment:
□ Take: ______ (short-acting beta$_2$-agonist) □ 2 or □ 4 puffs or □Nebulizer
□ Add: ______ (oral corticosteroid) mg per day For ______ (3-10) days
□ Call the doctor: ______ (phone) ,□before/□ within ______ hours after taking the oral corticosteroid.

RED ZONE

Medical Alert!
- Very short of breath, or
- Quick-relief medicines have not helped, or
- Cannot do usual activities, or
- Symptoms are same or get worse after 24 hours in Yellow Zone

-Or-
Peak flow: less than ______
(50% of my best peak flow)

Take this medicine:
□ ______ **(short-acting beta$_2$-agonist)** □ **4 or** □**6 puffs or** □ **Nebulizer**
□ ______ **(oral corticosteroid)** **mg**

Then call your doctor NOW. Go to the hospital or call an ambulance if:
- You are still in the red zone after 15 minutes AND
- You have not reached your doctor.

DANGER SIGNS
- **Trouble walking and talking due to shortness of breath**
- **Lips or fingernails are blue**

- **Take** □**4 or** □**6 puffs of your quick-relief medicine AND**
- **Go to the hospital or call for an ambulance** ______ **(phone) NOW!**

FIGURE 25-8. Asthma action plan. (Adapted from National Heart, Lung and Blood Institute (NHLBI). (2012). Asthma care quick reference: Diagnosing and managing asthma. NIH Publication No. 12-5075. Revised September 2012.)

purulent sputum, evidence of pneumonia, suspected bacterial sinusitis).

Despite insufficient data supporting or refuting the benefits of using a written asthma action plan as compared with medical management alone, it is recommend to use a written asthma action plan to educate patients about self-management (Fig. 25-8). Plans can be based on either symptoms or peak flow measurements. They should focus on daily management as well as the recognition and handling of worsening symptoms. Patient self-management and early recognition of problems lead to more efficient communication with health care providers about asthma exacerbations (GINA, 2015; NHLBI, 2012).

Peak Flow Monitoring

Peak flow meters measure the highest airflow during a forced expiration. Daily peak flow monitoring is recommended for patients who meet one or more of the following criteria: have moderate or severe persistent asthma, have poor perception of changes in airflow or worsening symptoms, have unexplained response to environmental or occupational exposures, or at the discretion of the clinician and patient (GINA, 2015). Peak flow monitoring helps measure asthma severity and, when added to symptom monitoring, indicates the current degree of asthma control.

The patient is instructed in the proper technique (see Fig. 25-9, Chart 25-6), particularly about using maximal effort; peak flows are monitored for 2 or 3 weeks after receipt of optimal asthma therapy. Then, the patient's "personal best" value is determined. The green (80% to 100% of personal best), yellow (60% to 80%), and red (less than 60%) zones are determined, and specific actions are delineated for each zone, enabling the patient to monitor and manipulate their own therapy after careful instruction (GINA, 2015; NHLBI, 2012).

GINA (2015) recommends that peak flow monitoring be considered as an adjunct to asthma management for patients with moderate to severe persistent asthma. Peak flow monitoring plans may enhance communication between the patient and health care providers and may increase the patient's awareness of disease status and control.

Nursing Management

The immediate nursing care of patients with asthma depends on the severity of symptoms. The patient may be treated successfully as an outpatient if asthma symptoms are relatively mild, or may require hospitalization and intensive care if symptoms are acute and severe. The patient and family are often frightened and anxious because of the patient's dyspnea. Therefore, a calm approach is an important aspect of care. The nurse assesses the patient's respiratory status by monitoring the severity of symptoms, breath sounds, peak flow, pulse oximetry, and vital signs.

The nurse generally performs the following interventions:

- Obtains a history of allergic reactions to medications before administering medications
- Identifies medications the patient is taking
- Administers medications as prescribed and monitors the patient's responses to those medications. These medications may include an antibiotic if the patient has an underlying respiratory infection
- Administers fluids if the patient is dehydrated

If the patient requires intubation because of acute respiratory failure, the nurse assists with the intubation procedure, continues close monitoring of the patient, and keeps the patient and family informed about procedures. (See Chapter 26 for discussion of intubation and mechanical ventilation.)

Promoting Home, Community-Based, and Transitional Care

Educating Patients About Self-Care

Implementation of basic asthma management principles at the community level is a major challenge. Strategies include education of health care providers, establishment of programs for asthma education (for patients and providers), the use of outpatient follow-up care for patients, and a focus on chronic management versus acute episodic care. Nurses are pivotal to achievement of all these objectives.

Patient education is a critical component of care for patients with asthma. Multiple inhalers, different types

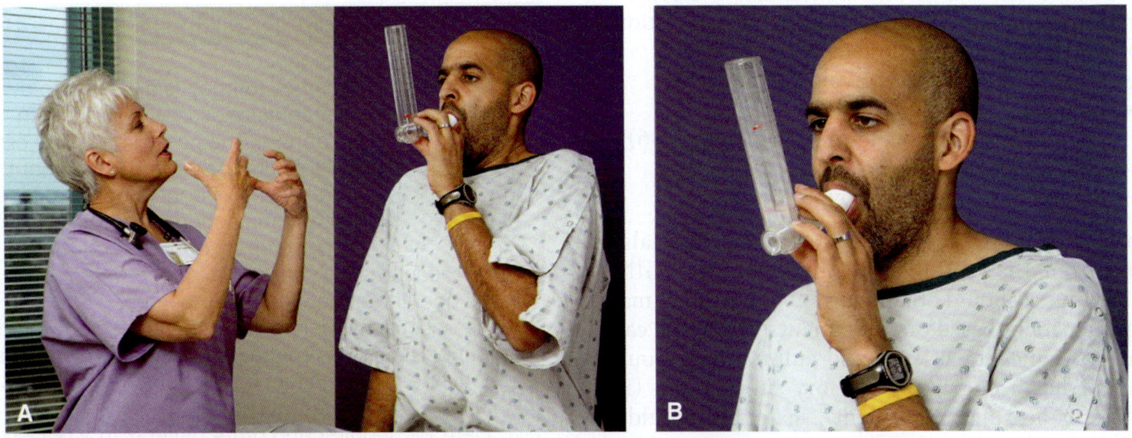

FIGURE 25-9. Peak flow meters measure the highest volume of airflow during a forced expiration. The patient takes a deep breath and places lips around the mouthpiece (**A**), and then exhales hard and fast (**B**). Volume may be measured in colour-coded zones: the green zone signifies 80% to 100% of personal best; yellow, 60% to 80%; and red, less than 60%. If peak flow falls below the red zone, the patient should take the appropriate actions prescribed by their primary provider.

CHART 25-6

HOME CARE CHECKLIST • Use of the Peak Flow Metre in Asthma Management

At the completion of education, the patient and/or caregiver will be able to:

- Describe the rationale for using a peak flow meter in asthma management
- Explain how peak flow monitoring is used along with symptoms to determine severity of asthma
- Demonstrate steps for using the peak flow meter correctly
- Move the indicator to the bottom of the numbered scale
- Stand up
- Take a deep breath, and fill the lungs completely
- Place mouthpiece in mouth, and close lips around mouthpiece. (Do not put tongue inside opening)
- Blow out hard and fast with a single blow
- Record the number achieved on the indicator. If patient coughs or a mistake is made in the process, do it again
- Repeat steps 1 to 5 two more times, and write the highest number in the asthma diary
- Explain how to determine the "personal best" peak flow reading
- Describe the significance of the colour zones for peak flow monitoring
- Demonstrate how to clean the peak flow meter
- Discuss how and when to contact the primary provider about changes or decreases in peak flow values

of inhalers, antiallergy therapy, antireflux medications, and avoidance measures are essential for long-term control. This complex therapy requires a partnership between the patient and the health care providers to determine the desired outcomes and to formulate a plan to achieve those outcomes. The patient then carries out daily therapy as part of self-care management, with input and guidance by the health care provider. Before a partnership can be established, the patient needs to understand the following:

- Nature of asthma as a chronic inflammatory disease
- Definitions of inflammation and bronchoconstriction
- Purpose and action of each medication
- Triggers to avoid and how to avoid them
- Proper inhalation technique
- How to perform peak flow monitoring (Chart 25-6)
- How to implement an asthma action plan
- When to seek assistance and how to do so

An assortment of excellent educational materials is available from the NHLBI and other sources (GINA, 2015). The nurse should obtain current educational materials for the patient based on the patient's diagnosis, causative factors, educational level, and cultural background. If a patient has a coexisting sensory impairment (i.e., vision loss or hearing impairment), materials should be provided in an alternative format.

Continuing and Transitional Care

Nurses who have contact with the patient in the hospital, clinic, school, or office use the opportunity to assess the patient's respiratory status and ability to manage self-care to prevent serious exacerbations. Nurses emphasize adherence to the prescribed therapy, preventive measures, and the need to keep follow-up appointments with health care providers. Home visits to assess the home environment for allergens may be indicated for the patient with recurrent exacerbations. Nurses refer patients to community support groups. In addition, nurses remind patients and families about the importance of health promotion strategies and recommended health screening.

Unfolding Patient Stories: Jennifer Hoffman • Part 1

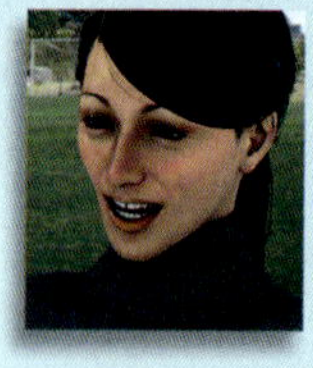

Jennifer Hoffman is a 33-year-old woman diagnosed with asthma in childhood. She has come to the clinic multiple times over the last 2 months complaining of continued symptoms. Her asthma action plan was adjusted by her primary provider last month. What measures can the nurse take to determine areas needing education reinforcement? How can the nurse ensure that Jennifer is accurately following the prescribed asthma regimen and monitoring medication effectiveness? (Jennifer Hoffman's story continues in Chapter 53.)

Care for Jennifer and other patients in a realistic virtual environment: ***vSim** for Nursing* (**thepoint.lww.com/vSimMedicalSurgical**). Practice documenting these patients' care in DocuCare (**thepoint.lww.com/DocuCareEHR**).

Status Asthmaticus

An asthma exacerbation can range from mild to severe with potential respiratory arrest (GINA, 2015). The term status asthmaticus is sometimes used to describe rapid onset, severe and persistent asthma that does not respond to conventional therapy. The attacks can occur with little or no warning and can progress rapidly to asphyxiation. Infection, anxiety, nebulizer abuse, dehydration, increased adrenergic blockage, and nonspecific irritants may contribute to these episodes. An acute episode may be precipitated by hypersensitivity to medications, such as aspirin, beta blockers, and nonsteroidal anti-inflammatory drugs (NSAIDs) (AAAAI, 2016b).

Pathophysiology

The basic characteristics of asthma (inflammation of bronchial mucosa, constriction of the bronchiolar smooth muscle, and thickened secretions) decrease the diameter of the bronchi and occur in status asthmaticus. The most common scenario is severe bronchospasm, with mucous plugging leading to asphyxia. A ventilation–perfusion abnormality results in hypoxemia. There is a reduced PaO_2 and initial respiratory alkalosis, with a decreased $PaCO_2$ and an increased pH. As status asthmaticus worsens, the $PaCO_2$ increases and the pH decreases, reflecting respiratory acidosis.

Clinical Manifestations

The clinical manifestations are the same as those seen in severe asthma; signs and symptoms include laboured breathing, prolonged exhalation, engorged neck veins, and wheezing. However, the extent of wheezing does not indicate the severity of the attack. As the obstruction worsens, the wheezing may disappear; this is frequently a sign of impending respiratory failure.

Assessment and Diagnostic Findings

The severity of an exacerbation may be evaluated by a general assessment of the patient (degree of breathlessness, ability to talk, positioning of patient, level of alertness or cognitive function), physical assessment (respiratory rate, the use of accessory muscles, presence of central cyanosis, auscultatory findings, pulse, and pulsus paradoxus), and laboratory evaluation (peak expiratory flow after a bronchodilator, PaO_2 and $PaCO_2$, and pulse oximetry). Pulmonary function studies are the most accurate means of assessing an acute, severe airway obstruction, though not practical to obtain during this type of an emergent situation. Arterial blood gas measurement and/or pulse oximetry are obtained if the patient cannot perform pulmonary function manoeuvres because of severe obstruction or fatigue or if the patient does not respond to treatment. Respiratory alkalosis (low $PaCO_2$) is the most common finding in patients with an ongoing asthma exacerbation and is due to hyperventilation.

> **NURSING ALERT**
>
> **In status asthmaticus, increasing $PaCO_2$ (to normal levels or levels indicating respiratory acidosis) is a danger sign signifying impending respiratory failure.**

Medical Management

Close monitoring of the patient and objective reevaluation for response to therapy are key in status asthmaticus. In the emergency setting, the patient is treated initially with a short-acting beta$_2$-adrenergic agonist and subsequently a short course of systemic corticosteroids, especially if the patient does not respond to the short-acting beta$_2$-adrenergic agonist. Corticosteroids are critical in the therapy of status asthmaticus and are used to decrease the intense airway inflammation and swelling. Short-acting inhaled beta$_2$-adrenergic agonists provide the most rapid relief from bronchospasm. An MDI with or without a spacer may be used for nebulization of the medications. However, more commonly, short-acting bronchodilators will be given via a nebulizer. A mouthpiece or face mask can be used and the bronchodilator is continuously given to the patient. The patient does not have to work to coordinate their breathing pattern, which can otherwise cause additional anxiety in this acute situation. The patient requires supplemental oxygen and IV fluids for hydration. Oxygen therapy is initiated to treat dyspnea, central cyanosis, and hypoxemia. High-flow supplemental oxygen is best delivered using a partial or complete nonrebreather mask. Sedatives are contraindicated. Magnesium sulphate, a calcium antagonist, may be given to induce smooth muscle relaxation; the magnesium can relax smooth muscle and hence cause bronchodilation by competing with calcium at calcium-mediated smooth muscle binding sites. IV magnesium sulphate is not recommended for routine use in asthma exacerbations; however, when given as a single 2 g infusion over 20 minutes, it may be helpful in treating patients who present with severely compromised pulmonary function, who have not responded to initial therapy, and with persistent hypoxemia (GINA, 2015). Adverse effects of magnesium sulphate may include facial warmth, flushing, tingling, nausea, central nervous system depression, respiratory depression, and hypotension.

If there is no response to repeated treatments, hospitalization is required. Other criteria for hospitalization include poor pulmonary function test results and deteriorating blood gas levels (respiratory acidosis), which may indicate that the patient is tiring and will require mechanical ventilation. Most patients do not need mechanical ventilation, but it is used for patients in respiratory failure, for those who tire and are too fatigued by the attempt to breathe, or for those whose condition does not respond to initial treatment.

For a very select group of patients with uncontrolled severe asthma, bronchial thermoplasty may be considered. Bronchial thermoplasty is the first nondrug therapy for the treatment of severe, uncontrolled asthma. It consists of controlled radiofrequency heating of the central airways through a bronchoscope. The thermal energy reduces the amount of smooth muscle involved in bronchospasm and potentially decreases the severity and frequency of symptoms. This therapy is invasive and relatively new; therefore, only select centres have the ability to perform this procedure, and it should only be considered in a select group of patients (GINA, 2015).

Death from asthma is associated with several risk factors, including the following (GINA, 2015):

- Past history of severe exacerbation (e.g., intubation or intensive care unit admission)
- Two or more hospitalizations for asthma within the past year
- Three or more emergency care visits for asthma in the past year
- Hospitalization or emergency care visit for asthma in the past month
- Use of more than two canisters of short-acting beta-agonist inhalers per month
- Difficulty in perceiving asthma symptoms or severity of exacerbations
- Lack of written asthma action plan
- Concurrent cardiovascular disease, COPD, or chronic psychiatric disease
- Low socioeconomic status or inner-city residence

Nursing Management

The main focus of nursing management is to actively assess the airway and the patient's response to treatment. The nurse should be prepared for the next intervention if the patient does not respond to treatment.

The nurse constantly monitors the patient for the first 12 to 24 hours or until the severe exacerbation resolves. The nurse also assesses the patient's skin turgor for signs of dehydration. Fluid intake is essential to combat dehydration, to loosen secretions, and to facilitate expectoration. Nurses administer IV fluids as prescribed, up to 3 to 4 L/day, unless contraindicated. Blood pressure and cardiac rhythm should be monitored continuously during the acute phase and until the patient stabilizes and responds to therapy. The patient's energy needs to be conserved, and his or her room should be quiet and free of respiratory irritants, including flowers, tobacco smoke, perfumes, or odours of cleaning agents. Nonallergenic pillows should be used. An asthma attack may also be precipitated or aggravated by exposure to latex if the patient has a latex allergy; therefore, this type of hypersensitivity must be identified and latex-free products used, as warranted. Once the exacerbation is resolved, the factors that precipitated the exacerbation should be identified and strategies for their future avoidance implemented. In addition, the patient's medication plan should be reviewed.

Cystic Fibrosis

CF is the most common fatal autosomal recessive disease among Caucasians. The majority of the Canadian CF population is Caucasian (92.8%). The 7.2% remaining who have an identified ethnicity are divided among First Nations, Black, Asian, South Asian, and Hispanic. A person must inherit a defective copy of the CF gene (one from each parent) to have CF. In 2016, 4,246 individuals with CF attended one of the 42 accredited CF clinics across Canada, with 122 of those being newly diagnosed. The total Canadian CF population has been steadily increasing and in the last two decades and has grown by 37.3%. In 2016, there were 2,580 (60.8%) individuals 18 years of age or older living with CF; 45.2% were females and 54.8% were males (Cystic Fibrosis Canada [CFC], 2016). Although CF was once considered a fatal childhood disease, in 2016, the median age of individuals with CF reported was 22.7 years, more than 7 years higher than it was two decades ago.

Although most patients are diagnosed by age 2 years, this disease may not be diagnosed until later in life (CFC, 2016). Approximately 59.1% of individuals with CF reported in 2016 were diagnosed by 1 year of age, and 92.4% had been diagnosed before the age of 18 years. Adults diagnosed after the 18 years of age accounted for only 7.6%.

Respiratory symptoms are frequently the major manifestation of CF when it is diagnosed later in life. However, many patients will not demonstrate the classic symptoms of CF, which may potentially cause a diagnostic dilemma.

Pathophysiology

CF is caused by mutations or dysfunction in the protein CF transmembrane conductance regulator (CFTR), which normally transports chloride ions across epithelial cell membranes. Gene mutations affect transport of these ions, leading to CF, which is characterized by thick, viscous secretions in the lungs, pancreas, liver, intestine, and reproductive tract as well as increased salt content in sweat gland secretions. The most common mutation is deltaF508; however, more than 2,000 mutations have been identified (Nakano, 2014; Pittman & Ferkol, 2015; CFC, 2016). Approximately 89.2% of patients in Canada with CF carry at least one copy of the deltaF508 mutation (CFC, 2016). The numerous mutations of the *CFTR* gene create multiple variations in the presentation and progression of the disease.

The ability to detect the common mutations of this gene allows for routine screening for CF and the detection of carriers of the disease. Genetic counselling is an important part of health care for couples at risk. People who are heterozygous for CF (i.e., have one defective gene and one normal gene) do not have the disease but can be carriers and pass the defective gene on to their children. If both parents are carriers, their risk of having a child with CF is one in four (25%) with each pregnancy. Genetic testing should be offered to adults with a positive family history of CF and to partners of people with CF who are planning a pregnancy or seeking prenatal counselling. The hallmark pathology of CF is bronchial mucus plugging, inflammation, and eventual bronchiectasis. Commonly, the bronchiectasis begins in the upper lobes and progresses to involve all lobes.

Clinical Manifestations

The pulmonary manifestations of CF include a productive cough, wheezing, hyperinflation of the lung fields on chest x-ray, and pulmonary function test results consistent with obstructive disease of the airways. Chronic respiratory inflammation and infection are caused by impaired mucus clearance. Colonization of the airways with pathogenic bacteria usually occurs early in life. *S. aureus* and *H. influenzae* are common organisms during early childhood. As the disease progresses, *P. aeruginosa* is ultimately isolated from the sputum of most patients (Katkin, 2016). Upper respiratory manifestations of the disease include sinusitis and nasal polyps.

Nonpulmonary manifestations include gastrointestinal problems (e.g., pancreatic insufficiency, recurrent abdominal pain, biliary cirrhosis, vitamin deficiencies, recurrent pancreatitis, and weight loss), CF-related diabetes, genitourinary problems (male and female infertility). (See Chapter 40 for a discussion of pancreatitis.)

Assessment and Diagnostic Findings

The diagnosis of CF requires a clinical picture consistent with the CF phenotype and laboratory evidence of CFTR dysfunction. Key assessment findings in adults include (Katkin, 2016):

- Chronic sinopulmonary disease as manifested by chronic cough and sputum production, persistent infection consistent with typical CF pathogens, and x-ray evidence of bronchiectasis and chronic sinusitis, often with nasal polyps
- Gastrointestinal tract and nutritional abnormalities (pancreatic insufficiency, recurrent pancreatitis, biliary cirrhosis and portal hypertension, CF-related diabetes)
- Male urogenital problems as manifested by congenital bilateral absence of the vas deferens; reduced female fertility

Medical Management

CF requires both acute and chronic therapy. Because chronic bacterial infection of the airways occurs in CF, control of infections is essential to treatment. For acute airway exacerbations, aggressive therapy involves airway clearance and antibiotics based on results of sputum cultures. The majority of patients are colonized with *P. aeruginosa;* however *S. aureus, methicillin-resistant S. aureus,* and *Burkholderia cepacia complex* may be found.

Chronic infection with *P. aeruginosa* is an independent risk factor for accelerated loss of lung function and decreased survival (Simon, 2016a). Routine cultures of respiratory secretions are used to identify organisms and guide antibiotic selection. Two IV antibiotics typically are chosen to treat a severe exacerbation of *P. aeruginosa.* Tobramycin (Nebcin), along with piperacillin-tazobactam (Zosyn), a third-generation cephalosporin (e.g., ceftizoxime [Cefizox], ceftazidime [Fortaz]), a carbapenem (e.g., meropenem [Merrem]), or aztreonam (Azactam) may be prescribed (Simon, 2016a). Dosing of antibiotics is determined on a case-by-case basis; some patients may require higher doses or an extended IV infusion. Careful monitoring is always required to minimize any side effects of the antibiotics.

Oral antibiotics such as dicloxacillin (Dynapen), amoxicillin-clavulanate or cephalexin (Keflex) may be appropriate to treat mild methicillin-sensitive *S. aureus* infection. For more serious exacerbations, oral linezolid (Zyvox) may be used (Simon, 2016a). Treatment is continued until the exacerbation has resolved and is usually a minimum of 10 days to as long as 3 weeks or more. Inhaled antibiotics may be used in severe exacerbations, bacterial resistance to all orally given antibiotics, or failure of oral antibiotics to resolve an exacerbation (Simon, 2016a).

In an acute exacerbation, airway clearance treatments may be used three to four times per day. The therapeutic options for chronic disease management of CF have undergone tremendous changes. Cornerstones of treatment include airway clearance measures, the mucolytic dornase alfa (Pulmozyme), nebulized antibiotics, antibiotic inhalation powder (tobramycin sulphate [TOBI Podhaler]), oral antibiotics, inhaled hypertonic saline, nutritional support, and exercise (Pittman & Ferkol, 2015).

Airway clearance is a key intervention, and various pulmonary techniques are used to enhance secretion clearance. Examples include manual postural drainage and chest physiotherapy; high-frequency chest wall oscillation; autogenic drainage (a combination of breathing techniques at different lung volume levels to move the secretions to where they can be huff-coughed out); and other devices that assist in airway clearance, such as masks that generate positive expiratory pressure (PEP masks) and "flutter devices" (devices that provide an oscillatory expiratory pressure pattern with PEP and assist with expectoration of secretions).

Dornase alfa is a nebulized medication given to degrade the large amount of deoxyribonucleic acid (DNA) that accumulates within CF mucus. This agent helps decrease the viscosity of the sputum and promotes expectoration of secretions. It is recommended for patients with moderate to severe disease (severity of lung disease classification is based on predicted FEV_1 percentage). In addition, inhaled hypertonic saline may be used in the chronic treatment of CF. Inhalations increase hydration of the airway surface liquid in patients with CF and improve airway clearance.

Nebulized and IV antibiotics or a combination may be used to treat chronic colonization of the lung. Nebulization provides high intrapulmonary drug concentrations and minimal systemic absorption. Inhaled tobramycin (TOBI) or aztreonam (AZLI) have been shown to decrease the frequency of pulmonary exacerbations. Acute infections are treated with a variety of IV antibiotics. Such infections remain a major cause of mortality related to pulmonary exacerbations in adults with CF.

Other therapeutic measures may be necessary as well. Anti-inflammatory agents may be used to treat inflammatory response in the airways. The CFF states that there is insufficient evidence for the use of routine inhaled or oral corticosteroids. IV corticosteroids are used during acute exacerbations and only for those patients with asthma-like symptoms (Simon, 2016b). Long-term use of high-dose nonsteroidal anti-inflammatory agents (ibuprofen) is recommended in children ages 6 to 17 years to slow the loss of lung function, but is not recommended for patients older than 13 years of age as there is no evidence to support this practice (Pittman & Ferkol, 2015; Simon, 2016b). Inhaled bronchodilators (e.g., salmeterol [Serevent Diskus], tiotropium bromide [Spiriva]) may be used in patients who have a significant bronchoconstrictive component; this is confirmed by spirometry before and after therapy is instituted. (Simon, 2016b).

Nearly 90% of patients with CF have pancreatic exocrine insufficiency and require oral pancreatic enzyme supplementation with meals (CFF, 2019). Given the fat malabsorption in CF and increased caloric needs due to the work of breathing, nutritional counseling and weight monitoring are extremely important. Supplements of fat-soluble vitamins A, D, E, and K are also used.

CFTR modulators are a new class of drugs and help to improve function of the defective CFTR protein (Simon, 2016b). Ivacaftor (Kalydeco) is approved by the FDA and Health Canada for adults and children ages 6 years of age and older. Ivacaftor is an oral CFTR potentiator designed to keep the proteins at the cell surface open more often to improve salt and water movement across the membrane (thus improving hydration and clearing of mucus from the airways). Only one gene mutation, G551D, is addressed by ivacaftor and this gene mutation occurs in approximately 4.4% of patients with CF (Simon, 2016b). The drug does not correct the gene mutation; it only helps in the movement of salt and water across the membrane.

Another CFTR drug, lumacaftor 200 mg/ivacaftor 125 mg (Orkambi), was approved by the FDA and Health Canada to treat CF in patients 12 years and older, who have the deltaF508 mutation. CF is the most common fatal genetic disease affecting Canadian children and young adults. Approximately one in 25 Canadians is a CF carrier, with one abnormal version of the gene responsible for this life-altering disease (Cystic Fibrosis Canada, 2019). These newer drugs for CF are extremely costly with some insurance companies reluctant to pay for these treatments.

As the pulmonary deterioration advances, supplemental oxygen is used to treat the progressive hypoxemia that occurs with CF. It helps correct the hypoxemia and may minimize the complications seen with chronic hypoxemia (pulmonary hypertension). Lung transplantation is an option for a small, selected population of patients with CF. A double-lung transplantation technique is used because of chronic infection of both lungs in end-stage CF. Because there is a long waiting list for lung transplants, many patients die while waiting for suitable lungs for transplantation.

Nursing Management

Nursing management is crucial to the interdisciplinary approach required for care of adults with CF. Nursing care includes helping patients manage pulmonary symptoms and prevent complications. Specific measures include strategies that promote removal of pulmonary secretions, chest physiotherapy (including postural drainage, chest percussion, and vibration), and breathing exercises (which are implemented and taught to the patient and family when the patient is very young). The patient is reminded of the need to reduce risk factors associated with respiratory infections (e.g., exposure to crowds or to people with known infections). In addition, the patient is taught the early signs and symptoms of respiratory infection and disease progression that indicate the need to notify the primary provider.

The nurse emphasizes the importance of an adequate fluid and dietary intake to promote removal of secretions and to ensure an adequate nutritional status. Because CF is a lifelong disorder, patients often have learned to modify their daily activities to accommodate their symptoms and treatment modalities. As the disease progresses, however, assessment of the home environment may be warranted to identify modifications required to address changes in the patient's needs, increasing dyspnea and fatigue, and nonpulmonary symptoms.

As with any chronic disease, palliative care and end-of-life issues and concerns need to be addressed with the patient when warranted. For the patient whose disease is progressing and who is developing increasing hypoxemia, preferences for end-of-life care should be discussed, documented, and honoured (see Chapter 15). Patients and family members need support as they face a shortened life span and an uncertain future.

Critical Thinking Exercises

1 In the ED, a 60-year-old man tells the triage nurse that he has limited medication insurance and does not have a primary provider because he has recently moved to a new community. He presents with a chief complaint of increased shortness of breath and a change in the quantity and colour of his sputum. He says he was diagnosed with COPD 6 years ago but continues to smoke 2 packs per day. He says he usually has little sputum in the morning and that it is clear, but in the last week it has become yellow in colour, continues all day, and is difficult to cough out. He is dyspneic at rest while sitting on the examination table and has difficulty completing a sentence without taking a breath. When asked if he has been on any medications, he told the nurse that he received a sample inhaler "for breathing" at a walk-in clinic, but that ran out a month ago. He does not know the name of the medication, but it did help him breathe better. What are your focused priorities with this patient? For instance, what additional questions would you ask him? What are some of the physical examination findings you might observe or assess? What other tests might be ordered to continue to evaluate this patient and why? What resources might be appropriate for this patient before he leaves the hospital?

2 A 37-year-old woman with a history of asthma presents to the clinic with tachypnea and acute shortness of breath with audible wheezing. She says that she has continued to take her prescribed inhaler with no relief in symptoms and symptoms have gotten worse over time. She admits she was taking her inhaler more frequently than she was supposed to do. She called her doctor a week ago but could not get an appointment until today. Physical examination reveals tachycardia at 110 bpm and tachypnea at 30 breaths/minute with signs of accessory muscle use. Auscultation reveals decreased breath sounds with inspiratory and expiratory wheezes. Her SaO_2 is 92% on room air. When you ask her what type of inhaler she uses, she says she has one for fast relief but did not bring it. She also could not afford the other one that that was prescribed 3 months ago. She never got it filled. The clinic is not equipped to give nebulizer treatments. What do you think the next step of care that may be needed with this

patient? What type of education and resources would benefit this patient? What type of follow-up is needed for this patient?

3 A 31-year-old woman with CF is admitted to your unit from the ED. She has been relatively free from exacerbations and started working about 3 months ago in an office setting. She obtains her CF care in a CF centre that is about 150 miles away from her home. She presently does not have a primary provider since she just moved to this city about 6 months ago. She lives alone. She has become progressively short of breath over the past week and has tried to manage her shortness of breath but finally came to the ED out of desperation. In short and choppy phrases, she tells you that she is extremely short of breath and that it has been getting worse; she is having paroxysms of coughing. You note that the cough is productive, with thick, yellow sputum, and that she is febrile. She does not know if she has lost any weight but has not been able to eat. She is extremely anxious and wants to see her "regular CF doctor" who is 150 miles away. She says he is the only one that understands CF. What are the pathophysiologic mechanisms that have caused these clinical manifestations? What evidence-based medical and nursing interventions might be used to decrease or alleviate these signs and symptoms? What is the strength of the evidence? How might you help in decreasing the anxiety and fear she has about not being seen by her CF specialist? What members of the health care team would you consult and why?

REFERENCES AND SELECTED READINGS

Books

Expert Panel Report 3. (2007). *Guidelines for the diagnosis and management of asthma*. National Asthma Education and Prevention Program. NIH Publication Number 08–5846. Bethesda, MD: U.S. Department of Health and Human Services, National Heart, Lung and Blood Institute.

National Heart, Lung and Blood Institute (NHLBI). (2012). *Asthma care quick reference: Diagnosing and managing asthma*. NIH Publication No. 12–5075. Revised September 2012.

Spiro, S. G., Sivestri, G. A., & Agusti, A. (2012). *Clinical Respiratory Medicine: Expert consult*. Philadelphia, PA: Elsevier Health Sciences.

Journals and Electronic Documents

American Academy of Allergy, Asthma and Immunology (AAAAI). (2016a). *Occupational asthma*. Retrieved January 10, 2016, from www.aaaai.org/conditions-and-treatments/library/at-a-glance/occupational-asthma

American Academy of Allergy, Asthma, and Immunology (AAAAI). (2016b). Medications that may trigger asthma symptoms. Retrieved May 18, 2016, from www.aaaai.org/conditions-and-treatments/library/asthma-library/medications-that-can-trigger-asthma-symptoms

American Liver Foundation. (2015). *Alpha-1 antitrypsin deficiency*. Retrieved December 1, 2015, from www.liverfoundation.org/abouttheliver/info/alphaone/

Barker, A. F. (2015a). Clinical manifestations and diagnosis of bronchiectasis in adults. *UpToDate*. Last updated December 10, 2015. Retrieved on May 18, 2016, from www.uptodate.com/contents/clinical-manifestations-and-diagnosis-of-bronchiectasis-in-adults

Barker, A. F. (2015b). *Treatment of bronchiectasis in adults. UpToDate*. Last updated December 15, 2015. Retrieved on 5/18/2016 at: www.uptodate.com/contents/treatment-of-bronchiectasis-in-adults

Bartlett, J. G., & Sethi, S. (2016). Management of infection in exacerbations of chronic obstructive pulmonary disease. *UpToDate*. Last updated March 17, 2016. Retrieved on May 18, 2016, from www.uptodate.com/contents/management-of-infection-in-exacerbations-of-chronic-obstructive-pulmonary-disease

Bellinger, C. R., & Peters, S. P. (2015). Outpatient chronic obstructive pulmonary disease management: going for the GOLD. *The Journal of Allergy and Clinical Immunology: In Practice*, *3*(4), 471–478.

British Columbia Medical association. (2017). *Chronic obstructive pulmonary disease (COPD): Diagnosis and management*. https://www2.gov.bc.ca/gov/content/health/practitioner-professional-resources/bc-guidelines/copd

Canadian Thoracic Society. (2012). *Cough: Etiology, evaluation and treatments*. Available at: http://www.respiratoryguidelines.ca

Centers for Disease Control and Prevention (CDC). (2015c). *Asthma: data, statistics and surveillance*. Atlanta, GA: National Center for Health Statistics. Retrieved on January 25, 2016, from www.cdc.gov/asthma/asthmadata.htm

Chapman, K. R., Boulet, L. P., Rea, R. M., et al. (2008). Suboptimal asthma control: Prevalence, detection and consequences in general practice. *European Respiratory Journal*, *31*(2), 320–325.

Cystic Fibrosis Canada. (2016). *The Canadian cystic fibrosis registry: 2016 annual data report*. Retrieved from https://www.cysticfibrosis.ca/uploads/2016%20Registry%20Annual%20Data%20Report.pdf

Cystic Fibrosis Canada. (2019). Retrieved from https://www.cysticfibrosis.ca/about-cf/living-with-cystic-fibrosis/resources

Cystic Fibrosis Foundation. (2015). *About cystic fibrosis*. Retrieved on January 25, 2016, from www.cff.org/AboutCF/

Cystic Fibrosis News Today. (2015). *Ivacaftor/lumacaftor (Orkambi)*. Retrieved on May 19, 2018, from cysticfibrosisnewstoday.com/orkambi-lumacaftor-ivacaftor-vertex/

Finkelstein, M. M., Chapman, K. R., McIvor, R. A., et al. (2011). Mortality among subjects with chronic obstructive pulmonary disease or asthma at two respiratory disease clinics in Ontario. *Canadian Respiratory Journal*, *18*(6), 327–332.

Global Initiative for Asthma (GINA). (2012). *Global strategy for asthma management and prevention*. Available at: http://www.ginasthma.org

Global Initiative for Chronic Obstructive Lung Disease (GOLD). (2019). *Global strategy for the diagnosis, management, and prevention of chronic obstructive pulmonary disease*. Available at: http://www.goldcopd.org/.

Global Strategy for Asthma Management and Prevention, Global Initiative for Asthma (GINA). (2015). Retrieved on January 25, 2015, from www.ginasthma.org/local/uploads/files/GINA_Report_2015_Aug11.pdf

Global Strategy for Asthma Management and Prevention (GINA). (2014). Available at: https://ginasthma.org/wp-content/uploads/2019/01/2014-GINA.pdf

Goodridge, D. (2006). People with chronic obstructive pulmonary disease at the end of life: A review of the literature. *International Journal of Palliative Nursing*, *12*(8), 390–396.

Government of Canada. (2018). *Public health infobase: Canadian Chronic Disease Surveillance System (CCDSS)*. Retrieved from https://infobase.phac-aspc.gc.ca/ccdss-scsmc/data-tool/

Health Canada. (2012). *Canadian tobacco use monitoring survey (CTUMS) 2012*. Available at: http://www.hc-sc.gc.ca/hc-ps/toba-tabac/research-recherche/stat/ctums-esutc_2012-eng.php

Hooley, J. (2015). Decoding the oxyhemoglobin dissociation curve. *American Nurse Today*, *10*(1), 18–23.

Ismaila, A. S., Sayani, A. P., Marin, M., et al. (2013). Clinical, economic, and humanistic burden of asthma in Canada: A systematic review. *BMC Pulmonary Medicine*, *13*, 70, 1471–2466. Available at: http://www.biomedcentral.com/1471-2466.

Jacobsen, R., Frelich, A., & Godtfredsen, N. S. (2012). Impact of exercise capacity on dyspnea and health-related quality of life in patients with chronic obstructive pulmonary disease. *Journal of Cardiopulmonary Rehabilitation and Prevention*, *32*, 92–100.

Katkin, J. P. (2016). Cystic fibrosis: Clinical manifestations and diagnosis. *UpToDate*. Last updated March 28, 2016. Retrieved on May 18, 2016, from www.uptodate.com/contents/cystic-fibrosis-clinical-manifestations-of-pulmonary-disease/contributors

Kaufman, G. (2012). Asthma update: Recommendations for diagnosis, treatment and management. *Primary Health Care*, *22*(4), 32–39.

Kaufman, G. (2013). The role of inhaled bronchodilators and inhaler devices in COPD management. *Primary Health Care*, *23*(8), 33–40.

Klomp, H., Lawson, J., Cockcroft, D., et al. (2008). Examining asthma quality of care using a population-based approach. *Canadian Medical Association Journal*, *178*(8), 1013–1021.

Lougheed, M. D., Lemiere, C., Ducharme, F. M., et al. (2012). Canadian thoracic society 2012 guideline update: Diagnosis and management of asthma in preschoolers, children, and adults. *Canadian Respiratory Journal, 19*(2), 127–164. Available at: http://www.respiratoryguidelines.ca

Marciniuk, D. D., Goodridge, D., Hernandez, P., et al. (2011). Managing dyspnea in patients with advanced chronic obstructive pulmonary disease: A Canadian Thoracic Society clinical practice guideline. *Canadian Respiratory Journal, 18*(2), 69–78. Available at: http://www.respiratoryguidelines.ca

Marciniuk, D. D., Hernandez, P., Balter, M., et al. (2012). Alpha-1 antititrypsin deficiency targeted testing and augmentation therapy: A Canadian Thoracic Society clinical practice guideline. *Canadian Respiratory Journal, 19*(2), 109–116. Available at: http://www.respiratoryguidelines.ca

McCarthy, B., Casey, D., Murphy, K., et al. (2015). Pulmonary rehabilitation for chronic obstructive pulmonary disease. *Cochrane Database Systematic Review, 23*(2), CD003793.

Mittmann, N., Kuramoto, L., Seung, S.J., et al. (2008). The cost of moderate and severe COPD exacerbations to the Canadian healthcare system. *Respir Med, 102*, 413–421.

Mogayzel, P., Naureckas, E. T., Robinson, K. A., et al. (2013). Cystic fibrosis pulmonary guidelines: Chronic medications for maintenance of lung health. *American Respiratory Critical Care Medicine, 187*(7), 680–689.

Nakano, S. J. (2014). Genomic breakthroughs in the diagnosis and treatment of cystic fibrosis. *American Journal of Nursing, 114*(6), 36–44.

O'Donnell, D., Hernandez, P., Kaplan, A., et al. (2008). Canadian Thoracic Society recommendations for management of chronic obstructive pulmonary disease—2008 update-highlights for primary care. *Canadian Respiratory Journal, 15*(Suppl A), 1A–8A.

Piers-Yfantouda, R., Absalom, G., & Clemens, F. (2013). Smoking cessation interventions for COPD: A review of the literature. *Respiratory Care, 58*(11), 1955–1962.

Pittman, J. E., & Ferkol, T. W. (2015). The evolution of cystic fibrosis care. *Chest, 148*(2), 533–542.

Public Health Agency of Canada. (2018a). *Asthma and chronic obstructive pulmonary disease (COPD) in Canada, 2018*. Retrieved from https://www.canada.ca/en/public-health/services/publications/diseases-conditions/asthma-chronic-obstructive-pulmonary-disease-canada-2018.html

Public Health Agency of Canada. (2018b). *Chronic obstructive pulmonary disease*. Retrieved from https://www.canada.ca/en/public-health/services/chronic-diseases/chronic-respiratory-diseases/chronic-obstructive-pulmonary-disease-copd.html

Public Health Agency of Canada [PHAC]. (2018c). *Public health infobase: Canadian Chronic Disease Surveillance System (CCDSS)*. Retrieved from https://infobase.phac-aspc.gc.ca/ccdss-scsmc/data-tool/

Regelmann, W. E., Schechter, M. S., Wagener, J. S., et al. (2013). Pulmonary exacerbations in cystic fibrosis: Young children with characteristic signs and symptoms. *Pediatric Pulmonology, 48*(7), 649–657.

Rocker, G. M., Simpson, A. C., & Horton, R. (2015). Palliative care in advanced lung disease: The challenge of integrating palliation into everyday care. *Chest, 143*(3), 801–809.

Ross, C., Williams, B. A., Low, G., et al. (2010). Perceptions about self-management among people with severe asthma. *Journal of Asthma, 47*, 330–336.

Scott, A. (2013). Cystic fibrosis. *Radiologic Technology, 84*(5), 493–518.

Shepherd, A. (2010). The nutritional management of COPD: An overview. *British Journal of Nursing, 19*(9), 559–562.

Simon, R. H. (2016a). *Cystic fibrosis: Antibiotic therapy for lung disease. UpToDate*. Last updated April 12, 2016. Retrieved on May 19, 2016, from www.uptodate.com/contents/cystic-fibrosis-antibiotic-therapy-for-lung-disease

Simon, R. H. (2016b). *Cystic fibrosis: Overview of the treatment of lung disease. UpToDate*. Last updated April 14, 2016. Retrieved on May 19, 2016, from www.uptodate.com/contents/cystic-fibrosis-overview-of-the-treatment-of-lung-disease

Simpson, E., & Jones, M. (2013). An exploration of self-efficacy and self-management in COPD patients. *British Journal of Nursing, 22*(19), 1105–1109.

Small, S. P., Eastlick Kushner, K., & Neufeld, A. (2012). Dealing with a latent danger: Parents communicating with their children about smoking. *Nursing Research and Practice, 2012*. doi:10.1155/2012/382075.

Statistics Canada. (2013). Asthma, by age group and sex. CANSIM, tables 105–0501, Catalogue no. 82-221-X. Available at: http://www.statcan.gc.ca/tables-tableaux/sum-som/l01/cst01/health49a-eng.htm

Statistics Canada. (2015). Retrieved from https://www150.statcan.gc.ca/n1/pub/82-624-x/2015001/article/14246-eng.htm#a2

Teva Respiratory, 2016. Retrieved from https://www.tevagenerics.com/products/product-search-result/

Vogelmeier, C. F., Criner, G. J., Martinez, F. J., et al. (2017). Global strategy for the diagnosis, management, and prevention of chronic obstructive lung disease 2017 report. GOLD executive summary. *American Journal of Respiratory and Critical Care Medicine, 195*(5), 557–582.

Wilson, D., Ross, C., Goodridge, D., et al. (2009). The care needs of community dwelling seniors suffering from advanced chronic obstructive pulmonary disease. *Canadian Journal on Aging, 27*(4), 347–358.

Resources

Agency for Healthcare Research and Quality: https://www.ahrq.gov/
Alpha-1 Association: http://www.alpha1.org
American Association of Cardiovascular and Pulmonary Rehabilitation: http://www.aacvpr.org
Canadian Council for Tobacco Control: http://9ncth.ca/program-description.php
Canadian Cystic Fibrosis Foundation (CCFF): http://www.cysticfibrosis.ca
Canadian Lung Association: http://www.lung.ca
Canadian Network for Asthma Care: http://www.cnac.net
Canadian Thoracic Society: https://bc.lung.ca/canadian-thoracic-society
Centers for Disease Control and Prevention: http://www.cdc.gov
Cystic Fibrosis Canada: https://www.cysticfibrosis.ca/about-cf/living-with-cystic-fibrosis/resources
Cystic Fibrosis Foundation: http://www.cff.org
Health Canada: http://www.hc-sc.gc.ca.
Health Canada's Tobacco Control Programme: http://www.hc-sc.gc.ca/hl-vs/tobac-tabac/about-apropos/programme/index-eng.php
National Heart, Lung and Blood Institute: http://www.nhlbi.nih.gov
Respiratory Nursing Society: http://www.respiratorynursingsociety.org
The Chief Public Health Officer's Report on the state of Public health in Canada 2013: http://www.phac-aspc.gc.ca/cphorsphc-respcacsp/2013/assets/pdf/2013-eng.pdf
World Allergy Organization: http://www.worldallergy.org

26 Respiratory Care Modalities

Adapted by Tanya Heuver

Learning Objectives

On completion of this chapter, the learner will be able to:

1. Describe the nursing management of patients receiving oxygen therapy, incentive spirometry, flutter valve therapy, small-volume nebulizer therapy, chest physiotherapy, and breathing retraining.
2. Discuss the patient education and transitions in care considerations for patients receiving oxygen therapy.
3. Describe the nursing care for a patient with an endotracheal tube and for a patient with a tracheostomy.
4. Use the nursing process as a framework for care of patients who are mechanically ventilated.
5. Describe the process of weaning the patient from mechanical ventilation.
6. Examine the significance of preoperative nursing assessment and patient teaching for the patient who is going to have thoracic surgery.
7. Explain the principles of chest drainage and the nursing responsibilities related to the care of the patient with a chest drainage system.
8. Utilize the nursing process as a framework for care of a patient who has had a thoracotomy.

Numerous treatment modalities are used when caring for patients with various respiratory conditions. The choice of modality is based on the oxygenation disorder and whether there is a problem with gas ventilation, diffusion, or both. Therapies range from simple and noninvasive (oxygen and nebulizer therapy, chest physiotherapy, breathing retraining) to complex and highly invasive treatments (intubation, mechanical ventilation, surgery). Assessment and management of the patient with respiratory disorders are best accomplished when the approach is multidisciplinary and collaborative.

NONINVASIVE RESPIRATORY THERAPIES

Oxygen Therapy

Oxygen therapy is the administration of oxygen at a concentration greater than that found in the environmental atmosphere. At sea level, the concentration of oxygen in room air is 21%. The goal of oxygen therapy is to provide adequate transport of oxygen in the blood while decreasing the work of breathing and reducing stress on the myocardium.

Oxygen transport to tissues depends on factors such as cardiac output, arterial oxygen content, concentration of hemoglobin, and metabolic requirements. These factors must be kept in mind when oxygen therapy is considered. (Respiratory physiology and oxygen transport are discussed in Chapter 22.)

Indications

A change in the patient's respiratory rate or pattern may be one of the earliest indicators of the need for oxygen therapy. These changes may result from hypoxemia or hypoxia. **Hypoxemia**, a decrease in the arterial oxygen tension in the blood, is manifested by changes in mental status (progressing through impaired judgment, agitation, disorientation, confusion, lethargy, and coma), dyspnea, increase in blood pressure, changes in heart rate, dysrhythmias, central cyanosis (late sign), diaphoresis, and cool extremities. Hypoxemia usually leads to **hypoxia**, a decrease in oxygen supply to the tissues, which can also be caused by problems outside the respiratory system. Severe hypoxia can be life threatening.

The signs and symptoms signalling the need for oxygen may depend on how suddenly this need develops. With rapidly developing hypoxia, changes occur in the central nervous system because the higher neurologic centres are very sensitive to oxygen deprivation. The clinical picture may resemble that of alcohol intoxication, with the patient

Glossary

airway pressure release ventilation (APRV): mode of mechanical ventilation that allows unrestricted, spontaneous breaths throughout the ventilatory cycle; on inspiration patient receives pre-set level of continuous positive airway pressure, and pressure is periodically released to aid expiration

assist–control ventilation (A/C): mode of mechanical ventilation in which the patient's breathing pattern may trigger the ventilator to deliver a pre-set tidal volume; in the absence of spontaneous breathing, the machine delivers a controlled breath at a pre-set minimum rate and tidal volume

bilevel positive airway pressure (BiPAP): noninvasive spontaneous breath mode of mechanical ventilation that allows for the separate control of inspiratory and expiratory pressures; given via a mask

chest drainage system: use of a chest tube and closed drainage system to re-expand the lung and to remove excess air, fluid, and blood

chest percussion: manually cupping over the chest wall to mobilize secretions by mechanically dislodging viscous or adherent secretions in the lungs

chest physiotherapy (CPT): therapy used to remove bronchial secretions, improve ventilation, and increase the efficiency of the respiratory muscles; types include postural drainage, chest percussion, and vibration

continuous mandatory (volume or pressure) ventilation (CMV): also referred to as assist–control (A/C) ventilation; mode of mechanical ventilation in which the patient's breathing pattern may trigger the ventilator to deliver a pre-set tidal volume or set pressure; in the absence of spontaneous breathing, the machine delivers a controlled breath at a pre-set minimum rate and tidal volume or set pressure

continuous positive airway pressure (CPAP): positive pressure applied throughout the respiratory cycle to a spontaneously breathing patient to promote alveolar and airway stability; may be administered with endotracheal or tracheostomy tube or by mask

controlled ventilation: mode of mechanical ventilation in which the ventilator completely controls the patient's ventilation according to pre-set tidal volumes and respiratory rate; because of problems with synchrony, it is rarely used except in paralyzed or anesthetized patients

endotracheal intubation: insertion of a breathing tube through the nose or mouth into the trachea

flutter valve: portable handheld mucous clearance device; consisting of a tube with an oscillating steel ball inside; upon expiration high-frequency oscillations facilitate mucous expectoration

fraction of inspired oxygen (FiO_2): concentration of oxygen delivered (1.0 = 100% oxygen)

hypoxemia: decrease in arterial oxygen tension in the blood

hypoxia: decrease in oxygen supply to the tissues and cells

incentive spirometry: method of deep breathing that provides visual feedback to help the patient inhale deeply and slowly and achieve maximum lung inflation

intermittent mandatory (volume or pressure) ventilation (IMV): mode of mechanical ventilation that provides a combination of mechanically assisted breaths at a pre-set volume or pressure and rate and spontaneous breaths

mechanical ventilator: a positive- or negative-pressure breathing device that supports ventilation and oxygenation

pneumothorax: partial or complete collapse of the lung due to positive pressure in the pleural space

positive end-expiratory pressure (PEEP): positive pressure maintained by the ventilator at the end of exhalation (instead of a normal zero pressure) to increase functional residual capacity and open collapsed alveoli; improves oxygenation with lower fraction of inspired oxygen

postural drainage: positioning the patient to allow drainage from all the lobes of the lungs and airways

pressure support ventilation (PSV): mode of mechanical ventilation in which pre-set positive pressure is delivered with spontaneous breaths to decrease work of breathing

proportional assist ventilation (PAV): mode of mechanical ventilation that provides partial ventilatory support in proportion to the patient's inspiratory efforts; decreases the work of breathing

respiratory weaning: process of gradual, systematic withdrawal or removal of ventilator, breathing tube, and oxygen

synchronized intermittent mandatory ventilation (SIMV): mode of mechanical ventilation in which the ventilator allows the patient to breathe spontaneously while providing a pre-set number of breaths to ensure adequate ventilation; ventilated breaths are synchronized with spontaneous breathing

thoracotomy: surgical opening into the chest cavity

tidal volume: volume of air inspired and expired with each breath

tracheostomy tube: indwelling tube inserted directly into the trachea to assist with ventilation

tracheotomy: surgical opening into the trachea

vibration: a type of massage administered by quickly tapping the chest with the fingertips or alternating the fingers in a rhythmic manner, or by using a mechanical device to assist in mobilizing lung secretions

CHART 26-1

Types of Hypoxia

Hypoxia can occur from either severe pulmonary disease (inadequate oxygen supply) or from extrapulmonary disease (inadequate oxygen delivery) affecting gas exchange at the cellular level. The four general types of hypoxia are hypoxemic hypoxia, circulatory hypoxia, anemic hypoxia, and histotoxic hypoxia.

Hypoxemic Hypoxia

Hypoxemic hypoxia is a decreased oxygen level in the blood resulting in decreased oxygen diffusion into the tissues. It may be caused by hypoventilation, high altitudes, ventilation–perfusion mismatch (as in pulmonary embolism), shunts in which the alveoli are collapsed and cannot provide oxygen to the blood (commonly caused by atelectasis), and pulmonary diffusion defects. It is corrected by increasing alveolar ventilation or providing supplemental oxygen.

Circulatory Hypoxia

Circulatory hypoxia is hypoxia resulting from inadequate capillary circulation. It may be caused by decreased cardiac output, local vascular obstruction, low-flow states such as shock, or cardiac arrest. Although tissue partial pressure of oxygen (PO_2) is reduced, arterial oxygen (PaO_2) remains normal. Circulatory hypoxia is corrected by identifying and treating the underlying cause.

Anemic Hypoxia

Anemic hypoxia is a result of decreased effective hemoglobin concentration, which causes a decrease in the oxygen-carrying capacity of the blood. It is rarely accompanied by hypoxemia. Carbon monoxide poisoning, because it reduces the oxygen-carrying capacity of hemoglobin, produces similar effects but is not strictly anemic hypoxia because hemoglobin levels may be normal.

Histotoxic Hypoxia

Histotoxic hypoxia occurs when a toxic substance, such as cyanide, interferes with the ability of tissues to use available oxygen.

exhibiting lack of coordination and impaired judgment. With long-standing hypoxia (as seen in chronic obstructive pulmonary disease [COPD] and chronic heart failure), fatigue, drowsiness, apathy, inattentiveness, and delayed reaction time may occur. The need for oxygen is assessed by arterial blood gas analysis, pulse oximetry, and clinical evaluation. More information about hypoxia is presented in Chart 26-1.

Complications

Oxygen is a medication, and as with other medications, the nurse should administer oxygen with caution and carefully assess its effects on each patient. In general, patients with respiratory conditions are given oxygen therapy only to increase the arterial oxygen pressure (PaO_2) back to the patient's normal baseline, which may vary from 60 to 95 mm Hg. In terms of the oxyhemoglobin dissociation curve (see Chapter 22), the blood at these levels is 80% to 98% saturated with oxygen; higher **fraction of inspired oxygen** (FiO_2) flow values add no further significant amounts of oxygen to the red blood cells or plasma. Instead of helping, increased amounts of oxygen may produce toxic effects on the lungs and central nervous system or may depress ventilation (see later discussion).

It is important to observe for subtle indicators of inadequate oxygenation when oxygen is administered by any method. Therefore, the nurse assesses the patient frequently for confusion, restlessness progressing to lethargy, diaphoresis, pallor, tachycardia, tachypnea, and hypertension. Intermittent or continuous pulse oximetry is used to monitor oxygen levels.

Oxygen Toxicity

Oxygen toxicity may occur when too high a concentration of oxygen (greater than 60%) is administered for an extended period (longer than 24 hours) (Sperlich, Zinner, Hauser, et al., 2017). It is caused by overproduction of oxygen-free radicals, which are by-products of cell metabolism. If oxygen toxicity is untreated, these radicals can severely damage or kill cells (Urden, Stacy, & Lough, 2014). Antioxidants such as vitamin E, vitamin C, and beta-carotene may help defend against oxygen-free radicals. Signs and symptoms of oxygen toxicity include substernal discomfort, paresthesia, dyspnea, restlessness, fatigue, malaise, progressive respiratory difficulty, refractory hypoxemia, alveolar atelectasis, and alveolar infiltrates evident on chest x-rays.

Prevention of oxygen toxicity is achieved by using the lowest amount of oxygen needed to maintain an acceptable PaO_2 level and treating the underlying condition. If high concentrations of oxygen are necessary, it is important to minimize the duration of administration and reduce its concentration as soon as possible. Often, **positive end-expiratory pressure (PEEP)** or **continuous positive airway pressure (CPAP)** is used with oxygen therapy to reverse or prevent microatelectasis, thus allowing a lower percentage of oxygen to be used. The level of PEEP that allows the best oxygenation without hemodynamic compromise is known as "best PEEP" or optimal PEEP (Cairo, 2014).

Absorption Atelectasis

An additional adverse effect of the administration of high concentrations of oxygen (greater than 50%) to patients who are sedated and breathing small **tidal volumes** of air (volume of air inspired and expired with each breath) is absorption atelectasis. Normally, 79% of room air is comprised of nitrogen. During inhalation, nitrogen, in addition to other gases, fills the alveoli and helps keep the alveoli open. With the administration of high concentrations of oxygen, nitrogen is diluted and replaced with oxygen. Oxygen in the alveoli is absorbed quickly into the bloodstream and not replaced rapidly enough in the alveoli to maintain patency. The alveoli collapse, causing atelectasis (Kacmarek, Stroller, & Huer, 2017).

Other Complications

Because oxygen supports combustion, there is always a danger of fire when it is used. It is important to post "No Smoking" signs when oxygen is in use. Oxygen therapy equipment is also a potential source of bacterial cross-infection; therefore, the tubing needs to be changed according to infection prevention policy, manufacturer's recommendations, and the type of oxygen delivery equipment.

Methods of Oxygen Administration

Oxygen is dispensed from a cylinder or a piped-in system. A reduction gauge is necessary to reduce the pressure to a working level, and a flow meter regulates the flow of oxygen in litres per minute. When oxygen is used at high flow rates, it should be moistened by passing it through a humidification system to prevent it from drying the mucous membranes of the respiratory tract.

The use of oxygen concentrators is another means of providing varying amounts of oxygen, especially in the home setting. These devices are relatively portable, easy to operate, and cost-effective. However, they require more maintenance than tank or liquid systems. These models can deliver oxygen flows from 1 to 10 L/min and provide an FiO_2 of about 40% (Cairo, 2014).

Many different oxygen devices are used, and all deliver oxygen if they are used as prescribed and maintained correctly (Table 26-1). The amount of oxygen delivered is expressed as a percentage concentration (e.g., 70%). The appropriate form of oxygen therapy is best determined by arterial blood gas levels, which indicate the patient's oxygenation status.

Oxygen delivery systems are classified as low-flow or high-flow delivery systems. Low-flow systems contribute partially to the inspired gas the patient breathes, which means that the patient breathes some room air along with the oxygen. These systems do not provide a constant or known concentration of inspired oxygen. The amount of inspired oxygen changes as the patient's breathing changes. Examples of low-flow systems include nasal cannula, oropharyngeal catheter, simple mask, partial-rebreather, and nonrebreather masks. In contrast, high-flow systems provide the total inspired air. A specific percentage of oxygen is delivered independent of the patient's breathing. High-flow systems are indicated for patients who require a constant and precise amount of oxygen. Examples of such systems include transtracheal catheters, Venturi masks, aerosol masks, tracheostomy collars, T-pieces, and face tents. See Table 26-1.

Nasal cannula is used when the patient requires a low to medium concentration of oxygen for which precise accuracy is not essential. This method is relatively simple and allows the patient to move about in bed, talk, cough, and eat without interrupting oxygen flow. Flow rates in excess of 6 to 8 L/min may lead to swallowing of air or may cause irritation and drying of the nasal and pharyngeal mucosa.

The oropharyngeal catheter is rarely used but may be prescribed for short-term therapy to administer low to

TABLE 26-1 Oxygen Administration Devices

Device	Suggested Flow Rate (L/min)	O_2 Percentage Setting	Advantages	Disadvantages
Low-Flow Systems				
Cannula	1–2 3–5 6	23–30 30–40 42	Lightweight, comfortable, inexpensive, continuous use with meals and activity	Nasal mucosal drying, variable FiO_2
Oropharyngeal catheter	1–6	23–42	Inexpensive, does not require a tracheostomy	Nasal mucosa irritation; catheter should be changed frequently to alternate nostril
Mask, simple	6–8	40–60	Simple to use, inexpensive	Poor fitting, variable FiO_2, must remove to eat
Mask, partial rebreather	8–11	50–75	Moderate O_2 concentration	Warm, poorly fitting, must remove to eat
Mask, nonrebreather	12	80–100	High O_2 concentration	Poorly fitting, must remove to eat
High-Flow Systems				
Transtracheal catheter	¼–4	60–100	More comfortable, concealed by clothing, less oxygen litres per minute needed than nasal cannula	Requires frequent and regular cleaning, requires surgical intervention
Mask, Venturi	4–6	24, 26, 28	Provides low levels of supplemental O_2	Must remove to eat
	6–8	30, 35, 40	Precise FiO_2, additional humidity available	
Mask, aerosol	8–10	30–100	Good humidity, accurate FiO_2	Uncomfortable for some
Tracheostomy collar	8–10	30–100	Good humidity, comfortable, fairly accurate FiO_2	
T-piece	8–10	30–100	Same as tracheostomy collar	Heavy with tubing
Face tent	8–10	30–100	Good humidity, fairly accurate FiO_2	Bulky and cumbersome
Oxygen Conserving Devices				
Pulse dose (or demand)	10–40 mL/breath		Deliver O_2 only on inspiration, conserve 50–75% of O_2 used	Must carefully evaluate function individually

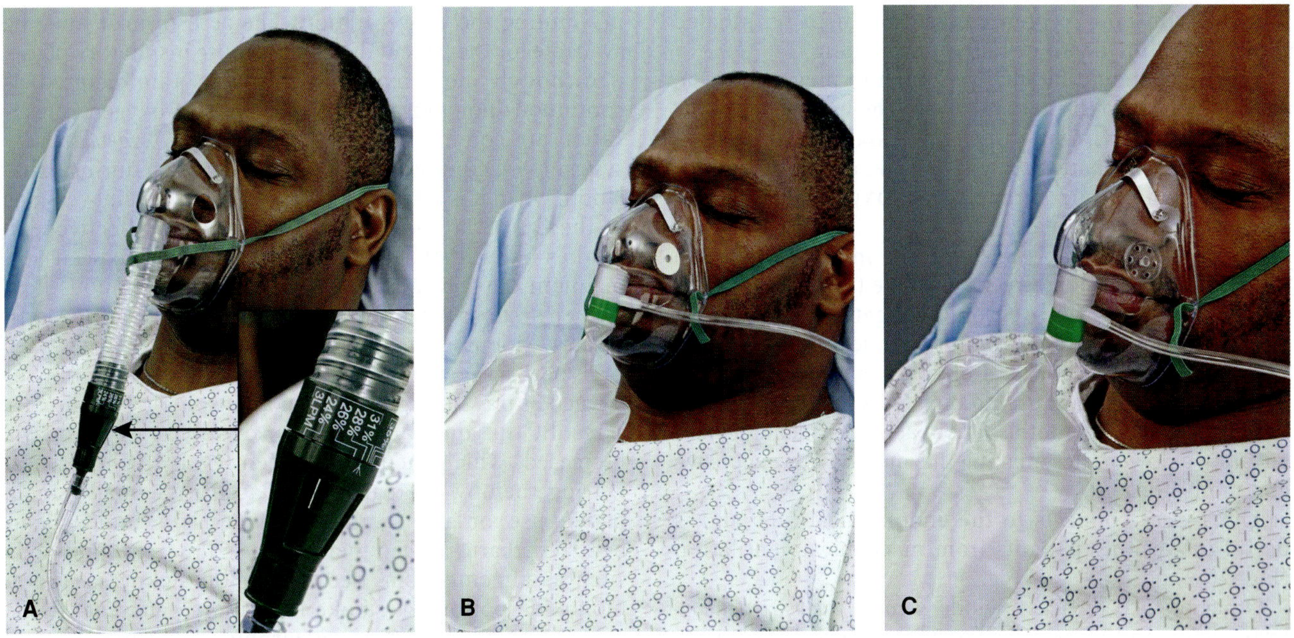

FIGURE 26-1. Types of oxygen masks used to deliver varying concentrations of oxygen. A. Venturi mask. B. Nonrebreathing mask. C. Partial-rebreathing mask.

moderate concentrations of oxygen. The catheter should be changed every 8 hours, alternating nostrils to prevent nasal irritation and infection.

When oxygen is administered via cannula or catheter, the percentage of oxygen reaching the lungs varies with the depth and rate of respirations, particularly if the nasal mucosa is swollen or if the patient is a mouth breather.

Oxygen masks come in several forms. Each is used for different purposes (Fig. 26-1). *Simple masks* are used to administer low to moderate concentrations of oxygen. The body of the mask itself gathers and stores oxygen between breaths. The patient exhales directly through openings or ports in the body of the mask. If oxygen flow ceases, the patient can draw air in through these openings around the mask edges. Although widely used, these masks cannot be used for controlled oxygen concentrations and must be adjusted for proper fit. They should not press too tightly against the skin because this can cause a sense of claustrophobia as well as skin breakdown; adjustable elastic bands are provided to ensure comfort and security.

Partial-rebreathing masks have a reservoir bag that must remain inflated during both inspiration and expiration. The nurse adjusts the oxygen flow to ensure that the bag does not collapse during inhalation. A high concentration of oxygen can be delivered because both the mask and the bag serve as reservoirs for oxygen. Oxygen enters the mask through small-bore tubing that connects at the junction of the mask and bag. As the patient inhales, gas is drawn from the mask, from the bag, and potentially from room air through the exhalation ports. As the patient exhales, the first third of the exhalation fills the reservoir bag. This is mainly dead space and does not participate in gas exchange in the lungs. Therefore, it has a high oxygen concentration. The remainder of the exhaled gas is vented through the exhalation ports. The actual percentage of oxygen delivered is influenced by the patient's ventilatory pattern (Cairo, 2014).

Nonrebreathing masks are similar in design to partial-rebreathing masks except that they have additional valves. A one-way valve located between the reservoir bag and the base of the mask allows gas from the reservoir bag to enter the mask on inhalation but prevents gas in the mask from flowing back into the reservoir bag during exhalation. One-way valves located at the exhalation ports prevent room air from entering the mask during inhalation. They also allow the patient's exhaled gases to exit the mask on exhalation. As with the partial-rebreathing mask, it is important to adjust the oxygen flow so that the reservoir bag does not completely collapse on inspiration. In theory, if the nonrebreathing mask fits the patient snugly and both side exhalation ports have one-way valves, it is possible for the patient to receive 100% oxygen, making the nonrebreathing mask a high-flow oxygen system. However, because it is difficult to get an exact fit from the mask on every patient, and some nonrebreathing masks have only one one-way exhalation valve, it is almost impossible to ensure 100% oxygen delivery, making it a low-flow oxygen system.

The *Venturi mask* is the most reliable and accurate method for delivering precise concentrations of oxygen through noninvasive means. The mask is constructed in a way that allows a constant flow of room air blended with a fixed flow of oxygen. It is used primarily for patients with COPD because it can accurately provide appropriate levels of supplemental oxygen, thus avoiding the risk of suppressing the hypoxic drive.

The Venturi mask uses the Bernoulli principle of air entrainment (trapping the air like a vacuum), which provides a high airflow with controlled oxygen enrichment. For each litre of oxygen that passes through a jet orifice, a fixed proportion of room air is entrained. A precise volume of oxygen can be delivered by varying the size of the jet orifice and adjusting the flow of oxygen. Excess gas leaves the mask through the two exhalation ports, carrying with it the exhaled carbon dioxide. This method allows a constant oxygen concentration to be inhaled regardless of the depth or rate of respiration.

The mask should fit snugly enough to prevent oxygen from flowing into the patient's eyes. The nurse checks the patient's skin for irritation. It is necessary to remove the mask so that the patient can eat, drink, and take medications, at which time supplemental oxygen is provided through a nasal cannula.

The *transtracheal oxygen catheter* is inserted through a small surgical incision directly into the trachea. It is indicated for patients with chronic oxygen therapy needs. These catheters are more comfortable, less dependent on breathing patterns, and less obvious than other oxygen delivery methods. Because no oxygen is lost into the surrounding environment, the patient achieves adequate oxygenation at lower rates, making this method less expensive and more efficient.

The *T-piece* connects to the endotracheal tube and is useful in weaning patients from mechanical ventilation (Fig. 26-2).

Other oxygen devices include *aerosol masks, tracheostomy collars*, and *face tents*, all of which are used with aerosol devices (nebulizers) that can be adjusted for oxygen concentrations from 27% to 100% (0.27 to 1). If the gas mixture flow falls below patient demand, room air is pulled in, diluting the concentration. The aerosol mist must be available for the patient during the entire inspiratory phase.

Although most oxygen therapy is administered as continuous-flow oxygen, new methods of oxygen conservation are coming into use. The *demand oxygen delivery system* (DODS) interrupts the flow of oxygen during exhalation, when it is otherwise mostly wasted. Several versions of the DODS are being evaluated for their effectiveness. Studies show that DODS models conserve oxygen and maintain oxygen saturation better than continuous-flow oxygen systems when the respiratory rate increases (Martí, Pajares, Morante, et al., 2013).

Hyperbaric oxygen therapy is the administration of oxygen at pressures greater than atmospheric pressure. As a result, the amount of oxygen dissolved in plasma is increased, which increases oxygen levels in the tissues. During therapy, the patient is placed in a small (single patient use) or large (multiple patient use) cylinder chamber. Hyperbaric oxygen therapy is used to treat conditions such as air embolism, decompression sickness, carbon monoxide poisoning, smoke inhalation, gangrene, tissue necrosis, and refractory anaerobic infections (Cairo, 2014). Potential side effects include ear trauma, central nervous system disorders, oxygen toxicity, and anxiety in patients with claustrophobia.

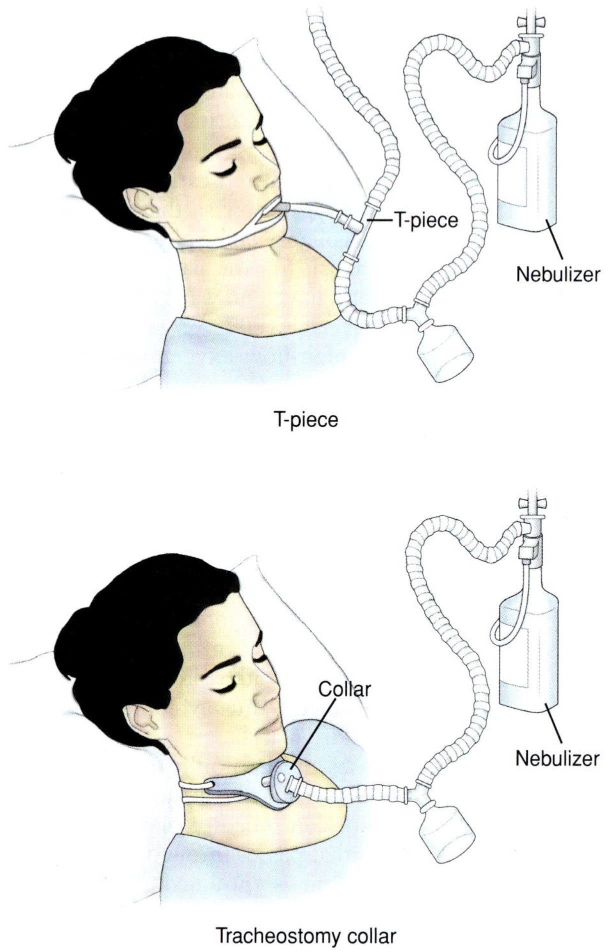

FIGURE 26-2. T-pieces and tracheostomy collars are devices used when weaning patients from mechanical ventilation.

Gerontologic Considerations

The respiratory system changes throughout the aging process, and it is important for nurses to be aware of these changes when assessing patients who are receiving oxygen therapy. As the respiratory muscles weaken and the large bronchi and alveoli become enlarged, the available surface area of the lungs decreases, resulting in reduced ventilation and respiratory gas exchange. The number of functional cilia is also reduced, decreasing ciliary action and the cough reflex. As a result of osteoporosis and calcification of the costal cartilages, chest wall compliance is decreased. Patients may display increased chest rigidity and respiratory rate and decreased PaO_2 and lung expansion. Nurses should be aware that the older adult is at risk for aspiration and infection related to these changes (Tabloski, 2014). In addition, patient education regarding adequate nutrition is essential because appropriate dietary intake can help diminish the excess buildup of carbon dioxide and maintain optimal respiratory functioning (Meiner, 2015).

Nursing Management

Promoting Home, Community-Based, and Transitional Care

Educating Patients About Self-Care

At times oxygen must be administered to the patient at home. The nurse instructs the patient or family in the methods for administering oxygen safely and informs the patient and family that oxygen is available in gas, liquid, and concentrated forms. The gas and liquid forms come in portable devices so that the patient can leave home while receiving oxygen therapy. Humidity must be provided while oxygen is used (except with portable devices) to counteract the dry, irritating effects of compressed oxygen on the airway (Chart 26-2).

CHART 26-2

HOME CARE CHECKLIST • Oxygen Therapy

At the completion of education, the patient and/or caregiver will be able to:

- State proper care of and administration of oxygen to patient:
  - State primary provider's prescription for oxygen and the manner in which it is to be used.
  - Indicate when a humidifier should be used.
  - Identify signs and symptoms indicating the need for change in oxygen therapy.
  - Describe precautions and safety measures to be used when oxygen is in use.
  - Know NOT to smoke or be around people who are smoking while using oxygen.
  - Post "No Smoking—Oxygen In Use" signs on doors.
  - Notify local fire department and electric company of oxygen use in home.
  - Never use paint thinners, cleaning fluids, gasoline, aerosol sprays, and other flammable materials while using oxygen.
  - Keep all methods of oxygen delivery at least 15 ft away from matches, candles, gas stove, or other source of flame, and 5 ft away from television, radio, and other appliances.
  - Keep oxygen tank out of direct sunlight.
  - When travelling in automobile, place oxygen tank on floor behind front seat.
  - If travelling by airplane, notify air carrier of need for oxygen at least 2 weeks in advance.
  - State how and when to place an order for more oxygen.

- Maintain and use equipment properly:
  - Identify when a portable oxygen delivery device should be used.
  - Demonstrate safe and appropriate use of and how to change from one oxygen delivery system to another (e.g., from oxygen concentrator to portable oxygen delivery)
  - Demonstrate correct adjustment of prescribed flow rate.
  - Describe how to clean and when to replace oxygen tubing.
  - Identify causes of malfunction of equipment and when to call for the replacement of equipment.
  - Describe the importance of determining that all electrical outlets are working properly.

Continuing and Transitional Care

Home visits by a home health nurse or respiratory therapist may be arranged based on the patient's status and needs. It is important to assess the patient's home environment, the patient's physical and psychological status, and the need for further teaching. The nurse reinforces the teaching points on how to use oxygen safely and effectively, including fire safety tips. To maintain a consistent quality of care and to maximize the patient's financial reimbursement for home oxygen therapy, the nurse ensures that the physician's prescription includes the diagnosis, the prescribed oxygen flow, and conditions for use (e.g., continuous use, nighttime use only). Because oxygen is a medication, the nurse reminds the patient receiving long-term oxygen therapy and the family about the importance of keeping follow-up appointments with the physician. The patient is instructed to see the physician every 6 months or more often, if indicated. Blood gas measurements and laboratory tests are repeated annually or more often if the patient's condition changes.

Incentive Spirometry (Sustained Maximal Inspiration)

Incentive spirometry is a method of deep breathing that provides visual feedback to encourage the patient to inhale slowly and deeply to maximize lung inflation and prevent or reduce atelectasis. The purpose of an incentive spirometer is to ensure that the volume of air inhaled is increased gradually as the patient takes deeper and deeper breaths.

Incentive spirometers are available in two types: volume or flow. In the volume type, the tidal volume is set using the manufacturer's instructions. The patient takes a deep breath through the mouthpiece, pauses at peak lung inflation, and then relaxes and exhales. Taking several normal breaths before attempting another with the incentive spirometer helps avoid fatigue. The volume is periodically increased as tolerated.

In the flow type, the volume is not pre-set. The spirometer contains a number of movable balls that are pushed up by the force of the breath and held suspended in the air while the patient inhales. The amount of air inhaled and the flow of the air are estimated by how long and how high the balls are suspended.

Indications

Incentive spirometry is used after surgery, especially thoracic and abdominal surgery, to promote the expansion of the alveoli and to prevent or treat atelectasis.

Nursing Management

Nursing management of the patient using incentive spirometry includes placing the patient in the proper position, teaching the technique for using the incentive spirometer, setting realistic goals for the patient, and recording the results of the therapy (Chart 26-3). Ideally, the patient assumes a sitting or semi-Fowler's position to enhance diaphragmatic excursion; however, this

CHART 26-3

Patient Education: Performing Incentive Spirometry

- The inspired air helps inflate the lungs. The ball or weight in the spirometer rises in response to the intensity of the intake of air. The higher the ball rises, the deeper the breath.

The nurse instructs the patient to:

- Assume a semi-Fowler's position or an upright position before initiating therapy.
- Use diaphragmatic breathing.
- Place the mouthpiece of the spirometer firmly in the mouth, breathe air in (inspire) through the mouth, and hold the breath at the end of inspiration for about 3 seconds. Exhale slowly through the mouthpiece.
- Cough during and after each session. Splint the incision when coughing postoperatively.
- Perform the procedure approximately 10 times in succession, repeating the 10 breaths with the spirometer each hour during waking hours.

CHART 26-4

Patient Education: Breathing Exercises

General Instructions

The nurse instructs the patient to:

- Breathe slowly and rhythmically to exhale completely and empty the lungs completely.
- Inhale through the nose to filter, humidify, and warm the air before it enters the lungs.
- If you feel out of breath, breathe more slowly by prolonging the exhalation time.
- Keep the air moist with a humidifier.

Diaphragmatic Breathing

Goal: To use and strengthen the diaphragm during breathing

The nurse instructs the patient to:

- Place one hand on the abdomen (just below the ribs) and the other hand on the middle of the chest to increase the awareness of the position of the diaphragm and its function in breathing.
- Breathe in slowly and deeply through the nose, letting the abdomen protrude as far as possible.
- Breathe out through pursed lips while tightening (contracting) the abdominal muscles.
- Press firmly inward and upward on the abdomen while breathing out.
- Repeat for 1 minute; follow with a rest period of 2 minutes.
- Gradually increase duration up to 5 minutes, several times a day (before meals and at bedtime).

Pursed-Lip Breathing

Goal: To prolong exhalation and increase airway pressure during expiration, thus reducing the amount of trapped air and the amount of airway resistance.

The nurse instructs the patient to:

- Inhale through the nose while slowly counting to 3—the amount of time needed to say "Smell a rose."
- Exhale slowly and evenly against pursed lips while tightening the abdominal muscles. (Pursing the lips increases intratracheal pressure; exhaling through the mouth offers less resistance to expired air.)
- Count to 7 slowly while prolonging expiration through pursed lips—the length of time to say "Blow out the candle."
- While sitting in a chair:
  Fold arms over the abdomen.
  Inhale through the nose while counting to 3 slowly.
  Bend forward and exhale slowly through pursed lips while counting to 7 slowly.
- While walking:
  Inhale while walking two steps.
  Exhale through pursed lips while walking four or five steps.

procedure may be performed with the patient in any position.

Small-Volume Nebulizer (Mini-Nebulizer) Therapy

The small-volume nebulizer is a handheld apparatus that disperses a moisturizing agent or medication, such as a bronchodilator or mucolytic agent, into microscopic particles and delivers it to the lungs as the patient inhales. The small-volume nebulizer is usually air driven by means of a compressor through connecting tubing. In some instances, the nebulizer is oxygen driven rather than air driven. To be effective, a visible mist must be available for the patient to inhale.

Indications

The indications for use of a mini-nebulizer include difficulty in clearing respiratory secretions, reduced vital capacity with ineffective deep breathing and coughing, and unsuccessful trials of simpler and less costly methods for clearing secretions, delivering aerosol, or expanding the lungs. The patient must be able to generate a deep breath. Diaphragmatic breathing (Chart 26-4) is a helpful technique to prepare for proper use of the mini-nebulizer. Mini-nebulizers are frequently used for patients with COPD to dispense inhaled medications, and they are commonly used at home on a long-term basis.

Nursing Management

The nurse instructs the patient to breathe through the mouth, taking slow, deep breaths, and then to hold the breath for a few seconds at the end of inspiration to increase intrapleural pressure and reopen collapsed alveoli, thereby increasing functional residual capacity. The nurse encourages the patient to cough and to monitor the effectiveness of the therapy. The nurse instructs the patient and family about the purpose of the treatment, equipment setup, medication additive, and proper cleaning and storage of the equipment.

Chest Physiotherapy

Chest physiotherapy (CPT) includes **postural drainage**, **chest percussion**, and **vibration**, and breathing retraining. In addition, teaching the patient effective coughing techniques is an important part of CPT. The goals of CPT are to remove bronchial secretions, improve ventilation, and increase the efficiency of the respiratory muscles.

Postural Drainage (Segmented Bronchial Drainage)

Postural drainage allows the force of gravity to assist in the removal of bronchial secretions. The secretions drain from the affected bronchioles into the bronchi and trachea and are removed by coughing or suctioning. Postural drainage is used to prevent or relieve bronchial obstruction caused by accumulation of secretions.

Because the patient usually sits in an upright position, secretions are likely to accumulate in the lower parts of the lungs. Several other positions (Fig. 26-3) are used so that

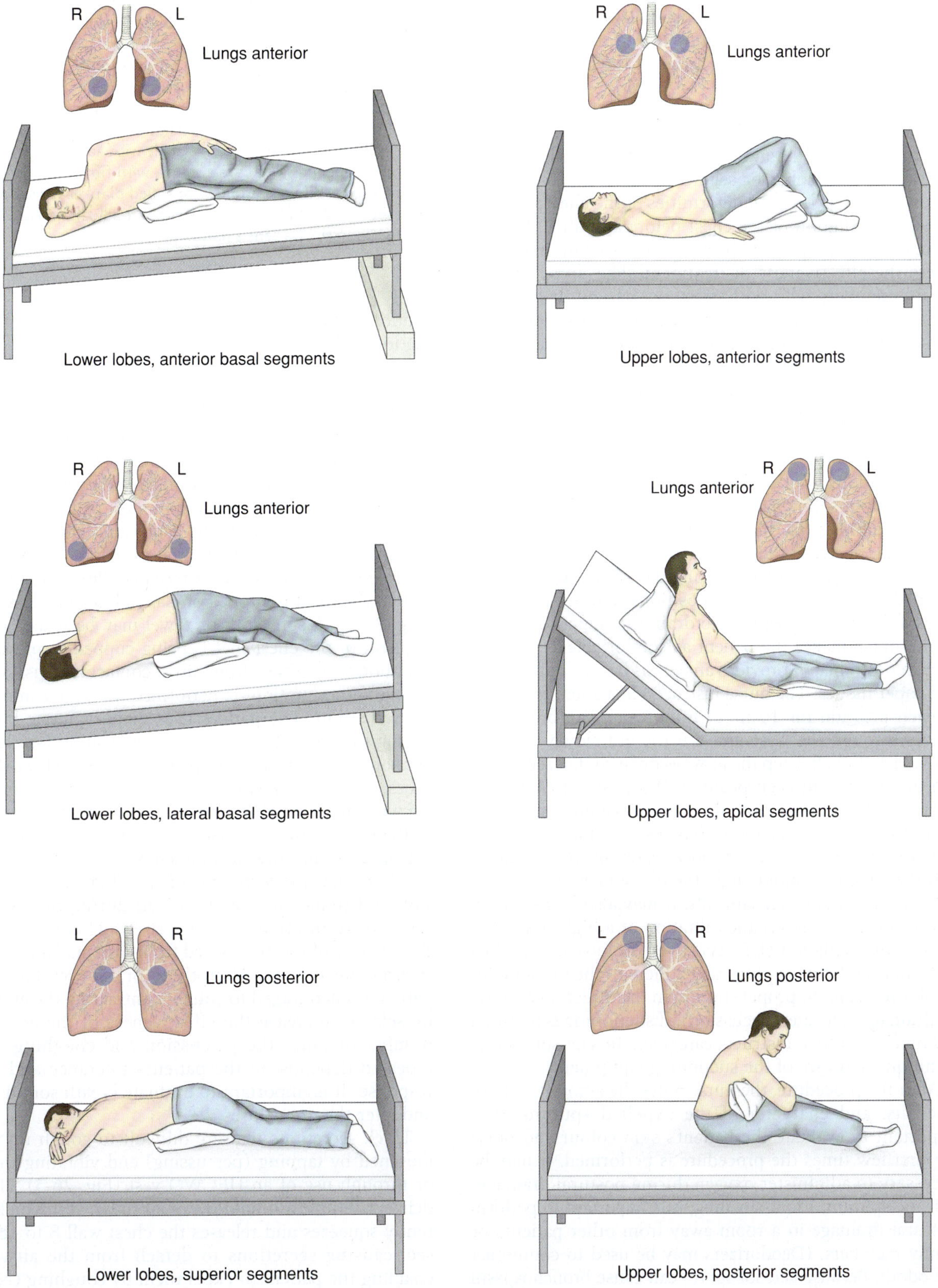

FIGURE 26-3. Postural drainage positions and the areas of lung drained by each position.

the force of gravity helps move secretions from the smaller bronchial airways to the main bronchi and trachea. Each position contributes to effective drainage of a different lobe of the lungs; lower and middle lobe bronchi drain more effectively when the head is down, while the upper lobe bronchi drain more effectively when the head is up. The secretions then are removed by coughing. The nurse instructs the patient to inhale bronchodilators and mucolytic agents, if prescribed, before postural drainage, because these medications improve drainage of the bronchial tree.

Nursing Management

The nurse should be aware of the patient's diagnosis as well as the lung lobes or segments involved, the cardiac status, and any structural deformities of the chest wall and spine. Auscultation of the chest before and after the procedure is used to identify the areas that need drainage and assess the effectiveness of treatment. The nurse teaches family members who will assist the patient at home to evaluate breath sounds before and after treatment. The nurse explores strategies that will enable the patient to assume the indicated positions at home. This may require the creative use of objects readily available at home, such as pillows, cushions, or cardboard boxes.

Postural drainage is usually performed two to four times daily, before meals (to prevent nausea, vomiting, and aspiration) and at bedtime. Prescribed bronchodilators, water, or saline may be nebulized and inhaled before postural drainage to dilate the bronchioles, reduce bronchospasm, decrease the thickness of mucus and sputum, and combat edema of the bronchial walls. The recommended sequence starts with positions to drain the lower lobes, followed by positions to drain the upper lobes.

The nurse makes the patient as comfortable as possible in each position and provides an emesis basin, sputum cup, and paper tissues. The nurse instructs the patient to remain in each position for 10 to 15 minutes and to breathe in slowly through the nose and breathe out slowly through pursed lips to help keep the airways open so that secretions can drain while in each position. If a position cannot be tolerated, the nurse helps the patient assume a modified position. When the patient changes position, the nurse explains how to cough and remove secretions (Chart 26-5).

If the patient cannot cough, the nurse may need to suction the secretions mechanically. It may also be necessary to use chest percussion and vibration or a high-frequency chest wall oscillation (HFCWO) vest to loosen bronchial secretions and mucus plugs that adhere to the bronchioles and bronchi and to propel sputum in the direction of gravity drainage (see later discussion). If suctioning is required at home, the nurse instructs caregivers in safe suctioning technique and care of the suctioning equipment.

After the procedure, the nurse notes the amount, colour, viscosity, and character of the expelled sputum. It is important to evaluate the patient's skin colour and pulse the first few times the procedure is performed. It may be necessary to administer oxygen during postural drainage.

If the sputum is foul-smelling, it is important to perform postural drainage in a room away from other patients or family members. (Deodorizers may be used to counteract the odour. Because aerosol sprays can cause bronchospasm and irritation, they should be used sparingly and with caution.) After the procedure, the patient may find it refreshing to brush the teeth and use a mouthwash before resting.

CHART 26-5

Patient Education: Effective Coughing Technique

The nurse instructs the patient to:

- Assume a sitting position and bend slightly forward. This upright position permits a stronger cough.
- Flex your knees and hips to promote relaxation and reduce the strain on the abdominal muscles while coughing.
- Inhale slowly through the nose and exhale through pursed lips several times.
- Cough twice during each exhalation while contracting (pulling in) the abdomen sharply with each cough.
- Splint the incisional area, if any, with firm hand pressure or support it with a pillow or rolled blanket while coughing (see Fig. 26-11). (The nurse can initially demonstrate this by using the patient's hands.)

Chest Percussion and Vibration

Chest percussion and vibration help dislodge mucus adhering to the bronchioles and bronchi. A scheduled program of coughing and clearing sputum, together with hydration, reduces the amount of sputum in most patients. Percussion is carried out by cupping the hands and lightly striking the chest wall in a rhythmic fashion over the lung segment to be drained. The wrists are alternately flexed and extended so that the chest is cupped or clapped in a painless manner (Fig. 26-4). A soft cloth or towel may be placed over the segment of the chest that is being cupped to prevent skin irritation and redness from direct contact. Percussion, alternating with vibration, is performed for 3 to 5 minutes for each position. The patient uses diaphragmatic breathing during this procedure to promote relaxation (see later discussion). As a precaution, percussion over chest drainage tubes, the sternum, spine, liver, kidneys, spleen, or breasts (in women) is avoided. Percussion is performed cautiously in the older adults because of their increased incidence of osteoporosis and risk of rib fracture.

Vibration is the technique of applying manual compression and tremor to the chest wall during the exhalation phase of respiration (see Fig. 26-4). This helps increase the velocity of the air expired from the small airways, thus freeing the mucus. After three or four vibrations, the patient is encouraged to cough, contracting the abdominal muscles to increase the effectiveness of the cough. The number of times the percussion and coughing cycle is repeated depends on the patient's tolerance and clinical response. It is important to evaluate breath sounds before and after the procedures.

Thick secretions that are difficult to cough up may be loosened by tapping (percussing) and vibrating the chest or through use of an HFCWO vest (Fig. 26-5). HFCWO delivers an intermittent flow of air into a vest which recurrently squeezes and releases the chest wall 8 to 18 times/sec, causing secretions to detach from the airway and enabling the patient to expel them by coughing (Nicolini, Cardini, Landucci, et al., 2013). Vest therapy is considered

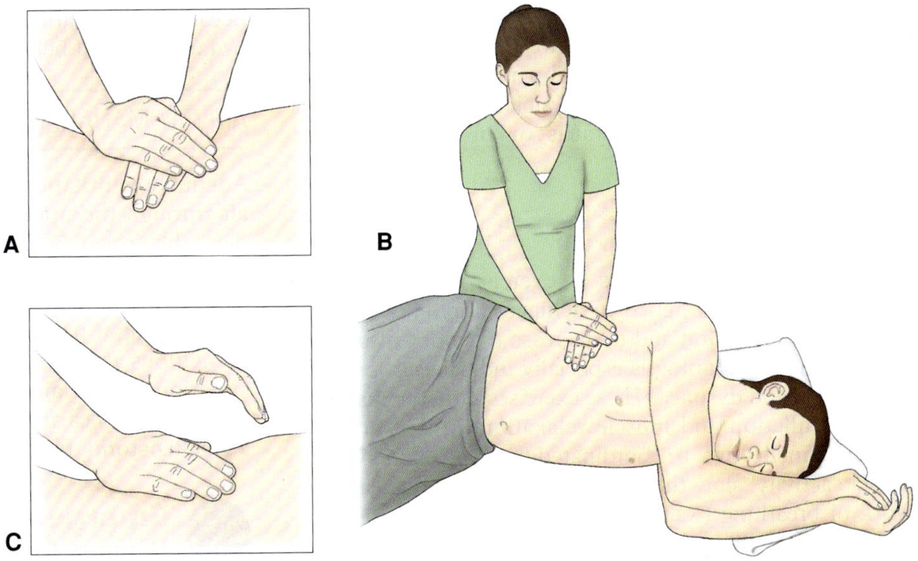

FIGURE 26-4. Percussion and vibration. A. Proper hand position for vibration. B. Proper technique for vibration. The wrists and elbows remain stiff; the vibrating motion is produced by the shoulder muscles. C. Proper hand position for percussion.

more effective than manual percussion because it is gentler and acts on all lobes of the lung simultaneously. Research has shown that the vest is equally effective to manual CPT, and some patients prefer it (Andrews, Sathe, Krishnaswami, et al., 2013; Hanlon, 2015; Main, Prasad, & van der Schans, 2013). The HFCWO vest has been used in individuals with a variety of diagnoses such as chronic obstructive pulmonary disease, asthma, cystic fibrosis, thoracic trauma, and neuromuscular diseases to improve central and peripheral mucus clearance (Nicolini et al., 2013).

To increase the effectiveness of coughing, a **flutter valve** is sometimes used, especially by people who have cystic fibrosis. The flutter valve looks like a pipe but has a cap covering the bowl, which contains a steel ball. When the patient exhales actively into the valve, movement of the ball causes pressure oscillations, thereby decreasing viscosity of the mucus, facilitating mucous clearance.

Nursing Management

When performing CPT, the nurse ensures that the patient is comfortable, is not wearing restrictive clothing, and has not just eaten. The nurse gives medication for pain, as prescribed, before percussion and vibration and splints any incision and provides pillows for support as needed. The positions are varied, but focus is placed on the affected areas. On completion of the treatment, the nurse assists the patient to assume a comfortable position.

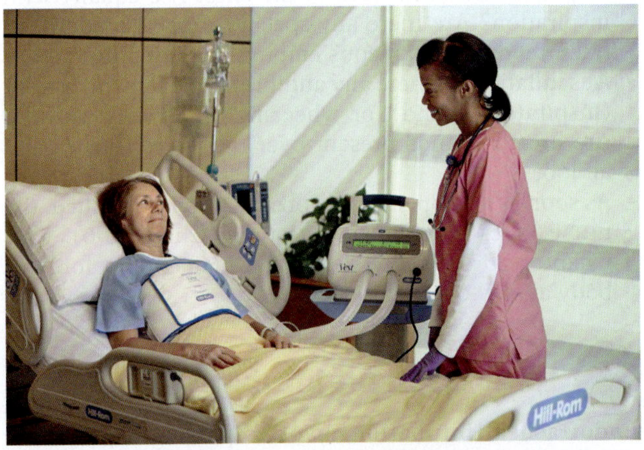

FIGURE 26-5. High-frequency chest wall oscillation vest. (© 2013 Hill-Rom Services, Inc. Reprinted with permission—all rights reserved.)

If an HFCWO vest is being used, the patient may assume whatever position is most comfortable and may even continue to perform light activity during therapy within the length of the compressed air hose. It is not necessary for the patient to assume specific positions for the vest to be effective.

Treatment should be stopped if any of the following occur: increased pain, increased shortness of breath, weakness, lightheadedness, or hemoptysis. Therapy is indicated until the patient has normal respirations, can mobilize secretions, and has normal breath sounds, and until the chest x-ray findings are normal.

Promoting Home, Community-Based, and Transitional Care

Educating Patients About Self-Care

CPT is frequently indicated at home for patients with COPD, bronchiectasis, or cystic fibrosis. The techniques are the same as described previously; however, gravity drainage is achieved by placing the hips over a box, a stack of magazines, or pillows. The nurse instructs the patient and family about the positions and techniques of percussion and vibration so that therapy can be continued in the home. In addition, the nurse instructs the patient to maintain an adequate fluid intake and air humidity to prevent secretions from becoming thick and tenacious. It is also important to teach the patient to recognize early signs of infection, such as fever and a change in the colour or character of sputum. Resting 5 to 10 minutes in each postural drainage position before CPT maximizes the amount of secretions obtained.

Continuing and Transitional Care

CPT may be carried out during visits by a home care nurse. The patient's physical status, understanding of the treatment plan, adherence with recommended therapy, and the effectiveness of therapy are assessed. Patient and family education is reinforced during these visits. The nurse reports to the patient's physician any deterioration in the patient's physical status or inability to clear secretions.

Breathing Retraining

Breathing retraining consists of exercises and breathing practices that are designed to achieve more efficient and **controlled ventilation** and to decrease the work of breathing. Breathing retraining is especially indicated in patients with COPD and dyspnea. These exercises promote maximal alveolar inflation and muscle relaxation; relieve anxiety; eliminate ineffective, uncoordinated patterns of respiratory muscle activity; slow the respiratory rate; and decrease the work of breathing (Kacmarek et al., 2017). Slow, relaxed, rhythmic breathing also helps to control the anxiety that occurs with dyspnea. Specific breathing exercises include diaphragmatic and pursed-lip breathing (see Chart 26-4).

Diaphragmatic breathing can become automatic with sufficient practice and concentration. Pursed-lip breathing, which improves oxygen transport, helps induce a slow, deep breathing pattern and assists the patient to control breathing, even during periods of stress. This type of breathing helps prevent airway collapse secondary to loss of lung elasticity in emphysema. The nurse instructs the patient in diaphragmatic breathing and pursed-lip breathing, as described in Chart 26-4. Breathing exercises should be practiced in several positions because air distribution and pulmonary circulation vary with the position of the chest.

Many patients require additional oxygen, using a low-flow method, while performing breathing exercises. Emphysema-like changes in the lung occur as part of the natural aging process of the lung; therefore, breathing exercises are appropriate for all older adult patients, whether hospitalized or not, who are sedentary, even without primary lung disease.

Nursing Management

The nurse instructs the patient to breathe slowly and rhythmically in a relaxed manner and to exhale completely to empty the lungs. The patient is instructed to always inhale through the nose because this filters, humidifies, and warms the air. If short of breath, the patient should be instructed to concentrate on prolonging the length of exhalation; this helps avoid initiating a cycle of increasing shortness of breath and panic. Minimizing the amount of dust or particles in the air and providing adequate humidification may also make it easier for the patient to breathe. Dust and particles in the air can be decreased by removing drapes and upholstered furniture, using air filters, and washing floors, dusting, and vacuuming frequently.

The nurse instructs the patient that an adequate dietary intake promotes gas exchange and increases energy levels. It is important to obtain adequate nutrition without overeating by consuming small, frequent meals and snacks. Having ready-prepared meals and favourite foods available helps encourage nutrient consumption. Gas-producing foods such as beans, legumes, broccoli, cabbage, and brussels sprouts should be avoided to prevent gastric distress. Because many patients lack the energy to eat, they should be taught to rest before and after meals to conserve energy.

AIRWAY MANAGEMENT

Adequate ventilation is dependent on free movement of air through the upper and lower airways. In many disorders, the airway becomes narrowed or blocked as a result of disease, bronchoconstriction (narrowing of airway by contraction of muscle fibres), a foreign body, or secretions. Maintaining a patent (open) airway is achieved through meticulous airway management, whether in an emergency situation such as airway obstruction or in long-term management, as in caring for a patient with an endotracheal or a **tracheostomy tube**.

Emergency Management of Upper Airway Obstruction

Upper airway obstruction has a variety of causes. Acute upper airway obstruction may be caused by food particles, vomitus, blood clots, or anything that obstructs the larynx or trachea. It may also occur from enlargement of tissue in the wall of the airway, as in epiglottitis, obstructive sleep apnea, laryngeal edema, laryngeal carcinoma, or peritonsillar abscess, or from thick secretions. Pressure on the walls of the airway, as occurs in retrosternal goitre, enlarged mediastinal lymph nodes, hematoma around the upper airway, and thoracic aneurysm, also may result in upper airway obstruction.

The patient with an altered level of consciousness from any cause is at risk for upper airway obstruction because of loss of the protective reflexes (cough and swallowing) and loss of the tone of the pharyngeal muscles, which causes the tongue to fall back and block the airway.

The nurse makes the following rapid observations to assess for signs and symptoms of upper airway obstruction:

- Inspection: Is the patient conscious? Is there any inspiratory effort? Does the chest rise symmetrically? Is there use or retraction of accessory muscles? What is the skin colour? Are there any obvious signs of deformity or obstruction (trauma, food, teeth, vomitus)? Is the trachea midline?
- Palpation: Do both sides of the chest rise equally with inspiration? Are there any specific areas of tenderness, fracture, or subcutaneous emphysema (crepitus)?
- Auscultation: Is there any audible air movement, stridor (inspiratory sound), or wheezing (expiratory sound)? Are breath sounds present over the lower trachea and all lobes?
- As soon as an upper airway obstruction is identified, the nurse takes emergency measures (Chart 26-6). (See Chapter 23 for more details on managing a foreign-body airway obstruction.)

Endotracheal Intubation

Endotracheal intubation involves passing an endotracheal tube through the mouth or nose into the trachea (Fig. 26-6). Intubation provides a patent airway when the

CHART 26-6

Clearing an Upper Airway Obstruction

Attempt to Open the Airway

Perform the head-tilt/chin-lift manoeuvre by placing one hand on the forehead and placing the fingers of the other hand underneath the jaw and lifting upward and forward. This action pulls the tongue away from the back of the pharynx.

Attempt to Clear the Airway

- Assess the patient by observing the chest and listening and feeling for the movement of air.
- Use a cross-finger technique to open the mouth and observe for obvious obstructions such as secretions, blood clots, or food particles.
- If no passage of air is detected, begin cardiopulmonary resuscitation (CPR).

Bag and Mask Resuscitation

- Apply the mask to the patient's face and create a seal by pressing the thumb of the nondominant hand on the bridge of the nose and the index finger on the chin.
- Using the rest of the fingers on that hand, pull on the chin and the angle of the mandible to maintain the head in extension.
- Use the dominant hand to inflate the lungs by squeezing the bag to its full volume.

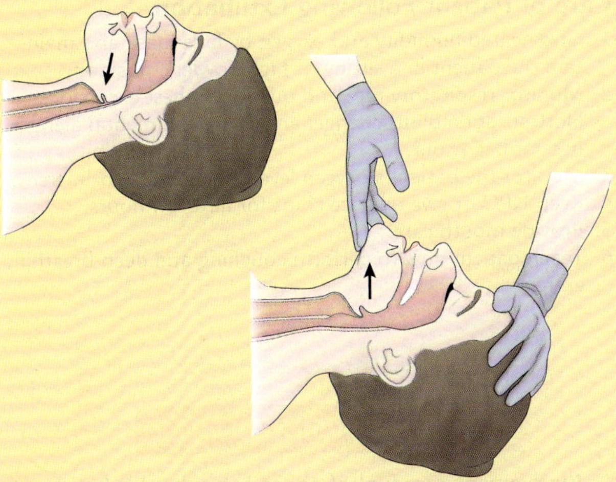

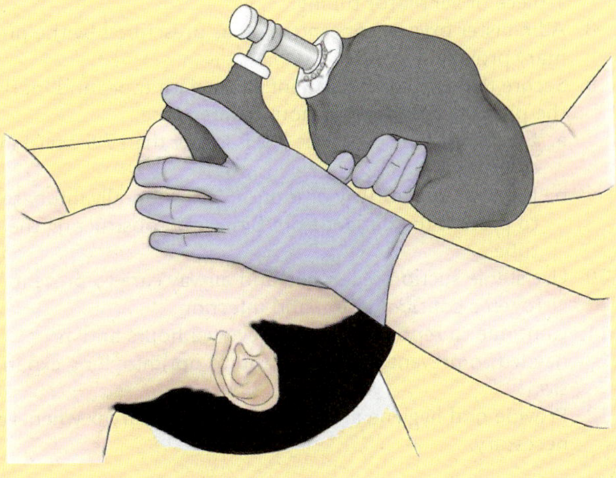

Adapted from American Heart Association. (2015). *Basic life support for healthcare providers: Student manual*. Dallas, TX: Author.

patient is having respiratory distress that cannot be treated with simpler methods and is the method of choice in emergency care. Endotracheal intubation is a means of providing an airway for patients who cannot maintain an adequate airway on their own (e.g., comatose patients, patients with upper airway obstruction), for patients needing mechanical ventilation, and for suctioning secretions from the pulmonary tree.

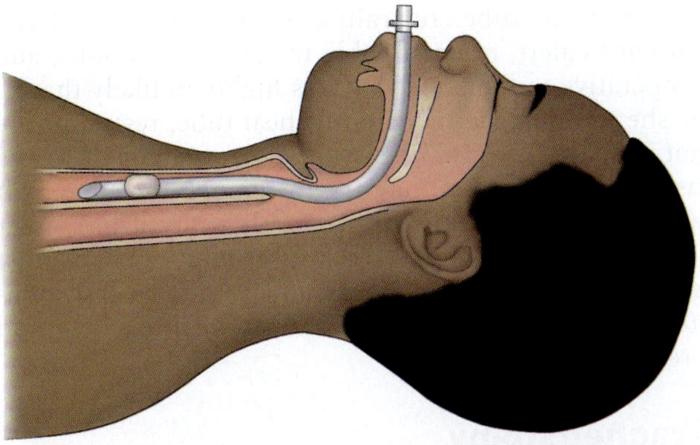

FIGURE 26-6. Endotracheal tube in place. The tube has been inserted using the oral route. The cuff has been inflated to maintain the tube's position and to minimize the risk of aspiration.

An endotracheal tube usually is passed with the aid of a laryngoscope by specifically trained medical, nursing, or respiratory therapy health care professionals. Once the tube is inserted, a cuff at the distal end of the tube is inflated to prevent air from leaking around the outer part of the tube to minimize the possibility of aspiration and to prevent movement of the tube. The position of the endotracheal tube is verified by checking end-tidal carbon dioxide levels and confirmed with chest x-ray. Chart 26-7 discusses the nursing care of the patient with an endotracheal tube.

Complications can occur from pressure exerted by the cuff on the tracheal wall. Cuff pressures should be maintained between 20 and 25 mm Hg (24 to 30 cm H_2O) because high cuff pressure can cause tracheal bleeding, ischemia, and pressure necrosis, whereas low cuff pressure can increase the risk of aspiration pneumonia (Bulamba, Kintu, Ayupo, et al., 2017). Routine deflation of the cuff is not recommended because of the increased risk of aspiration and hypoxia (Urden et al., 2014). Tracheobronchial secretions are suctioned through the tube. Warmed, humidified oxygen should always be introduced through

CHART 26-7

Care of the Patient With an Endotracheal Tube

Immediately After Intubation

1. Check symmetry of chest expansion.
2. Auscultate breath sounds of anterior and lateral chest bilaterally.
3. Obtain capnography or end-tidal CO_2 as indicated
4. Ensure chest x-ray obtained to verify proper tube placement.
5. Check cuff pressure every 6 to 8 hours.
6. Monitor for signs and symptoms of aspiration.
7. Ensure high humidity; a visible mist should appear in the T-piece or ventilator tubing.
8. Administer oxygen concentration as prescribed by the primary provider.
9. Secure the tube to the patient's face with tape, and mark the proximal end for position maintenance.
   a. Cut proximal end of tube if it is longer than 7.5 cm (3 in) to prevent kinking.
   b. Insert an oral airway or mouth device if orally intubated to prevent the patient from biting and obstructing the tube.
10. Use sterile suction technique and airway care to prevent iatrogenic contamination and infection.
11. Continue to reposition patient every 2 hours and as needed to prevent atelectasis and to optimize lung expansion.
12. Provide oral hygiene and suction the oropharynx whenever necessary.

Extubation (Removal of Endotracheal Tube)

1. Explain procedure.
2. Have self-inflating bag and mask ready in case ventilatory assistance is required immediately after extubation.
3. Suction the tracheobronchial tree and oropharynx, remove tape, and then deflate the cuff.
4. Give 100% oxygen for a few breaths, then insert a new, sterile suction catheter inside the tube.
5. Have the patient inhale. At peak inspiration remove the tube, suctioning the airway through the tube as it is pulled out.

Note: In some hospitals this procedure can be performed by respiratory therapists; in others, by nurses. Check hospital policy.

Care of Patient Following Extubation

1. Give heated humidity and oxygen by face mask and maintain the patient in a sitting or high-Fowler's position.
2. Monitor respiratory rate and quality of chest excursions. Note stridor, colour change, and change in mental alertness or behaviour.
3. Monitor the patient's oxygen level using a pulse oximeter.
4. Keep NPO or give only ice chips for next few hours.
5. Provide mouth care.
6. Teach patient how to perform coughing and deep-breathing exercises.

the tube, whether the patient is breathing spontaneously or is receiving ventilatory support. Endotracheal intubation may be used for no longer than 3 weeks, by which time a tracheostomy should be considered to decrease irritation of and trauma to the tracheal lining, to reduce the incidence of vocal cord paralysis (secondary to laryngeal nerve damage), and to decrease the work of breathing.

Endotracheal and tracheostomy tubes have several disadvantages. The tubes cause discomfort. The cough reflex is depressed because glottis closure is hindered. Secretions tend to become thicker because the warming and humidifying effect of the upper respiratory tract has been bypassed. The swallowing reflexes (glottic, pharyngeal, and laryngeal reflexes) are depressed because of prolonged disuse and the mechanical trauma produced by the endotracheal or tracheostomy tube, increasing the risk of micro aspiration, aspiration, and ventilator-associated pneumonia (Urden et al., 2014). In addition, ulceration and stricture of the larynx or trachea may develop. Of great concern to the patient is the inability to talk and to communicate needs.

Unintentional or premature removal of the tube is a potentially life-threatening complication of endotracheal intubation. Removal of the tube is a frequent problem in intensive care units and occurs mainly during nursing care or by the patient. It is important that nurses instruct and remind patients and family members about the purpose of the tube and the dangers of removing it. Baseline and ongoing assessment of the patient and of the equipment ensures effective care. Providing comfort measures, including opioid analgesia and sedation, can improve the patient's tolerance of the endotracheal tube.

NURSING ALERT

Inadvertent removal of an endotracheal tube can cause laryngeal swelling, hypoxemia, bradycardia, hypotension, and even death. Measures must be taken to prevent premature or inadvertent removal.

To prevent tube removal by the patient, the nurse should explain to the patient and family the purpose of the tube, distract the patient through one-to-one interaction or with television, and maintain comfort measures. If the patient cannot move the arms and hands to the endotracheal tube, restraints are not needed. If the patient is alert, oriented, able to follow directions, and cooperative to the point that it is highly unlikely that he or she will remove the endotracheal tube, restraints are not needed. However, if the nurse determines there is a risk that the patient may try to remove the tube, soft wrist restraints are appropriate with a physician's order (check agency policy). Discretion and caution must always be used before applying any restraint. Close monitoring of the patient is essential to ensure safety and prevent harm.

Tracheostomy

A **tracheotomy** is a surgical procedure in which an opening is made into the trachea. The indwelling tube inserted

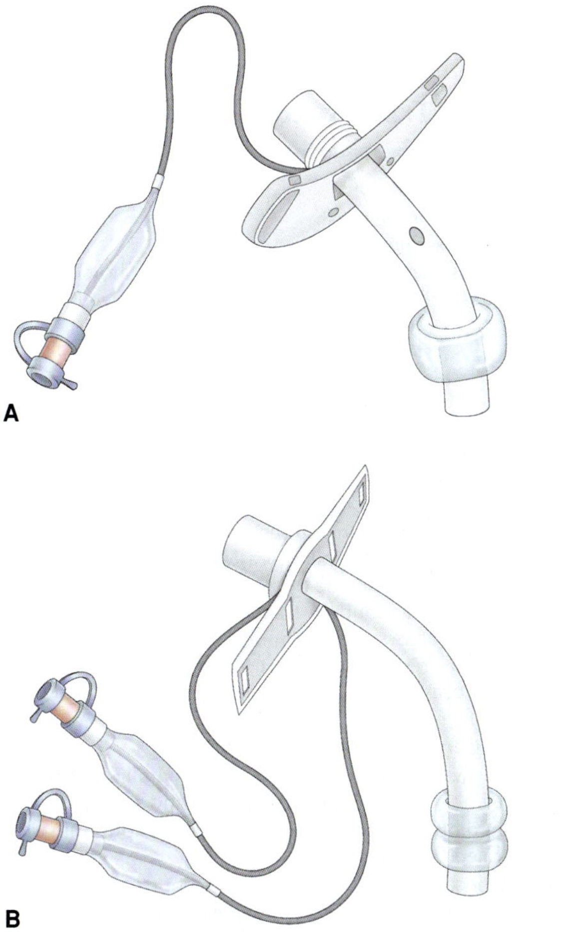

FIGURE 26-7. Tracheostomy tubes. A. Fenestrated tube, which allows patient to talk. B. Double-cuffed tube. Inflating the two cuffs alternately can help prevent tracheal damage.

into the trachea is called a tracheostomy tube (Fig. 26-7). A tracheostomy may be either temporary or permanent.

A tracheotomy is used to bypass an upper airway obstruction, to allow removal of tracheobronchial secretions, to permit the long-term use of mechanical ventilation, to prevent aspiration of oral or gastric secretions in the unconscious or paralyzed patient (by closing off the trachea from the esophagus), and to replace an endotracheal tube. Many disease processes and emergency conditions make a tracheotomy necessary.

Procedure

The surgical procedure is usually performed in the operating room or in an intensive care unit, where the patient's ventilation can be well controlled and optimal aseptic technique can be maintained. A surgical opening is made between the second and third tracheal rings. After the trachea is exposed, a cuffed tracheostomy tube of an appropriate size is inserted. The cuff is an inflatable attachment to the tracheostomy tube that is designed to occlude the space between the tracheal walls and the tube, to permit effective mechanical ventilation, and to minimize the risk of aspiration. See Figure 26-7 for the different types of tracheostomy tubes.

The tracheostomy tube is held in place by tapes fastened around the patient's neck. Usually a square of sterile gauze is placed between the tube and the skin to absorb drainage and reduce the risk for infection.

CHART 26-8

Preventing Complications Associated With Endotracheal and Tracheostomy Tubes

- Administer adequate warmed humidity.
- Maintain cuff pressure at appropriate level.
- Suction as needed per assessment findings.
- Maintain skin integrity. Change tape and dressing as needed or per protocol.
- Auscultate lung sounds.
- Monitor for signs and symptoms of infection, including temperature and white blood cell count.
- Administer prescribed oxygen and monitor oxygen saturation.
- Monitor for cyanosis.
- Maintain adequate hydration of the patient.
- Use sterile technique when suctioning and performing tracheostomy care.

Complications

Complications may occur early or late in the course of tracheostomy tube management. They may even occur years after the tube has been removed. Early complications include bleeding, **pneumothorax**, air embolism, aspiration, subcutaneous or mediastinal emphysema, recurrent laryngeal nerve damage, and posterior tracheal wall penetration. Long-term complications include airway obstruction from accumulation of secretions or protrusion of the cuff over the opening of the tube, infection, rupture of the innominate artery, dysphagia, tracheoesophageal fistula, tracheal dilation, tracheal ischemia, and necrosis. Tracheal stenosis may develop after the tube is removed. Chart 26-8 outlines measures nurses can take to prevent complications.

Nursing Management

The patient requires continuous monitoring and assessment. The newly made opening must be kept patent by proper suctioning of secretions. After the vital signs are stable, the patient is placed in a semi-Fowler's position to facilitate ventilation, promote drainage, minimize edema, and prevent strain on the suture lines. Analgesia and sedative agents must be administered with caution because of the risk of suppressing the cough reflex.

Major objectives of nursing care are to alleviate the patient's apprehension and to provide an effective means of communication. The nurse keeps paper and pencil or a whiteboard and the call light within the patient's reach at all times to ensure a means of communication. Chart 26-9 summarizes the care of the patient with a tracheostomy tube.

Suctioning the Tracheal Tube (Tracheostomy or Endotracheal Tube)

When a tracheostomy or endotracheal tube is in place, it is usually necessary to suction the patient's secretions

CHART 26-9

GUIDELINES for Care of the Patient With a Tracheostomy Tube

Equipment

- Sterile and clean gloves
- Hydrogen peroxide (used only if infection is present)
- Normal saline solution or sterile water
- Basin
- Cotton-tipped applicators
- Pipe cleaners or tube brush
- Split gauze dressing
- Tracheostomy ties (e.g., twill tape, Velcro tube holder)
- Type of tube prescribed, if the tube is to be changed

Implementation

ACTIONS	RATIONALE
1. Provide patient and family instruction on the key points for tracheostomy care, beginning with how to inspect the tracheostomy dressing for moisture or drainage. A cuffed tube (air injected into cuff) is required during mechanical ventilation. A low-pressure cuff is most commonly used. Patients requiring long-term use of a tracheostomy tube and who can breathe spontaneously commonly use an uncuffed, metal tube.	1. The tracheostomy dressing is changed as needed to keep the skin clean and dry. To prevent potential breakdown, moist or soiled dressings should not remain on the skin. A cuffed tube prevents air from leaking during positive-pressure ventilation and also prevents tracheal aspiration of gastric contents. An adequate seal is indicated by the disappearance of any air leakage from the mouth or tracheostomy or by the disappearance of the harsh, gurgling sound of air coming from the throat. Low-pressure cuffs exert minimal pressure on the tracheal mucosa and thus reduce the danger of tracheal ulceration and stricture.
2. Perform hand hygiene.	2. Hand hygiene reduces bacteria on hands.
3. Explain procedure to patient and family as appropriate.	3. A patient with a tracheostomy and their family may be apprehensive and require ongoing assurance and support.
4. Put on clean gloves; remove and discard the soiled dressing in a biohazard container.	4. Use of a biohazard container reduces cross-contamination from soiled dressings.
5. Prepare sterile supplies, including normal saline solution or sterile water, cotton-tipped applicators, pipe cleaners or tube brush, dressing, and twill ties or velcro tube holder.	5. Having necessary supplies and equipment readily available allows the procedure to be completed efficiently.
6. Put on sterile gloves. (Some primary providers approve clean technique for long-term tracheostomy patients in the home.)	6. Sterile equipment minimizes transmission of surface flora to the sterile respiratory tract. Clean technique may be used in the home because of decreased exposure to potential pathogens.
7. Cleanse the wound and the plate of the tracheostomy tube with sterile cotton-tipped applicators moistened with sterile saline solution or sterile water. Hydrogen peroxide is used if infection is present.	7. Cleansing the wound and plate will decrease the likelihood of pathogen transmission into the tube during the procedure.
8. Unlock and remove the inner cannula.	8. The inner cannula is locked and must be removed in order to be cleansed.
9. If nondisposable inner cannula: soak the inner cannula in sterile saline or sterile water, per manufacturer's instructions; clean the inner and outer cannula with a pipe cleaners or tube brush; rinse with sterile solution; and inspect to be sure all dried secretions have been removed. Dry and reinsert inner cannula.	9. Soaking loosens and removes secretions from the inner lumen of the tracheostomy tube. Retained secretions could harbour bacteria, leading to infection.
10. If disposable inner cannula: remove the inner cannula, discard, and replace with a new disposable inner cannula.	10. Inserting a new, clean inner cannula will decrease the likelihood of infection.
11. Place clean tracheostomy twill ties in position to secure the tracheostomy tube by inserting one end of the tie through the side opening of the outer cannula. Take the ties around the back of the patient's neck and thread them through the opposite opening of the outer cannula. Bring both ends around so that they meet on one side of the neck. Tighten the ties until only one finger can be comfortably inserted under them. Secure with a knot. A velcro tracheostomy tube holder may be used in place of twill ties. For a new tracheostomy, two people should assist with tie or holder changes. Remove soiled ties or holder after the new ties or holder is in place.	11. This anchoring technique is needed because the tracheostomy tube can be dislodged by movement or by a forceful cough if left unsecured. A dislodged tracheostomy tube is difficult to reinsert, and respiratory distress may occur. Dislodgement of the tube with a new tracheostomy is a medical emergency. Tracheostomy ties should not be changed for 24 hours following the tracheostomy procedure.

GUIDELINES for Care of the Patient With a Tracheostomy Tube (Continued)

ACTIONS	RATIONALE
12. Remove old tracheostomy ties and discard them in a biohazard container after the new ties are in place.	12. Tracheostomy ties with old secretions may harbor bacteria.
13. Although some long-term tracheostomies with healed stomas may not require a dressing, other tracheostomies do. In such cases, use a sterile tracheostomy dressing, fitting it securely under the tracheostomy ties and flange of tracheostomy tube so that the incision is covered, as shown below.	13. Healed tracheostomies with minimal secretions do not need a dressing. Dressings that will shred are not used around a tracheostomy because of the risk that pieces of material, lint, or thread may get into the tube, and eventually into the trachea, causing obstruction or abscess formation. Special dressings that do not have a tendency to shred are used.

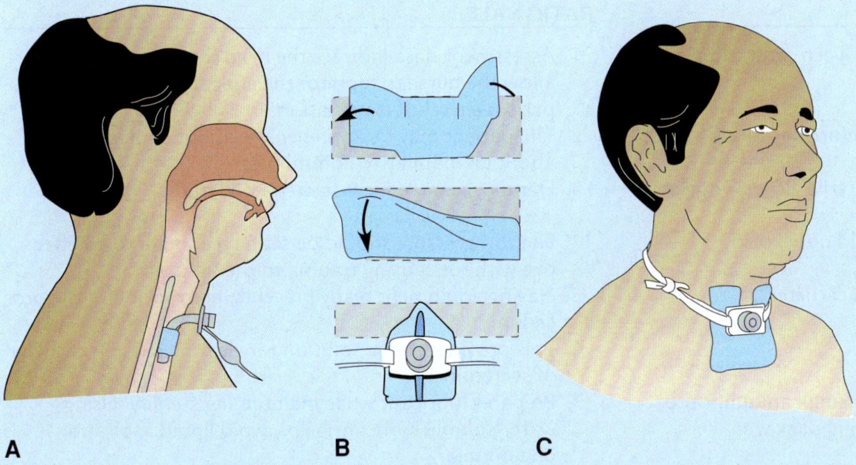

A. The cuff of the tracheostomy tube fits smoothly and snugly in the trachea in a way that promotes circulation but seals off the escape of secretions and air surrounding the tube. **B.** For a dressing change, a 4- × 4-in gauze pad may be folded (cutting would promote shredding, placing the patient at risk for aspiration) around the tracheostomy tube. **C.** The tracheostomy tube may then be stabilized by slipping the tracheostomy ties through the neck plate slots of the tracheostomy tube. The ties may be fastened to the side of the neck to eliminate the discomfort of lying on the knot.

Adapted from Kornusky, J. & Boling, B. (2016). Tracheostomy care: Providing. In D. Pravikoff (Ed.). *Nursing practice and skill*. Glendale, CA: CINAHL Information Systems.

because of the decreased effectiveness of the cough mechanism. Tracheal suctioning is performed when adventitious breath sounds are detected or whenever secretions are obviously present. Unnecessary suctioning can initiate bronchospasm and cause mechanical trauma to the tracheal mucosa.

All equipment that comes into direct contact with the patient's lower airway must be sterile to prevent sepsis. Chart 26-10 presents the procedure for suctioning a patient with a tracheostomy tube. In mechanically ventilated patients, an in-line suction catheter may be used to allow rapid suction when needed and to minimize cross-contamination by airborne pathogens. An in-line suction device allows the patient to be suctioned without being disconnected from the ventilator circuit. In-line suctioning (also called closed suctioning) decreases hypoxemia, sustains PEEP, and can decrease patient anxiety associated with suctioning. Because in-line suctioning protects staff from patient secretions, it can be performed without using personal protective gear.

Managing the Cuff

The cuff on an endotracheal or tracheostomy tube should be inflated if the patient requires mechanical ventilation or is at high risk for aspiration. The pressure within the cuff should be the lowest possible pressure (20 to 25 mm Hg) that allows delivery of adequate tidal volumes and prevents pulmonary aspiration (Urden et al., 2014). Cuff pressure must be monitored at least every 8 hours by attaching a handheld pressure gauge to the pilot balloon of the tube or by using the minimal leak volume or minimal occlusion volume technique.

Promoting Home, Community-Based, and Transitional Care

Educating Patients About Self-Care

If the patient is preparing to be discharged home with a tracheostomy tube, the nurse should ensure that suction and other appropriate equipment is in place in the home prior to discharge. The nurse should educate the patient and family about daily care, including techniques to prevent infection, as well as measures to take in an emergency. The nurse provides the patient and family with a list of community contacts for education and support needs.

Continuing and Transitional Care

A referral for home care is indicated for ongoing assessment of the patient and of the ability of the patient and family to provide appropriate and safe care. The nurse assesses the patient's and family's ability to cope with the physical changes and psychological challenges associated

CHART 26-10

GUIDELINES for Performing Tracheal Suction

Equipment

- Suction catheters (smallest diameter that will remove secretions effectively)
- Gloves (sterile and nonsterile), gown, mask, and goggles for eye protection
- Basin
- Sterile normal saline
- Water-soluble lubricant
- Manual resuscitation bag with supplemental oxygen
- Suction source

Implementation

ACTIONS	RATIONALE
1. Assess the patient's lung sounds and oxygen saturation via pulse oximeter.	1. Assessment data indicate the need for suctioning and allow the nurse to monitor the effect of suction on the patient's level of oxygenation.
2. Explain the procedure to the patient before beginning and offer reassurance during suctioning.	2. The patient may be apprehensive about choking and about an inability to communicate.
3. Performing hand hygiene. Put on nonsterile gloves, goggles, gown, and mask.	3. Hand hygiene reduces bacteria on hands.
4. Turn on suction source (pressure should not exceed 120 mm Hg).	4. Suction pressure should be set high enough to be effective without causing trauma to the tissues.
5. Using aseptic technique. Open suction catheter kit.	5. Having equipment ready prevents interruption of the procedure.
6. Fill basin with sterile water.	6. This provides sterile solution for clearing suction catheter of secretions.
7. Open water-soluble lubricant. Squeeze small amount onto sterile catheter package without touching package.	7. Prepares lubricant while maintaining sterility. Using water-soluble lubricant helps avoid lipoid aspiration pneumonia.
8. Put sterile glove on dominant hand.	8. Equipment that will contact the patient's lower airway must remain sterile to prevent infection.
9. Ventilate the patient with manual resuscitation bag and high-flow oxygen for about 30 seconds or turn on suction mode of ventilator (if available) to hyperoxygenate the patient. Instill normal saline solution into airway only if there are thick, tenacious secretions.	9. This prevents hypoxia during suctioning.
10. Instill normal saline solution into airway if there are thick, tenacious secretions.	10. Solution facilitates their removal.
11. Pick up suction catheter in sterile gloved hand and connect to suction.	11. Prevents contamination of sterile catheter.
12. Insert suction catheter at least as far as the end of the tube without applying suction, until you meet resistance or the patient coughs, then pull back 1 cm.	12. Inserting the catheter without applying suction permits insertion without causing trauma to the tissues.
13. Apply suction while withdrawing and gently rotating the catheter 360 degrees (no longer than 10 to 15 seconds).	13. Prolonged suctioning may result in hypoxia and dysrhythmias, leading to cardiac arrest.
14. Reoxygenate and inflate the patient's lungs for several breaths with manual resuscitation bag or allow ventilator to reoxygenate patient for several breaths using suction mode.	14. Prevents hypoxia during procedure and restores oxygen supply.
15. Rinse catheter by suctioning a few millilitres of sterile saline solution from the basin between suction attempts.	15. Keeps suction catheter patent.
16. Repeat steps 9 to 14 until the airway is clear.	16. This ensures removal of all tracheal secretions.
17. Suction oropharyngeal cavity after completing tracheal suctioning.	17. Avoids contamination of trachea with oropharyngeal secretions and organisms.
18. Rinse suction tubing and discard catheter, gloves, and basin appropriately.	18. Safe disposal of equipment avoids cross-contamination.
19. Assess the patient's lung sounds and oxygen saturation via pulse oximeter after the procedure.	19. Provides information about effectiveness of procedure.
20. Document the amount, colour, and consistency of secretions.	20. Documentation allows monitoring of patient's status over time.

Adapted from Perry, A., Potter, P., & Ostendorf, W. (Eds.). (2018). *Clinical nursing skills and techniques* (9th ed.). St. Louis, MO: Elsevier.

with having a tracheostomy. The nurse also identifies resources and makes referrals for appropriate services to assist the patient and family to manage the tracheostomy tube at home.

Mechanical Ventilation

Mechanical ventilation may be required for a variety of reasons: to control the patient's respirations during surgery, to oxygenate the blood when the patient's ventilatory efforts are inadequate, and to rest the respiratory muscles. Many patients placed on a ventilator can breathe spontaneously, but the effort needed to do so may be exhausting.

A **mechanical ventilator** is a positive- or negative-pressure breathing device that can maintain ventilation and oxygen delivery for a prolonged period. Caring for a patient on mechanical ventilation has become an integral part of nursing care in critical care or general medical-surgical units, extended care facilities, and the home. Nurses, physicians, and respiratory therapists must understand each patient's specific pulmonary needs and work together to set realistic goals. Positive patient outcomes depend on an understanding of the principles of mechanical ventilation and the patient's care needs as well as open communication among members of the health care team about the goals of therapy, weaning plans, and the patient's tolerance of changes in ventilator settings.

Indications

If a patient is unable to maintain the airway or has evidence of respiratory failure, endotracheal intubation and mechanical ventilation are indicated. Evidence of these indications may be seen with a continuous decrease in oxygenation (PaO_2), an increase in arterial carbon dioxide levels ($PaCO_2$), and/or a persistent acidosis (decreased pH). If the patient's clinical status shows rapid deterioration, then waiting for these lab results prior to ensuring adequate oxygenation and ventilation is imprudent (Amitai & Sinert, 2015). Conditions such as thoracic or abdominal surgery, drug overdose, neuromuscular disorders, inhalation injury, COPD, multiple trauma, shock, multisystem failure, and coma all may lead to respiratory failure and the need for mechanical ventilation. The criteria for mechanical ventilation guide the decision to place a patient on a ventilator (Chart 26-11).

CHART 26-11

Indications for Mechanical Ventilation

Laboratory Values

PaO_2 <55 mm Hg
$PaCO_2$ >50 mm Hg and pH <7.32
Vital capacity <10 mL/kg
Negative inspiratory force <25 cm H_2O
FEV_1 <10 mL/kg

Clinical Manifestations

Apnea or bradypnea
Respiratory distress with confusion
Increased work of breathing not relieved by other interventions
Confusion with need for airway protection
Circulatory shock
Controlled hyperventilation (e.g., patient with a severe head injury)

Adapted from Amitai, A., & Sinert, R. H. (2015). Introduction to ventilator management. *Medscape*. Retrieved May 7, 2016, from emedicine.medscape.com/article/810126-overview#a3

Classification of Ventilators

Mechanical ventilators were traditionally classified according to the method by which they supported ventilation. The two general categories are negative-pressure and positive-pressure ventilators. Negative-pressure ventilators (e.g., "iron lungs," chest cuirass) are older modes of ventilatory support that are rarely utilized today.

Positive-Pressure Ventilators

Positive-pressure ventilators inflate the lungs by exerting positive pressure on the airway, pushing air in, similar to a bellows mechanism, forcing the alveoli to expand during inspiration. Expiration occurs passively. Endotracheal intubation or tracheostomy is usually necessary. These ventilators are widely used in the hospital setting and are increasingly used in the home for patients with primary lung disease. Three types of positive-pressure ventilators are classified by the method of ending the inspiratory phase of respiration: volume-cycled, pressure-cycled, and high-frequency oscillatory support. The fourth type, noninvasive positive-pressure ventilation, does not require intubation (Cairo, 2014).

Volume-Cycled Ventilators

Volume-cycled ventilators deliver a pre-set volume of air with each inspiration. Once this pre-set volume is delivered to the patient, the ventilator cycles off and exhalation occurs passively. From breath to breath, the volume of air delivered by the ventilator is relatively constant, ensuring consistent, adequate breaths despite varying airway pressures. A major disadvantage to using volume-cycled ventilators is that patients may experience barotrauma because the pressures required to deliver the breaths may be excessive. This trauma causes damage to the alveolar capillary membrane and air to leak into the surrounding tissues.

Pressure-Cycled Ventilators

When the pressure-cycled ventilator cycles on, it delivers a flow of air (inspiration) until it reaches a pre-set pressure, and then cycles off, and expiration occurs passively. Its major limitation is that the volume of air or oxygen can vary as the patient's airway resistance or compliance changes. As a result, the tidal volume delivered may be inconsistent, possibly compromising ventilation.

High-Frequency Oscillatory Support Ventilators

These types of ventilators deliver very high respiratory rates (i.e., 180 to 900 breaths/min) that are accompanied by very low tidal volumes and high airway pressures (hence the name *high-frequency oscillatory support*) (see Fig. 26-5). These small pulses of oxygen-enriched air move down the centre of the airways, allowing alveolar air to exit the lungs along the margins of the airways. This ventilatory mode is used to open the alveoli in situations characterized by closed small airways, such as atelectasis and ARDS (see Chapter 24), and it is also thought to protect the lung from pressure injury (Cairo, 2014).

Noninvasive Positive-Pressure Ventilation

Noninvasive positive-pressure ventilation (NIPPV) is a method of positive-pressure ventilation that can be given via face masks that cover the nose and mouth, nasal masks, or other oral or nasal devices such as the nasal pillow (a small nasal cannula that seals around the nares to maintain the prescribed pressure). It eliminates the need for endotracheal intubation or tracheostomy and decreases the risk of nosocomial infections such as pneumonia. The most comfortable mode for the patient is pressure-controlled ventilation with pressure support. This eases the work of breathing and enhances gas exchange. The ventilator can be set with a minimum backup rate for patients with periods of apnea.

Patients are candidates for NIPPV if they have acute or chronic respiratory failure, acute pulmonary edema, COPD, chronic heart failure, or a sleep-related breathing disorder. The technique may also be used at home to improve tissue oxygenation and to rest the respiratory muscles while patients sleep at night. NIPPV is contraindicated for those who have experienced respiratory arrest, serious dysrhythmias, cognitive impairment, or head or facial trauma. NIPPV may also be used for obstructive sleep apnea, for patients at the end of life, and for those who do not want endotracheal intubation but may need short- or long-term ventilatory support (Amitai & Sinert, 2015).

CPAP provides positive pressure to the airways throughout the respiratory cycle. Although it can be used as an adjunct to mechanical ventilation with a cuffed endotracheal tube or tracheostomy tube to open the alveoli, it is also used with a leak-proof mask to keep alveoli open, thereby preventing respiratory failure. CPAP is an effective treatment for obstructive sleep apnea because the positive pressure acts as a splint, keeping the upper airway and trachea open during sleep. To use CPAP, the patient must be breathing independently.

Bilevel positive airway pressure (BiPAP) ventilation offers independent control of inspiratory and expiratory pressures while providing **pressure support ventilation (PSV)**. It delivers two levels of positive airway pressure provided via a nasal or oral mask, nasal pillow, or mouthpiece with a tight seal and a portable ventilator. Each inspiration can be initiated either by the patient or by the machine if it is programmed with a backup rate. The backup rate ensures that the patient receives a set number of breaths per minute. BiPAP is most often used for patients who require ventilatory assistance at night, such as those with severe COPD or sleep apnea. Tolerance is variable and is usually most successful with highly motivated patients.

Ventilator Modes

Ventilator mode refers to how breaths are delivered to the patient. The most commonly used modes are controlled mechanical ventilation, **assist–control ventilation (A/C)**, **intermittent mandatory (pressure or volume) ventilation (IMV)**, **synchronized intermittent mandatory ventilation (SIMV)**, PSV, and **airway pressure release ventilation (APRV)** (Fig. 26-8).

Controlled mechanical ventilation provides full ventilator support by delivering a pre-set tidal volume and respiratory rate. This mode of ventilation is indicated for patients who are apneic.

A/C ventilation provides full ventilatory support by delivering a pre-set tidal volume and respiratory rate. If the patient initiates a breath between the machine's breaths, the ventilator delivers at the pre-set volume (assisted breath). Therefore, every breath is the pre-set volume.

IMV provides a combination of mechanically assisted breaths and spontaneous breaths. Mechanical breaths are delivered at pre-set intervals and a preselected tidal volume, regardless of the patient's efforts. Although the patient can increase the respiratory rate by initiating inspiration between ventilator-delivered breaths, these spontaneous breaths are limited to the tidal volume generated by the patient. IMV allows patients to use their own muscles for ventilation to help prevent muscle atrophy. It lowers mean airway pressure, which can assist in preventing barotrauma. However, bucking the ventilator (trying to exhale when the ventilator is delivering a breath) may be increased.

SIMV also delivers a pre-set tidal volume and number of breaths per minute. Between ventilator-delivered breaths, the patient can breathe spontaneously with no assistance from the ventilator on those extra breaths. Because the ventilator senses patient breathing efforts and does not initiate a breath in opposition to the patient's efforts, bucking the ventilator is reduced. As the patient's ability to breathe spontaneously increases, the pre-set number of ventilator breaths is decreased, and the patient does more of the work of breathing. Like IMV, SIMV can be used to provide full or partial ventilatory support. Nursing interventions for patients receiving IMV or SIMV include monitoring progress by recording respiratory rate, minute volume, spontaneous and machine-generated tidal volume, FiO_2, and arterial blood gas levels.

PSV applies a pressure plateau to the airway throughout the patient-triggered inspiration to decrease resistance within the tracheal tube and ventilator tubing. Pressure support is reduced gradually as the patient's strength increases. An SIMV backup rate may be added for extra support. The nurse must closely observe the patient's respiratory rate and tidal volumes on initiation of PSV. It may be necessary to adjust the pressure support to avoid tachypnea or large tidal volumes.

APRV is a time-triggered, pressure-limited, time-cycled mode of mechanical ventilation that allows unrestricted, spontaneous breathing throughout the ventilatory cycle. The inflation period is long, and breaths may be initiated spontaneously as well as by the ventilator. APRV allows alveolar gas to be expelled through the lungs' natural recoil. Further research is needed on the effectiveness of this mode of mechanical ventilation, but it has been suggested that APRV has the important advantages of causing less ventilator-induced lung injury and fewer adverse effects on cardiocirculatory function and being associated with lower need for sedation and neuromuscular blockade (Cairo, 2014).

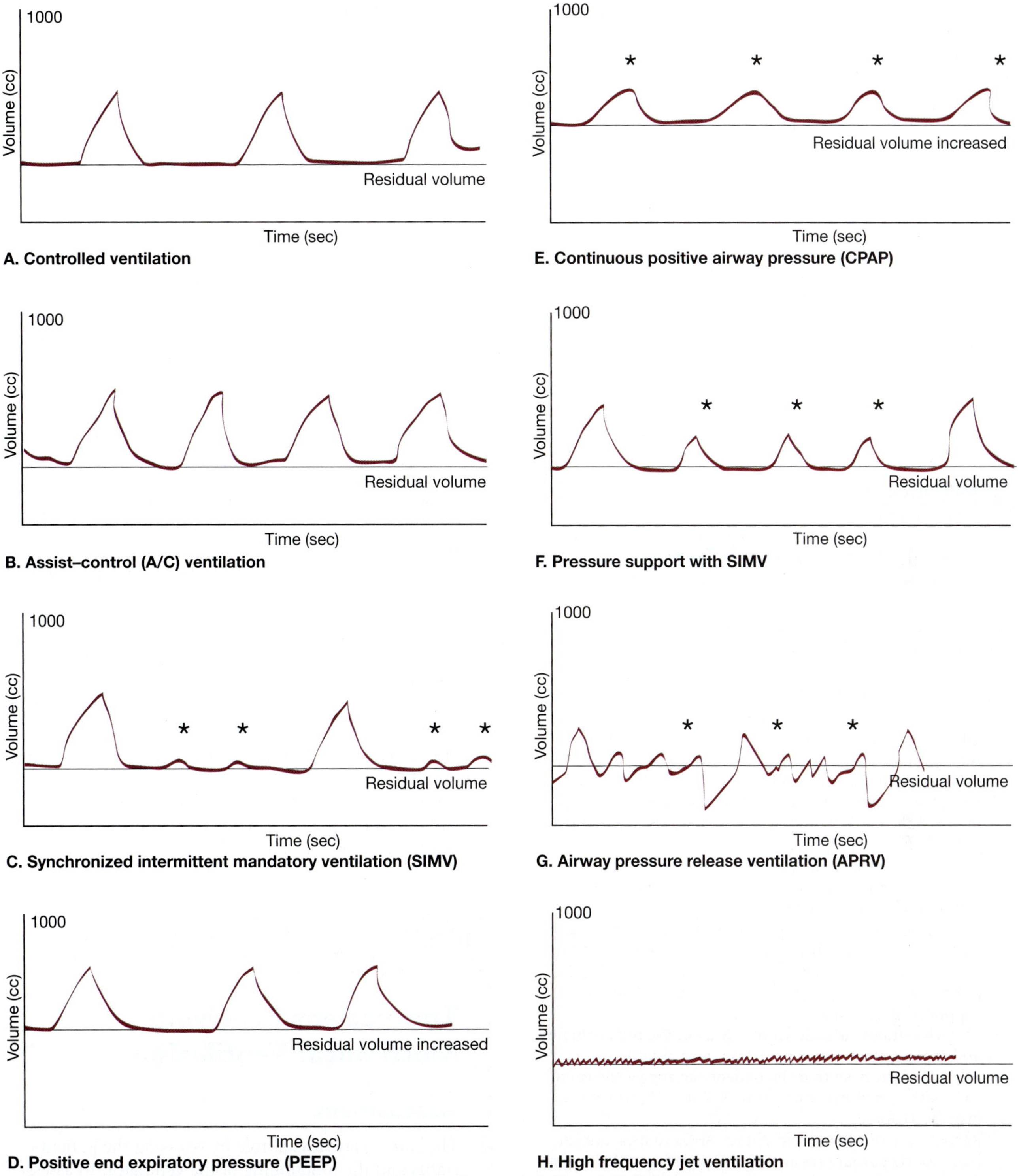

FIGURE 26-8. Modes of mechanical ventilation with airflow waveforms. Inhalations marked with an asterisk (*) are spontaneous.

A relatively new mode of support, **proportional assist ventilation (PAV)**, provides partial ventilatory support in which the ventilator generates pressure in proportion to the patient's inspiratory efforts. With every breath, the ventilator synchronizes with the patient's ventilatory efforts. The more inspiratory pressure the patient generates, the more pressure the ventilator generates, amplifying the patient's inspiratory effort without any specific preselected target pressure or volume. It generally adds "additional muscle" to the patient's effort; the depth and frequency of breaths are controlled by the patient (Cairo, 2014).

New modes of mechanical ventilation that incorporate computerized control of ventilation are being developed. In some of these modes, the ventilator constantly monitors many variables and adjusts gas delivery during individual breaths; these within-breath adjustment systems include automatic tube compensation, volume-ensured pressure support, and proportional support ventilation. In other modes, the ventilator evaluates gas delivery during one breath and uses that information to adjust the next breath; these between-breath adjustment systems can be made to ensure a pre-set tidal volume by adjusting pressure, up to a pre-set maximum, and include pressure volume support, pressure-regulated volume control, and adaptive support ventilation.

Adjusting the Ventilator

The ventilator is adjusted so that the patient is comfortable and breathes synchronously with the machine. Minimal alteration of normal cardiovascular and pulmonary dynamics is desired. If the volume ventilator is adjusted appropriately, the patient's arterial blood gas values will be satisfactory and there will be little or no cardiovascular compromise. Chart 26-12 describes initial ventilator settings.

CHART 26-12

Initial Ventilator Settings

The following guide is an example of the steps involved in operating a mechanical ventilator. The nurse, in collaboration with the respiratory therapist, always reviews the manufacturer's instructions, which vary according to the equipment, before beginning mechanical ventilation.

1. Set the machine to deliver the tidal volume required (6 to 10 mL/kg) or (4 to 8 mL/kg for patients with ARDS).
2. Adjust the machine to deliver the lowest concentration of oxygen to maintain normal PaO_2 (greater than 60 mm Hg) or an SpO_2 level greater than 92%. This setting may be high initially but will gradually be reduced based on arterial blood gas (ABG) results.
3. Record peak inspiratory pressure.
4. Set mode (**continuous mandatory (volume or pressure) ventilation** [**CMV**, also known as assist-control], or synchronized intermittent mandatory ventilation) and rate as prescribed by the primary provider. (See the glossary for definitions of modes of mechanical ventilation.) Set positive end-expiratory pressure (PEEP) and pressure support if prescribed.
5. Set sigh settings (usually set at 1.5 times the tidal volume and ranging from 1 to 3 per hour), if applicable.
6. Adjust sensitivity so that the patient can trigger the ventilator with a minimal effort (usually 2 mm Hg negative inspiratory force).
7. Record minute volume and obtain ABGs to measure carbon dioxide partial pressure ($PaCO_2$), pH, and PaO_2 after 20 minutes of continuous mechanical ventilation.
8. Adjust setting (FiO_2 and rate) according to results of ABG analysis to provide normal values or those set by the primary provider.
9. If there is poor coordination between the breathing rhythms of the patient and the ventilator (i.e., if the patient is "fighting" or "bucking the ventilator"), assess for hypoxia and manually ventilate on 100% oxygen with a resuscitation bag.

Adapted from Amitai, A., & Sinert, R. H. (2015). Introduction to ventilator management. *Medscape*. Retrieved May 7, 2016, from emedicine.medscape.com/article/810126-overview#a3

Monitoring the Equipment

The ventilator needs to be monitored to make sure that it is functioning properly and that the settings are appropriate. Although the nurse may not be primarily responsible for adjusting the settings on the ventilator or measuring ventilator parameters (these are usually responsibilities of the respiratory therapist), the nurse is responsible for the patient and therefore needs to evaluate how the ventilator affects the patient's overall status.

When monitoring the ventilator, the nurse notes the following:

- Controlling mode (e.g., controlled ventilation, A/C ventilation, SIMV)
- Tidal volume and rate settings (tidal volume is usually set at 6 to 12 mL/kg [ideal body weight]; rate is usually set at 12 to 16 breaths/min)
- FiO_2 setting may be set between 21% and 100% to maintain an optimal PaO_2 level or SpO_2 level
- Inspiratory pressure reached and pressure limit (normal is 15 to 20 cm H_2O; this increases if there is increased airway resistance or decreased compliance)
- Sensitivity (a 2-cm H_2O inspiratory force should trigger the ventilator)
- Inspiratory-to-expiratory ratio (usually 1:3 [1 second of inspiration to 3 seconds of expiration] or 1:2)
- Minute volume (tidal volume × respiratory rate, usually 6 to 8 L/min)
- Sigh settings (usually set at 1.5 times the tidal volume and ranging from 1 to 3 per hour), if applicable
- Water in the tubing, disconnection or kinking of the tubing
- Humidification (humidifier filled with water) and temperature
- Alarms (turned on and functioning properly)
- PEEP and pressure support level, if applicable (PEEP is usually set at 5 to 15 cm H_2O)

Nursing Process

The Patient Receiving Mechanical Ventilation

Assessment

The nurse plays a vital role in assessing the patient's status and the functioning of the ventilator. In assessing the patient, the nurse evaluates the patient's physiologic status and how he or she is coping with mechanical ventilation. Physical assessment includes systematic assessment of all body systems, with an in-depth focus on the respiratory system. Respiratory assessment includes vital signs, respiratory rate and pattern, breath sounds, evaluation of spontaneous ventilatory effort, and potential evidence of hypoxia (e.g., skin colour). Increased adventitious breath sounds may indicate a need for suctioning. The nurse maintains the patient's head of bed so that it is elevated 30 degrees higher unless contraindicated to prevent the risk of aspiration and ventilator-associated pneumonia. The nurse also evaluates the settings and functioning of the mechanical ventilator, as described previously.

Assessment also addresses the patient's neurologic status and effectiveness of coping with the need for assisted ventilation and the changes that accompany it (Hyzy, 2017). The nurse assesses the patient's comfort level and ability to communicate as well.

Nursing Priorities

Based on the assessment data, the patient's major nursing priorities may include:

- Impaired gas exchange
- Ineffective airway clearance
- Increased mucus production
- Trauma and infection from endotracheal intubation or tracheostomy
- Altered physical mobility
- Ventilator dependency
- Lack of verbal communication
- Powerlessness

Collaborative Problems/ Potential Complications

Based on the assessment data, potential complications may include the following (see Table 26-2):

- Ventilator problems (increase in peak airway pressure or decrease in pressure or loss of volume)
- Alterations in cardiac function
- Barotrauma (trauma to the trachea or alveoli secondary to positive pressure) and pneumothorax
- Pulmonary infection (see Chart 26-13)
- Sepsis
- Delirium

Planning and Goals

The major goals for the patient may include achievement of optimal gas exchange, maintenance of a patent airway, absence of trauma or infection, attainment of optimal mobility, adjustment to nonverbal methods of communication, acquisition of successful coping measures, and absence of complications.

Nursing Interventions

Nursing care of the mechanically ventilated patient requires expert technical and interpersonal skills. Nursing interventions are similar regardless of the setting; however, the frequency of interventions and the stability of the patient vary from setting to setting. Nursing interventions for the mechanically ventilated patient are not uniquely different from those for patients with other pulmonary disorders; but astute nursing assessment and a therapeutic nurse–patient relationship are critical. The specific interventions used by the nurse are determined by the underlying disease process and the patient's response.

TABLE 26-2 Troubleshooting Problems With Mechanical Ventilation

Problem	Cause	Solution
Ventilator Problems		
Increase in peak airway pressure	Coughing or plugged airway tube Patient "bucking" ventilator Decreasing lung compliance	Suction airway for secretions, empty condensation fluid from circuit Adjust sensitivity Manually ventilate patient Assess for hypoxia or bronchospasm Check arterial blood gas values Sedate only if necessary
	Tubing kinked Pneumothorax Atelectasis or bronchospasm	Check tubing; reposition patient; insert oral airway if necessary Manually ventilate patient; notify physician Clear secretions
Decrease in pressure or loss of volume	Increase in compliance Leak in ventilator or tubing; cuff on tube/humidifier not tight	None Check entire ventilator circuit for patency Correct leak
Patient Problems		
Cardiovascular compromise	Decrease in venous return due to application of positive pressure to lungs	Assess for adequate volume status by measuring heart rate, blood pressure, central venous pressure, pulmonary capillary wedge pressure, and urine output; notify physician if values are abnormal
Barotrauma/pneumothorax	Application of positive pressure to lungs; high mean airway pressures lead to alveolar rupture	Notify physician Prepare patient for chest tube insertion Avoid high pressure settings for patients with COPD, ARDS, or history of pneumothorax
Pulmonary infection	Bypass of normal defense mechanisms; frequent breaks in ventilator circuit; decreased mobility; impaired cough reflex	Use meticulous aseptic technique Provide frequent mouth care Optimize nutritional status

ARDS, acute respiratory distress syndrome; COPD, chronic obstructive pulmonary disease.

CHART 26-13

Collaborative Practice Interventions to Prevent Ventilator-Associated Pneumonia

Current best practices can include the implementation of specific evidence-based bundle interventions that, when used together (i.e., as a "bundle"), improve patient outcomes. This chart outlines specific parameters for the ventilator-bundled collaborative interventions that have been found to reduce ventilator-associated pneumonia (VAP).

What are the five key elements of the VAP bundle?

- Elevation of the head of the bed (30 to 45 degrees)
- Daily "sedation vacations" and assessment of readiness to extubate (see below)
- Peptic ulcer disease prophylaxis
- Deep venous thrombosis (DVT) prophylaxis (see below)
- Daily oral care with chlorhexidine (0.12% oral rinses)

What is meant by daily "sedation vacations," and how does this tie into assessing readiness to extubate?

- Protocols should be developed so that sedative doses are purposely decreased at a time of the day when it is possible to assess the patient's neurologic readiness for extubation.
- Vigilance must be employed during the time that sedative doses are lower to ensure that the patient does not self-extubate.

What effect does DVT prophylaxis have on preventing VAP?

- The exact relationship is unclear. However, when appropriate, evidence-based methods to ensure DVT prophylaxis are applied (see Chapter 31), then the rates of VAP also drop.

Adapted from Institute for Healthcare Improvement. (2012). *How-to guide: Prevent ventilator-associated pneumonia*. Cambridge, MA: Institute for Healthcare Improvements. Retrieved May 7, 2016, from www.ihi.org/resources/Pages/Tools/HowtoGuidePreventVAP.aspx

Two general nursing interventions that are important in the care of the mechanically ventilated patient are pulmonary auscultation and interpretation of arterial blood gas measurements. The nurse is often the first to note changes in physical assessment findings or significant trends in blood gases that signal the development of a serious problem (e.g., pneumothorax, tube displacement, pulmonary embolus).

Enhancing Gas Exchange

The purpose of mechanical ventilation is to optimize gas exchange by maintaining alveolar ventilation and oxygen delivery. The alteration in gas exchange may be caused by the underlying illness or by mechanical factors related to adjustment of the machine to the patient. The health care team, including the nurse, physician, and respiratory therapist, continually assesses the patient for adequate gas exchange, signs and symptoms of hypoxia, and response to treatment. Therefore, the nursing diagnosis of impaired gas exchange is, by its complex nature, multidisciplinary and collaborative. The team members must share goals and information freely. All other goals directly or indirectly relate to this primary goal.

Nursing interventions to promote optimal gas exchange include judicious administration of analgesic agents to relieve pain without suppressing the respiratory drive and frequent repositioning to diminish the pulmonary effects of immobility. The nurse also monitors for adequate fluid balance by assessing for the presence of peripheral edema, calculating daily intake and output, and monitoring daily weights. The nurse administers medications prescribed to control the primary disease and monitors for their side effects.

Promoting Effective Airway Clearance

Continuous positive-pressure ventilation increases the production of secretions regardless of the patient's underlying condition. The nurse assesses for the presence of secretions by lung auscultation at least every 2 to 4 hours. Measures to clear the airway of secretions include suctioning, CPT, frequent position changes, and increased mobility as soon as possible. Frequency of suctioning should be determined by patient assessment. If excessive secretions are identified by inspection or auscultation techniques, suctioning should be performed. Sputum is not produced continuously or every 1 to 2 hours but as a response to a pathologic condition. Therefore, there is no rationale for routine suctioning of all patients every 1 to 2 hours. Although suctioning is used to aid in the clearance of secretions, it can damage the airway mucosa and impair cilia action.

The sigh mechanism on the ventilator may be adjusted to deliver at least 1 to 3 sighs per hour at 1.5 times the tidal volume if the patient is receiving A/C ventilation. Periodic sighs prevent atelectasis and the further retention of secretions. Because of the risk for hyperventilation and trauma to pulmonary tissue from excess ventilator pressure (barotrauma, pneumothorax), the sigh feature is not used frequently. If the SIMV mode is being used, the mandatory ventilations act as sighs because they are of greater volume than the patient's spontaneous breaths.

Humidification of the airway via the ventilator is maintained to help liquefy secretions so that they are more easily removed. Bronchodilators may be administered to dilate the bronchioles and are classified as adrenergic or anticholinergic. Adrenergic bronchodilators (see Chapter 24) are mostly inhaled and work by stimulating the beta-receptor sites, mimicking the effects of epinephrine in the body. The desired effect is smooth muscle relaxation, which dilates the constricted bronchial tubes. Anticholinergic bronchodilators produce airway relaxation by blocking cholinergic-induced bronchoconstriction. Patients receiving bronchodilator therapy of either type should be monitored for adverse effects, including dizziness, nausea, decreased oxygen saturation, hypokalemia, increased heart rate, and urine retention. Mucolytic agents are administered to liquefy secretions so that they are more easily mobilized. Nursing management of patients receiving mucolytic therapy includes assessment for an adequate cough reflex, sputum characteristics, and (in patients not receiving mechanical ventilation) improvement in incentive spirometry. Side effects include nausea, vomiting, bronchospasm, stomatitis (oral ulcers), urticaria, and rhinorrhea (medicinenet.com, 2013).

Preventing Trauma and Infection

Maintaining the endotracheal or tracheostomy tube is an essential part of airway management. The nurse positions the ventilator tubing so that there is minimal pulling or distortion of the tube in the trachea, reducing the risk of trauma to the trachea. Cuff pressure is monitored every 6 to 8 hours to maintain the pressure at 20 to 25 mm Hg (Urden et al., 2014). The nurse assesses for the presence of a cuff leak at the same time.

Patients with an endotracheal or tracheostomy tube do not have the normal defenses of the upper airway. In addition, these patients frequently have multiple additional body system disturbances that lead to immunocompromise. Tracheostomy care is performed at least every 8 hours, and more frequently if needed, because of the increased risk for infection. The ventilator circuit tubing and in-line suction tubing are replaced periodically, according to infection control guidelines, to decrease the risk for infection.

The nurse administers oral hygiene frequently because the oral cavity is a primary source of contamination of the lungs in the intubated and compromised patient (Canadian Patient Safety Institute, 2016). The presence of a nasogastric tube in the intubated patient can increase the risk for aspiration, leading to nosocomial pneumonia. The nurse positions the patient with the head elevated above the stomach as much as possible.

Promoting Optimal Level of Mobility

Being connected to a ventilator limits the patient's mobility. Immobility in patients who are mechanically ventilated has been shown to result in decreased muscle strength, increased length of stay and increased mortality rates (Campbell, Fisher, Anderson, et al., 2015). The nurse helps the patient whose condition has become stable to get out of bed and move to a chair as soon as possible. Mobility and muscle activity are beneficial because they stimulate respirations and improve morale. If the patient is unable to get out of bed, the nurse encourages performance of active range-of-motion exercises every 6 to 8 hours. If the patient cannot perform these exercises, the nurse performs passive range-of-motion exercises every 8 hours to prevent contractures and venous stasis.

Promoting Optimal Communication

It is important to develop alternative methods of communication for the patient who is receiving mechanical ventilation. The nurse assesses the patient's communication abilities to evaluate for limitations. Questions to consider when assessing the ventilator-dependent patient's ability to communicate include the following:

- Is the patient conscious and able to communicate? Can the patient nod or shake his or her head?
- Is the patient's mouth unobstructed by the tube so that words can be mouthed?
- Is the patient's dominant hand strong and available for writing? For example, if the patient is right-handed, the intravenous (IV) line should be placed in the left arm if possible so that the right hand is free.
- Is the patient a candidate for a fenestrated tracheostomy tube or a one-way speaking valve that permit talking?

Once the patient's limitations are known, the nurse offers several appropriate communication approaches: lip or speech reading (use single key words), pad and pencil or whiteboard, communication board, gesturing, sign language, or electric larynx. The use of a "talking" or fenestrated tracheostomy tube or one-way valve may allow the patient to talk while on the ventilator. The nurse makes sure that the patient's eyeglasses, hearing aid, sign interpreter, and language translator are available if needed to enhance the patient's ability to communicate.

Some communication methods may be frustrating to the patient, family, and nurse; these need to be identified and minimized. A speech therapist can assist in determining the most appropriate method.

Promoting Coping Ability

Dependence on a ventilator is frightening to both the patient and the family and disrupts even the most stable families. Encouraging the family to verbalize their feelings about the ventilator, the patient's condition, and the environment in general is beneficial. Explaining procedures every time they are performed helps reduce anxiety and familiarizes the patient with ventilator procedures. To restore a sense of control, the nurse encourages the patient to participate in decisions about care, schedules, and treatment when possible (see Nursing Research Profile Chart 26-14: The Patient Receiving Mechanical Ventilation). The patient may become withdrawn or depressed while receiving mechanical ventilation, especially if its use is prolonged. To promote effective coping, the nurse informs the patient about progress when appropriate. It is important to provide diversions such as watching television, playing music, or taking a walk (if appropriate and possible). Stress reduction techniques (e.g., a back rub, relaxation measures) relieve tension and help the patient deal with anxieties and fears about both the condition and the dependence on the ventilator.

Monitoring and Managing Potential Complications

ALTERATIONS IN CARDIAC FUNCTION. Alterations in cardiac output may occur as a result of positive-pressure ventilation. The positive intrathoracic pressure during inspiration compresses the heart and great vessels, thereby reducing venous return and

NURSING RESEARCH PROFILE

Chart 26-14. The Patient Receiving Mechanical Ventilation

Fink, R. M., Makic, M. B. F., Poteet, A. W., et al. (2015). The ventilation patient's experience. *Dimensions of Critical Care Nursing, 34*(5), 301–308.

Purpose

Patients experience a variety of emotions while mechanically ventilated in the intensive care unit. Some patients have little or no recall of events while others have total recall. Limited studies have explored family recall of events or how these recollections correlate with the patient's experience. The purpose of this study was threefold: (1) to explore patient and family memories of pain, anxiety, distress, and dyspnea following mechanical ventilation, (2) to identify if a correlation exists among nurse documented pain assessment and patient-family reports of pain, and, (3) to explore patient and family satisfaction with mechanical ventilation care.

Design

This study was conducted using a mixed methods approach. Qualitative data were collected through individual semistructured interviews with each patient and family member or significant other. Quantitative data were collected from the medical record, and included patient demographics, medications given, and nurses' assessment of pain and sedation. The convenience sample consisted of 85 patients and 77 family members (32% were spouses); the mean ventilation time was 100.2 hours. Quantitative data were analyzed using descriptive statistics and tests of difference and association. Qualitative data were analyzed through qualitative content analysis, which gave rise to categories.

Findings

Findings from quantitative data revealed most patient and family members reported memories of symptom distress. Patients' memories of pain did not correlate with the nurses' assessment of pain; however, family members' memories of patients' pain did correlate. Both patients and family members were satisfied with the care they received. Through qualitative analysis, the researchers uncovered three main categories: pain/discomfort, sedation/sleeping, and communication difficulties. A source of major distress for patients was the lack of effective communication during the period of mechanical ventilation. Trying to talk and lack of a mechanism to communicate needs affected their pain management and sleeping schedule. Patients remembered being in pain.

Nursing Implications

These findings provide insight for nurses caring for patients who require mechanical ventilation and their families. These findings stress the importance of incorporating the input of family members in the plan of care. Moreover, nurses should strive to optimize communication techniques with patients requiring mechanical ventilation. Patients can benefit from frequent reorientation, use of communication boards, and a calming presence. These findings suggest that nurses should treat pain first and implement effective sedation management protocols second, in order to promote optimal patient outcomes and prevent complications.

cardiac output. This is usually corrected during exhalation when the positive pressure is off. The patient may have decreased cardiac output and resultant decreased tissue perfusion and oxygenation.

To evaluate cardiac function, the nurse first observes for signs and symptoms of hypoxia (restlessness, apprehension, confusion, tachycardia, tachypnea, pallor progressing to cyanosis, diaphoresis, transient hypertension, and decreased urine output). If a pulmonary artery catheter is in place, cardiac output, cardiac index, and other hemodynamic values can be used to assess the patient's status.

BAROTRAUMA AND PNEUMOTHORAX. Excessive positive pressure can cause lung damage, or barotrauma, which may result in a spontaneous pneumothorax, which may quickly develop into a tension pneumothorax, further compromising venous return, cardiac output, and blood pressure. The nurse considers any sudden changes in oxygen saturation or the onset of respiratory distress to be a life-threatening emergency requiring immediate action.

PULMONARY INFECTION. The patient is at high risk for infection. The nurse reports fever or a change in the colour or odour of sputum to the physician for follow-up. Subglottic secretions may increase the patients' risk for the development of ventilator-acquired pneumonia. Patients expected to be intubated for longer than 72 hours may benefit from the use of an endotracheal tube with a subglottic suction port. This extra port that is connected to continuous suction (20 to 30 cm H_2O) allows for the removal of secretions above the cuff (Urden et al., 2014).

DELIRIUM. Patients who are critically ill are at risk for delirium. The Awakening and Breathing Coordination, Delirium monitoring and management, Early mobility bundle (ABCDE) proposes an interdisciplinary process using evidence-based practice to manage delirium and weakness in the critically ill patient. The goal of this bundle is to (1) improve communication among members of the health care team, (2) standardize care related to the assessment and use of sedation, (3) provide nonpharmacologic interventions in the management of delirium, and (4) provide early exercise and ambulation (see Chart 26-15) (Balas, Vasilevskis, Burke, et al., 2012).

Promoting Home, Community-Based, and Transitional Care

Increasingly, patients are being cared for in extended care facilities or at home while receiving mechanical ventilation, with a tracheostomy tube, or receiving oxygen therapy. Patients receiving home ventilator

CHART 26-15

The ABCDE Bundle

The *A*wakening and *B*reathing *C*oordination, *D*elirium monitoring and management, *E*arly mobility bundle

Overview: Typically, patients on mechanical ventilators require some form of sedation or analgesia during their hospital stay. Recent studies suggest a correlation between the use of potent sedatives and analgesia and ICU acquired delirium, over sedation, and prolonged mechanical ventilation.

Key components of each of the three categories of the ABCDE Bundle include:

- *Awakening and spontaneous breathing trials*
  Using predefined criteria:
  - The nurse determines if it is safe to stop sedation.
  - If determined safe, the nurse will determine if patient tolerated the sedation interruption.
  - If the patient tolerated the interruption, the respiratory therapist will determine if the patient is a candidate for a breathing trial.
  - If the patient is a candidate for a breathing trial, the respiratory therapist and nurse will evaluate the patient's response.
- *Monitoring and management of delirium*
  - The patient will be assessed at least every 2 to 4 hours using a sedation assessment scale (e.g., the CAM-ICU).
- *Early Mobility*
  The patient will be assessed using the following criteria for mobility:
  - The patient is able to respond to verbal stimuli.
  - The patient is receiving less than 60% FiO_2 and less than 10 cm of PEEP.
  - The patient has no circulatory or central catheters or injuries that may contraindicate mobility.

ICU, intensive care unit; PEEP, positive end-expiratory pressure.
Adapted from Balas, M. C., Vasilevskis, E. E., Burke, W. J., et al. (2012). Critical care nurse's role in implementing the "ABCDE Bundle" into practice. *Critical Care Nurse, 32*(2), 35–48.

care usually have a chronic neuromuscular condition or COPD. Providing the opportunity for ventilator-dependent patients to return home to live with their families in familiar surroundings can be a positive experience. The ultimate goal of home ventilator therapy is to enhance the patient's quality of life, not simply to support or prolong life.

EDUCATING PATIENTS ABOUT SELF-CARE. Caring for the patient with mechanical ventilator support at home can be accomplished successfully. A home care team consisting of the nurse, physician, respiratory therapist, social service or home care agency, and equipment supplier is needed. The home is evaluated to determine whether the electrical equipment needed can be operated safely. Chart 26-16 summarizes the basic assessment criteria needed for successful home care.

Once the decision to initiate mechanical ventilation at home is made, the nurse prepares the patient and family for home care. The nurse teaches the patient and family about the ventilator, suctioning, tracheostomy care, signs of pulmonary infection, cuff inflation and deflation, and assessment of vital signs. Teaching begins in the hospital and continues at home. Nursing responsibilities include evaluating the patient's and family's understanding of the information presented.

The nurse teaches the family cardiopulmonary resuscitation, including mouth-to-tracheostomy tube (instead of mouth-to-mouth) breathing. The nurse also explains how to handle a power failure, which usually involves converting the ventilator from an electrical power source to a battery power source. Conversion is automatic in most types of home ventilators and lasts approximately 1 hour. The nurse instructs the family on the use of a manual self-inflation bag should it be necessary. Chart 26-17 lists some of the patient's and family's responsibilities. Chart 26-18 provides guidelines for caring for a patient with a tracheostomy tube and performing tracheal suction.

CONTINUING AND TRANSITIONAL CARE. A home care nurse monitors and evaluates how well the patient and family are adapting to providing care in the home. The nurse assesses the adequacy of the patient's ventilation and oxygenation as well as airway patency. The nurse addresses any unique adaptation problems the patient may have and listens to the patient's and family's anxieties and frustrations, offering support and encouragement where possible. The home care nurse helps identify and contact community resources that may assist in home management of the patient with mechanical ventilation. A respiratory therapist usually is assigned to the patient and makes frequent home

CHART 26-16

Criteria for Successful Home Ventilator Care

The decision to proceed with home ventilation therapy is usually based on the following parameters.

Patient Criteria

- The patient has a chronic underlying pulmonary or neuromuscular disorder.
- The patient's clinical pulmonary status is stable.
- The patient is willing to go home on mechanical ventilation.

Home Criteria

- The home environment is conducive to care of the patient.
- The electrical facilities are adequate to operate all equipment safely.
- The home environment is controlled, without drafts in cold weather and with proper ventilation in warm weather.
- Space is available for cleaning and storing ventilator equipment.

Family Criteria

- Family members are competent, dependable, and willing to spend the time required for proper training as primary caregivers.
- Family members understand the diagnosis and prognosis.
- Family has sufficient financial and supportive resources and can obtain professional support if necessary.

CHART 26-17

HOME CARE CHECKLIST • Ventilator Care

At the completion of education, the patient and/or caregiver will be able to:

- Name the procedure that was performed, as indicated, and how the patient's present status impacts physiologic functioning, ADLs, IADLs, relationships, and spirituality.
- State the name, dose, side effects, frequency, and schedule for all medications.
- State what types of changes are needed (if any) to maintain a clean home environment and prevent infection.
- State how to contact the primary provider, the team of home care professionals overseeing care, respiratory vendor and obtain supplies.
- Complete CPR training program for caregivers.
- Identify a plan for operation of ventilator and other devices during a power outage or other emergency.
- State proper care of patient on ventilator:
  - Observe physical signs such as colour, secretions, breathing pattern, and state of consciousness.
  - Perform physical care such as suctioning, postural drainage, and ambulation.
  - Observe the tidal volume and pressure manometer regularly. Intervene when they are abnormal (i.e., suction if airway pressure increases).
  - Provide a communication method for the patient (e.g., pad and pencil, electric larynx, talking tracheostomy tube, and sign language).
  - Monitor vital signs as directed.
  - Use a predetermined signal to indicate when feeling short of breath or in distress.
- Care for and maintain equipment properly:
  - Check the ventilator settings twice each day and whenever the patient is removed from the ventilator.
  - Adjust the volume and pressure alarms if needed.
  - Fill humidifier as needed and check its level three times a day.
  - Empty water in tubing as needed.
  - Use a clean humidifier when circuitry is changed.
  - Keep exterior of ventilator clean and free of any objects.
  - Change external circuitry once a week or more often as indicated.
  - Report malfunction or strange noises immediately.
- Identify caregiver support resources (e.g., backup caregivers, respite services, and support groups).

visits to evaluate the patient and perform a maintenance check of the ventilator.

Transportation services are identified in case the patient requires transportation in an emergency.

These arrangements must be made before an emergency arises.

Evaluation

Expected patient outcomes may include the following:

1. Exhibits adequate gas exchange, as evidenced by normal breath sounds, acceptable arterial blood gas levels, and vital signs
2. Demonstrates adequate ventilation with minimal mucus accumulation
3. Is free of injury or infection, as evidenced by normal temperature, white blood cell count, and clear sputum
4. Is mobile within limits of ability
   a. Gets out of bed to chair, bears weight, or ambulates as soon as possible
   b. Performs range-of-motion exercises every 6 to 8 hours
5. Communicates effectively through written messages, gestures, or other communication strategies
6. Copes effectively
   a. Verbalizes fears and concerns about condition and equipment
   b. Participates in decision making when possible
   c. Uses stress reduction techniques when necessary
7. Absence of complications
   a. Absence of cardiac compromise, as evidenced by stable vital signs and adequate urine output
   b. Absence of pneumothorax, as evidenced by bilateral chest excursion, normal chest x-ray, and adequate oxygenation
   c. Absence of pulmonary infection, as evidenced by normal temperature, clear pulmonary secretions, and negative sputum cultures
   d. Absence of delirium, as evidenced by not "fighting" the ventilator, and being oriented to person, place, and time

CHART 26-18

GUIDELINES for Performing Tracheal Suction

Equipment (as needed)

- Suction catheters
- Gloves (sterile and nonsterile), gown, mask, and goggles for eye protection
- Basin for sterile normal saline solution for irrigation
- Manual resuscitation bag with supplemental oxygen
- Suction device and source

Implementation

NURSING ACTIONS	RATIONALE
1. Assess the patient's lung sounds and oxygen saturation via pulse oximeter.	1. Assessment data indicate the need for suctioning and allow the nurse to monitor the effect of suction on the patient's level of oxygenation.
2. Explain the procedure to the patient before beginning and offer reassurance during suctioning.	2. The patient may be apprehensive about choking and about an inability to communicate.
3. Perform hand hygiene. Put on nonsterile gloves, goggles, gown, and mask.	3. Hand hygiene reduces bacteria on hands. Nonsterile gloves, goggles, gown, and mask serve as personal protective equipment (PPE) because they protect the clinician from becoming infected with pathogens.
4. Turn on suction source (pressure should not exceed 120 mm Hg for an open system and 160 mm Hg for a closed system).	4. Suction pressure should be set high enough to be effective without causing trauma to the tissues.
5. Open suction catheter kit.	5. Having equipment ready prevents interruption of the procedure.
6. Fill basin with sterile water.	6. This provides sterile solution for clearing suction catheter of secretions.
7. Put sterile glove on dominant hand.	7. Equipment that will contact the patient's lower airway must remain sterile to prevent infection.
8. Ventilate the patient with manual resuscitation bag and high-flow oxygen for about 30 seconds or turn on suction mode of ventilator (if available) to hyperoxygenate the patient. Ventilation or preoxygenation may not be required for a long-term tracheostomy patient who is not acutely ill.	8. This prevents hypoxia during suctioning.
9. Pick up suction catheter in sterile gloved hand and connect to suction.	9. This prevents contamination of sterile catheter.
10. Insert suction catheter at least as far as the end of the tube without applying suction, just far enough to stimulate the cough reflex.	10. Inserting the catheter without applying suction permits insertion without causing trauma to the tissues.
11. Apply suction while withdrawing and gently rotating the catheter 360 degrees (no longer than 10 seconds).	11. Prolonged suctioning may result in hypoxia and dysrhythmias, leading to cardiac arrest.
12. Reoxygenate and inflate the patient's lungs for several breaths with manual resuscitation bag, or allow ventilator to reoxygenate patient for several breaths using suction mode.	12. This prevents hypoxia during procedure and restores oxygen supply.
13. Rinse catheter by suctioning a few millilitres of sterile water solution from the basin between suction attempts.	13. This keeps suction catheter patent.
14. Repeat steps 8 to 13 until the airway is clear.	14. This ensures removal of all tracheal secretions.
15. Suction oropharyngeal cavity after completing tracheal suctioning.	15. This avoids contamination of trachea with oropharyngeal secretions and organisms.
16. Rinse suction tubing and discard catheter, gloves, and basin appropriately. Dispose of PPE as directed by facility's policies.	16. Safe disposal of equipment avoids cross-contamination.
17. Assess the patient's lung sounds and oxygen saturation via pulse oximeter after procedure.	17. Assessment provides information about effectiveness of procedure.
18. Document the amount, colour, and consistency of secretions.	18. Documentation allows monitoring of patient's status over time.

Adapted from Morris, L., Whitmer, A., & McIntosh, E. (2013). Tracheostomy care and complications in the intensive care unit. *Critical Care Nurse, 33*(5), 18–31; Woten, M., & Pilgrim, J. (2016). Tracheostomy tubes: Suctioning using an open system. In D. Pravikoff (Ed.). *Nursing practice and skill.* Glendale, CA: CINAHL Information Systems.

Weaning the Patient From the Ventilator

Respiratory weaning, the process of withdrawing the patient from dependence on the ventilator, takes place in three stages: the patient is gradually removed from the ventilator, then from the tube, and finally from oxygen. Weaning from mechanical ventilation is performed at the earliest possible time consistent with patient safety. The decision must be made from a physiologic rather than a mechanical viewpoint. A thorough understanding of the patient's clinical status is required in making this decision. Weaning is started when the patient is recovering from the acute stage of medical and surgical problems and when the cause of respiratory failure is sufficiently reversed (Kacmarek et al., 2017). Chart 26-19 presents information about patient care during weaning from mechanical ventilation.

Successful weaning involves collaboration among the physician, respiratory therapist, and nurse. Each health care provider must understand the scope and function of other team members in relation to patient weaning to conserve the patient's strength, use resources efficiently, and maximize successful outcomes.

Criteria for Weaning

Careful assessment is required to determine whether the patient is ready to be removed from mechanical ventilation. If the patient is stable and showing signs of improvement or reversal of the disease or condition that caused the need for mechanical ventilation, weaning indices should be assessed (see Chart 26-19).

Stable vital signs and arterial blood gases are also important predictors of successful weaning. Once readiness has been determined, the nurse records baseline measurements of weaning indices to monitor progress.

Patient Preparation

To maximize the chances of success of weaning, the nurse must consider the patient as a whole, taking into account factors that impair the delivery of oxygen and elimination of carbon dioxide as well as those that increase oxygen demand (e.g., sepsis, seizures, thyroid imbalances) or decrease the patient's overall strength (e.g., inadequate nutrition, neuromuscular disease). Adequate psychological preparation is necessary before and during the weaning process.

Methods of Weaning

Successful weaning depends on the combination of adequate patient preparation, available equipment, and an interdisciplinary approach to solve patient problems (see Chart 26-19). All usual modes of ventilation can be used for weaning.

When A/C ventilation is used, the control rate is decreased, so that the patient strengthens the respiratory muscles by triggering progressively more breaths. The nurse assesses the patient for signs of distress: rapid or shallow breathing, use of accessory muscles, reduced level of consciousness, increase in carbon dioxide levels, decrease in oxygen saturation, and tachycardia.

SIMV is indicated if the patient satisfies all the criteria for weaning but cannot sustain adequate spontaneous ventilation for long periods. As the patient's respiratory muscles become stronger, the rate is slowly decreased by 1 to 3 breaths/min until the patient is breathing spontaneously (Urden et al., 2014).

The PAV mode of partial ventilatory support allows the ventilator to generate pressure in proportion to the patient's efforts. With every breath, the ventilator synchronizes with the patient's ventilatory efforts. Nursing assessment includes careful monitoring of the patient's respiratory rate, arterial blood gases, tidal volume, minute ventilation, and breathing pattern.

CHART 26-19

Care of the Patient Being Weaned From Mechanical Ventilation

- Assess patient for weaning criteria:
  - Vital capacity: 10 to 15 mL/kg
  - Maximum inspiratory pressure (MIP) at least −20 cm H_2O
  - Tidal volume: 7 to 9 mL/kg
  - Minute ventilation: 6 L/min
  - Rapid/shallow breathing index: below 100 breaths/min/L; PaO_2 >60 mm Hg with FiO_2 less than 40%
- Monitor activity level, assess dietary intake, and monitor results of laboratory tests of nutritional status. Re-establishing independent spontaneous ventilation can be physically exhausting. It is crucial that the patient have enough energy reserves to succeed.
- Assess the patient's and family's understanding of the weaning process and address any concerns about the process. Explain that the patient may feel short of breath initially and provide encouragement as needed. Reassure the patient that he or she will be attended closely and that if the weaning attempt is not successful, it can be tried again later.
- Implement the weaning method prescribed: A/C ventilation, IMV, SIMV, PSV, PAV, CPAP, or T-piece.
- Monitor vital signs, pulse oximetry, ECG, and respiratory pattern constantly for the first 20 to 30 minutes and every 5 minutes after that until weaning is complete. Monitoring the patient closely provides ongoing indications of success or failure.
- Maintain a patent airway; monitor arterial blood gas levels and pulmonary function tests. Suction the airway as needed.
- In collaboration with the physician, terminate the weaning process if adverse reactions occur. These include a heart rate increase of 20 beats/min, systolic blood pressure increases of 20 mm Hg, a decrease in oxygen saturation to less than 90%, respiratory rate less than 8 or greater than 20 breaths/min, ventricular dysrhythmias, fatigue, panic, cyanosis, erratic or laboured breathing, paradoxical chest movement.
- If the weaning process continues, measure tidal volume and minute ventilation every 20 to 30 minutes; compare with the patient's desired values, which have been determined in collaboration with the physician.
- Assess for psychological dependence if the physiologic parameters indicate weaning is feasible and the patient still resists. Possible causes of psychological dependence include fear of dying and depression from chronic illness. It is important to address this issue before the next weaning attempt.

Adapted from Wiegand, D. J. L. (2016). *AACN procedure manual for critical care* (7th ed.). St. Louis, MO: Elsevier Saunders.

CPAP allows the patient to breathe spontaneously while applying positive pressure throughout the respiratory cycle to keep the alveoli open and promote oxygenation. Providing CPAP during spontaneous breathing also offers the advantage of an alarm system and may reduce patient anxiety if the patient has been taught that the machine is keeping track of breathing. It also maintains lung volumes and improves the patient's oxygenation status. CPAP is often used in conjunction with PSV. Nurses should carefully assess for tachypnea, tachycardia, reduced tidal volumes, decreasing oxygen saturations, and increasing carbon dioxide levels.

When the patient can breathe spontaneously, weaning trials using a T-piece or tracheostomy mask (see Fig. 26-2) are normally conducted with the patient disconnected from the ventilator, receiving humidified oxygen only and performing all work of breathing. Because patients do not have to overcome the resistance of the ventilator, they may find this mode more comfortable, or they may become anxious as they breathe with no support from the ventilator. During T-piece trials, the nurse monitors the patient closely and provides encouragement. This method of weaning is usually used when the patient is awake and alert, is breathing without difficulty, has good gag and cough reflexes, and is hemodynamically stable. During the weaning process, the patient is maintained on the same or a higher oxygen concentration than when receiving mechanical ventilation. While the patient is using the T-piece, he or she is observed for signs and symptoms of hypoxia, increasing respiratory muscle fatigue, or systemic fatigue. These include restlessness, increased respiratory rate (greater than 35 breaths/min), use of accessory muscles, tachycardia with premature ventricular contractions, and paradoxical chest movement (asynchronous breathing, chest contraction during inspiration and expansion during expiration). Fatigue or exhaustion is initially manifested by an increased respiratory rate associated with a gradual reduction in tidal volume; later there is a slowing of the respiratory rate.

If the patient appears to be tolerating the T-piece trial, a second set of arterial blood gas measurements is drawn 20 minutes after the patient has been on spontaneous ventilation at a constant FiO_2 PSV. (Alveolar–arterial equilibration takes 15 to 20 minutes to occur.)

Signs of exhaustion and hypoxia correlated with deterioration in the blood gas measurements indicate the need for ventilatory support. The patient is placed back on the ventilator each time signs of fatigue or deterioration develop.

If clinically stable, the patient usually can be extubated within 2 or 3 hours after weaning and allowed spontaneous ventilation by means of a mask with humidified oxygen. Patients who have had prolonged ventilatory assistance usually require more gradual weaning; it may take days or even weeks. They are weaned primarily during the day and placed back on the ventilator at night to rest.

Because patients respond in different manners to weaning methods, there is no definitive way to assess which method is best. Regardless of the weaning method being used, ongoing assessment of respiratory status is essential to monitor patient progress.

Successful weaning from the ventilator is supplemented by intensive pulmonary care. The following methods are used: oxygen therapy; arterial blood gas evaluation; pulse oximetry; bronchodilator therapy; CPT; adequate nutrition, hydration, and humidification; blood pressure measurement; and incentive spirometry. Daily spontaneous breathing trials may be used to evaluate the patient's ability to breathe without ventilatory support. If the patient is receiving IV sedatives (e.g., Propofol and midazolam), current guidelines recommend that the patient's sedative dose be decreased by 25% to 50% prior to weaning, called a *sedation vacation*. In order to decrease agitation in patients who do not tolerate withdrawal of sedation, dexmedetomidine (Precedex) may be initiated for spontaneous breathing trials without causing significant respiratory depression (Gupta, Singh, Sood, et al., 2015). A patient may still have borderline pulmonary function and need vigorous supportive therapy before his or her respiratory status returns to a level that supports activities of daily living.

Removal of the Tracheostomy Tube

Removal of the tube is considered when the patient can breathe spontaneously, maintain an adequate airway by effectively coughing up secretions, swallow, and move the jaw. If frequent suctioning is needed to clear secretions, tube weaning may be unsuccessful. Secretion clearance and aspiration risks are assessed to determine whether active pharyngeal and laryngeal reflexes are intact.

Once the patient can clear secretions adequately, a trial period of mouth breathing, or nose breathing is conducted. This can be accomplished by several methods. The first method requires changing to a smaller size tube to increase the resistance to airflow or plugging the tracheostomy tube (deflating the cuff first). The smaller tube is sometimes replaced by a cuffless tracheostomy tube, which allows the tube to be plugged at lengthening intervals to monitor patient progress. A second method involves changing to a fenestrated tube (a tube with an opening or window in its bend). This permits air to flow around and through the tube to the upper airway and enables talking. A third method involves switching to a smaller tracheostomy button (stoma button). A tracheostomy button is a plastic tube approximately 1 in long that helps keep the windpipe open after the larger tracheostomy tube has been removed. Finally, when the patient demonstrates the ability to maintain a patent airway, the tube can be removed. An occlusive dressing is placed over the stoma, which heals in several days to weeks.

Weaning From Oxygen

The patient who has been successfully weaned from the ventilator, cuff, and tube and has adequate respiratory function is then weaned from oxygen. The FiO_2 is gradually reduced until the PaO_2 is in the range of 70 to 100 mm Hg while the patient is breathing room air. If the PaO_2 is less than 70 mm Hg on room air, supplemental oxygen is recommended.

Nutrition

Success in weaning the long-term ventilator-dependent patient requires early and aggressive but judicious nutritional support. The respiratory muscles (diaphragm and especially intercostals) become weak or atrophied after just a few days of mechanical ventilation and may be catabolized for energy, especially if nutrition is inadequate. Compensation for inadequate nutrition must be undertaken with care; excessive intake can increase production of carbon dioxide and the demand for oxygen and lead to prolonged ventilator dependence and difficulty in weaning (Hess, 2012). Because the metabolism of fat produces less carbon dioxide than the metabolism of carbohydrates, it was once thought that a high-fat diet, in which 50% of daily kilocalories are from fat, would be best for patients; however, evidence-based findings do not supports its efficacy (McClave, Taylor, Martindale, et al., 2016). Adequate protein intake is important in increasing respiratory muscle strength. Protein intake should be approximately 25% of total daily kilocalories, or 1.2 to 1.5 g/kg/day. Daily nutrition should be closely monitored.

Soon after the patient is admitted, a consultation with a dietitian or nutrition support team should be arranged to plan the best form of nutritional replacement. Adequate nutrition may decrease the duration of mechanical ventilation and prevent other complications, especially sepsis. Sepsis can occur if bacteria enter the bloodstream and release toxins that, in turn, cause vasodilation and hypotension, fever, tachycardia, increased respiratory rate, and coma. Aggressive treatment of sepsis is essential to reverse this threat to survival and to promote weaning from the ventilator when the patient's condition improves.

THE PATIENT UNDERGOING THORACIC SURGERY

Assessment and management are particularly important for the patient undergoing thoracic surgery. Frequently, patients undergoing such surgery also have obstructive pulmonary disease or other chronic disease. Preoperative preparation and careful postoperative management are crucial for successful patient outcomes because these patients may have a narrow range between their physical tolerance for certain activities and their limitations, which, if exceeded, can lead to distress. Various types of thoracic surgical procedures are performed to relieve disease conditions such as lung abscesses, lung cancer, cysts, benign tumours, and emphysema (Chart 26-20). An exploratory **thoracotomy** (creation of a surgical opening into the thoracic cavity) may be performed to diagnose lung or chest disease. A biopsy may be performed in this procedure with a small amount of lung tissue removed for analysis; the chest incision is then closed.

The objectives of preoperative care for the patient undergoing thoracic surgery are to ascertain the patient's functional reserve, to determine whether the patient is likely to survive and recover from the surgery, and to ensure that the patient is in optimal condition for surgery.

Preoperative Management

Assessment and Diagnostic Findings

The nurse performs chest auscultation to assess breath sounds in all regions of the lungs (see Chapter 22). It is important to note whether breath sounds are normal, indicating a free flow of air in and out of the lungs. (In the patient with emphysema, the breath sounds may be markedly decreased or even absent on auscultation.) The nurse notes crackles and wheezes and assesses for hyperresonance and decreased diaphragmatic motion. Unilateral diminished breath sounds, and rhonchi can be the result of occlusion of the bronchi by mucus plugs. The nurse assesses for retained secretions during auscultation by asking the patient to cough. It is important to note any signs of rhonchi or wheezing. The patient history and assessment should include the following questions:

- What signs and symptoms (cough, sputum expectorated [amount and colour], hemoptysis, chest pain, dyspnea) are present?
- If there is a smoking history, how long has the patient smoked? Does the patient smoke currently? How many packs a day?
- What is the patient's cardiopulmonary tolerance while resting, eating, bathing, and walking?
- What is the patient's breathing pattern? How much exertion is required to produce dyspnea?
- Does the patient need to sleep in an upright position or with more than two pillows?
- What is the patient's general physiologic status (e.g., general appearance, mental alertness, behaviour, nutritional status)?
- What other medical conditions exist (e.g., allergies, cardiac disorders, diabetes)?

Numerous tests are performed to determine the patient's preoperative status and to assess the patient's physical assets and limitations. Many patients are seen by their surgeons in the office, and many tests and examinations are performed on an outpatient basis. The decision to perform any pulmonary resection is based on the patient's cardiovascular status and pulmonary reserve. Pulmonary function studies (especially lung volume and vital capacity) are performed to determine whether the planned resection will leave sufficient functioning lung tissue. Arterial blood gas values are assessed to provide a more complete picture of the functional capacity of the lung. Exercise tolerance tests are useful to determine whether the patient who is a candidate for pneumonectomy can tolerate removal of one of the lungs.

Preoperative studies are performed to provide a baseline for comparison during the postoperative period and to detect any unsuspected abnormalities. These studies may include a bronchoscopic examination (a lighted scope is inserted into the airways to examine the bronchi), chest x-ray, magnetic resonance imaging (MRI), electrocardiogram (ECG) for arteriosclerotic heart disease, conduction defects, nutritional assessment, determination of blood urea nitrogen and serum creatinine levels (to assess renal function), determination of glucose tolerance or blood glucose level, serum electrolytes and protein levels, blood volume determinations, and complete blood cell count.

Preoperative Nursing Management

Improving Airway Clearance

The underlying lung condition often is associated with increased respiratory secretions. Before surgery, the airway is cleared of secretions to reduce the possibility of postoperative atelectasis or infection. Chart 26-21 lists the risk

CHART 26-20

Thoracic Surgeries and Procedures

Pneumonectomy

The removal of an entire lung (pneumonectomy) is performed chiefly for cancer when the lesion cannot be removed by a less extensive procedure. It may also be performed for lung abscesses, bronchiectasis, or extensive unilateral tuberculosis. The removal of the right lung is more dangerous than the removal of the left, because the right lung has a larger vascular bed and its removal imposes a greater physiologic burden.

A posterolateral or anterolateral thoracotomy incision is made, sometimes with resection of a rib. The pulmonary artery and the pulmonary veins are ligated and severed. The main bronchus is divided, and the lung removed. The bronchial stump is stapled, and usually no drains are used because the accumulation of fluid in the empty hemithorax prevents mediastinal shift.

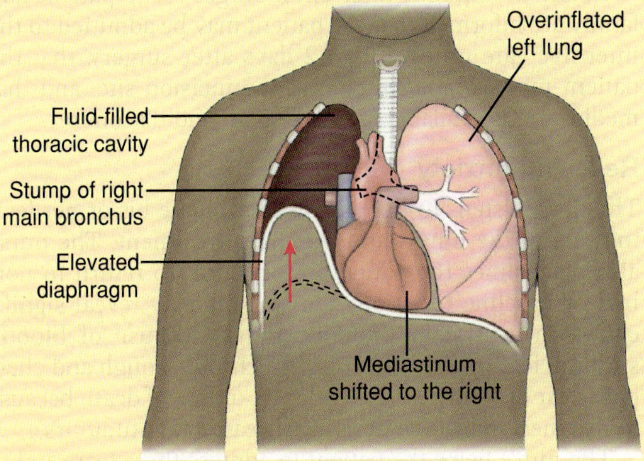

Pneumonectomy

Lobectomy

When the pathology is limited to one area of a lung, a lobectomy (removal of a lobe of a lung) is performed. Lobectomy, which is more common than pneumonectomy, may be carried out for bronchogenic carcinoma, giant emphysematous blebs or bullae, benign tumours, metastatic malignant tumours, bronchiectasis, and fungus infections.

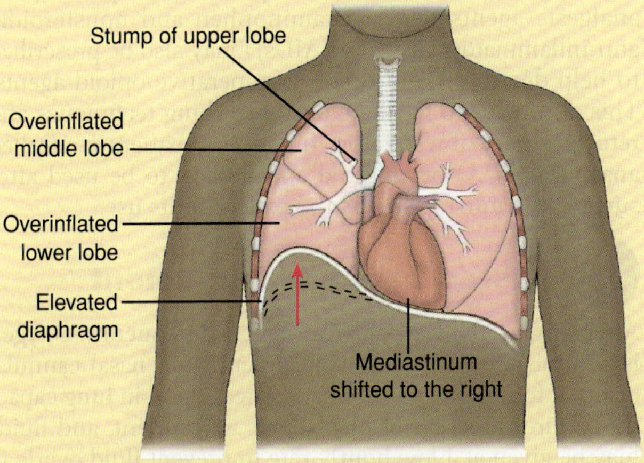

Lobectomy

The surgeon makes a thoracotomy incision: its exact location depends on the lobe to be resected. When the pleural space is entered, the involved lung collapses and the lobar vessels and the bronchus are ligated and divided. After the lobe is removed, the remaining lobes of the lung are re-expanded. Usually, two chest catheters are inserted for drainage. The upper tube is for air removal; the lower one is for fluid drainage. Sometimes, only one catheter is needed. The chest tube is connected to a chest drainage apparatus for several days.

Segmentectomy (Segmental Resection)

Some lesions are located in only one segment of the lung. Bronchopulmonary segments are subdivisions of the lung that function as individual units. They are held together by delicate connective tissue. Disease processes may be limited to a single segment. Care is used to preserve as much healthy and functional lung tissue as possible, especially in patients who already have limited cardiopulmonary reserve. Single segments can be removed from any lobe; the right middle lobe, which has only two small segments, invariably is removed entirely. On the left side, corresponding to a middle lobe, is a "lingular" segment of the upper lobe. This can be removed as a single segment or by lingulectomy. This segment frequently is involved in bronchiectasis.

Wedge Resection

A wedge resection of a small, well-circumscribed lesion may be performed without regard for the location of the intersegmental planes. The pleural cavity usually is drained because of the possibility of an air or blood leak. This procedure is performed for diagnostic lung biopsy and for the excision of small peripheral nodules.

Bronchoplastic or Sleeve Resection

Bronchoplastic resection is a procedure in which only one lobar bronchus, together with a part of the right or left bronchus, is excised. The distal bronchus is reanastomosed to the proximal bronchus or trachea.

Lung Volume Reduction

Lung volume reduction is a surgical procedure involving the removal of 20% to 30% of a patient's lung through a midsternal incision or video thoracoscopy. The diseased lung tissue is identified on a lung perfusion scan. This surgery leads to significant improvements in dyspnea, exercise capacity, quality of life, and survival of a subgroup of people with end-stage emphysema.

Video Thoracoscopy

A video thoracoscopy is an endoscopic procedure that allows the surgeon to look into the thorax without making a large incision. The procedure is performed to obtain specimens of tissue for biopsy, to treat recurrent spontaneous pneumothorax, and to diagnose either pleural effusions or pleural masses. Thoracoscopy has also been found to be an effective diagnostic and therapeutic alternative for the treatment of mediastinal disorders. Some advantages of video thoracoscopy are rapid diagnosis and treatment of some conditions, a decrease in postoperative complications, and a shortened hospital stay (see Chapter 21).

Adapted from Urden, L. D., Stacy, K. M., & Lough, M. E. (2014). *Critical care nursing: Diagnosis and management* (7th ed.). St. Louis: Elsevier Mosby.

CHART 26-21

Risk Factors: Surgery-Related Atelectasis and Pneumonia

Preoperative Risk Factors

- Increased age
- Obesity
- Poor nutritional status
- Smoking history
- Abnormal pulmonary function tests
- Pre-existing lung disease
- Emergency surgery
- History of aspiration
- Comorbid states
- Pre-existing disability

Intraoperative Risk Factors

- Thoracic incision
- Prolonged anesthesia

Postoperative Risk Factors

- Immobilization
- Supine position
- Decreased level of consciousness
- Inadequate pain management
- Prolonged intubation/mechanical ventilation
- Presence of nasogastric tube
- Inadequate preoperative education

factors for postoperative atelectasis and pneumonia. Strategies to reduce the risk for atelectasis and infection include humidification, postural drainage, and chest percussion after bronchodilators are administered, if prescribed. The nurse estimates the volume of sputum if the patient expectorates large amounts of secretions. Such measurements are carried out to determine whether and when the amount decreases. Antibiotics are administered as prescribed for infection, which can cause excessive secretions.

Educating the Patient

Increasingly, patients are admitted on the day of surgery, which does not provide much time for preoperative assessment or teaching. Nurses in all settings must take an active role in educating the patient and relieving anxiety. The nurse informs the patient what to expect, from administration of anesthesia to thoracotomy and the likely use of chest tubes and a drainage system in the postoperative period. The patient is also informed about the usual postoperative administration of oxygen to facilitate breathing and the possible use of a ventilator. It is essential to explain the importance of frequent turning to promote drainage of lung secretions. Instruction in the use of incentive spirometry begins before surgery to familiarize the patient with its correct use. The nurse teaches diaphragmatic and pursed-lip breathing, and the patient should begin practicing these techniques (see Charts 26-3).

Because a coughing schedule is necessary in the postoperative period to promote the clearance or removal of secretions, the nurse instructs the patient in the technique of coughing and warns the patient that the coughing routine may be uncomfortable. The nurse teaches the patient to splint the incision with the hands, a pillow, or a folded towel (see Chart 26-5).

Encouraging the use of forced expiratory techniques (FET) may be helpful for the patient with diminished expiratory flow rates or for the patient who refuses to cough because of severe pain. FET is the expulsion of air through an open glottis. This technique stimulates pulmonary expansion and assists in alveolar inflation (Kacmarek et al., 2017). The nurse instructs the patient as follows:

- Take a deep diaphragmatic breath and exhale forcefully against your hand in a quick, distinct pant, or huff.
- Practice doing small huffs and progress to one strong huff during exhalation.

Patients should be informed preoperatively that blood and other fluids may be administered, oxygen will be administered, and vital signs will be checked often for several hours after surgery. If a chest tube is needed, the patient should be informed that it will drain the fluid and air that normally accumulate after chest surgery. The patient and family are informed that the patient may be admitted to the intensive care unit for 1 to 2 days after surgery, that the patient may experience pain at the incision site, and that medication is available to relieve pain and discomfort.

Relieving Anxiety

The nurse listens to the patient to evaluate his or her feelings about the illness and proposed treatment. The nurse also determines the patient's motivation to return to normal or baseline function. The patient may reveal significant concerns: fear of hemorrhage because of bloody sputum, fear of discomfort from a chronic cough and chest pain, fear of ventilator dependence, or fear of death because of dyspnea and the underlying disease (e.g., tumours).

The nurse helps the patient to address these fears and to cope with the stress of surgery by correcting any misconceptions, supporting the patient's decision to undergo surgery, reassuring the patient that the incision will "hold," and dealing honestly with questions about pain and discomfort and the patient's treatment. The management and control of pain begin before surgery, when the nurse informs the patient that many postoperative problems can be overcome by following certain routines related to deep breathing, coughing, turning, and moving. Nonopioid pre-emptive analgesic agents (e.g., acetaminophen and nonsteroidal anti-inflammatory drugs [NSAIDs]) may also be prescribed to help decrease the dose of postoperative opioid agents. This also helps to facilitate deep-breathing techniques and return to normal respiratory function. If patient-controlled analgesia (PCA) or epidural analgesia is to be used after surgery, the nurse instructs the patient in its use.

Postoperative Management

After surgery, the vital signs are checked frequently. Oxygen is administered by a mechanical ventilator, nasal cannula, or mask for as long as necessary. A reduction in lung capacity requires a period of physiologic adjustment, and fluids may be given at a low hourly rate to prevent fluid overload and pulmonary edema. After the patient is conscious and the vital signs have stabilized, the head of the bed may be elevated 30 to 45 degrees. Careful positioning of the patient is important. After pneumonectomy, a patient is usually turned every hour from the back to the operative side and should not be completely turned to the unoperated side. This allows the fluid left in the space to consolidate and prevents the remaining lung and the heart from shifting (mediastinal shift) toward the operative side. The patient with a lobectomy may be turned to either side, and a patient with a segmental resection usually is not turned onto the operative side unless the surgeon prescribes this position.

Medication for pain is needed for several days after surgery; it is usually a combination of epidural analgesia, PCA, and scheduled or as-needed oral analgesics (Sole, Klein, Moseley, et al., 2013). Because coughing can be painful, the patient should be taught to splint the chest. Exercises are resumed early in the postoperative period to facilitate lung ventilation. The nurse assesses for signs of complications, including cyanosis, dyspnea, and acute chest pain. These may indicate atelectasis and should be reported immediately. Increased temperature or white blood cell count may indicate an infection, and pallor and increased pulse may indicate internal hemorrhage. Dressings are assessed for fresh bleeding.

Mechanical Ventilation

Depending on the nature of the surgery, the patient's underlying condition, the intraoperative course, and the depth of anesthesia, the patient may require mechanical ventilation after surgery. The physician is responsible for determining the ventilator settings and modes, as well as determining the overall method and pace of weaning. It is important to assess the patient's tolerance and weaning progress. Early extubation from mechanical ventilation can lead to earlier removal of arterial lines.

Chest Drainage

A crucial intervention for improving gas exchange and breathing in the postoperative period is the proper management of chest drainage and the **chest drainage system**. After thoracic surgery, chest tubes and a closed drainage system are used to re-expand the involved lung and to remove excess air, fluid, and blood. Chest drainage systems are also used in treatment of spontaneous pneumothorax and trauma resulting in pneumothorax. Table 26-3 describes and compares the main features of these systems, and Chart 26-22 explains the management of chest drainage systems. Chart 26-23 discusses actions that may prevent cardiopulmonary complications after thoracic surgery.

The normal breathing mechanism operates on the principle of negative pressure; that is, the pressure in the chest cavity normally is lower than the pressure of the atmosphere, causing air to move into the lungs during inspiration. Whenever the chest is opened, there is a loss of negative pressure, which results in collapse of the lung. The collection of air, fluid, or other substances in the chest can compromise cardiopulmonary function and can also cause the lung to collapse. Pathologic substances that collect in the pleural space include fibrin or clotted blood, liquids (serous fluids, blood, pus, chyle), and gases (air from the lung, tracheobronchial tree, or esophagus).

Chest tubes may be inserted to drain fluid or air from any of the three compartments of the thorax (the right and left pleural spaces and the mediastinum). The pleural space, located between the visceral and parietal pleura, normally contains 20 mL or less of fluid, which helps lubricate the visceral and parietal pleurae (Grossman & Porth, 2014). Air and fluid collect in the pleural space, restricting lung expansion and reducing gas exchange. Placement of a chest tube in the pleural space restores the negative intrathoracic pressure needed for lung re-expansion after surgery or trauma.

The mediastinal space is an extrapleural space that lies between the right and left thoracic cavities and contains the large blood vessels, heart, mainstem bronchus, and thymus gland. If fluid accumulates here, the heart can

TABLE 26-3 Comparison of Chest Drainage Systems[a]

Types of Chest Drainage Systems	Description	Comments
Traditional Water Seal		
Also referred to as wet suction	Has three chambers: a collection chamber, water seal chamber (middle chamber), and wet suction control chamber	Requires that sterile fluid be instilled into water seal and suction chambers Has positive- and negative-pressure release valves Intermittent bubbling indicates that the system is functioning properly Additional suction can be added by connecting system to a suction source
Dry Suction Water Seal		
Also referred to as dry suction	Has three chambers: a collection chamber, water seal chamber (middle chamber), and wet suction control chamber	Requires that sterile fluid be instilled in water seal chamber at 2-cm level No need to fill suction chamber with fluid Suction pressure is set with a regulator Has positive- and negative-pressure release valves Has an indicator to signify that the suction pressure is adequate Quieter than traditional water seal systems
Dry Suction		
Also referred to as one-way valve system	Has a one-way mechanical value that allows air to leave the chest and prevents air from moving back into the chest	No need to fill suction chamber with fluid; thus, can be set up quickly in an emergency Works even if knocked over, making it ideal for patients who are ambulatory

[a]If no fluid drainage is expected, a drainage collection device may not be needed.

CHART 26-22

GUIDELINES for Managing Chest Drainage Systems

Equipment

- Chest tube insertion tray (contains chest tube, scalpel, gloves)
- Antiseptic solution
- Local anesthetic agent
- Chest drainage system
- Adhesive tape

Implementation

ACTIONS	RATIONALE
1. Identify patient using two identifiers according to agency policy. Compare identifiers with information on patient's identification bracelet.	1. Ensures correct patient.
2. Check to ensure that the patient has provided informed consent.	2. Invasive medical procedures typically need informed consent.
3. Perform hand hygiene	3. Reduces possibility of contamination
4. If using a chest drainage system with a water seal, fill the water seal chamber with sterile water to the level specified by the manufacturer.	4. Water seal drainage allows air and fluid to escape into a drainage chamber. The water acts as a seal and keeps the air from being drawn back into the pleural space.
5. When using suction in chest drainage systems with a water seal, fill the suction control chamber with sterile water to the 20-cm level or as prescribed. In systems without a water seal, set the regulator dial at the appropriate suction level.	5. The water level regulator dial setting determines the degree of suction applied.
6. Attach the drainage catheter exiting the thoracic cavity to the tubing coming from the collection chamber. Tape securely with adhesive tape.	6. In chest drainage units, the system is closed. The only connection is the one to the patient's catheter.
7. If suction is used, connect the suction control chamber tubing to the suction unit. If using a wet suction system, turn on the suction unit and increase pressure until slow but steady bubbling appears in the suction control chamber. If using a chest drainage system with a dry suction control chamber, turn the regulator dial to 20 cm H_2O.	7. With a wet suction system, the degree of suction is determined by the amount of water in the suction control chamber and is not dependent on the rate of bubbling or the pressure gauge setting on the suction unit. With a dry suction control chamber, the regulator dial replaces the water.

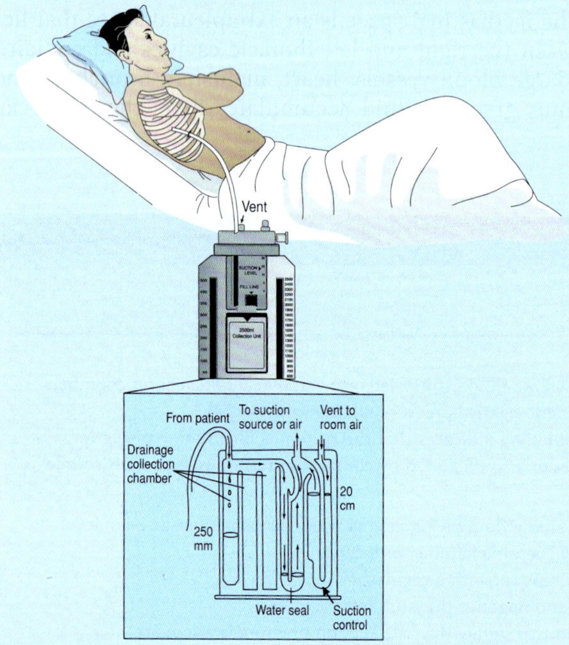

Example of a disposable chest drainage system.

ACTIONS	RATIONALE
8. Mark the drainage from the collection chamber with tape on the outside of the drainage unit. Mark hourly/daily increments (date and time) at the drainage level.	8. This marking shows the amount of fluid loss and how fast fluid is collecting in the drainage chamber. It serves as a basis for determining the need for blood replacement if the fluid is blood. Visibly bloody drainage will appear in the chamber in the immediate postoperative period but should gradually become serous.

GUIDELINES for Managing Chest Drainage Systems (Continued)

ACTIONS	RATIONALE
9. Ensure that the drainage tubing does not kink, loop, or interfere with the patient's movements.	9. Kinking, looping, or pressure on the drainage tubing can produce back-pressure, which may force fluid back into the pleural space or impede its drainage.
10. Encourage the patient to assume a comfortable position with good body alignment. With the lateral position, make sure that the patient's body does not compress the tubing. The patient should be turned and repositioned every 1.5 to 2 hours. Provide adequate analgesia.	10. Frequent position changes promote drainage. Proper positioning also helps breathing and promotes better air exchange. Analgesics may be needed to promote comfort.
11. Assist the patient with range-of-motion exercises for the affected arm and shoulder several times daily. Provide adequate analgesia.	11. Exercise helps to prevent ankylosis of the shoulder and to reduce postoperative pain and discomfort. Analgesics may be needed to relieve pain.
12. Make sure there is fluctuation ("tidaling") of the fluid level in the water seal chamber (in wet systems) or check the air leak indicator for leaks (in dry systems with a one-way valve). *Note:* Fluid fluctuations in the water seal chamber or air leak indicator area will stop when: a. The lung has re-expanded b. The tubing is obstructed by blood clots, fibrin, or kinks c. A loop of tubing hangs below the rest of the tubing d. Suction motor or wall suction is not working properly	12. Fluctuation of the water level in the water seal shows effective connection between the pleural cavity and the drainage chamber and indicates that the drainage system remains patent. Fluctuation is also a gauge of intrapleural pressure in systems with a water seal (wet and dry, but not with the one-way valve).
13. With a dry system, assess for the presence of the indicator (bellows or float device) when setting the regulator dial to the desired level of suction.	13. An air leak indicator shows changes in intrathoracic pressure in dry systems with a one-way valve. Bubbles will appear if a leak is present. The air leak indicator takes the place of fluid fluctuations in the water seal chamber.
14. Observe for air leaks in the drainage system; they are indicated by constant bubbling in the water seal chamber, or by the air leak indicator in dry systems with a one-way valve. Also assess the chest tube system for correctable external leaks. Notify the physician immediately of excessive bubbling in the water seal chamber not due to external leaks.	14. The indicator shows that the vacuum is adequate to maintain the desired level of suction. Leaking and trapping of air in the pleural space can result in tension pneumothorax.
15. When turning down the dry suction, depress the manual high-negativity vent, and assess for a rise in the water level of the water seal chamber.	15. A rise in the water level of the water seal chamber indicates high negative pressure in the system that could lead to increased intrathoracic pressure.
16. Observe and immediately report rapid and shallow breathing, cyanosis, pressure in the chest, subcutaneous emphysema, symptoms of hemorrhage, or significant changes in vital signs.	16. Many clinical conditions can cause these signs and symptoms, including tension pneumothorax, mediastinal shift, hemorrhage, severe incisional pain, pulmonary embolus, and cardiac tamponade. Surgical intervention may be necessary.
17. Encourage the patient to breathe deeply and cough at frequent intervals. Provide adequate analgesia. If needed, request an order for patient-controlled analgesia. Also teach the patient how to perform incentive spirometry.	17. Deep breathing and coughing help to raise the intrapleural pressure, which promotes drainage of accumulated fluid in the pleural space. Deep breathing and coughing also promote removal of secretions from the tracheobronchial tree, which in turn promotes lung expansion and prevents atelectasis.
18. If the patient is lying on a stretcher and must be transported to another area, place the drainage system below the chest level. If the tubing disconnects, place the end of the chest tube in a bottle of sterile water. Do *not* clamp the chest tube.	18. The drainage apparatus must be kept at a level lower than the patient's chest to prevent fluid from flowing backward into the pleural space. Clamping can result in a tension pneumothorax.
19. When assisting in the chest tube's removal, instruct the patient to perform a gentle Valsalva manoeuvre or to breathe quietly. The chest tube is then clamped and quickly removed. Simultaneously, a small bandage is applied and made airtight with petrolatum gauze covered by a 4 × 4-in gauze pad and thoroughly covered and sealed with nonporous tape.	19. The chest tube is removed as directed when the lung is re-expanded (usually 24 hours to several days), depending on the cause of the pneumothorax. During tube removal, the chief priorities are preventing air from entering the pleural cavity as the tube is withdrawn and preventing infection.

Adapted from Perry, A., Potter, P., & Ostendorf, W. (Eds.). (2018). *Clinical nursing skills and techniques* (9th ed.). St. Louis, MO: Elsevier.

CHART 26-23

Preventing Postoperative Cardiopulmonary Complications After Thoracic Surgery

Patient Management

- Auscultate lung sounds and assess for rate, rhythm, and depth.
- Monitor oxygenation with pulse oximetry.
- Monitor electrocardiogram for rate and rhythm changes.
- Assess capillary refill, skin colour, and status of the surgical dressing.
- Encourage and assist the patient to turn, cough, and take deep breaths.

Chest Drainage Management

- Verify that all connection tubes are patent and connected securely.
- Assess that the water seal is intact when using a wet suction system and assess the regulator dial in dry suction systems.
- Monitor characteristics of drainage including colour, amount, and consistency. Assess for significant increases or decreases in drainage output.
- Note fluctuations in the water seal chamber for wet suction systems and the air leak indicator for dry suction systems.
- Keep system below the patient's chest level.
- Assess suction control chamber for bubbling in wet suction systems.
- Keep suction at prescribed level.
- Maintain appropriate fluid in water seal for wet suction systems.
- Keep air vent open when suction is off.

become compressed and stop beating, causing death. Mediastinal chest tubes can be inserted either anteriorly or posteriorly to the heart to drain blood after surgery.

There are two types of chest tubes: small- and large-bore catheters. Small-bore catheters (7 Fr to 12 Fr) have a one-way valve apparatus to prevent air from moving back into the chest. They can be inserted through a small skin incision. Large-bore catheters, which range in size up to 40 Fr, are usually connected to a chest drainage system to collect any pleural fluid and monitor for air leaks. After the chest tube is positioned, it is sutured to the skin and connected to a drainage apparatus (Fig. 26-9) to remove the residual air and fluid from the pleural or mediastinal space. This results in the re-expansion of remaining lung tissue.

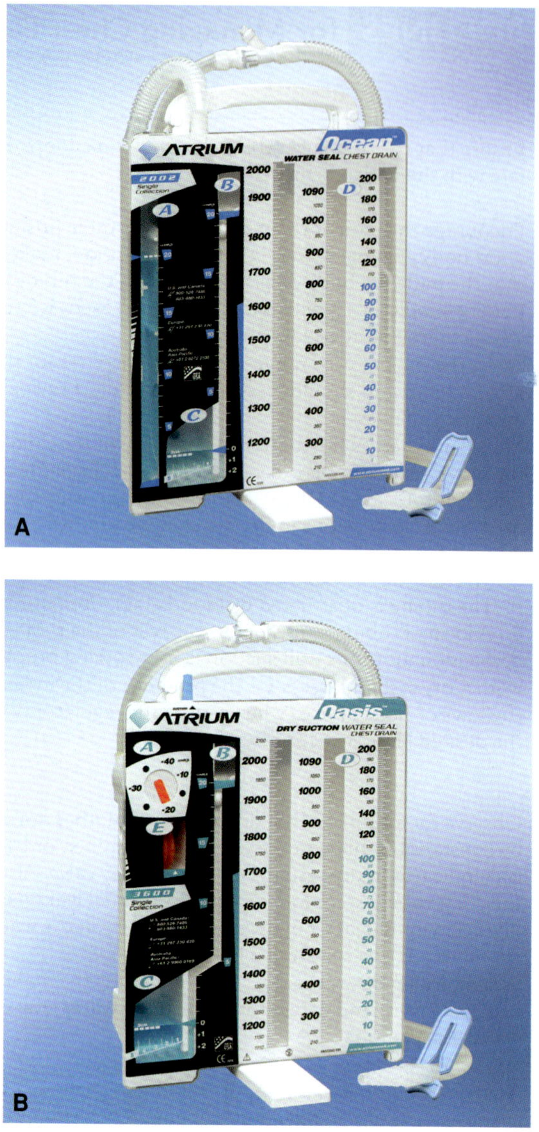

FIGURE 26-9. Chest drainage systems. **A.** The Atrium Ocean is an example of a water seal chest drain system composed of a drainage chamber and water seal chamber. The suction control is determined by the height of the water column in that chamber (usually 20 cm). (*A*, suction control chamber; *B*, water seal chamber; *C*, air leak zone; *D*, collection chamber.) **B.** The Atrium Oasis is an example of a dry suction water seal system that uses a mechanical regulator for vacuum control, a water seal chamber, and a drainage chamber. (*A*, dry suction regulator; *B*, water seal chamber; *C*, air leak monitor; *D*, collection chamber; *E*, suction monitor bellows.) (Photos used with permission from Atrium Medical Corporation, Hudson, NH.)

Chest Drainage Systems

Chest drainage systems have a suction source, a collection chamber for pleural drainage, and a mechanism to prevent air from re-entering the chest with inhalation. Various types of chest drainage systems are available for use in removal of air and fluid from the pleural space and re-expansion of the lungs. Chest drainage systems come with either wet (water seal) or dry suction control. In wet suction systems, the amount of suction is determined by the amount of water instilled in the suction chamber. The amount of bubbling in the suction chamber indicates how strong the suction is. Wet systems use a water seal to prevent air from moving back into the chest on inspiration. Dry systems use a one-way valve and may have a suction control dial in place of the water. Both systems can operate by gravity drainage, without a suction source.

NURSING ALERT

When the wall vacuum is turned off, the drainage system must be open to the atmosphere so that intrapleural air can escape from the system. This can be done by detaching the tubing from the suction port to provide a vent.

Water Seal Systems

The traditional water seal system (or wet suction) for chest drainage has three chambers: a collection chamber, a water seal chamber, and a wet suction control chamber. The collection chamber acts as a reservoir for fluid draining from the chest tube. It is graduated to permit easy measurement of drainage. Suction may be added to create negative pressure and promote drainage of fluid and removal of air. The suction control chamber regulates the amount of negative pressure applied to the chest. The amount of suction is determined by the water level. It is usually set at 20 cm H_2O; adding more fluid results in more suction. After the suction is turned on, bubbling appears in the suction chamber. A positive-pressure valve is located at the top of the suction chamber that automatically opens with increases in positive pressure within the system. Air is automatically released through a positive-pressure relief valve if the suction tubing is inadvertently clamped or kinked.

The water seal chamber has a one-way valve or water seal that prevents air from moving back into the chest when the patient inhales (Frazer, 2012). There is an increase in the water level with inspiration and a return to the baseline level during exhalation; this is referred to as tidaling. Intermittent bubbling in the water seal chamber is normal, but continuous bubbling can indicate an air leak. Bubbling and tidaling do not occur when the tube is placed in the mediastinal space; however, fluid may pulsate with the patient's heartbeat. If the chest tube is connected to gravity drainage only, suction is not used. The pressure is equal to the water seal only. Two-chamber chest drainage systems (water seal chamber and collection chamber) are available for use with patients who need only gravity drainage.

The water level in the water seal chamber reflects the negative pressure present in the intrathoracic cavity. A rise in the water level indicates negative pressure in the pleural or mediastinal space. Excessive negative pressure can cause trauma to tissue. Most chest drainage systems have an automatic means to prevent excessive negative pressure. By pressing and holding a manual high-negativity vent (usually located on the top of the chest drainage system) until the water level in the water seal chamber returns to the 2-cm mark, excessive negative pressure is avoided, preventing damage to tissue.

NURSING ALERT

If the chest tube and drainage system become disconnected, air can enter the pleural space, producing a pneumothorax. To prevent pneumothorax if the chest tube is inadvertently disconnected from the drainage system, a temporary water seal can be established by immersing the chest tube's open end in a bottle of sterile water.

Dry Suction Water Seal Systems

Dry suction water seal systems, also referred to as dry suction, have a collection chamber for drainage, a water seal chamber, and a dry suction control chamber. The water seal chamber is filled with water to the 2-cm level. Bubbling in this area can indicate an air leak. The dry suction control chamber contains a regulator dial that conveniently regulates vacuum to the chest drain. Water is not needed for suction in these systems. Without the bubbling in the suction chamber, the machine is quieter. However, if the container is knocked over, the water seal may be lost.

Once the tube is connected to the suction source, the regulator dial allows the desired level of suction to be set; the suction is increased until an indicator appears. The indicator has the same function as the bubbling in the traditional water seal system; that is, it indicates that the vacuum is adequate to maintain the desired level of suction. Some drainage systems use a bellows (a chamber that can be expanded or contracted) or an orange-coloured float device as an indicator of when the suction control regulator is set.

When the water in the water seal rises above the 2-cm level, intrathoracic pressure increases. Dry suction water seal systems have a manual high-negativity vent located on top of the drain. The manual high-negativity vent is pressed until the indicator appears (either a float device or bellows), and the water level in the water seal returns to the desired level, indicating that the intrathoracic pressure is decreased.

NURSING ALERT

The manual vent should not be used to lower the water level in the water seal when the patient is on gravity drainage (no suction) because intrathoracic pressure is equal to the pressure in the water seal.

Dry Suction Systems With a One-Way Valve

A third type of chest drainage system is dry suction with a one-way mechanical valve. This system has a collection chamber, a one-way mechanical valve, and a dry suction control chamber. The valve permits air and fluid to leave the chest but prevents their movement back into the pleural space. This model lacks a water seal chamber and therefore can be set up quickly in emergency situations, and the dry control drain still works even if it is knocked over. This makes the dry suction systems useful for the patient who is ambulating or being transported. However, without the water seal chamber, there is no way to tell by inspection whether the pressure in the chest has changed, even though an air leak indicator is present so that the system can be checked. If an air leak is suspected, 30 mL of water is injected into the air leak indicator or the container is tipped so that fluid enters the air leak detection chamber. Bubbles will appear if a leak is present.

If the chest tube has been inserted to re-expand a lung after pneumothorax, or if very little fluid drainage is expected, a one-way valve (Heimlich valve) may be connected to the chest tube. This valve may be attached to a collection bag (Fig. 26-10) or covered with a sterile dressing if no drainage is expected.

Postoperative Nursing Management

Postoperative nursing care of the patient who has undergone thoracic surgery addresses close monitoring of the patients respiratory and cardiovascular status, interventions to prevent complications, and the psychological reactions

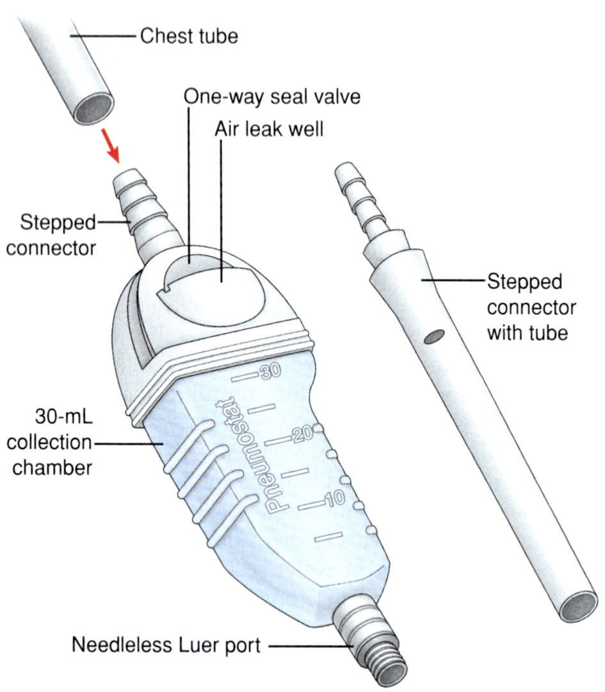

FIGURE 26-10. One-way (Heimlich) valve, a disposable, single-use chest drainage system with 30-mL collection volume. Used when minimal volume of chest drainage is expected.

that often occur in response to this major surgical procedure and the fears that it often engenders in patients and their families.

Monitoring Respiratory and Cardiovascular Status

The nurse monitors the heart rate and rhythm by auscultation and ECG because episodes of major dysrhythmias are common after thoracic and cardiac surgery. In the immediate postoperative period, an arterial line may be maintained to allow frequent monitoring of arterial blood gases, serum electrolytes, hemoglobin and hematocrit values, and arterial pressure. Central venous pressure may be monitored to detect early signs of fluid volume disturbances. Early extubation from mechanical ventilation can also lead to earlier removal of arterial lines (Urden et al., 2014). Another important component of postoperative assessment is to note the results of the preoperative evaluation of the patient's lung reserve by pulmonary function testing. A preoperative FEV_1 (the volume of air that the patient can forcibly exhale in 1 second) of more than 2 L or more than 70% of predicted value indicates a good lung reserve. Patients who have a postoperative FEV_1 of less than 40% of predicted value have decreased tidal volume, which places them at risk for respiratory failure, other morbidity, and death.

Improving Gas Exchange and Breathing

Gas exchange is determined by evaluating oxygenation and ventilation. In the immediate postoperative period, this is achieved by measuring vital signs (blood pressure, pulse, and respirations) at least every 15 minutes for the first 1 to 2 hours, and then less frequently as the patient's condition stabilizes. Pulse oximetry is used for continuous monitoring of the adequacy of oxygenation. Arterial blood gas measurements are obtained early in the postoperative period to establish a baseline to assess the adequacy of oxygenation and ventilation and the possible retention of carbon dioxide. The frequency with which postoperative arterial blood gases are measured depends on whether the patient is mechanically ventilated and whether he or she exhibits signs of respiratory distress; these measurements can help determine appropriate therapy. It is also a common practice for patients to have an arterial line in place to obtain blood for blood gas measurements and to monitor blood pressure closely. Hemodynamic monitoring may be used to assess hemodynamic stability (Urden et al., 2014).

Breathing techniques, such as diaphragmatic and pursed-lip breathing, taught prior to surgery should be performed by the patient every 2 hours to expand the alveoli and prevent atelectasis. Sustained maximal inspiration therapy or incentive spirometry promotes lung inflation, improves the cough mechanism, and allows early assessment of acute pulmonary changes. (See Chart 26-3 for more information.)

If the patient is oriented and blood pressure is stabilized, the head of the bed is elevated 30 to 40 degrees during the immediate postoperative period. This position facilitates ventilation, promotes chest drainage from the lower chest tube, and helps residual air to rise in the upper portion of the pleural space, where it can be removed through the upper chest tube.

The nurse consults with the surgeon about patient positioning to determine the best side-lying position. In general, the patient should be positioned from back to side frequently and moved from a flat to a semi upright position as soon as tolerated. Most commonly, the patient is instructed to lie on the operative side. However, the patient with unilateral lung pathology may not be able to turn well onto that side because of pain. In addition, positioning the patient with the "good lung" (the nonoperated lung) down allows a better match of ventilation and perfusion and therefore may actually improve oxygenation. The patient's position is changed from flat to semi upright as soon as possible because remaining in one position tends to promote the retention of secretions in the dependent portion of the lungs, and the upright position increases diaphragmatic excursion, enhancing lung expansion. After a pneumonectomy, the operated side should be dependent so that fluid in the pleural space remains below the level of the bronchial stump and the other lung can fully expand.

Improving Airway Clearance

Retained secretions are a threat to the patient after thoracotomy surgery. Trauma to the tracheobronchial tree during surgery, diminished lung ventilation, and diminished cough reflex all result in the accumulation of excessive secretions. If the secretions are retained, airway obstruction occurs. This, in turn, causes the air in the alveoli distal to the obstruction to become absorbed and the affected portion of the lung to collapse. Atelectasis, pneumonia, and respiratory failure may result.

To maintain a patent airway, secretions are suctioned from the tracheobronchial tree before the endotracheal tube is discontinued. Secretions continue to be removed by suctioning until the patient can cough up secretions effectively. Nasotracheal suctioning may be needed to stimulate a deep cough and aspirate secretions that the patient cannot clear by coughing. However, it should be used only after other methods to raise secretions have been unsuccessful (Chart 26-24).

CHART 26-24

GUIDELINES for Performing Nasotracheal Suction

Equipment

- Suction catheters
- Gloves (sterile and nonsterile), gown, mask, and goggles for eye protection
- Water-soluble lubricant gel
- Basin for sterile normal saline solution for irrigation
- Suction source
- Pulse oximeter
- Rubber nasal trumpet (if needed)
- Manual resuscitation bag and mask with supplemental oxygen (on standby, for use as needed)

Implementation

ACTIONS	RATIONALE
1. Assess the patient's lung sounds and oxygen saturation via pulse oximeter.	1. Assessment data indicate the need for suctioning and allow the nurse to monitor the effect of suction on the patient's level of oxygenation.
2. Explain procedure to the patient.	2. Explaining the procedure to the patient will help diminish anxiety.
3. Perform hand hygiene. Put on nonsterile gloves, goggles, gown, and mask.	3. Hand hygiene reduces bacteria on hands. Nonsterile gloves, goggles, gown, and mask serve as personal protective equipment (PPE) because they protect the clinician from becoming infected with pathogens.
4. Medicate patient for pain if necessary.	4. The procedure may be uncomfortable and premedication with analgesic agents may mitigate pain.
5. Place the patient in a sitting or semi-Fowler's position. Make sure the patient's head is not flexed forward. Remove excess pillows if necessary.	5. This position facilitates passage of the suction catheter.
6. Oxygenate the patient several minutes before initiating the suctioning procedure. Have oxygen source ready nearby during procedure.	6. Oxygenating the patient preprocedure should help to mitigate the loss of oxygen during suctioning.
7. Turn on suction source (pressure should not exceed 120 mm Hg for an open system and 160 mm Hg for a closed system).	7. Suction pressure should be set high enough to be effective without causing trauma to the tissues.
8. Open suction catheter kit.	8. Having equipment ready prevents interruption of the procedure.
9. Fill basin with sterile water.	9. This provides sterile solution for clearing suction catheter of secretions.
10. Put sterile glove on dominant hand. Pick up suction catheter in sterile gloved hand	10. The catheter may contact the patient's lower airway and therefore must remain sterile to prevent infection.
11. Lubricate catheter with water-soluble gel.	11. Lubrication will help to pass the catheter through the nasal passages minimizing trauma.
12. Gently pass catheter through the patient's nose to the pharynx. If it is difficult to pass the catheter, and repeated suctioning is expected, a soft rubber nasal trumpet may be placed nasopharyngeally to provide easier catheter passage. Check the position of the tip of the catheter by asking the patient to open the mouth to inspect it; the tip of the catheter should be in the lower pharynx.	12. Gentle passage is required to minimize trauma to the nasal passages and pharynx.
13. Instruct the patient to take a deep breath or stick out the tongue.	13. This action opens the epiglottis and promotes downward movement of the catheter.
14. Advance the catheter into the trachea only during inspiration. Listen for cough or for passage of air through the catheter.	14. Advancing the catheter during expiration may cause trauma to the airway.
15. Attach the catheter to suction apparatus. Apply intermittent suction while slowly withdrawing the catheter.	15. Suction will help to clear the lower and upper airway of obstructive secretions.
16. Do not suction for longer than 10 seconds.	16. Dysrhythmias, bradycardia, or cardiac arrest may occur in patients with borderline oxygenation.
17. If additional suctioning is needed, withdraw the catheter to the back of the pharynx. Reassure patient and oxygenate for several minutes before resuming suctioning.	17. Pausing the suction tip at the back of the pharynx will minimize the likelihood of trauma to the nasal passages.

Adapted from Schub, T., & Ashley, T. J. (2016). Nasotracheal suctioning: Performing. In D. Pravikoff (Ed.). *Nursing practice and skill*. Glendale, CA: CINAHL Information Systems.

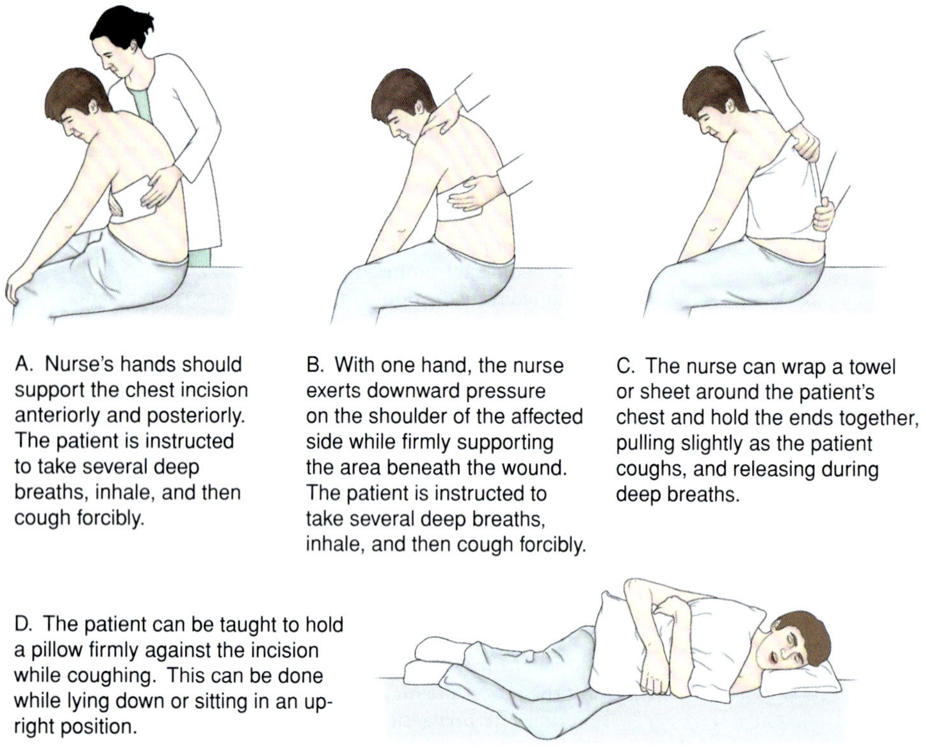

FIGURE 26-11. Techniques for supporting incision while a patient recovering from thoracic surgery coughs.

The patient is encouraged to cough effectively to maintain a patent airway; ineffective coughing results in exhaustion and retention of secretions (see Chart 26-5). To be effective, the cough must be low-pitched, deep, and controlled. Because it is difficult to cough in a supine position, the patient is helped to a sitting position on the edge of the bed, with the feet resting on a chair. The patient should cough at least every hour during the first 24 hours and when necessary thereafter. If audible crackles are present, it may be necessary to use chest percussion with the cough routine until the lungs are clear. Aerosol therapy is helpful in humidifying and mobilizing secretions so that they can easily be cleared with coughing. To minimize incisional pain during coughing, the nurse supports the incision or encourages the patient to do so (Fig. 26-11). If a patient is identified as being at high risk for postoperative pulmonary complications, then CPT is started immediately (perhaps even before surgery). The techniques of postural drainage, vibration, and percussion help loosen and mobilize the secretions so that they can be coughed up or suctioned.

Following the use of these measures, the nurse listens to both lungs, anteriorly and posteriorly, to determine whether there are any changes in breath sounds. Diminished breath sounds may indicate collapsed or hypoventilated alveoli.

Relieving Pain and Discomfort

Pain after a thoracotomy may be severe, depending on the type of incision and the patient's reaction and ability to cope with pain. Pain can impair the patient's ability to breathe deeply and cough. Immediately after the surgical procedure and before the incision is closed, the surgeon may perform a nerve block with a long-acting local anesthetic such as bupivacaine (Bottiger, Esper, & Stafford, 2014). Bupivacaine is titrated to relieve postoperative pain while allowing the patient to cooperate in deep breathing, coughing, and mobilization. An epidural catheter may be placed for continuous or PCA using a combination of a long-acting local anesthetic and an opioid, or a continuous epidural infusion may be combined with IV PCA using an opioid (Sole et al., 2013). Opioid analgesic agents such as morphine are commonly used in PCA, which allows the patient to control the frequency and total dosage. Pre-set limits on the pump avoid over dosage. With proper instruction, PCA is well tolerated and allows earlier mobilization and cooperation with the treatment regimen. (See Chapter 16 for a more extensive discussion of PCA and pain management.)

It is important to avoid depressing the respiratory system with excessive analgesia: the patient should not be so sedated as to be unable to cough. Inadequate treatment of pain, however, may also lead to hypoventilation and decreased coughing. Nurses are less confident in their ability to accurately assess pain for patients not able to self-report pain due to endotracheal intubation, level of consciousness or sedation (Rose et al., 2011).

NURSING ALERT

It is important not to confuse the restlessness of hypoxia with the restlessness caused by pain. Dyspnea, restlessness, increasing respiratory rate, increasing blood pressure, and tachycardia are warning signs of impending respiratory insufficiency. Pulse oximetry is used to monitor oxygenation and to differentiate causes of restlessness.

Lidocaine (Xylocaine) and prilocaine (Citanest) are local anesthetic agents that may be used to treat pain at the site of the chest tube insertion. These medications are administered as topical transdermal analgesics that penetrate the skin; they have also been found to be effective when used together. EMLA cream, which is a mixture of the two medications, may be effective in treating pain from chest tube removal. However, many physicians prefer not to use analgesia when removing chest tubes because the pain, although severe, is of short duration (usually less than a few minutes) and the analgesia might interfere with respiratory effort.

Promoting Mobility and Shoulder Exercises

Because large shoulder girdle muscles are transected during a thoracotomy, the arm and shoulder must be mobilized by full range of motion of the shoulder. As soon as physiologically possible, usually within 8 to 12 hours, the patient is helped to get out of bed. Although this may be painful initially, the earlier the patient moves, the sooner the pain will subside. In addition to getting out of bed, the patient begins arm and shoulder exercises to restore movement and prevent painful stiffening of the affected arm and shoulder as approved and recommended by the surgeon (Chart 26-25). Regular doses of acetaminophen can help relieve shoulder pain.

CHART 26-25

Patient Education: Performing Arm and Shoulder Exercises

Arm and shoulder exercises are performed after thoracic surgery to restore movement, prevent painful stiffening of the shoulder, and improve muscle power.

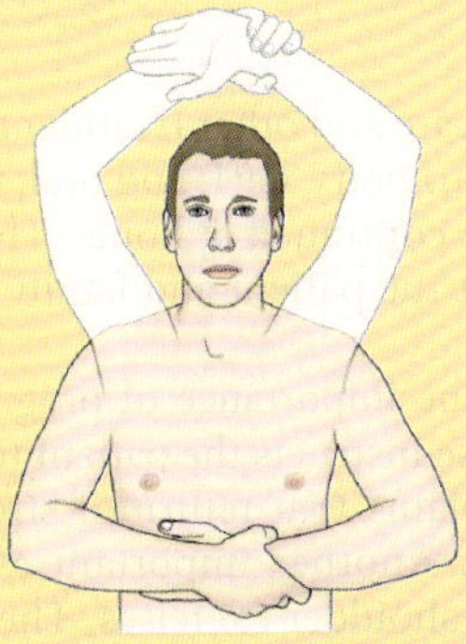

Hold hand of the affected side with the other hand, palms facing in. Raise the arms forward, upward, and then overhead, while taking a deep breath. Exhale while lowering the arms. Repeat five times.

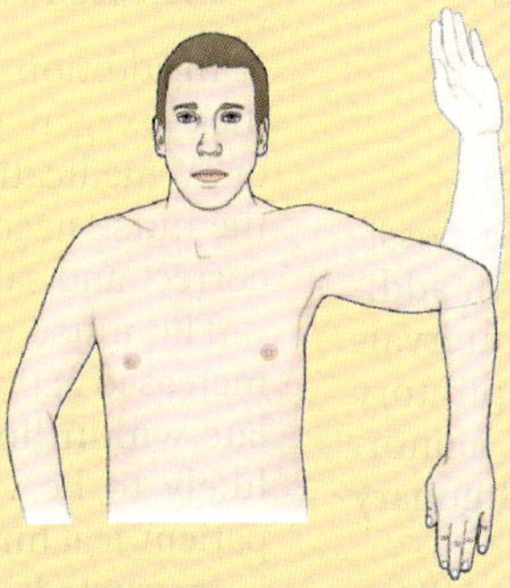

Raise arm sideward, upward, and downward in a waving motion

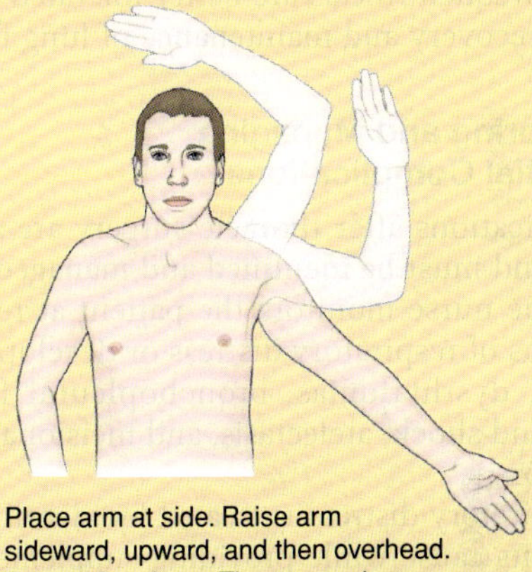

Place arm at side. Raise arm sideward, upward, and then overhead. Repeat five times. These exercises can also be performed while lying in bed.

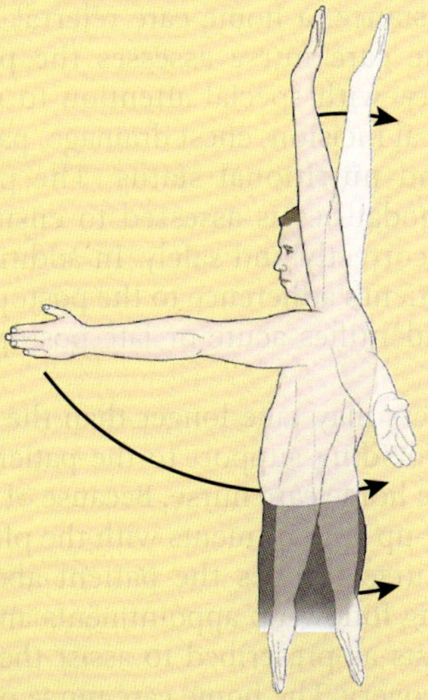

Extend the arm up and back, out to the side and back, down at the side, and back.

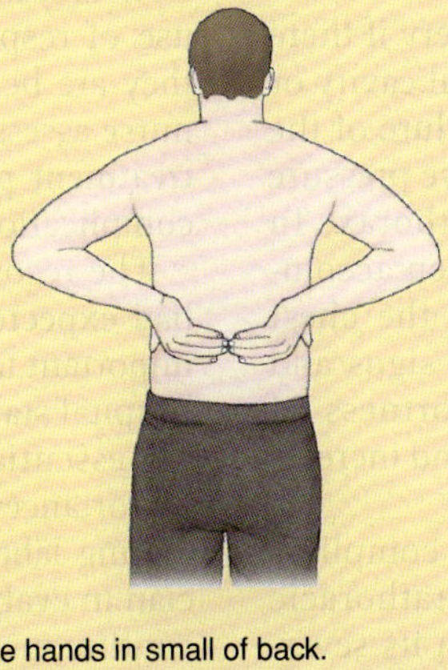

Place hands in small of back. Push elbows as far back as possible.

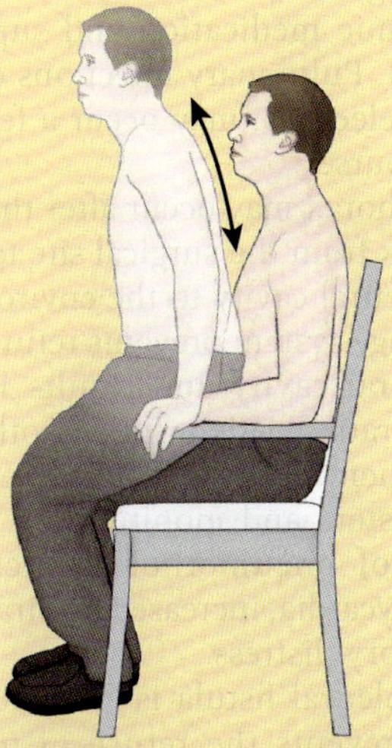

Sit erect in an armchair; place the hands on arms of the chair. Press down on hands, consciously pulling the abdomen in and stretching up from the waist. Inhale while raising the body until elbows are extended completely. Hold this position a moment, and begin exhaling while lowering the body slowly to the original position.

Maintaining Fluid Volume and Nutrition

During the surgical procedure or immediately after, the patient may receive a transfusion of blood products, followed by a continuous IV infusion. Because a reduction in lung capacity often occurs after thoracic surgery, a period of physiologic adjustment is needed. Fluids should be administered at a low hourly rate and titrated (as prescribed) to prevent overloading the vascular system and precipitating pulmonary edema. The nurse performs careful respiratory and cardiovascular assessments and monitors intake and output, vital signs, and jugular vein distention. The nurse also monitors the infusion site for signs of infiltration, including swelling, tenderness, and redness.

Patients undergoing thoracotomy may have poor nutritional status before surgery because of dyspnea, sputum production, and poor appetite. Therefore, it is especially important that adequate nutrition be provided. A liquid diet is provided as soon as bowel sounds return, and the patient is progressed to a full diet as soon as possible. Small, frequent meals are better tolerated and are crucial to the recovery and maintenance of lung function.

Monitoring and Managing Potential Complications

Complications after thoracic surgery are always a possibility and must be identified and managed early. In addition, the nurse monitors the patient at regular intervals for signs of respiratory distress or developing respiratory failure, dysrhythmias, bronchopleural fistula, hemorrhage and shock, atelectasis, and incisional or pulmonary infection.

Respiratory distress is treated by identifying and eliminating its cause while providing supplemental oxygen. If the patient progresses to respiratory failure, intubation and mechanical ventilation are necessary.

Dysrhythmias are often related to the effects of hypoxia or the surgical procedure. They are treated with antiarrhythmic medication and supportive therapy (see Chapter 28). Pulmonary infections or effusion, often preceded by atelectasis, may occur a few days into the postoperative course.

Pneumothorax may occur after thoracic surgery if there is an air leak from the surgical site to the pleural cavity or from the pleural cavity to the environment. Failure of the chest drainage system prevents return of negative pressure in the pleural cavity and results in pneumothorax. In the postoperative patient, pneumothorax is often accompanied by hemothorax. The nurse maintains the chest drainage system and monitors the patient for signs and symptoms of pneumothorax: increasing shortness of breath, tachycardia, increased respiratory rate, and increasing respiratory distress.

Bronchopleural fistula is a serious but rare complication that prevents the return of negative intrathoracic pressure and lung re-expansion. Depending on its severity, it is treated with closed chest drainage, mechanical ventilation, and possibly talc pleurodesis (described in Chapter 24).

Hemorrhage and shock are managed by treating the underlying cause, whether by reoperation or by administration of blood products or fluids. Pulmonary edema from over infusion of IV fluids is a significant danger. Early symptoms are dyspnea, crackles, bubbling sounds in the chest, tachycardia, and pink, frothy sputum. This constitutes an emergency and must be reported and treated immediately.

Promoting Home, Community-Based, and Transitional Care

Educating Patients About Self-Care

The nurse instructs the patient and family about postoperative care that will be continued at home. The nurse explains signs and symptoms that should be reported to the physician. These include the following:

- Change in respiratory status: increasing shortness of breath, fever, increased restlessness or other changes in mental or cognitive status, increased respiratory rate, change in respiratory pattern, change in amount or colour of sputum
- Bleeding or other drainage from the surgical incision or chest tube exit sites
- Increased chest pain

In addition, respiratory care and other treatment modalities (oxygen, incentive spirometry, CPT, and oral, inhaled, or IV medications) may be continued at home. Therefore, the nurse needs to instruct the patient and family in their correct and safe use.

The nurse emphasizes the importance of progressively increased activity. The nurse instructs the patient to ambulate within limits and explains that return of strength is likely to be very gradual. Another important aspect of patient teaching addresses shoulder exercises. The patient is instructed to do these exercises five times daily. Additional patient teaching is described in Chart 26-26.

Continuing and Transitional Care

Depending on the patient's physical status and the availability of family assistance, a home care referral may be indicated. The home care nurse assesses the patient's recovery from surgery, with special attention to respiratory status, the surgical incision, chest drainage, pain control, ambulation, and nutritional status. The patient's use of respiratory modalities is assessed to ensure that they are being used correctly and safely. In addition, the nurse assesses the patient's adherence to the postoperative treatment plan and identifies acute or late postoperative complications.

The recovery process may take longer than the patient had expected and providing support to the patient is an important task for the home care nurse. Because of shorter hospital stays, follow-up appointments with the physician are essential. The nurse teaches the patient about the importance of keeping follow-up appointments and completing laboratory tests as prescribed to assist the physician in evaluating recovery. The home care nurse provides continuous encouragement and education to the patient and family during the process. As recovery progresses, the nurse also reminds the patient and family about the importance of participating in health promotion activities and recommended health screening.

For a detailed plan of nursing care for the patient who has had a thoracotomy, see Chart 26-27.

CHART 26-26

HOME CARE CHECKLIST • The Patient With a Thoracotomy

At the completion of education, the patient and/or caregiver will be able to:

- Name the procedure that was performed and identify any permanent changes in anatomic structure or function as well as changes in ADLs, IADLs, roles, relationships, and spirituality.
- State the name, dose, side effects, frequency, and schedule for all medications.
- Identify interventions and strategies (e.g., durable medical equipment, oxygen, and adaptive equipment) used in adapting to any permanent changes in structure or function.
- Describe ongoing postoperative therapeutic regimen, including diet and activities to perform (e.g., walking and breathing exercises) and to limit or avoid (e.g., lifting weights, driving a car, and contact sports).
  - Alternate walking and other activities with frequent rest periods, expecting weakness and fatigue for the first 3 weeks.
  - Walk at a moderate pace, gradually and persistently extending walking time and distance.
  - Perform arm and shoulder exercises as prescribed
  - Perform breathing exercises several times daily for the first few weeks at home.
  - Avoid lifting >20 lb until complete healing has taken place; the chest muscles and incision may be weaker than normal for 3 to 6 months after surgery.
  - Use local heat and oral analgesia to relieve intercostal pain.
  - Immediately stop any activity that causes undue fatigue, increased shortness of breath, or chest pain.
  - Avoid bronchial irritants (smoke, fumes, air pollution, aerosol sprays).
  - Avoid others with known colds or lung infections.
- Describe signs and symptoms of complications (e.g., increased shortness of breath, fever, restlessness, mental status changes, change in rate or pattern of respiration, increased pain, or bleeding from incision).
- Relate how to reach primary provider with questions or complications.
- State time and date of follow-up appointments.
- Obtain an annual influenza vaccine, and discuss vaccination against pneumonia with the primary provider.
- State understanding of community resources and referrals (if any).
- Identify the need for health promotion (e.g., weight reduction, smoking cessation, and stress management), disease prevention and screening activities

ADL, activities of daily living; IADL, independent activities of daily living.

Plan of Nursing Care — Chart 26-27. Care of the Patient After Thoracotomy

NURSING INTERVENTIONS	RATIONALE	EXPECTED OUTCOMES
Nursing Priority: Altered gas exchange due to lung impairment and surgery **Goal:** Improvement of gas exchange and breathing		
1. Monitor pulmonary status as directed and as needed: a. Auscultate breath sounds. b. Check rate, depth, and pattern of respirations. c. Assess blood gases for signs of hypoxemia or CO_2 retention. d. Evaluate patient's colour for cyanosis.	1. Changes in pulmonary status indicate improvement or onset of complications.	• Lungs are clear on auscultation • Respiratory rate is within acceptable range with no episodes of dyspnea • Vital signs are stable • Dysrhythmias are not present or are under control • Demonstrates deep, controlled, effective breathing to allow maximal lung expansion

continued >

Plan of Nursing Care

Chart 26-27. Care of the Patient After Thoracotomy, *Continued*

NURSING INTERVENTIONS	RATIONALE	EXPECTED OUTCOMES
2. Monitor and record blood pressure, apical pulse, and temperature every 2 to 4 hours, central venous pressure (if indicated) every 2 hours.	2. Aid in evaluating effect of surgery on cardiac status.	• Uses incentive spirometer every 2 hours while awake • Demonstrates deep, effective coughing technique • Residual fluid and air is removed via the chest drainage system. • Lungs are expanded to capacity (evidenced by chest x-ray)
3. Monitor continuous electrocardiogram for pattern and dysrhythmias.	3. Dysrhythmias (especially atrial fibrillation and atrial flutter) are more frequently seen after thoracic surgery. A patient with total pneumonectomy is especially prone to cardiac irregularity.	
4. Elevate head of bed 30 to 40 degrees when patient is oriented and hemodynamic status is stable.	4. Maximum lung excursion is achieved when patient is as close to upright as possible.	
5. Encourage deep-breathing exercises (see section on Breathing Retraining) and effective use of incentive spirometer (sustained maximal inspiration).	5. Helps to achieve maximal lung inflation and to open closed airways.	
6. Encourage and promote an effective cough routine to be performed every 1 to 2 hours during first 24 hours.	6. Coughing is necessary to remove retained secretions.	
7. Assess and monitor the chest drainage system[a] a. Assess for leaks and patency as needed (see Chart 26-19). b. Monitor amount and character of drainage and document every 2 hours. Notify physician if drainage is 150 mL/hr or greater.	7. System is used to eliminate any residual air or fluid after thoracotomy.	

Nursing Priority: Decreased ability to clear airway
Goal: Improvement of airway clearance and achievement of a patent airway

NURSING INTERVENTIONS	RATIONALE	EXPECTED OUTCOMES
1. Maintain an open airway.	1. Provides for adequate ventilation and gas exchange.	• Airway is patent • Coughs effectively • Splints incision while coughing • Sputum is clear or colourless • Lungs are clear on auscultation
2. Perform endotracheal suctioning until patient can raise secretions effectively.	2. Endotracheal secretions are present in excessive amounts in post thoracotomy patients due to trauma to the tracheobronchial tree during surgery, diminished lung ventilation, and cough reflex.	
3. Assess and medicate for pain. Encourage deep-breathing and coughing exercises. Help splint incision during coughing.	3. Helps to achieve maximal lung inflation and to open closed airways. Coughing is painful; incision needs to be supported.	
4. Monitor amount, viscosity, colour, and odour of sputum. Notify physician if sputum is excessive or contains bright-red blood.	4. Changes in sputum suggest presence of infection or change in pulmonary status. Colourless sputum is not unusual; opacification or colouring of sputum may indicate dehydration or infection.	
5. Administer humidification and mininebulizer therapy as prescribed.	5. Secretions must be moistened and thinned if they are to be raised from the chest with the least amount of effort.	
6. Perform postural drainage, percussion, and vibration as prescribed. Do not percuss or vibrate directly over operative site.	6. Chest physiotherapy uses gravity to help remove secretions from the lung.	
7. Auscultate both sides of chest to determine changes in breath sounds.	7. Indications for tracheal suctioning are determined by chest auscultation.	

Plan of Nursing Care

Chart 26-27. Care of the Patient After Thoracotomy, *Continued*

NURSING INTERVENTIONS	RATIONALE	EXPECTED OUTCOMES
Nursing Priority: Pain due to surgical procedure **Goal:** Relief of pain and discomfort		
1. Evaluate location, character, quality, and severity of pain. Administer analgesic medication as prescribed and as needed. Observe for respiratory effect of opioid. Is patient too somnolent to cough? Are respirations depressed?	1. Pain limits chest excursions and thereby decreases ventilation.	• Asks for pain medication, but verbalizes that he or she expects some discomfort while deep breathing and coughing • Verbalizes that he or she is comfortable and not in acute distress • No signs of incisional infection evident
2. Maintain care postoperatively in positioning the patient: a. Place patient in semi-Fowler's position. b. Patients with limited respiratory reserve may not be able to turn on unoperated side. c. Assist or turn patient every 2 hours.	2. The patient who is comfortable and free of pain will be less likely to splint the chest while breathing. A semi-Fowler's position permits residual air in the pleural space to rise to upper portion of pleural space and be removed via the upper chest catheter.	
3. Assess incision area every 8 hours for redness, heat, induration, swelling, separation, and drainage.	3. These signs indicate possible infection.	
4. Request order for patient-controlled analgesia pump if appropriate for patient.	4. Allowing patient control over frequency and dose improves comfort and compliance with treatment regimen.	
Nursing Priority: Anxiety **Goal:** Reduction of anxiety to a manageable level		
1. Explain all procedures in understandable language.	1. Explaining what can be expected in understandable terms decreases anxiety and increases cooperation.	• States that anxiety is at a manageable level • Participates with health care team in treatment regimen • Uses appropriate coping skills (verbalization, pain relief strategies, use of support systems such as family, clergy) • Demonstrates basic understanding of technology used in care
2. Assess for pain and medicate, especially before potentially painful procedures.	2. Premedication before painful procedures or activities improves comfort and minimizes undue anxiety.	
3. Silence all *unnecessary* alarms on technology (monitors, ventilators).	3. *Unnecessary* alarms increase the risk of sensory overload and may increase anxiety. *Essential* alarms must be turned on at all times.	
4. Encourage and support patient while increasing activity level.	4. Positive reinforcement improves patient motivation and independence.	
5. Mobilize resources (family, clergy, social worker) to help patient cope with outcomes of surgery (diagnosis, change in functional abilities).	5. A multidisciplinary approach promotes the patient's strengths and coping mechanisms.	
Nursing Diagnosis: Decreased physical mobility of the upper extremities **Goal:** Increased mobility of the affected shoulder and arm		
1. Assist patient with normal range of motion and function of shoulder and trunk: a. Teach breathing exercises to mobilize thorax. b. Encourage skeletal exercises to promote abduction and mobilization of shoulder (see Chart 26-22). c. Assist out of bed to chair as soon as pulmonary and circulatory systems are stable (usually by evening of surgery).	1. Necessary to regain normal mobility of arm and shoulder and to speed recovery and minimize discomfort.	• Demonstrates arm and shoulder exercises and verbalizes intent to perform them on discharge • Regains previous range of motion in shoulder and arm

continued >

Plan of Nursing Care — Chart 26-27. Care of the Patient After Thoracotomy, *Continued*

NURSING INTERVENTIONS	RATIONALE	EXPECTED OUTCOMES
2. Encourage progressive activities according to level of fatigue.	2. Increases patient's use of affected shoulder and arm.	
Nursing Diagnosis: Risk for imbalanced fluid volume related to the surgical procedure **Goal:** Maintenance of adequate fluid volume		
1. Monitor and record hourly intake and output. Urine output should be at least >0.5 mL/kg/hr after surgery.	1. Fluid management may be altered before, during, and after surgery, and patient's response to and need for fluid management must be assessed.	• Patient is adequately hydrated, as evidenced by: • Urine output >0.5 mL/kg/hr • Vital signs stable, heart rate, and central venous pressure approaching normal • No excessive peripheral edema
2. Administer blood component therapy and parenteral fluids and/or diuretics as prescribed to restore and maintain fluid volume.	2. Pulmonary edema due to transfusion or fluid overload is an ever-present threat; after pneumonectomy, the pulmonary vascular system has been greatly reduced.	
Nursing Diagnosis: Deficient knowledge of home care procedures **Goal:** Increased ability to carry out care procedures at home		
1. Encourage patient to practice arm and shoulder exercises five times daily at home.	1. Exercise accelerates recovery of muscle function and reduces long-term pain and discomfort.	• Demonstrates arm and shoulder exercises • Verbalizes need to try to assume an erect posture • Verbalizes the importance of relieving discomfort, alternating walking and rest, performing breathing exercises, avoiding heavy lifting, avoiding undue fatigue, avoiding bronchial irritants, preventing colds or lung infections, getting influenza vaccine, keeping follow-up visits, and stopping smoking
2. Instruct patient to practice assuming a functionally erect position in front of a full-length mirror.	2. Practice will help restore normal posture.	
3. Instruct patient about home care (see Chart 26-3).	3. Knowing what to expect facilitates recovery.	

[a]A patient with a pneumonectomy usually does not have water seal chest drainage because it is desirable that the pleural space fill with an effusion, which eventually obliterates this space. Some surgeons do use a modified water seal system.

Critical Thinking Exercises

1 A 56-year-old man is admitted to a cardiopulmonary unit following a transbronchial lung biopsy for lung cancer. Shortly after arrival to the unit, the patient complains of excruciating pain in his upper right back, shortness of breath, and feeling anxious. Physical examination reveals tachycardia at 112 bpm, tachypnea at 28 breaths/min, and hypotension at 90/46 mm Hg. Auscultation reveals absence of breath sounds in the right mid and lower lobes. The patient is diaphoretic with an SpO_2 on room air of 88%. The physician prescribes emergent chest tube insertion with dry suction water seal chest drainage set up. What is the likely cause of the patient's clinical manifestations? What are your priority interventions? What is the primary difference between a traditional water seal chest drainage system and a dry suction water seal chest drainage system? Describe nursing responsibilities following chest tube insertion.

2 An 82-year-old man is admitted to an orthopedic unit following a total hip replacement for a right hip fracture, which occurred 2 days ago. Four hours after arrival to the unit, the patient complains of increasing shortness of breath and tachypnea with a respiratory rate of 38 breaths/min. Physical examination reveals tachycardia at 122 bpm, hypotension at 96/56 mm Hg, and SpO_2 of 84% on 4 L/min via nasal cannula. The nurse places the patient on a nonrebreather mask and notifies the physician. Arterial blood gases reveal pH 7.22, PO_2 48 mm Hg, PCO_2 52 mm Hg, and HCO_3 24 mEq/L. The patient's respiratory status continues to deteriorate and the physician emergently places an endotracheal tube. The patient is sedated and placed on mechanical ventilation. What is the likely cause of the patient's respiratory distress? How do you interpret the patient's blood gas values? Outline the nursing care of the patient on a

mechanical ventilator. Describe the essential components of the VAP bundle of evidence-based practice.

3 A 32-year-old woman is admitted to a general surgery unit following a thyroidectomy. Upon assessment of the patient, the nurse observes bleeding at the incision site, swelling of the neck, and harsh, high-pitched respiratory sounds. The nurse calls a rapid response and an emergent tracheostomy is performed at the bedside. The patient is transferred to the ICU. What are the priority nursing diagnoses for patients requiring a tracheostomy? Discuss nursing interventions to prevent complications following tracheostomy procedure. Describe the technique to suction an artificial airway.

REFERENCES AND SELECTED READINGS

Books

Cairo, J. M. (2012). *Pilbeam's mechanical ventilation: Physiological and clinical applications*. St. Louis, MO: Elsevier Mosby.

Cairo, J. M. (2014). *Mosby's respiratory care equipment* (9th ed.). St. Louis, MO: Elsevier Mosby.

Grossman, S., & Porth, C. M. (2014). *Pathophysiology: Concepts of altered health states* (9th ed.). Philadelphia, PA: Lippincott Williams & Williams.

Hess, D. (2012). *Respiratory care: Principles and practice*. Sudbury, ON: Jones & Bartlett Learning.

Hyzy, R. (2017). Weaning from mechanical ventilation. In A. Adegunsoye & J. Kress (Eds.). *Evidence-based critical care: A case study approach*. Springer.

Kacmarek, R. M., Stroller, J. K., & Huer, A. (2017). *Egan's fundamentals of respiratory care* (11th ed.). St. Louis, MO: Elsevier.

Meiner, S. E. (2015). *Gerontologic nursing* (5th ed.). St. Louis, MO: Elsevier Mosby.

Perry, G. A., Potter, P. A., & Ostendorf, W. (2018). *Clinical nursing skills and techniques* (9th ed.). St. Louis, MO: Elsevier.

Potter, P. A., Perry, A. G., Stockert, P., et al. (2018). *Canadian fundamentals of Nursing—Elsevier eBook on VitalSource* (6th ed.). Elsevier Health Sciences.

Sole, M. L., Klein, D. G., & Moseley, M. J. (2013). *Introduction to critical care nursing* (6th ed.). St. Louis, MO: Elsevier.

Tabloski, P. A. (2014). *Gerontological nursing* (3rd ed.). Boston, MA: Pearson.

Urden, L., Stacy, K., & Lough, M. (2014). *Critical care nursing: Diagnosis and management* (7th ed.). St. Louis, MO: Elsevier Mosby.

Wiegand, D. (2016). *AACN procedure manual for critical care* (7th ed.). St. Louis, MO: Elsevier Saunders.

Journals and Electronic Documents

Amitai, A., & Sinert, R. H. (2015). Introduction to ventilator management. *Medscape*. Retrieved May 7, 2016, from emedicine.medscape.com/article/810126-overview#a3

Andrews, J., Sathe, N. A., Krishnaswami, S., et al. (2013). Nonpharmacologic airway clearance techniques in hospitalized patients: A systematic review. *Respiratory Care*, *58*(12), 2160–2186.

Balas, M. C., Vasilevskis, E. E., Burke, W. J., et al. (2012). Critical care nurse's role in implementing the "ABCDE Bundle" into practice. *Critical Care Nurse*, *32*(2), 35–48.

Bennett, M. H., Stanford, R., & Turner, R. (2012). Hyperbaric oxygen therapy for promoting fracture healing and treating fracture nonunion. *Cochrane Database of Systematic Reviews*, *11*, CD004712.

Bottiger, B., Esper S., & Stafford-Smith, M. (2014). Pain management strategies for thoracotomy and thoracic pain syndromes. *Seminars in Cardiothoracic and Vascular Anesthesia*, *18*(1), 45–56.

Bulamba, F., Kintu, A., Ayupo, N., et al. (2017). Achieving the recommended endotracheal tube cuff pressure: A randomized control study comparing loss of resistance syringe to pilot balloon palpation. *Anesthesiology Research and Practice*, *2017*, 2032748.

Campbell, M. R., Fisher, J., Anderson, L., et al. (2015). Implementation of early exercise and progressive mobility: Steps to success. *Critical Care Nurse*, *35*(1), 82–88.

Chakravorty, I., Chahal, K., & Austin, G. (2013). A pilot study of the impact of high-frequency chest wall oscillation in chronic obstructive pulmonary disease patients with mucus hypersecretion. *International Journal of Chronic Obstructive Pulmonary Disease*, *6*, 693–699.

Chanques, G., Tarri, T., Ride, A., et al. (2017). Analgesia nociception index for the assessment of pain in critically ill patients: A diagnostic accuracy study. *BJA: British Journal of Anaesthesia*, *119*(4), 812–820.

Frazer, C. A. (2012). Managing chest tubes. *Academy of Medical-Surgical Nurses*, *21*(1),1, 10–12.

Gupta, S., Singh, D., Sood, D., et al. (2015). Role of dexmedetomidine in early extubation of the intensive care unit patients. *Journal of Anaesthesiology Clinical Pharmacology*, *31*(1), 92–98.

Hanlon, P. (2015). Secretion and airway clearance: Techniques and devices offer a range of treatment options. *RT: The Journal for Respiratory Care Practitioners*, *28*(8), 11–14.

Main, E., Prasad, A., & van der Schans, C. (2013). Conventional chest physiotherapy compared to other airway clearance techniques for cystic fibrosis. *Cochrane Database of Systematic Reviews*, 2, CD002911.

Martí, S., Pajares, V., Morante F., et al. (2013). Are oxygen-conserving devices effective for correcting exercise hypoxemia? *Respiratory Care*, *58*(10), 1606–1613.

McClave, S., Taylor, B., Martindale, R., et al., (2016). Guidelines for the provision and assessment of nutrition support therapy in the adult critically ill patient: Society of Critical Care Medicine (SCCM) and American Society for Parenteral and Enteral Nutrition (A.S.P.E.N.). *Journal of Parenteral and Enteral Nutrition*, *40*(2), 159–211.

McNarry, A. F., & Patel, A. (2017). The evolution of airway management—new concepts and conflicts with traditional practice. *BJA: British Journal of Anaesthesia*, *119*(suppl_1), i154–i166.

Medicinenet.com. (2013). Acetylcysteine—inhalation/oral. Retrieved from https://www.medicinenet.com/acetylcysteine-inhalationoral/article.htm

Nicolini, A., Cardini, F., Landucci, N., et al. (2013). Effectiveness of treatment with high-frequency chest wall oscillation in patients with bronchiectasis. *BMC Pulmonary Medicine*, *13*, 21.

Patient Safety Institute. (2016). Ventilator associated pneumonia. Retrieved from http://www.patientsafetyinstitute.ca/en/Topic/Pages/Ventilator-Associated-Pneumonia-(VAP).aspx

Rose, L., Haslam, L., Dale, C., et al. (2011). Survey of assessment and management of pain for critically ill adults. *Intensive and Critical Care Nursing*, *27*(3), 121–128.

Sperlich, B., Zinner, C., Hauser, A., et al. (2017). The impact of hyperoxia on human performance and recovery. *Sports Medicine*, *47*(3), 429–438.

Resources

Canadian Lung Association: http://www.lung.ca

National Heart, Lung and Blood Institute: http://www.nhlbi.nih.ov/index.htm

National Lung Health Education Program: http://www.nlhep.org

Registered Nurses' Association of Ontario: http://www.rnao.org

UNIT 6

Cardiovascular and Circulatory Function

Case Study

AVOIDING A NEAR MISS WITH ANTICOAGULATION THERAPY

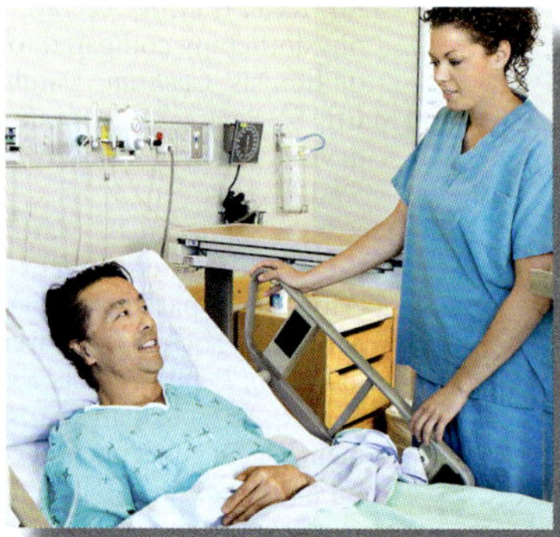

A 45-year-old patient is brought to the emergency department (ED) complaining of pain in his left lower leg, which is swollen and painful. Ultrasound reports reveal that he has a deep vein thrombosis (DVT). He is admitted to a general medical/surgical unit for anticoagulation therapy. He is begun on a weight-based heparin intravenous (IV) drip, with concomitant oral doses of warfarin (Coumadin). When the IV heparin arrives on the unit, the nurse notes that the prescribed order dose does not match the dose on the IV bag sent from the pharmacy. The nurse sends the bag back to the pharmacy, requesting that the correct dose be sent as soon as possible. The patient is anxious to begin the heparin therapy and asks the nurse why there is a delay in starting the heparin drip.

QSEN Competency Focus: Safety

The complexities inherent in today's health care system challenge nurses to demonstrate integration of specific interdisciplinary core competencies that are aimed at ensuring the delivery of safe and quality patient care (Institute of Medicine, 2003). The Quality and Safety Education for Nurses project (QSEN, 2017; Cronenwett, Sherwood, Barnsteiner, et al., 2007) provides a framework for the knowledge, skills, and attitudes (KSAs) required for nurses to demonstrate competency in these key areas, which include ***patient-centred care***, ***interdisciplinary teamwork and collaboration***, ***evidence-based practice***, ***quality improvement***, ***safety***, and ***informatics.***

Safety Definition: Minimizes risk of harm to patients and providers through both system effectiveness and individual performance.

SELECTED PRE-LICENSURE KSAs	APPLICATION AND REFLECTION
Knowledge	
Describe the factors that create a culture of safety (such as open communication strategies and organizational error–reporting systems).	Identify how medication errors may occur in hospitals. Identify the different points during the process, from the time a medication is prescribed to the time it is given to a patient that an error may occur. What system designs are in place in hospitals to prevent medication errors from occurring?
Skills	
Communicate observations or concerns related to hazards and errors to patients, families, and the health care team.	How and to whom should the nurse report this type of "near miss" event? Although a medication error was averted, the patient's treatment is delayed; describe how treatment delays such as these may also cause harm to patients. How should the nurse respond to the patient's question regarding his treatment delay? Should the nurse disclose that the wrong dose was sent to the unit by the pharmacy? Should others be involved in disclosing this "near miss" event to the patient?
Attitudes	
Value own role in preventing errors.	Reflect on how you would feel in this type of situation. Would you be pleased with yourself for discovering the error and inclined to blame the pharmacist? Or would you feel concerned that a flaw in the hospital's system design allowed this type of "near miss" event to occur, and frightened that you could have administered the wrong dose of medication to this patient? How could you engage in system-design advocacy so that this type of safety design flaw is rectified? How comfortable would you be in disclosing an error or potential error to a patient?

Cronenwett, L., Sherwood, G., Barnsteiner, J., et al. (2007). Quality and safety education for nurses. *Nursing Outlook*, *55*(3), 122–131; Institute of Medicine. (2003). *Health professions education: A bridge to quality*. Washington, DC: National Academies Press; and QSEN Institute. (2017). *QSEN competencies: Definitions and pre-licensure KSAs*. Retrieved June 12, 2019, from www.qsen.org/competencies/pre-licensure-ksas

27 Assessment of Cardiovascular Function

Adapted by Alice S.W. Khin

Learning Objectives

On completion of this chapter, the learner will be able to:

1. Explain cardiac physiology in relation to cardiac anatomy and the conduction system of the heart.
2. Incorporate assessment of cardiac risk factors into the health history and physical assessment of the patient with cardiovascular disease.
3. Discuss the clinical indications, patient preparation, and other related nursing implications for common tests and procedures used to assess cardiovascular function and diagnose cardiovascular diseases.
4. Compare the various methods of hemodynamic monitoring (e.g., central venous pressure, pulmonary artery pressure, and arterial pressure monitoring) with regard to indications for use, potential complications, and nursing responsibilities.

Introduction

Cardiovascular diseases (CVDs) such as heart disease and stroke represent two of the leading causes of death in Canada (Public Health Agency of Canada, 2015). Because of the prevalence of CVD, nurses practicing in any setting across the continuum of care, whether in the home, office, hospital, long-term care facility, or rehabilitation facility, must be able to assess the cardiovascular system. Key components of assessment include a health history, physical assessment, and monitoring of a variety of laboratory and diagnostic test results. This assessment provides the data necessary to identify nursing diagnoses, formulate an individualized plan of care, evaluate the response of the patient to the care provided, and revise the plan as needed.

Anatomic and Physiologic Overview

An understanding of the structure and function of the heart in health and in disease is essential to develop cardiovascular assessment skills.

Anatomy of the Heart

The heart is a hollow, muscular organ located in the centre of the thorax, where it occupies the space between the lungs (mediastinum) and rests on the diaphragm. It weighs approximately 300 g; the weight and size of the heart are influenced by age, gender, body weight, extent of physical exercise and conditioning, and heart disease. The heart pumps blood to the tissues, supplying them with oxygen and other nutrients.

The heart is composed of three layers (Fig. 27-1). The inner layer, or endocardium, consists of endothelial tissue and lines the inside of the heart and valves. The middle layer, or **myocardium**, is made up of muscle fibres and is responsible for the pumping action. The exterior layer of the heart is called the epicardium.

The heart is encased in a thin, fibrous sac called the pericardium, which is composed of two layers. Adhering to the epicardium is the visceral pericardium. Enveloping the visceral pericardium is the parietal pericardium, a tough fibrous tissue that attaches to the great vessels, diaphragm, sternum, and vertebral column and supports the heart in the mediastinum. The space between these two layers (pericardial space) is normally filled with about 20 mL of fluid, which lubricates the surface of the heart and reduces friction during systole.

Heart Chambers

The pumping action of the heart is accomplished by the rhythmic relaxation and contraction of the muscular walls of its four chambers. During the relaxation phase, called **diastole**, all four chambers relax simultaneously, which allows the ventricles to fill in preparation for contraction. Diastole is commonly referred to as the period of ventricular filling. **Systole** refers to the events in the heart during contraction of the two top chambers (atria) and two bottom chambers (ventricles). Unlike diastole, atrial and ventricular systole are not simultaneous events. Atrial systole occurs first, just at the end of diastole, followed by ventricular systole. This synchronization allows the ventricles to completely fill prior to ejection of blood from their chambers.

The right side of the heart, made up of the right atrium and right ventricle, distributes venous blood (deoxygenated blood) to the lungs via the pulmonary artery (pulmonary circulation) for oxygenation. The right atrium receives blood returning from the superior vena cava (head, neck, and upper extremities), inferior vena cava (trunk and lower extremities), and coronary sinus (coronary circulation). The left side of the heart, composed of the left atrium and left ventricle, distributes oxygenated blood to the remainder of the body via the aorta (systemic circulation). The left atrium receives oxygenated blood from the pulmonary circulation via four pulmonary veins. The

Glossary

acute coronary syndrome: refers to rupture of an atheromatous plaque in a diseased coronary artery, which rapidly forms an obstructive thrombus

afterload: the amount of resistance to ejection of blood from the ventricle

apical impulse (also called point of maximum impulse): impulse normally palpated at the fifth intercostal space, left midclavicular line; caused by contraction of the left ventricle

atrioventricular (AV) node: secondary pacemaker of the heart, located in the right atrial wall near the tricuspid valve

baroreceptors: nerve fibres located in the aortic arch and carotid arteries that are responsible for reflex control of the blood pressure

cardiac catheterization: an invasive procedure used to measure cardiac chamber pressures and assess patency of the coronary arteries

cardiac conduction system: specialized heart cells strategically located throughout the heart that are responsible for methodically generating and coordinating the transmission of electrical impulses to the myocardial cells

cardiac output: amount of blood pumped by each ventricle in litres per minute

cardiac stress test: a test used to evaluate the functioning of the heart during a period of increased oxygen demand

contractility: ability of the cardiac muscle to shorten in response to an electrical impulse

depolarization: electrical activation of a cell caused by the influx of sodium into the cell while potassium exits the cell

diastole: period of ventricular relaxation resulting in ventricular filling

ejection fraction: percentage of the end-diastolic blood volume ejected from the ventricle with each heartbeat

hemodynamic monitoring: use of pressure monitoring devices to directly measure cardiovascular function

hypertension: blood pressure that is persistently greater than 140/90 mm Hg

hypotension: a decrease in blood pressure to less than 100/60 mm Hg that compromises systemic perfusion

murmurs: sounds created by abnormal, turbulent flow of blood in the heart

myocardial ischemia: condition in which heart muscle cells receive less oxygen than needed

myocardium: muscle layer of the heart responsible for the pumping action of the heart

normal heart sounds: sounds produced when the valves close; normal heart sounds are S_1 (atrioventricular valves) and S_2 (semilunar valves)

opening snaps: abnormal diastolic sound generated during opening of a rigid AV valve leaflet

postural (orthostatic) hypotension: a significant drop in blood pressure (usually 10 mm Hg systolic or more) after an upright posture is assumed

preload: degree of stretch of the cardiac muscle fibres at the end of diastole

pulmonary vascular resistance: resistance to right ventricular ejection of blood

radioisotopes: unstable atoms that emit small amounts of energy in the form of gamma rays; used in cardiac nuclear medicine studies

repolarization: return of the cell to resting state, caused by reentry of potassium into the cell while sodium exits the cell

S_1: the first heart sound produced by closure of the atrioventricular (mitral and tricuspid) valves

S_2: the second heart sound produced by closure of the semilunar (aortic and pulmonic) valves

S_3: an abnormal heart sound detected early in diastole as resistance is met to blood entering either ventricle; most often due to volume overload associated with heart failure

S_4: an abnormal heart sound detected late in diastole as resistance is met to blood entering either ventricle during atrial contraction; most often caused by hypertrophy of the ventricle

sinoatrial (SA) node: primary pacemaker of the heart, located in the right atrium

stroke volume: amount of blood ejected from the ventricle per heartbeat

summation gallop: the abnormal sound created during tachycardia by the presence of an S_3 and S_4

systemic vascular resistance: resistance to left ventricle ejection

systole: period of ventricular contraction resulting in ejection of blood from the ventricles into the pulmonary artery and aorta

systolic click: abnormal systolic sound created by the opening of a calcified aortic or pulmonic valve during ventricular contraction

telemetry: the process of continuous electrocardiographic monitoring by the transmission of radio waves from a battery-operated transmitter worn by the patient

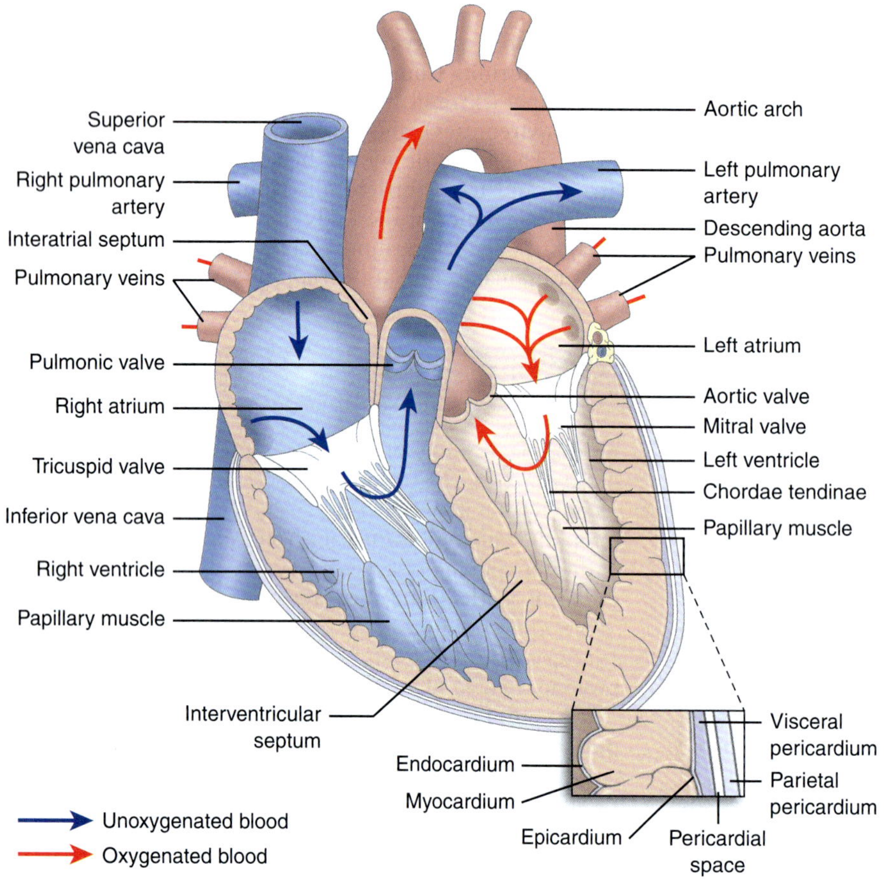

FIGURE 27-1. Structure of the heart. *Arrows* show course of blood flow through the heart chambers.

relationships among the four heart chambers are shown in Figure 27-1.

The varying thicknesses of the atrial and ventricular walls relate to the workload required by each chamber. The myocardial layer of both atria is much thinner than that of the ventricles because there is little resistance as blood flows out of the atria and into the ventricles during diastole. In contrast, the ventricular walls are much thicker than the atrial walls. During ventricular systole, the right and left ventricles must overcome resistance to blood flow from the pulmonary and systemic circulatory systems, respectively. The left ventricle is two-and-a-half times more muscular than the right ventricle. It must overcome high aortic and arterial pressures, whereas the right ventricle contracts against a low-pressure system within the pulmonary arteries and capillaries. Figure 27-2 identifies the pressures in each of these areas.

The heart lies in a rotated position within the chest cavity. The right ventricle lies anteriorly (just beneath the sternum) and the left ventricle is situated posteriorly. As a result of this close proximity to the chest wall, the pulsation created during normal ventricular contraction, called the **apical impulse (also called the point of maximal impulse [PMI])**, is easily detected. In the normal heart, the PMI is located at the intersection of the midclavicular line of the left chest wall and the fifth intercostal space.

Heart Valves

The four valves in the heart permit blood to flow in only one direction. The valves, which are composed of thin leaflets of fibrous tissue, open and close in response to the movement of blood and pressure changes within the chambers. There are two types of valves: atrioventricular and semilunar.

Atrioventricular Valves

The atrioventricular valves separate the atria from the ventricles. The tricuspid valve, so named because it is composed of three cusps or leaflets, separates the right atrium from the right ventricle. The mitral or bicuspid (two cusps) valve lies between the left atrium and the left ventricle (see Fig. 27-1).

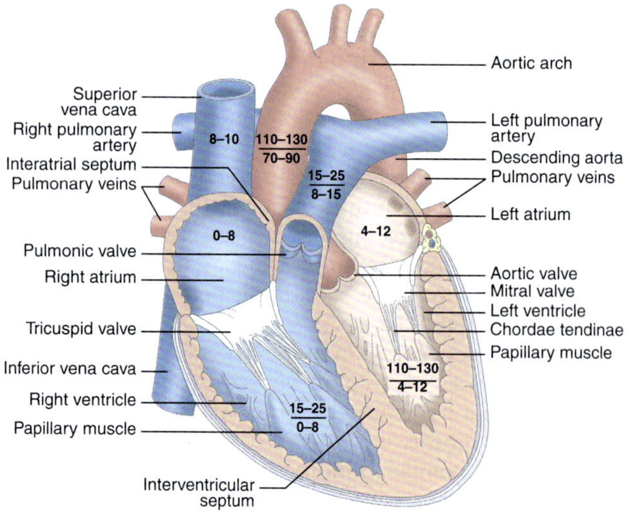

FIGURE 27-2. Great vessel and chamber pressures. Pressures are identified in mm Hg as mean pressure or systolic over diastolic pressure.

During diastole, the tricuspid and mitral valves are open, allowing the blood in the atria to flow freely into the relaxed ventricles. As ventricular systole begins, the ventricles contract and blood flows upward into the cusps of the tricuspid and mitral valves, causing them to close. As the pressure against these valves increases, two additional structures, the papillary muscles and the chordae tendineae, maintain valve closure. The papillary muscles, located on the sides of the ventricular walls, are connected to the valve leaflets by thin fibrous bands called chordae tendineae. During ventricular systole, contraction of the papillary muscles causes the chordae tendineae to become taut, keeping the valve leaflets approximated and closed. This action prevents backflow of blood into the atria (regurgitation) as blood is ejected out into the pulmonary artery and aorta.

Semilunar Valves

The two semilunar valves are composed of three leaflets, which are shaped like half-moons. The valve between the right ventricle and the pulmonary artery is called the pulmonic valve. The valve between the left ventricle and the aorta is called the aortic valve. The semilunar valves are closed during diastole. At this point, the pressure in the pulmonary artery and aorta decreases, causing blood to flow back toward the semilunar valves. This action fills the cusps with blood and closes the valves. The semilunar valves are forced open during ventricular systole as blood is ejected from the right and left ventricles into the pulmonary artery and aorta.

Coronary Arteries

The left and right coronary arteries and their branches supply arterial blood to the heart. These arteries originate from the aorta just above the aortic valve leaflets. The heart has high metabolic requirements, extracting approximately 70% to 80% of the oxygen delivered (other organs extract, on average, 25%). Unlike other arteries, the coronary arteries are perfused during diastole. With a normal heart rate of 60 to 80 bpm there is ample time during diastole for myocardial perfusion. However, as heart rate increases, diastolic time is shortened, which may not allow adequate time for myocardial perfusion. As a result, patients are at risk for **myocardial ischemia** (inadequate oxygen supply) during tachycardias (heart rate greater than 100), especially patients with CAD.

The left coronary artery has three branches. The artery from the point of origin to the first major branch is called the left main coronary artery. Two branches arise from the left main coronary artery: the left anterior descending artery, which courses down the anterior wall of the heart, and the circumflex artery, which circles around to the lateral left wall of the heart.

The right side of the heart is supplied by the right coronary artery, which leads to the inferior wall of the heart. The posterior wall of the heart receives its blood supply by an additional branch from the right coronary artery called the posterior descending artery (see Chapter 29).

Superficial to the coronary arteries are the coronary veins. Venous blood from these veins returns to the heart primarily through the coronary sinus, which is located posteriorly in the right atrium.

Myocardium

The myocardium is the middle, muscular layer of the atrial and ventricular walls. It is composed of specialized cells called myocytes, which form an interconnected network of muscle fibres. These fibres encircle the heart in a figure-of-eight pattern, forming a spiral from the base (top) of the heart to the apex (bottom). During contraction, this muscular configuration facilitates a twisting and compressive movement of the heart that begins in the atria and moves to the ventricles. The sequential and rhythmic pattern of contraction, followed by relaxation of the muscle fibres, maximizes the volume of blood ejected with each contraction. This cyclical pattern of myocardial contraction is controlled by the conduction system.

Function of the Heart

Cardiac Electrophysiology

The **cardiac conduction system** generates and transmits electrical impulses that stimulate contraction of the myocardium. Under normal circumstances, the conduction system first stimulates contraction of the atria and then the ventricles. The synchronization of the atrial and ventricular events allows the ventricles to fill completely before ventricular ejection, thereby maximizing **cardiac output**. Three physiologic characteristics of two types of specialized electrical cells, the nodal cells and the Purkinje cells, provide this synchronization:

Automaticity: ability to initiate an electrical impulse
Excitability: ability to respond to an electrical impulse
Conductivity: ability to transmit an electrical impulse from one cell to another

Both the **sinoatrial (SA) node** and the **atrioventricular (AV) node** are composed of nodal cells. The SA node, the primary pacemaker of the heart, is located at the junction of the superior vena cava and the right atrium (Fig. 27-3). The SA node in a normal resting adult heart has an inherent firing rate of 60 to 100 impulses per minute, but the rate changes in response to the metabolic demands of the body.

The electrical impulses initiated by the SA node are conducted along the myocardial cells of the atria via specialized

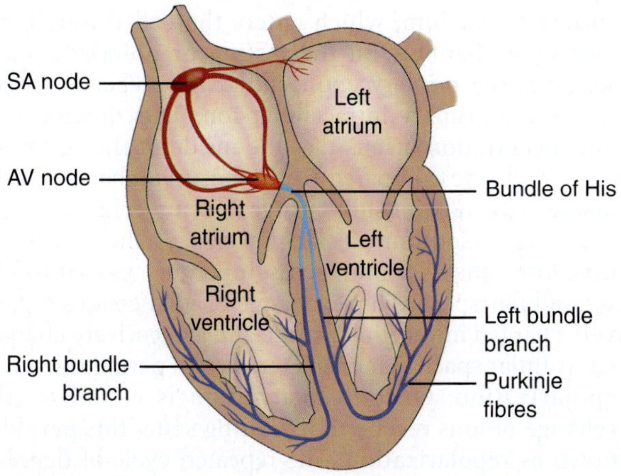

FIGURE 27-3. Cardiac conduction system. AV, atrioventricular; SA, sinoatrial.

tracts called internodal pathways. The impulses cause electrical stimulation and subsequent contraction of the atria. The impulses are then conducted to the AV node, which is located in the right atrial wall near the tricuspid valve (see Fig. 27-3). The AV node coordinates the incoming electrical impulses from the atria and after a slight delay (allowing the atria time to contract and complete ventricular filling) relays the impulse to the ventricles.

Initially, the impulse is conducted through a bundle of specialized conducting tissue, referred to as the bundle of His, which then divides into the right bundle branch (conducting impulses to the right ventricle) and the left bundle branch (conducting impulses to the left ventricle). To transmit impulses to the left ventricle, the largest chamber of the heart, the left bundle branch divides into the left anterior and left posterior bundle branches. Impulses travel through the bundle branches to reach the terminal point in the conduction system, called the Purkinje fibres. These fibres are composed of Purkinje cells, specialized to rapidly conduct the impulses through the thick walls of the ventricles. This is the point at which the myocardial cells are stimulated, causing ventricular contraction.

The heart rate is determined by the myocardial cells with the fastest inherent firing rate. Under normal circumstances, the SA node has the highest inherent rate (60 to 100 impulses per minute), the AV node has the second-highest inherent rate (40 to 60 impulses per minute), and the ventricular pacemaker sites have the lowest inherent rate (30 to 40 impulses per minute). If the SA node malfunctions, the AV node generally takes over the pacemaker function of the heart at its inherently lower rate. Should both the SA and the AV nodes fail in their pacemaker function, a pacemaker site in the ventricle will fire at its inherent bradycardic rate of 30 to 40 impulses per minute.

Cardiac Action Potential

The nodal and Purkinje cells (electrical cells) generate and transmit impulses across the heart, stimulating the cardiac myocytes (working cells) to contract. Stimulation of the myocytes occurs due to the exchange of electrically charged particles, called ions, across channels located in the cell membrane. The channels regulate the movement and speed of specific ions, namely, sodium, potassium, and calcium, as they enter and exit the cell. Sodium rapidly enters into the cell through sodium fast channels, in contrast to calcium, which enters the cell through calcium slow channels. In the resting or polarized state, sodium is the primary extracellular ion, whereas potassium is the primary intracellular ion. This difference in ion concentration means that the inside of the cell has a negative charge compared to the positive charge on the outside. This relationship changes during cellular stimulation, when sodium or calcium crosses the cell membrane into the cell and potassium ions exit into the extracellular space. This exchange of ions creates a positively charged intracellular space and a negatively charged extracellular space that characterizes the period known as **depolarization**. Once depolarization is complete, the exchange of ions reverts to its resting state; this period is known as **repolarization**. The repeated cycle of depolarization and repolarization is called the cardiac action potential.

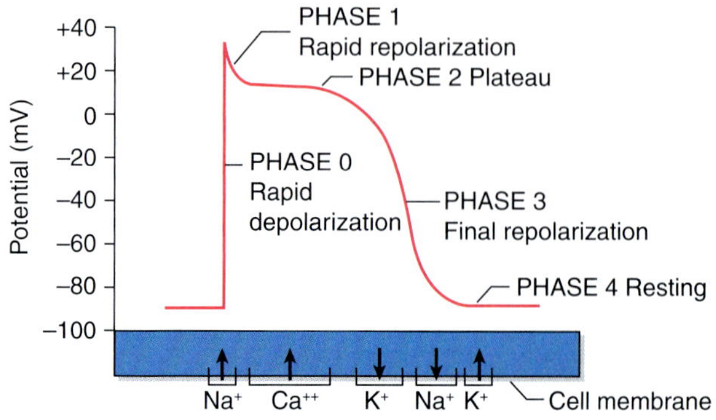

FIGURE 27-4. Cardiac action potential of a fast-response Purkinje fibre. The *arrows* indicate the approximate time and direction of movement of each ion influencing membrane potential. Ca^{++} movement out of the cell is not well defined but is thought to occur during phase 4.

As shown in Figure 27-4, the cardiac action potential has five phases:

- Phase 0: Cellular depolarization is initiated as positive ions influx into the cell. During this phase, the atrial and ventricular myocytes rapidly depolarize as sodium moves into the cells through sodium fast channels. The myocytes have a fast response action potential. In contrast, the cells of the SA and AV node depolarize when calcium enters these cells through calcium slow channels. These cells have a slow response action potential.
- Phase 1: Early cellular repolarization begins during this phase as potassium exits the intracellular space.
- Phase 2: This phase is called the plateau phase because the rate of repolarization slows. Calcium ions enter the intracellular space.
- Phase 3: This phase marks the completion of repolarization and return of the cell to its resting state.
- Phase 4: This phase is considered the resting phase before the next depolarization.

Refractory Periods

As reviewed previously, myocardial cells must completely repolarize before they can depolarize again. During this time, the cells are in what is called a refractory period. There are two phases of the refractory period, the effective (or absolute) refractory period and the relative refractory period. During the effective refractory period, the cell is completely unresponsive to any electrical stimulus; it is incapable of initiating an early depolarization. The effective refractory period corresponds with the time in phase 0 to the middle of phase 3 of the action potential. The relative refractory period corresponds with the short time at the end of phase 3. During the relative refractory period, if an electrical stimulus is stronger than normal, the cell may depolarize prematurely. Early depolarizations of the atrium or ventricle cause premature contractions, placing the patient at risk for dysrhythmias. Premature ventricular contractions in certain situations, such as the presence of myocardial ischemia, are of concern because these early ventricular depolarizations can trigger life-threatening dysrhythmias, including ventricular tachycardia or ventricular fibrillation. Several circumstances make the heart more susceptible to early depolarization during the relative refractory period, thus increasing the risk for serious dysrhythmias. These dysrhythmias and others are discussed in detail in Chapter 28.

Cardiac Hemodynamics

An important determinant of blood flow in the cardiovascular system is the principle that fluid flows from a region of higher pressure to one of lower pressure (see Fig. 27-2). The pressures responsible for blood flow in the normal circulation are generated during systole and diastole.

Cardiac Cycle

A cardiac cycle is composed of both systole and diastole. It refers to the events that occur in the heart from one heartbeat to the next. These events cause blood to flow through the heart due to changes in chamber pressures and valvular function during atrial and ventricular diastole and systole. During atrial and ventricular diastole, the heart chambers are relaxed. As a result, the AV valves are open, whereas the semilunar valves are closed. Pressures in all of the chambers are the lowest during diastole, which facilitates ventricular filling. Venous blood returns to the right atrium from the superior and inferior vena cava, then into the right ventricle. On the left side, oxygenated blood returns from the lungs via the four pulmonary veins into the left atrium and ventricle.

Toward the end of this diastolic period, atrial systole occurs as the atrial muscles contract in response to an electrical impulse initiated by the SA node. Atrial systole increases the pressure inside the atria, ejecting the remaining blood into the ventricles. Atrial systole augments ventricular blood volume by 15% to 25% and is sometimes referred to as the "atrial kick." At this point, ventricular systole begins in response to propagation of the electrical impulse that began in the SA node some milliseconds earlier.

Beginning with ventricular systole, the pressure inside the ventricles rapidly increases, forcing the AV valves to close. As a result, blood ceases to flow from the atria into the ventricles, and regurgitation (backflow) of blood into the atria is prevented. The rapid increase of pressure inside the right and left ventricles forces the pulmonic and aortic valves to open, and blood is ejected into the pulmonary artery and aorta, respectively. The exit of blood is at first rapid; then, as the pressure in each ventricle and its corresponding artery equalizes, the flow of blood gradually decreases. At the end of systole, pressure within the right and left ventricles rapidly decreases. As a result, pulmonary arterial and aortic pressures decrease, causing closure of the semilunar valves. These events mark the onset of diastole and the cardiac cycle is repeated.

Chamber pressures can be measured with the use of special monitoring catheters and equipment. This technique is called **hemodynamic monitoring**. Methods of hemodynamic monitoring are covered in more detail at the end of this chapter.

Cardiac Output

Cardiac output refers to the amount of blood pumped by each ventricle during a given period. The cardiac output in a resting adult is about 5 L/min but varies greatly depending on the metabolic needs of the body. Cardiac output is computed by multiplying the stroke volume by the heart rate. Stroke volume is the amount of blood ejected per heartbeat. The average resting **stroke volume** is about 70 mL, and the heart rate is 60 to 80 bpm. Cardiac output can be affected by changes in either stroke volume or heart rate.

EFFECT OF HEART RATE ON CARDIAC OUTPUT. Cardiac output must be responsive to changes in the metabolic demands of the tissues. For example, during exercise the total cardiac output may increase fourfold, to 20 L/min. This increase is normally accomplished by approximately doubling both the heart rate and the stroke volume. Changes in heart rate are accomplished by reflex controls mediated by the autonomic nervous system, including its sympathetic and parasympathetic divisions.

The parasympathetic impulses, which travel to the heart through the vagus nerve, can slow the cardiac rate, whereas sympathetic impulses increase it. These effects on heart rate result from action on the SA node, to either decrease or increase its inherent rate. The balance between these two reflex control systems normally determines the heart rate. The heart rate is increased by the sympathetic nervous system through an increased level of circulating catecholamines (secreted by the adrenal gland) and by excess thyroid hormone, which produces a catecholamine-like effect.

In addition, the heart rate is affected by central nervous system and baroreceptor activity. **Baroreceptors** are specialized nerve cells located in the aortic arch and in both right and left internal carotid arteries (at the point of bifurcation from the common carotid arteries). The baroreceptors are sensitive to changes in blood pressure (BP). During significant elevations in BP (**hypertension**), these cells increase their rate of discharge, transmitting impulses to the cerebral medulla. This initiates parasympathetic activity and inhibits sympathetic response, lowering the heart rate and the BP. The opposite is true during **hypotension** (low BP). Hypotension results in less baroreceptor stimulation, which prompts a decrease in parasympathetic inhibitory activity in the SA node, allowing for enhanced sympathetic activity. The resultant vasoconstriction and increased heart rate elevate the BP.

EFFECT OF STROKE VOLUME ON CARDIAC OUTPUT. Stroke volume is primarily determined by three factors: **preload**, **afterload**, and **contractility**.

Preload refers to the degree of stretch of the ventricular cardiac muscle fibres at the end of diastole. The end of diastole is the period when filling volume in the ventricles is the highest and the degree of stretch on the muscle fibres is the greatest. The volume of blood within the ventricle at the end of diastole determines preload, which directly affects stroke volume. Therefore, preload is commonly referred to as left ventricular end-diastolic pressure (LVEDP). As the volume of blood returning to the heart increases, muscle fibre stretch also increases (increased preload), resulting in stronger contraction and a greater stroke volume. This relationship, called the Frank–Starling (or Starling) law of the heart, is maintained until the physiologic limit of the muscle is reached.

The Frank–Starling law is based on the fact that, within limits, the greater the initial length or stretch of the cardiac muscle cells (sarcomeres), the greater the degree of shortening that occurs. This result is caused by increased interaction between the thick and thin filaments within the cardiac muscle cells. Preload is decreased by a reduction in the volume of blood returning to the ventricles. Diuresis, venodilating agents (e.g., nitrates), excessive loss of blood, or dehydration (excessive loss of body fluids from vomiting, diarrhea, or diaphoresis) reduce preload. Preload is increased by increasing the return of circulating blood volume to the ventricles. Controlling the loss of blood or body fluids and replacing fluids (i.e., blood transfusions and intravenous [IV] fluid administration) are examples of ways to increase preload.

Afterload, or resistance to ejection of blood from the ventricle, is the second determinant of stroke volume. The resistance of the systemic BP to left ventricular ejection is called **systemic vascular resistance**. The resistance of the pulmonary BP to right ventricular ejection is called **pulmonary vascular resistance**. There is an inverse relationship between afterload and stroke volume. For example, afterload is increased by arterial vasoconstriction, which leads to decreased stroke volume. The opposite is true with arterial vasodilation: Afterload is reduced because there is less resistance to ejection, and stroke volume increases.

Contractility refers to the force generated by the contracting myocardium. Contractility is enhanced by circulating catecholamines, sympathetic neuronal activity, and certain medications (e.g., digoxin [Lanoxin], dopamine [Intropin], or dobutamine [Dobutrex]). Increased contractility results in increased stroke volume. Contractility is depressed by hypoxemia, acidosis, and certain medications (e.g., beta-adrenergic blocking agents such as atenolol [Tenormin]).

The heart can achieve an increase in stroke volume (e.g., during exercise) if preload is increased (through increased venous return), if contractility is increased (through sympathetic nervous system discharge), and if afterload is decreased (through peripheral vasodilation with decreased aortic pressure).

The percentage of the end-diastolic blood volume that is ejected with each heartbeat is called the **ejection fraction**. The ejection fraction of the normal left ventricle is 55% to 65%. The right ventricular ejection fraction is rarely measured. The ejection fraction is used as a measure of myocardial contractility. An ejection fraction of less than 40% indicates that the patient has decreased left ventricular function and likely requires treatment for heart failure (HF) (refer to Chapter 30 for further discussion).

Gerontologic Considerations

Changes in cardiac structure and function are clearly observable in the aging heart. To understand the changes specifically related to aging, it is helpful to distinguish the normal aging process from changes related to CVD. The anatomic and functional changes in the aging heart are summarized in Table 27-1.

These changes lead to decreased myocardial contractility, increased left ventricular ejection time (prolonged systole), and delayed conduction. Therefore, stressful physical and emotional conditions, especially those that occur suddenly, may have adverse effects on the aged person. The heart cannot respond to such conditions with an adequate rate increase and needs more time to return to a normal resting rate after even a minimal increase in heart rate. In some patients, the added stress may precipitate HF.

Gender Considerations

Structural differences between the hearts of men and women have significant implications. The heart of a woman tends to be smaller than that of a man. The coronary arteries of a woman are also narrower in diameter than a man's arteries. When atherosclerosis occurs, these differences make procedures such as **cardiac catheterization** and angioplasty technically more difficult.

Women typically develop CAD 10 years later than men, as women have the benefit of the female hormone estrogen and its cardioprotective effects. The three major effects of estrogen are (1) an increase in high-density lipoprotein (HDL) that transports cholesterol out of arteries; (2) a reduction in low-density lipoprotein (LDL) that deposits cholesterol in the artery; and (3) dilatation of the blood vessels, which enhance blood flow to the heart. As women reach menopause, around 50 years of age, estrogen levels slowly disappear and place women at higher risk for CAD. By age 45 years for men and 55 years of age for women, the risk for CAD is equivalent (McSweeney, Rosenfeld, Abel, et al., 2016).

In the past, hormone therapy (HT) was routinely prescribed for postmenopausal women with the belief that it would deter the onset and progression of CAD. However, the AHA no longer recommends its use due to strong evidence that HT is not a beneficial CAD preventative strategy for women (McSweeney et al., 2016). In fact, recent studies report that HT after menopause can be harmful to women by putting them at increased risk for stroke and venous thromboembolic events (Boardman, Hartley, Eisinga, et al., 2015).

Assessment of the Cardiovascular System

The frequency and extent of the nursing assessment of cardiovascular function are based on several factors, including the severity of the patient's symptoms, the presence of risk factors, the practice setting, and the purpose of the assessment. An acutely ill patient with CVD who is admitted to the emergency department or coronary intensive care unit requires a very different assessment than a person who is being examined for a chronic stable condition. Although the key components of the cardiovascular assessment remain the same, the assessment priorities vary according to the needs of the patient. For example, an emergency department nurse performs a rapid and focused assessment of a patient in which **acute coronary syndrome** (ACS), rupture of an atheromatous plaque in a diseased coronary artery, is suspected. Diagnosis and treatment must be started within minutes of arrival to the emergency department. The physical assessment is ongoing and concentrates on evaluating the patient for ACS complications, such as dysrhythmias and HF, and determining the effectiveness of medical treatment.

Health History

The patient's ability to recognize cardiac symptoms and to know what to do when they occur is essential for effective self-care management. All too often, a patient's new symptoms or those of progressing cardiac dysfunction go

TABLE 27-1 Age-Related Changes of the Cardiac System

Cardiovascular Structure	Structural Changes	Functional Changes	History and Physical Findings
Atria	↑ Size of left atrium Thickening of the endocardium	↑ Atrial irritability	Irregular heart rhythm from atrial dysrhythmias
Left ventricle	Endocardial fibrosis Myocardial thickening (hypertrophy) Infiltration of fat into myocardium	Left ventricle stiff and less compliant Progressive decline in cardiac output ↑ Risk for ventricular dysrhythmias Prolonged systole	Fatigue ↓ Exercise tolerance Signs and symptoms of HF or ventricular dysrhythmias Point of maximal impulse palpated lateral to the midclavicular line ↓ Intensity S_1, S_2; split S_2 S_4 may be present
Valves	Thickening and rigidity of AV valves Calcification of aortic valve	Abnormal blood flow across valves during cardiac cycle	Murmurs may be present Thrill may be palpated if significant murmur is present
Conduction system	Connective tissue collects in SA node, AV node, and bundle branches ↓ Number of SA node cells ↓ Number of AV, bundle of His, and right and left bundle branch cells	Slower SA node rate of impulse discharge Slowed conduction across AV node and ventricular conduction system	Bradycardia Heart block ECG changes consistent with slowed conduction (↑ PR interval, widened QRS complex)
Sympathetic nervous system	↓ Response to beta-adrenergic stimulation	↓ Adaptive response to exercise: contractility and heart rate slower to respond to exercise demands Heart rate takes more time to return to baseline	Fatigue Diminished exercise tolerance ↓ Ability to respond to stress
Aorta and arteries	Stiffening of vasculature ↓ Elasticity and widening of aorta Elongation of aorta, displacing the brachiocephalic artery upward	Left ventricular hypertrophy	Progressive increase in systolic BP; slight ↑ in diastolic BP Widening pulse pressure Pulsation visible above right clavicle
Baroreceptor response	↓ Sensitivity of baroreceptors in the carotid artery and aorta to transient episodes of hypertension and hypotension	Baroreceptors unable to regulate heart rate and vascular tone, causing slow response to postural changes in body position	Postural blood pressure changes and reports of feeling dizzy, fainting when moving from lying to sitting or standing position

AV, atrioventricular; BP, blood pressure; ECG, electrocardiographic; HF, heart failure; SA, sinoatrial.

Adapted from Bickley, L. S. (2014). *Bates' guide to physical examination and history taking* (11th ed.). Philadelphia, PA: Lippincott Williams & Wilkins.

unrecognized. This results in prolonged delays in seeking lifesaving treatment. Major barriers to seeking prompt medical care include lack of knowledge about the symptoms of heart disease, attributing symptoms to a benign source, denying symptom significance, and feeling embarrassed about having symptoms (Gillis, Arslanian-Engoren, & Struble, 2014). Therefore, during the health history the nurse needs to determine if the patient and involved family members are able to recognize symptoms of an acute cardiac problem, such as ACS or HF, and seek timely treatment for these symptoms. Responses to this level of inquiry will help the nurse individualize the plan for patient and family education.

Common Symptoms

The signs and symptoms experienced by people with CVD are related to dysrhythmias and conduction problems (see Chapter 28); CAD (see Chapter 29); structural, infectious, and inflammatory disorders of the heart (see Chapter 30); and complications of CVD such as HF and cardiogenic shock (see Chapter 31). These disorders have many signs and symptoms in common; therefore, the nurse must be skillful at recognizing these signs and symptoms so that patients are given timely and often lifesaving care.

The following are the most common signs and symptoms of CVD, with related medical diagnoses in parentheses:

- Chest pain or discomfort (angina pectoris, ACS, dysrhythmias, valvular heart disease)
- Shortness of breath or dyspnea (ACS, cardiogenic shock, HF, valvular heart disease)
- Peripheral edema, weight gain, abdominal distention due to enlarged spleen and liver or ascites (HF)
- Palpitations (tachycardia from a variety of causes, including ACS, caffeine or other stimulants, electrolyte imbalances, stress, valvular heart disease, ventricular aneurysms)
- Vital fatigue, sometimes referred to as vital exhaustion (an early warning symptom of ACS, HF, or valvular heart disease, characterized by feeling unusually tired or fatigued, irritable, and dejected)
- Dizziness, syncope, or changes in level of consciousness (cardiogenic shock, cerebrovascular disorders, dysrhythmias, hypotension, postural hypotension, vasovagal episode)

Chest Pain

Chest pain and discomfort are common symptoms that may be caused by a number of cardiac and noncardiac problems. When a patient experiences chest symptoms, the nurse asks questions that aid in differentiating among these sources of chest symptoms. Table 27-2 summarizes the characteristics and patterns of the more common cardiac and noncardiac causes of chest symptoms. During the assessment the patient is asked to identify the quantity of pain using a 0 (no pain) to 10 (worst pain) scale. Next, the nurse asks the patient to describe the character or quality of the pain or discomfort and its location. The nurse needs to determine whether there is radiation to or discomfort in other areas and must assess for associated signs and symptoms such as diaphoresis or nausea. It is important to identify the events that precipitate the onset of symptoms, the duration of the symptoms, and measures that aggravate or relieve the symptoms.

The nurse should keep the following important points in mind when assessing patients reporting chest pain or discomfort:

- The location of chest symptoms is not well correlated with the cause of the pain. For example, substernal chest pain can result from a number of causes as outlined in Table 27-2.
- The severity or duration of chest pain or discomfort does not predict the seriousness of its cause. For example, a patient experiencing esophageal spasm may rate chest pain as a "10/10" (e.g., the worst pain the patient has ever felt), whereas a patient experiencing a myocardial infarction (MI) may report only mild to moderate chest pressure.
- More than one clinical cardiac condition may occur simultaneously. During an MI, patients may report chest pain from myocardial ischemia, shortness of breath from HF, and palpitations from dysrhythmias. Both HF and dysrhythmias can be complications of an acute MI.

TABLE 27-2 Assessing Chest Pain

Location	Character	Duration	Precipitating Events and Aggravating Factors	Alleviating Factors
Angina pectoris ***Acute coronary syndrome*** (ACS) (unstable angina, myocardial infarction [MI]) 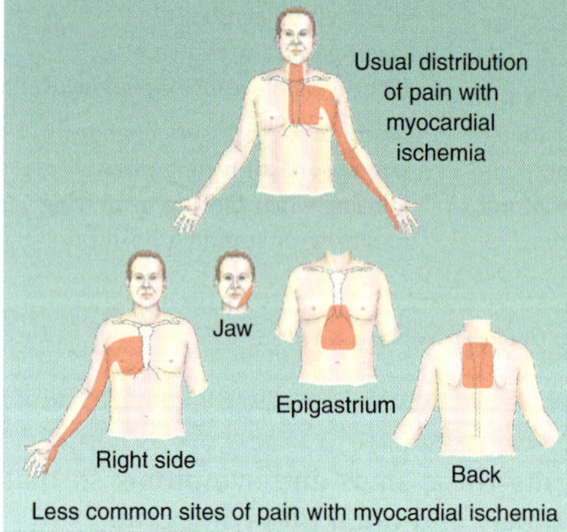 Less common sites of pain with myocardial ischemia	Angina: Uncomfortable pressure, squeezing, or fullness in substernal chest area Can radiate across chest to the medial aspect of one or both arms and hands, jaw, shoulders, upper back, or epigastrium Radiation to arms and hands, described as numbness, tingling, or aching	Angina: 5–15 minutes	Angina: Physical exertion, emotional upset, eating large meal, or exposure to extremes in temperature	Angina: Rest, nitroglycerin, oxygen
	ACS: Same as angina pectoris Pain or discomfort ranges from mild to severe Associated with shortness of breath, diaphoresis, palpitations, fatigue, and nausea or vomiting	ACS: >15 minutes	ACS: Emotional upset or unusual physical exertion occurring within 24 hours of symptom onset Can occur at rest or while asleep	ACS: Morphine, reperfusion of coronary artery with thrombolytic agent or percutaneous coronary intervention
Pericarditis 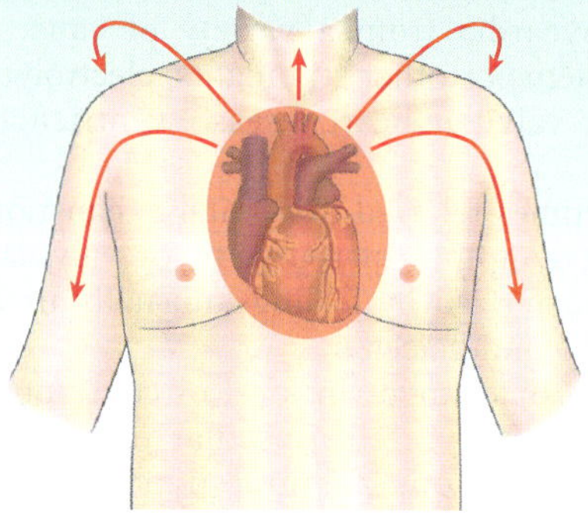	Sharp, severe substernal or epigastric pain Can radiate to neck, arms, and back Associated symptoms include fever, malaise, dyspnea, cough, nausea, dizziness, and palpitations	Intermittent	Sudden onset Pain increases with inspiration, swallowing, coughing, and rotation of trunk	Sitting upright, analgesia, anti-inflammatory medications

TABLE 27-2 Assessing Chest Pain (Continued)

Location	Character	Duration	Precipitating Events and Aggravating Factors	Alleviating Factors
Pulmonary disorders (pneumonia, pulmonary embolism) 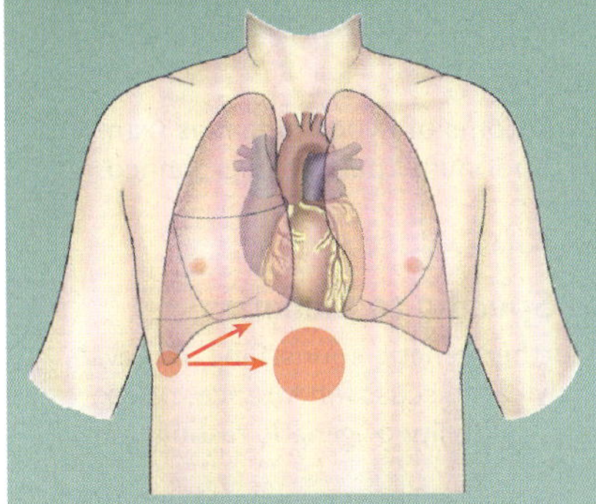	Sharp, severe substernal or epigastric pain arising from inferior portion of pleura (referred to as pleuritic pain). Patient may be able to localize the pain	≥30 minutes	Follows an infectious or noninfectious process (MI, cardiac surgery, cancer, immune disorders, uremia) Pleuritic pain increases with inspiration, coughing, movement, and supine positioning Occurs in conjunction with community-acquired or nosocomial lung infections (pneumonia) or deep vein thrombosis (pulmonary embolism)	Treatment of underlying cause
Esophageal disorders (hiatal hernia, reflux esophagitis or spasm) 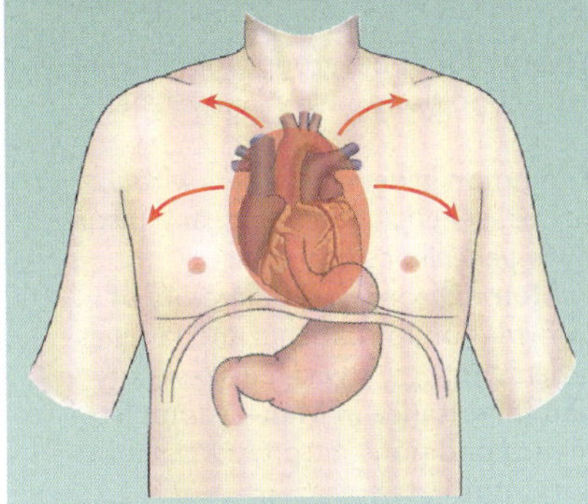	Substernal pain described as sharp, burning, or heavy Often mimics angina Can radiate to neck, arm, or shoulders	5–60 minutes	Recumbency, cold liquids, exercise	Food or antacid Nitroglycerin
Anxiety and panic disorders 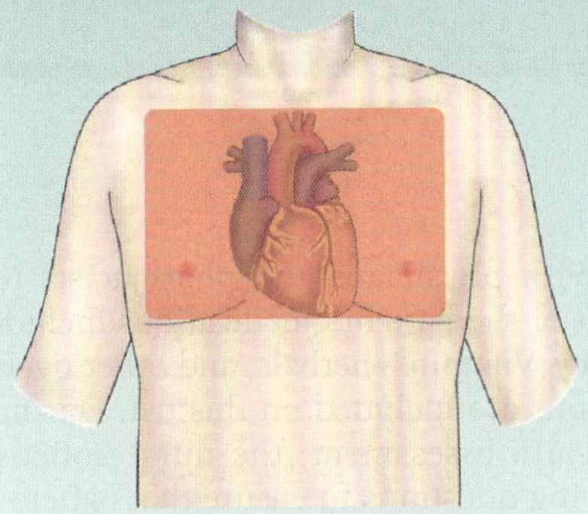	Pain described as stabbing to dull ache Associated with diaphoresis, palpitations, shortness of breath, tingling of hands or mouth, feeling of unreality, or fear of losing control	Peaks in 10 minutes	Can occur at any time including during sleep Can be associated with a specific trigger	Removal of stimulus, relaxation, medications to treat anxiety or underlying disorder
Musculoskeletal disorders (costochondritis) 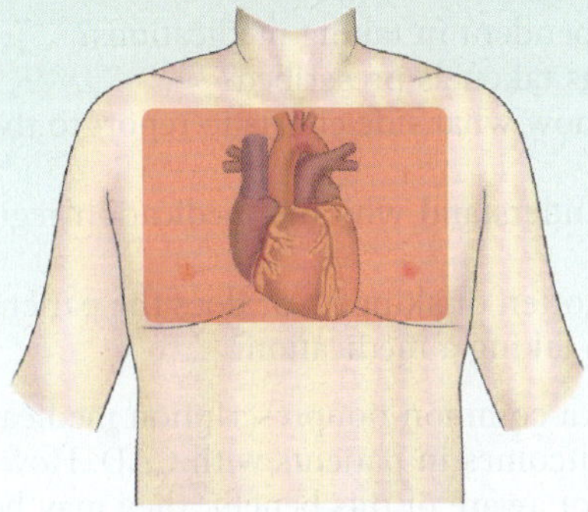	Sharp or stabbing pain localized in anterior chest Most often unilateral Can radiate across chest to epigastrium or back	Hours to days	Most often follows respiratory tract infection with significant coughing, vigorous exercise, or posttrauma Some cases are idiopathic Exacerbated by deep inspiration, coughing, sneezing, and movement of upper torso or arms	Rest, ice, or heat Analgesic or anti-inflammatory medications

Adapted from Bickley, L. S. (2014). *Bates' guide to physical examination and history taking* (11th ed.). Philadelphia, PA: Lippincott Williams & Wilkins; King, J. E., & Magdic, K. S. (2014). Chest pain: A time for concern? *AACN Advanced Critical Care*, *25*(3), 279–283; Woods, S. L., Froelicher, E. S., Motzer, S. A., et al. (2009). *Cardiac nursing* (6th ed.). Philadelphia, PA: Lippincott Williams & Wilkins.

GENETICS IN NURSING PRACTICE

Chart 27-1. Cardiovascular Disorders

Several cardiovascular disorders are associated with genetic abnormalities. Some examples are:

- Arrhythmogenic right ventricular dysplasia (ARVD)
- Brugada syndrome
- Familial hypercholesterolemia
- Hypertrophic cardiomyopathy
- Long QT syndrome
    - Jervell and Lange-Nielsen syndrome (autosomal recessive form)
    - Romano-Ward syndrome (autosomal dominant form)

Genetic connective tissue disorders that impact the cardiovascular system:

- Ehlers-Danlos syndrome
- Loeys-Dietz syndrome
- Marfan syndrome

Genetic blood disorders that can impair the function of the cardiovascular system:

- Factor V Leiden
- Hemochromatosis
- Sickle cell disease

Nursing Assessments

FAMILY HISTORY ASSESSMENT

- Assess all patients with cardiovascular symptoms for coronary artery disease (CAD), regardless of age (early-onset CAD occurs).
- Assess family history of sudden death in people who may or may not have been diagnosed with coronary disease (especially of early onset).
- Ask about sudden death in a previously asymptomatic child, adolescent, or adult.
- Ask about other family members with biochemical or neuromuscular conditions (e.g., hemochromatosis or muscular dystrophy).
- Assess whether DNA mutation or other genetic testing has been performed on an affected family member.

Patient Assessment

- Assess for signs and symptoms of hyperlipidemias (xanthomas, corneal arcus, abdominal pain of unexplained origin).
- Assess for muscular weakness.

Management Issues Specific to Genetics

- If indicated, refer for further genetic counselling and evaluation so that the family can discuss inheritance, risk to other family members, availability of genetic testing, and gene-based interventions.
- Offer appropriate genetic information and resources (e.g., Genetic Alliance website, Heart and Stroke Foundation of Canada).
- Provide support to families newly diagnosed with genetics-related cardiovascular disease.

Genetics Resources

Genetic Alliance—a directory of support groups for patients and families with genetic conditions, http://www.geneticalliance.org

Gene Tests—a listing of common genetic disorders with up-to-date clinical summaries, genetic counselling, and testing information, http://www.geneclinics.org

National Organization of Rare Disorders—a directory of support groups and information for patients and families with rare genetic disorders, http://www.rarediseases.org

OMIM: Online Mendelian Inheritance in Man—a complete listing of inherited genetic conditions, http://www.ncbi.nlm.nih.gov/omim/stats/html

Past Health, Family, and Social History

In an effort to determine how the patient perceives his or her current health status, the nurse must ask some of the following questions:

- How is your health? Have you noticed any changes from last year? From 5 years ago?
- Do you have a cardiologist or primary provider? How often do you go for checkups?
- What health concerns do you have?
- Do you have a family history of genetic disorders that place you at risk for CVD (see Chart 27-1)?
- What are your risk factors for CAD?
- What do you do to stay healthy and take care of your heart?

Patients who do not understand that their behaviours or diagnoses pose a threat to their health may be less motivated to make lifestyle changes or to manage their illness effectively. On the other hand, patients who perceive that their modifiable risk factors for heart disease affect their health and believe that they have the power to modify or change them may be more likely to change these behaviours.

Medications

Nurses collaborate with physicians and pharmacists to obtain a complete list of the patient's medications including dose and frequency. Vitamins, herbals, and other over-the-counter medications are included on this list. During this aspect of the health assessment, the nurse solicits answers to the following questions to ensure that patients are safely and effectively taking their medications.

- Is the patient independent in taking medications?
- Are the medications taken as prescribed?
- Does the patient know what side effects to report to the prescriber?
- Does the patient understand why the medication regimen is important?
- Are doses ever forgotten or skipped, or does the patient ever decide to stop taking a medication?

An aspirin a day is a common nonprescription medication that improves outcomes in patients with CAD. However, if patients are not aware of this benefit, they may be inclined to stop taking aspirin if they think it is a trivial medication. A careful medication history often uncovers common medication errors and causes for nonadherence to the medication regimen.

Nutrition

Dietary modifications, exercise, weight loss, and careful monitoring are important strategies for managing three major cardiovascular risk factors: hyperlipidemia, hypertension, and diabetes mellitus. Diets that are restricted in sodium, fat, cholesterol, or calories are commonly prescribed. The nurse obtains the following information:

- The patient's current height and weight (to determine body mass index [BMI]), waist measurement (assessment for obesity), BP, and any laboratory test results such as blood glucose, glycosylated hemoglobin (diabetes), total blood cholesterol, HDL and LDL levels, and triglyceride levels (hyperlipidemia)
- How often the patient self-monitors BP, blood glucose, and weight as appropriate to the medical diagnoses
- The patient's level of awareness regarding his or her target goals for each of the risk factors, and any problems achieving or maintaining these goals
- What the patient normally eats and drinks in a typical day and any food preferences (including cultural or ethnic preferences)
- Eating habits (canned or commercially prepared foods vs. fresh foods, restaurant cooking vs. home cooking, assessing for high-sodium foods, dietary intake of fats)
- Who shops for groceries and prepares meals

Elimination

Typical bowel and bladder habits need to be identified. Nocturia (awakening at night to urinate) is common in patients with HF. Fluid collected in gravity-dependent tissues (extremities) during the day (i.e., edema) redistributes into the circulatory system once the patient is recumbent at night. The increased circulatory volume is excreted by the kidneys (increased urine production).

When straining during defecation, the patient bears down (the Valsalva manoeuvre), which momentarily increases pressure on the baroreceptors. This triggers a vagal response, causing the heart rate to slow and resulting in syncope in some patients. Straining during urination can produce the same response.

Because many cardiac medications can cause gastrointestinal side effects or bleeding, the nurse asks about bloating, diarrhea, constipation, stomach upset, heartburn, loss of appetite, nausea, and vomiting. Patients taking platelet-inhibiting medications such as aspirin and clopidogrel (Plavix); platelet aggregation inhibitors such as abciximab (ReoPro), eptifibatide (Integrilin), and tirofiban (Aggrastat); and anticoagulants such as low–molecular-weight heparin (i.e., dalteparin [Fragmin], enoxaparin [Lovenox]), heparin, or warfarin (Coumadin) are screened for bloody urine or stools.

Activity and Exercise

As the nurse assesses the patient's activity and exercise history, it is important to note that decreases in activity tolerance are typically gradual and may go unnoticed by the patient. Therefore, the nurse needs to determine whether there has been a change in the activity pattern during the past 6 to 12 months. The patient's subjective response to activity is an essential assessment parameter. New symptoms or a change in the usual anginal symptoms during activity is a significant finding. Fatigue, associated with a low left ventricular ejection fraction (less than 40%) and certain medications (e.g., beta-adrenergic blocking agents), can result in activity intolerance. Patients with fatigue may benefit from having their medications adjusted and learning energy conservation techniques.

Additional areas to ask about include possible architectural barriers and challenges in the home, and what the patient does for exercise. If the patient exercises, the nurse asks additional questions: What is the intensity, duration, and frequency of exercise? Has the patient ever participated in a cardiac rehabilitation program? Functional levels are known to improve for almost all patients who participate in a cardiac rehabilitation program, and participation is highly recommended (Swift, Lavie, Johannsen, et al., 2013). Patients with disabilities may require an individually tailored exercise program.

Sleep and Rest

Clues to worsening cardiac disease, especially HF, can be revealed by sleep-related events. Determining where and how the patient sleeps or rests is important. Recent changes, such as sleeping upright in a chair instead of in bed, increasing the number of pillows used, awakening short of breath at night (paroxysmal nocturnal dyspnea [PND]), or awakening with angina (nocturnal angina), are all indicative of worsening HF.

Self-Perception and Self-Concept

Self-perception and self-concept are both related to the cognitive and emotional processes that people use to formulate their beliefs and feelings about themselves. Having a chronic cardiac illness, such as HF, or experiencing an acute cardiac event, such as an MI, can alter an individual's self-perception and self-concept. It is important for the nurse to understand that patients' beliefs and feelings about their health are key determinants in adherence to health regimen recommendations and recovery after an acute cardiac event. To reduce or minimize the reoccurrence of future cardiovascular-related health problems, patients are asked to make difficult lifestyle changes, such as quitting smoking. How well patients adhere to these recommendations is directly related to their health outcomes. Patients who do not understand the health consequences of their disease process and its management are at risk for noncompliance. On the contrary, patients with misperceptions about the consequences of their cardiac illness on their health may fail to return to their usual level of function, including work, despite being physically able. The health history is used to discover how patients perceive their health by asking questions that may include the following:

- What is your cardiac condition?
- How has this illness changed your feelings about your health?
- What do you think caused this illness?
- What consequences do you think this illness will have on your physical activity, work, social relationships, and role in your family?
- How much of an influence do you think you have on controlling this illness?

The patient's responses to these questions can guide the nurse in planning interventions to ensure that the patient is prepared to manage the illness and that adequate services are in place to support the patient's recovery and self-management needs.

Roles and Relationships

Hospital stays for cardiac disorders have shortened, with many invasive diagnostic cardiac procedures, such as cardiac catheterization and percutaneous coronary intervention (PCI), being performed as outpatient procedures.

To assess support systems, the nurse needs to ask: Who is the primary caregiver? With whom does the patient live? Are there adequate services in place to provide a safe home environment? The nurse also assesses for any significant effects the cardiac illness has had on the patient's role in the family. Are there adequate finances and health insurance? The answers to these questions help the nurse develop a plan to meet the patient's home care needs.

Sexuality and Reproduction

Although people recovering from cardiac illnesses or procedures are often concerned about sexual activity, they are unlikely to ask their nurse or other health care provider for information to help them resume their normal sex life. Therefore, the nurse needs to initiate a discussion about sexuality with the patient.

The most commonly cited reasons for changes in sexual activity are fear of another heart attack or sudden death; untoward symptoms such as angina, dyspnea, or palpitations; and problems with impotence or depression. In men, impotence may develop as a side effect of cardiac medications (e.g., beta-blockers); some men will stop taking their medication as a result. Other medications may be substituted, so patients should be encouraged to discuss this problem with their health care providers. Often, patients and their partners do not have adequate information about the physical demands related to sexual activity and ways in which these demands can be modified. The physiologic demands are greatest during orgasm, reaching 5 or 6 metabolic equivalents (METs). This level of activity is equivalent to walking 3 to 4 miles per hour on a treadmill. The METs expended before and after orgasm are considerably less, at 3.7 METs. Sharing this information may make the patient and his or her partner more comfortable about resuming sexual activity.

A reproductive history is necessary for women of childbearing age, particularly those with seriously compromised cardiac function. The reproductive history includes information about previous pregnancies, plans for future pregnancies, oral contraceptive use (especially in women older than 35 years of age who smoke), menopausal status, and use of HT.

Coping and Stress Tolerance

Anxiety, depression, and stress are known to influence both the development of and recovery from CAD and HF. High levels of anxiety are associated with an increased incidence of CAD and in-hospital complication rates after MI. Patients with a diagnosis of an acute MI and depression have an increased risk of rehospitalization, death, more frequent angina, more physical limitations, and poorer quality of life compared with patients without depression (Lichtman, Froelicher, Blumenthal, et al., 2014). Although the association between depression and CAD is not completely understood, both biologic factors (e.g., platelet abnormalities, inflammatory responses) and lifestyle factors may contribute to the development of CAD. Patients who are depressed are less motivated to adhere to recommended lifestyle changes and medical regimens necessary to prevent future cardiac events, such as an MI (Havranek et al., 2015; Lichtman et al., 2014).

Patients with CAD or HF should be assessed for depression. Patients who have depression exhibit common signs and symptoms, such as feelings of worthlessness or guilt, problems falling asleep or staying asleep, having little interest or pleasure in doing things that they usually enjoy, having difficulty concentrating, restlessness, and recent changes in appetite or weight. A quick and simple screening tool recommended by the AHA is the two-question Patient Health Questionnaire (PHQ-2) (Bigger & Glassman, 2010). The nurse asks the patient the following:

Over the past 2 weeks, how often have you been bothered by either of the following problems?

- *Little interest or pleasure in doing things*
- *Feeling down, depressed, or hopeless*

The nurse scores the patient's responses to each question by assigning 0 for "not at all," 1 for "several days," 2 for "more than half the days," or 3 for "nearly every day." The PHQ-2 score ranges from 0 to 6. Patients with a score of 3 or higher may be experiencing major depression and should be referred to their primary providers for further evaluation and treatment.

Stress initiates a variety of responses, including increased levels of catecholamines and cortisol, and has been strongly linked to cardiovascular events, such as an MI. Therefore, patients need to be assessed for sources of stress; the nurse asks about recent or ongoing stressors, previous coping styles and effectiveness, and the patient's perception of their current mood and coping ability. A widely used tool used to measure life stress is the Social Readjustment Rating Scale (Homes & Rahe, 1967). Examples of items on this scale include death of a spouse, divorce, and change in responsibilities at work. Each item is assigned a score of 11 to 100. Patients identify the items that happened to them in the previous year. Patients with a score less than 150 have a slight risk for future illness, whereas a score of 150 to 299 indicates a moderate risk. A score of 300 or higher indicates a high risk for future illness. Consultation with a psychiatric advanced practice nurse, psychologist, psychiatrist, or social worker is indicated for patients who are anxious or depressed or for patients who are having difficulty coping with their cardiac illness.

Physical Assessment

Physical assessment is conducted to confirm information obtained from the health history, establish the patient's current or baseline condition, and in subsequent assessments, evaluate the patient's response to treatment. Once the initial physical assessment is completed, the frequency of future assessments is determined by the purpose of the encounter and the patient's condition. For example, a focused cardiac assessment may be performed each time the patient is seen in the outpatient setting, whereas patients in the acute care setting may require a more extensive assessment at least every 8 hours. During the physical assessment, the nurse evaluates the cardiovascular system for any deviations from normal with regard to the following (examples of abnormalities are in parentheses):

- The heart as a pump (reduced pulse pressure, deviation of PMI from fifth intercostal space midclavicular line, gallop sounds, **murmurs**)
- Atrial and ventricular filling volumes and pressures (elevated jugular venous distention [JVD], peripheral edema, ascites, crackles, postural changes in BP)
- Cardiac output (reduced pulse pressure, hypotension, tachycardia, reduced urine output, lethargy, or disorientation)
- Compensatory mechanisms (peripheral vasoconstriction, tachycardia)

General Appearance

This part of the assessment evaluates the patient's level of consciousness (alert, lethargic, stuporous, comatose) and mental status (oriented to person, place, time; coherence). Changes in level of consciousness and mental status may be attributed to inadequate perfusion of the brain from a compromised cardiac output or thromboembolic event (stroke). Patients are observed for signs of distress, which include pain or discomfort, shortness of breath, or anxiety.

The nurse notes the size of the patient (normal, overweight, underweight, or cachectic). The patient's height and weight are measured to calculate BMI (weight in kilograms/square of the height in metres), as well as the waist circumference (refer to Chapter 5). These measures are used to determine if obesity (BMI greater than 30 kg/m^2) and abdominal fat (males: waist greater than 102 cm; females: waist greater than 88 cm) are placing the patient at risk for CAD.

Assessment of the Skin and Extremities

Examination of the skin includes all body surfaces, starting with the head and finishing with the lower extremities. Skin colour, temperature, and texture are assessed for acute and chronic problems with arterial or venous circulation. Table 27-3 summarizes common skin and extremity

TABLE 27-3 Common Assessment Findings Associated With Cardiovascular Disease

Assessment Findings	Associated Causes and Conditions
Clubbing of the fingers or toes (thickening of the skin under the fingers or toes)	Chronic hemoglobin desaturation most often due to congenital heart disease, advanced pulmonary diseases
Cool/cold skin and diaphoresis	Low cardiac output (e.g., cardiogenic shock, acute myocardial infarction) causing sympathetic nervous system stimulation with resultant vasoconstriction
Cold, pain, pallor of the fingertips or toes	Intermittent arteriolar vasoconstriction (Raynaud's disease). Skin may change in colour from white, blue, and red accompanied by numbness, tingling, and burning pain
Cyanosis, central (a bluish tinge observed in the tongue and buccal mucosa)	Serious cardiac disorders (pulmonary edema, cardiogenic shock, congenital heart disease) result in venous blood passing through the pulmonary circulation without being oxygenated
Cyanosis, peripheral (a bluish tinge, most often of the nails and skin of the nose, lips, earlobes, and extremities)	Peripheral vasoconstriction, allowing more time for the hemoglobin molecules to become desaturated. It can be caused by exposure to cold environment, anxiety, or ↓ cardiac output
Ecchymosis or bruising (a purplish-blue colour fading to green, yellow, or brown)	Blood leaking outside of the blood vessels Excessive bruising is a risk for patients on anticoagulants or platelet-inhibiting medications
Edema, lower extremities (collection of fluid in the interstitial spaces of the tissues)	Heart failure and vascular problems (PAD, chronic venous insufficiency, deep vein thrombosis, thrombophlebitis)
Hematoma (localized collection of clotted blood in the tissue)	Bleeding after catheter removal/tissue injury in patients on anticoagulant/antithrombotic agents
Pallor (↓ skin colour in fingernails, lips, oral mucosa, and lower extremities)	Anemia or ↓ arterial perfusion. Suspect PAD if feet develop pallor after elevating legs 60 degrees from a supine position
Rubor (a reddish-blue discolouration of the legs, seen within 20 seconds to 2 minutes after placing in a dependent position)	Filling of dilated capillaries with deoxygenated blood, indicative of PAD
Ulcers, feet and ankles: Superficial, irregular ulcers at medial malleolus. Red to yellow granulation tissue	Rupture of small skin capillaries from chronic venous insufficiency
Ulcers, feet and ankles: Painful, deep, round ulcers on feet or from exposure to pressure. Pale to black wound base	Prolonged ischemia to tissues due to PAD. Can lead to gangrene
Thinning of skin around a pacemaker or an implantable cardioverter defibrillator	Erosion of the device through the skin
Xanthelasma (yellowish, raised plaques observed along nasal portion of eyelids)	Elevated cholesterol levels (hypercholesterolemia)

assessment findings in patients with CVD. The most noteworthy changes include the following:

- Signs and symptoms of acute obstruction of arterial blood flow in the extremities, referred to as the 6 *P*'s, are *p*ain, *p*allor, *p*ulselessness, *p*aresthesia, *p*oikilothermia (coldness), and *p*aralysis. During the first few hours after invasive cardiac procedures (e.g., cardiac catheterization, PCI, or cardiac electrophysiology testing), affected extremities should be assessed frequently for these acute vascular changes.
- Major blood vessels of the arms and legs may be used for catheter insertion. During these procedures, systemic anticoagulation with heparin is necessary, and bruising or small hematomas may occur at the catheter access site. However, large hematomas are a serious complication that can compromise circulating blood volume and cardiac output. Patients who have undergone these procedures must have catheter access sites frequently observed until hemostasis is adequately achieved.
- Edema of the feet, ankles, or legs is called *peripheral edema*. Edema can be observed in the sacral area of patients on bed rest. The nurse assesses the patient for edema by using the thumb to place firm pressure over the dorsum of each foot, behind each medial malleolus, over the shins or sacral area for 5 seconds. *Pitting edema* is the term used to describe an indentation in the skin created by this pressure. The degree of pitting edema relies on the clinician's judgment of depth of edema and time the indentation remains after release of pressure. Pitting edema is graded as absent (0) or as present on a scale from slight (1+ = up to 2 mm) to very marked (4+ = more than 8 mm) (Weber & Kelley, 2014). It is important that clinicians use a consistent scale in order to ensure reliable clinical measurements and management. Peripheral edema is a common finding in patients with HF and peripheral vascular diseases, such as deep vein thrombosis or chronic venous insufficiency.
- Prolonged capillary refill time indicates inadequate arterial perfusion to the extremities. To test capillary refill time, the nurse compresses the nail bed briefly to occlude perfusion and the nail bed blanches. Then, the nurse releases pressure and determines the time it takes to restore perfusion. Normally, reperfusion occurs within 2 seconds, as evidenced by the return of colour to the nail bed. Prolonged capillary refill time indicates compromised arterial perfusion, a problem associated with cardiogenic shock and HF.
- Clubbing of the fingers and toes indicates chronic hemoglobin desaturation and is associated with congenital heart disease.
- Hair loss, brittle nails, dry or scaling skin, atrophy of the skin, skin colour changes, and ulcerations are indicative of chronically reduced oxygen and nutrient supply to the skin observed in patients with arterial or venous insufficiency (Weber & Kelley, 2014).

Blood Pressure

Systemic arterial BP is the pressure exerted on the walls of the arteries during ventricular systole and diastole. It is affected by factors such as cardiac output; distention of the arteries; and the volume, velocity, and viscosity of the blood. A normal BP in adults is considered a systolic BP less than 120 mm Hg over a diastolic BP less than 80 mm Hg. High BP or hypertension is defined by having a systolic BP that is consistently greater than 140 mm Hg or a diastolic BP greater than 90 mm Hg. Hypotension refers to an abnormally low systolic and diastolic BP that can result in lightheadedness or fainting (see Chapter 33 for additional definitions, measurement, and management).

Pulse Pressure

The difference between the systolic and the diastolic pressures is called the pulse pressure. It is a reflection of stroke volume, ejection velocity, and systemic vascular resistance. Pulse pressure, which normally is 30 to 40 mm Hg, indicates how well the patient maintains cardiac output. The pulse pressure increases in conditions that elevate the stroke volume (anxiety, exercise, bradycardia), reduce systemic vascular resistance (fever), or reduce distensibility of the arteries (atherosclerosis, aging, hypertension). Decreased pulse pressure reflects reduced stroke volume and ejection velocity (shock, HF, hypovolemia, mitral regurgitation) or obstruction to blood flow during systole (mitral or aortic stenosis). A pulse pressure of less than 30 mm Hg signifies a serious reduction in cardiac output and requires further cardiovascular assessment.

Postural (Orthostatic) Blood Pressure Changes

There is a gravitational redistribution of approximately 300 to 800 mL of blood into the lower extremities and the gastrointestinal system immediately upon standing. These changes reduce venous return to the heart, compromising preload that ultimately reduces stroke volume and cardiac output. As a consequence, the autonomic nervous system is activated. The sympathetic nervous system increases heart rate and enhances peripheral vasoconstriction, whereas parasympathetic activity of the heart via the vagus nerve is decreased. These compensatory mechanisms stabilize arterial BP (Arnold & Shibao, 2013).

Normal postural responses that occur when a person moves from a lying to a standing position include (1) a heart rate increase of 5 to 20 bpm above the resting rate; (2) an unchanged systolic pressure, or a slight decrease of up to 10 mm Hg; and (3) a slight increase of 5 mm Hg in diastolic pressure.

Postural (orthostatic) hypotension is a sustained decrease of at least 20 mm Hg in systolic BP or 10 mm Hg in diastolic BP within 3 minutes of moving from a lying or sitting to a standing position. It is usually accompanied by dizziness, lightheadedness, or syncope (Arnold & Shibao, 2013).

Postural hypotension in patients with CVD is most often due to a significant reduction in preload, which compromises cardiac output. Reduced preload, which is reflective of intravascular volume depletion, is caused by dehydration from overdiuresis, bleeding (due to antiplatelet or anticoagulant medications or postintravascular procedures), or medications that dilate the blood vessels (e.g., nitrates and antihypertensive agents). In these situations, the usual mechanisms needed to maintain cardiac output (increased heart rate and peripheral vasoconstriction) cannot compensate for the significant loss in intravascular volume. As a result, the BP drops and heart rate increases with changes from lying or sitting to upright positions (see Chart 27-2).

CHART 27-2

Assessment: Assessing Patients for Postural Hypotension

The following steps are recommended when assessing patients for postural hypotension:

- Position the patient supine for 10 minutes before taking the initial blood pressure (BP) and heart rate measurements.
- Reposition the patient to a sitting position with legs in the dependent position, wait 2 minutes, then reassess both BP and heart rate measurements.
- If the patient is symptom free or has no significant decreases in systolic or diastolic BP, assist the patient into a standing position, obtain measurements immediately, and recheck in 2 minutes; continue measurements every 2 minutes for a total of 10 minutes to rule out postural hypotension.
- Return the patient to a supine position if postural hypotension is detected or if the patient becomes symptomatic.
- Document heart rate and BP measured in each position (e.g., supine, sitting, and standing) and any signs or symptoms that accompany the postural changes.

Adapted from Woods, S. L., Froelicher, E. S., Motzer, S. A., et al. (2009). *Cardiac nursing* (6th ed.). Philadelphia, PA: Lippincott Williams & Wilkins.

The following is an example of BP and heart rate measurements in a patient with postural hypotension:

Supine: BP 120/70 mm Hg, heart rate 70 bpm
Sitting: BP 100/55 mm Hg, heart rate 90 bpm
Standing: BP 98/52 mm Hg, heart rate 94 bpm

Arterial Pulses

Factors to be evaluated in examining the pulse are rate, rhythm, quality, configuration of the pulse wave, and quality of the arterial vessel.

Pulse Rate

The normal pulse rate varies from a low of 50 bpm in healthy, athletic young adults to rates well in excess of 100 bpm after exercise or during times of excitement. Anxiety frequently raises the pulse rate during the physical examination. If the rate is higher than expected, it is appropriate to reassess it near the end of the physical examination, when the patient may be more relaxed.

Pulse Rhythm

The rhythm of the pulse is as important to assess as the rate. Minor variations in regularity of the pulse are normal. The pulse rate may increase during inhalation and slow during exhalation. This phenomenon, called sinus arrhythmia, occurs most commonly in children and young adults.

For the initial cardiac examination, or if the pulse rhythm is irregular, the heart rate should be counted by auscultating the apical pulse, located at the PMI, for a full minute while simultaneously palpating the radial pulse. Any discrepancy between contractions heard and pulses felt is noted. Disturbances of rhythm (dysrhythmias) often result in a pulse deficit, a difference between the apical pulse and the radial rate. Pulse deficits commonly occur with atrial fibrillation, atrial flutter, premature ventricular contractions, and varying degrees of heart block (see Chapter 28 for a detailed discussion of these dysrhythmias).

Pulse Amplitude

The quality, or amplitude, of the pulse can be described as absent, diminished, normal, or bounding. It should be assessed bilaterally. Scales can be used to rate the strength of the pulse. The following is an example of a 0 to 4 scale:

0: Not palpable or absent
+1: Diminished—weak, thready pulse; difficult to palpate; obliterated with pressure
+2: Normal—cannot be obliterated
+3: Moderately increased—easy to palpate, full pulse; cannot be obliterated
+4: Markedly increased—strong, bounding pulse; may be abnormal

The numerical classification is subjective; therefore, when documenting the pulse quality, it helps to specify a scale range (e.g., "left radial +3/+4").

Pulse Contour

The configuration (contour) of the pulse conveys important information. In patients with stenosis of the aortic valve, the valve opening is narrowed, reducing the amount of blood ejected into the aorta. The pulse pressure is narrow, and the pulse feels feeble. In aortic insufficiency, the aortic valve does not close completely, allowing blood to flow back from the aorta into the left ventricle. The rise of the pulse wave is abrupt and strong, and its fall is precipitous—a "collapsing" or "water hammer" pulse. The true configuration of the pulse is best appreciated by palpating over the carotid artery rather than the distal radial artery, because the dramatic characteristics of the pulse wave may be distorted when the pulse is transmitted to smaller vessels.

Palpation of Arterial Pulses

To assess peripheral circulation, the nurse locates and evaluates all arterial pulses. Arterial pulses are palpated at points where the arteries are near the skin surface and are easily compressed against bones or firm musculature. Pulses are detected over the right and left temporal, common carotid, brachial, radial, femoral, popliteal, dorsalis pedis, and posterior tibial arteries. A reliable assessment of the pulses depends on accurate identification of the location of the artery and careful palpation of the area. Light palpation is essential; firm finger pressure can obliterate the temporal, dorsalis pedis, and posterior tibial pulses and confuse the examiner. In approximately 10% of patients, the dorsalis pedis pulses are not palpable. In such circumstances, both are usually absent and the posterior tibial arteries alone provide adequate blood supply to the feet. Arteries in the extremities are often palpated simultaneously to facilitate comparison of quality.

NURSING ALERT

Do not simultaneously palpate both the temporal and carotid arteries, because it is possible to decrease the blood flow to the brain.

Jugular Venous Pulsations

Right-sided heart function can be estimated by observing the pulsations of the jugular veins of the neck and the central venous pressure (CVP), which reflects right atrial or right ventricular end-diastolic pressure (the pressure immediately preceding the contraction of the right ventricle).

Pulsations of the internal jugular veins are commonly assessed. If they are difficult to see, pulsations of the external jugular veins may be noted. These veins are more superficial and are visible just above the clavicles, adjacent to the sternocleidomastoid muscles. The external jugular veins are frequently distended while the patient lies supine on the examining table or bed. As the patient's head is elevated, distention of the veins normally disappears. The veins normally are not apparent if the patient's head is elevated more than 30 degrees.

Obvious distention of the veins with the patient's head elevated 45 to 90 degrees indicates an abnormal increase in the volume of the venous system. This occurs with right ventricular failure, pulmonary hypertension, and pulmonary stenosis; less commonly with obstruction of blood flow in the superior vena cava; and rarely with acute massive pulmonary embolism.

Heart Inspection and Palpation

The heart is examined by inspection, palpation, and auscultation of the chest wall. A systematic approach is used to examine the chest wall in the following six areas. Figure 27-5 identifies these important landmarks:

1. *Aortic area*—second intercostal space to the right of the sternum. To determine the correct intercostal space, the nurse first finds the angle of Louis by locating the bony ridge near the top of the sternum, at the junction of the body and the manubrium. From this angle, the second intercostal space is located by sliding one finger to the left or right of the sternum. Subsequent intercostal spaces are located from this reference point by palpating down the rib cage.
2. *Pulmonic area*—second intercostal space to the left of the sternum

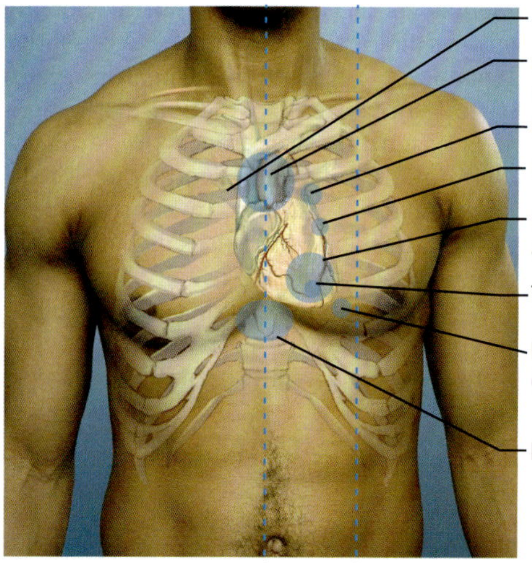

FIGURE 27-5. Areas of the precordium to be assessed when evaluating heart function. (Numerals identify ribs of adjacent intercostal spaces.)

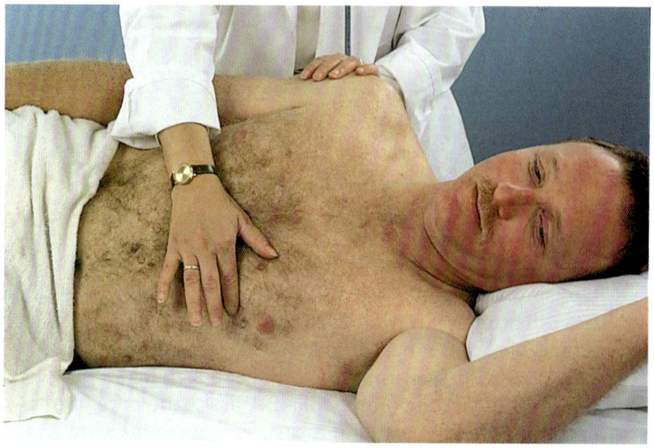

FIGURE 27-6. Locating and palpating the apical impulse (also called the point of maximal impulse [PMI]) in the left lateral position. The apical impulse normally is located at the fifth intercostal space to the left of the sternum at the midclavicular line. The nurse locates the impulse with the palm of the hand and palpates with the fingerpads. (Photo by B. Proud.)

3. *Erb's point*—third intercostal space to the left of the sternum
4. *Tricuspid area*—lower half of the sternum along the left parasternal area
5. *Mitral (apical) area*—left fifth intercostal space at the midclavicular line
6. *Epigastric area*—below the xiphoid process

For most of the examination, the patient lies supine, with the head of the bed slightly elevated. A right-handed examiner stands at the right side of the patient, a left-handed examiner at the left side.

Each area of the precordium is inspected and then palpated. Oblique lighting is used to assist the examiner in identifying subtle pulsations. The apical impulse is easier to discern in young patients and adults who have a thin chest wall, compared with patients who are obese or who have chest wall abnormalities.

In many cases, the apical impulse is palpable and is normally felt as a light pulsation, 1 to 2 cm in diameter. It is felt at the onset of the first heart sound and lasts for only half of ventricular systole (see the next section for a discussion of heart sounds). The nurse uses the palm of the hand to locate the apical impulse initially and the fingerpads to assess its size and quality. If the apical impulse cannot be palpated while the patient is supine, the patient is repositioned into the left lateral position as shown in Figure 27-6, to put the heart into closer contact with the chest wall and facilitate palpation of the apical impulse.

There are several abnormalities that the nurse may find during palpation of the precordium. Normally, the apical impulse is palpable in only one intercostal space; palpability in two or more adjacent intercostal spaces indicates left ventricular enlargement. An apical impulse below the fifth intercostal space or lateral to the midclavicular line usually denotes left ventricular enlargement from left ventricular failure. If the apical impulse can be palpated in two distinctly separate areas and the pulsation movements are paradoxical (not simultaneous), a ventricular aneurysm may be suspected. A broad and forceful apical impulse is known as a left ventricular heave or lift because it appears to lift the hand from the chest wall during palpation.

A vibration or purring sensation may be felt over areas where abnormal, turbulent blood flow is present. It is best detected by using the palm of the hand. This vibration is called a thrill and is associated with a loud murmur. Depending on the location of the thrill, it may be indicative of serious valvular heart disease, an atrial or ventricular septal defect (abnormal opening), or stenosis of a large artery, such as the carotid artery.

Heart Auscultation

A stethoscope is used to auscultate each of the locations identified in Figure 27-5, with the exception of the epigastric area. The purpose of cardiac auscultation is to determine heart rate and rhythm and evaluate heart sounds. The apical area is auscultated for 1 minute to determine the apical pulse rate and the regularity of the heartbeat. Normal and abnormal heart sounds detected during auscultation are described in the following section.

Normal Heart Sounds

Normal heart sounds, referred to as S_1 and S_2, are produced by closure of the AV valves and the semilunar valves, respectively. The period between S_1 and S_2 corresponds with ventricular systole (Fig. 27-7). When the heart rate is within the normal range, systole is much shorter than the period between S_2 and S_1 (diastole). However, as the heart rate increases, diastole shortens.

Normally, S_1 and S_2 are the only sounds heard during the cardiac cycle.

S_1—FIRST HEART SOUND. Tricuspid and mitral valve closure creates the first heart sound (S_1). The word "lub" is used to replicate its sound. S_1 is usually heard the loudest at the apical area. S_1 is easily identifiable and serves as the point of reference for the remainder of the cardiac cycle.

The intensity of S_1 increases during tachycardia or with mitral stenosis. In these circumstances, the AV valves are wide open during ventricular contraction. The accentuated S_1 occurs as the AV valves close with greater force than normal. Similarly, dysrhythmias can vary the intensity of S_1 from beat to beat due to lack of synchronized atrial and ventricular contraction.

S_2—SECOND HEART SOUND. Closure of the pulmonic and aortic valves produces the second heart sound (S_2), commonly referred to as the "dub" sound. The aortic component of S_2 is heard the loudest over the aortic and pulmonic areas. However, the pulmonic component of S_2 is a softer sound and is heard best over the pulmonic area.

Although these valves close almost simultaneously, the pulmonic valve lags slightly behind the aortic valve. In some individuals, it is possible to distinguish between the closure of the aortic and pulmonic valves. When this situation occurs, the patient is said to have a split S_2. Normal physiologic splitting of S_2 is accentuated on inspiration and disappears on expiration. During inspiration, there is a decrease in intrathoracic pressure and subsequent increase in venous return to the right atrium and ventricle. The right ventricle takes a little longer to eject this extra volume, which causes the pulmonic valve to close a little later than normal. Splitting of S_2 that remains constant during inspiration and expiration is an abnormal finding. Abnormal splitting of the second heart sound can be caused by a variety of disease states (valvular heart disease, septal defects, and bundle branch blocks). Splitting of S_2 is best heard over the pulmonic area.

Abnormal Heart Sounds

Abnormal sounds develop during systole or diastole when structural or functional heart problems are present. These sounds are called S_3, or S_4 gallops, **opening snaps**, **systolic clicks**, and murmurs. S_3 and S_4 gallop sounds are heard during diastole. These sounds are created by the vibration of the ventricle and surrounding structures as blood meets resistance during ventricular filling. The term *gallop* evolved from the cadence that is produced by the addition of a third or fourth heart sound, similar to the sound of a galloping horse. Gallop sounds are very low-frequency sounds and are heard with the bell of the stethoscope placed very lightly against the chest.

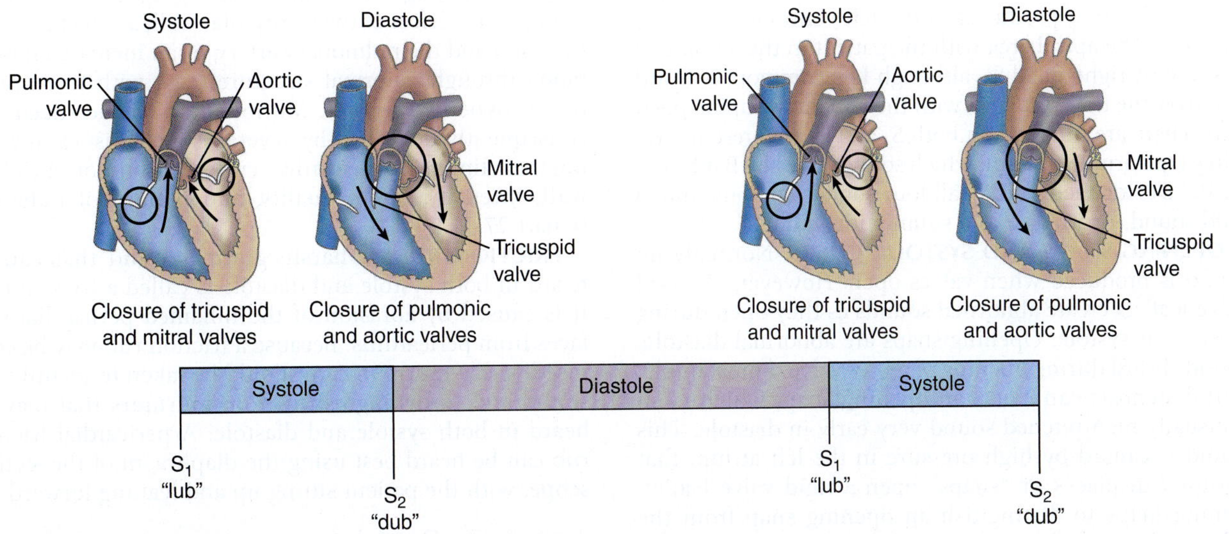

FIGURE 27-7. Normal heart sounds. The first heart sound (S_1) is produced by closure of the mitral and tricuspid valves ("lub"). The second heart sound (S_2) is produced by closure of the aortic and pulmonic valves ("dub"). *Arrows* represent the direction of blood flow.

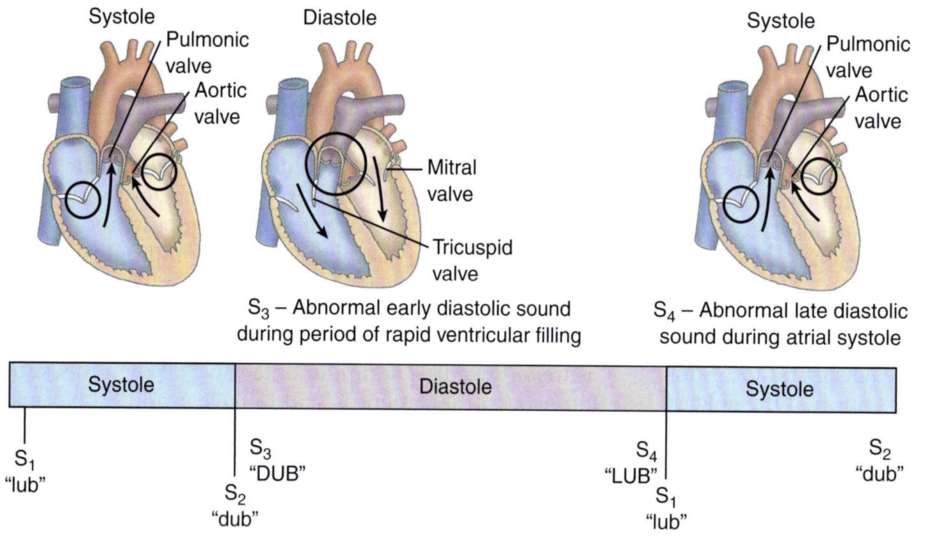

FIGURE 27-8. Gallop sounds. An S_3 ("DUB") is an abnormal sound heard immediately following S_2 (closure of semilunar valves). This sound is generated very early in diastole as blood flowing into the right or left ventricle is met with resistance. S_4 ("LUB") is an abnormal sound created during atrial systole as blood flowing into the right or left ventricle is met with resistance. *Arrows* represent the direction of blood flow.

S_3—THIRD HEART SOUND. An S_3 occurs early in diastole during the period of rapid ventricular filling. It is heard immediately after S_2. "Lub-dub DUB" (S_3) is used to imitate the sound of the beating heart with this gallop sound. It represents a normal finding in children and adults up to 35 or 40 years of age. In these cases, it is called a physiologic S_3 (Fig. 27-8). On the other hand, in older adults, it is a sign of significant pathophysiology, most commonly due to volume overload of one or both ventricles. It is a significant finding in patients with HF. If the right ventricle is involved, a right-sided S_3 is heard over the tricuspid area with the patient in a supine position. A left-sided S_3 is best heard over the apical area. Having the patient turn to the left lateral position may facilitate auscultation of an S_3 generated by the left ventricle.

S_4—FOURTH HEART SOUND. S_4 occurs late in diastole (see Fig. 27-8). An S_4 occurs just before S_1 and is generated during atrial contraction as blood forcefully enters a noncompliant ventricle. This resistance to blood flow is due to ventricular hypertrophy caused by hypertension, CAD, cardiomyopathies, aortic stenosis, and numerous other conditions. "LUB (S_4) lub-dub" is used to imitate this gallop sound. An S_4 produced in the left ventricle is auscultated over the apical area with the patient in the left lateral position. A right-sided S_4, although less common, is heard best over the tricuspid area with the patient in supine position. There are times when both S_3 and S_4 are present, creating a quadruple rhythm, which sounds like "LUB lub-dub DUB." During tachycardia, all four sounds combine into a loud sound, referred to as a **summation gallop**.

OPENING SNAPS AND SYSTOLIC CLICKS. Normally no sound is produced when valves open. However, diseased valve leaflets create abnormal sounds as they open during diastole or systole. Opening snaps are abnormal diastolic sounds heard during opening of an AV valve. For example, mitral stenosis can cause an opening snap, which is an unusually high-pitched sound very early in diastole. This sound is caused by high pressure in the left atrium that abruptly displaces or "snaps" open a rigid valve leaflet. Timing helps to distinguish an opening snap from the other gallop sounds. It occurs too long after S_2 to be mistaken for a split S_2 and too early in diastole to be mistaken for an S_3. The high-pitched, snapping quality of the sound is another way to differentiate an opening snap from an S_3. Hearing a murmur or the sound of turbulent blood flow is expected following the opening snap. An opening snap is heard best using the diaphragm of the stethoscope placed medial to the apical area and along the lower left sternal border.

In a similar manner, stenosis of one of the semilunar valves creates a short, high-pitched sound in early systole, immediately after S_1. This sound, called a systolic click, is the result of the opening of a rigid and calcified aortic or pulmonic valve during ventricular contraction. Mid- to late systolic clicks may be heard in patients with mitral or tricuspid valve prolapse, as the malfunctioning valve leaflet is displaced into the atrium during ventricular systole. Murmurs are expected to be heard following these abnormal systolic sounds. These sounds are the loudest in the areas directly over the malfunctioning valve.

Murmurs

Murmurs are created by turbulent flow of blood. The causes of the turbulence may be a critically narrowed valve, a malfunctioning valve that allows regurgitant blood flow, a congenital defect of the ventricular wall, a defect between the aorta and the pulmonary artery, or an increased flow of blood through a normal structure (e.g., with fever, pregnancy, hyperthyroidism). Murmurs are characterized and consequently described by several characteristics, including their timing in the cardiac cycle, location on the chest wall, intensity, pitch, quality, and pattern of radiation (Chart 27-3).

FRICTION RUB. A harsh, grating sound that can be heard in both systole and diastole is called a friction rub. It is caused by abrasion of the inflamed pericardial surfaces from pericarditis. Because a friction rub may be confused with a murmur, care should be taken to identify the sound and to distinguish it from murmurs that may be heard in both systole and diastole. A pericardial friction rub can be heard best using the diaphragm of the stethoscope, with the patient sitting up and leaning forward.

Auscultation Procedure

During auscultation, the patient remains supine and the examining room is as quiet as possible. A stethoscope with

CHART 27-3

Characteristics of Heart Murmurs

Heart murmurs are described in terms of location, timing, intensity, pitch, quality, and radiation. These characteristics provide information needed to determine the cause of the murmur and its clinical significance.

Location

Pinpointing the location of the murmur helps to determine the underlying structures that are involved in generating the abnormal sounds. The locations described in Figure 27-5 are used to identify where the loudest sounds are detected. It is helpful to include in the description the exact location from which the sound emanates, such as the location of the intercostal space and other important landmarks (right or left sternal border; midsternal, midclavicular, anterior axillary, or midaxillary lines). For example, a ventricular septal defect can be located at the left sternal border in the third and fourth intercostal spaces.

Timing

A murmur is described in terms of when it occurs during the cardiac cycle (systole or diastole). Murmurs are further differentiated by identifying exactly when during systole or diastole they are heard. A skilled clinician can detect that the murmur is occurring during early, mid, or late systole or diastole. Some murmurs have sounds that occur in both systole and diastole.

Intensity

A grading system is used to describe the intensity or loudness of a murmur.

Grade 1: very faint and difficult for the inexperienced clinician to hear

Grade 2: quiet, but readily perceived by the experienced clinician

Grade 3: moderately loud

Grade 4: loud and may be associated with a thrill

Grade 5: very loud; heard when stethoscope is partially off the chest; associated with a thrill

Grade 6: extremely loud; detected with the stethoscope off the chest; associated with a thrill

Pitch

Pitch is used to describe the sound frequency, identified as high, medium, or low pitched. High-pitched murmurs are heard best with the stethoscope's diaphragm, whereas low-pitched sounds are detected using the bell of the stethoscope placed lightly on the chest wall.

Quality

Quality is the term used to describe the sound that the murmur resembles. Murmurs can produce a rumbling, blowing, whistling, harsh, or musical sound. For example, murmurs caused by mitral or tricuspid regurgitation have a blowing quality, whereas mitral stenosis generates a rumbling sound.

Radiation

Radiation refers to the transmission of the murmur from the point of maximal intensity to other areas in the upper chest. The examiner determines if radiation is present by listening carefully to areas of the heart adjacent to the point where the murmur is the loudest. If radiation is present, the exact location is described. A murmur associated with aortic stenosis, for example, can radiate into the neck, down the left sternal border, and into the apical area.

both diaphragm and bell functions is necessary for accurate auscultation of the heart.

Using the diaphragm of the stethoscope, the examiner starts at the apical area and progresses upward along the left sternal border to the pulmonic and aortic areas. Alternatively, the examiner may begin the examination at the aortic and pulmonic areas and progress downward to the apex of the heart. Initially, S_1 is identified and evaluated with respect to its intensity and splitting. Next, S_2 is identified, and its intensity and any splitting are noted. After concentrating on S_1 and S_2, the examiner listens for extra sounds in systole and then in diastole.

Sometimes it helps to ask the following questions: Do I hear snapping or clicking sounds? Do I hear any high-pitched blowing sounds? Is this sound in systole, or diastole, or both? The examiner again proceeds to move the stethoscope to all of the designated areas of the precordium, listening carefully for these sounds. Finally, the patient is turned on the left side and the stethoscope is placed on the apical area, where an S_3, an S_4 and a mitral murmur are more readily detected.

Once an abnormality is heard, the entire chest surface is reexamined to determine the exact location of the sound and its radiation. The patient may be concerned about the prolonged examination and must be supported and reassured. The auscultatory findings, particularly murmurs, are documented by identifying the following characteristics (see Chart 27-3): location on chest wall, timing, intensity, pitch, quality, and radiation.

Interpretation of Heart Sounds

Interpreting heart sounds requires detailed knowledge of cardiac physiology and pathophysiology. However, all nurses should have adequate knowledge and skill to recognize normal heart sounds (S_1, S_2) and the presence of abnormal sounds. When assessment is at this very basic level of practice, abnormal findings are reported for further evaluation and treatment. More advanced skills are required of nurses caring for critically ill patients with CVD or those nurses functioning in advanced practice roles. Nurses in these roles readily identify abnormal heart sounds, recognize the diagnostic significance of their findings, and use their assessment skills to evaluate patients' responses to medical interventions. For example, these highly skilled nurses monitor heart sounds in patients with HF to detect the resolution of an S_3 after treatment with a diuretic.

Assessment of Other Systems

Lungs

The details of respiratory assessment are described in Chapter 22. Findings frequently exhibited by patients with cardiac disorders include the following:

Hemoptysis: Pink, frothy sputum is indicative of acute pulmonary edema.

Cough: A dry, hacking cough from irritation of small airways is common in patients with pulmonary congestion from HF.

Crackles: HF or atelectasis associated with bed rest, splinting from ischemic pain, or the effects of analgesic, sedative, or anesthetic agents often results in the development of crackles. Typically, crackles are first noted at the bases (because of gravity's effect on fluid accumulation and decreased ventilation of basilar tissue), but they may progress to all portions of the lung fields.

Wheezes: Compression of the small airways by interstitial pulmonary edema may cause wheezing. Beta-adrenergic blocking agents (beta-blockers), such as propranolol (Inderal), may cause airway narrowing, especially in patients with underlying pulmonary disease.

Abdomen

For the patient with a cardiovascular disorder, several components of the abdominal examination are relevant:

Abdominal distention: A protuberant abdomen with bulging flanks indicates ascites. Ascites develops in patients with right ventricular or biventricular HF (both right- and left-sided HF). In the failing right heart, abnormally high chamber pressures impede the return of venous blood. As a result, the liver and spleen become engorged with excessive venous blood (hepatosplenomegaly). As pressure in the portal system rises, fluid shifts from the vascular bed into the abdominal cavity. Ascitic fluid, found in the dependent or lowest points in the abdomen, will shift with position changes.

Hepatojugular reflux: This test is performed when right ventricular or biventricular HF is suspected. The patient is positioned so that the jugular venous pulse is visible in the lower part of the neck. While observing the jugular venous pulse, firm pressure is applied over the right upper quadrant of the abdomen for 30 to 60 seconds. An increase of 1 cm or more in jugular venous pressure is indicative of a positive hepatojugular reflux. This positive test aids in confirming the diagnosis of HF.

Bladder distention: Urine output is an important indicator of cardiac function. Reduced urine output may indicate inadequate renal perfusion or a less serious problem such as one caused by urinary retention. When urine output is decreased, the patient must be assessed for a distended bladder or difficulty voiding. The bladder may be assessed with an ultrasound scanner or the suprapubic area palpated for an oval mass and percussed for dullness, indicative of a full bladder.

Gerontologic Considerations

When performing a cardiovascular examination on an older adult patient, the nurse may note such differences as more readily palpable peripheral pulses because of decreased elasticity of the arteries and a loss of adjacent connective tissue. Palpation of the precordium in older adults is affected by the changes in the shape of the chest. For example, a cardiac impulse may not be palpable in patients with chronic obstructive pulmonary disease, because these patients usually have an increased anterior–posterior chest diameter. Kyphoscoliosis, a spinal deformity that occurs in many older adult patients, may move the cardiac apex downward so that palpation of the apical impulse is obscured.

Systolic BP increases with age, but diastolic BP usually plateaus after 50 years of age. Isolated systolic hypertension occurs most commonly among older adults and is associated with significant cardiovascular morbidity and mortality. Orthostatic hypotension may reflect decreased sensitivity of postural reflexes, which must be considered when medication therapy is prescribed.

An S_4 is heard in about 90% of older adult patients and is thought to be due to decreased compliance of the left ventricle. The S_2 is usually split. At least 60% of older adult patients have murmurs, the most common being a soft systolic ejection murmur resulting from sclerotic changes of the aortic leaflets (see Table 27-1).

Diagnostic Evaluation

Laboratory Tests

Laboratory tests may be performed for the following reasons:

- To assist in diagnosing the cause of cardiac-related signs and symptoms
- To determine baseline values before initiating therapeutic interventions
- To screen for modifiable CAD risk factors
- To ensure that therapeutic levels of medications (e.g., antiarrhythmic agents and warfarin) are maintained
- To evaluate the patient's response to the therapeutic regimen (e.g., effects of diuretics on serum potassium levels)
- To identify abnormalities that affect the prognosis of a patient with CVD

Normal values for laboratory tests may vary depending on the laboratory and the health care institution. This variation is due to the differences in equipment and methods of measurement across organizations.

Cardiac Biomarker Analysis

The diagnosis of MI is made by evaluating the history and physical examination, the 12-lead ECG, and results of laboratory tests that measure serum cardiac biomarkers. Myocardial cells that become necrotic from prolonged ischemia or trauma release–specific enzymes (creatine kinase [CK]), CK isoenzymes (CK-MB), and proteins (myoglobin, troponin T, and troponin I). These substances leak into the interstitial spaces of the myocardium and are carried by the lymphatic system into general circulation. As a result, abnormally high levels of these substances can be detected in serum blood samples. See Chapter 28 for further discussion of cardiac biomarker analysis.

Blood Chemistry, Hematology, and Coagulation Studies

Table 27-4 provides information about some common serum laboratory tests and the implications for patients with CVD. Discussion of lipid, brain (B-type) natriuretic peptide (BNP), C-reactive protein, and homocysteine measurements follows.

TABLE 27-4 Common Serum Laboratory Tests and Implications for Patients With Cardiovascular Disease (CVD)

Laboratory Test Reference Range	Implications
Blood Chemistries	
Blood urea nitrogen (BUN): 10–20 mg/dL	BUN and creatinine are end products of protein metabolism excreted by the kidneys. Elevated BUN reflects reduced renal perfusion from decreased cardiac output or intravascular fluid volume deficit as a result of diuretic therapy or dehydration.
Calcium (Ca^{++}): 8.5–10.5 mg/dL	Calcium is necessary for blood coagulability, neuromuscular activity, and automaticity of the nodal cells (sinus and atrioventricular nodes). *Hypocalcemia:* Decreased calcium levels slow nodal function and impair myocardial contractility. The latter effect increases the risk for heart failure. *Hypercalcemia:* Increased calcium levels can occur with the administration of thiazide diuretics because these medications reduce renal excretion of calcium. Hypercalcemia potentiates digitalis toxicity, causes increased myocardial contractility, and increases the risk for varying degrees of heart block and sudden death from ventricular fibrillation.
Creatinine: 0.7–1.4 mg/dL	Both BUN and creatinine are used to assess renal function, although creatinine is a more sensitive measure. Renal impairment is detected by an increase in both BUN and creatinine. A normal creatinine level and an elevated BUN suggest an intravascular fluid volume deficit.
Magnesium (Mg^{++}): 1.8–3.0 mg/dL	Magnesium is necessary for the absorption of calcium, maintenance of potassium stores, and metabolism of adenosine triphosphate. It plays a major role in protein and carbohydrate synthesis and muscular contraction. *Hypomagnesemia:* Decreased magnesium levels are due to enhanced renal excretion of magnesium from the use of diuretic or digitalis therapy. Low magnesium levels predispose patients to atrial or ventricular tachycardias. *Hypermagnesemia:* Increased magnesium levels are commonly caused by the use of cathartics or antacids containing magnesium. Increased magnesium levels depress contractility and excitability of the myocardium, causing heart block and, if severe, asystole.
Potassium (K^+): 3.5–5 mEq/L	Potassium has a major role in cardiac electrophysiologic function. *Hypokalemia:* Decreased potassium levels due to administration of potassium-excreting diuretics can cause many forms of dysrhythmias, including life-threatening ventricular tachycardia or ventricular fibrillation, and predispose patients taking digitalis preparations to digitalis toxicity. *Hyperkalemia:* Increased potassium levels can result from an increased intake of potassium (e.g., foods high in potassium or potassium supplements), decreased renal excretion of potassium, the use of potassium-sparing diuretics (e.g., spironolactone), or the use of angiotensin-converting enzyme inhibitors that inhibit aldosterone function. Serious consequences of hyperkalemia include heart block, asystole, and life-threatening ventricular dysrhythmias.
Sodium (Na^+): 135–145 mEq/L	Low or high serum sodium levels do not directly affect cardiac function. *Hyponatremia:* Decreased sodium levels indicate fluid excess and can be caused by heart failure or administration of thiazide diuretics. *Hypernatremia:* Increased sodium levels indicate fluid deficits and can result from decreased water intake or loss of water through excessive sweating or diarrhea.
Coagulation Studies	Injury to a vessel wall or tissue initiates the formation of a thrombus. This injury activates the coagulation cascade, the complex interactions among phospholipids, calcium, and clotting factors that convert prothrombin to thrombin. The coagulation cascade has two pathways: the intrinsic and extrinsic pathways. Coagulation studies are routinely performed before invasive procedures, such as cardiac catheterization, electrophysiology testing, and cardiac surgery.
Partial thromboplastin time (PTT): 60–70 seconds Activated partial thromboplastin time (aPTT): 20–39 seconds	PTT or aPTT measures the activity of the intrinsic pathway and is used to assess the effects of unfractionated heparin. A therapeutic range is 1.5–2.5 times baseline values. Adjustment of heparin dose is required for aPTT <50 seconds (↑ dose) or >100 seconds (↓ dose).
Prothrombin time (PT): 9.5–12 seconds	PT measures the extrinsic pathway activity and is used to monitor the level of anticoagulation with warfarin (Coumadin).
International normalized ratio (INR): 1	The INR, reported with the PT, provides a standard method for reporting PT levels and eliminates the variation of PT results from different laboratories. The INR, rather than the PT alone, is used to monitor the effectiveness of warfarin. The therapeutic range for INR is 2–3.5, although specific ranges vary based on diagnosis.
Hematologic Studies	
Complete blood count (CBC)	The CBC identifies the total number of white and red blood cells and platelets, and measures hemoglobin and hematocrit. The CBC is carefully monitored in patients with cardiovascular disease.

continued >

TABLE 27-4 Common Serum Laboratory Tests and Implications for Patients With Cardiovascular Disease (CVD) (Continued)

Laboratory Test Reference Range	Implications
Hematocrit *Male:* 42–52 %*Female:* 35–47 %Hemoglobin *Male:* 13–18 g/dL *Female:* 12–16 g/dL	The hematocrit represents the percentage of red blood cells found in 100 mL of whole blood. The red blood cells contain hemoglobin, which transports oxygen to the cells. Low hemoglobin and hematocrit levels have serious consequences for patients with cardiovascular disease, such as more frequent angina episodes or acute myocardial infarction.
Platelets: 150,000–450,000 (mm^3)	Platelets are the first line of protection against bleeding. Once activated by blood vessel wall injury or rupture of atherosclerotic plaque, platelets undergo chemical changes that form a thrombus. Several medications inhibit platelet function, including aspirin, clopidogrel (Plavix), and intravenous glycoprotein IIb/IIIa inhibitors (abciximab [ReoPro], eptifibatide [Integrilin], and tirofiban [Aggrastat]). When these medications are given, it is essential to monitor for thrombocytopenia (low platelet counts).
White blood cell (WBC) count: 4,500–11,000 (mm^3)	WBC counts are monitored in immunocompromised patients, including patients with heart transplants or in situations where there is concern for infection (e.g., after invasive procedures or surgery).

Adapted from Woods, S. L., Froelicher, E. S., Motzer, S. A., et al. (2009). *Cardiac nursing* (6th ed.). Philadelphia, PA: Lippincott Williams & Wilkins.

Lipid Profile

Cholesterol, triglycerides, and lipoproteins are measured to evaluate a person's risk of developing atherosclerotic disease, especially if there is a family history of premature heart disease, or to diagnose a specific lipoprotein abnormality. Cholesterol and triglycerides are transported in the blood by combining with plasma proteins to form lipoproteins. The lipoproteins are referred to as LDLs and HDLs. The risk of CAD increases as the ratio of LDL to HDL or the ratio of total cholesterol (LDL + HDL) to HDL increases. Although cholesterol levels remain relatively constant over 24 hours, the blood specimen for the lipid profile should be obtained after a 12-hour fast.

CHOLESTEROL LEVELS. Cholesterol is a lipid required for hormone synthesis and cell membrane formation. It is found in large quantities in brain and nerve tissue. Two major sources of cholesterol are diet (animal products) and the liver, where cholesterol is synthesized. Factors that contribute to variations in cholesterol levels include age, gender, diet, exercise patterns, genetics, menopause, tobacco use, and stress levels. Total cholesterol level is calculated by adding the HDL, LDL, and 20% of the triglyceride level.

New CAD prevention guidelines no longer focus on achieving specific cholesterol levels as there is inadequate evidence to support this practice. The mainstay of cholesterol-lowering therapy is lifestyle changes. Medical management focuses on determining an individual's 10-year risk for atherosclerotic vascular disease to identify those most likely to benefit from taking prescribed statins, a class of cholesterol-lowering medications (Stone, Robinson, Lichtenstein, et al., 2014).

LDL is the primary transporter of cholesterol and triglycerides into the cell. One harmful effect of LDL is the deposition of these substances in the walls of arterial vessels. HDL has a protective action because it transports cholesterol away from the tissue and cells of the arterial wall to the liver for excretion (Stone et al., 2014).

TRIGLYCERIDES. Triglycerides (normal range is 100 to 200 mg/dL), composed of free fatty acids and glycerol, are stored in the adipose tissue and are a source of energy. Triglyceride levels increase after meals and are affected by stress. Diabetes, alcohol use, and obesity can elevate triglyceride levels. These levels have a direct correlation with LDL and an inverse one with HDL.

Brain (B-Type) Natriuretic Peptide

Brain (B-type) natriuretic peptide (BNP) is a neurohormone that helps regulate BP and fluid volume. It is primarily secreted from the ventricles in response to increased preload with resulting elevated ventricular pressure. The level of BNP in the blood increases as the ventricular walls expand from increased pressure, making it a helpful diagnostic, monitoring, and prognostic tool in the setting of HF. Because this serum laboratory test can be quickly obtained, BNP levels are useful for prompt diagnosis of HF in settings such as the emergency department. Elevations in BNP can occur from a number of other conditions such as pulmonary embolus, MI, and ventricular hypertrophy. Therefore, the clinician correlates BNP levels with abnormal physical assessment findings and other diagnostic tests before making a definitive diagnosis of HF. A BNP level greater than 100 pg/mL is suggestive of HF.

C-Reactive Protein

High-sensitivity assay for C-reactive protein (hs-CRP) is a venous blood test that measures levels of CRP, a protein produced by the liver in response to systemic inflammation. Inflammation is thought to play a role in the development and progression of atherosclerosis. Therefore, hs-CRP is used as an adjunct to other tests to predict CVD risk, though its role as an independent risk factor for CVD is controversial. People with high levels of hs-CRP (3.0 mg/dL or greater) may be at greatest risk for CVD compared to people with moderate (1.0 to 3.0 mg/dL) or low (less than 1.0 mg/dL) levels of hs-CRP. In addition, an elevated hs-CRP may place patients with ACS at risk for recurrent cardiac events, including unstable angina and acute MI, higher mortality, and increased risk of restenosis of coronary arteries after PCI (Potts, 2013).

Homocysteine

Determining the homocysteine level enhances the clinician's ability to assess the patient's risk for CVD. Homocysteine, an amino acid, is linked to the development of atherosclerosis because it can damage the endothelial lining of arteries and promote thrombus formation. Therefore, an elevated blood level of homocysteine is thought to indicate a high risk for CAD, stroke, and peripheral vascular disease, although it is not an independent predictor of CAD. Genetic factors and a diet low in folic acid, vitamin B_6, and vitamin B_{12} are associated with elevated homocysteine levels. A 12-hour fast is necessary before drawing a blood sample for an accurate serum measurement. Test results are interpreted as optimal (less than 12 µmol/L), borderline (12 to 15 µmol/L), and high risk (greater than 15 µmol/L).

Chest X-Ray and Fluoroscopy

A chest x-ray is obtained to determine the size, contour, and position of the heart. It reveals cardiac and pericardial calcifications and demonstrates physiologic alterations in the pulmonary circulation. Although it does not help diagnose acute MI, it can help diagnose some complications (e.g., HF). Correct placement of pacemakers and pulmonary artery catheters is also confirmed by chest x-ray.

Fluoroscopy is an x-ray imaging technique that allows visualization of the heart on a screen. It shows cardiac and vascular pulsations and unusual cardiac contours. This technique uses a moveable x-ray source, which makes it a useful aid for positioning transvenous pacing electrodes and for guiding the insertion of arterial and venous catheters during cardiac catheterization and other cardiac procedures.

Electrocardiography

The ECG is a graphic representation of the electrical currents of the heart. The ECG is obtained by placing disposable electrodes in standard positions on the skin of the chest wall and extremities (see Chapter 28 for electrode placement). Recordings of the electrical current flowing between two electrodes is made on graph paper or displayed on a monitor. Several different recordings can be obtained by using a variety of electrode combinations, called leads. Simply stated, a lead is a specific view of the electrical activity of heart. The standard ECG is composed of 12 leads or 12 different views, although it is possible to record 15 or 18 leads.

The 12-lead ECG is used to diagnose dysrhythmias, conduction abnormalities, chamber enlargement, and myocardial ischemia, injury, or infarction. It can also suggest cardiac effects of electrolyte disturbances (high or low calcium and potassium levels) and the effects of antiarrhythmic medications. A 15-lead ECG adds three additional chest leads across the right precordium and is used for early diagnosis of right ventricular and left posterior (ventricular) infarction. The 18-lead ECG adds three posterior leads to the 15-lead ECG and is useful for early detection of myocardial ischemia and injury. To enhance interpretation of the ECG, the patient's age, gender, BP, height, weight, symptoms, and medications (especially digitalis and antiarrhythmic agents) are noted on the ECG requisition. The details of electrocardiography are presented in Chapter 28.

Continuous Electrocardiographic Monitoring

Continuous ECG monitoring is the standard of care for patients who are at high risk for dysrhythmias. This form of cardiac monitoring detects abnormalities in heart rate and rhythm. Many systems have the capacity to monitor for changes in ST segments, which are used to identify the presence of myocardial ischemia or injury (see Chapter 29). There are two types of continuous ECG monitoring techniques used in health care settings: hardwire cardiac monitoring, found in emergency departments, critical care units, and progressive care units; and **telemetry**, found in general nursing care units or outpatient cardiac rehabilitation programs. Hardwire cardiac monitoring and telemetry systems vary in sophistication; however, most systems have the following features in common:

- Monitor more than one lead simultaneously
- Monitor ST segments (ST-segment depression is a marker of myocardial ischemia; ST-segment elevation provides evidence of an evolving MI)
- Provide graded visual and audible alarms (based on priority, asystole merits the highest grade of alarm)
- Interpret and store alarms
- Trend data over time
- Print a copy of rhythms from one or more specific ECG leads over a set time (called a rhythm strip)

NURSING ALERT

Patients placed on continuous ECG monitoring must be informed of its purpose and cautioned that it does not detect shortness of breath, chest pain, or other ACS symptoms. Thus, patients are instructed to report new or worsening symptoms immediately.

Hardwire Cardiac Monitoring

Hardwire cardiac monitoring is used to continuously observe the heart for dysrhythmias and conduction disorders using one or two ECG leads. A real-time ECG is displayed on a bedside monitor and at a central monitoring station. In critical care units, additional components can be added to the bedside monitor to continuously monitor hemodynamic parameters (noninvasive BP, arterial pressures, pulmonary artery pressures) and respiratory parameters (respiratory rate, oxygen saturation).

Telemetry

In addition to hardwire cardiac monitoring, the ECG can be continuously observed by telemetry, the transmission of radio waves from a battery-operated transmitter to a central bank of monitors. The primary benefit of using telemetry is that the system is wireless, which allows patients to ambulate while one or two ECG leads are monitored. The patient has electrodes placed on the chest with a lead cable that connects to the transmitter. The transmitter can be placed in a disposable pouch and worn around

CHART 27-4

Applying Electrodes

The monitoring system requires an adequate electrical signal to analyze the patient's cardiac rhythm. When applying electrodes, the following recommendations should be followed to optimize skin adherence and conduction of the heart's electrical current:

- Débride the skin surface of dead cells with soap and water and dry well (or as recommended by the manufacturer).
- Clip (do not shave) hair from around the electrode site if needed.
- If the patient is diaphoretic (sweaty), apply a small amount of benzoin to the skin, avoiding the area under the centre of the electrode.
- Connect the electrodes to the lead wires prior to placing them on the chest (connecting lead wires when electrodes are in place may be uncomfortable for some patients).
- Peel the backing off the electrode and check to make sure the centre is moist with electrode gel.
- Locate the appropriate lead placement and apply the electrode to the skin, securing it in place with light pressure.
- Change the electrodes every 24 to 48 hours (or as recommended by the manufacturer), examine the skin for irritation, and apply the electrodes to different locations.
- If the patient is sensitive to the electrodes, use hypoallergenic electrodes.

Adapted from Sendelbach, S., & Jepsen, S. (2013). *AACN practice alert: Alarm management*. Retrieved January 25, 2016, from www.aacn.org/wd/practice/content/practicealerts/alarm-management-practice-alert.pcms?menu=practice

the neck, or simply secured to the patient's clothing. Most transmitter batteries are changed every 24 to 48 hours.

Lead Systems

The number of electrodes needed for hardwire cardiac monitoring and telemetry is dictated by the lead system used in the clinical setting. Electrodes need to be securely and accurately placed on the chest wall. Chart 27-4 provides helpful hints on how to apply these electrodes. There are three-, four-, or five-lead systems available for ECG monitoring. With a three-lead system, the nurse has only three lead options, whereas a four-lead system provides six possibilities. Newer monitoring systems have a five-lead system, which provides up to seven different lead selections. The advantage of the latter system is that it can more comprehensively monitor the activity of the anterior wall of the left ventricle (see Fig. 27-9 for electrode placement).

The two ECG leads most often selected for continuous ECG monitoring are leads II and V_1. Lead II provides the best visualization of atrial depolarization (represented by the P wave). Lead V_1 best records ventricular depolarization and is most helpful when monitoring for certain dysrhythmias (e.g., premature ventricular contractions, tachycardias, and bundle branch blocks) (see Chapter 28).

Ambulatory Electrocardiography

Ambulatory electrocardiography is a form of continuous ECG monitoring used for diagnostic purposes in the outpatient setting. Electrodes (number varies based on model used) are connected with lead wires to a cable that is inserted into a portable recorder (i.e., Holter monitor) that records the ECG onto a digital memory device. The patient wears the Holter monitor for 24 hours to detect dysrhythmias or myocardial ischemia that may occur during waking hours or sleep. The patient keeps a diary, noting the time of any symptoms or performance of unusual activities. Data from the digital memory device are uploaded into a computer for analysis, and rhythms that need further evaluation by a clinician are identified. Ambulatory electrocardiography is used to identify the etiology of symptoms (e.g., syncope, palpitations) that may be caused by dysrhythmias, to detect episodes of myocardial ischemia, and to evaluate effectiveness of cardiac medications (e.g., antiarrhythmic medications, nitrates) or pacemaker function.

Continuous Monitors

Commonly called Holter monitors, these small portable recorders are connected to chest electrodes (number varies based on model used) that record the ECG using several leads onto a digital memory device. The patient wears the

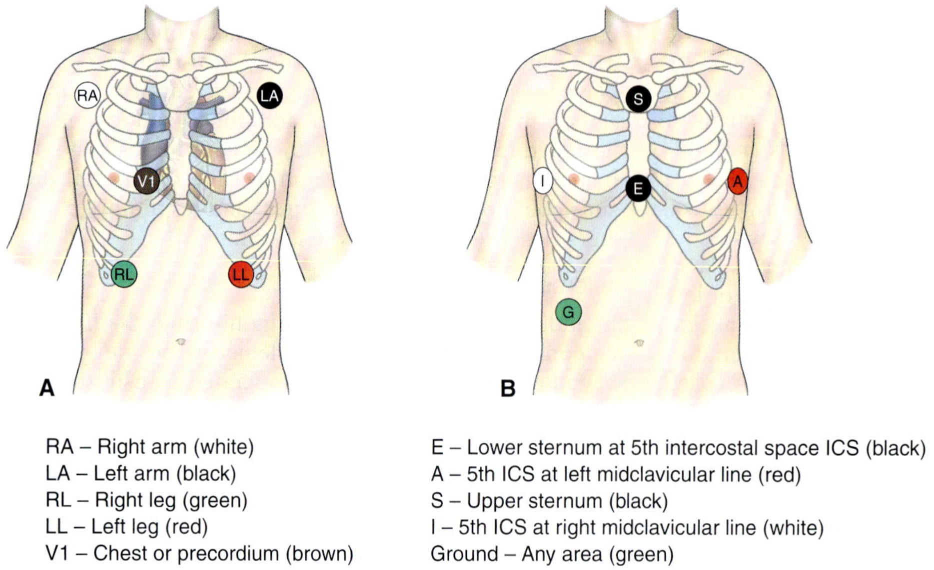

FIGURE 27-9. Electrode placement used in continuous electrocardiographic monitoring for (A) three-lead system, placement on RA, LA, and LL; four-lead system, placement on RA, LA, RL, and LL; five-lead system, placement on RA, LA, RL, LL, and V1; and (B) EASI-derived 12-lead ECG system.

recorder for 24 to 48 hours and in certain cases up to 2 weeks. If the patient experiences symptoms they are instructed to activate the event marker. The patient is also asked to keep a diary to note the date and time of symptoms or performance of unusual activities. The diary is used by the primary provider to correlate symptoms with detected dysrhythmias. Once monitoring is completed the patient returns the device to the primary provider's office. Data from the digital memory device are then uploaded into a computer for analysis, and rhythms that need further evaluation by the primary provider are identified. The effectiveness of this form of monitoring is dependent upon the patient's adherence with keeping a diary and marking events. Holter monitors do not provide real-time ECG recordings, which is another limitation.

A novel alternative to the use of the Holter monitor is ECG patch monitoring, which uses Bluetooth technology. An ECG patch with adhesive backing is placed over the left pectoral area, eliminating the need for multiple ECG electrodes, wires, and recorders. The patch is single use, waterproof, and easily concealed under clothing. The patient wears the patch for up to 14 days and then returns it to the manufacturer for analysis. These devices, which are available from several manufacturers, have one major limitation. The ECG patch is capable of monitoring just one ECG lead, which makes it less sensitive to dysrhythmia detection (Walsh, Topol, & Steinhubl, 2014).

Continuous Real-Time Monitors

This technology allows the ECG to be monitored continuously at a remote central monitoring station. The patient has three electrodes applied to the chest or wears an electrode belt that is attached to a small sensor. The sensor transmits each heartbeat to a small monitor. When a dysrhythmia is detected, the system automatically transmits the ECG to a monitoring centre either through the patient's telephone line when at home or through wireless communications systems when outside of the home. The patient can also trigger activation of ECG transmissions. The ECG is analyzed real time by technicians who communicate abnormal findings to the patient's primary provider. This method of monitoring enhances detection and early treatment of dysrhythmias that might otherwise be diagnosed only after the patient develops serious symptoms (Walsh et al., 2014).

Cardiac Event Recorders

Cardiac event recorders allow patients to record the electrical activity of the heart when they experience symptoms, such as palpitations, dizziness, or lightheadedness. Patients may need to record events for several days to a month. The recorded ECGs are transmitted to the primary provider by telephone. Newer technology has the capability of wireless transmission of the events automatically through the use of cellular networks. There are three main forms of recorders.

The symptom event monitor is used to record and store the ECG during only during times when the patient is experiencing symptoms. Patients activate the symptom event monitor by pressing a button for devices that are worn on the wrist or by placing a handheld device over the chest. The recorded event is then transmitted to the primary provider by telephone.

The continuous looping memory monitor, a small battery-operated device, can record and store the ECG for short periods of time. The monitor is attached to the patient with chest electrodes or a wrist band. Patients are instructed to activate ECG recordings by the push of a button. The device records the patient's ECG for a predetermined time before and after the device activation. Some of these devices are programmable to detect bradycardia, tachycardia, and irregular rhythms and do not require patient interaction. It is a preferred method over the symptom event monitor because it has more monitoring capabilities.

Real time smart phone monitoring is a novel approach to cardiac event recording. An adaptor, attached to the smart phone, converts the phone into a monitoring device. The patient places a finger in the device that digitally records lead I of the ECG. The ECG can be viewed immediately and also be sent as a PDF file via a secure server to the patient's primary provider (Walsh et al., 2014).

Cardiac Implantable Electronic Devices

Cardiac implantable electronic devices include pacemakers and ICDs. These lifesaving devices are used to manage patients with serious cardiac illnesses. The technology available today allows for remote wireless monitoring of these devices to determine battery life, pacing parameters and therapies, and occurrence of serious atrial and ventricular dysrhythmias. A transmitter, which is placed in the patient's home, sends device data to a secure data repository on a secure web portal. A unique feature of these implantable devices is that they have programmable alerts that automatically detect and transmit dysrhythmias without the need for patient interaction (Leahy & Davenport, 2015).

An implantable loop recorder is another type of a cardiac implantable electronic device. This small device, composed of a battery and microchips, is injected under the skin. Compared with event recorders described above, this device offers several advantages. It can record ECGs continuously for up to 3 years. It also can eliminate the patient's need to change electrodes and wear or carry the monitoring device. This type of monitoring is recommended for patients who have infrequent symptoms or require longer-term ECG monitoring (Romero, 2013).

Nursing Interventions for Inpatient Cardiac Monitoring

A body of evidence indicates that most alarms occurring during inpatient ECG monitoring are false alarms. Nurses dealing with excessive alarms become desensitized to these sounds and develop alarm fatigue. Alarm fatigue delays response time or results in missed alarms. Several nursing interventions facilitate acquisition of accurate data, reduce risk of alarm fatigue, and ensure patient safety when using various forms of cardiac monitoring (Hannibal, 2014; Sendelbach & Funk, 2013).

To minimize false alarms, the ECG recordings must be free of artifact, which is an abnormal ECG pattern caused by muscular activity, patient movement, electrical interference, or lead cable or electrode malfunction. Artifact can mimic dysrhythmias and cause unnecessary false alarms. Key to the elimination of artifact is using proper skin preparation before applying electrodes and changing the

NURSING RESEARCH PROFILE

Chart 27-5. Electrode Placement, Skin Preparation, and Alarm Fatigue

Walsh-Irwin, C. & Jurgens, C. Y. (2015). Proper skin preparation and electrode placement decreases alarms on a telemetry unit. *Dimensions of Critical Care Nursing*, *34*(3), 134–139.

Purpose

Electrocardiographic (ECG) monitoring in the inpatient setting is a common practice for patients at risk for cardiac dysrhythmias, ST-segment changes, or prolongation of the QT interval. It is used for the early detection and notification of an abnormality in the patient's ECG. When this situation occurs, the monitor sounds an alarm, which can vary in intensity and duration based on its clinical significance. Unfortunately, many things can cause the monitor to alarm inappropriately. Muscle tremors, patient movement, artifact from inadequate skin preparation, and improper ECG electrode placement are the most common reasons for these false alarms.

Nurses faced with excessive alarms become desensitized to these sounds, causing alarm fatigue. Alarm fatigue results in delayed responses to alarms and missing alarms, which may have serious life-threatening consequences for the patient. The Joint Commission has set a goal for 2017 that no patient should be harmed by false alarms. Therefore, the purpose of this study was to evaluate the effect of proper skin preparation and ECG electrode placement on alarm rates. The nurse researchers hypothesized that using proper techniques would reduce alarms on a telemetry unit.

Design

The conceptual framework for this study was the American Association of Critical Care Nurses *Synergy Model for Patient Care*. This model links competent nursing practice with positive patient outcomes. A prospective descriptive design was used to test the effect that proper skin preparation and ECG electrode placement had on the number of alarms on a telemetry unit in a suburban Veterans Affairs Medical Center. The hospital's Institutional review board ruled that the study was quality improvement and subjects were not required to provide consent to participate. After admission, the number of alarms was counted for 24 hours on 25 patients who had ECG electrodes placed using usual care. After 24 hours, the ECG electrodes were removed, the skin prepared (clipping hair if necessary, cleansing skin with soap and water, drying the skin with a wash cloth that causes mild skin abrasions), and reapplying the electrode using proper anatomic locations. The number of alarms was then recounted for 24 hours.

Findings

After the reapplication of ECG electrodes, nine patients were discharged before 24 hours and one patient refused to have his leads changed. Therefore, the final sample was composed of 15 men; the majority were white (93%) and had a mean age of 71.2 (±12.7) years. The initial alarm count for the first 24 hours was between 2 and 1341, compared with 1 and 992 alarms in the second 24 hours period. The mean number of alarms was significantly lower in patients after the second 24 hours, as compared with the first 24 hours. The use of proper skin preparation and lead placement was associated with a 44% reduction in the mean number of alarms.

Nursing Implications

The results of this study demonstrate that the use of guidelines for skin preparation and electrode placement recommended by the American Association of Critical Care Nurses results in safer and more effective ECG monitoring practices. The use of evidence-based ECG monitoring practices by nurses results in fewer false alarms and minimizes the risks to patients associated with alarm fatigue.

electrodes every 24 hours. During electrode changes, the skin should be assessed for allergic responses (itchy, reddened skin) to the adhesive or electrode gel. If present, the electrodes are replaced with hypoallergenic electrodes. Rotation of electrode placement on the skin will reduce the risk for skin breakdown (see Fig. 27-9). See Chart 27-5 for a Nursing Research Profile on electrode placement, skin preparation, and alarm fatigue.

Electrodes and lead connections need to be positioned correctly. Improper positioning can result in artifact that mimics ischemia or dysrhythmias. Two leads should be selected that provide the best tracing for dysrhythmia monitoring, which are usually lead II and the chest lead V_1. Electrical equipment in use around the patient should be inspected to be certain that it is functioning properly and has been recently checked by the medical engineering department per organization policy, because improperly functioning equipment may cause false alarms from artifact.

An effort should be made to individualize the ECG alarm parameters to meet the patient's monitoring needs. For example, if the patient has atrial fibrillation, it is appropriate to turn off the irregular heart rate alarm. Keeping it on will create unnecessary alarms, contributing to alarm fatigue. Similarly, the bradycardia and tachycardia alarms should be adjusted, slightly below or above the patient's underlying heart rate (Drew, Harris, Ze'gre-Hemsey, et al., 2014).

The nurse's role is to respond to and correct all monitor alarms immediately. Inoperative (inop) monitoring alarms—used to communicate that electrodes have fallen off, that leads are loose, or that the system's battery power is low (e.g., telemetry)—are just as significant as dysrhythmia alarms indicating that the patient is tachycardic, bradycardic, or experiencing another potentially life-threatening dysrhythmia. Timely responses to all alarms can prevent serious consequences, including death.

Hospital-acquired infections may be prevented by keeping lead wire cables and transmitter equipment clean, per organizational policy. A patient should never be connected to monitoring equipment that has not been thoroughly cleaned between patients. If a patient is scheduled for a device implant, such as a pacemaker, electrodes should not be placed over the planned incision site. Likewise, electrodes should never be placed over an incision, implanted device, open wounds, or inflamed skin.

Electrodes should be removed once monitoring is discontinued and skin cleansed to remove excess electrode gel and adhesive. Metal-containing electrodes must be removed before sending a patient for any magnetic resonance scan, including magnetic resonance angiography (MRA).

Telemetry transmitters and other monitoring equipment should be maintained according to the manufacturer's recommendations. Monitoring devices of any type should not be submerged in water. A monitoring device may break if dropped; therefore, it should be secured to the patient's gown or clothing.

Cardiac Stress Testing

Normally, the coronary arteries dilate to four times their usual diameter in response to increased metabolic demands for oxygen and nutrients. However, coronary arteries affected by atherosclerosis dilate less, compromising blood flow to the myocardium and causing ischemia. Therefore, abnormalities in cardiovascular function are more likely to be detected during times of increased demand, or "stress." The **cardiac stress test** procedures—the exercise stress test, the pharmacologic stress test, and the mental or emotional stress test—are noninvasive ways to evaluate the response of the cardiovascular system to stress. The stress test helps determine the following: (1) presence of CAD, (2) cause of chest pain, (3) functional capacity of the heart after an MI or heart surgery, (4) effectiveness of antianginal or antiarrhythmic medications, (5) dysrhythmias that occur during physical exercise, and (6) specific goals for a physical fitness program. Contraindications to stress testing include severe aortic stenosis, acute myocarditis or pericarditis, severe hypertension, suspected left main CAD, HF, and unstable angina. Because complications of stress testing can be life-threatening (MI, cardiac arrest, HF, and severe dysrhythmias), testing facilities must have staff and equipment ready to provide treatment, including advanced cardiac life support.

Stress testing is often combined with echocardiography or radionuclide imaging (discussed later). These techniques are performed during the resting state and immediately after stress testing.

Exercise Stress Testing

Procedure

During an exercise stress test, the patient walks on a treadmill (most common), pedals a stationary bicycle, or uses an arm crank. Exercise intensity progresses according to established protocols. The goal is to increase the heart rate to the "target heart rate," which is 80% to 90% of the maximum predicted heart rate based on the patient's age and gender. During the test, the following are monitored: two or more ECG leads for heart rate, rhythm, and ischemic changes; BP; skin temperature; physical appearance; perceived exertion; and symptoms, including chest pain, dyspnea, dizziness, leg cramping, and fatigue. The test is terminated when the target heart rate is achieved or when the patient experiences chest pain, extreme fatigue, a decrease in BP or pulse rate, serious dysrhythmias or ST-segment changes on the ECG, or other complications. When significant ECG abnormalities occur during the stress test (ST-segment depressions or elevations), the test result is reported as positive and further diagnostic testing such as a cardiac catheterization is required.

Nursing Interventions

In preparation for the exercise stress test, the patient is instructed to fast for 4 hours before the test and to avoid stimulants such as tobacco and caffeine. Medications may be taken with sips of water. The physician may instruct the patient not to take certain cardiac medications, such as beta-adrenergic blocking agents, before the test. Clothes and sneakers or rubber-soled shoes suitable for exercising are to be worn. The nurse prepares the patient for the stress test by describing how the stress test is performed, the type of monitoring equipment used, the rationale for having an IV catheter inserted, and what symptoms to report. The exercise method is reviewed and patients are asked to put forth their best exercise effort. If the test is to be performed with echocardiography or radionuclide imaging (described in the following section), this information is reviewed as well. After the test, the patient is monitored for 10 to 15 minutes. Once stable, patients may resume their usual activities.

Pharmacologic Stress Testing

Procedure

Patients who are physically disabled or deconditioned will not be able to achieve their target heart rate by exercising on a treadmill or bicycle. Two vasodilating agents, dipyridamole (Persantine) and adenosine (Adenocard), administered IV, are used to mimic the effects of exercise by maximally dilating the coronary arteries. The effects of dipyridamole last about 15 to 30 minutes. The side effects are related to its vasodilating action and include chest discomfort, dizziness, headache, flushing, and nausea. Adenosine has similar side effects, although patients report these symptoms as more severe. Adenosine has an extremely short half-life (less than 10 seconds), so any severe effects subside rapidly. Dipyridamole and adenosine are the agents of choice used in conjunction with radionuclide imaging techniques. Theophylline and other xanthines, such as caffeine, block the effects of dipyridamole and adenosine and must be avoided before these pharmacologic stress tests.

Dobutamine may also be used if the patient cannot exercise. Dobutamine, a synthetic sympathomimetic, increases heart rate, myocardial contractility, and BP, thereby increasing the metabolic demands of the heart. It is the agent of choice when echocardiography is used because of its effects on altering myocardial wall motion (due to enhanced contractility). Dobutamine is also used for patients who have bronchospasm or pulmonary disease and cannot tolerate having doses of theophylline withheld.

Nursing Interventions

In preparation for the pharmacologic stress test, the patient is instructed not to eat or drink anything for at least 4 hours before the test. This includes chocolate, caffeine, caffeine-free coffee, tea, carbonated beverages, or medications that contain caffeine (e.g., Anacin, Darvon). If caffeine is ingested before a dipyridamole or adenosine stress test, the test will have to be rescheduled. Patients taking aminophylline, theophylline, or dipyridamole are instructed to stop taking these medications for 24 to 48 hours before the test (if tolerated). The patient is informed about the transient sensations that may occur during infusion of the vasodilating agent, such as flushing or nausea, which will disappear quickly. The patient is instructed to report the occurrence of any other symptoms during the test to the cardiologist or nurse. The stress test may take about 1 hour, or up to 3 hours if imaging is performed.

Radionuclide Imaging

Radionuclide imaging studies are noninvasive tests that use **radioisotopes** to evaluate coronary artery perfusion, detect myocardial ischemia and infarction, and/or assess left ventricular function. Radioisotopes are unstable atoms that give off small amounts of energy in the form of gamma rays as they decay. When radioisotopes are injected into the bloodstream, the energy emitted can be detected by a gamma scintillation camera positioned over the body. These radioisotopes are called tracers.

Myocardial Perfusion Imaging

Myocardial perfusion imaging is performed using two types of techniques: single photon emission computed tomography (SPECT) or positron emission tomography (PET). It is commonly performed after an acute MI to determine if arterial perfusion to the heart is compromised during activity and to evaluate the extent of myocardial damage. It is also used to evaluate if myocardial ischemia from CAD is the cause of chest pain or other CAD-related symptoms.

These imaging techniques are performed in combination with stress testing to compare images obtained when the heart is resting to images of the heart in a stressed state resulting from exercise or medications. An area of the myocardium that shows no perfusion or reduced perfusion is said to have a "defect" present. Comparing resting images with images taken after the stress test help differentiate ischemic myocardium from infarct-related myocardium. A defect that does not change in size before and after stress is called a fixed defect. Fixed defects indicate that there is no perfusion in that area of the myocardium, which is the case after an MI. Defects that appear or that get larger after the stress test images are taken indicate reduced perfusion to that area of the heart. Because the defect disappears with rest, it is called a reversible defect. Reversible defects constitute positive stress test findings. Typically, cardiac catheterization is recommended after a positive test result to determine the severity of obstructions to blood flow caused by CAD.

The patient undergoing myocardial perfusion imaging with stress testing should be prepared for the type of stressor to be used (exercise or medication) and provided with details of what to expect during imaging. The imaging is performed in two stages. Usually, the resting images are taken first. An IV is inserted to administer the radioisotope, and electrodes are placed on the chest to monitor the heart rate and rhythm. Women who are nursing, pregnant or think they are pregnant should not undergo myocardial perfusion imaging. The nurse alerts the primary provider if any of these conditions are present.

Single Photon Emission Computed Tomography

SPECT is used most often because it is more widely available and is technically easier to perform than PET. In addition, the diagnostic and prognostic value of SPECT is better established than PET (Fletcher, Ades, Kligfield, et al., 2013).

Procedure

SPECT is a painless, noninvasive procedure that involves the injection of one of three commercially available tracers (technetium 99m (Tc^{99m}) sestamibi, Tc^{99m} tetrofosmin, or thallium 201).

During SPECT, patients are positioned supine on the table with their arms over their heads. The gamma camera circles around the chest area converting the signals from the traces into pictures of the heart. The procedure takes approximately 30 minutes. The second scan is repeated following the exercise or pharmacologic stress test.

Nursing Interventions

The nurse's primary role is to prepare the patient for SPECT and insert an IV catheter or assess an existing IV for patency and suitability. The IV is used to inject the tracer. The patient may be concerned about receiving a radioactive substance and needs to be reassured that these tracers are safe—the radiation exposure is similar to that of other diagnostic x-ray studies. No postprocedure radiation precautions are necessary.

Positron Emission Tomography

PET produces better pictures than SPECT, is faster, and uses lower doses of radiation. However, its use is limited because not all facilities have a PET scanner and the technical equipment needed to produce the tracers (Fletcher et al., 2013).

Procedure

During PET, tracers are given by injection; one compound is used to determine blood flow in the myocardium, and another determines the metabolic function. The PET camera provides detailed three-dimensional images of the distributed compounds. The viability of the myocardium is determined by comparing the extent of glucose metabolism in the myocardium to the degree of blood flow. For example, ischemic but viable tissue will show decreased blood flow and elevated metabolism. For a patient with this finding, revascularization through surgery or angioplasty will probably be indicated to improve heart function. Restrictions of food intake before the test vary among institutions, but because PET evaluates glucose metabolism, the patient's blood glucose level should be within the normal range before testing.

Nursing Interventions

The nurse instructs the patient to refrain from using alcohol and caffeine for 24 hours before undergoing PET because of the stimulating effects they may have on the heart. For patients with diabetes and who are taking insulin, the nurse needs to discuss insulin doses and food restrictions with the primary provider. The nurse assesses patients for fear of closed spaces or claustrophobia. Patients who have this condition are reassured that medications can be given to help them relax. The nurse also reassures patients that radiation exposure is at safe and acceptable levels, similar to those of other diagnostic x-ray studies.

To prepare the patient for PET, the nurse inserts an IV or assesses the existing IV catheter for patency and suitability, and then describes the procedure to the patient. The patient is positioned on a table with hands above the head. The table then slides into a doughnut-shaped scanner. While in the scanner, the patient must lie still so that clear images of the heart can be obtained. A baseline scan is performed, which takes about 30 minutes. Then a tracer is injected into the IV and the scan is repeated. The patient's glucose level is monitored throughout the procedure. The scan takes from 1 to 3 hours to complete.

Test of Ventricular Function and Wall Motion

Equilibrium radionuclide angiocardiography (ERNA), also known as multiple-gated acquisition (MUGA) scanning, is a common noninvasive technique that uses a conventional scintillation camera interfaced with a computer to record images of the heart during several hundred heartbeats. The computer processes the data and allows for sequential viewing of the functioning heart. The sequential images are analyzed to evaluate left ventricular function, wall motion, and ejection fraction.

The patient is reassured that there is no known radiation danger and is instructed to remain motionless during the scan.

Additional Imaging

Computed Tomography

Procedure

Cardiac CT scanning is a form of cardiac imaging that uses x-rays to provide accurate cross-sectional "virtual" slices of specific areas of the heart and surrounding structures. Complex mathematical and computer algorithms are used to analyze the slices to create three-dimensional images. Multidetector CT (MDCT) is a fast form of CT scanning that takes multiple slices at the same time. This technology helps to produce clear images by eliminating artifact created by the beating heart and respirations (Stone et al., 2014). There are two types of cardiac CT scanning that include coronary CT angiography and electron beam CT (EBCT) (for coronary calcium scoring).

Coronary CT angiography requires the use of an IV contrast agent to enhance the x-rays and improve visualization of cardiac structures. This test is used to evaluate coronary arteries for stenosis, the aorta for aneurisms or dissections, graft patency after coronary artery bypass grafting (CABG), pulmonary veins in patients with atrial fibrillation, and cardiac structures for congenital anomalies. Patients may receive beta-blockers prior to the scan to control heart rate and rhythm and reduce artifact. Another way to minimize artifact is to have patients hold their breath periodically throughout the scan. Coronary CT angiography is used with caution in patients with renal insufficiency. The contrast agent used during the CT scan is excreted through the kidneys; therefore, renal function should be assessed prior to the scan. It may be necessary to administer IV hydration before and after the scan to minimize the effect of the contrast on renal function. Patients will require premedication with corticosteroids and antihistamines if they experienced a reaction to a contrast agent in the past (Mervak, Davenport, Ellis, et al., 2015).

EBCT is used to calculate a coronary artery calcium score that is based on the amount of calcium deposits in the coronary arteries. This score is used to predict the likelihood of cardiac events, such as MI, or the need for a revascularization procedure in the future. Coronary artery calcium scoring is used for the evaluation of individuals without known CAD and offers limited incremental prognostic value for individuals with known CAD, such as those with stents and bypass grafts. Currently, EBCT is thought to be a reasonable test to consider in patients with low to intermediate risk for future CAD-related events. Results of the test may help to reclassify them to higher risk and thus intensify primary prevention measures (Lloyd-Jones, 2015).

Nursing Interventions

The nurse provides details of the procedure to help prepare the patient for the test. Patients need to be prepared to hold their breath at certain time during the procedure, so it is important for the nurse to practice with the patient before going for CT scan. The patient is positioned on a table, and the scanner rotates around the table during the test. The procedure is noninvasive and painless. However, to obtain adequate images, the patient must lie completely still during the scanning process. An IV is necessary if contrast is to be used to enhance the images. The patient should be told to expect transient flushing, metallic taste, nausea, or bradycardia during the contrast infusion.

Magnetic Resonance Angiography

Procedure

MRA is a noninvasive, painless technique that is used to examine both the physiologic and anatomic properties of the heart. MRA uses a powerful magnetic field and computer-generated pictures to image the heart and great vessels. It is valuable in diagnosing diseases of the aorta, heart muscle, and pericardium, as well as congenital heart lesions. The application of this technique to the evaluation of coronary artery anatomy is limited because the quality of the images are distorted by respirations, the beating heart, and certain implanted devices (stents and surgical clips). In addition, this technique cannot adequately visualize the small distal coronary arteries as accurately as conventional angiography performed during a cardiac catheterization.

Nursing Interventions

Because of the magnetic field used during MRA, patients must be screened for contraindications for its use. MRA cannot be performed on patients who have a pacemaker, metal plates, prosthetic joints, or other metallic implants that can become dislodged if exposed to MRA. Patients are instructed to remove any jewelry, watches, or other metal items (e.g., ECG leads). Transdermal patches that contain a heat-conducting aluminized layer (e.g., NicoDerm, Androderm, Transderm Nitro, Transderm Scop, Catapres-TTS) must be removed before MRA to prevent burning of the skin. During MRA, the patient is positioned supine on a table that is placed into an enclosed imager or tube containing the magnetic field. A patient who is claustrophobic may need to receive a mild sedative before undergoing an MRA. An intermittent clanking or thumping that can be annoying is generated by the magnetic coils, so the patient may be offered a headset to listen to music. The scanner is equipped with a microphone so that the patient can communicate with the staff. The patient is instructed to remain motionless during the scan.

Echocardiography

Traditional Echocardiography

Echocardiography is a noninvasive ultrasound test that is used to measure the ejection fraction and examine the size, shape, and motion of cardiac structures. It is particularly useful for diagnosing pericardial effusions; determining chamber size and the etiology of heart murmurs; evaluating the function of heart valves, including prosthetic heart valves; and evaluating ventricular wall motion.

Procedure

Echocardiography involves transmission of high-frequency sound waves into the heart through the chest wall and recording of the return signals. The ultrasound is generated by a handheld transducer applied to the front of the chest. The transducer picks up the echoes, converts them to electrical impulses, and transmits them for display on an oscilloscope and recording on a videotape. An ECG is recorded simultaneously to assist with interpreting the echocardiogram.

Two-dimensional or cross-sectional echocardiography creates a sophisticated, spatially correct image of the heart. Other techniques, such as Doppler and colour flow imaging echocardiography, show the direction and velocity of the blood flow through the heart.

Echocardiography may be performed with an exercise or pharmacologic stress test. Images are obtained at rest and then immediately after the target heart rate is reached. Myocardial ischemia from decreased perfusion during stress causes abnormalities in ventricular wall motion and is easily detected by echocardiography. A stress test using echocardiography is considered positive if abnormalities in ventricular wall motion are detected during stress but not during rest. These findings are highly suggestive of CAD and require further evaluation, such as a cardiac catheterization.

Nursing Interventions

Before echocardiography, the nurse informs the patient about the test, explaining that it is painless. Echocardiographic monitoring is performed while a transducer that emits sound waves is moved over the surface of the chest wall. Gel applied to the skin helps transmit the sound waves. Periodically, the patient is asked to turn onto the left side or hold a breath. The test takes about 30 to 45 minutes. If the patient is to undergo an exercise or pharmacologic stress test with echocardiography, information on stress testing is also reviewed with the patient.

Transesophageal Echocardiography

Procedure

A significant limitation of traditional echocardiography is the poor quality of the images produced. Ultrasound loses its clarity as it passes through tissue, lung, and bone. An alternate technique involves threading a small transducer through the mouth and into the esophagus. This technique, called transesophageal echocardiography (TEE), provides clearer images because ultrasound waves pass through less tissue. A topical anesthetic agent and moderate sedation are used during a TEE because of the discomfort associated with the positioning of the transducer in the esophagus (refer to Chapter 19 for further discussion of moderate sedation). Once the patient is comfortable, the transducer is inserted into the mouth and the patient is asked to swallow several times until it is positioned in the esophagus.

The high-quality imaging obtained during TEE makes this technique an important first-line diagnostic tool for evaluating patients with many types of CVD, including HF, valvular heart disease, dysrhythmias, and many other conditions that place the patient at risk for atrial or ventricular thrombi. Pharmacologic stress testing using dobutamine and TEE can also be performed. It is frequently used during cardiac surgery to continuously monitor the response of the heart to the surgical procedure (e.g., valve replacement or coronary artery bypass). Complications are uncommon during TEE, but if they do occur, they are serious. These complications are caused by sedation and impaired swallowing resulting from the topical anesthesia (respiratory depression and aspiration) and by insertion and manipulation of the transducer into the esophagus and stomach (vasovagal response or esophageal perforation). The patient must be assessed before TEE for a history of dysphagia or radiation therapy to the chest, which increases the likelihood of complications.

Nursing Interventions

Prior to the test the nurse provides preprocedure education and ensures that the patient has a clear understanding of what the test entails and why it is being performed, instructs the patient not to eat or drink anything for 6 hours prior to the study, and checks to make sure that informed consent has been obtained. The nurse also inserts an IV line or assesses an existing IV for patency and asks the patient to remove full or partial dentures. During the test, the nurse provides emotional support and monitors level of consciousness, BP, ECG, respiration, and oxygen saturation (SpO_2). During the recovery period, the patient must maintain bed rest with the head of the bed elevated to 45 degrees. Following the moderate sedation policy of the agency, the nurse monitors the patient for dyspnea and assesses vital signs, SpO_2, level of consciousness, and gag reflex as recommended. Food and oral fluids are withheld until the patient is fully alert and the effects of the topical anesthetic agent are reversed, usually 2 hours after the procedure; if gag reflex is intact, the nurse begins feeding with sips of water, and then advances to preprocedure diet. The patient is informed that a sore throat may be present for the next 24 hours; he or she is instructed to report the presence of a persistent sore throat, shortness of breath, or difficulty swallowing. If the procedure is performed in an outpatient setting, a family member or friend must be available to transport the patient home from the test site.

Cardiac Catheterization

Cardiac catheterization is a common invasive procedure used to diagnose structural and functional diseases of the heart and great vessels. The results guide treatment decisions including the need for revascularization (PCI or CABG) and other interventions to manage structural defects of the valves or septum.

This procedure involves the percutaneous insertion of radiopaque catheters into a large vein and an artery. Fluoroscopy is used to guide the advancement of the catheters through the right and left heart, referred to as right and left heart catheterization, respectively. In most situations, patients undergo both right and left heart catheterizations. However, right heart catheterization is performed without a left heart catheterization when patients only need myocardial biopsies or measurement of pulmonary artery pressures. Of note, left heart catheterization involves the use of a contrast agent. These agents are necessary to visualize patency of the coronary arteries and evaluate left ventricular function.

In preparation for the procedure, patients have blood tests performed to evaluate metabolic function (electrolytes and glucose) and renal function (blood urea nitrogen and creatinine level). Baseline coagulation studies (activated partial thromboplastin time [aPTT], international normalized ratio [INR] and prothrombin time [PT]) are obtained to guide dosing of anticoagulation during the procedure. Because bleeding and hematoma formation are procedural risks, a complete blood cell count (CBC; includes the hematocrit, hemoglobin, and platelets) is necessary to establish baseline values. Later these results are compared with postprocedure results to monitor for blood loss.

A health history is obtained to assess for previous reactions to a contrast agent and determine if the patient has any risk factors for contrast-induced nephropathy (CIN). This uncommon complication is a form of acute kidney injury that is usually reversible. Patients with chronic kidney disease or renal insufficiency, diabetes, HF, hypotension, dehydration, use of nephrotoxic medications, and advanced age are at risk for CIN. CIN is defined as an increase in the baseline serum creatinine by 25% or more or an absolute increase of 0.5 mg/dL within 48 to 72 hours after the procedure (Jorgensen, 2013).

During a cardiac catheterization, the patient has one or more IV catheters for administration of fluids, sedatives, heparin, and other medications. The patient is continuously monitored for chest pain or dyspnea and for changes in BP and ECG, which are indicative of myocardial ischemia, hemodynamic instability, or dysrhythmias. Resuscitation equipment must be readily available, and staff must be prepared to provide advanced cardiac life support measures as necessary.

Postprocedure, patients remain on bed rest for 2 to 6 hours before they are permitted to ambulate. Variations in time to ambulation are related to the size of the catheters used during the procedure, the site of catheter insertion (femoral or radial artery), the patient's anticoagulation status, and other factors (e.g., advanced age, obesity, and bleeding disorder). The use of smaller (4 or 6 Fr) arterial catheters is associated with shorter bed rest restrictions.

Cardiac catheterization may be performed in the ambulatory setting. Unless the results demonstrate the need for immediate treatment, patients are discharged home. Hospitalized patients undergoing cardiac catheterization for diagnostic and interventional purposes (PCI, valvuloplasty) are returned to their hospital rooms for recovery.

Right Heart Catheterization

Right heart catheterization usually precedes left heart catheterization. It involves the passage of a catheter from an antecubital or femoral vein into the right atrium, right ventricle, pulmonary artery, and pulmonary arterioles. Pressures and oxygen saturation levels from each of these areas are obtained and recorded. A biopsy of a small piece of myocardial tissue can also be obtained during a right heart catheterization. The results of the biopsy are used to diagnose the etiology of a cardiomyopathy (abnormality of myocardium) or heart transplant rejection. At the completion of the procedure, the venous catheter is removed and hemostasis of the affected vein is achieved using manual pressure.

Although right heart catheterization is considered relatively safe, potential complications include cardiac dysrhythmias, venous spasm, infection of the insertion site, cardiac perforation, and, rarely, cardiac arrest.

Left Heart Catheterization

Left heart catheterization is performed to evaluate the patency of the coronary arteries and the function of the left ventricle and the mitral and aortic valves. Potential complications include dysrhythmias, MI, perforation of the heart or great vessels, and systemic embolization. Left heart catheterization is performed by retrograde catheterization of the left ventricle. In this approach, the physician usually inserts the catheter into the right brachial artery or a femoral artery and advances it into the aorta and left ventricle. During a left heart catheterization, angiography is performed. Angiography is an imaging technique that involves the injection of the contrast agent into the arterial catheter. The contrast agent is filmed as it passes through the chambers of the left heart, aortic arch, and its major arteries. Coronary angiography is another technique used to observe the coronary artery anatomy and evaluate the degree of stenosis from atherosclerosis. To perform this test, a catheter is positioned into one of the coronary arteries. Once in position, the contrast agent is injected directly into the artery and images are obtained. The procedure is then repeated using the opposite coronary artery. Ventriculography is also performed to evaluate the size and function of the left ventricle. For this test, a catheter is positioned in the left ventricle and a large amount of contrast agent (30 mL) is rapidly injected into the ventricle.

The manipulation of catheters in the coronary arteries and left ventricle as well as injection of the contrast agent can cause intermittent myocardial ischemia. Vigilant monitoring throughout left heart catheterization is needed to detect myocardial ischemia, which can trigger chest pain and life-threatening dysrhythmias.

After the procedure, the catheter is carefully withdrawn and arterial hemostasis is achieved using manual pressure or other techniques previously described. If the physician performed an arterial or venous cutdown, the site is sutured and a sterile dressing is applied.

Nursing Interventions

Nursing responsibilities before cardiac catheterization include:

- Instructing the patient to fast, usually for 8 to 12 hours, before the procedure

- Informing the patient that if catheterization is to be performed as an outpatient procedure, a friend, family member, or other responsible person must transport the patient home
- Informing the patient about the expected duration of the procedure and advising that it will involve lying on a hard table for less than 2 hours
- Reassuring the patient that IV medications are given to maintain comfort
- Informing the patient about sensations that will be experienced during the catheterization. Knowing what to expect can help the patient cope with the experience. The nurse explains that an occasional pounding sensation (palpitation) may be felt in the chest because of extra heartbeats that almost always occur, particularly when the catheter tip touches the endocardium. The patient may be asked to cough and to breathe deeply, especially after the injection of the contrast agent. Coughing may help disrupt a dysrhythmia and clear the contrast agent from the arteries. Breathing deeply and holding the breath help lower the diaphragm for better visualization of heart structures. The injection of a contrast agent into either side of the heart may produce a flushed feeling throughout the body and a sensation similar to the need to void, which subsides in 1 minute or less.
- Encouraging the patient to express fears and anxieties. The nurse provides education and reassurance to reduce apprehension.

Nursing responsibilities after cardiac catheterization are dictated by hospital policy and primary provider preferences and may include:

- Observing the catheter access site for bleeding or hematoma formation and assessing peripheral pulses in the affected extremity (dorsalis pedis and posterior tibial pulses in the lower extremity, radial pulse in the upper extremity) every 15 minutes for 1 hour, every 30 minutes for 1 hour, and hourly for 4 hours or until discharge. BP and heart rate are also assessed during these same time intervals.
- Evaluating temperature, colour, and capillary refill of the affected extremity during these same time intervals. The patient is assessed for affected extremity pain, numbness, or tingling sensations that may indicate arterial insufficiency. The best technique to use is to compare the examination findings between the affected and unaffected extremities. Any changes are reported promptly.
- Screening carefully for dysrhythmias by observing the cardiac monitor or by assessing the apical and peripheral pulses for changes in rate and rhythm. A vasovagal reaction, consisting of bradycardia, hypotension, and nausea, can be precipitated by a distended bladder or by discomfort from manual pressure that is applied during removal of an arterial or venous catheter. The vasovagal response is reversed by promptly elevating the lower extremities above the level of the heart, infusing a bolus of IV fluid, and administering IV atropine to treat the bradycardia.
- Maintaining bed rest for 2 to 6 hours after the procedure. Duration of bed rest is dependent upon location of arterial approach, size of the catheter used during the procedure, and method used to maintain hemostasis. If manual pressure or a mechanical device was used during a femoral artery approach, the patient remains on bed rest for up to 6 hours with the affected leg straight and the head of the bed elevated no greater than 30 degrees. For comfort, the patient may be turned from side to side with the affected extremity straight. If a percutaneous vascular closure device or patch was deployed, the nurse checks local nursing care standards and anticipates that the patient will have fewer activity restrictions. The patient may be permitted to ambulate within 2 hours. If the radial artery was accessed, the patient remains on bed rest for 2 hours or until the effects of sedation have dissipated. The patient may sit up in bed. A hemostasis band or pressure dressing may be applied over the catheter access site. Patients are instructed to avoid sleeping on the affected arm for 24 hours and to avoid repetitive movement of the affected extremity for 24 to 48 hours (Rosendorff, 2013). Analgesic medication is given as prescribed for discomfort.
- Instructing the patient to report chest pain and bleeding or sudden discomfort from the catheter insertion sites promptly.
- Monitoring the patient for CIN by observing for elevations in serum creatinine levels. IV hydration is used to increase urinary output and flush the contrast agent from the urinary tract; accurate oral and IV intake and urinary output are recorded.
- Ensuring patient safety by instructing the patient to ask for help when getting out of bed the first time after the procedure. The patient is monitored for bleeding from the catheter access site and for orthostatic hypotension, indicated by complaints of dizziness or lightheadedness.

For patients being discharged from the hospital on the same day as the procedure, additional instructions are provided (see Chart 27-6).

Electrophysiologic Testing

The electrophysiology study (EPS) is an invasive procedure that plays a major role in the diagnosis and management of serious dysrhythmias. EPS may be indicated for patients with syncope, palpitations, or both, and for survivors of cardiac arrest from ventricular fibrillation (sudden cardiac death). EPS is used to distinguish atrial from ventricular tachycardias when the determination cannot be made from the 12-lead ECG, evaluate how readily a life-threatening dysrhythmia (e.g., ventricular tachycardia, ventricular fibrillation) can be induced, evaluate AV node function, evaluate the effectiveness of antiarrhythmic medications in suppressing the dysrhythmia, or determine the need for other therapeutic interventions, such as a pacemaker, implantable cardioverter-defibrillator, or radiofrequency ablation. See Chapter 28 for a detailed discussion of EPS.

Hemodynamic Monitoring

Critically ill patients require continuous assessment of their cardiovascular system to diagnose and manage their complex medical conditions. This type of assessment is achieved by the use of direct pressure monitoring systems, referred to as hemodynamic monitoring. Common forms include CVP, pulmonary artery pressure, and intra-arterial BP monitoring. Patients requiring hemodynamic monitoring are typically cared for in critical care units. Some

CHART 27-6

Patient Education: Self-Management After Cardiac Catheterization

After discharge from the hospital for cardiac catheterization, patients should follow these guidelines for self-care:

- *If the artery in your arm or wrist artery was used:* For the next 48 hours, avoid lifting anything heavier than 5 lb and avoid repetitive movement of your affected hand and wrist.
- *If the artery in your groin was used:* For the next 24 hours, do not bend at the waist, strain, or lift heavy objects.
- Do not submerge the puncture site in water. Avoid tub baths, but shower as desired.
- Talk with your primary provider about when you may return to work, drive, or resume strenuous activities.
- If bleeding occurs, sit (arm or wrist approach) or lie down (groin approach) and apply firm pressure to the puncture site for 10 minutes. Notify your primary provider as soon as possible and follow instructions. If there is a large amount of bleeding, call 911. Do not drive to the hospital.
- Call your primary provider if any of the following occur: swelling, new bruising or pain from your procedure puncture site, temperature of 101°F or more.
- If test results show that you have coronary artery disease, talk with your primary provider about options for treatment, including cardiac rehabilitation programs in your community.
- Talk with your primary provider about lifestyle changes to reduce your risk for further or future heart problems, such as quitting smoking, lowering your cholesterol level, initiating dietary changes, beginning an exercise program, or losing weight.
- Your primary provider may prescribe one or more new medications depending on your risk factors (medications to lower your blood pressure or cholesterol; aspirin or clopidogrel to prevent blood clots). Take all of your medications as instructed. If you feel that any of them are causing side effects, call your primary provider immediately. Do not stop taking any medications before talking to your primary provider.

Adapted from Woods, S. L., Froelicher, E. S., Motzer, S. A., et al. (2009). *Cardiac nursing* (6th ed.). Philadelphia, PA: Lippincott Williams & Wilkins.

progressive care units also admit stable patients with CVP or intra-arterial BP monitoring. To perform hemodynamic monitoring, a CVP, pulmonary artery, or arterial catheter is introduced into the appropriate blood vessel or heart chamber. It is connected to a pressure monitoring system that has several components, including:

- A flush system composed of IV solution (which may include heparin), tubing, stopcocks, and a flush device, which provides continuous and manual flushing of the system
- A pressure bag placed around the flush solution that is maintained at 300 mm Hg of pressure; the pressurized flush system delivers 3 to 5 mL of solution per hour through the catheter to prevent clotting and backflow of blood into the pressure monitoring system
- A transducer to convert the pressure coming from the artery or heart chamber into an electrical signal
- An amplifier or monitor, which increases the size of the electrical signal for display on an oscilloscope

Nurses caring for patients who require hemodynamic monitoring receive training prior to using this sophisticated technology. The nurse helps ensure safe and effective care by adhering to the following guidelines:

- Ensuring that the system is set up and maintained properly. For example, the pressure monitoring system must be kept patent and free of air bubbles.
- Checking that the stopcock of the transducer is positioned at the level of the atrium before the system is used to obtain pressure measurements. This landmark is referred to as the phlebostatic axis (see Fig. 27-10). The nurse uses a marker to identify this level on the chest wall, which provides a stable reference point for subsequent pressure readings.

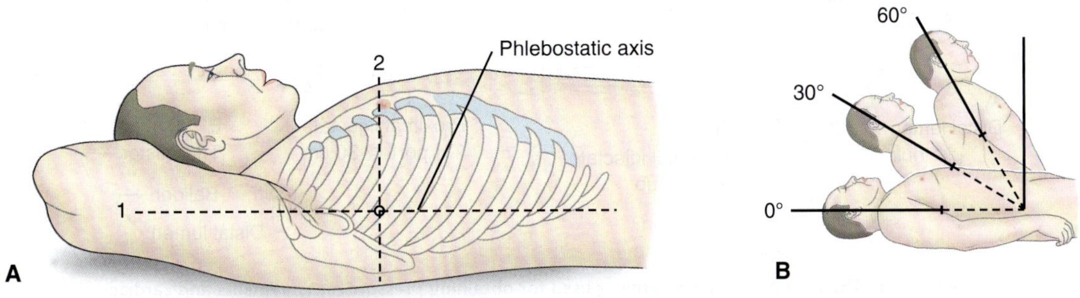

FIGURE 27-10. A. The phlebostatic axis is the reference point for the atrium when the patient is positioned supine. It is the intersection of two lines on the chest wall: (*1*) the midaxillary line drawn between the anterior and posterior surfaces of the chest and (*2*) the line drawn through the fourth intercostal space. Its location is identified with a skin marker. The stopcock of the transducer used in hemodynamic monitoring is "leveled" at this mark prior to taking pressure measurements. B. Measurements can be taken with the head of the bed (HOB) elevated up to 60 degrees. Note the phlebostatic axis changes as the HOB is elevated, so that the stopcock and transducer must be repositioned after each position change.

- Establishing the zero reference point in order to ensure that the system is properly functioning at atmospheric pressure. This process is accomplished by placing the stopcock of the transducer at the phlebostatic axis, opening the transducer to air, and activating the zero function key on the bedside monitor. Measurements of CVP, BP, and pulmonary artery pressures can be made with the head of the bed elevated up to 60 degrees; however, the system must be repositioned to the phlebostatic axis to ensure an accurate reading (Urden, Stacy, & Lough, 2014).

Complications from use of hemodynamic monitoring systems are uncommon and can include pneumothorax, infection, and air embolism. The nurse observes for signs of pneumothorax during the insertion of catheters using a central venous approach (CVP and pulmonary artery catheters). The longer any of these catheters are left in place (after 72 to 96 hours), the greater the risk of infection. Air emboli can be introduced into the vascular system if the stopcocks attached to the pressure transducers are mishandled during blood drawing, administration of medications, or other procedures that require opening the system to air. Therefore, nurses handling this equipment must demonstrate competence prior to independently caring for a patient requiring hemodynamic monitoring.

Central Venous Pressure Monitoring

CVP is a measurement of the pressure in the vena cava or right atrium. Since the pressure in the vena cava, right atrium, and right ventricle are equal at the end of diastole, the CVP also reflects the filling pressure of the right ventricle (preload). The normal CVP is 2 to 6 mm Hg. It is measured by positioning a catheter in the vena cava or right atrium and connecting it to a pressure monitoring system. The CVP is most valuable when it is monitored over time and correlated with the patient's clinical status. A CVP greater than 6 mm Hg indicates an elevated right ventricular preload. There are many problems that can cause an elevated CVP, but the most common is due to hypervolemia (excessive fluid circulating in the body) or right-sided HF. In contrast, a low CVP (less than 2 mm Hg) indicates reduced right ventricular preload, which is most often from hypovolemia. Dehydration, excessive blood loss, vomiting or diarrhea, and overdiuresis can result in hypovolemia and a low CVP. This diagnosis can be substantiated when a rapid IV infusion of fluid causes the CVP to increase.

Before insertion of a CVP catheter, the site is prepared by clipping excessive hair, if necessary, and by cleansing with an antiseptic solution. A local anesthetic agent is used. During this sterile procedure, the physician threads a single-lumen or multilumen catheter through the external jugular, antecubital, or femoral vein into the vena cava just above or within the right atrium.

Nursing Interventions

Once the CVP catheter is inserted, it is secured and a dry, sterile dressing is applied. Catheter placement is confirmed by a chest x-ray, and the site is inspected daily for signs of infection. The dressing and pressure monitoring system are changed according to hospital policy. In general, the dressing is kept dry and air occlusive. Dressing changes are performed using sterile technique. The frequency of CVP measurements is dictated by the patient's condition and the treatment plan. This catheter can also be used for infusing IV fluids, administering IV medications, and drawing blood specimens.

Pulmonary Artery Pressure Monitoring

Pulmonary artery pressure monitoring is used in critical care for assessing left ventricular function, diagnosing the etiology of shock, and evaluating the patient's response to medical interventions (e.g., fluid administration, vasoactive medications). A pulmonary artery catheter and a pressure monitoring system are used. A variety of catheters are available for cardiac pacing, oximetry, cardiac output measurement, or a combination of functions. Pulmonary artery catheters are balloon-tipped, flow-directed catheters that have distal and proximal lumens (Fig. 27-11). The distal lumen has a port that opens into the pulmonary artery. Once connected by its hub to the pressure monitoring system, it is used to measure continuous pulmonary

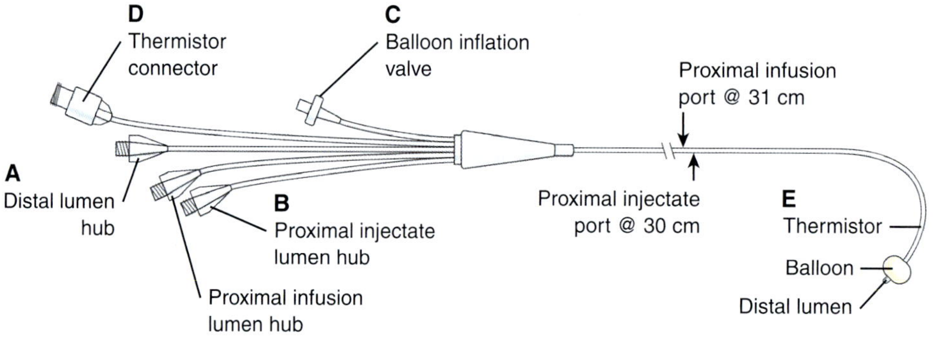

FIGURE 27-11. The pulmonary artery catheter used for obtaining pressure measurements and cardiac output. **A.** The pressure monitoring system is connected to the distal lumen hub. **B.** Intravenous solutions are infused through the proximal infusion and injectate lumen hubs. **C.** An air-filled syringe connected to the balloon inflation valve is used for balloon inflation during catheter insertion and pulmonary artery wedge pressure measurements. **D.** To obtain cardiac output, the thermistor connector is inserted into the cardiac output component of the bedside cardiac monitor and 5 to 10 mL of normal saline is injected in 4 seconds into the proximal injectate port. **E.** The thermistor located near the balloon is used to calculate the cardiac output. (Redrawn courtesy of Baxter Healthcare Corporation, Edwards Critical Care Division, Santa Ana, California.)

artery pressures. The proximal lumen has a port that opens into the right atrium. It is used to administer IV medications and fluids or to monitor right atrial pressures (i.e., CVP). Each catheter has a balloon inflation hub and valve. A syringe is connected to the hub, which is used to inflate or deflate the balloon with air (1.5-mL capacity). The valve opens and closes the balloon inflation lumen.

A pulmonary artery catheter with specialized capabilities has additional components. For example, the thermodilution catheter has three additional features that enable it to measure cardiac output: a thermistor connector attached to the cardiac output computer of the bedside monitor, a proximal injectate port used for injecting fluids when obtaining the cardiac output, and a thermistor (positioned near the distal port) (see Fig. 27-11).

The pulmonary artery catheter, covered with a sterile sleeve, is inserted into a large vein (subclavian, jugular, or femoral) through a sheath. The sheath is equipped with a side port for infusing IV fluids and medications. The catheter is then passed into the vena cava and right atrium. In the right atrium, the balloon tip is inflated, and the catheter is carried rapidly by the flow of blood through the tricuspid valve into the right ventricle, through the pulmonic valve, and into a branch of the pulmonary artery. When the catheter reaches the pulmonary artery, the balloon is deflated and the catheter is secured with sutures (Fig. 27-12). Fluoroscopy may be used during insertion to visualize the progression of the catheter through the right heart chambers to the pulmonary artery. This procedure can be performed in the operating room, in the cardiac catheterization laboratory, or at the bedside in the critical care unit. During insertion of the pulmonary artery catheter, the bedside monitor is observed for pressure and waveform changes, as well as dysrhythmias as the catheter progresses through the right heart to the pulmonary artery.

Once the catheter is in position, the following are measured: right atrial, pulmonary artery systolic, pulmonary artery diastolic, mean pulmonary artery, and pulmonary artery wedge pressures (see Fig. 27-2 for normal chamber pressures). Monitoring of the pulmonary artery diastolic and pulmonary artery wedge pressures is particularly important in critically ill patients because they are used to evaluate left ventricular filling pressures (i.e., left ventricular preload).

It is important to note that the pulmonary artery wedge pressure is achieved by inflating the balloon tip, which causes it to float more distally into a smaller portion of the pulmonary artery until it is wedged into position. This is an occlusive manoeuvre that impedes blood flow through that segment of the pulmonary artery. Therefore, the wedge pressure is measured immediately and the balloon is deflated promptly to restore blood flow.

NURSING ALERT

After measuring the pulmonary artery wedge pressure, the nurse ensures that the balloon is deflated and that the catheter has returned to its normal position. This important intervention is verified by evaluating the pulmonary artery pressure waveform displayed on the bedside monitor.

Nursing Interventions

Catheter site care is essentially the same as for a CVP catheter. Similar to CVP measurement, the transducer must be positioned at the phlebostatic axis to ensure accurate readings (see Fig. 27-10). Serious complications include pulmonary artery rupture, pulmonary thromboembolism, pulmonary infarction, catheter kinking, dysrhythmias, and air embolism.

Intra-Arterial Blood Pressure Monitoring

Intra-arterial BP monitoring is used to obtain direct and continuous BP measurements in critically ill patients who have severe hypertension or hypotension. Arterial catheters are also useful when arterial blood gas measurements and blood samples need to be obtained frequently.

Once an arterial site is selected, usually the radial artery, circulation to the involved extremity is assessed by the Allen test or an ultrasonic Doppler study because placing an arterial catheter can further impede perfusion to an area that has poor circulation. As a result, the tissue distal to the cannulated artery can become ischemic or necrotic. The Allen test is used to evaluate perfusion of the hand and fingers by the radial and ulnar arteries. To perform the Allen test, the hand is elevated and the patient is asked to make a fist for 30 seconds. The nurse compresses the radial and ulnar arteries simultaneously, causing the hand to blanch. After the patient opens the fist, the nurse releases the pressure on the ulnar artery. If blood flow is restored (hand turns pink) within 6 seconds, the circulation to the hand may be adequate enough to tolerate placement of a radial artery catheter. However, an ultrasonic Doppler is the most accurate method for assessing arterial perfusion of the hand.

Nursing Interventions

Site preparation and care are the same as for CVP catheters. The catheter flush solution is the same as for pulmonary artery catheters. A transducer is attached, and pressures are measured in mm Hg. The nurse monitors the patient for complications, which include local obstruction with distal ischemia, external hemorrhage, massive ecchymosis, dissection, air embolism, blood loss, pain, arteriospasm, and infection.

Minimally Invasive Cardiac Output Monitoring Devices

Monitoring cardiac output using the pulmonary artery catheter has been the standard of practice in critical care since its inception almost 50 years ago. Its use has diminished recently with the availability of new, less invasive devices. Several types of devices are commercially available. Selection of a specific device for clinical use is determined by availability, provider preferences, and the patient's clinical condition (Urden et al., 2014).

Pulse pressure analysis uses an arterial pressure waveform to continuously estimate the patient's stroke volume. One such device, the Edwards Lifesciences Vigileo monitoring system, is connected to an existing radial or femoral arterial line via its FloTrac transducer. Using age, gender, body surface area, and BP of the patient, this device calculates continuous cardiac output and other parameters used in the management of critically ill patients. The major drawback to this device is that in

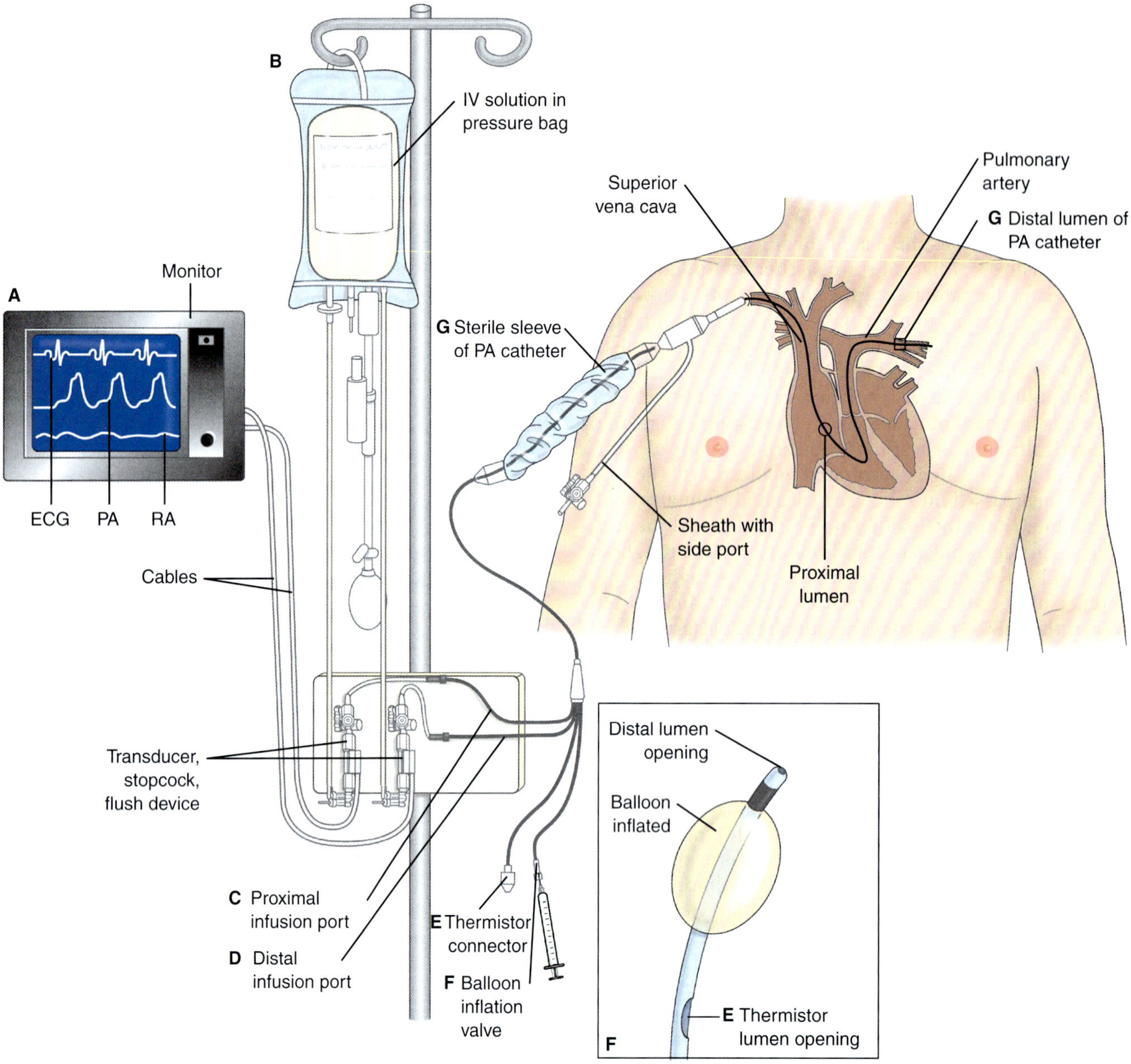

FIGURE 27-12. Pulmonary artery (PA) catheter and pressure monitoring systems. **A.** Bedside monitor that connects with cables to **(B)** the pressure monitoring systems (includes intravenous [IV] solution in a pressure bag, IV tubing, and two transducers with stopcocks and flush devices). This system connects to **(C)** the proximal infusion port that opens in the right atria and is used to infuse fluids or medications and monitor central venous pressures and **(D)** the distal infusion port. This port opens in the PA and is used to monitor PA pressures. **E.** The thermistor connector is attached to the bedside cardiac monitor to obtain cardiac output. **F.** An air-filled syringe is attached to the balloon inflation valve during catheter insertion and measurement of PA wedge pressure. **G.** PA catheter positioned in the pulmonary artery. Note the sterile sleeve over the PA catheter. The PA catheter is threaded through the sheath until it reaches the desired position in the PA. The side port on the sheath is used to infuse medications or fluids. ECG, electrocardiogram; RA, right atrium.

order for it to capture accurate data, it must first capture optimal arterial waveforms. Therefore, this type of device has limited usefulness in patients with poor waveform signals, various dysrhythmias, hemodynamic instability, and those who may be concomitantly using an intra-aortic balloon pump.

Esophageal Doppler probes are used to noninvasively estimate cardiac output. The esophageal probe measures blood flow velocity within a cross-sectional area of the descending aorta to calculate cardiac output. The use of this device in the perioperative setting has been shown to improve patient outcomes, including decreased lengths of hospital stay and an overall decrease in rates of complications (Urden et al., 2014).

In patients who are sedated, intubated, and on mechanical ventilation, the Fick principle, which uses carbon dioxide (CO_2) measures, is an additional method used to estimate cardiac output. To obtain cardiac output in this select patient population, a rebreathing loop is attached to the ventilator along with an infrared CO_2 sensor, an airflow sensor, and pulse oximeter. Continuous readings of cardiac output may be updated every 3 minutes with the use of this device.

Critical Thinking Exercises

1 Your patient is being admitted to the cardiac ICU directly from the chronic HF clinic with acute decompensated HF. He is a 74-year-old man with a history of several MIs and an ejection fraction of 28%. The clinic nurse tells you that he is not responding to diuretics due to poor renal function. The cardiologist is planning to insert a pulmonary artery catheter to monitor the patient's response to IV dobutamine, prescribed to strengthen myocardial contractility. What information will you need to gather during the admission history and physical assessment? What laboratory results will you review to determine the patient's renal function? Why is a pulmonary artery catheter indicated for monitoring this patient? What parameters will you monitor to determine the patient's response to dobutamine? How will you determine that the catheter remains in a stable position in the pulmonary artery?

2 After working on a medical nursing unit for a year, you are transferring to a new position in the diagnostic imaging department. As part of your responsibilities you provide preprocedure telephone calls to patients undergoing diagnostic cardiac catheterizations. How will you determine if patients are at risk for contrast agent allergies or CIN? What information will you include in your conversation with patients regarding what to expect during the procedure? What information will you teach the patient about pre- and postprocedure care? What is the strength of the evidence that guides your teaching strategies? How will you know your teaching was effective?

3 During morning cardiology rounds, the team tells your patient that he will be scheduled for a stress test with imaging the following day. As they leave the patient's bedside, the cardiologist asks you to prepare the patient for the stress test. What additional information do you need to discuss with the team before they leave the unit? What priority health history and physical assessment findings of the patient will be used to determine if a pharmacologic or exercise stress test is appropriate for this patient? Discuss the differences between these two stress tests. How do these differences affect patient preparation and education?

REFERENCES AND SELECTED READINGS

Books

Budoff, M. J., & Shinbane, J. S. (Eds.). (2016). *Cardiac CT imaging: Diagnosis of cardiovascular disease* (3rd ed.). Springer.

Chernecky, C., & Berger, B. J. (2013). *Laboratory tests and diagnostic procedures* (6th ed.). Philadelphia, PA: WB Saunders.

Herring, N., & Paterson, D. J. (2018). *Levick's introduction to cardiovascular physiology* (6th ed.). CRC Press.

Huff, J. (2012). *ECG workout: Exercises in arrhythmia interpretation* (6th ed.). Philadelphia, PA: Lippincott Williams & Wilkins.

Miller, C. (2012). *Nursing care of older adults: Theory and practice* (6th ed.). Philadelphia, PA: Lippincott Williams & Wilkins.

Pinkerman, C., Sander, P., Breeding, J. E., et al. (2013). *Institute for clinical systems improvement. Heart failure in adults*. Retrieved from https://www.icsi.org/_asset/50qb52/HeartFailure.pdf

Rosendorff, C. (2013). *Essential cardiology: Principles and practice* (3rd ed.). New York: Springer.

Stephen, T. C., Skillen, D. L., Day, R. A., et al. (2012). *Canadian Jensen's nursing health assessment: A best practice approach* (1st ed.). Philadelphia, PA: Wolters Kluwer Health/Lippincott Williams & Wilkins.

Urden, L. D., Stacy, K. M., & Lough, M. E. (2013). *Critical care nursing: Diagnosis and management (Thelans critical care nursing diagnosis)* (7th ed.). St. Louis, MO: Elsevier Mosby.

Weber, J. R., & Kelley, J. H. (2013). *Health assessment in nursing* (5th ed.). Philadelphia, PA: Lippincott Williams & Wilkins.

Zipes, D. P., Libby, P., Bonow, R. O., et al. (2018). *Braunwald's heart disease e-book: A textbook of cardiovascular medicine*. Elsevier Health Sciences.

Journals and Electronic Documents

Andrade, P. B., Mattos, L. A., Rinaldi, F. S., et al. (2017). Comparison of a vascular closure device versus the radial approach to reduce access site complications in non–ST-segment elevation acute coronary syndrome patients: The angio-seal versus the radial approach in acute coronary syndrome trial. *Catheterization and Cardiovascular Interventions, 89*(6), 976–982.

Araújo, C., Laszczyńska, O., Viana, M., et al. (2018). Sex differences in presenting symptoms of acute coronary syndrome: The EPIHeart cohort study. *BMJ Open, 8*(2), e018798.

Arnold, A. C., & Shibao, C. (2013). Current concepts in orthostatic hypotension management. *Current Hypertension Reports, 15*(4), 304–312.

Astin, F. (2018). Do patients take angioplasty seriously? *European Journal of Cardiovascular Nursing, 17*(3), 194–195.

Baird, D., Jackson, A. C., Higgins, R. O., et al. (2018). Screening, assessment and treatment for depression in patients with chronic heart failure. *British Journal of Cardiac Nursing, 13*(8), 386–393.

Bigger, J. T., & Glassman, A. H. (2010). The American Heart Association science advisory on depression and coronary heart disease: An exploration of the issues raised. *Cleveland Clinic Journal of Medicine, 77*(Suppl 3), S12–S19.

Boardman, H. M., Hartley, L., Eisinga, A., et al. (2015). Hormone therapy for preventing cardiovascular disease in post-menopausal women. *Cochrane Database of Systematic Review*, (3), CD002229.

Cowie, M. R., Anker, S. D., Cleland, J. G., et al. (2014). Improving care for patients with acute heart failure: Before, during and after hospitalization. *ESC Heart Failure, 1*(2), 110–145.

das Virgens, C. M. B., Lemos Jr, L., Noya-Rabelo, M., et al. (2017). Accuracy of gestalt perception of acute chest pain in predicting coronary artery disease. *World Journal of Cardiology, 9*(3), 241–247.

Dekker, R. L. (2014). Patient perspectives about depressive symptoms in heart failure: A review of the qualitative literature. *Journal of Cardiovascular Nursing, 29*(1), E9–E15.

Denn, P., Noonan, B., & Condon, C. (2017). Typical stable angina in a nurse-led chest pain assessment unit. *British Journal of Cardiac Nursing, 12*(2), 92–97.

Drew, B. J., Harris, P., Ze'gre-Hemsey, J. K., et al. (2014). Insights into the problem of alarm fatigue with physiologic monitor devices: A comprehensive observational study of consecutive intensive care unit patients. *PLoS ONE, 9*(10), e110274.

Fletcher, G. F., Ades, P. A., Kligfield, P., et al. (2013). Exercise standards for testing and training: A scientific statement from the American Heart Association. *Circulation, 128*(8), 873–934.

Gillis, N. K., Arslanian-Engoren, C., & Struble, L. (2014). Acute coronary syndromes in older adults: A review of literature. *Journal of Emergency Nursing, 40*(3), 270–275; quiz 292.

Hannibal, G. B. (2014). Cardiac monitoring and electrode placement revisited. *AACN Advanced Critical Care, 25*(2), 188–192.

Havranek, E. P., Mujahid, M. S., Barr, D. A., et al. (2015). Social determinants of risk and outcomes for cardiovascular disease: A scientific statement from the American Heart Association. *Circulation, 132*(9), 873–898.

Homes, T. H., & Rahe, R. H. (1967). The Social Readjustment Rating Scale. *Journal of Psychosomatic Research, 11*(2), 213–218.

Jorgensen, A. L. (2013). Contrast-induced nephropathy: Pathophysiology and preventive strategies. *Critical Care Nurse, 33*(1), 37–46.
Kilic, S., Hermanides, R. S., Ottervanger, J. P., et al; Zwolle Myocardial Infarction Study Group. (2017). Effects of radial versus femoral artery access in patients with acute myocardial infarction: A large centre prospective registry. *Netherlands Heart Journal, 25*(1), 33–39.
Kumar, A. J., Jones, L. E., Kollmeyer, K. R., et al. (2017). Radial artery access for peripheral endovascular procedures. *Journal of Vascular Surgery, 66*(3), 820–825.
Leahy, R. A., & Davenport, E. E. (2015). Home monitoring for cardiovascular implantable electronic devices: Benefits to patients and to their follow-up clinic. *AACN Advanced Critical Care, 26*(4), 343–355.
Lee, S., & Riegel, B. (2018). State of the science in heart failure symptom perception research: An integrative review. *Journal of Cardiovascular Nursing, 33*(3), 204–210.
Lichtman, J. H., Froelicher, E. S., Blumenthal, J. A., et al. (2014). Depression as a risk factor for poor prognosis among patients with acute coronary syndrome: Systematic review and recommendations: A scientific statement from the American Heart Association. *Circulation, 129*(12), 1350–1369.
Lloyd-Jones, D. M. (2015). Coronary artery calcium scoring. Are we there yet? *Journal of the American College of Cardiology, 66*(15), 1654–1656.
McDonnell, L. A., Turek, M., Coutinho, T., et al. (2018). Women's heart health: Knowledge, beliefs, and practices of Canadian physicians. *Journal of Women's Health, 27*(1), 72–82.
McSweeney, J. C., Rosenfeld, A. G., Abel, W. M., et al. (2016). Preventing and experiencing ischemic heart disease as a woman: State of the science: A scientific statement from the American Heart Association. *Circulation, 133*(13), 1302–1331.
Mervak, B. M., Davenport, M. S., Ellis, J. H., et al. (2015). Rates of breakthrough reactions in inpatients at high risk receiving premedication before contrast-enhanced CT. *American Journal of Roentgenology, 205*(1), 77–84.
Nielsen, C. G., Laut, K. G., Jensen, L. O., et al. (2017). Patient delay in patients with ST-elevation myocardial infarction: Time patterns and predictors for a prolonged delay. *European Heart Journal: Acute Cardiovascular Care, 6*(7), 583–591.
Pavlović, J., Greenland, P., Deckers, J. W., et al. (2018). Assessing gaps in cholesterol treatment guidelines for primary prevention of cardiovascular disease based on available randomised clinical trial evidence: The Rotterdam Study. *European Journal of Preventive Cardiology, 25*(4), 420–431.
Piepoli, M. F., Corrà, U., Abreu, A., et al. (2015). Challenges in secondary prevention of cardiovascular diseases: A review of the current practice. *International Journal of Cardiology, 180*, 114–119.
Potts, K. (2013). C-reactive protein and its role in coronary artery disease. *British Journal of Cardiac Nursing, 8*(4), 193–197.
Public Health Agency of Canada. (2015). Chronic Disease and Injury Indicator Framework—Quick Stats, 2015 Edition. *Health Promotion and Chronic Disease Prevention in Canada: Research, Policy and Practice, 35*(10), 194–195.
Romero, I. (2013). Ambulatory electrocardiology. *Cardiology in Review, 21*(5), 239–248.
Schlyter, M., Östman, M., Engström, G., et al. (2017). Personality factors and depression as predictors of hospital-based health care utilization following acute myocardial infarction. *European Journal of Cardiovascular Nursing, 16*(4), 318–325.
Sendelbach, S., & Funk, M. (2013). Alarm fatigue: A patient safety concern. *AACN Advanced Critical Care, 24*(4), 378–386.
Sendelbach, S., & Jepsen, S. (2013). AACN practice alert: Alarm management. Retrieved January 25, 2016, from www.aacn.org/wd/practice/content/practicealerts/alarm-management-practice-alert.pcms?menu=practice
Siegrist, P. T., & Sumitsuji, S. (2014). Chronic total occlusion: Current methods of revascularization. *Cardiovascular Medicine, 17*(12), 347–356.
Steinberg, J. S., Varma, N., Cygankiewicz, I., et al. (2017). 2017 ISHNE-HRS expert consensus statement on ambulatory ECG and external cardiac monitoring/telemetry. *Heart Rhythm, 14*(7), e55–e96.
Stone, J. A., Hauer, T., Haykowsky, M., et al. (2015). Exercise therapy for heart failure patients in Canada. *Heart Failure Clinics, 11*(1), 83–88.
Stone, N. J., Robinson, J., Lichtenstein, A. H., et al. (2014). 2013 ACC/AHA guideline on the treatment of blood cholesterol to reduce atherosclerotic cardiovascular risk in adults: A report of the American College of Cardiology/American Heart Association Task Force on Practice Guidelines. *Journal of the American College of Cardiology, 63*(25 Pt B), 2889–2934.
Swift, D. L., Lavie, C. J., Johannsen, N. M., et al. (2013). Physical activity, cardiorespiratory fitness, and exercise training in primary and secondary coronary prevention. *Circulation Journal, 77*(2), 281–292.
Tzikas, S., Palapies, L., Bakogiannis, C., et al. (2017). GDF-15 predicts cardiovascular events in acute chest pain patients. *PloS One, 12*(8), e0182314.
Walsh, J. A., Topol, E. J., & Steinhubl, R. S. (2014). Novel wireless devices for cardiac monitoring. *Circulation, 130*(7), 573–581.
White, K., Macfarlane, H., Hoffmann, B., et al. (2018). Consensus statement of standards for interventional cardiovascular nursing practice. *Heart, Lung and Circulation, 27*(5), 535–551.
You, B., Zhu, B., Su, X., et al. (2018). Gender differences among elderly patients with primary percutaneous coronary intervention. *Aging and Disease, 9*(5), 852–860.

Resources

Canadian Council of Cardiovascular Nurses: http://www.cccn.ca/index.php
Heart and Stroke Foundation of Canada: http://www.heartandstroke.com
Medi-Smart Cardiovascular Nursing Resources: http://www.medi-smart.com/cardiac.htm

28 Management of Patient With Dysrhythmias and Conduction Problems

Adapted by Colleen Norris and Nicole Tegg

Learning Objectives

On completion of this chapter, the learner will be able to:

1. Correlate the components of the normal electrocardiogram (ECG) with physiologic events of the heart.
2. Define the ECG as a waveform that represents the cardiac electrical event in relation to the lead (placement of electrodes).
3. Analyze elements of an ECG rhythm strip: ventricular and atrial rate, ventricular and atrial rhythm, QRS complex and shape, QRS duration, P wave and shape, PR interval, and P:QRS ratio.
4. Identify the ECG criteria, causes, and management of several dysrhythmias, including conduction disturbances.
5. Use the nursing process as a framework for care of patients with dysrhythmias.
6. Compare the different types of pacemakers, their uses, possible complications, and nursing implications.
7. Describe the nursing management of patients with implantable cardiac devices.
8. Describe the key points of using a defibrillator.
9. Describe the purpose of an implantable cardioverter defibrillator, the types available, and the nursing implications.
10. Describe invasive methods to diagnose and treat recurrent dysrhythmias and discuss the nursing implications.

Without a regular rate and rhythm, the heart may not perform efficiently as a pump to circulate oxygenated blood and other life-sustaining nutrients to all of the body's tissues and organs (including the heart itself). With an irregular or erratic rhythm, the heart is considered to be dysrhythmic (sometimes called arrhythmic). This is a potentially dangerous condition.

Nurses may encounter patients with dysrhythmias in all health care settings, including primary care settings, skilled nursing facilities, rehabilitation settings, and hospitals. Some dysrhythmias are acute and others chronic; some require emergent interventions, while others may not. Because patients with dysrhythmias are frequently encountered in many different types of settings, nurses must be able to identify and provide appropriate first-line treatment of dysrhythmias.

DYSRHYTHMIAS

Dysrhythmias are disorders of the formation or **conduction** (or both) of the electrical impulse within the heart. These disorders can cause disturbances of the heart rate, the heart rhythm, or both. Dysrhythmias may initially be evidenced by the hemodynamic effect they cause (e.g., a change in conduction may change the pumping action of the heart and cause decreased blood pressure). Dysrhythmias are diagnosed by analyzing the electrocardiographic (ECG) waveform. Their treatment is based on frequency and severity of symptoms produced. Dysrhythmias are named according to the site of origin of the impulse and the mechanism of formation or conduction involved. For example, an impulse that originates in the sinoatrial (SA) node and at a slow rate is called sinus bradycardia.

Normal Electrical Conduction

The electrical impulse that stimulates and paces the cardiac muscle normally originates in the SA node, an area located near the superior vena cava in the right atrium. Usually, the electrical impulse occurs at a rate of 60 to 100 times a minute in the adult. The electrical impulse quickly travels from the sinus node through the atria to the atrioventricular (AV) node (Fig. 28-1); this process is known as conduction. The electrical stimulation of the muscle cells of the atria causes them to contract. The structure of the AV node slows the electrical impulse, giving the atria time to contract and fill the ventricles with blood. This part of atrial contraction is frequently referred to as the "atrial kick" and accounts for nearly one third of the volume ejected during ventricular contraction (Fuster, Walsh, & Harrington, 2011). The electrical impulse then travels very quickly through the bundle of His to the right and left bundle branches and the Purkinje fibres, located in the ventricular muscle. The electrical stimulation of the muscle cells of the ventricles in turn causes the mechanical contraction of the ventricles (systole). The cells repolarize and the ventricles then relax (diastole). The electrical impulse causes the mechanical contraction of the heart muscle that follows.

The electrical stimulation is called **depolarization**, and the mechanical contraction is called systole. Electrical relaxation is called **repolarization**, and mechanical relaxation is called diastole. The process from sinus node electrical impulse generation through ventricular repolarization completes the electromechanical circuit, and the cycle

Glossary

ablation: purposeful destruction of heart muscle cells, usually in an attempt to control a dysrhythmia

antiarrhythmic medication: a medication that suppresses or prevents a dysrhythmia

automaticity: ability of the cardiac cells to initiate an electrical impulse

cardioversion: electrical current administered in synchrony with the patient's own QRS complex to stop a dysrhythmia

chronotropy: rate of impulse formation

conduction: transmission of electrical impulses from one cell to another

defibrillation: electrical current administered to stop a dysrhythmia, not synchronized with the patient's QRS complex

depolarization: process by which cardiac muscle cells change from a more negatively charged to a more positively charged intracellular state

dromotropy: conduction velocity

dysrhythmia: disorder of the formation or conduction (or both) of the electrical impulse within the heart, altering the heart rate, heart rhythm, or both and potentially causing altered blood flow (also referred to as arrhythmia)

elective replacement indicator (ERI): a signal produced by a pacemaker when it is interrogated to indicate a near-depleted battery

implantable cardioverter defibrillator (ICD): a device implanted into the chest to treat dysrhythmias

inhibited: in reference to pacemakers, term used to describe the pacemaker withholding an impulse (not firing)

inotropy: force of myocardial contraction

P wave: the part of an electrocardiogram (ECG) that reflects conduction of an electrical impulse through the atrium; atrial depolarization

PP interval: the duration between the beginning of one P wave and the beginning of the next P wave; used to calculate atrial rate and rhythm

PR interval: the part of an ECG that reflects conduction of an electrical impulse from the sinoatrial (SA) node through the atrioventricular (AV) node

proarrhythmic: an agent (e.g., a medication) that causes or exacerbates a dysrhythmia

QRS complex: the part of an ECG that reflects conduction of an electrical impulse through the ventricles; ventricular depolarization

QT interval: the part of an ECG that reflects the time from ventricular depolarization through repolarization

repolarization: process by which cardiac muscle cells return to a more negatively charged intracellular condition, their resting state

RR interval: the duration between the beginning of one QRS complex and the beginning of the next QRS complex; used to calculate ventricular rate and rhythm

sensitivity: the level that the intracardiac electrical activity must exceed in order to be sensed by a pacemaker

sinus rhythm: electrical activity of the heart initiated by the sinoatrial (SA) node

ST segment: the part of an ECG that reflects the end of the QRS complex to the beginning of the T wave

supraventricular tachycardia (SVT): a rhythm that originates in the conduction system above the ventricles

T wave: the part of an ECG that reflects repolarization of the ventricles

TP interval: the part of an ECG that reflects the time between the end of the T wave and the beginning of the next P wave; used to identify the isoelectric line

triggered: in reference to pacemakers, term used to describe the release of an impulse in response to some stimulus

U wave: the part of an ECG that may reflect Purkinje fibre repolarization; usually it is not seen unless a patient's serum potassium level is low

ventricular tachycardia (VT): a rhythm that originates in the ventricles

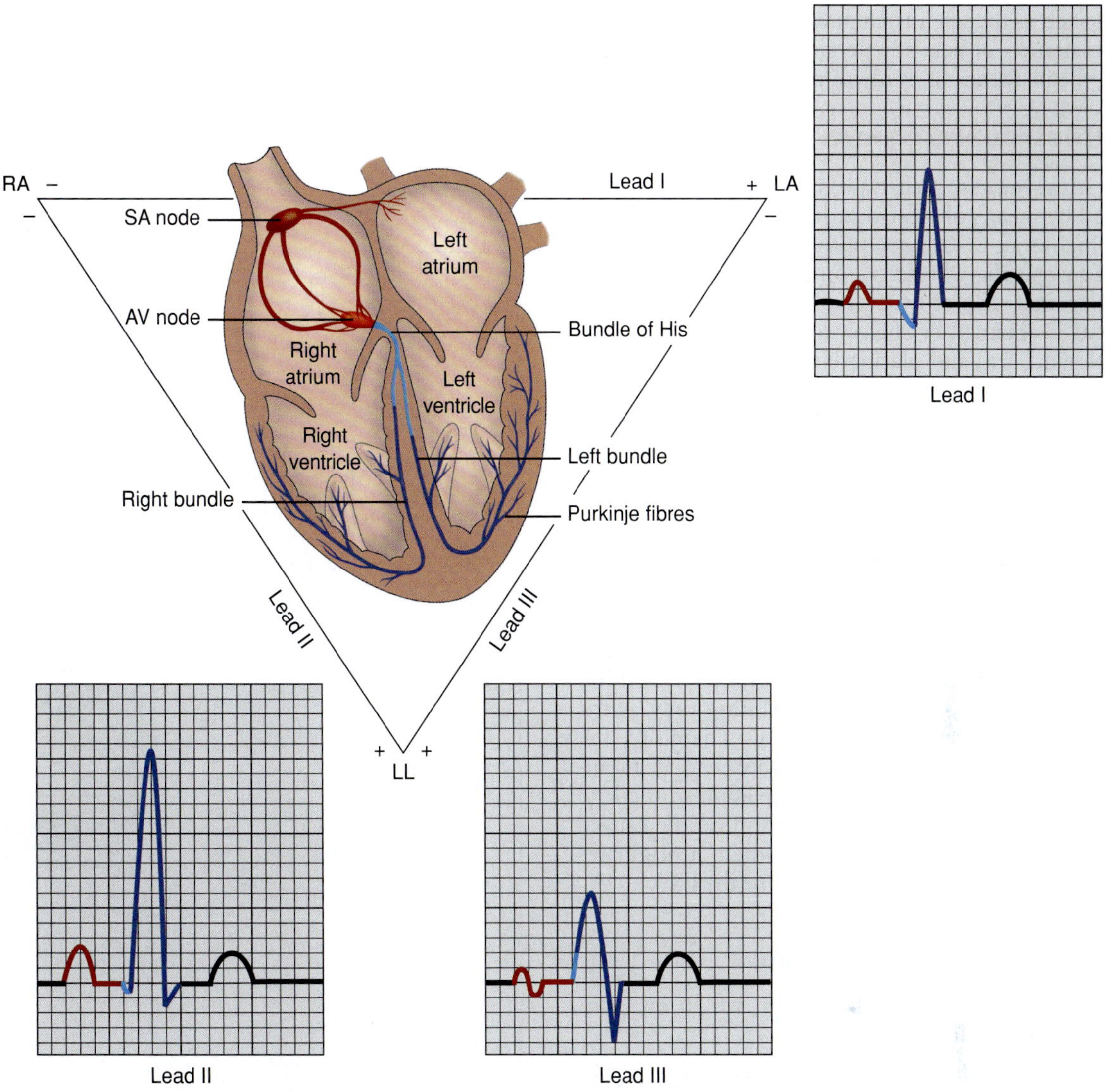

FIGURE 28-1. Relationship of ECG complex, lead system, and electrical impulse. The heart conducts electrical activity, which the ECG measures and shows. The configurations of electrical activity displayed on the ECG vary depending on the lead (or view) of the ECG and on the rhythm of the heart. Therefore, the configuration of a normal rhythm tracing from lead I will differ from the configuration of a normal rhythm tracing from lead II, lead II will differ from lead III, and so on. The same is true for abnormal rhythms and cardiac disorders. To make an accurate assessment of the heart's electrical activity or to identify where, when, and what abnormalities occur, the ECG needs to be evaluated from every lead, not just from lead II. Here the different areas of electrical activity are identified by colour. RA, right arm; LA, left arm; SA, sinoatrial; AV, atrioventricular; LL, left leg.

begins again. See Chapter 27 for a more complete explanation of cardiac function.

Influences on Heart Rate and Contractility

The heart rate is influenced by the autonomic nervous system, which consists of sympathetic and parasympathetic fibres. Sympathetic nerve fibres (also referred to as adrenergic fibres) are attached to the heart and arteries as well as several other areas in the body. Stimulation of the sympathetic system increases heart rate (positive **chronotropy**), conduction through the AV node (positive **dromotropy**), and the force of myocardial contraction (positive **inotropy**). Sympathetic stimulation also constricts peripheral blood vessels, therefore increasing blood pressure. Parasympathetic nerve fibres are also attached to the heart and arteries. Parasympathetic stimulation reduces the heart rate (negative chronotropy), AV conduction (negative dromotropy), and the force of atrial myocardial contraction. The decreased sympathetic stimulation results in dilation of arteries, thereby lowering blood pressure.

Manipulation of the autonomic nervous system may increase or decrease the incidence of dysrhythmias. Increased sympathetic stimulation (e.g., caused by exercise, anxiety, fever, or administration of catecholamines, such as dopamine [Intropin], aminophylline, or dobutamine [Dobutrex]) may increase the incidence of dysrhythmias. Decreased sympathetic stimulation (e.g., with rest, anxiety-reduction methods such as therapeutic communication or meditation, or administration of beta-adrenergic blocking agents) may decrease the incidence of dysrhythmias.

The Electrocardiogram

The electrical impulse that travels through the heart can be viewed by means of electrocardiography, the end product of which is an ECG. Each phase of the cardiac cycle is reflected by specific waveforms on the screen of a cardiac monitor or on a strip of ECG graph paper.

An ECG is obtained by slightly abrading the skin with a clean dry gauze pad and placing electrodes on the body at specific areas. Electrodes come in various shapes and sizes, but they all have two components: (1) an adhesive substance that attaches to the skin to secure the electrode in place and; (2) a substance that reduces the skin's electrical impedance and promotes detection of the electrical current.

The number and placement of the electrodes depend on the type of ECG needed. Most continuous monitors use 2 to 5 electrodes, usually placed on the limbs and the chest. These electrodes create an imaginary line, called a lead, that serves as a reference point from which the electrical activity is viewed. A lead is like an eye of a camera: It has a narrow peripheral field of vision, looking only at the electrical activity directly in front of it. Therefore, the ECG waveforms that appear on the paper or cardiac monitor represent the electrical current in relation to the lead (see Fig. 28-1). A change in the waveform can be caused by a change in the electrical current (where it originates or how it is conducted) or by a change in the lead.

Obtaining an Electrocardiogram

Electrodes are attached to cable wires, which are connected to one of the following:

- An ECG machine placed at the patient's side for an immediate recording (standard 12-lead ECG)
- A cardiac monitor at the patient's bedside for continuous reading; this kind of monitoring, usually called hardwire monitoring, is used in intensive care units
- A small box that the patient carries that continuously transmits the ECG information by radiowaves to a central monitor located elsewhere (called telemetry)
- A small, lightweight tape recorder–like machine (called ambulatory ECG monitoring or a Holter monitor) that the patient wears and that continuously records the ECG on a tape, which is later viewed and analyzed with a scanner

A patient may undergo an electrophysiology (EP) study in which electrodes are placed inside the heart in order to obtain an intracardiac ECG. This is used not only to diagnose the dysrhythmia, but also to determine the most effective treatment plan. However, because an EP study is invasive, it is performed in the hospital and may require that the patient be admitted. (A more in-depth discussion is found later in this chapter.)

The placement of electrodes for continuous monitoring, telemetry, or Holter monitoring varies with the type of technology, the purpose of monitoring, and the standards of the health care facility. For a standard 12-lead ECG, 10 electrodes (6 on the chest and 4 on the limbs) are

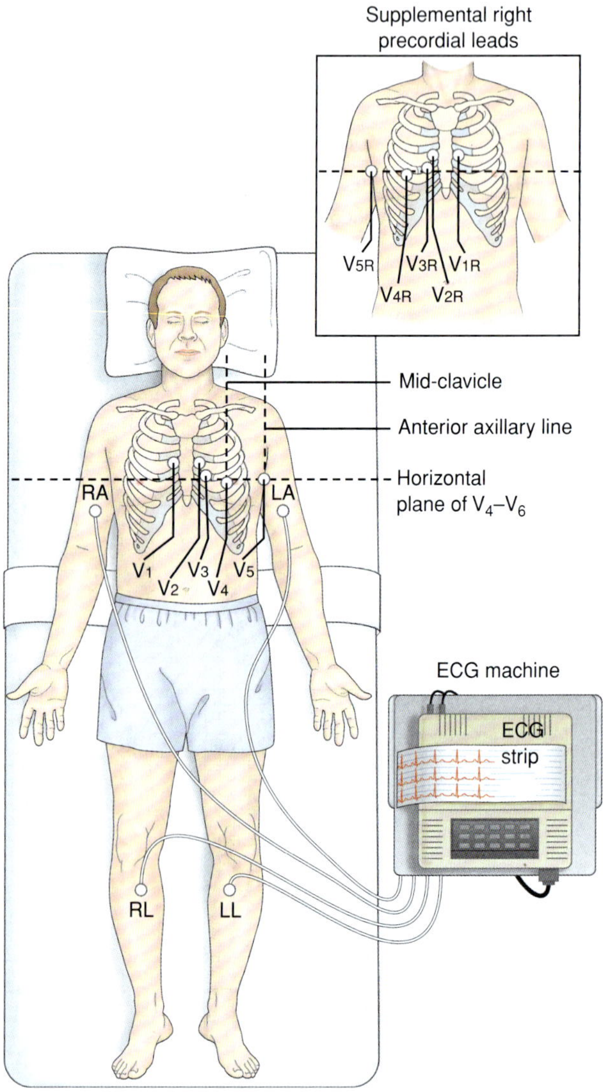

FIGURE 28-2. ECG electrode placement. The standard left precordial leads are V_1—4th intercostal space, right sternal border; V_2—4th intercostal space, left sternal border; V_3—diagonally between V_2 and V_4; V_4—5th intercostal space, left midclavicular line; V_5—same level as V_4, anterior axillary line; V_6 (not illustrated)—same level as V_4 and V_5, midaxillary line. The right precordial leads, placed across the right side of the chest, are the mirror opposite of the left leads. RA, right arm; LA, left arm; RL, right leg; LL, left leg. (Adapted from Molle, E. A., Kronenberger, J., West-Stack, C., et al. (2005). *Lippincott Williams & Wilkins's pocket guide to medical assisting* (2nd ed.). Philadelphia, PA: Lippincott Williams & Wilkins.)

placed on the body (Fig. 28-2). To prevent interference from the electrical activity of skeletal muscle, the limb electrodes are usually placed on areas that are not bony and that do not have significant movement. These limb electrodes provide the first six leads: leads I, II, III, aVR, aVL, and aVF. The six chest electrodes are applied to the chest at very specific areas. The chest electrodes provide the V or precordial leads, V_1 through V_6. To locate the 4th intercostal space and the placement of V_1, the sternal angle and then the sternal notch, which is about 3 or 5 cm below the sternal angle, are located. When the fingers are moved to the patient's immediate right, the 2nd rib can be palpated. The 2nd intercostal space is the indentation felt just below the 2nd rib.

Locating the specific intercostal space is critical for correct chest electrode placement. Errors in diagnosis can occur if electrodes are incorrectly placed. Sometimes, when the patient is in the hospital and needs to be monitored closely for ECG changes, the chest electrodes are left in place to ensure the same placement for follow-up ECGs.

A standard 12-lead ECG reflects the electrical activity primarily in the left ventricle. Placement of additional electrodes for other leads may be needed to obtain more complete information. For example, in patients with suspected right-sided heart damage, right-sided precordial leads are required to evaluate the right ventricle (see Fig. 28-2).

Components of the Electrocardiogram

The ECG waveform reflects the function of the heart's conduction system, which normally initiates and conducts the electrical activity, in relation to the lead. The ECG offers important information about the electrical activity of the heart. ECG waveforms are printed on graph paper that is divided by light and dark vertical and horizontal lines at standard intervals (Fig. 28-3). Time and rate are measured on the horizontal axis of the graph, and amplitude or voltage is measured on the vertical axis. When an ECG waveform moves toward the top of the paper, it is called a positive deflection. When it moves toward the bottom of the paper, it is called a negative deflection. When an ECG is reviewed, each waveform should be examined and compared with the others.

Waves, Complexes, and Intervals

The ECG is composed of waveforms (including the P wave, the QRS complex, the T wave, and possibly a U wave) and of segments and intervals (including the **PR interval**, the ST segment, and the QT interval) (see Fig. 28-3).

The **P wave** represents the electrical impulse starting in the sinus node and spreading through the atria. Therefore, the P wave represents atrial depolarization. It is normally 2.5 mm or less in height and 0.11 seconds or less in duration.

The **QRS complex** represents ventricular depolarization. Not all QRS complexes have all three waveforms. The Q wave is the first negative deflection after the P wave. The Q wave is normally less than 0.04 seconds in duration and less than 25% of the R-wave amplitude. The R wave is the first positive deflection after the P wave, and the S wave is the first negative deflection after the R wave. When a wave is less than 5 mm in height, small letters (q, r, s) are used; when a wave is taller than 5 mm, capital letters (Q, R, S) are used to label the waves. The QRS complex is normally less than 0.12 seconds in duration.

The **T wave** represents ventricular repolarization (when the cells regain a negative charge; also called the resting state). It follows the QRS complex and is usually the same direction as the QRS complex. Atrial repolarization also occurs but is not visible on the ECG because it occurs at the same time as the QRS.

The **U wave** is thought to represent repolarization of the Purkinje fibres, but it sometimes is seen in patients with hypokalemia (low potassium levels), hypertension, or heart disease. If present, the U wave follows the T wave and is usually smaller than the P wave. If tall, it may be mistaken for an extra P wave.

The PR interval is measured from the beginning of the P wave to the beginning of the QRS complex and represents the time needed for sinus node stimulation, atrial depolarization, and conduction through the AV node before ventricular depolarization. In adults, the PR interval normally ranges from 0.12 to 0.20 seconds in duration.

The **ST segment**, which represents early ventricular repolarization, lasts from the end of the QRS complex to the beginning of the T wave. The beginning of the ST segment is usually identified by a change in the thickness or angle of the terminal portion of the QRS complex. The

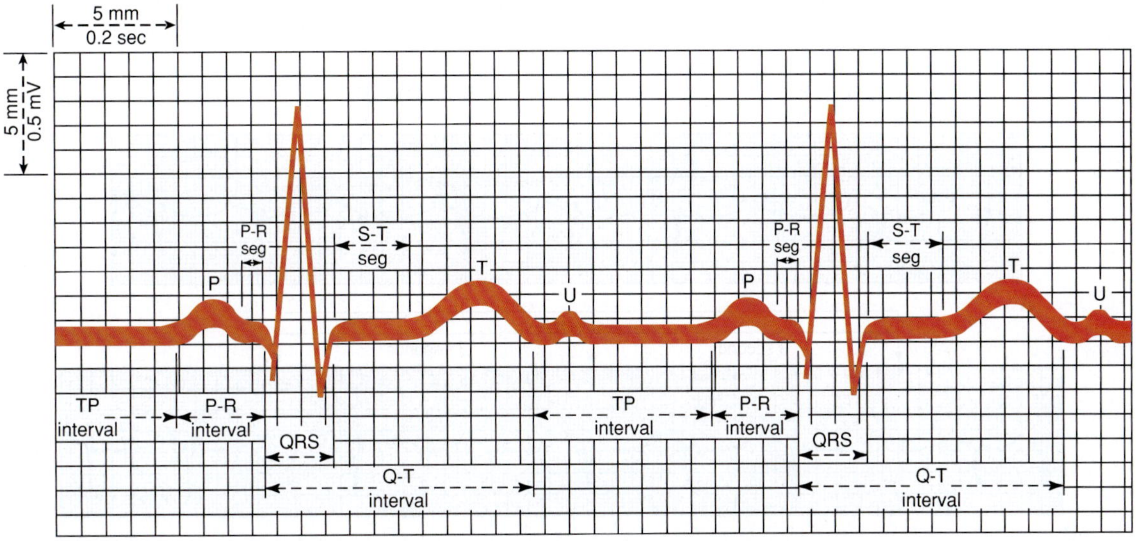

FIGURE 28-3. ECG graph and commonly measured components. Each small box represents 0.04 seconds on the horizontal axis and 1 mm or 0.1 mV on the vertical axis. The PR interval is measured from the beginning of the P wave to the beginning of the QRS complex; the QRS complex is measured from the beginning of the Q wave to the end of the S wave; the QT interval is measured from the beginning of the Q wave to the end of the T wave; and the TP interval is measured from the end of the T wave to the beginning of the next P wave.

end of the ST segment may be more difficult to identify because it merges into the T wave. The ST segment is normally isoelectric (see discussion of TP interval). It is analyzed to identify whether it is above or below the isoelectric line, which may be, among other signs and symptoms, a sign of cardiac ischemia (see Chapter 29).

The **QT interval**, which represents the total time for ventricular depolarization and repolarization, is measured from the beginning of the QRS complex to the end of the T wave. The QT interval varies with heart rate, gender, and age, and the measured interval needs to be corrected for these variables through specific calculations. Several ECG interpretation books contain charts for these calculations. The QT interval is usually 0.32 to 0.40 seconds in duration if the heart rate is 65 to 95 bpm (beats per minute). If the QT interval becomes prolonged, the patient may be at risk for a lethal ventricular dysrhythmia called torsades de pointes.

The **TP interval** is measured from the end of the T wave to the beginning of the next P wave, an isoelectric period (see Fig. 28-3). When no electrical activity is detected, the line on the graph remains flat; this is called the isoelectric line. The ST segment is compared with the TP interval to detect changes from the line on the graph during the isoelectric period.

The PP interval is measured from the beginning of one P wave to the beginning of the next. The **PP interval** is used to determine atrial rhythm and atrial rate. The **RR interval** is measured from one QRS complex to the next QRS complex. The RR interval is used to determine ventricular rate and rhythm.

Analyzing the Electrocardiogram Rhythm Strip

The ECG rhythm strip must be analyzed in a systematic manner to determine the patient's cardiac rate and rhythm, and to detect dysrhythmias and conduction disorders, as well as evidence of myocardial ischemia, injury, and infarction.

Determining Heart Rate From the Electrocardiogram

Heart rate can be obtained from the ECG strip by several methods. A 1-minute strip contains 300 large boxes and 1,500 small boxes. Therefore, an easy and accurate method of determining heart rate with a regular rhythm is to count the number of small boxes within an RR interval and divide 1,500 by that number. If, for example, there are 10 small boxes between two R waves, the heart rate is 1,500/10, or 150; if there are 25 small boxes, the heart rate is 1,500/25, or 60 (see Fig. 28-4A).

An alternative but less accurate method for estimating heart rate, which is usually used when the rhythm is irregular, is to count the number of RR intervals in 6 seconds and multiply that number by 10. The top of the ECG paper is usually marked at 3-second intervals, which is 15 large boxes horizontally (see Fig. 28-4B). The RR intervals are counted, rather than QRS complexes, because a computed heart rate based on the latter might be inaccurately high.

The same methods may be used for determining atrial rate, using the PP interval instead of the RR interval.

Determining Heart Rhythm From the Electrocardiogram

The rhythm is often identified at the same time the rate is determined. The RR interval is used to determine ventricular rhythm and the PP interval is used to determine atrial rhythm. If the intervals are the same or if the difference between the intervals is less than 0.8 seconds throughout the strip, the rhythm is called regular. If the intervals are different, the rhythm is called irregular (see Chart 28-1).

Normal Sinus Rhythm

Normal **sinus rhythm** occurs when the electrical impulse starts at a regular rate and rhythm in the sinus node and travels through the normal conduction pathway. Normal sinus rhythm has the following characteristics (Fig. 28-5):

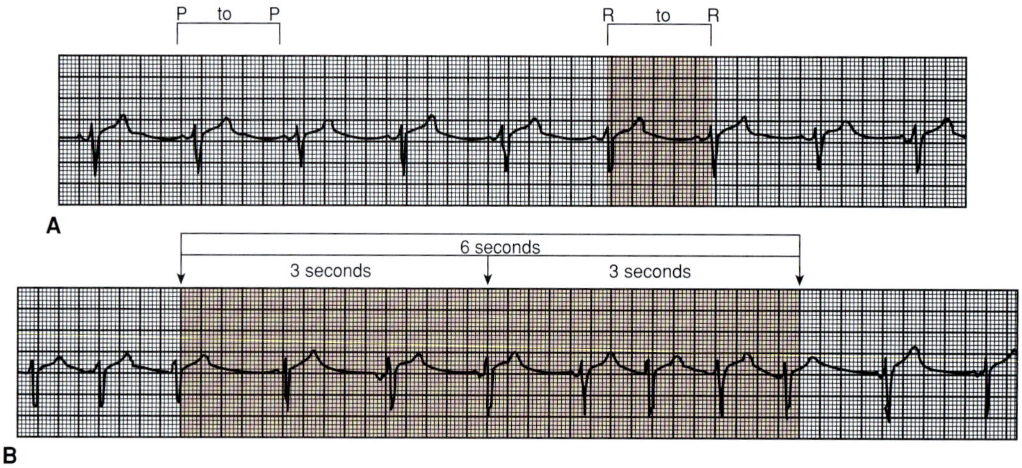

FIGURE 28-4. **A.** Ventricular and atrial heart rate determination with a regular rhythm: 1,500 divided by the number of small boxes between two P waves (atrial rate) or between two R waves (ventricular rate). In this example, there are 25 small boxes between both the R waves and the P waves, so the heart rate is 60 beats per minute. **B.** Heart rate determination if the rhythm is irregular. There are approximately seven RR intervals in 6 seconds, so there are about 70 RR intervals in 60 seconds ($7 \times 10 = 70$). The ventricular heart rate is 70 beats per minute.

CHART 28-1

Interpreting Dysrhythmias: Systematic Analysis of the Electrocardiogram

When examining an ECG rhythm strip to learn more about a patient's dysrhythmia:

1. Determine the ventricular rate.
2. Determine the ventricular rhythm.
3. Determine QRS duration.
4. Determine whether the QRS duration is consistent throughout the strip. If not, identify other duration.
5. Identify QRS shape; if not consistent, then identify other shapes.
6. Identify P waves; is there a P in front of every QRS?
7. Identify P-wave shape; identify whether it is consistent or not.
8. Determine the atrial rate.
9. Determine the atrial rhythm.
10. Determine each PR interval.
11. Determine if the PR intervals are consistent, irregular but with a pattern to the irregularity, or just irregular.
12. Determine how many P waves for each QRS (P:QRS ratio).

In many cases, the nurse may use a checklist and document the findings next to the appropriate ECG criterion.

Ventricular and atrial rate: 60 to 100 in the adult
Ventricular and atrial rhythm: Regular
QRS shape and duration: Usually normal, but may be regularly abnormal
P wave: Normal and consistent shape; always in front of the QRS
PR interval: Consistent interval between 0.12 and 0.20 seconds
P:QRS ratio: 1:1

Types of Dysrhythmias

Dysrhythmias include sinus, atrial, junctional, and ventricular dysrhythmias and their various subcategories.

Sinus Node Dysrhythmias

Sinus Bradycardia

Sinus bradycardia occurs when the sinus node creates an impulse at a slower-than-normal rate. Causes include lower metabolic needs (e.g., sleep, athletic training, hypothyroidism), vagal stimulation (e.g., from vomiting, suctioning, severe pain, extreme emotions), medications (e.g., calcium channel blockers, amiodarone, beta-blockers), idiopathic sinus node dysfunction, increased intracranial pressure (ICP), and myocardial infarction (MI), especially of the inferior wall. Other possible contributing factors in clinically significant bradycardia include what are referred to as the H's and the T's: hypovolemia, hypoxia, hydrogen ion (acidosis), hypokalemia or hyperkalemia, hypoglycemia, and hypothermia; toxins, tamponade (cardiac), tension pneumothorax, thrombosis (coronary or pulmonary), and trauma (hypovolemia, increased ICP) (Fuster et al., 2011). Sinus bradycardia has the following characteristics (Fig. 28-6):

Ventricular and atrial rate: Less than 60 in the adult
Ventricular and atrial rhythm: Regular
QRS shape and duration: Usually normal, but may be regularly abnormal
P wave: Normal and consistent shape; always in front of the QRS
PR interval: Consistent interval between 0.12 and 0.20 seconds
P:QRS ratio: 1:1

All characteristics of sinus bradycardia are the same as those of normal sinus rhythm, except for the rate. The patient is assessed to determine the hemodynamic effect and the possible cause of the dysrhythmia. If the decrease in heart rate results from stimulation of the vagus nerve, such as with bearing down during defecation or vomiting, attempts are made to prevent further vagal stimulation. If the bradycardia is caused by a medication such as a beta-blocker, the medication may be withheld. If the slow heart rate causes significant hemodynamic changes resulting in shortness of breath, acute alteration of mental status, angina, hypotension, ST-segment changes, or premature ventricular complexes (PVCs), treatment is directed toward increasing the heart rate. If the slow heart rate is due to sinus node dysfunction, which most often occurs in people older than 50 years of age, decreased exercise capacity, fatigue, unexplained confusion, or memory loss may result (Jensen, Gronroos, Chen, et al., 2014).

Medical Management

Management depends on the cause and symptoms. Resolving the causative factors may be the only treatment needed. If the bradycardia produces signs and symptoms of clinical instability (e.g., acute alteration in mental status, chest discomfort, or hypotension), 0.5 mg of atropine may be given rapidly as an intravenous (IV) bolus and repeated

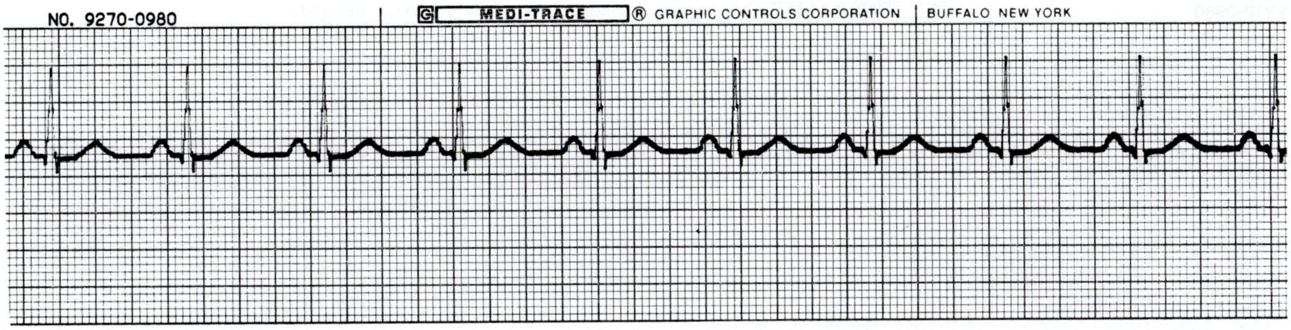

FIGURE 28-5. Normal sinus rhythm in lead II.

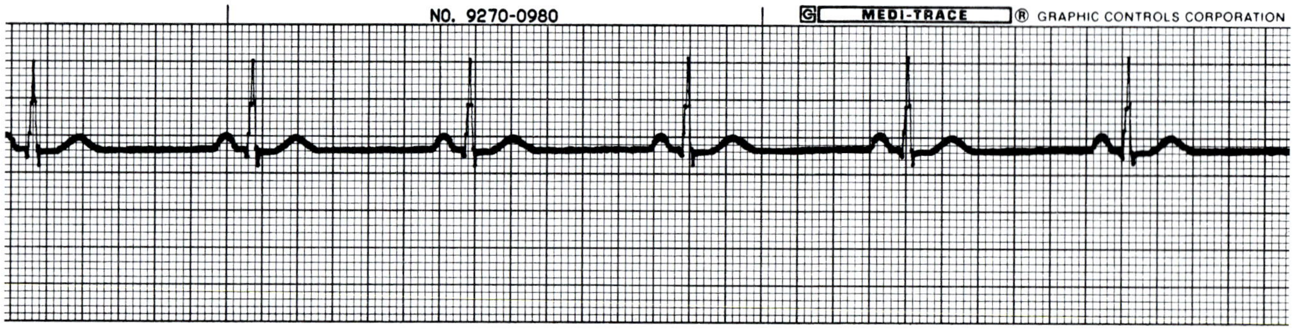

FIGURE 28-6. Sinus bradycardia in lead II.

every 3 to 5 minutes until a maximum dosage of 3 mg is given. Rarely if the bradycardia is unresponsive to atropine, emergency transcutaneous pacing can be instituted, or catecholamines, such as dopamine or epinephrine, are given (Link, Berkow, Kudenchuk, et al., 2015) (see later discussion in Pacemaker Therapy).

Sinus Tachycardia

Sinus tachycardia occurs when the sinus node creates an impulse at a faster-than-normal rate. Causes may include the following:

- Physiologic or psychological stress (e.g., acute blood loss, anemia, shock, hypervolemia, hypovolemia, heart failure, pain, hypermetabolic states, fever, exercise, anxiety)
- Medications that stimulate the sympathetic response (e.g., catecholamines, aminophylline, atropine), stimulants (e.g., caffeine, alcohol, nicotine), and illicit drugs (e.g., amphetamines, cocaine, Ecstasy)
- Enhanced **automaticity** of the SA node and/or excessive sympathetic tone with reduced parasympathetic tone, a condition called inappropriate sinus tachycardia
- Autonomic dysfunction, which results in a type of sinus tachycardia called postural orthostatic tachycardia syndrome (POTS). Patients with POTS have tachycardia without hypotension within 5 to 10 minutes of standing or with head-upright tilt testing (Sheldon, Grubb, Olshansky, et al., 2015).

Sinus tachycardia has the following characteristics (Fig. 28-7):

Ventricular and atrial rate: Greater than 100 in the adult, but usually less than 120
Ventricular and atrial rhythm: Regular
QRS shape and duration: Usually normal, but may be regularly abnormal
P wave: Normal and consistent shape; always in front of the QRS, but may be buried in the preceding T wave
PR interval: Consistent interval between 0.12 and 0.20 seconds
P:QRS ratio: 1:1

All aspects of sinus tachycardia are the same as those of normal sinus rhythm, except for the rate. Sinus tachycardia does not start or end suddenly (nonparoxysmal). As the heart rate increases, the diastolic filling time decreases, possibly resulting in reduced cardiac output and subsequent symptoms of syncope and low blood pressure. If the rapid rate persists and the heart cannot compensate for the decreased ventricular filling, the patient may develop acute pulmonary edema.

Medical Management

Medical management of sinus tachycardia is determined by the severity of symptoms and directed at identifying and abolishing its cause. If the tachycardia is persistent and causing hemodynamic instability, synchronized **cardioversion** is the treatment of choice (see later discussion). Otherwise, vagal maneuvers, such as carotid sinus massage, gagging, bearing down against a closed glottis (as if having a bowel movement), forceful and sustained coughing, and applying a cold stimulus to the face (such as immersing the face in ice water), or administration of adenosine (Adenocard) may be considered to interrupt the tachycardia. These increase parasympathetic stimulation, causing slower conduction through the AV node and blocking the reentry of the rerouted impulse (Smith, Fry, Taylor, et al., 2015). Beta-blockers (Class II antiarrhythmic) and calcium channel blockers (Class IV antiarrhythmic) (see Table 28-1),

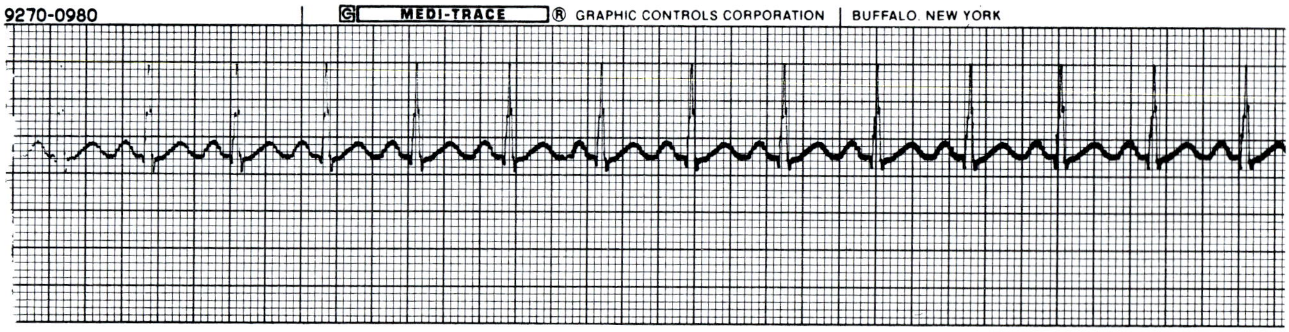

FIGURE 28-7. Sinus tachycardia in lead II.

TABLE 28-1 Summary of Antiarrhythmic Medications

Class[a]	Action	Drug Names	Side Effects	Nursing Interventions
IA	Moderate depression of depolarization; prolongs repolarization Treats and prevents atrial and ventricular dysrhythmias	Quinidine (Quinaglute, Quinidex, Cardioquin) Procainamide (Pronestyl, Procanbid, Disopyramide (Norpace)	Decreased cardiac contractility Prolonged QRS, QT Proarrhythmic Hypotension with IV administration Diarrhea with quinidine, constipation with disopyramide Cinchonism with quinidine Lupus-like syndrome with procainamide Anticholinergic effects: dry mouth, urinary hesitancy with disopyramide	Observe for HF Monitor BP with IV administration Monitor QRS duration for increase >50% from baseline Monitor for prolonged QT Monitor *N*-acetyl procainamide (NAPA) laboratory values during procainamide therapy. If given for atrial fibrillation, ensure that the patient has been pretreated with a medication to control AV conduction
IB	Minimal depression of depolarization; shortened repolarization Treats ventricular dysrhythmias	Lidocaine (Xylocaine, LidoPen)	CNS changes (e.g., confusion, lethargy) Bradycardia GI distress Tremors	Monitor for CNS changes and tremors. Discuss with the primary provider decreasing lidocaine dose in older adult patients and patients with cardiac/liver dysfunction
IC	Marked depression of depolarization; little effect on repolarization Treats atrial and ventricular dysrhythmias	Flecainide (Tambocor) Propafenone (Rythmol)	Proarrhythmic HF Dizziness, visual disturbances, dyspnea	Decrease dose with renal dysfunction and strict vegetarian diets Avoid use in patients with structural heart disease (e.g., coronary artery disease and heart failure)
II	Decreases automaticity and conduction Treats atrial and ventricular dysrhythmias	Acebutolol (Sectral)[c] Atenolol (Tenormin) Bisoprolol/HCTZ (Ziac, Zebeta) Esmolol (Brevibloc)[c] Labetalol (Trandate) Metoprolol (Lopressor, Toprol-XL) Nadolol (Corgard) Nebivolol (Bystolic) Propranolol (Inderal, InnoPran XL)[c] Sotalol (Betapace; Sorine; Sotylize also has class III actions)[c] Timolol (Blocadren)	Bradycardia, AV block Decreased contractility Bronchospasm Nausea Asymptomatic and symptomatic hypotension Masks hypoglycemia and thyrotoxicosis CNS disturbances (e.g., confusion, dizziness, fatigue, depression)	Monitor heart rate, PR interval, signs and symptoms of HF, especially in those also taking calcium channel blockers Monitor blood glucose level in patients with type 2 diabetes Caution the patient about abrupt withdrawal to avoid tachycardia, hypertension, and myocardial ischemia
III	Prolongs repolarization Amiodarone treats and prevents ventricular and atrial dysrhythmias, especially in patients with ventricular dysfunction. Dofetilide and ibutilide treat and prevent atrial dysrhythmias.	Amiodarone (Cordarone, Pacerone) Dofetilide (Tikosyn) Dronedarone (MULTAQ) Ibutilide (Corvert)	Pulmonary toxicity (amiodarone) Corneal microdeposits (amiodarone) Photosensitivity (amiodarone) Bradycardia Hypotension, especially with IV administration Polymorphic ventricular dysrhythmias (rare with amiodarone) Nausea and vomiting Potentiates digoxin (amiodarone) See beta-blockers above (sotalol)	Make sure that the patient is sent for baseline pulmonary function tests (amiodarone) Closely monitor the patient Assess for contraindications prior to administration Monitor QT duration Continuous ECG monitoring with initiation of dofetilide and ibutilide Monitor renal function
IV	Blocks calcium channel Treats and prevents paroxysmal atrial dysrhythmias[b]	verapamil (Calan, Covera-HS, Isoptin) Diltiazem (Cardizem, Dilacor, Tiazac, Diltia, Cartia)	Bradycardia, AV blocks Hypotension with IV administration HF, peripheral edema Constipation, dizziness, headache, nausea	Monitor heart rate, PR interval Monitor blood pressure closely with IV administration Monitor for signs and symptoms of HF Do not crush sustained-release medications

[a]Based on Vaughan–Williams classification.

[b]There are other calcium channel blockers, but they are not approved or used for dysrhythmias.

[c]Beta-blocker with labeled use for dysrhythmias.

IV, intravenous; HF, heart failure; BP, blood pressure; AV, atrioventricular; CNS, central nervous system; GI, gastrointestinal; HCTZ, hydrochlorothiazide; ECG, electrocardiogram.

Adapted from the American Society of Health System Pharmacists. (2012). *AHFS drug information*. Bethesda, MD: Author; Fuster, V., Walsh, R. A., & Harrington, R. A. (Eds.). (2011). *Hurst's the heart* (13th ed.). New York: McGraw-Hill.

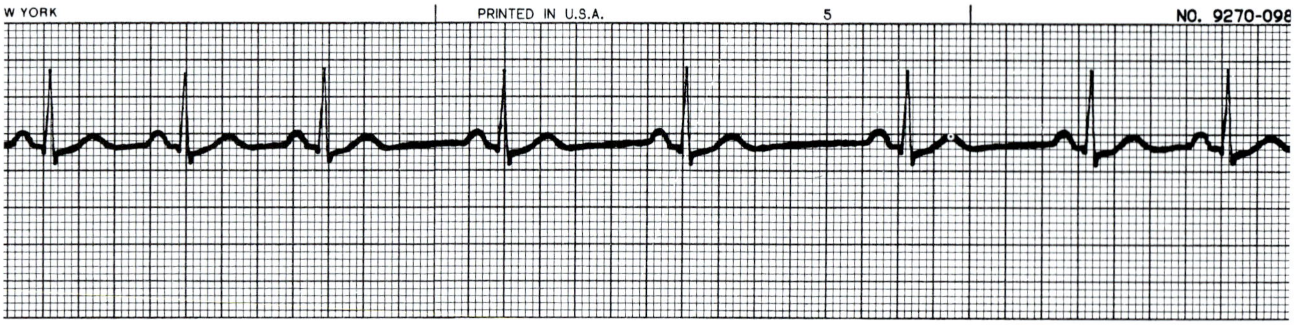

FIGURE 28-8. Sinus arrhythmia in lead II. Note irregular RR and PP intervals.

although rarely used, may also be considered in a narrow-QRS tachycardia. If the tachycardia has a wide QRS, then adenosine is considered only if the QRS is monomorphic (uniform shape) and the ventricular rhythm is regular. Otherwise, procainamide (Pronestyl), amiodarone, and sotalol (Betapace) are the options in wide QRS tachycardia (see later discussion of all of these medications). Catheter ablation (see later discussion in Atrial Fibrillation) of the SA node may be used in cases of persistent inappropriate sinus tachycardia unresponsive to other treatments. Treatment for POTS often involves a combination of approaches, with treatment targeted at the underlying problem. For example, patients with hypovolemia may be advised to increase their fluid and sodium intake, or use salt tablets if necessary (Sheldon et al., 2015).

Sinus Arrhythmia

Sinus arrhythmia occurs when the sinus node creates an impulse at an irregular rhythm; the rate usually increases with inspiration and decreases with expiration. Nonrespiratory causes include heart disease and valvular disease, but these are rare. Sinus arrhythmia has the following characteristics (Fig. 28-8):

Ventricular and atrial rate: 60 to 100 in the adult
Ventricular and atrial rhythm: Irregular
QRS shape and duration: Usually normal, but may be regularly abnormal
P wave: Normal and consistent shape; always in front of the QRS
PR interval: Consistent interval between 0.12 and 0.20 seconds
P:QRS ratio: 1:1

Sinus arrhythmia does not cause any significant hemodynamic effect and usually is not treated.

Atrial Dysrhythmias

Premature Atrial Complex

A premature atrial complex (PAC) is a single ECG complex that occurs when an electrical impulse starts in the atrium before the next normal impulse of the sinus node. The PAC may be caused by caffeine, alcohol, nicotine, stretched atrial myocardium (e.g., as in hypervolemia), anxiety, hypokalemia (low potassium level), hypermetabolic states (e.g., with pregnancy), or atrial ischemia, injury, or infarction. PACs are often seen with sinus tachycardia. PACs have the following characteristics (Fig. 28-9):

Ventricular and atrial rate: Depends on the underlying rhythm (e.g., sinus tachycardia)
Ventricular and atrial rhythm: Irregular due to early P waves, creating a PP interval that is shorter than the others. This is sometimes followed by a longer-than-normal PP interval, but one that is less than twice the normal PP interval. This type of interval is called a noncompensatory pause.
QRS shape and duration: The QRS that follows the early P wave is usually normal, but it may be abnormal

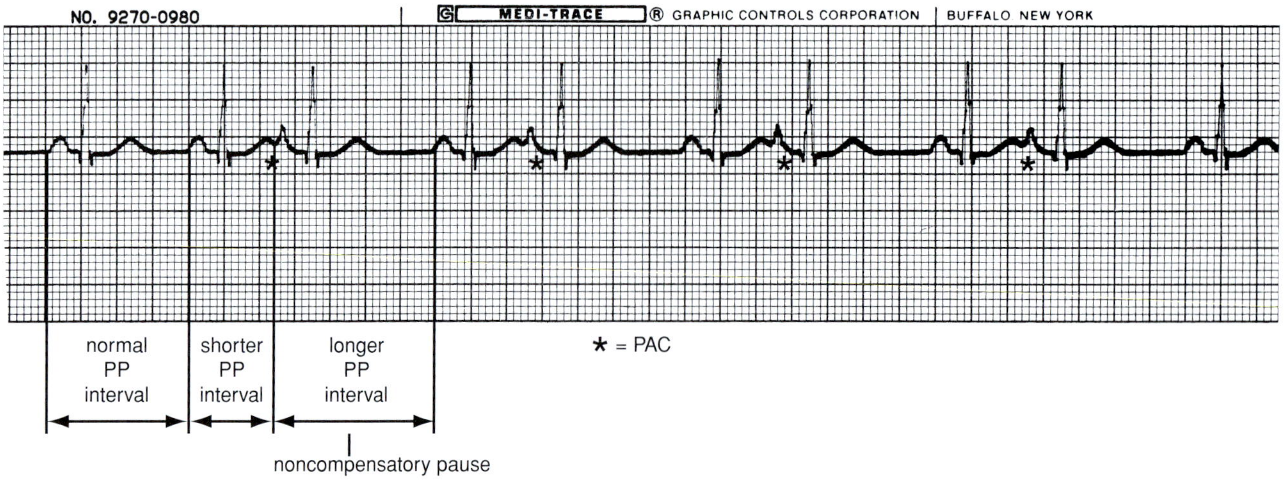

FIGURE 28-9. Premature atrial complexes (PACs) in lead II. Note that the pause following the PAC is longer than the normal PP interval but shorter than twice the normal PP interval.

(aberrantly conducted PAC). It may even be absent (blocked PAC).

P wave: An early and different P wave may be seen or may be hidden in the T wave; other P waves in the strip are consistent.

PR interval: The early P wave has a shorter-than-normal PR interval, but still between 0.12 and 0.20 seconds.

P:QRS ratio: usually 1:1

Medical Management

PACs are common in normal hearts. The patient may say, "My heart skipped a beat." A pulse deficit (a difference between the apical and radial pulse rate) may exist. If PACs are infrequent, no treatment is necessary. If they are frequent (more than 6 per minute), this may herald a worsening disease state or the onset of more serious dysrhythmias, such as atrial fibrillation. Medical management is directed toward treating the underlying cause (e.g., reduction of caffeine intake, correction of hypokalemia).

Atrial Flutter

Atrial flutter occurs because of a conduction defect in the atrium and causes a rapid, regular atrial rate, usually between 250 and 400 times per minute. Because the atrial rate is faster than the AV node can conduct, not all atrial impulses are conducted into the ventricle, causing a therapeutic block at the AV node. This is an important feature of this dysrhythmia. If all atrial impulses were conducted to the ventricle, the ventricular rate would also be 250 to 400, which could result in ventricular fibrillation, a life-threatening dysrhythmia. Atrial flutter often occurs in patients with chronic obstructive pulmonary disease, valvular disease, and thyrotoxicosis, as well as following open heart surgery and repair of congenital cardiac defects (Fuster et al., 2011).

Atrial flutter has the following characteristics (Fig. 28-10):

Ventricular and atrial rate: Atrial rate ranges between 250 and 400; ventricular rate usually ranges between 75 and 150

Ventricular and atrial rhythm: The atrial rhythm is regular; the ventricular rhythm is usually regular but may be irregular because of a change in the AV conduction

QRS shape and duration: Usually normal, but may be abnormal or may be absent

P wave: Saw-toothed shape; these waves are referred to as F waves

PR interval: Multiple F waves may make it difficult to determine the PR interval

P:QRS ratio: 2:1, 3:1, or 4:1

Vagal manoeuvres or administration of adenosine (Adenocard, Adenoscan), which causes sympathetic block and slowing of conduction in the AV node, may allow better visualization of flutter waves. Adenosine should be rapidly administered intravenously, followed by a 20-mL saline flush and elevation of the arm with the IV line to promote rapid circulation of the medication.

Medical Management

Atrial flutter can cause serious signs and symptoms, such as chest pain, shortness of breath, and low blood pressure. Medical management involves the use of vagal maneuvers (see previous discussion under Sinus Tachycardia) or a trial administration of adenosine, which causes sympathetic block and slowing of conduction through the AV node. This may terminate the tachycardia; optimally, it will facilitate visualization of flutter waves for diagnostic purposes. Adenosine is given intravenously by rapid administration, and immediately followed by a 20-mL saline flush and elevation of the arm with the IV line to promote rapid circulation of the medication.

Atrial flutter is treated with antithrombotic therapy, rate control, and rhythm control in the same manner as atrial fibrillation (January, Wann, Alpert, et al., 2014). Electrical cardioversion is often successful in converting atrial flutter to sinus rhythm (see later discussion of Electrical Cardioversion).

Atrial Fibrillation

Atrial fibrillation is the most common sustained dysrhythmia, affecting as many as 350,000 Canadians according to the Heart and Stroke Foundation of Canada. Atrial fibrillation causes electrophysiologic changes in the atrial myocardium (remodeling of the atrial electrical circuit) and structural remodeling (fibrosis), which provides the basis for continuance of the dysrhythmia (January et al., 2014; Stavrakis, Nakagawa, Po, et al., 2015). Atrial fibrillation can result from diverse pathophysiologic etiologies and risks (see Chart 28-2).

Atrial fibrillation results from abnormal impulse formation that occurs when structural or electrophysiologic abnormalities alter the atrial tissue causing a rapid, disorganized, and uncoordinated twitching of the atrial musculature (January et al., 2014). Both the extrinsic (central) and intrinsic cardiac autonomic nervous systems (CANS) are

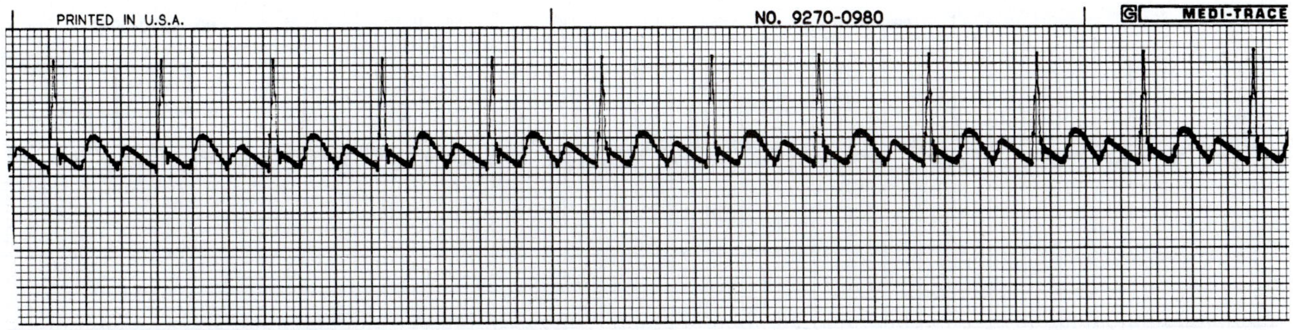

FIGURE 28-10. Atrial flutter in lead II.

CHART 28-2

Risk Factors: Atrial Fibrillation

- Increasing age
- Hypertension
- Diabetes
- Obesity
- Valvular heart disease
- Heart failure
- Obstructive sleep apnea
- Alcohol consumption—moderate (1 to 3 drinks/day) and high (>3 drinks/day)
- Hyperthyroidism
- Cardiac ischemia
- Cardiac inflammatory disease (pericarditis, myocarditis, amyloidosis)
- Myocardial hypertrophy, fibrosis, or dilation
- Atrial remodeling
- Postoperative cardiac surgery

Adapted from LaPar, D. J., Speir, A. M., Crosby, I. K., et al. (2014). Postoperative atrial fibrillation significantly increases mortality, hospital readmission, and hospital costs. *Annals of Thoracic Surgery*, *98*(2), 527–533; Larsson, S. C., Drca, N., & Wolk, A. (2014). Alcohol consumption and risk of atrial fibrillation: A prospective study and dose-response meta-analysis. *Journal of the American College of Cardiology*, *64*(3), 282–289; January, C. T., Wann, L. S., Alpert, J. S., et al. (2014). 2014 AHA/ACC/HRS guideline for the management of patients with atrial fibrillation: A report of the ACC/AHA Task Force on practice guidelines and the Heart Rhythm Society. *Circulation*, *130*(23), e199–e267; Shukla, A., Aizer, A., Holmes, D., et al. (2015). Effect of obstructive sleep apnea treatment on atrial fibrillation recurrence. *JACC: Clinical Electrophysiology*, *1*(1–2), 41–51.

CHART 28-3

Atrial Fibrillation Classification System

Type	Description
Paroxysmal	Sudden onset with termination that occurs spontaneously or after an intervention; lasts ≤7 days, but may recur
Persistent	Continuous, lasting >7 days
Long-standing persistent	Continuous, lasting >12 months
Permanent	Persistent, but decision has been made not to restore or maintain sinus rhythm
Nonvalvular	Absence of mitral stenosis, valve replacement or repair

Adapted from January, C. T., Wann, L. S., Alpert, J. S., et al. (2014). 2014 AHA/ACC/HRS guideline for the management of patients with atrial fibrillation: A report of the ACC/AHA Task Force on practice guidelines and the Heart Rhythm Society. *Circulation*, *130*(23), e199–e267.

thought to play an important role in the initiation and continuance of atrial fibrillation (Stavrakis et al., 2015). Separate from the extrinsic (central) nervous system, which includes the brain and spinal cord, the CANS consists of a highly interconnected network of autonomic ganglia and nerve cell bodies embedded within the epicardium, largely within the atrial myocardium and great vessels (pulmonary veins). Hyperactive autonomic ganglia in the CANS are thought to play a critical role in atrial fibrillation, resulting in impulses that are initiated from the pulmonary veins and conducted through to the AV node. The ventricular rate of response depends on the conduction of atrial impulses through the AV node, presence of accessory electrical conduction pathways, and therapeutic effect of medications.

Lack of consistency in describing patterns or types of atrial fibrillation has led to the use of numerous labels (e.g., paroxysmal [i.e., it has a sudden onset and terminates spontaneously], persistent, and permanent). The recommended classification system is noted in Chart 28-3. The use of the term "chronic atrial fibrillation" is no longer included in the classification system, due to a lack of consensus on what constitutes chronicity (January et al., 2014).

Atrial fibrillation has the following characteristics (Fig. 28-11):

Ventricular and atrial rate: Atrial rate is 300 to 600 bpm; ventricular rate is usually 120 to 200 bpm in untreated atrial fibrillation.
Ventricular and atrial rhythm: Highly irregular
QRS shape and duration: Usually normal, but may be abnormal
P wave: No discernible P waves; irregular undulating waves that vary in amplitude and shape are seen and referred to as fibrillatory or f waves
PR interval: Cannot be measured
P:QRS ratio: Many:1

Patients with atrial fibrillation are at increased risk of heart failure, myocardial ischemia, and embolic events such as stroke (January et al., 2014). A rapid and irregular ventricular response reduces the time for ventricular filling, resulting in a smaller stroke volume. Because atrial

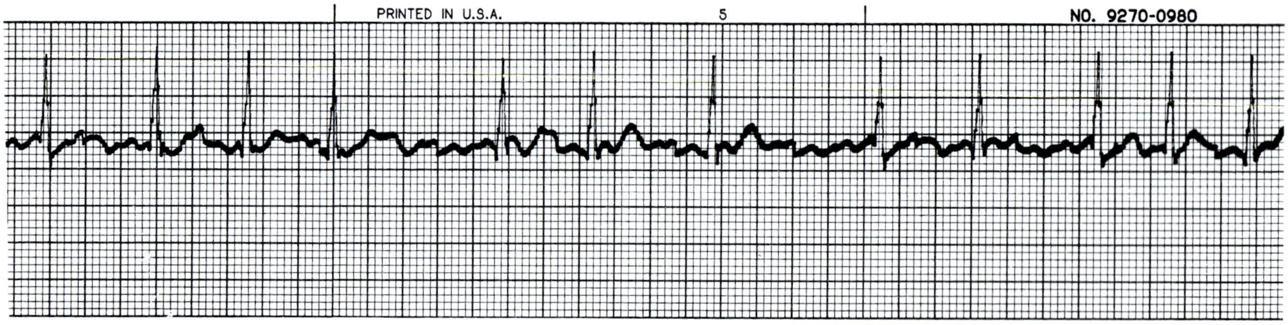

FIGURE 28-11. Atrial fibrillation in lead II.

fibrillation causes a loss in AV synchrony (the atria and ventricles contract at different times), the atrial kick (the last part of diastole and ventricular filling, which accounts for 25% to 30% of the cardiac output) is also lost. As a consequence, although some patients with atrial fibrillation are asymptomatic, others experience palpitations and clinical manifestations of heart failure (e.g., shortness of breath, hypotension, dyspnea on exertion, fatigue; see Chapter 28). In addition, a high ventricular rate of response during atrial fibrillation (greater than 80 bpm) can eventually lead to mitral valve dysfunction, mitral regurgitation, intraventricular conduction delays, and dilated ventricular cardiomyopathy.

Patients with atrial fibrillation may exhibit a pulse deficit—a numeric difference between apical and radial pulse rates. The shorter time in diastole reduces the time available for coronary artery perfusion, thereby increasing the risk of myocardial ischemia with the onset of anginal symptoms (see Chapter 29). Decreasing the ventricular rate may avoid and correct these effects.

The erratic nature of atrial contraction, alterations in ventricular ejection, and atrial myocardial dysfunction promote the formation of thrombi, especially within the left atrium, increasing the risk of an embolic event. The origin of embolisms resulting in stroke for patients with nonvalvular atrial fibrillation is most often the left atrial appendage (LAA) (Masoudi, Calkins, Kavinsky, et al., 2015). A therapeutic approach to addressing the role of the LAA in atrial fibrillation, left atrial appendage occlusion (LAAO), is discussed later in this chapter.

Assessment and Diagnostic Findings

The clinical evaluation of atrial fibrillation should include a history and physical examination that identifies the onset and nature of signs and symptoms, including their frequency, duration and any precipitating factors, and any response to medications. Whether or not the patient has a known history of heart disease or other risks is identified (see Chart 28-2). A 12-lead ECG is performed to verify the atrial fibrillation rhythm, as well as to identify the presence (or absence) of left ventricular (LV) hypertrophy, bundle branch block, prior myocardial ischemia, or other dysrhythmias. The RR, QRS, and QT intervals are analyzed to verify the effectiveness of any prescribed **antiarrhythmic medications** (January et al., 2014). A transthoracic echocardiogram (TEE) can identify the presence of valvular heart disease, provide information about LV and right ventricular (RV) size and function, RV pressures (to identify pulmonary hypertension, which may exist concomitant with atrial fibrillation), LV hypertrophy, and presence of left atrial thrombi (January et al., 2014).

Blood tests to screen for diseases that are known risks for atrial fibrillation (see Chart 28-2), including thyroid, renal, and hepatic function, are assessed in the patient with a new onset of atrial fibrillation, as well as when the ventricular rate is difficult to control (January et al., 2014). Additional tests may include a chest x-ray (to evaluate pulmonary vasculature in a patient suspected of having pulmonary hypertension), exercise stress test (to exclude myocardial ischemia or reproduce exercise-induced atrial fibrillation), Holter or event monitoring (see Chapter 27), and an EP study (January et al., 2014) (see later discussion).

Medical Management

Treatment of atrial fibrillation depends on the cause, pattern, and duration of the dysrhythmia, the ventricular response rate, as well as the presence of structural or valvular heart disease and other cardiac conditions such as coronary artery disease or heart failure. Strategies for both rhythm control (i.e., conversion to sinus rhythm) and rate control are dependent on shared clinical decision making between the patient and primary provider. In some cases, atrial fibrillation spontaneously converts to sinus rhythm within 24 to 48 hours and without treatment. However, in instances where atrial fibrillation is concomitant with significant other morbid conditions (e.g., severe heart failure), the atrial fibrillation may be classified as "permanent," meaning that the patient and primary provider have made a joint decision to stop further attempts to restore or maintain sinus rhythm. Therefore, management of atrial fibrillation may not only be different in different patients, but it also may change over time for any one patient.

Medical management revolves around preventing embolic events such as stroke with antithrombotic drugs, controlling the ventricular rate of response with antiarrhythmic agents, and treating the dysrhythmia as indicated so that it is converted to a sinus rhythm (i.e., *cardioversion*).

PHARMACOLOGIC THERAPY

Antithrombotic Medications. Antithrombotic drugs may include anticoagulants and antiplatelet drugs. Oral antithrombotic therapy is indicated for most patients with nonvalvular atrial fibrillation because it reduces the risk of stroke (Kovacs, Flaker, Saxonhouse, et al., 2015). Atrial fibrillation guidelines (January et al., 2014) recommend use of a scoring system to assist in assessment of stroke risk. Antithrombotic therapy is then selected based on risk factors outlined in the mnemonic CHA_2DS_2-VAS_C (see Chart 28-4) with each risk factor assigned points tallied for a total score that indicates an overall risk of stroke (Kovacs et al., 2015).

According to pharmacologic treatment guidelines (Kovacs et al., 2015):

- Patients with low stroke risk (i.e., CHA_2DS_2-VAS_C score of zero) may choose the option of no antithrombotic

CHART 28-4

Stroke Risk Assessment for the Patient With Atrial Fibrillation: The CHA_2DS_2-VAS_C Scoring System

	Risk Factor	Points
C	Congestive Heart Failure (left ventricular systolic dysfunction)	1
H	Hypertension (BP >140/90 mm Hg)	1
A_2	Age ≥75 years	2
D	Diabetes	1
S_2	Prior stroke or TIA	2
V	Vascular disease	1
A	Age 65–74 years	1
S_c	Sex category (female gender)	1

Adapted from Kovacs, R. J., Flaker, G. C., Saxonhouse, S. J., et al. (2015). Practical management of anticoagulation in patients with atrial fibrillation. *Journal of American College of Cardiology*, *65*(13), 1340–1360.

therapy or may be placed on aspirin therapy dosed at 75 to 325 mg daily.

- Patients with at least moderate risk (i.e., CHA_2DS_2-VAS_C score of one of higher) may choose either warfarin (Coumadin) or a direct-acting oral anticoagulant or Factor Xa inhibitor (e.g., dabigatran [Pradaxa], rivaroxaban [Xarelto], apixaban [Eliquis], edoxaban [Savaysa]).

Medication selection depends on patient characteristics, primary provider and patient preference, current medication regimen, and cost, as well as time required for therapeutic drug monitoring (Kovacs et al., 2015). For instance, treatment with warfarin will require weekly international normalized ratio (INR) testing during initiation of therapy, as well as ongoing monitoring (see Chapter 54 for further discussion). Home monitoring of therapy is an option in selected patients. Direct-acting oral anticoagulants and Factor Xa inhibitors require baseline assessment of hemoglobin and hematocrit, as well as liver and renal function, along with INR. Advantages of these medications include fewer drug–drug interactions and dietary limitations, as well as the elimination of frequent INR testing (Kovacs et al., 2015). For patients with mechanical heart valves, warfarin is recommended (January et al., 2014). If immediate or short-term anticoagulation is necessary, the patient may be placed on IV or low–molecular-weight heparin until warfarin therapy can be started and the INR level reaches a therapeutic range consistent with antithrombosis, usually defined as an INR between 2.0 and 3.0.

Medications That Control the Heart Rate. A strategy to control the ventricular rate of response so that the resting heart rate is less than 80 bpm is recommended in order to manage symptoms of atrial fibrillation (January et al., 2014). To decrease the ventricular rate in patients with paroxysmal, persistent, or permanent atrial fibrillation, a beta-blocker (Class II antiarrhythmic, see Table 28-1) or nondihydropyridine calcium channel blocker (Class IV antiarrhythmic, see Table 28-1) is generally recommended (January et al., 2014).

Medications That Convert the Heart Rhythm or Prevent Atrial Fibrillation. For patients with atrial fibrillation lasting 48 hours or longer, anticoagulation is recommended prior to attempts to restore sinus rhythm, which may be achieved through pharmacologic or electrical cardioversion (January et al., 2014). In the absence of therapeutic anticoagulation, TEE may be performed prior to cardioversion to identify left atrial thrombus formation, including in the LAA (January et al., 2014). If no thrombus is identified, cardioversion can proceed.

Medications that may be given to achieve pharmacologic cardioversion to sinus rhythm include flecainide (Tambocor), dofetilide (Tikosyn), propafenone (Rythmol), amiodarone, and IV ibutilide (Corvert) (January et al., 2014). These medications are most effective if given within 7 days of the onset of atrial fibrillation. It is recommended that patients who were prescribed dofetilide be hospitalized so that the QT interval and renal function both may be monitored. Despite a degree of risk, dofetilide is a preferred medication because it is highly effective at converting atrial fibrillation to sinus rhythm, has fewer drug–drug interactions, and is better tolerated by patients than other medications. Some patients with recurrent atrial fibrillation may be prescribed flecainide to self-administer at home, an approach referred to as "pill in the pocket" (January et al., 2014).

Prevention of atrial fibrillation following cardiac surgery is best achieved through administration of beta-blockers (see Table 28-1) for at least 24 hours prior to surgery (Shi, 2016). Cholesterol-lowering drugs such as the HMG-CoA reductase inhibitors (also called "statins," see Chapter 29) may also be prescribed for primary prevention of new-onset atrial fibrillation following cardiac surgery (January et al., 2014).

Therapy with angiotensin-converting enzyme (ACE) inhibitors and angiotensin receptor blockers (ARBs) (see Chapter 33) may decrease the incidence of atrial fibrillation for patients with concomitant hypertension, although the use of these drugs is not found to be beneficial as a primary prevention strategy for patients without hypertension (January et al., 2014).

If symptomatic, paroxysmal atrial fibrillation is refractory to at least one Class I or Class III antiarrhythmic medication (see Table 28-1), and rhythm control is desired, catheter ablation may be indicated (January et al., 2014) (see later discussion).

ELECTRICAL CARDIOVERSION FOR ATRIAL FIBRILLATION. Electrical cardioversion is indicated for patients with atrial fibrillation that is hemodynamically unstable (e.g., acute alteration in mental status, chest discomfort, hypotension) and does not respond to medications (January et al., 2014). Flecainide, propafenone, amiodarone, dofetilide, or sotalol may be given prior to cardioversion to enhance the success of cardioversion and maintain sinus rhythm (January et al., 2014).

NURSING ALERT

The patient with atrial fibrillation is at high risk for thrombus formation. When electrical cardioversion is indicated, the nurse may anticipate that a transesophageal echocardiogram may be performed to evaluate for possible atrial thrombi.

Because atrial function may be impaired for several weeks after cardioversion, warfarin is indicated for at least 4 weeks after the procedure (January et al., 2014). Repeated attempts at electrical cardioversion may be made, following administration of an antiarrhythmic medication (see later discussion on Electrical Cardioversion).

Cardiac Rhythm Therapies

Atrial fibrillation that does not respond to medications or electrical cardioversion may be treated by cardiac rhythm therapies, including catheter ablation, maze or mini-maze procedure, or convergent procedure.

CATHETER ABLATION THERAPY. Catheter **ablation** destroys specific cells that are the cause of a tachydysrhythmia. Catheter ablation is performed most often today for atrial fibrillation, although it may also be useful in treating AV nodal reentry tachycardia (AVNRT) and recurrent **ventricular tachycardia** (VT) (see later discussion of these dysrhythmias).

Recent evidence demonstrates that the pathogenesis of atrial fibrillation is associated with intrinsic cardiac autonomic nervous system activity to the pulmonary veins (Stavrakis et al., 2015). Ablation involves a procedure similar to a cardiac catheterization (see Chapter 27); however, in this instance, a special catheter is advanced at or near the origin of the dysrhythmia, where high-frequency, low-energy sound waves are passed through the catheter, causing thermal injury, localized cell destruction, and scarring. The tissue damage is more specific to the dysrhythmic tissue, with less trauma to the surrounding cardiac tissue. Ablation may also be accomplished using a special catheter to apply extremely cold temperature to destroy selected cardiac cells, called *cryoablation*. The goal of each of these ablation procedures is to eliminate the dysrhythmia, by preventing the ectopic activity arising from the pulmonary veins from reaching the atria, thereby stopping fibrillation (Stavrakis et al., 2015).

An EP study (see later discussion) may be performed to induce the dysrhythmia prior to the catheter ablation. During the ablation procedure, **defibrillation** pads, an automatic blood pressure cuff, and a pulse oximeter are used. The patient is usually given moderate sedation (see Chapter 19) and IV heparin to reduce the risk of periprocedural thromboembolism. Immediately postablation, the patient is monitored for another 30 to 60 minutes and then retested to ensure that the dysrhythmia does not recur. Successful ablation is achieved when the dysrhythmia cannot be induced. Major risks of catheter ablation include AV block, pericardial tamponade, phrenic nerve injury, stroke, hematoma, retroperitoneal bleeding, pulmonary vein stenosis, and atrioesophageal fistulas (January et al., 2014; Mann, Zipes, Libby, et al., 2015). Obstructive sleep apnea is one known risk factor associated with the recurrence of atrial fibrillation after catheter ablation (Shukla, Aizer, Holmes, et al., 2015).

Nursing Management. Postprocedural care on a step-down unit for the patient who has had ablation is similar to the nursing management of a patient who has had a cardiac catheterization (see Chapter 27); the patient is monitored closely to ensure recovery from sedation. Postprocedural nursing interventions include frequent monitoring for dysrhythmias and for signs and symptoms of a stroke, vascular access site complications (see Chapter 27), and fluid imbalance (Hoke & Steletsky, 2015). Because of the prolonged time required for the procedure as well as the time needed in bed to obtain hemostasis at the vascular access site, it is not unusual for the patient to have back discomfort. In addition to administering any pain medications, the nurse may help to alleviate this pain by placing rolled towels under the patient's knees and waist.

MAZE AND MINI-MAZE PROCEDURES. The maze procedure is an open heart surgical procedure for refractory atrial fibrillation. Small transmural incisions are made throughout the atria. The resulting formation of scar tissue prevents reentry conduction of the aberrant electrical impulse. Because the procedure requires significant time and cardiopulmonary bypass, its use is reserved only for those patients undergoing cardiac surgery for another reason (e.g., coronary artery bypass, see Chapter 29) (January et al., 2014). Some patients may need a permanent pacemaker after this surgery because of subsequent injury to the SA node.

A modification of the maze procedure, minimally invasive maze surgery, or mini-maze, may be performed by making small incisions between the ribs, through which video-guided instruments are inserted. The pulmonary veins are encircled with surgical incisions within the left atrium. This surgery eliminates the need for opening the sternum, heart–lung bypass, and the use of cardioplegia (see Chapter 29 for further discussion of cardiac surgery). This results in a shorter recovery time and a lower risk of infection (January et al., 2014).

CONVERGENT PROCEDURE. The convergent procedure utilizes a hybrid approach to ablation, requiring the skills of both a cardiothoracic surgeon and an electrophysiologist. The surgeon creates a few small incisions in the abdomen so that a special catheter that allows visualization can be inserted through the diaphragm and toward the posterior wall of the heart (Elrod, 2014). The surgeon performs ablation of the epicardial wall in the area around the pulmonary veins and the electrophysiologist performs ablation around the endocardial area of the pulmonary veins. Because of the incisions, the patient usually has a 3-day hospital length of stay (Elrod, 2014). The patient may experience mild dull chest pain that is caused by the resulting inflammation from the ablation that usually resolves within a few days (Elrod, 2014). This pain is usually alleviated by treatment with acetaminophen as needed. In addition, if the phrenic nerve was affected, the patient may experience shortness of breath that may take days to weeks to resolve (Elrod, 2014).

LAAO has been recently approved in Canada in 2016 as an alternative to warfarin for stroke prevention in patients with nonvalvular atrial fibrillation (Masoudi et al., 2015). As noted previously, the LAA is the area where the majority of stroke-causing blood clots form in patients with nonvalvular atrial fibrillation. However, concerns about the risk of long-term anticoagulant use and the risk of bleeding can complicate effective management (Alli, Asirvatham, & Holmes, 2015).

Candidates for LAAO include those patients with increased risk of stroke based on $CHA_2DS_2\text{-}VAS_C$ scores of one or higher (see Chart 28-4) and those patients seeking a nonpharmacologic alternative to warfarin (Masoudi et al., 2015). The device most commonly used is the WATCHMAN device; this device is typically inserted while the patient is under general anesthesia. Similar to a percutaneous coronary intervention (PCI) procedure (see Chapter 29), a small incision is made in the femoral area and a catheter is then inserted that guides the device into position. The parachute-shaped device is threaded through to the opening of the LAA, sealing it off and preventing it from releasing clots.

Patients typically stay in the hospital overnight after placement of a WATCHMAN device. The nursing management of patients who received this device is similar to that of patients post cardiac catheterization (see Chapter 27). Patients are prescribed aspirin and warfarin postprocedure; approximately 6 weeks postprocedure, they should return to the cardiology clinic for a TEE to confirm that the device has effectively occluded the LAA. If LAAO has occurred, then the patient may stop taking warfarin and is prescribed clopidogrel (Plavix), an antiplatelet medication. After 6 months, the patient may stop taking clopidogrel but must continue taking daily aspirin indefinitely.

Wolff–Parkinson–White Syndrome

In the patient with atrial fibrillation, if the QRS is wide and the ventricular rhythm is very fast and irregular, an accessory pathway should be suspected. An accessory pathway is typically congenital tissue between the atria, bundle of His, AV node, Purkinje fibres, or ventricular myocardium. This anomaly is known as Wolff–Parkinson–White (WPW) syndrome. Electrical cardioversion is the treatment of choice for atrial fibrillation in the presence of WPW syndrome that causes hemodynamic instability. Medications that block AV conduction (e.g., digoxin, diltiazem [Cardizem], and verapamil [Calan]) should be avoided in WPW because they can increase the ventricular rate. If the patient is hemodynamically stable, procainamide, propafenone, flecainide, and amiodarone are recommended to restore sinus rhythm (January et al., 2014). Catheter ablation is performed for long-term management (see previous discussion on Catheter Ablation Therapy).

Junctional Dysrhythmias

Premature Junctional Complex

A premature junctional complex is an impulse that starts in the AV nodal area before the next normal sinus impulse reaches the AV node. Premature junctional complexes are less common than PACs. Causes include digitalis toxicity, heart failure, and coronary artery disease. The ECG criteria for premature junctional complex are the same as for PACs, except for the P wave and the PR interval. The P wave may be absent, may follow the QRS, or may occur before the QRS but with a PR interval of less than 0.12 seconds. This dysrhythmia rarely produces significant symptoms. Treatment for frequent premature junctional complexes is the same as for frequent PACs.

Junctional Rhythm

Junctional or idionodal rhythm occurs when the AV node, instead of the sinus node, becomes the pacemaker of the heart. When the sinus node slows (e.g., from increased vagal tone) or when the impulse cannot be conducted through the AV node (e.g., because of complete heart block), the AV node automatically discharges an impulse. Junctional rhythm not caused by complete heart block has the following characteristics (Fig. 28-12):

Ventricular and atrial rate: Ventricular rate 40 to 60; atrial rate also 40 to 60 if P waves are discernible
Ventricular and atrial rhythm: Regular
QRS shape and duration: Usually normal, but may be abnormal
P wave: May be absent, after the QRS complex, or before the QRS; may be inverted, especially in lead II
PR interval: If the P wave is in front of the QRS, the PR interval is less than 0.12 seconds
P:QRS ratio: 1:1 or 0:1

Medical Management

Junctional rhythm may produce signs and symptoms of reduced cardiac output. If this occurs, the treatment is the same as for sinus bradycardia. Emergency pacing may be needed (see later discussion under Pacemaker Therapy).

Nonparoxysmal Junctional Tachycardia

Junctional tachycardia is caused by enhanced automaticity in the junctional area, resulting in a rhythm similar to junctional rhythm, except at a rate of 70 to 120. Although this rhythm generally does not have any detrimental hemodynamic effect, it may indicate a serious underlying condition, such as digitalis toxicity, myocardial ischemia, hypokalemia, or chronic obstructive pulmonary disease. Because junctional tachycardia is caused by increased automaticity, cardioversion is not an effective treatment; in fact, it causes an increase in the ventricular rate (Mann et al., 2015).

Atrioventricular Nodal Reentry Tachycardia

AVNRT is a common dysrhythmia that occurs when an impulse is conducted to an area in the AV node that causes the impulse to be rerouted back into the same area over and over again at a very fast rate. Each time the impulse is conducted through this area, it is also conducted down into the ventricles, causing a fast ventricular rate. AVNRT that has an abrupt onset and an abrupt cessation with a QRS of normal duration has been termed paroxysmal atrial tachycardia (PAT). AVNRT also occurs when the duration of the QRS complex is 0.12 seconds or greater and a block in the bundle branch is known to be present. This dysrhythmia may last for seconds or several hours. Factors associated with the development of AVNRT include caffeine, nicotine, hypoxemia, and stress. Underlying pathologies include coronary artery disease and cardiomyopathy; however, it occurs more often in females and not in association with underlying structural heart disease (Mann et al., 2015). AVNRT has the following characteristics (Fig. 28-13):

Ventricular and atrial rate: Atrial rate usually 150 to 250; ventricular rate usually 120 to 200

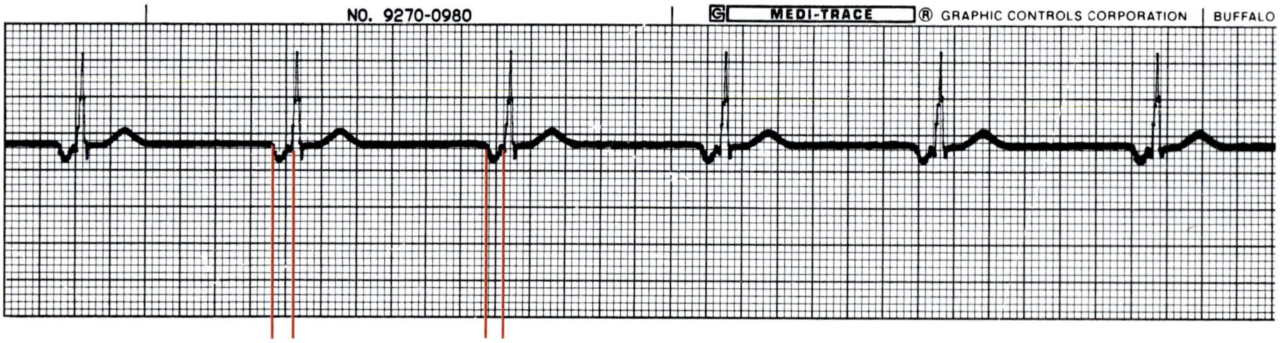

FIGURE 28-12. Junctional rhythm in lead II; note short PR intervals.

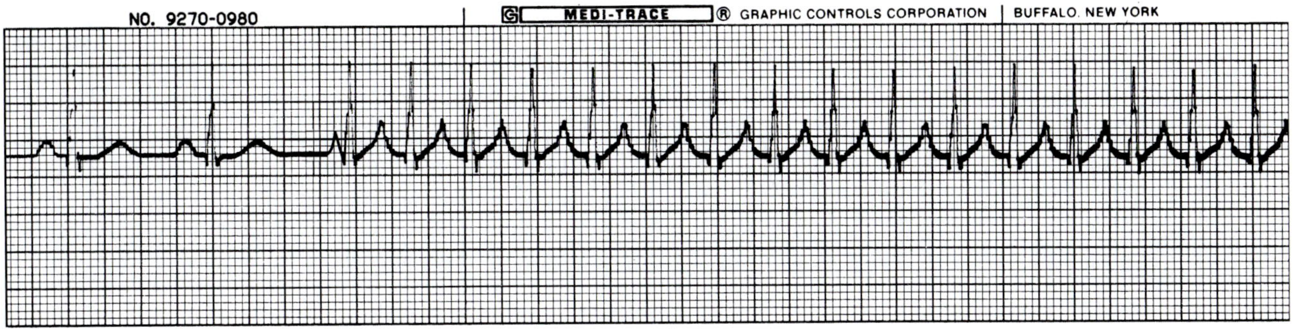

FIGURE 28-13. AV nodal reentry tachycardia in lead II.

Ventricular and atrial rhythm: Regular; sudden onset and termination of the tachycardia

QRS shape and duration: Usually normal, but may be abnormal

P wave: Usually very difficult to discern

PR interval: If the P wave is in front of the QRS, the PR interval is less than 0.12 seconds

P:QRS ratio: 1:1, 2:1

Medical Management

Because AVNRT is generally a benign dysrhythmia, the goal of medical management is to alleviate symptoms and improve quality of life. Patients who become significantly symptomatic and require emergency department visits to terminate the rhythm may want to initiate therapy immediately. However, those with minimum symptoms with an AVNRT that terminates spontaneously or with minimal treatment may choose just to be monitored and self-treat.

The aim of therapy is to break the reentry of the impulse. Catheter ablation is the initial treatment of choice and is used to eliminate the area that permits the rerouting of the impulse that causes the tachycardia (Mann et al., 2015) (see previous discussion of atrial fibrillation: Catheter Ablation Therapy). Vagal maneuvers (see previous discussion under Sinus Tachycardia) may be used to interrupt AVNRT. These techniques increase parasympathetic stimulation, causing slower conduction through the AV node and blocking the reentry of the rerouted impulse. Some patients use some of these methods to terminate the episode on their own. Because of the risk of a cerebral embolic event, carotid sinus massage, which may be performed by physicians, is contraindicated in patients with carotid artery disease.

PHARMACOLOGIC THERAPY. If the vagal maneuvers are ineffective, the patient may then receive a bolus of adenosine to correct the rhythm; this is nearly 100% effective in terminating AVNRT (Mann et al., 2015). Because the effect of adenosine is so short, AVNRT may recur; the first dose may be followed with a larger dose or with a calcium channel blocker, such as verapamil (Calan), followed by one or two additional boluses. If the patient is unstable or does not respond to the medications, electrical cardioversion is the treatment of choice (see later discussion). The patient who is unstable may be given adenosine while preparations for cardioversion are being made. For recurrent sustained AVNRT, treatment with calcium channel blockers such as verapamil and diltiazem, Class Ia antiarrhythmic agents such as procainamide and disopyramide (Norpace), Class Ic antiarrhythmic agents such as flecainide and propafenone, and Class III agents such as sotalol and amiodarone may prevent a recurrence. If the rhythm is infrequent and there is no underlying cardiac structural disorder, a single oral dose of flecainide or a combination of diltiazem and propranolol (Inderal) during an episode of tachycardia may be effective (Mann et al., 2015).

If P waves cannot be identified, the rhythm may be called **supraventricular tachycardia (SVT)**, or paroxysmal supraventricular tachycardia (PSVT) if it has an abrupt onset, until the underlying rhythm and resulting diagnosis is determined. SVT and PSVT indicate only that the rhythm is not VT. SVT could be atrial fibrillation, atrial flutter, or AVNRT, among others. Vagal maneuvers and adenosine may be used to convert the rhythm or at least slow conduction in the AV node to allow visualization of the P waves. If the ECG does not assist in the differentiation of the dysrhythmia, EP studies may be necessary to make the diagnosis (Mann et al., 2015) (see later discussion).

Ventricular Dysrhythmias

Premature Ventricular Complex

A PVC is an impulse that starts in a ventricle and is conducted through the ventricles before the next normal sinus impulse. PVCs can occur in healthy people, especially with intake of caffeine, nicotine, or alcohol. PVCs may be caused by cardiac ischemia or infarction, increased workload on the heart (e.g., heart failure, and tachycardia), digitalis toxicity, hypoxia, acidosis, or electrolyte imbalances, especially hypokalemia. The Sleep Heart Health Study found that those people with sleep disordered breathing (e.g., obstructive sleep apnea) had a significantly higher prevalence of complex ventricular ectopy and nonsustained VT during sleep. The implication of the presence of PVCs during and after exercise is not clear and remains controversial (Mann et al., 2015).

In a rhythm called bigeminy, every other complex is a PVC. In trigeminy, every third complex is a PVC, and in quadrigeminy, every fourth complex is a PVC. PVCs have the following characteristics (Fig. 28-14):

Ventricular and atrial rate: Depends on the underlying rhythm (e.g., sinus rhythm)

Ventricular and atrial rhythm: Irregular due to early QRS, creating one RR interval that is shorter than the others. PP interval may be regular, indicating that the PVC did not depolarize the sinus node.

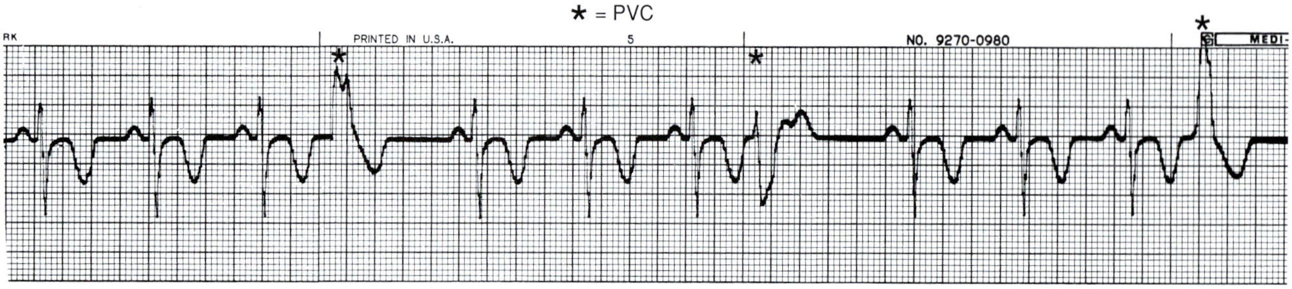

FIGURE 28-14. Multifocal premature ventricular complexes (PVCs) in quadrigeminy in lead V_1. Note regular PP interval (P wave within PVC).

QRS shape and duration: Duration is 0.12 seconds or longer; shape is bizarre and abnormal

P wave: Visibility of P wave depends on the timing of the PVC; may be absent (hidden in the QRS or T wave) or in front of the QRS. If the P wave follows the QRS, the shape of the P wave may be different.

PR interval: If the P wave is in front of the QRS, the PR interval is less than 0.12 seconds

P:QRS ratio: 0:1; 1:1

The patient may feel nothing or may say that the heart "skipped a beat." The effect of a PVC depends on its timing in the cardiac cycle and how much blood was in the ventricles when they contracted. Initial treatment is aimed at correcting the cause.

Medical Management

PVCs usually are not serious. PVCs that are frequent and persistent may be treated with amiodarone or sotalol, but long-term pharmacotherapy for only PVCs is not usually indicated. In patients with an acute MI, studies have found that PVCs are not associated with sudden cardiac death and do not warrant more aggressive therapy (Mann et al., 2015). PVCs are not considered a warning for ensuing VT. However, a recent study reported a higher frequency of PVCs preceded the development of cardiomyopathy, with an increased incidence of heart failure and increased mortality (Dukes, Dewland, Vittinghoff, et al., 2015).

Unfolding Patient Stories: Kenneth Bronson • Part 2

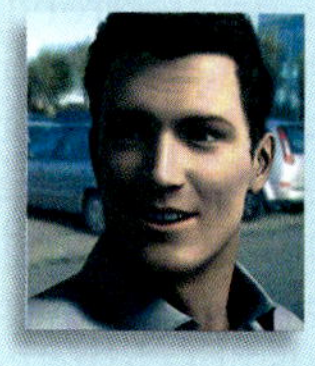

Recall from Chapter 24 Kenneth Bronson, who came to the Emergency Department with difficulty breathing after a week of flu-like symptoms, productive cough, and high fever. He was diagnosed with a right lower lobe pneumonia. Sinus tachycardia with occasional unifocal premature ventricular contractions (PVCs) is seen on the cardiac monitor. What are potential causes for the tachycardia and PVCs that the nurse should investigate when considering his age of 27 years, symptoms experienced over the last week, and the clinical manifestations associated with his diagnosis?

Care for Kenneth and other patients in a realistic virtual environment: ***vSim** for Nursing* (**thepoint.lww.com/vSimMedicalSurgical**). Practice documenting these patients' care in DocuCare (**thepoint.lww.com/DocuCareEHR**).

Ventricular Tachycardia

VT is defined as three or more PVCs in a row, occurring at a rate exceeding 100 bpm. The causes are similar to those of PVC. Patients with larger MIs and lower ejection fractions are at higher risk of lethal VT (see Chapter 31). VT is an emergency because the patient is usually (although not always) unresponsive and pulseless. VT has the following characteristics (Fig. 28-15):

Ventricular and atrial rate: Ventricular rate is 100 to 200 bpm; atrial rate depends on the underlying rhythm (e.g., sinus rhythm)

Ventricular and atrial rhythm: Usually regular; atrial rhythm may also be regular

QRS shape and duration: Duration is 0.12 seconds or more; bizarre, abnormal shape

P wave: Very difficult to detect, so atrial rate and rhythm may be indeterminable

PR interval: Very irregular, if P waves are seen

P:QRS ratio: Difficult to determine, but if P waves are apparent, there are usually more QRS complexes than P waves

Medical Management

Several factors determine the initial treatment, including the following: identifying the rhythm as monomorphic (having a consistent QRS shape and rate) or polymorphic (having varying QRS shapes and rhythms), determining the existence of a prolonged QT interval before the initiation of VT, any comorbidities, and ascertaining the patient's heart function (normal or decreased). If the patient is stable, continuing the assessment, especially obtaining a 12-lead ECG, may be the only action necessary.

However, the patient may need antiarrhythmic medications, antitachycardia pacing, or direct cardioversion or defibrillation. Procainamide may be used for monomorphic stable VT in patients who do not have acute MI or severe HF (Link et al., 2015). IV amiodarone is the medication of choice for a patient with impaired cardiac function or acute MI. Sotalol may also be considered for stable monomorphic VT. Although lidocaine had been the medication most commonly used for immediate, short-term therapy, especially for patients with impaired cardiac function, it has no proven short- or long-term efficacy in cardiac arrest (Link et al., 2015).

Cardioversion is the treatment of choice for monophasic VT in a symptomatic patient. Defibrillation is the treatment of choice for pulseless VT. Any type of VT in a patient who is unconscious and without a pulse is treated in the same manner as ventricular fibrillation: immediate

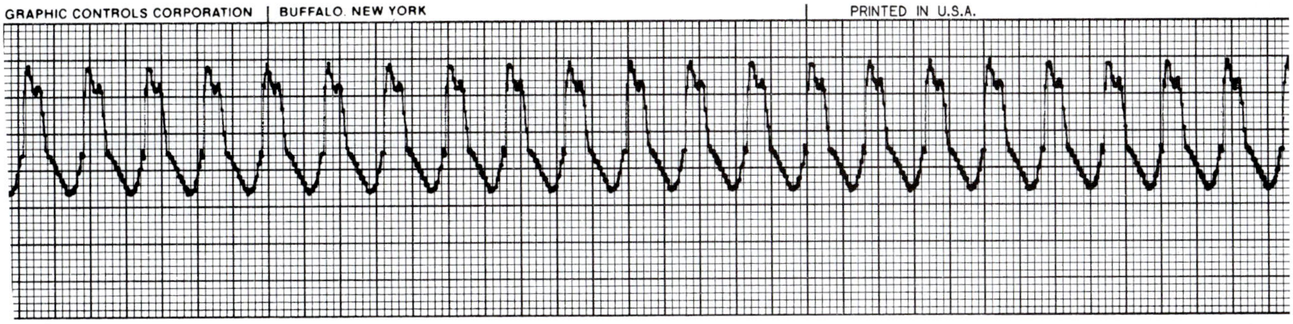

FIGURE 28-15. Ventricular tachycardia in lead V_1.

defibrillation is the action of choice (see later discussion on Cardioversion and Defibrillation).

For long-term management, patients with an ejection fraction less than 35% should be considered for an **implantable cardioverter defibrillator** (ICD) (see later discussion). Those with an ejection fraction greater than 35% may be managed with amiodarone. A small percentage of patients with VT have structurally normal hearts and respond well to medications and catheter ablation, and they have an excellent prognosis (Russo, Stainback, Bailey, et al., 2013). If the ventricular rate is above 200 bpm, then the presence of an accessory pathway should be suspected. If the ventricular rhythm is irregular, atrial fibrillation should be suspected and treated appropriately (Mann et al., 2015).

Torsades de pointes is a polymorphic VT preceded by a prolonged QT interval, which could be congenital or acquired. Common causes include central nervous system disease; certain medications (e.g., ciprofloxacin [Cipro], erythromycin [Zmax, Zithromax, Biaxin], haloperidol [Haldol], lithium [Eskalith, Lithobid], methadone [Dolophine, Methadose]); or low levels of potassium, calcium, or magnesium. Congenital QT prolongation is another cause. Because this rhythm is likely to cause the patient to deteriorate and become pulseless, immediate treatment is required and includes correction of any electrolyte imbalance, such as administration of IV magnesium, and with IV isoproterenol (Isuprel) or pacing if associated with bradycardia (Link et al., 2015).

Ventricular Fibrillation

The most common dysrhythmia in patients with cardiac arrest is ventricular fibrillation, which is a rapid, disorganized ventricular rhythm that causes ineffective quivering of the ventricles. No atrial activity is seen on the ECG. The most common cause of ventricular fibrillation is coronary artery disease and resulting acute MI. Other causes include untreated or unsuccessfully treated VT, cardiomyopathy, valvular heart disease, several **proarrhythmic** medications, acid–base and electrolyte abnormalities, and electrical shock. Another cause is Brugada syndrome, in which the patient (frequently of Asian descent) has a structurally normal heart, few or no risk factors for coronary artery disease, and a family history of sudden cardiac death (Aizawa, Takatsuki, Sano, et al., 2013; Tokioka, Kusano, Morita, et al., 2014). Ventricular fibrillation has the following characteristics (Fig. 28-16):

Ventricular rate: Greater than 300 per minute
Ventricular rhythm: Extremely irregular, without a specific pattern
QRS shape and duration: Irregular, undulating waves without recognizable QRS complexes

Medical Management

Ventricular fibrillation is always characterized by the absence of an audible heartbeat, a palpable pulse, and respirations. Because there is no coordinated cardiac activity, cardiac arrest and death are imminent if the dysrhythmia is not corrected. Early defibrillation is critical to survival, with administration of immediate bystander cardiopulmonary resuscitation (CPR) until defibrillation is available. For refractory ventricular fibrillation, administration of amiodarone and epinephrine may facilitate the return of a spontaneous pulse after defibrillation (Link et al., 2015) (see Chapter 31 for further discussion on interventions during cardiac arrest).

Idioventricular Rhythm

Idioventricular rhythm, also called ventricular escape rhythm, occurs when the impulse starts in the

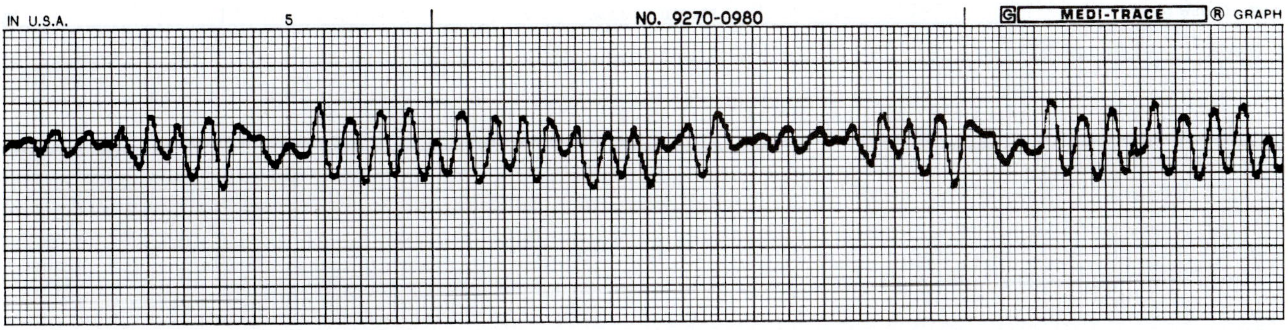

FIGURE 28-16. Ventricular fibrillation in lead II.

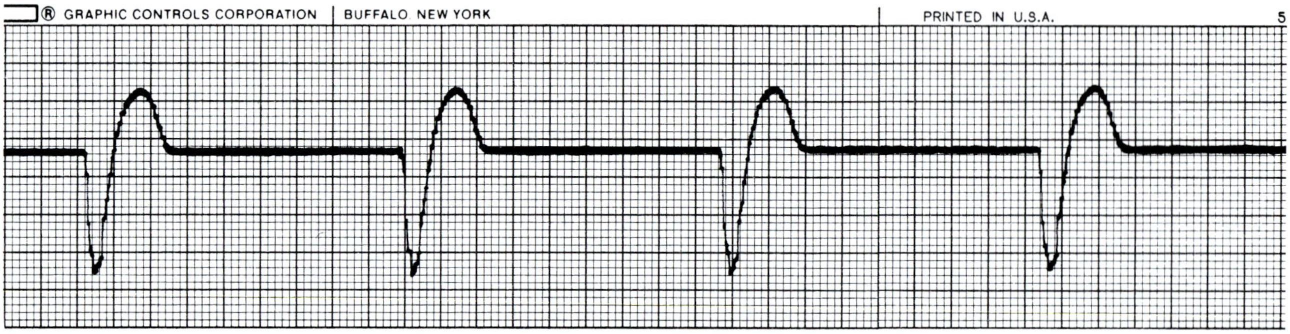

FIGURE 28-17. Idioventricular rhythm in lead V_1.

conduction system below the AV node. When the sinus node fails to create an impulse (e.g., from increased vagal tone) or when the impulse is created but cannot be conducted through the AV node (e.g., due to complete AV block), the Purkinje fibres automatically discharge an impulse. When idioventricular rhythm is not caused by AV block, it has the following characteristics (Fig. 28-17):

Ventricular rate: 20 and 40; if the rate exceeds 40, the rhythm is known as accelerated idioventricular rhythm (AIVR)
Ventricular rhythm: Regular
QRS shape and duration: Bizarre, abnormal shape; duration is 0.12 seconds or more

Medical Management

Idioventricular rhythm commonly causes the patient to lose consciousness and experience other signs and symptoms of reduced cardiac output. In such cases, the treatment is the same as for asystole and pulseless electrical activity (PEA) if the patient is in cardiac arrest or for bradycardia if the patient is not in cardiac arrest. Interventions include identifying the underlying cause; administering IV epinephrine, atropine, and vasopressor medications; and initiating emergency transcutaneous pacing. In some cases, idioventricular rhythm may cause no symptoms of reduced cardiac output.

Ventricular Asystole

Commonly called flatline, ventricular asystole (Fig. 28-18) is characterized by absent QRS complexes confirmed in two different leads, although P waves may be apparent for a short duration. There is no heartbeat, no palpable pulse, and no respiration. Without immediate treatment, ventricular asystole is fatal.

Medical Management

Ventricular asystole is treated the same as PEA, focusing on high-quality CPR with minimal interruptions and identifying underlying and contributing factors. The key to successful treatment is a rapid assessment to identify a possible cause, which is known as the Hs and Ts: hypoxia, hypovolemia, hydrogen ion (acid–base imbalance), hypo- or hyperglycemia, hypo- or hyperkalemia, hyperthermia, trauma, toxins, tamponade (cardiac), tension pneumothorax, or thrombus (coronary or pulmonary) (Link et al., 2015). After the initiation of CPR, intubation and establishment of IV access are the next recommended actions, with no or minimal interruptions in chest compressions (see Chapter 31 for interventions during cardiac arrest).

Conduction Abnormalities

When assessing the rhythm strip, the underlying rhythm is first identified (e.g., sinus rhythm, sinus arrhythmia). Then the PR interval is assessed for the possibility of an AV block. AV blocks occur when the conduction of the impulse through the AV nodal or His bundle area is decreased or stopped. These blocks can be caused by medications (e.g., digitalis, calcium channel blockers, beta-blockers), Lyme disease, myocardial ischemia and infarction, valvular disorders, cardiomyopathy, endocarditis, or myocarditis. If the AV block is caused by increased vagal tone (e.g., long-term athletic training, sleep, coughing, suctioning, pressure above the eyes or on large vessels, anal stimulation), it is commonly accompanied by sinus bradycardia. AV block may be temporary and resolve on its own, or it may be permanent and require permanent pacing.

The clinical signs and symptoms of a heart block vary with the resulting ventricular rate and the severity of any

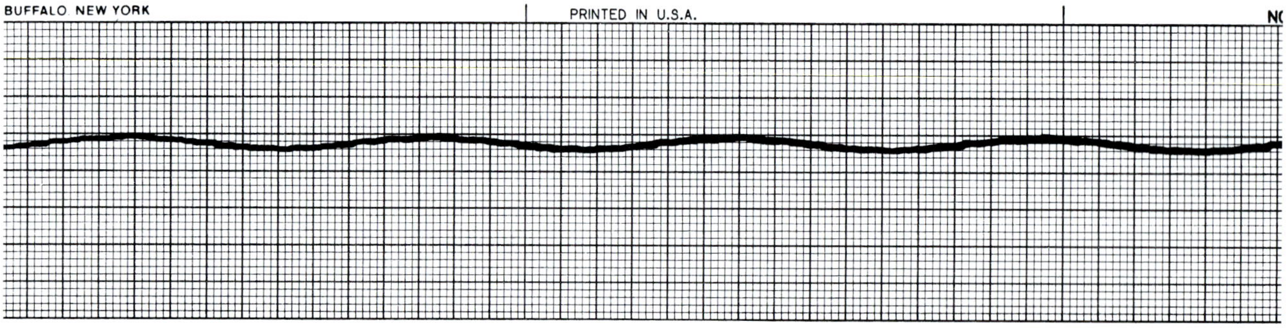

FIGURE 28-18. Asystole. Always check two different leads to confirm rhythm.

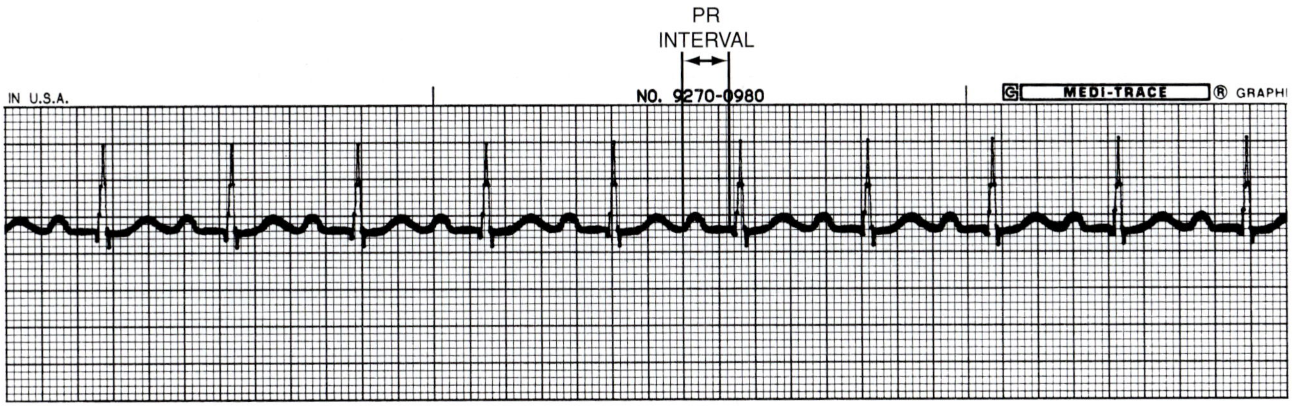

FIGURE 28-19. Sinus rhythm with first-degree AV block in lead II. Note that PR is constant but greater than 0.20 seconds.

underlying disease processes. Whereas first-degree AV block rarely causes any hemodynamic effect, the other blocks may result in decreased heart rate, causing a decrease in perfusion to vital organs, such as the brain, heart, kidneys, lungs, and skin. A patient with third-degree AV block caused by digitalis toxicity may be stable; another patient with the same rhythm caused by acute MI may be unstable. Health care providers must always keep in mind the need to treat the patient, not the rhythm. The treatment is based on the hemodynamic effect of the rhythm.

First-Degree Atrioventricular Block

First-degree AV block occurs when all the atrial impulses are conducted through the AV node into the ventricles at a rate slower than normal. This conduction disorder has the following characteristics (Fig. 28-19):

Ventricular and atrial rate: Depends on the underlying rhythm

Ventricular and atrial rhythm: Depends on the underlying rhythm

QRS shape and duration: Usually normal, but may be abnormal

P wave: In front of the QRS complex; shows sinus rhythm, regular shape

PR interval: Greater than 0.20 seconds; PR interval measurement is constant

P:QRS ratio: 1:1

Second-Degree Atrioventricular Block, Type I (Wenckebach)

Second-degree AV block, type I, occurs when there is a repeating pattern in which all but one of a series of atrial impulses are conducted through the AV node into the ventricles (e.g., every four of five atrial impulses are conducted). Each atrial impulse takes a longer time for conduction than the one before, until one impulse is fully blocked. Because the AV node is not depolarized by the blocked atrial impulse, the AV node has time to fully repolarize, so that the next atrial impulse can be conducted within the shortest amount of time. Second-degree AV block, type I, has the following characteristics (Fig. 28-20):

Ventricular and atrial rate: Depends on the underlying rhythm

Ventricular and atrial rhythm: The PP interval is regular if the patient has an underlying normal sinus rhythm;

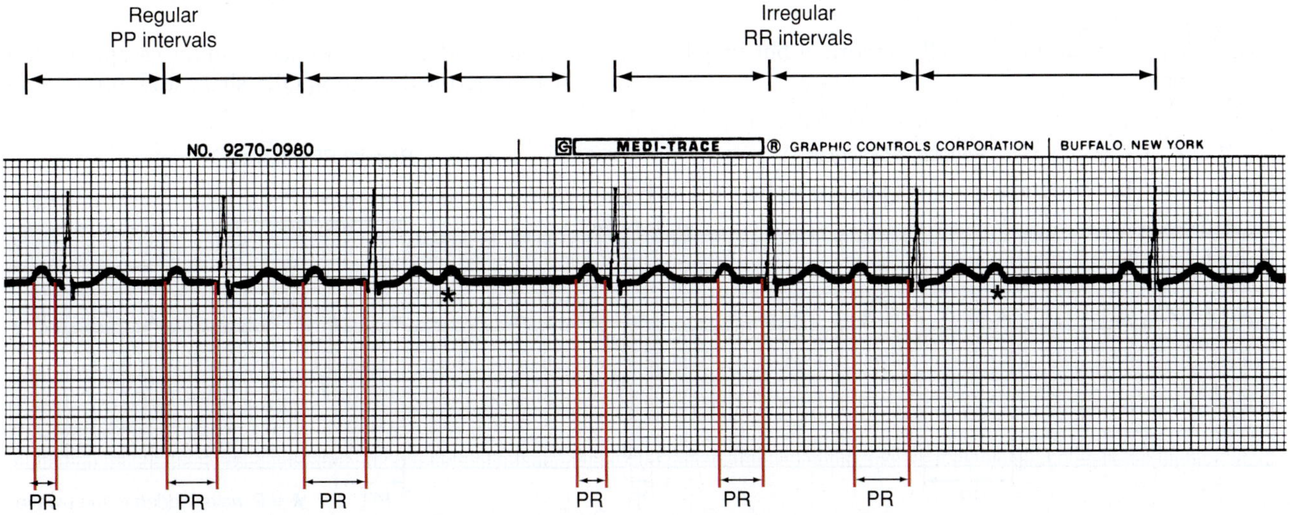

FIGURE 28-20. Sinus rhythm with second-degree AV block, type I in lead II. Note progressively longer PR durations until there is a nonconducted P wave, indicated by the *asterisk*.

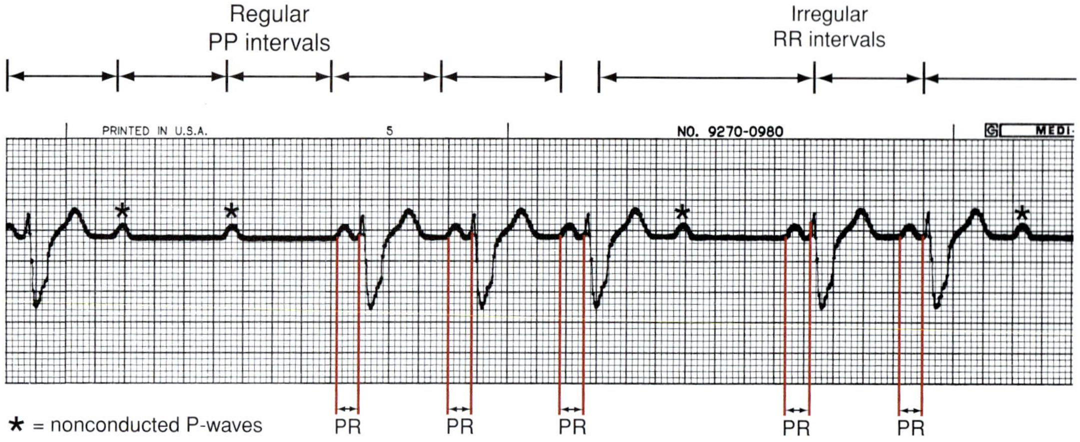

FIGURE 28-21. Sinus rhythm with second-degree AV block, type II in lead V_1; note constant PR interval and presence of more P waves than QRS complexes.

the RR interval characteristically reflects a pattern of change. Starting from the RR that is the longest, the RR interval gradually shortens until there is another long RR interval.

QRS shape and duration: Usually normal but may be abnormal

P wave: In front of the QRS complex; shape depends on underlying rhythm

PR interval: PR interval becomes longer with each succeeding ECG complex until there is a P wave not followed by a QRS. The changes in the PR interval are repeated between each "dropped" QRS, creating a pattern in the irregular PR interval measurements.

P:QRS ratio: 3:2, 4:3, 5:4, and so forth.

Second-Degree Atrioventricular Block, Type II

Second-degree AV block, type II, occurs when only some of the atrial impulses are conducted through the AV node into the ventricles. Second-degree AV block, type II, has the following characteristics (Fig. 28-21):

Ventricular and atrial rate: Depends on the underlying rhythm

Ventricular and atrial rhythm: The PP interval is regular if the patient has an underlying normal sinus rhythm. The RR interval is usually regular but may be irregular, depending on the P:QRS ratio.

QRS shape and duration: Usually abnormal but may be normal

P wave: In front of the QRS complex; shape depends on underlying rhythm

PR interval: PR interval is constant for those P waves just before QRS complexes

P:QRS ratio: 2:1, 3:1, 4:1, 5:1, and so forth

Third-Degree Atrioventricular Block

Third-degree AV block occurs when no atrial impulse is conducted through the AV node into the ventricles. In third-degree AV block, two impulses stimulate the heart: one stimulates the ventricles (e.g., junctional or ventricular escape rhythm), represented by the QRS complex, and one stimulates the atria (e.g., sinus rhythm or atrial fibrillation), represented by the P wave. P waves may be seen, but the atrial electrical activity is not conducted down into the ventricles to cause the QRS complex, the ventricular electrical activity. Having two impulses stimulate the heart results in a condition called AV dissociation, which may also occur during VT. Complete block (third-degree AV block) has the following characteristics (Fig. 28-22):

Ventricular and atrial rate: Depends on the escape rhythm and underlying atrial rhythm

Ventricular and atrial rhythm: The PP interval is regular and the RR interval is regular, but the PP interval is not equal to the RR interval

QRS shape and duration: Depends on the escape rhythm; with junctional rhythm, QRS shape and duration are

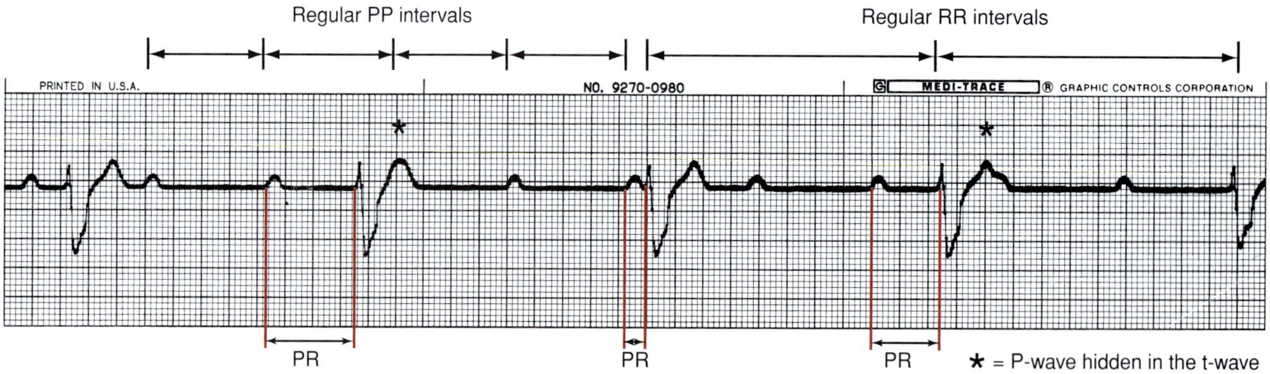

FIGURE 28-22. Sinus rhythm with third-degree AV block and idioventricular rhythm in lead V_1; note irregular PR intervals.

usually normal; with idioventricular rhythm, QRS shape and duration are usually abnormal

P wave: Depends on underlying rhythm

PR interval: Very irregular

P:QRS ratio: More P waves than QRS complexes

Medical Management of Conduction Abnormalities

Based on the cause of the AV block and the stability of the patient, treatment is directed toward increasing the heart rate to maintain a normal cardiac output. If the patient is stable and has no symptoms, no treatment may be indicated other than decreasing or eliminating the cause (e.g., withholding the medication or treatment). If the causal medication is necessary for treating other conditions and no effective alternative is available, pacemaker implantation may be indicated. The initial treatment of choice is an IV bolus of atropine, although it is not effective in second-degree AV block, type II, or third-degree AV block. If the patient does not respond to atropine, has advanced AV block, or has had an acute MI, temporary transcutaneous pacing may be started. If the patient has no pulse, treatment is the same as for ventricular asystole (Link et al., 2015). A permanent pacemaker may be necessary if the block persists.

Nursing Process

The Patient With a Dysrhythmia

Assessment

Major areas of assessment include possible causes of the dysrhythmia, contributing factors, and the dysrhythmia's effect on the heart's ability to pump an adequate blood volume. When cardiac output is reduced, the amount of oxygen reaching the tissues and vital organs is diminished. This diminished oxygenation produces the signs and symptoms associated with dysrhythmias. If these signs and symptoms are severe or if they occur frequently, the patient may experience significant distress and disruption of daily life.

A health history is obtained to identify any previous occurrences of decreased cardiac output, such as syncope (fainting), lightheadedness, dizziness, fatigue, chest discomfort, and palpitations. Coexisting conditions that could be possible causes of the dysrhythmia (e.g., heart disease, chronic obstructive pulmonary disease) may also be identified. All medications, prescribed and over-the-counter (including herbs and nutritional supplements), as well as the route of administration, are reviewed. If a patient is taking an antiarrhythmic medication, assessment for side effects, adverse reactions, and potential contraindications is necessary. For example, some medications (e.g., digoxin) can cause dysrhythmias. Laboratory results are reviewed to assess levels of medications as well as factors that could contribute to the dysrhythmia (e.g., anemia). A thorough psychosocial assessment is performed to identify the possible effects of the dysrhythmia, the patient's perception and understanding of the dysrhythmia and its treatment, and whether anxiety is a significant contributing factor.

The nurse conducts a physical assessment to confirm the data obtained from the history and to observe for signs of diminished cardiac output during the dysrhythmic event, especially changes in level of consciousness. The nurse assesses the patient's skin, which may be pale and cool. Signs of fluid retention, such as neck vein distention and crackles and wheezes auscultated in the lungs, may be detected. The rate and rhythm of apical and peripheral pulses are also assessed, and any pulse deficit is noted. The nurse auscultates for extra heart sounds (especially S_3 and S_4) and for heart murmurs, measures blood pressure, and determines pulse pressures. A declining pulse pressure indicates reduced cardiac output. Just one assessment may not disclose significant changes in cardiac output; therefore, the nurse compares multiple assessment findings over time, especially those that occur with and without the dysrhythmia.

Nursing Priorities

Based on assessment data, major nursing priorities of the patient may include:

- Reduced cardiac output
- Anxiety
- Lack of knowledge about the dysrhythmia and its treatment

Collaborative Problems/ Potential Complications

Potential complications that may develop include the following:

- Cardiac arrest (see Chapter 31)
- Heart failure (see Chapter 31)
- Thromboembolic event, especially with atrial fibrillation (see Chapter 31)

Planning and Goals

The major goals for the patient may include eliminating or decreasing the occurrence of the dysrhythmia (by decreasing contributory factors) to maintain cardiac output, minimizing anxiety, and acquiring knowledge about the dysrhythmia, tests used to diagnose the problem, and its treatment.

Nursing Interventions

Monitoring and Managing the Dysrhythmia

The nurse regularly evaluates the patient's blood pressure, pulse rate and rhythm, rate and depth of respirations, and breath sounds to determine the dysrhythmia's hemodynamic effect. The nurse also asks the patient about episodes of lightheadedness, dizziness, or fainting as part of the ongoing assessment. If a patient with a dysrhythmia is hospitalized, the nurse may obtain a

12-lead ECG, continuously monitor the patient, and analyze rhythm strips to track the dysrhythmia.

Control of the occurrence or the effect of the dysrhythmia, or both, is often achieved with antiarrhythmic medications. The nurse assesses and observes for the benefits and adverse effects of each medication. The nurse, in collaboration with the physician, also manages medication administration carefully so that a constant serum level of the medication is maintained. The nurse may also conduct a 6-minute walk test as prescribed, which is used to identify the patient's ventricular rate in response to exercise. The patient is asked to walk for 6 minutes, covering as much distance as possible. The nurse monitors the patient for symptoms. At the end, the nurse records the distance covered and the pre-exercise and postexercise heart rate as well as the patient's response.

The nurse assesses for factors that contribute to the dysrhythmia (e.g., oxygen deficits, acid–base and electrolyte imbalances, caffeine, or nonadherence to the medication regimen). The nurse also monitors for ECG changes (e.g., widening of the QRS, prolongation of the QT interval, increased heart rate) that increase the risk of a dysrhythmic event.

Minimizing Anxiety

When the patient experiences episodes of dysrhythmia, the nurse stays with the patient and provides assurance of safety and security while maintaining a calm and reassuring attitude. This assists in reducing anxiety (reducing the sympathetic response) and fosters a trusting relationship with the patient. The nurse seeks the patient's view of the events and discusses the emotional response to the dysrhythmia, encouraging verbalization of feelings and fears, providing supportive or empathetic statements, and assisting the patient to recognize feelings of anxiety, anger, or sadness. The nurse emphasizes successes with the patient to promote a sense of self-management of the dysrhythmia. For example, if a patient is experiencing episodes of dysrhythmia and a medication is administered that begins to reduce the incidence of the dysrhythmia, the nurse communicates that information to the patient. In addition, the nurse can help the patient develop a system to identify possible causative, influencing, and alleviating factors (e.g., keeping a diary). The nursing goal is to maximize the patient's control and to make the episode less threatening.

Promoting Home, Community-Based, and Transitional Care

EDUCATING PATIENTS ABOUT SELF-CARE. When educating patients about dysrhythmias, the nurse first assesses the patient's understanding, clarifies misinformation, and then shares needed information in terms that are understandable and in a manner that is not frightening or threatening. Research findings suggest that uncertainty about the cause of a dysrhythmia and when recurrence may occur is particularly disturbing among family members (Dalteg, Benzein, Sandgren, et al., 2014) (see Chart 28-5). The nurse clearly explains the etiology

NURSING RESEARCH PROFILE

Chart 28-5. Uncertainty Among Couples With Atrial Fibrillation

Dalteg, T., Benzein, E., Sandgren, A., et al. (2014). Managing uncertainty in couples living with atrial fibrillation. *Journal of Cardiovascular Nursing, 29*(3), e1–e10.

Purpose
Atrial fibrillation is a common dysrhythmia that has many root causes and morbid consequences. Patients diagnosed with atrial fibrillation have higher rates of morbidity and mortality than the general population. Atrial fibrillation is associated with symptoms that can include palpitations, chest pain, dizziness, and dyspnea, to name a few. Furthermore, patients with atrial fibrillation report diminished quality of life. Yet, little is known about the impact atrial fibrillation has on couples and their relationship. Therefore, the purpose of this study was to explore the main concerns that couples have when they live with atrial fibrillation.

Design
Classical grounded theory was chosen to discover couples' concerns relative to a diagnosis of atrial fibrillation. This study was conducted in a hospital in the south of Sweden among couples in a relationship where one member was admitted to the hospital with atrial fibrillation. Both members of the couple had to be at least 18 years of age and agreed to participate in the research. Twelve couples agreed to participate in the research and data collection process, which was conducted through interviews.

Findings
Participant couples living with atrial fibrillation voiced a common main concern that they lived with uncertainty. This uncertainty was grounded in not understanding what caused the atrial fibrillation and anxiety over its recurrence. Participant couples managed uncertainty through explicitly sharing their concerns with each other. They also managed uncertainty through implicitly sharing, which was conceptualized as keeping distance from each other as needed and through tacit understanding, or appreciating times when they would prefer to not talk through their feelings.

Nursing Implications
Findings from this study suggest that atrial fibrillation can have a profound effect on a couple's relationship because uncertainty becomes a part of their daily experience. Nurses can help alleviate stress experienced from uncertainty by explicitly sharing information with both members of couples confronted with a diagnosis of atrial fibrillation. Assessing their educational needs and providing them with information on the cause and rationale for treatment of atrial fibrillation can be helpful management strategies. Encouraging couples to give each other distance as needed may also be therapeutic.

of the dysrhythmia and treatment options to the patient and family. If necessary, the nurse explains the importance of maintaining therapeutic serum levels of antiarrhythmic medications so that the patient understands why medications should be taken regularly each day and the importance of regular blood testing. If the medication has the potential to alter the heart rate, the patient should be taught how to take their pulse before each dose and to notify the primary provider if the pulse is abnormal. In addition, the relationship between a dysrhythmia and cardiac output is explained so that the patient recognizes symptoms of the dysrhythmia and the rationale for the treatment regimen. The patient and family need to be educated about measures to take to decrease the risk of recurrence of the dysrhythmia. If the patient has a potentially lethal dysrhythmia, the nurse establishes with the patient and family a plan of action to take in case of an emergency and, if appropriate, encourages a family member to obtain CPR training.

The patient and family should also be educated about potential risks of the dysrhythmia and their signs and symptoms. For example, the patient with chronic atrial fibrillation should be educated about the possibility of an embolic event.

Continuing and Transitional Care

A referral for home, community-based, or transitional care usually is not necessary for the patient with a dysrhythmia unless the patient is hemodynamically unstable and has significant symptoms of decreased cardiac output. Home, community-based, or transitional care may be warranted if the patient has significant comorbidities, socioeconomic issues, or limited self-management skills that could increase the risk of nonadherence to the therapeutic regimen.

Evaluation

Expected patient outcomes may include:

1. Maintains cardiac output
   a. Demonstrates heart rate, blood pressure, respiratory rate, and level of consciousness within normal ranges
   b. Demonstrates no or decreased episodes of dysrhythmia
2. Experiences reduced anxiety
   a. Expresses a positive attitude about living with the dysrhythmia
   b. Expresses confidence in ability to take appropriate actions in an emergency
3. Expresses understanding of the dysrhythmia and its treatment
   a. Explains the dysrhythmia and its effects
   b. Describes the medication regimen and its rationale
   c. Explains the need to maintain a therapeutic serum level of the medication
   d. Describes a plan to eliminate or limit factors that contribute to the dysrhythmia
   e. States actions to take in the event of an emergency

ADJUNCTIVE MODALITIES AND MANAGEMENT

Dysrhythmia treatments depend on whether the disorder is acute or chronic as well as on the cause of the dysrhythmia and its actual or potential hemodynamic effects.

Acute dysrhythmias may be treated with medications or with external electrical therapy (emergency defibrillation, cardioversion, or pacing). Many antiarrhythmic medications are used to treat atrial and ventricular tachydysrhythmias (see Table 28-1). The choice of medication depends on the specific dysrhythmia and its duration, the presence of structural heart disease (e.g., heart failure), and the patient's response to previous treatment. The nurse is responsible for monitoring and documenting the patient's responses to the medication and for ensuring that the patient has the knowledge and ability to manage the medication regimen.

If medications alone are ineffective in eliminating or decreasing the dysrhythmia, certain adjunctive mechanical therapies are available. The most common therapies are elective cardioversion and defibrillation for acute tachydysrhythmia, and implantable devices (pacemakers for bradycardias and internal cardiodefibrillators for chronic tachydysrhythmias). Surgical treatments, although less common, are also available. The nurse is responsible for assessing the patient's understanding of and response to mechanical therapy, as well as the patient's self-management abilities. The nurse explains that the purpose of the device is to help the patient lead a life that is as active and productive as possible.

Cardioversion and Defibrillation

Cardioversion and defibrillation are used to treat tachydysrhythmias by delivering an electrical current that depolarizes a critical mass of myocardial cells. When the cells repolarize, the sinus node is usually able to recapture its role as the heart's pacemaker. One major difference between cardioversion and defibrillation is the timing of the delivery of electrical current. In cardioversion, the delivery of the electrical current is synchronized with the patient's electrical events; in defibrillation, the delivery of the current is immediate and unsynchronized.

The electrical current may be delivered externally through the skin with the use of paddles or with conductor pads. The paddles or pads may be placed on the front of the chest (Fig. 28-23) (standard placement), or one

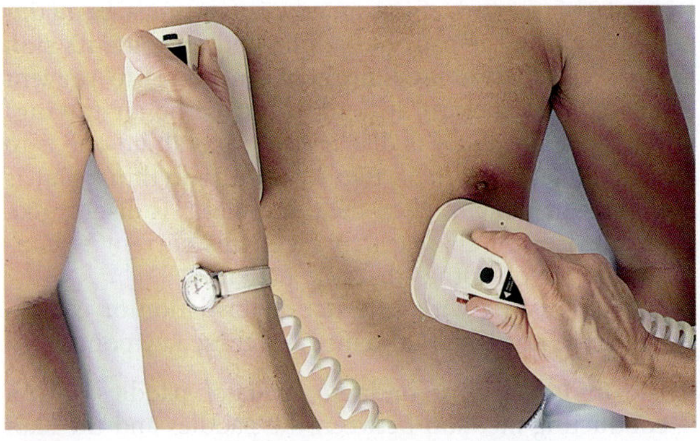

FIGURE 28-23. Standard paddle placement for defibrillation.

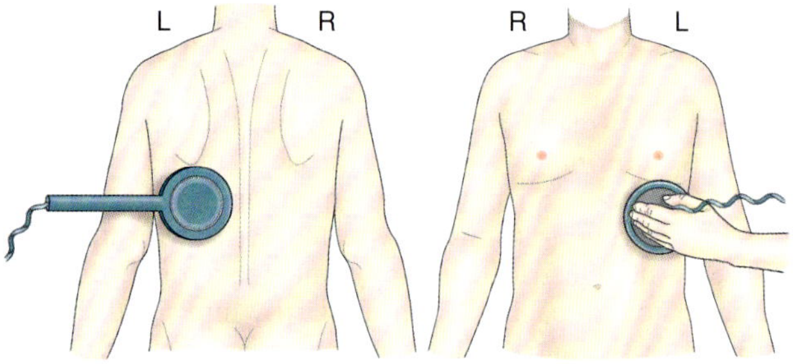

FIGURE 28-24. Anteroposterior paddle placement for defibrillation.

may be placed on the front of the chest and the other, using an adapter with a long handle if using paddles, placed under the patient's back just left of the spine (anteroposterior placement) (Fig. 28-24).

Defibrillator multifunction conductor pads contain a conductive medium and are connected to the defibrillator to allow for hands-off defibrillation. This method reduces the risk of touching the patient during the procedure and increases electrical safety. Automatic external defibrillators (AEDs), which are now found in public areas such as airports and grocery stores, use this type of delivery for the electrical current.

NURSING ALERT

One major difference between cardioversion and defibrillation is the timing of the delivery of electrical current. In cardioversion, the delivery of the electrical current is synchronized with the patient's electrical events; in defibrillation, the delivery of the current is immediate and unsynchronized.

NURSING ALERT

When using paddles, the appropriate conductant is applied between the paddles and the patient's skin. Any other type of conductant, such as ultrasound gel, should not be substituted.

Whether using pads or paddles, the nurse must observe two safety measures. First, good contact must be maintained between the pads or paddles and the patient's skin (with a conductive medium between them) to prevent electrical current from leaking through the air (arcing) when the defibrillator is discharged. Second, no one is to be in contact with the patient or with anything that is touching the patient when the defibrillator is discharged, to minimize the chance that electrical current is conducted to anyone other than the patient.

When assisting with external defibrillation or cardioversion, the nurse should remember these key points:

- Use multifunction conductor pads or paddles with a conducting medium between the paddles and the skin (the conducting medium is available as a sheet, gel, or paste). Do not use gels or pastes with poor electrical conductivity (e.g., ultrasound gel) (Link et al., 2015).
- Place paddles or pads so that they do not touch the patient's clothing or bed linen and are not near medication patches or direct oxygen flow.
- During cardioversion, ensure that the monitor leads are attached to the patient and that the defibrillator is in the synchronized mode ("in sync"). If defibrillating, ensure that the defibrillator is *not* in the synchronized mode (most machines default to the "not-sync" mode).
- If using paddles, exert 9 to 11 kg of pressure to ensure good skin contact.
- If using a manual discharge device, do not charge the device until ready to shock; then keep thumbs and fingers off the discharge buttons until paddles or pads are on the chest and ready to deliver the electrical charge.
- Before pressing the discharge button, call "Clear!" three times: As "Clear" is called the first time, ensure that you are not touching the patient, bed, or equipment; as "Clear" is called the second time, ensure that no one is touching the bed, the patient, or equipment, including the endotracheal tube or adjuncts; and as "Clear" is called the third time, perform a final visual check to ensure that you and everyone else are clear of the patient and anything touching the patient.
- Record the delivered energy.
- After the defibrillation, immediately resume CPR, starting with chest compressions.
- After five cycles (about 2 minutes) of CPR, check the cardiac rhythm and deliver another shock if indicated. Administer a vasoactive or antiarrhythmic medication as soon as possible after the rhythm check.

After the event is complete, inspect the skin under the pads or paddles for burns; if any are detected, consult with the physician or a wound care nurse about treatment.

Electrical Cardioversion

Electrical cardioversion involves the delivery of a "timed" electrical current to terminate a tachydysrhythmia. In cardioversion, the defibrillator is set to synchronize with the ECG on a cardiac monitor so that the electrical impulse discharges during ventricular depolarization (QRS complex). The synchronization prevents the discharge from occurring during the vulnerable period of repolarization (T wave), which could result in VT or ventricular fibrillation. The ECG monitor connected to the external defibrillator usually displays a mark or line that indicates sensing of a QRS complex. Sometimes the lead and the electrodes must be changed for the monitor to recognize the patient's QRS complex. When the synchronizer is on, no electrical current is delivered if the defibrillator does not discern a QRS complex. Therefore, it is important to ensure that the patient is connected to the monitor and to select a lead (not "paddles") that has the most appropriate sensing of the QRS. Because there may be a short delay until recognition of the QRS, the discharge buttons of an external manual defibrillator must be held down until the shock has been delivered. In most monitors, the synchronization mode must be reactivated if the initial cardioversion was ineffective and another cardioversion is needed (i.e., the device defaults to unsynchronized defibrillation mode).

If the cardioversion is elective and the dysrhythmia has lasted longer than 48 hours, anticoagulation for a few weeks before cardioversion may be indicated. Digoxin is usually withheld for 48 hours before cardioversion to ensure the resumption of sinus rhythm with normal conduction. The patient is instructed not to eat or drink for at least 4 hours before the procedure. Gel-covered paddles or conductor pads are positioned front and back (anteroposteriorly) for cardioversion. Before cardioversion, the patient receives moderate sedation IV as well as an analgesic medication or anesthesia. Respiration is then supported with supplemental oxygen delivered by a bag-mask-valve device with suction equipment readily available. Although patients rarely require intubation, equipment is nearby in case it is needed. The amount of voltage used varies from 50 to 360 J, depending on the defibrillator's technology, the type and duration of the dysrhythmia, and the size and hemodynamic status of the patient (Link et al., 2015). If ventricular fibrillation occurs after cardioversion, the defibrillator is used to defibrillate the patient (synchronization mode is *not* used).

Indications of a successful response are conversion to sinus rhythm, adequate peripheral pulses, and adequate blood pressure. Because of the sedation, airway patency must be maintained and the patient's state of consciousness assessed. Vital signs and oxygen saturation are monitored and recorded until the patient is stable and recovered from sedation and analgesic medications or anesthesia. ECG monitoring is required during and after cardioversion (Link et al., 2015).

Defibrillation

Defibrillation is used in emergency situations as the treatment of choice for ventricular fibrillation and pulseless VT, the most common cause of abrupt loss of cardiac function and sudden cardiac death. Defibrillation is not used for patients who are conscious or have a pulse. The sooner defibrillation is used, the better the survival rate: If it is used within 1 minute of the onset of VT or fibrillation, the survival rate is 90%; if it is delayed for 12 minutes, the survival rate is only 2% to 5%. Several studies have demonstrated that early defibrillation performed by lay people in a community setting can increase the survival rate. If immediate CPR is provided and defibrillation is performed within 5 minutes, more adults in ventricular fibrillation may survive with intact neurologic function (Link et al., 2015). A large multisite study found that the availability of AEDs in public places and their use shortened the interval from collapse to rhythm recognition and defibrillation, which significantly increased the number of survivors (Kronick, Kurz, Lin, et al., 2015). However, only a minority of prehospital arrests occur in public places, and prediction of the exact locations of future arrests is difficult. Therefore, although AEDs are clinically effective, money spent on AED equipment and training may be better spent on prevention interventions.

Defibrillation depolarizes a critical mass of myocardial cells all at once; when they repolarize, the sinus node usually recaptures its role as the pacemaker. The electrical voltage required to defibrillate the heart is usually greater than that required for cardioversion and may cause more myocardial damage. Defibrillators are classified as monophasic or biphasic. Monophasic defibrillators deliver current in only one direction and require increased energy loads. Newer biphasic defibrillators deliver the electrical charge to the positive paddle, which then reverses back to the originating paddle. This system allows for lower, possibly nonprogressive energy levels (e.g., 150 J with each defibrillation) with potentially less myocardial damage. If defibrillation was unsuccessful, CPR is immediately initiated and other advanced life support treatments are begun.

Epinephrine is administered after defibrillation to make it easier to convert the dysrhythmia to a normal rhythm with the next defibrillation. These medications may also increase cerebral and coronary artery blood flow. Antiarrhythmic medications such as amiodarone, lidocaine, or magnesium are administered if ventricular dysrhythmia persists (see Table 28-1). This treatment with continuous CPR, medication administration, and defibrillation continues until a stable rhythm resumes or until it is determined that the patient cannot be revived.

Electrophysiology Studies

An EP study is an invasive procedure used to evaluate and treat various chronic dysrhythmias that have caused cardiac arrest or significant symptoms. It also is indicated for patients with symptoms that suggest a dysrhythmia that has gone undetected and undiagnosed by other methods. Because an EP study is invasive, it is performed in the hospital and may require that the patient be admitted. An EP study is used to do the following:

- Identify the impulse formation and propagation through the cardiac electrical conduction system
- Assess the function or dysfunction of the SA and AV nodal areas
- Identify the location (called *mapping*) and mechanism of the dysrhythmogenic foci (the exact site where the dysrhythmia originates)
- Assess the effectiveness of antiarrhythmic medications and devices for the patient with a dysrhythmia
- Treat certain dysrhythmias through the destruction of the causative cells (ablation)

An EP procedure is a type of cardiac catheterization that is performed in a specially equipped cardiac catheterization laboratory by an electrophysiologist, who is a cardiologist with specialized training, assisted by other EP laboratory personnel. The patient is conscious but lightly sedated. Usually, a catheter with multiple electrodes is inserted through a small incision in the femoral vein, threaded through the inferior vena cava, and advanced into the heart; however, depending on the type of study and the information needed, a second catheter may be inserted into the femoral artery. The electrodes are positioned within the heart at specific locations—for instance, in the right atrium near the sinus node, in the coronary sinus, near the tricuspid valve, and at the apex of the right ventricle. The number and placement of electrodes depend on the type of study being conducted. These electrodes allow the electrical signal to be recorded from within the heart (intracardiogram).

The electrodes also allow the clinician to introduce a pacing stimulus to the intracardiac area at a precisely timed interval and rate, thereby stimulating the area (programmed stimulation). An area of the heart may be paced at a rate much faster than the normal rate of automaticity, the rate at which impulses are spontaneously formed (e.g., in the sinus node). This allows the pacemaker to become an artificial focus of automaticity and to assume control (overdrive suppression). Then, the pacemaker is stopped suddenly, and the time it takes for the sinus node to resume control is assessed. A prolonged time indicates dysfunction of the sinus node.

One of the main purposes of programmed stimulation is to assess the ability of the area surrounding the electrode to cause a reentry dysrhythmia. One or a series of premature impulses is delivered to an area in an attempt to cause the tachydysrhythmia. Because the precise location of the suspected area and the specific timing of the pacing needed are unknown, the electrophysiologist uses many different techniques to cause the dysrhythmia during the study. If the dysrhythmia can be reproduced by programmed stimulation, it is called *inducible*. Once a dysrhythmia is induced, a treatment plan is determined and implemented. If, on the follow-up EP study, the tachydysrhythmia cannot be induced, then the treatment is determined to be effective. Different medications may be given and combined with electrical devices (pacemaker, ICD) to determine the most effective treatment to suppress the dysrhythmia.

Patient care, patient education, and associated complications of an EP study are similar to those associated with cardiac catheterization (see Chapter 27). The study is usually about 2 hours in length; however, if the electrophysiologist conducts not only a diagnostic procedure but also treatment, the study can take up to 6 hours. During the procedure, patients benefit from a calm, reassuring approach.

Patients who are to undergo an EP study may be anxious about the procedure and its outcome. A detailed discussion involving the patient, the family, and the electrophysiologist usually occurs to ensure that the patient can give informed consent and to reduce the patient's anxiety about the procedure. Before the procedure, the patient should receive instructions about the procedure and its usual duration, the environment where the procedure is performed, and what to expect. Although an EP study is not painful, it does cause discomfort and can be tiring. It may also cause feelings that were experienced when the dysrhythmia occurred in the past. In addition, patients are educated about what will be expected of them (e.g., lying very still during the procedure, reporting symptoms or concerns).

The patient should also know that the dysrhythmia may occur during the procedure. It often stops on its own; if it does not, treatment is given to restore the patient's normal rhythm. The dysrhythmia may have to be terminated using cardioversion or defibrillation, but this is performed under more controlled circumstances than if performed in an emergency.

Postprocedural care is similar to that for cardiac catheterization, including restriction of activity to promote hemostasis at the insertion site (see Chapter 27). To identify any complications and to ensure healing, the patient's vital signs and the appearance of the insertion site are assessed frequently. Because an artery is not always used, there is a lower incidence of vascular complications than with other catheterization procedures. Cardiac arrest may occur, but the incidence is low (less than 1%) (Mann et al., 2015).

Pacemaker Therapy

A pacemaker is an electronic device that provides electrical stimuli to the heart muscle. Pacemakers are usually used when a patient has a permanent or temporary slower-than-normal impulse formation, or a symptomatic AV or ventricular conduction disturbance. They may also be used to control some tachydysrhythmias that do not respond to medication. Biventricular (both ventricles) pacing, also called resynchronization therapy, may be used to treat advanced heart failure that does not respond to medication. Pacemaker technology also may be used in an ICD (e.g., in patients with coronary artery disease and a reduced ejection fraction) (see Chapter 31 for further discussion of heart failure).

Pacemakers can be permanent or temporary. Temporary pacemakers are used to support patients until they improve or receive a permanent pacemaker (e.g., after acute MI or during open heart surgery). Temporary pacemakers are used only in hospital settings.

Pacemaker Design and Types

Pacemakers consist of two components: an electronic pulse generator and pacemaker electrodes, which are located on leads or wires. The generator contains the circuitry and batteries that determine the rate (measured in beats per minute) and the strength or output (measured in milliamperes [mA]) of the electrical stimulus delivered to the heart. The generator also has circuitry that can detect the intracardiac electrical activity to cause an appropriate response; this component of pacing is called **sensitivity** and is measured in millivolts (mV). Sensitivity is set at the level that the intracardiac electrical activity must exceed to be sensed by the device. Leads, which carry the impulse created by the generator to the heart, can be threaded by fluoroscopy through a major vein into the heart, usually the right atrium and ventricle (endocardial leads), or they can be lightly sutured onto the outside of the heart and brought through the chest wall during open heart surgery (epicardial wires). The epicardial wires are always temporary and are removed by a gentle tug a few days after surgery. The endocardial leads may be temporarily placed with catheters through a vein (usually the femoral, subclavian, or internal jugular vein [transvenous wires]), usually guided by fluoroscopy. The leads may also be part of a specialized pulmonary artery catheter (see Chapter 31). However, obtaining a pulmonary artery wedge pressure may cause the leads to move out of pacing position. The endocardial and epicardial wires are connected to a temporary generator, which is about the size of a small paperback book. The energy source for a temporary generator is a common household battery. Monitoring for pacemaker malfunctioning and battery failure is a nursing responsibility.

The endocardial leads also may be placed permanently, passed into the heart through the subclavian, axillary, or cephalic vein, and connected to a permanent generator. Most current leads have a fixation mechanism (e.g., a

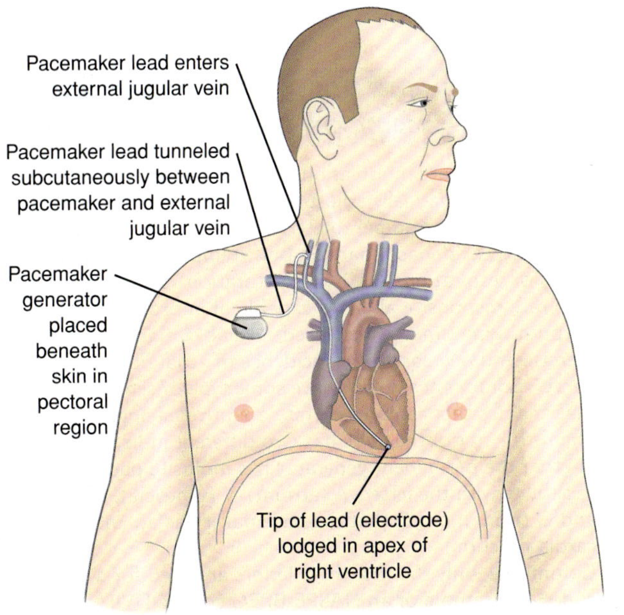

FIGURE 28-25. Implanted transvenous pacing lead (with electrode) and pacemaker generator.

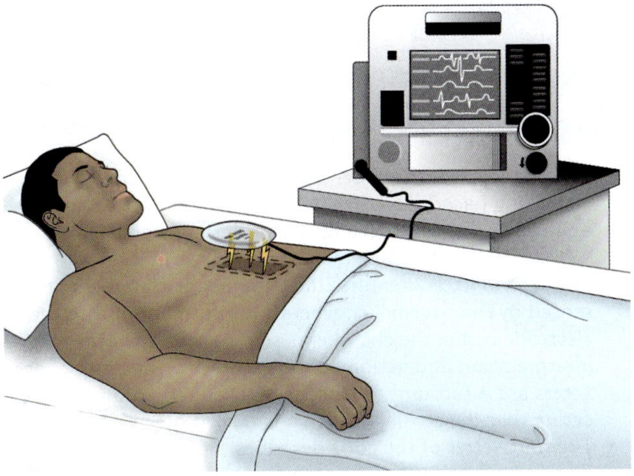

FIGURE 28-26. Transcutaneous pacemaker with electrode pads connected to the anterior and posterior chest walls.

screw) at the end of the lead that allows precise positioning and avoidance of dislodgement. The permanent generator, which often weighs less than 1 oz and is the size of a thick credit card, is usually implanted in a subcutaneous pocket created in the pectoral region, below the clavicle, or behind the breast, especially in young women (Fig. 28-25). This procedure usually takes about 1 hour, and it is performed in a cardiac catheterization laboratory using a local anesthetic and moderate sedation. Close monitoring of the respiratory status is needed until the patient is fully awake.

Permanent pacemaker generators are insulated to protect against body moisture and warmth and have filters that protect them from electrical interference from most household devices, motors, and appliances. Several different energy sources for permanent generators have been used and others have been investigated, but lithium cell units are most often used today. They last approximately 6 to 12 years, depending on the type of pacemaker, how it is programmed, and how often it is used. Most pacemakers have an **elective replacement indicator** (ERI), a signal that indicates when the battery is approaching depletion. The pacemaker continues to function for several months after the appearance of ERI to ensure that there is adequate time for a battery replacement. Although some batteries are rechargeable, most are not. Because the battery is permanently sealed in the pacemaker, the entire generator must be replaced. To replace a failing generator, the leads are disconnected, the old generator is removed, and a new generator is reconnected to the existing leads and reimplanted in the already existing subcutaneous pocket. Sometimes the leads are also replaced. Battery replacement is usually performed using a local anesthetic. Hospitalization is necessary for implantation or battery replacement; the patient usually can be discharged the next day.

If a patient suddenly develops a bradycardia, is symptomatic but has a pulse, and is unresponsive to atropine, emergency pacing may be started with transcutaneous pacing, which most defibrillators are now equipped to perform. AEDs are not yet able to do transcutaneous pacing. Large pacing ECG electrodes (sometimes the same conductive pads used for cardioversion and defibrillation) are placed on the patient's chest and back. The electrodes are connected to the defibrillator, which is the temporary pacemaker generator (Fig. 28-26). Because the impulse must travel through the patient's skin and tissue before reaching the heart, transcutaneous pacing can cause significant discomfort and is intended to be used only in emergencies. This type of pacing necessitates hospitalization. If the patient is alert, sedation and analgesia may be administered. Transcutaneous pacing is not indicated for pulseless bradycardia.

Pacemaker Generator Functions

Because of the sophistication and wide use of pacemakers, a universal code has been adopted to provide a means of safe communication about their function. The coding is referred to as the NASPE-BPEG code because it is sanctioned by the North American Society of Pacing and Electrophysiology and the British Pacing and Electrophysiology Group. The complete code consists of five letters; the fourth and fifth letters are used only with permanent pacemakers (Bernstein, Daubert, Fletcher, et al., 2002; Tracy, Epstein, Darbar, et al., 2012) (see Chart 28-6).

The pacemaker paces the atrium and then the ventricle when no ventricular activity is sensed for a period of time (the time is individually programmed into the pacemaker for each patient). A straight vertical line usually can be seen on the ECG when pacing is initiated. The line that represents pacing is called a *pacemaker spike.* The appropriate ECG complex should immediately follow the pacing spike; therefore, a P wave should follow an atrial pacing spike and a QRS complex should follow a ventricular pacing spike. Because the impulse starts in a different place than the patient's normal rhythm, the QRS complex or P wave that responds to pacing looks different from the patient's normal ECG complex. *Capture* is a term used to denote that the appropriate complex followed the pacing spike.

The type of pacemaker generator and the settings selected depend on the patient's dysrhythmia, underlying

CHART 28-6

North American Society of Pacing and Electrophysiology and the British Pacing and Electrophysiology Group Code (NASPE-BPEG Code) for Pacemaker Generator Function

- The first letter of the code identifies the chamber or chambers being paced (i.e., the chamber containing a pacing electrode). The letter characters for this code are A (atrium), V (ventricle), or D (dual, meaning both A and V).
- The second letter identifies the chamber or chambers being sensed by the pacemaker generator. Information from the electrode within the chamber is sent to the generator for interpretation and action by the generator. The letter characters are A (atrium), V (ventricle), D (dual), and O (indicating that the sensing function is turned off).
- The third letter of the code describes the type of response that will be made by the pacemaker to what is sensed. The letter characters used to describe this response are I (**inhibited**), T (**triggered**), D (dual—inhibited and triggered), and O (none). Inhibited response means that the response of the pacemaker is controlled by the activity of the patient's heart—that is, when the patient's heart beats, the pacemaker does not function, but when the heart does not beat, the pacemaker does function. In contrast, a triggered response means that the pacemaker responds (paces the heart) when it senses intrinsic heart activity.
- The fourth letter of the code is related to a permanent generator's ability to vary the heart rate. This ability is available in most current pacemakers. The possible letters are O, indicating no rate responsiveness, or R, indicating that the generator has rate modulation (i.e., the pacemaker has the ability to automatically adjust the pacing rate from moment to moment based on parameters, such as QT interval, physical activity, acid–base changes, body temperature, rate and depth of respirations, or oxygen saturation). A pacemaker with rate-responsive ability is capable of improving cardiac output during times of increased cardiac demand, such as exercise and decreasing the incidence of atrial fibrillation. All contemporary pacemakers have some type of sensor system that enables them to provide rate-adaptive pacing.
- The fifth letter of the code has two different indications: (1) that the permanent generator has multisite pacing capability with the letters A (atrium), V (ventricle), D (dual), and O (none); or (2) that the pacemaker has an antitachycardia function.
- Commonly, only the first three letters are used for a pacing code. An example of an NASPE-BPEG code is DVI:
  D: Both the atrium and the ventricle have a pacing electrode in place.
  V: The pacemaker is sensing the activity of the ventricle only.
  I: The pacemaker's stimulating effect is inhibited by ventricular activity—in other words, it does not create an impulse when the pacemaker senses that the patient's ventricle is active.

Adapted from Bernstein, A. D., Daubert, J. C., Fletcher, R. D., et al. (2002). The Revised NASPE/BPEG generic code for antibradycardia, adaptive-rate, and multisite pacing. *Journal of Pacing and Clinical Electrophysiology, 25*(2), 260–264; Gillis, A. M., Russo, A. M., Ellenbogen, K. A., et al. (2012). HRS/ACCF expert consensus statement on pacemaker device and mode selection. *Journal of American College of Cardiology, 60*(7), 682–703.

cardiac function, and age. Pacemakers are generally set to sense and respond to intrinsic activity, which is called *on-demand pacing* (see Fig. 28-27). If the pacemaker is set to pace but not to sense, it is called a *fixed* or *asynchronous pacemaker* (see Fig. 28-28); this is written in pacing code as AOO or VOO. The pacemaker paces at a constant rate, independent of the patient's intrinsic rhythm. VOO pacing may indicate battery failure.

VVI (V, paces the ventricle; V, senses ventricular activity; I, paces only if the ventricles do not depolarize) pacing causes loss of AV synchrony and atrial kick, which may cause a decrease in cardiac output and an increase in atrial distention and venous congestion. Pacemaker syndrome, causing symptoms such as chest discomfort, shortness of breath, fatigue, activity intolerance, and postural hypotension, is most common with VVI pacing (Tracy et al., 2012). Atrial pacing and dual-chamber (right atrial and RV) pacing have been found to reduce the incidence of atrial fibrillation, ventricular dysfunction, and heart failure (Tracy et al., 2012).

Single-chamber atrial pacing (AAI) or dual-chamber pacing (DDD) is recommended over VVI in patients with

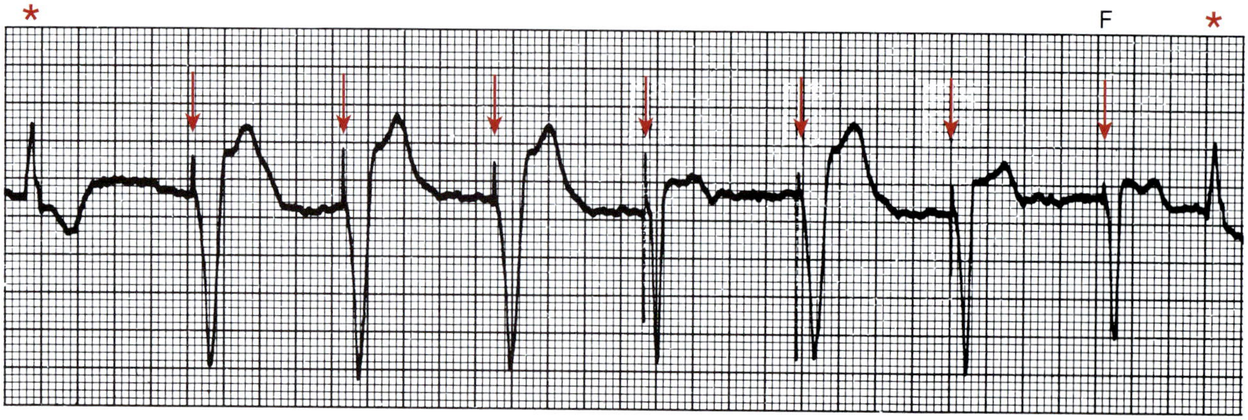

FIGURE 28-27. Pacing with appropriate sensing (on-demand pacing) in lead V_1. *Arrows* denote pacing spike. *Asterisk* denotes intrinsic (patient's own) beats; therefore, no pacing. F denotes a fusion beat, which is a combination of an intrinsic beat and a paced beat occurring at the same time.

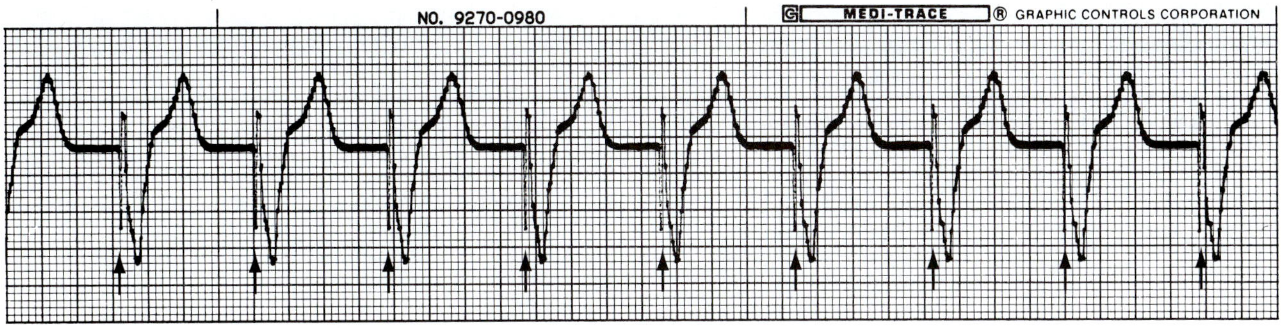

FIGURE 28-28. Fixed pacing or total loss of sensing pacing in lead V_1; *arrows* denote pacing spikes.

sinus node dysfunction (formerly called *sick sinus syndrome*), the most common cause of bradycardias requiring a pacemaker, and a functioning AV node (Tracy et al., 2012). AAI pacing ensures synchrony between atrial and ventricular stimulation (and therefore contraction), as long as the patient has no conduction disturbances in the AV node. Dual-chamber pacemakers are recommended as the treatment for patients with AV conduction disturbances (Tracy et al., 2012).

Synchronized biventricular pacing, also called *cardiac resynchronization therapy (CRT)*, has been found to modify the intraventricular, interventricular, and AV conduction defects identified with symptomatic moderate to severe left ventricular dysfunction and heart failure (New York Heart Association [NYHA] functional classes III and IV) (Cooper, 2015). CRT has also been implemented in patients with heart failure and atrial fibrillation and is associated with improved mortality rates (Gasparini, Leclercq, Lunati, et al., 2013). The generator for biventricular pacing has three leads: one for the right atrium; one for the right ventricle, as with most standard pacemaker generators; and one for the left ventricle, usually placed in the left lateral wall. This therapy improves cardiac function, resulting in decreased heart failure symptoms and an improved quality of life. Biventricular pacing may be used with an ICD.

Complications of Pacemaker Use

Complications associated with pacemakers relate to their presence within the body and improper functioning. The following complications may arise from a pacemaker:

- Local infection at the entry site of the leads for temporary pacing, or at the subcutaneous site for permanent generator placement. Prophylactic antibiotics and antibiotic irrigation of the subcutaneous pocket prior to generator placement has decreased the rate of infection to less than 2% (Fuster et al., 2011).
- Pneumothorax. However, the current procedure and use of safe sheaths reduce this risk.
- Bleeding and hematoma at the lead entry sites for temporary pacing or at the subcutaneous site for permanent generator placement. This usually can be managed with cold compresses and discontinuation of antiplatelet and antithrombotic medications.
- Hemothorax from puncture of the subclavian vein or internal mammary artery.
- Ventricular ectopy and tachycardia from irritation of the ventricular wall by the endocardial electrode.
- Movement or dislocation of the lead placed transvenously (perforation of the myocardium).
- Phrenic nerve, diaphragmatic (hiccupping may be a sign), or skeletal muscle stimulation if the lead is dislocated or if the delivered energy (mA) is set high. The occurrence of this complication is avoided by testing during device implantation.
- Cardiac perforation resulting in pericardial effusion and rarely, cardiac tamponade, which may occur at the time of implantation or months later. This condition can be recognized by the change in QRS complex morphology, diaphragmatic stimulation, or hemodynamic instability.
- Twiddler syndrome may occur when the patient manipulates the generator, causing lead dislodgement or fracture of the lead.

Pacemaker syndrome (hemodynamic instability caused by ventricular pacing and the loss of AV synchrony). This causes mild symptoms in more than 20% of ventricularly paced patients and severe symptoms in 5% to 7% of these patients (Fuster et al., 2011).

In the initial hours after a temporary or permanent pacemaker is inserted, the most common complication is dislodgment of the pacing electrode. Minimizing patient activity can help prevent this complication. If a temporary electrode is in place, the extremity through which the catheter has been advanced is immobilized. With a permanent pacemaker, the patient is instructed initially to restrict activity on the side of the implantation.

The ECG is monitored very carefully to detect pacemaker malfunction. Improper pacemaker function, which can arise from failure in one or more components of the pacing system, is outlined in Table 28-2. The following data should be noted on the patient's record: model of pacemaker, type of generator, date and time of insertion, location of pulse generator, stimulation threshold, and pacer settings (e.g., rate, energy output [mA], sensitivity [mV], and duration of interval between atrial and ventricular impulses [AV delay]). This information is important for identifying normal pacemaker function and diagnosing pacemaker malfunction.

A patient experiencing pacemaker malfunction may develop bradycardia as well as signs and symptoms of decreased cardiac output. The degree to which these symptoms become apparent depends on the severity of the malfunction, the patient's level of dependency on the pacemaker, and the patient's underlying condition. Pacemaker malfunction is diagnosed by analyzing the ECG. Manipulating the electrodes, changing the generator's settings, or replacing the pacemaker generator or leads (or both) may be necessary.

TABLE 28-2 Assessing Pacemaker Malfunction

Problem	Possible Cause	Intervention
Loss of capture-complex does *not* follow pacing spike	Inadequate stimulus Lead dislodgement Lead wire fracture Catheter malposition Battery depletion Electronic insulation break Medication change Myocardial ischemia	Check security of all connections; increase milliamperage Reposition extremity; turn patient to left side Change battery Change generator
Undersensing-pacing spike occurs at preset interval despite patient's intrinsic rhythm	Sensitivity too high Electrical interference (e.g., by a magnet) Faulty generator	Decrease sensitivity Eliminate interference Replace generator
Oversensing—loss of pacing artefact; pacing does not occur at preset interval despite lack of intrinsic rhythm	Sensitivity too low Electrical interference Battery depletion Change in medication	Increase sensitivity Eliminate interference Change battery
Loss of pacing—total absence of pacing spikes	Oversensing Battery depletion Loose or disconnected wires Perforation	Change battery Check security of all connections Apply magnet over permanent generator Obtain 12-lead ECG and portable chest x-ray Assess for murmur. Contact physician
Change in pacing QRS shape	Septal perforation	Obtain 12-lead ECG and portable chest x-ray Assess for murmur. Contact physician
Rhythmic diaphragmatic or chest wall twitching or hiccupping	Output too high Myocardial wall perforation	Decrease milliamperage Turn pacer off. Contact physician at once. Monitor closely for decreased cardiac output

Inhibition of permanent pacemakers or reversion to asynchronous fixed rate pacing can occur with exposure to strong electromagnetic fields (electromagnetic interference [EMI]). However, recent pacemaker technology allows patients to safely use most household electronic appliances and devices (e.g., microwave ovens, electric tools). Gas-powered engines should be turned off before working on them. Objects that contain magnets (e.g., the earpiece of a phone; large stereo speakers; mattresses, jewelry, and wraps) should not be near the generator for longer than a few seconds. Patients are advised to place digital cellular phones at least 15 to 30 centimeters away from (or on the side opposite of) the pacemaker generator and not to carry them in a shirt pocket. Large electromagnetic fields, such as those produced by magnetic resonance imaging, radio and television transmitter towers and lines, transmission power lines (not the distribution lines that bring electricity into a home), and electrical substations may cause EMI. Patients should be cautioned to avoid such situations or to simply move farther away from the area if they experience dizziness or a feeling of rapid or irregular heartbeats (palpitations). Welding and the use of a chain saw should be avoided. If such tools are used, precautionary steps such as limiting the welding current to a 60- to 130-A range or using electric rather than gasoline-powered chain saws are advised.

In addition, the metal of the pacemaker generator may trigger store and library antitheft devices as well as airport and building security alarms; however, these alarm systems generally do not interfere with the pacemaker function. Patients should walk through them quickly and avoid standing in or near these devices. The handheld screening devices used in airports may interfere with the pacemaker. Patients should be advised to ask security personnel to perform a hand search instead of using the handheld screening device. Patients also should be instructed to wear or carry medical identification to alert personnel to the presence of the pacemaker.

Pacemaker Surveillance

Pacemaker clinics have been established to monitor patients and to test pulse generators for impending pacemaker battery failure. A computerized device is held over the generator to "interrogate" it with painless radio signals; it detects the generator's settings, battery status and the presence of ERI, pacing threshold, sensing function, lead integrity, pacing data (e.g., number of pacing events), and other stored information. Several factors, such as lead fracture, muscle inhibition, and insulation disruption, also may be assessed depending on the type of pacemaker and the equipment available. If indicated, the pacemaker is turned off for a few seconds, using a magnet or a programmer, while the ECG is recorded to assess the patient's underlying cardiac rhythm. Transtelephonic transmission of the generator's information is another follow-up method. Special equipment is used to transmit information about the patient's pacemaker over the telephone to a receiving system at a pacemaker clinic. The information is converted into tones; equipment at the clinic converts these tones to an electronic signal and records them on an ECG strip. The pacemaker rate and other data concerning pacemaker function are obtained and evaluated by a cardiologist. This simplifies the diagnosis of a failing generator, reassures the patient, and improves management when the patient is physically remote from pacemaker testing facilities. The frequency of the pacemaker checks varies with the patient's age and underlying condition, the degree of pacemaker dependency, the age and type of the device, the results from previous pacemaker checks, and physician preference. A typical follow-up schedule is every 2 weeks during the first month, every 4 to 8 weeks for 3 years, and every 4 weeks thereafter.

Implantable Cardioverter Defibrillator

The ICD is an electronic device that detects and terminates life-threatening episodes of tachycardia or fibrillation, especially those that are ventricular in origin. Patients at high risk of VT or ventricular fibrillation and who would benefit from an ICD are those who have survived sudden cardiac death syndrome, which usually is caused by ventricular fibrillation, or have experienced spontaneous, symptomatic VT (syncope secondary to VT) not due to a reversible cause (called a *secondary prevention intervention*). Patients with coronary artery disease who are 40 days postacute MI with moderate to severe left ventricular dysfunction (ejection fraction less than or equal to 35%) are at risk of sudden cardiac death and therefore an ICD is indicated (called a *primary prevention intervention*) (Wilkoff, Fauchier, Stiles, et al., 2015). An ICD implantation is also recommended in patients who have been diagnosed with nonischemic dilated cardiomyopathy for at least 9 months and have functional NYHA Class II or III heart failure (Wilkoff et al., 2015). The American College of Cardiology, American Heart Association, and Society for Critical Care Medicine, in conjunction with other key clinical societies, developed appropriate use criteria (AUC) to be used as guides for cost-effective use of ICDs, with the caveat that AUC guidelines do not supersede clinical judgment (Russo et al., 2013). Indications for the use of ICDs continue to be refined (Kusumoto, Calkins, Boehmer, et al., 2014). In particular, use of ICDs for internal defibrillation in patients with symptomatic, recurrent, medication-refractory atrial fibrillation continues to be explored (Gerstenfeld & Everett, 2014).

Because there may be a waiting period for ICD implantation, especially those postacute MI, patients who are at risk for sudden cardiac death may be prescribed a wearable vest-like automated defibrillator, which works just like an AED in that a shock is delivered less than a minute after a life-threatening rhythm is detected (Epstein, Abraham, Bianco, et al., 2013). Prior to the delivery of the shock, the vest vibrates and issues an alarm to announce that a shock is imminent. The vest weighs about a pound, is worn under the patient's clothing, and is attached to a monitor with a battery that is worn in a holster or on a shoulder strap. The monitor automatically downloads information once a day, usually in the middle of the night. The vest must be worn at all times, even if the patient is admitted to the hospital and placed on an ECG monitor, and removed only when showering or bathing. The battery needs to be changed every day. Education is provided to the patient by the device manufacturer. However, the nurse should assess the patient's understanding of the education provided and explore any issues that may prevent the patient from wearing it.

An ICD has a generator about the size of a book of matches that is implanted in a subcutaneous pocket, usually in the upper chest wall. An ICD also has at least a RV lead that is implanted transvenously and can sense intrinsic electrical activity and deliver an electrical impulse. The implantation procedure, postimplantation care, and length of hospital stay are much like those for insertion of a pacemaker (see Fig. 28-29).

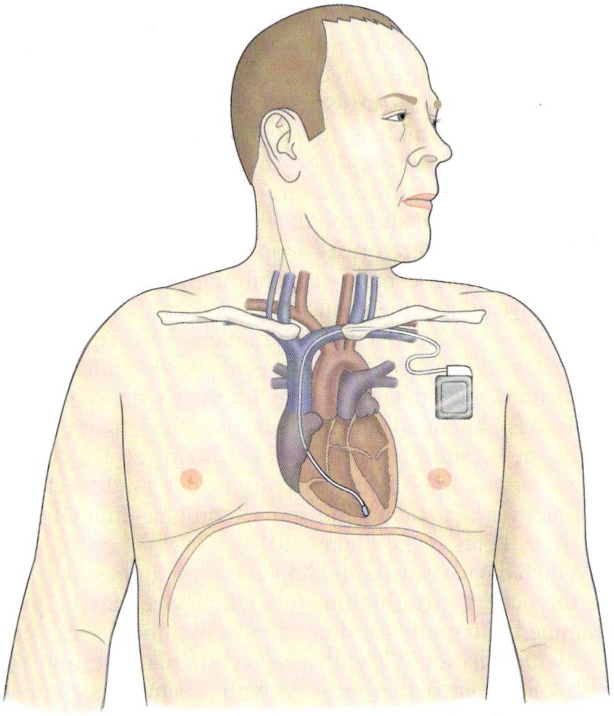

FIGURE 28-29. The implantable cardioverter defibrillator (ICD) consists of a generator and a sensing/pacing/defibrillating electrode.

ICDs are designed to respond to two criteria: a rate that exceeds a predetermined level and a change in the isoelectric line segments. When a dysrhythmia occurs, rate sensors require a set duration of time to sense the dysrhythmia. Then, the device automatically charges; after a second "look" confirms the dysrhythmia, it delivers the programmed charge through the lead to the heart. The time from dysrhythmia detection to electrical discharge depends on the charging time, which depends on the programmed energy level (Mann et al., 2015). However, in an ICD that has the capability of providing atrial therapies, the device can be programmed to be activated by the patient, giving the patient time to activate the charge at a time and place of their choosing. The life of the lithium battery is about 9 years but varies depending on the use of the ICD. ICD surveillance is similar to that of the pacemaker; however, it includes stored endocardial ECGs as well as information about the number and frequency of shocks that have been delivered.

Antiarrhythmic medication may be given with this technology to minimize the occurrence of a tachydysrhythmia and to reduce the frequency of ICD discharge.

Several types of devices are available. ICD, the generic name, is used as the abbreviation for these various devices. Each device offers a different delivery sequence, but all are capable of delivering high-energy (high-intensity) defibrillation to treat a tachycardia (atrial or ventricular). The device may deliver up to six shocks if necessary.

Some ICDs can respond with: (1) antitachycardia pacing, in which the device delivers electrical impulses at a fast rate in an attempt to disrupt the tachycardia; (2) low-energy (low-intensity) cardioversion; or (3) defibrillation; others may use all three techniques. Pacing is used to terminate tachycardias caused by a conduction disturbance called *reentry,* which is repetitive restimulation of the heart by the same impulse. An impulse or a series of impulses is delivered to the heart by the device at a fast rate to collide with and stop the heart's reentry conduction impulses, and therefore to stop the tachycardia. Some ICDs also have pacemaker capability if the patient develops bradycardia, which sometimes occurs after treatment of the tachycardia. Usually, the mode is VVI. Subcutaneous ICDs are now available; the generator is implanted in a subcutaneous pocket over the 5th intercostal space and the lead is implanted subcutaneously to the left and parallel to the sternum (Burke, Gold, Knight, et al., 2015). However, this technology does not include bradycardia or anti-tachycardia pacing and so currently has limited utility (Aziz, Leon, & El-Chami, 2014).

Which device is used and how it is programmed depend on the patient's dysrhythmia(s). The device may be programmed differently for different dysrhythmias (e.g., ventricular fibrillation, VT with a fast ventricular rate, and VT with a slow ventricular rate). As with pacemakers, there is an NASPE-BPEG code for communicating the functions of the ICDs (Bernstein et al., 2002; Wilkoff et al., 2015). The first letter represents the chamber or chambers shocked (O, none; A, atrium; V, ventricle; D, both atrium and ventricle). The second letter represents the chamber that can be antitachycardia paced (O, A, V, D, meaning the same as the first letter). The third letter indicates the method used by the generator to detect a tachycardia (E, electrogram; H, hemodynamics). The last letter represents the chambers that have antibradycardia pacing (O, A, V, D, meaning the same as the first and second letters of the ICD code).

Complications of ICD implantation are similar to those associated with pacemaker insertion. The primary complication is surgery-related infection; its risk increases with battery or lead replacement. Postimplantation mortality rates are higher when the procedure is done for reasons other than generator replacement, when the patient has advanced heart failure or renal dysfunction, and when it is performed as a consequence of an emergency admission (Dodson, Reynolds, Bao, et al., 2014). A few complications are associated with the technical aspects of the equipment, like those of pacemakers, such as premature battery depletion and dislodged or fractured leads. Inappropriate delivery of ICD therapy, usually due to oversensing or atrial and sinus tachycardias with a rapid ventricular rate response, is the most frequent long-term complication. This requires reprogramming of the device.

Nursing Management of the Patient With an Implantable Cardiac Device

After a permanent electronic device (pacemaker or ICD) is inserted, the patient's heart rate and rhythm are monitored by ECG. The device's settings are noted and compared with the ECG recordings to assess the device's function. For example, pacemaker malfunction is detected by examining the pacemaker spike and its relationship to the surrounding ECG complexes (Fig. 28-30). In addition, cardiac output and hemodynamic stability are assessed to identify the patient's response to pacing and

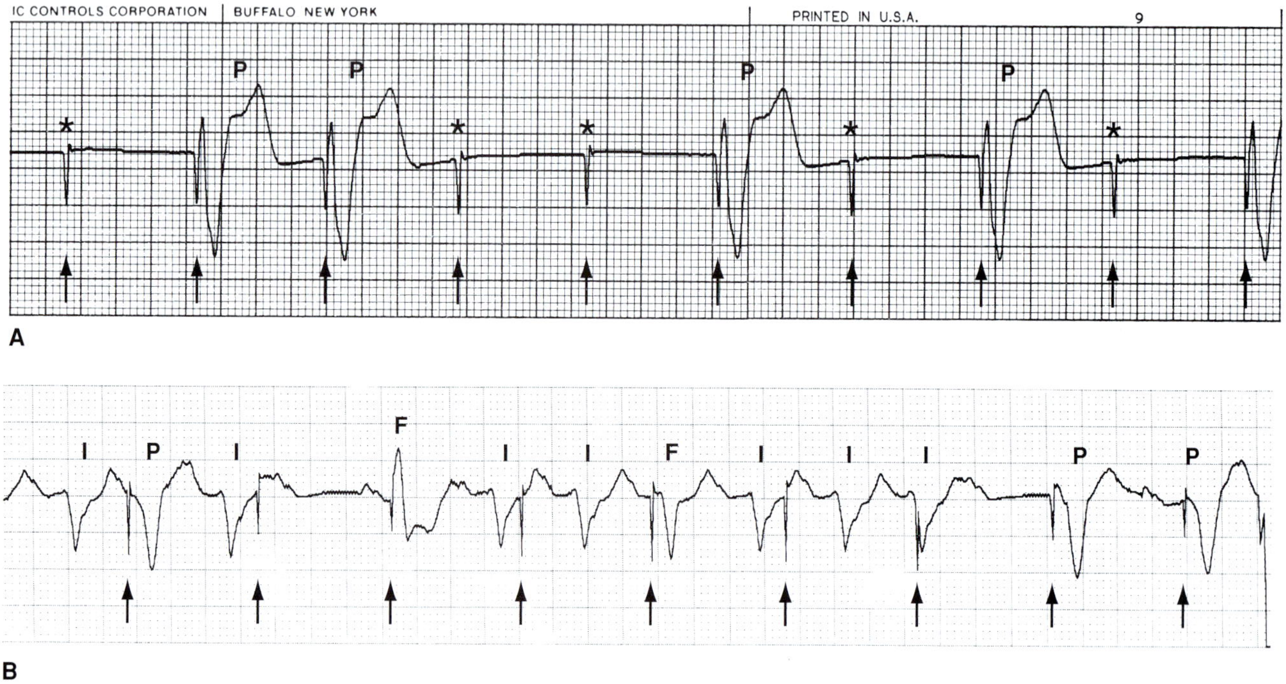

FIGURE 28-30. **A.** Ventricular pacing with intermittent loss of capture (a pacing spike not followed by a QRS complex). **B.** Ventricular pacing with loss of sensing (a pacing spike occurring at an inappropriate time). ↑, pacing spike; *, loss of capture; P, pacemaker-induced QRS complex; I, patient's intrinsic QRS complex; F, fusion (a QRS complex formed by a merging of the patient's intrinsic QRS complex and the pacemaker-induced QRS complex). Both in lead V_1.

the adequacy of pacing. The appearance or increasing frequency of dysrhythmia is observed and reported to the physician. If the patient has an ICD implanted and develops VT or ventricular fibrillation, the ECG should be recorded to note the time between the onset of the dysrhythmia and the onset of the device's shock or antitachycardia pacing.

The incision site where the generator was implanted is observed for bleeding, hematoma formation, or infection, which may be evidenced by swelling, unusual tenderness, drainage, and increased warmth. The patient may complain of continuous throbbing or pain. These symptoms are reported to the physician.

A chest x-ray is usually taken after the procedure and prior to discharge to document the position of leads in addition to ensuring that the procedure did not cause a pneumothorax. It is necessary to assess the function of the device throughout its lifetime and especially after changes in the patient's medication regimen. For example, antiarrhythmics, beta-blockers, and diuretics may increase the pacing threshold, whereas corticosteroids and alpha adrenergics may decrease the pacing threshold; the opposite effect occurs when the patient is taken off these medications.

The patient is also assessed for anxiety, depression, or anger, which may be symptoms of ineffective coping with the implantation. In addition, the level of knowledge and learning needs of the patient and family and the history of adherence to the therapeutic regimen should be identified. It is especially important to include the family when providing education and support.

In the perioperative and postoperative phases, the nurse carefully observes the patient's responses to the device and provides the patient and family with further teaching as needed (Chart 28-7). The nurse also assists the patient and family in addressing concerns and in making decisions about self-care and lifestyle changes necessitated by the dysrhythmia and resulting device implantation.

Preventing Infection

The nurse changes the dressing as needed and inspects the insertion site for redness, swelling, soreness, or any unusual drainage. Any change in wound appearance, an increase in the patient's temperature, or an increase in the patient's white blood cell count should be reported to the physician.

Promoting Effective Coping

The patient treated with an electronic device experiences not only lifestyle and physical changes but also emotional changes. At different times during the healing process, the patient may feel angry, depressed, fearful, anxious, or a combination of these emotions. Although each patient uses individual coping strategies (e.g., humour, prayer, communication with a significant other) to manage emotional distress, some strategies may work better than others. Signs that may indicate ineffective coping include social isolation, increased or prolonged irritability or depression, and difficulty in relationships.

To promote effective coping strategies, the nurse must recognize the patient's as well as the family's perceptions of the situation and their resulting emotional state and assist them to explore their reactions and feelings. Because of the unpredictable and possibly painful ICD discharge, patients with ICDs are most vulnerable to feelings of helplessness, leading to depression. The nurse can help the patient identify positive methods to deal with the actual or perceived limitations and manage any lifestyle changes needed. The nurse may help the patient identify changes (e.g., loss of ability to participate in contact sports), the emotional responses to the change (e.g., anger), and how the patient responds to that emotion (e.g., quickly becomes angry when talking with spouse). The nurse reassures the patient that the responses are normal and helps the patient identify realistic goals (e.g., develop interest in another activity) and develop a plan to attain these goals. The patient and family should be encouraged to talk about their experiences and emotions with each other and the health care team. The nurse may refer the patient and family to a hospital, community, or online support group. The nurse may also encourage the use of spiritual resources. The nurse also may teach the patient easy-to-use stress reduction techniques (e.g., deep-breathing exercises) to facilitate coping. Instructing the patient about the ICD may help the patient to cope with changes that occur as a result of device implantation (see Chart 28-7).

Promoting Home, Community-Based, and Transitional Care

After device insertion, the patient's hospital stay may be 1 day or less, and follow-up in an outpatient clinic or office is common. The patient's anxiety and feelings of vulnerability may interfere with the ability to learn information provided. The nurse needs to include caregivers in the teaching and provide printed materials for use by the patient and caregiver. The nurse establishes priorities for learning with the patient and caregiver. Teaching may include the importance of periodic device monitoring, promoting safety, surgical site care, and avoiding EMI (see Chart 28-7). In addition, the educational plan should include information about activities that are safe and those that may be dangerous. The nurse discusses with the patient and family what they are to do when a shock is delivered. The nurse may facilitate CPR training for the family.

Critical Thinking Exercises

1 Your aunt, who has a history of heart failure, calls to tell you that her primary provider told her that she has atrial fibrillation. She says that she has been prescribed warfarin and that she really doesn't want to take it because she knows it will stop her from clotting, and she is afraid of bleeding. What is the strength of the evidence that supports your aunt's continued adherence to warfarin therapy? What are the risks involved should she decide she will not take this drug as prescribed?

2 You answer a patient's call light on the medical/surgical unit where you work. The patient complains of a sudden onset of "palpitations" and "lightheadedness." Reviewing the bedside cardiac monitor, you see that the patient has

CHART 28-7

HOME CARE CHECKLIST • Educating the Patient With an Implantable Cardiac Device

At the completion of education, the patient and/or caregiver will be able to:

- State the impact of device implantation on physiologic functioning, ADLs, IADLs, self-image and roles, relationships (including sexuality), and spirituality
- State changes in lifestyle (e.g., diet, activity, mobility/driving restrictions) necessary to maintain health
- State the name, dose, side effects, frequency, and schedule for all medications
- For patients with pacemakers, check pulse daily. Report immediately any sudden slowing or increasing of the pulse rate. This may indicate pacemaker malfunction
- Avoid infection at the insertion site of the device:
  - Leave the incision uncovered and observe it daily for redness, increased swelling, and heat
  - Take temperature at same time each day; report any increase
  - Avoid wearing tight, restrictive clothing that may cause friction over the insertion site
  - Initially avoid soaking in the tub and lotion, creams, or powders in the area of the device
- Adhere to activity restrictions:
  - Restrict movement of arm until incision heals; do not raise arm above head for 2 weeks
  - Avoid heavy lifting for a few weeks
  - Discuss safety of activities (e.g., driving) with a primary provider
  - Recognize that although it may take up to 2 to 3 weeks to resume normal activities, physical activity does not usually have to be curtailed, with the exception of contact sports
- Electromagnetic interference: Understand the importance of the following:
  - Avoid large magnetic fields, such as those created by magnetic resonance imaging, large motors, arc welding, and electrical substations. Magnetic fields may deactivate the device, negating its effect on a dysrhythmia
  - At security gates at airports, government buildings, or other secured areas, show identification card and request a hand (not handheld device) search. Obtain and carry a letter from the primary provider about this requirement
  - Some electrical and small motor devices, as well as products that contain magnets (e.g., cellular phones), may interfere with the functioning of the cardiac device if the electrical device is placed very close to it. Avoid leaning directly over large electrical devices or motors, or ensure that contact is of brief duration; place cellular phone on opposite side of cardiac device
  - Household appliances (e.g., microwave ovens) should not cause any concern
- Describe precautions and safety measures to be used:
  - Describe what to do if symptoms occur, and notify the primary provider if any discharges seem unusual
  - Maintain a log that records discharges of an implantable cardioverter defibrillator (ICD). Record events that precipitate the sensation of shock. This provides important data for the primary provider to use in readjusting the medical regimen
  - Encourage family members to attend a cardiopulmonary resuscitation class
  - Call 911 for emergency assistance if feeling of dizziness occurs
  - Wear medical identification (e.g., Medic-Alert) that includes primary provider information
  - Avoid frightening family or friends with unexpected shocks from an ICD, which will not harm them. Inform family and friends that in the event they are in contact with the patient when a shock is delivered, they may also feel the shock. It is especially important to warn sexual partners that this may occur
  - Carry medical identification with the primary provider's name, type and model number of the device, manufacturer's name, and hospital where device was inserted
- Identify community resources for peer and caregiver/family support
- Adhere to appointments for follow-up care that are scheduled to monitor the electronic performance of the cardiac device. This is especially important during the first month after implantation and near the end of the battery life. Remember to take log of ICD discharges to review with the primary provider
- Identify the need for health promotion, disease prevention, and screening activities

ADL, activities of daily living; IADL, independent activities of daily living; ICD, implantable cardioverter defibrillator.

a new onset of atrial flutter with a heart rate of 145 bpm. Prior to contacting the primary provider, what other assessment information would you obtain? What interventions do you anticipate?

3 A 35-year-old mother of two grade school-aged children who is in the middle of a contentious divorce presents to the clinic where you work. She tells you that yesterday when she got home from work, she was bending over to put laundry in the washer and she suddenly felt her "heart racing, pounding" in her chest. She also tells you that her skin was cool and clammy. She rested and eventually her symptoms resolved. What are some possible causes of these symptoms? Identify other key factors that you would want to include in your assessment to help identify the cause of the dysrhythmia. What nursing interventions are needed?

REFERENCES AND SELECTED READINGS

Books

Fuster, V., Walsh, R. A., & Harrington, R. A. (Eds.). (2011). *Hurst's the heart* (13th ed.). New York: McGraw-Hill.

Mann, D. L., Zipes, D. P., Libby, P., et al. (2015). *Braunwald's heart disease: A textbook of cardiovascular medicine* (10th ed.). Philadelphia, PA: Elsevier.

McEvoy, G. K. (Ed.). (2014). *AHFS drug information*. Bethesda, MD: American Society of Health System Pharmacists.

Journals and Electronic Documents

Aizawa, Y., Takatsuki, S., Sano, M., et al. (2013). Brugada syndrome behind complete right bundle-branch block. *Circulation, 128*(10), 1048–1054.

Alli, O., Asirvatham, S., & Holmes, D. R. (2015). Strategies to incorporate left atrial appendage occlusion into clinical practice. *Journal of the American College of Cardiology, 65*(21), 2337–2344.

Aziz, S., Leon, A. R., & El-Chami, M. R. (2014). The subcutaneous defibrillator: A review of literature. *Journal of American College of Cardiology, 63*(15), 1473–1479.

Bernstein, A. D., Daubert, J. C., Fletcher, R. D., et al. (2002). The Revised NASPE/BPEG generic code for antibradycardia, adaptive-rate, and multisite pacing. *Journal of Pacing and Clinical Electrophysiology, 25*(2), 260–264.

Burke M. C., Gold, M. R., Knight, B. P., et al. (2015). Safety and efficacy of the totally subcutaneous implantable defibrillator. 2-year results from a pooled analysis of the IDE study and EFFORTLESS Registry. *Journal of American College of Cardiology, 65*(16), 1605–1615.

Cooper, K. L. (2015). Biventricular pacemakers in patients with heart failure. *Critical Care Nurse, 35*(2), 20–27.

Dalteg, T., Benzein, E., Sandgren, A., et al. (2014). Managing uncertainty in couples living with atrial fibrillation. *Journal of Cardiovascular Nursing, 29*(3), e1–e10.

Dodson, J. A., Reynolds, M. R., Bao, H., et al. (2014). Developing a risk model for in-hospital adverse events following implantable cardioverter-defibrillator implantation. A report from the NCDR, National Cardiovascular Data Registry. *Journal of American College of Cardiology, 63*(8), 788–796.

Dukes, J. W., Dewland, T. A., Vittinghoff, E., et al. (2015). Ventricular ectopy as a predictor of heart failure and death. *Journal of American College of Cardiology, 66*, 101–109.

Elrod, J. (2014). The convergent procedure: The CONVERGE IDE Clinical Trial. *EP Lab Digest, 14*(5). Retrieved July 10, 2016, from www.eplabdigest.com/articles/Convergent-Procedure-CONVERGE-IDE-Clinical-Trial

Epstein, A. E., Abraham, W. T., Bianco, N. R., et al. (2013). Wearable cardioverter-defibrillator use in patients perceived to be at high risk early post-myocardial infarction. *Journal of American College of Cardiology, 62*(21), 2000–2007.

Gasparini, M., Leclercq, C., Lunati, M., et al. (2013). Cardiac resynchronization therapy in patients with atrial fibrillation. The CERTIFY study (Cardiac Resynchronization Therapy in Atrial Fibrillation Patients Multinational Registry). *Journal of American College of Cardiology, 1*(6), 500–507.

Gerstenfeld, E. P., & Everett, T. H. (2014). Internal atrial defibrillation revisited. How long can we go? *Journal of American College of Cardiology, 62*(1), 49–51.

Gillis, A. M., Russo, A. M., Ellenbogen, K. A., et al. (2012). HRS/ACCF expert consensus statement on pacemaker device and mode selection. *Journal of American College of Cardiology, 60*(7), 682–703.

Hoke, L. M., & Steletsky, Y. (2015). Catheter ablations of atrial fibrillation. *American Journal of Nursing, 115*(10), 32–43.

January, C. T., Wann, L. S., Alpert, J. S., et al. (2014). 2014 AHA/ACC/HRS guideline for the management of patients with atrial fibrillation: A report of the ACC/AHA Task Force on practice guidelines and the Heart Rhythm Society. *Circulation, 130*(23), e199–e267.

Jensen, P. N., Gronroos, N. N., Chen, L. Y., et al. (2014). Incidence of and risk factors for sick sinus syndrome in the general population. *Journal of the American College of Cardiology, 64*(6), 531–538.

Kovacs, R. J., Flaker, G. C., Saxonhouse, S. J., et al. (2015). Practical management of anticoagulation in patients with atrial fibrillation. *Journal of American College of Cardiology, 65*(13), 1340–1360.

Kronick, S. L., Kurz, M. C., Lin, S., et al. (2015). Part 4: Systems of Care and Continuous Quality Improvement: 2015 American Heart Association Guidelines Update for Cardiopulmonary Resuscitation and Emergency Cardiovascular Care. *Circulation, 132*(18), S397–S413.

Kusumoto, F. M., Calkins, H., Boehmer, J., et al. (2014). HRS/ACC/AHA expert consensus statement on the use of implantable cardioverter-defibrillator therapy in patients who are not included or not well represented in clinical trials. *Journal of American College of Cardiology, 64*(11), 1143–1177.

LaPar, D. J., Speir, A. M., Crosby, I. K., et al. (2014). Postoperative atrial fibrillation significantly increases mortality, hospital readmission, and hospital costs. *Annals of Thoracic Surgery, 98*(2), 527–533.

Larsson, S. C., Drca, N., & Wolk, A. (2014). Alcohol consumption and risk of atrial fibrillation: A prospective study and dose-response meta-analysis. *Journal of the American College of Cardiology, 64*(3), 282–289.

Link, M. S., Berkow, L. C., Kudenchuk, P. J., et al. (2015). Part 7: Adult advanced cardiovascular life support: 2015 American Heart Association guidelines update for cardiopulmonary resuscitation and emergency cardiovascular care. *Circulation, 132*(18 Suppl 2), S444–S464.

Macle, L., Cairns, J., Leblanc, K., et al. (2016). 2016 focused update of the Canadian cardiovascular society guidelines for the management of atrial fibrillation. *Canadian Journal of Cardiology, 32*(10), 1170–1185.

Masoudi, F. A., Calkins, H., Kavinsky, C. J., et al. (2015). 2015 ACC/HRS/SCAI left atrial appendage occlusion device societal overview: A professional society overview from the American College of Cardiology, Heart Rhythm Society, and the Society for Cardiovascular Angiography and Interventions. *Heart Rhythm, 12*(10), e122–e136. Retrieved February 28, 2016, from dx.doi.org/10.1016/j.hrthm.2015.06.034

Matlock, D., Peterson, P., Wang, Y., et al. (2012). Variation in use of dual-chamber implantable cardioverter-defibrillators: Results from the national cardiovascular data registry. *Archives Of Internal Medicine, 172*(8), 634–641.

Mozaffarian, D., Benjamin, E. J., Go, A. S., et al. (2015). Heart disease and stroke statistics—2015 update: A report from the American Heart Association. *Circulation, 131*(1), e29–e322.

Page, R. L., Husain, S., White, L. Y., et al. (2013). Cardiac arrest at exercise facilities. Implications for placement of automated external defibrillators. *Journal of American College of Cardiology, 62*(22), 2102–2109.

Patel, N. J., Deshmukh, A., Pant, S., et al. (2014). Contemporary trends of hospitalization for atrial fibrillation in the United States, 2000 through 2010: Implications for healthcare planning. *Circulation, 129*(23), 2371–2379.

Pickham, D. (2013). Understanding and documenting QT intervals. *Critical Care Nurse, 33*(4), 73–75.

Russo, A. (2012). The reality of implantable cardioverter-defibrillator longevity: What can be done to improve cost-effectiveness? *Heart Rhythm, 9*(4), 520–521.

Russo, A. M., Stainback, R. F., Bailey, S. R., et al. (2013). ACCF/HRS/AHA/ASE/HFSA/SCAI/SCCT/SCMR 2013 appropriate use criteria for implantable cardioverter-defibrillators and cardiac resynchronization therapy. A report of the American College of Cardiology Foundation Appropriate Use Criteria Task Force, Heart Failure Society, American Heart Association, American Society of Echocardiography, Heart Failure Society of America, Society for Cardiovascular Angiography and Interventions, Society of Cardiovascular Computed Tomography and

Society for Cardiovascular Magnetic Resonance. *Journal of American College of Cardiology*, *61*(12), 1318–1368.

Sandau, K. E., Sendelbach, S., Fletcher, L., et al. (2015). Computer-assisted interventions to improve QTc documentation in patients receiving QT-prolonged drugs. *American Journal of Critical Care*, *24*(2), 6–14.

Sendelbach, S., & Jepsen, S. (2013). *American Association of Critical Care Nurses practice alert: Alarm management*. Retrieved September 22, 2015, from www.aacn.org/wd/practice/docs/practicealerts/alarm-management-practice-alert.pdf

Sheldon, R. S., Grubb, B. P., Olshansky, B., et al. (2015). 2015 Heart Rhythm Society Expert Consensus Statement on the diagnosis and treatment of postural tachycardia syndrome, inappropriate sinus tachycardia, and vasovagal syncope. *Heart Rhythm*, *12*(6), e41–e63.

Shi, X. (2016). Preventing postoperative atrial fibrillation. *Nursing Critical Care*, *11*(1), 5.

Shukla, A., Aizer, A., Holmes, D., et al. (2015). Effect of obstructive sleep apnea treatment on atrial fibrillation recurrence. *JACC: Clinical Electrophysiology*, *1*(1–2), 41–51.

Smith, G. D., Fry, M. M., Taylor, D., et al. (2015). Effectiveness of the Valsalva manoeuvre for reversion of supraventricular tachycardia. *Cochrane Database of Systematic Reviews*, 2, CD009502.

Stavrakis, S., Nakagawa, H., Po, S. S., et al. (2015). The role of the autonomic ganglia in atrial fibrillation. *JACC: Clinical Electrophysiology*, *1*(1–2), 1–13.

Tokioka, K., Kusano, K. F., Morita, H., et al. (2014). Electrocardiographic parameters and fatal arrhythmic evens in patients with Brugada syndrome. *Journal of American College of Cardiology*, *63*(20), 2131–2138.

Tracy, C. M., Epstein, A. E., Darbar, D., et al. (2012). ACCF/AHA/HRS focused update of the 2008 guidelines for device-based therapy of cardiac rhythm abnormalities: A report of the American College of Cardiology Foundation/American Heart Association Task Force on Practice Guidelines. *Journal of the American College of Cardiology*, *60*(14), 1297–1313.

Varma, N., Piccini, J. P., Snell, J., et al. (2015). Relationship between level of adherence to automatic wireless remote monitoring and survival in pacemaker and defibrillator patients. *Journal of American College of Cardiology*, *65*(24), 2601–2610.

Wilkoff, B. L., Fauchier, L., Stiles, M. K., et al. (2015). 2015 HRS/EHRA/APHRS/SOLAECE expert consensus statement on optimal implantable cardioverter-defibrillator programming and testing. *Journal of Arrhythmia*, *32*(1), 1–28.

Zielińska, D., Bellwon, J., Rynkiewicz, A., et al. (2013). Prognostic value of the six-minute walk test in heart failure patients undergoing cardiac surgery: A literature review. *Rehabilitation Research and Practice*, *2013*, 965494. doi:10.1155/2013/965494.

Resources

American Heart Association, National Center: http://www.american-heart.org

Canadian Association of Critical Care Nurses: http://caccn.ca/

Heart and Stroke Foundation: http://www.heartandstroke.com

29

Management of Patients With Coronary Vascular Disorders

Adapted by Karen Lynn Then and James A. Rankin

Learning Objectives

On completion of this chapter, the learner will be able to:

1. Describe the pathophysiology, clinical manifestations, and treatment of coronary atherosclerosis.
2. Describe the pathophysiology, clinical manifestations, and treatment of angina pectoris.
3. Use the nursing process as a framework for care of patients with angina pectoris.
4. Describe the pathophysiology, clinical manifestations, and treatment of myocardial infarction.
5. Use the nursing process as a framework for care of a patient with acute coronary syndrome.
6. Describe the percutaneous coronary interventional and coronary artery revascularization procedures.
7. Describe the nursing care of a patient who has had a percutaneous coronary interventional procedure for treatment of coronary artery disease.
8. Describe the nursing care of a patient who has undergone cardiac surgery.

Historically, identification and treatment of heart disease primarily focused on white, middle-aged men. Research now is more broadly focused and also includes the identification and treatment of cardiovascular disease in women, children, and people of diverse racial and ethnic backgrounds. Cardiovascular disease is the second most common cause of death in Canada and the leading cause of hospitalization (Statistics Canada, 2017). In 2014, 6% of Canadians 20 years and older were living with a cardiovascular disease (Statistics Canada, 2014). In 2016, 51,396 people died in Canada from a heart condition (19.2% of all deaths). Of the estimated 70,000 heart attacks that occur each year in Canada, about 16,000 Canadians die, most of whom die out of hospital (Statistics Canada, 2012).

Coronary Artery Disease

Coronary artery disease (CAD) is the most prevalent type of cardiovascular disease in adults, and contributes to hospitalizations, stress, chronic symptoms and disease, caregiver burden, and deaths. For these and other reasons, it is important for nurses to become familiar with various manifestations of coronary artery conditions and methods for assessing, preventing, and treating these disorders medically and surgically.

Coronary Atherosclerosis

The most common cause of cardiovascular disease in Canada is **atherosclerosis**, an abnormal accumulation of lipid, or fatty, substances and fibrous tissue in the lining of arterial blood vessel walls. These substances create blockages and narrow the coronary vessels in a way that reduces blood flow to the myocardium. It is now known that atherosclerosis involves a repetitious inflammatory response to injury to the artery wall and subsequent alteration in the structural and biochemical properties of the arterial walls. Ongoing research regarding the development of atherosclerosis has increased understanding of prevention and treatment of this progressive and potentially life-threatening process.

Pathophysiology

Atherosclerosis begins with inflammation and injury to the lining of the arterial wall. Fatty streaks of lipids are deposited in the **intima** of the arterial wall. These lesions commonly begin early in life, in childhood or adolescence. Genetics and environmental factors are involved in the progression of these lesions. The continued development of atherosclerosis involves an inflammatory response, which begins with injury to the vascular endothelium. The injury may be initiated by a variety of stimuli including: smoking, hypertension, diabetes, **metabolic syndrome**, and other inflammatory processes.

The presence of inflammation has multiple effects on the arterial wall, including the attraction of inflammatory cells (including macrophages) (Gimbrone & Garcia-Candena, 2016; Zipes, Libby, Bonow, et al., 2019). The macrophages infiltrate the injured vascular endothelium and ingest lipids, which turns them into what are called *foam cells*. Activated macrophages also release biochemical substances that can further damage the endothelium, attracting platelets, and initiating clotting.

Smooth muscle cells within the vessel wall subsequently proliferate and form a fibrous cap over a core filled with lipid and inflammatory infiltrate. These deposits, called **atheromas** or plaques, protrude into the lumen of the vessel, narrowing it and obstructing blood flow (Fig. 29-1). Plaque may be stable or unstable, depending on the degree of inflammation and consequent thickness of the fibrous cap. If the fibrous cap of the plaque is thick and the lipid pool remains relatively stable, it can resist the stress from blood flow and vessel movement. If the cap is thin and inflammation is ongoing, the lipid core may grow, causing it to rupture and hemorrhage into the plaque. A ruptured plaque is a focus for thrombus formation. The thrombus

Glossary

acute coronary syndrome (ACS): signs and symptoms that indicate unstable angina or acute myocardial infarction

afterload: amount of pressure against which the heart has to work to eject blood during systole

angina pectoris: chest pain brought about by myocardial ischemia—lack of oxygenation to the heart muscle

angiotensin-converting enzyme (ACE) inhibitors: medications that inhibit the angiotensin-converting enzyme

atheroma: fibrous cap composed of smooth muscle cells that forms over lipid deposits within arterial vessels and that protrudes into the lumen of the vessel, narrowing the lumen and obstructing blood flow; also called *plaque*

atherosclerosis: abnormal accumulation of lipid deposits and fibrous tissue within arterial walls and lumen

contractility: ability of the cardiac muscle to shorten in response to an electrical impulse

coronary artery bypass graft (CABG): a surgical procedure in which a blood vessel from another part of the body is grafted onto the occluded coronary artery below the occlusion in such a way that blood flow bypasses the blockage

creatine kinase (CK): an enzyme found in human tissues; one of the three types of CK is specific to heart muscle and may be used as an indicator of heart muscle injury

fibrinolytic: a medication that breaks down/lyses blood clots

high-density lipoprotein (HDL): a protein-bound lipid that transports cholesterol to the liver for excretion in the bile; composed of a higher proportion of protein to lipid than low-density lipoprotein; exerts a beneficial effect on the arterial wall

intima: inner lining of the arterial wall

ischemia: insufficient tissue oxygenation

low-density lipoprotein (LDL): a protein-bound lipid that transports cholesterol to tissues in the body; composed of a lower proportion of protein to lipid than high-density lipoprotein; exerts a harmful effect on the arterial wall

metabolic syndrome: a cluster of metabolic abnormalities that increase the risk of cardiovascular disease, including insulin resistance, abdominal obesity, dyslipidemia, and hypertension

myocardial infarction (MI): death of heart tissue caused by lack of oxygenated blood flow; if acute, abbreviated as AMI

NSTEMI—non-ST elevation myocardial infarction: myocardial infarction that does not cause ST-segment elevation on a 12-lead ECG

percutaneous coronary intervention (PCI): an invasive procedure in which a catheter is placed in a coronary artery, and one of several methods is employed to remove or reduce a blockage within the artery

percutaneous transluminal coronary angioplasty (PTCA): a type of percutaneous coronary intervention in which a balloon is inflated within a coronary artery to break an atheroma and open the vessel lumen, improving coronary artery blood flow

preload: amount of ventricular stretch at the end of diastole (left ventricular end-diastolic pressure [LVEDP])

primary prevention: interventions taken to prevent the development of coronary artery disease

secondary prevention: interventions taken to prevent the advancement of existing coronary artery disease

STEMI—ST-elevation myocardial infarction: myocardial infarction that causes ST-segment elevation on a 12-lead ECG

stent: a woven mesh that provides structural support to a coronary vessel, preventing its closure

sudden cardiac death: immediate cessation of effective heart activity resulting in loss of life

Troponin I, T and high sensitivity Troponin: myocardial proteins; biomarkers that are used to measure heart muscle damage

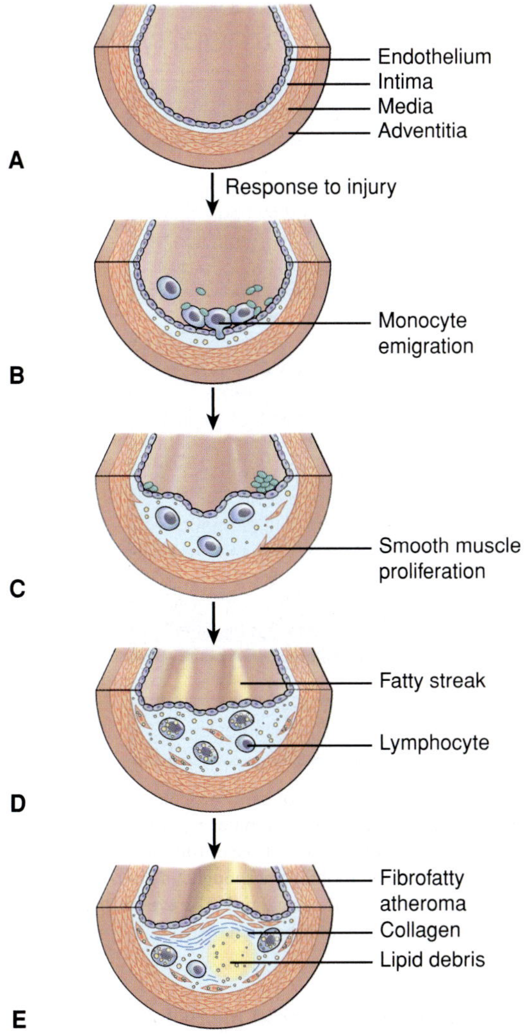

FIGURE 29-1. Atherosclerosis begins as monocytes and lipids enter the intima of an injured vessel (A, B). Smooth muscle cells proliferate within the vessel wall (C), contributing to the development of fatty accumulations and atheroma (D). As the plaque enlarges, the vessel narrows and blood flow decreases (E). The plaque may rupture and a thrombus might form, obstructing blood flow.

may then obstruct blood flow, leading to **sudden cardiac death** from dysrhythmias, or an acute **myocardial infarction (MI)**. When an MI occurs, a portion of the heart muscle no longer receives blood flow and becomes necrotic (dead).

The anatomic structure of the coronary arteries makes them particularly susceptible to the mechanisms of atherosclerosis. As Figure 29-2 shows, the three major coronary arteries have multiple branches. Atherosclerotic lesions most often form where the vessels branch, suggesting a hemodynamic component that favours their formation (Hannon & Porth, 2016). Although heart disease is most often caused by atherosclerosis of the coronary arteries, other phenomena may also decrease blood flow to the heart. Examples include vasospasm (sudden constriction or narrowing) of a coronary artery, myocardial trauma from internal or external forces, structural disease, congenital anomalies, decreased oxygen supply (e.g., from acute blood loss, anemia, or low blood pressure), and increased oxygen demand. An increased oxygen demand causing rapid heart rates can be seen in: thyrotoxicosis, or use of illicit drugs such as cocaine, amphetamines, methamphetamines (meth, crystal, ice) and 3,4-methylenedioxymethamphetamine (MDMA, ecstasy).

Clinical Manifestations

Coronary atherosclerosis produces symptoms and complications according to the location and degree of narrowing of the arterial lumen, thrombus formation, and obstruction of blood flow to the myocardium. This impediment to blood flow is usually progressive, causing an inadequate blood supply that deprives the cardiac muscle cells of oxygen needed for their survival. The condition is known as **ischemia**. **Angina pectoris** refers to chest pain that is brought about by myocardial ischemia. Angina pectoris usually is caused by significant coronary atherosclerosis. If the decrease in blood supply is great enough, of long enough duration, or both, irreversible damage and death of myocardial cells, or MI, may result. Over time, irreversibly damaged myocardium undergoes degeneration and is replaced by scar tissue,

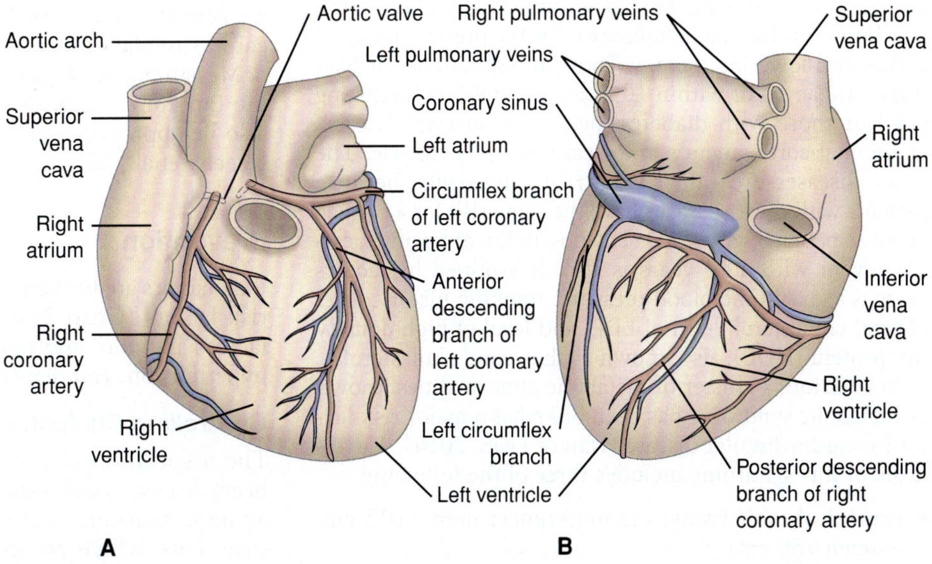

FIGURE 29-2. The coronary arteries supply the heart muscle with oxygenated blood, adjusting the flow according to metabolic needs. Anterior view (A), and posterior view (B) of the heart.

causing various degrees of myocardial dysfunction. Significant myocardial damage may result in persistently low cardiac output and heart failure, in which the heart cannot adequately maintain blood flow to meet the body's needs. A decrease in blood supply from CAD may even cause the heart to abruptly stop beating (sudden cardiac death). Sudden cardiac death affects men more than women and is responsible for approximately half of all heart disease deaths (Katritsis, Gersh, & Camm, 2016).

The most common manifestation of myocardial ischemia is acute onset of chest discomfort (burning, heaviness, squeezing). However, the classic epidemiologic study of people in Framingham, Massachusetts, showed that nearly 15% of men and women who had MIs were asymptomatic (Kannel, 1986). Older adults may present atypically and often wait the longest to be seen in the emergency department (Mnatzaganian, Braitberg, Hiller, et al., 2016).

Patients with myocardial ischemia may present to an emergency department or clinic with a variety of symptoms other than chest discomfort. Patients who are older or have a history of diabetes or heart failure may report symptoms such as shortness of breath. Many women have been found to have symptoms instead of or in addition to chest pain, including dyspnea, abdominal discomfort and indigestion, nausea, and weakness (Mehta, Beckie, Devon, et al., 2016). Prodromal symptoms may occur (i.e., angina a few hours to days before the acute episode), or a major cardiac event may be the first indication of coronary atherosclerosis.

Risk Factors

Epidemiologic studies point to several factors that increase the probability that heart disease will develop in a person. Major risk factors include elevated blood lipid levels, smoking, hypertension, diabetes, obesity, family history of premature cardiovascular disease (first-degree relative with cardiovascular disease at age 55 years or younger for men and at age 65 years or younger for women), and age (more than 45 years for men; more than 55 years for women). Some people do not have classic risk factors. The Canadian Cardiovascular Society (CCS) lists the clinical guidelines for cholesterol testing, **primary and secondary prevention** and management (Anderson, Grégoire, Pearson, et al., 2016). Elevated **low-density lipoprotein (LDL)** cholesterol, also known as the "bad cholesterol," is the primary target of cholesterol-lowering therapy. Those at highest risk for having a cardiac event within 10 years are those with existing CAD or those with diabetes, peripheral arterial disease, abdominal aortic aneurysm, or carotid artery disease. The latter diseases are called *CAD risk equivalents*, because patients with these diseases have the same risk for a cardiac event as patients with CAD. The possibility of having a cardiac event within 10 years is also determined by factors such as age; systolic blood pressure; smoking history; level of total cholesterol; level of LDL; and level of **high-density lipoprotein (HDL)**, also known as the "good cholesterol."

In addition, a cluster of metabolic abnormalities known as metabolic syndrome has been linked as a major risk factor for cardiovascular disease (Han & Lean, 2016). A diagnosis of this syndrome includes three of the following:

- central obesity (waist circumference: men >102 cm; women >88 cm)
- elevated triglycerides (≥150 mg/dL)
- diminished high-density lipoprotein (HDL) cholesterol (men <40 mg/dL; women <50 mg/dL);
- systemic hypertension (≥130/85 mm Hg);
- elevated fasting glucose (≥110 mg/dL).

Many people with type 2 diabetes fit this clinical picture. It is theorized that in patients with obesity, excessive adipose tissue may secrete mediators that lead to metabolic changes (Jung & Choi, 2014). Immune mechanisms are activated and contribute to atherogenic changes in the cardiovascular system (Fig. 29-3).

Measurement of lipoprotein(a) [Lp(a)] and homocysteine (an amino acid associated with cardiac disease) may also be appropriate in some people (Anderson, Gregoire, Hegele, et al., 2013).

Physiology/Pathophysiology

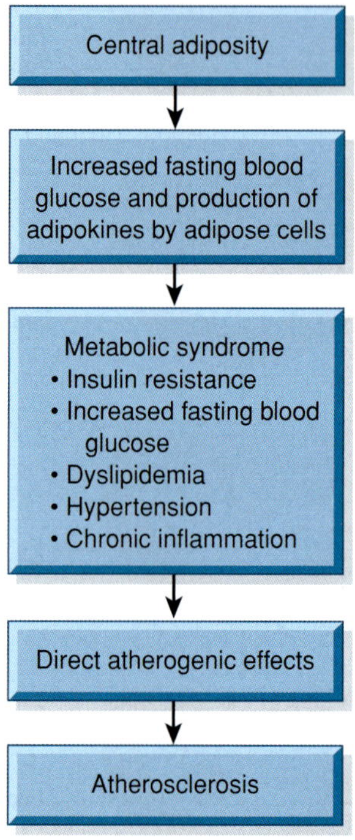

FIGURE 29-3. Pathophysiology of cardiovascular disease in metabolic syndrome. Central adiposity plays a major role in the development of metabolic syndrome. Adipokines released from fat cells along with other hormones and metabolites are thought to contribute to the development of metabolic abnormalities. The eventual effect of these processes is the promotion of atherosclerosis.

Prevention

Risk factors are broken into modifiable and nonmodifiable risk factors (Chart 29-1). The four main modifiable risk factors include: cholesterol abnormalities, tobacco use, hypertension, and diabetes.

Controlling Cholesterol Abnormalities

The association of a high blood cholesterol level with heart disease is well established. The metabolism of fats is an important contributor to the development of heart disease. Fats, which are insoluble in water, are encased in

CHART 29-1

Risk Factors: Coronary Artery Disease

A nonmodifiable risk factor is a circumstance over which a person has no control. A modifiable risk factor is one over which a person may exercise control, such as by changing a lifestyle or personal habit or by using medication. A risk factor may operate independently or in tandem with other risk factors. The more risk factors a person has, the greater the likelihood of coronary artery disease (CAD). Those at risk are advised to seek regular medical examinations and to engage in heart-healthy behaviour (a deliberate effort to reduce the number and extent of risks).

Nonmodifiable Risk Factors

Family history of CAD (first-degree relative with cardiovascular disease at 55 years of age or younger for men and at 65 years of age or younger for women)
Increasing age (more than 45 years for men; more than 55 years for women)
Gender (men develop CAD at an earlier age than women)
Race (higher incidence of heart disease in African Americans than in Caucasians)

Modifiable Risk Factors

Hyperlipidemia
Cigarette smoking, tobacco use
Hypertension
Diabetes
Metabolic syndrome
Obesity
Physical inactivity

Adapted from Mozaffarian, D., Benjamin, E. J., Go, A. S., et al. (2016). Heart disease and stroke statistics—2016 update: A report from the American Heart Association. *Circulation, 133*(4), e38–e360.

water-soluble lipoproteins that allow them to be transported within the circulatory system. The various lipoproteins are categorized by their protein content, which is measured in density. The density increases when more protein is present. Four elements of fat metabolism—total cholesterol, LDL, HDL, and triglycerides—affect the development of heart disease. Cholesterol is processed by the gastrointestinal tract into lipoprotein globules called *chylomicrons*. These are reprocessed by the liver as lipoproteins (Fig. 29-4). This is a physiologic process necessary for the formation of lipoprotein-based cell membranes and other important metabolic processes. When an excess of LDL is produced, LDL particles adhere to vulnerable points in the arterial endothelium. Here, macrophages ingest them, leading to the formation of foam cells and the beginning of plaque formation.

Canadian recommendations for regular screening of plasma lipids are dependent on numerous factors, including age and gender (over 40 years for both males and females), CVD risk factors, inflammatory or immune disease, and ethnicity (South Asian and First Nation ancestry are at higher risk) (Anderson et al., 2016). Patients who have had an acute event (e.g., MI), a **percutaneous coronary intervention (PCI)**, or a **coronary artery bypass graft (CABG)** require re-assessment of the LDL cholesterol level within a few months of the event or procedure, because LDL levels may be low immediately after the acute event or procedure.

LDL exerts a harmful effect on the coronary vasculature because the small LDL particles can be easily transported into the vessel lining. In contrast, HDL promotes the use of total cholesterol by transporting LDL to the liver, where it is biodegraded and then excreted. The goal is to have low LDL values and high HDL values. The desired level of LDL depends on the patient, and is part of managing other risk factors and promoting health behaviours (Anderson et al., 2016).

Canadian guidelines are routinely re-evaluated and the most current information and guidelines can always be found on the CCS Guidelines Library (see Resources section).

A high HDL level is a strong negative risk factor for heart disease (i.e., it protects against disease), whereas a low level is a risk factor. The level of HDL should exceed 1.0 mmol/L in males and 1.3 mmol/L in females. Smoking, excess weight, or being sedentary can decrease HDL levels, as can an increase in triglyceride levels (Anderson et al., 2013).

Triglyceride is another fatty substance, made up of fatty acids, that is transported through the blood by a lipoprotein. Although an elevated fasting triglyceride may be genetic in origin, it also can be caused by obesity; physical inactivity; excessive alcohol intake; high-carbohydrate diets; diabetes; kidney disease; and certain medications, such as oral contraceptives, corticosteroids, and beta-adrenergic blockers, when given in higher doses. Management of an elevated triglyceride level focuses on weight reduction, limiting fats, sugar and alcohol, smoking cessation, and increased physical activity. Medications such as nicotinic acid and fibric acids (e.g., fenofibrate [Tricor], clofibrate [Atromid-S]) may also be prescribed. The fasting triglyceride level should be ≤1.7 mmol/L.

Dietary Measures

Nutritional guidelines that focus on dietary patterns include the Mediterranean, DASH, or Portfolio diets (Anderson et al., 2016). The Mediterranean diet, which promotes vegetables and fish and restricts red meat, is reported to reduce mortality from cardiovascular disease (Anderson et al., 2016). People who adopt strict vegetarian diets can significantly reduce blood lipids, blood glucose, body mass index, and blood pressure. However, very intensive dietary programs such as these may not be acceptable to all patients who need to modify risk factors. The goal should be to maintain or achieve a healthy body weight, improve lipid profile and thereby reduce the risk of CV events. These general recommendations may need to be adjusted for the patient who has other nutritional needs, such as the patient who is pregnant or has diabetes. To assist in following the appropriate TLC diet (Table 29-1), the patient should be referred to a registered dietitian. Other TLC recommendations include weight loss, cessation of tobacco use, and increased physical activity.

Soluble dietary fibre may also help to reduce cholesterol levels. Soluble fibres, which are found in fresh fruit, cereal grains, vegetables, and legumes, enhance the excretion of metabolized cholesterol. The ability of fibre to reduce serum

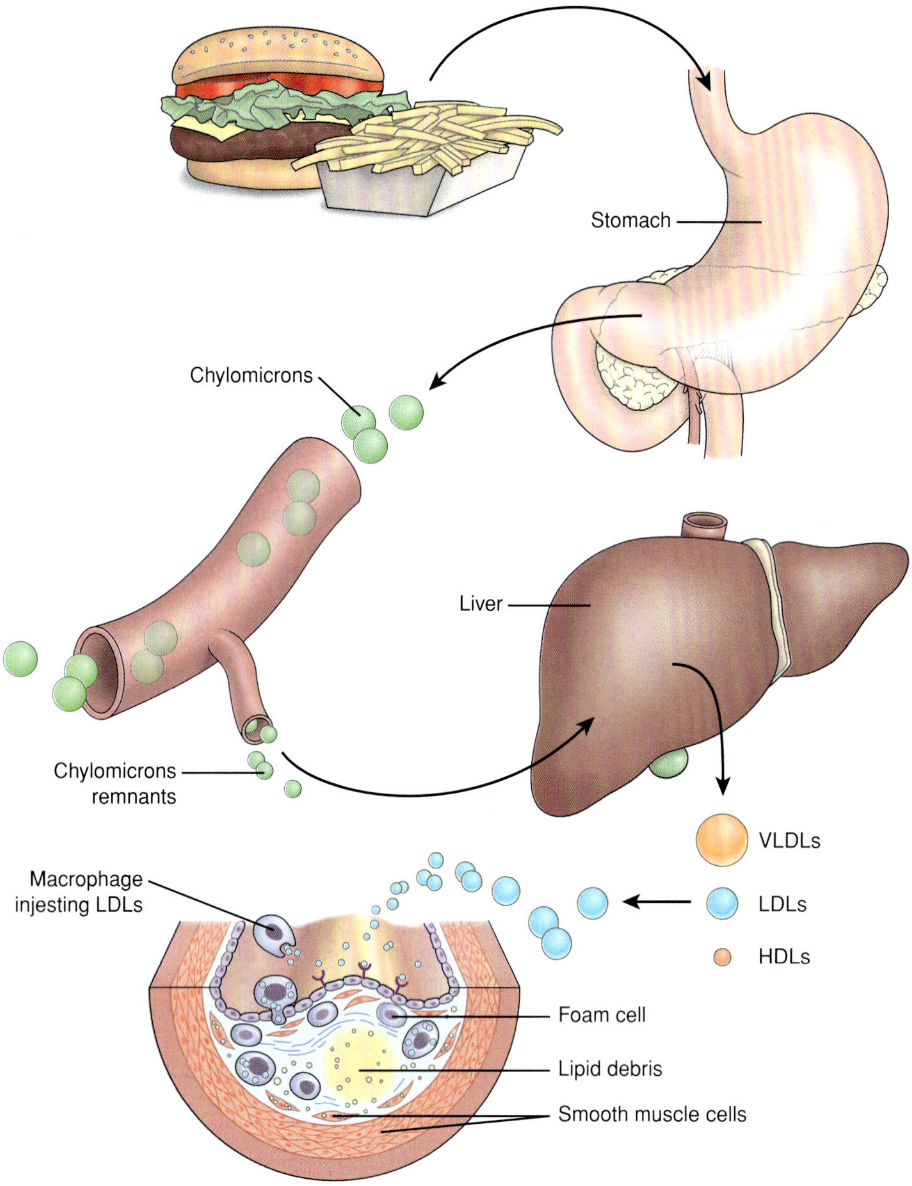

FIGURE 29-4. Lipoproteins and the development of atherosclerosis. As dietary cholesterol and saturated fat are processed by the gastrointestinal tract, chylomicrons enter the blood. They are broken down into chylomicron remnants in the capillaries. The liver processes them into lipoproteins. When these are released into the circulation, excess low-density lipoproteins (LDLs) adhere to receptors on the intimal wall. Macrophages also ingest LDLs and transport them into the vessel wall, beginning the process of plaque formation. VLDLs, very-low-density lipoproteins; HDLs, high-density lipoproteins.

cholesterol continues to be investigated. Intake of ≥30 g of fibre each day is recommended (Anderson et al., 2016).

Many resources are available to assist people to control their cholesterol levels, including the Heart and Stroke Foundation of Canada and the Canadian Diabetes Association as well as CAD support groups and reliable Internet sources. Cookbooks and recipes that include the nutritional contents of foods can be included as resources for patients. Dietary control has been made easier because food manufacturers are required to provide comprehensive nutritional data on product labels. The label information of interest to a person attempting to eat a heart-healthy diet is as follows:

- Serving size, expressed in household measures
- Amount of total fat per serving
- Amount of saturated fat and trans fat per serving
- Amount of cholesterol per serving
- Amount of fibre per serving

The effects of low-carbohydrate diets on blood lipid levels are under study; it is recommended that people decrease fats, sugars, and alcohol. The Mediterranean type diet has demonstrated effectiveness in decreasing lipid levels and mortality.

Physical Activity

Regular, moderate physical activity increases HDL levels and reduces triglyceride levels. The goal for the average person is a total of 150 minutes of moderate to vigorous aerobic activity per week in bouts of 10 minutes or more (Anderson et al., 2016). The nurse helps the patient set realistic goals for physical activity. For example, the inactive patient can start with activity that lasts 3 minutes, such as parking farther from a building to increase daily walking time. For sustained activity, patients should begin with a 5-minute warm-up period to stretch and prepare the body for exercise. They should end the exercise with a 5-minute cool-down period in which they gradually reduce the intensity of the activity to prevent a sudden decrease in cardiac output. Patients should be instructed to engage in an activity or variety of activities that interest

TABLE 29-1 Nutrient Content of the Therapeutic Lifestyle Changes Diet

Nutrient	Recommended Intake
Total calories[a]	Balance intake and expenditure to maintain desirable weight
Total fat	25–35% of total calories
Saturated fat[b]	<7% of total calories
Polyunsaturated fat	Up to 10% of total calories
Monounsaturated fat	Up to 20% of total calories
Carbohydrate[c]	50–60% of total calories
Dietary fibre	20–30 g/day
Protein	Approximately 15% of total calories
Cholesterol	<200 mg/day

[a]Daily energy expenditure should include at least moderate physical activity (contributing approximately 200 kcal/day).

[b]Trans-fatty acids are formed from the processing (manufacturing, hydrogenation) of vegetable oils into a more solid form. The effects of trans-fatty acids are similar to saturated fats (i.e., raising low-density lipoprotein and lowering high-density lipoprotein). Intake of trans-fatty acids should be minimized.

[c]Carbohydrates should be derived predominately from foods rich in complex carbohydrates, including grains, especially whole grains, fruits, and vegetables.

Adapted from the TLC Diet Regimen. Retrieved November 18, 2015, from tlcdiet.org/tlc-diet-regime/

them in order to maintain motivation. They should also be taught to exercise to an intensity that does not preclude their ability to talk; if they cannot have a conversation while exercising, they should slow down or switch to a less intensive activity. When the weather is hot and humid, the patient should exercise during the early morning, or indoors, and wear loose-fitting clothing. When the weather is cold, the patient should layer clothing and wear a hat. The nurse can also suggest walking in large stores or shopping malls in bad weather. The patient should stop any activity if chest pain, unusual shortness of breath, dizziness, lightheadedness, or nausea occurs.

Medications

If diet alone cannot normalize serum cholesterol levels, medications can have a synergistic effect with the prescribed diet and control cholesterol levels (see Table 29-2). Lipid-lowering medications can reduce CAD mortality in patients with elevated lipid levels and in at-risk patients with normal lipid levels (ICSI, 2013). The various types of lipid-lowering agents affect the lipid components somewhat differently; these types include 3-hydroxy-3-methylglutaryl coenzyme A (HMG-CoA) (or statins), fibric acids (or fibrates), bile acid sequestrants (or resins), cholesterol

TABLE 29-2 Medications Affecting Lipoprotein Metabolism

Medications	Therapeutic Effects	Considerations
HMG-CoA Reductase Inhibitors (Statins)		
Atorvastatin (Lipitor) Simvastatin (Zocor)	↓ Total cholesterol ↓ LDL ↑ HDL ↓ TGs Inhibit enzyme involved in lipid synthesis (HMG-CoA) Favourable effects on vascular endothelium, including anti-inflammatory and antithrombotic effects	Frequently given as initial therapy for significantly elevated cholesterol and LDL levels Myalgia and arthralgia are common adverse effects Myopathy and possible rhabdomyolysis are potential serious effects Monitor liver function tests Contraindicated in liver disease Check for drug interactions Indication for use now includes ACS and stroke Administer in evening
Fibric Acids (Fibrates)		
Fenofibrate (TriCor) Gemfibrozil (Lopid)	↑ HDL ↓ TGs ↓ Synthesis of TGs and other lipids	Adverse effects include diarrhea, flatulence, rash, myalgia Serious adverse effects include pancreatitis, hepatotoxicity, and rhabdomyolysis Contraindicated in severe renal and liver disease Use with caution in patients who are also taking statins
Bile Acid Sequestrants		
Cholestyramine (Questran) Colestipol (Colestid)	↓ LDL Slight ↑ HDL Oxidize cholesterol into bile acids, which ↓ fat absorption	Most often used as adjunct therapy when statins alone have not been effective in controlling lipid levels Side effects include constipation, abdominal pain, GI bleeding May decrease absorption of other drugs Taken before meals
Cholesterol Absorption Inhibitor		
Ezetimibe (Zetia)	↓ LDL Inhibits absorption of cholesterol in small intestine	Better tolerated than bile acid sequestrants Used in combination with other agents, such as statins Side effects include abdominal pain, arthralgia, myalgia Contraindicated in liver disease
Omega-3-Acid Ethyl Esters		
Fish oil capsules	↓ TGs Inhibit TG production in liver	May be used alone or in combination with other agents Side effects include GI distress, taste perversion, rash, and back pain

HMG-CoA, 3-hydroxy-3-methylglutaryl coenzyme A; ↓ decrease; ↑ increase; LDL, low-density lipoprotein; HDL, high-density lipoprotein; TGs, triglycerides; ACS, acute coronary syndrome; GI, gastrointestinal.

Adapted from Institute for Clinical Systems Improvement (ICSI). (2013). Lipid management in adults. Retrieved on November 18, 2015, from www.guideline.gov/content.aspx?id=47783&search=lipid+management+in+adult

absorption inhibitors, and omega-3-acid ethyl esters. A new class of lipid-lowering medications known as proprotein convertase subtilisin-kexin type 9 (PCSK9) agents has recently been approved by the U.S. Food and Drug Administration (FDA). Because of limited clinical trial evidence and their high cost, these PCSK9 agents are prescribed on a limited basis, but may be considered for more patients in the future (White, 2015).

- HMG-CoA reductase inhibitors or statins (e.g., simvastatin [Zocor], atorvastatin [Lipitor]); block cholesterol synthesis, lower LDL and triglyceride levels, and increase HDL levels. These medications are frequently the initial medication therapy for elevated cholesterol and LDL levels. Because of their effect on the liver, results of hepatic function tests are monitored.
- Nicotinic acids (niacin—Niacor, Niaspan) decrease lipoprotein synthesis, lower LDL and triglyceride levels, and increase HDL levels. The dose of niacin needs to be titrated weekly to achieve therapeutic dosage. Niacin may be used for minimally elevated cholesterol and LDL levels or as an adjunct to a statin when the lipid goal has not been achieved and triglycerides are elevated. Side effects include gastrointestinal upset, gout, and flushing. Because of the effect of niacin on the liver, hepatic function is monitored.
- Fibric acid or fibrates (e.g., fenofibrate [Tricor], clofibrate [Atromid-S]) decrease the synthesis of cholesterol, reduce triglyceride levels, and increase HDL levels. They have the potential to increase LDLs and may be used in patients with triglyceride levels above 7.6 mmol/L. Because of the risk of myopathy and acute renal failure, fibrates should be used with caution in patients who are also taking a statin.
- Bile acid sequestrants or resins (e.g., cholestyramine [LoCholest, Questran, Prevalite]) bind cholesterol in the intestine, increase its breakdown, and lower LDL levels with minimal effect on HDLs and no effect (or minimal increase) on triglyceride levels. These medications are more often used as adjunct therapy when statins alone have not been effective in controlling lipid levels and triglyceride levels are less than 3.8 mmol/L. Significant side effects, such as gastric distention and constipation, can occur with use of these medications.
- Ezetimibe is used to lower plasma cholesterol levels by decreasing cholesterol absorption in the small intestine. It is usually used in combination with an HMG-CoA reductase inhibitor (statin).
- Monoclonal antibody (Evolocumab/Repatha) is designed to be used when adequate lipid lowering is not achieved with other medications such as statins and ezetimibe. It can also be used in patients who are statin intolerant or those with familial hypercholesterolemia. Evolocumab binds PCSK9 and inhibits it from binding to LDL receptors in the liver, thereby allowing the liver to remove more LDL and triglycerides from the blood. It also can raise the levels of HDL cholesterol.

Medication therapy is reserved for at-risk patients and is not regarded as a substitute for dietary modification. Dietary modification should always be done simultaneously with the use of all lipid lowering medications.

Patients with elevated cholesterol levels should be monitored for adherence to the therapeutic plan, the effect of cholesterol-lowering medications, and the development of side effects. Lipid levels are obtained and adjustments made to the diet and medication every 6 weeks until the lipid goal or maximum dose is achieved.

Promoting Cessation of Tobacco Use

Cigarette smoking contributes to the development and severity of CAD in the following three ways:

- First, the inhalation of smoke increases the blood carbon monoxide level, and hemoglobin, the oxygen-carrying component of blood, combines more readily with carbon monoxide than with oxygen. A decreased amount of available oxygen may decrease the heart's ability to pump.
- Second, the nicotinic acid in tobacco triggers the release of catecholamines, which raise the heart rate and blood pressure. Nicotinic acid can also cause the coronary arteries to constrict. Smokers have a 10-fold increase in risk for sudden cardiac death. The increase in catecholamines may be a factor in sudden cardiac death.
- Third, use of tobacco causes a detrimental vascular response and increases platelet adhesion, leading to a higher probability of thrombus formation.

A person with increased risk for heart disease is encouraged to stop tobacco use through any means possible: educational programs, counselling, consistent motivation and reinforcement messages, support groups, and medications. Some people have found complementary therapies (e.g., acupuncture, guided imagery, hypnosis) to be helpful. People who stop smoking reduce their risk of heart disease by 30% to 50% within the first year, and the risk continues to decline as long as they refrain from smoking.

Exposure to other smokers' smoke (passive or secondhand smoke) is believed to cause heart disease in nonsmokers. Oral contraceptive use by women who smoke is inadvisable because these medications significantly increase the risk for CAD and sudden cardiac death. Other tobacco products such as electronic cigarettes (e-cigarettes or vapor cigarettes) and waterpipes (hookahs) are also thought to lead to health problems, but comprehensive research does not exist on the effects of these alternative smoking methods. There is concern that because these products expose people to tobacco and its toxins, they also may carry risk of lung disease, cancer, and cardiovascular disease.

Use of medications such as the nicotine patch (Nicotrol, NicoDerm CQ, Habitrol), Varenicline or the antidepressant bupropion (Zyban) may assist with stopping use of tobacco. Products containing nicotine have some of the same effects as smoking: catecholamine release (increasing heart rate and blood pressure) and increased platelet adhesion. Varenicline (Champix) works by reducing cravings and withdrawal symptoms and making tobacco smoking less satisfying. These medications should be used for a short time and at the lowest effective doses.

Managing Hypertension

Hypertension is defined as blood pressure measurements that repeatedly exceed 140/90 mm Hg. The risk of cardiovascular disease increases as blood pressure increases, and people with high risk of cardiovascular disease should be treated to a target pressure systolic <120 mm Hg (Nerenberg, Zarnke, Leung, et al., 2018). Blood pressure targets for patients with diabetes are <130/80 mm Hg. Long-standing elevated blood pressure may result in increased stiffness of the vessel walls, leading to vessel injury and a resulting inflammatory response within the intima. Inflammatory mediators then lead to the release of growth-promoting factors that cause vessel hypertrophy and hyperresponsiveness. These changes result in acceleration and aggravation of atherosclerosis. Hypertension also increases the work of the left ventricle, which must pump harder to eject blood into the arteries. Over time, the increased workload causes the heart to enlarge and thicken (i.e., hypertrophy) and may eventually lead to cardiac failure.

Early detection of high blood pressure and adherence to a therapeutic regimen can prevent the serious consequences associated with untreated elevated blood pressure. Hypertension is discussed in detail in Chapter 33.

Controlling Diabetes

The relationship between diabetes and heart disease has been confirmed. For 65% to 75% of patients with diabetes, cardiovascular disease is identified as the cause of death (Zipes et al., 2019). Hyperglycemia fosters dyslipidemia, increased platelet aggregation, and altered red blood cell function, which can lead to thrombus formation. It has been suggested that these metabolic alterations impair endothelial cell–dependent vasodilation and smooth muscle function. Treatment with insulin (e.g., Humalog, Humulin, Novolin) and metformin (Glucophage) to maintain lower blood sugars has shown improvement in endothelial function and improved endothelial-dependent dilation (Fysekidis, Cosson, Takbou, et al., 2018). Lifetime risk for CAD is higher in all patients with diabetes (Bertoluci & Rocha, 2017). Diabetes is discussed in detail in Chapter 41.

Gender

Because heart disease historically had been considered to primarily affect white men, the disease has not been as readily recognized and treated in women or other ethnic groups. However, in Canada, the number of women and men who die from cardiovascular disease is approximately the same at about 20% and the second cause of death (Statistics Canada, 2012). However, cardiovascular events occur an average of 10 years later in life for women than in men; women tend to have chronic disease, a higher incidence of complications, and a higher mortality. Women may not recognize the symptoms of MI as early as men or attribute them to heart disease, and therefore wait longer to report their symptoms and seek medical assistance (Mehta et al., 2016). In the past, women were less likely than men to be referred for coronary artery diagnostic procedures, to receive medical therapy (e.g., **fibrinolytic** therapy to break down the blood clots that cause acute MI, or nitroglycerin), and to be treated with invasive interventions (e.g., angioplasty). With better education of health care professionals and the general public, and improved diagnosis, gender differences now have less influence on diagnosis and treatment (Garcia, Mulvagh, Merz, et al., 2016).

In women younger than 55 years of age, the incidence of CAD remains significantly lower than in men. However, in women older than 55 years of age, the incidence of CAD is approximately equal to that in men. The age difference between women and men newly diagnosed with CAD was traditionally thought to be related to estrogen. It is now recognized that menopause is a milestone in the aging process during which risk factors tend to accumulate. Cardiovascular disease most likely will have been developing by the time of menopause, despite the supposed protective effects of estrogen (American Heart Association [AHA], 2015). It is likely that both aging and estrogen decline contribute to increased CAD risk. Although hormone therapy (HT)—formerly referred to as hormone replacement therapy (HRT)—for menopausal women was once promoted as preventive therapy for CAD, research studies do not support HT as an effective means of prevention. HT decreases menopausal symptoms and the risk for osteoporosis-related bone fractures, but HT also has been associated with an increased incidence of breast cancer, deep vein thrombosis, stroke, and pulmonary embolism. The evidence overall is controversial regarding HT and cardiovascular benefit. Although there are benefits such as lowering LDL cholesterol, increasing HDL cholesterol, and improving endothelial function, there are also adverse effects that can lead to pro-inflammatory responses (e.g., increase C-reactive protein) and pro-coagulant effects that can be detrimental. Both the CCS and the AHA (2015) current guidelines do not recommend HT for primary or secondary prevention of CAD.

Psychosocial Factors and Behaviour Patterns

There is now good evidence from large epidemiologic studies that stress, depression, and certain behaviours contribute to the pathogenesis of CAD and cardiac events (Anderson et al., 2013; Chauvet-Gelinier & Bonin, 2017; Dhar & Barton, 2016; Moudgil & Haddad, 2013). It has long been recognized that emotional stress can lead to a release of catecholamines and subsequent coronary ischemia. Nurses can assist by teaching cognitive restructuring and relaxation techniques. Because depression is associated with negative outcomes, patients should also be assessed for depression and appropriately treated.

Unfolding Patient Stories: Carl Shapiro • Part 1

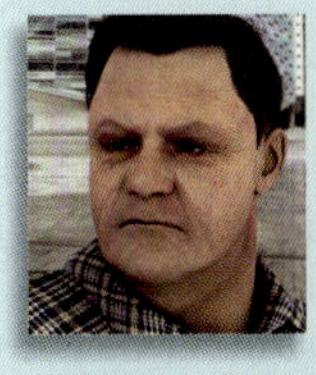

Carl Shapiro, who has a family history of atherosclerotic cardiovascular disease, is diagnosed with hypertension and hyperlipidemia during a routine visit to his primary provider. He is overweight, smokes a half pack of cigarettes per day, and describes his job as stressful. What questions can the nurse ask Carl Shapiro to help develop a plan for patient education? What topics are important for the nurse to address, and how can the information be presented? (Carl Shapiro's story continues in Chapter 73.)

Care for Carl and other patients in a realistic virtual environment: ***vSim** for Nursing* (**thepoint.lww.com/vSimMedicalSurgical**). Practice documenting these patients' care in DocuCare (**thepoint.lww.com/DocuCareEHR**).

Angina Pectoris

Angina pectoris is a clinical syndrome usually characterized by episodes or paroxysms of pain, discomfort, or pressure in the anterior chest. The cause is insufficient coronary blood flow, resulting in a decreased oxygen supply when there is increased myocardial demand for oxygen in response to physical exertion or emotional stress. In other words, the need for oxygen exceeds the supply. The severity of angina is based on the precipitating activity and its effect on activities of daily living, plus the underlying pathology of the arteries that are limiting blood flow.

Pathophysiology

Angina is usually caused by atherosclerotic disease. Almost invariably, angina is associated with an obstruction of a major coronary artery. Normally, the myocardium extracts a large amount of oxygen from the coronary circulation to meet its continuous demands. When there is an increase in demand, flow through the coronary arteries needs to be increased. When there is blockage in a coronary artery, flow cannot be increased and ischemia results. The types of angina are listed in Chart 29-2. Several factors are associated with typical anginal pain:

- Physical exertion, which can precipitate an attack by increasing myocardial oxygen demand
- Exposure to cold, which can cause vasoconstriction and elevated blood pressure, with increased oxygen demand
- Eating a heavy meal, which increases the blood flow to the mesenteric area for digestion, thereby reducing the blood supply available to the heart muscle. In a severely compromised heart, shunting of blood for digestion can be sufficient to induce anginal pain.
- Stress or any emotion-provoking situation, causing the release of catecholamines, which increases blood pressure, heart rate, and myocardial workload

Unstable angina can occur with or without physical exertion and can come on at rest. It can last longer and is more frequent than stable angina; rest or medicine (e.g., nitroglycerine) may not help relieve it. When unstable angina is diagnosed, it usually means that the blockages in the arteries of the heart have reached a critical level.

Clinical Manifestations

Ischemia of the heart muscle may produce pain or other symptoms, varying in severity from mild indigestion to a choking or heavy sensation in the upper chest that ranges from discomfort to agonizing pain accompanied by severe apprehension and a feeling of impending doom or death. The pain is often felt deep in the chest behind the sternum (retrosternal area). Typically, the pain or discomfort is poorly localized and may radiate to the neck, jaw, shoulders, and inner aspects of the upper arms, usually the left arm. The patient often feels tightness or a heavy, choking, or strangling sensation that has a viselike, insistent quality. The patient with diabetes may not have severe pain with angina because diabetic neuropathy can blunt nociceptors' transmission, dulling the perception of pain.

CHART 29-2

Types of Angina

- **Stable angina:** predictable and consistent pain that occurs on exertion and is relieved by rest and/or nitroglycerin
- **Unstable angina** (also called *preinfarction angina* or *crescendo angina*): symptoms increase in frequency and severity; may not be relieved with rest or nitroglycerin
- **Intractable or refractory angina:** severe incapacitating chest pain
- **Variant angina** (also called *Prinzmetal's angina*): pain at rest with reversible ST-segment elevation; thought to be caused by coronary artery vasospasm
- **Silent ischemia:** objective evidence of ischemia (such as electrocardiographic changes with a stress test), but patient reports no pain

A feeling of weakness or numbness in the arms, wrists, and hands, as well as shortness of breath, pallor, diaphoresis, dizziness or lightheadedness, and nausea and vomiting, may accompany the pain. Anxiety may occur with angina. An important characteristic of angina is that it usually subsides with rest or nitroglycerin. In many patients, anginal symptoms follow a stable, predictable pattern.

Unstable angina is characterized by attacks that increase in frequency and severity and are not relieved by rest and nitroglycerin. Patients with unstable angina require medical intervention as it indicates unstable plaque and platelet aggregation (see the Nursing Research Profile in Chart 29-3).

Gerontologic Considerations

The older person with angina may not exhibit the typical pain profile because of the diminished responses of neurotransmitters that occur with aging. Often, the presenting symptoms in the older adult are dyspnea, fatigue, or diaphoresis. Symptoms that do not include the typical symptom of chest discomfort are often termed angina equivalents (e.g., dyspnea). If pain occurs, it is often not chest pain, or pain that radiates to both arms rather than just the left arm. Sometimes, there are no symptoms ("silent" CAD), making recognition and diagnosis a clinical challenge. Older patients should be encouraged to recognize their chest pain–like symptom (e.g., weakness) as an indication that they should rest or take prescribed medications. Pharmacologic stress testing may be used to diagnose CAD in older patients because other conditions (e.g., peripheral vascular disease, arthritis, degenerative disk disease, physical disability, foot problems) may limit the patient's ability to exercise. Medications used in older adults with CVD have shown to clearly decrease cardiovascular mortality, but these medications must be used with caution. Aging may lead to impairment in absorption and excretion of some cardiac medications (Ayan, Pothineni, Siraj, et al., 2016). Some procedures might be considered to be too risky in older patients, but being older has not been found to be an independent predictor of complications of invasive procedures (e.g., PCI) (Hejazi,

NURSING RESEARCH PROFILE

Chart 29-3. Symptom Presentation in Acute Coronary Syndrome

O'Donnell, S., McKee, G., Mooney, M., et al. (2014). Slow-onset and fast-onset symptom presentations in acute coronary syndrome (ACS): New perspectives on prehospital delay in patients with ACS. *The Journal of Emergency Medicine*, *46*(4), 507–515.

Purpose

Patient decision delay is the main reason why many patients fail to receive timely medical intervention for symptoms of acute coronary syndrome (ACS). This study examines the validity of slow-onset and fast-onset ACS presentations and their influence on ACS prehospital delay times. A fast-onset ACS presentation is characterized by sudden, continuous, and severe chest pain, and slow-onset ACS pertains to all other ACS presentations.

Design

Baseline data pertaining to medical profiles, prehospital delay times, and ACS symptoms were recorded for all ACS patients who participated in a large multisite randomized control trial (RCT) in Dublin, Ireland. Patients were interviewed 2–4 days after their ACS event, and data were gathered using the ACS Response to Symptom Index.

Findings

Only baseline data from the RCT, $N = 893$ patients, were analyzed. A total of 65% ($N = 577$) of patients experienced slow-onset ACS presentation, whereas 35% ($N = 316$) experienced fast-onset ACS. Patients who experienced slow-onset ACS were significantly more likely to have longer prehospital delays than patients with fast-onset ACS (3.5 h vs. 2.0 h, respectively, $t = -5.63$, df 890, $p < 0.001$). A multivariate analysis of delay revealed that, in the presence of other known delay factors, the only independent predictors of delay were slow-onset and fast-onset ACS ($\beta = -0.096$, $p < 0.002$) and other factors associated with patient behaviour.

Nursing Implications

Slow-onset ACS and fast-onset ACS presentations are associated with distinct behavioural patterns that significantly influence prehospital time frames. As such, slow-onset ACS and fast-onset ACS are legitimate ACS presentation phenomena that nurses should be aware of when examining the factors associated with prehospital delay.

Iranirad, Doostali, et al., 2017). See Chart 29-4 for ethical considerations in older adults experiencing acute coronary syndrome.

Assessment and Diagnostic Findings

The diagnosis of angina begins with the patient's history related to the clinical manifestations of ischemia. A 12-lead electrocardiogram (ECG) and blood laboratory values help in making the diagnosis. In ischemia, a 12-lead ECG may show changes of T-wave inversion of ST-segment depression. The patient may undergo an exercise or pharmacologic stress test in which the heart is monitored by ECG, echocardiogram, or both. The patient may also be referred for a nuclear scan or invasive procedure (e.g., cardiac catheterization, coronary artery angiography).

Because CAD is believed to result from inflammation of the arterial endothelium, CRP, a marker for inflammation

CHART 29-4

Ethics and Related Issues

Should Aggressive Treatment Be Recommended for the Older With Acute Coronary Syndrome?

SITUATION

Many patients who present with acute coronary events are older. They often have chronic conditions such as diabetes or arthritis. Older patients have traditionally been managed conservatively with medications, but currently interventions such as cardiac catheterization may be recommended. These patients look to their family members for help with treatment decisions.

DILEMMA

An 80-year-old woman is hospitalized with unstable angina. The cardiologist discusses the situation with her two adult sons. He recommends cardiac catheterization with possible percutaneous transluminal coronary angioplasty and stent placement. The patient is oriented but lethargic. She defers to her sons regarding treatment decisions. One son worries that she will be subjected to an invasive procedure that is potentially high risk, painful, expensive, and possibly futile. The second son feels that if there is hope of success, she should have the procedure.

DISCUSSION

Research on the risks and benefits of treatment for acute coronary syndrome (ACS) now includes the older as a subgroup. One study reports that the older may benefit as much, if not more, than younger patients from coronary reperfusion procedures in terms of reduction of death or myocardial infarction (Bach, Cannon, Weintraub, et al., 2004).

1. What arguments would you offer that support or discourage aggressive treatment for ACS in the older?
2. What assistance can you offer to enhance the patient and family's autonomy regarding decision making as well as their sense of justice regarding the allocation of resources?

of vascular endothelium, may be measured. High blood levels of CRP have been associated with increased coronary artery calcification and risk of an acute cardiovascular event (e.g., MI), but are also indicative of other inflammatory states. CRP levels are not currently recommended as a routine test to evaluate risk (Anderson et al., 2013).

Medical Management

The objectives of the medical management of angina are to decrease the oxygen demand of the myocardium and to increase the oxygen supply. Medically, these objectives are met through pharmacologic therapy and control of risk factors. Alternatively, reperfusion procedures may be used to restore the blood supply to the myocardium. These include PCI procedures (e.g., **percutaneous transluminal coronary angioplasty [PTCA]**, and intracoronary stents) and coronary artery bypass graft (CABG).

Pharmacologic Therapy

Nitroglycerin

Nitrates are a standard treatment of angina pectoris. Nitroglycerine is a potent vasodilator that is administered to improve blood flow, thereby reducing myocardial oxygen consumption, which decreases ischemia and relieves pain. Nitroglycerin primarily dilates the veins and, to a lesser extent, the arteries. Dilation of the veins causes venous pooling of blood throughout the body. As a result, less blood returns to the heart, and filling pressure (**preload**) is reduced. If the patient is hypovolemic (does not have adequate circulating blood volume), the decrease in filling pressure can cause a significant decrease in cardiac output and blood pressure.

Nitrates in higher doses also relax the systemic arteriolar bed, lowering blood pressure, and decreasing **afterload**. These effects decrease myocardial oxygen requirements and increase oxygen supply, bringing about a more advantageous balance between supply and demand.

Nitroglycerin may be given by several routes: sublingual tablet or spray, oral capsule, topical agent, and intravenous (IV) administration. Sublingual nitroglycerin is generally placed under the tongue or in the cheek (buccal pouch) and alleviates the pain of ischemia within 3 minutes. Chart 29-5 provides more information on self-administration of sublingual nitroglycerin. If nitroglycerin spray is used, the nurse ensures that the patient can depress the spray container (e.g., patients with inflammatory conditions of the fingers and hands may not be able to depress the spray). Oral preparations and topical patches are used to provide sustained effects. The patches are often applied in the morning and removed at bedtime, or vice versa depending upon the individual. This regimen allows for a nitrate-free period to prevent the development of tolerance.

A continuous or intermittent IV infusion of nitroglycerin may be administered to the hospitalized patient with recurring signs and symptoms of ischemia or after a revascularization procedure. The amount of nitroglycerin administered is based on the patient's symptoms while avoiding side effects such as hypotension. It usually is not administered if the systolic blood pressure is 90 mm Hg or less and the patient is symptomatic. Generally, after the patient has no further angina, the nitroglycerin may be switched to an oral ortopical preparation within 24 hours. The most common side effect of nitroglycerine is headache, and this may limit the use of this medication in some patients.

CHART 29-5

Pharmacology: Self-Administration of Nitroglycerin

Most patients with angina pectoris must self-administer nitroglycerin on an as-needed basis. A key nursing role in such cases is educating patients about the medication and how to take it. Sublingual nitroglycerin comes in tablet and spray forms.

- Instruct the patient to make sure the mouth is moist, the tongue is still, and saliva is not swallowed until the nitroglycerin tablet dissolves. If the pain is severe, the patient can crush the tablet between the teeth to hasten sublingual absorption.
- Advise the patient to carry the medication at all times as a precaution. However, because nitroglycerin is very unstable, it should be carried securely in its original container (e.g., capped dark glass bottle); tablets should never be removed and stored in metal or plastic pillboxes.
- Explain that nitroglycerin is volatile and is inactivated by heat, moisture, air, light, and time. Instruct the patient to renew the nitroglycerin supply every 6 months.
- Inform the patient that the medication should be taken in anticipation of any activity that may produce pain. Because nitroglycerin increases tolerance for exercise and stress when taken prophylactically (i.e., before angina-producing activity, such as exercise, stair-climbing, or sexual intercourse), it is best taken before pain develops.
- Recommend that the patient note how long it takes for the nitroglycerin to relieve the discomfort. Advise the patient that if pain persists after taking three sublingual tablets at 5-minute intervals, emergency medical services should be called.
- Discuss possible side effects of nitroglycerin, including flushing, throbbing headache, hypotension, and tachycardia.
- Advise the patient to sit down for a few minutes when taking nitroglycerin to avoid hypotension and syncope.

Adapted from Burchum, J. R., & Rosenthal, L. D. (2016). *Lehne's pharmacology for nursing care* (9th ed.). St. Louis, MO: Elsevier.

Beta-Adrenergic Blocking Agents

Beta-blockers such as metoprolol (Lopressor, Toprol) and atenolol (Tenormin) reduce myocardial oxygen consumption by blocking beta-adrenergic sympathetic stimulation to the heart. The result is a reduction in heart rate, slowed conduction of impulses through the conduction system, decreased blood pressure, and reduced myocardial **contractility** (force of contraction). Because of these effects, beta-blockers balance the myocardial oxygen needs (demands) and the amount of oxygen available (supply). Beta-blockers reduce the incidence of recurrent angina, infarction, and cardiac mortality. The dose normally is titrated to achieve a resting heart rate of 50 to 60 beats/min.

Cardiac side effects and possible contraindications include hypotension, bradycardia, advanced atrioventricular block, and decompensated heart failure. If a beta-blocker is given IV for an acute cardiac event, the ECG, blood pressure, and heart rate are monitored closely after the medication has been administered. Beta-blockers that are not cardioselective (e.g., Propranolol, Carvedilol, Labetalol) also affect the beta-adrenergic receptors in the bronchioles, causing bronchoconstriction, and therefore are usually contraindicated in patients with significant pulmonary obstructive diseases, such as asthma. Other side effects include depression, fatigue, decreased libido, and masking of symptoms of hypoglycemia. Patients taking beta-blockers are cautioned not to stop taking them abruptly, because angina may worsen and an MI may occur. Beta-blocker therapy should be decreased gradually over several days before being discontinued. Patients with diabetes who take beta-blockers are instructed to monitor their blood glucose levels often and to observe for signs and symptoms of hypoglycemia.

Calcium Channel Blocking Agents

Calcium channel blockers (calcium ion antagonists) have a variety of effects on the ischemic myocardium. These agents decrease sinoatrial node automaticity and atrioventricular node conduction, resulting in a slower heart rate and a decrease in the strength of the heart muscle contraction (negative inotropic effect). These effects decrease the workload of the heart. Calcium channel blockers also relax the blood vessels, causing a decrease in blood pressure and an increase in coronary artery perfusion. Calcium channel blockers increase myocardial oxygen supply by dilating the smooth muscle wall of the coronary arterioles; they decrease myocardial oxygen demand by reducing systemic arterial pressure and the workload of the left ventricle.

The calcium channel blockers most commonly used are amlodipine (Norvasc) and diltiazem (Cardizem, Tiazac). They may be used by patients who cannot take beta-blockers, who develop significant side effects from beta-blockers or nitrates, or who still have pain despite beta-blocker and nitroglycerin therapy. In addition to their use to treat angina, they are commonly prescribed for hypertension. Calcium channel blockers are also used to prevent and treat vasospasm.

First-generation calcium channel blockers such as nifedipine should be avoided or used with great caution in people with heart failure, because they decrease myocardial contractility. Amlodipine and felodipine (Plendil) are the calcium channel blockers of choice for patients with heart failure. Hypotension may occur after the IV administration of any of the calcium channel blockers. Other side effects may include atrioventricular block, bradycardia, constipation, and gastric distress.

Antiplatelet and Anticoagulant Medications

Antiplatelet medications are administered to prevent platelet aggregation and subsequent thrombosis, which impedes blood flow through the coronary arteries.

ASPIRIN. Aspirin prevents platelet activation and reduces the incidence of MI and death in patients with CAD. A 160- to 325-mg dose of aspirin should be given to the patient with angina as soon as the diagnosis is made (e.g., in the emergency department or physician's office) and then continued with 81 to 325 mg daily. Although aspirin may be one of the most important medications in the treatment of CAD, it may be overlooked because of its low cost and common use. Patients should be advised to continue aspirin even if they concurrently take nonsteroidal anti-inflammatory drugs (NSAIDs) or other analgesics. Because aspirin may cause gastrointestinal upset and bleeding, the use of H_2-blockers (e.g., famotidine [Pepcid], ranitidine [Zantac]) or proton pump inhibitors (e.g., omeprazole [Prilosec]) may be considered to allow continued aspirin therapy in individuals experiencing these symptoms.

ADENOSINE DIPHOSPHATE RECEPTOR ANTAGONISTS ($P2Y_{12}$). Clopidogrel (Plavix) is given to patients who are allergic to aspirin or given in addition to aspirin in patients at high risk for MI, or post PCI. Unlike aspirin, these medications take a few days to achieve their antiplatelet effect. They also cause gastrointestinal upset. Newer agents such as Brilinta (Ticagrelor) may be used in place of Clopidogrel during coronary events and interventions. The benefit of Ticagrelor is that it does not require hepatic activation; therefore, can act faster than Clopidogrel.

HEPARIN. Unfractionated IV heparin is an anticoagulant and prevents the formation of new blood clots. Treating patients with unstable angina with heparin reduces the occurrence of MI. If the patient's signs and symptoms indicate a significant risk for a cardiac event, the patient is hospitalized and may be given an IV bolus of heparin and started on a continuous infusion. The amount of heparin administered is based on the results of the activated partial thromboplastin time (aPTT). Heparin therapy is usually considered therapeutic when the aPTT is 2.0 to 2.5 times the normal aPTT value.

A subcutaneous injection of low–molecular-weight heparin (LMWH; enoxaparin [Lovenox] or dalteparin [Fragmin]) may be used instead of IV unfractionated heparin to treat patients with unstable angina or non–ST-segment elevation MIs (Anderson, Adams, Antman, 2011). LMWH provides effective and stable anticoagulation, potentially reducing the risk of rebound ischemic events, and it eliminates the need to monitor aPTT results. LMWH may be beneficial before and during PCIs as well as for ACS. Enoxaparin is superior to UFH in reducing mortality in patients having a STEMI and undergoing PCI (Silvain, Beygui, Barthelemy, et al., 2012).

Because unfractionated heparin and LMWH increase the risk of bleeding, the patient is monitored for signs and symptoms of external and internal bleeding, such as low blood pressure, increased heart rate, and decreased serum hemoglobin and hematocrit. The patient receiving heparin is placed on bleeding precautions, which include the following:

- Applying pressure to the site of any needle puncture for a longer time than usual
- Avoiding intramuscular (IM) injections
- Avoiding tissue injury and bruising from trauma or use of constrictive devices (e.g., continuous use of an automatic blood pressure cuff)

A decrease in platelet count or evidence of thrombosis may indicate heparin-induced thrombocytopenia (HIT), an antibody-mediated reaction to heparin that may result in thrombosis (Frazer, 2013). Patients who have received heparin within the past 3 months and those who have been receiving unfractionated heparin for 5 to 15 days are at high risk for HIT (Greinacher, 2015).

GLYCOPROTEIN IIB/IIIA AGENTS. IV administration of glycoprotein (GP) IIb/IIIa agents (abciximab [ReoPro], tirofiban [Aggrastat], eptifibatide [Integrilin]) is indicated for hospitalized patients with unstable angina and as adjunct therapy for PCI. These agents prevent platelet aggregation by blocking the GPIIb/IIIa receptors on the platelets, preventing adhesion of fibrinogen and other factors that cross-link platelets to each other and thereby allow platelets to form a thrombus (clot). As with heparin, bleeding is the major side effect, and bleeding precautions should be initiated.

Oxygen Administration

Oxygen therapy is usually initiated at the onset of chest pain in an attempt to increase the amount of oxygen delivered to the myocardium and to decrease pain. The therapeutic effectiveness of oxygen is determined by observing the rate and rhythm of respirations. Blood oxygen saturation is monitored by pulse oximetry; the normal oxygen saturation (SpO_2) level is generally greater than 93%; targets are generally greater than 90% for patients with COPD. Routine use of supplemental oxygen in patients with MI who are do not have hypoxemia does not change mortality (Abuzaid, Fabrizio, Felpel, et al., 2018).

Nursing Process

PRACTICE & LEARN

The Patient With Angina Pectoris

Assessment

The nurse gathers information about the patient's symptoms and activities, especially those that precede and precipitate attacks of angina pectoris. Appropriate questions are listed in Chart 29-6. Other helpful questions may be asked: How long does the angina usually last? Does nitroglycerin relieve the angina? If so, how many tablets or sprays are needed to achieve relief? How long does it take for relief to occur?

The answers to these questions form a basis for designing an effective program of treatment and prevention. In addition to assessing angina pectoris or its equivalent, the nurse also assesses the patient's risk factors for CAD, the patient's response to angina, the patient and family's understanding of the diagnosis, and adherence to the current treatment plan.

CHART 29-6

Assessment: Assessing Symptoms Associated With Angina

Ask the following:

- "Where is the pain (or prodromal symptoms)? Can you point to it?"
- "Can you feel the pain anywhere else?"
- "How would you describe the pain?"
- "Is it like the pain you had before?"
- "Can you rate the pain on a 0–10 scale, with 10 being the most pain?"
- "When did the pain begin?"
- "How long does it last?"
- "What brings on the pain?"
- "What helps the pain go away?"
- "Do you have any other symptoms with the pain?"

Nursing Priorities

Based on the assessment data, major nursing priorities may include the following:

- Decreased myocardial perfusion
- Anxiety
- Lack of knowledge
- Difficulty with compliance

Collaborative Problems/ Potential Complications

Potential complications that may develop include the following, which are discussed in the chapters indicated:

- ACS (described later in this chapter)
- Dysrhythmias and cardiac arrest (see Chapters 28 and 31)
- Acute pulmonary edema (see Chapter 24)
- Heart failure (see Chapter 31)
- Cardiogenic shock (see Chapter 31)

Planning and Goals

Major patient goals include immediate and appropriate treatment when angina occurs, prevention of angina, reduction of anxiety, awareness of the disease process and understanding of the prescribed care, adherence to the self-care program, and absence of complications.

Nursing Interventions

Treating Angina

If the patient reports pain (or cardiac ischemia is suggested by prodromal symptoms, which may include sensations of indigestion or nausea, choking, heaviness, weakness or numbness in the upper extremities, dyspnea, or dizziness), the nurse takes immediate action. The patient experiencing angina is directed to stop all activities and sit or rest in bed in a semi-Fowler's position to reduce the oxygen requirements of the ischemic myocardium. The nurse assesses the patient's angina, asking questions to determine whether the angina is the same as the patient typically experiences. A change may indicate a worsening of the disease or a different cause. The nurse then continues to assess the patient, measuring vital signs and observing for signs of distress. If the patient is in the hospital, a 12-lead ECG is obtained and assessed for ST-segment and T-wave changes. If the patient has been placed on cardiac monitoring with continuous ST-segment monitoring, the ST segment is assessed for changes.

Nitroglycerin is administered sublingually, and the patient's response is assessed (relief of chest pain and effect on blood pressure and heart rate). If the chest pain is unchanged or is lessened but still present, nitroglycerin administration is repeated up to three doses. Each time, blood pressure, heart rate, and the ST segment (if the patient is on a monitor with ST-segment monitoring capability) are assessed. The nurse administers oxygen therapy if the patient's respiratory rate is increased or if the oxygen saturation level is decreased. Although oxygen is very beneficial in hypoxemic patients with acute myocardial infarction, it has not been shown to be beneficial in patients that are normoxemic. Some research suggests that oxygen use in patients who have normal oxygen saturation may actually have increased myocardial injury (Stub, 2017). If the pain is significant and continues after these interventions, the patient needs to be further evaluated for acute MI and may be transferred to a higher-acuity unit for further treatment (e.g., IV nitroglycerin).

Reducing Anxiety

Patients with angina often fear loss of their roles within society and the family. They may also fear that the discomfort and other symptoms may lead to an MI or death. Exploring the implications that the diagnosis has for the patient and providing information about the illness, its treatment, and methods of preventing its progression are important nursing interventions. Various stress reduction methods should be explored with the patient to reduce anxiety in patients. Addressing the spiritual needs of the patient and family may also assist in allaying anxieties and fears.

Preventing Pain

The nurse reviews the assessment findings, identifies the level of activity that causes the patient's discomfort or other symptoms, and plans the patient's activities accordingly. If the patient has pain frequently or with minimal activity, the nurse alternates the patient's activities with rest periods. Balancing activity and rest is an important aspect of the educational plan for the patient and family.

Promoting Home, Community-Based, and Transitional Care

Educating Patients About Self-Care

Learning about the modifiable risk factors that contribute to the development of CAD and resulting angina is essential. Exploring what the patient and family see as their priorities in managing the disease and developing a plan based on those priorities can assist with patient adherence to the therapeutic regimen. It is important to explore with the patient methods to avoid, modify, or adapt the triggers for anginal pain. The program for educating the patient with angina is designed so that the patient and family understand the illness, identify the symptoms of myocardial ischemia, state the actions to take when symptoms develop, and discuss methods to prevent chest pain and the advancement of CAD. The goals of the educational program are to reduce the frequency and severity of anginal attacks, to delay the progress of the underlying disease if possible, and to prevent complications. The factors outlined in Chart 29-7 are important in educating the patient with angina pectoris.

The self-care program is prepared in collaboration with the patient and family or friends. Activities should be planned to minimize the occurrence of angina episodes. The patient needs to understand that any pain unrelieved within 15 minutes by the usual methods, including nitroglycerin (Chart 29-8), should be treated at the closest emergency centre; the patient should call 911 for assistance.

CONTINUING AND TRANSITIONAL CARE. For patients with disabilities or special needs, arrangements are made for transitional, home, or community care when appropriate. The home care nurse can assist the patient with scheduling and keeping follow-up appointments. The patient may need reminders about follow-up monitoring, including periodic blood laboratory testing and ECGs. In addition, the home care nurse may monitor the patient's adherence to dietary restrictions and to prescribed antianginal medications, including nitroglycerin. If the patient has severe anginal symptoms, the nurse may assess the home environment and recommend modifications that diminish the occurrence of anginal episodes. For instance, if a patient cannot climb stairs without experiencing ischemia, the home care nurse may help the patient plan daily activities that minimize stair climbing. Some patients may benefit from moving the bedroom to a lower level in the home.

Evaluation

Expected patient outcomes may include the following:

1. Reports that pain is relieved promptly
   a. Recognizes symptoms
   b. Takes immediate action
   c. Seeks medical assistance if pain persists or changes in quality
2. Reports decreased anxiety
   a. Expresses understanding of the diagnosis
   b. Expresses control over choices within the medical regimen
   c. Does not exhibit signs and symptoms that indicate a high level of anxiety
3. Understands ways to avoid complications and is free of complications
   a. Describes the process of angina
   b. Explains reasons for measures to prevent complications (e.g., limiting strenuous exercise)
   c. Experiences no signs and symptoms of acute MI
4. Adheres to the self-care program
   a. Takes medications as prescribed
   b. Keeps health care appointments
   c. Implements a plan to reduce risk factors

CHART 29-7

HOME CARE CHECKLIST • Managing Angina Pectoris

At the completion of education, the patient and/or caregiver will be able to:

- State the impact of angina pectoris on physiologic functioning, ADLs, IADLs, roles, relationships, and spirituality.
- State changes in lifestyle (e.g., diet, activity) or home environment necessary to maintain health.
- Follow a diet low in saturated fat, high in fibre, and, if indicated, lower in calories.
- Reduce the probability of an episode of anginal pain by balancing rest with regular daily activities that do not produce chest discomfort, shortness of breath, or undue fatigue.
- Follow the prescribed exercise regimen.
  - Recognize that temperature extremes (particularly cold) may induce anginal pain; therefore, avoid exercise in temperature extremes.
- State the name, dose, side effects, frequency, and schedule for all medications.
- Take medications, especially aspirin and beta-blockers, as prescribed.
- Carry nitroglycerin at all times; state when and how to use it; identify its side effects.
- Avoid using medications or any over-the-counter substances (e.g., diet pills, nasal decongestants) that can increase the heart rate and blood pressure without first discussing with the primary provider.
- Use appropriate resources for support during emotionally stressful times (e.g., counsellor, nurse, clergy, physician).
- Stop smoking and the use of other forms of tobacco, and avoid secondhand smoke (because smoking increases the heart rate, blood pressure, and blood carbon monoxide levels).
- Achieve and maintain normal blood pressure.
- Achieve and maintain normal blood glucose levels.
- State how to reach primary provider with questions or complications.
  - Report increase in symptoms to the primary provider.
  - State time and date of follow-up appointments and testing.
- Identify the need for health promotion (e.g., weight reduction, smoking cessation, stress management), disease prevention, and screening activities.

ADL, activities of daily living; IADL, independent activities of daily living.

Acute Coronary Syndrome and Myocardial Infarction

Acute coronary syndrome (**ACS**) is an emergent situation characterized by an acute onset of myocardial ischemia that results in myocardial death (i.e., MI). (Although the terms *coronary occlusion*, *heart attack*, and *myocardial infarction* are used synonymously, the preferred term is *myocardial infarction*.) The spectrum of ACS includes unstable angina, **NSTEMI**, and ST-segment elevation myocardial infarction (**STEMI**).

Pathophysiology

In unstable angina, there is reduced blood flow in a coronary artery, which may be due to rupture of an atherosclerotic plaque. A clot begins to form on top of the coronary lesion, but the artery is not completely occluded. This is an acute situation that can result in chest pain and other symptoms that may be referred to as preinfarction angina because the patient will likely have an MI if prompt interventions do not occur.

In an MI, plaque rupture and subsequent thrombus formation result in complete occlusion of the artery, leading to injury and necrosis of the myocardium supplied by that artery. Other causes of MI include vasospasm (sudden constriction or narrowing) of a coronary artery, decreased oxygen supply (e.g., from acute blood loss, anemia, or low blood pressure), and increased demand for oxygen (e.g., from a rapid heart rate, thyrotoxicosis, or ingestion of cocaine). In each case, a profound imbalance exists between myocardial oxygen supply and demand.

The area of infarction develops over minutes to hours. As the cells are deprived of oxygen, ischemia develops, cellular injury occurs, and the lack of oxygen results in infarction (death of cells.) The expression "time is muscle" reflects the urgency of appropriate treatment to improve patient outcomes. Approximately every 7 minutes in Canada someone dies from heart disease or stroke seconds (Heart and Stroke Canada, 2017). Early recognition and treatment

CHART 29-8

Assessment: Assessing for Acute Myocardial Infarction or Acute Coronary Syndrome

Be on the alert for the following signs and symptoms:

Cardiovascular

- Chest pain or discomfort, palpitations. Heart sounds may include S_3, S_4, and new onset of a murmur.
- Increased jugular venous distention may be seen if the myocardial infarction (MI) has caused heart failure.
- Blood pressure may be elevated because of sympathetic stimulation or decreased because of decreased contractility, impending cardiogenic shock, or medications.
- Pulse deficit may indicate atrial fibrillation.
- In addition to ST-segment and T-wave changes, electrocardiogram may show tachycardia, bradycardia, or dysrhythmias.

Respiratory

Shortness of breath, dyspnea, tachypnea, and crackles if MI has caused pulmonary congestion. Pulmonary edema may be present.

Gastrointestinal

Nausea and vomiting.

Genitourinary

Decreased urinary output may indicate cardiogenic shock.

Skin

Cool, clammy, diaphoretic, and pale appearance due to sympathetic stimulation may indicate cardiogenic shock.

Neurologic

Anxiety, restlessness, and lightheadedness may indicate increased sympathetic stimulation or a decrease in contractility and cerebral oxygenation. The same symptoms may also herald cardiogenic shock.

Psychological

Fear with feeling of impending doom, or patient may deny that anything is wrong.

of patients presenting with an MI will improve their chances of survival.

Various descriptions are used to further identify an MI: the type (NSTEMI, STEMI), the location of the injury to the ventricular wall (anterior, septal inferior, posterior, right ventricle or lateral wall), and the point in time within the process of infarction (acute, age indeterminate, or old). The differentiation between NSTEMI and STEMI is determined by diagnostic tests and is explained later in this chapter. MI can also be classified into types (types 1 to 5) (Chapman, Adamson, & Mills, 2017).

The 12-lead ECG helps identify the type, location, and timing of the MI, while other indicators such as lab work (i.e., cardiac markers) and patient history identify the timing. Regardless of the location of the infarction of cardiac muscle, the goal of medical therapy is to prevent or minimize myocardial tissue death and to prevent complications. The pathophysiology of heart disease and the risk factors involved were discussed earlier in this chapter.

Clinical Manifestations

Chest pain/discomfort that occurs suddenly and continues despite rest and medication is the presenting symptom in most patients with an MI (Chart 29-8). Some of these patients have prodromal symptoms or a previous diagnosis of CAD, but others report experiencing no previous symptoms. Patients may present with a combination of symptoms, including chest discomfort, shortness of breath, indigestion, nausea, and anxiety. They may have cool, pale, and moist skin. Their heart rate and respiratory rate may be faster than normal. These signs and symptoms, which are caused by stimulation of the sympathetic nervous system, may be present for only a short time or may persist. In many cases, the signs and symptoms of MI cannot be distinguished from those of unstable angina, hence the development of the term acute coronary syndrome. Unstable angina, NSTEMI, and STEMI are on the continuum of ACS.

Assessment and Diagnostic Findings

The diagnosis of ACS is generally based on the presenting symptoms, the ECG, and laboratory test results (e.g., serial cardiac biomarkers). The prognosis depends on the severity of coronary artery obstruction and the extent of myocardial damage. Physical examination is always conducted, but the examination alone does not confirm the diagnosis.

Patient History

The patient history has two parts: the description of the presenting symptom (e.g., pain/discomfort) and the history of previous illnesses and family history of heart disease. Previous history should also include information about the patient's risk factors for heart disease. It is important to ask about chest discomfort rather than only chest pain as many individuals do not characterize their discomfort as pain (e.g., heaviness or burning instead of sharp).

Electrocardiogram

The 12-lead ECG provides information that assists in ruling out or diagnosing acute MI. It should be obtained within 10 minutes from the time a patient reports pain or arrives in the emergency department (ED). By monitoring serial ECG changes over time, the location, evolution, and resolution of an MI can be monitored.

The ECG changes that occur with an MI are seen in the leads that view the involved surface of the heart (reflecting leads). The classic ECG changes are T-wave inversion, ST-segment elevation, and development of an abnormal Q wave (Fig. 29-5). Because infarction evolves over time, the ECG also changes over time. The first ECG signs of an acute MI occur as a result of myocardial ischemia and

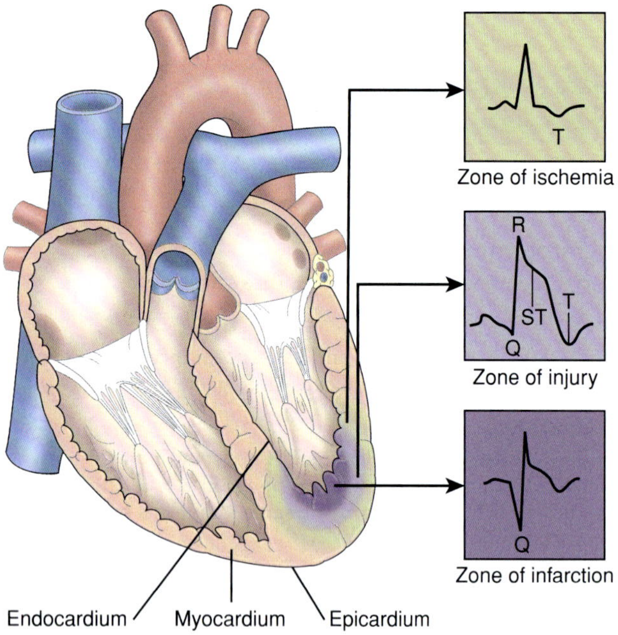

FIGURE 29-5. Effects of ischemia, injury, and infarction on an electrocardiogram recording. Ischemia causes inversion of the T wave because of altered repolarization. Cardiac muscle injury causes elevation of the ST segment and tall, symmetrical T waves. Later, Q waves develop because of the absence of depolarization current from the necrotic tissue and opposing currents from other parts of the heart.

injury. As the involved area becomes ischemic, myocardial repolarization is altered and delayed, causing the T wave to invert. Myocardial injury also causes ST-segment changes. Normally the ST segment is flat (isoelectric) on the ECG tracing (the area between the T wave and the next P wave is used as the reference for the isoelectric line). Depending on the extent of the injury, the ST segment may fall below or rise above the isoelectric line. The J point (junction) marks the interval between the QRS complex and the ST segment (Fig. 29-6). The injured myocardial cells depolarize normally but repolarize more rapidly than normal cells, causing the ST segment to rise

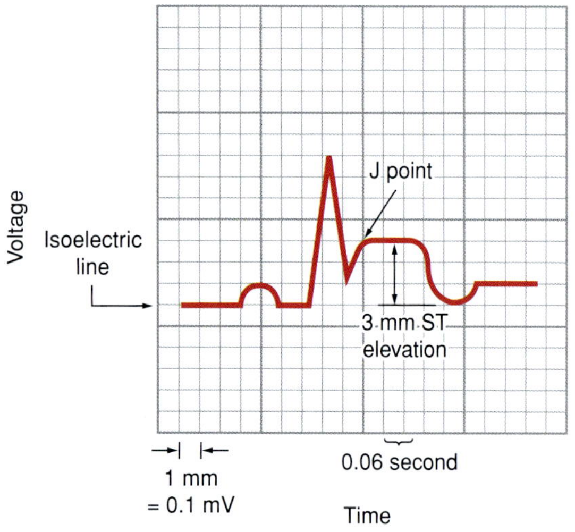

FIGURE 29-6. Using the electrocardiogram to diagnose acute myocardial infarction (MI). ST-segment elevation is measured 0.06 to 0.08 seconds after the J point. An elevation of more than 1 mm in contiguous leads is indicative of acute MI.

at least 1 mm above the isoelectric line. The change in the ST segment in two contiguous leads is a key diagnostic indicator for MI, classified as non–ST-elevated MI (depressed or normal ST) and ST-elevated MI.

The appearance of abnormal Q waves indicates the MI was transmural (involving the full thickness of the myocardium). Q waves can develop within hours of symptoms up until 48 hours in patients who experience a STEMI event. Q waves are a result of absence of electrical activity because there is no depolarization current conducted from necrotic tissue. A pathologic Q wave is >0.04 seconds (40 milliseconds) in duration and greater than ¼ to ⅓ height of the R-wave. An acute MI may also cause a significant decrease in the height of the R wave. During an acute MI, injury and ischemic changes are usually present. An abnormal Q wave on a 12-lead ECG may be present without ST-segment and T-wave changes, indicating an old, not acute, MI. For some patients, there are no persistent ECG changes, and the MI is diagnosed as an NSTEMI if cardiac biomarkers in the blood are elevated.

Using the above information, patients are diagnosed with one of the following forms of ACS:

- *Unstable angina:* The patient has clinical manifestations of coronary ischemia, but ECG or cardiac biomarkers show no evidence of acute MI.
- *Non–ST-segment elevation MI (NSTEMI):* The patient has elevated cardiac biomarkers but no definite ECG evidence of acute MI. In this type of MI, the damage is not transmural.
- *ST-segment elevation MI (STEMI):* The patient has ECG evidence of acute MI with characteristic changes in two contiguous leads on a 12-lead ECG. In this type of MI, there is significant damage to the myocardium.

During recovery from an MI, the ST segment often is the first ECG indicator to return to normal. The T wave goes through a process of inversion and then eventually normalizes. Q-wave alterations are usually permanent. An old STEMI is usually identified on an ECG by an abnormal Q wave or decreased height of the R wave without ST-segment and T-wave changes.

Echocardiogram

The echocardiogram is used to evaluate ventricular function. It may be used to assist in diagnosing an MI, especially when the ECG is nondiagnostic. The echocardiogram can detect hypokinetic and akinetic wall motion and can determine the ejection fraction (see Chapter 27).

Laboratory Tests

Laboratory tests called *cardiac biomarkers*, which include troponin, **creatine kinase (CK)**, and myoglobin, are used to diagnose an acute MI. Cardiac biomarkers can be analyzed rapidly, expediting an accurate diagnosis. These tests are based on the release of cellular contents into the circulation when myocardial cells die. Table 29-3 shows the time courses of cardiac biomarkers.

Troponin

Troponin, a protein found in the myocardial cells, regulates the myocardial contractile process. There are three isomers of troponin: C, I, and T. Troponins I and T are specific for cardiac muscle, and these tests are currently

TABLE 29-3 Biomarkers of Acute Myocardial Infarction

Serum Test	Earliest Increase (hours)	Test Running Time (minutes)	Peak (hours)	Return to Normal
Total CK	3–6	30–60	24–36	3 days
CK-MB: isoenzyme	4–8	30–60	12–24	3–4 days
mass assay	2–3	30–60	10–18	3–4 days
Myoglobin	1–3	30–60	4–12	12 hours
Troponin T or I	3–4	30–60	4–24	1–3 weeks

CK, creatine kinase; CK-MB, creatine kinase isoenzyme found in heart muscle.

recognized as reliable and critical markers of myocardial injury. An increase in the level of troponin in the serum can be detected within 6 hours during acute MI. It remains elevated for a long period, often as long as 2 weeks, and it therefore can be used to detect recent myocardial damage. Cardiac troponin levels may rise during inflammation, pulmonary embolism, sepsis, myocardial contusion, heart failure, end-stage renal disease and respiratory failure (Gibson & Morrow, 2018).

Creatine Kinase and Its Isoenzymes

There are three creatine kinase (CK) isoenzymes: CK-MM (skeletal muscle), CK-MB (heart muscle), and CK-BB (brain tissue). CK-MB is the cardiac-specific isoenzyme; CK-MB is found mainly in cardiac cells and therefore increases only when there has been damage to these cells. Elevated CK-MB assessed by mass assay is an indicator of acute MI; its level begins to increase within a few hours and peaks within 24 hours of an MI. If the area is reperfused (e.g., due to fibrinolytic therapy or PCI), it peaks earlier.

Myoglobin

Myoglobin is a heme protein that helps to transport oxygen. Like CK-MB enzyme, myoglobin is found in cardiac and skeletal muscle. The myoglobin level starts to increase within 1 to 3 hours and peaks within 12 hours after the onset of symptoms. An increase in myoglobin is not very specific in indicating an acute cardiac event; however, negative results are an excellent parameter for ruling out an acute MI.

Medical Management

The goal of medical management is to minimize myocardial damage, preserve myocardial function, and prevent complications. These goals are facilitated by the use of guidelines developed by the American College of Cardiology (ACC) and AHA (Chart 29-9). The goals for treating patients with acute MI may be achieved by interventions that reestablish coronary flow (antithrombotic medications, fibrinolytic medications, or by PCI). Minimizing myocardial damage is also accomplished by reducing myocardial oxygen demand and increasing oxygen supply with medications, oxygen administration, and bed rest. The resolution of pain and ECG changes indicate that demand and supply are in equilibrium; they may also indicate reperfusion. Visualization of blood flow through an open vessel in the catheterization laboratory is evidence of reperfusion.

Pharmacologic Therapy

The patient with suspected MI should immediately receive aspirin, nitroglycerin, and morphine. Oxygen should be given if the patient is hypoxemic. A beta-blocker may also be used if dysrhythmias occur. If a beta-blocker is not needed in the initial management period, it should be introduced within 24 hours of admission, once hemodynamics have stabilized and it is confirmed that the patient has no contraindications. Beta-blockers have been shown to slow heart rate and have a negative inotropic effect, leading to a reduction in myocardial oxygen consumption and improving short- and long-term mortality benefit (Noble & Roffi, 2017). Unfractionated heparin or LMWH

CHART 29-9

Treatment Guidelines for Acute Myocardial Infarction

- Use rapid transit to the hospital.
- Obtain 12-lead electrocardiogram to be read within 10 minutes.
- Obtain laboratory blood specimens of cardiac biomarkers, including troponin.
- Obtain other diagnostics to clarify the diagnosis.
- Begin routine medical interventions:
  - Supplemental oxygen
  - Nitroglycerin
  - Morphine
  - Aspirin
  - Beta-blocker
  - Angiotensin-converting enzyme inhibitor within 36 hours
  - Anticoagulation with heparin and platelet inhibitors
  - Statin
- Evaluate for indications for reperfusion therapy:
  - Percutaneous coronary intervention
  - Thrombolytic (fibrinolytic) therapy
- Continue therapy as indicated:
  - IV heparin, low-molecular-weight heparin, bivalirudin, or fondaparinux
  - Clopidogrel (Plavix)
  - Glycoprotein IIb/IIIa inhibitor
  - Bed rest for a minimum of 12–24 hours
  - Statin prescribed at discharge.

Adapted from O'Gara, P. T., Kushner, F. G., Ascheim, D. D., et al. (2013). 2013 ACCF/AHA guideline for the management of ST-elevation myocardial infarction: A report of the American College of cardiology Foundation/American Heart Association Task Force on practice guidelines. *Circulation, 127*(4), e362–e425.

may also be prescribed along with platelet-inhibiting agents to prevent further clot formation.

Thrombolytics (Fibrinolytics)

Thrombolytic (fibrinolytic) therapy is initiated when primary PCI is not available or the transport time to a PCI-capable hospital is too long and there is clear evidence of acute MI on the ECG. These agents are administered IV according to a specific protocol (see Chart 29-10). The thrombolytic (fibrinolytic) agents used most often are alteplase (Activase), reteplase (Retavase), and tenecteplase (TNKase). The purpose of thrombolytics (fibrinolytics) is to dissolve (i.e., lyse) the thrombus in a coronary artery (thrombolysis), allowing blood to flow through the coronary artery again (reperfusion), minimizing the size of the infarction and preserving ventricular function. However, although thrombolytics (fibrinolytics) may dissolve the thrombus, they do not affect the underlying atherosclerotic lesion. The patient should be referred for a cardiac catheterization and other invasive procedures following the use of thrombolytic (fibrinolytic) therapy. They should be ideally given within 30 minutes of presentation to the hospital. This is frequently referred to as door-to-needle time.

Thrombolytics (fibrinolytics) should not be used if the patient is bleeding or has a bleeding disorder. Fibrinolytics dissolve all clots, not just the one in the coronary artery. Thus, there are absolute and relative contraindications that must be considered prior to the administration of fibrinolytics. All patients who receive fibrinolytic therapy are placed on bleeding precautions to minimize the risk for bleeding. This means minimizing the number of punctures for inserting IV lines, avoiding IM injections, preventing tissue trauma, and applying pressure for longer than usual after any puncture.

Analgesics

The analgesic of choice for acute MI is morphine sulphate administered in IV boluses to reduce pain and anxiety. It reduces preload and afterload, which decreases the workload of the heart. Morphine also relaxes bronchioles to enhance oxygenation. The cardiovascular response to morphine is monitored carefully, as both blood pressure and respiratory rate, can be depressed.

Angiotensin-Converting Enzyme Inhibitors

Angiotensin-converting enzyme (ACE) inhibitors prevent the conversion of angiotensin I to angiotensin II. In the absence of angiotensin II, the blood pressure decreases and the kidneys excrete sodium and fluid (diuresis), decreasing the oxygen demand of the heart. Use of ACE inhibitors in patients after MI decreases mortality rates and prevents remodeling of myocardial cells that is associated with the onset of heart failure. It is important to ensure that the patient is not hypotensive, hyponatremic, hypovolemic, or hyperkalemic before administering ACE inhibitors. Blood pressure, urine output, and serum sodium, potassium, and creatinine levels need to be monitored closely. If an ACE inhibitor cannot be used because of side effects, an angiotensin receptor blocker (ARB) should be prescribed.

Inpatient Management

Following PCI or thrombolytic (fibrinolytic) therapy, continuous cardiac monitoring is indicated, preferably in a cardiac intensive care unit (CICU). Continuing pharmacologic management includes aspirin, a beta-blocker, an ACE inhibitor and a lipid lowering. ACE inhibitors prevent the conversion of angiotensin I to angiotensin II. In the absence of angiotensin II, the blood pressure decreases and the kidneys excrete sodium and fluid (diuresis), decreasing the oxygen demand of the heart. The use of ACE inhibitors in patients after MI decreases mortality rates and prevents remodeling of myocardial cells that is associated with the onset of heart failure. Blood pressure, urine output, and serum sodium, potassium, and creatinine levels need to be monitored closely. If an ACE inhibitor is not suitable, an ARB should be prescribed (Amsterdam, Wenger, Brindis, et al., 2014). Nicotine replacement therapy and smoking cessation counselling should also be initiated for smokers.

CHART 29-10

Pharmacology: Administration of Fibrinolytic Therapy

Indications

- Chest pain for longer than 20 minutes, unrelieved by nitroglycerin
- ST-segment elevation in at least two leads that face the same area of the heart
- Less than 6 hours from onset of pain

Absolute Contraindications

- Active bleeding
- Known bleeding disorder
- History of hemorrhagic stroke
- History of intracranial vessel malformation
- Recent major surgery or trauma
- Uncontrolled hypertension
- Pregnancy

Nursing Considerations

- Minimize the number of times the patient's skin is punctured.
- Avoid intramuscular injections.
- Draw blood for laboratory tests when starting the intravenous (IV) line.
- Start IV lines before fibrinolytic therapy; designate one line to use for blood draws.
- Avoid continual use of a noninvasive blood pressure cuff.
- Monitor for acute dysrhythmias and hypotension.
- Monitor for reperfusion: resolution of angina or acute ST-segment changes.
- Check for signs and symptoms of bleeding: decrease in hematocrit and hemoglobin values, decrease in blood pressure, increase in heart rate, oozing or bulging at invasive procedure sites, back pain, muscle weakness, changes in level of consciousness, complaints of headache.
- Treat major bleeding by discontinuing fibrinolytic therapy and any anticoagulants; apply direct pressure and notify the physician immediately.
- Treat minor bleeding by applying direct pressure if accessible and appropriate; continue to monitor.

Adapted from Urden, L. D., Stacy, K. M., & Lough, M. E. (2014). *Critical care nursing* (7th ed.). St. Louis, MO: Elsevier.

Emergent Percutaneous Coronary Intervention

The patient with STEMI is taken directly to the cardiac catheterization laboratory for an immediate PCI (if a cardiac catheterization laboratory is on site). PCI is used to open the occluded coronary artery and promote reperfusion to the area that has been deprived of oxygen. Superior outcomes have been reported with the use of PCI when compared to thrombolytic (Amsterdam et al., 2014) (also called *fibrinolytic*) agents; see the Thrombolytics (Fibrinolytics) section. Early PCI can be effective in patients of all ages, including those older than 75 years (Solhpour, Chang, Balan, et al., 2014). The choice between PCI and a fibrinolytic will depend in part on resources and access. Each is effective if initiated in a timely manner. PCI treats the underlying atherosclerotic lesion. Because the duration of oxygen deprivation is directly related to the number of cells that die, the time from the patient's arrival in the emergency department to the time PCI is performed should be less than 60 minutes (time is muscle). This is frequently referred to as *door-to-balloon time*. A cardiac catheterization laboratory and staff must be available if an emergent PCI is to be performed within this short time. The nursing care related to PCI is presented later in this chapter.

Cardiac Rehabilitation

After the MI patient is free of symptoms, an active rehabilitation program is initiated. Cardiac rehabilitation is an important program for patients with CAD that targets risk reduction by means of education, individual and group support, and physical activity. Large reviews have shown that cardiac rehabilitation can increase survival, reduce recurrent events and the need for interventional procedures, and improve the quality of life (Moe, Ezekowitz, O'Meara, et al., 2013). Cardiac rehabilitation programs are offered throughout Canada in both urban and rural settings. Patients eligible for programs may be diagnosed with angina or have had coronary artery bypass surgery. However, despite the potential benefits to this wide range of patients, internationally only around one third of patients who are eligible for cardiac rehabilitation programs participate (Moe et al., 2013).

The immediate objectives of cardiac rehabilitation are to limit the effects and progression of atherosclerosis, return the patient to work and pre-illness lifestyle, enhance the psychosocial and vocational status of the patient, and prevent another cardiac event. These objectives are accomplished by encouraging physical activity and physical conditioning, educating the patient and family, and providing counselling and behavioural interventions.

Throughout all phases of rehabilitation, the goals of activity and exercise tolerance are achieved through gradual physical conditioning, aimed at improving cardiac efficiency over time. Cardiac efficiency is achieved when work and activities of daily living can be performed at a lower heart rate and lower blood pressure, thereby reducing the heart's oxygen requirements and reducing cardiac workload.

Physical conditioning is achieved gradually over time. It is not unusual for patients to "overdo it" in an attempt to achieve their goals too rapidly. Patients are observed for chest pain, dyspnea, weakness, fatigue, and palpitations and are instructed to stop exercise if any of these develop. In a monitored program, they are also monitored for an increase in heart rate above the target heart rate, an increase in systolic or diastolic blood pressure of more than 20 mm Hg, a decrease in systolic blood pressure, onset or worsening of dysrhythmias, or ST-segment changes on the ECG.

The target heart rate during hospitalization is an increase of less than 10% from the resting heart rate, or 120 beats/min. Following discharge, the target heart rate is based on the patient's stress test results (usually 60% to 85% of the heart rate at which symptoms occurred), medications, and underlying condition. Oxygen saturation may also be assessed through pulse oximetry to ensure that it remains higher than 93%. If signs or symptoms occur, the patient is instructed to slow down or stop exercising. If the patient is exercising in an unmonitored program, he or she is cautioned to cease activity immediately if signs or symptoms occur and to seek appropriate medical attention.

Patients who are able to walk 5 to 6 km/hr (3 to 4 miles/hr) can usually resume sexual activities. The nurse recommends that the patient be well rested and in a familiar setting, wait at least 1 hour after eating or drinking alcohol, and use a comfortable position. Sexual dysfunction or cardiac symptoms should be reported to the health care provider.

Phases of Cardiac Rehabilitation

Cardiac rehabilitation occurs along the continuum of the disease. It is typically categorized in three phases.

Phase I begins with the diagnosis of atherosclerosis, which may occur when the patient is admitted to the hospital for ACS (e.g., unstable angina or acute MI). It consists of low-level activities and initial education for the patient and family. Because of today's brief hospital stays, mobilization occurs earlier and patient teaching focuses on the essentials of self-care, rather than instituting behavioural changes for risk reduction. Priorities for in-hospital teaching include the signs and symptoms that indicate the need to call 911 (seek emergency assistance), the medication regimen, rest–activity balance, and follow-up appointments with the physician. The nurse needs to reassure the patient that although CAD is a lifelong disease and must be treated as such, most patients can resume a normal life after an MI. This positive approach while in the hospital helps to motivate and teach the patient to continue the education and lifestyle changes that are usually needed after discharge. The amount of activity recommended at discharge depends on the age of the patient, his or her condition before the cardiac event, the extent of the disease, the course of the hospital stay, and the development of any complications.

Phase II occurs after the patient has been discharged. It usually lasts for 4 to 6 weeks but may last as long as 6 months. This outpatient program consists of supervised, often ECG-monitored, exercise training that is individualized based on the results of an exercise stress test. Moderate intensity exercise and strength training are introduced (Moe et al., 2013). Support and guidance related to the treatment of the disease and teaching and counselling related to lifestyle modification for risk factor reduction are a part of this phase. Short-term and long-range goals are collaboratively determined based on the patient's needs. At each session, the patient is assessed for the effectiveness of and adherence to the medical plan. To prevent complications and another hospitalization, the cardiac rehabilitation staff alerts the referring physician to any problems.

Outpatient cardiac rehabilitation programs are designed to encourage patients and families to support each other. Many programs offer support sessions for spouses and significant others while the patients exercise. The programs involve group educational sessions for both patients and families that are given by cardiologists, exercise physiologists, dietitians, nurses, and other health care professionals. These sessions may take place outside a traditional classroom setting. For instance, a dietitian may take a group of patients and their families to a grocery store to examine labels and meat selections or to a restaurant to discuss menu offerings for a "heart-healthy" diet.

Phase III (also called the *community-based phase*) focuses on maintaining cardiovascular stability and long-term conditioning. The patient is usually self-directed during this phase and does not require a supervised program, although it may be offered. The goals of each phase build on the accomplishments of the previous phase.

Nursing Process

The Patient With Acute Coronary Syndrome

Assessment

One of the most important aspects of care of the patient with an ACS is the assessment. It establishes the baseline for the patient so that any deviations may be identified, systematically identifies the patient's needs, and helps to determine the priority of those needs. Systematic assessment includes a careful history, particularly as it relates to symptoms: chest pain or discomfort, difficulty breathing (dyspnea), palpitations, unusual fatigue, faintness (syncope), or sweating (diaphoresis). Each symptom must be evaluated with regard to time, duration, and the factors that precipitate the symptom and relieve it and in comparison with previous symptoms (OPQRST of each symptom). A focused physical assessment is critical to detect complications and any change in patient status. Chart 29-8 identifies important assessments and possible findings.

Two IV lines are typically placed for any patient with ACS to ensure that access is available for administering emergency medications. Medications are administered intravenously to achieve rapid onset and to allow for timely adjustment. After the patient's condition stabilizes, IV lines may be changed to a saline lock to maintain IV access.

Nursing Priorities

Based on the clinical manifestations, history, and diagnostic assessment data, major nursing priorities may include the following:

- Altered Fluid volume balance
- Decreased peripheral perfusion
- Anxiety
- Lack of knowledge

Collaborative Problems/ Potential Complications

Based on the assessment data, potential complications that may develop include the following:

- Acute pulmonary edema (see Chapter 26)
- Heart failure (see Chapter 31)
- Cardiogenic shock (see Chapter 31)
- Dysrhythmias and cardiac arrest (see Chapters 28 and 31)
- Pericardial effusion and cardiac tamponade (see Chapter 30)

Planning and Goals

The major goals for the patient include relief of pain or ischemic signs and symptoms (e.g., ST-segment changes), prevention of further myocardial damage, absence of respiratory dysfunction, maintenance or attainment of adequate tissue perfusion by decreasing the heart's workload, reduced anxiety, adherence to the self-care program, and absence or early recognition of complications. Care of the patient with an uncomplicated ACS event is summarized in the Plan of Nursing Care (Chart 29-11).

Nursing Interventions

Relieving Pain and Other Signs and Symptoms of Ischemia

Balancing myocardial oxygen supply with demand (e.g., as evidenced by the relief of chest pain/discomfort) is the top priority in the care of the patient with an ACS. Although medication therapy is required to accomplish this goal, nursing interventions are also important. Collaboration among the patient, nurse, and physician is critical in assessing the patient's response to therapy and in altering the interventions accordingly.

The recommended treatment for acute MI is reperfusion, including fibrinolytic therapy or emergent PCI for patients who present to the health care facility immediately and who have no major contraindications. Use of a GPIIb/IIIa agent or PCI may be indicated for non-STEMIs. These therapies are important because in addition to relieving symptoms, they aid in minimizing or avoiding permanent injury to the myocardium. With or without reperfusion, administration of aspirin, an IV beta-blocker, and nitroglycerin is indicated. The nurse administers morphine to relieve pain and anxiety and to promote vasodilation, reducing preload and afterload.

Oxygen should be administered if the patient is hypoxemic along with medication therapy to assist with relief of symptoms. Administration of oxygen even in low doses raises the circulating level of oxygen to reduce pain associated with low levels of myocardial oxygen. The route of administration, usually

Plan of Nursing Care

Chart 29-11. Care of the Patient With an Uncomplicated Myocardial Infarction

Nursing Priority: Decreased myocardial perfusion
Goal: Relief of chest pain/discomfort

NURSING INTERVENTIONS	RATIONALE	EXPECTED PATIENT OUTCOMES
1. Initially assess, document, and report to the physician the following:	1. These data assist in determining the cause and effect of the chest discomfort and provide a baseline with which posttherapy symptoms can be compared	• Reports beginning relief of chest discomfort and symptoms • Appears comfortable and is free of pain and other signs or symptoms: Respiratory rate, cardiac rate, and blood pressure return to prediscomfort level Skin warm and dry • Adequate cardiac output as evidenced by stable/improving: Electrocardiogram (ECG) • Heart rate and rhythm Blood pressure Mentation Urine output Serum blood urea nitrogen (BUN) and creatinine Skin colour, temperature, and moisture
a. The patient's description of chest discomfort, including location, intensity, radiation, duration, and factors that affect it. Other symptoms such as nausea, diaphoresis, or complaints of unusual fatigue	a. There are many conditions associated with chest discomfort. There are characteristic clinical findings of ischemic pain and symptoms	
b. The effect of chest discomfort on cardiovascular perfusion—to the heart (e.g., change in blood pressure, heart sounds), to the brain (e.g., changes in level of consciousness), to the kidneys (e.g., decrease in urine output), and to the skin (e.g., colour, temperature)	b. Myocardial infarction (MI) decreases myocardial contractility and ventricular compliance and may produce dysrhythmias. Cardiac output is reduced, resulting in reduced blood pressure and decreased organ perfusion. The heart rate may increase as a compensatory mechanism to maintain cardiac output	
2. Obtain a 12-lead ECG recording during the symptomatic event, as prescribed, to determine extension of infarction	2. An ECG during symptoms may be useful in the diagnosis of an extension of MI	
3. Administer oxygen as prescribed	3. Oxygen therapy increases the oxygen supply to the myocardium if actual oxygen saturation is less than normal	
4. Administer medication therapy as prescribed and evaluate the patient's response continuously	4. Medication therapy (nitroglycerin, morphine, beta-blocker aspirin) is the first line of defense in preserving myocardial tissue. The side effects of these medications can be hazardous, and the patient's status must be assessed	
5. Ensure physical rest: use of the bedside commode with assistance; backrest elevated to promote comfort; diet as tolerated; arms supported during upper extremity activity; use of stool softener to prevent straining at stool. Provide a restful environment, and allay fears and anxiety by being supportive, calm, and competent. Individualize visitation, based on patient response	5. Physical rest reduces myocardial oxygen consumption. Fear and anxiety precipitate the stress response; this results in increased levels of endogenous catecholamines, which increase myocardial oxygen consumption. Also, with increased epinephrine, the pain threshold is decreased, and pain increases myocardial oxygen consumption	

continued >

Plan of Nursing Care

Chart 29-11. Care of the Patient With an Uncomplicated Myocardial Infarction, *Continued*

NURSING INTERVENTIONS	RATIONALE	EXPECTED PATIENT OUTCOMES
Nursing Priority: Decreased gas exchange **Goal:** Absence of respiratory difficulties		
1. Initially, every 4 hours, and with chest discomfort or symptoms, assess, document, and report to the physician abnormal heart sounds (particularly S_3 and S_4 gallops and the holosystolic murmur of left ventricular papillary muscle dysfunction), abnormal breath sounds (particularly crackles), and patient intolerance to specific activities	1. These data are useful in diagnosing left ventricular failure. Diastolic filling sounds (S_3 and S_4 gallop) result from decreased left ventricular compliance associated with MI. Papillary muscle dysfunction (from infarction of the papillary muscle) can result in mitral regurgitation and a reduction in stroke volume, leading to left ventricular failure. The presence of crackles (usually at the lung bases) may indicate pulmonary congestion from increased left heart pressures. The association of symptoms and activity can be used as a guide for activity prescription and a basis for patient teaching	• No shortness of breath, dyspnea on exertion, orthopnea, or paroxysmal nocturnal dyspnea • Respiratory rate less than 20 breaths/min with physical activity and 16 breaths/min with rest • Skin colour normal • PaO_2 and $PaCO_2$ within normal range • Heart rate less than 100 beats/min and greater than 60 beats/min, with blood pressure within patient's normal limits • Chest x-ray normal • Relief of chest discomfort • Appears comfortable • Appears rested • Respiratory rate, cardiac rate, and blood pressure return to pre-discomfort level • Skin warm and dry
2. Teach the patient: a. To adhere to the diet prescribed (e.g., explain low-sodium, low-calorie diet)	2. a. A low-sodium diet may reduce extracellular volume, thus reducing preload and afterload and thus myocardial oxygen consumption. In patients with obesity, weight reduction may decrease cardiac work and improve tidal volume	
b. To adhere to the activity prescription	b. The activity prescription is determined individually to maintain the heart rate and blood pressure within safe limits	
Nursing Priority: Decreased peripheral tissue perfusion **Goal:** Maintenance/attainment of adequate tissue perfusion		
1. Initially, every 4 hours, and with chest discomfort, assess, document, and report to the physician the following: a. Hypotension b. Tachycardia and other dysrhythmia c. Activity intolerance d. Mentation changes (use family input) e. Reduced urine output (less than 200 mL per 8 hours) f. Cool, moist, cyanotic extremities	1. These data are useful in determining a low cardiac output state. An ECG with pain may be useful in the diagnosis of an extension of myocardial ischemia, injury, and infarction and of variant angina	• Blood pressure within the patient's normal range • Ideally, normal sinus rhythm without dysrhythmia is maintained, or patient's baseline rhythm is maintained between 60 and 100 beats/min without further dysrhythmia. • No complaints of fatigue with prescribed activity • Remains fully alert and oriented and without cognitive or behavioural change • Appears comfortable • Urine output greater than 30 mL/hr • Extremities warm and dry with normal colour

Plan of Nursing Care Chart 29-11. Care of the Patient With an Uncomplicated Myocardial Infarction, *Continued*

NURSING INTERVENTIONS	RATIONALE	EXPECTED PATIENT OUTCOMES
Nursing Priority: Anxiety **Goal:** Reduction of anxiety		
1. Assess, document, and report to the physician the patient and family's level of anxiety and coping mechanisms	1. These data provide information about the psychological well-being and a baseline so that posttherapy symptoms can be compared. Causes of anxiety are variable and individual and may include acute illness, hospitalization, pain, disruption of activities of daily living at home and at work, changes in role and self-image due to illness, and financial concerns. Because anxious family members can transmit anxiety to the patient, the nurse must also identify strategies to reduce the family's fear and anxiety	• Reports less anxiety • Patient and family discuss their anxieties and fears about death • Patient and family appear less anxious • Appears restful, respiratory rate less than 16/min heart rate less than 100/min without ectopic beats, blood pressure within patient's normal limits, skin warm and dry • Participates actively in a progressive rehabilitation program • Practices stress reduction techniques
2. Assess the need for spiritual counselling and refer as appropriate	2. If a patient finds support in a religion, spiritual counselling may assist in reducing anxiety and fear	
3. Assess the need for social service referral	3. Social services can assist with post-hospital care and financial concerns	
4. Allow the patient (and family) to express anxiety and fear: a. By showing genuine interest and concern b. By facilitating communication (listening, reflecting, guiding) c. By answering questions	4. Unresolved anxiety (the stress response) increases myocardial oxygen consumption	
5. Use of flexible visiting hours allows the presence of a supportive family to assist in reducing the patient's level of anxiety	5. The presence of supportive family members may reduce patient and family's anxiety	
6. Encourage active participation in a cardiac rehabilitation program	6. Prescribed cardiac rehabilitation may help reduce anxiety, enhance feelings of well-being, and facilitate compliance with risk factor recommendations	
7. Teach stress reduction techniques	7. Stress reduction may help to reduce myocardial oxygen consumption and may enhance feelings of well-being	
Nursing Priority: Lack of knowledge **Goal:** Adheres to the home health care program Chooses lifestyle consistent with heart-healthy recommendations.		

See Chart 29-12, Promoting Health after MI and Other Acute Coronary Syndromes.

by nasal cannula, and the oxygen flow rate are documented. A flow rate of 2–4 L/min is usually adequate to maintain oxygen saturation levels of over 94% if no other disease is present.

Vital signs are assessed frequently as long as the patient is experiencing pain and other signs or symptoms of acute ischemia. Physical rest in bed with the backrest elevated or in a cardiac chair helps to decrease chest discomfort and dyspnea. Elevation of the head and torso is beneficial for the following reasons:

- Tidal volume improves because of reduced pressure from abdominal contents on the diaphragm and better lung expansion and gas exchange.
- Drainage of the upper lung lobes improves.
- Venous return to the heart (preload) decreases, reducing the work of the heart.

The pain associated with an acute MI reflects an imbalance in myocardial oxygen supply and demand or ineffective myocardial tissue perfusion. The pain also results in increases in heart rate, respiratory rate, and blood pressure. Promptly relieving the pain helps to reestablish this balance, thus decreasing the workload of the heart and minimizing damage to the myocardium. Relief of pain also helps to reduce the patient's anxiety level, which in turn reduces the sympathetic stress response, leading to a decrease in workload of the already stressed heart.

Improving Respiratory Function

Regular and careful assessment of respiratory function can help the nurse detect early signs of pulmonary complications. The nurse monitors fluid volume status to prevent fluid overload and encourages the patient to breathe deeply and change position frequently to maintain effective ventilation throughout the lungs. Pulse oximetry guides the use of oxygen therapy.

Promoting Adequate Tissue Perfusion

During the initial phase of treatment the patient should be limited to bed or chair rest as it reduces myocardial oxygen consumption. This limitation on mobility should remain until the patient is pain free and hemodynamically stable. Checking skin temperature and peripheral pulses frequently is important to monitor tissue perfusion.

Reducing Anxiety

Alleviating anxiety and decreasing fear are important nursing functions that reduce the sympathetic stress response. Decreased sympathetic stimulation decreases the workload of the heart, which may relieve pain and other signs and symptoms of ischemia.

The development of a trusting and caring relationship with the patient is critical in reducing anxiety. Providing information to the patient and family in an honest and supportive manner encourages the patient to be a partner in care and greatly assists in developing a positive relationship. Other nursing interventions that can be used to reduce anxiety include ensuring a quiet environment, preventing interruptions that disturb sleep, teaching the patient relaxation techniques, and providing spiritual support consistent with the patient's beliefs. The nurse should also provide opportunities for the patient to privately share concerns and fears. An atmosphere of acceptance helps the patient know that these concerns and fears are both realistic and normal. Music therapy is an effective method of reducing anxiety and managing stress (Bradt, Dileo, & Potvin, 2013). An alternative therapy, such as pet therapy, can assist certain patients by the providing emotional support and thereby reducing anxiety. Many hospitals have developed guidelines for the infection control and safety procedures pertaining to animals, their handlers, and the patients eligible for pet therapy.

Monitoring and Managing Potential Complications

Complications that can occur after an ACS are caused by the damage that occurs to the myocardium and the conduction system as a result of the reduced coronary blood flow. Because these complications can be life threatening, close monitoring for and early identification of their signs and symptoms are critical (see the Plan of Nursing Care).

The nurse monitors the patient closely for changes in cardiac rate and rhythm, heart sounds, blood pressure, chest pain, respiratory status, urinary output, skin colour and temperature, sensorium, 12-lead ECG changes, and laboratory values. Any changes in the patient's condition are reported promptly to the most responsible care provider, and emergency measures are instituted when necessary.

Promoting Home, Community-Based, and Transitional Care

EDUCATING PATIENTS ABOUT SELF-CARE. The most effective way to increase the probability that the patient will implement a self-care regimen after discharge is to identify the priorities as perceived by the patient, provide adequate education about heart-healthy living, and facilitate the patient's involvement in a cardiac rehabilitation program. Working with patients in developing plans to meet their specific needs further enhances the potential for an effective treatment plan (Chart 29-12).

CONTINUING AND TRANSITIONAL CARE. Depending on the patient's condition and the availability of family assistance, a referral for home, community-based, or transitional care may be indicated. The home care nurse assists the patient with scheduling and keeping follow-up appointments and with adhering to the prescribed cardiac rehabilitation regimen. The patient may need reminders about follow-up monitoring, including periodic blood laboratory testing and ECGs. In addition, the home care nurse may monitor the patient's adherence to dietary restrictions and to prescribed medications. If the patient is receiving home oxygen, the nurse ensures that the patient is using the oxygen as prescribed and that appropriate home safety measures are maintained. If the patient has evidence of heart failure secondary to the MI, appropriate home care guidelines for the patient with heart failure are followed (see Chapter 31).

Evaluation

Expected patient outcomes may include the following:

1. Experiences relief of angina
2. Has stable cardiac and respiratory status
3. Maintains adequate tissue perfusion
4. Reports decreased anxiety
5. Adheres to a self-care program
6. Reports no complications

CHART 29-12

Health Promotion: Promoting Health After Myocardial Infarction and Other Acute Coronary Syndromes

To extend and improve the quality of life, a patient who has had a myocardial infarction (MI) must learn to adjust his or her lifestyle to promote heart-healthy living. With this in mind, the nurse and patient develop a program to help the patient achieve desired outcomes.

Changing Lifestyle During Convalescence and Healing

Adaptation to an MI is an ongoing process and usually requires some modification of lifestyle. Some specific modifications include the following:

- Avoiding any activity that produces chest pain, extreme dyspnea, or undue fatigue
- Avoiding extremes of heat and cold and walking against the wind
- Losing weight, if indicated
- Stopping smoking and use of tobacco; avoiding secondhand smoke
- Using personal strengths to support lifestyle changes
- Developing heart-healthy eating patterns and avoiding large meals and hurrying while eating
- Modifying meals to align with the Mediterranean Diet, Dietary Approaches to Stopping Hypertension (DASH) diet, or the Therapeutic Lifestyle Changes (TLC)
- Adhering to the medical regimen, especially in taking medications
- Following recommendations that ensure blood pressure and blood glucose are in control
- Pursuing activities that relieve and reduce stress

Adopting an Activity Program

Additionally, the patient needs to undertake an *orderly* program of increasing activity and exercise for long-term rehabilitation as follows:

- Engaging in a regimen of physical conditioning with a gradual increase in activity duration and then a gradual increase in activity intensity
- Walking daily, increasing distance and time as prescribed
- Monitoring pulse rate during physical activity until the maximum level of activity is attained
- Avoiding activities that tense the muscles: isometric exercise, weightlifting, or any activity that requires sudden bursts of energy
- Avoiding physical exercise immediately after a meal
- Alternating activity with rest periods (some fatigue is normal and expected during convalescence)
- Participating in a daily program of exercise that develops into a program of regular exercise for a lifetime

Managing Symptoms

The patient must learn to recognize and take appropriate action for possible recurrences of symptoms as follows:

- Call 911 if chest pressure or pain (or anginal equivalent) is not relieved in 15 minutes by nitroglycerin
- Contact the physician if any of the following occur: shortness of breath, fainting, slow or rapid heartbeat, or swelling of feet and ankles

INVASIVE CORONARY ARTERY PROCEDURES

Methods to reperfuse ischemic myocardial tissue when patients are refractory to more conservative management methods include PCIs and CABG surgery, as noted previously. The following sections discuss specific indications for each of these and the nursing management of patients who are having either PCIs or CABGs.

Percutaneous Coronary Interventions

Invasive interventional procedures to treat angina and CAD include PTCA, intracoronary stent implantation. All of these procedures are classified as percutaneous coronary interventions (PCIs).

Types of Procedures

Percutaneous Transluminal Coronary Angioplasty

In PTCA, a balloon-tipped catheter is used to open blocked coronary vessels and resolve ischemia. It is used in patients with angina and as an intervention for acute MI. Catheter-based interventions can sometimes also be used to open blocked CABGs. The purpose of PTCA is to improve blood flow within a coronary artery by compressing the atheroma. The procedure is attempted when the cardiologist believes that PTCA can improve blood flow to the myocardium.

PTCA is carried out in the cardiac catheterization laboratory. Hollow catheters called *sheaths* are inserted, in the radial or femoral artery providing a conduit for other catheters. Catheters are then threaded through the artery, up through the aorta, and into the coronary arteries. Angiography is performed using injected radiopaque contrast agents (commonly called *dye*) to identify the location and extent of the blockage. A balloon-tipped dilation catheter is passed through the sheath and positioned over the lesion. The physician determines the catheter position by examining markers on the balloon that can be seen with fluoroscopy. When the catheter is properly positioned, the balloon is inflated with high pressure for several seconds and then deflated. The pressure compresses and possibly "cracks" the atheroma (Fig. 29-7). The media and adventitia of the coronary artery are also stretched.

Several inflations and several balloon sizes may be required to achieve the goal, usually defined as an improvement in blood flow and a residual stenosis of less than 30%. Other measures of the success of a PTCA are an increase in the artery's lumen and no clinically obvious arterial trauma. Because the blood supply to the coronary artery decreases while the balloon is inflated, the patient may complain of chest pain and the ECG may display significant ST-segment changes. Intracoronary stents are

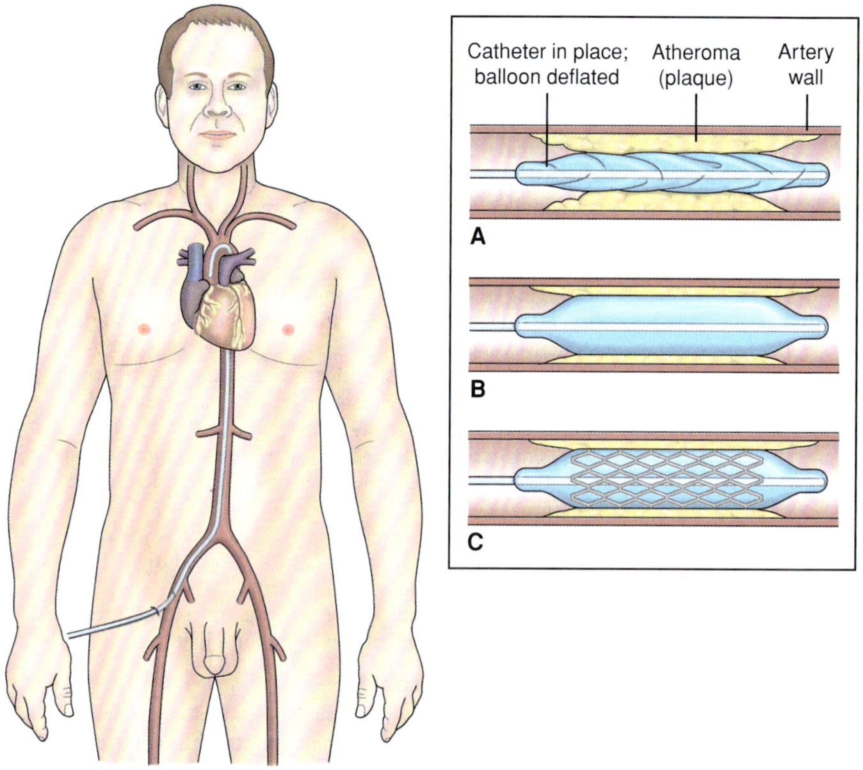

FIGURE 29-7. Percutaneous transluminal coronary angioplasty. **A.** A balloon-tipped catheter is passed into the affected coronary artery and placed across the area of the atheroma (plaque). **B.** The balloon is then rapidly inflated and deflated with controlled pressure. **C.** A stent is placed to maintain patency of the artery, and the balloon is removed.

usually positioned in the intima of the vessel to maintain patency after the balloon is withdrawn.

Coronary Artery Stent

After PTCA, the area that has been treated may close off partially or completely, a process called *restenosis*. The intima of the coronary artery has been injured and responds by initiating an acute inflammatory process. This process may include release of mediators that lead to vasoconstriction, clotting, and scar tissue formation. A coronary artery stent is placed to overcome these risks. A **stent** is a metal mesh that provides structural support to a vessel at risk of acute closure. The stent is positioned over the angioplasty balloon. When the balloon is inflated, the mesh expands and presses against the vessel wall, holding the artery open. The balloon is withdrawn, but the stent is left permanently in place within the artery (see Fig. 29-7). Eventually, endothelium covers the stent, and it is incorporated into the vessel wall. The original stents do not contain medications and are known as bare metal stents. Some stents are coated with medications, such as sirolimus (Rapamune) or paclitaxel (Taxol), which may minimize the formation of thrombi or scar tissue within the coronary artery lesion. These drug-eluting stents have increased the success of PCI (Palmerini, Benedetto, Biondi-Zoccai, et al., 2015). The patient receives antiplatelet medications (e.g., Clopidogrel [Plavix], or Brilinta [Ticagrelor] and lifetime use of aspirin) because of the risk of re-stenosis and thrombus formation in the stent.

The majority of PCIs in Canada involve implanting at least one stent to maintain perfusion. Stents are used most commonly in conjunction with PTCA, but may be used independently as a PCI. Care of the patient after coronary artery stent placement is the same as for a patient after PTCA.

Complications

Complications that can occur during a PCI procedure include dissection, perforation, abrupt closure, or vasospasm of the coronary artery; acute MI; acute dysrhythmias (e.g., ventricular tachycardia); and cardiac arrest. Some of these complications may require emergency surgical treatment (e.g., dissection). Complications after the procedure may include abrupt closure of the coronary artery and vascular complications, such as bleeding at the insertion site, retroperitoneal bleeding, hematoma, pseudo-aneurysm, arteriovenous fistula, or arterial thrombosis. In addition, there is a risk of acute kidney injury from the contrast agent used during the procedure (Ferreira, de Souza E Silva, & Salis, 2018) (see Table 29-4).

Postprocedure Care

Postprocedure patient care is similar to that for a cardiac catheterization (see Chapter 29). Many patients are admitted to the hospital on the day of the PCI. Those with no complications go home the next day. When the PCI is performed emergently to treat ACS, the patient will usually go to a CICU and stay in the hospital for a few days. During the PCI, patients receive IV heparin and are monitored closely for signs of bleeding. Patients may also receive a GPIIb/IIIa agent (e.g., eptifibatide [Integrilin]) for several hours following the PCI to prevent platelet aggregation and thrombus formation in the coronary artery. Hemostasis is achieved, and radial or femoral sheaths may be removed at the end of the procedure by using a vascular closure device (e.g., Angio-Seal, VasoSeal) or a device that sutures the vessels. Hemostasis after sheath removal may also be achieved by direct manual pressure, a mechanical

TABLE 29-4 Complications After Percutaneous Transluminal Coronary Angioplasty

Complication	Clinical Manifestations	Possible Causes	Nursing Actions
Myocardial ischemia	Chest pain Ischemic changes on ECG Dysrhythmias	Thrombosis Restenosis of coronary artery	Administer oxygen and nitroglycerin. Obtain 12-lead ECG. Notify cardiologist.
Bleeding and hematoma formation	Continuation of bleeding from vascular access site Swelling at site Formation of hard lump Pain with leg movement Possible hypotension and tachycardia	Anticoagulant therapy Vascular trauma Inadequate hemostasis Leg movement	Keep patient on bed rest. Apply manual pressure over sheath insertion site. Outline hematoma with marking pen. Notify primary provider if bleeding continues.
Retroperitoneal hematoma	Back, flank, or abdominal pain Hypotension Tachycardia Restlessness, agitation	Arterial leak of blood into the retroperitoneal space	Notify primary provider. Stop anticoagulants. Administer IV fluids. Anticipate diagnostic testing (e.g., computed tomography scan). Prepare patient for intervention.
Arterial occlusion	Lost/weakened pulse distal to sheath insertion site Extremity cool, cyanotic, painful	Arterial thrombus or embolus	Notify primary provider. Anticipate intervention.
Pseudoaneurysm formation	Swelling at vascular access site Pulsatile mass, bruit	Vessel trauma during the procedure	Notify primary provider. Anticipate intervention.
Arteriovenous fistula formation	Swelling at vascular access site Pulsatile mass, bruit	Vessel trauma during the procedure	Notify primary provider. Anticipate intervention.
Acute kidney injury	Decreased urine output Elevated BUN, serum creatinine	Nephrotoxic contrast agent	Monitor urine output, BUN, creatinine, electrolytes. Provide adequate hydration. Administer renal protective agents (acetylcysteine) before and after procedure as prescribed.

ECG, electrocardiogram; IV, intravenous; BUN, blood urea nitrogen.

Adapted from Urden, L. D., Stacy, K. M., & Lough, M. E. (2014). *Critical care nursing* (7th ed.). St. Louis, MO: Elsevier.

compression device (e.g., C-shaped clamp), or a pneumatic compression device (e.g., FemoStop).

The patient may return to the nursing unit with the large peripheral vascular access sheaths in place. The sheaths are removed after blood studies (e.g., activated clotting time) indicate that the heparin is no longer active and the clotting time is within an acceptable range. This usually takes a few hours, depending on the amount of heparin given during the procedure. The patient must remain flat in bed and keep the affected leg or arm straight until the sheaths are removed and then for a few hours afterward to maintain hemostasis. Because the immobility and bed rest may cause discomfort, treatment may include analgesics and sedation. Sheath removal and the application of pressure on the vessel insertion site may cause the heart rate to slow and the blood pressure to decrease (vasovagal response). An IV bolus of atropine may be given to treat this response.

Some patients with unstable lesions and at high risk for abrupt vessel closure are restarted on heparin after sheath removal, or they receive an IV infusion of a GPIIb/IIIa inhibitor. These patients are monitored more closely and may recover more slowly.

After hemostasis is achieved, a pressure dressing is applied to the site. Patients resume self-care and ambulate unassisted within a few hours of the procedure. The duration of immobilization depends on the size of the sheath inserted, the location of the sheath (radial or femoral), the amount and type of anticoagulant administered, the method of hemostasis, the patient's underlying condition, and the physician's preference. On the day after the procedure, the site is inspected and the dressing replaced with an adhesive bandage. The nurse teaches the patient to monitor the site for bleeding or development of a hard mass indicative of hematoma.

Surgical Procedures: Coronary Artery Revascularization

Advances in diagnostics, medical management, surgical and anesthesia techniques, as well as the care provided in critical care and surgical units, home care, and rehabilitation programs, have continued to make surgery a viable treatment option for patients with CAD. CAD has been treated by myocardial revascularization since the 1960s, and the most common CABG techniques have been performed for approximately 40 years. CABG is a surgical procedure in which a blood vessel is grafted to the occluded coronary artery so that blood can flow beyond the occlusion; it is also called a *bypass graft*.

The major indications for CABG are:

- Alleviation of angina that cannot be controlled with medication or PCI
- Treatment of left main coronary artery stenosis or multivessel CAD

- Prevention and treatment of MI, dysrhythmias, or heart failure
- Treatment for complications from an unsuccessful PCI

The recommendation for CABG is determined by a number of factors, including the number of diseased coronary vessels, the degree of left ventricular dysfunction, the presence of other health problems, the patient's symptoms, and any previous treatment. Studies have shown that CABG may be the preferred treatment for high-risk patients, such as those with severe triple-vessel CAD, ventricular dysfunction, and diabetes (Head & Kappetein, 2016; Nystrom, Sartipy, & Holzmann, 2018). Studies continue to compare clinical outcomes of CABG and PCI in patients with CAD (Ahn, Park, Lee, et al., 2017).

For a patient to be considered for CABG, the coronary arteries to be bypassed must have approximately a 70% occlusion (50% if in the left main coronary artery). If significant blockage is not present, the flow through the artery will compete with the flow through the bypass, and circulation to the ischemic area of myocardium may not be improved. It is also necessary that the artery be patent beyond the area of blockage, or the flow through the bypass will be impeded.

The most common used conduits in CABG are the left internal mammary artery (IMA) (Fig. 29-8) and the saphenous vein. Radial artery grafts can also be used if there is adequate flow from the ulnar artery. Recent studies demonstrate increased survival and freedom from cardiac-related events using bilateral IMA grafting (Davierwala & Mohr, 2015).

A vein commonly used for CABG is the greater saphenous vein, followed by the lesser saphenous vein (Fig. 29-9). The vein is removed from the leg (or arm) and grafted to the ascending aorta and to the coronary artery distal to the lesion. Some locations use endovascular methods of vein harvesting which reduce complications such as infection and wound dehiscence. Lower extremity edema continues to be a common adverse effect of vein removal. The degree of edema varies and usually diminishes over time. Within 5 to 10 years, atherosclerotic changes often develop in saphenous vein grafts.

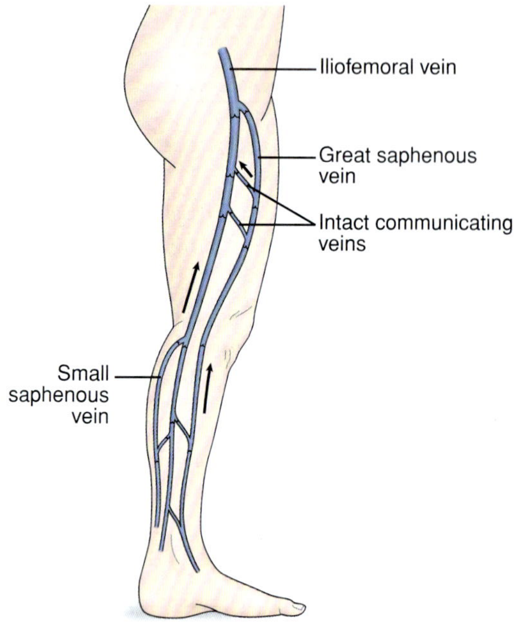

FIGURE 29-9. The greater and lesser saphenous veins are commonly used in bypass graft procedures.

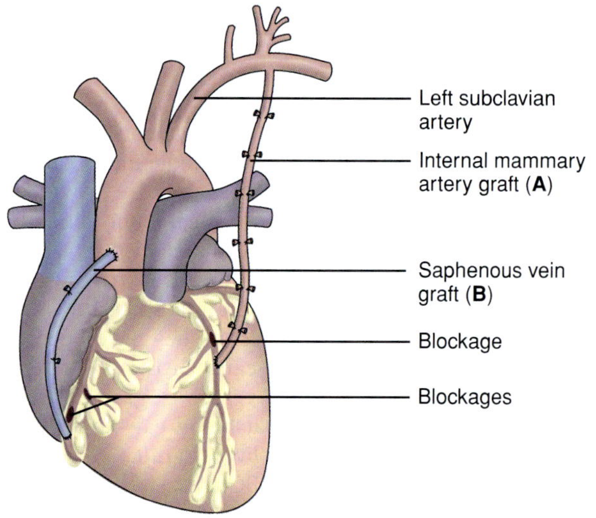

FIGURE 29-8. Coronary artery bypass grafts. One or more procedures may be performed using various veins and arteries. A. Left internal mammary artery, used frequently because of its functional longevity. B. Saphenous vein, also used as bypass graft.

The right and left IMAs and occasionally the radial arteries are also used for CABG. Arterial grafts are preferred to venous grafts because they do not develop atherosclerotic changes as quickly and remain patent longer. The surgeon leaves the proximal end of the mammary artery intact and detaches the distal end of the artery from the chest wall. This end of the artery is then grafted to the coronary artery distal to the occlusion. The IMAs may not be long enough to use for multiple bypasses. Because of this, many CABG procedures are performed with a combination of venous and arterial grafts.

Traditional Coronary Artery Bypass Graft

The traditional CABG procedure is performed with the patient under general anesthesia. The surgeon makes a median sternotomy incision and connects the patient to the cardiopulmonary bypass (CPB) machine. Next, a blood vessel from another part of the patient's body (e.g., saphenous vein, left IMA) is grafted distal to the coronary artery lesion, bypassing the obstruction (see Fig. 29-8). CPB is then discontinued, chest tubes and epicardial pacing wires are placed, and the incision is closed. The patient then is admitted to a critical care unit.

Cardiopulmonary Bypass

Many cardiac surgical procedures are possible because of CPB (i.e., extracorporeal circulation). The procedure mechanically circulates and oxygenates blood for the body while bypassing the heart and lungs. CPB maintains perfusion to body organs and tissues and allows the surgeon to complete the anastomoses in a motionless, bloodless surgical field.

CPB is accomplished by placing a cannula in the right atrium, vena cava, or femoral vein to withdraw blood from the body. The cannula is connected to tubing filled with an

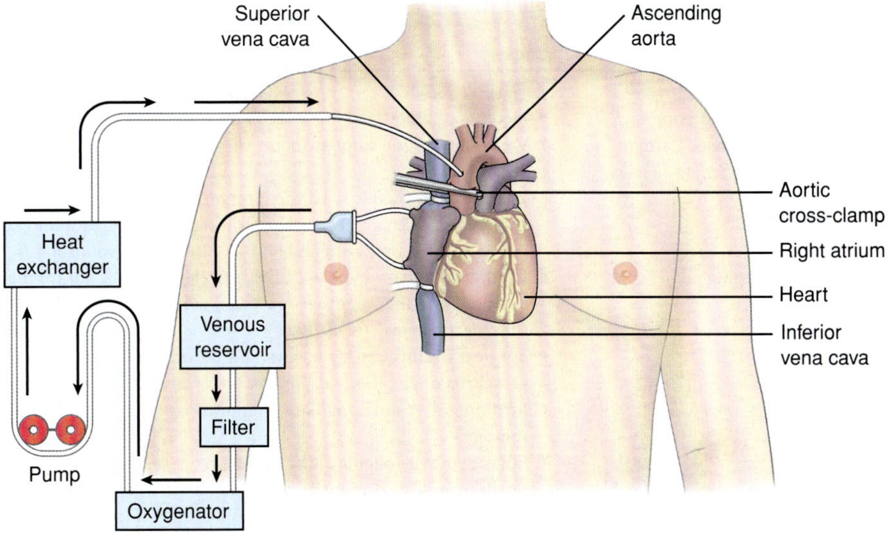

FIGURE 29-10. The cardiopulmonary bypass (CPB) system, in which cannulas are placed through the right atrium into the superior and inferior vena cavae to divert blood from the body and into the bypass system. The pump system creates a vacuum, pulling blood into the venous reservoir. The blood is cleared of air bubbles, clots, and particulates by the filter and then is passed through the oxygenator, releasing CO_2 and obtaining oxygen. Next, the blood is pulled to the pump and pushed out to the heat exchanger, where its temperature is regulated. The blood is then returned to the body via the ascending aorta.

isotonic crystalloid solution. Venous blood removed from the body by the cannula is filtered, oxygenated, cooled or warmed by the machine, and then returned to the body. The cannula used to return the oxygenated blood is usually inserted in the ascending aorta, or it may be inserted in the femoral artery (Fig. 29-10). The heart is stopped by the injection of cardioplegia solution, which is high in potassium, into the coronary arteries. The patient receives heparin to prevent clotting and thrombus formation in the bypass circuit when blood comes in contact with the foreign surfaces of the tubing. At the end of the procedure when the patient is disconnected from the bypass machine, protamine sulphate is administered to reverse the effects of heparin.

During the procedure, hypothermia is maintained, usually 28° to 32°C. The blood is cooled during CPB and returned to the body. The cooled blood slows the body's basal metabolic rate, thereby decreasing the demand for oxygen. Cooled blood usually has a higher viscosity, but the crystalloid solution used to prime the bypass tubing dilutes the blood. When the surgical procedure is completed, the blood is rewarmed as it passes through the CPB circuit. Urine output, arterial blood gases, electrolytes, and coagulation studies are monitored to assess the patient's status during CPB.

Alternative Coronary Artery Bypass Graft Techniques

A number of alternative CABG techniques have been developed that may have fewer complications for some groups of patients. Off-pump coronary artery bypass (OPCAB) graft surgery has been used successfully in many patients since the 1990s. OPCAB involves a standard median sternotomy incision, but the surgery is performed without CPB; surgery is done on a beating heart. A beta-adrenergic blocker may be used to slow the heart rate. The surgeon may use a myocardial stabilization device to hold the site still for the anastomosis of the bypass graft into the coronary artery while the heart continues to beat (Fig. 29-11). The potential benefits of OPCAB include a decrease in the incidence of stroke and other neurologic complications, renal failure, and other postoperative complications (Magee, Coombs, Peterson, et al., 2003). Comparison of this technique with traditional CABG has been found to be favourable in some patient groups, particularly in patients with hemodynamic instability, with regard to overall mortality as well as the incidence of stroke and MI and the need for repeat revascularization (Dhurandhar, Saxena, Parikh, et al., 2015).

Complications of Coronary Artery Bypass Graft

CABG may result in complications such as MI, dysrhythmias, and hemorrhage (Table 29-5). Although most patients improve symptomatically following surgery, CABG is not a cure for CAD, and angina, exercise intolerance, or other symptoms experienced before CABG may

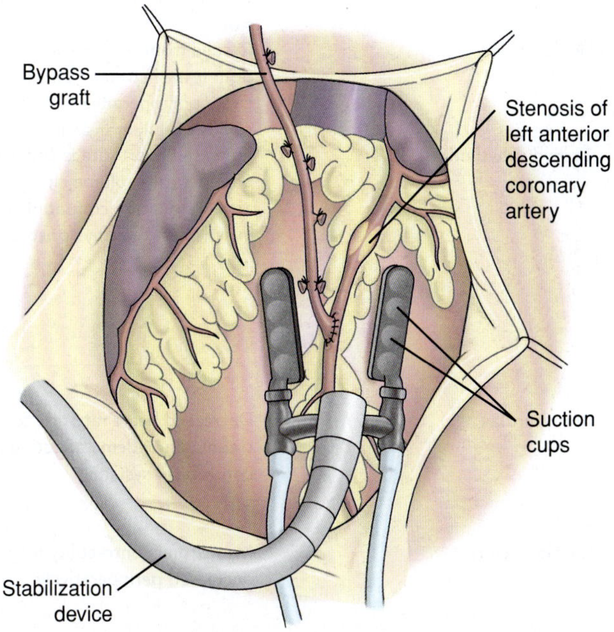

FIGURE 29-11. Stabilizer device for off-pump coronary artery bypass surgery.

TABLE 29-5 Potential Complications of Cardiac Surgery

Complication	Cause	Assessment and Management
Cardiac Complications		
Hypovolemia (most common cause of decreased cardiac output after cardiac surgery)	• Net loss of blood and intravascular volume • Vasodilation due to postoperative rewarming • Intravascular fluid loss to the interstitial spaces because surgery and anesthesia increase capillary permeability	• Arterial hypotension, tachycardia, low CVP, and low PAWP are often seen. • Fluid replacement may be prescribed. Replacement fluids include colloid (albumin), packed red blood cells, or crystalloid solution (normal saline, lactated Ringer's solution).
Persistent bleeding	• Cardiopulmonary bypass causes platelet dysfunction, and hypothermia alters clotting mechanisms. • Surgical trauma causes tissues and blood vessels to ooze bloody drainage. • Intraoperative anticoagulant (heparin) therapy • Postoperative coagulopathy may also result from liver dysfunction and depletion of clotting components.	• Accurate measurement of wound bleeding and chest tube blood is essential. Drainage should not exceed 200 mL/hr for the first 4–6 hours. Drainage should decrease and stop within a few days, while progressing from serosanguinous to serous. • Serial hemoglobin, hematocrit, and coagulation studies guide therapy. • Administration of blood products: packed red blood cells, fresh frozen plasma, platelet concentrate, recombinant factor VII • Protamine sulphate may be given to neutralize unfractionated heparin. • Administration of desmopressin acetate (DDAVP) to enhance platelet function • If bleeding persists, the patient may return to the operating room.
Cardiac tamponade	• Fluid and clots accumulate in the pericardial sac, which compress the heart, preventing blood from filling the ventricles.	• Signs and symptoms include arterial hypotension, tachycardia, decreased urine output, and ↑ CVP. Arterial pressure waveform may show pulsus paradoxus (decrease of >10 mm Hg systolic blood pressure during inspiration). • The chest drainage system is checked to eliminate possible kinks or obstructions in the tubing. • Chest x-ray may show a widening mediastinum. • Emergency medical management is required; may include return to surgery.
Fluid overload	• IV fluids and blood products increase circulating volume.	• High CVP and pulmonary artery pressures, as well as crackles, indicate fluid overload. • Diuretics are prescribed, and the rate of IV fluid administration is reduced. • Alternative treatments include continuous renal replacement therapy and dialysis.
Hypothermia	• Low body temperature leads to vasoconstriction, shivering, and arterial hypertension.	• Patient is rewarmed gradually after surgery, decreasing vasoconstriction.
Hypertension	• Results from postoperative vasoconstriction. It may stretch suture lines and cause postoperative bleeding. The condition is usually transient.	• Vasodilators (nitroglycerin [Tridil], nitroprusside [Nipride]) may be used to treat hypertension. Administer cautiously to avoid hypotension.
Tachydysrhythmias	• Increased heart rate is common with perioperative volume changes. Rapid atrial fibrillation commonly occurs during the first few days postoperatively.	• If a tachydysrhythmia is the primary problem, the heart rhythm is assessed and medications (e.g., amiodarone [Cordarone], diltiazem [Cardizem]) may be prescribed. Antidysrhythmic agents (e.g., beta-blockers) are often given before coronary artery bypass graft to minimize the risk. • Carotid massage may be performed by a primary provider to assist with diagnosing or treating the dysrhythmia. • Cardioversion and defibrillation are alternatives for symptomatic tachydysrhythmias.
Bradycardias	• Decreased heart rate due to surgical trauma and edema affecting the cardiac conduction system	• Many postoperative patients have temporary pacer wires that can be attached to an external pacemaker to stimulate the heart to beat faster. Less commonly, atropine or other medications may be used to increase heart rate.
Cardiac failure	• Myocardial contractility may be decreased perioperatively.	• The nurse observes for and reports signs of heart failure, including hypotension, ↑ CVP, ↑ PAWP, venous distention; laboured respirations; and edema. • Medical management includes diuretics and IV inotropic agents.

TABLE 29-5 Potential Complications of Cardiac Surgery (Continued)

Complication	Cause	Assessment and Management
MI (may occur intraoperatively or postoperatively)	• Portion of the cardiac muscle dies; therefore, contractility decreases. Impaired ventricular wall motion further decreases cardiac output. Symptoms may be masked by the postoperative surgical discomfort or the anesthesia–analgesia regimen.	• Careful assessment to determine the type of pain the patient is experiencing; MI is suspected if the mean blood pressure is low with normal preload. • Serial electrocardiograms and cardiac biomarkers assist in making the diagnosis (alterations may be due to the surgical intervention).
Pulmonary Complications		
Impaired gas exchange	• During and after anesthesia, patients require mechanical assistance to breathe. • Anesthetic agents stimulate production of mucus, and chest incision pain may decrease the effectiveness of ventilation. • Potential for postoperative atelectasis	• Pulmonary complications are detected during assessment of breath sounds, oxygen saturation levels, arterial blood gases, and ventilator readings. • Extended periods of mechanical ventilation may be required while complications are treated.
Neurologic Complications		
Neurologic changes; stroke	• Thrombi and emboli may cause cerebral infarction, and neurologic signs may be evident when patients recover from anesthesia.	• Inability to follow simple commands within 6 hours of recovery from anesthetic; weakness on one side of body or other neurologic changes may indicate stroke. • Patients who are older or who have renal or hepatic failure may take longer to recover from anesthesia.
Kidney Injury and Electrolyte Imbalance		
Acute kidney injury	• May result from hypoperfusion of the kidneys or from injury to the renal tubules by nephrotoxic drugs	• May respond to diuretics or may require continuous renal replacement therapy or dialysis • Fluids, electrolytes, and urine output are monitored frequently. • May result in chronic kidney injury and require ongoing dialysis
Electrolyte imbalance	• Postoperative imbalances in potassium, magnesium, sodium, calcium, and blood glucose are related to surgical losses, metabolic changes, and the administration of medications and IV fluids.	• Monitor electrolytes and basic metabolic studies frequently. • Implement treatment to correct electrolyte imbalance promptly (see Chapter 17).
Other Complications		
Hepatic failure	• Surgery and anesthesia stress the liver. Most common in patients with cirrhosis, hepatitis, or prolonged right-sided heart failure.	• The use of medications metabolized by the liver must be minimized. • Bilirubin and albumin levels are monitored, and nutritional support is provided.
Infection	• Surgery and anesthesia alter the patient's immune system. Multiple invasive devices used to monitor and support the patient's recovery may serve as a source of infection.	• Monitor for signs of possible infection: body temperature, white blood cell and differential counts, incision and puncture sites, urine (clarity, colour, and odor), bilateral breath sounds, sputum (colour, odor, amount). • Antibiotic therapy may be instituted or modified as necessary. • Invasive devices are discontinued as soon as they are no longer required. Institutional protocols for maintaining and replacing invasive lines and devices are followed to minimize the risk of infection.

CVP, central venous pressure; PAWP, pulmonary artery wedge pressure; ↑, increased; IV, intravenous; MI, myocardial infarction.

Adapted from Urden, L. D., Stacy, K. M., & Lough, M. E. (2014). *Critical care nursing* (7th ed.). St. Louis, MO: Elsevier.

recur. Medications (e.g., EcASA, BB, ACE, lipid lowering) required before surgery will need to be continued. Lifestyle modifications recommended before surgery remain important to treat the underlying CAD and for the continued viability of the newly implanted grafts.

Nursing Management

Preoperative Management

Comprehensive preoperative medical management prevents complications and improves outcomes. This is particularly important because patients undergoing CABG surgery tend to be older and often have multiple comorbidities. The use of aspirin, beta-blockers, and statins during the preoperative period, along with the assessment and management of glucose levels is associated with better outcomes (Chaisson, Sanford, Boss, et al., 2014). Preoperative use of aspirin is associated with a reduction in perioperative morbidity and mortality. Beta-blockers, when given at least 24 hours before CABG, reduce the incidence of postoperative atrial fibrillation.

Cardiac surgery patients have many of the same needs and require the same perioperative care as other surgical patients (see Chapters 19 through 21). These patients and their families are experiencing a major life crisis. The association of the heart with life and death intensifies their emotional and psychological needs.

Assessment

In routine, out-patient CABG surgery, patients frequently are admitted to the hospital on the day of the procedure. Therefore, preoperative teaching must take place at an earlier time, usually when the patient has preadmission testing. When patients are admitted to the hospital due to an ACS and end up requiring emergency surgery, they are at risk of being less prepared in terms of expectations and knowledge about the surgery.

Before surgery, physical and psychological assessments establish baselines for future reference. The patient's understanding of the surgical procedure, informed consent, and adherence to treatment protocols are evaluated. Helping the patient to cope, to understand the procedure, and to maintain dignity are nursing responsibilities.

A history and physical examination are performed by nursing and medical personnel. A chest x-ray, ECG, laboratory tests, blood typing and cross-matching, and autologous blood donation (patient's own blood) may also be performed. The nurse assesses the patient for disorders that could complicate or affect the postoperative course, such as diabetes, hypertension, pre-existing disabilities, and respiratory, gastrointestinal, and hematologic diseases.

The nurse clarifies how the medication regimen is to be altered before surgery, such as decreasing or discontinuing anticoagulants and maintaining medications for treatment of blood pressure, angina, diabetes, and dysrhythmias. The nurse also clarifies the need to maintain activity patterns, a healthy diet, healthful sleep habits, and cessation of smoking and alcohol to minimize the risks of surgery.

The patient and family's learning needs are identified and addressed as necessary. Of particular importance are the patient's usual functional level, coping mechanisms, and support systems. These are important because the support of the family or significant others affects the patient's postoperative course and rehabilitation. Discharge plans are influenced by the lifestyle demands of the home situation and the physical environment of the home.

Health History

The preoperative history and health assessment should be thorough and well documented because they provide a basis for postoperative comparison. A systematic assessment of all systems is performed, with emphasis on cardiovascular functioning.

The functional status of the cardiovascular system is determined by reviewing the patient's symptoms, including past and present experiences with chest pain, hypertension, palpitations, cyanosis, breathing difficulty (dyspnea), leg pain that occurs with walking (intermittent claudication), orthopnea, paroxysmal nocturnal dyspnea, and peripheral edema. Because alterations in cardiac output can affect renal, respiratory, gastrointestinal, integumentary, hematologic, and neurologic functioning, a history of these systems is also reviewed. The patient's history of major illnesses, previous surgeries, medication therapies, and use of drugs, alcohol, and tobacco is also obtained.

Physical Assessment

A complete physical examination is performed, with special emphasis on the following:

- General appearance and behaviour
- Vital signs
- Nutritional and fluid status, weight, and height
- Inspection and palpation of the heart, noting the point of maximal impulse, abnormal pulsations, and thrills
- Auscultation of the heart, noting pulse rate, rhythm, and quality; S_3 and S_4, snaps, clicks, murmurs, and friction rub
- Jugular venous pressure
- Carotid upstroke
- Peripheral pulses
- Peripheral edema

Psychosocial Assessment

The psychosocial assessment and the assessment of the patient and family's learning needs are also important. Anticipation of cardiac surgery is a source of great stress to the patient and family, and patients with high anxiety levels have poorer outcomes (Williams, Alexander, Morin, et al., 2013). Patients may be anxious and fearful and often have many unanswered questions. However, some anxiety is expected, and it is important to help patients identify priorities and find coping. Questions may be asked to obtain the following information:

- Knowledge and understanding of the surgical procedure, postoperative course, recovery and rehabilitation
- Fears and concerns regarding the surgery and future health status
- Coping mechanisms helpful to the patient
- Support systems available during and following hospitalization

Nursing Interventions

REDUCING FEAR AND ANXIETY. The nurse provides adequate time for the patient and family to express their fears. Topics of concern may include: pain, changes in body image, fear of the unknown, fear of pain, and fear of disability or death. It may be helpful to describe the sensations that the patient can expect, including the preoperative sedation, surgical anesthesia, and postoperative pain management. The nurse reassures the patient that the fear of pain is normal, that some pain will be experienced, that medication to relieve pain will be provided, and that the patient will be closely monitored. In addition, the nurse instructs the patient to request analgesic medication before the pain becomes severe. Positioning and relaxation often make the pain more tolerable. Patients who have concern about scarring from surgery are encouraged to discuss this concern, and misconceptions are corrected.

The patient and family may want to discuss their fear of the patient dying. They should be reassured that this fear is normal. After the fear is expressed, the nurse can help the patient and family explore their feelings.

By alleviating undue anxiety and fear, preparing the patient emotionally for surgery decreases the chance of preoperative problems, promotes smooth anesthesia induction, and enhances the patient's involvement in care and recovery after surgery. Preparing the family for the usual postoperative events helps them cope, support the patient, and participate in postoperative and rehabilitative care. For patients with extreme anxiety or fear and for whom emotional support and education are not successful, medication therapy may be helpful. The anxiolytic agents most commonly used before cardiac surgery are lorazepam (Ativan).

During the assessment, the nurse determines how much the patient and family know about the impending surgery and the expected postoperative events. They are encouraged to ask questions and to indicate how much information they wish to receive. Some patients prefer not to have detailed information, whereas others want to know as much as possible. Patients are approached as unique individuals with their own specific learning needs, learning styles, and levels of understanding.

Patients requiring emergency heart surgery may have cardiac catheterization and surgery within several hours of admission. The nurse has little opportunity to assess and meet their emotional and learning needs before surgery. As a result, patients require extra help after surgery to adjust to the situation.

MONITORING AND MANAGING POTENTIAL COMPLICATIONS. Angina may occur because of increased stress and anxiety related to the forthcoming surgery. The patient who develops angina usually responds to typical therapy for angina, most commonly nitroglycerin. Some patients require oxygen and IV nitroglycerin infusions. Physiologically unstable patients may require preoperative management in a critical care unit.

PROVIDING PATIENT EDUCATION. The major goals for the patient may include reducing fear, learning about the surgical procedure and postoperative course, and avoiding perioperative complications.

During the preoperative phase of cardiac surgery, the nurse develops a plan of care that includes emotional support and teaching for the patient and family. Establishing rapport, answering questions, listening to fears and concerns, clarifying misconceptions, and providing information about what to expect are interventions the nurse uses to prepare the patient and family emotionally for the surgery and the postoperative events.

Patient and family teaching is based on assessed learning needs. Prior to surgery, patients and their families are given specific instructions. This includes information on how the patient should take or stop specific medications, including anticoagulant agents, antihypertensive medications, and medications that control diabetes. Teaching also includes information about hospitalization, surgery (e.g., preoperative and postoperative care, length of surgery, pain and discomfort that can be expected, visiting hours and procedures in the critical care unit), the recovery phase (e.g., length of hospitalization; what to expect from home care and rehabilitation; when normal activities such as housework, shopping, and work can be resumed), and ongoing lifestyle habits. Any changes made in medical therapy and preoperative preparations need to be explained and reinforced.

The patient is instructed to shower with an antiseptic solution such as chlorhexidine gluconate. A sedative may be prescribed the night before and the morning of surgery. Most cardiac surgical teams use prophylactic antibiotic therapy, and this is initiated immediately before surgery.

Teaching the patient and family together may be most effective. Anxiety often increases with the admission process and impending surgery. Teaching the patient and family together capitalizes on their established support relationship.

The patient may be offered a tour of the critical care unit, the postanesthesia care unit (PACU), or both. (In some hospitals, the patient initially goes to the PACU.) The patient recovering from anesthesia may be reassured by having already seen the surroundings and having met someone from the unit. The patient and family are informed about the equipment, tubes, and lines that will be present after surgery and their purposes. They should know to expect monitors, several IV lines, chest tubes, and a urinary catheter. Explaining the purpose and the approximate time that these devices will be in place helps to reassure the patient. Most patients remain intubated and on mechanical ventilation for several hours after surgery. They should be aware that this prevents them from talking, and they should be reassured that the staff will be able to assist them with other means of communication.

The nurse takes care to answer the patient's questions about postoperative care and procedures. After the nurse explains deep breathing and coughing, the use of the incentive spirometer, and foot exercises, the nurse practices these procedures with the patient. The benefit of early and frequent ambulation is discussed. The family's questions at this time usually focus on the length of the surgery, who will discuss the results of the procedure with them after surgery and when this may occur, where to wait during the surgery, the visiting procedures for the critical care unit, and how they can support the patient before surgery and in the critical care unit.

Intraoperative Nursing Management

The perioperative nurse performs an assessment and prepares the patient for the operating room and recovery experience. Any changes in the patient's status and the need for changes in therapy are identified. Procedures are explained before they are performed, such as the application of electrodes and use of continuous monitoring, indwelling catheters, and an SpO_2 probe. IV lines are inserted to administer fluids, medications, and blood products. The patient receives general anesthesia, is intubated, and is placed on mechanical ventilation. In addition to assisting with the surgical procedures, perioperative nurses are responsible for the comfort and safety of the patient. Some of the areas of intervention include positioning, skin care, wound care, and emotional support of the patient and family.

Before the chest incision is closed, chest tubes are inserted to evacuate air and drainage from the mediastinum and the thorax. Temporary epicardial pacemaker electrodes may be implanted on the surface of the right atrium and the right ventricle. These epicardial electrodes can be connected to an external pacemaker if the patient has persistent bradycardia perioperatively. Possible intraoperative complications include low cardiac output, dysrhythmias, hemorrhage, MI, stroke, embolization, and organ failure from shock, embolus, or adverse drug reactions. Astute intraoperative patient assessment is critical to prevent, detect, and initiate prompt intervention for these complications.

Postoperative Nursing Management

Initial postoperative care focuses on achieving or maintaining hemodynamic stability and recovery from general anesthesia. Care may be provided in the PACU or CICU. The immediate postoperative period for the patient who has undergone cardiac surgery presents many challenges to the health care team. All efforts are made to facilitate the transition from the operating room to the critical care unit or PACU with minimal risk. Specific information about the surgical procedure and important factors about postoperative management are communicated by the surgical team and anesthesia personnel to the critical care nurse, who then assumes responsibility for the patient's care. Figure 29-12 presents an overview of the many aspects of postoperative care of the cardiac surgical patient.

After the patient's cardiac status and respiratory status are stable, the patient is transferred to a surgical progressive care unit with telemetry. Care in both the CICU and the progressive care unit focuses on the monitoring of cardiopulmonary status, pain management, wound care, progressive activity, and nutrition. Education about medications and risk factor modification is emphasized. Discharge from the hospital may occur 3 to 5 days after CABG in patients without complications (Chart 29-13).

(text continued on page 770)

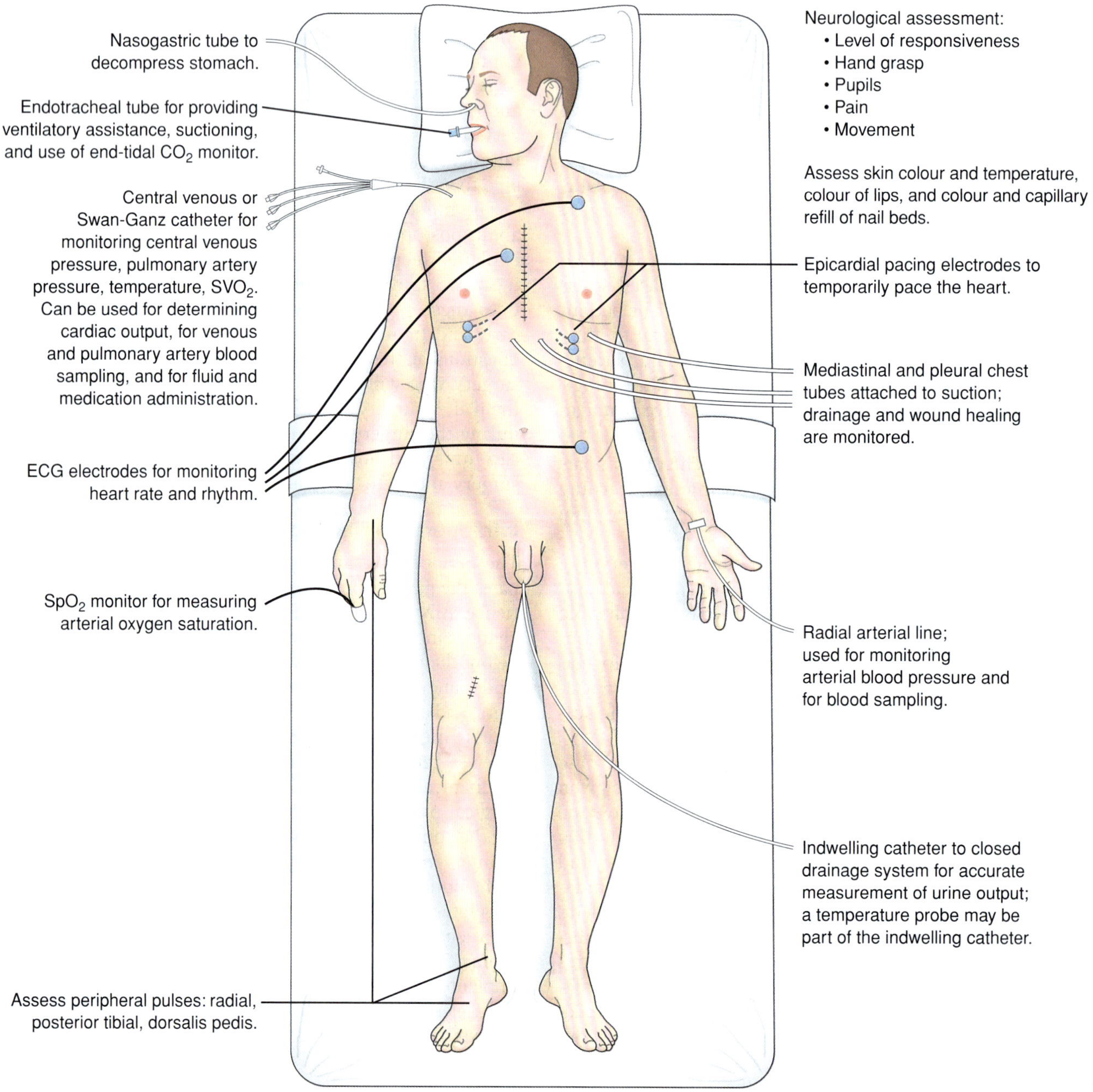

FIGURE 29-12. Postoperative care of the cardiac surgical patient requires the nurse to be proficient in interpreting hemodynamics, correlating physical assessments with laboratory results, sequencing interventions, and evaluating progress toward desired outcomes. CO_2, carbon dioxide; ECG, electrocardiogram; SvO_2, pulmonary artery oxygen saturation; SpO_2, percutaneous oxygen saturation.

Plan of Nursing Care — Chart 29-13. Care of the Patient After Cardiac Surgery

Nursing Priority: Reduced cardiac output
Goal: Restoration of cardiac output to maintain organ and tissue perfusion

NURSING INTERVENTIONS	RATIONALE	EXPECTED PATIENT OUTCOMES
1. Monitor cardiovascular status. Serial readings of blood pressures (arterial, pulmonary artery, pulmonary artery wedge pressure [PAWP], central venous pressure [CVP]), cardiac output/index, systemic and pulmonary vascular resistance, and cardiac rhythm and rate are obtained, recorded, and correlated with the patient's condition.	1. Effectiveness of cardiac output is determined by hemodynamic monitoring.	The following parameters are within the patient's normal ranges: • Arterial pressure • PAWP • Pulmonary artery pressures • CVP • Heart sounds • Pulmonary and systemic vascular resistance • Cardiac output and cardiac index • Peripheral pulses • Cardiac rate and rhythm • Cardiac biomarkers • Urine output • Skin and mucosal colour • Skin temperature
a. Assess arterial blood pressure every 15 minutes until stable; then arterial or cuff blood pressure every 1–4 hours × 24 hours; then every 8–12 hours until hospital discharge; then every visit.	a. Blood pressure is one of the most important physiologic parameters to follow; vasoconstriction after cardiopulmonary bypass may require treatment with an intravenous (IV) vasodilator.	
b. Auscultate for heart sounds and rhythm.	b. Auscultation provides evidence of cardiac tamponade (muffled distant heart sounds), pericarditis (precordial rub), and dysrhythmias.	
c. Assess peripheral pulses (pedal, tibial, radial).	c. Presence or absence and quality of pulses provide data about cardiac output as well as obstructive lesions.	
d. Measure pulmonary artery diastolic (PAD) pressure and PAWP to determine left ventricular end-diastolic volume and to assess cardiac output.	d. Rising pressures may indicate congestive heart failure or pulmonary edema. Low pressures may indicate need for volume replacement.	
e. Monitor PAWP, PAD, and CVP to assess blood volume, vascular tone, and pumping effectiveness of the heart. *Trends are more important than isolated readings*. Mechanical ventilation may alter hemodynamics.	e. High PAWP, PAD, or CVP may result from hypervolemia, heart failure, or cardiac tamponade. If blood pressure drop is due to low blood volume, PAWP, PAD, and CVP will show corresponding drop.	
f. Monitor electrocardiogram (ECG) pattern for cardiac dysrhythmias (see Chapter 28 for discussion of dysrhythmias).	f. Dysrhythmias may occur with coronary ischemia, hypoxia, alterations in serum potassium, edema, bleeding, acid–base or electrolyte disturbances, digitalis toxicity, and cardiac failure. ST-segment changes may indicate myocardial ischemia. Pacemaker capture and antiarrhythmic medications are used to maintain a heart rate and rhythm and to support stable blood pressures.	
g. Assess cardiac biomarker results when available.	g. Elevations may indicate myocardial infarction.	
h. Measure urine output every ½–1 hour at first, then with vital signs.	h. Urine output less than 25 mL/hr indicates decreased renal perfusion and may reflect decreased cardiac output.	
i. Observe buccal mucosa, nail beds, lips, earlobes, and extremities.	i. Duskiness and cyanosis may indicate decreased cardiac output.	
j. Assess skin; note temperature and colour.	j. Cool, moist skin indicates vasoconstriction and decreased cardiac output.	

continued >

Plan of Nursing Care Chart 29-13. Care of the Patient After Cardiac Surgery, *Continued*

NURSING INTERVENTIONS	RATIONALE	EXPECTED PATIENT OUTCOMES
2. Observe for persistent bleeding: steady, continuous drainage of blood; hypotension; low CVP; tachycardia. Prepare to administer blood products and/or IV solutions.	2. Bleeding can result from cardiac incisions, tissue fragility, trauma to tissues, and clotting defects.	• Less than 200 mL/hr of drainage through chest tubes during first 4–6 hours • Vital signs stable • CVP and other hemodynamic parameters within normal limits • Urinary output within normal limits • Skin colour normal • Respirations unlaboured, clear breath sounds • Pain limited to incision • ECG and cardiac biomarkers negative for ischemic changes
3. Observe for cardiac tamponade: hypotension; rising PAWP, PAD, CVP, or pulsus paradoxus; muffled heart sounds; weak, thready pulse; jugular vein distention; decreasing urinary output. Check for diminished amount of blood in chest drainage collection system. Prepare for reoperation.	3. Cardiac tamponade results from bleeding into the pericardial sac or accumulation of fluid in the sac, which compresses the heart and prevents adequate filling of the ventricles. Decrease in chest drainage may indicate that fluid and clots are accumulating in the pericardial sac.	
4. Observe for cardiac failure: hypotension, rising PAWP, PAD, CVP, tachycardia, restlessness, agitation, cyanosis, venous distention, dyspnea, moist crackles, ascites. Prepare to administer diuretics, digoxin, and/or IV inotropic agents.	4. Cardiac failure results from decreased pumping action of the heart; can cause deficient perfusion to vital organs.	
5. Observe for myocardial infarction: ST-segment elevations, T-wave changes, decreased cardiac output in the presence of normal circulating volume and filling pressures. Monitor serial ECGs and cardiac biomarkers. Differentiate myocardial pain from incisional pain.	5. Symptoms may be masked by the patient's level of consciousness and pain medication.	

Nursing Priority: Impaired gas exchange
Goal: Adequate gas exchange

NURSING INTERVENTIONS	RATIONALE	EXPECTED PATIENT OUTCOMES
1. Maintain mechanical ventilation until the patient is able to breathe independently.	1. Ventilatory support may be used to decrease work of the heart, to maintain effective ventilation, and to provide an airway in the event of complications.	• Airway patent • ABGs within normal range • Endotracheal tube correctly placed, as evidenced by x-ray • Breath sounds clear • Ventilator synchronous with respirations • Breath sounds clear after suctioning/coughing • Nail beds and mucous membranes pink • Mental acuity consistent with amount of sedatives and analgesics received • Oriented to person; able to respond yes and no appropriately • Able to be weaned successfully from ventilator
2. Monitor arterial blood gases, tidal volume, peak inspiratory pressure, and extubation parameters.	2. Arterial blood gases (ABGs) and ventilator parameters indicate effectiveness of the ventilator and changes that need to be made to improve gas exchange.	
3. Auscultate chest for breath sounds.	3. Crackles indicate pulmonary congestion; decreased or absent breath sounds may indicate pneumothorax, hemothorax, or dislodgement of tube.	
4. Suction tracheobronchial secretions as needed, using strict aseptic technique.	4. Retention of secretions leads to hypoxia and possible infection.	
5. Assist in weaning and endotracheal tube removal.	5. Decreased risk of pulmonary infections and enhanced ability of the patient to communicate without an endotracheal tube	
6. After extubation, promote deep breathing, coughing, and turning. Encourage use of the incentive spirometer and compliance with breathing treatments. Teach incisional splinting with a "cough pillow" to decrease discomfort.	6. Aids in keeping airway patent, preventing atelectasis, and facilitating lung expansion	

Plan of Nursing Care

Chart 29-13. Care of the Patient After Cardiac Surgery, *Continued*

Nursing Priority: Imbalanced fluid volume and electrolyte imbalance
Goal: Fluid and electrolyte balance

NURSING INTERVENTIONS	RATIONALE	EXPECTED PATIENT OUTCOMES
1. Maintain fluid and electrolyte balance.	1. Adequate circulating blood volume is necessary for optimal cellular activity; metabolic acidosis and electrolyte imbalance can occur after surgery.	• Fluid intake and output balanced • Hemodynamic assessment parameters negative for fluid overload or hypovolemia • Normal blood pressure with position changes • Absence of dysrhythmia • Stable weight • Blood pH 7.35–7.45 • Serum potassium 3.5–5.0 mEq/L (3.5–5.0 mmol/L) • Serum magnesium 1.3–2.3 mg/dL (0.62–0.95 mmol/L) • Serum sodium 135–145 mEq/L (135–145 mmol/L) • Serum calcium 8.6–10.2 mg/dL (2.15–2.55 mmol/L) • Serum glucose <110 mg/dL
a. Keep intake and output flow sheets; record urine volume every ½–4 hours while in critical care unit; then every 8–12 hours while hospitalized.	a. Provides a method to determine positive or negative fluid balance and fluid requirements	
b. Assess blood pressure, hemodynamic parameters, weight, electrolytes, hematocrit, jugular venous pressure, tissue turgor, breath sounds, urinary output, and nasogastric tube drainage.	b. Provides information about state of hydration	
c. Measure postoperative chest drainage (should not exceed 200 mL/hr for the first 4–6 hours); cessation of drainage may indicate kinked or blocked chest tube. Ensure patency and integrity of the drainage system. Maintain autotransfusion system, if in use.	c. Excessive blood loss from chest cavity can cause hypovolemia.	
d. Weigh daily. Notify physician if weight gain of 1 kg or more in 24 hours.	d. Indicator of fluid balance	
2. Be alert to changes in serum electrolyte levels.	2. A specific concentration of electrolytes is necessary in both extracellular and intracellular body fluids to sustain life.	
a. Hypokalemia (low potassium) *Effects:* dysrhythmias: premature ventricular complexes (PVCs), ventricular tachycardia. Observe for specific ECG changes. Administer IV potassium replacement as prescribed.	a. *Causes:* inadequate intake, diuretics, vomiting, excessive nasogastric drainage, stress from surgery	
b. Hyperkalemia (high potassium) *Effects:* ECG changes, tall peaked T waves, wide QRS, brachycardia. Be prepared to administer diuretic or an ion-exchange resin (sodium polystyrene sulfonate [Kayexalate]); IV sodium bicarbonate, or IV insulin and glucose.	b. *Causes:* increased intake, hemolysis from cardiopulmonary bypass/mechanical-assist devices, acidosis, renal insufficiency, tissue necrosis, adrenal cortical insufficiency The resin binds potassium and promotes intestinal excretion of it. IV sodium bicarbonate drives potassium into the cells from extracellular fluid. Insulin assists the cells with glucose and potassium absorption.	
c. Hypomagnesemia (low magnesium) *Effects:* dysrhythmias: PVCs, ventricular tachycardia, paresthesias, carpopedal spasm, muscle cramps, tetany, irritability, tremors, hyperexcitability, hyperreflexia, seizures. Be prepared to treat the cause. Magnesium supplements may be given (oral route preferred, IV administered with caution).	c. *Causes:* decreased intake, impaired absorption, increased excretion normal for 24 hours after major surgery and diuretic therapy	

continued >

Plan of Nursing Care

Chart 29-13. Care of the Patient After Cardiac Surgery, *Continued*

NURSING INTERVENTIONS	RATIONALE	EXPECTED PATIENT OUTCOMES
d. Hyponatremia (low sodium) *Effects:* weakness, fatigue, confusion, seizures, coma. Administer sodium or diuretics as prescribed.	d. *Causes:* reduction of total body sodium, or increased water intake causing dilution of sodium	
e. Hypocalcemia (low calcium) *Effects:* numbness and tingling; carpal spasm; muscle cramps; tetany, hypotension, dysrhythmias. Administer oral or IV replacement therapy as prescribed.	e. *Causes:* alkalosis, multiple blood transfusions of citrated blood products	
f. Hypercalcemia (high calcium) *Effects:* dysrhythmias Institute treatment as prescribed.	f. *Causes:* diuretic therapy, prolonged immobility	
g. Hyperglycemia (high blood glucose) *Effects:* increased urine output, thirst, metabolic acidosis. Administer insulin as prescribed.	g. *Cause:* stress response to surgery	
Nursing Priority: Disturbed sensory perception **Goal:** Reduction of symptoms of sensory perceptual imbalance; prevention of postcardiotomy delirium		
1. Use measures to prevent postcardiotomy delirium: a. Explain all procedures and the need for patient cooperation. b. Plan nursing care to provide for periods of uninterrupted sleep with patient's normal day–night pattern. c. Decrease sleep-preventing environmental stimuli as much as possible. d. Promote continuity of care. e. Orient to time and place frequently. Encourage family to visit. f. Assess for medications that may contribute to delirium. g. Teach relaxation techniques and diversions. h. Encourage self-care as much as tolerated to enhance self-control. Assess support systems and coping mechanisms.	1. Postcardiotomy delirium may result from anxiety, sleep deprivation, increased sensory input, and disorientation, to night and day. Normally, sleep cycles are at least 50 minutes long. The first cycle may be as long as 90–120 minutes and then shorten during successive cycles. Sleep deprivation results when the sleep cycles are interrupted or inadequate in number.	• Cooperates with procedures • Sleeps for long, uninterrupted intervals • Oriented to person, place, time • Experiences no perceptual distortions, hallucinations, disorientation, or delusions
2. Observe for perceptual distortions, hallucinations, disorientation, and paranoid delusions.		
Nursing Priority: Acute pain **Goal:** Relief of pain		
1. Record nature, type, location, intensity, and duration of pain.	1. Pain and anxiety increase pulse rate, oxygen consumption, and cardiac workload.	• States pain is decreasing in severity • Reports absence of pain • Restlessness decreased • Vital signs stable • Participates in deep-breathing and coughing exercises • Verbalizes fewer complaints of pain each day • Positions self; participates in care activities • Gradually increases activity
2. Assist patient to differentiate between surgical pain and anginal pain.	2. Anginal pain requires immediate assessment and treatment.	
3. Encourage routine pain medication dosing for the first 24–72 hours and observe for side effects of lethargy, hypotension, tachycardia, or respiratory depression.	3. Analgesia promotes rest, decreases oxygen consumption caused by pain, and aids patient in performing deep-breathing and coughing exercises; pain medication is more effective when taken before pain is severe.	

Plan of Nursing Care

Chart 29-13. Care of the Patient After Cardiac Surgery, *Continued*

NURSING INTERVENTIONS	RATIONALE	EXPECTED PATIENT OUTCOMES
Nursing Priority: Decreased renal perfusion **Goal:** Maintenance of adequate renal perfusion		
1. Assess renal function: a. Measure urine output every ½–4 hours in critical care, then every 8–12 hours until hospital discharge. b. Measure urine specific gravity. c. Monitor and report lab results: blood urea nitrogen (BUN), serum creatinine, urine and serum electrolytes.	1. Renal injury can be caused by deficient perfusion, hemolysis, low cardiac output, and use of vasopressor agents to increase blood pressure. a. Less than 30 mL/hr indicates decreased renal function. b. Indicates kidneys' ability to concentrate urine in renal tubules. c. Indicates kidneys' ability to excrete waste products.	• Urine output consistent with fluid intake; greater than 30 mL/hr • Urine specific gravity 1.020–1.030 • BUN, creatinine, electrolytes within normal limits
2. Prepare to administer rapid-acting diuretics or inotropic drugs (e.g., dobutamine).	2. Promotes renal function and increase cardiac output and renal blood flow.	
3. Prepare the patient for dialysis or continuous renal replacement therapy if indicated.	3. Provides patient with the opportunity to ask questions and prepare for the procedure.	
Nursing Priority: Ineffective thermoregulation **Goal:** Maintenance of normal body temperature		
1. Assess temperature every hour.	1. Fever can indicate an infectious or inflammatory process.	• Normal body temperature • Incisions are free of infection and are healing • Absence of symptoms of postpericardiotomy syndrome
2. Use aseptic technique when changing dressings or suctioning endotracheal tube; maintain closed systems for all IV and arterial lines and for indwelling urinary catheter.	2. Decreases risk of infection.	
3. Observe for symptoms of postpericardiotomy syndrome: fever, malaise, pericardial effusion, pericardial friction rub, arthralgia.	3. Occurs in approximately 10% of patients after cardiac surgery.	
4. Obtain cultures and other labwork (complete blood count [CBC], erythrocyte sedimentation rate [ESR]); administer antibiotics as prescribed.	4. Antibiotics treat documented infection.	
5. Administer anti-inflammatory agents as directed.	5. Relieves symptoms of inflammation (e.g., warm or flushed sensation, swelling, fullness, stiffness or aching sensation, and fatigue).	
Nursing Priority: Lack of knowledge **Goal:** Ability to perform self-care activities		
1. Develop teaching plan for the patient and family. Provide specific instructions for the following: • Diet and daily weights • Activity progression • Exercise	1. Each patient will have unique learning needs.	• Patient and family members explain and comply with the therapeutic regimen • Patient and family members identify necessary lifestyle changes

continued >

Plan of Nursing Care **Chart 29-13. Care of the Patient After Cardiac Surgery, *Continued***

NURSING INTERVENTIONS	RATIONALE	EXPECTED PATIENT OUTCOMES
• Deep breathing, coughing, lung expansion exercises • Temperature monitoring • Medication regimen • Pulse taking • Access to the emergency medical system • Need for MedicAlert identification		• Has copy of discharge instructions (in the patient's primary language and at appropriate reading level; has an alternate format if indicated) • Keeps follow-up appointments
2. Provide verbal and written instructions; provide several teaching sessions for reinforcement and answering questions.	2. Repetition promotes learning by allowing for clarification of misinformation. After cardiac surgery, patients have short-term memory difficulty; information written in the patient's primary language and appropriate reading level is essential because it can be used as a resource after discharge.	
3. Involve the family in teaching sessions.	3. Family members responsible for home care are usually anxious and require adequate time for learning.	
4. Provide contact information for the surgeon and cardiologist and instructions about follow-up visit with the surgeon.	4. Arrangements for contacts with health care personnel help to allay anxieties.	
5. Make appropriate referrals: home care agency, cardiac rehabilitation program, community support groups, Mended Hearts Club.	5. Learning and lifestyle changes continue after discharge from the hospital.	

Assessment

When the patient is admitted to the CICU or PACU, nursing and medical personnel perform a complete assessment of all systems at least every 4 hours. The following parameters are assessed:

Neurologic status: Level of responsiveness, pupil size and reaction to light, reflexes, facial symmetry, movement of the extremities, and hand grip strength

Cardiac status: Heart rate and rhythm, heart sounds, pacemaker status, arterial blood pressure, central venous pressure (CVP), pulmonary artery pressure, pulmonary artery wedge pressure (PAWP), waveforms from the invasive blood pressure lines, cardiac output or index, systemic and pulmonary vascular resistance, pulmonary artery oxygen saturation (SvO_2) (see Chapter 27 for a detailed description of hemodynamic monitoring)

Respiratory status: Chest movement, breath sounds, ventilator settings (e.g., rate, tidal volume, oxygen concentration, mode such as assist-control, positive end-expiratory pressure, pressure support), respiratory rate, peak inspiratory pressure, arterial oxygen saturation (SaO_2), percutaneous oxygen saturation (SpO_2), end-tidal carbon dioxide (CO_2), pleural chest tube drainage, arterial blood gases

Peripheral vascular status: Peripheral pulses; colour of skin, nail beds, mucosa, lips, and earlobes; skin temperature; edema; condition of dressings and invasive lines

Renal function: Urinary output; serum creatinine and electrolytes

Fluid and electrolyte status: Strict intake and output, including all IV fluids and blood products, output from all drainage tubes; clinical and laboratory indicators of imbalance

Pain: Nature, type, location, and duration; apprehension; response to analgesics

Assessment also includes observing all equipment and tubes to determine whether they are functioning properly: endotracheal tube, ventilator, end-tidal CO_2 monitor, SpO_2 monitor, pulmonary artery catheter, SvO_2 monitor, arterial and IV lines, IV infusion devices and tubing, cardiac monitor, pacemaker, chest tubes, and urinary drainage system.

As the patient regains consciousness and progresses through the postoperative period, the nurse also assesses indicators of psychological and emotional status. The patient may exhibit behaviour that reflects denial or depression or may experience postoperative delirium. Characteristic signs of delirium include transient perceptual illusions, visual and auditory hallucinations, disorientation, and paranoid delusions. Patients who have delirium after cardiac surgery have poorer outcomes than do similar patients without this complication (Mangusan, Hooper, Denslow, et al., 2015).

It is also necessary to assess the family's needs. The nurse ascertains how family members are coping with the situation; determines their psychological, emotional, and spiritual needs; and finds out whether they are receiving adequate information about the patient's condition.

Nursing Interventions

MONITORING FOR COMPLICATIONS. The patient is continuously assessed for indications of impending complications (see Table 29-5). The nurse and the surgeon function collaboratively to prevent complications, to identify early signs and symptoms of complications, and to institute measures to reverse their progression.

Decreased Cardiac Output. A decrease in cardiac output is always a threat to the patient who has had cardiac surgery. It can have a variety of causes:

- *Preload alterations:* Too little blood volume returning to the heart as a result of hypovolemia, persistent bleeding, or cardiac tamponade; or too much blood volume returning to the heart from fluid overload. Excessive postoperative bleeding can lead to decreased intravascular volume, hypotension, and low cardiac output. Bleeding problems are common after cardiac surgery because of the effects of CPB, trauma from the surgery, and anticoagulation. Preload can also decrease if there is a collection of fluid and blood in the pericardium (cardiac tamponade), which impedes cardiac filling. Cardiac output is also altered if too much volume returns to the heart, causing fluid overload.
- *Afterload alteration:* Constricted arteries from postoperative hypertension or hypothermic vasoconstriction impede left ventricular emptying, increasing the workload of the heart.
- *Heart rate alterations:* Too fast, too slow, or dysrhythmias can lead to decreased cardiac output.
- *Contractility alterations:* Contractility can be altered in cardiac failure, MI, electrolyte imbalances, hypoxia.

Fluid Volume and Electrolyte Imbalance. Fluid and electrolyte imbalance may occur after cardiac surgery. Nursing assessment for these complications includes monitoring of intake and output, weight, hemodynamic parameters, hematocrit levels, distention of neck veins, edema, liver size, breath sounds (e.g., fine crackles, wheezing), and electrolyte levels. Changes in serum electrolytes are reported promptly so that treatment can be instituted. Especially important are dangerously high or dangerously low levels of potassium, magnesium, sodium, and calcium. Elevated blood glucose levels (hyperglycemia) are common in the postoperative period due to the increased stress and are associated with increased morbidity and mortality. Administration of IV insulin may be required in patients both with and without diabetes to achieve the glycemic control necessary for promoting wound healing (Girish, Agarwal, Satsangi, et al., 2014). Implementing an insulin infusion protocol that targets moderate glycemic control has been demonstrated as effective in treating acute hyperglycemia following cardiac surgery while also decreasing the incidence of hypoglycemia (Hargraves, 2014).

Impaired Gas Exchange. Impaired gas exchange is another possible complication after cardiac surgery. All body tissues require an adequate supply of oxygen for survival. To decrease workload of breathing, optimize oxygen supply, and facilitate gas exchange, an endotracheal tube with ventilator assistance may be used for hours to days. The assisted ventilation is continued until the patient's blood gas measurements are acceptable and the patient demonstrates the ability to breathe independently. Patients who are stable after surgery may be extubated as early as 2 to 4 hours after surgery, which reduces their discomfort and anxiety regarding their limited ability to communicate, facilitates early ambulation, and decreases risk of ventilator-associated pneumonia.

While receiving mechanical ventilation, the patient is continuously assessed for signs of impaired gas exchange: restlessness, anxiety, cyanosis of mucous membranes and peripheral tissues, tachycardia, and fighting the ventilator. Breath sounds are assessed often to detect fluid in the lungs and monitor lung expansion. Arterial blood gases, SpO_2, and end-tidal CO_2 are assessed for decreased oxygen and increased CO_2. Following extubation, aggressive pulmonary interventions, such as turning, coughing, and deep breathing, are necessary to prevent atelectasis and pneumonia.

Impaired Cerebral Circulation. Hypoperfusion or microemboli during or following cardiac surgery may produce injury to the brain. Brain function depends on a continuous supply of oxygenated blood. The brain does not have the capacity to store oxygen and must rely on adequate continuous perfusion by the heart. It is important to observe the patient for any symptoms of hypoxia: restlessness, headache, confusion, dyspnea, hypotension, and cyanosis. An assessment of the patient's neurologic status includes level of consciousness, response to verbal commands and painful stimuli, pupil size and reaction to light, facial symmetry, movement of the extremities, hand grip strength, presence of pedal and popliteal pulses, and temperature and colour of extremities. Any indication of a change in status is documented and abnormal findings are reported to the surgeon, as they may signal the onset of a complication, such as a stroke.

MANAGING COMPLICATIONS. Based on the assessment data, potential complications that may develop include the following:

- *Cardiac complications:* Heart failure, MI, stunned myocardium, dysrhythmias, tamponade, cardiac arrest
- *Pulmonary complications:* Pulmonary edema, pulmonary emboli, pleural effusions, pneumothorax or hemothorax, respiratory failure, acute respiratory distress syndrome
- Hemorrhage/coagulopathy
- *Neurologic complications:* embolic or hemorrhagic stroke
- Renal failure
- Electrolyte imbalances
- Hepatic failure
- Infection/sepsis

MAINTAINING CARDIAC OUTPUT. To evaluate the patient's cardiac status, the nurse primarily determines the effectiveness of cardiac output through clinical observations and routine measurements: serial readings of blood pressure, heart rate, CVP, arterial pressure, and pulmonary artery pressures.

Renal function is related to cardiac function, as blood pressure and heart rate drive glomerular filtration; therefore, urinary output is measured and recorded. Urine output of less than 30 mL/hr may indicate a decrease in cardiac output. Urine output less than 0.5 mL/kg/hr may indicate a decrease in cardiac output or inadequate fluid volume. Urine specific gravity may also be assessed (normal is 1.010 to 1.025), as may urine osmolality. Inadequate fluid volume may be manifested by low urinary output and high specific gravity, whereas overhydration is manifested by high urine output and low specific gravity.

Body tissues depend on adequate cardiac output to provide a continuous supply of oxygenated blood to meet the changing demands of the organs and body systems. Because the buccal mucosa, nail beds, lips, and earlobes are sites with rich capillary beds, they should be observed for cyanosis or duskiness as possible signs of reduced cardiac output. Moist or dry skin may indicate vasodilation or vasoconstriction, respectively. Distention of the neck veins when the head of the bed is elevated to 30 degrees or more may signal right-sided heart failure. If cardiac output has decreased, the skin becomes cool, moist, and cyanotic or mottled.

Dysrhythmias may develop when perfusion of the heart is poor. The most common dysrhythmias encountered during the postoperative period are atrial fibrillation, bradycardias, tachycardias, and ectopic beats. Continuous observation of the cardiac monitor for dysrhythmias is essential. Temporary epicardial pacemaker wires are frequently inserted in surgery and then removed after the patient is stable.

Any indications of decreased cardiac output are reported promptly to the physician. These assessment data and results of diagnostic tests are used by the physician to determine the cause of the problem. After a diagnosis has been made, the physician and the nurse work collaboratively to restore cardiac output and prevent further complications. When indicated, the physician prescribes blood components, intravenous fluids, digitalis or other antidysrhythmics, diuretics, vasodilators, or vasopressors. Other interventions may include the insertion of an intra-aortic balloon pump, extracorporeal membrane oxygenation (ECMO) machine or ventricular assist device. If additional surgery is necessary, the patient and family are prepared for the procedure.

PROMOTING ADEQUATE GAS EXCHANGE. To ensure adequate gas exchange, the nurse assesses and maintains the patency of the endotracheal tube. Because a patent airway is essential for oxygen and CO_2 exchange, the endotracheal tube must be secured to prevent it from slipping into the right mainstem bronchus and occluding the left bronchus. Suctioning is necessary when crackles or coughing are present. Arterial blood gas determinations are compared with baseline data, and changes are reported to the physician promptly.

When the patient's condition stabilizes, body position is changed every 1 to 2 hours. Frequent changes of patient position provide for optimal pulmonary ventilation and perfusion by allowing the lungs to expand more fully. The nurse assesses breath sounds to detect crackles, wheezes, and fluid in the lungs.

Physical assessment and arterial blood gas results guide the process of weaning the patient from the ventilator. The nurse assists with the weaning process and eventually with removal of the endotracheal tube. Before being extubated, the patient should have cough and gag reflexes and stable vital signs. Deep breathing and coughing are encouraged at least every 1 to 2 hours after extubation to open the alveolar sacs and provide for increased ventilation and to clear secretions.

MAINTAINING FLUID AND ELECTROLYTE BALANCE. To promote fluid and electrolyte balance, the nurse carefully assesses intake and output. Flow sheets are used to determine positive or negative fluid balance. All fluid intake is recorded, including IV, nasogastric tube, and oral fluids. All output is recorded, including urine, nasogastric drainage, and chest drainage.

Hemodynamic parameters (i.e., blood pressure, CVP, PAWP) are correlated with intake, output, and weight to determine the adequacy of hydration and cardiac output. Serum electrolytes are monitored, and the patient is observed for signs of potassium, magnesium, sodium, or calcium imbalance.

Any indications of dehydration, fluid overload, or electrolyte imbalance are reported promptly, and the physician and nurse work collaboratively to restore fluid and electrolyte balance. The patient's response is monitored.

MINIMIZING CONFUSION. Some patients exhibit abnormal behaviours that occur with varying intensity and duration. The risk of delirium is high in cardiac surgery patients and increases with patients' age (O'Neal, Billings, Liu, et al., 2017). Advances in surgical techniques and in the delivery of anesthetic agents have decreased the incidence of postoperative delirium, however, all postoperative patients are at risk, particularly the older, and those with sensory impairments, alcohol abuse, or severe illness. Factors that contribute to delirium are sleep deprivation or disturbances, increased or decreased sensory input, medications (particularly benzodiazepines, opioids, anticholinergics, and antiarrhythmics), and physiologic problems such as pain, infection, hypoxemia, or electrolyte abnormalities (Alcover, Badenes, Montero, et al., 2013; Mangusan et al., 2015).

The delirium typically appears after a 2- to 5-day stay in an ICU. Patients are assessed for this problem with tools such as the Confusion Assessment Method for the ICU (CAM-ICU) (Brooks, Spillane, Dick, et al., 2014). The CAMU-ICU scale assesses for key indicators of delirium such as disorganized thinking and inattention. When this testing is positive, further assessment of the patient's physiologic and psychological status is required. Treatment includes correction of identified physiologic problems such as metabolic and electrolyte imbalances. In addition, behavioural interventions are used (e.g., frequent reorientation). Sedative medications such as haloperidol (Haldol) may help reduce agitation. The delirium often resolves after the patient is transferred from the unit, but nonetheless can be associated with negative outcomes including cognitive and functional decline, longer lengths of hospital stay, and higher mortality (Mangusan et al., 2015).

Basic comfort measures are used in conjunction with prescribed analgesics and sedatives to promote rest. Because of safety concerns, lines and tubes are discontinued as soon as possible. Patient care is coordinated to provide undisturbed periods of rest. As the patient's condition stabilizes and the patient is disturbed less frequently for monitoring and therapeutic procedures, rest periods can be extended. As much uninterrupted sleep as possible is provided, especially during the patient's normal hours of sleep.

Careful explanations of all procedures and of the need for cooperation help to keep the patient oriented throughout the postoperative course. Continuity of care is desirable; a familiar face and a nursing staff with a consistent approach help the patient feel safe. The patient's family should be welcomed at the bedside. A well-designed and individualized plan of nursing care can assist the nursing team in coordinating their efforts for the emotional well-being of the patient.

RELIEVING PAIN. Deep pain may not be felt in the peri-incisional area but may occur in a broader, more diffuse area. Patients who have had cardiac surgery experience pain caused by the interruption of intercostal nerves along the incision route and irritation of the pleura by the chest catheters. Incisional pain may also be experienced from peripheral vein or artery graft harvest sites.

It is essential to observe and listen to the patient for verbal and nonverbal clues about pain. The nurse accurately records the nature, type, location, and duration of the pain (chest incisional pain must be differentiated from anginal pain). To reduce the amount of pain, the nurse encourages the patient to accept medication on a regular basis. The addition of adjunctive pain relievers (anti-inflammatory agents, muscle relaxants) has decreased the amount of opioids required for pain relief and has increased patient comfort. Patients report the most pain during coughing, turning, and moving. Physical support of the incision with a folded bath blanket or small pillow during deep breathing and coughing helps to minimize pain. The patient should then be able to participate in respiratory exercises and increase self-care progressively. Patient comfort improves after removal of the chest tubes.

Pain produces distress, which may stimulate the central nervous system to release catecholamines, resulting in constriction of the arterioles and increased heart rate. This can cause increased afterload and decreased cardiac output. Opioids alleviate pain and induce sleep and feelings of euphoria, which reduces the metabolic rate and oxygen demands. After the administration of opioids, any observations indicating relief of apprehension and pain are documented in the patient's record. The patient is observed for any adverse effects of opioids, which may include respiratory depression, hypotension, ileus, or urinary retention. If serious side effects occur, an opioid antagonist (e.g., naloxone [Narcan]) may be used.

MAINTAINING ADEQUATE TISSUE PERFUSION. Peripheral pulses (e.g., pedal, tibial, femoral, radial, brachial) are routinely palpated to assess for arterial obstruction. If a pulse is absent in any extremity, the cause may be prior catheterization of that extremity or chronic peripheral vascular disease, or a thromboembolic obstruction. The nurse immediately reports newly identified absence of any pulse. Thromboembolic events can result from vascular injury, dislodging a clot from a damaged valve, loosening of mural thrombi, or coagulation problems. Air embolism can result from CPB or central venous cannulation. Symptoms of embolization vary according to site. The usual embolic sites are the lungs, coronary arteries, mesentery, spleen, extremities, kidneys, and brain. The patient is observed for onset of the following:

- Acute onset of chest pain and respiratory distress from pulmonary embolus or MI
- Abdominal or back pain from mesenteric emboli
- Pain, cessation of pulses, blanching, numbness, or coldness in an extremity
- Decreased urine output from renal emboli
- One-sided weakness and pupillary changes, as occur in stroke

All such symptoms are promptly reported to the physician.

Venous stasis, which can cause venous thromboembolism (e.g., deep vein thrombosis, pulmonary embolism), may occur after surgery. The following measures are taken to prevent venous stasis:

- Applying elastic compression stockings or elastic bandage wraps and sequential pneumatic compression wraps
- Discouraging crossing of legs
- Avoiding elevating the knees on the bed
- Omitting pillows in the popliteal space
- Instituting passive exercises followed by active exercises to promote circulation and prevent venous stasis

Inadequate renal perfusion can occur as a complication of cardiac surgery. One possible cause is low cardiac output. Trauma to blood cells during CPB can cause hemolysis of red blood cells, which then occlude the renal glomeruli. Use of vasopressor agents to increase blood pressure may constrict the renal arterioles and reduce blood flow to the kidneys.

Nursing management includes accurate measurement of urine output. An output of less than 30 mL/hr may indicate hypovolemia or renal insufficiency. Urine specific gravity can be monitored to determine the kidneys' ability to concentrate urine in the renal tubules. Fluids may be prescribed to increase cardiac output and renal blood flow. IV diuretics may be administered to increase urine output. The nurse should be aware of the patient's blood urea nitrogen, serum creatinine, and urine and serum electrolyte levels. Abnormal levels are reported promptly because it may be necessary to adjust fluids and the dose or type of medication administered. If efforts to maintain renal perfusion are ineffective, the patient may require continuous renal replacement therapy or dialysis (see Chapter 45).

MAINTAINING NORMAL BODY TEMPERATURE. Patients are usually hypothermic when admitted to the critical care unit following the cardiac surgical procedure. Because induced hypothermia from CPB and anesthesia lower the patient's core temperature, the patient must be gradually warmed to a normal temperature. This is accomplished partially by the patient's own basal metabolic processes and often with the assistance of heated air blanket systems. While the patient is hypothermic, shivering and hypertension are common. Lowering the blood pressure with a vasodilator may be necessary. These problems typically resolve as warming occurs.

After cardiac surgery, the patient is at risk for developing elevated body temperature as a result of tissue inflammation (postpericardiotomy syndrome) or infection (see Chart 29-13). The resultant increase in metabolic rate increases tissue oxygen demands and increases cardiac workload. Antipyretics and other measures are used to lower body temperature.

Common sites of infection include the lungs, urinary tract, incisions, and intravascular catheters. Meticulous care is used to prevent contamination at the sites of catheter and tube insertions. Aseptic technique is used when changing dressings and when providing endotracheal tube and catheter care. Clearance of pulmonary secretions is accomplished by frequent repositioning of the patient, suctioning, and chest physical therapy as well as teaching and encouraging the patient to breathe deeply and cough. All invasive equipment is discontinued as soon as possible after surgery.

Postpericardiotomy syndrome may occur in patients who undergo cardiac surgery (Hannon & Porth, 2016). The syndrome is characterized by fever, pericardial pain, pleural pain, dyspnea, pericardial effusion, pericardial friction rub, and arthralgia. Leukocytosis occurs, along with elevation of the erythrocyte sedimentation rate. These signs and symptoms may occur days to weeks after surgery, often after the patient has been discharged from the hospital.

It is necessary to differentiate postpericardiotomy syndrome from other postoperative complications (e.g., infection, incisional pain, MI, pulmonary embolus, bacterial endocarditis, pneumonia, atelectasis) (see Chart 29-13). Treatment depends on the severity of the symptoms. Anti-inflammatory agents may produce a dramatic improvement in symptoms.

PROMOTING HOME, COMMUNITY-BASED, AND TRANSITIONAL CARE

Educating Patients About Self-Care. Depending on the type of surgery and postoperative progress, the patient may be discharged from the hospital a few days after surgery. Following recovery from the surgery, patients can expect fewer symptoms from CAD and an improved quality of life. CABG has been shown to increase the lifespan of high-risk patients, including those with left main artery blockages and left ventricular dysfunction with multivessel blockages (Hlatky, Boothroyd, Baker, et al., 2013). Although the patient may be eager to return home, the patient and family usually are apprehensive about this transition. The family members often express the fear that they are not capable of caring for the patient at home or they are unprepared to handle complications that may occur.

The nurse helps the patient and family set realistic, achievable goals. A teaching plan that meets the patient's individual needs is developed with the patient and family. This is started before admission and reviewed each shift through the hospital stay or with each home care and rehabilitation contact. Specific instructions are provided about incision care; signs and symptoms of infection; diet; activity progression and exercise; deep breathing, incentive spirometry, and smoking cessation; weight and temperature monitoring; the medication regimen; and follow-up visits with home care nurses, the rehabilitation personnel, the surgeon, and the cardiologist or internist.

Some patients have difficulty learning and retaining information after cardiac surgery. Many patients have difficulties in cognitive function after cardiac surgery that do not occur after other types of major surgery. The patient may experience recent memory loss, short attention span, difficulty with simple math, poor handwriting, and visual disturbances. Patients with these difficulties often become frustrated when they try to resume normal activities and learn how to care for themselves at home. The patient and family are reassured that the difficulty is almost always temporary and will subside, usually in 6 to 8 weeks. In the meantime, instructions are given to the patient at a much slower pace than normal, and a family member assumes responsibility for making sure that the prescribed regimen is followed.

Continuing and Transitional Care. Arrangements are made for a home care nurse when appropriate. Because the hospital stay is relatively short, it is particularly important for the nurse to assess the patient and family's ability to manage care in the home. Teaching is continued by the home care nurse and at subsequent clinic visits. Vital signs and incisions are monitored, the patient is assessed for signs and symptoms of complications, and support for the patient and family is provided. Additional interventions may include dressing changes, IV antibiotic administration, diet counselling, and tobacco use cessation strategies. Patients and families need to know that cardiac surgery did not cure the patient's underlying heart disease. Lifestyle changes for risk factor reduction are essential, and medications taken before surgery to control problems such as blood pressure and hyperlipidemia will still be necessary.

Patient teaching does not end at the time of discharge from home health care. The patient is encouraged to contact the surgeon, cardiologist, general practitioner, or office with problems or questions. This provides the patient and family with reassurance that professional support is available. The patient is expected to have at least one follow-up visit with the surgeon.

Education does not end at the time of discharge from the hospital, transitional, or home health care. Many patients and families benefit from supportive programs such as cardiac surgery rehabilitation program. These programs provide exercise monitoring; instructions about diet and stress reduction; information about resuming exercise, work, driving, and sexual activity; assistance with tobacco use cessation; and support groups for patients and families.

Critical Thinking Exercises

1 You are working in a cardiology office, and you receive a phone call from a patient who had an MI 2 years ago. She reports that she is experiencing some shortness of breath and mild back pain. What evidence base is there to suggest that symptoms of an MI may be different for women than men? Discuss the strength of this evidence and its significance in determining assessment criteria to be used for women and men. What questions would you ask this patient? What would you instruct her to do? Provide rationale for your instructions.

2 You are taking over the care of a patient who returned from the catheterization laboratory 2 hours ago following a successful PCI. He was reported to be stable on bed rest, with no bleeding from the right femoral site. The patient appears very pale and complains of right flank pain. Identify the key parameters that need to be assessed. Describe the actions you would take, and state why.

3 You are caring for a patient who has been hospitalized awaiting CABG surgery. As you deliver his morning medications, he states that he is feeling "pressure" in the lower sternal area, but he thinks it is just "nerves." What questions would you ask, and what would you assess? What would be your next actions?

REFERENCES AND SELECTED READINGS

Books

Ackley, B. J., Ladwig, G. B., Msn, R. N., et al. (2019). *Nursing diagnosis handbook E-book: An evidence-based guide to planning care*. Mosby.

Hannon, R. A., & Porth, C. M. (2016). *Porth pathophysiology: Concepts of altered health states* (2nd Cdn ed.). Philadelphia, PA: Lippincott Williams & Wilkins.

Navarese, E. P., Kowalewski, M., & Kołodziejczak, M. (2015). Drug-eluting stents and coronary artery disease. In *Pathophysiology and pharmacotherapy of cardiovascular disease* (pp. 495–524). Adis, Cham.

Zipes, D. P., Libby, P., Bonow, R. O., et al. (2019). *Braunwald's heart disease: A textbook of cardiovascular medicine* (11th ed.). Philadelphia, PA: Saunders.

Journals and Electronic Documents

Abuzaid, A., Fabrizio, C., Felpel, K., et al. (2018). Oxygen therapy in patients with acute myocardial infarction: A systemic review and meta-analysis. *The American Journal of Medicine*, *131*, 693–701.

Ahn, J. M., Park, D. W., Lee, C. W., et al. (2017). Comparison of stenting versus bypass surgery according to the completeness of revascularization in severe coronary artery disease. *JACC: Cardiovascular Interventions*, *10*(14), 1415–1424.

Alcover, L., Badenes, R., Montero, M. J., et al. (2013). Postoperative delirium and cognitive dysfunction. *Trends in Anaesthesia and Critical Care*, *3*(4), 199–204.

Alves, A. J., Viana, J. L., Cavalcante, S. L., et al. (2016). Physical activity in primary and secondary prevention of cardiovascular disease: Overview updated. *World Journal of Cardiology*, *8*(10), 575.

American Heart Association (2015). Menopause and heart disease. Retrieved on November 18, 2015 at: www.heart.org/HEARTORG/Conditions/More/MyHeartandStrokeNews/Menopause-and-Heart-Disease_UCM_448432_Article.jsp

Amsterdam, E. A., Wenger, N. K., Brindis, R. G., et al. (2014). 2014 AHA/ACC Guideline for the management of patients with non–ST-elevation acute coronary syndromes. *Journal of the American College of Cardiology*, *64*(24), e139–e228.

Anderson, J. L., Adams, C. D., Antman, E. M., et al. (2011). 2011 ACCF/AHA Focused Update Incorporated Into the ACC/AHA 2007 Guidelines for the Management of Patients With Unstable Angina/Non–ST-Elevation Myocardial Infarction: A Report of the American College of Cardiology Foundation/American Heart Association Task Force on Practice Guidelines. *Circulation*, *123*(18), e426–e579.

Anderson, T. J., Grégoire, J., Hegele, R. A., et al. (2013). 2012 Update of the Canadian Cardiovascular Society Guidelines for the diagnosis and treatment of dyslipidemia for the prevention of cardiovascular disease in the adult. *Canadian Journal of Cardiology*, *29*(2), 151–167.

Anderson, T. J., Grégoire, J., Pearson, G. J., et al. (2016). 2016 Canadian Cardiovascular Society guidelines for the management of dyslipidemia for the prevention of cardiovascular disease in the adult. *Canadian Journal of Cardiology*, *32*(11), 1263–1282.

Appelman, Y., van Rijn, B. B., Monique, E., et al. (2015). Sex differences in cardiovascular risk factors and disease prevention. *Atherosclerosis*, *241*(1), 211–218.

Ayan, M., Pothineni, N. V., Siraj, A., et al. (2016). Cardiac drug therapy—considerations in the elderly. *Journal of Geriatric Cardiology*, *13*(12), 992–997.

Bach, R. G., Cannon, C. P., Weintraub, W. S., et al. (2004). The effect of routine, early invasive management on outcome for elderly patients with non–ST-segment elevation acute coronary syndromes. *Annals of Internal Medicine, 141*(3), 186–195.

Bertoluci, M. C., & Rocha, V. Z. (2017). Cardiovascular risk assessment in patients with diabetes. *Diabetology & Metabolic Syndrome*, *9*(25), 1–13.

Bradt, J., Dileo, C., & Potvin, N. (2013). Music for stress and anxiety reduction in coronary heart disease patients. *Cochrane Database of Systematic Reviews*, *12*, 1265–1858.

Brooks, P., Spillane, J. J., Dick, K., et al. (2014). Developing a strategy to identify and treat older patients with postoperative delirium. *AORN Journal*, *99*(2), 257–273.

Canto, J. G., Rogers, W. J., Goldberg, R. J., et al. (2012). Association of age and sex with myocardial infarction symptom presentation and in-hospital mortality. *The Journal of the American Medical Association*, *307*(8), 813–822.

Chaisson, K., Sanford, M., Boss, R. A., et al. (2014). Improving patients' readiness for coronary artery bypass graft surgery. *Critical Care Nurse*, *34*(6), 29–36.

Chapman, A. R., Adamson, P. D., & Mills, N. L. (2017). Assessment and classification of patients with myocardial injury and infarction in clinical practice. *Heart*, *103*, 10–18.

Chauvet-Gelinier, J., & Bonin, B. (2017). Stress, anxiety and depression in heart disease patients: A major challenge for cardiac rehabilitation. *Annals of Physical and Rehabilitation Medicine*, *60*(1), 6–12.

Clark, R. A., Conway, A., Poulsen, V., et al. (2015). Alternative models of cardiac rehabilitation: A systematic review. *European Journal of Preventive Cardiology*, *22*(1), 35–74.

Cutlip, D. E., Kereiakes, D. J., Mauri, L., et al. (2015). Thrombotic complications associated with early and late nonadherence to dual antiplatelet therapy. *JACC: Cardiovascular Interventions*, *8*(3), 404–410.

Davierwala, P. M., & Mohr, F. W. (2015). Bilateral internal mammary artery grafting: Rationale and evidence. *International Journal of Surgery*, *16*, 133–139.

Dhar, A. K., & Barton, D. A. (2016). Depression and the link with cardiovascular disease. *Front Psychiatry*, *7*(33), 1–9.

Dhurandhar, V., Saxena, A., Parikh, R., et al. (2015). Outcomes of on-pump versus off-pump coronary artery bypass graft surgery in the high risk (AusScore >5). *Geartm Kybg abd Curcykatuibm*, *24*(12), 1216–1224.

El Hussein, M., Hirst, S., & Salyers, V. (2015). Factors that contribute to underrecognition of delirium by registered nurses in acute care settings: A scoping review of the literature to explain this phenomenon. *Journal of Clinical Nursing*, *24*(7–8), 906–915.

Fernandez-Mendoza, J., He, F., LaGrotte, C., et al. (2017). Impact of the metabolic syndrome on mortality is modified by objective short sleep duration. *Journal of the American Heart Association*, *6*(5), e005479.

Ferreira, R. M., de Souza E Silva, N. A., & Salis, L. H. A. (2018). Complications after elective percutaneous coronary interventions: A comparison between public and private hospitals. *Indian Heart Journal*, *70*(1), 32–36.

Frazer, C. A. (2013). Heparin-induced thrombocytopenia. *MedSurg Nursing*, *22*(6), 399–401.

Fysekidis, M., Cosson, E., Takbou, K., et al. (2018). Effects of insulin analogs as an add-on to metformin on cutaneous microcirculation in type 2 diabetic patients. *Microvascular Research*, *116*, 6–14.

Garcia, M., Mulvagh, S. L., Merz, C. N., et al. (2016). Cardiovascular disease in women: Clinical perspectives. *Circulation Research*, *118*(8), 1273–1293.

Gibson, C. M., & Morrow, D. A. (2018). Elevated cardiac troponin concentration in the absence of an acute coronary syndrome. *UpToDate*. Retrieved from https://www.uptodate.com/contents/elevated-cardiac-troponin-concentration-in-the-absence-of-an-acute-coronary-syndrome

Gimbrone, M. A., & Garcia-Candena, G. (2016). Endothelial cell dysfunction and the pathobiology of atherosclerosis. *Circulation Research*, *118*(4), 620–626.

Girish, G., Agarwal, S., Satsangi, D. K., et al. (2014). Glycemic control in cardiac surgery: Rationale and current evidence. *Annals of Cardiac Anaesthesia*, *17*(3), 222–228.

Greer, A. E., Sui, X., Maslow, A. L., et al. (2015). The effects of sedentary behavior on metabolic syndrome independent of physical activity and cardiorespiratory fitness. *Journal of Physical Activity and Health*, *12*(1), 68–73.

Greinacher, A. (2015). Heparin-induced thrombocytopenia. *New England Journal of Medicine*, *373*, 252–261.

Han, T. S., & Lean, M. E. (2016). A clinical perspective of obesity, metabolic syndrome and cardiovascular disease. *JRSM Cardiovascular Disease*, *5*, 2048004016633371.

Hargraves, J. D. (2014). Glycemic control in cardiac surgery: Implementing an evidence-based insulin infusion protocol. *American Journal of Critical Care*, *23*(3), 250–258.

Head, S. J., & Kappetein, A. P. (2016). Coronary artery bypass grafting in diabetic patients: Do not bypass the pump! *European Journal of Cardio-Thoracic Surgery*, *49*(2), 418–419.

Heart and Stroke Canada. (2017). Getting to the heart of the matter. Retrieved from https://www.heartandstroke.ca/-/media/pdf-files/canada/2017-heart-month/heartandstroke-reportonhealth-2015.ashx?la=en&hash=5814B30179B3D77A960E57E7866D2B645B5BD960

Hejazi, S. F., Iranirad, L., Doostali, K., et al. (2017). In-hospital clinical outcomes and procedural complications of percutaneous coronary intervention in elderly patients. *Cardiology Research*, *8*(5), 199–205.

Hlatky, M. A., Boothroyd, D. B., Baker, L., et al. (2013). Comparative effectiveness of multivessel coronary bypass surgery and multivessel percutaneous coronary intervention: A cohort study. *Annals of Internal Medicine, 158*(10), 727–734.

Ho, J. E., Lyass, A., Courchesne, P., et al. (2018). Protein biomarkers of cardiovascular disease and mortality in the community. *Journal of the American Heart Association, 7*(14), e008108.

Jung, U. J., & Choi, M. S. (2014). Obesity and its metabolic complications: The role of adipokines and the relationship between obesity, inflammation, insulin resistance, dyslipidemia and nonalcoholic fatty liver disease. *International Journal of Molecular Sciences, 15*(4), 6184–6223.

Kachur, S., Chongthammakun, V., Lavie, C. J., et al. (2017). Impact of cardiac rehabilitation and exercise training programs in coronary heart disease. *Progress in Cardiovascular Diseases, 60*(1), 103–114.

Kannel, W. B. (1986). Silent myocardial ischemia and infarction: Insights from the Framingham Study. *Cardiology clinics, 4*(4), 583–591.

Katritsis, D. G., Gersh, B. J., & Camm, A. J. (2016). A clinical perspective on sudden cardiac death. *Arrhythmia Electrophysiology Review, 5*(3), 177–182.

Lubrano, V., & Balzan, S. (2015). Consolidated and emerging inflammatory markers in coronary artery disease. *World Journal of Experimental Medicine, 5*(1),21.

Magee, M. J., Coombs, L. P., Peterson, E. D., et al. (2003). Patient selection and current practice strategy for off-pump coronary artery bypass surgery. *Circulation, 108*(10_suppl_1), II-9.

Mangusan, R. F., Hooper, V., Denslow, S. A., et al. (2015). Outcomes associated with postoperative delirium after cardiac surgery. *American Journal of Critical Care, 24*(2), 156–163.

Mehta, P. K., Wei, J., & Merz, C. N. B. (2017). Angina in Patients with Evidence of Myocardial Ischemia and No Obstructive Coronary Artery Disease. Chronic Coronary Artery Disease: A Companion to Braunwald's Heart Disease, 374.

Mnatzaganian, G., Braitberg, G., Hiller, J. E., et al. (2016). Sex differences in in-hospital mortality following a first acute myocardial infarction: Symptomatology, delayed presentation, and hospital setting. *BMC Cardiovascular Disorders, 16*(1), 109.

Moe, G. W., Ezekowitz, J. A., O'Meara, E., et al. (2013). The 2013 Canadian Cardiovascular Society Heart Failure Management Guidelines Update: Focus on rehabilitation and exercise and surgical coronary revascularization. *Canadian Journal of Cardiology, 30*(3), 249–263.

Moudgil, R., & Haddad, H. (2013). Depression in heart failure. *Current Opinion in Cardiology, 28*(2), 249–258.

Nerenberg, K. A., Zarnke, K. B., Leung, A. A., et al. (2018). Hypertension Canada's 2018 guidelines for diagnosis, risk assessment, prevention, and treatment of hypertension in adults and children. *Canadian Journal of Cardiology, 34*(5), 506–525.

Noble, S., & Roffi, M. (2017). Routine beta-blocker administration following acute myocardial infarction: Why still an unsolved issue? *Journal of Thoracic Disease, 9*(11), 4191–4194.

Nystrom, T., Sartipy, U., & Holzmann, M. (2018). PCI or CABG in stable patients with multivessel CAD and diabetes. *American College of Cardiology*. Retrieved March 27, 2018, from https://www.acc.org/latest-in-cardiology/articles/2018/03/27/08/51/pci-or-cabg-in-stable-patients-with-multivessel-cad-and-diabetes

O'Gara, P. T., Kushner, F. G., Ascheim, D. D., et al. (2013). 2013 ACCF/AHA guideline for the management of ST-elevation myocardial infarction: A report of the American College of cardiology Foundation/American Heart Association Task Force on practice guidelines. *Circulation, 127*(4), e362–e425.

O'Neal, J. B., Billings, F. T., Liu, X., et al. (2017). Risk factors for delirium after cardiac surgery: An historical cohort study outlining the influence of cardiopulmonary bypass. *Canadian Journal of Anaesthesia, 64*(11), 1129–1137.

Oosterhouse, K. J., Vincent, C., Foreman, M. D., et al. (2016). Intensive care unit nurses' beliefs about delirium assessment and management. *AACN Advanced Critical Care, 27*(4), 379–393.

Palmerini, T., Benedetto, U., Biondi-Zoccai, G., et al. (2015). Long-term safety of drug-eluting and bare-metal stents. *Journal of the American College of Cardiology, 65*(23), 2496–2507.

Pantazi, E., Bejaoui, M., Folch-Puy, E., et al. (2016). Advances in treatment strategies for ischemia reperfusion injury. *Expert Opinion on Pharmacotherapy, 17*(2), 169–179.

Rosengren, A., Hawken, S., Ounpuu, S., et al. (2004). Association of psychosocial risk factors with risk of acute myocardial infarction in 11119 cases and 13648 controls from 52 countries (the INTERHEART study): Case-control study. *Lancet, 364*(9438), 953–962.

Shrivastava, A. K., Singh, H. V., Raizada, A., et al. (2015). C-reactive protein, inflammation and coronary heart disease. *The Egyptian Heart Journal, 67*(2), 89–97.

Silvain, J., Beygui, F., Barthelemy, O., et al. (2012). Efficacy and safety of enoxaparin versus unfractionated heparin during percutaneous coronary intervention: Systematic review and meta-analysis. *British Medical Journal, 344*, e553, 1–13.

Solhpour, A., Chang, K., Balan, P., et al. (2014). Comparison of outcomes for patients >=75 years of age treated with pre-hospital reduced-dose fibrinolysis followed by percutaneous coronary intervention versus percutaneous coronary intervention alone for treatment of ST-elevation myocardial infarction. *The American Journal of Cardiology, 113*(1), 60–63.

Statistics Canada. (2012). Tables by subject: Life expectancy and deaths. Retrieved January 23, from http://www.statcan.gc.ca/tables-tableaux/sum-som/l01/ind01/l3_2966_2979-eng.htm?hili_hlth36

Statistics Canada. (2014). Health Status of Canadians 2016: Report of the Chief Public Health Officer - How are we unhealthy? - Cardiovascular disease. Retrieved from https://www.canada.ca/en/public-health/corporate/publications/chief-public-health-officer-reports-state-public-health-canada/2016-health-status-canadians/page-17-how-are-we-unhealthy-cardiovascular-disease.html

Statistics Canada. (2017). Heart disease in Canada: Highlights from the Canadian Chronic Disease Surveillance System. Retrieved November 11, 2018, from https://www.canada.ca/en/public-health/services/publications/diseases-conditions/heart-disease-canada-fact-sheet.html

Stone, N. J., Robinson, J., Lichtenstein, A. H., et al. (2013). 2013 ACC/AHA Guideline on the treatment of blood cholesterol to reduce atherosclerotic cardiovascular risk in adults. A report of the American College of Cardiology/American Heart Association Task Force on Practice Guidelines. *Journal of the American College of Cardiology, 63*(25 Part B), 2889–2934.

Stub, D. (2017). Should patients with ACS routinely receive O2? *American College of Cardiology*. Retrieved from https://www.acc.org/latest-in-cardiology/articles/2017/05/15/08/34/should-patients-with-acs-routinely-receive-o2

Velazquez, E. J., Lee, K. L., Jones, R. H., et al. (2016). Coronary-artery bypass surgery in patients with ischemic cardiomyopathy. *New England Journal of Medicine, 374*(16), 1511–1520.

Vogel, B., Farhan, S., Hahne, S., et al. (2016). Sex-related differences in baseline characteristics, management and outcome in patients with acute coronary syndrome without ST-segment elevation. *European Heart Journal: Acute Cardiovascular Care, 5*(4), 347–353.

White, C. M. (2015). Therapeutic potential and critical analysis of the PCSK9 monoclonal antibodies evolocumab and alirocumab. *Annals of Pharmacology, 49*(12), 1327–1335.

Widmer, R. J., Flammer, A. J., Lerman, L. O., et al. (2015). The Mediterranean diet, its components, and cardiovascular disease. *The American Journal of Medicine, 128*(3), 229–238.

Williams, J. B., Alexander, K. P., Morin, J. F., et al. (2013). Preoperative anxiety as a predictor of mortality and major morbidity in patients >70 years of age undergoing cardiac surgery. *American Journal of Cardiology, 111*(1), 137–142.

Resources

American Dietetic Association, 216 West Jackson Boulevard, Chicago, IL 60606, (800) 366–1644: http://www.eatright.org.

American Heart Association, 7272 Greenville Avenue, Dallas, TX 75231, (800) AHA-USA1 242–8721: http://www.americanheart.org.

Canadian Cardiovascular Society (CCS). (2014). CCS Guideline Library: http://www.ccsguidelineprograms.ca/index.php?option=com_content&view=article&id=185&Itemid=107.

Healthy People 2010, Office of Disease Prevention and Health Promotion, U.S. Department of Health and Human Services, 200 Independence Avenue SW, Washington, DC 20201, (800) 877-696-6775: http://www.health.gov/healthypeople.

Heart and Stroke Foundation of Canada, 222 Queen Street, Suite 1402, Ottawa, ON K1P 5V9, (613) 569–4361: http://www.heartandstroke.com/site/c.ikIQLcMWJtE/b.2796497/k.BF8B/Home.htm?src=home.

Heartmates, PO Box 16202, Minneapolis, MN 55416, (952) 929–3331: http://www.heartmates.com.

National Heart, Lung and Blood Institute, National Institutes of Health, Building 31, Room 5A52, Bethesda, MD 20892, (301) 592–8593: http://www.nhlbi.nih.gov.

30 Management of Patients With Structural, Infections, and Inflammatory Cardiac Disorders

Adapted by Colleen Norris and Nicole Tegg

Learning Objectives

On completion of this chapter, the learner will be able to:

1. Define valvular disorders of the heart and describe the pathophysiology, clinical manifestations, and management of patients with mitral and aortic disorders.
2. Describe types of cardiac valve repair and replacement procedures used to treat valvular problems and the care needed by patients who undergo these procedures.
3. Describe the pathophysiology, clinical manifestations, and management of patients with intracardiac septal defects.
4. Describe the pathophysiology, clinical manifestations, and management of patients with cardiomyopathies.
5. Describe the pathophysiology, clinical manifestations, and management of patients with infections of the heart.

Structural, infectious, and inflammatory disorders of the heart present many challenges for the patient, family, and health care team. Problems with the heart valves, holes in the intracardiac septum, cardiomyopathies, and infectious diseases of the heart muscle alter cardiac output. Treatments for these disorders may be noninvasive, such as medication therapy and activity and dietary modification. Invasive treatments also may be used, such as valve repair or replacement, septal repair, ventricular assist devices (VADs), **total artificial hearts**, cardiac transplantation, and other procedures. Nurses have an integral role in the care of patients with structural, infectious, and inflammatory cardiac conditions.

VALVULAR DISORDERS

The valves of the heart control the flow of blood through the heart into the pulmonary artery and aorta by opening and closing in response to the blood pressure changes as the heart contracts and relaxes through the cardiac cycle.

The atrioventricular valves separate the atria from the ventricles and include the **tricuspid valve**, which separates the right atrium from the right ventricle, and the **mitral valve**, which separates the left atrium from the left ventricle. The tricuspid valve has three leaflets; the mitral valve has two. Both valves have **chordae tendineae** that anchor the valve leaflets to the papillary muscles of the ventricles.

The semilunar valves are located between the ventricles and their corresponding arteries. The **pulmonic valve** lies between the right ventricle and the pulmonary artery; the **aortic valve** lies between the left ventricle and the aorta. Figure 30-1 shows valves in the closed position.

When any of the heart valves do not close or open properly, blood flow is affected. When valves do not close completely, blood flows backward through the valve, a condition called **regurgitation**. When valves do not open completely, a condition called **stenosis**, the flow of blood through the valve is reduced.

Disorders of the mitral valve fall into the following categories: mitral valve **prolapse** (i.e., stretching of the valve leaflet into the atrium during systole), mitral regurgitation, and mitral stenosis. Disorders of the aortic valve are categorized as aortic regurgitation and aortic stenosis. These valvular disorders may require surgical repair or replacement of the valve to correct the problem, depending on severity of symptoms (Fig. 30-2). Tricuspid and pulmonic valve disorders also occur, usually with fewer symptoms and complications. Regurgitation and stenosis may occur at the same time in the same or different valves.

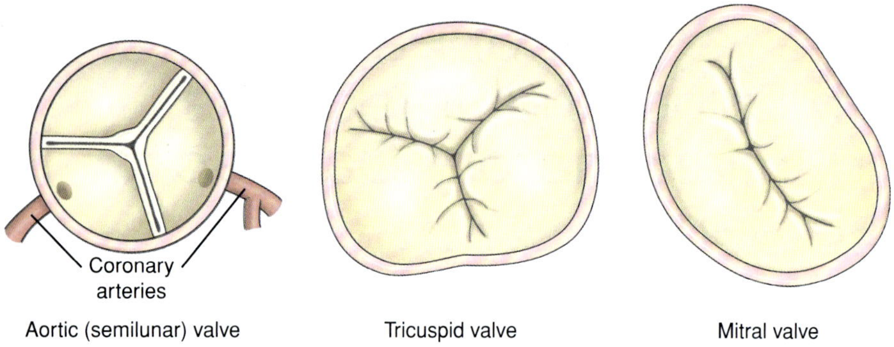

FIGURE 30-1. The valves of the heart (aortic or semilunar, tricuspid, and mitral) in the closed position.

Mitral Valve Prolapse

Mitral valve prolapse is a deformity that usually produces no symptoms. Rarely, it progresses and can result in sudden death. This condition occurs more frequently in women than in men and is being diagnosed more frequently than it once was, probably because of improved diagnostic methods (Delling & Vasan, 2014; Mann, Zipes, Bonow, et al., 2015). The cause is usually an inherited connective tissue disorder resulting in enlargement of one or both of the mitral valve leaflets. The annulus often dilates. The chordae tendineae and papillary muscles may elongate.

Pathophysiology

In mitral valve prolapse, a portion of one or both mitral valve leaflets balloons back into the atrium during systole. Rarely, the ballooning stretches the leaflet to the point that the valve does not remain closed during systole (i.e., ventricular contraction). Blood then regurgitates from the left ventricle back into the left atrium. About 15% of patients who develop murmurs eventually experience heart enlargement, atrial fibrillation, pulmonary hypertension, or heart failure (Fuster, Walsh, Harrington, et al., 2011).

Clinical Manifestations

Most people who have mitral valve prolapse never have symptoms. A few have symptoms of fatigue, shortness of breath, lightheadedness, dizziness, syncope, palpitations, chest pain, and anxiety (Mann, et al., 2015; Fuster et al., 2011). Fatigue may occur regardless of activity level and amount of rest or sleep. Shortness of breath is not correlated with activity levels or pulmonary function. Atrial or ventricular dysrhythmias may produce the

Glossary

allograft: heart valve replacement made from a human heart valve (synonym: homograft)
annuloplasty: repair of a cardiac valve's outer ring
aortic valve: semilunar valve located between the left ventricle and the aorta
autograft: heart valve replacement made from the patient's own heart valve (e.g., the pulmonic valve is excised and used as an aortic valve)
cardiomyopathy: disease of the heart muscle
chordae tendineae: nondistensible fibrous strands connecting papillary muscles to atrioventricular (mitral, tricuspid) valve leaflets
chordoplasty: repair of the chordae tendineae
commissurotomy: splitting or separating fused cardiac valve leaflets
heterograft: heart valve replacement made of tissue from an animal heart valve (synonym: xenograft)
homograft: heart valve replacement made from a human heart valve (synonym: allograft)
leaflet repair: repair of a cardiac valve's movable "flaps" (leaflets)
mitral valve: atrioventricular valve located between the left atrium and left ventricle
orthotopic transplantation: the recipient's heart is removed and a donor heart is grafted into the same site; the patient has one heart
prolapse (of a valve): stretching of an atrioventricular heart valve leaflet into the atrium during systole
pulmonic valve: semilunar valve located between the right ventricle and the pulmonary artery
regurgitation: backward flow of blood through a heart valve
stenosis: narrowing or obstruction of a cardiac valve's orifice
total artificial heart: mechanical device used to aid a failing heart, assisting the right and left ventricles
tricuspid valve: atrioventricular valve located between the right atrium and right ventricle
valve replacement: insertion of a device at the site of a malfunctioning heart valve to restore blood flow in one direction through the heart
valvuloplasty: repair of a stenosed or regurgitant cardiac valve by commissurotomy, annuloplasty, leaflet repair, or chordoplasty (or a combination of procedures)
ventricular assist device: mechanical device used to aid a failing right or left ventricle
xenograft: heart valve replacement made of tissue from an animal heart valve (synonym: heterograft)

Physiology/Pathophysiology

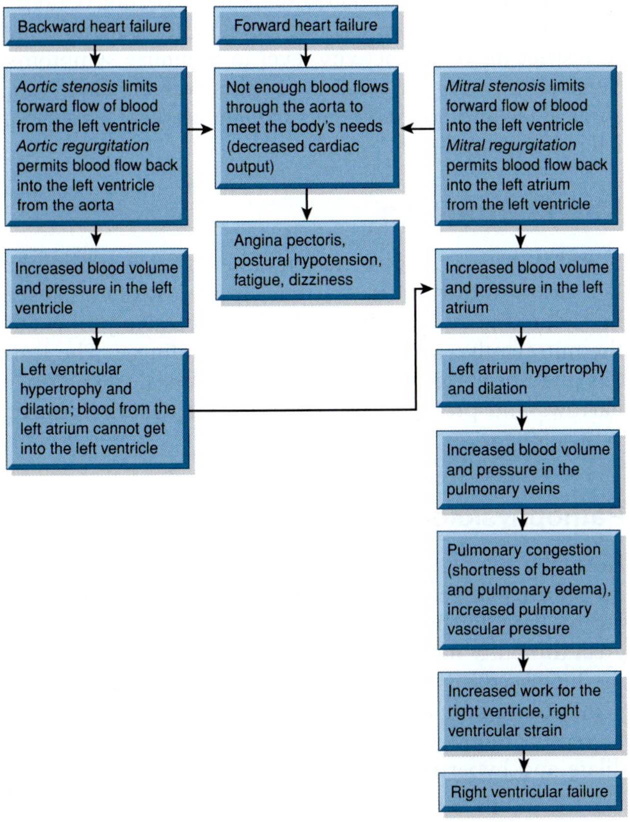

FIGURE 30-2. Pathophysiology: Left-sided heart failure as a result of aortic and mitral valvular heart disease and the development of right ventricular failure.

sensation of palpitations, but palpitations have been reported while the heart has been beating normally. Chest pain, which is often localized to the chest, is not correlated with activity and may last for days. Anxiety may be a response to the symptoms; however, some patients report anxiety as the only symptom. Some clinicians speculate that the symptoms may be explained by dysautonomia (a dysfunction of the autonomic nervous system that results in increased excretion of catecholamines). No consensus exists about the cause of the symptoms experienced by some patients (Mann et al., 2015; Runge, Stouffer, & Patterson, 2011).

Assessment and Diagnostic Findings

Often the first and only sign of mitral valve prolapse is identified when a physical examination of the heart reveals an extra heart sound, referred to as a mitral click. A systolic click is an early sign that a valve leaflet is ballooning into the left atrium. In addition to the mitral click, a murmur of mitral regurgitation may be heard if progressive valve leaflet stretching and regurgitation have occurred. A few patients experience signs and symptoms of heart failure if mitral regurgitation exists. Doppler echocardiography may be used to diagnose and monitor the progression of mitral valve prolapse (Mann et al., 2015).

Medical Management

Medical management is directed at controlling symptoms. If dysrhythmias are documented and cause symptoms, the patient is advised to eliminate caffeine and alcohol from the diet and to stop smoking. Most patients do not require any medications; prophylactic antibiotics are no longer recommended prior to dental or invasive procedures (Nishimura, Otto, Bonow, et al., 2014), although antiarrhythmic medications may be prescribed.

Chest pain that does not respond to nitrates may respond to calcium channel blockers or beta-blockers. Heart failure is treated the same as it would be for any other case of heart failure (see Chapter 31). In advanced stages of disease, mitral valve repair or replacement may be necessary (discussed later in this chapter).

Nursing Management

The nurse educates the patient about the diagnosis and the possibility that the condition is hereditary. First-degree relatives (e.g., parents, siblings) may be advised to have echocardiograms. Patients with mitral valve prolapse may be at risk for infectious endocarditis that results from bacteria entering the bloodstream and adhering to the abnormal valve structures. The nurse teaches the patient how to minimize this risk: practicing good oral hygiene, obtaining routine dental care, avoiding body piercing and body branding, and not using toothpicks or other sharp objects in the oral cavity.

Because most patients with mitral valve prolapse are asymptomatic, the nurse explains the need to inform the health care provider about any symptoms that may develop. To minimize symptoms, the nurse teaches the patient to avoid caffeine and alcohol. The nurse encourages the patient to read product labels, particularly on over-the-counter products such as cough medicine, because these products may contain alcohol, caffeine, ephedrine, and epinephrine, which may produce dysrhythmias and other symptoms. In addition, the nurse also explores possible diet, activity, sleep, and other lifestyle factors that may correlate with symptoms. Treatment of dysrhythmias, chest pain, heart failure, or other complications of mitral valve prolapse is described in Chapter 31. Women diagnosed with mitral valve prolapse without mitral regurgitation or other complications may complete pregnancies and have vaginal deliveries.

Mitral Regurgitation

Mitral regurgitation involves blood flowing back from the left ventricle into the left atrium during systole. Often the edges of the mitral valve leaflets do not close during systole. The leaflets cannot close completely because the leaflets and chordae tendineae have thickened and fibrosed, resulting in their contraction. The most common causes of mitral valve regurgitation in developed countries are degenerative changes of the mitral valve (e.g., mitral valve prolapse) and ischemia of the left ventricle (Fuster et al., 2011; Mann et al., 2015). The most common causes in developing countries are rheumatic heart disease and its sequelae (Fuster et al., 2011).

Other conditions that lead to mitral regurgitation include myxomatous changes, which enlarge and stretch the left atrium and ventricle, causing leaflets and chordae tendineae to stretch or rupture. Infective endocarditis may cause perforation of a leaflet, or the scarring following the infection may cause retraction of the leaflets or chordae tendineae. Collagen-vascular diseases (e.g., systemic lupus erythematosus), cardiomyopathy, and ischemic heart disease may also result in changes in the left ventricle, causing the papillary muscles, chordae tendineae, or leaflets to stretch, shorten, or rupture.

Pathophysiology

Mitral regurgitation may result from problems with one or more of the leaflets, the chordae tendineae, the annulus, or the papillary muscles. As previously stated, a mitral valve leaflet may shorten or tear, and the chordae tendineae may elongate, shorten, or tear. The annulus may be stretched by heart enlargement or deformed by calcification. The papillary muscle may rupture, stretch, or be pulled out of position by changes in the ventricular wall (e.g., scar from a myocardial infarction or ventricular dilation). The papillary muscles may be unable to contract because of ischemia. Regardless of the cause, blood regurgitates into the atrium during systole.

With each beat of the left ventricle, some of the blood is forced back into the left atrium, adding to the blood flowing in from the lungs. This causes the left atrium to stretch and eventually hypertrophy and dilate. The backward flow of blood from the ventricle diminishes the volume of blood flowing into the atrium from the lungs. As a result, the lungs become congested, eventually adding extra strain on the right ventricle.

Clinical Manifestations

Chronic mitral regurgitation is often asymptomatic, but acute mitral regurgitation (e.g., that resulting from a myocardial infarction) usually manifests as severe congestive heart failure. Dyspnea, fatigue, and weakness are the most common symptoms. Palpitations, shortness of breath on exertion, and cough from pulmonary congestion also occur.

Assessment and Diagnostic Findings

A systolic murmur is heard as a high-pitched, blowing sound at the apex (Mann et al., 2015; Weber & Kelley, 2014). The pulse may be regular and of good volume, or it may be irregular as a result of extrasystolic beats or atrial fibrillation. Doppler echocardiography is used to diagnose and monitor the progression of mitral regurgitation (Mann et al., 2015). Transesophageal echocardiography (TEE) provides the best images of the mitral valve.

Medical Management

Management of mitral regurgitation is the same as that for heart failure (see Chapter 31). Patients with mitral regurgitation and heart failure benefit from afterload reduction (arterial dilation) by treatment with angiotensin-converting enzyme (ACE) inhibitors, such as captopril (Capoten), enalapril (Vasotec), lisinopril (Prinivil, Zestril), ramipril (Altace), or hydralazine (Apresoline); angiotensin receptor blockers (ARBs), such as losartan (Cozar) or valsartan (Diovan); and beta-blockers, such as carvedilol (Coreg). Once symptoms of heart failure develop, the patient needs to restrict his or her activity level to minimize symptoms. Surgical intervention consists of mitral valvuloplasty (i.e., surgical repair of the valve) or **valve replacement** (discussed later) (Nishimura et al., 2014).

Mitral Stenosis

Mitral stenosis is an obstruction of blood flowing from the left atrium into the left ventricle. It is most often caused by rheumatic endocarditis, which progressively thickens the mitral valve leaflets and chordae tendineae. The leaflets often fuse together. Eventually, the mitral valve orifice narrows and progressively obstructs blood flow into the ventricle.

Pathophysiology

Normally, the mitral valve opening is as wide as the diameter of three fingers. In cases of marked stenosis, the opening narrows to the width of a pencil. The left atrium has great difficulty moving blood into the ventricle because of the increased resistance of the narrowed orifice. Poor left ventricular filling can cause decreased cardiac output. The increased blood volume in the left atrium causes it to dilate and hypertrophy. Because there is no valve to protect the pulmonary veins from the backward flow of blood from the atrium, the pulmonary circulation becomes congested. As a result, the right ventricle must contract against an abnormally high pulmonary arterial pressure and is subjected to excessive strain. Eventually, the right ventricle fails.

Clinical Manifestations

The first symptom of mitral stenosis is often dyspnea on exertion as a result of pulmonary venous hypertension. Symptoms usually develop after the valve opening is reduced by one third to one half its usual size. Patients are likely to show progressive fatigue as a result of low cardiac output. The enlarged left atrium may create pressure on the left bronchial tree, resulting in a dry cough or wheezing. Patients may expectorate blood (i.e., hemoptysis) or experience palpitations, orthopnea, paroxysmal nocturnal dyspnea (PND), and repeated respiratory infections.

Assessment and Diagnostic Findings

The pulse is weak and often irregular because of atrial fibrillation (caused by the strain on the atrium). A low-pitched, rumbling, diastolic murmur is heard at the apex (Mann et al., 2015; Weber & Kelley, 2014). As a result of the increased blood volume and pressure, the atrium dilates, hypertrophies, and becomes electrically unstable, and patients experience atrial dysrhythmias. Doppler echocardiography is used to diagnose mitral stenosis. Electrocardiography (ECG) and cardiac catheterization with angiography may be used to help determine the severity of the mitral stenosis.

Medical Management

Congestive heart failure is treated as described in Chapter 31. Patients with mitral stenosis may benefit from anticoagulants to decrease the risk for developing atrial thrombus and may also require treatment for anemia. Patients with mitral stenosis are advised to avoid strenuous activities and competitive sports, both of which increase the heart rate. Mitral stenosis decreases the amount of blood that can flow from the left atrium to the left ventricle during diastole. When the heart rate increases, diastole is shortened, and thus the amount of time for the forward flow of blood is less. Therefore, as the heart rate increases, cardiac output decreases and pulmonary pressures increase with the backup of blood from the left atrium into the pulmonary veins. Surgical intervention consists of valvuloplasty, usually a commissurotomy to open or rupture the fused commissures of the mitral valve. Percutaneous transluminal valvuloplasty or mitral valve replacement may be performed.

Aortic Regurgitation

Aortic regurgitation is the flow of blood back into the left ventricle from the aorta during diastole. It may be caused by inflammatory lesions that deform the leaflets of the aortic valve, preventing them from completely closing the aortic valve orifice. This valvular defect also may result from infective or rheumatic endocarditis, congenital abnormalities, diseases such as syphilis, a dissecting aneurysm that causes dilation or tearing of the ascending aorta, blunt chest trauma, or deterioration of an aortic valve replacement (Cohn, 2012; Fuster et al., 2011; Mann et al., 2015). In many cases, the cause is unknown and is classified as idiopathic.

Pathophysiology

Blood from the aorta returns to the left ventricle during diastole, in addition to the blood normally delivered by the left atrium. The left ventricle dilates in an attempt to accommodate the increased volume of blood. It also hypertrophies in an attempt to increase muscle strength to expel more blood with above-normal force, thus increasing systolic blood pressure. The arteries attempt to compensate for the higher pressures by reflex vasodilation; the peripheral arterioles relax, reducing peripheral resistance and diastolic blood pressure.

Clinical Manifestations

Aortic insufficiency develops without symptoms in most patients. Some patients are aware of a forceful heartbeat, especially in the head or neck. Marked arterial pulsations that are visible or palpable at the carotid or temporal arteries may be present as a result of the increased force and volume of the blood ejected from the hypertrophied left ventricle. Exertional dyspnea and fatigue follow. Signs and symptoms of progressive left ventricular failure include breathing difficulties (e.g., orthopnea, PND).

Assessment and Diagnostic Findings

A diastolic murmur is heard as a high-pitched, blowing sound at the 3rd or 4th intercostal space at the left sternal border (Weber & Kelley, 2014). The pulse pressure (i.e., difference between systolic and diastolic pressures) is considerably widened in patients with aortic regurgitation. One characteristic sign of the disease is the water-hammer (Corrigan) pulse, in which the pulse strikes the palpating finger with a quick, sharp stroke and then suddenly collapses. The diagnosis may be confirmed by Doppler echocardiography (preferably transesophageal), radionuclide imaging, ECG, magnetic resonance imaging (MRI), and cardiac catheterization (Mann et al., 2015; Pennell, Baksi, Kilner, et al., 2014). Patients with symptoms usually have echocardiograms every 4 to 6 months, and those without symptoms have echocardiograms every 2 to 3 years (Nishimura et al., 2014; Otto & Bonow, 2013).

Medical Management

The patient is advised to avoid physical exertion, competitive sports, and isometric exercise (Mann et al., 2015). Dysrhythmias and heart failure are treated as described in Chapters 28 and 31. There is no strong indication for medical therapy based on findings from clinical trials. Patients with aortic regurgitation and also hypertension should be treated with dihydropyridine calcium channel blockers (e.g., felodipine [Plendil], nifedipine [Adalat, Procardia]) or ACE inhibitors (e.g., captopril, enalapril, lisinopril, ramipril) to provide afterload reduction (Nishimura et al., 2014). Symptomatic patients should be instructed to restrict sodium intake to avoid volume overload (Mann et al., 2015; Nishimura et al., 2014). The treatment of choice is aortic valvuloplasty or valve replacement, preferably performed before left ventricular failure occurs. Surgery is recommended for any patient with left ventricular hypertrophy, regardless of the presence or absence of symptoms (Mann et al., 2015; Nishimura et al., 2014; Otto & Bonow, 2013).

Aortic Stenosis

Aortic valve stenosis is narrowing of the orifice between the left ventricle and the aorta. In adults, the stenosis is often a result of degenerative calcifications. Calcifications may be caused by inflammatory changes that occur in response to years of normal mechanical stress. Diabetes mellitus, hypercholesterolemia, hypertension, and low levels of high-density lipoprotein cholesterol may be risk factors for degenerative changes of the valve (Mann et al., 2015). Congenital leaflet malformations or an abnormal number of leaflets (i.e., one or two rather than three) may be involved. Rarely rheumatic endocarditis may cause adhesions or fusion of the commissures and valve ring, stiffening of the cusps, and calcific nodules on the cusps. However, the cause of cusp calcification may be unknown.

Pathophysiology

Progressive narrowing of the valve orifice occurs, usually over several years to several decades. The left ventricle overcomes the obstruction to circulation by contracting more slowly but with greater energy than normal, forcibly squeezing the blood through the smaller orifice. The obstruction to left ventricular outflow increases pressure on the left ventricle, and the ventricular wall thickens, or hypertrophies. When these compensatory mechanisms of the heart begin to fail, clinical signs and symptoms develop (Otto & Bonow, 2013).

Clinical Manifestations

Many patients with aortic stenosis are asymptomatic. When symptoms develop, patients usually first have exertional dyspnea, caused by increased pulmonary venous pressure due to left ventricular failure. Orthopnea, PND, and pulmonary edema may also occur, along with dizziness and syncope because of reduced blood flow to the brain. Angina pectoris is a frequent symptom; it results from the increased oxygen demands of the hypertrophied left ventricle, the decreased time in diastole for myocardial perfusion, and the decreased blood flow into the coronary arteries. Blood pressure is usually normal but may be low. Pulse pressure may be low (30 mm Hg or less) because of diminished blood flow.

Assessment and Diagnostic Findings

On physical examination, a loud, rough systolic murmur may be heard over the aortic area. The sound to listen for is a systolic crescendo–decrescendo murmur, which may radiate into the carotid arteries and to the apex of the left ventricle. The murmur is low-pitched, rough, rasping, and vibrating (Weber & Kelley, 2014). An S_4 sound may be heard. If the examiner rests a hand over the base of the heart (2nd intercostal space next to the sternum and above the suprasternal notch up along the carotid arteries), a vibration may be felt. The vibration is caused by turbulent blood flow across the narrowed valve orifice. By having the patient lean forward during auscultation and palpation, especially during exhalation, it is possible to accentuate the signs of aortic stenosis (Weber & Kelley, 2014).

Doppler echocardiography is used to diagnose and monitor the progression of aortic stenosis. Patients with symptoms usually have echocardiograms every 6 to 12 months, and those without symptoms have echocardiograms every 1 to 5 years (Fuster et al., 2011; Nishimura et al., 2014). Evidence of left ventricular hypertrophy may be seen on a 12-lead ECG and an echocardiogram. After stenosis progresses to the point that surgical intervention is considered, left-sided heart catheterization is necessary to measure the severity of the valvular abnormality and to evaluate the coronary arteries. Pressure tracings are taken from the left ventricle and from the base of the aorta. The systolic pressure in the left ventricle is considerably higher than that in the aorta during systole. Graded exercise studies (stress tests) are not usually prescribed for patients with aortic stenosis because of the high risk of precipitating ventricular tachycardia or fibrillation (Cohn, 2012; Mann et al., 2015; Nishimura et al., 2014).

Medical Management

Medications are prescribed to treat dysrhythmia or left ventricular failure (see Chapters 28 and 31). Definitive treatment for aortic stenosis is surgical replacement of the aortic valve. Patients who are symptomatic and are not surgical candidates may benefit from one-balloon or two-balloon percutaneous valvuloplasty procedures.

Nursing Management: Valvular Heart Disorders

The nurse teaches the patient with valvular heart disease about the diagnosis, the progressive nature of valvular heart disease, and the treatment plan. The patient is taught to report new symptoms or changes in symptoms to the health care provider. The nurse also teaches the patient that the infectious agent, usually a bacterium, is able to adhere to the diseased heart valve more readily than to a normal valve. Once attached to the valve, the infectious agent multiplies, resulting in endocarditis and further damage to the valve. In addition, the nurse teaches the patient how to minimize the risk of developing infectious endocarditis.

The nurse measures the patient's heart rate, blood pressure, and respiratory rate, compares these results with previous data, and notes any changes. Heart and lung sounds are auscultated and peripheral pulses palpated. The nurse assesses the patient with valvular heart disease for the following conditions:

- Signs and symptoms of heart failure, such as fatigue, dyspnea on exertion, an increase in coughing, hemoptysis, multiple respiratory infections, orthopnea, and PND (see Chapter 31)
- Dysrhythmias, by palpating the patient's pulse for strength and rhythm (i.e., regular or irregular) and asking whether the patient has experienced palpitations or felt forceful heartbeats (see Chapter 28)
- Symptoms such as dizziness, syncope, increased weakness, or angina pectoris (see Chapter 29)

The nurse collaborates with the patient to develop a medication schedule and teaches about the name, dosage, actions, adverse effects, and any drug–drug or drug–food interactions of the prescribed medications for heart failure, dysrhythmias, angina pectoris, or other symptoms. Specific precautions are emphasized, such as the risk to patients with aortic stenosis who experience angina pectoris and take nitroglycerin. The venous dilation that results from nitroglycerin decreases blood return to the heart, thus decreasing cardiac output and increasing the risk of syncope and decreased coronary artery blood flow. The nurse teaches the patient about the importance of attempting to relieve the symptoms of angina with rest and relaxation before taking nitroglycerin and to anticipate the potential adverse effects.

In addition, the nurse teaches the patient to weigh daily and report gains of 1 kg in 1 day or 2.25 kg in 1 week to the health care provider. The nurse may assist the patient with planning activity and rest periods to achieve an acceptable lifestyle. The patient may need to be advised to rest and sleep sitting in a chair or bed with the head elevated when experiencing symptoms of pulmonary congestion. Care of patients treated with valvuloplasty or surgical valve replacement is described later in this chapter.

SURGICAL MANAGEMENT: VALVE REPAIR AND REPLACEMENT PROCEDURES

Valvuloplasty

The repair, rather than replacement, of a cardiac valve is referred to as **valvuloplasty**. In general, valves that undergo valvuloplasty function longer than prosthetic valve replacements, and patients do not require continuous anticoagulation (Mann et al., 2015; Cohn, 2012; Otto & Bonow, 2013). The type of valvuloplasty depends on the cause and type of valve dysfunction. Repair may be made to the commissures between the leaflets in a procedure known as **commissurotomy**, to the annulus of the valve by annuloplasty, to the leaflets, or to the chordae by chordoplasty. TEE is usually performed at the conclusion of a valvuloplasty to evaluate the effectiveness of the procedure.

Most valvuloplasty procedures require general anesthesia and often require cardiopulmonary bypass. However, some procedures can be performed in the cardiac catheterization laboratory and do not always require general anesthesia or cardiopulmonary bypass. Percutaneous partial cardiopulmonary bypass is used in some cardiac catheterization laboratories. Cardiopulmonary bypass is achieved by inserting a large catheter (i.e., cannula) into two peripheral blood vessels, usually a femoral vein and an artery. Blood is diverted from the body through the venous catheter to the cardiopulmonary bypass machine (see Chapter 29) and returned to the patient through the arterial catheter.

Commissurotomy

The most common valvuloplasty procedure is commissurotomy. Each valve has leaflets; the site where the leaflets meet is called the commissure. The leaflets may adhere to one another and close the commissure (i.e., stenosis). Less commonly, the leaflets fuse in such a way that in addition to stenosis, the leaflets are also prevented from closing completely, resulting in a backward flow of blood (i.e., regurgitation). A commissurotomy is the procedure performed to separate the fused leaflets.

Closed Commissurotomy/Balloon Valvuloplasty

Closed commissurotomies do not require cardiopulmonary bypass. The valve is not directly visualized. Closed commissurotomies, in which a surgical technique is used, are performed in the operating room with the patient under general anesthesia; a midsternal incision is made, a small hole is cut into the heart, and the surgeon's finger or a dilator is used to open the commissure.

Percutaneous balloon valvuloplasty is the technique commonly performed in Canada for closed commissurotomy. Balloon valvuloplasty is beneficial for mitral valve stenosis in younger patients, for aortic valve stenosis in elderly patients, and for patients with complex medical conditions that place them at high risk for the complications of more extensive surgical procedures. Most often used for mitral and aortic valve stenosis, balloon valvuloplasty also has been used for tricuspid and pulmonic valve stenosis. The procedure is contraindicated for patients with left atrial or ventricular thrombus, severe aortic root dilation, significant mitral valve regurgitation, thoracolumbar scoliosis, rotation of the great vessels, and other cardiac conditions that require open heart surgery (Cohn, 2012; Fuster et al., 2011).

Balloon valvuloplasty (Fig. 30-3) is performed in the cardiac catheterization laboratory. The patient may receive light or moderate sedation or just a local anesthetic. Mitral

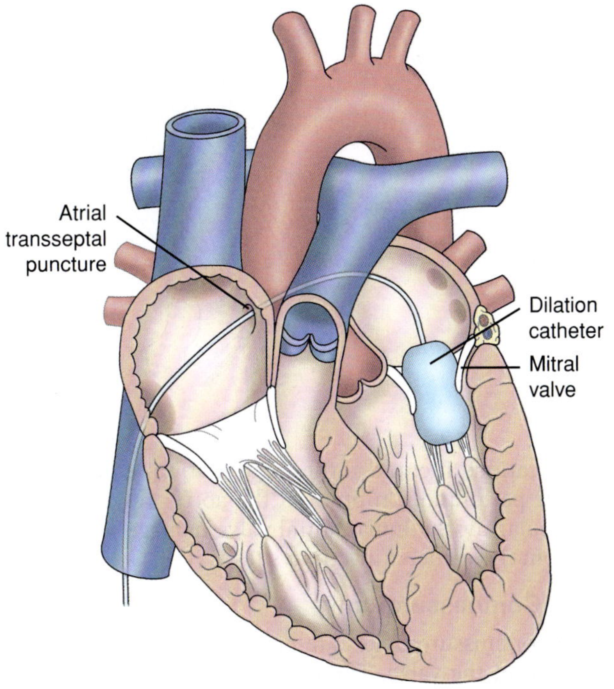

FIGURE 30-3. Balloon valvuloplasty: Cross-section of heart illustrating the guidewire and dilation catheter placed through an atrial transseptal puncture and across the mitral valve. The guidewire is extended out from the aortic valve into the aorta for catheter support.

balloon valvuloplasty involves advancing one or two catheters into the right atrium, through the atrial septum into the left atrium, across the mitral valve into the left ventricle, and out into the aorta. A guidewire is placed through each catheter, and the original catheter is removed. A large balloon catheter is then placed over the guidewire and positioned with the balloon across the mitral valve. The balloon is then inflated with a dilute angiographic solution. When two balloons are used, they are inflated simultaneously. The advantage of two balloons is that they are each smaller than the one large balloon often used, making smaller atrial septal defects. As the balloons are inflated, they usually do not completely occlude the mitral valve, thereby permitting some forward flow of blood during the inflation period. The balloons are usually inflated for 10 to 30 seconds. Multiple inflations are usually required to achieve the desired results.

All patients have some degree of mitral regurgitation after the procedure. Other possible complications include bleeding from the catheter insertion sites, emboli resulting in complications such as strokes, and rarely, left-to-right atrial shunts through an atrial septal defect caused by the procedure.

Aortic balloon valvuloplasty is performed most commonly by introducing a catheter through the aorta, across the aortic valve, and into the left ventricle, although it also may be performed by passing the balloon or balloons through the atrial septum. The one-balloon or the two-balloon technique can be used for treating aortic stenosis. Balloons are inflated for 15 to 60 seconds, and inflation is usually repeated multiple times. The aortic valve procedure is not as effective as the mitral valve procedure, and the rate of restenosis is approximately 50% in the first 6 months after the procedure (Mann et al., 2015). Possible

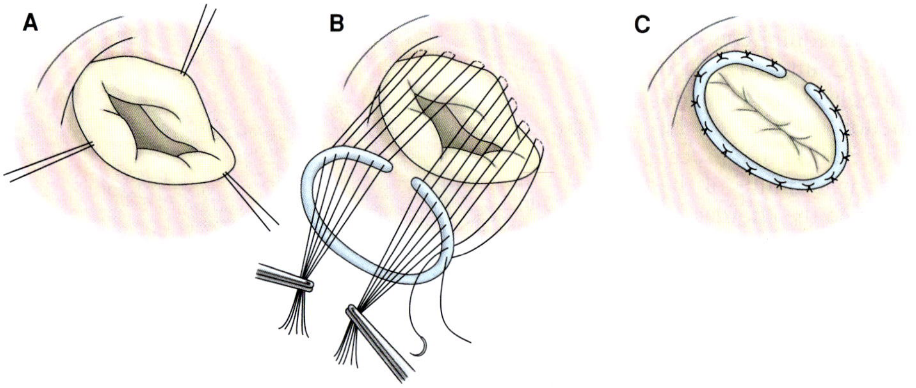

FIGURE 30-4. Annuloplasty ring insertion. **A.** Mitral valve regurgitation; leaflets do not close. **B.** Insertion of an annuloplasty ring. **C.** Completed valvuloplasty; leaflets close.

complications include aortic regurgitation, emboli, ventricular perforation, rupture of the aortic valve annulus, ventricular dysrhythmia, mitral valve damage, and bleeding from the catheter insertion sites.

Open Commissurotomy

Open commissurotomies are performed with direct visualization of the valve. The patient is under general anesthesia. A midsternal or left thoracic incision is made. Cardiopulmonary bypass is initiated and an incision is made into the heart. The valve is exposed and the surgeon uses a scalpel, finger, balloon, or dilator to open the commissures.

An added advantage of direct visualization of the valve is that thrombus and calcifications may be identified and removed. If the valve has chordae or papillary muscles, they may be inspected and surgically repaired as necessary.

Annuloplasty

Annuloplasty is the repair of the valve annulus (i.e., junction of the valve leaflets and the muscular heart wall). General anesthesia and cardiopulmonary bypass are required for all annuloplasties. The procedure narrows the diameter of the valve's orifice and is useful for the treatment of valvular regurgitation.

There are two annuloplasty techniques. One technique uses an annuloplasty ring (Fig. 30-4), which may be preshaped (rigid/semirigid) or flexible. The leaflets of the valve are sutured to a ring, creating an annulus of the desired size. When the ring is in place, the tension created by the moving blood and contracting heart is borne by the ring rather than by the valve or a suture line. Progressive regurgitation is prevented by the repair. The second technique involves tacking the valve leaflets to the atrium with sutures or taking tucks to tighten the annulus. Because the valve's leaflets and the suture lines are subjected to the direct forces of the blood and heart muscle movement, the repair may degenerate more quickly than one using an annuloplasty ring.

Leaflet Repair

Damage to cardiac valve leaflets may result from stretching, shortening, or tearing. **Leaflet repair** for elongated, ballooning, or other excess tissue leaflets is removal of the extra tissue. The elongated tissue may be folded over onto itself (i.e., tucked) and sutured (i.e., leaflet plication). A wedge of tissue may be cut from the middle of the leaflet and the gap sutured closed (i.e., leaflet resection) (Fig. 30-5). Short leaflets are most often repaired by chordoplasty. After the short chordae are released, the leaflets often unfurl and can resume their normal function (closing the valve during systole). A leaflet may be extended by suturing a piece of pericardium to it. A pericardial or synthetic patch may be used to repair holes in the leaflets.

Chordoplasty

Chordoplasty is repair of the chordae tendineae. The mitral valve is involved with chordoplasty (because it has chordae tendineae); the tricuspid valve seldom requires chordoplasty (Fuster et al., 2011). Stretched, torn, or shortened chordae tendineae may cause regurgitation. Stretched chordae tendineae can be shortened, transposed to the other leaflet, or replaced with synthetic chordae. Torn chordae can be reattached to the leaflet and shortened chordae can be elongated. Stretched papillary muscles, which may also cause regurgitation, can be shortened as well.

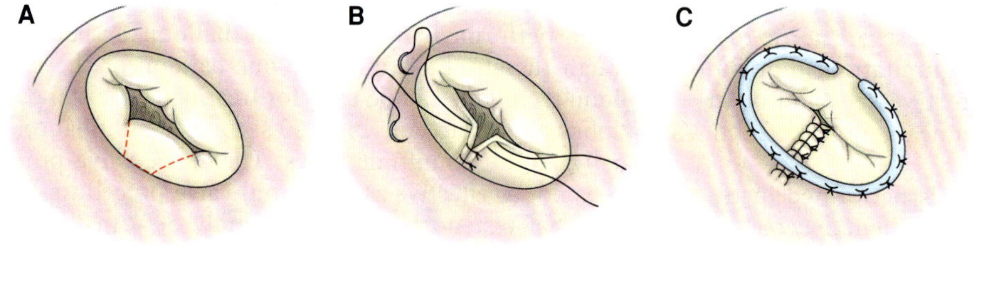

FIGURE 30-5. Valve leaflet resection and repair with a ring annuloplasty. **A.** Mitral valve regurgitation; the section indicated by dashed lines is excised. **B.** Approximation of edges and suturing. **C.** Completed valvuloplasty, leaflet repair, and annuloplasty ring.

Valve Replacement

When valvuloplasty is not a viable alternative (e.g., when the annulus or leaflets of the valve are immobilized by calcifications, severe fibrosis or fusion of leaflets, chordae tendineae, or papillary muscles), valve replacement is performed. Ideally, a multidisciplinary team (e.g., cardiologists, cardiac thoracic surgeons, structural valve interventionalists, anesthesiologists, and nurses) work together with the patient to determine candidacy for surgical versus more minimally invasive replacement (Nishimura et al., 2014). General anesthesia and cardiopulmonary bypass are used for most valve replacements. The standard surgical procedure is performed through a median sternotomy (i.e., incision through the sternum), although the mitral valve may be approached through a right thoracotomy incision.

Mitral, and more rarely aortic, valve replacements may be performed with minimally invasive techniques that do not involve cutting through the length of the sternum. Instead, a 2- to 4-in incision is made in only the upper or lower half of the sternum or between ribs, or performed percutaneously. Some minimally invasive procedures are robot assisted; surgical instruments are connected to a robot, and the surgeon, watching a video display, uses a joystick to control the robot and surgical instruments. With these procedures, patients have less bleeding, pain, risk of infection, and scarring. Hospital length of stay averages 5 days, and recovery may be as short as 3 to 4 weeks (Cohn, 2012; Holmes, Mack, Kaul, et al., 2012).

After the valve is visualized, leaflets of the aortic or pulmonic valve are removed, but some or all of the mitral valve structures (leaflets, chordae, and papillary muscles) are left in place to help maintain the shape and function of the left ventricle after mitral valve replacement. Sutures are placed around the annulus and then through the valve prosthesis. The replacement valve is slid down the suture into position and tied into place (see Fig. 30-6). The patient is weaned from cardiopulmonary bypass, the quality of the surgical repair is often assessed with colour flow Doppler TEE, and then surgery is completed.

Transcatheter aortic valve implantation (TAVI), a minimally invasive aortic valve replacement procedure, may be performed in a catheterization laboratory or hybrid room. It does not involve cardiopulmonary bypass or sternotomy (Hong, Hong, Ko, et al., 2014). TAVI is indicated for patients with aortic stenosis who are not candidates for surgical valve replacement or have a high surgical risk (Fuster et al., 2011; Holmes et al., 2012; Mann et al., 2015). With the patient under general anesthesia, a balloon valvuloplasty is performed. Then, a bioprosthetic (tissue) replacement valve attached to a catheter is inserted percutaneously, positioned at the aortic valve, and implanted (deployed). The MitraClip has been approved as a transcatheter procedure to treat degenerative forms of mitral regurgitation (Mann et al., 2015). This procedure is most beneficial for patients with severe symptomatic mitral regurgitation who have high surgical risk. The procedure creates a mechanical bridge between two leaflets; it has demonstrated decreased regurgitant flow, improvement of symptoms, and decreased rates of hospitalization for heart failure (Mann et al., 2015; Munkholm-Larsen, Wan, Tian, et al., 2014).

Before surgery, the heart gradually adjusted to the pathology; however, surgery abruptly "corrects" the way blood flows through the heart. Complications unique to valve replacement are related to the sudden changes in intracardiac blood pressures. All prosthetic valve replacements create a degree of stenosis when they are implanted in the heart. Usually, the stenosis is mild and does not affect heart function. If valve replacement was for a stenotic valve, blood flow through the heart is often improved. The signs and symptoms of backward heart failure resolve in a few hours or days. If valve replacement was for a regurgitant valve, it may take months for the chamber into which blood had been regurgitating to achieve its optimal postoperative function. Signs and symptoms of heart failure resolve gradually as heart function improves. Patients are at risk for many postoperative complications, such as bleeding, thromboembolism, infection, heart failure, hypertension, dysrhythmias, hemolysis, and mechanical obstruction of the valve.

Several types of mechanical and tissue valve prostheses may be used.

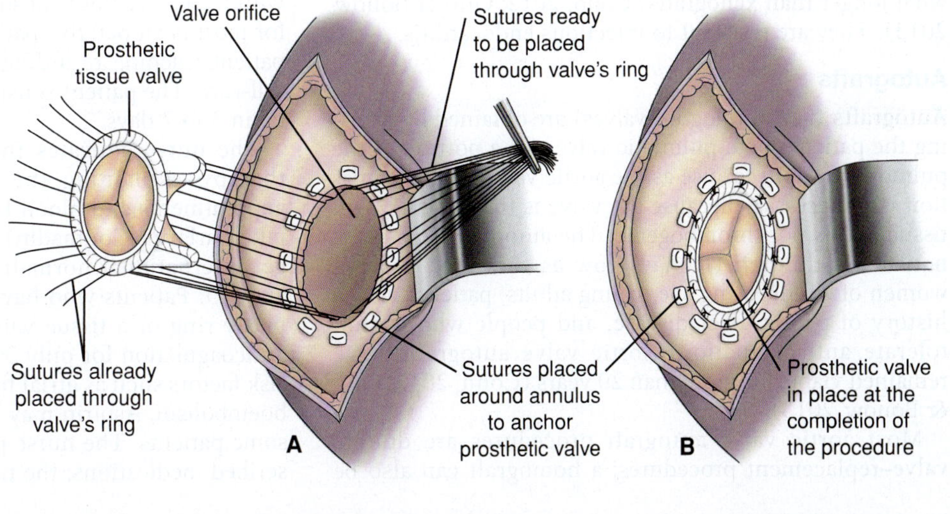

FIGURE 30-6. Valve replacement. **A.** The native valve is trimmed, and the prosthetic valve is sutured in place. **B.** Once all sutures are placed through the ring, the surgeon slides the prosthetic valve down the sutures and into the natural orifice. The sutures are then tied off and trimmed.

Mechanical Valves

Mechanical valves are of the bileaflet, ball-and-cage, or tilting-disk design and are thought to be more durable than tissue prosthetic valves; therefore, they are often used for younger patients. These valves are used for patients with renal failure, hypercalcemia, endocarditis, or sepsis who require valve replacement. The mechanical valves do not deteriorate or become infected as easily as the tissue valves used for patients with these conditions. Significant complications associated with mechanical valves are thromboemboli requiring long-term use of anticoagulants (Mann et al., 2015). Some amount of hemolysis also occurs with these valves; usually it is not clinically significant.

Tissue (Biologic) Valves

Tissue (i.e., biologic) valves are of three types: xenografts, homografts, and autografts. Tissue valves are less likely to generate thromboemboli, and long-term anticoagulation is not required. Tissue valves are not as durable as mechanical valves and require replacement more frequently.

Bioprostheses

Xenografts are tissue valves (e.g., bioprostheses, **heterografts**) that are used for tricuspid valve replacements. They are not thrombogenic, so patients do not need long-term anticoagulation therapy. They are used for women of childbearing age because the potential complications of long-term anticoagulation associated with menses, placental transfer to a fetus, and delivery of a child are avoided. They also are used for patients older than 70 years of age, patients with a history of peptic ulcer disease, and others who cannot tolerate long-term anticoagulation. Most xenografts come from pigs (porcine), but some come from cows (bovine). Viability is 7 to 15 years (Cohn, 2012; Fuster et al., 2011).

Homografts

Homografts, or **allografts** (i.e., human valves), are obtained from cadaver tissue donations and are used for aortic and pulmonic valve replacement. The aortic valve and a portion of the aorta or the pulmonic valve and a portion of the pulmonary artery are harvested and stored cryogenically. Homografts are not always available and are very expensive. They last for about 10 to 15 years, somewhat longer than xenografts (Cohn, 2012; Otto & Bonow, 2013). They are resistant to infectious endocarditis.

Autografts

Autografts (i.e., autologous valves) are obtained by excising the patient's own pulmonic valve and a portion of the pulmonary artery for use as the aortic valve. Anticoagulation is unnecessary because the valve is the patient's own tissue and is not thrombogenic. The autograft is an alternative for children (it may grow as the child grows), women of childbearing age, young adults, patients with a history of peptic ulcer disease, and people who cannot tolerate anticoagulation. Aortic valve autografts have remained viable for more than 20 years (Cohn, 2012; Otto & Bonow, 2013).

Most aortic valve autograft procedures are double valve–replacement procedures; a homograft can also be performed for pulmonic valve replacement. If pulmonary vascular pressures are normal, some surgeons elect not to replace the pulmonic valve. Patients can recover without a valve between the right ventricle and the pulmonary artery.

Nursing Management: Valvuloplasty and Replacement

The nurse assists the patient and family to prepare for the procedure, reinforces and supplements explanations provided by the physician, and provides psychosocial support. Care of the surgical patient is described in Chapters 19 through 21.

Patients who have undergone percutaneous balloon valvuloplasty procedures may be admitted to a telemetry or intensive care unit. The nurse assesses for signs and symptoms of heart failure and emboli (see Chapter 31), listens for any changes in heart sounds at least every 4 hours, and provides the patient with the same care as for postprocedure cardiac catheterization or percutaneous transluminal coronary angioplasty (PTCA) (see Chapter 29). After undergoing percutaneous balloon valvuloplasty, the patient usually remains in the hospital for 24 to 48 hours.

Patients who have undergone surgical valvuloplasty or valve replacements are admitted to the intensive care unit. Care focuses on recovery from anesthesia and hemodynamic stability. Vital signs are assessed every 5 to 15 minutes and as needed until the patient recovers from anesthesia or sedation, and then are assessed every 2 to 4 hours and as needed. Intravenous (IV) medications to increase or decrease blood pressure and to treat dysrhythmias or altered heart rates are administered and their effects monitored. The medications are gradually decreased until they are no longer required or the patient can take the needed medication by another route (e.g., oral, topical). Patient assessments are conducted every 1 to 4 hours and as needed, with particular attention to neurologic, respiratory, and cardiovascular systems. (See Chapter 29, Chart 29-13, which presents a plan of nursing care for a patient recovering from cardiac surgery.)

After the patient has recovered from anesthesia and sedation, is hemodynamically stable without IV medications, and has stable physical assessment parameters, he or she is usually transferred to a telemetry unit, typically within 24 to 72 hours of surgery. Nursing care continues as for most postoperative patients, including wound care and patient teaching regarding diet, activity, medications, and self-care. The patient is usually discharged from the hospital in 3 to 7 days.

The nurse educates the patient about anticoagulant therapy, explaining the need for frequent follow-up appointments and blood laboratory studies. Patients who take warfarin (Coumadin) usually have individualized target international normalized ratios (INRs) between 2.0 and 3.5. Patients who have been treated with an annuloplasty ring or a tissue valve replacement usually require anticoagulation for only 3 months, unless there are other risk factors such as atrial fibrillation or a history of thromboembolism. Aspirin may be prescribed with warfarin for some patients. The nurse provides teaching about all prescribed medications: the name of the medication, dosage, its actions, prescribed schedule, potential adverse effects, and any drug–drug or drug–food interactions.

Patients with a mechanical valve prosthesis (including annuloplasty rings and other prosthetic materials used in valvuloplasty) require education to prevent infective endocarditis. Patients may be at risk for infectious endocarditis that results from bacteria entering the bloodstream and adhering to the abnormal valve structures or prosthetic devices. The nurse teaches the patient how to minimize the risk of developing infectious endocarditis. Antibiotic prophylaxis is necessary before dental procedures involving manipulation of gingival tissue, the periapical area of the teeth, or perforation of the oral mucosa (not including routine anesthetic injections, placement of orthodontic brackets, or loss of deciduous teeth). Antibiotic therapy should also be used before invasive procedures involving the respiratory tract (e.g., biopsy of respiratory mucosa, tonsillectomy, and adenectomy).

Transitional, home care, and office or clinic nurses reinforce all new information and self-care instructions with patients and families for 4 to 8 weeks after the procedure. Doppler echocardiograms are often performed 3 to 4 weeks after discharge from the hospital to further evaluate the effects and results of the surgery. The echocardiogram also provides a baseline for future comparison if cardiac symptoms or complications develop. Doppler echocardiograms are usually repeated every 1 to 2 years.

Cardiomyopathy

Cardiomyopathy is a heart muscle disease associated with cardiac dysfunction. It is classified according to the structural and functional abnormalities of the heart muscle: dilated cardiomyopathy (DCM), hypertrophic cardiomyopathy (HCM), restrictive or constrictive cardiomyopathy (RCM), arrhythmogenic right ventricular cardiomyopathy (ARVC), and unclassified cardiomyopathy (Mann et al., 2015). A patient may have pathology representing more than one of these classifications, such as a patient with HCM developing dilation and symptoms of DCM. Ischemic cardiomyopathy is a term frequently used to describe an enlarged heart caused by coronary artery disease, which is usually accompanied by heart failure (see Chapter 31).

Pathophysiology

The pathophysiology of all cardiomyopathies is a series of events that culminate in impaired cardiac output. Decreased stroke volume stimulates the sympathetic nervous system and the renin–angiotensin–aldosterone response, resulting in increased systemic vascular resistance and increased sodium and fluid retention, which places an increased workload on the heart. These alterations can lead to heart failure (see Chapter 31).

Dilated Cardiomyopathy

DCM is the most common form of cardiomyopathy, with an incidence of 5 to 8 cases per 100,000 people per year (Mann & Felker, 2016). DCM is distinguished by significant dilation of the ventricles without simultaneous hypertrophy (i.e., increased muscle wall thickness) and systolic dysfunction (Fig. 30-7). The ventricles have elevated systolic and diastolic volumes but a decreased ejection fraction.

More than 75 conditions and diseases may cause DCM, including pregnancy, heavy alcohol intake, viral infection (e.g., influenza), chemotherapeutic medications (e.g., daunorubicin [Cerubidine], doxorubicin [Adriamycin]), and Chagas disease. When the causative factor cannot be identified, the diagnosis is idiopathic DCM, which accounts for approximately 25% of all heart failure cases. Because genetic factors may be involved, echocardiography and ECG should be used to screen all first-degree blood relatives (e.g., parents, siblings, children) for DCM (Bennett, 2014; Mann et al., 2015).

Microscopic examination of the muscle tissue shows diminished contractile elements (actin and myosin filaments) of the muscle fibres and diffuse necrosis of myocardial cells. The result is poor systolic function. The structural changes decrease the amount of blood ejected from the ventricle with systole, increasing the amount of blood remaining in the ventricle after contraction. Less blood is then able to enter the ventricle during diastole,

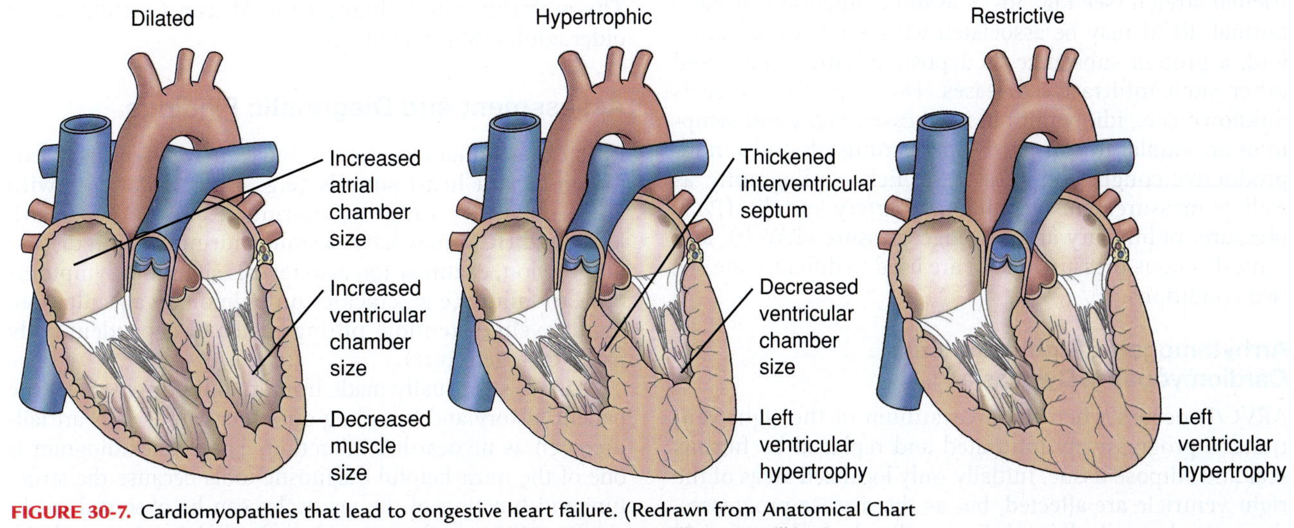

FIGURE 30-7. Cardiomyopathies that lead to congestive heart failure. (Redrawn from Anatomical Chart Company. (2010). *Atlas of pathophysiology* (3rd ed.). Ambler, PA: Lippincott Williams & Wilkins.)

increasing end-diastolic pressure and eventually increasing pulmonary and systemic venous pressures. Altered valve function, usually regurgitation, can result from an enlarged stretched ventricle. Poor blood flow through the ventricle may also cause ventricular or atrial thrombi, which may embolize to other locations in the body. Early diagnosis and treatment can prevent or delay significant symptoms and sudden death from DCM.

Hypertrophic Cardiomyopathy

HCM is a predominantly autosomal dominant condition occurring in 1 in 500 individuals affecting men, women, and children of all ethnic backgrounds (Jacoby, Depasquale, & McKenna, 2013). Echocardiograms may be performed every year from 12 to 18 years of age and then every 5 years from 18 to 70 years of age in susceptible individuals. Doppler echocardiography may also be used to detect the HCM and blood flow alterations (Mann et al., 2015). HCM also may be idiopathic (i.e., no known cause).

In HCM, the heart muscle asymmetrically increases in size and mass, especially along the septum (see Fig. 30-7). HCM often affects nonadjacent areas of the ventricle. The increased thickness of the heart muscle reduces the size of the ventricular cavities and causes the ventricles to take a longer time to relax after systole. During the first part of diastole it is more difficult for the ventricles to fill with blood. The atrial contraction at the end of diastole becomes critical for ventricular filling and systolic contraction.

Cardiac muscle cells normally lie parallel to and end-to-end with each other. The hypertrophied cardiac muscle cells are disorganized, oblique, and perpendicular to each other, decreasing the effectiveness of contractions and possibly increasing the risk of dysrhythmias such as ventricular tachycardia and ventricular fibrillation. In HCM the coronary arteriole walls are thickened, which decreases the internal diameter of the arterioles. The narrow arterioles restrict the blood supply to the myocardium, causing numerous small areas of ischemia and necrosis. The necrotic areas of the myocardium ultimately fibrose and scar, further impeding ventricular contraction.

Restrictive Cardiomyopathy

RCM is characterized by diastolic dysfunction caused by rigid ventricular walls that impair diastolic filling and ventricular stretch (see Fig. 30-7). Systolic function is usually normal. RCM may be associated with amyloidosis (amyloid, a protein substance, is deposited within cells) and other such infiltrative diseases. However, the cause is unknown (i.e., idiopathic) in most cases. Signs and symptoms are similar to constrictive pericarditis: dyspnea, nonproductive cough, and chest pain. Echocardiography, as well as measurement of pulmonary artery systolic (PAS) pressure, pulmonary artery wedge pressure (PAWP), and central venous pressure (CVP) are used to differentiate the two conditions.

Arrhythmogenic Right Ventricular Cardiomyopathy/Dysplasia

ARVC/D occurs when the myocardium of the right ventricle is progressively infiltrated and replaced by fibrous scar and adipose tissue. Initially, only localized areas of the right ventricle are affected, but as the disease progresses, the entire heart is affected. Eventually, the right ventricle dilates and develops poor contractility, right ventricular wall abnormalities, and dysrhythmias. The prevalence of ARVC/D is unknown because many cases are not recognized, however it is estimated to affect about 1 in 5,000 people (Rojas & Calkins, 2015; Fuster et al., 2011). Palpitations or syncope may develop between 15 and 40 years of age. ARVC/D should be considered in patients with ventricular tachycardia originating in the right ventricle (i.e., a left bundle branch block configuration on ECG) or sudden death, especially among young athletes (Mann et al., 2015). ARVC/D is genetic (i.e., autosomal dominant) (Corrado, Wichter, Link, et al., 2015; Fuster et al., 2011). First-degree blood relatives (e.g., parents, siblings, children) should be screened for the disease with a 12-lead ECG, Holter monitor, and echocardiography.

Unclassified Cardiomyopathies

Unclassified cardiomyopathies are different from or have characteristics of more than one of the previously described types. Examples of unclassified cardiomyopathies include fibroelastosis, noncompacted myocardium, systolic dysfunction with minimal dilation, and mitochondrial involvement (Mann et al., 2015).

Clinical Manifestations

Patients with cardiomyopathy may remain stable and without symptoms for many years. As the disease progresses, so do the symptoms. Frequently, dilated or restrictive cardiomyopathy is first diagnosed when the patient presents with signs and symptoms of heart failure (e.g., dyspnea on exertion, fatigue). Patients with cardiomyopathy may also report PND, cough (especially with exertion), and orthopnea, which may lead to a misdiagnosis of bronchitis or pneumonia. Other symptoms include fluid retention, peripheral edema, and nausea, which is caused by poor perfusion of the gastrointestinal system. The patient also may experience chest pain, palpitations, dizziness, nausea, and syncope with exertion. However, with HCM, cardiac arrest (i.e., sudden cardiac death) may be the initial manifestation in young people, including athletes (Mann et al., 2015).

Regardless of type and cause, cardiomyopathy may lead to severe heart failure, lethal dysrhythmias, and death. The mortality rate is highest for African Canadians and older adults (Mann et al., 2015).

Assessment and Diagnostic Findings

Physical examination at early stages may reveal tachycardia and extra heart sounds (e.g., S_3, S_4). Patients with DCM may have diastolic murmurs, and patients with DCM and HCM may have systolic murmurs. With disease progression, examination also reveals signs and symptoms of heart failure (e.g., crackles on pulmonary auscultation, jugular vein distention, pitting edema of dependent body parts, enlarged liver).

Diagnosis is usually made from findings disclosed by the patient history and by ruling out other causes of heart failure such as myocardial infarction. The echocardiogram is one of the most helpful diagnostic tools because the structure and function of the ventricles can be observed easily. Cardiac MRI may also be used, particularly to assist with the diagnosis of HCM (Mann et al., 2015; Mann & Felker, 2016; Semsarian, Ingles, Maron, et al., 2015). ECG demonstrates dysrhythmias (atrial fibrillation, ventricular dysrhythmias) and changes consistent with left ventricular hypertrophy (left axis deviation, wide QRS, ST changes, inverted T waves). In ARVC/D, there often is a small deflection, an epsilon wave, at the end of the QRS. The chest x-ray reveals heart enlargement and possibly pulmonary congestion. Cardiac catheterization is sometimes used to rule out coronary artery disease as a causative factor. Endomyocardial biopsy may be performed to analyze myocardial cells.

Medical Management

Medical management is directed toward identifying and managing possible underlying or precipitating causes; correcting the heart failure with medications, a low-sodium diet, and an exercise/rest regimen (see Chapter 31); and controlling dysrhythmias with antiarrhythmic medications and possibly with an implanted electronic device, such as an implantable cardioverter defibrillator (see Chapter 28). Systemic anticoagulation to prevent thromboembolic events is usually recommended. If the patient has signs and symptoms of congestion, fluid intake may be limited to 2 L each day. Patients with HCM should avoid dehydration and may need beta-blockers (atenolol [Tenormin], metoprolol [Lopressor], nadolol [Corgard], propranolol [Inderal]) to maintain cardiac output and minimize the risk of left ventricular outflow tract obstruction during systole. Patients with HCM or RCM may need to limit physical activity to avoid a life-threatening dysrhythmia. To date, amiodarone (Cordarone) is the only drug shown to reduce the incidence of arrhythmogenic sudden cardiac death (Corrado et al., 2015; Mann & Felker, 2016; Marcus & Abidov, 2012).

A pacemaker may be implanted to alter the electrical stimulation of the muscle and prevent the forceful hyperdynamic contractions that occur with HCM. Atrial-ventricular and biventricular pacing have been used to decrease symptoms and obstruction of the left ventricular outflow tract. For some patients with DCM and HCM, biventricular pacing increases the ejection fraction and reverses some of the structural changes in the myocardium.

Nonsurgical septal reduction therapy, also called alcohol septal ablation, has been used to treat obstructive HCM. In the cardiac catheterization laboratory, a percutaneous catheter is positioned in one or more of the septal coronary arteries. Once the position is verified, 1 to 5 mL of 96% to 98% ethanol (ethyl alcohol) is injected at a rate of about 1 mL/min to destroy the myocardial cells (Mann et al., 2015; Maron & Nishimura, 2014); it is believed that the ethanol causes dehydration of the cardiac cells (Jacoby et al., 2013). The slow rate of injection minimizes the risk of heart block and premature ventricular contractions. The procedure produces a septal myocardial infarction. The resulting scar is thinner than the living myocardium had been, so the obstruction is decreased. The patient may develop a left anterior hemibranch block or left bundle branch block. If the patient experiences pain, hydrocodone/acetaminophen (Vicodin) is usually administered. Nitrates and morphine are not used because coronary artery dilation is contraindicated.

Surgical Management

When heart failure progresses and medical treatment is no longer effective, surgical intervention, including heart transplantation, is considered. However, because of the limited number of organ donors, many patients die waiting for transplantation. In some cases, a left **ventricular assist device** is implanted to support the failing heart until a suitable donor heart becomes available.

Left Ventricular Outflow Tract Surgery

When patients with HCM become symptomatic despite medical therapy and a difference in pressure of 50 mm Hg or more exists between the left ventricle and the aorta, surgery is considered (Elliott et al., 2014; Mann et al., 2015). The most common procedure is a myectomy (sometimes referred to as a myotomy–myectomy), in which some of the heart tissue is excised. Septal tissue approximately 1-cm wide and deep is cut from the enlarged septum below the aortic valve. The length of septum removed depends on the degree of obstruction caused by the hypertrophied muscle.

Instead of a septal myectomy, the surgeon may open the left ventricular outflow tract to the aortic valve by mitral valvuloplasty involving the leaflets, chordae, or papillary muscles, or the patient's mitral valve may be replaced with a low-profile disk valve. The space taken up by the mitral valve is substantially reduced by the valvuloplasty or prosthetic valve, allowing blood to move around the enlarged septum to the aortic valve through the area the mitral valve once occupied. The primary complication of all the procedures is dysrhythmia. Additional complications include postoperative surgical complications such as pain, ineffective airway clearance, deep vein thrombosis, risk of infection, and delayed surgical recovery.

Heart Transplantation

Because of advances in surgical techniques and immunosuppressive therapies, heart transplantation is now a therapeutic option for patients with end-stage heart disease. Cyclosporine (Gengraf, Neoral, Sandimmune) is an immunosuppressant that greatly decreases the body's rejection of foreign proteins, such as transplanted organs. Unfortunately, cyclosporine also decreases the body's ability to resist infections, and a satisfactory balance must be achieved between suppressing rejection and avoiding infection.

Cardiomyopathy, ischemic heart disease, valvular disease, rejection of previously transplanted hearts, and congenital heart disease are the most common indications for transplantation (Lund et al., 2014). Typical candidates have severe symptoms uncontrolled by medical therapy, no other surgical options, and a prognosis of less than 2 years to live. A multidisciplinary team screens the candidate before recommending the transplantation procedure (Chart 30-1). The person's age, pulmonary status, other chronic health conditions, psychosocial status, family support, infections, history of other transplantations, compliance, and current health status are considered.

When a donor heart becomes available, a computer generates a list of potential recipients on the basis of ABO blood group compatibility, the body sizes of the donor and the potential recipient, age, severity of illness, length of

NURSING RESEARCH PROFILE

Chart 30-1. Living With a Total Artificial Heart: Patients' Perspectives

Savage, L. S., Salyer, J., Flattery, M. P., et al. (2014). Living with a total artificial heart: Patients' perspectives. *Journal of Cardiovascular Nursing, 29*(1), E1–E8.

Purpose

The purpose of this study was to describe the lived experience of patients currently supported by the total artificial heart (TAH-t) awaiting transplant.

Design

A qualitative method using Giorgi's modification of phenomenologic inquiry guided the investigation, which was conducted at a transplant centre located in the mid-Atlantic region of the United States. A purposive sample was selected to reflect participants currently supported by the TAH-t. All participants (9 men, 1 woman; mean age, 48.2 years; nonischemic etiology, 80%) were in-patients on the progressive care unit at the time of the interview and had been supported for at least 30 days. The mean length of device therapy was 84.7 days (range, 33 to 245 days).

Findings

Hope for the future was the overarching theme. Subthemes included reflections, for better or for worse, the secret club, and coping and adaptation. The patients reflected on severity of illness, progress, and expressed optimism. For better or for worse described how symptoms improved but were offset by restrictions imposed by the technology. The secret club described the support provided to help deal with their life situation. Coping and adaptation suggested that the patients came to terms with and accepted their circumstances.

Nursing Implications

Understanding how patients respond when faced with a life-changing situation such as the implant of the TAH-t can help nurses and other healthcare professionals better understand how to interact with and support them. Although this study found reliance on healthcare professionals was often because of their technical expertise, the patients became more confident as a consequence of their knowledge about the technology. This increased confidence may be due to patient and family education and the reassurance the patients received through interaction with health care professionals. This study also illustrates the suggested benefit of health care professionals encouraging relationships of patients with other recipients of the TAH-t. These opportunities can be enhanced through encouraging support groups that bring patients and clinicians together.

time on the waiting list, and the geographic locations of the donor and potential recipient. Distance is a factor because postoperative function depends on the heart being implanted within 4 hours of harvest from the donor. Some patients are candidates for more than one organ transplant (e.g., heart–lung, heart–kidney, heart–liver).

Orthotopic transplantation is the most common surgical procedure for cardiac transplantation (Fig. 30-8). The recipient's heart is removed, and the donor heart is implanted at the vena cava and pulmonary veins. Some surgeons prefer to remove the recipient's heart, leaving a portion of the recipient's atria (with the vena cava and pulmonary veins) in place. The donor heart, which usually has been preserved in ice, is prepared for implant by cutting away a small section of the atria that corresponds with the sections of the recipient's heart that were left in place. The donor heart is implanted by suturing the donor atria to the residual atrial tissue of the recipient's heart. After the venous or atrial anastomoses are complete, the recipient's pulmonary artery and aorta are sutured to those of the donor heart.

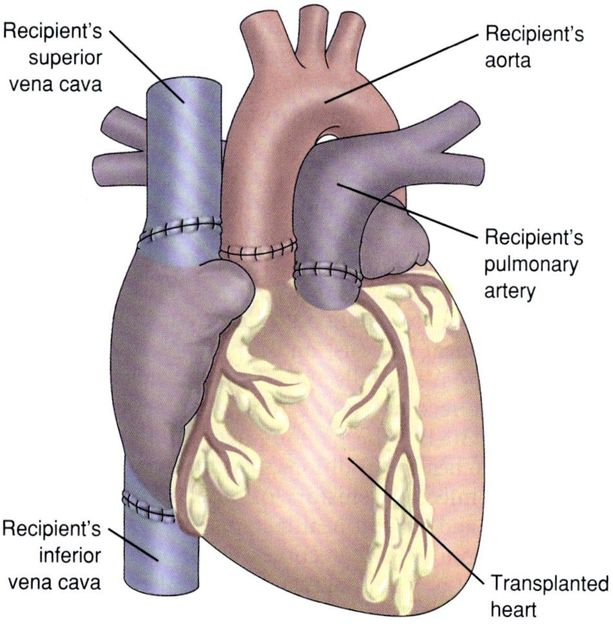

FIGURE 30-8. Orthotopic method of heart transplantation.

This technique has been modified to the *bicaval technique,* which includes removal of the recipient's heart, and the implantation of the donor heart with intact atria at the vena cava and pulmonary veins (Fuster et al., 2011; Mann & Felker, 2016). This newer approach is associated with decreased AV valve regurgitation, dysrhythmias, and conduction abnormalities.

Patients who have had heart transplants are constantly balancing the risk of rejection with the risk of infection. They must adhere to a complex regimen of diet, medications, activity, follow-up laboratory studies, biopsies of the transplanted heart (to diagnose rejection), and clinic visits. Most commonly, patients receive tacrolimus (Prograf) or cyclosporine, mycophenolate mofetil (CellCept) or azathioprine (Imuran), and corticosteroids (e.g., prednisone) to minimize rejection.

The transplanted heart has no nerve connections (i.e., denervated heart) to the recipient's body, so the sympathetic and vagus nerves do not affect the transplanted heart. The resting rate of the transplanted heart is approximately 70 to 90 bpm (beats per minute), but it increases gradually if catecholamines are in the circulation. Patients must gradually increase and decrease their exercise (i.e., extended warm-up and cool-down periods), because 20 to 30 minutes may be required to achieve the desired heart rate. Atropine does not increase the heart rate of transplanted hearts.

In addition to rejection and infection, complications may include accelerated atherosclerosis of the coronary arteries (i.e., cardiac allograft vasculopathy, accelerated graft atherosclerosis, transplant coronary artery disease). Both immunologic and nonimmunologic factors cause arterial injury and inflammation of the coronary arteries. The arterial smooth muscle proliferates and there is hyperplasia of the coronary artery intima, accelerating atherosclerosis along the entire length of the coronary arteries (Mann et al., 2015; Mann & Felker, 2016). Hypertension may occur in patients taking cyclosporine or tacrolimus; the cause has not been identified. Osteoporosis is a frequent side effect of the antirejection medications as well as pretransplantation dietary insufficiency and medications. Patients with a long-term sedentary lifestyle are at greater risk for osteoporosis.

Posttransplantation lymphoproliferative disease and cancer of the skin and lips are the most common malignancies after transplantation, possibly caused by immunosuppression. Weight gain; obesity; diabetes; dyslipidemias (e.g., hypercholesterolemia); hypotension; renal failure; and central nervous system, respiratory, and gastrointestinal disturbances may be adverse effects of the corticosteroids or other immunosuppressants. Toxicity from immunosuppressant medications may occur. The 1-year survival rate for patients with transplanted hearts is approximately 86%. At 10 years the survival rate decreases to approximately 62%, and at 20 years there is approximately a 36% survival rate (Fuster et al., 2011; Heart & Stroke Foundation of Canada, 2014).

In the first year after transplant, patients respond to the psychosocial stresses imposed by organ transplantation in various ways. Most report a better quality of life after transplantation. Some experience guilt that someone had to die for them to be able to live, have anxiety about the new heart, experience depression or fear about rejection, or have difficulty with family role changes before and after transplantation (Fuster et al., 2011; Mann et al., 2015; Mann & Felker, 2016). Adequate social support can improve health-related quality of life in patients post heart transplantation (White-Williams, Grady, Myers, et al., 2013).

Mechanical Assist Devices and Total Artificial Hearts

The use of cardiopulmonary bypass in cardiovascular surgery and the possibility of performing heart transplantation in patients with end-stage cardiac disease, as well as the desire for a treatment option for patients with such disease who are not transplant candidates, have increased the need for mechanical assist devices. Patients who cannot be weaned from cardiopulmonary bypass and patients in cardiogenic shock may benefit from a period of mechanical heart assistance. The most commonly used device is the intra-aortic balloon pump (see Chapter 30). This pump decreases the work of the heart during contraction but does not perform the actual work of the heart.

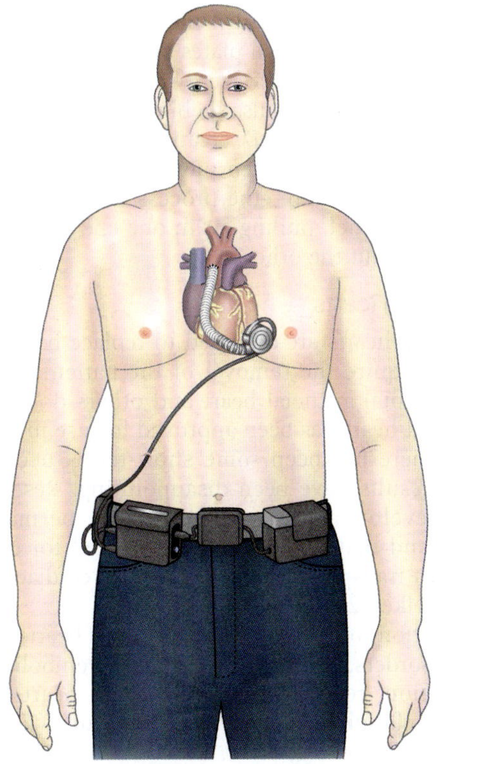

FIGURE 30-9. Left ventricular assist device.

Ventricular Assist Devices

More complex devices that actually perform some or all of the pumping function for the heart also are being used. These more sophisticated VADs can circulate as much blood per minute as the heart, if not more (Fig. 30-9). Each VAD is used to support one ventricle. Some VADs can be combined with an oxygenator; the combination is called extracorporeal membrane oxygenation (ECMO). The oxygenator–VAD combination is used for the patient whose heart cannot pump adequate blood through the lungs or the body.

VADs may be used as (1) a "bridge to recovery" for patients who require temporary assistance for reversible ventricular failure; (2) a "bridge to transplant" for patients with end-stage heart failure until a donor organ becomes available for transplant (most common); and (3) "destination therapy" for patients with end-stage heart failure who are not candidates for or decline heart transplantation. When VADs are used as destination therapy, patients are discharged from the hospital with the devices in place (Fuster et al., 2011; Mann & Felker, 2016).

VADs may be external, internal (i.e., implanted) with an external power source, or completely internal, and they may generate a pulsatile or continuous blood flow. There are three types of VADs: pneumatic, electric or electromagnetic, and axial flow. Pneumatic VADs are external or implanted pulsatile devices with a flexible reservoir housed in a rigid exterior. The reservoir usually fills with blood drained from the atrium or ventricle. The device then forces pressurized air into the rigid housing, compressing the reservoir and returning the blood to the circulation, usually into the aorta. Electric or electromagnetic VADs are similar to the pneumatic VADs, but instead of using pressurized air to return the blood to the circulation, one or more flat metal plates are pushed against the reservoir. Axial flow VADs use a rotary mechanism (an impeller) to create a nonpulsatile blood flow. The impeller spins rapidly within the VAD, creating a vacuum that pulls blood into the VAD and then pushes the blood out into the systemic circulation—the process is similar to a fan spinning in a tunnel, pulling air in one end of the tunnel and pushing it out the other.

Total Artificial Hearts

Total artificial hearts are designed to replace both ventricles. Some require the removal of the patient's heart to implant the total artificial heart and others do not. One total artificial heart has been approved for use in Canada. Although there has been some short-term success, the long-term results have been disappointing. Researchers hope to develop a device that can be permanently implanted and that will eliminate the need for donated human heart transplantation for end-stage cardiac disease (Mann & Felker, 2016).

Complications of VADs and total artificial hearts include bleeding disorders, hemorrhage, thrombus, emboli, hemolysis, infection, renal failure, right-sided heart failure, multisystem failure, and mechanical failure (Feldman, Pamboukian, Teuteberg, et al., 2013; Fuster et al., 2011; Mann et al., 2015; Starling, 2013). Nursing care of patients with these mechanical assist devices focuses on assessment for and minimization of these complications as well as providing emotional support and education about the device as well as the underlying cardiac disease.

Nursing Process

The Patient With Cardiomyopathy

Assessment

Nursing assessment for the patient with cardiomyopathy begins with a detailed history of the presenting signs and symptoms. The nurse identifies possible etiologic factors, such as heavy alcohol intake, recent illness or pregnancy, or history of the disease in immediate family members. If the patient reports chest pain, a thorough review of the pain, including its precipitating factors, is warranted. The review of systems includes the presence of orthopnea, PND, and syncope or dyspnea with exertion. The number of pillows needed to sleep, usual weight, any weight change, and limitations on activities of daily living are assessed. The patient's usual diet is evaluated to determine the need to reduce sodium intake, optimize nutrition, or supplement with vitamins.

Because of the chronicity of cardiomyopathy, the nurse conducts a careful psychosocial history, exploring the impact of the disease on the patient's role within the family and community. Identification of perceived stressors helps the patient and the health care team to implement activities to relieve anxiety related to changes in health status. Very early on, the patient's support systems are identified, and members are encouraged to become involved in the patient's care and therapeutic regimen. The assessment addresses the effect the diagnosis has had on the patient and members of his or her support system and the patient's emotional status. Depression is common in a patient with cardiomyopathy who has developed heart failure (Rustad, Stern, Hebert, et al., 2013).

The physical assessment focuses on signs and symptoms of heart failure. The baseline assessment includes such key components as:

- Vital signs
- Calculation of pulse pressure and identification of pulsus paradoxus
- Current weight and any weight gain or loss
- Detection by palpation of the point of maximal impulse, often shifted to the left
- Cardiac auscultation for a systolic murmur and S_3 and S_4 heart sounds
- Pulmonary auscultation for crackles
- Measurement of jugular vein distention
- Assessment of edema and its severity

Nursing Priorities

Based on the assessment data, major nursing priorities may include:

- Decreased cardiac output
- Impaired tissue perfusion
- Impaired gas exchange
- Activity intolerance
- Anxiety
- Powerlessness
- Noncompliance

Collaborative Problems/ Potential Complications

Based on the assessment data, potential complications include:

- Heart failure
- Ventricular dysrhythmias
- Atrial dysrhythmias
- Cardiac conduction defects
- Pulmonary or cerebral embolism
- Valvular dysfunction

These complications are discussed earlier in this chapter and in Chapters 28 and 31.

Planning and Goals

The major goals for patients include improvement or maintenance of cardiac output, increased activity tolerance, reduction of anxiety, adherence to the self-care program, increased sense of power with decision making, and absence of complications.

Nursing Interventions

Improving Cardiac Output

During a symptomatic episode, rest is indicated. Many patients with DCM find that sitting up with their legs down is more comfortable than lying down in a bed. This position is helpful in pooling venous blood in the periphery and reducing preload. Assessing the patient's oxygen saturation at rest and during activity may assist with determining a need for supplemental oxygen. Oxygen is usually administered through a nasal cannula when indicated.

Ensuring that medications are taken as prescribed is important to preserving adequate cardiac output. The nurse may assist the patient with planning a schedule for taking medications and identifying methods to remember to follow it, such as associating the time to take a medication with an activity (e.g., eating a meal, brushing teeth). It is important to ensure that patients with DCM avoid verapamil (Calan, Isoptin), patients with HCM avoid diuretics, and patients with RCM avoid nifedipine to maintain contractility. In patients with HCM, the inotropic action of digoxin may create or worsen left ventricular outflow track obstruction. Patients with RCM have increased sensitivity to digoxin, and the nurse must anticipate that low doses will be prescribed and assess for digoxin toxicity.

It is also important to ensure that the patient receives or chooses food selections that are appropriate for a low-sodium diet. One way to monitor a patient's response to treatment is to determine the patient's weight every day and identify any significant change. Another indication of the effect of treatment involves assessment of shortness of breath after activity and comparison to before treatment. Patients with low cardiac output may need assistance keeping warm and frequently changing position to stimulate circulation and reduce the possibility of skin breakdown. Patients with HCM must be taught to avoid dehydration. One guideline for patients to use for self-assessment is to anticipate the urge to void at least every 4 hours while awake; if the urge to void is not present or the urine is a deep yellow colour, more fluid intake is necessary.

Increasing Activity Tolerance

The nurse plans the patient's activities so that they occur in cycles, alternating rest with activity periods. This benefits the patient's physiologic status, and it helps teach the patient about the need for planned cycles of rest and activity. For example, after taking a bath or shower, the patient should plan to sit and read a newspaper or engage in other relaxing activities. Suggesting that the patient sit while chopping vegetables, drying his or her hair, or shaving helps the patient learn to balance rest with activity. The nurse also makes sure that the patient recognizes the symptoms indicating the need for rest and actions to take when the symptoms occur. Patients with HCM or RCM must avoid strenuous activity, isometric exercises, and competitive sports.

Reducing Anxiety

Spiritual, psychological, and emotional support may be indicated for patients, families, and significant others. Interventions are directed toward eradicating or alleviating perceived stressors. Patients receive appropriate information about cardiomyopathy and self-management activities. It is important to provide an atmosphere in which patients feel free to verbalize concerns and receive assurance that their concerns are legitimate. If the patient is awaiting transplantation or facing death, it is necessary to allow time to discuss these issues. Providing the patient with realistic hope helps reduce anxiety while he or she awaits a donor heart. The nurse helps the patient, family, and significant others with anticipatory grieving.

Decreasing the Sense of Powerlessness

Patients often go through a grieving process when cardiomyopathy is diagnosed. The patient is assisted in identifying the things in life that he or she has lost (e.g., foods that the patient enjoyed eating but are high in sodium, the ability to engage in an active lifestyle, the ability to play sports, the ability to lift grandchildren) and his or her emotional responses to the loss (e.g., anger, depression). The nurse assists the patient in identifying the amount of control that he or she still has over life, such as making food choices, managing medications, and working with health care providers to achieve the best possible outcomes. A diary in which the patient records food selections and weight may help with understanding the relationship between sodium intake and weight gain. Some patients can manage a self-titrating diuretic regimen in which they adjust the dose of diuretic to their symptoms.

Promoting Home, Community-Based, and Transitional Care

EDUCATING PATIENTS ABOUT SELF-CARE. A key part of the plan of nursing care involves teaching patients about the medication regimen, symptom monitoring, and symptom management. The nurse plays an integral role as the patient learns to balance lifestyle and work while accomplishing therapeutic activities. Helping patients cope with their disease status helps them adjust their lifestyles and implement a self-care program at home. Attainment of a goal, no matter how small, also promotes the patient's sense of well-being.

Continuing and Transitional Care

The nurse reinforces previous teaching and performs ongoing assessment of the patient's symptoms and progress. The nurse also assists the patient and family to adjust to lifestyle changes. Patients are taught to read nutrition labels, to maintain a record of daily weights and symptoms, and to organize daily activities to increase activity tolerance. In addition, the nurse assesses the patient's response to recommendations about diet and fluid intake and to the medication regimen and stresses the signs and symptoms that should be reported to the physician. Because of the risk of dysrhythmia, it may be necessary to teach the patient's family cardiopulmonary resuscitation. Women are often advised to avoid pregnancy, but each case is assessed individually. The nurse assesses the psychosocial needs of the patient and family on an ongoing basis. There may be concerns and fears about the prognosis, changes in lifestyle, effects of medications, and the possibility of others in the family having the same condition; these often increase the patient's anxiety and interfere with effective coping strategies. Establishing trust is vital to the nurse's relationship with these chronically ill patients and their families. This is particularly significant when the nurse is involved with a patient and family in discussions about end-of-life decisions. Patients who have significant symptoms of heart failure or other complications of cardiomyopathy may benefit from a home care referral. Transitional Care Models have now emerged to assist the patient's transition from the hospital to home while dealing with a chronic illness (Naylor, Bowles, McCauley, et al., 2013).

Evaluation

1. Maintains or improves cardiac function
   a. Exhibits heart and respiratory rates within normal limits
   b. Reports decreased dyspnea and increased comfort; maintains or improves gas exchange
   c. Reports no weight gain; appropriate weight for height
   d. Maintains or improves peripheral blood flow
2. Maintains or increases activity tolerance
   a. Carries out activities of daily living (e.g., brushes teeth, feeds self)
   b. Reports increased tolerance to activity
3. Is less anxious
   a. Discusses prognosis freely
   b. Verbalizes fears and concerns
   c. Participates in support groups if appropriate
4. Decreases sense of powerlessness
   a. Identifies emotional response to diagnosis
   b. Discusses control that he or she has
5. Adheres to self-care program
   a. Takes medications according to prescribed schedule
   b. Modifies diet to accommodate sodium and fluid recommendations
   c. Modifies lifestyle to accommodate activity and rest behaviour recommendations
   d. Identifies signs and symptoms to be reported to health care professionals

INFECTIOUS DISEASES OF THE HEART

Any of the heart's three layers may be affected by an infectious process. The infections are named for the layer of the heart most involved in the infectious process: infective endocarditis (endocardium), myocarditis (myocardium), and pericarditis (pericardium). Rheumatic endocarditis is a unique infective endocarditis syndrome. The diagnosis of infection is made primarily on the basis of the patient's symptoms and echocardiography. The ideal management for all infectious diseases is prevention. IV antibiotics are usually necessary once an infection has developed in the heart.

Rheumatic Endocarditis

Acute rheumatic fever, which occurs most often in school-age children, may develop after an episode of group A beta-hemolytic streptococcal pharyngitis (Chart 30-2). Patients with rheumatic fever may develop rheumatic heart disease as evidenced by a new heart murmur, cardiomegaly, pericarditis, and heart failure. Prompt treatment of "strep" throat with antibiotics can prevent the development of rheumatic fever. The streptococcus is spread by direct contact with oral or respiratory secretions. Although the bacteria are the causative agents, malnutrition, overcrowding, poor hygiene, and lower socioeconomic status may predispose individuals to rheumatic fever. The incidence of rheumatic fever in Canada and other developed countries generally has decreased (Josephson, 2014); but the exact incidence is difficult to determine because the infection may go unrecognized, and people may not seek treatment (Fuster et al., 2011). Clinical diagnostic criteria are not standardized, and autopsies are not routinely performed. Further information about rheumatic fever and rheumatic endocarditis can be found in pediatric nursing books.

Infective Endocarditis

Infective endocarditis is a microbial infection of the endothelial surface of the heart. It usually develops in people

CHART 30-2

Rheumatic Fever

Rheumatic fever is a preventable disease. Diagnosing and treating streptococcal pharyngitis can prevent rheumatic fever and, therefore, rheumatic heart disease. Signs and symptoms of streptococcal pharyngitis include:

- Fever 38.9°C to 40°C
- Chills
- Sore throat (sudden in onset)
- Diffuse redness of throat with exudate on oropharynx (may not appear until after the first day)
- Enlarged and tender lymph nodes
- Abdominal pain (more common in children)
- Acute sinusitis and acute otitis media (may cause or result from streptococcal pharyngitis)

If signs and symptoms of streptococcal pharyngitis are present, a throat culture is necessary to make an accurate diagnosis. All patients with throat cultures positive for streptococcal pharyngitis must adhere to the prescribed antibiotic treatment. Penicillin is the most common antibiotic prescribed. Completing the course of prescribed antibiotics minimizes the risk of developing rheumatic fever (and subsequent rheumatic heart disease).

Centers for Disease Control and Prevention. (2015). *Is it strep throat?* Retrieved on July 1, 2016, from www.cdc.gov/features/strepthroat.

CHART 30-3

Risk Factors: Infective Endocarditis

- Prosthetic cardiac valves or intracardiac devices
- History of bacterial endocarditis (even without heart disease)
- Congenital heart disease
- Unrepaired cyanotic congenital heart disease
- Chronic rheumatic heart disease
- Age-related degenerative valvular lesions
- Hemodialysis
- Coexisting conditions such as diabetes, human immunodeficiency virus infection, and intravenous drug use

Adapted from Nishimura, R. A., Otto, C. M., Bonow, R. O., et al. (2014). 2014 AHA/ACC guidelines for the management of patients with valvular heart disease. *Journal of the American College of Cardiology*, *63*(22), e57–e185.

with prosthetic heart valves or structural cardiac defects (e.g., valve disorders, HCM) (Chart 30-3). It is more common in older people (Josephson, 2014), who are more likely to have degenerative or calcific valve lesions, reduced immunologic response to infection, and the metabolic alterations associated with aging. Staphylococcal endocarditis infections of the valves in the right side of the heart are common among IV injection drug users. Hospital-acquired infective endocarditis occurs most often in patients with debilitating disease or indwelling catheters and in patients who are receiving hemodialysis or prolonged IV fluid or antibiotic therapy. Patients taking immunosuppressive medications or corticosteroids are more susceptible to fungal endocarditis.

Invasive procedures, particularly those involving mucosal surfaces, can cause a bacteremia, which rarely lasts for more than 15 minutes. However, if a patient has any anatomic cardiac defects, bacteremia can cause bacterial endocarditis. From 1950 to the mid-1980s, the incidence of infective endocarditis remained steady at about 3.6 cases per 100,000 patients. The incidence then increased, partially attributed to increased IV injection drug abuse and body piercing, especially oral, nasal, and nipple piercings (Fuster et al., 2011; Josephson, 2014; Mann et al., 2015).

Pathophysiology

A deformity or injury of the endocardium leads to accumulation on the endocardium of fibrin and platelets (clot formation). Infectious organisms, usually staphylococci, streptococci, enterococci, pneumococci, or chlamydia, invade the clot and endocardial lesion. Other causative microorganisms include fungi (e.g., *Candida, Aspergillus*) and Rickettsiae. The infection most frequently results in platelets, fibrin, blood cells, and microorganisms that cluster as vegetations on the endocardium. The vegetations may embolize to other tissues throughout the body. As the clot on the endocardium continues to expand, the infecting organism is covered by the new clot and concealed from the body's normal defenses. The infection may erode through the endocardium into the underlying structures (e.g., valve leaflets), causing tears or other deformities of valve leaflets, dehiscence of prosthetic valves, deformity of the chordae tendineae, or mural abscesses.

Usually the onset of infective endocarditis is insidious. The signs and symptoms develop from the toxic effect of the infection, from destruction of the heart valves, and from embolization of fragments of vegetative growths on the heart. Systemic emboli occur with left-sided heart infective endocarditis; pulmonary emboli occur with right-sided heart infective endocarditis (Fuster et al., 2011).

Clinical Manifestations

The primary presenting symptoms of infective endocarditis are fever and a heart murmur. The fever may be intermittent or absent, especially in patients who are receiving antibiotics or corticosteroids, in those who are elderly, or those who have heart failure or renal failure. A heart murmur may be absent initially but develops in almost all patients. Murmurs that worsen over time indicate progressive damage from vegetations or perforation of the valve or the chordae tendineae.

In addition to the fever and heart murmur, clusters of petechiae may be found on the body. Small, painful nodules (Osler nodes) may be present in the pads of fingers or toes. Irregular, red or purple, painless, flat macules (Janeway lesions) may be present on the palms, fingers, hands, soles, and toes. Hemorrhages with pale centres (Roth spots) caused by emboli may be observed in the fundi of the eyes. Splinter hemorrhages (i.e., reddish-brown lines and streaks) may be seen under the fingernails and toenails, and petechiae may appear in the conjunctiva and mucous membranes. Cardiomegaly, heart failure, tachycardia, or splenomegaly may occur.

Central nervous system manifestations of infective endocarditis include headache; temporary or transient cerebral ischemia; and strokes, which may be caused by emboli to the cerebral arteries. Embolization may be a presenting symptom, and it may occur at any time and may involve other organ systems. Embolic phenomena may occur, as discussed in the previous section on rheumatic endocarditis.

Heart failure, which may result from perforation of a valve leaflet, rupture of chordae, blood flow obstruction due to vegetations, or intracardiac shunts from dehiscence of prosthetic valves, indicates a poor prognosis with medical therapy alone and a higher surgical risk (Mann, et al., 2015). Valvular stenosis or regurgitation, myocardial damage, and mycotic (fungal) aneurysms are potential cardiac complications. First-degree, second-degree, and third-degree atrioventricular blocks may occur and are often a sign of a valve ring abscess. Emboli, immunologic responses, abscess of the spleen, mycotic aneurysms, cerebritis, and hemodynamic deterioration may cause complications in other organs.

Assessment and Diagnostic Findings

Although the previously described characteristics may indicate infective endocarditis, the signs and symptoms may indicate other diseases as well. Vague complaints of malaise, anorexia, weight loss, cough, and back and joint pain may be mistaken for influenza. The virulence of the causative organism usually correlates with the speed and degree of symptom development. A definitive diagnosis is made when a microorganism is found in two separate blood cultures, in a vegetation, or in an abscess. Three sets of blood cultures (with each set including one aerobic and one anaerobic culture) drawn over a 24-hour period (or every 30 minutes if the patient's condition is unstable) should be obtained before administration of any antimicrobial agents (Fuster et al., 2011; Mann et al., 2015; Nishimura et al., 2014). Negative blood cultures do not definitely rule out infective endocarditis. Patients may have elevated white blood cell (WBC) counts. In addition, patients may be anemic and have a positive rheumatoid factor and an elevated erythrocyte sedimentation rate (ESR) or C-reactive protein. Microscopic hematuria may be present on urinalysis.

Doppler echocardiography may assist in the diagnosis by demonstrating a mass on the valve, prosthetic valve, or supporting structures and by identifying vegetations, abscesses, new prosthetic valve dehiscence, or new regurgitation. The echocardiogram may reveal the development of heart failure. TEE may provide better data than transthoracic imaging (Fuster et al., 2011; Mann et al., 2015; Nishimura et al., 2014).

Prevention

Although rare, bacterial endocarditis may be life-threatening. A key strategy is primary prevention in high-risk patients (e.g., those with previous infective endocarditis, prosthetic heart valves). Antibiotic prophylaxis is recommended for high-risk patients immediately before and sometimes after dental procedures that involve manipulation of gingival tissue or periapical area of teeth or perforation of oral mucosa (except routine anesthetic injections through noninfected tissue, placement of orthodontic brackets, loss of deciduous teeth, bleeding from trauma to lips or oral mucosa, dental x-rays, adjustment of orthodontic appliances, and placement of removable prosthodontic or orthodontic appliances). Updated guidelines no longer recommend antibiotic prophylaxis for patients undergoing nondental procedures (Nishimura et al., 2014).

The type of antibiotic used for prophylaxis varies with the type of procedure and the degree of risk. Patients are usually instructed to take 2 g of amoxicillin (Amoxil) orally 1 hour before the procedure. If patients are allergic to penicillin, clindamycin (Cleocin), cephalexin (Keflex), cefazolin (Ancef, Kefzol), ceftriaxone (Rocephin), azithromycin (Zithromax), or clarithromycin (Biaxin) may be used (Fuster et al., 2011; Mann et al., 2015; Nishimura et al., 2014).

Equally important is ongoing good oral hygiene. Poor dental hygiene can lead to bacteremia, particularly in the setting of a dental procedure. The severity of oral inflammation and infection is a significant factor in the incidence and degree of bacteremia. Regular professional oral care combined with personal oral care may reduce the risk of bacteremia. Personal oral care includes using a soft toothbrush and toothpaste to brush the teeth, gums, tongue, and oral mucosa at least twice a day, as well as rinsing the mouth with an antiseptic mouthwash for 30 seconds intermittently between tooth brushing. Patients must be advised to avoid nail biting and to minimize outbreaks of acne and psoriasis. Female patients are advised not to use intrauterine devices (IUDs) and to avoid body piercing and branding.

Increased vigilance is also required in patients with IV catheters and during invasive procedures. To minimize the risk of infection, nurses must ensure meticulous hand hygiene, site preparation, and aseptic technique during insertion and maintenance procedures. All catheters, tubes, drains, and other devices are removed as soon as they are no longer needed or no longer function.

Medical Management

The objective of treatment is to eradicate the invading organism through adequate doses of an appropriate antimicrobial agent. Antibiotic therapy is usually administered parenterally in a continuous IV infusion for 2 to 6 weeks. Parenteral therapy is administered in doses that produce a high serum concentration for a significant period to ensure eradication of the dormant bacteria within the dense vegetations. This therapy is often delivered in the patient's home and is monitored by a home care nurse. Serum levels of the antibiotic are monitored. If there is insufficient bactericidal activity, increased dosages of the antibiotic are prescribed or a different antibiotic is used. Numerous antimicrobial regimens are in use, but penicillin is usually the medication of choice. Blood cultures are taken periodically to monitor the effect of therapy. In fungal endocarditis, an antifungal agent, such as amphotericin B (e.g., Abelcet, Amphocin, Fungizone), is the usual treatment.

In addition, the patient's temperature is monitored at regular intervals because the course of the fever is one indication of the effectiveness of treatment. However, febrile reactions also may occur as a result of medication. After adequate antimicrobial therapy is initiated, the infective organism is usually eliminated. The patient should begin to feel better, regain an appetite, and have less fatigue. During this time, patients require psychosocial support because although they feel well, they may find themselves confined to the hospital or home with restrictive IV therapy.

Surgical Management

Surgical intervention may be required if the infection does not respond to medications, the patient has a prosthetic heart valve endocarditis, has a vegetation larger than 1 cm, or develops complications such as a septal perforation (Fuster et al., 2011; Josephson, 2014; Mann et al., 2015; Nishimura et al., 2014). Surgical interventions include valve débridement or excision, débridement of vegetations, débridement and closure of an abscess, and closure of a fistula. Aortic or mitral valve débridement, excision, or replacement is required in patients who:

- Develop congestive heart failure despite adequate medical treatment
- Have more than one serious systemic embolic episode
- Develop a valve obstruction
- Develop a periannular (heart valve), myocardial, or aortic abscess
- Have uncontrolled infection, persistent or recurrent infection, or fungal endocarditis

Surgical valve replacement greatly improves the prognosis for patients with severe symptoms from damaged heart valves. The aortic valve may be best treated with an autograft, as previously described. Most patients who have prosthetic valve endocarditis (i.e., infected valve replacements) require valve replacement.

Nursing Management

The nurse monitors the patient's temperature. The patient may have a fever for weeks. Heart sounds are assessed. A new or worsening murmur may indicate dehiscence of a prosthetic valve, rupture of an abscess, or injury to valve leaflets or chordae tendineae. The nurse monitors for signs and symptoms of systemic embolization, or, for patients with right-sided heart endocarditis, for signs and symptoms of pulmonary infarction and infiltrates. In addition, the nurse assesses signs and symptoms of organ damage such as stroke (i.e., cerebrovascular accident or brain attack), meningitis, heart failure, myocardial infarction, glomerulonephritis, and splenomegaly.

Patient care is directed toward management of infection. Long-term IV antimicrobial therapy is often necessary; therefore, many patients have peripherally inserted central catheters or other long-term IV access. All invasive lines and wounds must be assessed daily for redness, tenderness, warmth, swelling, drainage, or other signs of infection. The patient and family are instructed about activity restrictions, medications, and signs and symptoms of infection. Patients with infective endocarditis are at high risk for another episode of infectious endocarditis. The nurse emphasizes the antibiotic prophylaxis previously described. If the patient has undergone surgical treatment, the nurse provides postoperative care and instructions.

As appropriate, the home care nurse supervises and monitors IV antibiotic therapy delivered in the home setting and educates the patient and family about prevention and health promotion. The nurse provides the patient and family with emotional support and facilitates coping strategies during the prolonged course of the infection and antibiotic treatment.

Myocarditis

Myocarditis, an inflammatory process involving the myocardium, can cause heart dilation, thrombi on the heart wall (mural thrombi), infiltration of circulating blood cells around the coronary vessels and between the muscle fibres, and degeneration of the muscle fibres themselves. Mortality varies with the severity of symptoms. Most patients with mild symptoms recover completely, but some patients develop cardiomyopathy and heart failure.

Pathophysiology

Myocarditis usually results from viral (e.g., coxsackievirus A and B, human immunodeficiency virus [HIV], influenza A), bacterial, rickettsial, fungal, parasitic, metazoal, protozoal (e.g., Chagas disease), or spirochetal infection. It also may be immune related, occurring after acute systemic infections such as rheumatic fever. It may develop in patients receiving immunosuppressive therapy or those with infective endocarditis, Crohn disease, or systemic lupus erythematosus (Mann et al., 2015; Mann & Felker, 2016).

Myocarditis may result from an inflammatory reaction to toxins such as pharmacologic agents used in the treatment of other diseases (e.g., anthracyclines for cancer therapy), ethanol, or radiation (especially to the left chest or upper back). It may begin in one small area of the myocardium and then spread throughout the myocardium. The degree of myocardial inflammation and necrosis determines the degree of interstitial collagen and elastin destruction. The greater the destruction, the greater the hemodynamic effect and resulting signs and symptoms. It is theorized that DCM and HCM are latent manifestations of myocarditis (Mann et al., 2015; Fuster et al., 2011). The most common pathogens involved in myocarditis tend to be viral, whereas in endocarditis they tend to be bacterial.

Clinical Manifestations

The symptoms of acute myocarditis depend on the type of infection, the degree of myocardial damage, and the capacity of the myocardium to recover. Patients may be asymptomatic, with an infection that resolves on its own. However, they may develop mild to moderate symptoms and seek medical attention, often reporting fatigue and dyspnea, palpitations, and occasional discomfort in the chest and upper abdomen. The most common symptoms are flu-like. Patients may also sustain sudden cardiac death or quickly develop severe congestive heart failure.

Assessment and Diagnostic Findings

Assessment of the patient may reveal no detectable abnormalities; as a result, the entire illness can go undiagnosed. Patients may be tachycardic or may report chest pain (with a subsequent cardiac catheterization demonstrating normal coronary arteries). Cardiac MRI with contrast may be diagnostic and can guide clinicians to sites for endocardial biopsies, which may be diagnostic for an organism or its genome, immune process, or a radiation reaction causing the myocarditis. Patients without any abnormal heart structure (at least initially) may suddenly develop dysrhythmias or ST–T-wave changes. If the patient has structural heart abnormalities (e.g., systolic dysfunction), a clinical assessment may disclose cardiac enlargement, faint heart sounds (especially S_1), a gallop rhythm, or a systolic murmur. The WBC count, ESR, leukocyte count, and C-reactive protein may be elevated (Mann et al., 2015; Mann & Felker, 2016; Marx, 2014).

Prevention

Prevention of infectious diseases by means of appropriate immunizations (e.g., influenza, hepatitis) and early treatment appears to be important in decreasing the incidence of myocarditis (Mann et al., 2015).

Medical Management

Patients are given specific treatment for the underlying cause if it is known (e.g., penicillin for hemolytic streptococci) and are placed on bed rest to decrease cardiac workload. Bed rest also helps decrease myocardial damage and the complications of myocarditis. In young patients with myocarditis, activities, especially athletics, should be limited for a 6-month period or at least until heart size and function have returned to normal. Physical activity is increased slowly, and the patient is instructed to report any symptoms that occur with increasing activity, such as a rapidly beating heart. If heart failure or dysrhythmia develops, management is essentially the same as for all causes of heart failure and dysrhythmias (see Chapters 28 and 31), except that beta-blockers are avoided because they decrease the strength of ventricular contraction (have a negative inotropic effect).

Nursing Management

The nurse assesses for resolution of tachycardia, fever, and any other clinical manifestations. The cardiovascular assessment focuses on signs and symptoms of heart failure and dysrhythmias. Patients with dysrhythmias should have continuous cardiac monitoring with personnel and equipment readily available to treat life-threatening dysrhythmias.

NURSING ALERT

Patients with myocarditis are sensitive to digitalis. Nurses must closely monitor these patients for digitalis toxicity, which is evidenced by dysrhythmia, anorexia, nausea, vomiting, headache, and malaise.

Antiembolism stockings and passive and active exercises should be used because embolization from venous thrombosis and mural thrombi can occur, especially in patients on bed rest.

Pericarditis

Pericarditis refers to an inflammation of the pericardium, the membranous sac enveloping the heart. It may be a primary illness or it may develop during various medical and surgical disorders. For example, pericarditis may occur after pericardiectomy (opening of the pericardium) following cardiac surgery. Pericarditis also may occur 10 days to 2 months after acute myocardial infarction (Dressler syndrome) (Curry, 2014; Mann et al., 2015). Pericarditis may be subacute, acute, or chronic. It is classified either as adhesive (constrictive), because the layers of the pericardium become attached to each other and restrict ventricular filling, or by what accumulates in the pericardial sac: serous (serum), purulent (pus), calcific (calcium deposits), fibrinous (clotting proteins), or sanguineous (blood). Pericarditis also may be described as exudative or noneffusive.

Pathophysiology

Causes underlying or associated with pericarditis are listed in Chart 30-4. The inflammatory process of pericarditis may lead to an accumulation of fluid in the pericardial sac (pericardial effusion) and increased pressure on the heart, leading to cardiac tamponade (see Chapter 30). Frequent or prolonged episodes of pericarditis may also lead to thickening and decreased elasticity of the pericardium, or scarring may fuse the visceral and parietal pericardium. These conditions restrict the heart's ability to fill with blood (constrictive pericarditis). The pericardium may become calcified, further restricting ventricular expansion during ventricular filling (diastole). With less filling, the ventricles pump less blood, leading to decreased cardiac output and signs and symptoms of heart failure. Restricted diastolic filling may result in increased systemic venous pressure, causing peripheral edema and hepatic failure.

CHART 30-4

Causes of Pericarditis

- Idiopathic or nonspecific causes
- Infection: usually viral (e.g., human immune deficiency virus, coxsackievirus, influenza); rarely bacterial (e.g., staphylococci, streptococci, meningococci, gonococci, gram-negative rods, *Borrelia* [Lyme disease], tuberculosis); mycotic (fungal); and parasitic
- Disorders of connective tissue: systemic lupus erythematosus, rheumatic fever, rheumatoid arthritis, polyarteritis, and scleroderma
- Sarcoidosis
- Hypersensitivity states: immune reactions, medication reactions, and serum sickness
- Disorders of adjacent structures: myocardial infarction, dissecting aneurysm, pleural and pulmonary disease (pneumonia)
- Neoplastic disease: caused by metastasis from lung or breast cancer, leukemia, and primary (mesothelioma) neoplasms
- Radiation therapy of chest and upper torso (peak occurrence 5 to 9 months after treatment)
- Trauma: chest injury, cardiac surgery, cardiac catheterization, implantation of pacemaker, or implantable cardioverter defibrillator
- Kidney injury and uremia

Adapted from Fuster, V., Walsh, R. A., Harrington, R. A., et al. (Eds.). (2011). *Hurst's the heart* (13th ed.). New York: McGraw-Hill.

Clinical Manifestations

Pericarditis may be asymptomatic. The most characteristic symptom of pericarditis is chest pain, although pain also may be located beneath the clavicle, in the neck, or in the left trapezius (scapula) region. The pain or discomfort usually remains fairly constant, but it may worsen with deep inspiration and when lying down or turning. It may be relieved with a forward-leaning or sitting position. The most characteristic sign of pericarditis is a creaky or scratchy friction rub heard most clearly at the left lower sternal border. Other signs may include a mild fever, increased WBC count, anemia, and an elevated ESR or C-reactive protein level. Patients may have a nonproductive cough or hiccough. Dyspnea and other signs and symptoms of heart failure may occur as the result of pericardial compression due to constrictive pericarditis or cardiac tamponade (Curry, 2014).

Assessment and Diagnostic Findings

The diagnosis is most often made on the basis of the history, signs, and symptoms. An echocardiogram may detect inflammation, pericardial effusion or tamponade, and heart failure. It may help confirm the diagnosis and may be used to guide pericardiocentesis (needle or catheter drainage of the pericardium). TEE may be useful in diagnosis but may underestimate the extent of pericardial effusions. Computed tomography (CT) may be the best diagnostic tool for determining the size, shape, and location of pericardial effusions and may be used to guide pericardiocentesis. MRI may assist with detection of inflammation and adhesions. Occasionally a video-assisted pericardioscope-guided biopsy of the pericardium or epicardium is performed to obtain tissue samples for culture and microscopic examination. Because the pericardial sac surrounds the heart, a 12-lead ECG may show concave ST elevations in many, if not all, leads (with no reciprocal changes) and may show depressed PR segments or atrial dysrhythmias (Curry, 2014; Mann et al., 2015).

Medical Management

The objectives of management of pericarditis are to determine the cause, administer therapy for treatment and symptom relief, and detect signs and symptoms of cardiac tamponade. When cardiac output is impaired, the patient is placed on bed rest until the fever, chest pain, and friction rub have subsided.

Analgesics and nonsteroidal anti-inflammatory drugs (NSAIDs) such as aspirin or ibuprofen (Motrin) may be prescribed for pain relief during the acute phase. These agents also hasten the reabsorption of fluid in patients with rheumatic pericarditis. Indomethacin (Indocin) is contraindicated because it may decrease coronary blood flow. Corticosteroids (e.g., prednisone) may be prescribed if the pericarditis is severe or if the patient does not respond to NSAIDs. Colchicine may also be used as alternative therapy (Curry, 2014; Imazio, Brucato, Cemin, et al., 2013; LeWinter, 2014; Mann et al., 2015; Marx, 2014).

Pericardiocentesis, a procedure in which some of the pericardial fluid is removed, is rarely necessary. It may be performed to assist in the identification of the cause or relieve symptoms, especially if there are signs and symptoms of heart failure or tamponade. Pericardial fluid is cultured if bacterial, tubercular, or fungal disease is suspected, and a sample is sent for cytology if neoplastic disease is suspected. A pericardial window, a small opening made in the pericardium, may be performed to allow continuous drainage into the chest cavity. Surgical removal of the tough encasing pericardium (pericardiectomy) may be necessary to release both ventricles from the constrictive and restrictive inflammation and scarring.

Nursing Management

Patients with acute pericarditis require pain management with analgesics, positioning, and psychological support. Patients with chest pain often benefit from education and reassurance that the pain is not due to a heart attack. To minimize complications, the nurse helps the patient with activity restrictions until the pain and fever subside. As the patient's condition improves, the nurse encourages gradual increases of activity. However, if pain, fever, or friction rub reappear, activity restrictions must be resumed. The nurse educates the patient and family about a healthy lifestyle to enhance the patient's immune system.

Nurses caring for patients with pericarditis must be alert to cardiac tamponade (see Chapter 31). The nurse monitors the patient for heart failure. Patients with hemodynamic instability or pulmonary congestion are treated as they would be if they had heart failure (see Chapter 31).

Nursing Process

The Patient With Pericarditis

Assessment

The primary symptom of the patient with pericarditis is pain, which is assessed by evaluating the patient in various positions. The nurse tries to identify whether the pain is influenced by respiratory movements, while holding an inhaled breath or holding an exhaled breath; by flexion, extension, or rotation of the spine, including the neck; by movements of the shoulders and arms; by coughing; or by swallowing. Recognizing the events that precipitate or intensify pain may help establish a diagnosis and differentiate the pain of pericarditis from the pain of myocardial infarction.

A pericardial friction rub occurs when the pericardial surfaces lose their lubricating fluid because of inflammation. The rub is audible on auscultation and is synchronous with the heartbeat. However, it may be elusive and difficult to detect.

NURSING ALERT

A pericardial friction rub is diagnostic of pericarditis. It has a creaky or scratchy sound and is louder at the end of exhalation. Nurses should monitor for the pericardial friction rub by placing the diaphragm of the stethoscope tightly against the thorax and auscultating the left sternal edge in the 4th intercostal space, the site where the pericardium comes into contact with the left chest wall. The rub may be heard best when a patient is sitting and leaning forward.

If there is difficulty in distinguishing a pericardial friction rub from a pleural friction rub, the patient is asked to hold his or her breath; a pericardial friction rub will continue.

The patient's temperature is monitored frequently. Pericarditis may cause an abrupt onset of fever in a patient who has been afebrile.

Nursing Priority

Based on the assessment data, the major nursing priority is pain likely due to the inflammatory process in the pericardium.

Collaborative Problems/ Potential Complications

Based on the assessment data, potential complications that may develop include:

- Pericardial effusion
- Cardiac tamponade

Planning and Goals

The patient's major goals may include relief of pain and absence of complications.

Nursing Interventions

Relieving Pain

Relief of pain is achieved by rest. Because sitting upright and leaning forward is the posture that tends to relieve pain, chair rest may be more comfortable. It is important to instruct the patient to restrict activity until the pain subsides. As the chest pain and friction rub abate, activities of daily living may be resumed gradually. If the patient is taking analgesics, antibiotics, or corticosteroids for the pericarditis, his or her responses are monitored and recorded. Patients taking NSAIDs are assessed for gastrointestinal adverse effects. If chest pain and friction rub recur, bed rest or chair rest is resumed.

Monitoring and Managing Potential Complications

PERICARDIAL EFFUSION. Fluid may accumulate between the pericardial linings (i.e., in the pericardial sac), a condition called pericardial effusion (see Chapter 31). Most patients have no effects or symptoms. However, enough fluid can accumulate to constrict the myocardium, impairing ventricular filling and the myocardium's ability to pump, a condition known as cardiac tamponade (discussed below) (Curry, 2014; Mann et al., 2015). Failure to identify and treat this problem can lead to death.

Cardiac Tamponade

The signs and symptoms of cardiac tamponade may begin with the patient reporting shortness of breath, chest tightness, or dizziness. The nurse may observe that the patient is becoming progressively more restless. Assessment of blood pressure may reveal a decrease of 10 mm Hg or more in the systolic blood pressure during inspiration (pulsus paradoxus). Usually, the systolic pressure decreases and the diastolic pressure remains stable; hence, the pulse pressure narrows. The patient usually has tachycardia, and the ECG voltage may be decreased or the QRS complexes may alternate in height (electrical alternans). Heart sounds may progress from distant to imperceptible. Blood continues to return to the heart from the periphery but cannot flow into the heart to be pumped back into the circulation. The patient develops neck vein distention and other signs of rising central venous pressure. Beck triad (hypotension, muffled heart sounds, and an elevated jugular venous pressure) is a useful diagnostic parameter of severe tamponade (Mann et al., 2015).

In such situations, the nurse notifies the physician immediately and prepares to assist with diagnostic echocardiography and pericardiocentesis (Mann et al., 2015) (see Chapter 31). The nurse stays with the patient and continues to assess and record signs and symptoms while intervening to decrease patient anxiety.

Promoting Home, Community-Based, and Transitional Care

Because patients, their family members, and their health care providers tend to focus on the most obvious needs and issues related to pericarditis, the nurse reminds them about the importance of continuing health promotion and screening practices. The nurse educates patients who have not been involved in these practices in the past about their importance and refers them to appropriate health care providers.

Evaluation

1. Freedom from pain
   a. Performs activities of daily living without pain, fatigue, or shortness of breath
   b. Temperature returns to normal range
   c. Exhibits no pericardial friction rub
2. Absence of complications
   a. Sustains blood pressure in normal range
   b. Has heart sounds that are strong and can be auscultated
   c. Shows absence of neck vein distention

Critical Thinking Exercises

1 A 19-year-old female college student presents to the student health clinic with recurrent tonsillitis. The physician on duty refers her to a surgeon for evaluation for tonsillectomy. Upon review of her medical history, the student reports an aortic valve replacement (prosthetic) as a child, but no other significant medical/surgical history. She remembers being told that she needs antibiotics before surgeries and asks if you agree. How would you respond to her questions? What complications are you focused on preventing? On what evidence do you base your response? What is the strength of your evidence?

2 Despite evidence-based medical management, a 57-year-old man with DCM continues to have significant functional limitations and is advised to consult with a cardiologist specializing in advanced heart failure therapy. The cardiologist recommends that the patient consider heart transplantation and begins the transplant workup. The patient expresses anxiety about what this entails and also fears about having "someone else's" heart. Based on what you know about transplant, how would you respond to these fears and anxiety?

3 A 47-year-old male presents to the emergency department complaining of malaise, fever, and painful nodules on the pads of his fingers. He admits to being an active IV drug abuser, while denying regular medical and dental care. Upon physical examination, the nurse notes a soft systolic murmur and small painful nodules on the pads of his fingers. Based upon these physical examination findings, the physician thinks that the patient may have infective endocarditis and prescribes antibiotics. What should the nurse ensure happens before the antibiotics are given? What are the care priorities for this patient?

4 A 39-year-old man presents to the cardiology clinic complaining of palpitations, fatigue, shortness of breath, and weakness over the last couple of weeks. On physical examination, you note a high-pitched systolic murmur and an irregular heartbeat. You suspect mitral regurgitation. What two diagnostic tests would be helpful in confirming your suspicion and directing treatment? What would you be concerned about for his future if this condition is not treated appropriately?

REFERENCES AND SELECTED READINGS

Books

Cohn, L. H. (2012). *Cardiac surgery in the adult* (4th ed.). New York: McGraw-Hill

Fuster, V., Walsh, R. A., Harrington, R. A., et al. (Eds.). (2011). *Hurst's the heart* (13th ed.). New York: McGraw-Hill.

Lynn-McHale Wiegand, D. J. (2010). *AACN procedure manual for critical care* (6th ed.). Philadelphia, PA: Elsevier.

Mann, D. L., & Felker, M. (2016). *Heart failure: A companion to Braunwald's heart disease* (3rd ed.). Philadelphia, PA: Elsevier Saunders.

Mann, D. L., Zipes, D. P., Bonow, R. O., et al. (Eds.). (2015). *Braunwald's heart disease: A textbook of cardiovascular medicine* (10th ed.). Philadelphia, PA: Elsevier Saunders.

Marx, J. A. (2014). *Rosen's emergency medicine: Concepts and clinical practice* (8th ed.). Philadelphia, PA: Elsevier Saunders.

Moser, D. K., & Riegel, B. (2008). *Cardiac nursing: A companion to Braunwald's heart disease*. St. Louis, MO: Elsevier Saunders.

Otto, C. M., & Bonow, R. O. (Eds.). (2013). *Valvular heart disease: A companion to Braunwald's heart disease* (4th ed.). Philadelphia, PA: Elsevier Saunders.

Runge, M. S., Stouffer, G. A., & Patterson, C. (Eds.). (2011). *Netter's cardiology* (2nd ed.). Philadelphia, PA: Elsevier Saunders.

Weber, J. R., & Kelley, J. H. (Eds.). (2014). *Health assessment in nursing* (5th ed.). Philadelphia, PA: Wolters Kluwer Health.

Woods, S. L., Bridges, E., Froelicher, E. S., et al. (2009). *Cardiac nursing* (6th ed.). Philadelphia, PA: Lippincott Williams & Wilkins.

Journals and Electronic Documents

Bennett, T. (2014). Treatment of dilated cardiomyopathy. *British Journal of Cardiac Nursing*, *9*(6), 297–302.

Corrado, D., Wichter, T., Link, M., et al. (2015). Treatment of arrhythmogenic right ventricular cardiomyopathy/dysplasia: An international task force consensus statement. *Circulation*, *132*, 441–453.

Curry, S. (2014). Acute pericarditis: An overview. *British Journal of Cardiac Nursing*, *9*(3), 124–131.

Delling, F. N., & Vasan, R. S. (2014). Epidemiology and pathophysiology of mitral valve prolapse. *Circulation*, *129*(21), 2158–2170.

Elliott, P. M., Anastasakis, A., Borger, M. A., et al. (2014). 2014 ESC guidelines on diagnosis and management of hypertrophic cardiomyopathy. *European Heart Journal*, *35*, 2733–2779.

Feldman, D., Pamboukian, S., Teuteberg, J., et al. (2013). The International Society of Heart and Lung Transplantation guidelines for mechanical circulatory support: Executive Summary. *The Journal of Heart and Lung Transplantation*, *32*(2), 157–187.

Heart & Stroke Foundation of Canada. (2014). Heart transplant surgery safe and effective: A Canadian retrospective spanning three decades finds survival now close to 90 per cent. Retrieved March 30, 2014, from http://www.heartandstroke.com/site/apps/nlnet/content2.aspx?c=ikIQLcMWJtE&b=7799765&ct=11300869.

Holmes, D. R., Mack, M. J., Kaul, S., et al. (2012). 2012 ACCF/AATS/SCAI/STS expert consensus document on transcatheter aortic valve replacement. *Annals of Thoracic Surgery*, *93*(4), 1340–1395.

Hong, S., Hong, M., Ko, Y., et al. (2014). Multidisciplinary team approach for identifying potential candidate for transcatheter aortic valve implantation. *Yonsei Medical Journal, 55*(5), 1246–1252.

Imazio, M., Brucato, A., Cemin, R., et al. (2013). A randomized trial of colchicine for acute pericarditis. *New England Journal of Medicine*, *369*(16), 1522–1528.

Jacoby, D., Depasquale, E., & McKenna, W. (2013). Hypertrophic cardiomyopathy: Diagnosis, risk stratification and treatment. *CMAJ: Canadian Medical Association Journal*, *185*(2), 127–134.

Josephson, L. (2014). Infective endocarditis: A review for nurses. *Dimensions of Critical Care Nursing*, *33*(6), 327–340.

LeWinter, M. M. (2014). Clinical practice. Acute pericarditis. *New England Journal of Medicine*, *371*(25), 2410–2416.

Lund, L. H., Edwards, L. B., Kucheryavaya, A. Y., et al. (2014). The registry of the International Society for Heart and Lung Transplantation: Thirty-first official adult heart transplant report 0 2014; focus theme: Retransplantation. *Journal of Heart Lung Transplantation*, *33*(10), 996–1008.

Marcus, F. I., & Abidov, A. (2012). Arrhythmogenic right ventricular cardiomyopathy 2012: Diagnostic challenges and treatment. *Journal of Cardiovascular Electrophysiology*, *23*(10), 1149–1153.

Maron, B. J., & Nishimura, R. A. (2014). Surgical septal myectomy versus alcohol septal ablation assessing the status of the controversy in 2014. *Circulation*, *130*, 1617–1624.

Maron, B. J., Towbin, J. A., Thiene, G., et al. (2006). Contemporary definitions and classification of the cardiomyopathies: An American Heart Association Scientific Statement from the Council on Clinical Cardiology, Heart Failure and Transplantation Committee; Quality of Care and Outcomes Research and Functional Genomics and Translational Biology Interdisciplinary Working Groups; and Council on Epidemiology and Prevention. *Circulation*, *113*(14), 1807–1816.

Martinez, G., & Valchanov, K. (2012). Infective endocarditis. Continuing Education in Anaesthesia, *Critical Care & Pain*, *12*(3), 134–139.

McRae, M. E. (2007). Myectomy for hypertrophic obstructive cardiomyopathy. *Canadian Journal of Cardiovascular Nursing*, *17*(2), 22–30.

Munkholm-Larsen, S., Wan, B., Tian, D. H., et al. (2014). A systematic review on the safety and efficacy of percutaneous edge-to-edge mitral valve repair with the MitraClip system for high surgical risk candidates. *Heart*, *100*(6), 473–478.

Naylor, M., Bowles, K., McCauley, K., et al. (2013). High-value transitional care: Translation of research into practice. *Journal of Evaluation in Clinic Practice*, *19*(5), 727–733.

Nishimura, R. A., Otto, C. M., Bonow, R. O., et al. (2014). 2014 AHA/ACC guidelines for the management of patients with valvular heart disease. *Journal of the American College of Cardiology*, *63*(22), e57–e185.

Pennell, D. J., Baksi, A. J., Kilner, P. J., et al. (2014). Review of The Journal of Cardiovascular Magnetic Resonance 2012. *Journal of Cardiovascular Magnetic Resonance*, *16*(1), 100.

Rojas, L., & Calkins, H. (2015). Present understanding of the relationship between exercise and arrhythmogenic right ventricular dysplasia/cardiomyopathy. *Trends in Cardiovascular Medicine*, *25*(3), 181–188.

Rustad, J., Stern, T., Hebert, K., et al. (2013). Diagnosis and treatment of depression in patients with congestive heart failure: A review of the literature. *The Primary Care Companion for CNS Disorders, 15*(4), PCC.13r01511.
Savage, L. S., Salyer, J., Flattery, M. P., et al. (2014). Living with a total artificial heart: Patients' perspectives. *Journal of Cardiovascular Nursing, 29*(1), E1–E8.
Semsarian, C., Ingles, J., Maron, M., et al. (2015). New perspectives on the prevalence of hypertrophic cardiomyopathy. *Journal of the American College of Cardiology, 65*(12), 1249–1254.
Starling, R. C. (2013). Advanced heart failure: Transplantation, LVADs, and beyond. *Cleveland Clinic Journal of Medicine, 80*(1), 33–40.
Statistics Canada. (2014). Table 102-0529—Deaths, by cause, Chapter IX: Diseases of the circulatory system (I00 to I99), age group and sex, Canada, annual (2014), CANSIM (Death database). Retrieved from http://www5.statcan.gc.ca/cansim/a26?lang=eng&retrLang=eng&id=1020529&tabMode=dataTable&srchLan=-1&p1=-1&p2=9
White-Williams, C., Grady, K. L., Myers, S., et al. (2013). The relationships among satisfaction with social support, quality of life, and survival 5 to 10 years after heart transplantation. *Journal of Cardiovascular Nursing, 28*(5), 407–416.

Resources

Cardiomyopathy Association: http://www.cardiomyopathy.org
Heart and Stroke Foundation of Canada: http://www.heartandstroke.com
Heartmates: http://www.heartmates.com

31 Management of Patients With Complications From Heart Disease

Adapted by Karen Lynn Then and James A. Rankin

Learning Objectives

On completion of this chapter, the learner will be able to:

1. Describe the etiology, pathophysiology, and clinical manifestations of heart failure.
2. Describe the management of patients with heart failure.
3. Use the nursing process as a framework for care of patients with heart failure.
4. Develop a teaching plan for patients with heart failure.
5. Identify the etiology, pathophysiology, and clinical manifestations of pulmonary edema.
6. Describe the management of patients with pulmonary edema.
7. Describe the management of patients with complications from heart disease including thromboembolism, pericardial effusion, and sudden cardiac death.

Today, it is possible to help the patient with heart disease to live longer and achieve a high quality of life. Advances in diagnostic procedures, treatments, technologies, and pharmacotherapies allow earlier and more accurate diagnoses, and treatment that can begin well before significant debilitation occurs. However, heart disease remains a chronic condition, which often progresses. It also is associated with serious complications. This chapter outlines the most common complications associated with heart diseases and the treatment options available to treat these complications.

Cardiac Hemodynamics

The basic function of the heart is to pump blood. The heart's ability to pump is evaluated by **cardiac output (CO)**, the amount of blood pumped per minute. CO is determined by measuring the heart rate (HR) and multiplying it by the **stroke volume (SV)**, the amount of blood pumped out of the ventricle with each contraction. CO usually is calculated using the equation CO = HR × SV.

The HR is primarily controlled by the autonomic nervous system, that is, by the sympathetic and parasympathetic nervous systems. When the sympathetic nervous system is stimulated, both HR and SV increase. When the parasympathetic system is stimulated, HR decreases. HR is easily measured, but SV is more difficult to measure. SV depends on three factors: preload, afterload, and contractility (Fig. 31-1). Evaluation of these factors requires hemodynamic monitoring.

Preload is the amount of blood within the ventricle just before systole. It increases pressure in the ventricle, which stretches the ventricular wall. Like a rubber band, the ventricular muscle fibres need to be stretched (by blood volume) to produce optimal ejection of blood. Too little or too much muscle fibre stretch decreases the volume of blood ejected. The major factor that determines preload is venous return, the volume of blood that enters the ventricle during diastole. Another factor that determines preload is ventricular **compliance**, the elasticity or amount of "give" when blood enters the ventricle. Elasticity is decreased when the muscle thickens, as in hypertrophic cardiomyopathy (see Chapter 30) or when there is increased fibrotic tissue within the ventricle. Fibrotic tissue replaces dead myocardial cells, such as after a myocardial infarction (MI) (see Chapter 29). Fibrotic tissue has little compliance, making the ventricle stiff. Given the same volume of blood, a noncompliant ventricle has a higher intraventricular pressure than a compliant one. Higher pressure increases the workload of the heart and can lead to heart failure (HF) if it is sustained.

Afterload refers to the amount of resistance to the ejection of blood from the ventricle. To eject blood, the ventricle must overcome the resistance caused by tension in the aorta and systemic vessels. Afterload is inversely related to SV, and an increase in afterload causes the ventricle to work harder and may decrease the amount of blood ejected. The major factors that determine afterload are the diameter and distensibility of the great vessels (aorta and pulmonary artery) and the opening and competence of the semilunar valves (pulmonic and aortic valves). When the valves open easily, resistance is lower. If the patient has significant vasoconstriction, hypertension, or a narrowed valvular opening from stenosis, resistance (afterload) increases. When afterload increases, the workload of the heart must increase to overcome the resistance and eject blood.

Contractility, the force of contraction, is related to the status of the myocardium. Catecholamines, released by sympathetic stimulation during exercise or from administration of positive inotropic medications, can increase contractility and SV. MI causes necrosis and subsequent fibrosis of some myocardial cells, shifting the workload to the remaining cells. Significant loss of myocardial cells can decrease contractility and cause HF. Afterload can be reduced by medications to match the lower contractility and maintain adequate CO.

Noninvasive Assessment of Cardiac Hemodynamics

Several noninvasive assessment findings can indicate cardiac hemodynamic status, although the findings do not directly correlate to preload, afterload, or contractility. Right ventricular preload may be estimated by measuring jugular venous distention (JVD). Elevated right ventricular preload may be identified by a positive hepatojugular test. Mean arterial blood pressure is an approximate indicator of left ventricular (LV) afterload. Activity tolerance may be used as an indicator of overall cardiac functioning. These assessments are described in more detail later in this chapter.

Invasive Assessment of Cardiac Hemodynamics

An important tool for evaluating the components of SV in a hemodynamically unstable patient is the pulmonary artery catheter, which is used to obtain the hemodynamic data essential for diagnosis and treatment (see Chapter 27). Measurements of intracardiac pressures, pulmonary artery

Glossary

afterload: the amount of resistance to ejection of blood from a ventricle

anuria: urine output of less than 50 mL/24 hours

ascites: an accumulation of serous fluid in the peritoneal cavity

cardiac output (CO): the amount of blood pumped out of the heart in 1 minute

cardiac resynchronization therapy (CRT): a treatment for heart failure in which a device paces both ventricles to synchronize contractions

compliance: the elasticity or amount of "give" when blood enters the ventricle

congestive heart failure (CHF): a fluid overload condition (congestion) associated with heart failure

contractility: the force of ventricular contraction; related to the number and state of myocardial cells

diastolic heart failure: the inability of the heart to pump sufficiently because of an alteration in the ability of the heart to fill; current term used to describe a type of heart failure

dyspnea on exertion (DOE): shortness of breath that occurs with exertion

ejection fraction (EF): percentage of blood volume in the ventricles at the end of diastole that is ejected during systole; a measurement of contractility

heart failure (HF): the inability of the heart to pump sufficient blood to meet the needs of the tissues for oxygen and nutrients; signs and symptoms of pulmonary and systemic congestion may or may not be present

implantable cardioverter defibrillator (ICD): a device implanted in patients with ventricular dysrhythmias that detects and treats dysrhythmias

left-sided heart failure (left ventricular failure): inability of the left ventricle to fill or pump (empty) sufficient blood to meet the needs of the tissues for oxygen and nutrients; traditional term used to describe patient's symptoms of heart failure

oliguria: diminished urine output; less than 400 mL/24 hours

orthopnea: shortness of breath when lying flat

paroxysmal nocturnal dyspnea (PND): shortness of breath that occurs suddenly during sleep

pericardiocentesis: procedure that involves aspiration of fluid from the pericardial sac

pericardiotomy: surgically created opening of the pericardium

preload: the amount of myocardial stretch just before systole caused by the volume of blood presented to the ventricle

pulmonary edema: abnormal accumulation of fluid in the interstitial spaces or in the alveoli of the lungs

pulseless electrical activity (PEA): condition in which electrical activity is present but there is not an adequate pulse or blood pressure because of ineffective cardiac contraction or circulating blood volume

pulsus paradoxus: systolic blood pressure of more than 10 mm Hg higher during exhalation than during inspiration; difference is normally less than 10 mm Hg

right-sided heart failure (right ventricular failure): inability of the right ventricle to fill or pump (empty) sufficient blood to the pulmonary circulation

stroke volume (SV): the amount of blood pumped out of the ventricle with each contraction

systolic heart failure: the inability of the heart to pump sufficiently because of an alteration in the ability of the heart to contract; current term used to describe a type of heart failure

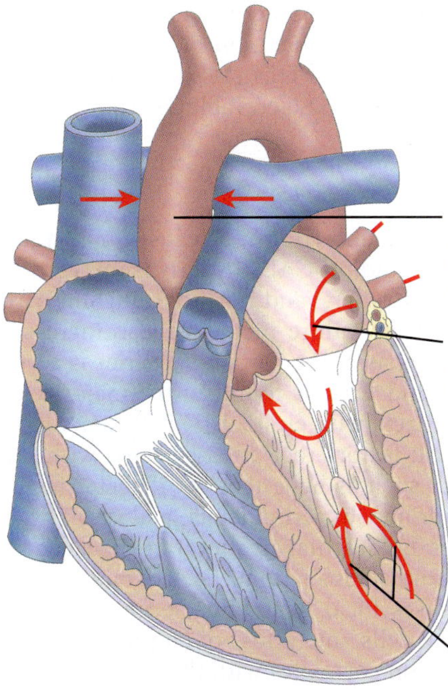

FIGURE 31-1. The determinants of stroke volume (SV). The SV is determined by the amount of preload presented to the ventricle, the amount of afterload or resistance to ventricular ejection, and the strength of cardiac contractility. The CO is the product of SV and HR. (Redrawn from Porth, C. M. (2005). *Pathophysiology: Concepts of altered health states* (7th ed.). Philadelphia, PA: Lippincott Williams & Wilkins.)

pressures, and CO are made at intervals. Therapy, especially intravenous (IV) medication, is adjusted based on the assessment and diagnostic findings. The patient with an invasive hemodynamic catheter is usually managed in a critical care environment because of the need for frequent nursing assessments and interventions.

Heart Failure

Heart failure (HF) is a clinical syndrome resulting from structural or functional cardiac disorders that impair the ability of the ventricles to fill or eject blood (Yancy, Jessup, Bozkurt, et al., 2013). In the past, HF was often referred to as **congestive heart failure (CHF)**, because many patients experience pulmonary or peripheral congestion with edema. Currently, HF is recognized as a clinical syndrome characterized by signs and symptoms of fluid overload or inadequate tissue perfusion. Fluid overload and decreased tissue perfusion result when the heart cannot generate CO sufficient to meet the body's demands for oxygen and nutrients. The term *heart failure* indicates myocardial disease in which impaired contraction of the heart (systolic dysfunction) or filling of the heart (diastolic dysfunction) may cause pulmonary or systemic congestion. Some cases of HF are reversible, depending on the cause. Most often, HF is a chronic, progressive condition that is managed with lifestyle changes and medications to prevent episodes of **acute decompensated heart failure.** These episodes are characterized by increased symptoms, decreased CO, and low perfusion (Pinkerman, Sander, Breeding, et al., 2013). These episodes are also associated with increased hospitalizations, increased health care costs, and decreased quality of life.

Chronic Heart Failure

As with coronary heart disease, the incidence of HF increases with age. Overall, although the mortality rate of coronary artery disease (CAD) is decreasing, just the opposite is true for HF. Over 669,600 (3.6%) of Canadians aged 40 years and older live with HF, and approximately 92,900 Canadians aged 40 years and older received a new diagnosis of heart failure in 2012/13 (Government of Canada, 2017). HF is the leading cause of hospitalizations, and although there have been significant improvements in the diagnosis and treatment of HF, the readmission rate exceeds 20% within 30 days of discharge and the mortality rate is approximately 30% at a year after diagnosis (Virani, Bains, Code, et al., 2017). HF at present is responsible for more than $2.8 billion dollars per year in direct health care costs. Although HF can affect people of all ages, it is most common in people older than 75 years. As the Canadian and North American population ages, HF has become an epidemic that challenges the country's health care resources.

The prevalence of HF is expected to increase in the coming decades in Canada since there are significant cardiovascular risk factors among young and middle-aged adults, as well as an increasingly aging population. Subsequently, there will be increasing demand for acute care admissions, emergency visits, specialty clinics, and home care services (Virani, Bains, Code, et al., 2017). Rates of HF are higher in rural settings, in part because HF is more prevalent in older adults and the proportion of older adults in rural places is slightly higher. The increase in the incidence of HF reflects both the increased number of older people and improvements in treatment of cardiac diseases, resulting in increased survival rates. Many hospitalizations could be prevented by appropriate outpatient management. Prevention, early intervention, and outpatient specialty heart failure programs are essential to arrest the progression of HF and are major health initiatives in Canada.

Heart failure is classified into categories based on ejection fraction as identified by echocardiogram. **Ejection fraction (EF)** is measured in percentages and is the volume of blood that the LV ejects out with each contraction. EF, is calculated by subtracting the amount of blood at the end of systole from the amount at the end of diastole and calculating the percentage of blood that is ejected. A normal EF is 55% to 65% of the ventricular volume; the ventricle does not completely empty between contractions. The EF is normal in diastolic HF but severely reduced in systolic HF.

- HFpEF refers to HF with preserved ejection fraction: Left ventricle ejection fraction (LVEF) >50%
- HFmEF refers to HF with a midrange ejection fraction: LVED 41% to 49%
- HFrEF refers to HF with reduced ejection fraction: LVEF <40%

(Ezekowitz, O'Meara, McDonald, et al., 2017)

HFpEF, also known as **diastolic heart failure,** can be a result of aging, diabetes, or hypertension. It occurs when the ventricles are still and do not relax (noncompliant), thereby making it difficult for the ventricle to fill. HFrEF, **systolic heart failure,** occurs when the heart muscle is weak and is not able to contract adequately; therefore,

TABLE 31-1 New York Heart Association Classification of Heart Failure

Classification	Signs and Symptoms
I	No limitation of physical activity Ordinary activity does not cause undue fatigue, palpitation, or dyspnea
II	Slight limitation of physical activity Comfortable at rest, but ordinary physical activity causes fatigue, palpitation, or dyspnea
III	Marked limitation of physical activity Comfortable at rest, but less than ordinary activity causes fatigue, palpitation, or dyspnea
IV	Unable to carry out any physical activity without discomfort Symptoms of cardiac insufficiency at rest If any physical activity is undertaken, discomfort is increased

Adapted from Yancy, C. W., Jessup, M., Bozkurt, B., et al. (2013). 2013 ACCF/AHA Guideline for the management of heart failure. A report of the American College of Cardiology Foundation/American Heart Association Task Force on Practice Guidelines. *Circulation, 128*(16), e240–e327.

there is a lower than adequate blood flow of oxygen-rich blood into the systemic system.

Although a low EF is a hallmark of HF, the severity of HF is frequently classified according to the patient's symptoms. The New York Heart Association (NYHA) Classification is described in Table 31-1, and the causes are explained in subsequent sections of this chapter. The American College of Cardiology and the American Heart Association (ACC/AHA) proposed another classification system which takes into consideration the natural history and progressive nature of HF. This classification includes four stages: stage A to stage D (see Table 31-2).

Etiology

Myocardial dysfunction and HF can be caused by a number of conditions, including CAD, hypertension, cardiomyopathy, valvular disorders, and renal dysfunction with volume overload. Heart failure incidence also increases with age. Atherosclerosis of the coronary arteries is a primary cause of HF, and CAD is found in the majority of patients with HF (Ezekowitz et al., 2017). Patients with CAD often have risk factors that are associated with the development of HF such as hypertension, diabetes mellitus, metabolic syndrome, hyperlipidemia, and smoking.

Ischemia causes myocardial dysfunction because of resulting hypoxia and acidosis from the accumulation of lactic acid. MI causes focal heart muscle necrosis, the death of myocardial cells, and a loss of contractility; the extent of the infarction correlates with the severity of HF. Revascularization of the coronary artery by a percutaneous coronary intervention (PCI) or by coronary artery bypass surgery (coronary artery bypass graft [CABG]) and appropriate medical management may improve myocardial oxygenation and ventricular function and prevent more extensive myocardial necrosis that can lead to HF.

Cardiomyopathy is a disease of the myocardium. There are four types of cardiomyopathy: dilated, hypertrophic, restrictive, and arrhythmogenic right ventricular dysplasia

TABLE 31-2 American College of Cardiology and American Heart Association Classification of Heart Failure

Classification	Criteria	Patient Characteristics	Treatment Recommendations for Appropriate Patients
Stage A	Patients at high risk for developing left ventricular dysfunction but without structural heart disease or symptoms of HF	Hypertension Atherosclerotic disease Diabetes Metabolic syndrome	Heart healthy lifestyle Risk factor control of hypertension, lipids, diabetes, obesity
Stage B	Patients with left ventricular dysfunction or structural heart disease who have not developed symptoms of HF	History of myocardial infarction Left ventricular hypertrophy Low ejection fraction	Implement stage A recommendations, plus: • ACE inhibitor or ARB for low EF or history of MI • Beta-blocker • Statin
Stage C	Patients with left ventricular dysfunction or structural heart disease with current or prior symptoms of heart disease	Shortness of breath Fatigue Decreased exercise tolerance	Implement stage A and B recommendations, plus: • Diuretics • Aldosterone antagonist • Sodium restriction • Implantable defibrillator • Cardiac resynchronization therapy

Stage D	Patients with refractory end-stage HF requiring specialized interventions	Symptoms despite maximal medical therapy
		Recurrent hospitalizations
			Implement stage A, B, and C recommendations, plus:
			• Fluid restriction
			• End-of-life care
			• Extraordinary measures:
			  • Inotropes
			  • Cardiac transplantation
			  • Mechanical support

ACE, angiotensin-converting enzyme; ARB, angiotensin receptor blocker; EF, ejection fraction; HF, heart failure; MI, myocardial infarction.

Adapted from Yancy, C. W., Jessup, M., Bozkurt, B., et al. (2013). 2013 ACCF/AHA Guideline for the management of heart failure. A report of the American College of Cardiology Foundation/American Heart Association Task Force on Practice Guidelines. *Circulation, 128*(16), e240–e327.

(see Chapter 30). Dilated cardiomyopathy, the most common type of cardiomyopathy, causes diffuse cellular necrosis and fibrosis, leading to decreased contractility (systolic failure) and HF. Dilated cardiomyopathy can be idiopathic (unknown cause), or it can result from an inflammatory process, such as myocarditis, or from a cytotoxic agent, such as alcohol or certain antineoplastic drugs. Hypertrophic cardiomyopathy and restrictive cardiomyopathy lead to decreased distensibility and ventricular filling (diastolic failure). Arrhythmogenic right ventricular dysplasia is a problem that results when the proteins that hold heart muscle cells together are replaced with fibrous scar tissue and fatty cells. Usually, HF due to cardiomyopathy becomes chronic and progressive. However, cardiomyopathy and HF may improve or resolve following removal of the causative agent, such as with the cessation of alcohol ingestion. Systemic or pulmonary hypertension (e.g., pulmonary artery hypertension, obstructive pulmonary disease) increases afterload (resistance to ejection), which increases the workload of the heart and leads to hypertrophy of myocardial muscle fibres; this can be considered a compensatory mechanism because it increases contractility. However, sustained hypertension eventually leads to changes that impair the heart's ability to fill properly during diastole, and the hypertrophied ventricles may dilate and fail.

Valvular heart disease is also a cause of HF. The valves ensure that blood flows in one direction. With valvular dysfunction, blood has increasing difficulty moving forward, increasing pressure within the heart and increasing cardiac workload, leading to HF. See Chapter 30 for discussion of the effects of valvular heart disease.

Several systemic conditions contribute to the development and severity of HF, including increased metabolic rate (e.g., fever, thyrotoxicosis), iron overload (e.g., from hemochromatosis), hypoxia, severe anemia (serum hematocrit less than 25%), and progressive renal failure. All of these conditions require an increase in CO to satisfy the systemic oxygen demand. Hypoxia or anemia also may decrease the supply of oxygen to the myocardium. More than 40% of patients with chronic HF have impaired renal function. The term *cardiorenal syndrome* defines disorders of the heart and kidneys in which acute or chronic decompensation in one organ may cause acute or chronic decompensation of the other. In addition, cardiac dysrhythmias such as atrial fibrillation may cause or result from HF. The altered electrical stimulation from the dysrhythmia impairs myocardial contraction and decreases the overall efficiency of myocardial function. Other factors, such as hypoxia, acidosis (respiratory or metabolic), electrolyte abnormalities, and antiarrhythmic medications may also worsen myocardial function.

Pathophysiology

The pathophysiology of HF results in similar changes and clinical manifestations, regardless of the etiology. Significant myocardial dysfunction usually occurs before the patient experiences signs and symptoms of HF such as shortness of breath, edema, or fatigue. Many patients with HF have comorbidities, complicating both diagnosis and management.

As HF develops, the body activates neurohormonal compensatory mechanisms. These mechanisms represent the body's attempt to cope with the HF and are responsible for the signs and symptoms that eventually develop. Understanding these mechanisms is important because these mechanisms eventually contribute to the worsening of heart function and of HF.

Systolic HF results in decreased blood volume being ejected from the ventricle. The decreased vascular stretch is sensed by baroreceptors in the aortic and carotid. The sympathetic nervous system is then stimulated to release epinephrine and norepinephrine (Fig. 31-2). The purpose of this initial response is to increase HR and contractility and support the failing myocardium, but the continued response has multiple negative effects. Sympathetic stimulation causes vasoconstriction of the skin, gastrointestinal tract, and kidneys. A decrease in renal perfusion due to low CO and vasoconstriction then causes the release of renin by the kidney. Renin converts the plasma protein angiotensinogen to angiotensin I, which then circulates to the lungs. Angiotensin-converting enzyme (ACE), primarily located in the lumen of pulmonary blood vessels, converts angiotensin I to angiotensin II, a potent vasoconstrictor, which then increases the blood pressure and afterload. Angiotensin II also stimulates the release of aldosterone from the adrenal cortex, resulting in sodium and fluid retention by the renal tubules and stimulation of the thirst centre. This leads to the fluid retention and potential volume overload commonly seen in HF. Angiotensin, aldosterone, and other neurohormones (e.g., endothelin, prostacyclin) lead to an increase in preload and afterload, which increases stress on the ventricular wall, causing an increase in the workload of the heart. A counter-regulatory mechanism is attempted through the release of natriuretic peptides. Atrial natriuretic peptide (ANP) and brain (B-type) natriuretic peptide (BNP) are released from the overdistended cardiac chambers. These substances promote vasodilation and diuresis. However, as chronic heart failure progresses, their effects are not strong enough to overcome the negative effects of the other mechanisms.

As the heart's workload increases, contractility of the myocardial muscle fibres decreases. Decreased contractility results in an increase in end-diastolic blood volume in the ventricle, stretching the myocardial muscle fibres and increasing the size of the ventricle (ventricular dilation). The increased size of the ventricle further increases the stress on the ventricular wall, adding to the workload of the heart. One way the heart compensates for the increased workload is to increase the thickness of the heart muscle (ventricular hypertrophy). However, hypertrophy results in an abnormal proliferation of ineffective myocardial cells, a process known as ventricular remodelling. Under the influence of neurohormones (e.g., norepinephrine, angiotensin II), enlarged myocardial cells are produced that are dysfunctional and die early (a process called *apoptosis*), leaving the other normal myocardial cells to struggle to maintain CO.

As cardiac cells die and the heart muscle becomes fibrotic, diastolic HF can develop, leading to further dysfunction. Diastolic HF develops because of continued increased workload on the heart, which responds by increasing the number and size of myocardial cells (i.e., ventricular

Physiology/Pathophysiology

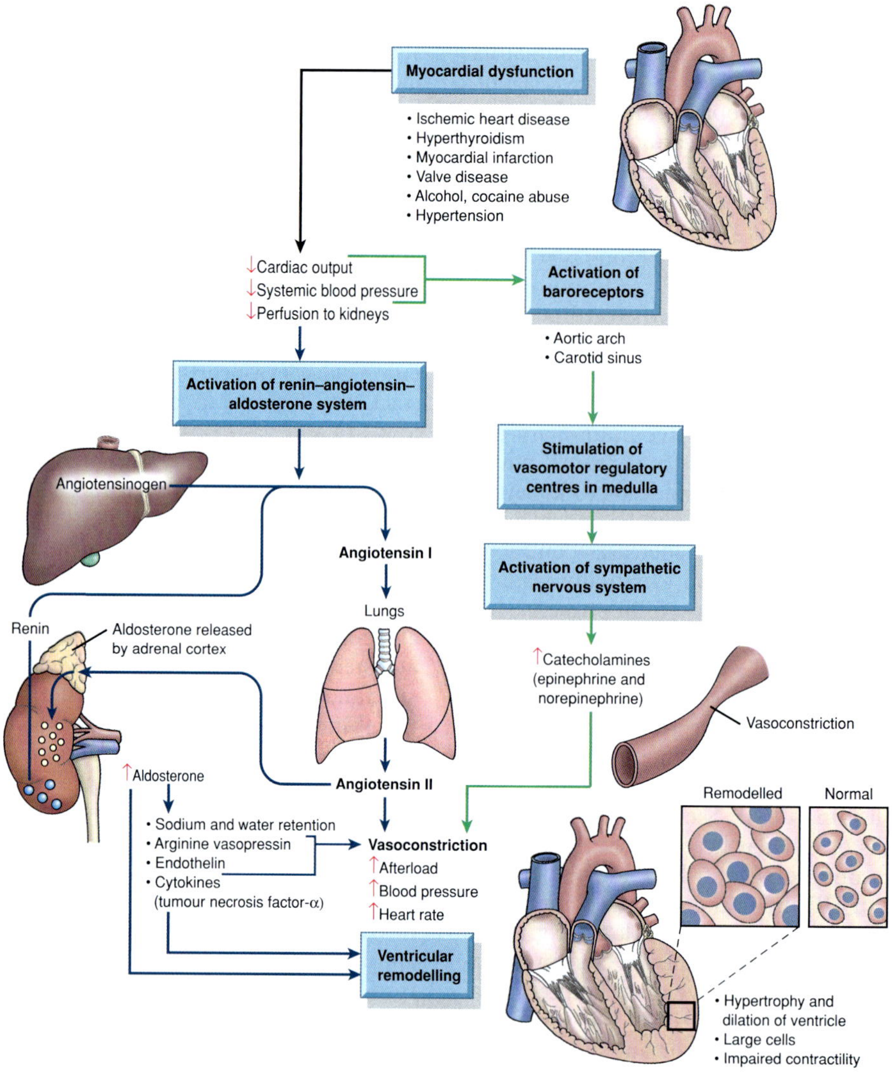

FIGURE 31-2. The pathophysiology of heart failure. A decrease in CO activates multiple neurohormonal mechanisms that ultimately result in the signs and symptoms of HF.

hypertrophy and altered cellular functioning). These responses cause resistance to ventricular filling, which increases ventricular filling pressures despite a normal or reduced blood volume. A stiff ventricle resists filling, and less blood in the ventricles causes a further decrease in CO. The low CO and high ventricular filling pressures can cause the same neurohormonal responses as described for systolic HF. The compensatory mechanisms of HF have been called the *vicious cycle of HF* because the heart does not pump sufficient blood to the body, which causes the body to stimulate the heart to work harder; the heart cannot respond, and failure becomes worse.

Clinical Manifestations

Clinical manifestations associated with HF are presented in Chart 31-1. These signs and symptoms are related to congestion and poor perfusion. The signs and symptoms of HF can also be related to the ventricle that is most affected. **Left-sided heart failure (left ventricular failure)** causes different manifestations than **right-sided heart failure (right ventricular failure).** In chronic HF, patients may have both left and right ventricular failure and subsequent signs and symptoms. In either left- or right-sided HF, the patient may have fatigue due to poor CO.

Left-Sided Heart Failure

Pulmonary congestion occurs when the LV cannot effectively pump blood out of the ventricle into the aorta and the systemic circulation. The increased LV end-diastolic blood volume increases the LV end-diastolic pressure, which decreases blood flow from the left atrium into the LV during diastole. The blood volume and pressure in the left atrium increases, which decreases blood flow from the pulmonary vessels into the left atrium. Pulmonary venous blood volume and pressure increase in the lungs, forcing fluid from the pulmonary capillaries into the pulmonary tissues and alveoli, causing pulmonary interstitial edema

CHART 31-1

Assessment: Heart Failure

Be alert for the following signs and symptoms:

Congestion

- Dyspnea
- Orthopnea
- Paroxysmal nocturnal dyspnea
- Cough (recumbent or exertional)
- Pulmonary crackles that do not clear with cough
- Weight gain (rapid)
- Dependent edema
- Abdominal bloating or discomfort
- Ascites
- Jugular venous distention
- Sleep disturbance (anxiety or air hunger)
- Fatigue

Poor Perfusion/Low Cardiac Output

- Decreased exercise tolerance
- Muscle wasting or weakness
- Anorexia or nausea
- Unexplained weight loss
- Light-headedness or dizziness
- Unexplained confusion or altered mental status
- Resting tachycardia
- Daytime oliguria with recumbent nocturia
- Cool or vasoconstricted extremities
- Pallor or cyanosis

Adapted from Pinkerman, C., Sander, P., Breeding, J. E., et al. (2013). *Heart failure in adults, Institute for Clinical Systems Improvement*. Retrieved November 29, 2015, from www.guidelines.gov/content.aspx?id=47030&search=heart+failure

and impaired gas exchange. The clinical manifestations of pulmonary congestion include dyspnea, cough, fatigue, pulmonary crackles, and low oxygen saturation levels. The patient may even become light-headed, anxious, or confused. An extra heart sound, the S_3, or "ventricular gallop," may be detected on auscultation. It is caused by abnormal ventricular filling in which a large volume of fluid enters the ventricle at the beginning of diastole. In contrast, the S_4, or "atrial gallop," occurs when the atrium contract into a stiff ventricle, such as in systolic failure post MI.

Dyspnea, or shortness of breath, may be precipitated by minimal to moderate activity (**dyspnea on exertion [DOE]**; **shortness of breath on exertion** [SOBE]); dyspnea also can occur at rest. The patient may report **orthopnea**, difficulty breathing when lying flat. Patients with orthopnea usually prefer not to lie flat and they may use pillows to prop themselves up in bed, or they may sit in a chair and even sleep sitting up. Some patients have sudden attacks of dyspnea at night, a condition known as **paroxysmal nocturnal dyspnea (PND)**. Fluid that has accumulated in the dependent extremities during the day begins to be reabsorbed into the circulating blood volume when the patient lies down. Because the impaired LV cannot eject the increased circulating blood volume, the pressure in the pulmonary circulation increases, causing further shifting of fluid into the alveoli. The fluid-filled alveoli cannot exchange oxygen and carbon dioxide. Without sufficient oxygen, the patient experiences dyspnea and has difficulty sleeping.

The cough associated with LV failure is initially dry and nonproductive as fluid collects in the very small airways in the bases of the lungs. Most often, patients complain of a dry hacking cough that may be mislabelled as asthma or chronic obstructive pulmonary disease (COPD). The cough may become moist over time. Large quantities of frothy sputum, which is sometimes pink (blood tinged), may be produced, indicating acute decompensated HF with pulmonary edema. Acute pulmonary edema if not treated promptly may become life threatening.

Adventitious or added breath sounds may be heard in various areas of the lungs. In the early phase of LV failure, crackles (that do not clear with coughing) are heard bilaterally late in inspiration in the dependent portions of the lungs. As the failure worsens and pulmonary congestion increases, crackles may be auscultated throughout all lung fields. At this point, oxygen saturation may decrease.

In addition to increased pulmonary pressures that cause decreased oxygenation, the amount of blood ejected from the LV decreases and can lead to inadequate tissue perfusion. The diminished CO has widespread manifestations because not enough blood reaches all the tissues and organs (low perfusion) to provide the necessary oxygen. The decrease in SV can also lead to stimulation of the sympathetic nervous system to release catecholamines, which further impedes perfusion to many organs, including the kidneys.

Blood flow to the kidneys decreases, causing decreased perfusion and reduced urine output (**oliguria**). Renal perfusion pressure falls, and the renin–angiotensin–aldosterone system is stimulated to increase blood pressure and intravascular volume. However, when the patient is lying down, the CO is increased, improving renal perfusion, which may lead to frequent urination at night (nocturia). As HF progresses, decreased CO may cause other symptoms. Decreased gastrointestinal perfusion causes altered digestion. Decreased brain perfusion causes dizziness, light-headedness, confusion, restlessness, and anxiety due to decreased oxygenation and blood flow. As anxiety increases, so does dyspnea, increasing anxiety and creating a vicious cycle. Stimulation of the sympathetic system also causes the peripheral blood vessels to constrict, so the skin appears pale or ashen and feels cool and clammy. Cyanosis may be present due to low oxygen saturation, peripheral vasoconstriction, or both.

A decrease in SV causes the sympathetic nervous system to increase the HR (tachycardia) and dysrhythmias may occur, often causing the patient to complain of palpitations. The peripheral pulses as a result of the tachycardia may become weak and thready. Without adequate CO, the body cannot respond to increased energy demands, and the patient becomes easily fatigued and has decreased activity tolerance. Fatigue also results from the increased energy expended in breathing and the insomnia that results from respiratory distress, coughing, and nocturia.

Right-Sided Heart Failure

When the right ventricle fails, congestion in the peripheral tissues and the viscera predominates. This occurs because the right side of the heart cannot eject blood and cannot accommodate all of the blood that normally returns to it from the venous circulation. Increased venous pressure leads to increased jugular venous pressure (JVP) and increased hydrostatic pressure throughout the venous system.

Systemic clinical manifestations include edema of the lower extremities (dependent edema), hepatomegaly (enlargement of the liver), pleural effusion (fluid accumulation in the pleural space), **ascites** (accumulation of fluid in the peritoneal cavity), anorexia and nausea (congestion in the gut), weakness, and weight gain due to retention of fluid.

Edema usually affects the feet and ankles, which worsens when the patient stands or dangles the legs, and decreases when the legs are elevated. The edema can gradually progress up the legs and thighs and eventually into the external genitalia and lower trunk. Edema in the abdomen, as evidenced by increased abdominal girth, may accompany lower body edema or may be the only edema present. Sacral edema is common in patients who are on bed rest, because the sacral area is dependent. Pitting edema, in which indentations in the skin remain after even slight compression with the fingertips (Fig. 31-3), is obvious only after retention of at least 4.5 kg of fluid (4.5 L).

Hepatomegaly and tenderness in the right upper quadrant of the abdomen result from venous engorgement of the liver. The increased pressure may interfere with the liver's ability to function (secondary liver dysfunction). As hepatic dysfunction progresses, increased pressure within the portal vessels may force fluid into the abdominal cavity, causing ascites. Ascites may increase pressure on the stomach and intestines and cause gastrointestinal distress. Hepatomegaly may also increase pressure on the diaphragm, causing respiratory distress.

Anorexia (loss of appetite), nausea, or abdominal pain results from the venous engorgement and venous stasis within the abdominal organs. The weakness that accompanies right-sided HF results from reduced CO, impaired circulation, and inadequate removal of catabolic waste products from the tissues. Cachexia is a potential complication of chronic end-stage heart failure, which has many factors: cellular (inflammatory mediators, cytokines and toxins), illness and intervention side effects (medications, depression, dietary restrictions, hospitalizations), and nutritional (alterations in appetite, digestion and absorption of the gastrointestinal system) (Andre, Santos, & Neto, 2017).

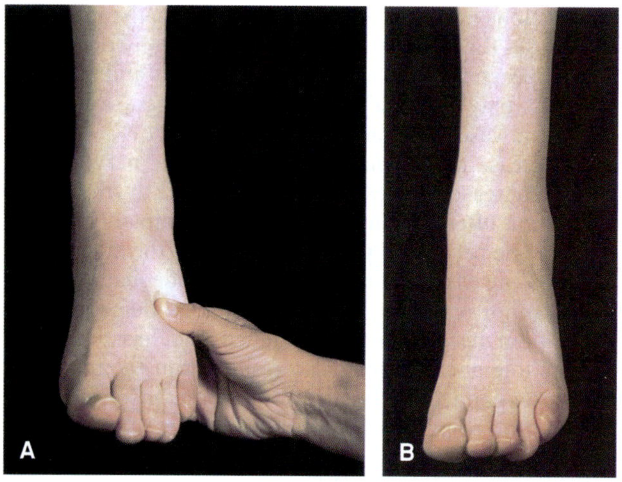

FIGURE 31-3. Example of pitting edema. **A.** The nurse applies thumb pressure over the dorsum of the foot for at least 5 seconds. **B.** When the pressure is released, an indentation remains in the edematous tissue. (From Bickley, L. S. [2017]. *Bates' guide to physical examination and history taking* [12th ed.]. Philadelphia, PA: Lippincott Williams & Wilkins.)

Assessment and Diagnostic Findings

HF may go undetected until the patient presents with signs and symptoms of pulmonary and peripheral edema. Some of the physical signs that suggest HF may also occur with other diseases, such as renal failure, liver failure, oncologic conditions, and COPD, therefore, further assessment and diagnostic testing is essential to confirm a diagnosis of HF.

Assessment of ventricular function is an essential part of the initial diagnostic workup. An echocardiogram is usually performed to confirm the diagnosis of HF; help identify the underlying cause; and determine the EF, which helps to identify anatomic features such as structural abnormalities and valve malfunction, and confirm the diagnosis of HF. This information may also be obtained noninvasively by radionuclide ventriculography or invasively by ventriculography as part of a cardiac catheterization procedure. Differential identification of systolic and diastolic HF is important, as treatment differs.

A thorough history, chest x-ray, and an electrocardiogram (ECG) are obtained to assist in the diagnosis and to determine the underlying cause of HF (e.g., MI). Laboratory studies usually completed in the initial workup include serum electrolytes, blood urea nitrogen (BUN), creatinine, thyroid-stimulating hormone, complete blood cell count, BNP, liver function tests, and routine urinalysis. The BNP level is a key diagnostic indicator of HF. High levels of BNP are a sign of high cardiac filling pressure and can aid in the diagnosis of HF, worsened episodes, as well as exclude HF when levels are low (Roberts, Ludman, Dworzynski, et al., 2015). The results of these laboratory studies assist in determining the underlying cause and can also be used to establish a baseline to assess effects of treatment. Cardiac stress testing or cardiac catheterization may be performed to determine whether CAD and cardiac ischemia are causing the HF.

Medical Management

The overall goals of management of HF are to relieve patient symptoms, improve functional status and quality of life, and extend survival. Management is based on the type, severity, and cause of HF. Specific objectives of guideline-directed patient management include the following:

- Eliminate or reduce any etiologic contributory factors, especially those that may be reversible (e.g., hypertension, ischemia, atrial fibrillation, excessive alcohol ingestion)
- Reduce the workload on the heart by reducing afterload and preload
  - Improvement of cardiac function with optimal pharmacologic management

- Reduction of symptoms and improvement of functional status
- Stabilization of patient condition and lowering of the risk of hospitalization
- Delay of the progression of HF and extension of life expectancy
- Promotion of a lifestyle conducive to cardiac health

Treatment options vary according to the severity of the patient's condition and may include oral and IV pharmacologic management; major lifestyle changes; supplemental oxygen; implantation of assistive devices; and surgical approaches, including cardiac transplantation. Canada, as has many other countries, has committed resources to development of best practices based on evidence, including guidelines and educational tools.

Managing the patient with HF includes providing comprehensive education and counselling to the patient and family. It is essential that the patient and family understand the nature of HF and the importance of their participation in the treatment regimen. Lifestyle recommendations include restriction of dietary sodium; avoidance of excessive fluid and alcohol intake and smoking; weight reduction when indicated; regular exercise as tolerated; and daily weigh if fluid is retained. The patient must know how to recognize signs and symptoms that need to be reported to the health care professional.

Pharmacologic Therapy

Several medications are routinely prescribed for systolic HF, including ACE inhibitors, beta-blockers, diuretics, and vasodilators. Many of these medications, particularly ACE inhibitors and beta-blockers, improve symptoms and extend survival. Others, such as diuretics, improve symptoms but may not affect survival. Target doses for these medications are identified in the ACC/AHA guidelines, and nurses and physicians work collaboratively toward achieving effective dosing of these medications (Yancy et al., 2013). Medications for diastolic failure depend on the underlying condition, such as hypertension (see Chapter 33) or valvular dysfunction (see Chapter 30).

Angiotensin-Converting Enzyme Inhibitors

ACE inhibitors play a pivotal role in the management of systolic HF. They have been found to relieve the signs and symptoms of HF, decrease ventricular remodelling, and significantly decrease mortality and morbidity, especially in patients with an LVEF less than 35%. ACE inhibitors slow the progression of HF, improve exercise tolerance, and decrease the number of hospitalizations for HF (Ezekowitz et al., 2017; Shah, Gandhi, Srivastava, et al., 2017). ACE inhibitors promote vasodilation and diuresis by decreasing afterload and preload. Vasodilation reduces resistance to LV ejection of blood, diminishing the heart's workload and improving ventricular emptying. In promoting diuresis, ACE inhibitors decrease the secretion of aldosterone, a hormone that causes the kidneys to retain sodium and water. ACE inhibitors also promote renal excretion of sodium and fluid (while retaining potassium), thereby reducing LV filling pressure and decreasing pulmonary congestion. ACE inhibitors may be the first medication prescribed for patients in mild failure—patients with fatigue or DOE but without signs of fluid overload and pulmonary congestion. These agents are also recommended for prevention of HF in patients at risk due to vascular disease and diabetes (Ezekowitz et al., 2017).

ACE inhibitors are started at a low dose that is gradually increased until the optimal dose is achieved. The final maintenance dose depends on the patient's blood pressure, fluid status, renal status, and the severity of the HF.

Patients receiving ACE inhibitors are monitored for hypotension, hypovolemia, hyperkalemia (increased potassium in the blood), and alterations in renal function, especially if they are also receiving diuretics.

When to observe for these effects and for how long depends on the onset, peak, and duration of the medication. Table 31-3 identifies several types of ACE inhibitors

TABLE 31-3 Angiotensin-Converting Enzyme Inhibitors

	Pharmacokinetics			
ACE Inhibitor	**Onset**	**Peak (hours)**	**Duration (hours)**	**Nursing Considerations**
benazepril (Lotensin)	Within 1 hour	2–4	24	Monitor blood pressure, urine output, and electrolyte levels.
captopril (Capoten)	15–60 minutes	1–1.5	6–12[a]	
enalapril (Vasotec)	1 hour	4–6	24	Monitor serum creatinine and urine creatinine clearance.
enalaprilat (Vasotec IV)	15 minutes	1–4	6	
fosinopril (Monopril)	Within 1 hour	2–6	24	Monitor for development of cough that is resistant to cough suppressants.
lisinopril (Prinivil, Zestril)	1 hour	6	24	
moexipril (Univasc)	1 hour	3–6	24	Teach patient to change positions gradually and to report signs of dizziness or lethargy.
quinapril (Accupril)	Within 1 hour	2–4	Up to 24[a]	
perindopril (Coversyl)	1–2 hours	3–7	Up to 24	
ramipril (Altace)	1–2 hours	4–6	24	Instruct patient to weigh self daily and to report rapid weight gain and significant feet and hand swelling.
trandolapril (Mavik)	Within 30 minutes	2–4	>8 days	

[a]Duration of effect is related to the dose.

ACE, angiotensin-converting enzyme.

and their pharmacokinetics. Hypotension is most likely to develop from ACE inhibitor therapy in patients older than 75 years of age and in those with a systolic blood pressure of 100 mm Hg or less, a serum sodium level of lower than 135 mEq/L, or severe HF. Adjusting the dose or type of diuretic in response to the patient's blood pressure and renal function may allow for continued increases in the dosage.

Because ACE inhibitors cause the kidneys to retain potassium, the patient who is also receiving a diuretic may not need to take oral potassium supplements. However, patients receiving potassium-sparing diuretics (which do not cause potassium loss with diuresis) must be carefully monitored for hyperkalemia. Before the initiation of the ACE inhibitor, hyperkalemic and hypovolemic states must be corrected. ACE inhibitors may be discontinued if the potassium level remains greater than 5 mEq/L or if the serum creatinine rises more than 30% from the patient's baseline.

Other side effects of ACE inhibitors include a dry, persistent cough that may not respond to cough suppressants. The reason for the cough needs to be determined as it could indicate a worsening of ventricular function and failure. Rarely, ACE inhibitors can cause an allergic reaction accompanied by angioedema. If angioedema affects the oropharyngeal area and impairs breathing, the ACE inhibitor must be stopped immediately and emergency care provided.

If the patient cannot continue taking an ACE inhibitor because of development of cough, an elevated creatinine level, or hyperkalemia, an angiotensin II receptor blocker (ARB) or a combination of hydralazine and isosorbide dinitrate (Dilatrate) is prescribed.

Angiotensin II Receptor Blockers

Although the specific action of ARBs is different from that of ACE inhibitors, the overall mechanism is to decrease the activation of angiotensin II. Therefore, ARBs (e.g., irbesartan [Avapro]) have similar hemodynamic effects: decreased blood pressure, decreased systemic vascular resistance, and improved CO. Whereas ACE inhibitors block the conversion of angiotensin I to angiotensin II, ARBs block the effects of angiotensin II at the angiotensin II receptor. ACE inhibitors and ARBs also have similar side effects: hyperkalemia, hypotension, and renal dysfunction. ARBs are usually prescribed as an alternative to ACE inhibitors, especially when patients cannot tolerate ACE inhibitors because of cough.

Beta-Blockers

Beta-blockers are also considered first-line therapy and are routinely prescribed in addition to ACE inhibitors. These agents block the adverse effects of the sympathetic nervous system. They relax blood vessels, lower blood pressure, decrease afterload, and decrease cardiac workload. Beta-blockers, such as carvedilol (Coreg) and metoprolol (Lopressor, Toprol), have been found to reduce mortality and morbidity in patients with NYHA class II or III HF by reducing the adverse effects from the constant stimulation of the sympathetic nervous system. Beta-blockers are recommended for all patients with an EF of less than 40% (Ezekowitz et al., 2017). The therapeutic effects of these drugs may not be seen for several weeks or even months.

Beta-blockers may produce many side effects and may exacerbate symptoms of HF. Side effects are most common in the initial few weeks of treatment. The most frequent side effects are dizziness, hypotension, and bradycardia. Beta-blockers should not be started during acute decompensated heart failure due to their side effects and should only be started after the patient is stabilized and euvolemic (e.g., state of normal volume). The dose is titrated slowly (every few weeks), with close monitoring at each increase. If symptoms of HF increase during the titration phase, treatment options include increasing the dose of the diuretic, reducing the dose of the ACE inhibitor, or decreasing the dose of the beta-blocker.

An important nursing role during titration is educating the patient about the potential worsening of symptoms during the early phase of treatment and stressing that improvement may take several weeks. It is very important for nurses to provide support to patients going through this symptom-provoking phase of treatment. Because beta-blockade can cause bronchiole constriction, these drugs are used with caution in patients with a history of bronchospastic diseases such as asthma. If a $beta_1$-selective beta-blocker (i.e., one that primarily blocks the beta-adrenergic receptor sites in the heart) is prescribed for a patient with asthma, the patient needs to be monitored closely for increased asthma symptoms, as even cardioselective beta-blockers retain some modest $beta_2$ effects.

Ivabradine

Ivabradine (Corlanor) is used in addition to beta-blockers for HR control in patients with stable angina and chronic heart failure (Ezekowitz et al., 2017; Shah et al., 2017). It is used in patients with HFrEF with an EF of 35% or less and a resting HR that is greater than 70 beats per minute.

Diuretics

Diuretics are prescribed to remove excess extracellular fluid by increasing the rate of urine produced in patients with signs and symptoms of fluid overload. The most common types of diuretics prescribed for patients with edema from HF include the following: thiazide, loop, and potassium-sparing diuretics. These medications are classified according to their site of action in the kidney and their effects on renal electrolyte excretion and reabsorption.

Loop diuretics, such as furosemide (Lasix), inhibit sodium and chloride reabsorption mainly in the ascending loop of Henle. HF patients with severe volume overload are generally treated with a loop diuretic first. Thiazide diuretics, such as metolazone (Zaroxolyn), inhibit sodium and chloride reabsorption mainly in the early distal tubules. Both of these classes of diuretics increase potassium excretion; therefore, patients treated with these medications must have their serum potassium levels closely monitored. Diuretics help alleviate symptoms but it is unclear whether or not they improve mortality (Casu & Merella, 2015). Both a loop and a thiazide diuretic may be used for patients in severe HF who are unresponsive to a single diuretic. These medications may not be necessary if the patient responds to activity recommendations, avoids excessive fluid intake (e.g., more than 2 L/day), and adheres to a low-sodium diet (e.g., 2 g/day). In moderate to severe heart failure, these lifestyle modifications may become insufficient, and a diuretic required.

Aldosterone antagonists such as spironolactone (Aldactone) are potassium-sparing diuretics that block the effects of aldosterone in the distal tubule and collecting duct. They can effectively reduce mortality and morbidity in patients with moderate to severe HF (Shah et al., 2017). Serum creatinine and potassium levels are monitored frequently (e.g., within the first week and then every 4 weeks) when this medication is first administered. These drugs are not prescribed for patients with an elevated serum creatinine.

Side effects of diuretics include electrolyte imbalances, symptomatic hypotension (especially with overdiuresis), hyperuricemia (causing gout), orthostatic hypotension, ototoxicity, and kidney injury (Shah et al., 2017). The dose depends on the indications, patient age, clinical signs and symptoms, and renal function. Careful patient monitoring and dose adjustments are necessary to balance the effectiveness of these medications with the side effects (Chart 31-2). Diuretics are administered IV for exacerbations of HF when rapid diuresis is necessary. Diuretics tend to improve the patient's symptoms, provided that renal function is adequate (Ezekowitz et al., 2017; Shah et al., 2017).

CHART 31-2

Pharmacology: Administering and Monitoring Diuretic Therapy

When nursing care involves diuretic therapy for conditions such as heart failure, the nurse needs to administer the medication and monitor the patient's response carefully, as follows:

- Administer the diuretic at a time conducive to the patient's lifestyle; for example, early in the day to avoid nocturia.
- Give supplementary potassium with thiazide and loop diuretics as prescribed to replace potassium loss.
- Check laboratory results for electrolyte depletion, especially potassium, magnesium, and sodium; and for electrolyte elevation, especially potassium with potassium-sparing agents.
- Monitor daily weights, intake, and output to assess response. Monitor serum blood urea nitrogen and creatinine. Notify health care provider if renal impairment is suspected.
- Assess lung sounds, jugular vein distention, daily weight, and peripheral, abdominal, or sacral edema to identify response to therapy.
- Monitor for adverse reactions, such as nausea and gastrointestinal distress, vomiting, diarrhea, weakness, headache, fatigue, anxiety or agitation, and cardiac dysrhythmias.
- Assess for signs of volume depletion, such as postural hypotension, dizziness, and balance problems.
- Monitor for glucose intolerance in patients with and without diabetes mellitus who are receiving thiazide diuretics.
- Monitor for potential ototoxicity in patients, especially those with renal failure, who are receiving a loop diuretic.
- Advise patients to avoid prolonged exposure to the sun because of the risk of photosensitivity.
- Monitor for elevated serum uric acid levels and the development of gout.
- Implement nursing actions to facilitate effect of medication, such as positioning patient supine after dose is taken.

Hydralazine and Isosorbide Dinitrate

A combination of hydralazine (Apresoline) and isosorbide dinitrate (Dilatrate SR, Isordil, Sorbitrate) may be another alternative for patients who cannot take ACE inhibitors. Nitrates (e.g., isosorbide dinitrate) cause venous dilation, which reduces the amount of blood return to the heart and lowers preload. Hydralazine lowers systemic vascular resistance and LV afterload. This combination of medications is also recommended for black Canadians with low EF (Ezekowitz et al., 2017; Shah et al., 2017).

Digitalis

For many years, digitalis (digoxin) was considered an essential agent for the treatment of HF, but with the advent of new medications, it is not prescribed as often. Digoxin increases the force of myocardial contraction and slows conduction through the atrioventricular node. It improves contractility, increasing LV output. The effect of a given dose of digoxin depends on the state of the myocardium, electrolyte and fluid balance, and renal function. Although the use of digitalis does not result in decreased mortality rates among patients with HF, it may decrease symptoms and reduce hospitalizations in a subset of patients (Shah et al., 2017).

A key concern associated with digitalis therapy is digitalis toxicity, particularly because toxic effects may occur within the therapeutic dose and symptoms easily missed. Chart 31-3 summarizes the actions and uses of digoxin along with the nursing surveillance required when it is administered. Clinical manifestations of toxicity include anorexia, nausea, visual disturbances, confusion, and bradycardia. Patients with renal dysfunction and older patients should receive smaller doses of digoxin, as it is excreted through the kidneys. The serum potassium level is measured at intervals, because diuresis may cause hypokalemia and subsequent digoxin toxicity. Other risks for toxicity that require monitoring, including digoxin levels, are alterations in renal function, dehydration, older adults, and low body weight.

Calcium Channel Blockers

First-generation calcium channel blockers, such as verapamil (Calan, Isoptin), nifedipine (Adalat, Procardia), and diltiazem (Cardizem, Tiazac), are contraindicated in patients with systolic dysfunction, although they may be used in patients with diastolic dysfunction or patient with rapid ventricular rates. Amlodipine (Norvasc) and felodipine (Plendil), which are dihydropyridine calcium channel blockers, cause vasodilation, reducing systemic vascular resistance. They may be used to improve symptoms, especially in patients with nonischemic cardiomyopathy.

Intravenous Infusions

Medications are delivered via the IV route when rapid improvement of the symptoms of HF is required. Intermittent or continuous IV furosemide is the first line of therapy for pulmonary or venous congestion.

IV inotropes (milrinone [Primacor], dobutamine [Dobutrex]) increase the force of myocardial contraction; as such, they may be indicated for hospitalized patients with acute

CHART 31-3

Pharmacology: Digoxin Use and Toxicity in Heart Failure

Digoxin, a cardiac glycoside derived from digitalis, is used for patients with systolic heart failure (HF), atrial fibrillation, and atrial flutter. Digoxin improves cardiac function as follows:

- Increases the force of myocardial contraction
- Slows cardiac conduction through the atrioventricular (AV) node and therefore slows the ventricular rate in instances of supraventricular dysrhythmias
- Increases cardiac output by enhancing the force of ventricular contraction
- Promotes diuresis by increasing cardiac output

The therapeutic level is usually 0.5 to 2 ng/mL. Blood samples are usually obtained and analyzed to determine digitalis concentration at least 6 to 10 hours after the last dose. Toxicity may occur despite normal serum levels, and recommended dosages vary considerably.

Preparations

DIGOXIN

- Tablets: 0.125, 0.25, 0.5 mg (Lanoxin)
- Capsules: 0.05, 0.1, 0.2 mg (Lanoxicaps)
- Elixir: 0.05 mg/mL (Lanoxin Pediatric elixir)
- Injection: 0.25 mg/mL, 0.1 mg/mL (Lanoxin)

Digoxin Toxicity

A serious complication of digoxin therapy is toxicity. Diagnosis of digoxin toxicity is based on the patient's clinical symptoms, which include the following:

- Anorexia, nausea, vomiting, fatigue, depression, and malaise (early effects of digitalis toxicity)
- Changes in heart rate or rhythm; onset of irregular rhythm
- Electrocardiogram changes indicating sinoatrial (SA) or AV block; new onset of irregular rhythm indicating ventricular dysrhythmias; and atrial tachycardia with block, junctional tachycardia, and ventricular tachycardia

Reversal of Toxicity

Digoxin toxicity is treated by holding the medication while monitoring the patient's symptoms and serum digoxin level. If the toxicity is severe, digoxin immune FAB (Digibind) may be prescribed. Digibind binds with digoxin and makes it unavailable for use. The Digibind dosage is based on the digoxin level and the patient's weight. Serum digoxin values are not accurate for several days after administration of Digibind, because they do not differentiate between bound and unbound digoxin. Because Digibind quickly decreases the amount of available digoxin, an increase in ventricular rate due to atrial fibrillation and worsening of symptoms of HF may ensue shortly after its administration.

Nursing Considerations and Actions

1. Assess the patient's clinical response to digoxin therapy by evaluating relief of symptoms such as dyspnea, orthopnea, crackles, hepatomegaly, and peripheral edema.
2. Monitor the patient for factors that increase the risk of toxicity:
   - Decreased potassium level (hypokalemia), which may be caused by diuretics. Hypokalemia increases the action of digoxin and predisposes patients to digoxin toxicity and dysrhythmias.
   - Use of medications that enhance the effects of digoxin, including oral antibiotics and cardiac drugs that slow AV conduction and can further decrease heart rate.
   - Impaired renal function, particularly in patients age 65 years and older. Because digoxin is eliminated by the kidneys, renal function (serum creatinine) is monitored and doses of digoxin are adjusted accordingly.
3. Before administering digoxin, it is standard nursing practice to assess apical heart rate. When the patient's rhythm is atrial fibrillation and the heart rate is less than 60, or the rhythm becomes regular, the nurse may withhold the medication and notify the physician, because these signs indicate the development of AV conduction block. Although withholding digoxin is a common practice, the medication does not need to be withheld for a heart rate of less than 60 if the patient is in sinus rhythm, because digoxin does not affect SA node automaticity. Measuring the PR interval for a patient with cardiac monitoring is more important than the apical pulse in determining whether digoxin should be held.
4. Monitor for gastrointestinal side effects: anorexia, nausea, vomiting, and abdominal pain and distention.
5. Monitor for neurologic side effects: headache, malaise, nightmares, forgetfulness, social withdrawal, depression, agitation, confusion, paranoia, hallucinations, decreased visual acuity, yellow or green halo around objects (especially lights), or "snowy" vision.

decompensated HF. These agents are used for patients who do not respond to routine pharmacologic therapy and are reserved for patients with severe ventricular dysfunction (Ezekowitz et al., 2017). They are used with caution, as some studies have associated their use with increased mortality. IV vasodilators such as nitroprusside (Nipride), nitroglycerin, or nesiritide (Natrecor) may also be used in patients with severe decompensated HF (Ezekowitz et al., 2017). Patients usually require admission to the cardiac intensive care unit (CICU) and may also have hemodynamic monitoring with a pulmonary artery catheter or alternative technology (see Chapter 27). Hemodynamic data are used to assess cardiac function and volume status and to guide therapy with inotropes, vasodilators, and diuretics. Patients with end-stage HF who cannot be weaned from IV inotropes may be candidates for continuous or intermittent therapy at home.

MILRINONE. Milrinone is a phosphodiesterase inhibitor that leads to an increase in intracellular calcium within myocardial cells, increasing their contractility (O'Donovan, 2014). This agent also promotes vasodilation, resulting in decreased preload and afterload and reduced cardiac workload. Milrinone is administered IV to patients with severe HF, including patients who are waiting for heart transplantation. Because the drug causes vasodilation, the patient's blood pressure is monitored prior to administration; if the patient is hypovolemic, the blood pressure could drop quickly. The major side effects are new-onset ventricular arrhythmias, symptomatic hypotension, and chest pain (Tariq & Aronow, 2015). Blood pressure and

ECG are monitored closely during and following infusions of milrinone.

DOBUTAMINE. Dobutamine, a catecholamine with $beta_1$- and $beta_2$-adrenergic agonist properties, can be used to improve myocardial contractility in patients with acute decompensated heart failure. Dobutamine works by decreasing LV end-diastolic pressure and increasing CO, thereby increasing blood pressure (Tariq & Aronow, 2015). However, dobutamine can increase the HR and can precipitate ectopic beats and tachydysrhythmias.

Medications for Diastolic Dysfunction

Patients with predominant diastolic dysfunction and preserved LVEF are treated differently than those with systolic dysfunction. Contributing causes of diastolic dysfunction, such as hypertension and ischemic heart disease, are evaluated and treated. Patients with diastolic dysfunction do not tolerate tachycardia, as it does not allow time for ventricular filling. Beta-blockers may be used to treat atrial tachycardias. Other pharmacologic therapies include ACE inhibitors or ARBs, and diuretics.

Other Medications

Anticoagulants may be prescribed, especially if the patient has a history of an embolic event or atrial fibrillation or a mural thrombus is present. Antiarrhythmic drugs such as amiodarone (Cordarone) may be prescribed for patients with dysrhythmias, along with evaluation for device therapy with an **implantable cardioverter defibrillator (ICD)** (see Chapter 28). Other medications, such as antianginal medications, may be administered to treat the underlying cause of HF. Medications that manage hyperlipidemia (e.g., statins) are also routinely prescribed. Omega-3 polyunsaturated fatty acids might also be beneficial in HF patients, especially those who have dilated cardiomyopathy (Wang, Xiong, & Huang, 2017). Nonsteroidal anti-inflammatory drugs (NSAIDs) such as ibuprofen (Aleve, Advil, Motrin), and cyclooxygenase-2 inhibitors should be avoided because they increase systemic vascular resistance and decrease renal perfusion, especially in the older patient. For similar reasons, use of decongestants should be avoided.

Nutritional Therapy

A low-sodium (2 g/day) diet and avoidance of excessive amounts of fluid are usually recommended. Dietary restriction of sodium reduces fluid retention and the symptoms of peripheral and pulmonary congestion. The purpose of sodium restriction is to decrease the amount of circulating blood volume, which would decrease the need for the heart to pump that volume. A balance needs to be achieved between the ability of the patient to comply with the diet and the recommended dietary restriction. Any change in diet needs to be made with consideration of good nutrition as well as the patient's likes, dislikes, and cultural food patterns. Patient compliance is important because dietary indiscretions may result in severe exacerbations of HF requiring hospitalization. However, behavioural changes in this area are difficult for many patients (Chart 31-4).

NURSING ALERT

Grapefruit (fresh and juice) is a good dietary source of potassium but has serious drug–food interactions. Patients are advised to consult their physician or pharmacist before including grapefruit in their diet.

Additional Therapy

Supplemental Oxygen

Oxygen therapy may become necessary as HF progresses. However, supplemental oxygen has a risk of harm when used in excess and should be used cautiously. Therefore, oxygen therapy is used for patients with hypoxemia and

NURSING RESEARCH PROFILE

Chart 31-4. Helping Patients With Heart Failure Adhere to a Low-Sodium Diet

Chung, M. L., Lennie, T. A., Mudd-Martin, G., et al. (2015). Adherence to a low-sodium diet in patients with heart failure is best when family members also follow the diet. *Journal of Cardiovascular Nursing, 30*(1), 44–50.

Purpose

Excess dietary sodium is associated with increased clinical manifestations of HF and an increased rate of hospitalization. Inadequate family support is one of the barriers to a patient's ability to follow a low-sodium diet (LSD). The purpose of this study was to evaluate the effect of family members' adherence to an LSD on the patient's ability to follow the diet.

Design

The study used data from 370 patients with HF. A 24-hour urinary sodium excretion was measured in each patient as an indicator of dietary sodium intake. A questionnaire on whether their family members followed the diet was also completed by the patients.

Findings

Patients whose family members followed the LSD had lower urine sodium levels, indicating adherence to the diet, when compared with patients whose family members did not. It did not make a difference whether the family member was a spouse or whether family members lived with the patient.

Nursing Implications

Strong support from family members can help patients effectively manage many aspects of their HF, including the important aspect of sodium restriction. Nursing interventions aimed at increasing adherence to an LSD should include encouraging family members to also follow the diet.

titrated to an oxygen saturation of between 90% and 94%. Some patients require supplemental oxygen only during activity.

Other Interventions

A number of procedures and surgical approaches may benefit patients with HF. If the patient has underlying CAD, coronary artery revascularization with PCI or coronary artery bypass surgery (see Chapter 29) may be considered. Ventricular function may improve in some patients when coronary flow is increased.

Patients with HF are at high risk for dysrhythmias. The most common dysrhythmia is atrial fibrillation, which is not life threatening but contributes to numerous symptoms and risk of adverse events, including stroke (Ezekowitz et al., 2017). Sudden cardiac death accounts for many HF deaths, most commonly by ventricular dysrhythmias, which may be prevented by placement of an implantable cardioverter defibrillator (ICD) (Ezekowitz et al., 2017). Candidates for an ICD include those with an EF less than 30% (Ezekowitz et al., 2017).

Cardiac resynchronization therapy (CRT) is another treatment that may be beneficial for patients in sinus rhythm with altered electrical conduction to the ventricles and low EF. CRT involves the use of a biventricular pacemaker to treat electrical conduction defects. CRT has been shown to improve morbidity and mortality in certain patients with HFrEF (Sun, Li, Guo, et al., 2016).

Use of a pacing device with leads placed in the right atrium, right ventricle, and LV cardiac vein can synchronize the contractions of the right and left ventricles. This intervention has been shown to improve CO, optimize myocardial energy consumption, reduce mitral regurgitation, and slow the ventricular remodelling process. For selected patients, this results in fewer symptoms and increased functional status, but with little evidence to recommend for other groups. For patients who would benefit from CRT and an ICD, combination devices are available. See Chapter 28 for further discussion of care of patients with pacemakers and ICDs.

Ultrafiltration is an alternative intervention for patients with severe fluid overload. It is generally reserved for patients with advanced HF who are resistant to diuretic therapy or for patients with inadequate diuresis (Costanzo, Ronco, Abraham, et al., 2017). A dual-lumen central IV catheter is placed, and the patient's blood is circulated through a small bedside filtration machine. Litres of excess fluid and plasma are removed slowly from the patient's intravascular circulating volume over a number of hours. The patient's output of filtration fluid, blood pressure, and hemoglobin (analyzed for hemoconcentration) are monitored as indicators of volume status. Research continues regarding the effectiveness of ultrafiltration (Costanzo et al., 2017).

For some patients with severe or end-stage HF, cardiac transplantation is one of the few options for long-term survival. Patients with NYHA class III to IV HF who are eligible are referred for consideration of transplantation. Patients may require mechanical circulatory assistance with an implanted ventricular assist device (VAD) as a bridge therapy to cardiac transplantation (see Chapter 30). Research continues toward perfection of a totally implantable artificial heart that may be used as an alternative to transplantation. For others with end-stage HF, the focus of care shifts from active management of the disease to active management of the symptoms, support for the person and family, and alleviation of suffering (McIlvennan & Allen, 2016). It is important that nurses and other health professionals both initiate and follow up and discuss wishes, goals, and values about care early in their illness, not just at end of life.

Gerontologic Considerations

Several normal age-related changes increase the frequency of HF: decreased LV function, sinus node dysfunction, LV hypertrophy (increased LV wall thickness), increased systolic blood pressure, atrial hypertrophy and dilation, and increased myocardial fibrosis (Steenman & Lande, 2017). Older adults may not always detect or accurately interpret common symptoms of HF such as shortness of breath, or they may have atypical symptoms such as weakness and somnolence. In addition, older adults often also have other comorbidities and the symptoms they have may be assumed to be related to the other conditions. Decreased renal function can make the older patient resistant to diuretics and more sensitive to changes in volume. Older men may have bladder distention caused by urethral obstruction from an enlarged prostate gland—benign prostatic hyperplasia (BPH). Urinary frequency and urgency may be particularly stressful to older patients, as many have arthritis and limited mobility. Frailty, reduced physical activity, depression, anxiety, and cognitive impairment are all related to worse clinical outcomes for older patients who have HF (Diez-Villanueva & Alfonso, 2016).

Nursing Management

In both inpatient and outpatient settings, nursing interventions for the patient with HF include the following:

- Administer medications and assess the patient's response to the pharmacologic regimen, and understanding of medications including beneficial and adverse effects
- Assess sodium, potassium, and fluid balance, including intake and output, with a goal of optimizing electrolyte and volume status
- Evaluate patient/family understanding of lifestyle changes, including signs and symptoms of fluid retention, sodium intake, weight loss, physical activity, and provide education and support
- Weigh the patient daily at the same time and on the same scale, usually in the morning after urination; monitor for a 1- to 1.50-kg gain in a day or 2.25-kg gain in a week; educate patient/family on taking weights on regular intervals
- Auscultate lung sounds to assess for adventitia (e.g., pulmonary crackles)
- Determine the degree of JVP
- Identify and evaluate the severity of dependent edema; educate patient regarding maintaining skin integrity
- Examine skin turgor and mucous membranes for signs of dehydration
- Monitor pulse rate and blood pressure; check for postural hypotension due to dehydration and medications and educate patient on strategies to prevent dizziness
- Assess for symptoms of fluid overload (e.g., orthopnea, PND, and DOE) and evaluate changes

- Assess symptoms related to medication side effects, illness experience, and quality of life (e.g., fatigue, dyspnea, depression, lower sexual activity)
- Provide patients and families education, strategies, and resources (e.g., home care support, exercise, smoking cessation)
- Discuss goals, wishes, values, and preferences for care (advance care planning)

Monitoring and Managing Potential Complications

Many potential problems associated with HF therapy relate to the use of diuretics:

- Diuresis can lead to hypokalemia (i.e., potassium depletion). Signs include ventricular dysrhythmias, hypotension, muscle weakness, diminished deep tendon reflexes, and generalized weakness. Hypokalemia poses problems for the patient with HF because it markedly weakens cardiac contractions. In patients receiving digoxin, hypokalemia can lead to digitalis toxicity. Digitalis toxicity and hypokalemia increase the likelihood of dangerous dysrhythmias. Patients with HF may also develop low levels of magnesium, which can add to the risk of dysrhythmias.
- Hyperkalemia may occur, especially with the use of ACE inhibitors, ARBs, or spironolactone.
- Prolonged diuretic therapy may produce hyponatremia (deficiency of sodium in the blood), which results in disorientation, apprehension, weakness, fatigue, malaise, and muscle cramps.
- Other problems associated with diuretic administration are hyperuricemia (excessive uric acid in the blood) and gout, plus volume depletion from excessive fluid loss.

NURSING ALERT

The sources of sodium should be specified in describing the regimen, rather than simply saying "low salt" or "salt free," and the quantity should be indicated in milligrams. Salt is not 100% sodium; there are 393 mg of sodium in 1 g (1,000 mg) of salt. Suggest patients and their family members look in their fridges, cupboards, or pantry as many packaged, processed, and canned foods use sodium as a preservative.

Nursing Process

The Patient With Heart Failure

Despite advances in medical and surgical approaches to HF, mortality remains high. Nurses have a major impact on outcomes for patients with HF, especially in the areas of patient education and monitoring.

Assessment

The nursing assessment for the patient with HF focuses on observing for effectiveness of therapy and for the patient's ability to understand and implement self-management strategies. Signs and symptoms of pulmonary and systemic fluid overload are recorded and reported so that adjustments can be made in therapy. Assessment should also include how patients feel that they are doing and the challenges they are encountering. Since HF is often a chronic and progressive condition, it can affect the patient's feeling of well-being and can cause distress and depression. Appropriate discussion and referrals will help patients negotiate the challenges HF poses to their biopsychosocial and spiritual well-being.

Health History

The health history focuses on the signs and symptoms of HF, such as dyspnea, shortness of breath, fatigue, cough, edema and weight gain. Sleep disturbances, particularly sleep suddenly interrupted by shortness of breath, may be reported. The nurse also asks about the number of pillows needed for sleep (an indication of orthopnea), edema, abdominal symptoms, altered mental status, activities of daily living, and the activities that cause fatigue. Nurses need to be aware of the variety of clinical manifestations that may indicate worsening HF and assess the patient accordingly. While obtaining the patient's history, the nurse assesses the patient's understanding of HF, self-management strategies, and the desire to adhere to those strategies. The nurse helps patients identify the impact the illness has had on their quality of life and successful coping skills that they have used. Family and significant others are often included in these discussions.

Physical Examination

Sensorium and level of consciousness must be evaluated. As the volume of blood ejected by the heart decreases, so does the amount of oxygen transported to the brain. The patient is observed for restlessness and anxiety that might suggest hypoxia from pulmonary congestion. The patient's level of consciousness is also evaluated for any changes, as low CO can decrease the flow of oxygen to the brain.

The rate and depth of respirations are assessed along with the effort required for breathing. The lungs are auscultated to detect crackles and wheezes. Fine crackles are produced by the sudden opening of small airways and alveoli that have been collapsed by fluid, or exudate. Crackles that do not clear with coughing indicate abnormal fluid in the lungs. Wheezing may also be heard in some patients who have bronchospasm along with pulmonary congestion.

The blood pressure is carefully evaluated, because HF patients may present with hypotension or hypertension. Patients may be assessed for orthostatic hypotension, especially if they report light-headedness, dizziness, or syncope. The heart is auscultated for an S_3 heart sound, which is a sign that there is increased blood volume within the ventricle. Heart rate and rhythm are also documented, and patients are often placed on continuous ECG monitoring in the hospital setting. The pulse is taken and rate, rhythm, and volume are documented. When the heart rate is rapid or very slow, the CO decreases and potentially worsens the HF. When the HR is rapid, the SV decreases because the ventricle has less time to fill. This in turn produces increased pressure in the atria and eventually in the pulmonary vascular bed. An irregular pulse may indicate dysrhythmias.

JVD is assessed with the patient sitting at a 30- to 45-degree angle. Distention greater than 3 cm above the sternal angle is considered abnormal. This is an estimate, not a precise measurement, of central venous pressure, and pressure or volume within the right ventricle. Hepatojugular reflex (HJR) or abdominojugular reflex (AJR) can be assessed while assessing the JVP. These tests are helpful in diagnosing right ventricular dysfunction. The patient is asked to breathe normally while manual pressure is applied over the right upper quadrant (HJR) or the abdomen (AJR) for 10 seconds for at least three respiratory cycles. Normally the JVP will rise temporarily when the pressure is applied but then normalizes. A positive result is defined as a sustained elevation in the JVP.

The nurse assesses peripheral pulses and rates their volume on a scale from 0 (not palpable) to 4+ (bounding). The skin is also assessed for colour and temperature. The nurse assesses dependent parts of the patient's body for perfusion and edema. With significant decreases in SV, there is a decrease in perfusion to the periphery, causing the skin to feel cool and appear pale, mottled, or cyanotic. The feet, lower legs, and sacrum are examined for edema. The upper extremities (hands, fingers) may also become edematous in some patients. Edema is typically rated on a scale from 0 (no edema) to 4+ (severe pitting edema).

The abdomen is examined for tenderness and hepatomegaly or splenomegaly. The presence of firmness, distention, and possible ascites is noted.

If the patient is hospitalized, acute intake and output is evaluated to help establish the effectiveness of diuretic therapy. It is important to know whether the patient has ingested more fluid than he or she has excreted (positive fluid balance), which is then correlated with a gain in weight. The goal is to have a negative fluid balance while on diuretics. The intake and output is then compared with changes in weight. Although diuresis is expected, the patient with HF must be monitored for oliguria (diminished urine output, less than 0.5 mL/kg/hr) or **anuria** (urine output less than 50 mL/24 hours) because of the risk of renal dysfunction.

The patient is weighed daily in the hospital or at home, at the same time of day, with the same type of clothing, and on the same scale. If there is a significant change in weight (i.e., 1- to 1.50-kg increase in a day or 2.25-kg increase in a week), the patient is instructed to notify the primary provider or heart failure team or to adjust the medications as directed (e.g., the diuretic dose is increased).

Nursing Priorities

Based on the assessment data, major nursing priorities for the patient with HF may include the following:

- Fatigue and limitation in activity
- Hypervolemia due to excess fluid or sodium intake
- Anxiety due to breathlessness
- Inability to perform role responsibilities
- Lack of sleep
- Risk for break in skin integrity related to edema and decreased tissue perfusion

Collaborative Problems/ Potential Complications

Based on the patient, potential complications that may develop include the following:

- Hypotension, poor perfusion, and cardiogenic shock (see Chapter 18)
- Dysrhythmias (see Chapter 28)
- Thromboembolism (see Chapter 32)
- Pericardial effusion and cardiac tamponade (see Chapters 30 and 31)

Planning and Goals

Major goals for the patient may include promoting activity and reducing fatigue, relieving fluid overload symptoms, decreasing the incidence of anxiety or increasing the patient's ability to manage anxiety, encouraging the patient to verbalize his or her ability to make decisions and influence outcomes, and educating the patient and family about health management.

Nursing Interventions

Promoting Activity Tolerance

Reduced physical activity caused by HF symptoms leads to physical deconditioning that worsens the patient's symptoms and exercise tolerance. Prolonged inactivity, which may be self-imposed, should be avoided because of its deconditioning effects and risks such as pressure ulcers (especially in edematous patients), venous and pulmonary thromboembolism. An acute illness that exacerbates HF symptoms or that requires hospitalization may be an indication for temporary bed rest. Otherwise, a daily individualized physical activity regime should be encouraged (Van Craenenbroeck, 2017). Exercise training has many favourable effects for HF, including increasing functional capacity and decreasing dyspnea and improved quality of life. The exercise regimen might include 10 to 15 minutes of warm-up activities, followed by about 30 minutes of exercise at the prescribed intensity level. A typical program for a patient with HF might include a daily walking regimen, with duration increased over a 6-week period. The primary provider, nurse, and patient collaborate to develop a schedule that promotes pacing and prioritization of activities. The schedule should alternate activities with periods of rest and avoid having two significant energy-consuming activities occur on the same day or in immediate succession. Before undertaking physical activity, the patient should consult with their health care provider. Because some patients may be severely debilitated, they may need to limit physical activities to only 3 to 5 minutes at a time, one to four times per day. The patient should increase the duration of the activity, then the frequency, before increasing the intensity of the activity.

Exercise Safety Guidelines:

Before undertaking physical activity, the patient should be given the following safety guidelines:

- Begin with a few minutes of warm-up activities.
- Avoid performing physical activities outside in extreme hot, cold, or humid weather.
- Ensure that you are able to talk during the physical activity; if you cannot do so, decrease the intensity of activity.
- Wait 2 hours after eating a meal before performing the physical activity.
- Stop the activity if severe shortness of breath, pain, or dizziness develops.
- End with cool-down activities and a cool-down period.

Barriers to performing other activities are identified, and methods of adjusting an activity are discussed. For example, vegetables can be chopped or peeled while sitting at the kitchen table rather than standing at the kitchen counter. Small, frequent meals decrease the amount of energy needed for digestion while providing adequate nutrition. The nurse helps the patient identify peak and low periods of energy, planning energy-consuming activities for peak periods. For example, the patient may prepare the meals for the entire day in the morning. Pacing and prioritizing activities help maintain the patient's energy to allow participation in regular physical activity.

The patient's response to activities needs to be monitored. If the patient is hospitalized, vital signs and oxygen saturation level are monitored before, during, and immediately after an activity to identify whether they are within the desired range. Heart rate should return to baseline within 3 minutes following the activity. If the patient is at home, the degree of fatigue felt after the activity can be used to assess the response. If the patient tolerates the activity, short- and long-term goals can be developed to gradually increase the intensity, duration, and frequency of activity.

Adherence to exercise training is essential if the patient is to benefit from it, but it may be difficult for patients with multiple other conditions (e.g., arthritis, COPD, and longer duration of HF). Referral to a cardiac rehabilitation program is recommended, especially for HF patients with recent MI, or recent open heart surgery. A supervised program may also benefit those who need a structured environment, significant educational support, regular encouragement, and interpersonal contact.

Managing Fluid Volume

Patients with severe HF may receive IV diuretic therapy; however, patients with less severe symptoms are typically prescribed oral diuretics (see Table 31-4 for a summary of common diuretics). Oral diuretics should be administered early in the morning, and midafternoon if given twice daily, so that diuresis does not interfere with the patient's nighttime rest. Discussing the timing of medication administration is especially important for older patients who may have urinary urgency or incontinence. A single dose of a diuretic may cause the patient to excrete a large volume of fluid shortly after its administration.

The patient's fluid status is monitored closely by auscultating the lungs, monitoring daily body weight, and assisting the patient to adhere to a low-sodium diet by reading food labels and avoiding high-sodium foods such as canned, processed, and convenience foods (Chart 31-5). If the diet includes fluid restriction, the nurse can assist the patient to plan fluid intake throughout the day while respecting the patient's dietary preferences. If the patient is receiving IV fluids and medications, the amount of fluid needs to be monitored closely, and consideration given to maximizing the amount of medication in the lowest volume of IV fluid (e.g., double concentrating to decrease the fluid volume administered).

The patient is positioned or taught how to assume a position that facilitates breathing. The number of pillows may be increased, the head of the bed may be elevated, or the patient may sit in a recliner. In these positions, the venous return to the heart (preload) is reduced, pulmonary congestion is alleviated, and pressure on the diaphragm is minimized. The lower arms are supported with pillows to eliminate the fatigue caused by the constant pull of their weight on the shoulder muscles, and to decrease dependent edema to the hands and fingers.

Because decreased circulation in edematous areas increases the risk of skin injury and pressure ulcers, the nurse assesses for skin breakdown and institutes preventive measures. Frequent changes of position, positioning to avoid pressure, the use of graduated compression stockings, and leg exercises may help to prevent skin injury.

Controlling Anxiety

Patients with HF may exhibit signs and symptoms of anxiety. Complex medical interventions such as implantation of an ICD can provoke anxiety in patients and families. These sources of anxiety include living with the threat of shocks, role changes, and concerns about the patient's ability to carry out activities of daily living. Symptoms of anxiety may intensify at night and interfere with sleep. In addition to psychosocial sources of anxiety, the physiologic compensatory mechanisms include activation of neurohormones including catecholamines. Emotional stress or exertion stimulates the sympathetic nervous system, which causes vasoconstriction, elevated arterial pressure, and increased HR. This sympathetic response increases the cardiac

TABLE 31-4 Diuretic Medications Used to Treat Heart Failure

Diuretic	Usual Adult Dose	Onset (hours)	Peak (hours)	Duration (hours)
Thiazide Diuretics				
bendroflumethiazide (Naturetin)	2.5–20 mg in single or divided dose, once a day, once every other day, or once a day for 3–5 d/wk	2	4	12–16
benzthiazide (Exna)	12.5–200 mg in single or divided dose	2	4–6	16–18
chlorothiazide (Diuril)	Oral: 0.25–2 g as single or divided dose; may be given on alternate days	2	4	16–18
	Intravenous (IV): 0.5–1 g in single or divided dose (Note: Avoid extravasation)	15 minutes	30 minutes	
chlorthalidone (Hygroton)	12.5–200 mg once a day, once every other day, or once a day for 3 d/wk	2	2–6	24–72
hydrochlorothiazide (HydroDIURIL, Esidrix, Oretic)	12.5–200 mg as single or divided dose once a day, once every other day, or once a day for 3–5 d/wk	2	4–6	12–16
hydroflumethiazide (Diucardin, Saluron)	25–200 mg as single or divided dose once a day, once every other day, or once a day for 3–5 d/wk	2	4	12–16
methyclothiazide (Enduron)	2.5–10 mg once a day	2	6	24
metolazone (Zaroxolyn, Mykrox)	Zaroxolyn: 2.5–20 mg once a day Mykrox: 0.5–1 mg once a day	1	2	12–24
polythiazide (Renese)	1–4 mg once a day, once every other day, or once a day for 3–5 d/wk	2	6	24–28
quinethazone (Hydromox)	25–100 mg as single or divided dose; rarely, 200 mg once a day	2	6	18–24
trichlormethiazide (Metahydrin, Naqua)	1–4 mg once or twice a day	2	6	24
Loop Diuretics				
bumetanide (Bumex)	0.5–2 mg once, twice, or three times/day; may be given on alternate days or once every 3 days	30–60 minutes	1–2	4–6
	0.5–1 mg over 2 minutes; repeat every 2–3 hours; a continuous infusion may be given at a rate of 1 mg/hr	5–10 minutes	15–30 minutes	½–1
ethacrynic acid (Edecrin)	50–400 mg as single or divided dose	<30 minutes	2	6–8
	0.5–1 mg/kg (max 100 mg) over several minutes; may be repeated within 2–6 hours; repeat every hour in emergencies	<5 minutes	15–30 minutes	2
furosemide (Lasix)	20–600 mg as single daily dose, divided daily dose, as a dose given every other day or given once a day for 2–4 d/wk	<1	1–2	6–8
	20–200 mg (max 6 mg/kg) given at a rate of 4 mg/min; after response obtained, given once or twice a day	<5 minutes	30 minutes	2
torsemide (Demadex)	5–200 mg as a daily single dose	<1	1–2	6–8
	IV and oral doses are equivalent; give IV over 2 minutes	<10 minutes	<1	6–8
Potassium-Sparing Diuretics				
amiloride (Midamor)	5–20 mg daily as single dose	2	6–10	24
spironolactone (Aldactone)	25–400 mg as single dose or divided up to four doses	24–48	48–72	48–72
triamterene (Dyrenium)	50–300 mg as single dose	2–4	6–8	12–16

workload. By decreasing anxiety, the patient's cardiac workload also is decreased. Oxygen may be administered if the patient is hypoxic to increase the oxygen saturation, diminish the work of the heart, and increase the patient's comfort.

When the patient exhibits anxiety, the nurse takes steps to promote physical comfort and psychological support. In many cases, a family member's presence provides reassurance. Patients with HF rely on their families for many aspects of care; therefore, nurses should assess the needs of family caregivers and provide support to them as well. To help decrease the patient's anxiety, the nurse should speak in a slow, calm, and confident manner and maintain eye contact.

Once the patient is comfortable, the nurse can educate the patient and family about techniques for controlling and avoiding anxiety-provoking situations. This includes how to identify factors that contribute to anxiety and how to use relaxation techniques to

CHART 31-5

Facts About Dietary Sodium

Although the major source of sodium in the average American diet is salt, many types of natural foods contain varying amounts of sodium. Even if no salt is added in cooking and if salty foods are avoided, the daily diet will still contain about 2,000 mg of sodium.

Additives in Food

In general, food prepared at home is lower in sodium than restaurant or processed foods. Added food substances (additives), such as sodium alginate, which improves food texture, sodium benzoate, which acts as a preservative, and disodium phosphate, which improves cooking quality in certain foods, increase the sodium intake when included in the daily diet. Therefore, patients on low-sodium diets should be advised to check labels carefully for such words as "salt" or "sodium," especially on canned foods. For example, without looking at the sodium content per serving found on the nutrition labels, when given a choice between a serving of potato chips and a cup of canned cream of mushroom soup, most would think that soup is lower in sodium. However, when the labels are examined, the lower sodium choice is found to be the chips. Note: Potato chips are *not* recommended in a low-sodium diet; this example illustrates that it is important to read food labels to determine both sodium content and serving size.

Nonfood Sodium Sources

Sodium is also contained in municipal water. Patients on sodium-restricted diets should be cautioned against using nonprescription medications such as antacids, cough syrups, and laxatives. Salt substitutes may be allowed, but it is recognized that they are high in potassium. Over-the-counter medications should not be used without first consulting the physician.

Promoting Dietary Adherence

If patients find food unpalatable because of the dietary sodium restrictions and/or the taste disturbances caused by the medications, they may refuse to eat or to comply with the dietary regimen. For this reason, severe sodium restrictions should be avoided, and the amount of medication should be balanced with the patient's ability to restrict dietary sodium. A variety of flavouring, such as lemon juice, vinegar, and herbs, may be used to improve the taste of the food and increase acceptance of the diet. The patient's food preferences should be taken into account—diet counselling and educational handouts can be geared to individual and ethnic preferences. It is very important to involve the family in the dietary teaching.

manage these situations. Lack of sleep may increase anxiety, which may prevent adequate rest. Other contributing factors may include misinformation, lack of information, or poor nutritional status. As the patient's anxiety decreases, cardiac function may improve and symptoms of HF may decrease, with overall improved relaxation.

In cases of confusion and anxiety reactions that affect the patient's safety, the use of restraints should be avoided. Restraints are likely to be resisted, and resistance inevitably increases the cardiac workload. The patient who insists on getting out of bed at night can be seated comfortably in an armchair. As cerebral and systemic circulation improves, the degree of anxiety decreases and the quality of sleep improves.

In addition to anxiety, patients with HF have a high incidence of depression and should be screened for this condition as they may hesitate to report their symptoms and it is easily missed or overlooked (Mbakwem, Aina, & Amadi, 2016). Patients may have a history of depression before their HF or acquire it afterward. Factors that contribute to depression are anxiety, social isolation, medications (e.g., beta-blockers), decrease in activity, and physiologic factors (e.g., mediators). Depression is related in part to physiologic changes associated with HF such as the presence of increased inflammatory mediators. Because these depressive symptoms are known to increase as the disease worsens, patients with HF need to be screened for depression so that it can be appropriately treated. It is important to identify and manage depression as it contributes to higher morbidity and mortality, and a lower quality of life (Mbakwem et al., 2016).

Minimizing Powerlessness

Patients with HF may feel overwhelmed with their diagnosis and treatment regimen, leading to feelings of powerlessness. Patients need to recognize that they are not helpless and that they can influence the direction of their lives and the outcomes of treatment. Contributing factors may include lack of knowledge and lack of opportunities to make decisions, particularly if health care providers and family members do not encourage the patient to participate in the treatment decision-making process.

Nurses should help patients recognize their choices, and that they can positively influence the outcomes of their diagnosis and treatment. Taking time to listen actively to patients often encourages them to express their concerns and ask questions. Other strategies include providing the patient with decision-making opportunities, such as when activities are to occur, or encouraging food and fluid choices consistent with the dietary restrictions. Encouragement is provided, progress is identified, and the patient is assisted to differentiate between factors that can and cannot be controlled.

In some cases, the nurse may want to review hospital policies and standards that tend to promote powerlessness and advocate for their elimination or change (e.g., limited visiting hours, prohibition of food from home).

Promoting Home, Community-Based, and Transitional Care

EDUCATING PATIENTS ABOUT SELF-CARE. The nurse provides education and involves the patient and family in the therapeutic regimen to promote understanding and adherence to the plan. When the patient recognizes that the diagnosis of HF can be successfully managed with lifestyle changes and medications, recurrences of acute HF lessen, unnecessary hospitalizations decrease, and life expectancy increases. Patients and their families are taught to follow the medication regimen as prescribed, maintain a low-sodium diet, perform and record daily weights, engage in routine physical activity, and recognize and report symptoms that indicate worsening HF. Ensuring that patients and their family have an accurate understanding of HF and what they need to do promotes adherence and improved outcomes. A summary of teaching points for the patient with HF is presented in Chart 31-6. It is helpful for patients to have

CHART 31-6

HOME CARE CHECKLIST • The Patient With Heart Failure

At the completion of education, the patient and/or caregiver will be able to:

- Identify heart failure as a chronic disease that can be managed with medications and specific self-management behaviours.
- State the impact of heart failure on physiologic functioning, ADLs, IADLs, roles, relationships, and spirituality.
- State the name, dose, side effects, frequency, and schedule for all medications.
- Take or administer medications daily, exactly as prescribed.
- Monitor effects of medication such as changes in breathing and edema.
- Know signs and symptoms of orthostatic hypotension and how to prevent it.
- Weigh self daily at the same time with same clothes.
- Restrict sodium intake to no more than 2 g/day:
  - Adapt diet by examining nutrition labels to check sodium content per serving.
  - Avoid canned or processed foods, eating fresh or frozen foods.
  - Consult the written diet plan and the list of permitted and restricted foods.
  - Avoid salt use.
  - Avoid excesses in eating and drinking.
- Participate in prescribed activity program.
  - Participate in a daily exercise program.
  - Increase walking and other activities gradually, provided they do not cause unusual fatigue or dyspnea.
  - Conserve energy by balancing activity with rest periods.
  - Avoid activity in extremes of heat and cold, which increase the work of the heart.
  - Recognize that air-conditioning may be essential in a hot, humid environment.
- Develop methods to manage and prevent stress.
  - Avoid tobacco.
  - Avoid alcohol.
  - Engage in social and diversional activities.
- Identify community resources for peer and caregiver/family support:
  - Identify sources of support (e.g., friends, relatives, faith community).
  - Identify phone numbers of support groups for people with heart failure and their caregivers/families.
  - State meeting locations and times.
- Report immediately to the primary provider or clinic any of the following:
  - Gain in weight of 2 to 3 lb (0.9 to 1.4 kg) in 1 day, or 5 lb (2.3 kg) in 1 week
  - Unusual shortness of breath with activity or at rest
  - Increased swelling of ankles, feet, or abdomen
  - Persistent cough
  - Loss of appetite
  - Development of restless sleep; increase in number of pillows needed to sleep
  - Profound fatigue
- State how to reach primary provider with questions or complications.
  - State time and date of follow-up appointments and diagnostic tests.
- Identify the need for health promotion, disease prevention, and screening activities.

ADLs, activities of daily living; IADLs, independent activities of daily living.

access to a variety of learning opportunities (face to face, written materials, specific web sites, and apps).

The patient and family members are supported and encouraged to ask questions so that information can be clarified and understanding enhanced. The patient's readiness to learn and potential barriers to learning are assessed. Older adult patients with HF and cognitive impairment are more likely to be readmitted to hospital for worsening HF and an identified caregiver is essential (Agarwal, Kazim, Xu, et al., 2016). An effective treatment plan incorporates both the patient's goals and those of the health care providers. The nurse must consider cultural factors and adapt the education plan accordingly. Patients and their families need to be informed that the progression of the disease is influenced in part by choices made about treatment options and their ability to follow the recommendations. They also need to be informed that health care providers are there to assist them in reaching their health care goals.

Continuing and Transitional Care

Successful management of HF requires adherence to a complex medical regimen and multiple lifestyle changes for the patient. It is recognized that lifestyle changes can be difficult and assistance may be provided through a variety of options to optimize evidence-based recommendations for HF management. These may include home care, an HF clinic, or telehealth management. Depending on the patient's physical status, the availability of family assistance, and the geographical location and services, a home care referral may be indicated for a patient who has been hospitalized. Older patients and those who have long-standing heart disease with compromised physical stamina often require assistance with the transition to home after hospitalization for an acute episode of HF. It is important for the home care nurse to assess the physical environment of the home. Suggestions for adapting the home environment to meet the patient's activity limitations are important. If stairs are a concern, the patient can plan the day's activities so that stair climbing is minimized; for some patients, a temporary bedroom may be set up on the main level of the home as long as there is a bathroom on this level. The home care nurse works with the patient and family to maximize the benefits of these changes.

The home care nurse also reinforces and clarifies information about dietary changes and fluid restrictions, the need to monitor symptoms and daily body weights, and the importance of obtaining follow-up care with the primary provider. Assistance may be given in scheduling and keeping appointments as well. The patient is encouraged to gradually increase his or her self-care and responsibility for accomplishing the therapeutic regimen.

Evidence-based HF guidelines also recommend patient referral to HF clinics (Ezekowitz et al., 2017). HF clinics offer a multidisciplinary approach to disease management strategies for patients with HF. Referral to an HF clinic gives the patient access to continuing education, professional staff, and individualized treatment regimens. HF clinics can also provide outpatient treatment (e.g., IV diuretics, laboratory monitoring) as an alternative to hospitalization. Because of the additional support and coordination of care, patients managed through HF clinics have fewer exacerbations of HF, fewer hospitalizations, decreased costs of medical care, and increased quality of life (Mirra, Vitulano, Virtuoso, et al., 2015).

Other disease management programs are carried out through telemonitoring, using telephones or computers to maintain contact with patients and to obtain patient data. This enables nurses and others to assess and manage patients on a frequent basis, without requiring patients to make frequent visits to health care providers. A variety of techniques ranging from simple telephone monitoring to sophisticated computer and video connections that monitor symptoms, daily weight, vital signs, heart sounds, and breath sounds may be used. Patient data may also include hemodynamics and other parameters transmitted from implantable devices. Studies have shown that telehealth management for remote rural areas can decrease all-cause mortality and HF-related hospital admission, and improve quality of life (Koehler, Koehler, Deckwart, et al., 2018).

End-of-Life Considerations

Since HF is a chronic and often progressive condition, patients and families need to consider issues related to the end of life and when palliative or hospice care should be considered (McIlvennan & Allen, 2016). Although the prognosis in patients with HF may be uncertain, issues often arise related to the patient's thoughts and possible concerns about the use of complex treatment options (e.g., implantation of an ICD or a ventricular assist device [VAD]). VADs are an option for some patients with HF who have failed medical therapy and who are not candidates for cardiac transplantation. Discussions concerning the use of technology, preferences for end-of-life care, and advance directives should take place while the patient is able to participate and express preferences. For example, with the expanded use of ICDs in the HF population, patients with ICDs, their families, and their primary providers should receive instructions for ICD deactivation at the end of life to prevent inappropriate discharges. See Chapter 15 for further discussion of end-of-life care.

Evaluation

Expected patient outcomes may include the following:

1. Demonstrates tolerance for increased activity
   a. Describes adaptive methods for usual activities
   b. Identifies factors that contribute to activity intolerance and takes actions to avoid them
   c. Establishes priorities for activities
   d. Schedules activities to conserve energy and to reduce fatigue and dyspnea

   e. Maintains vital signs (pulse, blood pressure, respiratory rate, and pulse oximetry) within the targeted range
2. Maintains fluid balance
   a. Exhibits decreased peripheral and sacral edema
   b. Verbalizes understanding of fluid intake and diuretic use
3. Decreased anxiety
   a. Avoids situations that produce stress
   b. Sleeps comfortably at night
   c. Reports decreased stress and anxiety
   d. Denies symptoms of depression
4. Makes sound decisions regarding care and treatment
   a. Demonstrates ability to influence outcomes
5. Adheres to self-care regimen
   a. Performs and records daily weights
   b. Ensures dietary intake includes no more than 2 g of sodium per day
   c. Takes medications as prescribed
   d. Reports any symptoms of worsening HF
   e. Makes and keeps appointments for follow-up care

NURSING ALERT

Periodic assessment of the patient's electrolyte levels alerts health team members to hypokalemia, hypomagnesemia, and hyponatremia. Serum levels are assessed frequently when the patient starts diuretic therapy and then usually every 3 to 12 months. It is important to remember that serum potassium levels do not always indicate the total amount of potassium within the body.

NURSING ALERT

Cerebral hypoxia with superimposed carbon dioxide retention may be a problem in HF, causing the patient to react to sedative–hypnotic medications with confusion and increased anxiety. Hepatic congestion may slow the liver's metabolism of medication, leading to toxicity. Sedative–hypnotic medications must be administered with caution.

Pulmonary Edema (Acute Heart Failure)

Pulmonary edema is the abnormal accumulation of fluid in the interstitial spaces and alveoli of the lungs. It is a critical diagnosis and if not treated in a timely manner can lead to acute respiratory failure and death.

Pathophysiology

Pulmonary edema is an acute event that results from HF. It can occur acutely, such as with MI, or it can occur as an exacerbation of chronic HF. Myocardial scarring as a result of ischemia can limit the distensibility of the ventricle and render it vulnerable to a sudden increase in workload. With increased resistance to LV filling, blood backs up into the pulmonary circulation, causing pulmonary interstitial edema. Blood volume overload in the lungs can occur quickly in some patients and is referred to as *flash pulmonary edema*. Pulmonary edema can also develop slowly, especially when it is caused by noncardiac disorders that cause fluid overload such as renal failure, liver failure, and oncologic conditions. The pathophysiology is similar to that seen in HF, in that the left ventricle cannot handle the volume overload and blood volume and pressure buildup in the left atrium. The rapid increase in atrial pressure results in an acute increase in pulmonary venous pressure, which produces an increase in hydrostatic pressure that forces fluid out of the pulmonary capillaries into the interstitial spaces and alveoli.

Impaired lymphatic drainage also contributes to the accumulation of fluid in the lung tissues. The fluid within the alveoli mixes with air, creating "bubbles" that are expelled from the mouth and nose, producing the classic symptom of pulmonary edema: frothy pink (blood-tinged) sputum. Because of the fluid within the alveoli, air cannot enter and gas exchange is impaired. The result is hypoxemia, which is often severe. The onset may be preceded by premonitory symptoms of pulmonary congestion, but it also may develop quickly in the patient with a ventricle that has little reserve to meet increased oxygen needs.

Clinical Manifestations

As a result of decreased cerebral oxygenation, the patient becomes increasingly restless and anxious. Along with a sudden onset of breathlessness and a sense of suffocation, the patient is tachypneic with noisy, moist breathing and low oxygen saturation rates. The patient's hands become cold and moist, the nail beds become cyanotic (bluish), and the skin turns ashen (grey). The pulse is weak and rapid (tachycardia), and the neck veins (JVP) are distended. Incessant coughing may occur, producing increasing quantities of pink foamy sputum. As pulmonary edema progresses, the patient's anxiety and restlessness increase; the patient becomes confused, then stuporous. The patient is literally drowning by suffocation from their own secretions. The situation demands emergent action.

Assessment and Diagnostic Findings

The patient's airway and breathing are assessed to determine the severity of respiratory distress, along with vital signs. The patient is placed on a cardiac monitor, and IV access is confirmed or established for administration of drugs. The diagnosis is made by evaluating the clinical manifestations resulting from pulmonary congestion. Laboratory tests are obtained, including arterial blood gases, electrolytes, BUN, and creatinine. A chest x-ray is obtained to confirm the extent of pulmonary edema in the lung fields. Abrupt onset of signs of left-sided HF (e.g., crackles on auscultation of the lungs, flash pulmonary edema, sudden decrease in oxygen saturation) may occur without evidence of right-sided HF (e.g., no JVD, no dependent edema).

Prevention

Like most complications, pulmonary edema is easier to prevent than to treat. Patient and family education is important to provide for prevention and early recognition in the home setting. To recognize it in its early stages, the nurse auscultates the lung fields and heart sounds, measures JVD, and assesses the degree of peripheral edema and the severity of breathlessness. A dry, hacking cough; fatigue; weight gain; development or worsening of edema; and decreased activity tolerance may be early indicators of developing pulmonary edema.

In an early stage, the condition may be alleviated by increasing dosages of diuretics and by implementing other interventions to decrease preload. For instance, placing the patient in an upright position with the feet and legs dependent, eliminating overexertion, and minimizing emotional stress reduce LV workload. The treatment regimen and the patient's understanding of and adherence to it are reexamined. The long-range approach to preventing pulmonary edema must be directed at identifying and managing its precipitating factors.

Management

Clinical management of a patient with acute pulmonary edema due to LV failure is directed toward reducing volume overload, improving ventricular function, decreasing afterload, and increasing respiratory exchange. These goals are accomplished through a combination of oxygen and ventilatory support, IV medications, and nursing interventions.

Oxygen Therapy

Oxygen is administered in concentrations adequate to relieve hypoxemia and dyspnea. Usually, a facemask or nonrebreathing mask is initially used. If respiratory failure is severe or persists, noninvasive positive pressure ventilation (BiPAP) is recommended. For some patients, endotracheal intubation and mechanical ventilation are required. The ventilator provides positive end-expiratory pressure, which is effective in reducing venous return, decreasing fluid movement from the pulmonary capillaries to the alveoli, and improving oxygenation. Oxygenation is monitored by pulse oximetry and by measurement of arterial blood gases.

Morphine

Morphine is titrated IV in small doses (e.g., 2 to 5 mg IV prn) to reduce peripheral resistance and venous return so that blood can be redistributed from the pulmonary circulation to other parts of the body. This decreases pressure in the pulmonary capillaries and seepage of fluid into the lung tissue. The effect of morphine in decreasing anxiety is also beneficial.

Diuretics

Diuretics promote the excretion of sodium and water by the kidneys and decrease the amount of blood returning to the heart. Furosemide (Lasix), a loop diuretic, is administered IV push or as a continuous infusion to produce a rapid diuretic effect. The blood pressure is closely monitored as the urine output increases, because it is possible for the patient to become hypotensive as intravascular volume decreases. The intake and output, daily weights, serum electrolytes, and creatinine are carefully monitored. As the clinical manifestations stabilize, the patient is transitioned to oral diuretics. Furosemide is the first line of therapy and the recommended diuretic by the Canadian Cardiovascular Society (Ezekowitz et al., 2017).

Intravenous Infusions

Vasodilators such as IV nitroglycerin or nesiritide may enhance symptom relief in pulmonary edema. Nitroglycerin is titrated to relieve dyspnea, improve oxygenation, and support cardiac function. Hemodynamically unstable patients (e.g., SBP less than 90 to 100 mm Hg) may require a positive inotrope to improve contractility.

Nitroglycerin acts directly on the vascular cells to dilate the peripheral vasculature (both veins and arteries at high doses), which decreases preload and afterload. Nesiritide (Natrecor) is a recombinant BNP which binds to vascular smooth muscle and endothelial cells, causing dilation of arteries and veins. It also suppresses the neurohormones responsible for fluid retention, thus promoting diuresis.

Dobutamine and milrinone increase contractility within the heart muscle and decrease afterload by vasodilation of the arteries, however they act by different mechanisms. Milrinone (Primacor) is a phosphodiesterase inhibitor that alters release and uptake of calcium from intracellular reservoirs in the myocardium and arterial muscle cells. This increases contractility in the heart and vasodilation of the systemic arteries, resulting in decreased afterload, improved SV, yet reduced cardiac workload. The major side effects are hypotension (usually asymptomatic), gastrointestinal dysfunction, increased ventricular dysrhythmias, and, rarely, decreased platelet counts. Dobutamine (Dobutrex) is a synthetic catecholamine that stimulates the $beta_1$- and $beta_2$-adrenergic receptors. Its major action is to increase cardiac contractility; however, it also results in some vasodilation of the systemic and pulmonary arteries.

Patients receiving continuous IV infusions of any of these vasoactive medications are routinely monitored continuously via ECG, and their vital signs are assessed frequently.

Nursing Management

Positioning the Patient to Promote Circulation

Proper positioning can help reduce venous return to the heart. The patient is positioned upright in bed or a reclining chair. This has the immediate effect of decreasing venous return, lowering the output of the right ventricle and decreasing lung congestion.

Providing Psychological Support

As the ability to breathe decreases, the patient's fear and anxiety rise proportionately, making the condition more severe. Reassuring the patient and providing skillful anticipatory nursing care are integral parts of the therapy. Because the patient feels a sense of impending doom and has an unstable condition, the nurse must remain with the patient. The nurse gives the patient simple, concise information in a reassuring voice about what is being done to treat the condition and the expected results. The nurse also identifies any anxiety-inducing factors (e.g., a pet left alone at home, presence of an unwelcome family member at the bedside, a wallet full of money) and initiates strategies to eliminate the concern or reduce its effect.

Monitoring Medications

The patient receiving morphine is observed for respiratory depression, hypotension, and vomiting; a morphine antagonist, such as naloxone hydrochloride (Narcan), is kept available and given to the patient who exhibits any serious respiratory adverse effects.

The patient receiving diuretic therapy may excrete a large volume of urine within minutes after a potent diuretic is administered. A bedside commode may be used to decrease the energy required by the patient and to reduce the resultant increase in cardiac workload induced by getting on and off a bedpan. If frequent monitoring of urine output is necessary, an indwelling urinary catheter may be inserted.

The patient receiving continuous IV infusions of vasoactive drugs requires ECG monitoring and frequent measurement of vital signs. These patients are usually managed in an ICU setting.

OTHER COMPLICATIONS

Cardiogenic Shock

Cardiogenic shock occurs when decreased CO leads to inadequate tissue perfusion and initiation of the shock syndrome. Cardiogenic shock most commonly occurs following MI when a large area of myocardium becomes ischemic, necrotic, and hypokinetic. It also can occur as a result of end-stage HF, cardiac tamponade, pulmonary embolism, cardiomyopathy, metabolic disturbances, and dysrhythmias. Cardiogenic shock is a life-threatening condition with a high mortality rate (for further detailed information, see Chapter 18).

Pathophysiology

The signs and symptoms of cardiogenic shock reflect the circular nature of the pathophysiology of HF. The degree of shock is proportional to the extent of LV dysfunction. The heart muscle loses its contractile power, resulting in a marked reduction in SV and CO. The decreased CO in turn reduces arterial blood pressure and tissue perfusion in the vital organs (heart, brain, lung, kidneys). Flow to the coronary arteries is reduced, resulting in decreased oxygen supply to the myocardium, which increases ischemia and further reduces the heart's ability to pump. Inadequate emptying of the ventricle also leads to increased pulmonary pressures, pulmonary congestion, and pulmonary edema, exacerbating the hypoxia, causing ischemia of vital organs, and setting a vicious cycle in motion (Fig. 31-4).

Physiology/Pathophysiology

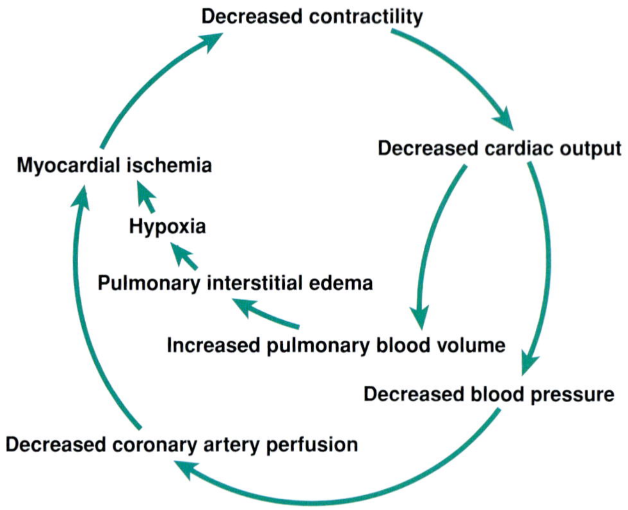

FIGURE 31-4. Pathophysiology of cardiogenic shock.

Clinical Manifestations

The classic signs of cardiogenic shock are those of tissue hypoperfusion and result from HF and the overall shock state. They include cerebral hypoxia (restlessness, confusion, agitation), low blood pressure, rapid (tachycardia) and weak pulse, cold and clammy skin, tachypnea with respiratory crackles, and decreased urinary output. Initially, arterial blood gas analysis may show respiratory alkalosis. Both atrial and ventricular dysrhythmias are common in cardiogenic shock and result from myocardial ischemia.

Assessment and Diagnostic Findings

The patient with cardiogenic shock is managed in an ICU. A pulmonary artery catheter may be inserted to measure CO and other hemodynamic parameters that are used to assess the severity of the problem and to guide patient management. The pulmonary artery wedge pressure is elevated and the CO is decreased as the left ventricle loses its ability to pump. The systemic vascular resistance is elevated because of the sympathetic nervous system stimulation that occurs as a compensatory response to the decrease in blood pressure. The decreased blood flow to the kidneys causes a hormonal response (i.e., activation of the renin–angiotensin–aldosterone system) that causes fluid retention and further vasoconstriction. Increases in HR, circulating volume, and vasoconstriction occur to maintain circulation to the brain, heart, kidneys, and lungs, but at a cost—an increase in the workload of the heart.

The reduction in blood volume delivered to the tissues results in an increase in the amount of oxygen extracted from the blood that is delivered to the tissues (to try to meet the cellular demand for oxygen). The increased systemic oxygen extraction results in decreased venous (mixed and central) oxygen saturation. When the cellular oxygen needs cannot be met, anaerobic metabolism and buildup of lactic acid occur. Continuous central venous oximetry and measurement of blood lactic acid (lactate) levels may help to assess the severity of the shock as well as the effectiveness of treatment.

Continued cellular hypoperfusion eventually results in organ failure. The patient becomes unresponsive; severe hypotension ensues; and the patient develops shallow respirations, and cold, cyanotic, or mottled skin. Arterial blood gas analysis shows metabolic acidosis, and all laboratory test results indicate progression to multisystem organ dysfunction. Chapter 18 presents more detail about the pathophysiology and management of cardiogenic shock.

Medical Management

The most important approach to treating cardiogenic shock is to correct the underlying problem (e.g., opening the blocked coronary artery), reduce preload and afterload to decrease cardiac workload, improve oxygenation, and restore tissue perfusion. Major dysrhythmias are corrected because they may have caused or contributed to the shock. If the patient has hypervolemia, diuresis is indicated. Diuretics, vasodilators, and mechanical therapies, such as continuous renal replacement therapy, have been used to reduce the circulating blood volume. If hypovolemia (low intravascular volume) is suspected or detected through hemodynamic pressure readings, the patient is given IV volume expanders (e.g., normal saline solution, lactated Ringer's solution) to increase the amount of circulating fluid. If the patient has hypoxemia, as detected by pulse oximetry or arterial blood gas analysis, oxygen administration is increased, often under positive pressure when regular flow is insufficient to meet tissue demands. Intubation and sedation may be necessary to maintain oxygenation. The settings for mechanical ventilation are adjusted according to the patient's oxygenation status and the need for conserving energy. In addition to standard critical care support with ventilatory and pharmacologic interventions, patients may require mechanical circulatory assistance.

Pharmacologic Therapy

Medication therapy is selected and guided according to CO, other cardiac parameters, and mean arterial blood pressure. Because of the decreased perfusion to the gastrointestinal system and the need to adjust the dosage quickly, most medications are administered IV.

Diuretics may be administered to decrease preload and afterload, reducing the workload of the heart. They are administered carefully to avoid worsening tissue hypoperfusion. Vasodilators reduce the volume returning to the heart, decrease blood pressure, and decrease cardiac workload. They cause the arteries and veins to dilate, thereby shunting much of the intravascular volume to the periphery and causing a reduction in preload and afterload.

Positive inotropic medications are administered to increase myocardial contractility. Milrinone (Primacor) and dobutamine (Dobutrex) have great effect on contractility than HR, so are the first recommendations. Dopamine (Intropin) and epinephrine (Adrenalin) can each cause tachydysrhythmias because they increase automaticity in addition to contractility with increasing dosage. Therefore, monitoring baseline HR is important. As the baseline HR increases, so does the risk of developing tachydysrhythmias.

Vasopressors, or pressor agents, are used to increase blood pressure by vasoconstriction. Many pressor medications are catecholamines, such as norepinephrine (Levophed) and high-dose dopamine (Intropin). Their purpose is to promote perfusion to the heart and brain, but they compromise circulation to other organs (e.g., kidney). They also tend to increase the workload of the heart by increasing oxygen demand; thus, they are not administered early in cardiogenic shock or only in small dosages that are carefully titrated and monitored.

Other Treatments

Other therapeutic modalities for cardiogenic shock include use of circulatory assist devices. The most frequently used mechanical support device is the intra-aortic balloon pump (IABP). The IABP is a catheter with an inflatable balloon at the end. The catheter is usually inserted through the femoral artery, and the balloon is positioned in the descending thoracic aorta (Fig. 31-5). The IABP uses internal counterpulsation through the regular inflation and deflation of the balloon to augment the pumping action of the heart. It inflates during diastole, increasing the pressure in the aorta during diastole and therefore increasing blood flow through the coronary and peripheral arteries. It deflates just before systole, lessening the pressure within the aorta before LV contraction, decreasing the amount of resistance the heart has to overcome to eject blood and therefore decreasing the amount of work the heart must put forth to eject blood. The device is connected to a console that synchronizes the inflation and deflation of the balloon with the ECG or the arterial pressure (as indicators for systole and diastole). Hemodynamic monitoring is essential to determine the patient's response to the IABP.

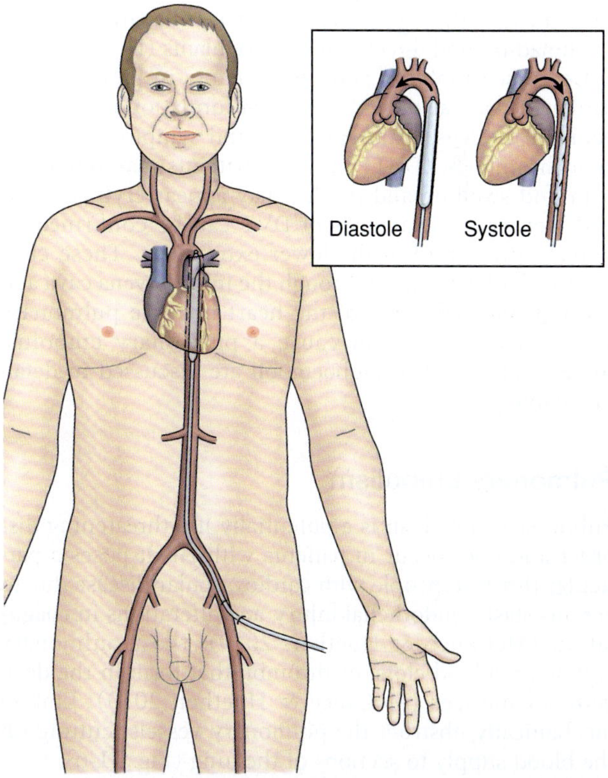

FIGURE 31-5. The intra-aortic balloon pump inflates at the beginning of diastole, which results in increased perfusion of the coronary and peripheral arteries. It deflates just before systole, which results in a decrease in afterload (resistance to ejection) and in the left ventricular workload.

The IABP provides short-term (days) support for the failing myocardium. Other VADs for long-term support of the failing heart are described in Chapter 30.

Nursing Management

The patient in cardiogenic shock requires constant monitoring. Because of the frequency of nursing interventions and the technology required for effective patient management, the patient is treated in an intensive care unit. The critical care nurse must carefully assess the patient, observe the cardiac rhythm, monitor hemodynamic parameters, monitor fluid status, and adjust medications and therapies based on the assessment data. The patient is continuously evaluated for responses to the medical interventions and for the development of complications so that problems can be addressed immediately.

Thromboembolism

Patients with cardiovascular disorders are at risk for the development of arterial and venous thromboemboli. Intracardiac thrombi can form in patients with atrial fibrillation because the atria do not contract forcefully, resulting in slow and turbulent flow, and increasing the likelihood of thrombus formation. Mural thrombi can also form on ventricular walls when contractility is poor. Intracardiac thrombi can break off and travel through the circulation to other structures, including the brain, where they cause a stroke (i.e., cerebrovascular accident). Clots within the cardiac chambers can be detected by an echocardiogram and treated with anticoagulant agents, such as heparin, warfarin (Coumadin), and direct oral anticoagulants (DOACs).

Decreased mobility and other factors in patients with cardiac disease also can lead to clot formation in the deep veins of the legs. Although signs and symptoms of deep vein thrombosis (DVT) can vary, patients may report leg pain and swelling and the leg may appear erythematous and feel warm. Diagnosis of DVT can be confirmed by duplex ultrasound of the lower extremities. These clots can break off and travel through the inferior vena cava and through the right side of the heart into the pulmonary artery, where they can cause a pulmonary embolus. Adverse effects of thromboemboli are discussed in detail in Chapter 32.

Pulmonary Embolism

Pulmonary embolism is a potentially life-threatening disorder and does occur in patients with HF. It poses a particular threat to people with cardiovascular disease due to venous stasis, endothelial injury, and alterations in coagulation (McCance & Huether, 2019). Most pulmonary emboli are blood clots, or thrombi, that form in the deep veins of the legs (McCance & Huether, 2019). Emboli mechanically obstruct the pulmonary vessels, cutting off the blood supply to sections of the lung (Fig. 31-6).

Clinical indicators of pulmonary embolism can vary depending on the size of the thrombus, but typically include dyspnea, tachypnea, chest pain, hemoptysis, tachycardia, and symptoms of deep venous thrombosis. Diagnostic tests may include a chest x-ray, lower limb compression ultrasound, ventilation–perfusion lung scan, pulmonary angiogram, or high-resolution CT scan. A blood D-dimer assay although not specific to pulmonary emboli can be helpful to determine whether fibrinolysis of clots is taking place somewhere in the body.

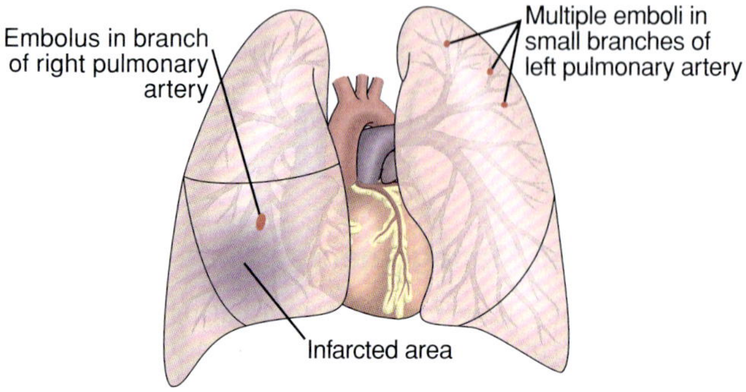

FIGURE 31-6. Pulmonary emboli may be single or multiple.

Patient management begins with cardiopulmonary assessment and intervention. Emboli can cause hypoxic vasoconstriction and the release of inflammatory mediators in the pulmonary vessels, which can ultimately lead to right HF and respiratory failure (McCance & Huether, 2019). Anticoagulant therapy with unfractionated IV heparin or low–molecular-weight heparin is started when pulmonary embolism is suspected. Thrombolytic therapy may be used in patients with massive pulmonary emboli accompanied by hypotension and shock. Following initial therapy, patients are placed on an oral anticoagulant (e.g., DOAC or warfarin [Coumadin]) for at least 3 to 6 months. Prevention of DVT and pulmonary emboli is an important aspect of patient management. Both pharmacologic and mechanical means (e.g., pneumatic compression devices) have proven effective in at-risk patients. Care for patients with pulmonary embolism is further discussed in Chapter 24.

Pericardial Effusion and Cardiac Tamponade

Pathophysiology

Pericardial effusion (accumulation of fluid in the pericardial sac) may accompany pericarditis (see Chapter 30), advanced HF, metastatic carcinoma, cardiac surgery, or trauma. Normally, the pericardial sac contains up to 20 mL of fluid, which is needed to decrease friction for the beating heart. An increase in pericardial fluid raises the pressure within the pericardial sac and compresses the heart. This has the following effects:

- Increased right and left ventricular end-diastolic pressures
- Decreased venous return
- Inability of the ventricles to distend and fill adequately

NURSING ALERT

Cardiac tamponade is a life-threatening situation, demanding immediate intervention.

Pericardial fluid may accumulate slowly without causing noticeable symptoms until a large amount accumulates (1 to 2 L). However, a rapidly developing effusion (e.g., hemorrhage into the pericardial sac from chest trauma, postcardiac surgery) can stretch the pericardium to its maximum size and cause acute compromise. As pericardial fluid increases, pericardial pressure increases, reducing venous return to the heart and decreasing CO. This can result in cardiac tamponade (e.g., compression of the heart), which causes low CO and obstructive shock.

Clinical Manifestations

The signs and symptoms of pericardial effusion can vary according to whether the problem develops quickly or slowly. In acute cardiac tamponade, the patient suddenly develops chest pain, tachypnea, and dyspnea. JVP increases (engorges neck veins) from poor right atrial filling and increased venous pressure. The subacute presentation of a pericardial effusion is less dramatic. The patient may report a feeling of fullness within the chest or may have substantial or ill-defined pain. The feeling of pressure in the chest may result from stretching of the pericardial sac. These patients also develop dyspnea, JVD, and hypotension over time. Hypotension occurs from low CO, and heart sounds are often muted.

Patients with cardiac tamponade typically have tachycardia in response to low CO. In addition to hypotension, patients with cardiac tamponade may develop **pulsus paradoxus**, a systolic blood pressure that is markedly lower during inhalation. The difference in systolic pressure between the point that it is heard during exhalation and the point that it is heard during inhalation is measured. Pulsus paradoxus exceeding 10 mm Hg is abnormal. This difference is caused by the variation in cardiac filling that occurs with changes in intrathoracic pressure during breathing. The cardinal signs of cardiac tamponade are falling systolic blood pressure, narrowing pulse pressure, rising venous pressure (increased JVD), and distant (muffled) heart sounds (Chart 31-7).

CHART 31-7

Assessing for Cardiac Tamponade

Assessment findings in cardiac tamponade resulting from pericardial effusion include feelings of faintness, shortness of breath, anxiety, and pain from decreased cardiac output, cough from pressure created in the trachea from swelling of the pericardial sac, distended neck veins from rising venous pressure, paradoxical pulse, and muffled or distant heart sounds.

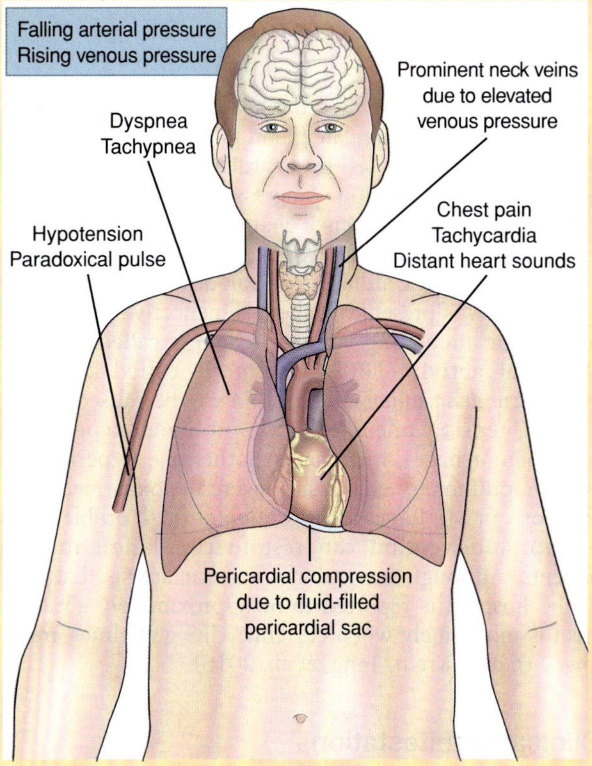

Assessment and Diagnostic Findings

An echocardiogram is performed to confirm the diagnosis and quantify the amount of pericardial fluid. A chest x-ray may show an enlarged cardiac silhouette due to pericardial effusion, but an x-ray is not used to diagnose a pericardial effusion. The ECG shows tachycardia and may also show low voltage (York, Kane, & Smith, 2018). See Chapter 27 for discussion of the significance of ECG abnormalities.

Medical Management

Pericardiocentesis

If cardiac function becomes seriously impaired, **pericardiocentesis** (puncture of the pericardial sac to aspirate pericardial fluid) is performed to remove fluid from the pericardial sac. The major goal is to prevent cardiac tamponade, which restricts normal heart filling and contraction.

Catheter pericardiocentesis is performed using echocardiography to guide placement of the drainage catheter (York et al., 2018). During the procedure, the patient is monitored by ECG and hemodynamic pressure measurements. Emergency resuscitation equipment should be readily available. If a peripheral IV line is not already in place, one is inserted and a slow IV infusion is started in case it becomes necessary to administer emergency medications or blood products.

A resulting decrease in central venous pressure and an associated increase in blood pressure after withdrawal of pericardial fluid indicate that the cardiac tamponade has been relieved. The patient almost always feels immediate relief. If there is a substantial amount of pericardial fluid, a small catheter may be left in place to drain recurrent accumulation of blood or fluid. Pericardial fluid is sent to the laboratory for examination for tumour cells, bacterial culture, chemical and serologic analysis, and differential blood cell count.

Complications of pericardiocentesis include ventricular or coronary artery puncture, dysrhythmias, pleural laceration, gastric puncture, and myocardial trauma. After pericardiocentesis, the patient's heart rhythm, blood pressure, venous pressure, and heart sounds are monitored to detect possible recurrence of cardiac tamponade. A follow-up echocardiogram is also performed. If it recurs, repeated aspiration is necessary. Cardiac tamponade may require treatment by open pericardial drainage (pericardiotomy) (see Chapter 24).

Pericardiotomy

Recurrent pericardial effusions, usually associated with neoplastic disease, may be treated by a **pericardiotomy** (pericardial window). Under general anesthesia, a portion of the pericardium is excised to permit the pericardial fluid to drain into the lymphatic system. The nursing care is the same as that for other cardiac surgery (see Chapter 29).

Cardiac Arrest

Cardiac arrest occurs when the heart ceases to produce an effective pulse and circulate blood to the body's organs and tissues. It is often caused by a cardiac electrical event such as ventricular fibrillation, progressive profound bradycardia, or asystole (i.e., absence of any cardiac electrical activity and heart muscle contraction). Cardiac arrest may follow respiratory arrest. Cardiac arrest can also occur when electrical activity is present but there is ineffective cardiac contraction or circulating volume, which is called **pulseless electrical activity (PEA).** Formerly called *electrical–mechanical dissociation* (EMD), PEA can be caused by tamponade, tension pneumothorax, profound hypovolemia (e.g., hemorrhage), hypoxia, hypothermia, hyperkalemia, massive pulmonary embolism, severe hypoxia, medication overdose, or MI. Rapid identification of these problems and prompt intervention can restore circulation in some patients. Although survival after cardiac arrests that occur in the hospital is reported to be approximately 23%, survival is more likely when current ACLS guidelines are followed (Chan, Krein, Tang, et al., 2016).

Clinical Manifestations

In cardiac arrest, consciousness, pulse, and blood pressure are lost almost immediately. Breathing usually ceases, but ineffective respiratory gasping may occur. The pupils of the eyes begin dilating in less than a minute, and seizures may occur. Pallor (dusky or grey) and cyanosis are seen in the skin and mucous membranes.

NURSING ALERT

The most reliable sign of cardiac arrest is the absence of a pulse. In the adult and the child, the carotid pulse is assessed. In an infant, the brachial pulse is assessed. Valuable time should not be wasted taking the blood pressure, listening for the heartbeat, or checking proper contact of electrodes.

The risk of irreversible brain damage and death increases with every minute from the time that circulation ceases. The interval varies with the age and underlying condition of the patient. As soon as possible, the diagnosis of cardiac arrest must be made, and measures must be taken immediately to restore circulation.

Emergency Assessment and Management: Cardiopulmonary Resuscitation

Cardiopulmonary resuscitation (CPR) provides blood flow to vital organs until effective circulation can be reestablished. Following the recognition of unresponsiveness, a protocol for basic life support is initiated. The 2015 AHA Guidelines Update for Cardiopulmonary Resuscitation and Emergency Cardiovascular Care direct the current protocols (Neumar, Shuster, Callaway, et al., 2015). The resuscitation process begins with the immediate assessment of the patient and action to call for assistance, as CPR can be performed most effectively with the addition of more health care providers and equipment (e.g., defibrillator). The four basic steps in CPR are as follows:

1. *Recognition of sudden cardiac arrest.* The patient is checked for responsiveness and breathing.
2. *Activation of the Emergency Response System (ERS).* Within a medical facility, a call is made to alert the emergency response team, often called the "Code 4" or "Code Blue" team. Outside of a medical facility, 911 is called to activate the Emergency Medical Service (EMS).
3. *Performance of high-quality CPR.* If no carotid pulse is detected and no defibrillator is yet available, chest compressions are initiated. Rescue breathing may be added by a health care provider in a ratio of 30 compressions to 2 ventilations.
4. *Rapid cardiac rhythm analysis and defibrillation as soon as it is available.* Patients in ventricular fibrillation must be defibrillated as soon as possible.

Outcomes following CPR are improved by high-quality CPR (Meaney, Bobrow, Mancini, et al., 2013). Compressions are performed with the patient on a firm surface such as the floor or a cardiac board. The provider, facing the patient's side, places one hand in the centre of the chest on the lower half of the sternum and positions the other hand on top of the first hand (see Fig. 31-7). The chest is compressed 2 in at a rate of 100 to 120 compressions per minute. Complete recoil of the chest is allowed between compressions. Interruptions in CPR to switch providers or check for a pulse are minimized. It is recommended that providers switch every 2 minutes due to the exertion of delivering effective compressions.

Maintaining Airway and Breathing

Rescue breathing is no longer recommended unless health care providers are present; if that is the case, it is then started after chest compressions. When establishing an airway, obvious material in the mouth or throat should be removed, but no blind sweeps should be done. The airway should be opened using a head-tilt chin-lift manoeuvre or a jaw thrust if trauma is suspected. The rescuer no longer "looks, listens, and feels" for air movement. An oropharyngeal airway is inserted if available. Ventilation is provided using a bag-mask or mouth-mask device (Fig. 31-8). Excessive ventilation is avoided by the 30 to 2 ratio of compressions to ventilations.

An obstructed airway should be suspected when the rescuer cannot give the initial ventilations, and the Heimlich manoeuvre or abdominal thrusts should be administered to relieve the obstruction. If the patient is in the hospital,

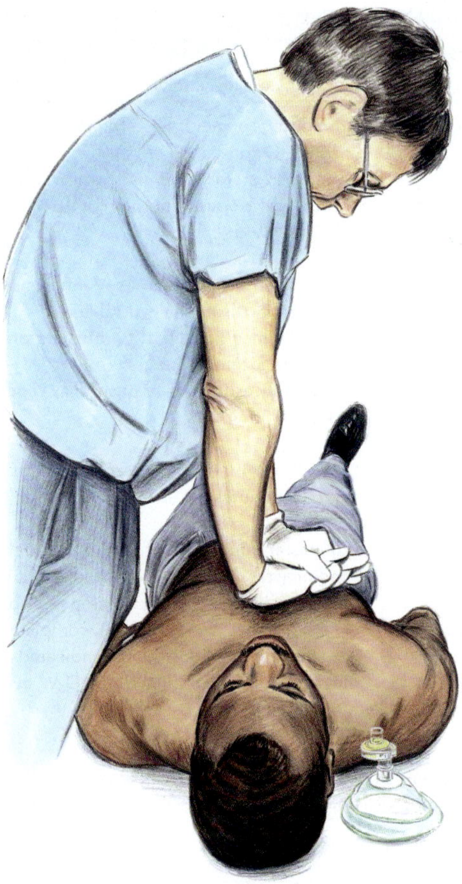

FIGURE 31-7. Chest compressions in cardiopulmonary resuscitation (CPR) are performed by placing the heel of one hand in the centre of the chest over the sternum and the other hand on top of the first hand. Elbows are kept straight and body weight is used to apply forceful compressions to the lower sternum. The patient should be on a hard surface such as a cardiac board. (From Field, J. M., Kudenchuk, P. J., O'Connor, R. E., et al. [2009]. *The textbook of emergency cardiovascular care and CPR*. Philadelphia, PA: Lippincott Williams & Wilkins.)

endotracheal intubation may be performed by a physician, nurse practitioner, or respiratory therapist during a resuscitation procedure (also called a *code*) to ensure an adequate airway and ventilation. The resuscitation bag device is then connected directly to the endotracheal tube (ET).

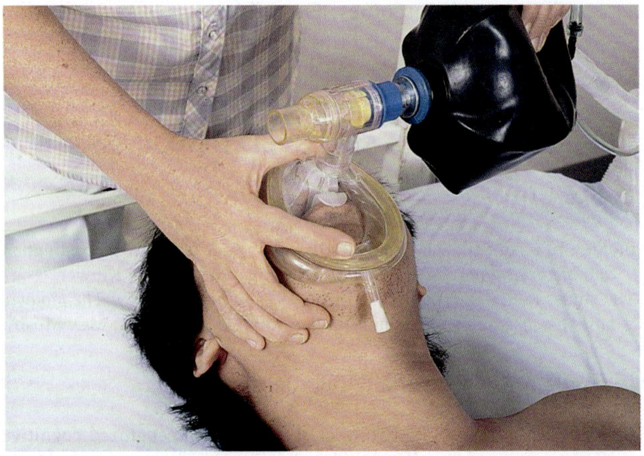

FIGURE 31-8. The chin-lift and bag-and-mask technique for ventilating patients who need cardiopulmonary resuscitation.

Because of the risk of unrecognized esophageal intubation or dislodgement of the ET, tracheal intubation must be confirmed by two different methods: a primary method (visualization of the ET through the vocal cords, auscultation of breath sounds in five areas on the chest, or bilateral chest expansion) and a secondary method (carbon dioxide detector). A chest x-ray, which is frequently obtained after ET placement, is helpful in determining whether the ET is too high or too low in the trachea. However, a chest x-ray cannot definitively confirm placement of an ET. An ET in the esophagus or the trachea produces the same appearance on the x-ray. Arterial blood gas levels are measured to guide oxygen therapy.

Defibrillation

As soon as a monitor/defibrillator is available, monitor electrodes are applied to the patient's chest and the heart rhythm is analyzed. When an automated external defibrillator (AED) is used, the device is turned on, the pads are applied to the patient's chest, and the rhythm is analyzed by the defibrillator to determine whether a shock is indicated. When the ECG shows ventricular fibrillation or pulseless ventricular tachycardia, immediate defibrillation is the treatment of choice. The survival time decreases for every minute that defibrillation is delayed. Following defibrillation, high-quality CPR is resumed immediately. Survival after cardiac arrest has been improved by extensive education of health care providers and by the use of AEDs.

Advanced Cardiovascular Life Support

Additional care may be indicated for patients in cardiac arrest. Placement of an advanced airway such as an ET tube may be performed by a qualified provider during resuscitation to ensure a patent airway and adequate ventilation. Because of the risk of unrecognized esophageal intubation or dislodgement of the ET tube, tracheal intubation must be confirmed by assessment of specific parameters: auscultation of breath sounds, observation of chest expansion, and a carbon dioxide detector. A chest x-ray is always obtained after ET tube placement to confirm that the tube is in the proper position within the trachea. Arterial blood gases may also be obtained to assess ventilation and oxygenation.

Specific subsequent advanced support interventions depend on the assessment of the patient's condition and response to therapy. For example, if asystole is detected on the monitor, CPR is continued while IV epinephrine is given and an attempt is made to determine the cause of the arrest, such as severe hypovolemia or hypoxia. Selected medications (Table 31-5) may be used during and after resuscitation.

Follow-Up Monitoring and Care

The care provided to the patient following resuscitation is another determinant of survival (Heart and Stroke Foundation of Canada—Resuscitation Guidelines). The patient normally will be transferred to an ICU for close monitoring. Following resuscitation and return of spontaneous circulation (ROSC), patients may benefit from therapeutic hypothermia protocols. Although there is not clear evidence, it is recommended that patients be cooled to 32° to 34°C (Howes, Gray, Brooks, et al., 2016). Continuous ECG monitoring and frequent blood pressure

TABLE 31-5 Medications Used in Cardiopulmonary Resuscitation

Agent and Action	Indications	Nursing Considerations
Epinephrine—vasopressor used to optimize BP and cardiac output; improves perfusion and myocardial contractility	Given to patients in cardiac arrest caused by asystole, pulseless electrical activity, pulseless VT or VF	Administer 1 mg every 3–5 minutes by IV push or via IO route Follow peripheral IV administration with 20-mL flush and elevate extremity for 10–20 seconds
Vasopressin—increases systemic vascular resistance and BP	An alternative to epinephrine	Give 40 U IV one time only
Norepinephrine—vasopressor given to increase BP	Given for hypotension and shock	Give 0.1–0.5 mcg/kg/min as IV infusion, preferably through a central line
Dopamine—vasopressor given to increase BP and contractility	Given for hypotension and shock	Give 5–10 mcg/kg/min as IV infusion, preferably through a central line
Atropine—blocks parasympathetic action; increases SA node automaticity and AV conduction	Given to patients with symptomatic bradycardia (i.e., hemodynamically unstable with hypotension)	Give rapidly as 0.5-mg IV push; may repeat to dose of 3 mg
Amiodarone—acts on sodium-potassium and calcium channels to prolong action potential and refractory period	Used to treat pulseless VT and VF unresponsive to shock delivery	Give 300 mg IV; may give second dose of 150 mg in 3–5 minutes
Sodium bicarbonate ($NaHCO_3$)—corrects metabolic acidosis	Given to correct metabolic acidosis that is refractory to standard advanced cardiac life support interventions (cardiopulmonary resuscitation, intubation, and respiratory management)	Administer initial dose of 1 mEq/kg IV; then administer dose based on base deficit Recognize that to prevent development of rebound metabolic alkalosis, complete correction of acidosis is not indicated
Magnesium sulphate—promotes adequate functioning of cellular sodium–potassium pump	Given to patients with torsade de pointes, a type of VT	May give 1–2 g diluted in 10 mL D_5W over 5–20 minutes

BP, blood pressure; VT, ventricular tachycardia; VF, ventricular fibrillation; IV, intravenous; IO, intraosseous; SA, sinoatrial; AV, atrioventricular; D_5W, dextrose 5% in water.
Adapted from Heart and Stroke Foundation of Canada. Retrieved from https://www.heartandstroke.ca/-/media/pdf-files/cpr/new-pdfs/highlightsofthe2018focusedupdatestoguidelinesforcprandeccadvancedcardiovascularlifesupportandpediatr.ashx

assessments are essential until hemodynamic stability is reestablished. Etiologic factors that precipitated the arrest, such as metabolic or rhythm abnormalities, must be identified and treated. Possible contributing factors, such as electrolyte or acid–base imbalances, need to be identified and corrected.

Critical Thinking Exercises

1 You are assessing a 72-year-old woman with a 3-year history of HF. Her medications include carvedilol, valsartan, furosemide, and potassium. She reports two episodes of severe dizziness. What are possible causes of dizziness in this patient? What questions would you include in your assessment? What medical and nursing interventions would be appropriate for each possible cause?

2 On an inpatient progressive care unit, you are assigned to care for a 60-year-old man who has been readmitted for the third time with severe HF and widespread edema. According to the patient's chart, he has a history of not taking his medications regularly or following his low-sodium and low-cholesterol diet. What are your immediate priorities and short-term goals for this patient? What medical interventions are indicated? Develop an evidence-based plan of care for this patient in the future. Describe your planned interaction with the patient (i.e., communication technique, behaviours) that would encourage the patient to participate in the plan.

3 On an inpatient progressive care unit, you receive a 55-year-old man who has just been transferred from the cardiac intensive care unit (CICU). You realize that he is at risk of complications after a large anterior wall MI, which was treated with emergent cardiac catheterization and percutaneous coronary intervention (PCI). His medications include aspirin, clopidogrel, metoprolol, and lisinopril. During your initial assessment, you notice that the patient appears weak and pale. You have trouble hearing his blood pressure but think you hear a systolic pressure of about 80 mm Hg. List the possible complications that this patient may be experiencing. What assessment parameters would you check next? Discuss the strength of the evidence that supports priority nursing interventions and expected outcomes. Describe your communication with the patient during the interventions.

REFERENCES AND SELECTED READINGS

Books

Bickley, L. S., & Szilagyi, P. G. (2016). *Bates' guide to physical examination and history taking* (12th ed.). Philadelphia, PA: Wolters Kluwer.
McCance, K. L., & Huether, S. E. (2019). *Pathophysiology: The biologic basis for disease in adults and children* (8th ed.). St. Louis, MO: Mosby.

Journals and Electronic Documents

Agarwal, K. S., Kazim, R., Xu, J., et al. (2016). Unrecognized cognitive impairment and its effect on heart failure readmissions of elderly adults. *Journal of the American Geriatrics Society*, *64*, 2296–2301. https://doi.org/10.1111/jgs.14471

American Heart Association (AHA). (2015). *Heart disease and stroke statistics—2015 update*. Retrieved September 24, 2015, from professional.heart.org/professional/ScienceNews/UCM_480113_Heart-Disease-and-Stroke-Statistics—2015-Update.jsp
American Heart Association (AHA). (2016a). *Adult advanced cardiovascular life support*. Retrieved March 31, 2016, from cpr.heart.org/AHAECC/CPRAndECC/Training/HealthcareProfessional/Advanced-CardiovascularLifeSupportACLS/UCM_473186_Advanced-Cardiovascular-Life-Support-ACLS.jsp
American Heart Association (AHA). (2016b). *Shaking the salt habit*. Retrieved March 31, 2016, from www.heart.org/HEARTORG/Conditions/HighBloodPressure/PreventionTreatmentofHighBloodPressure/Shaking-the-Salt-Habit_UCM_303241_Article.jsp#.Vzy9eNe3BK8
Anderson, M. L., Nichol, G., Dai, D., et al. (2016). Association between hospital process composite performance and patient outcomes after in-hospital cardiac arrest care. *JAMA Cardiology*, *1*, 37–45. Retrieved March 1, 2016, from www.medscape.com/viewarticle/859491
Andre, T. R., Santos, A. L., & Neto, I. G. (2017). Cardiac cachexia syndrome. *European Medical Journal of Cardiology*, *5*(1), 101–107.
Casu, G., & Merella, P. (2015). Diuretic therapy in heart failure—current approaches. *European Cardiology Review*, *10*(1), 42–47. https://doi.org/10.15420/ecr.2015.10.01.42
Chan, P. S., Krein, S. L., Tang, F., et al. (2016). Resuscitation practices associated with survival after in-hospital cardiac arrest: A nation\wide survey. *Journal of the American Medical Association—Cardiology*, *1*(2), 189–197.
Costanzo, M. R., Ronco, C., Abraham, W. T., et al. (2017). Extracorporeal ultrafiltration for fluid overload in heart failure: Current status and prospects for further research. *Journal of the American College of Cardiology*, *69*(19), 2428–2445. http://dx.doi.org/10.1016/j.jacc.2017.03.528
Creber, R. M., Patey, M., Lee, C. S., et al. (2016). Motivational interviewing to improve self-care for patients with chronic heart failure: MITI-HF randomized controlled trial. *Patient Education and Counseling*, *99*(2), 256–264.
Diez-Villanueva, P., & Alfonso, F. (2016). Heart failure in the elderly. *Journal of Geriatric Cardiology*, *13*(12), 115–117.
Ezekowitz, J. A., O'Meara, E., McDonald, M. A., et al. (2017). 2017 Comprehensive update of the Canadian Cardiovascular Society guidelines for the management of heart failure. *Canadian Journal of Cardiology*, *33*, 1342–1433.
Government of Canada. (2017). *Heart disease in Canada: Highlights from the Canadian Chronic Disease Surveillance System*. Retrieved from https://www.canada.ca/en/public-health/services/publications/diseases-conditions/heart-disease-canada-fact-sheet.html
Howes, D., Gray, S. H., Brooks, S. C., et al. (2016). Canadian guidelines for the use of targeted temperature management (therapeutic hypothermia) after cardiac arrest: A joint statement from The Canadian Critical Care Society (CCCS), Canadian Neurocritical Care Society (CNCCS), and the Canadian Critical Care Trials Group (CCCTG). *Resuscitation*, *98*(2016), 48–63.
Koehler, F., Koehler, K., Deckwart, O., et al. (2018). Efficacy of telemedical interventional management in patients with heart failure (TIM-HR2): A randomized, controlled, parallel-group, unmasked trial. *The Lancet*, *392*, 1047–1057.
Mbakwem, A., Aina, F., & Amadi, C. (2016). Expert opinion-depression in patients with heart failure: Is enough being done? *Cardiac Failure Review*, *2*(2), 110–112.
Mcllvennan, C. K., & Allen, L. A. (2016). Palliative care in patients with heart failure. *British Medical Journal*, *353*, 1–13. https://doi.org/10.1136/bmj.i1010
Meaney, P. A., Bobrow, B. J., Mancini, M. E., et al. (2013). Cardiopulmonary resuscitation quality: Improving cardiac resuscitation outcomes both inside and outside the hospital. A consensus statement from the American Heart Association. *Circulation*, *128*(4), 417–435.
Mirra, M., Vitulano, G., Virtuoso, N., et al. (2015). Heart failure in a dedicated outpatient clinic: Results after 58 month follow-up. Can I be enough? *Translational Medicine UniSa*, *11*, 59–62.
Neumar, R. W., Shuster, M., Callaway, C. W., et al. (2015). Part 1. Executive summary: 2015 American Heart Association guidelines update for cardiopulmonary resuscitation and emergency cardiovascular care. *Circulation*, *132*(18), S315–S367.
Pinkerman, C., Sander, P., Breeding, J. E., et al. (2013). Heart failure in adults, Institute for Clinical Systems Improvement. Retrieved November 29, 2015, from www.guidelines.gov/content.aspx?id=47030&search=heart+failure
Roberts, E., Ludman, A. J., Dworzynski, K., et al.; NICE Guideline Development Group for Acute Heart Failure. (2015). The diagnostic accuracy of the natriuretic peptides in heart failure: Systematic review and diagnostic meta-analysis in the acute care setting. *The British Medical Journal*, *350*, h910, 1–16.
Shah, A., Gandhi, D., Srivastava, S., et al. (2017). Heart failure: A class review of pharmacotherapy. *Pharmacology and Therapeutics*, *42*(7), 464–472.
Steenman, M., & Lande, G. (2017). Cardiac aging and heart disease in humans. *Biophysical Reviews*, *9*(2), 131–137.
Sun, W. P., Li, C. L., Guo, J. C., et al. (2016). Long-term efficacy of implantable cardiac resynchronization therapy plus defibrillator for primary prevention of sudden cardiac death in patients with mild heart failure: An updated meta-analysis. *Heart Failure Reviews*, *21*(4), 447–453.
Tariq, S., & Aronow, W. S. (2015). Use of inotropic agents in treatment of systolic heart failure. *International Journal of Molecular Sciences*, *16*(12), 29060–29068.
Van Craenenbroeck, E. M. (2017). Exercise training as therapy for chronic heart failure. *European Society of Cardiology: E-Journal of Cardiology Practice*, *14*(43). Retrieved April 12, 2017, from https://www.escardio.org/Journals/E-Journal-of-Cardiology-Practice/Volume-14/Exercise-training-as-therapy-for-chronic-heart-failure
Virani, S. A., Bains, M., Code, J., et al. (2017). The need for heart failure advocacy in Canada, *Canadian Journal of Cardiology*, *33*(11), 1450–1454. doi: 10.1016/j.cjca.2017.08.024.
Wang, C., Xiong, B., & Huang, J. (2017). The role of Omega-3 polyunsaturated fatty acids in heart failure: A meta-analysis of randomized controlled trials. *Nutrients*, *9*(1), 1–16.
Yancy, C. W., Jessup, M., Bozkurt, B., et al. (2013). 2013 ACCF/AHA Guideline for the management of heart failure. A report of the American College of Cardiology Foundation/American Heart Association Task Force on Practice Guidelines. *Circulation*, *128*(16), e240–e327.
York, N. L., Kane, C., & Smith, C. S. (2018). Identification and management of acute cardiac tamponade. *Dimensions of Critical Care Nursing*, *37*(3), 130–134.

Resources

American Heart Association: http://www.americanheart.org
Canadian Association of Cardiovascular Prevention and Rehabilitation: http://www.cacr.ca/about/index.cfm
Canadian Cardiovascular Society: http://www.ccs.ca
Canadian Council of Cardiovascular Nurses: http://www.cccn.ca
Heart and Stroke Foundation of Canada: http://www.heartandstroke.ca/
Heart Failure Society of America: http://www.abouthf.org

32 Assessment and Management of Patients With Vascular Disorders and Peripheral Circulation Concerns

Adapted by Alice S.W. Khin

Learning Objectives

On completion of this chapter, the learner will be able to:

1. Identify anatomic and physiologic factors that affect peripheral blood flow and tissue oxygenation.
2. Use appropriate parameters for assessment of peripheral circulation.
3. Use the nursing process as a framework of care for patients with vascular insufficiency of the extremities.
4. Compare the various diseases of the arteries and their causes, pathophysiologic changes, clinical manifestations, management, and prevention.
5. Describe the prevention and management of venous thromboembolism.
6. Compare strategies to prevent venous insufficiency, leg ulcers, and varicose veins.
7. Use the nursing process as a framework of care for patients with leg ulcers.
8. Describe the relationship between lymphangitis and lymphedema.
9. Describe the medical and nursing management of lymphatic disorders.

Conditions of the vascular system include arterial disorders, venous disorders, lymphatic disorders, and cellulitis. Nursing management depends on an understanding of the vascular system.

Assessment of Vascular Function

Adequate perfusion ensures oxygenation and nourishment of body tissues, and it depends in part on a properly functioning cardiovascular system. Adequate blood flow depends on the efficiency of the heart as a pump, the patency and responsiveness of the blood vessels, and the adequacy of circulating blood volume. Nervous system activity, blood viscosity, and the metabolic needs of tissues influence the rate and adequacy of blood flow.

Anatomic and Physiologic Overview

The vascular system consists of two interdependent systems. The right side of the heart pumps blood through the lungs to the pulmonary circulation, and the left side of the heart pumps blood to all other body tissues through the systemic circulation. The blood vessels in both systems channel the blood from the heart to the tissues and back to the heart (Fig. 32-1). Contraction of the ventricles is the driving force that moves blood through the vascular system.

Arteries distribute oxygenated blood from the left side of the heart to the tissues, whereas the veins carry deoxygenated blood from the tissues to the right side of the heart. Capillary vessels located within the tissues connect the arterial and venous systems. These vessels permit the exchange of nutrients and metabolic wastes between the circulatory system and the tissues. Arterioles and venules immediately adjacent to the capillaries, together with the capillaries, make up the microcirculation.

The lymphatic system complements the function of the circulatory system. Lymphatic vessels transport lymph (a fluid similar to plasma) and tissue fluids (containing proteins, cells, and cellular debris) from the interstitial space to systemic veins.

Anatomy of the Vascular System

Arteries and Arterioles

Arteries are thick-walled structures that carry blood from the heart to the tissues. The aorta, which has a diameter of

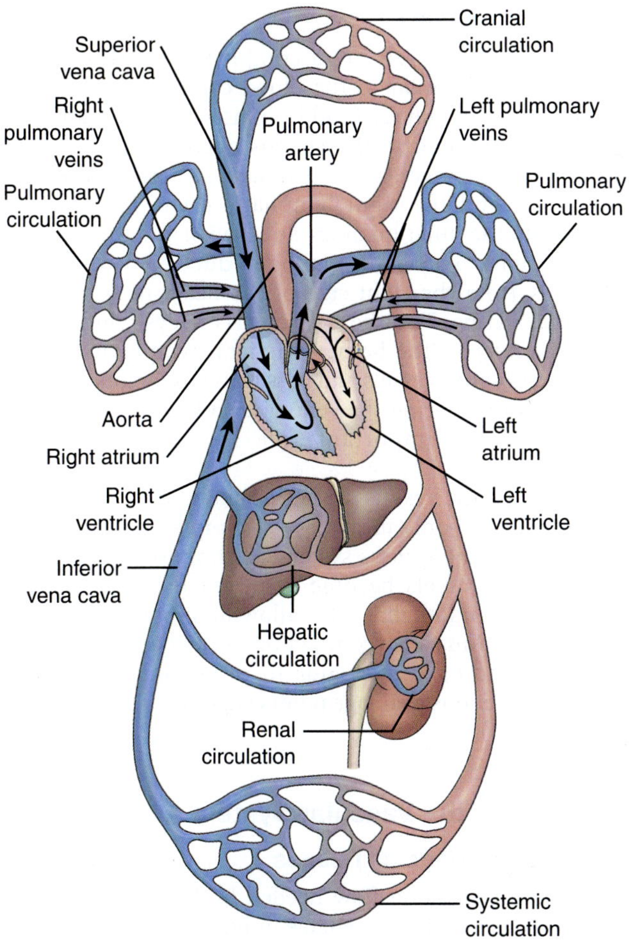

FIGURE 32-1. Systemic and pulmonary circulation. Oxygen-rich blood from the pulmonary circulation is pumped from the left heart into the aorta and the systemic arteries to the capillaries, where the exchange of nutrients and waste products takes place. The deoxygenated blood returns to the right heart by way of the systemic veins and is pumped into the pulmonary circulation.

approximately 25 mm in the average-sized adult, gives rise to numerous branches, which continue to divide into progressively smaller arteries that are 4 mm in diameter. The vessels divide further, diminishing in size to approximately 30 μm in diameter. These smallest arteries, called the arterioles, are generally embedded within the tissues (Grossman & Porth, 2014).

The walls of the arteries and arterioles are composed of three layers: the intima, an inner endothelial cell layer; the media, a middle layer of smooth muscle and elastic tissue; and the adventitia, an outer layer of connective tissue. The intima, a very thin layer, provides a smooth surface for contact with the flowing blood. The media makes up most of the vessel wall in the aorta and other large arteries of the body. This layer is composed chiefly of elastic and connective tissue fibres that give the vessels considerable strength and allow them to constrict and dilate to accommodate the blood ejected from the heart during each cardiac cycle (stroke volume) and maintain an even, steady flow of blood. The adventitia is a layer of connective tissue that anchors the vessel to its surroundings. There is much less elastic tissue in the smaller arteries and arterioles, and the media in these vessels is composed primarily of smooth muscle (Grossman & Porth, 2014). Smooth muscle controls the diameter of the vessels by contracting and relaxing. Chemical, hormonal, and neuronal factors influence the activity of smooth muscle. Because arterioles offer resistance to blood flow by altering their diameter, they are often referred to as *resistance vessels*. Arterioles regulate the volume and pressure in the arterial system and the rate of blood flow to the capillaries. Because of the large amount of smooth muscle in the media, the walls of the arteries are relatively thick, accounting for approximately 25% of the total diameter of the artery.

The intima and the inner third of the smooth muscle layer of the media are in such close contact with the blood that the blood vessels receive their nourishment by direct diffusion. The adventitia and the outer media layers have

Glossary

anastomosis: junction of two vessels

aneurysm: a localized sac or dilation of an artery formed at a weak point in the vessel wall

angioplasty: an invasive procedure that uses a balloon-tipped catheter to dilate a stenotic area of a blood vessel

ankle-brachial index (ABI) or ankle-arm index (AAI): ratio of the ankle systolic pressure to the arm systolic pressure; an objective measurement of arterial disease that provides quantification of the degree of stenosis

arteriosclerosis: diffuse process whereby the muscle fibres and the endothelial lining of the walls of small arteries and arterioles thicken

atherosclerosis: inflammatory process involving the accumulation of lipids, calcium, blood components, carbohydrates, and fibrous tissue on the intimal layer of a large- or medium-sized artery

bruit: sound produced by turbulent blood flow through an irregular, tortuous, stenotic, or dilated vessel

dissection: separation of the weakened elastic and fibromuscular elements in the medial layer of an artery

duplex ultrasonography: combines B-mode grey-scale imaging of tissue, organs, and blood vessels with capabilities of estimating velocity changes by use of a pulsed Doppler

intermittent claudication: a muscular, cramplike pain in the extremities consistently reproduced with the same degree of exercise or activity and relieved by rest

ischemia: deficient blood supply

rest pain: persistent pain in the foot or digits when the patient is resting, indicating a severe degree of arterial insufficiency

rubor: reddish blue discolouration of the extremities; indicative of severe peripheral arterial damage in vessels that remain dilated and unable to constrict

stenosis: narrowing or constriction of a vessel

a limited vascular system for nourishment and require their own blood supply to meet metabolic needs.

Capillaries

The walls of the capillaries, which lack smooth muscle and adventitia, are composed of a single layer of endothelial cells. This thin-walled structure permits rapid and efficient transport of nutrients to the cells and removal of metabolic wastes. The diameter of capillaries ranges from 5 to 10 μm; this means that red blood cells must alter their shape to pass through these vessels. Changes in a capillary's diameter are passive and are influenced by contractile changes in the blood vessels that carry blood to and from a capillary. The capillary's diameter also changes in response to chemical stimuli. In some tissues, a cuff of smooth muscle, called the precapillary sphincter, is located at the arteriolar end of the capillary and is responsible, along with the arteriole, for controlling capillary blood flow (Grossman & Porth, 2014).

Some capillary beds, such as those in the fingertips, contain arteriovenous anastomoses, through which blood passes directly from the arterial to the venous system. These vessels are believed to regulate heat exchange between the body and the external environment.

The distribution of capillaries varies with the type of tissue. For example, skeletal tissue, which has high metabolic requirements, has a denser capillary network than cartilage, which has low metabolic needs.

Veins and Venules

Capillaries join to form larger vessels called venules, which join to form veins. The venous system is therefore structurally analogous to the arterial system; venules correspond to arterioles, veins to arteries, and the vena cava to the aorta. Analogous types of vessels in the arterial and venous systems have approximately the same diameters (Fig. 32-1).

The walls of the veins, in contrast to those of the arteries, are thinner and considerably less muscular. In most veins, the wall makes up only 10% of the diameter, in contrast to 25% in most arteries. In veins, the walls are composed of three layers, like those of arteries, although in veins, these layers are not as well defined.

The thin, less muscular structure of the vein wall allows these vessels to distend more than arteries. Greater distensibility and compliance permit large volumes of blood to remain in the veins under low pressure. For this reason, veins are referred to as *capacitance vessels*. Approximately 75% of total blood volume is contained in the veins. The sympathetic nervous system, which innervates the vein musculature, can stimulate the veins to constrict (venoconstriction), thereby reducing venous volume and increasing the volume of blood in the general circulation. Contraction of skeletal muscles in the extremities creates the primary pumping action to facilitate venous blood flow back to the heart (Grossman & Porth, 2014).

Some veins, unlike arteries, are equipped with valves. In general, veins that transport blood against the force of gravity, as in the lower extremities, have one-way bicuspid valves that prevent blood from seeping backward as it is propelled toward the heart. Valves are composed of endothelial leaflets, the competency of which depends on the integrity of the vein wall.

Lymphatic Vessels

The lymphatic vessels are a complex network of thin-walled vessels similar to the blood capillaries. This network collects lymphatic fluid from tissues and organs and transports the fluid to the venous circulation. The lymphatic vessels converge into two main structures: the thoracic duct and the right lymphatic duct. These ducts empty into the junction of the subclavian and the internal jugular veins. The right lymphatic duct conveys lymph primarily from the right side of the head, neck, thorax, and upper arms. The thoracic duct conveys lymph from the remainder of the body. Peripheral lymphatic vessels join larger lymph vessels and pass through regional lymph nodes before entering the venous circulation. The lymph nodes play an important role in filtering foreign particles.

The lymphatic vessels are permeable to large molecules and provide the only means by which interstitial proteins can return to the venous system. With muscular contraction, lymph vessels become distorted to create spaces between the endothelial cells, allowing protein and particles to enter. Muscular contraction of the lymphatic walls and surrounding tissues aids in propelling the lymph toward the venous drainage points (Zaleska, Olszewski, & Durlik, 2014).

Function of the Vascular System

Circulatory Needs of Tissues

The amount of blood flow needed by body tissues constantly changes. The percentage of blood flow received by individual organs or tissues is determined by the rate of tissue metabolism, the availability of oxygen, and the function of the tissues. When metabolic requirements increase, blood vessels dilate to increase the flow of oxygen and nutrients to the tissues. When metabolic needs decrease, vessels constrict and blood flow to the tissues decreases. Metabolic demands of tissues increase with physical activity or exercise, local heat application, fever, and infection. Reduced metabolic requirements of tissues accompany rest or decreased physical activity, local cold application, and cooling of the body. If the blood vessels fail to dilate in response to the need for increased blood flow, tissue **ischemia** (deficient blood supply to a body part) results. The mechanism by which blood vessels dilate and constrict to adjust for metabolic changes ensures that normal arterial pressure is maintained (Grossman & Porth, 2014).

As blood passes through tissue capillaries, oxygen is removed and carbon dioxide is added. The amount of oxygen extracted by each tissue differs. For example, the myocardium tends to extract about 50% of the oxygen from arterial blood in one pass through its capillary bed, whereas the kidneys extract only about 7% of the oxygen from the blood that passes through them. The average amount of oxygen removed collectively by all of the body tissues is about 25%. This means that the blood in the vena cava contains about 25% less oxygen than aortic blood. This is known as the *systemic arteriovenous oxygen difference* (Grossman & Porth, 2014). This difference becomes greater when less oxygen is delivered to the tissues than they need.

Blood Flow

Blood flow through the cardiovascular system always proceeds in the same direction: left side of the heart to the aorta, arteries, arterioles, capillaries, venules, veins, vena cava, and right side of the heart. This unidirectional flow is caused by a pressure difference that exists between the arterial and venous systems. Because arterial pressure (approximately 100 mm Hg) is greater than venous pressure (approximately 40 mm Hg) and fluid always flows from an area of higher pressure to an area of lower pressure, blood flows from the arterial to the venous system.

The pressure difference (ΔP) between the two ends of the vessel propels the blood. Impediments to blood flow offer the opposing force, which is known as resistance (R). The rate of blood flow is determined by dividing the pressure difference by the resistance:

$$\text{Flow rate} = \Delta P/R$$

This equation clearly shows that when resistance increases, a greater driving pressure is required to maintain the same degree of flow (Hannon et al., 2017). In the body, an increase in driving pressure is accomplished by an increase in the force of contraction of the heart. If arterial resistance is chronically elevated, the myocardium hypertrophies (enlarges) to sustain the greater contractile force.

In most long smooth blood vessels, flow is laminar or streamlined, with blood in the centre of the vessel moving slightly faster than the blood near the vessel walls. Laminar flow becomes turbulent when the blood flow rate increases, when blood viscosity increases, when the diameter of the vessel becomes greater than normal, or when segments of the vessel are narrowed or constricted (Krishna, Moxon, & Golledge, 2015). Turbulent blood flow creates a sound, called a **bruit**, which can be heard with a stethoscope.

Blood Pressure

Chapter 33 provides more information on the physiology and measurement of blood pressure.

Capillary Filtration and Reabsorption

Fluid exchange across the capillary wall is continuous. This fluid, which has the same composition as plasma without the proteins, forms the interstitial fluid. The equilibrium between hydrostatic and osmotic forces of the blood and interstitium, as well as capillary permeability, determines the amount and direction of fluid movement across the capillary. Hydrostatic force is a driving pressure that is generated by the blood pressure. Osmotic pressure is the pulling force created by plasma proteins. Normally, the hydrostatic pressure at the arterial end of the capillary is relatively high compared with that at the venous end. This high pressure at the arterial end of the capillaries tends to drive fluid out of the capillary and into the tissue space. Osmotic pressure tends to pull fluid back into the capillary from the tissue space, but this osmotic force cannot overcome the high hydrostatic pressure at the arterial end of the capillary. However, at the venous end of the capillary, the osmotic force predominates over the low hydrostatic pressure, and there is a net reabsorption of fluid from the tissue space back into the capillary (Grossman & Porth, 2014).

Except for a very small amount, fluid that is filtered out at the arterial end of the capillary bed is reabsorbed at the venous end. The excess filtered fluid enters the lymphatic circulation. These processes of filtration, reabsorption, and lymph formation aid in maintaining tissue fluid volume and removing tissue waste and debris. Under normal conditions, capillary permeability remains constant.

Under certain abnormal conditions, the fluid filtered out of the capillaries may greatly exceed the amounts reabsorbed and carried away by the lymphatic vessels. This imbalance can result from damage to capillary walls and subsequent increased permeability, obstruction of lymphatic drainage, elevation of venous pressure, or a decrease in plasma protein osmotic force. Accumulation of excess interstitial fluid that results from these processes is known as *edema*.

Hemodynamic Resistance

The most important factor that determines resistance in the vascular system is the vessel radius. Small changes in vessel radius lead to large changes in resistance. The predominant sites of change in the calibre or width of blood vessels, and therefore in resistance, are the arterioles and the precapillary sphincter. Peripheral vascular resistance is the opposition to blood flow provided by the blood vessels. This resistance is proportional to the viscosity or thickness of the blood and the length of the vessel and is influenced by the diameter of the vessels. Under normal conditions, blood viscosity and vessel length do not change significantly, and these factors do not usually play an important role in blood flow. However, a large increase in hematocrit may increase blood viscosity and reduce capillary blood flow.

Peripheral Vascular Regulating Mechanisms

Even at rest, the metabolic needs of body tissues are continuously changing. Therefore, an integrated and coordinated regulatory system is necessary so that blood flow to individual tissues is maintained in proportion to the needs of those tissues. This regulatory mechanism is complex and consists of central nervous system influences, circulating hormones and chemicals, and independent activity of the arterial wall itself.

Sympathetic (adrenergic) nervous system activity, mediated by the hypothalamus, is the most important factor in regulating the calibre and therefore the blood flow of peripheral blood vessels. All vessels are innervated by the sympathetic nervous system except the capillary and precapillary sphincters. Stimulation of the sympathetic nervous system causes vasoconstriction. The neurotransmitter responsible for sympathetic vasoconstriction is norepinephrine (Grossman & Porth, 2014). Sympathetic activation occurs in response to physiologic and psychological stressors. Diminution of sympathetic activity by medications or sympathectomy results in vasodilation.

Other hormones affect peripheral vascular resistance. Epinephrine, released from the adrenal medulla, acts like norepinephrine in constricting peripheral blood vessels in most tissue beds. However, in low concentrations, epinephrine causes vasodilation in skeletal muscles, the heart, and the brain. Angiotensin I, which is formed from the interaction of renin (synthesized by the kidney) and angiotensinogen, a circulating serum protein, is then converted to angiotensin II by an enzyme secreted by the pulmonary vasculature, called angiotensin-converting enzyme (ACE). Angiotensin II is a potent vasoconstrictor, particularly of the arterioles. Although the amount of angiotensin II concentrated in the blood is usually small, its profound vasoconstrictive effects are important in certain abnormal states, such as heart failure and hypovolemia (Grossman & Porth, 2014).

Alterations in local blood flow are influenced by various circulating substances that have vasoactive properties. Potent vasodilators include nitric oxide, prostacyclin, histamine, bradykinin, prostaglandin, and certain muscle metabolites. A reduction in available oxygen and nutrients and changes in local pH also affect local blood flow. Thromboxane A_2 and serotonin are substances liberated from platelets that aggregate at the site of damaged vessels, causing arteriolar vasoconstriction and continued platelet aggregation at the site of injury (Favero, Paganelli, Buffoli, et al., 2014).

The application of hot to parts of the body surface causes local vasodilation, whereas the application of cold causes vasoconstriction.

Pathophysiology of the Vascular System

Reduced blood flow through peripheral blood vessels characterizes all peripheral vascular diseases. The physiologic effects of altered blood flow depend on the extent to which tissue demands exceed the supply of oxygen and nutrients available. If tissue needs are high, even modestly reduced blood flow may be inadequate to maintain tissue integrity. Tissues then fall prey to ischemia, become malnourished, and ultimately die unless adequate blood flow is restored.

Pump Failure

Inadequate peripheral blood flow occurs when the heart's pumping action becomes inefficient. Left-sided heart failure (left ventricular failure) causes an accumulation of blood in the lungs and a reduction in forward flow or cardiac output, which results in inadequate arterial blood flow to the tissues. Right-sided heart failure (right ventricular failure) causes systemic venous congestion and a reduction in forward flow (see Chapter 31).

Alterations in Blood and Lymphatic Vessels

Intact, patent, and responsive blood vessels are necessary to deliver adequate amounts of oxygen to tissues and to remove metabolic wastes. Arteries can become damaged or obstructed as a result of atherosclerotic plaque, thromboemboli, chemical or mechanical trauma, infections or inflammatory processes, vasospastic disorders, and congenital malformations. A sudden arterial occlusion causes profound and often irreversible tissue ischemia and tissue death. When arterial occlusions develop gradually, there is less risk of sudden tissue death because collateral circulation may develop, giving that tissue the opportunity to adapt to gradually decreased blood flow.

Venous blood flow can be reduced by a thromboembolus obstructing the vein, by incompetent venous valves, or by a reduction in the effectiveness of the pumping action of surrounding muscles. Decreased venous blood flow results in increased venous pressure, a subsequent increase in capillary hydrostatic pressure, net filtration of fluid out of the capillaries into the interstitial space, and subsequent edema. Edematous tissues cannot receive adequate nutrition from the blood and consequently are more susceptible to breakdown, injury, and infection. Obstruction of lymphatic vessels also results in edema. Lymphatic vessels can become obstructed by a tumour or by damage from mechanical trauma or inflammatory processes.

Circulatory Insufficiency of the Extremities

Although many types of peripheral vascular diseases exist, most result in ischemia and produce some of the same symptoms: pain, skin changes, diminished pulse, and possible edema. The type and severity of symptoms depend in part on the type, stage, and extent of the disease process and on the speed with which the disorder develops. Table 32-1 highlights the distinguishing features of arterial and venous insufficiency. In this chapter, peripheral vascular disease is categorized as arterial, venous, or lymphatic.

TABLE 32-1 Characteristics of Arterial and Venous Insufficiency and Resulting Ulcers

Characteristic	Arterial	Venous
General Characteristics		
Pain	Intermittent claudication to sharp, unrelenting, constant	Aching, cramping
Pulses	Diminished or absent	Present, but may be difficult to palpate through edema
Skin characteristics	Dependent rubor—elevation pallor of foot; dry, shiny skin; cool-to-cold temperature; loss of hair over toes and dorsum of foot; nails thickened and ridged	Pigmentation in gaiter area (area of medial and lateral malleolus), skin thickened and tough, may be reddish blue, frequently associated with dermatitis
Ulcer Characteristics		
Location	Tip of toes, toe webs, heel or other pressure areas if confined to bed	Medial malleolus; infrequently lateral malleolus or anterior tibial area
Pain	Very painful	Minimal pain if superficial or may be very painful
Depth of ulcer	Deep, often involving joint space	Superficial
Shape	Circular	Irregular border
Ulcer base	Pale to black and dry gangrene	Granulation tissue—beefy red to yellow fibrinous in chronic long-term ulcer
Leg edema	Minimal unless extremity kept in dependent position constantly to relieve pain	Moderate to severe

Gerontologic Considerations

Aging produces changes in the walls of the blood vessels that affect the transport of oxygen and nutrients to the tissues. The intima thickens as a result of cellular proliferation and fibrosis. Elastin fibres of the media become calcified, thin, and fragmented, and collagen accumulates in the intima and the media. These changes cause the vessels to stiffen, which results in increased peripheral resistance, impaired blood flow, and increased left ventricular workload.

Assessment

Health History

The nurse obtains an in-depth description from the patient of any pain and its precipitating factors. A muscular, cramp-type pain in the extremities consistently reproduced with the same degree of exercise or activity and relieved by rest is experienced by patients with peripheral arterial insufficiency. Referred to as **intermittent claudication**, this pain is caused by the inability of the arterial system to provide adequate blood flow to the tissues in the face of increased demands for nutrients and oxygen during exercise. As the tissues are forced to complete the energy cycle without adequate nutrients and oxygen, muscle metabolites and lactic acid are produced. Pain is experienced as the metabolites aggravate the nerve endings of the surrounding tissue. Typically, about 50% of the arterial lumen or 75% of the cross-sectional area must be obstructed before intermittent claudication is experienced. When the patient rests and thereby decreases the metabolic needs of the muscles, the pain subsides. The progression of the arterial disease can be monitored by documenting the amount of exercise or the distance the patient can walk before pain is produced. Persistent pain in the forefoot (i.e., the anterior portion of the foot) when the patient is resting indicates a severe degree of arterial insufficiency and a critical state of ischemia. Known as **rest pain**, this discomfort is often worse at night and may interfere with sleep. This pain frequently requires that the extremity be lowered to a dependent position to improve perfusion to the distal tissues.

The site of arterial disease can be deduced from the location of claudication, because pain occurs in muscle groups distal to the diseased vessel. Calf pain may accompany reduced blood flow through the superficial femoral or popliteal artery, whereas pain in the hip or buttock may result from reduced blood flow in the abdominal aorta or the common iliac or hypogastric arteries.

Physical Assessment

A thorough assessment of the patient's skin colour and temperature and the character of the peripheral pulses are important in the diagnosis of arterial disorders.

Inspection of the Skin

Adequate blood flow warms the extremities and gives them a rosy colouring. Inadequate blood flow results in cool and pale extremities. Further reduction of blood flow to these tissues, which occurs when the extremity is elevated, for example, results in an even whiter or more blanched appearance (e.g., pallor). **Rubor**, a reddish-blue discolouration of the extremities, may be observed within 20 seconds to 2 minutes after the extremity is placed in the dependent position. Rubor suggests severe peripheral arterial damage in which vessels that cannot constrict remain dilated. Even with rubor, the extremity begins to turn pale with elevation. Cyanosis, a bluish tint of the skin, is manifested when the amount of oxygenated hemoglobin contained in the blood is reduced.

Additional changes resulting from a chronically reduced nutrient supply include loss of hair, brittle nails, dry or scaling skin, atrophy, and ulcerations. Edema may be apparent bilaterally or unilaterally and is related to the affected extremity's chronically dependent position because of severe rest pain. Gangrenous changes appear after prolonged, severe ischemia and represent tissue necrosis.

Palpation of Pulses

Determining the presence or absence, as well as the quality, of peripheral pulses is important in assessing the status of peripheral arterial circulation (Fig. 32-2). Palpation of pulses is subjective, and the examiner may mistake his or her own pulse for that of the patient. To prevent this, the examiner should use light touch and avoid using only the index finger for palpation because this finger has the strongest arterial pulsation of all the fingers. The thumb should not be used for the same reason. Absence of a pulse may indicate that the site of **stenosis** (narrowing or constriction) is proximal to that location. Occlusive arterial disease impairs blood flow and can reduce or obliterate palpable pulsations in the extremities. Pulses should be palpated bilaterally and simultaneously, comparing both sides for symmetry in rate, rhythm, and quality.

Gerontologic Considerations

In older adults, symptoms of peripheral arterial disease (PAD) may be more pronounced than in younger people. In older adult patients who are inactive, gangrene may be the first sign of disease. These patients may have adjusted their lifestyle to accommodate the limitations imposed by the disease and may not walk far enough to develop symptoms of claudication. Circulation is decreased, but this is not apparent to the patient until trauma occurs. At this point, gangrene develops when minimal arterial flow is impaired further by edema formation resulting from the traumatic event.

Intermittent claudication may occur after walking only one half to one block or after walking up a slight incline. Any prolonged pressure on the foot can cause pressure areas that become ulcerated, infected, and gangrenous. The outcomes of arterial insufficiency can include reduced mobility and activity as well as a loss of independence. Older adults with reduced mobility are less likely to remain in the community setting, have higher rates of hospitalizations, and experience a poorer quality of life.

Diagnostic Evaluation

Various tests may be performed to identify and diagnose abnormalities that can affect the vascular structures (arteries, veins, and lymphatics).

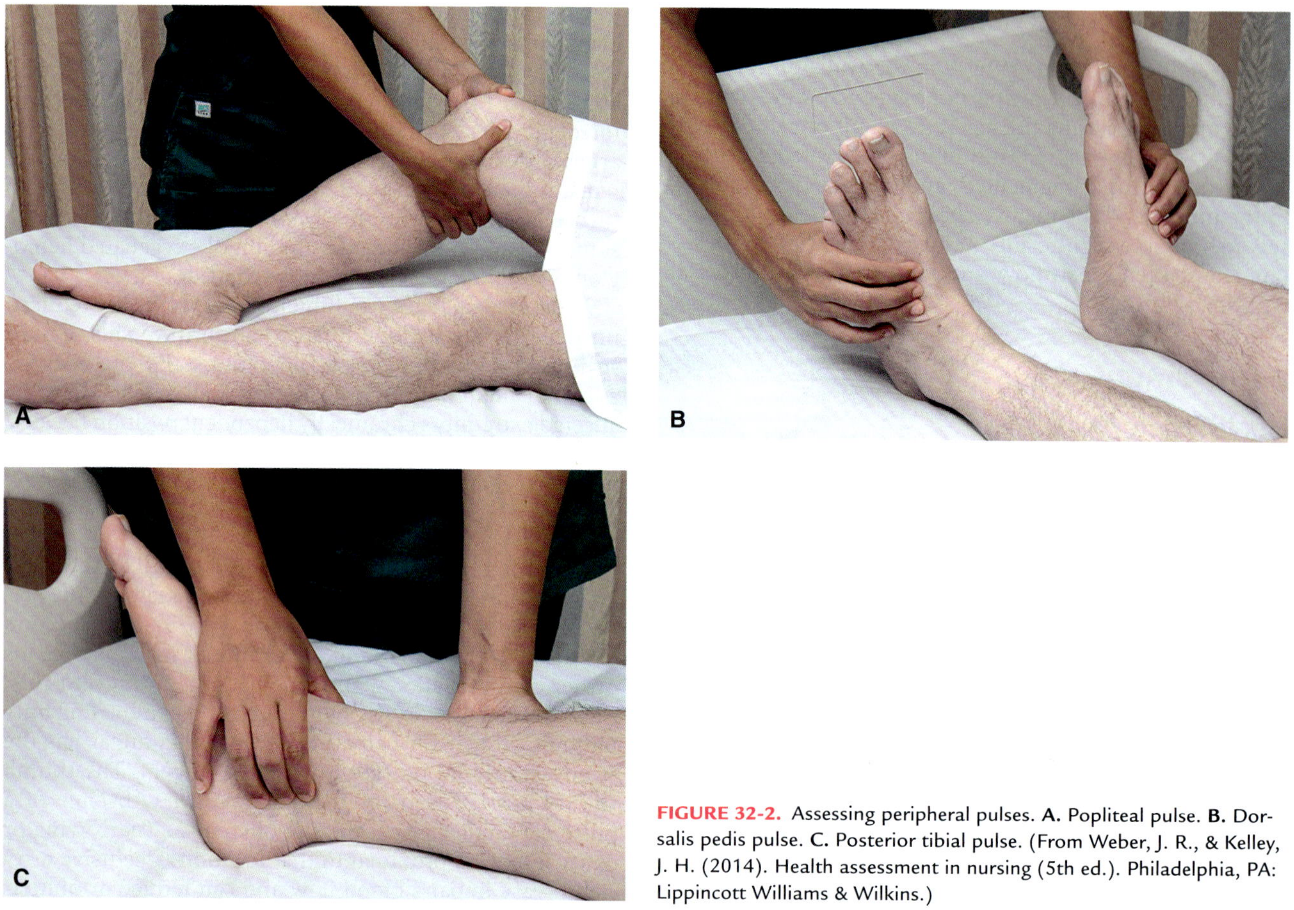

FIGURE 32-2. Assessing peripheral pulses. A. Popliteal pulse. B. Dorsalis pedis pulse. C. Posterior tibial pulse. (From Weber, J. R., & Kelley, J. H. (2014). Health assessment in nursing (5th ed.). Philadelphia, PA: Lippincott Williams & Wilkins.)

Doppler Ultrasound Flow Studies

When pulses cannot be reliably palpated, a handheld continuous wave (CW) Doppler ultrasound device may be used to hear (insonate) the blood flow in vessels. This handheld device emits a continuous signal through the patient's tissues. The signals are reflected by ("echo off") the moving blood cells and are received by the device. The filtered-output Doppler signal is then transmitted to a loudspeaker or headphones, where it can be heard for interpretation. Because CW Doppler emits a continuous signal, all vascular structures in the path of the sound beam are insonated, and differentiating arterial from venous flow and detecting the site of a stenosis may be difficult. The depth at which blood flow can be detected by Doppler is determined by the frequency (in megahertz [MHz]) it generates. The lower the frequency, the deeper the tissue penetration; a 5- to 10-MHz probe may be used to evaluate the peripheral arteries.

To evaluate the lower extremities, the patient is placed in the supine position with the head of the bed elevated 20 to 30 degrees; the legs are externally rotated, if possible, to permit adequate access to the medial malleolus. Acoustic gel is applied to the patient's skin to permit uniform transmission of the ultrasound wave. The tip of the Doppler transducer is positioned at a 45- to 60-degree angle over the expected location of the artery and angled slowly to identify arterial blood flow. Excessive pressure is avoided because severely diseased arteries can collapse with even minimal pressure.

Because the transducer can detect blood flow in advanced arterial disease states, especially if collateral circulation has developed, identifying a signal documents only the presence of blood flow. The patient's provider must be notified of the absence of a signal if one had been detected previously.

CW Doppler is more useful as a clinical tool when combined with ankle blood pressures, which are used to determine the **ankle-brachial index (ABI)**, also called the **ankle-arm index (AAI)**. The ABI is the ratio of the systolic blood pressure in the ankle to the systolic blood pressure in the arm. It is an objective indicator of arterial disease that allows the examiner to quantify the degree of stenosis. With increasing degrees of arterial narrowing, there is a progressive decrease in systolic pressure distal to the involved sites.

The first step in determining the ABI is to have the patient rest in a supine position (not seated) for approximately 5 minutes. An appropriate-sized blood pressure cuff (typically, a 10-cm cuff) is applied to the patient's ankle above the malleolus. After identifying an arterial signal at the posterior tibial and dorsalis pedis arteries, the systolic pressures are obtained in both ankles. Diastolic pressures in the ankles cannot be measured with a Doppler. If pressure in these arteries cannot be measured, pressure can be measured in the peroneal artery, which can also be assessed at the ankle (Fig. 32-3).

Doppler ultrasonography is used to measure brachial pressures in both arms. Both arms are evaluated because the patient may have an asymptomatic stenosis in the subclavian artery, causing brachial pressure on the affected side to

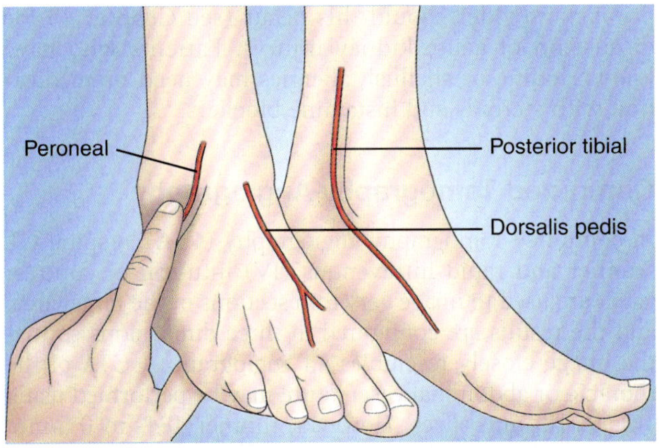

FIGURE 32-3. Location of peroneal artery; lateral malleolus.

be 20 mm Hg or more lower than systemic pressure. The abnormally low pressure should not be used for assessment.

To calculate ABI, the ankle systolic pressure for each foot is divided by the higher of the two brachial systolic pressures (Chart 32-1). The ABI can be computed for a patient with the following systolic pressures:

Right brachial: 160 mm Hg
Left brachial: 120 mm Hg
Right posterior tibial: 80 mm Hg
Right dorsalis pedis: 60 mm Hg
Left posterior tibial: 100 mm Hg
Left dorsalis pedis: 120 mm Hg

The highest systolic pressure for each ankle (80 mm Hg for the right, 120 mm Hg for the left) would be divided by the highest brachial pressure (160 mm Hg):

Right: 80/160 mm Hg = 0.50 ABI
Left: 120/160 mm Hg = 0.75 ABI

In general, systolic pressure in the ankle of a healthy person is the same or slightly higher than the brachial systolic pressure, resulting in an ABI of about 1.0 (no arterial insufficiency). Patients with claudication usually have an ABI of 0.95 to 0.50 (mild to moderate insufficiency); patients with ischemic rest pain have an ABI of less than 0.50; and patients with severe ischemia or tissue loss have an ABI of 0.40 or less (Zierler & Dawson, 2015).

CHART 32-1

Avoiding Common Errors in Calculating Ankle-Brachial Index

Take the following precautions to ensure an accurate ankle-brachial index (ABI) calculation:

- *Use correctly sized blood pressure (BP) cuffs.* To obtain accurate BP measurements, use a cuff with a bladder width at least 40% and length at least 80% of the limb circumference.
- *On the nursing plan of care, document the BP cuff sizes used* (e.g., "12-cm adult BP cuff used for brachial pressures; 10-cm pediatric BP cuff used for ankle pressures"). This minimizes the risk of shift-to-shift discrepancies in ABIs.
- *Use sufficient BP cuff inflation.* To ensure complete closure of the artery and the most accurate measurements, inflate cuffs 20 to 30 mm Hg beyond the point at which the last arterial signal is detected.
- *Do not deflate BP cuffs too rapidly.* Try to maintain a deflation rate of 2 to 4 mm Hg/s for patients without dysrhythmias and 2 mm Hg/s or slower for patients with dysrhythmias. Deflating the cuff more rapidly may miss the patient's highest pressure and result in recording an erroneous (low) BP measurement.
- *Suspect medial calcific sclerosis any time an ABI is 1.20 or greater or ankle pressure is more than 250 mm Hg.* Medial calcific sclerosis is associated with diabetes, chronic kidney disease, and hyperparathyroidism. It produces falsely elevated ankle pressures by hardening the media of the arteries, making the vessels noncompressible.
- *Be suspicious of arterial pressures recorded at less than 40 mm Hg.* This may mean the venous signal has been mistaken for the arterial signal. If the arterial pressure, which is normally 120 mm Hg, is measured at less than 40 mm Hg, ask a colleague to double-check the findings before recording this as an arterial pressure.

Nursing Implications

Nurses should perform a baseline ABI on any patient with decreased pulses or any patient 70 years or older, especially patients with a history of diabetes or use of tobacco products (Conte, Pomposelli, Clair, et al., 2015). Patients who undergo an arterial interventional procedure or surgery should have ABIs performed per their institution's protocols. In addition, if there is a change in the clinical status of a patient, such as a sudden cold or painful limb, an ABI should be performed.

Prior to the procedure, nurses should educate patients about the indications for ABI and what to expect. Patients should be instructed to avoid use of tobacco products or drinking caffeinated beverages for at least 2 hours prior to testing (if it is done on a nonurgent basis). There may be some discomfort involved when the cuffs are inflated.

Exercise Testing

Exercise testing is used to determine how long a patient can walk and to measure the ankle systolic blood pressure in response to walking. The patient walks on a treadmill at 2.5 km/hr with a 10% incline for a maximum of 5 minutes. Most patients can complete the test unless they have severe cardiac, pulmonary, or orthopedic problems or a physical disability. A normal response to the test is little or no drop in ankle systolic pressure after exercise. However, in a patient with true vascular claudication, the ankle pressure drops. Combining this hemodynamic information with the walking time helps the clinician determine whether intervention is necessary.

Duplex Ultrasonography

Duplex ultrasonography involves B-mode grey-scale imaging of the tissue, organs, and blood vessels (arterial and venous) and permits estimation of velocity changes by use of a pulsed Doppler (Fig. 32-4). Colour flow techniques, which can identify vessels, may be used to shorten the examination time. The procedure primarily helps determine the level and extent of venous disease. The technique makes it possible to image and assess blood flow, evaluate flow of the distal vessels, locate the disease (stenosis vs. occlusion), and determine anatomic morphology and the

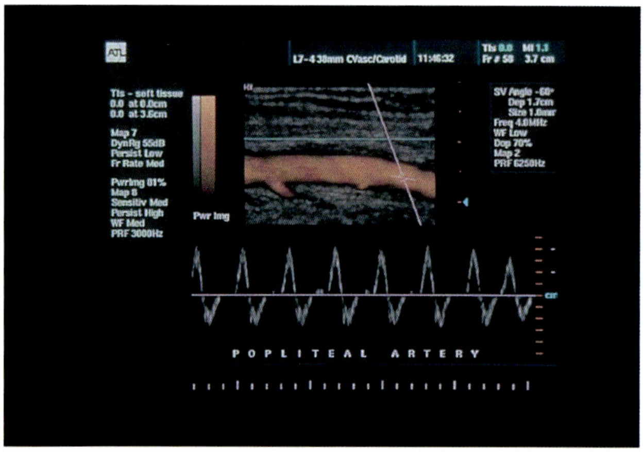

FIGURE 32-4. Colour flow duplex image of popliteal artery with normal triphasic Doppler flow.

hemodynamic significance of plaque causing stenosis. Duplex ultrasound findings help in planning therapy and monitoring its outcomes. The test is noninvasive and usually requires no patient preparation. The equipment is portable, making it useful anywhere for initial diagnosis, screening, or follow-up evaluations.

Computed Tomography Scanning

Computed tomography (CT) scanning provides cross-sectional images of soft tissue and visualizes the area of volume changes to an extremity and the compartment where changes take place. CT of a lymphedematous arm or leg, for example, demonstrates a characteristic honeycomb pattern in the subcutaneous tissue. In multidetector-computed tomography (MDCT), a spiral CT scanner and rapid intravenous (IV) infusion of contrast agent are used to image very thin sections of the target area, and the results are configured in three dimensions so that the image can be rotated and viewed from multiple angles. The scan head moves circumferentially around the patient as the patient passes through the scanner, creating a series of overlapping images that are connected to one another in a continuous spiral. Scan times are short. However, the patient is exposed to x-rays, and a contrast agent is injected to visualize the blood vessels. The high volume of contrast agent injected into a peripheral vein may contraindicate the use of MDCT in children and patients with significantly impaired renal function (Conte et al., 2015).

Nursing Implications

Patients with impaired renal function scheduled for MDCT may require preprocedural treatment to prevent contrast-induced nephropathy. This may include oral or IV hydration 6 to 12 hours preprocedure or administration of sodium bicarbonate, which alkalinizes urine and protects against free radical damage. Meta-analysis of research studies that used oral and IV N-acetylcysteine do not support its use for protection against contrast-induced nephropathy (Sadat, 2013). The nurse should monitor the patient's urinary output postprocedurally, which should be at least 0.5 mL/kg/hr. Contrast-induced acute kidney injury may occur within 48 to 96 hours postprocedure; therefore, the nurse should follow up with the patient's primary provider should this occur (see Chapter 45 for discussion of acute kidney injury). Patients who have known iodine or shellfish allergies may need premedication with steroids and histamine blockers.

Computed Tomography Angiography

In computed tomography angiography (CTA), a spiral CT scanner and rapid intravenous (IV) infusion of contrast agent are used to image very thin sections of the target area, and the results are configured in three dimensions so that the image closely resembles an angiogram. A CTA of the thoracic or abdominal vasculature may be performed using 1.0- to 1.5-mm slices. However, thinner, 0.4- to 0.6-mm slices may be needed to evaluate small vessels such as those in the brain, kidney, upper extremity, or below-knee lower extremity. Achieving this increased resolution requires a higher radiation dose; therefore, this test is justified only if there is a potentially significant diagnostic gain. The high volume of contrast agent injected into a peripheral vein limits the usefulness of CTA in children and patients with significantly impaired renal function.

Angiography

An arteriogram produced by angiography may be used to confirm the diagnosis of occlusive arterial disease when surgery or other interventions are considered. It involves injecting a radiopaque contrast agent directly into the arterial system to visualize the vessels. The location of a vascular obstruction or an **aneurysm** (abnormal dilation of a blood vessel) and the collateral circulation can be demonstrated. Typically, the patient experiences a temporary sensation of warmth as the contrast agent is injected, and local irritation may occur at the injection site. Infrequently, a patient may have an immediate or delayed allergic reaction to the iodine contained in the contrast agent. Manifestations include dyspnea, nausea and vomiting, sweating, tachycardia, and numbness of the extremities. Any such reaction must be reported to the interventionalist at once; treatment may include the administration of epinephrine, antihistamines, or corticosteroids. Additional risks include vessel injury, acute arterial occlusion, bleeding, or contrast nephropathy.

Magnetic Resonance Angiography

Magnetic resonance angiography (MRA) is performed with a standard magnetic resonance imaging (MRI) scanner and special software programmed to isolate the blood vessels. The resulting images can be rotated and viewed from multiple angles (Conte et al., 2015).

Nursing Implications

MRA is contraindicated in patients with any metal implants or devices such as pacemakers, including old tattoos, which may contain trace elements (newer materials used in tattoos such as nitinol and titanium are MRI compatible). The nurse should educate the patient regarding what to expect during and after the procedure. The patient should be prepared to lie on a cold, hard table that slides into an enclosed small tube. The nurse should instruct the patient that he or she will hear noises, including banging and popping sounds that will occur periodically. Patients with a history of claustrophobia may be prescribed a sedative prior to the procedure. Patients should be instructed to close their eyes before entering the tube, and to keep them closed, as this may decrease claustrophobic symptoms. Patients should be reassured that they will be provided with a panic button that they may press if they feel a need to stop the procedure. MRA procedures require the use of IV contrast dye; therefore, nursing implications following MRA are the same as those for MDCT (discussed in CT section).

Air Plethysmography

Air plethysmography is used to quantify venous reflux and calf muscle pump ejection. Changes in leg volumes are measured with the patient's legs elevated, with the patient supine and standing, and after the patient performs toe-ups (the patient extends the ankle while standing; stands on his or her toes) by an air-filled device wrapped around the feet and legs. Air plethysmography provides information about venous filling time, functional venous volume, ejected volume, and residual volume. It is useful in evaluating patients with suspected valvular incompetence or chronic venous insufficiency but is not used for diagnosis of deep vein thrombosis (DVT).

Contrast Phlebography (Venography)

Also known as venography, contrast phlebography involves injecting a radiopaque contrast agent into the venous system. If a thrombus exists, the x-ray image reveals an unfilled segment of vein in an otherwise completely filled vein. Injection of the contrast agent may cause brief but painful inflammation of the vein. The test is generally performed if the patient is to undergo thrombolytic therapy; however, duplex ultrasonography is considered the standard for diagnosing lower extremity venous thrombosis (Zierler & Dawson, 2015). The nurse should instruct the patient anticipating a contrast venogram that he or she will receive contrast dye through a peripheral vein and will be monitored for 2 hours post venogram for access site oozing or hematoma. The guidelines for nursing care following venogram are the same as those for MDCT (see earlier discussion).

Lymphangiography

Lymphangiography provides a way of detecting lymph node involvement resulting from metastatic carcinoma, lymphoma, or infection in sites that are otherwise inaccessible to the examiner except by surgery. In this test, a lymphatic vessel in each foot (or hand) is injected with contrast agent. A series of x-rays is taken at the conclusion of the injection, 24 hours later, and periodically thereafter, as indicated. The failure to identify subcutaneous lymphatic collection of contrast agent and the persistence of contrast agent in the tissue for days afterward help confirm a diagnosis of lymphedema.

Lymphoscintigraphy

Lymphoscintigraphy is a reliable alternative to lymphangiography. A radioactively labelled colloid is injected subcutaneously in the second interdigital space. The extremity is then exercised to facilitate the uptake of the colloid by the lymphatic system, and serial images are obtained at preset intervals.

Nursing Implications

The nurse should educate the patient regarding what to expect. For instance, the blue dye typically used for this procedure may stain the injection site. If the patient has a lymphatic leak, as can occur with groin incisions, there may be blue drainage from the incision until the dye clears from the system, which may take several days.

ARTERIAL DISORDERS

Arteriosclerosis and Atherosclerosis

Arteriosclerosis is the most common disease of the arteries; the term means "hardening of the arteries." It is a diffuse process whereby the muscle fibres and the endothelial lining of the walls of small arteries and arterioles become thickened. **Atherosclerosis** involves a different process, affecting the intima of the large and medium-sized arteries. These changes consist of the accumulation of lipids, calcium, blood components, carbohydrates, and fibrous tissue on the intimal layer of the artery. These accumulations are referred to as atheromas or plaques.

Although the pathologic processes of arteriosclerosis and atherosclerosis differ, rarely does one occur without the other, and the terms are often used interchangeably. Atherosclerosis is a generalized disease of the arteries, and when it is present in the extremities, it is usually present elsewhere in the body.

Pathophysiology

The most common direct results of atherosclerosis in arteries include narrowing (stenosis) of the lumen, obstruction by thrombosis, aneurysm, ulceration, and rupture. Its indirect results are malnutrition and the subsequent fibrosis of the organs that the sclerotic arteries supply with blood. All actively functioning tissue cells require an abundant supply of nutrients and oxygen and are sensitive to any reduction in the supply of these nutrients. If such reductions are severe and permanent, the cells undergo ischemic necrosis (death of cells due to deficient blood flow) and are replaced by fibrous tissue, which requires much less blood flow.

Atherosclerosis can develop at any point in the body, but certain sites are more vulnerable, such as regions where arteries bifurcate or branch into smaller vessels. In the proximal lower extremity, these include the distal abdominal aorta, the common iliac arteries, the orifice of the superficial femoral and profunda femoris arteries, and the superficial femoral artery in the adductor canal, which is particularly narrow. Distal to the knee, atherosclerosis can occur anywhere along the artery.

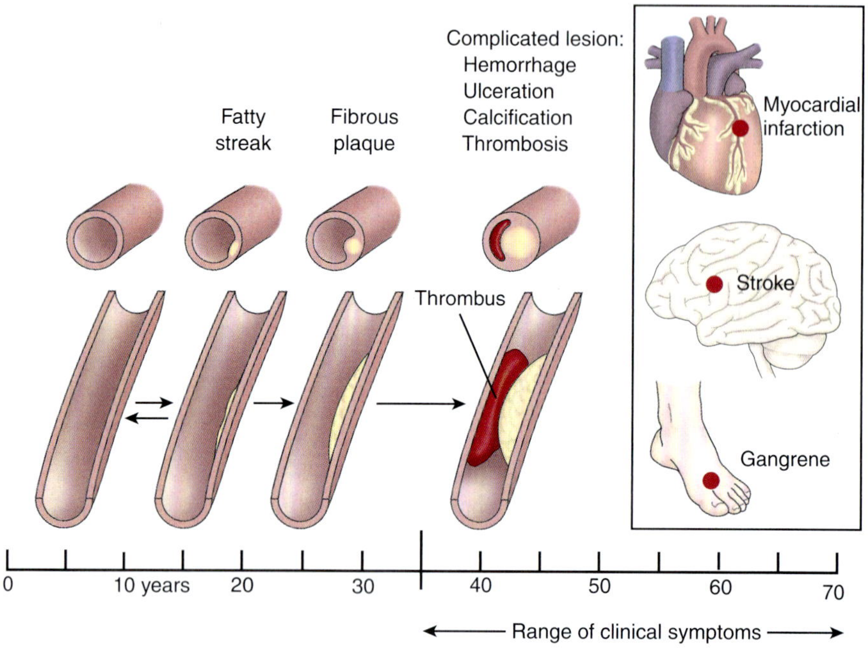

FIGURE 32-5. Schematic concept of the progression of atherosclerosis. Fatty streaks constitute one of the earliest lesions of atherosclerosis. Many fatty streaks regress, whereas others progress to fibrous plaques and eventually to atheroma, which may be complicated by hemorrhage, ulceration, calcification, or thrombosis and may produce myocardial infarction, stroke, or gangrene.

Although many theories exist about the development of atherosclerosis, no single theory explains the pathogenesis completely; however, tenets of several theories are incorporated into the reaction-to-injury theory. According to this theory, vascular endothelial cell injury results from prolonged hemodynamic forces, such as shearing stresses and turbulent flow, irradiation, chemical exposure, or chronic hyperlipidemia. Injury to the endothelium increases the aggregation of platelets and monocytes at the site of the injury. Smooth muscle cells migrate and proliferate, allowing a matrix of collagen and elastic fibres to form (Puranik, Dawson, & Peppas, 2013).

Atherosclerotic lesions are of two types: fatty streaks and fibrous plaque:

- Fatty streaks are yellow and smooth, protrude slightly into the lumen of the artery, and are composed of lipids and elongated smooth muscle cells. These lesions have been found in the arteries of people of all age groups, including infants. It is not clear whether fatty streaks predispose a person to the formation of fibrous plaques or whether they are reversible. They do not usually cause clinical symptoms.
- Fibrous plaques are composed of smooth muscle cells, collagen fibres, plasma components, and lipids. They are white to white-yellow and protrude in various degrees into the arterial lumen, sometimes completely obstructing it. These plaques are found predominantly in the abdominal aorta and the coronary, popliteal, and internal carotid arteries, and they are believed to be progressive lesions (Fig. 32-5).

Gradual narrowing of the arterial lumen stimulates the development of collateral circulation (Fig. 32-6). Collateral circulation arises from pre-existing vessels that enlarge to reroute blood flow around a hemodynamically significant stenosis or occlusion. Collateral flow allows continued perfusion to the tissues, but it is often inadequate to meet increased metabolic demand, and ischemia results.

Risk Factors

Many risk factors are associated with atherosclerosis (Chart 32-2). Although it is not entirely clear whether modification of these risk factors prevents the development of cardiovascular disease, evidence indicates that it may slow the disease process. Recent studies have reported the prevalence of atherosclerosis in women is the same, if not higher, than in men, and that female gender is an independent risk factor for PAD (Barochiner, Aparicio, & Waisman, 2014).

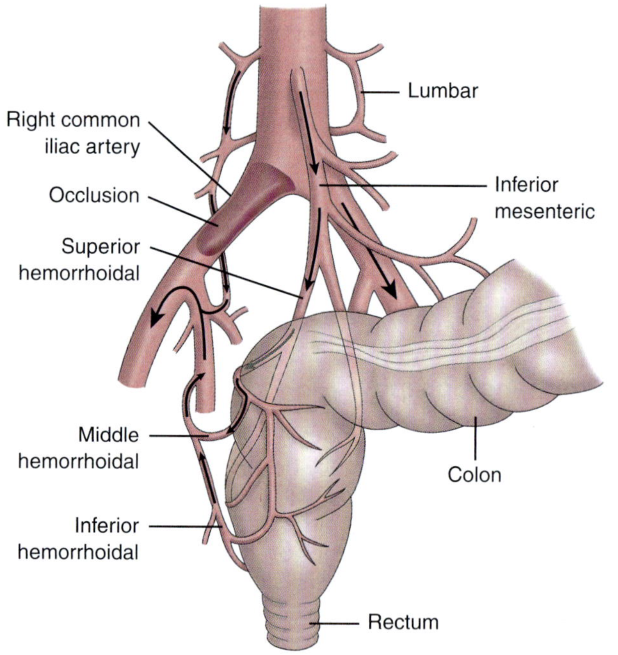

FIGURE 32-6. Development of channels for collateral blood flow in response to occlusion of the right common iliac artery and the terminal aortic bifurcation.

CHART 32-2

Risk Factors: Atherosclerosis and Peripheral Arterial Disease

Modifiable Risk Factors

- Nicotine use (i.e., tobacco product such as cigarettes, e-cigarettes, or chewing tobacco)
- Diet (contributing to hyperlipidemia)
- Hypertension
- Diabetes (speeds the atherosclerotic process by thickening the basement membranes of both large and small vessels)
- Hyperlipidemia
- Stress
- Sedentary lifestyle
- Elevated C-reactive protein
- Hyperhomocysteinemia

Nonmodifiable Risk Factors

- Increasing age
- Female gender
- Familial predisposition/genetics

Adapted from Cronenwett, J. L., & Johnston, K. W. (2014). *Rutherford's vascular surgery* (8th ed., Vols. 1 and 2). Philadelphia, PA: W. B. Saunders.

The use of tobacco products may be one of the most important risk factors in the development of atherosclerotic lesions. Nicotine in tobacco decreases blood flow to the extremities and increases heart rate and blood pressure by stimulating the sympathetic nervous system, causing vasoconstriction. It also increases the risk of clot formation by increasing the aggregation of platelets. Carbon monoxide, a toxin produced by burning tobacco, combines more readily with hemoglobin than oxygen, depriving the tissues of oxygen. There is evidence that smoking decreases high-density lipoprotein (HDL) levels and alters the ratios between HDL and low-density lipoprotein (LDL), HDL and triglycerides, and HDL and total cholesterol levels (see Chapter 27 for discussion of HDL and LDL and their association with atherosclerosis). The amount of tobacco used—inhaled in traditional or e-cigarette form, or chewed—is directly related to the extent of the disease, and cessation of any type of tobacco product use reduces the risks (Barochiner et al., 2014).

Diabetes increases the overall risk of PAD two- to fourfold, with amputation rates five to ten times higher than in patients without diabetes. Patients with diabetes show an earlier onset and more rapid progression of PAD than patients without diabetes; furthermore, they also exhibit a different anatomical distribution of pathology, with a greater severity of disease in the profunda femoris and in all segments below the knee (Conte et al., 2015). How diabetes affects the onset and progression of atherosclerosis is multifactorial and includes incitation of inflammatory processes, derangement of various cell types within vessel walls, promotion of coagulation, and inhibition of fibrinolysis (Thiruvoipati, Kielhorn, & Armstrong, 2015). Black race has been reported to increase the risk of developing PAD by over twofold and is also associated with higher rates of hypertension (Krishna et al., 2015). Many other factors, such as obesity, stress, and lack of exercise, have been identified as contributing to the disease process.

C-reactive protein (CRP) is a sensitive marker of cardiovascular inflammation, both systemically and locally. Slight increases in serum CRP levels are associated with an increased risk of damage in the vasculature, especially if these increases are accompanied by other risk factors, including increasing age, female gender, hypertension, hypercholesterolemia, obesity, elevated blood glucose levels, smoking, or a positive family history of cardiovascular disease (Krishna et al., 2015). There is also a positive association between PAD and the hemostatic or inflammatory markers fibrinogen and D-dimer.

Hyperhomocysteinemia has been positively correlated with the risk of peripheral, cerebrovascular, and coronary artery disease as well as venous thromboembolism (VTE). Homocysteine is a protein that promotes coagulation by increasing factor V and factor XI activity while depressing protein C activation and increasing the binding of lipoprotein(a) in fibrin. These processes increase thrombin formation and the propensity for thrombosis. Folic acid and vitamin B_{12} have been reported to reduce serum homocysteine levels but there are no data demonstrating this therapy reduces adverse cardiovascular events (Conte et al., 2015).

Prevention

Intermittent claudication is a symptom of generalized atherosclerosis and may be a marker of occult coronary artery disease. Because it is suspected that a high-fat diet contributes to atherosclerosis, it is reasonable to measure serum cholesterol and to begin disease prevention efforts that include diet modification. The Canadian Cardiovascular Society recommends reducing the amount of fat ingested in a healthy diet, substituting unsaturated fats for saturated fats, and decreasing cholesterol intake to reduce the risk of cardiovascular disease.

Certain medications that supplement dietary modification and exercise are used to reduce blood lipid levels. The medications classified as HMG-CoA reductase inhibitors or "statins," including but not limited to atorvastatin, lovastatin, pravastatin, simvastatin, fluvastatin, and rosuvastatin, are commonly used for secondary prevention and cardiovascular risk reduction (Armstrong, Chen, Westin, et al., 2014). Several other classes of medications used to reduce lipid levels include bile acid sequestrants (cholestyramine, colesevelam, colestipol) and nicotinic acid. Patients receiving long-term therapy with these medications require close monitoring.

Hypertension, which may accelerate the rate at which atherosclerotic lesions form in high-pressure vessels, can lead to a stroke, ischemic renal disease, severe PAD, or coronary artery disease. Hypertension is a major risk factor for the development of PAD and may be a more significant risk factor for women than men based upon research findings from the classic Framingham Heart Study and a similar study performed in Europe (Barochiner et al., 2014). The majority of patients with hypertension require more than two antihypertensive agents to reach goal blood pressure, and at least one third require more than three antihypertensive agents to achieve effective blood pressure control (Cooper, Murphy, Cutlip, et al., 2014). See Chapter 33 for further discussion of hypertension.

Although no single risk factor has been identified as the primary contributor to the development of atherosclerotic cardiovascular disease, it is clear that the greater the number of risk factors, the greater the risk of atherosclerosis. Elimination of all controllable risk factors, particularly the use of nicotine products, is strongly recommended.

Clinical Manifestations

The clinical signs and symptoms resulting from atherosclerosis depend on the organ or tissue affected. Coronary atherosclerosis (heart disease), angina, and acute myocardial infarction are discussed in Chapter 29. Cerebrovascular diseases, including transient cerebral ischemic attacks and stroke, are discussed in Chapter 64. Atherosclerosis of the aorta, including aneurysm, and atherosclerotic lesions of the extremities are discussed later in this chapter. Renovascular disease (renal artery stenosis and end-stage renal disease) is discussed in Chapter 45.

Medical Management

The management of atherosclerosis involves modification of risk factors, a controlled exercise program to improve circulation and its functioning capacity, medication therapy, and interventional or surgical graft procedures.

Surgical Management

Vascular surgical procedures are divided into two groups: inflow procedures, which improve blood supply from the aorta into the femoral artery, and outflow procedures, which provide blood supply to vessels below the femoral artery. Inflow surgical procedures are described with diseases of the aorta and outflow procedures with peripheral arterial occlusive disease.

Radiologic Interventions

Several interventional radiologic techniques are important adjunctive therapies to surgical procedures. If an isolated lesion or lesions are identified during the arteriogram, angioplasty, also called percutaneous transluminal angioplasty (PTA), may be performed. After the patient receives a local anesthetic agent, a balloon-tipped catheter is manoeuvred across the area of stenosis. Although some clinicians theorize that PTA improves blood flow by overstretching (and thereby dilating) the elastic fibres of the nondiseased arterial segment, most believe that the procedure widens the arterial lumen by "cracking" and flattening the plaque against the vessel wall (see Chapter 29). Complications from PTA include hematoma formation, embolus, **dissection** (separation of the intima) of the vessel, acute arterial occlusion, and bleeding. To decrease the risk of reocclusion, stents (small, mesh tubes made of nitinol, titanium, or stainless steel) may be inserted to support the walls of blood vessels and prevent collapse immediately after balloon inflation (Fig. 32-7). A variety of stents and stent grafts may be used for short-segment stenoses. Complications associated with stent or stent graft use include distal embolization, intimal damage (dissection), and dislodgment. The advantage of angioplasty, stents, and stent grafts is the decreased length of hospital stay required for the treatment; many of the procedures are performed on an outpatient basis.

Nursing Management

An overview of the care of a patient with peripheral arterial problems is provided in the Plan of Nursing Care: The Patient With Peripheral Vascular Problems (Chart 32-3).

Improving Peripheral Arterial Circulation

Arterial blood supply to a body part can be enhanced by positioning the part below the level of the heart. For the lower extremities, this is accomplished by elevating the head of the patient's bed or by having the patient use a reclining chair or sit with the feet resting on the floor.

For patients with PAD, blood flow to the lower extremities needs to be enhanced; therefore, the nurse encourages keeping the lower extremities in a neutral or dependent position. In contrast, for patients with venous insufficiency, blood return to the heart needs to be enhanced, so the lower extremities are elevated.

The nurse can assist the patient with walking or other moderate or graded isometric exercises that may be prescribed to promote blood flow and encourage the development of collateral circulation. The nurse instructs the

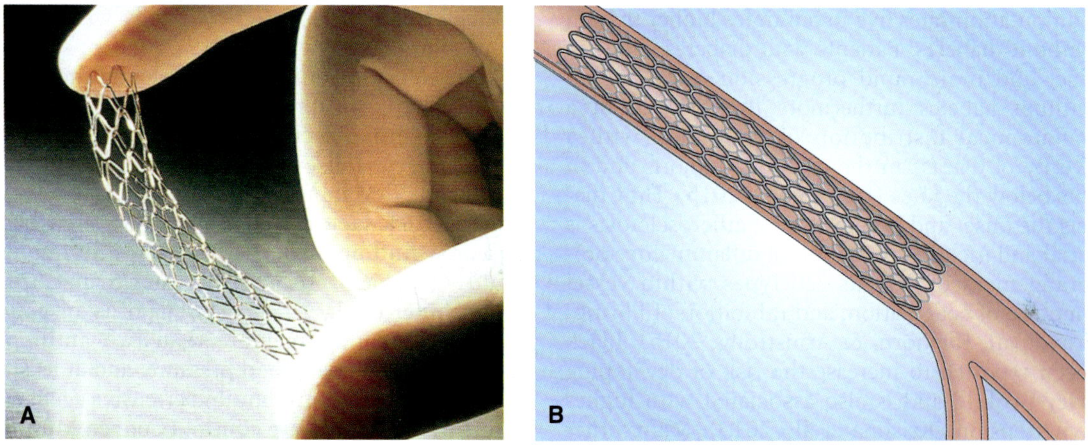

FIGURE 32-7. A. Flexible stent. (Courtesy of Medtronics, Peripheral Division, Santa Rosa, California.) B. Representation of a common iliac artery with a Wallstent.

Plan of Nursing Care — Chart 32-3. The Patient With Peripheral Vascular Problems

NURSING INTERVENTIONS	RATIONALE	EXPECTED OUTCOMES
Nursing Priority: Peripheral tissue perfusion **Goal:** Increased arterial blood supply to extremities		
1. Lower the extremities below the level of the heart (if condition is arterial in nature).	1. Dependency of lower extremities enhances arterial blood supply.	• Has extremities warm to touch • Has extremities with improved colour
2. Encourage moderate amount of walking or graded extremity exercises if no contraindications exist.	2. Muscular exercise promotes blood flow and the development of collateral circulation.	• Experiences decreased muscle pain with exercise
Goal: Decrease in venous congestion		
1. Elevate extremities above heart level (if condition is venous in nature).	1. Elevation of extremities counteracts gravity, promotes venous return, and prevents venous stasis.	• Elevates lower extremities as prescribed • Has decreased edema of extremities
2. Discourage standing still or sitting for prolonged periods.	2. Prolonged standing still or sitting promotes venous stasis.	• Avoids prolonged standing still or sitting
3. Encourage walking.	3. Walking promotes venous return by activating the "muscle pump."	• Gradually increases walking time daily
Goal: Promotion of vasodilation and prevention of vascular compression		
1. Maintain warm temperature and avoid chilling.	1. Warmth promotes arterial flow by preventing the vasoconstriction effects of chilling.	• Protects extremities from exposure to cold
2. Discourage use of tobacco products.	2. Nicotine in all tobacco products causes vasospasm, which impedes peripheral circulation.	• Avoids all tobacco products • Uses stress management program to minimize emotional upset
3. Counsel in ways to avoid emotional upsets; stress management.	3. Emotional stress causes peripheral vasoconstriction by stimulating the sympathetic nervous system.	• Avoids constricting clothing and accessories • Avoids crossing legs • Takes medication as prescribed
4. Encourage avoidance of constrictive clothing and accessories.	4. Constrictive clothing and accessories impede circulation and promote venous stasis.	
5. Encourage avoidance of crossing the legs.	5. Crossing the legs causes compression of vessels with subsequent impediment of circulation, resulting in venous stasis.	
6. Administer vasodilator medications and adrenergic blocking agents as prescribed, with appropriate nursing considerations.	6. Vasodilators relax smooth muscle; adrenergic blocking agents block the response to sympathetic nerve impulses or circulating catecholamines.	
Nursing Priority: Chronic pain management **Goal:** Relief of pain		
1. Promote increased circulation.	1. Enhancement of peripheral circulation increases the oxygen supplied to the muscle and decreases the accumulation of metabolites that cause muscle spasms.	• Uses measures to increase arterial blood supply to extremities • Uses analgesic agents as prescribed
2. Administer analgesic agents as prescribed, with appropriate nursing considerations.	2. Analgesic agents help reduce pain and allow the patient to participate in activities and exercises that promote circulation.	
Nursing Priority: Skin Care **Goal:** Attainment/maintenance of tissue integrity		
1. Instruct in ways to avoid trauma to extremities.	1. Poorly nourished tissues are susceptible to trauma and bacterial invasion; healing of wounds is delayed or inhibited due to poor tissue perfusion.	• Inspects skin daily for evidence of injury or ulceration • Avoids trauma and irritation to skin • Wears protective shoes

Plan of Nursing Care

Chart 32-3. The Patient With Peripheral Vascular Problems, *Continued*

NURSING INTERVENTIONS	RATIONALE	EXPECTED OUTCOMES
2. Encourage wearing protective shoes and padding for pressure areas; wear new shoes for short period of time and inspect feet for signs of injury.	2. Protective shoes and padding prevent foot injuries and blisters.	• Adheres to meticulous hygiene regimen • Eats a healthy diet that contains adequate protein and vitamins A and C
3. Encourage meticulous hygiene: bathing with neutral soaps, applying lotions, and carefully trimming nails.	3. Neutral soaps and lotions prevent drying and cracking of skin; avoid lotion between toes as the increased moisture can lead to maceration of tissue.	
4. Caution to avoid scratching or vigorous rubbing.	4. Scratching and rubbing can cause skin abrasions and bacterial invasion.	
5. Promote good nutrition; adequate intake of vitamins A and C, protein, and zinc; and control of obesity.	5. Good nutrition promotes healing and prevents tissue breakdown.	
Nursing Priority: Deficient knowledge **Goal:** Adherence to the self-care program		
1. Include family/significant others in teaching program.	1. Adherence to the self-care program is enhanced when the patient receives support from family and from appropriate self-help groups and agencies.	• Practices frequent position changes as prescribed • Practices postural exercises as prescribed • Takes medications as prescribed • Avoids vasoconstrictors • Uses measures to prevent trauma • Uses stress management program • Accepts condition as chronic but amenable to therapies that will decrease symptoms
2. Provide written instructions about foot care, leg care, and exercise program.	2. Written instructions serve as reminder and reinforcement of information.	
3. Assist to obtain properly fitting clothing, shoes, and stockings.	3. Constrictive clothing and accessories impede circulation and promote venous stasis.	
4. Refer to self-help groups as indicated, such as smoking cessation clinics or stress management, weight management, and exercise program.	4. Reducing risk factors may reduce symptoms or slow disease progression.	

patient to walk to the point of pain, rest until the pain subsides, and then resume walking so that endurance can be increased as collateral circulation develops. Pain can serve as a guide in determining the appropriate amount of exercise. The onset of pain indicates that the tissues are not receiving adequate oxygen, signalling the patient to rest before continuing activity. A regular exercise program can result in increased walking distance before the onset of claudication. The amount of exercise a patient can tolerate before the onset of pain is determined to provide a baseline for evaluation.

Not all patients with peripheral vascular disease should exercise. Before recommending any exercise program, the patient's primary health care provider should be consulted. Conditions that worsen with exercise include leg ulcers, cellulitis, gangrene, or acute thrombotic occlusions.

Promoting Vasodilation and Preventing Vascular Compression

Arterial dilation promotes increased blood flow to the extremities and is therefore a goal for patients with PAD. However, if the arteries are severely sclerosed, inelastic, or damaged, dilation is not possible. For this reason, measures to promote vasodilation, such as medications or surgery, may be only minimally effective.

Nursing interventions may involve applications of warmth to promote arterial flow and instructions to the patient to avoid exposure to cold temperatures, which causes vasoconstriction. Adequate clothing and warm temperatures protect the patient from chilling. If chilling occurs, a warm bath or drink is helpful. A hot water bottle or heating pad may be applied to the patient's abdomen, causing vasodilation throughout the lower extremities.

NURSING ALERT

Patients are instructed to test the temperature of bath water and to avoid using hot water bottles and heating pads on the extremities. It is safer to apply a hot water bottle or a heating pad to the abdomen; this can cause reflex vasodilation in the extremities.

In patients with vasospastic disorders (e.g., Raynaud's disease), heat may be applied directly to ischemic extremities using a warmed or electric blanket; however, the temperature of the heat source must not exceed body temperature. Even at low temperatures, trauma to the tissues can occur in ischemic extremities.

NURSING ALERT

Excess heat may increase the metabolic rate of the extremities and increase the need for oxygen beyond that provided by the reduced arterial flow through the diseased artery. Heat must be used with great caution!

Nicotine from tobacco products causes vasospasm and can thereby dramatically reduce circulation to the extremities. Tobacco smoke also impairs transport and cellular use of oxygen and increases blood viscosity. Patients with arterial insufficiency who smoke or chew tobacco must be fully informed of the effects of nicotine on circulation and are encouraged to stop.

Emotional upsets stimulate the sympathetic nervous system, resulting in peripheral vasoconstriction. Emotional stress can be minimized to some degree by avoiding stressful situations when possible or by consistently following a stress management program. Counselling services or relaxation training may be indicated for people who cannot cope effectively with situational stressors.

Constrictive clothing and accessories such as tight socks or shoelaces may impede circulation to the extremities and promote venous stasis and therefore should be avoided. Crossing the legs for more than 15 minutes at a time should be discouraged because it compresses vessels in the legs.

Relieving Pain

Frequently, the pain associated with peripheral arterial insufficiency is chronic, continuous, and disabling. It limits activities, affects work and responsibilities, disturbs sleep, and alters the patient's sense of well-being. Patients are often depressed, irritable, and unable to exert the energy necessary to execute prescribed therapies, making pain relief even more difficult. Analgesic agents such as oxycodone (OxyContin) plus acetylsalicylic acid (Aspirin), or oxycodone plus acetaminophen (Tylenol) may be helpful in reducing pain so that the patient can participate in therapies that can increase circulation and ultimately relieve pain more effectively.

Maintaining Tissue Integrity

Poorly perfused tissues are susceptible to damage and infection. When lesions develop, healing may be delayed or inhibited because of the poor blood supply to the area. Infected, nonhealing ulcerations of the extremities can be debilitating and may require prolonged and often expensive treatments. Amputation of an ischemic limb may eventually be necessary. Measures to prevent these complications must be a high priority and vigorously implemented.

Trauma to the extremities must be avoided. Advising the patient to wear sturdy, well-fitting shoes or slippers to prevent foot injury and blisters may be helpful, and recommending neutral soaps and body lotions may prevent drying and cracking of skin. However, it is important to instruct the patient not to apply lotion between the toes because the increased moisture can lead to maceration of tissue. Scratching and vigorous rubbing can abrade skin and create sites for bacterial invasion; therefore, feet should be patted dry. Stockings should be clean and dry. Fingernails and toenails should be carefully trimmed straight across and sharp corners filed to follow the contour of the nail. If the nails cannot be trimmed safely, it is necessary to consult a podiatrist, who can also remove corns and calluses. Special shoe inserts may be needed to prevent calluses from recurring. All signs of blisters, ingrown toenails, infection, or other problems should be reported to health care professionals for treatment and follow-up. Patients with diminished vision and those with disabilities that limit mobility of the arms or legs may require assistance in periodically examining the lower extremities for trauma or evidence of inflammation or infection.

Good nutrition promotes healing and prevents tissue breakdown and is therefore included in the overall therapeutic program for patients with peripheral vascular disease. Eating a diet that contains adequate protein and vitamins is necessary for patients with arterial insufficiency. Key nutrients play specific roles in wound healing. However, a meta-analysis of randomized controlled trials found no evidence to support that supplementation with vitamins and antioxidants prevents vascular diseases (Myung, Ju, Cho, et al., 2013). Vitamin C is essential for collagen synthesis and capillary development. Vitamin A enhances epithelialization. Zinc is necessary for cell mitosis and cell proliferation. Obesity strains the heart, increases venous congestion, and reduces circulation; therefore, a weight reduction plan may be necessary for some patients. A diet low in lipids may be indicated for patients with atherosclerosis.

Gerontologic Considerations

In older adults, symptoms of PAD may be more pronounced than in younger people. In older patients who are inactive, limb ischemia or gangrene may be the first sign of disease (Walker, Bunch, Cavros, et al., 2015). These patients may have adjusted their lifestyle to accommodate the limitations imposed by the disease and may not walk far enough to develop symptoms of claudication due to other comorbid conditions such as chronic obstructive pulmonary disease (COPD) or congestive heart failure. Circulation is decreased, although this is not apparent to the patient until trauma occurs. At this point, gangrene develops when minimal arterial flow is impaired further by edema formation resulting from the traumatic event.

Intermittent claudication may occur after walking only one half to one block or after walking up a slight incline. Any prolonged pressure on the foot can cause pressure areas that become ulcerated, infected, and gangrenous. The outcomes of arterial insufficiency can include reduced mobility and activity as well as a loss of independence. Older adults with reduced mobility are less likely to remain in the community setting, have higher rates of hospitalizations, and experience a poorer quality of life (Walker et al., 2015).

CHART 32-4

HOME CARE CHECKLIST • Foot and Leg Care in Peripheral Vascular Disease

At the completion of education, the patient and/or caregiver will be able to:

- Describe the rationale for proper foot and leg care in managing peripheral vascular disease.
- Demonstrate daily foot bathing: Wash between toes with mild soap and lukewarm water, then rinse thoroughly and pat rather than rub dry.
- Recognize the dangers of thermal injury.
  - Wear clean, loose, soft cotton socks (they are comfortable, allow air to circulate, and absorb moisture)
  - In cold weather, wear extra socks in extra-large shoes.
  - Avoid heating pads, whirlpools, and hot tubs.
  - Avoid sunburn.
- Identify safety concerns.
  - Inspect feet daily with a mirror for redness, dryness, cuts, blisters, and so forth.
  - Always wear soft shoes or slippers when out of bed.
  - Trim nails straight across after showering.
  - Consult podiatrist to trim nails if vision is decreased and for care of corns, blisters, and ingrown nails.
  - Clear pathways in house to prevent injury.
  - Avoid wearing thong sandals.
  - Use lamb's wool between toes if they overlap or rub each other.
- Demonstrate the use of comfort measures.
  - Wear leather shoes with an extra-depth toe box. Synthetic shoes do not allow air to circulate.
  - If feet become dry and scaly, use cream with lanolin. Never put cream between toes.
  - Avoid scratching or vigorous rubbing which could cause abrasions.
  - If feet perspire, especially between toes, use powder daily and/or lamb's wool between toes to promote drying.
- Demonstrate strategies to decrease risk of constricting blood vessels.
  - Avoid circular compression around feet or knees—e.g., by applying knee-high stockings or tight socks.
  - Do not cross legs at knees.
  - Stop using all tobacco products (i.e., smoking or chewing) because nicotine causes vasoconstriction and vasospasm.
  - Avoid applying tight, constricting bandages.
  - Participate in a regular walking exercise program to stimulate circulation.
- Recognize when to seek medical attention.
  - Contact health care provider at the onset of skin breakdown such as abrasions, blisters, fungus infection (athlete's foot), or pain.
  - Do not use any medication on feet or legs unless prescribed.
  - Avoid using iodine, alcohol, corn/wart-removing compound, or adhesive products before checking with primary provider.
- State understanding of community resources and referrals (if any).

Promoting Home, Community-Based, and Transitional Care

The self-care program is planned with the patient so that activities that promote arterial and venous circulation, relieve pain, and promote tissue integrity are acceptable. The patient and family are helped to understand the reasons for each aspect of the program, the possible consequences of nonadherence, and the importance of keeping follow-up appointments. Long-term care of the feet and legs is of prime importance in the prevention of trauma, ulceration, and gangrene. Chart 32-4 provides detailed patient instructions for foot and leg care.

Peripheral Arterial Occlusive Disease

Arterial insufficiency of the extremities occurs most often in men and is a common cause of disability. The legs are most frequently affected; however, the upper extremities may be involved. The age of onset and the severity are influenced by the type and number of atherosclerotic risk factors (Chart 32-2). In PAD, obstructive lesions are predominantly confined to segments of the arterial system extending from the aorta below the renal arteries to the popliteal artery (Fig. 32-8). Distal occlusive disease is frequently seen in patients with diabetes mellitus and in older adult patients (Conte et al., 2015).

Clinical Manifestations

The hallmark symptom is intermittent claudication. This pain may be described as aching, cramping, or inducing fatigue or weakness that occurs with the same degree of exercise or activity and is relieved with rest. The pain commonly occurs in muscle groups distal to the area of stenosis or occlusion. As the disease progresses, the patient may

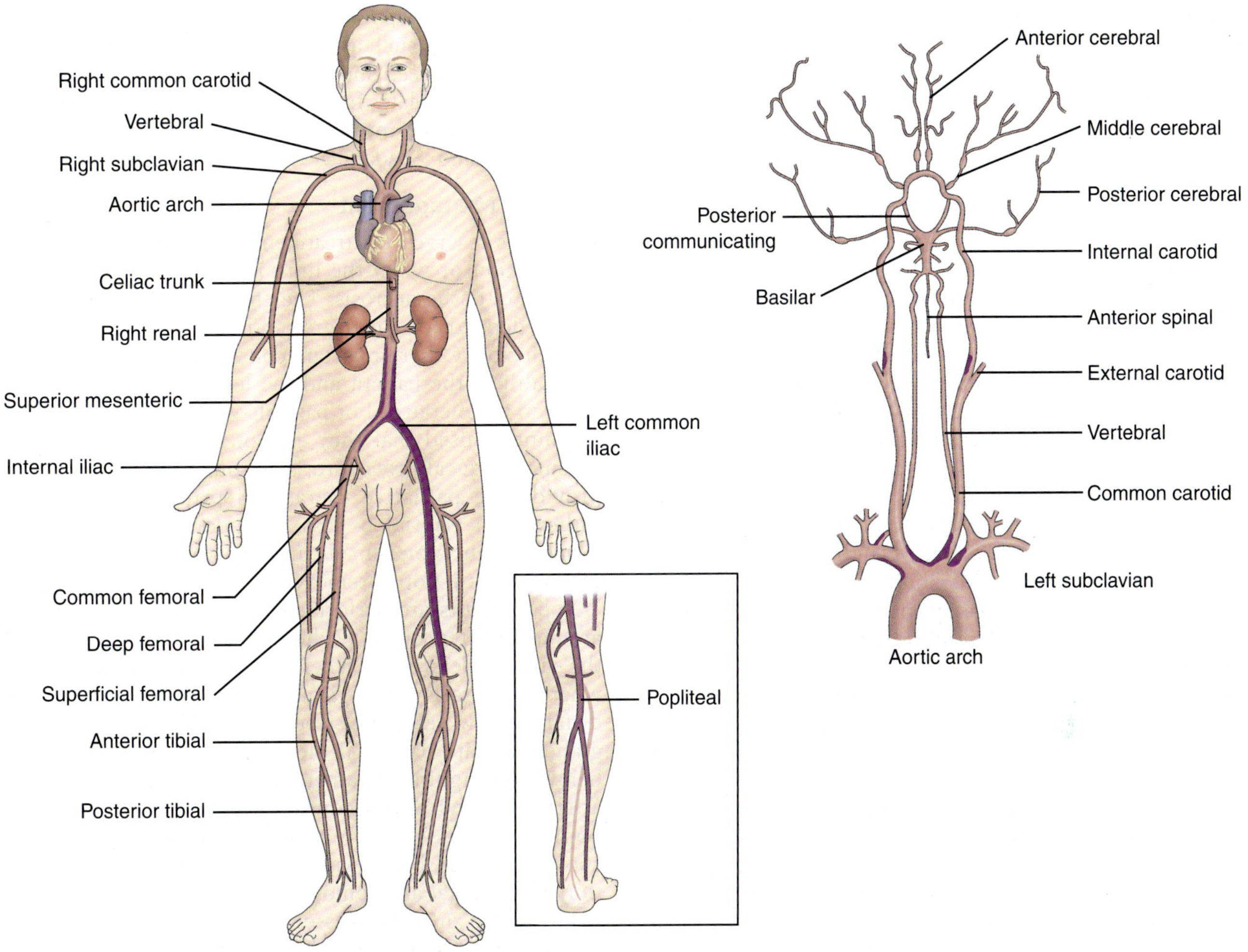

FIGURE 32-8. Common sites of atherosclerotic obstruction in major arteries.

have a decreased ability to walk the same distance as previously or may notice increased pain with ambulation. When the arterial insufficiency becomes severe, the patient has rest pain. This pain is associated with critical ischemia of the distal extremity and is persistent, aching, or boring; it may be so excruciating that it is unrelieved by opioids and is disabling. Ischemic rest pain is usually worse at night and often wakes the patient. Elevating the extremity or placing it in a horizontal position increases the pain, whereas placing the extremity in a dependent position reduces the pain. Some patients sleep with the affected leg hanging over the side of the bed. Some patients sleep in a reclining chair in an attempt to prevent or relieve the pain.

Assessment and Diagnostic Findings

A sensation of coldness or numbness in the extremities may accompany intermittent claudication and is a result of reduced arterial flow. The extremity is cool and pale when elevated or ruddy and cyanotic when placed in a dependent position. Skin and nail changes, ulcerations, gangrene, and muscle atrophy may be evident. Bruits may be auscultated with a stethoscope. Peripheral pulses may be diminished or absent.

Examination of the peripheral pulses is an important part of assessing arterial occlusive disease. Unequal pulses between extremities or the absence of a normally palpable pulse is a sign of PAD.

The presence, location, and extent of arterial occlusive disease are determined by a careful history of the symptoms and by physical examination. The colour and temperature of the extremity are noted and the pulses palpated. The nails may be thickened and opaque, and the skin may be shiny, atrophic, and dry, with sparse hair growth. The assessment includes comparison of the right and left extremities.

The diagnosis of peripheral arterial occlusive disease may be made using CW Doppler and ABIs, treadmill testing for claudication, duplex ultrasonography, or other imaging studies previously described.

Medical Management

Generally, patients feel better and have fewer symptoms of claudication after they participate in an exercise program. Unsupervised walking exercise programs are attractive for many patients with PAD as they may not have access to a supervised exercise program, their insurance will not cover a supervised exercise program, or they like the independence that an unsupervised program gives them. Two recent trials of unsupervised walking exercise in patients with PAD found similar findings between the supervised and unsupervised groups, suggesting no greater therapeutic benefit for those who engage in supervised walking programs (McDermott, 2013). These findings suggest that home-based programs may be a viable and efficacious option for patients unable to participate in a structured, on-site, supervised exercise program. If a walking program is combined with weight reduction and cessation of tobacco use, patients often can further improve their activity tolerance. Patients should not be promised that their symptoms will be relieved if they stop tobacco use, however, because claudication may persist, and they may lose their motivation to stop using tobacco. In addition to these interventions, arm-ergometer exercise training effectively improves physical fitness, central cardiorespiratory function, and walking capacity in patients with PAD claudication symptoms (McDermott, 2013).

Pharmacologic Therapy

Pentoxifylline (Trental) and cilostazol (Pletal) are approved for the treatment of symptomatic claudication. Pentoxifylline increases erythrocyte flexibility, lowers blood fibrinogen concentrations, and has antiplatelet effects. Cilostazol, a phosphodiesterase III inhibitor, is a vasodilator that inhibits platelet aggregation. Despite its physiologic effects, however, there has been no positive effect on ABIs at rest or postexercise in multiple trials; therefore, its usefulness is questionable in treatment of PAD (Conte et al., 2015).

Antiplatelet agents such as aspirin or clopidogrel (Plavix) prevent the formation of thromboemboli, which can lead to myocardial infarction and stroke. Aspirin has been shown to reduce the risk of cardiovascular events (e.g., myocardial infarction, stroke, and cardiovascular death) in patients with vascular disease; however, adverse events associated with aspirin use include gastrointestinal upset or bleeding. In a study conducted with a large, international registry of outpatients with known PAD, the 1-year rate for a cardiovascular event was high. The rate depended on whether the patient had risk factors (2.2%) alone or also symptomatic coronary or cerebrovascular disease (9.2%), suggesting that atherothrombosis is a type of global arterial disease.

Statins improve endothelial function in patients with PAD. Studies suggest that statins improve symptoms of intermittent claudication and also increase walking distance to the onset of claudication (Barochiner et al., 2014). These medications have beneficial effects on vascular inflammation, plaque stabilization, endothelial dysfunction, and thrombosis, and have been linked to decreased rates of repeat peripheral interventions, amputations, and major adverse cardiovascular events up to 3 years postprocedure (Armstrong et al., 2014).

Endovascular Management

Radiologic interventional (endovascular) management can include a balloon angioplasty, stent, stent graft, or an atherectomy. These revascularization procedures are less invasive than conventional surgery; their objective is to establish adequate inflow to the distal vessels. A recent meta-analysis reported that the efficacy and safety of all of these endovascular procedures are comparable to surgical interventions. Some stents that may be selected are drug eluting. Although costly, these are particularly efficacious in patients who have recurrent disease. By releasing antiproliferative drugs such as paclitaxel, drug-eluting balloons and stents have been shown to reduce the risk of restenosis. Eligible candidates for drug-eluting stents must be able to take antiplatelet medications for 6 months post procedure (Di Minno, Spadarella, Cafaro, et al., 2014).

Surgical Management

Surgery is reserved for treatment of severe and disabling claudication or when the limb is at risk for amputation because of tissue necrosis. The choice of the surgical procedure depends on the degree and location of the stenosis or occlusion. Other important considerations are the overall health of the patient and the length of the procedure that can be tolerated. For patients whose overall health is so compromised that they cannot tolerate an extensive vascular surgical procedure, it is sometimes necessary to provide the palliative therapy of primary amputation rather than arterial bypass. If endarterectomy is performed, an incision is made into the artery and the atheromatous obstruction is removed.

Bypass grafts are performed to reroute the blood flow around the stenosis or occlusion. Before bypass grafting, the surgeon determines where the distal **anastomosis** (site where the vessels are surgically joined) will be placed. The distal outflow vessel must be at least 50% patent for the graft to remain patent. If the atherosclerotic occlusion is below the inguinal ligament in the superficial femoral artery, the surgical procedure of choice is the femoral-to-popliteal graft. This procedure is further classified as above-knee and below-knee grafts, referring to the location of the distal anastomosis.

Lower leg or ankle vessels with occlusions may also require grafts. Occasionally, the popliteal artery is completely occluded and only collateral vessels maintain perfusion. The distal anastomosis may be made onto any of the tibial arteries (posterior tibial, anterior tibial, or peroneal arteries) or the dorsalis pedis or plantar artery. The distal anastomosis site is determined by the ease of exposure of the vessel in surgery and by which vessel provides the best flow to the distal limb. These grafts require the use of native vein (i.e., autologous; the patient's own vein) to ensure patency. The greater or lesser saphenous vein or a combination of one of the saphenous veins and an upper extremity vein such as the cephalic vein is used to provide the required length.

How long the graft remains patent is determined by several factors, including the size of the graft, graft location, and development of intimal hyperplasia at anastomosis sites. Bypass grafts may be synthetic or use autologous vein. Several synthetic materials are available for use as a peripheral bypass graft: woven or knitted Dacron or expanded polytetrafluoroethylene (ePTFE, such as Gore-Tex or Impra). Cryopreserved saphenous veins and umbilical veins are also available. Infection can be a problem that threatens survival of the graft and almost always requires its removal.

If a vein graft is the surgical choice, care must be taken in the operating room not to damage the vein after harvesting (removing the vein from the patient's body). The vein is occluded at one end and inflated with a heparinized solution to check for leakage and competency. The graft is then placed in a heparinized solution to keep it from becoming dry and brittle.

Nursing Management

Nursing care for patients with peripheral vascular disease is reviewed in Chart 30-3. Nursing care for the patient who has had endovascular revascularization procedures mostly mirrors the care of patients who have had endovascular repair to aortic aneurysms (see later section). The patient who has had an endovascular procedure may be discharged home the day of the procedure, or by the following day.

Maintaining Circulation

The primary objective in the postoperative period is to maintain adequate circulation through the arterial repair. Pulses, Doppler assessment, colour and temperature, capillary refill, and sensory and motor function of the affected extremity are checked and compared with those of the other extremity; these values are recorded initially every 15 minutes and then at progressively longer intervals if the patient's status remains stable. Doppler evaluation of the vessels distal to the bypass graft should be performed for all postoperative vascular patients because it is more sensitive than palpation for pulses. The ABI is monitored at least once every 8 hours for the first 24 hours and then once each day until discharge (not usually assessed with pedal artery bypasses). An adequate circulating blood volume should be established and maintained. Disappearance of a pulse that was present may indicate thrombotic occlusion of the graft; the surgeon is immediately notified.

Monitoring and Managing Potential Complications

Continuous monitoring of urine output, central venous pressure, mental status, and pulse rate and volume permits early recognition and treatment of fluid imbalances. Bleeding can result from the heparin administered during surgery or from an anastomotic leak. A hematoma may form as well.

Leg crossing and prolonged extremity dependency are avoided to prevent thrombosis. Edema is a normal postoperative finding; however, elevating the extremities and encouraging the patient to exercise the extremities while in bed reduces edema. Graduated compression or antiembolism stockings may be prescribed for some patients, but care must be taken to avoid compressing distal vessel bypass grafts. Severe edema of the extremity, pain, and decreased sensation of toes or fingers can be an indication of compartment syndrome (see Chapter 72).

Promoting Home, Community-Based, and Transitional Care

Discharge planning includes assessing the patient's ability to manage activities of daily living (ADLs) independently. The nurse determines whether the patient has a network of family and friends to assist with ADLs. The patient is encouraged to make the lifestyle changes necessitated by the onset of a chronic disease, including pain management and modifications in diet, activity, and hygiene (skin care). The nurse ensures that the patient has the knowledge and ability to assess for any postoperative complications such as infection, occlusion of the artery or graft, and decreased blood flow. The nurse assists the patient in developing and implementing a plan to stop using tobacco.

Nursing care for patients with peripheral vascular disease is reviewed in Chart 32-3.

Upper Extremity Arterial Occlusive Disease

Arterial occlusions occur less frequently in the upper extremities (arms) than in the legs and cause less severe symptoms because the collateral circulation is significantly better in the arms. The arms also have less muscle mass and are not subjected to the workload of the legs.

Clinical Manifestations

Stenosis and occlusions in the upper extremity result from atherosclerosis or trauma. The stenosis usually occurs at the origin of the vessel proximal to the vertebral artery, setting up the vertebral artery as the major contributor of flow. The patient typically complains of arm fatigue and pain with exercise (forearm claudication), inability to hold or grasp objects (e.g., combing hair, placing objects on shelves above the head), and occasionally difficulty driving.

The patient may develop a "subclavian steal" syndrome characterized by reverse flow in the vertebral and basilar artery to provide blood flow to the arm. This syndrome may cause vertebrobasilar (cerebral) symptoms, including vertigo, ataxia, syncope, or bilateral visual changes.

Assessment and Diagnostic Findings

Assessment findings include coolness and pallor of the affected extremity, decreased capillary refill, and a difference in arm blood pressures of more than 20 mm Hg. Noninvasive studies performed to evaluate for upper extremity arterial occlusions include upper and forearm blood pressure determinations and duplex ultrasonography to identify the anatomic location of the lesion and to evaluate the hemodynamics of the blood flow. Transcranial Doppler evaluation is performed to evaluate the intracranial circulation and to detect any siphoning of blood flow from the posterior circulation to provide blood flow to the affected arm. If a surgical or interventional procedure is planned, a diagnostic arteriogram may be necessary.

Medical Management

If a short, focal lesion is identified in an upper extremity artery, a PTA with possible stent or stent graft placement may be performed. If the lesion involves the subclavian artery with documented siphoning of blood flow from the intracranial circulation and an interventional radiologic procedure is not possible, a surgical bypass may be performed.

Nursing Management

Nursing assessment involves bilateral comparison of upper arm blood pressures (obtained by stethoscope and Doppler); radial, ulnar, and brachial pulses; motor and sensory function; temperature; colour changes; and capillary refill every 2 hours. Disappearance of a pulse or Doppler flow that had been present may indicate an acute occlusion of the vessel, and the physician is notified immediately.

After surgery, the arm is kept at heart level or elevated, with the fingers at the highest level. Pulses are monitored with Doppler assessment of the arterial flow every hour for 4 hours and then every shift. Blood pressure (obtained by stethoscope and Doppler) is also assessed every hour for 4 hours and then every shift. Motor and sensory function, warmth, colour, and capillary refill are monitored with each arterial flow (pulse) assessment.

NURSING ALERT

Before and for 24 hours after surgery, the patient's arm is kept at heart level and protected from cold, venipunctures or arterial sticks, tape, and constrictive dressings.

Discharge planning is similar to that for the patient with peripheral arterial occlusive disease. Chart 32-3 describes nursing care for patients with peripheral vascular disease.

Thromboangiitis Obliterans (Buerger's Disease)

Buerger's disease is characterized by recurring inflammation of the intermediate and small arteries and veins of the lower and upper extremities. It results in thrombus formation and segmental occlusion of the vessels. It is differentiated from other vessel diseases by its microscopic appearance. In contrast to atherosclerosis, Buerger's disease is believed to be an autoimmune vasculitis that results in occlusion of distal vessels.

Buerger's disease occurs most often in men between 20 and 35 years of age, and it has been reported in all races and in many areas of the world. There is considerable evidence that heavy smoking or chewing of tobacco is a causative or an aggravating factor (Ketha & Cooper, 2013).

Clinical Manifestations

Pain is the outstanding symptom of Buerger's disease, which is generally bilateral and symmetric with focal lesions. Superficial thrombophlebitis may be present. The patient complains of foot cramps, especially of the arch (instep claudication), after exercise. The pain is relieved by rest; often, a burning pain is aggravated by emotional disturbances, nicotine, or chilling. Cold sensitivity of the Raynaud's type is found in half the patients and is frequently confined to the hands. Digital rest pain is constant, and the characteristics of the pain do not change between activity and rest.

Physical signs include intense rubor (reddish-blue discolouration) of the foot and absence of the pedal pulse, but with normal femoral and popliteal pulses. If the upper extremities are involved, the radial and ulnar artery pulses are absent or diminished. Various types of paresthesias may develop.

As the disease progresses, definite redness or cyanosis of the part appears when the extremity is in a dependent position. Involvement is generally bilateral, but colour changes may affect only one extremity or only certain digits. Colour changes may progress to ulceration, and ulceration with gangrene eventually occurs.

Assessment and Diagnostic Findings

Segmental limb blood pressures are taken to demonstrate the distal location of the lesions or occlusions. Duplex ultrasonography is used to document patency of the proximal vessels and to visualize the extent of distal disease. Contrast angiography is used to identify the diseased portion of the anatomy.

Although Buerger's disease is different from atherosclerosis, it may be accompanied by atherosclerosis of the larger vessels. The patient's ability to walk may be severely limited. Patients are at higher risk for nonhealing wounds because of impaired circulation.

Medical Management

The treatment of Buerger's disease is essentially the same as that for atherosclerotic PAD. The main objectives are to improve circulation to the extremities, prevent the progression of the disease, and protect the extremities from trauma and infection. Treatment of ulceration and gangrene is directed toward minimizing infection and conservative débridement of necrotic tissue. Tobacco use is highly detrimental, and patients are strongly advised to completely stop using tobacco. Symptoms are often relieved by cessation of tobacco use.

Vasodilators are rarely prescribed because these medications cause dilation of only healthy vessels; vasodilators may divert blood away from the partially occluded vessels, thus exacerbating the manifestations of the disease. A regional sympathetic block or ganglionectomy may be useful in some instances to produce vasodilation and increase blood flow.

If gangrene of a toe develops as a result of arterial occlusive disease in the leg, it is unlikely that toe amputation or even transmetatarsal amputation will be sufficient; often, a below-knee amputation or occasionally an above-knee amputation is necessary. The indications for amputation include gangrene, especially if the infected area is moist; severe rest pain; or severe sepsis.

Nursing Management

The patient is assisted in developing and implementing a plan to stop using tobacco and to manage pain. The patient may need to be encouraged to make the lifestyle changes necessary to adequately manage a chronic disease, including modifications in diet, activity, and hygiene (skin care). The nurse determines whether the patient has a network of family and friends to assist with ADLs. The nurse ensures that the patient has the knowledge and ability to assess for any postoperative complications such as infection and decreased blood flow. Chart 32-3 describes nursing care for patients with peripheral vascular disease. Nursing management during the immediate postoperative phase after amputation and through the rehabilitation phase is described in Chapter 72.

Aortoiliac Disease

If collateral circulation has developed, patients with a stenosis or occlusion of the aortoiliac segment may be asymptomatic, or they may complain of buttock or low back discomfort associated with walking. Men may experience impotence. These patients may have decreased or absent femoral pulses.

Medical Management

The treatment of aortoiliac disease is essentially the same as that for atherosclerotic peripheral arterial occlusive disease. The surgical procedure of choice is the aortoiliac graft. If possible, the distal graft is anastomosed to the iliac artery, and the entire surgical procedure is performed within the abdomen. If the iliac vessels are diseased, the distal anastomosis is made to the femoral arteries (aortobifemoral graft). Bifurcated woven or knitted Dacron grafts are preferred for this surgical procedure.

Nursing Management

Preoperative assessment, in addition to the standard parameters (see Chapter 19), includes evaluating the brachial, radial, ulnar, femoral, posterior tibial, and dorsalis pedis pulses to establish a baseline for follow-up after arterial lines are placed and postoperatively. Patient teaching includes an overview of the procedure to be performed, the preparation for surgery, and the anticipated postoperative plan of care. Sights, sounds, and sensations that the patient may experience are discussed.

Postoperative care includes monitoring for signs of thrombosis in arteries distal to the surgical site. The nurse assesses colour and temperature of the extremity, capillary refill time, sensory and motor function, and pulses by palpation and Doppler initially every 15 minutes and then at progressively longer intervals if the patient's status remains stable. Any dusky or bluish discolouration, coldness, decrease in sensory or motor function, or decrease in pulse quality is reported immediately to the physician.

Postoperative care also includes monitoring urine output and ensuring that output is at least 30 mL/hr. Renal function may be impaired as a result of hypoperfusion from hypotension, ischemia to the renal arteries during the surgical procedure, hypovolemia, or embolization of the renal artery or renal parenchyma. Vital signs, pain, and intake and output are monitored with the pulse and extremity assessments. Results of laboratory tests are monitored and reported to the physician. Abdominal assessment for bowel sounds and paralytic ileus is performed at least every 8 hours. Bowel sounds may not return before the third postoperative day. The absence of bowel sounds, absence of flatus, and abdominal distention are indications of paralytic ileus. Manual manipulation of the bowel during surgery may have caused bruising, resulting in decreased peristalsis. Nasogastric suction may be necessary to decompress the bowel until peristalsis returns. A liquid bowel movement before the third postoperative day may indicate bowel ischemia, which may occur when the mesenteric blood supply (celiac, superior mesenteric, or inferior mesenteric arteries) is occluded. Ischemic bowel usually causes increased pain and a markedly elevated white blood cell count (20,000 to 30,000 cells/mm^3).

Aneurysms

An aneurysm is a localized sac or dilation formed at a weak point in the wall of the artery. It may be classified by its shape or form. The most common forms of aneurysms are saccular and fusiform. A saccular aneurysm projects from only one side of the vessel. If an entire arterial segment becomes dilated, a fusiform aneurysm develops. Very small aneurysms due to localized infection are called mycotic aneurysms.

Historically, the cause of abdominal aortic aneurysm, the most common type of degenerative aneurysm, has been attributed to atherosclerotic changes in the aorta. Other causes of aneurysm formation are listed in Chart 32-5. Aneurysms are serious because they can rupture, leading to hemorrhage and death.

Thoracic Aortic Aneurysm

Approximately 85% of all cases of thoracic aortic aneurysm are caused by atherosclerosis. They occur most frequently in men between the ages of 40 and 70 years. The thoracic area is the most common site for a dissecting aneurysm. Untreated thoracic aortic aneurysms are potentially lethal. Without intervention half of the patients dies within 48 hours, and 75% of patients within 2 weeks (Rylski, Hoffmann, Beyersdorf, et al., 2014).

CHART 32-5

Etiologic Classification of Arterial Aneurysms

Congenital: Primary connective tissue disorders (Marfan's syndrome, Ehlers–Danlos syndrome) and other diseases (focal medial agenesis, tuberous sclerosis, Turner's syndrome, Menkes' syndrome)

Mechanical (hemodynamic): Poststenotic and arteriovenous fistula and amputation related

Traumatic (pseudoaneurysms): Penetrating arterial injuries, blunt arterial injuries, pseudoaneurysms

Inflammatory (noninfectious): Associated with arteritis (Takayasu's disease, giant cell arteritis, systemic lupus erythematosus, Behçet's syndrome, Kawasaki's disease) and periarterial inflammation (i.e., pancreatitis)

Infectious (mycotic): Bacterial, fungal, spirochetal infections

Pregnancy-related degenerative: Nonspecific, inflammatory variant

Anastomotic (postarteriotomy) and graft aneurysms: Infection, arterial wall failure, suture failure, graft failure

Adapted from Cronenwett, J. L., & Johnston, K. W. (2014). *Rutherford's vascular surgery* (8th ed., Vols. 1 and 2). Philadelphia, PA: W. B. Saunders.

Clinical Manifestations

Symptoms are variable and depend on how rapidly the aneurysm dilates and how the pulsating mass affects surrounding intrathoracic structures. Some patients are asymptomatic. In most cases, pain is the most prominent symptom. The pain is usually constant and boring but may occur only when the person is supine. Other conspicuous symptoms are dyspnea, the result of pressure of the aneurysm sac against the trachea, a main bronchus, or the lung itself; cough, frequently paroxysmal and with a brassy quality; hoarseness, stridor, or weakness or complete loss of the voice (aphonia), resulting from pressure against the laryngeal nerve; and dysphagia (difficulty in swallowing) due to impingement on the esophagus by the aneurysm.

Assessment and Diagnostic Findings

When large veins in the chest are compressed by the aneurysm, the superficial veins of the chest, neck, or arms become dilated, and edematous areas on the chest wall and cyanosis are often evident. Pressure against the cervical sympathetic chain can result in unequal pupils. Diagnosis of a thoracic aortic aneurysm is principally made by chest x-ray, CTA, and transesophageal echocardiography (TEE).

Medical Management

Treatment is based on whether the aneurysm is symptomatic, is expanding in size, is caused by an iatrogenic injury, contains a dissection, and involves branch vessels. General measures such as controlling blood pressure and correcting risk factors may be helpful. It is important to control blood pressure in patients with dissecting aneurysms. Preoperatively, the systolic pressure is maintained at approximately 100 to 120 mm Hg with a beta-blocker such as esmolol or metoprolol. Occasionally, antihypertensives such as hydralazine are used for this purpose. Sodium nitroprusside (Nipride) may be used by continuous IV drip to emergently lower the blood pressure. The goal of surgery is to repair the aneurysm and restore vascular continuity with a vascular graft (Fig. 32-9). Intensive monitoring is usually required after this type of surgery, and the patient is cared for in the critical care unit.

Repair of thoracic aneurysms using endovascular grafts placed percutaneously in an interventional suite (e.g., interventional radiology, cardiac catheterization laboratory) or an operating room may decrease postoperative recovery time and decrease complications compared with traditional surgical techniques. Thoracic endografts are made of similar materials as aortic endografts, such as Gore-Tex or PTFE material reinforced with nitinol or titanium stents. These endovascular grafts are inserted into the thoracic aorta via various vascular access routes, usually the brachial or femoral artery. Because a large surgical incision is not necessary to gain vascular access, the overall patient recovery time tends to be shorter than with open surgical repair. To decrease the chances of paraplegia, spinal drains are usually placed in patients undergoing an endovascular repair of thoracic aortic aneurysms. Cerebral spinal drainage is performed to decrease the arterial to cerebral spinal fluid gradient, thereby improving spinal perfusion. What appears to be most important in preventing neurologic deficit is to maintain the blood pressure 20 mm Hg above baseline and to keep the mean arterial pressure greater than 90 mm Hg for the first 48 hours postoperatively.

Abdominal Aortic Aneurysm

The most common cause of abdominal aortic aneurysm is atherosclerosis. This condition affects men two to six times more often than women, is two to three times more

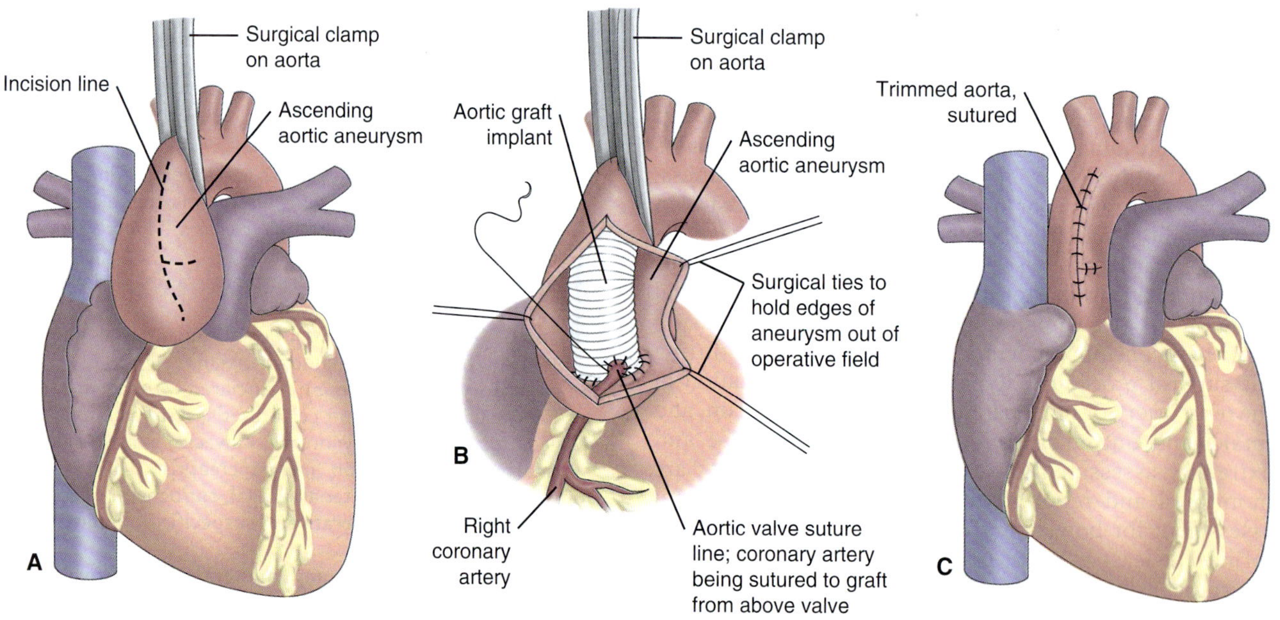

FIGURE 32-9. Repair of an ascending aortic aneurysm and aortic valve replacement. A. Incision into aortic aneurysm. B. Aortic valve replacement with aortic graft implant to repair ascending aortic aneurysm. C. Aortic aneurysm trimmed and closed over graft.

common in Caucasian versus black men, and is most prevalent in patients older than 65 years of age (Kuivaniemi, Ryer, Elmore, et al., 2014). Most of these aneurysms occur below the renal arteries (infrarenal aneurysms). Untreated, the eventual outcome may be rupture and death.

Pathophysiology

All aneurysms involve a damaged media layer of the vessel. This may be caused by congenital weakness, trauma, or disease. After an aneurysm develops, it tends to enlarge. Risk factors include genetic predisposition, tobacco use, and hypertension; more than half of patients with aneurysms have hypertension.

Clinical Manifestations

Only about 40% of patients with abdominal aortic aneurysms have symptoms. Some patients complain that they can feel their heart beating in their abdomen when lying down, or they may say they feel an abdominal mass or abdominal throbbing. If the abdominal aortic aneurysm is associated with thrombus, a major vessel may be occluded or smaller distal occlusions may result from emboli. Small cholesterol, platelet, or fibrin emboli may lodge in the interosseous or digital arteries, causing cyanosis and mottling of the toes.

Assessment and Diagnostic Findings

The most important diagnostic indication of an abdominal aortic aneurysm is a pulsatile mass in the middle and upper abdomen. About 80% of these aneurysms can be palpated. A systolic bruit may be heard over the mass. Duplex ultrasonography or CTA is used to determine the size, length, and location of the aneurysm. When the aneurysm is small, ultrasonography is conducted at 6-month intervals until the aneurysm reaches a size so that surgery to prevent rupture is of more benefit than the possible complications of a surgical procedure. Some aneurysms remain stable over many years of monitoring.

Gerontologic Considerations

Most abdominal aortic aneurysms occur in patients between 60 and 90 years of age. Rupture is likely with coexisting hypertension and with aneurysms more than 6 cm wide. In most cases at this point, the chances of rupture are greater than the chance of death during surgical repair. If the older adult patient is considered at moderate risk of complications related to surgery or anesthesia, the aneurysm is not repaired until it is at least 5.5 cm wide (De Martino, Goodney, Nolan, et al., 2013).

Medical Management

Pharmacologic Therapy

If the aneurysm is stable in size based on serial duplex ultrasound scans, the blood pressure is closely monitored over time, because there is an association between increased diastolic blood pressure (above 100 mm Hg) and aneurysm rupture (Kuivaniemi et al., 2014). Antihypertensive agents, including diuretics, beta-blockers, ACE inhibitors, angiotensin II receptor antagonists, and calcium channel blockers, are frequently prescribed to maintain the patient's blood pressure within acceptable limits (see Chapter 33).

Endovascular and Surgical Management

An expanding or enlarging abdominal aortic aneurysm is likely to rupture. When an abdominal aortic aneurysm measured at least 5.5 cm (2 in) wide or was enlarging, the standard treatment had been open surgical repair of the aneurysm by resecting the vessel and sewing a bypass graft in place. However, endovascular aortic repair has become a mainstay of therapy for treating an infrarenal abdominal aortic aneurysm and involves the transluminal placement and attachment of a sutureless aortic graft prosthesis across an aneurysm (see Fig. 32-10). This procedure can be performed under local or regional anesthesia. Endovascular grafting of abdominal aortic aneurysms may be performed if the patient's abdominal aorta and iliac arteries are not extremely tortuous, small, calcified, or filled with thrombi. Results from multiple, prospective studies suggest comparable mortality rates among patients with aneurysms treated by endovascular grafting and those treated with surgical repair, with similar 5-year survival rates (De Martino et al., 2013). Potential complications include bleeding, hematoma, or wound infection at the arterial insertion site; distal ischemia or embolization; dissection or perforation of the aorta; graft thrombosis or infection; break of the attachment system; graft migration; proximal or distal graft leaks; delayed rupture; and bowel ischemia.

Nursing Management

Before surgery, nursing assessment is guided by anticipating a rupture and by recognizing that the patient may have

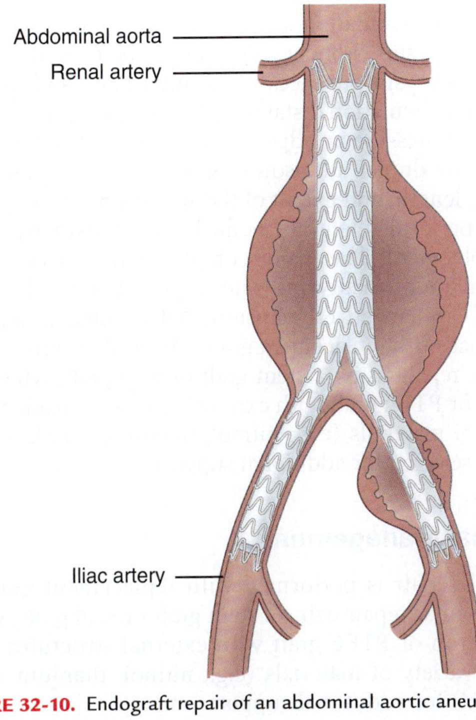

FIGURE 32-10. Endograft repair of an abdominal aortic aneurysm.

cardiovascular, cerebral, pulmonary, and renal impairment from atherosclerosis. The functional capacity of all organ systems should be assessed. Medical therapies designed to stabilize physiologic function should be promptly implemented.

Signs of impending rupture include severe back or abdominal pain, which may be persistent or intermittent. Abdominal pain is often localized in the middle or lower abdomen to the left of the midline. Low back pain may be present because of pressure of the aneurysm on the lumbar nerves. Indications of a rupturing abdominal aortic aneurysm include constant, intense back pain; falling blood pressure; and decreasing hematocrit. Rupture into the peritoneal cavity is rapidly fatal. A retroperitoneal rupture of an aneurysm may result in hematomas in the scrotum, perineum, flank, or penis. Signs of heart failure or a loud bruit may suggest a rupture into the vena cava. If the aneurysm adheres to the adjacent vena cava, the vena cava may become damaged when rupture or leak of the aneurysm occurs. Rupture into the vena cava results in higher-pressure arterial blood entering the lower-pressure venous system and causing turbulence, which is heard as a bruit. The high blood pressure and increased blood volume returning to the right side of the heart from the vena cava may cause right-sided heart failure.

Postoperative care requires frequent monitoring of pulmonary, cardiovascular, renal, and neurologic status. Possible complications of surgery include arterial occlusion, hemorrhage, infection, ischemic bowel, renal failure, and impotence.

Other Aneurysms

Aneurysms may also arise in the peripheral vessels, most often as a result of atherosclerosis. These may involve such vessels as the subclavian artery, renal artery, femoral artery, or (most frequently) popliteal artery. Between 50% and 60% of popliteal aneurysms are bilateral; the true incidence is unknown but has been reported to be between 0.1% and 3% of the adult population and is associated with abdominal aortic aneurysms (Ronchey, Pecoraro, Alberti, et al., 2015).

The aneurysm produces a pulsating mass and disturbs peripheral circulation distal to it. Pain and swelling develop because of pressure on adjacent nerves and veins. Diagnosis is made by duplex ultrasonography or CTA to determine the size, length, and extent of the aneurysm. Arteriography may be performed to evaluate the level of proximal and distal involvement. The major complication associated with popliteal artery aneurysms is not rupture but distal embolization (Cronenwett & Johnston, 2014). Surgical repair is performed with replacement grafts. As an alternative, endovascular repair using a stent graft or wall graft, which is a Dacron or PTFE graft with external structures made from a variety of materials (e.g., nitinol, titanium, stainless steel) may be selected for additional support.

Medical Management

Surgical repair is performed with replacement grafts or endovascular repair using a stent graft or wall graft, which is a Dacron or PTFE graft with external structures made from a variety of materials (e.g., nitinol, titanium, stainless steel) for additional support.

Nursing Management

The patient who has had an endovascular repair must lie supine for 6 hours; the head of the bed may be elevated up to 45 degrees after 2 hours. The patient needs to use a bedpan or urinal while on bed rest, or an indwelling urinary catheter may be used. Vital signs and Doppler assessment of peripheral pulses are performed initially every 15 minutes and then at progressively longer intervals if the patient's status remains stable. The access site (usually the femoral or iliac artery) is assessed when vital signs and pulses are monitored. The nurse assesses for bleeding, pulsation, swelling, pain, and hematoma formation. Skin changes of the lower extremity, lumbar area, or buttocks that might indicate signs of embolization, such as extremely tender, irregularly shaped, cyanotic areas, as well as any changes in vital signs, pulse quality, bleeding, swelling, pain, or hematoma, are immediately reported to the physician.

The patient's temperature should be monitored every 4 hours, and any signs of postimplantation syndrome should be reported. Postimplantation syndrome typically begins within 24 hours of stent graft placement and consists of a spontaneously occurring fever, leukocytosis, and, occasionally, transient thrombocytopenia. This condition has been attributed to complex immunologic changes, although the exact etiology is unknown. The symptoms are thought to be related to the activation of cytokines (Arnaoutoglou, Kouvelos, Koutsoumpelis, et al., 2015). They can be managed with mild analgesic or anti-inflammatory agents, such as acetaminophen (Tylenol) or ibuprofen (Motrin) and usually subside within a week.

Because of the increased risk of hemorrhage, the physician is also notified of persistent coughing, sneezing, vomiting, or systolic blood pressure greater than 180 mm Hg. Most patients can resume their preprocedure diet and are encouraged to drink fluids. An IV infusion may be continued until the patient can drink normally. Fluids are important to maintain blood flow through the arterial repair site and to assist the kidneys with excreting IV contrast agent and other medications used during the procedure. Six hours after the procedure, the patient may be able to roll from side to side and may be able to ambulate with assistance to the bathroom. Once the patient can take adequate fluids orally, the IV infusion may be discontinued and the IV access converted to a saline lock.

Dissecting Aorta

Occasionally, in an aorta diseased by arteriosclerosis, a tear develops in the intima or the media degenerates, resulting in a dissection. Arterial dissections are three times more common in men than in women and occur most commonly in the 50- to 70-year-old age group (Bergmark, Sobieszczyk, Gravereaux, et al., 2013).

Pathophysiology

Arterial dissections (separations) are commonly associated with poorly controlled hypertension, blunt chest trauma, and cocaine use. The profound increase in sympathetic response caused by cocaine use creates an increase in the force of left ventricular contraction that causes heightened shear forces upon the aortic wall. Dissection is caused by rupture in the intimal layer. A rupture may occur through adventitia or into the lumen through the intima, allowing blood to reenter the main channel and resulting in chronic dissection (e.g., pseudoaneurysm) or occlusion of branches of the aorta.

As the separation progresses, the arteries branching from the involved area of the aorta shear and occlude. The tear occurs most commonly in the region of the aortic arch, with the highest mortality rate associated with ascending aortic dissection. The dissection of the aorta may progress backward in the direction of the heart, obstructing the openings to the coronary arteries or producing hemopericardium (effusion of blood into the pericardial sac) or aortic insufficiency, or it may extend in the opposite direction, causing occlusion of the arteries supplying the gastrointestinal tract, kidneys, spinal cord, and legs.

Clinical Manifestations

Onset of symptoms is usually sudden. Severe and persistent pain, described as tearing or ripping, may be reported. The pain is in the anterior chest or back and extends to the shoulders, epigastric area, or abdomen. Aortic dissection may be mistaken for an acute myocardial infarction, which could confuse the clinical picture and initial treatment. Cardiovascular, neurologic, and gastrointestinal symptoms are responsible for other clinical manifestations, depending on the location and extent of the dissection. The patient may appear pale. Sweating and tachycardia may be detected. Blood pressure may be elevated or markedly different from one arm to the other if dissection involves the orifice of the subclavian artery on one side. Because of the variable clinical picture associated with this condition, early diagnosis is usually difficult.

Assessment and Diagnostic Findings

Arteriography, CTA, TEE, duplex ultrasonography, and MRA aid in the diagnosis.

Medical Management

The medical or surgical treatment of a dissecting aorta depends on the type of dissection present and follows the general principles outlined for the treatment of thoracic aortic aneurysms.

Nursing Management

A patient with a dissecting aorta requires the same nursing care as a patient with an aortic aneurysm requiring surgical intervention, as described earlier in this chapter. Interventions described in Chart 32-3 are also appropriate.

Arterial Embolism and Arterial Thrombosis

Acute vascular occlusion may be caused by an embolus or acute thrombosis. Acute arterial occlusions may result from iatrogenic injury, which can occur during insertion of invasive catheters such as those used for arteriography, PTA or stent placement, or an intra-aortic balloon pump, or it may occur as a result of IV drug abuse. Other causes include trauma from a fracture, crush injury, and penetrating wounds that disrupt the arterial intima. The accurate diagnosis of an arterial occlusion as embolic or thrombotic in origin is necessary to initiate appropriate treatment.

Pathophysiology

Arterial emboli arise most commonly from thrombi that develop in the chambers of the heart as a result of atrial fibrillation, myocardial infarction, infective endocarditis, or chronic heart failure. These thrombi become detached and are carried from the left side of the heart into the arterial system, where they lodge in and obstruct an artery that is smaller than the embolus. Emboli may also develop in advanced aortic atherosclerosis because the atheromatous plaques ulcerate or become rough. Acute thrombosis frequently occurs in patients with pre-existing ischemic symptoms.

Clinical Manifestations

The symptoms of arterial emboli depend primarily on the size of the embolus, the organ involved, and the state of the collateral vessels. The immediate effect is cessation of distal blood flow. The blockage can progress distal and proximal to the site of the obstruction. Secondary vasospasm can contribute to the ischemia. The embolus can fragment or break apart, resulting in occlusion of distal vessels. Emboli tend to lodge at arterial bifurcations and areas narrowed by atherosclerosis. Cerebral, mesenteric, renal, and coronary arteries are often involved in addition to the large arteries of the extremities.

The symptoms of acute arterial embolism in extremities with poor collateral flow are acute, severe pain, and a gradual loss of sensory and motor function. The six *Ps* associated with acute arterial embolism are *p*ain, *p*allor, *p*ulselessness, *p*aresthesia, *p*oikilothermia (coldness), and *p*aralysis. Eventually, superficial veins may collapse because of decreased blood flow to the extremity. Because of ischemia, the part of the extremity distal to the occlusion is markedly colder and paler than the part proximal to the occlusion.

Arterial thrombosis can also acutely occlude an artery. A thrombosis is a slowly developing clot that usually occurs where the arterial wall has become damaged, generally as a result of atherosclerosis. Thrombi may also develop in an arterial aneurysm. The manifestations of an acute thrombotic arterial occlusion are similar to those described for embolic occlusion. However, treatment is more difficult with a thrombus because the arterial occlusion has occurred in a degenerated vessel and requires more extensive reconstructive surgery to restore flow than is required with an embolic event.

Assessment and Diagnostic Findings

An arterial embolus is usually diagnosed on the basis of the sudden nature of the onset of symptoms and an apparent source for the embolus. Two-dimensional transthoracic echocardiography or TEE, chest x-ray, and electrocardiography (ECG) may reveal underlying cardiac disease. Noninvasive duplex and Doppler ultrasonography can determine the presence and extent of underlying atherosclerosis, and arteriography may be performed.

Medical Management

Management of arterial thrombosis depends on its cause. Management of acute embolic occlusion usually requires surgery because time is of the essence. Because the onset of the event is acute, collateral circulation has not developed, and the patient quickly moves through the list of six *P*s to paralysis, the most advanced stage. Heparin therapy is initiated immediately to prevent further development of emboli and to prevent the extension of existing thrombi. Typically, an initial IV bolus of 5,000 units or 60 units/kg body weight is administered, followed by a continuous infusion of 12 units/kg/hr until the patient undergoes surgery.

Surgical Management

Emergency embolectomy is the procedure of choice if the involved extremity is viable. Arterial emboli are usually treated by insertion of an embolectomy catheter. The catheter is passed through a groin incision into the affected artery and advanced past the occlusion. The catheter balloon is inflated with sterile saline solution, and the thrombus is extracted as the catheter is withdrawn. This procedure involves incising the vessel and removing the clot.

Endovascular Management

Percutaneous mechanical thrombectomy devices may also be used for the treatment of an acute thrombosis. All endovascular devices necessitate obtaining access to the patient's arterial system and inserting a catheter into the patient's artery to obtain access to the thrombus. The approach is similar to that used for angiograms in that it is made through the groin to the femoral artery. Some devices require that a small incision be made into the patient's artery. These devices may use (1) a jet of fluid to disrupt the thrombus and then aspirate the particles; (2) a rotating, sinusoidal-shaped wire that mixes a thrombolytic agent that simultaneously dissolves the clot; or (3) high-frequency, low-energy ultrasound to dissolve an occlusive thrombus. Complications arising from the use of any of the endovascular devices may include arterial dissection or distal artery embolization.

Pharmacologic Therapy

When the patient has collateral circulation, treatment may include IV anticoagulation with heparin, which can prevent the thrombus from spreading and reduce muscle necrosis. Intra-arterial thrombolytic medications are used to dissolve the embolus. Fibrin-specific thrombolytic medications (e.g., tissue plasminogen activator [t-PA, alteplase, Activase] and single-chain urokinase-type plasminogen activator [scu-PA, prourokinase]) do not deplete circulating fibrinogen and plasminogen, which prevents the development of systemic fibrinolysis. Other thrombolytic medications are reteplase (r-PA, Retavase), tenecteplase (TNKase), and staphylokinase (Harter, Levine, & Henderson, 2015). Although these agents differ in their pharmacokinetics, they are administered in a similar manner: A catheter is advanced under x-ray visualization to the clot, and the thrombolytic agent is infused.

Thrombolytic therapy should not be used when there are known contraindications to therapy or when the extremity cannot tolerate the several additional hours of ischemia that it takes for the agent to lyse (disintegrate) the clot. Contraindications to peripheral thrombolytic therapy include active internal bleeding, cerebrovascular hemorrhage, recent major surgery, uncontrolled hypertension, and pregnancy.

Nursing Management

Before surgery, the patient remains on bed rest with the affected extremity level or slightly dependent (15 degrees). The affected part is kept at room temperature and protected from trauma. Heating and cooling pads are contraindicated because ischemic extremities are easily traumatized by alterations in temperature. If possible, tape and ECG electrodes should not be used on the extremity; sheepskin and foot cradles are used to protect an affected leg from mechanical trauma (Klein & Guha, 2014).

If the patient is treated with thrombolytic therapy, the dose is based on the patient's weight. The patient is admitted to a critical care unit for continuous monitoring. Vital signs are taken initially every 15 minutes and then at progressively longer intervals if the patient's status remains stable. The patient is closely monitored for bleeding. The nurse minimizes the number of punctures for inserting IV lines and obtaining blood samples, avoids intramuscular injections, prevents any possible tissue trauma, and applies pressure at least twice as long as usual after any puncture is performed. If t-PA is used for the treatment, heparin is usually administered to prevent another thrombus from forming at the site of the lesion. The t-PA activates plasminogen on the thrombus, but it does not decrease the clotting factors as much as other thrombolytic therapies, so patients receiving t-PA can make new thrombi more readily than if they receive other thrombolytics.

During the postoperative period, the nurse collaborates with the surgeon about the patient's appropriate activity level based on the patient's condition. Generally, every effort is made to encourage the patient to move the extremity to stimulate circulation and prevent stasis. Anticoagulant therapy may be continued after surgery to prevent thrombosis of the affected artery and to diminish the development of subsequent thrombi at the initiating site. The nurse assesses for evidence of local and systemic hemorrhage, including mental status changes, which can occur when anticoagulants are administered. Pulses, Doppler signals, ABI, and motor and sensory function are assessed every hour for the first 24 hours, because significant changes may indicate reocclusion. Metabolic abnormalities, renal failure, and compartment syndrome may be complications after an acute arterial occlusion.

Raynaud's Phenomenon and Other Acrosyndromes

Raynaud's phenomenon is a form of intermittent arteriolar vasoconstriction that results in coldness, pain, and pallor of the fingertips or toes. There are two forms of this disorder. Primary or idiopathic Raynaud's (Raynaud's disease) occurs in the absence of an underlying disease. Secondary Raynaud's (Raynaud's syndrome) occurs in association with an underlying disease, usually a connective tissue disorder, such as systemic lupus erythematosus, rheumatoid arthritis, or scleroderma; trauma; or obstructive arterial lesions. Symptoms may result from a defect in basal heat production that eventually decreases the ability of cutaneous vessels to dilate. Episodes may be triggered by emotional factors or by unusual sensitivity to cold. Raynaud's phenomenon is five times more common in women with the typical onset before age 30 (Ratchford & Evans, 2015). Acrocyanosis has been thought to be a variant of Raynaud's phenomenon because both are aggravated by cold and emotional stress and both present with blue discoloration of the fingers and hyperhidrosis (excessive sweating).

The prognosis for patients with Raynaud's phenomenon varies; some slowly improve, some become progressively worse, and others show no change. Raynaud's symptoms may be mild so that treatment is not required. However, secondary Raynaud's is characterized by vasospasm and fixed blood vessel obstructions that may lead to ischemia, ulceration, and gangrene. Acrocyanosis is a poorly understood phenomenon that may be benign and require little or no treatment, or the patient may have chronic pain and ulcerations.

Clinical Manifestations

The classic clinical picture reveals pallor brought on by sudden vasoconstriction. The skin then becomes bluish (cyanotic) because of pooling of deoxygenated blood during vasospasm. As a result of exaggerated reflow (hyperemia) due to vasodilation, a red colour (rubor) is produced when oxygenated blood returns to the digits after the vasospasm stops. The characteristic sequence of colour change of Raynaud's phenomenon is described as white, blue, and red. Numbness, tingling, and burning pain occur as the colour changes. The manifestations tend to be bilateral and symmetric and may involve toes and fingers.

Acrocyanosis is differentiated from Raynaud's by a relative persistence of skin colour changes, symmetry, and an absence of the paroxysmal pallor that is found with Raynaud's. Almost all patients with acrocyanosis have marked clamminess and hyperhidrosis of their hands and feet, which tend to worsen in warmer temperatures while the colour changes improve. Finger colour normalizes when the hands are transferred from the dependent to horizontal position (Das & Maiti, 2013).

Medical Management

Avoiding the particular stimuli (e.g., cold, tobacco) that provoke vasoconstriction is a primary factor in controlling Raynaud's phenomenon. Calcium channel blockers (nifedipine [Procardia], amlodipine [Norvasc]) may be effective in relieving symptoms. Sympathectomy (interrupting the sympathetic nerves by removing the sympathetic ganglia or dividing their branches) may help some patients.

Avoidance of exposure to cold and trauma and implementing measures to improve local circulation are the primary focus of treatment for acrocyanosis. Calcium channel blockers have not been effective in treating acrocyanosis (Das & Maiti, 2013).

Nursing Management

The nurse teaches the patient to avoid situations that may be stressful or unsafe. Stress management classes may be helpful. Exposure to cold must be minimized, and in areas where the fall and winter months are cold, the patient should wear layers of clothing when outdoors. Hats and mittens or gloves should be worn at all times when outside. Fabrics specially designed for cold climates (e.g., Thinsulate) are recommended. Patients should warm up their vehicles before getting in so that they can avoid touching a cold steering wheel or door handle, which could elicit an attack. During summer, a sweater should be available when entering air-conditioned rooms.

Patients are often concerned about serious complications, such as gangrene and amputation, but these complications are uncommon unless the patient has another underlying disease causing arterial occlusions. Patients should avoid all forms of nicotine; nicotine gum or patches used to help people quit smoking may induce attacks.

Patients should be cautioned to handle sharp objects carefully to avoid injuring their fingers. Patients should be informed about the postural hypotension that may result from medications, such as calcium channel blockers, used to treat Raynaud's phenomenon.

VENOUS DISORDERS

Venous Thromboembolism

DVT and pulmonary embolism (PE) collectively make up the condition called VTE. The annual incidence of VTE is estimated at 1 to 2 per 1,000 population (Barnes, Kanthi, & Froehlich, 2015). The incidence of VTE is 10% to 20% in general medical patients and up to 80% in critically ill patients. Autopsy studies detected PE in 7% to 27% of critically ill patients; of these, only one third were clinically suspected (Minet, Potton, Bonadona, et al., 2015). VTE is frequently not diagnosed because DVT and PE are often clinically silent. It is estimated that as many as 30% of patients hospitalized with VTE develop long-term postthrombotic complications. The majority of symptomatic thromboembolic complications in surgical patients occur after hospital discharge due to short lengths of stay.

Pathophysiology

Superficial veins, such as the greater saphenous, lesser saphenous, cephalic, basilic, and external jugular veins, are thick-walled muscular structures that lie just under the skin. Deep veins are thin walled and have less muscle in the media. They run parallel to arteries and bear the same names as the arteries. Deep and superficial veins have valves that permit unidirectional flow back to the

CHART 32-6

Risk Factors: Deep Vein Thrombosis and Pulmonary Embolism

Endothelial Damage
- Trauma
- Surgery
- Pacing wires
- Central venous catheters
- Dialysis access catheters
- Local vein damage
- Repetitive motion injury

Venous Stasis
- Bed rest or immobilization
- Obesity
- History of varicosities
- Spinal cord injury
- Age (>65 years)

Altered Coagulation
- Cancer
- Pregnancy
- Oral contraceptive use
- Protein C deficiency
- Protein S deficiency
- Antiphospholipid antibody syndrome
- Factor V Leiden defect
- Prothrombin G20210A defect
- Hyperhomocysteinemia
- Elevated factors II, VIII, IX, XI
- Antithrombin III deficiency
- Polycythemia
- Septicemia

Adapted from Heit, J. A. (2015). Epidemiology of venous thromboembolism. *Nature Reviews in Cardiology*, *12*(8), 464–474.

heart. The valves lie at the base of a segment of the vein that is expanded into a sinus. This arrangement permits the valves to open without coming into contact with the wall of the vein, permitting rapid closure when the blood starts to flow backward. Other kinds of veins are known as perforating veins. These vessels have valves that allow one-way blood flow from the superficial system to the deep system.

Although the exact cause of VTE remains unclear, three factors, known as Virchow's triad, are believed to play a significant role in its development: endothelial damage, venous stasis, and altered coagulation (see Chart 32-6). Damage to the intimal lining of blood vessels creates a site for clot formation. Direct trauma to the veins may occur with fractures or dislocation, diseases of the veins, and chemical irritation of the vein from IV medications or solutions. Venous stasis occurs when blood flow is reduced, as in heart failure or shock; when veins are dilated, as an effect of some medication therapies; and when skeletal muscle contraction is reduced, as in immobility, paralysis of the extremities, or anesthesia. Altered coagulation occurs most commonly in patients for whom anticoagulant medications have been abruptly withdrawn. Oral contraceptive use, elevated CRP levels (Piazza, 2015), and several blood dyscrasias (abnormalities) also can lead to hypercoagulability, with prevalence depending on the ethnicity of the patient. Pregnancy is also considered a hypercoagulable state, as it is accompanied by an increase in clotting factors that may not return to baseline until longer than 6 weeks postpartum, increasing the risk of thrombosis. In addition, there is a 50% decrease in venous outflow due to hormonally decreased venous capacitance and reduced venous outflow due to compression from the uterus (Lucania, Camiolo, Carmina, et al., 2014).

Formation of a thrombus frequently accompanies phlebitis, which is an inflammation of the vein walls. When a thrombus develops initially in the veins as a result of stasis or hypercoagulability but without inflammation, the process is referred to as phlebothrombosis. Venous thrombosis can occur in any vein, but it occurs more often in the veins of the lower extremities. The superficial and deep veins of the extremities may be affected.

Upper extremity venous thrombosis is not as common as lower extremity thrombosis. Upper extremity venous thrombosis is more common in patients with IV catheters or in patients with an underlying disease that causes hypercoagulability. Internal trauma to the vessels may result from pacemaker leads, chemotherapy ports, dialysis catheters, or parenteral nutrition lines. The lumen of the vein may be decreased as a result of the catheter or from external compression, such as by neoplasms or an extra cervical rib. Effort thrombosis of the upper extremity is caused by repetitive motion (e.g., in competitive swimmers, tennis players, and construction workers) that irritates the vessel wall, causing inflammation and subsequent thrombosis.

Venous thrombi are aggregates of platelets attached to the vein wall that have a tail-like appendage containing fibrin, white blood cells, and many red blood cells. The "tail" can grow or can propagate in the direction of blood flow as successive layers of the thrombus form. A propagating venous thrombosis is dangerous because parts of the thrombus can break off and occlude the pulmonary blood vessels. Fragmentation of the thrombus can occur spontaneously as it dissolves naturally, or it can occur with an elevated venous pressure, such as when a person stands suddenly or engages in muscular activity after prolonged inactivity. After an episode of acute DVT, recanalization (i.e., reestablishment of the lumen of the vessel) typically occurs. The time required for complete recanalization is an important determinant of venous valvular incompetence, which is one complication of venous thrombosis. Other complications of venous thrombosis are listed in Chart 32-7.

Clinical Manifestations

A major challenge in recognizing DVT is that the signs and symptoms are nonspecific. The exception is phlegmasia cerulea dolens (massive iliofemoral venous thrombosis), in which the entire extremity becomes massively swollen, tense, painful, and cool to the touch. The large DVT

CHART 32-7

Complications of Venous Thrombosis

Chronic venous occlusion
Pulmonary emboli from dislodged thrombi
Valvular destruction:
- Chronic venous insufficiency
- Increased venous pressure
- Varicosities
- Venous ulcers

Venous obstruction:
- Increased distal pressure
- Fluid stasis
- Edema
- Venous gangrene

Adapted from Kahn, S. R., Comerota, A. J., Cushman, M., et al; American Heart Association Council on Peripheral Vascular Disease, Council on Clinical Cardiology, and Council on Cardiovascular and Stroke Nursing. (2014). The postthrombotic syndrome: Evidence-based prevention, diagnosis, and treatment strategies. A scientific statement from the American Heart Association. *Circulation, 130*, 1636–1661.

creates severe and sudden venous hypertension that leads to tissue ischemia with resultant translocation of fluid into the interstitial space. Venous gangrene occurs in 20% to 50% of cases and is associated with a poor prognosis for survival (Hu, Cai, Wang, et al., 2014).

Deep Veins

With obstruction of the deep veins comes edema and swelling of the extremity because the outflow of venous blood is inhibited. The amount of swelling can be determined by measuring the circumference of the affected extremity at various levels with a tape measure and comparing one extremity with the other at the same level to determine size differences. If both extremities are swollen, a size difference may be difficult to detect. The affected extremity may feel warmer than the unaffected extremity, and the superficial veins may appear more prominent.

Tenderness, which usually occurs later, is produced by inflammation of the vein wall and can be detected by gently palpating the affected extremity. Homans' sign (pain in the calf after the foot is sharply dorsiflexed) is *not* a reliable sign for DVT because it can be elicited in any painful condition of the calf and has no clinical value in assessment for DVT. In some cases, signs and symptoms of a pulmonary embolus are the first indication of DVT.

Superficial Veins

Thrombosis of superficial veins produces pain or tenderness, redness, and warmth in the involved area. The risk of the superficial venous thrombi becoming dislodged or fragmenting into emboli is very low because most of them dissolve spontaneously. This condition can be treated at home with bed rest, elevation of the leg, analgesic agents, and possibly anti-inflammatory medication.

Assessment and Diagnostic Findings

Careful assessment is invaluable in detecting early signs of venous disorders of the lower extremities. Patients with a history of varicose veins, hypercoagulation, neoplastic disease, cardiovascular disease, or recent major surgery or injury are at high risk. Other patients at high risk include patients with obesity, older adults, and women taking oral contraceptives.

When performing the nursing assessment, key concerns include limb pain, a feeling of heaviness, functional impairment, ankle engorgement, and edema; differences in leg circumference bilaterally from thigh to ankle; increase in the surface temperature of the leg, particularly the calf or ankle; and areas of tenderness or superficial thrombosis (i.e., cordlike venous segment).

Prevention

VTE can be prevented, especially if patients who are considered at high risk are identified and preventive measures are instituted without delay. Preventive measures include the application of graduated compression stockings, the use of intermittent pneumatic compression devices, and encouragement of early mobilization and leg exercises. An additional method to prevent venous thrombosis in surgical patients is administration of subcutaneous unfractionated or low–molecular-weight heparin (LMWH). Patients should be advised to make lifestyle changes as appropriate, which may include weight loss, smoking cessation, and regular exercise.

Medical Management

The objectives of treatment for DVT are to prevent the thrombus from growing and fragmenting (thus risking PE), recurrent thromboemboli, and postthrombotic syndrome (discussed later in the chapter) (Bonner & Johnson, 2012). Anticoagulant therapy (administration of a medication to delay the clotting time of blood, prevent the formation of a thrombus in postoperative patients, and forestall the extension of a thrombus after it has formed) can meet these objectives. However, anticoagulants cannot dissolve a thrombus that has already formed. Combining anticoagulation therapy with thrombolytic therapy may eliminate venous obstruction, maintain venous patency, and prevent postthrombotic syndrome caused by early removal of the thrombus (Jenkins & Michael, 2014).

Pharmacologic Therapy

Measures for preventing or reducing blood clotting within the vascular system are indicated in patients with thrombophlebitis, recurrent embolus formation, and persistent leg edema from heart failure. They are also indicated in older adult patients with a hip fracture that may result in lengthy immobilization. Contraindications for anticoagulant therapy are noted in Chart 32-8.

Unfractionated Heparin

Unfractionated heparin is given subcutaneously to prevent development of DVT, or by intermittent or continuous IV infusion using weight-adjusted dosing guidelines along with a vitamin K antagonist (e.g., warfarin [Coumadin]) for 5 to 7 days to prevent the extension of a thrombus and the development of new thrombi (Jenkins & Michael, 2014). Medication dosage is regulated by monitoring the

CHART 32-8

Pharmacology: Contraindications to Anticoagulant Therapy

- Lack of patient cooperation
- Bleeding from the following systems:
  - Gastrointestinal
  - Genitourinary
  - Respiratory
  - Reproductive
- Hemorrhagic blood dyscrasias
- Aneurysms
- Severe trauma
- Alcoholism
- Recent or impending surgery of the eye, spinal cord, or brain
- Severe hepatic or renal disease
- Recent cerebrovascular hemorrhage
- Infections
- Open ulcerative wounds
- Occupations that involve a significant hazard for injury
- Recent childbirth

activated partial thromboplastin time (aPTT), the international normalized ratio (INR), and the platelet count.

Low-Molecular-Weight Heparin

Subcutaneous LMWHs that may include medications such as dalteparin and enoxaparin are effective treatments for some cases of DVT. These agents have longer half-lives than unfractionated heparin, so doses can be given in one or two subcutaneous injections each day. Doses are adjusted according to weight. LMWHs prevent the extension of a thrombus and development of new thrombi, and they are associated with fewer bleeding complications and lower risks of heparin-induced thrombocytopenia (HIT) than unfractionated heparin. Because there are several preparations, the dosing schedule must be based on the product used and the protocol at each institution. The cost of LMWH is higher than that of unfractionated heparin; however, LMWH may be used safely in pregnant women, and patients who take it may be more mobile and have an improved quality of life.

Oral Anticoagulants

Warfarin is a vitamin K antagonist that is indicated for extended anticoagulant therapy. Routine coagulation monitoring is essential to ensure that a therapeutic response is obtained and maintained over time. Interactions with a range of other medications can reduce or enhance the anticoagulant effects of warfarin, as can variable intake of foods containing vitamin K. Warfarin has a narrow therapeutic window, and there is a slow onset of action. Treatment is initially supported with concomitant parenteral anticoagulation with heparin until the warfarin demonstrates anticoagulant effectiveness.

Factor Xa and Direct Thrombin Inhibitors

Fondaparinux (Arixtra) selectively inhibits factor Xa. This agent is given daily subcutaneously at a fixed dose, has a half-life of 17 hours, and is excreted unchanged via the kidneys (and therefore must be used with caution in patients with renal insufficiency). It has no effect on routine tests of coagulation, such as the aPTT or activated clotting time (ACT), so routine coagulation monitoring is unnecessary. Fondaparinux is approved for prophylaxis during major orthopedic surgery, such as hip or knee arthroplasties, and has been found to be effective for the treatment of VTE. Rivaroxaban (Xarelto) is an oral factor Xa inhibitor available for DVT prophylaxis and treatment that may be taken orally once daily; it is not indicated in patients with an estimated creatinine clearance less than 30 mL/min. Apixaban (Eliquis) is another oral factor Xa inhibitor available for DVT prophylaxis and treatment and is taken twice daily. Clinical trials have reported patients treated with apixaban had a lower risk of VTE recurrence without significantly increased risk of bleeding. Apixaban is not indicated in patients with an estimated creatinine clearance of less than 25 mL/min (Barnes et al., 2015). Dabigatran (Pradaxa), a direct thrombin inhibitor, which was FDA approved to reduce the risk of stroke and systemic embolism in patients with nonvalvular atrial fibrillation is also approved for acute and extended therapy for patients with VTE (Barnes et al., 2015). Dabigatran should be given twice daily but is not advised for patients with an estimated creatinine clearance of less than 30 mL/min. There is no need for routine coagulation laboratory monitoring or laboratory test–guided dosage adjustments; however, if measured, aPTT levels may be prolonged approximately 1.5 to 2 times (Skeik, Murphy, & Porten, 2014).

Thrombolytic Therapy

Unlike the heparins, catheter-directed thrombolytic (fibrinolytic) therapy lyses and dissolves thrombi in at least 50% of patients. Thrombolytic therapy (e.g., alteplase) is given within the first 3 days after acute thrombosis. Therapy initiated beyond 14 days after the onset of symptoms is significantly less effective. The advantages of thrombolytic therapy include less long-term damage to the venous valves and a reduced incidence of postthrombotic syndrome and chronic venous insufficiency. However, thrombolytic therapy results in a threefold greater incidence of bleeding than heparin. If bleeding occurs and cannot be stopped, the thrombolytic agent is discontinued.

Endovascular Management

Endovascular management is necessary for DVT when anticoagulant or thrombolytic therapy is contraindicated (Chart 32-8), the danger of pulmonary embolism is extreme, or venous drainage is so severely compromised that permanent damage to the extremity is likely. A thrombectomy may be necessary. This mechanical method of clot removal may involve using intraluminal catheters with a balloon or other devices. Some of these spin to break the clot, and others use oscillation to break up the clot to facilitate removal. A vena cava filter may be placed at the time of the thrombectomy; this filter traps large emboli and prevents pulmonary emboli (see Chapter 24).

Nursing Management

If the patient is receiving anticoagulant therapy, the nurse must frequently monitor the aPTT, prothrombin time (PT), INR, ACT, hemoglobin and hematocrit values, platelet count, and fibrinogen level, depending on which medication is being given. Close observation is also required to detect bleeding; if bleeding occurs, it must be reported immediately and anticoagulant therapy discontinued.

Assessing and Monitoring Anticoagulant Therapy

To prevent inadvertent infusion of large volumes of unfractionated heparin, which could cause hemorrhage, unfractionated heparin is administered by continuous IV infusion using an electronic infusion device. Dosage calculations are based on the patient's weight, and any possible bleeding tendencies are detected by a pretreatment clotting profile. If renal insufficiency exists, lower doses of heparin are required. Periodic coagulation tests and hematocrit levels are obtained. Heparin is in the effective, or therapeutic, range when the aPTT is 1.5 times the control.

Oral anticoagulants, such as warfarin, are monitored by the PT or the INR. Because the full anticoagulant effect of warfarin is delayed for 3 to 5 days, it is usually administered concurrently with heparin until desired anticoagulation has been achieved (i.e., when the PT is 1.5 to 2 times normal or the INR is 2.0 to 3.0).

Monitoring and Managing Potential Complications

Bleeding

The principal complication of anticoagulant therapy is spontaneous bleeding. Bleeding from the kidneys is detected by microscopic examination of the urine and is often the first sign of excessive dosage. Bruises, nosebleeds, and bleeding gums are also early signs. To promptly reverse the effects of heparin, IV injections of protamine sulphate may be administered. Risks of protamine administration include bradycardia and hypotension, which can be minimized by slow administration. Protamine sulphate can be used to reverse the effects of LMWH, but it is less effective with LMWH than with unfractionated heparin. Reversing the anticoagulation effects of warfarin is more difficult, but effective measures that may be prescribed include administration of vitamin K and/or infusion of fresh frozen plasma or prothrombin concentrate. Oral and low-dose IV vitamin K significantly reduces the INR within 24 hours (Dobesh & Fanikos, 2014).

Idarucizumab (Praxbind) is a humanized monoclonal antibody fragment that has been approved as a reversal agent for dabigatran (Pradaxa). It is administered IV at dosages of 5 g, provided as two separate infusions of 2.5 g/50 mL. At this time, there are no specific antidotes for the factor Xa inhibitors, although they are under development. The only option for reversal is by withholding the drugs, which have a relatively rapid rate of systemic clearance. It is recommended that activated charcoal be given within 1 to 2 hours following a dose. PCC may be used for patients with major bleeding, but its use carries the risk of disseminated intravascular coagulation (DIC) (Mohanty, Looser, Gokanapudy, et al., 2014).

Thrombocytopenia

A complication of heparin therapy may be HIT, which is defined as a sudden decrease in the platelet count by at least 30% of baseline levels. Patients at greatest risk are those who receive unfractionated heparin for a long period of time (i.e., several days or weeks). Therefore, it is preferable not to use unfractionated heparin over the long term. The administration of LMWH is less frequently associated with HIT. Beginning warfarin concomitantly with unfractionated heparin can provide a stable INR or PT by day 5 of heparin treatment, at which time the heparin may be discontinued.

The thrombocytopenia associated with HIT is thought to result from an autoimmune mechanism that causes destruction of platelets. If the process is not arrested, platelets may aggregate, initiating inappropriate clotting, and thrombosis may occur. This serious complication results in thromboembolic manifestations known as HIT with thrombosis (HITT), and the prognosis is extremely guarded.

Prevention of thrombocytopenia depends on regular monitoring of platelet counts. Early signs include a decreasing platelet count, the need for increasing doses of heparin to maintain the therapeutic level, and thromboembolic or hemorrhagic complications (appearance of skin necrosis, either at the site of injection or at distal sites where thromboses occur; skin discolouration consisting of large hemorrhagic areas; hematomas; purpura; and blistering) (Gauer & Braun, 2012). If thrombocytopenia does occur, platelet aggregation studies are performed, the heparin is discontinued, and alternate anticoagulant therapy is rapidly initiated because the continued prothrombotic state poses an ongoing threat of continuous clot development.

Lepirudin and argatroban are direct thrombin inhibitors approved for treatment of HIT. Lepirudin has a half-life of 1.3 hours, is excreted by the kidneys, and can be monitored using the aPTT. An initial IV bolus infusion followed by a continuous infusion with subsequent adjustments to maintain the aPTT between 1.5 and 2.5 times baseline is recommended. Strict dosage adjustment in renal failure is required, because the clearance of lepirudin is proportional to the patient's creatinine clearance. Argatroban has a half-life of 30 to 45 minutes, is metabolized by the liver, and is unaffected by renal function. The anticoagulant effect of argatroban is predictable, with low variability between patients, but it is dose dependent and requires monitoring with either the aPTT or ACT.

Drug Interactions

Because oral anticoagulants (i.e., warfarin) interact with many other medications and herbal and nutritional supplements, close monitoring of the patient's medication schedule is necessary. Many medications and supplements potentiate or inhibit oral anticoagulants; it is always wise to check to see if any medications or supplements are contraindicated with warfarin (see Chart 34-15). Contraindications to anticoagulant therapy are summarized in Chart 32-8.

Providing Comfort

Elevation of the affected extremity, graduated compression stockings, and analgesic agents for pain relief are adjuncts to therapy. They help improve circulation and increase comfort. Warm, moist packs applied to the affected extremity reduce the discomfort associated with DVT. The patient is encouraged to walk once anticoagulation therapy has been initiated. The nurse should instruct the patient that walking is better than standing or sitting for long periods. Bed exercises, such as repetitive dorsiflexion of the foot, are also recommended.

Stockings

Graduated compression stockings usually are prescribed for patients with venous insufficiency. The amount of pressure gradient is determined by the amount and severity of venous disease. For example, a 20 to 30 mm Hg pressure gradient is prescribed for patients with asymptomatic varicose veins, whereas at least a 40 mm Hg pressure gradient is prescribed for patients with venous stasis ulceration. These stockings should not be confused with antiembolism stockings (i.e., TED stockings) that provide less compression (12 to 20 mm Hg). Graduated compression stockings are designed to apply 100% of the prescribed pressure gradient at the ankle and pressure that decreases as the stocking approaches the thigh, reducing the calibre of the superficial veins in the leg and increasing flow in the deep veins. These stockings may be knee high, thigh high, or pantyhose.

NURSING ALERT

Any type of stocking can inadvertently become a tourniquet if applied incorrectly (i.e., rolled tightly at the top). In such instances, the stockings produce rather than prevent stasis. For ambulatory patients, graduated compression stockings are removed at night and reapplied before the legs are lowered from the bed to the floor in the morning.

When the stockings are off, the skin is inspected for signs of irritation, and the calves are examined for tenderness. Any skin changes or signs of tenderness are reported. Stockings are contraindicated in patients with severe pitting edema because they can produce severe pitting at the knee.

GERONTOLOGIC CONSIDERATIONS. Because of decreased strength and manual dexterity, older adult patients may be unable to apply graduated compression stockings properly. If this is the case, a family member or friend should be taught to assist the patient to apply the stockings so that they do not cause undue pressure on any part of the feet or legs. Frames have been designed to assist patients with applying stockings, and if there is any concern regarding patients' physical abilities, they should be referred to a stocking vendor that can provide examples and training of stocking assistance devices.

External Compression Devices and Wraps

Short stretch elastic wraps may be applied from the toes to the knee in a 50% spiral overlap. These wraps are available in a two-layer system, which includes an inner layer of soft padding. These wraps are rectangular and become squares on stretching, indicating the appropriate degree of stretch and reducing the possibility of wrapping a leg too loosely or too tightly. Three- and four-layer systems are also available (e.g., Profore, Dyna-Care), but these may be used only once compared with the two-layer system, which can be used multiple times.

Other types of compression are available. The Unna boot, which consists of a paste bandage impregnated with zinc oxide, glycerin, gelatin, and sometimes calamine, is applied without tension in a circular fashion from the base of the toes to the tibial tuberosity with a 50% spiral overlap. It is important to keep the foot dorsiflexed at a 90-degree angle to the leg, thus avoiding excess pressure or trauma to the anterior ankle area. Once the bandage dries, it provides a constant and consistent compression of the venous system. This type of compression may remain in place for as long as 1 week, although it may be too heavy for debilitated patients to handle.

The CircAid, a nonelastic leg wrap with a series of overlapping, interlocking Velcro straps, augments the effect of muscle while the patient is walking. The CircAid is usually worn during the day. Patients may find the CircAid easier to apply and wear than the Unna boot because it is lighter; they can remove it to shower, and it is adjustable. This readily adjustable feature may also be problematic; patients may be tempted to loosen the straps, and the compression achieved may not be adequate.

Intermittent Pneumatic Compression Devices

These devices can be used with elastic or graduated compression stockings to prevent DVT. They consist of an electric controller that is attached by air hoses to plastic knee-high or thigh-high sleeves. The leg sleeves are divided into compartments, which sequentially fill to apply pressure to the ankle, calf, and thigh at 35 to 55 mm Hg of pressure. These devices can increase blood velocity beyond that produced by the stockings. Nursing measures include ensuring that prescribed pressures are not exceeded, assessing for patient comfort, and ensuring compliance to therapy.

Positioning the Body and Encouraging Exercise

When the patient is on bed rest, the feet and lower legs should be elevated periodically above the level of the heart. This position allows the superficial and tibial veins to empty rapidly and to remain collapsed. Active and passive leg exercises, particularly those involving calf muscles, should be performed to increase venous flow. Early ambulation is most effective in preventing venous stasis. Deep breathing exercises are beneficial because they produce increased negative pressure in the thorax, which assists in emptying the large veins. Once ambulatory, the patient is instructed to avoid sitting for more than an hour at a time. The goal is to walk at least 10 minutes every 1 to 2 hours. The patient is also instructed to perform active and passive leg exercises as frequently as necessary when he or she cannot ambulate, such as during long car, bus, train, and plane trips.

Promoting Home, Community-Based, and Transitional Care

In addition to teaching the patient how to apply graduated compression stockings and explaining the importance of elevating the legs and exercising adequately, the nurse teaches about the prescribed anticoagulant, its purpose, and the need to take the correct amount at the specific times prescribed (Chart 32-9). The patient should also be aware that periodic blood tests are necessary to determine if a change in medication or dosage is required. If the patient fails to adhere to the therapeutic regimen, continuation of the medication therapy should be questioned. A person who

CHART 32-9

Patient Education: Taking Anticoagulant Medications

The nurse instructs the patient to:

- Take the anticoagulant medication at the same time each day, usually between 8:00 and 9:00 AM.
- Wear or carry identification indicating the anticoagulant medication being taken.
- Keep all appointments for blood tests.
- Because other medications affect the action of the anticoagulant medication do not take any of the following medications or supplements without consulting with the primary health care provider: vitamins, cold medicines, antibiotics, aspirin, mineral oil, and anti-inflammatory agents, such as ibuprofen (Motrin) and similar medications or herbal or nutritional supplements. The primary health care provider should be contacted before taking any over-the-counter drugs.
- Avoid alcohol, because it may change the body's response to an anticoagulant medication.
- Avoid food fads, crash diets, or marked changes in eating habits.
- Do not take warfarin (Coumadin) unless directed.
- Do not stop taking warfarin (when prescribed) unless directed.
- When seeking treatment from a physician, dentist, podiatrist, or another health care provider, be sure to inform the caregiver that you are taking an anticoagulant medication.
- Contact your primary health care provider before having dental work or elective surgery.
- If any of the following signs appear, report them immediately to the primary health care provider:
  - Faintness, dizziness, or increased weakness
  - Severe headaches or abdominal pain
  - Reddish or brownish urine
  - Any bleeding—for example, cuts that do not stop bleeding
  - Bruises that enlarge, nosebleeds, or unusual bleeding from any part of the body
  - Red or black bowel movements
  - Rash
- Avoid injury that can cause bleeding.
- For women: Notify the primary health care provider if you suspect pregnancy.

refuses to discontinue the use of alcohol should not receive anticoagulants because chronic alcohol use decreases their effectiveness. In patients with liver disease, the potential for bleeding may be exacerbated by anticoagulant therapy.

Chronic Venous Insufficiency/Postthrombotic Syndrome

Venous insufficiency results from obstruction of the venous valves in the legs or a reflux of blood through the valves. Superficial and deep leg veins can be involved. Resultant venous hypertension can occur whenever there has been a prolonged increase in venous pressure, such as occurs with DVT. Because the walls of veins are thinner and more elastic than the walls of arteries, they distend readily when venous pressure is consistently elevated. In this state, leaflets of the venous valves are stretched and prevented from closing completely, causing a backflow or reflux of blood in the veins. Duplex ultrasonography confirms the obstruction and identifies the level of valvular incompetence. From 20% to 50% of patients who are post-DVT when the valves in the deep veins become incompetent suffer from postthrombotic syndrome (Fig. 32-11) (Kahn, Comerota, Cushman, et al., 2014).

Clinical Manifestations

Postthrombotic syndrome is characterized by chronic venous stasis, resulting in edema, altered pigmentation, pain, and stasis dermatitis. The patient may notice the symptoms less in the morning and more in the evening. Obstruction or poor calf muscle pumping in addition to valvular reflux must be present for the development of severe postthrombotic syndrome and stasis ulcers. Superficial veins may be dilated. The disorder is long-standing, difficult to treat, and often disabling (Kahn et al., 2014).

Stasis ulcers develop as a result of the rupture of small skin veins and subsequent ulcerations. When these vessels rupture, red blood cells escape into surrounding tissues and then degenerate, leaving a brownish discolouration of the tissues. The pigmentation and ulcerations usually occur in the lower part of the extremity, in the area of the medial malleolus of the ankle. The skin becomes dry, cracks, and itches; subcutaneous tissues fibrose and atrophy. The risk of injury and infection of the extremities is increased.

Complications

Venous ulceration is the most serious complication of chronic venous insufficiency and can be associated with other conditions affecting the circulation of the lower

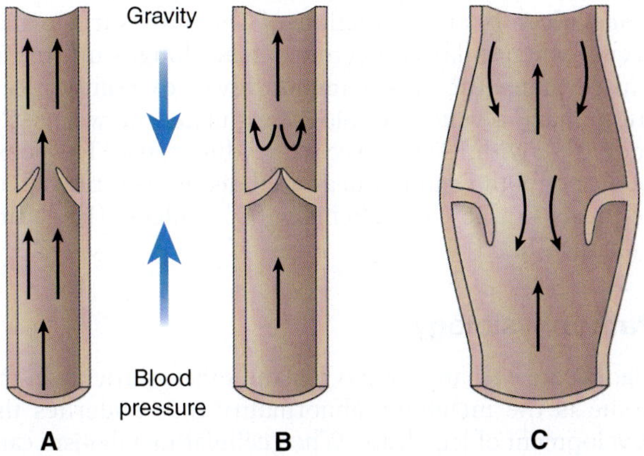

FIGURE 32-11. Competent valves showing blood flow patterns when the valve is open (A) and closed (B), allowing blood to flow against gravity. C. With faulty or incompetent valves, the blood cannot move toward the heart.

extremities. Cellulitis or dermatitis may complicate the care of chronic venous insufficiency and venous ulcerations.

Medical and Nursing Management

Management of the patient with venous insufficiency is directed at reducing venous stasis and preventing ulcerations. Measures that increase venous blood flow are antigravity activities, such as elevating the leg, and compression of superficial veins with graduated compression stockings.

Elevating the legs decreases edema, promotes venous return, and provides symptomatic relief. The legs should be elevated frequently throughout the day (at least 15 to 30 minutes every 2 hours). At night, the patient should sleep with the foot of the bed elevated about 15 cm. Prolonged sitting or standing in one position is detrimental; walking should be encouraged. When sitting, the patient should avoid placing pressure on the popliteal spaces, as occurs when crossing the legs or sitting with the legs dangling over the side of the bed. Constricting garments, especially socks that are too tight at the top or that leave marks on the skin, should be avoided.

Compression of the legs with graduated compression stockings reduces the pooling of venous blood, enhances venous return to the heart, and is recommended for people with venous insufficiency. There are no single standards for graduated compression stockings but low compression refers to pressure of less than 20 mm Hg or class 1; medium compression to pressure of 20 to 30 mm Hg or class 2; and high compression to pressure of greater than 30 mm Hg, or class 3 or higher (Sim Lim & Davies, 2014). Each stocking should fit so that pressure is greater at the foot and ankle and then gradually declines to a lesser pressure at the knee or groin. If the top of the stocking is too tight or becomes twisted, a tourniquet effect is created, which worsens venous pooling. Stockings should be applied after the legs have been elevated for a period, when the amount of blood in the leg veins is at its lowest.

Extremities with venous insufficiency must be carefully protected from trauma; the skin is kept clean, dry, and soft. Signs of ulceration are immediately reported to the health care provider for treatment and follow-up.

Leg Ulcers

A leg ulcer is an excavation of the skin surface that occurs when inflamed necrotic tissue sloughs off. In the United States the most common lower extremity ulcerations have a venous etiology (estimated between 45% and 90%), with PAD the second leading cause. The coexistence of both venous and arterial disease is estimated to be present in 26% of patients with leg ulcers (Hedayati, Carson, Chi, et al., 2015).

Pathophysiology

Inadequate exchange of oxygen and other nutrients in the tissue is the metabolic abnormality that underlies the development of leg ulcers. When cellular metabolism cannot maintain energy balance, cell death (necrosis) results. Alterations in blood vessels at the arterial, capillary, and venous levels may affect cellular processes and lead to the formation of ulcers.

Clinical Manifestations

The characteristics of leg ulcers are determined by the cause of the ulcer. Most ulcers, especially in older adults, have more than one cause. The symptoms depend on whether the problem is arterial or venous in origin (Table 32-1). The severity of the symptoms depends on the extent and duration of the vascular insufficiency. The ulcer itself appears as an open, inflamed sore. The area may be draining or covered by eschar (dark, hard crust).

Arterial Ulcers

Chronic arterial disease is characterized by intermittent claudication, which is pain caused by activity and relieved after a few minutes of rest. The patient may also complain of digital or forefoot pain at rest. If the onset of arterial occlusion is acute, ischemic pain is unrelenting and rarely relieved even with opioids. Typically, arterial ulcers are small, circular, deep ulcerations on the tips of toes or in the web spaces between the toes. Ulcers often occur on the medial side of the hallux or lateral fifth toe and may be caused by a combination of ischemia and pressure (Fig. 32-12).

Venous Ulcers

Chronic venous insufficiency is characterized by pain described as aching or heavy. The foot and ankle may be edematous. Ulcerations are in the area of the medial or lateral malleolus (gaiter area) and are typically large,

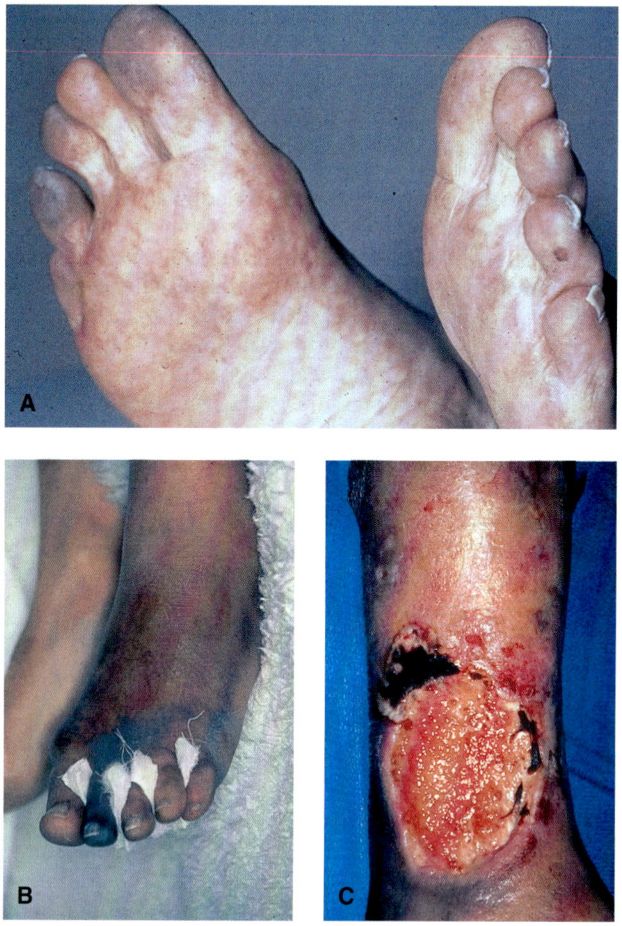

FIGURE 32-12. A. Ulcers resulting from arterial emboli. B. Gangrene of the toes resulting from severe arterial ischemia. C. Ulcer from venous stasis.

superficial, and highly exudative. Venous hypertension causes extravasation of blood, which discolours the area (Fig. 32-12). Patients with neuropathy frequently have ulcerations on the side of the foot over the metatarsal heads. These ulcers are painless and are described in further detail in Chapter 72.

Assessment and Diagnostic Findings

Because ulcers have many causes, the cause of each ulcer needs to be identified so appropriate therapy can be prescribed. The history of the condition is important in determining venous or arterial insufficiency. The pulses of the lower extremities (femoral, popliteal, posterior tibial, and dorsalis pedis) are carefully examined. More conclusive diagnostic aids are Doppler and duplex ultrasound studies, arteriography, and venography. Cultures of the ulcer bed may be necessary to determine whether an infecting agent is the primary cause of the ulcer.

Medical Management

Patients with ulcers can be effectively managed by advanced practice nurses or wound–ostomy–continence nurses in collaboration with physicians. All ulcers have the potential to become infected.

Pharmacologic Therapy

Antibiotic therapy is prescribed when the ulcer is infected; the specific antibiotic agent is based on culture and sensitivity test results. Oral antibiotics usually are prescribed because topical antibiotics have not proven to be effective for leg ulcers.

Compression Therapy

Adequate compression therapy involves the application of external or counterpressure to the lower extremity to facilitate venous return to the heart. The pressure should be applied in a gradient or graduated fashion with the pressure being somewhat higher at the ankle. Graduated compression stockings are one option; some of these are custom-made to the patient's anatomic specifications. The patient should be instructed to wear the stockings at all times except at night and to reapply the stockings in the morning before getting out of bed. Short stretch elastic wraps, Unna boots, and CircAids may be other effective options. (See Venous Thromboembolism, Compression Therapy.)

Débridement

To promote healing, the wound is kept clean of drainage and necrotic tissue. The usual method is to flush the area with normal saline solution or clean it with a noncytotoxic wound-cleansing agent (Saf-Clens, Biolex, Restore). If this is unsuccessful, débridement may be necessary. Débridement is the removal of nonviable tissue from wounds. Removing the dead tissue is important, particularly in instances of infection. Débridement can be accomplished by several different methods:

- Surgical débridement is the fastest method and can be performed by a physician, skilled advanced practice nurse, or wound–ostomy–continence nurse in collaboration with the physician.
- Nonselective débridement can be accomplished by applying isotonic saline dressings of fine-mesh gauze to the ulcer. When the dressing dries, it is removed (dry), along with the debris adhering to the gauze. Pain management is usually necessary.
- Enzymatic débridement with the application of enzyme ointments may be prescribed to treat the ulcer. The ointment is applied to the lesion but not to normal surrounding skin. Most enzymatic ointments are covered with saline-soaked gauze that has been thoroughly wrung out. A dry gauze dressing and a loose bandage are then applied. The enzymatic ointment is discontinued when the necrotic tissue has been débrided, and an appropriate wound dressing is applied.
- Calcium alginate dressings may be used for débridement when absorption of exudate is needed. These dressings are changed when the exudate seeps through the cover dressing or at least every 7 days. The dressing can also be used on areas that are bleeding, because the material helps stop the bleeding. As the dry fibres absorb exudate, they become a gel that can be painlessly removed from the ulcer bed. Calcium alginate dressings should not be used on dry or nonexudative wounds.
- Foam dressings may be an option for exudative wounds because they absorb exudate into the foam, keeping the wound moist.

Arterial insufficiency may result in gangrene of the toe (digital gangrene), which usually is caused by trauma. The toe is stubbed and then turns black (see Fig. 32-12). Usually, patients with this problem are older people without adequate circulation to provide revascularization. Débridement is contraindicated in these instances. Although the toe is gangrenous, it is dry. Managing dry gangrene is preferable to débriding the toe and causing an open wound that will not heal because of insufficient circulation. If the toe were to be amputated, the lack of adequate circulation would prevent healing and might make further amputation necessary—a below-knee or an above-knee amputation. A higher-level amputation in an older adult could result in a loss of independence and possibly the need for institutional care. Dry gangrene of the toe in an older adult with poor circulation is usually left undisturbed. The nurse keeps the toe clean and dry until it separates (without creating an open wound).

Topical Therapy

A variety of topical agents can be used in conjunction with cleansing and débridement therapies to promote healing of leg ulcers. The goals of treatment are to remove devitalized tissue and to keep the ulcer clean and moist while healing takes place. The treatment should not destroy developing tissue. For topical treatments to be successful, adequate nutritional therapy must be maintained.

Wound Dressing

After the circulatory status has been assessed and determined to be adequate for healing (ABI of more than 0.5), surgical dressings can be used to promote a moist environment. Semiocclusive or occlusive wound dressings prevent evaporative water loss from the wound and retain warmth; these factors favour healing. When determining the appropriate dressing to apply, the following should be considered: simplicity of application, frequency of required dressing changes, ability to absorb wound drainage, expense, and patient comfort. Available options that promote the growth of granulation tissue and reepithelialization include the hydrocolloids (e.g., Comfeel, DuoDERM CGF, Restore, Tegasorb). These materials also provide a barrier for protection because they adhere to the wound bed and surrounding tissue. Semipermeable film dressings (e.g., Bioclusive, OpSite, Tegaderm) may be selected because they keep the wound moist and are impervious to bacteria while allowing some gas exchange. However, they may not be effective treatment for deep wounds and infected wounds (Sood, Granick, & Tomaselli, 2014).

Growth factor dressings (e.g., OASIS, becaplermin [Regranex], keratinocyte lysate, collagen matrix Promogran) may directly provide a growth factor, or they may stimulate important growth substances within the wound. Guidelines published by the Society of Vascular Surgery and American Venous Forum note no benefit in venous ulcer healing from using silver impregnated dressings (Chi & Raffetto, 2015). Calcium alginate, hydrofiber, and hydroconductive dressings are used for wounds with moderate to high amount of exudate. The hydroconductive dressings (Levafiber) provide a capillary action that lifts and moves exudate away from a wound into the core of the dressing from where it disperses into a second layer. These dressings can be left in place for up to 7 days (Sood et al., 2014).

Knowledge deficit, frustration, fear, and depression can decrease the patient's and family's compliance with the prescribed therapy; therefore, patient and family education is necessary before beginning and throughout the wound care program.

Stimulated Healing

Tissue-engineered human skin equivalent (e.g., Apligraf [Graftskin]) is a skin product cultured from human dermal fibroblasts and keratinocytes used in combination with therapeutic compression. When applied, it interacts with the patient's cells within the wound to stimulate the production of growth factors. Application is not difficult, no suturing is involved, and the procedure is painless. PriMatrix is a bioactive and regenerative extracellular matrix that binds with the patient's own cells and growth factors. PriMatrix has been used successfully for tunnelling wounds, as well as wounds with exposed tendon and bone, in which Apligraf cannot be used. Dermagraft, which is a human fibroblast-derived dermal replacement, demonstrates efficacy similar to Apligraf (Chi & Raffetto, 2015).

Hyperbaric Oxygenation

Hyperbaric oxygenation (HBO) may be beneficial as an adjunct treatment in patients with diabetes with no signs of wound healing after 30 days of standard wound treatment. HBO is accomplished by placing the patient into a chamber that increases barometric pressure while the patient is breathing 100% oxygen. The process by which HBO is thought to work involves several factors. The edema in the wound area is decreased because high oxygen tension facilitates vasoconstriction and enhances the ability of leukocytes to phagocytize and kill bacteria. In addition, HBO is thought to increase diffusion of oxygen to the hypoxic wound, thereby enhancing epithelial migration and improving collagen production. The two most common adverse effects of HBO are middle-ear barotrauma and confinement anxiety. The benefit from this therapy on wound healing in patients without diabetes is unclear (Gould, Abadir, Brem, et al., 2015).

Negative Pressure Wound Therapy

Research findings suggest that negative pressure wound therapy using vacuum-assisted closure (VAC) devices decreases time to healing in complex wounds that have not healed in a 3-week period. Groin incisions, common in vascular surgery, may be complicated by wound dehiscence, lymphatic fistula, or infections in 5% to 10% of patients. Wound VAC therapy has been found to be effective in treating patients who develop postoperative groin wound infections, decreasing hospital lengths of stay, rates of graft infection, and likelihood of limb loss (Ingargiola, Daniali, & Lee, 2013). Patients who are ambulatory may be given the small, portable VAC devices, giving patients the freedom to perform their ADLs. Research is underway to evaluate the bacterial load and changes in the bacterial spectrum in wounds while using a VAC device (Patmo, Krijnen, Tuinebreijer, et al., 2014).

Nursing Process

The Patient With Leg Ulcers

Assessment

A careful nursing history and assessment are important. The extent and type of pain are carefully assessed, as are the appearance and temperature of the skin of both legs. The quality of all peripheral pulses is assessed, and the pulses in both legs are compared. The legs are checked for edema. If the extremity is edematous, the degree of edema is determined. Any limitation of mobility and activity that results from vascular insufficiency is identified. The patient's nutritional status is assessed, and a history of diabetes, collagen disease, or varicose veins is obtained.

Nursing Priorities

Based on the assessment data, major nursing priorities for the patient may include:

- Skin care
- Mobility
- Nutrition

Collaborative Problems/ Potential Complications

Based on the assessment data, potential complications that may develop include:

- Infection
- Gangrene

Planning and Goals

The major goals for the patient may include restoration of skin integrity, improved physical mobility, adequate nutrition, and absence of complications.

Nursing Interventions

The nursing challenge in caring for these patients is great, whether the patient is in the hospital, in a long-term care facility, or at home. The physical problem is often a long-term and disabling one that causes a substantial drain on the patient's physical, emotional, and economic resources.

Restoring Skin Integrity

To promote wound healing, measures are used to keep the area clean. Cleansing requires very gentle handling, a mild soap, and lukewarm water. Positioning of the legs depends on whether the ulcer is of arterial or venous origin. If there is arterial insufficiency, the patient should be referred for evaluation for vascular reconstruction. If there is venous insufficiency, dependent edema can be avoided by elevating the lower extremities. A decrease in edema promotes the exchange of cellular nutrients and waste products in the area of the ulcer, promoting healing.

Avoiding trauma to the lower extremities is imperative in promoting skin integrity. Protective boots may be used (e.g., Rooke Vascular boot); they are soft and provide warmth and protection from injury and displace tissue pressure to prevent ulcer formation. If the patient is on bed rest, it is important to relieve pressure on the heels to prevent pressure ulcerations. When the patient is in bed, a bed cradle can be used to relieve pressure from bed linens and to prevent anything from touching the legs. When the patient is ambulatory, all obstacles are moved from the patient's path so that the patient's legs are not bumped. Heating pads, hot water bottles, or hot baths are avoided, because they increase the oxygen demands and thus the blood flow demands of the already compromised tissue. The patient with diabetes mellitus suffers from neuropathy with decreased sensation, and heating pads may produce injury before the patient is aware of being burned.

Improving Physical Mobility

Generally, physical activity is initially restricted to promote healing. When infection resolves and healing begins, ambulation should resume gradually and progressively. Activity promotes arterial flow and venous return and is encouraged after the acute phase of the ulcer process. Until full activity is resumed, the patient is encouraged to move about when in bed, to turn from side to side frequently, and to exercise the upper extremities to maintain muscle tone and strength. Meanwhile, diversional activities are encouraged. Consultation with an occupational therapist may be helpful if prolonged immobility and inactivity are anticipated.

If pain limits the patient's activity, analgesic agents may be prescribed. The pain of peripheral vascular disease is typically chronic and often disabling. Analgesic agents may be taken before scheduled activities to help the patient participate more comfortably.

Promoting Adequate Nutrition

Nutritional deficiencies are common, requiring dietary alterations to remedy deficiencies. A diet that is high in protein, vitamins C and A, iron, and zinc is encouraged to promote healing. Many patients with peripheral vascular disease are older adults. Particular consideration should be given to their iron intake, because many older adults are anemic. After a dietary plan has been developed that meets the patient's nutritional needs and promotes healing, diet instruction is provided to the patient and family.

Promoting Home, Community-Based, and Transitional Care

The self-care program is planned with the patient so that activities that promote arterial and venous circulation, relieve pain, and promote tissue integrity are encouraged. Reasons for each aspect of the program are explained to the patient and family. Leg ulcers are often chronic and difficult to heal; they frequently recur, even when the patient rigorously follows the plan of care. Long-term care of the feet and legs to promote healing of wounds and prevent recurrence of ulcerations is the primary goal. Leg ulcers increase the patient's risk of infection, may be painful, and may limit mobility, necessitating lifestyle changes. Participation of family members and home health care providers may be necessary for treatments such as dressing changes, reassessments, reinforcement of instruction, and evaluation of the effectiveness of the plan of care. Regular follow-up with a primary health care provider is necessary.

Evaluation

Expected patient outcomes may include:

1. Demonstrates restored skin integrity
   a. Exhibits absence of inflammation
   b. Exhibits absence of drainage; negative wound culture
   c. Avoids trauma to the legs
2. Increases physical mobility
   a. Progresses gradually to optimal level of activity
   b. Reports that pain does not impede activity
3. Attains adequate nutrition
   a. Selects foods high in protein, vitamins, iron, and zinc
   b. Discusses with family members dietary modifications that need to be made at home
   c. Plans, with the family, a diet that is nutritionally sound

Varicose Veins

Varicose veins (varicosities) are abnormally dilated; tortuous, superficial veins caused by incompetent venous valves (Fig. 32-11). Most commonly, this condition occurs in the lower extremities, the saphenous veins, or the lower trunk, but it can occur elsewhere in the body, such as the esophagus (e.g., esophageal varices).

Up to 20% of the Canadian population is affected by varicose veins (Dooner, 2013). Varicose-Veins. The condition is most common in women and in people whose occupations require prolonged standing, such as salespeople, hair stylists, teachers, nurses and ancillary medical personnel, and construction workers. A hereditary weakness of the vein wall may contribute to the development of varicosities, and it commonly occurs in several members of the same family. Varicose veins are rare before puberty. Pregnancy may cause varicosities because of hormonal effects related to decreased venous outflow, increased pressure by the gravid uterus, and increased blood volume (Costantine, 2014).

Pathophysiology

Varicose veins may be primary (without involvement of deep veins) or secondary (resulting from obstruction of deep veins). A reflux of venous blood in the veins results in venous stasis. If only the superficial veins are affected, the person may have no symptoms but may be troubled by their appearance.

Clinical Manifestations

Symptoms, if present, may include dull aches, muscle cramps, increased muscle fatigue in the lower legs, ankle edema, and a feeling of heaviness of the legs. Nocturnal cramps are common. When deep venous obstruction results in varicose veins, the patient may develop the signs and symptoms of chronic venous insufficiency: edema, pain, pigmentation, and ulcerations. Susceptibility to injury and infection is increased.

Assessment and Diagnostic Findings

Diagnostic tests for varicose veins include the duplex ultrasound scan, which documents the anatomic site of reflux and provides a quantitative measure of the severity of valvular reflux. Air plethysmography measures the changes in venous blood volume. Venography is not routinely performed to evaluate for valvular reflux. However, when it is used, it involves injecting a radiopaque contrast agent into the leg veins so that the vein anatomy can be visualized by x-ray studies during various leg movements.

Prevention

The patient should avoid activities that cause venous stasis, such as wearing socks that are too tight at the top or that leave marks on the skin, crossing the legs at the thighs, and sitting or standing for long periods. Changing position frequently, elevating the legs when they are tired, and getting up to walk for several minutes of every hour promote circulation. The patient is encouraged to walk 1.5 or 3 km each day if there are no contraindications. Walking up the stairs rather than using the elevator or escalator is helpful, and swimming is good exercise.

Graduated compression stockings, especially knee-high stockings, are useful. The overweight patient should be encouraged to begin a weight reduction plan.

Medical Management

Ligation and Stripping

Surgery for varicose veins requires that the deep veins be patent and functional. The saphenous vein is ligated and divided. The vein is ligated high in the groin, where the saphenous vein meets the femoral vein. Also, the vein may be removed (stripped). After the vein is ligated, an incision is made 2 to 3 cm below the knee, and a metal or plastic wire is passed the full length of the vein to the point of ligation. The wire is then withdrawn, pulling (removing, stripping) the vein as it is removed. Pressure and elevation minimize bleeding during surgery.

If there are superficial varicose veins that are close to the surface, a micro phlebectomy may be performed. This procedure involves removal of a superficial varicosity using anywhere from 1 to 20 small incisions. There can be extensive bruising and risk of infection with this procedure.

Thermal Ablation

Thermal ablation is a nonsurgical approach using thermal energy. Radiofrequency ablation uses an electrical contact inside the vein. As the device is withdrawn, the vein is sealed. Laser ablation uses a laser fibre tip that seals the vein (decompressed). Topical gel may be used first to numb the skin along the course of the saphenous vein. To protect the surrounding tissue, several small punctures are made along the vein, and 100 to 200 mL of dilute lidocaine is delivered to the perivenous space using ultrasound guidance. The goal of this tumescent anesthesia (i.e., anesthesia that causes localized swelling) is to provide analgesia, thermal protection (the cuff of fluid surrounds the veins and accompanying nerves), and extrinsic compression of the vein (Joh, Kim, Jung, et al., 2014). The saphenous vein is entered percutaneously near the knee using ultrasound guidance. A catheter is introduced into the saphenous vein and advanced to the saphenofemoral junction. The device is then activated and withdrawn, sealing the vein. Small bandages and graduated compression stockings are applied after the procedure. The patient is asked not to remove the stockings for at least 24 hours and then to rewrap the legs and wear the compression stockings while ambulatory for at least 1-week postprocedure. A simultaneous micro phlebectomy of branch varicosities may be performed at the same time; this is associated with a lower incidence of thrombophlebitis. This is also associated with quality-of-life improvements such as decreased leg swelling, pain, skin changes and healing of ulcerations, because all symptomatic veins may be treated at one time (Jarjous, Jarjous, & Nahhas, 2015). Patients are ambulatory prior to being discharged from the outpatient facility and have no activity restrictions, except that strenuous exercise, such as weight lifting, bicycle riding, or swimming is discouraged for 2 weeks. Nonsteroidal anti-inflammatory medications such as ibuprofen (Motrin) and cool compresses are used as needed for pain. The patient is informed that bruising may occur along the course of the saphenous vein and that he or she may experience leg cramps for a few days and may find it difficult to straighten the knees for up to 1.5 weeks.

Cyanoacrylate embolization for varicose veins has recently been approved for the treatment of an incompetent greater saphenous vein. Cyanoacrylate adhesive has been used for the treatment of arteriovenous malformations and a modified cyanoacrylate adhesive was developed that has rapid polymerization on contact with blood and tissue, flexibility sufficient to tolerate dynamic movements in the legs without generation of symptoms or be perceptible by the patient, and has a high viscosity to decrease the risk of propagation or embolization into the deep veins (Morrison, Gibson, McEnroe, et al., 2015). During this procedure, a sheath is placed into the greater saphenous vein (guided by ultrasound). A catheter is advanced to the proximal saphenous vein and injections of cyanoacrylate are given, followed by local compression, and then repeated injections with repeated compression until the entire length of the target vein segment is treated. Cyanoacrylate embolization has been associated with less procedural ecchymosis because heat is not needed during this procedure.

Sclerotherapy

Sclerotherapy involves injection of an irritating chemical into a vein to produce localized phlebitis and fibrosis, thereby obliterating the lumen of the vein. This treatment may be performed alone for small varicosities or may follow vein ablation, ligation, or stripping. Sclerotherapy is typically performed in an examination or procedure room and does not require sedation. After the sclerosing agent is injected, graduated compression stockings are applied to the leg and are worn for approximately 7 days after the procedure. Ultrasound-guided foam sclerotherapy has been found to be more effective in achieving closure of the branch veins. It is also associated with decreased symptoms of leg aching, itching, and edema, less skin changes and ulcerations, and patient satisfaction in excess of 70% (Jarjous et al., 2015; Piazza, 2014). After sclerotherapy, walking activities are encouraged as prescribed to maintain blood flow in the leg.

Nursing Management

Ligation and stripping can be performed in an outpatient setting, or the patient can be admitted to the hospital on the day of surgery and discharged the next day if a bilateral procedure is to be performed and the patient is at high risk for postoperative complications. If the procedure is performed in an outpatient setting, nursing measures are the same as if the patient were hospitalized. Bed rest is discouraged and the patient is encouraged to become ambulatory as soon as sedation has worn off. The patient is instructed to walk every hour for 5 to 10 minutes while awake for the first 24 hours if he or she can tolerate the discomfort, and then to increase walking and activity as tolerated. Graduated compression stockings are worn continuously for about 1 week after vein stripping. The nurse assists the patient to perform exercises and move the legs. The foot of the bed should be elevated. Standing and sitting are discouraged.

Promoting Comfort and Understanding

Analgesic agents are prescribed to help the patient move the affected extremities more comfortably. Dressings are inspected for bleeding, particularly at the groin, where the risk of bleeding is greatest. The nurse is alert for reported sensations of "pins and needles." Hypersensitivity to touch in the involved extremity may indicate a temporary or permanent nerve injury resulting from surgery, because the saphenous vein and nerve are close to each other in the leg.

Usually, the patient may shower after the first 24 hours. The patient is instructed to dry the incisions well with a clean towel using a patting technique, rather than rubbing. Alternatively, the patient may be instructed to dry the area using a blow-dryer. Application of skin lotion is avoided until the incisions are completely healed to avoid infection. The patient is instructed to apply sunscreen or zinc oxide to the incisional area prior to sun exposure; otherwise, hyperpigmentation of the incision, scarring, or both may occur.

If the patient underwent sclerotherapy, a burning sensation in the injected leg may be experienced for 1 or 2 days. The nurse may encourage the use of a mild analgesic medication as prescribed and walking to provide relief.

Promoting Home, Community-Based, and Transitional Care

Long-term venous compression is essential after discharge, and the patient needs to obtain adequate supplies of graduated compression stockings or elastic bandages. Exercise of the legs is necessary; the development of an individualized plan requires consultation with the patient and the health care team.

LYMPHATIC DISORDERS

The lymphatic system consists of a set of vessels that spread throughout most of the body. These vessels start as lymph capillaries that drain unabsorbed plasma from the interstitial spaces (spaces between the cells). The lymphatic capillaries unite to form the lymph vessels, which pass through the lymph nodes and then empty into the large thoracic duct that joins the jugular vein on the left side of the neck.

The fluid drained from the interstitial space by the lymphatic system is called lymph. The flow of lymph depends on the intrinsic contractions of the lymph vessels, the contraction of muscles, respiratory movements, and gravity. The lymphatic system of the abdominal cavity maintains a steady flow of digested fatty food (chyle) from the intestinal mucosa to the thoracic duct. In other parts of the body, the lymphatic system's function is regional; the lymphatic vessels of the head, for example, empty into clusters of lymph nodes located in the neck, and those of the extremities empty into nodes of the axillae and the groin.

Lymphangitis and Lymphadenitis

Lymphangitis is an acute inflammation of the lymphatic channels. It arises most commonly from a focus of infection in an extremity. Usually, the infectious organism is a hemolytic streptococcus. The characteristic red streaks that extend up the arm or the leg from an infected wound outline the course of the lymphatic vessels as they drain.

The lymph nodes located along the course of the lymphatic channels also become enlarged, red, and tender (acute lymphadenitis). They can also become necrotic and form an abscess (suppurative lymphadenitis). The nodes involved most often are those in the groin, axilla, or cervical region.

Because these infections are nearly always caused by organisms that are sensitive to antibiotics, it is unusual to see abscess formation. Recurrent episodes of lymphangitis are often associated with progressive lymphedema. After acute attacks, a graduated compression stocking should be worn on the affected extremity for several months to prevent long-term edema.

Lymphedema and Elephantiasis

Lymphedema may be primary (congenital malformations) or secondary (acquired obstructions). Tissue swelling occurs in the extremities because of an increased quantity of lymph that results from obstruction of lymphatic vessels. It is especially marked when the extremity is in a dependent position. Initially, the edema is soft and pitting. As the condition progresses, the edema becomes firm, nonpitting, and unresponsive to treatment. The most common type is congenital lymphedema (lymphedema praecox), which is caused by hypoplasia of the lymphatic system of the lower extremity. This disorder is usually seen in women and first appears before age 35 (Brouillard, Boon, & Vikkula, 2014).

The obstruction may be in the lymph nodes and the lymphatic vessels. Sometimes, it is seen in the arm after an axillary node dissection (e.g., for breast cancer) and in the leg in association with varicose veins or chronic thrombophlebitis. In the latter case, the lymphatic obstruction usually is caused by chronic lymphangitis. Lymphatic obstruction caused by a parasite (filaria) is most frequently seen in the tropics. When chronic swelling is present, there may be frequent bouts of acute infection characterized by high fever and chills and increased residual edema after the inflammation has resolved. These lead to chronic fibrosis, thickening of the subcutaneous tissues, and hypertrophy of the skin. This condition, in which chronic swelling of the extremity recedes only slightly with elevation, is referred to as elephantiasis. There are an estimated 120 million people in the world infected by lymph-dwelling filarial parasites; of these, 40 million have lymphedema and secondary infections, creating an enormous global burden (Mortimer & Rockson, 2014).

Medical Management

The goal of therapy is to reduce and control the edema and prevent infection. Active and passive exercises assist in moving lymphatic fluid into the bloodstream. External compression devices milk the fluid proximally from the foot to the hip or from the hand to the axilla. When the patient is ambulatory, custom-fitted graduated compression stockings or sleeves are worn; those with the highest compression strength (exceeding 40 mm Hg) are suggested; however, many patients cannot tolerate the pressure. When the leg is affected, continuous bed rest with the leg elevated may aid in mobilizing the fluids. Manual lymphatic drainage performed by specially trained therapists is a technique designed to direct or shift the congested lymph through functioning lymphatics that have preserved drainage. Manual lymphatic drainage is incorporated in a sequential treatment approach used in combination with multilayer compression bandages, exercises, skin care, pressure gradient sleeves, and pneumatic pumps, depending on the severity and stage of the lymphedema (Zaleska et al., 2014).

Pharmacologic Therapy

As initial therapy, the diuretic furosemide (Lasix) may be prescribed to prevent fluid overload due to mobilization of extracellular fluid. Diuretics have also been used along with elevation of the leg and the use of graduated compression stockings or sleeves. However, the use of diuretics alone has little benefit because their main action is to limit capillary filtration by decreasing the circulating blood volume. If lymphangitis or cellulitis is present, antibiotic therapy is initiated. Lymphedema carries a 71-fold enhancement of risk for cellulitis; therefore, the patient is taught to inspect the skin for evidence of infection (Mortimer & Rockson, 2014).

Surgical Management

Surgery is performed if the edema is severe and uncontrolled by medical therapy, if mobility is severely compromised, or if infection persists. One surgical approach involves the excision of the affected subcutaneous tissue and fascia, with skin grafting to cover the defect. Another procedure involves the surgical relocation of superficial lymphatic vessels into the deep lymphatic system, also known as lymph node transfer, by means of a buried dermal flap to provide a conduit for lymphatic drainage (Ciudad, Orfaniotis, Socas, et al., 2015). Lymphaticovenous bypasses also are performed with anastomosing the end of the lymphatic vessels to the side of veins to reduce lymphatic flow in the limbs (Qiu, Chen, & Cheng, 2014).

Nursing Management

After surgery, the management of skin grafts and flaps is the same as when these therapies are used for other conditions. Antibiotics may be prescribed for 5 to 7 days. Constant elevation of the affected extremity and observation for complications are essential. Complications may include flap necrosis, hematoma or abscess under the flap, and cellulitis. The nurse instructs the patient or caregiver to inspect the dressing daily. Unusual drainage or any inflammation around the wound margin suggests infection and should be reported to the surgeon. The patient is informed that there may be a loss of sensation in the skin graft area. The patient is also instructed to avoid the application of heating pads or exposure to sun to prevent burns or trauma to the area.

CELLULITIS

Cellulitis is the most common infectious cause of limb swelling. Cellulitis can occur as a single isolated event or a series of recurrent events. It is sometimes misdiagnosed as recurrent thrombophlebitis or chronic venous insufficiency.

Pathophysiology

Cellulitis occurs when an entry point through normal skin barriers allows bacteria to enter and release their toxins in the subcutaneous tissues.

Clinical Manifestations

The acute onset of swelling, localized redness, and pain is frequently associated with systemic signs of fever, chills, and sweating. The redness may not be uniform and often skips areas. Regional lymph nodes may also be tender and enlarged (Horseman & Bowman, 2013).

NURSING ALERT

Cellulitis needs to be differentiated from lymphangitis. With cellulitis, the swelling and redness is localized and anatomically nonspecific. With lymphangitis, characteristic red streaks appear denoting the outline of the lymphatic vessels that are affected.

Medical Management

Mild cases of cellulitis can be treated on an outpatient basis with oral antibiotic therapy. If the cellulitis is severe, the patient is treated with IV antibiotics. The key to preventing recurrent episodes of cellulitis lies in adequate antibiotic therapy for the initial event and in identifying the site of bacterial entry. Cracks and fissures that occur in the skin between the toes must be examined as potential sites of bacterial entry. Other locations include drug use injection sites, contusions, abrasions, ulceration, ingrown toenails, and hangnails.

Nursing Management

The patient is instructed to elevate the affected area above heart level and apply warm, moist packs to the site every 2 to 4 hours. Patients with sensory and circulatory deficits, such as those caused by diabetes and paralysis, should use caution when applying warm packs because burns may occur; it is advisable to use a thermometer or have a caregiver ensure that the temperature is not more than lukewarm. Education should focus on preventing a recurrent episode. The patient with peripheral vascular disease or diabetes mellitus should receive education or reinforcement about skin and foot care.

Critical Thinking Exercises

1 A 55-year-old female presents to the emergency department with 4- to 6-hour history of chest and back pain, hoarse voice, and difficulty swallowing. She is taking apixaban (Eliquis) for atrial fibrillation and has renal insufficiency (creatinine of 2.2 mg/dL) as a complication of poorly managed diabetes. Her blood glucose is 420 mg/dL and you note her blood pressure is 200/102 mm Hg. She admits to using methamphetamines today but insists she hasn't taken any other drugs. What additional assessment and vital signs need to be obtained? What are your priority assessments for this patient? Is the methamphetamine impacting the diagnosis and treatment? How would you triage and prioritize your nursing care for this patient?

2 A 22-year-old female college student presents to campus health care with complaints of left upper extremity edema and a generalized ache of her shoulder and upper arm that is worse at the end of the day. She noted the onset of the symptoms 2 months ago after joining an intramural volleyball team. She is concerned as she has noted new veins across her left shoulder and upper chest wall. There is a positive maternal family history for DVT. What further diagnostic studies should be performed? Are there any labs that should be drawn? At the time of her clinic visit she mentions that she would like to begin taking birth control pills. What is the strength of the evidence that supports the best method of contraception for her, assuming she is at risk for thromboembolism? What additional information should you obtain? What risks should you discuss with this patient? Should she be given birth control pills at this visit?

3 A 54-year-old man presents to the community clinic. He needs a physical examination prior to beginning a job as a cashier at a local grocery store. The patient is found to have a history of diabetes that has not been consistently managed, and has a 38-year history of smoking a pack of cigarettes each day. Physical examination reveals blood pressure of 162/104 mm Hg, absent anterior tibial and posterior tibial artery pulses, bilateral varicose veins, and 1+ pitting ankle edema. What additional information is needed as part of the history and physical examination? What risk factor modifications would you want to address with this patient?

REFERENCES AND SELECTED READINGS

Books

Cronenwett, J. L., & Johnston, K. W. (2014). *Rutherford's vascular surgery.* (8th ed., *Vols. I and II*). Philadelphia, PA: W. B. Saunders.

Grossman, S., & Porth, C. M. (2014). *Porth's pathophysiology: Concepts of altered health states.* (9th ed.). Philadelphia, PA: Lippincott Williams & Wilkins.

Hannon, R. A. (2017). *Porth pathophysiology: Concepts of altered health states.* Philadelphia, PA: Wolters Kluwer.

Weber, J. R., & Kelley, J. H. (2014). *Health assessment in nursing* (5th ed.). Philadelphia, PA: Lippincott Williams & Wilkins.

Zierler, R. E., & Dawson, D. L. (2015). *Strandness's duplex scanning in vascular disorders.* (5th ed.). Philadelphia, PA: Lippincott Williams & Wilkins.

Journals and Electronic Documents

Armstrong, E. J., Chen, D. C., Westin, G. G., et al. (2014). Adherence to guideline-recommended therapy is associated with decreased major adverse cardiovascular events and major adverse limb events among patients with peripheral arterial disease. *Journal of the American Heart Association, 3*, e000697.

Arnaoutoglou, E., Kouvelos, G., Koutsoumpelis, A., et al. (2015). An update on the inflammatory response after endovascular repair for abdominal aortic aneurysm. *Mediators of Inflammation, 2015*, 945035. Hindawi Publishing Corporation, Article ID 945035, 6 pages, dx.doi.org/10.1155/2015/945035.

Barnes, G. D., Kanthi, Y., & Froehlich, J. B. (2015). Venous thromboembolism: Predicting recurrence and the need for extended anticoagulation. *Vascular Medicine, 20*(2), 143–152.

Barochiner, J., Aparicio, L. S., & Waisman, G. D. (2014). Challenges associated with peripheral arterial disease in women. *Vascular Health and Risk Management, 10*, 115–128.

Bergmark, B. A., Sobieszczyk, P., Gravereaux, E. C., et al. (2013). Acute dissection of the descending aorta: A case report and review of the literature. *Cardiology and Therapy, 2*, 199–213.

Birn, J., & Vedantham, S. (2015). May-Thurner syndrome and other obstructive iliac vein lesions: Meaning, myth, and mystery. *Vascular Medicine, 20*, 74–83.

Bonner, L., & Johnson, J. (2014). Deep vein thrombosis: Diagnosis and treatment. *Nursing standard, 28*(21).

Bremme, K., Hamad, R. R., Berg, E., et al. (2012). The APC-PCI concentration as an early marker of activation of blood coagulation. A study of women on combined oral contraceptives. *Thrombosis Research, 130*, 636–639.

Brouillard, P., Boon, L., & Vikkula, M. (2014). Genetics of lymphatic anomalies. *The Journal of Clinical Investigation, 124*(3), 898–904.

Chi, Y. W., & Raffetto, J. D. (2015). Venous leg ulceration pathophysiology and evidence based treatment. *Vascular Medicine, 20*(2), 168–181.

Ciudad, P., Orfaniotis, G., Socas, J., et al. (2015). Technical considerations to avoid microvascular complications during groin lymph node free flap transfer. *Archives of Plastic Surgery, 42*(5), 650–652.

Conte, M. S., Pomposelli, F. B., Clair, D. G., et al. (2015). Society for vascular surgery practice guidelines for atherosclerotic occlusive disease of the lower extremities: Management of asymptomatic disease and claudication. *Journal of Vascular Surgery, 61*(3 Suppl), 2S–41S.

Cooper, C. J., Murphy, T. P., Cutlip, D. E., et al; CORAL Investigators. (2014). Stenting and medical therapy for atherosclerotic renal-artery stenosis. *The New England Journal of Medicine, 370*(1), 13–22.

Costantine, M. M. (2014). Physiologic and pharmacokinetic changes in pregnancy. *Frontiers in Pharmacology*, *5*, 65.

Das, S., & Maiti, A. (2013). Acrocyanosis: An overview. *Indian Journal of Dermatology*, *58*(6), 417–420.

De Martino, R. R., Goodney, P. P., Nolan, B. W., et al; Vascular Study Group of New England. (2013). Optimal selection of patients for elective abdominal aortic aneurysm repair based on life expectancy. *Journal of Vascular Surgery*, *58*(3), 589–595.

Di Minno, G., Spadarella, G., Cafaro, G., et al. (2014). Systematic reviews and meta-analyses for more profitable strategies in peripheral artery disease. *Annals of Medicine*, *46*(7), 475–489.

Dobesh, P. P., & Fanikos, J. (2014). New oral anticoagulants for the treatment of venous thromboembolism: Understanding differences and similarities. *Drugs*, *74*, 2015–2032.

Favero, G., Paganelli, C., Buffoli, B., et al. (2014). Endothelium and its alterations in cardiovascular diseases: Life style intervention. *BioMed Research International*, *2014*, 801896.

Fernandes, J., Arts, J., Dimond, E., et al. (2013). Dietary factors are associated with coronary heart disease risk factors in college students. *Nutrition Research*, *33*, 647–652.

Gauer, R. L., & Braun, M. M. (2012). Thrombocytopenia. *American Family Physician, 85*(6).

Gould, L., Abadir, P., Brem, H., et al. (2015). Chronic wound repair and healing in older adults: current status and future research. *Wound Repair and Regeneration, 23*(1), 1–13.

Harter, K., Levine, M., & Henderson, S. O. (2015). Anticoagulation drug therapy: A review. *Western Journal of Emergency Medicine*, *16*(1), 11–17.

Hedayati, N., Carson, J. G., Chi, Y. W., et al. (2015). Management of mixed arterial venous lower extremity ulceration: A review. *Vascular Medicine*, *20*(5), 479–486.

Horseman, M., & Bowman, J. D. (2013). Is community-acquired methicillin-resistant Staphylococcus aureus coverage needed for cellulitis?. *Infectious Diseases and Therapy*, 2, 175–185.

Hu, H., Cai, Y., Wang, C., et al. (2014). Successful treatment of posttraumatic phlegmasia cerulea dolens by reconstructing the external iliac vein: A case report. *Journal of Medical Case Reports*, *8*, 149.

Ingargiola, M. J., Daniali, L. N., & Lee, E. S. (2013). Does the application of incisional negative pressure therapy to high-risk wounds prevent surgical site complications? A systematic review. *Eplasty*, *13*, e49. Retrieved on October 26, 2015, from www.eplasty.com

Jarjous, F., Jarjous, R., & Nahhas, G. (2015). One-step approach to treating venous insufficiency. *Journal of Clinical Medicine Research*, *7*(9), 681–684.

Jenkins, J. S., & Michael, P. (2014). Deep venous thrombosis: An interventionalist's approach. *The Ochsner Journal*, *14*, 633–640.

Joh, J. H., Kim, W. S., Jung, I. M., et al; Consensus Working Group. (2014). Consensus for the treatment of varicose vein with radiofrequency ablation. *Vascular Specialist International*, *30*(4), 105–112.

Kahn, S. R., Comerota, A. J., Cushman, M., et al; American Heart Association Council on Peripheral Vascular Disease, Council on Clinical Cardiology, and Council on Cardiovascular and Stroke Nursing. (2014). The postthrombotic syndrome: Evidence-based prevention, diagnosis, and treatment strategies: A scientific statement from the American Heart Association. *Circulation*, *130*, 1636–1661.

Ketha, S. S., & Cooper, L. T. (2013). The role of autoimmunity in thromboangiitis obliterans (Buerger's disease). *Annals of the New York Academy of Sciences*, *1285*, 15–25.

Klein, K. C., & Guha, S. C. (2014). Cutaneous wound healing: Current concepts and advances in wound care. *Indian Journal of Plastic Surgery*, *47*(3), 303–317.

Krishna, S. M., Moxon, J. V., & Golledge, J. (2015). A review of the pathophysiology and potential biomarkers for peripheral artery disease. *International Journal of Molecular Sciences*, *16*, 11294–11322.

Kuivaniemi, H., Ryer, E. J., Elmore, J. R., et al. (2014). Update on abdominal aortic aneurysm research: From clinical to genetic studies. *Scientifica*, *2014*, 564734.

Lim, M. Y., & Moll, S. (2015). Thrombophilia. *Vascular Medicine*, *20*(2), 193–196.

Lucania, G., Camiolo, E., Carmina, M. G., et al. (2014). Multidisciplinary approach in pregnancy-associated thrombotic thrombocytopenic purpura: A case report. *Blood Transfusion*, *12*(Suppl 1), s137–s140.

McDermott, M. M. (2013). Functional impairment in peripheral artery disease and how to improve it in 2013. *Current Cardiology Reports*, *15*(4), 347.

Minet, C., Potton, L., Bonadona, A., et al. (2015). Venous thromboembolism in the ICU: Main characteristics, diagnosis and thromboprophylaxis. *Critical Care*, *19*, 287.

Mohanty, B. D., Looser, P. M., Gokanapudy, L. R., et al. (2014). Controversies regarding the new oral anticoagulants for stroke prevention in patients with atrial fibrillation. *Vascular Medicine*, *19*(3), 190–204.

Morrison, N., Gibson, K., McEnroe, S., et al. (2015). Randomized trial comparing cyanoacrylate embolization and radiofrequency ablation for incompetent great saphenous veins (VeClose). *Journal of Vascular Surgery*, *61*(4), 985–994.

Mortimer, P. S., & Rockson, S. G. (2014). New developments in clinical aspects of lymphatic disease. *The Journal of Clinical Investigation*, *124*(3), 915–921.

Myung, S. K., Ju, W., Cho, B., et al. (2013). Efficacy of vitamin and antioxidant supplements in prevention of cardiovascular disease: Systematic review and meta-analysis of randomised controlled trials. *British Medical Journal*, *346*, f10.

Patmo, A. S., Krijnen, P., Tuinebreijer, W. E., et al. (2014). The effect of vacuum-assisted closure on the bacterial load and type of bacteria: A systematic review. *Advances in Wound Care*, *3*(5), 383–389.

Piazza, G. (2014). Varicose veins. *Circulation*, *130*, 582–587.

Piazza, G. (2015). Beyond Virchow's triad: Does cardiovascular inflammation explain the recurrent nature of venous thromoembolism?. *Vascular Medicine*, *20*(2), 102–104.

Prete, M., Fatone, M. C., Favoino, E., et al. (2014). Raynaud's phenomenon: From molecular pathogenesis to therapy. *Autoimmunity Reviews*, *13*, 655–667.

Puranik, A. S., Dawson, E. R., & Peppas, N. A. (2013). Recent advances in drug eluting stents. *International Journal of Pharmaceutics*, *441*(1–2), 665–679.

Qiu, S. S., Chen, H. Y., & Cheng, M. H. (2014). Vascularized lymph node flap transfer and lymphovenous anastomosis for Klippel-Trenaunay syndrome with congenital lymphedema. *Plastic and Reconstructive Surgery Global Open*, *2*, e167.

Ratchford, E. V., & Evans, N. S. (2015). Raynaud's phenomenon. *Vascular Medicine*, *20*(3), 269–271.

Ronchey, S., Pecoraro, F., Alberti, V., et al. (2015). Popliteal artery aneurysm repair in the endovascular era. Fourteen-years single center experience. *Medicine (Baltimore)*, *94*(30), e1130. Retrieved on November 14, 2015, from www.md-journal.com

Rylski, B., Hoffmann, I., Beyersdorf, F., et al. (2014). Acute aortic dissection type A: Age-related management and outcomes reported in the German registry for acute aortic dissection Type A (GERAADA) of over 2000 patients. *Annals of Surgery*, *259*(3), 598–604.

Sadat, U. (2013). Radiographic contrast-media-induced acute kidney injury: Pathophysiology and prophylactic strategies. *ISRN Radiology*, *2013*, 496438.

Sim Lim, C., & Davies, A. H. (2014). Graduated compression stockings. *Canadian Medical Association Journal*, *186*(10), E391–E398.

Skeik, N., Murphy, C. J., & Porten, B. R. (2014). The role of novel anticoagulants in the management of venous thromboembolism. *Vascular Medicine*, *19*(3), 205–214.

Sood, A., Granick, M. S., & Tomaselli, N. L. (2014). Wound dressings and comparative effectiveness data. *Advances in Wound Care (New Rochelle)*, *3*(8), 511–529.

Thiruvoipati, T., Kielhorn, C. E., & Armstrong, E. J. (2015). Peripheral artery disease in patients with diabetes: Epidemiology, mechanisms, and outcomes. *World Journal of Diabetes*, *6*(7), 961–969.

Walker, C. M., Bunch, F. T., Cavros, N. G., et al. (2015). Multidisciplinary approach to the diagnosis and management of patients with peripheral arterial disease. *Clinical Interventions in Aging*, *10*, 1147–1153.

Zaleska, M., Olszewski, W. L., & Durlik, M. (2014). The effectiveness of intermittent pneumatic compression in long-term therapy of lymphedema of lower limbs. *Lymphatic Research and Biology*, *12*(2), 103–109.

Ziganshin, B. A., Dumfarth, J., & Elefteriades, J. A. (2014). Natural history of type B aortic dissection: Ten tips. *Annals of Cardiothoracic Surgery*, *3*(3), 247–254.

Resources

Canadian Cardiovascular Society: http://www.ccs.ca

Canadian Healthcare Association: Guide to Canadian Healthcare Facilities: http://www.cha.ca

Canadian Society for Vascular Surgery: http://www.csvs.vascularweb.org

Centre for Chronic Disease Prevention and Control, Cardiovascular Disease, Public Agency of Canada: http://www.phacaspc.gc.ca

Dooner, J. 2013: https://canadianvascular.ca/Varicose-Veins

Vascular Disease Foundation: http://www.vdf.org

Vascular Web: http://www.vascularweb.org

33 Assessment and Management of Patients With Hypertension

Adapted by Kelly Power-Kean

Learning Objectives

On completion of this chapter, the learner will be able to:

1. Define normal blood pressure and categories of abnormal pressures.
2. Identify risk factors for hypertension.
3. Explain the differences between normal blood pressure and hypertension and discuss the significance of hypertension.
4. Describe treatment approaches for hypertension, including lifestyle modification and medication therapy.
5. Use the nursing process as a framework for care of the patient with hypertension.
6. Describe hypertensive crises and their treatments.

Hypertension is a chronic medical condition in which blood pressure in the arteries is elevated and remains above the goal set for blood pressures. Hypertension is one of the most common chronic diseases affecting Canadians (Nerenberg, Zarnke, Leung, et al., 2018). It is identified as the leading risk factor for premature death, disability, and overall disease burden worldwide because it may lead to myocardial infarction, heart failure, stroke, and chronic kidney disease when not appropriately treated (Mozaffarian, Benjamin, Go, et al., 2016). The overall risk of developing these cardiovascular and renal disorders is low among patients with blood pressures (BPs) that are consistently stable around 115/75 mm Hg; however, each increase of 20 mm Hg in the systolic BP or 10 mm Hg in the diastolic BP doubles the risk for having a cardiovascular event (e.g., heart attack or stroke) (Weber, Schiffrin, White, et al., 2014). Most patients with hypertension may lower their blood pressure, thereby significantly modifying these risks (see Chart 33-1), through lifestyle changes (e.g., diet, exercise, smoking cessation) and adhering to appropriate medication regimens. This chapter presents an overview of hypertension and how it is classified and managed so that nurses may appropriately assess, monitor, educate, and intervene with patients with hypertension.

Hypertension

Nerenberg et al. (2018), in association with Hypertension Canada (2018a), have established comprehensive guidelines for the diagnosis and treatment of hypertension. Hypertension in persons without diabetes is defined as an automated office blood pressure (AOBP) 135/85 mm Hg or higher or non-AOBP ≥140/90 mm Hg or higher. For those patients diagnosed with diabetes, hypertension is defined as an AOBP or non-AOBP 130/80 mm Hg or higher. These findings are assessed using a stepwise approach with measurements obtained over one to five visits, and a diagnosis of hypertension is made contingent upon the degree of blood pressure elevation.

Patients diagnosed with hypertension are encouraged to adopt lifestyle changes while being treated with medications and regularly seen by their primary provider until their blood pressure goal is reached.

In Canada, 7.5 million people are living with hypertension and an additional 7.4 million people are at risk of hypertension. It is estimated that nine in 10 adults will develop hypertension if they live a normal lifespan (Hypertension Canada, 2018a). It is estimated that 68% of those diagnosed with hypertension are controlled. A considerable number of Canadians with hypertension have not been diagnosed and therefore remain untreated. Hypertension affects one in five adults and, in people over 60, one in two (Dasgupta, Quinn, Zarnke, et al., 2014). In Canadians who have diabetes, the prevalence of hypertension is 67.1%, with 60.1% of those cases controlled (Padwal, Bienek, McAlister, et al., 2016). The prevalence and incidence of hypertension is highest in the Atlantic region of Canada and lowest in the west and north (Yukon, Northwest Territories, and British

CHART 33-1

Risk Factors: Hypertension

- Family history
- Advancing age
- Cigarette smoking
- Obesity
- Heavy alcohol consumption
- Gender (men greater than women before age 55; women greater than men after 55)
- Being of African descent (see Chart 33-2)
- Being of indigenous descent
- Immigration-related change in socioeconomic status
- High dietary sodium intake
- Low dietary intake of potassium, calcium, magnesium
- Glucose intolerance

Source: El-Hussein, M. T., Power-Kean, K., & Zettle, S. (2019). *Understanding Pathophysiology*. Milton, ON: Elsevier.

Columbia). The risk of hypertension increases with age, comorbidities, and the presence of other risk factors. Adults of South Asian, indigenous, and African ancestry (see Chart 33-2) are identified as higher-risk populations (Heart Research Institute, 2017; The Canadian Task Force on Preventative Health Care, 2012). In Canada, age-specific prevalence rates were similar between men and women for those under age 55, however, rates for women were increasingly higher than men from age 55 onward (Robitaille, Dai, Waters, et al., 2012). Immigration-related change in socioeconomic status and cultural changes have also been associated with hypertension in this population (Sanou, O'Reilly, Ngnie-Teta, et al., 2014).

About 95% of patients with high blood pressure have **primary hypertension** (also called *essential hypertension*), which is defined as high blood pressure from an unidentified cause. The remaining 5% percent have secondary hypertension, which occurs when a cause for the high blood pressure can be identified (Weber et al., 2014). These causes include chronic kidney disease, renal artery stenosis, hyperaldosteronism (mineralocorticoid hypertension), pheochromocytoma, and sleep apnea (Weber et al., 2014). High blood pressure can also occur with pregnancy; women who experience high blood pressure during pregnancy are at increased risk of ischemic heart disease, heart attacks, strokes, kidney disease, diabetes, and death from heart attack (Männistö, Mendola, Vääräsmäki, et al., 2013).

Hypertension is sometimes called the *silent killer* because people who are affected are often symptom free. Once identified, elevated blood pressure requires monitoring at regular intervals because hypertension is a lifelong condition.

High blood pressure can be viewed as a sign, as a risk factor for atherosclerotic cardiovascular disease, or as a disease. As a sign, blood pressure is used by nurses and other health care professionals to monitor a patient's clinical status. Elevated pressure may indicate an excessive dose of vasoconstrictive medication, stress, or other problems. As a risk factor, hypertension contributes to the rate at which atherosclerotic plaque accumulates within arterial walls. As a disease, hypertension is a major contributor to death related to cardiac, cerebrovascular, kidney, and peripheral vascular disease.

Hypertension often accompanies other risk factors for atherosclerotic heart disease, such as **dyslipidemia** (abnormal blood lipid levels, including high total, low-density lipoprotein [LDL], and triglyceride levels as well as low high-density lipoprotein [HDL] levels), obesity, diabetes, a family history of early cardiovascular events, metabolic syndrome, a sedentary lifestyle, and obstructive sleep apnea (Weber et al., 2014). The prevalence is also higher in patients who have other cardiovascular conditions, including heart failure, coronary artery disease, and a history of stroke. Cigarette smoking does not cause high blood pressure; however, if a patient with hypertension smokes, their risk of dying of a cardiovascular event increases significantly (Weber et al., 2014). Excess sodium intake increases the risk for hypertension, whereas sodium restriction lowers blood pressure.

Prolonged blood pressure elevation gradually damages blood vessels throughout the body, particularly in target organs such as the heart, kidneys, brain, and eyes. The typical outcomes of prolonged, uncontrolled hypertension are myocardial infarction, heart failure, chronic kidney disease, strokes, and impaired vision. Hypertrophy (enlargement) of the left ventricle of the heart may occur

Glossary

dyslipidemia: abnormal blood lipid levels, including high total, low-density lipoprotein, and triglyceride levels as well as low high-density lipoprotein levels

hypertensive emergency: a marked elevation in blood pressure in the presence of acute symptoms or progressive target organ damage

hypertensive urgency: a situation in which blood pressure is severely elevated but there is no evidence of impending or target organ damage

isolated systolic hypertension: a condition most commonly seen in older adults in which the systolic pressure is greater than 140 mm Hg and the diastolic pressure is less than 90 mm Hg

monotherapy: medication therapy with a single agent

primary hypertension: denotes high blood pressure from an unidentified cause; also called *essential hypertension*

rebound hypertension: blood pressure that is controlled with medication and that becomes uncontrolled (abnormally high) with the abrupt discontinuation of medication

secondary hypertension: high blood pressure from an identified cause, such as renal disease

white coat hypertension: white coat hypertension is a condition characterized by blood pressure that is elevated in the health care provider's office or clinic but normal elsewhere

NURSING RESEARCH PROFILE

Chart 33-2. Perceptions of Hypertension and Health Behaviours Among African American Women

Stallings, D. T. (2016). Illness perceptions and health behaviours of black women. *Journal of Cardiovascular Nursing, 31*(6), 492–499.

Purpose

African American women have the highest prevalence of hypertension in the world. Despite a plethora of research findings that indicate that health behaviours, including physical activity and diet, can influence hypertension and deter its morbid complications, many African American women who are at risk make poor diet choices and are physically inactive. The aim of this study was to analyze the relationships between perceptions of hypertension and self-reported health behaviours, specifically physical activity and fruit and vegetable consumption, among African American women with hypertension.

Design

This descriptive correlational study recruited African American women from five churches and a hair salon in Tennessee and Mississippi. Eligible participants were 18 to 65 years of age, able to read, write, and speak English, and self-reported that they had been diagnosed with hypertension. Participants ($n = 204$) completed a demographic form, the Illness Perception Questionnaire, a 7-day Physical Activity Recall, and the Fruit and Vegetable Quick Food Scan. In addition, they had their blood pressures and body mass indices measured by the investigators.

Findings

Most participants were married ($n = 108$; 52.9%), college-educated ($n = 102$; 50%) and were middle-aged (average age of 48.12 years of age ±10.3 years). In this sample, the mean systolic blood pressure was 138.4 mm Hg (SD = 14.9 mm Hg), the mean diastolic blood pressure was 83.4 mm Hg (SD = 9.9 mm Hg), and the mean body mass index was 34.14 kg/m^2 (SD = 8.00 kg/m^2). Hierarchical multiple regression analyses revealed that perceiving hypertension as chronic ($\beta = -0.149$; $P = 0.05$) and as caused by environmental factors ($\beta = -0.25$; $P = 0.05$) were both inversely associated with self-reported moderate-intensity physical activity. Emotional responses to hypertension, such as fear or anxiety, were positively correlated with moderate-intensity physical activity ($\beta = 0.32$; $P = 0.05$) and with fruit and vegetable consumption ($\beta = 0.28$; $P = 0.01$).

Nursing Implications

In this study, African American women with hypertension who saw hypertension as a chronic disease caused by environmental factors reported less moderate physical activity. This may imply that knowledge of the chronicity of hypertension may not be sufficient to motivate them to modify their health behaviours. However, fear and anxiety about hypertension seemed to motivate physical activity and fruit and vegetable consumption. Engaging in health coaching behaviours with African American women with hypertension that empowers them to cope and adapt to health challenges may assist them in self-managing hypertension. In particular, nurses who care for African American women with hypertension should assess their perceptions of hypertension, clarify any misperceptions, cultivate healthy coping skills, and motivate them to self-manage hypertension.

as it works to pump blood against the elevated pressure. See Chapter 30 for discussion of ventricular hypertrophy.

Pathophysiology

CONCEPTS IN ACTION

Primary Hypertension

Blood pressure is the product of cardiac output multiplied by peripheral resistance. Cardiac output is the product of the heart rate multiplied by the stroke volume. Each time the heart contracts, pressure is transferred from the contraction of the heart muscle to the blood and then pressure is exerted by the blood as it flows through the blood vessels. Hypertension can result from increases in cardiac output, increases in peripheral resistance (constriction of the blood vessels), or both. Increases in cardiac output are often related to an expansion in vascular volume. Although no precise cause can be identified for most cases of hypertension, it is understood that hypertension is a multifactorial condition. Because hypertension can be a sign, it is most likely to have many causes, just as fever has many causes.

For hypertension to occur there must be a change in one or more factors affecting peripheral resistance or cardiac output. In addition, there must also be a problem with the body's control systems that monitor or regulate pressure (see Fig. 33-1). More than 40 single-gene mutations associated with hypertension have been identified, but most types of hypertension are thought to be polygenic (i.e., mutations in more than one gene) (Ehret & Caulfield, 2013). The tendency to develop hypertension is inherited; however, genetic profiles alone cannot predict who will and will not develop hypertension. In fact, researchers estimate that genetics play a role in explaining blood pressure variation between individuals in 30% to 70% of cases (Ehret & Caulfield, 2013).

Many causes of hypertension have been suggested (Schiffrin, 2014):

- Increased sympathetic nervous system activity related to dysfunction of the autonomic nervous system
- Increased renal reabsorption of sodium, chloride, and water related to a genetic variation in the pathways by which the kidneys handle sodium
- Increased activity of the renin–angiotensin–aldosterone system, resulting in expansion of extracellular fluid volume and increased systemic vascular resistance
- Decreased vasodilation of the arterioles related to dysfunction of the vascular endothelium
- Resistance to insulin action, which may be a common factor linking hypertension, type 2 diabetes, hypertriglyceridemia, obesity, and glucose intolerance

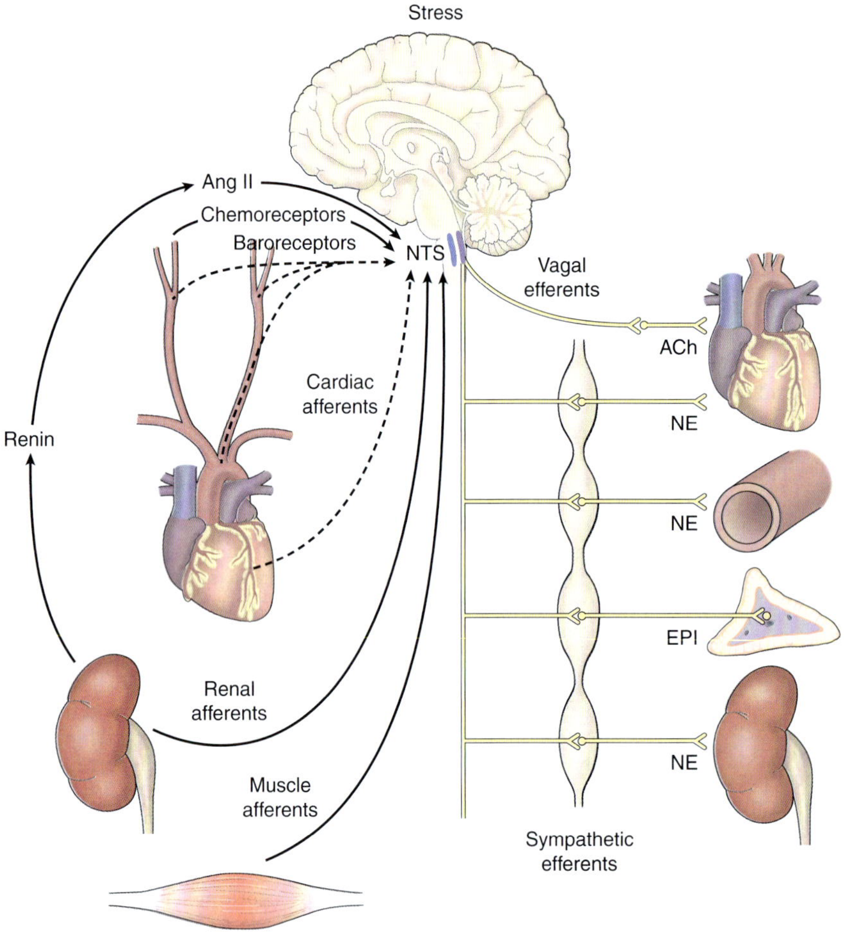

FIGURE 33-1. Central and reflex mechanisms involved in the neural control of blood pressure. *Dotted arrows* represent inhibitory neural influences, and *solid arrows* represent excitatory neural influences on sympathetic outflow. EPI, epinephrine; NTS, nucleus tractus solitarius; NE, norepinephrine; ACh, acetylcholine; Ang II, angiotensin II. (Adapted from Kaplan, N. M., & Victor, R. G. (2015). *Kaplan's clinical hypertension* (11th ed.). Philadelphia, PA: Lippincott Williams & Wilkins.)

Activation of the innate and adaptive components of the immune response that may contribute to renal inflammation and dysfunction.

Secondary Hypertension

Secondary hypertension is high blood pressure that occurs from an identified underlying disease process or medication. A number of conditions may lead to secondary hypertension (El-Hussein, Power-Kean, & Zettle, 2019; Weber et al., 2014):

- Primary renal disease: Both acute and chronic kidney diseases, particularly with glomerular or vascular disorders.
- Oral contraceptives: Oral contraceptives often raise the blood pressure within the expected range but can also induce overt hypertension.
- Pharmaceuticals: Chronic nonsteroidal anti-inflammatory agents and many antidepressants can induce hypertension.
- Alcohol: Chronic alcohol intake and alcohol abuse can raise blood pressure.
- Pheochromocytoma: About one half of patients with pheochromocytoma have paroxysmal hypertension, whereas most of the rest have what appears to be primary hypertension.
- Primary aldosteronism: The presence of primary mineralocorticoid excess, primarily aldosterone, should be suspected in any patient with the triad of hypertension, unexplained hypokalemia, and metabolic alkalosis. However, some patients have a normal plasma potassium concentration. The prevalence of primary aldosteronism should also be considered in people with resistant hypertension.
- Renovascular disease: Renovascular disease is a common disorder occurring primarily in patients with generalized atherosclerosis.
- Cushing syndrome: Hypertension is a major cause of morbidity and death in patients with Cushing syndrome.
- Other endocrine disorders: Hypothyroidism, hyperthyroidism, and hyperparathyroidism may also induce hypertension.
- Obstructive sleep apnea: Disordered breathing during sleep appears to be an independent risk factor for systemic hypertension.
- Coarctation of the aorta: Coarctation of the aorta is one of the major causes of secondary hypertension in young children.

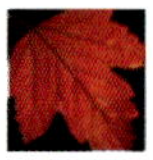

Gerontologic Considerations

Structural and functional changes in the heart, blood vessels, and kidneys contribute to increases in blood pressure that occur with aging. These changes include accumulation of atherosclerotic plaque, fragmentation of arterial elastins, increased collagen deposits, impaired vasodilation, and renal dysfunction. The result of these changes is decreased elasticity or stiffening of the major blood vessels, particularly the aorta, and volume expansion (Aronow, Fleg, Pepine, et al., 2011; Weber et al., 2014). Consequently, the aorta and large arteries are less able to accommodate the volume of blood pumped out by the heart (stroke volume), and the energy that would have stretched the vessels instead elevates the SBP, resulting in an elevated systolic pressure without a change in diastolic pressure. This condition, known as **isolated systolic hypertension**, is more common in older adults and is associated with significant cardiovascular and cerebrovascular morbidity and mortality (Weber et al., 2014).

White Coat Hypertension

White coat hypertension (Cobos, Haskard-Zolnierek, & Howard, 2015) is a condition characterized by blood pressure that is elevated in the doctor's office or clinic but normal elsewhere. It is found in 10% to 30% of patients with suspected hypertension. Most studies contend that these patients face no higher risk of cardiovascular complications than other patients and do not require treatment, other than the adoption of a healthy lifestyle. It is possible, however, that white coat hypertension is the precursor to sustained hypertension. In fact, observations in specialized units have shown that 50% of patients with normal ambulatory blood pressure and elevated clinic blood pressure develop hypertension over a period of 5 years.

White Coat Effect

The white coat effect is a phenomenon that is also seen in patients with confirmed sustained hypertension who are undergoing treatment. In these patients, clinic blood pressure readings are significantly higher than those measured outside of the office.

Masked Hypertension

In masked hypertension, a patient will have high blood pressure that is undetected in the clinic setting. This condition is characterized by readings of less than 140/90 mm Hg in the health care provider's office and mean daytime ambulatory blood pressure readings or readings at home that exceed 135/85 mm Hg. This condition is more common in older men and in people who smoke, drink alcohol, are overweight, or are affected by psychosocial factors such as anxiety and workplace stress.

Population studies have shown the negative impact of masked hypertension on all-cause mortality and cardiovascular mortality. This phenomenon also occurs in people treated for hypertension. A relationship between masked hypertension and target organ damage has also been documented (Hannine, Niiranen, Puukka, et al., 2013). Furthermore, increased left ventricular mass index and microalbuminuria are more commonly found in people with masked hypertension. It is therefore recommended that all people with hypertension measure their blood pressure at home. If the reading is high-normal (systolic BP 135 to 139 or diastolic BP 85 to 89 mm Hg) or higher than the office reading, alternate blood pressure monitoring should be done to confirm the diagnosis of masked hypertension.

Clinical Manifestations

Physical examination may reveal no abnormalities other than elevated blood pressure. Occasionally, retinal changes such as hemorrhages, exudates (fluid accumulation), arteriolar narrowing, and cotton-wool spots (small infarctions) occur. In severe hypertension, papilledema (swelling of the optic disc) may be seen. People with hypertension may be asymptomatic and remain so for many years. However, when specific signs and symptoms appear, they usually indicate vascular damage, with specific manifestations related to the organs served by the involved vessels. Coronary artery disease with angina and myocardial infarction are common consequences of hypertension. Left ventricular hypertrophy occurs in response to the increased workload placed on the ventricle as it contracts against higher systemic pressure. When heart damage is extensive, heart failure follows. Pathologic changes in the kidneys (indicated by increased blood urea nitrogen [BUN] and serum creatinine levels) may manifest as nocturia. Cerebrovascular involvement may lead to a transient ischemic attack (TIA) or stroke, manifested by alterations in vision or speech, dizziness, weakness, a sudden fall, or transient or permanent paralysis on one side (hemiplegia). Cerebral infarctions account for most of the strokes in patients with hypertension.

Complications of Hypertension

Hypertension is associated with a number of serious adverse effects. The likelihood of developing these complications varies with the blood pressure. The increase in risk begins as the blood pressure rises above 115/75 mm Hg in all age groups. However, this relationship does not prove causality, which can only be demonstrated by randomized trials showing benefit from blood pressure reduction.

The increase in cardiovascular risk associated with hypertension is importantly affected by the presence or absence of other risk factors:

- Hypertension is quantitatively the major risk factor for premature cardiovascular disease, other risk factors are cigarette smoking, dyslipidemia, and diabetes. In older patients, systolic pressure and pulse pressure are more powerful determinants of risk than diastolic pressure.
- The risk of heart failure increases with the degree of blood pressure elevation.
- Left ventricular hypertrophy is a common finding in patients with hypertension and is associated with an enhanced incidence of heart failure, ventricular arrhythmias, death following myocardial infarction, and sudden cardiac death.
- Hypertension is the most common and most important risk factor for ischemic stroke, the incidence of which can be markedly reduced by effective antihypertensive therapy.
- Hypertension is the most important risk factor for the development of intracerebral hemorrhage.
- Hypertension is a risk factor for chronic kidney disease and end-stage renal disease.

It can both directly cause kidney disease and accelerate the progression of a variety of underlying renal diseases.

- Marked elevations in blood pressure can be an acute, life-threatening emergency.

Assessment and Diagnostic Findings

The latest 2018 recommendations from the Hypertension Canada feature an algorithm for expediting the diagnosis of hypertension.

For patients with urgent cases of hypertension or who are in hypertensive crisis, hypertension can be diagnosed during the patient's initial visit, where hypertension becomes the focus of a complete evaluation (Nerenberg et al., 2018). Hypertension urgency is a situation in which blood pressure must be lowered within a few hours. Taking the blood pressure every 5 minutes is required. Nurses monitor for a rapid drop in blood pressure which requires immediate action to restore the blood pressure to an acceptable level.

See https://guidelines.hypertension.ca/diagnosis-assessment/supplementary-tables/#suptbl3 for examples of hypertensive urgent situations and emergencies, which includes asymptomatic diastolic blood pressure (DBP) of 130 mm Hg or higher (Hypertension Canada, 2018b).

A thorough health history and physical examination are necessary. The retinas are examined, and laboratory studies are performed to assess possible target organ damage. Routine laboratory tests include urinalysis, blood chemistry (i.e., analysis of sodium, potassium, creatinine, fasting glucose and/or glycated hemoglobin [A1c], and serum total cholesterol, low-density lipoprotein, high-density lipoprotein [HDL], non-HDL cholesterol, and triglycerides), and a standard 12-lead electrocardiogram. Patients with diabetes should have their urinary albumin excretion assessed. All treated hypertensive patients should also be monitored according to the current Diabetes Canada guidelines for the new appearance of diabetes. Finally, during the maintenance phase of hypertension management, tests (including those for electrolytes, creatinine, and fasting lipids) should be repeated with a frequency reflecting the clinical situation (Nerenberg et al., 2018).

A risk factor assessment is needed to classify and guide the treatment of those with hypertension who are at risk for cardiovascular damage. Risk factors for hypertension are presented in Chart 33-1.

For examples of target organ damage, see https://guidelines.hypertension.ca/diagnosis-assessment/supplementary-tables/#suptbl3.

If during the first visit the mean AOBP or non-AOBP is high (see thresholds outlined in Hypertension Canada guidelines) a history and physical examination is performed and, if clinically indicated, diagnostic tests for target organ damage and associated cardiovascular risk factors should be arranged within two visits. Other factors that could induce or aggravate hypertension should be assessed and eliminated if possible. The second visit should be scheduled within 1 month (Hypertension Canada, 2018a).

Prior history of clinically overt atherosclerotic disease indicates a very high risk for a recurrent atherosclerotic event (e.g., peripheral arterial disease, stroke, or TIA).

Hypertension Canada (2018a) recognizes four procedures that have been validated for diagnosing hypertension: AOBP, office blood pressure measurement (non-AOBP), home blood pressure measurement, and ambulatory pressure monitoring.

Since both the diagnosis of hypertension and decisions on initiating and adjusting treatment depend upon blood pressure levels, precise blood pressure readings are critical, not only for identifying, classifying, and treating individuals, but also for evaluating populations during health studies. Normal, high-normal, and grade 1 hypertension are differentiated by systolic and diastolic differences of as little as 10 and 5 mm Hg, respectively, and errors as slight as 5 mm Hg can significantly affect the reliability of this classification.

Accurate readings are important not only for classification purposes, but also, and especially, for clinical care. Labelling a patient as "hypertensive" is not without consequences, as imprecise readings can lead to diagnostic errors or inappropriate treatments. In addition, individual blood pressure values are inherently variable: There is little chance that two consecutive readings will be the same. This is why multiple readings are strongly recommended. Even then, blood pressure measurement is subject to multiple sources of variability or errors attributable to the patient, instrument, observer, or the technique itself.

Do not assume that every health care professional knows how to take an accurate blood pressure reading. Adequate training with an experienced observer is required.

AOBP is the preferred method of performing in-office BP measurement. When using AOBP a displayed mean SBP ≥135 mm Hg is high, or DBP ≥85 mm Hg is high. When using non-AOBP, a mean SBP ≥140 mm Hg or DBP ≥90 mm Hg is high, and SBP between 130 and 139 mm Hg and/or a DBP between 85 and 89 mm Hg is high-normal.

Using ambulatory BP monitoring, patients can be diagnosed as hypertensive if the mean awake SBP is ≥135 mm Hg or the DBP is ≥85 mm Hg or if the mean 24-hour SBP is ≥130 mm Hg or the DBP is ≥80 mm Hg.

Using home BP monitoring patients can be diagnosed as hypertensive if the mean SBP is ≥135 mm Hg or the DBP is ≥85 mm Hg. If the office BP measurement is high and the mean home BP is ≤135/85 mm Hg, it is advisable to either repeat home monitoring to confirm the home BP is ≤135/85 mm Hg or perform 24-hour ABPM to confirm that the mean 24-hour ABPM IS ≤130/80 mm Hg and the mean awake ABPM is ≤135/85 mm Hg before diagnosing white coat hypertension.

It has been established that blood pressure measurements procedures conducted outside the health care providers office are just as effective if not more so in evaluating the diagnostic importance of elevations in blood pressure. Hypertension Canada (2018a) states the out-of-office BP measurement allows for earlier and accurate diagnosis of hypertension. An earlier diagnosis can assist in faster BP control and reductions in cardiovascular events.

To be effective, these technologies, including ambulatory and home monitoring of blood pressure, must be carried out by people who are properly trained (practitioners for ambulatory blood pressure monitoring (ABPM) or patients for home blood pressure monitoring [HBPM]), and the equipment must be validated and accurately calibrated.

In recent years, most hospitals have installed automated oscillometric devices that can assess blood pressure. These devices can perform repeated measurements using preset intervals and number of measurements, although not all

TABLE 33-1 Classification of Blood Pressure According to the World Health Organization

Category	Systolic (mm Hg)		Diastolic (mm Hg)
Optimal	<120	and/or	<80
Normal	<130	and/or	<85
High-normal	130–139	and/or	85–89
Grade 1	140–159	and/or	90–99
Grade 2	160–179	and/or	100–109
Grade 3	≥180	and/or	≥110
Isolated systolic hypertension	>140	and	<90

Source: Mancia, G., Fagard, R., Narkiewicz, K., et al. (2013). 2013 ESH/ESC Guidelines for the management of arterial hypertension: The Task Force for the management of arterial hypertension of the European Society of Hypertension (ESH) and of the European Society of Cardiology (ESC). *Journal of Hypertension, 31*(7), 1281–1357.

devices average the values obtained (see Hypertension Canada guidelines).

Investigations into secondary causes of hypertension should be initiated in patients with suggestive clinical and/or laboratory features.

Table 33-1 demonstrates the classifications of blood pressure by WHO.

Medical Management

The goal of hypertension treatment is to prevent complications and death by achieving and maintaining the arterial blood pressure lower than 135/85 mm Hg (AOBP) or lower than 140/90 mm Hg (non-AOBP). Hypertension Canada recommended more aggressive blood pressure management in patients with hypertension who also have diabetes to a target lower than 135/90 mm Hg (AOBP or non-AOBP). See additional clinical management suggestions by Hypertension Canada.

TABLE 33-3 The Dietary Approaches to Stop Hypertension (DASH) Diet

Food Group	Number of Servings/Day
Grains and grain products	7 or 8
Vegetables	4 or 5
Fruits	4 or 5
Low-fat or fat-free dairy foods	2 or 3
Lean meat, fish, and poultry	≤2
Nuts, seeds, and dry beans	4 or 5 weekly

Note: The diet is based on 2,000 calories/day.

Adapted from U.S. Department of Health and Human Services. (2003). *Your guide to lowering your blood pressure with DASH: DASH eating plan.* Retrieved on November 27, 2015, from www.nhlbi.nih.gov/health/public/heart/hbp/dash/new_dash.pdf

If blood pressure is found to be high-normal, annual follow-up is recommended.

The management options for hypertension include lifestyle modifications and pharmacologic therapy. Table 33-2 summarizes recommended lifestyle modifications. Research findings demonstrate that weight loss, reduced alcohol and sodium intake, and regular physical activity are effective lifestyle adaptations to reduce blood pressure (Coxson, Cook, Joffres, et al., 2013; Eckel, Jakicic, Ard, et al., 2014; Knight, 2012; Weber et al., 2014).

Diets high in fruits, vegetables, and low-fat dairy products can prevent the development of hypertension and lower elevated blood pressure. Table 33-3 shows the Dietary Approaches to Stop Hypertension (DASH) diet, which has been shown to lower blood pressure in people who follow it (Eckel et al., 2014).

Pharmacologic Therapy

The antihypertensive medications used for treating hypertension decrease peripheral resistance, blood volume, or the strength and rate of myocardial contraction (see Table 33-4).

(text continued on page 887)

TABLE 33-2 Lifestyle Modifications to Prevent and Manage Hypertension[a]

Modification	Recommendation	Goal of SBP Reduction (Range)[b]
Weight reduction	Maintain normal body weight (body mass index 18.5–24.9 kg/m^2)	5–20 mm Hg/10 kg
Adopt DASH eating plan	Consume a diet rich in fruits, vegetables, and low-fat dairy products with a reduced content of saturated and total fat	8–14 mm Hg
Dietary sodium reduction	Reduce dietary sodium intake to ≤2,400 mg sodium daily. Further reduction to no more than 1,500 mg sodium daily is better, as it is associated with an even greater reduction in blood pressure. Reduce overall sodium intake from baseline by at least 1,000 mg daily, even if goal of ≤2,400 mg is not achievable; that reduction from baseline is associated with blood pressure reduction	2–8 mm Hg
Physical activity	Engage in regular aerobic physical activity such as brisk walking (≥30 min/day, most days of the week)	4–9 mm Hg
Moderation of alcohol consumption	Limit consumption to ≤2 drinks (e.g., 24 oz beer, 10 oz wine, or 3 oz 80-proof whiskey) per day in most men and to ≤1 drink per day in women and lighter-weight people	2–4 mm Hg

[a]For overall cardiovascular risk reduction, stop smoking.

[b]The effects of implementing these modifications are dose and time dependent and could be greater for some individuals.

SBP, systolic blood pressure; DASH, dietary approaches to stop hypertension.

Adapted from Chobanian, A. V., Bakris, G. L., Black, H. R., et al. (2003b). Seventh Report of the Joint National Committee on prevention, detection, evaluation, and treatment of high blood pressure. *Hypertension, 42*(6), 1206–1252; Go, A. S., Bauman, M. A., Coleman King, S. M., et al. (2014). An effective approach to high blood pressure control: A science advisory from the American Heart Association, the American College of Cardiology, and the Centers for Disease Control and Prevention. *Journal of the American College of Cardiology, 63*(12), 1230–1238.

TABLE 33-4 Medication Therapy for Hypertension

Medications	Major Action	Advantages and Contraindications	Effects and Nursing Considerations
Diuretics and Related Drugs			
Thiazide Diuretics			
Chlorothiazide (Diuril) Chlorthalidone (Hygroton) Hydrochlorothiazide (Hydrodiuril) Indapamide (Lozol) Methyclothiazide (Enduron) Metolazone (Zaroxolyn)	Decrease of blood volume, renal blood flow, and cardiac output Depletion of extracellular fluid Negative sodium balance (from natriuresis), mild hypokalemia Directly affects vascular smooth muscle	Relatively inexpensive Effective orally Effective during long-term administration Mild side effects Enhances other antihypertensive medications Counters sodium retention effects of other antihypertensive medications *Contraindications:* Gout, known sensitivity to sulfonamide-derived medications, severely impaired kidney function, and history of hyponatremia	Side effects include dry mouth, thirst, weakness, drowsiness, lethargy, muscle aches, muscular fatigue, tachycardia, GI disturbance Postural hypotension may be potentiated by alcohol, barbiturates, opioids, or hot weather Because thiazides cause loss of sodium, potassium, and magnesium, monitor for signs of electrolyte imbalance Encourage intake of potassium-rich foods (i.e., fruits) *Gerontologic considerations:* Risk of postural hypotension is significant because of volume depletion; measure blood pressure in three positions; caution patient to rise slowly
Loop Diuretics			
Bumetanide (Bumex) Ethacrynic acid (Edecrin) Furosemide (Lasix) Torsemide (Demadex)	Volume depletion Blocks reabsorption of sodium, chloride, and water in kidney	Action rapid Potent Used when thiazides fail or patient needs rapid diuresis *Contraindications:* Same as for thiazides	There is risk of volume and electrolyte depletion from the profound diuresis that can occur Fluid and electrolyte replacement may be required *Gerontologic considerations:* Same as for thiazides
Potassium-Sparing Diuretics			
Amiloride (Midamor) Triamterene (Dyrenium)	Blocks sodium reabsorption Acts on distal tubule independently of aldosterone	Causes potassium retention *Contraindications:* Kidney disease, azotemia, severe hepatic disease, hyperkalemia	Drowsiness, lethargy, headache Monitor for hyperkalemia if given with ACE inhibitor or angiotensin receptor blocker Diarrhea and other GI symptoms—administer medication after meals
Aldosterone Receptor Blockers			
Eplerenone (Inspra) Spironolactone (Aldactone)	Competitive inhibitors of aldosterone binding	Indicated for patients with a history of myocardial infarction or symptomatic ventricular dysfunction *Contraindications:* Hyperkalemia and impaired renal function Eplerenone is contraindicated in diabetes with microalbuminuria	Drowsiness, lethargy, headache Monitor for hyperkalemia if given with ACE inhibitor or angiotensin receptor blocker Diarrhea and other GI symptoms—administer medication after meals Avoid the use of potassium supplements or salt substitutes Educate patients, families, and caregivers about the signs and symptoms of hyperkalemia Spironolactone may cause gynecomastia
Central Alpha$_2$-Agonists and Other Centrally Acting Drugs			
Clonidine (Catapres) Clonidine patch (Catapres-TTS)	Exact mode of action is not understood, but acts through the central nervous system, apparently through centrally mediated alpha-adrenergic stimulation in the brain, producing blood pressure reduction	Little or no orthostatic effect; moderately potent, and sometimes is effective when other medications fail to lower blood pressure. *Contraindications:* Severe coronary artery disease, pregnancy	Dry mouth, drowsiness, sedation, and occasional headaches and fatigue. Anorexia, malaise, and vomiting with mild disturbance of liver function have been reported Rebound or withdrawal hypertension is relatively common; monitor blood pressure when stopping medication Common side effects include dry mouth, dizziness, sleepiness, fatigue, headache, constipation, and impotence

TABLE 33-4 Medication Therapy for Hypertension (Continued)

Medications	Major Action	Advantages and Contraindications	Effects and Nursing Considerations
Guanfacine (Tenex)	Stimulates central $alpha_2$-adrenergic receptors	Reduces heart rate and causes vasodilation. Serious adverse reactions are uncommon; use with caution in persons with diminished liver function, recent myocardial infarction, or known cardiovascular disease	If taking concurrent with another antihypertensive medication, administer at bedtime to avoid excessive sleepiness Do not administer extended-release tablet formulation with high fat meal
Methyldopa (Aldomet)	Dopa decarboxylase inhibitor; displaces norepinephrine from storage sites	Drug of choice for pregnant women with hypertension Useful in patients with chronic kidney disease or prostate disease Does not decrease cardiac output or renal blood flow Does not induce oliguria *Contraindications:* Liver disease	Drowsiness, dizziness Dry mouth; nasal congestion (troublesome at first but then tends to disappear) Use with caution with kidney disease *Gerontologic considerations:* May produce mental and behavioural changes in the older adult
Beta-Blockers			
Atenolol (Tenormin) Betaxolol (Kerlone) Bisoprolol (Zebeta) Metoprolol (Lopressor) Metoprolol extended release (Toprol-XL) Nadolol (Corgard) Propranolol (Inderal) Propranolol long acting (Inderal LA) Timolol (Blocadren)	Blocks the sympathetic nervous system (beta-adrenergic receptors), especially the sympathetics to the heart, producing a slower heart rate and lowered blood pressure	Reduces pulse rate in patients with tachycardia and blood pressure elevation Indicated for patients who also have stable angina pectoris and silent ischemia *Contraindications:* Bronchial asthma, allergic rhinitis, right ventricular failure from pulmonary hypertension, heart failure, depression, diabetes, dyslipidemia, heart block, peripheral vascular disease, heart rate <60 bpm	Mental depression manifested by insomnia, lassitude, weakness, and fatigue Avoid sudden discontinuation. Lightheadedness and occasional nausea, vomiting, and epigastric distress Check heart rate before giving *Gerontologic considerations:* Risk of toxicity is increased for older adult patients with decreased renal and liver function. Take blood pressure in three positions, and observe for hypotension
Beta-Blockers With Intrinsic Sympathomimetic Activity			
Acebutolol (Sectral) Penbutolol (Levatol) Pindolol (Visken)	Block both cardiac beta-1 and beta-2 receptors Also have antiarrhythmic activity by slowing atrioventricular conduction	Similar to beta-blockers *Contraindications:* Similar to beta-blockers	Avoid sudden discontinuation Withhold if bradycardia or heart block is present Use with caution with COPD, diabetes Similar to beta-blockers
Beta-Blocker With Cardioselective and Vasodilatory Activity			
Nebivolol (Bystolic)	Blocks beta-1 adrenergic receptors	Similar to other beta-blockers with additional capacity for vasodilation *Contraindications:* Similar to beta-blockers but with greater risk of severe bradycardia, heart block, cardiogenic shock, decompensated cardiac failure, sick sinus syndrome, severe hepatic impairment	Avoid sudden discontinuation. FDA warns that drug has not been shown to be more effective than any other beta-blocker
$Alpha_1$-Blockers			
Doxazosin (Cardura) Prazosin (Minipress) Terazosin (Hytrin)	Peripheral vasodilator acting directly on the blood vessel; similar to hydralazine (see discussion of Vasodilators)	Acts directly on the blood vessels and are effective agents in patients with adverse reactions to hydralazine *Contraindications:* Angina pectoris and coronary artery disease; induces tachycardia if not preceded by administration of propranolol and a diuretic	Occasional vomiting and diarrhea, urinary frequency, and cardiovascular collapse, especially if given in addition to hydralazine without lowering the dose of the latter. Patients occasionally experience drowsiness, lack of energy, and weakness
Combined Alpha- and Beta-Blockers			
Carvedilol (Coreg) Labetalol (Trandate)	Block alpha- and beta-adrenergic receptors; cause peripheral dilation and decrease peripheral vascular resistance	Fast acting No decrease in renal blood flow *Contraindications:* Asthma, cardiogenic shock, severe tachycardia, heart block	Orthostatic hypotension, tachycardia

continued >

TABLE 33-4 Medication Therapy for Hypertension (Continued)

Medications	Major Action	Advantages and Contraindications	Effects and Nursing Considerations
Vasodilators			
Hydralazine (Apresoline)	Decreases peripheral resistance but concurrently elevates cardiac output Acts directly on smooth muscle of blood vessels	Not used as initial therapy; used in combination with other medications Used also in pregnancy-induced hypertension *Contraindications:* Angina or coronary disease, heart failure, hypersensitivity	Headache, tachycardia, flushing, and dyspnea may occur—can be prevented by pretreating with reserpine Peripheral edema may require diuretics May produce lupus erythematosus–like syndrome Tachycardia, angina pectoris, ECG changes, edema
Minoxidil (Loniten)	Direct vasodilatory action on arteriolar vessels, causing decreased peripheral vascular resistance; reduces systolic and diastolic pressures	Hypotensive effect more pronounced than with hydralazine No effect on vasomotor reflexes, so does not cause postural hypotension *Contraindications:* Pheochromocytoma	Take blood pressure and apical pulse before administration Monitor intake and output and daily weights Causes hirsutism Dizziness, headache, nausea, edema, tachycardia, palpitations
Nitroprusside (Nitropress) Nitroglycerin	Peripheral vasodilation by relaxation of smooth muscle	Fast acting Used only in hypertensive emergencies *Contraindications:* Sepsis, azotemia, high intracranial pressure	Can cause thiocyanate and cyanide intoxication
ACE Inhibitors			
Benazepril (Lotensin) Captopril (Capoten) Enalapril (Vasotec) Enalaprilat (Vasotec IV) Fosinopril (Monopril) Lisinopril (Prinivil) Moexipril (Univasc) Perindopril (Aceon) Quinapril (Accupril) Ramipril (Altace) Trandolapril (Mavik)	Inhibit conversion of angiotensin I to angiotensin II Lower total peripheral resistance	Fewer cardiovascular side effects Can be used with thiazide diuretic and digitalis Hypotension can be reversed by fluid replacement Angioedema is a rare but potentially life-threatening complication *Contraindications:* Renal impairment, pregnancy	*Gerontologic considerations:* Requires reduced dosages and the addition of loop diuretics when there is renal dysfunction
Angiotensin II Receptor Blockers			
Azilsartan (Edarbi) Candesartan (Atacand) Eprosartan (Teveten) Irbesartan (Avapro) Losartan (Cozaar) Olmesartan (Benicar) Telmisartan (Micardis) Valsartan (Diovan)	Blocks the effects of angiotensin II at the receptor Reduces peripheral resistance	Minimal side effects *Contraindications:* Pregnancy, lactation, renovascular disease, hypersensitivity reaction to other ARBs	Monitor for hyperkalemia
Calcium Channel Blockers			
Nondihydropyridines			
Diltiazem extended release (Cardizem CD, Dilacor XR, Tiazac) Diltiazem long acting (Cardizem LA)	Inhibits calcium ion influx Reduces cardiac afterload	Inhibits coronary artery spasm not controlled by beta-blockers or nitrates *Contraindications:* Sick sinus syndrome, AV block, hypotension, heart failure	Do not discontinue suddenly Observe for hypotension Report irregular heartbeat, dizziness, edema Instruct on regular dental care because of potential gingivitis
Verapamil immediate release (Calan, Isoptin) Verapamil long acting (Calan SR, Isoptin SR) Verapamil (Covera-HS, Verelan PM)	Inhibits calcium ion influx Slow velocity of conduction of cardiac impulse	Effective antiarrhythmic Rapid IV onset Blocks SA and AV node channels *Contraindications:* Sinus or AV node disease, severe heart failure, severe hypotension	Administer on empty stomach or before meal Do not discontinue suddenly Depression may subside when medication is discontinued To relieve headaches, reduce noise, monitor electrolytes Decrease dose for patients with liver or kidney disease

TABLE 33-4 Medication Therapy for Hypertension (Continued)

Medications	Major Action	Advantages and Contraindications	Effects and Nursing Considerations
Dihydropyridines			
Amlodipine (Norvasc) Felodipine (Plendil) Isradipine (Dynacirc CR) Nicardipine (Cardene) Nifedipine long acting (Procardia XL, Adalat CC) Nisoldipine (Sular)	Inhibits calcium ion influx across membranes Vasodilatory effects on coronary arteries and peripheral arteriole Decreases cardiac work and energy consumption, increases delivery of oxygen to myocardium	Rapid action Effective by oral or sublingual route No tendency to slow SA nodal activity or prolong AV node conduction Isolated systolic hypertension *Contraindications:* None (except heart failure for nifedipine)	Administer on empty stomach Use with caution in patients with diabetes Small frequent meals if nausea develops Muscle cramps, joint stiffness, sexual difficulties may disappear when dose decreased Report irregular heartbeat, constipation, shortness of breath, edema May cause dizziness
Clevidipine (Cleviprex)	Calcium channel antagonist causing rapid vasodilation	*Advantages:* Rapid acting with additional capacity for vasodilation; given IV *Contraindications:* Allergies to soybeans, soy products, eggs or egg products; impaired lipid metabolism as might be seen with pancreatitis and other hyperlipidemias; severe aortic stenosis	Monitor carefully for hypotension and tachycardia; there is risk of rebound hypertension, so careful monitoring after cessation of treatment is indicated
Direct Renin Inhibitors			
Aliskiren (Tekturna)	Blocks the conversion of angiotensinogen to angiotensin I by inhibiting the activity of the enzyme renin	Given once daily for mild-to-moderate high blood pressure with minimal side effects Headaches, dizziness, and diarrhea are most frequent side effects Angioedema is a rare but potentially life-threatening complication Contraindicated in pregnancy; has not been studied in persons with diminished renal function	Monitor for hyperkalemia and hypotension

GI, gastrointestinal; ACE, angiotensin-converting enzyme; COPD, chronic obstructive pulmonary disease; FDA, U.S. Food and Drug Administration; IV, intravenous; ECG, electrocardiogram; ARBs, angiotensin receptor blockers; AV, atrioventricular; SA, sinoatrial.

Adapted from Karch, A. (2014). *2015 Lippincott's nursing drug guide*. Philadelphia, PA: Lippincott Williams & Wilkins; U.S. Food and Drug Administration. (2016). *Drug approvals and databases*. Retrieved on October 29, 2016, from www.fda.gov/Drugs/InformationOnDrugs

Hypertension Canada (2018d) suggests that antihypertensive therapy should be prescribed for average DBP measurements of ≥100 mm Hg or average SBP measurements of ≥160 mm Hg in patients without macrovascular target organ damage or other cardiovascular risk factors. In addition, antihypertensive therapy should be strongly considered for average DBP readings ≥90 mm Hg or for average SBP readings ≥140 mm Hg in the presence of macrovascular target organ damage or other independent cardiovascular risk factors (see Table 33-4).

Hypertension Canada (2018e) has also offered comprehensive guidelines for the choice of therapy for adults with diastolic and/or systolic hypertension without compelling indications for specific agents.

See Table 33-4 for a list of medication therapy available for the treatment of hypertension.

In addition, Hypertension Canada (2018b) offers a list of possible reasons for poor response to antihypertensive therapy.

Global Vascular Protection Therapy

Hypertension Canada (2018f) has also suggested guidelines surrounding the global vascular protection therapy for adults with hypertension without compelling indications for specific agents.

Gerontologic Considerations

DBP tends to plateau in late middle age. However, age-related changes in the great vessels, related to an increase in collagen and decrease in elastin, cause them to stiffen. These age-related changes are associated with progressive increases in SBP, but do not have the same effects on the DBP (Aronow et al., 2011). Isolated systolic hypertension is the most common type of hypertension in adults older than 50 years of age (Busko, 2015). Isolated systolic hypertension is associated with increased risk of death, stroke, and heart failure, and treatment reduces this risk (Rosendorff, Lackland, Allison, et al., 2015). Like younger patients, older patients should begin treatment with lifestyle modifications.

More than 75% of adults older than 75 years of age have hypertension, and yet, there has been less research on hypertension treatment and appropriate goals in this population than in younger adults. Furthermore, studies conducted to date have yielded contradictory results, with some showing a reduction in morbidity and mortality, whereas other studies have found either no benefit or increased risk associated with treatment. For instance, the Systolic Blood Pressure Intervention Trial (SPRINT) found that among 2,636 ambulatory participants (mean age of 79.9 years) with hypertension, those whose SBPs were treated to less than 120 mm Hg had significantly lower rates of death and cardiovascular morbidity than those whose SBPs were managed to less than 140 mm Hg (Williamson, Supiano, Applegate, et al., 2016). However, another cohort-based study (Tinetti, Han, McAvay, et al., 2014) found that antihypertensive treatment, including high-intensity antihypertensive treatment, was associated with lower rates of death, but not cardiovascular morbidity, in a sample of 4,961 community-dwelling participants (mean age of 80.1 years). A parallel study in this same cohort found that antihypertensive treatment was associated with an increased risk of falls, particularly among those participants who had previously reported falls (Tinetti et al., 2014). One possible explanation for these discrepant results may be the health of the study participants. Odden, Peralta, Haan, et al. (2012) found that adults older than 65 years of age who were able to walk briskly (faster than 0.8 m/s) benefited from hypertension treatment. Survey participants who walked more slowly or who could not complete a walk test of 20 ft actually benefited from having elevated blood pressures, and blood pressure treatment did not reduce mortality (Odden et al., 2012).

If medications are needed to achieve the blood pressure goal of less than 150/90 mm Hg in the older adult patient, the starting dose should be the lowest available and then gradually increased with a second medication from a different class added if control is difficult to achieve. As older adults often have other comorbid conditions, awareness of possible drug interactions is critical. In addition, older adults are at increased risk for the side effects of hyperkalemia and orthostatic hypotension, putting them at increased risk for falls and fractures (Tinetti et al., 2014).

Follow-Up

If at the last diagnostic visit, the patient is not diagnosed as hypertensive and has no evidence of macrovascular target organ damage, the patient's blood pressure should be reassessed at yearly intervals.

If blood pressure is found to be high-normal annual follow-up is recommended.

Patients with hypertension receiving lifestyle modification advice alone (nonpharmacologic treatment) should receive follow-up assessment at 3- to 6-month intervals. Shorter intervals (every 1 or 2 months) are needed for patients with higher blood pressures.

Patients on antihypertensive drug treatment should be seen monthly or every 2 months, depending on their blood pressure levels, until readings on two consecutive visits are below target values (see Table 33-4).

Shorter intervals between visits will be needed for symptomatic patients and those with severe hypertension, intolerance to antihypertensive drugs, or target organ damage. Once target blood pressure has been reached, patients should be seen every 3 to 6 months.

For more information, consult the complete version of the Canadian Hypertension Education Program's recommendations found in Hypertension Canada website.

Some tools have been developed to help health professionals with patient education. They include reminders about proper blood pressure measurement technique, home blood pressure log sheet, and educational leaflets. To ensure easy understanding, they are all written in laymen's terms. This material can be downloaded freely from the Hypertension Canada.

Assessment of Cardiovascular Risk

The risk of cardiovascular complications is not only a function of the number of risk factors, but also of their intensity (Daskalopoulou et al., 2015). Several models for predicting cardiovascular risk have been developed, based on epidemiologic studies. These models are drawn or derived from cohorts that excluded symptomatic subjects or subjects having extreme risk factors (e.g., SBP >180 mm Hg). As a result, these tables apply only to individuals with no history or evidence of cardiovascular disease. The nurse should consider informing patients of their global risk to improve the effectiveness of risk factor modification. The nurse may also consider using analogies that describe comparative risk such as "cardiovascular age," "vascular age," or "heart age" to inform patients of their risk status.

Helping Patients Understand Cardiovascular Risk

The purpose of evaluating individual cardiovascular risk is to improve care management for high-risk individuals. Yet very few studies have measured the effectiveness of using risk scores in cardiovascular disease primary prevention. Until recently, there was no evidence that clinicians' risk assessments had any influence on clinical outcomes.

Several authors have stated that the complexity of these tables may reduce their value as tools for health education, within a framework of shared decision making. It is true that a great deal of attention has been focused on creating a risk assessment tool that is as accurate as possible, while little attention has been paid to how well the information provided by the tool is communicated to patients. A thorough understanding of risk should help the patient understand the importance of reducing his or her risk factors and adhering to treatment, including adopting a healthy lifestyle. Recent theories stress that health professionals should adopt a more patient-oriented, personalized attitude. Therapeutic decisions should be made collaboratively and should allow patients to take responsibility for their own health in a more enlightened way, thus easing pressure on health professionals.

The concept of making patients aware of risk fits well with a process of shared decision making, an idea that has been often studied in the field of chronic disease and cancer management. Not only can a shared decision-making approach favourably affect clinical outcomes, but it can also have a positive effect on patients' levels of satisfaction and their feeling of being in control of their condition. The goal of this approach is to obtain an informed consent from the patient, so that he or she will adopt the proposed care plan without being needlessly alarmed by a poor understanding of risk levels or by errors in perception. The clinician's role is to communicate a clear message, one that neither trivializes the risks involved nor needlessly alarms the patient.

The risk evaluation approach offers an excellent opportunity for opening a dialogue with the patient: It can help both health professionals and patients discuss the situation and encourage them to take preventive or therapeutic measures that take risk levels adequately into account. This takes time, however, and may prolong consultations. That is why the manner in which risk is explained must be as clear and effective as possible, while at the same time ensuring that the patient understands and has correctly interpreted his or her risk level. It is also true that any discussion of risk will call upon not only the patient's intellect, but also his or her emotions; the latter may weigh heavily in the balance, depending upon the patient's value system and beliefs. For example, the short-term risk of drug-related side effects may outweigh the risk of complications in the form of a cardiovascular event in the distant future.

Evaluating and explaining the concept of risk, and providing this with follow-up and support strategies, are crucial components for any therapeutic approach. Informing patients about risk and discussing it with them enhances communication and interaction and has an impact on motivation for action and behaviour change, on the part of both patients and their health care professionals.

Explaining risk to patients using the concept of vascular age can bring home the stakes to patients and encourage them to adopt therapeutic recommendations; it can help patients comply with guidelines more fully and over longer periods of time. Enough persuasive evidence exists to justify recommending an explanation of risk using the concept of vascular age; this technique should be part of the risk assessment procedure for all patients.

Nursing Process

The Patient With Hypertension

Assessment

When hypertension is initially detected, nursing assessment involves carefully monitoring the blood pressure at frequent intervals and then at routinely scheduled intervals. When the patient begins an antihypertensive treatment regimen, blood pressure assessments are needed to determine the effectiveness of medication therapy and to detect any changes in blood pressure that may indicate the need for a modification in the treatment plan.

The ASH and ISH have defined the standards for blood pressure measurement, including conditions required before measurements are made, equipment specifications, and techniques for measuring blood pressure to obtain accurate and reliable readings (Coogan, Marra, & Lomonaco, 2015; Weber et al., 2014).

A complete history is obtained to assess for other cardiovascular risk factors and for signs and symptoms that indicate target organ damage (i.e., whether specific tissues are damaged by the elevated blood pressure). Manifestations of target organ damage may include angina; shortness of breath; alterations in speech, vision, or balance; nosebleeds; headaches; dizziness; or nocturia. The patient's partner may be helpful in identifying whether the patient may be experiencing obstructive sleep apnea.

During the physical examination, the nurse must also pay specific attention to the rate, rhythm, and character of the apical and peripheral pulses to detect the effects of hypertension on the heart and blood vessels. A thorough assessment can yield valuable information about the extent to which the hypertension has affected the body and any other personal, social, or financial factors. For example, a patient's ability to adhere to an antihypertensive medication regimen may be influenced by the patient's financial resources to buy the medication and also by limited health insurance (Iuga & McGuire, 2014). Furthermore, patients' perceptions about the diagnosis of hypertension can affect whether they engage in key health behaviours, including exercising and modifying dietary habits (Stallings, 2016).

Nursing Priorities

Based on the assessment data, nursing priorities may include the following:

- Deficient knowledge
- Nonadherence to therapy

Collaborative Problems/ Potential Complications

Potential complications may include the following:

- Left ventricular hypertrophy
- Myocardial infarction
- Heart failure
- TIA
- Cerebrovascular disease (stroke or brain attack)
- Renal insufficiency and chronic kidney disease
- Retinal hemorrhage

Planning and Goals

The major goals for the patient include understanding of the disease process and its treatment, participation in a self-care program, and absence of complications.

Nursing Interventions

The objective of nursing care for patients with hypertension focuses on lowering and controlling the blood pressure without adverse effects and without undue cost. To achieve these goals, the nurse's role is to support and educate the patient about the treatment regimen, including making lifestyle changes, taking medications as prescribed, and scheduling regular follow-up appointments with the patient's primary provider to monitor progress or identify and treat any complications of disease or therapy.

Increasing Knowledge

The patient needs to understand the disease process and how lifestyle changes and medications can control hypertension. The nurse needs to emphasize the concept of controlling hypertension rather than curing it. The nurse can encourage the patient to consult a dietitian to help develop a plan for improving nutrient intake or for weight loss. The program usually consists of restricting sodium and fat intake, increasing intake of fruits and vegetables, and implementing regular physical activity. Explaining that it takes 2 to 3 months for the taste buds to adapt to changes in salt intake may help the patient adjust to reduced salt intake. The patient should be advised to limit alcohol intake (see Chart 33-3 for specific recommendations), and tobacco should be avoided because anyone with high blood pressure is already at increased risk for heart disease, and smoking amplifies this risk.

Promoting Adherence to the Therapeutic Regimen

Deviation from the therapeutic program is a significant problem for people with hypertension and other chronic conditions requiring lifetime management. An estimated 50% of patients discontinue their medications within 1 year of beginning to take them. Blood pressure control is achieved by only 54% (Valderrama, Gillespie, King, et al., 2012). Adherence to the therapeutic regimen increases, however, when patients actively participate in self-care, including self-monitoring of blood pressure and diet, possibly because patients receive immediate feedback and have a greater sense of control. Nurse-led wellness programs that are tailored to take into account patients' behaviours and eating and exercise practices are more effective than generic programs. Patients with hypertension must make considerable effort to adhere to recommended lifestyle modifications (see Chart 33-3) and to take regularly prescribed medications (Table 33-4).

CHART 33-3

Measuring Blood Pressure

Equipment

FOR THE PATIENT AT HOME

- Automatic or semiautomatic device with digital display of readings

FOR THE PRACTITIONER

- Preferably, a validated electronic device; if not available, a mercury sphygmomanometer, recently calibrated aneroid manometer
- Appropriately sized arm cuff

Instructions for the Patient

- Avoid smoking cigarettes or drinking caffeine for 30 minutes before blood pressure (BP) is measured
- Empty bladder
- Sit quietly for 5 minutes before the measurement
- Sit comfortably, with back supported, with the forearm supported at heart level on a firm surface, with both feet on the ground; avoid talking while the measurement is being taken

Instructions for the Practitioner

- Select the size of the cuff based on the size of the patient. (The cuff size should have a bladder width of at least 40% of limb circumference and length at least 80% of limb circumference.) The average adult cuff is 12 to 14 cm wide and 30 cm long. Using a cuff that is too small will give a higher BP measurement, and using a cuff that is too large results in a lower BP measurement compared to one taken with a properly sized cuff
- Wrap the cuff firmly around the arm. Centre the cuff bladder directly over the brachial artery
- Position the patient's arm at the level of the heart
- If a mercury sphygmomanometer is used, palpate the systolic pressure before auscultating. This technique helps to detect the presence of an auscultatory gap more readily
- Ask the patient to sit quietly while the BP is measured, because the BP can increase when the patient is engaged in conversation
- Initially, record BP results of both arms and take subsequent measurements from the arm with the higher BP. Normally, the BP should vary by no more than 5 mm Hg between arms
- Take two readings 1 to 2 minutes apart and use the average of these measurements
- Record the site where the BP was measured and the position of the patient (i.e., right arm)
- Inform the patient of their BP value and what it means. Emphasize the need for periodic reassessment, and encourage patients who measure BP at home to keep a written record of readings

Interpretation

Assessment is based on the average of at least two readings. (If two readings differ by more than 5 mm Hg, additional readings are taken and an average reading is calculated from the results.)

Adapted from Coogan, N., Marra, A., & Lomonaco, E. A. (2015). Assessing accurate BP measurement: Size and technique matter!. *Nursing, 45*(4), 16–18; Weber, M. A., Schiffrin, D. L., White, W. B., et al. (2014). Clinical practice guidelines for the management of hypertension in the community: A statement by the American Society of Hypertension and the International Society of Hypertension. *The Journal of Clinical Hypertension (Greenwich), 16*(1), 14–26.

The effort needed to follow the therapeutic plan may seem unreasonable to some, particularly when they have no symptoms without medications but do have side effects with medications. Continued education and encouragement are usually needed to enable patients to formulate an acceptable plan that helps them live with their hypertension and adhere to the treatment plan. Compromises may have to be made about some aspects of therapy to achieve higher-priority goals.

The nurse can assist with behaviour change by supporting patients in making small changes with each visit that moves them toward their goals. Another important factor is following up at each visit to see how the patient has progressed with the plans made at the prior visit. If the patient has had difficulty with a particular aspect of the plan, the patient and nurse can work together to develop an alternative or modification to the plan that the patient believes will be more successful. Support groups for weight control, smoking cessation, and stress reduction may be beneficial for some patients; others can benefit from the support of family and friends. The nurse assists the patient to develop and adhere to an appropriate exercise regimen, because regular activity is a significant factor in weight reduction and a blood pressure–reducing intervention in the absence of any loss in weight (Weber et al., 2014).

Promoting Home, Community-Based, and Transitional Care

Blood pressure screenings with the sole purpose of case finding are not recommended by the National High Blood Pressure Education Program because approximately 83% of people with hypertension are already aware of their blood pressure levels (Mozaffarian et al., 2016). If asked to participate in a blood pressure screening program, the nurse should ensure that proper blood pressure measurement technique is being used, that validated electronic devices are used or, if sphygmomanometers are used, that they are properly calibrated, and that provision has been made to provide follow-up for any person identified as having an elevated blood pressure level. Adequate time should also be allowed to educate each person screened about what the blood pressure numbers mean. Each person should be given a written record of their blood pressure at the screening.

Educating Patients About Self-Care

The therapeutic regimen is the responsibility of the patient in collaboration with the primary provider. The nurse can help the patient achieve blood pressure control through education about managing blood pressure (see earlier discussion), setting goal blood pressures, and providing assistance with social support. Involving family members in education programs enables them to support the patient's efforts to control hypertension. Hypertension Canada provides printed and electronic patient education materials (see Chart 33-4).

Providing written information about the expected effects and side effects of medications is important. When side effects occur, patients need to understand the importance of reporting them and to whom they should be reported. Patients need to be informed that rebound hypertension (i.e., abnormally high blood pressure) can occur if antihypertensive medications are suddenly stopped. Thus, patients should be advised to have an adequate supply of medication, particularly

CHART 33-4

Patient Education: Treatment for High Blood Pressure

Hypertension is the medical term for high blood pressure. Untreated hypertension increases the strain on the heart and arteries, eventually causing organ damage. Hypertension increases the risk of heart failure, heart attack (myocardial infarction), kidney failure leading to dialysis, and stroke. Fortunately, treatments to lower blood pressure are usually easy to take and can help prevent health problems.

This topic will review the treatment of primary hypertension. Primary hypertension does not have a known underlying cause. Other topics about hypertension are also available.

Lifestyle Changes

Making lifestyle changes is an important first step in the treatment of high blood pressure. In some patients, lowering sodium and alcohol intake, keeping weight in the ideal range, engaging in regular aerobic exercise, and stopping smoking may be sufficient to control high blood pressure. As an example, most professional societies suggest that sodium intake should be less than 2.3 g (2,300 mg) per day. Such lifestyle changes can lower blood pressure as effectively as therapy with one blood pressure–lowering drug.

However, many patients also require one or more medications to lower the blood pressure. The following is an overview of the different types of drugs that may initially be prescribed.

High Blood Pressure Medications

There are various medications that are commonly used to treat high blood pressure.

Some people will respond well to one drug but not to another. Therefore, it may take time to determine the right drug or drugs and proper dose to effectively lower blood pressure with a minimum of side effects.

Although generally well tolerated, high blood pressure medications can cause side effects; the side effects depend on the specific drug given, the dose, and other factors. Some side effects result from lowering of the blood pressure, usually if it is abrupt, and therefore can be caused by any high blood pressure medication. These include dizziness, drowsiness, light-headedness, or feeling tired. They usually subside after a few weeks when the body has adapted to the lower blood pressure.

when traveling and in case of emergencies such as natural disasters. If traveling by airplane, patients should pack the medication in their carry-on luggage. All patients should be informed that some medications, such as beta-blockers, might cause sexual dysfunction and that other medications are available if problems with sexual function or satisfaction occur. The nurse can encourage and educate patients to measure their blood pressure at home. This practice involves patients in their own care and emphasizes that failing to take medications may result in an identifiable rise in blood pressure. Patients need to know that blood pressure varies continuously and that the range within which their pressure varies should be monitored.

Gerontologic Considerations

Adherence to the therapeutic program may be more difficult for older adults. The medication regimen can be difficult to remember, and the expense can be a challenge (see Table 33-4).

Monotherapy (treatment with a single agent), if appropriate, may simplify the medication regimen and make it less expensive. Special care must be taken to ensure that the older adult patient understands the regimen and can see and read instructions, open the medication container, and get the prescription refilled. The older adult's family or caregivers should be included in the educational program so that they understand the patient's needs, can encourage adherence to the treatment plan, and know when and whom to call if problems arise or information is needed.

Continuing and Transitional Care

Regular follow-up care is imperative so that the disease process can continue to be optimally assessed and treated, as shown in Table 33-5. A history and physical examination should be completed at each clinic visit. The history should include all data pertaining to any potential problem, specifically medication-related problems such as postural (orthostatic) hypotension (experienced as dizziness or lightheadedness on standing).

NURSING ALERT

The patient and caregivers should be cautioned that antihypertensive medications might cause hypotension. Low blood pressure or postural hypotension should be reported immediately. Older adults have impaired cardiovascular reflexes and thus are more sensitive to the extracellular volume depletion caused by diuretics and to the sympathetic inhibition caused by adrenergic antagonists. The nurse educates patients to change positions slowly when moving from a lying or sitting position to a standing position. The nurse also counsels older adult patients to use supportive devices such as handrails and walkers as necessary to prevent falls that could result from dizziness.

TABLE 33-5 Recommendations for Follow-Up Based on Initial Blood Pressure Measurements for Adults Without Acute End-Organ Damage

Initial BP (mm Hg)[a]	Follow-Up Recommended[b]
Normal	Recheck in 2 years
Prehypertension	Recheck in 1 year[c]
Stage 1 hypertension	Confirm within 1 month[c]
Stage 2 hypertension	Evaluate or refer to source of care within 1 month For those with higher pressures (e.g., >180/100 mm Hg), evaluate and treat immediately or within 1 week, depending on clinical situation and complications

[a]If systolic and diastolic values fall into different categories, follow recommendations for shorter follow-up (e.g., 160/86 mm Hg should be evaluated or referred to source of care within 1 month).

[b]Modify the scheduling of follow-up according to reliable information about past BP measurements, other cardiovascular risk factors, or target organ disease.

[c]Provide advice about lifestyle modifications.

BP, blood pressure.

Adapted from Weber, M. A., Schiffrin, E. L., White, W. B., et al. (2014). Clinical practice guidelines for the management of hypertension in the community: A statement by the American Society of Hypertension and the International Society of Hypertension. *The Journal of Clinical Hypertension (Greenwich), 16*(1), 14–26.

Monitoring and Managing Potential Complications

Symptoms suggesting that hypertension is progressing to the extent that target organ damage is occurring must be detected early so that appropriate treatment can be initiated. When the patient returns for follow-up care, all body systems must be assessed to detect any evidence of vascular damage. An eye examination with an ophthalmoscope is particularly important because retinal blood vessel damage indicates similar damage elsewhere in the vascular system. The patient is questioned about blurred vision, spots in front of the eyes, and diminished visual acuity. The heart, nervous system, and kidneys are also carefully assessed. Any significant findings are promptly reported to determine whether additional diagnostic studies are required. Based on the findings, medications may be changed to improve blood pressure control.

Evaluation

Expected patient outcomes may include:

1. Reports knowledge of disease management sufficient to maintain adequate tissue perfusion
   a. Maintains blood pressure at less than 140/90 mm Hg (or less than 150/90 mm Hg for adults older than 60 years of age) with lifestyle modifications, medications, or both
   b. Demonstrates no symptoms of angina, palpitations, or vision changes
   c. Has stable BUN and serum creatinine levels
   d. Has palpable peripheral pulses

2. Adheres to the self-care program
   a. Adheres to the dietary regimen as prescribed: reduces calorie, sodium, and fat intake; increases fruit and vegetable intake
   b. Exercises regularly
   c. Takes medications as prescribed and reports any side effects
   d. Measures blood pressure routinely
   e. Abstains from tobacco and excessive alcohol intake
   f. Keeps follow-up appointments
3. Has no complications
   a. Reports no changes in vision
   b. Exhibits no retinal damage on vision testing
   c. Maintains pulse rate and rhythm and respiratory rate within normal ranges
   d. Reports no dyspnea or edema
   e. Maintains urine output consistent with intake
   f. Has renal function test results within normal range
   g. Demonstrates no motor, speech, or sensory deficits
   h. Reports no headaches, dizziness, weakness, changes in gait, or falls

Hypertensive Crises

Two classes of hypertensive crisis that require immediate intervention include hypertensive emergency and hypertensive urgency (pressures above 180 mm Hg systolic and/or above 120 mm Hg diastolic). Hypertensive emergencies and urgencies may occur in patients whose hypertension has been poorly controlled, whose hypertension has been undiagnosed, or in those who have abruptly discontinued their medications. Once the hypertensive crisis has been managed, a complete evaluation is performed to review the patient's ongoing treatment plan and strategies to minimize the occurrence of subsequent hypertensive crises are implemented (Hopkins, 2015).

A **hypertensive emergency** is a situation in which blood pressures are extremely elevated and must be lowered quickly (not necessarily to less than 140/90 mm Hg) to halt or prevent damage to the target organs (Monnet & Marik, 2015). Assessment will reveal actual or developing clinical dysfunction of the target organ. Conditions associated with a hypertensive emergency include hypertension of pregnancy, acute myocardial infarction, dissecting aortic aneurysm, and intracranial hemorrhage. Hypertensive emergencies are acute, life-threatening blood pressure elevations that require prompt treatment in an intensive care setting because of the serious target organ damage that may occur. The therapeutic goals are reduction of the mean blood pressure by 20% to 25% within the first hour of treatment, a further reduction to a goal pressure of about 160/100 mm Hg over a period of up to 6 hours, and then a more gradual reduction in pressure over a period of days. The exceptions to these goals are the treatment of ischemic stroke (in which there is no evidence of benefit from immediate pressure reduction) and treatment of aortic dissection (in which the goal is to lower systolic pressure to less than 100 mm Hg if the patient can tolerate the reduction) (Chobanian, Bakris, Black, et al., 2003a).

The medications of choice in hypertensive emergencies are those that have an immediate effect. Intravenous vasodilators, including sodium nitroprusside (Nitropress), nicardipine (Cardene), clevidipine (Cleviprex), enalaprilat (Vasotec), and nitroglycerin have immediate actions that are short-lived (minutes to 4 hours), and they are therefore frequently used for initial treatment. Nicardipine and labetalol (Trandate) have demonstrated safety and effectiveness in treating hypertensive crises, with nicardipine demonstrating more predictability in controlling blood pressure (Monnet & Marik, 2015) (see Table 33-4). Experts also recommend assessing the patient's fluid volume status. If there is volume depletion secondary to natriuresis caused by the elevated blood pressure, then volume replacement with normal saline can prevent large sudden drops in blood pressure when antihypertensive medications are given (Monnet & Marik, 2015).

Hypertensive urgency describes a situation in which blood pressure is very elevated but there is no evidence of impending or progressive target organ damage (Bisognano, 2015). Elevated blood pressures associated with severe headaches, nosebleeds, or anxiety are classified as urgencies. In these situations, oral agents can be given with the goal of normalizing blood pressure within 24 to 48 hours (Monnet & Marik, 2015). Oral doses of fast-acting agents such as beta-adrenergic blockers (i.e., labetalol [Trandate]), ACE inhibitors (i.e., captopril [Capoten]), or alpha2-agonists (i.e., clonidine [Catapres]) are recommended for the treatment of hypertensive urgencies (see Table 33-4).

Extremely close hemodynamic monitoring of the patient's blood pressure and cardiovascular status is required during treatment of hypertensive emergencies and urgencies (see Chapter 27). The exact frequency of monitoring is a matter of clinical judgment and varies with the patient's condition. Taking vital signs every 5 minutes is appropriate if the blood pressure is changing rapidly; taking vital signs at 15- or 30-minute intervals in a more stable situation may be sufficient. A precipitous drop in blood pressure can occur that would require immediate action to restore blood pressure to an acceptable level.

Critical Thinking Exercises

1 You are working as a nurse in a clinic that serves both an assisted living and skilled nursing facility. One of the patients is an 80-year-old woman who is a new resident of the facility. When you take her blood pressure, you note that it is 120/88 mm Hg. While talking with her, you find that she reports episodes of dizziness and has fallen twice in the past 2 weeks. She tells you that she takes her medications as prescribed and has had no other concerns. What additional assessment data do you plan to gather from this patient? What is your priority plan of action?

2 You are employed as an occupational health nurse in a manufacturing facility. A 32-year-old man who operates

a forklift presents to be treated after scraping his forearm on a piece of equipment. During your assessment, he tells you he takes a beta-blocker for his hypertension; you find that his blood pressure is 120/76 mm Hg. While dressing his wound, he tells you he is dedicated to staying healthy, by taking his meds and going to the gym, but he can't seem to get his heart rate up and feels tired all the time. What further follow-up would you recommend? Discuss the evidence that supports specific strategies aimed at treating hypertension.

3 You are working at the student health centre at the local community college and a 28-year-old man comes into the office complaining of a headache and blurry vision. While obtaining assessment information, you discover his blood pressure to be 150/96 mm Hg. You continue to obtain assessment information and discover that he has been staying up late to get his assignments completed by drinking caffeinated energy drinks. What additional assessment data would you gather from this patient? What is your priority plan of action?

REFERENCES AND SELECTED READINGS

Books

El-Hussein, M. T., Power-Kean, K., & Zettle, S. (2019). *Understanding Pathophysiology*. Milton, ON: Elsevier.

Kaplan, N. M., & Victor, R. G. (2015). *Kaplan's clinical hypertension* (11th ed.). Philadelphia, PA: Lippincott Williams & Wilkins.

Karch, A. (2014). *2015 Lippincott's nursing drug guide*. Philadelphia, PA: Lippincott Williams & Wilkins.

Journals and Electronic Documents

Aronow, W. S., Fleg, J. L., Pepine, C. J., et al. (2011). ACCF/AHA 2011 expert consensus document on hypertension in the elderly: A report of the American College of Cardiology Foundation Task Force on clinical expert consensus documents developed in collaboration with the American Academy of Neurology, American Geriatrics Society, American Society for Preventive Cardiology, American Society of Hypertension, American Society of Nephrology, Association of Black Cardiologists, and European Society of Hypertension. *Journal of the American College of Cardiology, 57*(20), 2037–2114.

Bisognano, J. D. (2015). Malignant hypertension. *Medscape*. Retrieved on October 27, 2016, from emedicine.medscape.com/article/241640-overview

Busko, M. (2015). Isolated systolic hypertension in young adults ups CVD risk. *Medscape*. Retrieved from www.medscape.com/viewarticle/838941

The Canadian Task Force on Preventative Health Care. (2012). Hypertension: Summary of recommendations for clinicians and policy-makers. Retrieved from https://canadiantaskforce.ca/guidelines/published-guidelines/hypertension/

Chobanian, A. V., Bakris, G. L., Black, H. R., et al. (2003a). The Seventh Report of the Joint National Committee on Prevention, Detection, Evaluation, and Treatment of High Blood Pressure: The JNC 7 report. *The Journal of the American Medical Association, 289*(19), 2560–2572.

Chobanian, A. V., Bakris, G. L., Black, H. R., et al; National High Blood Pressure Education Program Coordinating Committee. (2003b). Seventh Report of the Joint National Committee on prevention, detection, evaluation, and treatment of high blood pressure. *Hypertension, 42*(6), 1206–1252.

Cobos, B., Haskard-Zolnierek, K., & Howard, K. (2015). White coat hypertension: Improving the patient-care practitioner relationship. *Psychology Research and Behaviour Management, 8*, 133–141.

Coogan, N., Marra, A., & Lomonaco, E. A. (2015). Assessing accurate BP measurement: Size and technique matter!. *Nursing, 45*(4), 16–18.

Coxson, P. G., Cook N. R., Joffres, M., et al. (2013). Mortality benefits from US population-wide reduction in sodium consumption: Projections from 3 modeling approaches. *Hypertension, 61*(3), 564–570.

Daskalopoulou, S. S., Rabi, D. M., Zarnke, K. B., et al. (2015). The 2015 Canadian Hypertension Education Program recommendations for blood pressure measurement, diagnosis, assessment of risk, prevention, and treatment of hypertension. *Canadian Journal of Cardiology, 31*(5), 549–568.

Dasgupta, K., Quinn, R. R., Zarnke, K. B., et al. (2014). The 2014 Canadian Hypertension Education Program recommendations for blood pressure measurement, diagnosis, assessment of risk, prevention, and treatment of hypertension. *Canadian Journal of Cardiology, 30*(5), 485–501.

Eckel, R. H., Jakicic, J. M., Ard, J. D., et al. (2014). 2013 AHA/ACC guideline on lifestyle management to reduce cardiovascular risk. A report of the American College of Cardiology/American Heart Association Task Force on Practice Guidelines. *Journal of the American College of Cardiology, 63*(25 Pt B), 2961–2984.

Egan, B. M., Zhao, Y., & Axon, R. N. (2010). US trends in prevalence, awareness, treatment, and control of hypertension, 1988–2008. *The Journal of the American Medical Association, 303*, 2043–2050.

Ehret, G. B., & Caulfield, M. J. (2013). Genes for blood pressure: An opportunity to understand hypertension. *European Heart Journal, 34*(13), 951–961.

Elmer, P. J., Obarzanek, E., Vollmer, W. M., et al. (2006). Effects of comprehensive lifestyle modification on diet, weight, physical fitness, and blood pressure control: 18-month results of a randomized trial. *Annals of Internal Medicine, 144*(7), 485–495.

Franklin, S. S., Larson, M. G., Khan, S. A., et al. (2001). Does the relation of blood pressure to coronary heart disease risk change with aging? The Framingham Heart Study. *Circulation, 103*, 1245–1249.

Hanninen, M. R., Niiranen, T. J., Puukka, P. J., et al. (2013). Target organ damage and masked hypertension in the general population: The Finn-home study. *Journal of Hypertension, 31*(6), 1131–1143.

Heart Research Institute. (2017). First nations people and heart disease. Retrieved from http://www.hricanada.org/about-heart-disease/first-nations-people-and-heart-disease

Hopkins, C. (2015). Hypertensive emergencies. *Medscape*. Retrieved on October 27, 2016, from emedicine.medscape.com/article/1952052-overview

Hypertension Canada. (2016). Hypertension prevention and control in Canada: A strategic approach to save lives, improve quality of life and reduce health care costs. Retrieved from https://hypertension.ca/wp-content/uploads/2017/11/Hypertension-Framework-Update-2015_Oct_26.pdf

Hypertension Canada. (2018a). Criteria for diagnosis of Hypertension and guidelines for follow-up. Retrieved from https://guidelines.hypertension.ca/diagnosis-assessment/diagnosis/

Hypertension Canada. (2018b). Supplementary tables. Retrieved from https://guidelines.hypertension.ca/diagnosis-assessment/supplementary-tables/#suptbl3

Hypertension Canada. (2018c). Health behaviour management: Prevention and treatment. Retrieved from https://guidelines.hypertension.ca/prevention-treatment/health-behaviour-management/

Hypertension Canada. (2018d). Indications for drug therapy for adults with hypertension without compelling indications for specific agents. Retrieved from https://guidelines.hypertension.ca/prevention-treatment/uncomplicated-hypertension/

Hypertension Canada. (2018e). Choice of therapy for adults with hypertension without compelling indications for specific agents. Retrieved from https://guidelines.hypertension.ca/prevention-treatment/uncomplicated-hypertension-therapy/

Hypertension Canada. (2018f). Global vascular protection therapy for adults with hypertension without compelling indications for specific agents. Retrieved from https://guidelines.hypertension.ca/prevention-treatment/uncomplicated-hypertension-vascular-protection/

Iuga, A. O., & McGuire, M. J. (2014). Adherence and health care costs. *Risk Management and Health Care Policy, 7*, 35–44.

Jackson, R., Lawes, C. M., Bennett, D. A., et al. (2005). Treatment with drugs to lower blood pressure and blood cholesterol based on an individual's absolute cardiovascular risk. *Lancet, 365*(6457), 434–441.

Knight, J. A. (2012). Physical inactivity: Associated diseases and disorders. *Annals of Clinical & Laboratory Science, 42*(3), 320–337.

Mancia, G., Fagard, R., Narkiewicz, K., et al. (2013). 2013 ESH/ESC Guidelines for the management of arterial hypertension: The Task Force for the management of arterial hypertension of the European Society of Hypertension (ESH) and of the European Society of Cardiology (ESC). *Journal of Hypertension, 31*(7), 1281–1357.

Männistö, T., Mendola, P., Vääräsmäki, M., et al. (2013). Elevated blood pressure in pregnancy and subsequent chronic disease risk. *Circulation, 127*(6), 681–690.

Monnet, X., & Marik, P. E. (2015). What's new with hypertensive crises?. *Intensive Care Medicine, 41*(1), 127–130.

Mozaffarian, D., Benjamin, E. J., Go, A. S., et al. (2016). Heart Disease and Stroke Statistics—2016 Update: A report from the American Heart Association. *Circulation, 133*(4), e38–e360.

Nerenberg, K. A., Zarnke, K. B., Leung, A. A., et al; Hypertension Canada. (2018). Hypertension Canada's 2018 guidelines for diagnosis, risk assessment, prevention, and treatment of hypertension in adults and children. *Canadian Journal of Cardiology, 34*(5), 506–525.

Odden, M. C., Peralta, C. A., Haan, M. N., et al. (2012). Rethinking the association of high blood pressure with mortality in elderly adults: The impact of frailty. *Archives of Internal Medicine, 172*(15), 1162–1168.

Padwal, R. S., Bienek, A., McAlister, F. A., et al. (2016). Epidemiology of hypertension in Canada: An update. *Canadian Journal of Cardiology, 32*(5), 687–694.

Robitaille, C., Dai, S., Waters, C., et al. (2012). Diagnosed hypertension in Canada: Incidence, prevalence and associated mortality. *Canadian Medical Association Journal, 184*(1), E49–E56.

Rosendorff, C., Lackland, D. T., Allison, M., et al. (2015). Treatment of hypertension in patients with coronary artery disease. A scientific statement from the American Heart Association, American College of Cardiology, and American Society of Hypertension. *Journal of the American Society of Hypertension, 9*(6), 453–498.

Sanou, D., O'Reilly, E., Ngnie-Teta, I., et al. (2014). Acculturation and nutritional health of immigrants in Canada: A scoping review. *Journal of Immigrant and Minority Health, 16*(1), 24–34.

Schiffrin, E. L. (2014). Immune mechanisms in hypertension and vascular injury. *Clinical Science (London), 126*(4), 267–274.

Stallings, D. T. (2016). Illness perceptions and health behaviors of black women. *Journal of Cardiovascular Nursing, 31*(6), 492–499.

Tinetti, M. E., Han, L., McAvay, G. J., et al. (2014). Anti-hypertensive medications and cardiovascular events in older adults with multiple chronic conditions. *PLoS One, 9*(3), e90733.

Valderrama, A. L., Gillespie, C., King, S. C., et al. (2012). Vital signs: Awareness and treatment of uncontrolled hypertension among adults—United States, 2003–2010. *Morbidity and Mortality Weekly Report, 61*(35).

Weber, M. A., Schiffrin, E. L., White, W. B., et al. (2014). Clinical practice guidelines for the management of hypertension in the community: A statement by the American Society of Hypertension and the International Society of Hypertension. *The Journal of Clinical Hypertension (Greenwich), 16*(1), 14–26.

Williamson, J. D., Supiano, M. A., Applegate, W. B., et al; SPRINT Research Group. (2016). Intensive versus standard blood pressure control and cardiovascular disease outcomes in adults aged ≥75 years: A randomized clinical trial. *Journal of the American Medical Association, 315*(24), 2673–2682.

Wilson, P. W. (1994). Established risk factors and coronary artery disease: The Framingham Study. *American Journal of Hypertension*, 7, 7S–12S.

Resources

Canadian Council of Cardiovascular Nurses: http://www.cccn.ca.

Canadian Stroke Network: http://canadianstrokenetwork.ca/en/

Centers for Disease Control and Prevention (CDC), Cardiovascular Health Program: https://www.cdc.gov/heartdisease/index.htm

Heart and Stroke Foundation of Canada: https://www.heartandstroke.ca/

Hypertension Canada: https://hypertension.ca/

World Health Organization (WHO), Cardiovascular diseases: https://www.who.int/cardiovascular_diseases/en/

UNIT 7

Digestive and Gastrointestinal Function

Case Study

PROMOTING SELF-CARE IN THE PATIENT WITH A NEW OSTOMY

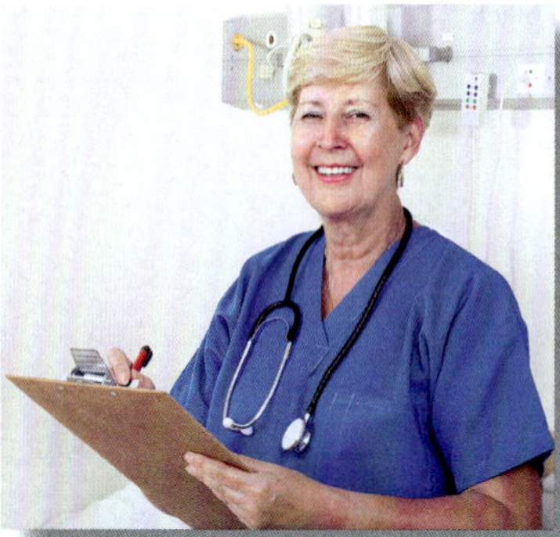

A 64-year-old woman with a long history of ulcerative colitis is admitted to a surgical unit following a total colectomy and an ileostomy. The patient had a preoperative evaluation with a wound–ostomy–continence (WOC) nurse, who had an educational session with the patient. The WOC nurse taught the patient basic principles of stoma care and recommended strategies for involvement in self-care in the postoperative period. It is now 4 days postoperative and the patient has had a good physical recovery without complications, but she refuses to participate in any ostomy care or even look at the stoma.

QSEN Competency Focus: Evidence-Based Practice

The complexities inherent in today's health care system challenge nurses to demonstrate integration of specific interdisciplinary core competencies that are aimed at ensuring the delivery of safe and quality patient care (Institute of Medicine, 2003). The Quality and Safety Education for Nurses project (QSEN, 2017; Cronenwett, Sherwood, Barnsteiner, et al., 2007) provides a framework for the knowledge, skills, and attitudes (KSAs) required for nurses to demonstrate competency in these key areas, which include ***patient-centred care***, ***interdisciplinary teamwork and collaboration***, ***evidence-based practice***, ***quality improvement***, ***safety***, and ***informatics.***

The College of Nurses Ontario (CNO) outlines entry-level practice expectations of the registered nurse. These competencies include self-regulation, professional responsibility and accountability, knowledge-based practice, service to the public, and ethical practice. According to CNO (2014), these competencies are not tasks, but behavioural outcomes "that require the registered nurse to utilize a depth and breadth of knowledge, skill, and judgement that allow them safely practise and competently adapt to changes in the health care environment" (CNO, 2014).

Evidence-Based Practice Definition: Integrate best current evidence with clinical expertise and patient/family preferences and values for delivery of optimal health care.

SELECTED PRE-LICENSURE KSAs	APPLICATION AND REFLECTION
Knowledge	
Discriminate between valid and invalid reasons for modifying evidence-based clinical practice based on clinical expertise or patient/family preferences.	What is the strength of the evidence that suggests that patients should be involved in their ostomy care? What do you think are this patient's reasons for not participating in her care? What is the psychological process patients go through after a disfiguring surgery?
Skills	
Consult with clinical experts before deciding to deviate from evidence-based protocols.	Identify members of the health care team you would consult with to help you craft the most appropriate, individualized plan of care for this patient.
Attitudes	
Acknowledge own limitations in knowledge and clinical expertise before determining when to deviate from evidence-based best practices.	Reflect on the complex interrelationships between the physical and psychological aspects of this patient's condition. Think about your own desire for this patient to accept her ostomy. How might your desire for her acceptance hamper the care you provide?

College of Nurses of Ontario (CNO). (2014). *Entry to practice competencies for Registered Nurses*. Retrieved June 13, 2019, from https://www.cno.org/globalassets/docs/reg/41037_entrytopracitic_final.pdf; Cronenwett, L., Sherwood, G., Barnsteiner, J., et al. (2007). Quality and safety education for nurses. *Nursing Outlook, 55*(3), 122–131; Institute of Medicine. (2003). *Health professions education: A bridge to quality*. Washington, DC: National Academies Press; and QSEN Institute. (2017). *QSEN competencies: Definitions and pre-licensure KSAs*. Retrieved June 12, 2019, from www.qsen.org/competencies/pre-licensure-ksas

34 Assessment of Digestive and Gastrointestinal Function

Adapted by Pamela Cawley

Learning Objectives

On completion of this chapter, the learner will be able to:

1. Describe the structure and function of the organs of the gastrointestinal (GI) tract.
2. Describe the mechanical and chemical processes involved in digesting and absorbing foods and eliminating waste products.
3. Use assessment parameters appropriate for determining the status of GI function.
4. Describe the appropriate preparation, teaching, and follow-up care for patients who are undergoing diagnostic testing of the GI tract.

Abnormalities of the gastrointestinal (GI) tract are numerous and represent every type of major pathology that can affect other organ systems, including bleeding, perforation, obstruction, inflammation, and cancer. Congenital, inflammatory, infectious, traumatic, and neoplastic lesions are encountered in every portion and at every site along the length of the GI tract. As with all other organ systems, the GI tract is subject to circulatory disturbances, faulty nervous system control, and aging.

Apart from the many organic diseases to which the GI tract is susceptible, many extrinsic factors can interfere with its normal function and produce symptoms. Stress and anxiety, for example, often find their chief expression in indigestion, anorexia, or motor disturbances of the intestines, sometimes producing constipation or diarrhea. In addition to the state of mental health, physical factors such as fatigue and an inadequate or abruptly changed dietary intake can markedly affect the GI tract. When assessing and instructing the patient, the nurse should consider the variety of mental and physical factors that affect the function of the GI tract.

Anatomic and Physiologic Overview

Anatomy of the Gastrointestinal System

The GI tract is a 7- to 7.9-m (23- to 26-foot) long pathway that extends from the mouth to the **esophagus**, **stomach**, small and **large intestines**, and rectum to the terminal structure, the **anus** (Fig. 34-1). The esophagus is located in the mediastinum anterior to the spine and posterior to the trachea and heart. This hollow muscular tube, which is approximately 25 cm (10 in) in length, passes through the diaphragm at an opening called the *diaphragmatic hiatus*.

The remaining portion of the GI tract is located within the peritoneal cavity. The stomach is situated in the left upper portion of the abdomen under the left lobe of the liver and the diaphragm; overlaying most of the pancreas (see Fig. 34-1). A hollow muscular organ with a capacity of approximately 1,500 mL (1.58 qt), the stomach stores food during eating, secretes digestive fluids, and propels the partially digested food, or **chyme**, into the **small intestine**. The gastroesophageal junction is the inlet to the stomach. The stomach has four anatomic regions: the cardia (entrance), fundus, body, and pylorus (outlet). Circular smooth muscle in the wall of the pylorus forms the pyloric sphincter and controls the opening between the stomach and the small intestine.

The small intestine is the longest segment of the GI tract, accounting for about two thirds of the total length. It folds back and forth on itself, providing approximately 7,000 cm/70 m (230 ft) of surface area for **secretion** and **absorption**, the process by which nutrients enter the bloodstream through the intestinal walls. It has three sections: The most proximal section is the duodenum, the middle section is the jejunum, and the distal section is the ileum. The ileum terminates at the ileocecal valve. This valve, or sphincter, controls the flow of digested material from the ileum into the cecal portion of the large intestine

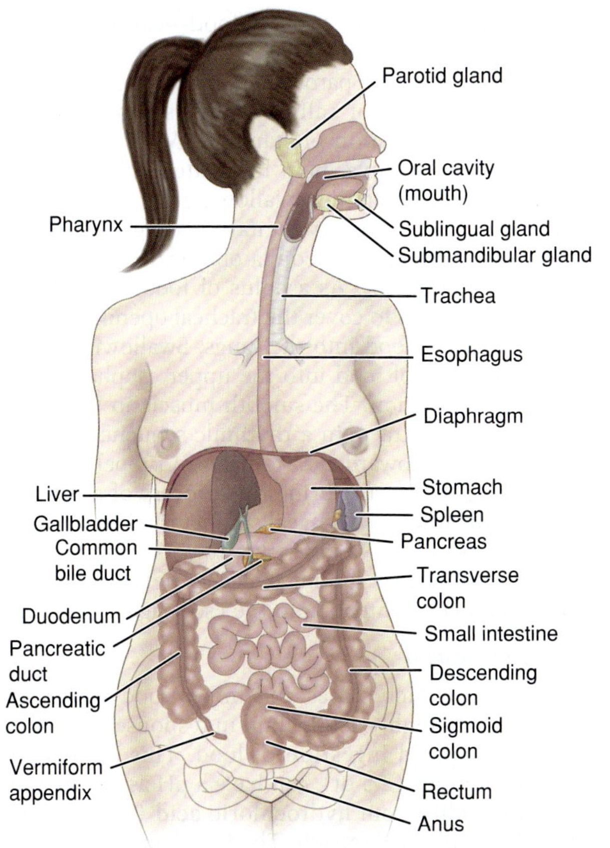

FIGURE 34-1. Organs of the digestive system and associated structures.

and prevents reflux of bacteria into the small intestine. Attached to the cecum is the vermiform appendix, an appendage that has little or no physiologic function. Emptying into the duodenum at the ampulla of Vater is the common bile duct, which allows for the passage of both bile and pancreatic secretions.

The large intestine consists of an ascending segment on the right side of the abdomen, a transverse segment that extends from right to left in the upper abdomen, and a descending segment on the left side of the abdomen. The sigmoid colon, the rectum, and the anus complete the terminal portion of the large intestine. A network of striated muscle that forms both the internal and the external anal sphincters regulates the anal outlet.

The GI tract receives blood from arteries that originate along the entire length of the thoracic and abdominal aorta and veins that return blood from the digestive organs and the spleen. This portal venous system is composed of five large veins: the superior mesenteric, inferior mesenteric, gastric, splenic, and cystic veins, which eventually form the vena portae that enters the liver. Once in the liver, the blood distributes through the liver and collects in the hepatic veins that then terminate in the inferior vena cava. Of particular importance are the gastric artery and the superior and inferior mesenteric arteries. The gastric artery supplies oxygen and nutrients to the stomach and to the intestine by the mesenteric arteries (Fig. 34-2). Venous blood returns from the small intestine, cecum, and ascending and transverse portions of the colon by the superior mesenteric vein, which corresponds with the

Glossary

absorption: phase of the digestive process that occurs when small molecules, vitamins, and minerals pass through the walls of the small and large intestine and into the bloodstream

achalasia: absence of peristalsis of the lower esophagus resulting in difficulty swallowing, regurgitation, and sometimes pain

amylase: an enzyme that aids in the digestion of starch

anus: last section of the GI tract; outlet for waste products from the system

chyme: mixture of food with saliva, salivary enzymes, and gastric secretions that is produced as the food passes through the mouth, esophagus, and stomach

digestion: phase of the digestive process that occurs when digestive enzymes and secretions mix with ingested food and when proteins, fats, and sugars are broken down into their component smaller molecules

dyspepsia: indigestion; upper abdominal discomfort associated with eating

elimination: phase of digestive process that occurs after digestion and absorption, when waste products are evacuated from the body

esophagus: collapsible tube connecting the mouth to the stomach, through which food passes as it is ingested

fibroscopy (gastrointestinal): intubation of a part of the GI system with a flexible, lighted tube to assist in diagnosis and treatment of diseases of that area

hydrochloric acid: acid secreted by the glands in the stomach; mixes with chyme to break it down into absorbable molecules and to aid in the destruction of bacteria

ingestion: phase of the digestive process that occurs when food is taken into the GI tract via the mouth and esophagus

intrinsic factor: a gastric secretion that combines with vitamin B_{12} so that the vitamin can be absorbed

large intestine: the portion of the GI tract into which waste material from the small intestine passes as absorption continues and elimination begins; consists of several parts—ascending segment, transverse segment, descending segment, sigmoid colon, and rectum

lipase: an enzyme that aids in the digestion of fats

pepsin: a gastric enzyme that is important in protein digestion

small intestine: longest portion of the GI tract, consisting of three parts—duodenum, jejunum, and ileum—through which food mixed with all secretions and enzymes passes as it continues to be digested and begins to be absorbed into the bloodstream

stomach: distensible pouch into which the food bolus passes to be digested by gastric enzymes

trypsin: enzyme that aids in the digestion of protein

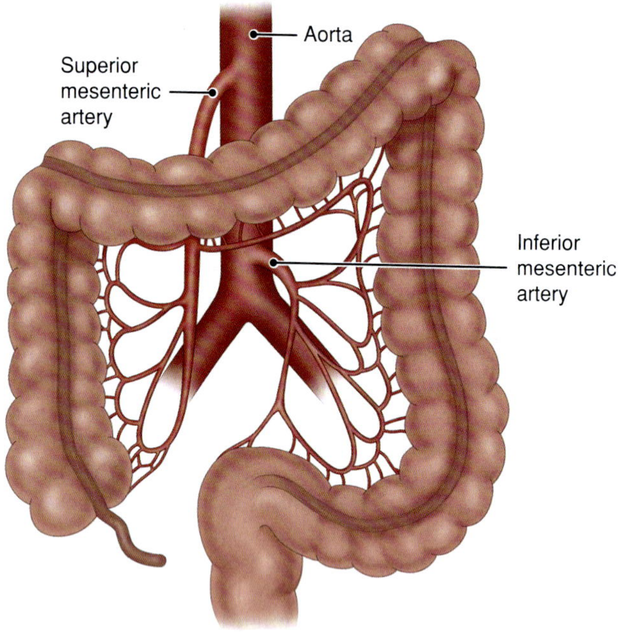

FIGURE 34-2. Anatomy and blood supply of the large intestine.

distribution of the branches of the superior mesenteric artery. Blood flow to the GI tract is about 20% of the total cardiac output and increases significantly after eating.

Both the sympathetic and parasympathetic portions of the autonomic nervous system innervate the GI tract. In general, sympathetic nerves exert an inhibitory effect on the GI tract, decreasing gastric secretion and motility and causing the sphincters and blood vessels to constrict. Parasympathetic nerve stimulation causes peristalsis and increases secretory activities. The sphincters relax under the influence of parasympathetic stimulation except for the sphincter of the upper esophagus and the external anal sphincter, which are under voluntary control (Grossman & Porth, 2014).

Function of the Digestive System

All cells of the body require nutrients. These nutrients are derived from the intake of food that contains proteins, fats, carbohydrates, vitamins, minerals, and cellulose fibres and other vegetable matter, some of which has no nutritional value. The primary functions of the GI tract are the following:

- The breakdown of food particles into the molecular form for **digestion**
- The absorption into the bloodstream of small nutrient molecules produced by digestion
- The **elimination** of undigested unabsorbed foodstuffs and other waste products

After food is ingested, it is propelled through the GI tract, and comes in contact with a wide variety of secretions that aid in its digestion, absorption, or elimination from the GI tract.

Chewing and Swallowing

The process of digestion begins with the act of chewing, in which food is broken down into small particles that are swallowed and mixed with digestive enzymes. Eating—or even the sight, smell, or taste of food—can cause reflex salivation. Approximately 1.5 L (1.58 qt) of saliva is secreted daily from the parotid, submaxillary, and sublingual glands. Ptyalin, or salivary **amylase**, is an enzyme that begins the digestion of starches. Water and mucus, also contained in saliva, help lubricate the food as it is chewed, thereby facilitating swallowing.

Swallowing begins as a voluntary act regulated by the swallowing centre in the medulla oblongata of the central nervous system (CNS). As a bolus of food is swallowed, the epiglottis moves to cover the tracheal opening and prevent aspiration of food into the lungs. Swallowing, which propels the bolus of food into the upper esophagus, thus ends as a reflex action. The smooth muscle in the wall of the esophagus contracts in a rhythmic sequence from the upper esophagus toward the stomach to propel the bolus of food along the tract. During this process of esophageal peristalsis, the lower esophageal sphincter relaxes and permits the bolus of food to enter the stomach. Subsequently, the lower esophageal sphincter closes tightly to prevent reflux of stomach contents into the esophagus.

Gastric Function

The stomach, which stores and mixes food with secretions, secretes a highly acidic fluid in response to the presence or anticipated **ingestion** of food. This fluid, which can total 2.4 L/day (2.5 qt), can have a pH as low as 1 and derives its acidity from **hydrochloric acid** (HCl) secreted by the glands of the stomach. The function of this gastric secretion is twofold: to break down food into more absorbable components and to aid in the destruction of most ingested bacteria. **Pepsin**, an important enzyme for protein digestion, is the end product of the conversion of pepsinogen from the chief cells (Table 34-1). **Intrinsic factor**, also secreted by the gastric mucosa, combines with dietary vitamin B_{12} so that the vitamin can be absorbed in the ileum. In the absence of intrinsic factor, vitamin B_{12} cannot absorb, and pernicious anemia results (see Chapter 54).

Peristaltic contractions in the stomach propel the stomach's contents toward the pylorus. Because large food particles cannot pass through the pyloric sphincter, they churn back into the body of the stomach. In this way, food in the stomach is mechanically broken down into smaller particles. Food remains in the stomach for a variable length of time, from 30 minutes to several hours, depending on the volume, osmotic pressure, and chemical composition of the gastric contents. Peristalsis in the stomach and contractions of the pyloric sphincter allow the partially digested food to enter the small intestine at a rate that permits efficient absorption of nutrients. Chyme is partially digested food mixed with gastric secretions. Hormones, neuroregulators, and local regulators found in the gastric secretions control the rate of gastric secretions and influence gastric motility (Table 34-2).

Small Intestine Function

The digestive process continues in the duodenum. Duodenal secretions come from the accessory digestive organs—the pancreas, liver, and gallbladder—and the glands in the wall of the intestine itself. These secretions contain digestive enzymes: amylase, **lipase**, and bile. Pancreatic secretions have an alkaline pH due to their high concentration

TABLE 34-1 The Major Digestive Enzymes and Secretions

Enzyme/Secretion	Enzyme Source	Digestive Action
Action of Enzymes That Digest Carbohydrates		
Ptyalin (salivary amylase)	Salivary glands	Starch → dextrin, maltose, glucose
Amylase	Pancreas and intestinal mucosa	Starch → dextrin, maltose, glucose Dextrin → maltose, glucose
Maltase	Intestinal mucosa	Maltose → glucose
Sucrase	Intestinal mucosa	Sucrose → glucose, fructose
Lactase	Intestinal mucosa	Lactose → glucose, galactose
Action of Enzymes/Secretions That Digest Protein		
Pepsin	Gastric mucosa	Protein → polypeptides
Trypsin	Pancreas	Proteins and polypeptides → polypeptides, dipeptides, amino acids
Aminopeptidase	Intestinal mucosa	Polypeptides → dipeptides, amino acids
Dipeptidase	Intestinal mucosa	Dipeptides → amino acids
Hydrochloric acid	Gastric mucosa	Protein → polypeptides, amino acids
Action of Enzymes Secretions That Digest Fat (Triglyceride)		
Pharyngeal lipase	Pharynx mucosa	Triglycerides → fatty acids, diglycerides, monoglycerides
Steapsin	Gastric mucosa	Triglycerides → fatty acids, diglycerides, monoglycerides
Pancreatic lipase	Pancreas	Triglycerides → fatty acids, diglycerides, monoglycerides
Bile	Liver and gallbladder	Fat emulsification

of bicarbonate. This alkalinity neutralizes the acid entering the duodenum from the stomach. Digestive enzymes secreted by the pancreas include **trypsin**, which aids in digesting protein; amylase, which aids in digesting starch; and lipase, which aids in digesting fats. These secretions drain into the pancreatic duct, which empties into the common bile duct at the ampulla of Vater. Bile, secreted by the liver and stored in the gallbladder, aids in emulsifying ingested fats, making them easier to digest and absorb. The sphincter of Oddi, found at the confluence of the

TABLE 34-2 The Major Gastrointestinal Regulatory Substances

Substance	Stimulus for Production	Target Tissue	Effect on Secretions	Effect on Motility
Neuroregulators				
Acetylcholine	Sight, smell, chewing food, stomach distention	Gastric glands, other secretory glands, gastric and intestinal muscle	Increased gastric acid	Generally increased; decreased sphincter tone
Norepinephrine	Stress, other various stimuli	Secretory glands, gastric and intestinal muscle	Generally inhibitory	Generally decreased; increased sphincter tone
Hormonal Regulators				
Gastrin	Stomach distention with food	Gastric glands	Increased secretion of gastric juice, which is rich in HCl	Increased motility of stomach, decreased time required for gastric emptying Relaxation of ileocecal sphincter Excitation of colon Constriction of gastroesophageal sphincter
Cholecystokinin	Fat in duodenum	Gallbladder Pancreas Stomach	Release of bile into duodenum Increased production of enzyme-rich pancreatic secretions	
Secretin	pH of chyme in duodenum below 4–5	Stomach Pancreas	Inhibits gastric secretion somewhat Increased production of bicarbonate-rich pancreatic juice	
Local Regulator				
Histamine	Unclear; substances in food	Gastric glands	Increased gastric acid production	Inhibits stomach contractions

common bile duct and duodenum, controls the flow of bile. Hormones, neuroregulators, and local regulators found in these intestinal secretions control the rate of intestinal secretions and influence GI motility. Intestinal secretions total approximately 1 L/day (approximately 33 oz) of pancreatic juice, 0.5 L/day (approximately 17 oz) of bile, and 3 L/day (approximately 66 oz) of secretions from the glands of the small intestine. Table 34-1 gives further information about the actions of digestive enzymes and GI regulatory substances.

Two types of contractions occur regularly in the small intestine: segmentation contractions and intestinal peristalsis. *Segmentation contractions* produce mixing waves that move the intestinal contents back and forth in a churning motion. *Intestinal peristalsis* propels the contents of the small intestine toward the colon. Chyme stimulates both movements.

Food, ingested as fats, proteins, and carbohydrates, is broken down into absorbable particles (constituent nutrients) by the process of digestion. Carbohydrates are broken down into disaccharides (e.g., sucrose, maltose, galactose) and monosaccharides (e.g., glucose, fructose). Glucose is the major carbohydrate that tissue cells use as fuel. Proteins are a source of energy after they are broken down into amino acids and peptides. Ingested fats become monoglycerides and fatty acid through emulsification, which makes them smaller and easier to absorb. Chyme stays in the small intestine for 3 to 6 hours, allowing for continued breakdown and absorption of nutrients.

Small, fingerlike projections called *villi* line the entire intestine and function to produce digestive enzymes as well as to absorb nutrients. Absorption is the primary function of the small intestine. Vitamins and minerals are absorbed essentially unchanged. Absorption begins in the jejunum accomplished by active transport and diffusion across the intestinal wall into the circulation. Nutrients are absorbed at specific locations in the small intestine and duodenum, whereas fats, proteins, carbohydrates, sodium, and chloride are absorbed in the jejunum. Vitamin B_{12} and bile salts are absorbed in the ileum. Magnesium, phosphate, and potassium are absorbed throughout the small intestine.

Colonic Function

Within 4 hours after eating, residual waste material passes into the terminal ileum and slowly into the proximal portion of the right colon through the ileocecal valve. With each peristaltic wave of the small intestine, the valve opens briefly and permits some of the contents to pass into the colon.

Bacteria, a major component of the contents of the large intestine, assist in completing the breakdown of waste material, especially of undigested or unabsorbed proteins and bile salts. Two types of colonic secretions add to the residual material: an electrolyte solution and mucus. The electrolyte solution is chiefly a bicarbonate solution that acts to neutralize the end products formed by the colonic bacterial action, whereas the mucus protects the colonic mucosa from the intraluminal contents and provides adherence for the fecal mass.

Slow, weak peristalsis moves the colonic contents along the tract. This slow transport allows for efficient reabsorption of water and electrolytes, which is the primary function of the colon. Intermittent strong peristaltic waves propel the contents for considerable distances. After the ingestion of another meal, intestine-stimulating hormones release. The waste materials from a meal eventually reach and distend the rectum, usually in about 12 hours. As much as one fourth of the waste materials from a meal may still be in the rectum 3 days after meal ingestion.

Waste Products of Digestion

Feces consist of undigested foodstuffs, inorganic materials, water, and bacteria. Fecal matter is about 75% fluid and 25% solid material (Grossman & Porth, 2014). The composition is relatively unaffected by alterations in diet because a large portion of the fecal mass is of nondietary origin, derived from the secretions of the GI tract. The brown colour of the feces results from the breakdown of bile by the intestinal bacteria. Chemicals formed by intestinal bacteria are responsible in large part for the fecal odour. Gases formed contain methane, hydrogen sulphide, and ammonia, among others. The GI tract normally contains approximately 150 mL (approximately 5 oz) of these gases, which are either absorbed into the portal circulation and detoxified by the liver or expelled from the rectum as flatus.

Elimination of stool begins with distention of the rectum, which initiates reflex contractions of the rectal musculature and relaxes the normally closed internal anal sphincter. The autonomic nervous system controls the internal sphincter; the external sphincter is under the conscious control of the cerebral cortex. During defecation, the external anal sphincter voluntarily relaxes to allowing expulsion of colonic contents. Normally, the external anal sphincter is in a tonic state of tonic contraction. Thus, defecation is seen to be a spinal reflex (involving the parasympathetic nerve fibres) that inhibited voluntarily by keeping the external anal sphincter closed. Contracting the abdominal muscles (straining) facilitates emptying of the colon. The average frequency of defecation in humans is once daily, but this varies among individuals.

Gerontologic Considerations

Although an increased prevalence of several common GI disorders occurs in the elderly population, aging per se appears to have minimal direct effect on most GI functions, in large part because of the functional reserve of the GI tract. Table 34-3 identifies normal physiologic changes of the GI system occurring with age. Careful assessment and monitoring of signs and symptoms related to these changes are imperative. Although irritable bowel symptoms decrease with aging, there seems to be an increase in many GI disorders of function and motility. The gastroenterologist frequently encounters elderly patients who report dysphagia, anorexia, **dyspepsia**, and disorders of colonic function (Eliopoulos, 2018; Khan, Ghaffar, & Khan, 2015; Malhi, 2016; Tsutsumimotoa, Takehiko, Hyuma, et al., 2017).

Assessment of the Gastrointestinal System

Health History

A focused GI assessment begins with a complete history. This includes information about abdominal pain, dyspepsia, gas, nausea and vomiting, diarrhea, constipation, fecal

TABLE 34-3 Age-Related Changes in the Gastrointestinal System

Structural Changes	Implications
Oral Cavity and Pharynx	
• Injury/loss or decay of teeth • Atrophy of taste buds • ↓ Saliva production • Reduced ptyalin and amylase in saliva	Difficulty chewing and swallowing
Esophagus	
• Motility and emptying • Weakened gag reflex • ↓ Resting pressure of lower esophageal sphincter	Reflux and heartburn
Stomach	
• Degeneration and atrophy of gastric mucosal surfaces with ↓ production of HCl • ↓ Secretion of gastric acids and most digestive enzymes • ↓ Gastric motility and emptying	Food intolerances, malabsorption, or decrease in vitamin B_{12} absorption
Small Intestine	
• Atrophy of muscle and mucosal surfaces • Thinning of villi and epithelial cells	↓ Motility and transit time, which lead to complaints of indigestion and constipation
Large Intestine	
• ↓ Mucus secretion • ↓ Elasticity of rectal wall • ↓ Tone of internal anal sphincter • Slower and duller nerve impulses in rectal area	↓ Motility and transit time, which lead to complaints of indigestion and constipation ↓ Absorption of nutrients (dextrose, fats, calcium, and iron) Fecal incontinence

↓, decreased; HCl, hydrochloric acid.

incontinence, jaundice, and previous GI disease (Weber & Kelley, 2017).

Common Symptoms

Pain

Pain can be a major symptom of GI disease. The character, duration, pattern, frequency, location, distribution of referred pain (Fig. 34-3), and time of the pain vary greatly depending on the underlying cause. Other factors such as meals, rest, activity, and defecation patterns may directly affect this pain.

Dyspepsia

Dyspepsia, upper abdominal discomfort associated with eating (commonly called *indigestion*), is the most common symptom of patients with GI dysfunction affecting 25% to 40% of individuals over a lifetime (Overland, 2014). Indigestion is an imprecise term that refers to a host of upper abdominal or epigastric symptoms such as pain, discomfort, fullness, bloating, early satiety, belching, heartburn, or regurgitation; it occurs in approximately 25% of the adult population (Achem & DeVault, 2014; Grossman & Porth, 2014). Typically, fatty foods cause the most discomfort because they remain in the stomach for digestion longer than proteins or carbohydrates. Salads and coarse vegetables as well as highly seasoned foods may also cause considerable GI distress.

Intestinal Gas

The accumulation of gas in the GI tract may result in belching (expulsion of gas from the stomach through the mouth) or flatulence (expulsion of gas from the rectum). Usually, gases in the small intestine pass into the colon and release as flatus. Patients often complain of bloating, distention, or feeling "full of gas" with excessive flatulence as a symptom of food intolerance or gallbladder disease.

Nausea and Vomiting

Nausea is a vague, uncomfortable sensation of sickness or "queasiness" that may or may not be followed by vomiting. Triggers may include odour, activity, medications, or food intake. The emesis, or vomitus, may vary in colour and

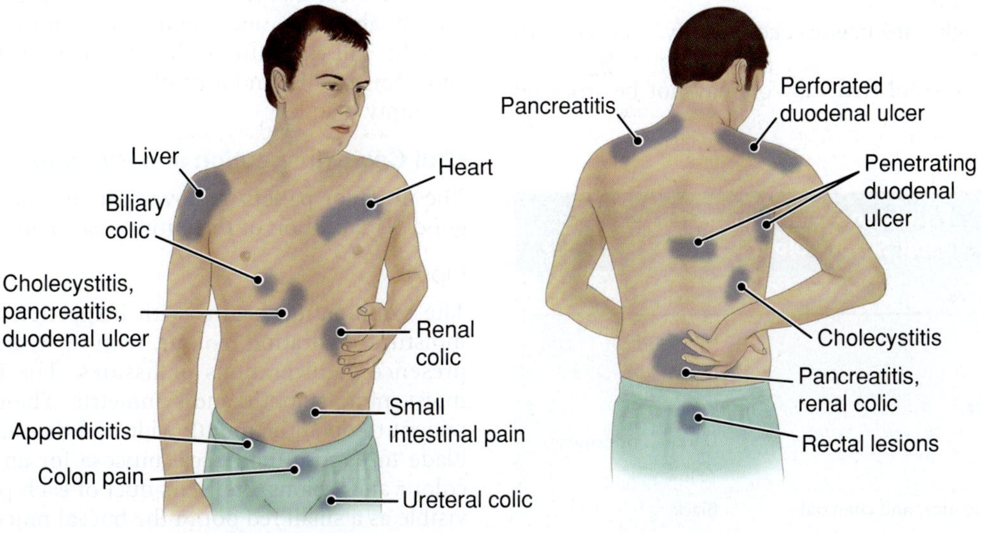

FIGURE 34-3. Common sites of referred abdominal pain.

content and may contain undigested food particles, blood (hematemesis), or bilious material mixed with gastric juices. The causes of nausea and vomiting are many; they may result from (1) visceral afferent stimulation (i.e., dysmotility, peritoneal irritation, infections, hepatobiliary or pancreatic disorders, mechanical obstruction); (2) CNS disorders (i.e., vestibular disorders, increased intracranial pressure, infections, psychogenic disorder); or (3) irritation of the chemoreceptor trigger zone from radiation therapy, systemic disorders, and antitumour chemotherapy medications (Grossman & Porth, 2014).

Change in Bowel Habits and Stool Characteristics

Changes in bowel habits may signal colonic dysfunction or disease. Diarrhea, an abnormal increase in the frequency and liquidity of the stool or in daily stool weight or volume, commonly occurs when the contents move so rapidly through the intestine and colon that there is inadequate time for the GI secretions and oral contents to be absorbed. This physiologic function is typically associated with abdominal pain or cramping and nausea or vomiting. Constipation, a decrease in the frequency of stool, or stools that are hard, dry, and of smaller volume than normal, may be associated with anal discomfort and rectal bleeding. See Chapter 38 for further discussion of diarrhea and constipation.

The characteristics of the stool can vary greatly. Stool is normally light to dark brown; however, specific disease processes and ingestion of certain foods and medications may change the appearance of stool (Table 34-4). Blood in the stool can present in various ways and must be investigated. If blood sheds in sufficient quantities into the upper GI tract, it produces a tarry-black colour (melena), whereas blood entering the lower portion of the GI tract or passing rapidly through it will appear bright or dark red. Lower rectal or anal bleeding is suspected if there is streaking of blood on the surface of the stool or if blood is noted on toilet tissue. Other common abnormalities in stool characteristics described by the patient may include:

- Bulky, greasy, foamy stools that are foul in odour and may or may not float
- Light-grey or clay-coloured stool, caused by a decrease or absence of conjugated bilirubin
- Stool with mucous threads or pus that may be visible on gross inspection of the stool
- Small, dry, rock-hard masses occasionally streaked with blood
- Loose, watery stool that may or may not be streaked with blood

TABLE 34-4 Foods and Medications That Alter Stool Colour

Altering Substance	Colour
Meat protein	Dark brown
Spinach	Green
Carrots and beets	Red
Cocoa	Dark red or brown
Senna	Yellow
Bismuth, iron, licorice, and charcoal	Black
Barium	Milky white

CHART 34-1

Health Promotion: Denture Care

- Brush dentures twice a day.
- Remove dentures at night and soak them in water or a denture product. (Never put dentures in hot water, because they may warp.)
- Rinse mouth with warm salt water in the morning, after meals, and at bedtime.
- Clean well under partial dentures, where food particles tend to get caught.
- Consume nonsticky foods that have been cut into small pieces; chew slowly.
- See dentist regularly to assess and adjust fit.

Past Health, Family, and Social History

The nurse asks about the patient's normal brushing and flossing routine; frequency of dental visits; awareness of any lesions or irritated areas in the mouth, tongue, or throat; recent history of sore throat or bloody sputum; discomfort caused by certain foods; daily food intake; use of alcohol and tobacco, including smokeless chewing tobacco; and the need to wear dentures or a partial plate. For information about denture care, see Chart 34-1.

Past and current medication use and any previous diagnostic studies, treatments, or surgery is noted. The nurse assesses current nutritional status via history; laboratory tests (complete metabolic panel including liver function studies, triglycerides, iron studies, and complete blood count [CBC]) are obtained. History of tobacco and alcohol use includes details about type, amount, length of use, and the date of discontinuation, if any. The nurse and patient discuss changes in appetite or eating patterns and any unexplained weight gain or loss over the past year. It is also important to include questions about psychosocial, spiritual, or cultural factors that may be affecting the patient.

Physical Assessment

The physical examination includes assessment of the mouth, abdomen, and rectum and requires a good source of light, full exposure of the abdomen, warm hands with short fingernails, and a comfortable, relaxed patient with an empty bladder.

Oral Cavity Inspection and Palpation

The nurse or patient removes patient's dentures to allow good visualization of the entire oral cavity.

Lips

The examination begins with inspection of the lips for moisture, hydration, colour, texture, symmetry, and the presence of ulcerations or fissures. The lips should be moist, pink, smooth, and symmetric. The nurse instructs patient to open the mouth wide and then inserts a tongue blade to expose the buccal mucosa for an assessment of colour and lesions. Stensen's duct of each parotid gland is visible as a small red dot in the buccal mucosa next to the upper molars.

Gums

The nurse inspects gums for inflammation, bleeding, retraction, and discolouration. The odour of the breath is also noted. The nurse examines hard palate for colour and shape.

Tongue

The nurse inspects the dorsum (back) of the tongue for texture, colour, and lesions. A thin white coat and large, vallate papillae in a "V" formation on the distal portion of the dorsum of the tongue are normal findings. The nurse instructs patient to protrude the tongue and move it laterally. This provides the examiner with an opportunity to estimate the tongue's size as well as its symmetry and strength (to assess the integrity of the 12th cranial nerve [hypoglossal]).

Further inspection of the ventral surface of the tongue and the floor of the mouth is accomplished by asking the patient to touch the roof of the mouth with the tip of the tongue. The nurse assesses for any lesions of the mucosa or any abnormalities involving the frenulum or superficial veins on the undersurface of the tongue for location, size, colour, and pain. This is a common area for oral cancer, which presents as a white or red plaque, an indurated ulcer, or a warty growth (Weber & Kelley, 2017).

The nurse uses a tongue blade to depress the tongue for adequate visualization of the pharynx, pressing firmly beyond the midpoint of the tongue (proper placement avoids a gagging response). The nurse tells patient to tip head back, open the mouth wide, take a deep breath, and say "ah." Often this flattens the posterior tongue and briefly allows a full view of the tonsils, uvula, and posterior pharynx. The nurse inspects these structures for colour, symmetry, and evidence of exudate, ulceration, or enlargement. Normally, the uvula and soft palate rise symmetrically with a deep inspiration or "ah"; this indicates an intact vagus nerve (10th cranial nerve).

A complete assessment of the oral cavity is essential because many disorders, such as cancer, diabetes, and immunosuppressive conditions resulting from medication therapy or acquired immunodeficiency syndrome (AIDS), can manifest by changes in the oral cavity, including stomatitis.

Abdominal Inspection, Auscultation, Palpation, and Percussion

WATCH & LEARN

The patient lies supine with knees flexed slightly for inspection, auscultation, palpation, and percussion of the abdomen. For the purposes of examination and documentation, the abdomen is divided into either four quadrants or nine regions (Fig. 34-4).

Consistent use of one of these mapping methods results in a thorough evaluation of the abdomen and appropriate documentation. The four-quadrant method involves the use of an imaginary line drawn vertically from the sternum to the pubis through the umbilicus and a horizontal line drawn across the abdomen through the umbilicus. The nurse performs inspection first, noting skin changes, nodules, lesions, scarring, discolouration, inflammation, bruising, or striae. Lesions are of particular importance, because GI diseases often produce skin changes. The nurse identifies and notes the contour and symmetry of the abdomen, and identifies any localized bulging, distention, or peristaltic waves. Expected contours of the anterior abdominal wall are described as flat, rounded, or scaphoid.

Auscultation always precedes percussion and palpation because they may alter sounds. The nurse uses auscultation to determine the character, location, and frequency of bowel sounds and to identify vascular sounds. The nurse assesses bowel sounds in all four quadrants using the diaphragm of the stethoscope for high-pitched and gurgling sounds (Weber & Kelley, 2017). The frequency and character of the sounds are usually heard as clicks and gurgles that occur irregularly and range from 5 to 35 per minute. The terms *normal* (sounds heard about every 5 to 20 seconds), *hypoactive* (one or two sounds in 2 minutes), *hyperactive* (five to six sounds heard in less than 30 seconds), or *absent* (no sounds in 3 to 5 minutes) are frequently used in documentation, but these assessments are highly subjective (Li, Wang, & Ma, 2012). Using the bell of the stethoscope, any bruits in the aortic, renal, iliac, and femoral arteries are noted. Friction rubs are high-pitched and heard over the liver and spleen during respiration. Borborygmi or "stomach growling" is heard as a loud prolonged gurgle.

Percussion is used to assess the size and density of the abdominal organs and to detect the presence of air-filled, fluid-filled, or solid masses. The nurse uses percussion either independently or concurrently with palpation because it can validate palpation findings. Light palpation is appropriate for identifying areas of tenderness or muscular resistance, and deep palpation to identify masses. The nurse percusses all quadrants for overall tympani and dullness. Tympani is the sound that results from the

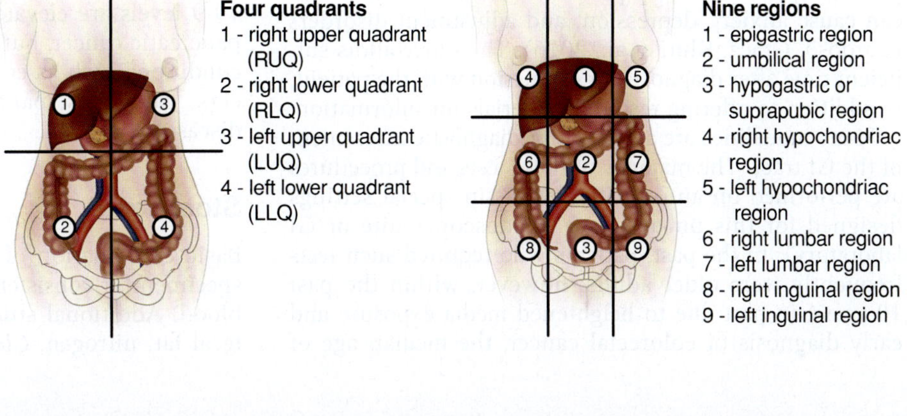

FIGURE 34-4. Division of the abdomen into four quadrants or nine regions.

presence of air in the stomach and small intestines; dullness is heard over organs and solid masses. Many examiners do not perform testing for rebound tenderness because it can cause severe pain; the nurse should use light percussion instead to produce a mild localized response when peritoneal irritation is present.

Rectal Inspection and Palpation

The final part of the examination is evaluation of the terminal portions of the GI tract, rectum, perianal region, and anus. The anal canal is approximately 2.5 to 4 cm (1 to 1.6 in) in length and opens into the perineum. Concentric rings of muscle, the internal and external sphincters, normally keep the anal canal securely closed. Gloves, water-soluble lubrication, a penlight, and drapes are necessary tools for the evaluation. Although the rectal examination is generally uncomfortable and often embarrassing for the patient, it is a mandatory part of every thorough examination.

For women, the rectal examination may be part of the gynecologic examination. Positions for the rectal examination include knee–chest, left lateral with hips and knees flexed, or standing with hips flexed and upper body supported by the examination table. Most patients are comfortable on the right side with knees brought up to the chest.

External examination includes inspection for lumps, rashes, inflammation, excoriation, tears, scars, pilonidal dimpling, and tufts of hair at the pilonidal area. The discovery of tenderness, inflammation, or both should alert the examiner to the possibility of a pilonidal cyst, perianal abscess, or anorectal fistula or fissure.

The patient's buttocks are carefully spread and visually inspected until the patient has relaxed the external sphincter control. The nurse asks patient to bear down, thus allowing the ready appearance of fistulas, fissures, rectal prolapse, polyps, and internal hemorrhoids. The nurse performs internal examination with a lubricated index finger inserted into the anal canal while the patient bears down. Note the tone of the sphincter and any nodules or irregularities of the anal ring. Because this is an uncomfortable part of the examination for most patients, the patient is encouraged to focus on deep breathing and visualization of a pleasant setting during the brief examination.

Diagnostic Evaluation

GI diagnostic studies can confirm, rule out, stage, or diagnose disease. The diagnosis and treatment of cancer brings psychological distress to patients and their families and can cause anxiety, depression, and adjustment disorders (Cardoso, Graca, Klut, et al., 2016). The nurse allots sufficient time after diagnosis for discussion with the patient, in addition to offering resource materials for information.

Many modalities are available for diagnostic assessment of the GI tract. The majority of these tests and procedures are performed on an outpatient basis in special settings designed for this purpose (e.g., endoscopy suite or GI laboratory). In the past, patients who required such tests frequently were older adults; however, within the past 10 years, in part due to heightened media exposure and early diagnosis of colorectal cancer, the median age of patients evaluated for colorectal cancer has decreased significantly.

Preparation for many of these studies includes clear liquid diet, fasting, ingestion of a liquid bowel preparation, the use of laxatives or enemas, and ingestion or injection of a contrast agent or a radiopaque dye. Measures may be poorly tolerated by some patients and are especially problematic in older adults or patients with comorbidities due to alterations in the internal fluid and electrolyte balance. If required after an outpatient procedure, a patient is admitted to hospital for further assessment or treatment.

Specific nursing interventions for each test are provided later in this chapter. General nursing interventions for the patient who is undergoing a GI diagnostic evaluation include:

- Establishing the nursing diagnosis
- Providing needed information about the test and the activities required of the patient
- Providing instructions about postprocedure care and activity restrictions
- Providing health information and procedural teaching to patients and significant others
- Helping the patient cope with discomfort and alleviating anxiety
- Informing the primary care provider of known medical conditions or abnormal laboratory values that may affect the procedure
- Assessing for adequate hydration before, during, and immediately after the procedure, and providing education about maintenance of hydration

Serum Laboratory Studies

Initial diagnostic tests begin with serum laboratory studies, including but not limited to CBC, complete metabolic panel, prothrombin time/partial thromboplastin time, triglycerides, liver function tests, amylase, and lipase. Studies such as carcinoembryonic antigen (CEA) and cancer antigen (CA) 19-9 that have sensitivity for colorectal cancer, and alpha-fetoprotein that has sensitivity for liver cancer may be performed. CEA is a protein that is normally not detected in the blood of a healthy person; therefore, when detected, it indicates that cancer is present, but not what type of cancer is present. Practitioners can use CEA results to determine the stage and extent of the disease and the prognosis for those with cancer, especially GI and, in particular, colorectal cancer (Chin & Chen, 2017). CA 19-9 is also a protein that exists on the surface of certain cells and shed by tumour cells, making it useful as a tumour marker to follow the course of the cancer. CA 19-9 levels are elevated in most patients with advanced pancreatic cancer, but they may also be elevated in other conditions such as colorectal, lung, and gallbladder cancers; gallstones; pancreatitis; cystic fibrosis; and liver disease.

Stool Tests

Basic examination of the stool includes inspecting the specimen for consistency, colour, and occult (not visible) blood. Additional studies, including fecal urobilinogen, fecal fat, nitrogen, *Clostridium difficile*, fecal leukocytes, calculation of stool osmolar gap, parasites, pathogens, food residues, and other substances, require laboratory evaluation.

Stool samples are usually collected on a random basis unless a quantitative study (e.g., fecal fat, urobilinogen) is to be performed. The nurse sends random specimens promptly to the laboratory for analysis; however, the quantitative 24- to 72-hour collections must be kept refrigerated until transported to the laboratory. Some stool collections require the patient to follow a specific diet or refrain from taking certain medications before the collection. Thorough and accurate patient education regarding a specific stool study prior to collection greatly increases the accuracy of study results.

Fecal occult blood testing (FOBT) is one of the most commonly performed stool tests. It can be useful in initial screening for several disorders, although used most frequently in early cancer detection programs. FOBT can be performed at the bedside, in the laboratory, or at home. Probably the most widely used in-office or at-home occult blood test is the Hemoccult II. It is inexpensive, is noninvasive, and carries minimal risk to the patient. However, the nurse should not perform when there is hemorrhoidal bleeding. In the past, patients were advised to avoid ingesting red meats, aspirin, nonsteroidal anti-inflammatory drugs, turnips, and horseradish for 72 hours prior to the study because it was thought that these were associated with false-positive results; likewise, patients were advised to avoid ingesting vitamin C from supplements or foods as it was believed that this was associated with false-negative results. However, these restrictions are no longer advised as their actual effects on test results have not been established; plus, they unnecessarily restricted patient participation in screening (Garborg, 2015).

The nurse applies a small amount of the specimen to the guaiac-impregnated paper slide. If the test is performed at home, the patient mails the slide to the physician in an envelope provided for that purpose. Other occult blood tests that may yield more specific and more sensitive readings include Hematest II SENSA and HemoQuant.

Fecal immunologic tests use monoclonal or polyclonal antibodies to detect the globin protein in human hemoglobin. There is no reaction with nonhuman hemoglobin or with foods that contain peroxidase activity; these tests are therefore more specific than guaiac tests (Le Pimpec, Moutel, Piette, et al., 2017). Dietary restrictions are not required prior to submission of the stool specimen (Wong, Ching, Chan, et al., 2015). Since only one fecal stool sample is required, it is associated with improved screening participation (Garborg, 2015). Hemoporphyrin assays detect the broadest range of blood derivatives, but a strict dietary protocol is essential. Quantitative fecal immunochemical tests may be more accurate than guaiac testing and useful for patients who refuse invasive testing (Goede, Rabeneck, van Ballegooijen, et al., 2017).

The stool DNA test is a relatively new test to detect certain DNA related to colon cancer. More research is needed to determine how often the test needs to be performed. The stool DNA test does not require any dietary or medication restrictions and can detect neoplasia anywhere in the colon. The stool sample can be collected at home (Rutten, Jacobsen, Wilson, et al., 2017).

Breath Tests

The hydrogen breath test developed to evaluate carbohydrate absorption, in addition to aiding in the diagnosis of bacterial overgrowth in the intestine and short bowel syndrome. This test determines the amount of hydrogen expelled in the breath after production in the colon (on contact of galactose with fermenting bacteria) and absorbed into the blood.

Urea breath tests detect the presence of *Helicobacter pylori*, the bacteria that can live in the mucosal lining of the stomach and cause peptic ulcer disease. After the patient ingests a capsule of carbon-labeled urea, a breath sample is obtained 10 to 20 minutes later. Because *H. pylori* metabolizes urea rapidly, the labeled carbon is absorbed quickly and measured as carbon dioxide in the expired breath to determine whether *H. pylori* is present. The patient is instructed to avoid antibiotics or loperamide (Pepto-Bismol) for 1 month before the test; sucralfate (Carafate) and omeprazole (Prilosec) for 1 week before the test; and cimetidine (Tagamet), famotidine (Pepcid), and ranitidine (Zantac) for 24 hours before the test. Also, *H. pylori* is detected by assessing serum antibody levels without requiring medication therapy adjustments (Overland, 2014).

Abdominal Ultrasonography

Ultrasonography is a noninvasive diagnostic technique in which high-frequency sound waves pass into internal body structures with the ultrasonic echoes recorded on an oscilloscope as they strike tissues of different densities. It is particularly useful in the detection of an enlarged gallbladder or pancreas, the presence of gallstones, an enlarged ovary, an ectopic pregnancy, or appendicitis. Recently this technique has proven useful in diagnosing acute colonic diverticulitis (Tomizawa, Shinozaki, Hsaegawa, et al., 2017).

Advantages of abdominal ultrasonography include an absence of ionizing radiation, no noticeable side effects, relatively low cost, and almost immediate results. It cannot be used to examine structures that lie behind bony tissue because bone prevents sound waves from traveling into deeper structures. Gas and fluid in the abdomen or air in the lungs also prevents transmission of ultrasound. An ultrasound produces no ill effects. However, some patients, typically pregnant women, have concerns regarding the energy emitted by the probe.

Endoscopic ultrasonography (EUS) is a specialized enteroscopic procedure that aids in the diagnosis of GI disorders by providing direct imaging of a target area. A small high-frequency ultrasonic transducer mounted at the tip of the fibreoptic scope displays an image that enables tumour staging and visualization of marginal structures. The resulting images have higher-quality resolution and definition than regular ultrasound imaging. EUS may be used to evaluate submucosal lesions, specifically their location and depth of penetration. Moderate sedation is typically indicated (Fischbach & Dunning, 2015). In addition, EUS may aid in the evaluation of Barrett's esophagus, portal hypertension, chronic pancreatitis, suspected pancreatic neoplasm, biliary tract disease, and changes in the bowel wall due to ulcerative colitis. EUS is a safe and accurate test to use to select patients suspected of having biliary obstructive disease for therapeutic endoscopic retrograde cholangiopancreatography (ERCP) (Yi, Lu, Chujun, et al., 2017). Intestinal gas, bone, and thick layers of adipose tissue, which hamper conventional ultrasonography, are not problems when EUS is used.

Nursing Interventions

The nurse instructs patient to fast for 8 to 12 hours before the test to decrease the amount of gas in the bowel. If gallbladder studies are performed, the patient should eat a fat-free meal the evening before the test. If barium studies are performed, they should be scheduled after ultrasonography; otherwise, the barium could interfere with the transmission of the sound waves. Patients who receive moderate sedation are observed for about 1 hour to assess for level of consciousness, orientation, and ability to ambulate. Patients treated on an outpatient basis are given instructions regarding diet, activity, and how to monitor for complications.

DNA Testing

Researchers have refined methods for genetic risk assessment, preclinical diagnosis, and prenatal diagnosis to identify people who are at risk for certain GI disorders (e.g., gastric cancer, lactose deficiency, inflammatory bowel disease, colon cancer) (Chart 34-2). In some cases, DNA testing allows clinicians to prevent (or minimize) disease, by intervening before its onset, and to improve therapy (Simard & Hall, 2013). People identified as at risk for certain GI disorders may choose to have genetic counselling to learn about the disease and options for preventing and treating the disease and to receive support in coping with the situation.

Imaging Studies

Numerous minimally invasive and noninvasive imaging studies, including x-ray and contrast studies, computed tomography (CT), three-dimensional CT, magnetic resonance imaging (MRI), positron emission tomography (PET), scintigraphy (radionuclide imaging), and virtual colonoscopy, are available today.

GENETICS IN NURSING PRACTICE

Chart 34-2. Digestive and Gastrointestinal Disorders

Several digestive and gastrointestinal disorders are associated with genetic abnormalities. Some examples include:

Autosomal dominant:
- Hereditary diffuse gastric cancer
- Hereditary nonpolyposis colorectal cancer (Lynch's syndrome)
- Hirschsprung's disease (aganglionic megacolon)

Autosomal recessive:
- Glucose galactose malabsorption
- Glycogen storage disease (von Gierke's disease)
- Pompe's disease
- Zellweger's syndrome

Inheritance pattern includes autosomal dominant and autosomal recessive:
- Familial adenomatous polyposis

X-linked:
- Fabry's disease

Inheritance pattern is not distinct; however, there is a genetic predisposition for the disease:
- Crohn's disease
- Type 1 diabetes
- Celiac disease
- Pancreatic cancer

Other genetic disorders that will impact the digestive and gastrointestinal system:
- Cleft lip and/or palate
- Cystic fibrosis

Nursing Assessments

FAMILY HISTORY ASSESSMENT RELATED TO DIGESTIVE AND GASTROINTESTINAL DISORDERS
- Careful family history assessment for other family members with a similar condition (e.g., cleft lip/palate, pyloric stenosis).
- Assess for other family members in several generations with early-onset colorectal cancer.
- Inquire about other family members with inflammatory bowel disease.
- Assess family history for other cancers (e.g., endometrial, ovarian, kidney).

PATIENT ASSESSMENT SPECIFIC TO DIGESTIVE AND GASTROINTESTINAL DISORDERS
- Ask about bowel pattern and color of stool.
- Assess if patient experiences episodes of abdominal cramping, diarrhea, or dehydration.
- Assess for unexplained weight loss.
- Identify intolerance to specific foods (e.g., gluten, high fat foods, lactose).
- Assess for prior history of liver disorders.

Assess for presence of other clinical conditions:
- With clefting—congenital heart defect, other birth defects suggestive of a genetic syndrome.
- With familial adenomatous polyposis—congenital hypertrophy of retinal pigment epithelium.

Genetics Resources

Cancer.Net, www.cancer.net
Celiac Support Association, www.csaceliacs.org
Crohn's & Colitis Foundation of America, www.ccfa.org

Upper Gastrointestinal Tract Study

An upper GI fluoroscopy delineates the entire GI tract after the introduction of a contrast agent. A radiopaque liquid (e.g., barium sulphate) is commonly used; however, thin barium, Hypaque, and at times water are used due to their low associated risks. The GI series enables the examiner to detect or exclude anatomic or functional disorders of the upper GI organs or sphincters. It also aids in the diagnosis of ulcers, varices, tumours, regional enteritis, and malabsorption syndromes. The procedure can extend to examine the duodenum and small bowel (small bowel follow-through). As the barium descends into the stomach, the position, patency, and calibre of the esophagus is visualized, enabling the examiner to detect or exclude any anatomic or functional derangement of that organ. Fluoroscopic examination next extends to the stomach as its lumen fills with barium, allowing observation of stomach motility, thickness of the gastric wall, the mucosal pattern, patency of the pyloric valve, and the anatomy of the duodenum. The procedure produces multiple x-ray films, and additional images may be taken at intervals for up to 24 hours to evaluate the rate of gastric emptying. Small bowel x-rays taken while the barium is passing through that area allow for observation of the motility of the small bowel. Also, potentially detected are obstructions, ileitis, and diverticula.

Variations of the upper GI study include double-contrast studies and enteroclysis. The double-contrast method of examining the upper GI tract involves administration of a thick barium suspension to outline the stomach and esophageal wall, and a following administration of tablets that release carbon dioxide in the presence of water. This technique has the advantage of showing the esophagus and stomach in finer detail, permitting noting of signs of early superficial neoplasms.

Enteroclysis is a very detailed, double-contrast study of the entire small intestine that involves the continuous infusion, through a duodenal tube, of 500 to 1,000 mL (17 to 34 oz) of a thin barium sulphate suspension; after this, the nurse infuses methylcellulose through the tube. The barium and methylcellulose fill the intestinal loops and are observed continuously by fluoroscopy and viewed at frequent intervals as they progress through the jejunum and the ileum. This process (even with normal motility) can take up to 6 hours and can be quite uncomfortable for the patient. The procedure aids in the diagnosis of partial small bowel obstructions or diverticula. The value of these x-ray screening studies has diminished as better technology has emerged including magnetic resonance enteroclysis (Mansoori, Delaney, Willis, et al., 2016; Melamud, Colip, & Soto, 2016).

Nursing Interventions

Education regarding dietary changes prior to the study should include a clear liquid diet, with nothing by mouth (NPO) from midnight the night before the study; however, each physician may prefer a specific bowel preparation for specific studies. The nurse advises against smoking, chewing gum, and using mints because they can stimulate gastric motility and salivation (Bontrager & Lampignano, 2014). Typically, oral morning medications are withheld on day of study, and resumed in evening. However, each patient's medication regimen is evaluated individually. When a patient with insulin-dependent diabetes is NPO, his or her insulin requirements are adjusted accordingly.

The nurse provides follow-up care after the upper GI procedure to ensure that the patient has eliminated most of the ingested barium. Increasing fluids may facilitate evacuation of stool and barium, if not contraindicated.

Lower Gastrointestinal Tract Study

Barium instilled in the lower GI tract permits visualization. The barium enema is used to detect the presence of polyps, tumours, or other lesions of the large intestine and demonstrate any anatomic abnormalities or malfunctioning of the bowel. After proper preparation and evacuation of the entire colon, each portion of the colon may be readily observed. The procedure usually takes about 15 to 30 minutes, including obtaining x-ray images. Other means for visualizing the colon include double-contrast studies and a water-soluble contrast study. Although these tests are still used due to their relative cost and simplicity, new studies indicate a move to other imaging modalities (Joshi & Wang, 2016; Royle, Ferguson, Mak, et al., 2013). A double-contrast or air-contrast barium enema involves the instillation of a thicker barium solution, followed by the instillation of air. The patient may feel some cramping or discomfort during this process. This test provides a contrast between the air-filled lumen and the barium-coated mucosa, allowing easier detection of smaller lesions.

If active inflammatory disease, fistulas, or perforation of the colon is suspected, a water-soluble iodinated contrast agent (e.g., Gastrografin) can be used. The procedure is the same as for a barium enema, but the nurse assesses the patient for allergic reactions to iodine or contrast agents. The contrast agent eliminates readily after the procedure, so there is no need for postprocedure laxatives. Some diarrhea may occur in a few patients until the contrast agent is eliminated.

Nursing Interventions

Preparation of the patient includes emptying and cleansing the lower bowel. This often necessitates a low-residue diet 1 to 2 days before the test (the preparation required by different x-ray departments may vary); a clear liquid diet and a laxative the evening before; NPO after midnight; and cleansing enemas until returns are clear the following morning. The nurse ensures that if ordered the barium enema is scheduled before any upper GI studies. If the patient has active inflammatory disease of the colon, enemas are contraindicated. Barium enemas also are contraindicated in patients with signs of perforation or obstruction; instead, a water-soluble contrast study is performed. Active GI bleeding may prohibit the use of laxatives and enemas.

Postprocedural patient education includes information about increasing fluid intake; evaluating bowel movements for evacuation of barium; and noting increased number of bowel movements, because barium, due to its high osmolarity, may draw fluid into the bowel, thus increasing the intraluminal contents and resulting in greater output.

Computed Tomography

CT provides cross-sectional images of abdominal organs and structures. In a CT, multiple images taken from numerous angles are digitized, reconstructed, and then viewed on a computer monitor. The use of CT has increased over the years as the sensitivity and specificity of CT has improved. Volume CT scanners (i.e., helical or spiral scanning) provide more accurate reconstruction of patient data into alternate planes, require shorter scan times, and have less artefact when compared to single slice scanning (Bontrager & Lampignano, 2014).

CT is a valuable tool for detecting and localizing many inflammatory conditions in the colon, such as appendicitis, diverticulitis, regional enteritis, and ulcerative colitis, as well as evaluating the abdomen for diseases of the liver, spleen, kidney, pancreas, and pelvic organs, and structural abnormalities of the abdominal wall. As the adequacy of detail in the test depends on the presence of fat, this diagnostic tool is not useful for very thin, cachectic patients. The procedure is painless, but radiation doses are considerable. A CT scan may be performed with or without oral or intravenous (IV) contrast, but the enhancement of the study is greater with the use of a contrast agent. For those patients who may be at risk for complications from use of contrast (see later discussion), the use of contrast should be contraindicated if the suspected pathology can be visualized from a non–contrast-enhanced study (Rawson & Pelletier, 2013). Continuous-motion (helical or spiral), three-dimensional CT that provides very detailed pictures of the GI organs and vasculature is available (Wampole, Kairys, Mitchell, et al., 2013).

Nursing Interventions

CT may be performed with or without oral or IV contrast, but the enhancement of the study is greater with use of a contrast agent. Any allergies to contrast agents, iodine, or shellfish; the patient's current serum creatinine level; and urine human chorionic gonadotropin must be determined before administration of a contrast agent. Patients allergic to the contrast agent may be premedicated with IV prednisone 24 hours, 12 hours, and 1 hour before the scan.

In addition, renal protective measures include the administration of IV sodium bicarbonate 1 hour before and 6 hours after IV contrast and oral acetyl cysteine (Mucomyst) before or after the study. Both sodium bicarbonate and Mucomyst are free radical scavengers that sequester the contrast byproducts that are destructive to renal cells (Zhang, Ding, Li, et al., 2017).

Magnetic Resonance Imaging

MRI supplements ultrasound and CT in gastroenterology. MRI, a noninvasive technique using magnetic fields and radio waves, produces images of the area under examination (Melamud et al., 2016). The use of oral contrast agents to enhance the image has increased the application of this technique for the diagnosis of GI diseases. It is useful in evaluating abdominal soft tissues as well as blood vessels, abscesses, fistulas, neoplasms, and other sources of bleeding.

The physiologic artefacts of heartbeat, respiration, and peristalsis may create a less-than-clear image, but newer, fast-imaging MRI techniques help eliminate these physiologic motion artefacts. MRIs are not totally safe for all people. Any ferromagnetic objects (metals that contain iron) can be attracted to the magnet and cause injury. Items that can be problematic or dangerous include jewellery, pacemakers, dental implants, paperclips, pens, keys, IV poles, clips on patient gowns, and oxygen tanks.

> **NURSING ALERT**
>
> **MRI is contraindicated for patients with permanent pacemakers, artificial heart valves and defibrillators, implanted insulin pumps, or implanted transcutaneous electrical nerve stimulation devices, because the magnetic field could cause malfunction. MRI is also contraindicated for patients with internal metal devices (e.g., aneurysm clips), intraocular metallic fragments, or cochlear implants. Foil-backed skin patches (e.g., NicoDerm, nitroglycerin [Transderm-Nitro], scopolamine [Transderm-Scop], clonidine [Catapres-TTS]) are removed before an MRI due to the risk of burns. The patient's physician requires consultation prior to patch removal to determine if an alternate form of the medication should be provided.**

Nursing Interventions

Prestudy patient education includes NPO status 6 to 8 hours before the study and removal of all jewellery and other metals. The nurse informs the patient and family that the study may take 60 to 90 minutes. During the study the technician will instruct the patient to take deep breaths at specific intervals. The close-fitting scanners used in many MRI facilities may induce feelings of claustrophobia, and the machine will make a knocking sound during the procedure. Patients may choose to wear a headset and listen to music or to wear a blindfold during the procedure. Open MRIs that are less close fitting eliminate the claustrophobia experienced by many patients.

Positron Emission Tomography

PET scans produce images of the body by detecting the radiation emitted from radioactive substances. The radioactive substances injected into the body by IV are usually tagged with a radioactive atom, such as carbon-11, fluorine-18, oxygen-15, or nitrogen-13 (Bontrager & Lampignano, 2014). The atoms decay quickly, do not harm the body, have lower radiation levels than a typical x-ray or CT scan, and eliminate in the urine or feces. The scanner essentially "captures" where the radioactive substances are in the body, transmits information to a scanner, and produces a scan with "hot spots" for evaluation by the radiologist or oncologist.

Scintigraphy

Scintigraphy (radionuclide testing) relies on the use of radioactive isotopes (i.e., technetium, iodine, and indium) to reveal displaced anatomic structures, changes in organ size, and the presence of neoplasms or other focal lesions, such as cysts or abscesses. Also, scintigraphic scanning is used to measure the uptake of tagged red blood cells and leukocytes. Tagging of red blood cells and leukocytes by injection of a radionuclide is performed to define areas of inflammation, abscess, blood loss, or neoplasm. A sample of blood is removed, mixed with a radioactive substance, and reinjected into the patient. Abnormal concentrations of blood cells are then detected at 24- and 48-hour intervals. Tagged red cell studies are useful in determining the source of internal bleeding when all other studies have returned a negative result.

Gastrointestinal Motility Studies

Radionuclide testing is used to assess gastric emptying and colonic transit time. During gastric emptying studies, the liquid and solid components of a meal (typically scrambled eggs) are tagged with radionuclide markers (Kar, Jones, Horowitz, et al., 2015). After ingestion of the meal, the patient is positioned under a scintiscanner, which measures the rate of passage of the radioactive substance from the stomach. This is useful in diagnosing disorders of gastric motility, diabetic gastroparesis, and dumping syndrome.

Colonic transit studies are used to evaluate colonic motility and obstructive defecation syndromes. The patient is administered a capsule containing 20 radionuclide markers and instructed to follow a regular diet and normal daily activities. Abdominal x-rays are taken every 24 hours until all markers pass. This process usually takes 4 to 5 days, but in the presence of severe constipation, it may take as long as 10 days. Patients with chronic diarrhea may be evaluated at 8-hour intervals. The amount of time that it takes for the radioactive material to move through the colon indicates colonic motility.

Endoscopic Procedures

Endoscopic procedures used in GI tract assessment include **fibroscopy**/esophagogastroduodenoscopy (EGD), small bowel enteroscopy, colonoscopy, sigmoidoscopy, proctoscopy, anoscopy, and endoscopy through an ostomy.

Upper Gastrointestinal Fibroscopy/ Esophagogastroduodenoscopy

Fibroscopy of the upper GI tract allows direct visualization of the esophageal, gastric, and duodenal mucosa through a lighted endoscope (gastroscope) (Fig. 34-5).

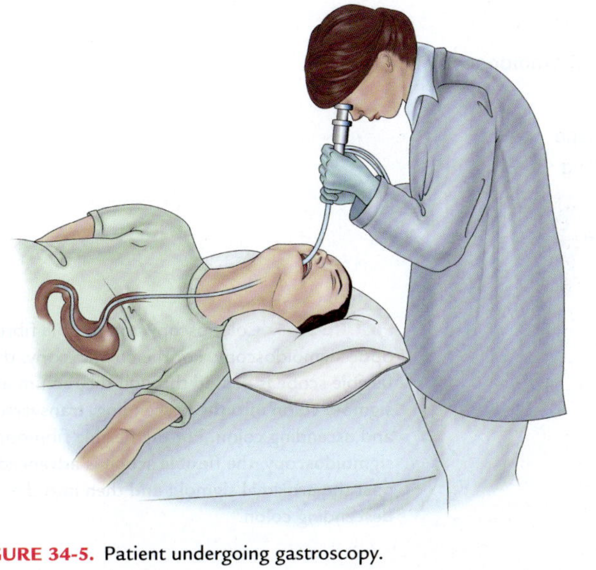

FIGURE 34-5. Patient undergoing gastroscopy.

EGD is valuable for suspected esophageal, gastric, or duodenal disorders or inflammatory, neoplastic, or infectious processes. This procedure is also used to evaluate esophageal and gastric motility and to collect secretions and tissue specimens for further analysis.

In EGD, the gastroenterologist views the GI tract through a viewing lens and can obtain images through the scope to document findings. Electronic video endoscopes also are available that attach directly to a video processor, converting the electronic signals into pictures on a television screen. This allows larger and continuous viewing capabilities, as well as the simultaneous recording of the procedure.

PillCam ESO2, a pill-sized instrument equipped with two cameras and combined with flexible spectral imaging colour enhancement (FICE), is advancing as a diagnostic technique. The ESO2 camera takes seven photographs per second and transmits them wirelessly to a nearby storage device. The colour enhancing technique allows for visualizations of lesions not seen or not detectable in earlier ESO versions. This technique is advancing rapidly as a more comfortable, convenient alternative to traditional endoscopy. Previous major drawbacks to this method of endoscopy such as only evaluating the esophagus and lodging of the instrument in previously anastomosed section of bowel are being overcome by combining ESO2 with enhanced visualization techniques such as FICE (Sharma & Rana, 2016). ERCP uses the endoscope in combination with x-rays to view the ductal structures of the biliary tract (Laing & Adler, 2012). The side-viewing flexible scopes are used to visualize the common bile duct and the pancreatic and hepatic ducts through the ampulla of Vater in the duodenum. ERCP is helpful in evaluating jaundice, pancreatitis, pancreatic tumours, common bile duct stones, and biliary tract disease. ERCP is described further in Chapter 40.

Upper GI fibroscopy also can be a therapeutic procedure when combined with other procedures. Therapeutic endoscopy is used to remove common bile duct stones, dilate strictures, and treat gastric bleeding and esophageal varices. Laser-compatible scopes are used to provide laser therapy for upper GI neoplasms. Sclerosing solutions can be injected through the scope in an attempt to control upper GI bleeding.

After the patient is sedated, the endoscope is lubricated with a water-soluble lubricant and passed smoothly and slowly along the back of the mouth and down into the esophagus. The gastroenterologist views the gastric wall and the sphincters, and then advances the endoscope into the duodenum for further examination. Biopsy forceps to obtain tissue specimens or cytology brushes to obtain cells for microscopic study can be passed through the scope. The procedure usually takes about 30 minutes.

The patient may experience nausea, gagging, or choking. Use of topical anesthetic agents and moderate sedation makes it important to monitor and maintain the patient's oral airway during and after the procedure. An oximeter placed either on a finger or an ear monitors oxygen saturation, with supplemental oxygen administered if needed. Precautions must be taken to protect the scope, because the fibreoptic bundles can be broken if the scope is bent at an acute angle. The patient wears a mouth guard to keep from biting the scope.

Nursing Interventions

The patient is NPO for 8 hours prior to the examination. Before the introduction of the endoscope, a local anesthetic gargle or spray is given to the patient. Midazolam (Versed), a sedative that provides moderate sedation and relieves anxiety during the procedure, may be administered. Atropine may be administered to reduce secretions, and glucagon may be administered to relax smooth muscle. The patient is positioned in the left lateral position to facilitate clearance of pulmonary secretions and provide smooth entry of the scope.

After gastroscopy, assessment includes level of consciousness, vital signs, oxygen saturation, pain level, and monitoring for signs of perforation (i.e., pain, bleeding, unusual difficulty swallowing, and rapidly elevated temperature). After the patient's gag reflex has returned, lozenges, saline gargle, and oral analgesic agents may be offered to relieve minor throat discomfort. Patients sedated for the procedure must remain in bed until fully alert. After moderate sedation, the patient is discharged with a responsible accompanying adult if the procedure was performed on an outpatient basis. A responsible adult should stay with the patient until the morning after the procedure to help the patient with mobilization and to mitigate the potential for falls that may result from the action of sedation. Because of sedation, many patients will not remember postprocedure instructions. For this reason, discharge and follow-up instructions are provided to the responsible adult accompanying the patient home, as well as to the patient. In addition, many endoscopy suites provide follow-up with a nurse, who contacts the patient the morning after the procedure to find out if the patient has any concerns or questions related to the procedure.

Fibreoptic Colonoscopy

Historically, direct visualization of the bowel was the only means to evaluate the colon, but virtual colonoscopy (also known as CT colonography) has brought a more patient-friendly approach to this study. Virtual colonoscopy provides a computer-simulated endoluminal perspective of the air-filled distended colon using conventional spiral or helical CT scanning (Spada, Stoker, Alarcon, et al., 2015).

Direct visual inspection of the large intestine (anus, rectum, sigmoid, transcending and ascending colon) is possible by means of a flexible fibreoptic colonoscope (Fig. 34-6). These scopes have the same capabilities as those used for EGD but are larger in diameter and longer. Still and video recordings can be used to document the procedure and findings.

This procedure is used commonly as a diagnostic aid and screening device and is most frequently used for cancer screening and for surveillance in patients with previous colon cancer or polyps. In addition, tissue biopsies can be obtained as needed, and polyps can be removed and evaluated. Other uses of colonoscopy include the evaluation of patients with diarrhea of unknown cause, occult bleeding, or anemia; further study of abnormalities detected on barium enema; and diagnosis, clarification, and determination of the extent of inflammatory or other bowel disease.

Therapeutically, the procedure can be used to remove all visible polyps with a special snare and cautery through the colonoscope. Many colon cancers begin with adenomatous polyps of the colon; therefore, one goal of colonoscopic polypectomy is early detection and prevention of colorectal cancer. This procedure also is used to treat areas of bleeding or stricture. Use of bipolar and unipolar coagulators, use of heater probes, and injections of sclerosing agents or vasoconstrictors are all possible during this procedure. Laser-compatible scopes provide laser therapy for bleeding lesions or colonic neoplasms. Bowel decompression (removal of intestinal contents to prevent gas and fluid from distending the coils of the intestine) can also be completed during the procedure.

Colonoscopy is performed with the patient lying on the left side, legs drawn up toward the chest. The patient's position may be changed during the test to facilitate advancement of the scope. Biopsy forceps or a cytology brush may be passed through the scope to obtain specimens for histology and cytology examinations. Complications during and after the procedure can include cardiac dysrhythmias and respiratory depression resulting from the medications administered; vasovagal reactions; and circulatory overload or hypotension resulting from overhydration or underhydration during bowel preparation.

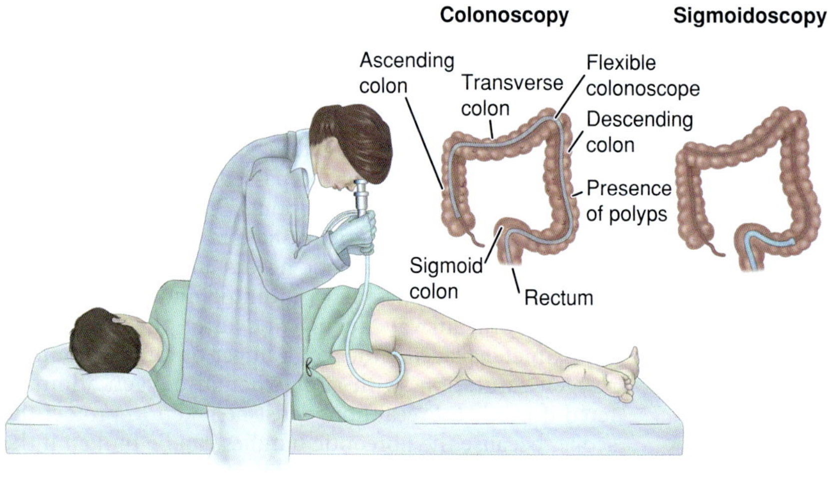

FIGURE 34-6. Colonoscopy and flexible fibreoptic sigmoidoscopy. For the colonoscopy, the flexible scope is passed through the rectum and sigmoid colon into the descending, transverse, and ascending colon. For the flexible fibreoptic sigmoidoscopy, the flexible scope is advanced past the proximal sigmoid and then into the descending colon.

The patient's cardiac and respiratory function and oxygen saturation are monitored continuously, with supplemental oxygen used as necessary. Typically, the procedure takes about 1 hour, and postprocedure discomfort results from instillation of air to expand the colon and insertion and movement of the scope during the procedure.

Capsule colonoscopy is another option for patients who cannot tolerate colonoscopy. This minimally invasive test consists of an ingestible capsule with a two-sided camera (similar to the PillCam ESO). This test requires that the patient completes the same type of extensive bowel preparation as for a colonoscopy. In addition, the patient must ingest a lot of fluids to ensure that the capsule transits through the colon (Garborg, 2015).

Nursing Interventions

The success of the procedure depends on how well the colon is prepared and on adequate sedation (Chen, Athilingam, Saloum, et al., 2015). Adequate colon cleansing provides optimal visualization and decreases the time needed for the procedure. Cleansing of the colon is accomplished in various ways. The physician may prescribe a laxative for 2 nights before the examination and a Fleet's or saline enema until the return is clear the morning of the test. However, more commonly, polyethylene glycol electrolyte lavage solutions (Go-LYTELY, CoLyte, and Nu-Lytely) are used as intestinal lavages for effective cleansing of the bowel. Current recommendations support the use of 2-L PEG split-dose regimen in low- or no-risk patients, and 4-L split-dose with sodium picosulphate plus bisacodyl in patients with comorbidities such as diabetes, chronic constipation, or current history of opioid use, or with a history of problematic colonoscopies (Chen et al., 2015). The patient maintains a clear liquid diet starting at noon the day before the procedure. Then the patient ingests the lavage solution orally at intervals over 3 to 4 hours. If necessary, the nurse can give the solution through a feeding tube if the patient cannot swallow. Patients with a colostomy can receive this same bowel preparation. The use of lavage solutions is contraindicated in patients with intestinal obstruction or inflammatory bowel disease.

A sodium phosphate tablet (Osmoprep, Visicol) can be used for colon cleansing prior to colonoscopy. Dosing consists of 32 tablets: 20 tablets (4 tablets every 15 minutes) with 8 ounces of any clear liquid (water, any clear carbonated beverage, or juice) on the evening prior to the examination and 12 tablets (taken in the same manner) on the morning of the examination. Same-day preparations and minimal bowel cleansing preparations are being studied in patients' groups (Pollentine, Mortimer, & Archer, 2012), however this is not yet a standard practice.

With the use of lavage solutions, bowel cleansing is fast (rectal effluent is clear in about 4 hours) and is tolerated fairly well by most patients. Side effects of the electrolyte solutions include nausea, bloating, cramps or abdominal fullness, fluid and electrolyte imbalance, and hypothermia (patients are often told to drink the preparation as cold as possible to make it more palatable). The side effects are especially problematic for older adult patients, and sometimes they have difficulty ingesting the required volume of solution. Monitoring older adult patients after a bowel prep is especially important because their physiologic ability to compensate for fluid loss is diminished. Many older people take multiple medications each day; therefore, the nurse's knowledge of their daily medication regimen can prompt assessment for and prevention of potential problems and early detection of physiologic changes.

Additionally, the nurse advises the patient with diabetes to consult with his or her physician about medication adjustment to prevent hyperglycemia or hypoglycemia resulting from the dietary modifications required in preparing for the test. The nurse also instructs all patients, especially the older adults, to maintain adequate fluid, electrolyte, and caloric intake while undergoing bowel cleansing.

Special precautions must be taken for some patients. Implantable defibrillators and pacemakers are at high risk of malfunction if electrosurgical procedures (i.e., polypectomy) are performed in conjunction with colonoscopy. A cardiologist should be consulted before the test is performed, and the defibrillator should be turned off. These patients require careful cardiac monitoring during the procedure.

Colonoscopy cannot be performed if there is a suspected or documented colon perforation, acute severe diverticulitis, or fulminant colitis. Patients with prosthetic heart valves or a history of endocarditis require prophylactic antibiotics before the procedure.

Informed consent is obtained by the practitioner before the patient is sedated. Before the examination, an opioid analgesic or sedative agent (e.g., midazolam [Versed]) is administered to provide moderate sedation and relieve anxiety during the procedure. Glucagon may be administered, if needed, to relax the colonic musculature and to reduce spasm during the test. Older adults or debilitated patients may require a reduced dosage of the analgesic or sedative agent to decrease the risks of oversedation and cardiopulmonary complications.

During the procedure, the patient is monitored for changes in oxygen saturation, vital signs, colour and temperature of the skin, level of consciousness, abdominal distention, vagal response, and pain intensity. After the procedure, patients are maintained on bed rest until fully alert. Some patients have abdominal cramps caused by increased peristalsis stimulated by the air insufflated into the bowel during the procedure.

Immediately after the test, the patient is monitored for signs and symptoms of bowel perforation (e.g., rectal bleeding, abdominal pain or distention, fever, focal peritoneal signs). Because of the amnesic effects of midazolam, it is important to provide written instructions, because the patient may be unable to recall verbal information. If the procedure is performed on an outpatient basis, someone must transport the patient home. After a therapeutic procedure, the nurse instructs the patient to report any bleeding to the physician.

Anoscopy, Proctoscopy, and Sigmoidoscopy

Endoscopic examination of the anus, rectum, and sigmoid and descending colon is used to evaluate chronic diarrhea, fecal incontinence, ischemic colitis, and lower GI hemorrhage and to observe for ulceration, fissures, abscesses, tumour, polyps, or other pathologic processes.

Flexible scopes have largely replaced the rigid scopes used in the past for routine examinations. The flexible fibreoptic sigmoidoscope (see Fig. 34-6) permits the colon to be examined up to 40 to 50 cm (16 to 20 in) from the anus, much more than the 25 cm (10 in) that can be visualized with the rigid sigmoidoscope (Cox, 2016). It has many of the same capabilities as the scopes used for the upper GI study, including the use of still or video images to document findings.

For flexible scope procedures, the patient assumes a comfortable position on the left side with the right leg bent and placed anteriorly. It is important to keep the patient informed throughout the examination and to explain the sensations associated with it. Biopsies and polypectomies can be performed during this procedure. Biopsy is performed with small biting forceps introduced through the endoscope; one or more small pieces of tissue may be removed. If polyps are present, they may be removed with a wire snare, which is used to grasp the pedicle, or stalk. An electrocoagulating current is then used to sever the polyp and prevent bleeding. It is extremely important that all excised tissue be placed immediately in moist gauze or in an appropriate receptacle, labeled correctly, and delivered without delay to the pathology laboratory for examination (Cox, 2016).

Nursing Interventions

These examinations require only limited bowel preparation, including a warm tap water or Fleet's enema until returns are clear. Dietary restrictions usually are not necessary, and sedation usually is not required. During the procedure, the nurse monitors vital signs, skin colour and temperature, pain tolerance, and vagal response. After the procedure, the nurse monitors the patient for rectal bleeding and signs of intestinal perforation (i.e., fever, rectal drainage, abdominal distention, and pain). On completion of the examination, the patient can resume his or her regular activities and diet.

Small Bowel Enteroscopy

There are several methods available for visualization of the small intestine, including capsule endoscopy and double-balloon endoscopy. Capsule endoscopy allows the noninvasive visualization of the mucosa throughout the entire small intestine. It is particularly useful in the evaluation of obscure GI bleeding. The technique consists of the patient swallowing a capsule that has embedded in it a wireless miniature camera, a light source, and an image transmission system. The capsule is the size of a large vitamin pill (26 mm long, 11 mm wide, and 3.7 g in weight). It is propelled through the intestine by peristalsis. Images are transmitted from the end of the capsule to a recording device worn on a belt. Typically the capsule passes from the rectum in 1 or 2 days. This diagnostic procedure is limited by its inability to allow for obtaining tissue samples for histology and for providing endoscopic therapy (Li, Gui, Zhao, et al., 2018).

Double-balloon enteroscopy (DBE), also known as push-and-pull enteroscopy, has made it possible to visualize the mucosa of the entire small bowel as well as carry out diagnostic and therapeutic interventions (Lu, Qi, Weng, et al., 2017). This endoscope is composed of two balloons, one that is attached to the distal end of the scope and the other that is attached to the transparent overtube that slides over the endoscope. The endoscope is advanced using a push-and-pull technique that involves alternately inflating and deflating the balloons, causes telescoping of the small intestine onto the overtube. As a result of this telescoping, the endoscope can visualize much more of the small intestine than the length of the scope itself. The procedure takes between 1 and 3 hours and requires moderate sedation.

Endoscopy Through Ostomy

Endoscopy through an ostomy stoma is useful for visualizing a segment of the small or large intestine and may be indicated to evaluate the anastomosis for recurrent disease, or to visualize and treat bleeding in a segment of the bowel. Nursing interventions are similar to those for other endoscopic procedures.

Manometry and Electrophysiologic Studies

Manometry and electrophysiologic studies are methods for evaluating patients with GI motility disorders. The manometry test measures changes in intraluminal pressures and the coordination of muscle activity in the GI tract with the pressures transmitted to a computer analyzer.

Esophageal manometry is used to detect motility disorders of the esophagus and the upper and lower esophageal sphincters. Also known as esophageal motility studies, these studies are very helpful in the diagnosis of **achalasia**, diffuse esophageal spasm, scleroderma, and other esophageal motor disorders. The patient must refrain from eating or drinking for 8 to 12 hours before the test. Medications that could have a direct effect on motility (e.g., calcium channel blockers, anticholinergic agents, sedatives) are withheld for 24 to 48 hours. A pressure-sensitive catheter is inserted through the nose and is connected to a transducer and a video recorder. The patient then swallows small amounts of water while the resultant pressure changes are recorded. Evaluation of a patient for gastroesophageal reflux disease (GERD) typically includes esophageal manometry (Peixoto et al., 2017).

Gastroduodenal, small intestine, and colonic manometry procedures are used to evaluate delayed gastric emptying and gastric and intestinal motility disorders such as irritable bowel syndrome or atonic colon. This is often an ambulatory outpatient procedure lasting 24 to 72 hours. Anorectal manometry measures the resting tone of the internal anal sphincter and the contractibility of the external anal sphincter (Peixoto et al., 2017). It is helpful in evaluating patients with chronic constipation or fecal incontinence and is useful in biofeedback for the treatment of fecal incontinence. It can be performed in conjunction with rectal sensory functioning tests. Phospho-Soda or a saline cleansing enema is administered 1 hour before the test, and positioning for the test is either the prone or the lateral position (Peixoto et al., 2017).

Rectal sensory function studies are used to evaluate rectal sensory function and neuropathy. A catheter and balloon are passed into the rectum, with increasing balloon inflation until the patient feels distention. Then the tone and pressure of the rectum and anal sphincter are measured. The results are especially helpful in the evaluation of patients with chronic constipation, diarrhea, or incontinence.

Electrogastrography, an electrophysiologic study, also may be performed to assess gastric motility disturbances and can be useful in detecting motor or nerve dysfunction in the stomach. Electrodes are placed over the abdomen, and gastric electrical activity is recorded for up to 24 hours. Patients may exhibit rapid, slow, or irregular waveform activity.

Defecography measures anorectal function and is performed with very thick barium paste instilled into the rectum (Nogueira et al., 2016). Fluoroscopy is used to assess the function of the rectum and anal sphincter while the patient attempts to expel the barium. The test requires no preparation.

Gastric Analysis, Gastric Acid Stimulation Test, and pH Monitoring

Analysis of the gastric juice yields information about the secretory activity of the gastric mucosa and the presence or degree of gastric retention in patients thought to have pyloric or duodenal obstruction. It is also useful for diagnosing Zollinger–Ellison syndrome, or atrophic gastritis.

The patient is NPO for 8 to 12 hours before the procedure. Any medications that affect gastric secretions are withheld for 24 to 48 hours before the test. Smoking is not allowed on the morning of the test because it increases gastric secretions. A small nasogastric tube with a catheter tip marked at various points is inserted through the nose. When the tube is at a point slightly less than 50 cm (21 in), it should be within the stomach, lying along the greater curvature. Once in place, the tube is secured to the patient's cheek and the patient is placed in a semireclining position. The entire stomach contents are aspirated by gentle suction into a syringe, and gastric samples are collected every 15 minutes for the next hour.

Important diagnostic information to be gained from gastric analysis includes the ability of the mucosa to secrete HCl. This ability is altered in various disease states, including:

- Pernicious anemia—patients with this disease secrete no acid under basal conditions or after stimulation.
- Severe chronic atrophic gastritis or gastric cancer—patients with these diseases secrete little or no acid.
- Peptic ulcer—patients with this disease secrete some acid.
- Duodenal ulcers—patients with this disease usually secrete an excess amount of acid.

The gastric acid stimulation test usually is performed in conjunction with gastric analysis. Histamine or pentagastrin is administered subcutaneously to stimulate gastric secretions. It is important to inform the patient that this injection may produce a flushed feeling. The nurse monitors the patient's blood pressure and pulse frequently to detect hypotension. Gastric specimens are collected after the injection every 15 minutes for 1 hour and are labeled to indicate the time of specimen collection after histamine injection. The volume and pH of the specimen are measured; in certain instances, cytologic study by the Papanicolaou technique may be used to determine the presence or absence of malignant cells.

Esophageal reflux of gastric acid may be diagnosed by ambulatory pH monitoring (Liu, Xu, Ming, et al., 2017). The patient is NPO for 6 hours before the test, and all medications affecting gastric secretions are withheld for 24 to 36 hours before the test. A probe that measures pH is inserted through the nose and into position about 5 in above the lower esophageal sphincter. It is connected to an external recording device and is worn for 24 hours while the patient continues normal daily activities. The end result is a computer analysis and graphic display of the results. This test allows for the direct correlation between chest pain and reflux episodes. The Bravo pH monitoring system offers the advantage of pH monitoring of the esophagus without the transnasal catheter. The clinician, by means of endoscopy, attaches a capsule (approximately the size of a gel cap) to the patient's esophageal wall. Data related to pH are transmitted from the capsule to a pager-sized receiver that the patient wears. Data are collected for up to 48 hours and then downloaded and analyzed. The capsule spontaneously detaches from the esophagus in 7 to 10 days and then is passed through the patient's digestive system. The accuracy of this method of pH testing is greater than methods in which a catheter is used because the patient can eat normally and continue normal activities during the testing. The system reliably distinguishes reflux conditions from functional conditions if the study is performed with the patient off medications.

Laparoscopy (Peritoneoscopy)

With the tremendous advances in minimally invasive surgery, diagnostic laparoscopy is efficient, cost-effective, and useful in the diagnosis of GI disease. After a pneumoperitoneum (injecting carbon dioxide into the peritoneal cavity to separate the intestines from the pelvic organs) is created, a small incision is made lateral to the umbilicus, allowing for the insertion of the fibreoptic laparoscope. This permits direct visualization of the organs and structures within the abdomen, permitting visualization and identification of any growths, anomalies, and inflammatory processes. In addition, biopsy samples can be taken from the structures and organs as necessary. This procedure can be used to evaluate peritoneal disease, chronic abdominal pain, abdominal masses, and gallbladder and liver disease. However, laparoscopy has not become an important diagnostic modality in patients with acute abdominal pain, because less invasive tools (e.g., CT and MRI) are readily available. Laparoscopy usually requires general anesthesia and sometimes requires that the stomach and bowel be decompressed. Gas (usually carbon dioxide) is insufflated into the peritoneal cavity to create a working space for visualization. One of the benefits of this procedure is that after visualization of a problem, excision (e.g., removal of the gallbladder) can then be performed at the same time, if appropriate.

Critical Thinking Exercises

1 You are caring for a 60-year-old man with a history of diabetes, pancreatitis, alcohol abuse, and abdominal pain associated with meals. He states that he sometimes has nausea and vomiting after eating dinner. Identify questions that should be asked when taking the patient's history. What assessment parameters would be addressed? What diagnostic tests would you expect to be ordered?

2 **ebp** You are working in a medical internist's office. A 56-year-old female patient comes into the office for a routine examination. She states that she did not get her recommended colonoscopy examination because no one in her family has colon cancer and she did not understand the instructions. How would you assess educational needs to determine what education you would provide for this patient? What is the evidence base that supports the education? Discuss the strength of the evidence for the education. Identify the criteria used to evaluate the strength of the evidence.

REFERENCES AND SELECTED READINGS

Books

Bickley, L. S. (2016). *Bates' guide to physical examination and history taking* (12th ed.). Philadelphia, PA: Lippincott Williams & Wilkins.

Bontrager, K., & Lampignano, J. (2014). *Textbook of radiographic positioning and related anatomy* (8th ed.). St. Louis, MO: Elsevier.

Eliopoulos, C. (2018). *Gerontological nursing* (9th ed.). Philadelphia, PA: Lippincott Williams & Wilkins.

Fischbach, F., & Dunning, M. (2015). *A manual of laboratory and diagnostic tests* (9th ed.). Philadelphia, PA: Wolters Kluwer Health.

Grossman, S., & Porth, C. (2014). *Porth's pathophysiology. Concepts of altered health states* (9th ed.). Philadelphia, PA: Lippincott Williams & Wilkins.

Weber, J., & Kelley, J. (2017). *Health assessment in nursing* (6th ed.). Philadelphia, PA: Lippincott Williams & Wilkins.

Journals and Electronic Documents

Achem, S. R., & DeVault, K. R. (2014). Gastroesophageal reflux disease and the elderly. *Gastroenterology Clinics of North America, 43*(1), 147–160.

Ahnen, D. J., Wade, S. W., Jones, W. F., et al. (2014). The increasing incidence of young-onset colorectal cancer: A call to action. *Mayo Clinic Proceedings, 89*(2), 216–224.

Andreucci, M. (2017). Iodinated contrast-induced acute kidney injury. Pathophysiology and prevention. *Giornale di Tecniche Nefrologiche e Dialitiche, 29*(1), 11–19.

Benson, M., Pier, J., Kraft, S., et al. (2012). Optical colonoscopy and virtual colonoscopy numbers after initiation of a CT colonography program: Long term data. *Journal of Gastrointestinal and Liver Diseases, 21*(4), 391–395.

Bradbury, P. A., Morris, D. G., Nicholas, G., et al. (2018). Canadian Cancer Trials Group (CCTG) IND211: A randomized trial of pelareorep (Reolysin) in patients with previously treated advanced or metastatic non-small cell lung cancer receiving standard salvage therapy. *Lung Cancer, 120*, 142–148.

Brenner, D. R., Ruan, Y., Shaw, E., et al. (2017). Increasing colorectal cancer incidence trends among younger adults in Canada. *Preventive Medicine, 105*, 345–349.

Cardoso, G., Graca, J., Klut, C., et al. (2016). Depression and anxiety symptoms following cancer diagnosis: A cross-sectional study. *Psychology, Health & Medicine, 21*(5), 562–570.

Carethers, J. M. (2012). Proteomics, genomics, and molecular biology in the personalized treatment of colorectal cancer. *Journal of Gastrointestinal Surgery, 16*(9), 1648–1650.

Carey, M., Sanson-Fisher, R., Macrae, F., et al. (2012). Improving adherence to surveillance and screening recommendations for people with colorectal cancer and their first degree relatives: A randomized controlled trial. *BMC Cancer, 12*, 62.

Cash, B., Riddle, M., Bhattacharya, I., et al. (2012). CT colonography of a Medicare-age population: Outcomes observed in an analysis of more than 1400 patients. *American Journal of Roentgenology, 199*, W27–W34.

Chander, B., Hanley-Williams, N., Deng, Y., et al. (2012). 24 versus 48-hour bravo pH monitoring. *Journal of Clinical Gastroenterology, 46*(3), 197–200.

Chen, J., Athilingam, P., Saloum, Y., et al. (2015). Enhancing bowel preparation for screening colonoscopy: An evidence-based literature review. *The Journal for Nurse Practitioners, 11*(5), 519–525.

Chin, S. W., & Chen, Y. K. (2017). High CFA levels in a case of resected colorectal cancer: Delayed diagnosis of metachronous medullary thyroid cancer. *World Journal of Surgical Oncology, 15*(4), 230.

Chu, C., Du, Q., Li, C., et al. (2017). Ambulatory 24-hour multichannel intraluminal impedance-pH monitoring and high resolution endoscopy distinguish patients with non-erosive reflux disease from those with functional heartburn. *PLos One, 12*(4), 1–12.

Cox, B. (2016). Flexible sigmoidoscopy is the best approach for a national bowel screening programme. *The New Zealand Medical Journal (Online), 129*(1430), 14–17.

de Sa Goncalves, A. N., Sala, M. A. S., Bruno, R. C., et al. (2016). Defecography by digital radiography: Experience in clinical practice. *Radiologia Brasileira, 49*(6), 376–381.

Ekkelenkamp, V. E., Koch, A. D., de Man, R. A., et al. (2016). Training and competence assessment in GI endoscopy: A systematic review. *Gut, 65*, 607–615.

Foronda, C. L., Alfes, C. M., Dev, P., et al. (2017). Virtually nursing: Emerging technologies in nursing education. *Nurse Educator, 42*(1), 14–17.

Garborg, K. (2015). Colorectal cancer screening. *The Surgical Clinics of North America, 95*(5), 979–989.

Goede, S. L., Rabeneck, L., van Ballegooijen, M., et al. (2017). Harms, benefits and costs of fecal immunochemical testing versus guaiac fecal occult blood testing for colorectal cancer screening. *PLos One, 12*(3), e0172864.

Joshi, B., & Wang, T. (2016). Gastrointestinal imaging in 2015: Emerging trends in endoscopic imaging. *Nature Reviews Gastroenterology & Hepatology, 13*(2), 72–73.

Kar, P., Jones, K. L., Horowitz, M., et al. (2015). Measurement of gastric emptying in the critically ill. *Clinical Nutrition, 34*(4), 557–564.

Keefer, L., Palsson, O. S., & Pandolfino, J. E. (2018). Best practice update: Incorporating psycho-gastroenterology into management of digestive disorders. *Gastroenterology, 154*, 1249–1257.

Khan, S., Ghaffar, T., & Khan, I. (2015). Dyspepsia; frequency of common upper gastrointestinal endoscopic findings in elderly patients with iron deficiency anemia. *Professional Medical Journal, 22*(7), 871–875.

Laing, P., & Adler, D. (2012). Diagnosis and management of biliary obstruction. *Journal of Clinical Outcomes Management, 19*(10), 465.

Lawrance, I., Willert, R., & Murray, K. (2013). A validated bowel-preparation tolerability questionnaire and assessment of three commonly used bowel-cleansing agents. *Digestive Diseases and Sciences, 58*(4), 926–935.

Lee, Y. J., Kim, E. S., Park, K. S., et al. (2015). Education for ward nurses influences the quality of inpatient's bowel preparation for colonoscopy. *Medicine, 94*(34).

Le Pimpec, F., Moutel, G., Piette, C., et al. (2017). Fecal immunological blood tests is more appealing than the guaiac-based test for colorectal cancer screening. *Digestive and Liver Disease, 49*(11), 1267–1272.

Li, B., Wang, J., & Ma, Y. (2012). Bowel sounds and monitoring gastrointestinal motility in critically ill patients. *Clinical Nurse Specialist, 26*(1), 29–34.

Li, X., Gui, Y., Shen, F., et al. (2018). The application value of capsule endoscopy in diagnosing small intestinal carcinoma. *Journal of Cancer Research and Therapeutics, 14*, 57–60.

Liu, S., Xu, M., Yang, J., et al. (2017). Research on gastroesophageal reflux disease based on dynamic features of ambulatory 24-hour esophageal pH monitoring. *Computational and Mathematical Methods in Medicine, 2017*, 1–7.

Lu, Z, Qi, Y., Weng, J., et al. (2017). Efficacy and safety of single-balloon versus double-balloon enteroscopy: A single-center retrospective analysis. *Medical Science Monitor, 23*, 1933–1939.

Malhi, H. (2016). Dysphagia: Warning signs and management. *British Journal of Nursing, 25*(16), 546–549.

Mansoori, B., Delaney, C., Willis, J., et al. (2016). Magnetic resonance enterography/enteroclysis in acquired small bowel diverticulitis and small bowel diverticulosis. *European Radiology, 26*(9), 2881–2891.

Malfertheiner, P. (2017). STW 5 (Iberogast) Therapy in gastrointestinal functional disorders. *Digestive Diseases*, *35*(Suppl 1), 25–29.

Melamud, K., Colip, C., & Soto, J. A. (2016). MR in the small bowel: Applications, techniques, and imaging findings. *Applied Radiology*, *19*(6), 24–30.

Nagata, K., Endo, S., Honda, T., et al. (2017). Accuracy of CT colonography for detection of polypoid and nonpolypoid neoplasia by gastroenterologists and radiologists: A nationwide multicenter study in Japan. *The American Journal of Gastroenterology*, *112*(1), 163.

Nam, S. J., Lee, H. S., & Lim, Y. J. (2018). Evaluation of gastric disease with capsule endoscopy. *Clinical Endoscopy*, *51*(4), 323.

Overland, M. (2014). Dyspepsia. *Medical Clinics of North America*, *98*(3), 549–564.

Park, E., Choi, M., Baeg, M., et al. (2013). The value of early wireless esophageal pH monitoring in diagnosing functional heartburn in refractory gastroesophageal reflux disease. *Digestive Diseases and Sciences*, *58*(10), 2933–2939.

Park, J., Cho, Y. K., & Kim, J. H. (2018). Current and future use of esophageal capsule endoscopy. *Clinical Endoscopy*, *51*(4), 317.

Peixoto, A., Morais, R., Silva, M., et al. (2017). Conventional esophageal manometry in clinical practice: Current impact of its use on patient management. *Clinics and Research in Hepatology and Gastroenterology*, *41*(6), e91–e92.

Pollentine, A., Mortimer, A., McCoubrie, P., et al. (2012). Evaluation of two minimal-preparation regimes for CT colonography: Optimising image quality and patient acceptability. *The British Journal of Radiology*, *85*(1016), 1085–1092.

Pu, K., Shi, J. H., Xu Wang, Q. T., et al. (2017). Diagnostic accuracy of transient elastography (FibroScan) in detection of esophageal varices in patients with cirrhosis: A meta-analysis. *World Journal of Gastroenterology*, *23*(2), 345.

Rawson, J., & Pelletier, A. (2013). When to order contrast-enhanced CT. *American Family Physician*, *88*(5), 312–316.

Rey, J. (2013). The future of capsule endoscopy. *The Keio Journal of Medicine*, *62*(2), 41–46.

Royle, T., Ferguson, H., Mak, T., et al. (2013). Same-day assessment and management of urgent (2-week wait) colorectal referrals: An analysis of the outcome of 1606 patients attending an endoscopy unit-based colorectal clinic. *Colorectal Disease*, *16*(5), O176–O181.

Rutten, L., Jacobsen, R., Wilson, P., et al. (2017). Early adoption of multitarget stool DNA test for colorectal cancer screening. *Mayo Clinic Proceedings*, *92*(5), 726–733.

Sakai, E., Endo, H., Kato, S., et al. (2012). Capsule endoscopy with flexible spectral imaging color enhancement reduces the bile pigment effect and improves the detectability of small bowel lesions. *BMC Gastroenterology*, *12*, 83.

Sali, L., Grazzini, G., Carozzi, F., et al. (2013). Screening for colorectal cancer with FOBT, virtual colonoscopy and optical colonoscopy: Study protocol for a randomized controlled trial in the Florence district (SAVE study). *Trials*, *14*, 74.

Saltzman, J. R., Cash, B. D., Pasha, S. F., et al. (2015). Bowel preparation before colonoscopy. *Gastrointestinal Endoscopy*, *81*(4), 781–794.

Sami, S. S., Iyer, P. G., Pophali, P., et al. (2018). Acceptability, accuracy and safety of disposable transnasal capsule endoscopy for Barrett's esophagus screening. *Clinical Gastroenterology and Hepatology*, S1542–3565(18), 30743–2. doi:10.1016/j.cgh.2018.07.019

Sharma, V., & Rana, S. (2016). Capsule endoscopy: Coming of age! *Journal of Digestive Endoscopy*, *7*(4), 163–165.

Simard, J., & Hall, P. (2013). Lessons learned and challenges posed in cancer genetics. *Journal of Internal Medicine*, *274*(5), 396–398.

Spada, C., Stoker, J., Alarcon, O., et al. (2015). Clinical indications for computed tomographic colonography: European Society of Gastrointestinal Endoscopy (ESGE) and European Society of Gastrointestinal and Abdominal Radiology (ESGAR) Guideline. *European Radiology*, *25*(2), 331–345.

Tomizawa, M., Shinozaki, F., Hsaegawa, R., et al. (2017). Abdominal ultrasonography for patients with abdominal pain as a first-line diagnostic imaging modality. *Experimental and Therapeutic Medicine*, *13*(5), 1932–1936.

Tsutsumimotoa, K., Takehiko, D., Hyuma, M., et al. (2017). The association between anorexia of aging and physical frailty: Results from the national center for geriatrics and gerontology's study of geriatric syndromes. *Maturitas*, *97*, 32–37.

Wampole, M., Kairys, J., Mitchell, E., et al. (2013). Consistent surgeon evaluations of three-dimensional rendering of PET/CT scans of the abdomen of a patient with a ductal pancreatic mass. *PLoS One*, *8*(9), e75237.

Wong, M., Ching, J., Chan, V., et al. (2015). Factors associated with false-positive and false-negative fecal immunochemical test results for colorectal cancer screening. *Gastrointestinal Endoscopy*, *81*(3), 596–607.

Yi, L., Lu, C., Chujun, L., et al. (2017). Diagnostic utility of endoscopic ultrasonography-elastography in the evaluation of solid pancreatic masses: A meta-analysis and systematic review. *Medical Ultrasonography*, *19*(2), 150–158.

Zhang, Y., Ding, S., Li, C., et al. (2017). Effects of N-acetylcysteine treatment in acute respiratory distress syndrome: A meta-analysis. *Experimental and Therapeutic Medicine*, *14*(4), 2863–2868.

35 Management of Patients With Oral and Esophageal Disorders

Adapted by Pamela Cawley

Learning Objectives

On completion of this chapter, the learner will be able to:

1. Describe the nursing management of patients with conditions of the oral cavity.
2. Describe the relationship of dental hygiene and dental problems to nutrition.
3. Describe the nursing management of patients with abnormalities of the lips, gums, teeth, mouth, and salivary glands.
4. Describe the nursing management of patients with cancer of the oral cavity.
5. Identify the physical and psychosocial long-term needs of patients with oral cancer.
6. Use the nursing process as a framework for care of patients undergoing neck dissection.
7. Use the nursing process as a framework for care of patients with various conditions of the esophagus.
8. Describe the various conditions of the esophagus and their clinical manifestations and management.

Because digestion begins in the mouth, adequate nutrition is related to good dental health and the general condition of the mouth. Any discomfort or adverse condition in the oral cavity can affect a person's nutritional status. Changes in the oral cavity can influence the type and amount of food ingested as well as the degree to which food particles are properly mixed with salivary enzymes. Disease of the mouth or tongue can interfere with speech and thus affect communication and self-image. Esophageal problems related to swallowing can also adversely affect food and fluid intake, thereby jeopardizing general health and well-being. Given the close relationship between adequate nutritional intake and the structures of the upper gastrointestinal tract (lips, mouth, teeth, pharynx, and esophagus), health teaching can help prevent disorders associated with these structures (Fig. 35-1).

DISORDERS OF THE ORAL CAVITY

Oral health is a very important component of a person's physical and psychological sense of well-being. About 62% of Canadians have private dental insurance and 32% have no coverage. Approximately six million people avoid seeing the dentist yearly due to cost (Canadian Academy of Health Sciences, 2014). Fifty-three percent of the population age 60 to 79 years of age do not have dental insurance (Canadian Academy of Health Sciences, 2014) with similar statistics for other vulnerable populations including First Nations' children and adolescents. Table 35-1 reviews common abnormalities of the oral cavity, their possible causes, and nursing management. Figure 35-2 illustrates structures of the oral cavity.

Dental Plaque and Caries

Tooth decay is an erosive process that begins with the action of bacteria on fermentable carbohydrates in the mouth, which produces acids that dissolve tooth enamel. Tooth enamel is the hardest substance in the human body, but dental erosion occurs for several reasons. Contributing factors include nutrition, soft drink consumption, and

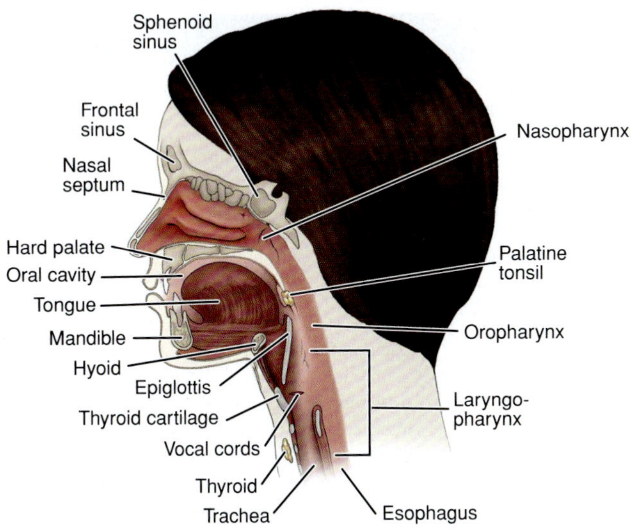

FIGURE 35-1. Anatomy of the head and neck.

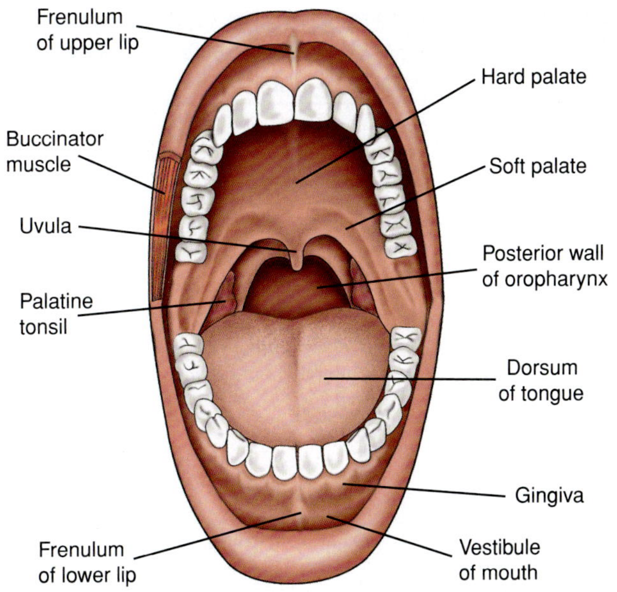

FIGURE 35-2. Structures of the mouth, including the tongue and palate.

genetic predisposition. In addition, the extent of damage to the teeth may be related to the following:

- The presence of dental plaque. Dental plaque is a gluey, gelatinlike substance that adheres to the teeth. The initial action that causes damage to a tooth occurs under dental plaque.
- The length of time acids are in contact with the teeth.
- The strength of acids and the ability of the saliva to neutralize them.
- The susceptibility of the teeth to decay.

Dental decay begins with a small hole, usually in a fissure (a break in the tooth's enamel) or in an area that is hard to clean. Left unchecked, the decay extends into the dentin. Because dentin is not as hard as enamel, decay progresses more rapidly and in time reaches the pulp of the tooth.

Dentists can determine the extent of damage and the type of treatment needed using x-ray studies. Treatment for dental caries includes fillings, dental implants, or extraction, if necessary. In general, dental decay can occur in anyone. Contributing factors can be as simple as not brushing teeth on a regular basis to an improper diet. Older adults are subject to decay from drug-induced or age-related oral dryness (Chart 35-1).

(text continued on page 922)

Glossary

achalasia: absent or ineffective peristalsis (wavelike contraction) of the distal esophagus accompanied by failure of the esophageal sphincter to relax in response to swallowing
Boerhaave's syndrome: spontaneous esophageal rupture due to forceful vomiting or straining
dysphagia: difficulty swallowing
dysplasia: abnormal change in cells
esophagogastroduodenoscopy (EGD): passage of a fibreoptic tube through the mouth and throat into the digestive tract for visualization of the esophagus, stomach, and small intestine; biopsies can be performed
Frey's syndrome: a rare syndrome characterized by undesirable sweating and flushing occurring on the cheek, temporal region, and behind the ears after eating certain foods; also called auriculotemporal syndrome
gastroesophageal reflux: backflow of gastric or duodenal contents into the esophagus
gastroesophageal reflux disease (GERD): disorder marked by backflow of gastric or duodenal contents into the esophagus that causes troublesome symptoms and/or mucosal injury to the esophagus
hernia: protrusion of an organ or part of an organ through the wall of the cavity that normally contains it
lithotripsy: use of shock waves to break up or disintegrate stones
odynophagia: pain on swallowing
parotitis: inflammation of the parotid gland
periapical abscess: abscessed tooth
pyrosis: heartburn
sialadenitis: inflammation of the salivary glands
stomatitis: inflammation of the oral mucosa
temporomandibular disorders: a group of conditions that cause pain or dysfunction of the temporomandibular joint (TMJ) and surrounding structures
vagotomy syndrome: dumping syndrome; gastrointestinal symptoms, such as diarrhea and abdominal cramping, resulting from rapid gastric emptying
xerostomia: dry mouth

TABLE 35-1 Disorders of the Lips, Mouth, and Gums

Condition	Signs and Symptoms	Possible Causes and Sequelae	Nursing Considerations
Abnormalities of the Lips			
Actinic cheilitis	Irritation of lips associated with scaling, crusting, fissure; white overgrowth of horny layer of epidermis (hyperkeratosis) Considered a premalignant squamous cell skin cancer	Exposure to sun; more common in fair-skinned people and in those whose occupations involve sun exposure, such as farmers Chronic inflammatory lesion that may lead to squamous cell cancer of the lip	Educate patient on importance of protecting lips from the sun by using protective ointment such as sun block Instruct patient to have a periodic checkup by primary provider.
Chancre	Reddened circumscribed lesion that ulcerates and becomes crusted	Primary lesion of syphilis	Use comfort measures such as cold soaks to lip, mouth care Administer antibiotics as prescribed Instruct patient regarding contagion Use topical over-the-counter agents (e.g., Blistex, Carmex) or antiviral agents (e.g., acyclovir, penciclovir) as prescribed
Contact dermatitis (i.e., allergic contact cheilitis)	Red area or rash; itching	Allergic reaction to lipstick, cosmetic ointments, or toothpaste	Instruct patient to avoid possible causes Administer corticosteroids as prescribed
Herpes simplex virus-1 (cold sore or fever blister)	Symptoms may be delayed up to 20 days after exposure; singular or clustered, irregular, painful vesicles throughout the oral cavity and lips that may rupture	An opportunistic infection; frequently seen in patients who are immunosuppressed May recur with menstruation, fever, or sun exposure	Use acyclovir ointment or systemic medications as prescribed Administer analgesic agents as prescribed. Instruct patient to avoid irritating foods
Abnormalities of the Mouth			
Leukoplakia	White patches; may be hyperkeratotic; usually in buccal mucosa; typically painless	Fewer than 2% are malignant, but may progress to cancer (premalignant) Common among tobacco users	Instruct patient to see the primary provider if leukoplakia persists >2 weeks Eliminate risk factors, such as cigarettes, smokeless tobacco
Oral hairy leukoplakia	White patches with rough hairlike projections; typically found on lateral border of the tongue	Possibly viral Related to smoking and the use of tobacco Associated with HIV infection	Instruct patient to see the primary provider if condition persists >2 weeks
Lichen planus	Radiating white striations on the tongue and buccal mucosa; often association with painful ulcerations and erythema	Chronic inflammatory condition of unknown cause Recurrences are common May lead to a malignant process	Apply topical corticosteroids such as fluocinolone acetonide gel Avoid foods that irritate Administer corticosteroids systemically or intralesionally as prescribed Instruct the patient of need for follow-up if condition is chronic
Candidiasis (moniliasis/thrush)	Cheesy white plaque that looks like milk curds; when rubbed off, it leaves an erythematous and often bleeding base	*Candida albicans* fungus; predisposing factors include diabetes, antibiotic therapy, and immunosuppression	Antifungal medications such as nystatin or clotrimazole may be prescribed as suspensions or troche; when used as a suspension, instruct the patient to swish vigorously for at least 1 minute and then swallow If these treatments fail, oral agents such as fluconazole may be prescribed
Aphthous stomatitis (canker sore) (Classified as *major* or *minor* depending upon size)	Shallow ulcer with a white or yellow centre and typically a well-defined red border; seen on the inner side of the lip and cheek or on the tongue; it begins with a burning or tingling sensation and slight swelling; painful; usually lasts 7–10 days (*minor*) and heals without a scar	Immune-mediated inflammatory disorder associated with HIV infection Associated with emotional or mental stress, fatigue, hormonal factors, minor trauma (e.g., biting), allergies, acidic foods and juices, and dietary deficiencies May recur	Instruct the patient in comfort measures (e.g., saline rinses) and a soft or bland diet Antibiotics or corticosteroids may be prescribed Use over-the-counter benzocaine as indicated
Nicotine stomatitis (smoker's patch)	Two stages—begins as a red stomatitis; over time, the tongue and mouth become covered with a creamy, thick, white mucous membrane, which may slough, leaving a beefy red base	Chronic irritation by tobacco	Cessation of tobacco use; if condition exists >2 weeks, a primary provider should be consulted and a biopsy may be needed

TABLE 35-1 Disorders of the Lips, Mouth, and Gums (Continued)

Condition	Signs and Symptoms	Possible Causes and Sequelae	Nursing Considerations
Erythroplakia	Red patch on the oral mucous membrane	Nonspecific inflammation; more frequently seen in older adults	
Kaposi's sarcoma	Appears first on the oral mucosa as a red, purple, or blue lesion; may be singular or multiple; may be flat or raised Lesions can occur in other parts of the body: skin, lymph nodes, lungs, digestive tract	Cancer that develops from the cells that line the blood vessels and lymph system Associated with HIV infection (AIDS), men who are HIV negative and who have sex with men, organ transplantation, and geographic region (Mediterranean, Africa)	Instruct patient regarding side effects of planned treatment for HIV
Stomatitis	Mild erythema and edema; severe forms include painful ulcerations, bleeding, and secondary infection	Inflammation of the mucous lining of the mouth Associated with chemotherapy; radiation therapy; severe drug allergy; myelosuppression (bone marrow depression)	Prophylactic mouth care, including brushing, flossing, and rinsing, for any patient receiving chemotherapy or radiation therapy Educate patient about proper oral hygiene, including the use of a soft-bristled toothbrush and nonabrasive toothpaste; for painful ulcers, oral swabs with spongelike applicators can be used in place of a toothbrush; avoid alcohol-based mouth rinses and hot or spicy foods Apply topical anti-inflammatory, antibiotic, and anesthetic agents as prescribed
Abnormalities of the Gums			
Gingivitis	Painful, inflamed, swollen gums; usually, the gums bleed in response to light contact	Reversible form of inflammation of the gingiva (i.e., mild form of periodontal disease) Associated with poor oral hygiene: food debris, bacterial plaque, and calculus (tartar) accumulate Gums may also swell in response to normal processes such as puberty and pregnancy, with certain medications (phenytoin [Dilantin], calcium channel blockers, cyclosporine [Neoral]), or with a deficiency in the immune system (i.e., AIDS) or nutritional status	Educate patient about proper oral hygiene; tooth-brushing, flossing, rinsing (i.e., chlorhexidine), dental appointments every 3–6 mo Remove causal agents as appropriate—medications, smoking, dental appliances
Necrotizing gingivitis (trench mouth)	Gray-white pseudomembranous ulcerations affecting the edges of the gums, mucosa of the mouth, tonsils, and pharynx; halitosis; painful, bleeding gums; swallowing and talking are painful	Progressive, painful bacterial infection Related to poor oral hygiene, lack of access to dental care, inadequate rest, overwork, emotional stress, smoking, and poor nutrition	Educate patient about proper oral hygiene; see Chart 35-2 Irrigate with 2–3% hydrogen peroxide or normal saline solution Avoid irritants such as smoking and spicy foods
Herpetic gingivostomatitis	Burning sensation with the appearance of small vesicles 24–48 h later; vesicles may rupture, forming sore, shallow ulcers covered with a gray membrane	Herpes simplex viral infection Occurs most frequently in people who are immunosuppressed; may occur in other infectious processes such as streptococcal pneumonia, meningococcal meningitis, and malaria	Apply topical anesthetics as prescribed; may need opioids if pain is severe Saline or 2–3% hydrogen peroxide irrigations Antiviral agents such as acyclovir may be prescribed
Periodontitis	Little discomfort at onset; may have bleeding, infection, gum recession, and loosening of teeth; later in the disease, tooth loss may occur	Deep, chronic inflammation of the gingiva May result from untreated gingivitis Poor or inadequate dental hygiene and inadequate diet contribute to development	Instruct patient in proper oral hygiene, chlorhexidine rinses Instruct patient to consult a dentist or periodontist for antibiotic prescription, deep root scaling

AIDS, acquired immunodeficiency syndrome; HIV, human immunodeficiency virus.

Adapted from American Cancer Society (ACS). (2016). Kaposi sarcoma. Retrieved on June 6, 2016 at: www.cancer.org/cancer/kaposisarcoma/detailedguide/kaposi-sarcoma-whatis-kaposi-sarcoma; Anderson, W. D., Treister, N. S., Mayeaux, E. J., et al. (2015). Oral lesions you can't afford to miss. *Journal of Family Practice, 64*(7), 392–399; O'Gorman, S. M., & Torgerson, R. R. (2016). Contact allergy in cheilitis. *International Journal of Dermatology, 55*(7), 386–391; Silk, H. (2014). Disease of the mouth. *Primary Care, 41*(1), 75–90.

CHART 35-1

Gerontologic Considerations: Oral Conditions in the Older Adult

Many medications taken by older adults cause dry mouth, which is uncomfortable, impairs communication, and increases the risk of oral infection. These medications include the following:

- Diuretics
- Antihypertensive medications
- Anti-inflammatory agents
- Antidepressant medications

Poor dentition can exacerbate problems of aging, such as:

- Decreased food intake
- Loss of appetite
- Social isolation
- Increased susceptibility to systemic infection (from periodontal disease)
- Trauma to the oral cavity secondary to thinner, less vascular oral mucous membranes

Prevention

Measures used to prevent and control dental caries include practicing effective mouth care, reducing the intake of starches and sugars (refined carbohydrates), applying fluoride to the teeth or drinking fluoridated water, refraining from smoking, controlling diabetes, and using pit and fissure sealants. Regular dental visits are another method of preventive dental maintenance.

Mouth Care

Healthy teeth must be conscientiously and effectively cleaned on a daily basis. Brushing and flossing are particularly effective in mechanically breaking up the bacterial plaque that collects around teeth. Caring for the teeth and gums is important because of the physiological and mechanical pathways between the oral cavity and lung tissue. Poor oral health practices put hospital patients at risk for nonventilator hospital-acquired pneumonia (Quinn, Baker, Cohen, et al., 2014).

Mastication (chewing) and the flow of saliva also aid greatly in keeping the teeth clean. Because many ill patients do not eat adequate amounts of food, they produce less saliva, which in turn reduces this natural tooth-cleaning process. The nurse may need to assume the responsibility for brushing the patient's teeth. Merely wiping the patient's mouth and teeth with a swab is ineffective. The most effective method is mechanical cleansing (brushing). If brushing is impossible, it is better to wipe the teeth with a gauze pad, and then have the patient swish an antiseptic mouthwash several times before expectorating into an emesis basin. A soft-bristled toothbrush is more effective than a sponge or foam stick. To prevent drying, the lips may be coated with a water-soluble gel.

Diet

Dental caries may be prevented by decreasing the amount of sugar and starch in the diet. Patients who snack should be encouraged to choose less cariogenic alternatives, such as fruits, vegetables, nuts, cheeses, or plain yogurt. In addition, frequent brushing, especially after meals, is necessary. Flossing should be performed daily.

Fluoridation

Fluoridation of public water supplies has been found to decrease dental caries. Some areas of the country have natural fluoridation; other communities have added fluoride to public water supplies. As of 2017, 38.7% of Canadians were living in areas with fluoridated water (Government of Canada, 2017), with the highest levels of fluoridations in Ontario (71.1%). Fluoridation may also be achieved by having a dentist apply a concentrated gel or solution to the teeth; adding fluoride to home water supplies; using fluoridated toothpaste or mouth rinse; or using sodium fluoride tablets, drops, or lozenges. Studies suggest that by instituting a community water fluoridation program, tooth decay is reduced by 25% in both children and adults (Weno, 2015).

Pit and Fissure Sealants

The occlusal surfaces of the teeth have pits and fissures, areas that are prone to caries. Some dentists apply a special coating to fill and seal these areas from potential exposure to cariogenic processes. These sealants can last 5 to 10 years, depending on how dry the tooth surface is prior to application. Recently, fluoride varnish, a relatively easy-to-apply treatment, was found to be as effective as sealant and at lower cost (Chestnutt, Hutchings, Playle, et al., 2017).

Dental Health and Disease

Studies are ongoing that show the link between oral health and chronic disease such as diabetes, heart disease, low birth weight, premature births, and stroke. As early as 1989, it was posited that bacteria, specifically gram-negative bacteria, were the culprits that link periodontal disease to other systemic diseases, specifically coronary artery disease, including myocardial infarction, and stroke. More recently, it was confirmed that these bacteria cause an inflammatory response that initiates an increase in inflammatory markers such as C-reactive protein, white blood cells, and fibrinogen. These markers are associated with an increased risk of cardiovascular disease. Although research has not proven periodontal disease to be a direct cause of cardiovascular disease, data from short-term studies suggest that if periodontal disease is treated, systemic inflammation and endothelial dysfunction are reduced (Papapanou, 2015).

The World Health Organization (WHO) Global Oral Health Programme (2015) espouses a global focus on oral health promotion and disease prevention, with an emphasis on policy and guideline development to support equitable implementation of evidence-based practices in global communities. The Programme supports an emphasis on addressing modifiable risk factors (e.g., diet, nutrition, tobacco, alcohol, oral hygiene), water sanitation, and fluoride initiatives (WHO, 2015).

Periapical Abscess

Periapical abscess, more commonly referred to as an abscessed tooth, involves a collection of pus in the apical dental periosteum (fibrous membrane supporting the tooth structure) and the tissue surrounding the apex of the tooth (where it is suspended in the jaw bone). The abscess may be acute or chronic. Acute periapical abscess is usually secondary to a suppurative pulpitis (a pus-producing inflammation of the dental pulp) that arises from an infection extending from dental caries. The infection of the dental pulp extends through the apical foramen of the tooth to form an abscess around the apex.

Chronic dentoalveolar abscess is a slowly progressive infectious process. In contrast to the acute form, a fully formed abscess may occur without the patient's knowledge. The infection eventually leads to a "blind dental abscess," which is actually a periapical granuloma. It may enlarge to as much as 1 cm in diameter. It is often discovered on x-ray films and is treated by extraction or root canal therapy, often with apicectomy (excision of the apex of the tooth root).

Clinical Manifestations

The abscess produces a dull, gnawing, continuous pain, often with a surrounding cellulitis and edema of the adjacent facial structures, and mobility of the involved tooth. The gum opposite the apex of the tooth is usually swollen on the cheek side. Swelling and cellulitis of the facial structures may make it difficult for the patient to open the mouth. There may also be a systemic reaction, fever, and malaise.

Medical Management

In the early stages of an infection, a dentist or oral surgeon may perform a needle aspiration or drill an opening into the pulp chamber to relieve pressure and pain and to provide drainage. Usually, the infection will have progressed to a periapical abscess. Drainage is provided by an incision through the gingiva down to the jawbone. Purulent material escapes under pressure. This procedure may be performed in the dentist's office, an outpatient surgery centre, or a same-day surgery department. After the inflammatory reaction has subsided, the tooth may be extracted or root canal therapy performed. Antibiotics and opioids may be prescribed (Robertson, Keys, Rautemaa-Richardon, et al., 2015).

Nursing Management

The nurse assesses the patient for bleeding after treatment and instructs the patient to use a warm saline or warm water mouth rinse to keep the area clean. The patient is also instructed to take antibiotics and analgesics as prescribed, to advance from a liquid diet to a soft diet as tolerated, and to keep follow-up appointments.

DISORDERS OF THE JAW

Abnormal conditions affecting the mandible (jaw) and of the temporomandibular joint (TMJ) (which connects the mandible to the temporal bone at the side of the head in front of the ear) include congenital malformation, fracture, chronic dislocation, cancer, and syndromes characterized by pain and limited motion. Temporomandibular disorders and jaw surgery (a treatment common in many structural abnormalities or cancer of the jaw) are presented in this section.

Temporomandibular Disorders

Temporomandibular disorders are categorized as follows (Canadian Dental Association, 2019):

- Myofascial pain: a discomfort in the muscles controlling jaw function and in neck and shoulder muscles
- Internal derangement of the joint: a dislocated jaw, a displaced disk, or an injured condyle
- Degenerative joint disease: rheumatoid arthritis or osteoarthritis in the jaw joint

Recent work related to the diagnosis and treatment of temporomandibular disorders produced the first evidence-based set of criteria related to the diagnosis of temporomandibular disorders (Schiffman, Ohrbach, Truelove, et al., 2014). Temporomandibular disorders are thought to affect about 10% to 15% of people in Canada. Misalignment of the joints in the jaw and other problems associated with the ligaments and muscles of mastication are thought to result in tissue damage and muscle tenderness (Gil-Martinez, Lopez-de-Uralde-Villanueva, Lopez, et al., 2016). Suggested causes include arthritis of the jaw, head injury, trauma or injury to the jaw or joint, stress, and malocclusion (although research does not support malocclusion as a cause).

Clinical Manifestations

Patients have jaw pain ranging from a dull ache to throbbing, debilitating pain that can radiate to the ears, teeth, neck muscles, and facial sinuses. They often have restricted jaw motion and locking of the jaw. There also may be a sudden change in the way the upper and lower teeth fit together. The patient may hear clicking, popping, and grating sounds when the mouth is opened, and chewing and swallowing may be difficult. Symptoms such as headaches, earaches, dizziness, and hearing problems may sometimes be related to temporomandibular disorders (Gil-Martinez et al., 2016; National Institute of Dental and Craniofacial Research [NIDCR], 2013b).

Assessment and Diagnostic Findings

Diagnosis is based on the patient's report of pain, limitations in range of motion, **dysphagia**, difficulty chewing, difficulty with speech, or hearing difficulties. Magnetic resonance imaging and x-ray studies are generally only used for severe or chronic symptoms.

Medical Management

Signs and symptoms improve over time for the majority of patients with TMJ disorders, with or without treatment. Some practitioners think the role of stress in these disorders is overrated, but patient education in stress management may be helpful (to reduce grinding and clenching of teeth). Patients may also benefit from range-of-motion exercises. Pain management measures may include nonsteroidal anti-inflammatory drugs (NSAIDs), with the possible addition of opioids, muscle relaxants, or mild antidepressants. Occasionally, intraoral orthotics (a plastic guard worn over the upper and lower teeth) may be worn to reposition the condyle head in the joint space to a more usual position, which in turn relieves the stress and pressure on the tissues of the joint (Gauer & Semidey, 2015; Reid & Greene, 2013).

This allows the tissues to heal. Conservative and reversible treatment is recommended (Reid & Greene, 2013). If irreversible surgical options are recommended, patients are encouraged to seek a second opinion.

Jaw Disorders Requiring Surgical Management

Correction of mandibular structural abnormalities may require surgery involving repositioning or reconstruction of the jaw. Simple fractures of the mandible without displacement, resulting from a blow on the chin, and planned surgical interventions, as in the correction of long or short jaw syndrome, may require treatment by these means. Jaw reconstruction may be necessary in the aftermath of trauma from a severe injury or cancer, both of which can cause tissue and bone loss. New research supports screening for concussion (see Chapter 65) with mandibular fractures associated with high-force impacts (Sobin, Kopp, Walsh, et al., 2016).

Mandibular fractures are usually closed fractures. Rigid plate fixation (insertion of metal plates and screws into the bone to approximate and stabilize the bone) is the current treatment of choice in many cases of mandibular fracture and in some mandibular reconstructive surgery procedures. Current research revolves around the use of various types of reconstruction plates and fixation devices, quality of life after specific instrumentation, and device choice (van den Bergh, de Mol van Otterloo, van der Ploeg, et al., 2015), as well as surgical advances such as the use of endoscopic-assisted positioning of the fixator and surgical reduction (Belli, Liberatore, Elidon, et al., 2015). Bone grafting may be performed to replace structural defects using bones from the patient's own ilium, ribs, or cranial sites.

Nursing Management

Depending on the fracture, surgical reduction, and extent of maxillomandibular fixation (referred to as "wiring the jaw shut"), patients may have various levels of diet restrictions (Haggerty, 2015). A liquid or soft diet may be recommended for up to 4 to 6 weeks; if this is the case, dietary counselling should be obtained to ensure optimal caloric and protein intake. Nutritional supplements may be recommended. The patient needs specific guidelines for mouth care and feeding. Any irritated areas in the mouth should be reported to the primary provider. The importance of keeping scheduled appointments to assess the stability of the fixation appliance is emphasized.

Promoting Home and Community-Based Care

The patient needs specific guidelines for mouth care and feeding. Any irritated areas in the mouth should be reported to the physician. The importance of keeping scheduled appointments to assess the stability of the fixation appliance is emphasized.

Consultation with a dietitian may be indicated so that the patient and family can learn about foods that are high in essential nutrients and ways in which these foods can be prepared so that they can be consumed through a straw or spoon while remaining palatable. Nutritional supplements may be recommended.

DISORDERS OF THE SALIVARY GLANDS

The salivary glands consist of the parotid glands, one on each side of the face below the ear; the submandibular and sublingual glands, both in the floor of the mouth; and the buccal gland, beneath the lips. About 1,200 mL of saliva are produced daily and swallowed. The glands' primary functions are lubrication, protection against harmful bacteria, and digestion.

Parotitis

Parotitis (inflammation of the parotid gland) is the most common inflammatory condition of the salivary glands, although inflammation can occur in the other salivary glands as well. Mumps (epidemic parotitis), a communicable disease caused by viral infection and most commonly affecting children, is an inflammation of a salivary gland, usually the parotid.

Older adults, acutely ill, or debilitated people with decreased salivary flow from general dehydration or medications are at high risk for parotitis. The infecting organisms travel from the mouth through the salivary duct. The organism is usually *Staphylococcus aureus* (except in mumps). The onset of this complication is sudden, with an exacerbation of both fever and the symptoms of the primary condition. The gland swells and becomes tense and tender. The patient feels pain in the ear, and swollen glands interfere with swallowing. The swelling increases rapidly, and the overlying skin soon becomes red and shiny.

Medical management includes maintaining adequate nutritional and fluid intake, good oral hygiene, and discontinuing medications (e.g., tranquilizers, diuretics) that can diminish salivation. Antibiotic therapy is necessary, and analgesics may be prescribed to control pain. If antibiotic therapy is not effective, the gland may need to be drained by a surgical procedure known as parotidectomy. This procedure may be necessary to treat chronic parotitis. The patient is advised to have any necessary dental work performed prior to surgery.

Sialadenitis

Sialadenitis (inflammation of the salivary glands) may be caused by dehydration, radiation therapy, stress, malnutrition, salivary gland calculi (stones), or improper oral hygiene. The inflammation is associated with infection by *S. aureus*, *Streptococcus viridans*, or *pneumococci*. In hospitalized or institutionalized patients, the infecting organism may be methicillin-resistant *S. aureus* (MRSA). Symptoms include pain, swelling, and purulent discharge. Antibiotics are used to treat infections. Massage, hydration, warm compresses, and corticosteroids frequently cure the condition. Chronic sialadenitis with uncontrolled pain is treated by surgical drainage of the gland or excision of the gland and its duct. Rarely, subacute necrotizing sialadenitis (SANS) develops, requiring excision, treatment, and follow up (Almeida, Fernandes, Ortega, et al., 2017).

Salivary Calculus (Sialolithiasis)

Sialolithiasis, or salivary calculi (stones), usually occurs in the submandibular gland (Sigismund, Zenk, Koch, et al., 2015). Salivary gland ultrasonography or sialography (x-ray studies filmed after the injection of a radiopaque substance into the duct) may be required to demonstrate obstruction of the duct by stenosis. Salivary calculi are formed mainly from calcium phosphate. If located within the gland, the calculi are irregular and vary in diameter from 3 to 35 mm (Sigismund et al., 2015). Calculi in the duct are small and oval.

Calculi within the salivary gland itself cause no symptoms unless infection arises; however, a calculus that obstructs the gland's duct causes sudden, local, and often colicky pain, which is abruptly relieved by a gush of saliva. This characteristic symptom is often disclosed in the patient's health history. On physical assessment, the gland is swollen and quite tender, the stone itself can be palpable, and its shadow may be seen on x-ray films.

The calculus can be extracted fairly easily from the duct in the mouth. Sometimes, enlargement of the ductal orifice permits the stone to pass spontaneously. Occasionally **lithotripsy**, a procedure that uses shock waves to disintegrate the stone, may be used instead of surgical extraction for parotid stones and smaller submandibular stones. Lithotripsy requires no anesthesia, sedation, or analgesia. Side effects can include local hemorrhage and swelling. Surgery may be necessary to remove the gland if symptoms and calculi recur repeatedly.

Neoplasms

Although they are uncommon, neoplasms (tumours or growths) of almost any type may develop in the salivary gland; 50% of these are benign, with 70% to 80% of all salivary neoplasms beginning in the parotid gland. Neoplasm accounts for more than 0.5% of all malignancies and 3% to 5% of all head and neck cancers (National Cancer Institute [NCI], 2014). Risk factors include prior exposure to radiation to the head and neck, older age, and specific carcinogens introduced in specific work environments (asbestos, plumbing, and woodworking). Most patients with a benign tumour present with painless swelling of the glands; patients with a malignancy tend to have neurologic symptoms (weakness or numbness) and persistent facial pain. Diagnosis is based on the health history, physical examination, and the results of fine-needle aspiration biopsy.

Management of salivary gland tumours may involve partial excision of the gland, along with the tumour and a wide margin of surrounding tissue. Dissection is carefully performed to preserve the seventh cranial nerve (facial nerve), although it may not be possible to do so if the tumour is extensive. Complications from surgery may involve facial nerve dysfunction and Frey's syndrome. **Frey's syndrome**, also known as auriculotemporal syndrome, involves facial sweating and flushing in the general location of the (removed) parotid gland that occurs while eating. Frey's syndrome may be successfully treated with botulinum toxin type A injections (Dutta, Passi, Singh, et al., 2016). If the tumour is malignant, radiation therapy may follow surgery. Radiation therapy alone may be a treatment choice for tumours that are thought to be localized or if there is risk of facial nerve damage from surgical intervention. Chemotherapy is usually used for palliative purposes. Local recurrences are common, and the recurrence rate can be as high as 25% (Son, Panwar, Mosher, et al., 2018). Recurrent tumours usually are more aggressive than initial tumours. Tumours of the salivary gland lead to an increased incidence of second primary cancers, which may be due to inadequate excision of the original tumour.

CANCER OF THE ORAL CAVITY AND PHARYNX

Cancers of the oral cavity, and pharynx which can occur in any part of the mouth or throat, are curable if discovered early. Risk factors for cancer of the oral cavity, larynx, and esophagus include cigarette, cigar, and pipe smoking; use of smokeless tobacco; and excessive use of alcohol (Foulkes, 2013). Oral cancers are often associated with the combined use of alcohol and tobacco; these substances have a synergistic carcinogenic effect. Patient education directed toward avoiding high-risk behaviours is critical to prevent oral cancers.

The incidence of cancers of the oral cavity, larynx, and esophagus is greatest in men older than 50 years of age. In general, it is almost twice as high in men as it is in women. Cancers of the oral cavity, esophagus, and larynx, occur more often in African Canadians than in Caucasians.

Approximately 4,640 new cases of cancer of the oral cavity (3,196 males and 1,444 females), 2,269 cases of cancer of the esophagus (1,753 males and 516 females), and 1,134 cases of cancer of the larynx (928 males and 206 females) were predicted for Canadians in 2017 (Canadian Cancer Society's Advisory Committee on Cancer Statistics [CCSACCS], 2017). Rates for new cases of diagnoses of noted cancers were increased between 10% and 14% over reported 2013 rates (CCSACCS, 2017).

Of the noted cancers, the incident rates of laryngeal cancer decreased significantly from 1992 to 2013 for both males (decreasing 3.2% per year) and females (decreasing 3.4% per year). As cancer of the larynx is most strongly associated with smoking and alcohol, the decreasing trends in smoking may have contributed to the declines in incidence rates (CCSACCS, 2017). As of 2017, projected deaths from all cancers were 42,600 (males)/38,200 (females); of those deaths, 3.9% (males)/1.3% (females) were projected for cancer of the esophagus, 2.0% (males)/1.0% (females) for oral cancer, and 0.8% (males)/0.2 (females) for cancer of the larynx (CCSACCS, 2017).

Pathophysiology

Malignancies of the oral cavity are usually squamous cell carcinomas (Steinau, Saraiya, Goodman, et al., 2014).

Any area of the oropharynx can be a site of malignant growths, but the lips, the lateral aspects of the tongue, and the floor of the mouth are most commonly affected. HPV is known to be associated with the development of cervical and other forms of cancer. A recent study retrospectively examined tumour tissue samples from patients diagnosed with oropharyngeal cancer from 1995 to 2005 to determine the prevalence of HPV infection before the HPV vaccine became readily available. More than 72% of the sample had some type of the HPV virus, with 60.5% testing positive for HPV-16 (Steinau et al., 2014).

Clinical Manifestations

Many oral cancers produce few or no symptoms in the early stages. Later, the most frequent symptom is a painless sore or mass that does not heal. It may bleed easily and it may present as a red or white patch that persists (Canadian Cancer Society, 2017). A typical lesion in oral cancer is a painless indurated (hardened) ulcer with raised edges. As the cancer progresses, the patient may report tenderness; difficulty in chewing, swallowing, or speaking; coughing of blood-tinged sputum; or enlarged cervical lymph nodes.

Assessment and Diagnostic Findings

Diagnostic evaluation consists of an oral examination as well as an assessment of the cervical lymph nodes to detect possible metastases. Biopsies are performed on suspicious lesions (those that have not healed in 2 weeks). In people who use snuff or smoke cigars or pipes, high-risk areas include the buccal mucosa and gingiva. In those who smoke cigarettes and drink alcohol, high-risk areas include the floor of the mouth, the ventrolateral tongue, and the soft palate complex (soft palate, anterior and posterior tonsillar area, uvula, and the area behind the molar and tongue junction).

Human Papillomavirus Prevention

HPV vaccine is generally recommended for all children ages 11 or 12, up to the age of 26 years for women and 21 years for men. Men who have sex with men may receive the vaccine up to 26 years of age. These vaccines protect against HPV-16, which is associated with oropharyngeal cancer (Steinau et al., 2014).

Medical Management

In patients diagnosed with oropharyngeal cancer, management varies with the nature of the lesion, the preference of the physician, and patient choice. Surgical resection and radiation therapy are standard treatment. Chemotherapy may be useful for advanced disease (American Cancer Society [ACS], 2015).

In cancer of the lip, small lesions are usually excised liberally. Radiation therapy may be more appropriate for larger lesions involving more than one third of the lip because of superior cosmetic results. The choice depends on the extent of the lesion and what is necessary to cure the patient while preserving the best appearance. Tumours larger than 4 cm often recur.

In cancer of the tongue, treatment with radiation therapy and chemotherapy may preserve function and maintain quality of life. A combination of radioactive interstitial implants (surgical implantation of a radioactive source into the tissue adjacent to or at the tumour site) and external-beam radiation may be used. Surgical procedures include hemiglossectomy (surgical removal of half of the tongue) and total glossectomy (removal of the tongue). Glossectomy remains the principal treatment of advanced stage or cancers at the base of the tongue; long-term data on functional outcomes following these procedures are being studied (Lin, Yarlagadda, Sethi, et al., 2015).

Often, cancer of the oral cavity has metastasized through the extensive lymphatic channel in the neck region, requiring a neck dissection and reconstructive surgery of the oral cavity. Reconstructive techniques involve the use of a free (cut and removed) or pedicled (attached and tunnelled) tissue flap (graft of tissue with its own blood supply) most commonly obtained from the pectoralis major, rectus abdominis, or radial forearm (Rihani, Lee, Lee, et al., 2013). Laryngeal preservation is associated with better speech and verbal communication (Lin et al., 2015).

Nursing Management

The nurse assesses the patient's nutritional status preoperatively, and a dietary consultation may be necessary. The patient may require enteral (through the gastrointestinal tract) or parenteral (intravenous [IV]) feedings before and after surgery to maintain adequate nutrition. Continual assessment and reevaluation are necessary. If a radial graft is to be performed, an Allen's test on the donor arm must be performed to ensure that the ulnar artery is patent and can provide blood flow to the hand after removal of the radial artery. Allen's test is performed by asking the patient to make a fist and then manually compressing the ulnar artery. The patient is then asked to open the hand into a relaxed, slightly flexed position. The palm is pale. Pressure on the ulnar artery is released. If the ulnar artery is patent, the palm flushes within about 3 to 5 seconds.

Verbal communication may be impaired by radical surgery for oral cancer. It is therefore vital to assess the patient's ability to communicate in writing before surgery. Pen and paper are provided postoperatively to patients who can use them to communicate. A communication board with commonly used words or pictures is obtained preoperatively and given after surgery to patients who cannot write so that they may point to needed items. A speech therapist is also consulted postoperatively.

Postoperatively, the nurse assesses for a patent airway. The patient may be unable to manage oral secretions, making suctioning necessary. If grafting was part of the surgery, suctioning must be performed with care to prevent damage to the graft. The graft is assessed postoperatively for viability. Although colour should be assessed (white may indicate arterial occlusion, and blue mottling may indicate venous congestion), it can be difficult to assess the graft by looking into the mouth. A Doppler ultrasound device may be used to locate the radial pulse at the graft site and to assess graft perfusion.

NURSING MANAGEMENT OF THE PATIENT WITH CONDITIONS OF THE ORAL CAVITY

Promoting Mouth Care

The nurse instructs the patient about the importance and techniques of preventive mouth care. If a patient cannot tolerate brushing or flossing, an irrigating solution of 1 tsp of baking soda to 8 oz of warm water (5 cc to 240 cc), half-strength hydrogen peroxide, or normal saline solution is recommended. The nurse reinforces the need to perform oral care and provides such care to patients who cannot provide it for themselves.

If a bacterial or fungal infection is present, the nurse administers the prescribed medications and instructs the patient how to administer the medications at home. The nurse monitors the patient's physical and psychological response to treatment.

Xerostomia (dryness of the mouth) is a frequent sequela of oral cancer, particularly when the salivary glands have been exposed to radiation or major surgery. It is also seen in patients who are receiving psychopharmacologic agents, patients who are taking multiple medications, patients who use drugs recreationally, patients with rheumatic diseases, patients with eating disorders (Villa, Nordio, & Gohel, 2015), patients with human immune deficiency virus (HIV) infection, and patients who cannot close the mouth and as a result, breathe through the mouth instead of the nose. To minimize this problem, the patient is advised to avoid dry, bulky, and irritating foods and fluids, as well as alcohol and tobacco. The patient is also encouraged to increase intake of fluids (when not contraindicated) and to use a humidifier while sleeping. The use of synthetic saliva, a moisturizing antibacterial gel, or a saliva production stimulant such as Salagen may be helpful (Miranda-Rius, Brunet-Llobet, Lahor-Soler, et al., 2015).

Stomatitis, a type of oral mucositis, which involves inflammation and breakdown of the oral mucosa, is often a side effect of chemotherapy or radiation therapy. Prophylactic mouth care is started when the patient begins receiving treatment; however, mucositis may become so severe that a break in treatment is necessary. Current evidence recommends benzydamine mouthwash, a type of NSAID, be used to prevent oral mucositis (Lalla, Bowen, Barasch, et al., 2014). Other options that may be recommended include solutions that contain diphenhydramine (Benadryl), aluminum-magnesium hydroxide (Maalox) lidocaine (Xylocaine), and on occasion an oral antifungal or antibiotic. These solutions are known by various names such as magic mouthwash, Pink Lady and Noll's solution (Hoven, 2014).

(See Chapter 68 for more information about stomatitis.)

Ensuring Adequate Food and Fluid Intake

The patient's weight, age, and level of activity are recorded to determine whether nutritional intake is adequate. A daily calorie count may be necessary to determine the exact quantity of food and fluid ingested. The frequency and pattern of eating are recorded to determine whether any psychosocial or physiologic factors are affecting ingestion. Based on the disorder and the patient's preferences, the nurse recommends changes in the consistency of foods and the frequency of eating. Consultation with a dietitian may be helpful (Bossola, 2015). The goal is to help the patient attain and maintain desirable body weight and level of energy, as well as to promote the healing of tissue.

Supporting a Positive Self-Image

A patient who has a disfiguring oral condition or has undergone disfiguring surgery may experience an alteration in self-image. The patient is encouraged to verbalize the perceived change in body appearance and to realistically discuss actual changes or losses. The nurse offers support while the patient verbalizes fears and negative feelings (withdrawal, depression, anger). The nurse listens attentively and determines the patient's needs and individualizes the plan of care. The patient's strengths and achievements are reinforced.

The nurse determines the patient's anxieties concerning relationships with others. Referral to support groups, a psychiatric liaison nurse, a social worker, or a spiritual advisor may be useful in helping the patient to cope with anxieties and fears. The patient's progress toward development of positive self-esteem is documented. The nurse should be alert to signs of grieving and should document emotional changes. By providing acceptance and support, the nurse encourages the patient to verbalize feelings.

Minimizing Pain and Discomfort

Oral lesions can be painful. Strategies to reduce pain and discomfort include avoiding foods that are spicy, hot, or hard (e.g., pretzels, nuts). A soft or liquid diet may be preferred. The patient is instructed about mouth care. Using a soft tooth brush may prevent secondary trauma. It may be necessary to provide the patient with an analgesic such as viscous lidocaine (Xylocaine Viscous 2%) or opioids, as prescribed. Topical medications such as sucralfate (Carafate) and aluminum–magnesium liquid antacids may provide relief. The nurse can reduce the patient's fear of pain by providing information about pain control methods.

Preventing Infection

Leukopenia (a decrease in white blood cells) may result from radiation, chemotherapy, acquired immunodeficiency syndrome (AIDS), and some medications used to treat HIV infection. Leukopenia reduces defense mechanisms, increasing the risk of infections. Malnutrition, which is also common among these patients, may further decrease resistance to infection. If the patient has diabetes, the risk of infection is further increased.

Laboratory results should be evaluated frequently and the patient's temperature checked every 4 to 8 hours for an elevation that may indicate infection. Visitors who might transmit microorganisms are prohibited if the patient's immunologic system is depressed. Sensitive skin tissues are protected from trauma to maintain skin integrity and prevent infection. Aseptic technique is necessary when changing dressings. Desquamation (shedding of the epidermis) is a reaction to radiation therapy that causes dryness and itching and can lead to a break in skin integrity and subsequent infection.

Signs of wound infection (redness, swelling, drainage, and tenderness) are reported to the physician. Antibiotics may be prescribed prophylactically.

Promoting Home and Community-Based Care

Educating Patients About Self-Care

The patient who is recovering from treatment of an oral condition is instructed about mouth care, nutrition, prevention of infection, and signs and symptoms of complications (Chart 35-2). Methods of preparing nutritious foods that are seasoned according to the patient's preference and at the preferred temperature are explained to the patient and family. For some patients, it may be more convenient (but also more expensive) to use commercial baby foods than to prepare liquid and soft diets. The patient who cannot take foods orally may receive enteral or parenteral nutrition; the administration of these feedings is explained and demonstrated to the patient and the caregiver.

For patients with oral cancer, instructions are provided in the use and care of any dentures. The importance of keeping dressings clean and the need for conscientious oral hygiene are emphasized.

Continuing and Transitional Care

The need for ongoing care in the home depends on the patient's condition. The patient, the family members, and others responsible for home care (e.g., nurse, speech therapist, dietitian, psychologist) work together to prepare an individual plan of care.

If suctioning of the mouth or tracheostomy tube is required, the necessary equipment is obtained and the patient and caregivers are taught how to use it. Considerations include the control of odours and humidification of the home to keep secretions moist. The patient and caregivers are taught how to assess for obstruction, hemorrhage, and infection and what actions to take if they occur. The home care nurse may provide physical care, monitor for changes in the patient's physical status (e.g., skin integrity, nutritional status, respiratory function), and assess the adequacy of pain control measures. The nurse also assesses the patient's and family's ability to manage incisions, drains, and feeding tubes and the use of recommended strategies for communication. The ability of the patient and family to accept physical, psychological, and role changes is assessed and addressed.

Follow-up visits to the physician are important to monitor the patient's condition and to determine the need for

CHART 35-2

HOME CARE CHECKLIST • **The Patient With an Oral Disorder**

At the completion of education, the patient and/or caregiver will be able to:

- State the impact of the oral disorder and treatment on communication and other physiologic functioning, ADLs, IADLs, body image, roles, relationships, and spirituality.
- Identify modification of home environment, interventions, and strategies (e.g., durable medical equipment, home health aide) used in safely adapting to changes in structure or function and promote effective recovery and rehabilitation.
- Describe ongoing therapeutic regimen, including diet and activities to perform (e.g., oral care, suctioning) and to limit or avoid (e.g., oral foods if NPO).
  - Identify foods or therapies necessary to meet caloric needs and dietary needs (e.g., change in consistency, seasoning limitations, supplements, enteral or parenteral therapy).
  - Participate in prescribed therapy (e.g., speech therapy) to promote recovery and rehabilitation.
  - Demonstrate the use of suction equipment if indicated.
  - Demonstrate the use of humidification if indicated.
  - Demonstrate effective oral hygiene.
  - Demonstrate care of incision as appropriate.
- State the name, dose, side effects, frequency, and schedule for all medications.
  - Describe approaches to controlling pain (e.g., take analgesics as prescribed; use nonpharmacologic interventions).
- Identify possible complications and interventions.
- Relate how to reach primary provider with questions or complications.
- State time and date of follow-up medical/dental appointments, therapy, and testing.
- Identify sources of support (e.g., friends, relatives, faith community, cancer support, caregiver support).
- Identify the need for health promotion, disease prevention, and screening activities.

ADL, activities of daily living; IADL, independent activities of daily living; NPO, nothing by mouth.

modifications in treatment and general care. Because patients and their family members, as well as health care providers, tend to focus on the most obvious needs and issues, the nurse reminds the patient and family about the importance of continuing health promotion and screening practices and refers them to appropriate practitioners. The nurse also reinforces instructions in an effort to promote the patient's self-care and comfort.

NECK DISSECTION

Malignancies of the head and neck include those of the oral cavity, oropharynx, hypopharynx, nasopharynx, nasal cavity, paranasal sinus, and larynx. (Laryngeal cancer is presented in Chapter 23.) These cancers account for 6.6% of all cancers (CCSACCS, 2017). Depending on the location and stage, treatment may consist of radiation therapy, chemotherapy, surgery, or a combination of these modalities. Deaths from malignancies of the head and neck are primarily attributable to local–regional metastasis to the cervical lymph nodes in the neck. This often occurs by way of the lymphatics before the primary lesion has been treated. This local–regional metastasis is not amenable to surgical resection and responds poorly to chemotherapy and radiation therapy. The cervical lymph nodes are classified as anterior or posterior and divided into regions for classification (Grègoire, Ang, Budach, et al., 2014).

A radical neck dissection involves removal of all cervical lymph nodes (Fig. 35-3) from the mandible to the clavicle and removal of the sternocleidomastoid muscle, internal jugular vein, and spinal accessory muscle on one side of the neck. The associated complications include shoulder drop and poor cosmesis (visible neck depression). Modified radical neck dissection, which preserves one or more of the nonlymphatic structures, is used more often. A selective neck dissection (in comparison to a radical dissection) preserves one or more of the lymph node groups, the internal jugular vein, the sternocleidomastoid muscle, and the spinal accessory nerve (Fig. 35-4).

Reconstructive techniques may be performed with a variety of grafts. A cutaneous flap (skin and subcutaneous tissue), such as the deltopectoral flap, may be used. A myocutaneous flap (subcutaneous tissue, muscle, and skin) is a more frequently used graft; the pectoralis major muscle is usually used. For large grafts, a microvascular free flap may be used. This involves the transfer of muscle, skin, or bone with an artery and vein to the area of reconstruction, using micro-instrumentation (Fang, Zhang, Chen, et al., 2016). Areas used for a free flap include the scapula, the radial area of the forearm, or the fibula. The fibula, which provides a larger bone area, may be used if mandibular reconstruction is involved.

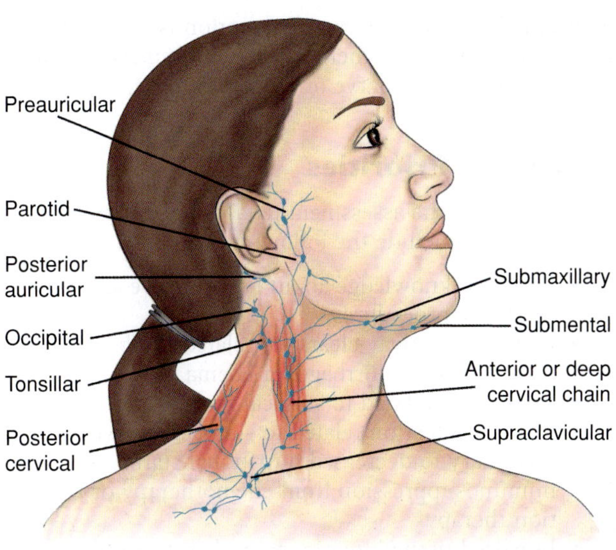

FIGURE 35-3. Lymphatic drainage of the head and neck.

Nursing Process

The Patient Undergoing a Neck Dissection

Assessment

Preoperatively, the patient's physical and psychological preparation for major surgery is assessed, along with his or her knowledge of the preoperative and postoperative procedures. Postoperatively, the patient is assessed for complications such as altered respiratory status, wound infection, and hemorrhage. As

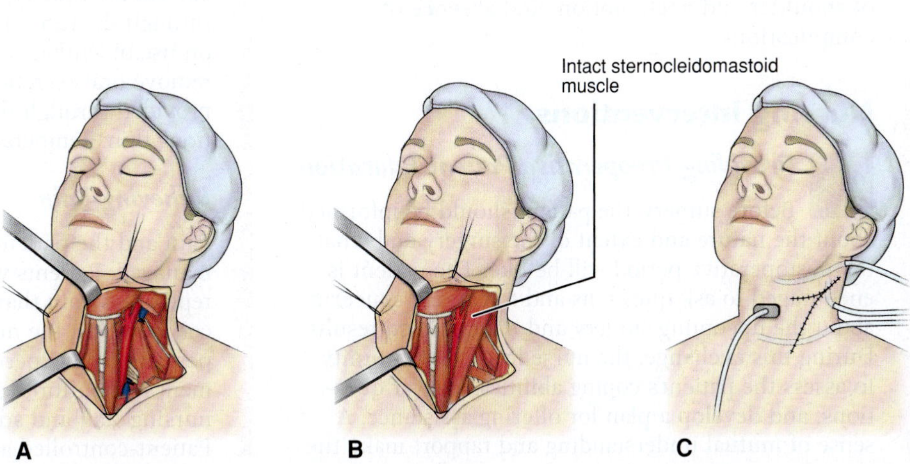

FIGURE 35-4. A. A classic radical neck dissection in which the sternocleidomastoid and smaller muscles are removed. All tissues are removed, from the ramus of the jaw to the clavicle. The jugular vein has also been removed. **B.** The selective neck dissection is similar but preserves the sternocleidomastoid muscle, internal jugular vein, and spinal accessory nerve. **C.** The wound is closed, and portable suction drainage tubes are in place.

healing occurs, neck range of motion is assessed to determine whether there has been a decrease in range of motion due to nerve or muscle damage.

Nursing Priorities

Based on all the assessment data, major nursing priorities may include the following:

- Deficient knowledge about preoperative and postoperative procedures
- Ineffective airway clearance related to obstruction by mucous, hemorrhage, or edema
- Acute pain related to surgical incision
- Risk for infection related to surgical intervention secondary to decreased nutritional status, or immunosuppression from chemotherapy or radiation therapy
- Impaired tissue integrity secondary to surgery and grafting
- Imbalanced nutrition, less than body requirements, related to disease process or treatment
- Situational low self-esteem related to diagnosis or prognosis
- Impaired verbal communication secondary to surgical resection
- Impaired physical mobility secondary to nerve injury

Collaborative Problems/Potential Complications

Potential postoperative complications that may develop include the following:

- Hemorrhage
- Chyle fistula
- Nerve injury

Planning and Goals

The major goals for the patient include participation in the treatment plan, maintenance of respiratory status, attainment of comfort, absence of infection, viability of the graft, maintenance of adequate intake of food and fluids, effective coping strategies, effective communication, maintenance of shoulder and neck motion, and absence of complications.

Nursing Interventions

Providing Preoperative Patient Education

Before surgery, the patient should be informed about the nature and extent of the surgery and what the postoperative period will be like. The patient is encouraged to ask questions and to express concerns about the upcoming surgery and the expected results. During this exchange, the nurse has an opportunity to assess the patient's coping abilities, answer questions, and develop a plan for offering assistance. A sense of mutual understanding and rapport make the postoperative experience less traumatic for the patient. The patient's expressions of concern, anxieties, and fears guide the nurse in providing support postoperatively.

Providing General Postoperative Care

The general postoperative nursing interventions are similar to those presented in Chapter 21 and are directed toward the identified nursing diagnoses and goals.

Maintaining the Airway

After the endotracheal tube or airway has been removed and the effects of the anesthesia have worn off, the patient may be placed in Fowler's position to facilitate breathing and promote comfort. This position also increases lymphatic and venous drainage, facilitates swallowing, decreases venous pressure on the skin flaps, and prevents regurgitation and aspiration of stomach contents. Signs of respiratory distress, such as dyspnea, cyanosis, changes in mental status, and changes in vital signs, are assessed because they may suggest edema, hemorrhage, inadequate oxygenation, or inadequate drainage.

NURSING ALERT

In the immediate postoperative period, the nurse assesses for stridor (coarse, high-pitched sound on inspiration) by listening frequently over the trachea with a stethoscope. This finding must be reported immediately because it indicates obstruction of the airway.

Pneumonia may occur in the postoperative phase if pulmonary secretions are not removed. To aid in the removal of secretions, coughing and deep breathing are encouraged. With the nurse supporting the neck, the patient should assume a sitting position so that excessive secretions can be coughed up and expectorated. If this is ineffective, the patient's respiratory tract may have to be suctioned. Care is taken to protect the suture lines during suctioning. If a tracheostomy tube is in place, suctioning is performed through the tube. The patient may also be instructed on use of Yankauer suction (tonsil tip suction) to remove oral secretions. Humidified air or oxygen is provided through the tracheostomy to keep secretions thin. Temperature should not be taken orally.

Relieving Pain

Pain and the patient's fear of pain are assessed and managed. Patients with head and neck cancer often report less pain than patients with other types of cancer; however, the nurse needs to be aware that each person's pain experience is individual. Pain management is monitored on a continual basis by the nursing staff and adjusted on an individual basis. Patient-controlled analgesia may be prescribed for postoperative pain management, thereby reducing the wait time for pain relief.

Providing Wound Care

Wound drainage tubes are usually inserted during surgery to prevent the collection of fluid subcutaneously. The drainage tubes are connected to a portable suction device (e.g., Jackson–Pratt), and the container is emptied periodically. Between 80 and 120 mL of serosanguineous secretions may drain over the first 24 hours. Excessive drainage may be indicative of a chyle fistula or hemorrhage (see later discussion). Dressings are reinforced as needed and are observed for evidence of hemorrhage and constriction, which impairs respiration and perfusion of the graft. A graft, if present, is assessed for colour and temperature and for the presence of a pulse, if applicable, to determine viability. The graft should be pale pink and warm to the touch. The surgical incisions are also assessed for signs of infection (purulent, malodorous drainage), which are reported immediately. Prophylactic antibiotics may be prescribed in the early postoperative period. Aseptic technique is used when cleansing skin around the drains; dressings are changed as prescribed by the surgeon, usually on the second through the fifth postoperative days. Care should be taken to not apply excessive pressure to the surgical site in order to not impair flap perfusion and viability (Carr, 2016).

Maintaining Adequate Nutrition

Nutritional status is assessed preoperatively; early intervention to correct nutritional imbalances may decrease the risk of postoperative complications. Frequently, nutrition is less than optimal because of inadequate intake, and the patient often requires enteral or parenteral supplements preoperatively and postoperatively to attain and maintain a positive nitrogen balance. Supplements (e.g., Ensure, Sustacal, Glucerna, Boost) that are nutritionally dense may help reestablish a positive nitrogen balance. They may be taken enterally by mouth, by nasogastric feeding tube, or by gastrostomy feeding tube.

The patient who can chew may take food by mouth; the patient's chewing ability determines whether some diet modification (e.g., soft, puréed, or liquid foods) is necessary. Food preferences should also be discussed with the patient. Oral care before eating may enhance the patient's appetite, and oral care after eating is important to prevent infection and dental caries. Most patients can maintain and gain weight.

Supporting Patient Self-Esteem and the Needs of Caregivers

Preoperatively, information about the planned surgery is given to the patient and family. Any questions are answered as accurately as possible. It is important for the health care provider to pay attention to nonverbal behaviour that may indicate something different from what the patient is able to articulate. Postoperatively, psychological nursing interventions are aimed at supporting the patient who has had a change in body image or who has major concerns related to the prognosis. The patient may have difficulty communicating and may be concerned about his or her ability to breathe and swallow normally. The nurse supports the patient's family in encouraging and reassuring the patient that adjusting to the results of this surgery will take time. The nurse is also sensitive to the needs of family caregivers who are often responsible for both the physical and psychosocial care of the patient (Fronczek, 2015).

The person who has had extensive neck surgery often is sensitive about his or her appearance. This can occur when the operative area is covered by bulky dressings, when the incision line is visible, or later after healing has occurred and the appearance of the neck and possibly the lower face has been significantly altered. If the nurse accepts the patient's appearance and expresses a positive, optimistic attitude, the patient is more likely to be encouraged. The patient also needs an opportunity to express fears and concerns regarding the success of the surgery and the prognosis. The Canadian Cancer Society (CCS) may be a resource to provide a volunteer who meets with the patient either preoperatively or postoperatively and shares his or her own experience about the diagnosis, treatment, and recovery. The "Look Good, Feel Better" programs of the CCS also are a source of information about clothing and cosmetics that can be used to deemphasize physical defects.

People with cancer of the head and neck frequently have used alcohol or tobacco before surgery; postoperatively, they are encouraged to abstain from these substances. Alternative methods of coping need to be explored. A referral to Alcoholics Anonymous, a smoking cessation program, and family counselling may be appropriate.

Promoting Effective Communication

Communication begins preoperatively, when the patient and family determine which method of communication will be the best postoperatively. Useful communication methods for the patient who has undergone a laryngectomy include Magic Slates, writing materials, pictorial guides, computer aids, and hand signals. During the postoperative period, the call bell must be readily accessible to the patient at all times.

The nurse obtains a consultation with a speech therapist. Alternative speech techniques, such as an electrolarynx (a mechanical device held against the neck) or esophageal speech, may be taught by a speech therapist. The most widely used technique for creating laryngeal speech is tracheoesophageal puncture. A surgically created fistula extends from the superior wall of the tracheal stoma into the proximal esophageal wall. A voice prosthesis is then inserted into the fistula to assist with speech (see Chapter 23).

Maintaining Physical Mobility

Excision of muscles and nerves results in weakness at the shoulder that can cause shoulder drop, a forward

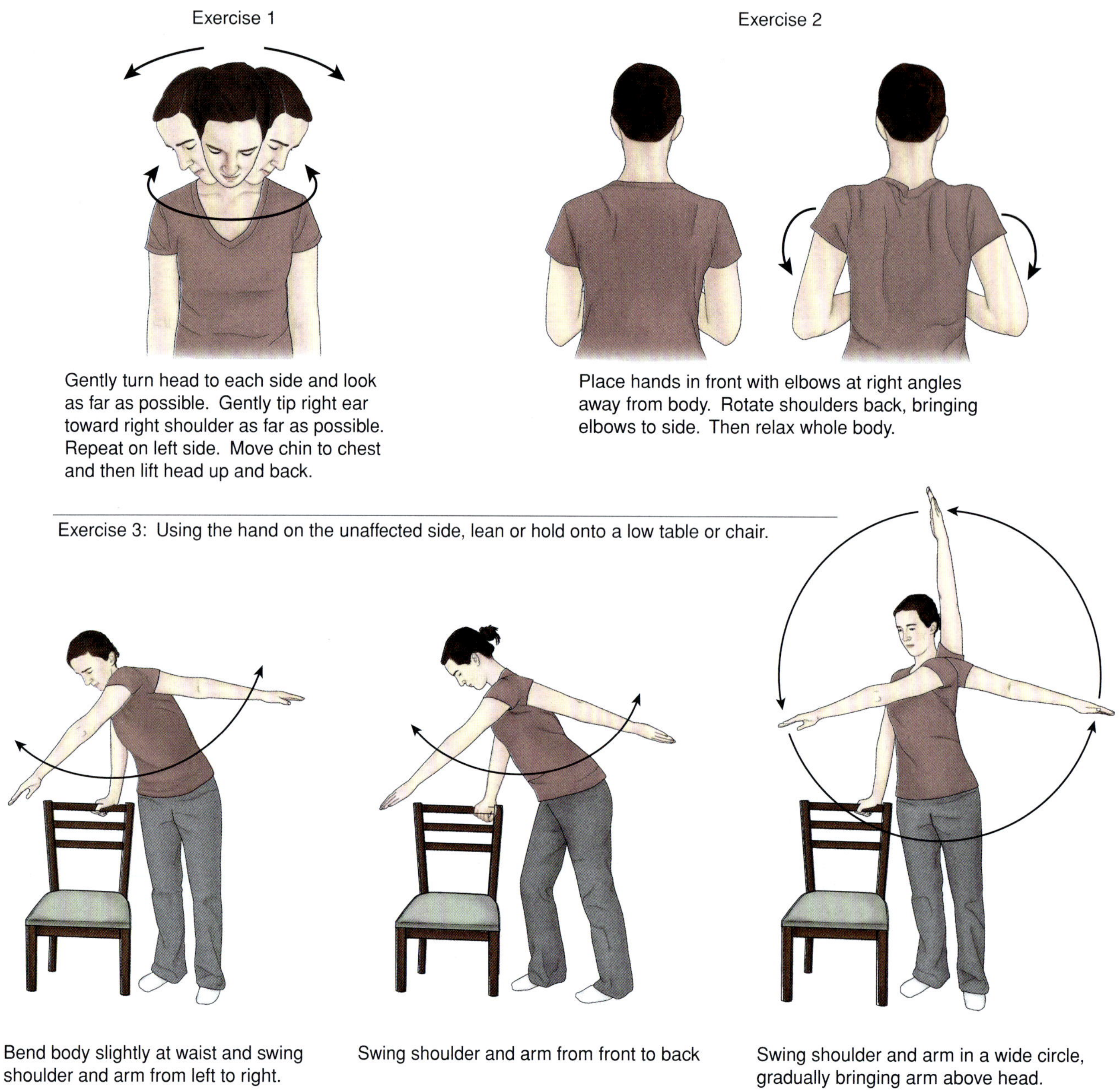

FIGURE 35-5. Three rehabilitation exercises after head and neck surgery. The objective is to regain maximum shoulder function and neck motion after neck surgery. (From Exercise for radical neck surgery patients. Head and Neck Service, Department of Surgery, Memorial Hospital, New York, NY.)

curvature of the shoulder. Many problems can be avoided with a conscientious exercise program. These exercises are usually started after the drains have been removed and the neck incision is sufficiently healed. The purpose of the exercises depicted in Figure 35-5 is to promote maximal shoulder function and neck motion after surgery. Physical therapists and occupational therapists can assist patients in performing these exercises.

Monitoring and Managing Potential Complications

HEMORRHAGE. Hemorrhage may occur from carotid artery rupture as a result of necrosis of the graft or damage to the artery itself from tumour or infection. The following measures are indicated:

- Vital signs are assessed frequently (every 1 to 2 hours or every 15 minutes if the patient is critical). Once the patient is stabilized, assessment is increased to every 4 hours. Tachycardia, tachypnea, and hypotension may indicate hemorrhage and impending hypovolemic shock.
- The patient is instructed to avoid the Valsalva manoeuvre to prevent stress on the graft and carotid artery.
- Signs of impending rupture, such as high epigastric pain or discomfort, are reported.
- Dressings and wound drainage are observed for excessive bleeding.

- If hemorrhage occurs, assistance is summoned immediately.
- Hemorrhage requires the continuous application of pressure to the bleeding site or major associated vessel.
- Although some clinicians advocate placing the patient in the modified Trendelenburg position to maintain blood pressure, others recommend that the head of the patient's bed be elevated to maintain airway patency and prevent aspiration.
- A controlled, calm manner allays the patient's anxiety.
- The surgeon is notified immediately, because a vascular or ligature tear requires surgical intervention.

CHYLE FISTULA. A chyle fistula (milk-like drainage from the thoracic duct into the thoracic cavity) may develop as a result of damage to the thoracic duct during surgery. Although not very common (1% to 2.5% of cases), this complication is serious and life-threatening (Swanson, Hudson, Bhandari, et al., 2015). The diagnosis of chyle fistula is made in case of excessive output into the chest tube drainage. The output should have 3% fat content and a specific gravity of 1.012 or greater. Treatment of a small leak (500 mL or less) requires a diet of medium-chain fatty acids or parenteral nutrition, although there is emerging support for the use of IV or subcutaneous administration of octreotide (Sandostatin) in conservative management (Swanson et al., 2015). Octreotide, a synthetic analog of the natural hormone somatostatin, works primarily by decreasing the absorption of triglycerides and inhibiting gastrointestinal circulation and motility, thereby reducing lymph flow and decreasing the chyle flow (Swanson et al., 2015). Surgical intervention may be needed to repair the damaged duct (Tessier, 2019).

NERVE INJURY. Nerve injury can occur if the cervical plexus or spinal accessory nerves are severed during surgery. Because lower facial paralysis may occur as a result of injury to the facial nerve, this complication is observed for and reported. Likewise, if the superior laryngeal nerve is damaged, the patient may have difficulty swallowing liquids and food because of the partial lack of sensation of the glottis. Speech therapy may be indicated to assist with the problems related to nerve injury.

Promoting Home and Community-Based Care

EDUCATING PATIENTS ABOUT SELF-CARE. The patient and caregiver require instructions about management of the wound, the dressing, and any drains that remain in place. Patients who require oral suctioning or who have a tracheostomy may be very anxious about their care at home; the transition to home can be eased if the caregiver is given several opportunities to demonstrate the ability to meet the patient's needs (Chart 35-3).

CHART 35-3

HOME CARE CHECKLIST • The Patient Recovering From Neck Surgery

At the completion of education, the patient and/or caregiver will be able to:

- Name the procedure that was performed and identify any permanent changes in anatomic structure or function as well as changes in communication, ADLs, IADLs, roles, body image, relationships, and spirituality.
- Identify modification of home environment, interventions, and strategies (e.g., durable medical equipment, home health aide) used in safely adapting to changes in structure or function and promote effective recovery and rehabilitation.
- Describe ongoing therapeutic regimen, including diet and activities to perform (e.g., oral care, suctioning) and to limit or avoid (e.g., lifting weights, driving a car, contact sports).
  - Identify foods or therapies necessary to meet caloric needs and dietary needs (e.g., change in consistency, seasoning limitations, supplements, enteral or parenteral therapy).
  - Participate in prescribed therapy (e.g., speech therapy, PT, OT) to promote recovery and rehabilitation.
  - Demonstrate the use of tracheostomy care and suctioning if indicated.
  - Demonstrate the use of humidification if indicated.
  - Demonstrate effective oral hygiene.
  - Demonstrate care of incision and drains.
- State the name, dose, side effects, frequency, and schedule for all medications.
  - Describe approaches to controlling pain (e.g., take analgesics as prescribed; use nonpharmacologic interventions).
- Identify possible complications (e.g., bleeding, respiratory distress) and interventions.
- Relate how to reach primary provider with questions or complications.
- State time and date of follow-up medical/dental appointments, therapy, and testing.
- Identify sources of support (e.g., friends, relatives, faith community, cancer support, caregiver support).
- Identify the need for health promotion, disease prevention, and screening activities.

ADL, activities of daily living; IADL, independent activities of daily living; PT, physical therapy; OT, occupational therapy.

The patient and caregiver are also instructed about possible complications such as bleeding and respiratory distress and when to notify the health care provider of signs and symptoms of these complications.

If the patient cannot take food by mouth, detailed instructions and demonstration of enteral or parenteral feedings will be required. Education in techniques of effective oral hygiene is also important.

CONTINUING AND TRANSITIONAL CARE. A referral for home care nursing may be necessary in the early period after discharge. The nurse assesses healing, ensures that feedings are being administered properly, and monitors for any complications. The nurse also assesses the patient's adjustment to changes in physical appearance and status and ability to communicate and eat normally. Physical and speech therapy also are likely to be continued at home.

The patient is given information regarding local support groups such as "I Can Cope" or "New Voice Club," if indicated. The local chapter of the CCS may be contacted for information and equipment needed for the patient.

Evaluation

Expected patient outcomes may include:

1. Discusses expected course of treatment
2. Demonstrates adequate respiratory exchange
   a. Lungs are clear to auscultation
   b. Breathes easily with no shortness of breath
   c. Demonstrates ability to use suction effectively
3. Remains free of infection
   a. Maintains usual laboratory values
   b. Is afebrile
4. Graft is pink and warm to touch
5. Maintains adequate intake of foods and fluids
   a. Accepts altered route of feeding
   b. Is well hydrated
   c. Maintains or gains weight
6. Demonstrates ability to cope
   a. Discusses emotional responses to the diagnosis
   b. Attends support group meetings
7. Verbalizes comfort
8. Attains maximal mobility
   a. Adheres to physical therapy exercises
   b. Attains maximal range of motion
9. Exhibits no complications
   a. Vital signs stable
   b. No excessive bleeding or discharge
   c. Able to move muscles of lower face

DISORDERS OF THE ESOPHAGUS

The esophagus is a mucus-lined, muscular tube that carries food from the mouth to the stomach. It begins at the base of the pharynx and ends about 4 cm below the diaphragm. Its ability to transport food and fluid is facilitated by two sphincters. The upper esophageal sphincter, also called the *hypopharyngeal sphincter*, is located at the junction of the pharynx and the esophagus. The lower esophageal sphincter, also called the *gastroesophageal sphincter* or *cardiac sphincter* is located at the junction of the esophagus and the stomach. An incompetent lower esophageal sphincter allows reflux (backward flow) of gastric contents. There is no serosal layer of the esophagus; therefore, if surgery is necessary, it is more difficult to perform suturing or anastomosis.

Disorders of the esophagus include motility disorders (**achalasia**, diffuse spasm), hiatal **hernias**, diverticula, perforation, foreign bodies, chemical burns, **gastroesophageal reflux disease (GERD)**, Barrett's esophagus (BE), benign tumours, and carcinoma. Dysphagia (difficulty swallowing), the most common symptom of esophageal disease, may vary from an uncomfortable feeling that a bolus of food is caught in the upper esophagus to acute pain on swallowing (**odynophagia**). Obstruction of food (solid and soft) and even liquids may occur anywhere along the esophagus. Often the patient can indicate that the problem is located in the upper, middle, or lower third of the esophagus.

Achalasia

Achalasia is absent or ineffective peristalsis of the distal esophagus, accompanied by failure of the esophageal sphincter to relax in response to swallowing. Narrowing of the esophagus just above the stomach results in a gradually increasing dilation of the esophagus in the upper chest. Achalasia may progress slowly and occurs most often in people 40 years of age or older.

Clinical Manifestations

The primary symptom is difficulty in swallowing both liquids and solids. The patient has a sensation of food sticking in the lower portion of the esophagus. As the condition progresses, food is commonly regurgitated either spontaneously or intentionally by the patient to relieve the discomfort produced by prolonged distention of the esophagus by food that will not pass into the stomach. The patient may also report chest pain and heartburn (**pyrosis**) that may or may not be associated with eating. Secondary pulmonary complications may result from aspiration of gastric contents.

Assessment and Diagnostic Findings

X-ray studies show esophageal dilation above the narrowing at the gastroesophageal junction. Barium swallow, computed tomography (CT) of the chest, and endoscopy may be used for diagnosis; however, manometry, a process in which the esophageal pressure is measured by a radiologist or gastroenterologist, confirms the diagnosis.

Management

The patient is instructed to eat slowly and to drink fluids with meals. As a temporary measure, calcium channel blockers and nitrates have been used to decrease esophageal pressure and improve swallowing. Injection of botulinum toxin (Botox) into quadrants of the esophagus via endoscopy has been helpful because it inhibits the

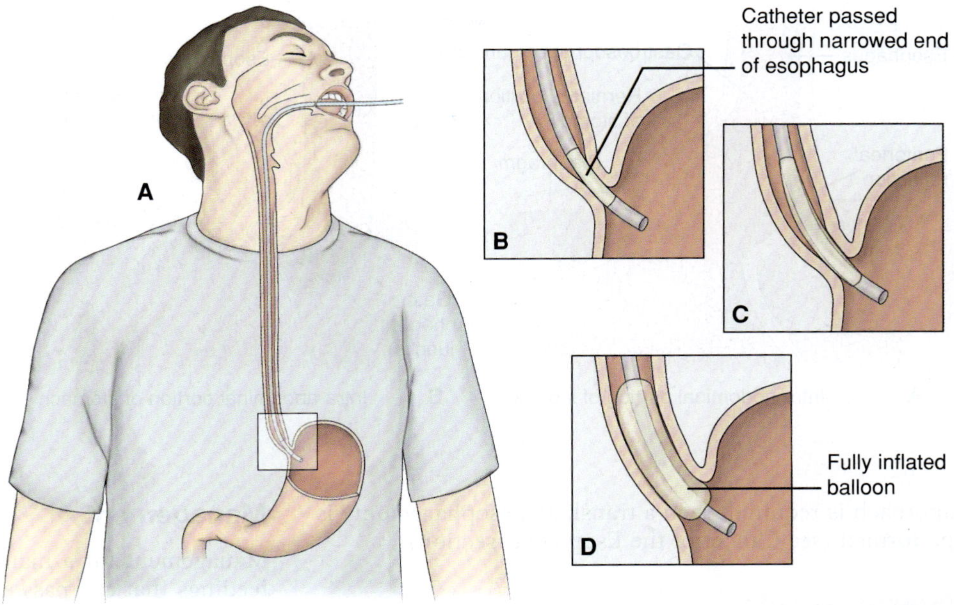

FIGURE 35-6. Treatment of achalasia by pneumatic dilation. A–C. The dilator is passed, guided by a previously inserted guide wire. D. When the balloon is in proper position, it is distended by pressure sufficient to dilate the narrowed area of the esophagus.

contraction of smooth muscle. Periodic injections are required to maintain remission (Pandolfino & Gawron, 2015).

Achalasia may be treated conservatively by pneumatic dilation to stretch the narrowed area of the esophagus (Fig. 35-6). Pneumatic dilation has a high success rate. Although perforation is a potential complication, its incidence is low. The procedure can be painful; therefore, moderate sedation in the form of an analgesic or tranquilizer, or both, is administered for the treatment. The patient is monitored for perforation. Abdominal tenderness and fever may indicate perforation (see later discussion).

Achalasia may be treated surgically by esophagomyotomy, which involves cutting the esophageal muscle fibres. The procedure is usually performed laparoscopically, either with a complete lower esophageal sphincter myotomy and an antireflux procedure or without an antireflux procedure. A new technique, an endoscopic myotomy (per-oral endoscopic myotomy [POEM]), may provide an alternative procedure (Pandolfino & Gawron, 2015).

Esophageal Spasm

The two types of esophageal spasm include diffuse esophageal spasm (DES) and hypertensive peristalsis, also known as nutcracker esophagus (NE). In DES, the spasms are normal in amplitude, but are uncoordinated, move quickly, or occur at various places in the esophagus at once. In NE, peristalsis is coordinated, but the amplitude is very high. Hypercontractile esophagus, also known as jackhammer esophagus, is an extreme form of NE in which the contractions involve the entire esophagus and occur over a prolonged period (Khan, Kumbhari, Ngamruengphong, et al., 2017). NE is more common in women and usually manifests in middle age. The cause is unknown, but stress may be a factor. There may also be a relationship between NE and psychiatric disorders or psychotropic medications (Lufrano, Heckman, Diehl, et al., 2015).

Clinical Manifestations

Diffuse spasm is characterized by difficulty (dysphagia) or pain (odynophagia) on swallowing and by chest pain similar to that of coronary artery spasm. Dysphagia is more common in DES from the noncoordinated peristalsis.

Assessment and Diagnostic Findings

Esophageal manometry, which measures the motility of the esophagus and the pressure within the esophagus, indicates that simultaneous contractions of the esophagus occur irregularly. Diagnostic x-ray studies after ingestion of barium show separate areas of spasm.

Management

Conservative therapy includes administration of sedatives and long-acting nitrates to relieve pain. Calcium channel blockers (e.g., nifedipine [Procardia], verapamil [Calan]) have also been used to manage diffuse spasm. Small, frequent feedings and a soft diet are usually recommended to decrease the esophageal pressure and irritation that lead to spasm. Dilation performed by bougienage (use of progressively sized flexible dilators), pneumatic dilation, or esophagomyotomy may be necessary if the pain becomes intolerable.

If none of the conservative approaches is successful in managing symptoms, surgery may be considered. A POEM or an esophageal Heller myotomy (a surgical procedure in which the cardiac sphincter is cut, allowing food and liquids to pass into the stomach) is considered to be a minimally invasive approach and is considered first with positive results (Khan et al., 2017). If an open surgical

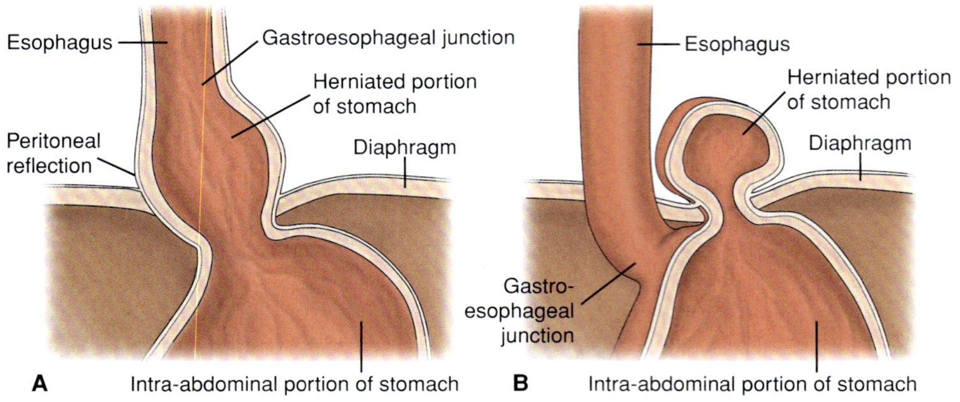

FIGURE 35-7. **A.** Sliding esophageal hernia. The upper stomach and gastroesophageal junction have moved upward and slide in and out of the thorax. **B.** Paraesophageal hernia. All or part of the stomach pushes through the diaphragm next to the gastroesophageal junction.

approach is required, then a transhiatal esophagectomy is performed (see Cancer of the Esophagus section).

Hiatal Hernia

In the condition known as hiatus (or hiatal) hernia, the opening in the diaphragm through which the esophagus passes becomes enlarged, and part of the upper stomach tends to move up into the lower portion of the thorax. Hiatal hernia occurs more often in women than in men. There are two types of hiatal hernias: sliding and paraesophageal. Sliding, or type I, hiatal hernia occurs when the upper stomach and the gastroesophageal junction are displaced upward and slide in and out of the thorax (Fig. 35-7A). About 90% of patients with esophageal hiatal hernia have a sliding hernia. A paraesophageal hernia occurs when all or part of the stomach pushes through the diaphragm beside the esophagus (see Fig. 35-7B). Paraesophageal hernias are further classified as types II, III, or IV, depending on the extent of herniation. Type IV has the greatest herniation, with other intra-abdominal viscera such as the colon, spleen, or small bowel evidencing displacement into the chest along with the stomach (Oleynikov & Jolley, 2015).

Clinical Manifestations

The patient with a sliding hernia may have heartburn, regurgitation, and dysphagia, but at least 50% of patients are asymptomatic. Sliding hiatal hernia is often implicated in reflux. The patient with a paraesophageal hernia usually feels a sense of fullness or chest pain after eating, or there may be no symptoms. Reflux usually does not occur, because the gastroesophageal sphincter is intact. Hemorrhage, obstruction, and strangulation can occur with any type of hernia (Oleynikov & Jolley, 2015).

Assessment and Diagnostic Findings

Diagnosis is typically confirmed by x-ray studies; barium swallow; **esophagogastroduodenoscopy** (EGD), which is the passage of a fibreoptic tube through the mouth and throat into the digestive tract for visualization of the esophagus, stomach, and small intestine; esophageal manometry; or chest CT scan (Kohn, Price, DeMeester, et al., 2013; Weijenborg, van Hoeij, Smout, et al., 2015).

Management

Management for a hiatal hernia includes frequent, small feedings that can pass easily through the esophagus. The patient is advised not to recline for 1 hour after eating, to prevent reflux or movement of the hernia, and to elevate the head of the bed on 10- to 20-cm blocks to prevent the hernia from sliding upward. Surgery is indicated in about 15% of patients. Medical and surgical management of a paraesophageal hernia is similar to that for **gastroesophageal reflux**; however, people with paraesophageal hernias may require emergency surgery to correct torsion (twisting) of the stomach or other body organ that leads to restriction of blood flow to that area.

Up to 50% of patients may experience early postoperative dysphagia; therefore, the nurse advances the diet slowly from liquids to solids, while managing nausea and vomiting, tracking nutritional intake, and monitoring weight. The nurse also monitors for postoperative belching, vomiting, gagging, abdominal distension, and epigastric chest pain, which may indicate the need for surgical revision; these should be reported immediately to the primary provider. Surgical repair is often reserved for patients with more extreme cases that involve gastric outlet obstruction or suspected gastric strangulation, which may result in ischemia, necrosis, or perforation of the stomach (Kohn et al., 2013).

Diverticulum

A diverticulum is an outpouching of mucosa and submucosa that protrudes through a weak portion of the musculature. Diverticula may occur in one of the three areas of the esophagus—the pharyngoesophageal or upper area of the esophagus, the midesophageal area, or the epiphrenic or lower area of the esophagus—or they may occur along the border of the esophagus intramurally.

The most common type of diverticulum, which is found three times more frequently in men than in women, is Zenker's diverticulum (also known as pharyngoesophageal pulsion diverticulum or a pharyngeal pouch) (Smith, 2015). Located in the pharyngoesophageal area, Zenker's diverticula are caused by a dysfunctional sphincter that fails to open, which leads to increased pressure that forces the mucosa and submucosa to herniate through the esophageal musculature (called a pulsion diverticulum).

It is usually seen in people older than 60 years of age. Other types of diverticula include midesophageal, epiphrenic, and intramural diverticula.

Midesophageal diverticula are uncommon. Symptoms are less acute, and usually the condition does not require surgery. Epiphrenic diverticula are usually larger diverticula in the lower esophagus just above the diaphragm. They may be related to the improper functioning of the lower esophageal sphincter or to motor disorders of the esophagus. Intramural diverticulosis is the occurrence of numerous small diverticula associated with a stricture in the upper esophagus.

Clinical Manifestations

Symptoms experienced by the patient with a pharyngoesophageal pulsion diverticulum include difficulty swallowing, fullness in the neck, belching, regurgitation of undigested food, and gurgling noises after eating. The diverticulum, or pouch, becomes filled with food or liquid. When the patient assumes a recumbent position, undigested food is regurgitated, and coughing may be caused by irritation of the trachea. Halitosis and a sour taste in the mouth are also common because of the decomposition of food retained in the diverticulum (Smith, 2015).

Symptoms produced by midesophageal diverticula are less acute. One third of patients with epiphrenic diverticula are asymptomatic, and the remaining two thirds report dysphagia and chest pain. Dysphagia is the most common symptom of patients with intramural diverticulosis.

Assessment and Diagnostic Findings

A barium swallow may determine the exact nature and location of a diverticulum. Manometric studies are often performed for patients with epiphrenic diverticula to rule out a motor disorder. Esophagoscopy usually is contraindicated because of the danger of perforation of the diverticulum, with resulting mediastinitis (inflammation of the organs and tissues that separate the lungs). Blind insertion of a nasogastric tube should be avoided.

Management

Because pharyngoesophageal pulsion diverticulum is progressive, the only means of cure is surgical removal of the diverticulum. During surgery, care is taken to avoid trauma to the common carotid artery and internal jugular veins. The sac is dissected free and amputated flush with the esophageal wall. In addition to a diverticulectomy, a myotomy of the cricopharyngeal muscle is often performed to relieve spasticity of the musculature, which otherwise seems to contribute to a continuation of the previous symptoms. A nasogastric tube may be inserted at the time of surgery. Postoperatively, the surgical incision must be observed for evidence of leakage from the esophagus and a developing fistula. Food and fluids are withheld until x-ray studies show no leakage at the surgical site. The diet begins with liquids and is progressed as tolerated.

Advances in technology include the minimally invasive endoscopic stapling diverticulotomy, which expedites oral intake and discharge, reduces the risk of fistula formation, and does not require an NG tube. Patients who are not good candidates for this endoscopic procedure include those with a stiff or short neck, poor mouth opening, prominent teeth, large tongue, and with larger diverticula (Yuan, Zhao, Hu, et al., 2013).

Surgery is indicated for epiphrenic and midesophageal diverticula only if the symptoms are troublesome and becoming worse. Treatment consists of a diverticulectomy and long myotomy. Intramural diverticula usually regress after the esophageal stricture is dilated.

Perforation

Esophageal perforation is a surgical emergency. It may result from iatrogenic causes, such as endoscopy or intraoperative injury, or from spontaneous perforation associated with forceful vomiting or severe straining (**Boerhaave's syndrome**), foreign-body ingestion, trauma, and malignancy. Immediate diagnosis and treatment are essential to minimize mortality. A delay of more than 24 hours is associated with higher mortality (27%) when compared to rapid recognition and treatment (14%). Perforation can occur at the cervical, thoracic, or abdominal portion of the esophagus (Watson & Peyre, 2019).

Clinical Manifestations

The patient has excruciating retrosternal pain followed by dysphagia. Infection, fever, leukocytosis, and severe hypotension may be noted. In addition, mediastinal sepsis can occur with Boerhaave's syndrome, which may be accompanied by pneumothorax and subcutaneous emphysema.

Assessment and Diagnostic Findings

X-ray studies and fluoroscopy by either a barium swallow or esophagram (noninvasive test), or a chest CT scan may be used to identify the site and scope of the injury.

Management

Esophageal perforation requires immediate treatment. Treatment includes having the patient remain NPO (nothing by mouth), beginning IV fluid therapy, administering broad-spectrum antibiotics (ampicillin-sulbactam [Unasyn], piperacillin-tazobactam [Zosyn], or a carbapenem [e.g., imipenem{Primaxin}]), considering the need for antifungal therapy (if the patient is immunosuppressed, has HIV infection, or shows no improvement with antibiotics), supportive monitoring and care (intensive care unit level-of-care often required), and evaluating and preparing the patient for surgery (Watson & Peyre, 2019). Surgical repair of the perforation site is performed in most cases, even if the diagnosis is made after 24 hours. If surgical repair of the perforation is not possible due to the clinical status of the patient, then drainage, diversion, stent placement, or an esophagostomy (removal of the esophagus) may be performed (Watson & Peyre, 2019).

Postoperative nutritional status is a major concern. The patient remains NPO for approximately 7 days, so enteral (e.g., jejunal feeding) or parenteral nutrition is started on postoperative day 2 or 3 (see Chapter 21). The nurse uses water to moisten the patient's mouth for comfort measures only. A repeat esophagram is obtained on postoperative day 7 to verify there is no leak or ileus before the NG tube is removed and oral intake is permitted. It is common for broad-spectrum antibiotics to continue for 7 to 10 days postoperatively (Watson & Peyre, 2019).

Foreign Bodies

Many swallowed foreign bodies pass through the gastrointestinal tract without the need for medical intervention. However, some swallowed foreign bodies (e.g., dentures, fish bones, pins, small batteries, items containing mercury or lead) may injure the esophagus or obstruct its lumen and must be removed. Pain and dysphagia may be present, and dyspnea may occur as a result of pressure on the trachea. The foreign body may be identified by x-ray. Perforation may have occurred (see earlier discussion).

Glucagon, because of its relaxing effect on the esophageal muscle, may be injected intramuscularly. An endoscope (with a covered hood or overtube) may be used to remove the impacted food or object from the esophagus. A mixture consisting of sodium bicarbonate and tartaric acid may be prescribed to increase intraluminal pressure by the formation of a gas. Caution must be used with this treatment because of the risk of perforation.

NURSING ALERT

The nurse performs an initial and ongoing respiratory (airway-focused) assessment of a patient with a foreign body in the esophagus. Intubation may be required to protect the airway.

Chemical Burns

Chemical burns of the esophagus occur most often when a patient, either intentionally (67% adults) or unintentionally (33% children), swallows a strong acid or base (e.g., lye), with alkaline agents most common (Byard, 2015). This patient is emotionally distraught as well as in acute physical pain. Chemical burns of the esophagus may also be caused by undissolved medications in the esophagus. This occurs more frequently in older adults than it does among the general adult population. A chemical burn may also occur after swallowing of a battery, which may release a caustic alkaline. An acute chemical burn of the esophagus may be accompanied by severe burns of the lips, mouth, and pharynx, with pain on swallowing. There may be difficulty in breathing due to either edema of the throat or a collection of mucus in the pharynx.

The patient, who may be profoundly toxic, febrile, and in shock, is treated immediately for shock, pain, and respiratory distress. Esophagoscopy and barium swallow are performed as soon as possible to determine the extent and severity of damage. The patient is given NPO, and IV fluids are administered. A nasogastric tube may be inserted by the physician. Vomiting and gastric lavage are avoided to prevent further exposure of the esophagus to the caustic agent. Recently, the administration of omeprazole (a protein pump inhibitor) immediately post burn has been found effective in initial studies (Cakal, Akbal, Köklü, et al., 2013). Antibiotics are used post trauma, although the use of corticosteroids to reduce inflammation and minimize subsequent scarring and stricture formation is not found to be clearly linked in evidence-based research (De Lusong, Timbol, & Tuazon, 2017).

After the acute phase has subsided, the patient may need nutritional support via enteral or parenteral feedings. The patient may require further treatment to prevent or manage strictures of the esophagus. Dilation by bougienage may be sufficient but may need to be repeated periodically. (In bougienage, cylindrical rubber tubes of different sizes, called bougies, are advanced into the esophagus via the oral cavity. Progressively larger bougies are used to dilate the esophagus. The procedure usually is performed in the endoscopy suite or clinic by the gastroenterologist.) Some strictures require rigid dilators, such as Savary dilators. These dilators are used in the same fashion as bougies but may be more successful for opening difficult strictures. For strictures that do not respond to either method of dilation, surgical management may be necessary. Reconstruction may be accomplished by esophagectomy and colon interposition to replace the portion of esophagus removed. This surgery is quite complex and should be considered only when other options have failed.

Gastroesophageal Reflux Disease

GERD is a fairly common disorder marked by backflow of gastric or duodenal contents into the esophagus that causes troublesome symptoms and/or mucosal injury to the esophagus. Excessive reflux may occur because of an incompetent lower esophageal sphincter, pyloric stenosis, hiatal hernia, or a motility disorder. The incidence of GERD seems to increase with aging and is seen in patients with irritable bowel syndrome and obstructive airway disorders (asthma, COPD, cystic fibrosis) (Robinson & DiMango, 2014), BE (see later discussion), peptic ulcer disease, and angina. GERD is associated with tobacco use, coffee drinking, alcohol consumption, and gastric infection with *Helicobacter pylori*.

Clinical Manifestations

Symptoms may include pyrosis (heartburn, more commonly described as a burning sensation in the esophagus), dyspepsia (indigestion), regurgitation, dysphagia or odynophagia (pain on swallowing), hypersalivation, and esophagitis. The symptoms may mimic those of a heart attack. GERD can result in dental erosion, ulcerations in the pharynx and esophagus, laryngeal damage, esophageal strictures, adenocarcinoma, and pulmonary complications (Hart, 2013).

Assessment and Diagnostic Findings

The patient's history aids in obtaining an accurate diagnosis. Diagnostic testing may include an endoscopy or barium swallow to evaluate damage to the esophageal mucosa (Hart, 2013). Ambulatory 12- to 36-hour esophageal pH monitoring is used to evaluate the degree of acid reflux. Esophageal pH monitoring was historically an uncomfortable procedure, but the advent of wireless capsule pH monitoring is better tolerated and quite accurate (Singhal & Khaitan, 2015).

TABLE 35-2 Pharmacologic Management of GERD

Key Examples	Actions/Class	Key Nursing Considerations
Antacids/Acid neutralizing agents • Calcium carbonate (Tums) • Aluminum hydroxide, magnesium, hydroxide, and simethicone (Maalox)	**Neutralize acid** *Therapeutic and Pharmacologic class*—Antacid	• Potential risk of gastric acid suppression is the loss of protective flora and an increased risk of infection, especially *Clostridium difficile*
Histamine-2 (H_2) receptor antagonists • Famotidine (Pepcid) • Ranitidine (Zantac) • Cimetidine (Tagamet)	**Decrease gastric acid production** *Therapeutic class*—Antiulcer drugs *Pharmacologic class*—H_2-receptor antagonists	• Potential risk of gastric acid suppression is the loss of protective flora and an increased risk of infection, especially *Clostridium difficile* • For direct injection (IVP), dilute 2 mL (20 mg) with compatible solution to a total volume of either 5 or 10 mL; administer over at least 2 minutes • Monitor for QT-interval prolongation in patients with kidney injury
Prokinetic agents Metoclopramide (Reglan)	**Accelerate gastric emptying** *Therapeutic class*—GI stimulants *Pharmacologic class*—Dopamine antagonist	• May cause tardive dyskinesia • Typically used short term
Proton pump inhibitors (PPIs) • Pantoprazole (Protonix) • Omeprazole (Prilosec) • Esomeprazole (Nexium) • Lansoprazole (Prevacid) • Rabeprazole (AcipHex) • Dexlansoprazole (Dexilant)	**Decrease gastric acid production** *Therapeutic class*—Antiulcer drugs *Pharmacologic class*—Proton pump inhibitors	• Potential risk of gastric acid suppression is the loss of protective flora and an increased risk of infection, especially *Clostridium difficile* • For a 2-minute infusion (IVP), give the reconstituted vials (4 mg/mL) over at least 2 minutes • May increase the risk of hip fractures and interfere with some vitamin and mineral absorption (B_{12}, iron, magnesium) • Interact with commonly prescribed medications such as diuretics and clopidogrel
Reflux inhibitors Bethanechol chloride (Urecholine)	**Stimulates parasympathetic** *Therapeutic and Pharmacologic class*—Cholinergic	• Primary use is for urinary retention • Do not use with possible GI obstruction or peptic ulcer
Surface Agents/Alginate-based barriers • Sucralfate	**Preserve mucosal barrier** *Therapeutic class*—Antiulcer drugs *Pharmacologic class*—GI protectants	• Give on an empty stomach hour before or 2 h after meals • Separate from doses of antacid by 30 minutes

Adapted from Frandsen, G., & Pennington, S. S. (2014). *Abrams' clinical drug therapy: Rationales for nursing practice* (10th ed.). Philadelphia, PA: Wolters Kluwer Health/Lippincott Williams & Wilkins; Garg, S. K., & Gurusamy, K. S. (2015). Laparoscopic fundoplication surgery versus medical management for gastro-oesophageal reflux disease (GORD) in adults. *Cochrane Database Systematic Reviews, 11*, CD003243; Hart, A. M. (2013). Evidence-based recommendations for GERD treatment. *The Nurse Practitioner, 38*(8), 26–34.

Management

Management begins with teaching the patient to avoid situations that decrease lower esophageal sphincter pressure or cause esophageal irritation. The patient is instructed to eat a low-fat diet; to avoid caffeine, tobacco, beer, milk, foods containing peppermint or spearmint, and carbonated beverages; to avoid eating or drinking 2 hours before bedtime; to maintain an appropriate body weight; to avoid tight-fitting clothes; to elevate the head of the bed on 15- to 20-cm blocks; and to elevate the upper body on pillows. If reflux persists, antacids or H_2 receptor antagonists, such as famotidine (Pepcid), nizatidine (Axid), or ranitidine (Zantac), may be prescribed. Proton pump inhibitors (medications that decrease the release of gastric acid, such as lansoprazole [Prevacid], rabeprazole [AcipHex], esomeprazole [Nexium], omeprazole [Prilosec], and pantoprazole [Protonix]) may be used; however, these products may increase intragastric bacterial growth and the risk of infection. In addition, the patient may receive prokinetic agents, which accelerate gastric emptying. These agents include bethanechol (Urecholine), domperidone (Motilium), and metoclopramide (Reglan). Because metoclopramide can have extrapyramidal side effects that are increased in certain neuromuscular disorders, such as Parkinson's disease, it should be used only if no other option exists, and the patient should be monitored closely.

If medical management is unsuccessful, surgical intervention may be necessary. Surgical management involves a Nissen fundoplication (wrapping of a portion of the gastric fundus around the sphincter area of the esophagus). A Nissen fundoplication can be performed by the open method or by laparoscopy. See Table 35-2.

Barrett's Esophagus

BE is a condition in which the lining of the esophageal mucosa is altered. It typically occurs in association with GERD; indeed, longstanding untreated GERD may lead to BE. Commonly cited risk factors for Barrett's Esophagus are age over 50 years, male, European descent, obesity, smoking, a family History of BE or esophageal adenocarcinoma (EAC), in addition to a diet low in fruits and vegetables (Domper Arnal, 2015). Reflux eventually causes changes in the cells lining the lower esophagus. The cells that are laid to cover the exposed area are no longer squamous in origin. These precancerous cells initiate the healing process and can be a precursor to EAC.

Clinical Manifestations

The patient reports symptoms of GERD, notably frequent heartburn. The patient may also describe symptoms related to peptic ulcers or esophageal stricture, or both.

Assessment and Diagnostic Findings

An EGD is performed. This usually reveals an esophageal lining that is red rather than pink. Biopsies are performed, and high-grade **dysplasia** (HGD) is evidenced by the squamous mucosa of the esophagus replaced by columnar epithelium that resembles that of the stomach or intestines. HGD has been found to be associated with a 30% risk of development of cancer (Guarner-Argente, Buoncristiano, Furth, et al., 2013).

Management

Monitoring varies depending on the extent of cell changes. Follow-up endoscopy is performed within 6 months if there are minor cell changes. Treatment is individualized for each patient. The options include intensive surveillance with biopsies, endoscopic ablation therapy (e.g., photodynamic therapy), and esophagectomy, each of which has been found to result in similar outcomes (Guarner-Argente et al., 2013).

Benign Tumours of the Esophagus

Benign tumours are rare but can arise anywhere along the esophagus. The most common lesion is a leiomyoma (tumour of the smooth muscle), which can occlude the lumen of the esophagus and cause dysphagia, pain, and pyrosis. Half of patients with benign tumours are asymptomatic and the other half present with multiple symptoms that have been present for a long period of time. The diagnosis may be made incidentally and is confirmed by endoscopy and needle biopsy. Due to the slow growth of most of these tumours, monitoring and minimally invasive techniques (endoscopic, thoracic, or laparoscopic resections) tend to be indicated rather than surgical resection (Ha, Regan, Cetindag, et al., 2015).

Nursing Process

The Patient With a Noncancerous Condition of the Esophagus

Assessment

Emergency conditions of the esophagus (perforation, chemical burns) usually occur in the home or away from medical help and require emergency medical care. The patient is treated for shock and respiratory distress and transported as quickly as possible to a health care facility. Foreign bodies in the esophagus do not pose an immediate threat to life unless pressure is exerted on the trachea, resulting in dyspnea or interfering with respiration, or unless there is leakage of caustic alkali from a battery or exposure to another corrosive agent. Educating the public to prevent inadvertent swallowing of foreign bodies or corrosive agents is a major health goal.

For nonemergency symptoms, a complete health history may reveal the nature of the esophageal disorder. The nurse asks about the patient's appetite. Has it remained the same? Increased? Or decreased? Is there any discomfort with swallowing? If so, does it occur only with certain foods? Is it associated with pain? Does a change in position affect the discomfort? The patient is asked to describe the pain. Does anything aggravate it? Are there any other symptoms that occur regularly, such as regurgitation, nocturnal regurgitation, eructation (belching), heartburn, substernal pressure, a sensation that food is sticking in the throat, a feeling of fullness after eating a small amount of food, nausea, vomiting, or weight loss? Are the symptoms aggravated by emotional upset? If the patient reports any of these symptoms, the nurse asks about when they occur, their relationship to eating, and factors that relieve or aggravate them (e.g., position change, belching, antacids, vomiting) (Bickley, 2016).

This history also includes questions about past or present causative factors, such as infections and chemical, mechanical, or physical irritants; alcohol and tobacco use; and the amount of daily food intake. The nurse determines whether the patient appears emaciated and auscultates the patient's chest to assess for pulmonary complications (Bickley, 2016).

Nursing Priorities

Based on the assessment data, the nursing priorities may include the following:

- Imbalanced nutrition, less than body requirements, related to impaired swallowing
- Risk for aspiration related to impaired swallowing or to tube feeding
- Acute pain related to impaired swallowing, ingestion of an abrasive agent, tumour, or frequent episodes of gastric reflux
- Deficient knowledge about the esophageal disorder, diagnostic studies, medical management, surgical intervention, and rehabilitation

Planning and Goals

The major goals for the patient may include attainment of adequate nutritional intake, avoidance of respiratory compromise from aspiration, relief of pain, and increased knowledge level.

Nursing Interventions

Encouraging Adequate Nutritional Intake

The patient is encouraged to eat slowly and to chew all food thoroughly so that it can pass easily into the stomach. Small, frequent feedings of nonirritating foods are recommended to promote digestion and to prevent tissue irritation. Sometimes liquid swallowed with food helps the food pass through the esophagus, but usually liquids should be consumed between meals. Food should be prepared in an appealing manner to help stimulate the appetite. Irritants such as tobacco and alcohol should be avoided. A baseline weight is obtained, and daily weights are recorded. The patient's intake of nutrients is assessed.

Decreasing Risk of Aspiration

The patient who has difficulty swallowing or difficulty handling secretions should be kept in at least a semi-Fowler's position to decrease the risk of aspiration. The patient is instructed in the use of oral suction to decrease the risk of aspiration further.

Relieving Pain

Small, frequent feedings (six to eight per day) are recommended because large quantities of food overload the stomach and promote gastric reflux. The patient is advised to avoid any activities that increase pain and to remain upright for 1 to 4 hours after each meal to prevent reflux. The head of the bed should be placed on 10- to 20-cm blocks. Eating before bedtime is discouraged.

The patient is advised that excessive use of over-the-counter antacids can cause rebound acidity. Antacid use should be directed by the primary care professional, who can recommend the daily, safe dose needed to neutralize gastric juices and prevent esophageal irritation. H_2 antagonists are administered as prescribed to decrease gastric acid irritation.

Providing Patient Education

The patient is prepared physically and psychologically for diagnostic tests, treatments, and possible surgery. The principal nursing interventions include reassuring the patient and explaining the procedures and their purposes. Some disorders of the esophagus evolve over time, whereas others are the result of trauma (e.g., chemical burns, perforation). In instances of trauma, the emotional and physical preparation for treatment is more difficult because of the short time available and the circumstances of the injury. Treatment interventions must be evaluated continually, and the patient is given sufficient information to participate in care and diagnostic tests. If endoscopic diagnostic methods are used, the patient is instructed regarding the moderate sedation that will be used during the procedure. If outpatient procedures are performed with the use of moderate sedation, someone must be available to drive the patient home after the procedure. If surgery is required, immediate and long-term evaluation is similar to that for a patient undergoing thoracic surgery.

Promoting Home and Community-Based Care

EDUCATING PATIENTS ABOUT SELF-CARE. The self-care required of the patient depends on the nature of the disorder and on the surgery or treatment measures used (e.g., diet, positioning, medications). If an ongoing condition exists, the nurse helps the patient plan for needed physical and psychological adjustments and for follow-up care (Chart 35-4).

Special equipment, such as suction or enteral or parenteral feeding devices, may be required. The patient may need assistance in planning meals, using medications as prescribed, and resuming activities. Education about nutritional requirements and how to measure the adequacy of nutrition is important. Older patients and patients who are debilitated in particular often need assistance and education about ways they can adjust to their limitations and resume activities that are important to them.

CONTINUING AND TRANSITIONAL CARE. Patients with chronic esophageal conditions require an individualized approach to their management at home. Foods may need to be prepared in a special way (blenderized foods, soft foods), and the patient may need to eat more frequently (e.g., six to eight small servings per day). The medication schedule is adjusted to the patient's daily activities as much as possible. Analgesic medications and antacids can usually be taken as needed every 3 to 4 hours.

Postoperative home care focuses on nutritional support, management of pain, and respiratory function. Some patients are discharged from the hospital with enteral feeding by means of a gastrostomy or jejunostomy tube or parenteral nutrition. The patient and caregiver need specific instructions regarding management of the equipment and treatments. Home care visits by a nurse may be necessary to assess the patient and the caregiver's ability to provide the necessary care. (See Chapter 37 for more information about parenteral nutrition and management of the patient with a gastrostomy.) For some patients, a multidisciplinary team that includes a dietitian, a social worker, and family members is helpful. Hospice care and consideration of end-of-life issues are appropriate for some patients.

Evaluation

Expected patient outcomes may include:

1. Achieves an adequate nutritional intake
   a. Eats small, frequent meals
   b. Drinks small sips of water with small servings of food
   c. Avoids irritants (alcohol, tobacco, very hot beverages)
   d. Maintains desired weight
2. Does not aspirate or develop pneumonia
   a. Maintains upright position during feeding
   b. Uses oral suction equipment effectively

CHART 35-4

HOME CARE CHECKLIST • The Patient With an Esophageal Disorder

At the completion of education, the patient and/or caregiver will be able to:

- State the impact of the esophageal disorder and treatment on physiologic functioning, ADLs, IADLs, body image, roles, relationships, and spirituality.
- Identify modification of home environment, interventions, and strategies (e.g., durable medical equipment, home health aide) used in safely adapting to changes in structure or function and promote effective recovery and rehabilitation.
- Describe ongoing therapeutic regimen, including diet and activities to perform (e.g., suctioning) and to limit or avoid (e.g., oral foods if NPO).
    - Identify foods or therapies necessary to meet caloric needs and dietary needs (e.g., change in consistency, seasoning limitations, supplements, enteral or parenteral therapy).
    - Participate in prescribed therapy (e.g., speech therapy) to promote recovery and rehabilitation.
    - Demonstrate the use of suction equipment if indicated.
    - Demonstrate care of incision if indicated.
- State the name, dose, side effects, frequency, and schedule for all medications.
    - Describe approaches to controlling pain (e.g., take analgesics as prescribed; use nonpharmacologic interventions).
- Identify possible complications (e.g., difficulty swallowing, pain, respiratory distress) and interventions.
- Relate how to reach primary provider with questions or complications.
- State time and date of follow-up medical appointments, therapy, and testing.
- Identify sources of support (e.g., friends, relatives, faith community, cancer support, caregiver support).
- Identify the need for health promotion, disease prevention, and screening activities.

ADL, activities of daily living; IADL, independent activities of daily living; NPO, nothing by mouth.

3. Is free of pain or able to control pain within a tolerable level
    a. Avoids large meals and irritating foods
    b. Takes medications as prescribed and with adequate fluids (at least 4 oz), and remains upright for at least 10 minutes after taking medications
    c. Maintains an upright position after meals for 1 to 4 hours
    d. Reports that there is less eructation and chest pain
4. Increases knowledge level of esophageal condition, treatment, and prognosis
    a. States cause of condition
    b. Discusses rationale for medical or surgical management and diet or medication regimen
    c. Describes treatment program
    d. Practices preventive measures so injuries are avoided

Cancer of the Esophagus

The incidence of EACs in Canada has doubled in the past 20 years, while a decline has been observed for esophageal squamous cell carcinoma (SCC) (Otterstatter, Brierley, De, et al., 2012). Given the geographic distribution of subtypes and increasing incidence of EAC in Canada, esophageal cancer has a lower incidence than other cancers, but a high mortality rate. Esophageal cancer is the 13th most common cancer in men and 19th most common in women, but the 6th and 14th most common cause of cancer deaths, respectively (CCSACCS, 2015). In 2015, there were an estimated 2,200 cases of esophageal cancer newly diagnosed in Canada, and 2,100 deaths from the disease (CCSACCS, 2015). Between 1986 and 2006, the incidence of EAC in Canada increased from 1.8 to 3.5 per 100,000 in men, and 0.2 to 0.5 per 100,000 in women; the incidence of EAC is projected to increase by 40% in men and 50% in women by 2026 (Otterstatter et al., 2012).

Pathophysiology

Esophageal cancer can be of two cell types: adenocarcinoma and squamous cell carcinoma. The rate of adenocarcinoma is rapidly increasing in the United States as well as in other Western countries. It is found primarily in the distal esophagus and gastroesophageal junction (CCSACCS, 2015).

Risk factors for esophageal cancer include chronic esophageal irritation. In Canada, cancer of the esophagus has been associated with ingestion of alcohol and the use of tobacco. There is an apparent association between GERD and adenocarcinoma of the esophagus. People with BE (which is caused by chronic irritation of the mucous membranes due to reflux of gastric and duodenal contents) have a higher incidence of esophageal cancer

(CCSACCS, 2015). Risk factors for squamous cell carcinoma of the esophagus include chronic ingestion of hot liquids or foods, nutritional deficiencies, poor oral hygiene, exposure to nitrosamines in the environment or food, cigarette smoking or chronic alcohol exposure, and some esophageal medical conditions such as caustic injury.

Tumour cells of adenocarcinoma and of squamous cell carcinoma may spread beneath the esophageal mucosa or directly into, through, and beyond the muscle layers into the lymphatics. In the latter stages, obstruction of the esophagus is noted, with possible perforation into the mediastinum and erosion into the great vessels.

Clinical Manifestations

Many patients have an advanced ulcerated lesion of the esophagus before symptoms are manifested. Symptoms include dysphagia, initially with solid foods and eventually with liquids; a sensation of a mass in the throat; painful swallowing; substernal pain or fullness; and, later, regurgitation of undigested food with foul breath and hiccups. The patient first becomes aware of intermittent and increasing difficulty in swallowing. As the tumour grows and the obstruction becomes nearly complete, even liquids cannot pass into the stomach. Regurgitation of food and saliva occurs, hemorrhage may take place, and progressive loss of weight and strength occurs from inadequate nutrition. Later symptoms include substernal pain, persistent hiccups, respiratory difficulty, and foul breath.

The delay between the onset of early symptoms and the patient seeking medical advice is often 12 to 18 months. Any person having swallowing difficulties should be encouraged to consult a physician immediately.

Assessment and Diagnostic Findings

Currently, diagnosis is confirmed most often by EGD with biopsy and brushings (95% to 100% sensitivity), although the double-contrast esophagography also has a sensitivity of more than 95% (Levine & Rubesin, 2012). The biopsy can be used to determine the presence of disease and cell differentiation. At presentation, most patients have moderately differentiated tumours.

Several imaging techniques may provide useful diagnostic information. CT of the chest and abdomen is beneficial for detecting any metastatic disease, especially of the lungs, liver, and kidney. Positron emission tomography (PET) may help detect metastasis with more sensitivity than CT. Endoscopic ultrasound is used to determine whether the cancer has spread to the lymph nodes and other mediastinal structures; it can also determine the size and invasiveness of the tumour. Exploratory laparoscopy is the best method for finding positive lymph nodes in patients with distal lesions.

Future diagnostic techniques that may serve as predictors for dysplastic progression in patients with BE involve molecular markers. The usefulness of molecular markers in treating esophageal cancer is being researched. Research also includes the development of medications that target the pathways of various molecular markers (Paterson, Shannon, Lao-Sirieix, et al., 2013).

Medical Management

If esophageal cancer is detected at an early stage, treatment goals may be directed toward cure; however, it is often detected in late stages, making relief of symptoms the only reasonable goal of therapy. Treatment may include surgery, radiation, chemotherapy, or a combination of these modalities, depending on the type of cancer cell, the extent of the disease, and the patient's condition. A standard treatment plan for a person who is newly diagnosed with esophageal cancer includes the following: preoperative combination chemotherapy and radiation therapy for 4 to 6 weeks; followed by a period of no medical intervention for 4 weeks; and, finally, surgical resection of the esophagus (NCI, 2014).

Standard surgical management includes a total resection of the esophagus (esophagectomy) with removal of the tumour plus a wide tumour-free margin of the esophagus and the lymph nodes in the area. The surgical approach may be through the thorax or the abdomen, depending on the location of the tumour. When tumours occur in the cervical or upper thoracic area, esophageal continuity may be maintained by a free jejunal graft transfer, in which the tumour is removed and the area is replaced with a portion of the jejunum (Fig. 35-8). A segment of the colon may be used, or the stomach can be elevated into the chest and the proximal section of the esophagus anastomosed to the stomach (Kitagawa, Namikawa, Iwabu, et al., 2018).

Tumours of the lower thoracic esophagus are more amenable to surgery than are tumours located higher in the esophagus. Gastrointestinal tract integrity is maintained by anastomosing the lower esophagus to the stomach (Fig. 35-9).

Surgical resection of the esophagus has a relatively high mortality rate because of infection, pulmonary complications, or leakage through the anastomosis. Postoperatively, the patient has a nasogastric tube in place that should not be manipulated. The patient is given NPO until x-ray studies confirm that the anastomosis is free from an

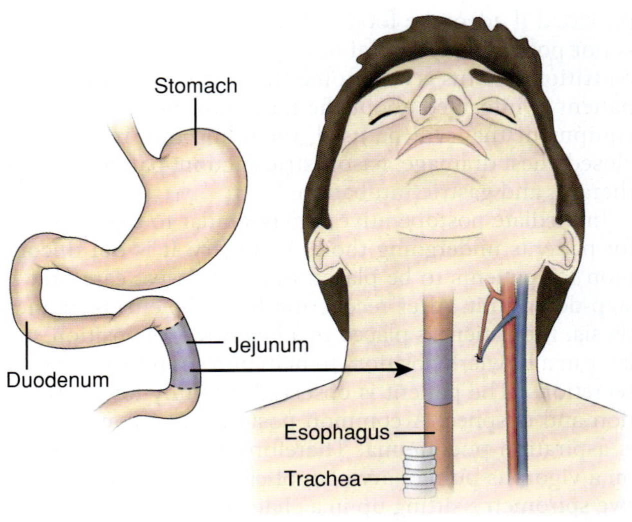

FIGURE 35-8. Esophageal reconstruction with free jejunal transfer. A portion of the jejunum is grafted between the esophagus and pharynx to replace the abnormal portion of the esophagus. The vascular structures are also anastomosed.

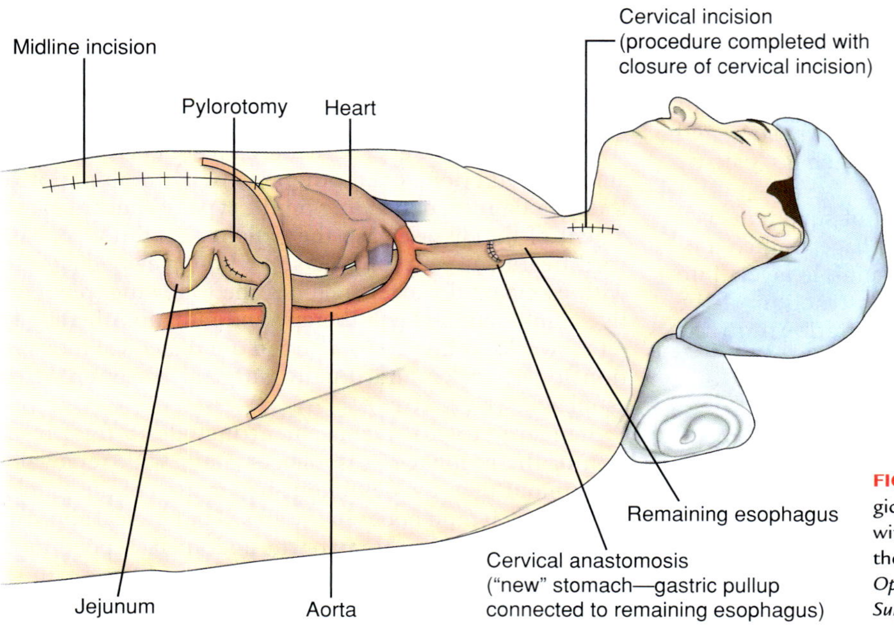

FIGURE 35-9. Transhiatal esophagectomy: surgical removal of tumour of the lower esophagus with anastomosis of the remaining esophagus to the stomach. (Redrawn with permission from *Operative Techniques in Thoracic and Cardiovascular Surgery, 4*(3), 263 © 1999 Elsevier Inc.)

esophageal leak, there is no obstruction, and there is no evidence of pulmonary aspiration.

Palliative treatment may be necessary to keep the esophagus open, to assist with nutrition, and to control saliva. Palliation may be accomplished with dilation of the esophagus, laser therapy, placement of an endoprosthesis (stent) via EGD, radiation, or chemotherapy.

Nursing Management

Preoperative nursing management is directed toward improving the patient's nutritional and physical status in preparation for surgery, radiation therapy, or chemotherapy. A program to promote weight gain based on a high-calorie and high-protein diet, in liquid or soft form, is provided if adequate food can be taken by mouth. If this is not possible, parenteral or enteral nutrition is initiated. Nutritional status is monitored throughout treatment. The patient is informed about the nature of the postoperative equipment that will be used, including that required for closed chest drainage, nasogastric suction, parenteral fluid therapy, and gastric intubation.

Immediate postoperative care is similar to that provided for patients undergoing thoracic surgery. It is not uncommon for patients to be placed in an intensive care unit or step-down unit. After recovering from the effects of anesthesia, the patient is placed in a low Fowler's position, and later in a Fowler's position, to help prevent reflux of gastric secretions. The patient is observed carefully for regurgitation and dyspnea. A common postoperative complication is aspiration pneumonia. Therefore, the patient is placed on a vigorous pulmonary plan of care that includes incentive spirometry, sitting up in a chair, and, if necessary, nebulizer treatments. Chest physiotherapy is avoided due to the risk of aspiration. The patient's temperature is monitored to detect any elevation that may indicate aspiration or seepage of fluid through the operative site into the mediastinum, which would indicate an esophageal leak. Drainage from the cervical neck wound, usually saliva, is evidence of an early esophageal leak. Typically, no treatment other than NPO and parenteral or enteral support is warranted.

Cardiac complications include atrial fibrillation, which occurs due to irritation of the vagus nerve at the time of surgery. Typical medical management includes digitalization or use of beta blockers, depending on the patient's response. Rarely, cardioversion may be used.

During surgery, a nasogastric tube is inserted and taped in place. It is connected to low intermittent suction. The nasogastric tube is not manipulated; if displacement occurs, it is not replaced, because damage to the anastomosis may occur. The nasogastric tube is removed 5 to 7 days after surgery; before the patient is allowed to eat, a barium swallow is performed to assess for any anastomotic leak.

Once feeding begins, the nurse encourages the patient to swallow small sips of water. Eventually, the diet is advanced as tolerated to a soft, mechanical diet. When the patient can increase his or her food and fluid intake to an adequate amount, parenteral fluids are discontinued. After each meal, the patient remains upright for at least 2 hours to allow the food to move through the gastrointestinal tract. It is a challenge to encourage the patient to eat because the appetite is usually poor. Family involvement and home-cooked favourite foods may help the patient to eat. Antacids may help patients with gastric distress. Metoclopramide is useful in promoting gastric motility.

If chemotherapy and radiation are part of the therapy, the patient's appetite will be further depressed, and esophagitis may occur, causing pain when food is eaten. Liquid supplements may be more easily tolerated. However, supplements such as Boost and Ensure (although no sugar supplements such as Glucerna are recommended) should be avoided because they promote **vagotomy syndrome** (dumping syndrome), which can occur with each meal or approximately 20 minutes to 2 hours after eating. The vagotomy syndrome occurs due to interruption of vagal nerve fibres, which in turn causes an alteration in the storage function of the stomach and the pyloric emptying mechanism. As a result, large amounts of solids and liquids rapidly "dump" into the duodenum. The patient experiences severe abdominal cramping, followed by a liquid bowel movement that may or may not be associated with diaphoresis, rapid heart rate or rapid respirations, or both. It can be quite disabling but typically resolves without incident, and the patient is left feeling extremely tired. The vagotomy syndrome is common following esophageal surgery, but as the patient's recovery progresses and the patient begins to eat soft foods and remains in an upright position for 2 hours after eating, the frequency and severity of episodes decrease.

Often, in either the preoperative or the postoperative period, an obstructed or nearly obstructed esophagus causes difficulty with excess saliva, and drooling becomes a problem. Oral suction may be used if the patient cannot handle oral secretions, or wick-type gauze may be placed at the corner of the mouth to direct secretions to a dressing or emesis basin. The possibility that the patient may aspirate saliva into the tracheobronchial tree and develop pneumonia is of significant concern.

When the patient is ready to go home, the family is instructed about how to promote nutrition, what observations to make, what measures to take if complications occur, how to keep the patient comfortable, and how to obtain needed physical and emotional support.

Critical Thinking Exercises

1 ebp A 52-year-old female patient presents to a primary care clinic with a mostly painless, but sometimes sore, hardened white patch in her oral cavity. What questions should the nurse ask her? What are the primary risk factors for oral cancer? If she is diagnosed with oral cancer, what treatment protocol would likely be recommended?

2 pq You are a nurse working on an inpatient oncology unit and have been assigned a postoperative patient who has had a modified radical neck resection due to cancer. What are the primary differences between a radical, modified, and selective neck dissection? You learn that the patient's internal jugular vein is intact, but that the sternocleidomastoid muscle and the spinal accessory nerve have both been impacted by the surgery. Based on this information, what are the key priority nursing interventions that will prevent long-term complications in this patient?

3 A patient diagnosed with esophageal cancer undergoes the standard treatment of chemoradiation prior to an esophagostomy. After the esophagostomy, the patient receives enteral nutrition through an NG tube. Although several days have passed, the patient remains disengaged from the staff and his family, making little eye contact, admitting to extreme pain only when asked, and refusing to engage in postoperative care. What are your two major nursing diagnoses for this patient? Identify three expected outcomes and interventions that address each of these diagnoses.

REFERENCES AND SELECTED READINGS

Books

American Cancer Society (ACS). (2015). *Cancer facts and figures*. Atlanta, GA: Author.

Bickley, L. S. (2016). *Bates' guide to physical examination and history taking* (12th ed.). Philadelphia, PA: Wolters Kluwer Health/Lippincott Williams & Wilkins.

Canadian Academy of Health Sciences. (2014). *Improving access to oral health care: For vulnerable people living in Canada*. Ottawa, Ontario: Canadian Academy of Health Sciences.

Canadian Cancer Society's Advisory Committee on Cancer Statistics (CCSACCS). (2015). *Canadian Cancer Statistics 2015*. Toronto, ON. Canadian Cancer Society.

Canadian Cancer Society's Advisory Committee on Cancer Statistics (CCSACCS). (2017). *Canadian Cancer Statistics 2013*. Toronto, ON: Canadian Cancer Society.

Carr, E. (2016). Head and neck cancers. In J. K. Itano (Ed.). *Core curriculum for oncology nursing* (5th ed.). St. Louis, MO: Elsevier Inc.

Haggerty, C. J. (2015). Mandibular fractures. In C. J. Haggerty, & R. M. Laughlin (Eds.). *Atlas of operative oral and maxillofacial surgery*. Ames, Iowa: John Wiley & Sons, Inc.

Levine, M., & Rubesin, S. (2012). Radiology of the pharynx and esophagus. In D. O. Castell, & J. E. Richter (Eds.). *The esophagus* (5th ed.). Philadelphia, PA: Lippincott Williams & Wilkins.

Watson, T. J., & Peyre, C. G. (2019). Etiology and Management of Esophageal Perforation. In C. J. Yeo (Ed.). *Shackelford's Surgery of the Alimentary Tract* (8th ed.). 2 Volume Set (pp. 526–535). Elsevier Inc.

Journals and Electronic Documents

Almeida, L. Y., Fernandes, D., Ortega, M., et al. (2017). Nodular swelling of the buccal mucosa. *Oral Surgery, Oral Medicine, Oral Pathology and Oral Radiology*, *123*, 150–156.

Belli, E., Liberatore, G., Elidon, M., et al. (2015). Surgical evolution in the treatment of mandibular condyle fractures. *BMC Surgery*, *15*(16), 1–6.

Boonekamp, C., Voruz, F., & Fehlmann, C. (2018). Case Report: Accidental aspiration of a solid tablet of sodium hypochlorite. *BMJ Case Reports*, *2018*.

Bossola, M. (2015). Nutritional interventions in head and neck cancer patients undergoing chemoradiotherapy: A narrative review. *Nutrients*, *7*(1), 265–276.

Byard, R. (2015). Caustic ingestion: A forensic overview. *Journal of Forensic Sciences*, *60*(3), 812–815.

Cakal, B., Akbal, E., Köklü, S., et al. (2013). Acute therapy with intravenous omeprazole on caustic esophageal injury: A prospective case series. *Diseases of the Esophagus*, *26*(1), 22–26.

Chestnutt, I., Hutchings, S., Playle, R., et al. (2017). Seal or Varnish? A randomised controlled trial to determine the relative cost and effectiveness of pit and fissure sealant and fluoride varnish in preventing dental decay. *Health Technology Assessment*, *21*(21), 1–256.

De Lusong, M., Timbol, A., & Tuazon, D. (2017). Management of esophageal caustic injury. *World Journal of Gastrointestinal Pharmacology and Therapeutics*, *8*(2), 90–98.

Domper Arnal M., Fernandez Arenas, A., & Lanas Arbeloa, A. (2015). Esophageal cancer: Risk factors, screening and endoscopic treatment in Western and Eastern countries. *World Journal of Gastroenterology: WJG*, *21*(26), 7933.

Dutta, S. R., Passi, D., Singh, M., et al. (2016). Botulinum toxin the poison that heals: A brief review. *National Journal of Maxillofacial Surgery*, *7*(1), 10–16.

Fang, S. L., Zhang, D. M., Chen, W. L., et al. (2016). Reconstruction of full-thickness cheek defects with a folded extended supraclavicular fasciocutaneous island flap following ablation of advanced oral cancer. *Journal of Cancer Research and Therapeutics*, *12*(2), 888–891.

Foulkes, M. (2013). Oral cancer: Risk factors, treatment and nursing care. *Nursing Standard*, *28*(8), 49–57.

Fronczek, A. (2015). A phenomenological study of family caregivers of patients with head and neck cancers. *Oncology Nursing Forum*, *42*(6), 593–600.

Gauer, R., & Semidey, M. (2015). Diagnosis and treatment of temporomandibular disorders. *American Family Physician*, *91*(6), 378–386.

Gil-Martínez, A., Grande-Alonso, M., López-de-Uralde-Villanueva, I., et al. (2016). Chronic temporomandibular disorders: Disability, pain intensity and fear of movement. *The Journal of Headache and Pain*, *17*(1), 103.

Government of Canada. (2018). *Public Health Agency of Canada: Community Water Fluoridation in Canada, 2017*. Retrieved from: https://www.canada.ca/en/public-health/services/fluoride-water-map-canada.html

Grègoire, V., Ang, K., Budach, W., et al. (2014). Delineation of the neck node levels for head and neck tumors: A 2013 update. DAHANCA, EORTC, HKNPCSG, NCIC CTG, NCRI, RTOG, TROG consensus guidelines. *Radiotherapy and Oncology*, *110*(1), 172–181.

Guarner-Argente, C., Buoncristiano, T., Furth, E., et al. (2013). Long-term outcomes of patients with Barrett's esophagus and high-grade dysplasia or early cancer treated with endoluminal therapies with intention to complete eradication. *Gastrointestinal Endoscopy*, *77*(2), 190–199.

Ha, C., Regan, J., Cetindag, I., et al. (2015). Benign esophageal tumors. *Surgical Clinics of North America*, *95*(3), 491–514.

Hart, A. (2013). Evidence-based recommendations for GERD treatment. *The Nurse Practitioner*, *38*(8), 26–34.

Hoven, A. (2014). Magic mouthwash explained. *Family Practice Oncology Network Journal, Fall*. Retrieved from: http://www.bccancer.bc.ca/managing-symptoms-site/Documents/magic%20mouthwash%20excerpt%20from%202014%20Fall%20FPON%20journal.pdf

Khan, M., Kumbhari, V., Ngamruengphong, S., et al. (2017). Is POEM the answer for management of spastic esophageal disorders? A systematic review and meta-analysis. *Digestive Diseases and Sciences*, *62*(1), 35–44.

Kitagawa, H., Namikawa, T., Iwabu, J., et al. (2018). Outcomes of abdominal esophageal cancer patients who were treated with esophagectomy. *Molecular and Clinical Oncology*, *8*(2), 286–291.

Kohn, G. P., Price, R. R., DeMeester, S. R., et al. (2013). Guidelines for the management of hiatal hernia. *Surgical Endoscopy*, *27*(12), 4409–4428.

Lalla, R., Bowen, J., Barasch, A., et al. (2014). MASCC/ISOO clinical practice guidelines for the management of mucositis secondary to cancer therapy. *Cancer*, *120*(10), 1453–1461.

Lin, D., Yarlagadda, B., Sethi, R., et al. (2015). Long-term functional outcomes of total glossectomy with or without total laryngectomy. *JAMA Otolaryngol Head & Neck Surgery*, *141*(9), 797–803.

Lufrano, R., Heckman, M., Diehl, N., et al. (2015). Nutcracker esophagus: Demographic, clinical features, and esophageal tests in 115 patients. *Diseases of the Esophagus*, *28*(1), 11–18.

Miranda-Rius, J., Brunet-Llobet, L., Lahor-Soler, E., et al. (2015). Salivary secretory disorders, inducing drugs, and clinical management. *International Journal of Medical Sciences*, *12*(10), 811–824.

National Cancer Institute (NCI). (2014). A snapshot of esophageal cancer. Retrieved from: www.cancer.gov/research/progress/snapshots/esophageal

National Institute of Dental and Craniofacial Research (NIDCR). (2013b). *TMJ (temporomandibular joint and muscle disorders)*. Retrieved from: www.nidcr.nih.gov/oralhealth/Topics/TMJ/TMJDisorders.htm

Oleynikov, D., & Jolley, J. (2015). Paraesophageal hernia. *Surgical Clinics of North America*, *95*(3), 555–565.

Otterstatter, M., Brierley, J., De, P., et al. (2012). Esophageal cancer in Canada: Trends according to morphology and anatomical location. *Canadian Journal of Gastroenterology and Hepatology*, *26*(10), 723–727.

Pandolfino, J., & Gawron, A. (2015). Achalasia: A systematic review. *Journal of the American Medical Association*, *313*(18), 1841–1852.

Papapanou, P. (2015). Systemic effects of periodontitis: Lessons learned from research on atherosclerotic vascular disease and adverse pregnancy outcomes. *International Dental Journal*, *65*(6), 283–291.

Paterson, A., Shannon, N., Lao-Sirieix, P., et al. (2013). A systematic approach to therapeutic target selection in oesophago-gastric cancer. *Gut*, *62*(10), 1415–1424.

Quinn, B., Baker, D., Cohen, S., et al. (2014). Basic nursing care to prevent nonventilator hospital-acquired pneumonia. *Journal of Nursing Scholarship*, *46*(1), 11–19.

Reid, K., & Greene, C. (2013). Diagnosis and treatment of temporomandibular disorders: An ethical analysis of current practices. *Journal of Oral Rehabilitation*, *40*, 546–561.

Rihani, J., Lee, M., Lee, T., et al. (2013). Flap selection and functional outcomes in total glossectomy with laryngeal preservation. *Otolaryngology Head and Neck Surgery*, *149*(4), 547–553.

Robertson, D., Keys, W., Rautemaa-Richardon, R., et al. (2015). Management of severe acute dental infections. *British Medical Journal*, *350*, h1300.

Robinson, N., & DiMango, E. (2014). Prevalence of gastroesophageal reflux in cystic fibrosis and implications for lung disease. *Annals of the American Thoracic Society*, *11*(6), 964–968.

Sigismund, P., Zenk, J., Koch, M., et al. (2015). Nearly 3,000 salivary stones: Some clinical and epidemiologic aspects. *The Laryngoscope*, *125*(8), 1879–1882.

Schiffman, E., Ohrbach, R., Truelove, E., et al. (2014). Diagnostic criteria for temporomandibular disorders (DC/TMD) for clinical and research applications: recommendations of the International RDC/TMD Consortium Network and Orofacial Pain Special Interest Group. *Journal of Oral & Facial Pain and Headache*, *28*(1), 6.

Singhal, V., & Khaitan, L. (2015). Preoperative evaluation of gastroesophageal reflux disease. *Surgical Clinics of North America*, *95*(3), 615–627.

Smith, C. (2015). Esophageal strictures and diverticula. *Surgical Clinics of North America*, *95*(3), 669–681.

Sobin, L., Kopp, R., Walsh, R., et al. (2016). Incidence of concussion in patients with isolated mandible fractures. *JAMA Facial Plastic Surgery*, *18*(1), 15–18.

Son, E., Panwar, A., Mosher, C., et al. (2018). Cancers of the major salivary gland. *Journal of Oncology Practice*, *14*(2), 99–109.

Steinau, M., Saraiya, M., Goodman, M., et al. (2014). Human papillomavirus prevalence in oropharyngeal cancer before vaccine introduction, United States. *Emerging Infectious Diseases*, *20*(5), 822–828.

Swanson, M., Hudson, R., Bhandari, N., et al. (2015). Use of octreotide for the management of chyle fistula following neck dissection. *JAMA Otolaryngology Head & Neck Surgery*, *141*(8), 723–727.

van den Bergh, B., de Mol van Otterloo, J. J., van der Ploeg, T., et al. (2015). IMF-screws or arch bars as conservative treatment for mandibular condyle fractures: Quality of life aspects. *Journal of Cranio-Maxillo-Facial Surgery*, *43*(7), 1004–1009.

Villa, A., Nordio, F., & Gohel, A. (2015). A risk prediction model for xerostomia: A retrospective cohort study. *Gerodontology*, *33*(4), 562–568.

Weijenborg, P., van Hoeij, F., Smout, A., et al. (2015). Accuracy of hiatal hernia detection with esophageal high-resolution manometry. *Neurogastroenterology & Motility*, *27*(2), 293–299.

Weno, K. (2015). *Statement on the evidence supporting the safety and effectiveness of community water fluoridation*. Atlanta, GA: Centers for Disease Control and Prevention. Retrieved from: www.cdc.gov/fluoridation/pdf/statement-cwf-6-8-2015.pdf

World Health Organization (WHO). (2015). *Strategies for oral disease prevention and health promotion*. Retrieved from: www.who.int/oral_health/strategies/en/

Yuan, Y., Zhao, Y., Hu, Y., et al. (2013). Surgical treatment of Zenker's diverticulum. *Digestive Surgery*, *30*(3), 207–218.

Resources

Canadian Cancer Society: http://cancer.ca

Canadian Dental Association: http://www.cd-adc.ca

Canadian Dental Association: https://www.cda-adc.ca/en/oral_health/talk/complications/temporomandibular_disorder/

Government of Canada: https://www.canada.ca/en/services/health/publications/healthy-living/community-water-fluoridation-across-canada-2017.html

Tessier: https://emedicine.medscape.com/article/190025-overview

36 Gastrointestinal Intubation and Special Nutritional Modalities

Adapted by Pamela Cawley

Learning Objectives

On completion of this chapter, the learner will be able to:

1. Describe the purposes and types of gastrointestinal intubation.
2. Discuss nursing management of the patient who has a nasogastric or nasoenteric tube.
3. Use the nursing process as a framework for care of the patient receiving an enteral feeding.
4. Explain the preoperative and postoperative care of the patient with a gastrostomy.
5. Use the nursing process as a framework for care of the patient with a gastrostomy.
6. Identify the purposes and uses of parenteral nutrition.
7. Use the nursing process as a framework for care of the patient receiving parenteral nutrition.
8. Describe the nursing measures used to prevent complications from parenteral nutrition.

Nurses encounter patients using digestive and gastrointestinal (GI) treatment modalities across many practice settings. This chapter presents several topics related to GI intubation. Nursing management topics relate to managing the care of patients with **nasogastric (NG) tubes**, nasoenteric tubes, and gastrostomies; providing tube feedings; and teaching points concerning home health care and nutritional therapy. In addition, **parenteral nutrition (PN)** is presented, including general indications for this nutritional modality and nursing care of patients receiving these support measures.

Gastrointestinal Intubation

GI intubation is the insertion of a flexible tube into the stomach beyond the pylorus into the duodenum (the first section of the small intestine) or the jejunum (the second section of the small intestine). The tube may be inserted through the mouth, the nose, or the abdominal wall. The tubes are of various lengths, depending on their intended use. GI intubation may be performed to:

- Decompress the stomach and remove gas and fluid
- Lavage the stomach and remove ingested toxins
- Diagnose disorders of GI motility and other disorders
- Administer medications and feedings
- Treat an obstruction
- Compress a bleeding site
- Aspirate gastric contents for analysis

A variety of tubes are used for **decompression**, aspiration, and lavage. Orogastric tubes are large-bore tubes with wide proximal outlets for removal of gastric contents; they are primarily used in emergency departments or in intensive care settings (see Chapter 35). The Sengstaken–Blakemore tube is a type of NG tube used to treat bleeding esophageal varices (see Chapter 39). Various other tubes are used to administer feedings and medications. The tubes are made of various materials (rubber, polyurethane, silicone); polyurethane catheters are more resistant to deterioration. They also vary in length (90 cm to 3 m), in size (6 to 18 French [Fr]), in purpose, and in placement in the GI tract (stomach, duodenum, jejunum) (Table 36-1). Any solution administered through a tube is poured through a syringe or delivered by a drip mechanism by gravity or regulated by an electric pump. **Aspiration** (suctioning) to remove gas and fluids is accomplished with the use of a syringe, an electric suction machine, or a wall suction outlet.

TABLE 36-1 Selected Gastric and Enteric Tubes

Tube Type	Length (cm)	Size (French)	Lumen	Other Characteristics
Gastric Tubes				
Levin (plastic or rubber)	125	14–18	Single	Circular markings at intervals along the tube serve as guidelines for insertion
Salem Sump (plastic)	120	12–18	Double	Smaller lumen acts as a vent
Moss	90	12–16	Triple	Contains both a gastric decompression lumen and a duodenal lumen for postoperative feedings
Sengstaken–Blakemore (rubber)			Triple	Two lumens are used to inflate the gastric and esophageal balloons, and one tube is reserved for suction or drainage
Enteric Feeding Tube				
Dobhoff or EnteraFlo (polyurethane or silicone rubber)	160–175	8–12	Single	Tungsten-weighted tip, radiopaque, stylet

Gastric Tubes

Gastric Tubes for Decompression, Drainage, Aspiration, and Lavage

A variety of tubes are used for decompression, drainage, aspiration (removal of substances by suction), and **lavage** of the stomach. Gastric tubes may also be labelled by their point of origin and end points. For instance, an orogastric tube is a large-bore tube inserted through the mouth into the stomach that contains a wide outlet for removal of gastric contents. Gastric tubes, commonly called **NG tubes**, are introduced through the nose into the stomach, often before or during surgery or at the bedside, to remove fluid and gas from the upper GI tract by the process known as decompression (gastric/intestinal). Other tubes, such as the Sengstaken–Blakemore and the Minnesota tube, are used to treat bleeding esophageal varices. Commonly used gastric tubes include the Levin and the Salem Sump tube.

Glossary

antireflux valve: valve that prevents return or backward flow of fluid

aspiration: removal of substance by suction; breathing of fluids or foods into the trachea and lungs

bolus: a feeding administered into the stomach in large amounts and at designated intervals

central venous access device (CVAD): a device designed and used for long-term administration of medications and fluids into central veins

cyclic feeding: periodic feeding/infusion given over a short period (8 to 12 hours)

decompression (intestinal): removal of intestinal contents to prevent gas and fluid from distending the coils of the intestine

dumping syndrome: rapid emptying of the stomach contents into the small intestine; characterized by sweating and weakness

duodenum: first part of the small intestine, which connects with the pylorus of the stomach and extends to the jejunum

gastrostomy: surgical creation of an opening into the stomach for the purpose of administering foods and fluids

intravenous fat emulsion (IVFE, intralipids): an oil-in-water emulsion of oils, egg phospholipids, and glycerin

jejunum: second portion of the small intestine, extending from the duodenum to the ileum

lavage: flushing of the stomach via the gastric tube with water or other fluids to clear it

low-profile gastrostomy device (LPGD, G-button): an enteral feeding access device that is flush with the skin and is used for long-term feeding

nasoduodenal tube: tube inserted through the nose into the beginning of the small intestine (duodenum)

nasogastric (NG) tube: tube inserted through the nose into the stomach

nasojejunal tube: tube inserted through the nose into the second portion of the small intestine (jejunum)

osmolality: ionic concentration of fluid

osmosis: passage of solvent through a semi-permeable membrane; the solvent, usually water, passes through the membrane from a region of low concentration of solute to that of a higher concentration of solute

parenteral nutrition (PN): method of supplying nutrients to the body by an intravenous route

percutaneous endoscopic gastrostomy (PEG): an endoscopic procedure for inserting a feeding tube into the stomach in order to provide long-term nutritional support

peripherally inserted central catheter (PICC): a device used for intermediate-term intravenous therapy

peristalsis: wave-like movement that occurs involuntarily in the alimentary canal

pH: the degree of acidity or alkalinity of a substance or solution

stoma: artificially created opening between a body cavity (e.g., intestine) and the body surface

total nutrient admixture (TNA): an admixture of lipid emulsions, proteins, carbohydrates, electrolytes, vitamins, trace minerals, and water

Levin Tube

The Levin tube has a single lumen (the hollow part of the tube), ranges from 14 to 18 Fr in size, and is made of plastic or rubber with openings near its tip. It is 125 cm long. Circular markings at specific points on the tube serve as guides for insertion. A marking is made on the tube to indicate the midpoint. The tube is advanced cautiously until this marking reaches the patient's nostril, suggesting that the tube is in the stomach. Placement is checked by observing the characteristics of the aspirate and by testing the **pH** (which varies according to the source of the aspirate). Visualizing the tube's placement on x-ray is the only definitive way to verify its location. The Levin tube is connected to low intermittent suction (30 to 40 mm Hg). Intermittent suction is used to avoid erosion or tearing of the stomach lining, which can result from constant adherence of the tube's lumen to the mucosal lining of the stomach.

Gastric Sump (Salem Sump)

The gastric sump (Salem) tube is a radiopaque (easily seen on x-ray), clear plastic, double-lumen NG tube used to decompress the stomach and keep it empty. It is 120 cm long and is passed into the stomach in the same way as the Levin tube. The inner, smaller tube vents the larger suction-drainage tube to the atmosphere by means of an opening at the distal end of the tube. The sump tube can protect gastric suture lines because when used properly, it maintains the force of suction at the drainage openings, or outlets, at less than 25 mm Hg, which is the level of capillary fragility. The small vent tube (known as the blue pigtail or port) controls this action. Gastric sump tubes are connected to low continuous suction. The suction lumen is irrigated as prescribed to maintain patency.

To prevent reflux of gastric contents through the vent lumen (blue pigtail), the vent lumen is kept above the patient's waist; otherwise, it will act as a siphon. A one-way **antireflux valve** seated in the blue pigtail can prevent the reflux of gastric contents out of the vent lumen. The valve is removed after irrigation of the suction lumen, and 20 mL of air is injected to reestablish a buffer of air between the gastric contents and the valve.

Enteric Tubes

Nasoenteric tubes are used for feeding. Feeding tubes placed in the **duodenum** are 160 cm long and called *nasoduodenal tubes*; feeding tubes placed in the **jejunum** (the portion of the small intestine distal to the duodenum) are 175 cm long. They can be inserted before or during surgery, by interventional radiologists assisted by fluoroscopy, or at the bedside. If the tube is inserted at the bedside, placement is verified by an x-ray study. After insertion, the tip of the tube is initially placed in the stomach; it usually takes 24 hours for the tube to pass through the stomach and into the intestines by **peristalsis**. Surgically placed enteric tubes are inserted directly into the jejunum.

Polyurethane or silicone rubber feeding tubes have narrow diameters (6 to 12 Fr) and tungsten tips (rather than mercury-filled bags), and some have a water-activated lubricant that makes it easier to insert the tube. The tubing may kink when a stylet is not used, particularly if the patient is uncooperative or unable to swallow. Feeding tubes with a stylet are inserted with caution in patients predisposed to esophageal puncture, such as patients who are older or frail or who have thin tissues. These tubes are advanced in the same way as an NG tube (i.e., with the patient in the Fowler's position). If this is not possible, the patient is placed on the right side.

Nursing Management

Nursing interventions include the following:

- Explaining to the patient the purpose of the tube and the procedure required for inserting and advancing it
- Describing the sensations to be expected during tube insertion
- Inserting the NG tube and assisting with insertion of the nasoenteric tube
- Confirming the placement of the NG tube
- Advancing the nasoenteric tube
- Monitoring the patient and maintaining tube function
- Providing oral and nasal hygiene and care
- Monitoring for potential complications
- Removing the tube

Preparing the Patient

Before the patient is intubated, the nurse explains the purpose of the tube; this information may assist the patient to be cooperative and tolerant of what is often an unpleasant procedure. The general activities related to inserting the tube are then reviewed, including the fact that the patient may have to breathe through the mouth and that the procedure may cause gagging until the tube has passed the area of the gag reflex.

Inserting the Tube

Before inserting the tube, the nurse determines the length of tubing that will be needed to reach the stomach or the small intestine. A mark is made on the tube to indicate the desired length. This length is determined by measuring the distance from the tip of the nose to the earlobe and from the earlobe to the xiphoid process for NG placement (Fig. 36-1). If an intestinal placement is needed, add 20 to 25 cm from the xiphoid process.

While the tube is being inserted, the patient usually sits upright with a towel or some type of protective barrier spread bib-fashion over the chest. Tissue wipes are made available. Privacy and adequate light are provided. The physician may swab the nostril and spray the oropharynx with benzocaine/butamben/tetracaine (Cetacaine) to numb the nasal passage and suppress the gag reflex (Lor, Shih, Chen, et al., 2018). This makes the entire procedure more tolerable. Having the patient gargle with a liquid anesthetic or hold ice chips in the mouth for a few minutes can have a similar effect. Encouraging the patient to breathe through the mouth or to pant often helps, and (if permitted) swallow water.

A polyurethane tube may need to be warmed to make it more pliable. To make the tube easier to insert, it should be lubricated with a water-soluble lubricant unless it has a dry coating (called *hydromer*), which when moistened provides its own lubrication. The nurse wears gloves during the procedure.

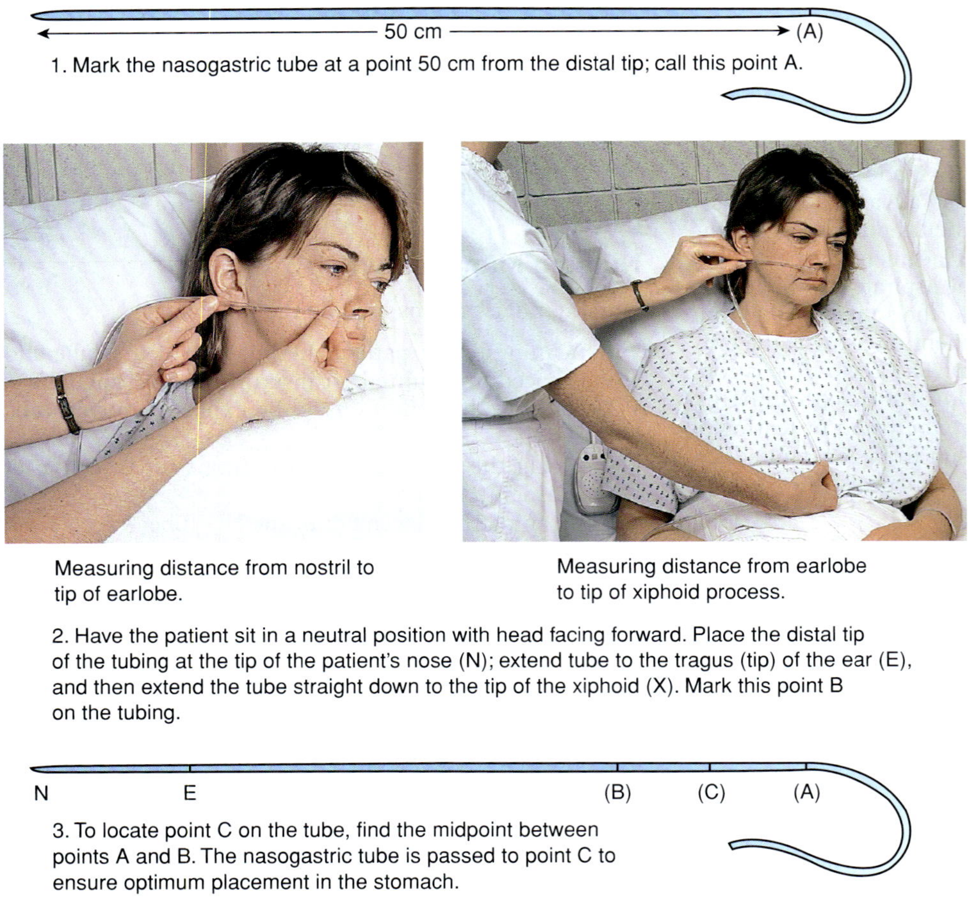

FIGURE 36-1. Measuring length of nasogastric tube for placement into stomach.

The patient is placed in the Fowler's position, and the nostrils are inspected for any obstruction. The more patent nostril is selected for use. The tip of the patient's nose is tilted, and the tube is aligned to enter the nostril. When the tube reaches the nasopharynx, the patient is instructed to lower the head slightly and to begin to swallow as the tube is advanced. The patient may also sip water through a straw to facilitate advancement of the tube. The oropharynx is inspected to ensure that the tube has not coiled in the pharynx or mouth.

Confirming Placement

To ensure patient safety, it is essential to confirm that the tube has been placed correctly. The tube may be inadvertently inserted in the lungs, and this may go undetected in high-risk patients (e.g., those with decreased levels of consciousness, confused mental states, poor or absent cough and gag reflexes, or agitation during insertion). The presence of an endotracheal tube or the recent removal of an endotracheal tube also increases the risk of inadvertent placement of the tube in the lung (Santos, Woith, Freitas, et al., 2016). Initially, an x-ray study should be used to confirm tube placement. However, each time liquids or medications are administered, and once per shift for continuous feedings, the tube must be checked to ensure that it remains properly placed. The traditional recommendation has been to inject air through the tube while auscultating the epigastric area with a stethoscope to detect air insufflation. However, studies indicate that this auscultatory method is not absolutely accurate in determining whether the tube has been inserted into the stomach, intestines, or respiratory tract (Santos et al., 2016). Instead of the auscultation method, a combination of three methods is recommended:

- Measurement of tube length
- Visual assessment of aspirate
- pH measurement of aspirate

After the tube is inserted, the exposed portion of the tube is measured, and the length is documented. The nurse measures the exposed tube length every shift and compares it with the original measurement. An increase in the length of exposed tube may indicate dislodgement or a leaking or ruptured balloon if the tube has a balloon.

Visual assessment of the colour of the aspirate may help to identify tube placement. Gastric aspirate is most frequently cloudy and green, tan or off-white, or bloody or brown. Intestinal aspirate is primarily clear and yellow to bile coloured. Pleural fluid is usually pale yellow and serous and tracheobronchial secretions are usually tan or off-white mucus. The appearance of the aspirate may be helpful in distinguishing between gastric and intestinal placement but is of little value in ruling out respiratory placement. Visual inspection is less helpful when the patient is receiving continuous tube feedings, because the gastric or intestinal aspirate often looks like the formula being used for the feeding (Ni, Huddy, Priest, et al., 2017; Eveleigh, Law, Pullyblank, et al., 2011). Determining the pH of the tube aspirate is a more accurate method of confirming tube placement than maintaining tube length or visually assessing tube aspirate. The pH method can also be used to monitor the advancement of the tube into the small intestine. The pH of gastric aspirate is acidic (1 to 5). The pH of intestinal aspirate is approximately 6 or higher, and the pH of respiratory aspirate is more alkaline (7 or greater). pH testing is best suited for distinguishing between gastric and intestinal placement. A pH sensor enteral tube that does not require fluid aspirate to obtain pH values is available and can be useful in distinguishing gastric from small intestinal placement of the tube. The pH method is less helpful with continuous feedings, because tube feedings have a pH value of 6.6 and neutralize the GI pH (Ni et al., 2017).

Ensuring bedside placement of postpyloric feeding tubes into the duodenum can be a challenge. If a gastroenterologist inserts the feeding tube using fibreoptic endoscopy, appropriate confirmation is ensured. However, this method of placement is relatively costly. Other placement methods are less invasive and less costly for the health care system. For instance, external magnets can sometimes be used to help guide a postpyloric feeding tube that has a magnet inserted in the tip. Metoclopramide (Reglan), a prokinetic agent, is administered intravenously and facilitates GI peristalsis, thereby encouraging movement of the feeding tube into the duodenum. Insufflating (e.g., administering) 100 to 500 mL of air into the feeding tube once its placement in the stomach is confirmed may also be a useful method of ensuring eventual postpyloric placement. Findings from research suggest that the air insufflation method results in quicker postpyloric placement, particularly among patients who also receive opioid agents (Wong, Chan, Wong, et al., 2017). Typical guidelines for all of these bedside methods require that the patient be placed on his or her right side (Leckey, Davis, & Raphael-Grimm, 2017).

Using gastric aspiration to verify the correct placement of the NG tube may be a problem because of the characteristic properties and diameter of the tubes. Aspiration may be performed more easily with polyurethane tubes and tubes with a size 10 Fr diameter or larger. If it is difficult to aspirate fluid from small-bore or large-bore feeding tubes, 20 mL of air is injected through the tube with a large syringe (30 to 60 mL) and then the plunger is pulled back. If this is ineffective, another 20 mL of air is injected, the large syringe is replaced with a smaller one (10 mL), and aspiration is attempted. The patient's position is changed, and aspiration is again attempted. If these measures are unsuccessful, the physician is notified.

Cola and cranberry juice have historically been recommended as effective, noninvasive means of declogging tubes, but evidence indicates that a mixture of pancreatic enzymes and water is superior in restoring the patency of feeding tubes (Rahnemai-Azar, Rahnemaiazar, Naghshizadian, et al., 2014). However, correct placement of the NG tube must be confirmed before any mixture is injected to declog the tube (Shipley, Gallo, & Fields, 2016).

Securing the Tube

After the correct position of the tip of the tube has been confirmed, the NG tube is secured to the nose (Fig. 36-2). A liquid skin barrier should be applied to the skin where the NG tube will be secured. The prepared area is covered with a strip of hypoallergenic tape or Op-Site, and the tube is then placed over the tape and secured with a second piece of tape. Instead of tape, a feeding tube attachment device (Hollister) can be used to secure the tube. This device adheres to the nose and uses an adjustable clip to hold the tube in place.

Monitoring the Patient and Maintaining Tube Function

If the NG tube is used for decompression, it is attached to suction. If it is used for enteral nutrition, the end of the tube is plugged between feedings. The nurse confirms tube placement by measuring tube length and comparing the length to the baseline before any fluids or medications are instilled and once per shift for continuous feedings. Displacement of the tube may be caused by tension on the tube (when the patient moves around in the bed or room), coughing, tracheal or nasotracheal suctioning, or airway intubation. If the NG tube is removed inadvertently in a patient who has undergone esophageal or gastric surgery, it is usually replaced under fluoroscopy by the physician to avoid trauma to the suture line.

It is important to keep an accurate record of all fluid intakes, feedings, and irrigations. To maintain patency, the tube is irrigated every 4 to 6 hours with water or normal saline to avoid electrolyte loss through gastric drainage. The nurse records the amount, colour, and type of all drainage every 8 hours.

When double- or triple-lumen tubes are used, each lumen is labelled according to its intended use: aspiration, feeding, or balloon inflation. To avoid tension on the tube, the portion of the tube from the nose to the drainage unit is fixed in position, either with a safety pin or with adhesive tape loops that are pinned to the patient's pajamas or

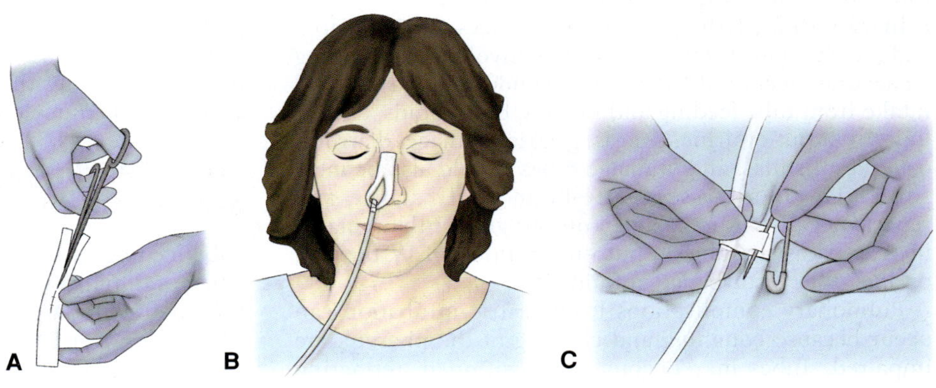

FIGURE 36-2. Securing nasogastric (NG) tubes. **A.** The NG tube is secured to the nose with tape to prevent injury to the nasopharyngeal passages. **B, C.** The tubing is secured to the patient's gown with either an elastic band or tape attached to a safety pin to prevent tension on the line during movement of the patient.

gown. The tube must be looped loosely to prevent tension and dislodgement (see Fig. 36-2).

Providing Oral and Nasal Hygiene

Regular and conscientious oral and nasal hygiene is a vital part of patient care, because the tube causes discomfort and pressure and may be in place for several days. Moistened cotton-tipped swabs can be used to clean the nose, followed by cleansing with a water-soluble lubricant. Frequent mouth care is comforting for the patient. The nasal tape is changed every 2 to 3 days, and the nose is inspected for skin irritation. If the nasal and pharyngeal mucosae are excessively dry, steam or cool vapor inhalations may be beneficial. Throat lozenges, an ice collar, chewing gum, or sucking on hard candies (if permitted) and limiting talking also assist in relieving patient discomfort. These activities keep the mucous membranes moist and help to prevent inflammation of the parotid glands.

Monitoring and Managing Potential Complications

Patients with NG or nasoenteric intubation are susceptible to a variety of issues, including fluid volume deficit, pulmonary complications, and tube-related irritations. These potential complications require careful ongoing assessment.

The Institute for Safe Medication Practices (ISMP) has reported significant errors with inadvertent administration of liquid enteral medications into intravenous (IV) lines. To create a safer environment, a new industry-wide standard for enteral feeding connectors (which are incompatible with Luer-lock or small-bore syringes) known as the ENFit is in the process of being fully implemented for use in all feeding tubes, feeding syringes, and feeding administration sets (ISMP, 2015; Joint Commission, 2014).

Symptoms of fluid volume deficit include dry skin and mucous membranes, decreased urinary output, lethargy, and increased heart rate. Assessment of fluid volume deficit involves maintaining an accurate record of intake and output (I&O). This includes measuring NG drainage, fluid instilled by irrigation of the NG tube, water taken by mouth, vomitus, water administered with tube feedings, and IV fluids. Laboratory values, particularly blood urea nitrogen and creatinine, are monitored. The nurse assesses 24-hour fluid balance and reports negative fluid balance, increased NG output, interruption of IV therapy, or any other disturbance in fluid intake or output.

The nurse should be vigilant for symptoms of fluid volume deficit in patients receiving enteral nutrition. These can include dry skin and mucous membranes, decreased urinary output, lethargy, lightheadedness, hypotension, and increased heart rate. Assessment involves maintaining an accurate record of I&O. This includes measuring fluid intake from tube feeding and flushes, oral liquids, and IV fluids. Output of urine, emesis, gastric drainage, diarrhea, ostomies, fistulas, and drainage tubes should also be measured. The nurse assesses 24-hour fluid balance and reports negative fluid balance (output greater than intake, increased gastric tube output, interruption of IV therapy, or any other disturbance in fluid I&O).

Pulmonary complications from gastric intubation can occur because coughing and clearing of the pharynx are impaired. Tubes may become malpositioned, retracting the distal end above the esophagogastric sphincter. Aspiration pneumonia occurs when regurgitated stomach contents or enteral feedings from an improperly positioned feeding tube are instilled into the pharynx or the trachea or when oral secretions are aspirated. Feeding patients through tubes placed beyond the pylorus or using prokinetic agents (e.g., erythromycin, metoclopramide) can decrease the frequency of feeding regurgitation and aspiration. In addition, feedings and medications should always be given with the patient in the semi-Fowler's position, and the patient's head should be elevated at least 30 to 45 degrees to reduce the risk of reflux and pulmonary aspiration. This position is maintained at least 1 hour after completion of an intermittent tube feeding and is maintained whenever possible for patients receiving continuous tube feedings. A reverse Trendelenburg position can be considered when it is not possible or advisable to elevate the head of the patient's bed.

Patients at risk for aspiration pneumonia include those older than 70 years of age, unable to protect their airways, with altered mental status or other neurologic deficits, receiving mechanical ventilation, with gastric or enteral tubes, and in the supine position (McClave, Taylor, Martindale, et al., 2016). Although it has been thought that enteral feedings should be withheld when patients receiving mechanical ventilation are repositioned, research findings question the advisability of this practice (DiLibero, Lavieri, O'Donoghue, et al., 2015) (see Chart 36-1).

Signs and symptoms of pulmonary complications include coughing during the administration of foods or medications, difficulty clearing the airway, tachypnea, and fever. Assessment includes regular auscultation of lung sounds and monitoring of vital signs and laboratory values. The nurse also carefully confirms the proper placement of the tube with a variety of methods before instilling any fluids or medications. If tube position is ever in question, radiographic confirmation is essential (Metheny, 2016).

Removing the Tube

Before removing a tube, the nurse may intermittently clamp and unclamp it for a trial period of several hours to ensure that the patient does not experience nausea, vomiting, or distention. Before the tube is removed, it is flushed with 10 mL of water or normal saline to ensure that it is free of debris and away from the gastric lining; then, the balloon (if present) is deflated. Gloves are worn to remove the tube. The tube is withdrawn gently and slowly for 15 to 20 cm until the tip reaches the esophagus; the remainder is withdrawn rapidly from the nostril. If the tube does not come out easily, force should not be used, and the problem should be reported to the physician. As the tube is withdrawn, it is concealed in a towel to prevent secretions from soiling the patient or nurse. After the tube is removed, the nurse provides oral hygiene.

Tube Feedings With Nasogastric and Nasoenteric Devices

Tube feedings are given to meet nutritional requirements when oral intake is inadequate or not possible and the GI tract is functioning normally. Tube feedings have several advantages over PN: they are low in cost, safe, well tolerated by the patient, and easy to use both in extended care

NURSING RESEARCH PROFILE

Chart 36-1. Enteral Feedings During Repositioning and the Incidence of Aspiration

DiLibero, J., Lavieri, M., O'Donoghue, S., et al. (2015). Withholding or continuing enteral feedings during repositioning and the incidence of aspiration. *American Journal of Critical Care, 24*(3), 258–261.

Purpose

The practice of continuing or withholding enteral feedings during repositioning of patients who are critically ill and mechanically ventilated varies among nurses, and is not necessarily research based. The purpose of this study was to see if there were differences in the incidence of aspiration between patients receiving mechanical ventilation and enteral feedings whose enteral feedings were either continued or stopped during repositioning.

Design

Twenty-three adult patients who were intubated and mechanically ventilated in medical or surgical intensive care units and who were receiving enteral feedings at rates of at least 50 mL/hour comprised the study sample. Participants were required to tolerate backrest elevation of at least 30 degrees and maintain gastric residual volumes less than 200 mL. A crossover design was utilized, which allowed each patient to serve as their own control. Two samples of subglottal secretions were obtained on each participant, one during repositioning when feedings were withheld, and another during repositioning when feedings were continued ($N = 46$). The specimens were tested for presence of pepsin, which would indicate aspiration.

Findings

Of the 23 patients, 13 were admitted to medical intensive care units and 10 were admitted to surgical intensive care units. Patients were 31 to 91 years old (median, 64 years). Enteral feeding rates were 30 to 75 mL/hour (mean; 52 mL/hour; SD, 12.3 mL/hour). Feeding rates did not change between the time of collection of the first and second set of subglottal specimens.

There was no significant difference between the incidence of aspiration during repositioning when enteral feedings were withheld or when they were continued.

Nursing Implications

Results from this study suggest that precautionary withholding of enteral feedings during repositioning does not seem to reduce the incidence of aspiration in patients who are mechanically ventilated. However, further research is needed to provide definitive evidence for optimal enteral feeding practices.

facilities and in the patient's home. Tube feedings have other advantages, such as they:

- Preserve GI integrity by delivery of nutrients and medications intraluminally
- Preserve the usual sequence of intestinal and hepatic metabolism
- Maintain fat metabolism and lipoprotein synthesis
- Maintain appropriate insulin/glucagon ratios

Tube feedings are delivered to the stomach (in the case of NG intubation or gastrostomy) or to the distal duodenum or proximal jejunum (in the case of nasoduodenal or **nasojejunal tube** feeding). Nasoduodenal or nasojejunal feeding is indicated when the esophagus and stomach need to be bypassed or when the patient is at risk for aspiration. For long-term feedings (longer than 4 weeks), gastrostomy or jejunostomy tubes are preferred for administration of medications or food. The numerous conditions requiring enteral nutrition are summarized in Table 36-2.

Osmosis and Osmolality

Osmolality is an important consideration for patients receiving tube feedings through the duodenum or jejunum because feeding formulas with a high osmolality may lead to undesirable effects, such as dumping syndrome (described later).

Fluid balance is maintained by **osmosis**, the process by which water moves through membranes from a dilute solution of lower osmolality (ionic concentration) to a more concentrated solution of higher osmolality until both

TABLE 36-2 Conditions That May Require Enteral Therapy

Condition or Need	Examples
Preoperative bowel preparation	—
Gastrointestinal issues	Fistula, short-bowel syndrome, mild pancreatitis, Crohn's disease, ulcerative colitis, nonspecific maldigestion or malabsorption
Cancer therapy	Radiation, chemotherapy
Convalescent care	Surgery, injury, severe illness
Coma, semi-consciousness[a]	Stroke, head injury, neurologic disorder, neoplasm
Hypermetabolic conditions	Burns, trauma, multiple fractures, sepsis, AIDS, organ transplantation
Alcoholism, chronic depression, anorexia nervosa[a]	Chronic illness, psychiatric, or neurologic disorder
Debilitation[a]	Disease or injury
Maxillofacial or cervical surgery	Disease or injury
Oropharyngeal or esophageal paralysis[a]	Disease or injury, neoplasm, inflammation, trauma, respiratory failure

[a]Because some of these patients are at risk for regurgitating or vomiting and aspirating administered formula, each condition must be considered individually.
AIDS, acquired immunodeficiency syndrome.

solutions are of nearly equal osmolality. The osmolality of body fluids is approximately 300 mmol/kg. The body attempts to keep the osmolality of the contents of the stomach and intestines at approximately this level.

Highly concentrated solutions and certain foods can upset the usual fluid balance in the body. Individual amino acids and carbohydrates are small particles that have great osmotic effect. Proteins are extremely large particles and therefore have less osmotic effect. Fats are not water soluble and do not enter into a solution in water; thus, they have no osmotic effect. Electrolytes, such as sodium and potassium, are comparatively small particles; they have a great effect on osmolality and consequently on the patient's ability to tolerate a given solution.

When a concentrated solution of high osmolality is taken in large amounts, water moves to the stomach and intestines from fluid surrounding the organs and the vascular compartment. The patient has a feeling of fullness, nausea, and diarrhea; this causes dehydration, hypotension, and tachycardia, collectively termed the ***dumping syndrome*** (Berg & McCallum, 2016). It is generally believed that starting with a more dilute commercial formula and increasing the concentration over several days may alleviate this problem. However, there is a lack of research data supporting the dilution of formula with water to relieve dumping syndrome (Gagnon & Kawawacki Sheff, 2012). Patients vary in the degree to which they tolerate the effects of high osmolality; usually, patients who are debilitated are less tolerant. The nurse needs to be knowledgeable about the osmolality of the patient's formula and needs to observe for and take steps to prevent undesired effects.

Tube-Feeding Formulas

The choice of formula to be delivered by tube feeding is influenced by the status of the GI tract and the nutritional needs of the patient. The formula characteristics that are considered prior to selection include the chemical composition of the nutrient source (protein, carbohydrates, fat), caloric density, osmolality, residue, bacteriologic safety, vitamins, minerals, and cost.

Various major formula types for tube feedings are available commercially. Blenderized formulas can be made by the patient's family or obtained in a ready-to-use form that is carefully prepared according to directions. Commercially prepared polymeric formulas (formulas with high-molecular weight) are composed of protein, carbohydrates, and fats in a high-molecular weight form (e.g., Ensure, Isosource, Osmolite HN). Chemically defined formulas (e.g., Vivonex) contain predigested and easy-to-absorb nutrients. Modular products contain only one major nutrient, such as protein (Beneprotein). Disease-specific formulas are available for various conditions. For patients with renal failure, a formula such as Nepro that is high in calories and low in electrolytes is ideal because it is formulated to maintain electrolyte and fluid balance. For patients with severe chronic obstructive pulmonary disease, a formula such as Pulmocare may be selected because it is high in fat and low in carbohydrates, has a high density (1.5 calories/mL) that helps maintain fluid restriction, and reduces carbon dioxide production. Fibre is added to some formulas (e.g., Jevity) to decrease the occurrence of diarrhea in some at-risk patients. Some feedings are given as supplements, and others are designed to meet the patient's total nutritional needs. Dietitians collaborate with physicians and nurses to determine the best formula for the patient.

NURSING ALERT

Commercial formulas frequently present issues because the composition is fixed and some patients cannot tolerate certain ingredients, such as sodium, protein, or potassium. Modular products may be substituted, and the critical constituents of sodium, potassium, and fat can be added. Attention is given to including all essential minerals and vitamins. Total intake of calories, nutrients, and fluids must be assessed when there is a reduction in total intake or excessive dilution of feedings.

Tube-Feeding Administration Methods

Many patients do not tolerate NG and nasoenteric tube feedings well. Often, a medium- or fine-bore Silastic nasoenteric tube is better tolerated than a plastic or rubber tube. The finer-bore tube requires a finely dispersed formula to ensure that the tube remains patent. For long-term tube-feeding therapy, a gastrostomy or jejunostomy tube is often used (see later discussion).

The tube-feeding method chosen depends on the location of the tube in the GI tract, patient tolerance, convenience, and cost. Intermittent **bolus** feedings are administered into the stomach (usually by gastrostomy tube [G tube]) in large amounts at designated intervals and may be given four to eight times per day. The intermittent gravity drip, another method for administering tube feedings into the stomach, is commonly used when the patient is at home. In this instance, the tube feeding is administered over 30 minutes at designated intervals. Both of these tube-feeding methods are practical and inexpensive. However, the feedings delivered at variable rates may be poorly tolerated and time consuming.

Continuous feeding is the delivery of feedings incrementally by a slow infusion over long periods. Slow drip feedings may reduce aspiration rates, distention, nausea, vomiting, and diarrhea in patients with poor gastric emptying or who are receiving hypertonic feeding solutions, as well as patients with severe reflux or altered mental status (Blumenstein, Shastri, & Stein, 2014). This method may also be used to administer tube feedings into the small intestine. Enteral feeding pumps control the delivery rate of the formula (see Fig. 36-3). They allow for a constant flow rate and can infuse a viscous formula through a small-diameter feeding tube. However, they do not allow the patient as much flexibility as intermittent feedings. Portable lightweight enteral pumps are available for home use. In addition, feeding pumps have built-in alarms that signal when the bag is empty, the battery is low, or the tube is occluded. The patient and caregiver need to be aware of these alarms and know how to "troubleshoot" the pump.

An alternative to the continuous infusion method is **cyclic feeding**, in which the infused feeding is given by an enteral feeding pump over 8 to 18 hours. Feedings may be

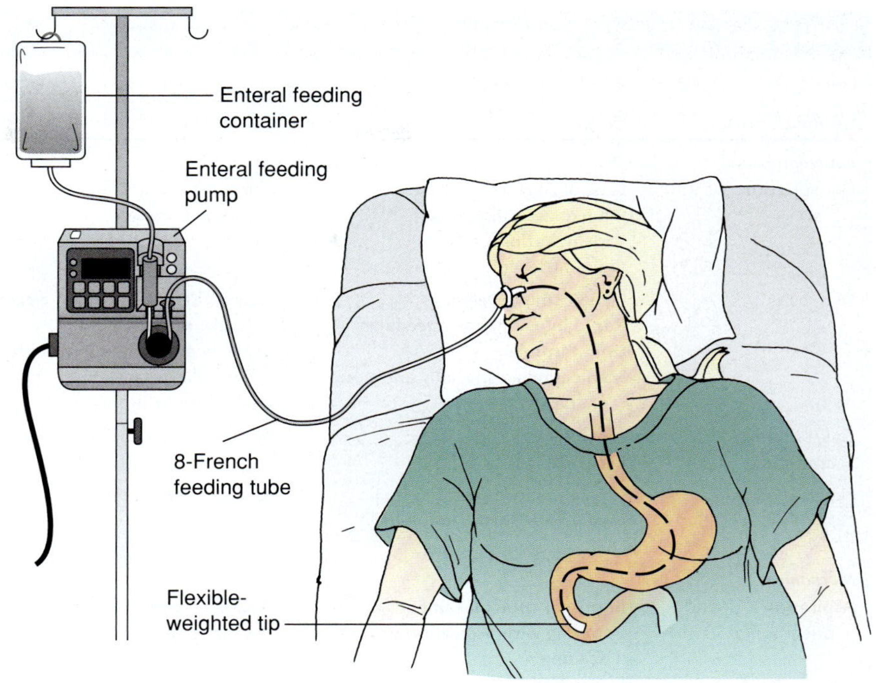

FIGURE 36-3. Nasoenteric tube feeding by continuous controlled pump. The head of the bed should be elevated to prevent aspiration.

infused at night to avoid interrupting the patient's lifestyle. Cyclic infusions may be appropriate for patients who are being weaned from tube feedings to an oral diet, for patients who cannot eat enough and need supplements, and for patients at home who need daytime hours free from the pump.

Tube-feeding solutions vary in terms of required preparation, consistency, and the number of calories and vitamins they contain. The choice of solution depends on the size and location of the tube in the GI tract, the patient's nutritional needs, the type of nutritional supplement, the method of delivery, and the convenience for the patient at home. A wide variety of containers, feeding tubes and catheters, delivery systems, and pumps are available for use with tube feedings.

Nursing Process

The Patient Receiving a Tube Feeding

Assessment

A preliminary assessment of the patient who requires a tube feeding includes several considerations:

- What is the patient's nutritional status, as judged by current physical appearance, dietary history, and history of recent weight loss?
- Are there any existing chronic illnesses or factors that will increase metabolic demands on the body (e.g., surgical stress, fever)?
- What is the patient's hydration status? Are fluid requirements (i.e., 30 to 40 mL/kg body weight) being met?
- Is the patient's digestive tract functioning?
- Are the patient's kidneys functioning effectively? What are the patient's electrolyte levels?
- What medications and other therapies is the patient receiving that may affect nutritional intake and function of the digestive system?
- Does the dietary prescription fulfill the patient's needs?

In addition, a more elaborate assessment is performed for patients who require extensive nutritional therapy. A team that includes the nurse, advanced practice nurse, physician, and dietitian conducts this assessment. In addition to the history and physical examination (which includes anthropometric measurements), a nutritional assessment is performed. This consists of recording any weight change; determining albumin, prealbumin, and transferrin levels; measuring total lymphocyte count; and evaluating muscle function. (See Chapter 5 for a detailed description of nutritional assessment.)

Nursing Priorities

Based on the assessment data, the major nursing priorities may include the following:

- Nutrition
- Risk for diarrhea
- Airway clearance
- Fluid and electrolyte balance
- Coping and discomfort
- Treatment management and adherence
- Patient teaching

TABLE 36-3 Potential Complications of Enteral Therapy

Complications	Causes	Selected Nursing Interventions: *Therapeutic*	Selected Nursing Interventions: *Preventive*
Gastrointestinal			
Constipation	Lack of fibre Inadequate fluid intake/dehydration Opioid use	Check fibre and water content; report findings	Administer adequate amount of hydration as flushes. Consider a cathartic
Diarrhea	Hyperosmolar feedings Rapid infusion/bolus feedings Cold formula Medications, especially antibiotic therapy	Assess fluid balance and electrolyte levels; report findings Implement changes in tube-feeding formula or rate Review medications	Appropriate rate of infusion and temperature of formula Avoid multiple elixirs and prokinetic medications
Gas/bloating/cramping	Air in tube Excess fibre	Notify primary provider if persistent	Keep tubing free of air
Nausea/vomiting	Change in formula or rate Inadequate gastric emptying	Review medications	Check residuals; if ≥200 mL, reinstill and recheck; report if residual is consistently high
Mechanical			
Aspiration pneumonia	Improper tube placement Vomiting with aspiration of tube feeding Flat in bed	Assess respiratory status and notify primary provider	Implement reliable method for checking tube placement Keep head of bed elevated at 30 degrees
Nasopharyngeal irritation	Tube position/improper taping Use of large tubes	Assess nasopharyngeal mucous membranes every 8 hours	Tape tube to prevent pressure on nares Reposition tape
Tube displacement	Excessive coughing/vomitus Tension on the tube or unsecured tube Tracheal suctioning Airway intubation	Stop feeding, and notify primary provider	Check tube placement before administering feeding
Tube obstruction	Inadequate flushing/formula rate Inadequate crushing of medications and flushing after administration	Follow policy for declogging feeding tubes (see procedural guidelines on feeding tube care)	Obtain liquid medications when possible Flush tube and crush medications adequately
Metabolic			
Dehydration and azotemia (excessive urea in the blood)	Hyperosmolar feedings with insufficient fluid intake	Report signs and symptoms of dehydration Implement changes in tube-feeding formula, rate, or ratio to water	Provide adequate hydration through flushes
Hyperglycemia	Glucose intolerance High carbohydrate content of the feeding	Check blood glucose levels routinely Dietary consult to reevaluate feeding regimen	

Adapted from Blumenstein, I., Shastri, Y. M., & Stein, J. (2014). Gastroenteric tube feeding: Techniques, problems, and solutions. *World Journal of Gastroenterology*, *20*(26), 8505–8524.

Collaborative Problems/Potential Complications

Complications of NG and nasoenteric tube-feeding therapy are classified into three types—GI, mechanical, and metabolic. Table 36-3 summarizes complications, possible causes, and appropriate interventions.

Planning and Goals

The major goals for the patient may include nutritional balance, usual bowel elimination pattern, reduced risk of aspiration, adequate hydration, individual coping, knowledge and skill in self-care, and prevention of complications.

Nursing Interventions

Maintaining Feeding Equipment and Nutritional Balance

The temperature and volume of the feeding, the flow rate, and the patient's total fluid intake are important factors to consider when tube feedings are given. The schedule of tube feedings, including the correct quantity and frequency, is maintained. The nurse must carefully monitor the drip rate and avoid administering fluids too rapidly.

For patients receiving tube feedings, measuring gastric residual volumes (GRVs) by removing gastric contents with a large syringe at routine intervals has been a commonly prescribed practice; however, the usefulness of measuring GRVs has not been validated by research (Reignier, Mercier, Le Gouge, et al., 2013; Williams, Leslie, Mills, et al., 2013). Previously, GRV in excess of 250 to 500 mL had been thought to indicate feeding intolerance. Other measures of feeding tolerance that the nurse may employ include physical assessment findings such as abdominal distention, patient reports of discomfort, vomiting, changes in passing flatus, and presence of diarrhea (McClave et al., 2016). The most recent guidelines for assessment and provision of nutrition in the patient who is critically ill, authored by the Society of Critical Care Medicine (SCCM) and the American Society for Parenteral and Enteral Nutrition (ASPEN), do not advocate using GRVs to monitor tolerance of enteral feedings (McClave et al., 2016). Recent research shows that GRVs between 250 and 500 mL did not increase the incidence of vomiting, aspiration, or pneumonia (McClave et al., 2016). Growing evidence supports moving away from routine assessment of GRVs.

Maintaining tube function is an ongoing responsibility of the nurse, patient, primary provider, and caregiver. To ensure patency and to decrease the chance of bacterial growth, sludge build-up, or occlusion of the tube, at least 30 mL of water is given in each of the following instances (Blumenstein et al., 2014):

- Before and after intermittent tube feeding and medication administration (with at least 5 mL of water in between each individual medication)
- After checking for gastric residuals and gastric pH
- Every 4 hours with continuous feedings
- When the tube feeding is discontinued or interrupted for any reason
- When the tube is not being used, where a minimum of once daily flushing is recommended

Water used to irrigate these tubes must be recorded as fluid intake. Sterile water or sterile saline should be used for patients who are immunocompromised or to flush postpyloric nasoduodenal and jejunostomy tubes (Blumenstein et al., 2014). While various studies show different results on flushing solutions, current research recommends distilled water (Blumenstein et al., 2014).

Potential complications of enteral therapy are noted in Table 36-3.

Providing Medications by Tube

When different types of medications are administered, each type is given separately, using a bolus method that is compatible with the medication's preparation (Table 36-4). The tube is flushed with 30 to 50 mL of water after each dose, and this fluid is recorded as intake. If a liquid form of a medication is not available and the medication can be crushed, it must first be reduced to a fine powder or the tube will become clogged. Devices are available that crush and dissolve tablets with water. Medications are not mixed with each other or with the feeding formula. When small-bore feeding tubes for continuous infusion are irrigated after medication administration, a 30-mL or larger syringe is used because the pressure generated by smaller syringes could rupture the tube. Administering medications through postpyloric enteric tubes may adversely affect their absorption; therefore, this should be avoided if possible.

TABLE 36-4 Preparing Medication for Delivery by Feeding Tube

Medication Form	Preparation
Liquid	None
Simple compressed tablets	Crush and dissolve in water
Buccal or sublingual tablets	Administer as prescribed
Soft gelatin capsules filled with liquid	Make an opening in capsule, and squeeze out contents
Enteric-coated tablets	Do not crush; change in form is required
Timed-release tablets	Do not crush tablets, because doing so may release too much drug too quickly (overdose); check with pharmacist for alternative formulation
Timed-release capsules or sustained-release capsules	Some can be opened and contents added to tube-feeding formula; *always* check with pharmacist before doing this

NURSING ALERT

Administering medications through postpyloric enteric tubes may adversely affect their absorption; therefore, this should be avoided if possible. In addition, to avoid nutrient and drug interactions, medications should not be mixed with the feeding formulas.

Maintaining Delivery Systems

Tube-feeding formula is delivered to patients by either an open or a closed system. The open system is packaged as a liquid or a powder to be mixed with water that is either poured into a feeding container or given by a large syringe. The feeding container (which is hung on a pole) and the tubing used with the open system should be changed every 24 hours. The open system can be used for bolus feedings, intermittent feedings, or continuous drip feedings and can be delivered by push (with a syringe and plunger), gravity (syringe with plunger removed or gravity bag with roller clamp), or pump. To avoid bacterial contamination, the formula hang time in the bag at room temperature should never exceed what the formula manufacturer recommends, which is usually no more than 4 to 8 hours. Closed delivery systems use a prefilled, sterile container of about 1 L of formula that is spiked with enteral tubing and allows a hang time of 24 to 48 hours at room

CHART 36-2

Assessment: Assessing Patients Receiving Tube Feedings

Be alert for the following assessment findings:

- Tube placement, patient's position (head of bed elevated 30 to 45 degrees), and formula flow rate
- Patient's ability to tolerate the formula; observe for fullness, bloating, distention, nausea, vomiting, and stool pattern
- Clinical responses, as noted in laboratory findings (blood urea nitrogen, serum protein, prealbumin, electrolytes, kidney function, hemoglobin, hematocrit)
- Signs of dehydration (dry mucous membranes, thirst, decreased urine output)
- Amount of formula actually taken in by the patient
- Elevated blood glucose level, decreased urinary output, sudden weight gain, and periorbital or dependent edema
- Infection control practices: Replace any formula given by an open system every 4 to 8 hours with fresh formula; change tube-feeding container and tubing every 24 hours
- Check gastric residual volume before each feeding or, in the case of continuous feedings, every 4 hours; return the aspirate to the stomach
- Intake and output
- Weekly weights
- Recommendations made on dietitian consult

Adapted from McClave, S. A., Taylor, B. E., Martindale, R. G., et al. (2016). Guidelines for the provision and assessment of nutrition support therapy in the adult critically ill patient: Society of Critical Care Medicine (SCCM) and American Society for Parenteral and Enteral Nutrition (ASPEN). *Journal of Parenteral and Enteral Nutrition*, *40*(2), 159–211.

temperature. The closed delivery system must always use a pump to control formula rate in order to avoid dispensing a large formula volume in a short period of time.

The tube-feeding regimen must be assessed frequently to evaluate its effectiveness and avoid complications (Chart 36-2).

Maintaining Normal Bowel Elimination Pattern

Patients receiving gastric or enteric tube feedings can experience diarrhea or constipation. Possible causes of diarrhea include:

- Malnutrition: A decrease in the intestinal absorptive area can cause diarrhea.
- Medication therapy:
  - Elixir-based medications—often contain sorbitol, which can act as a cathartic
  - Magnesium—acts as a cathartic
  - Antibiotics—thought to alter normal intestinal flora, allowing pathogenic bacteria to flourish
- *Clostridium difficile* (*C. difficile*) colitis: Can result after antibiotic use alters normal intestinal flora and promotes the abnormal growth of this potentially dangerous microbe. *C. difficile* colitis occurs most commonly in hospitalized older adult patients treated with antibiotics and causes significant, potentially lethal diarrhea (Gupta & Khanna, 2014).
- Zinc deficiency: Zinc is lost with diarrhea, and zinc deficiency can then cause continued diarrhea.
- Concomitant lactose intolerance
- Concomitant hyperthyroidism
- Dumping syndrome: Formula is infused into the small intestine quickly or formula bypasses the stomach too readily into the small intestine and causes expansion of the intestinal wall. This leads to bloating, cramping, diarrhea, dizziness, diaphoresis, and weakness. Measures for managing the GI symptoms associated with dumping syndrome are presented in Chart 36-3.
- Contamination of the formula and feeding equipment with diarrhea-causing pathogens

Possible causes of constipation include:

- Inadequate water intake: Tube feedings typically do not meet total fluid needs and additional water needs to be given.
- Administration of fibre-free tube-feeding formulas
- Concomitant use of opioids

CHART 36-3

Preventing Symptoms of Dumping Syndrome

The following strategies may help to prevent some of the uncomfortable symptoms of dumping syndrome related to tube feeding:

- Slow the formula instillation rate to provide time for carbohydrates and electrolytes to be diluted.
- Administer feedings at room temperature, because temperature extremes stimulate peristalsis.
- Administer feeding by continuous drip (if tolerated) rather than by bolus to prevent sudden distention of the intestine.
- Advise the patient to remain in a semi-Fowler's position for 1 hour after the feeding; this position prolongs intestinal transit time by decreasing the effect of gravity.
- Instill the minimal amount of water needed to flush the tubing before and after a feeding, because fluid given with a feeding increases intestinal transit time.

Reducing the Risk for Aspiration

Aspiration pneumonia occurs when stomach contents or enteral feedings are regurgitated and aspirated or when an NG tube is improperly positioned and feedings are instilled into the pharynx or the trachea. Feeding patients through nasoenteric tubes placed beyond the pylorus has helped to decrease the frequency of regurgitation and aspiration.

NURSING ALERT

To prevent aspiration, the nurse must verify the correct tube placement before every feeding, each time medications are administered, and once every shift if the tube feeding is continuous.

Feedings and medications should always be administered with the patient in the proper position to prevent regurgitation. The semi-Fowler's position is necessary for an NG feeding, with the patient's head elevated at least 30 to 45 degrees to reduce the risk for reflux and pulmonary aspiration. This position is maintained at least 1 hour after completion of an intermittent tube feeding and is maintained at all times for patients receiving continuous tube feedings. Another prevention strategy is to monitor the residual volume and notify the physician and stop the feedings if the residual volume is excessive, as discussed previously.

NURSING ALERT

If aspiration is suspected, the feeding is stopped immediately, the pharynx and trachea are suctioned, and the patient is placed on the right side with the head of the bed down. The physician is notified immediately.

Maintaining Adequate Hydration

The nurse carefully monitors hydration, because in many cases the patient cannot communicate the need for water. Water is given every 4 to 6 hours and after feedings to prevent hypertonic dehydration. At the beginning of administration, the feeding is given in continuous drip administration. This gradual administration allows assessment of residual volume and helps the patient develop tolerance, especially for hyperosmolar solutions. Key nursing interventions include observing for signs of dehydration (e.g., dry mucous membranes, thirst, decreased urine output); administering water routinely and as needed; and monitoring intake, output, residual volume, and fluid balance (24-hour intake vs. output).

Promoting Coping Ability

The psychosocial goal of nursing care is to support and encourage the patient to accept physical changes and to convey hope that daily progressive improvement is possible. If the patient is having difficulty adjusting to the treatment, the nurse intervenes by encouraging self-care (e.g., recording daily weight and intake and output) within the parameters of the patient's activity level. In addition, the nurse reinforces an optimistic approach by identifying indicators of progress (daily weight trends, electrolyte balance, absence of nausea and diarrhea).

Promoting Home, Community-Based, and Transitional Care

EDUCATING PATIENTS ABOUT SELF-CARE. Patients who require long-term tube feedings may have had recent surgery, dysphagia due to a neuromuscular disease, radiation or other types of trauma to the throat, an obstruction of the upper GI tract, or decreased level of consciousness. For a patient to be considered for tube feeding at home, the patient should:

- Be medically stable and successfully tolerating at least 60% to 70% of the feeding regimen
- Be capable of self-care or have a caregiver willing to assume the responsibility
- Have access to supplies and interest in learning how to administer tube feedings at home

Preparation of the patient for home administration of enteral feedings begins while the patient is still hospitalized. The nurse should educate the patient and caregiver while administering the feedings so that they can observe the mechanics and participate in the procedure, ask questions, and express any concerns. Before discharge, the nurse provides information about the equipment needed, formula purchase and storage, and administration of the feedings and water flushes (frequency, quantity, rate of instillation).

Family members who will be active in the patient's home care are encouraged to participate in all teaching sessions. Available printed information about the equipment, the formula, and the procedure is reviewed. The nurse encourages the patient and caregiver to learn the basic process with the supervision of the nurse. Arrangements are made for the caregiver to obtain the equipment and formula and have it ready for use before the patient's discharge (Providence Health Care, 2018).

CONTINUING AND TRANSITIONAL CARE. Referral to a home care agency is important so that a nurse can supervise and provide support during the first feeding at home. Additional visits will depend on the skill and comfort of the patient or caregiver in administering the feedings. During all visits, the nurse monitors the patient's physical status (weight, vital signs, activity level) and the ability of the patient and family to administer the tube feedings correctly. In addition, the nurse assesses for any complications (dumping syndrome, nausea or vomiting, weight loss, lethargy, confusion, excessive thirst). The patient or caregiver is encouraged to keep a diary to record times and amounts of feedings and any symptoms that occur. The nurse can review the diary with the patient and caregiver during home visits.

Evaluation

Expected patient outcomes may include the following:

1. Attains or maintains nutritional balance
   a. Has a positive nitrogen balance
   b. Maintains laboratory values within expected limits (i.e., blood urea nitrogen, hemoglobin, hematocrit, prealbumin, serum protein)
   c. Attains or maintains hydration of body tissue
   d. Attains or maintains desired body weight
2. Is free of episodes of diarrhea
   a. Has fewer than three watery stools a day
   b. Does not have a bowel movement after a bolus feeding
   c. Reports no intestinal cramping
   d. Has usual bowel sounds

3. Avoids aspiration
   a. Lungs are clear to auscultation
   b. Exhibits expected heart rate and respiratory rate
4. Attains or maintains hydration of body tissue
   a. Has a balanced fluid intake and output every 24 hours
   b. Does not have dry skin or dry mucous membranes
5. Copes effectively with tube-feeding regimen
6. Demonstrates skill in managing tube-feeding regimen
7. Experiences no complications
   a. Has no GI disturbances
   b. Tube remains intact and patent for duration of therapy
   c. Maintains metabolic balance within normal limits

Gastrostomy and Jejunostomy

A **gastrostomy** is a procedure in which an opening is created into the stomach either for the purpose of administering nutrition, fluids, and medications via a feeding tube, or for gastric decompression in patients with gastroparesis, gastroesophageal reflux disease, or intestinal obstruction. A gastrostomy is preferred over a nasally inserted tube to deliver enteral nutrition support longer than 4 weeks (Blumenstein et al., 2014). Gastrostomy is also preferred over NG or orogastric feedings in the patient who is comatose because the gastroesophageal sphincter remains intact, making regurgitation and aspiration less likely. Recent research demonstrates an early emergence of percutaneous transesophageal gastrotubing as an alternative in patients where gastrostomy or jejunostomy may not be feasible (advanced gastric cancer, severe herniations of gastric walls, severe ascites, etc.) (Yoon & Nishihara, 2017).

Balloon and nonballoon G tubes may be placed surgically, endoscopically, or fluoroscopically (Fig. 36-4). Each technique requires an abdominal incision, and either a permanent gastric **stoma** (an artificially created opening) is created surgically that can be accessed with a feeding tube (Janeway gastrostomy), or a gastric stoma is established that remains open as long as it remains intubated (i.e., a tube remains in place).

Different types of feeding gastrostomies may be used, including the Stamm (temporary and permanent), Janeway (permanent), and **percutaneous endoscopic gastrostomy** (PEG; temporary) systems. The Stamm and Janeway gastrostomies require either an upper abdominal midline incision or a left upper quadrant transverse incision. The Stamm procedure requires the use of concentric purse-string sutures to secure the tube to the anterior gastric wall. To create the gastrostomy, an exit wound is created in the left upper abdomen. The Janeway procedure necessitates the creation of a tunnel (called a *gastric tube*) that is brought out through the abdomen to form a permanent stoma.

Insertion of a PEG requires the services of two physicians (or a physician and a nurse with specialty skills). After administering a local anesthetic, one physician inserts a cannula into the stomach through an abdominal incision and then threads a nonabsorbable suture through the cannula; the second physician inserts an endoscope via the patient's upper GI tract and uses the endoscopic snare to grasp the end of the suture and guide it up through the patient's mouth. The suture is knotted to the dilator tip at the end of the PEG tube. The endoscopist then advances the dilator tip through the patient's mouth while the first physician pulls the suture through the cannula site. The attached PEG tube is guided down the esophagus, into the stomach, and out through the abdominal incision (Fig. 36-4A). The mushroom catheter tip and internal crossbar secure the tube against the stomach wall. An external retention bolster (crossbar, circular, or star shaped) is threaded down the tube and positioned snug to the skin. The tension between the external and internal fixation bolsters keeps the tube in place. G tubes can also be placed fluoroscopically by a skilled provider when an endoscope cannot be passed through a strictured or obstructed esophagus (DeLegge, 2015).

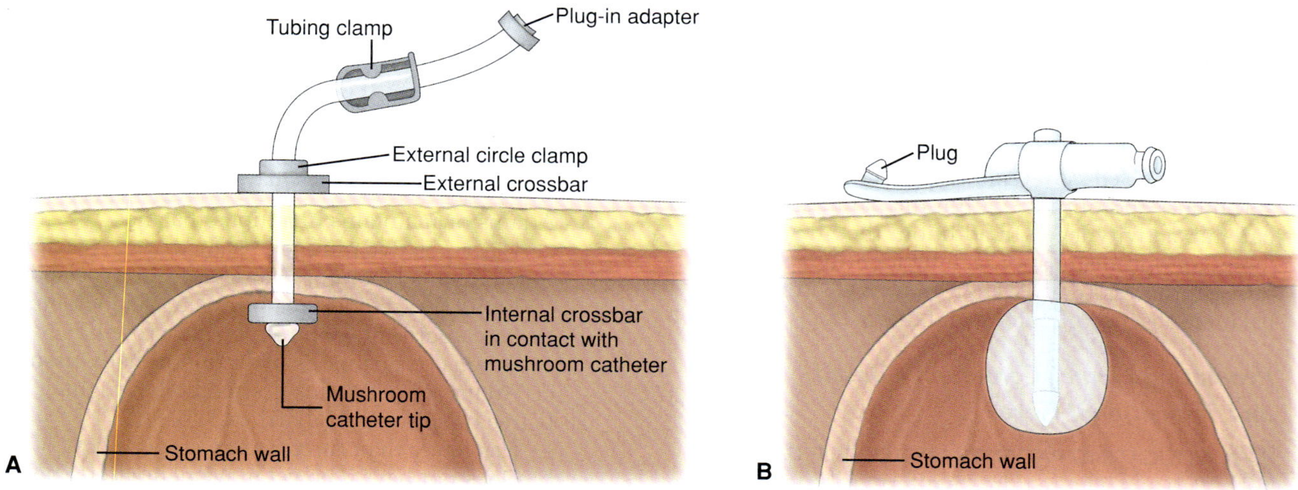

FIGURE 36-4. **A.** A detail of the abdomen and the percutaneous endoscopic gastrostomy (PEG) tube, showing catheter fixation. **B.** A detail of the abdomen and the nonobturated low-profile gastrostomy device (LPGD), showing balloon fixation.

feedings typically is not forced to give up usual dietary patterns, which may prove to be psychologically more acceptable. In addition, near-normal bowel function is promoted because the fibre and residue are similar to those of a usual diet.

If the tube has been placed for gastric drainage, it can be connected to either a low intermittent suction or to a gravity drainage bag. This drainage should be measured and recorded because it is a significant indicator of GI function. A decrease in the amount of drainage may indicate that the tube can be clamped for periods of time, allowing greater freedom of movement. High output can result in significant fluid and electrolyte losses.

Providing Tube Care and Preventing Infection

A small dressing can be applied over the tube insertion site, and the gastrostomy tube can be held in place by a thin strip of adhesive tape that is first placed around the tube and then firmly attached to the abdomen. The dressing protects the skin around the incision from seepage of gastric acid and spillage of feedings.

The nurse verifies the tube's placement, assesses residuals, and gently manipulates the tube or stabilizing disk once daily to prevent skin breakdown. Some gastrostomy tubes have balloons that are inflated with water to anchor the tube in the stomach. Balloon integrity is checked weekly by deflating and reinflating the balloon using a Luer-tip syringe.

Preventing Infection and Providing Skin Care

The skin surrounding a gastrostomy or jejunostomy requires special care because it may become irritated from the enzymatic action of gastric or intestinal juices that may leak around the tube. Left untreated, the skin becomes macerated and painful. The nurse washes the area around the tube under the bumper with soap and water or 2% chlorhexidine gluconate daily and as needed to remove any encrustation. If soap and water is used, the area is rinsed well with water and patted dry. If chlorhexidine is used, the area is allowed to air dry. A protective skin barrier may be applied. Skin at the exit site is evaluated daily for signs of breakdown, irritation, excoriation, and the presence of drainage, bleeding or hypertrophic tissue growth or scattered, raised red papules that could indicate a yeast or candidal infection. Candida may appear in warm moist areas of the body; the area beneath the G tube external retention bolster is a common location for it to develop and spread. The nurse encourages the patient and family members to participate in this evaluation and in hygiene activities

A thin gauze or foam dressing is applied, if needed, under the external bumper. Dressings placed under the bumper may exert excessive tension on the tube tract (DeLegge, 2015). A tube stabilizer may also be used to anchor the G tube (Miller, McClave, Kiraly, et al., 2014).

It is normal to see scant serous drainage at the site for a few days post insertion. After this drainage ceases, the site may be left open to air. The nurse rotates the tube once daily to prevent skin breakdown and *buried bumper syndrome*. Buried bumper syndrome can occur when there is excessive traction on the G tube from the external retention bolster to the extent that the internal fixation bolster becomes embedded in the gastric mucosa. This causes pain during tube feedings and can lead to tube obstruction and peritonitis (DeLegge, 2015).

Enhancing Body Image

The patient with a gastrostomy has experienced a major assault to body image. Eating, a physiologic and social function, can no longer be taken for granted. The patient is also aware that gastrostomy as a therapeutic intervention is performed only in the presence of a major, chronic, or perhaps terminal illness.

Calm discussion of the purposes and routines of gastrostomy feeding can help to keep the patient from feeling overwhelmed. Talking with a person who has had a gastrostomy can also help the patient accept the expected changes. Adjusting to a change in body image takes time and requires family support and acceptance. Evaluating the existing family support system is necessary.

Monitoring and Managing Potential Complications

During the postoperative course, the nurse monitors the patient for potential complications. The most common complications are wound infection and other wound problems, including cellulitis at the exit site and abscesses in the abdominal wall. Because many patients who receive tube feedings are debilitated and have compromised nutritional status, any signs of infection are promptly reported to the physician so that appropriate therapy can be instituted.

Bleeding from the insertion site in the stomach may also occur. The nurse closely monitors the patient's vital signs and observes all drainage from the operative site, vomitus, and stool for evidence of bleeding. Any signs of bleeding are reported promptly.

Premature removal of the tube, whether it is done inadvertently by the patient or by the caregiver, is another complication. If the tube is removed prematurely, the skin is cleansed and a sterile dressing is applied; the nurse immediately notifies the physician. The tract will close within 4 to 6 hours if the tube is not replaced promptly.

Promoting Home, Community-Based, and Transitional Care

EDUCATING PATIENTS ABOUT SELF-CARE. The patient with a G or J tube in the home setting must be capable of maintaining patency of the tube or have a caregiver who can do so. The nurse assesses the

patient's level of knowledge and interest in learning about the tube, as well as an ability to understand how to flush, provide site care, and administer feedings or facilitate decompression and drainage. Education is similar to that described earlier. To facilitate self-care, the nurse encourages the patient to participate in flushing the tube, administering medications and tube feedings during hospitalization, and establishing as normal a routine as possible.

Adapters are available that can be secured to the end of the tube to create a "Y" site for ease of flushing, suction, or medication delivery. The flushing equipment is cleaned with warm, soapy water and rinsed after each use. The tube can be marked at skin level to provide the patient with a baseline for later comparison. The patient or caregiver should be advised to monitor the tube's length and to notify the primary provider or home care nurse if the segment of the tube outside the body becomes shorter or longer.

Demonstration of the tube feeding begins by showing the patient how to check for residual gastric contents before the feeding. The patient then learns how to check and maintain the patency of the tube by administering room temperature water before and after the feeding. This establishes patency before the feeding and then clears the tube of food particles, which could decompose if allowed to remain in the tube. All feedings are given at room temperature or near body temperature.

For a bolus feeding, the nurse shows the patient how to introduce the liquid into the catheter by using a funnel or the barrel of a syringe. The receptacle is tilted to allow air to escape while the liquid is being instilled initially. As the funnel or syringe fills with liquid, the feeding is allowed to flow into the stomach by gravity by holding the barrel or syringe perpendicular to the abdomen (Fig. 36-5). Raising or lowering the receptacle to no higher than 45 cm above the abdominal wall regulates the rate of flow.

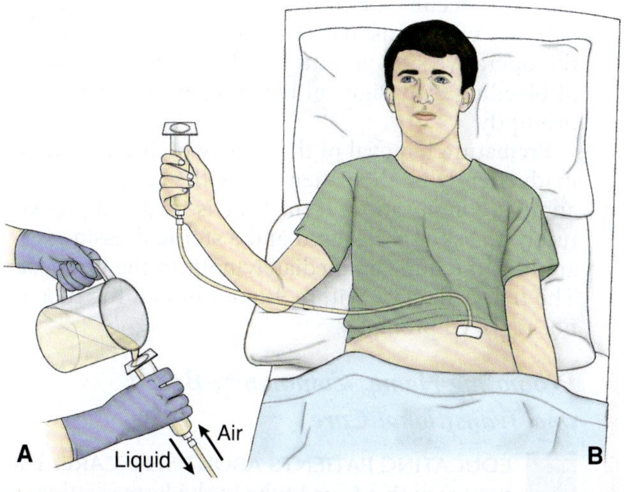

FIGURE 36-5. Bolus gastrostomy feeding by gravity. **A.** Feeding is instilled at an angle so that air does not enter the stomach. **B.** Syringe is raised perpendicular to the abdomen so that feeding can enter by gravity.

A bolus feeding of 300 to 500 mL usually is given for each meal and requires 10 to 15 minutes to complete. The amount is often determined by the patient's reaction. If the patient feels full, it may be desirable to give smaller amounts more frequently.

The patient and caregiver must understand that keeping the head of the bed elevated a minimum of 45 degrees for at least 1 hour after feeding facilitates digestion and decreases the risk of aspiration. Any obstruction requires that the feeding be stopped and the physician notified.

The patient or caregiver is instructed to flush the tube with 30 to 50 mL of water after each bolus or medication administration and to also flush the tube daily to keep it patent. Adaptors are available that can be secured to the end of the tube to create a "Y" site for ease of flushing or medication delivery. The flushing equipment is cleaned with warm, soapy water and rinsed after each use.

The patient and caregiver are made aware that the tube is marked at skin level to provide the patient with a baseline for later comparison. They are advised to monitor the tube's length and to notify the physician or home care nurse if the segment of the tube outside the body becomes shorter or longer.

If the patient is to use an intermittent or continuous-pressure feeding pump at home, instruction in the use of the particular type of pump is essential. Most feeding pumps have built-in alarms that signal when the bag is empty, when the battery is low, or when the tube is occluded. The patient and caregiver need to be aware of these alarms and how to troubleshoot the pump.

CONTINUING AND TRANSITIONAL CARE. Referral to home, community-based, or transitional care is important to ensure initial supervision and support for the patient and caregiver. The home care nurse assesses the patient's status and progress and evaluates the techniques used in administering the tube feeding. Further instruction and supervision in the home setting may be required to help the patient and caregiver adapt to a physical environment and equipment that are different from the hospital setting (Chart 36-5). The nurse also reviews with the patient and caregiver complications to report (e.g., dumping syndrome, nausea and vomiting, infection of the skin at the insertion site of the tube).

The home care nurse assists the patient and family in establishing as normal a routine as possible. The patient or caregiver is encouraged to keep a diary to record the times and amounts of feedings and any symptoms that occur. The nurse reviews the diary during home visits. In addition, the patient or caregiver must be taught how to replace the tube.

Evaluation

Expected patient outcomes may include the following:

1. Achieves an adequate intake of nutrients
   a. Tolerates quantity and frequency of tube feedings
   b. Has 100 mL or less of residual gastric content before each feeding

CHART 36-5

HOME CARE CHECKLIST • The Patient Receiving Tube Feeding

At the completion of education, the patient and/or caregiver will be able to:

- Name the procedure that was performed and identify any permanent changes in anatomic structure or function as well as changes in ADLs, IADLs, roles, relationships, and spirituality.
- State what types of changes are needed (if any) to maintain a clean home environment and prevent infection.
- State how to contact the primary provider, the team of home care professionals overseeing care, and tube-feeding supply vendor.
  - List emergency phone numbers.
- State how to obtain medical supplies and carry out dressing changes, site care, and other prescribed regimens.
- Demonstrate how to perform site care.
- Demonstrate how to prepare tube feeding.
- Demonstrate how to deliver tube feeding via prescribed method (e.g., bolus method, intermittent drip method, continuous feeding).
  - When indicated, demonstrate how to operate, disconnect, and clean the tube-feeding pump.
  - When indicated, demonstrate tube maintenance functions.
    - Flush before and after bolus and intermittent feeding and medication administration
    - Flush every 4 hours with continuous feeding
    - Flush once daily if tube is not being used
- Demonstrate how to record all fluid intake and output.
- Identify a plan for operation of tube-feeding pump during a power outage or other emergencies.
- State the name, dose, side effects, frequency, and schedule for all medications.
- Demonstrate medication preparation and administration via bolus method, with flushing before, after and between medications.
- Identify possible tube-feeding complications and interventions.
- Relate how to reach primary provider with questions or complications.
- State time and date of follow-up appointments and testing.
- State understanding of community resources and referrals (if any).
- Identify the need for health promotion (e.g., weight reduction, smoking cessation, stress management), disease prevention, and screening activities.

ADL, activities of daily living; IADL, independent activities of daily living.

   c. Has no diarrhea
   d. Maintains or gains weight
   e. Has expected electrolyte values
2. Is free from infection and skin breakdown
   a. Is afebrile
   b. Has no drainage from the incision
   c. Demonstrates intact skin surrounding the exit site
   d. Inspects exit site daily
3. Adjusts to change in body image
   a. Is able to discuss expected changes
   b. Verbalizes concerns
4. Demonstrates skill in managing feeding regimen
   a. Helps to prepare prescribed formula or blenderized feeding
   b. Handles equipment competently
   c. Helps to administer the feeding or does so independently
   d. Demonstrates how to maintain tube patency
   e. Cleans tubing as needed
   f. Keeps an accurate record of intake
   g. If indicated, can remove and reinsert tube as appropriate and needed for feedings
5. Avoids complications
   a. Exhibits adequate wound healing
   b. Has no abnormal bleeding from puncture site
   c. Tube remains intact for duration of therapy

Parenteral Nutrition

PN is a method of providing nutrients to the body by an IV route. The nutrients are a complex admixture containing proteins, carbohydrates, fats, electrolytes, vitamins, trace minerals, and sterile water in a single container. The goals of PN are similar to the goals of enteral feedings; namely, to improve nutritional status, establish a positive nitrogen balance, maintain muscle mass, promote weight maintenance or gain, and enhance the healing process.

Establishing Positive Nitrogen Balance

When a patient's intake of protein and nutrients is significantly less than that required by the body to meet energy expenditures, a state of negative nitrogen balance results. In response, the body begins to convert the protein found in muscles into carbohydrates to be used to meet energy needs. The result is muscle wasting, weight loss, fatigue, and, if left uncorrected, death. The goal for patients receiving nutrition support is to achieve positive nitrogen balance (Dickerson, Pitts, Maish, et al., 2012).

The average postoperative adult patient requires approximately 1,500 calories/day to keep the body from using its own store of protein. Traditional IV fluids do not provide sufficient calories or nitrogen to meet the body's daily requirements. PN solutions, which supply nutrients such as dextrose, amino acids, electrolytes, vitamins, minerals, and fat emulsions, provide enough calories and nitrogen to meet the patient's daily nutritional needs. In general, PN usually provides 25 to 35 kcal/kg of ideal body weight and 1.0 to 1.5 g of protein/kg of ideal body weight.

The patient with fever, trauma, burns, major surgery, or hyper metabolic disease requires additional daily calories. The volume of fluid necessary to provide these calories would surpass fluid tolerance and lead to pulmonary edema or heart failure. To provide the required calories in a small volume, it is necessary to increase the concentration of nutrients and use a route of administration (i.e., a large, high-flow vein such as the subclavian) that rapidly dilutes incoming nutrients to the proper levels of body tolerance.

When highly concentrated dextrose is administered, caloric requirements are satisfied and the body uses amino acids for protein synthesis rather than for energy. Additional potassium is added to the solution to maintain correct electrolyte balance and to transport glucose and amino acids across cell membranes. To prevent deficiencies and fulfill requirements for tissue synthesis, other elements, such as calcium, phosphorus, magnesium, and sodium chloride, are added.

Clinical Indications

The indications for PN include an inability to ingest adequate oral food or fluids within a 7- to 10-day timeframe (McClave et al., 2016). Enteral nutrition should be considered before parenteral support since it assists in maintaining gut mucosal integrity (Silander, Jacobsson, Bertéus-Forslund, et al., 2013). In both the home and hospital setting, PN is indicated in the following situations:

- The patient's intake is insufficient to maintain an anabolic state (e.g., severe burns, malnutrition, short bowel syndrome, acquired immunodeficiency syndrome [AIDS], sepsis, cancer).
- The patient's ability to ingest food orally or by tube is impaired (e.g., paralytic ileus, Crohn's disease with obstruction, postradiation enteritis, severe hyperemesis gravidarum in pregnancy).
- The patient is unwilling or unable to ingest adequate nutrients (e.g., anorexia nervosa, postoperative older patients).
- The underlying medical condition precludes being fed orally or by tube (e.g., acute pancreatitis, high enterocutaneous fistula).
- Preoperative and postoperative nutritional needs are prolonged (e.g., extensive bowel surgery).

Formulas

A total of 1 to 3 L of solution is given over a 24-hour period. The label of the solution is verified with the prescription. **IV fat emulsions (IVFEs or lipids)** may be infused simultaneously with PN through a Y connector close to the infusion site and should not be filtered. The PN solution is not to be piggybacked into the IVFE. Usually, 500 mL of a 10% IVFE or 250 mL of 20% IVFE is given over 6 to 12 hours, one to three times a week. IVFEs can provide up to 30% of the total daily calorie intake.

NURSING ALERT

Before PN infusion is given, the solution must be inspected for separation, oily appearance (also known as a "cracked solution"), or any precipitate (which appears as white crystals). If any of these are present, it is not used.

IVFEs can be admixed with other components of PN to create a "three-in-one formulation" commonly called a ***total nutrient admixture*** (TNA) (Gervasio, 2015). All the parenteral nutrient components are mixed in one container and administered to the patient over a 24-hour period. A special final filter (1.5-μ filter) is used with this solution. Before administration, the solution is observed for oil droplets that have separated from the solution, forming a noticeable layer ("cracking of lipid emulsion"); such a solution should be discarded. Advantages of the TNA over PN are cost savings in preparation and equipment, decreased risk of catheter or nutrient contamination, decreased pharmacy preparation time, less nursing time, and increased patient convenience and satisfaction (see Chart 36-6). Ideally, the pharmacist, dietitian, and physician collaborate to determine the specific formula needed.

NURSING RESEARCH PROFILE

Chart 36-6. Interventions to Improve Professional Adherence to Guidelines for Prevention of Device-Related Infections

Flodgren, G., Conterno, L. O., Mayhew, A., et al. (2013). Interventions to improve professional adherence to guidelines for prevention of device-related infections. *The Cochrane Database of Systematic Reviews*, (3), CD006559.

Purpose

Health care-related infections (HAIs) are a major threat to patients, with mortality rates of 5% to 35%. The purpose of this Cochrane Systematic Review was to examine the breakdown of aseptic technique particularly during insertion, on-going care of the devices, and length of time the devices were used.

Design

Electronic databases were searched for studies up to June, 2012. In the end, 13 studies including randomized control trials, nonrandomized control trials, interrupted time series, and before and after studies; all related to preventing device-related infections were included. The research studies involved "40 hospitals, 51 intensive care units (ICUs), 27 wards, and more than 3,504 patients and 1,406 health care professionals." (p. 2).

Findings

Due to the low quality of the evidence included in this study, it is difficult to know which interventions were most effective in which situations. Where changes occurred after an intervention, it was not always sustained. The best effects occurred in studies to decrease ventilator-associated pneumonia, where the effect was sustained up to 12 months.

Nursing Implications

Nurses need to be very aware of the need for excellent sterile technique when caring for patients with a variety of inserted devices.

Initiating Therapy

PN solutions are initiated slowly and advanced gradually each day to the desired rate as the patient's fluid and glucose tolerance permits. The patient's laboratory test results and response to PN therapy are monitored on an ongoing basis by the physician, dietitian, and nurse. Standing orders are initiated for weighing the patient; monitoring intake, output, and blood glucose; and baseline and periodic monitoring of complete blood count, platelet count, and chemistry panel, including serum carbon dioxide, magnesium, phosphorus, triglycerides, and prealbumin. A 24-hour urine nitrogen determination may be performed for analysis of nitrogen balance. In most hospitals, the physician prescribes PN solutions on a daily standard PN order form. The formulation of the PN solutions is calculated carefully each day to meet the complete nutritional needs of the individual patient.

NURSING ALERT

Formulations with dextrose concentrations of more than 10% should not be given through peripheral veins because they irritate the intima (innermost walls) of small veins, causing chemical phlebitis.

Administration Methods

Various vascular access devices are used to administer PN solutions in clinical practice. PN may be administered through either peripheral or central IV lines, depending on the patient's condition and the anticipated length of therapy. In all cases attention must be paid to avoid infection (see Chart 36-6).

Peripheral Method

To supplement oral intake, peripheral parenteral nutrition (PPN) may be prescribed. PPN is given through a peripheral vein; this is possible because the solution is less hypertonic than a full-calorie PN solution. PPN formulas are not nutritionally complete because of their low dextrose content. Lipids are given simultaneously to buffer the PPN and to protect the peripheral vein from irritation. The usual length of therapy using PPN is 5 to 7 days.

Central Method

Because central parenteral nutrition (CPN) solutions have five or six times the solute concentration of blood (and exert an osmotic pressure of about 2,000 mOsm/L), they are given into the vascular system through a catheter inserted into a high-flow, large blood vessel (e.g., ideally at the superior vena cava/right atriocaval junction). Concentrated solutions are then very rapidly diluted to isotonic levels by the blood in this vessel.

Several types of **central venous access devices (CVADs)** are available: percutaneous (or nontunnelled), **peripherally inserted central catheters (PICCs)**, surgically placed (or tunnelled) catheters, and implanted vascular access ports.

Four types of CVADs are available—nontunnelled (or percutaneous) central catheters, PICCs, tunnelled catheters, and implanted ports. Whenever one of these catheters is inserted, catheter tip placement should be confirmed by x-ray studies before PN therapy is initiated. The optimal position is the mid-proximal third of the superior vena cava at the junction of the right atrium.

Percutaneous (Nontunnelled) Central Catheters

Percutaneous (nontunnelled) central catheters are used for short-term (less than 6 weeks) IV therapy in acute care, long-term care, and home care settings. The physician inserts these catheters. Examples of nontunnelled central

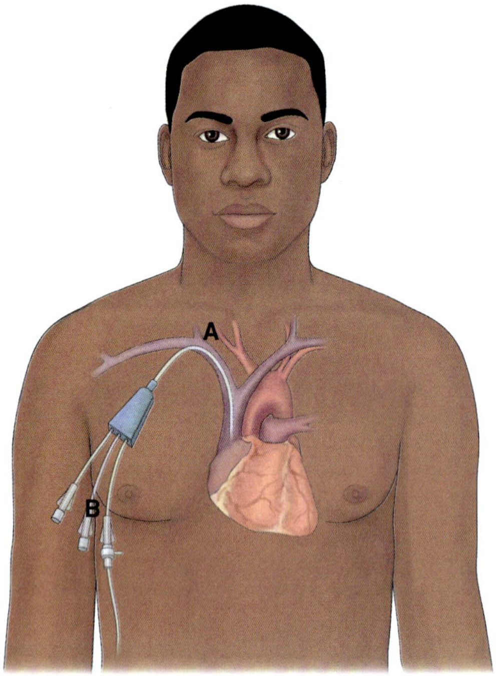

FIGURE 36-6. Subclavian triple-lumen catheter used for parenteral nutrition and other adjunctive therapies. **A.** The catheter is threaded through the subclavian vein into the vena cava. **B.** Each lumen is an avenue for solution administration. The lumens are secured with threaded needleless adapters or Luer-lock–type caps when the device is not in use.

catheters are Vas Cath, percutaneous subclavian Arrow, and Hohn catheters. The subclavian vein is the most common vessel used, because the subclavian area provides a stable insertion site to which the catheter can be anchored, allows the patient freedom of movement, and provides easy access to the dressing site. The jugular vein should only be used as a last resort and then only for 1 to 2 days. Single-, double-, and triple-lumen central catheters are available for central lines, but single-lumen catheters should be used for TNA whenever practicable. The femoral vein should be avoided for this purpose and should only be used as a last resort because of concerns about infection (Gorski, Hadaway, Hagle, et al., 2016). To ensure accessibility in a patient with limited IV access, a triple-lumen subclavian catheter can be used because it offers three ports for various uses (Fig. 36-6). The 16-gauge distal lumen can be used to infuse blood or other viscous fluids. The 18-gauge middle lumen is reserved for PN infusion. The 18-gauge proximal port can be used for administration of blood or medications. A port not being used for fluid administration can be used for obtaining blood specimens, if indicated.

If a single-lumen central catheter is used for administering PN, various restrictions apply. Blood cannot be drawn from the catheter and transfusions of blood products cannot be given through the main line, because red blood cells may coat the lumen of the catheter, thereby reducing the flow of the nutritional solution. Medications also cannot be administered through it, because the medication may be incompatible with the components of the nutritional solution (insulin is an exception). If medications must be given, they must be infused through a separate peripheral IV line, not by piggyback into the PN line.

INSERTION. The procedure is explained so that the patient understands the importance of not touching the catheter insertion site and is aware of what to expect during the insertion procedure. The patient is placed supine in the Trendelenburg position (to produce dilation of neck and shoulder vessels, which makes entry easier and prevents air embolus). The area is shaved if necessary, and the skin is prepared with acetone and alcohol to remove surface oils. Final skin preparation includes cleaning with tincture of 2% iodine or chlorhexidine. To afford maximal accuracy in the placement of the catheter, the patient is instructed to turn the head away from the site of venipuncture and to remain motionless while the catheter is inserted and the wound is dressed. The preferred insertion route is the subclavian vein, which leads into the superior vena cava. The external jugular route can be used, but usually only in emergency situations. Because a nontunnelled central catheter is always a potential source of serious infection, the insertion site should be changed every 4 to 6 weeks or as recommended by latest guidelines.

Full-length sterile drapes are applied. Procaine or lidocaine is injected to anesthetize the skin and underlying tissues. The target area is the inferior border at the midpoint of the clavicle. A large-bore needle on a syringe is inserted and moved parallel to and beneath the clavicle until it enters the vein. The syringe is then detached, and a radiopaque wire is inserted through the needle into the vein. The catheter is then advanced over the wire, the needle is withdrawn, and the hub of the catheter is attached to the IV tubing. Until the syringe is detached from the needle and the catheter is inserted, the patient may be asked to perform the Valsalva manoeuvre. (To do this, the patient is instructed to take a deep breath, hold it, and bear down with mouth closed. Compression of the abdomen may also accomplish the manoeuvre.) The Valsalva manoeuvre is performed to produce a positive phase in central venous pressure, thereby lessening the possibility of air being drawn into the circulatory system (air embolism). The physician sutures the catheter to the skin to avoid inadvertent removal.

A chlorhexidine-impregnated disc or gel with a semipermeable transparent dressing is applied using strict sterile technique (Marschall, Mermel, Fakih, et al., 2014). An isotonic IV solution, such as dextrose 5% in water (D_5W), is administered to keep the vein patent.

The position of the tip of the catheter is checked with x-ray or fluoroscopy to confirm its location in the superior vena cava and to rule out a pneumothorax resulting from inadvertent puncture of the pleura. Once the catheter's position is confirmed, the prescribed PN solution is started. The initial rate of infusion is usually 50 mL/hour, and the rate is gradually increased to the maintenance rate or predetermined dose (e.g., 100 to 125 mL/hour). An infusion pump is always used for administration of PN.

An injection site cap is attached to the end of each central catheter lumen, creating a closed system. IV infusion tubing is connected to the insertion site cap of the central catheter with a threaded needleless adapter or Luer-lock device. Each lumen is labelled according to location (proximal, middle, distal). To ensure patency, all lumens are flushed with a diluted heparin flush initially, daily when not in use, after each intermittent infusion, after blood drawing, and whenever an infusion is disconnected. Force is never used to flush the catheter. If resistance is met, aspiration may restore lumen patency; if this is not effective, the physician is notified. Low-dose tissue plasminogen activator (alteplase) may be prescribed to dissolve a clot or fibrin sheath. If attempts to clear the lumen are ineffective, the lumen is labelled as "clotted off" and not used again.

Peripherally Inserted Central Catheters

PICCs are used for intermediate-term (several days to months) IV therapy in the hospital, long-term care, or home setting. These catheters may be inserted at the bedside or in the outpatient setting by a specially prepared nurse (Walker & Todd, 2013). The basilic or cephalic vein is accessed through the antecubital space, and the catheter is threaded to a designated location, depending on the type of solution to be infused (superior vena cava for PN). Taking of blood pressure and blood specimens from the extremity with the PICC is avoided (see Fig. 36-6).

Surgically Placed (Tunnelled) Central Catheters

Surgically placed central catheters are for long-term use and may remain in place for many years. These catheters are cuffed and can have single or double lumens; examples are the Hickman, Groshong, and Permacath. These catheters are inserted surgically. They are threaded under the skin (reducing the risk of ascending infection) to the subclavian vein, and the distal end of the catheter is advanced into the superior vena cava (Povoski, 2016).

Implanted Vascular Access Ports

Implanted vascular access ports are also used for long-term home IV therapy; examples include the Port-A-Cath, Mediport, Hickman Port, and P.A.S. Port. Instead of exiting from the skin, as do the Hickman and Groshong catheters, the end of the catheter is attached to a small chamber that is placed in a subcutaneous pocket, either on the anterior chest wall or on the forearm. The subcutaneous port requires minimal care and allows the patient complete freedom of activity. Implanted ports are more expensive than the external catheters, and access requires passing a special noncoring needle (Huber-tipped) through the skin into the chamber to initiate IV therapy. Taking of blood pressure and blood specimens from the extremity with the port system should be avoided.

Discontinuing Parenteral Nutrition

The PN solution is discontinued gradually to allow the patient to adjust to decreased levels of glucose. If the PN solution is abruptly terminated, isotonic dextrose is administered for 1 to 2 hours to protect against rebound hypoglycemia. Providing oral carbohydrates shortens the tapering time. Specific symptoms of rebound hypoglycemia include weakness, faintness, sweating, shakiness, feeling cold, confusion, and increased heart rate. Once all IV therapy is completed, the nurse (with a physician's order) removes the nontunnelled central venous catheter or PICC and applies an occlusive dressing to the exit site. Surgically placed central catheters and implanted vascular access ports are removed only by the physician.

In cases of serious illness when death is imminent, some patients or families may request that PN be discontinued. This situation poses many ethical questions, some of which are discussed in Chart 36-4.

Nursing Process

The Patient Receiving Parenteral Nutrition

Assessment

The nurse assists in identifying patients who may be candidates for PN. Indicators include any significant weight loss (10% or more of usual weight), a decrease in oral food intake for more than 1 week, any significant sign of protein loss (serum albumin levels less than 32 g/L, muscle wasting, decreased tissue healing, or abnormal urea nitrogen excretion), and persistent vomiting and diarrhea. The nurse carefully monitors the patient's hydration status, electrolyte levels, and calorie intake.

Nursing Priorities

Based on the assessment data, the major nursing priorities may include the following:

- Nutrition
- Infection prevention
- Fluid and electrolyte balance
- Managing immobility
- Adhering to treatment regimen

Collaborative Problems/ Potential Complications

The most common complications are pneumothorax, air embolism, a clotted or displaced catheter, sepsis, hyperglycemia, rebound hypoglycemia, and fluid overload. These problems and the associated collaborative interventions are described in Table 36-5.

Planning and Goals

The major goals for the patient may include optimal level of nutrition, absence of infection, adequate fluid volume, optimal level of activity (within individual limitations), knowledge of and skill in self-care, and absence of complications.

Nursing Interventions

Maintaining Optimal Nutrition

A continuous, uniform infusion of PN solution over a 24-hour period is desired. However, in some cases (e.g., home care patients), cyclic PN may be

TABLE 36-5 Potential Complications of Parental Nutrition

		Nursing Actions and Collaborative Interventions	
Complications	**Cause**	***Treatment***	***Prevention***
Pneumothorax	Improper catheter placement and inadvertent puncture of the pleura	Place patient in Fowler position Offer reassurance Monitor vital signs Prepare for thoracentesis or chest tube insertion	Assist patient to remain still in Trendelenburg position during catheter insertion
Air embolism	Disconnected tubing Cap missing from port Blocked segment of vascular system	Replace tubing immediately and notify primary provider Replace cap and notify primary provider Turn patient on left side and place in the head-low position. Notify primary provider	Examine all tubing connection sites for their security
Clotted catheter line	Inadequate/infrequent saline/heparin flushes Disruption of infusion	At direction of primary provider, flush with thrombolytic medication as prescribed	Flush lines per established protocols Monitor infusion rate hourly and inspect integrity of the line
Catheter displacement and contamination	Excessive movement, possibly with a nonsecured catheter Separation of tubing and contamination	Stop the infusion, and notify the primary provider	Examine all tubing connection sites Avoid interrupting the main line or piggybacking other lines
Sepsis	Separation of dressings Contaminated solution Infection at insertion site of catheter	Reinforce or change dressing quickly using aseptic technique Discard. Notify pharmacist Notify primary provider. Monitor vital signs	Maintain sterile technique when changing tubing, dressing, or PN bag. Scrub the hub for 15 seconds prior to accessing line for any reason; air dry prior to use
Hyperglycemia	Glucose intolerance	Notify primary provider; addition of insulin to PN solution may be prescribed	Monitor glucose levels (blood and urine) Monitor urine output Observe for stupor, confusion, or lethargy
Fluid overload	Fluid infusing rapidly	Decrease infusion rate Monitor vital signs Notify primary provider Treat respiratory distress by sitting patient upright and administering oxygen as needed, if prescribed	Use infusion pump Verify correct infusion rate ordered
Rebound hypoglycemia	Feedings stopped too abruptly	Monitor for symptoms (weakness, tremors, diaphoresis, headache, hunger, and apprehension); notify primary provider	Gradually wean patient from PN

PN, parenteral nutrition.

Adapted from McClave, S. A., Taylor, B. E., Martindale, R. G., et al. (2016). Guidelines for the provision and assessment of nutrition support therapy in the adult critically ill patient: Society of Critical Care Medicine (SCCM) and American Society for Parenteral and Enteral Nutrition (ASPEN). *Journal of Parenteral and Enteral Nutrition*, *40*(2), 159–211.

appropriate. With cyclic PN, there is a set time during a 24-hour period when PN is infused and a set time when it is not. The time periods for infusion are sufficient to meet the patient's nutritional and pharmacologic needs. Ideally, cyclic PN is infused over a 10- to 15-hour period during the night.

The patient is weighed daily (this may be decreased to two or three times per week) at the same time of the day under the same conditions for accurate comparison. Under the PN regimen (without additional energy expenditure), satisfactory weight maintenance or gain is usually achieved. It is important to keep accurate intake and output records and calculations of fluid balance. A calorie count is kept of any oral nutrients. Trace elements (copper, zinc, chromium, manganese, and selenium) are included in PN solutions and are individualized for each patient. The PN solutions are prescribed daily by the physician form based on laboratory results and patient tolerance.

Preventing Infection

The high dextrose and fat content of PN solutions makes them an ideal culture medium for bacterial and fungal growth, and CVADs provide a port of entry. Gram-positive cocci, gram-negative bacilli, and *Candida* species are frequently isolated as causes of CLABSI. Common organisms include *Staphylococcus aureus, Staphylococcus epidermidis, Pseudomonas aeruginosa, Acinetobacter* species, and *Klebsiella pneumoniae.*

NURSING ALERT

Meticulous aseptic technique is essential to prevent infection any time the IV line setup is manipulated.

The primary sources of microorganisms for catheter-related infections are the skin and the catheter hub. The catheter site is covered with an occlusive gauze dressing that is usually changed every 2 days with opaque or transparent dressing (Gorski et al., 2016). It is recommended that CVAD dressings only if they are damp, bloody, loose, or soiled. The dressings are changed using sterile technique. The nurse and patient wear masks during dressing changes to reduce the possibility of airborne contamination. The area is checked for leakage; bloody or purulent drainage; a kinked catheter; and skin reactions such as inflammation, redness, swelling, or tenderness. The nurse wears sterile gloves and cleanses the area with 70% alcohol, tincture of 2% iodine, or a chlorhexidine gluconate solution on sterile gauze is recommended. The site is cleaned thoroughly using a circular motion from the site outward to approximately 7.5 cm; this procedure is repeated two times. Then, the same cleaning procedure is performed, using 5 × 5-cm gauze pads moistened with sterile water or saline solution (alcohol is used to remove iodine). Next, the catheter ports are cleaned from the exit site to the distal end with an alcohol wipe. The insertion site is covered with an occlusive gauze pad or transparent dressing centred over the area.

The advantages of using a transparent dressing instead of a gauze pad are that it allows frequent examination of the catheter site without changing the dressing, it adheres well, and it is more comfortable for the patient. When an extension set is used with a central catheter, it is considered an extension of the catheter itself. It is not routinely changed with dressing or tubing changes. The connection (hub) between the catheter and extension tubing is secured with adhesive tape to prevent separation and exposure to air. Mainline IV tubing and filters are changed every 72 to 96 hours, and all connections are taped securely to avoid breaks in the integrity of the system. The dressing and tubing are labelled with the date, time of insertion, time of dressing change, and initials of the person who carried out the procedure; this information is also documented in the patient's medical record.

The catheter is another major source of colonization and infection. Studies have been conducted on the use of catheters with antiseptic coatings, antimicrobial coatings, and impregnated antimicrobial cuffs with varying conclusions (Freixas, Bella, Limón, et al., 2013). Prophylactic antibiotic therapy, antibiotic locks, use of antithrombolytics, various exit-site dressings, and the use of various disinfectants for cleansing catheter exit sites have also been proposed (Touré, Lauverjat, Peraldi, et al., 2012).

Maintaining Fluid Balance

An infusion pump is necessary for PN to maintain an accurate rate of administration. A designated rate is set in milliliters per hour, and the rate is checked every 3 to 4 hours. An alarm signals a problem. The infusion rate should not be increased or decreased to compensate for fluids that have infused too quickly or too slowly. If the solution runs out, 10% dextrose and water is infused until the next PN solution is available from the pharmacy.

If the rate is too rapid, hyperosmolar diuresis occurs. Excess glucose is excreted by the renal tubules, pulling large volumes of water into the tubules via osmosis, resulting in higher than normal urine output and intravascular fluid volume deficit. If the hyperosmolar diuresis is severe enough, it can cause dehydration of brain cells resulting in intractable seizures, coma, and death. Symptoms of rapid hypertonic fluid intake include headache, nausea, fever, chills, and increasing lethargy.

If the flow rate is too slow, the patient does not receive the maximal benefit of calories and nitrogen. Intake and output are recorded every 8 hours so that fluid imbalance can be readily detected. The patient is weighed two or three times a week; ideally, the patient shows neither weight loss nor significant weight gain. The nurse assesses for signs of dehydration (e.g., thirst, decreased skin turgor, decreased central venous pressure) and reports these findings to the physician immediately. It is essential to monitor blood glucose levels, because hyperglycemia can cause diuresis and excessive fluid loss.

Encouraging Activity

Activities and ambulation are encouraged when the patient is physically able. With a catheter in the subclavian vein, the patient is free to move the extremities, and activity should be encouraged to maintain good muscle tone. If applicable, the teaching and exercise program initiated in the occupational and physical therapy departments is reinforced.

Promoting Home, Community-Based, and Transitional Care

EDUCATING PATIENTS ABOUT SELF-CARE. Successful home PN requires teaching the patient and family specialized skills using an intensive training program and follow-up supervision in the home. This is best accomplished through a team effort. The financial costs of such programs, although high, are less than those incurred in a hospital. Initiation of a home program may be the only way the patient can be discharged from the hospital.

Ideal candidates for home PN are patients who have a reasonable life expectancy after return home, have a limited number of illnesses other than the one that has resulted in the need for PN, and are highly motivated and fairly self-sufficient. In addition, ability to learn, availability of family interest and support, adequate finances, and the physical plan of the home are factors that must be

CHART 36-7

Assessment: Assessing for Home Nutrition Support

Be alert to the following assessment findings:

- *Water:* Water is necessary for hand hygiene and cleaning of work areas.
- *Electricity:* A reliable power source is needed to provide proper lighting and charging of pumps.
- *Refrigeration:* Refrigeration must be adequate for accommodation of several bags of parenteral nutrition solution.
- *Telephone:* A telephone is necessary for contacting home health personnel, arranging for prompt delivery of supplies, and for emergency purposes.
- *Environment:*
  - Should be free of rodents and insects
  - Should have storage that is not accessible to pets and small children
  - Should be assessed for stairs, carpets, and inaccessible areas, which can limit mobility with infusion pumps if the patient has a disability

Adapted from Durfee, S. M., Adams, S. C., Arthur, E., et al.; Home and Alternate Site Care Task Force and the American Society for Parenteral and Enteral Nutrition (ASPEN). (2014). ASPEN standards for nutrition support: Home and alternate site care. *Nutrition in Clinical Practice*, *29*(4), 542–555.

assessed when the decision about home PN is made (Chart 36-7).

Home health care agencies sponsoring home PN programs have developed teaching brochures and videos for every aspect of treatment, including catheter and dressing care, use of an infusion pump, administration of fat emulsions, and instillation of heparin flushes. Teaching begins in the hospital and continues in the home or in an ambulatory infusion centre. If the patient or assisting family member has a disability (motor or sensory deficit, vision or hearing loss), alternate formats of educational materials are needed to ensure adequate preparation and self-management (Tsang & Carey, 2015).

CONTINUING AND TRANSITIONAL CARE. The home, community-based, or transitional care nurse should be aware that the typical patient needs several instruction sessions for assessment of learning and reinforcement. For more information about home patient education, see Charts 36-8 and 36-9. Special considerations for patients who are older and who go home with nutrition support are presented in Chart 36-10.

Evaluation

Expected patient outcomes may include the following:

1. Attains or maintains nutritional balance
2. Is free of infection at catheter site
   a. Is afebrile
   b. Has no purulent drainage from catheter insertion site
   c. Has intact IV access
3. Is hydrated, as evidenced by good skin turgor
4. Achieves an optimal level of activity, within limitations
5. Demonstrates skill in managing PN regimen
6. Prevents complications
   a. Maintains proper catheter and equipment function
   b. Has no symptoms of sepsis
   c. Maintains metabolic balance within appropriate limits
   d. Shows improved and stabilized nutritional status

CHART 36-8

Educating Patients About Home Parenteral Nutrition

An effective home care teaching program prepares the patient to manage the appropriate form of parenteral nutrition (PN): how to store solutions, set up the infusion, flush the line with heparin, change the dressings, and troubleshoot for problems. The most common complication is sepsis. Strict aseptic technique is taught for hand hygiene, handling equipment, changing the dressing, and preparing the solution.

Troubleshooting Mechanical Difficulties

Mechanical problems usually arise from technical complications in the infusion pump or catheter site. The patient needs to know how to measure the length of the external portion of the catheter; this measurement is used as a comparison if the line is pulled or if dislodgement is suspected. The patient also needs to know how to recognize catheter problems (e.g., leakage, loose cap, blood clot, dislodgement) and should receive a list of instructions explaining what to do for each problem.

Recognizing Metabolic Complications

The patient is given a list of signs and symptoms that indicate metabolic complications (neuropathies, mentation changes, diarrhea, nausea, skin changes, decreased urine output) and directions on how to contact the home health care nurse or physician if any of these complications occurs. The patient is instructed to have routine serum chemistry and hematology tests as well.

Obtaining Psychosocial Support

The psychosocial aspects of home PN are as important as the physiologic and technical concerns. Patients must cope with the loss of eating and with changes in lifestyle brought on by sleep disturbances (frequent urination during infusions, usually two or three times during the night).

Major psychosocial reactions include depression, anger, withdrawal, anxiety, and impaired self-image. A successful home PN program depends on the patient's and family's motivation, emotional stability, and technical competence. Patients and families need to know which support groups are available in the community to help them cope with the transition and to minimize disruption of lifestyle.

CHART 36-9

HOME CARE CHECKLIST • The Patient Receiving Parenteral Nutrition

At the completion of education, the patient and/or caregiver will be able to:

- State the goal and purpose of parenteral nutrition (PN) therapy and any impact on physiologic functioning, ADLs, IADLs, roles, relationships, and spirituality.
- State what types of changes are needed (if any) to support home PN therapy and maintain a clean home environment and prevent infection.
- State how to contact the primary provider, the team of home care professionals overseeing care, and parental nutrition supply vendor.
  - List emergency phone numbers
- State how to obtain medical supplies and carry out catheter and dressing care, and other prescribed regimens.
- Demonstrate how to perform catheter and dressing care.
- Discuss basic components of PN solution and **intravenous fat emulsions**.
- State the name, dose, side effects, frequency, and schedule for all medications.
- Demonstrate accurate and safe administration of medications.
- Demonstrate how to handle solutions and medications correctly.
- Demonstrate correct administration of PN
  - Operate infusion pump
  - Prime tubing and filter
  - Connect and disconnect PN infusion
  - Flush central line
  - Clean and maintain pump
  - Change tubing and filters as directed
- Discuss pump warning signals and how to address these signals.
- Identify possible PN complications and interventions.
- Relate how to reach primary provider with questions or complications.
- Identify a plan for refrigeration of PN solutions and operation of parental nutrition pump during a power outage or other emergency.
- State time and date of follow-up appointments and testing.
- Identify the need for health promotion, disease prevention and screening activities.

ADL, activities of daily living; IADL, independent activities of daily living.

CHART 36-10

The Older Adult Patient and Home Parenteral and Enteral Nutrition

Age-related conditions that affect home nutrition support goals include the following:

- *Arthritis:* Possible decreased hand dexterity and fine motor coordination
- *Sensory impairment:* Inability to hear pump alarms; vision loss may affect ability to see pump menus or fill syringes
- *Constipation:* Decreased overall bowel tone, which can cause intolerance of enteral feedings; increasing water flushes and assessing fibre needs may help
- *Dehydration:* Decreased sensation of thirst, which may require close clinical management of fluid needs
- *Obesity:* Decreased basal metabolic rate increases tendency toward weight gain; may require a reduction in overall kilocalorie intake to compensate
- *Diabetes:* Increased insulin resistance, which makes glucose control during parenteral nutrition infusion more challenging
- *Depression/dementia*: Mood and memory disorders, which may present as low motivation to learn and adhere to the nutrition support regimen
- *Multiple medications:* Conversion to an appropriate intravenous or enteral route, if possible, is required

Adapted from Durfee, S. M., Adams, S. C., Arthur, E., et al.; Home and Alternate Site Care Task Force and the American Society for Parenteral and Enteral Nutrition (ASPEN). (2014). ASPEN standards for nutrition support: Home and alternate site care. *Nutrition in Clinical Practice*, *29*(4), 542–555.

Critical Thinking Exercises

1 A patient with a small bowel obstruction needs a central intravenous catheter for parenteral nutrition. Outline the steps you will take to assist the primary provider during insertion of the central line, including evidence-based infection prevention measures. A patient who is receiving gastrostomy tube feedings is to be discharged from the hospital to return home within the next few days. The patient has many questions regarding the equipment that he will need. What is the strength of the evidence that leads you to espouse the advantages of a simple bolus regimen of tube feeding versus around-the-clock pump feeding? For this ambulatory patient, what is the evidence base that assists you in advising him to select an optimal regimen of administration?

2 A patient has just been diagnosed with small bowel strictures from Crohn's disease and requires preoperative TNA for at least 1 week. The patient does not want a central access catheter placed and prefers to continue with simple IV fluids. What can you tell her about the nutritional advantages of TNA when compared with simple hydration fluids? With strict adherence to protocols for IV line management and dressing care, what complications can be avoided?

3 You are preparing to administer a gravity bolus enteral tube feeding to a patient assigned to your care on a general medicine inpatient unit. You find the patient lying on his side in the bed with the tape no longer around the tube but still adhered to his outer nares. Before proceeding with the feeding, what is the strength of the evidence you will consider when you determine optimal positioning of this patient to prevent complications such as regurgitation and aspiration? What is the evidence base that guides you in determining appropriate placement of the feeding tube?

REFERENCES AND SELECTED READINGS

Books

Brantley, S. L., & Mills, M. E. (2012). Chapter 10: Overview of enteral nutrition. In C. M. Mueller (Ed.). *The ASPEN nutrition support core curriculum* (2nd ed.). Silver Springs, MD: American Society for Parenteral and Enteral Nutrition.

Gangadharan, S. P. (2015). Jejunal feeding tube complications. In T. M. Pawlick, S. K. Maithel, & N. B. Merchant (Eds.). *Gastrointestinal surgery*. New York: Springer.

Journals and Electronic Documents

Arora, G., & Lukens, F. J. (2015). Percutaneous endoscopic gastrostomy (PEG) tube placement. In D. A. Sherwinter (Ed.): *Medscape News and Perspective*. Retrieved from: www.emedicine.medscape.com/article/149665-overview#a9.

American Nurses Association (ANA). (2011). *Forgoing nutrition and hydration*. Retrieved from: www.nursingworld.org/MainMenuCategories/EthicsStandards/Ethics-Position-Statements/prtetnutr14451.pdf

Gastrostomies, Nasogastric, and Nasoenteric Intubation and Feeding

Berg, P., & McCallum, R. (2016). Dumping syndrome: A review of the current concepts of pathophysiology, diagnosis, and treatment. *Digestive Diseases and Sciences*, *61*(1), 11–18.

Blumenstein, I., Shastri, Y. M., & Stein, J. (2014). Gastroenteric tube feeding: Techniques, problems, and solutions. *World Journal of Gastroenterology*, *20*(26), 8505–8524.

DeLegge, M. H. (2015). Gastrostomy tubes: Placement and routine care. In J. R. Saltzman, T. O. Lipman, & A. C. Travis (Eds.). *UpToDate*. Waltham, MA: UpToDate. Retrieved from www.uptodate-com.medjournal.hmc.psu.edu.

Dickerson, R. N., Pitts, S. L., Maish, G. O, 3rd., et al. (2012). A reappraisal of nitrogen requirements for patients with critical illness and trauma. *Journal of Trauma and Acute Care Surgery*, *73*(3), 549–557.

DiLibero, J., Lavieri, M., O'Donoghue, S., et al. (2015). Withholding or continuing enteral feedings during repositioning and the incidence of aspiration. *American Journal of Critical Care*, *24*(3), 258–261.

Eveleigh, Law, Pullyblank, et al., (2011). Nasograstric feeding tube placement: Changing culture. *Nursing Times*, *107*(41), 14–16.

Flodgren, G., Conterno, L., Mayhew, A., et al. (2013). Interventions to improve professional adherence to guidelines for prevention of device-related infections. *The Cochrane Database of Systematic Reviews*, (3), CD006559.

Freixas, N., Bella, F., Limón, E., et al. (2013). Impact of a multimodal intervention to reduce bloodstream infections related to vascular catheters in non-ICU wards: A multicentre study. *Clinical Microbiology and Infection*, *19*(9), 838–844.

Fujita, T., Tanabe, M., Kobayashi, T., et al. (2013). Percutaneous gastrostomy tube placement using a balloon catheter in patients with head and neck cancer. *Journal of Parenteral and Enteral Nutrition*, *37*(1), 117–122.

Gagnon, L. E., & Kawawacki Sheff, E. J. (2012). Outcomes and complications after bariatric surgery. *American Journal of Nursing*, *112*(9), 26–36.

Gervasio, J. (2015). Total nutrient admixtures (3-in-1) pros vs cons for adults. *Nutrition in Clinical Practice*, *30*(3), 331–335.

Gorski, L., Hadaway, L., Hagle, M. E., et al. (2016). Infusion therapy standards of practice. *Journal of Infusion Nursing (Supplement)*, *39*(1S), S1–S159.

Gupta, A., & Khanna, S. (2014). Community-acquired *Clostridium difficile* infection: An increasing public health threat. *Infectious Drug Resistance Journal, 7*, 63–72. doi: 10.2147/IDR.S46780.

Headley, C. M. (2012). Deadly Diarrhea: Clostridium difficile infection. *Nephrology Nursing Journal*, *39*(6), 459–468.

Institute for Safe Medication Practices (ISMP). (2015). *Update on implementation of the new ENFit enteral connectors*. Retrieved from www.ismp.org/newsletters/acutecare/showarticle.aspx?id = 114.

Joint Commission (2014). Managing risk during transition to new ISO tubing connector standards. *Joint Commission Sentinel Event Alert*. Issue 53. Retrieved on 06/20/2016 at www.jointcommission.org/assets/1/6/SEA_53_Connectors_8_19_14_final.pdf

Leckey, J., Davis, S., & Raphael-Grimm, T. (2017). Nursing assessment of patients requiring enteral and gastric feeding tubes: An exploratory approach. *Gastroenterology Nursing*, *40*(6), 469–483.

Lor, Y. C., Shih, P. C., Chen, H. H., et al. (2018). The application of lidocaine to alleviate the discomfort of nasogastric tube insertion: A systematic review and meta-analysis. *Medicine (Baltimore)*, *97*(5), e9746.

Marschall, J., Mermel, L. A., Fakih, M., et al. (2014). Strategies to prevent central line-associated bloodstream in acute care hospitals: 2014 update. *Infection Control and Hospital Epidemiology*, *35*(7), 753–771.

McClave, S. A., Taylor, B. E., Martindale, R. G., et al. (2016). Guidelines for the provision and assessment of nutrition support therapy in the adult critically ill patient: Society of Critical Care Medicine (SCCM) and American Society for Parenteral and Enteral Nutrition (ASPEN). *Journal of Parenteral and Enteral Nutrition*, *40*(2), 159–211.

Metheny, N. (2016). AACN practice alert: Initial and ongoing verification of feeding tube placement in adults. *Critical Care Nurse*, *36*(2), e8–e13.

Miller, K. R., McClave, S. A., Kiraly, L. N., et al. (2014). A tutorial on enteral access in adult patients in the hospitalized setting. *Journal of Parenteral and Enteral Nutrition*, *38*(3), 282–295.

Ni, M. Z., Huddy, J. R., Priest, O. H., et al. (2017). Selecting pH cut-offs for the safe verification of nasogastric feeding tube placement: A decision analytical modelling approach. *BMJ Open*, *7*, e018128.

Povoski, S. (2016). Long-term central venous access. *Cancer Management*. Retrieved May 27, 2018, from http://www.cancernetwork.com/cancer-management/long-term-central-venous-access.

Providence Health Care. (2018). *Tube feeding at home: A guidebook for patients, families, and caregivers. Catalogue no. BB.210.T79, Vancouver, BC: Vancouver Coastal Health*. Retrieved May 27, 2018, from https://vch.eduhealth.ca/pdfs/bb/bb.210.t79.pdf

Rahnemai-Azar, A. A., Rahnemaiazar A. A., Naghshizadian, R., et al. (2014). Percutaneous endoscopic gastrostomy: Indications, technique, complications and management. *World Journal of Gastroenterology, 20*(24), 7739–7751.

Reignier, J., Mercier, E., Le Gouge, A., et al. (2013). Effect of not monitoring residual gastric volume on risk of ventilator-associated pneumonia in adults receiving mechanical ventilation and early enteral feeding: A randomized controlled study. *Journal of American Medical Association, 309*(3), 249–256.

Santos, S. C., Woith, W., Freitas, M. I., et al. (2016). Methods to determine the internal length of nasogastric feeding tubes: An integrative review. *International Journal of Nursing Studies, 61*, 95–103.

Shipley, K., Gallo, A. M., & Fields, W. (2016). Is your feeding tube clogged? maintenance of gastrostomy and gastrojejunostomy tubes. *Medsurg Nursing, 25*(4), 224–228.

Silander, E., Jacobsson, I., Bertéus-Forslund, H., et al. (2013). Energy intake and sources of nutritional support in patients with head and neck cancer: A randomised longitudinal study. *European Journal of Clinical Nutrition, 67*(1), 47–52.

Staes, C., Jacobs, J., Mayer, J., et al. (2013). Description of outbreaks of health-care-associated infections related to compounding pharmacies, 2000–12. *American Journal of Health-System Pharmacy, 70*(15), 1301–1312.

Styles, E. (2013). Providing artificial nutrition and hydration in palliative care. *Nursing Standard, 27*(20), 35–42.

Touré, A., Lauverjat, M., Peraldi, C., et al. (2012). Taurolidine lock solution in the secondary prevention of central venous catheter-associated bloodstream infection in home parenteral nutrition patients. *Clinical Nutrition, 31*(4), 567–570.

Tsang, P. Y., & Carey, S. (2015). Impact of home parenteral nutrition on daily life: A qualitative study of eight patients. *Nutrition & Dietetics, 72*(1), 16–21.

Walker, G., & Todd, A. (2013). Nurse-led PICC insertion: Is it cost effective?. *British Journal of Nursing, 22*(19), S9–S15.

Williams, T. A., Leslie, G., Mills, L., et al. (2013). Frequency of aspirating gastric tubes for patients receiving enteral nutrition in the ICU: A randomized controlled trial. *Journal of Parenteral and Enteral Nutrition, 38*(7), 809–816.

Wong, K., Chan, H., Wong, C., et al. (2017). Using color flow detection of air insufflation to improve accuracy in verifying nasogastric tube position. *The American Journal of Emergency Medicine, 35*(2), 333–336.

Yoon, E., & Nishihara, K. (2017). Percutaneous transesophageal gastrotubing (PTEG) as an alternative long-term tube feeding procedure when gastrostomy is not feasible. *Therapeutic Advances in Gastroenterology, 10*(12), 911–917.

Resources

American Cancer Society: http://www.cancer.org
American Society for Nutrition: http://www.nutrition.org/
American Society for Gastrointestinal Endoscopy: http://www.asge.org
American Society for Parenteral and Enteral Nutrition (ASPEN): http://www.nutritioncare.org
Canadian Cancer Society, National Office: http://www.cancer.ca
Canadian Parenteral-Enteral Nutrition Association: http://www.cpena.ca
Canadian Society for Clinical Nutrition: http://www.cscn-scnc.ca
Canadian Society of Intestinal Research: http://www.badgut.com
Health Canada, Drug Product Database (DPD): http://www.hc-sc.gc.ca/dhp-mps/prodpharma/databasdon/index-eng.php/
Society of Gastroenterology Nurses and Associates, Inc.: http://www.sgna.org

37 Management of Patients With Gastric and Duodenal Disorders

Adapted by Pamela Cawley

Learning Objectives

On completion of this chapter, the learner will be able to:

1. Compare the etiology, clinical manifestations, and management of acute gastritis, chronic gastritis, and peptic ulcer.
2. Describe nursing management of patients with gastritis.
3. Use the nursing process as a framework for care of patients with peptic ulcer.
4. Describe the dietary, pharmacologic, and surgical treatment of peptic ulcer.
5. Describe the nursing management of patients who undergo surgical procedures to treat obesity.
6. Use the nursing process as a framework for care of patients with gastric cancer.
7. Use the nursing process as a framework for care of patients undergoing gastric surgery.
8. Identify the complications of gastric surgery and their prevention and management.
9. Describe the home health care needs of the patient who has had gastric surgery.

A person's nutritional status depends not only on the type and amount of intake, but also on the functioning of the gastric and intestinal portions of the gastrointestinal (GI) system. According to the Canadian Digestive Health Foundation, more than 20 million Canadians experience a digestive health challenge or disorder (Canadian Digestive Health Foundation, 2018). This chapter describes disorders of the stomach and **duodenum**, their treatment, and related nursing care.

Gastritis

Gastritis (inflammation of the **gastric** or stomach mucosa) is a common GI concern. Gastritis may be acute, lasting several hours to a few days, or chronic, resulting from repeated exposure to irritating agents or recurring episodes of acute gastritis.

Acute gastritis is often caused by dietary indiscretion—a person eats food that is irritating, too highly seasoned, or contaminated with disease-causing microorganisms. Other causes of acute gastritis include overuse of aspirin and other nonsteroidal anti-inflammatory drugs (NSAIDs), excessive alcohol intake, bile reflux, and radiation therapy. A more severe form of acute gastritis is caused by the ingestion of strong acid or alkali, which may cause the mucosa to become gangrenous or to perforate. Scarring can occur, resulting in pyloric stenosis or obstruction. Acute gastritis also may develop in acute illnesses, especially when the patient has had major traumatic injuries; burns; severe infection; hepatic, renal, or respiratory failure; or major surgery. Gastritis may be the first sign of an acute systemic infection.

Chronic gastritis and prolonged inflammation of the stomach may be caused either by benign or malignant ulcers of the stomach or by the bacteria ***Helicobacter pylori***. Chronic gastritis is sometimes associated with autoimmune diseases such as pernicious anemia; dietary factors such as caffeine; the use of medications such as NSAIDs or bisphosphonates (e.g., alendronate [Fosamax], risedronate [Actonel], ibandronate [Boniva]); alcohol; smoking; or chronic reflux of pancreatic secretions and bile into the stomach.

Pathophysiology

In gastritis, the gastric mucous membrane becomes edematous and hyperemic (congested with fluid and blood) and undergoes superficial erosion (Fig. 37-1). It secretes a scanty amount of gastric juice, containing very little acid but much mucus. Superficial ulceration may occur and can lead to hemorrhage.

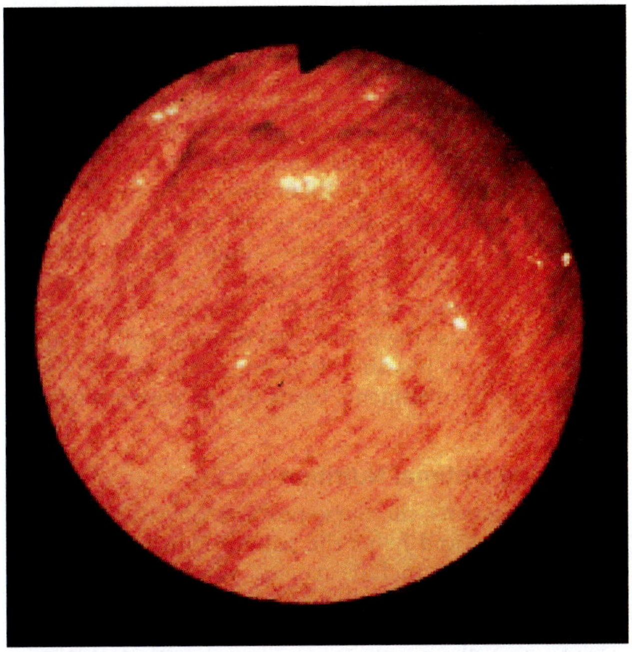

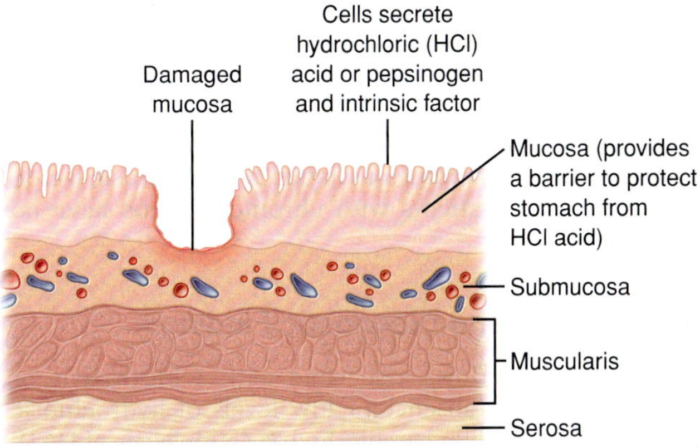

FIGURE 37-1. Endoscopic view of erosive gastritis (**left**). Damage from irritants (**right**) results in increased intracellular pH, impaired enzyme function, disrupted cellular structures, ischemia, vascular stasis, and tissue death. (Reproduced with permission from Porth, C. M., & Matfin, G. (2009). *Pathophysiology: Concepts of altered health states* (8th ed.). Philadelphia, PA: Lippincott Williams & Wilkins.)

Glossary

achlorhydria: lack of hydrochloric acid in digestive secretions of the stomach

antrectomy: removal of the pyloric (antrum) portion of the stomach with anastomosis (surgical connection) to the duodenum (gastroduodenostomy or Billroth I) or anastomosis to the jejunum (gastrojejunostomy or Billroth II)

dumping syndrome: physiologic response to rapid emptying of gastric contents into the jejunum, manifested by nausea, weakness, sweating, palpitations, syncope, and possibly diarrhea; occurs in patients who have had partial gastrectomy and gastrojejunostomy

duodenum: first portion of the small intestine, between the stomach and the jejunum

enteroclysis: fluoroscopic x-ray of the small intestine; a tube is placed from the nose or mouth through the esophagus and the stomach to the duodenum, a barium-based liquid contrast material is infused through the tube, and x-rays are taken as it travels through the duodenum

gastric: refers to the stomach

gastric outlet obstruction: any condition that mechanically impedes usual gastric emptying; there is obstruction of the channel of the pylorus and duodenum through which the stomach empties

gastritis: inflammation of the stomach

Helicobacter pylori: a spiral-shaped gram-negative bacterium that colonizes the gastric mucosa; is involved in most cases of peptic ulcer disease

hematemesis: vomiting of blood: histamine-2 (H_2) receptor antagonist: a pharmacologic agent that inhibits histamine action at the H_2 receptors of the stomach, resulting in inhibition of gastric acid secretion

melena: tarry or black stools; indicative of blood in stools

omentum: fold of the peritoneum that surrounds the stomach and other organs of the abdomen

peritoneum: thin membrane that lines the inside of the wall of the abdomen and covers all the abdominal organs

proton pump inhibitors: pharmacologic agents that block acid secretion by irreversibly binding to and inhibiting the hydrogen–potassium adenosine triphosphatase pump system at the secretory surface of gastric parietal cells; most potent inhibitors of gastric acid secretion

pyloroplasty: surgical procedure to increase the opening of the pyloric orifice

pylorus: opening between the stomach and the duodenum

pyrosis: heartburn

serosa: thin membrane that covers the outer surface of the stomach; visceral peritoneum covering the outer surface of the stomach

stenosis: narrowing or tightening of an opening or passage in the body

Clinical Manifestations

The patient with acute gastritis may have a rapid onset of symptoms, such as abdominal discomfort, headache, lassitude, nausea, anorexia, vomiting, and hiccupping, which can last from a few hours to a few days. The patient with chronic gastritis may report anorexia, heartburn after eating, belching, a sour taste in the mouth, or nausea and vomiting. Some patients may have only mild epigastric discomfort or report intolerance to spicy or fatty foods or slight pain that is relieved by eating. Patients with chronic gastritis from vitamin deficiency usually have evidence of malabsorption of vitamin B_{12} caused by the production of antibodies that interfere with the binding of vitamin B_{12} to intrinsic factor. However, some patients with chronic gastritis have no symptoms.

Assessment and Diagnostic Findings

Gastritis is sometimes associated with **achlorhydria** or hypochlorhydria (absence or low levels of hydrochloric acid [HCl]) or with hyperchlorhydria (high levels of HCl). Diagnosis can be determined by an upper GI x-ray series or endoscopy and histologic examination of a tissue specimen obtained by biopsy. Diagnostic measures for detecting *H. pylori* infection may be used and are discussed in the section on peptic ulcers.

Medical Management

The gastric mucosa is capable of repairing itself after an episode of gastritis. As a rule, the patient recovers in about 1 day, although the appetite may be diminished for an additional 2 or 3 days. Acute gastritis is also managed by instructing the patient to refrain from alcohol and food until symptoms subside. When the patient can take nourishment by mouth, a nonirritating diet is recommended. If the symptoms persist, intravenous (IV) fluids may need to be administered. If bleeding is present, management is similar to the procedures used to control upper GI tract hemorrhage discussed later in this chapter.

If gastritis is caused by ingestion of strong acids or alkalis, emergency treatment consists of diluting and neutralizing the offending agent. To neutralize acids, common antacids (e.g., aluminum hydroxide) are used; to neutralize an alkali, diluted lemon juice or diluted vinegar is used. If corrosion is extensive or severe, emetics and lavage are avoided because of the danger of perforation and damage to the esophagus.

Therapy is supportive and may include nasogastric (NG) intubation, analgesic agents and sedatives, antacids, and IV fluids. Fibreoptic endoscopy may be necessary. In extreme cases, emergency surgery may be required to remove gangrenous or perforated tissue. A gastric resection or a gastrojejunostomy (anastomosis of jejunum to stomach to detour around the pylorus) may be necessary to treat pyloric obstruction, a narrowing of the pyloric orifice, which cannot be relieved by medical management.

Chronic gastritis is managed by modifying the patient's diet, promoting rest, reducing stress, recommending avoidance of alcohol and NSAIDs, and initiating pharmacotherapy. *H. pylori* may be treated with selected drug combinations (Table 37-1) (Guo-Xing & Jun, 2018).

Nursing Management

Reducing Anxiety

If the patient has ingested acids or alkalis, emergency measures may be necessary. The nurse offers supportive therapy to the patient and family during treatment and after the ingested acid or alkali has been neutralized or diluted. In some cases, the nurse may need to prepare the patient for additional diagnostic studies (endoscopies) or surgery. The patient may be anxious because of pain and planned treatment modalities. The nurse uses a calm approach to assess the patient and to answer all questions as completely as possible. It is important to explain all procedures and treatments based on the patient's level of understanding.

Promoting Optimal Nutrition

For acute gastritis, the nurse provides physical and emotional support and helps the patient manage the symptoms, which may include nausea, vomiting, heartburn, and fatigue. The patient should take no foods or fluids by mouth—possibly for a few days—until the acute symptoms subside, thus allowing the gastric mucosa to heal. If IV therapy is necessary, the nurse monitors fluid intake and output along with serum electrolyte values. After the symptoms subside, the nurse may offer the patient ice chips followed by clear liquids. Introducing solid food as soon as possible may provide adequate oral nutrition, decrease the need for IV therapy, and minimize irritation to the gastric mucosa. As food is introduced, the nurse evaluates and reports any symptoms that suggest a repeat episode of gastritis.

The nurse discourages the intake of caffeinated beverages, because caffeine is a central nervous system stimulant that increases gastric activity and pepsin secretion. It is also important to discourage alcohol use. Discouraging cigarette smoking is important because nicotine reduces the secretion of pancreatic bicarbonate, which inhibits the neutralization of gastric acid in the duodenum (Nordenstedt, Graham, Kramer, et al., 2013). When appropriate, the nurse initiates and refers the patient for alcohol counselling and smoking cessation programs.

Promoting Fluid Balance

Daily fluid intake and output are monitored to detect early signs of dehydration (minimal fluid intake of 1.5 L/day, minimal output of 30 mL/hour). If food and oral fluids are withheld, IV fluids (3 L/day) usually are prescribed and a record of fluid intake plus caloric value (1 L of 5% dextrose in water = 170 calories of carbohydrate) needs to be maintained. Electrolyte values (sodium, potassium, chloride) are assessed every 24 hours to detect any imbalance.

The nurse must always be alert for any indicators of hemorrhagic gastritis, which include **hematemesis** (vomiting of blood), tachycardia, and hypotension. If these occur, the physician is notified and the patient's vital signs are monitored as the patient's condition warrants. Guidelines for managing upper GI tract bleeding are discussed later in this chapter.

Relieving Pain

Measures to help relieve pain include instructing the patient to avoid foods and beverages that may be irritating to the gastric mucosa and instructing the patient about the

TABLE 37-1 Selected Pharmacotherapy for Peptic Ulcer Disease and Gastritis

Pharmacologic Agent	Major Action	Key Nursing Considerations
Antibiotics		
Amoxicillin (Amoxil)	A bactericidal antibiotic that assists with eradicating *H. pylori* bacteria in the gastric mucosa	• May cause diarrhea • Should not be used in patients allergic to penicillin
Clarithromycin (Biaxin)	Exerts bactericidal effects to eradicate *H. pylori* bacteria in the gastric mucosa	• May cause GI upset, headache, altered taste • Many drug–drug interactions (e.g., cisapride, colchicine, lovastatin, warfarin [Coumadin])
Metronidazole (Flagyl)	A synthetic antibacterial and antiprotozoal agent that assists with eradicating *H. pylori* bacteria in the gastric mucosa when administered with other antibiotics and proton pump inhibitors	• Should be administered with meals to decrease GI upset; may cause anorexia and metallic taste • Patient should avoid alcohol; Flagyl increases blood-thinning effects of warfarin (Coumadin)
Tetracycline	Exerts bacteriostatic effects to eradicate *H. pylori* bacteria in the gastric mucosa	• May cause photosensitivity reaction; warn patient to use sunscreen • May cause GI upset • Must be used with caution in patients with renal or hepatic impairment • Milk or dairy products may reduce effectiveness
Antidiarrheal		
Bismuth subsalicylate (Pepto-Bismol)	Suppresses *H. pylori* bacteria in the gastric mucosa and assists with healing of mucosal ulcers	• Given concurrently with antibiotics to eradicate *H. pylori* infection • Should be taken on empty stomach
Histamine-2 (H_2) Receptor Antagonists		
Cimetidine (Tagamet)	Decreases amount of HCl produced by stomach by blocking action of histamine on histamine receptors of parietal cells in the stomach	• Least expensive of H_2 receptor antagonists • May cause confusion, agitation, or coma in older adults or those with renal or hepatic insufficiency • Long-term use may cause diarrhea, dizziness, gynecomastia • Many drug–drug interactions (e.g., amiodarone, amitriptyline, benzodiazepines, metoprolol, nifedipine, phenytoin, warfarin [Coumadin])
Famotidine (Pepcid)	Same as for cimetidine	• Best choice for critically ill patient because it is known to have the least risk of drug–drug interactions; does not alter liver metabolism • Prolonged half-life in patients with renal insufficiency • Short-term relief for GERD
Nizatidine (Axid)	Same as for cimetidine	• Used for treatment of ulcers and GERD • Prolonged half-life in patients with renal insufficiency • May cause headache, dizziness, diarrhea, nausea/vomiting, GI upset as well as urticaria
Ranitidine (Zantac)	Same as for cimetidine	• Prolonged half-life in patients with renal and hepatic insufficiency • Causes fewer side effects than cimetidine • May cause headache, dizziness, constipation, nausea and vomiting, or abdominal discomfort
Proton Pump Inhibitors of Gastric Acid (PPIs)		
Esomeprazole (Nexium)	Decreases gastric acid secretion by slowing the hydrogen–potassium adenosine triphosphatase (H^+, K^+-) pump on the surface of the parietal cells of the stomach	• Used mainly for treatment of duodenal ulcer disease and *H. pylori* infection • A delayed-release capsule that is to be swallowed whole and taken before meals
Lansoprazole (Prevacid)	Decreases gastric acid secretion by slowing the H^+, K^+-ATPase pump on the surface of the parietal cells	• A delayed-release capsule that is to be swallowed whole and taken before meals
Omeprazole (Prilosec)	Same as for lansoprazole	• A delayed-release capsule that is to be swallowed whole and taken before meals • May cause diarrhea, nausea, constipation, abdominal pain, vomiting, headache, or dizziness
Pantoprazole (Protonix)	Same as for lansoprazole	• A delayed-release capsule that is to be swallowed whole and taken before meals • May cause diarrhea and hyperglycemia, headache, abdominal pain, and abnormal liver function tests

continued >

TABLE 37-1 Selected Pharmacotherapy for Peptic Ulcer Disease and Gastritis (Continued)

Pharmacologic Agent	Major Action	Key Nursing Considerations
Rabeprazole (AcipHex)	Same as for lansoprazole	• A delayed-release tablet to be swallowed whole • May cause abdominal pain, diarrhea, nausea, and headache • Drug–drug interactions with digoxin, iron, and warfarin (Coumadin)
Prostaglandin E_1 Analogue		
Misoprostol (Cytotec)	Synthetic prostaglandin; protects the gastric mucosa from agents that cause ulcers; also increases mucous production and bicarbonate levels	• Used to prevent ulceration in patients using NSAIDs • Administer with food • May cause diarrhea and cramping (including uterine cramping) • Used mainly for the treatment of duodenal ulcers
Sucralfate (Carafate)	Creates a viscous substance in the presence of gastric acid that forms a protective barrier, binding to the surface of the ulcer, and prevents digestion by pepsin	• Should be taken without food but with water • Other medications should be taken 2 hours before or after this medication • May cause constipation or nausea

GERD, gastroesophageal reflux disease; GI, gastrointestinal; NSAID, nonsteroidal anti-inflammatory drug.

Adapted from Karch, A. M. (2014). *Lippincott nursing drug guide*. Philadelphia, PA: Lippincott Williams & Wilkins.

correct use of medications to relieve chronic gastritis. The nurse must regularly assess the patient's level of pain and the extent of comfort achieved through the use of medications and avoidance of irritating substances.

Promoting Home, Community-Based, and Transitional Care

Educating Patients About Self-Care

The nurse evaluates the patient's knowledge about gastritis and develops an individualized teaching plan that includes information about stress management, diet, and medications (Chart 37-1). Dietary instructions take into account the patient's daily caloric needs, food preferences, and pattern of eating. The nurse and patient review foods and other substances to be avoided (e.g., spicy, irritating, or highly seasoned foods; caffeine; nicotine; alcohol). Consultation with a dietitian may be recommended.

Providing information about prescribed antibiotics, bismuth salts, medications to decrease gastric secretion, and medications to protect mucosal cells from gastric secretions may help the patient to better understand why these medications assist in recovery and prevent recurrence. The importance of completing the medication regimen as prescribed to eradicate *H. pylori* infection must be reinforced to the patient and any caregivers.

Continuing and Transitional Care

The nurse reinforces previous teaching and conducts ongoing assessment of the patient's symptoms and progress. Patients with malabsorption of vitamin B_{12} need information about lifelong vitamin B_{12} injections; the nurse may

CHART 37-1

HOME CARE CHECKLIST • The Patient With Gastritis

At the completion of education, the patient and/or caregiver will be able to:

- State the impact of gastritis on physiologic functioning, ADLs, IADLs, roles, relationships, and spirituality.
  - State need for vitamin B_{12} injections if patient has pernicious anemia.
- Explain the importance of and necessity for adherence with prescribed medication regimen.
- Demonstrate methods of keeping track of the medication regimen and storage of the prescribed medications, and use reminders such as beepers and/or pillboxes.
- State the name, dose, side effects, frequency, and schedule for all medications.
- Identify foods and other substances that may cause gastritis (e.g., spicy, highly seasoned foods, caffeine, nicotine, alcohol).
- Identify side effects and complications (e.g., increased or return of abdominal discomfort, inability to ingest adequate solids and liquids) that should be reported to primary provider.
- State how to reach primary provider with questions or complications.
- State time and date of follow-up appointments and testing.

ADL, activities of daily living; IADL, independent activities of daily living.

instruct a family member or caregiver how to administer the injections or make arrangements for the patient to receive the injections from a health care professional. Finally, the nurse emphasizes the importance of keeping follow-up appointments with health care professionals.

Peptic Ulcer Disease

A peptic ulcer may be referred to as a gastric, duodenal, or esophageal ulcer, depending on its location. A peptic ulcer is an excavation (hollowed-out area) that forms in the mucosal wall of the stomach, in the **pylorus** (the opening between the stomach and the duodenum), in the duodenum (the first part of the small intestine), or in the esophagus. Erosion of a circumscribed area of mucous membrane is the cause (Fig. 37-2). This erosion may extend as deeply as the muscle layers or through the muscle to the **peritoneum**. It is estimated that there are 1.3 million Canadians with peptic ulcer disease, and that 1 in 10 Canadians will develop the disease in their lifetime (Canadian Digestive Health Foundation, 2018).

Peptic ulcers are more likely to occur in the duodenum than in the stomach. As a rule they occur alone, but they may occur in multiples. Chronic gastric ulcers tend to occur in the lesser curvature of the stomach, near the pylorus. Table 37-2 compares the features of gastric and duodenal ulcers. Esophageal ulcers occur as a result of the backward flow of HCl from the stomach into the esophagus (gastroesophageal reflux disease [GERD]).

Peptic ulcer disease occurs with the greatest frequency in people between 40 and 60 years of age. It is relatively uncommon in women of childbearing age, but it has been observed in children and even in infants. After menopause, the incidence of peptic ulcers in women is almost equal to that in men. Peptic ulcers in the body of the stomach can occur without excessive acid secretion.

In the past, stress and anxiety were thought to be causes of ulcers, but research has documented that peptic ulcers result from infection with the gram-negative bacteria *H. pylori*, which may be acquired through ingestion of food and water. Person-to-person transmission of the bacteria also occurs through close contact and exposure to emesis.

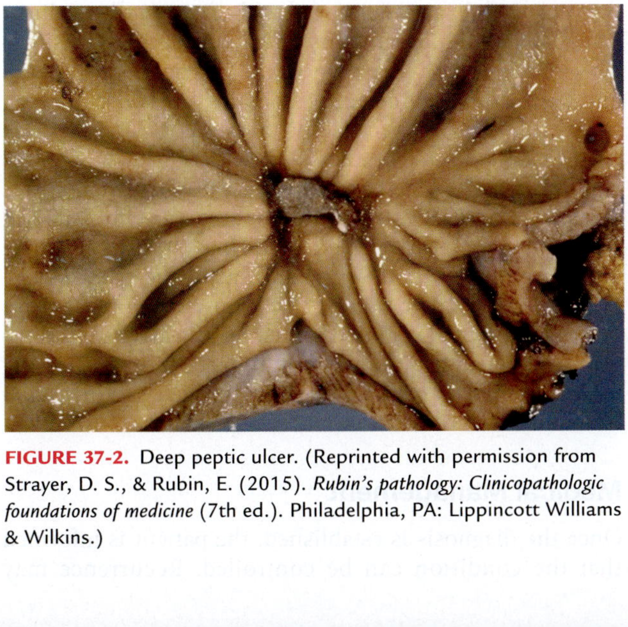

FIGURE 37-2. Deep peptic ulcer. (Reprinted with permission from Strayer, D. S., & Rubin, E. (2015). *Rubin's pathology: Clinicopathologic foundations of medicine* (7th ed.). Philadelphia, PA: Lippincott Williams & Wilkins.)

TABLE 37-2 Comparison of Duodenal and Gastric Ulcers

Gastric Ulcer	Incidence
Age 30–60	Usually 50 and over
Male:female = 2–3:1	Male:female = 1:1
80% of peptic ulcers are duodenal	15% of peptic ulcers are gastric
Signs, Symptoms, and Clinical Findings	
Hypersecretion of stomach acid (HCl)	Normal–hyposecretion of stomach acid (HCl)
May have weight gain	Weight loss may occur
Pain occurs 2–3 hours after a meal; often awakened 1–2 AM; ingestion of food relieves pain	Pain occurs ½–1 hour after a meal; rarely occurs at night; may be relieved by vomiting; ingestion of food does not help, sometimes increases pain
Vomiting uncommon	Vomiting common
Hemorrhage less likely than with gastric ulcer, but if present, melena more common than hematemesis	Hemorrhage more likely to occur than with duodenal ulcer; hematemesis more common than melena
More likely to perforate than gastric ulcers	
Malignancy Possibility	
Rare	Occasionally
Risk Factors	
H. pylori, alcohol, smoking, cirrhosis, stress	*H. pylori*, gastritis, alcohol, smoking, use of NSAIDs, stress

NSAID, nonsteroidal anti-inflammatory drug.

Adapted from https://emedicine.medscape.com/article/181753-clinical.

Although *H. pylori* infection is common in Canada, most infected people do not develop ulcers. It is not known why *H. pylori* infection does not cause ulcers in all people, but most likely the predisposition to ulcer formation depends on certain factors, such as the type of *H. pylori* and other as yet unknown factors (Lacy, Talley, Locke, et al., 2012; Smolovic, Stanisavljevic, Golubovic, et al., 2014; Fashner & Gitu, 2015).

In addition, excessive secretion of HCl in the stomach may contribute to the formation of peptic ulcers, and stress may be associated with its increased secretion. The ingestion of milk and caffeinated beverages, smoking, and alcohol also may increase HCl secretion. Stress and eating spicy foods may make peptic ulcers worse.

Familial tendency also may be a significant predisposing factor. People with blood type O are more susceptible to peptic ulcers than are those with blood type A, B, or AB. There is also an association between peptic ulcers and chronic pulmonary disease or chronic renal disease. Other predisposing factors associated with peptic ulcer include chronic use of NSAIDs, alcohol ingestion, and excessive smoking.

Peptic ulcers are found in rare cases in patients with tumours that cause secretion of excessive amounts of the hormone gastrin. The Zollinger–Ellison syndrome (ZES) consists of severe peptic ulcers, extreme gastric hyperacidity, and gastrin-secreting benign or malignant tumours of the pancreas (Tooker & Dexter, 2017).

Pathophysiology

Peptic ulcers occur mainly in the gastroduodenal mucosa because this tissue cannot withstand the digestive action of gastric acid (HCl) and pepsin. The erosion is caused by the increased concentration or activity of acid–pepsin or by decreased resistance of the mucosa. A damaged mucosa cannot secrete enough mucus to act as a barrier against HCl. The use of NSAIDs inhibits the secretion of mucus that protects the mucosa. Patients with duodenal ulcers secrete more acid than usual, whereas patients with gastric ulcers tend to secrete usual or decreased levels of acid. Damage to the gastroduodenal mucosa results in decreased resistance to bacteria, and thus infection from *H. pylori* bacteria may occur.

ZES is suspected when a patient has several peptic ulcers or an ulcer that is resistant to standard medical therapy. It is identified by the following: hypersecretion of gastric juice, duodenal ulcers, and gastrinomas (islet cell tumours) in the pancreas. Ninety percent of tumours are found in the "gastric triangle," which encompasses the cystic and common bile ducts, the second and third portions of the duodenum, and the junction of the head and body of the pancreas. Approximately one third of gastrinomas are malignant. Diarrhea and steatorrhea (unabsorbed fat in the stool) may be evident. The patient may have coexisting parathyroid adenomas or hyperplasia and may therefore exhibit signs of hypercalcemia. The most common symptom is epigastric pain. *H. pylori* is not a risk factor for ZES (Epelboym & Mazeh, 2014).

Stress ulcer is the term given to the acute mucosal ulceration of the duodenal or gastric area that occurs after physiologically stressful events, such as burns, shock, severe sepsis, and multiple organ traumas. These ulcers, which are clinically different from peptic ulcers, are most common in ventilator-dependent patients after trauma or surgery. Fibreoptic endoscopy within 24 hours of trauma or surgery reveals shallow erosions of the stomach wall; by 72 hours, multiple gastric erosions are observed. As the stressful condition continues, the ulcers spread. When the patient recovers, the lesions are reversed. This pattern is typical of stress ulceration.

Differences of opinion exist as to the actual cause of mucosal ulceration in stress ulcers. Usually, the ulceration is preceded by shock; this leads to decreased gastric mucosal blood flow and to reflux of duodenal contents into the stomach. In addition, large quantities of pepsin are released. The combination of ischemia, acid, and pepsin creates an ideal climate for ulceration (Epelboym & Mazeh, 2014).

Stress ulcers should be distinguished from Cushing's ulcers and Curling's ulcers, two other types of gastric ulcers. Cushing's ulcers are common in patients with head injury and brain trauma. They may occur in the esophagus, stomach, or duodenum and are usually deeper and more penetrating than stress ulcers. Curling's ulcer is frequently observed about 72 hours after extensive burns and involves the antrum of the stomach or the duodenum.

Clinical Manifestations

Symptoms of an ulcer may last for a few days, weeks, or months and may disappear only to reappear, often without an identifiable cause. Many people with ulcers have no symptoms, and perforation or hemorrhage may occur in 20% to 30% of patients who had no preceding manifestations (Satoh, Yoshino, Akamatsu, et al., 2016).

As a rule, the patient with an ulcer reports dull, gnawing pain or a burning sensation in the midepigastrium or the back. It is believed that the pain occurs when the increased acid content of the stomach and duodenum erodes the lesion and stimulates the exposed nerve endings. Another theory suggests that contact of the lesion with acid stimulates a local reflex mechanism that initiates contraction of the adjacent smooth muscle. Pain is usually relieved by eating, because food neutralizes the acid, or by taking alkali; however, once the stomach has emptied or the alkali's effect has decreased, the pain returns. Sharply localized tenderness can be elicited by applying gentle pressure to the epigastrium at or slightly to the right of the midline.

Other symptoms include pyrosis (heartburn), vomiting, constipation or diarrhea, and bleeding. **Pyrosis** is a burning sensation in the stomach and esophagus that moves up to the mouth. Heartburn is often accompanied by sour eructation, or burping, which is common when the patient's stomach is empty.

Although vomiting is rare in uncomplicated duodenal ulcer, it may be a symptom of a complication of an ulcer. It results from obstruction of the pyloric orifice, caused by either muscular spasm of the pylorus or mechanical obstruction from scarring or acute swelling of the inflamed mucous membrane adjacent to the ulcer. Vomiting may or may not be preceded by nausea; usually it follows a bout of severe pain and bloating, which is relieved by vomiting. Emesis often contains undigested food eaten many hours earlier. Constipation or diarrhea may occur, probably as a result of diet and medications.

Fifteen percent of patients with peptic ulcer experience bleeding. Patients may present with GI bleeding as evidenced by the passage of **melena** (tarry stools). A small portion of patients who bleed from an acute ulcer have only very mild symptoms or none at all (Al Dhahab, Mc-Nabb Baltar, Al-Taweel, et al., 2013).

Assessment and Diagnostic Findings

A physical examination may reveal pain, epigastric tenderness, or abdominal distention. A barium study of the upper GI tract may show an ulcer; however, endoscopy is the preferred diagnostic procedure because it allows direct visualization of inflammatory changes, ulcers, and lesions. Through endoscopy, a biopsy of the gastric mucosa and of any suspicious lesions can be obtained. Endoscopy may reveal lesions that, because of their size or location, are not evident on x-ray studies.

Stools may be tested periodically until they are negative for occult blood. Gastric secretory studies are of value in diagnosing achlorhydria and ZES. *H. pylori* infection may be determined by endoscopy and histologic examination of a tissue specimen obtained by biopsy, or a rapid urease test of the biopsy specimen. Other less invasive diagnostic measures for detecting *H. pylori* include serologic testing for antibodies against the *H. pylori* antigen, stool antigen test, and urea breath test.

Medical Management

Once the diagnosis is established, the patient is informed that the condition can be controlled. Recurrence may develop; however, peptic ulcers treated with antibiotics to eradicate *H. pylori* have a lower recurrence rate than those not treated with antibiotics. The goals are to eradicate *H. pylori* and to manage gastric acidity. Methods used include medications, lifestyle changes, and surgical intervention.

Pharmacologic Therapy

Currently, the most commonly used therapy for peptic ulcers is a combination of antibiotics, **proton pump inhibitors**, and bismuth salts that suppress or eradicate *H. pylori*. Recommended therapy for 10 to 14 days includes triple therapy with two antibiotics (e.g., metronidazole [Flagyl] or amoxicillin [Amoxil] and clarithromycin [Biaxin]) plus a proton pump inhibitor (e.g., lansoprazole [Prevacid], omeprazole [Prilosec], or rabeprazole [Aciphex]), or quadruple therapy with two antibiotics (metronidazole and tetracycline) plus a proton pump inhibitor and bismuth salts (Pepto-Bismol). Research is being conducted to develop a vaccine against *H. pylori* (Guo, Liu, Zhao, et al., 2013; Sjökvist, Jeverstam, Yrlid, et al., 2016).

Histamine-2 (H_2) receptor antagonists and proton pump inhibitors are used to treat NSAID-induced ulcers and other ulcers not associated with *H. pylori* infection. Table 37-3 provides information about the medication regimens used for peptic ulcer disease. (Table 37-1 presents details about specific medications.)

The patient is advised to adhere to and complete the medication regimen to ensure complete healing of the ulcer. Because most patients become symptom-free within a week, the nurse stresses to the patient the importance of following the prescribed regimen so that the healing process can continue uninterrupted and the return of chronic ulcer symptoms can be prevented. Rest, sedatives, and tranquilizers may be added for the patient's comfort and are prescribed as needed. Maintenance dosages of H_2 receptor antagonists are usually recommended for 1 year.

For patients with ZES, hypersecretion of acid may be controlled with high doses of H_2 receptor antagonists. These patients may require twice the usual dose, and dosages usually need to be increased with prolonged use. Octreotide (Sandostatin), a medication that suppresses gastrin levels, also may be prescribed.

Patients at risk for stress ulcers (e.g., patients with head injury or extensive burns) may be treated prophylactically with IV H_2 receptor antagonists and cytoprotective agents (e.g., misoprostol, sucralfate) because of the risk of upper GI tract hemorrhage.

Stress Reduction and Rest

Reducing environmental stress requires physical and psychological modifications on the patient's part as well as the aid and cooperation of family members and significant others. The nurse assists the patient to identify situations that are stressful or exhausting. A hectic lifestyle and an irregular schedule may aggravate symptoms and interfere with regular meals taken in relaxed settings along with the regular administration of medications. The patient may benefit from regular rest periods during the day, at least during the acute phase of the disease. Biofeedback, hypnosis, behaviour modification, massage, or acupuncture may be helpful.

Smoking Cessation

Studies have shown that smoking decreases the secretion of bicarbonate from the pancreas into the duodenum, resulting in increased acidity of the duodenum. Research indicates that continued smoking may significantly inhibit ulcer repair (Nordenstedt et al., 2013). Therefore, the patient is strongly encouraged to stop smoking.

TABLE 37-3 Drug Regimens for Peptic Ulcer Disease

Indications	Drug Regimen	Nursing Considerations
Ulcer healing	**H_2 receptor antagonists:** Ranitidine 150 mg bid or 300 mg at bedtime Cimetidine 400 mg bid or 800 mg at bedtime Famotidine 20 mg bid or 40 mg at bedtime Nizatidine 150 mg bid or 300 mg at bedtime	Should be used for 6–8 weeks for complete peptic ulcer healing; patients who are at high risk require a maintenance dose for 1 year
	PPIs: Omeprazole 20 mg daily Lansoprazole 30 mg daily Rabeprazole 20 mg daily Pantoprazole 40 mg daily Esomeprazole 40 mg daily	Should be used for 4–8 weeks for complete peptic ulcer healing; patients who are at high risk require a maintenance dose for 1 year
H. pylori infection	*Triple therapy* with a PPI bid, plus clarithromycin 500 mg bid, plus amoxicillin 1,000 mg bid (or metronidazole 500 mg bid) for 10–14 days *Quadruple therapy* with bismuth subsalicylate 525 mg qid, plus tetracycline 500 mg qid, plus metronidazole 250 mg qid, plus a PPI daily for 10–14 days	Efficacy of therapy is approximately 85% qid dosing may decrease adherence to the regimen
Prophylactic therapy for NSAID ulcers	Peptic ulcer healing doses of PPIs (above) Misoprostol 100–200 mcg qid	Prevents recurrent ulceration in approximately 80–90% of patients; qid dosing may decrease adherence to the regimen

H_2, histamine-2; bid, two times a day; PPIs, proton pump inhibitors; qid, four times a day; NSAID, nonsteroidal anti-inflammatory drug.

Adapted from Anand, B. S. (2015). Peptic ulcer disease. *Medscape*. Retrieved on May 3, 2016, from emedicine.medscape.com/article/181753.

Dietary Modification

The intent of dietary modification for patients with peptic ulcers is to avoid oversecretion of acid and hypermotility in the GI tract. These can be minimized by avoiding extremes of temperature of food and beverage and overstimulation from consumption of meat extracts, alcohol, coffee (including decaffeinated coffee, which also stimulates acid secretion) and other caffeinated beverages, and diets rich in milk and cream (which stimulate acid secretion). In addition, an effort is made to neutralize acid by eating three regular meals a day. Small, frequent feedings are not necessary as long as an antacid or a histamine blocker is taken. Diet compatibility becomes an individual matter: The patient eats foods that are tolerated and avoids those that produce pain.

Surgical Management

The introduction of antibiotics to eradicate *H. pylori* and of H_2 receptor antagonists as treatment for ulcers has greatly reduced the need for surgical intervention. However, surgery is usually recommended for patients with intractable ulcers (those that fail to heal after 12 to 16 weeks of medical treatment), life-threatening hemorrhage, perforation, or obstruction and for those with ZES that is unresponsive to medications (Griffiths, Devitt, Bright, et al., 2013). Surgical procedures include vagotomy, with or without **pyloroplasty** (transecting nerves that stimulate acid secretion and opening the pylorus), and **antrectomy**, which is removal of the pyloric (antrum) portion of the stomach with anastomosis (surgical connection) to either the duodenum (gastroduodenostomy or Billroth I) or jejunum (gastrojejunostomy or Billroth II) (Table 37-4; see also the section on gastric surgery later in this chapter).

Patients who require surgery may have had a long illness. They may be discouraged and have had interruptions in their work and pressures in their family life that affect their outlook on surgery and resolution of their disease.

Follow-Up Care

Recurrence of peptic ulcer disease within 1 year may be prevented with the prophylactic use of H_2 receptor antagonists taken at a reduced dose. Not all patients require maintenance therapy; it may be prescribed only for those with two or three recurrences per year, those who have had a complication such as bleeding or **gastric outlet obstruction**, or those who are candidates for gastric surgery but for whom it poses too high a risk. The likelihood of recurrence is reduced if the patient avoids smoking, coffee (including decaffeinated coffee) and other caffeinated beverages, alcohol, and ulcerogenic medications (e.g., NSAIDs).

Nursing Process

The Patient With Peptic Ulcer Disease

Assessment

The nurse asks the patient to describe the pain and strategies used to relieve it (e.g., food, antacids). The patient usually describes peptic ulcer pain as burning or gnawing; it occurs about 2 hours after a meal and frequently awakens the patient between midnight and 3 AM. Taking antacids, eating, or vomiting often relieves the pain. If the patient reports a recent history of vomiting, the nurse determines how often emesis has occurred and notes important characteristics of the vomitus: Is it bright red, does it resemble coffee grounds, or is there undigested food from previous meals? Has the patient noted any bloody or tarry stools?

The nurse also asks the patient to list his or her usual food intake for a 72-hour period and to describe food habits (e.g., speed of eating, regularity of meals, preference for spicy foods, use of seasonings, use of caffeinated beverages and decaffeinated coffee). Lifestyle and other habits are a concern as well. Does the patient use irritating substances? For example, does he or she smoke cigarettes? If yes, how many? Does the patient ingest alcohol? If yes, how much and how often? Are NSAIDs used? The nurse inquires about the patient's level of anxiety and his or her perception of current stressors. How does the patient express anger or cope with stressful situations? Is the patient experiencing occupational stress or problems within the family? Is there a family history of ulcer disease?

TABLE 37-4 Surgical Procedures for Peptic Ulcer Disease

Operation	Description	Adverse Effects
Vagotomy 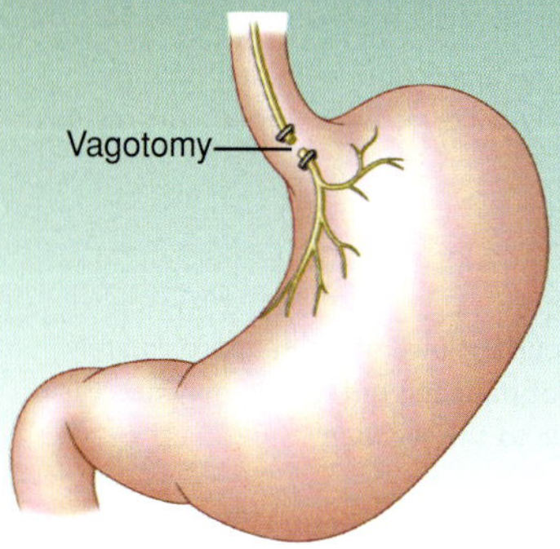	Severing of the vagus nerve. Decreases gastric acid by diminishing cholinergic stimulation to the parietal cells, making them less responsive to gastrin. May be performed via an open surgical approach or laparoscopy. May be performed to reduce gastric acid secretion. A drainage type of procedure (see pyloroplasty) is usually performed to assist with gastric emptying (because there is total denervation of the stomach)	Some patients experience problems with feeling of fullness, dumping syndrome, diarrhea, and gastritis

TABLE 37-4 Surgical Procedures for Peptic Ulcer Disease (Continued)

Operation	Description	Adverse Effects
Truncal vagotomy	Severs the right and left vagus nerves as they enter the stomach at the distal part of the esophagus; most commonly used to decrease acid secretions	Some patients experience problems with feeling of fullness, dumping syndrome, diarrhea, or constipation
Selective vagotomy	Severs vagal innervation to the stomach but maintains innervation to the rest of the abdominal organs	Fewer associated adverse effects than with truncal vagotomy
Proximal (parietal cell) gastric vagotomy without drainage	Denervates acid-secreting parietal cells but preserves vagal innervation to the gastric antrum and pylorus	No associated dumping syndrome
Pyloroplasty 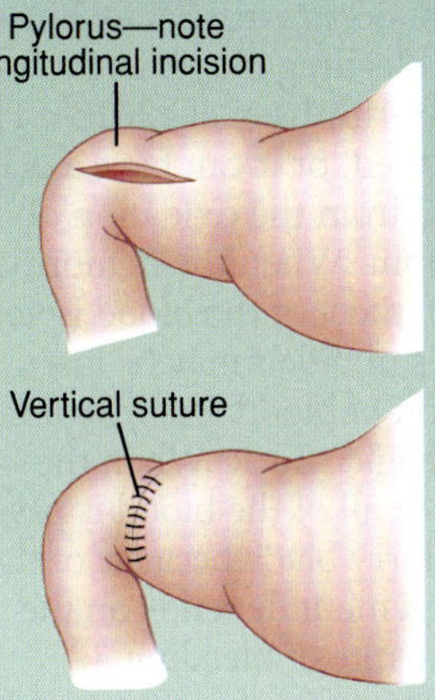	Longitudinal incision is made into the pylorus and transversely sutured closed to enlarge the outlet and relax the muscle; usually accompanies truncal and selective vagotomies	See adverse effects associated with truncal and selective vagotomies, as appropriate
Antrectomy Billroth I (gastroduodenostomy) 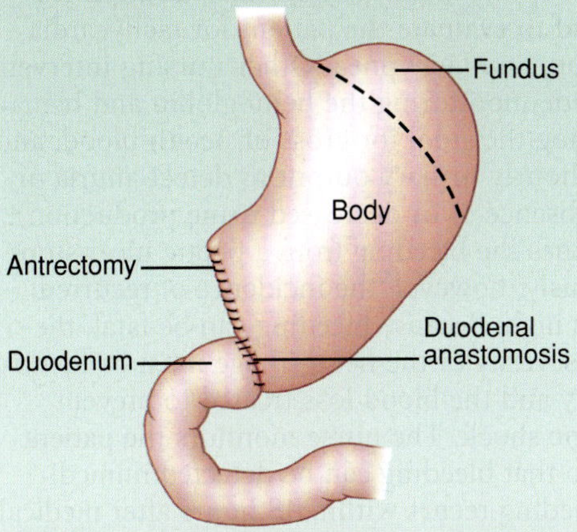	Removal of the lower portion of the antrum of the stomach (which contains the cells that secrete gastrin) as well as a small portion of the duodenum and pylorus. The remaining segment is anastomosed to the duodenumMay be performed in conjunction with a truncal vagotomy	Patients may have problems with feeling of fullness, dumping syndrome, and diarrhea
Billroth II (gastrojejunostomy) 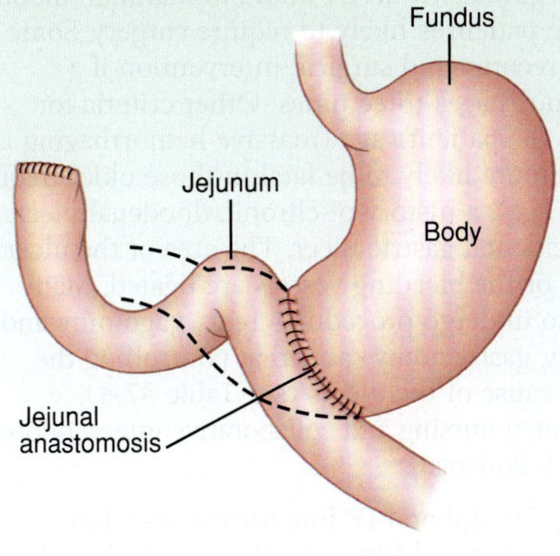	Removal of lower portion (antrum) of stomach with anastomosis to jejunum. Dotted lines show portion removed (antrectomy). A duodenal stump remains and is oversewn	Patients frequently have associated dumping syndrome, anemia, weight loss, and malabsorption

The nurse assesses the patient's vital signs and reports tachycardia and hypotension, which may indicate anemia from GI bleeding. The stool is tested for occult blood, and a physical examination, including palpation of the abdomen for localized tenderness, is performed.

Nursing Priorities

Based on the assessment data, the patient's nursing priorities may include the following:

- Acute pain due to damaged tissue
- Anxiety
- Nutrition and diet
- Lack of knowledge

Collaborative Problems/ Potential Complications

Potential complications may include the following:

- Hemorrhage
- Perforation
- Penetration
- Pyloric obstruction (gastric outlet obstruction)

Planning and Goals

The goals for the patient may include relief of pain, reduced anxiety, maintenance of nutritional requirements, knowledge about the management and prevention of ulcer recurrence, and absence of complications.

Nursing Interventions

Relieving Pain

Pain relief can be achieved with prescribed medications. The patient should avoid aspirin, foods and beverages that contain caffeine, and decaffeinated coffee. In addition, meals should be eaten at regularly paced intervals in a relaxed setting. Some patients benefit from learning relaxation techniques to help manage stress and pain.

Reducing Anxiety

The nurse assesses the patient's level of anxiety. Patients with peptic ulcers are usually anxious, but their anxiety is not always obvious. Appropriate information is provided at the patient's level of understanding, all questions are answered, and the patient is encouraged to express fears openly. Explaining diagnostic tests and administering medications as scheduled also help reduce anxiety. The nurse interacts with the patient in a relaxed manner, helps identify stressors, and explains various coping techniques and relaxation methods, such as biofeedback, hypnosis, or behaviour modification. The patient's family is also encouraged to participate in care and to provide emotional support (Taha, Lipsitz, Galea, et al., 2014).

Maintaining Optimal Nutritional Status

The nurse assesses the patient for malnutrition and weight loss. After recovery from an acute phase of peptic ulcer disease, the patient is advised about the importance of complying with the medication regimen and dietary restrictions.

Monitoring and Managing Potential Complications

HEMORRHAGE. Gastritis and hemorrhage from peptic ulcer are the two most common causes of upper GI tract bleeding (which may also occur with esophageal varices, as discussed in Chapter 39). Hemorrhage, the most common complication, occurs in 10% to 20% of patients with peptic ulcers. Bleeding may be manifested by hematemesis or melena (Griffiths et al., 2013). The vomited blood can be bright red, or it can have a dark "coffee grounds" appearance from the oxidation of hemoglobin to methemoglobin. When the hemorrhage is large (2,000 to 3,000 mL), most of the blood is vomited. Because large quantities of blood may be lost quickly, immediate correction of blood loss may be required to prevent hemorrhagic shock. When the hemorrhage is small, much or all of the blood is passed in the stools, which appear tarry black because of the digested hemoglobin. Management depends on the amount of blood lost and the rate of bleeding.

The nurse assesses the patient for faintness or dizziness and nausea, which may precede or accompany bleeding. It is important to monitor vital signs frequently and to evaluate the patient for tachycardia, hypotension, and tachypnea. Other nursing interventions include monitoring the hemoglobin and hematocrit, testing the stool for gross or occult blood, and recording hourly urinary output to detect anuria or oliguria (absence of or decreased urine production).

Many times the bleeding from a peptic ulcer stops spontaneously; however, the incidence of recurrent bleeding is high. Because bleeding can be fatal, the cause and severity of the hemorrhage must be identified quickly and the blood loss treated to prevent hemorrhagic shock. The nurse monitors the patient carefully so that bleeding can be detected immediately. If bleeding recurs within 48 hours after medical therapy has begun, or if more than 6 to 10 units of blood are required within 24 hours to maintain blood volume, the patient is likely to require surgery. Some physicians recommend surgical intervention if a patient hemorrhages three times. Other criteria for surgery are the patient's age (massive hemorrhaging is three times more likely to be fatal in those older than 60 years of age), a history of chronic duodenal ulcer, and a coincidental gastric ulcer. The area of the ulcer is removed or the bleeding vessels are ligated. Many patients also undergo procedures (e.g., vagotomy and pyloroplasty, gastrectomy) aimed at controlling the underlying cause of the ulcers (see Table 37-4).

Other related nursing and collaborative interventions include the following:

- Inserting a peripheral IV line for the infusion of saline or lactated Ringer's solution and blood

products. The nurse may need to assist with the placement of a central venous catheter for rapid infusion of large amounts of blood and fluids as well as hemodynamic monitoring. Blood component therapy is initiated if there are signs of shock (e.g., tachycardia, sweating, coldness of the extremities).
- Inserting an NG tube to distinguish fresh blood from "coffee grounds" material, to aid in the removal of clots and acid, to prevent nausea and vomiting, and to provide a means of monitoring further bleeding
- Monitoring oxygen saturation and administering oxygen therapy
- Placing the patient in the recumbent position with the legs elevated to prevent hypotension, or placing the patient on the left side to prevent aspiration from vomiting
- Treating hemorrhagic shock (described in Chapter 18)

If bleeding cannot be managed by the measures described, other treatment modalities such as endoscopy may be used to halt bleeding and avoid surgical intervention. There is debate regarding how soon endoscopy should be performed. Some clinicians believe endoscopy should be performed within the first 24 hours after hemorrhaging has ceased. Others believe endoscopy may be performed during acute bleeding, as long as the esophageal or gastric area can be visualized (blood may decrease visibility).

For patients who are unable to undergo surgery, selective embolization may be used. This procedure involves forcing emboli of autologous blood clots with or without Gelfoam (absorbable gelatin sponge) through a catheter in the artery to a point above the bleeding lesion. This procedure is performed by an interventional radiologist (George, Manousos-George, Dimitrios, et al., 2012; Mine, Murata, Nakazawa, et al., 2013).

PERFORATION AND PENETRATION. Perforation is the erosion of the ulcer through the gastric **serosa** into the peritoneal cavity without warning. It is an abdominal catastrophe and requires immediate surgery. Penetration is erosion of the ulcer through the gastric serosa into adjacent structures such as the pancreas, biliary tract, or gastrohepatic **omentum**. Symptoms of penetration include back and epigastric pain not relieved by medications that were effective in the past. Like perforation, penetration usually requires surgical intervention (Saverio, Bassi, Smerieri, et al., 2014).

Signs and symptoms of perforation include the following:

- Sudden, severe upper abdominal pain (persisting and increasing in intensity); pain may be referred to the shoulders, especially the right shoulder, because of irritation of the phrenic nerve in the diaphragm
- Vomiting
- Collapse (fainting)
- Extremely tender and rigid (board-like) abdomen
- Hypotension and tachycardia, indicating shock

Because chemical peritonitis develops within a few hours of perforation and is followed by bacterial peritonitis, the perforation must be closed as quickly as possible and the abdominal cavity lavaged of stomach or intestinal contents. In some patients, it may be safe and advisable to perform surgery to treat the ulcer disease in addition to suturing the perforation.

During surgery and postoperatively, the stomach contents are drained by means of an NG tube. The nurse monitors fluid and electrolyte balance and assesses the patient for localized infection or peritonitis (increased temperature, abdominal pain, paralytic ileus, increased or absent bowel sounds, abdominal distention). Antibiotic therapy is administered parenterally as prescribed.

PYLORIC OBSTRUCTION (GASTRIC OUTLET OBSTRUCTION). Pyloric obstruction, also called gastric outlet obstruction (GOO), occurs when the area distal to the pyloric sphincter becomes scarred and stenosed from spasm or edema or from scar tissue that forms when an ulcer alternately heals and breaks down. The patient may have nausea and vomiting, constipation, epigastric fullness, anorexia, and, later, weight loss.

In treating the patient with pyloric obstruction, the first consideration is to insert an NG tube to decompress the stomach. Confirmation that obstruction is the cause of the discomfort is accomplished by assessing the amount of fluid aspirated from the NG tube. A residual of more than 400 mL strongly suggests obstruction. Usually an upper GI study or endoscopy is performed to confirm pyloric obstruction. Decompression of the stomach and management of extracellular fluid volume and electrolyte balances may improve the patient's condition and avert the need for surgical intervention. A balloon dilation of the pylorus via endoscopy may be beneficial. If the obstruction is unrelieved by medical management, surgery (in the form of a vagotomy and antrectomy or gastrojejunostomy and vagotomy) may be required.

Promoting Home, Community-Based, and Transitional Care

EDUCATING PATIENTS ABOUT SELF-CARE. The nurse instructs the patient about the factors that relieve and those that aggravate the condition. The nurse reviews information about medications to be taken at home, including name, dosage, frequency, and possible side effects, stressing the importance of continuing to take medications even after signs and symptoms have decreased or subsided (Chart 37-2). The nurse instructs the patient to avoid certain medications and foods that exacerbate symptoms as well as substances that have acid-producing potential (e.g., alcohol; caffeinated and decaffeinated beverages such as coffee, tea, and colas). It is important to counsel the patient to eat meals at regular times and in a relaxed setting and to avoid overeating. If relevant, the nurse also informs the patient about the irritant effects of smoking on the ulcer and provides information about smoking cessation programs.

CHART 37-2

HOME CARE CHECKLIST • The Patient With Peptic Ulcer Disease

At the completion of education, the patient and/or caregiver will be able to:

- State the impact of peptic ulcer disease on physiologic functioning, ADLs, IADLs, roles, relationships, and spirituality.
- Explain the importance of and necessity for adherence with prescribed medication regimen.
- Demonstrate methods of keeping track of the medication regimen and storage of the prescribed medications, and use reminders such as beepers and/or pillboxes.
- State the name, dose, side effects, frequency, and schedule for all medications.
- Identify foods and other substances to avoid (e.g., food and drinks with extreme temperatures, coffee and other caffeinated beverages, alcohol, foods that were not tolerated in the past).
- Identify side effects and complications that should be reported to primary provider:
  - Hemorrhage—cool skin, confusion, increased heart rate, laboured breathing, blood in stool (either bright red or tarry black)
  - Penetration and perforation—severe abdominal pain, rigid and tender abdomen, vomiting, elevated temperature, increased heart rate
  - Gastric outlet obstruction—nausea and vomiting, distended abdomen, abdominal pain
- State how to reach primary provider with questions or complications.
- State time and date of follow-up appointments and testing.
- Identify the need for health promotion (e.g., cessation of use of tobacco products, stress management), disease prevention and screening activities.

ADL, activities of daily living; IADL, independent activities of daily living.

NURSING ALERT

The nurse reviews with the patient and family the signs and symptoms of complications to be reported. These complications include hemorrhage (cool skin, confusion, increased heart rate, laboured breathing, and blood in the stool), penetration and perforation (severe abdominal pain, rigid and tender abdomen, vomiting, elevated temperature, and increased heart rate), and pyloric obstruction (nausea, vomiting, distended abdomen, and abdominal pain).

CONTINUING AND TRANSITIONAL CARE. The nurse reinforces the importance of follow-up care for approximately 1 year, the need to report recurrence of symptoms, and the need for treating possible problems that occur after surgery, such as intolerance to dairy products and sweet foods. The nurse also reminds the patient and family of the importance of participating in health promotion activities and recommended health screening.

Evaluation

Expected patient outcomes may include the following:

1. Reports freedom from pain between meals and at night
2. Reports feeling less anxiety
3. Maintains weight
4. Demonstrates knowledge of self-care activities
   a. Avoids irritating foods and beverages (alcohol) and medications (NSAIDs)
   b. Takes medications as prescribed
5. No evidence of complications (e.g., hemorrhage, perforation or penetration, gastric outlet obstruction)

Gastric Cancer

Although the incidence of gastric or stomach cancer continues to decrease in Canada, it still accounts for 3,300 cases (2,100 males and 1,200 females). Predicted deaths from stomach cancer in Canada were 1,260 deaths in men and 794 deaths in women (Canadian Cancer Society's Advisory Committee on Cancer Statistics [CCSACCS], 2013). The typical patient with gastric cancer is between 40 and 70 years of age, but gastric cancer can occur in people younger than 40 years of age. Men have a higher incidence of gastric cancer than women. First Nations, Inuit and Metis, Hispanic Canadians, and African Canadians are twice as likely as Caucasian Canadians to develop gastric cancer. The incidence of gastric cancer is much greater in Japan, which has instituted mass screening programs for earlier diagnosis. Diet appears to be a significant factor: A diet high in smoked, salted, or pickled foods and low in fruits and vegetables may increase the risk of gastric cancer. Other factors include chronic inflammation of the stomach, *H. pylori* infection, pernicious anemia, smoking, achlorhydria, gastric ulcers, previous subtotal gastrectomy (more than 20 years ago), and genetics. The prognosis is generally poor; the diagnosis is usually made late because most patients are asymptomatic during the early stages of the disease. Most cases of gastric cancer are discovered only after local invasion has advanced, or metastases are present (Di, Wu, Zhu, et al., 2017).

Pathophysiology

Most gastric cancers are adenocarcinomas; they can occur anywhere in the stomach. The tumour infiltrates the surrounding mucosa, penetrating the wall of the stomach and adjacent organs and structures. The liver, pancreas, esophagus, and duodenum are often already affected at the time of diagnosis. Metastasis through lymph to the peritoneal cavity occurs later in the disease.

Clinical Manifestations

Symptoms of early disease, such as pain relieved by antacids, resemble those of benign ulcers and are seldom definitive, because most gastric tumours begin on the lesser curvature of the stomach, where they cause little disturbance of gastric function. Symptoms of progressive disease include dyspepsia (indigestion), early satiety, weight loss, abdominal pain just above the umbilicus, loss or decrease in appetite, bloating after meals, nausea and vomiting, and symptoms similar to those of peptic ulcer disease.

Assessment and Diagnostic Findings

The physical examination is usually not helpful in detecting the cancer because most early gastric tumours are not palpable. Advanced gastric cancer may be palpable as a mass. Ascites and hepatomegaly (enlarged liver) may be apparent if the cancer cells have metastasized to the liver. Palpable nodules around the umbilicus, called Sister Mary Joseph's nodules, are a sign of a GI malignancy, usually a gastric cancer. Esophagogastroduodenoscopy for biopsy and cytologic washings is the diagnostic study of choice, and a barium x-ray examination of the upper GI tract may also be performed. Endoscopic ultrasound is an important tool to assess tumour depth and any lymph node involvement. Computed tomography (CT) completes the diagnostic studies, particularly to assess for surgical resectability of the tumour before surgery is scheduled. CT of the chest, abdomen, and pelvis is valuable in staging gastric cancer.

Medical Management

There is no successful treatment for gastric carcinoma except removal of the tumour. If the tumour can be removed while it is still localized to the stomach, the patient may be cured. If the tumour has spread beyond the area that can be excised, cure is less likely. In many patients, effective palliation to prevent discomfort caused by obstruction or dysphagia may be obtained by resection of the tumour (see Gastric Surgery). A diagnostic laparoscopy may be the initial surgical approach to evaluate the gastric tumour, obtain tissue for pathologic diagnosis, and detect metastasis. The patient with a tumour that is deemed resectable undergoes an open surgical procedure to resect the tumour and appropriate lymph nodes. The patient with an unresectable tumour and advanced disease undergoes chemotherapy. Some success is being reported with new laparoscopic techniques for minimally invasive open surgeries for gastric cancer (Liu, Huang, & Chen, 2017).

A total gastrectomy may be performed for a resectable cancer in the midportion or body of the stomach. The entire stomach is removed along with the duodenum, the lower portion of the esophagus, supporting mesentery, and lymph nodes. Reconstruction of the GI tract is performed by anastomosing the end of the jejunum to the end of the esophagus, a procedure called an esophagojejunostomy. A radical subtotal gastrectomy is performed for a resectable tumour in the middle and distal portions of the stomach. A Billroth I or a Billroth II operation (see Table 37-4) is performed. The Billroth I involves a limited resection and offers a lower cure rate than the Billroth II. The Billroth II procedure is a wider resection that involves removing approximately 75% of the stomach and decreases the possibility of lymph node spread or metastatic recurrence. A proximal subtotal gastrectomy may be performed for a resectable tumour located in the proximal portion of the stomach or cardia. A total gastrectomy or an esophagogastrectomy is usually performed in place of this procedure to achieve a more extensive resection.

Common issues of advanced gastric cancer that often require surgery include pyloric obstruction, bleeding, and severe pain. Gastric perforation is an emergency situation requiring surgical intervention. A gastric resection may be the most effective palliative procedure for advanced gastric cancer. Palliative procedures such as gastric or esophageal bypass, gastrostomy, or jejunostomy may temporarily alleviate symptoms such as nausea and vomiting. Palliative rather than radical surgery may be performed if there is metastasis to other vital organs, such as the liver, or to achieve a better quality of life.

If surgical treatment does not offer cure, treatment with chemotherapy may offer further control of the disease or palliation. Commonly used single-agent chemotherapeutic medications include 5-fluorouracil (5-FU), cisplatin (Platinol), doxorubicin (Adriamycin), etoposide (Etopophos), and mitomycin-C (Mutamycin). For improved response rates it is more common to administer combination therapy, primarily 5-FU–based therapy, with other agents. Studies are being conducted to assess the use of chemotherapy before surgery. Radiation therapy is mainly used for palliation in patients with obstruction, GI bleeding secondary to tumour, and significant pain. Assessment of tumour markers (blood analysis for antigens indicative of cancer) such as carcinoembryonic antigen (CEA), carbohydrate antigen (CA 19-9), and CA 50 may help determine the effectiveness of treatment. If these values were elevated before treatment, they should decrease if the tumour is responding to the treatment (Shimada, Noie, Ohashi, et al., 2014).

Gerontologic Considerations

Despite the decreased incidence of gastric cancer, the number of older patients (75 years of age and older) with gastric cancer is increasing (Hu, Fang, & Xiao, 2013). Sixty percent of cancer-related deaths occur in people 65 years of age and older. Confusion, agitation, and restlessness may be the only symptoms seen in older adult patients, who may have no gastric symptoms until their tumours are well advanced. At this time, they present with reduced functional ability and other signs and symptoms of malignancy.

Surgery is more hazardous for older adults, and the risk increases with age. When gastric cancer is treated with traditional surgery in older patients, the survival rate does not differ from that of younger patients (Tural, Selcukbiricik, Serdengecti, et al., 2012). As noted previously, minimally invasive surgical techniques are in early research as alternatives to traditional surgeries (Liu et al., 2017). Patient education is important to prepare older patients with cancer for treatment, to help them manage adverse effects, and to face the challenges that cancer and aging present.

Nursing Process

The Patient With Gastric Cancer

Assessment

The nurse obtains a dietary history from the patient, focusing on recent nutritional intake and status. Has the patient lost weight? If so, how much and over what period of time? Can the patient tolerate a full diet? If not, what foods can he or she eat? What other changes in eating habits have occurred? Does the patient have an appetite? Does the patient feel full after eating a small amount of food? Is the patient in pain? Do foods, antacids, or medications relieve the pain, make no difference, or worsen the pain? Is there a history of infection with *H. pylori*? Other health information to obtain includes the patient's smoking and alcohol history and family history (e.g., any first- or second-degree relatives with gastric or other cancers). A psychosocial assessment, including questions about social support, individual and family coping skills, and financial resources, helps the nurse plan for care in acute and community settings.

After the interview, the nurse performs a complete physical examination, carefully assesses the patient's abdomen for tenderness or masses, and palpates and percusses the abdomen to detect ascites (Roach, 2012).

Nursing Priorities

Based on the assessment data, the patient's major nursing priorities may include the following:

- Anxiety
- Lack of nutrition due to early satiety or anorexia
- Acute pain
- Grieving
- Lack of knowledge regarding symptom identification and management of condition

Planning and Goals

The major goals for the patient may include reduced anxiety, optimal nutrition, relief of pain, and adjustment to the diagnosis and anticipated lifestyle changes.

Nursing Interventions

Reducing Anxiety

A relaxed, nonthreatening atmosphere is provided so the patient can express fears, concerns, and possibly anger about the diagnosis and prognosis. The nurse encourages the family or significant other to support the patient, offering reassurance and supporting positive coping measures. The nurse advises the patient about any procedures and treatments so that the patient knows what to expect.

Promoting Optimal Nutrition

The nurse encourages the patient to eat small, frequent portions of nonirritating foods to decrease gastric irritation. Food supplements should be high in calories, as well as vitamins A and C and iron, to enhance tissue repair. If the patient is unable to eat adequately prior to surgery to meet nutritional requirements, parenteral nutrition may be necessary. Because the patient may develop dumping syndrome when enteral feeding resumes after gastric resection, the nurse explains ways to prevent and manage it (six small feedings daily that are low in carbohydrates and sugar; fluids between meals rather than with meals) and informs the patient that symptoms often resolve after several months. If a total gastrectomy is performed, injection of vitamin B_{12} will be required for life, because intrinsic factor, secreted by parietal cells in the stomach, binds to vitamin B_{12} to get absorbed in the ileum. This deficiency of intrinsic factor—and in turn, vitamin B_{12} absorption—can result in pernicious anemia. Weight loss is a common occurrence in the postoperative period following gastric surgery; research findings suggest that individualizing dietary interventions based on patient preferences can improve outcomes (Kim, Suh, Lee, et al., 2014) (see Chart 37-3). The nurse monitors the IV therapy and nutritional status and records intake, output, and daily weights to ensure that the patient is maintaining or gaining weight. The nurse assesses for signs of dehydration (thirst, dry mucous membranes, poor skin turgor, tachycardia, decreased urine output) and reviews the results of daily laboratory studies to note any metabolic abnormalities (sodium, potassium, glucose, blood urea nitrogen). Anti-emetics are administered as prescribed.

Relieving Pain

The nurse administers analgesic agents as prescribed. A continuous IV infusion of an opioid may be necessary for postoperative or severe pain. The nurse routinely assesses the frequency, intensity, and duration of the pain to determine the effectiveness of the analgesic agent. The nurse works with the patient to help manage pain by suggesting nonpharmacologic methods for pain relief, such as position changes, imagery, distraction, relaxation exercises (using relaxation audiotapes), back rubs, massage, and periods of rest and relaxation.

NURSING RESEARCH PROFILE

Chart 37-3. The Effects of a Dietary Intervention on Patients With Gastrectomy

Kim, H., Suh, E. E., Lee, H. J., et al. (2014). The effects of patient participation-based dietary intervention on nutritional and functional status for patients with gastrectomy. *Cancer Nursing, 37*(2), E10–E20.

Purpose

Patients undergoing a gastrectomy for gastric cancer often have poor oral intake, which may lead to weight loss, malnutrition, and poor treatment outcomes. Previous researchers have not examined the effectiveness of a patient participation-based dietary intervention (PPDI) that was individualized based upon patient preferences and motivated patients in this population to monitor their own food tolerance and dietary intake. The purpose of this nursing research was to develop a PPDI and evaluate its effects on nutritional and functional status in patients following a partial or total gastrectomy for gastric cancer.

Design

This study used a true experimental design. Participants were recruited using convenience sampling techniques from one cancer center in South Korea. Participants were randomly assigned to either the control group or experimental group. The control group received standard care. The experimental group received the PPDI, which included two face-to-face and two telephone interventional sessions within 6 weeks of hospital discharge. Study data were collected from participants in both groups on the day before hospital discharge and again 12 weeks later.

The intervention (PPDI) included individualized nutritional assessments and interventions guided by the acronym CANCER (conversation, assessment, nutrition plan, complications, evaluation, and reassurance or removal). During PPDI sessions, participants worked with nurse researchers to develop a dietary plan that was tailored to their food preferences. All dietary plans were approved by a clinical dietician. Participants were also provided two educational booklets and encouraged to closely monitor and record their dietary plan, food intake, and any food tolerances/negative dietary symptoms.

Findings

Forty-eight participants, of the 56 participants recruited, completed the study. Participants were primarily middle-aged, married adults, from a socioeconomically middle class with higher than a high school education. Participants in the intervention (PPDI) group demonstrated a statistically significant reduction in adverse dietary symptoms and statistically significant improvements in functional status, dietary intake, performance status, adherence to dietary guidelines, dietary knowledge, and satisfaction as compared with participants in the control group over time. The researchers concluded that PPDI is a promising approach to individualize and motivate patients to participate in a dietary intervention program. However, the researchers cautioned that additional research is needed to determine the effects of the PPDI in a more diverse population of patients with gastric cancer undergoing a gastrectomy.

Nursing Implications

This study highlights the value of using a patient-centered approach to enhance motivation and incorporate patient perspectives and opinions into dietary interventions following a gastrectomy for gastric cancer, which may contribute to improved patient outcomes and quality of nursing care.

Providing Psychosocial Support

The nurse helps the patient express fears, concerns, and grief about the diagnosis. It is important to answer the patient's questions honestly and to encourage the patient to participate in treatment decisions. Some patients mourn the loss of a body part and perceive their surgery as a type of mutilation. Some express disbelief and need time and support to accept the diagnosis.

The nurse offers emotional support and involves family members and significant others whenever possible. This includes recognizing mood swings and defense mechanisms (e.g., denial, rationalization, displacement, regression) and reassuring the patient, family members, and significant others that emotional responses are usual and expected. The services of clergy, psychiatric clinical nurse specialists, psychologists, social workers, and psychiatrists are made available, if needed. The nurse projects an empathetic attitude and spends time with the patient. Many patients may begin to participate in self-care activities after they have acknowledged their loss.

Promoting Home, Community-Based, and Transitional Care

EDUCATING PATIENTS ABOUT SELF-CARE. Self-care activities depend on the type of treatments used—surgery, chemotherapy, radiation, or palliative care. Patient and family teaching include information about diet and nutrition, treatment regimens, activity and lifestyle changes, pain management, and possible complications (Chart 37-4). Consultation with a dietitian is essential to determine how the patient's nutritional needs can best be met at home. The nurse teaches the patient or caregiver about administration of enteral or parenteral nutrition. If chemotherapy or radiation is prescribed, the nurse provides explanations to the patient and family about what to expect, including the length of treatments, the expected side effects (e.g., nausea, vomiting, anorexia, fatigue, neutropenia), and the need for transportation to appointments for treatment. Psychological counselling may also be helpful.

CONTINUING AND TRANSITIONAL CARE. The need for ongoing care in the home depends on the patient's condition and treatment. The home care nurse reinforces nutritional counselling and supervises the

CHART 37-4

HOME CARE CHECKLIST • The Patient With Gastric Cancer

At the completion of education, the patient and/or caregiver will be able to:

- State the impact of cancer and treatment on physiologic functioning, ADLs, IADLs, roles, relationships, and spirituality.
- Identify modification of home environment, interventions, and strategies (e.g., durable medical equipment, home health aide) used in safely adapting to changes in structure or function and promote effective recovery and rehabilitation.
- Identify foods or therapies necessary to meet caloric needs and dietary needs (e.g., change in consistency, seasoning limitations or other dietary restrictions, supplements, enteral or parenteral therapy).
  - Demonstrate safe management of enteral or parenteral feedings, if applicable.
- State the name, dose, side effects, frequency, and schedule for all medications.
  - Describe approaches to controlling pain (e.g., take analgesics as prescribed; use nonpharmacologic interventions).
- When indicated, list possible side effects of chemotherapeutic agents and suggested management approaches.
- When indicated, list possible side effects of radiation therapy and suggested management approaches.
- Identify possible complications (e.g., infection, bleeding, obstruction, perforation or worsening pain or other symptoms) and interventions.
- Relate how to reach primary provider with questions or complications.
- State time and date of follow-up medical appointments, therapy, and testing.
- Identify sources of support (e.g., friends, relatives, faith community, cancer support, caregiver support).
- Identify the need for health promotion, disease prevention, and screening activities.
- Make decisions about end-of-life care as appropriate.

ADL, activities of daily living; IADL, independent activities of daily living.

administration of any enteral or parenteral feedings; the patient or caregiver must become skillful in administering the feedings and in detecting and preventing untoward effects or complications related to the feedings (see Chapter 36 to review management of enteral and parenteral feedings). The nurse teaches the patient or caregiver to record the patient's daily intake, output, and weight and explains strategies to manage pain, nausea, vomiting, or other symptoms. The nurse also teaches the patient or caregiver to recognize and report signs and symptoms of complications that require immediate attention, such as bleeding, obstruction, perforation, or any symptoms that become progressively worse. It is important to explain the chemotherapy or radiation therapy regimen. The patient and family or significant other need to understand the care that will be needed during and after treatments (see Chapter 68). Because the prognosis for gastric cancer is poor, the nurse may need to assist the patient, family, or significant other with decisions regarding end-of-life care and make referrals as warranted.

Evaluation

Expected patient outcomes may include the following:

1. Reports less anxiety
   a. Expresses fears and concerns about surgery
   b. Seeks emotional support
2. Attains optimal nutrition
   a. Eats small, frequent meals high in calories, iron, and vitamins A and C
   b. Complies with enteral or parenteral nutrition as needed
3. Has decreased pain
4. Performs self-care activities and adjusts to lifestyle changes
   a. Resumes usual activities within 3 months
   b. Alternates periods of rest and activity
   c. Manages enteral feedings
5. Verbalizes knowledge of disease management
   a. Acknowledges disease process
   b. Reports control of symptoms
   c. Verbalizes fears and concerns about dying; involves family/caregiver in discussions
   d. Completes advance directives for health care, a will, and other appropriate documents

Gastric Surgery

Gastric surgery may be performed on patients with peptic ulcers who have life-threatening hemorrhage, obstruction, perforation, or penetration or whose condition does not respond to medication. It may also be indicated for patients with gastric cancer or trauma. Surgical procedures include a vagotomy and pyloroplasty, a partial gastrectomy, or a total gastrectomy (see Table 37-4).

Nursing Management

Before surgery, the nurse assesses the patient's and family's knowledge of preoperative and postoperative surgical routines and the rationale for surgery. The nurse also assesses the patient's nutritional status: Has the patient lost weight? How much? Over how much time? Does the patient have nausea and vomiting? Has the patient had hematemesis? The nurse assesses for the presence of bowel sounds and palpates the abdomen to detect masses or tenderness (Skillen, 2012).

After surgery, the nurse assesses the patient for complications secondary to the surgical intervention, such as hemorrhage, infection, abdominal distention, atelectasis, or impaired nutritional status (see Chapter 21).

In addition to the complications to which all postoperative patients are subject, the patient undergoing gastric surgery is at increased risk for:

- Hemorrhage
- Dietary deficiencies
- Bile reflux
- Dumping syndrome

Reducing Anxiety

An important part of the preoperative nursing care involves allaying the patient's fears and anxieties about the impending surgery and its implications. The nurse encourages the patient to verbalize fears and concerns and answers the patient's and family's questions. If the patient has an acute obstruction, a perforated bowel, or an active GI hemorrhage, adequate psychological preparation may not be possible. In this event, the nurse caring for the patient after surgery should anticipate the concerns, fears, and questions that are likely to surface and should be available for support and further explanations.

Relieving Pain

After surgery, analgesic agents are administered as prescribed to relieve pain and discomfort. It is important to provide adequate pain relief so the patient can perform pulmonary care activities (deep breathing and coughing) and leg exercises, turn from side to side, and ambulate. The nurse assesses the effectiveness of analgesic intervention and consults with other members of the health care team if pain is not adequately controlled. Positioning the patient in Fowler's position promotes comfort and allows emptying of the stomach after gastric surgery.

The nurse maintains functioning of the NG tube to prevent distention and secures the tube to prevent dislocation, which may result in increased pain and tension on the suture line. Normally, the amount of NG drainage after a total gastrectomy is minimal, because there is no reservoir where secretions can collect.

Increasing Knowledge

The nurse explains routine preoperative and postoperative procedures to the patient, which include preoperative medications, NG intubation, IV fluids, abdominal dressings, the possible need for a feeding tube, pain management, and pulmonary care. These explanations need to be reinforced after surgery, especially if the patient had emergency surgery.

Resuming Enteral Intake

The patient's nutritional status is evaluated before surgery. If surgery is performed for gastric cancer, the patient is often malnourished and may require preoperative enteral or, more often, parenteral nutrition (see Chapter 36). After surgery, parenteral nutrition may be continued to meet caloric needs, to replace fluids lost through drainage and vomiting, and to support the patient metabolically until oral intake is adequate.

After the return of bowel sounds and removal of the NG tube, the nurse may give fluids, followed by food in small portions. Foods are gradually added until the patient is able to eat six small meals a day and drink 120 mL of fluid between meals. The key to increasing the dietary content is to offer food and fluids gradually as tolerated and to recognize that each patient's tolerance is different.

Recognizing Obstacles to Adequate Nutrition

Dysphagia and Gastric Retention

Dysphagia may occur in patients who have had a truncal vagotomy, a surgical procedure that may result in trauma to the lower esophagus. Gastric retention may be evidenced by abdominal distention, nausea, and vomiting. Regurgitation may also occur if the patient has eaten too much or too quickly. It also may indicate that edema along the suture line is preventing fluids and food from moving into the intestinal tract. If gastric retention occurs, it may be necessary to reinstate NPO (nothing by mouth) status and NG suction; pressure must be low in the remaining portion of the stomach to avoid disrupting the sutures.

Bile Reflux

Bile reflux gastritis and esophagitis may occur with the removal of the pylorus, which acts as a barrier to the reflux of duodenal contents. Burning epigastric pain and vomiting of bilious material manifest this condition. Eating or vomiting does not relieve the situation. Agents that bind with bile acid, such as cholestyramine (Questran), may be helpful. Aluminum hydroxide gel (an antacid) and metoclopramide hydrochloride (Reglan) have been used with limited success.

Dumping Syndrome

Dumping syndrome is an unpleasant set of vasomotor and GI symptoms that sometimes occur in patients who have had gastric surgery or a form of vagotomy. It may be the mechanical result of surgery in which a small gastric remnant is connected to the jejunum through a large opening. Foods high in carbohydrates and electrolytes must be diluted in the jejunum before absorption can take place, but the passage of food from the stomach remnant into the jejunum is too rapid to allow this to happen. The hypertonic intestinal contents draw extracellular fluid from the circulating blood volume into the jejunum to dilute the high concentration of electrolytes and sugars. The ingestion of fluid at mealtime also causes the stomach contents to empty rapidly into the jejunum.

Early symptoms include a sensation of fullness, weakness, faintness, dizziness, palpitations, diaphoresis, cramping pains, and diarrhea. These symptoms resolve once the intestine has been evacuated. Later, there is a rapid elevation of blood glucose, followed by increased insulin secretion. This results in a reactive hypoglycemia, which also is unpleasant for the patient. Vasomotor symptoms that occur 10 to 90 minutes after eating are pallor, perspiration, palpitations, headache, and feelings of warmth, dizziness, and even drowsiness. Anorexia may also be a result of the dumping syndrome, because the person may be reluctant to eat.

Steatorrhea (fatty stools) also may occur in the patient with gastric surgery. It is partially the result of rapid gastric emptying, which prevents adequate mixing with pancreatic and biliary secretions. In mild cases, reducing the intake of fat and administering an antimotility medication (e.g., loperamide [Imodium]) may control steatorrhea.

Vitamin and Mineral Deficiencies

Other dietary deficiencies that the nurse should be aware of include malabsorption of organic iron, which may require supplementation with oral or parenteral iron, and a low serum level of vitamin B_{12}, which may require supplementation by the intramuscular route. Total gastrectomy results in lack of intrinsic factor, a gastric secretion required for the absorption of vitamin B_{12} from the GI tract. Unless this vitamin is supplied by parenteral injection after gastrectomy, the patient inevitably suffers vitamin B_{12} deficiency, which eventually leads to a condition identical to pernicious anemia. All manifestations of pernicious anemia, including macrocytic anemia and combined system disease (neurologic disorders of the central and peripheral nervous systems), may be expected to develop within a period of 5 years or less; they progress in severity thereafter and, in the absence of therapy, are fatal. This complication is avoided by the regular monthly intramuscular injection of vitamin B_{12}. This regimen should be started without delay after gastrectomy. Weight loss is a common long-term concern because the patient experiences early fullness, which suppresses the appetite (Kreykes, Choxi, Rothberg, 2017).

Teaching Dietary Self-Management

Because the patient may experience any of the described conditions affecting nutrition, nursing intervention includes proper dietary instruction. The following teaching points are emphasized:

- To delay stomach emptying and dumping syndrome, the patient should assume a low Fowler's position during mealtime and then remain in that position for 20 to 30 minutes.
- Antispasmodics, as prescribed, also may aid in delaying the emptying of the stomach.
- Fluid intake with meals is discouraged; instead, fluids may be consumed up to 1 hour before or 1 hour after mealtime.
- Meals should contain more dry items than liquid items.
- The patient can eat fat as tolerated but should keep carbohydrate intake low and avoid concentrated sources of carbohydrates.
- The patient should eat smaller but more frequent meals.
- Dietary supplements of vitamins and medium-chain triglycerides and injections of vitamin B_{12} and iron may be prescribed.

The nurse also gives instructions regarding enteral or parenteral supplementation if it is needed.

Monitoring and Managing Potential Complications

Occasionally hemorrhage complicates gastric surgery. The patient has the usual signs of rapid blood loss and shock (see Chapter 18) and may vomit considerable amounts of bright red blood. The nurse assesses NG drainage for type and amount; some bloody drainage for the first 12 hours is expected, but excessive bleeding should be reported. The nurse also assesses the abdominal dressing for bleeding. Because this situation is upsetting to the patient and family, the nurse needs to remain calm. The nurse performs emergency measures, such as NG lavage and administration of blood and blood products, along with vigilant hemodynamic monitoring.

Promoting Home, Community-Based, and Transitional Care

Educating Patients About Self-Care

Patient teaching is based on the assessment of the patient's physical and psychological readiness to participate in self-care. The nurse provides information about nutrition, enteral or parenteral nutrition if required, nutritional supplements, pain management, and the symptoms of dumping syndrome and measures to prevent or minimize these symptoms (Chart 37-5). It is important to emphasize the continued need for vitamin B_{12} injections.

Continuing and Transitional Care

The patient and caregivers benefit from a team approach to discharge planning. The team members include the patient and caregiver along with the nurse, physician, dietitian, and social worker. Written or video instructions about meals, activities, medications, and follow-up care are helpful. After the patient is discharged from the hospital, the home care nurse helps with the transition to home by supervising the administration of any enteral or parenteral feedings and emphasizing information about detection and prevention of untoward effects or complications related to feedings. Information about community support groups and end-of-life care is provided to the patient, family, or significant other when indicated.

Duodenal Tumours

Tumours of the duodenum are uncommon and are usually benign and asymptomatic. They are most often discovered at autopsy. Malignant tumours are more likely to cause specific signs and symptoms leading to diagnosis. Unfortunately, malignant tumours are often not discovered until they have metastasized to distant sites. Benign tumours may place patients at an increased risk for malignancy. The relative rarity of tumours of the duodenum and the nonspecific nature of their manifestations complicate their diagnosis and treatment.

Clinical Manifestations

Duodenal tumours often present insidiously with vague, nonspecific symptoms. Most benign tumours are discovered incidentally on an x-ray study, during surgery, or at autopsy. When the patient is symptomatic, benign tumours often present with intermittent pain. The next most

CHART 37-5

HOME CARE CHECKLIST • The Patient Undergoing Gastric Surgery

At the completion of education, the patient and/or caregiver will be able to:

- Demonstrate enteral or parenteral feedings as applicable
- State necessary dietary changes
- Use nutritional supplements as appropriate
- Relieve pain with pharmacologic or nonpharmacologic interventions
- Identify available support groups
- Explain medication regimen
- Identify the need for continued vitamin B_{12} injections
- Identify signs and symptoms of complications
- State schedule of follow-up appointments

common presentation is occult bleeding. Malignant tumours often result in symptoms that lead to their diagnosis, although these symptoms may reflect advanced disease. Most patients have sustained weight loss and are malnourished at diagnosis. Bleeding and pain are common. Perforation of the bowel occurs in approximately 10% of patients (Saito, Ueno, Ota, et al., 2013; Smyth & Cunningham, 2012).

Assessment and Diagnostic Findings

An upper GI x-ray series with small bowel follow-through using oral water-insoluble contrast with frequent and detailed x-rays to follow the contrast through the small bowel is the traditional approach to diagnosis. A more sensitive examination is an **enteroclysis**, in which an NG tube is advanced into the small bowel to a position above the area in question; the area is then studied by single-contrast and double-contrast techniques. Abdominal CT is used to determine the extent of disease outside the lumen of the duodenum.

Management

Benign tumours of the duodenum include adenomas, lipomas, hemangiomas, and hamartomas (a focal malformation that resembles a neoplasm, but unlike a neoplasm does not result in compression of adjacent tissue). These tumours may be treated endoscopically by excision/resection or electrocautery if the patient is symptomatic. Routine monitoring is recommended to assess for malignant transformation.

The most common primary malignant tumour of the duodenum is adenocarcinoma; the second and third portions of the duodenum are most often involved. These tumours may present with bleeding or duodenal obstruction. If the tumour is located at the ampulla of Vater, obstructive jaundice is likely. Other rare malignant tumours of the duodenum include carcinoid tumours, lymphoma, and gastrointestinal stromal tumours. Abdominal surgery may be required to remove these rare tumours. Chemotherapy and radiation therapy may also be part of the treatment regimen.

The nursing process related to the care of the patient with a duodenal tumour is similar to that of the patient with gastric cancer. Each patient requires specialized care, astute assessment for complications, prompt interventions, and individualized teaching for self-care.

Critical Thinking Exercises

1 A 70-year-old woman is diagnosed with chronic *H. pylori* gastritis after experiencing fatigue, mild epigastric discomfort, anorexia, and occasional nausea for several months. She is started on treatment for *H. pylori* with triple therapy, including amoxicillin (Amoxil), clarithromycin (Biaxin), and omeprazole (Prilosec). The patient asks you if taking these medications will be successful in treating her infection. How would you respond to this patient? On what evidence do you base your response?

2 A 55-year-old female patient returns to your unit following a partial gastrectomy for the treatment of gastric cancer. Upon admission, she is awake, alert, and oriented. Her pain level is 2 (on a 0 to 10 numeric pain scale). She denies nausea. Her blood pressure is 128/78 mm Hg, heart rate is 98 bpm, respiratory rate is 16 breaths/minute and regular, and temperature is 36.7°C (98.1°F). Her nasogastric (NG) tube is patent and draining scant amounts of bloody secretions. Two hours later, you observe that her NG tube has drained 200 mL of bright red blood. What is your first nursing action? Describe the priorities of care for this patient.

3 You are caring for a 67-year-old man with chronic lower back pain who was recently diagnosed with peptic ulcer disease. As you are providing discharge education, the patient asks if he can continue to take ibuprofen (Motrin) to manage his lower back pain. How would you respond to this patient? On what evidence do you base your response?

REFERENCES AND SELECTED READINGS

Books

Bickley, L. S. (2016). *Bates's guide to physical examination and history taking*, (12th ed.). Philadelphia, PA: Wolters Kluwer.

Roach, S. (2012). Abdominal assessment. In T. C. Stephen, D. L. Skillen, R. A. Day, et al. (Eds.). *Canadian Jensen's nursing health assessment: A best practice approach* (1st ed., pp. 602–644). Philadelphia, PA: Wolters Kluwer Health/Lippincott Williams & Wilkins.

Skillen, D. L., (2012). Head-to-Toe Assessment of the Adult. In T. C. Stephen, D. L. Skillen, R. A. Day, et al. (Eds.). *Canadian Jensen's nursing health assessment*. (1st ed., pp. 959–980). Philadelphia, PA: Wolters Kluwer, Lippincott Williams & Wilkins.

Journals and Electronic Documents

Gastric Cancer

Bray, F., Ferlay, J., Soerjomataram, I., et al. (2018). Global cancer statistics 2018: GLOBOCAN estimates of incidence and mortality worldwide for 36 cancers in 185 countries. *CA: A Cancer Journal for Clinicians*, *68*(6), 394–424.

Canadian Cancer Society's Advisory Committee on Cancer Statistics (2013). *Canadian Cancer Statistics 2013*. Toronto. ON: Canadian Cancer Society.

Carioli, G., Malvezzi, M., Rodriguez, T., et al. (2017). Trends and predictions to 2020 in breast cancer mortality in Europe. *The Breast*, *36*, 89–95.

Di, L., Wu, H., Zhu, R., et al (2017). Multi-disciplinary team for early gastric cancer diagnosis improves the detection rate of early gastric cancer. *BMC Gastroenterology*, *17*(1), 147.

Hu, Y., Fang, J., & Xiao, S. (2013). Can the incidence of gastric cancer be reduced in the new century? *Journal of Digestive Diseases*, *14*(1), 11–15.

Ingram, S. (2017). Taking a comprehensive health history: Learning through practice and reflection. *British Journal of Nursing*, *26*(18), 1033–1037.

Jemal, A., Bray, F., Center, M. M., et al. (2011). Global cancer statistics. *CA: A Cancer Journal for Clinicians*, *61*(2), 69–90.

Kreykes, A., Choxi, H., & Rothberg, A. (2017). Post-bariatric surgery patients: Your role in their long-term care. *Journal of Family Practice*, *66*(6), 356–363.

Liu, C. A., Huang, K. H., Chen, M. H., et al. (2017). Comparison of the surgical outcomes of minimally invasive and open surgery for octogenarian and older compared to younger gastric cancer patients: A retrospective cohort study. *BMC Surgery*, *17*(1), 68.

Lochhead, P., & El-Omar, E. M. (2007). Helicobacter pylori infection and gastric cancer. *Best Practice & Research Clinical Gastroenterology*, *21*(2), 281–297.

Shimada H., Noie, T., Ohashi, M., et al. (2014). Clinical significance of serum tumor markers for gastric cancer: A systematic review of literature by the Task Force of the Japanese Gastric Cancer Association. *Gastric Cancer*, *17*(1), 26–33.

Siegel, R. L., Miller, K. D., & Jemal, A. (2017). Cancer statistics, 2017. *CA: A Cancer Journal for Clinicians*, *67*(1), 7–30.

Tural, D., Selcukbiricik, F., Serdengecti, S., et al. (2012). A comparison of patient characteristics, prognosis, treatment modalities, and survival according to age group in gastric cancer patients. *World Journal of Surgical Oncology*, *10*(1), 234–241.

Peptic Ulcers and Gastritis

Al Dhahab, H., Mc-Nabb Baltar, J., Al-Taweel, T., et al. (2013). State-of-the-art management of acute bleeding peptic ulcer disease. *Saudi Journal of Gastroenterology*, *19*(5), 195–204.

Di Saverio, S., Bassi, M., Smerieri, N. et al. (2014). Diagnosis and treatment of perforated or bleeding ulcers: 2013 WSES position paper. *World Journal of Emergency Surgery*, *9*(45). https://www.ncbi.nlm.nih.gov/pmc/articles/PMC4127969/

Epelboym, I., & Mazeh, H. (2014). Zollinger-Ellison syndrome: Classical considerations and current controversies. *Oncologist*, *19*(1), 44–50.

Fashner, J., & Gitu, A. C. (2015). Diagnosis and treatment of peptic ulcer disease and H. pylori infection. *American Family Physician*, *91*(4), 236–242.

George, V., Manousos-George, P., Dimitrios, R., et al. (2012). Selective embolization for massive upper gastrointestinal bleeding deriving from gastric angiodysplasia. *Journal of Surgical Case Reports*, *2012*(3), 1–4.

Griffiths, E. A., Devitt, P. G., Bright, T., et al. (2013). Surgical management of peptic ulcer bleeding by Australian and New Zealand upper gastrointestinal surgeons. *ANZ Journal of Surgery*, *83*(3), 104–108.

Guo, L., Liu, K., Zhao, W., et al. (2013). Immunological features and efficacy of the reconstructed epitope vaccine CtUBE against Helicobacter pylori infection in BALB/c mice model. *Applied Microbiology and Biotechnology*, *97*(6), 2367–2378.

Guo-Xing, Y., & Jun, Z. (2018). Clinical effect of health education intervention in chronic gastritis nursing. *Biomedical Research (0970-938X)*, *29*(1), 99-102.

Kim, H., Suh, E. E., Lee, H. J., et al. (2014). The effects of patient participation-based dietary intervention on nutritional and functional status for patients with gastrectomy. *Cancer Nursing*, *37*(2), E10–E20.

Lacy, B., Talley, N., Locke, G., et al. (2012). Review article: Current treatment options and management of functional dyspepsia. *Alimentary Pharmacology and Therapeutics*, *36*(1), 3–15.

Mine, T., Murata, S., Nakazawa, K., et al. (2013). Glue embolization for gastroduodenal ulcer bleeding: Contribution to hemodynamics and healing process. *Acta Radiologica (Stockholm, Sweden: 1987)*, *54*(8), 934–938.

Nordenstedt, H., Graham, D. Y., Kramer, J. R., et al. (2013). Helicobacter pylori-negative gastritis: Prevalence and risk factors. *The American Journal of Gastroenterology*, *108*(1), 65–71.

Satoh, K., Yoshino, J., Akamatsu, T., et al (2016). Evidence-based clinical practice guidelines for peptic ulcer disease 2015. *Journal of Gastroenterology*, *51*(3), 177–194.

Sjökvist Ottsjö, L., Jeverstam, F., Yrlid, L., et al. (2017). Induction of mucosal immune responses against Helicobacter pylori infection after sublingual and intragastric route of immunization. *Immunology*, *150*(2), 172–183.

Smolović, B., Stanisavljević, D., Golubović, M., et al. (2014). Bleeding gastroduodenal ulcers in patients without Helicobacter pylori infection and without exposure to non-steroidal anti-inflammatory drugs. *Vojnosanitetski Pregled*, *71*(2):183–190.

Taha, F., Lipsitz, J. D., Galea, S., et al. (2014). Anxiety disorders and risk of self-reported ulcer: A 10-year longitudinal study among US adults. *General Hospital Psychiatry*, *36*, 674–679.

Tooker, L. B., & Dexter, K. (2017). Zollinger-Ellison Syndrome: Not your average peptic ulcer disease. *Clinician Reviews*, *27*(7), 32–34.

Duodenal Tumours

Saito, T., Ueno, M., Ota, Y., et al. (2013). Histopathological and clinical characteristics of duodenal gastrointestinal stromal tumors as predictors of malignancy. *World Journal of Surgical Oncology*, *11*(1), 1–7.

Smyth, E., & Cunningham, D. (2012). Gastrointestinal oncology—What you need to know. *Clinical Medicine*, *12*(6), 575–579.

Resources

Canadian Digestive Health Foundation (2018). Canadian statistics of digestive disease. Retrieved from: http://www.cdhf.ca/en/statistics.

38 Management of Patients With Intestinal and Rectal Disorders

Adapted by Pamela Cawley

Learning Objectives

On completion of this chapter, the learner will be able to:

1. Identify the health care learning needs of patients with constipation or diarrhea.
2. Compare the conditions of malabsorption with regard to their pathophysiology, clinical manifestations, and management.
3. Use the nursing process as a framework for care of patients with diverticular disease.
4. Compare Crohn's disease (regional enteritis) and ulcerative colitis with regard to their pathophysiology; clinical manifestations; diagnostic evaluation; and medical, surgical, and nursing management.
5. Apply the nursing process as a framework for care of the patient with inflammatory bowel disease.
6. Describe the responsibilities of the nurse in meeting the needs of the patient with an intestinal diversion.
7. Describe the various types of intestinal obstructions and their management.
8. Use the nursing process as a framework for care of the patient with cancer of the colon or rectum.
9. Explain nursing management of the patient with an anorectal condition.

The types of diseases and disorders that affect the lower gastrointestinal (GI) tract are many and varied. Approximately 20 million Canadians are affected by a type of disease of the GI tract (Canadian Digestive Health Foundation, 2018). These diseases account for more than 12% of all hospital admissions annually.

In all age groups, lifestyle, high levels of stress, irregular eating habits, insufficient intake of fibre and water, and lack of daily exercise contribute to GI disorders. There is a growing understanding of the biopsychosocial implications of GI disease. Nurses can have an impact on these GI disorders by identifying behaviour patterns that put patients at risk, by educating the public about prevention and management, and by helping those affected to improve their condition and prevent complications.

ABNORMALITIES OF FECAL ELIMINATION

Changes in patterns of fecal elimination are symptoms of functional disorders or diseases of the GI tract. The most common changes seen are constipation, diarrhea, and fecal incontinence. The nurse is aware of the causes and therapeutic management of these disorders and of nursing management techniques. Education is important for patients with these conditions.

Constipation

Constipation is an abnormal infrequency or irregularity of defecation, abnormal hardening of stools that makes their passage difficult and sometimes painful, a decrease in stool volume, or retention of stool in the rectum for a prolonged period often with a sense of incomplete evacuation after defecation. Any variation from usual habits may be considered a concern. The Canadian Digestive Health Foundation (2014) estimates that one in four Canadians experiences constipation symptoms. Rates for women in all age groups are twice that of men in Canada and North America, and higher in lower income groups (Canadian Digestive Health Foundation, 2014). Constipation increases with age, and because life spans are increasing, this health challenge will increase.

Constipation can be caused by certain medications (i.e., tranquilizers, anticholinergics, antidepressants, antihypertensives, bile acid sequestrants, diuretics, opioids, aluminum-based antacids, iron preparations, selected antibiotics, and muscle relaxants); rectal or anal disorders (e.g., hemorrhoids, fissures); obstruction (e.g., bowel tumours); metabolic, neurologic, and neuromuscular conditions (e.g., Hirschsprung's disease, Parkinson's disease, multiple sclerosis); endocrine disorders (e.g., hypothyroidism, pheochromocytoma); lead poisoning; and connective tissue disorders (e.g., scleroderma, systemic lupus erythematosus). Constipation is a major issue for patients taking opioids for pain. Diseases of the colon commonly associated with constipation include irritable bowel syndrome (IBS) and diverticular disease. Constipation can also occur with an acute disease process in the abdomen (e.g., appendicitis).

Other causes of constipation may include weakness, immobility, debility, fatigue, and an inability to increase intra-abdominal pressure to facilitate the passage of stools, as may occur in patients with emphysema or spinal cord injury, for instance. Many people develop constipation because they do not take the time to defecate or they ignore the urge to defecate. Constipation is also a result of dietary habits (i.e., low consumption of fibre and inadequate fluid intake), lack of regular exercise, and a stress-filled life. Fibre is particularly important to bowel health because it increases the bulk of stool, generally easing the passage. More importantly, it also promotes optimal fermentation, providing good bowel wall health (McRorie, 2015).

The perception or understanding of constipation can be an issue. This subjective problem occurs when a person's bowel elimination pattern is not consistent with what he or she considers "normal." Chronic laxative use may contribute to this problem and is a major health issue in Canada. Researchers (Mitsuhashi et al., 2018) studied self-reports of normal bowel patterns in the United States. The study upheld the concept that the minimum normal was 3 bowel movements per week but found that 95.9% of the sample reported between 3 and 21 bowel movements per week.

"Normal" bowel function varies substantially from three bowel movements a day to three times per week.

Pathophysiology

The pathophysiology of constipation is not well understood, but it is thought to include interference with one of the three major functions of the colon: mucosal transport (i.e., mucosal secretions facilitate the movement of colon contents), myoelectric activity (i.e., mixing of the rectal mass and propulsive actions), or the processes of defecation (e.g., pelvic floor dysfunction). Any of the causative

Glossary

abscess: localized collection of purulent material surrounded by inflamed tissues, typically associated with signs of infection

borborygmus: rumbling noise caused by the movement of gas through the intestines

colostomy: surgical opening into the colon by means of a stoma to allow drainage of bowel contents; one type of fecal diversion

constipation: subjectively described infrequency or irregularity of defecation, with or without an abnormal hardening of feces that makes their passage difficult and sometimes painful, with or without a decrease in fecal volume

diverticulitis: inflammation of a diverticulum from obstruction (by fecal matter), resulting in abscess formation

diverticulosis: presence of several diverticula in the intestine; common in middle age

diverticulum: saclike outpouching of the lining of the bowel protruding through the muscle of the intestinal wall, usually caused by high intraluminal pressure

fecal incontinence: involuntary passage of feces

fissure: normal or abnormal fold, groove, or crack in body tissue

fistula: anatomically abnormal tract that arises between two internal organs or between an internal organ and the body surface

hemorrhoids: dilated portions of the anal veins; can occur internal or external to the anal sphincter

ileostomy: surgical opening into the ileum by means of a stoma to allow drainage of bowel contents; one type of fecal diversion

inflammatory bowel disease (IBD): group of chronic disorders (most common are ulcerative colitis and Crohn's disease) that result in inflammation or ulceration (or both) of the bowel lining; associated with abdominal pain, diarrhea, fever, and weight loss

irritable bowel syndrome (IBS): functional disorder that affects frequency of defecation and consistency of stool; is associated with no specific structural or biochemical alterations; associated with cramping abdominal pain and bloating

Kock pouch: type of continent ileal reservoir created surgically by making an internal pouch with a portion of the ileum and placing a nipple valve flush with the stoma

malabsorption: impaired transport across the mucosa

peritonitis: inflammation of the lining of the abdominal cavity, usually as a result of a bacterial infection of an area in the gastrointestinal tract with leakage of contents into the abdominal cavity

steatorrhea: excess of fatty wastes in the feces or the urine

tenesmus: ineffective and sometimes painful straining to eliminate either feces or urine

Valsalva manoeuvre: forcible exhalation against a closed glottis followed by a rise in intrathoracic pressure and subsequent possible dramatic rise in arterial pressure; may occur during straining at stool

wound–ostomy–continence (WOC) nurse: nurse specially educated in the appropriate management of fecal and urinary diversions; guides patients, their families, surgeons, and nurses by recommending appropriate use of skin, wound, ostomy, and continence products; formerly called enterostomal therapist factors previously identified can interfere with any of these three processes. There are three classes of constipation, based upon their underlying pathophysiologic mechanisms (Grossman & Porth, 2014):

- Functional constipation, which involves normal transit mechanisms of mucosal transport. This type of constipation is most common and can be successfully treated by increasing intake of fibre and fluids.
- Slow-transit constipation, which is caused by inherent disorders of the motor function of the colon (e.g., Hirschsprung's disease), and is characterized by infrequent bowel movements.
- Defecatory disorders, which are caused by dysfunctional motor coordination between the pelvic floor and anal sphincter. This can cause not only constipation but also fecal incontinence (see later discussion).

The urge to defecate is stimulated usually by rectal distention that initiates a series of four actions: stimulation of the inhibitory rectoanal reflex, relaxation of the internal sphincter muscle, relaxation of the external sphincter muscle and muscles in the pelvic region, and increased intra-abdominal pressure. Interference with any of these processes can lead to constipation.

If all organic causes are eliminated, idiopathic constipation is diagnosed. When the urge to defecate is ignored, the rectal mucous membrane and musculature become insensitive to the presence of fecal masses, and consequently a stronger stimulus is required to produce the necessary peristaltic rush for defecation. The initial effect of fecal retention is to produce irritability of the colon, which at this stage frequently goes into spasm, especially after meals, giving rise to colicky midabdominal or low abdominal pains. After several years of this process, the colon loses muscular tone and becomes essentially unresponsive to usual stimuli (similar to an overstretched balloon). Atony or decreased muscle tone occurs with aging. This also leads to constipation because the stool is retained for longer periods.

Clinical Manifestations

Clinical manifestations of constipation include fewer than three bowel movements per week; abdominal distention; pain and pressure; decreased appetite; headache; fatigue; indigestion; a sensation of incomplete evacuation; straining at stool; and the elimination of small-volume, lumpy, hard, dry stools. To make diagnosis more efficient, an international committee developed the Rome criteria (Mearin et al., 2016).

Assessment and Diagnostic Findings

Chronic constipation is usually considered idiopathic, but secondary causes should be excluded. In patients with severe, intractable constipation, further diagnostic testing is needed (Basson, 2015a). The diagnosis of constipation is based on the patient's history, physical examination, possibly the results of a barium enema or sigmoidoscopy, and stool testing for occult blood. These tests are used to determine whether this symptom results from spasm or narrowing of the bowel. Anorectal manometry (i.e., pressure studies such as a balloon expulsion test) may be performed to assess malfunction of the sphincter. Defecography and colonic transit studies can also assist in the diagnosis because they permit assessment of active anorectal function (see Chapter 34). Newer tests such as pelvic floor magnetic resonance imaging (MRI) may identify occult pelvic floor defects (Basson, 2015a; Cerro et al., 2017).

Complications

Complications of constipation include hypertension, fecal impaction, **hemorrhoids** (dilated portions of anal veins), **fissures** (tissue folds), and megacolon. Increased arterial pressure can occur with defecation. Straining at stool, which results in the **Valsalva manoeuvre** (i.e., forcibly exhaling with the glottis closed), has a striking effect on arterial blood pressure. During active straining, the flow of venous blood in the chest is temporarily impeded because of increased intrathoracic pressure. This pressure tends to collapse the large veins in the chest. The atria and the ventricles receive less blood, and consequently less blood is ejected by the left ventricle. Cardiac output is decreased, and there is a transient drop in arterial pressure. Almost immediately after this period of hypotension, an increase in arterial pressure occurs; the pressure is elevated momentarily to a point far exceeding the original level (i.e., rebound phenomenon). In patients with hypertension, this compensatory reaction may be exaggerated greatly, and the peak pressure attained may be dangerously high—sufficient to rupture a major artery in the brain or elsewhere. Orthostasis, dizziness, or syncope may occur (Grossman & Porth, 2014).

Fecal impaction occurs when an accumulated mass of dry feces cannot be expelled. The mass may be palpable on digital examination, may produce pressure on the colonic mucosa that results in ulcer formation, and frequently causes seepage of liquid stools. Treatment can be embarrassing and painful, because impaction usually involves digital dislodgement and enema administration (NIDDK, 2014c).

Hemorrhoids and anal fissures can develop as a result of constipation. Hemorrhoids develop as a result of perianal vascular congestion caused by straining. Anal fissures may result from the passage of the hard stool through the anus, tearing the lining of the anal canal (NIDDK, 2014c).

Megacolon is a dilated and atonic colon caused by a fecal mass that obstructs the passage of colon contents. Symptoms include constipation, liquid fecal incontinence, and abdominal distention. Megacolon can lead to perforation of the bowel (Grossman & Porth, 2014).

Gerontologic Considerations

Physician visits for treatment of constipation are most common in people 65 years and older (Bailes & Reeve, 2013; Eliopoulos, 2018). The most common concern they voice is the need to strain at stool. People who have loose-fitting dentures or have lost their teeth have difficulty chewing and frequently choose soft, processed foods that are low in fibre. Older adults tend to have decreased food intake, reduced mobility, and weak abdominal and pelvic muscles, and they are more likely to have multiple chronic illnesses requiring multiple medications (polypharmacy) that often cause constipation (Gallegos-Orozco et al., 2012). Low-fibre convenience foods are widely used by people who have lost interest in eating. Some older people reduce their fluid intake if they are not eating regular meals. Depression, weakness, and prolonged bed rest also contribute to constipation by decreasing intestinal motility and anal sphincter tone. Nerve impulses are dulled, and there is a decreased urge to defecate. Many older people overuse laxatives in an attempt to have a daily bowel movement and become dependent on them. Chronic constipation cannot be underestimated as a health condition that significantly affects health and quality of life (QOL; Bailes & Reeve, 2013; Eliopoulos, 2018).

Medical Management

Treatment targets the underlying cause of constipation and aims to prevent recurrence. It includes education, bowel habit training, increased fibre and fluid intake, and judicious use of laxatives. Management may also include discontinuing laxative abuse or replacing medications with nonconstipating medications (Mearin et al., 2016). Patients can be educated to sit on the toilet with legs supported and to utilize the gastrocolic reflex (peristaltic movements of the large bowel occurring five to six times daily that are triggered by distention of the stomach) by attempting to defecate following a meal and a warm drink. Routine exercise to strengthen abdominal muscles is encouraged.

Routine exercise to strengthen abdominal muscles is encouraged. Biofeedback is a technique that can be used to help patients learn to relax the sphincter mechanism to expel stool. It is considered first-line therapy once anorectal structural lesions have been excluded as the cause for constipation (Collins et al., 2014). Daily dietary intake of 25 to 30 g/day of fibre (soluble and bulk forming) is recommended, especially for the treatment of constipation in older adults. If laxative use is necessary, one of the following may be prescribed: bulk-forming agents, saline and osmotic agents, lubricants, stimulants, or fecal softeners. The physiologic action and patient education information related to these laxatives are presented in Table 38-1.

If laxative use is necessary, one of the following may be prescribed: bulk-forming agents (fibre laxatives), saline and osmotic agents, lubricants, stimulants, or fecal softeners. Enemas and rectal suppositories are generally not recommended for treating constipation unless other medications have failed; then, glycerin suppositories may be tried (Bailes & Reeve, 2013).

Specific medications may be prescribed to enhance colonic transit by increasing propulsive motor activity. These may include cholinergic agents (e.g., bethanechol [Urecholine]), cholinesterase inhibitors (e.g., neostigmine [Prostigmin]), or prokinetic agents (e.g., metoclopramide [Reglan]). Newer prokinetic agents include serotonin receptors such as tegaserod (Zelnorm) and prostones such as lubiprostone (Amitiza). They should be used only for patients with unremitting constipation (Gardiner & Hilton, 2014).

Nursing Management

The nurse elicits information about the onset and duration of constipation, current and past elimination patterns, the patient's expectation of normal bowel elimination, and lifestyle information (e.g., exercise and activity level, occupation, food and fluid intake, and stress level) during the health history interview. Past medical and surgical history, current medications, and laxative and enema use are important, as is information about the sensation of rectal pressure or fullness, abdominal pain, excessive straining at defecation, and flatulence.

Patient education and health promotion are important functions of the nurse (Chart 38-1). After the health history is obtained, the nurse sets specific goals for teaching. Goals for the patient include restoring or maintaining a regular pattern of elimination by responding to the urge to defecate, ensuring adequate intake of fluids and high-fibre foods, and learning about methods to avoid constipation, relieving anxiety about bowel elimination patterns, and avoiding complications.

CHART 38-1

Patient Education: Preventing Constipation

The nurse instructs the patient to:

- Recognize the physiology of defecation and the importance of responding to the urge to defecate.
- Understand the normal variations in patterns of defecation.
- Establish a bowel routine, and be aware that having a regular time for defecation (e.g., best time is after a meal) may aid in initiating the reflex.
- Ensure proper dietary habits, such as eating high-residue, high-fibre foods (e.g., fruits, vegetables); adding bran daily (must be introduced gradually); and increasing fluid intake (unless contraindicated) to help prevent constipation.
- Increase muscle strength through an exercise regimen, increased ambulation, and abdominal muscle toning to help propel colon contents.
- Perform abdominal toning exercises, including contracting abdominal muscles 4 times daily and leg-to-chest lifts 10–20 times each day.
- Use the normal position (semisquatting) to maximize the use of abdominal muscles and force of gravity.
- Avoid overuse or long-term use of stimulant laxatives.

Diarrhea

Diarrhea is an increased frequency of bowel movements (more than three per day), an increased amount of stool (more than 200 g/day), and altered consistency (i.e., increased liquidity) of stool. It is usually associated with urgency, perianal discomfort, incontinence, or a combination of these factors. Any condition that causes increased intestinal secretions, decreased mucosal absorption, or altered motility can produce diarrhea. IBS, inflammatory bowel disease (IBD), and lactose intolerance are frequently the underlying disease processes that cause diarrhea.

Diarrhea can be acute or chronic. Acute diarrhea is most often associated with infection and is usually self-limiting, lasting up to 7 to 14 days; chronic diarrhea persists for more than 2 to 3 weeks and may return sporadically. Diarrhea can be caused by certain medications (e.g., thyroid hormone replacement, stool softeners and laxatives, prokinetic agents,

TABLE 38-1 Selected Laxative Medications

Classification/Medications	Action	Patient Education
Bulk Forming		
Methylcellulose (Citrucel), psyllium (Metamucil), wheat dextrin (Benefiber)	Polysaccharides and cellulose and wheat derivatives mix with intestinal fluids, swell, and stimulate peristalsis.	Take with 8-oz water and follow with 8-oz water; do not take dry. Report abdominal distention or unusual amount of flatulence.
Saline Agent		
Magnesium hydroxide (milk of magnesia)	Nonabsorbable magnesium ions alter stool consistency by drawing water into the intestines by osmosis; peristalsis is stimulated. Action occurs within 2 hours.	Be aware that the liquid preparation is more effective than the tablet form. Note that only short-term use is recommended because of toxicity (central nervous system or neuromuscular depression, electrolyte imbalance). Do not take magnesium laxatives with renal insufficiency.
Lubricant		
Mineral oil, glycerin suppository	Nonabsorbable hydrocarbons soften fecal matter by lubricating the intestinal mucosa; the passage of stool is facilitated. Action occurs within 6–8 hours for mineral oil and within 30 minutes for glycerin suppository.	Do not take mineral oil with meals, because it can impair the absorption of fat-soluble vitamins and delay gastric emptying. Swallow carefully, because drops of oil that gain access to the pharynx can produce a lipid pneumonia. Insert glycerin suppositories fully and retain.
Stimulant		
Bisacodyl (Dulcolax), Senna (Senokot)	Irritates the colonic epithelium by stimulating sensory nerve endings and increasing mucosal secretions and decreasing large intestinal water absorption. Action occurs within 6–8 hours.	Be aware that catharsis may cause fluid and electrolyte imbalance, especially in the older adult. Do not swallow, crush, or chew tablets. Avoid milk or antacids within 1 hour of taking medication, because the enteric coating may dissolve prematurely. Note that stimulant laxatives are *not* indicated for long-term use.
Fecal Softener		
Docusate (Colace)	Hydrates the stool by its surfactant action on the colonic epithelium (increases the wetting efficiency of intestinal water); aqueous and fatty substances are mixed. Does *not* exert a laxative action.	Note that this can be used safely by patients who should avoid straining (cardiac patients, patients with anorectal disorders). Be aware that this will not evacuate hard stool because it is not a true laxative.
Osmotic Agent		
Polyethylene glycol (PEG) and electrolytes (CoLyte, GoLYTELY)	Cleanses colon rapidly and induces diarrhea	Note that because this is a large-volume product, it takes time to consume it safely. Recognize that it can cause considerable nausea and bloating. Know that it has high level of research evidence support.
Chloride Channel Activator		
Lubiprostone (Amitiza)	Stimulates chloride channels in the colonic mucosa, causing passive passage of sodium and fluid into the colon.	Avoid pregnancy during treatment, keep in mind that it may cause increased flatulence and loose stools. Do not use for more than 4 weeks.

Adapted from Bailes, B. K., & Reeve, K. (2013). Constipation in older adults. *The Nurse Practitioner*, *38*(8), 21–25.

antibiotics, chemotherapy, antiarrhythmics, antihypertensives, magnesium-based antacids), certain tube-feeding formulas, metabolic and endocrine disorders (e.g., diabetes, Addison's disease, thyrotoxicosis), and viral or bacterial infectious processes (e.g., dysentery, shigellosis, food poisoning, Norwalk virus). Other disease processes associated with diarrhea include nutritional and malabsorptive disorders (e.g., celiac disease), anal sphincter defect, Zollinger–Ellison syndrome, paralytic ileus, intestinal obstruction, and acquired immunodeficiency syndrome (AIDS) (NIDDK, 2014d).

Clostridium difficile is the most commonly identified agent in antibiotic-associated diarrhea in the hospital (Levy et al., 2015). Moreover, it is the most common health care–associated infection in Canada, with an estimated 37,900 episodes in 2012, and $281 million in cost (Levy et al., 2015).

Pathophysiology

Types of diarrhea include secretory, osmotic, malabsorptive, infectious, and exudative. Secretory diarrhea is usually high-volume diarrhea. Often associated with bacterial toxins and neoplasms, it is caused by increased production and secretion of water and electrolytes by the intestinal mucosa into the intestinal lumen. Osmotic diarrhea occurs when water is pulled into the intestines by the osmotic pressure of unabsorbed particles, slowing the reabsorption of water. It can be caused by lactase deficiency, pancreatic dysfunction, or intestinal hemorrhage. Malabsorptive diarrhea combines mechanical and biochemical actions, inhibiting effective absorption of nutrients manifested by markers of malnutrition that include hypoalbuminemia. Low serum albumin levels lead to intestinal mucosa swelling and liquid stool. Infectious diarrhea results from infectious agents invading the intestinal mucosa. *C. difficile* is the most commonly identified agent in antibiotic-associated diarrhea in the hospital. Exudative diarrhea is caused by changes in mucosal integrity, epithelial loss, or tissue destruction by radiation or chemotherapy. Diarrhea may also be caused by laxative misuse (Grossman & Porth, 2014).

Clinical Manifestations

In addition to the increased frequency and fluid content of stools, the patient usually has abdominal cramps, distention, intestinal rumbling (i.e., **borborygmus**), anorexia, and thirst. Painful spasmodic contractions of the anus and ineffective straining (i.e., **tenesmus**) may occur with defecation. Other symptoms depend on the cause and severity of the diarrhea but are related to dehydration and to fluid and electrolyte imbalances.

Watery stools are characteristic of disorders of the small bowel, whereas loose, semisolid stools are associated more often with disorders of the large bowel. Voluminous, greasy stools suggest intestinal malabsorption, and the presence of blood, mucus, and pus in the stools suggests inflammatory enteritis or colitis. Oil droplets on the toilet water are almost always diagnostic of pancreatic insufficiency. Nocturnal diarrhea may be a manifestation of diabetic neuropathy. The possibility of *C. difficile* infection should be considered in all patients with unexplained diarrhea who are taking or have recently taken antibiotics (Murray, 2016).

Assessment and Diagnostic Findings

When the cause of the diarrhea is not obvious, the following diagnostic tests may be performed: complete blood cell count; serum chemistries; urinalysis; routine stool examination; and stool examinations for infectious or parasitic organisms, bacterial toxins, blood, fat, electrolytes, and white blood cells. Endoscopy or barium enema may assist in identifying the cause (NIDDK, 2014d).

Complications

Complications of diarrhea include the potential for cardiac dysrhythmias because of significant fluid and electrolyte loss (especially loss of potassium). Urinary output of less than 30 mL per hour for 2 to 3 consecutive hours, muscle weakness, paresthesia, hypotension, anorexia, and drowsiness with a potassium level of less than 3.5 mEq/L (3.5 mmol/L) must be reported. Chronic diarrhea can also result in skin care issues related to irritant dermatitis (NIDDK, 2014d), which can be prevented by cleansing with a wet wipe, drying the skin, and then applying barrier cream (Voegeli, 2012).

Gerontologic Considerations

Older patients can become dehydrated quickly and develop low potassium levels (i.e., hypokalemia) as a result of diarrhea. The nurse observes for clinical manifestations of muscle weakness, dysrhythmias, or decreased peristaltic motility that may lead to paralytic ileus. The older patient taking digitalis (e.g., digoxin [Lanoxin]) must be aware of how quickly dehydration and hypokalemia can occur with diarrhea. The nurse teaches the patient to recognize the symptoms of hypokalemia because low levels of potassium potentiate the action of digitalis, leading to digitalis toxicity (Eliopoulous, 2018).

The skin of an older person is more sensitive to excoriation due to decreased turgor and reduced subcutaneous fat layers. Gentle cleansing with a perineal cleansing solution (i.e., wet wiping method) and the use of a barrier cream or a liquid skin sealant will prevent and/or treat the excoriation (Eliopoulos, 2018).

Medical Management

Primary management is directed at controlling symptoms, preventing complications, and eliminating or treating the underlying disease. Certain medications (e.g., antibiotics, anti-inflammatory agents) and antidiarrheals (e.g., loperamide [Imodium], diphenoxylate [Lomotil]) may be used to reduce the severity of the diarrhea and treat the underlying disease (Barr & Smith, 2014). In most cases, loperamide is the medication of choice because it has fewer side effects than diphenoxylate. Recent research has discouraged the use of antidiarrheal medications in favour of hydration, indicating inconclusive results and possible harmful effects from these drugs (Guandalini, Frye, & Tamer, 2017). Some research supports the use of probiotics (live organisms given to a host) in some forms of diarrhea. These organisms consist of *Saccharomyces boulardii* (yeast) or lactic acid bacteria such as *Lactobacillus* species (Avadhani & Steefel, 2015).

Nursing Management

The nurse's role includes assessing and monitoring the characteristics and pattern of diarrhea. A health history should address the patient's medication therapy, medical and surgical history, and dietary patterns and intake. Reports of recent exposure to an acute illness or recent travel to another geographic area are important (Moore, 2015). Assessment includes abdominal auscultation and palpation for tenderness. Inspection of the abdomen (Ford & Roach, 2014), mucous membranes, and skin (Stephen et al., 2012) is important to determine hydration status. Stool samples are obtained for testing. It is also necessary to assess the perianal area. Position the patient either standing and bending forward on the exam table or lying on left side with left leg extended and right leg flexed (Sims position). Spread the buttocks apart and have the patient bear down. Look for anal lesions, hemorrhoids, warts, or rectal fissures (Day, 2013).

During an episode of acute diarrhea, the nurse encourages bed rest and intake of liquids and foods low in bulk until the acute attack subsides. When the patient is able to tolerate food intake, the nurse recommends a bland diet of semisolid and solid foods. The patient should avoid caffeine, carbonated beverages, and very hot and very cold foods, because they stimulate intestinal motility (NIDDK, 2014d). It may be necessary to restrict milk products, fat, whole-grain products, fresh fruits, and vegetables for several days. The nurse administers antidiarrheal medications such as diphenoxylate or loperamide as prescribed. Intravenous (IV) fluid therapy may be necessary for rapid rehydration in some patients, especially in older patients and in patients with pre-existing GI conditions (e.g., IBD). It is important to monitor serum electrolyte levels closely. The nurse immediately reports evidence of dysrhythmias or a change in patient's level of consciousness.

The perianal area may become excoriated because diarrheal stool contains digestive enzymes that can irritate the skin. The patient should follow a perianal skin care routine to decrease irritation and excoriation (see Chapters 14,58). The skin of an older person is very sensitive because of decreased turgor and reduced subcutaneous fat layers.

Fecal Incontinence

Fecal incontinence describes the recurrent involuntary passage of stool from the rectum for at least 3 months. Factors that influence this disorder include the ability of the rectum to sense and accommodate stool, the amount and consistency of stool, the integrity of the anal sphincters and musculature, and rectal motility. Fecal incontinence can have a substantially negative impact on QOL (Rao et al., 2016; Wald et al., 2014).

Pathophysiology

Fecal incontinence has many causes and risk factors and may be a symptom of an underlying condition. In general, it results from conditions that interrupt or disrupt the structure or function of the anorectal unit (Price & Bradley, 2013). Common causes include anal sphincter weakness, both traumatic (e.g., after surgical procedures involving the rectum) and nontraumatic (e.g., scleroderma); neuropathies both peripheral (e.g., pudendal) and generalized (e.g., diabetes); disorders of the pelvic floor (e.g., rectal prolapse); inflammation (radiation proctitis, IBD); central nervous system disorders (e.g., dementia, stroke, spinal cord injury, multiple sclerosis); diarrhea; fecal impaction with overflow; and behavioural disorders. It is less commonly a long-term consequence of vaginal childbirth injuries than in years past, most likely because of improved delivery methods. It is more common with advancing age (i.e., weakness or loss of anal or rectal muscle tone) (Rao et al., 2016; Wald et al., 2014).

Clinical Manifestations

Patients may have minor soiling, occasional urgency and loss of control, or complete incontinence. Patients may also experience poor control of flatus, diarrhea, or constipation. Passive incontinence occurs without warning; whereas, patients with urge incontinence have the sensation of the urge to defecate but cannot reach the toilet in time (Rao et al., 2016).

Assessment and Diagnostic Findings

Diagnostic studies are necessary because the treatment of fecal incontinence depends on the cause. A rectal examination and endoscopic examination such as a flexible sigmoidoscopy are performed to rule out tumours, inflammation, or fissures. X-ray studies such as barium enema, computed tomography (CT), anorectal manometry, and transit studies may be helpful in identifying alterations in intestinal mucosa and muscle tone or in detecting other structural or functional problems (Rao et al., 2016; Wald et al., 2014).

Medical Management

Medical management of fecal incontinence is directed at correcting the underlying cause. If fecal incontinence is related to diarrhea, the incontinence may disappear when diarrhea is successfully treated. Fecal incontinence secondary to a fecal impaction may cease after the impaction is removed and the rectum is cleansed. If the fecal incontinence is related to the use of contributory drugs (e.g., laxatives, antacids containing magnesium), the incontinence may improve or cease when the drug regimen is altered. When fecal incontinence is related to other disorders, treatments targeted at correcting the underlying disorder are initiated. Some patients benefit from the addition of psyllium (Metamucil) as a fibre supplement. In addition, administering loperamide 30 minutes prior to meals can be an effective intervention in some patients. Biofeedback therapy with pelvic floor muscle training can be of assistance if the problem is decreased sensory awareness or sphincter control. Bowel training programs can also be effective (Rao et al., 2016; Wald et al., 2014). Sacral nerve stimulation, provided by implanting a subcutaneous stimulator that delivers low amplitude electrical stimulation to the sacral nerve, may be an option for some patients refractory to other interventions (Yong, 2016). Surgical procedures include surgical reconstruction or repair of anal sphincter, artificial sphincter implantation, anal sphincter bulking by injection of synthetic agents, sacral nerve stimulation, or fecal diversion (Rao et al., 2016; Wald et al., 2014).

Nursing Management

The nurse obtains a thorough health history, including information about previous surgical procedures, chronic illnesses, dietary patterns, bowel habits and problems, and current medication regimen. Stool charts (e.g., Bristol Stool Form, see later discussion) may help with identifying frequency, volume, and consistency of the feces. The nurse also completes an examination of the rectal area (Stephen et al., 2012). If a fecal impaction is noted, it must be removed before instituting any preventive therapies (Gump & Schmelzer, 2016).

The nurse initiates a bowel training program that involves setting a schedule to establish bowel regularity. The goal is to help the patient achieve fecal continence. If this is not possible, the goal should be to manage the problem so the patient can have predictable, planned elimination. Sometimes it is necessary to use suppositories to stimulate the anal reflex. After the patient has achieved a regular schedule, the suppository can be discontinued. Biofeedback can be used in conjunction with these therapies to help the patient improve sphincter contractility and rectal sensitivity. Bowel regulation also involves the therapeutic use of diet and fibre. Foods that thicken stool (e.g., applesauce) and fibre products (e.g., psyllium) help improve continence (Gump & Schmelzer, 2016).

Fecal incontinence can also cause problems with perineal skin integrity. Maintaining skin integrity is a priority, especially in the debilitated or older patient. Incontinence briefs or adult diapers, although helpful in containing the fecal material, permit increased skin contact with feces and may cause skin excoriation. In general, incontinence briefs are to be used only for brief periods of time. The nurse encourages and teaches meticulous skin hygiene and uses perineal skin cleansers and skin protection products to protect perineal skin (Ness, 2018). In particular, participants enrolled in a randomized controlled trial who took psyllium supplements had less frequent stools and improved stool consistency than participants who took other fibre supplements, such as carboxymethylcellulose (MCM) or gum Arabic (GA) (Bliss et al., 2014). Conversely, foods that loosen stool (e.g., rhubarb, figs, prunes, plums) should be avoided. Some patients with fecal incontinence may benefit from the use of antidiarrheal medications (Gump & Schmelzer, 2016). Loperamide and diphenoxylate with atropine can be used; loperamide is the preferred medication because it does not cause central nervous system adverse effects (Rao et al., 2016).

Some patients may benefit from occasional use of foam anal plugs. However, many people find them unacceptable (Gump & Schmelzer, 2016).

Continence sometimes cannot be achieved, and the nurse assists the patient and family to accept and cope with this chronic situation. Patients with dementia may benefit from toileting assistance, including prompted or timed voiding and habit training, which is the setting of a regular time to go to the bathroom (e.g., after breakfast to have a bowel movement) (Gump & Schmelzer, 2016). The patient can use fecal incontinence devices, which include external collection devices and internal drainage systems. External devices are special rectal pouches, called fecal incontinence collectors, which are drainable. They are attached to a synthetic adhesive skin barrier specially designed to conform to the buttocks. Internal drainage systems can be used to eliminate fecal skin contact and are especially useful when there is extensive excoriation or skin breakdown. New fecal and bowel management systems (e.g., Flexi-Seal Fecal Management System) are available. These systems, which consist of a tube with a low-pressure balloon that conforms to the internal rectal area, may be used for up to 29 consecutive days (Fig. 38-1). Compared with rectal catheters, the newer bowel management systems are associated with improved patient safety; therefore, the former are now generally contraindicated (Pittman et al., 2012). However cases of hemorrhage have been reported with newer fecal management systems, and therefore careful assessment of clients receiving anticoagulation treatment is recommended prior to instituting these systems (Girard & Ousey, 2015; Gump & Schmelzer, 2016; Mulhall & Jindal, 2013).

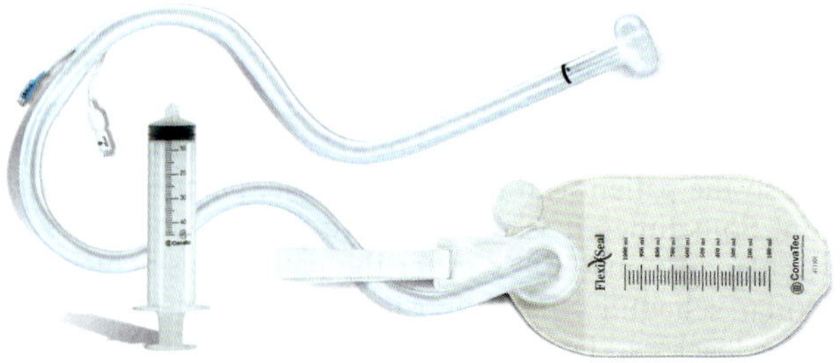

FIGURE 38-1. Flexi-Seal Fecal Management System. (Courtesy of Convatec, Inc., © Skillman, NJ.)

Irritable Bowel Syndrome

IBS is one of the most common GI conditions. Approximately 12% of adults in Canada report classic symptoms of IBS (Anastasi, Capili, & Chang, 2013; Chey, Kurlander, & Eswaran, 2015). IBS accounts for 3.5 million office visits and is a leading cause of workforce absenteeism (de Graaf et al., 2012). It occurs more commonly in women than in men, and the cause remains unknown (Surdea-Blaga & Dumitrascu, 2013). Although no anatomic or biochemical abnormalities have been found that account for its common symptoms, various factors are associated with the syndrome: heredity, psychological stress, or conditions such as depression and anxiety, a diet high in fat and stimulating or irritating foods, alcohol consumption, and smoking. The diagnosis is made only after tests confirm the absence of structural or other disorders (Surdea-Blaga & Dumitrascu, 2013).

Pathophysiology

IBS results from a functional disorder of intestinal motility. The change in motility may be related to neuroendocrine dysregulation, especially if there are changes in serotonin signalling, which regulates intestinal motility. Changes in intestinal motility may also result from infections or other inflammatory disorders or vascular or metabolic disturbances. The peristaltic waves are affected at specific segments of the intestine and in the intensity with which they propel the fecal matter forward. There is no evidence of inflammation or tissue changes in the intestinal mucosa (Mearin et al., 2016).

Clinical Manifestations

Symptoms can vary widely, ranging in intensity and duration from mild and infrequent to severe and continuous. The main symptom is an alteration in bowel patterns: constipation (classified as IBS-C), diarrhea (classified as IBS-D), or a combination of both (classified as IBS-M for "mixed"). The few patients with IBS who do not fit any of these three categories of IBS-C, IBS-D, or IBS-M, are classified as IBS-U for "unknown." Pain, bloating, and abdominal distention often accompany changes in bowel pattern. The abdominal pain is sometimes precipitated by eating and is frequently relieved by defecation. IBS frequently occurs concomitant with other GI disorders, including gastroesophageal reflux disease (GERD) and with a variety of non-GI functional disorders, including chronic fatigue syndrome, chronic pelvic pain, fibromyalgia, interstitial cystitis, migraine headaches, anxiety, and depression (Mearin et al., 2016; NIDDK, 2015).

Assessment and Diagnostic Findings

The clinical manifestations of IBS must be present sometime during the last 3 months with onset for at least 6 months prior to diagnosis. These manifestations include recurrent abdominal pain for at least 1 day weekly that is associated with two or more of the following (Mearin et al., 2016):

- Abdominal pain related to defecation;
- Abdominal pain associated with a change in frequency of stool;
- Abdominal pain associated with a change in form/appearance of stool.

A definite diagnosis of IBS also necessitates testing to confirm the absence of structural or other disorders. Results from a CBC and C-reactive protein or fecal calprotectin can rule out IBD (see later discussion) for patients who may have IBS-D or IBS-M, as well as serologic tests for celiac disease (see later discussion). Stool studies and colonoscopy may be performed to rule out other colon diseases (e.g., colorectal cancer, colitis) (Mearin et al., 2016).

Recording the quality and quantity of bowel movements in a stool diary such as the Bristol Stool Form Scale can be useful in determining the category of IBS (Mearin et al., 2016).

A definite diagnosis requires tests that confirm the absence of structural or other disorders. Stool studies, contrast x-ray studies, and proctoscopy may be performed to rule out other colon diseases (Mearin et al., 2016). Results from CBC and C-reactive protein or fecal calprotectin can rule out IBD. Barium enema and colonoscopy may reveal spasm, distention, or mucus accumulation in the intestine (Fig. 38-2). Manometry and electromyography (EMG) are used to study intraluminal pressure changes generated by spasticity.

Medical Management

The goals of treatment are relieving abdominal pain, controlling the diarrhea or constipation, and reducing stress. Restriction and then gradual reintroduction of foods that are possibly irritating may help determine what types of food are acting as irritants (e.g., beans, caffeinated products, corn, wheat, dairy lactose, fried foods, alcohol, spicy foods, aspartame). A high-fibre diet is prescribed to help control the diarrhea and constipation. Exercise can assist in reducing anxiety and increasing intestinal motility. Patients often find it helpful to participate in a stress reduction or behaviour modification program. Hydrophilic colloids (i.e., bulk) and antidiarrheal agents (e.g., loperamide) may be given to control the diarrhea and fecal urgency. Loperamide has not been found effective in reducing abdominal pain but is effective as an antidiarrheal agent (Chang, Lembo, & Sultan, 2014). Peppermint oil, a complementary medication, has proven effective in diminishing abdominal discomfort (Mearin et al., 2016).

Antidepressants can assist in treating underlying anxiety and depression but also have secondary benefits. They may affect serotonin levels, thus slowing intestinal transit time and improving diarrhea and abdominal comfort. Anticholinergics or antispasmodics (e.g., propantheline [Pro-Banthine]) may be prescribed to decrease smooth muscle spasm, cramping, and constipation.

Other alternatives for IBS management include probiotics and alternative medicines. Probiotics are bacteria that include *Lactobacillus* and *Bifidobacterium* that can be administered to help decrease abdominal bloating and gas. Complementary medicine approaches to treatment of IBS include artichoke leaf extract, peppermint oil, and caraway oil. They reputedly diminish IBS symptoms; however, formal studies are needed to examine their effectiveness (Mearin et al., 2016; Usher et al., 2013).

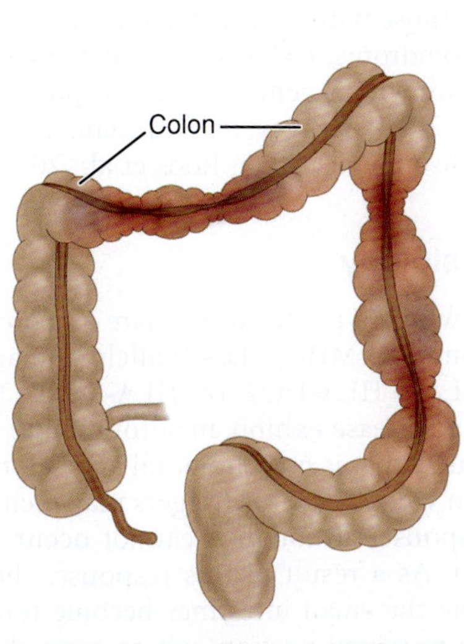

FIGURE 38-2. In irritable bowel syndrome (IBS), the spastic contractions of the bowel can be seen on x-ray contrast studies.

Nursing Management

The nurse's role is to provide patient and family education and encourage self-care activities (Ghiyasvandian et al., 2016) (Chart 38-2). The nurse may provide education on the appropriate use of a bowel habit diary, such as the Bristol Stool Form Scale. The nurse emphasizes and reinforces good sleep habits and good dietary habits (e.g., avoidance of food triggers). A good way to identify problem foods is to keep a 1- to 2-week food diary. Patients are encouraged to eat at regular times and to avoid food triggers. They should understand that although adequate fluid intake is necessary, fluid should not be taken with meals because this results in abdominal distention. Alcohol use and cigarette smoking are discouraged. Stress management via relaxation techniques, cognitive-behavioural therapy, yoga, and exercise can be recommended (Ghiyasvandian et al., 2016; Skrastins & Fletcher, 2016).

DISORDERS OF MALABSORPTION

The inability of the digestive system to absorb one or more of the major vitamins (especially A and B_{12}), minerals (i.e., iron and calcium), and nutrients (i.e., carbohydrates, fats, and proteins) occurs in disorders of **malabsorption**. Interruptions in the complex digestive process may occur anywhere in the digestive system and cause decreased absorption (Goebel, 2014; Grossman & Porth, 2014). The

NURSING RESEARCH PROFILE

Chart 38-2. The Efficacy of a Self-Care Program on Symptoms and Quality of Life of Patients With Irritable Bowel Syndrome

Ghiyasvandian, S., Ghorbani, M., Zakermoghadam, M., et al. (2016). The effects of a self-care program on the severity of symptoms and quality of life of patients with irritable bowel syndrome. *Gastroenterology Nursing*, *39*(5), 359–365.

Purpose

Patients with irritable bowel syndrome (IBS) experience abdominal pain, bloating, flatulence, and disordered bowel movements that can include diarrhea, constipation, or a combination of both. These symptoms can lead to embarrassment, anxiety, and depression, and negatively affect overall quality of life. Nurses can educate patients in self-care activities, including treatment, diet, and stress management activities, which can mitigate the effects of IBS. The purpose of this study was to examine the effects of a nurse-led self-care management program on the severity of symptoms and quality of life (QOL) of patients with IBS.

Design

This study was a randomized controlled trial that enrolled patients diagnosed with mild to moderate IBS who were treated in gastroenterology clinics in Arak, Iran. Criteria for participation included being between 18 and 65 years of age, able to read the training booklet, and able to complete the questionnaire. Sixty participants were randomized into the experimental group, and 59 participants were randomized into the control group. All participants received usual treatment of IBS by a gastroenterologist. Participants in the experimental group were educated in the self-care program, which consisted of a series of individual and group sessions that included education on the causes and treatment of IBS and the role of stress management, medications, and complementary medicine on alleviating IBS symptoms. Two follow-up phone calls were made to receive feedback on the effectiveness of the education. QOL was measured by having all participants complete the IBS-QOL questionnaire before and 2 months after the intervention. IBS symptom severity was measured by having all participants complete the IBS Symptom Severity Scale (IBS-SSS) during those same two intervals.

Findings

Independent *t* tests for the experimental and control groups preintervention showed no significant differences in either severity of symptoms or QOL. Paired *t* tests showed no difference in either severity of symptoms or QOL from preintervention to postintervention in the control group. However, paired *t* tests in the experimental group demonstrated significant differences from preintervention to postintervention in terms of both severity of symptoms ($p < 0.0001$) and QOL ($p < 0.0001$).

Nursing Implications

Findings from this study confirm that a nurse-led self-care intervention with patients with mild to moderate IBS can significantly improve symptom severity and overall QOL. Designing a specific training booklet, mixing individual and group education sessions, and scheduling follow-up phone calls appear to ensure successful delivery of this type of intervention. This self-care intervention can be modified and replicated for use in patients with other chronic disorders that adversely affect QOL.

conditions that cause malabsorption can be grouped into the following categories (Grossman & Porth, 2014):

- Mucosal (transport) disorders causing generalized malabsorption (e.g., celiac disease, Crohn's disease, radiation enteritis)
- Luminal disorders causing malabsorption (e.g., bile acid deficiency, Zollinger–Ellison syndrome, pancreatic insufficiency, small bowel bacterial overgrowth, or chronic pancreatitis)
- Lymphatic obstruction, interfering with transport of fat by-products of digestion into the systemic circulation (e.g., neoplasms, surgical trauma)

Table 38-2 lists the clinical and pathologic aspects of selected malabsorptive disorders. Chart 38-3 provides an education plan for a patient with lactose intolerance, a common malabsorptive disorder caused by a deficiency in lactase.

Celiac Disease

Celiac disease is a disorder of malabsorption caused by an autoimmune response to consumption of products that contain the protein gluten. Gluten is most commonly found in wheat, barley, rye, and other grains, malt, dextrin, and brewer's yeast. Celiac disease has become more common in the past decade, with an estimated prevalence of 1% in Canada (Canadian Celiac Association, 2018). Women are afflicted twice as often as men. This disease is more common among Caucasians, although the rates of celiac disease are on the rise among non-Caucasians. Celiac disease also has a familial risk component, particularly among first-degree relatives. Others at heightened risk include those with type 1 diabetes, Down syndrome, and Turner syndrome. Celiac disease may manifest at any age in a person who is genetically predisposed (Ferrara & Saccomano, 2015; Heavey & Stoltman, 2016; NIDDK, 2016a; Robinson et al., 2015; Roos et al., 2013).

Pathophysiology

Individuals who are predisposed share a major histocompatibility complex (MHC) class II allele human leukocyte antigen (HLA), HLA-DQ2 or HLA-DQ8. Those who develop celiac disease exhibit an autoimmune response to gluten products that is both humoral and cell mediated. It is not known what trigger or triggers may incite this autoimmune response, although it cannot occur if gluten is not ingested. As a result of this response, the epithelial cells that line the small intestines become inflamed, particularly the proximal portion, where most absorption of nutrients occurs. Eventually, the mucosal villi of the small

TABLE 38-2 Selected Disorders of Malabsorption

Diseases/Disorders	Pathophysiology	Clinical Features
Gastric resection with gastrojejunostomy	Decreased pancreatic stimulation because of duodenal bypass; poor mixing of food, bile, pancreatic enzymes; decreased intrinsic factor	Weight loss, moderate steatorrhea, anemia (combination of iron deficiency, vitamin B_{12} malabsorption, folate deficiency)
Pancreatic insufficiency (chronic pancreatitis, pancreatic carcinoma, pancreatic resection, cystic fibrosis)	Reduced intraluminal pancreatic enzyme activity, with maldigestion of lipids and proteins	History of abdominal pain followed by weight loss; marked steatorrhea, azotorrhea (excess of nitrogenous matter in the feces or urine); also frequent glucose intolerance (70% in pancreatic insufficiency)
Ileal dysfunction (resection or disease)	Loss of ileal absorbing surface leads to reduced bile-salt pool size and reduced vitamin B_{12} absorption; bile in colon inhibits fluid absorption	Diarrhea, weight loss with steatorrhea, especially when greater than 100 cm resection, decreased vitamin B_{12} absorption
Stasis syndromes (surgical strictures, blind loops, enteric fistulas, multiple jejunal diverticula, scleroderma)	Overgrowth of intraluminal intestinal bacteria, especially anaerobic organisms, to greater than 10^6/mL results in deconjugation of bile salts, leading to decreased effective bile-salt pool size, also bacterial utilization of vitamin B_{12}	Weight loss, steatorrhea; low vitamin B_{12} absorption; may have low D-xylose absorption
Zollinger–Ellison syndrome	Hyperacidity in duodenum inactivates pancreatic enzymes	Ulcer diathesis, steatorrhea
Lactose intolerance	Deficiency of intestinal lactase results in high concentration of intraluminal lactose with osmotic diarrhea	Varied degrees of diarrhea and cramps after ingestion of lactose-containing foods; positive lactose intolerance test, decreased intestinal lactase
Celiac disease (gluten-sensitive enteropathy)	Toxic response to a gluten fraction gliadin by surface epithelium results in destruction of absorbing surface of intestine	Weight loss, diarrhea, bloating, anemia (low iron, folate), osteomalacia, steatorrhea, azotorrhea, low D-xylose absorption; folate and iron malabsorption
Tropical sprue	Unknown toxic factor results in mucosal inflammation, partial villous atrophy	Weight loss, diarrhea, anemia (low folate, vitamin B_{12}); steatorrhea; low D-xylose absorption, low vitamin B_{12} absorption
Whipple's disease	Bacterial invasion of intestinal mucosa	Arthritis, hyperpigmentation, lymphadenopathy, serous effusions, fever, weight loss, steatorrhea, azotorrhea
Certain parasitic diseases (giardiasis, strongyloidiasis, coccidiosis, capillariasis)	Damage to or invasion of surface mucosa	Diarrhea, weight loss; steatorrhea; organism may be seen on jejunal biopsy or recovered in stool
Immunoglobulinopathy	Decreased local intestinal defences, lymphoid hyperplasia, lymphopenia	Frequent association with *Giardia:* hypogammaglobulinemia or isolated IgA deficiency

Adapted from Goebel, S. U. (2014). *Malabsorption*. Medscape. Retrieved December 27, 2016, from emedicine.medscape.com/article/180785-overview; Grossman, S. C., & Porth, C. M. (2014). *Porth's pathophysiology: Concepts of altered health states* (9th ed.). Philadelphia, PA: Wolters Kluwer.

intestine become denuded and cannot function. This results in loss of ability to absorb both micronutrients and macronutrients, causing systemic nutritional deficits (Ferrara & Saccomano, 2015; Grossman & Porth, 2014).

Clinical Manifestations

The most common GI clinical manifestations of celiac disease include diarrhea, steatorrhea, abdominal pain, abdominal distention, flatulence, and weight loss. However, these manifestations are more common among children than adults. Adults can present with non-GI signs and symptoms of celiac disease, which are highly variable and can include fatigue, general malaise, depression, hypothyroidism, migraine headaches, osteopenia, anemia, seizures, paresthesias in the hands and feet, and a red, shiny tongue. Some adults and children may evidence ridges in the enamel of their adult teeth, as well as discoloration or yellowing. Dermatitis herpetiformis is a rash that is frequently associated with celiac disease in adults; it manifests as clusters of erythematous macules that develop into itchy papules and vesicles on the forearms, elbows, knees, face, or buttocks (Heavy & Stoltman, 2016; NIDDK, 2016a).

Assessment and Diagnostic Findings

A comprehensive assessment of the patient's presenting signs and symptoms, as well as a family history and risk factor assessment, may provide the first clues that the patient may have celiac disease. The definitive diagnosis is based upon a series of serologic tests and endoscopic biopsy. It is important that the patient continues to consume gluten products during testing, or there could be a false-negative serologic finding. The first serologic test is the immunoglobulin A (IgA) antitissue transglutaminase (tTG), which is 90% sensitive and 95% specific to celiac disease. Findings are confirmed with upper endoscopy

CHART 38-3

Patient Education: Managing Lactose Intolerance

The nurse instructs the patient to:

- Recognize that deficiency of lactase, a digestive enzyme essential for the digestion and absorption of lactose ("milk sugar") from the intestines, results in an intolerance to milk.
- Prevent symptoms by eliminating milk and milk substances.
- Eliminate processed foods that have fillers, such as dried milk, added to them; recognizing this can help determine which foods may need to be eliminated.
- Reduce symptoms by pretreating foods with lactase preparations (e.g., Lactaid drops) before ingestion or by ingesting lactase enzyme tablets with the first bite of food.
- Understand that most people can tolerate 1 to 2 cups of milk or milk products daily without major problems; they are best tolerated if ingested in small amounts during the day.
- Be aware that lactase activity of yogurt with "active cultures" helps the digestion of lactose within the intestine better than lactase preparations.
- Recognize that milk and milk products are rich sources of calcium and vitamin D; elimination of milk from the diet may result in calcium and vitamin D deficiencies; decreased intake without supplements can lead to osteoporosis.

CHART 38-4

Patient Education: Foods That Contain Gluten

The nurse instructs the patient to avoid consuming the following:

- Foods that contain gluten-containing grains, including wheat, barley, bran, durum, spelt, faro, khorasan, rye, seitan, bulgur, graham, semolina, farina, emmer, and triticale; these generally include[a]:
  - Cakes, pastries, cookies
  - Breads, pastas, rolls, pizza, crackers
- Brewer's yeast; this generally includes beer, ale, and porter
- Malt, malt extract, and malt flavouring
- Modified food starch made from wheat (commonly contained in sour cream)

The nurse instructs the patient to exercise caution and carefully read the labels before consuming the following:

- Candies
- Caramel-coloured foods
- Oat products not specifically labelled as produced in gluten-free facilities
- Processed lunch meats and "shaped" foods (e.g., cheese sticks)
- Salad dressings, condiments, soy sauce, seasonings
- Soft drinks

[a]Some foods are specifically labelled "gluten free."

Adapted from Heavey, E., & Stoltman, J. (2016). Caring for hospitalized patients with celiac disease. *Nursing 2016*, *46*(11), 50–55; Robinson, B. L., Davis, S. C., Vess, J., et al. (2015). Primary care management of celiac disease. *The Nurse Practitioner*, *40*(2), 28–34.

with biopsies of the proximal small intestine (Heavey & Stoltman, 2016; Robinson et al., 2015).

Medical Management

Celiac disease is a chronic, noncurable, lifelong disease. There are no drugs that induce remission; the treatment is to refrain from exposure to gluten in foods and other products (see later discussion). A consult with a dietician may be advisable. The patient should be advised that it will likely take time before bothersome signs and symptoms resolve; indeed, it will take a full year before the integrity of the intestinal villi can be restored. Other manifestations of celiac disease may require specific, targeted treatment. For instance, patients who present with anemia may require folate, cobalamin, or iron supplements (see Chapter 54). Patients with osteopenia may require treatment for osteoporosis (see Chapter 71) (Ferrara & Saccomano, 2015; Heavey & Stoltman, 2016; Robinson et al., 2015).

Nursing Management

The nurse provides patient and family education regarding adherence to a gluten-free diet (see Chart 38-4), and how to avoid other gluten products. For instance, oats are not contraindicated in gluten-free diets; however, many oat products are produced in facilities that are cross-contaminated with wheat or other contraindicated grains. Likewise, gluten-free foods prepared in restaurants or dining areas that share preparatory space can become gluten contaminated. For instance, gluten-free toast prepared in a toaster that is also used for wheat-based toast can become gluten contaminated. Patients must become vigilant in asking restaurant and dining hall staff about how gluten-free foods are prepared.

Products that are not foods can also contain gluten. Many generic and over-the-counter drugs can be prepared with gluten gels. Toothpastes, communion wafers, and some cosmetics (e.g., lipsticks) and art supplies (e.g., modelling clay) can also contain gluten. Patients must understand how to carefully read labels on both food and nonfood products to determine if they contain gluten. Since 2013, the U.S. Food and Drug Administration (FDA) has regulated and monitored the appropriate application of gluten-free labels (Heavey & Stoltman, 2016; Robinson et al., 2015).

ACUTE ABDOMEN

An acute abdomen, sometimes called a *surgical abdomen* is characterized by an acute onset of abdominal pain that does not have a traumatic etiology and most typically requires swift surgical intervention to prevent peritonitis, sepsis, and septic shock. Disorders of the lower GI tract that may cause similar initial presenting clinical manifestations, causing acute abdominal pain and an acute abdomen include appendicitis, severe diverticulitis, and intestinal obstruction, all of which may lead to **peritonitis**, which is an inflammation of the lining of the abdominal cavity (Ansari, 2014; Saccomano & Ferrara, 2013).

Appendicitis

The appendix is a small, vermiform (i.e., wormlike) appendage about 8 to 10 cm (3 to 4 in) long that is attached to the cecum just below the ileocecal valve. The appendix fills with by-products of digestion and empties regularly into the cecum. Because it empties inefficiently and its lumen is small, the appendix is prone to obstruction and is particularly vulnerable to infection (i.e., appendicitis). Appendicitis, the most frequent cause of acute abdomen in the United States, is the most common reason for emergency abdominal surgery. Although it can occur at any age, it typically occurs between the ages of 10 and 30 years. Its incidence is slightly higher among males and there is a familial predisposition (Craig, 2015; NIDDK, 2014a).

Pathophysiology

The appendix becomes inflamed and edematous as a result of becoming kinked or occluded by a fecalith (i.e., hardened mass of stool), lymphoid hyperplasia (secondary to inflammation or infection), or rarely, foreign bodies (e.g., fruit seeds) or tumours. The inflammatory process increases intraluminal pressure, causing edema and obstruction of the orifice. Once obstructed, the appendix becomes ischemic, bacterial overgrowth occurs, and eventually gangrene or perforation occurs (Craig, 2015; Saccomano & Ferrara, 2013).

Clinical Manifestations

Vague epigastric or periumbilical pain (i.e., visceral pain that is dull and poorly localized) progresses to right lower quadrant pain (i.e., parietal pain that is sharp, discrete, and well localized) and is usually accompanied by a low-grade fever and nausea and sometimes by vomiting. Loss of appetite is common. In up to 50% of presenting cases, local tenderness is elicited at McBurney's point when pressure is applied (Fig. 38-3). Rebound tenderness (i.e., production or intensification of pain when pressure is released) may be present. The extent of tenderness and muscle spasm and the existence of constipation or diarrhea depend not so much on the severity of the appendiceal infection as on the location of the appendix. If the appendix curls around behind the cecum, pain and tenderness may be felt in the lumbar region. If its tip is in the pelvis, these signs may be elicited only on rectal examination. Pain on defecation suggests that the tip of the appendix is resting against the rectum; pain on urination suggests that the tip is near the bladder or impinges on the ureter. Some rigidity of the lower portion of the right rectus muscle may occur. Rovsing's sign may be elicited by palpating the left lower quadrant; this paradoxically causes pain to be felt in the right lower quadrant (see Fig. 38-3). If the appendix has ruptured, the pain becomes more diffuse; abdominal distention develops as a result of paralytic ileus, and the patient's condition worsens (Craig, 2015; Saccomano & Ferrara, 2013).

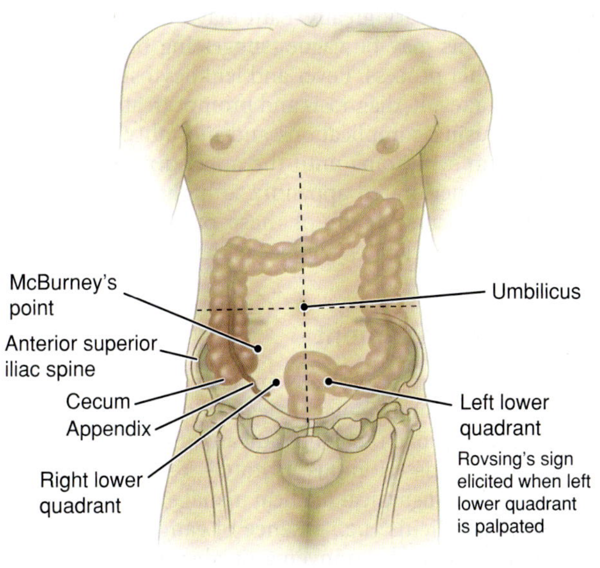

FIGURE 38-3. When the appendix is inflamed, tenderness can be noted in the right lower quadrant at McBurney's point, which is between the umbilicus and the anterior superior iliac spine. Rovsing's sign is pain felt in the right lower quadrant after the left lower quadrant has been palpated.

Constipation can also occur with appendicitis. Laxatives administered in this instance may result in perforation of the inflamed appendix. In general, a laxative or cathartic should never be given when a person has fever, nausea, and abdominal pain.

Assessment and Diagnostic Findings

Diagnosis is based on results of a complete physical examination and on laboratory findings and imaging studies. The complete blood cell count demonstrates an elevated white blood cell count with an elevation of the neutrophils. Abdominal x-ray films, ultrasound studies, and CT scans may reveal a right lower quadrant density or localized distention of the bowel. A pregnancy test may be performed for women of childbearing age to rule out ectopic pregnancy and before x-rays are obtained. A diagnostic laparoscopy may be used to rule out acute appendicitis in equivocal cases (Ansari, 2014).

Complications

The major complication of appendicitis is perforation of the appendix, which can lead to peritonitis, **abscess** formation (collection of purulent material), or portal pylephlebitis, which is septic thrombosis of the portal vein caused by vegetative emboli that arise from septic intestines. Perforation generally occurs 24 hours after the onset of pain. Symptoms include a fever of 37.7°C or greater, a toxic appearance, and continued abdominal pain or tenderness (Craig, 2015; Saccomano & Ferrara, 2013).

Gerontologic Considerations

Acute appendicitis is uncommon in the older population. When it does occur, classic signs and symptoms are altered and may vary greatly. Pain may be absent or minimal. Symptoms may be vague, suggesting bowel obstruction or another process. Fever and leukocytosis may not be present. As a result, diagnosis and prompt treatment may be delayed, causing complications and mortality. The patient may have no symptoms until the appendix ruptures. The incidence of perforated appendix is higher in the elderly population because many of these patients do not seek health care as quickly as younger patients.

Medical Management

Immediate surgery is typically indicated if appendicitis is diagnosed, although newer research is indicating that a nonsurgical approach may be indicated in early uncomplicated appendicitis (Horattas, Horattas, & Vasiliou, 2018). Conservative nonsurgical medical management for uncomplicated appendicitis (i.e., absence of gangrene or perforation of the appendix, empyema or abscess formation, or peritonitis) has been instituted in some instances with a reduced risk of complications and similar hospital length of stay as appendectomy (Salminen et al., 2015). To correct or prevent fluid and electrolyte imbalance, dehydration, and sepsis, antibiotics and IV fluids are administered until surgery is performed. Appendectomy (i.e., surgical removal of the appendix) is performed as soon as possible to decrease the risk of perforation. It may be performed using general or spinal anesthesia with a low abdominal incision (laparotomy) or by laparoscopy. Both laparotomy and laparoscopy are safe and effective in the treatment of appendicitis with perforation. However, recovery after laparoscopic surgery is generally quicker (Andersson, 2014; Bozkurt et al., 2015). Consequently, laparoscopic appendectomy is more common.

For complicated appendicitis (e.g., with gangrene or perforation), the patient is typically treated with a 3- to 5-day course of antibiotics postoperatively (van Rossem et al., 2014). Although it had been common practice for the surgeon to place a surgical drain, recent research findings suggest there is no improvement in outcomes but longer hospital lengths of stay when drains are used (Cheng et al., 2015).

Some patients may have abscess formation that involves the cecum and/or terminal ileum. In these selected cases, appendectomy may be deferred until the mass is drained. Most commonly, these abscesses are drained percutaneously or surgically. The patient continues to receive treatment with antibiotics. After the abscess is drained and there is no further evidence of infection, an appendectomy is then performed (Ansari, 2014; Craig, 2015).

Nursing Management

Goals include relieving pain, preventing fluid volume deficit, reducing anxiety, eliminating infection due to the potential or actual disruption of the GI tract, maintaining skin integrity, and attaining optimal nutrition.

The nurse prepares the patient for surgery, which includes an IV infusion to replace fluid loss and promote adequate renal function, antibiotic therapy to prevent infection, and administration of analgesic agents for pain (Saccomano & Ferrara, 2013). An enema is not given because it can lead to perforation. After surgery, the nurse places the patient in a high Fowler position. This position reduces the tension on the incision and abdominal organs, helping to reduce pain. It also promotes thoracic expansion, diminishing the work of breathing, and decreasing the likelihood of atelectasis. The patient is educated on the use of an incentive spirometer and encouraged to use it at least every 2 hours while awake. A parenteral opioid (e.g., morphine) is typically prescribed to relieve pain; this is switched to an oral agent when the patient is able to tolerate oral fluids and foods. Any patient who was dehydrated before surgery receives IV fluids. When tolerated, oral fluids are given. Food is provided as desired and tolerated on the day of surgery when bowel sounds are present. The nurse auscultates for the return of bowel sounds and queries the patient for passing of flatus. Urine output is monitored to ensure that the patient is not hampered by postoperative urinary retention and to ensure that hydration status is adequate. The patient is encouraged to ambulate the day of surgery to reduce risks of atelectasis and venous thromboemboli (VTE) formation.

The patient may be discharged on the day of surgery if the temperature is within expected limits, there is no undue discomfort in the operative area, and the appendectomy was uncomplicated. Discharge teaching for the patient and family is imperative. The nurse instructs the patient to make an appointment to have the surgeon remove the sutures between the fifth and seventh days after surgery (Evans & Curtin, 2014). Incision care and activity guidelines are discussed; heavy lifting is to be avoided postoperatively, although usual activities can usually be resumed within 2 to 4 weeks.

If there is a possibility of peritonitis, a drain is left in place at the area of the incision. Patients at risk for this complication may be kept in the hospital for several days and are monitored carefully for signs of intestinal obstruction or secondary hemorrhage. Secondary abscesses may form in the pelvis, under the diaphragm, or in the liver, causing elevation of the temperature, pulse rate, and white blood cell count.

When the patient is ready for discharge, the patient and family are taught to care for the incision and perform dressing changes and irrigations as prescribed. A home care nurse may be needed to assist with this care and to monitor the patient for complications and wound healing. Other complications of appendectomy are listed in Table 38-3.

Diverticular Disease

A **diverticulum** is a saclike herniation of the lining of the bowel that extends through a defect in the muscle layer. Diverticula may occur anywhere in the small intestine or colon but most commonly occur in the sigmoid colon (at least 95%) (DiMarino, 2013; Shahedi et al., 2016). However, persons of Asian heritage tend to develop diverticula in the right colon, probably because of genetic differences (Shahedi et al., 2016).

Diverticulosis exists when multiple diverticula are present without inflammation or symptoms. Diverticular disease of the colon is very common in developed countries, and its prevalence increases with age; indeed, it is present in half of all adults over 65 years of age, and nearly all adults by 90 years of age (DiMarino, 2013). Diverticulosis

TABLE 38-3 Potential Complications and Nursing Interventions After Appendectomy

Complication	Nursing Interventions
Peritonitis	Monitor for abdominal tenderness, fever, vomiting, abdominal rigidity, and tachycardia. Employ constant nasogastric suction. Correct dehydration as prescribed.
Pelvic abscess	Administer antibiotic agents as prescribed. Evaluate for anorexia, chills, fever, and diaphoresis. Observe for diarrhea, which may indicate pelvic abscess. Prepare patient for rectal examination. Prepare patient for surgical drainage procedure.
Subphrenic abscess (abscess under the diaphragm)	Assess patient for chills, fever, and diaphoresis. Prepare for x-ray examination. Prepare for surgical drainage of abscess.
Ileus (paralytic and mechanical)	Assess for bowel sounds. Employ nasogastric intubation and suction. Replace fluids and electrolytes by intravenous route as prescribed. Prepare for surgery, if diagnosis of mechanical ileus is established.

is the most common pathologic incidental finding on colonoscopy. Approximately 80% of patients with diverticulosis never develop any complications or symptoms of disease.

A low intake of dietary fibre is considered a risk factor, as well as obesity, a history of cigarette smoking, regular use of nonsteroidal anti-inflammatory drugs (NSAIDs) and acetaminophen (Tylenol), and a positive family history. Although there is an equal prevalence of diverticulosis between men and women, complications related to diverticulosis more commonly happen in men younger than 44 years of age, and in women older than 54 years of age (Razik & Nguyen, 2015).

Diverticulitis results when food and bacteria retained in a diverticulum produce infection and inflammation that can impede drainage and lead to perforation or abscess formation. At least 10% of patients with diverticulosis have diverticulitis at some point. A congenital predisposition is suspected when the disorder occurs in those younger than 40 years. Diverticulitis may occur as an acute attack or may persist as a continuing, smoldering infection. The symptoms manifested generally result from complications: abscess, **fistula** (abnormal tract) formation, obstruction, perforation, peritonitis, and hemorrhage (DiMarino, 2013).

Pathophysiology

Diverticula form when the mucosa and submucosal layers of the colon herniate through the muscular wall because of high intraluminal pressure, low volume in the colon (i.e., fibre-deficient contents), and decreased muscle strength in the colon wall (i.e., muscular hypertrophy from hardened fecal masses). Bowel contents can accumulate in the diverticulum and decompose, causing inflammation and infection. The diverticulum can also become obstructed and then inflamed if the obstruction continues. The inflammation of the weakened colonic wall of the diverticulum can cause it to perforate, giving rise to irritability and spasticity of the colon (i.e., diverticulitis). In addition, abscesses develop and may eventually perforate, leading to peritonitis and erosion of the arterial blood vessels, resulting in bleeding. When symptoms of diverticulitis have developed, microperforation of the colon may also take place (DiMarino, 2013; Shahedi et al., 2016).

Clinical Manifestations

Chronic constipation often precedes the development of diverticulosis by many years. Frequently, no problematic symptoms occur with diverticulosis. Signs and symptoms of diverticulosis are relatively mild and include bowel irregularity with intervals of diarrhea, nausea and anorexia, and bloating or abdominal distention (Shahedi et al., 2016).

With repeated local inflammation of the diverticula, the large bowel may narrow with fibrotic strictures, leading to cramps, narrow stools, and increased constipation or at times intestinal obstruction. Weakness, fatigue, and anorexia are common symptoms. With diverticulitis, the patient reports an acute onset of mild to severe pain in the left lower quadrant, accompanied by nausea, vomiting, fever, chills, and leukocytosis (acute infection with more than 10,000 leukocytes [white blood cells]). The condition, if untreated, can lead to peritonitis and septicemia (DiMarino, 2013; Shahedi et al., 2016).

Assessment and Diagnostic Findings

Diverticulosis is typically diagnosed by colonoscopy, which permits visualization of the extent of diverticular disease and allows the physician to biopsy tissue to rule out other diseases. Until recently, barium enema had been the preferred diagnostic test, but it is now used less frequently than colonoscopy. If there are symptoms of peritoneal irritation when the diagnosis is diverticulitis, barium enema is contraindicated because of the potential for perforation.

CT with contrast agent is the diagnostic test of choice if the suspected diagnosis is diverticulitis; it can also reveal abscesses. Abdominal x-rays may demonstrate free air under the diaphragm if a perforation has occurred from the diverticulitis. Results from these radiologic tests confirm whether or not the patient has uncomplicated diverticulitis or complicated diverticulitis that could require surgical intervention. The Hinchey classification is used as a guide to determine treatment (DiMarino, 2013; Shahedi et al., 2016), see Table 38-4. Laboratory tests that assist in diagnosis include a complete blood cell count, revealing an elevated white blood cell count, and elevated erythrocyte sedimentation rate (ESR).

Complications

Complications of diverticulitis include peritonitis, abscess formation, fistulas, and bleeding. If an abscess develops, the associated findings are tenderness, a palpable mass,

TABLE 38-4 Hinchey Classification: Staging of Acute, Complicated Diverticulitis

Hinchey Stage	Complication of Acute Diverticulitis
I	Localized pericolic or mesenteric abscess
II	Walled-off pelvic, intra-abdominal, or retroperitoneal abscess
III	Generalized purulent peritonitis
IV	Generalized fecal peritonitis

Adapted from Hinchey, E. J., Schaal, P. G., & Richards, G. K. (1978). Treatment of perforated diverticular disease of the colon. *Advances in Surgery*, *12*, 85–109.

fever, and leukocytosis. An inflamed diverticulum that perforates results in abdominal pain localized over the involved segment, usually the sigmoid; local abscess or peritonitis follows. Abdominal pain, a rigid boardlike abdomen, loss of bowel sounds, and signs and symptoms of shock occur with peritonitis. On occasion, the diverticular inflammation creates an abnormal passage between body structures such as a colovesical fistula (between bowel and bladder). Noninflamed or slightly inflamed diverticula may erode areas adjacent to arterial branches, causing massive rectal bleeding.

Gerontologic Considerations

The incidence of diverticular disease increases with age because of degeneration and structural changes in the circular muscle layers of the colon and because of cellular hypertrophy. The symptoms are less pronounced in older adults. Older adults do not have abdominal pain until infection occurs. They may delay reporting symptoms because they fear surgery or are afraid that they may have cancer (Eliopoulos, 2018). Blood in the stool is overlooked frequently, especially in older patients, because of a failure to examine the stool or the inability to see changes if vision is impaired.

Medical Management

Dietary and Pharmacologic Management

Diverticulitis can usually be treated on an outpatient basis with diet and medication (Balasubramanian et al., 2017). When symptoms occur, rest, analgesics, and antispasmodics are recommended. Initially, a clear liquid diet is consumed until the inflammation subsides; then a high-fibre, low-fat diet is recommended. This type of diet helps increase stool volume, decrease colonic transit time, and reduce intraluminal pressure. Antibiotics are prescribed for 7 to 10 days. A bulk-forming laxative is also prescribed.

In acute cases of diverticulitis with significant symptoms, hospitalization is required. Hospitalization is often indicated for those who are older, immunocompromised, or taking corticosteroids. Withholding oral intake, administering IV fluids, and instituting nasogastric suctioning if vomiting or distention occurs are used to rest the bowel. Broad-spectrum antibiotics are prescribed for 7 to 10 days. An opioid (e.g., meperidine [Demerol]) is prescribed for pain relief. Morphine is contraindicated because it can increase intraluminal pressure in the colon, exacerbating symptoms (Tursi, 2012). Oral intake is increased as symptoms subside. A low-fibre diet may be necessary until signs of infection decrease.

Antispasmodics such as propantheline bromide and oxyphencyclimine (Daricon) may be prescribed. Often it is not possible for patients to consume the 20 to 30 g of daily fibre that is recommended. Usual stools can be achieved by supplementing dietary fibre by using bulk preparations (psyllium) or stool softeners (docusate), by instilling warm oil into the rectum, or by inserting an evacuant suppository (bisacodyl). Such a prophylactic plan can reduce the bacterial flora of the bowel, diminish the bulk of the stool, and soften the fecal mass so that it moves more easily through the area of inflammatory obstruction.

Surgical Management

Although acute diverticulitis usually subsides with medical management, immediate surgical intervention is necessary if complications (e.g., perforation, peritonitis, hemorrhage, obstruction) occur. In particular, patients with Hinchey Stage III or IV diverticulitis are considered surgical candidates (Shahedi et al., 2016). In cases of abscess formation without peritonitis, hemorrhage, or obstruction, CT-guided percutaneous drainage may be performed to drain the abscess, and IV antibiotics are administered. After the abscess is drained and the acute episode of inflammation has subsided (after approximately 6 weeks), surgery may be recommended to prevent repeated episodes. Two types of surgery are typically considered either to treat acute complications or prevent further episodes of inflammation:

- One-stage resection, in which the inflamed area is removed and a primary end-to-end anastomosis is completed
- Multiple-stage procedures for complications such as obstruction or perforation (Fig. 38-4)

The type of surgery performed depends on the extent of complications found during surgery. When possible, the

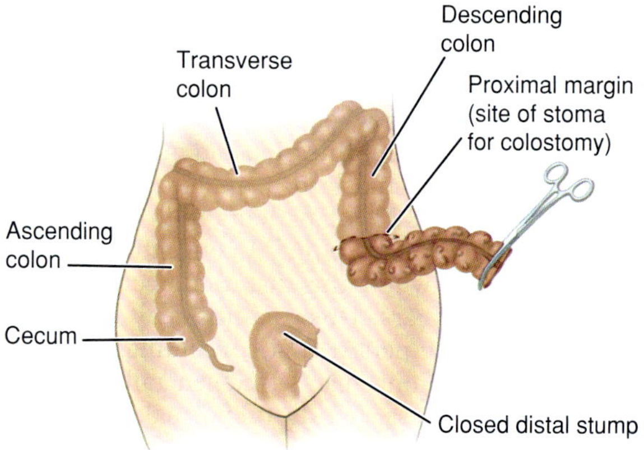

FIGURE 38-4. The Hartmann's procedure for diverticulitis: Primary resection for diverticulitis of the colon. The affected segment (clamp attached) has been divided at its distal end. In a primary anastomosis, the proximal margin (*dotted line*) is transected and the bowel attached end to end. In a two-stage procedure, a colostomy is constructed at the proximal margin with the distal stump oversewn (Hartmann's procedure, as shown) and the stump is left in the pelvis. The distal stump may be brought to the surface as a mucous fistula if there is concern about blood supply. The second stage consists of colostomy takedown and anastomosis.

area of diverticulitis is resected and the remaining bowel is joined end-to-end (i.e., primary resection and end-to-end anastomosis). This is performed using traditional surgical or laparoscopically assisted colectomy. More primary anastomoses are completed because surgeons are now able to perform intraoperative colonic lavage to decrease intestinal bacterial load. A two-stage resection may be performed in which the diseased colon is resected (as in a one-stage procedure) but no anastomosis is performed. In this procedure, one end of the bowel is brought out to the abdominal wall and the distal end is closed over and left in the abdomen (Hartmann's procedure) or if the blood supply to the distal colon is questionable, both ends of the bowel are brought out to the abdominal wall (double barrel) (McDermott et al., 2014). Both Hartmann's and double-barrel colostomies are usually reanastomosed at a later time. Fecal diversion procedures are discussed later in this chapter.

Nursing Process

The Patient With Diverticulitis

Assessment

When obtaining the health history, the nurse asks the patient about the onset and duration of pain and about past and present elimination patterns. The nurse reviews dietary habits to determine fibre intake and asks the patient about straining at stool, history of constipation with periods of diarrhea, tenesmus, abdominal bloating, and distention.

Assessment includes auscultation for the presence and character of bowel sounds and palpation for left lower quadrant pain, tenderness, or firm mass. The stool is inspected for pus, mucus, or blood. Temperature, pulse, and blood pressure are monitored for abnormal variations.

Nursing Priorities

Based on the assessment data, the nursing priorities may include the following:

- Constipation related to narrowing of the colon
- Acute pain as a result of inflammation and infection

Collaborative Problems/ Potential Complications

Potential complications that may develop include the following:

- Peritonitis
- Abscess formation
- Bleeding

Planning and Goals

The major goals for the patient may include attainment and maintenance of normal elimination patterns, pain relief, and absence of complications.

Nursing Interventions

Maintaining Normal Elimination Patterns

The nurse recommends a fluid intake of 2 L per day (within limits of the patient's cardiac and renal reserve) and suggests foods that are soft but have increased fibre, such as prepared cereals or soft-cooked vegetables, to increase the bulk of the stool and facilitate peristalsis, thereby promoting defecation. An individualized exercise program is encouraged to improve abdominal muscle tone. It is important to review the patient's daily routine to establish a schedule for meals and a set time for defecation and to assist in identifying habits that may have suppressed the urge to defecate. The nurse encourages daily intake of bulk laxatives such as psyllium, which helps propel feces through the colon. Stool softeners are administered as prescribed to decrease straining at stool, which decreases intestinal pressure. Oil retention enemas may be prescribed to soften the stool, making it easier to pass. Some people with diverticulosis may have food triggers such as nuts and popcorn that bring on an attack of diverticulitis. Patients should be urged to identify these triggers and avoid them.

Relieving Pain

Opioid analgesics (e.g., meperidine) to relieve the pain of diverticulitis and antispasmodic agents to decrease intestinal spasm are administered as prescribed (Tursi, 2012). The nurse records the intensity, duration, and location of pain to determine whether the inflammatory process worsens or subsides.

Monitoring and Managing Potential Complications

The major nursing focus is to prevent complications by identifying patients at risk and managing their symptoms as needed. The nurse assesses for the following signs and symptoms of perforation: increased abdominal pain and tenderness accompanied by abdominal rigidity, elevated white blood cell count, elevated ESR, increased temperature, tachycardia, and hypotension. Perforation is a surgical emergency. The clinical manifestations of perforation and peritonitis and the care of the patient with peritonitis are presented in the next section. The nurse monitors vital signs and urine output and administers IV fluids to replace volume loss as needed.

Promoting Home and Community-Based Care

Because patients and their family members and health care providers tend to focus on the most obvious needs and issues, the nurse reminds the patient and family about the importance of continuing health promotion and screening practices. The nurse educates patients who have not been involved in these practices in the past about their importance and refers the patients to appropriate health care providers.

Evaluation

Expected patient outcomes may include the following:

1. Attains a normal pattern of elimination
   a. Reports less abdominal cramping and pain
   b. Reports the passage of soft, formed stool without pain
   c. Adds unprocessed bran to foods
   d. Drinks at least 10 glasses of fluid each day (if fluid intake is tolerated)
   e. Exercises daily
2. Reports decreased pain
   a. Requests analgesics as needed
   b. Adheres to a low-fibre diet during acute episodes
3. Recovers without complications
   a. Is afebrile
   b. Has normal blood pressure
   c. Has a soft, nontender abdomen with normal bowel sounds
   d. Maintains adequate urine output
   e. Has no blood in the stool

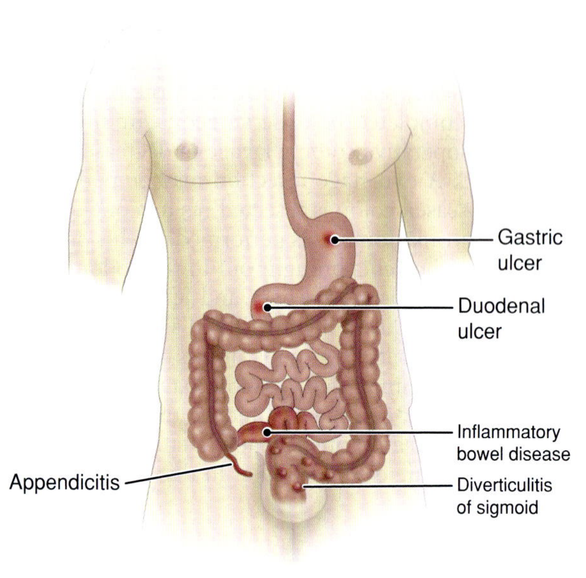

FIGURE 38-5. Common gastrointestinal causes of peritonitis.

Peritonitis

Peritonitis is inflammation of the peritoneum, which is the serous membrane lining the abdominal cavity and covering the viscera. Usually, it is a result of bacterial infection but may occur secondary to a fungal or mycobacterial infection; the organisms come from diseases or disorders of the GI tract or, in women, from the internal reproductive organs (e.g., fallopian tube). The most common bacteria implicated are *Escherichia coli* and *Klebsiella, Proteus, Pseudomonas*, and *Streptococcus* species. Peritonitis can also result from external sources such as abdominal surgery or trauma (e.g., gunshot wound, stab wound) or an inflammation that extends from an organ outside the peritoneal area, such as the kidney, or from continuous ambulatory peritoneal dialysis (CAPD) (see Chapter 45) (Ansari, 2014; Daley, 2015). Peritonitis can be categorized as (Daley, 2015):

- Primary peritonitis, also called *spontaneous bacterial peritonitis* (*SBP*), occurs as a spontaneous bacterial infection of ascitic fluid. This occurs most commonly in adult patients with liver failure (see Chapter 39).
- Secondary peritonitis occurs secondary to perforation of abdominal organs with spillage that infects the serous peritoneum. The most common causes include a perforated appendix (see later discussion), perforated peptic ulcer (see Chapter 37), perforated sigmoid colon caused by severe diverticulitis (see later discussion), volvulus of the colon (see later discussion), and strangulation of the small intestine (see later discussion). The major focus of this section is on secondary peritonitis.
- Tertiary peritonitis occurs as a result of a suprainfection in a patient who is immunocompromised. Tuberculous peritonitis in a patient with AIDS is an example of tertiary peritonitis; these are rare causes of peritonitis.

Pathophysiology

Secondary peritonitis is caused by leakage of contents from abdominal organs into the abdominal cavity, usually as a result of inflammation, infection, ischemia, trauma, or tumour perforation. Bacterial proliferation occurs. Edema of the tissues results, and exudation of fluid develops in a short time. Fluid in the peritoneal cavity becomes turbid with increasing amounts of protein, white blood cells, cellular debris, and blood. The immediate response of the intestinal tract is hypermotility, soon followed by paralytic ileus with an accumulation of air and fluid in the bowel (Daley, 2015; Grossman & Porth, 2014). (See Fig. 38-5 for common causes of peritonitis.)

Clinical Manifestations

Symptoms depend on the location and extent of the inflammation. The early clinical manifestations of peritonitis frequently are the signs and symptoms of the disorder causing the condition (e.g., manifestations of infection). At first, pain is diffuse but then becomes constant, localized, and more intense over the site of the pathologic process (site of maximal peritoneal irritation). Movement usually aggravates it. The affected area of the abdomen becomes extremely tender and distended, and the muscles become rigid. Rebound tenderness may be present. Usually, anorexia, nausea, and vomiting occur and peristalsis is diminished, followed by paralytic ileus. An initial temperature of 37.8° to 38.3°C (100° to 101°F) can be expected, along with an increased pulse rate. With progression of the condition, patients may become hypotensive. Without swift and decisive intervention, clinical manifestations will mirror those of sepsis and septic shock (Ansari, 2014; Daley, 2015; Saccomano & Ferrara, 2013) (see Chapter 18).

Assessment and Diagnostic Findings

The white blood cell count is elevated and may demonstrate a relative increase in the immature neutrophils (i.e., bands), consistent with bacterial infection. The hemoglobin and hematocrit levels may be low if blood loss has occurred. Serum electrolyte studies may reveal altered levels of potassium, sodium, and chloride.

An abdominal x-ray may show air and fluid levels as well as distended bowel loops. Abdominal ultrasound may reveal **abscesses** (localized collection of purulent material surrounded by inflamed tissues) and fluid collections, and ultrasound-guided aspiration may assist in easier placement of drains. A CT scan of the abdomen may show abscess formation. Peritoneal aspiration and culture and sensitivity studies of the aspirated fluid may reveal infection and identify the causative organisms. MRI may be used for diagnosis of intra-abdominal abscesses (Daley, 2015).

Complications

The inflammation is most commonly not localized, and the entire abdominal cavity shows evidence of widespread infection. Sepsis is the major cause of death from peritonitis. Shock may result from septicemia or hypovolemia. The inflammatory process may cause intestinal obstruction, primarily from the development of bowel adhesions.

Medical Management

Fluid, colloid, and electrolyte replacement is the major focus of medical management. The administration of several litres of an isotonic solution is prescribed. Hypovolemia occurs because massive amounts of fluid and electrolytes move from the intestinal lumen into the peritoneal cavity and deplete the fluid in the vascular space.

Analgesic medications are prescribed for pain. Antiemetic agents are given as prescribed for nausea and vomiting. Intestinal intubation and suction assist in relieving abdominal distention and in promoting intestinal function. Fluid in the abdominal cavity can cause pressure that restricts expansion of the lungs and causes respiratory distress. Oxygen therapy by nasal cannula or mask generally promotes adequate oxygenation, but airway intubation and ventilator assistance occasionally are required.

Antibiotic therapy is initiated early in the treatment of peritonitis. Large doses of a broad-spectrum antibiotic are given IV until the specific organism causing the infection is identified and appropriate antibiotic therapy can be initiated.

The main focus of treatment in secondary peritonitis is to identify the source of infection and eradicate it. Surgical treatment is directed toward excision (e.g., appendix), resection with or without anastomosis (e.g., intestine), repair (e.g., perforation), and drainage (e.g., abscess). With extensive sepsis, a fecal diversion may need to be created (see later discussions). In selected instances, ultrasound-guided and CT-guided peritoneal drainage of abdominal and extraperitoneal abscesses has allowed for avoidance or delay of surgical therapy until the acute septic process has subsided (Ansari, 2014; Daley, 2015; Saccomano & Ferrara, 2013). Antibiotics are continued postoperatively; a systematic review of antibiotic regimens noted that no one regimen of antibiotics is superior to another in terms of improving outcomes (Wong et al., 2012).

Nursing Management

Intensive care is needed for the patient with septic shock. Signs indicating that peritonitis is subsiding include a decrease in temperature and pulse rate, softening of the abdomen, return of peristaltic sounds, passing of flatus, and bowel movements. The nurse increases fluid and food intake gradually and reduces parenteral fluids as prescribed. A worsening clinical condition may indicate a complication, and the nurse must prepare the patient for emergency surgery. The nursing management of a patient treated for secondary peritonitis is based upon the patient's primary diagnosis and treatment (see discussions of Nursing Management of patients with Appendicitis, Diverticular Disease, and Intestinal Obstruction).

Signs that indicate that peritonitis is subsiding include a decrease in temperature and pulse rate, softening of the abdomen, return of peristaltic sounds, passing of flatus, and bowel movements. The nurse increases fluid and food intake gradually and reduces parenteral fluids as prescribed. A worsening clinical condition may indicate a complication, and the nurse then prepares the patient for emergency surgery.

Drains are frequently inserted during the surgical procedure, and the nurse monitors and records the character of the drainage postoperatively. Care must be taken when moving and turning the patient to prevent the drains from being dislodged. It is also important for the nurse to prepare the patient and family for discharge by teaching the patient to care for the incision and drains if the patient will be sent home with the drains still in place. Referral for home care may be indicated for further monitoring and patient and family teaching.

INFLAMMATORY BOWEL DISEASE

IBD refers to two chronic inflammatory GI disorders: Crohn's disease (i.e., regional enteritis) and ulcerative colitis. Both disorders have striking similarities but also several differences, which are compared in Table 38-5.

The incidence of IBD in the Canadian population has increased in the past century and affects 1 out of every 140 Canadians (Crohn's and Colitis Canada, 2018). People between 15 and 30 years of age are at the greatest risk of developing IBD, followed by people between 50 and 70 years of age. Women and men tend to be equally affected, and family history appears to predispose people to IBD, particularly if a first-degree relative has the disease. Some genetic linkage exists, and in fact, a positive family history is the largest independent risk factor for IBD. Crohn's disease and ulcerative colitis are more prevalent in Jewish people, especially North American Jews of eastern European descent, than in any other ethnic group with recent advances in phenotyping examining overall population patterns (Ananthakrishnan et al., 2014; Basso, Zambon, & Plebani, 2014). It was previously believed that psychological conditions such as anxiety or depression predisposed certain people to IBD; however, this theory has been discarded.

Despite extensive research, the cause of IBD is still unknown. Researchers theorize that it is triggered by environmental agents such as pesticides, food additives, tobacco, and radiation (Basso et al., 2014). NSAIDs have been found

TABLE 38-5 Comparison of Crohn's Disease and Ulcerative Colitis

Factor	Crohn's Disease	Ulcerative Colitis
Course	Prolonged, variable	Exacerbations, remissions
Pathology		
Early	Transmural thickening	Mucosal ulceration
Late	Deep, penetrating granulomas	Minute, mucosal ulcerations
Clinical Manifestations		
Location	Ileum, ascending colon (usually)	Rectum, descending colon
Bleeding	Usually not, but if it occurs, tends to be mild	Common–severe
Perianal involvement	Common	Rare–mild
Fistulas	Common	Rare
Rectal involvement	About 20%	Almost 100%
Diarrhea	Less severe	Severe
Abdominal mass	Common	Rare
Diagnostic Study Findings		
Barium series	Regional, discontinuous skip lesions Narrowing of colon Thickening of bowel wall Mucosal edema Stenosis, fistulas	Diffuse involvement No narrowing of colon No mucosal edema Stenosis rare Shortening of colon
Sigmoidoscopy	May be unremarkable unless accompanied by perianal fistulas	Abnormal inflamed mucosa
Colonoscopy	Distinct ulcerations separated by relatively normal mucosa in ascending colon	Friable mucosa with pseudopolyps or ulcers in descending colon
Therapeutic Management	Corticosteroids, sulfonamide (sulfasalazine [Azulfidine]) Antibiotics Parenteral nutrition Partial or complete colectomy, with ileostomy or anastomosis Rectum can be preserved in some patients Recurrence common	Corticosteroids, sulphonamides; sulfasalazine useful in preventing recurrence Bulk hydrophilic agents Antibiotics Proctocolectomy, with ileostomy Rectum can be preserved in only a few patients "cured" by colectomy
Systemic Complications	Small bowel obstruction Right-sided hydronephrosis Nephrolithiasis Cholelithiasis Arthritis Retinitis, iritis Erythema nodosum	Toxic megacolon Perforation Hemorrhage Malignant neoplasms Pyelonephritis Nephrolithiasis Cholangiocarcinoma Arthritis Retinitis, iritis Erythema nodosum

to exacerbate IBD. Allergies and immune disorders have also been suggested as causes. Abnormal response to dietary or bacterial antigens has been studied extensively, and genetic factors also are being studied. There is a high prevalence of coexistent IBS, which complicates the overall symptom presentation.

Crohn's Disease (Regional Enteritis)

Crohn's disease is usually first diagnosed in adolescents or young adults but can appear at any time of life. The incidence has risen over the past 30 years. Crohn's disease is seen more often in smokers than in nonsmokers (Nunes et al., 2013).

Pathophysiology

Crohn's disease is a subacute and chronic inflammation of the GI tract wall that extends through all layers (i.e., transmural lesion). Although its characteristic histopathological changes can occur anywhere in the GI tract, it most commonly occurs in the distal ileum and, to a lesser degree, the ascending colon. It is characterized by periods of remission and exacerbation. The disease process begins with edema and thickening of the mucosa. Ulcers begin to appear on the inflamed mucosa. These lesions are not in continuous contact with one another and are separated by normal tissue. Hence, these clusters of ulcers tend to take on a classic "cobblestone" appearance. Fistulas, fissures, and abscesses form as the inflammation extends into the peritoneum. Granulomas occur in 50% of patients. As the disease advances, the bowel wall thickens and becomes fibrotic, and the intestinal lumen narrows. Diseased bowel loops sometimes adhere to other loops surrounding them. Approximately 35% of patients have only ileal involvement (ileitis), 45% have diseased ileum and colon (ileocolitis), and 20% have only colon involvement (granulomatous colitis) (Walfish, 2016).

Clinical Manifestations

The onset of symptoms is usually insidious in Crohn's disease, with prominent right lower quadrant abdominal pain and diarrhea unrelieved by defecation. Scar tissue and the formation of granulomas interfere with the ability of the intestine to transport products of upper intestinal digestion through the constricted lumen, resulting in cramping abdominal pains. There is abdominal tenderness and spasm. Because eating stimulates intestinal peristalsis, the cramping pains occur after meals. To avoid these bouts of cramping pain, the patient tends to limit food intake, reducing the amounts and types of food to such a degree that expected nutritional requirements are often not met. As a result, weight loss, malnutrition, and secondary anemia occur (NIDDK, 2016b). Ulcers in the membranous lining of the intestine and other inflammatory changes result in a weeping, edematous intestine that continually empties an irritating discharge into the colon. Disrupted absorption causes chronic diarrhea and nutritional deficits. The result is a person who is thin and emaciated from inadequate food intake and constant fluid loss. In some patients, the inflamed intestine may perforate, leading to intra-abdominal and anal abscesses. Fever and leukocytosis occur. Chronic symptoms include diarrhea, abdominal pain, **steatorrhea** (i.e., excessive fat in the feces), anorexia, weight loss, and nutritional deficiencies.

Abscesses, fistulas, and fissures are common. Manifestations may extend beyond the GI tract and can include joint disorders (e.g., arthritis), skin lesions (e.g., erythema nodosum), ocular disorders (e.g., conjunctivitis), and oral ulcers. The clinical course and symptoms can vary; in some patients, periods of remission and exacerbation occur, but in others, the disease follows a fulminating course. When intestinal symptoms worsen, extraintestinal manifestations often worsen also. Both usually improve simultaneously (Basso et al., 2014).

Assessment and Diagnostic Findings

A proctosigmoidoscopy is usually performed initially to determine whether the rectosigmoid area is inflamed. A stool examination is also performed; the result may be positive for occult blood and steatorrhea. The most conclusive diagnostic aid for Crohn's disease is a barium study of the upper GI tract that shows the classic "string sign" on an x-ray film of the terminal ileum, indicating the constriction of a segment of intestine. Endoscopy, colonoscopy, and intestinal biopsies may be used to confirm the diagnosis. A barium enema may show ulcerations (the cobblestone appearance described earlier), fissures, and fistulas. A CT scan may show bowel wall thickening and fistula formation.

A complete blood cell count is performed to assess hematocrit and hemoglobin levels (usually decreased) as well as the white blood cell count (may be elevated). The ESR is usually elevated. Albumin and protein levels may be decreased, indicating malnutrition.

Complications

Complications of Crohn's disease include intestinal obstruction or stricture formation, perianal disease, fluid and electrolyte imbalances, malnutrition from malabsorption, and fistula and abscess formation. The most common type of small bowel fistula caused by Crohn's disease is the enterocutaneous fistula (i.e., an abnormal opening between the small bowel and the skin). Abscesses can be the result of an internal fistula that results in fluid accumulation and infection. Patients with Crohn's disease are also at increased risk of colon cancer (NIDDK, 2016a; Walfish, 2016).

Ulcerative Colitis

Ulcerative colitis is a recurrent ulcerative and inflammatory disease of the mucosal and submucosal layers of the colon and rectum. The prevalence of ulcerative colitis is highest in Caucasians and people of Jewish heritage (Basso et al., 2014). It is typically accompanied by systemic complications and a high mortality rate. Approximately 5% of patients with ulcerative colitis develop colon cancer (Harris & Jelemensky, 2014; Walfish, 2016).

Pathophysiology

Ulcerative colitis affects the superficial mucosa of the colon and is characterized by multiple ulcerations, diffuse inflammations, and desquamation or shedding of the colonic epithelium. Bleeding occurs as a result of the ulcerations. The mucosa becomes edematous and inflamed. The lesions are contiguous, occurring one after the other. Abscesses form, and infiltrate is seen in the mucosa and submucosa, with clumps of neutrophils found in the lumens of the crypts (i.e., crypt abscesses) that line the intestinal mucosa. The disease process usually begins in the rectum and spreads proximally to involve the entire colon. Eventually, the bowel narrows, shortens, and thickens because of muscular hypertrophy and fat deposits. Because the inflammatory process is not transmural (i.e., it affects the inner lining only), fistulas, obstruction, and fissures are uncommon (Basso et al., 2014; Harris & Jelemensky, 2014; Walfish, 2016).

Clinical Manifestations

The clinical course is usually one of exacerbations and remissions. The predominant symptoms of ulcerative colitis include diarrhea, passage of mucus and pus, left lower quadrant abdominal pain, intermittent tenesmus, and rectal bleeding. The bleeding may be mild or severe, and pallor, anemia, and fatigue result. The patient may have anorexia, weight loss, fever, vomiting, and dehydration, as well as cramping, the feeling of an urgent need to defecate, and the passage of 10 to 20 liquid stools each day. The disease is classified as mild, severe, or fulminant, depending on the severity of the symptoms. Hypoalbuminemia, electrolyte imbalances, and anemia frequently develop. Rebound tenderness may occur in the right lower quadrant. Extraintestinal manifestations include skin lesions (e.g., erythema nodosum), eye lesions (e.g., uveitis), joint abnormalities (e.g., arthritis), and liver disease (Harris & Jelemensky, 2014; NIDDK, 2014e; Walfish, 2016).

Assessment and Diagnostic Findings

The patient should be assessed for tachycardia, hypotension, tachypnea, fever, and pallor. Other assessments address the level of hydration and nutritional status. The abdomen is examined for bowel sounds, distention, and tenderness. These findings assist in determining the severity of the disease (Basson, 2015b).

Abdominal x-ray studies are useful for determining the cause of symptoms. Free air in the peritoneum and bowel dilation or obstruction should be excluded as a source of the presenting symptoms. Colonoscopy is the definitive screening test that can distinguish ulcerative colitis from other diseases of the colon with similar symptoms. It may reveal friable, inflamed mucosa with exudate and ulcerations and it assists in defining the extent and severity of the disease Biopsies are typically taken to determine histologic characteristics of the colonic tissue and extent of disease. CT scanning, MRI, and ultrasound studies can identify abscesses and perirectal involvement.

The stool is positive for blood, and laboratory test results reveal low hematocrit and hemoglobin levels in addition to an elevated white blood cell count, low albumin levels, and an electrolyte imbalance. Elevated antineutrophil cytoplasmic antibody levels are common (Basso et al., 2014). A barium enema may show mucosal irregularities, focal strictures or fistulas, shortening of the colon, and dilation of bowel loops. Leukocyte tagging (see Chapter 38) is useful when severe colitis prohibits the use of colonoscopy to determine the extent of inflammation.

Careful stool examination for parasites and other microbes is performed to rule out dysentery caused by common intestinal organisms, especially *Entamoeba histolytica, C. difficile, Campylobacter*, *Salmonella*, *Shigella*, and *Cryptospora* (Basson, 2015b).

Complications

Complications of ulcerative colitis include toxic mega colon, perforation, and bleeding as a result of ulceration, vascular engorgement, and highly vascular granulation tissue. In toxic megacolon, the inflammatory process extends into the muscularis, inhibiting its ability to contract and resulting in colonic distention. Symptoms include fever, abdominal pain and distention, vomiting, and fatigue. If the patient with toxic mega colon does not respond within 24 to 72 hours to medical management with nasogastric suction, IV fluids with electrolytes, corticosteroids, and antibiotics, surgery is required. A subtotal colectomy may be performed if bowel perforation has not occurred. Otherwise, colectomy is indicated; it is ultimately needed in up to one third of patients with severe ulcerative colitis (Walfish, 2016). For many patients, surgery becomes necessary to relieve the effects of the disease and to treat these serious complications; an ileostomy usually is performed. The surgical procedures involved and the care of patients with this type of fecal diversion are discussed later in this chapter.

Patients with ulcerative colitis also have a significantly increased risk of osteoporotic fractures due to decreased bone mineral density. Corticosteroid therapy may also contribute to the diminished bone density. Patients with ulcerative colitis area are also at increased risk for colon cancer. It is estimated that 20 years post diagnosis, approximately 7% to 10% of patients with extensive ulcerative colitis (i.e., not contained to the rectum) will have colon cancer (Walfish, 2016).

Medical Management of Chronic Inflammatory Bowel Disease

Most patients have long periods of well-being interspersed with short intervals of illness (Katz, 2013). Management depends on the disease location, severity, and complications (Harris & Jelemensky, 2014; Walfish, 2016).

Nutritional Therapy

Oral fluids and a low-residue, high-protein, high-calorie diet with supplemental vitamin therapy and iron replacement are prescribed to meet nutritional needs, reduce inflammation, and control pain and diarrhea. Fluid and electrolyte imbalances from dehydration caused by diarrhea are corrected by IV therapy as necessary if the patient is hospitalized or by oral fluids if the patient is managed at home. Any foods that exacerbate diarrhea are avoided. Milk may contribute to diarrhea in those with lactose intolerance. Cold foods and smoking are avoided because both increase intestinal motility. Parenteral nutrition may be indicated (see Chapter 36).

Pharmacologic Therapy

Sedatives and antidiarrheal and antiperistaltic medications are used to minimize peristalsis to rest the inflamed bowel. They are continued until the patient's stools approach normal frequency and consistency.

Aminosalicylates such as sulfasalazine (Azulfidine) are often effective for mild or moderate inflammation and are used to prevent or reduce recurrences in long-term maintenance regimens. Corticosteroids are used to treat severe and fulminant disease and can be administered orally (e.g., prednisone [Deltasone]) in outpatient treatment or parenterally (e.g., hydrocortisone [Solu-Cortef]) in hospitalized patients. Topical (i.e., rectal administration) corticosteroids (e.g., budesonide [Entocort EC]) are also widely used in the treatment of distal colon disease. When the dosage of corticosteroids is reduced or stopped, the symptoms of disease may return. If corticosteroids are continued, numerous adverse sequelae may ensue; these are discussed in Chapter 43 and summarized in Table 43-6. Antibiotics (e.g., metronidazole [Flagyl]) are used for complications such as abscesses or fistula formation (Walfish, 2016).

Immunomodulators (e.g., azathioprine [Imuran], mercaptopurine [6-MP], methotrexate [MTX], cyclosporine [Neoral]) have been used to alter the immune response. The exact mechanism of action of these medications in treating IBD is unknown. They are used in patients with severe disease who have not responded favourably to other therapies—in maintenance regimens to prevent relapses. Among the newer biologic therapies using monoclonal antibodies are natalizumab (Tysabri) for Crohn's disease (Walfish, 2016)) and infliximab (Remicade) for ulcerative colitis (Walfish, 2016). Clinical outcomes associated with the use of both biologic agents are promising), although adverse effects may seriously limit their usefulness. Other biologic therapies recently tested in Crohn's disease include anticytokine therapy using anti-interleukin–type drugs (e.g., anti-IL-12), which has thus far demonstrated a satisfactory safety profile. It is hoped that newer gut specific drugs will improve therapy over time, with particular focus on efficacy and safety.

A major issue associated with appropriate pharmacological treatment of IBD is noncompliance. Patients who are noncompliant may suffer a greater chance of disease relapse that can be severe. However, recent studies indicate that those clients who undertake both complementary and alternative therapies may be more compliant in overall treatment (Weizman et al., 2012).

Surgical Management

When nonsurgical measures fail to relieve the severe symptoms of IBD, surgery may be necessary. Nearly one third of patients with severe ulcerative colitis and between 60% and 70% of patients with Crohn's disease require surgery (NIDDK, 2016b; Walfish, 2016). The most common indications for surgery are medically intractable disease, poor QOL, or complications from the disease or its treatment. Recurrence of inflammation and disease after surgery in Crohn's disease is inevitable (Mosli et al., 2014). Common indications for surgery in patients with ulcerative colitis include the presence of colon cancer or colonic dysplasia/polyps (see later discussion); megacolon; severe, intractable bleeding; or perforation (NIDDK, 2014e; Walfish, 2016). Common indications for surgery in patients with Crohn's disease include recurrent partial intestinal obstructions; complete intestinal obstructions; intractable fistulas; or intractable abscesses (NIDDK, 2016b; Walfish, 2016). Furthermore, patients with either ulcerative colitis or Crohn's disease may require surgery to relieve strictures, or to correct underlying pathology in disease not responsive to long-term use of corticosteroids (NIDDK, 2014e; NIDDK, 2016b; Walfish, 2016).

A common procedure performed for strictures of the small intestines is laparoscope-guided strictureplasty, in which the blocked or narrowed sections of the intestines are widened, leaving the intestines intact. In some cases, a small bowel resection is performed and diseased segments of the small intestines are resected and the remaining portions of the intestines are anastomosed. Surgical removal of up to 50% of the small bowel usually can be tolerated. In cases of severe Crohn's disease of the colon, a total colectomy and ileostomy may be the procedure of choice.

Surgical cure is not possible with Crohn's disease; however, nearly 50% of patients with Crohn's disease who require surgical intervention will eventually require additional future surgery (Walfish, 2016).

A newer surgical procedure developed for patients with severe Crohn's disease is intestinal transplant (Dunn et al., 2014). This technique is now available to children and to young and middle-aged adults who have lost intestinal function from disease. It may provide improvement in QOL for some patients. The associated technical and immunologic problems remain formidable, and the costs and mortality rates continue to be high. At this time surgical cure is not possible with Crohn's disease; nearly 50% of patients with Crohn's disease who require surgical intervention will eventually require additional future surgery (Walfish, 2016). Ultimately, achievement of remission depends on medical therapy (Shaffer & Wexner, 2013).

At least 25% of patients with ulcerative colitis eventually have total colectomies. When the colon is surgically removed, the patient is considered "cured" in that extraintestinal manifestations subside and the disease process is otherwise limited to the colon. Indications for surgery include lack of improvement and continued deterioration, profuse bleeding, perforation, continued stricture formation, and cancer. Surgical excision usually improves QOL. Proctocolectomy with ileostomy (i.e., complete excision of colon, rectum, and anus) is recommended when the rectum is severely diseased. If the rectum can be preserved, restorative proctocolectomy with ileal pouch anal anastomosis (IPAA) is the procedure of choice. Although IPAA is not "perfect," it generally leads to a good to excellent QOL (Fazio et al., 2013; Francone & Champagne, 2013).

Total Colectomy With Ileostomy

An **ileostomy**, the surgical creation of an opening into the ileum or small intestine (usually by means of an ileal stoma on the abdominal wall), is commonly performed after a total colectomy (i.e., excision of the entire colon). It allows for drainage of fecal matter (i.e., effluent) from the ileum to the outside of the body. The drainage is liquid to unformed and occurs at frequent intervals. Nursing management of the patient with an ileostomy is discussed later in this chapter.

Continent Ileostomy

Another procedure involves the creation of a continent ileal reservoir (i.e., **Kock pouch**) by diverting a portion of the distal ileum to the abdominal wall and creating a stoma. This procedure eliminates the need for an external fecal collection bag. Approximately 30 cm of the distal ileum is reconstructed to form a reservoir with a nipple valve that is created by pulling a portion of the terminal ileal loop back into the ileum. GI effluent can accumulate in the pouch for several hours and then be removed by means of a catheter inserted through the nipple valve. In many patients, a total colectomy is also performed with the Kock pouch. Possible indications for a total colectomy with Kock pouch placement (rather than a restorative proctocolectomy with IPAA) include a badly diseased rectum, lack of rectal sphincter tone, or inability to achieve fecal continence post-IPAA (Crawshaw, Williams, & Woodhouse, 2014).

The major problem with the Kock pouch is malfunction of the nipple valve, which often requires additional corrective surgery. Kock pouches are used less commonly because they have greater complication rates than does restorative proctocolectomy with IPAA (Crawshaw et al., 2014).

Research is currently focused on developing valves that may fail less frequently than the nipple valve.

Restorative Proctocolectomy With Ileal Pouch Anal Anastomosis

A restorative proctocolectomy with IPAA is the surgical procedure of choice in cases where the rectum can be preserved in that it eliminates the need for a permanent ileostomy. It establishes an ileal reservoir that functions as a "new" rectum, and anal sphincter control of elimination is retained. The procedure involves connecting the ileum to the anal pouch (made from a small intestine segment), and the surgeon connects the pouch to the anus in conjunction with removing the colon and the rectal mucosa (i.e., total abdominal colectomy and mucosal proctectomy) (Fig. 38-6). A temporary diverting loop ileostomy that promotes healing of the surgical anastomoses is constructed at the time of surgery and closed about 3 months later (Francone & Champagne, 2013).

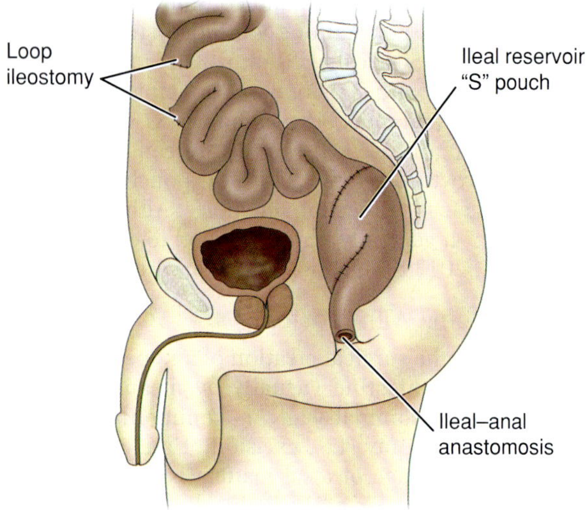

FIGURE 38-6. A mucosal proctectomy precedes anastomosis of the ileal reservoir. A temporary loop ileostomy diverts effluent for several months to allow healing.

With IPAA or restorative proctocolectomy, the diseased colon and rectum are removed, voluntary defecation is maintained, and anal continence is preserved. The ileal reservoir decreases the number of bowel movements by 50%, from approximately 14 to 20 per day to 7 to 10 per day. Nighttime elimination is gradually reduced to one bowel movement. Complications of ileoanal anastomosis include irritation of the perianal skin from leakage of fecal contents, stricture formation at the anastomosis site, small bowel obstruction, and "pouchitis" (inflammation of the ileoanal pouch due to altered microbial levels) (Francone & Champagne, 2013). For patients with IBD history, dietary intolerances may persist after the IPAA is formed. Increased stool output, flatulence, and perineal irritation are associated with consumption of nuts, corn, chocolate, spicy foods, onions, and citrus fruits. Consequently, some patients may need to alter their diet to avoid complications and perineal breakdown (Perrin, 2013).

Nursing Process

Management of the Patient With Chronic Inflammatory Bowel Disease

PRACTICE & LEARN

Assessment

The nurse obtains a health history to identify the onset, duration, and characteristics of abdominal pain; the presence of diarrhea or fecal urgency, straining at stool (tenesmus), nausea, anorexia, or weight loss; and family history of IBD. It is important to discuss dietary patterns, including the amounts of alcohol, caffeine, and nicotine-containing products used daily and weekly. The nurse asks about patterns of bowel elimination, including character, frequency, and presence of blood, pus, fat, or mucus. It is important to note allergies and food intolerance, especially milk (lactose) intolerance. The patient may identify sleep disturbances if diarrhea or pain occurs at night.

Nursing Priorities

Based on the assessment data, the nursing priorities may include the following:

- Management of diarrhea
- Acute pain
- Fluid and electrolyte balance
- Imbalanced nutrition
- Activity intolerance
- Anxiety
- Ineffective coping
- Risk for impaired skin integrity
- Risk for ineffective therapeutic regimen management

Collaborative Problems/ Potential Complications

Potential complications that may develop include the following:

- Electrolyte imbalance
- Cardiac dysrhythmias related to electrolyte imbalances
- GI bleeding with fluid volume loss
- Perforation of the bowel

Planning and Goals

The major goals for the patient include attainment of normal bowel elimination patterns, relief of abdominal pain and cramping, prevention of fluid volume deficit, maintenance of optimal nutrition and weight, avoidance of fatigue, reduction of anxiety, promotion of effective coping, absence of skin breakdown, increased knowledge about the disease process and therapeutic regimen, and avoidance of complications.

Nursing Interventions

Maintaining Normal Elimination Patterns

The nurse provides ready access to a bathroom, commode, or bedpan and keeps the environment clean and odour free. It is important to administer antidiarrheal medications as prescribed, to record the frequency and consistency of stools after therapy is initiated, and to encourage bed rest to decrease peristalsis.

Relieving Pain

The character of the pain is described as dull, burning, or cramping. It is important to ask about its onset. Does it occur before or after meals, during the night, or before elimination? Is the pattern constant or intermittent? Is it relieved with medications? The nurse administers anticholinergic medications 30 minutes before a meal as prescribed to decrease intestinal motility and administers analgesics as prescribed for pain. Position changes, local application of heat (as prescribed), diversional activities, and prevention of fatigue also are helpful for reducing pain.

Maintaining Fluid Intake

To detect fluid volume deficit, the nurse keeps an accurate record of oral and IV fluids and maintains a record of output (i.e., urine, liquid stool, vomitus, and wound or fistula drainage). The nurse monitors daily weights for fluid gains or losses and assesses the patient for signs of fluid volume deficit (i.e., dry skin and mucous membranes, decreased skin turgor, oliguria, fatigue, decreased temperature, increased hematocrit, elevated urine specific gravity, and hypotension). It is important to encourage oral intake of fluids and to monitor the flow rate of any IV fluids. The nurse initiates measures to decrease diarrhea (e.g., dietary restrictions, stress reduction, antidiarrheal agents).

Maintaining Optimal Nutrition

Parenteral nutrition is used when the symptoms of IBD are severe. With parenteral nutrition, the nurse maintains an accurate record of fluid intake and output as well as the daily weight. The patient should gain 0.5 kg daily during parenteral nutrition therapy. Because parenteral nutrition is very high in glucose and can cause hyperglycemia, blood glucose levels are monitored every 6 hours. Once the symptoms of IBD exacerbation have diminished and the patient has gained or stabilized weight, parenteral nutrition is stopped and the patient is advanced on oral elemental feedings. Elemental feedings are high in protein and low in fat and residue. They are digested primarily in the jejunum, do not stimulate intestinal secretions, and allow the bowel to continue to rest. The nurse notes intolerance if the patient exhibits nausea, vomiting, diarrhea, or abdominal distention.

If oral foods are tolerated, small, frequent, low-residue feedings are given to avoid over distending the stomach and stimulating peristalsis. It is important that the patient restrict activity to conserve energy, reduce peristalsis, and reduce caloric requirements.

Promoting Rest

The nurse recommends intermittent rest periods during the day and schedules or restricts activities to conserve energy and reduce the metabolic rate. It is important to encourage activity within the limits of the patient's capacity. The nurse suggests bed rest for a patient who is febrile, has frequent diarrheal stools, or is bleeding. However, the patient on bed rest should perform active exercises to maintain muscle tone and prevent thromboembolic complications. If the patient cannot perform these active exercises, the nurse performs passive exercises and joint range of motion. Activity restrictions are modified as needed on a day-to-day basis.

Reducing Anxiety

The patient may be labile because of the consequences of the disease and the uncertainty of exacerbations with complications. The nurse tailors information about possible impending surgery to the patient's level of understanding and desire for detail. If surgery is planned, pictures and illustrations help explain the surgical procedure and help the patient visualize what a stoma looks like.

Enhancing Coping Measures

Any patient suffering the discomforts of frequent bowel movements and rectal soreness is anxious, discouraged, and depressed. It is important to develop a relationship with the patient that supports all attempts to cope with these stressors. Stress reduction measures that may be used include relaxation techniques, visualization, breathing exercises, and biofeedback. Professional counselling may be needed to help the patient and family manage issues associated with chronic illness and resulting disability.

Preventing Skin Breakdown

The nurse examines the patient's skin frequently, especially the perianal skin. Perianal care, including the use of a skin barrier (e.g., petroleum ointment [Vaseline]), is important after each bowel movement. The nurse gives immediate attention to reddened or irritated areas over bony prominences and uses pressure-relieving devices to prevent skin breakdown. Consultation with a wound–ostomy–continence nurse (WOC nurse, or WOCN) (a nurse specially educated in the management of a variety of fecal and urinary diversions) is often helpful.

Monitoring and Managing Potential Complications

Serum electrolyte levels are monitored daily, and electrolyte replacements are administered as prescribed. It is important to report evidence of dysrhythmias or changes in level of consciousness immediately.

The nurse carefully monitors rectal bleeding and administers blood component therapy and volume expanders as prescribed to prevent hypovolemia. It is important to monitor the blood pressure for hypotension and to obtain coagulation profiles and hemoglobin and hematocrit levels frequently. Vitamin K may be prescribed to increase clotting factors.

The nurse closely monitors the patient for indications of perforation (i.e., acute increase in abdominal pain, rigid abdomen, vomiting, or hypotension) and obstruction and toxic megacolon (i.e., abdominal distention, decreased or absent bowel sounds, change in mental status, fever, tachycardia, hypotension, dehydration, and electrolyte imbalances).

Promoting Home, Community-Based, and Transitional Care

EDUCATING PATIENTS ABOUT SELF-CARE. The nurse assesses the patient's understanding of the

CHART 38-5

HOME CARE CHECKLIST • The Patient With Inflammatory Bowel Disease

At the completion of education, the patient and/or caregiver will be able to:

- State the impact of inflammatory bowel disease on physiologic functioning, ADLs, IADLs, roles, relationships, and spirituality.
- Discuss nutritional management: bland, low-residue, high-protein, high-vitamin diet; identify foods to include and foods to be avoided.
- Explain the importance of and necessity for adherence with prescribed medication regimen.
- Demonstrate methods of keeping track of the medication regimen, storing the prescribed medications, and using reminders such as beepers and/or pillboxes.
- State the name, dose, side effects, frequency, and schedule for all medications.
- Identify measures to be used to treat exacerbation of symptoms, to include rest, dietary modifications, and medications.
- Identify measures to be used to promote fluid and electrolyte balance during acute exacerbations.
- Demonstrate management of parenteral nutrition therapy, if applicable; identify possible complications and interventions.
- State how to reach primary provider with questions or complications.
- State time and date of follow-up appointments, testing.
- Verbalize ways to cope with stress successfully, plans for regular exercise, and rationale for obtaining adequate rest.
- Identify the need for health promotion (e.g., cessation of use of tobacco products, alcohol avoidance), disease prevention and screening activities.

ADL, activities of daily living; IADL, independent activities of daily living.

disease process and his or her need for additional information about medical management (e.g., medications, diet) and surgical interventions. The nurse provides information about nutritional management; a bland, low-residue, high-protein, high-calorie, and high-vitamin diet relieves symptoms and decreases diarrhea. It is important to explain the rationale for the use of corticosteroids and anti-inflammatory, antibacterial, antidiarrheal, and antispasmodic medications. The nurse emphasizes the importance of taking medications as prescribed and not abruptly discontinuing them (especially corticosteroids) to avoid development of serious medical problems (Chart 38-5). The nurse reviews ileostomy care as necessary (see Nursing Management of the Patient Requiring an Ileostomy). Patient education information can be obtained from the Crohn's and Colitis Foundation of Canada.

CONTINUING AND TRANSITIONAL CARE. Patients with chronic IBD are managed at home with follow-up care by their physician or through an outpatient clinic. Those whose nutritional status is compromised and who are receiving parenteral nutrition need home care nursing to ensure that their nutritional requirements are being met and that they or their caregivers can follow through with the instructions for parenteral nutrition. Patients who are undergoing medical treatment need to understand that their disease can be controlled and that they can lead a healthy life between exacerbations. Control implies management based on an understanding of the disease and its treatment. Patients in the home setting need information about their medications (i.e., name, dose, side effects, and frequency of administration) and need to take medications on schedule. Medication reminders such as containers that separate pills according to day and time or daily checklists are helpful.

During a flare-up, the nurse encourages the patient to rest as needed and to modify activities according to his or her energy level. Patients should limit tasks that impose strain on the lower abdominal muscles. They should sleep in a room close to the bathroom because of the frequent diarrhea (10 to 20 times per day); quick access to a toilet helps alleviate worry about having an "accident." Room deodorizers help control odours.

Dietary modifications can control but do not cure the disease; the nurse recommends a low-residue, high-protein, high-calorie diet, especially during an acute phase. It is important to encourage the patient to keep a record of the foods that irritate the bowel and to avoid them and to drink at least eight glasses of water each day.

The prolonged nature of the disease has an impact on the patient and often strains his or her family life and financial resources. Family support is vital; however, some family members may be resentful, or feel guilty, tired, or unable to cope with the emotional demands of the illness and the physical demands of providing care. Some patients with IBD do not socialize for fear of being embarrassed. Many prefer to eat alone. Because they have lost control over elimination, they may fear losing control over other aspects of their lives. They need time to express their fears and frustrations. Individual and family counselling may be helpful.

Evaluation

Expected patient outcomes may include the following:

1. Reports a decrease in the frequency of diarrheal stools
   a. Complies with dietary restrictions; maintains bed rest
   b. Takes medications as prescribed
2. Has reduced pain
3. Maintains fluid volume balance
   a. Drinks 1 to 2 L of oral fluids daily
   b. Has normal body temperature
   c. Displays adequate skin turgor and moist mucous membranes
4. Attains optimal nutrition; tolerates small, frequent feedings without diarrhea
5. Avoids fatigue
   a. Rests periodically during the day
   b. Adheres to activity restrictions
6. Is less anxious
7. Copes successfully with diagnosis
   a. Verbalizes feelings freely
   b. Uses appropriate stress reduction behaviours
8. Maintains skin integrity
   a. Cleans perianal skin after defecation
   b. Uses lotion or ointment as skin barrier
9. Acquires an understanding of the disease process
   a. Modifies diet appropriately to decrease diarrhea
   b. Adheres to medication regimen as prescribed
10. Recovers without complications
    a. Electrolytes within expected ranges
    b. Normal sinus or baseline cardiac rhythm
    c. Maintains fluid balance
    d. Experiences no perforation or rectal bleeding

NURSING MANAGEMENT OF THE PATIENT REQUIRING AN OSTOMY

Some patients with IBD eventually require a permanent fecal diversion with creation of an ileostomy to manage symptoms and to treat or prevent complications. The Plan of Nursing Care summarizes care for the patient requiring an ostomy (Chart 38-6).

Providing Preoperative Care

A period of preparation with intensive replacement of fluid, blood, and protein is necessary prior to surgery. Antibiotics may be prescribed. If the patient has been taking corticosteroids, they will be continued during the surgical phase to prevent steroid-induced adrenal insufficiency. Usually, the patient is given a low-residue diet, provided in frequent, small feedings. All other preoperative measures are similar to those for general abdominal surgery. The patient must have a thorough understanding of the surgery to be performed and what to expect after surgery. Preoperative teaching includes management of drainage from the stoma; the nature of drainage; and the need for nasogastric intubation, parenteral fluids, and possibly perineal packing.

The abdomen is marked for the proper placement of the stoma by the surgeon or the **wound–ostomy–continence** (WOC) nurse (Hendren et al., 2015). Care is taken to ensure that the stoma is conveniently placed—usually in the right lower quadrant about 2 in below the waist, in an area away from previous scars, bony prominences, skin folds, or fistulas. It is essential that the stoma site be visible to the patient.

Providing Postoperative Care

General abdominal surgery wound care is required. The nurse observes the stoma for colour and size. It should be pink to bright red and shiny. Typically, a temporary plastic bag (i.e., appliance or pouch) with an adhesive facing is placed over the ileostomy in the operating room and firmly pressed onto the surrounding skin. The nurse monitors the ileostomy for fecal drainage, which should begin about 24 to 48 hours after surgery. The drainage is a continuous liquid from the small intestine because the stoma does not have a controlling sphincter. The contents drain into the pouch and are thus kept from coming into contact with the skin. They are collected, measured, and discarded when the pouch becomes full. If a continent ileal reservoir was created, as described for the Kock pouch, continuous drainage is provided by an indwelling reservoir catheter for 2 to 3 weeks after surgery. This allows the suture lines to heal.

Because these patients lose large fluid volumes in the early postoperative period, an accurate record of fluid intake, urinary output, and fecal discharge is necessary to help gauge the fluid needs of the patient. There may be 1,000 to 2,000 mL of fluid lost each day in addition to expected fluid loss through urine, perspiration, respiration, and other sources. With this loss, sodium and potassium are depleted. The nurse monitors laboratory values and administers electrolyte replacements as prescribed. Replacement fluids are administered intravenously for 4 to 5 days.

Nasogastric suction is also a part of the immediate postoperative care, with the tube requiring frequent irrigation, as prescribed. The purpose of nasogastric suction is to prevent a buildup of gastric contents while the intestines are not functioning. After the tube is removed, the nurse offers sips of clear liquids and gradually progresses the diet. It is important to report nausea and abdominal distention, which may indicate intestinal obstruction, immediately.

By the end of the first week, rectal packing is removed. Because this procedure may be uncomfortable, the nurse may administer an analgesic an hour before the removal. After the packing is removed, the perineum is irrigated two or three times daily until full healing takes place.

Providing Emotional Support

The patient may think that everyone is aware of the ileostomy and may view the stoma as a mutilation compared with other abdominal incisions that heal and are hidden. Due to the loss of a body part and a major change in

(text continued on page 1026)

Plan of Nursing Care

Chart 38-6. The Patient Undergoing Ostomy Surgery

Nursing Priority: Patient Education
Goal: Understands the surgical process and the necessary preoperative preparations

Preoperative Care

NURSING INTERVENTIONS	RATIONALE	EXPECTED OUTCOMES
1. Ascertain whether the patient has had a previous surgical experience and ask for recollections of positive and negative impressions.	1. Fear of a repeated negative experience increases anxiety. Talking about the experience with a nurse helps clarify misconceptions and helps the patient ventilate any repressed emotions. Positive experiences are reinforced.	• Expresses anxieties and fears about the surgical process • Projects a positive attitude toward the surgical procedure • Repeats in own words information given by the surgeon • Identifies normal anatomy and physiology of gastrointestinal tract and how it will be altered; can point to expected location of abdominal wound and stoma; describes stoma appearance and size • Adheres to "bowel prep" regimen of antimicrobials or mechanical cleansing • Tolerates the presence of nasogastric/nasoenteric tube
2. Determine what information the surgeon gave the patient and family and whether it was understood. Clarify and elaborate as necessary. Determine whether the stoma is permanent or temporary. Be aware of the patient's prognosis if carcinoma exists.	2. Clarification prevents misunderstandings and alleviates anxiety.	
3. Use pictures or drawings to illustrate the location and appearance of the surgical wounds (abdominal, perineal) and the stoma if the patient is receptive.	3. Knowledge, for some, alleviates anxiety because fear of the unknown is decreased. Others choose not to know because it makes them more anxious.	
4. Explain that oral/parenteral antimicrobials will be administered to cleanse the bowel preoperatively. Mechanical cleansing may also be required.	4. Antimicrobials and mechanical cleansing (e.g., laxatives, enemas) reduce intestinal bacterial flora.	
5. Assist the patient during nasogastric/nasoenteric intubation. Measure drainage from the tube.	5. Nasoenteral intubation is used for decompression and drainage of gastrointestinal contents before surgery.	

Nursing Priority: Altered body image
Goal: Attainment of a positive self-concept

NURSING INTERVENTIONS	RATIONALE	EXPECTED OUTCOMES
1. Encourage the patient to verbalize feelings about the stoma. Offer to be present when the stoma is first viewed and touched.	1. Free expression of feelings allows the patient the opportunity to verbalize and identify concerns. Expressed concerns can be therapeutically addressed by health care team members.	• Freely expresses concerns and fears • Accepts support • Seeks help as needed • States is willing to talk with another patient with a stoma
2. Suggest that the spouse or significant other view the stoma.	2. Helps patient to overcome fears about partner's response.	
3. Offer counselling, if desired.	3. Provides opportunity for additional support.	
4. Arrange for a visit or a phone call with another patient with a stoma.	4. People with stomas can offer support and share mutual feelings and experiences.	

Nursing Priority: Anxiety
Goal: Reduction of anxiety

Postoperative Care

NURSING INTERVENTIONS	RATIONALE	EXPECTED OUTCOMES
1. Provide information about expected bowel function: a. Characteristics of effluent. b. Frequency of discharge.	1. Emotional adjustment is facilitated if adequate information is provided at the level of the learner.	• Expresses interest in learning about altered bowel function • Handles equipment correctly • Changes the appliance unassisted • Irrigates colostomy successfully • Progresses toward a regular schedule of elimination

Plan of Nursing Care

Chart 38-6. The Patient Undergoing Ostomy Surgery, *Continued*

NURSING INTERVENTIONS	RATIONALE	EXPECTED OUTCOMES
2. Teach the patient how to prepare the appliance for an adequate fit.	2. Adequate fit is necessary for successful use of the appliance.	
a. Choose the drainage appliance that will provide a secure fit around the stoma. Measure the stoma size with a measuring guide provided by the ostomy equipment manufacturer and compare with the opening on the pouch. The barrier opening should be sized to "hug" the stoma and cover the peristomal skin. *Note:* Newer wafer barriers can be pulled or molded to the size of the stoma.	a. The appliance opening should be larger than the stoma for an adequate fit. Available brands come in different sizes to fit the stoma. Adjustments are made as necessary.	
b. Remove any plastic covering that protects the appliance adhesive. *Note:* The pouch is applied by pressing the adhesive for 30 seconds to the skin or skin barrier.	b. The appliance is ready to apply directly to the skin or skin protector.	
3. Demonstrate how to change the appliance or empty the pouch before leakage occurs. Be aware that the older person may have diminished vision and difficulty handling equipment.	3. Manipulation of the appliance is a learned motor skill that requires practice and positive reinforcement.	
4. When appropriate, demonstrate how to irrigate the colostomy (usually on the 4th or 5th day). Recommend that irrigation be performed at a consistent time, depending on the type of colostomy.	4. Colostomy irrigation is used to regulate the passage of fecal material; alternatively the bowel can be allowed to evacuate naturally. Irrigation is not routinely indicated.	

Nursing Priority: Risk for impaired skin integrity
Goal: Maintenance of skin integrity

NURSING INTERVENTIONS	RATIONALE	EXPECTED OUTCOMES
1. Provide information about signs and symptoms of irritated or inflamed skin. Use pictures if possible.	1. Peristomal skin should be slightly pink without abrasions and similar to that of the entire abdomen.	• Describes appearance of healthy skin • Correctly cleanses the skin • Successfully applies a skin barrier • Gently removes the drainage appliance without skin damage • Demonstrates intact skin around the colostomy stoma
2. Teach patient how to cleanse the peristomal skin gently.	2. Mild friction with warm water and a gentle soap cleanses the skin and minimizes irritation and possible abrasions. After rinsing the soap, patting the skin dry prevents tissue trauma.	
3. Demonstrate how to apply a skin barrier (powder, gel, paste, wafer).	3. Skin barriers protect the peristomal skin from enzymes and bacteria.	
4. Demonstrate how to remove the pouch.	4. Gently separate adhesive from the skin to avoid irritation. Never pull!	

Nursing Priority: Potential for imbalanced nutrition
Goal: Achievement of an optimal nutritional intake

NURSING INTERVENTIONS	RATIONALE	EXPECTED OUTCOMES
1. Conduct a complete nutritional assessment to identify any foods that may increase peristalsis by irritating the bowel.	1. Patients react differently to certain foods because of individual sensitivity.	• Modifies diet to avoid offensive foods yet maintains adequate nutritional intake • Avoids cellulose-based foods such as peanuts • Modifies intake of certain fruits
2. Advise the patient to avoid food products with a cellulose or hemicellulose base (nuts, seeds).	2. Cellulose food products are the nondigestible residue of plant foods. They hold water, provide bulk, and stimulate elimination.	
3. Recommend moderation in intake of certain irritating fruits such as prunes, grapes, and bananas.	3. These fruits tend to increase the quantity of effluent.	

continued >

Plan of Nursing Care — Chart 38-6. The Patient Undergoing Ostomy Surgery, *Continued*

NURSING INTERVENTIONS	RATIONALE	EXPECTED OUTCOMES
Nursing Priority: Sexual dysfunction **Goal:** Attainment of satisfactory sexual performance		
1. Encourage the patient to verbalize concerns and fears. The sexual partner is welcomed to participate in the discussion.	1. Expressed needs help the therapist develop a plan of care.	• Expresses fears and concerns • Discusses alternative sexual positions • Accepts services of a professional counsellor
2. Recommend alternative sexual positions.	2. Avoid patient embarrassment with the visual appearance of the stoma. Avoid peristomal skin irritation or stomal trauma secondary to friction.	
3. Seek assistance from a sexual therapist or wound-ostomy-continence (WOC) nurse.	3. Some patients need professional sexual counselling.	
Nursing Priority: Risk for fluids and electrolyte imbalances **Goal:** Attainment of fluid balance		
1. Estimate fluid intake and output: a. Strict intake and output b. Daily weights	1. Provides indication of fluid balance. a. An early indicator of fluid imbalance is a daily, significant difference between intake and output. The average person ingests (food, fluids) and loses (urine, feces, lungs) about 2 L of fluid every 24 hours. b. A gain/loss of 1 L of fluid is reflected in a body weight change of 2.2 lb.	• Maintains fluid balance • Maintains expected serum and urinary values for sodium and potassium • Usual skin turgor • Surface of tongue is pink, with a moist mucous membrane
2. Assess serum and urinary values of sodium and potassium.	2. Sodium is the major electrolyte regulating water balance. Vomiting results in decreased urinary and serum sodium levels. Urinary sodium values, in contrast to serum values, reflect early, sensitive changes in sodium balance. Sodium works in conjunction with potassium, which is also decreased with vomiting. A significant deficiency in potassium is associated with a decrease in intracellular potassium bicarbonate, which leads to acidosis and compensatory hyperventilation.	
3. Observe and record skin turgor and the appearance of the tongue.	3. Adequate hydration is reflected by the skin's ability to return to its usual shape after being grasped between the fingers. *Note:* In the older person, it is usual for the return to be delayed. Changes in the mucous membrane covering the tongue are accurate and early indicators of hydration status.	

anatomy and function, the patient may experience the phases of grief—denial, anger, bargaining, depression, and acceptance. Nursing support through these phases is important, and understanding of the patient's emotional state should determine the approach taken. For example, education may be ineffective until the patient is ready to learn. Concern about body image may lead to questions related to family relationships, sexual function, and, for women, the ability to become pregnant and to deliver a baby (Watson et al., 2013). Patients need to know that someone understands and cares about them. A calm, nonjudgmental attitude exhibited by the nurse aids in gaining the patient's confidence. It is important to recognize that treatment of a possibly terminal illness (e.g., cancer) makes patients irritable, anxious, and unhappy. The nurse can coordinate patient care needs, including needs for emotional support, through meetings attended by consultants such as the physician, psychologist, psychiatrist, social worker, WOC nurse, and dietitian. The team approach is important in facilitating the often complex care of the patient.

Conversely, a surgical procedure to create an ileostomy can produce dramatic positive changes in patients who have suffered from IBD for several years. After the discomfort of the disease has decreased and the patient learns how to take care of the ileostomy, he or she often develops a more positive outlook. Until the patient progresses to this phase, an empathetic and tolerant approach by the nurse plays an important part in recovery. The sooner the patient masters the physical care of the ileostomy, the sooner he or she will psychologically accept it (Perrin, 2013).

Support from other people with ostomies is also helpful. The United Ostomy Associations of Canada (UOAC) is dedicated to the rehabilitation of people with ostomies. This organization gives patients useful information about living with an ostomy through an educational program of literature, lectures, and exhibits. Local associations offer visiting services by qualified members who provide hope and rehabilitation services to patients with new ostomies.

Managing Skin and Stoma Care

The patient with a traditional ileostomy cannot establish regular bowel habits because the contents of the ileum are fluid and are discharged continuously. The patient must wear a pouch at all times. Stomal size and pouch size vary initially; the stoma should be rechecked 3 weeks after surgery, when the edema has subsided. The final size and type of appliance is selected in 3 months, after the patient's weight has stabilized and the stoma shrinks to a stable shape.

The incidence of complications related to a **colostomy** is usually less than that of an ileostomy. Postoperatively, the stoma is examined for swelling (slight edema from surgical manipulation is normal), colour (a healthy stoma is pink or red), discharge (a small amount of oozing is normal), and bleeding (an abnormal sign if bright red or more than trace amounts) (Watson et al., 2013).

The location and length of the stoma are significant to the management of the ileostomy by the patient. The surgeon positions the stoma as close to the midline as possible and at a location where even an obese patient with a protruding abdomen can see it and can care for it easily. Usually, the ileostomy stoma is about 2.5 cm long, which makes it convenient for the attachment of an appliance.

Skin excoriation around the stoma can be a persistent problem. Peristomal skin integrity may be compromised by several factors, such as an allergic reaction to the ostomy appliance, skin barrier, or paste; chemical irritation from the effluent; mechanical injury from the removal of the appliance; and infection. If irritation and yeast growth occur, nystatin powder (Mycostatin) is dusted lightly on the peristomal skin and a pouch with skin barrier is applied over the affected area (Watson et al., 2013).

Changing an Appliance

A regular schedule for changing the pouch before leakage occurs needs to be established for those with a traditional ileostomy. The patient can be taught to change the pouch in a manner similar to that described in Chart 38-7.

The amount of time a person can keep the appliance sealed to the body surface depends on the location of the stoma and on body structure. The usual wearing time, which also depends on the type of skin barrier, is 5 to 10 days. The appliance is emptied every 4 to 6 hours, or at the same time the patient empties the bladder. An emptying spout at the bottom of the appliance is closed with a special clip or Velcro closure.

Most pouches are disposable and odour proof. Foods such as spinach and parsley act as deodorizers in the intestinal tract; foods that cause odours include asparagus, cabbage, onions, and fish. Bismuth subcarbonate tablets, which may be prescribed and taken orally three or four times each day, are effective in reducing odour. Oral diphenoxylate atropine (Lomotil) can be prescribed to diminish intestinal motility, thereby thickening the stool and assisting in odour control. Foods such as rice, mashed potatoes, and applesauce may also thicken stool.

Irrigating a Colostomy

The purpose of irrigating a colostomy is to empty the colon of gas, mucus, and feces so that the patient can go about social and business activities without fear of fecal drainage. A stoma does not have voluntary muscular control and may empty at irregular intervals. Regulating the passage of fecal material is achieved by irrigating the colostomy or allowing the bowel to evacuate naturally without irrigations. This choice depends on the person and the type of the colostomy (i.e., descending or sigmoid colostomies). By irrigating the stoma at a regular time, there is less gas and retention of the irrigant. The time for irrigating the colostomy should be consistent with the schedule that the person will follow after leaving the hospital.

Colostomy irrigation is not recommended for persons with extensive pelvic irradiation because it carries a risk of perforation. Likewise, it is contraindicated in patients currently receiving chemotherapy, those with IBS, Crohn's disease, diverticulitis, and peristomal hernias (Bauer, Arnold-Long, & Kent, 2016).

As soon as the patient with a descending or sigmoid colostomy has established a routine for evacuation with irrigations, pouches may be dispensed with, and a closed ostomy appliance or a stoma cap is used to cover the stoma. Except for gas and a slight amount of mucus, nothing escapes from the colostomy opening between irrigations. New assistive devices and ostomy care algorithms are available to help nurses learn ostomy assessment and ostomy product selection.

Irrigating a Continent Ileostomy

For a continent ileostomy (i.e., Kock pouch), the nurse teaches the patient to drain the pouch, as described in Chart 38-8. A catheter is inserted into the reservoir to drain the fluid. The length of time between drainage periods is gradually increased until the reservoir needs to be drained only every 4 to 6 hours and irrigated once each day. A pouch is not necessary; instead, most patients wear a small dressing over the opening.

When the fecal discharge is thick, water can be injected through the catheter to loosen and soften it. The consistency of the effluent is affected by food intake. At first,

CHART 38-7

GUIDELINES for Changing an Ostomy Appliance

Equipment

- Mild soap
- Clean cloths or towels
- Skin barrier (e.g., Stomahesive)
- Cutting guide
- Appliance pouch
- Barrier powder, antifungal spray or powder, barrier washer (optional equipment)

Implementation

NURSING ACTIONS	RATIONALE
1. Promote patient comfort and involvement in the procedure. Perform hand hygiene. a. Have the patient assume a relaxed position. b. Provide privacy. c. Explain details of the procedure. d. Expose the ileostomy area; remove the ileostomy belt (if worn).	1. Providing a relaxed atmosphere and adequate explanations help the patient to become an active participant in the procedure; hand hygiene is necessary before any intervention to decrease the likelihood of transmitting a hospital-associated infection.
2. Remove the appliance. a. Have the patient sit on the toilet or on a chair facing the toilet. A patient who prefers to stand should face the toilet. b. The appliance (pouch) can be removed by gently pushing the skin away from the adhesive.	2. These positions facilitate disposal or drainage.
3. Cleanse the skin. a. Wash the skin gently with a soft cloth moistened with tepid water and mild soap; the patient may prefer to bathe before putting on a clean appliance. b. Rinse the soap off and dry the skin thoroughly after cleansing.	3. The patient may shower with or without the pouch. a. Micropore or waterproof tape applied to the sides of the faceplate keeps it secure during bathing. b. Moisture or soap residue interferes with appliance adhesion.

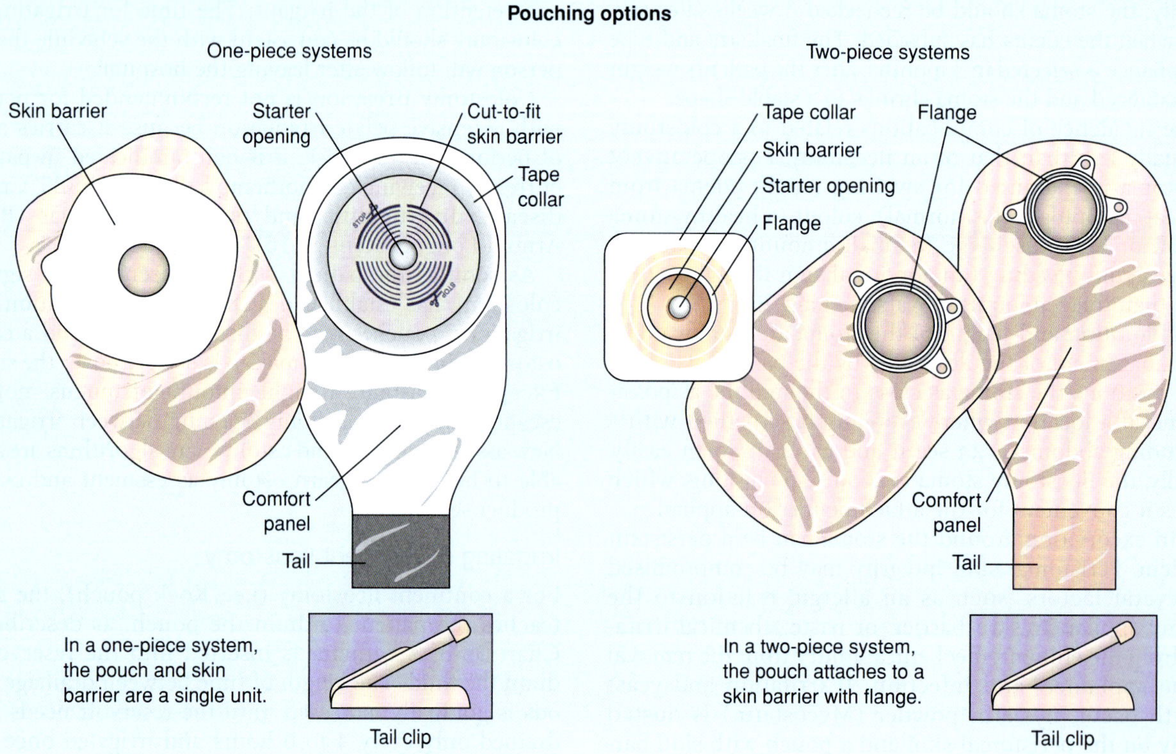

GUIDELINES for Changing an Ostomy Appliance (Continued)

NURSING ACTIONS	RATIONALE
4. Apply appliance. When there is no skin irritation: a. Apply an appropriate skin barrier to the peristomal skin before the appliance is applied. b. Remove cover from adherent surface of disk of disposable plastic appliance, and apply directly to the skin. c. Press firmly in place for 30 seconds to ensure adherence.	4. Many appliances have a built-in skin barrier. The skin should be thoroughly dried before applying the appliance.
When there is skin irritation: a. Cleanse the skin thoroughly but gently; pat dry. Apply barrier powder.	a. Cleansing removes debris and protects irritated skin under wafer.
b. If more irritation develops, apply triamcinolone aerosol (Kenalog spray); blot excess moisture with a cotton pledget and dust lightly with nystatin (Mycostatin) powder.	b. The corticosteroid preparation (triamcinolone) helps decrease inflammation. The antifungal agent (nystatin) treats those types of infections that are common around stomas. A prescription is required for either medication. A skin barrier is a substance that facilitates healing of excoriated skin. It adheres well even to moist, irritated skin.
c. Apply a wafer or barrier (e.g., Stomahesive), which is commercially available. The opening in the wafer should be the same size as the stoma; use a cutting guide (supplied with appliance as indicated). The wafer is applied directly to the skin. If using a moldable barrier, stretch it to the size of the stoma. Barrier powder can be used to dry irritated skin before barrier application. OR Another alternative is to apply a special barrier washer (e.g., Eakin Seals). The special barrier adheres well to irritated skin.	c. A special barrier protects skin from effluent, promotes healing and helps with adherence.
d. The pouch is then applied to the treated skin.	d. This allows skin to heal while the appliance is in place.
5. Check the pouch bottom for closure; use clamp, Velcro closure, or clip provided.	5. Proper closure controls leakage.

Adapted from Burch, J. (2014). Caring for a stoma: Making the right choices. *Nursing and Residential Care, 16*(9), 495–500.

drainage is only 60 to 80 mL, but as time goes on, the amount increases significantly. The internal Kock pouch stretches, eventually accommodating 500 to 1,000 mL. The patient learns to use the sensation of pressure in the pouch as a gauge to determine how often the pouch should be drained.

Managing Dietary and Fluid Needs

A low-residue diet is followed for the first 6 to 8 weeks. Strained fruits and vegetables are given. These foods are important sources of vitamins A and C. Later, there are few dietary restrictions, except for avoiding foods that are high in fibre or hard-to-digest kernels, such as celery, popcorn, corn, poppy seeds, caraway seeds, and coconut, which may result in a stomal obstruction (food blockage) for the person with an ileostomy. Foods are reintroduced one at a time. The nurse assesses the patient's tolerance for these foods and reminds him or her to chew food thoroughly.

Fluids may be a problem during the summer, when fluid lost through perspiration adds to the fluid loss through the ileostomy. Fluids such as Gatorade are helpful in maintaining electrolyte balance. If the fecal discharge is too watery, fibrous foods (e.g., whole-grain cereals, fresh fruit skins, beans, corn, nuts) are restricted. If the effluent is excessively dry, salt intake is increased. Increased intake of water or fluid does not increase the effluent, because excess water is excreted in the urine.

Preventing Complications

Monitoring for complications is an ongoing activity for the patient with an ileostomy. Peristomal skin irritation, which results from leakage of effluent, is the most common complication of an ileostomy. A drainable pouching system that does not fit well is often the cause. Components of the drainable pouching system include the pouch, a solid skin barrier, and adhesive. The WOC nurse typically recommends the appropriate drainable pouching system. The solid skin barrier is the component of this system that is most important in ensuring healthy peristomal skin. Solid skin barriers are typically shaped as rectangular or elliptical wafers and are composed of polymers and hydrocolloids. They protect the skin around the stoma from effluent from the stoma and provide a stable interface between the stoma and the pouch. It is critical that the barrier be sized appropriately to "hug" the stoma (up to the stoma but not touching) and not expose peristomal skin.

Other common complications include diarrhea, stomal stenosis, urinary calculi, and cholelithiasis. Even in the presence of a properly fitted drainable pouching system, diarrhea can be problematic. Diarrhea, manifested by very

CHART 38-8

GUIDELINES for Draining a Continent Ileostomy (Kock Pouch)

A continent ileostomy is the surgical creation of a pouch of small intestine that can serve as an internal receptacle for fecal and urinary discharge; a nipple valve is constructed at the outlet. Postoperatively, a catheter extends from the stoma and is attached to a closed drainage suction system. To ensure patency of the catheter, 10–20 mL of normal saline is instilled gently into the pouch usually every 3 hours; return flow is not aspirated but is allowed to drain by gravity.

After approximately 2 weeks, when the healing process has progressed to the point at which the catheter is removed from the stoma, the patient is taught to drain the pouch. A catheter is inserted into the reservoir to drain the fluid. The length of time between drainage periods is gradually increased until the reservoir needs to be drained only every 4 to 6 hours and irrigated once each day. A pouch is not necessary; instead, most patients wear a small dressing over the opening.

When the fecal discharge is thick, water can be injected through the catheter to loosen and soften it. The consistency of the effluent is affected by food intake. At first, drainage is only 60 to 80 mL, but as time goes on, the amount increases significantly. The internal Kock pouch stretches, eventually accommodating 500 to 1,000 mL. The patient learns to use the sensation of pressure in the pouch as a gauge to determine how often the pouch should be drained.

The following procedure is used to drain the pouch; the patient is helped to participate in this procedure to learn to perform it unassisted.

Equipment

- Catheter
- Tissues
- Water-soluble lubricant
- Gauze squares
- Syringe
- Irrigating solution in a bowl
- Emesis or receiving basin

Implementation

NURSING ACTIONS	RATIONALE
1. Perform hand hygiene.	1. Hand hygiene is necessary before any intervention to decrease the likelihood of transmitting a hospital-associated infection.
2. Lubricate the catheter and gently insert it about 5 cm (2 in), at which point some resistance may be felt at the valve or nipple.	2. When gentle pressure is used, the catheter usually enters the pouch.
3. If there is much resistance, fill a syringe with 20 mL of air or water and inject it through the catheter, while still exerting some pressure on the catheter.	3. This permits the catheter to enter the pouch.
4. Place the other end of the catheter in a drainage basin held below the level of the stoma. Later, this process can be carried out at the toilet with drainage delivered into the toilet bowl.	4. Gravity facilitates drainage. Drainage may include flatus as well as effluent.
5. After drainage, the catheter is removed and the area around the stoma is gently washed with warm water. Pat dry and apply an absorbent pad over the stoma. Fasten the pad with hypoallergenic tape.	5. The entire procedure requires about 5 to 10 minutes; at first, it is performed every 3 hours. The time between procedures is gradually lengthened until irrigation is only required once daily.

Adapted from Chapman, G. M., Sinclair, L., & Langevin, J. M. (2009). *Ileoanal reservoir guide*. United Ostomy Associations of America: Author.

irritating effluent that rapidly fills the pouch (every hour or sooner), can quickly lead to dehydration and electrolyte losses. Supplemental water, sodium, and potassium are administered to prevent hypovolemia and hypokalemia. Antidiarrheal agents are administered. Stenosis is caused by circular scar tissue that forms at the stoma site. The scar tissue must be surgically released. Urinary calculi may occur in patients with ileostomies and are at least partly attributed to dehydration from decreased fluid intake. Intense lower abdominal pain that radiates to the legs, hematuria, and signs of dehydration indicate that the urine should be strained. Fluid intake is encouraged. Sometimes, small stones are passed during urination; treatment that crushes or removes larger stones is necessary (see Chapter 46).

Cholelithiasis (i.e., gallstones) occurs more commonly in patients with an ileostomy than in members of the general population because of changes in the absorption of bile acids that occur postoperatively. Spasm of the gallbladder causes severe upper right abdominal pain that can radiate to the back and right shoulder (see Chapter 40).

Promoting Home, Community-Based, and Transitional Care

EDUCATING PATIENTS ABOUT SELF-CARE. The partner and family should be familiar with the adjustments that will be necessary when the patient returns home. They need to know why it is necessary for the patient to occupy the bathroom for 10 minutes or more at certain times of the day and why certain equipment is needed. Their understanding is necessary to reduce tension; a relaxed patient tends to have fewer problems. Visits from a WOC nurse may be arranged to ensure

CHART 38-9

HOME CARE CHECKLIST • Managing Ostomy Care

At the completion of education, the patient and/or caregiver will be able to:

- Name the procedure that was performed and identify changes in anatomic structure or function as well as changes in ADLs, IADLs, roles, relationships, and spirituality.
  - Describe the frequency and character of effluent.
- Identify sources for obtaining ostomy care/appliance supplies.
- State the name, dose, side effects, frequency, and schedule for all medications.
- Demonstrate ostomy care, including wound cleansing, irrigation, and appliance changing.
- Describe the importance of assessing and maintaining peristomal skin integrity.
- Identify dietary restrictions (foods that can cause diarrhea and constipation), process for reintroduction of foods, as well as foods that may be encouraged.
- Identify measures to be used to promote fluid and electrolyte balance.
- Describe potential complications and necessary actions to be taken if complications occur.
- Relate how to reach primary provider with questions or complications.
  - Identify how to contact wound-ostomy-continence or home health nurse.
- State time and date of follow-up medical appointments, therapy, and testing.
- Identify sources of support (e.g., friends, relatives, faith community, ostomy support, caregiver support).
- Identify the need for health promotion, disease prevention, and screening activities.

ADL, activities of daily living; IADL, independent activities of daily living.

that the patient is progressing as expected and to provide additional guidance and teaching as needed.

CONTINUING AND TRANSITIONAL CARE. The patient needs to know the commercial name of the drainable pouching system to be used so that he or she can obtain a ready supply and should know how to obtain other supplies. The names and contact information of a local WOC nurse and local self-help groups are often helpful. Any restrictions on driving or working also need to be reviewed. The nurse teaches the patient about common postoperative complications and how to recognize and report them (Chart 38-9).

Intestinal Obstruction

Intestinal obstruction exists when blockage prevents the usual flow of intestinal contents through the intestinal tract. Two types of processes can impede this flow:

- *Mechanical obstruction:* An intraluminal obstruction or a mural obstruction from pressure on the intestinal wall occurs. Examples are intussusception, polypoid tumours and neoplasms, stenosis, strictures, adhesions, hernias, and abscesses (Ansari, 2014).
- *Functional obstruction:* The intestinal musculature cannot propel the contents along the bowel. Examples are amyloidosis, muscular dystrophy, endocrine disorders such as diabetes mellitus, or neurologic disorders such as Parkinson's disease. The blockage also can be temporary and the result of the manipulation of the bowel during surgery (Grossman & Porth, 2014).

The obstruction can be partial or complete. Its severity depends on the region of bowel affected, the degree to which the lumen is occluded, and especially the degree to which the vascular supply to the bowel wall is disturbed (Ansari, 2014).

Most bowel obstructions occur in the small intestine. Adhesions are the most common cause of small bowel obstruction, followed by hernias and neoplasms (Ansari, 2014; Nobie, 2015). Other causes include intussusception, volvulus (i.e., twisting of the bowel), and paralytic ileus. Most obstructions in the large bowel occur in the sigmoid colon. The most common causes are carcinoma, diverticulitis, inflammatory bowel disorders, benign tumours, and fecal impaction (Ansari, 2014; Hopkins, 2016). Table 38-6 and Figure 38-7 list mechanical causes of obstruction and describe how they occur.

Small Bowel Obstruction

Pathophysiology

Intestinal contents, fluid, and gas accumulate above the intestinal obstruction. The abdominal distention and retention of fluid reduce the absorption of fluids and stimulate more gastric secretion. With increasing distention, pressure within the intestinal lumen increases, causing a decrease in

TABLE 38-6 Mechanical Causes of Intestinal Obstruction

Cause	Course of Events	Result
Adhesions	Loops of intestine become adherent to areas that heal slowly or scar after abdominal surgery; occurs most commonly in small intestine.	After surgery, adhesions produce a kinking of an intestinal loop.
Intussusception	One part of the intestine slips into another part located below it (like a telescope shortening); occurs more commonly in infants than adults.	The intestinal lumen becomes narrowed and blood supply becomes strangulated.
Volvulus	Bowel twists and turns on itself and occludes the blood supply. Protrusion of intestine through a weakened area in the abdominal muscle or wall.	Intestinal lumen becomes obstructed. Gas and fluid accumulate in the trapped bowel. Intestinal flow may be completely obstructed. Blood flow to the area may be obstructed as well.
Tumour	A tumour that exists within the wall of the intestine extends into the intestinal lumen, or a tumour outside the intestine causes pressure on the wall of the intestine. Most common type is colorectal adenocarcinoma.	Intestinal lumen becomes partially obstructed; if the tumour is not removed, complete obstruction results.

venous and arteriolar capillary pressure. This causes edema, congestion, necrosis, and eventual rupture or perforation of the intestinal wall, with resultant peritonitis (Ansari, 2014; Nobie, 2015; Saccomano & Ferrara, 2013).

Clinical Manifestations

The initial symptom is usually cramping pain that is wave-like and colicky due to persistent peristalsis both above and below the blockage. The patient may pass blood and mucus but no fecal matter and no flatus. Vomiting occurs. If the obstruction is complete, the peristaltic waves initially become extremely vigorous and eventually assume a reverse direction, with the intestinal contents propelled toward the mouth instead of toward the rectum. If the obstruction is in the ileum, fecal vomiting takes place. First, the patient vomits the stomach contents, then the bile-stained contents of the duodenum and the jejunum, and finally, with each paroxysm of pain, the darker, fecal-like contents of the ileum. The signs of dehydration become evident: intense thirst, drowsiness, generalized malaise, aching, and a parched tongue and mucous membranes. The abdomen becomes distended. The lower the obstruction is in the GI tract, the more marked the abdominal distention. If the obstruction continues uncorrected, hypovolemic shock occurs from dehydration and loss of plasma volume.

Reflux vomiting results in loss of hydrogen ions and potassium from the stomach, leading to reduction of chloride and potassium in the blood and to metabolic alkalosis. Dehydration and acidosis develop from loss of water and sodium. With acute fluid losses, hypovolemic shock may occur; septic shock may also occur (Ansari, 2014; Nobie, 2015; Saccomano & Ferrara, 2013) (see Chapter 18).

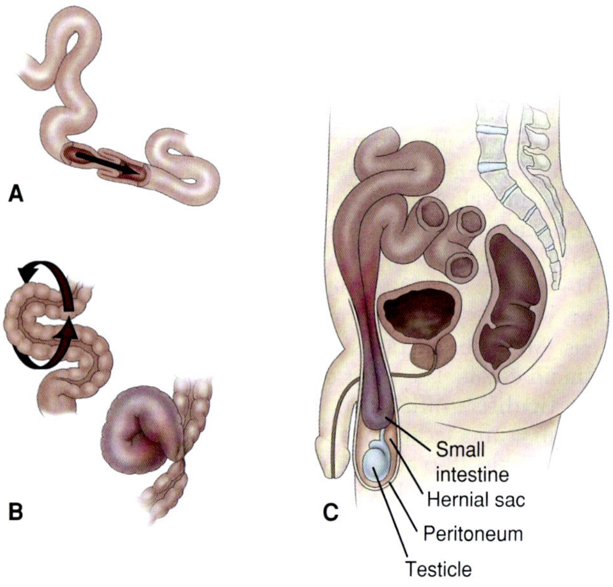

FIGURE 38-7. Three causes of intestinal obstruction. **A.** Intussusception; invagination or shortening of the colon caused by the movement of one segment of bowel into another. **B.** Volvulus of the sigmoid colon; the twist is counterclockwise in most cases. Note the edematous bowel. **C.** Hernia (inguinal). The sac of the hernia is a continuation of the peritoneum of the abdomen. The hernial contents are intestine, omentum, or other abdominal contents that pass through the hernial opening into the hernial sac.

Assessment and Diagnostic Findings

Diagnosis is based on the symptoms described previously and on imaging studies. Abdominal x-ray and CT findings include abnormal quantities of gas, fluid, or both in the intestines. Laboratory studies (i.e., electrolyte studies and a complete blood cell count) reveal a picture of dehydration, loss of plasma volume, and possible infection (Ansari, 2014; Nobie, 2015; Saccomano & Ferrara, 2013).

Medical Management

Decompression of the bowel through a nasogastric tube (see Chapter 36) is successful in most cases (Nobie, 2015). When the bowel is completely obstructed, the possibility of strangulation and tissue necrosis (i.e., tissue death) warrants surgical intervention. Before surgery, IV fluids are necessary to replace the depleted water, sodium, chloride, and potassium.

Surgical Management

The surgical treatment of intestinal obstruction depends on the cause of the obstruction. For the most common causes of obstruction, such as hernia and adhesions, the surgical procedure involves repairing the hernia or dividing the adhesion to which the intestine is attached. In some instances, the portion of affected bowel may be removed and an anastomosis performed. The complexity of the surgical procedure depends on the duration of the intestinal obstruction and the condition of the intestine. Laparoscopy has become increasingly common because it can facilitate diagnosis and is easily converted to open laparotomy if warranted (Nobie, 2015).

Nursing Management

Nursing management of the nonsurgical patient with a small bowel obstruction includes maintaining the function of the nasogastric tube, assessing and measuring the nasogastric output, assessing for fluid and electrolyte imbalance, monitoring nutritional status, and assessing improvement (e.g., return of usual bowel sounds, decreased abdominal distention, subjective improvement in abdominal pain and tenderness, passage of flatus or stool). The nurse reports discrepancies in intake and output, worsening of pain or abdominal distention, and increased nasogastric output. If the patient's condition does not improve, the nurse prepares him or her for surgery. Nursing care of the patient after surgical repair of a small bowel obstruction is similar to that for other abdominal surgeries (see Chapter 21).

Large Bowel Obstruction

Pathophysiology

As in small bowel obstruction, large bowel obstruction results in an accumulation of intestinal contents, fluid, and gas proximal to the obstruction. It can lead to severe distention and perforation unless some gas and fluid can flow back through the ileal valve. Large bowel obstruction, even if complete, may be undramatic if the blood supply to the colon is not disturbed. However, if the blood supply is cut off, intestinal strangulation and necrosis occur; this condition is life threatening. In the large intestine, dehydration occurs more slowly than in the small intestine because the colon can absorb its fluid contents and can distend to a size considerably beyond its usual full capacity.

Adenocarcinoid tumours account for the majority of large bowel obstructions. Most tumours occur beyond the splenic flexure, making them accessible with a flexible sigmoidoscope (Hopkins, 2016).

Clinical Manifestations

Large bowel obstruction differs clinically from small bowel obstruction in that the symptoms develop and progress relatively slowly. In patients with obstruction in the sigmoid colon or the rectum, constipation may be the only symptom for months. The shape of the stool is altered as it passes the obstruction that is gradually increasing in size. Blood loss in the stool may result in iron deficiency anemia. The patient may experience weakness, weight loss, and anorexia. Eventually, the abdomen becomes markedly distended, loops of large bowel become visibly outlined through the abdominal wall, and the patient has cramping lower abdominal pain. Finally, fecal vomiting develops. Symptoms of shock may occur.

Assessment and Diagnostic Findings

Diagnosis is based on symptoms and on imaging studies. Abdominal x-ray and abdominal CT or MRI findings reveal a distended colon and pinpoint the site of the obstruction. Barium studies are contraindicated (Hopkins, 2016).

Medical Management

Restoration of intravascular volume, correction of electrolyte abnormalities, and nasogastric aspiration and decompression are instituted immediately. A colonoscopy may be performed to untwist and decompress the bowel. A cecostomy, in which a surgical opening is made into the cecum, may be performed in patients who are poor surgical risks and urgently need relief from the obstruction. The procedure provides an outlet for releasing gas and a small amount of drainage. A rectal tube may be used to decompress an area that is lower in the bowel. As an alternative, a metal colonic stent may be used as either a palliative intervention or as a bridge to definitive surgery. The colonic stent is placed endoscopically with the assistance of an image intensifier, which creates a fluoroscopic image (Hopkins, 2016). However, the usual treatment is surgical resection to remove the obstructing lesion. A temporary or permanent colostomy may be necessary. An ileoanal anastomosis may be performed if removal of the entire large bowel is necessary (Ansari, 2014; Hopkins, 2016).

Nursing Management

The nurse's role is to monitor the patient for symptoms that indicate that the intestinal obstruction is worsening and to provide emotional support and comfort. The nurse administers IV fluids and electrolytes as prescribed. If the patient's condition does not respond to nonsurgical treatment, the nurse prepares the patient for surgery. This preparation includes preoperative teaching as the patient's condition indicates. After surgery, general abdominal wound care and routine postoperative nursing care are provided.

COLORECTAL NEOPLASMS

Colorectal Cancer

Tumours of the colon and rectum are relatively common; the colorectal area (the colon and rectum combined) is now the third most common site of new cancer cases in Canada for women and second most common for men. Colorectal cancer is a disease of Western cultures. In Canada, 26,800 new cases (13% of all new cases) and 9,400 deaths (12% of all cancer deaths) from colorectal cancer were predicted for 2013 (Canadian Cancer Society Advisory Committee on Cancer Statistics [CCSACCS], 2017). Colorectal cancer is the second leading cause of cancer death for men and the third cause for women (CCSACCS, 2017). The lifetime risk of developing colorectal cancer is 1 in 13 for Canadian men and 1 in 16 for

CHART 38-10

Risk Factors: Colorectal Cancer

- Cigarette smoking
- Family history of colon cancer (Lynch syndrome) or polyps (familial adenomatous polyposis)
- High consumption of alcohol (i.e., >2 drinks daily in men, >1 drink daily in women)
- High-fat, high-protein (with high intake of beef), low-fibre diet
- History of genital cancer (e.g., endometrial cancer, ovarian cancer) or breast cancer (in women)
- History of inflammatory bowel disease
- History of type 2 diabetes
- Increasing age
- Male gender
- Overweight or obesity
- Previous colon cancer or adenomatous polyps
- Racial/ethnic background: African American or Ashkenazi Jewish

Adapted from American Cancer Society (ACS). (2016). *Cancer facts and figures 2016*. Atlanta, GA: American Cancer Society; Bibbins-Domingo, K., Grossman, D. C., Curry, S. J., et al. (2016). Screening for colorectal cancer: U.S. Preventive Services Task Force Recommendation Statement. *JAMA, 315*(23), 2564–2575; and National Cancer Institute (NCI). (2016a). Colorectal cancer prevention: Who is at risk? Retrieved January 1, 2017, from www.cancer.gov/types/colorectal/hp/colorectal-prevention-pdq

Canadian women (CCSACCS, 2017). Incidence increases with age (the incidence is highest in people older than 85 years) and is higher in people with a family history of colon cancer and those with IBD or polyps. The exact cause of colon and rectal cancer is still unknown, but risk factors have been identified (Chart 38-10).

Improved screening strategies have helped reduce the number of deaths from colon cancer in recent years. Early diagnosis and prompt treatment could save almost three of every four people. Survival rates after late diagnosis are very low. Most people are asymptomatic for long periods and seek health care only when they notice a change in bowel habits or rectal bleeding. Prevention and early screening are key to detection and reduction of mortality rates (Saldana-Ruiz et al., 2013).

Hereditary colon cancer accounts for about 20% of all colon cancers. Early diagnosis helps target treatment and screening for clients and family members (Gomy & Estevez, 2013). Genetic counsellors are trained to help patients and their family members understand the significance of genetics information (Gomy & Estevez, 2013). If patients are found to have a genetic susceptibility to cancer, they should be offered counselling and follow-up to ensure that care is consistent with current standards (Gomy & Estevez, 2013).

Pathophysiology

Cancer of the colon and rectum is predominantly (95%) adenocarcinoma (i.e., arising from the epithelial lining of the intestine) (NCI, 2016b). It may start as a benign polyp but may become malignant, invade and destroy normal tissues, and extend into surrounding structures. Cancer cells may migrate away from the primary tumour and spread to other parts of the body (most often to the liver, peritoneum, and lungs) (NCI, 2016b).

Clinical Manifestations

The symptoms are greatly determined by the location of the tumour, the stage of the disease, and the function of the affected intestinal segment. The most common presenting symptom is a change in bowel habits. The passage of blood in or on the stools is the second most common symptom. Symptoms may also include unexplained anemia, anorexia, weight loss, and fatigue (Canadian Cancer Society, 2018).

The symptoms most commonly associated with right-sided lesions are dull abdominal pain and melena (i.e., black, tarry stools). The symptoms most commonly associated with left-sided lesions are those associated with obstruction (i.e., abdominal pain and cramping, narrowing stools, constipation, distention), as well as bright-red blood in the stool. Symptoms associated with rectal lesions are tenesmus (i.e., ineffective, painful straining at stool), rectal pain, the feeling of incomplete evacuation after a bowel movement, alternating constipation and diarrhea, and bloody stool. In many instances, symptoms do not develop until colorectal cancer is at an advanced stage (Livstone, 2014).

Assessment and Diagnostic Findings

Along with an abdominal and rectal examination, the most important diagnostic procedures for cancer of the colon are fecal occult blood testing, barium enema, proctosigmoidoscopy, and colonoscopy (see Chapter 34).

A stool test checks for hidden (occult) blood in the stool. Cancerous tumours and other growths in the lining of the colon or rectum (such as polyps) have blood vessels on their surface that can release a small amount of blood into the stool. Stool tests help identify adenomas (adenomatous polyps) early, before they become cancerous.

There are two types of stool tests used to screen for colorectal cancer in Canada.

- **gFOBT (guaiac-based fecal occult blood test)** is the original type of stool test. It uses a chemical reaction on a paper card to find blood in the stool from adenomatous polyps or tumours.
- **FIT (fecal immunochemical test)** uses specific antibodies for human blood to find blood in the stool. FIT is being used by most screening programs in Canada.

Follow-up may include a colonoscopy, flexible sigmoidoscopy, or a double barium enema along with biopsy or cytology smears (colonoscopy; sigmoidoscopy).

Carcinoembryonic antigen (CEA) studies may also be performed. Although CEA may not be a highly reliable indicator in diagnosing colon cancer because not all lesions secrete CEA, studies show that CEA levels are reliable prognostic predictors. With complete excision of the tumour, the elevated levels of CEA should return to expected values within 48 hours. Elevations of CEA at a later date suggest recurrence (Canadian Cancer Society, 2018a).

Complications

Tumour growth may cause partial or complete bowel obstruction. Extension of the tumour and ulceration into the surrounding blood vessels result in hemorrhage. Each of these complications is treated surgically. Obstruction may be resected without anastomosis (e.g., Hartmann's procedure) or with anastomosis (e.g., colectomy or partial colectomy). Perforation typically carries a grim prognosis; it is typically treated with an ostomy. Acute hemorrhage is a rare complication; when it occurs, it is most effectively treated with surgical resection (Chang, Kaiser, Mills, et al., 2012).

Gerontologic Considerations

The incidence of carcinoma of the colon and rectum increases with age. These cancers are considered common malignancies in advanced age. In men, only the incidence of prostate cancer and lung cancer exceeds that of colorectal cancer. In women, only the incidence of breast and lung cancer exceeds that of colorectal cancer (CCSACCS, 2017; Logan et al., 2012). Symptoms are often insidious. Patients with colorectal cancer usually report fatigue, which is caused primarily by iron deficiency anemia. In early stages, minor changes in bowel patterns and occasional bleeding may occur. The later symptoms most commonly reported by older people are abdominal pain, obstruction, tenesmus, and rectal bleeding.

Colon cancer in older people has been closely associated with dietary carcinogens. Lack of fibre is a major causative factor because the passage of feces through the intestinal tract is prolonged, which extends exposure to possible carcinogens. Excess dietary fat, high alcohol consumption, and smoking all increase the incidence of colorectal tumours. Physical activity and dietary folate have protective effects (Kushi et al., 2012).

Prevention

Several primary prevention strategies might thwart the onset of colorectal cancer. Use of tobacco products is implicated in one third of all cancers, including colorectal cancer. Physical activity, diet, and weight reduction strategies mirror those for other cancers (Greenwald, 2015b). In addition to these strategies, it is recommended that adults between the ages of 50 and 59 who are also at risk for developing cardiovascular disease, and who have no contraindication to aspirin, take daily or alternate-day aspirin (dosage ≥75 mg) for 5 to 10 years, as an effective primary prevention strategy for both cardiovascular disease and colorectal cancer (Chubak et al., 2015). In addition, some evidence shows that patients with a diagnosis of colorectal cancer may benefit from aspirin therapy; however, these benefits may be specific to the genetic subtype of the tumour (Liao et al., 2012). To date, there is no expert consensus guideline that advocates routine prescription of aspirin postcolorectal cancer diagnosis.

Medical Management

The patient with symptoms of intestinal obstruction is treated with IV fluids and nasogastric suction. If there has been significant bleeding, blood component therapy may be required.

Treatment for colorectal cancer depends on the stage of the disease (Chart 38-11) and consists of surgery to remove the tumour, supportive therapy, and adjuvant therapy. Patients who receive some form of adjuvant therapy, which may include chemotherapy, radiation therapy, immunotherapy, or multimodality therapy, typically demonstrate delays in tumour recurrence and increases in survival time (Chang et al., 2012).

Adjuvant Therapy

Patients diagnosed with colorectal cancer are referred to a medical oncologist for further management after they are discharged from the hospital after surgery. Patients at the lowest risk for recurrence (i.e., those with Stage 0 or I disease) do not require chemotherapy or radiation therapy. Those with Stage 0 disease do not require specific follow-up. Patients with Stage I colorectal cancer should have follow-up colonoscopies 1-year postoperatively, then again in another 3 years, and then every 5 years (Benson et al., 2013).

Most patients with Stage II disease do not require any adjuvant chemotherapy. However, some patients with Stage II tumours have mutations in their DNA mismatch repair genes (MMR) that are classified as proficient (MMR-P). Patients in this subset have improved survival and less disease recurrence if they take the antimetabolite chemotherapeutic drug capecitabine (Xeloda) for 6 months. In order to screen for the MMR-P gene, the tumour should be analyzed by a multigene assay (i.e., genetic test). Patients with Stage II disease who may also benefit from capecitabine are those who had inadequately sampled lymph nodes, with T4-sized tumours, or with poorly differentiated tumours (Benson et al., 2013). Capecitabine is equivalent to the dual chemotherapeutic drugs 5-fluorouracil and leucovorin. It may be given either orally or intravenously. The most common adverse effects of capecitabine include anemia, neutropenia, fatigue, diarrhea, and palmar–plantar erythrodysesthesia (PPE; hand–foot syndrome), which manifests by reddening, pain, and swelling of the palms of the hands and soles of the feet (NCI, 2016b).

Patients with Stage III tumours are typically prescribed the combination chemotherapeutic drug of 5-fluorouracil, leucovorin, and oxaliplatin, called FOLFOX. This combination chemotherapeutic drug must be administered IV in 2-week cycles over 6 months. The adverse effects mirrors that of capecitabine, plus patients frequently experience paresthesias of their hands and feet, which typically cease after the chemotherapy is completed (NCI, 2016b).

Patients with Stage II or Stage III tumours should have routine follow-ups and CEA testing every 3 to 6 months for 5 years. CT scans of the abdomen and chest should be done each year for 3 years. Colonoscopy should also be done 1-year postoperatively, and then every 5 years (Meyerhardt et al., 2013).

Patients with Stage IV or recurrent colorectal tumours have metastases to distant organs. The treatment is highly variable and individualized, based upon the extent of the tumour mass(es), and the health status and wishes of the patient. Treatment might consist of targeted therapy aimed at possible cure, or palliative care. Chemotherapeutic drugs that might be tried include those previously described for

CHART 38-11

Staging of Colorectal Cancer: American Joint Committee on Cancer (AJCC) Stage Groupings

Stage	TNM	Description
Stage 0	Tis, N0, M0	Tis: Carcinoma in situ; intraepithelial or invasion of lamina propria N0: No regional lymph node metastasis M0: No distant metastasis
Stage I	T1, N0, M0 T2, N0, M0	T1: Tumour invades submucosa T2: Tumour invades muscularis propria
Stage IIA	T3, N0, M0	T3: Tumour invades through the muscularis propria into pericolorectal tissues
Stage IIB	T4a, N0, M0	T4a: Tumour penetrates to the surface of the visceral peritoneum
Stage IIC	T4b, N0, M0	T4b: Tumour directly invades or is adherent to other organs or structures
Stage IIIA	T1–T2, N1–N1c, M0 T1, N2a, M0	N1: Metastases in 1–3 regional lymph nodes N1a: Metastasis in 1 regional lymph node N1b: Metastases in 2–3 regional lymph nodes N1c: Tumour deposit(s) in the subserosa, mesentery, or nonperitonealized pericolic or perirectal tissues without regional nodal metastasis N2: Metastases in ≥4 regional lymph nodes N2a: Metastases in 4–6 regional lymph nodes
Stage IIIB	T3–T4a, N1–N1c, M0 T2–T3, N2a, M0 T1–T2, N2b, M0	N2b: Metastases in ≥7 regional lymph nodes
Stage IIIC	T4a, N2a, M0 T3–T4a, N2b, M0 T4b, N1–N2, M0	
Stage IVA	Any T, Any N, M1a	M1a: Metastasis confined to 1 organ or site (e.g., liver, lung, ovary, nonregional node)
Stage IVB	Any T, Any N, M1b	M1b: Metastasis in >1 organ/site or the peritoneum

T, primary tumour; N, regional lymph nodes; M, distant metastasis.

Adapted from National Cancer Institute (NCI). (2016b). Stage information for colon cancer. Retrieved January 1, 2017, from www.cancer.gov/types/colorectal/hp/colon-treatment-pdq#link/_331

Note: This is based upon AJCC and National Cancer Institute (NCI) recommendations that at least 12 regional lymph nodes are examined in patients with colorectal cancer to confirm staging.

treating Stage II or Stage III disease, as well as other categories of agents, including monoclonal antibodies (e.g., cetuximab, bevacizumab), and antivascular endothelial growth factor (anti-VEGF) agents (e.g., aflibercept), to name a few. When metastasis occurs, the liver is implicated half the time. Therapy targeted to treat metastases to the liver can include surgical resection, radiofrequency ablation, and intra-arterial chemotherapy (NCI, 2016b). Surveillance for patients with Stage IV disease is also individualized, and is done on an ongoing basis (Steele et al., 2015).

Surgical Management

Surgery is the mainstay of treatment for colorectal cancer. It may be curative or palliative. Advances in surgical techniques can enable the patient with rectal cancer to have sphincter-sparing devices that restore continuity of the GI tract. The type of surgery recommended depends on the location and size of the tumour; in up to 10% of patients with new diagnoses of colorectal cancer, there is more than one tumour, which is known as a synchronous tumour (Chang et al., 2012).

Patients who have Stage 0 tumours typically have endoscopic or laparoscopic excision of their tumours (NCI, 2016b). Laparoscopic surgery for Stage I, II, and III colorectal tumours achieves equivalent oncologic outcomes to surgery done by traditional open laparotomy (Chang et al., 2012). In addition, laparoscopic surgery is associated with shorter hospital lengths of stay, fewer postoperative complications, improved pain control, and earlier progression to a normal diet (Kapritsou, Korkolis, & Konstantinou, 2013).

Possible surgical procedures include the following (note that only segmental resections with anastomoses may be done by laparoscope):

- Segmental resection with anastomosis (i.e., removal of the tumour and portions of the bowel on either side of the growth, as well as the blood vessels and lymphatic nodes) (Fig. 38-8)
- Abdominoperineal resection with permanent sigmoid colostomy (i.e., removal of the tumour and a portion of the sigmoid and all of the rectum and anal sphincter, also called *Miles resection*) (Fig. 38-9)
- Temporary colostomy followed by segmental resection and anastomosis and subsequent reanastomosis of the colostomy, allowing initial bowel decompression and bowel preparation before resection
- Permanent colostomy or ileostomy for palliation of unresectable obstructing lesions
- Construction of a coloanal reservoir called a *colonic J-pouch*, which is performed in two steps. A temporary loop ileostomy is constructed to divert intestinal flow, and the newly constructed J-pouch (made from

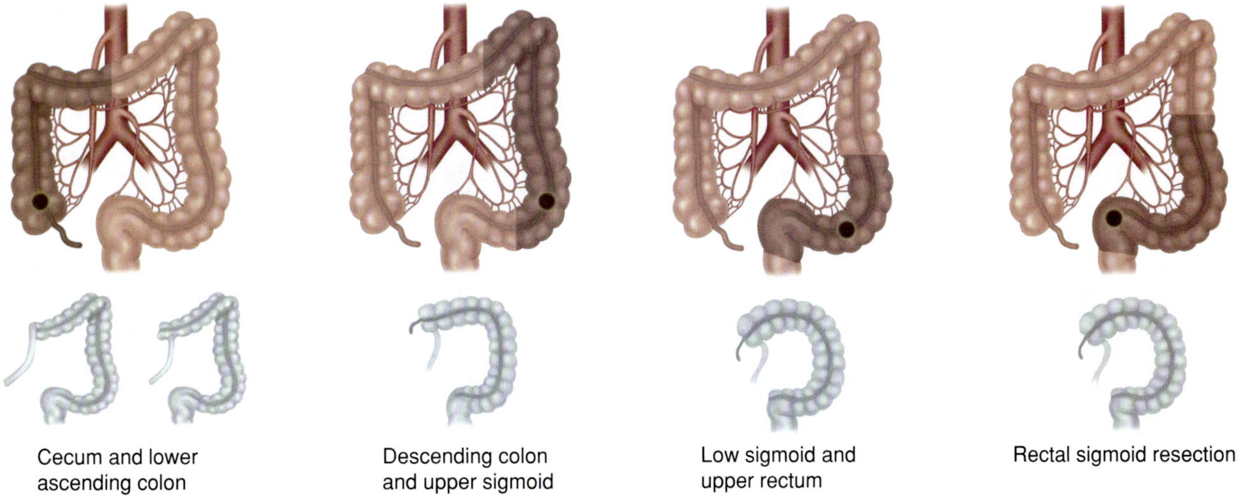

FIGURE 38-8. Examples of areas where cancer can occur, the area that is removed, and how the anastomosis is performed (*small diagrams*).

6 to 10 cm of colon) is reattached to the anal stump. About 3 months after the initial stage, the ileostomy is reversed and intestinal continuity is restored. The anal sphincter and therefore continence are preserved

The colostomy can be created as a temporary or permanent fecal diversion. It allows the drainage or evacuation of colon contents to the outside of the body. The consistency of the drainage is related to the placement of the colostomy, which is dictated by the location of the tumour and the extent of invasion into surrounding tissues (Fig. 38-10).

Gerontologic Considerations

Older adults are at increased risk of complications after surgery and may have difficulty managing colostomy

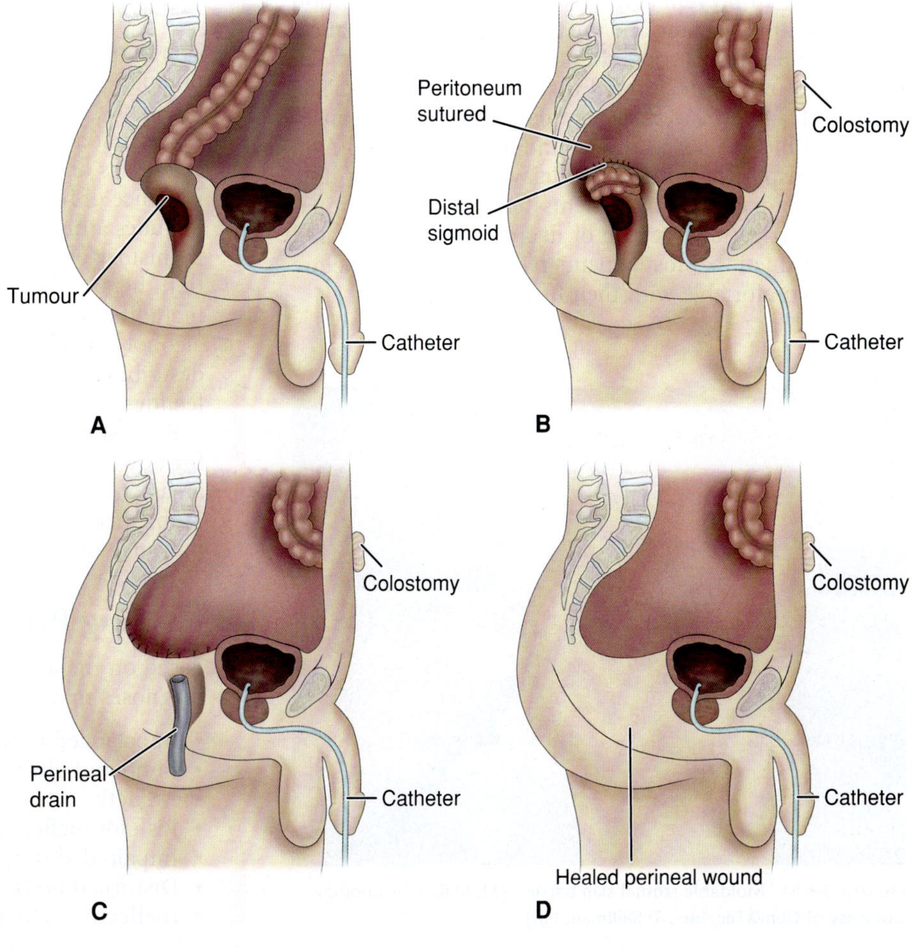

FIGURE 38-9. Abdominoperineal resection for carcinoma of the rectum. **A.** Prior to surgery. Note tumour in rectum. **B.** During surgery, the sigmoid is removed and the colostomy is established. The distal bowel is dissected free to a point below the pelvic peritoneum, which is sutured over the closed end of the distal sigmoid and rectum. **C.** Perineal resection includes removal of the rectum and free portion of the sigmoid from below. A perineal drain is inserted. **D.** The final result after healing. Note the healed perineal wound and the permanent colostomy.

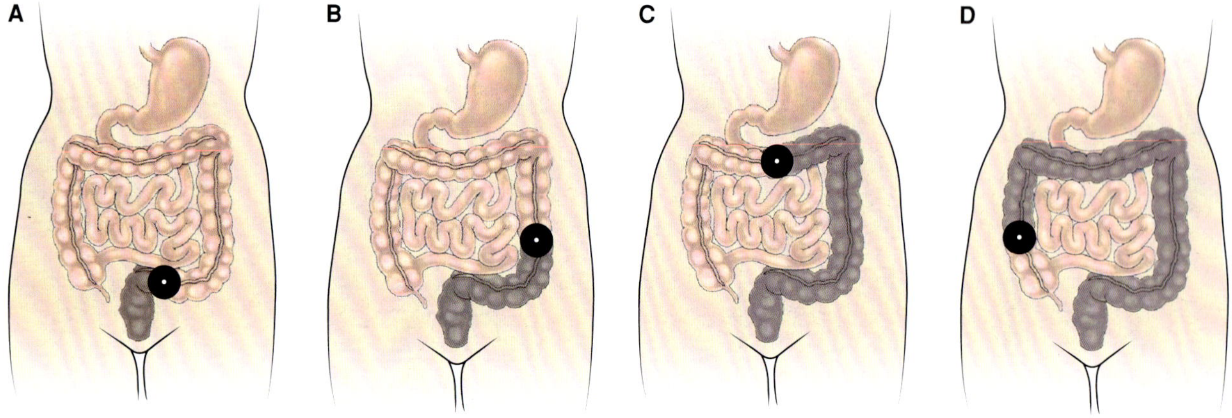

FIGURE 38-10. Placement of permanent colostomies. The nature of the discharge varies with the site. Shaded areas show sections of bowel removed. **A.** With a sigmoid colostomy, the feces are formed. **B.** With a descending colostomy, the feces are semiformed. **C.** With a transverse colostomy, the feces are unformed. **D.** With an ascending colostomy, the feces are fluid.

care. Some older patients may have decreased vision, impaired hearing, and difficulty with fine motor coordination. It may be helpful for patients to handle ostomy equipment and simulate cleaning the peristomal skin and irrigating the stoma before surgery. Skin care is a major concern in older patients with a colostomy because of the skin changes that occur with aging—the epithelial and subcutaneous fatty layers become thin, and the skin is irritated easily. To prevent skin breakdown, special attention is paid to skin cleansing and the proper fit of an appliance. Newer stoma skin barriers do not have to be cut but can be molded into shape around the stoma (e.g., ConvaTec; Fig. 38-11). Arteriosclerosis may also be an issue; it causes decreased blood flow to the wound and stoma site. As a result, transport of nutrients is delayed and healing time may be prolonged. Some patients have delayed elimination after irrigation because of decreased peristalsis and mucus production. Most patients require 6 months before they feel comfortable with their ostomy care.

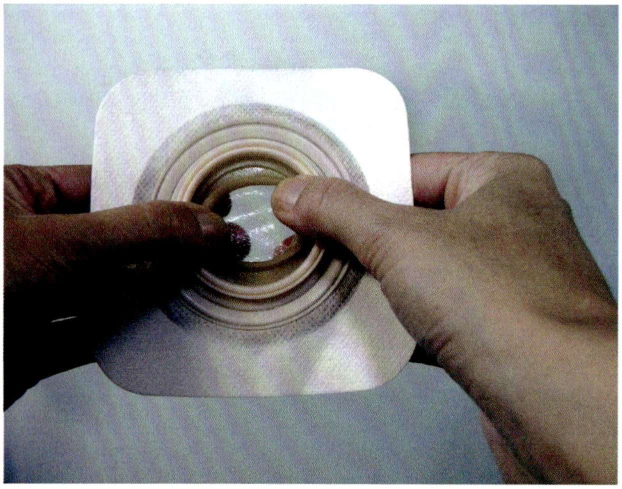

FIGURE 38-11. Moldable stomal skin barrier. (Moldable Technology, Courtesy of ConvaTec, Inc., © Skillman, NJ.)

Nursing Process

The Patient With Colorectal Cancer

Assessment

The nurse obtains a health history about the presence of fatigue, abdominal or rectal pain (e.g., location, frequency, duration, association with eating or defecation), past and present elimination patterns, and characteristics of stool (e.g., colour, odour, consistency, presence of blood or mucus). Additional information includes a history of IBD or colorectal polyps, a family history of colorectal disease, and current medication therapy. The nurse assesses dietary patterns, including fat and fibre intake, as well as amounts of alcohol consumed and history of smoking. The nurse describes and documents a history of weight loss and feelings of weakness and fatigue.

Assessment includes auscultation of the abdomen for bowel sounds and palpation of the abdomen for areas of tenderness, distention, and solid masses. Stool specimens are inspected for character and presence of blood.

Nursing Priorities

Based on the assessment data, the major nursing diagnoses may include the following:

- Imbalanced nutrition
- Fluid and electrolyte balance
- Anxiety
- Risk for ineffective therapeutic regimen management
- Impaired skin integrity
- Disturbed body image
- Ineffective sexuality patterns

Collaborative Problems/ Potential Complications

Potential complications that may develop include the following:

- Intraperitoneal infection
- Complete large bowel obstruction
- GI bleeding
- Bowel perforation
- Peritonitis, abscess, and sepsis

Planning and Goals

The major goals for the patient may include attainment of optimal level of nutrition; maintenance of fluid and electrolyte balance; reduction of anxiety; learning about the diagnosis, surgical procedure, and self-care after discharge; maintenance of optimal tissue healing; protection of peristomal skin; learning how to irrigate the colostomy (done only with sigmoid colostomies) and change the appliance; expressing feelings and concerns about the colostomy and the impact on self; and avoidance of complications.

Nursing Interventions

Preparing the Patient for Surgery

The patient awaiting surgery for colorectal cancer has many concerns, needs, and fears. He or she may be physically debilitated and emotionally distraught with concerns about lifestyle changes after surgery, prognosis, ability to perform in established roles, and finances. Priorities for nursing care include preparing the patient physically for surgery; providing information about postoperative care, including stoma care if a colostomy is to be created; and supporting the patient and family emotionally. Ideally, a WOC nurse or surgeon should identify the stoma site preoperatively to ensure that its placement is visible and accessible to the patient.

Physical preparation for surgery involves building the patient's stamina in the days preceding surgery and cleansing and sterilizing the bowel the day before surgery. If the patient's condition permits, the nurse recommends a diet high in calories, protein, and carbohydrates and low in residue for several days before surgery to provide adequate nutrition and minimize cramping by decreasing excessive peristalsis. A full liquid diet may be prescribed for 24 to 48 hours before surgery to decrease bulk. If the patient is hospitalized in the days preceding surgery, parenteral nutrition may be required to replace depleted nutrients, vitamins, and minerals. In some instances, parenteral nutrition is administered at home before surgery. Antibiotics such as kanamycin (Kantrex), neomycin (Mycifradin), and cephalexin (Keflex) are administered orally the day before surgery to reduce intestinal bacteria. The bowel is cleansed with laxatives, enemas, or colonic irrigations the evening before and the morning of surgery.

For the patient who is very ill and hospitalized, the nurse measures and records intake and output, including vomitus, to provide an accurate record of fluid balance. The patient's intake of oral food and fluids may be restricted to prevent vomiting. The nurse administers antiemetics as prescribed. Full or clear liquids may be tolerated, or the patient may be allowed nothing by mouth. A nasogastric tube may be inserted to drain accumulated fluids and prevent abdominal distention. The nurse monitors the abdomen for increasing distention, loss of bowel sounds, and pain or rigidity, which may indicate obstruction or perforation. It is also important to monitor IV fluids and electrolytes. Monitoring serum electrolyte levels can detect the hypokalemia and hyponatremia that occur with GI fluid loss. The nurse observes for signs of hypovolemia (e.g., tachycardia, hypotension, decreased pulse volume); assesses hydration status; and reports decreased skin turgor, dry mucous membranes, and concentrated urine.

The nurse assesses the patient's knowledge about the diagnosis, prognosis, surgical procedure, and expected level of functioning after surgery. It is important to include information about the physical preparation for surgery, the expected appearance and care of the wound, the technique of ostomy care (if applicable), dietary restrictions, pain control, and medication management in the teaching plan (see the Plan of Nursing Care in Chart 38-6). If the patient is admitted on the day of surgery, the physician's office may arrange for the patient to be seen by a WOC nurse in the days preceding surgery. The WOC nurse helps determine the optimal site for the stoma and provides teaching about care. If the patient is hospitalized before the day of surgery, the WOC nurse is involved in the preoperative teaching. All procedures are explained in a language the patient can understand.

Providing Emotional Support

Patients anticipating bowel surgery for colorectal cancer may be very anxious. They may grieve about the diagnosis, the impending surgery, and possible permanent colostomy. Patients undergoing surgery for a temporary colostomy may express fears and concerns similar to those of a person with a permanent stoma. All members of the health care team, including the WOC nurse, should be available for assistance and support. The nurse's role is to assess the patient's anxiety level and coping mechanisms and suggest methods for reducing anxiety, such as deep-breathing exercises and visualizing a successful recovery from surgery and cancer. The nurse can arrange a meeting with a spiritual advisor if the patient desires or with the physician if the patient wishes to discuss the treatment or prognosis.

The patient undergoing a colostomy may find the anticipated changes in body image and lifestyle profoundly disturbing. Because the stoma is located on the abdomen, the patient may think that everyone will be aware of the ostomy. The nurse helps reduce this fear by presenting facts about the surgical procedure and the creation and management of the ostomy. If the patient is receptive, the nurse can use diagrams, photographs, and appliances to explain and clarify. Because the patient is experiencing emotional stress, the nurse will likely need to repeat some of the information. Consultation with a WOC nurse during the preoperative period can be extremely helpful, as can speaking with a person who is successfully managing a colostomy. The Canadian Cancer Society provides visiting services by qualified members and rehabilitation services for patients with new ostomies.

Providing Postoperative Care

Postoperative nursing care for patients undergoing colon resection or colostomy is similar to nursing care for any abdominal surgery patient (see Chapter 21), including pain management during the immediate postoperative period. The nurse assesses the abdomen for returning peristalsis and assesses the initial stool characteristics. It is important to help patients with a colostomy get out of bed on the first postoperative day and to encourage them to begin participating in managing the colostomy.

MAINTAINING OPTIMAL NUTRITION. The nurse teaches all patients undergoing surgery for colorectal cancer about the health benefits to be derived from consuming a healthy diet. The diet is individualized as long as it is nutritionally sound and does not cause diarrhea or constipation. The return to usual diet is rapid.

A complete nutritional assessment (Pasia, 2017) is important for the patient with a colostomy. The patient avoids foods that cause excessive odour and gas, including foods in the cabbage family, eggs, asparagus, fish, beans, and high-cellulose products such as peanuts. It is important to determine whether the elimination of specific foods is causing any nutritional deficiency. Nonirritating foods are substituted for those that are restricted so that deficiencies are corrected. The nurse advises the patient to experiment with an irritating food several times before restricting it, because an initial sensitivity may decrease with time. The nurse can help the patient identify any foods or fluids that may be causing diarrhea, such as fruits, high-fibre foods, coffee, tea, pop, or other carbonated beverages. Diphenoxylate with atropine may be prescribed as needed to control the diarrhea. For constipation, prune or apple juice or a mild laxative is effective. The nurse suggests fluid intake of at least 2 L per day.

PROVIDING WOUND CARE. The nurse frequently examines the abdominal dressing during the first 24 hours after surgery to detect signs of hemorrhage. It is important to help the patient splint the abdominal incision during coughing and deep breathing to lessen tension on the edges of the incision. The nurse monitors temperature, pulse, and respiratory rate for elevations that may indicate an infectious process. If the patient has a colostomy, the stoma is examined for swelling (slight edema from surgical manipulation is expected), colour (a healthy stoma is pink or red), discharge (a small amount of oozing is usual), and bleeding (an abnormal sign if bright red or beyond trace amounts).

If the malignancy has been removed using the perineal route, the perineal wound is observed for signs of hemorrhage. This wound may contain a drain or packing that is removed gradually. Bits of tissue may slough off for a week. This process is hastened by mechanical irrigation of the wound or with sitz baths performed two or three times each day initially. The condition of the perineal wound and any bleeding, infection, or necrosis is documented.

MONITORING AND MANAGING COMPLICATIONS. The patient is observed for signs and symptoms of complications. It is important to frequently assess the abdomen, including bowel sounds and abdominal girth, to detect bowel obstruction. The nurse monitors vital signs for increased temperature, pulse, and respirations and for decreased blood pressure that may indicate an intra-abdominal infectious process. It is important to report rectal bleeding immediately because it indicates hemorrhage. The nurse monitors hemoglobin and hematocrit levels and administers blood component therapy as prescribed. Any abrupt change in abdominal pain is reported promptly. Elevated white blood cell counts and temperature or symptoms of shock are reported because they may indicate sepsis. The nurse administers antibiotics as prescribed.

Pulmonary complications are always a concern with abdominal surgery; patients older than 50 years are at risk, especially if they are or have been receiving sedatives or are being maintained on bed rest for a prolonged period. Two major pulmonary complications are pneumonia and atelectasis. Frequent activity (e.g., turning the patient from side to side every 2 hours), deep breathing, coughing, and early ambulation can reduce the risk for these complications. Table 38-7 lists postoperative complications.

The incidence of complications related to the colostomy is usually less than that of an ileostomy. Some common complications are prolapse of the stoma, parastomal hernia, perforation (from improper stoma irrigation), stoma retraction, mucocutaneous separation, and skin irritation. Leakage from an anastomotic site can occur if the remaining bowel segments are diseased or weakened. Leakage from an intestinal anastomosis causes peritonitis with abdominal distention and rigidity, temperature elevation, and signs of shock. Surgical repair is necessary.

Removing and Applying the Colostomy Appliance

The colostomy begins to function 3 to 6 days after surgery. The nurse manages the colostomy and teaches the patient about its care until the patient can take over its management. The nurse teaches skin care and how to apply, empty, and remove the drainage pouch. Care of the peristomal skin is an ongoing concern because excoriation or ulceration can develop quickly. The presence of such irritation makes adhering the ostomy appliance difficult, and

TABLE 38-7 Potential Complications and Nursing Interventions After Intestinal Surgery

Complications	Nursing Interventions
General Complications	
Mechanical obstruction	Initiate or continue nasogastric intubation as prescribed. Prepare patient for x-ray study. Ensure adequate fluid and electrolyte replacement. Administer prescribed antibiotics if patient has symptoms of peritonitis. Assess patient for intermittent colicky pain, nausea, and vomiting.
Intra-Abdominal Septic Conditions	
Peritonitis	Evaluate patient for nausea, hiccups, chills, spiking fever, tachycardia, boardlike abdomen. Administer antibiotics as prescribed. Prepare patient for drainage procedure. Administer parenteral fluid and electrolyte therapy as prescribed. Prepare patient for surgery if condition deteriorates.
Abscess formation	Administer antibiotics as prescribed. Apply warm compresses as prescribed. Prepare for surgical drainage.
Surgical Wound Complications	
Infection	Monitor temperature; report temperature elevation. Observe for redness, tenderness, hardening (induration), and pain around the surgical wound. Assist in establishing local drainage. Obtain specimen of drainage material for culture and sensitivity studies.
Wound disruption	Observe for sudden drainage of profuse serous fluid from wound. Cover wound area with sterile moist dressings supported with binder or similar method. Prepare patient immediately for surgery.
Intraperitoneal infection and abdominal wound infection	Monitor for evidence of constant or generalized abdominal pain, rapid pulse, and elevation of temperature. Prepare for tube decompression of bowel. Administer fluids and electrolytes by IV route as prescribed. Administer antibiotics as prescribed.
Anastomotic Complications	
Dehiscence of anastomosis	Prepare patient for surgery.
Fistulas	Prepare for tube decompression of bowel. Administer parenteral fluids as prescribed to correct fluid and electrolyte deficits.

adhering the ostomy appliance to irritated skin can worsen the skin condition. The effluent discharge and the degree to which it is irritating vary with the type of ostomy. With a transverse colostomy, the stool is soft and unformed and irritating to the skin. With a descending or sigmoid colostomy, the stool is fairly solid and less irritating to the skin. Other skin problems include yeast infections and allergic dermatitis. If the patient wants to bathe or shower before putting on a clean appliance, micropore tape applied to the sides of the pouch keeps it secure during bathing. Refer to Chart 38-7 for guidelines on changing an ostomy appliance.

Colostomy appliances are not always necessary for some patients who have end-sigmoid colostomies and who irrigate them. As soon as the patient has learned a routine for evacuation, pouches may be dispensed with, and a closed ostomy appliance or a stoma cap is used to cover the stoma. Except for gas and a slight amount of mucus, nothing escapes from the colostomy opening between irrigations.

Irrigating the Colostomy

The purpose of irrigating a colostomy is to empty the colon of gas, mucus, and feces so that the patient can go about social and business activities without fear of fecal drainage. A stoma does not have voluntary muscular control and may empty at irregular intervals. Regulating the passage of fecal material is achieved by irrigating the colostomy or allowing the bowel to evacuate naturally without irrigations. This choice depends on the person and the type of the colostomy (i.e., descending or sigmoid colostomies). By irrigating the stoma at a regular time, there is less gas and retention of the irrigant. The time for irrigating the colostomy should be consistent with the schedule the person will follow after leaving the hospital. Chart 38-12 describes the irrigating procedure.

Colostomy irrigation is not recommended for persons with extensive pelvic irradiation because it carries a risk of perforation (Grant et al., 2012).

Supporting a Positive Body Image

The patient is encouraged to verbalize feelings and concerns about altered body image and to discuss the surgery and the stoma (if one was created). If applicable, the patient must learn colostomy care and begin to plan for incorporating stoma care into daily life. The nurse helps the patient overcome aversion to the stoma or fear of self-injury by providing care and teaching in an open, accepting manner and by encouraging the patient to talk about his or her feelings about the stoma.

CHART 38-12

GUIDELINES for Irrigating a Colostomy

A colostomy is irrigated to empty the colon of feces, gas, or mucus, cleanse the lower intestinal tract, and establish a regular pattern of evacuation so that normal life activities may be pursued. A suitable time for the irrigation is selected that is compatible with the patient's posthospital pattern of activity (preferably after a meal). Irrigation should be performed at the same time each day.

Before the procedure, the patient sits on a chair in front of the toilet or on the toilet itself. An irrigating reservoir containing 500 to 1,500 mL of lukewarm tap water is hung 45–50 cm (18–20 in) above the stoma (shoulder height when the patient is seated). The dressing or pouch is removed. The following procedure is used; the patient is helped to participate in the procedure so that he or she can learn to perform it unassisted.

Equipment

- Irrigating sleeve or sheath
- Irrigating catheter or cone and tubing
- Lubricant
- Clamp
- Mild soap
- Cloth or towel
- New colostomy dressing or appliance

Implementation

NURSING ACTIONS	RATIONALE
1. Perform hand hygiene; then, apply an irrigating sleeve or sheath to the stoma. Place the end in the commode.	1. Hand hygiene is necessary before any intervention to decrease the likelihood of transmitting a hospital-associated infection. Application of the sleeve or sheath helps control odour and splashing and allows feces and water to flow directly into the commode.
2. Allow some of the solution to flow through the tubing and catheter/cone.	2. Air bubbles in the setup are released so that air is not introduced into the colon, which would cause crampy pain.
3. Lubricate the irrigating cone and gently insert it into the stoma (Fig. A). Insert the cone into the stoma and hold it gently, but firmly, against the stoma to prevent backflow of water.	3. Lubrication permits ease of insertion of the cone. A cone is used to prevent internal damage if a catheter is used.
4. Allow water to flow slowly while advancing catheter (Fig. B).	4. A slow rate of flow helps to relax the bowel.
5. Allow tepid fluid to enter the colon slowly. If cramping occurs, clamp off the tubing and allow the patient to rest before progressing. Water should flow in over a 5- to 10-minute period.	5. Painful cramps usually are caused by too rapid a flow or by too much solution; 300 mL of fluid may be all that is needed to stimulate evacuation. Volume may be increased with subsequent irrigations to 500, 1,000, or 1,500 mL as needed by the patient for effective results.
6. Hold the cone in place 10 seconds after the water has been instilled, then gently remove it (Fig. C).	6. This minimizes or eliminates spillage of water.

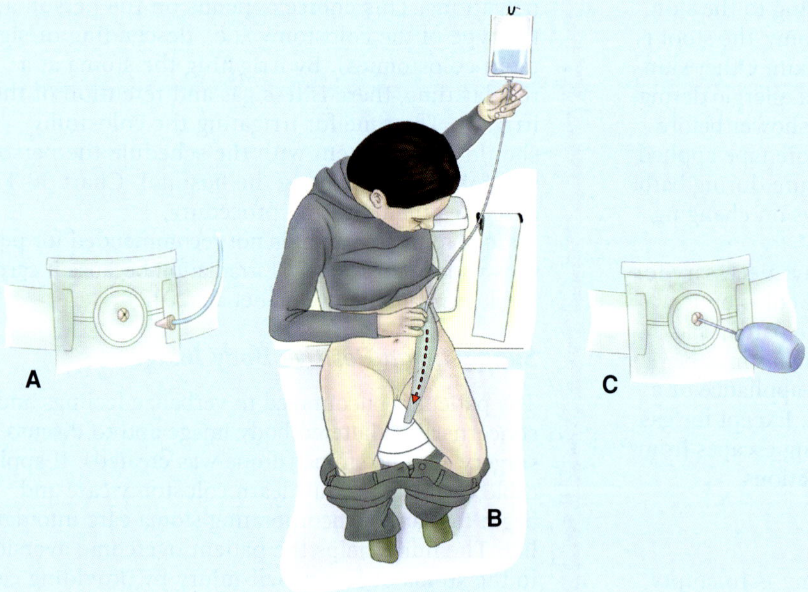

GUIDELINES for Irrigating a Colostomy (Continued)

NURSING ACTIONS	RATIONALE
7. Allow 10–15 minutes for most of the return; then, dry the bottom of the sleeve/sheath and attach it to the top, or apply the appropriate clamp to the bottom of the sleeve.	7. Most of the water, feces, and flatus will be expelled in 10–15 minutes.
8. Leave the sleeve/sheath in place for 30–45 minutes while the patient gets up and moves around.	8. Ambulation stimulates peristalsis and completion of the irrigation return.
9. Cleanse the area with a mild soap and water; pat the area dry.	9. Cleanliness and dryness will provide the patient with hours of comfort.
10. Replace the colostomy dressing or appliance.	10. The patient should use an appliance until the colostomy is sufficiently controlled. A dressing may then be all that is needed.

Adapted from Bauer, C., Arnold-Long, M., & Kent, D. J. (2016). Colostomy irrigation to maintain continence: An old method revived. *Nursing, 46*(8), 59–62.

Discussing Sexuality Issues

The nurse encourages the patient to discuss feelings about sexuality and sexual function. The nurse can say, "Many people after surgery wonder how this will affect their role as a sexual partner. Do you have concerns about that?" (Anaraki et al., 2012; Williams, 2012). Some patients may initiate questions about sexual activity directly or give indirect clues about their fears. Some may view the surgery as mutilating and a threat to their sexuality; some fear impotence. Others may express worry about odour or leakage from the pouch during sexual activity. Although the appliance presents no deterrent to sexual activity, some patients wear silk or cotton covers and smaller pouches during sex. Alternative sexual positions are recommended, as well as alternative methods of stimulation to satisfy sexual drives. The nurse assesses the patient's needs and attempts to identify specific concerns. If the nurse is uncomfortable with this or if the patient's concerns seem complex, the nurse may seek assistance from a WOC nurse, sex counsellor or therapist, or advanced practice nurse (Williams, 2012).

Promoting Home, Community-Based, and Transitional Care

EDUCATING PATIENTS ABOUT SELF-CARE. Patient education and discharge planning require the combined efforts of the physician, nurse, WOC nurse, social worker, and dietitian. Patients are given specific information, individualized to their needs, about ostomy care and signs and symptoms of potential complications. Dietary instructions are essential to help patients identify and eliminate irritating foods that can cause diarrhea or constipation. It is important to teach patients about their prescribed medications (i.e., action, purpose, and possible side and toxic effects).

The nurse reviews treatments (e.g., irrigations, wound cleansing) and dressing changes and encourages the family to participate. Because the hospital stay is short, the patient may not become proficient in all stoma care techniques before discharge home. However, it is critical that the patient or family member learn how to empty and change the pouch before leaving the hospital. Many patients need referral to a home care agency and the telephone number of the local chapter of the Canadian Cancer Society. The home care nurse provides further care and teaching and assesses the patient's and family's adjustment to the colostomy. The home environment is assessed for adequacy of resources that allow the patient to manage self-care activities. A family member may assume responsibility for purchasing the equipment and supplies needed at home.

Patients need very specific directions about when to call the physician. They need to know which complications require prompt attention (i.e., bleeding, abdominal distention and rigidity, diarrhea, fever, wound drainage, and disruption of suture line). If radiation therapy is planned, the possible side effects (i.e., anorexia, vomiting, diarrhea, fatigue) are reviewed.

CONTINUING AND TRANSITIONAL CARE. Ongoing care of the patient with cancer and a colostomy often extends well beyond the initial hospital stay. Home care nurses manage ostomy follow-up care, manage the assessment and care of the debilitated patient, and coordinate adjuvant therapy. The home visits also provide an opportunity to assess the patient's physical and emotional status and the patient's and family's ability to carry out recommended care strategies. Visits from a WOC nurse are available to the patient and family as they learn to care for the ostomy and work through their feelings about it, the diagnosis of cancer, and the future. Some patients are interested in and can benefit from involvement in an ostomy support group.

Evaluation

Expected patient outcomes may include the following:

1. Consumes a healthy diet
   a. Avoids foods and fluids that cause diarrhea, constipation, and obstruction
   b. Substitutes nonirritating foods and fluids for those that are restricted

2. Maintains fluid balance
    a. Experiences no vomiting or diarrhea
    b. Experiences no signs or symptoms of dehydration
3. Feels less anxious
    a. Expresses concerns and fears freely
    b. Uses coping measures to manage stress
4. Acquires information about diagnosis, surgical procedure, preoperative preparation, and self-care after discharge
    a. Discusses the diagnosis, surgical procedure, and postoperative self-care
    b. Demonstrates techniques of ostomy care
5. Maintains clean incision, stoma, and perineal wound
6. Expresses feelings and concerns about self
    a. Gradually increases participation in stoma and peristomal skin care
    b. Discusses feelings related to changed appearance
7. Discusses sexuality in relation to ostomy and to changes in body image
8. Recovers without complications
    a. Is afebrile
    b. Regains regular bowel activity
    c. Exhibits no signs and symptoms of perforation or bleeding
    d. Identifies signs and symptoms that should be reported to health care professional

Polyps of the Colon and Rectum

A polyp is a mass of tissue that protrudes into the lumen of the bowel. Polyps can occur anywhere in the intestinal tract and rectum. They can be classified as neoplastic (i.e., adenomas and carcinomas) or nonneoplastic (i.e., mucosal and hyperplastic). Nonneoplastic polyps, which are benign epithelial growths, are common in the Western world. They occur more commonly in the large intestine than in the small intestine. Although most polyps do not develop into invasive neoplasms, they must be identified and followed closely (Livstone, 2014). Adenomatous polyps are more common in men. The proportion of these polyps arising in the proximal part of the colon increases with age (after 50 years of age). Prevalence rates vary from 25% to 60%, depending on age. Nonneoplastic polyps occur in 80% of the population, and their frequency increases with age. Up to two thirds of people older than 65 years are at risk for colonic adenomas (Papadakis, McPhee, & Rabow, 2013).

Clinical manifestations depend on the size of the polyp and the amount of pressure it exerts on intestinal tissue. The most common symptom is rectal bleeding. Lower abdominal pain may also occur. If the polyp is large enough, symptoms of obstruction occur. The diagnosis is based on history and digital rectal examination, barium enema studies, sigmoidoscopy, or colonoscopy (Livstone, 2014; NIDDK, 2014b).

After a polyp is identified, it should be removed. Several methods are used: colonoscopy with the use of special equipment (i.e., biopsy forceps and snares), laparoscopy, or colonoscopic excision with laparoscopic visualization. The latter technique enables immediate detection of potential problems and allows laparoscopic resection and repair of the major complications of perforation and bleeding that may occur with polypectomy. Microscopic examination of the polyp then identifies the type of polyp and indicates what further surgery is required, if any (Livstone, 2014; NIDDK, 2014b).

DISORDERS OF THE ANORECTUM

Anorectal disorders are common, and the majority of the population will experience one at some time during their lives. Patients with anorectal disorders seek medical care primarily because of pain, rectal bleeding, or change in bowel habits. Other common concerns are protrusion of hemorrhoids, anal discharge, perianal itching, swelling, anal tenderness, stenosis, and ulceration. Constipation results from delaying defecation because of anorectal pain.

There has been a steady increase in the prevalence of sexually transmitted infections (STIs) in recent decades, leading to the identification of new anorectal syndromes. The prevalence of these conditions is increasing. These syndromes include STIs such as syphilis, gonorrhea, herpes, chlamydia, and candidiasis, and they are most commonly seen in male homosexuals who practice anorectal intercourse.

Proctitis

Three infectious syndromes that are related to STIs have been identified: proctitis, proctocolitis, and enteritis. Proctitis refers to inflammation of the mucosa of the rectum, which may be secondary to infection, IBD, or radiation. Infectious diseases are the most frequent cause of proctitis; these etiologies may be either from enteric organism (e.g., *Shigella, Salmonella*) or from STIs (also called *sexually transmitted diseases,* or STDs).

Proctitis secondary to an STI may occur in any gender but is more prevalent among homosexual men who practice anorectal intercourse. It is commonly associated with recent anal-receptive intercourse with an infected partner. Symptoms include mucopurulent discharge or bleeding, rectal pain, and diarrhea. The pathogens most frequently involved are *Neisseria gonorrhoeae, Chlamydia trachomatis,* herpes simplex virus, and *Treponema pallidum*. These infections may progress into proctocolitis and enteritis. Proctocolitis involves the rectum and lowest portion of the descending colon. Symptoms are similar to proctitis but may also include watery or bloody diarrhea, cramps, pain, and bloating. Enteritis involves more of the descending colon, and symptoms include watery, bloody diarrhea; abdominal pain; and weight loss. The most common pathogens causing enteritis are *E. histolytica, Giardia lamblia, and Shigella,* and *Campylobacter* species.

Sigmoidoscopy is performed to identify portions of the anorectum involved. Samples are taken with rectal swabs, and cultures are obtained to identify the pathogens involved. Antibiotics (i.e., ceftriaxone [Rocephin] or cefixime [Suprax], doxycycline [Vibramycin], and penicillin G) are the treatment of choice for bacterial infections. Acyclovir (Zovirax) is given to patients with viral infections.

Antiamebic therapy (i.e., metronidazole) is appropriate for infections with *E. histolytica* and *G. lamblia*. Ciprofloxacin (Cipro) is effective for *Shigella*. The antibiotics erythromycin and ciprofloxacin are the treatment of choice for *Campylobacter* infection (Ansari, 2014; Irizarry & Yade, 2014).

Anorectal Abscess

An anorectal abscess is caused by obstruction of an anal gland, resulting in retrograde infection. People with Crohn's disease or immunosuppressive conditions such as AIDS are particularly susceptible to these infections. Many of these abscesses result in fistulas.

An abscess may occur in a variety of spaces in and around the rectum. It often contains a quantity of foul-smelling pus and is painful. If the abscess is superficial, swelling, redness, and tenderness are observed. A deeper abscess may result in severe lower abdominal pain and fever.

Palliative therapy consists of sitz baths and analgesics. However, prompt surgical treatment to incise and drain the abscess is the treatment of choice. When a deeper infection exists with the possibility of a fistula, the fistulous tract must be excised. If possible, the fistula is excised when the abscess is incised and drained, or a second procedure may be necessary to do so. The wound may be packed with an absorptive dressing (e.g., calcium alginate or hydrofibre) and allowed to heal by granulation.

Anal Fistula

An anal fistula is a tiny, tubular, fibrous tract that extends into the anal canal from an opening located beside the anus in the perianal skin (Fig. 38-12A). Fistulas usually result from an infection. They may also develop from trauma, fissures, or Crohn's disease (up to 25% of patients with Crohn's disease develop a perianal fistula). Purulent drainage or stool may leak constantly from the cutaneous opening. Other symptoms may be the passage of flatus or feces from the vagina or bladder, depending on the location of the fistula tract. Untreated fistulas may cause systemic infection with related symptoms (Prosst et al., 2012).

Medical therapy includes antibiotics or anti-inflammatory–type agents (e.g., azathioprine, infliximab, cyclosporine). Fistula recurrence is common (Simpson et al., 2012). Surgery is recommended because few fistulas heal spontaneously. A fistulectomy (i.e., excision of the fistulous tract) is the recommended surgical procedure. The lower bowel is evacuated thoroughly with several prescribed enemas. The fistula is dissected out or laid open by an incision from its rectal opening to its outlet. The wound is packed with gauze.

Anal Fissure

An anal fissure is a longitudinal tear or ulceration in the lining of the anal canal (see Fig. 38-12B). Fissures are usually caused by the trauma of passing a large, firm stool or from persistent tightening of the anal canal because of stress and anxiety (leading to constipation). Other causes include childbirth, trauma, and overuse of laxatives.

Extremely painful defecation, burning, and bleeding characterize fissures. Bright-red blood may be seen on the toilet tissue after a bowel movement. Most of these fissures heal if treated by conservative measures that include dietary modification with addition of fibre supplements, stool softeners and bulk agents, an increase in water intake, sitz baths, and emollient suppositories. A suppository combining an anesthetic with a corticosteroid helps relieve the discomfort. Anal dilation under anesthesia may be required. A novel therapy, perianal or intra-anal application of nitroglycerin ointment, has increased the rate of healing and lowered pain levels in chronic anal fissures. The ointment is believed to increase blood supply to the wound and relax the anal sphincter (Sajid et al., 2013).

If fissures do not respond to conservative treatment, surgery is indicated. Most surgeons consider the procedure of choice to be the tailored lateral internal sphincterotomy with excision of the fissure and a VY advancement flap (Magdy et al., 2012).

Hemorrhoids

Hemorrhoids are dilated portions of veins in the anal canal. They are very common; by 50 years of age, about 50% of people have hemorrhoids (Evans, Manley, & Rooney, 2016). Shearing of the mucosa during defecation results in the sliding of the structures in the wall of the anal canal,

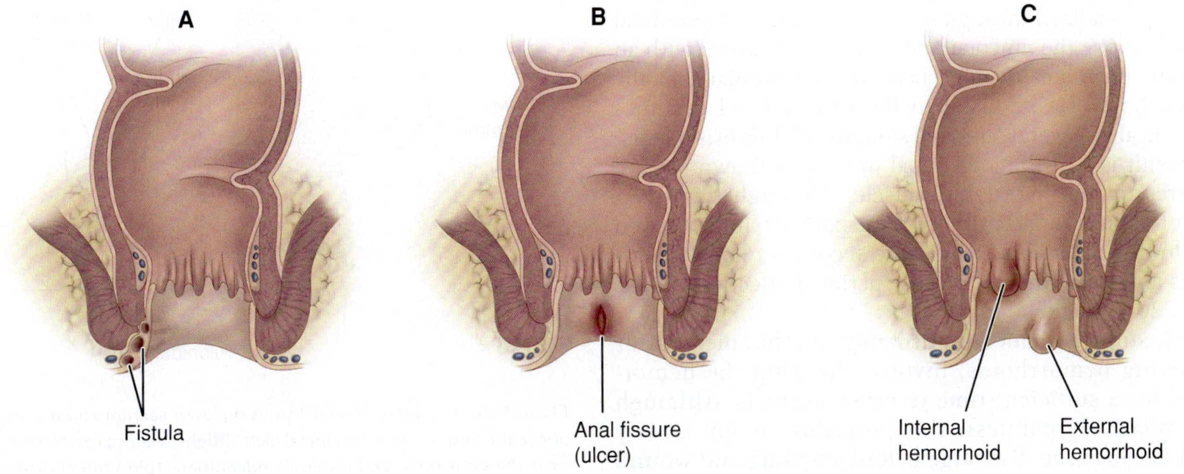

FIGURE 38-12. Various types of anal lesions. **A.** Fistula. **B.** Fissure. **C.** External and internal hemorrhoids.

including the hemorrhoidal and vascular tissues. Increased pressure in the hemorrhoidal tissue due to pregnancy may initiate hemorrhoids or aggravate existing ones. Hemorrhoids are classified as one of the two types: those above the internal sphincter are called internal hemorrhoids, and those appearing outside the external sphincter are called external hemorrhoids (see Fig. 38-12C) (Ansari, 2014). Internal hemorrhoids are also classified by degree of prolapse (Thornton, Rosh, & Perry, 2015):

- First degree—do not prolapse and protrude into anal canal
- Second degree—prolapse outside the anal canal during defecation but reduce spontaneously
- Third degree—prolapsed to the extent that they require manual reduction
- Fourth degree—prolapsed to the extent that they may not be reduced

Hemorrhoids cause itching and pain and are the most common cause of bright-red bleeding with defecation. External hemorrhoids are associated with severe pain from the inflammation and edema caused by thrombosis (i.e., clotting of blood within the hemorrhoid). This may lead to ischemia of the area and eventual necrosis. Internal hemorrhoids are not usually painful until they bleed or prolapse when they become enlarged.

Hemorrhoid symptoms and discomfort can be relieved by good personal hygiene and by avoiding excessive straining during defecation. A high-residue diet that contains fruit and bran along with an increased fluid intake may be all the treatment that is necessary to promote the passage of soft, bulky stools to prevent straining. If this treatment is not successful, the addition of hydrophilic bulk-forming agents such as psyllium may help. Warm compresses, sitz baths, analgesic ointments and suppositories, astringents (e.g., witch hazel), and bed rest reduce engorgement (Ansari, 2014; Wald et al., 2014).

There are several types of nonsurgical treatments for hemorrhoids. Infrared photocoagulation, bipolar diathermy, and laser therapy are used to affix the mucosa to the underlying muscle. Sclerotherapy involves injecting a sclerosing agent (5% phenol in saline) into the base of the hemorrhoid to cause blood vessel thrombosis. These procedures help prevent prolapse (Wald et al., 2014).

A conservative surgical treatment of internal hemorrhoids is the rubber-band ligation procedure. The hemorrhoid is visualized through the anoscope, and its proximal portion above the mucocutaneous lines is grasped with an instrument. A small rubber band is then slipped over the hemorrhoid. Tissue distal to the rubber band becomes necrotic after several days and sloughs off. Fibrosis occurs; the result is that the lower anal mucosa is drawn up and adheres to the underlying muscle. Although this treatment has been satisfactory for some patients, it has proven painful for others and may cause secondary hemorrhage. It has also been known to cause perianal infection (Evans et al., 2016; Wald et al., 2014).

Cryosurgical hemorrhoidectomy, another method for removing hemorrhoids, involves freezing the hemorrhoid for a sufficient time to cause necrosis. Although it is relatively painless, this procedure is not widely used because the discharge is foul smelling and wound healing is prolonged. The Nd:YAG laser is useful in excising hemorrhoids, particularly external hemorrhoidal tags. The treatment is quick and relatively painless. Hemorrhage and abscess are rare postoperative complications.

The previously described methods of treating hemorrhoids are not effective for advanced thrombosed veins, which must be treated by more extensive surgery. Stapled hemorrhoidopexy, a newer procedure, uses surgical staples to treat prolapsing hemorrhoids and is associated with less postoperative pain and fewer complications (Lin et al., 2012). If it is not successful, hemorrhoidectomy, or surgical excision, may be performed to remove all the redundant tissues involved in the process. During surgery, the rectal sphincter is usually dilated digitally, and the hemorrhoids are removed with a clamp and cautery or are ligated and then excised. After the surgical procedures are completed, a small tube may be inserted through the sphincter to permit the escape of flatus and blood; pieces of Gelfoam or Oxycel gauze may be placed over the anal wounds.

Pilonidal Sinus or Cyst

A pilonidal sinus or cyst is found in the intergluteal cleft on the posterior surface of the lower sacrum (Fig. 38-13). Current theories suggest that it results from local trauma, causing penetration of hairs into the epithelium and subcutaneous tissue. It may also be formed congenitally by an infolding of epithelial tissue beneath the skin, which may communicate with the skin surface through one or several small sinus openings. Hair frequently is seen protruding from these openings, and this gives the cyst its name, *pilonidal* (i.e., a nest of hair). The cysts rarely cause symptoms until adolescence or early adult life, when infection produces an irritating drainage or an abscess. Perspiration and friction easily irritate this area (Ansari, 2014; Koyfman & Long, 2016).

In the early stages of the inflammation, the infection may be controlled by antibiotic therapy, but after an abscess has formed, surgery is indicated. The abscess is incised and drained under local anesthesia. After the acute

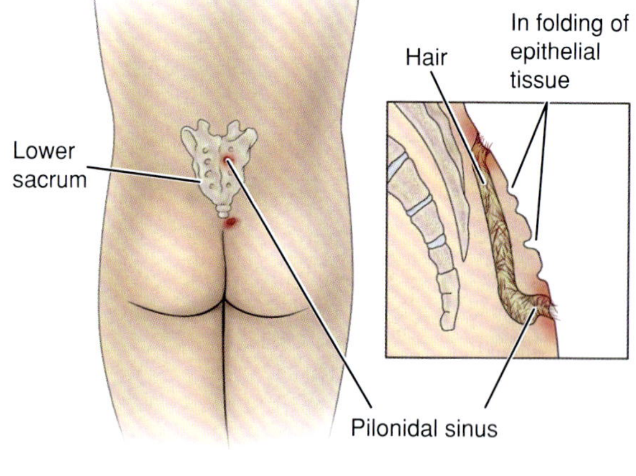

FIGURE 38-13. (**Left**) Pilonidal sinus on lower sacrum about 5 cm (2 in) above the anus in the intergluteal cleft. (**Right**) Hair particles emerge from the sinus tract, and localized indentations (pits) can appear on the skin near the sinus openings.

process resolves, further surgery is performed to excise the cyst and the secondary sinus tracts. The wound is allowed to heal by granulation. Absorptive dressings are placed in the wound to keep its edges separated while healing occurs.

Nursing Management of Patients With Anorectal Conditions

Promoting Home, Community-Based, and Transitional Care

Educating Patients About Self-Care

Most patients with anorectal conditions are not hospitalized. Those who undergo surgical procedures to correct the condition often are discharged directly from the outpatient surgical centre. If they are hospitalized, it is for a short time, usually only 24 hours. Patient teaching is essential to facilitate recovery at home.

The nurse instructs the patient to keep the perianal area as clean as possible by gently cleansing with warm water and then drying with absorbent cotton wipes. The patient should avoid rubbing the area with toilet tissue. Instructions are provided about how to take a sitz bath and how to test the temperature of the water.

During the first 24 hours after rectal surgery, painful spasms of the sphincter and perineal muscles may occur. The nurse instructs the patient that ice and analgesic ointments may decrease the pain. Warm compresses may promote circulation and soothe irritated tissues. Sitz baths taken three or four times each day can relieve soreness and pain by relaxing sphincter spasm. Twenty-four hours after surgery, topical anesthetic agents may be beneficial in relieving local irritation and soreness. Medications may include topical anesthetics (i.e., suppositories), astringents, antiseptics, tranquilizers, and antiemetics. Patients are more compliant and less apprehensive if they are free of pain.

Wet dressings saturated with equal parts of cold water and witch hazel help relieve edema. When wet compresses are being used continuously, petrolatum is applied around the anal area to prevent skin maceration. The patient is instructed to assume a prone position at intervals because this position reduces edema of the tissue.

Continuing and Transitional Care

Sitz baths may be given in the bathtub or plastic sitz bath unit three or four times each day. Sitz baths should follow each bowel movement for 1 to 2 weeks after surgery. The nurse encourages intake of at least 2 L of water daily to provide adequate hydration and recommends high-fibre foods to promote bulk in the stool and to make it easier to pass fecal matter through the rectum. Bulk laxatives such as psyllium may be recommended and stool softeners (e.g., docusate) may be prescribed. The patient is advised to set aside a time for bowel movements and to heed the urge to defecate as promptly as possible. The nurse encourages the patient to respond quickly to the urge to defecate to prevent constipation. The diet is modified to increase fluids and fibre. Moderate exercise is encouraged, and the patient is taught about the prescribed diet, the significance of proper eating habits and exercise, and the laxatives that can be taken safely.

Critical Thinking Exercises

1 A 92-year-old woman in a long-term care facility is a patient assigned to your care. With visible discomfort, she tells you that she has noticed blood in the toilet bowl with her last several bowel movements and she has had blood on her underwear. What other questions should you ask this woman to clarify potential causes of this problem? Explain how the patient's age might affect your focused assessment.

2 A fellow nursing student enrolled in your pharmacology class shares with you that she has been feeling poorly for the past 2 weeks. She has been tired, has lost 10 lb recently, and has had recurrent abdominal pain. She appears pale to you. She is very worried about her success on the final examination that is scheduled for next week. This student casually mentions that she hopes that she does not develop ulcerative colitis like her sister. What further questions might you ask? What is the strength of the evidence that suggests she may be at risk for ulcerative colitis? What advice would you give to your classmate? What further workup do you think should be recommended?

3 A 40-year-old female teacher is admitted to the outpatient surgery clinic with reports of anorectal swelling. You note in this patient's health history that her swelling has worsened over the past 2 weeks, and today there is purulent drainage from the anus. A surgeon examines the patient and schedules immediate surgery in the adjacent operating room suite. The patient asks you, "Why can't I just get an antibiotic?" Given the likely pathophysiology involved in her condition, explain to this patient why surgical intervention is indicated. Identify essential actions you must take before she is taken to the operating room. After your interventions, this patient decides to undergo surgery. Later that afternoon, she is prepared for discharge. Design a discharge plan for her for the next 2 weeks, and include the principles of care that you should teach her so that she may understand the reasons for her home care routine.

4 You work in a family practice clinic. A 25-year-old female patient presents to the clinic with iron deficiency anemia. After a thorough workup, she is diagnosed with celiac disease. How might her anemia have been caused by her celiac disease? Describe the education plan you would devise for this patient. What foods and other products must she learn to avoid?

REFERENCES AND SELECTED READINGS

Books

Canadian Cancer Society Advisory Committee on Cancer Statistics (CCSACCS). (2017). *Canadian Cancer Statistics Publication*. Retrieved from https://www.google.com/search?q=canadian+cancer+society%27s+advisory+committee+on+cancer+statistics+canada+cancer+statistics+2017&rlz=1C1GGRV_enCA756CA756&oq=Canadian+Cancer+Society+Advisory+Committee+on+Cancer+Statistics&aqs=chrome.4.69i57j0l4.6666j0j8&sourceid=chrome&ie=UTF-8

Chubak, J., Kamineni, A., Buist, D. S., et al. (2015). *Aspirin use for the prevention of colorectal cancer: An updated systematic evidence review for the U.S. Preventive Services Task Force. Evidence Synthesis No. 133.*

AHRQ Publication No. 15-05228-EF-1. Rockville, MD: Agency for Healthcare Research and Quality.

Day, R. A. (2013). Nutritional assessment. In T. C. Stephen, D. L. Skillen, R. A. Day, et al. (Eds.), *Canadian Jensen's nursing health assessment: A best practice approach* (1st ed., pp. 152–184). Philadelphia, PA: Wolters Kluwer Health/Lippincott Williams & Wilkins.

Eliopoulos, C. (2018). *Gerontological nursing* (9th ed.). Philadelphia, PA: Wolters Kluwer.

Ford, S. M., & Roach, S. S. (2014). *Roach's introductory clinical pharmacology* (10th ed.). Philadelphia, PA: Wolters Kluwer Health/Lippincott Williams & Wilkins.

Grossman, S. C., & Porth, C. M. (2014). *Porth's pathophysiology: Concepts of altered health states* (9th ed.). Philadelphia, PA: Wolters Kluwer.

Papadakis, M., McPhee, S., & Rabow, M. (2013). *Current medical diagnosis and treatment, 2013* (52nd ed.). New York: McGraw-Hill Medical.

Pasia, M. (2017). *Ostomy nutrition guide*. United Ostomy Association. From https://www.ostomy.org/wp-content/uploads/2018/01/Ostomy-NutritionGuide.pdf

Stephen, T. C., Skillen, D. L., Day, R. A., et al. (2012). *Canadian Jensen's nursing health assessment: A best practice approach*. Philadelphia, PA: Wolters Kluwer Health/Lippincott Williams & Wilkins.

Journals and Electronic Documents

Ansari, P. (2014). *Acute abdomen and surgical gastroenterology. Merck Manual: Professional Version*. Retrieved December 28, 2016, from www.merckmanuals.com/professional/gastrointestinal-disorders/acute-abdomen-and-surgical-gastroenterology/introduction-to-acute-abdomen-and-surgical-gastroenterology

Avadhani, A., & Steefel, L. (2015). Probiotics: A review for NPs. *The Nurse Practitioner, 40*(8), 50–54.

Bailes, B. K., & Reeve, K. (2013). Constipation in older adults. *The Nurse Practitioner*, *38*(8), 21–25.

Barr, W., & Smith, A. (2014). Acute diarrhea. *American Family Physician*, *89*(3), 180–189.

Basson, M. D. (2015a). *Constipation treatment and management. MedScape*. Retrieved December 25, 2016, from emedicine.medscape.com/article/184704-overview

Bauer, C., Arnold-Long, M., & Kent, D. J. (2016). Colostomy irrigation to maintain continence: An old method revived. *Nursing 2018*, *46*(8), 59–62.

Benson, A. B., Bekaii-Saab, T., Chan, E., et al. (2013). Localized colon cancer, version 3.2013: Featured updates to the NCCN Guidelines. *Journal of the National Comprehensive Cancer Network*, *11*(5), 519–528.

Bliss, D. Z., Savak, K., Jung, H. J., et al. (2014). Dietary fiber supplementation for fecal incontinence: A randomized clinical trial. *Research in Nursing and Health*, *37*(5), 367–378.

Brownawell, A., Caers, W., Gibson, G., et al. (2012). Prebiotics and the health benefits of fiber: Current regulatory status, future research, and goals. *The Journal of Nutrition*, *142*(5), 962–974.

Canadian Cancer Society. (2018a). Carcinoembryonic antigen. Retrieved June 3, 2018, from http://www.cancer.ca/en/cancer-information/diagnosis-and-treatment/tests-and-procedures/carcinoembryonic-antigen-cea/?region=on

Canadian Cancer Society. (2018b). *Screening*. Retrieved June 3, 2018, from http://www.cancer.ca/en/cancer-information/cancer-type/colorectal/screening/?region=on

Canadian Cancer Society. (2018c). *Signs and symptoms of colo-rectal cancer*. Retrieved June 3, 2018, from www.cancer.ca/en/cancer-information/cancer-type/colorectal/signs-and-symptoms/?region=on

Canadian Celiac Association. (2018). *Myths and facts*. Retrieved from https://www.celiac.ca/living-gluten-free/myths-facts/

Canadian Digestive Health Foundation. (2014). *Canadian statistics of digestive disease*. Retrieved from http://www.cdhf.ca/en/statistics

Canadian Digestive Health Foundation. (2018). *Canadian statistics of digestive disease*. Retrieved from http://www.cdhf.ca/en/statistics

Cerro, C. R., Franco, E. M., Santoro, G. A., et al. (2017). Residual defects after repair of obstetric anal sphincter injuries and pelvic floor muscle strength are related to anal incontinence symptoms. *International Urogynecology Journal*, *28*(3), 455–460.

Chang, G. J., Kaiser, A. M., Mills, S., et al. (2012). Practice parameters for the management of colon cancer. *Diseases of the Colon and Rectum*, *55*(8), 831–843.

Collins, E., Hibberts, F., Lyons, M., et al. (2014). Outcomes in non-surgical management for bowel dysfunction. *British Journal of Nursing*, *23*(14), 776–780.

Craig, S. (2015). *Appendicitis. MedScape*. Retrieved December 28, 2016, from emedicine.medscape.com/article/773895-overview

Crohn's and Colitis Canada. (2018). *About Crohn's and colitis*. Retrieved from http://crohnsandcolitis.ca/

Evans, L., Manley, K., & Rooney, L. (2016). A technical note regarding hemorrhoid banding. *The Nurse Practitioner*, *41*(5), 18–21.

Ferrara, L. R., & Saccomano, S. J. (2015). Celiac disease: A case of unresolved anemia. *The Nurse Practitioner*, *40*(3), 20–22.

Gallegos-Orozco, J., Foxx-Orenstein, A., Sterler, S., et al. (2012). Chronic constipation in the elderly. *The American Journal of Gastroenterology*, *107*(1), 18–25.

Gardiner, A., & Hilton, A. (2014). The management of constipation in adults. *Nurse Prescribing*, *12*(3), 128–133.

Girard, N. J., & Ousey, K. (2015). An easily forgotten tube. *AORN Journal*, *101*(6), 718–719.

Gomy, I., & Diz, M. D. P. E. (2013). Hereditary cancer risk assessment: Essential tools for a better approach. *Hereditary Cancer in Clinical Practice*, *11*(1), 16.

Greenwald, B. (2015b). Reducing the risk for colon cancer with healthy food choices and physical activity. *Gastroenterology Nursing*, *38*(4), 307–310.

Guandalini, S., Frye, R., & Tamer, M. (2017). *Diarrhea. Medscape*. Retrieved May 30, 2018, from https://emedicine.medscape.com/article/928598-overview

Gump, K., & Schmelzer, M. (2016). Gaining control over fecal incontinence. *Medsurg Nursing*, *25*(2), 97–103.

Heavey, E., & Stoltman, J. (2016). Caring for hospitalized patients with celiac disease. *Nursing*, *46*(11), 50–55.

Hebra, A. (2016). *Anorectal abscess. MedScape*. Retrieved December 30, 2016, from emedicine.medscape.com/article/191975-overview#showall

Hoogenboom, F. J., Bosker, R. I., Groen, H., et al. (2014). Laparoscopic and open subtotal colectomies have similar short-term results. *Digestive Surgery*, *30*(4–6), 265–269.

Koyfman, A., & Long, B. J. (2016). *Pilonidal cyst and sinus. MedScape*. Retrieved December 30, 2016, from emedicine.medscape.com/article/788127-overview

Kushi, L. H., Doyle, C., McCullough, M., et al. (2012). American Cancer Society Guidelines on nutrition and physical activity for cancer prevention: Reducing the risk of cancer with healthy food choices and physical activity. *CA: A Cancer Journal for Clinicians*, *62*(1), 30–67.

Levy, A. R., Szabo, S. M., Lozano-Ortega, G., et al. (2015). Incidence and costs of Clostridium difficile infections in Canada. *Open Forum Infectious Diseases*, 2(3), ofv076.

Liao, X., Lochhead, P., Nichihara, R., et al. (2012). Aspirin use, tumor PIK3CA mutation, and colorectal-cancer survival. *New England Journal of Medicine*, *367*(17), 1596–1606.

Lin, H. C., Ren, D. L., He, Q. L., et al. (2012). Partial stapled hemorrhoidopexy versus circular stapled hemorrhoidopexy for grade III-IV prolapsing hemorrhoids: A two-year prospective controlled study. *Techniques in Coloproctology*, *16*(5), 337–343.

Livstone, E. M. (2014). *Colorectal cancer. Merck Manual: Professional Version*. Retrieved December 29, 2016, from www.merckmanuals.com/professional/gastrointestinal-disorders/tumors-of-the-gi-tract/colorectal-cancer

Logan, R. F., Patnick, J., Nickerson, C., et al. (2012). Outcomes of the Bowel Cancer Screening Programme (BCSP) in England after the first 1 million tests. *Gut*, *61*(10), 1439–1446.

Magdy, A., El Nakeeb, A., Fouda, E., et al. (2012). Comparative study of conventional lateral internal sphincterotomy, V-Y anoplasty, and tailored lateral internal sphincterotomy with V-Y anoplasty in the treatment of chronic anal fissure. *Journal of Gastrointestinal Surgery: Official Journal of the Society for Surgery of the Alimentary Tract*, *16*(10), 1955–1962.

McRorie, J. W. (2015). Evidence-based approach to fiber supplements and clinically meaningful health benefits, Part 2: What to look for and how to recommend an effective fiber therapy. *Nutrition Today*, *50*(2), 90–97.

Mearin, F., Lacy, B. E., Chang, L., et al (2016). Bowel disorders. *Gastroenterology*, pii, S0016-5085(16)00222-5.

Meyerhardt, J. A., Mangu, P. B., Flynn, P. J., et al. (2013). Follow-up care, surveillance protocol, and secondary prevention measures for survivors of colorectal cancer: American Society of Clinical Oncology Clinical Practice Guideline Endorsement. *Journal of Clinical Oncology*, *31*(35), 4465–4470.

Mitsuhashi, S., Ballou, S., Jiang, Z., et al. (2018). Characterizing normal bowel frequency and consistency in a representative sample of adults in the United States (NHANES). *The American Journal of Gastroenterology*, *113*(1), 115–123.

Moore, K. S. (2015). Traveler's diarrhea: Risk reduction and management. *The Nurse Practitioner*, *40*(11), 1–5.

Mulhall, A. M., & Jindal, S. K. (2013). Massive gastrointestinal hemorrhage as a complication of the Flexi-Seal fecal management system. *American Journal of Critical Care*, *22*(6), 537–543.

Murray, K. (2016). Cracking down on C. diff. *Nursing Management*, *47*(7), 56.

National Cancer Institute (NCI). (2016b). *Stage information for colon cancer*. Retrieved January 1, 2017, from www.cancer.gov/types/colorectal/hp/colon-treatment-pdq#link/_331

National Institute of Diabetes and Digestive and Kidney Diseases (NIDDK). (2014a). *Appendicitis*. Retrieved December 28, 2016, from www.niddk.nih.gov/health-information/digestive-diseases/appendicitis

National Institute of Diabetes and Digestive and Kidney Diseases (NIDDK). (2014b). *Colon polyps*. Retrieved January 3, 2017, from www.niddk.nih.gov/health-information/digestive-diseases/colon-polyps/treatment

National Institute of Diabetes and Digestive and Kidney Diseases (NIDDK). (2014c). *Constipation*. Retrieved December 25, 2016, from www.niddk.nih.gov/health-information/digestive-diseases/constipation

National Institute of Diabetes and Digestive and Kidney Diseases (NIDDK). (2014d). *Diarrhea*. Retrieved December 26, 2016, from https://www.niddk.nih.gov/health-information/digestive-diseases/diarrhea

National Institute of Diabetes and Digestive and Kidney Diseases (NIDDK). (2014e). *Ulcerative colitis*. Retrieved December 31, 2016, from www.niddk.nih.gov/health-information/digestive-diseases/ulcerative-colitis

National Institute of Diabetes and Digestive and Kidney Diseases (NIDDK). (2015). *Irritable bowel syndrome*. Retrieved December 27, 2016, from www.niddk.nih.gov/health-information/digestive-diseases/irritable-bowel-syndrome

National Institute of Diabetes and Digestive and Kidney Diseases (NIDDK). (2016a). *Celiac disease*. Retrieved December 28, 2016, from www.niddk.nih.gov/health-information/digestive-diseases/celiac-disease

National Institute of Diabetes and Digestive and Kidney Diseases (NIDDK). (2016b). *Crohn's disease*. Retrieved December 31, 2016, from www.niddk.nih.gov/health-information/digestive-diseases/crohns-disease

Ness, W. (2018). Managing faecal incontinence. *British Journal of Nursing*, *27*(7), 378–381.

Pittman, J., Beeson, T., Terry, C., et al. (2012). Methods of bowel management in critical care: A randomized controlled trial. *Journal of Wound, Ostomy and Continence Nursing*, *39*(6), 633–639.

Price, R. O., & Bradley, R. (2013). Assessing and treating faecal incontinence. *Nursing Older People*, *25*(7), 16–23.

Prosst, R. L., Herold, A. A., Joos, A. K., et al. (2012). The anal fistula claw: The OTSC clip for anal fistula closure. *Colorectal Disease*, *14*(9), 1112–1117.

Rao, S. S., Bharucha, A. E., Chiaroni, G., et al. (2016). Anorectal disorders. *Gastroenterology*, *150*(6), 1430–1442.

Razik, R., & Nguyen, G. C. (2015). Diverticular disease: Changing epidemiology and management. *Drugs and Aging*, *32*(5), 349–360.

Robinson, B. L., Davis, S. C., Vess, J., et al. (2015). Primary care management of celiac disease. *The Nurse Practitioner*, *40*(2), 28–34.

Roos, S., Hellstrom, I., Hallert, C., et al. (2013). Everyday life for women with celiac disease. *Gastroenterology Nursing*, *36*(4), 266–273.

Sajid, M. S., Whitehouse, P. A., Sains, P. P., et al. (2013). Systematic review of the use of topical diltiazem compared with glyceryltrinitrate for the nonoperative management of chronic anal fissure. *Colorectal Disease*, *15*(1), 19–26.

Saldana-Ruiz, N., Clouston, S. A., Rubin, M. S., et al. (2013). Fundamental causes of colorectal cancer mortality in the United States: Understanding the importance of socioeconomic status in creating inequality in mortality. *American Journal of Public Health*, *103*(1), 99–104.

She, W. H., Poon, J. T., Fan, J. K., et al. (2013). Outcome of laparoscopic colectomy for cancer in elderly patients. *Surgical Endoscopy*, *27*(1), 308–312.

Simpson, A., Baneriea, J., Howard, A., et al. (2012). Management of anal fistulas. *British Medical Journal*, *345*(779), 3–41.

Steele, S. R., Chang, G. J., Hendren, S., et al. (2015). Practice guideline for the surveillance of patients after curative treatment of colon and rectal cancer. *Diseases of the Colon and Rectum*, *58*(8), 713–725.

Thompson, C., & Williams, J. (2013). Who should be treating rectal cancer in 2013? *British Journal of Hospital Medicine (London, England: 2005)*, *74*(7), 372–376.

Thornton, S. C., Rosh, A. J., & Perry, K. R. (2015). *Hemorrhoids*. *MedScape*. Retrieved December 30, 2016, from emedicine.medscape.com/article/775407-overviewvan

Voegeli, D. (2012). Understanding the main principles of skin care in older adults. *Nursing Standard*, *27*(11), 59–68.

Wald, A., Bharucha, A. E., Cosman, B. C., et al. (2014). ACG clinical guideline: Management of benign anorectal disorders. *The American Journal of Gastroenterology*, *109*(8), 1141–1157.

Wolthuis, A. M., Penninckx, F., Fieuws, S., et al. (2012). Outcomes for case-matched single-port colectomy are comparable with conventional laparoscopic colectomy. *Colorectal Disease: The Official Journal of the Association of Coloproctology of Great Britain and Ireland*, *14*(5), 634–641.

Yong, J. (2016). What's new in neuromodulation for anorectal dysfunction. *Australian-New Zealand Continence Journal*, *22*(4), 93–94.

Inflammatory Bowel Disease

Ananthakrishnan, A. N., Huang, H., Nguyen, D. D., et al. (2014). Differential effect of genetic burden on disease phenotypes in Crohn's disease and ulcerative colitis: Analysis of a North American cohort. *American Journal of Gastroenterology*, *109*(3), 395–400.

Anaraki, F., Vafaie, M., Behboo, R., et al. (2012). Quality of life outcomes in patients living with stoma. *Indian Journal of Palliative Care*, *18*(3), 176–180.

Anastasi, J. K., Capili, B., & Chang, M. (2013). Managing irritable bowel syndrome. *American Journal of Nursing*, *113*(7), 42–52.

Andersson, R. E. (2014). Short-term complications and long-term morbidity of laparoscopic and open appendectomy in a national cohort. *British Journal of Surgery*, *101*(9), 1135–1142.

Balasubramanian, I., Fleming, C., Mohan, H. M., et al. (2017). Outpatient management of mild or uncomplicated diverticulitis: A systematic review. *Digestive Surgery*, *34*(2), 151–160.

Basso, D., Zambon, C., & Plebani, M. (2014). Inflammatory bowel diseases: From pathogenesis to laboratory testing. *Clinical Chemistry and Laboratory Medicine*, *52*(4), 471–481.

Basson, M. D. (2015b). *Ulcerative colitis workup*. *MedScape*. Retrieved December 31, 2016, from emedicine.medscape.com/article/183084-workup#showall

Bozkurt, M. A., Unsal, M. G., Kapan, S., et al. (2015). Is laparoscopic appendectomy going to be standard procedure for acute appendicitis; a 5-year single center experience with 1,788 patients. *European Journal of Emergency Surgery*, *41*(1), 87–89.

Chang, L., Lembo, A., & Sultan, S. (2014). American Gastroenterological Association Institute technical review on the pharmacological management of irritable bowel syndrome. *Gastroenterology*, *147*(5), 1149–1172.

Cheng, Y., Zhou, S., Zhou, R., et al. (2015). Abdominal drainage to prevent intra-peritoneal abscess for complicated appendicitis. *Cochrane Database of Systematic Reviews*, (2), CD010168.

Chey, W. D., Kurlander, J., Eswaran, S. (2015). Irritable bowel syndrome: a clinical review. *JAMA*, *313*(9), 949–958.

Craig, S. (2015). *Appendicitis*. *MedScape*. Retrieved December 28, 2016, from emedicine.medscape.com/article/773895-overview

Crawshaw, A., Williams, J., & Woodhouse, F. (2014). The Kock pouch reconsidered: An alternative surgical technique. *British Journal of Nursing*, *23*(17), S26–S29.

Daley, B. J. (2015). *Peritonitis and abdominal sepsis*. *MedScape*. Retrieved December 30, 2016, from emedicine.medscape.com/article/180234-overview

de Graaf, R., Tuithof, M., van Dorsselaer, S., et al. (2012). Comparing the effects on work performance of mental and physical disorders. *Social Psychiatry and Psychiatric Epidemiology*, *47*(11), 1873–1883.

DiMarino, M. C. (2013). *Diverticular disease*. *Merck Manual: Professional Version*. Retrieved December 28, 2016, from www.merckmanuals.com/professional/gastrointestinal-disorders/diverticular-disease/definition-of-diverticular-disease

Dunn, P., Greenstein, S. M., Prowse, O., et al. (2014). *Intestinal transplant*. *MedScape*. Retrieved January 1, 2017, from emedicine.medscape.com/article/1013245-overview

Evans, M. M., & Curtin, M. (2014). Acute appendicitis: A case study describing standards of care. *Medsurg Nursing*, *23*(6), 3, 15.

Fazio, V. W., Kiran, R. P., Remzi, F. H., et al. (2013). Ileal pouch anastomosis: Analysis of outcome and quality of life in 3707 patients. *Annals of Surgery*, *257*(4), 679–785.

Ford, A. C., Quigley, E. M., Lacy, B. E., et al. (2014). Effect of antidepressants and psychological therapies, including hypnotherapy, in irritable bowel syndrome: Systematic review and meta-analysis. *The American Journal of Gastroenterology*, *109*(9), 1350–1365.

Francone, T. D., & Champagne, B. (2013). Considerations and complications in patients undergoing ileal pouch anal anastomosis. *Surgical Clinics of North America*, *93*(1), 107–143.

Ghiyasvandian, S., Ghorbani, M., Zakermoghadam, M., et al. (2016). The effects of a self-care program on the severity of symptoms and quality of life of patients with irritable bowel syndrome. *Gastroenterology Nursing, 39*(5), 359–365.

Goebel, S. U. (2014). *Malabsorption. Medscape*. Retrieved December 27, 2016, from emedicine.medscape.com/article/180785-overview

Grant, M., Mcmullen, C. K., Altschuler, A., et al. (2012). Irrigation practices in long-term survivors of colorectal cancer with colostomies. *Clinical Journal of Oncology Nursing, 16*(5), 514–519.

Harris, H., & Jelemensky, L. (2014). Managing the ups and downs of ulcerative colitis. *Nursing, 44*(8), 36–42.

Hendren, S., Hammond, K., Glasgow, S. C., et al. (2015). Clinical practice guidelines for ostomy surgery. *Diseases of the Colon and Rectum, 58*(4), 375–387.

Hopkins, C. (2016). *Large-bowel obstruction. MedScape*. Retrieved December 29, 2016, from emedicine.medscape.com/article/774045-overview

Horattas, M. C., Horattas, I. K., & Vasiliou, E. M. (2018). Early uncomplicated appendicitis—who can we treat nonoperatively? *The American Surgeon, 84*(2), 174–180.

Kapritsou, M., Korkolis, D. P., & Konstantinou, E. A. (2013). Open or laparoscopic surgery for colorectal cancer: a retrospective comparative study. *Gastroenterology Nursing, 36*(1), 37–41.

Katz, S. (2013). My treatment approach to the management of ulcerative colitis. *Mayo Clinic Proceedings, 88*(8), 841–853.

Kent, D., Arnold-Long, M., & Bauer, C. (2016). Revisiting colostomy irrigation: A viable option for persons with permanent descending and sigmoid colostomies. *Journal of Wound Ostomy and Continence Nursing, 42*(2), 162–164.

Margulies, S. L., Kurian, D., Elliott, M. S., et al. (2015). Vitamin D deficiency in patients with intestinal malabsorption syndromes—think in and outside the gut. *Journal of Digestive Diseases, 16*(11), 617–633.

McDermott, F. D., Collins, D., Heeney, A., et al. (2014). Minimally invasive and surgical management strategies tailored to the severity of acute diverticulitis. *The British Journal of Surgery, 101*(1), e90–e99.

Mosli, M., Al Beshir, M., Al-Judaibi, B., et al. (2014). Advances in the diagnosis and management of inflammatory bowel disease: Challenges and uncertainties. *Saudi Journal of Gastroenterology, 20*(2), 81–101.

Nobie, B. A. (2015). *Small-bowel obstruction. MedScape*. Retrieved December 29, 2016, from emedicine.medscape.com/article/774140-overview

Nunes, T., Etchevers, M. J., Domènech, E., et al. (2013). Smoking does influence disease behaviour and impacts the need for therapy in Crohn's disease in the biologic era. *Alimentary Pharmacology & Therapeutics, 38*(7), 752–760.

Perrin, A. (2013). Quality of life after ileo-anal pouch formation: Patient perceptions. *Gastrointestinal Nursing, 11*(3), 35–44.

Saccomano, S. J., & Ferrara, L. R. (2013). Evaluation of acute abdominal pain. *The Nurse Practitioner, 38*(11), 46–53.

Salminen, P., Paajanen, H., Rautio, T., et al. (2015). Antibiotic therapy vs appendectomy for treatment of uncomplicated acute appendicitis: The APPAC randomized clinical trial. *JAMA, 313*(23), 2340–2348.

Shaffer, V., & Wexner, S. (2013). Surgical management of Crohn's disease. *Langenbeck's Archives of Surgery, 398*(1), 13–27.

Shahedi, K., Dea, S. K., Chudasama, Y. N., et al. (2016). *Diverticulitis. MedScape*. Retrieved December 29, 2016, from emedicine.medscape.com/article/173388-overview

Skrastins, O., & Fletcher, P. C. (2016). "One flare at a time": Adaptive and maladaptive behaviors of women coping with inflammatory bowel disease and irritable bowel syndrome. *Clinical Nurse Specialist, 30*(5), e1–e11.

Surdea-Blaga, T., & Dumitrascu, D. L. (2013). An expert system for the diagnosis of irritable bowel syndrome. *Clujul Medical, 86*(3), 208–212.

Tursi, A. (2012). Advances in the management of colonic diverticulitis. *CMAJ: Canadian Medical Association Journal/Journal de L'association Medicale Canadienne, 184*(13), 1470–1476.

Tursi, A. (2014). Efficacy, safety, and applicability of outpatient treatment for diverticulitis. *Drug, Healthcare and Patient Safety, 6*, 29–36.

Usher, L., Fox, P., Lafarge, C., et al. (2013). Factors associated with complementary and alternative medicine use in irritable bowel syndrome: A literature review. *Psychology, Community & Health, 2*(3), 346–361.

van Rossem, C. C., Schreinemacher, M. H., Treskes, K., et al. (2014). Duration of antibiotic treatment after appendicectomy for acute complicated appendicitis. *British Journal of Surgery, 101*(6), 715–719.

Walfish, A. E. (2016). *Inflammatory bowel disease. Merck Manual: Professional Version*. Retrieved December 29, 2016, from www.merckmanuals.com/professional/gastrointestinal-disorders/inflammatory-bowel-disease-ibd

Watson, A. J., Nicol, L., Donaldson, S., et al. (2013). Complications of stomas: Their aetiology and management. *British Journal of Community Nursing, 18*(3), 111–112, 114–116.

Weizman, A. V., Ahn, E. E., Thanabalan, R. R., et al. (2012). Characterisation of complementary and alternative medicine use and its impact on medication adherence in inflammatory bowel disease. *Alimentary Pharmacology & Therapeutics, 35*(3), 342–349.

Williams, J. (2012). Stoma care: Intimacy and body image issues. *Practice Nursing, 23*(2), 91–93.

Wong, P. F., Gilliam, A. D., Kumar, S., et al. (2012). Antibiotic regimens for secondary peritonitis of gastrointestinal origin in adults. *Cochrane Database of Systematic Reviews, (2)*, CD00453939.

Resources

American Cancer Society: http://www.cancer.org
Canadian Association for Enterostomal Therapy: http://www.caet.ca
Canadian Cancer Society: http://www.cancer.ca
Canadian Cancer Society Research Institute: http://www.ncic.cancer.ca
Canadian Digestive Health Foundation: http://www.cdhf.ca
Canadian Society of Gastroenterology Nurses & Associates: http://www.csgna.com
Canadian Society of Intestinal Research: http://www.badgut.com
Colon Cancer Alliance: http://www.ccalliance.org
Colorectal Cancer Screening Initiative Foundation: http://www.screencolons.ca/
Crohn's and Colitis Foundation of Canada: http://www.ccfc.ca
International Foundation for Functional Gastrointestinal Disorders: http://www.iffgd.org
Medicine Online: Colon Cancer Information Library: http://www.meds.com/colon/colon.html
National Association for Continence: http://www.nafc.org
National Digestive Disease Information Clearinghouse: http://www.digestive.niddk.nih.gov
STOP Colon/Rectal Cancer Foundation: http://www.coloncancerprevention.org
United Ostomy Associations of Canada, Inc.: http://www.ostomyCanada.ca
Wound, Ostomy, Continence Nurses Society: http://www.wocn.org

39 Assessment and Management of Patients With Hepatic Disorders

Adapted by Lisa McKendrick-Calder

Learning Objectives

On completion of this chapter, the learner will be able to:

1. Identify the metabolic functions of the liver and the alterations in these functions that occur with liver disease.
2. Explain liver function tests and the clinical manifestations of liver dysfunction in relation to pathophysiologic alterations of the liver.
3. Relate jaundice, portal hypertension, ascites, varices, nutritional deficiencies, and hepatic coma to pathophysiologic alterations of the liver.
4. Describe the medical, surgical, and nursing management of patients with esophageal varices.
5. Compare the various types of hepatitis and their causes, prevention, clinical manifestations, management, prognosis, and home health care needs.
6. Use the nursing process as a framework for care of the patient with cirrhosis of the liver.
7. Compare the nonsurgical and surgical management of patients with cancer of the liver.
8. Describe the postoperative nursing care of the patient undergoing liver transplantation.

Liver function is complex, and liver dysfunction affects all body systems. For this reason, the nurse must understand how the liver functions and must have expert clinical assessment and management skills to care for patients undergoing complex diagnostic and treatment procedures. The nurse also must understand technologic advances in the management of liver disorders. Liver disorders are common, as one in four Canadians may be affected by them (Canadian Liver Foundation, n.d.). They may result from genetic factors, a virus, obesity, insulin resistance, a tumour, or exposure to toxic substances such as alcohol.

ASSESSMENT OF THE LIVER

Anatomic and Physiologic Overview

The liver, the largest gland of the body, manufactures, stores, alters, and excretes a large number of substances involved in metabolism (Hall, 2015). The location of the liver is essential in this function because it receives nutrient-rich blood directly from the gastrointestinal (GI) tract and then either stores or transforms these nutrients into chemicals that are used elsewhere in the body for metabolic needs. The liver is especially important in the regulation of glucose and protein metabolism. The liver manufactures and secretes bile, which has a major role in the digestion and absorption of fats in the GI tract. The liver removes waste products from the bloodstream and secretes them into the bile. The bile is stored temporarily in the gallbladder until it is needed for digestion, at which time the gallbladder empties and bile enters the intestine (Fig. 39-1).

Anatomy of the Liver

The liver is a large, highly vascular organ located behind the ribs in the upper right portion of the abdominal cavity. It weighs between 1,200 and 1,500 g and is divided into

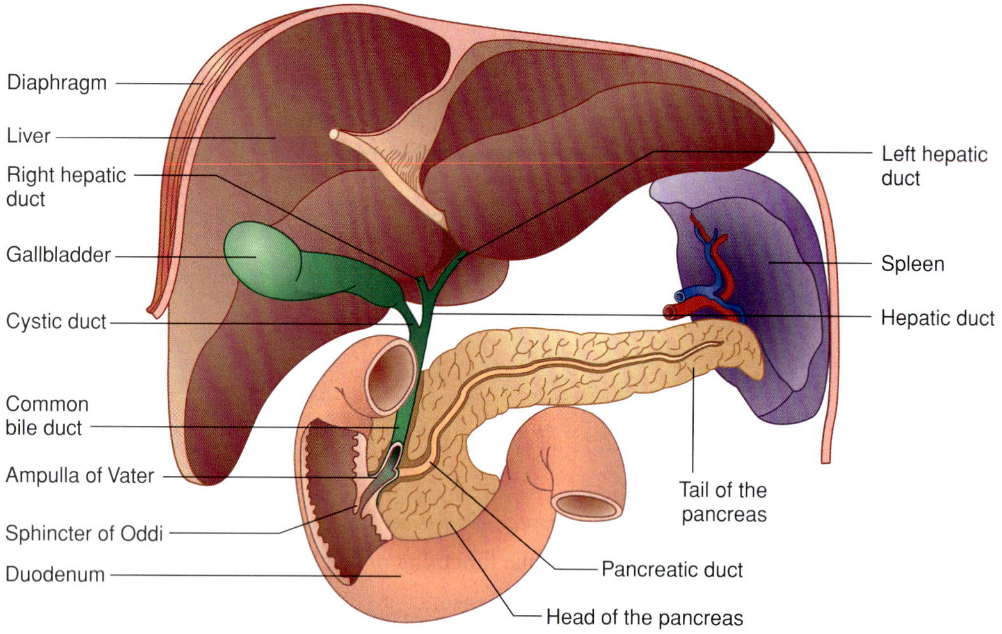

FIGURE 39-1. The liver and biliary system. (From Grossman, S. C., & Porth, C. M. (2014). *Pathophysiology: Concepts of altered health states* (9th ed.). Philadelphia, PA: Lippincott Williams & Wilkins.)

four lobes. A thin layer of connective tissue surrounds each lobe, extending into the lobe itself and dividing the liver mass into small, functional units called lobules (Fullwood & Purushothaman, 2014).

The blood that perfuses the liver comes from two sources. Approximately 75% of the blood supply comes from the portal vein, which drains the GI tract and is rich in nutrients but lacks oxygen (Fullwood & Purushothaman, 2014). The remainder of the blood supply enters by way of the hepatic artery and is rich in oxygen. Terminal branches of these two blood vessels join to form common capillary beds, which constitute the sinusoids of the liver (Fig. 39-2). Thus, a mixture of venous and arterial blood bathes the liver cells (hepatocytes). The sinusoids empty into venules that occupy the centre of each liver lobule and are called the central veins. The central veins join to form the hepatic vein, which constitutes the venous drainage from the liver and empties into the inferior vena cava, close to the diaphragm (Fullwood & Purushothaman, 2014).

In addition to hepatocytes, phagocytic cells called Kupffer cells belonging to the reticuloendothelial system are present in the liver (Hall, 2015). As the most common phagocyte in the human body, their main function is to

Glossary

ascites: an albumin-rich fluid accumulation in the peritoneal cavity

asterixis: involuntary flapping movements of the hands

cirrhosis: a chronic liver disease characterized by fibrotic changes, the formation of dense connective tissue within the liver, subsequent degenerative changes, and loss of functioning cells

constructional apraxia: inability to draw figures in two or three dimensions

endoscopic variceal ligation (EVL): procedure that uses a modified endoscope loaded with an elastic rubber band passed through an overtube directly onto the varix (or varices) to be banded to ligate the area and stop bleeding

fetor hepaticus: sweet, slightly fecal odour to the breath, presumed to be of intestinal origin; prevalent with the extensive collateral portal circulation in chronic liver disease

fulminant hepatic failure: sudden, severe onset of acute liver failure that occurs within 8 weeks after the first symptoms of jaundice

hepatic encephalopathy: central nervous system dysfunction frequently associated with elevated ammonia levels that produce changes in mental status, altered level of consciousness, and coma

jaundice: condition where the body tissues, including the sclerae and the skin, become tinged yellow or greenish-yellow, due to high bilirubin levels

orthotopic liver transplantation (OLT): grafting of a donor liver into the normal anatomic location, with removal of the diseased native liver

portal hypertension: elevated pressure in the portal circulation resulting from obstruction of venous flow into and through the liver

sclerotherapy: the injection of substances into or around esophagogastric varices to cause constriction, thickening, and hardening of the vessel and stop bleeding

xenograft: transplantation of organs from one species to another

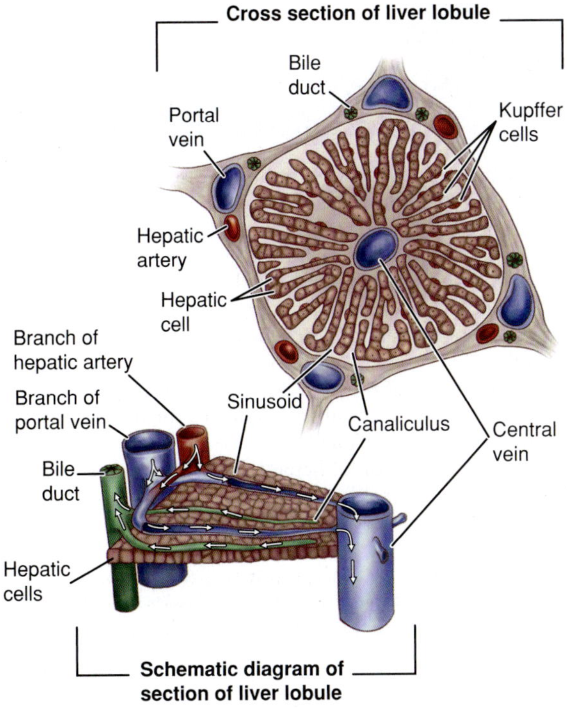

FIGURE 39-2. A section of liver lobule showing the location of hepatic veins, hepatic cells, liver sinusoids, and branches of the portal vein and hepatic artery.

engulf particulate matter (e.g., bacteria) that enters the liver through the portal blood.

The smallest bile ducts, called canaliculi, are located between the lobules of the liver. The canaliculi receive secretions from the hepatocytes and carry them to larger bile ducts, which eventually form the hepatic duct. The hepatic duct from the liver and the cystic duct from the gallbladder join to form the common bile duct, which empties into the small intestine. The sphincter of Oddi, located at the junction where the common bile duct enters the duodenum, controls the flow of bile into the intestine.

Functions of the Liver

Glucose Metabolism

The liver plays a major role in the metabolism of glucose and the regulation of blood glucose concentration. After a meal, glucose is taken up from the portal venous blood by the liver and converted into glycogen, which is stored in the hepatocytes. Subsequently, the glycogen is converted back to glucose (glycogenolysis) and released as needed into the bloodstream to maintain normal levels of blood glucose. However, this process provides a limited amount of glucose. Additional glucose can be synthesized by the liver through a process called gluconeogenesis. For this process, the liver uses amino acids from protein breakdown or lactate produced by exercising muscles. This process occurs in response to hypoglycemia (Hall, 2015).

Ammonia Conversion

Use of amino acids from protein for gluconeogenesis results in the formation of ammonia as a byproduct. The liver converts this metabolically generated ammonia into urea. Ammonia produced by bacteria in the intestines is also removed from portal blood for urea synthesis. In this way, the liver converts ammonia, a potential toxin, into urea, a compound that is excreted in the urine (Grossman, 2013; Hall, 2015; Lee & Moreau, 2015).

Protein Metabolism

The liver also plays an important role in protein metabolism. It synthesizes almost all of the plasma proteins (except gamma-globulin), including albumin, alpha-globulins and beta-globulins, blood clotting factors, specific transport proteins, and most of the plasma lipoproteins. Vitamin K is required by the liver for synthesis of prothrombin and some of the other clotting factors. Amino acids are used by the liver for protein synthesis (Grossman, 2013; Hall, 2015; Lee & Moreau, 2015).

Fat Metabolism

The liver is also active in fat metabolism. Fatty acids can be broken down for the production of energy and ketone bodies. Ketone bodies are small compounds that can enter the bloodstream and provide a source of energy for muscles and other tissues. Breakdown of fatty acids into ketone bodies occurs primarily when the availability of glucose for metabolism is limited, as in starvation or in uncontrolled diabetes. Fatty acids and their metabolic products are also used for the synthesis of cholesterol, lecithin, lipoproteins, and other complex lipids (Grossman, 2013; Hall, 2015; Lee & Moreau, 2015).

In some conditions, lipids may accumulate in the hepatocytes, resulting in the abnormal condition called fatty liver.

Vitamin and Iron Storage

Vitamins A, B, and D and several of the B-complex vitamins are stored in large amounts in the liver. Certain substances, such as iron and copper, are also stored in the liver. Because the liver is rich in these substances, liver extracts have been used for therapy for more than a century for a wide range of nutritional disorders; however, the U.S. Food and Drug Administration (FDA) has urged caution regarding the use of any animal organ extract because of possible risk of exposure to pathogenic organisms (Hall, 2015).

Bile Formation

Bile is continuously formed by the hepatocytes and collected in the canaliculi and bile ducts. It is composed mainly of water and electrolytes such as sodium, potassium, calcium, chloride, and bicarbonate, and it also contains significant amounts of lecithin, fatty acids, cholesterol, bilirubin, and bile salts. The functions of bile are excretory, as in the excretion of bilirubin; bile also serves as an aid to digestion through the emulsification of fats by bile salts.

Bile salts are synthesized by the hepatocytes from cholesterol. After conjugation or binding with amino acids, bile salts are excreted into the bile. The bile salts, together with cholesterol and lecithin, are required for emulsification of fats in the intestine, which is necessary for efficient digestion and absorption. Bile salts are then reabsorbed, primarily in the distal ileum, into portal blood for return to the liver and are again excreted into the bile. This pathway from hepatocytes to bile to intestine and back to the hepatocytes is called the enterohepatic circulation. Because of the enterohepatic circulation, only a small fraction of the bile salts that enter the intestine are excreted in the feces. This decreases the need for active synthesis of bile salts by the liver cells (Grossman, 2013; Hall, 2015).

Bilirubin Excretion

Bilirubin is a pigment derived from the breakdown of hemoglobin by cells of the reticuloendothelial system, including the Kupffer cells of the liver. Hepatocytes remove bilirubin from the blood and chemically modify it through conjugation to glucuronic acid, which makes the bilirubin more soluble in aqueous solutions. The conjugated bilirubin is secreted by the hepatocytes into the adjacent bile canaliculi and is eventually carried in the bile into the duodenum.

In the small intestine, bilirubin is converted into urobilinogen, which is partially excreted in the feces and partially absorbed through the intestinal mucosa into the portal blood. Much of this reabsorbed urobilinogen is removed by the hepatocytes and secreted into the bile once again (enterohepatic circulation). Some of the urobilinogen enters the systemic circulation and is excreted by the kidneys in the urine. Elimination of bilirubin in the bile represents the major route of its excretion.

The bilirubin concentration in the blood may be increased in the presence of liver disease, if the flow of bile is impeded (e.g., by gallstones in the bile ducts), or if there is excessive destruction of red blood cells. With bile duct obstruction, bilirubin does not enter the intestine; as a consequence, urobilinogen is absent from the urine and decreased in the stool (Grossman, 2013).

Drug Metabolism

The liver metabolizes many medications, such as barbiturates, opioids, sedatives, anesthetics, and amphetamines (Goldman & Schafer, 2015; Hall, 2015). Metabolism generally results in drug inactivation, although activation may also occur. One of the important pathways for medication metabolism involves conjugation (binding) of the medication with a variety of compounds, such as glucuronic acid or acetic acid, to form more soluble substances. These substances may be excreted in the feces or urine, similar to bilirubin excretion. Bioavailability is the fraction of the administered medication that actually reaches the systemic circulation. The bioavailability of an oral medication (absorbed from the GI tract) can be decreased if the medication is metabolized to a great extent by the liver before it reaches the systemic circulation; this is known as first-pass effect. Some medications have such a large first-pass effect that their use is essentially limited to the parenteral route, or oral doses must be substantially larger than parenteral doses to achieve the same effect.

CHART 39-1

Age-Related Changes of the Hepatobiliary System

- Atypical clinical presentation of biliary disease
- Decreases in the following:
  - Clearance of hepatitis B surface antigen
  - Drug metabolism and clearance capabilities
  - Intestinal and portal vein blood flow
  - Gallbladder contraction after a meal
  - Rate of replacement and or repair of liver cells after injury
  - Size and weight of the liver, particularly in women
- Increased prevalence of gallstones due to the increase in cholesterol secretion in bile
- More rapid progression of hepatitis C infection and lower response rate to therapy
- More severe complications of biliary tract disease

Adapted from Townsend, C. M., Beauchamp, R. D., Evers, B. M., et al. (2016). *Sabiston's textbook of surgery: The biological basis of modern surgical practice*. Philadelphia, PA: Elsevier.

Gerontologic Considerations

Chart 39-1 summarizes age-related changes in the liver. In the older adult, the most common change in the liver is a decrease in size and weight, accompanied by a decrease in total hepatic blood flow. In general, these decreases are proportional to the decreases in body size and weight seen in normal aging. Results of liver function tests do not normally change.

Metabolism of medications by the liver decreases in the older adult, but such changes are usually accompanied by changes in intestinal absorption, renal excretion, and altered body distribution of some medications secondary to changes in fat deposition. These alterations necessitate careful medication administration and monitoring; if appropriate, reduced dosages or increased time intervals between administrations may be needed to prevent medication toxicity.

Assessment

Health History

If liver function test results are abnormal, the patient is evaluated for liver disease. In such cases, the health history focuses on risk factors and previous exposure of the patient to hepatotoxic substances or infectious agents. When looking for hepatotoxic risk factors the patient's occupational, recreational, and travel history may assist in identifying exposure to hepatotoxins (e.g., industrial chemicals, other toxins). The patient's history of alcohol and drug use, including but not limited to the use of intravenous (IV) or injection drugs, provides additional information about exposure to toxins and infectious agents. Because many medications (including acetaminophen, ketoconazole, and valproic acid) contribute to hepatic dysfunction and disease, a thorough medication history should address all current and past prescription medications, over-the-counter medications, herbal remedies, and dietary supplements.

Lifestyle behaviours that contribute to fatty liver disease or behaviours that increase the risk for exposure to infectious agents are identified. Dietary and lifestyle factors like exercise are taken into consideration along with BMI and other health history. IV or injection drug use, sexual practices, and foreign travel are all potential risk factors for

GENETICS IN NURSING PRACTICE

Chart 39-2. Hepatic Disorders

A number of hepatic disorders have an underlying genetic cause. However, other genetic disorders associated with metabolic, gastrointestinal, or bleeding disorders will also impact the function of the liver. Some examples of hepatic disorders caused by genetic abnormalities include:

Autosomal Dominant:
- Alagille syndrome
- Hereditary coproporphyria
- Polycystic liver disease

Autosomal Recessive:
- Crigler–Najjar syndrome
- Dublin–Johnson syndrome
- Hemochromatosis
- Progressive familial intrahepatic cholestasis
- Thalassemia
- Wilson disease

Inheritance Pattern is not distinct; however, there is a genetic predisposition for the disorder:
- Biliary atresia
- Gilbert syndrome

Other genetic disorders that impact the hepatic system:
- Alpha-1 antitrypsin deficiency
- Cystic fibrosis
- Glycogen storage disease
- Lysosomal storage disease
- Polycystic kidney disease
- Zellweger syndrome

Nursing Assessments

FAMILY HISTORY ASSESSMENT RELATED TO HEPATIC DISORDERS
- Collect family history for three generations of maternal and paternal relatives in the patient's family
- Assess family history for relatives with early-onset hepatic disease

PATIENT ASSESSMENT RELATED TO GENETIC HEPATIC DISORDERS
- Assess for physical signs or history of the following:
  - Abdominal bloating, and constipation
  - Changes to skin colour or yellow hue to sclera
  - Enlarged liver, spleen, or abdomen
  - Episodes of nausea and vomiting
  - Hemorrhoids, esophageal varices, or gallstones
  - Intolerance to fatty foods or alcohol
  - Pale-coloured stools
  - Presence and frequency of indigestion or reflux
  - Unexplained weight loss
- Assess for associated nervous system disorders such as depression and mood changes especially anger and irritability (Wilson disease).
- Assess for associated blood sugar problems such as hypoglycemia
- Inquire about and assess for abnormal bleeding or bruising
- Obtain and review laboratory values: Liver function tests, ammonia, bilirubin, fat soluble vitamins (e.g., vitamins A, D, E, K)

Genetics Resources

American Liver Foundation: www.liverfoundation.org
Canadian Liver Foundation: www.liver.ca
See Chapter 11, Chart 11.7 for components of genetic counselling.

liver disease. The amount and type of alcohol consumption are identified. Men who consume 60 to 80 g/day of alcohol (approximately four glasses of beer, wine, or mixed drinks) and women whose alcohol intake is 40 to 60 g/day are considered at high risk for liver alterations and **cirrhosis**.

The history also includes an evaluation of the patient's past medical history to identify risk factors for the development of liver disease. Current and past medical conditions, including those of a psychological or psychiatric nature, are identified. The family history includes questions about familial liver disorders that may have their origin in alcohol abuse or gallstone disease, as well as other familial or genetic diseases, such as hemochromatosis, Wilson's disease, or alpha$_1$-antitrypsin disease (see Chart 39-2).

The history also addresses symptoms that suggest liver disease. Symptoms that may have their origin in liver disease but are not specific to hepatic dysfunction include **jaundice**, malaise, weakness, fatigue, pruritus, abdominal pain, joint pain, fever, anorexia, weight gain, edema, increasing abdominal girth, hematemesis, melena, hematochezia (passage of bloody stools), easy bruising, changes in mental acuity, personality changes, sleep disturbances, and decreased libido in men and secondary amenorrhea in women.

Physical Assessment

The nurse assesses the patient for physical signs that may occur with liver dysfunction, including the pallor often seen with chronic illness and jaundice. The skin, mucosa, and sclerae are inspected for jaundice, and the extremities are assessed for muscle atrophy, edema, and skin excoriation secondary to scratching. The nurse observes the skin for petechiae or ecchymotic areas (bruises), spider angiomas (see Fig. 39-3), and palmar erythema. The male patient is assessed for unilateral or bilateral gynecomastia and testicular atrophy due to hormonal changes. The patient's cognitive status (recall, memory, abstract thinking) and neurologic status are assessed. The nurse observes for general tremor, **asterixis**, weakness, and slurred speech. These symptoms are discussed later.

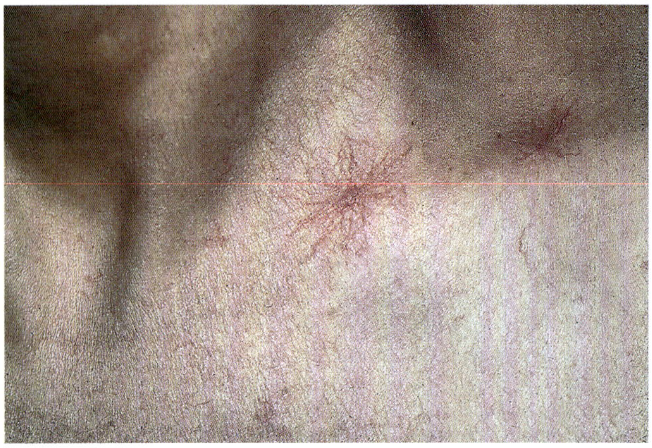

FIGURE 39-3. Spider angioma. This vascular (arterial) spider appears on the skin. Beneath the elevated centre and radiating branches, the blood vessels are looped and tortuous.

Nonalcoholic fatty liver disease (NAFLD) and nonalcoholic steatohepatitis (NASH) are two diseases within the spectrum of fatty liver to fibrosis and cirrhosis that are strongly associated with obesity (Lee & Moreau, 2015). Two preliminary studies further suggest that being overweight and drinking too much alcohol can cause severe harm to the liver (European Association for the Study of the Liver, 2013). One study found that overweight and obese women who were heavy drinkers had a significantly increased risk of developing and dying of chronic liver disease. The other study found an increased risk of liver cancer in people with alcoholic cirrhosis who also have fatty liver disease, type 2 diabetes, and are overweight or obese. In patients who are overweight, obese, or have high alcohol intake, the nurse observes for signs of associated liver dysfunction.

The nurse assesses for the presence of an abdominal fluid wave (discussed later). The abdomen is palpated to assess liver size and to detect any tenderness over the liver. A palpable liver presents as a firm, sharp ridge with a smooth surface (Fig. 39-4). The nurse estimates the size of the liver by percussing its upper and lower borders. If the liver is not palpable but tenderness is suspected, tapping the lower right thorax briskly may elicit tenderness. For comparison, the nurse then performs a similar manoeuvre on the left lower thorax (Lee & Moreau, 2015).

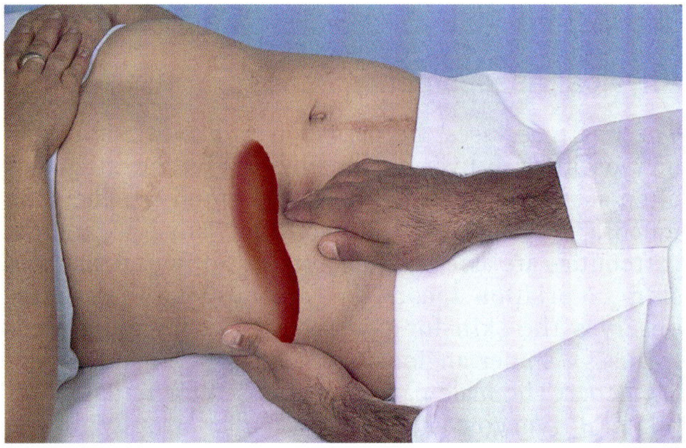

FIGURE 39-4. Technique for palpating the liver. The examiner places one hand under the right lower rib cage and presses downward with light pressure with the other hand. (From Bickley, L. S. (2017). *Bates' guide to physical examination and history taking* (12th ed.). Philadelphia, PA: Lippincott Williams & Wilkins.)

If the liver is palpable, the examiner notes and records its size, its consistency, any tenderness, and whether its outline is regular or irregular. If the liver is enlarged, the degree to which it descends below the right costal margin is recorded to provide some indication of its size. The examiner determines whether the liver's edge is sharp and smooth or blunt and whether the enlarged liver is nodular or smooth. The liver of a patient with cirrhosis is small and hard; whereas the liver of a patient with acute hepatitis is soft, and the hand easily moves the edge. Stages of liver disease and cirrhosis are not evident in physical examination alone but can provide some clues as to the extent of the illness and guide diagnostic care.

Tenderness of the liver indicates recent acute enlargement with consequent stretching of the liver capsule. The absence of tenderness may imply that the enlargement is of long-standing duration. The liver of a patient with viral hepatitis is tender; whereas that of a patient with alcoholic hepatitis is not. Enlargement of the liver is an abnormal finding that requires evaluation (Lee & Moreau, 2015).

Diagnostic Evaluation

A wide range of diagnostic studies may be performed in patients with hepatic disorders, both for diagnostic purposes and to monitor the status of the liver in those with chronic hepatic alterations. The nurse should educate the patient about the purpose, what to expect, and any possible side effects related to these examinations prior to testing. The nurse should note trends in results because they provide information about disease progression as well as the patient's response to therapy.

Liver Function Tests

More than 70% of the parenchyma of the liver may be damaged before liver function test results become abnormal. Function is generally measured in terms of serum enzyme activity (i.e., serum aminotransferases, alkaline phosphatase, lactic dehydrogenase) and serum concentrations of proteins (albumin and globulins), bilirubin, ammonia, clotting factors, and lipids (Lee & Moreau, 2015). Several of these tests may be helpful for assessing patients with liver disease. However, the nature and extent of hepatic dysfunction cannot be determined by these tests alone, because other disorders can affect test results. The pattern of serum blood abnormalities may be useful in determining the type of liver injury or alteration the patient is experiencing and provide guidance to clinicians in terms of the diagnostic pathway.

Serum aminotransferases are sensitive indicators of injury to or inflammation of the liver cells and are useful in detecting acute liver disease such as hepatitis. Alanine aminotransferase (ALT), aspartate aminotransferase (AST), and gamma-glutamyl transferase (GGT) are the most frequently used tests of liver damage. ALT levels

TABLE 39-1 Common Laboratory Tests to Assess Liver Function

Test	Normal	Clinical Functions
Pigment Studies		
Serum bilirubin, direct	0.1–0.4 mg/dL (1.7–3.7 mcmol/L)	These studies measure the ability of the liver to conjugate and excrete bilirubin. Results are abnormal in liver and biliary tract disease and are associated with jaundice clinically.
Serum bilirubin, total	0.3–1 mg/dL (5–17 mcmol/L)	
Urine bilirubin	<0.25 mg/24 hr (<0.42 mcmol/24 hr)	
Urine urobilinogen	(Urine urobilinogen) 0.05–2.5 mg/24 hr (0.5–4 Ehrlich U/24 hr)	
Fecal urobilinogen (infrequently used)	(Fecal urobilinogen) 50–300 mg/24 hr (100–400 Ehrlich U/100 g)	
Protein Studies		
Total serum protein	7–7.5 g/dL (70–75 g/L)	Proteins are manufactured by the liver. Their levels may be affected in a variety of liver impairments: albumin is affected in cirrhosis, chronic hepatitis, edema; and ascites; globulins are affected in cirrhosis, liver disease, chronic obstructive jaundice, and viral hepatitis.
Serum albumin	3.5–5.5 g/dL (40–55 g/L)	
Serum globulin	2.3–3.5 g/dL (23–35 g/L)	
Serum protein electrophoresis		
Albumin	4–6 g/dL (40–60 g/L)	
α_1-Globulin	0.15–0.25 g/dL (1.5–2.5 g/L)	
α_2-Globulin	0.43–0.75 g/dL (4.3–7.5 g/L)	
β-Globulin	0.5–1 g/dL (5–10 g/L)	
γ-Globulin	0.6–1.3 g/dL (6–13 g/L)	
A/G ratio	A > G or 1.5:1–2.5:1	A/G ratio is reversed in chronic liver disease (decreased albumin and increased globulin).
Prothrombin Time	100% or 12–16 seconds	Prothrombin time may be prolonged in liver disease. It will not return to normal with vitamin K in severe liver cell damage.
Serum Alkaline Phosphatase	Varies with method: *Adults:* 30–120 U/L	Serum alkaline phosphatase is manufactured in bones, liver, kidneys, and intestine and excreted through biliary tract. In the absence of bone disease, it is a sensitive measure of biliary tract obstruction. Results may vary because this test is temperature and lab method dependent.
Serum Aminotransferase Studies		
AST	10–40 U/mL (0.34–0.68 U/L)	The studies are based on release of enzymes from damaged liver cells. These enzymes are elevated in liver cell damage. Normal values may differ in men and women.
ALT	8–40 U/mL (0.14–0.68 U/L)	
GGT, GGTP	0–30 U/L IU/L	Values are elevated in alcohol abuse and markers for biliary cholestasis.
LDH	100–200 units (100–225 U/L)	
Ammonia (plasma)	15–45 mcg/dL (11–32 mcmol/L)	Liver converts ammonia to urea. Ammonia level rises in liver failure.
Cholesterol		
Ester	60–70% of total cholesterol, fraction of total cholesterol 0.60–0.70	Cholesterol levels are elevated in biliary obstruction and decreased in parenchymal liver disease.
HDL	*Male:* 35–70 mg/dL; *Female:* 35–85 mg/dL	
LDL	<130 mcg/dL	

A/G, albumin/globulin; AST, aspartate aminotransferase; ALT, alanine aminotransferase; GGT, gamma-glutamyl transferase; GGTP, gamma-glutamyl transpeptidase; LDH, lactate dehydrogenase; HDL, high-density lipoprotein; LDL, low-density lipoprotein.

Adapted from Alldredge, B. K., Corelli, R. L., Ernst, M. E., et al. (Eds.). (2013). *Koda-Kimble & Young's applied therapeutics: The clinical use of drugs*. Philadelphia, PA: Lippincott Williams & Wilkins.

increase primarily in liver disorders and may be used to monitor the course of hepatitis or cirrhosis or the effects of treatments that may be toxic to the liver. AST is present in tissues that have high metabolic activity; therefore, the level may be increased if there is damage to or death of tissues of organs such as the heart, liver, skeletal muscle, and kidney. Although not specific to liver disease, levels of AST may be increased in cirrhosis, hepatitis, and liver cancer. Increased GGT levels are associated with cholestasis but can also be due to alcoholic liver disease. Although the kidney has the highest level of the enzyme, the liver is considered the source of normal serum activity. The test determines liver cell dysfunction and is a sensitive indicator of cholestasis. Its main value in liver disease is confirming the hepatic origin of an elevated alkaline phosphatase level. Common liver function tests are summarized in Table 39-1.

Liver Biopsy

Liver biopsy is the removal of a small amount of liver tissue, usually through needle aspiration. It permits examination of liver cells and evaluation of diffuse disorders of the parenchyma and diagnosis of space-occupying lesions.

Liver biopsy is especially useful when clinical findings and laboratory tests are not diagnostic. Bleeding and bile peritonitis after liver biopsy are the major complications; therefore, coagulation studies are obtained, their values are noted, and abnormal results are treated before liver biopsy is performed (Feldman, Friedman, & Brandt, 2015). Other techniques for liver biopsy are preferred if **ascites** or coagulation abnormalities exist. A liver biopsy can be performed percutaneously with ultrasound guidance or transvenously through the right internal jugular vein to right hepatic vein under fluoroscopic control. Liver biopsy can also be performed laparoscopically. Nursing responsibilities related to percutaneous liver biopsy are summarized in Chart 39-3.

Other Diagnostic Tests

Ultrasonography, computed tomography (CT), and magnetic resonance imaging (MRI) are used to identify normal structures and abnormalities of the liver and biliary tree. A radioisotope liver scan may be performed to assess liver size and hepatic blood flow and obstruction. A fibroscan is a noninvasive ultrasound based vibration used to measure levels of fibrosis and degree of elasticity in the liver tissue. Studies have shown it to be as effective as biopsy for monitoring disease severity (Wilder & Patel, 2014). Because fibroscan machines are newer, they are not available in all locations; additionally they require a specially trained operator to use them. Fibroscans can provide diagnostic information in a matter of minutes. Across Canada, many hepatology offices and departments use this tool for outpatient appointments and follow ups. Emerging technologies like these mean patients with chronic liver disease are having less invasive biopsy procedures.

Laparoscopy (insertion of a fibreoptic endoscope through a small abdominal incision) is used to examine the liver and other pelvic structures. It is also used to perform guided liver biopsy, to determine the cause of ascites, and to diagnose and stage tumours of the liver and other abdominal organs.

MANIFESTATIONS OF HEPATIC DYSFUNCTION

Hepatic dysfunction results from damage to the liver's parenchymal cells, directly from primary liver diseases, or indirectly from either obstruction of bile flow or derangements of hepatic circulation. Liver dysfunction may be acute or chronic; the latter is far more common.

It is estimated that one in four Canadians may be impacted by liver disease (Canadian Liver Foundation, 2017). There are over 100 forms of liver disease, and chronic liver disease and cirrhosis remain high contributors to the mortality of Canadians. Each of these liver diseases has its own pathophysiology, treatment, and management. The Canadian Liver Foundation (www.liver.ca) is an excellent source of information on these various types of liver diseases and compiles clinical practice guidelines, statistics, and research.

The rate of chronic liver disease for men is twice that for women, and chronic liver disease is more common in Asian and African countries than it is in Europe and the

CHART 39-3

GUIDELINES for Assisting With Percutaneous Liver Biopsy

Equipment

- Antiseptic solution
- Liver biopsy tray (contains needles, scalpel, specimen tubes, etc.)
- Local anesthetic
- Nonlatex sterile gloves
- Sphygmomanometer to monitor blood pressure
- Sterile dressing

Implementation

NURSING ACTIONS	RATIONALE
Preprocedure	
1. Ascertain that results of coagulation tests (prothrombin time, partial thromboplastin time, and platelet count) are available and that compatible donor blood is available.	1. Many patients with liver disease have clotting defects and are at risk for bleeding.
2. Check for signed consent; confirm that informed consent has been provided. Confirm patient identity using two identifiers.	2. Ensures that the patient consents to this invasive procedure. Correctly identifies the patient.
3. Perform hand hygiene, and put on disposable nonlatex gloves.	3. Asepsis is essential to prevent infection. The use of nonlatex gloves prevents exposure of nurse to patient's blood and of patient and nurse to latex.
4. Measure and record the patient's pulse, respirations, and blood pressure immediately before biopsy.	4. Prebiopsy values provide a basis on which to compare the patient's vital signs and evaluate status after the procedure.
5. Describe the following to the patient in advance: steps of the procedure, sensations expected, after-effects anticipated, restrictions of activity and monitoring procedures to follow.	5. Explanations allay fears and ensure cooperation.

GUIDELINES for Assisting With Percutaneous Liver Biopsy (Continued)

NURSING ACTIONS	RATIONALE
Procedure	
1. Support the patient during the procedure.	1. Encouragement and support of the nurse enhance comfort and promote a sense of security.
2. Expose the right side of the patient's upper abdomen (right hypochondriac).	2. The skin at the site of penetration will be cleansed, and a local anesthetic will be infiltrated.
3. Instruct the patient to inhale and exhale deeply several times, finally to exhale, and to hold breath at the end of expiration. The physician promptly introduces the biopsy needle by way of the transthoracic (intercostal) or transabdominal (subcostal) route, penetrates the liver, aspirates, and withdraws.	3. Holding the breath immobilizes the chest wall and the diaphragm; penetration of the diaphragm thereby is avoided, and the risk of lacerating the liver is minimized.
4. Instruct the patient to resume breathing.	4. The patient often continues holding his or her breath because of anxiety.

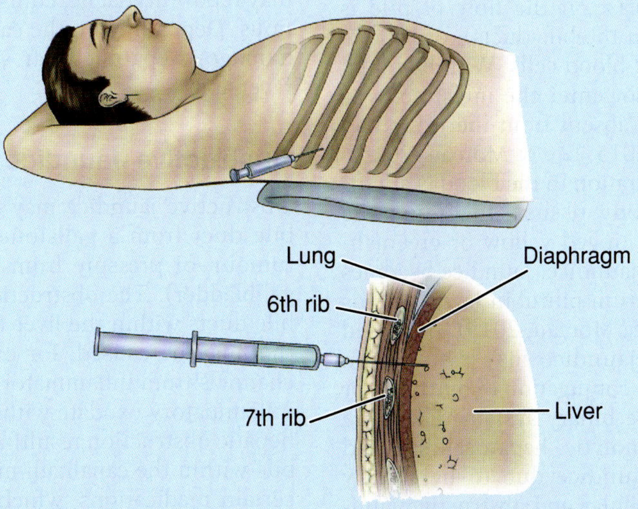

NURSING ACTIONS	RATIONALE
Postprocedure	
1. Immediately after the biopsy, assist the patient to turn on to the right side; place a pillow under the costal margin, and caution the patient to remain in this position, recumbent and immobile, for several hours. Instruct the patient to avoid coughing or straining.	1. In this position, the liver capsule at the site of penetration is compressed against the chest wall, and the escape of blood or bile through the perforation is prevented.
2. Measure and record the patient's pulse, respiratory rate, and blood pressure at 10–15-minute intervals for the first hour, then every 30 minutes for the next 3–4 hours or until the patient's condition stabilizes.	2. Changes in vital signs may indicate bleeding, severe hemorrhage, or bile peritonitis, which are potential complications of liver biopsy. Most cases of hemorrhage occur within 3–4 hours.
3. If the patient is discharged after the procedure, instruct the patient to avoid heavy lifting and strenuous activity for 1 week.	3. Activity restriction reduces the risk of bleeding at the biopsy puncture site.

Adapted from Beddoe, A. M, & Caple, C. (2016). Liver biopsy: Assisting with. In D. Pravikoff (Ed.). *Nursing practice and skill*. Glendale, CA: CINAHL Information Systems.

United States. Approximately 80% of patients diagnosed with cirrhosis compensate and remain asymptomatic for the next 10 years (Fox, 2014; Nusrat, Khan, Fazili, et al., 2014). Liver disease is still highly associated with alcoholism, but fatty liver disease is now the most common alteration. Liver disease continues to be stigmatized with assumptions of alcoholism.

Disease processes that lead to hepatocellular dysfunction may be caused by infectious agents such as bacteria and viruses and by anoxia, metabolic disorders, toxins and medications, nutritional deficiencies, and hypersensitivity states. The most common cause of parenchymal damage is malnutrition, especially that related to alcoholism (Fialla, Israelsen, Hamberg, et al., 2015).

The parenchymal cells respond to most noxious agents by replacing glycogen with lipids, producing fatty infiltration with or without cell death or necrosis. This is commonly associated with inflammatory cell infiltration and growth of fibrous tissue. Cell regeneration can occur if the disease process is not too toxic to the cells. The result of chronic parenchymal disease is the shrunken, fibrotic liver seen in cirrhosis. In some conditions, lipids may accumulate in the hepatocytes, resulting in the abnormal condition called *fatty liver disease*.

The consequences of liver disease are numerous and varied. Their ultimate effects are often incapacitating or life threatening, and their presence is ominous. Among the most common and significant manifestations of liver disease are jaundice, **portal hypertension**, ascites and varices, nutritional deficiencies (resulting from the inability of damaged liver cells to metabolize certain vitamins), and **hepatic encephalopathy** or coma. Treatment of liver disease varies with the type of alteration but it can be difficult to manage.

Jaundice

The bilirubin concentration in the blood may be increased in the presence of liver disease, if the flow of bile is impeded (e.g., by gallstones in the bile ducts), or if there is excessive destruction of red blood cells. With bile duct obstruction, bilirubin does not enter the intestine; as a consequence, urobilinogen is absent from the urine and decreased in the stool (Hall, 2015; Lee & Moreau, 2015).

When the bilirubin concentration in the blood is abnormally elevated, all of the body tissues, including the sclerae and the skin, become tinged yellow or greenish-yellow, a condition known as jaundice. Jaundice becomes clinically evident when the serum bilirubin level exceeds 2.0 mg/dL (34 mmol/L) (Lee & Moreau, 2015). Increased serum bilirubin levels and jaundice may result from impairment of hepatic uptake, conjugation of bilirubin, or excretion of bilirubin into the biliary system. There are several types of jaundice: hemolytic, hepatocellular, and obstructive jaundice, and jaundice due to hereditary hyperbilirubinemia. Hepatocellular and obstructive jaundice are the two types commonly associated with liver disease.

Hemolytic Jaundice

Hemolytic jaundice is the result of an increased destruction of the red blood cells, the effect of which is to flood the plasma with bilirubin so rapidly that the liver, although functioning normally, cannot excrete the bilirubin as quickly as it is formed. This type of jaundice is encountered in patients with hemolytic transfusion reactions and other hemolytic disorders. In these patients, the bilirubin in the blood is predominantly unconjugated or free. Fecal and urine urobilinogen levels are increased, but the urine is free of bilirubin. Patients with this type of jaundice, do not experience symptoms or complications as a result of the jaundice. However, prolonged jaundice, even if mild, predisposes to the formation of pigment stones in the gallbladder, and extremely severe jaundice (levels of free bilirubin exceeding 300 to 400 μmol/L) poses a risk for central nervous system effects.

Hepatocellular Jaundice

Hepatocellular jaundice is caused by the inability of damaged liver cells to clear normal amounts of bilirubin from the blood. The cellular damage may be caused by hepatitis viruses, other viruses that affect the liver (e.g., yellow fever virus, Epstein–Barr virus), medications or chemical toxins (e.g., chloroform, arsenicals, certain medications), or alcohol. Cirrhosis of the liver may produce jaundice. It is usually associated with excessive alcohol intake, but it may also be a late result of liver cell necrosis caused by viral infection, inflammation, and a variety of other etiologies. In prolonged obstructive jaundice, cell damage eventually develops, so that both types of jaundice (i.e., obstructive and hepatocellular jaundice) appear together.

Patients with hepatocellular jaundice may be mildly or severely ill, with lack of appetite, nausea, malaise, fatigue, weakness, and possible weight loss. In some cases of hepatocellular disease, jaundice may not be obvious. The serum bilirubin concentration and the urine urobilinogen level may be elevated. In addition, AST and ALT levels may be increased, indicating cellular necrosis. The patient may report headache, chills, and fever if the cause is infectious. Depending on the cause and extent of the liver cell damage, hepatocellular jaundice may be completely reversible.

Obstructive Jaundice

Obstructive jaundice may be caused by occlusion of the bile duct from a gallstone, an inflammatory process, a tumour, or pressure from an enlarged organ (e.g., liver, gallbladder). The obstruction may also involve the small bile ducts within the liver (i.e., intrahepatic obstruction); this may be caused, for example, by pressure on these channels from inflammatory swelling of the liver or by an inflammatory exudate within the ducts themselves. Intrahepatic obstruction resulting from stasis and thickening of bile within the canaliculi may occur after the ingestion of certain medications, which are referred to as cholestatic agents. These agents include phenothiazines, antithyroid medications, tricyclic antidepressant agents, androgens, and estrogens.

Regardless of whether the obstruction is intrahepatic or extrahepatic, and regardless of its cause, bile cannot flow normally into the intestine and becomes backed up into the liver substance. It is then reabsorbed into the blood and carried throughout the entire body, staining the skin, mucous membranes, and sclerae. It is excreted in the urine, which becomes deep orange and foamy. Because of the decreased amount of bile in the intestinal tract, the stools become light or clay-coloured. The skin may itch intensely, requiring repeated soothing baths. Dyspepsia and intolerance to fatty foods may develop because of impaired fat digestion in the absence of intestinal bile. In general, AST, ALT, and GGT levels rise only moderately, but bilirubin and alkaline phosphatase levels are elevated.

Liver diseases that lead to obstruction generally include the name cholangitis within them (such as primary sclerosing cholangitis or primary biliary cholangitis).

Hereditary Hyperbilirubinemia

Increased serum bilirubin levels (hyperbilirubinemia), resulting from any of several inherited disorders, can also produce jaundice. Gilbert's syndrome is a familial disorder characterized by an increased level of unconjugated bilirubin that causes jaundice. Although serum bilirubin levels are increased, liver histology and liver function test results are normal, and there is no hemolysis. This syndrome affects 3% to 8% of the population, predominantly males (Bope & Kellerman, 2015).

Other conditions that are probably caused by inborn errors of biliary metabolism include Dubin–Johnson syndrome (chronic idiopathic jaundice, with pigment in the liver) and Rotor's syndrome (chronic familial conjugated hyperbilirubinemia, without pigment in the liver); the "benign" cholestatic jaundice of pregnancy, with retention of conjugated bilirubin, probably secondary to unusual sensitivity to the hormones of pregnancy; and benign recurrent intrahepatic cholestasis.

Portal Hypertension

Portal hypotension is the increased pressure throughout the portal venous system that results from obstruction of blood flow through the damaged liver. Commonly associated with hepatic cirrhosis, it can also occur with noncirrhotic liver disease. Although splenomegaly (enlarged spleen) with possible hypersplenism is a common manifestation of portal hypertension, the two major consequences of portal hypertension are ascites and varices.

Ascites

Pathophysiology

The mechanisms responsible for the development of ascites are not completely understood. Portal hypertension and the resulting increase in capillary pressure and obstruction of venous blood flow through the damaged liver are contributing factors. The vasodilation that occurs in the splanchnic circulation (the arterial supply and venous drainage of the GI system from the distal esophagus to the midrectum including the liver and spleen) is also a suspected causative factor. The failure of the liver to metabolize aldosterone increases sodium and water retention by the kidney. Sodium and water retention, increased intravascular fluid volume, increased lymphatic flow, and decreased synthesis of albumin by the damaged liver all contribute to the movement of fluid from the vascular system into the peritoneal space. The process becomes self-perpetuating; loss of fluid into the peritoneal space causes further sodium and water retention by the kidney in an effort to maintain the vascular fluid volume.

As a result of liver damage, large amounts of albumin-rich fluid, 20 L or more, may accumulate in the peritoneal cavity as ascites (Hall, 2015; Lee & Moreau, 2015). With the movement of albumin from the serum to the peritoneal cavity, the osmotic pressure of the serum decreases. This, combined with increased portal pressure, results in movement of fluid into the peritoneal cavity (Fig. 39-5).

Physiology/Pathophysiology

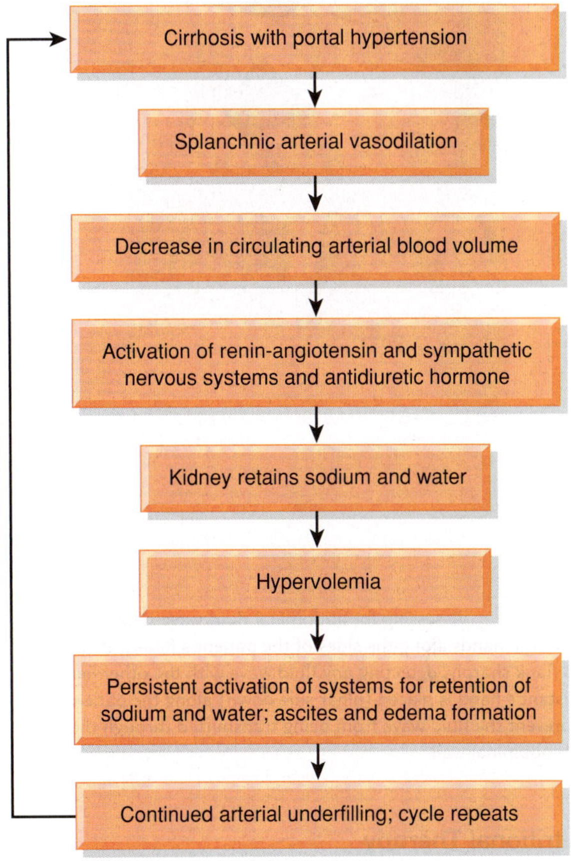

FIGURE 39-5. Pathogenesis of ascites (arterial vasodilation theory).

Clinical Manifestations

Increased abdominal girth and rapid weight gain are common presenting symptoms of ascites. The patient may be short of breath and uncomfortable from the enlarged abdomen, and striae and distended veins may be visible over the abdominal wall. Umbilical hernias also occur frequently in those patients with cirrhosis. Fluid and electrolyte imbalances are common.

Assessment and Diagnostic Findings

The presence and extent of ascites can be assessed by percussion of the abdomen. When fluid has accumulated in the peritoneal cavity, the flanks bulge when the patient assumes a supine position. The presence of fluid can be confirmed either by percussing for shifting dullness or by detecting a fluid wave (Fig. 39-6) (Lee & Moreau, 2015; Weber & Kelley, 2014). A fluid wave is likely to be found only if a large amount of fluid is present. The ballottement technique is a palpation technique performed to identify a mass or enlarged organ within an abdomen with ascites (Weber & Kelley, 2009). Ballottement can be performed in two different ways: single handed or bimanually. Daily measurement and recording of abdominal girth and body weight are essential to assess the progression of ascites and its response to treatment.

Medical Management

The medical management of the patient with ascites includes dietary modifications, pharmacologic therapy, bed rest, paracentesis, the use of shunts, and other therapies.

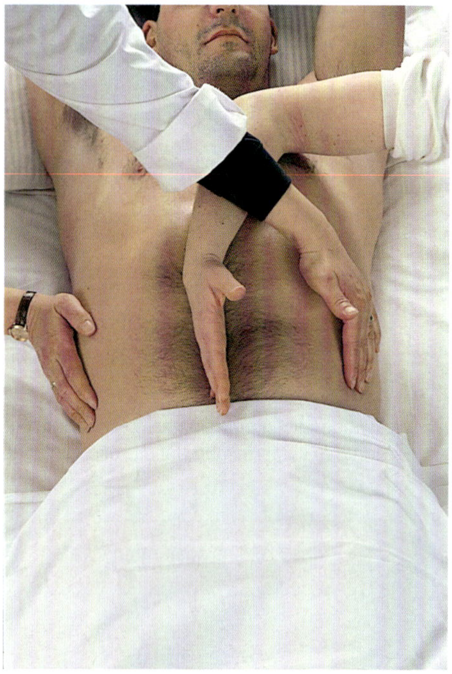

FIGURE 39-6. Assessing for abdominal fluid wave. The examiner places the hands along the sides of the patient's flanks, then strikes one flank sharply, detecting any fluid wave with the other hand. An assistant's hand is placed (ulnar side down) along the patient's midline to prevent the fluid wave from being transmitted through the tissues of the abdominal wall.

Nutritional Therapy

The goal of treatment for the patient with ascites is a negative sodium balance to reduce fluid retention. Table salt, salty foods, salted butter and margarine, and all ordinary canned and frozen foods that are not specifically prepared for low-sodium diets should be avoided (Lee & Moreau, 2015). It may take 2 to 3 months for the patient's taste buds to adjust to unsalted foods. In the meantime, the taste of unsalted foods can be improved by using salt substitutes such as lemon juice, oregano, and thyme. Commercial salt substitutes need to be approved by the physician, because those that contain ammonia could precipitate hepatic encephalopathy and potential for coma. Many salt substitutes contain potassium and should be avoided if the patient has impaired renal function. The patient should make liberal use of powdered, low-sodium milk and milk products. If fluid accumulation is not controlled with this regimen, the daily sodium allowance may be reduced to 500 mg, and diuretics may be administered. However, most patients will not accept such a severe sodium restriction as 500 mg, so clinicians often will not recommend it (Lee & Moreau, 2015).

Dietary control of ascites via strict sodium restriction is difficult to achieve at home. The likelihood that the patient will follow even a 2-g sodium diet increases if the patient and the person preparing meals understand the rationale for the diet and receive periodic guidance about selecting and preparing appropriate foods. Approximately 10% of patients with ascites respond to these measures alone (Lee & Moreau, 2015). Nonresponders and those who find sodium restriction difficult will usually require diuretic therapy.

Pharmacologic Therapy

Use of diuretics along with sodium restriction is successful in 90% of patients with ascites (Goldman & Schafer, 2015; Lee & Moreau, 2015). Spironolactone an aldosterone-blocking agent, is most often the first-line therapy in patients with ascites from cirrhosis. When used with other diuretics, spironolactone helps prevent potassium loss. Oral diuretics such as furosemide may be added but should be used cautiously, because long-term use may induce severe sodium depletion (hyponatremia).

Ammonium chloride and acetazolamide are contraindicated because of the possibility of precipitating hepatic encephalopathy. Daily weight loss should not exceed 1 to 2 kg in patients with ascites and peripheral edema or 0.5 to 0.75 kg in patients without edema. Fluid restriction is not attempted unless the serum sodium concentration is very low.

Possible complications of diuretic therapy include fluid and electrolyte disturbances (including hypovolemia, hypokalemia, hyponatremia, and hypochloremic alkalosis) and encephalopathy. Encephalopathy may be precipitated by dehydration and hypovolemia. In addition, when potassium stores are depleted, the amount of ammonia in the systemic circulation increases, which may cause impaired cerebral functioning and encephalopathy.

Bed Rest

In patients with ascites, an upright posture is associated with activation of the renin–angiotensin–aldosterone system and sympathetic nervous system (Grossman, 2013). This causes reduced renal glomerular filtration and sodium excretion and a decreased response to loop diuretics. Therefore, bed rest may be a useful therapy, especially for patients whose condition is refractory to diuretics.

Paracentesis

Paracentesis is the removal of fluid (ascites) from the peritoneal cavity through a puncture or a small surgical incision through the abdominal wall under sterile conditions (Goldman & Schafer, 2015). Coagulation studies should be performed to verify safety of the procedure prior to undertaking it, and ultrasound guidance may be indicated in some patients who are at high risk for bleeding because of an abnormal coagulation profile and in those who have had previous abdominal surgery and may have adhesions.

Paracentesis was once considered a routine form of treatment for ascites. However, it is now performed primarily for diagnostic examination of ascitic fluid; for treatment of massive ascites that is resistant to nutritional and diuretic therapy and that is causing severe problems to the patient; and as a prelude to diagnostic imaging studies, peritoneal dialysis, or surgery. A sample of the ascitic fluid may be sent to the laboratory for cell count, albumin and total protein levels, culture, and other tests.

Large-volume (5 to 6 L) paracentesis has been shown to be a safe method for treating patients with severe ascites. The use of this therapeutic intervention should not be restricted to patients in whom diuretic therapy has failed but should be considered the treatment of choice for all patients with large-volume ascites (Lee & Moreau, 2015). This technique, in combination with the IV infusion of salt-poor albumin or other colloid, has become a standard management strategy yielding an immediate effect.

Refractive, massive ascites is unresponsive to multiple diuretics and sodium restriction for 2 weeks or more and can result in severe sequelae such as respiratory distress, which requires rapid intervention. Albumin infusions help to correct decreases in effective arterial blood volume that lead to sodium retention. Use of this colloid reduces the incidence of postparacentesis circulatory dysfunction with renal dysfunction, hyponatremia, and rapid reaccumulation of ascites associated with decreased effective arterial volume (Lee & Moreau, 2015).

The beneficial effects of albumin administration on hemodynamic stability and renal functional status may be related to an improvement in cardiac function as well as a decrease in the degree of arterial vasodilation. Although the patient with cirrhosis has a greatly increased extracellular blood volume, the kidney incorrectly senses that the effective volume has decreased. The renin–angiotensin–aldosterone axis is stimulated, and sodium is reabsorbed (Lee & Moreau, 2015; Nusrat et al., 2014). In addition, antidiuretic hormone (ADH) secretion increases, which leads to increased retention of free water and sometimes to the development of dilutional hyponatremia. Therapeutic paracentesis provides only temporary removal of fluid; ascites rapidly recurs, necessitating repeated fluid removal. Nursing care of the patient undergoing paracentesis is presented in Chart 39-4.

Transjugular Intrahepatic Portosystemic Shunt

Transjugular intrahepatic portosystemic shunt (TIPS) is a method of treating ascites in which a cannula is threaded into the portal vein by the transjugular route (Fig. 39-7). To reduce portal hypertension, an expandable stent is inserted to serve as an intrahepatic shunt between the portal circulation and the hepatic vein (Lee & Moreau, 2015; Nusrat et al., 2014). TIPS is the treatment of choice for refractive ascites. It is extremely effective in decreasing sodium retention, improving the renal response to diuretic therapy, and preventing recurrence of fluid accumulation (Lee & Moreau, 2015; Nusrat et al., 2014).

Because the development of ascites in patients with cirrhosis is associated with a 50% mortality rate, any patient who is considered a candidate for liver transplantation should be referred for TIPS.

CHART 39-4

GUIDELINES for Assisting With a Paracentesis

Equipment

- Paracentesis tray (contains trocar, syringe, needles, drainage tube)
- Nonlatex sterile gloves
- Antiseptic solution
- Local anesthetic
- Sterile dressing
- Drainage collection bottles, receptacles
- Sphygmomanometer to monitor blood pressure

Implementation

NURSING ACTIONS	RATIONALE
Preprocedure	
1. Confirm that informed consent has been provided and identify the patient using two identifiers.	1. Ensures that patient has agreed to procedure. Correctly identifies the patient.
2. Prepare the patient by providing the necessary information and education and by offering reassurance.	2. Education increases the patient's understanding of the procedure and the reason for it.
3. Instruct the patient to void.	3. An empty bladder minimizes the risk of inadvertent puncture of the bladder and minimizes discomfort from a full bladder.
4. Gather appropriate sterile equipment and collection receptacles.	4. Sterility of equipment is essential to minimize risk of infection; having equipment available enables the procedure to be performed smoothly.
5. Place the patient in upright position on the edge of the bed or in a chair with feet supported on a stool. Fowler's position should be used by the patient confined to bed.	5. An upright position results in movement of the peritoneal fluid close to the abdominal wall and promotes easier puncture and removal of fluid.
6. Perform hand hygiene, and put on disposable nonlatex gloves.	6. Asepsis is essential to prevent infection. The use of nonlatex gloves prevents exposure of nurse to patient's blood and of patient and nurse to latex.
7. Place the sphygmomanometer cuff around patient's arm.	7. This allows the nurse to monitor the patient's blood pressure during procedure.
Procedure	
1. The primary provider, using aseptic technique, inserts the trocar through a puncture below the umbilicus. The trocar or needle is connected to a drainage tube, the end of which is inserted into a collecting receptacle.	1. Sterile technique minimizes the risk of infection. Bleeding at the puncture site is minimal at this location. The fluid drains by gravity or mild siphon into the container.
2. Help the patient maintain position throughout the procedure.	2. The patient who is fatigued or weak may have difficulty maintaining an optimal position for drainage of fluid.

continued >

GUIDELINES for Assisting With a Paracentesis (Continued)

NURSING ACTIONS	RATIONALE
3. Measure and record blood pressure at frequent intervals throughout the procedure.	3. Decreased blood pressure may occur with vascular collapse, which can result from removal of the fluid from the peritoneal cavity and fluid shifts.
4. Monitor the patient closely for signs of vascular collapse: pallor, increased pulse rate, or decreased blood pressure.	4. Vascular collapse (hypovolemia) may occur as fluid moves from the vascular system to replace fluid drained from peritoneal cavity.

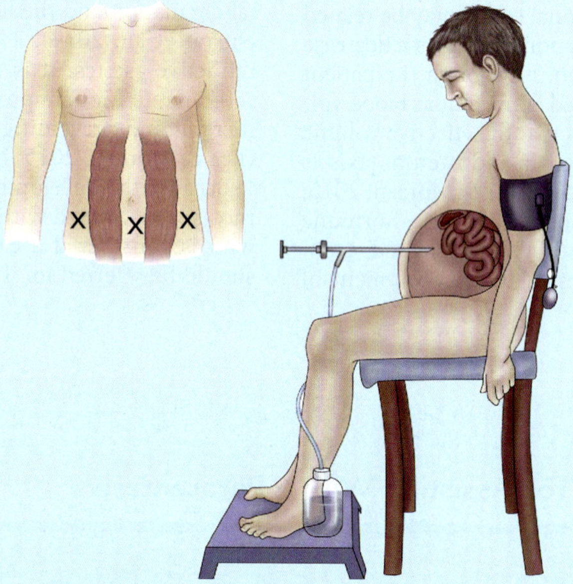

Figure on left shows possible sites for insertion of trocar.

Postprocedure

1. Return the patient to bed or to a comfortable sitting position.	1. The weak or fatigued patient may have difficulty resuming a comfortable position without assistance.
2. Measure, describe, and record the fluid collected.	2. The volume of fluid removed may range from small to very large, and its removal may affect fluid and vascular status; volume should be included in input and output records. The characteristics of the fluid (clear vs. cloudy, red vs. colorless) may be helpful in diagnostic evaluation.
3. Label samples of fluid and send to laboratory.	3. Peritoneal fluid is analyzed as part of the diagnostic workup.
4. Monitor vital signs every 15 minutes for 1 hour, every 30 minutes for 2 hours, every hour for 2 hours, and then every 4 hours.	4. Vital signs (blood pressure, pulse rate) may change as fluid shifts occur after removal of fluid, especially if a large volume of fluid has been removed.
5. Measure the patient's temperature.	5. An elevated temperature is a sign of infection and should be reported to the patient's primary provider.
6. Assess for hypovolemia, electrolyte shifts, changes in mental status, and encephalopathy.	6. Changes in fluid and electrolyte states and mental and cognitive status may occur with removal of fluid and fluid shifts, and should be reported.
7. When taking vital signs, check puncture site for leakage or bleeding.	7. Leakage of fluid may occur because of changes in abdominal pressure and may contribute to further loss of fluid if undetected. Leakage suggests a possible site for infection, and bleeding may occur in patients with altered clotting secondary to liver disease.
8. Provide patient education regarding need to monitor for bleeding or excessive drainage from puncture site, importance of avoiding heavy lifting or straining for 1 week, the need to change position slowly, and frequency of monitoring for fever.	8. The patient (or family members) needs to monitor the puncture site for bleeding and excessive drainage if the patient is discharged home after the procedure. Heavy lifting or straining is avoided to enable the puncture site to close. Slow changes in position are recommended because of the risk of hypovolemia related to fluid removal. Monitoring for fever is needed to detect infection.

Adapted from Smith, N., & Caple, C. (2016). Paracentesis: Assisting with. In D. Pravikoff (Ed.). *Nursing practice and skill*. Glendale, CA: CINAHL Information Systems.

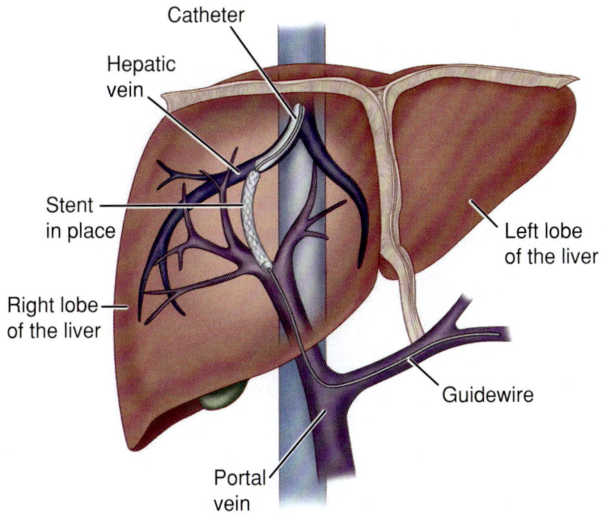

FIGURE 39-7. Transjugular intrahepatic portosystemic shunt (TIPS). A stent is inserted via catheter to the portal vein to divert blood flow and reduce portal hypertension.

Other Methods of Treatment

Ascites can also be treated by the insertion of a peritoneovenous shunt to redirect ascitic fluid from the peritoneal cavity into the systemic circulation (Chen, Ge, Huang, et al., 2014; Lee & Moreau, 2015). However, this procedure is rarely used due to the availability of newer, more effective therapies such as TIPS.

Nursing Management

If a patient with ascites from liver dysfunction is hospitalized, nursing measures include assessment and documentation of intake and output, abdominal girth, and daily weight to assess fluid status. The nurse monitors serum ammonia and electrolyte levels to assess electrolyte balance, response to therapy, and indicators of encephalopathy.

Promoting Home, Community-Based, and Transitional Care

Educating Patients About Self-Care

The patient treated for ascites is likely to be discharged with some ascites still present. During the hospital stay, the nurse teaches the patient and family about the treatment plan, including the need to avoid all alcohol intake, adhere to a low-sodium diet, take medications as prescribed, and check with the physician before taking any new medications (Chart 39-5). Additional patient and family teaching addresses skin care and the need to weigh the patient daily and to watch for and report signs and symptoms of complications.

Continuing and Transitional Care

A referral for transitional, home, or community-based care may be warranted, especially if the patient lives alone or cannot provide self-care. The home visit enables the nurse to assess changes in the patient's condition and weight, abdominal girth, skin, and cognitive and emotional status. The home care nurse assesses the home environment and the availability of resources needed to adhere to the treatment plan (e.g., a scale to obtain daily weights, facilities to prepare and store appropriate foods, resources to purchase needed medications). It is important to assess the patient's adherence to the treatment plan and the ability to buy, prepare, and eat appropriate foods. The nurse reinforces previous teaching and emphasizes the need for regular follow-up and the importance of keeping scheduled health care appointments.

Esophageal Varices

Esophageal varices are present in 30% of patients with compensated cirrhosis and 60% of patients with decompensated cirrhosis at the time of diagnosis (Lee & Moreau, 2015; Satapathy & Sanyal, 2014). Varices are varicosities that develop from elevated pressure in the veins that drain into the portal system. They are prone to rupture and often are the source of massive hemorrhages from the upper GI tract and the rectum. In addition, blood clotting abnormalities, often seen in patients with severe liver disease, increase the likelihood of bleeding and significant blood loss.

Once esophageal varices form, they increase in size and eventually bleed (Wang, Hu, Dong, et al., 2014); in cirrhosis, they are the most significant source of bleeding. Most patients with cirrhosis will develop esophageal varices over their life time and the mortality rate still remains high (20% to 35%) (Wang et al., 2014).

Pathophysiology

Esophageal varices are dilated, tortuous veins that are usually found in the submucosa of the lower esophagus but may develop higher in the esophagus or extend into the stomach. This condition is almost always caused by portal hypertension, which results from obstruction of the portal venous circulation within the damaged liver.

Because of increased obstruction of the portal vein, venous blood from the intestinal tract and spleen seeks an outlet through collateral circulation (new pathways for return of blood to the right atrium). The effect is increased pressure, particularly in the vessels in the submucosal layer of the lower esophagus and upper part of the stomach. These collateral vessels are not very elastic; rather, they are tortuous and fragile, and they bleed easily (Fig. 39-8). Less common causes of varices are abnormalities of the circulation in the splenic vein or superior vena cava and hepatic venothrombosis.

Bleeding esophageal varices can result in hemorrhagic shock that produces decreased cerebral, hepatic, and renal perfusion. In turn, there is an increased nitrogen load from bleeding into the GI tract and an increased serum ammonia level, increasing the risk of encephalopathy. Usually the dilated veins cause no symptoms. However, if the portal pressure increases sharply and the mucosa or supporting structures become thin, massive hemorrhaging occurs.

Factors that contribute to hemorrhage are muscular exertion from lifting heavy objects; straining at stool; sneezing, coughing, or vomiting; esophagitis; irritation of vessels by poorly chewed foods or irritating fluids; and reflux of stomach contents (especially alcohol). Salicylates and any medication that erodes the esophageal mucosa or

CHART 39-5

HOME CARE CHECKLIST • Management of Ascites

At the completion of education, the patient and/or caregiver will be able to:

- State the impact of ascites and treatment on physiologic functioning, ADLs, IADLs, roles, relationships, and spirituality.
- State the name, dose, side effects, frequency, and schedule for all medications.
- Describe effects, side effects, and monitoring parameters for diuretic therapy.
- Discuss importance of avoiding nonsteroidal anti-inflammatory agents, medications (e.g., cough mixtures) containing alcohol, antibiotics, or antacids containing salt.
- Make appropriate dietary choices consistent with dietary prescription and recommendations.
  - Explain the use of salt substitutes must be approved by primary provider.
- State the importance of weighing self-daily and keeping a daily record of weight.
  - Maintain record of daily weight, and identify daily weight-loss goals.
  - List weight changes (loss or gain) that should be reported to the primary provider.
- Identify rationale for fluid restrictions (if needed) monitoring and keeping a daily record intake and output.
  - Maintain a record of daily intake and output.
  - Identify changes in output that should be reported to primary provider (e.g., decreasing urine output).
- Identify need to stop all alcohol intake as critical to well-being.
- Explain how to contact Alcoholics Anonymous or alcohol counsellors in related organizations if indicated.
- Demonstrate how to inspect and care for skin, alleviate pressure over bony prominences by turning when in bed or chair, and decrease edema by position changes.
- Identify early signs and symptoms of complications (encephalopathy, spontaneous bacterial peritonitis, dehydration, electrolyte abnormalities, azotemia).
- Relate how to reach primary provider with questions or complications.
- State time and date of follow-up medical appointments, therapy, and testing.
- Identify sources of support (e.g., friends, relatives, faith community, support groups, caregiver support).
- Identify the need for health promotion, disease prevention, and screening activities.

ADL, activities of daily living; IADL, independent activities of daily living.

interferes with cell replication also may contribute to bleeding and should be avoided in general by patients with liver disease and cirrhosis.

Clinical Manifestations

The patient with bleeding esophageal varices may present with hematemesis, melena, or general deterioration in mental or physical status and often has a history of liver disease or alcohol abuse. Signs and symptoms of shock (cool clammy skin, hypotension, tachycardia) may be present. Patients with more advanced liver disease may undergo routine endoscopy to find smaller bleeds and may not present with as advanced findings.

Assessment and Diagnostic Findings

Endoscopy is used to identify the bleeding site, along with ultrasonography, CT scanning, and angiography. Another diagnostic tool, the endoscopic video capsule, can detect esophageal varices but does not substitute for endoscopy unless this test cannot be performed. Standard endoscopy is superior to video capsule for the diagnosis of esophageal varices (Goldman & Schafer, 2015; Lee & Moreau, 2015). Because varices are present in 50% of patients with cirrhosis, it is recommended that patients who have been diagnosed with cirrhosis undergo screening endoscopy. If no varices are detected on initial endoscopy, the test should be repeated in 2 to 3 years in an effort to identify and treat large varices, which are the ones most likely to bleed. If small varices are identified on initial endoscopy, the test should be repeated in 1 to 2 years (Feldman et al., 2015; Lee & Moreau, 2015). Small varices can be treated with **sclerotherapy** or banded during these endoscopic procedures to prevent them from bleeding.

Endoscopy

Immediate endoscopy (see Chapter 34) is indicated to identify the cause and the site of bleeding as the bleed can be life threatening. Approximately 40% of patients with

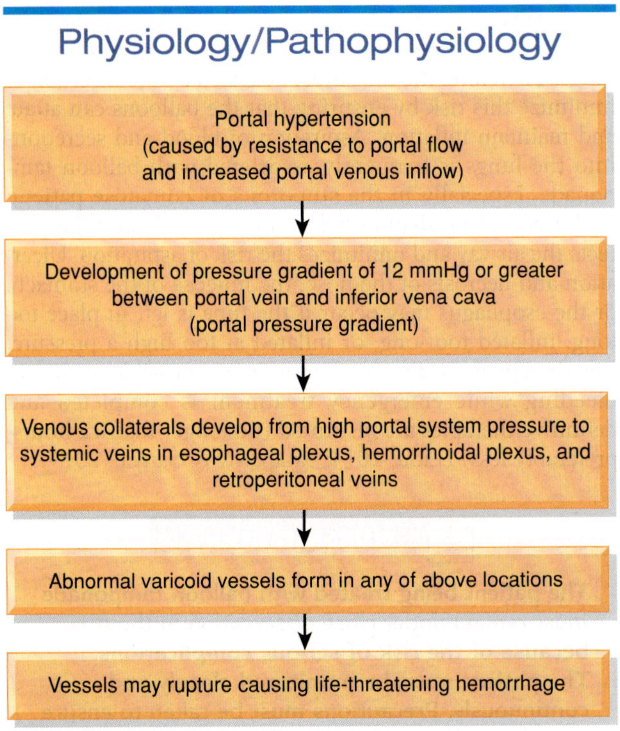

FIGURE 39-8. Pathogenesis of bleeding esophageal varices.

suspected bleeding from esophageal varices are actually bleeding from another source (gastritis, ulcer) (Lee & Moreau, 2015). Nursing support is essential during this often stressful experience. Careful monitoring can detect early signs of cardiac dysrhythmias, perforation, and hemorrhage.

After the examination, fluids are not given until the patient's gag reflex returns. If the patient is actively bleeding, oral intake will not be permitted, and the patient will be prepared for further diagnostic and therapeutic procedures.

Portal Hypertension Measurements

Portal hypertension may be suspected if dilated abdominal veins and hemorrhoids are detected. A palpable enlarged spleen (splenomegaly) and ascites may also be present. Portal venous pressure can be measured directly or indirectly. Indirect measurement of the hepatic vein pressure gradient is the most common procedure. The measurement requires insertion of a catheter with a balloon into the antecubital or femoral vein. The catheter is advanced under fluoroscopy to a hepatic vein. Fluid is infused once the catheter is in position to inflate the balloon. A "wedged" pressure (similar to pulmonary artery wedge pressure) is obtained by occluding the blood flow in the blood vessel; pressure in the unoccluded vessel is also measured and the hepatic venous pressure gradient (HVPG) is obtained. An HVPG of over 10 mmHg is indicative of clinically significant portal hypertension (Abraldes, Sarlieve, & Tandon, 2014). Although the values obtained may underestimate portal pressure, this measurement may be taken several times to evaluate the results of therapy (Bloom, Kemp, & Lubel, 2015).

Direct measurement of portal vein pressure can be obtained by several methods. One direct measurement requires insertion of a catheter into the portal vein or one of its branches (Bloom et al., 2015). Endoscopic measurement of pressure within varices is used only in conjunction with endoscopic sclerotherapy.

Laboratory Tests

Laboratory tests may include various liver function tests, such as serum aminotransferases, bilirubin, alkaline phosphatase, and serum proteins. Splenoportography, which involves serial or segmental x-rays, is used to detect extensive collateral circulation in esophageal vessels, which would indicate varices. Other tests are hepatoportography and celiac angiography. These are usually performed in the operating room or x-ray department.

Medical Management

Bleeding from esophageal varices is an emergency that can quickly lead to hemorrhagic shock. The patient is critically ill, requiring aggressive medical care and expert nursing care, and is usually transferred to the intensive care unit (ICU) for close monitoring and management. See Chapter 18 for a discussion of care of the patient in shock.

The extent of bleeding is evaluated, and vital signs are monitored continuously if hematemesis and melena are present. Signs of potential hypovolemia are noted, such as cold clammy skin, tachycardia, a drop in blood pressure, decreased urine output, restlessness, and weak peripheral pulses. The volume of circulating blood is estimated and monitored with a central venous catheter or pulmonary artery catheter. Blood pressure is monitored via an arterial catheter. Oxygen is administered to prevent hypoxia and to maintain adequate blood oxygenation.

Because patients with bleeding esophageal varices have intravascular volume depletion and are subject to electrolyte imbalance, IV fluids with electrolytes and volume expanders are provided to restore fluid volume and replace electrolytes. Transfusion of blood components also may be required.

Caution must be taken with volume resuscitation so that overhydration does not occur, because this would raise portal pressure and increase bleeding. An indwelling urinary catheter is usually inserted to permit frequent monitoring of urine output.

Although a variety of pharmacologic, endoscopic, and surgical approaches are used to treat bleeding esophageal varices, none is ideal, and most are associated with considerable risk to the patient. Nonsurgical treatment of bleeding esophageal varices is preferable because of the high mortality rate of emergency surgery to control bleeding esophageal varices and because of the poor physical condition that is typical of the patient with severe liver dysfunction.

Pharmacologic Therapy

In suspected variceal bleeding, vasoactive drugs need to be given as soon as possible and before endoscopy (Satapathy & Sanyal, 2014). In an actively bleeding patient, medications are given initially because they can be obtained and given more quickly than other therapies. Octreotide (Sandostatin), a synthetic analog of the hormone somatostatin, is effective in decreasing bleeding from esophageal varices, and lacks the vasoconstrictive effects of vasopressin. Because of this safety and efficacy profile, octreotide is considered the preferred treatment regimen for immediate control of variceal bleeding. These medications cause selective splanchnic vasoconstriction by inhibiting glucagon release and are used mainly in the management of active hemorrhage. Adverse effects are rare with octreotide but mild hypoglycemia and abdominal cramping can occur (Satapathy & Sanyal, 2014).

Vasopressin may be the initial mode of therapy in urgent situations because it produces constriction of the splanchnic arterial bed and decreases portal pressure. Vasopressin constricts distal esophageal and proximal gastric veins, thus reducing the inflow into the portal system and therefore the portal pressure. Vital signs and the presence or absence of blood in the gastric aspirate indicate the effectiveness of vasopressin. Monitoring of fluid intake and output and electrolyte levels is necessary because hyponatremia may develop and vasopressin may have an antidiuretic effect.

Coronary artery disease is a contraindication to the use of vasopressin because coronary vasoconstriction is a side effect that may precipitate myocardial infarction. The combination of vasopressin with nitroglycerin (administered by the IV, sublingual, or transdermal route) has been effective in reducing or preventing the side effects (constriction of coronary vessels and angina) caused by vasopressin alone. Side effects include myocardial and extremity ischemia as well as cardiac dysrhythmias; therefore, vasopressin is used only in urgent situations and with close monitoring (Satapathy & Sanyal, 2014).

Somatostatin and octreotide have been reported to be effective in decreasing bleeding from esophageal varices, and they lack the vasoconstrictive effects of vasopressin. These medications cause selective splanchnic vasoconstriction and are used mainly in the management of active hemorrhage. Propranolol and nadolol, beta-blocking agents that decrease portal pressure, are the most common medications used both to prevent a first bleeding episode in patients with known varices and to prevent rebleeding (James & Liou, 2015; Lee & Moreau, 2015; Liou, 2014; Tripathi & Hayes, 2014). Beta-blockers have been shown to effectively reduce the risk of variceal bleeding and its associated mortality (Barrera, Zuniga, & Arrese, 2015). Beta-blockers should not be used in acute variceal hemorrhage, but they are effective prophylaxis against such an episode. Nitrates such as isosorbide (Isordil) lower portal pressure by venodilation and decreased cardiac output and may be used in combination with beta-blockers to reduce the risk of variceal bleeding (Bloom et al., 2015; Lee & Moreau, 2015).

Balloon Tamponade

Although used infrequently today, balloon tamponade therapy may be used to temporarily control hemorrhage and to stabilize a patient with massive bleeding prior to other definitive management (Feldman et al., 2015; Liou, 2014; Satapathy & Sanyal, 2014).

When indicated, balloon tamponade can be successful; however, there are risks. Displacement of the tube and the inflated balloon into the oropharynx can cause life-threatening obstruction of the airway and asphyxiation. This may occur if the patient pulls on the tube because of confusion or discomfort. It may also result from rupture of the gastric balloon, which causes the esophageal balloon to move into the oropharynx. Sudden rupture of the balloon causes airway obstruction and aspiration of gastric contents into the lungs. Therefore, the tube must be tested before insertion to minimize this risk by ensuring that the balloons can attain and maintain inflation. Aspiration of blood and secretions into the lungs is frequently associated with balloon tamponade, especially in the stuporous or comatose patient. Endotracheal intubation before insertion of the tube protects the airway and minimizes the risk of aspiration. Ulceration and necrosis of the nose, the mucosa of the stomach, or the esophagus may occur if the tube is left in place too long, inflated too long, or inflated at too high a pressure. The therapy is used for as short a time as possible to control bleeding while emergency treatment is completed and definitive therapies are instituted (no longer than 12 hours, preferably less) (Liou, 2014; Satapathy & Sanyal, 2014).

NURSING ALERT

The patient being treated with balloon tamponade must remain under close observation in the ICU because of the risk of serious complications. The patient must be monitored closely and continuously. Precautions must be taken to ensure that the patient does not pull on or inadvertently displace the tube.

Nursing measures include frequent mouth and nasal care. For secretions that accumulate in the mouth, tissues should be within easy reach of the patient. Oral suction may be necessary to remove oral secretions.

The patient with esophageal hemorrhage is usually extremely anxious and frightened. Knowing that the nurse is nearby and ready to respond immediately can help alleviate some of this anxiety. Tube insertion is uncomfortable and never pleasant. Careful explanation during the procedure and while the tube is in place may be reassuring to the patient. Sedation may be prescribed.

Although balloon tamponade stops the bleeding in 90% of patients, bleeding recurs in 60% to 70%, necessitating other treatment modalities, such as sclerotherapy or banding (Wang et al., 2014). Once the balloons are deflated or the tube is removed, the patient must be assessed frequently because of the high risk of recurrent bleeding.

Endoscopic Therapies

In endoscopic sclerotherapy (Fig. 39-9), also referred to as injection sclerotherapy, a sclerosing agent is injected

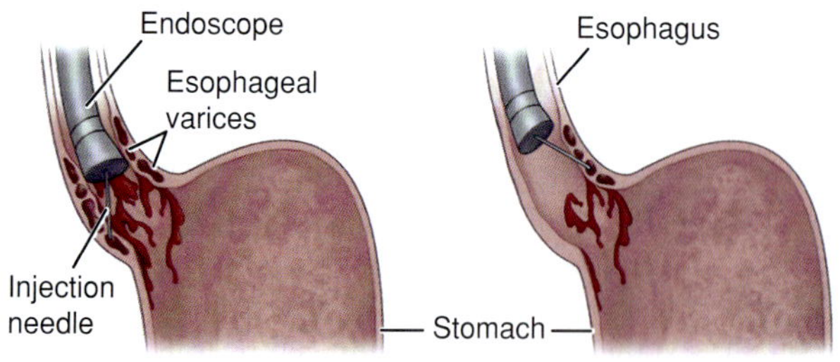

FIGURE 39-9. Endoscopic or injection sclerotherapy. Injection of sclerosing agent into esophageal varices through an endoscope promotes thrombosis and eventual sclerosis, thereby obliterating the varices.

through a fibreoptic endoscope into the bleeding esophageal varices to promote thrombosis and eventual sclerosis. The process of sclerotherapy causes inflammation of the involved vein with eventual thrombosis and loss of the lumen of the vessel. The procedure has been used successfully to treat acute GI hemorrhage but is not recommended for prevention of first and subsequent variceal bleeding episodes where **endoscopic variceal ligation** (EVL), also known as esophageal banding therapy (discussed later), is the first-line treatment (Lee & Moreau, 2015).

After treatment for acute hemorrhage, the patient must be observed for bleeding, perforation of the esophagus, aspiration pneumonia, and esophageal stricture. Antacids, histamine-2 antagonists such as cimetidine, or proton pump inhibitors such as pantoprazole may be administered after the procedure to counteract the chemical effects of the sclerosing agent on the esophagus and the acid reflux associated with the therapy.

Esophageal Banding Therapy (Variceal Band Ligation)

In variceal banding (Fig. 39-10), a modified endoscope loaded with an elastic rubber band is passed through an overtube directly onto the varix (or varices) to be banded. After the bleeding varix is suctioned into the tip of the endoscope, the rubber band is slipped over the tissue, causing necrosis, ulceration, and eventual sloughing of the varix.

Variceal banding is comparable to endoscopic sclerotherapy in its effectiveness in controlling acute bleeding. Compared with sclerotherapy, variceal banding also significantly reduces the rebleeding rate, mortality, procedure-related complications, and the number of sessions needed to eradicate varices. Esophageal band ligation has replaced sclerotherapy as the treatment of choice in the management of esophageal varices. Complications include superficial ulceration and dysphagia, transient chest discomfort, and, rarely, esophageal strictures. Band ligation in combination with pharmacologic therapy may be more effective than monotherapy (i.e., a single mode of therapy) in the treatment of acute hemorrhage. Band litigation is recommended for patients who have experienced variceal bleeding while receiving beta-blocker therapy and for those who cannot tolerate beta-blocking agents (Wang et al., 2014).

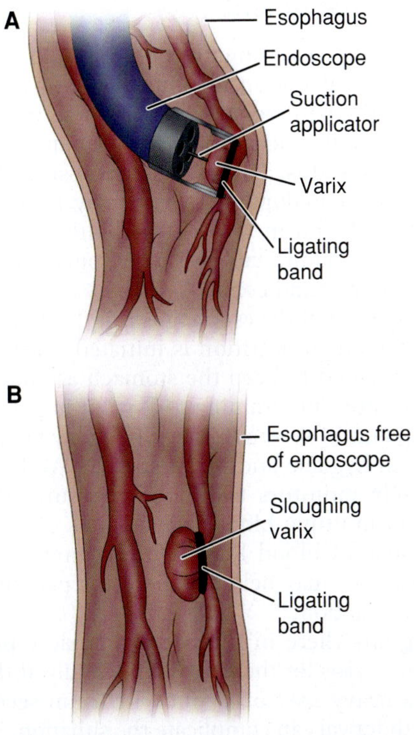

FIGURE 39-10. Esophageal banding. **A.** A rubber band–like ligature is slipped over an esophageal varix via an endoscope. **B.** Necrosis results, and the varix eventually sloughs off.

Transjugular Intrahepatic Portosystemic Shunting

A TIPS procedure (see Fig. 39-7) is indicated for the treatment of an acute episode of variceal bleeding refractory to pharmacologic or endoscopic therapy. In 10% to 20% of patients for whom urgent band ligation or sclerotherapy and medications are not successful in eradicating bleeding, a TIPS procedure can effectively control acute variceal hemorrhage by rapidly lowering portal pressure. TIPS is also indicated for those patients who rebleed after pharmacologic or endoscopic prophylaxis has failed (Lee & Moreau, 2015). In addition, this technique is used as a bridge to liver transplantation. Potential complications include bleeding, sepsis, heart failure, organ perforation, shunt thrombosis, and progressive liver failure.

Additional Therapies

The use of endoscopically placed tissue adhesives and fibrin glue has been successful in the treatment of gastric and esophageal varices. Coated expandable stents (placed via endoscope) have also been used effectively for the same purpose. These developing technologies require further study to determine their role in the management of bleeding esophageal varices (Lee & Moreau, 2015; Liou, 2014).

Surgical Management

Several surgical procedures have been developed to treat esophageal varices and to minimize rebleeding, but these procedures are often accompanied by significant risk. Procedures that may be used for esophageal varices are direct surgical ligation of varices; splenorenal, mesocaval, and portacaval venous shunts to relieve portal pressure; and esophageal transection with devascularization. Use of these procedures is controversial, and studies regarding their effectiveness and outcomes continue. What is known thus far is that these procedures are very effective in controlling variceal bleeding. They may be considered as second-line management (rescue therapy) for those patients for whom all other treatments have failed, those who are not candidates for liver transplantation, and those who require a bridge to transplantation. There is a high incidence of encephalopathy after the surgical shunting procedures, and morbidity and mortality statistics remain high (Lee & Moreau, 2015). The TIPS procedure has largely replaced the use of surgical decompressive shunts and ligation procedures.

Surgical Bypass Procedures

Surgical decompression of the portal circulation can prevent variceal bleeding if the shunt remains patent. Although effective in eradicating bleeding, survival statistics and encephalopathy are worse than other preventative measures such as a TIPS procedure when this method is employed for prophylaxis, and shunt surgery for this purpose has largely been abandoned worldwide (Lee & Moreau, 2015; Nusrat et al., 2014).

One of the various surgical shunting procedures (Fig. 39-11) is the distal splenorenal shunt, which is made between the splenic vein and the left renal vein after splenectomy. A mesocaval shunt is created by anastomosing the superior mesenteric vein to the proximal end of the vena cava or to the side of the vena cava using grafting material. The goal of distal splenorenal and mesocaval shunts is to decrease portal pressure by draining only a portion of venous blood from the portal bed; therefore, they are considered selective shunts. The liver continues to receive some portal flow, and the incidence of encephalopathy may be reduced. Portacaval shunts are considered nonselective shunts because they divert all portal flow to the vena cava via end-to-side or side-to-side approaches.

These procedures are extensive and are not always successful because of secondary thrombosis in the veins used for the shunt and because of complications (e.g., encephalopathy). The effectiveness of these procedures has been studied extensively. All shunt procedures are equally effective in preventing recurrent variceal bleeding but may cause further impairment of liver function and encephalopathy. Partial portacaval shunts with interposition grafts are as effective as other shunts but are associated with a lower rate of encephalopathy (Doherty, 2015; Townsend, Beauchamp, Evers, et al., 2016). The severity of the disease and the potential for future liver transplantation guide the treatment decision. If the cause of portal hypertension is the rare Budd–Chiari syndrome or other venous obstructive disease, a portacaval or a mesoatrial shunt may be performed (see Fig. 39-11). The mesoatrial shunt is required when the infrahepatic vena cava is thrombosed and must be bypassed.

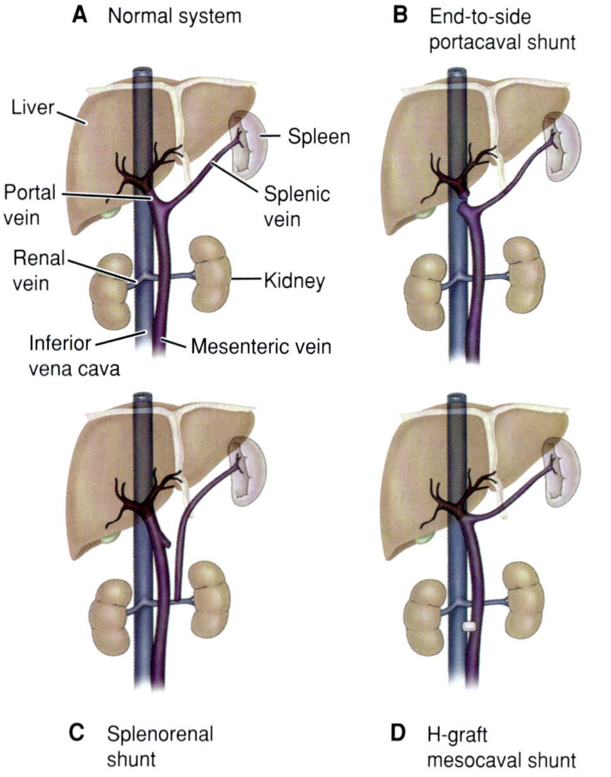

FIGURE 39-11. Portal systemic shunts. **A.** Normal portal system. **B–D.** Examples of portal shunts to reduce portal pressure.

Devascularization and Transection

Devascularization and staple-gun transection procedures to separate the bleeding site from the high-pressure portal system have been used in the emergency management of variceal bleeding. The lower end of the esophagus is reached through a small gastrostomy incision; a staple gun permits anastomosis of the transected ends of the esophagus. Rebleeding is a risk, and the outcomes of these procedures vary among patient populations.

NURSING ALERT

The surgical procedures used to treat esophageal varices do not alter the course of the progressive liver disease, and bleeding may recur as new collateral vessels develop. The risk of complications (hypovolemic or hemorrhagic shock, hepatic encephalopathy, electrolyte imbalance, metabolic and respiratory alkalosis, alcohol withdrawal syndrome, and seizures) is high.

Nursing Management

Overall nursing assessment includes monitoring the patient's physical condition and evaluating emotional responses and cognitive status. The nurse monitors and records vital signs and assesses the patient's nutritional and neurologic status. This assessment assists in identifying hepatic encephalopathy, which may result from the breakdown of blood in the GI tract with a rising serum ammonia level. Manifestations range from drowsiness and confusion to profound coma.

If complete rest of the esophagus is indicated because of bleeding, parenteral nutrition is initiated. Gastric suction usually is initiated to keep the stomach as empty as possible and to prevent straining and vomiting. The patient often complains of severe thirst, which may be relieved by frequent oral hygiene and moist sponges to the lips. The nurse closely monitors the blood pressure. Vitamin K therapy and multiple blood transfusions often are indicated because of blood loss. A quiet environment and calm reassurance may help to relieve the patient's anxiety and reduce agitation.

Bleeding anywhere in the body is anxiety provoking, resulting in a crisis for the patient and family. If the patient has been a heavy user of alcohol, delirium secondary to alcohol withdrawal can complicate the situation. The nurse provides support and explanations about medical and nursing interventions. Close monitoring of the patient helps in detecting and managing complications. Management

TABLE 39-2 Select Modalities and Nursing Care for the Patient With Bleeding Esophageal Varices

Treatment Modality[a]	Nursing Interventions
Nonsurgical Modalities	
Pharmacologic agents	Observe response to therapy.
Propranolol (Inderal)/nadolol (Corgard)	Monitor for side effects: *propranolol* and *nadolol*—decreased pulse pressure, impaired cardiovascular response to hemorrhage; *vasopressin*—angina (nitroglycerin may be prescribed to prevent or treat angina).
Vasopressin (Pitressin)	
Octreotide (Sandostatin)	Support patient during treatment.
Injection sclerotherapy	Observe for aspiration, perforation of the esophagus, and recurrence of bleeding after treatment.
Endoscopic variceal ligation	Observe for recurrence of bleeding, esophageal perforation.
Transjugular intrahepatic portosystemic shunt	Observe for rebleeding and signs of infection.
Balloon tamponade	Explain procedure to patient briefly to obtain cooperation with insertion and maintenance of esophageal/gastric tamponade tube and reduce patient's fear of the procedure. Monitor closely to prevent inadvertent removal or displacement of tube, subsequent airway obstruction, and aspiration. Provide frequent oral hygiene.
Surgical Modalities	
Portal-systemic shunt	Observe for development of portal-systemic encephalopathy (altered mental status, neurologic dysfunction), hepatic failure, and rebleeding. Requires intensive, expert nursing care for prolonged period.
Surgical ligation of varices	Observe for rebleeding.
Esophageal transection and devascularization	Observe for rebleeding. Provide postthoracotomy care.

[a]Several modalities may be used concurrently or in sequence.

Adapted from Feldman, M., Friedman, L. S., & Brandt, L. J. (2015). *Sleisinger & Fordtran's gastrointestinal & liver disease* (10th ed.). Philadelphia, PA: Saunders Elsevier.

modalities and nursing care of the patient with bleeding esophageal varices are summarized in Table 39-2.

Hepatic Encephalopathy and Coma

Hepatic encephalopathy, or portosystemic encephalopathy (PSE), is a life-threatening complication of liver disease that occurs with profound liver failure. Patients with this condition have no overt signs of the illness but do have abnormalities on neuropsychologic testing (Ellul, Gholkar, & Cross, 2015; Lee & Moreau, 2015; Nusrat et al., 2014). Hepatic encephalopathy is the neuropsychiatric manifestation of hepatic failure associated with portal hypertension and the shunting of blood from the portal venous system into the systemic circulation (Ellul et al., 2015; Lee & Moreau, 2015). This reversible metabolic form of encephalopathy can improve with recovery of liver function. The onset is often insidious and subtle, and initially the disease is termed subclinical or minimal hepatic encephalopathy.

Table 39-3 presents the stages of hepatic encephalopathy, common signs and symptoms, and potential nursing diagnoses for each stage.

Pathophysiology

Despite the frequency with which hepatic encephalopathy occurs, the precise pathophysiology is not fully defined (Ellul et al., 2015). Two major alterations underlie its development in acute and chronic liver disease. First,

TABLE 39-3 Stages of Hepatic Encephalopathy and Possible Nursing Priorities

Stage	Clinical Symptoms	Clinical Signs and EEG Changes	Selected Potential Nursing Priority
1	Normal level of consciousness with periods of lethargy and euphoria; reversal of day–night sleep patterns	Asterixis; impaired writing and ability to draw line figures. Normal EEG	Activity intolerance Self-care deficit Disturbed sleep pattern
2	Increased drowsiness; disorientation; inappropriate behaviour; mood swings; agitation	Asterixis; fetor hepaticus. Abnormal EEG with generalized slowing	Social interaction Role performance Injury
3	Stuporous; difficult to rouse; sleeps most of time; marked confusion; incoherent speech	Asterixis; increased deep tendon reflexes; rigidity of extremities. EEG markedly abnormal	Nutrition Mobility Verbal communication
4	Comatose; may not respond to painful stimuli	Absence of asterixis; absence of deep tendon reflexes; flaccidity of extremities. EEG markedly abnormal	Aspiration Gas exchange Tissue integrity Sensory perception

hepatic insufficiency may result in encephalopathy because of the inability of the liver to detoxify toxic byproducts of metabolism. Second, portal-systemic shunting, in which collateral vessels develop as a result of portal hypertension, allows elements of the portal blood (laden with potentially toxic substances usually extracted by the liver) to enter the systemic circulation (Ellul et al., 2015; Lee & Moreau, 2015). Ammonia is considered the major etiologic factor in the development of encephalopathy. It enters the brain and excites peripheral benzodiazepine-type receptors on astrocyte cells, thus increasing neurosteroid synthesis; this then stimulates gamma-aminobutyric acid (GABA) neurotransmission. GABA causes depression of the central nervous system (Ellul et al., 2015; Lee & Moreau, 2015). Ammonia inhibits neurotransmission and synaptic regulation, producing sleep and behaviour patterns associated with hepatic encephalopathy.

Circumstances that increase serum ammonia levels tend to aggravate or precipitate hepatic encephalopathy. The largest source of ammonia is the enzymatic and bacterial digestion of dietary and blood proteins in the GI tract. Ammonia from these sources increases as a result of GI bleeding (i.e., bleeding esophageal varices, chronic GI bleeding), a high-protein diet, bacterial infection, or uremia. The ingestion of ammonium salts also increases the blood ammonia level. In the presence of alkalosis or hypokalemia, increased amounts of ammonia are absorbed from the GI tract and from the renal tubular fluid. Conversely, serum ammonia is decreased by elimination of protein from the diet and by the administration of antibiotic agents, such as neomycin sulfate (which reduce the number of intestinal bacteria capable of converting urea to ammonia (Ellul et al., 2015; Lee & Moreau, 2015).

Other factors unrelated to increased serum ammonia levels that can cause hepatic encephalopathy in susceptible patients include excessive diuresis, dehydration, infections, surgery, fever, and some medications (sedatives, tranquilizers, analgesics, and diuretics that cause potassium loss). Additional causes include elevated levels of serum manganese (Ellul et al., 2015; Romero-Gomez, Mantagnese, & Jalan, 2015) as well as changes in the types of circulating amino acids, mercaptans, and levels of dopamine and other neurotransmitters in the central nervous system. Mercaptans are toxic metabolites of sulphur-containing compounds that are excreted by the liver under normal conditions. Mercaptans and these other so-called "false" neurotransmitters may be generated from an intestinal source or from metabolism of protein by the liver and, with defective hepatic clearance, may precipitate encephalopathy.

Clinical Manifestations

The earliest symptoms of hepatic encephalopathy include minor mental changes and motor disturbances. The patient appears slightly confused and unkempt and has alterations in mood and sleep patterns. The patient tends to sleep during the day and has restlessness and insomnia at night. As hepatic encephalopathy progresses, the patient may become difficult to awaken and completely disoriented with respect to time and place. With further progression, the patient lapses into frank coma and may have seizures.

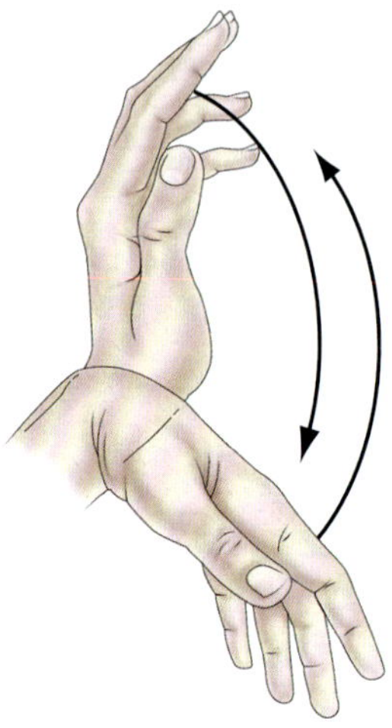

FIGURE 39-12. Asterixis or "liver flap" may occur in hepatic encephalopathy. The patient is asked to hold the arm out with the hand held upward (dorsiflexed). Within a few seconds, the hand falls forward involuntarily and then quickly returns to the dorsiflexed position.

Asterixis (flapping tremor of the hands) may be seen in stage II encephalopathy (Fig. 39-12). Simple tasks, such as handwriting, become difficult. A handwriting or drawing sample (e.g., star figure), taken daily, may provide graphic evidence of progression or reversal of hepatic encephalopathy. Inability to reproduce a simple figure is referred to as **constructional apraxia**. In the early stages of hepatic encephalopathy, the deep tendon reflexes are hyperactive; with worsening of the encephalopathy, these reflexes disappear and the extremities may become flaccid. It is vital for the nurse to understand the four stages of hepatic encephalopathy and common signs and symptoms. These key points, as well as selected nursing priorities, are summarized in Table 39-3.

Occasionally, **fetor hepaticus**, a sweet, slightly fecal odour to the breath that is presumed to be of intestinal origin, may be noticed. The odour has also been described as similar to that of freshly mowed grass, acetone, or old wine. Fetor hepaticus is prevalent with extensive collateral portal circulation in chronic liver disease.

Assessment and Diagnostic Findings

Several diagnostic algorithms and a variety of psychometric tests are used in determining the presence and severity of hepatic encephalopathy. The electroencephalogram shows generalized slowing, an increase in the amplitude of brain waves, and characteristic triphasic waves. The survival rate after a first episode of overt hepatic encephalopathy in patients with cirrhosis is approximately 40% at 1 year. Eligible patients should be referred for liver transplantation after this initial episode (Ellul et al., 2015; Lee & Moreau, 2015; Romero-Gomez et al., 2015).

Medical Management

Medical management focuses on identifying and eliminating the precipitating cause, if possible, initiating ammonia-lowering therapy, minimizing potential medical complications of cirrhosis and depressed consciousness, and reversing the underlying liver disease, if possible.

Correction of the possible reasons for the deterioration such as bleeding, electrolyte abnormalities, sedation, or azotemia is essential (Feldman et al., 2015; Lee & Moreau, 2015). Lactulose (Cephulac) is given to reduce serum ammonia levels. It acts by trapping and expelling the ammonia in the feces (Poordad, 2015; Romero-Gomez et al., 2015). Two or three soft stools per day are desirable; this indicates that lactulose is performing as intended.

NURSING ALERT

The patient receiving lactulose is monitored closely for the development of watery diarrheal stools, because they indicate a medication overdose.

Possible side effects of lactulose include intestinal bloating and cramps, which usually disappear within a week. To mask the sweet taste, which some patients dislike, it can be diluted with fruit juice. The patient is closely monitored for hypokalemia and dehydration. Other laxatives are not prescribed during lactulose administration because their effects disturb dosage regulation. Lactulose may be administered by nasogastric tube or enema for patients who are comatose or for those in whom oral administration is contraindicated or impossible (Poordad, 2015; Romero-Gomez et al., 2015).

Other management strategies include IV administration of glucose to minimize protein breakdown, administration of vitamins to correct deficiencies, and correction of electrolyte imbalances (especially potassium). Antibiotics may also be added to the treatment regimen. Neomycin, metronidazole (Flagyl), and rifaximin (Xifaxan) have been used to reduce levels of ammonia-forming bacteria in the colon. However, no benefit has been shown for long-term treatment with these antibiotics (Poordad, 2015; Romero-Gomez et al., 2015). Additional principles of management of hepatic encephalopathy include the following:

- Neurologic status is assessed frequently.
- Mental status is monitored by keeping a daily record of handwriting and arithmetic performance.
- Fluid intake and output and body weight are recorded each day.
- Vital signs are measured and recorded every 4 hours.
- Potential sites of infection (peritoneum, lungs) are assessed frequently, and abnormal findings are reported promptly.
- Serum ammonia level is monitored daily.
- Protein intake is moderately restricted in patients who are comatose or who have encephalopathy that is refractory to lactulose and antibiotic therapy (Chart 39-6). Long-term restriction of dietary protein to less than 1 g/kg daily should be avoided. If animal protein precipitates encephalopathy, vegetable or dairy proteins may be used as most patients can tolerate a diet of vegetable protein up to 120 g/day.
- Patients and families are advised about foods that are high in protein (e.g., meat, eggs), which may need to be eliminated from the diet for the short term to reduce production of ammonia.

CHART 39-6

Nutritional Management of Hepatic Encephalopathy

- Minimize the formation and absorption of toxins, principally ammonia, from the intestine.
- Keep daily protein intake between 1.2 and 1.5 g/kg body weight per day.
- Avoid protein restriction if possible, even in those with encephalopathy.
- For patients who are truly protein intolerant, provide additional nitrogen in the form of an amino acid supplement. The use of branched-chain amino acids should be a consideration in patients with cirrhosis. It has improved outcomes in varied populations with the disease.
- Provide small, frequent meals and 3 small snacks per day in addition to a late-night snack before bed.

Adapted from Mueller, C. M. (2012). *The A.S.P.E.N. adult nutrition support core curriculum* (2nd ed.). Silver Spring, MD: American Society for Parenteral and Enteral Nutrition; Fialla, A. D., Israelsen, M., Hamberg, O., et al. (2015). Nutritional therapy in cirrhosis or alcoholic hepatitis: A systematic review and meta-analysis. *Liver International*, *35*(9), 2072–2078.

- Enteral feeding is provided for patients whose encephalopathic state persists.
- Reduction in the absorption of ammonia from the GI tract is accomplished by the use of gastric suction, enemas, or oral antibiotics.
- Electrolyte status is monitored and corrected if abnormal.
- Sedatives, tranquilizers, and analgesic medications are discontinued.
- Benzodiazepine antagonists such as flumazenil may be administered to improve encephalopathy. This action may have short-term efficacy because patients with hepatic encephalopathy have an increased concentration of benzodiazepine receptors.

Nursing Management

The nurse is responsible for maintaining a safe environment to prevent injury, bleeding, and infection. The nurse administers the prescribed treatments and monitors the patient for the numerous potential complications. The potential for respiratory compromise is great given the patient's depressed neurologic status. The nurse encourages deep breathing and position changes to prevent the development of atelectasis, pneumonia, and other respiratory complications. Despite aggressive pulmonary care, patients may develop respiratory compromise. They may require intubation and mechanical ventilation to protect the airway, and they are frequently admitted to the ICU.

The nurse communicates with the patient's family to inform them about the patient's status and supports them by explaining the procedures and treatments that are part of the patient's care. If the patient recovers from hepatic encephalopathy and coma, rehabilitation is likely to be prolonged. Therefore, the patient and family will require assistance to understand the causes of this severe complication and to recognize that it may recur.

Promoting Home, Community-Based, and Transitional Care

Educating Patients About Self-Care

If the patient has recovered from hepatic encephalopathy and is to be discharged home, the nurse educates the family about subtle signs of recurrent encephalopathy. The goals for caloric intake and protein intake should be 35 to 40 kcal/kg body weight per day and 1.2 to 1.5 g/kg body weight per day (see Chart 39-6) (Ellul et al., 2015; Poordad, 2015). Protein intake should not be limited too severely, because doing so worsens nutritional status and increases mortality (Ellul et al., 2015; Poordad, 2015). Continued use of lactulose after discharge is not uncommon, and the patient and family should closely monitor its efficacy and side effects. They should also be cautioned that constipation can precipitate encephalopathy and should be prevented through the prescribed use of lactulose, which is crucial in preventing constipation.

Continuing and Transitional Care

Referral for transitional, home, or community-based care is warranted for the patient who returns home after recovery from hepatic encephalopathy. The nurse assesses the patient's physical and mental status and collaborates closely with the physician. The home visit also provides an opportunity for the nurse to assess the home environment and the ability of the patient and family to monitor signs and symptoms and to follow the treatment regimen. It is important to evaluate the patient's fluid volume status and be alert for changes indicative of hypovolemia due to decreased intake and for decreased urine output associated with hepatorenal syndrome. Monitoring of laboratory values continues to be important, and the home care nurse must obtain physician orders to correct abnormalities, especially electrolyte imbalances, which also can worsen encephalopathy.

The safety of the home environment is also assessed closely to identify areas of risk for falls and other injuries. Home care visits are especially important if the patient lives alone because encephalopathy may affect the patient's ability to remember or follow the treatment regimen. The nurse reinforces previous teaching and reminds the patient and family about the importance of dietary restrictions, close monitoring, and follow-up. In addition, the nurse must observe the patient for subtle behaviour changes of worsening hepatic encephalopathy. Patients with all types and stages of hepatic encephalopathy should have periodic neurologic evaluations to determine their cognitive function so that they do not engage in potentially harmful activities. Even subtle neuropsychiatric abnormalities may preclude patients from driving, operating machinery, or participating in other activities that require psychomotor coordination.

Patients and families may need additional education and support during those times that the patient exhibits mood disturbances and sleep disorders. Patients should be as active as possible during the day and develop a normal sleep–wake pattern. Sedating medications should be avoided because they may precipitate encephalopathy. Patients and families may require assistance in developing plans to cope with changes in mood and mental status changes. This plan should identify support persons to attend to the patient in the home situation if needed. Social workers and case managers may make appropriate referrals for assistance with physical and psychosocial support and care. Referrals to other experts such as psychologists, psychiatric liaison nurses, case managers, social workers, or therapists may assist family members with coping. Spiritual advisors may also provide another outlet for communication and guidance. If alcohol played a role in the development of the liver disease and encephalopathy, referral to Alcoholics Anonymous or Al-Anon may provide needed support and education.

Other Manifestations of Hepatic Dysfunction

Edema and Bleeding

Many patients with liver dysfunction develop generalized edema caused by hypoalbuminemia due to decreased hepatic production of albumin. The production of blood clotting factors by the liver is also reduced, leading to an increased incidence of bruising, epistaxis, bleeding from wounds, and, as described previously, GI bleeding. Abnormalities in the number and effectiveness of platelets also contribute to the bleeding in liver dysfunction. Congestion of the spleen secondary to portal hypertension causes increased pooling of platelets in the organ (hypersplenism). The resultant thrombocytopenia generally correlates with spleen size. In patients who are alcoholics, suppression of bone marrow by the acute toxic effects of alcohol or folate deficiency may contribute to the thrombocytopenia (Goldman & Schafer, 2015). These factors predispose patients to easy bruising, petechiae formation, and bleeding from a variety of sources such as the GI or genitourinary tract (Goldman & Schafer, 2015).

Vitamin Deficiency

Decreased production of several clotting factors may be partially due to deficient absorption of vitamin K from the GI tract. This probably is caused by the inability of liver cells to use vitamin K to make prothrombin. Absorption of the other fat-soluble vitamins (vitamins A, D, and E) as well as dietary fats may also be impaired because of decreased secretion of bile salts into the intestine.

Another group of problems common to patients with severe chronic liver dysfunction results from inadequate intake of sufficient vitamins. These include the following:

- Vitamin A deficiency, resulting in night blindness and eye and skin changes
- Thiamine deficiency, leading to beriberi, polyneuritis, and Wernicke–Korsakoff psychosis
- Riboflavin deficiency, resulting in characteristic skin and mucous membrane lesions
- Pyridoxine deficiency, resulting in skin and mucous membrane lesions and neurologic changes
- Vitamin C deficiency, resulting in the hemorrhagic lesions of scurvy
- Vitamin K deficiency, resulting in hypoprothrombinemia, characterized by spontaneous bleeding and ecchymoses
- Folic acid deficiency, resulting in macrocytic anemia

Because of these deficiencies, the diet of every patient with chronic liver disease (especially if alcohol related) should be supplemented with vitamins A, B complex, C, K, and folic acid.

Metabolic Abnormalities

Abnormalities of glucose metabolism also occur; the blood glucose level may be abnormally high shortly after a meal (a diabetic-type glucose tolerance test result), but hypoglycemia may occur during fasting because of decreased hepatic glycogen reserves and decreased gluconeogenesis. Medications must be used cautiously and in reduced dosages because the ability to metabolize medications is decreased in the patient with liver failure.

Many endocrine abnormalities also occur with liver dysfunction because the liver cannot properly metabolize hormones, including androgens and sex hormones. Failure of the damaged liver to inactivate estrogens normally can cause gynecomastia, amenorrhea, testicular atrophy, loss of pubic hair in the male, menstrual irregularities in the female, and other disturbances of sexual function and sex characteristics.

Pruritus and Other Skin Changes

Patients with liver dysfunction resulting from biliary obstruction commonly develop severe pruritus due to retention of bile salts. Patients may develop vascular (or arterial) spider angiomas (see Fig. 39-3) on the skin, usually above the waistline. These are numerous small vessels resembling a spider's legs. They are most often associated with cirrhosis and more advanced liver disease but not always. Patients may also develop reddened palms ("liver palms" or palmar erythema). There is no evidenced based practice on management of pruritus but medications exist that have some success.

VIRAL HEPATITIS

Viral hepatitis is a systemic, viral infection in which necrosis and inflammation of liver cells produce a characteristic cluster of clinical, biochemical, and cellular changes. To date, five definitive types of viral hepatitis have been identified: hepatitis A, B, C, D, and E. Hepatitis A and E are similar in mode of transmission (fecal–oral route), whereas hepatitis B, C, and D share many other characteristics.

Hepatitis is easily transmitted and causes high morbidity and prolonged loss of time from school or employment. In Canada, about 600,000 people are living with hepatitis B virus (HBV) and/or hepatitis C virus (HCV) (Public Health Agency of Canada, 2012). The occurrence rate has been decreasing steadily since 1990, largely because of the use of hepatitis A and B vaccines as well as public health education regarding high-risk behaviours (Dan, Moses-Eisenstein, & Valdiserri, 2015; Goldman & Schafer, 2015). It is estimated that 60% to 90% of viral hepatitis cases go unreported. The occurrence of subclinical cases, failure to recognize mild cases, and misdiagnosis are thought to contribute to the underreporting. Table 39-4 compares the major forms of viral hepatitis.

TABLE 39-4 Comparison of Major Forms of Viral Hepatitis

Previous Names	Hepatitis A Infectious Hepatitis	Hepatitis B Serum Hepatitis	Hepatitis C Non-A, Non-B Hepatitis	Hepatitis D	Hepatitis E
Epidemiology					
Cause	Hepatitis A virus (HAV)	Hepatitis B virus (HBV)	Hepatitis C virus (HCV)	Hepatitis D virus (HDV)	Hepatitis E virus (HEV)
Immunity	*Average:* 30 days Homologous	*Average:* 70–80 days Homologous	*Average:* 50 days Second attack may indicate weak immunity or infection with another agent.	*Average:* 35 days Homologous	*Average:* 31 days Unknown
Nature of Illness					
Signs and symptoms	May occur with or without symptoms; flu-like illness *Preicteric phase:* Headache, malaise, fatigue, anorexia, fever *Icteric phase:* Dark urine, jaundice of sclera and skin, tender liver	May occur without symptoms May develop arthralgias, rash	Similar to HBV; less severe and anicteric	Similar to HBV	Similar to HAV; very severe in pregnant women
Outcome	Usually mild with recovery. No carrier state or increased risk of chronic hepatitis, cirrhosis, or hepatic cancer.	May be severe. Carrier state possible. Increased risk of chronic hepatitis, cirrhosis, and hepatic cancer.	Frequent occurrence of chronic carrier state and chronic liver disease. Increased risk of hepatic cancer.	Similar to HBV but greater likelihood of carrier state, chronic active hepatitis, and cirrhosis	Similar to HAV except very severe in pregnant women

Adapted from Kumar, V., Abbas, A. K., Fausto, N., et al. (2014). *Robbins and Cotran pathologic basis of disease* (9th ed.). Philadelphia, PA: Saunders Elsevier.

Hepatitis A Virus

Hepatitis A virus (HAV) accounts for 20% to 25% of cases of clinical hepatitis in developed countries. Hepatitis A is caused by an RNA virus of the Enterovirus family. Persons at increased risk of HVA include travellers to HVA endemic countries (44% to 55% of reported cases are linked to travel), illicit drug users, men who have sex with men (Public Health Agency of Canada, 2013). Age-specific incidence is highest among those 5 to 9 years old (2.1 per 100,000) followed by those aged 1 to 4 (1.5 per 100,000) (Public Health Agency of Canada, 2013). This form of hepatitis is transmitted primarily through the fecal–oral route, by the ingestion of food or liquids infected by the virus. It is more prevalent in countries with overcrowding and poor sanitation. The virus has been found in the stool of infected patients before the onset of symptoms and during the first few days of illness.

Typically, a child or a young adult acquires the infection at school through poor hygiene, hand-to-mouth contact, or close contact during play. The virus is carried home, where haphazard sanitary habits spread it through the family. An infected food handler can spread the disease, and people can contract it by consuming water or shellfish from sewage-contaminated waters. Outbreaks have occurred in day care centres and institutions as a result of poor hygiene among people with developmental disabilities. Hepatitis A can be transmitted during sexual activity; this is more likely with oral–anal contact or anal intercourse and with multiple sex partners (Dan et al., 2015; Goldman & Schafer, 2015). It is rarely, if ever, transmitted by blood transfusions.

The incubation period is estimated to be between 2 and 6 weeks, with a mean of approximately 4 weeks (CDC, 2013). The illness may be prolonged, lasting 4 to 8 weeks. It usually lasts longer and is more severe in those older than 40 years of age. Most patients recover from hepatitis A; it rarely progresses to acute liver necrosis or fulminant hepatitis resulting in cirrhosis of the liver or death. The mortality rate of hepatitis A is approximately 0.5% for those younger than 40 years of age and 1% to 2% for older people. In patients with underlying chronic liver disease, morbidity and mortality are increased in the presence of an acute hepatitis A infection. No carrier state exists, and no chronic hepatitis is associated with hepatitis A. The virus is present only briefly in the serum; by the time jaundice occurs, the patient is likely to be noninfectious. Although hepatitis A confers immunity against itself, the person may contract other forms of hepatitis.

Clinical Manifestations

Many patients are anicteric (without jaundice) and symptomless. When symptoms appear, they resemble those of a mild, flulike upper respiratory tract infection, with low-grade fever. Anorexia, an early symptom, is often severe. It is thought to result from release of a toxin by the damaged liver or from failure of the damaged liver cells to detoxify an abnormal product. Later, jaundice and dark urine may become apparent. Indigestion is present in varying degrees, marked by vague epigastric distress, nausea, heartburn, and flatulence. The patient may also develop a strong aversion to the taste of cigarettes or the presence of cigarette smoke and other strong odours (Papadakis & McPhee, 2016). These symptoms tend to clear as soon as the jaundice reaches its peak, perhaps 10 days after its initial appearance. Symptoms may be mild in children; in adults, they may be more severe and the course of the disease prolonged.

Assessment and Diagnostic Findings

The liver and spleen are often moderately enlarged for a few days after onset; other than jaundice, there are few other physical signs. Hepatitis A antigen may be found in the stool 7 to 10 days before illness and for 2 to 3 weeks after symptoms appear. HAV antibodies are detectable in the serum, but usually not until symptoms appear. Analysis of subclasses of immunoglobulins can help determine whether the antibody represents acute or past infection.

Prevention

A number of strategies exist to prevent transmission of HAV. Patients and their families are encouraged to follow general precautions that can prevent transmission of the virus (Chart 39-7). Scrupulous handwashing, safe water supplies, and proper control of sewage disposal are just a few of these prevention strategies.

Effective (95% to 100% after two to three doses) and safe HAV vaccines include Havrix and Vaqta (Mandell, Bennett, & Dolin, 2014). It is recommended that the two-dose vaccine be given to adults 18 years of age or older, with the second dose given 6 to 12 months after the first. Protection against hepatitis A develops within several weeks after the first dose of the vaccine. Children and adolescents 2 to 18 years of age receive three doses; the second dose is given 1 month after the first, and the third dose is given 6 to 12 months later. Hepatitis A routine immunization of young children has proved effective in reducing disease incidence and maintaining very low incidence levels among vaccine recipients and across all age groups in many settings (Goldman & Schafer, 2015). Hepatitis A vaccine is recommended for people travelling to locations where sanitation and hygiene are unsatisfactory. Vaccination is also recommended for those from high-risk groups, such as homosexual men, IV or injection drug users, staff of day care centres, and health care personnel. The vaccine has also been used to interrupt community-wide outbreaks. As with other vaccinations, precautions must be taken to ensure prevention, detection, and treatment of hypersensitivity reactions to the vaccine.

For people who have not been previously vaccinated, hepatitis A can be prevented by intramuscular administration of globulin during the incubation period, if given within 2 weeks of exposure. This bolsters the person's antibody production and provides 6 to 8 weeks of passive immunity. Immune globulin may suppress overt symptoms of the disease; the resulting subclinical case of hepatitis A would produce immunity to subsequent episodes of the virus.

Immune globulin is also recommended for household members and sexual contacts of people with hepatitis A. Susceptible people in the same household as the patient are usually also infected by the time the diagnosis is made

CHART 39-7

Health Promotion: Prevention of Hepatitis

Hepatitis A

- Educate patients regarding safe practices for preparing and dispensing food.
- Encourage conscientious individual hygiene.
- Encourage proper community and home sanitation.
- Facilitate mandatory reporting of viral hepatitis to local health departments.
- Promote community health education programs.
- Promote vaccination to interrupt community-wide outbreaks.
- Recommend pre-exposure vaccination for all children 12–23 months of age. Continue existing immunization programs for children 1–18 years of age.
- Recommend vaccination for travellers to developing countries, illegal drug users (injection and noninjection drug users), men who have sex with men, people with chronic liver disease, people who work with HAV-infected animals or work with HAV in research facilities and recipients (e.g., hemophiliacs) of pooled plasma products for clotting factor disorders.
- Support effective health supervision of schools, dormitories, extended care facilities, barracks, and camps.

Hepatitis B

- Advise avoidance of high-risk behaviours.
- Avoid multidose vials in patient care settings.
- Monitor cleaning, disinfection, and sterilization of reusable devices in patient care settings.
- Recommend vaccination for international travellers to regions with high or intermediate levels of endemic hepatitis B virus infection and for persons with chronic liver disease or with human immune deficiency virus infection.
- Recommend vaccination for persons at risk for infection by sexual exposure, by percutaneous or mucosal exposure to blood.
- Recommend vaccination of all infants in the United States regardless of the mother's hepatitis B.
- Use barrier precautions in situations of contact with blood or body fluids.
- Use needleless IV and injection systems in health care.
- Use standard precautions in clinical care.

Hepatitis C

- Advise avoidance of high-risk behaviours such as IV drug use.
- Avoid multidose vials in patient care settings.
- Monitor cleaning, disinfection, and sterilization of reusable devices in patient care settings.
- Use barrier precautions in situations of contact with blood or body fluids.
- Use needleless IV and injection systems in health care.
- Use standard precautions in clinical care.

Adapted from Ferri, F. F. (Ed.). (2014). *Practical guide to the care of the medical patient* (9th ed.). Philadelphia, PA: Mosby Elsevier.

and should receive immune globulin. Institutional contacts of patients with hepatitis A should also receive post-exposure prophylaxis with immune globulin. Prophylaxis is not necessary for casual contacts of an infected person, such as classmates, coworkers, or hospital employees (Dan et al., 2015; Mandell et al., 2014). Although they are rare, systemic reactions to immune globulin do occur. Caution is required when anyone who has previously had angioedema, hives, or other allergic reactions is treated with any human immune globulin. Epinephrine should be available in case of systemic, anaphylactic reaction. The vaccine has also been used to interrupt community-wide outbreaks.

Pre-exposure prophylaxis is recommended for those travelling to developing countries or settings with poor or uncertain sanitation conditions who do not have sufficient time to acquire protection by administration of hepatitis A vaccine (Mandell et al., 2014).

Medical Management

Bed rest during the acute stage and a diet that is both acceptable to the patient and nutritious are part of the treatment and nursing care. During the period of anorexia, the patient should receive frequent small feedings, supplemented if necessary by IV fluids with glucose. Because the patient often has an aversion to food, gentle persistence and creativity may be required to stimulate appetite. Optimal food and fluid levels are necessary to counteract weight loss and to speed recovery. Even before the icteric phase, however, many patients recover their appetites (Chart 39-8).

The patient's sense of well-being and laboratory test results is generally appropriate guides to bed rest and

CHART 39-8

Dietary Management of Hepatitis

- Advise patient to avoid substances (medications, herbs, illicit drugs, and toxins) that may affect liver function, such as St. John's wort in patients taking hepatitis C virus protease inhibitors.
- Be aware that that enteral feedings may be necessary if anorexia, nausea, and vomiting persist.
- Carefully monitor fluid balance.
- Instruct patient to abstain from alcohol during acute illness and for at least 6 months after recovery.
- Provide intake of 25–30 kcal/day.
- Provide protein intake of 1.2–1.5 g/kg/day.
- Recommend small, frequent meals; minimize periods without food intake.

Adapted from Mueller, C. M. (2012). *The A.S.P.E.N. adult nutrition support core curriculum* (2nd ed.). Silver Spring, MD: American Society for Parenteral and Enteral Nutrition; Fialla, A.D., Israelsen, M., Hamberg, et al. (2015). Nutritional therapy in cirrhosis or alcoholic hepatitis: A systematic review and meta-analysis. *Liver International*, *35*(9), 2072–2078.

restriction of physical activity. Gradual but progressive ambulation seems to hasten recovery, provided the patient rests after activity and does not participate in activities to the point of fatigue (Wu, Wu, Lien, et al., 2012).

Nursing Management

Management usually occurs in the home unless symptoms are severe. Therefore, the nurse assists the patient and family in coping with the temporary disability and fatigue that are common in hepatitis and instructs them to seek additional health care if the symptoms persist or worsen. The patient and family also need specific guidelines about diet, rest, follow-up blood work, and the importance of avoiding alcohol, as well as sanitation and hygiene measures (particularly handwashing) to prevent spread of the disease to other family members.

Specific teaching to patients and families about reducing the risk of contracting hepatitis A includes good personal hygiene, stressing careful handwashing (after bowel movements and before eating) and environmental sanitation (safe food and water supply, effective sewage disposal). A combined hepatitis A and B vaccine (Twinrix) is available for vaccination of people 18 years of age and older with indications for both hepatitis A and B vaccination. Vaccination consists of three doses, given on the same schedule as that used for single-antigen hepatitis B vaccine.

Hepatitis B Virus

Unlike HAV, the HBV is transmitted primarily through blood (percutaneous and permucosal routes). HBV can be found in blood, saliva, semen, and vaginal secretions and can be transmitted through mucous membranes and breaks in the skin. HBV is also transferred from carrier mothers to their infants, especially in areas with a high incidence (e.g., Southeast Asia). The infection usually is not transmitted via the umbilical vein but from the mother at the time of birth and during close contact afterward. Hepatitis B rates are not as high in Canada as many places in the world; in 2014 there were 178 new reported cases in Canada (Public Health Agency of Canada, 2014).

HBV has a long incubation period. It replicates in the liver and remains in the serum for relatively long periods, allowing transmission of the virus. Risk factors for HBV infection are summarized in Chart 39-9. Screening of blood donors has greatly reduced the occurrence of hepatitis B after blood transfusion.

Most people (more than 90%) who contract HBV infection develop antibodies and recover spontaneously in 6 months. The mortality rate from hepatitis B has been reported to be as high as 10%. Another 10% of patients who have hepatitis B progress to a carrier state or develop chronic hepatitis with persistent HBV infection and hepatocellular injury and inflammation. It remains a major worldwide cause of cirrhosis and hepatocellular carcinoma (HCC).

Gerontologic Considerations

The older adult patient who contracts hepatitis B has a serious risk of severe liver cell necrosis or **fulminant hepatic failure**, particularly if other illnesses are present.

CHART 39-9

Risk Factors: Hepatitis B

- Close contact with carrier of hepatitis B virus
- Frequent exposure to blood, blood products, or other body fluids
- Health care workers: hemodialysis staff, oncology and chemotherapy nurses, personnel at risk for needlesticks, operating room staff, respiratory therapists, surgeons, dentists
- Hemodialysis
- IV/injection drug use
- Male homosexual and bisexual activity
- Mother-to-child transmission
- Multiple sexual partners
- Receipt of blood or blood products (e.g., clotting factor concentrate)
- Recent history of sexually transmitted infection
- Tattooing
- Travel to or residence in area with uncertain sanitary conditions

Adapted from Bope, E. T., & Kellerman, R. D. (Eds.). (2015). *Conn's current therapy*. Philadelphia, PA: Saunders.

Because the patient is seriously ill and the prognosis is poor, efforts should be undertaken to eliminate other factors (e.g., medications, alcohol) that may affect liver function.

The immune system is altered in the aged. A less responsive immune system may be responsible for the increased incidence and severity of hepatitis B among older people and the increased incidence of liver abscesses secondary to decreased phagocytosis by the Kupffer cells. With the advent of hepatitis B vaccine as the standard for prevention, the incidence of hepatic diseases may decrease in the future.

Clinical Manifestations

Clinically, the disease closely resembles hepatitis A, but the incubation period is much longer (1 to 6 months). Signs and symptoms of hepatitis B may be insidious and variable. Fever and respiratory symptoms are rare; some patients have arthralgias and rashes. The patient may have loss of appetite, dyspepsia, abdominal pain, generalized aching, malaise, and weakness. Jaundice may or may not be evident. If jaundice occurs, light-coloured stools and dark urine accompany it. The liver may be tender and enlarged to 12 to 14 cm vertically. The spleen is enlarged and palpable in a few patients; the posterior cervical lymph nodes may also be enlarged. Subclinical episodes also occur frequently.

Assessment and Diagnostic Findings

HBV is a DNA virus composed of the following antigenic particles:

- HBcAg—hepatitis B core antigen (antigenic material in an inner core)
- HBsAg—hepatitis B surface antigen (antigenic material on the viral surface, a marker of active replication and infection)

- HBeAg—an independent protein circulating in the blood
- HBxAg—gene product of X gene of HBV DNA

Each antigen elicits its specific antibody and is a marker for different stages of the disease process:

- anti-HBc—antibody to core antigen of HBV; persists during the acute phase of illness; may indicate continuing HBV in the liver
- anti-HBs—antibody to surface determinants on HBV; detected during late convalescence; usually indicates recovery and development of immunity
- anti-HBe—antibody to hepatitis B e-antigen; usually signifies reduced infectivity
- anti-HBxAg—antibody to the hepatitis B x-antigen; may indicate ongoing replication of HBV

HBsAg appears in the circulation in 80% to 90% of infected patients 1 to 10 weeks after exposure to HBV and 2 to 8 weeks before the onset of symptoms or an increase in transferase levels. Patients with HBsAg that persists for 6 months or longer after acute infection are considered to be HBsAg carriers (McMahon, 2014). HBeAg is the next antigen of HBV to appear in the serum. It usually appears within 1 week of the appearance of HBsAg but before changes in aminotransferase levels; it disappears from the serum within 2 weeks. HBV DNA, detected by polymerase chain reaction testing, appears in the serum at about the same time as HBeAg. HBcAg is not always detected in the serum in HBV infection.

Prevaccination screening for anti-HBs is not recommended except for high-risk adults who may have already been exposed to the disease. According to the government of Canada in 2014, there were 4,058 cases of chronic HBV reported in addition to a total of 178 cases of acute hepatitis B.

Prevention

Preventing Transmission

Continued screening of blood donors for the presence of hepatitis B antigens further decreases the risk of transmission by blood transfusion. The use of disposable syringes, needles, and lancets and the introduction of needleless IV administration systems have reduced the risk of spreading this infection from one patient to another or to health care personnel during the collection of blood samples or the administration of parenteral therapy. Good personal hygiene is fundamental to infection control. In the clinical laboratory, work areas should be disinfected daily. Gloves are worn when handling all blood and body fluids, as well as HBAg-positive specimens, or when there is potential exposure to blood (e.g., blood drawing) or to patients' secretions. Eating and smoking are prohibited in the laboratory and in other areas exposed to secretions, blood, or blood products. Patient education regarding the nature of the disease, its infectiousness, and prognosis is a critical factor in preventing transmission and protecting contacts.

Active Immunization: Hepatitis B Vaccine

Universal childhood vaccination for hepatitis B prevention has been instituted in all provinces and territories of Canada. The age at vaccination differs across regions but occurs most commonly in fourth grade. The efficacy of the vaccine (98% in childhood) declines with age. Active immunization is recommended for people who are at high risk for hepatitis B (e.g., health care personnel, hemodialysis patients). In addition, people with hepatitis C and other chronic liver diseases should receive the vaccine. A yeast-recombinant hepatitis B vaccine (Recombivax HB) is used to provide active immunity and has shown rates of protection greater than 90% in healthy people (Chan, Wong, Qin, et al., 2016; Dan et al., 2015; Mandell et al., 2014). Although antibody levels may become low or undetectable, immunologic memory may remain intact for at least 5 to 10 years. Measurable levels of antibodies may not be essential for protection. In general, in those with normal immune systems, booster doses are not required, and no data support the use of booster doses of hepatitis B vaccine among immunocompetent people who have responded to the vaccination series. However, booster doses are recommended for people who are immunocompromised (Chan et al., 2016; Mandell et al., 2014). Additional information is required to determine if booster injections are needed for adults 15 years or more after initial vaccination as well as those at high risk for HBV infection.

A hepatitis B vaccine prepared from plasma of humans chronically infected with HBV is used only rarely in patients who are immunodeficient or allergic to recombinant yeast-derived vaccines.

Both forms of the hepatitis B vaccine are administered intramuscularly in three doses; the second and third doses are given 1 and 6 months, respectively, after the first dose. The third dose is very important in producing prolonged immunity. Hepatitis B vaccination should be administered to adults in the deltoid muscle. Antibody response may be measured by anti-HBs levels 1 to 3 months after completion of the basic course of vaccine, but this testing is not routine and is not currently recommended. People who do not respond may benefit from one to three additional doses (Mandell et al., 2014).

People who are at high risk, including nurses and other health care personnel exposed to blood or blood products, should receive active immunization. Health care workers who have had frequent contact with blood are screened for anti-HBs to determine whether immunity is already present from previous exposure. The vaccine produces active immunity to HBV in 90% of healthy people (Dan et al., 2015). It does not provide protection to those already exposed to HBV, and it provides no protection against other types of viral hepatitis. Side effects of immunization are infrequent; soreness and redness at the injection site are the most common complaints.

Because hepatitis B infection is frequently transmitted sexually, hepatitis B vaccination is recommended for all unvaccinated people being evaluated for a sexually transmitted infection (STI). It is also recommended for those with a history of an STI, people with multiple sex partners, people who have sex with IV or injection drug users, and sexually active men who have sex with other men (Dan et al., 2015; Feldman et al., 2015; Mandell et al., 2014; Public Health Agency of Canada, 2013).

Universal childhood vaccination for hepatitis B prevention has been instituted in Canada, and universal vaccination of all infants is encouraged. Catch-up vaccination is recommended for all children and prepubertal adolescents up to the age of 19 years who have not been previously immunized (Public Health Agency of Canada, 2013). Development of chronic carrier states has not been reported in adult responders to the vaccine.

Passive Immunity: Hepatitis B Immune Globulin

Hepatitis B immune globulin (HBIG) provides passive immunity to hepatitis B and is indicated for people exposed to HBV who have never had hepatitis B and have never received hepatitis B vaccine. Specific indications for postexposure vaccine with HBIG include (1) inadvertent exposure to HBAg-positive blood through percutaneous (needlestick) or transmucosal (splashes in contact with mucous membrane) routes, (2) sexual contact with people positive for HBAg, and (3) perinatal exposure (infants born to HBV-infected mothers should receive HBIG within 12 hours after delivery). HBIG is prepared from plasma selected for high titers of anti-HBs. Prompt immunization with HBIG (within hours to a few days after exposure to hepatitis B) increases the likelihood of protection. Both active and passive immunization are recommended for people who have been exposed to hepatitis B through sexual contact or through the percutaneous or transmucosal routes. If HBIG and hepatitis B vaccine are administered at the same time, separate sites and separate syringes should be used. There has been no evidence that human immunodeficiency virus (HIV) infection can be transmitted by HBIG (Chan et al., 2016).

Medical Management

The goals of treatment are to minimize infectivity and liver inflammation and decrease symptoms. Of all the agents that have been used to treat chronic type B viral hepatitis, alpha-interferon as the single modality of therapy that offers the most promise. A regimen of 5 million units daily or 10 million units three times weekly for 16 to 24 weeks results in remission of disease in approximately one third of patients (Chan et al., 2016; Ferri, 2014; Ghaziani, Sendi, Shahraz, et al., 2014). A prolonged course of treatment may also have additional benefits and is currently under study. Interferon must be administered by injection and has significant side effects, including fever, chills, anorexia, nausea, myalgias, and fatigue. Delayed side effects are more serious and may necessitate dosage reduction or discontinuation. These include bone marrow suppression, thyroid dysfunction, alopecia, and bacterial infections. Several recombinant forms of alpha-interferon are also available, including the pegylated form, with once-weekly dosing (Ferri, 2014).

Two antiviral agents, entecavir (ETV) and tenofovir (TDF), which are oral nucleoside analogs, have been approved for use in chronic hepatitis B in the United States. They are the currently recommended agents for patients with HBV-related decompensated cirrhosis. Either of these agents may be indicated for use in combination with peginterferon (Cholongitas, Tziomalos, & Pipili, 2015; Govan, Wu, Xin, et al., 2015). Studies have revealed improved seroconversion rates and loss of detectable virus, improved liver function, and reduced progression to cirrhosis with ETV and TDF. These agents can also be used for patients with decompensated cirrhosis who are awaiting liver transplantation (Chan et al., 2016; Cholongitas et al., 2015; Ferri, 2014). Patients with decompensated cirrhosis have such severely damaged liver parenchyma that normal liver function severely deteriorates, resulting in life-threatening ascites, encephalopathy, or variceal hemorrhage (Chan et al., 2016; Feldman et al., 2015).

Bed rest may be recommended, regardless of other treatment, until the symptoms of hepatitis have subsided. Activities are restricted until the hepatic enlargement and levels of serum bilirubin and liver enzymes have decreased. Gradually increased activity is then allowed.

Adequate nutrition should be maintained. Proteins are restricted if symptoms indicate that the liver's ability to metabolize protein byproducts is impaired. Measures to control the dyspeptic symptoms and general malaise include the use of antacids and antiemetics, but all medications should be avoided if vomiting occurs. If vomiting persists, the patient may require hospitalization and fluid therapy. Because of the mode of transmission, the patient is evaluated for other bloodborne diseases (e.g., HIV infection).

Nursing Management

Convalescence may be prolonged, with complete symptomatic recovery sometimes requiring 3 to 4 months or longer. During this stage, gradual resumption of physical activity is encouraged after the jaundice has resolved.

The nurse identifies psychosocial issues and concerns, particularly the effects of separation from family and friends if the patient is hospitalized during the acute and infective stages. Even if not hospitalized, the patient will be unable to work and must avoid sexual contact. Planning is required to minimize social isolation. Planning that includes the family helps to reduce their fears and anxieties about the spread of the disease.

Promoting Home, Community-Based, and Transitional Care

EDUCATING PATIENTS ABOUT SELF-CARE. Because of the prolonged period of convalescence, the patient and family must be prepared for home care. Provision for adequate rest and nutrition must be ensured. The nurse informs family members and friends who have had intimate contact with the patient about the risks of contracting hepatitis B and makes arrangements for them to receive hepatitis B vaccine or hepatitis B immune globulin as prescribed. Those at risk must be made aware of the early signs of hepatitis B and of ways to reduce risk by avoiding all modes of transmission. Patients with all forms of hepatitis should avoid drinking alcohol and eating raw shellfish.

Continuing Care and Transitional Care

Follow-up visits by a transitional or home care nurse may be needed to assess the patient's progress and answer family members' questions about disease transmission. During a home visit, the nurse assesses the patient's physical and psychological status and confirms that the patient and family understand the importance of adequate rest and nutrition. The nurse also reinforces previous instructions. Because of the risk of transmission through sexual intercourse, strategies to prevent exchange of body fluids are recommended, such as abstinence or the use of condoms. The nurse emphasizes the importance of keeping follow-up appointments and participating in other health promotion activities and recommended health screenings.

Hepatitis C Virus

A significant proportion of cases of viral hepatitis are neither hepatitis A, hepatitis B, nor hepatitis D, and are classified as hepatitis C. Whereas blood transfusions and sexual contact once accounted for most cases of hepatitis C in the United States, other parenteral means, such as sharing of contaminated needles by IV or injection drug users and unintentional needlesticks and other injuries in health care workers now account for a significant number of cases. About 250,000 people in Canada (0.8% of the population) are infected with the HCV, making it the most common chronic bloodborne infection nationally. However, it is difficult to fully ascertain rates as there is not a universal reporting of hepatitis C in Canada in relation to acute and chronic states; the reporting guidance is evolving to allow for better information (Public Health Agency of Canada, 2014). The highest prevalence of hepatitis C is in males over the age of 40 years. HCV is the underlying cause of about one third of cases of HCC, and it is the most common reason for liver transplantation (Public Health Agency of Canada, 2014).

People who are at particular risk for hepatitis C include IV or injection drug users, sexually active people with multiple partners, patients receiving frequent transfusions, those who require large volumes of blood, and health care personnel (Chart 39-10).

The incubation period is variable and may range from 15 to 160 days. The clinical course of acute hepatitis C is similar to that of hepatitis B; symptoms are usually mild. However, a chronic carrier state occurs frequently, and there is an increased risk of chronic liver disease, including cirrhosis or liver cancer, after hepatitis C. Small amounts of alcohol taken regularly appear to cause progression of the disease. Therefore, alcohol and medications that may affect the liver should be avoided.

There is no benefit from rest, diet, or vitamin supplements. A combination of two antiviral agents, peginterferon and ribavirin (Rebetol), was effective in producing improvement in patients with hepatitis C and in treating relapses (Papadakis & McPhee, 2016). In the United States, this combination therapy was the standard treatment beginning in 2001. However, this treatment regimen is no longer employed in the United States for most genotypes of HCV since new antivirals agents are now recommended. Simeprevir (Olysio) plus sofosbuvir (Sovaldi), ledipasvir-sofosbuvir (Harvoni) and ombitasvir-paritaprevir-ritonavir packaged with dasabuvir (Viekira Pak) have fewer side effects, shorter treatment durations and higher cure rates than the previously recommended antiviral agents (Chan et al., 2016; Dan et al., 2015). Peginterferon (Pegasys) and ribavirin are now used only for genotype 5 HCV and in countries which have not approved the newest antiviral drugs (American Association for the Study of Liver Diseases [AASLD], 2014; Dan et al., 2015). There are HCV treatments in development that are expected to be more effective in curing the disease and better tolerated with fewer adverse effects and contraindications (Dan et al., 2015). As a result of the rapidly changing landscape for treatment of viral infections, it is important to monitor related websites for the most up-to-date recommendations (AASLD, 2014).

Screening of blood has reduced the incidence of hepatitis C associated with blood transfusion, and public health programs are helping to reduce the number of cases associated with shared needles in IV or injection drug use.

CHART 39-10

Risk Factors: Hepatitis C

- Children born to women infected with hepatitis C virus
- Health care and public safety workers after needlestick injuries or mucosal exposure to blood
- Multiple contacts with a hepatitis C virus–infected person
- Multiple sex partners, history of sexually transmitted infection, unprotected sex
- Past/current illicit IV/injection drug use
- Recipient of blood products or organ transplant before 1992 or clotting factor concentrates before 1987

Adapted from Kumar, V., Abbas, A. K., Fausto, N., et al. (2014). *Robbins and Cotran pathologic basis of disease* (9th ed.). Philadelphia, PA: Saunders Elsevier.

Hepatitis D Virus

Hepatitis D virus (delta agent) infection occurs in some cases of hepatitis B. Because the virus requires hepatitis B surface antigen for its replication, only people with hepatitis B are at risk for hepatitis D. Anti-delta antibodies in the presence of HBAg on testing confirm the diagnosis. Hepatitis D is common among IV or injection drug users, hemodialysis patients, and recipients of multiple blood transfusions. Sexual contact with those with hepatitis B is considered to be an important mode of transmission of hepatitis B and D. The incubation period varies between 30 and 150 days (Feldman et al., 2015).

The symptoms of hepatitis D are similar to those of hepatitis B, except that patients are more likely to develop fulminant hepatitis and to progress to chronic active hepatitis and cirrhosis. Treatment is similar to that of other forms of hepatitis; interferon as a specific treatment for hepatitis D is under investigation.

Hepatitis E Virus

It is believed that hepatitis E virus (HEV) is transmitted by the fecal–oral route, principally through contaminated water in areas with poor sanitation. The incubation period is variable, estimated to range between 15 and 65 days. In general, hepatitis E resembles hepatitis A. It has a self-limited course with an abrupt onset. Jaundice is almost always present. Chronic forms do not develop.

Avoiding contact with the virus through good hygiene, including handwashing, is the major method of prevention of hepatitis E. The effectiveness of immune globulin in protecting against HEV is uncertain.

Hepatitis G Virus and GB Virus-C

It has long been believed that there is another non-A–E agent causing hepatitis in humans. The incubation period for posttransfusion hepatitis is 14 to 145 days, too long for hepatitis B or C. In the United States, about 5% of chronic liver disease remains cryptogenic (i.e., does not appear to be autoimmune or viral in origin), and 50% of these patients have received blood transfusions before developing disease. Therefore, another form of hepatitis, called hepatitis G virus (HGV) or GB virus-C (GBV-C), has been described; these are thought to be two different isolates of the same virus. Autoantibodies are absent.

The clinical significance of this virus remains uncertain. Risk factors are similar to those for hepatitis C. There is no clear relationship between HGV/GBV-C infection and progressive liver disease. Persistent infection does occur but does not affect the clinical course.

NONVIRAL HEPATITIS

Certain chemicals have toxic effects on the liver and produce acute liver cell necrosis or toxic hepatitis when inhaled, injected parenterally, or are taken by mouth. The chemicals most commonly implicated in this disease are carbon tetrachloride, phosphorus, chloroform, and gold compounds. These substances are true hepatotoxins. Many medications can induce hepatitis but are only sensitizing rather than toxic. Drug-induced hepatitis is similar to acute viral hepatitis, but parenchymal destruction tends to be more extensive. Medications that can lead to hepatitis include isoniazid, halothane, acetaminophen, methyldopa, and certain antibiotics, antimetabolites, and anesthetic agents. Autoimmune hepatitis is a nonviral form of hepatitis where the body's immune system begins attacking the liver causing inflammation and cellular damage.

Toxic Hepatitis

At the onset of disease, toxic hepatitis resembles viral hepatitis. Obtaining a history of exposure to hepatotoxic chemicals, medications, botanical agents, or other toxic agents assists in early treatment and removal of the causative agent. Anorexia, nausea, and vomiting are the usual symptoms; jaundice and hepatomegaly are noted on physical assessment. Symptoms are more intense for the more severely toxic patient.

Recovery from acute toxic hepatitis is rapid if the hepatotoxin is identified early and removed or if exposure to the agent has been limited. Recovery is unlikely if there is a prolonged period between exposure and onset of symptoms. There are no effective antidotes. The fever rises; the patient becomes toxic and prostrated. Vomiting may be persistent, with the emesis containing blood. Clotting abnormalities may be severe, and hemorrhages may appear under the skin. The severe GI symptoms may lead to vascular collapse. Delirium, coma, and seizures develop, and within a few days the patient may die of fulminant hepatic failure (discussed later) unless he or she receives a liver transplant.

Short of liver transplantation, few treatment options are available. Therapy is directed toward restoring and maintaining fluid and electrolyte balance, blood replacement, and comfort and supportive measures. A few patients recover from acute toxic hepatitis only to develop chronic liver disease. If the liver heals, there may be scarring, followed by postnecrotic cirrhosis.

Drug-Induced Hepatitis

Drug-induced liver disease is the most common cause of acute liver failure, accounting for more than 50% of all cases in the United States (Lancaster, Hiatt, & Zarrinpar, 2015; Singanayagam & Bernal, 2015). Manifestations of sensitivity to a medication may occur on the first day of its use or not until several months later. Usually, the onset is abrupt, with chills, fever, rash, pruritus, arthralgia, anorexia, and nausea. Later, there may be jaundice, dark urine, and an enlarged and tender liver. After the offending medication is withdrawn, symptoms may gradually subside. However, reactions can be severe, or even fatal, even if the medication is stopped. If fever, rash, or pruritus occurs from any medication, its use should be stopped immediately.

Although any medication can affect liver function, use of acetaminophen (found in many over-the-counter medications used to treat fever and pain) has been identified as the leading cause of acute liver failure (Lancaster et al., 2015; Singanayagam & Bernal, 2015). Other mechanisms commonly associated with liver injury include many anesthetic agents, medications used to treat rheumatic and musculoskeletal disease, antidepressants, psychotropic medications, anticonvulsants, and antituberculosis agents (Whitehouse & Wendon, 2013).

A short course of high-dose corticosteroids may be used in patients with severe hypersensitivity reactions, although its efficacy is uncertain. Liver transplantation is an option for drug-induced hepatitis, but outcomes may not be as successful as with other causes of liver failure.

FULMINANT HEPATIC FAILURE

Fulminant hepatic failure is the clinical syndrome of sudden and severely impaired liver function in a previously healthy person. According to the original and generally accepted definition, fulminant hepatic failure develops within 8 weeks after the first symptoms of jaundice (Feldman et al., 2015; Singanayagam & Bernal, 2015).

Patterns of the progression from jaundice to encephalopathy have been identified and have led to proposals of time-based classifications. However, no agreement as to these classifications has been reached. Three categories are frequently cited: hyperacute, acute, and subacute liver failure. In hyperacute liver failure, the duration of jaundice before the onset of encephalopathy is 0 to 7 days; in acute liver failure, it is 8 to 28 days; and in subacute liver failure, it is 28 to 72 days. The prognosis for fulminant hepatic failure is much worse than for chronic liver failure. However, in fulminant failure, the hepatic lesion is potentially reversible, and survival rates are approximately 20% to 50%, depending greatly on the cause of liver failure. Those who do not survive die of massive hepatocellular injury and necrosis (Feldman et al., 2015; Singanayagam & Bernal, 2015).

Viral hepatitis is a common cause of fulminant hepatic failure; other causes include toxic medications (e.g., acetaminophen) and chemicals (e.g., carbon tetrachloride), metabolic disturbances (e.g., Wilson's disease, a hereditary syndrome with deposition of copper in the liver), and structural changes (e.g., Budd–Chiari syndrome, an obstruction to outflow in major hepatic veins) (Whitehouse & Wendon, 2013).

Jaundice and profound anorexia may be the initial reasons the patient seeks health care. Fulminant hepatic failure is often accompanied by coagulation defects, renal failure and electrolyte disturbances, cardiovascular abnormalities, infection, hypoglycemia, encephalopathy, and cerebral edema (Whitehouse & Wendon, 2013).

The key to optimized treatment is rapid recognition of acute liver failure and intensive intervention. Supporting the patient in the ICU and assessing the indications for and feasibility of liver transplantation are hallmarks of management of this population. The use of antidotes for certain conditions may be indicated such as *N*-acetylcysteine for acetaminophen toxicity and penicillin for mushroom poisoning. Treatment modalities may include plasma exchanges (plasmapheresis) to correct coagulopathy and to stabilize the patient awaiting liver transplantation and prostaglandin therapy to enhance hepatic blood flow; however, more clinical trials are needed to determine the effects or outcomes of these treatments (Feldman et al., 2015; Siddiqui & Stravitz, 2014; Singanayagam & Bernal, 2015). Hepatocytes within synthetic fibre columns have been tested as liver support systems (liver assist devices) to provide a bridge to transplantation.

Research into interventions for acute liver failure has begun to focus on techniques that combine the efficacy of a whole liver with the convenience and biocompatibility of hemodialysis. The acronyms ELAD (*e*xtracorporeal *l*iver *a*ssist *d*evices) and BAL (*b*io*a*rtificial *l*iver) have been used to describe these hybrid devices. These short-term devices, which remain experimental, may help patients survive until transplantation is possible. The BAL device exposes separated plasma to a cartridge containing porcine liver cells after the plasma has flowed through a charcoal column that removes substances toxic to hepatocytes. The ELAD exposes whole blood to cartridges containing human hepatoblastoma cells, resulting in removal of toxic substances. In the near future, similar extracorporeal circuits using **xenografts** may be studied as a bridge to liver transplantation. These approaches appear promising and have had success in animal studies. In human clinical application, the use of various BAL systems has resulted in improved neurologic and biochemical parameters. Adding albumin to the dialysate is effective in removing protein-bound toxins and is potentially useful in unstable patients with fulminant liver failure (Banares, Catalina, & Vaquero, 2014; Papadakis & McPhee, 2016; Romero-Gomez et al., 2015; Singanayagam & Bernal, 2015).

In patients who have fulminant liver failure with stage 4 encephalopathy, there is a high risk of cerebral edema, a life-threatening complication. The cause is not fully understood, although disruption of the blood–brain barrier and plasma leakage into the cerebrospinal fluid may be one cause. An increase in the intracellular osmolarity within cerebral astrocyte cells, possibly related to increased sodium and glutamine in these cells, may be another (Singanayagam & Bernal, 2015). These patients require intracranial pressure monitoring. Measures to promote adequate cerebral perfusion include careful fluid balance and hemodynamic assessments, a quiet environment, and diuresis with mannitol, an osmotic diuretic.

The use of pharmacologic neuromuscular blockade (NMB) and sedation is indicated to prevent surges in intracranial pressure related to agitation. Other support measures include monitoring for and treating hypoglycemia, coagulopathies, and infection. Despite these treatment modalities, the mortality rate remains high. Consequently, liver transplantation (discussed later) has become the treatment of choice for fulminant hepatic failure.

HEPATIC CIRRHOSIS

Cirrhosis is a chronic disease characterized by replacement of normal liver tissue with diffuse fibrosis that disrupts the structure and function of the liver. There are three types of cirrhosis or scarring of the liver:

- Alcoholic cirrhosis, in which the scar tissue characteristically surrounds the portal areas. This is most frequently caused by chronic alcoholism and is the most common type of cirrhosis.
- Postnecrotic cirrhosis, in which there are broad bands of scar tissue. This is a late result of a previous bout of acute viral hepatitis.
- Biliary cirrhosis, in which scarring occurs in the liver around the bile ducts. This type of cirrhosis usually results from chronic biliary obstruction and infection (cholangitis); it is much less common than the other two types.

The portion of the liver chiefly involved in cirrhosis consists of the portal and the periportal spaces, where the bile canaliculi of each lobule communicate to form the liver bile ducts. These areas become the sites of inflammation, and the bile ducts become occluded with inspissated (thickened) bile and pus. The liver attempts to form new bile channels; hence, there is an overgrowth of tissue made up largely of disconnected, newly formed bile ducts and surrounded by scar tissue.

Pathophysiology

Although several factors have been implicated in the etiology of cirrhosis, alcohol consumption is considered the major causative factor. Cirrhosis occurs with greatest frequency among people with alcoholism. Although nutritional deficiency with reduced protein intake contributes to liver destruction in cirrhosis, excessive alcohol intake is the major causative factor in fatty liver and its consequences. However, cirrhosis has also occurred in people who do not consume alcohol and in those who consume a normal diet and have a high alcohol intake.

Some people appear to be more susceptible than others to this disease, whether or not they have alcoholism or are malnourished. Other factors may play a role, including exposure to certain chemicals (carbon tetrachloride, chlorinated naphthalene, arsenic, or phosphorus) or infectious schistosomiasis. Twice as many men as

TABLE 39-5 Modified Child–Pugh Classification of the Severity of Liver Disease[a]

Parameter	Points Assigned 1	2	3
Ascites	Absent	Slight	Moderate
Bilirubin (mg/dL)	≤2	2–3	>3
Albumin (g/dL)	>3.5	2.8–3.5	<2.8
Prothrombin time (seconds over control)	1–3	4–6	>6
Encephalopathy	None	Grade 1–2	Grade 3–4

Total score of 5–6, grade A; 7–9, grade B; 10–15, grade C.

Adapted from Feldman, M., Friedman, L. S., & Brandt, L. J. (2015). *Sleisinger & Fordtran's gastrointestinal & liver disease* (10th ed.). Philadelphia, PA: Saunders Elsevier.

women are affected, although, for unknown reasons, women are at greater risk for development of alcohol-induced liver disease. Most patients are between 40 and 60 years of age.

Alcoholic cirrhosis is characterized by episodes of necrosis involving the liver cells, which sometimes occur repeatedly throughout the course of the disease. The destroyed liver cells are gradually replaced by scar tissue. Eventually, the amount of scar tissue exceeds that of the functioning liver tissue. Islands of residual normal tissue and regenerating liver tissue may project from the constricted areas, giving the cirrhotic liver its characteristic hobnail appearance. The disease usually has an insidious onset and a protracted course, occasionally proceeding over a period of 30 or more years.

The prognoses for different forms of cirrhosis caused by various liver diseases have been investigated in several studies. Of the many prognostic indicators, the Child–Pugh classification seems most useful in predicting the outcome of patients with liver disease (Table 39-5). It is also used in choosing management approaches.

Clinical Manifestations

Signs and symptoms of cirrhosis increase in severity as the disease progresses. Their severity is used to categorize the disorder as compensated or decompensated cirrhosis (Chart 39-11). Compensated cirrhosis, with its less severe, often vague symptoms, may be discovered secondarily at a routine physical examination. The hallmarks of decompensated cirrhosis result from failure of the liver to synthesize proteins, clotting factors, and other substances and manifestations of portal hypertension (see earlier sections of this chapter for clinical manifestations and management of portal hypertension, ascites, varices, and hepatic encephalopathy).

Liver Enlargement

Early in the course of cirrhosis, the liver tends to be large, and the cells are loaded with fat. The liver is firm and has a sharp edge that is noticeable on palpation. Abdominal pain may be present because of recent, rapid enlargement of the liver, which produces tension on the fibrous covering of the liver (Glisson's capsule). Later in the disease, the liver decreases in size as scar tissue contracts the liver tissue. The liver edge, if palpable, is nodular.

Portal Obstruction and Ascites

Portal obstruction and ascites, late manifestations of cirrhosis, are caused partly by chronic failure of liver function and partly by obstruction of the portal circulation. Almost all of the blood from the digestive organs is collected in the portal veins and carried to the liver. Because a cirrhotic liver does not allow free blood passage, blood backs up into the spleen and the GI tract, and these organs become the seat of chronic passive congestion; that is, they are stagnant with blood and therefore cannot function properly. Indigestion and altered bowel function result. Fluid rich in protein may accumulate in the peritoneal cavity, producing ascites. This can be detected through percussion for shifting dullness or a fluid wave (see Fig. 39-6).

Infection and Peritonitis

Bacterial peritonitis may develop in patients with cirrhosis and ascites in the absence of an intra-abdominal source of infection or an abscess. This condition is referred to as spontaneous bacterial peritonitis (SBP). Bacteremia due to translocation of intestinal flora is believed to be the most likely route of infection. Clinical signs may be absent, necessitating paracentesis for diagnosis. Antibiotic therapy is effective in the treatment and prevention of recurrent episodes of SBP. The most severe complication of SBP is hepatorenal syndrome, a form of renal failure unresponsive

CHART 39-11

Assessment: Assessing for Cirrhosis

Be alert for the following signs and symptoms:

Compensated

- Intermittent mild fever
- Vascular spiders
- Palmar erythema (reddened palms)
- Unexplained epistaxis
- Ankle edema
- Vague morning indigestion
- Flatulent dyspepsia
- Abdominal pain
- Firm, enlarged liver
- Splenomegaly

Decompensated

- Ascites
- Jaundice
- Weakness
- Muscle wasting
- Weight loss
- Continuous mild fever
- Clubbing of fingers
- Purpura (due to decreased platelet count)
- Spontaneous bruising
- Epistaxis
- Hypotension
- Sparse body hair
- White nails
- Gonadal atrophy

Adapted from Lee, S. S., & Moreau, R. (2015). *Cirrhosis: A practical guide to management* (1st ed.). Hoboken, NJ: John Wiley & Sons, Ltd.

to administration of fluid or diuretics. This type of renal failure is characterized by a lack of pathologic changes in the kidney; there is no evidence of dehydration or obstruction of the urinary tract or any other renal disorder.

Gastrointestinal Varices

The obstruction to blood flow through the liver caused by fibrotic changes also results in the formation of collateral blood vessels in the GI system and shunting of blood from the portal vessels into blood vessels with lower pressures. As a result, the patient with cirrhosis often has prominent, distended abdominal blood vessels, which are visible on abdominal inspection (caput medusae) and distended blood vessels throughout the GI tract. The esophagus, stomach, and lower rectum are common sites of collateral blood vessels. These distended blood vessels form varices or hemorrhoids, depending on their location (see Fig. 39-8).

Because these vessels were not intended to carry the high pressure and volume of blood imposed by cirrhosis, they may rupture and bleed. Therefore, assessment must include observation for occult and frank bleeding from the GI tract.

Edema

Another late symptom of cirrhosis is edema, which is attributed to chronic liver failure. A reduced plasma albumin concentration predisposes the patient to the formation of edema. Although edema is generalized, it often affects the lower extremities, the upper extremities, and the presacral area. Facial edema is not typical. Overproduction of aldosterone occurs, causing sodium and water retention and potassium excretion.

Vitamin Deficiency and Anemia

Because of inadequate formation, use, and storage of certain vitamins (notably vitamins A, C, and K), signs of deficiency are common, particularly hemorrhagic phenomena associated with vitamin K deficiency. Chronic gastritis and impaired GI function, together with inadequate dietary intake and impaired liver function, account for the anemia that is often associated with cirrhosis. The patient's anemia, poor nutritional status, and poor state of health result in severe fatigue, which interferes with the ability to carry out routine activities of daily living (ADLs).

Mental Deterioration

Additional clinical manifestations include deterioration of mental and cognitive function with impending hepatic encephalopathy and hepatic coma, as previously described. Neurologic assessment is indicated, including assessment of the patient's general behaviour, cognitive abilities, orientation to time and place, and speech patterns.

Assessment and Diagnostic Findings

The extent of liver disease and the type of treatment are determined after review of the laboratory findings. The functions of the liver are complex, and many diagnostic tests provide information about liver function (see Table 39-1). The patient needs to know why these tests are being performed and how to cooperate.

In severe parenchymal liver dysfunction, the serum albumin level tends to decrease, and the serum globulin level rises. Enzyme tests indicate liver cell damage: serum alkaline phosphatase, AST, ALT, and GGT levels increase, and the serum cholinesterase level may decrease. Bilirubin tests are performed to measure bile excretion or retention; increased levels of bilirubin can occur with cirrhosis and other liver disorders. Prothrombin time is prolonged.

Ultrasound scanning is used to measure the difference in density of parenchymal cells and scar tissue. CT, MRI, and radioisotope liver scans give information about liver size and hepatic blood flow and obstruction. Diagnosis is confirmed by liver biopsy. Arterial blood gas analysis may reveal a ventilation–perfusion imbalance and hypoxia.

Medical Management

The management of the patient with cirrhosis is usually based on the presenting symptoms. For example, antacids or histamine-2 (H_2) antagonists are prescribed to decrease gastric distress and minimize the possibility of GI bleeding. Vitamins and nutritional supplements promote healing of damaged liver cells and improve the patient's general nutritional status. Potassium-sparing diuretics such as spironolactone or triamterene (Dyrenium) may be indicated to decrease ascites, if present; these diuretics are preferred because they minimize the fluid and electrolyte changes commonly seen with other agents. An adequate diet and avoidance of alcohol are essential. Although the fibrosis of the cirrhotic liver cannot be reversed, its progression may be halted or slowed by such measures.

Preliminary studies indicate that colchicine, an anti-inflammatory agent used to treat the symptoms of gout, may increase survival time in patients with mild to moderate cirrhosis. Many medications have been shown to possess antifibrotic activity for the treatment of cirrhosis. Some of these medications include angiotensin system inhibitors, statins, diuretics, immunosuppressants, and glitazones. These medications have reasonable safety profiles, but their long-term safety and efficacy in patients with cirrhosis has yet to be demonstrated (Lee & Moreau, 2015; Poordad, 2015).

Many patients who have end-stage liver disease (ESLD) with cirrhosis use the herb milk thistle (*Silybum marianum*) to treat jaundice and other symptoms. This herb has been used for centuries because of its healing and regenerative properties for liver disease. Silymarin from milk thistle has anti-inflammatory and antioxidant properties that may have beneficial effects, especially in hepatitis. The natural compound, SAM-e (s-adenosylmethionine), may improve outcomes in liver disease by improving liver function, possibly through enhancing antioxidant function. Primary biliary cirrhosis (now renamed to primary biliary cholangitis) has been treated with ursodeoxycholic acid (Actigall, Urso) to improve liver function and halt the progression of the disease. For patients with primary biliary cholangitis that are nonresponders to this, obeticholic acid (oclavia) has just been approved in the United States and Canada for use in this population.

Nursing Management

Nursing management for the patient with cirrhosis of the liver is described in detail in the Plan of Nursing Care for the Patient with Impaired Liver Function (Chart 39-12).

(text continued on page 1093)

Plan of Nursing Care — Chart 39-12. The Patient With Impaired Liver Function

NURSING INTERVENTIONS	RATIONALE	EXPECTED OUTCOMES
Nursing Priority: Activity intolerance **Goal:** Patient reports decrease in fatigue and reports increased ability to participate in activities		
1. Assess level of activity tolerance and degree of fatigue, lethargy, and malaise when performing routine activities of daily living.	1. Provides baseline for further assessment and criteria for assessment of effectiveness of interventions.	• Exhibits increased interest in activities and events. • Participates in activities and gradually increases exercise within physical limits.
2. Assist with activities and hygiene when fatigued.	2. Promotes exercise and hygiene within patient's level of tolerance.	• Reports increased strength and well-being.
3. Encourage rest when fatigued or when abdominal pain or discomfort occurs.	3. Conserves energy and protects the liver.	• Reports absence of abdominal pain and discomfort.
4. Assist with selection and pacing of desired activities and exercise.	4. Stimulates patient's interest in selected activities.	• Plans activities to allow ample periods of rest.
5. Provide diet high in carbohydrates with protein intake consistent with liver function.	5. Provides calories for energy and protein for healing.	• Takes vitamins as prescribed.
6. Administer supplemental vitamins (A, B complex, C, and K).	6. Provides additional nutrients.	
Nursing Priority: Imbalanced nutrition **Goal:** Positive nitrogen balance, no further loss of muscle mass; meets nutritional requirements		
1. Assess dietary intake and nutritional status through diet history and diary, daily weight measurements, and laboratory data.	1. Identifies deficits in nutritional intake and adequacy of nutritional state.	• Exhibits improved nutritional status by increased weight (without fluid retention) and improved laboratory data.
2. Provide diet high in carbohydrates with protein intake consistent with liver function.	2. Provides calories for energy, sparing protein for healing.	• States rationale for dietary modifications.
3. Assist patient in identifying low-sodium foods.	3. Reduces edema and ascites formation.	• Identifies foods high in carbohydrates and within protein requirements (moderate to high protein in cirrhosis and hepatitis, low protein in hepatic failure).
4. Elevate the head of the bed during meals.	4. Reduces discomfort from abdominal distention and decreases sense of fullness produced by pressure of abdominal contents and ascites on the stomach.	• Reports improved appetite. • Participates in oral hygiene measures. • Reports increased appetite; identifies rationale for smaller, frequent meals.
5. Provide oral hygiene before meals and pleasant environment for meals at meal time.	5. Promotes positive environment and increased appetite; reduces unpleasant taste.	• Demonstrates intake of high-calorie diet; adheres to protein restriction. • Identifies foods and fluids that are nutritious and permitted on diet.
6. Offer smaller, more frequent meals (6 per day).	6. Decreases feeling of fullness, bloating.	• Gains weight without increased edema or ascites formation.
7. Encourage patient to eat meals and supplementary feedings.	7. Encouragement is essential for the patient with anorexia and gastrointestinal discomfort.	• Reports increased appetite and well-being.
8. Provide attractive meals and an aesthetically pleasing setting at meal time.	8. Promotes appetite and sense of well-being.	• Excludes alcohol from diet. • Takes medications for gastrointestinal disorders as prescribed.
9. Eliminate alcohol.	9. Eliminates "empty calories" and further damage from alcohol.	• Reports normal gastrointestinal function with regular bowel function.
10. Apply an ice collar for nausea.	10. May reduce incidence of nausea.	
11. Administer medications prescribed for nausea, vomiting, diarrhea, or constipation.	11. Reduces gastrointestinal symptoms and discomforts that decrease the appetite and interest in food.	
12. Encourage increased fluid intake and exercise if the patient reports constipation.	12. Promotes normal bowel pattern and reduces abdominal discomfort and distention.	

Plan of Nursing Care — Chart 39-12. The Patient With Impaired Liver Function, *Continued*

Nursing Priority: Impaired skin integrity
Goal: Decrease potential for pressure ulcer development; breaks in skin integrity

NURSING INTERVENTIONS	RATIONALE
1. Assess degree of discomfort related to pruritus and edema.	1. Assists in determining appropriate interventions.
2. Note and record degree of jaundice and extent of edema.	2. Provides baseline for detecting changes and evaluating effectiveness of interventions.
3. Keep patient's fingernails short and smooth.	3. Prevents skin excoriation and infection from scratching.
4. Provide frequent skin care; avoid use of soaps and alcohol-based lotions.	4. Removes waste products from skin while preventing dryness of sin.
5. Massage every 2 hours with emollients; turn every 2 hours.	5. Promotes mobilization of edema.
6. Initiate use of alternating-pressure mattress or low air loss bed.	6. Minimizes prolonged pressure on bony prominences susceptible to breakdown.
7. Recommend avoiding use of harsh detergents.	7. May decrease skin irritation and need for scratching.
8. Assess skin integrity every 4–8 hours. Instruct patient and family in this activity.	8. Edematous skin and tissue have compromised nutrient supply and are vulnerable to pressure and trauma.
9. Restrict sodium as prescribed.	9. Minimizes edema formation.
10. Perform range of motion exercises every 4 hours; elevate edematous extremities whenever possible.	10. Promotes mobilization of edema.

EXPECTED OUTCOMES

- Exhibits intact skin without redness, excoriation, or breakdown.
- Reports relief from pruritus.
- Exhibits no skin excoriation from scratching.
- Uses nondrying soaps and lotions. States rationale for use of nondrying soaps and lotions.
- Turns self periodically. Exhibits reduced edema of dependent parts of the body.
- Exhibits no areas of skin breakdown.
- Exhibits decreased edema; normal skin turgor.

Nursing Priority: High risk for injury related due to impaired clotting mechanisms and decreased level of consciousness
Goal: Reduced risk of injury

NURSING INTERVENTIONS	RATIONALE
1. Assess level of consciousness and cognitive level.	1. Assists in determining patient's ability to protect self and comply with required self-protective actions; may detect deterioration of hepatic function.
2. Provide safe environment (pad side rails, remove obstacles in room, prevent falls).	2. Minimizes falls and injury if falls occur.
3. Provide frequent surveillance to orient patient and avoid use of restraints.	3. Protects patient from harm while stimulating and orienting patient; use of restraints may disturb patient further.
4. Replace sharp objects (razors) with safer items.	4. Avoids cuts and bleeding.
5. Observe each stool for colour, consistency, and amount.	5. Permits detection of bleeding in gastrointestinal tract.
6. Be alert for symptoms of anxiety, epigastric fullness, weakness, and restlessness.	6. May indicate early signs of bleeding and shock.
7. Test each stool and emesis for occult blood.	7. Detects early evidence of bleeding.
8. Observe for hemorrhagic manifestations: ecchymosis, epistaxis, petechiae, and bleeding gums.	8. Indicates altered clotting mechanisms.
9. Record vital signs at frequent intervals, depending on patient acuity (every 1–4 hours).	9. Provides baseline and evidence of hypovolemia, and hemorrhagic shock.

EXPECTED OUTCOMES

- Is oriented to time, place, and person.
- Exhibits no hallucinations, and demonstrates no efforts to get up unassisted or to leave hospital.
- Exhibits no ecchymoses (bruises), cuts, or hematoma.
- Uses electric razor rather than sharp-edged razor.
- Exhibits absence of frank bleeding from gastrointestinal tract.
- Exhibits absence of restlessness, epigastric fullness, and other indicators of hemorrhage and shock.
- Exhibits negative results of test for occult gastrointestinal bleeding.

continued >

Plan of Nursing Care

Chart 39-12. The Patient With Impaired Liver Function, *Continued*

NURSING INTERVENTIONS	RATIONALE	EXPECTED OUTCOMES
10. Keep patient quiet and limit activity.	10. Minimizes risk of bleeding and straining.	• Is free of ecchymotic areas or hematoma formation. • Exhibits normal vital signs. • Maintains rest and remains quiet if active bleeding occurs. • Identifies rationale for blood transfusions and measures to treat bleeding. • Uses measures to prevent trauma (e.g., uses soft toothbrush, blows nose gently, avoids bumps and falls, avoids straining during defecation). • Experiences no side effects of medications. • Takes all medications as prescribed. • Identifies rationale for precautions with use of all medications. • Cooperates with treatment modalities.
11. Assist physician in passage of tube for esophageal balloon tamponade, if its insertion is indicated.	11. Promotes nontraumatic insertion of tube in anxious and combative patient for immediate treatment of bleeding.	
12. Observe during blood transfusions.	12. Permits detection of transfusion reactions (risk is increased with multiple blood transfusions needed for active bleeding from esophageal varices).	
13. Measure and record nature, time, and amount of vomitus.	13. Assists in evaluating extent of bleeding and blood loss.	
14. Maintain patient in fasting state, if indicated.	14. Reduces risk of aspiration of gastric contents and minimizes risk of further trauma to esophagus and stomach by preventing vomiting.	
15. Administer vitamin K as prescribed.	15. Promotes clotting by providing fat-soluble vitamin necessary for clotting.	
16. Remain with patient during episodes of bleeding.	16. Reassures anxious patient and permits monitoring and detection of further needs of the patient.	
17. Offer cold liquids by mouth when bleeding stops (if prescribed).	17. Minimizes risk of further bleeding by promoting vasoconstriction of esophageal and gastric blood vessels.	
18. Institute measures to prevent trauma:	18. Promotes safety of patient	
a. Maintain safe environment.	a. Minimizes risk of trauma and bleeding by avoiding falls and cuts, etc.	
b. Encourage *gentle* blowing of nose.	b. Reduces risk of nosebleed (epistaxis) secondary to trauma and decreased clotting.	
c. Provide soft toothbrush and avoid use of toothpicks.	c. Prevents trauma to oral mucosa while promoting good oral hygiene.	
d. Encourage intake of foods with high content of vitamin C.	d. Promotes healing.	
e. Apply cold compresses where indicated.	e. Minimizes bleeding into tissues by promoting local vasoconstriction.	
f. Record location of bleeding sites.	f. Permits detection of new bleeding sites and monitoring of previous sites of bleeding.	
g. Use small-gauge needles for injections.	g. Minimizes oozing and blood loss from repeated injections.	
19. Administer medications carefully; monitor for side effects.	19. Reduces risk of side effects secondary to damaged liver's inability to detoxify (metabolize) medications normally.	

Plan of Nursing Care — Chart 39-12. The Patient With Impaired Liver Function, *Continued*

Nursing Priority: Disturbed body image and sexual dysfunction
Goal: Patient verbalizes feelings consistent with improvement of body image and self-esteem

NURSING INTERVENTIONS	RATIONALE
1. Assess changes in appearance and the meaning these changes have for patient and family.	1. Provides information for assessing impact of changes in appearance, sexual function, and role on the patient and family.
2. Encourage patient to verbalize reactions and feelings about these changes.	2. Enables patient to identify and express concerns; encourages patient and significant others to share these concerns.
3. Assess patient's and family's previous coping strategies.	3. Permits encouragement of those coping strategies that are familiar to patient and have been effective in the past.
4. Assist and encourage patient to maximize appearance (such as strategies to limit the appearance of jaundice and ascites through careful selection of colours and type of clothing) and explore alternatives to previous sexual and role functions.	4. Encourages patient to continue safe roles and functions while encouraging exploration of alternatives.
5. Assist patient in identifying short-term goals.	5. Accomplishing these goals serves as positive reinforcement and increases self-esteem.
6. Encourage and assist patient in decision making about care.	6. Promotes patient's control of life and improves sense of well-being and self-esteem.
7. Identify with patient resources to provide additional support (counsellor, spiritual advisor).	7. Assists patient in identifying resources and accepting assistance from others when indicated.
8. Assist patient in identifying previous practices that may have been harmful to self (alcohol and drug abuse). Involve patient in goal-setting and provide positive feedback for accomplishments.	8. Recognition and acknowledgement of the harmful effects of these practices are necessary for identifying a healthier lifestyle.

EXPECTED OUTCOMES

- Verbalizes concerns related to changes in appearance, life, and lifestyle.
- Shares concerns with significant others.
- Identifies past coping strategies that have been effective.
- Uses past effective coping strategies to deal with changes in appearance, life, and lifestyle.
- Maintains good grooming and hygiene.
- Identifies short-term goals and strategies to achieve them.
- Takes an active role in decision making about self and care.
- Identifies resources that are not harmful.
- Verbalizes that some of previous lifestyle practices have been harmful.
- Uses healthy expressions of frustration, anger, and anxiety.

Nursing Priority: Chronic pain and due to enlarged tender liver and ascites
Goal: Increased level of comfort

NURSING INTERVENTIONS	RATIONALE
1. Maintain bed rest when patient experiences abdominal discomfort.	1. Reduces metabolic demands and protects the liver.
2. Administer antispasmodic and analgesic agents as prescribed.	2. Reduces irritability of the gastrointestinal tract and decreases abdominal pain and discomfort.
3. Observe, record, and report presence and character of pain and discomfort.	3. Provides baseline to detect further deterioration of status and to evaluate interventions.
4. Reduce sodium and fluid intake if prescribed.	4. Minimizes further formation of ascites.
5. Prepare patient and assist with paracentesis.	5. Removal of ascites fluid may decrease abdominal discomfort.
6. Encourage the use of distracting activities such as music, reading, or meditation.	6. Distraction may limit the perception of pain.

EXPECTED OUTCOMES

- Reports pain and discomfort if present.
- Maintains bed rest and decreases activity in presence of pain.
- Takes antispasmodic and analgesics as indicated and as prescribed.
- Reports decreased pain and abdominal discomfort.
- Reduces sodium and fluid intake to prescribed levels if indicated to treat ascites.
- Exhibits decreased abdominal girth and appropriate weight changes.
- Reports decreased discomfort after paracentesis.

continued >

Plan of Nursing Care — Chart 39-12. The Patient With Impaired Liver Function, *Continued*

NURSING INTERVENTIONS | **RATIONALE** | **EXPECTED OUTCOMES**

Nursing Priority: Ascites and edema formation
Goal: Restoration of normal fluid volume

Nursing Interventions

1. Restrict sodium and fluid intake if prescribed.
2. Administer diuretics, potassium, and protein supplements as prescribed.
3. Record intake and output every 1–8 hours depending on response to interventions and on patient acuity.
4. Measure and record abdominal girth and weight daily.
5. Explain rationale for sodium and fluid restriction.
6. Prepare patient and assist with paracentesis.

Rationale

1. Minimizes formation of ascites and edema.
2. Promotes excretion of fluid through the kidneys and maintenance of normal fluid and electrolyte balance.
3. Indicates effectiveness of treatment and adequacy of fluid intake.
4. Monitors changes in ascites formation and fluid accumulation.
5. Promotes patient's understanding of restriction and cooperation with it.
6. Paracentesis will temporarily decrease amount of ascites present.

Expected Outcomes

- Consumes diet low in sodium and within prescribed fluid restriction.
- Takes diuretics, potassium, and protein supplements as indicated without experiencing side effects.
- Exhibits increased urine output.
- Exhibits decreasing abdominal girth.
- Exhibits no rapid increase in weight.
- Identifies rationale for sodium and fluid restriction.
- Shows a decrease in ascites with decreased weight.

Nursing Priority: Altered thought processes and mental deterioration due to decreased liver function and increased serum ammonia level
Goal: Improved mental status; safety maintained; ability to cope with cognitive and behavioural changes

Nursing Interventions

1. Restrict dietary protein as prescribed for transient period.
2. Give frequent, small feedings of carbohydrates.
3. Protect from infection.
4. Keep environment warm and draft-free.
5. Pad the side rails of the bed.
6. Limit visitors.
7. Provide careful nursing surveillance to ensure patient's safety.
8. Avoid opioids and barbiturates.
9. Awaken at intervals (every 2–4 hours) to assess cognitive status.
10. Identify subtle changes in behaviour or sleep–wake pattern (consistent staff caring for the patient enhances this assessment as they become familiar with patient's baseline).
11. Assess handwriting or drawing skill daily as indication of cognitive ability.

Rationale

1. Reduces source of ammonia (protein foods).
2. Promotes consumption of adequate carbohydrates for energy requirements and spares protein from breakdown for energy.
3. Minimizes risk for further increase in metabolic requirements.
4. Minimizes shivering, which would increase metabolic requirements.
5. Provides protection for the patient should hepatic coma and seizure activity occur.
6. Minimizes patient's activity and metabolic requirements.
7. Provides close monitoring of new symptoms and minimizes trauma to the confused patient.
8. Prevents masking of symptoms of hepatic coma and prevents drug overdose secondary to reduced ability of the damaged liver to metabolize opioids and barbiturates. Prevents respiratory depression.
9. Provides stimulation to the patient and opportunity for observing the patient's level of consciousness.

10/11. These changes may herald worsening of encephalopathy which requires rapid intervention including medication.

Expected Outcomes

- Adheres to protein restriction.
- Demonstrates an interest in events and activities in environment.
- Demonstrates normal attention span.
- Follows and participates in conversation appropriately.
- Is oriented to person, place, and time.
- Remains in bed when indicated.
- Reports no urinary or fecal incontinence.
- Experiences no seizures.
- No neurologic or respiratory depression.
- Develops no cognitive impairments but if they develop they are quickly identified and treated enhancing the potential of recovery.
- Patient and family describe adequate feelings of coping and lowered anxiety. They demonstrate ability to listen and to make decisions as able.
- Patient and family communicate their feelings and their needs in a secure and caring environment.

Plan of Nursing Care

Chart 39-12. The Patient With Impaired Liver Function, *Continued*

NURSING INTERVENTIONS	RATIONALE	EXPECTED OUTCOMES
12. Encourage patient and family to participate in therapeutic strategies to enhance coping with episodes of mental deterioration.	12. Promoting activities such as listening to music, relaxation techniques, or preillness coping strategies can reduce anxiety.	
13. Encourage patient and family to discuss feeling of fear, powerlessness, or emotional distress related to patient's mental deterioration.	13. Actively listening demonstrates caring and concern.	

Nursing Priority: Imbalanced body temperature and hyperthermia secondary to the inflammatory processes of cirrhosis or hepatitis

Goal: Maintenance of normal body temperature, free from infection

NURSING INTERVENTIONS	RATIONALE	EXPECTED OUTCOMES
1. Record temperature regularly (every 4 hours).	1. Provides baseline to detect fever and to evaluate interventions.	• Exhibits normal temperature and reports absence of chills or sweating.
2. Encourage fluid intake.	2. Corrects fluid loss from perspiration and fever and increases patient's level of comfort.	• Demonstrates adequate intake of fluids.
3. Apply cool sponges or ice bag for elevated temperature.	3. Promotes reduction of fever and increases patient's comfort.	• Exhibits no evidence of local or systemic infection.
4. Administer antibiotics as prescribed.	4. Ensures appropriate serum concentration of antibiotics to treat infection.	• Develops no nosocomial infections related to invasive procedures/lines.
5. Avoid exposure to infections.	5. Minimizes risk of further infection and further increases in body temperature and metabolic rate.	
6. Keep patient at rest while temperature is elevated.	6. Reduces metabolic rate.	
7. Assess for abdominal pain, tenderness.	7. May occur with bacterial peritonitis.	
8. Use sterile technique for all invasive procedures.	8. Many evidence-based practice guidelines (e.g., central venous catheter care) recommend the use of sterile technique to prevent nosocomial infections.	

Nursing Priority: Ineffective breathing pattern

Goal: Improved respiratory status

NURSING INTERVENTIONS	RATIONALE	EXPECTED OUTCOMES
1. Elevate head of bed to at least 30 degrees.	1. Reduces abdominal pressure on the diaphragm and permits fuller thoracic excursion and lung expansion.	• Experiences improved respiratory status.
2. Conserve patient's strength by providing rest periods and assisting with activities.	2. Reduces metabolic and oxygen requirements.	• Reports decreased shortness of breath.
3. Change position every 2 hours.	3. Promotes expansion and oxygenation of all areas of the lungs.	• Reports increased strength and sense of well-being.
4. Assist with paracentesis or thoracentesis.	4. Paracentesis and thoracentesis (performed to remove fluid from the abdominal and thoracic cavities, respectively) may be frightening to the patient.	• Exhibits normal respiratory rate (12–18/min) with no adventitious sounds.
		• Exhibits full thoracic excursion without shallow respirations.
		• Exhibits normal arterial blood gases.
		• Exhibits adequate oxygen saturation by pulse oximetry.
a. Explain procedure and its purpose to patient.	a. Helps obtain patient's cooperation with procedures.	• Experiences absence of confusion or cyanosis.
b. Have patient void before paracentesis.	b. Prevents inadvertent bladder injury.	
c. Support and maintain position during procedure.	c. Prevents inadvertent organ or tissue injury.	
d. Record both the amount and the character of fluid aspirated.	d. Provides record of fluid removed and indication of severity of limitation of lung expansion by fluid.	
e. Observe for evidence of coughing, increasing dyspnea, or pulse rate.	e. Indicates irritation of the pleural space and evidence of pneumothorax or hemothorax.	

continued >

Plan of Nursing Care — Chart 39-12. The Patient With Impaired Liver Function, *Continued*

Collaborative Problem: Gastrointestinal bleeding and hemorrhage
Goal: Absence of episodes of gastrointestinal bleeding and hemorrhage

NURSING INTERVENTIONS	RATIONALE	EXPECTED OUTCOMES
1. Assess patient for evidence of gastrointestinal bleeding or hemorrhage. If bleeding does occur: a. Monitor vital signs (blood pressure, pulse, respiratory rate) every 4 hours or more frequently, depending on acuity. b. Assess skin temperature, level of consciousness every 4 hours or more frequently, depending on acuity. c. Monitor gastrointestinal secretions and output (emesis, stool for occult or obvious bleeding). Test emesis for blood once per shift and with any colour change. Hematest each stool. d. Monitor hematocrit and hemoglobin for trends and changes.	1. Allows early detection of signs and symptoms of bleeding and hemorrhage.	• Experiences no episodes of bleeding and hemorrhage. • Vital signs are within acceptable range for patient. • No evidence of bleeding from gastrointestinal tract. • Hematocrit and hemoglobin levels within acceptable limits. • Turns and moves without straining and increasing intra-abdominal pressure. • No straining with bowel movements. • No further bleeding episodes if aggressive treatment of bleeding and hemorrhage was needed. • Patient and family state rationale for treatments. • Patient and family identify supports available to them. • Patient and family describe signs and symptoms of a recurrent bleeding episode and identify needed action.
2. Avoid activities that increase intra-abdominal pressure (straining, turning). a. Avoid coughing/sneezing. b. Assist patient to turn. c. Keep all needed items within easy reach. d. Use measures to prevent constipation such as adequate fluid intake; stool softeners. e. Ensure small meals.	2. Minimizes increases in intra-abdominal pressure that could lead to rupture and bleeding of esophageal or gastric varices.	
3. Have equipment (Blakemore tube, medications, IV fluids) available if indicated.	3. Equipment, medications, and supplies will be readily available if patient experiences bleeding from ruptured esophageal or gastric varices.	
4. Assist with procedures and therapy needed to treat gastrointestinal bleeding and hemorrhage.	4. Gastrointestinal bleeding and hemorrhage require emergency measures (e.g., insertion of Blakemore tube, administration of fluids and medications).	
5. Monitor respiratory status every hour and minimize risk of respiratory complications if balloon tamponade is needed.	5. The patient is at high risk for respiratory complications, including asphyxiation if gastric balloon of tamponade tube ruptures or migrates upward.	
6. Prepare patient physically and psychologically for other treatment modalities if needed.	6. The patient who experiences hemorrhage is very anxious and fearful; minimizing anxiety assists in control of hemorrhage.	
7. Monitor patient for recurrence of bleeding and hemorrhage.	7. Risk of rebleeding is high with all treatment modalities used to halt gastrointestinal bleeding.	
8. Keep family informed of patient's status.	8. Family members are likely to be anxious about the patient's status; providing information will reduce their anxiety level and promote more effective coping.	
9. Once recovered from bleeding episode, provide patient and family with information regarding signs and symptoms of gastrointestinal bleeding.	9. Risk of rebleeding is high. Subtle signs may be more quickly identified.	

Plan of Nursing Care

Chart 39-12. The Patient With Impaired Liver Function, *Continued*

NURSING INTERVENTIONS	RATIONALE	EXPECTED OUTCOMES
Collaborative Problem: Hepatic encephalopathy **Goal:** Absence of changes in cognitive status and of injury		
1. Assess cognitive status every 4–8 hours: a. Assess patient's orientation to person, place, and time. b. Monitor patient's level of activity, restlessness, and agitation. Assess for presence of flapping hand tremors (asterixis). c. Obtain and record daily sample of patient's handwriting or ability to construct a simple figure (e.g., star). d. Assess neurologic signs (deep tendon reflexes, ability to follow instructions).	1. Data will provide baseline of patient's cognitive status and enable detection of changes.	• Remains awake, alert, and aware of surroundings. • Is oriented to time, place, and person. • Exhibits no restlessness or agitation. • Record of handwriting demonstrates no deterioration in cognitive function. • States rationale for treatment used to prevent or treat hepatic encephalopathy. • Demonstrates stable serum ammonia level within acceptable limits. • Consumes adequate caloric intake and adheres to protein restriction. • Takes medications as prescribed. • Breath sounds are normal without adventitious sounds. • Skin and tissue intact without evidence of pressure or breaks in integrity. • Verbalizes understanding of need for treatments and procedures to promote recovery.
2. Monitor medications to prevent administration of those that may precipitate hepatic encephalopathy (sedatives, hypnotics, analgesics).	2. Medications are a common precipitating factor in development of hepatic encephalopathy in patients at risk.	
3. Monitor laboratory data, especially serum ammonia level.	3. Increases in serum ammonia level are associated with hepatic encephalopathy and coma.	
4. Notify physician of even subtle changes in patient's neurologic assessment, cognitive function, sleep pattern, or mood.	4. Allows early initiation of treatment of hepatic encephalopathy and prevention of hepatic coma.	
5. Limit sources of protein from diet if indicated.	5. Reduces breakdown and conversion of protein to ammonia.	
6. Administer medications prescribed to reduce serum ammonia level (e.g., lactulose, antibiotics, glucose, benzodiazepine antagonist [Flumazenil] if indicated).	6. Reduces serum ammonia level.	
7. Assess respiratory status and initiate measures to prevent complications.	7. The patient who develops hepatic coma is at risk for respiratory complications (i.e., pneumonia, atelectasis, infection).	
8. Protect patient's skin and tissue from pressure and breakdown.	8. The patient in coma is at risk for skin breakdown and pressure ulcer formation.	
9. Provide support and active listening for patient and family as patient's mental status deteriorates.	9. The patient with hepatic encephalopathy can experience episodes of mental deterioration due to liver failure. This can produce feelings of fear and anxiety.	

Nursing interventions are directed toward promoting patient's rest, improving nutritional status, providing skin care, reducing risk of injury, and monitoring and managing potential complications.

Promoting Rest

The patient with cirrhosis requires rest and other supportive measures to permit the liver to reestablish its functional ability. If the patient is hospitalized, weight and fluid intake and output are measured and recorded daily. The nurse adjusts the patient's position in bed for maximal respiratory efficiency, which is especially important if ascites is marked, because it interferes with adequate thoracic excursion. Oxygen therapy may be required in liver failure to oxygenate the damaged cells and prevent further cell destruction.

Rest reduces the demands on the liver and increases the liver's blood supply. Because the patient is susceptible to the hazards of immobility, efforts to prevent respiratory, circulatory, and vascular disturbances are initiated. These measures may help prevent such problems as pneumonia, thrombophlebitis, and pressure ulcers. After nutritional status improves and strength increases, the nurse encourages the patient to increase activity gradually. Activity and mild exercise, as well as rest, are planned.

Improving Nutritional Status

The patient with cirrhosis without ascites, edema, or signs of impending hepatic coma should receive a nutritious, high-protein diet, if tolerated, supplemented by vitamins of the B complex, as well as A, C, and K. The nurse encourages the patient to eat. If ascites is present, small, frequent meals may be better tolerated than three large meals because of the abdominal pressure exerted by ascites. Patient preferences are considered. Patients with prolonged or severe anorexia and those who are vomiting or eating poorly for any reason may receive nutrients by the enteral or parenteral route.

The use of probiotics for the management of hepatic encephalopathy is currently the topic of ongoing research. Imbalance of the intestinal flora is not uncommon. Some research suggests that the oral ingestion of 1 cup of probiotic yogurt three times a day reduces intestinal flora imbalance by decreasing *Escherichia coli* counts and promoting the growth of non–urease-producing bacteria. This strategy is thought to then reduce ammonia levels and improve mental status (Nusrat et al., 2014).

Patients with fatty stools (steatorrhea) should receive water-soluble forms of fat-soluble vitamins A, D, and E. Folic acid and iron are prescribed to prevent anemia. If the patient shows signs of impending or advancing coma, the amount of protein in the diet is decreased temporarily. Protein is restricted if encephalopathy develops. Incorporating vegetable protein to meet protein needs may decrease the risk for encephalopathy. Sodium restriction is also indicated to prevent ascites.

Providing Skin Care

Providing careful skin care is important because of subcutaneous edema, the patient's immobility, jaundice, and increased susceptibility to skin breakdown and infection. Frequent changes in position are necessary to prevent pressure ulcers. Irritating soaps and the use of adhesive tape are avoided to prevent trauma to the skin. Lotion may be soothing to irritated skin; the nurse takes measures to minimize scratching by the patient.

Reducing Risk of Injury

The nurse protects the patient with cirrhosis from falls and other injuries. The side rails should be in place and padded with blankets or other materials in case the patient becomes agitated or restless. To minimize agitation, the nurse orients the patient to time and place and explains all procedures. The nurse instructs the patient to ask for assistance to get out of bed. The nurse carefully evaluates any injury because of the possibility of internal or external bleeding and the potential for prolonged clotting times.

Because of the risk for bleeding from abnormal clotting, the patient should use an electric razor rather than a safety razor. A soft-bristled toothbrush helps minimize bleeding gums, and pressure applied to all venipuncture sites helps minimize bleeding.

Monitoring and Managing Potential Complications

A major role of the nurse is monitoring of the patient with cirrhosis for complications.

Bleeding and Hemorrhage

The patient is at increased risk for bleeding and hemorrhage because of decreased production of prothrombin and decreased ability of the diseased liver to synthesize the necessary substances for blood coagulation. This was discussed earlier in the section on esophageal varices.

Hepatic Encephalopathy

As previously described, hepatic encephalopathy and coma, complications of cirrhosis, may manifest as deteriorating mental status and dementia or as physical signs such as abnormal voluntary and involuntary movements. Hepatic encephalopathy was discussed earlier in the chapter in detail and in Chart 39-12.

Monitoring is an essential nursing function to identify early deterioration in mental status. The nurse monitors the patient's mental status closely and reports changes so that treatment of encephalopathy can be initiated promptly. An extensive neurologic evaluation is key to identify progression through the four stages of encephalopathy.

Each advancing stage demands more intensive nursing interventions aimed at providing for patient safety and prevention and early identification of life-threatening complications such as respiratory failure and cerebral edema, which would necessitate interventions in an ICU. Because electrolyte disturbances can contribute to encephalopathy, serum electrolyte levels are carefully monitored and corrected if abnormal. Oxygen is administered if oxygen desaturation occurs. The nurse monitors for fever or abdominal pain, which may signal the onset of bacterial peritonitis or other infection (see earlier discussion of hepatic encephalopathy).

Fluid Volume Excess

Patients with advanced chronic liver disease develop cardiovascular abnormalities. These occur due to an increased cardiac output and decreased peripheral vascular resistance, possibly resulting from the release of vasodilators. A hyperdynamic circulatory state develops in patients with cirrhosis, and plasma volume increases. This increase in circulating plasma volume is probably multifactorial, but some studies have implicated excess production of nitrous oxide, like that seen in sepsis, as one causative factor (Nusrat et al., 2014). The greater the degree of hepatic decompensation, the more severe the hyperdynamic state. Close assessment of cardiovascular and respiratory status is of key importance for the care of patients with this disorder. Pulmonary compromise, which is always a potential complication of ESLD because of plasma volume excess, makes prevention of pulmonary complications an important role for the nurse. Administering diuretics, implementing fluid restrictions, and enhancing patient positioning can optimize pulmonary function. Fluid retention may be noted in the development of ascites, lower extremity swelling, and dyspnea. Monitoring of intake and output, daily weight changes, changes in abdominal girth, and edema formation is part of nursing assessment in the hospital or in the home setting. Patients are also monitored for nocturia and, later, for oliguria, because these states indicate increasing severity of liver dysfunction (Nusrat et al., 2014).

Promoting Home, Community-Based, and Transitional Care

Educating Patients About Self-Care

During the hospital stay, the nurse and other health care providers prepare the patient with cirrhosis for discharge, focusing on dietary instruction. Of greatest importance is the exclusion of alcohol from the diet. The patient may need referral to Alcoholics Anonymous, psychiatric care, or counselling or may benefit from support from a spiritual advisor. The patient should also avoid the consumption of raw shellfish.

Sodium restriction will continue for a considerable time, if not permanently. The patient will require written instructions, teaching, reinforcement, and support from the staff as well as family members.

Successful treatment depends on convincing the patient of the need to adhere completely to the therapeutic plan. This includes rest, lifestyle changes, adequate dietary intake, and the elimination of alcohol. The nurse also instructs the patient and family about symptoms of impending encephalopathy, possible bleeding tendencies, and susceptibility to infection.

Recovery is neither rapid nor easy; there are frequent setbacks and apparent lack of improvement. Many patients find it difficult to refrain from using alcohol for comfort or escape. The nurse has a significant role in offering support and encouragement to the patient and in providing positive feedback when the patient experiences success.

Continuing Care and Transitional

Referral for transitional or home care may assist the patient in dealing with the transition from hospital to home. The use of alcohol may have been an important part of normal home and social life in the past. The home care nurse assesses the patient's progress at home and the manner in which the patient and family are coping with the elimination of alcohol and the dietary restrictions. The nurse also reinforces previous teaching and answers questions that may not have occurred to the patient or family until the patient is back home and trying to establish new patterns of eating, drinking, and lifestyle.

CANCER OF THE LIVER

Hepatic tumours may be malignant or benign. Benign liver tumours were uncommon until oral contraceptives were in widespread use. Now benign liver tumours occur most frequently in women in their reproductive years who are taking oral contraceptives (Greenberger et al., 2015). In 2017 in Canada, approximately 2,500 people were diagnosed with liver cancer (Canadian Cancer Society, 2018).

Primary Liver Tumours

Few cancers originate in the liver. Primary liver tumours usually are associated with chronic liver disease, hepatitis B and C infections, and cirrhosis. HCC is the most common type of primary liver cancer, with more than half a million cases diagnosed each year on a worldwide basis. HCC is the third leading cause of cancer-related mortality worldwide. It is rare in the United States and Northern Europe, accounting for less than 5 cases per 100,000 inhabitants (James & Liou, 2015; Nusrat et al., 2014). Other types of primary liver cancer include cholangiocellular carcinoma and combined hepatocellular and cholangiocellular carcinoma. HCC is usually nonresectable because of rapid growth and metastasis. If found early, resection of primary liver cancer may be possible, but early detection is unlikely.

Cirrhosis, chronic infection with hepatitis B and C, and exposure to certain chemical toxins (e.g., vinyl chloride, arsenic) have been implicated as causes of HCC. Cigarette smoking has also been identified as a risk factor, especially when combined with alcohol use. Some evidence suggests that aflatoxin, a metabolite of the fungus *Aspergillus flavus*, may be a risk factor for HCC. This is especially true in areas where HCC is endemic (i.e., Asia and Africa). Aflatoxin and other similar toxic molds can contaminate food such as ground nuts and grains and may act as cocarcinogens with hepatitis B (Greenberger et al., 2015; Salgia & Singal, 2014). The risk of contamination is greatest when these foods are stored unrefrigerated in tropical or subtropical climates.

Liver Metastases

Metastases from other primary sites, particularly the digestive system, breast, and lung, are found in the liver 2.5 times more frequently than tumours due to primary liver cancers. Malignant tumours are likely to reach the liver eventually, by way of the portal system or lymphatic channels, or by direct extension from an abdominal tumour. Moreover, the liver apparently is an ideal place for these malignant cells to thrive. Often the first evidence of cancer in an abdominal organ is the appearance of liver metastases; unless exploratory surgery or an autopsy is performed, the primary tumour may never be identified.

Clinical Manifestations

The early manifestations of malignancy of the liver include pain—a continuous dull ache in the right upper quadrant, epigastrium, or back. Weight loss, loss of strength, anorexia, and anemia may also occur. The liver may be enlarged and irregular on palpation. Jaundice is present only if the larger bile ducts are occluded by the pressure of malignant nodules in the hilum of the liver. Ascites develops if such nodules obstruct the portal veins or if tumour tissue is seeded in the peritoneal cavity.

Assessment and Diagnostic Findings

The diagnosis of liver cancer is based on clinical signs and symptoms, the history and physical examination, and the results of laboratory and x-ray studies. Increased serum levels of bilirubin, alkaline phosphatase, AST, GGT, and lactic dehydrogenase may occur. Leukocytosis (increased white blood cells), erythrocytosis (increased red blood cells), hypercalcemia, hypoglycemia, and hypocholesterolemia may also be seen on laboratory assessment.

The serum level of alpha-fetoprotein (AFP), which serves as a tumour marker, is elevated in 30% to 40% of patients with primary liver cancer (Feldman et al., 2015; Salgia & Singal, 2014). The level of carcinoembryonic antigen (CEA), a marker of advanced cancer of the digestive tract, may be elevated. These two markers together are useful to distinguish between metastatic liver disease and primary liver cancer.

Many patients have metastases from the primary liver tumour to other sites by the time the diagnosis is made; metastases occur primarily to the lung but may also occur to regional lymph nodes, adrenals, bone, kidneys, heart, pancreas, or stomach.

X-rays, liver scans, CT scans, ultrasound studies, MRI, arteriography, and laparoscopy may be part of the diagnostic workup and may be performed to determine the extent of the cancer. Positive emission tomogram (PET) scans are used to evaluate a wide range of metastatic tumours of the liver.

Confirmation of a tumour's histology can be made by biopsy under imaging guidance (CT scan or ultrasound) or laparoscopically. Local or systemic dissemination of the tumour by needle biopsy or fine-needle biopsy can occur but is rare. Some clinicians believe that these procedures should not be performed if the tumour is thought to be resectable; rather, primary HCC diagnosis should be confirmed by frozen section at the time of laparotomy in those patients with resectable lesions detected by imaging studies.

Medical Management

Although surgical resection of the liver tumour is possible in some patients, the underlying cirrhosis is so prevalent in cancer of the liver that it increases the risks associated with surgery. Radiation therapy and chemotherapy have been used to treat cancer of the liver with varying degrees of success. Although these therapies may prolong survival and improve quality of life by reducing pain and discomfort, their major effect is palliative.

Radiation Therapy

The use of external beam radiation for the treatment of liver tumours has been limited by the radiosensitivity of normal hepatocytes and the risk of destruction of normal liver parenchyma. More effective methods of delivering radiation to tumours of the liver include (1) IV or intra-arterial injection of antibodies tagged with radioactive isotopes that specifically attack tumour-associated antigens and (2) percutaneous placement of a high-intensity source for interstitial radiation therapy (delivery of radiation directly to the tumour cells). Internal radiotherapy can result in reduction in tumour size, but its effect on survival is yet to be determined.

Chemotherapy

Typically, studies of patients with advanced cases of liver cancer have shown that the use of systemic chemotherapeutic agents leads to poor outcomes. For patients with stable hepatic function (Child class A), a targeted molecular therapy, sorafenib (Nexavar), has been developed and approved for use and has shown some degree of improvement in treating patients with HCC (Nusrat et al., 2014). Systemic chemotherapy may be used to treat metastatic liver lesions. Embolization of tumour vessels with chemotherapy (a process known as transarterial chemoembolization or TACE) produces anoxic necrosis with high concentrations of trapped chemotherapeutic agents. This therapy has begun to show some promising results. An implantable pump has been used to deliver a high concentration of chemotherapy by constant infusion to the liver through the hepatic artery in cases of metastatic disease. This method has shown a moderate response rate (Feldman et al., 2015).

Percutaneous Biliary Drainage

Percutaneous biliary or transhepatic drainage is used to bypass biliary ducts obstructed by liver, pancreatic, or bile duct tumours in patients who have inoperable tumours or are considered poor surgical risks. Under fluoroscopy, a catheter is inserted through the abdominal wall and past the obstruction into the duodenum. Such procedures are used to reestablish biliary drainage, relieve pressure and pain from the buildup of bile behind the obstruction, and decrease pruritus and jaundice. As a result, the patient is made more comfortable and quality of life and survival are improved.

For several days after its insertion, the catheter is opened to external drainage. The bile is observed closely for amount, colour, and presence of blood and debris. Complications of percutaneous biliary drainage include sepsis, leakage of bile, hemorrhage, and reobstruction of the biliary system by debris in the catheter or by encroaching tumour. Therefore, the patient is observed for fever and chills, bile drainage around the catheter, changes in vital signs, and evidence of biliary obstruction, including increased pain or pressure, pruritus, and recurrence of jaundice.

Other Nonsurgical Treatments

Laser hyperthermia has been used to treat hepatic metastases. Heat has been directed to tumours through several methods to cause necrosis of the tumour cells while sparing normal tissue. In radiofrequency thermal ablation, a needle electrode is inserted into the liver tumour under imaging guidance. Radiofrequency energy passes through to the noninsulated needle tip, causing heat and tumour cell death from coagulation necrosis.

Immunotherapy is another treatment modality under investigation. In this therapy, lymphocytes with antitumour reactivity are administered to the patient with hepatic cancer. Tumour regression has been demonstrated in patients with metastatic cancer for whom standard treatment has failed.

Transcatheter arterial embolization interrupts the arterial blood flow to small tumours by injecting small particulate embolic or chemotherapeutic agents (as previously described) into the artery supplying the tumour. As a result, ischemia and necrosis of the tumour occur.

For multiple small lesions, ultrasound-guided injection of alcohol promotes dehydration of tumour cells and tumour necrosis (Feldman et al., 2015; Salgia & Singal, 2014).

Surgical Management

Surgical resection is the treatment of choice when HCC is confined to one lobe of the liver and the function of the remaining liver is considered adequate for postoperative recovery. In the case of metastasis, hepatic resection can be performed if the primary site can be completely excised and the metastasis is limited. However, metastases to the liver are rarely limited or solitary. Capitalizing on the regenerative capacity of the liver cells, some surgeons have successfully removed 90% of the liver. However, the presence of cirrhosis limits the ability of the liver to regenerate. Staging of liver tumours aids in predicting the likelihood of surgical cure.

In preparation for surgery, the patient's nutritional, fluid, and general physical status are assessed, and efforts are undertaken to ensure the best physical condition possible. Extensive diagnostic studies may be performed. Specific studies may include liver scan, liver biopsy, cholangiography, selective hepatic angiography, percutaneous needle biopsy, peritoneoscopy, laparoscopy, ultrasound, CT scan, PET scan, MRI, and blood tests, particularly determinations of serum alkaline phosphatase, AST, and GGT and its isoenzymes.

Lobectomy

Removal of a lobe of the liver is the most common surgical procedure for excising a liver tumour. If it is necessary to restrict blood flow from the hepatic artery and portal vein for longer than 15 minutes, it is likely that hypothermia will be used. For a right-liver lobectomy or an extended right lobectomy (including the medial left lobe), a thoracoabdominal incision is used. An extensive abdominal incision is made for a left lobectomy.

Local Ablation

In patients who are not candidates for resection or transplantation, ablation of HCC may be accomplished by chemicals such as ethanol or by physical means such as radiofrequency ablation or microwave coagulation. These techniques may be performed under ultrasound or CT guidance laparoscopically or percutaneously. Radiofrequency ablation is becoming a standard mode of treatment; a tumour up to 5 cm in size can be destroyed in one session. The most common complications following ablation are local pain or bleeding. Serious complications are rare (Feldman et al., 2015; Salgia & Singal, 2014).

Immunotherapy with interferon has been under study as an adjuvant after liver resection or ablation of HCC. When patients have developed HCC related to hepatitis B or C, interferon may prevent recurrence of the lesion.

Liver Transplantation

Liver transplantation offers good patient outcomes. Candidates with liver cancer meet stringent selection criteria, including having small, early-stage lesions (Nusrat et al., 2014). The Milan criteria have been developed to limit transplantation to patients who are most likely to have better outcomes. The Milan criteria include that the patient must have a single tumour measuring less than 5 cm, or have three or fewer lesions with none over 3 cm in size (Nusrat et al., 2014). This treatment involves removing the liver and replacing it with a healthy donor organ. Studies report decreased recurrence rates of the primary liver malignancy after transplantation, with improvement in 4-year survival rates to approximately 85% (Nusrat et al., 2014). Metastasis and recurrence may be enhanced by the immunosuppressive therapy that is needed to prevent rejection of the transplanted liver. In patients with small (less than 5 cm), single lesions, liver transplantation has been shown to be beneficial, but its use is limited by organ shortages. The increasing use of living donor transplantation may improve this situation and decrease the waiting time and tumour proliferation that is characteristic of patients with liver cancer (see later discussion).

Nursing Management

For the surgical patient, support, explanation, and encouragement are provided to help the patient prepare psychologically for the surgery. After surgery, potential problems related to cardiopulmonary involvement may include vascular complications and respiratory and liver dysfunction. Metabolic abnormalities require careful attention. A constant infusion of 10% glucose may be required in the first 48 hours to prevent a precipitous fall in the blood glucose level that results from decreased gluconeogenesis. Because extensive blood loss may occur as well, the patient receives infusions of blood and IV fluids. The patient requires constant, close monitoring and care for the first 2 or 3 days, similar to postsurgical abdominal and thoracic nursing care.

If the patient is to receive chemotherapy or radiation therapy in an effort to relieve symptoms, he or she may be discharged home while still receiving one or both of these therapies. The patient may also go home with a biliary drainage system or hepatic artery catheter in place. In most cases, the hepatic artery catheter has been inserted surgically and has a prefilled infusion pump that delivers a continuous chemotherapeutic dose until completed. An hepatic artery port may also be inserted to provide access for intermittent chemotherapy infusion. This port dwells under the skin, but, because it provides direct arterial access, it is not used for continuous infusion therapy in the home environment; the access line is discontinued once the chemotherapeutic agent has infused. The patient and family require teaching about care of the biliary catheter and the effects and side effects of hepatic artery chemotherapy. This teaching is necessary because of participation of the patient and family in patient care in the home setting.

Promoting Home, Community-Based, and Transitional Care

Educating Patients About Self-Care

The nurse instructs the patient to recognize and report the potential complications and side effects of the chemotherapy and the desirable and undesirable effects of the specific chemotherapy regimen. The nurse also emphasizes the importance of follow-up visits to assess the patient and the tumour's response to chemotherapy and radiation therapy. In addition, if the patient is receiving chemotherapy on an outpatient basis, the nurse explains the patient's and family's role in managing the chemotherapy infusion and in assessing the infusion or insertion site. The nurse encourages the patient to resume routine activities as soon as possible, while cautioning about activities that may damage the infusion pump or site.

The family of as well as the patient at home with a biliary drainage system in place typically fear that the catheter will become dislodged. Reassurance and instruction can help reduce their fear that the catheter will fall out easily. The patient and family also require instruction on catheter care. The family and the patient need to learn how to keep the catheter site clean and dry and how to assess the catheter and its insertion site. Irrigation of the catheter with sterile normal saline solution or water may be prescribed to keep the catheter patent and free of debris. The patient and caregivers are taught proper technique to avoid introducing bacteria into the biliary system or catheter during irrigation. They are instructed not to aspirate or draw back on the syringe during irrigation, to prevent entry of irritating duodenal contents into the biliary tree or catheter. The patient and caregivers are also instructed about the signs of complications and are encouraged to notify the nurse or physician if problems or questions arise.

Patients with implantable ports are instructed about the chemotherapy regimen, types of medications, effects and side effects that may occur, and appropriate management strategies if problems occur. If a hepatic artery port is inserted for intermittent chemotherapy, patients and their families are provided the same educational content. Such a port has an internal one-way valve; therefore, it is not aspirated for a blood return before the infusion is initiated. The patient is instructed to assess the port site between infusions and to note and report any sign of infection or inflammation.

Continuing and Transitional Care

In many cases, referral for transitional or home care enables the patient with liver cancer to be at home in a familiar environment with family and friends. Because of the poor prognosis associated with liver cancer, the home care nurse serves a vital role in assisting the patient and family to cope with the symptoms that may occur and the prognosis. The home care nurse assesses the patient's physical and psychological status, adequacy of pain relief, nutritional status, and presence of symptoms indicating complications of treatment or progression of disease. During home visits, the nurse assesses the function of the chemotherapy pump, the infusion site, and the biliary drainage system, if indicated. The nurse collaborates with the other members of the health care team, the patient, and the family to ensure effective pain management and to manage potential problems, which include weakness, pruritus, inadequate dietary intake, jaundice, and symptoms associated with metastasis to other sites. The home care nurse also assists the patient and family in making decisions about hospice care and assists with initiation of referrals. The patient is encouraged to discuss preferences for end-of-life care with family members and health care providers.

LIVER TRANSPLANTATION

Liver transplantation is used to treat life-threatening ESLD for which no other form of treatment is available. The transplantation procedure involves total removal of the diseased liver and replacement with a healthy liver in the same anatomic location (**orthotopic liver transplantation [OLT]**). Removal of the liver creates a space for the new liver and permits anatomic reconstruction of the hepatic vasculature and biliary tract as close to normal as possible.

The success of liver transplantation depends on successful immunosuppression. Immunosuppressant agents currently used include cyclosporine (Neoral), tacrolimus (Prograf), corticosteroids, azathioprine (Imuran), mycophenolate mofetil (CellCept), sirolimus (formerly known as rapamycin [Rapamune]), everolimus (Afinitor), antithymocyte globulin (Thymoglobulin), basiliximab (Simulect), and daclizumab (Zenapax). There is no one, accepted, optimal immunosuppressive regimen. Most transplant centres have developed their own therapeutic practices, largely based on experience. Multiple immunosuppressive strategies can be used to prevent transplanted organ rejection. Most strategies involve the use of more than one agent but current recommendations advise the minimization of immunosuppression in order to avoid toxicity (Gotthardt, Bruns, Weiss, et al., 2014). Using multiple immunosuppressive agents has the effect of blocking multiple targets in the immune response cascade. This allows the use of lower doses of each drug, thus avoiding toxicity associated with high doses of these powerful drugs. Some patients are treated with "triple therapy" using corticosteroids, a calcineurin inhibitor such as tacrolimus or cyclosporine, and either an antiproliferative agent (mycophenolate mofetil) or a TOR (target of rapamycin) inhibitor such as sirolimus and everolimus (Doherty, 2015; Gotthardt et al., 2014). Some transplant centres also prescribe steroid-free immunosuppressant regimens after liver transplantation. This regimen has been found to be a safe alternative. Still other transplant centres advocate monotherapy with a calcineurin inhibitor alone to provide long-term immunosuppression (Doherty, 2015; Gotthardt et al., 2014; Townsend et al., 2016). In order to prevent acute rejection in the early, high-risk months after liver transplantation, some centres employ induction therapy, which is the use of prophylactic, perioperative course of immunosuppressant drugs that suppress the body's response to the foreign, transplanted tissue and may improve graft survival by reducing the risk of acute cellular rejection (Gotthardt et al., 2014). Medications used for induction include basiliximab and a lymphocyte immune globulin (Atgam). Over time, withdrawal of all immunosuppressants is possible but rare; randomized, prospective studies are needed before this clinical practice is accepted (Gotthardt et al., 2014).

Despite the success of immunosuppression in reducing the incidence of rejection of transplanted organs, liver transplantation is not routine and may be accompanied by complications related to the lengthy surgical procedure, immunosuppressive therapy, infection, and the technical difficulties encountered in reconstructing the blood vessels and biliary tract. Long-standing systemic problems resulting from the primary liver disease may complicate the preoperative and postoperative course. Previous surgery of the abdomen, including procedures to treat complications of advanced liver disease (i.e., shunt procedures used to treat portal hypertension and esophageal varices) increase the complexity of the transplantation procedure.

The indications for liver transplantation are not as limited today as they were when the procedure was first introduced because of advances in immunosuppressive therapy, improvements in biliary tract reconstruction, and, in some cases, the use of venovenous bypass. General indications for liver transplantation include irreversible advanced chronic liver disease, fulminant hepatic failure, metabolic liver diseases, and some hepatic malignancies. Examples of disorders that are indications for liver transplantation include hepatocellular liver diseases (e.g., viral hepatitis, drug-induced or alcohol-induced liver disease, fatty liver, Wilson's disease) and cholestatic diseases (primary biliary cirrhosis, sclerosing cholangitis, and biliary atresia).

The patient being considered for liver transplantation frequently has many systemic problems that influence preoperative and postoperative care. Because transplantation is more difficult if the patient has developed severe GI bleeding and hepatic coma, efforts are made to perform the procedure before the disease progresses to this stage. The patient must undergo a thorough evaluation of hepatic reserve and general health. Part of this evaluation includes classification of the degree of medical need, an objective determination known as the model of end-stage liver disease (MELD) classification, which stratifies the level of illness of those awaiting a liver transplant. The MELD score is derived from a complex formula incorporating bilirubin levels, prothrombin time (reported as international normalized ratio [INR]), creatinine, and the cause of the liver disease (i.e., cholestatic, alcoholic, or other). This system has replaced the Child–Pugh classification and other related scoring systems for prioritizing patients on the liver transplantation list (Fox, 2014). Although the Child–Pugh score classifies the severity of liver disease and stratifies patients into levels for varied treatment regimens, the MELD score is an indicator of short-term mortality for those with ESLD. Organs are allocated using the MELD score in an effort to provide transplants to the most severely ill patients.

Because liver transplantation is now an established therapeutic modality, rather than an experimental procedure, the number of liver transplantation centres is increasing. Patients requiring transplantation are often referred from distant hospitals to these centres. To prepare the patient and family for liver transplantation, nurses in all settings must understand the processes and procedures of liver transplantation.

Many ethical issues arise concerning liver transplantation, particularly concerning the allocation of organs. The way in which some persons contracted liver disease (e.g., alcohol use; hepatitis) leads others to question allocation of organs to them, and some believe that preference should be given to people who need liver transplants but do not have a history of socially unacceptable behaviour. Even more controversy exists when a patient requires a second transplant operation because of a return to alcohol or drug use or failure to follow immunosuppressive regimens (Chart 39-13). These are difficult issues with no easy solutions. Transplant recipients must go through a rigorous selection and preparation process that includes counselling and education to aid them in making critical choices for their improved health. Nurses and other health care providers need to be aware of and confront their own biases and work toward improved understanding and acceptance.

CHART 39-13

Ethical Dilemma

What Ethical Principles Apply When a Candidate for a Second Liver Transplantation Continues His Drug Use?

SITUATION

A 34-year-old man received a liver transplant a year ago for end-stage liver disease due to hepatitis C (with a history of IV or injection use) and alcoholic liver disease. He experienced a difficult postoperative course with many complications. His liver function has now deteriorated to the point that he is listed to receive a second organ. He is in the hospital, where he is quite ill and in pain. Although he denies further use of alcohol and drug use following his first liver transplant, several bottles of opioids and sedatives are found in his bedside table.

What ethical implications exist in this case? What actions should be taken by the transplant team? What should the nurse document concerning this situation? What factors should be considered when deciding how to proceed in this case?

DILEMMA

This patient has already received one liver transplant, and he will not survive unless he receives another one. He is on the list for a second transplant. Because of the limited availability of livers for transplantation and the fact that there is a strong likelihood of his continued use of drugs, questions have been raised about the appropriateness of a second transplant.

DISCUSSION

1. What ethical principles are involved in this situation?
2. What are the competing issues in this case that must be considered in this man's case?
3. How does the nurse respond if the patient asks about the likelihood of his receiving a second liver transplant?

Surgical Procedure

During the procedure, the donor liver is freed from other structures, the bile is flushed from the gallbladder to prevent damage to the walls of the biliary tract, and the liver is perfused with a preservative and cooled. Before the donor liver is placed in the recipient, it is flushed with cold lactated Ringer's solution to remove potassium and air bubbles. The presence of portal hypertension increases the difficulty of the procedure. To minimize this problem, many centres use venovenous bypass, which decompresses the venous system below the diaphragm by temporarily shunting blood to the superior vena cava via the axillary vein (Rai, 2013).

Anastomoses (connections) of the blood vessels and bile duct are performed between the donor liver and the recipient liver. There are two types of biliary anastomoses. Biliary reconstruction is performed with an end-to-end anastomosis of the donor and recipient common bile ducts; a stented T-tube may be inserted for external drainage of bile. In patients with biliary disease such as primary sclerosing cholangitis or if the recipient's bile duct is not suitable for anastomosis for other reasons, a biliary-enteric end-to-side anastomosis with a 40 to 50 cm Roux-en-Y loop of jejunum is created for biliary drainage (Fig. 39-13A); in this case, bile drainage is internal, and a T-tube is not inserted

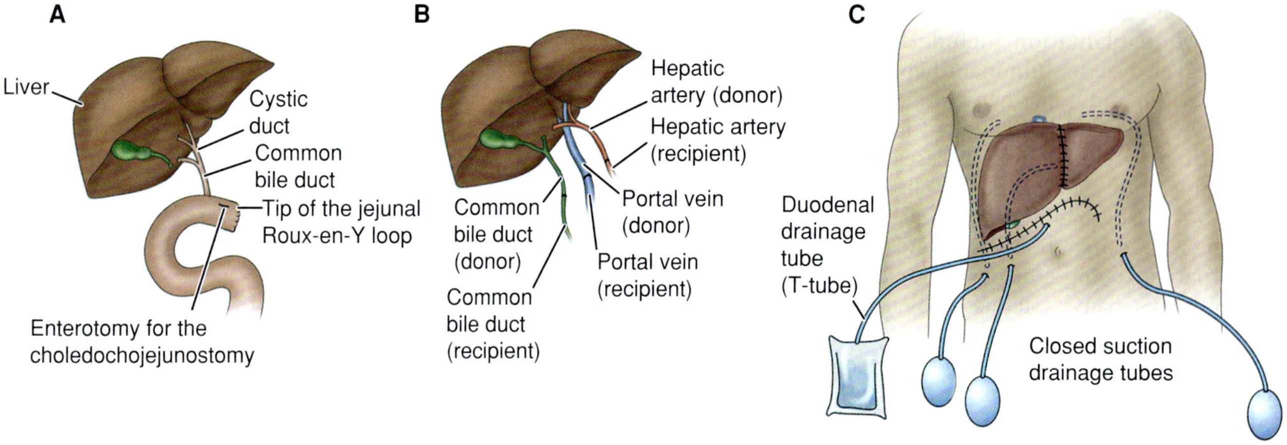

FIGURE 39-13. A. Some transplant recipients have diseases or conditions that cause their bile ducts to be unusable for anastomosis to the donor liver bile duct. In this case, a loop of jejunum is used as a bridge from the donor liver bile duct to the recipient's small bowel for biliary continuity and drainage. This procedure is termed a Roux-en-Y hepaticojejunostomy. **B.** Final appearance of implanted liver graft with an end-to-end biliary anastomosis. **C.** Final closure and drain placement after liver transplantation with an end-to-end biliary anastomosis and T-tube placement.

(Townsend et al., 2016). Figure 39-13B and C illustrates the final appearance of the grafted liver and final closure and drain placement.

Several additional techniques have been developed to expand the donor pool for liver transplantation. In a split-liver transplant, a single organ is used to provide grafts for two individuals with ESLD, with the smaller patient receiving the smaller left lobe. This procedure has resulted in a higher complication rate and lower survival rate than traditional liver transplantation. Living donor transplantation is being increasingly performed from adult to adult using full right lobes, although it is controversial because it is a major surgical procedure for the donor, and some donor deaths have occurred.

Living donor liver transplantation (LDLT) is considered for patients who have a high potential for mortality while awaiting a cadaveric liver donor, such as those patients with HCC or those with severe complications of cirrhosis including GI bleeding or hepatic encephalopathy (Townsend et al., 2016). The results thus far have indicated that this procedure is most successful when donor and recipient are appropriately selected using careful screening criteria (Townsend et al., 2016). The option of LDLT decreases the waiting list mortality and produces positive recipient outcomes with a low risk of morbidity and mortality for the donor. The LDLT procedure involves transplantation of the right hepatic lobe from an adult donor to the recipient. Potential donors are evaluated by a donor advocate team. Donors must be completely healthy and have hepatic size and anatomy compatible with right lobe transplantation (Townsend et al., 2016). There is an extensive informed consent process for live liver donors. The donor advocate ensures that the concern for donor safety is paramount, especially in the intra- and postoperative period when complications can occur. The clear separation of donor and recipient teams ensures that the donor is treated without ulterior motives, which might occur if the same team cared for both the donor and recipient (Townsend et al., 2016).

Complications

The postoperative complication rate is high, primarily because of technical complications or infection. Immediate postoperative complications may include bleeding, infection, and rejection. Disruption, infection, obstruction of the biliary anastomosis, and impaired biliary drainage may occur. Vascular thrombosis and stenosis are other potential complications. These complications occur in patients receiving either a cadaver or live donor organ. Despite the development of some complications, the 1-year patient survival rate approaches 90% and the 5-year patient survival rate is approximately 80% (Townsend et al., 2016; Wong & Pagalilauan, 2015).

Bleeding

Bleeding is common in the postoperative period and may result from coagulopathy, portal hypertension, and fibrinolysis caused by ischemic injury to the donor liver. Hemodynamic instability and transient hypotension may occur in this phase, secondary to blood loss, loss of vasomotor tone, and vasodilatation due to rewarming the hypothermic patient or due to pre-existing cardiac conditions such as cardiomyopathy (Goldman & Schafer, 2015; Wong & Pagalilauan, 2015). Administration of platelets, fresh-frozen plasma, or other blood products may be necessary.

Hypertension

Hypertension may co-occur postoperatively but is more common later in the postoperative phase, although its cause is uncertain. Currently available hypertension guidelines do not have specific recommendations for management in the liver transplant population. However, calcium channel blockers such as nifedipine or amlodipine are frequently used for their vasodilatory effects. These drugs also are preferable due to their low interaction level with the cytochrome P450 enzyme system with resultant minimal risk of disruption of immunosuppressant levels. Angiotensin-converting enzyme inhibitors and angiotensin receptor blockers are not first-line drugs for the treatment of hypertension during the first year after transplant due to low levels of renin during this time period. Thiazide diuretics are reserved for patients requiring more than one medication for blood pressure control (Wong & Pagalilauan, 2015). Blood pressure elevation that is significant or sustained is also managed with lifestyle modifications, a low-sodium diet, and an exercise regimen.

Infection

Infection is the leading cause of death after liver transplantation. Pulmonary and fungal infections are common; susceptibility to infection is increased by the immunosuppressive therapy that is needed to prevent rejection (Wong & Pagalilauan, 2015). Therefore, precautions must be taken to prevent health care–associated infections. The nurse uses strict asepsis when manipulating central venous catheters, arterial lines, and urine, bile, and other drainage systems; obtaining specimens; and changing dressings. Meticulous hand hygiene is crucial. In the ICU, the nurse vigilantly monitors for early clinical manifestations of sepsis (see Chapter 55, Charts 55-5 and 55-6) and uses evidence-based practice guidelines (or bundles) developed by the Institute for Healthcare Improvement (IHI) in the care of the postoperative liver transplant patient. Some of these care guidelines include prevention of sepsis through prevention of central line–associated bloodstream infections and its rapid treatment (see Chart 55-2) and prevention of ventilator-associated pneumonia (VAP) (see Chapter 55, Chart 55-6).

Rejection

Rejection is a primary concern. A transplanted liver is perceived by the immune system as a foreign antigen. This triggers an immune response, leading to the activation of T lymphocytes that attack and destroy the transplanted liver. Immunosuppressive agents are used as long-term therapy to prevent this response and rejection of the transplanted liver. These agents inhibit the activation of immunocompetent T lymphocytes to prevent the production of effector T cells.

Although the 1- and 5-year survival rates have increased dramatically with the use of new immunosuppressive therapies, these advances are not without major side effects. A major side effect of cyclosporine, which was widely used in transplantation, is nephrotoxicity; this problem seems to be dose related. Cyclosporine-related side effects have caused many centres to use tacrolimus as first-line therapy because of its efficacy and lower side-effect profile.

Corticosteroids, azathioprine, mycophenolate mofetil, sirolimus, antithymocyte globulin, basiliximab, and daclizumab are also used in various regimens of immunosuppression. These agents may be used as the initial therapy to prevent rejection or used later to treat rejection. Liver biopsy and ultrasound may be required to evaluate suspected episodes of rejection.

Retransplantation is usually attempted if the transplanted liver fails, but the success rate of retransplantation does not approach that of initial transplantation.

Complications of the LDLT Donor

Improved surgical techniques have made the LDLT procedure an increasingly safe one; however, complications do occur for donors as well. The most frequently occurring complications include pulmonary emboli, portal vein thrombosis, bile duct injury, and liver insufficiency secondary to a resection that is too extensive (Townsend et al., 2016).

Nursing Management

The patient considering transplantation, together with the family, must make difficult choices about treatment, use of financial resources, and relocation to another area to be closer to the medical centre. They must also be aware of the risks and benefits of the procedure and its consequences. In addition, they must also cope with the patient's long-standing health problems and any social and family problems associated with behaviours that may have caused the patient's liver failure if this is applicable. As a result, considerable emotional stress occurs while the patient and family consider liver transplantation and wait for an available liver.

If the patient and family are considering undergoing a live donor liver transplant, they are subject to additional stressors. Both the patient and the potential donor must undergo a thorough and exhaustive physical and psychological workup to ensure that all involved parties are physically and emotionally prepared. Often, but not always, the donor is a close family member. Coercion must be excluded as influencing the decision to donate a portion of one's liver to another. The potential donor must be aware of the risks associated with the procedure.

If the patient and family believe that liver transplantation may be appropriate, the nurse, surgeon, hepatologist, and other health care team members provide the patient and family with full explanations about the procedure, the chances of success, and the risks, including the side effects of long-term immunosuppression. The need for close follow-up and lifelong compliance with the therapeutic regimen, including immunosuppression, is emphasized to the patient and family.

Preoperative Nursing Interventions

Once the patient has been accepted as a candidate, he or she is placed on a waiting list at the transplant centre, and patient information is entered into the United Network for Organ Sharing (UNOS) computer system. The UNOS system uses the MELD score to determine organ allocation priorities so that the patient with the highest MELD score will receive the first available organ. Candidates may be matched with appropriate organs as they become available. MELD scores provide the necessary information regarding medical need.

Except in the case of segmental liver transplantation from a living donor, a liver becomes available for transplantation only with the death of another person, usually someone who had been healthy except for severe brain injury and brain death. Therefore, the patient and family undergo a stressful waiting period, and the nurse is often their major source of support. The patient must be accessible at all times in case an appropriate liver becomes available. During this time, liver function may deteriorate further, and the patient may experience other complications from the primary liver disease. Because of the shortage of donor organs, many patients die awaiting transplantation.

Malnutrition, massive ascites, and fluid and electrolyte disturbances are treated before surgery to increase the likelihood of a successful outcome. If the patient's liver dysfunction has a very rapid onset, as in fulminant hepatic failure, there is little time or opportunity for the patient to consider and weigh options and their consequences; often this patient is in a coma, and the decision to proceed with transplantation is made by the family.

The nurse coordinator is an integral member of the transplant team and plays an important role in preparing the patient for liver transplantation. The nurse serves as an advocate for the patient and family and assumes the important role of liaison between the patient and the other members of the transplant team. The nurse also serves as a resource to other nurses and health care team members involved in evaluating and caring for the patient.

Postoperative Nursing Interventions

The patient is maintained in an environment as free from bacteria, viruses, and fungi as possible, because immunosuppressive medications reduce the body's natural defenses. In the immediate postoperative period, cardiovascular, pulmonary, renal, neurologic, and metabolic functions are monitored continuously. Mean arterial and pulmonary artery pressures are also monitored continuously. Cardiac output, central venous pressure, pulmonary capillary wedge pressure, arterial and mixed venous blood gases, oxygen saturation, oxygen demand and delivery, urine output, heart rate, and blood pressure are used to evaluate the patient's hemodynamic status and intravascular fluid volume. Liver function tests, electrolyte levels, the coagulation profile, chest x-ray, electrocardiogram, and fluid output (including urine, bile from the T-tube, and drainage from Jackson–Pratt tubes) are monitored closely. Because the liver is responsible for the storage of glycogen and the synthesis of protein and clotting factors, these substances need to be monitored and replaced in the immediate postoperative period.

There is a high risk of atelectasis and an altered ventilation–perfusion ratio caused by insult to the diaphragm during the surgical procedure, prolonged anesthesia, immobility, and postoperative pain. The patient will have an endotracheal tube in place and will require mechanical ventilation during the initial postoperative period. Suctioning is performed as required, and sterile humidification is provided. Evidence-based practice guidelines are implemented to prevent the development of VAP in the postoperative liver transplant recipient. Actions such as keeping the head of the bed elevated at least 30 degrees and performing frequent oral suctioning and cleansing are effective in preventing VAP.

As the patient's condition stabilizes, efforts are made to promote recovery from the trauma of this complex surgery. After removal of the endotracheal tube, the nurse encourages the patient to use an incentive spirometer to decrease the risk of atelectasis. Following extubation, the patient is assisted to get out of bed, to ambulate as tolerated, and to participate in self-care to prevent the complications associated with immobility. Close monitoring for signs and symptoms of liver dysfunction and rejection continue throughout the hospital stay. Plans are made for close follow-up after discharge as well. Teaching is initiated during the preoperative period and continues after surgery.

Promoting Home, Community-Based, and Transitional Care

Educating Patients About Self-Care

Teaching the patient and family about long-term measures to promote health is crucial for the success of transplantation and is an important role of the nurse. The patient and family must understand why they need to adhere closely to the therapeutic regimen, with special emphasis on the methods of administration, rationale, and side effects of the prescribed immunosuppressive agents. The nurse provides written as well as verbal instructions about how and when to take the medications. To avoid running out of medication or skipping a dose, the patient must make sure that an adequate supply of medication is available. Instructions are also provided about the signs and symptoms that indicate problems necessitating consultation with the transplant team. The patient with a T-tube in place must be taught how to manage the tube, drainage, and skin care.

Continuing and Transitional Care

The nurse emphasizes the importance of follow-up blood tests and appointments with the transplant team. Trough blood levels of immunosuppressive agents are obtained, along with other blood tests that assess the function of the liver and kidneys. During the first months, the patient is likely to require blood tests two or three times a week. As the patient's condition stabilizes, blood studies and visits to the transplant team are less frequent. The importance of routine ophthalmologic examinations is emphasized because of the increased incidence of cataracts and glaucoma associated with the long-term corticosteroid therapy used with transplantation. Regular oral hygiene and follow-up dental care, with administration of prophylactic antibiotics before dental examinations and treatments, are recommended because of the immunosuppression.

The nurse reminds the patient that preventing rejection and infection is essential and increases the chances for survival and a more normal life than before transplantation. Many patients have lived successful and productive lives after receiving a liver transplant. In fact, pregnancy can be considered 1 year after transplantation. Although successful outcomes have been reported, these pregnancies are considered high risk for both mother and infant. Transplant recipients should be advised about birth control. The 1-year waiting period allows time to establish good health, stable liver function, and lower maintenance levels of immunosuppressive therapy (Feldman et al., 2015; Wong & Pagalilauan, 2015).

LIVER ABSCESSES

Two categories of liver abscess have been identified: amebic and pyogenic. Amebic liver abscesses are most commonly caused by *Entamoeba histolytica*. Most amebic liver abscesses occur in the developing countries of the tropics and subtropics because of poor sanitation and hygiene. Pyogenic liver abscesses are much less common, but they are more common in developed countries than the amebic type (Townsend et al., 2016).

Pathophysiology

Whenever an infection develops anywhere along the biliary or GI tract, infecting organisms may reach the liver through the biliary system, portal venous system, or hepatic arterial or lymphatic system. Most bacteria are destroyed promptly, but occasionally some gain a foothold. The bacterial toxins destroy the neighbouring liver cells, and the resulting necrotic tissue serves as a protective wall for the organisms.

Meanwhile, leukocytes migrate into the infected area. The result is an abscess cavity full of a liquid containing living and dead leukocytes, liquefied liver cells, and bacteria. Pyogenic abscesses of this type may be either single or multiple and small. Examples of causes of pyogenic liver abscess include cholangitis (usually related to benign or malignant obstruction of the biliary tree) and abdominal trauma.

Clinical Manifestations

The clinical picture is one of sepsis with few or no localizing signs. Fever with chills and diaphoresis, malaise, anorexia, nausea, vomiting, and weight loss may occur. The patient may complain of dull abdominal pain and tenderness in the right upper quadrant of the abdomen. Hepatomegaly, jaundice, anemia, and pleural effusion may develop. Sepsis and shock may be severe and life-threatening. In the past, the mortality rate was 100% because of the vague clinical symptoms, inadequate diagnostic tools, and inadequate surgical drainage of the abscess. With the aid of ultrasound, CT, MRI, and liver scans, early diagnosis and surgical drainage of abscesses have greatly reduced the mortality rate.

Assessment and Diagnostic Findings

Although blood cultures are obtained, the organism may not be identified. Aspiration of the liver abscess, guided by ultrasound, CT, or MRI, may be performed to assist in diagnosis and to obtain cultures of the organism. Percutaneous drainage of pyogenic abscesses is carried out to evacuate the abscess material and promote healing. A catheter may be left in place for continuous drainage; the patient must be instructed about its management.

Medical Management

Treatment includes IV antibiotic therapy; the specific antibiotic used in treatment depends on the organism identified. Continuous supportive care is indicated because of the serious condition of the patient. Open surgical drainage may be required if antibiotic therapy and percutaneous drainage are ineffective.

Nursing Management

Although the manifestations of liver abscess vary with the type of abscess, most patients appear acutely ill. Others appear to be chronically ill and debilitated. The nursing management depends on the patient's physical status and the medical management that is indicated. For patients who undergo evacuation and drainage of an abscess, monitoring of the drainage and skin care are imperative. Strategies must be implemented to contain the drainage and to protect the patient from other sources of infection. Vital signs are monitored to detect changes in the patient's physical status. Deterioration in vital signs or the onset of new symptoms such as increasing pain, which may indicate rupture or extension of the abscess, is reported promptly. The nurse administers IV antibiotic therapy as prescribed. The white blood cell count and other laboratory test results are monitored closely for changes consistent with worsening infection. The nurse prepares the patient for discharge by providing instruction about symptom management, signs and symptoms that should be reported to the physician, management of drainage, and the importance of taking antibiotics as prescribed.

Critical Thinking Exercises

1 A 56-year-old woman is at high risk for hepatitis B and C due to a history of IV drug abuse. What laboratory testing is likely to be done first for this patient? If laboratory testing is positive for either or both diseases, what invasive and noninvasive testing is warranted next? Describe the education a nurse working with this patient should provide about these tests.

2 A 68-year-old man is admitted to the hospital with a diagnosis of ESLD with hepatic encephalopathy. What is the evidence base for meeting the nutritional needs of this patient? What are the most appropriate caloric and protein intake recommendations? Identify the criteria used to evaluate the strength of the evidence for the treatment practices you have identified.

3 A 66-year-old man underwent an orthotopic liver transplant for decompensated cirrhosis. He is placed on an immunosuppressant regimen including corticosteroids, mycophenolate mofetil, and tacrolimus. On day 10 postoperatively, he develops an acute change in mental status with confusion and severe extremity tremors. As this patient's nurse, you are in attendance when the patient appears to have a generalized clonic seizure. Identify the priorities, approach, and techniques you would use to provide immediate interventions for this patient. What are your concerns regarding the potential causes of these neurologic abnormalities? What testing would you anticipate? Could his medication regimen have a role in the symptomatology? What laboratory testing would be important in identifying a cause for the seizure?

4 A 44-year-old woman with obesity is diagnosed with NAFLD and is symptomatic with jaundice and fatigue. What are the best risk reduction tactics for this patient? How should the nurse prepare and educate the patient to achieve specific evidence-based management goals and potentially control the disease?

REFERENCES AND SELECTED READINGS

Books

Aqel, B. A. (2016). *Practical gastroenterology and hepatology board review toolkit*. John Wiley & Sons.

Bateson, M. C., & Bouchier, I. A. (2017). Gastrointestinal bleeding. In *Clinical investigations in gastroenterology* (pp. 103–108). Cham: Springer.

Benjamin, I., Griggs, R. C., & Wing, E. J., et al. (2015). *Andreoli and Carpenter's Cecil essentials of medicine e-book*. Elsevier Health Sciences.

Feldman, M., Friedman, L. S., & Brandt, L. J. (Eds.). (2015). *Sleisenger and Fordtran's gastrointestinal and liver disease: Pathophysiology, diagnosis, management*. Elsevier Health Sciences.

Goldman, L., & Schafer, A. I. (2015). *Goldman's Cecil medicine* (25th ed.). Philadelphia, PA: Saunders Elsevier.

Grossman, S. (2013). *Porth's pathophysiology: Concepts of altered health status* (9th ed.). Philadelphia, PA: Lippincott Williams & Wilkins.

Koppula, R., & Haskal, Z. J. (2018). Transjugular intrahepatic portosystemic shunt (TIPS) and portal hypertension. In *IR Playbook* (pp. 419–427). Cham: Springer.

Public Health Agency of Canada. (2012). *Hepatitis*. Ottawa, ON: Author.

Public Health Agency of Canada. (2013). *Canadian immunization guide*. Ottawa, ON: Author.

Public Health Agency of Canada. (2014). *Hepatitis C in Canada: 2005–2010 surveillance report*. Ottawa, ON: Author.

Public Health Agency of Canada. (2017). *Report on hepatitis B and C in Canada: 2014*. Ottawa, ON: Author.

Ross, A. C., Caballero, B., Cousins, R. J., et al. (Eds). (2012). *Modern nutrition in health and disease* (11th ed.). Philadelphia, PA: Lippincott Williams & Wilkins.

Schiff, E. R., Maddrey, W. C., & Sorrell, M. F. (Eds.). (2012). *Schiff's diseases of the liver* (11th ed.). Philadelphia, PA: Lippincott Williams & Wilkins.

Standring, S. (Ed.). (2015). *Gray's anatomy e-book: The anatomical basis of clinical practice*. Elsevier Health Sciences.

Townsend, C. M., Beauchamp, R. D., Evers, B. M., et al. (2016). *Sabiston's textbook of surgery: The biological basis of modern surgical practice*. Philadelphia, PA: Elsevier.

Journals and Electronic Documents

Abraldes, J. G., Sarlieve, P., & Tandon, P. (2014). Measurement of portal pressure. *Clinics in Liver Disease*, *18*(4), 779–792.

American Association for the Study of Liver Diseases Society of America, International Antiviral Society—USA. (2014). Recommendations for testing, managing and treating hepatitis C. Alexandria, VA. Retrieved December 1, 2015, from www.hcvguidelines.org.

Banares, R., Catalina, M. V., & Vaquero, J. (2014). Molecular adsorbent recirculating system and bioartificial devices for liver failure. *Clinics in Liver Disease*, *18*(4), 945–956.

Barrera, F., Zuniga, P., & Arrese, M. (2015). Prediction of esophageal variceal bleeding in liver cirrhosis: Is there a role for hemostatic factors? *Seminars in Thrombosis and Hemostasis*, *41*(5), 481–487.

Bloom, S., Kemp, W., & Lubel, J. (2015). Portal hypertension: Pathophysiology, diagnosis and management. *Internal Medicine Journal*, *45*(1), 16–26.

Bonder, A., Tapper, E. B., & Afdhal, N. H. (2015). Contemporary assessment of hepatic fibrosis. *Clinics in Liver Disease*, *19*(1), 123–134.

Bope, E. T., & Kellerman, R. D. (2015). Conn's current therapy 2016. Philadelphia, PA: Elsevier Health Sciences.

Cameron, A. M. (2015). Screening for viral hepatitis and hepatocellular carcinoma. *Surgical Clinics of North America*, *95*(5), 1013–1021.

Canadian Liver Foundation. (2017). Retrieved from https://www.liver.ca/patients-caregivers/liver-diseases/

Centers for Disease Control and Prevention (CDC), Division of Viral Hepatitis. (2013). Viral hepatitis surveillance—United States, 2013. Retrieved December 1, 2015, from www.cdc.gov/hepatitis/Statistics/2010Surveillance/index.htm

Chalasani, N., Younossi, Z., Lavine, J. E., et al. (2018). The diagnosis and management of nonalcoholic fatty liver disease: Practice guidance from the American Association for the Study of Liver Diseases. *Hepatology*, *67*(1), 328–357.

Chan, S. L., Wong, V. W., Qin, S., et al. (2016). Infection and cancer: The case of hepatitis B. *Journal of Clinical Oncology*, *34*(1), 83–90.

Chen, R. P., Zhu Ge, X. J., Huang, Z. M., et al. (2014). Prophylactic use of transjugular intrahepatic portosystemic shunt aids in treatment of refractory ascites: Metaregression and trial sequential meta-analysis. *Journal of Clinical Gastroenterology*, *48*(3), 290–299.

Cholongitas, E., Tziomalos, K., & Pipili, C. (2015). Management of patients with hepatitis B in special populations. *World Journal of Gastroenterology*, *21*(6), 1738–1748.

Dan, C., Moses-Eisenstein, M., & Valdiserri, R. O. (2015). Viral hepatitis: New US screening recommendations, assessment tools, and treatments. *American Journal of Nursing*, *115*(7), 26–36; quiz 36, 48.

Doherty, G. (2015). Current diagnosis and treatment: Surgery (14th ed.). New York, NY: McGraw-Hill.

Ellul, M. A., Gholkar, S. A., & Cross, T. J. (2015). Hepatic encephalopathy due to liver cirrhosis. *British Medical Journal*, *351*, 26–30.

European Association for the Study of the Liver. (2013). Too much drinking, weight may harm liver. News release, April 25, 2013. Retrieved on November 28, 2015, from www.easl.eu

Fabrellas, N., Alemany, M., Urquizu, M., et al. (2013). Using transient elastography to detect chronic liver diseases in a primary care nurse consultancy. *Nursing Research*, *62*(6), 450–454.

Ferri, F. F. (Ed.). (2014). Practical guide to the care of the medical patient (9th ed.). Philadelphia, PA: Mosby Elsevier.

Fialla, A. D., Israelsen, M., Hamberg, O., et al. (2015). Nutritional therapy in cirrhosis or alcoholic hepatitis: A systematic review and meta-analysis. *Liver International*, *35*(9), 2072–2078.

Fox, R. K. (2014). When to consider liver transplantation during the management of chronic liver disease. *Medical Clinics of North America*, *98*(1), 153–168.

Fullwood, D., & Purushothaman, A. (2014). Managing ascites in patients with chronic liver disease. *Nursing Standard*, *28*(23), 51–58; quiz 60.

Ghaziani, T., Sendi, H., Shahraz, S., et al. (2014). Hepatitis B and liver transplantation: Molecular and clinical features that influence recurrence and outcome. *World Journal of Gastroenterology*, *20*(39), 14142–14155.

Gotthardt, D. N., Bruns, H., Weiss, K. H., et al. (2014). Current strategies for immunosuppression following liver transplantation. *Langenbeck's Archives of Surgery*, *399*(8), 981–988.

Govan, L., Wu, O., Xin, Y., et al. (2015). Comparative effectiveness of antiviral treatment for hepatitis B: A systematic review and Bayesian network meta-analysis. *European Journal of Gastroenterology and Hepatology*, *27*(8), 882–894.

Government of Canada. Retrieved from https://www.canada.ca/en/services/health/publications/diseases-conditions/report-hepatitis-b-c-canada-2014.html

Greenberger, N. J., Blumberg, R. S., & Burakoff, R. (Eds.). (2015). Current diagnosis and treatment: Gastroenterology, hepatology & endoscopy. New York, NY: McGraw-Hill.

Hall, J. E. (2015). *Guyton & Hall textbook of medical physiology* (13th ed.). Philadelphia, PA: Saunders Elsevier.

James, J., & Liou, I. W. (2015). Comprehensive care of patients with chronic liver disease. *Medical Clinics of North America*, *99*(5), 913–933.

Karvellas, C. J., Durand, F., & Nadim, M. K. (2015). Acute kidney injury in cirrhosis. *Critical Care Clinics*, *31*(4) 737–750.

Kathpalia, P., & Ahn, J. (2015). Assessment of jaundice in the hospitalized patient. *Clinics in Liver Disease*, *19*(1), 155–170.

Lancaster, E. M., Hiatt, J. R., & Zarrinpar, A. (2015). Acetaminophen hepatotoxicity: An updated review. *Archives of Toxicology*, *89*(2), 193–199.

Lardiere-Deguelte, S., Ragot, E., Amroun, K., et al. (2015). Hepatic abscess: Diagnosis and management. *Journal of Visceral Surgery*, *152*(4), 231–243.

Lee, S. G. (2015). A complete treatment of adult living donor liver transplantation: A review of surgical technique and current challenges to expand indication of patients. *American Journal of Transplantation*, *15*(1), 17–38.

Lee, S. S., & Moreau, R. (2015). Cirrhosis: A practical guide to management (1st ed.). Hoboken, NJ: John Wiley & Sons, Ltd.

LeFevre, M. L.; U.S. Preventive Services Task Force. (2014). Screening for hepatitis B virus infection in nonpregnant adolescents and adults: U.S. Preventive Services Task Force recommendation statement. *Annals of Internal Medicine*, *16*(1), 58–66.

Lim, J. K., Flamm, S. L., Singh, S., et al. (2017). American Gastroenterological Association Institute guideline on the role of elastography in the evaluation of liver fibrosis. *Gastroenterology*, *152*(6), 1536–1543.

Liou, I. W. (2014). Management of end-stage liver disease. *Medical Clinics of North America*, *98*(1), 119–152.

Madrigal-Santillan, E., Madrigal-Bujaidair, E., Alvarez-Gonzalez, I., et al. (2014). Review of natural products with hepatoprotective effects. *World Journal of Gastroenterology*, *20*(40), 14787–14804.
Mandell, G. L., Bennett, J. E., & Dolin, R. (2014). Mandell, Douglas and Bennett's principles and practice of infectious diseases (8th ed.). Philadelphia, PA: Elsevier.
Mastron, J. K., Siveen, K. S., Sethi, G., et al. (2015). Silymarin and hepatocellular carcinoma: A systematic, comprehensive and critical review. *Anti-Cancer Drugs*, *26*(5), 475–486.
McMahon, B. J. (2014). Chronic hepatitis B virus infection. *Medical Clinics of North America*, *98*(1), 39–54.
Moyer, V. A.; U.S. Preventive Services Task Force. (2013). Screening for hepatitis C virus infection in adults: U.S. Preventive Services Task Force recommendation statement. *Annals of Internal Medicine*, *159*(5), 349–357.
Neong, S. F., Adebayo, D., & Wong, F. (2018). An update on the pathogenesis and clinical management of cirrhosis with refractory ascites. *Expert Review of Gastroenterology & Hepatology*, 1–13.
Nusrat, S., Khan, M. S., Fazili, J., et al. (2014). Cirrhosis and its complications: Evidence-based treatment. *World Journal of Gastroenterology*, *20*(18), 5442–5460.
Ohri, N., Dawson, L. A., Krishnan, S., et al. (2016). Radiotherapy for hepatocellular carcinoma: New indications and directions for future study. *JNCI: Journal of the National Cancer Institute*, *108*(9), September 2016, djw133.
Organ Procurement and Transplant Network (OPTN): U.S. Department of Health and Human Services (HHS). (2016). Split versus whole liver transplantation. Retrieved December 3, 2016, from optn.transplant.hrsa.gov/resources/ethics/split-versus-whole-liver-transplantation
Papadakis, M. A., & McPhee, S. J. (Eds.). (2016). Current medical diagnosis and treatment (55th ed.). New York, NY: McGraw-Hill.
Poordad, F. F. (2015). Presentation and complications associated with cirrhosis of the liver. *Current Medical Research & Opinion*, *31*(5), 925–937.
Rai, R. (2013). Liver transplantatation-an overview. *Indian Journal of Surgery*, *75*(3), 185–191.
Romero-Gomez, M., Mantagnese, S., & Jalan, R. (2015). Hepatic encephalopathy in patients with acute decompensation of cirrhosis and acute-on-chronic liver failure. *Journal of Hepatology*, *62*(2), 437–467.
Rude, M. K., & Crippen, J. S. (2015). Liver transplantation for hepatocellular carcinoma. *Current Gastroenterology Reports*, *17*(3), 11–15.
Salgia, R., & Singal, A. G. (2014). Hepatocellular carcinoma and other liver lesions. *Medical Clinics of North America*, *98*(1), 103–118.
Satapathy, S. K., & Sanyal, A. J. (2014). Nonendoscopic management strategies for acute esophagogastric variceal bleeding. *Gastroenterology Clinics of North America*, *43*(4), 819–833.
Siddiqui, M. S., & Stravitz, R. T. (2014). Intensive care unit management of patients with liver failure. *Clinics in Liver Disease*, *18*(4), 957–978.
Singanayagam, A., & Bernal, W. (2015). Update on acute liver failure. *Current Opinion in Critical Care*, *21*(2), 134–141.
Trieu, H., Lee, E. W., & Kee, S. T. (2017). Transjugular Intrahepatic Portosystemic Shunt in Ascites: Updates. *Digestive Disease Interventions*, *1*(04), 254–258.
Tripathi, D., & Hayes, P. C. (2014). Beta-blockers in portal hypertension: New developments and controversies. *Liver International*, *34*(5), 655–667.
Wang, L., Hu, J., Dong, S., et al. (2014). Noninvasive prediction of large esophageal varices in liver cirrhosis patients. *Clinical and Investigative Medicine*, *37*(1), E38–E46.
Weber, J., & Kelley, J. (2009). Health assessment in nursing (4th ed.). Philadelphia, PA: Lippincott, Williams & Wilkins.
Weber, J., & Kelley, J. (2014). Health assessment in nursing (5th ed.). Philadelphia, PA: Lippincott, Williams & Wilkins.
Whitehouse, T., & Wendon, J. (2013). Acute liver failure. *Best Practice & Research in Clinical Gastroenterology*, *27*(5), 757–769.
Wilder, J., & Patel, K. (2014). The clinical utility of FibroScan® as a noninvasive diagnostic test for liver disease. Medical Devices (Auckland, NZ), 7, 107.
Wong, C. J., & Pagalilauan, G. (2015). Primary care of the solid organ transplant recipient. *Medical Clinics of North America*, *99*(5), 1075–1103.
Woreta, T. A., & Alqahtani, S. A. (2014). Evaluation of abnormal liver tests. *Medical Clinics of North America*, *98*(1), 1–16.
Wu, L. J., Wu, M. S., Lien, G. S., et al. (2012). Fatigue and physical activity levels in patients with liver cirrhosis. *Journal of Clinical Nursing*, *21*(1), 129–138.
Yantiss, R. K. (2015). Gastrointestinal pathology and its clinical implications. *American Journal of Clinical Pathology*, *143*(3), 462.

Resources

Alcoholics Anonymous World Services: http://aa.org
Canadian Cancer Society: https://www.cancer.ca/en/about-us/news/national/2018/?region=on
Canadian Liver Foundation: http://www.liver.ca/
Hepatitis Foundation International: http://www.hepfi.org

40 Assessment and Management of Patients With Biliary Disorders

Adapted by Lisa McKendrick-Calder

Learning Objectives

On completion of this chapter, the learner will be able to:

1. Compare approaches to management of cholelithiasis.
2. Use the nursing process as a framework for care of patients with cholelithiasis and those undergoing laparoscopic or open cholecystectomy.
3. Differentiate between acute and chronic pancreatitis.
4. Describe nursing management of patients with acute pancreatitis.
5. Describe the nutritional and metabolic effects of surgical treatment of tumours of the pancreas.

Disorders of the biliary tract and pancreas are common and include gallbladder stones and pancreatic dysfunction. An understanding of the structure and function of the biliary tract and pancreas is essential, along with an understanding of how biliary tract disorders are closely linked with liver disease. Patients with acute or chronic biliary tract or pancreatic disease require care from nurses who are knowledgeable about the diagnostic procedures and interventions that are used in the management of gallbladder and pancreatic disorders.

ANATOMIC AND PHYSIOLOGIC OVERVIEW

The Gallbladder

The gallbladder, a pear-shaped, hollow, saclike organ, is 7.5 to 10 cm in length. It lies in a shallow depression on the inferior surface of the liver, to which it is attached by loose connective tissue. The capacity of the gallbladder is approximately 50 mL of bile (Mahadevan, 2014). Its wall is composed largely of smooth muscle and is connected to the common bile duct by the cystic duct (Fig. 40-1).

The gallbladder functions as a storage depot for bile (Mahadevan, 2014). Between meals, when the sphincter of Oddi is closed, bile produced by the hepatocytes enters the gallbladder. During storage, a large portion of the water in bile is absorbed through the walls of the gallbladder making the bile in the gallbladder 5 to 10 times more concentrated than that originally secreted by the liver. When food enters the duodenum, the gallbladder contracts and the sphincter of Oddi (located at the junction of the common bile duct with the duodenum) relaxes. Relaxation of this sphincter allows the bile to enter the intestine. This response is mediated by secretion of the hormone cholecystokinin-pancreozymin (CCK-PZ) from the intestinal wall (Ferri, 2014; Marx, Hockberger, & Walls, 2013). Bile is composed of water and electrolytes (sodium, potassium, calcium, chloride, and bicarbonate) along with significant amounts of lecithin, fatty acids, cholesterol, bilirubin, and bile salts. The bile salts, together with cholesterol, assist in emulsification of fats in the distal ileum. They are then reabsorbed into the portal blood for return to the liver, after which they are once again excreted into the bile. This pathway from hepatocytes to bile to intestine and back to the hepatocytes is called the enterohepatic circulation. Because of this circulation, only a small fraction of the bile salts that enter the intestine are excreted in the feces. This decreases the need for active synthesis of bile salts by the liver cells.

Approximately half of the bilirubin, a pigment derived from the breakdown of red blood cells, is a component of bile. It is converted by the intestinal flora into urobilinogen, a highly soluble substance. Urobilinogen is either excreted in the feces or returned to the portal circulation, where it is reexcreted into the bile. About 5% is usually absorbed into the general circulation and then excreted by the kidneys (Feldman, Friedman, & Brandt, 2015; Goldman & Schafer, 2015).

If the flow of bile is impeded (e.g., by gallstones in the bile ducts), bilirubin does not enter the intestine. As a result, blood levels of bilirubin increase. This causes increased renal excretion of urobilinogen, which results from conversion of bilirubin in the small intestine, and

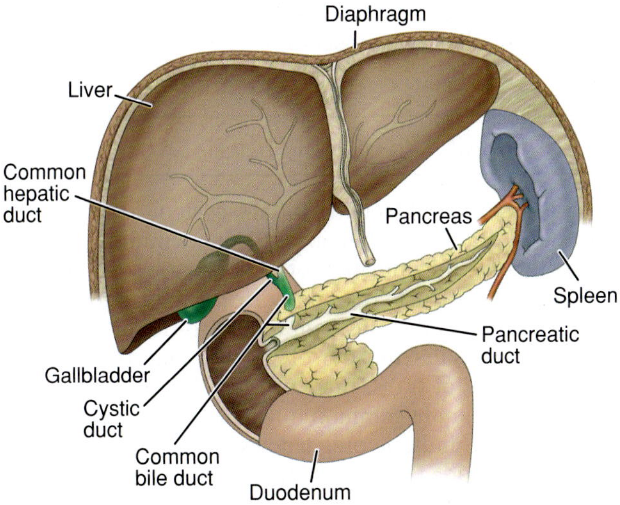

FIGURE 40-1. The liver, biliary system, and pancreas.

decreased excretion in the stool. These changes produce many of the signs and symptoms seen in gallbladder disorders.

The Pancreas

The pancreas, located in the upper abdomen, has **endocrine** as well as **exocrine** functions (see Fig. 40-1). The exocrine functions include secretion of pancreatic enzymes into the gastrointestinal (GI) tract through the pancreatic duct. The endocrine functions include secretion of insulin, glucagon, and somatostatin directly into the bloodstream.

The Exocrine Pancreas

The secretions of the exocrine portion of the pancreas are collected in the pancreatic duct, which joins the common bile duct and enters the duodenum at the ampulla of Vater. Surrounding the ampulla is the sphincter of Oddi, which partially controls the rate at which secretions from the pancreas and the gallbladder enter the duodenum.

The secretions of the exocrine pancreas are digestive enzymes high in protein content and an electrolyte-rich fluid and are needed for digestion of a meal with carbohydrates, proteins, and fat. The secretions, which are very alkaline because of their high concentration of sodium bicarbonate, are capable of neutralizing the highly acidic gastric juice that enters the duodenum. The enzyme secretions include **amylase**, which aids in the digestion of carbohydrates; **trypsin**, which aids in the digestion of proteins; and **lipase**, which aids in the digestion of fats. Other enzymes that promote the breakdown of more complex foodstuffs are also secreted. If production of pancreatic enzymes decreases to lower than 10% of usual levels, or if flow of pancreatic juice is physically obstructed, nutrition is impaired.

Hormones originating in the GI tract stimulate the secretion of these exocrine pancreatic juices. **Secretin** is the major stimulus for increased bicarbonate secretion from the pancreas, and the major stimulus for digestive enzyme secretion is the hormone CCK-PZ. The vagus nerve also influences exocrine pancreatic secretion.

The Endocrine Pancreas

The islets of Langerhans, the endocrine part of the pancreas, are collections of cells embedded in the pancreatic tissue. They are composed of alpha, beta, and delta cells. The hormone produced by the beta cells is called insulin, the alpha cells secrete glucagon, and the delta cells secrete somatostatin.

Insulin

A major action of insulin is to lower blood glucose by permitting entry of glucose into the cells of the liver, muscle, and other tissues, where it is either stored as glycogen or used for energy. Insulin also promotes the storage of fat

Glossary

amylase: pancreatic enzyme; aids in the digestion of carbohydrates
cholecystectomy: removal of the gallbladder
cholecystitis: inflammation of the gallbladder, which can be acute or chronic
cholecystojejunostomy: anastomosis of the jejunum to the gallbladder to divert bile flow
cholecystokinin-pancreozymin (CCK-PZ): hormone; major stimulus for digestive enzyme secretion; stimulates contraction of the gallbladder
cholecystostomy: surgical opening and drainage of the gallbladder
choledochostomy: opening into the common bile duct
cholelithiasis: calculi in the gallbladder
dissolution therapy: the use of medications to break up/dissolve gallstones
endocrine: secreting internally; hormonal secretion of a ductless gland
endoscopic retrograde cholangiopancreatography (ERCP): procedure using fibreoptic technology to visualize the biliary system
exocrine: secreting externally; hormonal secretion from excretory ducts
lipase: pancreatic enzyme; aids in the digestion of fats
lithotripsy: disintegration of gallstones by shock waves
pancreatitis: inflammation of the pancreas; may be acute or chronic
secretin: hormone responsible for stimulating bicarbonate secretion from the pancreas; also used as an aid in diagnosing pancreatic exocrine disease
steatorrhea: frothy, foul-smelling stools with a high fat content; results from impaired digestion of proteins and fats due to a lack of pancreatic juice in the intestine
trypsin: pancreatic enzyme; aids in the digestion of proteins
Zollinger–Ellison syndrome: hypersecretion of gastric acid that produces peptic ulcers as a result of a non-beta-cell tumour of the pancreatic islets

in adipose tissue and the synthesis of proteins in various body tissues. In the absence of insulin, glucose cannot enter the cells and is excreted in the urine. This condition, called diabetes, can be diagnosed by high levels of glucose in the blood. In diabetes, stored fats and protein are used for energy instead of glucose, causing loss of body mass. (Diabetes is discussed in detail in Chapter 41.) The level of glucose in the blood usually regulates the rate of insulin secretion from the pancreas.

Glucagon

The effect of glucagon (opposite to that of insulin) is chiefly to raise the blood glucose by converting glycogen to glucose in the liver. Glucagon is secreted by the pancreas in response to a decrease in the level of blood glucose.

Somatostatin

Somatostatin exerts a hypoglycemic effect by interfering with the release of growth hormone from the pituitary and glucagon from the pancreas, both of which tend to raise blood glucose levels.

Endocrine Control of Carbohydrate Metabolism

Glucose required for energy is derived by metabolism of ingested carbohydrates and also from proteins by the process of gluconeogenesis. Glucose can be stored temporarily in the form of glycogen in the liver, muscles, and other tissues. The endocrine system controls the level of blood glucose by regulating the rate at which glucose is synthesized, stored, and moved to and from the bloodstream. Through the action of hormones, blood glucose is maintained at less than 5.5 mmol/L. Insulin is the primary hormone that lowers the blood glucose level. Hormones that raise the blood glucose level are glucagon, epinephrine, adrenocorticosteroids, growth hormone, and thyroid hormone.

The endocrine and exocrine functions of the pancreas are interrelated. The major exocrine function is to facilitate digestion through secretion of enzymes into the proximal duodenum. Secretin and CCK-PZ are hormones from the GI tract that aid in the digestion of food substances by controlling the secretions of the pancreas. Neural factors also influence pancreatic enzyme secretion. Considerable dysfunction of the pancreas must occur before enzyme secretion decreases and protein and fat digestion becomes impaired. Pancreatic enzyme secretion is usually 1,500 to 2,500 mL/day.

Gerontologic Considerations

There is little change in the size of the pancreas with age. However, there is an increase in fibrous material and some fatty deposition in the normal pancreas in people older than 70 years of age. Some localized arteriosclerotic changes occur with age. There is also a decreased rate of pancreatic secretion (decreased lipase, amylase, and trypsin) and decreased bicarbonate output in older people. Some impairment of normal fat absorption occurs with increasing age, possibly because of delayed gastric emptying and pancreatic insufficiency. Decreased calcium absorption may also occur. These changes require care in interpreting diagnostic test results in the older patient and in providing dietary counselling.

DISORDERS OF THE GALLBLADDER

Several disorders affect the biliary system and interfere with usual drainage of bile into the duodenum. These disorders include inflammation of the biliary system and carcinoma that obstructs the biliary tree. Gallbladder disease with gallstones is the most common disorder of the biliary system and occurs in 20% of women and 10% of men before the age of 60 (Canadian Liver Foundation, n.d.). Gallstones are more common in women, particularly those who have had multiple pregnancies. Other risk factors for gallstones include family history, weight loss, diet (high fat and high carbohydrate), and obesity (Beckingham, 2017). Additionally, in Canada, up to 70% to 80% of the First Nations population is afflicted with gallstones, which may suggest or support a genetic component of the disease (Canadian Liver Foundation). Although not all occurrences of gallbladder inflammation (**cholecystitis**) are related to gallstones (**cholelithiasis**), more than 90% of patients with acute cholecystitis have gallstones. Many people with gallstones are asymptomatic (no pain) and are unaware of the presence of stones. Up to 90% of people on postmortem review with gallstones present had no known symptoms prior (Beckingham, 2017).

Cholecystitis

Cholecystitis, acute inflammation of the gallbladder, causes pain, tenderness, and rigidity of the upper right abdomen that may radiate to the midsternal area or right shoulder and is associated with nausea, vomiting, and the usual signs of an acute inflammation (Beckingham, 2017). An empyema infection of the gallbladder develops if the gallbladder becomes filled with purulent fluid (pus).

Calculous cholecystitis is the cause of more than 90% of cases of acute cholecystitis (Feldman et al., 2015; Rakel & Rakel, 2015). In calculous cholecystitis, a gallbladder stone obstructs bile outflow. Bile remaining in the gallbladder initiates a chemical reaction; autolysis and edema occur; and the blood vessels in the gallbladder are compressed, compromising its vascular supply. Gangrene of the gallbladder with perforation may result. Bacteria play a minor role in acute cholecystitis; however, secondary infection of bile occurs in approximately 50% of cases. The organisms involved are generally enteric (usually live in the GI tract) and include *Escherichia coli*, *Klebsiella* species, and *Streptococcus* (Katabathina, Zafar, & Suri, 2015). Bacterial contamination is not believed to stimulate the actual onset of acute cholecystitis (Feldman et al., 2015).

Acalculous cholecystitis describes acute gallbladder inflammation in the absence of obstruction by gallstones. Acalculous cholecystitis occurs after major surgical procedures, severe trauma, or burns. Other factors associated with this type of cholecystitis include torsion, cystic duct obstruction, primary bacterial infections of the gallbladder, and multiple blood transfusions. It is speculated that acalculous cholecystitis is caused by alterations in fluids

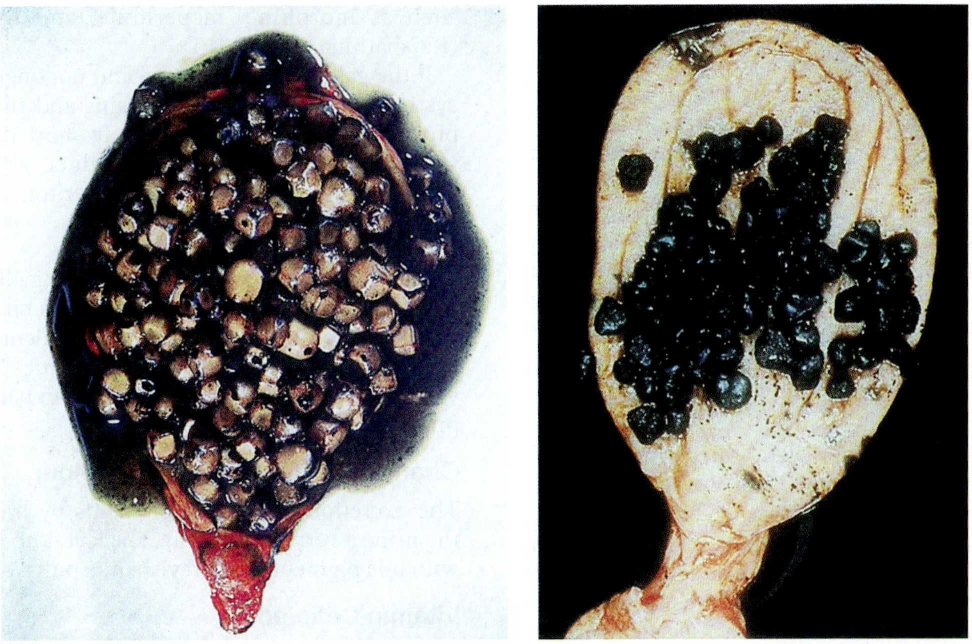

FIGURE 40-2. Examples of cholesterol gallstones (**left**) made up of a coalescence of multiple small stones and pigment gallstones (**right**) composed of calcium bilirubinate. (From Strayer, D. S., & Rubin, E. [2015]. *Rubin's pathology* [7th ed.]. Philadelphia, PA: Lippincott Williams & Wilkins.)

and electrolytes and alterations in regional blood flow in the visceral circulation. Bile stasis (lack of gallbladder contraction) and increased viscosity of the bile are also thought to play a role. The occurrence of acalculous cholecystitis with major surgical procedures or trauma makes its diagnosis difficult.

Cholelithiasis

Calculi, or gallstones, usually form in the gallbladder from the solid constituents of bile; they vary greatly in size, shape, and composition (Fig. 40-2).

Pathophysiology

There are two major types of gallstones: those composed predominantly of pigment and those composed primarily of cholesterol. Pigment stones probably form when unconjugated pigments in the bile precipitate to form stones; these stones (black or brown) account for about 20% of cases in Canada (Porth, 2010). The risk of developing such stones is increased in patients with cirrhosis, hemolysis, and infections of the biliary tract. Pigment stones require surgical removal as they cannot be dissolved.

Cholesterol stones account for most of the remaining 80% of cases of gallbladder disease in Canada. Cholesterol, a constituent of bile, is insoluble in water. Its solubility depends on bile acids and lecithin (phospholipids) in bile. In gallstone-prone patients, there is decreased bile acid synthesis and increased cholesterol synthesis in the liver, resulting in bile supersaturated with cholesterol, which precipitates out of the bile to form stones (Hall, 2015). The cholesterol-saturated bile predisposes to the formation of gallstones and acts as an irritant that produces inflammatory changes in the gallbladder (Feldman et al., 2015; Lee, Keane, & Pereira, 2015).

Stone formation is more frequent in women who use oral contraceptives, estrogen, or clofibrate; these medications are known to increase biliary cholesterol saturation (Feldman et al., 2015; Kumar, Abbas, Fausto, et al., 2014). The incidence of stone formation increases with age as a result of increased hepatic secretion of cholesterol and decreased bile acid synthesis (Greenberger, Blumberg, & Burakoff, 2015; Kumar et al., 2014). In addition, there is an increased risk because of malabsorption of bile salts in patients with GI disease or T-tube fistula and in those who have undergone ileal resection or bypass. The incidence is also greater in people with diabetes (Chart 40-1).

CHART 40-1

Risk Factors: Cholelithiasis

- Obesity
- Women, especially those who have had multiple pregnancies or who are of First Nations, Inuit, or Metis ethnicity
- Frequent changes in weight
- Rapid weight loss (leads to rapid development of gallstones and high risk of symptomatic disease)
- Treatment with high-dose estrogen (e.g., in prostate cancer)
- Low-dose estrogen therapy—a small increase in the risk of gallstones
- Ileal resection or disease
- Cystic fibrosis
- Diabetes

Adapted from Lee, J. Y. J., Keane, M. G., & Pereira, S. (2015). Diagnosis and treatment of gallstone disease. *Practitioner*, *259*(1783), 15–19; Greenberger, N. J., Blumberg, R. S., & Burakoff, R. (Eds.). (2015). *Current diagnosis and treatment: Gastroenterology, hepatology & endoscopy*. New York: McGraw-Hill.

Clinical Manifestations

Gallstones may be silent, producing no pain and only mild GI symptoms. Such stones may be detected incidentally during surgery or evaluation for unrelated problems.

The patient with gallbladder disease resulting from gallstones may develop two types of symptoms: those due to disease of the gallbladder itself and those due to obstruction of the bile passages by a gallstone. The symptoms may be acute or chronic. Epigastric distress, such as fullness, abdominal distension, and vague pain in the right upper quadrant of the abdomen, may occur. This distress may follow a meal rich in fried or fatty foods.

Pain and Biliary Colic

If a gallstone obstructs the cystic duct, the gallbladder becomes distended, inflamed, and eventually infected (acute cholecystitis). The patient develops a fever and may have a palpable abdominal mass. The patient may have what is described as biliary colic with excruciating upper right abdominal pain that radiates to the back or right shoulder. Biliary colic is usually associated with nausea and vomiting, and it is noticeable several hours after a heavy meal (Beckingham, 2017). The patient often moves about restlessly and is unable to find a comfortable position. In many patients, pain is constant and not colicky (intermittent).

Such a bout of biliary colic is caused by contraction of the gallbladder, which cannot release bile because of obstruction by the stone. When distended, the fundus of the gallbladder comes in contact with the abdominal wall in the region of the right 9th and 10th costal cartilages. This produces marked tenderness in the right upper quadrant on deep inspiration and prevents full inspiratory excursion.

The pain of acute cholecystitis may be so severe that analgesics are required. Nonsteroidal anti-inflammatory medications have shown effectiveness in speeding recovery (Beckingham, 2017). These anti-inflammatory medications should be utilized as first-line therapy with opiates such as morphine, meperidine, and hydromorphone (Katabathina et al., 2015).

If the gallstone is dislodged and no longer obstructs the cystic duct, the gallbladder drains and the inflammatory process subsides after a relatively short time. If the gallstone continues to obstruct the duct, abscess, necrosis, and perforation with generalized peritonitis may result.

Jaundice

Jaundice occurs in a few patients with gallbladder disease, usually with obstruction of the common bile duct. The bile, which is no longer carried to the duodenum, is absorbed by the blood and gives the skin and mucous membranes a yellow colour. This is frequently accompanied by marked pruritus (itching) of the skin.

Changes in Urine and Stool Colour

The excretion of the bile pigments by the kidneys gives the urine a very dark colour. The feces, no longer coloured with bile pigments, are greyish, like putty, or clay coloured.

Vitamin Deficiency

Obstruction of bile flow interferes with absorption of the fat-soluble vitamins A, D, E, and K. Patients may exhibit deficiencies of these vitamins if biliary obstruction has been prolonged. For example, a patient may have bleeding caused by vitamin K deficiency (vitamin K is necessary for blood clotting).

Assessment and Diagnostic Findings

Blood tests may show inflammatory changes that may assist with diagnosis and management. White blood cell counts (WBC), erythrocyte sedimentation rate (ESR), and C-reactive protein (CRP) may be elevated. Liver function tests should also be checked as they may also be altered due to the inflammation and a potential compression of the common bile duct (Beckingham, 2017).

Table 40-1 identifies various procedures and their diagnostic uses.

TABLE 40-1 Studies Used in the Diagnosis of Biliary Tract and Pancreatic Disease

Studies	Diagnostic Uses
Magnetic resonance cholangiopancreatography (MRCP)	Visualizes the biliary tree and capable of detecting biliary tract obstruction
Cholecystogram, cholangiogram	Visualize gallbladder and bile duct
Celiac axis arteriography	Visualizes liver and pancreas
Laparoscopy	Visualizes anterior surface of liver, gallbladder, and mesentery through a trocar
Ultrasonography	Shows size of abdominal organs and presence of masses
Helical computed tomography and magnetic resonance imaging	Detect neoplasms; diagnose cysts, pseudocysts, abscess, and hematomas; determine severity of pancreatitis based on the presence of necrosis and/or peripancreatic fluid collections
Endoscopic retrograde cholangiopancreatography	Visualizes biliary structures and pancreas via endoscopy
Endoscopic ultrasound	Identifies small tumours and facilitates fine-needle aspiration biopsy of tumours or lymph nodes for diagnosis
Serum alkaline phosphatase	In absence of bone disease, to measure biliary tract obstruction
Gamma-glutamyl, gamma-glutamyl transpeptidase, lactate dehydrogenase	Markers for biliary stasis; also elevated in alcohol abuse
Cholesterol levels	Elevated in biliary obstruction; decreased in parenchymal liver disease

Abdominal X-Ray

If gallbladder disease is suspected, an abdominal x-ray is obtained to exclude other causes of symptoms. However, only 15% to 20% of gallstones are calcified sufficiently to be visible on such x-ray studies.

Ultrasonography

Ultrasonography has replaced cholecystography (discussed later) as the diagnostic procedure of choice because it is rapid and accurate and can be used in patients with liver dysfunction and jaundice. It does not expose patients to ionizing radiation. The procedure is most accurate if the patient fasts overnight so that the gallbladder is distended. Ultrasonography can detect calculi in the gallbladder or a dilated common bile duct with 81% to 82% sensitivity and specificity with a variety of different potential findings that are suggestive of acute cholecystitis (Katabathina et al., 2015).

Radionuclide Imaging or Cholescintigraphy

Cholescintigraphy is used successfully in the diagnosis of acute cholecystitis or blockage of a bile duct. In this procedure, a radioactive agent, ^{99m}Tc-hepatic iminodiacetic acid (HIDA), is administered intravenously (IV). It is taken up by the hepatocytes and excreted rapidly through the biliary tract. The biliary tract is then scanned, and images of the gallbladder and biliary tract are obtained. This test is more expensive than ultrasonography, takes longer to perform, exposes the patient to radiation, and cannot detect gallstones. It is often used when ultrasonography is not conclusive. It has the highest sensitivity (96%) and specificity (90%) of all the diagnostic tests (Katabathina et al., 2015). It can be referred to as a HIDA scan.

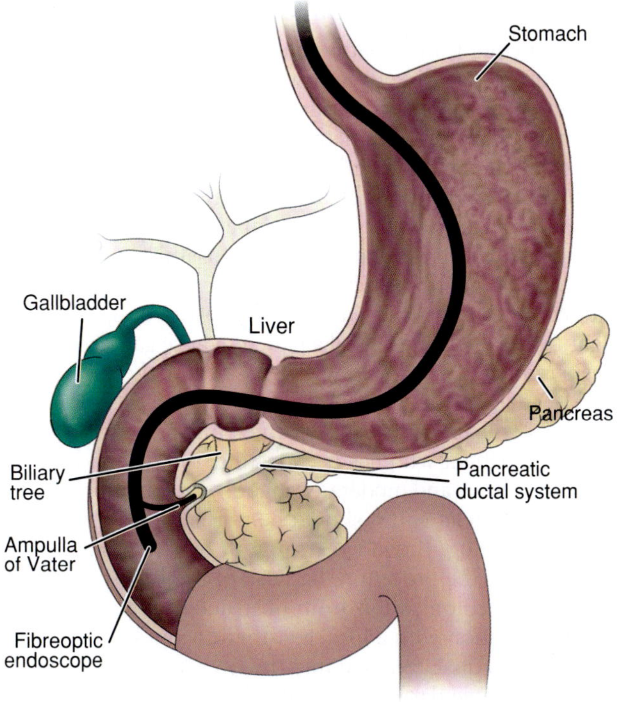

FIGURE 40-3. Endoscopic retrograde cholangiopancreatography (ERCP). A fibreoptic duodenoscope, with side-viewing apparatus, is inserted into the duodenum. The ampulla of Vater is catheterized, and the biliary tree is injected with contrast agent. The pancreatic ductal system is also assessed, if indicated. This procedure is of special value in visualizing neoplasms of the ampulla area and extracting a biopsy specimen.

Cholecystography

Oral cholecystography is used if ultrasound equipment is not available or if the ultrasound results are inconclusive. This study may be performed to detect gallstones and to assess the ability of the gallbladder to fill, concentrate its contents, contract, and empty. If the patient is not allergic to iodine or seafood, an iodide-containing contrast agent that is excreted by the liver and concentrated in the gallbladder is given 10 to 12 hours before the x-ray study (Feldman et al., 2015; Marx et al., 2013). The normal gallbladder fills with this radiopaque substance. If gallstones are present, they appear as shadows on the x-ray image.

Oral cholecystography may be used as part of the evaluation of patients who have been treated with gallstone **dissolution therapy** (the use of medications to break up/dissolve gallstones) or **lithotripsy** (disintegration of gallstones by shock waves).

Endoscopic Retrograde Cholangiopancreatography

Endoscopic retrograde cholangiopancreatography (ERCP) permits direct visualization of structures that previously could be seen only during laparotomy. The examination of the hepatobiliary system is carried out via a side-viewing flexible fibre optic endoscope inserted through the esophagus to the descending duodenum (Fig. 40-3). Multiple position changes are required to pass the endoscope during the procedure, beginning in the left semiprone position.

Fluoroscopy and multiple x-rays are used during ERCP to evaluate the presence and location of ductal stones. Careful insertion of a catheter through the endoscope into the common bile duct is the most important step in sphincterotomy (division of the muscles of the biliary sphincter) for gallstone extraction via this technique (see later discussion).

Nursing Implications

The procedure requires a cooperative patient to permit insertion of the endoscope without damage to the GI tract structures, including the biliary tree. Before the procedure, the patient is given an explanation of the procedure and his or her role in it. The patient takes nothing by mouth for several hours before the procedure. Moderate sedation is used, and the sedated patient must be monitored closely. It may be necessary to administer medications, such as glucagon or anticholinergics, to make cannulation easier by decreasing duodenal peristalsis. The nurse observes closely for signs of respiratory and CNS depression, hypotension, oversedation, and vomiting (if glucagon is administered). During ERCP, the nurse monitors IV fluids, administers medications, and positions the patient.

After the procedure, the nurse monitors the patient's condition, observing vital signs and monitoring for signs of perforation or infection. The nurse also monitors the patient for side effects of any medications received during the procedure and for return of the gag and cough reflexes after the use of local anesthetics.

Percutaneous Transhepatic Cholangiography

Percutaneous transhepatic cholangiography involves the injection of dye directly into the biliary tract. Because of the relatively large concentration of dye that is introduced into the biliary system, including the hepatic ducts within the liver, the entire length of the common bile duct, the cystic duct, and the gallbladder is outlined clearly.

This procedure can be carried out even in the presence of liver dysfunction and jaundice. It is useful for (1) distinguishing jaundice caused by liver disease (hepatocellular jaundice) from that caused by biliary obstruction, (2) investigating the GI symptoms of a patient whose gallbladder has been removed, (3) locating stones within the bile ducts, and (4) diagnosing cancer involving the biliary system.

This sterile procedure is performed under moderate sedation on a patient who has been fasting; the patient receives local anesthesia and moderate sedation. Coagulation parameters and platelet count should be normal to minimize the risk of bleeding. Broad-spectrum antibiotics are administered during the procedure because of the high prevalence of bacterial colonization from obstructed biliary systems. After infiltration with a local anesthetic agent has occurred, a flexible needle is inserted into the liver from the right side in the midclavicular line immediately beneath the right costal margin. Successful entry of a duct is noted when bile is aspirated or on injection of a contrast agent. Ultrasound can be used to guide puncture of the duct. Bile is aspirated and samples are sent for bacteriology and cytology. A water-soluble contrast agent is injected to fill the biliary system. The fluoroscopy table is tilted and the patient is repositioned to allow x-rays to be taken in multiple projections. Delayed x-ray views can identify abnormalities of more distant ducts and determine the length of a stricture or multiple strictures. Before the needle is removed, as much dye and bile as possible are aspirated to forestall subsequent leakage into the needle tract and eventually into the peritoneal cavity, thus minimizing the risk of bile peritonitis.

Nursing Implications

Although the complication rate after this procedure is low, the nurse must closely observe the patient for symptoms of bleeding, peritonitis, and septicemia. The nurse assesses the patient for pain and indications of these complications and reports them promptly to the physician. Antibiotic agents are often prescribed to minimize the risk of sepsis and septic shock.

Medical Management

The major objectives of medical therapy are to reduce the incidence of acute episodes of gallbladder pain and cholecystitis by supportive and dietary management and, if possible, to remove the cause of cholecystitis by pharmacologic therapy, endoscopic procedures, or surgical intervention. Although nonsurgical approaches eliminate risks associated with surgery, these approaches are associated with persistent symptoms or recurrent stone formation. Most of the nonsurgical approaches, including lithotripsy and dissolution of gallstones, provide only temporary solutions to gallstone problems and are infrequently used in Canada. In some instances, other treatment approaches may be indicated; these are described later.

Removal of the gallbladder (**cholecystectomy**) through traditional surgical approaches was the standard treatment for more than 100 years. It has largely been replaced by **laparoscopic cholecystectomy** (removal of the gallbladder through a small incision through the umbilicus). As a result, surgical risks have decreased, along with the length of hospital stay and the long recovery period required after standard surgical cholecystectomy. In relatively rare instances, a standard surgical procedure may be necessary.

Nutritional and Supportive Therapy

Approximately 80% of the patients with acute gallbladder inflammation achieve remission with rest, IV fluids, nasogastric suction, analgesia, and antibiotic agents. Unless the patient's condition deteriorates, surgical intervention is delayed just until the acute symptoms subside (usually within a few days). At this time, the patient undergoes a laparoscopic cholecystectomy (Goldman & Schafer, 2015; Michetti, Griffen, Tran, et al., 2015).

The diet required immediately after an episode is usually limited to low-fat liquids. These can include powdered supplements high in protein and carbohydrate stirred into skim milk. Cooked fruits, rice or tapioca, lean meats, mashed potatoes, non–gas-forming vegetables, bread, coffee, or tea may be added as tolerated. The patient should avoid eggs, cream, pork, fried foods, cheese, rich dressings, gas-forming vegetables, and alcohol. It is important to remind the patient that fatty foods may induce an episode of cholecystitis. Dietary management may be the major mode of therapy in patients who have had only dietary intolerance to fatty foods and vague GI symptoms (Dudek, 2013). Once a patient has had one episode of acute cholecystitis, the recurrence rate is 38% to 50% per annum (Beckingham, 2017); so dietary changes need to be maintained long term.

Pharmacologic Therapy

Ursodeoxycholic acid (UDCA [URSO, Actigall]) and chenodeoxycholic acid (chenodiol or CDCA [Chenix]) have been used to dissolve small, radiolucent gallstones composed primarily of cholesterol. UDCA has fewer side effects than chenodiol and can be administered in smaller doses to achieve the same effect. It acts by inhibiting the synthesis and secretion of cholesterol, thereby desaturating bile. Treatment with UDCA can reduce the size of existing stones, dissolve small stones, and prevent new stones from forming. Six to twelve months of therapy are required in many patients to dissolve stones, and monitoring of the patient for recurrence of symptoms or the occurrence of side effects (e.g., GI symptoms, pruritus, headache) is required during this time. The effective dose of medication depends on body weight. This method of treatment is generally indicated for patients who refuse surgery or for whom surgery is considered too risky.

Patients with significant, frequent symptoms; cystic duct occlusion; or pigment stones are not candidates for therapy with UDCA. Laparoscopic or open cholecystectomy is more appropriate for symptomatic patients with acceptable operative risk.

Nonsurgical Removal of Gallstones

Dissolving Gallstones

Several methods have been used to dissolve gallstones by infusion of a solvent (monooctanoin or methyl tertiary butyl ether [MTBE]) into the gallbladder. The solvent can be infused through the following routes: through a tube or catheter inserted percutaneously directly into the gallbladder; through a tube or drain inserted through a T-tube tract to dissolve stones not removed at the time of surgery; endoscopically with ERCP; or via a transnasal biliary catheter.

In the latter procedure, the catheter is introduced through the mouth and inserted into the common bile duct. The upper end of the tube is then rerouted from the mouth to the nose and left in place. This enables the patient to eat and drink while passage of stones is monitored or chemical solvents are infused to dissolve the stones. This method of dissolution of stones is not widely used.

Stone Removal by Instrumentation

Several nonsurgical methods are used to remove stones that were not removed at the time of cholecystectomy or have become lodged in the common bile duct (Fig. 40-4A,B). A catheter and instrument with a basket attached are threaded through the T-tube tract or fistula formed at the time of T-tube insertion; the basket is used to retrieve and remove the stones lodged in the common bile duct.

A second procedure involves the use of the ERCP endoscope (Fig. 40-4C). After the endoscope is inserted, a cutting instrument is passed through the endoscope into the ampulla of Vater of the common bile duct. It may be used to cut the submucosal fibres, or papilla, of the sphincter of Oddi, enlarging the opening, which may allow the lodged stones to pass spontaneously into the duodenum. Another instrument with a small basket or balloon at its tip may be inserted through the endoscope to retrieve the stones (Fig. 40-4D–F). The patient is observed closely for bleeding, perforation, and the development of pancreatitis or sepsis.

The ERCP procedure is particularly useful in diagnosis and treatment of patients who have symptoms after biliary tract surgery, patients with intact gallbladders, and patients for whom surgery is particularly hazardous.

Surgical Management

Surgical treatment of gallbladder disease and gallstones is carried out to relieve persistent symptoms, to remove the cause of biliary colic, and to treat acute cholecystitis. Surgery may be delayed until the patient's symptoms have subsided, or it may be performed as an emergency procedure, if necessitated by the patient's condition.

Preoperative Measures

Chest x-ray, electrocardiogram (ECG), and liver function tests may be performed in addition to studies of the gallbladder. Vitamin K may be administered if the prothrombin level is low. Nutritional requirements are considered, and, if the nutritional status is suboptimal, it may be necessary to provide IV glucose with protein supplements to aid wound healing and help prevent liver damage.

Preparation for gallbladder surgery is similar to that for any upper abdominal laparotomy or laparoscopy. Instructions and explanations are given before surgery with regard to turning and deep breathing. Postoperative pneumonia and atelectasis can be avoided by deep-breathing exercises and frequent turning. The patient is informed that drainage tubes and a nasogastric tube and suction might be required during the immediate postoperative period if an open cholecystectomy is performed.

Laparoscopic Cholecystectomy

Laparoscopic cholecystectomy (Fig. 40-5) has dramatically changed the approach to the management of cholecystitis. It has become the new standard for therapy of symptomatic gallstones. Of the patients requiring surgery for removal of the gallbladder, 80% to 90% of them are candidates for laparoscopic cholecystectomy (Doherty, 2015; Feldman

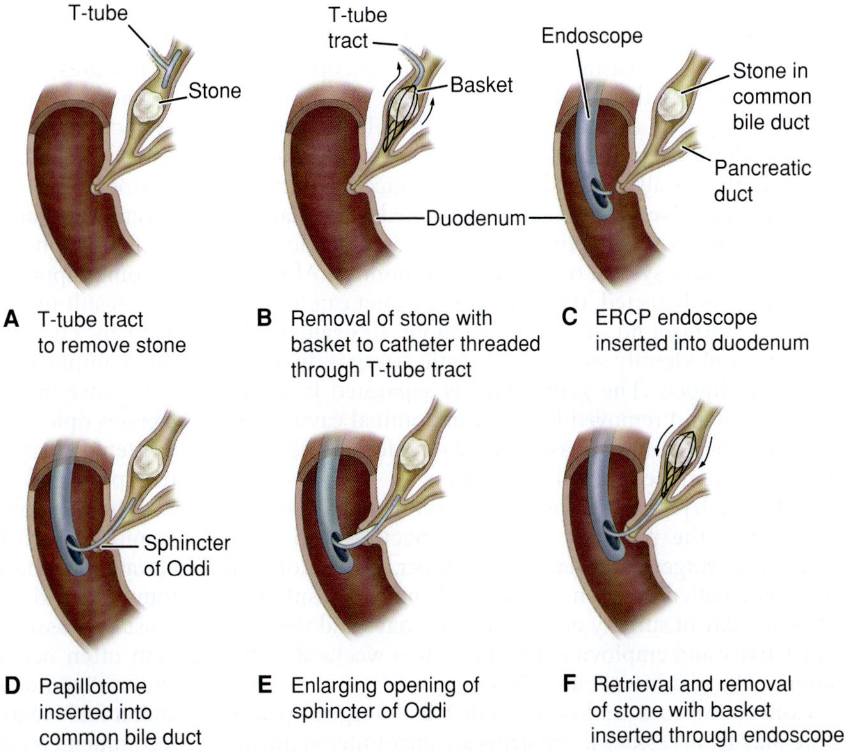

FIGURE 40-4. A–F. Nonsurgical techniques for removing gallstones.

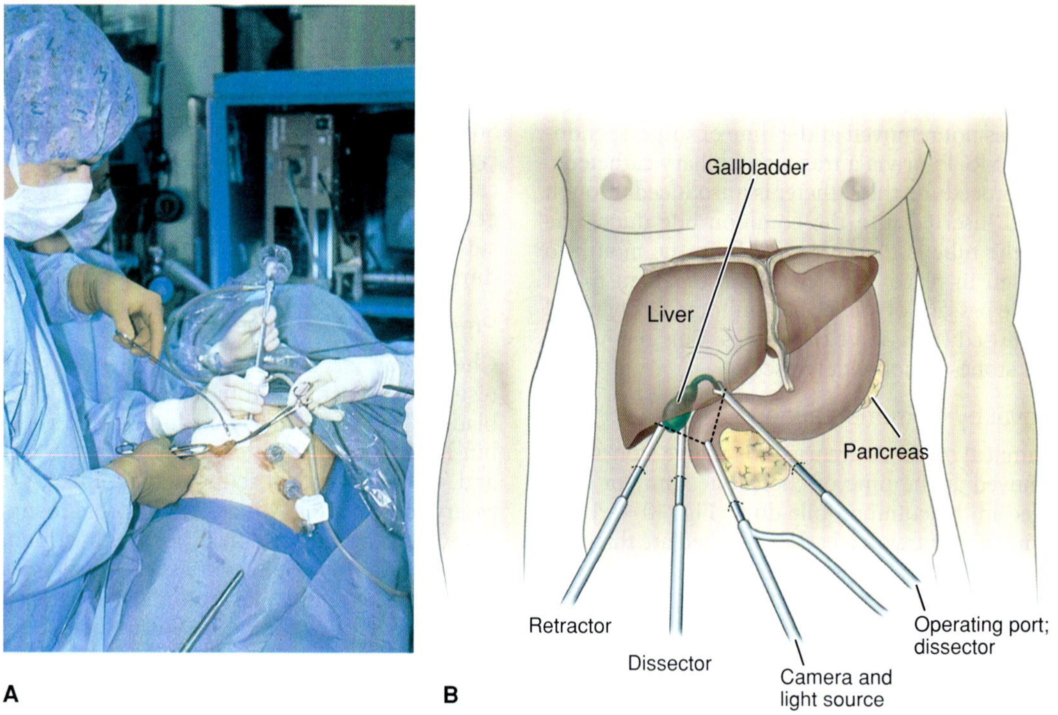

FIGURE 40-5. **A.** In laparoscopic cholecystectomy, the surgeon makes four small incisions (less than one half in each) in the abdomen. **B.** Inserts a laparoscope with a miniature camera through the umbilical incision. The camera apparatus displays the gallbladder and adjacent tissues on a screen, allowing the surgeon to visualize the sections of the organ for removal.

et al., 2015). If the common bile duct is thought to be obstructed by a gallstone, an ERCP with sphincterotomy may be performed to explore the duct before laparoscopy (Goldman & Schafer, 2015; Lee et al., 2015).

Before the procedure, the patient is informed that an open abdominal procedure may be necessary, and general anesthesia is administered. Laparoscopic cholecystectomy is performed through a small incision or puncture made through the abdominal wall at the umbilicus. The abdominal cavity is insufflated with carbon dioxide (pneumoperitoneum) to assist in inserting the laparoscope and to aid in visualizing the abdominal structures. The fibreoptic scope is inserted through the small umbilical incision. Several additional punctures or small incisions are made in the abdominal wall to introduce other surgical instruments into the operative field. A camera attached to the laparoscope permits the surgeon to view the intra-abdominal field and biliary system on a television monitor. After the cystic duct is dissected, the common bile duct can be visualized by ultrasound or cholangiography to evaluate the anatomy and identify stones. The cystic artery is dissected free and clipped. The gallbladder is separated from the hepatic bed and removed from the abdominal cavity after bile and small stones are aspirated. Stone forceps also can be used to remove or crush larger stones.

With the laparoscopic procedure, the patient does not experience the paralytic ileus that occurs with open abdominal surgery and has less postoperative abdominal pain. The patient is often discharged from the hospital on the same day of surgery or within 1 or 2 days and resumes full activity and employment within 2 to 4 weeks after the surgery (Katabathina et al., 2015).

Conversion to a traditional abdominal surgical procedure may be necessary if problems are encountered during the laparoscopic procedure; this occurs in very few cases in Canada. Conversion to an open procedure occurs if there is inflammation in and around the gallbladder making safe dissection of the porta hepatis difficult (Feldman et al., 2015). (The porta hepatis is the fissure of the liver where the portal vein and the hepatic artery enter and the hepatic ducts exit the liver.) Careful screening of patients and identification of those at low risk for complications limit the frequency of conversion to an open abdominal procedure. However, with increasing use of laparoscopic procedures, the number of such conversions may increase.

The most serious complication after laparoscopic cholecystectomy is a bile duct injury, which may be identified and corrected at the time of the procedure. Patients with a postoperative bile leak may not develop symptoms until several days after the procedure, and some have an even more prolonged period before injury to the bile duct becomes apparent (Cuschieri & Hanna, 2014). A bile leak may result in fluid collections, which can usually be managed by endoscopic stent placement. Bile peritonitis, a rare complication, may result in serious illness or death.

Because of the short hospital stay with uncomplicated laparoscopic cholecystectomies, it is important to provide written and verbal instructions about managing postoperative pain and reporting signs and symptoms of intra-abdominal complications, including loss of appetite, vomiting, pain, distension of the abdomen, and temperature elevation. Although recovery from laparoscopic cholecystectomy is rapid, patients are drowsy afterward. The patient must have assistance at home during the first 24 to 48 hours. Pain often occurs in the right shoulder or scapular area (from migration of the carbon dioxide used to insufflate the abdominal cavity during the procedure), so the nurse may recommend a heating pad for 15 to 20 minutes hourly.

Open Cholecystectomy

In cholecystectomy, the gallbladder is removed through an abdominal incision (usually right subcostal) after the cystic duct and artery are ligated. The procedure is performed for acute and chronic cholecystitis. In some patients, a drain is placed close to the gallbladder bed and brought out through a puncture wound if there is a bile leak. The drain type is chosen based on the physician's preference. A small leak should close spontaneously in a few days, with the drain preventing accumulation of bile. Usually only a small amount of serosanguineous fluid drains in the initial 24 hours after surgery; afterward, the drain is removed. The drain is typically maintained if there is excess oozing or bile leakage. Insertion of a T-tube into the common bile duct during the open procedure is now uncommon; it is used only in the setting of a complication (i.e., retained common bile duct stone). Bile duct injury is a serious complication of cholecystectomy, but it occurs less frequently with the laparoscopic approach, which has largely replaced traditional surgical cholecystectomy.

Small-Incision Cholecystectomy

Mini-cholecystectomy is a surgical procedure in which the gallbladder is removed through a small incision. If needed, the surgical incision is extended to remove larger gallbladder stones. Drains may or may not be used. The cost savings resulting from the short hospital stay have been identified as a major reason for pursuing this type of procedure. However, the procedure is controversial because it limits exposure to all the involved biliary structures.

Choledochostomy

Choledochostomy is reserved for the patient with acute cholecystitis who may be too ill to undergo a surgical procedure. It involves making an incision in the common duct, usually for removal of stones (choledochostomy). After the stones have been evacuated, a tube is usually inserted into the duct for drainage of bile until edema subsides. This tube is connected to gravity drainage tubing; the patient is monitored closely, and a laparoscopic cholecystectomy is planned for a future date after acute inflammation has resolved.

Surgical Cholecystostomy

Cholecystostomy is performed when the patient's condition precludes more extensive surgery or when an acute inflammatory reaction is severe. The gallbladder is surgically opened, stones and the bile or the purulent drainage are removed, and a drainage tube is secured with a purse-string suture. The drainage tube is connected to a drainage system to prevent bile from leaking around the tube or escaping into the peritoneal cavity. After recovery from the acute episode, the patient may return for subsequent laparoscopic cholecystectomy. Despite its lower risk, surgical cholecystostomy has a high mortality rate (reported to be as high as 20% to 30%) because of the underlying disease process.

Percutaneous Cholecystostomy

Percutaneous cholecystostomy has been used in the treatment and diagnosis of acute cholecystitis in patients who are poor risks for any surgical procedure or for general anesthesia. These may include patients with sepsis or severe cardiac, renal, pulmonary, or liver failure. Under local anesthesia, utilizing a transhepatic or transperitoneal approach, a fine needle is inserted through the abdominal wall and liver edge into the gallbladder under the guidance of ultrasound or computed tomography (CT). Bile is aspirated to ensure adequate placement of the needle, and a catheter is inserted into the gallbladder to decompress the biliary tract. Almost immediate relief of pain and resolution of signs and symptoms of sepsis and cholecystitis have been reported with this procedure. Antibiotic agents are administered before, during, and after the procedure. Patients who do not respond to this nonsurgical approach should be sent for cholecystectomy (Katabathina et al., 2015).

Gerontologic Considerations

Surgical intervention for disease of the biliary tract is the most common operative procedure performed in older adults. Cholesterol saturation of bile increases with age because of increased hepatic secretion of cholesterol and decreased bile acid synthesis.

Although the incidence of gallstones increases with age, the older patient may not exhibit the typical symptoms of fever, pain, chills, and jaundice. Symptoms of biliary tract disease in the older patient may be accompanied or preceded by those of septic shock, which include oliguria, hypotension, changes in mental status, tachycardia, and tachypnea.

While surgery in the older patient presents a risk because of pre-existing associated diseases, the mortality rate from serious complications of biliary tract disease itself is also high. The risk of death and complications is increased in the older patient who undergoes emergency surgery for life-threatening disease of the biliary tract. As a result, patients requiring the procedure are seen in later stages of the disease. At the same time, patients undergoing surgery are increasingly older than 60 years of age and may have complicated acute cholecystitis. Despite chronic illness in many older patients, elective cholecystectomy is usually well tolerated and can be carried out with low risk if expert assessment and care are provided before, during, and after the surgical procedure. The higher risk of complications and shorter hospital stay make it essential that older patients and their family members receive specific information about signs and symptoms of complications and measures to prevent them.

Nursing Process

The Patient Undergoing Surgery for Gallbladder Disease

Assessment

The patient who is to undergo surgical treatment of gallbladder disease is often admitted to the hospital or same-day surgery unit on the morning of surgery. Preadmission testing is often completed a week or longer before admission. At that time, the nurse instructs the patient about the need to avoid smoking, to enhance pulmonary recovery postoperatively, and to avoid respiratory complications. It is also important to instruct the patient to avoid the use of aspirin and other agents (over-the-counter medications and herbal remedies) that can alter coagulation and other biochemical processes.

Assessment focuses on the patient's respiratory status. If a traditional surgical approach is planned, the high abdominal incision required during surgery may interfere with full respiratory excursion. The nurse notes a history of smoking, previous respiratory conditions, shallow respirations, a persistent or ineffective cough, and the presence of adventitious breath sounds. Nutritional status is evaluated through a dietary history and a general examination performed at the time of preadmission testing. The nurse also reviews previously obtained laboratory results to obtain information about the patient's nutritional status.

Nursing Priorities

Based on all the assessment data, the major postoperative nursing priorities for the patient undergoing surgery for gallbladder disease may include the following:

- Acute pain due to surgical incision
- Impaired gas exchange due to high abdominal surgical incision
- Breakdown in skin integrity related to altered biliary drainage after surgical intervention (if a T-tube was inserted because of retained stones in the common bile duct or another drainage device was employed)
- Imbalanced nutrition, due to inadequate bile secretion
- Lack of knowledge about self-care activities
- Nausea related to anesthesia

Collaborative Problems/ Potential Complications

Based on assessment data, potential complications may include the following:

- Bleeding
- GI symptoms (may be related to biliary leak or injury to the bowel)
- Vomiting related to anesthesia and opioids

Planning and Goals

The goals for the patient include relief of pain, adequate ventilation, intact skin and improved biliary drainage, optimal nutritional intake, absence of complications, absence of nausea and/or vomiting, and understanding of self-care routines.

Postoperative Nursing Interventions

After recovery from anesthesia, the patient is placed in the low Fowler's position. Fluids may be administered intravenously, and nasogastric suction (a nasogastric tube was probably inserted immediately before surgery for a non-laparoscopic procedure) may be instituted to relieve abdominal distension. Water and other fluids are administered within hours after laparoscopic procedures. A soft diet is started after bowel sounds return, which is usually the next day if the laparoscopic approach is used.

Relieving Pain

The location of the subcostal incision in non-laparoscopic gallbladder surgery often causes the patient to avoid turning and moving, to splint the affected site, and to take shallow breaths to prevent pain. Because full expansion of the lungs and gradually increased activity are necessary to prevent postoperative complications, the nurse administers analgesic agents as prescribed to relieve the pain and to promote well-being in addition to helping the patient turn, cough, breathe deeply, and ambulate as indicated. Use of a pillow or binder over the incision may reduce pain during these manoeuvres.

Improving Respiratory Status

Patients undergoing biliary tract surgery are especially prone to pulmonary complications, as are all patients with upper abdominal incisions. Therefore, the nurse reminds the patient to take deep breaths and cough every hour to expand the lungs fully and prevent atelectasis. The early and consistent use of incentive spirometry also helps improve respiratory function. Early ambulation prevents pulmonary complications as well as other complications, such as thrombophlebitis. Pulmonary complications are more likely to occur in patients who are older, with obesity, and with pre-existing pulmonary disease.

Maintaining Skin Integrity and Promoting Biliary Drainage

In patients who have undergone a cholecystostomy or choledochostomy, the drainage tube must be connected immediately to a drainage receptacle. The nurse should fasten the tubing to the dressings or to the patient's gown, with enough leeway for the patient to move without dislodging or kinking the tube. Because a drainage system remains attached when the patient is ambulating, the drainage bag may be placed in a bathrobe pocket or fastened so that it is below the waist or common duct level. If a Penrose drain is used, the nurse changes the dressings as required and observes the skin integrity more closely.

After these surgical procedures, the patient is observed for indications of infection, leakage of bile into the peritoneal cavity, and obstruction of bile drainage. If bile is not draining properly, an obstruction is probably causing bile to be forced back into the liver and bloodstream. This may lead to jaundice, so the nurse assesses the colour of the sclerae to observe for this. The nurse should note and report right upper quadrant abdominal pain, nausea and vomiting, bile drainage around any drainage tube, clay-coloured stools, and a change in vital signs.

Bile may continue to drain from the drainage tract in considerable quantities for some time, necessitating frequent changes of the outer dressings and protection of the skin from irritation (bile is corrosive to the skin). To prevent total loss of bile, the physician may want the drainage tube or collection receptacle elevated above the level of the abdomen so that the bile drains externally only if pressure develops in the duct system. Every 24 hours, the nurse measures the bile collected and records the amount, colour, and character of the drainage. After several days of drainage, the tube may be clamped for 1 hour before and after each meal to deliver bile to the duodenum to aid in digestion. Within 7 to 14 days, the drainage tube is removed. The patient who goes home with a drainage tube in place requires instruction and reassurance about the function and care of the tube.

In all patients with biliary drainage, the nurse (or the patient, if at home) observes the colour of stools daily. Urine and stool specimens may be sent to the laboratory for examination for bile pigments. In this way, it is possible to determine whether the bile pigment is disappearing from the blood and is draining again into the duodenum. Maintaining a careful record of fluid intake and output is important.

Improving Nutritional Status

The nurse encourages the patient to eat a diet that is low in fats and high in carbohydrates and proteins immediately after surgery. At the time of hospital discharge there are usually no special dietary instructions other than to maintain a nutritious diet and avoid excessive fats. Fat restriction usually is lifted in 4 to 6 weeks, when the biliary ducts dilate to accommodate the volume of bile once held by the gallbladder and when the ampulla of Vater again functions effectively. After this time, when the patient eats fat, adequate bile will be released into the GI tract to emulsify the fats and allow their digestion. This is in contrast to the condition before surgery, when fats may not have been digested completely or adequately and flatulence may have occurred. One purpose of gallbladder surgery is to allow a normal diet.

Monitoring and Managing Potential Complications

Bleeding may occur as a result of inadvertent puncture or injury to a major blood vessel. Postoperatively, the nurse closely monitors vital signs and inspects the surgical incisions and any drains for bleeding. The nurse also assesses the patient for increased tenderness and rigidity of the abdomen. If these signs and symptoms occur, they are reported to the surgeon. The nurse instructs the patient and family to report any change in the colour of stools, because this may indicate complications. GI symptoms, although not common, may occur with manipulation of the intestines during surgery. The nurse should assess for nausea and use antiemetics as ordered to prevent vomiting postoperatively, which may impact wound healing. Patients are at risk of vomiting due to anesthesia and the use of opioids for pain management.

After laparoscopic cholecystectomy, the nurse assesses the patient for anorexia, vomiting, pain, abdominal distension, and temperature elevation. These may indicate infection or disruption of the GI tract and are reported to the surgeon promptly. Because the patient is discharged soon after laparoscopic surgery, the patient and family are instructed verbally and in writing about the importance of reporting these symptoms promptly.

Promoting Home, Community-Based, and Transitional Care

EDUCATING PATIENTS ABOUT SELF-CARE. The nurse instructs the patient about the medications that are prescribed (vitamins, anticholinergics, and antispasmodics) and their actions. It also is important to inform the patient and family about symptoms that should be reported to the physician, including jaundice, dark urine, pale-coloured stools, pruritus, and signs of inflammation and infection, such as pain or fever.

Some patients report one to three bowel movements a day, which is a result of a continual trickle of bile through the choledochoduodenal junction after cholecystectomy. Usually, such frequency diminishes over a period of a few weeks to several months.

If a patient is discharged from the hospital with a drainage tube still in place, the patient and family need instructions about its management. The nurse instructs them in proper care of the drainage tube and the importance of reporting promptly any changes in the amount or characteristics of drainage. Assistance in securing the appropriate dressings reduces the patient's anxiety about going home with the drain or tube still in place. See Chart 40-2 for additional details.

CONTINUING AND TRANSITIONAL CARE. With sufficient support at home, most patients recover quickly from a cholecystectomy. However, older or frail patients and those who live alone may require a referral for home care. During home visits, the nurse assesses the patient's physical status, especially wound healing, and progress toward recovery. Assessing the patient for adequacy of pain relief and pulmonary exercises is also important. If the patient has a drainage system in place, the nurse assesses it for patency and appropriate management by the patient and family. Assessing for signs of infection and teaching the patient about the signs and symptoms of infection are also important nursing interventions. The patient's understanding of the therapeutic regimen (medications, gradual return to usual activities) is assessed, and previous teaching is reinforced. The nurse emphasizes the importance of keeping follow-up appointments and reminds the patient and family of the importance of participating in health promotion activities and recommended health screening.

CHART 40-2

Patient Education: Managing Self-Care After Laparoscopic Cholecystectomy

Resuming Activity

- Begin light exercise (walking) immediately.
- Take a shower or bath after 1 or 2 days.
- Drive a car after 3 or 4 days.
- Avoid lifting objects exceeding 2.25 kg (5 lb) after surgery, usually for 1 week.
- Resume sexual activity when desired.

Caring for the Wound

- Check puncture site daily for signs of infection.
- Wash puncture site with mild soap and water.
- Allow special adhesive strips on the puncture site to fall off. Do not pull them off.

Resuming Eating

- Resume your usual diet.
- If you had fat intolerance before surgery, gradually add fat back into your diet in small increments.

Managing Pain

- You may experience pain or discomfort in your right shoulder from the gas used to inflate your abdominal area during surgery. Sitting upright in bed or a chair, walking, or use of a heating pad may ease the discomfort.
- Take analgesics as needed and as prescribed. Report to surgeon if pain is unrelieved even with analgesic use.

Managing Follow-up Care

- Make an appointment with your surgeon for 7 to 10 days after discharge.
- Call your surgeon if you experience any signs or symptoms of infection at or around the puncture site: redness, tenderness, swelling, heat, or drainage.
- Call your surgeon if you experience a fever of 37.7°C (100°F) or more for 2 consecutive days.
- Call your surgeon if you develop nausea, vomiting, or abdominal pain.

Evaluation

Expected patient outcomes may include the following:

1. Reports decrease in pain
   a. Splints abdominal incision to decrease pain
   b. Avoids foods that cause pain
   c. Uses postoperative analgesia as prescribed
2. Demonstrates appropriate respiratory function
   a. Achieves full respiratory excursion, with deep inspiration and expiration
   b. Coughs effectively, using pillow to splint abdominal incision
   c. Uses postoperative analgesia as prescribed
   d. Exercises as prescribed (e.g., turns, ambulates)
3. Exhibits intact skin integrity around biliary drainage site (if applicable)
   a. Is free of fever, abdominal pain, change in vital signs, and presence of bile, foul-smelling drainage, or pus around drainage tube
   b. Demonstrates correct management of drainage tube (if applicable)
   c. Identifies signs and symptoms of biliary obstruction to be noted and reported
   d. Has serum bilirubin level within expected range
4. Obtains relief from dietary intolerance
   a. Maintains adequate dietary intake and avoids foods that cause gastrointestinal symptoms
   b. Reports decreased or absent nausea, vomiting, diarrhea, flatulence, and abdominal discomfort
5. Absence of complications
   a. Has usual vital signs (blood pressure, pulse, respiratory rate and pattern, and temperature)
   b. Reports absence of bleeding from GI tract and from biliary drainage tube or catheter (if present) and no evidence of bleeding in stool
   c. Reports return of appetite and no evidence of nausea, vomiting, abdominal distension, or pain
   d. Lists symptoms that should be reported to surgeon promptly and demonstrates an understanding of self-care, including wound care

DISORDERS OF THE PANCREAS

Pancreatitis (inflammation of the pancreas) is a serious disorder and one of the most common GI reasons for hospitalization. Acute pancreatitis affects more than 600,000 Canadians, and chronic pancreatitis affects more than 300,000 Canadians (Canadian Digestive Health Foundation, n.d.).

The most basic classification system used to describe or categorize the various stages and forms of pancreatitis divides the disorder into acute and chronic forms. Acute pancreatitis can be a medical emergency associated with a high risk of life-threatening complications and mortality, whereas chronic pancreatitis often goes undetected until 80% to 90% of the exocrine and endocrine tissue is destroyed. Acute pancreatitis does not usually lead to chronic pancreatitis unless complications develop. However, chronic pancreatitis can be characterized by acute episodes, and 20% to 30% of patients with acute pancreatitis develop recurrences (Cenci et al., 2017).

Although the mechanisms causing pancreatic inflammation are unknown (Cenci et al., 2017), pancreatitis is commonly described as autodigestion of the pancreas. It is believed that the pancreatic duct becomes temporarily obstructed (often with stones), accompanied by hypersecretion of the exocrine enzymes of the pancreas. These enzymes enter the bile duct, where they are activated and, together with bile, back up (reflux) into the pancreatic duct, causing pancreatitis.

Acute Pancreatitis

PRACTICE & LEARN · INTERACTIVE TUTORIALS

Acute pancreatitis ranges from a mild, self-limited disorder to a severe, rapidly fatal disease that does not respond to any treatment. Approximately 20% of patients with acute pancreatitis will have a severe form. Mild acute pancreatitis is characterized by edema and inflammation confined to the pancreas.

These two main types of acute pancreatitis (mild and severe) are classified as interstitial edematous pancreatitis and necrotizing pancreatitis, respectively. Interstitial pancreatitis affects the majority of patients. It is characterized by a lack of pancreatic or peripancreatic parenchymal necrosis with diffuse enlargement of the gland due to inflammatory edema (Wu & Banks, 2013). The edema and inflammation in interstitial pancreatitis are confined to the pancreas itself. Minimal organ dysfunction is present, and return to regular function usually occurs within 6 months. Although this is considered the milder form of pancreatitis, the patient is acutely ill and at risk for hypovolemic shock, fluid and electrolyte disturbances, and sepsis.

A more widespread and complete enzymatic digestion of the gland characterizes severe acute pancreatitis. This type can be sterile or infected; if the parenchyma is involved this is a marker for more severe disease (Lankisch, Apte, & Banks, 2015; Wu & Banks, 2013). The tissue may become necrotic, with damage extending into the retroperitoneal tissues. Local complications include pancreatic cysts or abscesses and acute fluid collections in or near the pancreas. Patients who develop systemic complications with organ failure, such as pulmonary insufficiency with hypoxia, shock, renal failure, and GI bleeding, are also characterized as having severe acute pancreatitis.

Gerontologic Considerations

Acute pancreatitis affects people of all ages, but the mortality rate associated with acute pancreatitis increases with advancing age (Wu & Banks, 2013). In addition, the pattern of complications changes with age. Younger patients tend to develop local complications; the incidence of multiple organ dysfunction syndrome (MODS) increases with age, possibly as a result of progressive decreases in physiologic function of major organs with increasing age. Close monitoring of major organ function (i.e., lungs, kidneys) is essential, and aggressive treatment is necessary to reduce mortality from acute pancreatitis in older adults.

Pathophysiology

Self-digestion of the pancreas by its own proteolytic enzymes, principally trypsin, causes acute pancreatitis. Eighty percent of patients with acute pancreatitis have biliary tract disease or a history of long-term alcohol abuse. These patients usually have had undiagnosed chronic pancreatitis before their first episode of acute pancreatitis. Gallstones have a strong correlation with acute pancreatitis, with estimates of 60% of cases of acute pancreatitis being associated with gallstones. Gallstones enter the common bile duct and lodge at the ampulla of Vater, obstructing the flow of pancreatic juice or causing a reflux of bile from the common bile duct into the pancreatic duct, thus activating the powerful enzymes within the pancreas. Usually, these remain in an inactive form until the pancreatic secretions reach the lumen of the duodenum. Activation of the enzymes can lead to vasodilation, increased vascular permeability, necrosis, erosion, and hemorrhage (Fagenholz & de Moya, 2014; Townsend, Beauchamp, Evers, et al., 2016).

Other less common causes of pancreatitis include bacterial or viral infection, with pancreatitis occasionally developing as a complication of mumps virus. Spasm and edema of the ampulla of Vater, caused by duodenitis, can probably produce pancreatitis. Blunt abdominal trauma, peptic ulcer disease, ischemic vascular disease, hyperlipidemia, hypercalcemia, and the use of corticosteroids, thiazide diuretics, oral contraceptives, and other medications have also been associated with an increased incidence of pancreatitis. Acute pancreatitis may develop after surgery on or near the pancreas or after instrumentation of the pancreatic duct. Acute idiopathic pancreatitis accounts for up to 10% of the cases of acute pancreatitis. Some experts postulate that these cases may be related to occult microlithiasis (small stones in the bile) (Cuschieri & Hanna, 2014). In addition, there is a small incidence of hereditary pancreatitis. Obesity is also a known risk factor for pancreatitis, and it is anticipated that with growing obesity rates, a higher prevalence of pancreatitis will be seen.

The overall mortality rate of patients with acute pancreatitis is high (10% to 30%) due to associated shock, anoxia, hypotension, or fluid and electrolyte imbalances. This mortality rate may also be related to the 20% of patients with severe acute disease characterized by pancreatic and peripancreatic necrosis (De Waele, 2014; Townsend et al., 2016). Attacks of acute pancreatitis may result in complete recovery, may recur without permanent damage, or may progress to chronic pancreatitis. The patient who is admitted to the hospital with a diagnosis of pancreatitis is acutely ill and needs expert nursing and medical care.

The severity of acute alcoholic pancreatitis and its outcomes can be predicted based on clinical and laboratory data (Chart 40-3).

CHART 40-3

Criteria for Predicting Severity of Pancreatitis[a]

Criteria on Admission to Hospital

Age >55 years
WBC >16,000 mm^3
Serum glucose >11.1 mmol/L
Serum LDH >350 U/L
AST >120 U/L

Criteria Within 48 Hours of Hospital Admission

Fall in hematocrit >10% (>0.10)
BUN increase >1.7 mmol/L
Serum calcium <2.0 mmol/L
Base deficit >4 mmol/L
Fluid retention or sequestration >6 L
PO_2 <60 mm Hg
Two or fewer signs, 1% mortality; 3 or 4 signs, 15% mortality; 5 or 6 signs, 40% mortality; >6 signs, 100% mortality.

[a]The more risk factors a patient has, the greater the severity and likelihood of complications or death.
Adapted from Ranson, J. H., Rifkind, K. M., Roses, D. F., et al. (1974). Prognostic signs and the role of operative management in acute pancreatitis. *Surgery, Gynecology & Obstetrics, 139*(1), 69–81.

Clinical Manifestations

Severe abdominal pain is the major symptom of pancreatitis that causes the patient to seek medical care. Abdominal pain and tenderness and back pain result from irritation and edema of the inflamed pancreas. Increased tension on the pancreatic capsule and obstruction of the pancreatic ducts also contribute to the pain. Typically, the pain occurs in the midepigastrium. Pain is frequently acute in onset, occurring 24 to 48 hours after a very heavy meal or alcohol ingestion, and it may be diffuse and difficult to localize. It is generally more severe after meals and is unrelieved by antacids. Pain may be accompanied by abdominal distension, a poorly defined, palpable abdominal mass; decreased peristalsis; and vomiting that fails to relieve the pain or nausea.

The patient appears acutely ill. Abdominal guarding is present. A rigid or boardlike abdomen may develop and is generally an ominous sign, usually indicating peritonitis. Ecchymosis (bruising) in the flank or around the umbilicus may indicate severe pancreatitis. Nausea and vomiting are common in acute pancreatitis. The emesis is usually gastric in origin but may also be bile stained. Fever, jaundice, mental confusion, and agitation may also occur.

Hypotension is typical and reflects hypovolemia and shock caused by the loss of large amounts of protein-rich fluid into the tissues and peritoneal cavity. In addition to hypotension, the patient may develop tachycardia, cyanosis, and cold, clammy skin. Acute kidney injury is common.

Respiratory distress and hypoxia are common, and the patient may develop diffuse pulmonary infiltrates, dyspnea, tachypnea, and abnormal blood gas values. Myocardial depression, hypocalcemia, hyperglycemia, and disseminated intravascular coagulation may also occur with acute pancreatitis.

Assessment and Diagnostic Findings

The diagnosis of acute pancreatitis is based on a history of abdominal pain, the presence of known risk factors, physical examination findings, and diagnostic findings. Serum amylase and lipase levels are used in making the diagnosis of acute pancreatitis with lipase being the measurement of choice for acute pancreatitis (Cenci et al., 2017). Serum lipase will rise within 4 to 8 hours and stay elevated for 8 to 14 days. A lipase level over five times the upper limit of testing is indicative of acute pancreatitis. Serum amylase is usually elevated within 24 hours and returns to usual within 48 to 72 hours, but serum lipase levels may remain elevated for a longer period, often days longer than amylase. Urinary amylase levels also become elevated and remain elevated longer than serum amylase levels. The WBC is usually elevated; hypocalcemia is present in many patients and correlates well with the severity of pancreatitis. Transient hyperglycemia and glucosuria and elevated serum bilirubin levels occur in some patients with acute pancreatitis.

X-ray studies of the abdomen and chest may be obtained to differentiate pancreatitis from other disorders that can cause similar symptoms and to detect pleural effusions. Ultrasound and contrast-enhanced CT scans are used to identify an increase in the diameter of the pancreas and to detect pancreatic cysts, abscesses, or pseudocysts. Ultrasound is useful in the initial diagnosis of acute pancreatitis and also to monitor for potential complications such as abscesses, necrosis, peripancreatic fluid, pseudocysts, abscesses, and vascular disease (Cenci et al., 2017).

Hematocrit and hemoglobin levels are used to monitor the patient for bleeding. Peritoneal fluid, obtained through paracentesis or peritoneal lavage, may contain increased levels of pancreatic enzymes. ERCP is rarely used in the diagnostic evaluation of acute pancreatitis, because the patient is acutely ill; however, it may be valuable in the treatment of gallstone pancreatitis.

Medical Management

Management of acute pancreatitis is directed toward relieving symptoms and preventing or treating complications. All oral intakes are withheld to inhibit stimulation of the pancreas and its secretion of enzymes. Parenteral nutrition plays an important role in the nutritional support of patients with severe acute pancreatitis, particularly in those who are debilitated and those with a prolonged paralytic ileus (more than 48 to 72 hours) (Cuschieri & Hanna, 2014). Ongoing research has shown positive outcomes with the use of enteral feedings. The current recommendation is that, whenever possible, the enteral route should be used to meet nutritional needs in patients with pancreatitis (McClave, 2013; Zerem, 2014). This strategy also has been found to prevent infectious complications, safely and cost effectively (Cuschieri & Hanna, 2014). It is now thought that enteral feedings should be started early in the course of acute pancreatitis. Patients who do not tolerate enteral feeding require parenteral nutrition. In some cases nasogastric suction may be used to relieve nausea and vomiting and to decrease painful abdominal distension and paralytic ileus, but research data do not support the routine use of nasogastric tubes to remove gastric secretions in an effort to limit pancreatic secretion. Histamine-2 (H_2) antagonists such as cimetidine (Tagamet) and ranitidine (Zantac) may be prescribed to decrease pancreatic activity by inhibiting secretion of gastric acid. Proton pump inhibitors such as pantoprazole (Protonix) may be used for patients who do not tolerate H_2 antagonists or for whom this therapy is ineffective.

Pain Management

Adequate administration of analgesia is essential during the course of acute pancreatitis to provide sufficient pain relief and to minimize restlessness, which may stimulate pancreatic secretion further. Pain relief may require parenteral opioids such as morphine, fentanyl (Sublimaze), or hydromorphone (Dilaudid). The use of morphine was avoided in the past because of concern that it could cause painful spasms of the sphincter of Oddi and worsen pancreatitis; however, all opioids stimulate this sphincter to some degree. There is no clinical evidence to support the use of meperidine for pain relief in pancreatitis, and in fact, accumulation of its metabolites can cause CNS irritability and possibly seizures. The current recommendation for pain management is the use of opioids, with assessment for their effectiveness and altering therapy if pain is not controlled or increased. More research is needed to identify the best option for pain management in the patient with acute pancreatitis. Antiemetic agents may be prescribed to prevent vomiting.

Intensive Care

Correction of fluid and blood loss and low albumin levels is necessary to maintain fluid volume and prevent renal failure. The patient is usually acutely ill and is monitored in the intensive care unit, where hemodynamic monitoring and arterial blood gas monitoring are initiated. Antibiotic agents may be prescribed if infection is present. The role of prophylactic antibiotics is controversial and still under study. Insulin may be required if hyperglycemia occurs. Intensive insulin therapy (continuous infusion) in the critically ill patient has undergone much study and has shown promise in terms of positive patient outcomes when compared with intermittent insulin dosing. Glycemic control with usual or near usual blood glucose levels improves patient outcomes.

Respiratory Care

Aggressive respiratory care is indicated because of the high risk of elevation of the diaphragm, pulmonary infiltrates and effusion, and atelectasis. Hypoxemia occurs in a significant number of patients with acute pancreatitis, even with normal x-ray findings. Respiratory care may range from close monitoring of arterial blood gases to use of humidified oxygen to intubation and mechanical ventilation (see Chapter 22 for further discussion).

Biliary Drainage

Placement of biliary drains (for external drainage) and stents (indwelling tubes) in the pancreatic duct through endoscopy has been performed to reestablish drainage of the pancreas. This has resulted in decreased pain and increased weight gain.

Surgical Intervention

Although surgery is often risky because the acutely ill patient is a poor surgical risk, it may be performed to assist in the diagnosis of pancreatitis (diagnostic laparotomy), to establish pancreatic drainage, or to resect or débride a necrotic pancreas. The patient who undergoes pancreatic surgery may have multiple drains in place postoperatively, as well as a surgical incision that is left open for irrigation and repacking every 2 to 3 days to remove necrotic debris (Fig. 40-6).

Postacute Management

Antacids may be used after acute pancreatitis begins to resolve. Oral feedings that are low in fat and protein are initiated gradually. Caffeine and alcohol are eliminated from the diet. If the episode of pancreatitis occurred during treatment with thiazide diuretics, corticosteroids, or oral contraceptives, these medications are discontinued. Follow-up may include ultrasound, x-ray studies, or ERCP to determine whether the pancreatitis is resolving and to assess for abscesses and pseudocysts. ERCP may also be used to identify the cause of acute pancreatitis if it is in question and for endoscopic sphincterotomy and removal of gallstones from the common bile duct.

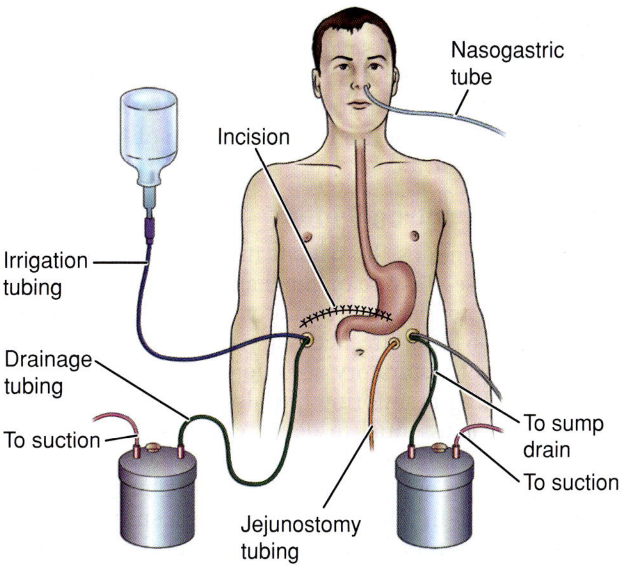

FIGURE 40-6. Multiple sump tubes are used after pancreatic surgery. Triple-lumen tubes consist of ports that provide tubing for irrigation, air venting, and drainage.

Nursing Management

Relieving Pain and Discomfort

Because the pathologic process responsible for pain is autodigestion of the pancreas, the objectives of therapy are to relieve pain and decrease secretion of pancreatic enzymes. The pain of acute pancreatitis is often very severe, necessitating the liberal use of analgesics. The current recommendation for pain management in this population is parenteral opioids, including morphine, hydromorphone, or fentanyl via patient-controlled analgesia or bolus. In critically ill patients, a continuous infusion may be needed. Because most opioids stimulate spasm of the sphincter of Oddi to some degree, consensus has not been reached on the most effective agent. Ensuring patient comfort, regardless of the opioid prescribed, is the most essential aspect of care. The nurse frequently assesses the pain and the effectiveness of the pharmacologic (and nonpharmacologic) interventions. Changes may be needed in the regimen for pain management based on the achievement of pain control. Pain assessment tools (see Chapter 16) are available for the nurse to ensure an accurate rating of pain. Nonpharmacologic interventions such as proper positioning, music, distraction, and imagery may be effective in reducing pain when used along with medications.

In some patients requiring intensive care, oral feedings are withheld to decrease the secretion of secretin. Parenteral fluids and electrolytes are prescribed to restore and maintain fluid balance. Nasogastric suction may be used to relieve nausea and vomiting or to treat abdominal distension and paralytic ileus. The nurse provides frequent oral hygiene and care to decrease discomfort from the nasogastric tube and relieve dryness of the mouth.

The acutely ill patient is maintained on bed rest to decrease the metabolic rate and reduce the secretion of pancreatic and gastric enzymes. If the patient experiences increasing severity of pain, the nurse reports this to the physician because the patient may be experiencing hemorrhage of the pancreas or the dose of analgesic may be inadequate.

The patient with acute pancreatitis often has a clouded sensorium because of severe pain, fluid and electrolyte disturbances, and hypoxia. Therefore, the nurse provides frequent and repeated but simple explanations about the need for withholding fluids, maintenance of gastric suction, and bed rest.

Improving Breathing Pattern

The nurse maintains the patient in a semi-Fowler's position to decrease pressure on the diaphragm by a distended abdomen and to increase respiratory expansion. Frequent changes of position are necessary to prevent atelectasis and pooling of respiratory secretions. Pulmonary assessment, including monitoring of pulse oximetry or arterial blood gases, is essential to detect changes in respiratory status so that early treatment can be initiated. The nurse instructs the patient in techniques of coughing and deep breathing and in the use of incentive spirometry to improve respiratory function and assists the patient to perform these activities every hour.

Improving Nutritional Status

Oral food or fluid intake is not permitted. However, it is important to assess the patient's nutritional status and to note factors that alter the patient's nutritional requirements (e.g., temperature elevation, surgery, drainage). Laboratory test results and daily weights are useful to monitor the nutritional status.

Enteral or parenteral nutrition may be prescribed. In addition to administering enteral or parenteral nutrition, the nurse monitors serum glucose levels every 4 to 6 hours. As the acute symptoms subside, oral feedings are gradually reintroduced. Between acute attacks, the patient receives a diet that is low in fats and proteins (Dudek, 2013). The patient should avoid heavy meals and alcoholic beverages.

Maintaining Skin Integrity

The patient is at risk for skin breakdown because of poor nutritional status, enforced bed rest, and restlessness, which may result in pressure ulcers and breaks in tissue integrity. In addition, the patient who has undergone surgery may have multiple drains or an open surgical incision and is at risk for skin breakdown and infection. The nurse carefully assesses the wound, drainage sites, and skin for signs of infection, inflammation, and breakdown. The nurse carries out wound care as prescribed and takes precautions to protect intact skin from contact with drainage. Consultation with a wound-ostomy-continence (WOC) nurse is often helpful in identifying appropriate skin care devices and protocols. It is important to turn the patient every 2 hours; use of specialty beds may be indicated to prevent skin breakdown.

Monitoring and Managing Potential Complications

Fluid and electrolyte disturbances are common complications because of nausea, vomiting, movement of fluid from the vascular compartment to the peritoneal cavity, diaphoresis, fever, and the use of gastric suction. The nurse assesses the patient's fluid and electrolyte status by noting skin turgor and moistness of mucous membranes. The nurse weighs the patient daily and carefully measures fluid intake and output, including urine output, nasogastric secretions, and diarrhea. In addition, it is important to assess for other factors that may affect fluid and electrolyte status, including increased body temperature and wound drainage. The nurse assesses the patient for ascites and measures abdominal girth daily if ascites is suspected.

Fluids are administered IV and may be accompanied by infusion of blood or blood products to maintain the blood volume and to prevent or treat hypovolemic shock. It is important to keep emergency medications readily available because of the risk of circulatory collapse and shock. The nurse promptly reports decreased blood pressure and reduced urine output, which indicate hypovolemia and shock or renal failure. Low serum calcium and magnesium levels may occur and require prompt treatment.

Pancreatic necrosis is a major cause of morbidity and mortality in patients with acute pancreatitis because of resulting hemorrhage, septic shock, and multiple organ failure. The patient may undergo diagnostic procedures for confirmation of pancreatic necrosis, for surgical débridement, or for insertion of multiple drains. Percutaneous or endoscopic catheter drainage is the first step of what is known as the "Step-Up Approach." Here, catheters are placed via the left or right retroperitoneal approach to drain the infection. This intervention, coupled with appropriate, targeted antibiotic therapy may be the only necessary treatment for some patients (da Costa, Boerma, van Santvoort, et al., 2014; Lankisch et al., 2015; Martin & Hein, 2013). These procedures are considered first-line approaches with surgery reserved for patients for whom these interventions do not work. Prophylactic antibiotics are not indicated (Lankisch et al., 2015; Zerem, 2014). The patient with pancreatic necrosis is usually critically ill and requires expert medical and nursing management, including hemodynamic monitoring in the intensive care unit.

In addition to carefully monitoring vital signs and other signs and symptoms, the nurse is responsible for administering prescribed fluids, medications, and blood products; assisting with supportive management, such as use of a ventilator; preventing additional complications; and providing physical and psychological care.

Shock and multiple organ failure may occur with acute pancreatitis. Hypovolemic shock may occur as a result of hypovolemia and sequestering of fluid in the peritoneal cavity. Hemorrhagic shock may occur with hemorrhagic pancreatitis. Septic shock may occur with bacterial infection of the pancreas. Cardiac dysfunction may occur as a result of fluid and electrolyte disturbances, acid–base imbalances, and release of toxic substances into the circulation.

The nurse closely monitors the patient for early signs of neurologic, cardiovascular, renal, and respiratory dysfunction. The nurse must be prepared to respond quickly to rapid changes in the patient's status, treatments, and therapies. In addition, it is important to inform the family about the status and progress of the patient and to allow them to spend time with the patient. (Management of shock is discussed in detail in Chapter 18.)

Promoting Home, Community-Based, and Transitional Care

Educating Patients About Self-Care

The patient who has survived an episode of acute pancreatitis has been acutely ill. A prolonged period is needed to regain strength and return to the previous level of activity. The patient is often still weak and debilitated for weeks or months after an acute episode of pancreatitis. Because of the severity of the acute illness, the patient may not recall many of the explanations and instructions given during the acute phase. Teaching often needs to be repeated and reinforced. The nurse instructs the patient about the factors implicated in the onset of acute pancreatitis and about the need to avoid high-fat foods, heavy meals, and alcohol. It is important to give the patient and family verbal and written instructions about signs and symptoms of acute pancreatitis and possible complications that should be reported promptly to the physician.

If acute pancreatitis is a result of biliary tract disease, such as gallstones and gallbladder disease, additional explanations are needed about required dietary modifications. If the pancreatitis is a result of alcohol use, the nurse reinforces the need to avoid all alcohol.

Continuing and Transitional Care

A referral for home care is often indicated. This enables the nurse to assess the patient's physical and psychological status and adherence to the therapeutic regimen. The nurse also assesses the home situation and reinforces instructions about fluid and nutrition intake and, if appropriate, the avoidance of alcohol. After the acute attack has subsided, some patients with alcoholism may be inclined to return to their previous drinking habits. The nurse provides specific information about resources and support groups that may be of assistance in avoiding alcohol in the future. Referral to Alcoholics Anonymous or other appropriate support groups is essential. See the accompanying plan of nursing care in Chart 40-4 for the patient with acute pancreatitis.

Chronic Pancreatitis

Chronic pancreatitis is an inflammatory disorder characterized by progressive destruction of the pancreas. As cells are replaced by fibrous tissue with repeated attacks of pancreatitis, pressure within the pancreas increases. The result is obstruction of the pancreatic and common bile ducts and the duodenum. In addition, there is atrophy of the epithelium of the ducts, inflammation, and destruction of the secreting cells of the pancreas.

Alcohol consumption in Western societies and malnutrition worldwide are the major causes of chronic pancreatitis. The median age of patients diagnosed with chronic pancreatitis has been reported to be 62 years (Muniraj, Aslanian, Farrell, et al., 2014). Frequently, at that age, patients already report a long history of alcohol abuse. Excessive and prolonged consumption of alcohol accounts for approximately 70% to 80% of all cases of chronic pancreatitis (Cuschieri & Hanna, 2014). The incidence of pancreatitis is 50 times greater in people with alcoholism than in those who do not abuse alcohol. Long-term alcohol consumption causes hypersecretion of protein in pancreatic secretions, resulting in protein plugs and calculi within the pancreatic ducts. Alcohol also has a direct toxic effect on the cells of the pancreas. Damage to these cells is more likely to occur and to be more severe in patients whose diets are poor in protein content and either very high or very low in fat. Smoking is another factor in the development of chronic pancreatitis and patients with it should refrain from smoking.

Clinical Manifestations

Chronic pancreatitis is characterized by recurring episodes of severe upper abdominal and back pain, accompanied by vomiting. Attacks are often so painful that opioids, even in large doses, do not provide relief. The risk of opioid dependence is increased in pancreatitis because of the chronic nature and severity of the pain. As the disease progresses, recurring attacks of pain are more severe, more frequent, and of longer duration. Some patients experience continuous severe pain, and others have dull, nagging constant pain. Periods of well-being sometimes follow the episodes of pain (Muniraj et al., 2014). In some patients, chronic pancreatitis is painless. The natural history of abdominal pain (character, timing, severity) is variable, and many studies have documented a decrease in pain ("burnout") over time in a majority of patients (Muniraj et al., 2014).

Weight loss is a major issue in chronic pancreatitis: Most patients experience significant weight loss, which is usually caused by decreased dietary intake secondary to anorexia or fear that eating will precipitate another attack. Malabsorption occurs late in the disease, when as little as 10% of pancreatic function remains (Bope & Kellerman, 2015). As a result, digestion, especially of proteins and fats, is impaired. The stools become frequent, frothy, and foul smelling because of impaired fat digestion, which results in stools with a high fat content. This is referred to as **steatorrhea**. As the disease progresses, calcification of the gland may occur, and calcium stones may form within the ducts.

Assessment and Diagnostic Findings

ERCP is the most useful study in the diagnosis of chronic pancreatitis. It provides details about the anatomy of the pancreas and the pancreatic and biliary ducts. It is also helpful in obtaining tissue for analysis and differentiating pancreatitis from other conditions, such as carcinoma. Various imaging procedures, including magnetic resonance imaging (MRI), CT scans, and ultrasound, are used in the diagnostic evaluation of patients with suspected pancreatic disorders. A CT scan or ultrasound study is also helpful to detect pancreatic cysts.

A glucose tolerance test evaluates pancreatic islet cell function and provides necessary information for making decisions about surgical resection of the pancreas. An abnormal glucose tolerance test may indicate the presence of diabetes associated with decreased pancreatic function from chronic pancreatitis and cellular destruction. Acute exacerbations of chronic pancreatitis may result in increased serum amylase levels. Steatorrhea is best confirmed by laboratory analysis of fecal fat content.

Medical Management

The management of chronic pancreatitis depends on its probable cause in each patient. Treatment is directed

(text continued on page 1126)

Plan of Nursing Care

Chart 40-4. Care of the Patient With Acute Pancreatitis

Nursing Priority: Pain
Goal: Relief of pain and discomfort

NURSING INTERVENTIONS	RATIONALE	EXPECTED OUTCOMES
1. Using a pain scale, assess pain level at baseline, before and after administration of analgesic medications.	1. Baseline assessment and control of pain are important because restlessness increases the body's metabolism, which stimulates the secretion of pancreatic and gastric enzymes.	• Patient rates pain using pain scale • Reports relief of pain, discomfort, and abdominal cramping • Moves and turns without increasing pain and discomfort • Rests comfortably and sleeps for increasing periods • Reports increased feelings of well-being and security with the health care team
2. Administer morphine, fentanyl, or hydromorphone frequently, as prescribed, to achieve level of pain acceptable to patient.	2. Morphine, fentanyl, and hydromorphone act by depressing the central nervous system and thereby increasing the patient's pain threshold. Meperidine (Demerol) is avoided because it has failed acute pain studies and possesses toxic metabolites.	
3. Maintain the patient NPO (nothing by mouth) as prescribed.	3. Pancreatic secretion is increased by food and fluid intake.	
4. Maintain the patient on bed rest.	4. Bed rest decreases body metabolism and thus reduces pancreatic and gastric secretions.	
5. Maintain continuous nasogastric drainage if paralytic ileus or nausea and vomiting, abdominal distension are present.	5. Nasogastric suction relieves nausea, vomiting, and abdominal distension. Decompression of the intestines (if intestinal intubation is used) also assists in relieving respiratory distress.	
6. Measure gastric secretions at specified intervals.	6. Pain may increase pancreatic enzymes and may also indicate pancreatic hemorrhage.	
7. Observe and record colour and viscosity of gastric secretions.	7. Frequent turning relieves pressure and assists in preventing pulmonary and vascular complications.	
8. Ensure that the nasogastric tube is patent to permit free drainage.	8. The use of nonpharmacologic methods will enhance the effects of analgesic medications.	
9. Report unrelieved pain or increasing intensity of pain.	9. Demonstration of caring can help to decrease anxiety.	
10. Assist patient to assume positions of comfort; turn and reposition every 2 hours.		
11. Use nonpharmacologic interventions for relieving pain (e.g., relaxation, focused breathing, diversion).		
12. Listen to patient's expression of pain experience.		

Nursing Priority: Management of NG tube discomfort
Goal: Relief of discomfort associated with nasogastric intubation used to treat ileus, vomiting, distension

NURSING INTERVENTIONS	RATIONALE	EXPECTED OUTCOMES
1. Use water-soluble lubricant around external nares.	1. Prevents irritation of nares.	• Exhibits intact skin and tissue of nares at site of nasogastric tube insertion • Reports no pain or irritation of nares or oropharynx • Exhibits moist, clean mucous membranes of mouth and nasopharynx • States that thirst is relieved by oral hygiene • Identifies rationale for nasogastric tube and suction
2. Turn patient at intervals; avoid pressure or tension on nasogastric tube.	2. Relieves pressure of tube on esophageal and gastric mucosa	
3. Provide oral hygiene and gargling solutions without alcohol.	3. Relieves dryness and irritation of oropharynx.	
4. Explain rationale for the use of nasogastric drainage.	4. Assists patient to cooperate with the drainage, nasogastric tube, and suction.	

Plan of Nursing Care — Chart 40-4. Care of the Patient With Acute Pancreatitis, *Continued*

Nursing Priority: Nutrition
Goal: Improvement in nutritional status

NURSING INTERVENTIONS	RATIONALE
1. Assess current nutritional status and increased metabolic requirements.	1. Alteration in pancreatic secretions interferes with normal digestive processes. Acute illness, infection, and fever increase metabolic needs.
2. Monitor serum glucose levels and administer insulin as prescribed.	2. Impairment of endocrine function of the pancreas leads to increased serum glucose levels.
3. Administer IV fluid and electrolytes, enteral or parenteral nutrition as prescribed.	3. Parenteral administration of fluids and electrolytes, and enteral or parenteral nutrients are essential to provide fluids, calories, electrolytes, and nutrients when oral intake is prohibited.
4. Provide high-carbohydrate, low-protein, low-fat diet when tolerated.	4. These foods increase caloric intake without stimulating pancreatic secretions beyond the ability of the pancreas to respond.
5. Instruct patient to eliminate alcohol, and refer to Alcoholics Anonymous, if indicated.	5. Alcohol intake produces further damage to pancreas and precipitates attacks of acute pancreatitis.
6. Counsel patient to avoid excessive use of coffee and spicy foods.	6. Coffee and spicy foods increase pancreatic and gastric secretions.
7. Monitor daily weights.	7. This provides a baseline and a means to measure weight gain or weight loss.

EXPECTED OUTCOMES

- Maintains normal body weight
- Demonstrates no additional weight loss
- Maintains normal serum glucose levels
- Reports decreasing episodes of vomiting and diarrhea
- Reports return of normal stool characteristics and bowel pattern
- Consumes foods high in carbohydrates, low in fat and protein
- Explains rationale for high-carbohydrate, low-fat, low-protein diet
- Eliminates alcohol from diet
- Explains rationale for limiting coffee intake and avoiding spicy foods
- Participates in Alcoholics Anonymous as appropriate or other counselling approach
- Returns to and maintains desirable weight

Nursing Priority: Breathing
Goal: Improvement in respiratory function

NURSING INTERVENTIONS	RATIONALE
1. Assess respiratory status (rate, pattern, breath sounds), pulse oximetry, and arterial blood gases.	1. Acute pancreatitis produces retroperitoneal edema, elevation of the diaphragm, pleural effusion, and inadequate lung ventilation. Intra-abdominal infection and labored breathing increase the body's metabolic demands, which further decreases pulmonary reserve and leads to respiratory failure.
2. Maintain semi-Fowler position.	2. Decreases pressure on diaphragm and allows greater lung expansion.
3. Instruct and encourage patient to take deep breaths and to cough every hour.	3. Taking deep breaths and coughing will clear the airways and reduce atelectasis.
4. Assist patient to turn and change position every 2 hours.	4. Changing position frequently assists aeration and drainage of all lobes of the lungs.
5. Reduce the excessive metabolism of the body. a. Administer antibiotics as prescribed. b. Place patient in an air-conditioned room. c. Administer nasal oxygen as required for hypoxia. d. Use a hypothermia blanket if necessary.	5. Pancreatitis produces a severe peritoneal and retroperitoneal reaction that causes fever, tachycardia, and accelerated respirations. Placing the patient in an air-conditioned room and supporting the patient with oxygen therapy decrease the workload of the respiratory system and the tissue utilization of oxygen. Reduction of fever and pulse rate decreases the metabolic demands on the body.

EXPECTED OUTCOMES

- Demonstrates normal respiratory rate and pattern and full lung expansion
- Demonstrates normal breath sounds and absence of adventitious breath sounds
- Demonstrates normal arterial blood gases and pulse oximetry
- Maintains semi-Fowler position when in bed
- Changes position in bed frequently
- Coughs and takes deep breaths at least every hour
- Demonstrates normal body temperature
- Exhibits no signs or symptoms of respiratory infection or impairment
- Is alert and responsive to environment

continued >

Plan of Nursing Care

Chart 40-4. Care of the Patient With Acute Pancreatitis, *Continued*

Collaborative Problem: Hypovolemia and alteration in fluid and electrolytes levels
Goal: Improvement in fluid and electrolyte status, prevention of hypovolemia and shock

NURSING INTERVENTIONS	RATIONALE	EXPECTED OUTCOMES
1. Assess fluid and electrolyte status (skin turgor, mucous membranes, urine output, vital signs, hemodynamic parameters).	1. The amount and type of fluid and electrolyte replacement are determined by the status of the blood pressure, the laboratory evaluations of serum electrolyte and blood urea nitrogen levels, the urinary volume, and the assessment of the patient's condition.	• Exhibits moist mucous membranes and normal skin turgor • Exhibits normal blood pressure without evidence of postural (orthostatic) hypotension • Excretes adequate urine volume • Exhibits normal, not excessive, thirst • Maintains normal pulse and respiratory rate • Remains alert and responsive • Exhibits normal arterial pressures and blood gases • Exhibits normal electrolyte levels • Exhibits no signs or symptoms of calcium deficit (e.g., tetany, carpopedal spasm) • Exhibits no additional losses of fluids and electrolytes through vomiting, diarrhea, or diaphoresis • Reports stabilization of weight • Demonstrates no increase in abdominal girth • Demonstrates no fluid wave on palpation of the abdomen • Demonstrates stable organ function without manifestations of failure
2. Assess sources of fluid and electrolyte loss (vomiting, diarrhea, nasogastric drainage, excessive diaphoresis).	2. Electrolyte losses occur from nasogastric suctioning, severe diaphoresis, and emesis, and as a result of the patient being in a fasting state.	
3. Combat shock if present. a. Administer corticosteroids as prescribed if patient does not respond to conventional treatment. b. Evaluate the amount of urinary output. Attempt to maintain this at ≥0.5 mL/kg/hour.	3. Extensive acute pancreatitis may cause peripheral vascular collapse and shock. Blood and plasma may be lost into the abdominal cavity; therefore, there is a decreased blood and plasma volume. The toxins from the bacteria of a necrotic pancreas may cause shock.	
4. Administer blood products, fluids, and electrolytes (sodium, potassium, chloride) as prescribed.	4. Patients with hemorrhagic pancreatitis lose large amounts of blood and plasma, which decreases effective circulation and blood volume.	
5. Administer plasma and blood products as prescribed.	5. Replacement with blood, plasma, or albumin assists in ensuring effective circulating blood volume.	
6. Keep a supply of IV calcium gluconate or calcium chloride readily available.	6. Calcium may be prescribed to prevent or treat tetany, which may result from calcium losses into retroperitoneal (peripancreatic) exudate.	
7. Assess abdomen for ascites formation. a. Measure abdominal girth daily. b. Weigh patient daily. c. Assess abdomen for ascites (see Fig. 49-6)	7. During acute pancreatitis, plasma may be lost into the abdominal cavity, which diminishes the blood volume.	
8. Monitor for manifestations of multiple organ dysfunction syndrome: neurologic, cardiovascular, renal, and respiratory dysfunction.	8. All body systems may fail if pancreatitis is severe and treatment is ineffective.	

toward preventing and managing acute attacks, relieving pain and discomfort, and managing exocrine and endocrine insufficiency of pancreatitis.

Nonsurgical Management

Nonsurgical approaches may be indicated for the patient who refuses surgery, who is a poor surgical risk, or whose disease and symptoms do not warrant surgical intervention. Endoscopy to remove pancreatic duct stones, correct strictures with stenting, and drain cysts may be effective in selected patients to manage pain and relieve obstruction via ERCP (Muniraj et al., 2015; Talukdar & Nageshwar, 2014).

Management of abdominal pain and discomfort is similar to that of acute pancreatitis; however, the focus is usually on the use of nonopioid methods to manage pain and the implementation of the World Health Organization's (WHO) three-step ladder for the treatment of chronic pain. This involves initiating monotherapy and, if ineffective, instituting combination therapy with peripherally acting and centrally acting medications. Pain management in the early stages may respond to nonopioid analgesics, but if the pain becomes more constant or debilitating, introduction of opioid analgesics is appropriate. The abuse of opioids is possible in these patients, and may be more likely in patients with depression, higher pain intensity, and alcohol use (Gupte & Forsmark, 2014). Adjunct means of pain modulation, such as use of antioxidants, antidepressants, and nonnarcotic agents as well as avoidance of smoking and alcohol, are recommended before starting opioids for pain control (Gupte & Forsmark, 2014). Antioxidants have shown effect in the relief of pain and in improving quality of life and are often given to patients with chronic pancreatitis (Gupte & Forsmark, 2014). An endoscopic ultrasound (EUS)–guided placement of a celiac nerve block is a potential option for chronic, unrelieved pain of this disease (D'Haese, Ceyhan, Demir, et al., 2014). Yoga and other mindfulness-based therapies may be effective nonpharmacologic methods for pain reduction and for relief of other coexisting symptoms of chronic pancreatitis. Persistent, unrelieved pain is often the most difficult aspect of management (Gupte & Forsmark, 2014; Muniraj et al., 2015). The primary provider, nurse, and dietitian emphasize to the patient and family the importance of avoiding alcohol and foods that have produced abdominal pain and discomfort in the past. The health care team stresses to the patient that no other treatment is likely to relieve pain if the patient continues to consume alcohol.

Diabetes resulting from dysfunction of the pancreatic islet cells is treated with diet, insulin, or oral antidiabetic agents. The hazard of severe hypoglycemia with alcohol consumption is stressed to the patient and family. Pancreatic enzyme replacement is indicated for the patient with malabsorption and steatorrhea.

Surgical Management

Chronic pancreatitis is not often managed by surgery. However, surgery may be indicated to relieve persistent abdominal pain and discomfort, restore drainage of pancreatic secretions, and reduce the frequency of acute attacks of pancreatitis and hospitalization (D'Haese et al., 2014; Gupte & Forsmark, 2014; Muniraj et al., 2015). The type of surgery performed depends on the anatomic and functional abnormalities of the pancreas, including the location of disease within the pancreas, the presence of diabetes, exocrine insufficiency, biliary stenosis, and pseudocysts of the pancreas. Other considerations for surgery selection include the patient's likelihood for continued use of alcohol and the likelihood that the patient will be able to manage the endocrine or exocrine changes that are expected after surgery.

Pancreaticojejunostomy (also referred to as Roux-en-Y), with a side-to-side anastomosis or joining of the pancreatic duct to the jejunum, allows drainage of the pancreatic secretions into the jejunum. Pain relief occurs within 6 months in more than 85% of the patients who undergo this procedure, but pain returns in a substantial number of patients as the disease progresses (D'Haese et al., 2014; Gupte & Forsmark, 2014).

Other surgical procedures may be performed for different degrees and types of underlying disorders. These procedures include revision of the sphincter of the ampulla of Vater, internal drainage of a pancreatic cyst into the stomach (see later discussion), insertion of a stent, and wide resection or removal of the pancreas. A Whipple's resection (pancreaticoduodenectomy) can be carried out to relieve the pain of chronic pancreatitis. In an effort to provide permanent pain relief and avoid endocrine and exocrine insufficiency that ensue with major resections of the pancreas, surgeons have designed new procedures that combine limited resection of the head of the pancreas with a pancreaticojejunostomy. These procedures, known as the Beger or Frey operations, remove most of the head of the pancreas except for a shell of pancreatic tissue posteriorly (D'Haese et al., 2014; Gupte & Forsmark, 2014).

When chronic pancreatitis develops as a result of gallbladder disease, surgery is performed to explore the common duct and remove the stones; usually, the gallbladder is removed at the same time. In addition, an attempt is made to improve the drainage of the common bile duct and the pancreatic duct by dividing the sphincter of Oddi, a muscle that is located at the ampulla of Vater (this surgical procedure is known as a sphincterotomy). A T-tube usually is placed in the common bile duct, requiring a drainage system to collect the bile postoperatively. Nursing care after such surgery is similar to that indicated after other biliary tract surgery.

Approximately two thirds of all patients with chronic pancreatitis can be managed with endoscopic or laparoscopic intervention (D'Haese et al., 2014; Gupte & Forsmark, 2014; Muniraj et al., 2015). Endoscopic and laparoscopic procedures such as distal pancreatectomy, longitudinal decompression of the pancreatic duct, nerve denervation, and stenting have been performed in patients with jaundice or recurrent inflammation and are being refined. Minimally invasive procedures to treat chronic pancreatitis may prove to be successful adjuncts in the management of this complex disorder (D'Haese et al., 2014; Gupte & Forsmark, 2014).

Patients who undergo surgery for chronic pancreatitis may experience weight gain and improved nutritional status; this may result from reduction in pain associated with eating rather than from correction of malabsorption. However, morbidity and mortality after these surgical procedures are high because of the complexity and poor physical condition of the patient before surgery and frequently the concomitant presence of cirrhosis and other comorbidities.

Pancreatic Cysts

As a result of the local necrosis that occurs at the time of acute pancreatitis, collections of fluid may form close to the pancreas. These fluid collections become walled off by fibrous tissue and are called pancreatic pseudocysts. They are the most common type of pancreatic cyst. Less common cysts occur as a result of congenital anomalies or secondary to chronic pancreatitis or trauma to the pancreas.

Diagnosis of pancreatic cysts and pseudocysts is made by ultrasound, CT scan, and ERCP. ERCP may be used to define the anatomy of the pancreas and evaluate the patency of pancreatic drainage. Pancreatic pseudocysts may be of considerable size. When pancreatic pseudocysts enlarge, they impinge on and displace the adjacent stomach or the colon because of the location of pseudocysts behind the posterior peritoneum. Eventually, through pressure or secondary infection, they produce symptoms and require drainage.

Drainage into the GI tract or through the skin and abdominal wall may be established. In the latter instance, the drainage is likely to be profuse and destructive to tissue because of the enzyme contents. Hence, steps (including application of skin ointment) must be taken to protect the skin near the drainage site from excoriation. A suction apparatus may be used to continuously aspirate digestive secretions from the drainage tract so that skin contact with the digestive enzymes is avoided. Expert nursing attention is required to ensure that the suction tube does not become dislodged and suction is not interrupted. Consultation with a WOC nurse is indicated to identify appropriate strategies for maintaining drainage and protecting the skin.

Cancer of the Pancreas

Pancreatic cancer is the fourth leading cause of cancer death in both men and women in Canada because of its low survival rate. In 2017, approximately 5,500 Canadians were diagnosed with pancreatic cancer and 4,800 died from it (Canadian Cancer Society, n.d.). It is very rare before the age of 45 years, and the majority of patients present in or beyond the sixth decade of life (Feldman et al., 2015; Papadakis & McPhee, 2016; Yeo, 2015). The incidence of pancreatic cancer increases with age, peaking in the seventh and eighth decades for both men and women (Canadian Cancer Society's Advisory Committee on Cancer Statistics [CCSACCS], 2013). The frequency of pancreatic cancer has decreased slightly over the past 25 years among non-Caucasian men. Cigarette smoking, exposure to industrial chemicals or toxins in the environment, and a diet high in fat and meat are all associated with pancreatic cancer, although their roles are not completely clear.

The risk of pancreatic cancer increases as the extent of cigarette smoking increases and is twice as high in smokers than nonsmokers (Yeo, 2015). Diabetes, chronic pancreatitis, and hereditary pancreatitis are also associated with pancreatic cancer. The pancreas can also be the site of metastasis from other tumours.

Cancer may develop in the head (60%), body (10%), or tail (5%) of the pancreas and diffusely spread throughout the pancreas. Clinical manifestations vary depending on the site and whether functioning insulin-secreting pancreatic islet cells are involved. The majority of pancreatic cancers originate in the head of the pancreas and give rise to a distinctive clinical picture (Feldman et al., 2015). Functioning islet cell tumours, whether benign (adenoma) or malignant (carcinoma), are responsible for the syndrome of hyperinsulinism. The symptoms are typically nonspecific, and patients usually do not seek medical attention until late in the disease. Only about 7% of cases are diagnosed in early stages; 80% to 85% of patients have advanced, unresectable tumour when first detected. As a result, pancreatic carcinoma has only an 8% survival rate at 5 years regardless of the stage of disease at diagnosis or treatment (CCSACCS, 2013). The number of new cases estimated for 2013 were 2,300 males and 2,400 females (CCSACCS, 2013).

Clinical Manifestations

Pain, jaundice, or both are present in more than 80% of patients and, along with weight loss, are considered classic signs of pancreatic carcinoma (Feldman et al., 2015). However, they often do not appear until the disease is far advanced. Other signs include rapid, profound, and progressive weight loss as well as vague upper or midabdominal pain or discomfort that is unrelated to any GI function and is often difficult to describe. Such discomfort radiates as a boring pain in the midback and is unrelated to posture or activity. It is often progressive and severe, requiring the use of opioids. It is often more severe at night and is accentuated when lying supine. Relief may be obtained by sitting up and leaning forward.

Malignant cells from pancreatic cancer are often shed into the peritoneal cavity, increasing the likelihood of metastasis. The formation of ascites is common. An important sign, if it is present, is the onset of symptoms of insulin deficiency: glucosuria, hyperglycemia, and abnormal glucose tolerance. Therefore, diabetes may be an early sign of carcinoma of the pancreas. Meals often aggravate epigastric pain, which usually occurs before the appearance of jaundice and pruritus.

Assessment and Diagnostic Findings

Spiral (helical) CT is more than 85% to 90% accurate in the diagnosis and staging of pancreatic cancer and is currently the most useful preoperative imaging technique. MRI may also be used. ERCP is also used in the diagnosis of pancreatic carcinoma. EUS is useful in identifying small tumours and in performing fine-needle aspiration biopsy of the primary tumour or lymph nodes (Goldman & Schafer, 2015; Papadakis & McPhee, 2016). Cells obtained during ERCP are sent to the laboratory for analysis. GI x-ray findings may demonstrate deformities in adjacent organs caused by the impinging pancreatic mass.

A histologic diagnosis is not usually required in patients who are candidates for surgery. The tissue diagnosis is made at the time of the surgical procedure. Percutaneous fine-needle aspiration biopsy of the pancreas, which is used to diagnose pancreatic tumours, is also used to confirm the diagnosis in patients whose tumours are not resectable so that a palliative plan of care can be determined. This may eliminate the stress and postoperative pain of ineffective surgery. In this procedure, a needle is inserted through the anterior abdominal wall into the pancreatic mass, guided by CT, ultrasound, ERCP, or other imaging techniques. The aspirated material is examined for malignant cells. Although percutaneous biopsy is a valuable diagnostic tool, it has some potential drawbacks: a false-negative result if small tumours are missed and the risk of seeding of cancer cells along the needle track. Low-dose radiation to the site may be used before the biopsy to reduce this risk.

Percutaneous transhepatic cholangiography is another procedure that may be performed to identify obstructions of the biliary tract by a pancreatic tumour. Several tumour markers (e.g., cancer antigen [CA] 19-9, carcinoembryonic antigen [CEA], DU-PAN-2) may be used in the diagnostic workup, but they are nonspecific for pancreatic carcinoma. These tumour markers are useful as indicators of disease progression.

Angiography, CT scans, and laparoscopy may be performed to determine whether the tumour can be removed surgically. Intraoperative ultrasonography has been used to determine whether there is metastatic disease to other organs.

Medical Management

If the tumour is resectable and localized (typically tumours in the head of the pancreas), the surgical procedure to remove it is usually extensive (see later discussion). However, total excision of the lesion often is not possible for two reasons: (1) extensive growth of tumour before diagnosis and (2) probable widespread metastases (especially to the liver, lungs, and bones). More often, treatment is limited to palliative measures.

Although pancreatic tumours may be resistant to standard radiation therapy, the patient may be treated with radiation and chemotherapy (5-fluorouracil [5-FU, Adrucil], leucovorin [Wellcovorin], gemcitabine [Gemzar], irinotecan [Camptosar], oxaliplatin [Eloxatin]) (Canadian Cancer Society, n.d.). Currently, gemcitabine is the standard of care for patients with metastatic pancreatic cancer and has been found to lengthen survival (American Cancer Society [ACS], 2015; Feldman et al., 2015). The targeted anticancer drug erlotinib (Tarceva) has demonstrated a slight improvement in advanced pancreatic cancer survival when used in combination with gemcitabine (ACS, 2015). Clinical trials with new agents such as S-1 (an oral fluoropyrimidine), Folfirinox, or the use of nanoparticle albumin-bound paclitaxel (nab-paclitaxel) with gemcitabine therapy, combined with radiation and/or surgery may also result in improved survival (ACS, 2015; Kamisawa, Wood, Itoi, et al., 2016). If the patient undergoes surgery, intraoperative radiation therapy (IORT) may be used to deliver a high dose of radiation to the tumour with minimal injury to other tissues; this may also be helpful in relief of pain. Interstitial implantation of radioactive sources has also been used, although the rate of complications is high. A large biliary stent inserted percutaneously or by endoscopy may be used to relieve jaundice.

Nursing Management

Pain management and attention to nutritional requirements are important nursing measures that improve the level of patient comfort. Skin care and nursing measures are directed toward relief of pain and discomfort associated with jaundice, anorexia, and profound weight loss. Specialty mattresses are beneficial and protect bony prominences from pressure. Pain associated with pancreatic cancer may be severe and may require liberal use of opioids; patient-controlled analgesia should be considered for the patient with severe, escalating pain.

Because of the poor prognosis and likelihood of short survival, end-of-life preferences are discussed and honoured. If appropriate, the nurse refers the patient to hospice care. (See Chapter 15 for care of the patient with cancer and end-of-life care.)

Promoting Home, Community-Based, and Transitional Care

Educating Patients About Self-Care

The specific teaching for the patient and family varies with the stage of disease and the treatment choices made by the patient. If the patient elects to receive chemotherapy or radiation, the nurse focuses teaching on prevention of side effects and complications of the agents used. If surgery is performed to relieve obstruction and establish biliary drainage, teaching addresses management of the drainage system and monitoring for complications. The nurse instructs the family about changes in the patient's status that should be reported to the physician.

Continuing and Transitional Care

A referral for home care is indicated to help the patient and family deal with the physical problems and discomforts associated with pancreatic cancer and the psychological impact of the disease. The home care nurse assesses the patient's physical status, fluid and nutritional status, skin integrity, and the adequacy of pain management. The nurse teaches the patient and family strategies to prevent skin breakdown and relieve pain, pruritus, and anorexia. It is important to discuss and arrange palliative care (hospice services) in an effort to relieve patient discomfort, assist with care, and comply with the patient's end-of-life decisions and wishes.

Tumours of the Head of the Pancreas

Sixty percent of pancreatic tumours occur in the head of the pancreas (Muniraj et al., 2014; Yeo, 2015). Tumours in this region of the pancreas obstruct the common bile duct where the duct passes through the head of the pancreas to join the pancreatic duct and empty at the ampulla of Vater into the duodenum. The tumours producing the obstruction may arise from the pancreas, the common bile duct, or the ampulla of Vater.

Clinical Manifestations

The obstructed flow of bile leads to jaundice, clay-coloured stools, and dark urine. Malabsorption of nutrients and fat-soluble vitamins may result if the tumour obstructs the entry of bile to the GI tract. Abdominal discomfort or pain and pruritus may be noted, along with anorexia, weight loss, and malaise. If these signs and symptoms are present, cancer of the head of the pancreas should be suspected.

The jaundice of this disease must be differentiated from that due to a biliary obstruction caused by a gallstone in the common duct. Jaundice caused by a gallstone is usually intermittent and appears typically in patients with obesity, who are most often women, and who have had previous symptoms of gallbladder disease.

Assessment and Diagnostic Findings

Diagnostic studies may include duodenography, angiography by hepatic or celiac artery catheterization, pancreatic scanning, percutaneous transhepatic cholangiography, ERCP, and percutaneous needle biopsy of the pancreas. Results of a biopsy of the pancreas may aid in the diagnosis.

Medical Management

Before extensive surgery can be performed, a fairly long period of preparation is often necessary, because the patient's nutritional status and physical condition are often quite compromised. Various liver and pancreatic function studies are performed. A diet high in protein along with pancreatic enzymes is often prescribed. Preoperative preparation includes adequate hydration, correction of prothrombin deficiency with vitamin K, and treatment of anemia to minimize postoperative complications. Parenteral nutrition and blood component therapy are frequently required.

A biliary drainage procedure may be performed, usually with a catheter via percutaneous access, to relieve the jaundice and, perhaps, to provide time for a thorough diagnostic evaluation. Total pancreatectomy (removal of the pancreas) may be performed if there is no evidence of direct extension of the tumour to adjacent tissues or regional lymph nodes. A pancreaticoduodenectomy (Whipple's procedure or resection) is used for potentially resectable cancer of the head of the pancreas (Fig. 40-7) (Alemi et al., 2015; Li et al., 2015). This procedure involves removal of the gallbladder, a portion of the stomach, duodenum, proximal jejunum, head of the pancreas, and distal common bile duct. Reconstruction involves anastomosis of the remaining pancreas and stomach to the jejunum (Townsend et al., 2016). A pylorus-preserving pancreaticojejunostomy (PPPD) may also be performed for tumours of the head of the pancreas and may reduce postgastrectomy symptoms and improve overall GI function (Feldman et al., 2015). The result of these procedures is removal of the tumour, allowing flow of bile into the jejunum. If the tumour cannot be excised, the jaundice may be relieved by diverting the bile flow into the jejunum by anastomosing the jejunum to the gallbladder, a procedure known as **cholecystojejunostomy**.

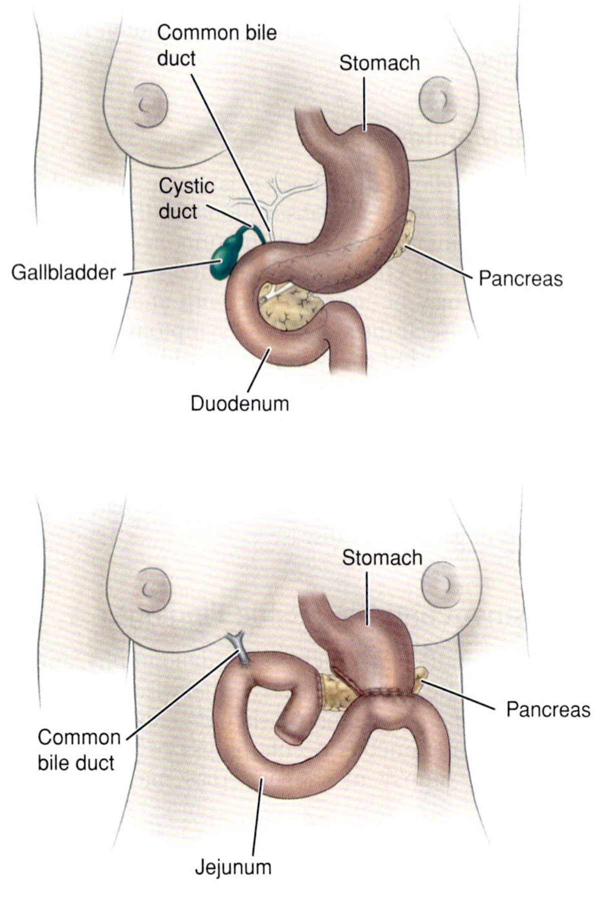

FIGURE 40-7. Pancreaticoduodenectomy (Whipple's procedure or resection). End result of resection of carcinoma of the head of the pancreas or the ampulla of Vater. The common duct is sutured to the side of the jejunum (choledochojejunostomy), and the remaining portion of the pancreas and the end of the stomach are sutured to the side of the jejunum.

The postoperative management of patients who have undergone a pancreatectomy or a pancreaticoduodenectomy is similar to the management of patients after extensive GI or biliary surgery. The patient's physical status is often suboptimal, increasing the risk of postoperative complications. Hemorrhage, vascular collapse, and hepatorenal failure remain the major postoperative complications. The mortality rate associated with these procedures has decreased because of advances in nutritional support and improved surgical techniques. A nasogastric tube with suction and parenteral nutrition allow the GI tract to rest while promoting adequate nutrition.

Nursing Management

Preoperatively and postoperatively, nursing care is directed toward promoting patient comfort, preventing complications, and assisting the patient to return to and maintain as normal and comfortable a life as possible. The nurse closely monitors the patient in the intensive care unit after surgery; in the immediate postoperative period, multiple IV and arterial lines are used for fluid and blood replacement and hemodynamic monitoring, and a mechanical ventilator may be used. It is important to note and report changes in vital signs, arterial blood gases and pressures, pulse oximetry, laboratory values, and urine output. The nurse must also consider the patient's compromised nutritional status and risk of bleeding. Depending on the type of surgical procedure performed, malabsorption syndrome and diabetes are likely; the nurse addresses these issues during acute and long-term patient care.

Although the patient's physiologic status is the focus of the health care team in the immediate postoperative period, the patient's psychological and emotional states must be considered, along with that of the family. The patient has undergone a major high-risk surgery and is critically ill; anxiety and depression may affect recovery. The immediate and long-term outcomes of this extensive surgical resection are uncertain, and the patient and family require emotional support and understanding in the critical and stressful pre- and postoperative periods.

Promoting Home, Community-Based, and Transitional Care

Educating Patients About Self-Care

The patient who has undergone this extensive surgery requires careful and thorough preparation for self-care at home. The nurse instructs the patient and family about the need for modifications in the diet because of malabsorption and hyperglycemia resulting from the surgery. It is important to instruct the patient and family about the continuing need for pancreatic enzyme replacement, a low-fat diet, and vitamin supplementation.

The nurse teaches the patient and family strategies to relieve pain and discomfort, along with strategies to manage drains, if present, and to care for the surgical incision. The patient and family members may require instruction about use of patient-controlled analgesia, parenteral nutrition, wound care, skin care, and management of drainage. It is important to describe, verbally and in writing, the signs and symptoms of complications and to teach the patient and family about indicators of complications that should be reported promptly.

Discharge of the patient to a long-term care or rehabilitation facility may be warranted after surgery as extensive as pancreatectomy or pancreaticoduodenectomy, particularly if the patient's preoperative status was not optimal. Information about the teaching that has been provided is shared with the long-term care staff so that instructions can be clarified and reinforced. During the recovery or long-term phase of care, the patient and family receive further instructions about self-care in the home.

Continuing and Transitional Care

A referral for home care may be indicated when the patient returns home. The home care nurse assesses the patient's physical and psychological status and the ability of the patient and family to manage needed care. The home care nurse provides needed physical care and monitors the adequacy of pain management. In addition, it is important to assess the patient's nutritional status and monitor the use of enteral or parenteral nutrition, if used. The nurse discusses the use of hospice services with the patient and family and makes a referral if indicated.

Pancreatic Islet Tumours

The pancreas contains the islets (islands) of Langerhans, small nests of cells that secrete hormones directly into the bloodstream and therefore are part of the endocrine system. The hormone insulin is essential for the metabolism of glucose. Diabetes (see Chapter 41) is the result of deficient insulin secretion. At least two types of tumours of the pancreatic islet cells are known: those that secrete insulin (insulinoma) and those in which insulin secretion is not increased (nonfunctioning islet cell cancer). All of these types of tumours combined are termed *neuroendocrine tumours* (NETs). Insulinomas produce hypersecretion of insulin and cause an excessive rate of glucose metabolism. The resulting hypoglycemia may produce symptoms of weakness, mental confusion, and seizures. These symptoms may be relieved almost immediately by oral or IV administration of glucose. The 5-hour glucose tolerance test is helpful to diagnose insulinoma and to distinguish this diagnosis from other causes of hypoglycemia.

Surgical Management

If a tumour of the islet cells has been diagnosed, surgical treatment with removal of the tumour is usually recommended (Canadian Cancer Society, n.d.). The tumours may be benign adenomas or they may be malignant. Complete removal usually results in almost immediate relief of symptoms. In some patients, symptoms may be produced by simple hypertrophy of this tissue rather than a tumour of the islet cells. In such cases, a partial pancreatectomy (removal of the tail and part of the body of the pancreas) is performed. Additionally, drug therapy and radiation may be utilized (Canadian Cancer Society, n.d.).

Nursing Management

In preparing the patient for surgery, the nurse must be alert for symptoms of hypoglycemia and be ready to administer glucose as prescribed if symptoms occur. Postoperatively, the nursing management is the same as after other upper abdominal surgical procedures, with special emphasis on monitoring serum glucose levels. Patient teaching is determined by the extent of surgery and alterations in pancreatic function.

Hyperinsulinism

Hyperinsulinism is caused by overproduction of insulin by the pancreatic islets. Symptoms resemble those of excessive doses of insulin and are attributable to the same mechanism: an abnormal reduction in blood glucose levels. Clinically it is characterized by episodes during which the patient experiences unusual hunger, nervousness, sweating, headache, and faintness; in severe cases, seizures and episodes of unconsciousness may occur. The findings at the time of surgery or at autopsy may indicate hyperplasia (overgrowth) of the islets of Langerhans or a benign or malignant tumour involving the islets that is capable of producing large amounts of insulin (see preceding discussion). Occasionally, tumours of nonpancreatic origin produce an insulin-like material that can cause severe hypoglycemia and may be responsible for seizures coinciding with blood glucose levels that are too low to sustain normal brain function (i.e., lower than 30 mg/dL [1.6 mmol/L]) (Bope & Kellerman, 2015; Goldman & Schafer, 2015).

All the symptoms that accompany spontaneous hypoglycemia are relieved by the oral or parenteral administration of glucose. Surgical removal of the hyperplastic or neoplastic tissue from the pancreas is the only successful method of treatment. About 15% of patients with spontaneous or functional hypoglycemia eventually develop diabetes.

Ulcerogenic Tumours

Some tumours of the islets of Langerhans are associated with hypersecretion of gastric acid that produces ulcers in the stomach, duodenum, and jejunum. This is referred to as **Zollinger–Ellison syndrome**. The hypersecretion is so excessive that even after partial gastric resection enough acid is produced to cause further ulceration. If a marked tendency to develop gastric and duodenal ulcers is noted, an ulcerogenic tumour of the islets of Langerhans is considered (Dacha, Razvi, Massaad, et al., 2015).

These tumours, which may be benign or malignant, are treated by excision, if possible. Frequently, however, removal is not possible because of extension beyond the pancreas. In many patients, a total gastrectomy may be necessary to reduce the secretion of gastric acid sufficiently to prevent further ulceration. This procedure is also indicated to treat gastric carcinoid tumours that may arise from the effect of prolonged hypersecretion of gastric acids (Dacha, Razvi, Massaad, et al., 2015).

Critical Thinking Exercises

1 A 77-year-old man underwent a right total hip replacement. His clinical course was initially stable but on day 4 postoperatively he became nauseated and began vomiting. He also complained of right upper quadrant pain and was hypotensive and tachycardic. His urine output has decreased to 10 mL/hour. What are the initial priorities of care for this patient? An abdominal ultrasound and abdominal CT scan were performed and revealed marked thickening of the gallbladder wall and pericholecystic effusion but no gallstones were identified. He was determined to have acalculous cholecystitis. What would be the initial treatment the nurse would expect to implement? If the patient continued to deteriorate with worsening pain and signs of systemic inflammation and hypovolemia, what additional interventions should the nurse be prepared to implement?

2 A 58-year-old man presents to the emergency department with complaints of severe midepigastric pain. He is also nauseated and vomiting. His vital signs reveal hypotension and tachycardia and he is febrile. His history is significant for alcohol abuse and hypertension. What laboratory and imaging studies do you expect to be performed? His CT scan revealed pancreatic necrosis and multiple fluid collections. An evidence-based approach for managing infected pancreatic necrosis was implemented. What first-line intervention would you expect to be implemented in this case? What classification of pancreatitis is this patient experiencing?

3 A 55-year-old woman has been experiencing upper abdominal pain for several weeks. She believes that she has gallbladder disease but is concerned because her mother died from pancreatic cancer. She visits her physician who prescribes a CT scan and initial laboratory screening studies. Which laboratory tests would you expect to be assessed? The CT scan revealed no masses but did show dilatation of the pancreatic duct. The woman grew more concerned due to her family history even though her initial laboratory tests were normal. Her physician shared her concern and prescribed an MRI, which revealed a small mass at the head of the pancreas. The woman was referred to a surgeon who began an assessment to determine if the patient was a candidate for potentially curative resection. What testing is needed to assess if the mass was cancerous and if it may have metastasized? The patient is determined to be a candidate for surgery. List two postoperative nursing interventions that can be effective in preventing complications. What education will the nurse provide the patient to enhance comfort, nutrition, and quality of life after discharge?

REFERENCES AND SELECTED READINGS

Books

Bope, E. T., & Kellerman, R. D. (Eds.). (2015). *Conn's current therapy*. Philadelphia, PA: Saunders.

Canadian Cancer Society's Advisory Committee on Cancer Statistics (CCSACCS). (2013). *Canadian cancer statistics 2013*. Toronto, ON: Canadian Cancer Society.

Cuschieri, A., & Hanna, G. (2014). *Higher surgical training in general surgery* (5th ed.). London, UK: Hodder.

Dawson, P. A. (2018). Bile formation and the enterohepatic circulation. In H. M. Said (Ed.). *Physiology of the gastrointestinal tract* (6th ed., pp. 931–956). Irvine, CA, United States: Academic Press.

Dudek, S. (2013). *Nutrition essentials for nursing practice* (7th ed.). Philadelphia, PA: Wolters Kluwer Health/Lippincott Williams & Wilkins.

Feldman, M., Friedman, L. S., & Brandt, L. J. (2015). *Sleisenger & Fordtran's gastrointestinal & liver disease* (10th ed.). Philadelphia, PA: Saunders Elsevier.

Ferri, F. F. (Ed.). (2014). *Practical guide to the care of the medical patient* (9th ed.). Philadelphia, PA: Mosby Elsevier.

Goldman, L., & Schafer, A. I. (2015). *Goldman's cecil medicine* (25th ed.). Philadelphia, PA: Saunders Elsevier.

Greenberger, N. J., Blumberg, R. S., & Burakoff, R. (Eds.). (2015). *Current diagnosis and treatment: Gastroenterology, hepatology & endoscopy*. New York: McGraw-Hill.

Hall, J. E. (2015). *Guyton & Hall textbook of medical physiology* (13th ed.). Philadelphia, PA: Saunders Elsevier.

Kumar, V., Abbas, A. K., Fausto, N., et al. (2014). *Robbins and Cotran pathologic basis of disease* (9th ed.). Philadelphia, PA: Saunders Elsevier.

Lefkowitch, J. H. (2018). Anatomy and function. In J. S. Dooley, A. S. Lok, G. Garcia-Tsao, et al. (Eds.). *Sherlock's diseases of the liver and biliary system* (13th ed., pp. 1–19). Hoboken, NJ: Wiley-Blackwell.

Marx, J., Walls, R., & Hockberger, R. (2013). *Rosen's Emergency Medicine-Concepts and Clinical Practice E-Book*. Elsevier Health Sciences.

Papadakis, M. A., & McPhee, S. J. (Eds.). (2016). *Current medical diagnosis and treatment* (55th ed.). New York: McGraw-Hill.

Porth, C. (2010). Disorders of hepatocbiliary and excocrine pancreas function. *Porth pathophysiology: Concepts of altered health status* (1st Canadian ed.), 911–942.

Rakel, R. E., & Rakel, D. P. (Eds.). (2015). *Textbook of family medicine* (9th ed.). Philadelphia, PA: Saunders Elsevier.

Sun, C. K. (2018). ERCP for pancreatic disorders. In K. H. Lai, L. R. Mo, & H. P. Wang (Eds.). *Biliopancreatic endoscopy* (pp. 97–105). Singapore: Springer.

Townsend, C. M., Beauchamp, R. D., Evers, B. M., et al. (2016). *Sabiston's textbook of surgery: The biological basis of modern surgical practice*. Philadelphia, PA: Elsevier.

Journals and Electronic Documents

Gallbladder Disease

Beckingham, I. (2017). Gallstones. *Surgery, 35*(12), 682–691.

Ekwenife, C. N., & Ofoegbu, J. I. (2013). Isolated gallbladder perforation following blunt abdominal trauma: A missed diagnosis. *Nigerian Journal of Clinical Practice, 16*(3), 392–394.

Fagenholz, P. J., & de Moya, M. A. (2014). Acute inflammatory surgical disease. *Surgical Clinics of North America, 94*(1), 1–30.

Huang, H. S., Chuang, C. H., & Yang, P. J. (2013). Abnormal gas in the gall bladder: Emphysematous cholecystitis. *Journal of Emergency Medicine, 45*(2), 254–255.

Joafr, G., Persson, G., Svennblad, B., et al. (2014). Outcomes of antibiotic prophylaxis in acute cholecystectomy in a population-based gallstone surgery registry. *British Journal of Surgery, 101*(2), 69–73.

Katabathina, V. S., Zafar, A. M., & Suri, R. (2015). Clinical presentation, imaging, and management of acute cholecystitis. *Techniques in Vascular and Interventional Radiology, 18*(4), 256–265.

Kaur, J., Rana, S. V., Gupta, R., et al. (2014). Prolonged orocecal transit time entrains serum bile acids through bacterial overgrowth, contributing factor to gallstone disease. *Journal of Clinical Gastroenterology, 48*(4), 365–369.

Khan, M. L., Abbasi, M. R., Jawed, M., et al. (2014). Male gender and sonographic gallbladder wall thickness: Important predictable factors for empyema and gangrene in acute cholecystitis. *Journal of Pakistani Medical Association, 64*(2), 159–162.

Lee, J. Y., Keane, M. G., & Pereira, S. (2015). Diagnosis and treatment of gallstone disease. *Practitioner, 259*(1783), 15–19.

Mahadevan, V. (2014). Anatomy of the gallbladder and bile ducts. *Surgery*. https://doi.org/10.1016/j.mpsur.2014.10.003

Michetti, C. P., Griffen, M., Tran, H. T., et al. (2015). Laparoscopic cholecystectomy performed by acute care surgeons and general surgeons. *American Surgeon, 81*(5), E220–E221.

Niknahad, H., Jamshidzadeh, A., Heidari, R., et al. (2017). Ammonia-induced mitochondrial dysfunction and energy metabolism disturbances in isolated brain and liver mitochondria, and the effect of taurine administration: Relevance to hepatic encephalopathy treatment. *Clinical and Experimental Hepatology*, *3*(3), 141.

Pajak, C., Lee, S. V., Konkin, D., et al. (2018). Early surgical management of acute cholecystitis: A quality improvement initiative. *British Columbia Medical Journal*, *60*(7), 352–357.

Pancreatic Disorders

American Cancer Society (ACS). (2015). *Cancer facts & figures 2015*. Retrieved December 12, 2015, from www.cancer.org/Research/CancerFactsFigures.

Campbell-Thompson, M., Wasserfall, C., Kaddis, J., et al. (2012). Network for pancreatic organ donors with diabetes (NPOD): Developing a tissue biobank for type 1 diabetes. *Diabetes/Metabolism Research and Reviews*, *28*, 608–617.

Carlise, D. (2013). The artificial pancreas. *Nursing Standard*, *27*(52), 22–23.

Cayón-Blanco, M., García-Figueras-Mateos, C., García-Martínez, A., et al. (2018). Complications related to parenteral nutrition in patients with bilio-pancreatic disorders. *Clinical Nutrition*, *37*, S187.

Chaen, R. P., Zhu Ge, X. J., Huang, Z. M., et al. (2014). Prophylactic use of transjugular intrahepatic portosystematic shunt aids in the treatment of refractory ascites: Metaregression and trial sequential met-analysis. *Journal of Clinical Gastroenterology*, *48*(5), 290–299.

da Costa, D. W., Boerma, D., van Santvoort, H. C., et al. (2014). Staged multidisciplinary step-up management for necrotizing pancreatitis. *British Journal of Surgery*, *10*(1), e65–e79.

Dacha, S., Razvi, M., Massaad, J., et al. (2015). Hypergastrinemia. *Gastroenterology Report*, *3*(3), 201–208.

De Waele, J. J. (2014). Acute pancreatitis. *Current Opinion in Critical Care*, *20*(2), 189–195.

Desai, A. P., Satoskar, R., Appanagari, A., et al. (2014). Co-management between hospitals and hepatologist improves the quality of care of inpatients with chronic liver disease. *Journal of Clinical Gastroenterology*, *48*(4), e30–e36.

D'haese, J. G., Ceyhan, G. O., Demir, I. E., Tieftrunk, E., & Friess, H. (2014). Treatment options in painful chronic pancreatitis: a systematic review. *HPB*, *16*(6), 512–521.

Gupte, A. R., & Forsmark, C. E. (2014). Chronic pancreatitis. *Current opinion in gastroenterology*, *30*(5), 500–505.

Jinjuvadia, R., Liangpunsakul, S., & Antaki, F. (2014). Past exposure to Hepatitis B: A risk factor for increase in mortality? *Journal of Clinical Gastroenterology*, *48*(5), 267–271.

Kamisawa, T., Wood, L. D., Itoi, T., et al. (2016). Pancreatic cancer. *The Lancet*, *388*(10039), 73–85.

Lankisch, P. G., Apte, M., & Banks, P. A. (2015). Acute pancreatitis. *The Lancet*, *386*(9988), 85–96.

Martin, R. F., & Hein, A. R. (2013). Operative management of acute pancreatitis. *Surgical Clinics of North America*, *93*(3), 595–610.

Masamune, A., & Shimosegawa, T. (2018). Epidemiology and pathophysiology of alcoholic chronic pancreatitis. *The Pancreas: An Integrated Textbook of Basic Science, Medicine, and Surgery*, 342–348.

McClave, S. A. (2013). Nutrition in pancreatitis. *World Review of Nutrition & Dietetics*, *105*, 160–168.

Mocci, E., & Klein, A. P. (2018). Epidemiology of pancreatic cancer. *The Pancreas: An Integrated Textbook of Basic Science, Medicine, and Surgery*, 665–672.

Muniraj, T., Aslanian, H. R., Farrell, J., et al. (2014). Chronic pancreatitis, a comprehensive review and update. Part I: Epidemiology, etiology, risk factors, genetics, pathophysiology, and clinical features. *Disease-A-Month*, *60*(12), 530–550.

Muniraj, T., Aslanian, H. R., Farrell, J., et al. (2015). Chronic pancreatitis, a comprehensive review and update. Part II: Diagnosis, complications, and management. *Disease-A-Month*, *61*(1), 5–37.

Rickels, M. R. (2012). Recovery of endocrine function after islet and pancreas transplant. *Current Diabetes Reports*, *12*(5), 587–596.

Sarkaria, S., Sethi, A., Rondon, C., et al. (2014). Pancreatic necrosectomy using covered esophageal stents: A novel approach. *Journal of Clinical Gastroenterology*, *48*(4), 145–152.

Scherer, J., Singh, V., Pitchumoni, C. S., et al. (2013). Issues in hypertriglyceridemic pancreatitis: An update. *Journal of Clinical Gastroenterology*, *48*(4), 195–203.

Sikkens, E. C., Cahen, D. L., deWit, J., et al. (2014). A prospective assessment of the natural cause of the exocrine pancreatic function in patients with a pancreatic head tumor. *Journal of Clinical Gastroenterology*, *48*(1), 43–46.

Talukdar, R., & Nageshwar, R. D. (2014). Endoscopic therapy for chronic pancreatitis. *Current Opinion in Gastroenterology*, *30*(5), 484–489.

Vege, S. S., DiMagno, M. J., Forsmark, C. E., et al. (2018). Initial medical treatment of acute pancreatitis: American Gastroenterological Association Institute technical review. *Gastroenterology*, *154*(4), 1103–1139.

Weinmann, A., Koch, S., Niederle, I. M., et al. (2014). Trends in epidemiology, treatment, and survival of hepatocellular carcinoma patients between 1998 and 2009: An analysis of 1,066 cases of a German HCC registry. *Journal of Clinical Gastroenterology*, *48*(5), 279–289.

Weir, M. R., Bartlett, S. T., & Drachenberg, C. B. (2012). Eosinophilia as an early indicator of pancreatic allograft rejection. *Clinical Transplantation*, *26*, 238–241.

Wu, B. U., & Banks, P. A. (2013). Clinical management of patients with acute pancreatitis. *Gastroenterology*, *144*(6), 1272–1281.

Yeo, T. P. (2015). Demographics, epidemiology, and inheritance of pancreatic ductal adenocarcinoma. *Seminars in Oncology*, *42*(1), 8–18.

Zerboni, G., Signoretti, M., Crippa, S., et al. (2019). Systematic review and meta-analysis: Prevalence of incidentally detected pancreatic cystic lesions in asymptomatic individuals. *Pancreatology*, *19*(1), 2–9.

Zerem, E. (2014). Treatment of severe acute pancreatitis and its complications. *World Journal of Gastroenterology*, *20*(38), 13879–13892.

Zhang, H., Chen, L., Gu, Z., et al. (2013). Clinical observation and nursing care on the prevention of abdominal organ cluster transplantation rejection. *Journal of Clinical Nursing*, *22*(11–12), 1599–1603.

Resources

Canadian Association of Gastroenterology: http://www.cag-acg.org

Canadian Cancer Society/Société Canadienne du Cancer: http://www.cancer.ca

Canadian Digestive Health Foundation: http://www.cdhf.ca

Endocrine Society: http://www.endo-society.org

National Digestive Diseases Information Clearing House: https://www.niddk.nih.gov/

The National Pancreas Foundation: http://www.pancreasfoundation.org

UNIT 8

Metabolic and Endocrine Function

Case Study ENSURING OPEN COMMUNICATION AND APPROPRIATE DELEGATION

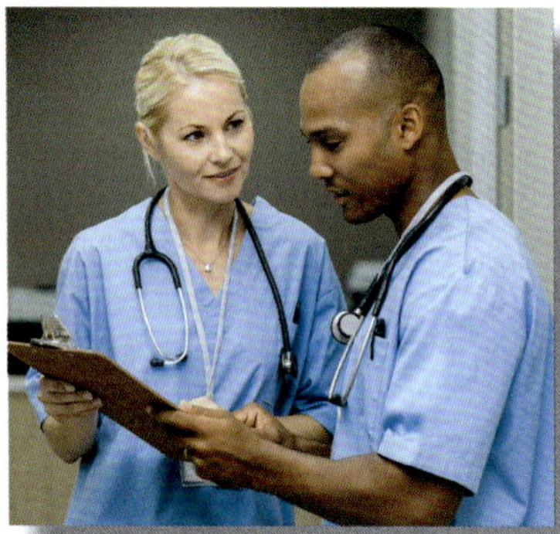

A nurse has just started a 12-hour day shift on a medical unit. The assignment includes five patients; a 24-year-old male with a new diagnosis of type 1 diabetes; a 45-year-old female admitted last night with diabetic ketoacidosis; a 55-year-old male with cancer of the liver who is scheduled for chemotherapy today; a 65-year-old female patient with a diagnosis of hepatitis B; and a 66-year-old male with acute pancreatitis receiving total parenteral nutrition through a central line. The nurse requests a “huddle” with the unlicensed assistant assigned to the team for the day. How can the nurse foster open communication, mutual respect, and shared decision making with her team to achieve quality patient care for these five patients?

Teamwork and Collaboration

The complexities inherent in today's health care system challenge nurses to demonstrate integration of specific interdisciplinary core competencies. These competencies are aimed at ensuring the delivery of safe, quality patient care (Institute of Medicine, 2003). The Quality and Safety Education for Nurses project (QSEN, 2017; Cronenwett, Sherwood, Barnsteiner, et al., 2007) provides a framework for the knowledge, skills, and attitudes (KSAs) required for nurses to demonstrate competency in these key areas, which include ***patient-centred care***, ***interdisciplinary teamwork and collaboration***, ***evidence-based practice***, ***quality improvement***, ***safety***, and ***informatics.***

Teamwork and Collaboration Definition: Function effectively within nursing and interprofessional teams, fostering open communication, mutual respect, and shared decision making to achieve quality patient care.

SELECTED PRE-LICENSURE KSAs	APPLICATION AND REFLECTION
Knowledge	
Examine strategies for improving systems to support team functioning.	Discuss what should happen during the beginning of the shift "huddle" in this busy medical unit. What tasks can the nurse delegate to the aide? Are there other resources within the hospital the nurse can draw on to help support these five patients?
Skills	
Participate in designing systems that support effective teamwork.	Give examples of checklists or other tools that may be used so that consistent processes are followed during a "huddle."
Attitudes	
Value the influence of system solutions in achieving effective team functioning.	How can a team approach to job completion assure best outcomes, generally speaking? Why is teamwork and collaboration of such great importance in assuring best patient outcomes?

Cronenwett, L., Sherwood, G., Barnsteiner, J., et al. (2007). Quality and safety education for nurses. *Nursing Outlook, 55*(3), 122–131; Institute of Medicine. (2003). *Health professions education: A bridge to quality*. Washington, DC: National Academies Press; and QSEN Institute. (2017). *QSEN Competencies: Definitions and pre-licensure KSAs*. Retrieved March 1, 2017, from www.qsen.org/competencies/pre-licensure-ksas

41 Assessment and Management of Patients With Diabetes Mellitus

Adapted by Rhonda Roedler

Learning Objectives

On completion of this chapter, the learner will be able to:

1. Differentiate between type 1 and type 2 diabetes.
2. Describe etiologic factors associated with diabetes.
3. Relate the clinical manifestations of diabetes to the associated pathophysiologic alterations.
4. Identify the diagnostic and clinical significance of blood glucose tests.
5. Explain the dietary modifications used for management of people with diabetes.
6. Describe the relationship between diet, exercise, and medication (i.e., insulin or oral hypoglycemic agents) for people with diabetes.
7. Develop a plan for teaching insulin self-administration.
8. Identify the role of oral and injectable antihyperglycemic agents in therapy.
9. Differentiate between diabetic ketoacidosis and hyperosmolar hyperglycemic syndrome.
10. Describe management strategies for a person with diabetes to use during "sick days."
11. Describe the major macrovascular, microvascular, and neuropathic complications of diabetes and the self-care behaviours important in their prevention.
12. Identify the teaching aids and community support groups available for people with diabetes.
13. Use the nursing process as a framework for care of the patient with diabetes.

Diabetes is a condition in which the body either cannot produce **insulin** or cannot effectively use the insulin it produces (Diabetes Canada, 2018a). Diabetes mellitus is a group of metabolic diseases characterized by elevated levels of glucose in the blood (hyperglycemia) (American Diabetes Association [ADA], 2016a). Glucose levels in the blood are normally well controlled in the body. The major sources of this glucose are from absorption of ingested food in the gastrointestinal (GI) tract and formation of glucose by the liver (and to a lesser extent the kidney) through the processes of glycogenolysis and gluconeogenesis.

Insulin, a hormone produced by the pancreas, controls the level of glucose in the blood by regulating the production and storage of glucose. In the diabetic state, the cells may stop responding to insulin or the pancreas may stop producing insulin entirely. This leads to hyperglycemia, which may result in acute metabolic complications such as **diabetic ketoacidosis** (DKA) and **hyperglycemic hyperosmolar syndrome (HHS)**. Long-term effects of hyperglycemia may contribute to macrovascular complications (coronary artery disease, cerebrovascular disease, and peripheral vascular disease), chronic microvascular complications (kidney and eye disease), and neuropathic complications (diseases of the nerves).

According to Diabetes Canada (2018a), about 11 million Canadians are currently living with diabetes or prediabetes, and it is suspected that up to 1 million of those

Glossary

alpha-glucosidase inhibitor (acarbose): oral agent used in the treatment of type 2 diabetes that delays the absorption of carbohydrate, resulting in lower postprandial blood glucose levels

biguanide (metformin): class of oral antihyperglycemic agents that improve sensitivity to insulin

continuous subcutaneous insulin infusion (CSII): an insulin pump which delivers rapid-acting insulin hourly as a basal dose and is also programmed by the patient to deliver a bolus dose before eating a meal in an attempt to mimic normal pancreatic function

diabetes: group of metabolic diseases characterized by hyperglycemia resulting from defects in insulin secretion, insulin action, or both (formerly known as diabetes mellitus)

diabetic ketoacidosis (DKA): metabolic derangement that results from a deficiency of insulin, which most commonly occurs in patients with type 1 diabetes. Highly acidic ketone bodies are formed, resulting in acidosis; usually requires hospitalization for treatment and is usually caused by multiple factors including nonadherence to the insulin regimen, concurrent illness, medications, or infection.

dipeptidyl dipeptidase 4 (DPP-4) inhibitors (alogliptin, saxagliptin, linagliptin, sitagliptin): oral antihyperglycemic that inhibits the dipeptidyl dipeptidase enzyme, responsible for the degradation of glucagon-like peptides, leading to increased insulin secretion and feelings of satiety

fasting plasma glucose (FPG): blood glucose determination obtained in the laboratory after fasting for more than 8 hours. Although plasma levels are specified in diagnostic criteria, blood glucose levels, which are slightly higher than plasma levels, are more commonly used

glucagon-like peptide (GLP-1) receptor agonists (liraglutide, exenatide, dulaglutide): injectable antihyperglycemics that mimic the action of glucagon-like peptide, a neuroendocrine hormone, causing insulin secretion and feelings of satiety

glycated hemoglobin (A1C): long-term measure of glucose control that is a result of glucose irreversibly attaching to hemoglobin in the red blood cell (attaches for up to 120 days). The goal A1C for a patient is determined by multiple factors including comorbidities, age, and occurrence of hypoglycemia

hyperglycemia: elevated blood glucose level—fasting level greater than 6.1 mmol/L; 2-hour postprandial level greater than 7.8 mmol/L

hyperglycemic hyperosmolar syndrome (HHS): metabolic disorder of type 2 diabetes resulting from a relative insulin deficiency initiated by an intercurrent illness that raises the demand for insulin; associated with polyuria and severe dehydration

hypoglycemia: blood glucose level less than or equal to 3.9 mmol/L

impaired fasting glucose (IFG): classified as a fasting plasma glucose of 6.1 to 6.9 mmol/L and used as diagnostic criteria for prediabetes

impaired glucose tolerance (IGT): classified as a blood glucose result of 7.8 to 11.0 mmol/L 2 hours following a 75-g oral glucose tolerance test; used as diagnostic criteria for prediabetes

insulin: hormone secreted by the beta cells of the islets of Langerhans of the pancreas that is necessary for the metabolism of carbohydrates, proteins, and fats; a deficiency of insulin results in diabetes

islet cell transplant: investigational procedure in which purified islet cells from cadaver donors are injected into the portal vein of the liver, with the goal of having these cells secrete insulin for better control of diabetes

ketone: highly acidic substance formed when the liver breaks down free fatty acids in the absence of insulin. Large amounts of ketones in the blood may lead to diabetic ketoacidosis

nephropathy: long-term complication of diabetes in which the kidney cells are damaged; characterized by microalbuminuria in early stages and progressing to end-stage renal disease

neuropathy: long-term complication of diabetes resulting from damage to the nerve cell due to hyperglycemia

retinopathy: long-term complication of diabetes in which the microvascular system of the eye is damaged due to hyperglycemia

self-monitoring of blood glucose (SMBG): method of capillary blood glucose testing in which the patient pricks his or her finger and applies a drop of blood to a test strip that is read by a meter

sodium glucose transporter 2 (SGLT2) inhibitors (empagliflozin, dapagliflozin, canagliflozin): classification of oral antihyperglycemic agent

sulfonylurea (glyburide, gliclazide, glimepiride, chlorpropamide, tolbutamide): classification of oral antihyperglycemic medication for treating type 2 diabetes that enhances insulin secretion and insulin action

thiazolidinedione (rosiglitazone, pioglitazone): class of oral antidiabetic medications that reduce insulin resistance in target tissues, enhancing insulin action without directly stimulating insulin secretion

type 1 diabetes: metabolic disorder characterized by an absence of insulin production and secretion from autoimmune destruction of the beta cells of the islets of Langerhans in the pancreas. Formerly called *insulin-dependent, juvenile diabetes*, or *type I diabetes*

type 2 diabetes: metabolic disorder characterized by the relative deficiency of insulin production and a decreased insulin action and increased insulin resistance. Formerly called *non–insulin-dependent diabetes, adult-onset diabetes*, or *type II diabetes* living with this condition may have undiagnosed **type 2 diabetes**. The prevalence of diabetes among obese Canadians was 13.2% in 2016, compared with 6.6% among overweight Canadians and 3.6% among those classified as having a normal weight (Diabetes Canada, 2018a). According to the Canadian Institute for Health Information's (CIHI) report, International Comparisons: A Focus on Diabetes, just over 9% of Canadians have diabetes, that's more than 3 million Canadians living with diabetes. Of these Canadians, approximately 10% of the population have been diagnosed with **type 1 diabetes** and the remaining 90% have been diagnosed with type 2 diabetes. A third classification, gestational diabetes mellitus, occurs in approximately 3.5% to 3.8% of non-Aboriginal populations and 8.0% to 18.0% of Aboriginal populations during pregnancy. Aboriginal people are three to five times more likely to develop type 2 diabetes than the general population. Canadians who are of Hispanic, Asian, South Asian, or African descent also have a greater risk of developing type 2 diabetes. There is an increase in the incidence of type 2 diabetes occurring in children from high-risk groups; risk factors include ethnicity or the presence of obesity (Diabetes Canada, 2018a). Chart 41-1 summarizes other risk factors of diabetes mellitus.

The far-reaching and devastating physical, social, and economic consequences of diabetes are as follows:

- Diabetes is a leading cause of non-traumatic amputations and blindness among working-age adults, and end-stage kidney disease (ESKD).
- There is a high rate of cardiovascular disease (myocardial infarction, stroke, and peripheral vascular disease) among people with diabetes.
- In Canada, diabetes is now the sixth leading cause of death, causing 3.4% of all deaths in 2016 (Statistics Canada, 2018a).
- According to The Public Health Agency of Canada (PHAC) (2018), the overall prevalence of diabetes is higher among males (8.7%) than females (7.6%). In 2017, almost 3 million Canadians (8.1%) were living with diabetes and about 20% of diabetes cases remain undiagnosed.
- People of Aboriginal descent are three to five times more likely than the general population to develop type 2 diabetes.
- Hospitalization rates for people with diabetes are three times greater for adults and about six times greater for children than for the general population.
- Although only 3.4% of all deaths in Canada were attributed to diabetes in 2017. Diabetes itself does not typically lead directly to death, but the complications associated with diabetes do (PHAC, 2018).
- At every age group, individuals with diabetes experienced mortality rates at least two times higher than those without. This results in noticeable decreases in life expectancy as well as health-adjusted life expectancy (PHAC, 2018).
- "The predicted 10-year risk of developing diabetes for the Canadian population in 2011/12 was 9.98%, corresponding to 2.16 million new cases, and total health care costs attributable to diabetes during this period were $7.55 billion for females and $7.81 billion for males ($15.36 billion total)" (Anja & Laura, 2017).

The economic cost of diabetes continues to rise because of increasing health care costs and an aging population. Annual per capita health care costs are estimated to be three to four times greater in a population with diabetes compared to a population without the disease. This higher cost is due to more frequent visits to family physicians, increased trips to specialists, and an increased likelihood of hospitalization for patients with diabetes.

The primary goals of treatment for patients with diabetes include maintaining blood glucose levels within normal range and preventing acute and long-term complications. Thus, the nurse who cares for patients with diabetes must work with them to develop self-care management skills.

CHART 41-1

Risk Factors: Diabetes

- Family history of diabetes (e.g., parents or siblings with diabetes)
- Obesity (i.e., ≥20% over desired body weight or body mass index ≥30 kg/m^2)
- Race/ethnicity (e.g., African Americans, Hispanic Americans, Native Americans, Asian Americans, Pacific Islanders)
- Age equal to or greater than 45 years
- Previously identified impaired fasting glucose or impaired glucose tolerance
- Hypertension (≥140/90 mm Hg)
- High-density lipoprotein (HDL) cholesterol level ≤35 mg/dL (0.90 mmol/L) and/or triglyceride level ≥250 mg/dL (2.8 mmol/L)
- History of gestational diabetes or delivery of a baby over 9 lb

Adapted from American Diabetes Association (ADA). (2016b). Standards of medical care in diabetes—2016. Classification and diagnosis of diabetes. *Diabetes Care, 39*(Suppl 1), S13–S24.

Classification of Diabetes

The major classifications of diabetes are type 1 diabetes, type 2 diabetes, gestational diabetes, latent autoimmune diabetes of adults (LADA), and diabetes associated with other conditions or syndromes (ADA, 2016b). The different types of diabetes vary in cause, clinical course, and treatment (see Table 41-1). The classification system is dynamic in two ways. First, research findings suggest many differences among individuals within each category. Second, except for people with type 1 diabetes, patients may move from one category to another. For example, a woman with gestational diabetes may, after delivery, move into type 2 diabetes. Prediabetes is classified as **impaired glucose tolerance (IGT)** or **impaired fasting glucose (IFG)** and refers to a condition in which blood glucose concentrations fall between normal levels and those considered diagnostic for diabetes (CDC, 2014).

Overview

The terms *insulin-dependent diabetes* and *non–insulin-dependent diabetes* and their acronyms (IDDM and NIDDM,

TABLE 41-1 Classification of Diabetes and Related Glucose Intolerances

Current Classification	Clinical Characteristics and Clinical Implications
Type 1 (5% of all diabetes; previously classified as juvenile diabetes, juvenile-onset diabetes, ketosis-prone diabetes, brittle diabetes, and insulin-dependent diabetes mellitus [IDDM])	Onset any age, but usually young (<30 years) Usually thin at diagnosis; recent weight loss Etiology includes genetic, immunologic, and environmental factors (e.g., virus) Often have islet cell antibodies Often have antibodies to insulin even before insulin treatment Little or no endogenous insulin Need exogenous insulin to preserve life Ketosis prone when insulin absent Acute complication of hyperglycemia: diabetic ketoacidosis
Type 2 (95% of all diabetes: obese—80% of type 2, nonobese—20% of type 2; previously classified as adult-onset diabetes, maturity-onset diabetes, ketosis-resistant diabetes, stable diabetes, and non-insulin-dependent diabetes mellitus [NIDDM])	Onset any age, usually >30 years Usually obese at diagnosis Causes include obesity, heredity, and environmental factors No islet cell antibodies Decrease in endogenous insulin, or increased with insulin resistance Most patients can control blood glucose through weight loss if obese Oral antidiabetic agents may improve blood glucose levels if dietary modification and exercise are unsuccessful May need insulin on a short- or long-term basis to prevent hyperglycemia Ketosis uncommon, except in stress or infection Acute complication: hyperglycemic hyperosmolar syndrome
Diabetes associated with other conditions or syndromes (previously classified as secondary diabetes)	Accompanied by conditions known or suspected to cause the disease: pancreatic diseases, hormonal abnormalities, medications such as corticosteroids and estrogen-containing preparations Depending on the ability of the pancreas to produce insulin, the patient may require treatment with oral antidiabetic agents or insulin
Gestational diabetes	Onset during pregnancy, usually in the second or third trimester Because of hormones secreted by the placenta, which inhibit the action of insulin Above-normal risk for perinatal complications, especially macrosomia (abnormally large babies) Treated with diet and, if needed, insulin to strictly maintain normal blood glucose levels Occurs in about 18% of pregnancies Glucose intolerance transitory but may recur: • In subsequent pregnancies • 35–60% will develop diabetes (usually type 2) within 10–20 years, especially if obese Risk factors include obesity, age >30 years, family history of diabetes, previous large babies (>9 lb) Screening tests (glucose challenge test) should be performed on all pregnant women between 24 and 28 weeks of gestation Should be screened for diabetes periodically
Prediabetes (previously classified as previous abnormality of glucose tolerance)	Previous history of hyperglycemia (e.g., during pregnancy or illness) Current normal glucose metabolism Impaired glucose tolerance or impaired fasting glucose screening after age 40 years if there is a family history of diabetes or if symptomatic Encourage ideal body weight, because loss of 10–15 lb may improve glycemic control

Adapted from American Diabetes Association (ADA). (2016b). Standards of medical care in diabetes—2016. Classification and diagnosis of diabetes. *Diabetes Care, 39*(Suppl 1), S13–S24; American Diabetes Association (ADA). (2016c). Standards of medical care in diabetes—2016; Management of diabetes in pregnancy. *Diabetes Care, 39*(Suppl 1), S94–S98.

respectively) are no longer used because they have resulted in classification of patients on the basis of the treatment of their diabetes rather than the underlying etiology. Use of roman numerals (type I and type II) to distinguish between the two types has been changed to type 1 and type 2 to reduce confusion.

Approximately 10% of people with diabetes have type 1 diabetes, in which the insulin-producing pancreatic beta cells are destroyed by an autoimmune process. As a result, they produce little or no insulin and require insulin injections to control their blood glucose levels. Type 1 diabetes is characterized by an acute onset, usually before age 30 years (Diabetes Canada, 2018a).

Approximately 90% of people with diabetes have type 2 diabetes (Diabetes Canada, 2018a), which results from decreased sensitivity to insulin (called *insulin resistance*) and impaired beta cell functioning resulting in decreased insulin production. Type 2 diabetes may first be treated with diet and exercise, but medications may be needed at diagnosis. If elevated glucose levels persist, diet and exercise are supplemented with oral hypoglycemic agents. In some individuals with type 2 diabetes, oral agents do not control **hyperglycemia**, and insulin injections are required. In addition, some individuals whose type 2 diabetes can usually be controlled with diet, exercise, and oral agents may require insulin injections during periods of acute physiologic stress (e.g., illness or surgery). The development of type 2 diabetes is insidious, and it usually develops in people older than 30 years who have increased amounts of visceral fat.

Prediabetes, defined as a state which places individuals at a higher risk of developing diabetes and its consequential complications, is diagnosed by the following criteria:

fasting plasma glucose of 6.1 to 6.9 mmol/L, 2-hour plasma glucose of 7.8 to 11.0 mmol/L following a 75-g oral glucose tolerance test (OGTT), or a **glycated hemoglobin** of 6.0% to 6.4% (Diabetes Canada, 2018b). Regardless of the treatment used (oral or injectable antihyperglycemics, insulin, or lifestyle changes), all patients diagnosed with diabetes are at risk for developing complications. It is important for the nurse to emphasize to these individuals that they *do* have diabetes and not a borderline problem with sugar (glucose). Previously, patients were diagnosed with borderline diabetes; however, this classification has now changed to **impaired glucose tolerance** (**IGT**) or **impaired fasting glucose** (**IFG**) and refers to a condition in which blood glucose levels fall above normal levels and below levels considered diagnostic for diabetes.

Table 41-1 summarizes the major classifications of diabetes, current terminology, old labels, and major clinical characteristics. This classification system is dynamic in two ways. First, research findings suggest many differences among individuals within each category. Second, with the exception of those with type 1 diabetes, patients may move from one category to another. For example, a woman with gestational diabetes may, after delivery, develop type 2 diabetes. These types also differ in their etiology, clinical course, and management.

Chart 41-2 outlines the diagnosis of diabetes using laboratory testing. In the case of symptomatic hyperglycemia, the diagnosis has been made and a confirmatory test is not required before a patient's treatment is initiated. In the absence of symptomatic hyperglycemia, a laboratory test is required in order to diagnose the patient with diabetes and a repeat confirmatory laboratory test must be performed on another day. Usually, the same test is repeated, but a random PG in the diabetes range in an asymptomatic individual should be confirmed with an alternate test. If the results of two different tests are above the diagnostic cutpoints, the diagnosis of diabetes is confirmed. For individuals in whom type 1 diabetes is likely, patients who are younger, lean, or show symptomatic hyperglycemia, confirmatory testing should not delay initiation of treatment to avoid the rapid deterioration of their health.

CHART 41-2

Diagnosis of Diabetes—Diabetes Canada (2018a)

FPG ≥7.0 mmol/L
Fasting = no caloric intake for at least 8 hours
or
A1C ≥6.5% (in adults)
Using a standardized, validated assay in the absence of factors that affect the accuracy of the A1C and not for suspected type 1 diabetes (see text)
or
2hPG in a 75-g OGTT ≥11.1 mmol/L
or
Random PG ≥11.1 mmol/L
Random = any time of the day, without regard to the interval since the last meal

In the absence of symptomatic hyperglycemia, if a single laboratory test result is in the diabetes range, a repeat confirmatory laboratory test (FPG, A1C, 2hPG in a 75-g OGTT) must be done on another day. It is preferable that the same test be repeated (in a timely fashion) for confirmation, but a random PG in the diabetes range in an asymptomatic individual should be confirmed with an alternate test. In the case of symptomatic hyperglycemia, the diagnosis has been made and a confirmatory test is not required before treatment is initiated. In individuals in whom type 1 diabetes is likely (younger or lean or symptomatic hyperglycemia, especially with ketonuria or ketonemia), confirmatory testing should not delay initiation of treatment to avoid rapid deterioration. If results of two different tests are available and both are above the diagnostic cutpoints, the diagnosis of diabetes is confirmed.

2hPG, 2-hour plasma glucose; *A1C*, glycated hemoglobin; *FPG*, fasting plasma glucose; *OGTT*, oral glucose tolerance test; *PG*, plasma glucose.

Pathophysiology

Insulin is a hormone secreted by beta cells, which are one of four types of cells in the islets of Langerhans in the pancreas (Grossman & Porth, 2014). Insulin is an anabolic, or storage, hormone. When a person eats a meal, insulin secretion increases and moves glucose from the blood into muscle, liver, and fat cells. In those cells, insulin has the following actions:

- Transports and metabolizes glucose for energy
- Stimulates storage of glucose in the liver and muscle (in the form of glycogen)
- Signals the liver to stop the release of glucose
- Enhances storage of dietary fat in adipose tissue
- Accelerates transport of amino acids (derived from dietary protein) into cells
- Inhibits the breakdown of stored glucose, protein, and fat

During fasting periods (between meals and overnight), the pancreas continuously releases a small amount of insulin (basal insulin); another pancreatic hormone called *glucagon* (secreted by the alpha cells of the islets of Langerhans) is released when blood glucose levels decrease, which stimulates the liver to release stored glucose. The insulin and the glucagon together maintain a constant level of glucose in the blood by stimulating the release of glucose from the liver.

Initially, the liver produces glucose through the breakdown of glycogen (glycogenolysis). After 8 to 12 hours without food, the liver forms glucose from the breakdown of noncarbohydrate substances, including amino acids (gluconeogenesis).

Type 1 Diabetes

Type 1 diabetes affects approximately 5% of adults with the disease (CDC, 2014). It is characterized by the destruction of the pancreatic beta cells (Grossman & Porth, 2014). Combined genetic, immunologic, and possibly environmental (e.g., viral) factors are thought to contribute to beta-cell destruction. Although the events that lead to beta-cell destruction are not fully understood, it is generally accepted that a genetic susceptibility is a common underlying factor in the development of type 1 diabetes. People do not inherit type 1 diabetes itself but rather a genetic predisposition, or tendency, toward the development of type 1 diabetes. This genetic tendency has been found in people with certain human leukocyte antigen types. There is also evidence of an autoimmune response in type 1 diabetes. This is an abnormal response in which antibodies are directed against normal tissues of the body, responding to these tissues as if they were foreign. Autoantibodies against islet cells and against endogenous (internal) insulin have been detected in people at the time of diagnosis and even several years before the development of clinical signs of type 1 diabetes. In addition to genetic and immunologic components, environmental factors such as viruses or toxins that may initiate destruction of the beta cell continue to be investigated.

Regardless of the specific etiology, the destruction of the beta cells results in decreased insulin production, unchecked glucose production by the liver, and fasting hyperglycemia. In addition, glucose derived from food cannot be stored in the liver but instead remains in the bloodstream and contributes to postprandial (after meal) hyperglycemia. If the concentration of glucose in the blood exceeds the renal threshold for glucose, usually 9.9 to 11.1 mmol/L, the kidneys may not reabsorb all of the filtered glucose; the glucose then appears in the urine (glucosuria). When excess glucose is excreted in the urine, it is accompanied by excessive loss of fluids and electrolytes. This is called *osmotic diuresis*.

Because insulin usually inhibits glycogenolysis (breakdown of stored glucose) and gluconeogenesis (production of new glucose from amino acids and other substrates), these processes occur in people with insulin deficiency in an unrestrained fashion and contribute further to hyperglycemia. In addition, when there is a deficiency in the presence of insulin, the stored fat is broken down to provide a source of energy, resulting in the production of **ketone** bodies, which can lead to the development of ketosis.

NURSING ALERT

Ketone bodies are acids that disturb the acid–base balance of the body when they accumulate in excessive amounts. The resulting diabetic ketoacidosis (DKA) may cause signs and symptoms such as abdominal pain, nausea, vomiting, hyperventilation, a fruity breath odour, and, if left untreated, altered level of consciousness, coma, and death. Initiation of fluid treatment, along with insulin and electrolytes as needed, is essential to treat hyperglycemia and DKA and rapidly improves the metabolic abnormalities.

Type 2 Diabetes

Type 2 diabetes differs from type 1 diabetes in many different ways (Fig. 41-1). The onset of type 1 diabetes is more abrupt, whereas the development of hyperglycemia in type 2 diabetes may take years before the person experiences symptoms. There is no autoimmune destruction of the islet cells of the pancreas in type 2 diabetes, so the production of insulin continues. As the disease progresses over time, however, there is loss of function of the pancreatic beta cells. Although there is a strong genetic predisposition to type 2 diabetes, it is not linked to HLA markers on the sixth chromosome. Genetic predisposition coupled with environmental factors, such as the presence of visceral/abdominal obesity and a sedentary lifestyle, seem to be the major contributors to the development of insulin resistance, which is the most salient characteristic of type 2 diabetes. In Canada, an estimated 80% to 90% of individuals with type 2 diabetes are overweight or obese, and the increased body mass index (BMI) in people with diabetes is associated with increased mortality (Diabetes Canada, 2018a).

Physiology/Pathophysiology

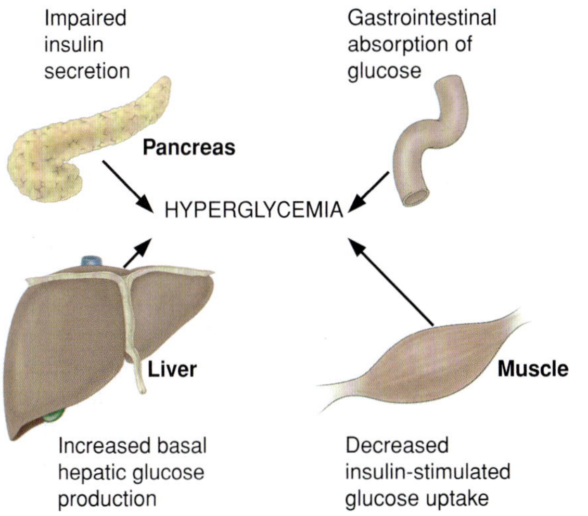

FIGURE 41-1. Pathogenesis of type 2 diabetes.

The pathogenesis of insulin resistance is complex. There are numerous coexisting signs that are associated with the development of insulin resistance. These include: hypertension (blood pressure of 130/85 mm Hg or greater), fasting blood glucose of 6.1 mmol/L or higher, triglycerides of 1.7 mmol/L or higher, high-density lipoprotein (HDL) of less than 1.0 mmol/L for men or 1.3 mmol/L for women, and the presence of visceral or abdominal obesity (defined as a waist circumference of 102 cm or greater for men and 88 cm or greater for women) (Diabetes Canada, 2018a). This constellation of abnormal signs is often referred to as metabolic syndrome or syndrome X. Over the years, there have been many criteria that have been put forward by various groups on what constitutes metabolic syndrome. Most recently, there is a growing body of data about ethnic variability of waist circumference that may see changes to more ethnic-specific measurements in the upcoming criteria and guidelines. Other concomitant illnesses, such as Cushing's syndrome or polycystic ovarian syndrome (PCOS), may also lead to the development of type 2 diabetes. Another major difference between type 1 and 2 diabetes is that those with type 2 diabetes are not as likely to develop DKA because insulin is still being produced endogenously. The insulin produced prevents lipids from being broken down and used as an alternative energy source; therefore, no ketone by-products are produced. Patients with type 2 diabetes who rely solely on insulin to treat their diabetes (insulin-deficient patients) may be at risk of developing DKA.

The symptoms experienced around the time patients are diagnosed with type 2 diabetes may include fatigue, irritability, polyuria, polydipsia, skin wounds that heal poorly, vaginal infections, or blurred vision (if glucose levels are very high).

For most patients (approximately 75%), type 2 diabetes is detected incidentally (e.g., when routine laboratory tests or ophthalmoscopic examinations are performed). One consequence of undetected diabetes is that long-term diabetes complications (e.g., eye disease, peripheral **neuropathy**, and peripheral vascular disease) may have developed before the actual diagnosis of diabetes is made (ADA, 2016b). It is recommended to screen for these complications as close to diagnosis as possible.

Because insulin resistance is associated with abdominal obesity, the primary treatment of type 2 diabetes is weight loss. Exercise is also important in enhancing the effectiveness of endogenously produced insulin. Oral antidiabetic agents may be added if diet and exercise are not successful in controlling blood glucose levels. Insulin may be added to certain oral agent regimens, or patients may move to insulin therapy entirely. Some patients require insulin on an ongoing basis, and others may require insulin on a temporary basis during periods of acute physiologic stress, such as illness or surgery.

A recent report has demonstrated that the development of type 2 diabetes can be reduced or delayed in persons at high risk for the disease through weight reduction and increased participation in moderate exercise (Diabetes Canada, 2018a). Intensive and structured lifestyle modifications that result in a loss of approximately 5% of the patient's initial body weight can reduce the risk of progression of IFG or IGT to type 2 diabetes by about 60% (Diabetes Canada, 2018a). Progression from prediabetes to type 2 diabetes can also be reduced by pharmacologic therapy with metformin or resulting in a 30% reduction of risk.

Metformin, one of the antidiabetic agents, has also prevented or delayed the onset of type 2 diabetes but to a lesser degree. The findings of this study support the role that weight reduction and exercise have in reducing the risk of developing type 2 diabetes.

Gestational Diabetes

Gestational diabetes is any degree of glucose intolerance with its onset during pregnancy. Hyperglycemia develops during pregnancy because of the secretion of placental hormones, which may cause insulin resistance. For women who meet one or more of the following criteria, selective screening for diabetes during pregnancy is now being recommended between the 24th and 28th weeks of gestation: previous history of gestational diabetes mellitus, delivery of a macrosomic (abnormally large) infant, age 35 years or older, presence of obesity (BMI greater than 30), member of a group with a high prevalence of diabetes (e.g., Hispanic, Aboriginal, South Asian, Asian, or African descent), polycystic ovary syndrome and/or hirsutism, acanthosis nigricans, or corticosteroid use.

Gestational diabetes is any degree of glucose intolerance with its onset during pregnancy. Hyperglycemia develops during pregnancy because of the secretion of placental hormones, which causes insulin resistance. Gestational diabetes occurs in as many as 18% of pregnant women and increases their risk for hypertensive disorders during pregnancy (CDC, 2014; Wu, Nien, Kuo, et al., 2016).

NURSING ALERT

Initial management includes dietary modification and blood glucose monitoring.

Oral antidiabetic agents should not be used during pregnancy, although there is some evidence to indicate metformin may be used. Goals for blood glucose levels during pregnancy are 5.3 mmol/L (preprandial) or less, 7.8 mmol/L (1 hour after meal) or less, or 6.7 mmol/L (2 hours after meal) or less.

After delivery of the infant, blood glucose levels in the woman with gestational diabetes return to normal. However, women who have had gestational diabetes may develop type 2 diabetes later in life.

Approximately 35% to 60% of women who have had gestational diabetes develop diabetes in the next 10 to 20 years (CDC, 2014; Wu et al., 2016).

Latent Autoimmune Diabetes of Adults (LADA)

In adults, LADA is a subtype of diabetes in which the progression of autoimmune beta-cell destruction in the pancreas is slower than in types 1 and 2 diabetes (Deng, Xiang, Tan, et al., 2016). Patients with LADA are not insulin dependent in the initial 6 months of disease onset. Clinical manifestation of LADA shares the features of types 1 and 2 diabetes (Deng et al., 2016). The emergence of this subtype has led some to propose the diabetes classification scheme should be revised to reflect changes in the beta cells in the pancreas (Schwartz, Epstein, Corkey, et al., 2016).

Clinical Manifestations

Clinical manifestations depend on the patient's level of hyperglycemia. Classic clinical manifestations of diabetes include the "three Ps": polyuria, polydipsia, and polyphagia. Polyuria (increased urination) and polydipsia (increased thirst) occur as a result of the excess loss of fluid associated with osmotic diuresis. Patients also experience polyphagia (increased appetite) that results from the catabolic state induced by insulin deficiency and the breakdown of proteins and fats (Grossman & Porth, 2014). Other symptoms include fatigue and weakness, sudden vision changes, tingling or numbness in hands or feet, dry skin, skin lesions or wounds that are slow to heal, and recurrent infections. The onset of type 1 diabetes may also be associated with sudden weight loss or nausea, vomiting, or abdominal pains, if DKA has developed.

Assessment and Diagnostic Findings

The diagnosis of diabetes is based on elevated plasma glucose levels with or without symptoms. Based on the Diabetes Canada's 2018b Clinical Practice Guidelines,

CHART 41-3

Assessing the Patient With Diabetes

History

Symptoms related to the diagnosis of diabetes:
- Symptoms of hyperglycemia
- Symptoms of hypoglycemia
  - Frequency, timing, severity, and resolution

Results of blood glucose monitoring

Status, symptoms, and management of chronic complications of diabetes
- Eye, kidney, nerve, genitourinary and sexual, bladder, and gastrointestinal
- Cardiac, peripheral vascular, foot complications associated with diabetes

Adherence to/ability to follow prescribed dietary management plan

Adherence to prescribed exercise regimen

Adherence to/ability to follow prescribed pharmacologic treatment (e.g., insulin, oral antidiabetic agents, enteric-coated aspirin)

Use of tobacco, alcohol, and prescription and over-the-counter medications

Lifestyle, cultural, psychosocial, and economic factors that may affect diabetes treatment

Effects of diabetes or its complications on functional status (e.g., mobility, vision)

Physical Examination

Blood pressure (sitting and standing to detect orthostatic changes)

Body mass index (height and weight)

Fundoscopic examination and visual acuity

Foot examination (lesions, signs of infection, pulses)

Skin examination (lesions and insulin-injection sites)

Neurologic examination
- Vibratory and sensory examination using monofilament
- Deep tendon reflexes

Oral examination

Laboratory Examination

$HgbA_{1C}$ (A1C)

Fasting lipid profile

Test for microalbuminuria

Serum creatinine level

Urinalysis

Electrocardiogram

Need for Referrals

Ophthalmology/Optometrist

Cardiology

Nephrology

Podiatry

Dietitian

Diabetes educator

Psychologist

Social worker

Others if indicated

a fasting plasma glucose (FPG) level of 7.0 mmol/L or more, a glycated hemoglobin (A1C) of 6.5% or more, a level of 11.1 mmol/L or more following a 75-g OGTT or random plasma glucose level of 11.1 mmol/L or more with symptoms constitute the diagnosis of diabetes. See Chart 41-2 for the diagnostic criteria for diabetes.

In addition to the assessment and diagnostic evaluation performed to diagnose diabetes, ongoing specialized assessment of patients with known diabetes and evaluation for complications in patients with newly diagnosed diabetes are important components of care. Parameters that should be regularly assessed are presented in Chart 41-3.

Screening for diabetes in adults should be considered every 1 to 2 years in Aboriginal individuals with more than one risk factor. Screening every 2 years should be considered in patients starting at 10 years of age or those children in puberty with more than one risk factors, including exposure to diabetes in utero. Screening for type 1 diabetes is currently not recommended. Screening for type 2 diabetes when using an FPG level and/or a glycated hemoglobin level (A1C) should be performed every 3 years in individuals above the age of 40 or in individuals at a high risk for developing the disease (Diabetes Canada, 2018b).

Gerontologic Considerations

Diabetes is particularly prevalent in older adults. In fact, type 2 diabetes is the seventh leading cause of death and affects approximately 20% of older adults (Eliopoulos, 2018). There is a high prevalence among African Americans and those who are 65 to 74 years of age (Eliopoulos, 2018).

Early detection is important but may be challenging because symptoms may be absent or nonspecific. A glucose tolerance test is more effective in diagnosis than urine testing for glucose in older patients due to the higher renal threshold for glucose (Eliopoulos, 2018).

What causes age-related changes in carbohydrate metabolism is unresolved. Possibilities include: poor diet, physical inactivity, a decreased in the lean body mass in which ingested carbohydrate may be stored, altered insulin secretion, and increase in fat tissue, which may increases insulin resistance.

Medical Management

The main goal of diabetes treatment is to normalize insulin activity and blood glucose levels to reduce the development of micro- and macrovascular complications. The importance of tight blood glucose control was demonstrated by the Diabetes Control and Complications Trial (DCCT), a 10-year prospective clinical trial conducted from 1983 to 1993 (DCCT Research Group, 1993). The trial investigated the impact of intensive glucose control on the development and progression of complications such as **retinopathy**, **nephropathy**, and neuropathy. A cohort of 1,441 people with type 1 diabetes were randomly assigned to conventional treatment (one or two insulin injections per day) or intensive treatment (three or four insulin injections per day or insulin pump therapy plus frequent blood glucose monitoring and weekly contacts with diabetes educators). Results demonstrated that the risk for developing retinopathy, neuropathy, and early signs of nephropathy (microalbuminuria and albuminuria) was dramatically reduced. The reduction was attributed to control of blood glucose levels to normal or near-normal levels. The ADA now recommends that all patients with diabetes strive for glucose control ($HgbA_{1C}$ less than 7%) to reduce their risk of complications (ADA, 2016a).

The major adverse effect of intensive therapy was a threefold increase in the incidence of severe **hypoglycemia** (defined as a hypoglycemic incident requiring the assistance of another person for treatment) coma, or seizure. Because of these adverse effects, intensive therapy must be initiated with caution and must be accompanied by thorough education of the patient and family and by responsible behaviour of the patient. Careful screening of patients is a key step in initiating intensive therapy. (For situations that preclude the initiation of very tight blood glucose control, see the discussion of insulin regimens in this chapter.)

Therefore, the therapeutic goal for diabetes management is to achieve normal blood glucose levels (euglycemia) without hypoglycemia and without seriously disrupting the patient's usual lifestyle and activity. There are five components of diabetes management:

- Nutrition
- Exercise
- Monitoring
- Pharmacologic therapy
- Education

Treatment varies because of changes in lifestyle and physical and emotional status as well as advances in treatment methods. Therefore, diabetes management involves constant assessment and modification of the treatment plan by health professionals in conjunction with the patient. Education of the patient and/or family/caregivers is an essential component of diabetes treatment.

Nutrition

Nutrition, weight control, and exercise are the foundation of diabetes management. According to Diabetes Canada (2018a), the most important objective in the dietary and nutritional management of diabetes is control of total caloric intake to attain or maintain a reasonable body weight and control of blood glucose levels. Success of this alone is often associated with reversal of hyperglycemia in patients with type 2 diabetes. However, achieving this goal is not always easy. Because nutritional management of diabetes is so complex, a registered dietitian who understands diabetes management has the major responsibility for this aspect of the therapeutic plan. However, the nurse and all other members of the health care team need to be knowledgeable about nutritional therapy and supportive of the patient who needs to implement dietary and lifestyle changes. Nutritional management of the patient with diabetes includes the following goals:

- Providing all of the essential food constituents (e.g., vitamins, minerals) necessary for optimal nutrition
- Meeting energy needs
- Achieving and maintaining a reasonable weight
- Preventing wide daily fluctuations in blood glucose levels, with blood glucose levels as close to normal as is safe and practical to prevent or reduce the risk for complications
- Decreasing serum lipid levels, if elevated, to reduce the risk for macrovascular disease

For patients who require fixed doses of insulin to help control blood glucose levels, maintaining consistency in the amount of calories and carbohydrates ingested at mealtimes is essential. In addition, consistency in the approximate time intervals between meals, with the addition of snacks if necessary, helps prevent hypoglycemic reactions and maintain overall blood glucose control.

For patients with diabetes who are overweight or who have obesity (especially those with type 2 diabetes), weight loss is one aspect of treatment. (Weight loss also may help to prevent the development of type 2 diabetes.) In general, a BMI of 25.0 to 29.9 is classified as overweight, and a BMI of 30.0 or greater is classified as obese (Diabetes Canada, 2018a).

Nutrition therapy can reduce glycated hemoglobin (A1C) by 1.0% to 2.0% and, when used with other components of diabetes care, can further improve clinical and metabolic outcomes (Diabetes Canada, 2018a).

Because the location of the adipose tissue is of critical importance in the development of type 2 diabetes, it is also important to consider the waist circumference of the individual. A waist circumference of more than 102 cm for men and 88 cm for women is indicative of visceral or abdominal obesity (Diabetes Canada, 2018b). (See Chapter 42 for how to measure waist circumference and calculate BMI.) Obesity is associated with an increased resistance to insulin; it is also a main factor in type 2 diabetes. Some patients who have obesity and have type 2 diabetes and who require insulin or oral agents to control blood glucose levels may be able to reduce or eliminate the need for medication through weight loss; a weight loss as small as 5% to 10% of total weight may significantly improve blood glucose levels, insulin sensitivity, hypertension, and dyslipidemia. For patients with diabetes who do not take insulin, consistent meal content or timing is not as critical. Rather, decreasing the overall caloric intake assumes more importance for those who are overweight or obese. However, meals should not be skipped. Pacing food intake throughout the day places more manageable demands on the pancreas.

Long-term adherence to the meal plan is one of the most challenging aspects of diabetes management. For patients who are overweight or obese, it may be more realistic to restrict calories only moderately. For those who have lost weight, maintaining the weight loss may be difficult. To help these patients incorporate new dietary habits into their lifestyles, diet education, behavioural therapy, group support, and ongoing nutrition counselling are encouraged.

Meal Planning and Related Education

According to the Diabetes Canada (2018a), it is important for individuals with diabetes to receive nutrition counselling from a registered dietitian to lower A1C levels for those with type 2 diabetes [Grade B, Level 2 (1)], Grade D

Consensus for type 1 diabetes, and to reduce hospitalization rates [Grade C, Level 3 (2)].

Because of limited evidence to support one dietary prescription over another, meal planning for all patients with diabetes must consider the patient's food preferences, lifestyle, usual eating times, ethnic and cultural background, and readiness to change (Diabetes Canada, 2018a). For patients using intensive insulin therapy, there may be greater flexibility in the timing and content of meals by allowing adjustments in insulin dosage for changes in eating and exercise habits. Advances in insulin management (new insulin analogues, insulin algorithms, insulin pumps) permit greater flexibility of schedules than previously possible. This is in contrast to the older concept of maintaining a constant dose of insulin and requiring the patient to adjust his or her schedule to the actions and duration of the insulin.

The first step in preparing a meal plan is a thorough review of the patient's diet history to identify his or her eating habits and lifestyle. A thorough assessment of the patient's need for weight loss, gain, or maintenance is also undertaken. In most instances, the person with type 2 diabetes requires weight reduction.

In teaching about meal planning, the clinical dietitian uses various educational tools, materials, and approaches. Initial education addresses the importance of consistent eating habits, the relationship of food and insulin, and the provision of an individualized meal plan. In-depth follow-up education then focuses on management skills, such as eating at restaurants, reading food labels, and adjusting the meal plan for exercise, illness, and special occasions. The nurse plays an important role in communicating pertinent information to the dietitian and reinforcing the patient's understanding. Nutrition education is effective when delivered in either a small group or a one-on-one setting [Grade B, Level 2 (3)]. Group education should incorporate adult education principles, such as hands-on activities, problem solving, role playing, and group discussions [Grade B, Level 2 (4)] (Diabetes Canada, 2018a).

For some patients, certain aspects of meal planning may be difficult to learn. This may be related to limitations in the patient's intellectual level or to emotional issues, such as difficulty accepting the diagnosis of diabetes, or feelings of deprivation and undue restriction in eating. In any case, it helps to emphasize that eating a variety of healthy foods each day provides a way of thinking about food (Health Canada, 2019). It is also important to simplify information as much as possible and to provide opportunities for the patient to practice and repeat activities and information.

CALORIC REQUIREMENTS. Calorie-controlled diets are planned by first calculating the individual's energy needs and caloric requirements based on the patient's age, gender, height, and weight. An activity element is then factored in to provide the actual number of calories required for weight maintenance. To promote a 0.5 to 1.0 kg weight loss per week, 500 to 1,000 calories are subtracted from the daily total.

The priority for a young patient with type 1 diabetes, for example, should be a diet with enough calories to maintain normal growth and development. Some patients may be underweight at the onset of type 1 diabetes because of rapid weight loss from severe hyperglycemia. The goal with these patients initially may be to provide a higher-calorie diet to regain lost weight. The calories are distributed into carbohydrates, proteins, and fats, and a meal plan is then developed.

CALORIC DISTRIBUTION. A reduction in caloric intake to achieve and maintain a healthier body weight is a recommended treatment goal for those who are overweight or obese and have diabetes. A diabetic meal plan also focuses on the percentage of calories to come from carbohydrates, proteins, and fats. In adults with diabetes, the macronutrient distribution as a percentage of total energy can range from 45% to 60% carbohydrate, 15% to 20% protein, and 20% to 35% fat. This allows for the individualization of nutrition therapy based on patient preferences and treatment goals [Grade D, Consensus] (Diabetes Canada, 2018a). In general, carbohydrate foods have the greatest effect on blood glucose levels because they are more quickly digested than other foods and are converted into glucose rapidly.

Carbohydrates. Consistent carbohydrate intake, spacing, and regularity in meal consumption may help control blood glucose and weight (Diabetes Canada, 2018a). The caloric distribution currently recommended is higher in carbohydrates than in fats and protein. Carbohydrates consist of sugars and starches, which are essential to provide fuel for our bodies. There is much debate about the amount, source, and type of carbohydrates a person with diabetes should consume. Diabetes Canada's clinical practice guidelines on nutrition therapy recommend that people with diabetes choose carbohydrates that have the lowest postprandial response (a low glycemic index) to optimize blood glucose control. Also, counting the number of carbohydrates the person consumes at each meal is recommended.

Replacing high glycemic index carbohydrates with low glycemic index carbohydrates in mixed meals has a clinically significant benefit for glycemic control in people with type 1 and type 2 diabetes (Diabetes Canada, 2018a).

Carbohydrate counting is a nutritional tool used for blood glucose management. This method provides flexibility in food choices, and allows more accurate management with multiple daily injections (insulin before each meal). However, if carbohydrate counting is not used with other meal-planning techniques, weight gain can result. A variety of methods are used to count carbohydrates. When developing a diabetic meal plan using carbohydrate counting, all food sources should be considered. Once digested, 100% of carbohydrates are converted to glucose. However, approximately 50% of protein foods (meat, fish, and poultry) are also converted to glucose.

One method of carbohydrate counting includes counting grams of carbohydrates. If target goals are not reached by counting carbohydrates alone, protein will be factored into the calculations. This is especially true if the meal consists of only meat, fish, and non-starchy vegetables.

An alternative to counting grams of carbohydrate is measuring servings or choices. This method is used more often by people with type 2 diabetes. It emphasizes portion control of total servings of carbohydrate at meals and snacks. One carbohydrate serving is equivalent to 15 g of carbohydrate. Examples of one serving are an apple, a 250-mL glass of milk, or one slice of bread.

Fats. The recommendations regarding fat content of the diabetic diet include both reducing the total percentage of calories from fat sources to less than 30% of the total calories and limiting the amount of saturated fats and trans-fatty acids to 10% of total calories. Adults with diabetes should consume no more than 7% of total daily energy from saturated fats [Grade D, Consensus] and should limit intake of trans fatty acids to a minimum [Grade D, Consensus] (Diabetes Canada, 2018a). Meal plans should favour foods rich in omega-3 fatty acids and plant oils. This approach may help to reduce risk factors such as elevated serum cholesterol levels, which are associated with the development of coronary artery disease—the leading cause of death and disability among people with diabetes (ADA, 2016d; Evert, Boucher, Cypress, et al., 2013).

Protein. The meal plan may include the use of some non-animal sources of protein (e.g., legumes and whole grains) to help reduce saturated fat and cholesterol intake. In addition, the amount of protein intake may be reduced in patients with early signs of renal disease.

Fibre. The addition of fibre to the diet has received increased attention as researchers study the effects of a high-carbohydrate, high-fibre diet on diabetes. This type of diet plays a role in lowering total cholesterol and low-density lipoprotein (LDL) cholesterol in the blood. Increasing fibre in the diet may also improve blood glucose levels and decrease the need for exogenous insulin.

There are two types of dietary fibres: soluble and insoluble. Soluble fibre—in foods such as legumes, oats, and some fruits—plays more of a role in lowering blood glucose and lipid levels than does insoluble fibre, although the clinical significance of this effect is probably small (ADA, 2016d). Soluble fibre is thought to be related to the formation of a gel in the GI tract. This gel slows stomach emptying and the movement of food through the upper digestive tract. The potential glucose-lowering effect of fibre may be caused by the slower rate of glucose absorption from foods that contain soluble fibre. Insoluble fibre is found in whole-grain breads and cereals and in some vegetables. This type of fibre plays more of a role in increasing stool bulk and preventing constipation. Both insoluble and soluble fibre increase satiety, which may be helpful for weight loss.

Patients that increase their fibre intake suddenly may develop issues with abdominal fullness, nausea, diarrhea, increased flatulence, and constipation if fluid intake is inadequate. If fibre is added to or increased in the meal plan, it should be done gradually and in consultation with a dietitian. Occasionally, increasing the fibre intake may require adjusting the dosage of insulin or oral agents to prevent hypoglycemia due to changes in stomach emptying.

FOOD CLASSIFICATION SYSTEMS. To teach diet principles and to help patients in meal planning, several systems have been developed in which foods are organized into groups with common characteristics, such as number of calories, composition of foods (i.e., amount of carbohydrate, protein, or fat in the food), or effect on blood glucose levels.

Eating a Variety of Healthy Food Each Day. The dietary goal for patients diagnosed with diabetes is to maintain their blood glucose levels within normal limits to reduce or prevent the occurrence of complications. They must therefore learn to balance the carbohydrates, protein, and fats they ingest to control the amount of glucose that enters their bloodstream. Improvement in glycemic control can be monitored through regular readings of the diabetic individual's glycosylated hemoglobin (A1C). To achieve sustained metabolic control through lifestyle and behavioural changes, the nutritional therapy must be based on the individual's needs and preferences and should be regularly re-evaluated and reinforced.

Generally, individuals with diabetes should follow the new Canada food guide (see Eating a Variety of Healthy foods Each day; Health Canada, 2019) (see Chapter 42). These guidelines encourage the selection of a variety of foods from four food groups: grain products, fruits and vegetables, milk products, and meat or alternatives. Using these guidelines, the individual should plan his or her total daily caloric or energy intake.

Healthy Food Choices. An alternative to counting grams of carbohydrate is measuring servings or choices. This method is used more often by people with type 2 diabetes. It is similar to the food exchange list and emphasizes portion control of total servings of carbohydrate at meals and snacks. One carbohydrate serving is equivalent to 15 g of carbohydrate. Examples of one serving are an apple 2 in in diameter and one slice of bread. Vegetables and meat are counted as one third of a carbohydrate serving. This system works well for those who have difficulty with more complicated systems.

Glycemic Index. One of the main goals of diet therapy in diabetes is to avoid sharp, rapid increases in blood glucose levels after food is eaten. The term *glycemic index* is used to describe how much a given food increases the blood glucose level compared with an equivalent amount of glucose. The effects of the use of the glycemic index on blood glucose levels and on long-term patient outcomes are unclear, but it may be beneficial (ADA, 2016e). Although more research is necessary, the following guidelines may be helpful when making dietary recommendations:

- Combining starchy foods with protein- and fat-containing foods tends to slow their absorption and lower the glycemic index.
- In general, eating foods that are raw and whole results in a lower glycemic index than eating chopped, puréed, or cooked foods (except meat).
- Eating whole fruit instead of drinking juice decreases the glycemic index, because fibre in the fruit slows absorption.
- Adding foods with sugars to the diet may result in a lower glycemic index if these foods are eaten with foods that are more slowly absorbed.

Patients can create their own glycemic index by monitoring their blood glucose level after ingestion of a particular food. This can help improve blood glucose control through individualized manipulation of the diet. Many patients who use frequent monitoring of blood glucose levels can use this information to adjust their insulin doses in accordance with variations in food intake.

Other Dietary Concerns

ALCOHOL CONSUMPTION. Patients with diabetes do not need to give up alcoholic beverages entirely, but patients and primary providers must be aware of the potential adverse effects of alcohol specific to diabetes. Alcohol is absorbed before other nutrients and does not require insulin for absorption. Large amounts can be converted to fats, increasing the risk for DKA. In general, the same precautions regarding the use of alcohol by people without diabetes should be applied to patients with diabetes. Moderation is recommended. A major danger of alcohol consumption by the patient with diabetes is hypoglycemia, especially for patients who take insulin or insulin secretagogues (medications that increase the secretion of insulin by the pancreas). Alcohol may decrease the normal physiologic reactions in the body that produce glucose (gluconeogenesis). Therefore, if a patient with diabetes consumes alcohol on an empty stomach, there is an increased likelihood of hypoglycemia. In addition, excessive alcohol intake may impair the patient's ability to recognize and treat hypoglycemia or to follow a prescribed meal plan to prevent hypoglycemia. To reduce the risk of hypoglycemia, the patient should be cautioned to consume food along with the alcohol; however, carbohydrate consumed with alcohol may raise blood glucose.

Alcohol consumption may lead to excessive weight gain (from the high caloric content of alcohol), hyperlipidemia, and elevated glucose levels (especially with mixed drinks and liqueurs). Patient education regarding alcohol intake must emphasize moderation in the amount of alcohol consumed. Moderate intake is considered to be one alcoholic beverage per day for women and two per day for men. Lower-calorie or less-sweet drinks (e.g., light beer, dry wine) and food intake along with alcohol consumption are advised (ADA, 2016e). Patients with type 2 diabetes who wish to control their weight should incorporate the calories from alcohol into the overall meal plan.

SWEETENERS. Using sweeteners is acceptable for patients with diabetes, especially if it assists in overall dietary adherence. Moderation in the amount of sweetener used is encouraged to avoid potential adverse effects. There are two main types of sweeteners: nutritive and nonnutritive. The nutritive sweeteners contain calories, and the nonnutritive sweeteners have few or no calories in the amounts usually used.

Nutritive sweeteners include fructose (fruit sugar), sorbitol, and xylitol. They are not calorie-free; they provide calories in amounts similar to those in sucrose (table sugar). They cause less elevation in blood sugar levels than sucrose and are often used in "sugar-free" foods. Sweeteners containing sorbitol may have a laxative effect.

Nonnutritive sweeteners have minimal or no calories. They are used in food products and are also available for table use. They produce minimal or no elevation in blood glucose levels and have been approved by Health Canada as safe for people with diabetes. Saccharin contains no calories and is only available in pharmacies and is not added to packaged foods or beverages; its use should be avoided in pregnancy. Cyclamate (Sweet'N Low, SugarTwin), another nonnutritive sweetener, is available in different forms, but the flavour may change when heated. It also should be avoided during pregnancy and not be added to packaged foods and beverages. Aspartame (NutraSweet, Equal) is packaged with dextrose; it contains 4 calories per packet and also loses sweetness with heat. Acesulfame-K (Ace-K) is added by only the manufacturer to packaged foods and beverages and contains 1 calorie per packet. Sucralose (Splenda) is a newer nonnutritive, high-intensity sweetener that is about 600 times sweeter than sugar. It has been approved for use in baked goods, nonalcoholic beverages, chewing gum, coffee, confections, frostings, and frozen dairy products. Aspartame, acesulfame-K, and sucralose are all safe for use during pregnancy.

MISLEADING FOOD LABELS. Foods labelled "sugarless" or "sugarfree," if they are made with nutritive sweeteners, may still provide the same amount of calories as the equivalent sugar-containing products. Thus, for weight loss, these products may not always be useful. In addition, patients must not consider them "free" foods to be eaten in unlimited quantity, because they may elevate blood glucose levels.

Foods labelled "dietetic" are not necessarily reduced-calorie foods. They may be lower in sodium or have other special dietary uses. Patients are advised that foods labelled dietetic may still contain significant amounts of sugar or fat.

It is also important to read the labels of "health foods"—especially snacks—because they often contain carbohydrates such as honey, brown sugar, and corn syrup. In addition, these supposedly healthy snacks frequently contain saturated vegetable fats (e.g., coconut or palm oil), hydrogenated vegetable fats, or animal fats, which may be contraindicated in patients with elevated blood lipid levels.

Exercise

Benefits

Exercise is extremely important in managing diabetes because of its effects on lowering blood glucose and reducing cardiovascular risk factors. Exercise lowers the blood glucose level by increasing the uptake of glucose by body muscles and by improving insulin utilization. It also improves circulation and muscle tone. Resistance (strength) training, such as weight lifting, can increase lean muscle mass, thereby increasing the resting metabolic rate. These effects are useful in diabetes in relation to losing weight, easing stress, and maintaining a feeling of well-being. Exercise also alters blood lipid levels, increasing levels of HDL and decreasing total cholesterol and triglyceride levels. This is especially important to the person with diabetes because of the increased risk of cardiovascular disease (Tomlin & Asimakopoulou, 2014). General guidelines for exercise in diabetes are presented in Chart 41-4.

Recommendations

Ideally, a person with diabetes should engage in regular exercise. Exercise recommendations must be altered as necessary for patients with diabetic complications, such as retinopathy, autonomic neuropathy, sensorimotor neuropathy, and cardiovascular disease (ADA, 2016b). Increased blood pressure associated with exercise may aggravate diabetic retinopathy and increase the risk of a hemorrhage into the vitreous or retina.

In general, a slow, gradual increase in the exercise period is encouraged. For many patients, walking is a safe and beneficial form of exercise that requires no special equipment (except for proper shoes) and can be performed anywhere. People with diabetes should discuss an exercise program with their primary provider and undergo

CHART 41-4

General Considerations for Exercise in Patients With Diabetes

The nurse instructs the patient to:

- Exercise three times each week with no more than 2 consecutive days without exercise.
- Perform resistance training twice a week if you have type 2 diabetes.
- Exercise at the same time of day (preferably when blood glucose levels are at their peak) and for the same duration each session.
- Use proper footwear and, if appropriate, other protective equipment (i.e., helmets for cycling).
- Avoid trauma to the lower extremities, especially if you have numbness due to peripheral neuropathy.
- Inspect feet daily after exercise.
- Avoid exercise in extreme heat or cold.
- Avoid exercise during periods of poor metabolic control.
- Stretch for 10 to 15 minutes before exercising.

Adapted from American Diabetes Association (ADA). (2016b). Standards of medical care in diabetes—2016. Classification and diagnosis of diabetes. *Diabetes Care, 39*(Suppl 1), S13–S24.

a careful medical evaluation with appropriate diagnostic studies before beginning a program (ADA, 2016f).

For patients who are older than 30 years and who have two or more risk factors for heart disease, an exercise stress test is recommended prior to starting an exercise program (ADA, 2016f). Risk factors for heart disease include hypertension, obesity, high cholesterol levels, abnormal resting electrocardiogram (ECG), sedentary lifestyle, smoking, male gender, and a family history of heart disease. An abnormal stress test may indicate cardiac ischemia. Typically, an abnormal stress test is followed by a cardiac catheterization and, in some cases, with an intervention such as angioplasty, stent placement, or cardiac surgery.

Exercise Precautions

Patients who have blood glucose levels exceeding (14 mmol/L) and who have ketones in their urine should not begin exercising until the urine test results are negative for ketones and the blood glucose level is closer to normal. Exercising with elevated blood glucose levels increases the secretion of glucagon, growth hormone, and catecholamines. The liver then releases more glucose, and the result is an increase in the blood glucose level (ADA, 2016b).

The physiologic decrease in circulating insulin that normally occurs with exercise cannot occur in patients treated with insulin. Initially, patients who require insulin should be taught to eat a 15-g carbohydrate snack (a fruit exchange) or a snack of complex carbohydrates with a protein before engaging in moderate exercise to prevent unexpected hypoglycemia. The exact amount of food needed varies from person to person and should be determined by blood glucose monitoring.

Another concern for patients who take insulin is hypoglycemia that occurs many hours after exercise. To avoid post-exercise hypoglycemia, especially after strenuous or prolonged exercise, the patient may need to eat a snack at the end of the exercise session and at bedtime and monitor the blood glucose level more frequently. Patients who are capable, knowledgeable, and responsible can learn to adjust their own insulin doses by working closely with a diabetes educator. Others need specific instructions on what to do when they exercise.

Patients taking insulin and participating in extended periods of exercise should test their blood glucose levels before, during, and after the exercise period, and they should snack on carbohydrates as needed to maintain blood glucose levels. Other participants or observers should be aware that the person exercising has diabetes, and they should know what assistance to give if severe hypoglycemia occurs.

In people with type 2 diabetes who are overweight or obese, exercise in addition to dietary management both improves glucose metabolism and enhances loss of body fat. Exercise coupled with weight loss improves insulin sensitivity and may decrease the need for insulin or oral antidiabetic agents (ADA, 2016b). Eventually, the patient's glucose tolerance may return to normal. Patients with type 2 diabetes who are not taking insulin or an oral agent may not need extra food before exercise.

Gerontologic Considerations

Physical activity that is consistent and realistic is beneficial to older adults with diabetes. Physical fitness in the older adult population with diabetes may lead to improved glycemic control, decreased risk for chronic vascular disease, and an improved quality of life (Eliopoulos, 2018; Weinger, Beverly, & Smaldone, 2014). Advantages of exercise in this population include a decrease in hyperglycemia, a general sense of well-being, and better use of ingested calories, resulting in weight reduction. Because there is an increased incidence of cardiovascular problems in older adults, a physical examination and exercise stress test may be warranted before an exercise program is initiated. A pattern of gradual, consistent exercise, including a combination of stretching, aerobic exercise, and resistance training, should be planned that does not exceed the patient's physical capacity. Physical impairment because of other chronic diseases must also be considered. In some cases, a physical therapy evaluation may be indicated, with the goal of determining exercises specific to the patient's needs and abilities. Tools such as the armchair fitness videos or the Go4life fitness booklet and video may be helpful (see resource section at the end of this chapter for links).

Monitoring Glucose Levels and Ketones

Blood glucose monitoring is a cornerstone of diabetes management, and **self-monitoring of blood glucose (SMBG)** levels by patients has dramatically altered diabetes care. Frequent SMBG enables people with diabetes to adjust the treatment regimen to obtain optimal blood glucose control, allowing for detection and prevention of hypoglycemia and hyperglycemia. Overall, monitoring plays a crucial role in normalizing blood glucose levels, which in turn may reduce the risk of long-term diabetic complications.

Various SMBG methods are available. Most involve obtaining a drop of blood from the fingertip, applying the blood to a special reagent strip, and allowing the blood to stay on the strip for the amount of time specified by the

CHART 41-5

Age-Related Changes That May Affect Diabetes and Its Management

Sensory Changes
Decreased vision
Decreased smell
Taste changes
Decreased proprioception
Diminished thirst

Gastrointestinal Changes
Dental problems
Appetite changes
Delayed gastric emptying
Decreased bowel motility

Activity/Exercise Pattern Changes
More sedentary

Renal Function Changes
Decreased function
Decreased drug clearance

Affective/Cognitive Changes
Medications/meals omitted or taken erratically

Socioeconomic Factors
Fad diets
Loneliness/Living alone
Lack of money/Lack of support system

Chronic Diseases
Hypertension
Arthritis
Neoplasms
Acute/chronic infections

Potential Drug Interactions
Use of another person's medications
Consulting multiple prescribers for different illnesses
Alcohol use/abuse

manufacturer (usually 5 to 30 seconds). The meter gives a digital readout of the blood glucose value. Advantages of the newer meters include less blood needed on the strips for an accurate reading and the ability to connect to a smartphone via Bluetooth. Other meters have audio components that are helpful for those with visual impairments. In addition, meters are available to check both blood glucose and blood ketone levels.

Advantages and Disadvantages of Self-Monitoring Systems

The monitoring method used by the patient must match his or her skill level. Factors affecting SMBG performance include visual acuity, fine motor coordination, cognitive ability, comfort with technology, willingness, and cost.

A potential hazard of all SMBG methods is that the patient may obtain and report erroneous blood glucose values as a result of using incorrect techniques. Some common sources of error include the following:

- Improper application of blood (e.g., drop too small)—there are meters that allow for a second application of blood
- Improper meter cleaning and maintenance (e.g., allowing dust or blood to accumulate on the optic window). This is not an issue in the biosensor type of meter.
- Damage to the reagent strips by heat or humidity; use of outdated strips
- Not washing hands prior to testing

The nurse plays an important role in providing initial teaching about SMBG techniques. Equally important is evaluating the techniques of patients who are experienced in self-monitoring. Every 12 months, patients should conduct a comparison of their meter with a simultaneous laboratory-measured blood glucose level at their local lab. There should not be any more than 15% difference between the two readings.

CANDIDATES FOR SELF-MONITORING. For everyone with diabetes, SMBG is useful for managing self-care. It is a key component of treatment for any intensive insulin therapy regimen (including two to four injections per day or insulin pumps) and for diabetes management during pregnancy. It is also recommended for patients with the following:

- Unstable diabetes
- A tendency for severe ketosis or hypoglycemia
- Hypoglycemia without warning symptoms

For patients not taking insulin, SMBG is helpful for monitoring the effectiveness of exercise, diet, and oral or injectable antihyperglycemic agents. It can also help in motivating patients to continue with treatment. For patients with type 2 diabetes, SMBG is recommended during periods of suspected hyperglycemia (e.g., illness) or hypoglycemia (e.g., unusual increased activity levels) (Diabetes Canada, 2018b).

FREQUENCY OF SELF-MONITORING. For most patients who require insulin, SMBG is recommended two to four times daily (usually before meals and at bedtime). For patients who take insulin before each meal, SMBG is required at least three times daily before meals to determine each dose (AADE, 2014; ADA, 2016d). Those not receiving insulin may be instructed to assess their blood glucose levels at least two or three times per week, including a 2-hour postprandial test. For all patients, testing is recommended whenever hypoglycemia or hyperglycemia is suspected; with changes in medications, activity, or diet; and with stress or illness.

RESPONDING TO SELF-MONITORING RESULTS. Patients are instructed to keep a record or logbook of blood glucose levels so that they can detect patterns. Testing is done at the peak action time of the medication to evaluate the need for dosage adjustments. To evaluate basal insulin and determine bolus insulin doses, testing is performed before meals. To determine efficacy of bolus insulin doses of short- or rapid-acting insulin, testing is done 2 hours after meals. Patients with type 2 diabetes are encouraged to test immediately before and 2 hours after the largest meal of the day. Patients who take insulin at bedtime or who are on an insulin infusion pump may be required to test at 3 AM periodically to ensure that the blood glucose level is remaining stable throughout the night. If a patient is unwilling or cannot afford to test frequently, then once or twice a day may be sufficient if the patient varies the time of day to test (e.g., before breakfast one day, before lunch the next day).

A tendency to discontinue SMBG is more likely to occur when patients do not receive instruction about using the results to alter their treatment regimen. Instructions vary according to the patient's understanding and the health care provider's philosophy of diabetes management. At the very least, patients should be given parameters for calling their health care provider. Patients using intensive insulin therapy regimens may be instructed in the use of insulin to carbohydrate ratios and/or insulin sensitivity factors to adjust doses of bolus insulin. Or the patient may elect to keep a fixed dose of insulin and eat a consistent number of carbohydrates at each meal. Baseline patterns should be established by SMBG for 1 to 2 weeks.

Using a Continuous Glucose Monitoring System

A continuous glucose monitoring system (CGMS) can be used to monitor blood glucose levels. A sensor attached to an infusion set, which is similar to an insulin pump infusion set, is inserted subcutaneously in the abdomen and connected to the device worn on the patient's clothing or placed in a pocket. After 120 to 168 hours, the data from the device are downloaded, and blood glucose readings are analyzed. Although the CGMS cannot be used for making decisions about specific insulin doses, it can be used to determine whether treatment is adequate over a 24-hour period. This device is most useful in patients with type 1 diabetes (ADA, 2016d).

Testing for Glycosylated Hemoglobin

Glycated hemoglobin (also referred to as glycosylated hemoglobin, $HgbA_{1C}$, or A1C) is a measure of glucose control for the past 3 months (ADA, 2016e). When blood glucose levels are elevated, glucose molecules attach to hemoglobin in red blood cells. The longer the amount of glucose in the blood remains above normal, the more glucose binds to hemoglobin and the higher the glycated hemoglobin level becomes. This complex (hemoglobin attached to the glucose) is permanent and lasts for the life of an individual red blood cell, approximately 120 days. If near-normal blood glucose levels are maintained, with only occasional increases, the overall value will not be greatly elevated. However, if the blood glucose values are consistently high, then the test result is also elevated. If the patient reports mostly normal SMBG results but the glycated hemoglobin is high, there may be errors in the methods used for glucose monitoring, errors in recording results, or frequent elevations in glucose levels at times during the day when the patient is not usually monitoring blood sugar levels. Normal values typically range from 4% to 6% and indicate consistently near-normal blood glucose concentrations. The target range for people with diabetes is less than 7% (ADA, 2016e).

Testing for Ketones

Ketones (or ketone bodies) in the urine signal that control of type 1 diabetes is deteriorating and the risk of DKA is high. When there is almost no effective insulin available, the body starts to break down stored fat for energy. Ketone bodies are by-products of this fat breakdown, and they accumulate in the blood and urine. Urine testing is the most common method used for self-testing of ketone bodies by patients. A meter that enables testing of blood for ketones is available and is more accurate than urine testing, but this method of testing is not widely used.

Most commonly, patients use a urine dipstick (Ketostix or Chemstrip uK) to detect ketonuria. The reagent pad on the strip turns purplish when ketones are present. (One of the ketone bodies is called *acetone*, and this term is frequently used interchangeably with the term *ketones*.) Other strips are available for measuring both urine glucose and ketones (Keto-Diastix or Chemstrip uGK). Large amounts of ketones may depress the colour response of the glucose test area.

Urine ketone testing should be performed whenever patients with type 1 diabetes have glucosuria or persistently elevated blood glucose levels (more than 14.0 mmol/L for two testing periods in a row) and during illness, in pregnancy with pre-existing diabetes, and in gestational diabetes (AADE, 2014; ADA, 2016e).

Pharmacologic Therapy

As stated previously, insulin is secreted by the beta cells of the islets of Langerhans and works to lower the blood glucose level after meals by facilitating the uptake and utilization of glucose by muscle, fat, and liver cells. In the absence of adequate secretion and/or response to insulin, pharmacologic therapy is essential.

Insulin Therapy and Insulin Preparations

Because the body loses the ability to produce insulin in type 1 diabetes, exogenous insulin must be administered for life. In type 2 diabetes, insulin may be necessary on a long-term basis to control glucose levels if diet and oral/injectable agents fail. In addition, some patients in whom type 2 diabetes is usually controlled by diet alone or by diet and an oral/injectable agent may require insulin temporarily during illness, infection, pregnancy, surgery, or some other stressful event. In many cases, insulin injections are administered two or more times daily to control the blood glucose level. Because the insulin dose required by the individual patient is determined by the level of glucose in the blood, accurate monitoring of blood glucose levels is essential; thus, SMBG has become a cornerstone of insulin therapy. A number of insulin preparations are available. They vary according to three main characteristics: time course of action, species (source), and manufacturer.

TIME COURSE OF ACTION. Insulins may be grouped into several categories based on the onset, peak, and duration of action (Table 41-2). Human insulin preparations have a shorter duration of action than insulin from animal sources because the presence of animal proteins triggers an immune response that results in the binding of animal insulin, which slows its availability.

TABLE 41-2 Selected Categories of Insulin

Time Course	Agent	Onset	Peak	Duration	Indications
Rapid acting	lispro (Humalog) aspart (NovoLog) glulisine (Apidra)	10–15 minutes 5–15 minutes 5–15 minutes	1 hour 40–50 minutes 30–60 minutes	2–4 hours 2–4 hours 2 hours	Used for rapid reduction of glucose level, to treat postprandial hyperglycemia, and/or to prevent nocturnal hypoglycemia
Short acting	regular (Humulin R, Novolin R, Iletin II Regular)	30–60 minutes	2–3 hours	4–6 hours	Usually given 20–30 minutes before a meal; may be taken alone or in combination with longer-acting insulin
Intermediate acting	NPH (neutral protamine Hagedorn)	2–4 hours	4–12 hours	16–20 hours	Usually taken after food
	(Humulin N, Iletin II Lente, Iletin II NPH, Novolin N [NPH])	3–4 hours	4–12 hours	16–20 hours	
Very long acting	glargine (Lantus) detemir (Levemir) glargine (Toujeo)	1 hour 6 hours	Continuous (no peak)	24 hours 24–36 hours	Used for basal dose
Rapid-acting inhaled insulin	Afrezza	<15 minutes	~50 minutes	2–3 hours	Used as rapid-acting insulin

Rapid-acting analogue (clear) insulins such as insulin lispro (Humalog), insulin glulisine (Apidra) and insulin aspart (NovoRapid) are blood glucose–lowering agents that produce a more rapid effect that is of shorter duration than regular insulin. These insulins have an onset of 10 to 15 minutes, a peak action of 60 to 90 minutes after injection, and a duration of 4 to 5 hours. Because of their rapid onset, patients should be instructed to eat within 10 to 15 minutes after injection. Insulin aspart (FiAsp), which has a slightly faster onset of action, is also available. Because of the short duration of action of these insulin analogues, patients with type 1 diabetes and some patients with type 2 or gestational diabetes also require a long-acting insulin to maintain glucose control. Basal insulin is necessary to maintain blood glucose levels irrespective of meals. A constant level of insulin is required at all times. Intermediate-acting insulins function as basal insulins but may have to be split into two injections to achieve 24-hour coverage.

Short-acting (clear) insulins have an onset of 30 minutes to 1 hour, a peak action of 2 to 4 hours, and a duration of 5 to 8 hours. They are usually administered 20 to 30 minutes before a meal, either alone or in combination with a longer-acting insulin. Humulin R and Novolin ge Toronto are examples of this type of insulin.

Intermediate-acting (cloudy) insulins, called *neutral protamine Hagedorn* (NPH) *insulin*, have an onset of 1 to 3 hours, a peak of 5 to 8 hours, and a duration of 18 hours. Intermediate-acting insulins, which are similar in their time course of action, appear white and cloudy and must be resuspended prior to injection. If NPH insulin is taken alone, it is not crucial that it be taken 30 minutes before the meal. Humulin N and Novolin ge NPH, are examples of these insulins.

"Peakless" basal insulin, insulin glargine (Lantus or Basaglar), is absorbed very slowly over 24 hours and can be given once a day. It is also available in a higher concentration (300 u/mL) as Toujeo, which is ideal for patients on high doses of glargine. Because insulin glargine is in a suspension with a pH of 4, it cannot be mixed with other insulins as a precipitate may form. It is generally given once a day at bedtime or in the morning, depending on the patient's preference. Another basal insulin analogue is insulin detemir (Levemir), and its duration of action is up to 24 hours depending on dosage; this insulin can be administered once or twice daily depending on the patient's need.

Insulin degludec (Tresiba) is a new peakless insulin available on the Canadian market with a long duration of action (42 hours). It is administered once daily and is ideal for patients at high risk of hypoglycemia, those that work shift work, and those that travel frequently.

NURSING ALERT

When administering insulin, it is very important to read the label carefully and to be sure that the correct type of insulin is administered.

The nurse may find that different sources list differing numbers of hours for the onset, peak, and duration of action of the main types of insulin, and patient responses may vary (i.e., larger doses prolong onset, duration, and peak). The nurse should focus on which meals—and snacks—are being "covered" by which insulin doses. In general, the rapid- and short-acting insulins are expected to cover the rise in glucose levels after meals, immediately after the injection; the intermediate-acting insulins are expected to cover subsequent meals; and the long-acting insulins provide a relatively constant level of insulin and act as a basal insulin. Use of both rapid/short-acting and intermediate- and long-acting insulins mimics the physiologic release of insulin by the pancreas.

INSULIN REGIMENS. Insulin regimens vary from one to four injections per day. Usually, there is a combination of a short-acting insulin and a longer-acting insulin. The normally functioning pancreas continuously secretes small amounts of insulin during the day and night. In addition, whenever blood glucose rises after ingestion of food, there is a rapid burst of insulin secretion in proportion to the glucose-raising effect of the food. The goal of all but the simplest, one-injection insulin regimens is to mimic this usual physiologic pattern of insulin secretion in response to food intake and activity patterns. Table 41-3 depicts several insulin regimens and the advantages and disadvantages of each.

Patients can learn to use SMBG results and carbohydrate counting to vary the insulin doses. This allows patients more flexibility in the timing and content of meals and exercise periods. However, complex insulin regimens require a strong level of commitment, intensive education, and close follow-up by the health care team. In addition, patients aiming for normal blood glucose levels may run the risk of more hypoglycemic reactions.

The type of regimen used by any particular patient varies. For example, patient knowledge, willingness, goals, health status, and finances all may affect decisions regarding insulin treatment. There are two general approaches to insulin therapy: conventional and intensive.

Conventional Regimen. One approach to insulin therapy is to simplify the insulin regimen as much as possible, with the aim of avoiding the acute complications of diabetes (hypoglycemia and symptomatic hyperglycemia). With this type of simplified regimen (e.g., one or more injections of a mixture of short- and intermediate-acting insulins per day), patients may frequently have blood glucose levels above normal. The exception is the patient who never varies meal patterns and activity levels. This approach would be appropriate for the terminally ill, the older adult who is frail with limited self-care abilities, or any patient who is unwilling or unable to engage in the self-management activities that are part of a more complex insulin regimen.

Intensive Regimen. The second approach is to use a more complex insulin regimen to achieve as much control over blood glucose levels as is safe and practical. A more complex insulin regimen allows the patient more flexibility to change the insulin doses from day to day in accordance with changes in eating and activity patterns, with stress and illness, and as needed for variations in the prevailing glucose level.

While intensive treatment (three or four injections of insulin per day) reduces the risk of complications, not all people with diabetes are candidates for very tight control of blood glucose. The risk of severe hypoglycemia increases threefold in patients receiving intensive treatment (ADA, 2016d). Patients who have received a kidney transplant because of nephropathy and chronic kidney failure should follow an intensive insulin regimen to preserve function of the new kidney.

Those who are not candidates include those with:

- Nervous system disorders rendering them unaware of hypoglycemic episodes (e.g., those with autonomic neuropathy)
- Recurring severe hypoglycemia
- Irreversible diabetic complications, such as blindness or ESKD
- Severe cerebrovascular or cardiovascular disease
- Ineffective self-care skills
- Limited life expectancy

An exception is the patient who has received a kidney transplant because of nephropathy and chronic renal failure; this patient should be on an intensive regimen to preserve function of the transplanted kidney.

The patient needs to be involved in the decision regarding which insulin regimen to use. Patients need to compare the potential benefits of different regimens with the potential costs (e.g., time involved, number of injections or finger sticks for glucose testing, amount of record keeping). There are no set guidelines as to which insulin regimen should be used for which patients. It must not be assumed that an older patient or a patient with visual impairment should automatically be given a simplified regimen. Likewise, it must not be assumed that all people will want to be involved in a complex treatment regimen. Nurses play an important role in educating patients about the different approaches to insulin therapy. Nurses should refer patients to diabetes specialists or diabetes education centres, when available, for further training and education in the various insulin treatment regimens.

COMPLICATIONS OF INSULIN THERAPY

Local Allergic Reactions. A local allergic reaction (redness, swelling, tenderness, and induration or a 2- to 4-cm wheal) may appear at the injection site 1 to 2 hours after the administration of insulin. Reactions usually resolve in a few hours or days. If they do not resolve, another type of insulin can be prescribed (Comerford, 2015).

Systemic Allergic Reactions. Systemic allergic reactions to insulin are rare. When they do occur, there is an immediate local skin reaction that gradually spreads into generalized urticaria (hives). The treatment is desensitization, with small doses of insulin administered in gradually increasing amounts using a desensitization kit. These rare reactions are occasionally associated with generalized edema or anaphylaxis.

Insulin Lipodystrophy. Lipodystrophy refers to a localized reaction, in the form of either lipoatrophy or lipohypertrophy, occurring at the site of insulin injections. Lipoatrophy is loss of subcutaneous fat and appears as slight dimpling or more serious pitting of subcutaneous fat. The use of human insulin has almost eliminated this disfiguring complication.

Lipohypertrophy, the development of fibrofatty masses at the injection site, is caused by the repeated use of an injection site. If insulin is injected into scarred areas, absorption may be delayed. To prevent this, it is imperative that the patient rotates injection sites each time an insulin injection is administered. The patient should avoid injecting insulin into these areas until the hypertrophy disappears.

Insulin Resistance. Most patients, regardless if they have type 1 or type 2 diabetes, may have some degree of insulin resistance. This may occur for various reasons, including the use of certain medications, such as corticosteroids and protease inhibitors, obesity, and disorders of cellular mechanisms. Some patients with diabetes taking insulin may develop antibodies to insulin, decreasing the amount

TABLE 41-3 Insulin Regimens

Schematic Representation	Description	Advantages	Disadvantages
Normal pancreas 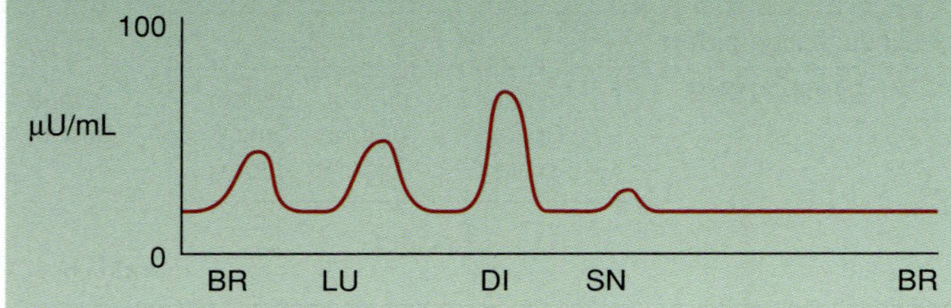	Insulin release increases when blood glucose levels rise and continues at a low steady rate between meals		
1 injection per day 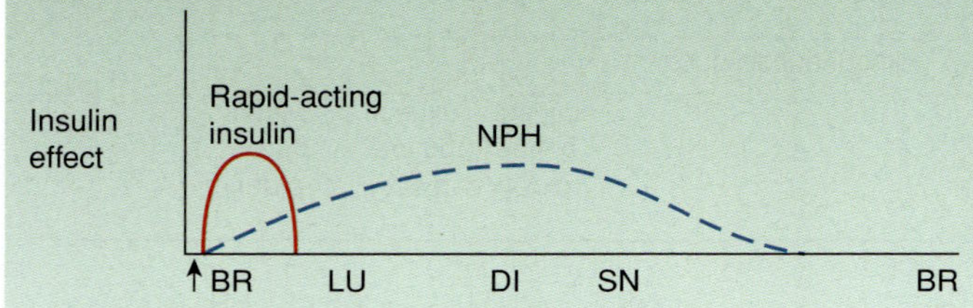	Before breakfast: • NPH or • NPH with rapid-acting insulin	Simple regimen	Difficult to control fasting blood glucose if effects of NPH do not last Afternoon hypoglycemia may result from attempts to control fasting glucose level by increasing NPH dose
2 injections per day–mixed 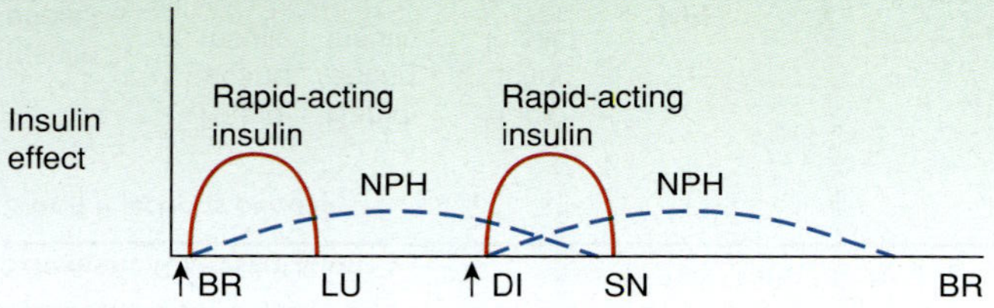	Before breakfast and dinner: • NPH or • NPH with rapid-acting insulin or • Premixed (rapid-acting insulin) insulin	Simplest regimen that attempts to mimic normal pancreas	Need relatively fixed schedule of meals and exercise Cannot independently adjust NPH or regular if premixed insulin is used

continued >

TABLE 41-3 Insulin Regimens (Continued)

Schematic Representation	Description	Advantages	Disadvantages
3 or 4 injections per day 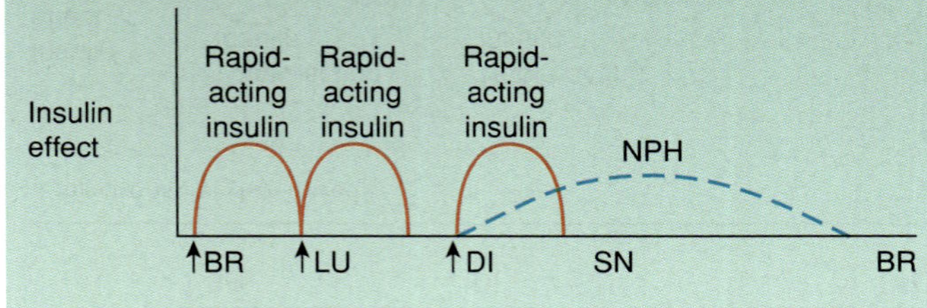	Rapid-acting insulin before each meal with: • NPH at dinner or • NPH at bedtime or • Long-acting insulin one or two times a day	More closely mimics normal pancreas than 3-injection regimen Each premeal dose of regular insulin decided independently More flexibility with meals and exercise	Requires more injections than other regimens Requires multiple blood glucose tests on a daily basis Requires intensive education and follow-up
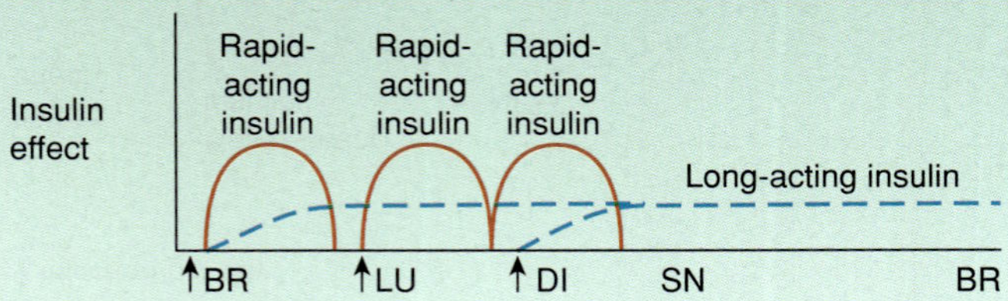			
Insulin pump 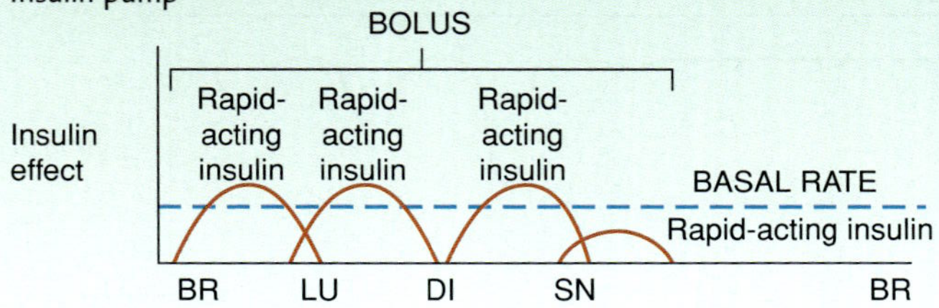	Uses ONLY rapid-acting insulin infused at continuous, low rate called *basal rate* (commonly 0.5–1.5 units/h) and premeal *bolus doses* activated by pump wearer	Most closely mimics normal pancreas Decreases unpredictable peaks of intermediate- and long-acting insulins Increases meal and exercise flexibility	Requires intensive training and frequent follow-up Potential for mechanical problems Requires multiple blood glucose tests on a daily basis Potential increase in expenses (depending on insurance coverage)

Note: Rapid-acting insulin—lispro, aspart, or glulisine (Apidra).

BR, breakfast; LU, lunch; DI, dinner; SN, snack; NPH, neutral protamine Hagedorn; regular; ↑, insulin injections.

Adapted from Comerford, K. C. (2015). *Nursing 2015 drug handbook*. Philadelphia, PA: Wolters Kluwer; U.S. Food and Drug Administration (FDA). (2014). FDA approves Afrezza to treat diabetes. Retrieved on June 21, 2016, from www.fda.gov/newsevents/newsroom/pressannouncements/ucm403122.htm

of insulin available for use. This is more prevalent with the animal insulins, although human insulins may cause this to a lesser degree. Clinical insulin resistance has been defined as a daily insulin requirement of 200 units or more. Highly concentrated insulin U500 (Entuzity), Lispro 200 u/mL (Humalog), Glargine 300 u/mL (Toujeo) are available to help reduce the volume of insulin taken in patients requiring more than 200 units per day.

Morning Hyperglycemia. An elevated blood glucose level upon arising in the morning may be caused by an insufficient level of insulin due to several causes: the Dawn phenomenon, the Somogyi effect, or insulin waning. The dawn phenomenon is characterized by a relatively normal blood glucose level until approximately 3 AM, when blood glucose levels begin to rise, due to the physiologic release of counterregulatory hormones such as cortisone, growth hormone, glucagon and norepinephrine. It must be distinguished from insulin waning (the progressive increase in blood glucose from bedtime to morning) or the Somogyi effect (nocturnal hypoglycemia followed by rebound hyperglycemia). Insulin waning is frequently seen if the evening NPH dose is administered before dinner and may be prevented by moving the evening dose of NPH insulin to bedtime.

It may be difficult to tell from the patient's history which of these causes is responsible for morning hyperglycemia. To determine the cause, the patient should test their blood glucose levels at bedtime, at 3 AM, and upon awakening to provide information that can be used in making adjustments in insulin to avoid morning hyperglycemia. Table 41-4 provides a summary of the differences among insulin waning, the dawn phenomenon, and the Somogyi effect.

METHODS OF INSULIN DELIVERY

Insulin Pens. Insulin pens use small (150- to 300-unit) prefilled insulin cartridges that are loaded into a penlike holder. A disposable needle is attached to the device for insulin injection. Insulin is delivered by dialing in a dose or pushing a button for every 1- or 2-unit increment given. People using these devices still need to insert the needle for each injection (see Fig. 41-2); however, they do not need to carry insulin bottles or draw up insulin before each injection. These devices are most useful for patients who need to inject only one type of insulin at a time (e.g., premeal rapid-acting insulin three times a day and bedtime NPH insulin) or who can use the premixed insulins. These pens are convenient for those who administer insulin before dinner if eating out or travelling. They are also useful for patients with impaired manual dexterity, vision, or cognitive function, which makes the use of traditional syringes difficult.

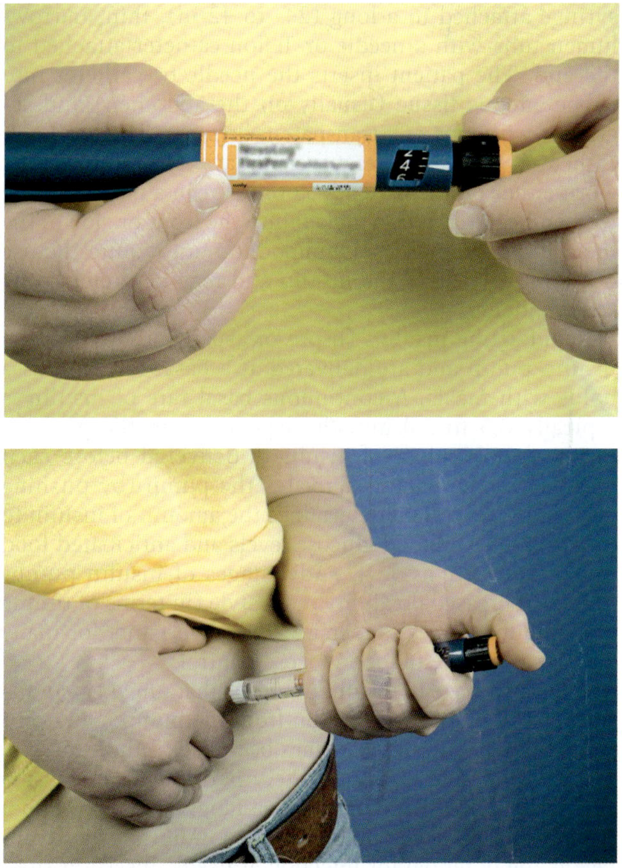

FIGURE 41-2. Prefilled insulin syringe.

TABLE 41-4 Causes of Morning Hyperglycemia

Characteristic	Treatment
Insulin Waning	
Progressive rise in blood glucose from bedtime to morning	Increase evening (predinner or bedtime) dose of intermediate- or long-acting insulin, or institute a dose of insulin before the evening meal if one is not already in use.
Dawn Phenomenon	
Relatively normal blood glucose until about 3 AM, when the level begins to rise	Change time of injection of evening intermediate-acting insulin from dinnertime to bedtime.
Somogyi Effect	
Normal or elevated blood glucose at bedtime, a decrease at 2–3 AM to hypoglycemic levels, and a subsequent increase caused by the production of counterregulatory hormones	Decrease evening (predinner or bedtime) dose of intermediate- or long-acting insulin, or increase bedtime snack.

Jet Injectors. As an alternative to needle injections, jet injection devices deliver insulin through the skin under pressure in an extremely fine stream. These devices are more expensive than other alternative devices mentioned previously and require thorough training and supervision when first used. In addition, patients should be cautioned that absorption rates, peak insulin activity, and insulin levels may be different when changing to a jet injector. (Insulin administered by jet injector is usually absorbed faster.) Bruising has occurred in some patients with use of the jet injector.

Insulin Pumps. **Continuous subcutaneous insulin infusion** involves the use of small, externally worn devices (insulin pumps) that closely mimic the functioning of the normal pancreas (ADA, 2016f). Insulin pumps contain a 3-mL syringe attached to a long (24- to 42-in), thin, narrow-lumen tube with a needle or Teflon catheter attached to the end. The patient inserts the needle or catheter into subcutaneous tissue (usually on the abdomen) and secures it with tape or a transparent dressing. The needle or catheter is changed at least every 3 days. The pump is then worn either on the patient's clothing or in a pocket. Some women keep the pump tucked into the front or side of the bra. Pumps such as the Omnipod, do not require the use of tubing to deliver the insulin and may be preferred by some patients.

Rapid-acting insulins (lispro or aspart) are used in the insulin pump and are delivered at a basal rate and as a bolus with meals. A continuous basal rate of insulin is typically 0.5 to 2.0 units/h, depending on the patient's needs. A bolus dose of insulin is delivered before each meal when the patient activates the pump (by pushing buttons). The patient determines the amount of insulin to infuse based on blood glucose levels and anticipated food intake and activity level. Advantages of insulin pumps include increased flexibility in lifestyle (in terms of timing and amount of meals, exercise, and travel) and, for many patients, improved blood glucose control.

A disadvantage of insulin pumps is that unexpected disruptions in the flow of insulin from the pump may occur if the tubing or needle becomes occluded, if the supply of insulin runs out, or if the battery is depleted, increasing the risk of DKA. Patients must be taught to troubleshoot to prevent the development of DKA. Another disadvantage is the potential for infection at needle insertion sites. Hypoglycemia may occur with insulin pump therapy; however, this is usually related to the lowered blood glucose levels that many patients achieve rather than to a specific problem with the pump itself.

Some patients find that wearing the pump for 24 hours each day is an inconvenience. However, the pump can easily be disconnected, per patient preference, for limited periods (e.g., for showering, exercise, or sexual activity).

Insulin pump candidates must be willing to assess blood glucose levels multiple times daily. Most important, patients using insulin pumps must have extensive education in the use of the insulin pump and in self-management of blood glucose and insulin doses. They must work closely with a team of health care professionals who are experienced in insulin pump therapy—specifically, an endocrinologist, a dietitian, and a certified diabetes educator.

Transplantation of Pancreatic Cells. Transplantation of the whole pancreas or a segment of the pancreas is being performed on a limited population (mostly diabetic patients receiving kidney transplantations simultaneously). One main issue regarding pancreatic transplantation is weighing the risks of antirejection medications against the advantages of pancreas transplantation.

Another approach is the implantation of insulin-producing pancreatic islet cells (Diabetes Canada, 2018a). This latter approach involves a less extensive surgical procedure and a potentially lower incidence of immunogenic problems. However, thus far, independence from exogenous insulin declines with time from 70% at 1 year to 10% at 5 years after transplantation of islet cells. A recent study of patients with **islet cell transplants** using less toxic antirejection drugs has shown promise (the Edmonton Protocol) (Shapiro, Ryan, & Lakey, 2001).

Oral/Injectable Antihyperglycemic Agents

Oral/injectable antihyperglycemic agents may be effective for patients who have type 2 diabetes that cannot be treated by diet and exercise alone; however, they cannot be used during pregnancy. In Canada, oral antihyperglycemic agents include the sulfonylureas/meglitinides, **biguanides**, **alpha-glucosidase inhibitors**, **thiazolidinediones** (TZDs), **dipeptidyl-dipeptidase 4 (DPP-4) inhibitors**, and **sodium glucose cotransporter 2 (SGLT-2) inhibitors**. Injectable antihyperglycemics include the **glucagon-like peptide 1 (GLP-1) receptor agonists**.

Sulfonylureas/Meglitinides

Sulfonylureas and meglitinides are considered insulin secretagogues because their action increases the secretion of insulin by the pancreatic beta cells.

The sulfonylureas exert their primary action by directly stimulating the pancreas to secrete insulin. Therefore, a functioning pancreas is necessary for these agents to be effective, and they cannot be used in patients with type 1 diabetes. These agents improve insulin action at the cellular level and may also directly decrease glucose production by the liver.

The sulfonylureas can be divided into first- and second-generation categories. First-generation **sulfonylureas** include **tolbutamide** and **chlorpropamide** and are very rarely used. Second-generation sulfonylureas include **glyburide** (Diabeta), **gliclazide** (Diamicron/Diamicron MR) and **Glimepiride** (Amaryl). Second-generation sulfonylureas have the advantage of a shorter half-life and excretion by both the kidney and the liver. This makes these medications safer to use in older people, in whom accumulation of the medication can cause recurring hypoglycemia.

Meglitinides have a very similar mechanism of action to the sulfonylureas. Repaglinide (Gluconorm) is the only medication available in this class and binds to the sulfonylurea receptor on the beta cell and stimulates the release of insulin. Therefore, its effectiveness also depends on the presence of functioning beta cells, so is contraindicated in patients with type 1 diabetes. Repaglinide has a fast action and a short duration. It should be taken before each meal to stimulate the release of insulin in response to that meal. It is also indicated for use in combination with metformin in patients whose hyperglycemia cannot be controlled by exercise, diet, and either metformin or repaglinide alone.

The most common side effects of these medications are GI symptoms and dermatologic reactions. Hypoglycemia may occur when an excessive dose of a sulfonylurea is used or when the patient omits or delays meals, reduces food intake, or increases activity. Because of the prolonged hypoglycemic effects of these agents (especially chlorpropamide), some patients need to be hospitalized for treatment of oral agent–induced hypoglycemia. Another side effect of chlorpropamide is a disulfiram type of reaction when alcohol is ingested (see Alcohol Consumption section for more information). Some medications may directly interact with sulfonylureas, potentiating their hypoglycemic effects (e.g., sulfonamide antibiotics). In addition, certain medications may independently affect blood glucose levels, thereby indirectly interfering with these agents. Medications that may increase glucose levels include non–potassium sparing diuretics, corticosteroids, estrogen compounds, and phenytoin. Medications that may cause hypoglycemia include salicylates, propranolol, monoamine oxidase inhibitors, and pentamidine.

Biguanides

The biguanide class includes metformin (Glucophage) and produces its antihyperglycemic effects by facilitating insulin's action on peripheral receptor sites. Therefore, it can be used only in the presence of insulin. Biguanides have no effect on pancreatic beta cells. Biguanides used with a sulfonylurea may enhance the glucose-lowering effect more than either medication used alone. Lactic acidosis is a rare and serious complication of biguanide therapy in patients with renal impairment; the patient must be monitored closely when therapy is initiated or when dosage changes. Medications that may interact with biguanides include anticoagulants, corticosteroids, diuretics, and oral contraceptives. Metformin should be used with caution in patients with renal impairment (creatinine clearance of less than 30 mL/min). Metformin should not be administered for 2 days before any diagnostic testing that may require use of a contrast agent. These situations increase the risk for lactic acidosis.

Alpha-Glucosidase Inhibitors

Acarbose (Glucobay) is an oral alpha-glucosidase inhibitor used in type 2 diabetes management. It works by delaying the absorption of glucose in the intestinal system, resulting in a lower postprandial blood glucose level. As a consequence of plasma glucose reduction, A1C levels drop (approximately 0.5'% to 1.0%). In contrast to the sulfonylureas, acarbose does not enhance insulin secretion. It can be used alone with dietary treatment as monotherapy or in combination with sulfonylureas, TZDs, or meglitinides. When this medication is used in combination with sulfonylureas or meglitinides, hypoglycemia may occur. The patient must be advised that if hypoglycemia occurs, sucrose absorption will be blocked and treatment for hypoglycemia should be in the form of glucose, such as glucose tablets. The advantage of an oral alpha-glucosidase inhibitor is that it is not systemically absorbed and is safe to use. The side effects are diarrhea and flatulence. These effects may be minimized by starting at a very low dose and increasing the dose gradually. Because acarbose affects food absorption, it must be taken immediately before a meal, making therapeutic adherence a potential problem.

Thiazolidinediones (TZDs)

Rosiglitazone (Avandia) and pioglitazone (Actos) are oral diabetes medications categorized as **TZDs**. They are indicated for patients with type 2 diabetes but are not recommended for use with insulin injections or in those whose blood glucose control is inadequate (A1C level greater than 8.5%). They have also been approved as first-line agents to treat type 2 diabetes, in combination with diet. TZDs enhance insulin action at the receptor site without increasing insulin secretion from the beta cells of the pancreas. These medications may take up to 3 months to exert their effect.

These medications may affect liver function; therefore, liver function studies must be performed at baseline and at frequent intervals (monthly for the first 12 months of treatment and quarterly thereafter). Women should be informed that TZDs can cause resumption of ovulation in perimenopausal anovulatory women, making pregnancy a possibility.

Although TZDs are very effective in their blood glucose lowering capabilities, their use has fallen out of favour due to side effects. Pioglitazone has been associated with an increased risk of bladder cancer, especially in those with a family history of bladder cancer and myocardial infarction. Since the time this article was released, many practitioners have switched and employ alternative oral agents to attempt to achieve glycemic control in their patients.

Dipeptidyl Peptidase IV (DPP-4) Inhibitors

Dipeptidyl peptidase IV inhibitors (gliptins) are a new class of oral agents. These agents block the enzyme dipeptidyl peptidase 4, which in turn prevents the inactivation of glucagon-like peptide (GLP), an incretin hormone released when nutrients are ingested. GLP, one type of incretin hormone, is responsible for many metabolic effects that regulate glucose hemostasis, including suppression of glucagon secretion, enhancement of glucose disposal, and slowing of gastric emptying. In Canada, there are four DPP-4 inhibitors currently available: **sitagliptin** (Januvia), **alogliptin** (Nesina), **linagliptin** (Trajenta), and **saxagliptin** (Onglyza). These medications can be used as monotherapy or in combination with metformin.

Sodium Glucose Cotransporter 2 (SGLT-2) Inhibitors

The SGLT-2 inhibitors include **canagliflozin** (Invokana), **dapagliflozin** (Forxiga), and **empagliflozin** (Jardiance). They work by inhibiting the **sodium glucose transporter** protein within the kidney that works to reabsorb the glucose from the filtered blood. As a result, the glucose is excreted through the urine. Empagliflozin and canagliflozin have shown beneficial cardiovascular outcomes through the EMPA-REG and CANVAS trials.

Side effects of the SGLT-2 inhibitors may include urinary tract infections, yeast infections of the male and female genitalia and hypoglycemia, when used in combination with other medications. As well, there is an increased risk of euglycemic diabetic ketoacidosis (DKA), especially in those patients who have been using insulin on an ongoing basis. Patients who develop this have all the symptoms of DKA (increased anion gap, nausea and vomiting and ketones, but have normal to slightly elevated blood glucose levels). There have also been reports of increased toe amputations and acute kidney injury with these medications. These agents are not recommended for use in patients with type 1 diabetes at this time.

Glucagon-Like Peptide (GLP-1) Receptor agonists

Glucagon-like peptide is an incretin hormone that is released from the intestine in response to food intake. The hormone works to increase insulin secretion, decrease glucagon release, increase satiety and slow gastric emptying. Medications available in this class include liraglutide

(Victoza), exenatide (Byetta, Bydureon), dulaglutide (Trulicity), lixisenatide (Adlyxine), and semaglutide (Ozempic). These medications are administered as subcutaneous injections. In addition to helping to lower blood glucose levels, the GLP-1 agonists have also been noted to aid in weight loss, which may lower insulin resistance.

The major side effects of these medications are mainly GI in nature including nausea and diarrhea. They should be titrated to effect slowly in order to lessen the GI effects.

General Considerations for Oral Agents

In individuals with type 2 diabetes, if glycemic targets are not achieved using lifestyle management within 2 to 3 months, an antihyperglycemic agent should be initiated [Grade A, Level 1A (1)]. This therapy should begin concomitantly with initial lifestyle management if A1C is greater than or equal to 8.5%. Additionally, initiating combination therapy with two agents, one of which may be insulin, should be considered, especially if symptomatic hyperglycemia and metabolic decompensation is noted [Grade D, Consensus].

Metformin is recommended as the initial medication of choice in patients with type 2 diabetes. If additional therapy is needed, any other agent may be added second line; however, if the patient has a history of cardiovascular disease, a GLP-1 agonist or SGLT-2 inhibitor should be considered. These adjustments to and/or additions of antihyperglycemic agents should be made in order to attain target A1C within 3 to 6 months.

When basal insulin is added to antihyperglycemic agents, long-acting analogues (detemir or glargine) may be used instead of intermediate-acting NPH to reduce the risk of nocturnal and symptomatic hypoglycemia [Grade A, Level 1A (4–6)]. When bolus insulin is added, rapid-acting analogues may be used instead of regular insulin to improve glycemic control [Grade B, Level 2 (7)] and to reduce the risk of hyperglycemia [Grade D, Consensus].

The choice of pharmacologic treatment agents should be individualized, taking into consideration patient characteristics including degree of hyperglycemia, presence of comorbidities, patient preference (and ability to access treatments). In addition, the properties of treatment, including blood glucose lowering capacity, risk of hypoglycemia, effects on body weight, side effects, and contraindications should be taken into consideration when choosing therapy. All individuals with type 2 diabetes currently using or starting therapy with insulin or insulin secretagogues should be counselled about the prevention, recognition, and treatment of drug-induced hypoglycemia.

Patients need to understand that oral/injectable agents are prescribed as an addition to, not as a substitute for, other treatment modalities such as diet and exercise. The use of oral/injectable antihyperglycemic medications may need to be halted temporarily and insulin prescribed if hyperglycemia develops that is attributable to infection, trauma, or surgery.

In time, oral/injectable antihyperglycemic agents may no longer be effective in controlling the patient's diabetes. In such cases, the patient is treated with insulin. Approximately half of all patients who initially use oral/injectable antihyperglycemic agents eventually require insulin. This is referred to as a secondary failure. Primary failure occurs when the blood glucose level remains high a month after initial medication use.

Because the mechanisms of action vary (Fig. 41-3), the blood glucose lowering effect may be enhanced by using multiple medications. Using a combination of oral/injectable agents with insulin may help to lower the dose of insulin needed, which in turn may prevent weight gain in patients with type 2 diabetes.

Nursing Management

Nursing management of the patient with diabetes can involve treatment of a wide variety of physiologic disorders, depending on the patient's health status and whether the patient is newly diagnosed or seeks care for an unrelated health problem. Nursing management of the newly diagnosed patient and the patient with diabetes as a

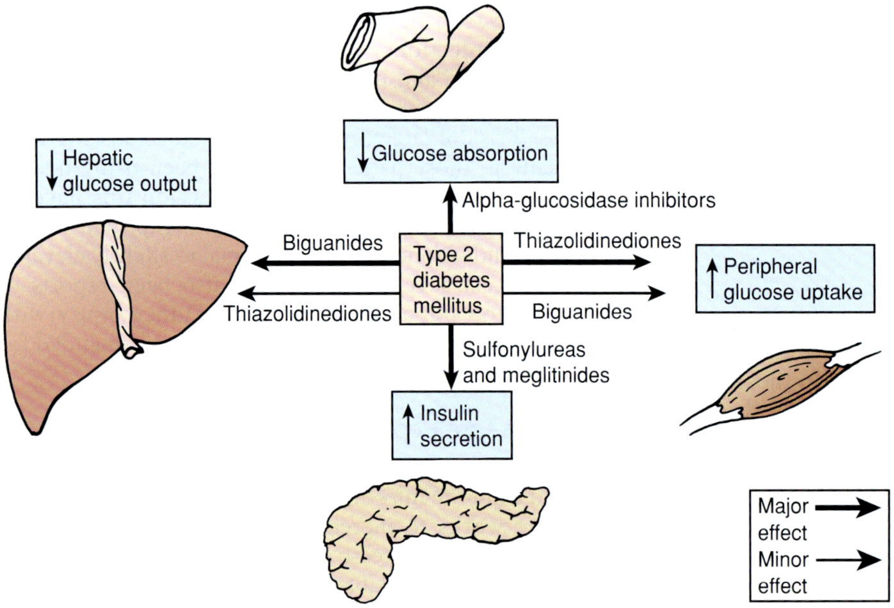

FIGURE 41-3. Sites of action of oral antidiabetic medications.

NURSING RESEARCH PROFILE

Chart 41-6. Impact of Community Diabetes Education

Gaillard, T., Amponsah, G., & Osei, K. (2015). Patient-centered community diabetes education program improves glycemic control in African American patients with poorly controlled type 2 diabetes: Importance of point of care metabolic measurements. *Journal of the National Black Nurses Association*, *26*(1), 51–58.

Purpose

The purpose of this study was to evaluate the benefits of a 6-month patient-centred, intensive lifestyle and diabetes self-management education support (DSMES) program on improving glycemic control as assessed by point-of-care (POC) A1C testing, body weight, blood pressure, and lipids and lipoprotein levels in African Americans with poorly controlled type 2 diabetes compared to standard diabetes cares.

Design

This was a single-centre randomized clinical trial of participants with poorly controlled type 2 diabetes (A1C >7.0%) residing in the inner city. Participants were randomized to DSMES ($n = 58$) or to standard diabetes care ($n = 38$). Participants in the DSMES group received intensive lifestyle and behavioural program that included didactic lectures provided by the Diabetes Care Team at 1- to 2-week intervals for 6 months. A community health worker, trained in diabetes self-management, provided support in the form of weekly phone calls and information about community resources. At the end of each didactic session, goals from the prior week, barriers, and challenges were discussed. The group then discussed alternate strategies for goal attainment. Participants were provided with quarterly POC testing (A1C, blood pressure, cholesterol, weight) and were reminded of targets. Emphasis was placed on how lifestyle changes could assist in meeting targets/goals. Participants in the standard care group attended the initial orientation, but did not attend the didactic nor intensive self-management lectures. General diabetes topics were discussed to increase group participation. POC testing was done in both groups at baseline, 3 and 6 months.

Findings

At 6 months, the DSMES group had significant reduction in A1C ($8.2 \pm 1.4\%$ vs. $7.5 \pm 1.5\%$, $p = 0.02$) and random glucose (190.4 ± 77.6 vs. 160.6 ± 59.8 mg/dL, $p = 0.03$) when compared with the standard care group. However, there were no changes in body weight, blood pressure, or lipids/lipoprotein levels. In addition, participants in the DSMES verbalized enjoying meeting with the group to discuss strategies and challenges faced with controlling type 2 diabetes.

Nursing Implications

Nurses need to encourage patients with diabetes and prediabetes to attend diabetes self-management, education, and support groups. In addition, these programs should be culturally sensitive, located in the community, and offered at times that are convenient to participants. Finally, the addition of POC testing allows individuals to reconcile their results with goals of therapy and provides immediate feedback and suggestions for change.

secondary diagnosis is presented in subsequent sections of this chapter. Because all patients with diabetes must master the concepts and skills necessary for long-term management of diabetes and its potential complications, a solid educational foundation is necessary for competent self-care and is an ongoing focus of nursing care. See Nursing Research Profile Chart 41-6.

Managing Glucose Control in the Hospital Setting

Hyperglycemia can prolong lengths of stay and increase infection rates and mortality; thus, nurses need to address glucose management in all hospital patients (Seggelke & Everhart, 2013). Hyperglycemia occurs most often in patients with known diabetes (i.e., type 1, type 2, gestational) and in those newly diagnosed with diabetes or stress hyperglycemia. Nursing management of hyperglycemia in the hospital uses the following principles (ADA, 2016g):

- Blood glucose targets are 7 to 10 mmol/L or according to stated target by the medical team.
- Insulin (subcutaneous or IV) is preferred to oral antidiabetic agents to manage hyperglycemia.
- Hospital insulin protocols or order sets should minimize complexity, ensure adequate staff training, include standardized hypoglycemic treatment, and make guidelines available for glycemic goals and insulin dosing.
- Appropriate timing of blood glucose checks, meal consumption, and insulin dose are all crucial for glucose control and to avoid hypoglycemia.

Providing Patient Education

Diabetes mellitus is a chronic illness requiring a lifetime of special self-management behaviours. Because diet, physical activity, and physical and emotional stress affect control of blood glucose levels, patients need to learn to balance a multitude of factors. They must learn daily self-care skills to prevent acute fluctuations in blood glucose, and they must also incorporate preventive behaviour into their lifestyle for avoidance of long-term complications of diabetes. Patients with diabetes must become knowledgeable about nutrition, medication effects and side effects, exercise, disease progression, prevention strategies, blood glucose monitoring techniques, and medication adjustment. In addition, they need to learn the skills associated with monitoring and managing diabetes and how to incorporate many new activities into their daily routines. Taking a broad perspective in understanding what is most important to the patient with diabetes in planning patients' education can help the nurse/practitioner in providing effective patient education and counselling (Bartol, 2012).

Developing an Education Plan for Patients With Diabetes

Changes in the health care delivery system as a whole have had a major impact on diabetes education and training (Chart 41-6). Patients with new-onset type 1 diabetes have much shorter hospital stays or may be managed completely on an outpatient basis; patients with new-onset type 2 diabetes are rarely hospitalized for initial care. There has been a proliferation of outpatient diabetes education and training programs in both institutional and community settings. For some patients, however, exposure to diabetes education during hospitalization may be the only opportunity for learning self-management skills and preventing complications.

Many hospitals employ nurses who specialize in diabetes education and management. However, because of the large number of patients with diabetes who are admitted to every unit of a hospital for reasons other than diabetes or its complications, the staff nurse plays a vital role in identifying diabetic patients, assessing self-care skills, providing basic education, reinforcing the teaching provided by the specialist, and referring patients for follow-up care after discharge.

Unfolding Patient Stories: Skyler Hansen • Part 2

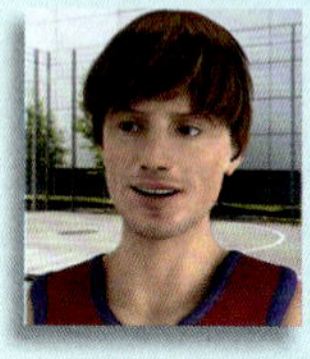

Recall from Chapter 9 Skyler Hansen, a high school student recently diagnosed with type 1 diabetes. Outline a diabetes education plan for Skyler and his parents. What are important patient education topics, resources, and methods for the nurse to consider? How would the nurse evaluate whether the patient and his family understand the education provided?

Care for Skyler and other patients in a realistic virtual environment: ***vSim** for Nursing* (**thepoint.lww.com/vSimMedicalSurgical**). Practice documenting these patients' care in DocuCare (**thepoint.lww.com/DocuCareEHR**).

ORGANIZING INFORMATION. There are various strategies for organizing and prioritizing the vast amount of information that must be taught to diabetic patients. In addition, many hospitals and outpatient diabetes centres have devised written guidelines, care plans, and forms (often based on guidelines from the Diabetes Canada) that may be used to document and evaluate teaching. A general approach is to organize information and skills into two main types: (a) basic, initial, or "survival" skills and information and (b) in-depth (advanced) or continuing education.

EDUCATING PATIENTS ABOUT BASIC SKILLS. Basic skills must be learned by all patients with newly diagnosed type 1 or type 2 diabetes and all patients receiving insulin for the first time. Basic information that patients must know is included in Chart 41-7.

For patients with newly diagnosed type 2 diabetes, emphasis is initially placed on meal planning and exercise. Those who are starting to take oral antidiabetic agents need to know about detecting, preventing, and treating hypoglycemia. If diabetes has gone undetected for many years, the patient may already be experiencing some chronic complications from diabetes. Therefore, for some patients with newly diagnosed type 2 diabetes, basic diabetes education must include information on preventive skills, such as foot care (Fisher, 2016) and eye care (e.g., planning yearly or more frequent complete [dilated eye] examinations by an ophthalmologist, understanding that retinopathy is largely asymptomatic until advanced stages).

CHART 41-7

Patient Education: Basic Skills for People With Diabetes

The nurse includes the following basic information in education:

1. Pathophysiology
   a. Basic definition of diabetes (having a high blood glucose level)
   b. Normal blood glucose ranges and target blood glucose levels
   c. Effect of insulin and exercise (decrease glucose)
   d. Effect of food and stress, including illness and infections (increase glucose)
   e. Basic treatment approaches
2. Treatment modalities
   a. Administration of insulin and oral antidiabetes medications
   b. Meal planning (food groups, timing of meals)
   c. Monitoring of blood glucose and urine ketones
3. Recognition, treatment, and prevention of acute complications
   a. Hypoglycemia
   b. Hyperglycemia
4. Pragmatic information
   a. Where to buy and store insulin, syringes, and glucose monitoring supplies
   b. When and how to contact the primary provider

Patients also need to realize that once they master the basic skills and information, diabetes education is a lifelong process. Acquiring in-depth and advanced diabetes knowledge occurs both formally through programs of continuing education and informally through experience and sharing of information with other people with diabetes.

PLANNING IN-DEPTH AND CONTINUING EDUCATION. The planning of in-depth and continuing education involves teaching more detailed information related to survival skills (e.g., learning to vary diet and insulin and preparing for travel) as well as learning preventive measures for avoiding long-term diabetic complications. Preventive measures include the following:

- Foot care
- Eye care
- General hygiene (e.g., skin care, oral hygiene)
- Risk factor management (e.g., control of blood pressure and blood lipid levels, normalizing blood glucose levels)

More advanced continuing education may include alternative methods for insulin delivery, such as the insulin pump, and algorithms or rules for evaluating and adjusting insulin doses. For example, patients can be taught to increase or decrease insulin doses based on a several-day pattern of blood glucose levels. The degree of advanced diabetes education to be provided depends on the patient's interest and ability. However, learning preventive measures (especially foot care and eye care) is mandatory for reducing the occurrence of amputations and blindness in patients with diabetes.

Assessing Readiness to Learn

Before initiating diabetes education, the nurse needs to assess the patient and family's current readiness to learn, previous education, level of confidence and self-management skills (Bartol, 2012). When patients are first diagnosed with diabetes (or first told of their need for insulin), they often go through various stages of the grieving process. These stages may include shock and denial, anger, depression, negotiation, and acceptance. The amount of time it takes for patients and family members to work through the grieving process varies from patient to patient. They may experience helplessness, guilt, altered body image, loss of self-esteem, and concern about the future. The nurse assesses the patient's coping strategies and reassures patients and families that feelings of depression and shock are expected. A referral may be needed to a member of the psychosocial team (psychologist or social worker) in order to help the patient develop coping skills for dealing with a chronic disease.

Asking the patient and family about their major concerns or fears is an important way to learn about any misinformation that may be contributing to anxiety.

After dispelling misconceptions or answering questions that concern the patient the most, the nurse focuses attention on concrete survival skills. Because of the immediate need for multiple new skills, teaching is initiated as soon as possible after diagnosis. Nurses whose patients are in the hospital rarely have the luxury of waiting until the patient feels ready to learn; short hospital stays necessitate initiation of survival skill education as early as possible. This gives the patient the opportunity to practice skills with supervision by the nurse before discharge. Follow-up by home care nurses or in an ambulatory setting is often necessary for reinforcement of basic skills.

Determining Education Methods

Maintaining flexibility with regard to education approaches is important. Providing education on skills and information in a logical sequence is not always the most helpful for patients. For example, many patients fear the injection. Before they learn how to draw up, purchase, store, and mix insulins, they should be taught to insert the needle and inject insulin (or practice with saline solution). Numerous demonstrations by the nurse or practice injections before the patient (or family) gives the first injection may actually increase the patient's anxiety and fear of self-injection. Once patients have actually performed the injection, most are more prepared to hear and comprehend other information. (They may want to continue to practice using a pillow or an orange.) Thus, having patients self-inject first or having patients perform a finger stick for glucose monitoring first may enhance learning to draw up the insulin or to operate the glucose meter. Ample opportunity should be provided for the patient and family to practice skills under supervision (including self-injection, self-testing, meal selection, verbalization of symptoms, and treatment of hypoglycemia). Once skills have been mastered, participation in ongoing support groups may assist patients in incorporating new habits and maintaining adherence to the treatment regimen.

Various tools can be used to complement education. Many of the companies that manufacture products for diabetes self-care also provide booklets and videotapes to assist in patient teaching. It is important to use a variety of written handouts that match the patient's learning needs (including different languages, low-literacy information or large print). Patients can continue learning about diabetes care by participating in activities sponsored by local hospitals and diabetes organizations. In addition, magazines with information on all aspects of diabetes management are available for people with diabetes.

Educating Experienced Patients

Nurses need to continue to assess the skills and self-care behaviours of patients who have had diabetes for many years. Assessment of these patients must include direct observation of skills, not just the patient's self-report of self-care behaviours. In addition, these patients must be fully aware of preventive measures related to foot care, eye care, and risk factor management. Those experiencing long-term complications from diabetes for the first time may go through the grieving process again. Some patients may have a renewed interest in diabetes self-care in the hope of delaying further complications. Others may have guilt and depression. The patient is encouraged to discuss feelings and fears related to complications. Meanwhile, the nurse provides appropriate information regarding complications from diabetes.

Educating Patients to Self-Administer Insulin

Insulin injections are self-administered into the subcutaneous tissue with the use of special insulin syringes. Basic information includes explanations of the equipment, insulins, and syringes and how to mix insulin, if necessary.

STORING INSULIN. Cloudy insulins should be thoroughly mixed by gently inverting the vial or rolling it between the hands before drawing the solution into a syringe or a pen. The vial should not be shaken vigorously to avoid denaturing the insulin structure.

Whether insulin is the short- or long-acting preparation, the vials not in use should be refrigerated and extremes of temperature should be avoided; insulin should not be allowed to freeze and should not be kept in direct sunlight or in a hot car. The insulin vial in use should be kept at room temperature to reduce local irritation at the injection site, which may occur when cold insulin is injected. Once a vial of insulin has been punctured, it is only good for 30 days regardless if it is kept at room temperature or in the refrigerator. Patients should be instructed to always have a spare vial of the type or types of insulin they use.

Insulin bottles should also be inspected for flocculation, which is a frosted, whitish coating inside the bottle of intermediate- or long-acting insulins. This occurs most commonly with human insulins that are not refrigerated. If a frosted, adherent coating is present, some of the insulin is bound and should not be used.

SELECTING SYRINGES. Syringes must be matched with the insulin concentration (e.g., U-100). Currently, three sizes of U-100 insulin syringes are available:

- 1-mL (cc) syringes that hold 100 units
- 0.5-mL syringes that hold 50 units
- 0.3-mL syringes that hold 30 units

The concentration of insulin used in Canada is U-100; that is, there are 100 units per millilitre (or cubic centimetre). Syringe size varies. Small syringes allow patients who require small amounts of insulin to measure and draw up the amount of insulin accurately. Patients who require large amounts of insulin would use larger syringes.

PREPARING THE INJECTION: MIXING INSULINS. When rapid- or short-acting insulins are to be given simultaneously with longer-acting insulins, they are usually mixed together in the same syringe; the longer-acting insulins must be mixed thoroughly before use. There is some question as to whether the two insulins are stable if the mixture is kept in the syringe for more than 5 to 15 minutes. This may depend on the ratio of the insulins as well as the time between mixing and injecting. When regular insulin is mixed with long-acting insulin, there is a binding reaction that slows the action of the regular insulin. Patients are advised to consult their health care provider for advice on this matter. The most important issue is that patients be consistent in how they prepare their insulin injections from day to day. Only NPH can be mixed with rapid- or short-acting insulins; glargine and detemir should not be mixed with other insulins.

While there are varying opinions regarding which type of insulin (short or longer acting) should be drawn up into the syringe first when they are going to be mixed, the Diabetes Canada recommends that the regular insulin be drawn up first. The most important issues are, again, that patients be consistent in technique so as not to draw up the wrong dose accidentally or the wrong type of insulin and that patients not inject one type of insulin into the bottle containing a different type of insulin.

For patients who have difficulty mixing insulins, two options are available: They may use a premixed insulin, or they may have prefilled syringes prepared or insulin pens. For patients who can inject insulin but who have difficulty drawing up a single or mixed dose, syringes can be prefilled with the help of home care nurses or family and friends. A 3-week supply of insulin syringes may be prepared and kept in the refrigerator. The prefilled syringes should be stored with the needle in an upright position to avoid clogging of the needle.

WITHDRAWING INSULIN. There is ongoing increased interest among diabetic patients to use insulin pens and cartridges for their insulin injection, in which case new needles are put on, and patients may need to prime the cartridge by expelling 2 units of insulin afterwards. Most (if not all) of the printed materials available on insulin dose preparation for those clients using insulin syringes and needles instruct patients to inject air into the bottle of insulin equivalent to the number of units of insulin to be withdrawn. The rationale for this is to prevent the formation of a vacuum inside the bottle, which would make it difficult to withdraw the proper amount of insulin. Some nurses who specialize in diabetes report that some patients (who have been taking insulin for many years) have stopped injecting air before withdrawing the insulin. These patients have found that the extra step was not necessary for accurately drawing up the insulin dose. Most patients find it easier to withdraw the insulin by eliminating the step and report no difficulty in preparing the proper insulin dose.

Eliminating this step, or alternating it by, for instance, injecting a syringe full of air into the vial once per week, facilitates the teaching process for some patients learning to draw up insulin for the first time. Some patients become confused with the sequence of steps involved in injecting air into two separate bottles in two different amounts before drawing up a mixed dose. For many individuals, including older ones, simplifying the procedure for preparing insulin injections may help them maintain independence in daily living.

As with other variations in insulin injection technique, the most important factors are that the patient maintains consistency in the procedure and that the nurse is flexible when teaching new patients or assessing the skills of experienced patients.

SELECTING AND ROTATING THE INJECTION SITE. The four main areas for injection are the abdomen, arms (posterior surface), thighs (anterior surface), and hips (Fig. 41-4). Insulin is absorbed faster in some areas of the body than others. The abdomen provides the most consistent absorption rate of the various sites. The arms and thighs are the most variable and are influenced by the level of activity in which they are involved.

Systematic rotation of injection sites within an anatomic area is recommended to prevent localized changes in fatty tissue (lipodystrophy). In addition, to promote consistency in insulin absorption, patients should be encouraged to use all available injection sites within one area rather than randomly rotating sites from area to area (Diabetes Canada, 2018a). For example, some patients almost exclusively use the abdominal area, administering each injection 1 to 2 cm away from the previous injection. They can also divide the abdomen into quadrants and inject into one quadrant per week or at a predetermined interval depending on the number of injections to be given. Another approach to rotation is always to use the same

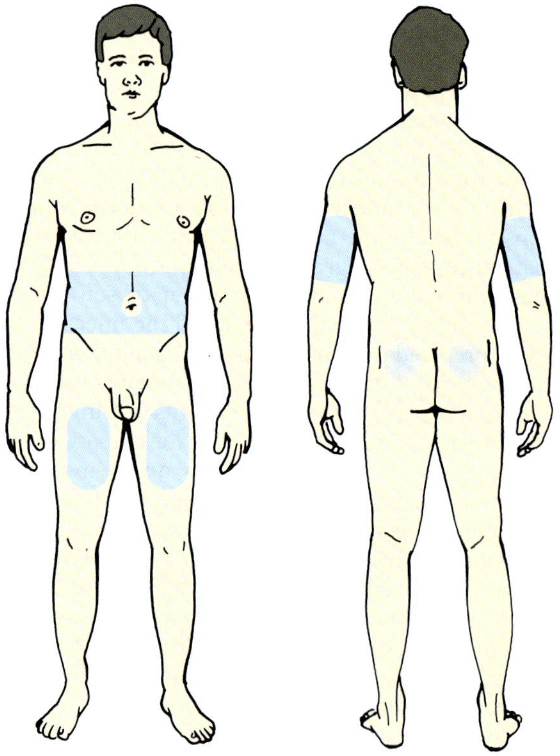

FIGURE 41-4. Suggested areas (*shading*) for insulin injection.

area at the same time of day. For example, patients may inject morning doses into the abdomen and evening doses into the arms or legs. If using the thighs for injection, the needle used should be no longer than 6 mm.

A few general principles apply to all rotation patterns. First, patients should try not to use the same site more than once in 2 to 3 weeks. In addition, if the patient is planning to exercise, insulin should not be injected into the limb that will be exercised, as it will be absorbed faster, and this may result in hypoglycemia.

In the past, patients were taught to rotate injections from one area to the next (e.g., injecting once in the right arm, then once in the right abdomen, then once in the right thigh). Patients who still use this system must be taught to avoid repeated injections into the same site within an area. However, as stated previously, it is preferable for the patient to use the same anatomic area at the same time of day consistently; this reduces day-to-day variation in blood glucose levels because of different absorption rates.

PREPARING THE SKIN. The use of alcohol to cleanse the skin is not recommended, but patients who have learned this technique often continue to use it. They should be cautioned to allow the skin to dry after cleansing with alcohol. If the skin is not allowed to dry before the injection, the alcohol may be carried into the tissues, resulting in a localized reddened area.

INSERTING THE NEEDLE. There are varying approaches to inserting the needle for insulin injections. The correct technique is based on the need for the insulin to be injected into the subcutaneous tissue. Injection that is too deep (e.g., intramuscular) or too shallow may affect the rate of absorption of the insulin. Aspiration (inserting the needle and then pulling back on the plunger to assess for blood being drawn into the syringe) is generally not recommended with self-injection of insulin. Many patients who have been using insulin for an extended period have eliminated this step from their insulin injection routine with no apparent adverse effects.

Promoting Home, Community-Based, and Transitional Care

Educating the Patient About Self-Care

If poor glucose control or preventable complications occur, the nurse needs to assess the reasons for the patient's ineffective management of the treatment regimen. It should not be assumed that problems with diabetes management are related to the patient's decision to ignore self-management. The patient may have forgotten or may have never learned certain information, or there may be cultural or religious beliefs that interfere with adherence. The problem may be correctable simply through providing complete information and ensuring that the patient understands the information. The focus of diabetes education should be patient empowerment. Patient education must address behaviour change, self-efficacy, and health beliefs.

If knowledge deficit is not the issue, physical or emotional factors may be impairing the patient's ability to perform self-care skills. For example, decreased visual acuity may impair the patient's ability to administer insulin accurately, measure the blood glucose level, or inspect the skin and feet. In addition, decreased joint mobility (especially in older adults) or pre-existing disability may impair the patient's ability to inspect the bottom of the feet. Denial of the diagnosis or depression may impair the patient's ability to carry out multiple daily self-care measures. The patient whose family, personal, or work problems may be of higher priority may benefit from assistance in establishing priorities. The nurse must also assess the patient for infection or emotional stress, which may lead to elevated blood glucose levels despite adherence to the treatment regimen.

The following approaches are helpful for promoting self-care management skills:

- Address any underlying factors (e.g., knowledge deficit, self-care deficit, illness) that may affect control of diabetes.
- Simplify the treatment regimen if it is too difficult for the patient to follow.
- Adjust the treatment regimen to meet patient requests (e.g., adjust diet or insulin schedule to allow increased flexibility in meal content or timing).
- Establish a specific plan or contract with each patient with simple, measurable goals.
- Provide positive reinforcement of self-care behaviours performed instead of focusing on behaviours that were neglected (e.g., positively reinforce blood glucose tests that were performed instead of focusing on the number of missed tests).
- Help the patient identify personal motivating factors rather than focusing on wanting to please primary providers.
- Encourage the patient to pursue life goals and interests, and discourage an undue focus on diabetes.

Continuing and Transitional Care

As discussed, continuing care of the patient with diabetes is critical in managing and preventing complications. The degree to which the client interacts with health care providers to obtain ongoing care depends on many factors. Age, socioeconomic status, existing complications, type of diabetes, and comorbid conditions may dictate the frequency of follow-up visits. Many patients with diabetes may be seen by home health nurses for education, wound care, insulin preparation, or assistance with glucose monitoring. Even patients who achieve excellent glucose control and have no complications can expect to see their primary health care provider at least twice a year for ongoing evaluation.

In addition to follow-up care with health professionals, participation in support groups is encouraged for those who have had diabetes for many years as well as those who are newly diagnosed. Such participation may assist the patient and family in coping with changes in lifestyle that occur with the onset of diabetes and with its complications. Those who participate in support groups often have an opportunity to share valuable information and experiences and to learn from others. Support groups provide an opportunity for discussion of strategies to deal with diabetes and its management and to clarify and verify information with the nurse or other health care professionals. Participation in support groups may help patients and their families become more knowledgeable about diabetes and its management and may promote adherence to the management plan. Another very important role of the nurse is to remind the patient about the importance of participating in other health promotion activities and recommended health screening.

ACUTE COMPLICATIONS OF DIABETES

There are three major acute complications of diabetes related to short-term imbalances in blood glucose levels: hypoglycemia, diabetic ketoacidosis (DKA), and HHS.

Hypoglycemia (Insulin Reactions)

Hypoglycemia (abnormally low blood glucose level) occurs when the blood glucose falls to less than 3.7 mmol/L. It can be caused by too much insulin or oral/injectable antihyperglycemic agents, inadequate food intake, or excessive physical activity. Hypoglycemia may occur at any time of the day or night. It often occurs before meals, especially if meals are delayed or snacks are omitted. For example, midmorning hypoglycemia may occur when the morning regular or rapid insulin is peaking, whereas hypoglycemia that occurs in the late afternoon may coincide with the peak of the morning NPH insulin. Middle-of-the-night hypoglycemia may occur because of peaking evening or pre-dinner NPH insulins, especially in patients who have not eaten a bedtime snack.

Clinical Manifestations

The clinical manifestations of hypoglycemia may be grouped into two categories: adrenergic symptoms and central nervous system (CNS) symptoms. In mild hypoglycemia, as the blood glucose level falls, the sympathetic nervous system is stimulated, resulting in a surge of epinephrine and norepinephrine. This causes symptoms such as sweating, tremor, tachycardia, palpitations, nervousness, and hunger.

In moderate hypoglycemia, the fall in blood glucose level deprives the brain cells of needed fuel for functioning. Signs of impaired function of the CNS may include inability to concentrate, headache, lightheadedness, confusion, memory lapses, numbness of the lips and tongue, slurred speech, impaired coordination, emotional changes, irrational or combative behaviour, double vision and drowsiness. Any combination of these symptoms (in addition to adrenergic symptoms) may occur with moderate hypoglycemia.

In severe hypoglycemia, CNS function is so impaired that the patient needs the assistance of another person for treatment of hypoglycemia. Symptoms may include disoriented behaviour, seizures, difficulty arousing from sleep, or loss of consciousness.

Assessment and Diagnostic Findings

Hypoglycemic symptoms can occur suddenly and unexpectedly. The combination of symptoms varies considerably from person to person. To some degree, this may be related to the actual level to which the blood glucose drops or to the rate at which it is dropping. For example, patients who usually have a blood glucose level in the hyperglycemic range (e.g., 10.5 mmol/L or greater) may feel hypoglycemic (adrenergic) symptoms when their blood glucose quickly drops into the normal range (4.0–7.0 mmol/L). Conversely, patients who frequently have low blood glucose levels (<4.0 mmol/L) and ignore the symptoms may not notice any symptoms until their blood glucose levels drop to less than 2.0 mmol/L (hypoglycemia unawareness).

Another factor contributing to altered hypoglycemic symptoms is a decreased hormonal (adrenergic) response to hypoglycemia. This occurs in some patients who have had diabetes for many years. It may be related to autonomic neuropathy, one of the chronic complications of diabetes (see the section regarding Hypoglycemia Unawareness). As the blood glucose level falls, the normal surge in epinephrine does not occur. The patient does not feel the usual adrenergic symptoms, such as sweating and shakiness. The hypoglycemia may not be detected until moderate or severe CNS impairment occurs. These patients must perform SMBG on a frequent regular basis, especially before driving or engaging in other potentially dangerous activities.

Gerontologic Considerations

In the older diabetic patient, hypoglycemia is a particular concern for many reasons:

- Older people frequently live alone and may not recognize the symptoms of hypoglycemia.
- With decreasing kidney function, it takes longer for oral antihyperglycemic agents to be excreted by the kidneys.
- Skipping meals may occur because of decreased appetite or financial limitations.
- Decreased visual acuity may lead to errors in insulin administration.

Management

Immediate treatment must be given when hypoglycemia occurs. The usual recommendation is for 15 g of a fast-acting concentrated source of carbohydrate such as the following, given orally:

- Three or four commercially prepared glucose tablets (check glucose content)
- 125 mL of fruit juice or regular soft drink
- 6 Lifesavers
- 10 jellybeans
- 15 mL (3 teaspoons or 1 tablespoon) of sugar or honey
- 3 hard candies

It is not necessary to add sugar to juice, even if it is labelled as unsweetened, as the fruit sugar in juice contains enough carbohydrate to raise the blood glucose level. Adding table sugar to juice may cause a sharp increase in the blood glucose level, and the patient may experience hyperglycemia for hours after treatment.

The blood glucose level should be retested in 15 minutes and retreated if it is less than 4.0 mmol/L. If the symptoms persist more than 10 to 15 minutes after initial treatment, the treatment is repeated even if blood glucose testing is not possible. Once the symptoms resolve, a snack containing protein and starch (e.g., milk or cheese and crackers) is recommended unless the patient plans to eat a regular meal or snack within 30 to 60 minutes.

Initiating Emergency Measures

For patients who are unconscious and cannot swallow, an injection of glucagon 1 mg can be administered either subcutaneously or intramuscularly. Glucagon is a hormone produced by the alpha cells of the pancreas that stimulates the liver to release glucose (through the breakdown of glycogen, the stored glucose). Injectable glucagon is packaged as a powder in 1-mg vials and must be mixed with a diluent before being injected. After injection of glucagon, it may take up to 20 minutes for the patient to regain consciousness. A concentrated source of carbohydrate followed by a snack should be given to the patient on awakening to prevent recurrence of hypoglycemia (onset of action is 5 to 15 minutes and its duration of action is 10 to 40 minutes) and to replenish hepatic stores of glucose. Some patients experience nausea after the administration of glucagon; if this occurs, the patient should be turned to the side to prevent aspiration. The patient should be instructed to notify the physician or health care provider after severe hypoglycemia has occurred.

Glucagon is sold by prescription only and should be part of the emergency supplies kept available by patients with diabetes who require insulin. Family members, neighbours, or coworkers should be instructed about the use of glucagon. This is especially true for patients who receive little or no warning of hypoglycemic episodes.

In the hospital or emergency department, patients who are unconscious or cannot swallow may be treated with 25 to 50 mL of 50% dextrose in water ($D_{50}W$) administered intravenously. The effect is usually seen within minutes. Patients may complain of a headache and pain at the injection site. Assuring patency of the intravenous (IV) line used for injection of 50% dextrose is essential because hypertonic solutions such as 50% dextrose are very irritating to the vein.

Providing Patient Education

Hypoglycemia is prevented by a consistent pattern of eating, administering insulin, and exercising. Between-meal and bedtime snacks may be needed to counteract the maximum insulin effect. In general, the patient should cover the time of peak activity of insulin by eating a snack and by taking additional food when physical activity is increased. Routine blood glucose tests are performed so that changing insulin requirements may be anticipated and the dosage adjusted. Because unexpected hypoglycemia may occur, all patients treated with insulin should wear an identification bracelet or tag stating that they have diabetes.

Patients and family members must be instructed about the symptoms of hypoglycemia. Family members in particular must be made aware that any subtle (but unusual) change in behaviour may be an indication of hypoglycemia. They should be taught to encourage and even insist that the person with diabetes assess blood glucose levels if hypoglycemia is suspected. Some patients (when hypoglycemic) become very resistant to testing or eating and become angry at family members trying to treat the hypoglycemia. Family members must be taught to persevere and to understand that the hypoglycemia can cause irrational behaviour, due to low supply of glucose to the brain.

Some patients with autonomic neuropathy or those taking beta-blockers (e.g., metoprolol, bisoprolol, atenolol) to treat hypertension or cardiac dysrhythmias may not experience the typical symptoms of hypoglycemia. It is very important for these patients to perform blood glucose tests on a frequent and regular basis. Patients who have type 2 diabetes and who take oral sulfonylurea agents may also develop hypoglycemia (especially those taking glyburide, a long-lasting oral hypoglycemic agent).

It is important for patients with diabetes, especially those receiving insulin, to learn that they must carry some form of simple sugar with them at all times (Diabetes Canada, 2018b). There are many different commercially prepared glucose tablets and gels that patients may find convenient to carry.

Patients are advised to refrain from eating high-calorie, high-fat dessert foods (e.g., cookies, cakes, doughnuts, chocolate, ice cream) to treat hypoglycemia. The high fat content of these foods may slow the absorption of the glucose, and the hypoglycemic symptoms may not resolve as quickly as they would with the intake of carbohydrates. The patient may subsequently eat more of the foods when symptoms do not resolve rapidly. This in turn may cause very high blood glucose levels for several hours after the reaction and may also contribute to weight gain.

Patients who feel unduly restricted by their meal plan may view hypoglycemic episodes as a time to reward themselves with desserts. It may be more prudent to teach these patients to incorporate occasional desserts into the meal plan. This may make it easier for them to limit their treatment of hypoglycemic episodes to simple (low-calorie) carbohydrates such as juice or glucose tablets.

Diabetic Ketoacidosis

DKA is caused by an absence or markedly inadequate amount of insulin. This deficit in available insulin results in disorders in the metabolism of carbohydrate, protein, and fat. The following are the three main clinical features of DKA:

- Hyperglycemia
- Dehydration and electrolyte loss
- Acidosis

Pathophysiology

Without insulin, the amount of glucose entering the cells is reduced, and the liver increases glucose production. Both factors lead to hyperglycemia. In an attempt to rid the body of the excess glucose, the kidneys excrete the glucose along with water and electrolytes (e.g., sodium and potassium). This osmotic diuresis, which is characterized by excessive urination (polyuria), leads to dehydration and marked electrolyte loss. Patients with severe DKA may lose up to 6.5 L of water and up to 400 to 500 mmol/L each of sodium, potassium, and chloride over a 24-hour period.

Another effect of insulin deficiency or deficit is the breakdown of fat (lipolysis) into free fatty acids and glycerol. The free fatty acids are converted into ketone bodies by the liver. In DKA, there is excessive production of ketone bodies because of the lack of insulin that would normally prevent this from occurring. Ketone bodies are acids; their accumulation in the circulation leads to metabolic acidosis.

The three main causes of DKA are a decreased or missed dose of insulin, illness or infection, and undiagnosed and untreated diabetes (DKA may be the initial manifestation of diabetes). An insulin deficit may result from an insufficient dosage of insulin prescribed or from insufficient insulin being administered by the patient. Errors in insulin dosage may be made by patients who are ill and who assume that if they are eating less or if they are vomiting, they must decrease their insulin doses. (Because illness, especially infections, may cause increased blood glucose levels, patients do not need to decrease their insulin doses to compensate for decreased food intake when ill and may even need to increase their insulin dose.)

Other potential causes of decreased insulin include patient error in drawing up or injecting insulin (especially in patients with visual impairments), intentional skipping of insulin doses (especially in adolescents with diabetes who are having difficulty coping with diabetes or other aspects of their lives), or equipment problems (e.g., occlusion of insulin pump tubing).

Illness and infections are associated with insulin resistance. In response to physical (and emotional) stressors, there is an increase in the level of "stress" hormones—glucagon, epinephrine, norepinephrine, cortisol, and growth hormone. These hormones promote glucose production by the liver and interfere with glucose utilization by muscle and fat tissue, counteracting the effect of insulin. If insulin levels are not increased during times of illness and infection, hyperglycemia may progress to DKA in patients with type 1 diabetes.

CHART 41-8

Patient Education: Guidelines to Follow During Periods of Illness ("Sick Day" Rules)

The nurse instructs the patient to:

- Take insulin or oral/injectable antihyperglycemic agents as usual.
- Test blood glucose and test urine ketones every 3–4 hours.
- Report elevated glucose levels (greater than 16.6 mmol/L or as otherwise specified) or urine ketones to the physician or health care provider.
- Insulin-requiring patients may need supplemental doses of regular insulin every 3–4 hours.
- If the usual meal plan cannot be followed, substitute soft foods (e.g., regular gelatin, cream soup, custard graham crackers) six to eight times per day.
- If vomiting, diarrhea, or fever persists, take liquids with carbohydrate if your blood sugar is less than 12 mmol/L (e.g., regular pop or juice or Gatorade) or liquids without carbohydrate if your blood sugar level is greater than 12 mmol/L (e.g., broth, water, sugar-free gelatin, tea, coffee) every ½ to 1 hour to prevent dehydration and to provide calories.
- Report nausea, vomiting, and diarrhea to the physician or health care provider, because extreme fluid loss may be dangerous.
- For patients with type 1 diabetes, the inability to retain oral fluids may warrant hospitalization to avoid diabetic ketoacidosis and possibly coma.

Prevention

For prevention of DKA related to illness, patients must be taught "sick day" rules for managing their diabetes when ill (Chart 41-8). The most important issue to teach patients is not to eliminate insulin doses when nausea and vomiting occur. Rather, they should take their usual insulin dose (or previously prescribed special "sick day" doses) and then attempt to consume frequent small portions of carbohydrates (including foods usually avoided, such as juices, regular sodas, and gelatin). Drinking fluids every hour is important to prevent dehydration. Blood glucose and urine ketones must be assessed every 3 to 4 hours.

If the patient cannot take fluids without vomiting, or if elevated glucose or ketone levels persist, the physician or health care provider must be contacted. Patients are taught to have available foods for use on sick days. In addition, a supply of urine test strips (for ketone testing) and blood glucose test strips should be available.

Diabetes self-management skills (including insulin administration and blood glucose testing) should be assessed to ensure that an error in insulin administration or blood glucose testing did not occur. Psychological counselling is recommended for patients and family members if an intentional alteration in insulin dosing was the cause of the DKA.

Clinical Manifestations

The signs and symptoms of DKA are listed in Figure 41-5. The hyperglycemia of DKA leads to polyuria and polydipsia (increased thirst). In addition, patients may experience blurred vision, weakness, and headache. Patients with marked intravascular volume depletion may have orthostatic hypotension (drop in systolic blood pressure of 20 mm Hg or more upon standing). Volume depletion may also lead to frank hypotension with a weak, rapid pulse.

The ketosis and acidosis of DKA lead to GI symptoms such as anorexia, nausea, vomiting, and abdominal pain. The abdominal pain and physical findings on examination can be so severe that they resemble an acute abdominal disorder that requires surgery. Patients may have acetone breath (a fruity odour), which occurs with elevated ketone levels. In addition, hyperventilation (with very deep, but not laboured, respirations) may occur. These Kussmaul respirations represent the body's attempt to decrease the acidosis, counteracting the effect of the ketone buildup. In addition, mental status changes in DKA vary widely from patient to patient. Patients may be alert, lethargic, or comatose, most likely depending on the plasma osmolarity (concentration of osmotically active particles).

Assessment and Diagnostic Findings

Blood glucose levels may vary from 16.6 to 44.4 mmol/L. Some patients have lower glucose values, and others have

Physiology/Pathophysiology

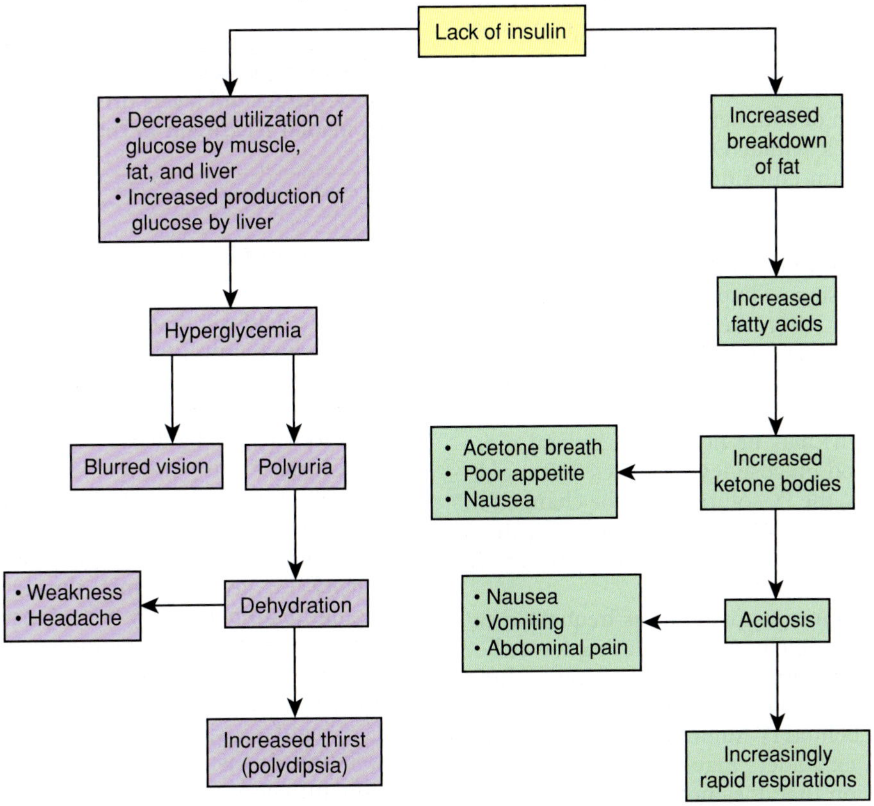

FIGURE 41-5. Abnormal metabolism that causes signs and symptoms of diabetic ketoacidosis. (Redrawn from Pearce, M. A., Rosenberg, C. S., & Davidson, M. D. (2003). Patient education. In M. B. Davidson (Ed.). *Diabetes mellitus: Diagnosis and treatment*. New York: Churchill Livingstone.)

values of 55.5 mmol/L or more (usually depending on the degree of dehydration). The severity of DKA is not necessarily related to the blood glucose level. Some patients may have severe acidosis with modestly elevated blood glucose levels, whereas others may have no evidence of DKA despite very high blood glucose levels. A new recommendation suggests point-of-care capillary beta-hydroxybutyrate may be measured in the hospital in patients with type 1 diabetes with capillary glucose level greater than 14.0 mmol/L in order to screen for DKA. Also, a beta-hydroxybutyrate level greater than 1.5 mmol/L warrants further testing for DKA.

Some patients may not have elevations in blood glucose levels and have all the other features of DKA (anion gap, presence of ketones, nausea and vomiting). This is diagnosed as euglycemic DKA and may occur in patients who are taking SGLT-2 inhibitors.

Evidence of ketoacidosis is reflected in low serum bicarbonate (0 to 15 mmol/L) and low pH (6.8 to 7.3) values. A low PCO_2 level (10 to 30 mm Hg) reflects respiratory compensation (Kussmaul respirations) for the metabolic acidosis. Accumulation of ketone bodies (which precipitates the acidosis) is reflected in blood and urine ketone measurements.

Sodium and potassium levels may be low, normal, or high, depending on the amount of water loss (dehydration). Despite the plasma concentration, there has been a marked total body depletion of these (and other) electrolytes. Ultimately, these electrolytes will need to be replaced.

Elevated levels of creatinine, blood urea nitrogen (BUN), hemoglobin, and hematocrit may also be seen with dehydration. After rehydration, continued elevation in the serum creatinine and BUN levels will be present in the patient with underlying renal insufficiency.

Medical Management

In addition to treating hyperglycemia, management of DKA is aimed at correcting dehydration, electrolyte loss, and acidosis.

In adult patients with DKA, it is recommended that a protocol be followed that incorporates the following principles of treatment:

- fluid resuscitation
- avoidance of hypokalemia
- insulin administration
- avoidance of rapidly falling serum osmolality
- search for precipitating cause

[Grade D, Consensus]

Rehydration

In dehydrated patients, rehydration is important for maintaining tissue perfusion. In addition, fluid replacement enhances the excretion of excessive glucose by the kidneys. Patients may need up to 6 to 10 L of IV fluid to replace fluid losses caused by polyuria, hyperventilation, diarrhea, and vomiting. In individuals with DKA, IV 0.9% sodium chloride should be administered initially at 500 mL/h for 4 hours, then 250 mL/h for 4 hours [Grade B, Level 2 (7)] with consideration of a higher initial rate (1 to 2 L/h) in the presence of shock [Grade D, Consensus].

Initially, 0.9% sodium chloride (normal saline [NS]) solution is given at a rapid rate, usually 0.5 to 1 L/h for 2 to 3 hours. Half-strength NS (0.45%) solution (also known as hypotonic saline solution) may be used for patients with hypertension or hypernatremia and those at risk for heart failure. After the first few hours, half-strength NS solution is the fluid of choice for continued rehydration, provided the blood pressure is stable and the sodium level is not low. Moderate to high rates of infusion (200 to 500 mL/h) may be needed for several more hours. When the blood glucose level reaches 300 mg/dL (16.6 mmol/L) or less, the IV solution may be changed to dextrose 5% in water (D_5W) to prevent a precipitous decline in the blood glucose level (Umpeirrez & Korytkowski, 2016).

Monitoring fluid volume status involves frequent measurements of vital signs (including monitoring for orthostatic changes in blood pressure and heart rate), lung assessment, and monitoring intake and output. Initial urine output will lag behind IV fluid intake as dehydration is corrected. Plasma expanders may be necessary to correct severe hypotension that does not respond to IV fluid treatment. Monitoring for signs of fluid overload is especially important for older patients, those with renal impairment, or those at risk for heart failure.

Restoring Electrolytes

The major electrolyte of concern during treatment of DKA is potassium. Although the initial plasma concentration of potassium may be low, normal, or even high, there is a major loss of potassium from body stores and an intracellular to extracellular shift of potassium. Further, the serum level of potassium drops during the course of treatment of DKA as potassium reenters the cells; therefore, it must be monitored frequently. Some of the factors related to treating DKA that reduce the serum potassium concentration include the following:

- Rehydration, which leads to increased plasma volume and subsequent decreases in the concentration of serum potassium. Rehydration also leads to increased urinary excretion of potassium.
- Insulin administration, which enhances the movement of potassium from the extracellular fluid into the cells.

Cautious but timely potassium replacement is vital to avoid dysrhythmias that may occur with hypokalemia. Up to 40 mmol/L/h may be needed for several hours. Because extracellular potassium levels drop during DKA treatment, potassium must be infused even if the plasma potassium level is normal.

Frequent (every 2 to 4 hours initially) ECGs and laboratory measurements of potassium are necessary during the first 8 hours of treatment. Potassium replacement is withheld only if hyperkalemia is present or if the patient is not urinating.

NURSING ALERT

Because a patient's serum potassium level may drop quickly as a result of rehydration and insulin treatment, potassium replacement must begin once potassium levels drop to normal and prior to insulin treatment in the patient with DKA.

Reversing Acidosis

Ketone bodies (acids) accumulate as a result of fat breakdown. The acidosis that occurs in DKA is reversed with insulin, which inhibits fat breakdown, thereby ending ketone production and acid buildup. Insulin is usually infused IV at a slow, continuous rate (e.g., 5 units per hour). Hourly blood glucose values must be measured. IV fluid solutions with higher concentrations of glucose, such as NS solution (e.g., D_5NS, $D_5.45NS$), are given when blood glucose levels reach 250 to 300 mg/dL (13.8 to 16.6 mmol/L) to avoid too rapid a drop in the blood glucose level (i.e., hypoglycemia) during treatment.

Regular insulin, the only type of insulin approved for IV use, may be added to IV solutions. The nurse must convert hourly rates of insulin infusion (frequently prescribed as units per hour) to IV drip rates. For example, if 100 units of regular insulin are mixed into 500 mL of 0.9% NS, then 1 unit of insulin equals 5 mL; therefore, an initial insulin infusion rate of 5 units per hour would equal 25 mL/h. The insulin is often infused separately from the rehydration solutions to allow frequent changes in the rate and content of the latter.

Insulin must be infused continuously until subcutaneous administration of insulin can be resumed. Any interruption in administration may result in the reaccumulation of ketone bodies and worsening acidosis. Even if blood glucose levels are decreasing and returning to normal, the insulin drip must not be stopped until subcutaneous insulin therapy has been started. Rather, the rate or concentration of the dextrose infusion may be increased to prevent hypoglycemia. Blood glucose levels are usually corrected before the acidosis is corrected. Therefore, IV insulin may be continued for 12 to 24 hours, until the serum bicarbonate level increases (to at least 15 to 18 mEq/L) and until the patient can eat. In general, bicarbonate infusion to correct severe acidosis is avoided during treatment of DKA because it precipitates further, sudden (and potentially fatal) decreases in serum potassium levels. Continuous insulin infusion is usually sufficient for reversal of DKA (Noble-Bell & Cox, 2014; Umpeirrez & Korytkowski, 2016).

NURSING ALERT

When mixing the insulin drip, it is important to flush the insulin solution through the entire IV infusion set and to discard the first 50 mL of fluid. Insulin molecules adhere to the inner surface of IV infusion sets; thus, the initial fluid may contain a decreased concentration of insulin.

Nursing Management

Nursing care of the patient with DKA focuses on monitoring fluid and electrolyte status as well as blood glucose levels; administering fluids, insulin, and other medications; and preventing other complications such as fluid overload. Urine output is monitored to ensure adequate renal function before potassium is administered to prevent hyperkalemia. The ECG is monitored for dysrhythmias indicating abnormal potassium levels. Vital signs, arterial blood gases, and other clinical findings are recorded on a flow sheet. The nurse documents the patient's laboratory values and the frequent changes in fluids and medications that are prescribed and monitors the patient's responses. As DKA resolves and the potassium replacement rate is decreased, the nurse ensures the following:

- There are no signs of hyperkalemia on the ECG (tall, peaked [or tented] T waves).
- The laboratory values of potassium are normal or low.
- The patient is urinating (i.e., no renal shutdown).

As the patient recovers, the nurse reassesses the factors that may have led to DKA and teaches the patient and family about strategies to prevent its recurrence. If indicated, the nurse initiates a referral for home care to ensure the patient's continued recovery.

Hyperglycemic Hyperosmolar Syndrome

HHS is a metabolic disorder of type 2 diabetes resulting from a relative insulin deficiency initiated by an illness that raises the demand for insulin. This is a serious condition in which hyperosmolarity and hyperglycemia predominate, with alterations of the sensorium (sense of awareness). At the same time, ketosis is usually minimal or absent. The basic biochemical defect is the lack of effective insulin (i.e., insulin resistance). Persistent hyperglycemia causes osmotic diuresis, which results in losses of water and electrolytes. To maintain osmotic equilibrium, water shifts from the intracellular fluid space to the extracellular fluid space. With glycosuria and dehydration, hypernatremia and increased osmolarity occur. Table 41-5 compares DKA and HHS.

This condition occurs most often in older people (ages 50 to 70 years) with no known history of diabetes or with mild type 2 diabetes. HHS can be traced to a precipitating event such as an acute illness (e.g., pneumonia or stroke), medications that exacerbate hyperglycemia (thiazide diuretics), or treatments such as dialysis. The history includes days to weeks of polyuria with adequate fluid intake. What distinguishes HHS from DKA is that ketosis and acidosis do not occur in HHS partly because of differences in insulin levels. In DKA, no insulin is present, and this promotes the breakdown of stored glucose, protein, and fat, which leads to the production of ketone bodies and ketoacidosis. In HHS, the insulin level is too low to prevent hyperglycemia (and subsequent osmotic diuresis), but it is high enough to prevent fat breakdown. Patients with HHS do not have the ketosis-related GI symptoms that lead them to seek medical attention. Instead, they may tolerate polyuria and polydipsia until neurologic changes or an underlying illness (or family members or others) prompts them to seek treatment. Because of possible delays in therapy, hyperglycemia, dehydration, and hyperosmolality may be more severe in HHS.

Clinical Manifestations

The clinical picture of HHS is one of hypotension, profound dehydration (dry mucous membranes, poor skin turgor), tachycardia, and variable neurologic signs (e.g., alteration of sensorium, seizures, hemiparesis). The mortality rate ranges from 10% to 40%, usually related to an underlying illness.

Assessment and Diagnostic Findings

Diagnostic assessment includes a range of laboratory tests, including blood glucose, electrolytes, BUN, complete blood count, serum osmolality, and arterial blood gas analysis. The blood glucose level and the osmolality are excep-

TABLE 41-5 Comparison of Diabetic Ketoacidosis and Hyperglycemic Hyperosmolar Syndrome

Characteristics	DKA	HHS
Patients most commonly affected	Can occur in type 1 or type 2 diabetes; more common in type 1 diabetes	Can occur in type 1 or type 2 diabetes; more common in type 2 diabetes, especially older patients with type 2 diabetes
Precipitating event	Omission of insulin; physiologic stress (infection, surgery, stroke, MI)	Physiologic stress (infection, surgery, stroke, MI)
Onset	Rapid (<24 hours)	Slower (over several days)
Blood glucose levels	Usually >250 mg/dL (>13.9 mmol/L)	Usually >600 mg/dL (>33.3 mmol/L)
Arterial pH level	<7.3	Normal
Serum and urine ketones	Present	Absent
Serum osmolality	300–350 mOsm/L	>350 mOsm/L
Plasma bicarbonate level	<15 mEq/L	Normal
BUN and creatinine levels	Elevated	Elevated
Mortality rate	1–5%	10–20%

DKA, diabetic ketoacidosis; HHS, hyperglycemic hyperosmolar syndrome; MI, myocardial infarction; BUN, blood urea nitrogen.

Adapted from Umpeirrez, G., & Korytkowski, M. (2016). Diabetic emergencies—ketoacidosis, hyperglycaemic hyperosmolar state and hyperglycemia. *Nature Reviews. Endocrinology*, *12*, 222–232.

tionally high. Electrolyte and BUN levels are consistent with the clinical picture of severe dehydration. Mental status changes, focal neurologic deficits, and hallucinations are common secondary to the cerebral dehydration that results from extreme hyperosmolality. Postural hypotension may accompany the dehydration as a result of fluid loss.

Management

The overall approach to the treatment of HHS is similar to that of DKA: fluid replacement, correction of electrolyte imbalances, and insulin administration. Because patients with HHS are typically older, close monitoring of volume and electrolyte status is important for prevention of fluid overload, heart failure, and cardiac dysrhythmias. Fluid treatment is started with 0.9% or 0.45% NS, depending on the patient's sodium level and the severity of volume depletion. Central venous or hemodynamic pressure monitoring guides fluid replacement. Potassium is added to IV fluids when urinary output is adequate and is guided by continuous ECG monitoring and frequent laboratory determinations of potassium (Noble-Bell & Cox, 2014; Umpeirrez & Korytkowski, 2016).

Extremely elevated blood glucose concentrations decrease as the patient is rehydrated. Insulin plays a less important role in the treatment of HHS because it is not needed for reversal of acidosis, as in DKA. Nevertheless, insulin is usually given at a continuous low rate to treat hyperglycemia, and replacement IV fluids with dextrose are given (as in DKA) after the glucose level has decreased to the range of 250 to 300 mg/dL (13.8 to 16.6 mmol/L) (Noble-Bell & Cox, 2014; Umpeirrez & Korytkowski, 2016).

Other therapeutic modalities are determined by the underlying illness and the results of continuing clinical and laboratory evaluation. It may take 3 to 5 days for neurologic symptoms to clear, and treatment of HHS usually continues well after metabolic abnormalities have resolved. After recovery from HHS, many patients can control their diabetes with MNT alone or with MNT and oral antidiabetic medications. Insulin may not be needed once the acute hyperglycemic complication is resolved. Frequent SBGM is important in prevention of recurrence of HHS.

After recovery from HHS, many patients can control their diabetes with diet alone or with diet and oral/injectable antihyperglycemic agents. Insulin may not be needed once the acute hyperglycemic complication is resolved.

Nursing Management

Nursing care of the patient with HHS includes close monitoring of vital signs, fluid status, and laboratory values. In addition, strategies are implemented to maintain safety and prevent injury related to changes in the patient's sensorium secondary to HHS. Fluid status and urine output are closely monitored because of the high risk for renal failure secondary to severe dehydration. In addition, the nurse must direct nursing care to the condition that may have precipitated the onset of HHS. Because HHS tends to occur in older patients, the physiologic changes that occur with aging make careful assessment of cardiovascular, pulmonary, and renal function important throughout the acute and recovery phases of HHS.

Nursing Process

The Patient Newly Diagnosed With Diabetes

Assessment

The history and physical assessment of the patient with newly diagnosed diabetes first focus on the signs and symptoms of prolonged hyperglycemia. In addition, there should be a focus on the physical, social, and emotional factors that may affect the patient's ability to learn and perform diabetes self-care activities. The patient is asked to describe symptoms that preceded the diagnosis of diabetes, such as polyuria, polydipsia, polyphagia, skin dryness, blurred vision, weight loss, genital itching, and non-healing ulcers. Blood glucose and urine ketone (for patients with type 1 diabetes) levels are measured.

Patients with type 1 diabetes are assessed for signs of DKA, including ketonuria, Kussmaul respirations, orthostatic hypotension, and lethargy upon presentation. The patient is questioned about symptoms of DKA, such as nausea, vomiting, and abdominal pain. Laboratory values are monitored for metabolic acidosis (i.e., decreased pH and decreased bicarbonate level) and electrolyte imbalance. Patients with type 2 diabetes are assessed for signs of HHS, including hypotension, altered sensorium, seizures, and decreased skin turgor. Laboratory values are monitored for hyperosmolality and electrolyte imbalance.

If the patient exhibits signs and symptoms of DKA or HHS, nursing care first focuses on treatment of these acute complications, as outlined in previous sections. Once these complications begin to resolve, nursing care then focuses on long-term management of diabetes, as discussed in this section.

The patient is assessed for physical factors that may impair his or her ability to learn or perform self-care skills, such as the following:

- Visual deficits (the patient is asked to read numbers or words on the insulin pen, a menu, a newspaper, or written teaching materials)
- Deficits in motor coordination (the patient is observed eating or performing other tasks or handling a syringe or finger-lancing device)
- Neurologic deficits (e.g., due to stroke, other neurologic disorders, or other disabling conditions; the patient is assessed for aphasia or decreased ability to follow simple commands)
- The nurse evaluates the patient's social situation for factors that may influence the treatment and education plan, such as the following:
  - Low literacy level (may be evaluated while assessing for visual deficits by having patient read from teaching materials)
  - Limited financial resources
  - Presence or absence of family support

- Typical daily schedule (patient is asked about timing and number of usual daily meals, work and exercise schedule, plans for travel)

The patient's emotional status is assessed by observing general demeanour (e.g., withdrawn, anxious) and body language (e.g., avoids eye contact). The patient is asked about major concerns and fears about diabetes; this allows the nurse to assess for any misconceptions or misinformation regarding diabetes. Coping skills are assessed by asking how the patient has dealt with difficult situations in the past.

Nursing Priorities

Based on the assessment data, the patient's major priorities may include the following:

- Fluid volume deficit
- Nutrition
- Patient education
- Self-care approaches
- Anxiety

Collaborative Problems/ Potential Complications

Based on assessment data, potential complications may include the following:

- Fluid overload, pulmonary edema, or heart failure
- Hypokalemia
- Hyperglycemia and ketoacidosis
- Hypoglycemia
- Cerebral edema

Planning and Goals

The major goals for the patient may include maintenance of fluid and electrolyte balance, optimal control of blood glucose levels, reversal of weight loss, ability to perform diabetes basic skills and self-care activities, decreased anxiety, and absence of complications.

Nursing Interventions

Maintaining Fluid and Electrolyte Balance

Intake and output are measured. IV fluids and electrolytes are administered as prescribed, and oral fluid intake is encouraged when it is permitted. Laboratory values of serum electrolytes (especially sodium and potassium) are monitored. Vital signs are monitored for signs of dehydration (tachycardia, orthostatic hypotension).

Improving Nutritional Intake

The diet is planned with control of glucose as the primary goal. It must take into consideration the patient's lifestyle, cultural background, activity level, and food preferences. An appropriate caloric intake allows the patient to achieve and maintain the desired body weight. The patient is encouraged to eat full meals and snacks as prescribed with portion control in mind. It is important for the nurse to ensure that insulin orders are altered as needed for delays in eating because of diagnostic and other procedures or for increased physical activity.

Reducing Anxiety

The nurse provides emotional support and sets aside time to talk with the patient who wishes to express feelings, cry, or ask questions about this new diagnosis. Any misconceptions the patient or family may have regarding diabetes are dispelled. The patient and family are assisted to focus on learning self-care behaviours. The patient is encouraged to perform the skills that are feared most and must be reassured that once a skill such as self-injection or lancing a finger for glucose monitoring is performed for the first time, anxiety will decrease. Positive reinforcement is given for the self-care behaviours attempted, even if the technique is not yet completely mastered.

Improving Self-Care

Patient teaching (discussed earlier in the Nursing Management section and below) is the major strategy used to prepare the patient for self-care. Special equipment may be needed for instruction on diabetes survival skills, such as a magnifying glass for insulin preparation or an injection-aid device for insulin injection. Low-literacy information and literature in other languages can be obtained from the ADA. The family is also taught so that they can assist in diabetes management by preparing and administering doses or monitoring the blood glucose level. The diabetes educator is consulted regarding various blood glucose monitors and other equipment for use by patients with physical impairments. The patient is assisted in identifying community resources for education and supplies as needed. Other members of the health care team are informed about variations in the timing of meals and the work schedule (e.g., if the patient works night or evening shifts and sleeps during the day) so that the diabetes treatment regimen can be adjusted accordingly.

Monitoring and Managing Potential Complications

FLUID OVERLOAD. Fluid overload can occur because of the administration of a large volume of fluid at a rapid rate that is often required to treat the patient with DKA or HHS. This risk is increased in older patients and in those with pre-existing cardiac disease. To avoid fluid overload and resulting congestive heart failure and pulmonary edema, the nurse monitors the patient closely during treatment by measuring vital signs at frequent intervals. Central venous pressure monitoring and hemodynamic monitoring may be initiated to provide additional measures of the fluid status. Physical examination focuses on assessment of cardiac rate and rhythm, breath sounds, venous distention, skin turgor, and urine output. The nurse monitors fluid intake and keeps careful records of IV and other fluid intake, along with urine output measurements.

HYPOKALEMIA. As described previously, hypokalemia is a potential complication during the treatment of DKA as potassium is depleted from body stores. Low serum potassium levels may result from rehydration, increased urinary excretion of potassium, and movement of potassium from the extracellular fluid into the cells with insulin administration. Prevention of hypokalemia includes cautious replacement of potassium; before its administration, however, it is important to ensure that the patient's kidneys are functioning properly. Because of the adverse effects of hypokalemia on cardiac function, monitoring of the cardiac rate, cardiac rhythm, ECG, and serum potassium levels is essential.

HYPERGLYCEMIA AND KETOACIDOSIS. Although the hyperglycemia and ketoacidosis that may have led to the new diagnosis of diabetes may be resolved, the patient is at risk for their subsequent recurrence. Therefore, blood glucose levels and urine ketones are monitored, and medications (insulin, oral/injectable antihyperglycemic agents) are administered as prescribed. The patient is monitored for signs and symptoms of impending hyperglycemia and ketoacidosis; if they occur, insulin and IV fluids are administered.

HYPOGLYCEMIA. Hypoglycemia may occur if the patient skips or delays meals, does not follow the prescribed diet, or greatly increases the amount of exercise without modifying diet and/or insulin. Also, the hospitalized patient or outpatient who fasts in preparation for diagnostic testing is at risk for hypoglycemia. Juice, pop, honey, or glucose tablets are used for treatment of hypoglycemia. The patient is encouraged to eat full meals and snacks as prescribed per the diabetic diet. If hypoglycemia is a recurrent problem, the total therapeutic regimen should be re-evaluated.

Because of the risk of hypoglycemia, especially with intensive insulin regimens, it is important for the nurse to review with the patient its signs and symptoms, possible causes, and measures for prevention and treatment.

CEREBRAL EDEMA. Although the cause of cerebral edema is unknown, it is thought to be caused by rapid correction of hyperglycemia, resulting in fluid shifts. Cerebral edema can be prevented by gradual reduction in the blood glucose level (ADA, 2004d). An hourly flow sheet is used to enable close monitoring of the blood glucose level, serum electrolyte levels, urine output, mental status, and neurologic signs. Precautions are taken to minimize activities that could increase intracranial pressure.

Promoting Home, Community-Based, and Transitional Care

EDUCATING PATIENTS ABOUT SELF-CARE. The patient is taught basic skills, including simple pathophysiology, treatment modalities (insulin administration, monitoring of blood glucose, ketones [for patients with type 1 diabetes] and diet) recognition, treatment, and prevention of acute complications (hypoglycemia and hyperglycemia) and practical information (where to obtain supplies, when to call a health care provider). If the patient has signs of long-term diabetes complications at the time of diagnosis of diabetes, teaching about appropriate preventive behaviours (e.g., foot care or eye care) should be included at this time (Chart 41-9).

CONTINUING AND TRANSITIONAL CARE. Follow-up education is arranged with a home care nurse or an outpatient diabetes education centre. This is particularly important for the patient who has had difficulty coping with the diagnosis, the patient who has limitations that may affect his or her ability to learn or to carry out the management plan, or the patient without any family or social supports. Referral to social services and community resources (e.g., centres for the visually impaired) may be needed, depending on the patient's financial circumstances and physical limitations. The importance of self-monitoring and of monitoring and follow-up by primary health care providers is reinforced, and the patient is reminded about the importance of attending follow-up appointments. The patient who is newly diagnosed with diabetes is also reminded about the importance of participating in other health promotion activities and health screening. Chart 41-10 is a checklist of home care skills.

Evaluation

Expected patient outcomes may include the following:

1. Achieves fluid and electrolyte balance
    a. Demonstrates intake and output balance
    b. Exhibits electrolyte values within normal limits
    c. Exhibits vital signs that remain stable with resolution of orthostatic hypotension and tachycardia
2. Achieves metabolic balance
    a. Avoids extremes of glucose levels (hypoglycemia or hyperglycemia)
    b. Demonstrates rapid resolution of hypoglycemic episodes
    c. Avoids further weight loss (if applicable) and begins to approach desired weight
3. Demonstrates/verbalizes diabetes survival skills
    a. Defines diabetes as a condition in which high blood glucose levels are present
    b. States normal and target blood glucose ranges
    c. Identifies factors that cause the blood glucose level to fall (insulin, exercise, some oral/injectable antihyperglycemic medications)
    d. Identifies factors that cause the blood glucose level to rise (food, illness, stress, and infections)
    e. Describes the major treatment modalities: diet, exercise, monitoring, medication, and education
    f. Demonstrates proper technique for administration of insulin
    g. States dose and timing of injections, peak action, duration, and adverse effects of insulin
    h. Verbalizes plan for rotating insulin injection sites.
    i. States dose, timing, peak action, and duration of prescribed oral/injectable antihyperglycemic agents
    j. Verbalizes understanding of foods containing carbohydrate and their effect on blood glucose levels

CHART 41-9

Patient Education: Foot Care Tips

The nurse instructs the patient to:

1. Take care of your diabetes.
   - Work with your health care team to keep your blood glucose level within a normal range.
2. Inspect your feet every day.
   - Look at your bare feet every day for cuts, blisters, red spots, and swelling.
   - Use a mirror to check the bottoms of your feet, or ask a family member for help if you have trouble seeing.
   - Check for changes in temperature.
3. Wash your feet every day.
   - Wash your feet in warm, not hot, water.
   - Dry your feet well. Be sure to dry between the toes.
   - Do not soak your feet.
   - Do not check water temperature with your feet; use a thermometer or elbow.
4. Keep the skin soft and smooth.
   - Rub a thin coat of skin lotion over the tops and bottoms of your feet but not between your toes.
5. Smooth corns and calluses gently.
   - Use a pumice stone to smooth corns and calluses.
6. Trim your toenails each week or when needed.
   - Trim your toenails straight across, and file the edges with an emery board or nail file.
7. Wear shoes and socks at all times.
   - Never walk barefoot.
   - Wear comfortable shoes that fit well and protect your feet.
   - Feel inside your shoes before putting them on each time to make sure the lining is smooth and there are no objects inside.
8. Protect your feet from hot and cold.
   - Wear shoes at the beach or on hot pavement.
   - Wear socks at night if your feet get cold.
9. Keep the blood flowing to your feet.
   - Put your feet up when sitting.
   - Wiggle your toes and move your ankles up and down for 5 minutes, two or three times a day.
   - Do not cross your legs for long periods of time.
   - Do not smoke.
10. Check with your doctor or health care provider.
    - Have your doctor/health care provider check your bare feet and find out whether you are likely to have serious foot problems. Remember that you may not feel the pain of an injury.
    - Call your doctor right away if a cut, sore, blister, or bruise on your foot does not begin to heal after 1 day.
    - Follow your doctor/health care provider's advice about foot care.
    - Do not self-medicate or use home remedies or over-the-counter agents to treat foot problems.

Adapted from National Institute of Diabetes and Digestive and Kidney Diseases (NIDDK). (2013b). *Diabetic neuropathies: The nerve damage of diabetes.* Retrieved on June 21, 2016, from www.niddk.nih.gov/health-information/health-topics/Diabetes/diabetic-neuropathies-nerve-damage-diabetes/Pages/diabetic-neuropathies-nerve-damage.aspx; Fisher T. (2016). Your annual comprehensive foot exam. Diabetes Self Management. AACE/ ACE Consensus Statement. *Endocrine Practice*, *22*(1), 84–102.

k. Verbalizes appropriate schedule for eating snacks and meals, orders appropriate foods on menus, identifies foods that may be substituted for one another on the meal plan

l. Demonstrates proper technique for monitoring blood glucose, including using finger-lancing device, obtaining a drop of blood, applying blood properly to strip, obtaining value of blood glucose, and recording blood glucose value. Also, is able to, change batteries and identify alarms and warnings on meter

m. Demonstrates proper technique for disposing of lancets and needles used for blood glucose monitoring and insulin injections (discarding them into a hard plastic container such as an empty bleach or detergent container or medical waste container)

n. Demonstrates proper technique for urine ketone testing (for patients with type 1 diabetes) and verbalizes appropriate times to assess for ketones (when ill or when blood glucose test results are repeatedly and inexplicably more than 14.0 mmol/L)

o. Identifies community outpatient resources for obtaining further diabetes education

p. Identifies acute complications (hypoglycemia and hyperglycemia)

q. Verbalizes symptoms of hypoglycemia (shakiness, sweating, headache, hunger, numbness or tingling of lips or fingers, weakness, fatigue, difficulty concentrating, change of mood) and dangers of untreated hypoglycemia (seizures and coma)

r. Identifies appropriate treatment of hypoglycemia, including 15 g of simple carbohydrate (e.g., four glucose tablets, 125-mL juice or soft drinks, 15-g sugar, or 6 Lifesavers to 10 jelly beans) followed by a snack of protein and carbohydrate (e.g., cheese and crackers or milk) or a regularly scheduled meal

s. States potential causes of hypoglycemia (too much insulin, delayed or decreased food intake, increased physical activity) and verbalizes preventive behaviours, such as frequent monitoring of blood glucose when daily schedule is changed and eating a snack or reducing insulin before exercise

t. Verbalizes importance of wearing medical identification and carrying a source of simple carbohydrate at all times

u. Verbalizes symptoms of prolonged hyperglycemia (increased thirst and urination)

v. Verbalizes rules for sick day management

CHART 41-10

HOME CARE CHECKLIST • The Person With Newly Diagnosed Diabetes

At the completion of education, the patient and/or caregiver will be able to:

- State the importance of diabetes survival skills.
- Explain the underlying pathology of diabetes.
- State the normal range of blood glucose.
- Identify factors that cause hyper- and hypoglycemia.
- Describe the major modalities used to control diabetes (diet, exercise, monitoring, medication, education).
- Demonstrate proper technique for drawing up and injecting insulin (including mixing two types of insulin if necessary) or using insulin pens.
- State the dose and timing of injections and peak action and duration of insulin.
- Explain the insulin injection rotation plan and its rationale.
- State the dose, timing, peak action, and duration of prescribed oral agents.
- Describe where to purchase and store insulin pens, syringes, and glucose monitoring supplies.
- Identify the foods that contain carbohydrate and their effect on blood glucose levels.
- State the appropriate schedule for eating snacks and meals.
- Select appropriate foods on menus, and identify foods that may be substituted for one another on the meal plan.
- Demonstrate proper technique for monitoring blood glucose.
- Describe treatment for hypoglycemia.
- Use proper technique for disposing of lancets used for blood glucose monitoring and equipment used for insulin injections.
- Demonstrate proper technique for urine/blood ketone testing (for patients with type 1 diabetes or patients on SGLT2 inhibitors), and verbalize the appropriate times to assess for ketones.
- Identify community outpatient resources for obtaining further diabetes education.
- Identify signs and symptoms of hypoglycemia.
- Describe the appropriate treatment of hypoglycemia.
- Identify factors that may cause hypoglycemia.
- State strategies that minimize the risk for hypoglycemia.
- State the rationale for wearing medical identification and carrying a source of simple carbohydrate at all times.
- Identify the signs and symptoms of hyperglycemia.
- Describe the appropriate treatment of hyperglycemia.
- Identify factors that may cause hyperglycemia.
- Identify rules for sick-day management.
- Identify the appropriate circumstances for contacting the physician.

w. Describes where to purchase and store insulin, pens, and glucose monitoring supplies

x. Identifies appropriate circumstances for calling the physician or health care provider (when ill, when glucose levels repeatedly exceed a certain level [per guidelines], or when skin wounds fail to heal) and also identifies name of physician (or other health care team member) and 24-hour phone number

4. Absence of complications
   a. Exhibits normal cardiac rate and rhythm and normal breath sounds

b. Exhibits jugular venous pressure and distention within normal limits
c. Exhibits blood glucose and urine ketone levels within normal limits
d. Exhibits no manifestations of hypoglycemia or hyperglycemia
e. Shows improved mental status without signs of cerebral edema
f. States measures to prevent complications

LONG-TERM COMPLICATIONS OF DIABETES

There has been a steady decline in the number of deaths of patients with diabetes attributable to ketoacidosis and infection but an alarming rise in the number of deaths from cardiovascular and renal complications. Long-term complications are becoming more common as more people with diabetes live longer. The long-term complications of diabetes can affect almost every organ system of the body. In Canada, hospitalization rates are more than double (18% compared to 8% admitted each year) among adults who have diabetes compared with adults who do not have diabetes (Diabetes Canada, 2018a). The general categories of chronic complications of diabetes are macro- and microvascular diseases.

The specific causes and pathogenesis of each type of complication are still being investigated. It appears, however, that increased levels of blood glucose may play a role in neuropathic disease, microvascular complications, and risk factors contributing to macrovascular complications. Hypertension may also be a major contributing factor, especially in macro- and microvascular diseases.

Long-term complications are seen in patients with both type 1 and type 2 diabetes but usually do not occur within the first 5 to 10 years of the diagnosis. However, evidence of these complications may be present at the time of diagnosis of type 2 diabetes, as the patient may have had undiagnosed diabetes for many years. Renal (microvascular) disease is more prevalent among patients with type 1 diabetes, and cardiovascular (macrovascular) complications are more prevalent among older patients with type 2 diabetes.

Macrovascular Complications

Macrovascular complications of diabetes result from changes in the medium to large blood vessels. Blood vessel walls thicken, sclerose, and become occluded by plaque that adheres to the vessel walls. Eventually, blood flow is blocked. These atherosclerotic changes are indistinguishable from atherosclerotic changes in people without diabetes, but they tend to occur more often and at an earlier age in patients with diabetes. Coronary artery disease, cerebrovascular disease, and peripheral vascular disease are the three main types of macrovascular complications that occur more frequently in the population with diabetes.

Myocardial infarction is twice as common in men with diabetes and three times as common in women with diabetes. There is also an increased risk for complications resulting from myocardial infarction and an increased likelihood of a second myocardial infarction. Coronary artery disease may account for 50% to 60% of all deaths in patients with diabetes. One unique feature of coronary artery disease in patients with diabetes is that the typical ischemic symptoms may be absent. Thus, patients may not experience the early warning signs of decreased coronary blood flow and may have "silent" myocardial infarctions. These silent myocardial infarctions may be discovered only as changes on the ECG. A new recommendation suggests that a repeat resting ECG should be performed every 3 to 5 years in patients with diabetes rather than just in individuals at high risk for cardiovascular (CV) events (Diabetes Canada, 2018c). This lack of ischemic symptoms may be secondary to autonomic neuropathy (see below).

Cerebral blood vessels are similarly affected by accelerated atherosclerosis. Occlusive changes or the formation of an embolus elsewhere in the vasculature that lodges in a cerebral blood vessel can lead to transient ischemic attacks and strokes. People with diabetes have twice the risk of developing cerebrovascular disease, and studies suggest that there may be a greater likelihood of death from cerebrovascular disease in patients with diabetes. In addition, recovery from a stroke may be impaired in patients who have elevated blood glucose levels at the time of and immediately after a stroke. Because symptoms of cerebrovascular disease may be similar to symptoms of acute complications of diabetes (HHS or hypoglycemia), it is very important to rapidly assess the blood glucose level (and treat abnormal levels) in patients reporting these symptoms so that testing and treatment of cerebrovascular disease (stroke) can be initiated if indicated.

Atherosclerotic changes in the large blood vessels of the lower extremities are responsible for the increased incidence of occlusive peripheral arterial disease in patients with diabetes (two to three times higher than in people without diabetes). Signs and symptoms of peripheral vascular disease include diminished peripheral pulses and intermittent claudication (pain in the buttock, thigh or calf during walking). The severe form of arterial occlusive disease in the lower extremities is largely responsible for the increased incidence of gangrene and subsequent amputation in patients with diabetes. Neuropathy and impairments in wound healing also play a role in diabetic foot disease (see below).

Role of Diabetes in Macrovascular Diseases

Researchers continue to investigate the relationship between diabetes and macrovascular diseases. The main feature unique to diabetes is elevated blood glucose; however, a direct link has not been found between hyperglycemia and atherosclerosis. Although it may be tempting to attribute the increased prevalence of macrovascular diseases to the increased prevalence of certain risk factors (e.g., obesity, increased triglyceride levels, hypertension) in patients with diabetes, there is a higher-than-expected rate of macrovascular diseases among patients with diabetes compared with patients without diabetes who have the same risk factors (ADA, 2016d). Therefore, diabetes itself is seen as an independent risk factor for accelerated atherosclerosis. Other potential factors that may play a role in diabetes-related atherosclerosis include platelet and clotting factor abnormalities, decreased flexibility of red blood cells, decreased oxygen release, changes in the arterial wall related to hyperglycemia, and possibly hyperinsulinemia.

1. All individuals with diabetes (type 1 or type 2) should follow a comprehensive, multifaceted approach to reduce cardiovascular risk, including:
   a. Achievement and maintenance of healthy body weight
   b. Healthy diet
   c. Regular physical activity
   d. Smoking cessation
   e. Optimal glycemic control (usually A1C ≤7%)
   f. Optimal blood pressure control (<130/80 mm Hg)
   g. Additional vascular protective medications in the majority of adult patients (see recommendations below) [Grade D, Consensus, for those with type 1 diabetes; Grade D, Consensus, for children/adolescents; Grade A, Level 1 (8,9), for those with type 2 diabetes age >40 years with microalbuminuria]
2. Statin therapy should be used to reduce cardiovascular risk in adults with type 1 or type 2 diabetes with any of the following features:
   a. Clinical macrovascular disease [Grade A, Level 1 (50)]
   b. Age ≥40 years [Grade A Level 1 (50,51), for type 2 diabetes; Grade D, Consensus for type 1 diabetes]
   c. Age <40 years and 1 of the following:
      - Diabetes duration >15 years and age >30 years [Grade D, Consensus]
      - Microvascular complications [Grade D, Consensus]
      - Warrants therapy based on the presence of other risk factors according to the 2012 Canadian Cardiovascular Society Guidelines for the Diagnosis and Treatment of Dyslipidemia (53). [Grade D, Consensus]
3. ACE inhibitor or ARB, at doses that have demonstrated vascular protection, should be used to reduce cardiovascular risk in adults with type 1 or type 2 diabetes with any of the following:
   a. Clinical macrovascular disease [Grade A, Level 1 (43,45)]
   b. Age ≥55 years [Grade A, Level 1 (43,45), for those with an additional risk factor or end-organ damage; Grade D, Consensus, for all others]
   c. Age <55 years and microvascular complications [Grade D, Consensus]

   Note: Among women with childbearing potential, angiotensin-converting enzyme (ACE) inhibitors, angiotensin receptor blockers (ARBs) or statins should only be used if there is reliable contraception.
4. ASA should not be routinely used for the primary prevention of cardiovascular disease in people with diabetes [Grade A, Level 2 (36)]. ASA may be used in the presence of additional cardiovascular risk factors [Grade D, Consensus].
5. Low-dose ASA therapy (81 to 325 mg) may be used for secondary prevention in people with established cardiovascular disease [Grade D, Consensus].
6. Clopidogrel 75 mg may be used in people unable to tolerate ASA [Grade D, Consensus].

All individuals with diabetes (type 1 or 2), should follow a comprehensive, multifaceted approach to reducing cardiovascular risk, including achievement and maintenance of a healthy body weight with a healthy diet and regular physical activity, smoking cessation, optimal glycemic control, optimal blood pressure control, and additional vascular protective medications in the majority of adult patients (see recommendations below) [Grade D, Consensus, for type 1 diabetes; Grade D, Consensus, for children/adolescents; Grade A, Level 1 (8,9), for those with type 2 diabetes age >40 years with microalbuminuria].

Statin therapy should be used to reduce cardiovascular risk in adults with type 1 or type 2 diabetes who have clinical macrovascular disease or are 40 years of age or older. Statin therapy also applies to individuals who are less than 40 years of age and have either had diabetes for less than 15 years and are under the age of 30 [Grade D, Consensus], have microvascular complications [Grade D, Consensus], or exhibit the presence of other risk factors according to the 2012 Canadian Cardiovascular Society Guidelines for the Diagnosis and Treatment of Dyslipidemia [Grade D, Consensus (53)].

Use of an ACE inhibitor or ARB at doses that have demonstrated vascular protection should be used to reduce cardiovascular risk in adults with type 1 or type 2 diabetes and exhibit any of the following: clinical macrovascular disease [Grade A, Level 1 (43, 350)], are 55 or older and have additional risk factors or end-organ damage [Grade D, Consensus], or are under 55 years of age and have microvascular complications [Grade D, Consensus]. However, among women with childbearing potential, ACE inhibitors, ARBs, or statins should only be used if there is reliable contraconception.

Acetylsalicylic acid (ASA) should not be routinely used for the primary prevention of cardiovascular disease in people with diabetes [Grade A, Level 2 (36)]. However, ASA may be used in the presence of additional cardiovascular risk factors [Grade D, Consensus]. Low-dose ASA therapy (81 to 325 mg) may be used for secondary prevention in people with established cardiovascular disease [Grade D, Consensus]. Individuals who may need ASA therapy but are unable to tolerate it can use 75 mg of Clopidogrel [Grade D, Consensus].

Management

Management of macrovascular complications involves prevention and treatment of the commonly accepted risk factors for atherosclerosis. Diet and exercise are important in managing obesity, hypertension, and hyperlipidemia. In addition, the use of medications to control hypertension and hyperlipidemia may be indicated. Smoking cessation is essential. Control of blood glucose levels may reduce triglyceride levels and can significantly reduce the incidence of complications.

When macrovascular complications do occur, treatment is the same as with nondiabetic patients. In addition, patients may require increased amounts of insulin or may need to switch from oral antidiabetic agents to insulin during illnesses.

Microvascular Complications and Diabetic Retinopathy

Although macrovascular atherosclerotic changes are seen in both diabetic and nondiabetic patients, the microvascular changes are unique to diabetes. Microvascular disease of diabetes (or microangiopathy) is characterized by capillary basement membrane thickening. The basement membrane surrounds the endothelial cells of the capillary. Researchers believe that increased blood glucose levels react through a series of biochemical responses to thicken the basement membrane to several times its normal thickness. The retinas and the kidneys are affected by these changes. According to the Canadian National Institute for the Blind (2014), diabetic retinopathy is the leading cause of vision loss in Canadians younger than 50 years. After 20 years of diabetes, nearly all patients with type 1 diabetes and over 60% of patients with type 2 diabetes have some degree of retinopathy. Similarly, about one in every four individuals starting dialysis has nephropathy caused by diabetes.

People with diabetes are subject to multiple visual complications (Table 41-6). The eye pathology referred to as diabetic retinopathy is caused by changes in the small blood vessels in the retina, the area of the eye that receives images and sends information about the images to the brain (Fig. 41-6). The retina is richly supplied with blood vessels of all kinds: small arteries and veins, arterioles, venules, and capillaries. There are three main stages of retinopathy: non-proliferative (background) retinopathy, pre-proliferative retinopathy, and proliferative retinopathy.

Changes in the microvasculature may include microaneurysms, intraretinal hemorrhage, hard exudates, and focal capillary closure. Although most patients do not develop visual impairment, it can be devastating if it occurs. A complication of non-proliferative retinopathy, macular edema, occurs in approximately 10% of people with type 1 or type 2 diabetes and may lead to visual distortion and loss of central vision.

An advanced form of background retinopathy, pre-proliferative retinopathy, is considered a precursor to the more serious proliferative retinopathy. In pre-proliferative retinopathy, there are more widespread vascular changes and loss of nerve fibres. Epidemiologic evidence suggests that 10% to 50% of patients with pre-proliferative retinopathy will develop proliferative retinopathy within a short time (possibly as little as 1 year). As with background retinopathy, if visual changes occur during the pre-proliferative stage, they are usually caused by macular edema.

Proliferative retinopathy represents the greatest threat to vision. It is characterized by the proliferation of new blood vessels growing from the retina into the vitreous humour. These new vessels are prone to bleeding. The visual loss associated with proliferative retinopathy is caused by vitreous hemorrhage and/or retinal detachment. The vitreous humour is usually clear, allowing light to be transmitted to the retina. When there is a hemorrhage, the vitreous humour becomes clouded and cannot transmit light, resulting in loss of vision. Another consequence of hemorrhage into the vitreous humour is that resorption of

TABLE 41-6 Ocular Complications of Diabetes

Eye Disorder	Characteristics
Retinopathy	Deterioration of the small blood vessels that nourish the retina
Background	Early stage, asymptomatic retinopathy. Blood vessels within the retina develop microaneurysms that leak fluid, causing swelling and forming deposits (exudates). In some cases, macular edema causes distorted vision.
Pre-proliferative	Represents increased destruction of retinal blood vessels.
Proliferative	Abnormal growth of new blood vessels on the retina. New vessels rupture, bleeding into the vitreous and blocking light. Ruptured blood vessels in the vitreous form scar tissue, which can pull on and detach the retina.
Cataracts	Opacity of the lens of the eye; cataracts occur at an earlier age in patients with diabetes.
Lens changes	The lens of the eye can swell when blood glucose levels are elevated. For some patients, visual changes related to lens swelling may be the first symptoms of diabetes. It may take up to 2 months of improved blood glucose control before hyperglycemic swelling subsides and vision stabilizes. Therefore, patients are advised not to change eyeglass prescriptions during the 2 months after discovery of hyperglycemia.
Extraocular muscle palsy	This may occur as a result of diabetic neuropathy. The involvement of various cranial nerves responsible for ocular movements may lead to double vision. This usually resolves spontaneously.
Glaucoma	Results from occlusion of the outflow channels by new blood vessels. Glaucoma may occur with slightly higher frequency in the population with diabetes.

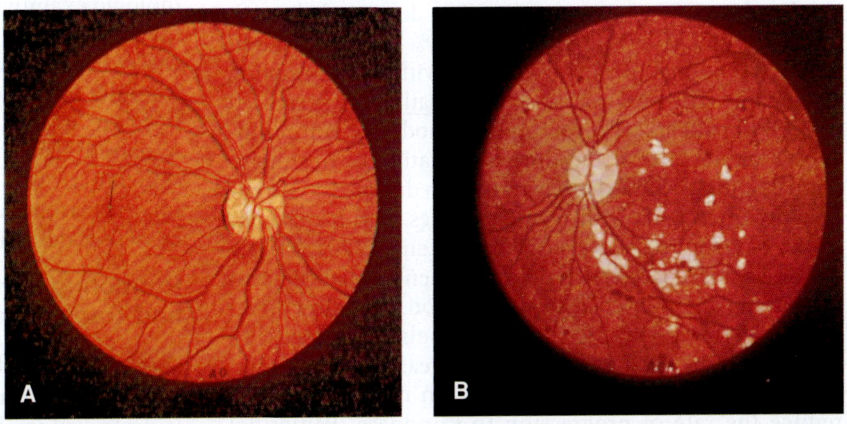

FIGURE 41-6. Diabetic retinopathy. **A.** In this fundus photograph of a normal eye, the light circular area over which a number of blood vessels converge is the optic disc, where the optic nerve meets the back of the eye. **B.** The fundus photograph of a patient with diabetic retinopathy shows characteristic waxy-looking retinal lesions, microaneurysms of the vessels, and hemorrhages. (Courtesy of American Optometric Association.)

the blood leads to the formation of fibrous scar tissue. This scar tissue may place traction on the retina, resulting in retinal detachment and subsequent visual loss.

Clinical Manifestations

Retinopathy is a painless process. In non-proliferative and pre-proliferative retinopathy, blurry vision secondary to macular edema occurs in some patients, although many patients are asymptomatic. Even patients with a significant degree of proliferative retinopathy and some hemorrhaging may not experience major visual changes. However, symptoms indicative of hemorrhaging include floaters or cobwebs in the visual field, sudden visual changes including spotty or hazy vision, or complete loss of vision.

Assessment and Diagnostic Findings

Diagnosis is by direct visualization with an ophthalmoscope or with a technique known as fluorescein angiography. Fluorescein angiography can document the type and activity of the retinopathy. Dye is injected into an arm vein and is carried to various parts of the body through the blood, but especially through the vessels of the retina. This technique allows the ophthalmologist, using special instruments, to see the retinal vessels in bright detail and gives useful information that cannot be obtained with an ophthalmoscope.

Side effects of this diagnostic procedure may include nausea during the dye injection, yellowish, fluorescent discolouration of the skin and urine lasting 12 to 24 hours and occasional allergic reactions, usually manifested by hives or itching. Generally, however, it is a safe diagnostic procedure. Patient preparation includes an explanation of the following:

- The steps of the procedure
- The fact that the procedure is painless
- The potential side effects
- The type of information the technique can provide
- That the flash of the camera may be slightly uncomfortable for a short time

Medical Management

The first focus of management is on primary and secondary prevention. The results of the DCCT demonstrated that maintenance of blood glucose to a normal or near-normal level in patients with type 1 diabetes through intensive insulin therapy and patient education decreased the risk for development of retinopathy by 76% when compared with conventional therapy in patients without pre-existing retinopathy. The progression of retinopathy was decreased by 54% in patients with very mild to moderate non-proliferative retinopathy at the time of initiation of treatment. Similarly, the UKPDS demonstrated a reduced risk of retinopathy in patients with type 2 diabetes with better control of blood glucose levels (Diabetes Canada, 2018b).

For advanced cases, the main treatment of diabetic retinopathy is argon laser photocoagulation. The laser treatment destroys leaking blood vessels and areas of neovascularization. For patients at increased risk for hemorrhaging, panretinal photocoagulation may significantly reduce the rate of progression to blindness. Panretinal photocoagulation involves the systematic application of multiple (more than 1,000) laser burns throughout the retina (except in the macular region). This stops the widespread growth of new vessels and hemorrhaging of damaged vessels. The role of "mild" panretinal photocoagulation (with only one third to one half as many laser burns) in the early stages of proliferative retinopathy or in patients with pre-proliferative changes is being investigated. For macular edema, focal photocoagulation is used to apply smaller laser burns to specific areas of microaneurysms in the macular region. This may reduce the rate of visual loss from macular edema by 50%.

Photocoagulation treatments are usually performed on an outpatient basis, and most patients can return to their usual activities by the next day. For some patients, limitations may be placed on activities involving weight bearing or bearing down. For most patients, the treatment does not cause intense pain, although they may report varying degrees of discomfort. Usually, an anesthetic eye drop is all that is needed during the treatment. A few patients may experience slight visual loss, loss of peripheral vision, or impairments in adaptation to the dark. For most patients, however, the risk of slight visual changes from the laser treatment itself is much less than the potential for loss of vision from progression of retinopathy.

When a major hemorrhage into the vitreous humour occurs, the vitreous fluid becomes mixed with blood and prevents light from passing through the eye, which may lead to blindness. A vitrectomy is a surgical procedure in which vitreous humour filled with blood or fibrous tissue is removed with a special drill-like instrument and replaced with saline or another liquid. A vitrectomy is performed on patients who already have visual loss and in whom the vitreous hemorrhage has not cleared on its own after 6 months. The purpose is to restore useful vision; recovery to near-normal vision is not usually expected. Other strategies that may slow the progression of diabetic retinopathy include the following:

- Control of hypertension
- Control of blood glucose
- Cessation of smoking

Nursing Management

Nursing management of patients with diabetic retinopathy or other eye disorders involves implementing the individual plan of care and providing patient education. Education focuses on prevention through regular ophthalmologic examinations and blood glucose control and self-management of eye care regimens. The effectiveness of early diagnosis and prompt treatment is emphasized in teaching the patient and family. If vision loss occurs, nursing care must also address the patient's adjustment to impaired vision and use of adaptive devices for diabetes self-care as well as activities of daily living. Nursing care for the patient with low vision or loss of vision is discussed in detail in Chapter 60.

Promoting Home, Community-Based, and Transitional Care

Educating Patients About Self-Care

In all forms of therapy for retinopathy, something is destroyed in the process of saving vision, and the facts must be presented to the patient and family as honestly as possible. The course of the retinopathy may be long and stressful. In teaching and counselling the patient, it is important to stress the following:

- Retinopathy may appear after many years of diabetes, and its appearance does not necessarily mean that the diabetes is getting worse.
- The odds for maintaining vision are in the patient's favour, especially with adequate control of glucose levels and blood pressure.
- Frequent eye examinations are the best way to preserve vision, because they allow for the detection of any retinopathy.

Some additional points to keep in mind when the patient with diabetes has some type of visual impairment include the following:

- Visual impairment can be a shock. The person's response to vision loss depends on personality, self-concept, and coping mechanisms. Support may be needed.
- As in any loss, acceptance of blindness by the patient occurs in stages; some patients may learn to accept blindness quickly and others may not.
- Although retinopathy occurs bilaterally, the severity may differ between eyes.
- Many of the chronic complications of diabetes occur simultaneously. For example, a patient who is blind due to diabetic retinopathy may also have peripheral neuropathy and may experience impairment of manual dexterity and tactile sensation.

Continuing and Transitional Care

Continuing care for the patient with impaired vision due to diabetic changes depends on the severity of the impairment and the effectiveness of the patient's coping in response to the impairment. The importance of careful diabetes management is emphasized as one means of slowing the progression of visual changes. The patient is reminded of the need to see the ophthalmologist regularly. If eye changes are progressive and unrelenting, the patient needs to be prepared for inevitable blindness. Therefore, consideration is given to making referrals for teaching the patient Braille and for training with a guide dog. Referral to provincial/territorial agencies should be made to ensure that the patient receives services for the blind. Family members are also taught how to assist the patient to remain as independent as possible despite decreasing visual acuity.

Referral for home care may be indicated for some patients, particularly those who live alone, those not coping well, and those who have other health problems or complications of diabetes that may interfere with their ability to perform self-care. During home visits, the nurse can assess the patient's home environment and ability to manage diabetes despite visual impairments. Medical management and nursing care of patients with visual disturbances are discussed in detail in Chapter 60.

Nephropathy

Nephropathy, or renal disease secondary to diabetic microvascular changes in the kidney, is a common complication of diabetes. Fifty percent of people with diabetes have chronic kidney disease (CKD), which when associated with diabetes is the leading cause of kidney failure in Canada (Diabetes Canada, 2018b).

Patients with type 1 diabetes frequently show initial signs of renal disease after 10 to 15 years, whereas patients with type 2 diabetes develop renal disease within 10 years of the diagnosis of diabetes. Many patients with type 2 diabetes have had diabetes for many years before it was diagnosed and treated. Therefore, they may have evidence of nephropathy at the time of diagnosis.

There is no reliable method to predict whether a person will develop renal disease. The DCCT results showed that intensive treatment of diabetes with a goal of achieving an A1C level as close to the target range as possible reduced the occurrence of early signs of nephropathy, such as microalbuminuria by 39% and albuminuria by 54%. Similarly, the UKPDS demonstrated a reduced incidence of overt nephropathy in type 2 diabetes with control of blood glucose levels.

Soon after the onset of diabetes, and especially if the blood glucose levels are elevated, the kidney's filtration mechanism is stressed, allowing blood proteins to leak into the urine. As a result, the pressure in the blood vessels of the kidney increases. It is thought that the elevated pressure serves as the stimulus for the development of nephropathy. Various medications and diets are being tested to prevent these complications.

Clinical Manifestations

Most of the signs and symptoms of renal dysfunction in the patient with diabetes are similar to those seen in patients without diabetes. (Refer to Chapter 45 for the management of patients with renal disorders.) Also, as renal failure progresses, the catabolism (breakdown) of both exogenous and endogenous insulin decreases, and frequent hypoglycemic episodes may result. Insulin needs change as a result of changes in the catabolism of insulin and also as a result of changes in diet related to the treatment of nephropathy. The stress of renal disease affects self-esteem, family relationships, marital relations, and virtually all aspects of daily life. As renal function decreases, the patient commonly has multiple-system failure (e.g., declining visual acuity, impotence, foot ulcerations, heart failure, and nocturnal diarrhea).

Assessment and Diagnostic Findings

One of the most important blood proteins that leaks into the urine is albumin. Small amounts may leak undetected for years. Of the patients with microalbuminuria, clinical nephropathy eventually develops in more than 85%. However, if microalbuminuria is not present, nephropathy develops in fewer than 5%. Early microalbuminuria can be discovered by testing a random urine sample for the albumin to creatinine ratio (ACR) along with a urine dipstick test to rule out nondiabetic renal disease. If the urinary albumin is 30 to 300 mg/day (ACR is 2.0 to 20.0 mg/mmol for both men and women), two more random urine tests are required between 1 week and 2 months apart. Nephropathy is diagnosed if two of the three urine specimens show an ACR greater than 2.0 mg/mmol (Diabetes Canada, 2018b).

When a urine dipstick test reads consistently positive for significant amounts of albumin, serum creatinine and BUN levels are obtained. At this point in the development of renal disease, diagnostic testing for cardiac or other systemic problems may also be required. Some of the tests involve injection of special dyes that are not easily cleared by the damaged kidney, so the value of the diagnostic test must be weighed against the potential risks.

Hypertension often develops in patients (both diabetic and nondiabetic) who are in the early stages of renal disease. However, essential hypertension occurs in up to 50% of all individuals with diabetes (for unknown reasons). Thus, it should not be assumed that someone with diabetes who has hypertension also has renal disease; other diagnostic criteria must also be present.

Medical Management

In addition to achieving and maintaining near-normal blood glucose levels, management for all patients with diabetes should include careful attention to the following:

- Control of hypertension (the use of ACE inhibitors, such as perindopril, because control of hypertension may also decrease or delay the onset of early proteinuria)
- Prevention or vigorous treatment of urinary tract infections
- Avoidance of nephrotoxic substances
- Adjustment of medications as renal function changes
- Low-sodium diet
- Low-protein diet

If the patient has already developed microalbuminuria an ACE inhibitor should be prescribed. ACE inhibitors lower blood pressure and reduce microalbuminuria, protecting the kidney. Alternatively, ARB agents may be prescribed. This preventive strategy should be part of the standard of care for the person with diabetes. Carefully designed low-protein diets also appear to reverse early leakage of small amounts of protein from the kidney (Diabetes Canada, 2018b).

In chronic or end-stage renal failure, two types of treatment are available: dialysis (hemodialysis or peritoneal dialysis) and transplantation from a relative or a cadaver. Hemodialysis for the patient with diabetes is similar to that for patients without the disease (see Chapter 45). Because hemodialysis creates additional stress for patients with cardiovascular disease, it may not be appropriate for certain patients. In addition, it is extremely intrusive to a patient's life.

Continuous ambulatory peritoneal dialysis is being used by an increasing number of patients with diabetes, mainly because of the independence it allows patients. In addition, insulin can be mixed into the dialysate, which may result in better blood glucose control and end the need for insulin injections. However, these patients may require more insulin because the dialysate contains glucose. Major risks of peritoneal dialysis are infection and peritonitis. The mortality rate for diabetic patients undergoing dialysis is higher than that in patients without diabetes undergoing dialysis and is closely related to the severity of cardiovascular problems.

Renal disease is frequently accompanied by advancing retinopathy that may require laser treatments and surgery. Severe hypertension also worsens eye disease because of the additional stress it places on the blood vessels. Patients being treated with hemodialysis who require eye surgery may be changed to peritoneal dialysis and have their hypertension aggressively controlled for several weeks before surgery. The rationale for this change is that hemodialysis requires anticoagulants that can increase the risk of bleeding after the surgery, and peritoneal dialysis minimizes pressure changes in the eyes.

The success rate for kidney transplantation in patients with diabetes has improved. In medical centres performing large numbers of transplants, the chances are 75% to 80% that the transplanted kidney will continue to function in the patient with diabetes for at least 5 years. Like the original kidneys, transplanted kidneys in patients with diabetes can eventually be damaged if blood glucose levels are consistently high after the transplantation. Therefore, monitoring blood glucose levels frequently and adjusting insulin levels in patients with diabetes and transplanted kidneys are essential for long-term success. Pancreas transplants are sometimes attempted when a kidney transplant is performed. Pancreatic transplants have not been successful enough to be performed alone because of the risks associated with immunosuppression.

Diabetic Neuropathies

Diabetic neuropathy refers to a group of diseases that affect all types of nerves, including peripheral (sensorimotor), autonomic, and spinal nerves. The disorders appear to be clinically diverse and depend on the location of the affected nerve cells. The prevalence increases with the age of the patient and the duration of the disease and may be as high as 40% to 50% in patients who have had diabetes for 10 years. For people with type 1 diabetes, neuropathy rarely occurs within the first 5 years from diagnosis. However, for those with type 2 diabetes, neuropathy may be present very soon after onset (Diabetes Canada, 2018b).

Elevated blood glucose levels over a period of years have been implicated in the etiology of neuropathy. The pathogenesis of neuropathy may be attributed to either a vascular or a metabolic mechanism or both, but their relative contributions have yet to be determined. Capillary basement membrane thickening and capillary closure may be present. In addition, there may be demyelinization of the nerves, which is thought to be related to hyperglycemia. Nerve conduction is disrupted when there are aberrations of the myelin sheaths. Control of blood glucose levels to normal or near-normal levels was shown in the DCCT to decrease the incidence of neuropathy by 60%.

The two most common types of diabetic neuropathy are sensorimotor polyneuropathy and autonomic neuropathy. Cranial mononeuropathies—for example, those affecting the oculomotor nerve—also occur in diabetes, especially among older persons.

Sensorimotor polyneuropathy is a diabetic neuropathy that is also called *peripheral neuropathy*. It most commonly affects the distal portions of the nerves, especially the nerves of the lower extremities. It affects both sides of the body symmetrically and may spread in a proximal direction.

Peripheral Neuropathy

Clinical Manifestations

Initial symptoms include paresthesias (prickling, tingling, or heightened sensation) and burning sensations (especially at night). As the neuropathy progresses, the feet become numb. In addition, a decrease in proprioception (awareness of posture and movement of the body and of position and weight of objects in relation to the body) and a decreased sensation of light touch may lead to an unsteady gait. Decreased sensations of pain and temperature place patients with neuropathy at increased risk for injury and undetected foot infections. Deformities of the foot may also occur, with neuropathy-related joint changes producing Charcot joints. These joint deformities result from the abnormal weight distribution on joints due to lack of proprioception.

On physical examination, a decrease in deep tendon reflexes and vibratory sensation is found. For patients who have few or no symptoms of neuropathy, these physical findings may be the only indication of neuropathic changes. For patients with signs or symptoms of neuropathy, it is important to rule out other possible neuropathies, including alcohol-induced or vitamin-deficiency neuropathies.

Management

The results of the DCCT demonstrate that intensive insulin therapy and control of blood glucose levels delay the onset and slow the progression of neuropathy. Pain, particularly of the lower extremities, is a disturbing symptom in some people with neuropathy secondary to diabetes. For some patients, neuropathic pain spontaneously resolves within 6 months. For other patients, pain persists for many years. Various approaches to pain management can be tried. These include analgesics (preferably non-opioid); tricyclic antidepressants; phenytoin, carbamazepine, or gabapentin (anticonvulsant medications); mexiletine (antiarrhythmic); or transcutaneous electrical nerve stimulation (TENS).

The topical medication capsaicin (Capsaicin cream) has been shown in preliminary reports to decrease lower extremity neuropathic pain. Studies of the role of this topical medication in neuropathy continue.

Autonomic Neuropathies

Neuropathy of the autonomic nervous system results in a broad range of dysfunctions affecting almost every organ system of the body.

Clinical Manifestations

The manifestations of autonomic neuropathy are related to the cardiac, GI, and renal systems. Cardiovascular symptoms range from a fixed, slightly tachycardic heart rate, orthostatic hypotension, and silent, or painless, myocardial ischemia, and infarction. Delayed gastric emptying may occur with the typical symptoms of early satiety, bloating, nausea, and vomiting. In addition, there may be unexplained wide swings in blood glucose levels related to inconsistent absorption of the glucose from ingested foods secondary to the inconsistent gastric emptying. "Diabetic" constipation or diarrhea (especially nocturnal diarrhea) may occur as a result.

Urinary retention, a decreased sensation of bladder fullness, and other urinary symptoms of neurogenic bladder result from autonomic neuropathy. Patients with a neurogenic bladder are predisposed to developing urinary tract infections due to inability to completely empty the bladder. This is especially true in patients with poorly controlled diabetes, because hyperglycemia impairs resistance to infection.

Hypoglycemia Unawareness

Autonomic neuropathy of the adrenal medulla is responsible for diminished or absent adrenergic symptoms of hypoglycemia. Patients may report that they no longer feel the typical shakiness, sweating, nervousness, and palpitations associated with hypoglycemia. Strict blood glucose monitoring, including frequent SMBG, is recommended for these patients. Their inability to detect and treat the warning signs of hypoglycemia puts patients at risk for developing dangerously low blood glucose levels. Therefore, their goals for blood glucose levels may need to be adjusted to reduce the risk for hypoglycemia. The patient and family need to be taught to recognize subtle signs and symptoms of hypoglycemia.

Sudomotor Neuropathy

Sudomotor neuropathy is a condition that refers to a decrease or absence of sweating (anhidrosis) of the extremities, with a compensatory increase in upper body sweating. Dryness of the feet increases the risk for the development of foot ulcers.

Sexual Dysfunction

Sexual dysfunction, especially impotence in men, is a complication of diabetes. The effects of autonomic neuropathy on female sexual functioning are not well documented. Reduced vaginal lubrication has been mentioned as a possible neuropathic effect; other possible changes in sexual function in women with diabetes include decreased libido and lack of orgasm. Vaginal infection (especially candida [yeast]), which is increased in incidence in women with diabetes, may be associated with decreased lubrication and vaginal itching and tenderness. Urinary tract infections and vaginitis may also affect sexual function.

Impotence (inability of the penis to become rigid and sustain an erection adequate for penetration) occurs with greater frequency in men with diabetes than in men without diabetes of the same age. However, diabetic neuropathy is not the only cause of impotence in men with diabetes. Medications such as antihypertensive agents, psychological factors, and other medical conditions (e.g., vascular insufficiency) that may affect men without diabetes also play a role in impotence in men with diabetes.

Some men with autonomic neuropathy have normal erectile function and can experience orgasm but do not ejaculate. Retrograde ejaculation occurs, meaning that seminal fluid is propelled backward through the posterior urethra and into the urinary bladder. Examination of the urine confirms the diagnosis due to the large number of active sperm present. Fertility counselling is necessary for couples attempting conception.

Management

Management strategies depend on the symptoms. There is no treatment for painless cardiac ischemia, and the prognosis is poor. Detection, however, is important so that education about avoiding strenuous exercise can be provided. Orthostatic hypotension may respond to a diet high in sodium, the discontinuation of medications that impede autonomic nervous system responses, the use of sympathomimetics and other agents (e.g., caffeine) that stimulate an autonomic response and the use of lower body elastic garments that maximize venous return and prevent pooling of blood in the extremities.

Treatment of delayed gastric emptying includes a low-fat diet, frequent small meals, tight blood glucose control, and use of agents that increase gastric motility (e.g., metoclopramide, bethanechol, domperidone). Treatment of diabetic diarrhea may include bulk-forming laxatives or antidiarrheal agents. Constipation is treated with a high-fibre diet and adequate hydration; medications, laxatives, and enemas may be necessary when constipation is severe. Management of the patient with a neurogenic bladder is discussed in Chapter 46.

Treatment of sudomotor dysfunction focuses on education about skin care and heat intolerance. Erectile dysfunction is discussed in Chapter 50.

Foot and Leg Problems

From 50% to 75% of lower extremity amputations are performed on people with diabetes. More than 50% of these amputations are thought to be preventable, provided patients are taught foot care measures and practice them on a daily basis. Complications of diabetes that contribute to the increased risk of foot infections include the following:

- *Neuropathy:* Sensory neuropathy leads to loss of pain and pressure sensation, and autonomic neuropathy leads to increased dryness and fissuring of the skin (secondary to decreased sweating). Motor neuropathy results in muscular atrophy, which may lead to changes in the shape of the foot.
- *Peripheral vascular disease:* Poor circulation of the lower extremities contributes to poor wound healing and the development of gangrene.
- *Immunocompromise:* Hyperglycemia impairs the ability of specialized leukocytes to destroy bacteria. Thus, in poorly controlled diabetes, there is a lowered resistance to certain infections.

The typical sequence of events in the development of a diabetic foot ulcer begins with a soft tissue injury of the foot, formation of a fissure between the toes or in an area of dry skin, or formation of a callus (Fig. 41-7). Injuries are not felt by the patient with an insensitive foot and may be thermal (e.g., from using heating pads, walking barefoot on hot concrete, or testing bath water with the foot), chemical (e.g., burning the foot while using caustic agents on calluses, corns, or bunions), or traumatic (e.g., injuring skin while cutting nails, walking with an undetected foreign object in the shoe, or wearing ill-fitting shoes and socks).

If the patient is not in the habit of thoroughly inspecting both feet on a daily basis, the injury or fissure may go unnoticed until a serious infection has developed. Drainage, swelling, redness (from cellulitis) or gangrene may be the first sign of foot problems that the patient notices. Treatment of foot ulcers involves bed rest, antibiotics, and debridement. In addition, controlling glucose levels, which tend to increase when infections occur, is important for promoting wound healing. In patients with peripheral vascular disease, foot ulcers may not heal because of the decreased ability of oxygen, nutrients, and antibiotics to reach the injured tissue. Amputation may be necessary to prevent the spread of infection.

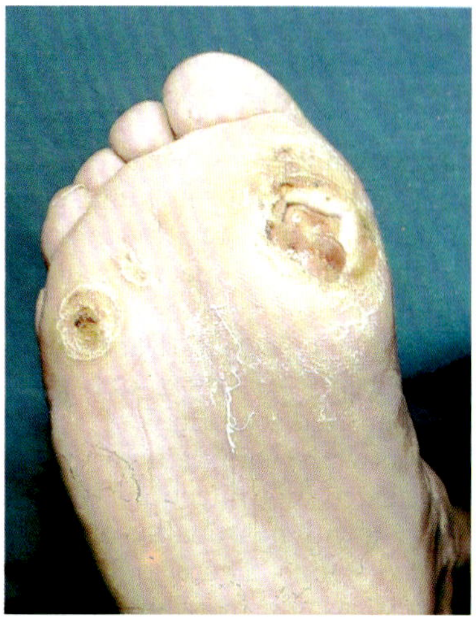

FIGURE 41-7. Neuropathic ulcers occur on pressure points in areas with diminished sensation in diabetic polyneuropathy. Pain is absent (and therefore the ulcer may go unnoticed).

Foot assessment and foot care instructions are most important when caring for patients who are at high risk for developing foot infections. Some of the high-risk characteristics include the following:

- Duration of diabetes more than 10 years
- Age older than 40 years
- History of smoking
- Decreased peripheral pulses
- Decreased sensation
- Anatomic deformities or pressure areas (e.g., bunions, calluses, hammertoes)
- History of previous foot ulcers or amputation

Management

Teaching patients proper foot care is a nursing intervention that can prevent costly, painful, and debilitating complications. Preventive foot care begins with careful daily assessment of the feet. The feet must be inspected on a daily basis for any redness, blisters, fissures, calluses, ulcerations, changes in skin temperature, and the development of foot deformities (i.e., hammertoes, bunions). For patients with visual impairment or decreased joint mobility (especially older adults), the use of a mirror to inspect the bottom of the feet or the help of a family member in foot inspection may be necessary. The interior surfaces of shoes should be inspected for any rough spots or foreign objects.

In addition to the daily visual and manual inspection of the feet, the feet should be examined during every health care visit or at least once per year (more often if there is an increase in the patient's risk) by a podiatrist, physician, or nurse. Patients with neuropathy should also undergo evaluation of neurologic status using a monofilament device by an experienced examiner. Patients with pressure areas, such as calluses, or thick toenails should see the podiatrist routinely for treatment of calluses and trimming of nails.

Additional aspects of preventive foot care that are taught to the patient and family include the following:

- Properly bathing, drying, and lubricating the feet, taking care not to allow moisture (water or lotion) to accumulate between the toes.
- Wearing closed-toe shoes that fit well. Podiatrists can provide patients with inserts (orthotics) to remove pressure from pressure points on the foot. New shoes should be broken in slowly (i.e., worn for 1 to 2 hours initially, with gradual increases in the length of time worn) to avoid blister formation. Patients with bony deformities may need extra-wide or extra-depth shoes. High-risk behaviours should be avoided, such as walking barefoot, using heating pads on the feet, wearing open-toed shoes, soaking the feet, and shaving calluses.
- Trimming toenails straight across and filing sharp corners to follow the contour of the toe. If patients have visual deficits or thickened toenails, a podiatrist should cut the nails.
- Reducing risk factors, such as smoking and elevated blood lipids, that contribute to peripheral vascular disease.
- Avoiding self-medicating with home remedies or over-the-counter agents to treat foot problems.

Blood glucose control is important for avoiding decreased resistance to infections and for preventing diabetic neuropathy. The patient may be referred by the physician to a wound care centre for managing persistent wounds of the feet or legs. Many wound care centres provide diabetes education; however, the patient needs to discuss recommendations for treating wounds and diabetes management with his or her own physician/health care provider as well.

SPECIAL ISSUES IN DIABETES CARE

Patients With Diabetes Undergoing Surgery

During periods of physiologic stress such as surgery, blood glucose levels tend to rise as a result of an increase in the level of stress hormones (epinephrine, norepinephrine, glucagon, cortisol, and growth hormone). If hyperglycemia is not controlled during surgery, the resulting osmotic diuresis may lead to excessive loss of fluids and electrolytes. Patients with type 1 diabetes also risk developing ketoacidosis during periods of stress. The perioperative glycemic targets have been simplified to 5.0 to 10.0 mmol/L for most surgical situations.

Hypoglycemia is also a concern in patients with diabetes undergoing surgery. This is especially a concern during the preoperative period if surgery is delayed beyond the morning in a patient who received a morning injection of intermediate-acting insulin.

There are various approaches to managing glucose control during the perioperative period. Frequent capillary glucose monitoring is essential throughout the preoperative and postoperative periods, regardless of the method used for glucose control. Examples of these approaches are described in Chart 41-11, although the use of IV insulin and dextrose has become widespread with the increased availability of meters for intraoperative glucose monitoring.

During the postoperative period, patients with diabetes must also be closely monitored for cardiovascular complications because of the increased prevalence of atherosclerosis in patients with diabetes, wound infections, and skin breakdown (especially in the patient with decreased pain sensation in the extremities due to neuropathy). Maintaining adequate nutrition and blood glucose control promotes wound healing.

Management of Hospitalized Patients With Diabetes

For the majority of non-critically ill patients, preprandial blood glucose targets of 5.0 to 10.0 mmol/L are suggested. For most medical or surgical critically ill patients with hyperglycemia using a continuous intravenous insulin infusion, glucose levels of 8.0 to 10.0 mmol/L are suggested.

At any one time, 10% to 20% of general medical-surgical patients in the hospital have diabetes. This number will increase as older patients make up a greater proportion of the population. Although some hospitals may have a specialized endocrinology unit, typically patients with diabetes are admitted throughout the hospital.

Often, diabetes is not the primary medical diagnosis, yet problems with the control of diabetes frequently result from changes in the patient's normal routine or from surgery or illness. Some of the main issues pertinent to nursing care of the hospitalized patient with diabetes are presented in the following section.

Self-Care Issues

All patients admitted to the hospital must relinquish control of some aspects of their daily care to the hospital staff. For the patient with diabetes who is actively involved in diabetes self-management (especially insulin dose adjustment), relinquishing control over meal timing, insulin timing, and insulin dosage may be particularly difficult. The patient may fear hypoglycemia and express much concern over possible delays in receiving attention from the nurse if hypoglycemic symptoms occur.

It is important for the nurse to acknowledge the patient's concerns and to involve the patient as much as possible in the plan of care. If the patient disagrees with certain aspects of the nursing or medical care related to diabetes, the nurse must communicate this to other members of the health care team and, where appropriate, make changes in the plan to meet the patient's needs. The nurse and other health care providers need to pay particular attention to patients who are successful in managing self-care, assess their self-care management skills, and encourage them to continue their self-care management if correct and appropriate.

CHART 41-11

Approaches to Management of Glucose Control During the Perioperative Period

- For those with a diagnosis of diabetes:
  - Monitor blood glucose levels frequently (every 1 to 2 hours).
- For patients taking insulin:
  - The morning of surgery, all subcutaneous insulin doses are withheld (unless the blood glucose level is elevated—e.g., more than 11.1 mmol/L, in which case a small dose of subcutaneous regular/rapid insulin may be prescribed). The blood glucose level is controlled during surgery with the IV infusion of regular insulin, which is balanced by an infusion of dextrose. The insulin and dextrose infusion rates are adjusted according to frequent (hourly) capillary glucose determinations. After surgery, the insulin infusion may be continued until the patient can eat. If IV insulin is discontinued, subcutaneous regular insulin may be administered at set intervals (every 4 to 6 hours) or intermediate- or long-acting insulin may be administered every 12 to 24 hours with supplemental regular insulin as necessary until the patient is eating and the usual pattern of insulin dosing is resumed. The nurse caring for a patient with diabetes who is receiving IV insulin must carefully monitor the insulin infusion rate and blood glucose levels. IV insulin has a much shorter duration of action than subcutaneous insulin. Thus, if the infusion is interrupted or discontinued, hyperglycemia will develop rapidly (within 1 hour in patients with type 1 diabetes and within a few hours in patients with type 2 diabetes). The nurse must ensure that subcutaneous insulin is administered 30 minutes before discontinuing the IV insulin infusion.
  - One half to two thirds of the patient's usual morning dose of insulin (intermediate- or long-acting insulin alone) is administered subcutaneously in the morning before surgery. The patient's regular regimen of insulin is resumed following surgery once the patient is eating.
  - Patients with type 2 diabetes who do not usually take insulin may require insulin during the perioperative period to control blood glucose elevations. Most oral/injectable antihyperglycemic agents are held the morning of surgery. Some of these patients may resume their usual regimen of diet and oral agent during the recovery period. Other patients (whose diabetes was not well controlled with diet and an oral/injectable antihyperglycemic agent before surgery) need to continue with insulin injections after discharge.
  - For patients with type 2 diabetes who are undergoing minor surgery but who do not normally take insulin, glucose levels may remain stable provided no dextrose is infused during the surgery. After surgery, they may require small doses of regular/rapid insulin until the usual diet and oral agent are resumed.

Adapted from Comerford, K. C. (2015). *Nursing 2015 drug handbook*. Philadelphia, PA: Wolters Kluwer.

Hyperglycemia During Hospitalization

Individuals with diabetes should maintain their prehospitalization oral/injectable antihyperglycemic agents or insulin regimens provided that their medical conditions, dietary intake, and glycemic control are acceptable. For hospitalized patients with diabetes treated with insulin, a proactive approach that includes basal, bolus, and correction (supplemental) insulin along with pattern management should be used to reduce adverse events and improve glycemic control instead of the reactive sliding-scale insulin approach that uses only short- or rapid-acting insulin [Grade B, Level 2 (1,2)].

For the majority of non-critically ill patients treated with insulin, preprandial BG targets should be 5.0 to 10.0 mmol/L in conjunction with random BG values less than 10.0 mmol/L as long as these targets can safely be achieved [Grade D, Consensus].

For most medical-surgical critically ill patients with hyperglycemia, a continuous IV of insulin infusion should be used to maintain glucose levels between 8 and 10 mmol/L [Grade D, Consensus].

Perioperative glycemic levels should be maintained between 5.0 and 10.0 mmol/L for most surgical situations with an appropriate protocol and trained staff to ensure the safe and effective implementation of therapy to minimize the likelihood of hypoglycemia. To maintain intraoperative glycemic levels between 5.0 and 10.0 mmol/L for patients with diabetes undergoing coronary artery bypass grafting, a continuous IV insulin infusion protocol administered by trained staff should be used [Grade C, Level 3 (3–5)].

In hospitalized patients, hypoglycemia should be avoided. Protocols for hypoglycemia avoidance, recognition, and management should be implemented with nurse-initiated treatment. Patients at risk for hypoglycemia should have ready access to an appropriate source of glucose, oral or IV, at all times. For example, when IV access is not readily available, the nurse should use glucagon for severe hypoglycemia [Grade D, Consensus].

Hyperglycemia may occur in the hospitalized patient as a result of the original illness that led to the need for hospitalization. In addition, a number of other factors may contribute to hyperglycemia, such as the following:

- Changes in the usual treatment regimen (e.g., increased food, decreased insulin, decreased activity)
- Medications (e.g., glucocorticoids such as prednisone or hydrocortisone, which are used in the treatment of a variety of inflammatory disorders)
- IV dextrose, which may be part of the maintenance fluids or may be used for the administration of antibiotics and other medications
- Overly vigorous treatment of hypoglycemia
- Mismatched timing of meals and insulin (e.g., postprandial hyperglycemia may occur if short-acting insulin is administered immediately before or even after meals)

Nursing actions to correct some of these factors are important for avoiding hyperglycemia. Assessment of the patient's usual home routine is important. The nurse should try to maintain the home schedule of insulin, meals, and activities as much as possible. Monitoring blood glucose levels has been identified by the ADA as an additional "vital sign" essential in assessing the patient's status. The results of blood glucose monitoring provide information needed to obtain orders for extra doses of insulin (at times when insulin is usually taken by the patient), an important nursing function. The insulin doses must not be withheld when blood glucose levels are normal.

Short- or rapid-acting insulin is usually needed to avoid postprandial hyperglycemia (even in the patient with normal pre-meal glucose levels), and NPH insulin does not peak until many hours after the dose is given. It is important to avoid overly vigorous treatment of hypoglycemia, which may lead to hyperglycemia. Treatment of hypoglycemia should be based on the established hospital protocol (usually 15 g of carbohydrate in the form of juice/pop, glucose tablets, or, if necessary, ½ to 1 ampule of 50% dextrose administered intravenously). Extra sugar should not be added to the juice. If the initial treatment does not increase the glucose level adequately after 15 minutes, the same treatment may be repeated.

Hypoglycemia During Hospitalization

Hypoglycemia in a patient who is hospitalized is usually the result of too much insulin, increased activity (physiotherapy sessions), or delays in eating. Specific examples include the following:

- Overuse of "sliding scale" short/long-acting insulin, particularly as a supplement to regularly scheduled, twice-daily short/rapid- and intermediate/long-acting insulins
- Lack of dosage change when dietary intake is changed (e.g., in the patient taking nothing by mouth [NPO])
- Overly vigorous treatment of hyperglycemia (e.g., giving too-frequent successive doses of regular insulin before the time of peak insulin activity is reached) so that there is an accumulated effect
- Delaying the meal after administration of lispro, glulisine, or aspart insulin (patient should eat within 15 minutes of administration)

Nurses must assess the pattern of glucose values and adjust the doses of insulin that repeatedly lead to hypoglycemia. Successive doses of subcutaneous rapid/short-acting insulin should be administered no more frequently than every 3 to 4 hours. To avoid hypoglycemic reactions caused by delayed food intake, the nurse should arrange for a snack to be given to the patient if meals are going to be delayed because of procedures, physical therapy, or other activities.

Common Alterations in Diet

Dietary modifications common during hospitalization require special consideration in the patient with diabetes.

Nothing by Mouth

For the patient who must be NPO in preparation for diagnostic or surgical procedures, the nurse must ensure that the usual insulin dosage has been changed. These changes may include eliminating the short- or rapid-acting insulin and giving a decreased amount (e.g., half to three quarters of the usual dose) of intermediate- or long-acting insulin. IV dextrose may be administered to provide calories and to avoid hypoglycemia.

Even when no food is taken, glucose levels may rise as a result of hepatic glucose production, especially in patients with type 1 diabetes and lean patients with type 2 diabetes. Further, in type 1 diabetes, elimination of the basal insulin dose may lead to the development of DKA. Thus, administering basal insulin to the patient with type 1 diabetes who is NPO is an important nursing action.

For patients with type 2 diabetes who are taking insulin, DKA does not normally develop when insulin doses are eliminated because the patient's pancreas produces some insulin. However, for patients with type 2 diabetes who have been receiving insulin for an extended period of time (e.g., 5 years), they may be classified as insulin deficient and are at risk of DKA if insulin is stopped.

For patients who are NPO for extended periods, glucose testing and insulin administration should be performed at regular intervals, usually two to four times per day. Insulin regimens for the patient who is NPO for an extended period may include NPH, or detemir insulin every 12 hours or glargine insulin daily (in addition to short- or rapid-acting insulin if needed) or short-acting insulin only every 4 to 6 hours. These patients should receive dextrose infusions to provide some calories and limit ketosis.

To prevent these problems resulting from the need to withhold food, diagnostic tests and procedures and surgery should be scheduled early in the morning if possible.

Clear Liquid Diet

When the diet is advanced to include clear liquids, the patients with diabetes will be receiving more simple carbohydrate foods, such as juice and gelatin desserts, than are usually included in the diabetic diet. It is important for hospitalized patients to maintain their nutritional status as much as possible to promote healing. Thus, the use of reduced-calorie substitutes such as diet soft drinks or diet gelatin desserts would not be appropriate when the only source of calories is clear liquids. Simple carbohydrates, when eaten alone, cause a rapid rise in blood glucose levels; thus, it is important to try to match peak times of insulin with peaks in glucose. If a patient was receiving insulin at regular intervals while NPO, the scheduled times for glucose tests and insulin injections must be changed to match meal times.

Enteral Tube Feedings

Tube feeding formulas contain more simple carbohydrates and less protein and fat than the typical diabetic diet. This results in increased levels of glucose in the patient with diabetes receiving tube feedings. It is important that insulin doses be administered at regular intervals (e.g., NPH, detemir or glargine every 12 hours or short-acting insulin every 4 to 6 hours) when tube feedings are administered at a continuous rate. If insulin is administered at routine (pre-breakfast and pre-dinner) times, hypoglycemia during the day may result from patients receiving more insulin without more calories, and hyperglycemia may occur during the night when feedings continue but insulin action decreases.

A common cause of hypoglycemia in patients receiving continuous tube feedings and insulin is inadvertent or purposeful discontinuation of the feeding. The nurse must discuss with the medical team any plans for temporarily discontinuing the tube feeding (e.g., when the patient is away from the unit or to avoid medication interactions). Planning ahead may allow alterations to be made in the insulin dose, or it may allow for IV dextrose to be administered. In addition, if problems with the tube feeding develop unexpectedly (e.g., the patient pulls out the tube, the tube clogs, or the feeding is discontinued when residual gastric contents are found), the nurse must notify the physician, assess blood glucose levels more frequently, and administer IV dextrose if indicated.

Parenteral Nutrition

If the patient is receiving continuous parenteral nutrition, the blood glucose level should be monitored and insulin administered at regular intervals. If the parenteral nutrition is infused over a limited number of hours, subcutaneous insulin should be administered so that peak times of insulin action coincide with times of parenteral nutrition infusion.

Hygiene

The nurse caring for a hospitalized patient with diabetes must focus attention on oral hygiene and skin care. Because patients with diabetes are at increased risk for periodontal disease, it is important for the nurse to assist patients with daily dental care. The patient may also require assistance in keeping the skin clean and dry, especially in areas of contact between two skin surfaces (e.g., groin, axilla, skin folds in those with obesity, and under the breasts in women), where chafing and fungal infections tend to occur.

For the patient with diabetes who is confined to bed, nursing care must emphasize the prevention of skin breakdown at pressure points. The heels are particularly susceptible to breakdown because of loss of sensation of pain and pressure associated with sensory neuropathy.

Feet should be cleaned, dried, lubricated with lotion (but not between the toes), and inspected frequently. If the patient is in the supine position, pressure on the heels can be alleviated by elevating the lower legs on a pillow, with the heels positioned over the edge of the pillow. When the patient is seated in a chair, the feet should be positioned so that pressure is not placed on the heels. If the patient has a foot ulcer, it is important to provide preventive foot care to the unaffected foot as well as to carry out special care of the affected foot (offloading).

As always, every opportunity should be taken to teach the patient about diabetes self-management, including daily oral, skin, and foot care. Female patients with diabetes should also be instructed about measures for the avoidance of vaginal infections, which occur more frequently when blood glucose levels are elevated. Patients often take their cues from the nurse and realize the importance of daily personal hygiene if this is emphasized during their hospitalization.

Stress

As mentioned previously, physiologic stress, such as infections and surgery, contributes to hyperglycemia and may precipitate DKA or HHS. Emotional stress may have a negative impact on control of diabetes as well. An increase in stress hormones leads to an increase in glucose levels, especially when the intake of food and insulin remains unchanged. In addition, during periods of emotional stress, the person with diabetes may alter the usual pattern of meals, exercise, and medication. This contributes to hyperglycemia or even hypoglycemia (e.g., in the patient taking insulin or oral/injectable antihyperglycemic agents who stops eating in response to stress).

People who have diabetes must be made aware of the potential deterioration in diabetic control that can accompany emotional stress. They are encouraged to try to adhere to the diabetes treatment plan as much as possible during times of stress. In addition, learning strategies for minimizing stress and coping with stress when it does occur are important aspects of diabetes education.

Gerontologic Considerations

People with diabetes are living longer; therefore, both type 1 and type 2 diabetes are seen more frequently in the older population. Regardless of the type or duration of diabetes, the goals of diabetes treatment may need to be altered when caring for older adults. The focus is on quality-of-life issues, such as maintaining independent functioning and promoting general well-being. Although striving for strict blood glucose control may not be safe or appropriate, prolonged symptomatic hyperglycemia should be avoided.

While some older patients cannot manage a detailed diabetes treatment plan, the nurse should not assume that all patients older than a certain age can adhere only to the simplest regimen. Although the goal may be simply to avoid hypoglycemia and symptomatic hyperglycemia, certain patients may prefer more complex regimens that allow more flexibility in meals and daily schedule. As with all people with diabetes, individualization of the treatment plan with frequent follow-up by the health care team is important.

Some of the barriers to learning and self-care that may be seen in older people include decreased vision, hearing loss, memory deficits, decreased mobility, fine motor coordination, increased tremors, depression and loneliness, decreased financial resources, and limitations related to other medical illnesses. Assessing patients for these barriers as well as discussing any misconceptions or "folk beliefs" regarding the cause and treatment of diabetes is important in setting up a diabetes treatment plan and educational activities. Presenting brief, simplified instructions with ample opportunity for practice of skills is important. The use of special devices such as a magnifier, an insulin pen, or a mirror for foot inspection is helpful. If necessary, family members and other community resources are called on to assist with diabetes basic skills. It is preferable to teach patients or family members to test blood glucose at home; the choice of meter should be tailored to the patient's visual and cognitive status and dexterity. Frequent evaluation of self-care skills (insulin administration, blood glucose monitoring, foot care, diet planning) is essential, especially in patients with deteriorating vision and memory.

Dietary adherence is difficult for some older patients because of decreased appetite, poor dentition, and decreased physical and financial ability to prepare meals. In addition, patients may be unwilling to change long-standing dietary habits. Altering the meal plan to incorporate these eating habits or other limitations may be necessary.

NURSING ALERT

Careful monitoring for diabetes complications must not be neglected in older patients. Hypoglycemia is especially dangerous because it may go undetected and result in falls. Dehydration is a concern in patients who have chronically elevated blood glucose levels. Assessment for long-term complications, especially eye and foot problems, is important. Avoiding blindness and amputation through early detection and treatment of retinopathy and foot ulcers may mean the difference between institutionalization and continued independent living for the older person with diabetes.

Nursing Process

The Patient With Diabetes as a Secondary Diagnosis

People with diabetes frequently seek medical attention for problems not directly related to blood glucose control. However, during the course of treatment for the primary medical diagnosis, blood glucose control may worsen. In addition, the only opportunity for some patients with diabetes to update their knowledge about diabetes self-care and prevention of complications is during hospitalization. Therefore, it is important for the nurse caring for the patient with diabetes to focus attention on diabetes, regardless of the primary problem. Further, control of blood glucose levels is important because hyperglycemia impairs resistance to certain infections and impedes wound healing.

Assessment

Assessment of the patient with diabetes with a primary problem such as cardiac disease, renal disease, cerebrovascular disease, peripheral vascular disease, surgery or any other type of illness is the same as that for a patient without diabetes and is described in other chapters. In addition to nursing assessment for the primary problem, assessment of the patient with diabetes must also focus on hypoglycemia and hyperglycemia, skin breakdown, and diabetes self-care skills, including survival skills and measures for prevention of long-term complications. In addition, the patient is asked about use of alternative or complementary therapies; studies have demonstrated that patients with diabetes are twice as likely as other patients to use these therapies, and some may be harmful.

The patient is assessed for hypoglycemia and hyperglycemia with frequent blood glucose monitoring (usually prescribed before meals and at bedtime) and with monitoring for signs and symptoms of hypoglycemia or prolonged hyperglycemia (including DKA or HHS), as described in previous sections.

Careful assessment of the skin, especially at pressure points and on the lower extremities, is important. The skin is assessed for dryness, cracks, skin breakdown, and redness. The patient is asked about symptoms of neuropathy, such as tingling and pain or numbness of the feet. Deep tendon reflexes are assessed.

Assessment of diabetes self-care skills is performed as early as possible to determine whether the patient requires further diabetes teaching. The nurse observes the patient preparing and injecting the insulin, monitoring blood glucose, and performing foot care. (Simply questioning the patient about these skills without actually observing performance of the skills is not sufficient.) Knowledge about diet can be assessed with the help of the dietitian through direct questioning and review of patient choices on the menu. The patient is questioned regarding signs, treatment, and prevention of hypoglycemia and hyperglycemia. The patient's knowledge of risk factors for macrovascular disease, including hypertension, increased lipids, and smoking is assessed. The patient is asked the date of the last eye examination (including dilation of the pupils). It is also important to assess the patient's use of preventive health measures: annual influenza vaccination (flu shot), date of pneumonia vaccine daily dose of aspirin (unless contraindicated) and smoking cessation.

Nursing Priorities

Based on the assessment data, the patient's major nursing priorities may include the following:

- Nutrition
- Risk for pressure injuries
- Education for self-care and medical care

Collaborative Problems/ Potential Complications

Based on the assessment data, potential complications may include the following:

- Inadequate control of blood glucose levels (hyperglycemia, hypoglycemia)
- DKA and HHS

Planning and Goals

The major goals for the patient may include improved nutritional status, maintenance of skin integrity, ability to perform basic diabetes self-care skills as well as preventive care for the avoidance of chronic complications from diabetes, and absence of complications.

Nursing Interventions

Improving Nutritional Status

The patient's diet is planned with the primary goal of glucose control; however, the dietary prescription must also consider the patient's primary health problem in addition to lifestyle, cultural background, activity level, and food preferences. If alterations are needed in the patient's diet because of the primary health problem (e.g., GI problems), alternative strategies to ensure adequate nutritional intake must be implemented. The patient's nutritional intake is monitored carefully along with blood glucose, urine ketones (as needed), and daily weight. Blood glucose records are assessed for patterns of hypoglycemia and hyperglycemia at the same time of day, and findings are reported to the physician for alteration in insulin orders. In the patient with elevated blood glucose levels that are prolonged, laboratory values and the patient's physical condition are monitored for signs of DKA or HHS.

Maintaining Skin Care

The skin is assessed daily for dryness or breaks. The feet are cleaned with warm water and soap. Excessive soaking of the feet is avoided. The feet are dried thoroughly, especially between the toes, and lotion is applied to the entire foot except between the toes. For bedridden patients (especially those with a history of neuropathy), the heels are elevated off the bed with a pillow placed under the lower legs and the heels resting over the edge of the pillow. Dermal ulcers are treated as indicated and prescribed. The nurse promotes optimal blood glucose control in patients with skin breakdown.

Addressing Knowledge Deficits

Hospital admission of the patient with diabetes provides an ideal opportunity for the nurse to assess the patient's level of knowledge about diabetes and its management. The nurse uses this opportunity to assess the patient's understanding of diabetes management, including blood glucose monitoring, administration of medications (i.e., insulin, oral/injectable antihyperglycemic agents), dietary requirements, exercise, and strategies to prevent long- and short-term complications of diabetes. The nurse also assesses the adjustment of the patient and family to diabetes and its management and identifies any misconceptions they have.

Monitoring and Managing Potential Complications

Inadequate control of blood glucose levels may hinder recovery from the immediate health problem. Blood glucose levels are monitored, and insulin is administered as prescribed. It is important for the nurse to ensure that insulin prescribed is modified as needed to compensate for changes in the patient's schedule or eating pattern. Treatment is given for hypoglycemia (with oral glucose) or hyperglycemia (with supplemental short- or rapid-acting insulin no more often than every 3 to 4 hours). Blood glucose records are assessed for patterns of hypoglycemia and hyperglycemia at the same time of day, and findings are reported to the physician for modification in insulin orders. In the patient with prolonged elevated blood glucose levels, laboratory values and the patient's physical condition are monitored for signs of DKA or HHS.

Development of acute complications of diabetes secondary to inadequate control of blood glucose levels may be associated with other health care problems because of changes in activity level and diet and physiologic alterations related to the primary health problem itself. Therefore, the patient must be monitored for acute complications (hyperglycemia, hypoglycemia) and measures must be implemented for their prevention and early treatment.

Promoting Home, Community-Based, and Transitional Care

EDUCATING PATIENTS ABOUT SELF-CARE. Even if the patient has had diabetes for many years, it is important to assess his or her knowledge and adherence to the plan of care. It may be necessary to plan and implement a teaching plan that includes basic information about diabetes, its cause and symptoms, and acute and chronic complications and their treatment. The nurse asks the patient to give repeated return demonstrations of skills that were not performed correctly during the initial assessment. The patient is taught self-care activities for the prevention of long-term complications, including foot care, eye care, and risk factor management. The nurse also reminds the patient and family about the importance of health promotion activities and recommended health screening.

CONTINUING AND TRANSITIONAL CARE. The patient who is hospitalized for another health problem may require referral for home care for that problem or if gaps in knowledge about self-care are uncovered. In either case, the home care nurse can use this opportunity to assess the patient's knowledge about diabetes management and the patient and family's ability to carry out that management. Teaching provided in the hospital, clinic, office, or diabetes education centre is reinforced by the nurse. The home care environment is assessed to determine its adequacy for self-care and safety.

During home care visits, the nurse assesses the patient for signs and symptoms of long-term complications and assesses the patient and family's techniques in blood glucose monitoring, insulin administration, and food selection. In addition, the patient and family are reminded of the importance of participating in health promotion activities as well as recommended health screening.

Evaluation

Expected patient outcomes may include the following:

1. Achieves optimal control of blood glucose
   a. Avoids extremes of hypoglycemia and hyperglycemia
   b. Takes steps to resolve rapidly any hypoglycemic episodes
2. Maintains skin integrity
   a. Demonstrates intact skin without dryness and cracking
   b. Avoids ulcers caused by pressure and neuropathy
3. Demonstrates/verbalizes diabetes survival skills and preventive care
4. Understands treatment modalities
   a. Demonstrates proper technique for administering insulin or oral/injectable antihyperglycemic medications and assessing blood glucose
   b. Demonstrates appropriate knowledge of diet through proper menu selections and identification of pattern used for selecting foods at home
   c. Verbalizes signs, appropriate treatment, and prevention of hypoglycemia and hyperglycemia
5. Demonstrates proper foot care
   a. Inspects feet (using mirror if necessary to see bottom of foot), including inspection for cracks or fungal infections between toes
   b. Washes feet with warm water and soap; dries feet thoroughly
   c. Applies lotion to entire foot except between toes
   d. Verbalizes behaviours that decrease the risk of foot ulcers, including wearing shoes at all times, using hand or elbow, not foot, to test temperature of bathwater, avoiding use of heating pad on feet, avoiding constrictive shoes, wearing new shoes for brief periods, avoiding home remedies for treatment of corns and calluses, having feet examined at every appointment with the physician, and consulting a podiatrist for regular nail care if necessary
6. Takes steps to prevent eye disease
   a. Verbalizes need for yearly or more frequent thorough dilated eye examinations by an ophthalmologist (starting at 5 years after diagnosis for type 1 diabetes or the year of diagnosis for type 2 diabetes)
   b. Verbalizes that retinopathy usually does not cause change in vision until serious damage to the retina has occurred
   c. States that early laser treatment along with good control of blood glucose and blood pressure may prevent visual loss from retinopathy
   d. Identifies hypoglycemia and hyperglycemia as two causes of temporary blurred vision
7. States measures to control macrovascular risk factors
   a. Smoking cessation
   b. Limitation of fats and cholesterol
   c. Control of hypertension
   d. Exercise
   e. Regular monitoring of renal function
8. Reports absence of acute complications
   a. Maintains blood glucose and urine ketones within normal limits
   b. Experiences no signs or symptoms of hypoglycemia or hyperglycemia
   c. Identifies signs and symptoms of hypoglycemia or hyperglycemia
   d. Reports appearance of symptoms so that treatment can be initiated

Critical Thinking Exercises

1 A patient is newly diagnosed with type 1 diabetes. Identify the major nursing assessment issues and nursing interventions in each of the following situations: (a) the patient is in the first trimester of pregnancy, (b) the patient refuses to use insulin, and (c) the patient is developmentally disabled and able to understand only simple instructions.

2 A patient with type 2 diabetes is scheduled for major abdominal surgery. What modifications in nursing assessment and care before, during, and after surgery are indicated because of the diagnosis of type 2 diabetes? How would these differ if the patient had type 1 diabetes?

3 A 57-year-old patient is brought to the emergency department by his daughter because he has become drowsy and has developed slurred speech over the last hour. His daughter, who lives out of town, tells you that he has recently been diagnosed with diabetes and has been depressed ever since. She does not know how the diabetes is being managed. What assessment data would you initially obtain? What diagnostic tests and treatments would you anticipate? Provide the rationale for those tests and treatments.

4 A 28-year-old patient is newly diagnosed with type 1 diabetes. Identify the major nursing assessment issues and nursing interventions in each of the following situations: (a) the patient has a phobia about use of needles, (b) the patient has been blind from birth, and (c) the patient speaks very little English.

5 You are caring for a patient with diabetes, and blood glucose monitoring is recommended. Identify teaching approaches to instruct the patient about blood glucose monitoring. What is the evidence base for the teaching approach or strategy that you selected? What is the strength of the evidence, and what criteria do you use to select the approach? How would you evaluate the effectiveness of your teaching to this patient? Explain how the results of monitoring are used in the management of type 1 and type 2 diabetes.

REFERENCES AND SELECTED READINGS

Books

Bader, M. K., Littlejohns, L. R., & Olson, D. M. (2016). *AANN core curriculum for neuroscience nursing* (6th ed.). Chicago, IL: American Association of Neuroscience Nurses.

Bartol, T. (2012). Improving the treatment experience for patients with type 2 diabetes: Role of the nurse practitioner. *Journal of the American Academy of Nurse Practitioners, 24*(suppl 1), 270–276.

Comerford, K. C. (2015). *Nursing 2015 drug handbook*. Philadelphia, PA: Wolters Kluwer.

Dudek, S. G. (2014). *Nutrition essentials for nursing practice* (7th ed.). Philadelphia, PA: Lippincott Williams & Wilkins.

Eliopoulos, C. (2018). *Gerontological nursing* (9th ed.). Philadelphia, PA: Lippincott Williams & Wilkins.

Fischbach, F. T., & Dunning, M. B. (2015). *A manual of laboratory and diagnostic tests* (9th ed.). Philadelphia, PA: Lippincott Williams & Wilkins.

Grossman, S. C., & Porth, C. M. (2014). *Pathophysiology: Concepts of altered health states* (9th ed.). Philadelphia, PA: Lippincott Williams & Wilkins.

Journals and Electronic Documents

General

American Association of Diabetes Educators (AADE). (2014). AADE7 self-care behaviors. Retrieved on June 20, 2016, from www.diabeteseducator.org/patient-resources/aade7-self-care-behaviors

American Diabetes Association (ADA). (2016a). Standards of medical care in diabetes—2016. *Diabetes Care, 39*(Suppl 1), S1–S2.

American Diabetes Association (ADA). (2016b). Standards of medical care in diabetes—2016. Classification and diagnosis of diabetes. *Diabetes Care, 39*(Suppl 1), S13–S24.

American Diabetes Association (ADA). (2016c). Standards of medical care in diabetes—2016. Management of diabetes in pregnancy. *Diabetes Care, 39*(Suppl 1), S94–S98.

American Diabetes Association (ADA). (2016d). Standards of medical care in diabetes—2016. Foundations of care and comprehensive medical evaluation. *Diabetes Care, 39*(Suppl 1), S23–S35.

American Diabetes Association (ADA). (2016e). Standards of medical care in diabetes—2016. Glycemic targets. *Diabetes Care, 39*(Suppl 1), S39–S47.

American Diabetes Association (ADA). (2016f). Standards of medical care in diabetes—2016. Cardiovascular disease and risk management. *Diabetes Care, 39*(Suppl 1), S60–S71.

American Diabetes Association (ADA). (2016g). Standards of medical care in diabetes—2016. Diabetes care in the hospital. *Diabetes Care, 39*(Suppl 1), S99–S104.

Anja, B., & Laura, R. (2017). The cost of diabetes in Canada over 10 years: applying attributable care costs to a diabetes incidence prediction model. *Health Promotion, Chronic Disease Prevention in Canada, 37*(2), 49–53.

Centers for Disease Control and Prevention (CDC). (2014). Diabetes report card. Retrieved on June 17, 2016, from www.cdc.gov/diabetes/pdfs/library/diabetesreportcard2014.pdf

Centers for Disease Control and Prevention (CDC). (2018). About diabetes. Retrieved from https://www.cdc.gov/diabetes/basics/diabetes.html

Deng, C., Xiang, Y., Tan, T., et al. (2016). Altered peripheral b-lymphocyte subsets in type 1 diabetes and latent autoimmune diabetes in adults. *Diabetes Care, 39*(3), 434–440.

Diabetes Canada. (2018a). Types of diabetes. Retrieved from https://www.diabetes.ca/about-diabetes/types-of-diabetes

Diabetes Canada. (2018b). Clinical practice guidelines. Retrieved from http://guidelines.diabetes.ca/docs/CPG-2018-full-EN.pdf

Diabetes Canada. (2018c). Screening for the presence of cardiovascular disease. Retrieved from http://guidelines.diabetes.ca/cpg/chapter24

Evert, A. B., Boucher, J. L., Cypress, M., et al. (2013). Nutrition therapy recommendation for the management of adults with diabetes. *Diabetes Care, 36*(11), 3821–3842.

Fisher, T. (2016). Your annual comprehensive foot exam. Diabetes self management. AACE/ACE Consensus Statement. *Endocrine Practice, 22*(1), 84–102.

Gaillard, T., Amponsah, G., & Osei, K. (2015). Patient-centered community diabetes education program improves glycemic control in African American patients with poorly controlled type 2 diabetes: Importance of point of care metabolic measurements. *Journal of the National Black Nurses Association, 26*(1), 51–58.

Government of Canada. (2019). Eating a variety of healthy food each day. Retrieved from: https://food-guide.canada.ca/

Noble-Bell, G., & Cox, A. (2014). Management of diabetic ketoacidosis in adults. *Nursing Times, 110*(10), 14–17.

Public Health Agency of Canada (PHAC). (2018). Diabetes in Canada. Retrieved from https://www.canada.ca/en/public-health/services/publications/diseases-conditions/diabetes-canada-highlights-chronic-disease-surveillance-system.html

Schwartz, S. S., Epstein, S., Corkey, B. E., et al. (2016). The time is right for a new classification system for diabetes: Rationale and implications of the β-cell-centric classification schema. *Diabetes Care, 39*(2), 179–186.

Seggelke, S., & Everhart, B. (2013). Management of type 2 diabetes. *Nurse Practioner, 38*(6), 13–16.

Shapiro, A. M., Ryan, E. A., & Lakey, J. R. (2001). Clinical islet transplant—state of the art. *Transplant Proceedings, 33*(7–8), 3502–3505.

Statistics Canada. (2018). Leading causes of death, total population, by age group. Retrieved from https://www.canada.ca/en/public-health/services/publications/diseases-conditions/diabetes-canada-highlights-chronic-disease-surveillance-system.html

The DCCT Research Group. (1993). The effect of intensive treatment of Diabetes on the development and progression of long term complications in insulin dependent diabetes mellitus. *The New England Journal of Medicine, 329*(14), 977–986.

Tomlin, A., & Asimakopoulou, K. (2014). Supporting behavior change in older people with type 2 diabetes. *British Journal of Community Nursing, 19*(1), 22–27.

Umpeirrez, G., & Korytkowski, M. (2016). Diabetic emergencies—ketoacidosis, hyperglycaemic hyperosmolar state and hyperglycemia. *Nature Reviews. Endocrinology, 12*, 222–232.

Weinger, K., Beverly, E. A., & Smaldone, A. (2014). Diabetes self-care and the older adult. *Western Journal of Nursing Research, 36*(9), 1272–1298.

World Health Organization (WHO). (2015a). Diabetes. Fact Sheet No. 312. Retrieved on June 17, 2016, from www.who.int/mediacentre/factsheets/fs312/en/

World Health Organization (WHO). (2015b). *Obesity and overweight*. Retrieved on June 17, 2016, from www.who.int/mediacentre/factsheets/fs311/en/

Wu, E. T., Nien, F. J., Kuo, C. H., et al. (2016). Diagnosis of more gestational diabetes lead to better pregnancy outcomes: Comparing the International Association of the Diabetes and Pregnancy Study Group Criteria, and the Carpenter and Coustan criteria. *Journal of Diabetes Investigation, 7*(1), 121–126.

Resources

American Association of Diabetes Educators: http://www.diabeteseducator.org/
American Diabetes Association (ADA): http://www.diabetes.org
American Dietetic Association: http://www.eatright.org
American Foundation for the Blind: http://www.afb.org
ArmChair Fitness Videos: http://www.armchairfitness.com/
Canadian Diabetes Association: info@diabetes.ca; http://www.diabetes.ca
Canadian National Institute for the Blind: info@cnib.ca; http://cnib.ca/
Centers for Disease Control and Prevention: http://www.cdc.gov/diabetes//pubs/factsheet.htm
Dietitians of Canada: http://www.dietitians.ca
Health Canada: Eating a variety of healthy food each day: https://food-guide.canada.ca/
Juvenile Diabetes Foundation International: http://www.jdrf.org
MedicAlert Foundation International: http://www.medicalert.org
National Diabetes Information Clearinghouse: http://www.niddk.nih.gov
National Institute on aging at NIH: https://go4life.nia.nih.gov/
National Library Services for the Blind and Physically Handicapped (NLSBPH), Library of Congress: http://www.lcweb.loc.gov/nls
Nutrition Labelling Education Centre: http://www.healthyeatingisinstore.ca

42 Assessment and Management of Patients With Obesity

Written by Jennifer Densmore

Learning Objectives

On completion of this chapter, the learner will be able to:

1. Discuss the incidence of obesity worldwide.
2. List risk factors associated with obesity.
3. List obesity-related comorbidities.
4. Discuss the incidence of obesity in children and adults in Canada.
5. Describe the impact of obesity on the health care system.
6. Describe the causes, classifications, and diseases and disorders associated with obesity.
7. Identify strategies aimed at preventing and treating obesity, including lifestyle modification, pharmacologic therapy, and nonsurgical interventions.
8. Explain nursing management considerations for the patient with obesity using nonsurgical interventions.
9. Compare and contrast surgical modalities indicated to treat patients with obesity in terms of preoperative, postoperative, and long-term management and complications.
10. Use the nursing process as a framework for care of patients who undergo bariatric surgical procedures.

The rates of **obesity** in Canada and globally have reached pandemic proportions. Given the high prevalence of obesity, nurses will encounter adults with obesity in every inpatient and outpatient clinical setting. This chapter describes the etiology, clinical manifestations, management, and related nursing care of the patient with obesity. The management of patients with obesity using both nonsurgical and surgical treatments is discussed.

Obesity is an expanding public health problem worldwide, creating a global health epidemic. Over the last 20 years, it has become the **most** prevalent nutritional problem in the world and the most significant contributor to ill health and mortality. It is a key risk factor for many chronic conditions and is currently one of the most prevalent noncommunicable diseases (Kushner, 2018). According to the World Health Organization (WHO), worldwide obesity has tripled since 1975, with more than 1.9 billion adults considered to have obesity in 2016 (WHO, 2019).

- In the United States, the prevalence of obesity was 39.8% in 2015–2016; obesity affected 93.3 million people at that time (CDC, 2018).
- In Australia, 63% of the adult population is considered to have obesity, while 10% are considered to have severe obesity (AIHW, 2016).
- In 2015, 57.3 million people in China were identified as having obesity (GBD, 2017).

The WHO (2014) describes obesity as one of the most visible, yet most neglected, public health problems that threatens to overwhelm both more and less developed countries. The problems of being overweight and having obesity have achieved global recognition only during the past 10 years, in contrast to malnutrition, infectious diseases, and being underweight which have always dominated thinking. WHO now accepts a **body mass index (BMI)** of 25 or higher as abnormal; the overweight category is classified as obese when the BMI is 30 or more. The risks of diabetes,

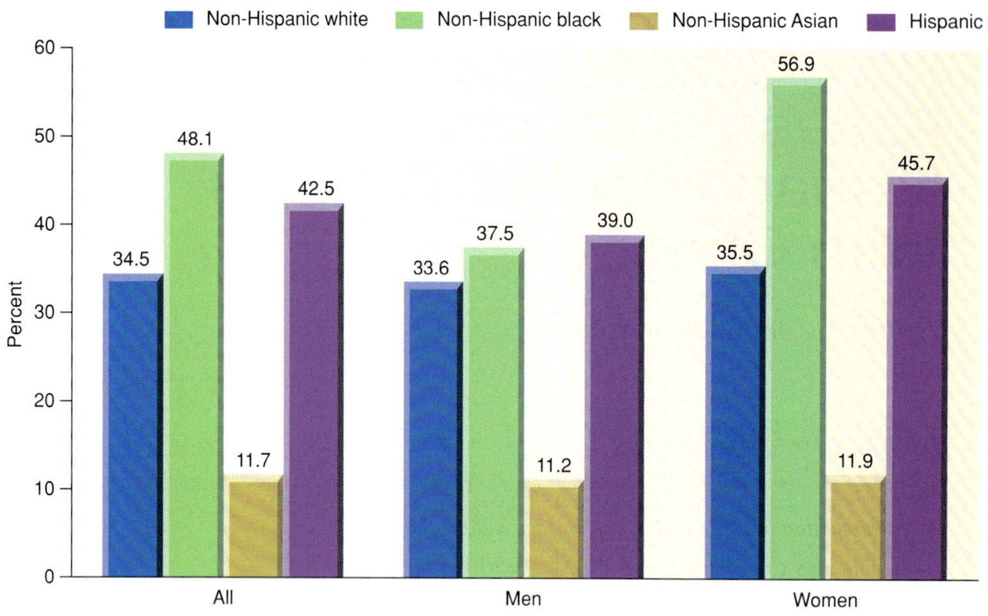

FIGURE 42-1. Prevalence of obesity among adults aged 20 and older, by gender and race/ethnicity in the United States (2011 to 2014). (Adapted from Ogden, C. L., Carroll, M. D., Fryar, C. D., et al. (2015). *Prevalence of obesity among adults and youth: United States, 2011–2014.* NCHS data brief, no 219. Hyattsville, MD: National Center for Health Statistics.)

hypertension, and dyslipidemia increase from a BMI of about 21, thereby reducing life expectancy and greatly increasing the health and societal economic burden; excess bodyweight is now the sixth most important risk factor contributing to the overall burden of disease worldwide (WHO, 2014).

In Canada, according to the most recent estimates from the 2013 Canadian Community Health Survey (Rao, Kropac, Do, et al., 2016), 59% of the adult population is overweight. The large number of people who are overweight and who are obese identify a public health problem that shows no signs of improving in the near future. What is more alarming is the issue of obesity among children and adolescents in Canada, which is advancing at an even quicker pace than obesity among adults. A Canadian Health Measures survey conducted in 2012–2013 indicated that 8.8% of children aged 5 to 11 years old had obesity; 16.5% of children aged 12 to 17 years had obesity; and 26.4% of adults had obesity (Chang, Chaput, Roberts, et al., 2018). This increase is of concern, since there is a tendency for children with obesity to have obesity as adults. Obesity-related health problems are now occurring at an earlier age and continue to progress into adulthood. Therefore, the prevalence of obesity among adults will likely continue to increase as the current generation of children enters adulthood. It has been estimated that about 1 in 10 premature deaths among Canadian adults 20 to 64 years of age is directly attributable to overweight and obesity. The increased health risks translate into an increased burden on the health care system. The cost of obesity in Canada has been estimated to be close to 11.08 billion dollars (Tran, Nair, Kuhule, et al., 2013). Therefore, the continuing epidemic of obesity in Canada is taking a huge toll on the health of the population.

Obesity Risks

The causes of obesity are complex and multifactorial, and include behavioural, environmental, physiologic, and genetic factors. While there are certain demographic groups who seem to be at risk for obesity (see Fig. 42-1)

Glossary

adiposopathy: dysfunction of adipose tissue that causes chronic inflammation and disease

bariatric: relating to obesity; term derives from two Greek words meaning "weight" and "treatment"

body mass index (BMI): a simple index of weight-for-height that is commonly used to classify overweight and obesity in adults. It is defined as a person's weight in kilograms divided by the square of his/her height in metres (kg/m^2). BMI provides the most useful population-level measure of overweight and obesity as it is the same for both sexes and for all ages of adults. However, it should be considered a rough guide because it does not provide information regarding an individual's percentage of body fat.

dumping syndrome: physiologic response to rapid emptying of gastric contents into the jejunum, manifested by nausea, weakness, sweating, palpitations, syncope, and possibly diarrhea

dysphagia: difficulty swallowing

genome: the total complement of individual genes in an organism

microbiome: the collective genome of all microbes in a microbiota

microbiota: the complement of microbes in a given environment

obesity: BMI greater than or equal to 30

obesogenic: a factor that promotes weight gain and obesity

orexigenic: a factor that stimulates appetite

recidivism: regaining of lost weight due to a return to poor eating habits

satiety: feeling of having eaten sufficient quantities of food

CHART 42-1

Patient Education: Health Risks of Having Obesity

What does it mean to be have obesity?—Doctors use a special measure called "body mass index," or BMI, to decide who is underweight, at a healthy weight, overweight, or who has obesity. A person with obesity weighs way too much for his or her height.

Your BMI will tell you whether your weight is appropriate for your height.

Having obesity is a problem, because it increases the risks of many different health problems. It can also make it hard for you to move, breathe, and do other things that people who are at a healthy weight can do easily. Plus, having obesity can be emotionally difficult, because it can make you feel ashamed or like you don't fit in.

What are the health risks of having obesity?—Having obesity increases a person's risk of developing many health problems. Here are just a few examples:

- Diabetes
- High blood pressure
- High cholesterol
- Heart disease (including heart attacks)
- Stroke (rain attack)
- Sleep apnea (a disorder in which you stop breathing for short periods while asleep)
- Asthma
- Cancer

Does having obesity shorten a person's life?—Yes. Studies show that people with obesity die younger than people who are a healthy weight. They also show that the risk of death goes up the heavier a person is. The degree of increased risk depends on how long the person has had obesity, and on what other medical problems he or she has.

Should I see a health care provider?—Yes. If you are overweight or have obesity, see your health care provider. He or she might have suggestions on ways to lose weight.

Are there medical treatments that can help me lose weight?—Yes. There are medicines and surgery to help with weight loss. But those treatments are only for people with severe obesity who have not been able to lose weight through diet and exercise. Also, weight loss treatments do not take the place of diet and exercise. People who have those treatments must also change how they eat and how active they are.

What can I do to prevent the problems caused by having obesity?—The obvious answer is that you can lose weight. But even if weight loss is not possible, you can improve your health and reduce your risk if you:

- Become more active—Many types of physical activity can help, including walking. You can start with a few minutes a day and add more as you get stronger.
- Improve your diet—No single diet turns out to be better than any other. It is healthy to have regular meal times and smaller portions, and not to skip meals. Avoid sweets and processed snack foods, and increase vegetables and fruit intake.
- Quit smoking (if you smoke).
- Limit alcohol—Drink no more than one drink a day if you are woman, and no more than two drinks a day if you are a man.

What increases a person's risk of having obesity? The thing that increases a person's risk the most is having an unhealthy lifestyle. Most people have obesity because they simply eat too much and move too little. That's especially true of people who watch too much TV. But there are also a number of other factors that seem to increase the risk of obesity that many people do not know about. Here are some things that might affect a person's chance of having obesity:

- Mom's habits during pregnancy—Women who eat a lot of calories, have diabetes, or smoke during pregnancy have a higher chance of having babies who grow up to be obese.
- Formula feeding—Babies who are fed formula are more likely than babies who are breastfed to grow up to have obesity.
- Habits and weight gain during childhood—People who are overweight or have obesity as children or as teens are more likely to be obese as adults.
- Sleeping too little—People who do not get enough sleep are more likely to have obesity than people who sleep enough.
- Taking certain medicines—Long-term use of certain medicines, such as some medicines to treat depression, can cause a lot of weight gain.

There are also hormonal conditions that can increase the risk of having obesity, but those conditions are to blame for only a tiny fraction of cases of obesity.

What if I want to have children?—If you want to have children, you should know that having obesity can make it hard for a woman to conceive. It can also impair a man's ability to have sex, especially if the man has high blood pressure or diabetes. Also, children born to parents with obesity have a high risk of have obesity themselves.

What if my child has obesity?—In children, obesity has many of the same risks as it does in adults. For example, it can increase the risk of diabetes, high blood pressure, asthma, and sleep apnea. It can also cause added problems related to childhood. For example, obesity can make children grow faster than expected and speed up sexual development in girls.

and while there are notable familial patterns of obesity, identification of risk factors that specify odds of being diagnosed with obesity are not as clearly elucidated as those for other diseases (Centers for Disease Control and Prevention [CDC], 2016a), such as coronary artery disease (see Chapter 29) and cerebrovascular disease (see Chapter 64) (see Chart 42-1).

What is abundantly clear, however, is that obesity incurs a greater overall risk of mortality. Obesity is associated with a 6- to 20-year decrease in overall life expectancy (Moyer, LeFevre, Siu, et al., 2012). Furthermore, obesity is associated with morbidity and mortality from numerous other diseases (see Fig. 42-2 and Chart 42-2). For instance, as BMI increases, so does the overall risk of cancer and risk for death from cancer. Having obesity increases the likelihood of having type 2 diabetes by 10-fold and the likelihood of having either asthma or hypertension by nearly fourfold. Adults with obesity are twice as likely to eventually be diagnosed with Alzheimer's disease as those adults who maintain a normal weight (Mozaffarian, Benjamin, Go, et al., 2016).

CHART 42-2

Diseases and Disorders Associated With Obesity

Alzheimer's disease
Anxiety and depression
Asthma
Cancers (breast, cervical, colorectal, endometrial, esophageal, gallbladder, liver, ovarian, non-Hodgkin lymphoma, pancreatic, prostate, kidney, thyroid)
Chronic low back pain
Coronary artery disease (angina, acute coronary syndrome, myocardial infarction)
Diabetes (type 2)
Gallbladder disease (cholecystitis, cholelithiasis)
Gastroesophageal Reflux Disease (GERD)
Gout
Heart failure
Hypercholesterolemia
Hypertension
Nonalcoholic fatty liver disease
Obstructive sleep apnea
Osteoarthritis
Respiratory infections
Stroke

Adapted from American Society for Metabolic and Bariatric Surgery (ASMBS). (2015b). The impact of obesity on your body and health. Retrieved November 19, 2015, from asmbs.org/patients/impact-of-obesity; Centers for Disease Control and Prevention (CDC). (2016a). *Adult obesity causes and consequences*. Retrieved January 8, 2017, from www.cdc.gov/obesity/adult/causes.html

Pathophysiology

Obesity is a chronic, relapsing disease characterized by an excessive accumulation of body fat and weight gain (ASMBS, 2015a). These increases in body fat cause **adiposopathy** (i.e., dysfunction of adipose tissue), which promotes the development of metabolic, biomechanical, and psychosocial diseases and disorders (Bays, Jones, Jacobson, et al., 2016). Dysfunctional adipose tissue cells release biochemical mediators that cause chronic inflammatory changes, which can lead to a multitude of diseases, including heart disease, hypertension, and type 2 diabetes (ASMBS, 2013b).

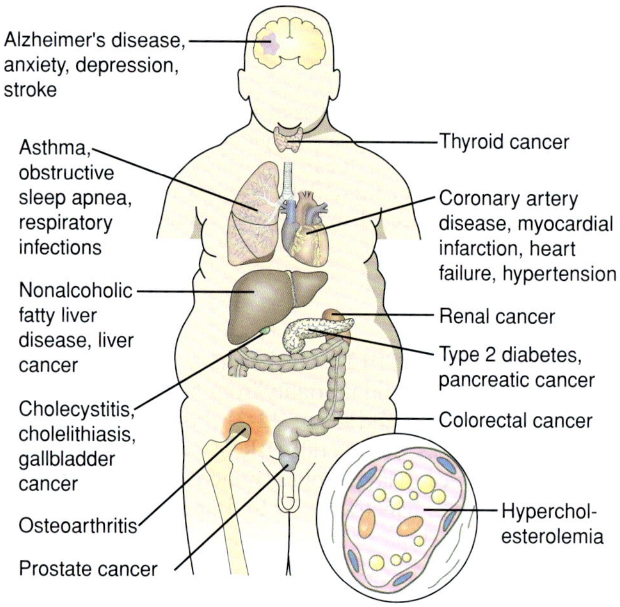

FIGURE 42-2. Morbid diseases and disorders associated with obesity.

At the most fundamental level, obesity results from a metabolic imbalance, characterized by an excess of caloric consumption relative to caloric expenditures. That is, too many foods are consumed and too little physical activity is conducted over the long term, resulting in weight gain (Grossman & Porth, 2014). According to the "thrifty gene" hypothesis, the human **genome** (i.e., the total complement of genes in humans) was sequenced during times when finding and storing food sources expended more energy than during contemporary times. Hunting for scarce food sources during prehistoric times consumed a lot of energy, and food sources were not abundant. Storing fat to provide energy sources during times of food scarcity was a physiologic adaptive response to these environmental challenges (Budd & Peterson, 2014).

The "thrifty gene" hypothesis has come under scrutiny in recent years, however, as human genome sequencing research findings suggest that a far more complex genetic explanation may be responsible for the recent global obesity pandemic. Research findings suggest that having at least one of over 25 different genetic mutations can strongly predispose people who have ready access to food sources to having obesity (Kolata, 2016). For instance, the presence of a variant mutation of the *FTO* gene is associated with more daily meals, snacks, and fat and sweet intake (Budd & Peterson, 2014). However, these types of single genetic mutations are relatively rare occurrences, and therefore cannot account for the high prevalence of obesity. Most people who are predisposed to obesity are thought to have a collection of several genetic mutations from more than 300 possible mutated genes that each can contribute to several pounds of additional body fat (Kolata, 2016).

The types and quantities of foods consumed affect complex digestive and metabolic pathways. Certain processed and high caloric foods that contain fructose corn syrup, simple sugars, or trans fats, are hypothesized to be obesogenic (i.e., promote weight gain) because they are associated with food cravings consonant with other type of addictive cravings (Budd & Peterson, 2014).

Multiple hormones that control food cravings and feelings of fullness could be affected by individual genes. In response to periods of fasting, the hormone ghrelin is secreted by the stomach and the hormone neuropeptide Y (NPY) is secreted by the small intestines. These hormones are orexigenic, meaning that they stimulate appetite through central nervous system (CNS) pathways that lead to the hypothalamus, signalling higher neural pathways that lead to eating behaviours. Once eating occurs, multiple hormones are released throughout the gastrointestinal (GI) tract that promote satiety, including somatostatin, cholecystokinin (CCK), and insulin, to name a few. CCK also slows gastric motility and emptying, stimulates gallbladder contraction and release of bile into the duodenum, and stimulates the release of pancreatic digestive enzymes, all of which serve to enhance the digestive process. Somatostatin also slows gastric emptying but has other effects that are in opposition to CCK, such as decreasing the secretion of bile, depending on foods consumed and metabolic needs (Bays, Kothari, Azagury, et al., 2016).

Increases in fat stores, or adipose tissue, result in increases in the hormone leptin, which is secreted by fat cells. Leptin also has the effect of signalling satiety in the hypothalamus. Patients with obesity who lose weight are thought to also have drops in leptin levels that persist for the long term, creating persistent feelings of hunger, which may partially explain why many patients with obesity who lose weight tend to regain it (Budd & Peterson, 2014).

The GI tract **microbiota**, which is the complement of microbes within the gut, has been found to contain up to 100 trillion microbes, or 10 times the cells present in the human body (Davis, 2016). The collective genome of the microbiota, or the gut **microbiome**, has more than 100 times more genes than in the human genome (Davis, 2016). It has long been known that gut microbes perform numerous digestive, metabolic, and immunologic functions. The composition and diversity of these microbes may very well be tied in with obesity. For instance, patients with obesity tend to have less diverse microbiota than patients who are lean. In turn, these patients with obesity who have less diverse microbiota typically also have dyslipidemia, impaired glucose metabolism, and low-grade generalized inflammatory disorders. The effects of "Western-style diets," high in processed foods, fat, and sugars, and low in fibre, is thought to not only negatively affect the diversity of the gut microbiota, but also negatively affect the complement of *Bacteroidetes* species microbes, which are associated with a leaner type of microbiome (Davis, 2016). Whether or not it is possible to regulate the composition of the gut microbiota and prevent or treat obesity is the focus of ongoing research (Davis, 2016).

Assessment and Diagnostic Findings

Patient height and weight is measured to determine the BMI. The BMI is the definitive measure used to determine whether or not a patient is overweight or has obesity; this is based upon a ratio of body weight in kilograms and height in meters. Patients identified as overweight or pre-obese have a BMI of 25 to 29.9 kg/m^2 and those with obesity have a BMI that exceeds 30 kg/m^2. Those with a BMI exceeding 40 kg/m^2 are considered to have severe or extreme obesity (previously referred to as morbid obesity) (WHO, 2015) (see Fig. 42-3 and Table 42-1).

Patients with obesity may also have their waist circumferences assessed. Women with waist circumferences more than 35 in and men with waist circumferences more than 40 in have greater risks for obesity-related morbidity than those with smaller waistlines (Fitch, Everling, Fox, et al., 2013). The hip may also be measured and the waist-to-hip ratio assessed. Women with waist-to-hip ratios greater

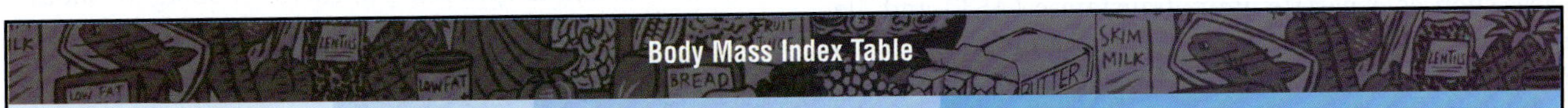

	Normal						Overweight					Obese										Extreme Obesity														
BMI	**19**	**20**	**21**	**22**	**23**	**24**	**25**	**26**	**27**	**28**	**29**	**30**	**31**	**32**	**33**	**34**	**35**	**36**	**37**	**38**	**39**	**40**	**41**	**42**	**43**	**44**	**45**	**46**	**47**	**48**	**49**	**50**	**51**	**52**	**53**	**54**
Height (inches)	**Body Weight (pounds)**																																			
58	91	96	100	105	110	115	119	124	129	134	138	143	148	153	158	162	167	172	177	181	186	191	196	201	205	210	215	220	224	229	234	239	244	248	253	258
59	94	99	104	109	114	119	124	128	133	138	143	148	153	158	163	168	173	178	183	188	193	198	203	208	212	217	222	227	232	237	242	247	252	257	262	267
60	97	102	107	112	118	123	128	133	138	143	148	153	158	163	168	174	179	184	189	194	199	204	209	215	220	225	230	235	240	245	250	255	261	266	271	276
61	100	106	111	116	122	127	132	137	143	148	153	158	164	169	174	180	185	190	195	201	206	211	217	222	227	232	238	243	248	254	259	264	269	275	280	285
62	104	109	115	120	126	131	136	142	147	153	158	164	169	175	180	186	191	196	202	207	213	218	224	229	235	240	246	251	256	262	267	273	278	284	289	295
63	107	113	118	124	130	135	141	146	152	158	163	169	175	180	186	191	197	203	208	214	220	225	231	237	242	248	254	259	265	270	278	282	287	293	299	304
64	110	116	122	128	134	140	145	151	157	163	169	174	180	186	192	197	204	209	215	221	227	232	238	244	250	256	262	267	273	279	285	291	296	302	308	314
65	114	120	126	132	138	144	150	156	162	168	174	180	186	192	198	204	210	216	222	228	234	240	246	252	258	264	270	276	282	288	294	300	306	312	318	324
66	118	124	130	136	142	148	155	161	167	173	179	186	192	198	204	210	216	223	229	235	241	247	253	260	266	272	278	284	291	297	303	309	315	322	328	334
67	121	127	134	140	146	153	159	166	172	178	185	191	198	204	211	217	223	230	236	242	249	255	261	268	274	280	287	293	299	306	312	319	325	331	338	344
68	125	131	138	144	151	158	164	171	177	184	190	197	203	210	216	223	230	236	243	249	256	262	269	276	282	289	295	302	308	315	322	328	335	341	348	354
69	128	135	142	149	155	162	169	176	182	189	196	203	209	216	223	230	236	243	250	257	263	270	277	284	291	297	304	311	318	324	331	338	345	351	358	365
70	132	139	146	153	160	167	174	181	188	195	202	209	216	222	229	236	243	250	257	264	271	278	285	292	299	306	313	320	327	334	341	348	355	362	369	376
71	136	143	150	157	165	172	179	186	193	200	208	215	222	229	236	243	250	257	265	272	279	286	293	301	308	315	322	329	338	343	351	358	365	372	379	386
72	140	147	154	162	169	177	184	191	199	206	213	221	228	235	242	250	258	265	272	279	287	294	302	309	316	324	331	338	346	353	361	368	375	383	390	397
73	144	151	159	166	174	182	189	197	204	212	219	227	235	242	250	257	265	272	280	288	295	302	310	318	325	333	340	348	355	363	371	378	386	393	401	408
74	148	155	163	171	179	186	194	202	210	218	225	233	241	249	256	264	272	280	287	295	303	311	319	326	334	342	350	358	365	373	381	389	396	404	412	420
75	152	160	168	176	184	192	200	208	216	224	232	240	248	256	264	272	279	287	295	303	311	319	327	335	343	351	359	367	375	383	391	399	407	415	423	431
76	156	164	172	180	189	197	205	213	221	230	238	246	254	263	271	279	287	295	304	312	320	328	336	344	353	361	369	377	385	394	402	410	418	426	435	443

Adapted from *Clinical Guidelines on the Identification, Evaluation, and Treatment of Overweight and Obesity in Adults: The Evidence Report.*

FIGURE 42-3. Body mass index table. (Adapted from National Heart, Lung, and Blood Institute (NHLBI) of the National Institutes of Health. (2016a). Aim for a healthy weight: Body mass index table. Retrieved March 2, 2017, from www.nhlbi.nih.gov/health/educational/lose_wt/BMI/bmi_tbl.pdf)

TABLE 42-1 Body Mass Index (BMI) Classification for Overweight and Obesity

Classification	BMI Range (kg/m^2)
Overweight/Preobese	25–29.9
Class I Obesity	30–34.9
Class II Obesity	35–39.9
Class III (also called "extreme" or "severe") Obesity	≥40

Adapted from Centers for Disease Control and Prevention (CDC). (2016b). Defining adult overweight and obesity. Retrieved January 24, 2017, from www.cdc.gov/obesity/adult/defining.html

than 0.80 and men with waist-to-hip ratios greater than 0.90 are presumed to have proportionally more visceral (i.e., abdominal) fat stores. This morphologic appearance is called android obesity, and is sometimes referenced as an "apple-shaped" appearance. Patients with android obesity have greater risk for developing hypertension, coronary artery disease, stroke, and type 2 diabetes, than patients who have gynoid obesity, also called the "pear-shaped" body (Weber & Kelley, 2014) (see Fig. 42-4).

Patients with obesity or who are overweight may have other diagnostic laboratory studies done to screen for cardiovascular diseases, such as cholesterol and triglycerides (see Chapter 27), for type 2 diabetes, such as fasting blood glucose and glycosylated hemoglobin (hemoglobin A1c) (see Chapter 41), or for nonalcoholic fatty liver disease, such as aspartate aminotransferase (AST) and alanine aminotransferase (ALT) (Orringer, Harrison, Nichani, et al., 2016).

In some instances, obesity may be secondary to other diseases or disorders, such as hypothyroidism or Cushing syndrome (see Chapter 43). In those particular cases, the diagnostic workup follows that prescribed for the primary disease or disorder, and, when the therapeutic regimen is implemented, the patient may lose weight and the obesity may even resolve (Orringer et al., 2016). In addition, some patients who are overweight or have obesity may develop secondary diseases or disorders (see Chart 42-2) and may be prescribed medications aimed at treating those secondary diseases or disorders that can exacerbate weight gain (see Chart 42-3). Other patients may not have had a previous history of being overweight or having obesity, but may gain weight after being prescribed specific medications associated with weight gain. A history of weight gain that parallels the timeframe of commencing treatment with specific prescriptive medications may suggest that the medication has a key role in promoting weight gain. In some instances, prescription medication dosages may be adjusted or another medication may be prescribed. For instance, patients with type 2 diabetes and obesity may reap the dual benefits of achieving better glycemic control and weight loss by taking the prescription drug metformin (Glucophage) (Apovian, Aronne, Bessesen, et al., 2015).

Medical Management

Treatment of obesity generally includes lifestyle modification, pharmacologic management, and nonsurgical or surgical interventions.

Lifestyle Modification

The first approach used to treat obesity consists of lifestyle modification aimed at weight loss and then weight maintenance. All adults with BMIs in excess of 30 kg/m^2 should be advised to engage in multicomponent behavioural interventions that include (Moyer et al., 2012):

- Setting weight-loss goals
- Improving diet habits
- Increasing physical activity
- Addressing barriers to change, and
- Self-monitoring and strategizing ongoing lifestyle changes aimed at a healthy weight

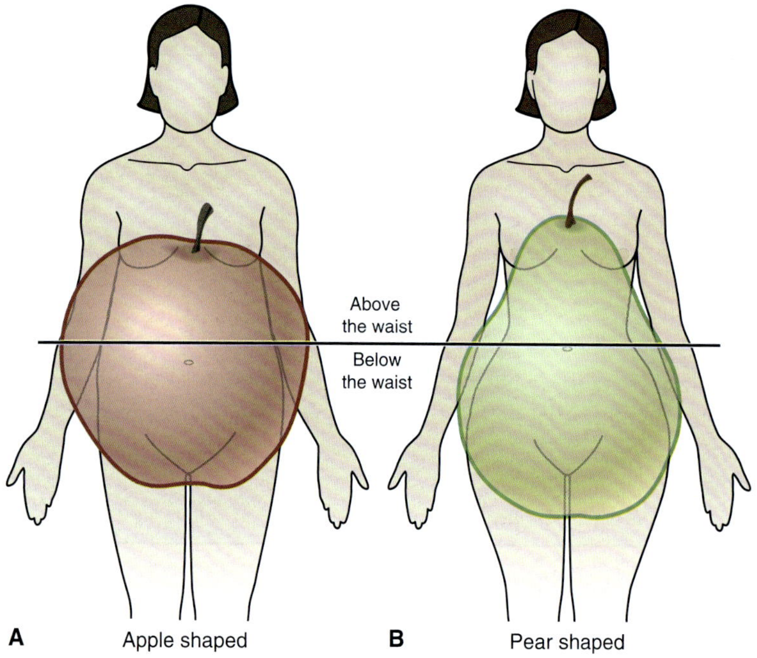

FIGURE 42-4. **A.** Android obesity, with greater visceral/abdominal fat stores. **B.** Gynoid obesity. (Reprinted with permission from Weber, J. R., & Kelley, J. H. (2014). *Health assessment in nursing* (5th ed.). Philadelphia, PA: Lippincott Williams & Wilkins.)

CHART 42-3

Pharmacology: Selected Medications That Affect Body Weight

Many medications prescribed to treat a variety of chronic diseases and disorders have the untoward side effect of weight gain, whereas others are associated with weight loss. The following list contains some examples of each of these.

Medications Associated With Weight Gain

Anticonvulsant Medications:

- Carbamazepine (Tegretol)
- Gabapentin (Neurontin)
- Pregabalin (Lyrica)[a]
- Valproate (Depakote)[b]

Antidepressant Medications:

- Selective serotonin reuptake inhibitors (SSRIs) (Note—these tend to be associated with early weight loss followed by gain within 6 months in some patients):
  - Citalopram (Celexa)
  - Fluvoxamine (Luvox)
  - Paroxetine (Paxil)
  - Sertraline (Zoloft)
- Tricyclic Antidepressants:
  - Amitriptyline (Elavil)
  - Doxepin (Sinequan)
  - Imipramine (Tofranil, Tofranil PM)
  - Mirtazapine (Remeron)
  - Nortriptyline (Aventyl)
  - Trimipramine (Surmontil)

Antihistamines:

- Cetirizine (Zyrtec)
- Diphenhydramine (Benadryl)

Antihypertensive Medications:

- Beta Blockers:
  - Atenolol (Tenormin)
  - Metoprolol (Lopressor, Toprol)
  - Propranolol (Inderal)
- Dihydropyridine calcium channel blockers:
  - Amlodipine (Norvasc)
  - Felodipine (Plendil)
  - Nifedipine (Procardia, Procardia XL)

Antipsychotic Medications:

- Asenapine (Saphris)
- Chlorpromazine (Thorazine)
- Clozapine (Clozaril)[c]
- Iloperidone (Fanapt)
- Olanzapine (Zyprexa)[d]
- Paliperidone (Invega)
- Quetiapine (Seroquel)
- Risperidone (Risperdal)

Diabetes Medications:

- Insulins:
  - Insulin aspart (Novolog)
  - Insulin glulisine (Apidra)
  - Insulin lispro (Humalog)
- Meglitinides:
  - Nateglinide (Starlix)
  - Repaglinide (Prandin)
- Sulfonylureas:
  - Chlorpropamide (Amaryl)
  - Glimepiride (Glynase)
  - Glipizide (Glucotrol, Glucotrol XL)
  - Glyburide (Diabeta, Micronase)
  - Tolbutamide (Diabinese)
- Thiazolidinediones:
  - Pioglitazone (Actos)

Hormones:

- Corticosteroids:
  - Prednisone
  - Budesonide (Pulmicort)
- Hormonal contraceptives:
  - Medroxyprogesterone (Depo-Provera)
- *Mood Stabilizers:*
  - Lithium (Lithobid)
  - Vigabatrin (Sabril)

Medications Associated With Weight Loss

Anticonvulsant Medications:

- Lamotrigine (Lamictal)
- Topiramate (Topamax)
- Zonisamide (Zonegran)

Antidepressant Medications:

- Bupropion (Wellbutrin, Zyban)

Diabetes Medications:

- Metformin (Glucophage)

[a]Medications associated with significant weight gain.
[b]Medications associated with significant weight gain.
[c]Medications associated with significant weight gain.
[d]Medications associated with significant weight gain.

Adapted from Bays, H. E., Seger, J. C., Primack, C., et al. (2016). Obesity algorithm presented by the Obesity Medicine Association. Retrieved January 7, 2017, from www.obesityalgorithm.org; Budd, G. M., & Peterson, J. A. (2015). The obesity epidemic, part 2: Nursing assessment and intervention. *American Journal of Nursing, 115*(1), 38–46; Kyle, T., & Kuehl, B. (2017). Prescription medications and weight gain—What you need to know. Retrieved January 7, 2017, from www.obesityaction.org/educational-resources/resource-articles-2/general-articles/prescription-medications-weight-gain

The most effective behavioural interventions are those considered high intensity; that is, they consist of 12 to 26 sessions annually, which may include individual counselling sessions between the primary provider and patient, group nutrition education sessions, and physical activity sessions, to name a few (Moyer et al., 2012). The US Preventive Services Task Force notes that modest weight loss of 5% total body weight can be associated with significant clinical improvements and benefits to patients with obesity (Moyer et al., 2012).

A patient with obesity should be counselled to plan a caloric deficit of between 500 and 1,000 calories daily from baseline, in order to achieve a 5% to 10% reduction in weight within about 6 months. This can be achieved

CHART 42-4

Patient Education: Weight Loss (The Basics)

How do I know if I am overweight and by how much?—Doctors use a special measure called "body mass index," or BMI, to decide who is underweight, normal weight, or overweight. Your BMI will tell you whether your weight is appropriate for your height.

Should I see a doctor or nurse?—If you are overweight or have obesity, see your doctor or nurse. He or she might have suggestions on ways to lose weight.

People with obesity are more likely than people of normal weight to get diabetes, heart disease, cancer, and lots of other health problems. That's why it's important to try to keep your weight in the expected range.

What's the best way to lose weight on my own?—To lose weight, you have to eat less or move more. Doing both is even better.

Studies have compared different diets such as the Atkins diet, the Zone diet, and the Weight Watchers diet. No single diet turns out to be better than any other. Any diet that reduces the number of calories you eat can help you lose weight—as long as you stick with it.

Physical activity works the same way. You can walk, dance, garden, or even just move your arms while sitting. What's important is that you increase the number of calories you burn by moving more. And you have to keep doing the extra activity.

If you go on a diet for a short time, or increase your activity for a while, you might lose weight. But you will regain the weight if you go back to your old habits. Weight loss is about changing your habits for good.

The best way to start is to make small changes and stick with them. Then, little by little, you can add new changes that you also stick with.

Are there medical treatments that can help me lose weight?—There are medicines and surgery to help with weight loss. But those treatments are only for people with extreme weight problems who have not been able to lose weight through diet and exercise. What's more, weight loss treatments do not take the place of diet and exercise. People who have those treatments must also change how they eat and how active they are.

How do weight loss medicines work?—Weight loss medicines work by reducing your appetite or by changing how you absorb food. They are appropriate only for people who:

- Have a BMI of 30 or greater; or
- Have a BMI between 27 and 30 and also have medical problems, such as diabetes, heart disease, or high blood pressure

How does weight loss surgery work?—Weight loss surgery works by making your stomach smaller. Some types of surgery also change the path food takes through your gut so that fewer calories and nutrients get absorbed. Weight loss surgery is appropriate only for people who:

- Have a BMI greater than 40; or
- Have a BMI between 35 and 40 and also have medical problems, such as diabetes, heart disease, or high blood pressure

How do I decide if weight loss treatment is right for me?—If your doctor suggests weight loss treatment, ask these questions:

- About how much weight can I expect to lose and how long will that take? Many people are surprised to learn that even with surgery, most people never become thin.
- What are the risks of treatment for someone like me? Medicines can have side effects. Surgery can lead to infections, bleeding, the need for other operations, and even death. To reduce the risk of these problems, make sure your surgeon is very experienced and that you are treated at an accredited institution.
- What changes will I need to make to my diet and lifestyle? Weight loss treatments are not "short-cuts" that get you out of making lifestyle changes. People getting treated must also change how they eat and how active they are. No weight loss treatment works on its own. Sometimes people can get surgery only after they prove they can make lifestyle changes—by losing some weight on their own.
- Will I be able to process food normally? Some types of surgery leave people unable to get all the nutrients they need from food. People who have this problem must take vitamin and mineral supplements for the rest of their lives.

through increasing physical activity and decreasing caloric dietary intake (Orringer et al., 2016).

Increasing physical activity through promotion of an exercise regimen is a key recommendation that can burn calories and result in weight loss (Chart 42-4). Physical activity recommendations for all adults (those with and without obesity) include at least 150 minutes of moderate-intensity aerobic exercise weekly or 75 minutes of vigorous-intensity aerobic exercise weekly. In addition, muscle strengthening exercises that engage all major muscle groups should be done at least twice weekly (Fitch et al., 2013; Orringer et al., 2016). Patients with obesity who were previously sedentary and deconditioned may not be able to achieve this at the start; however, as little as 10 minutes of daily physical activity can result in weight loss and improved exercise tolerance (Fitch et al., 2013).

Patients with obesity should be counselled that reducing dietary caloric intake is a necessary component of weight loss therapy. This must also include a change in dietary habits in order for weight loss to be sustained over the long term. It is important to identify current dietary patterns and typical daily caloric intake in order to recommend an appropriate diet plan. Assessing food records or 24-hour recalls or conducting dietary interviews are all effective methods to gather baseline dietary information from patients (see Chapter 5). There are a plethora of commercial diets that patients may select (see Chart 42-5). To date, there have not been sufficiently rigorous longitudinal studies to determine which diet plans are superior to others in terms of achieving long-term weight loss (Katz & Meller, 2014).

Patients need not purchase commercial diet plans in order to achieve weight loss and embrace healthy diet habits. Most nutritionists advocate that healthy diets include few processed foods, sugars, and trans fats, and are heavy in plant-based foods (Katz & Meller, 2014). The Dietary Approaches to Stop Hypertension (DASH) diet is an example of a superior healthy noncommercial diet. Although initially promoted to manage hypertension, the DASH diet also provides a solid foundation for achieving

CHART 42-5

Select Popular Commercial Diets

Atkins Diet: www.atkins.com
eDiets: www.ediets.com
Jenny Craig: www.jennycraig.com
Medifast: www.medifast1.com/index.jsp
Nutrisystem: www.nutrisystem.com/jsps_hmr/home/index.jsp
Optifast: www.optifast.com/Pages/index.aspx
South Beach Diet: www.southbeachdiet.com/home/index.jsp
The Biggest Loser Diet: www.biggestloserclub.com
Weight Watchers: www.weightwatchers.com/us/
Zone Diet: www.zonediet.com

CHART 42-6

Patient Education: Healthy Eating Strategies

The nurse instructs the patient about the healthy eating strategies outlined below.

Limit or eliminate the following:
- Processed foods with limited nutritional value (e.g., packaged cakes, cookies, chips)
- High-caloric beverages (sugar-sweetened, juices, cream-enhanced)
- Fast foods
- Vending machine foods
- Foods high in sugars (e.g., candies) and saturated fats (e.g., fried foods, hot dogs)

Track the following:
- Daily food intake (food journals, diaries, smartphone, and tablet applications)
- Nutritional value and caloric content on food labels

Encourage the following:
- Reduce portions; use smaller plates and measure foods
- Schedule and plan meals and snacks in advance for each day; prepack lunches and snacks when you are out of the home (e.g., for work)
- Eat at home more often than you would eat outside the home; when eating out, avoid fried foods and choose lean meats and vegetables and salads with condiments on the side
- Eat breakfast
- Limit snacks
- Eat a variety of nutritious foods; monitoring quality of foods consumed is as important as the quantity of foods consumed
- Drink plenty of water
- Stay within your daily caloric intake plan; do not become discouraged if one day you do not adhere to your plan

Adapted from Fruh, S. M., Mulekar, M. S., & Dierking, J. (2013). Guiding patients to safe weight loss. *The Nurse Practitioner*, *38*(10), 1–7; Orringer, K. A., Harrison, A. V., Nichani, S. S., et al. (2016). University of Michigan Health System Clinical Alignment and Performance Excellence Guideline: Obesity prevention and management. Retrieved January 25, 2017, from www.med.umich.edu/1info/FHP/practiceguides/obesity/obesity.pdf

and maintaining weight loss (Goldstein, Aoun, Gaar, et al., 2014) (see Chapter 33). Other healthy diet plans that may form a basis for weight loss, though not specifically designed for this purpose, include the Mediterranean Diet and the Therapeutic Lifestyle Changes (TLC) Diet (see Chapter 29 for description of both diets) Patient education tips for managing ongoing healthy eating strategies are noted in Chart 42-6.

In addition to promoting healthy exercise and diet habits, ensuring healthy sleep habits is an additional lifestyle strategy that is associated with weight loss and maintenance of a healthy weight. It is posited that sleep deprivation can cause changes in cortisol levels that promote weight gain (Orringer et al., 2016). Advising patients with sleep disturbances to plan to be in bed with lights out at least 7 hours prior to wake-up time, to create a dark, relaxing bedroom environment, to avoid activities that can cause arousal around bedtime (e.g., texting), and to avoid beverages with caffeine after lunchtime can all be helpful strategies aimed at ensuring a restful night's sleep that is consonant with weight reduction (Orringer et al., 2016).

Pharmacologic Therapy

Patients who are not successful at meeting weight loss goals from lifestyle modification alone may be prescribed antiobesity medications. Some patients may exhibit initial success with lifestyle modifications, but be stymied with attempts to maintain a lower BMI over the long term. These patients may also benefit from antiobesity medications. Patients who are prescribed antiobesity medications should be counselled that these prescriptions are meant to supplement, not supplant diet modification and exercise (Yanovski & Yanovksi, 2014). Indications for antiobesity medications include a BMI >30 kg/m^2 or a BMI >27 kg/m^2 with concomitant morbidity that is related to being overweight (e.g., type 2 diabetes, hypertension) (Apovian et al., 2015; Bays, Seger, Primack, et al., 2016).

Today, there are about five antiobesity medications that may be prescribed over the long term to assist in decreasing and then maintaining a lower BMI. Of these, only one, orlistat (Xenical), was FDA approved prior to 2012 (Bendich, 2013) (see Table 42-2). It is thought that concerns about the safety of antiobesity medications coupled with the relatively recent FDA approval of safe and effective antiobesity medications likely account for the relative dearth of these prescriptions (Yanovski & Yanovski, 2014).

Antiobesity medications work by either inhibiting GI absorption of fats, or by altering central brain receptors to enhance satiety or reduce cravings (National Institute of Diabetes and Digestive and Kidney Diseases [NIDDK], 2016). Each of these medications has distinct side effects and contraindications; therefore, selection of these agents is very individualized. The patient is monitored while taking the selected medication; if the patient does not lose at least 5% body weight after 12 weeks, the prescription may need to be changed, or the patient may be referred for other weight-reduction therapy (e.g., **bariatric** surgery) (NIDDK, 2016).

The class of antiobesity medications known as the sympathomimetic amines have been FDA approved for many years. However, they are only supposed to be prescribed for short-term use (i.e., no longer than 12 weeks). They have many side effects (see Table 42-2), and patients do tend to

TABLE 42-2 Medications Prescribed to Treat Obesity

Medication	Adverse Effects	Nursing Considerations[a]
Gastrointestinal Lipase Inhibitor		
Mechanism of action: Diminishes intestinal absorption and metabolism of fats, particularly triglycerides		
Orlistat (Xenical) *Note: Also available in lower dosages over-the-counter under the trade name of Alli*	Diarrhea Flatus Oily stools Fecal incontinence	Patients may have associated problems with malabsorption of nutrients; advise them to take a concomitant daily multivitamin Caution in patients with known history of renal insufficiency, liver disease, or gallbladder disease as concomitant use is associated with renal calculi, liver failure, and cholelithiasis Do not administer with cyclosporine (Neoral)
Selective Serotonergic 5-HT2C Receptor Agonist		
Mechanism of action: Stimulates central 5-HT2C receptors, causing appetite suppression		
Lorcaserin (Belviq)	Fatigue Dizziness Nausea Headaches Cough Dry mouth Constipation	Can be associated with deficits in attention or memory; administer with caution in patients who drive or work with hazardous equipment when first prescribed until effects are realized Can cause hypoglycemia in patients with diabetes Patients concomitantly taking antidepressants or migraine medications can have synergistic effects Discontinue in patients who express suicidal ideation Rarely, serotonin syndrome may develop—be alert for high fevers, brisk reflexes, agitation, and diarrhea; notify primary provider immediately and hold medication if these occur
GLP-1 Receptor Agonists		
Mechanism of action: Mimics the effects of incretins, resulting in delayed gastric emptying, thus curbing appetite		
Liraglutide (Saxenda) *Note: Also available in lower dosages under the trade name of Victoza to treat type 2 diabetes*	Nausea Diarrhea or constipation Headache Tachycardia	Must be given subcutaneously on a daily basis in the abdomen, thigh, or upper arm. Dosage increases weekly until week 5 Discontinue in patients who express suicide ideation May be associated with pancreatitis; also associated with thyroid tumours in animal models
Sympathomimetic Amines		
Mechanism of Action: Stimulate central noradrenergic receptors, causing appetite suppression		
Phentermine (Adipex-P, Fastin) Benzphetamine (Didrex) Diethylpropion (Tenuate) Phendimetrazine (Bontril)	Palpitations and tachycardia Tremors Hypertension Dizziness Insomnia Diarrhea or constipation Mouth dryness Restlessness Alterations in taste	These are only FDA-approved for short-term use (i.e., no more than 12 weeks) Contraindications include heart disease, uncontrolled hypertension, hyperthyroidism, and glaucoma Caution patients to not drink alcohol while taking one of these medications
Dual Agents		
Mechanism of action: Each of these medications combines two medications with known antiobesity effects; when taken together, the effects are synergistic		
Phentermine/topiramate-ER (Qsymia) Mechanism of action: combines the effectiveness of phentermine (see above) and topiramate, an anticonvulsant, which stimulates central GABA receptors and inhibits central glutamate receptors, suppressing appetite	Paresthesias Dizziness Insomnia Mouth dryness Alterations in taste Insomnia Constipation Tachycardia	Same contraindications apply as for phentermine (see above). May need to monitor electrolytes, as hypokalemia and metabolic acidosis are possible Monitor creatinine and watch for manifestations of renal calculi
Naltrexone/bupropion (Contrave) Mechanism of action: inhibits central opioid receptors and inhibits reuptake of dopamine and norepinephrine selectively, resulting in diminished appetite and cravings	Constipation or diarrhea Nausea Vomiting Insomnia Dizziness Mouth dryness Hypertension Tachycardia	Contraindications include uncontrolled hypertension, epilepsy, history of eating disorder such as anorexia nervosa or bulimia, and history of alcohol abuse of illicit drug abuse Discontinue in patients who express suicidal ideation

[a]All antiobesity medications may be teratogenic; pregnancy is a contraindication to all of these agents.

FDA, U.S. Food and Drug Administration.

Adapted from Bays, H. E., Seger, J. C., Primack, C., et al. (2016). Obesity algorithm presented by the Obesity Medicine Association. Retrieved January 7, 2017, from www.obesityalgorithm.org; National Institute of Diabetes and Digestive and Kidney Diseases (NIDDK). (2016). Prescription medications to treat overweight and obesity. Retrieved January 7, 2017, from www.niddk.nih.gov/health-information/health-topics/weight-control/prescription-medications-treat-overweight-obesity/Pages/facts.aspx; Yanovski, S. Z., & Yanovski, J. A. (2014). Long-term drug treatment for obesity: A systematic and clinical review. *JAMA*, *311*(1), 74–86.

regain weight once they are no longer taking these medications (NIDDK, 2016).

Nonsurgical Interventions

Adult patients with obesity that does not respond to lifestyle interventions or antiobesity medications and who have either Class III/severe/extreme obesity (i.e., BMI in excess of 40 kg/m^2) or Class II obesity (BMI 35 to 39.9 kg/m^2) with obesity-related diseases or disorders (e.g., obstructive sleep apnea [OSA], type 2 diabetes) may be candidates for bariatric surgical interventions (see later discussion). Some patients may pursue minimally invasive interventions, such as vagal blocking (i.e., neurometabolic modulation) or intragastric balloon therapy (Ali, Moustarah, Kim, et al., 2015; Papasavas, El Chaar, Kothari, et al., 2016).

Vagal blocking therapy involves placement of a pacemaker-like device (vBloc) into the subcutaneous tissue in the lateral thoracic cavity with two leads that are laparoscopically implanted at the point where the vagus nerve truncates, at the gastroesophageal junction. A preprogrammed, pulsating signal is delivered for 12 hours daily. This signal causes intermittent "blocking" of the vagus nerve. Vagal blocking results in diminished gastric contraction and emptying, limited ghrelin secretion, and diminished pancreatic enzyme secretion; these cause increased satiety, decreased cravings, and diminished absorption of calories, all of which lead to weight loss (Papasavas et al., 2016). Results from a randomized controlled trial found greater initial and 18-month sustained weight loss with participants with obesity who received vagal blocking versus control sham device implantation (Ikramuddin, Blackstone, Brancatisano, et al., 2014; Shikora, Wolfe, Apovian, et al., 2015). There are few adverse effects noted with use of this device, which include GI symptoms (e.g., heartburn, belching). Patients must be educated to recharge the device twice weekly for about an hour with an external coil device.

Intragastric balloon therapy involves endoscopic placement of a saline-filled balloon (ORBERA) or a saline-filled dual balloon (ReShape) into the stomach. The mechanism by which these devices result in weight loss is poorly understood, but thought to be related to increased feelings of satiety and decreased gastric emptying. Postinsertion, the intragastric balloon(s) remain in place for 3 to 6 months, and are then deflated and removed. Studies suggest greater weight loss with these than with sham therapy or with lifestyle interventions alone (Ali et al., 2015). Early adverse effects include complaints of nausea and vomiting, which are generally transient and do not require balloon removal. Balloon rupture can occur over the long term, however, which may infrequently lead to intestinal obstruction. In order to monitor for this serious complication, it is recommended that the balloons be impregnated with methylene blue preinsertion so that patients with silent ruptures can report the presence of green urine to their primary providers and receive timely interventions to remove the deflated balloons before they cause obstruction. Patients who seem unlikely to return for follow-up appointments should not be candidates for intragastric balloons. Balloons should be removed within 6 months of placement; longer placement periods are associated with increased likelihood of rupture and intestinal obstruction (Ali et al., 2015).

Gerontologic Considerations

As adults age, lean skeletal mass decreases and adipose tissue increases. Adipose tissue does not burn calories as efficiently as lean skeletal mass; furthermore, basal metabolism drops by 2% for each additional decade of adult life. Therefore, older adults are more likely to gain weight unless they either increase activity levels or decrease their caloric intake (Eliopoulos, 2018).

Research suggests that older adults with obesity are at risk for complications that may negatively affect their quality of life. In particular, older adults with obesity may be at greater risk of falls (Joen, 2013) and mobility impairments (Murphy, Reinders, Register, et al., 2014). More older adults with obesity are admitted to nursing homes than normal weight older adults (Felix, Bradway, Chisholm, et al., 2015). One study found that older adults with obesity had lower resting hemoglobin–oxygen saturation levels (i.e., SpO_2 levels), which presumably could lead to hypoxemia, dyspnea, and ischemic complications (e.g., myocardial infarction) (Kapur, Wilsdon, Au, et al., 2013). Another study found that in one long-term care facility, more older adult residents who were overweight had indwelling urinary catheters than their counterparts who were leaner, which presumably could lead to urosepsis (Felix, Thostenson, Bursac, et al., 2013).

There is some evidence that older adults with an overweight body mass (i.e., between 25 and 29.9 kg/m^2) have reasonably good health outcomes; therefore, overweight older adults are not necessarily counselled to lose weight (Orringer et al., 2016). However, older adults with obesity (i.e., with BMIs in excess of 30 kg/m^2) should be encouraged to engage in lifestyle modifications, including diet and exercise, much as younger adults (Orringer et al., 2016). Along with decreasing dietary caloric intake, older adult patients should be counselled that the quality of calories consumed should be the focus of the daily diet (see Chapter 14). Fats should be limited to less than 30% of total calories, while proteins should comprise 10% to 20% of the daily diet. Intake of soluble fibres (e.g., oats, pectin) is particularly important since these can lower cholesterol levels and prevent cardiovascular diseases and cancers. Fewer than one third of older adults consume the recommended five servings of fruits and vegetables daily (Eliopoulos, 2018). Identifying barriers to consumption of these important sources of nutrients may help the older adult patient with obesity lose weight and adopt healthier eating habits. For instance, the older adult who has difficulty chewing raw fruits may enjoy fruit smoothies.

Whether or not older adult patients with obesity should be candidates for bariatric surgery (see later discussion) has been a point of contention. Study findings suggest that many older adults with obesity benefit from bariatric surgery, although their weight loss tends to be less than that of younger adults who have bariatric surgery (Caceres, Moskowitz, & O'Connell, 2015). At present, there are no guidelines that identify the profile of which older adult patients with obesity can most benefit from bariatric surgery.

Nursing Management

Patients with obesity report feeling socially marginalized, judged, and unsupported by society at large. Many times, patients with obesity report that they suffer stigmatization by their health care providers, including nurses (Buxton & Snethen, 2013; Gilmartin, 2013; Puhl, Phelan, Nadglowski, et al., 2016). The bias that nurses may have against patients with obesity may not directly affect their nursing care; however, indirectly, the consequences of this stigmatization can lead to poor health outcomes. Patients with obesity who feel stigmatized by their health care providers report increased depression, low self-esteem, and avoidance of health care appointments and health maintenance activities (e.g., diet and exercise) (Budd & Peterson, 2015).

Nurses need to approach patients with obesity with the same respectful, courteous, and empathetic behaviour that they extend to patients without obesity. Confronting their own attitudes and beliefs about patients with obesity may help to mitigate biases. For instance, using patient-first language for all patients with diagnosed diseases, including the disease of obesity, can be an effective way to dispel bias. By referencing *the patient with obesity,* the nurse is effectively noting that the patient, not the disease, is the central point of concern and that the disease is amenable to treatment. On the other hand, referencing *the patient with obesity* tends to define the person by having obesity, which can lead to subliminal impressions that the patient is somehow responsible for having obesity. Research studies report that many health care providers, including nurses, hold negative attitudes toward patients with obesity and believe that they are indulgent, lazy, and lack willpower (Puhl et al., 2016).

The patient with obesity who requires medical/surgical nursing care, whether it is because the patient is admitted to the hospital, needs home care, or is admitted to a transitional care setting, merits special considerations. Obesity can adversely affect the mechanics of ventilation and circulation, pharmacokinetics and pharmacodynamics, skin integrity, and body mechanics and mobility. These adverse effects are more common with higher BMIs; thus, the patient with Class III obesity (BMI in excess of 40 kg/m^2) is particularly vulnerable.

Obesity can result in anatomical remodelling, including compression of the oropharynx and increased neck circumference and chest diameter. These changes can predispose the patient with obesity to OSA (see Chapter 23), respiratory failure (see Chapter 26), and obesity hypoventilation syndrome. Obesity hypoventilation syndrome is characterized by daytime hypoventilation with hypercapnia (i.e., $PaCO_2$ >45 mm Hg) and hypoxemia (i.e., PaO_2 <80 mm Hg), and sleep-disordered breathing. Potential adverse effects of obesity hypoventilation syndrome can be mitigated by maintaining the patient in the low Fowler's position, which maximizes diaphragmatic chest expansion. Continuous pulse oximetry monitoring may be advisable, as well as supplemental oxygen therapy (see Chapter 26) and frequent respiratory assessments (at least every shift). For the patient with a known diagnosis of OSA, ensuring that the patient utilizes prescribed therapy (e.g., oral appliance, continuous positive airway pressure [CPAP]) if newly hospitalized or in a different transitional care environment is important in order to ensure breathing effectiveness and avert respiratory failure (Berrios, 2016; Dambaugh & Ecklund, 2016; Sturman-Floyd, 2013).

The patient with obesity may have central and peripheral circulatory compromise. Heart failure is more commonplace among patients with obesity (see Chapter 31). Hypertension is also more prevalent; the nurse must use appropriately sized blood pressure cuffs to obtain valid blood pressure readings (see Chapter 33). Peripheral blood flow can be compromised for the patient with obesity, resulting in stasis of blood flow, one of three components of Virchow triad, which are the broad categories of risk for venous thromboembolism (VTE) (see Chapter 32). Peripheral circulatory compromise not only can increase the risk for VTE formation (e.g., pulmonary embolism [PE] and deep vein thrombosis [DVT]), but it can also make finding venous access difficult when the patient with obesity requires intravenous (IV) therapy. Finding appropriate venous access can be exacerbated by the presence of increased adipose tissue in the extremities. Ultrasound guidance may be required in order to successfully gain IV access and place an IV cannula in the patient with obesity (Berrios, 2016; Dambaugh & Ecklund, 2016).

The patient with obesity may have differences in both pharmacokinetics (i.e., the movement of drug metabolites within the body) and pharmacodynamics (i.e., how drugs are metabolized and the effects of drugs) that can affect drug dosages, drug effectiveness, and patient safety. The effectiveness of many drugs is affected by the ratio of lean skeletal muscle mass to adipose tissue. The active metabolites of many drugs are protein bound in the plasma. In patients with greater adipose tissue, more of these active metabolites can be unbound in plasma, or free, and exert greater effects. Some drugs readily bind to adipose tissue, which may either inactivate them or prolong their effects. In addition, increased adiposity can have indirect effects on metabolic pathways within the liver, resulting in changes in drug metabolic pathways, which can result in either increased or decreased drug metabolism, depending upon the drug and the affected metabolic pathway. In other words, some drugs have enhanced effects while others have diminished effects with patients with obesity compared to patients of normal weight. For instance, one research study found that patients with obesity who were critically ill required proportionally lower dosages of IV drip norepinephrine, which is typically given based upon weight-based calculation, than patients with normal weight (Radosevich, Patanwala, & Erstad, 2016). On the other hand, patients with obesity who require opioid agents to treat pain many times require higher dosages of opioid agents to achieve pain relief, but are more likely to have serious adverse effects of sedation and respiratory depression (D'Arcy, 2015). The nurse should be cognizant that weight-based calculations of drug dosages for patients with obesity may need to be altered, depending upon the patient and the drug, and should consult with clinical pharmacologists and the patient's primary provider as needed to ensure optimal drug effectiveness and patient safety (Berrios, 2016).

Patients with obesity are particularly vulnerable to developing pressure ulcers. Increased adipose tissue can diminish the supply of blood, oxygen, and nutrients to peripheral tissue. The presence of more folds in the skin is associated with more skin moisture and increased skin friction, which are pressure ulcer risks. Moreover, skin folds may be present in uncommon areas, including under the breasts, under the lower abdomen, within gluteal folds, and at the nape of the neck (Berrios, 2016; Dambaugh &

NURSING RESEARCH PROFILE

Chart 42-7. Pressure Ulcers Among Critically Ill Patients With Extreme Obesity

Hyun, S., Li, X., Vermillion, B., et al. (2014). Body mass index and pressure ulcers: Improved predictability of pressure ulcers in intensive care patients. *American Journal of Critical Care, 23*(6), 494–500.

Purpose

The Braden Scale is a validated tool used to assess pressure ulcer risk among multiple populations of patients at risk for pressure ulcers and is commonly used in hospitals in the United States in a variety of settings. Patients who are admitted to intensive care units are at heightened risk for pressure ulcers. Those patients who are critically ill and who also have obesity are presumably at even higher risk for pressure ulcers, because they have heightened immobility problems as a consequence of their weight. This study sought to investigate whether or not body mass index (BMI) could serve as an additional predictor for pressure ulcer development that could complement Braden Scale Scores among patients who are critically ill who also had obesity.

Design

This retrospective study examined electronic health record data from adult patients admitted to the adult critical care units in one Midwest academic health centre over a 3-year period. Patients were sorted into four groups; underweight, with a BMI less than 19 kg/m^2; normal weight, with a BMI between 19 and 25 kg/m^2; obese, with a BMI between 25 and 40 kg/m^2; and extremely obese, with a BMI greater than 40 kg/m^2. Patient demographics, the incidence of pressure ulcers, and Braden Scale Scores were compared and analyzed between groups.

Findings

Data gathering yielded information on 2,632 patients admitted to both medical and surgical intensive care units. The incidence of pressure ulcers in the underweight cohort was 8.6%, in the normal weight cohort was 5.5%, in the obese cohort was 2.8%, and in the extremely obese cohort was 9.9%. Logistic regression analysis revealed that patients who were underweight or who had extreme obesity were more likely to develop pressure ulcers. The odds of pressure ulcer development based upon BMI cohort groups was not more predictive than Braden Scale Scores, however.

Nursing Implications

Results from this study validated that the Braden Scale is a useful tool for predicting pressure ulcer risk among adults who are critically ill and who have obesity. BMI scores, although not more predictive of risk than Braden Scale Scores, may be roughly equivalent measures of ascertaining pressure ulcer risk. In particular, findings from this study suggest that patients who are critically ill and who have extreme obesity (i.e., with BMIs in excess of 40 kg/m^2) are at high risk for developing pressure ulcers. This is particularly concerning, since 26% of this study sample of adults who were critically ill had extreme obesity. Additional nursing considerations for patients with extreme obesity who are critically ill are needed so that pressure ulcers may be prevented. These considerations may include the use of specialty lifts, turning devices, and other safe patient handling devices so that these patients may be appropriately mobilized to prevent pressure ulcers.

Ecklund, 2016; Sturman-Floyd, 2013). In addition, patients with obesity many times have more limitations in mobility than patients of normal weight. Immobility is another risk for pressure ulcer development (Hyun, Li, Vermillion, et al., 2014) (see Chart 42-7). Consultation with a wound–ostomy–continence (WOC) nurse may be advisable to ensure that pressure ulcer risks for the patient with obesity are minimized.

The nurse must ensure that the appropriate specialty equipment is utilized as needed so that the patient with obesity who is immobilized is turned and mobilized as indicated to prevent pressure ulcers. The typical nursing protocol is that the patient who is immobilized and bedfast should be turned every 2 hours to prevent pressure ulcers (Berrios, 2016). Nurses should be familiar with and comfortable using specialized durable medical bariatric equipment (e.g., lifts, transport equipment, commodes) so that the patient with obesity receives necessary care. It is also important to enforce and implement safe patient handling protocols so that the nurse does not incur musculoskeletal injury (Berrios, 2016).

Surgical Management

Bariatric surgery, or surgery for obesity, is typically performed after other nonsurgical attempts at weight control have failed. Insurance coverage for bariatric surgery varies widely, but most insurance companies will consider surgery as a treatment if the patient has Class III obesity or Class II obesity with a related medical condition (e.g., type 2 diabetes, OSA) (Obesity Action Coalition [OAC], 2015a).

The Canadian Institute for Health Information (CIHI, 2014) reports that in 2012–2013, there were about 6,000 bariatric surgeries performed in Canada, and this is almost 4 times the number performed in 2006–2007. Bariatric surgical procedures work by restricting a patient's ability to eat (restrictive procedure), interfering with ingested nutrient absorption (malabsorptive procedures), or both. The different types of bariatric surgical procedures require unique lifestyle modifications. In order to optimize their success, patients should be well informed about the specific lifestyle changes, eating habits, and bowel habits that may result from each type of procedure.

Bariatric surgery typically results in a weight loss of 10% to 35% of total body weight within 2 to 3 years postoperatively (Colquitt, Pickett, Loveman, et al., 2014; OAC, 2015b), with the majority of weight loss occurring within the first year (Courcoulas, Christian, Belle, et al., 2013). Comorbid conditions such as type 2 diabetes, hypertension, and OSA may resolve; and dyslipidemia improves (ASMBS, 2013a; Courcoulas, Belle, Neiberg,

CHART 42-8

Selection Criteria for Bariatric Surgery

BMI ≥40 kg/m^2 without excessive surgical risk
Patients with BMI ≥35 kg/m^2 and one or more severe obesity-associated comorbid conditions (e.g., hyperlipidemia, obstructive sleep apnea, obesity hypoventilation syndrome, nonalcoholic fatty liver disease, hypertension, asthma, debilitating arthritis, or considerably impaired quality of life)
Patients with *BMI* ≥30 kg/m^2 with type 2 diabetes or metabolic syndrome
Ability to perform activities of daily living and self-care
Presence of a support network of family and friends
Failure of previous nonsurgical attempts at weight loss, including nonprofessional programs
Expectation that patient will adhere to postoperative care, follow-up visits, and recommended medical management, including the use of dietary supplements

Exclusions

Reversible endocrine or other disorders that can cause obesity
Current drug or alcohol abuse
Uncontrolled, severe psychiatric illness
Lack of comprehension of risks, benefits, expected outcomes, alternatives, and lifestyle changes required with bariatric surgery

Adapted from Mechanick, J. I., Youdim, A., Jones, D. B., et al. (2013). Clinical practice guidelines for the perioperative nutritional, metabolic, and nonsurgical support of the bariatric surgery patient—2013 update: Cosponsored by the American Association of Clinical Endocrinologists, the Obesity Society, and American Society for Metabolic and Bariatric Surgery. *Surgery for Obesity and Related Diseases*, *9*(2), 159–191.

et al., 2015). Bariatric surgery has been extended to carefully selected adolescents with severe obesity and comorbidity because of the positive results it has achieved in adults (Michalsky, Reichard, Inge, et al., 2012).

Patient selection is critical, and the preliminary process may necessitate months of counselling, education, and evaluation by a multidisciplinary team, including social workers, dietitians, a nurse counsellor, a psychologist or psychiatrist, and a bariatric surgeon. The selection criteria for patients has changed considerably since the advent of bariatric surgery, with patients with BMIs as low as 30 kg/m^2 now considered candidates for surgical intervention if they have comorbid conditions that may demonstrably improve post weight loss (e.g., type 2 diabetes) (Mechanick, Youdim, Jones, et al., 2013) (see Chart 42-8).

Because bariatric surgery involves a drastic change in the functioning of the digestive system, patients need counselling before and after the surgery. Guidelines have been developed to assist in the care of patients having bariatric surgery (Broome, Ayala, Georgeson, et al., 2015; Mechanick et al., 2013).

Roux-en-Y gastric bypass (RYGB), gastric banding, sleeve gastrectomy, and biliopancreatic diversion with duodenal switch are the current bariatric procedures of choice. These procedures may be performed by laparoscopy or by an open surgical technique. The RYGB and the sleeve gastrectomy are the two most commonly used procedures (ASMBS, 2014); a systematic review found that outcomes were equally favourable between RYGB and sleeve gastrectomy, and generally better than outcomes with gastric banding (Colquitt et al., 2014). Biliopancreatic diversion with duodenal switch tends to result in the most postoperative weight loss, and is therefore more commonly indicated for patients with very high BMIs (Colquitt et al., 2014).

The RYGB is a combined restrictive and malabsorptive procedure. The gastric banding and sleeve gastrectomy are restrictive procedures, and the biliopancreatic diversion with duodenal switch combines gastric restriction with intestinal malabsorption. Figure 42-5A–D provides additional details about these procedures.

Nursing Process

The Patient Undergoing Bariatric Surgery

Assessment

Preoperatively, the nurse assesses for contraindications to major abdominal surgery. Previous attempts at losing weight are also assessed, including strategies such as nutritional counselling, dieting, or exercise programs. The nurse ensures the patient has received education and counselling regarding the possible risks and benefits of bariatric surgery including the complications, postsurgical outcomes, dietary changes, and the need for lifelong follow-up. The nurse also confirms that the patient has been screened for behavioural disorders that may interfere with postsurgical outcomes. Dietary counselling is initiated preoperatively to prepare for postoperative dietary changes (Mechanick et al., 2013; OAC, 2015b).

The nurse ensures that preoperative screening tests are obtained and scrutinizes the results. Typical laboratory tests include a complete blood cell count CBC, electrolytes, blood urea nitrogen (BUN), and creatinine. Patients with obesity may have OSA, gastroesophageal reflux disease (GERD), heart disease, nonalcoholic fatty liver disease, diabetes (or prediabetes), and vitamin and mineral deficiencies; thus, other screening tests that may be obtained include a sleep study, upper endoscopy, electrocardiogram (ECG), lipid panel, AST, ALT, glucose, and hemoglobin A1c, as well as iron, vitamin B_{12}, thiamine, folate, vitamin D, and calcium levels.

Postoperatively, the nurse assesses the patient to ensure that goals for recovery are met and that the patient exhibits absence of complications secondary to the surgical intervention. See Chapter 21 for general assessment of the postoperative patient.

Nursing Priorities

Based on the assessment data, major nursing priorities may include the following:

- Deficient knowledge
- Anxiety

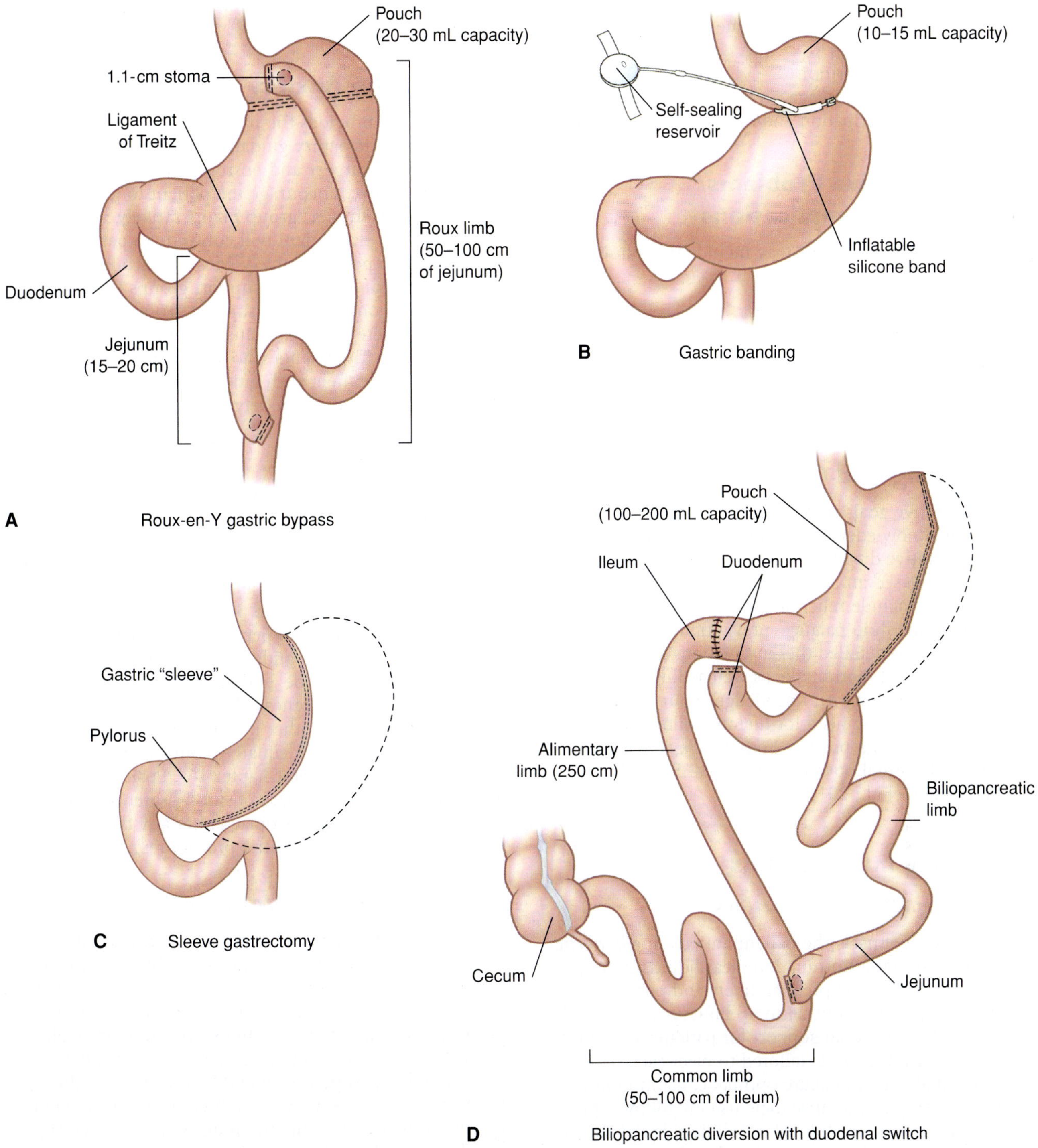

FIGURE 42-5. Bariatric surgical procedures. **A.** Roux-en-Y gastric bypass. A horizontal row of staples across the fundus of the stomach creates a pouch with a capacity of 20 to 30 mL. The jejunum is divided distal to the ligament of Treitz, and the distal end is anastomosed to the new pouch. The proximal segment is anastomosed to the jejunum. **B.** Gastric banding. A prosthetic device is used to restrict oral intake by creating a small pouch of 10 to 15 mL that empties through the narrow outlet into the remainder of the stomach. **C.** Sleeve gastrectomy. The stomach is incised vertically and up to 85% of the stomach is surgically removed, leaving a "sleeve"-shaped tube that retains intact nervous innervation and does not obstruct or decrease the size of the gastric outlet. **D.** Biliopancreatic diversion with duodenal switch (also called *sleeve gastrectomy with duodenal switch*). Half of the stomach is removed, leaving a small area that holds about 60 mL. The entire jejunum is excluded from the rest of the gastrointestinal tract. The duodenum is disconnected and sealed off. The ileum is divided above the ileocecal junction, and the distal end of the jejunum is anastomosed to the first portion of the duodenum. The distal end of the biliopancreatic limb is anastomosed to the ileum.

- Acute pain
- Risk for deficient fluid volume
- Risk for infection
- Imbalanced nutrition
- Disturbed body image
- Risk for constipation and/or diarrhea

Collaborative Problems/ Potential Complications

Potential complications may include the following:

- Hemorrhage
- Venous thromboembolism
- Bile reflux
- Dumping syndrome
- Dysphagia
- Bowel or gastric outlet obstruction

Planning and Goals

Preoperative goals include that the patient will become knowledgeable about the preoperative and postoperative dietary routine/restrictions and will have decreased anxiety about the surgery. Postoperative goals include relief of pain, maintenance of homeostatic fluid balance, prevention of infection, adherence to detailed diet instructions to include progression of food intake as well as fluid intake (to prevent dehydration), knowledge about vitamin supplements and the need for lifelong follow-up, achievement of a positive body image, and maintenance of normal bowel habits (ASMBS, 2013a; Mechanick et al., 2013).

Nursing Interventions

Ensuring Dietary Restrictions

The nurse counsels the patient anticipating bariatric surgery to ingest nothing but clear liquids for a specified period of time preoperatively and postoperatively (typically about 24 to 48 hours before and after surgery). Nutritional support for patients scheduled for bariatric surgery is tailored to meet each patient's individual need to ensure optimal consumption of micronutrients. Bariatric diets usually follow a progression from clear liquids to full liquids to soft solids and eventually solid foods. This slow progression is necessary to maximize weight loss, and to prevent complications such as nausea, vomiting, bile reflux, and diarrhea.

The patient's diet will be limited upon discharge from the hospital; because of this, patients scheduled for bariatric surgery are given guidelines prior to surgery on which foods and liquids they may consume postoperatively so that they may stock up on these items at home before they are admitted to the hospital. These typically include sugar-free drinks, gelatins and puddings, flavoured electrolyte drinks, fat-free milk, protein drinks, sugar-free applesauce, and low-fat soups (Cole, Beckman, & Earthman, 2014; Isom, Andromalos, Ariagno, et al., 2014; Mechanick et al., 2013).

Reducing Anxiety

The nurse provides the patient preparing for bariatric surgery anticipatory guidance as to what to expect during the surgery and postoperatively. In addition, the nurse may encourage the patient to join a bariatric surgery support group preoperatively, with the intent that the patient will continue to participate in this group postoperatively. Most bariatric surgery centres sponsor patient support groups that meet in person or online. These support groups provide a forum where patients contemplating bariatric surgery may talk with patients who have had the surgery and may provide them with guidance and tips that can help to lessen their anxiety (Mechanick et al., 2013).

Relieving Pain

After surgery, analgesic agents may be given as prescribed to relieve pain and discomfort. Patients are usually prescribed opioid agents via patient-controlled analgesia (PCA) pumps; the nurse should educate the patient about its use and monitor its effectiveness. It is especially important to provide adequate pain relief so that the patient can perform pulmonary care activities (deep breathing and coughing) and leg exercises, turn from side to side, and ambulate. The nurse assesses the effectiveness of analgesic intervention and consults with other members of the health care team if pain is not adequately controlled (Patil & Melander, 2015) (see Chapter 16). Positioning the patient in a low Fowler's position promotes comfort and emptying of the stomach after any type of gastric surgery, including bariatric procedures).

Ensuring Fluid Volume Balance

Patients who have had bariatric surgery usually receive intravenous (IV) fluids for the first several hours postoperatively. Once they are awake and alert on the surgical unit, they are encouraged to begin intake of sugar-free oral fluids. Introducing small volumes of these liquids is believed to stimulate GI peristalsis and perfusion and thwart gastric reflux. Sugar-free fluids are preferred because they are not implicated in causing dumping syndrome (see later discussion). With a typical regimen, patients are encouraged to slowly sip 30 mL of these fluids every 15 minutes. Patients should stop ingesting fluids, however, if they feel nauseated or full. Antiemetic agents may be prescribed to relieve nausea and prevent vomiting, which could cause strain on the surgical site and cause either a hemorrhage or anastomotic leak (Mechanick et al., 2013).

Preventing Infection/ Anastomotic Leak

Disruption at the site of anastomosis (i.e., surgically resected site) may cause leakage of gastric contents into the peritoneal cavity, causing infection and possible sepsis. Patients at risk for this particular complication tend to be older, male, and with greater body mass. In addition, anastomotic leak is more commonly associated with open rather than laparoscopic procedures. Patients with anastomotic leaks typically exhibit nonspecific signs and symptoms that include fever, abdominal pain, tachycardia, and leukocytosis. This may progress to sepsis and possibly septic shock if not recognized and treated early (see Chapter 18). The nurse must be astute in recognizing these manifestations and alerting the patient's primary provider should they occur (Dunham, 2013; Patil & Melander, 2015).

A patient suspected of having an anastomotic leak may have an upper GI series that includes follow-up computed tomography (CT) scan with contrast dye, which may find leaking contrast dye, thus confirming the diagnosis. Treatment varies depending on the timing (early or late postoperatively) and severity of the leak. CT-guided drainage of the area may be appropriate for a less severe leak in the later postoperative phase of recovery, but an early or severe leak requires immediate open surgical intervention to repair the leak (Jacobsen, Nergard, Leifsson, et al., 2014).

Ensuring Adequate Nutritional Status

After bowel sounds have returned and oral intake is resumed, six small feedings consisting of a total of 600 to 800 calories per day are provided, and consumption of fluids between meals is encouraged to prevent dehydration. The nurse instructs the patient to eat slowly and stop when feeling full. Eating too much or too fast or eating high-calorie liquids and soft foods can result in vomiting or painful esophageal distention. Gastric retention may be evidenced by abdominal distention, nausea, and vomiting. A nutritionist is typically consulted to assist with diet restrictions and diet progression (Mechanick et al., 2013) (see Chart 42-9).

Common dietary deficiencies in patients who have had bariatric surgery include malabsorption of organic iron, which may require supplementation with oral or parenteral iron, and a low serum level of vitamin B_{12}; the patient may be prescribed monthly vitamin B_{12} intramuscular injections to prevent pernicious anemia (Dunham, 2013; Isom et al., 2014) (see Chapter 54 for further discussion).

Supporting Body Image Changes

Most patients post bariatric surgery report greatly improved perceptions of their body image, as well as improved quality of life. However, some patients report lingering dissatisfaction with their body images. In particular, some patients may report dissatisfaction related to loose skin folds and may eventually seek elective body-contouring surgical options (e.g., breast reductions, breast lifts, abdominoplasty). The nurse provides support to the patient who reports dissatisfaction with body image post weight

CHART 42-9

Patient Education: Dietary Guidelines for the Patient Who Has Had Bariatric Surgery

The nurse instructs the patient to:

- Eat smaller but more frequent meals that contain protein and fibre; each meal size should not exceed 1 cup
- Eat only foods high in nutrients (e.g., peanut butter, cheese, chicken, fish, beans)
- Consume fat as tolerated
- Ensure a low carbohydrate intake; in particular, avoid concentrated sources of carbohydrates (e.g., candy)
- Eat two protein snacks daily; animal protein may be poorly tolerated after Roux-en-Y gastric bypass, however patients are encouraged to diversify their source of dietary protein, and this should include animal proteins if tolerated
- Eat slowly and chew thoroughly
- Assume a low Fowler's position during mealtime and then remain in that position for 20 to 30 minutes after mealtime—this delays stomach emptying and decreases the likelihood of dumping syndrome
- Know that antispasmodic agents, as prescribed, also may aid in delaying the emptying of the stomach
- Do not drink fluid with meals; instead, consume fluids up to 30 minutes before a meal and 30 to 60 minutes after mealtime
- Do drink plenty of water; refrain from drinking liquid calories (e.g., alcoholic beverages, fruit drinks, nondiet sodas)
- Take prescribed dietary supplements of vitamins and medium-chain triglycerides
- Follow-up with primary provider for monthly injections of vitamin B_{12} and iron as prescribed
- Walk for at least 30 minutes daily

Adapted from Mechanick, J. I., Youdim, A., Jones, D. B., et al. (2013). Clinical practice guidelines for the perioperative nutritional, metabolic, and nonsurgical support of the bariatric surgery patient—2013 update: Cosponsored by the American Association of Clinical Endocrinologists, the Obesity Society, and American Society for Metabolic & Bariatric Surgery. *Surgery for Obesity and Related Diseases*, *9*(2), 159–191.

loss by acknowledging the patient's feelings as real, sharing that these perceptions are not unusual, and providing links to live or online supports groups or counsellors, as necessary (Gilmartin, 2013; Pfeil, 2014; Schauer, Woodruff, Hotz, et al., 2014).

Ensuring Maintenance of Bowel Habits

Patients may complain of either diarrhea or constipation postoperatively. Diarrhea is more common an occurrence postbariatric surgery, particularly after malabsorptive procedures (Mechanick et al., 2013). Both may be prevented if the patient consumes a nutritious diet that is high in fibre. Steatorrhea also may occur as a result of rapid gastric emptying, which prevents adequate mixing with pancreatic and biliary secretions (Mechanick et al., 2013). In mild cases, reducing the intake of fat and administering an antimotility medication (e.g., loperamide [Imodium]) may control symptoms. Persistent diarrhea or steatorrhea may warrant further diagnostic testing, such as an upper endoscopy or colonoscopy with biopsies to rule out the presence of additional pathology, such as celiac diseases or *Clostridium difficile* infection (Mechanick et al., 2013) (see Chapter 38).

Monitoring and Managing Potential Complications

After surgery, the nurse assesses the patient for complications from the bariatric surgery, such as hemorrhage, venous thromboembolism, bile reflux, dumping syndrome, dysphagia, and bowel or gastric outlet obstruction.

Hemorrhage

Postoperative hemorrhage may be a complication following bariatric surgery. Intra-abdominal hemorrhage may be evident by frank, bright red oral or rectal bleeding, tarry melena, bloody output from the wound or drains, if present, as well as typical clinical manifestations of severe bleeding and hemorrhagic shock (e.g., tachycardia, hypotension, syncope) (see Chapter 18). Bleeding within the first 72 hours postoperatively is most likely caused by disruption in a staple or suture. Bleeding 72 hours to 30 days postoperatively is most likely from formation of a gastric or duodenal ulcer (Patil & Melander, 2015) (see Chapter 37).

Venous Thromboembolism

Patients who have bariatric surgery are at moderate to high risk of VTE, including both PE and DVT. Patients who are older, have higher BMIs, and have a prior history of a VTE or coagulation defect are at higher risk (Brethauer, 2013). ASMBS guidelines for VTE prevention specify that in the immediate postoperative period, patients who have had bariatric surgery should be prescribed mechanical compression (e.g., intermittent pneumatic compression devices) and prophylactic anticoagulation with subcutaneous low–molecular-weight heparin (LMWH) agents (e.g., dalteparin [Fragmin], enoxaparin [Lovenox]). The duration of time that mechanical compression and anticoagulation should continue postoperatively are not described, however, and are left to the discretion of the patient and primary provider. In addition to implementing this prescribed therapy, nurses caring for patients post bariatric surgery should encourage them to begin early ambulation to further deter the advent of VTE (Brethauer, 2013).

Bile Reflux

Bile reflux may occur with procedures that manipulate or remove the pylorus, which acts as a barrier to the reflux of duodenal contents. Reflux of bile can cause inflammation of the stomach (i.e., gastritis) or esophagus (i.e., esophagitis). Burning epigastric pain and vomiting of bilious material manifest this condition. Eating or vomiting does not relieve the symptoms. Bile reflux may be managed with proton pump inhibitors (e.g., omeprazole [Prilosec]) (Sifrim, 2013).

Dumping Syndrome

Dumping syndrome is an unpleasant set of vasomotor and GI symptoms that commonly occurs in patients who have had bariatric surgery. For many years, it had been theorized that the hypertonic gastric food boluses that quickly transit into the intestines drew extracellular fluid from the circulating blood volume into the small intestines to dilute the high concentration of electrolytes and sugars, resulting in symptoms. Now, it is thought that this rapid transit of the food bolus from the stomach into the small intestines instead causes a rapid and exuberant release of metabolic peptides that are responsible for the symptoms of dumping syndrome (Patil & Melander, 2015).

Symptoms of dumping syndrome typically occur 15 minutes to 2 hours after eating and include tachycardia, dizziness, sweating, nausea, vomiting, bloating, abdominal cramping, and diarrhea (Patil & Melander, 2015). These symptoms typically resolve once the intestine has been evacuated (i.e., with defecation). Later, blood glucose rises rapidly, followed by increased insulin secretion. This results in a reactive hypoglycemia, which also is unpleasant for the patient. Vasomotor symptoms that occur 10 to 90 minutes after eating are pallor, perspiration, palpitations, headache, and feelings of warmth, dizziness, and even drowsiness. Anorexia may also result from dumping syndrome, because the patient may be reluctant to eat (Patil & Melander, 2015).

NURSING ALERT

Dumping syndrome is a physiologic response to the rapid emptying of gastric contents into the jejunum. The rapid transit of the food bolus from the stomach into the small intestines causes a rapid and exuberant release of metabolic peptides that are responsible for the symptoms of dumping syndrome.

Dysphagia

Dysphagia, or difficulty swallowing, may occur in patients who have had any type of restrictive bariatric procedure. If it occurs, it tends to be most severe 4 to 6 weeks postoperatively and may persist for up to 6 months after surgery. Dysphagia may be prevented by educating patients to eat slowly, to chew food thoroughly, and to avoid eating tough foods such as steak or dry chicken or doughy bread. Patients with severe dysphagia who have had gastric banding may benefit from having their bands adjusted. Patients who have had other restrictive procedures may experience relief of symptoms after having stomal strictures relieved endoscopically (Mechanick et al., 2013).

Bowel and Gastric Outlet Obstruction

Bowel or gastric outlet obstruction may occur as a complication of bariatric surgery. The typical manifestations and treatments of gastric outlet obstruction are described in Chapter 38; however, there is a key difference in the treatment of a patient who has undergone bariatric surgery with a gastric outlet obstruction. It is contraindicated to insert a nasogastric (NG) tube in patients that have had bariatric surgery, even if they have a gastric outlet obstruction. Alternative treatment options may include endoscopic procedures aimed at relieving the obstruction, such as balloon dilation, or surgical revisions (Patil & Melander, 2015).

NURSING ALERT

Insertion of NG tubes is contraindicated in the patient postbariatric surgery. This procedure may disrupt the surgical suture line and cause anastomotic leak or hemorrhage.

Promoting Home, Community-Based, and Transitional Care

Patients are usually discharged from the hospital within 4 days postoperatively (this may be within 24 to 72 hours for patients who have had laparoscopic procedures) with detailed dietary instructions (see Chart 42-9) as well as instructions about how to either begin or resume an appropriate exercise regimen. Instructions on making follow-up appointments with the bariatric surgeon for routine postoperative visits or for complications are shared with the patient (Mechanick et al., 2013).

Educating Patients About Self-Care

The nurse provides education with the patient about nutrition, nutritional supplements, pain management, the importance of physical activity, and the symptoms of dumping syndrome and measures to prevent or minimize these symptoms. Patients who undergo laparoscopic or open RYGB procedures may have one or more Jackson–Pratt drains, which may remain in place after discharge. The nurse educates the patient or caregiver about how to empty, measure, and record the amount of drainage. Patients should be instructed to avoid taking nonsteroidal anti-inflammatory drugs (NSAIDs) (e.g., ibuprofen [Motrin]) postdischarge, as they have been implicated in development of stomach ulcers (Mechanick et al., 2013). The nurse must emphasize the continued need for follow-up (even after weight-loss goals are met) and continued support group participation (Wykowski & Krouse, 2013).

Continuing and Transitional Care

After bariatric surgery, all patients require lifelong monitoring of weight, comorbidities, metabolic and nutritional status, and dietary and activity behaviours because they are at risk for developing malnutrition or weight gain. Women of childbearing age who have bariatric surgery are advised to use contraceptives for at least 18 months after surgery to avoid pregnancy until their weight stabilizes. After weight loss, the patient may elect additional surgical interventions for body contouring. These may include breast reductions, lipoplasty to remove fat deposits, or a panniculectomy or abdominoplasty to remove excess abdominal skin folds (Mechanick et al., 2013; OAC, 2015b; Wykowski & Krouse, 2013).

Evaluation

Expected patient outcomes may include the following:

1. Relief of pain
   a. Reports relief of pain
   b. Engages in early mobilization activities as prescribed
2. Maintenance of fluid balance
   a. Able to tolerate progressive fluid intake without complaints of nausea or gastric reflux
   b. Voids 0.5 mL/kg/hr
3. Maintenance of asepsis
   a. No evidence of infection (e.g., no fever, no leukocytosis, no complaints of abdominal pain)
4. Achievement of nutritional balance
   a. Able to consume small, frequent meals as prescribed
   b. Adheres to prescribed intake of vitamins and supplements
   c. Achieves and maintains weight reduction goals
5. Promotion of positive body image
   a. Verbalizes continued satisfaction with weight reduction plan and its effect on body image
6. Maintenance of usual bowel habits
   a. No evidence of diarrhea
   b. No evidence of constipation
7. Has no complications (e.g., no bleeding, VTE, bile reflux, dumping syndrome, dysphagia, or bowel or gastric outlet obstruction)

Critical Thinking Exercises

1 You work as a staff nurse in a women's health clinic. A 20-year-old woman presents to the clinic for her annual screening physical examination and is requesting a prescription refill for "birth control." You note that her height is 64 in and she weighs 163 lb. You note on her electronic health record that she weighed 152 lb last year. What is her BMI? She says to you "I would really like to lose some weight before I go on my vacation in 6 weeks. What diet do you think will help me to quickly lose the most weight?" Describe what other information you may gather from her that might help guide her to a healthier lifestyle. What is the strength of the evidence suggesting that any given commercial or other diet plan may offer her the healthiest weight loss outcomes?

2 A 51-year-old male patient is just over 24-hours postcoronary artery bypass graft surgery and is a patient on your progressive care unit. You note on his electronic health record that his BMI is 42 kg/m^2. His BP is 124/72 mm Hg, HR 112 bpm, RR 22 breaths/min, T 100.9°F and his SpO_2 is 90%. Describe your priority nursing assessments for this patient. What nursing interventions would you implement first?

3 Your friend's mother is 9 months post bariatric surgery. She tells you that she is doing well and has been successful in reaching her weight loss goal. She says she does not feel the need to follow up with her nutritional counsellor, primary provider, or support group, as she is "handling it on her own." What reasons would you give her for continuing with these follow-up appointments? On what evidence do you base your answer?

REFERENCES AND SUGGESTED READINGS

Books

Eliopoulos, C. (2018). *Gerontological nursing* (9th ed.). Philadelphia, PA: Lippincott Williams & Wilkins.

Fitch, A., Everling, L., Fox, C., et al. (2013). *Prevention and management of obesity for adults*. Bloomington, MN: Institute for Clinical Systems Improvement. Retrieved January 25, 2017, from www.icsi.org/_asset/s935hy/ObesityAdults.pdf

Goldstein, M., Aoun, A., Gaar, E., et al. (2014). *VA/DoD clinical practice guideline for screening and management of overweight and obesity*. Washington, DC: Department of Veterans Affairs. Retrieved January 25, 2017, from guideline.gov/summaries/summary/48461/vadod-clinical-practice-guideline-for-screening-and-management-of-overweight-and-obesity?q=obesity

Grossman, S. C., & Porth, C. M. (2014). *Porth's pathophysiology: Concepts of altered health states* (9th ed.). Philadelphia, PA: Lippincott Williams & Wilkins.

Hypertension Canada (2014). *Sodium key messages. Beyond the salt shaker key messages for health professionals*. Markham ON: Canadian Hypertension Education Program, Hypertension Canada. Retrieved from https://www.hypertension.ca/images/2014_EducationalResources/2014_SodiumKeyMessages_EN_HCP1012.pdf

Ogden, C. L., Carroll, M. D., Fryar, C. D., et al. (2015). *Prevalence of obesity among adults and youth: United States, 2011–2014*. NCHS data brief, no 219. Hyattsville, MD: National Center for Health Statistics.

Weber, J. R., & Kelley, J. H. (2014). *Health assessment in nursing* (5th ed.). Philadelphia, PA: Lippincott Williams & Wilkins.

Journals and Electronic Documents

AIHW. (2016). *Australia's health 2016: We're a mostly healthy bunch, but we have room to improve*. Retrieved March 26, 2019, from https://www.aihw.gov.au/news-media/news/2016/september/australia-s-health-2016-we-re-a-mostly-healthy-bun

Ali, M. R., Moustarah, F., Kim, J. J., et al. (2015). *ASMBS position statement on intragastric balloon therapy endorsed by SAGES*. Retrieved January 6, 2017, from asmbs.org/resources/position-statement-on-intragastric-balloon-therapy-endorsed-by-sages

American Medical Association (AMA) House of Delegates. (2013). Recognition of obesity as a disease. *Resolution: 420 (A-13)*; received 5/16/13. AMA: Author.

American Society for Metabolic and Bariatric Surgery (ASMBS). (2013a). Medical and bariatric surgery: Medical outcomes of bariatric surgery. Retrieved November 19, 2015, from asmbs.org/resources/metabolic-and-bariatric-surgery

American Society for Metabolic and Bariatric Surgery (ASMBS). (2013b). Obesity in America: Fact sheet. Retrieved January 22, 2017, from asmbs.org/wp/uploads/2014/06/Obesity-in-America-1.pdf

American Society for Metabolic and Bariatric Surgery (ASMBS). (2014). New procedure estimates for bariatric surgery: What the numbers reveal. Retrieved November 19, 2015, from connect.asmbs.org/may-2014-bariatric-surgery-growth.html

American Society for Metabolic and Bariatric Surgery (ASMBS). (2015a). Disease of obesity. Retrieved November 19, 2015, from asmbs.org/patients/disease-of-obesity (Accessed 11/19/15)

American Society for Metabolic and Bariatric Surgery (ASMBS). (2015b). The impact of obesity on your body and health. Retrieved November 19, 2015, from asmbs.org/patients/impact-of-obesity

Amianto, F., Ottone, L., Daga, G. A., et al. (2015). Binge-eating disorder diagnosis and treatment: A recap in front of DSM-5. *BAC Psychiatry*, *15*(17). 1—22.

Apovian, C. M., Aronne, L. J., Bessesen, D. H., et al. (2015). Pharmacological management of obesity: An Endocrine Society Clinical Practice Guideline. *Journal of Clinical Endocrinology and Metabolism*, *100*(2), 342–362.

Bays, H. E., Jones, P. H., Jacobson, T. A., et al. (2016). Lipids and bariatric procedures part 1 of 2: Scientific statement from the National Lipid Association, American Society for Metabolic and Bariatric Surgery, and Obesity Medicine Association: Executive summary. *Journal of Clinical Lipidology*, *10*(1), 15–32.

Bays, H. E., Kothari, S. N., Azagury, D. E., et al. (2016). Lipids and bariatric procedures part 2 of 2: Scientific statement from the National Lipid Association, American Society for Metabolic and Bariatric Surgery, and Obesity Medicine Association. *Surgery for Obesity and Related Diseases*, *12*(3), 468–495.

Bays, H. E., Seger, J. C., Primack, C., et al. (2016). Obesity algorithm presented by the Obesity Medicine Association. Retrieved January 7, 2017, from www.obesityalgorithm.org

Bendich, A. (2013). Prescription and over-the-counter options for weight loss. *Nutrition Today*, *48*(2), 76–78.

Berrios, L. A. (2016). The ABCDs of managing morbidly obese patients in intensive care units. *Critical Care Nurse*, *36*(5), 17–26.

Bray, G. A., Fruhbeck, G., Ryan, D. H., et al. (2016). Management of obesity. *The Lancet*, *387*(10031). 1947–1956.

Brethauer, S. A. (2013). ASMBS updated position statement on prophylactic measures to reduce the risk of venous thromboembolism in bariatric surgery patients. *Surgery for Obesity and Related Diseases*, *9*(4), 493–497.

Broome, C. A., Ayala, E. M., Georgeson, K. A., et al. (2015). Nursing care of the super bariatric patient: Challenges and lessons learned. *Rehabilitation Nursing*, *40*(2), 92–99.

Budd, G. M., & Peterson, J. A. (2014). The obesity epidemic, part 1: Understanding the origins. *American Journal of Nursing*, *114*(12), 40–46.

Budd, G. M., & Peterson, J. A. (2015). The obesity epidemic, part 2: Nursing assessment and intervention. *American Journal of Nursing*, *115*(1), 38–46.

Buxton, B. K., & Snethen, J. (2013). Obese women's perceptions and experiences of healthcare and primary care providers: A phenomenological study. *Nursing Research*, *62*(4), 252–259.

Caceres, B. A., Moskowitz, D., & O'Connell, T. (2015). A review of the safety and efficacy of bariatric surgery in adults over the age of 60: 2002–2013. *Journal of the American Association of Nurse Practitioners*, *27*(7), 403–410.

Centers for Disease Control and Prevention (CDC). (2016a). *Adult obesity causes & consequences*. Retrieved January 8, 2017, from www.cdc.gov/obesity/adult/causes.html

Centers for Disease Control and Prevention (CDC). (2016b). *Defining adult overweight and obesity*. Retrieved January 24, 2017, from www.cdc.gov/obesity/adult/defining.html

CDC (2018). Adult obesity facts. Retrieved November 2018 from https://www.cdc.gov/obesity/data/adult.html

Chang, V. C., Chaput, J. P., Roberts, K. C., et al. (2018). Original quantitative research—Factors associated with sleep duration across life stages: Results from the Canadian health measures survey. *Health Promotion and Chronic Disease Prevention in Canada: Research, Policy and Practice*, *38*(11), 404.

CIHI (2014). *Bariatric Surgery in Canada*. Retrieved from https://secure.cihi.ca/free_products/Bariatric_Surgery_in_Canada_EN.pdf

Cole, A. J., Beckman, L. M., & Earthman, C. P. (2014). Vitamin D status following bariatric surgery: Implications and recommendations. *Nutrition in Clinical Practice*, *29*(6), 751–758.

Colquitt, J. L., Pickett, K., Loveman, E., et al. (2014). Surgery for weight loss in adults. *Cochrane Database of Systematic Reviews*, *8*, CD003641.

Courcoulas, A. P., Belle, S. H., Neiberg, R. H., et al. (2015). Three-year outcomes of bariatric surgery vs lifestyle intervention for type 2 diabetes mellitus treatment: A randomized controlled trial. *JAMA Surgery*, *150*(10), 931–940.

Courcoulas, A. P., Christian, N. J., Belle, S. H., et al. (2013). Weight changes and health outcomes at three years after bariatric surgery among individuals with severe obesity. *JAMA, 310*(22), 2416–2425.

Dambaugh, L. A., & Ecklund, M. M. (2016). Progressive care of obese patients. *Critical Care Nurse, 36*(4), 58–63.

D'Arcy, Y. (2015). Managing pain in obese patients: Meeting weighty challenges. *Nursing, 45*(2), 42–49.

Davis, C. D. (2016). The gut microbiome and its role in obesity. *Nutrition Today, 51*(4), 167–174.

Dimick, J. B., Nicholas, L. H., Ryan, A. M., et al. (2013). Bariatric surgery complications before vs after implementation of a national policy restricting coverage to Centers of Excellence. *JAMA, 309*(8), 792–799.

Dunham, M. (2013). Caring for patients undergoing bariatric surgery. *American Journal of Nursing, 43*(10), 45–50.

Felix, H. C., Bradway, C., Chisholm, L., et al. (2015). Prevalence of moderate to severe obesity among U.S. nursing home residents, 2000–2010. *Research in Gerontological Nursing, 8*(4), 173–178.

Felix, H. C., Thostenson, J. D., Bursac, Z., et al. (2013). Effect of weight on indwelling catheter use among long-term care facility residents. *Urologic Nursing, 33*(4), 194–200.

Fruh, S. M., Mulekar, M. S., & Dierking, J. (2013). Guiding patients to safe weight loss. *The Nurse Practitioner, 38*(10), 1–7.

Gilmartin, J. (2013). Body image concerns amongst massive weight loss patients. *Journal of Clinical Nursing, 22*(9–10), 1299–1309.

Global Burden of Disease (GBD) Obesity Collaboration. (2017). Health effects of overweight and obesity in 195 countries over 25 years. *New England Journal of Medicine, 377*(1), 13–27.

Gloy, V. L., Briel, M., Bhatt, D. L., et al. (2013). Bariatric surgery versus non-surgical treatment for obesity: A systematic review and meta-analysis of randomized controlled trials. *British Medical Journal, 347*, 15934.

Hyun, S., Li, X., Vermillion, B., et al. (2014). Body mass index and pressure ulcers: Improved predictability of pressure ulcers in intensive care patients. *American Journal of Critical Care, 23*(6), 494–500.

Ikramuddin, S., Blackstone, R. P., Brancatisano, A., et al. (2014). Effect of reversible intermittent intra-abdominal vagal nerve blockade on morbid obesity: The ReCharge randomized clinical trial. *JAMA, 312*(9), 915–922.

International Association for the Study of Obesity (IASO). (2014). World map of obesity. Retrieved from http://www.worldobesity.org/aboutobesity/world-map-obesity/

Isom, K. A., Andromalos, L., Ariagno, M., et al. (2014). Nutrition and metabolic support recommendations for the bariatric patient. *Nutrition in Clinical Practice, 29*(6), 718–739.

Jääskeläinen, A., Schwab, U., Kolehmainen, M., et al. (2013). Associations of meal frequency and breakfast with obesity and metabolic syndrome traits in adolescents of Northern Finland Birth Cohort 1986. *Nutrition, Metabolism, and Cardiovascular Diseases, 23*(10), 1002–1009.

Jacobsen, H. J., Nergard, B. J., Leifsson, B. G., et al. (2014). Management of suspected anastomotic leak after bariatric laparoscopic Roux-en-Y gastric bypass. *British Journal of Surgery, 101*(4), 417–423.

Joen, B. Y. (2013). The effects of obesity on fall efficacy in elderly people. *Journal of Physical Therapy Science, 25*(11), 1485–1489.

Kapur, V. K., Wilsdon, A. G., Au, D., et al. (2013). Obesity is associated with lower resting oxygen saturation in the ambulatory elderly: Results from the cardiovascular health study. *Respiratory Care, 58*(5), 831–837.

Katz, D. L., & Meller, S. (2014). Can we say what diet is best for health? *Annual Reviews of Public Health, 35*, 83–103.

Katzmarzyk, P. T., Reeder, B. A., Elliot, S., et al. (2014). Body mass index and risk of cardiovascular disease, cancer and all-cause mortality. *Canadian Journal of Public Health, 103*(2). 147–151.

Kolata, G. (2016). *One weight loss approach fits all? No, not even close.* New York Times, Health Section, published on 12/12/2016. Retrieved January 22, 2017, from www.nytimes.com/2016/12/12/health/weight-loss-obesity.html

Kusher, R. F. (2018). Weight loss strategies for treatment of obesity: Lifestyle management and pharmacotherapy. *Progress in Cardiovascular Disease, 61*, 246–252.

Kyle, T., & Kuehl, B. (2017). *Prescription medications & weight gain—What you need to know.* Retrieved January 7, 2017, from www.obesityaction.org/educational-resources/resource-articles-2/general-articles/prescription-medications-weight-gain

Levi, J., Segal, L. M., St. Laurent, R., et al. (2014). *The state of obesity: 2014 – Better policies for a healthier America.* Robert Wood Johnson Foundation. Retrieved January 6, 2017, from healthyamericans.org/assets/files/TFAH-2014-ObesityReport%20FINAL.pdf

Loos, R. J. (2012). Genetic determinants of common obesity and their value in prediction. *Best Practice & Research. Clinical Endocrinology & Metabolism, 26*(2), 211–226.

Mechanick, J. I., Youdim, A., Jones, D. B., et al. (2013). Clinical practice guidelines for the perioperative nutritional, metabolic, and nonsurgical support of the bariatric surgery patient—2013 update: Cosponsored by the American Association of Clinical Endocrinologists, the Obesity Society, and American Society for Metabolic & Bariatric Surgery. *Surgery for Obesity and Related Diseases, 9*(2), 159–191.

Michalsky, M., Reichard, K., Inge, T., et al. (2012). ASMBS pediatric committee best practice guidelines. *Surgery for Obesity and Related Diseases, 8*(1), 1–7.

Moyer, V. A., LeFevre, M. L., Siu, A. L., et al. (2012). Screening for and management of obesity in adults: U.S. Preventive Services Task Force recommendation statement. *Annals of Internal Medicine, 157*(5), 373–378.

Mozaffarian, D., Benjamin, E. J., Go, A. S., et al. (2016). Heart disease and stroke statistics—2016 update: A report from the American Heart Association. *Circulation, 133*(4), e38–3360.

Murphy, R. A., Reinders, I., Register, T. C., et al. (2014). Associations of BMI and adipose tissue area and density with incident mobility limitation and poor performance in older adults. *American Journal of Clinical Nutrition, 99*(5), 1059–1065.

National Heart, Lung, and Blood Institute (NHLBI) of the National Institutes of Health. (2016a). *Aim for a healthy weight: Body mass index table.* Retrieved March 2, 2017, from www.nhlbi.nih.gov/health/educational/lose_wt/BMI/bmi_tbl.pdf

National Heart, Lung, and Blood Institute (NHLBI) of the National Institutes of Health. (2016b). *Serving sizes and portions.* Retrieved January 22, 2017, from www.nhlbi.nih.gov/health/educational/wecan/eat-right/distortion.htm

National Institute of Diabetes and Digestive and Kidney Diseases (NIDDK). (2016). *Prescription medications to treat overweight and obesity.* Retrieved January 7, 2017, from www.niddk.nih.gov/health-information/health-topics/weight-control/prescription-medications-treat-overweight-obesity/Pages/facts.aspx.

Obesity Action Coalition (OAC). (2015a). *OAC insurance guide.* Retrieved November 19, 2015, from www.obesityaction.org/educational-resources/brochures-and-guides/oac-insurance-guide/reviewing-your-insurance-policy-or-employer-sponsored-medical-benefits-plan

Obesity Action Coalition (OAC). (2015b). *Obesity treatments: Bariatric surgery (severe obesity).* Retrieved November 19, 2015, from www.obesityaction.org/obesity-treatments/bariatric-surgery

Ogden, C. L., Carroll, M. D., Kit, B. K., et al. (2014). Prevalence of childhood and adult obesity in the United States, 2011–2012. *JAMA, 311*(8), 806–814.

Orringer, K. A., Harrison, A. V., Nichani, S. S., et al. (2016). *University of Michigan Health System Clinical Alignment and Performance Excellence Guideline: Obesity prevention and management.* Retrieved January 25, 2017, from www.med.umich.edu/1info/FHP/practiceguides/obesity/obesity.pdf

Papasavas, P., El Chaar, M., Kothari, S. N., et al. (2016). American Society for Metabolic and Bariatric Surgery position statement on vagal blocking therapy for obesity. *Surgery for Obesity and Related Diseases, 12*(3), 460–461.

Patil, R., & Melander, S. (2015). Postoperative complications and emergency care for patients following bariatric surgery. *MEDSURG Nursing, 24*(4), 243–248.

Pfeil, M. (2014). Patients' perception of the nursing contribution to gastric band surgery. *British Journal of Nursing, 23*(2), 95–99.

Puhl, R. M., Phelan, S. M., Nadglowski, J., et al. (2016). Overcoming weight bias in the management of patients with diabetes and obesity. *Clinical Diabetes Journals, 34*(1), 44–50.

Radosevich, J. J., Patanwala, A. E., & Erstad, B. L. (2016). Norepinephrine dosing in obese and nonobese patients with septic shock. *American Journal of Critical Care, 25*(1), 27–32.

Rao, D., Kropac, E., Do, M. T., et al. (2016). Childhood overweight and obesity trends in Canada. *Health Promotion and Chronic Disease Prevention in Canada, 36*(9), 194–198.

Rimm, A. A., Verner, L. H., Yserloo, B. V., et al. (1975). Relationship of obesity and disease in 73,532 weight-conscious women. *Public Health Reports, 90*, 44–54.

Schauer, G. L., Woodruff, R. C., Hotz, J., et al. (2014). A qualitative inquiry about weight counseling practices in community health centers. *Patient Education and Counseling, 97*(1), 82–87.

Segal, L. M., Rayburn, J., & Martin, A. (2016). *The state of obesity: 2016—Better policies for a healthier America.* Robert Wood Johnson

Foundation. Retrieved January 21, 2017, from stateofobesity.org/files/stateofobesity2016.pdf

Shikora, S. A., Wolfe, B. M., Apovian, D. M., et al. (2015). Sustained weight loss with vagal nerve blockade but not with sham: 18-month results of the ReCharge trial. *Journal of Obesity*, *2015*, 365604.

Sifrim, D. (2013). Management of bile reflux. *Gastroenterology and Hepatology*, *9*(3), 179–180.

Sturman-Floyd, M. (2013). Moving and handling: Supporting bariatric residents. *Nursing and Residential Care*, *15*(6), 432–437.

Tran, B. X., Nair, A. V., Kuhle, S., et al. (2013). Cost analysis of obesity in Canada: scope, quality and implications. *Cost Effectiveness and Resourse Allocation*, *11*(1), 3. doi: 10.1186/1478-7547-11-3.

Wharton, S. (2016). Current perspectives on long-term obesity pharmotherapy. *Canadian Journal of Diabetes*, *40*, 184–191.

World Health Organization. (2014). Obesity. Retrieved from http://www.who.int/topics/obesity/en/

World Health Organization (WHO). (2015). 10 facts on obesity. Retrieved November 19, 2015 from www.who.int/features/factfiles/obesity/facts/en/index1.html

World Health Organization (WHO). (2016). Obesity and overweight: Fact sheet. Retrieved January 21, 2017, from www.who.int/mediacentre/factsheets/fs311/en/

World Health Organization (WHO) (2019). Obesity facts. Retrieved March 26, 2019, from www.who.int/features/factfiles/obesity/facts

Wykowski, K., & Krouse, H. J. (2013). Self-care predictors for success post-bariatric surgery. *Gastroenterology Nursing*, *36*(2), 129–135.

Yanovski, S. Z., & Yanovski, J. A. (2014). Long-term drug treatment for obesity: A systematic and clinical review. *JAMA*, *311*(1), 74–86.

Resources

American Society for Metabolic and Bariatric Surgery (ASMBS): www.asmbs.org

Centers for Disease Control and Prevention (CDC): www.cdc.gov/obesity/

DASH Diet for Healthy Eating: dashdiet.org

National Heart, Lung, and Blood Institute of the National Institutes of Health, Aim for a Healthy Weight: www.nhlbi.nih.gov/health/educational/lose_wt/index.htm

National Institute of Diabetes and Digestive and Kidney Diseases, Weight Management: www.niddk.nih.gov/health-information/weight-management

Obesity Action Coalition: www.obesityaction.org

Obesity Medicine Association: www.obesitymedicine.org

Obesity Society: www.obesity.org

Robert Wood Johnson Foundation the State of Obesity: Better Policies for a Healthier America: stateofobesity.org

Rudd Center for Food Policy and Obesity: www.uconnruddcenter.org

Therapeutic Lifestyle Changes (TLC) Diet: TLCdiet.org

US Preventive Services Task Force. https://www.uspreventiveservicestaskforce.org/Page/Document/RecommendationStatementFinal/obesity-in-adults-interventions1

43 Assessment and Management of Patients With Endocrine Disorders

Adapted by Joanne Bouma

Learning Objectives

On completion of this chapter, the learner will be able to:

1. Describe the functions of each of the endocrine glands and their hormones.
2. Identify the diagnostic tests used to determine alterations in function of each of the endocrine glands.
3. Compare hypothyroidism and hyperthyroidism: their causes, clinical manifestations, management, and nursing interventions.
4. Develop a plan of nursing care for the patient undergoing thyroidectomy.
5. Compare hyperparathyroidism and hypoparathyroidism: their causes, clinical manifestations, management, and nursing interventions.
6. Compare Addison disease with Cushing syndrome: their causes, clinical manifestations, management, and nursing interventions.
7. Describe nursing management of patients with adrenal insufficiency.
8. Use the nursing process as a framework for care of patients with Cushing syndrome.
9. Identify the teaching needs of patients requiring corticosteroid therapy.

The **endocrine** system plays a vital role in orchestrating cellular interactions, metabolism, growth, reproduction, aging, and response to adverse conditions (Porth, 2015). This interconnected network of glands is closely linked with the nervous and immune systems, regulating the functions of multiple body organs. Disorders of the endocrine system are common and are manifested as hyperfunction and hypofunction.

Nursing interventions are essential in the management of patients with endocrine disorders. This chapter focuses on the anatomy and physiology of the endocrine system; the most common endocrine disorders of the pituitary, thyroid, parathyroid, and adrenal glands; clinical manifestations; diagnostic studies; medical management; and nursing interventions. The unique endocrine and **exocrine** functions of the pancreas, pancreatic function, and associated pancreatic disorders are discussed in Chapters 41 and 42, and reproductive structures, including the ovaries and testes, are discussed in Chapters 47 and 50.

ASSESSMENT OF THE ENDOCRINE SYSTEM

Anatomic and Physiologic Overview

The endocrine system involves the release of chemical substances known as **hormones** to regulate and integrate body functions by acting on local or distant target sites. Generally, these hormones are produced by the endocrine glands, but some are also produced by other tissues. The gastrointestinal (GI) mucosa produces hormones (e.g., gastrin, enterogastrone, secretin, cholecystokinin) that are important in the digestive process; the kidneys produce erythropoietin, a hormone that stimulates the bone marrow to produce red blood cells; and the white blood cells produce cytokines (hormone like proteins) that actively participate in inflammatory and immune responses.

The endocrine system has a unique relationship with the immune and the nervous systems. Chemicals such as neurotransmitters (e.g., epinephrine) released by the nervous

Glossary

acromegaly: disease process resulting from excessive secretion of somatotropin; causes progressive enlargement of peripheral body parts

addisonian crisis: acute adrenocortical insufficiency; characterized by hypotension, cyanosis, fever, nausea/vomiting, and classic signs of shock; precipitated by stress or abrupt withdrawal of therapeutic glucocorticoids

Addison disease: chronic adrenocortical insufficiency secondary to destruction of the adrenal glands

adrenalectomy: surgical removal of one or both adrenal glands

adrenocorticotropic hormone (ACTH): hormone secreted by the anterior pituitary, essential for growth and development

adrenogenital syndrome: masculinization in women, feminization in men, or premature sexual development in children; result of abnormal secretion of adrenocortical hormones, especially androgens

androgens: hormones secreted by the adrenal cortex; stimulate activity of accessory male sex organs and development of male sex characteristics

basal metabolic rate: chemical reactions occurring when the body is at rest

calcitonin: hormone secreted by the parafollicular cells of the thyroid gland; participates in calcium regulation

Chvostek sign: spasm of the facial muscles produced by sharply tapping over the facial nerve in front of the parotid gland and anterior to the ear; suggestive of latent tetany in patients with hypocalcemia

corticosteroids: hormones produced by the adrenal cortex or their synthetic equivalents; also referred to as adrenal-cortical hormone and adrenocorticosteroid; consist of glucocorticoids, mineralocorticoids, and androgens

cretinism: stunted body growth and mental development appearing during the first year of life as a result of congenital hypothyroidism

Cushing syndrome: group of symptoms produced by an excess of free circulating cortisol from the adrenal cortex; characterized by truncal obesity, "moon face," acne, abdominal striae, and hypertension

diabetes insipidus: condition in which abnormally large volumes of dilute urine are excreted as a result of deficient production of vasopressin

dwarfism: generalized limited growth resulting from insufficient secretion of growth hormone during childhood

endocrine: secreting internally; hormonal secretion of a ductless gland

euthyroid: state of normal thyroid hormone production

exocrine: secreting externally; hormonal secretion from excretory ducts

exophthalmos: abnormal protrusion of one or both eyeballs

glucocorticoids: steroid hormones secreted by the adrenal cortex in response to ACTH; produce a rise of liver glycogen and blood glucose

goitre: enlargement of the thyroid gland; usually caused by an iodine-deficient diet

Graves' disease: a form of hyperthyroidism; characterized by a diffuse goitre and exophthalmos

hormones: chemical transmitter substances produced in one organ or part of the body and carried by the bloodstream to other cells or organs on which they have a specific regulatory effect; produced mainly by endocrine glands

hypophysectomy: removal or destruction of all or part of the pituitary gland

mineralocorticoid: steroid of the adrenal cortex

myxedema: severe hypothyroidism; can be with or without coma

negative feedback: regulating mechanism in which an increase or decrease in the level of a substance decreases or increases the function of the organ producing the substance

oxytocin: hormone secreted by the posterior pituitary; causes myometrial contraction at term and milk release during lactation

pheochromocytoma: chromaffin cell tumour, usually benign, located in the adrenal medulla; characterized by secretion of catecholamines resulting in hypertension, severe headache, profuse sweating, visual blurring, anxiety, and nausea

syndrome of inappropriate antidiuretic hormone (SIADH) secretion: excessive secretion of antidiuretic hormone (ADH) from the pituitary gland despite low serum osmolality level

thyroidectomy: surgical removal of all or part of the thyroid gland

thyroiditis: inflammation of the thyroid gland; may lead to chronic hypothyroidism or may resolve spontaneously

thyroid-stimulating hormone: released from the pituitary gland; causes stimulation of the thyroid, resulting in release of T3 and T4

thyroid storm: severe life-threatening hyperthyroidism precipitated by stress; characterized by high fever, extreme tachycardia, and altered mental state

thyrotoxicosis: condition produced by excessive endogenous or exogenous thyroid hormone

thyroxine (T_4): thyroid hormone; active iodine compound formed and stored in the thyroid; deiodinated in peripheral tissues to form triiodothyronine; maintains body metabolism in a steady state

triiodothyronine (T_3): thyroid hormone; formed and stored in the thyroid; released in smaller quantities, biologically more active and with faster onset of action than T_4; widespread effect on cellular metabolism

Trousseau's sign: carpopedal spasm induced when blood flow to the arm is occluded using a blood pressure cuff or tourniquet, causing ischemia to the distal nerves; suggestive sign for latent tetany in hypocalcemia

vasopressin: ADH secreted by the posterior pituitary; causes contraction of smooth muscle, particularly blood vessels

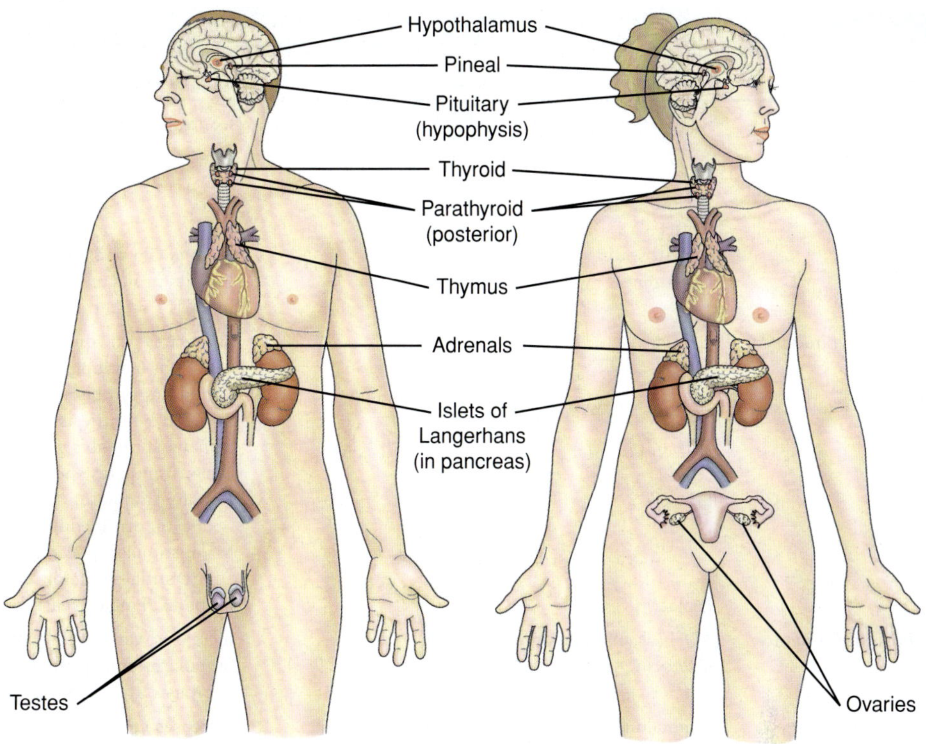

FIGURE 43-1. Major hormone-secreting glands of the endocrine system.

system can also function as hormones when needed. The immune system responds to the introduction of foreign agents by means of chemical messengers (cytokines), and is also subject to regulation by adrenal corticosteroid hormones (Porth, 2015).

Glands of the Endocrine System

The endocrine system is composed of several glands: the pituitary, the thyroid gland, parathyroid glands, adrenal glands, pancreatic islets, ovaries, and testes (Fig. 43-1). Most hormones secreted from endocrine glands are released directly into the bloodstream. Exocrine glands, such as sweat glands, secrete their products through ducts onto epithelial surfaces or into the GI tract.

Function and Regulation of Hormones

Hormones help regulate organ function in concert with the nervous system. This dual regulatory system, in which rapid action by the nervous system is balanced by slower hormonal action, permits precise control of organ functions in response to varied changes within and outside the body. Table 43-1 lists the major hormones, their target tissues, and some of their properties.

The endocrine glands are composed of secretory cells arranged in minute clusters known as acini. No ducts are present, but the glands have a rich blood supply, so the hormones they produce enter the bloodstream rapidly. In the healthy physiologic state, hormone concentration in the bloodstream is maintained at a relatively constant level. **Negative feedback** is the mechanism for regulating hormone concentration in the bloodstream. When the hormone concentration increases, further production of that hormone is inhibited. Conversely, when the hormone concentration decreases, the rate of production of that hormone increases.

Hormones are either water soluble or lipid soluble. They are generally transported in body fluids and the amount of specific hormones circulating at any given time depends on the body's needs. Some hormones may affect different tissues in different ways or at times several may be necessary for the regulation of a certain body function.

Classification and Action of Hormones

Hormones are classified into four categories according to their structure: (1) amines and amino acids (e.g., epinephrine, norepinephrine, and thyroid hormones); (2) peptides, polypeptides, proteins, and glycoproteins (e.g., thyrotropin-releasing hormone [TRH], follicle-stimulating hormone [FSH], and growth hormone [GH]); (3) steroids (e.g., **corticosteroids**, which are hormones produced by the adrenal cortex or their synthetic equivalents); and (4) fatty acid derivatives (e.g., eicosanoid, retinoids) (Porth, 2015). Although most hormones released by endocrine glands can be transported to distant target sites for action, some hormones never enter the bloodstream. Some hormones act locally in the area where they are released; this is called **paracrine action** (e.g., the effect of sex hormones on the ovaries). Others may act on the actual cells from which they were released; this is called **autocrine action** (e.g., the effect of insulin from pancreatic beta cells on those cells) (Lazar & Birnbaum, 2016).

Hormones can alter the function of the target tissue by interacting with chemical receptors located either on the cell membrane or in the interior of the cell. For example, *peptide and protein hormones* interact with receptor sites on the cell surface, resulting in stimulation of the intracellular enzyme adenyl cyclase. This causes increased production

TABLE 43-1 Major Action and Source of Selected Hormones

Source	Hormone	Major Action
Hypothalamus	Releasing and inhibiting hormones	Controls the release of pituitary hormones
	CRH	
	TRH	
	GHRH	
	GnRH	
	Somatostatin	Inhibits GH and TSH
	Dopamine	Inhibits prolactin release from the pituitary
		Inhibits FSH and LH
Anterior pituitary	GH	Stimulates growth of bone and muscle, promotes protein synthesis and fat metabolism, decreases carbohydrate metabolism
	ACTH	Stimulates synthesis and secretion of adrenal cortical hormones
	TSH	Stimulates synthesis and secretion of thyroid hormone
	FSH	Female: stimulates growth of ovarian follicle, ovulation
		Male: stimulates sperm production
	LH	Female: stimulates development of corpus luteum, release of oocyte, production of estrogen and progesterone
		Male: stimulates secretion of testosterone, development of interstitial tissue of testes
	Prolactin	Prepares female breast for breast-feeding
Posterior pituitary	ADH (arginine vasopressin [AVP])	Increases water reabsorption by kidney
	Oxytocin	Stimulates contraction of pregnant uterus, milk ejection from breasts after childbirth
Adrenal cortex	Mineralocorticosteroids, mainly aldosterone	Increases sodium absorption, potassium loss by kidney
	Glucocorticoids, mainly cortisol	Affects metabolism of all nutrients; regulates blood glucose levels, affects growth, has anti-inflammatory action, and decreases effects of stress
	Adrenal androgens, mainly dehydroepiandrosterone (DHEA) and androstenedione	Have minimal intrinsic androgenic activity; they are converted to testosterone and dihydrotestosterone (DHT) in the periphery
Adrenal medulla	Epinephrine	Serve as neurotransmitters for the sympathetic nervous system
	Norepinephrine	
Thyroid (follicular cells)	Thyroid hormones: triiodothyronine (T_3), thyroxine (T_4)	Increase the metabolic rate; increase protein and bone turnover; increase responsiveness to catecholamines; necessary for fetal and infant growth and development
	Calcitonin	Lowers blood calcium and phosphate levels
Parathyroid glands	Parathyroid hormone (PTH)	Regulates serum calcium
Pancreatic islet cells	Insulin	Lowers blood glucose by facilitating glucose transport across cell membranes of muscle, liver, and adipose tissue
	Glucagon	Increases blood glucose concentration by stimulation of glycogenolysis and glyconeogenesis
	Somatostatin	Delays intestinal absorption of glucose
Kidney	1,25-Dihydroxyvitamin D	Stimulates calcium absorption from the intestine
Ovaries	Estrogen	Affects development of female sex organs and secondary sex characteristics
	Progesterone	Influences menstrual cycle; stimulates growth of uterine wall; maintains pregnancy
Testes	Androgens, mainly testosterone	Affect development of male sex organs and secondary sex characteristics; aid in sperm production

CRH, corticotropin-releasing hormone; TRH, thyrotropin-releasing hormone; GHRH, growth hormone–releasing hormone; GnRH, gonadotropin-releasing hormone; GH, growth hormone; ACTH, adrenocorticotropic hormone; TSH, thyroid-stimulating hormone; FSH, follicle-stimulating hormone; LH, luteinizing hormone; ADH, antidiuretic hormone.

Reprinted with permission from Grossman, S. C., & Porth, C. M. (2014). *Pathophysiology: Concepts of altered health states* (9th ed.). Philadelphia, PA: Lippincott Williams & Wilkins.

of cyclic 3′,5′-adenosine monophosphate (AMP). The cyclic AMP inside the cell alters enzyme activity. Thus, cyclic AMP is the "second messenger" that links the peptide hormone at the cell surface to a change in the intracellular environment. Some protein and peptide hormones also act by changing membrane permeability and act within seconds or minutes. The mechanism of action for *amine hormones* is similar to that for peptide hormones (Porth, 2015).

Steroid hormones, because of their smaller size and **higher lipid solubility**, penetrate cell membranes and interact with intracellular receptors. The steroid–receptor complex modifies cell metabolism and the formation of messenger ribonucleic acid (mRNA) from deoxyribonucleic acid (DNA).

The mRNA then stimulates protein synthesis within the cell. Steroid hormones require several hours to exert their effects, because they exert their action by the modification of protein synthesis.

Assessment

Health History

Although specific endocrine disorders are often accompanied by specific clinical symptoms, more general manifestations may also occur. Some common signs and symptoms of endocrine imbalances include changes in energy level, tolerance to heat or cold, weight, fat and fluid distribution, secondary sexual characteristics, sexual dysfunction, memory, concentration, sleep patterns, and mood. The health history should include information regarding (1) the severity of these changes, (2) the length of time the patient has experienced these changes, (3) the way in which these changes have affected the patient's ability to carry out activities of daily living, and (4) the effect of the changes on the patient's self-perception. Specific symptoms of various endocrine disorders are discussed with each disorder. Possible genetics-related issues may also be important (Chart 43-1).

Physical Assessment

The physical examination should include vital signs; head-to-toe inspection; and palpation of skin, hair, and thyroid. Current findings should be compared with previous findings, if available. Physical, psychological, and behavioural changes should be noted. Examples of changes in physical characteristics on examination may include appearance of facial hair in women, "moon face," "buffalo hump," **exophthalmos** (abnormal protrusion of one or both eyeballs), vision changes, edema, thinning of the skin, obesity of the trunk, thinness of the extremities, increased size of the feet and hands, edema, and hypo- or hyperreflexia. The patient may also exhibit changes in mood and behaviour such as nervousness, lethargy, and fatigue (Weber & Kelley, 2014).

Diagnostic Evaluation

Blood Tests

Blood tests determine the levels of circulating hormones, the presence of autoantibodies, and the effect of a specific hormone on other substances (e.g., the effect of insulin on blood glucose levels). The serum levels of a specific hormone may provide information to determine the presence of hypofunction or hyperfunction of the endocrine system and the site of dysfunction. Radioimmunoassays are radioisotope-labelled antigen tests that are commonly indicated blood tests used to measure the levels of hormones or other substances (Sluss & Hayes, 2016).

Urine Tests

Urine tests are used to measure the amount of hormones or the end products of hormones excreted by the kidneys. One-time specimens or, in some disorders, 24-hour urine specimens are collected to measure hormones or their metabolites. For example, urinary levels of free catecholamines (norepinephrine, epinephrine, and dopamine) may be measured in patients with suspected tumours of

GENETICS IN NURSING PRACTICE

Chart 43-1. Metabolic and Endocrine Disorders

Metabolic and endocrine disorders that are influenced by genetic factors are complex and typically impact multiple body systems. Some examples of genetic metabolic and endocrine disorders include:

- Diabetes
- Disorders in amino acids (e.g., phenylketonuria, homocystinuria, maple syrup urine disease)
- Disorders of carbohydrate metabolism (e.g., galactosemia)
- Disorders of fatty acid oxidation (e.g., medium-chain acyl-CoA dehydrogenase deficiency)
- Disorders of glycogen storage (e.g., Pompe's disease, Von Gierke's disease, Danon's disease, Cori's disease, Anderson's disease, McArdle's disease)
- Disorders of lysosomal storage disease (e.g., Tay–Sachs, Gaucher's, Niemann-Pick's, Fabry's diseases)
- Disorders of mucopolysaccharides (e.g., Hurler's syndrome, Hunter's disease, Morquio's syndrome)
- Disorders in urea cycle (e.g., ornithine transcarbamylase deficiency)
- Hemochromatosis
- McCune–Albright syndrome
- Multiple endocrine neoplasia type I and type II

Nursing Assessments

FAMILY HISTORY ASSESSMENT

- Assess family history for relatives with early-onset hepatic, pancreatic, or endocrine disease.
- Inquire about family members with diabetes and their ages at onset.
- Assess family history of other related genetic conditions such as cystic fibrosis, alpha-1 antitrypsin deficiency, and hereditary hemochromatosis.

PATIENT ASSESSMENT

- Assess for physical symptoms such as mucosal neuromas, hypertrophied lips, skeletal abnormalities, and marfanoid appearance.
- Assess for signs of arthritis and bronze pigmentation of the skin (hemochromatosis).
- Assess for history of seizures, sweet smell to urine, jaundice, lethargy, vomiting, dehydration, acidosis, neutropenia, hepatomegaly, high ammonia levels

Genetics Resources

Society for Inherited Metabolic Disorders: www.simd.org
Association for Glycogen Storage Disease: www.agsdus.org
See Chapter 11 for components of genetic counselling.

the adrenal medulla (**pheochromocytoma**). Several disadvantages related to urine tests that must be considered are that patients may be unable to urinate at scheduled intervals and that some medications or disease states may affect the test results (Porth, 2015).

Additional Diagnostic Studies

Stimulation tests are used to confirm hypofunction of an endocrine organ. The tests determine how an endocrine gland responds to the administration of stimulating hormones that are normally produced or released by the hypothalamus or pituitary gland. If the endocrine gland responds to this stimulation, the specific disorder may be in the hypothalamus or pituitary. Failure of the endocrine gland to respond to this stimulation helps identify the problem as being in the endocrine gland itself.

Suppression tests are used to detect hyperfunction of an endocrine organ. They determine if the organ is not responding to the negative feedback mechanisms that normally control secretion of hormones from the hypothalamus or pituitary gland. Suppression tests measure the effect of a given exogenous dose of the hormone on the endogenous secretion of the hormone or on the secretion of stimulation hormones from the hypothalamus or pituitary gland.

Imaging studies include radioactive scanning, magnetic resonance imaging (MRI), computed tomography (CT), ultrasonography, positron emission tomography (PET), and dual-energy x-ray absorptiometry (DEXA) (Porth, 2015).

Genetic screening is increasingly becoming more routine in the assessment of endocrine disorders (see Chart 43-1). DNA testing can be used for the identification of specific genes associated with endocrine disorders, selective targeting for drug development, and increased understanding of the function of the endocrine system. Genetic screening is used to determine the presence of a gene mutation that may predispose an individual to a certain condition. The implications of genetic screening must be considered carefully by the primary provider and patient (Majithia, Altshuler, & Hirschhorn, 2016; Rosenthal, 2014).

THE PITUITARY GLAND

Anatomic and Physiologic Overview

The pituitary gland, or hypophysis, is commonly referred to as the master gland because of the influence it has on secretion of hormones by other endocrine glands (Porth, 2015) (Fig. 43-2). The round structure, about 1.27 cm in diameter, is located on the inferior aspect of the brain and is divided into anterior and posterior lobes. It is controlled by the hypothalamus, which is an adjacent area of the brain that is connected to the pituitary by the pituitary stalk.

Anterior Pituitary

The major hormones of the anterior pituitary gland are FSH, luteinizing hormone (LH), prolactin (PRL), **adrenocorticotropic hormone** (ACTH), **thyroid-stimulating hormone (TSH)**, and GH (also referred to as somatotropin). The secretion of these major hormones is controlled by releasing factors secreted by the hypothalamus. These releasing factors reach the anterior pituitary by way of the bloodstream in a special circulation called the *pituitary portal blood system*. Other hormones include melanocyte-stimulating hormone and beta-lipotropin; the function of lipotropin is poorly understood.

The hormones released by the anterior pituitary enter the general circulation and are transported to their target organs. The main function of TSH, ACTH, FSH, and LH is the release of hormones from other endocrine glands. PRL acts on the breast to stimulate milk production. Hormones that stimulate other organs and tissues are discussed in conjunction with their target organs.

GH, the most abundant anterior pituitary hormone, regulates growth in children and energy and metabolism in adults. GH increases protein synthesis in many tissues, increases the breakdown of fatty acids in adipose tissue, and increases blood glucose levels. Other hormones, such as thyroid hormone and insulin, are required for the GH system to function as well. Secretion of GH is increased by deep sleep, stress, exercise, fasting, malnutrition, hypoglycemia, trauma, hypovolemic shock, and sepsis, and is decreased in the presence of obesity, depression, and hypothyroidism (Kaiser & Ho, 2016).

Posterior Pituitary

The important hormones secreted by the posterior lobe of the pituitary gland are **vasopressin**, also called antidiuretic hormone (ADH), and **oxytocin**. These hormones are synthesized in the hypothalamus and travel from the hypothalamus to the posterior pituitary gland for storage. Vasopressin controls the excretion of water by the kidney; its secretion is stimulated by an increase in the osmolality of the blood or by a decrease in blood pressure. Oxytocin secretion is stimulated during pregnancy and at childbirth. It facilitates milk ejection during lactation and increases the force of uterine contractions during labour and delivery.

Pathophysiology

Abnormalities of pituitary function are caused by oversecretion or undersecretion of any of the hormones produced or released by the gland. Abnormalities of the anterior and posterior portions of the gland may occur independently. Hypofunction of the pituitary gland (hypopituitarism) can result from disease of the pituitary gland itself or disease of the hypothalamus; the result is essentially the same. Hypopituitarism can result from radiation therapy to the head and neck area. The total destruction of the pituitary gland by trauma, tumour, or vascular lesion removes all stimuli that are normally received by the thyroid, the gonads, and the adrenal glands. The result is extreme weight loss, emaciation, atrophy of all endocrine glands and organs, hair loss, impotence, amenorrhea, hypometabolism, and hypoglycemia. Coma and death occur if the missing hormones are not replaced.

Anterior Pituitary

Oversecretion (hypersecretion) of the anterior pituitary gland most commonly involves ACTH or GH and results in **Cushing syndrome** (group of symptoms produced by an

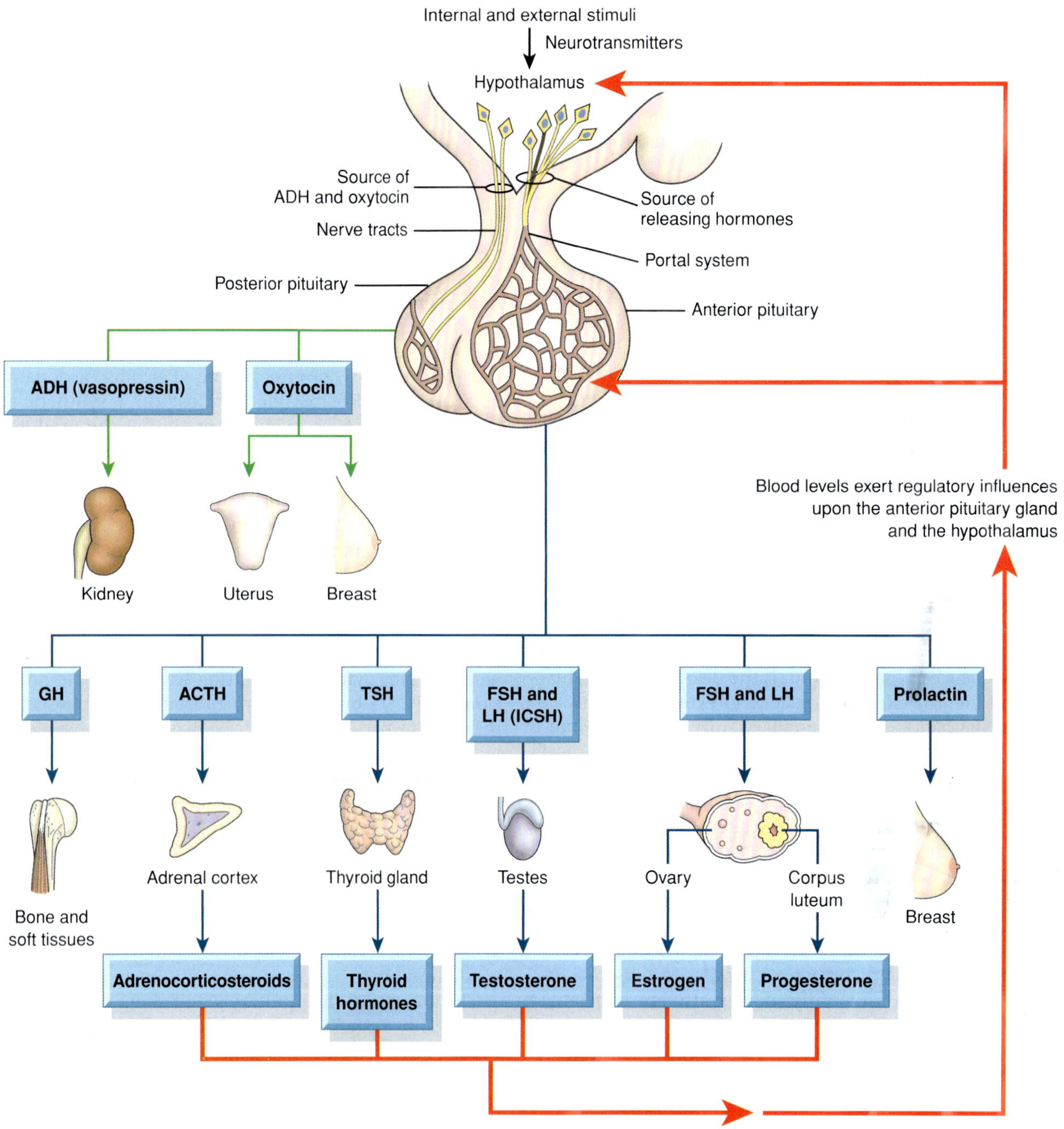

FIGURE 43-2. The pituitary gland, the relationship of the brain to pituitary action, and the hormones secreted by the anterior and posterior pituitary lobes. ACTH, adrenocorticotropic hormone; ADH, antidiuretic hormone; FSH, follicle-stimulating hormone; GH, growth hormone; ICSH, interstitial cell-stimulating hormone; LH, luteinizing hormone; TSH, thyroid-stimulating hormone.

oversecretion of ACTH) or **acromegaly**, respectively. Acromegaly, a disorder caused by an excess of GH in adults, results in enlargement of peripheral body parts and soft tissue, after the fusion of the epiphyseal plates has occurred, without an increase in height (Woodworth, Lakhani, Aleryani, et al., 2014). It occurs in approximately four cases per 1 million people per year (Katznelson, Laws, Melmed, et al., 2014). Although rare, oversecretion of GH in children before the fusion of epiphyseal growth plates result in pituitary gigantism; a person may grow to be 7 or even 8 ft tall. Conversely, insufficient secretion of GH during childhood can result in generalized limited growth and pituitary **dwarfism** (Eugster, 2017). Undersecretion (hyposecretion) commonly involves all of the anterior pituitary hormones and is termed *panhypopituitarism*. In this condition, the thyroid gland, the adrenal cortex, and the gonads atrophy (shrink) because of loss of the tropic-stimulating hormones. Hypopituitarism may result from destruction of the anterior lobe of the pituitary gland.

Posterior Pituitary

The most common disorder related to posterior lobe dysfunction is **diabetes insipidus** (DI), a condition in which

abnormally large volumes of dilute urine are excreted as a result of deficient production of vasopressin. DI may occur following surgical treatment of a brain tumour, secondary to nonsurgical brain tumours, traumatic brain injury, infections of the nervous system, post **hypophysectomy**, failure of renal tubules to respond to ADH, and the use of specific medications (Kaiser & Ho, 2016).

Pituitary Tumours

Almost all pituitary tumours are benign. The tumours may be primary or secondary and functional or nonfunctional (Porth, 2015). Functional tumours secrete pituitary hormones, whereas nonfunctional tumours do not. The location and effects of these tumours on hormone production by target organs can have life-threatening effects. Three principal types of pituitary tumours represent an overgrowth of (1) eosinophilic cells, (2) basophilic cells, or (3) chromophobic cells (i.e., cells with no affinity for either eosinophilic or basophilic stains).

Clinical Manifestations

Eosinophilic tumours that develop early in life result in gigantism. The affected person may be more than 2.1 m tall and large in all proportions, yet so weak and lethargic that he or she can hardly stand. If the disorder begins during adult life, the excessive skeletal growth occurs only in the feet, the hands, the superciliary ridge, the molar eminences, the nose, and the chin, giving rise to the clinical picture called **acromegaly**. However, enlargement involves all tissues and organs of the body (Porth, 2015). Many of these patients suffer from severe headaches and visual disturbances because the tumours exert pressure on the optic nerves (Porth, 2015). Assessment of central vision and visual fields may reveal loss of colour discrimination, diplopia (double vision), or blindness in a portion of a field of vision. Decalcification of the skeleton, muscular weakness, and endocrine disturbances, similar to those occurring in patients with hyperthyroidism, also are associated with this type of tumour.

Basophilic tumours give rise to Cushing syndrome with features largely attributable to hyperadrenalism, including masculinization and amenorrhea in females, truncal obesity, hypertension, osteoporosis, and polycythemia.

Chromophobic tumours represent 90% of pituitary tumours. These tumours usually produce no hormones but destroy the rest of the pituitary gland, causing hypopituitarism. People with this disease are often obese and somnolent and exhibit fine, scanty hair; dry, soft skin; a pasty complexion; and small bones. They also experience headaches, loss of libido, and visual defects progressing to blindness. Other signs and symptoms include polyuria, polyphagia, a lowering of the **basal metabolic rate** (chemical reactions occurring when the body is at rest), and a subnormal body temperature.

Assessment and Diagnostic Findings

Diagnostic evaluation requires a careful history and physical examination, including assessment of visual acuity and visual fields. CT and MRI scans are used to diagnose the presence and extent of pituitary tumours. Serum levels of pituitary hormones may be obtained along with measurements of hormones of target organs (e.g., thyroid, adrenal) to assist in diagnosis.

Medical Management

Surgical removal of the pituitary gland (hypophysectomy) through a transsphenoidal approach is the usual treatment. Stereotactic radiation therapy, which requires the use of a neurosurgery-type stereotactic frame, may be used to deliver external-beam radiation therapy precisely to the pituitary tumour with minimal effect on normal tissue (see Chapter 17). Other treatments include conventional radiation therapy, bromocriptine (Parlodel, a dopamine antagonist), and octreotide (Sandostatin, a synthetic analogue of GH). These medications inhibit the production or release of GH and may bring about marked improvement of symptoms (Mercado, 2016). Octreotide and lanreotide (Somatuline Depot, a somatostatin analogue) may also be used preoperatively to improve the patient's clinical condition and to shrink the tumour (Comerford, 2015).

Surgical Management

Hypophysectomy is the treatment of choice in patients with Cushing syndrome resulting from excessive production of ACTH by a pituitary tumour. Hypophysectomy may also be performed on occasion as a palliative measure to relieve bone pain secondary to metastasis of malignant lesions of the breast and prostate.

Several approaches are used to remove or destroy the pituitary gland, including surgical removal by transfrontal, subcranial, or oronasal–transsphenoidal approaches; irradiation; and cryosurgery. (The transsphenoidal approach and the nursing management of a patient undergoing cranial surgery are discussed in Chapter 63.) Features or symptoms of acromegaly are unaffected by surgical removal of the tumour.

The absence of the pituitary gland alters the function of many body systems. Menstruation ceases and infertility occurs after total or near-total ablation of the pituitary gland. Replacement therapy with corticosteroids and thyroid hormone is necessary; therefore, patient teaching is imperative (see later discussion).

Diabetes Insipidus

DI is the most common disorder of the posterior lobe of the pituitary gland and is characterized by a deficiency of ADH (vasopressin). Excessive thirst (polydipsia) and large volumes of dilute urine are manifestations of the disorder. It may occur secondary to head trauma, brain tumour, or surgical ablation or irradiation of the pituitary gland (Kaiser & Ho, 2016). It may also occur with infections of the central nervous system (meningitis, encephalitis, tuberculosis) or with tumours (e.g., metastatic disease, lymphoma of the breast or lung). Another cause of DI is failure of the renal tubules to respond to ADH; this nephrogenic form may be related to hypokalemia, hypercalcemia, and a variety of medications (e.g., lithium, demeclocycline [Declomycin]).

NURSING ALERT

It is important to distinguish between DI, a disorder of insufficient output of pituitary ADH, and diabetes, a metabolic disorder characterized by hyperglycemia caused by deficient insulin secretion or action (or both).

Clinical Manifestations

Without the action of ADH on the distal nephron of the kidney, an enormous daily output (greater than 250 mL per hour) of very dilute urine with a specific gravity of 1.001 to 1.005 occurs (John & Day, 2012). The urine contains no abnormal substances such as glucose or albumin. Because of the intense thirst, the patient tends to drink 2 to 20 L of fluid daily and craves cold water. In adults, the onset of DI may be insidious or abrupt.

The disease cannot be controlled by limiting fluid intake, because the high-volume loss of urine continues even without fluid replacement. Attempts to restrict fluids cause the patient to experience an insatiable craving for fluid and to develop hypernatremia and severe dehydration.

Assessment and Diagnostic Findings

The fluid deprivation test is carried out by withholding fluids for 8 to 12 hours or until 3% to 5% of the body weight is lost. The patient is weighed frequently during the test. Plasma and urine osmolality studies are performed at the beginning and end of the test. The inability to increase the specific gravity and osmolality of the urine is characteristic of DI. The patient continues to excrete large volumes of urine with low specific gravity and experiences weight loss, increasing serum osmolality, and elevated serum sodium levels. The patient's condition needs to be monitored frequently during the test, and the test is terminated if tachycardia, excessive weight loss, or hypotension develops.

Other diagnostic procedures include concurrent measurements of plasma levels of ADH and plasma and urine osmolality as well as a trial of desmopressin (synthetic vasopressin) therapy and intravenous (IV) infusion of hypertonic saline solution. If the diagnosis is confirmed and the cause (e.g., head injury) is not obvious, the patient is carefully assessed for tumours that may be causing the disorder.

Medical Management

The objectives of therapy are (1) to replace ADH (which is usually a long-term therapeutic program), (2) to ensure adequate fluid replacement, and (3) to identify and correct the underlying intracranial pathology. Nephrogenic causes require different management approaches (John & Day, 2012).

Pharmacologic Therapy

Desmopressin (DDAVP), a synthetic vasopressin without the vascular effects of natural ADH, is particularly valuable because it has a longer duration of action and fewer adverse effects than other preparations previously used to treat the disease. It is given intranasally; the patient sprays the solution into the nose through a flexible calibrated plastic tube. One or two administrations daily (i.e., every 12 to 24 hours) usually control the symptoms (McPhee, Rabow, & Papadakis, 2016). Vasopressin causes vasoconstriction; thus, it must be used cautiously in patients with coronary artery disease.

Chlorpropamide (Diabinese) and thiazide diuretics are also used in mild forms of the disease because they potentiate the action of vasopressin (Comerford, 2015). Hyperglycemia is possible.

If the DI is renal in origin, the previously described treatments are ineffective. Thiazide diuretics, mild salt depletion, and prostaglandin inhibitors (ibuprofen [Advil, Motrin], indomethacin [Indocin], and aspirin) are used to treat the nephrogenic form of DI.

Nursing Management

Physical assessment and patient education are the pillars of skilled nursing management of the patient with a diagnosis of DI. The nurse is responsible to educate the patient, family, and other caregivers about the medication, follow-up care, prevention of complications, and emergency measures. It is also necessary to provide information regarding the signs and symptoms of hyponatremia. The nurse should demonstrate and observe a return demonstration of medication administration. The patient should be advised to wear a medical identification bracelet and carry required medication and information about DI at all times.

Syndrome of Inappropriate Antidiuretic Hormone Secretion

The **syndrome of inappropriate antidiuretic hormone (SIADH) secretion** includes excessive ADH secretion from the pituitary gland even in the face of subnormal serum osmolality. Patients with SIADH cannot excrete a dilute urine, retain fluids, and develop a sodium deficiency known as dilutional hyponatremia. SIADH is often of nonendocrine origin; for instance, the syndrome may occur in patients with bronchogenic carcinoma in which malignant lung cells synthesize and release ADH. SIADH has also occurred in patients with severe pneumonia, pneumothorax, and other disorders of the lungs, as well as malignant tumours that affect other organs (Kaiser & Ho, 2016; Porth, 2015).

Disorders of the central nervous system, such as head injury, brain surgery or tumour, and infection, are thought to produce SIADH by direct stimulation of the pituitary gland (Kaiser & Ho, 2016). Some medications (e.g., vincristine [Oncovin], phenothiazines, tricyclic antidepressants, thiazide diuretics) and nicotine have been implicated in SIADH; they either directly stimulate the pituitary gland or increase the sensitivity of renal tubules to circulating ADH.

Interventions include eliminating the underlying cause, if possible, and restricting fluid intake (John & Day, 2012). Because retained water is excreted slowly through the kidneys, the extracellular fluid volume contracts and the serum sodium concentration gradually increases toward normal. Diuretic agents such as furosemide (Lasix) may be used along with fluid restriction if severe hyponatremia is present.

Nursing Management

Close monitoring of fluid intake and output, daily weight, urine and blood chemistries, and neurologic status is indicated for the patient at risk for SIADH. Supportive measures and explanations of procedures and treatments assist the patient in managing this disorder.

THE THYROID GLAND

The thyroid gland is a butterfly-shaped organ located in the lower neck, anterior to the trachea (Fig. 43-3). It consists of two lateral lobes connected by an isthmus. The gland is about 5 cm long and 3 cm wide and weighs about 30 g. The blood flow to the thyroid is very high (about 5 mL/min per gram of thyroid tissue), approximately five times the blood flow to the liver. This reflects the high metabolic activity of the thyroid gland. The thyroid gland produces three hormones: **thyroxine (T_4)**, **triiodothyronine (T_3)**, and **calcitonin**.

Anatomic and Physiologic Overview

Various hormones and chemicals are responsible for thyroid function. Key among them are thyroid hormone, calcitonin, and iodine.

Thyroid Hormone

Thyroid hormone is composed of T_4 and T_3, two separate hormones produced by the thyroid gland. Both are amino acids that contain iodine molecules bound to the amino acid structure; T_4 contains four iodine atoms in each molecule, and T_3 contains three. These hormones are synthesized and stored bound to proteins in the cells of the thyroid gland until needed for release into the bloodstream. Three thyroid-binding hormones—thyroxine-binding globulin (TBG), transthyretin (formerly known as thyroid-binding prealbumin), and albumin—bind and transport T_3 and T_4 (Porth, 2015).

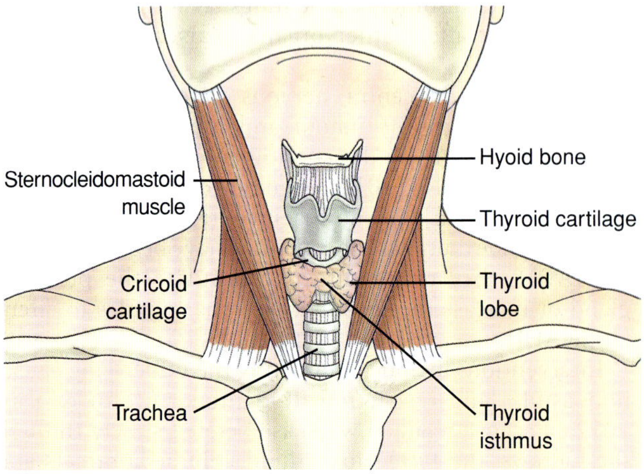

FIGURE 43-3. The thyroid gland and surrounding structures.

Synthesis of Thyroid Hormone

Iodine is essential to the thyroid gland for synthesis of its hormones. The major use of iodine in the body is by the thyroid, and the major derangement in iodine deficiency is alteration of thyroid function. Iodide is ingested in the diet and absorbed into the blood in the GI tract. The thyroid gland is extremely efficient at taking up iodide from the blood and concentrating it within the cells, where iodide ions are converted to iodine molecules, which react with tyrosine (an amino acid) to form the thyroid hormones (Salvatore, Davies, Sclumberger, et al., 2016).

Regulation of Thyroid Hormone

The secretion of T_3 and T_4 by the thyroid gland is controlled by TSH (also called thyrotropin) from the anterior pituitary gland. TSH controls the rate of thyroid hormone release through a negative feedback mechanism. In turn, the level of thyroid hormone in the blood determines the release of TSH. If the thyroid hormone concentration in the blood decreases, the release of TSH increases, which causes increased output of T_3 and T_4. The term **euthyroid** refers to thyroid hormone production that is within usual limits.

Thyrotropin-releasing hormone (TRH), secreted by the hypothalamus, exerts a modulating influence on the release of TSH from the pituitary. Environmental factors, such as a decrease in temperature, may lead to increased secretion of TRH, resulting in elevated secretion of thyroid hormones. Figure 43-4 shows the hypothalamic–pituitary–thyroid axis, which regulates thyroid hormone production.

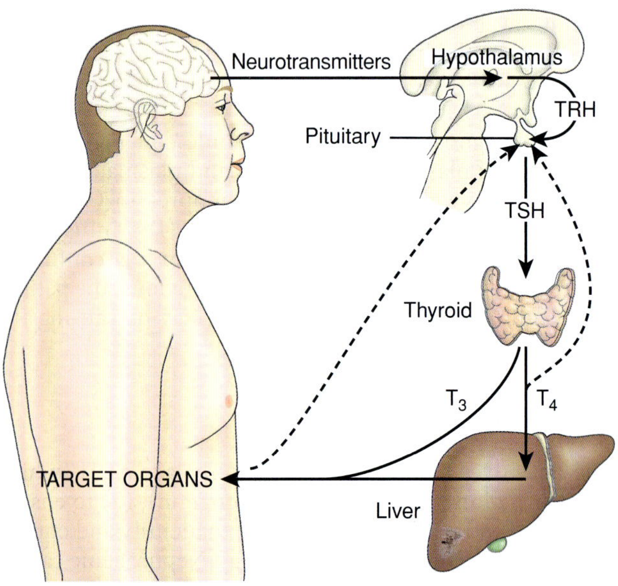

FIGURE 43-4. The hypothalamic–pituitary–thyroid axis. Thyroid-releasing hormone (TRH) from the hypothalamus stimulates the pituitary gland to secrete thyroid-stimulating hormone (TSH). TSH stimulates the thyroid to produce thyroid hormone (triiodothyronine [T_3] and thyroxine [T_4]). High circulating levels of T_3 and T_4 inhibit further TSH secretion and thyroid hormone production through a negative feedback mechanism (*dashed lines*).

Function of Thyroid Hormone

The main function of thyroid hormone is to control cellular metabolic activity. T_4, a relatively weak hormone, maintains body metabolism in a steady state. T_3 is about five times as potent as T_4 and has a more rapid metabolic action. These hormones accelerate metabolic processes by increasing the level of specific enzymes that contribute to oxygen consumption and altering the responsiveness of tissues to other hormones. The thyroid hormones influence cell replication and are important in brain development. Thyroid hormone is also necessary for normal growth. Thyroid hormones affect virtually every major organ system and tissue function, including the basal metabolic rate, tissue thermogenesis, serum cholesterol levels, and vascular resistance (Porth, 2015).

Calcitonin

Calcitonin, or thyrocalcitonin, is another important hormone secreted by the thyroid gland. It is secreted in response to high plasma levels of calcium, and it reduces the plasma level of calcium by increasing its deposition in bone.

Pathophysiology

Inadequate secretion of thyroid hormone during fetal and neonatal development results in intellectual disability and stunted physical growth (**congenital hypothyroidism**) because of general depression of metabolic activity (LaFranchi, 2016). In adults, hypothyroidism manifests as lethargy, slow mentation, weight gain, constipation, cold intolerance, and generalized slowing of body functions (Surks, 2016a).

Oversecretion of thyroid hormones (hyperthyroidism) is manifested by a greatly increased metabolic rate. Many of the other characteristics of hyperthyroidism result from the increased response to circulating catecholamines (epinephrine and norepinephrine). Oversecretion of thyroid hormones is usually associated with an enlarged thyroid gland known as a **goitre**. Goitre also commonly occurs with iodine deficiency. In this latter condition, lack of iodine results in low levels of circulating thyroid hormones, which causes increased release of TSH; the elevated TSH causes overproduction of thyroglobulin (a precursor of T_3 and T_4) and hypertrophy of the thyroid gland.

Assessment

Physical Examination

The thyroid gland is inspected and palpated routinely in all patients. Inspection begins with identification of landmarks. The lower neck region between the sternocleidomastoid muscles is inspected for swelling or asymmetry. The patient is instructed to extend the neck slightly and swallow. Thyroid tissue rises normally with swallowing. The thyroid is then palpated for size, shape, consistency, symmetry, and the presence of tenderness (Weber & Kelley, 2014).

The thyroid may be examined from an anterior or a posterior position. In the posterior position, both hands encircle the patient's neck. The thumbs rest on the nape of the neck, while the index and middle fingers palpate for the thyroid isthmus and the anterior surfaces of the lateral lobes. When palpable, the isthmus is perceived as firm and of a rubber-band consistency.

The left lobe is examined by positioning the patient so that the neck flexes slightly forward and to the left. The thyroid cartilage is then displaced to the left with the fingers of the right hand. This manoeuvre displaces the left lobe deep into the sternocleidomastoid muscle, where it can be more easily palpated. The left lobe is then palpated by placing the left thumb deep into the posterior area of the sternocleidomastoid muscle, while the index and middle fingers exert opposite pressure in the anterior portion of the muscle. Having the patient swallow during the manoeuvre may assist the examiner to locate the thyroid as it ascends in the neck. The procedure is reversed to examine the right lobe. The isthmus is the only portion of the thyroid that is normally palpable. If a patient has a very thin neck, two thin, smooth, nontender lobes may also be palpable.

If palpation discloses an enlarged thyroid gland, both lobes are auscultated using the diaphragm of the stethoscope. Auscultation identifies the localized audible vibration of a bruit. This is indicative of increased blood flow through the thyroid gland associated with hyperthyroidism and necessitates referral to a primary provider. Other abnormal findings that require referral for further evaluation may include a soft texture (**Graves' disease**), firmness (Hashimoto's thyroiditis or malignancy), and tenderness (**thyroiditis**) (see Table 43-2) (Weber & Kelley, 2014).

Diagnostic Evaluation

Assessment measures in addition to palpation and auscultation include thyroid function tests, such as laboratory measurement of thyroid hormones, thyroid scanning, biopsy, and ultrasonography. Thyroid-stimulating hormone (TSH) is the most sensitive and specific test for the investigation and management of primary thyroid dysfunction (Canadian Medical Association; Toward Optimized Practice [TOP] Endocrine Working Group, 2014 April). Free T_4 levels correlate with metabolic status; they are elevated in hyperthyroidism and decreased in hypothyroidism. Ultrasound, CT, and MRI may be used to clarify or confirm the results of other diagnostic studies.

Thyroid Tests

Serum Thyroid-Stimulating Hormone

Measurement of the serum TSH concentration is the single best screening test of thyroid function in outpatients because of its high sensitivity. The ability to detect minute changes in serum TSH makes it possible to distinguish subclinical thyroid disease from euthyroid states in patients with low or high normal values. Measurement of TSH is also used for monitoring thyroid hormone replacement therapy and for differentiating between disorders of the thyroid gland itself and disorders of the pituitary or hypothalamus. Current recommendations for testing are adults and children with suspected or primary thyroid dysfunction and women who used thyroid replacement therapy prior to pregnancy due to the increased demand for thyroxine during pregnancy. Achieving euthyroidism

TABLE 43-2 Summary of Findings on Physical Examination of the Thyroid Gland

Physical Finding	Differential Diagnosis	Special Features
Single nodule	Autonomously functioning adenoma	Opposite lobe not palpable
	Adenoma or adenomatous nodule	Rubbery, firm; tenderness suggests recent hemorrhage or infarction
	Cancer	Usually hard; may have associated lymph node enlargement or vocal cord palsy
	Hyperplasia secondary to unilobar agenesis	Opposite lobe not palpable
Multiple nodules	Multinodular goitre Hashimoto's thyroiditis	Firm lobes or irregular surface may be misinterpreted as multiple nodules
Diffuse goitre	Graves' disease	Bruit or thrill; pyramidal lobe
	Hashimoto's thyroiditis	Irregular surface; pyramidal lobe; rubbery or firm; occasionally tender; fibrous variant may be hard
	Thyroid lymphoma	Rapidly growing goitre particularly in setting of pre-existing Hashimoto's thyroiditis
	Multinodular goitre	Nodules may be hidden within gland and may become apparent with thyroid hormone suppression
Tenderness	Subacute thyroiditis	Unilateral or bilateral; tenderness often severe
	Hemorrhagic or infarcted adenoma	Discrete nodule with tenderness
	Hashimoto's thyroiditis	Mild tenderness
	Cancer	Irregular, firm thyroid nodule with chronic tenderness

prior to pregnancy is ideal. Exclusion recommendations include neonatal and asymptomatic, nonpregnant, seemingly healthy individuals having a periodic exam (Canadian Medical Association; TOP Endocrine Working Group, 2014 April).

Serum Free T_4

Serum free T_4 is a direct measurement of free (unbound) thyroxine, the only metabolically active fraction of T_4. The range of free T_4 in serum is normally 0.9 to 1.7 ng/dL (11.5 to 21.8 pmol/L). When measured by the dialysis method, free T_4 is not affected by variations in protein binding and is the procedure of choice for monitoring the changes in T_4 secretion during treatment for hyperthyroidism.

Serum T_3 and T_4

Measurement of total T_3 or T_4 includes protein-bound and free hormone levels that occur in response to TSH secretion. T_4 is 70% bound to TBG; T_3 is bound less firmly. Only 0.03% of T_4 and 0.3% of T_3 are unbound. Serious systemic illnesses, medications (e.g., oral contraceptives, corticosteroids, carbamazepine [Tegretol], salicylates), and protein wasting as a result of nephrosis or the use of **androgens** may interfere with accurate test results (Fischbach & Dunning, 2015). Normal range for T_4 is 5.4 to 11.5 µg/dL (57 to 148 nmol/L) (Fischbach & Dunning, 2015). Although serum T_3 and T_4 levels generally increase or decrease together, the T_3 level appears to be a more accurate indicator of hyperthyroidism or severity of the disorder, as T_4 levels are often within normal range. The normal range for serum T_3 is 80 to 200 ng/dL (1.2 to 3.1 nmol/L) (Fischbach & Dunning, 2015).

T_3 Resin Uptake Test

The T_3 resin uptake test is an indirect measure of unsaturated TBG. Its purpose is to determine the amount of thyroid hormone bound to TBG and the number of available binding sites. This provides an index of the amount of thyroid hormone already present in the circulation. Normally, TBG is not fully saturated with thyroid hormone, and additional binding sites are available to combine with radioiodine-labelled T_3 added to the blood specimen. The normal T_3 uptake value is 25% to 35% (relative uptake fraction, 0.25 to 0.35), which indicates that about one third of the available sites of TBG are occupied by thyroid hormone (Fischbach & Dunning, 2015). If the number of free or unoccupied binding sites is low, as in hyperthyroidism, the T_3 uptake is greater than 35% (0.35). If the number of available sites is high, as occurs in hypothyroidism, the test result is less than 25% (0.25).

T_3 uptake is useful in evaluating thyroid hormone levels in patients who have received diagnostic or therapeutic doses of iodine. The test results may be altered by the use of estrogens, androgens, salicylates, phenytoin, anticoagulants, or corticosteroids.

Thyroid Antibodies

Autoimmune thyroid diseases include both hypothyroid and hyperthyroid conditions. Results of testing by immunoassay techniques for antithyroid antibodies are positive in chronic autoimmune thyroid disease (90%), Hashimoto's thyroiditis (100%), Graves' disease (80%), and other organ-specific autoimmune diseases, such as systemic lupus erythematosus (SLE) and rheumatoid arthritis. Antithyroid antibody titres are normally present in 5% to 10% of the population and increase with age.

Radioactive Iodine Uptake

The radioactive iodine uptake test measures the rate of iodine uptake by the thyroid gland. The patient is administered a tracer dose of iodine 123 (^{123}I) or another radionuclide, and a count is made over the thyroid gland with a scintillation counter, which detects and counts the gamma rays released from the breakdown of ^{123}I in the thyroid. It measures the proportion of the administered dose that is present in the thyroid gland at a specific time after its administration. It is a simple test and provides reliable results. It is affected by the patient's intake of iodide or thyroid hormone; therefore, a careful preliminary clinical history is essential in evaluating results. Normal values vary from one geographic region to another and with the intake of iodine. Patients with hyperthyroidism exhibit a high uptake of the ^{123}I (in some patients, as high as 90%), whereas patients with hypothyroidism exhibit a very low uptake.

Fine-Needle Aspiration Biopsy

Use of a small-gauge needle to sample the thyroid tissue for biopsy is a safe and accurate method of detecting malignancy. It is often the initial test for evaluation of thyroid masses. Results are reported as (1) negative (benign), (2) positive (malignant), (3) indeterminate (suspicious), and (4) inadequate (nondiagnostic) (Dhyani, Faquin, Lubitz, et al., 2013).

Thyroid Scan, Radioscan, or Scintiscan

In a thyroid scan, a scintillation detector or gamma camera moves back and forth across the area to be studied in a series of parallel tracks, and a visual image is made of the distribution of radioactivity in the area being scanned. The most commonly used isotopes of iodine are ^{123}I and iodine 131 (^{131}I) (Fischbach & Dunning, 2015).

Scans are helpful in determining the location, size, shape, and anatomic function of the thyroid gland, particularly when thyroid tissue is substernal or large (Fischbach & Dunning, 2015). Identifying areas of increased function ("hot" areas) or decreased function ("cold" areas) can assist in diagnosis. Although most areas of decreased function do not represent malignancies, lack of function increases the likelihood of malignancy, particularly if only one nonfunctioning area is present. Scanning of the entire body, to obtain the total body profile, may be carried out in a search for a functioning thyroid metastasis (i.e., a lesion that produces thyroid hormones).

Serum Thyroglobulin

Thyroglobulin (Tg) can be measured reliably in the serum by radioimmunoassay. Clinically, it is used to detect persistence or recurrence of thyroid carcinoma.

Nursing Implications

When thyroid tests are scheduled, it is necessary to determine if the patient is allergic to iodine (shellfish) and whether the patient has taken medications or agents that contain iodine, because these may alter the test results (Fischbach & Dunning, 2015). Obvious sources of iodine-containing medications include contrast agents and those used to treat thyroid disorders such as radioactive iodine. Less obvious sources of iodine are topical antiseptics; multivitamin preparations; food supplements that may contain kelp and seaweed (frequently found in health food stores); and amiodarone (Cordarone), an antiarrhythmic agent (Surks, 2016b). Other medications that may affect test results are estrogens, salicylates, amphetamines, chemotherapeutic agents, antibiotics, corticosteroids, and diuretics. This information should be documented in the patient's medical record and the laboratory requisition. Chart 43-2 gives a list of selected medications that may interfere with accurate testing of thyroid gland function.

Hypothyroidism

Hypothyroidism results from suboptimal levels of thyroid hormone. Thyroid deficiency can affect all body functions and can range from mild, subclinical forms to **myxedema** (severe deficiency discussed later), an advanced life-threatening form (Ross, 2016a). The most common cause of hypothyroidism in adults is autoimmune thyroiditis (Hashimoto's disease), in which the immune system attacks the thyroid gland. Symptoms of hyperthyroidism may later be followed by those of hypothyroidism and myxedema. Hypothyroidism also commonly occurs in patients with previous hyperthyroidism that has been treated with radioiodine or antithyroid medications or **thyroidectomy** (surgical removal of all or part of the thyroid gland). In addition, there is an increased incidence of thyroid cancer in men who have undergone radiation therapy for head and neck cancer. Therefore, testing of thyroid function is recommended for all patients who receive such treatment. Other causes of hypothyroidism are presented in Chart 43-3.

More than 95% of patients with hypothyroidism have primary or thyroidal hypothyroidism, which refers to dysfunction of the thyroid gland itself. If the cause of the thyroid dysfunction is failure of the pituitary gland, the hypothalamus, or both, the hypothyroidism is known as central hypothyroidism. If the cause is entirely a pituitary

CHART 43-2

Pharmacology: Selected Medications That May Alter Thyroid Test Results

amiodarone (Cordarone)
aspirin
cimetidine (Tagamet)
diazepam (Valium)
furosemide (Lasix)
heparin
lithium (Lithotabs)
phenytoin (Dilantin) and other anticonvulsants
propranolol (Inderal)

Adapted from Fischbach, F., & Dunning, M. B. (2015). *A manual of laboratory and diagnostic tests* (9th ed.). Philadelphia, PA: Lippincott Williams & Wilkins.

CHART 43-3

Causes of Hypothyroidism

- Autoimmune disease (Hashimoto's thyroiditis, post-Graves' disease)
- Atrophy of thyroid gland with aging
- Therapy for hyperthyroidism
  - Radioactive iodine (^{131}I)
  - Thyroidectomy
- Medications
  - Lithium
  - Iodine compounds
  - Antithyroid medications
- Radiation to head and neck for treatment of head and neck cancers, lymphoma
- Infiltrative diseases of the thyroid (amyloidosis, scleroderma, lymphoma)
- Iodine deficiency and iodine excess

disorder, it may be referred to as pituitary or secondary hypothyroidism. If the cause is a disorder of the hypothalamus resulting in inadequate secretion of TSH due to decreased stimulation of TRH, it is referred to as hypothalamic or tertiary hypothyroidism. If thyroid deficiency is present at birth, it is referred to as neonatal hypothyroidism. In such instances, the mother may also have thyroid deficiency. The term *myxedema* refers to the accumulation of mucopolysaccharides in subcutaneous and other interstitial tissues. Although myxedema occurs in long-standing hypothyroidism, the term is used appropriately only to describe the extreme symptoms of severe hypothyroidism (Ross, 2016a).

Clinical Manifestations

Extreme fatigue makes it difficult for the person to complete a full day's work or participate in usual activities. Reports of hair loss, brittle nails, and dry skin are common, and numbness and tingling of the fingers may occur. On occasion, the voice may become husky, and the patient may complain of hoarseness. Hypothyroidism affects women five to eight times more frequently than men and occurs most often between 40 and 70 years of age (Visser, Visser, & Peeters, 2013). Menstrual disturbances such as menorrhagia or amenorrhea occur, in addition to loss of libido. The prevalence of the disease increases with increasing age; however, experts question if the standard reference range for serum TSH levels (0.4 to 4.5 mU/L) should be used for diagnosis in the older adult. Women and older adults may exhibit different symptoms (Dunn & Turner, 2016; Harman, 2016; Visser et al., 2013).

Severe hypothyroidism results in a subnormal body temperature and pulse rate. The patient usually begins to gain weight even without an increase in food intake, although he or she may be cachectic. The skin becomes thickened because of an accumulation of mucopolysaccharides in the subcutaneous tissues. The hair thins and falls out, and the face becomes expressionless and masklike. The patient often complains of being cold even in a warm environment.

At first, the patient may be irritable and may complain of fatigue, but as the condition progresses, the emotional responses are subdued. The mental processes become dulled, and the patient appears apathetic. Speech is slow, the tongue enlarges, the hands and feet increase in size, and deafness may occur. The patient frequently reports constipation.

Advanced hypothyroidism may produce personality and cognitive changes characteristic of dementia. Inadequate ventilation and sleep apnea can occur with severe hypothyroidism (Morgan & Tsai, 2015). Pleural effusion, pericardial effusion, and respiratory muscle weakness may also occur.

Severe hypothyroidism is associated with an elevated serum cholesterol level, atherosclerosis, coronary artery disease, and poor left ventricular function. The patient with advanced hypothyroidism is hypothermic and abnormally sensitive to sedative, opioid, and anesthetic agents, which must be given with extreme caution.

Patients with unrecognized hypothyroidism who are undergoing surgery are at increased risk for intraoperative hypotension, postoperative heart failure, and altered mental status.

Myxedema coma is a rare life-threatening condition. It is the decompensated state of severe hypothyroidism in which the patient is hypothermic and unconscious (Ross, 2016a). This condition may develop with undiagnosed hypothyroidism and may be precipitated by infection or other systemic disease or by use of sedatives or opioid analgesic agents. Patients may also experience myxedema coma if they forget to take their thyroid replacement medication. The condition occurs most often among older women in the winter months and appears to be precipitated by cold. However, the disorder can affect any age group.

In myxedema coma, the patient may initially show signs of depression, diminished cognitive status, lethargy, and somnolence (Ross, 2016a). Increasing lethargy may progress to stupor. The patient's respiratory drive is depressed, resulting in alveolar hypoventilation, progressive carbon dioxide retention, narcosis, and coma. In addition, patients with myxedema coma can also exhibit hyponatremia, hypoglycemia, hypoventilation, hypotension, bradycardia, and hypothermia. These symptoms, along with cardiovascular collapse and shock, require aggressive and intensive supportive and hemodynamic therapy if the patient is to survive. Although there has been a decline in mortality rates over the past two decades due to early intervention and improved therapies, the mortality rate remains high at 30% to 40%. Patients at greatest risk are older adults, individuals with cardiac complications, reduced consciousness, persistent hypothermia, and sepsis (Ross, 2016a).

Medical Management

The objectives in the management of hypothyroidism are to restore a normal metabolic state by replacing the missing hormone, as well as prevention of disease progression and complications.

Pharmacologic Therapy

Synthetic levothyroxine (Synthroid or Levothroid) is commonly prescribed for treating hypothyroidism and suppressing nontoxic goitres (Jonklaas, Bianco, Bauer, et al., 2014). The dosage is based on the patient's serum TSH concentration. If replacement therapy is adequate, the symptoms of myxedema disappear and normal metabolic activity is resumed. Although rare, if the disease progresses to myxedema coma, IV administration of T_4 and T_3 are recommended rather than T_4 alone. T_4 is administered IV until the patient is able to safely take T_4 in oral form. T_3 is administered IV until the patient is stable (Ross, 2016a).

Administration of high-dose **glucocorticoids** (hydrocortisone) every 8 to 12 hours for 24 hours followed by low-dose therapy is recommended until coexisting adrenal insufficiency is ruled out (Ross, 2016a). Serum levels of T_4, TSH, and cortisol should be obtained before and after administration of ACTH and before administration of glucocorticoid and thyroid hormone therapies. Associated conditions such as infection, GI bleeding, hyponatremia, hypotension, bradycardia, hypoglycemia, and hypothermia will also require appropriate pharmacologic management (Ross, 2016a).

Prevention of Cardiac Dysfunction

Any patient who has had hypothyroidism for a long period is almost certain to have elevated serum cholesterol, atherosclerosis, and coronary artery disease. As long as metabolism is subnormal and the tissues, including the myocardium, require relatively little oxygen, a reduction in blood supply is tolerated without overt symptoms of coronary artery disease. When thyroid hormone is administered, the oxygen demand increases, but oxygen delivery cannot be increased unless, or until, the atherosclerosis improves. This occurs very slowly, if at all. The occurrence of angina and acute coronary syndrome (ACS) is the signal that the oxygen needs of the myocardium exceed its blood supply. Angina or dysrhythmias can occur when thyroid replacement is initiated because thyroid hormones enhance the cardiovascular effects of catecholamines.

> **NURSING ALERT**
>
> **The nurse must monitor for signs and symptoms of ACS, which can occur in response to therapy in patients with severe, long-standing hypothyroidism or myxedema coma, especially during the early phase of treatment. ACS must be aggressively treated at once to avoid morbid complications (e.g., myocardial infarction).**

Obviously, if angina or dysrhythmias occur, thyroid hormone administration must be discontinued immediately. Later, when it can be resumed safely, it should be prescribed cautiously at a lower dosage and under the close observation of the physician and the nurse.

Prevention of Medication Interactions

Oral thyroid hormones interact with many other medications. There is a decrease in thyroid hormone absorption when patients are also taking magnesium-containing antacids. Thyroid hormones may also decrease the pharmacologic effects of digitalis glycosides. Doses of anticoagulant agents need to be decreased when beginning thyroid replacement because of the increased risk of bleeding (Comerford, 2015).

Even in small IV doses, hypnotic and sedative agents may induce profound somnolence, lasting far longer than anticipated and leading to narcosis (stupor-like condition). Furthermore, they are likely to cause respiratory depression, which can easily be fatal because of decreased respiratory reserve and alveolar hypoventilation. The dose of these medications should be one half or one third of that typically prescribed for patients of similar age and weight with normal thyroid function.

Supportive Therapy

Severe hypothyroidism and myxedema coma require prompt, aggressive management to maintain vital functions. Arterial blood gases may be measured to determine carbon dioxide retention and to guide the use of assisted ventilation to combat hypoventilation. Oxygen saturation levels should be monitored using pulse oximetry. Fluids are given cautiously because of the danger of water intoxication. Passive rewarming with a blanket is recommended versus active rewarming such as application of external heat (e.g., heating pads) (Ross, 2016a). The latter should be avoided to prevent increased oxygen demands and hypotension. If myxedema has progressed to myxedema coma, refer to the current recommendations stated in the previous Pharmacologic Therapy section.

Nursing Management

Nursing care of the patient with hypothyroidism and myxedema is summarized in the plan of nursing care in Chart 43-4. In patients with hypothyroidism, the effects of analgesic, sedative, and anesthetic agents are prolonged. The nurse should carefully monitor patients who are prescribed these agents for adverse effects. Older patients are at increased risk because of age-related changes in liver and renal function.

> **NURSING ALERT**
>
> **Medications are administered to the patient with hypothyroidism with extreme caution because of the potential for altered metabolism and excretion as well as depressed metabolic rate and respiratory status.**

Promoting Home, Community-Based, and Transitional Care

Educating Patients About Self-Care

The patient and family require education and support to manage this complex disorder at home. Verbal and written instructions should be provided regarding the following:

- Desired actions and side effects of medications
- Correct medication administration ("Take first thing in the morning with a full glass of water.")
- Importance of continuing to take the medications as prescribed even after symptoms improve
- When to seek medical attention
- Importance of nutrition and diet to promote weight loss and normal bowel patterns
- Importance of periodic follow-up testing

The patient and family should be informed that many of the symptoms observed during the course of the disorder will disappear with effective treatment (Chart 43-5).

Continuing Care and Transitional Care

If indicated, a referral is made for home, community-based or transitional care. The nurse monitors the patient's recovery and ability to cope with the recent changes, along with the patient's physical and cognitive status and the patient's and family's understanding of previous education. The nurse documents and reports to the patient's primary health care professional subtle signs and symptoms that may indicate either inadequate or excessive thyroid hormone.

(text continued on page 1230)

Plan of Nursing Care

Chart 43-4. Care of the Patient With Hypothyroidism

Nursing Priorities: Intolerance to activity
Goal: Increased participation in activities and increased independence

NURSING INTERVENTIONS	RATIONALE	EXPECTED OUTCOMES
1. Promote independence in self-care activities.	1. Encouragement needed in patients with decreased energy	• Participates in self-care activities • Reports increased level of energy • Displays interest and awareness in environment • Participates in activities and events in environment • Participates in family events and activities • Reports no chest pain, increased fatigue, or breathlessness with increased level of activity
a. Space activities to promote rest and exercise as tolerated.	a. Encourages activities while allowing time for adequate rest	
b. Assist with self-care activities when patient is fatigued.	b. Permits patient to participate to the extent possible in self-care activities	
c. Provide stimulation through conversation and nonstressful activities.	c. Promotes interest without stressing the patient	
d. Monitor patient's response to increasing activities.	d. Guards against over- and under-exertion by the patient	

Nursing Priority: Imbalanced body temperature
Goal: Maintenance of normal body temperature

NURSING INTERVENTIONS	RATIONALE	EXPECTED OUTCOMES
1. Provide extra layer of clothing or extra blanket.	1. Minimizes heat loss	• Experiences relief of discomfort and cold intolerance • Maintains baseline body temperature • Reports adequate feeling of warmth and lack of chilling • Uses extra layer of clothing or extra blanket • Explains rationale for avoiding external heat source
2. Avoid and discourage the use of external heat source (e.g., heating pads, electric or warming blankets).	2. Reduces risk of peripheral vasodilation and vascular collapse	
3. Monitor patient's body temperature and report decreases from patient's baseline value.	3. Detects decreased body temperature and onset of myxedema coma	
4. Protect from exposure to cold and drafts.	4. Increases patient's level of comfort and decreases further heat loss	

Nursing Priority: Constipation
Goal: Return of normal bowel function

NURSING INTERVENTIONS	RATIONALE	EXPECTED OUTCOMES
1. Encourage increased fluid intake within limits of fluid restriction.	1. Promotes passage of soft stools	• Reports normal bowel function • Identifies and consumes foods high in fibre • Drinks recommended amount of fluid each day • Participates in gradually increasing exercises • Uses laxatives as prescribed and avoids excessive dependence on laxatives and enemas
2. Provide foods high in fibre.	2. Increases bulk of stools and more frequent bowel movements	
3. Instruct patient about foods with high water content.	3. Provides rationale for patient to increase fluid intake	
4. Monitor bowel function.	4. Permits detection of constipation and return to normal bowel pattern	
5. Encourage increased mobility within patient's exercise tolerance.	5. Promotes evacuation of the bowel	
6. Encourage patient to use laxatives and enemas sparingly.	6. Minimizes patient's dependence on laxatives and enemas and encourages normal pattern of bowel evacuation	

Nursing Priority: Lack of knowledge
Goal: Knowledge and acceptance of the prescribed therapeutic regimen

NURSING INTERVENTIONS	RATIONALE	EXPECTED OUTCOMES
1. Explain rationale for thyroid hormone replacement.	1. Provides rationale for patient to use thyroid hormone replacement as prescribed	• Describes therapeutic regimen correctly • Explains rationale for thyroid hormone replacement • Identifies positive outcomes of thyroid hormone replacement • Administers medication to self as prescribed
2. Describe desired effects of medication to patient.	2. Provides encouragement to patient by identifying improved physical status and well-being that will occur with thyroid hormone therapy and return to a euthyroid state	

Plan of Nursing Care — Chart 43-4. Care of the Patient With Hypothyroidism, *Continued*

NURSING INTERVENTIONS	RATIONALE	EXPECTED OUTCOMES
3. Assist patient to develop schedule and checklist to ensure self-administration of thyroid replacement.	3. Increases chances that medication will be taken as prescribed	• Identifies adverse side effects that should be reported promptly to primary provider: recurrence of symptoms of hypothyroidism and occurrence of symptoms of hyperthyroidism • Restates need for periodic/long-term follow-up visits to primary provider
4. Describe signs and symptoms of over- and underdose of medication.	4. Serves as check for patient to determine if therapeutic goals are met	
5. Explain the necessity for long-term follow-up to patient and family.	5. Increases likelihood that hypo- or hyperthyroidism will be detected and treated	

Nursing Priority: Altered breathing pattern
Goal: Improved respiratory status and maintenance of normal breathing pattern

NURSING INTERVENTIONS	RATIONALE	EXPECTED OUTCOMES
1. Monitor respiratory rate, depth, pattern, pulse oximetry, and arterial blood gases.	1. Identifies patient's baseline to monitor further changes and evaluate effectiveness of interventions	• Shows improved respiratory status and maintenance of normal breathing pattern • Demonstrates normal respiratory rate, depth, and pattern • Takes deep breaths, coughs, and uses incentive spirometry when encouraged • Demonstrates normal breath sounds without adventitious sounds on auscultation • Explains rationale for cautious use of medications • Cooperates with suction procedure and ventilator support when necessary
2. Encourage deep breathing, coughing, and the use of incentive spirometry.	2. Prevents atelectasis and promotes adequate ventilation	
3. Administer medications (hypnotics and sedatives) with caution.	3. Patients with hypothyroidism are very susceptible to respiratory depression with the use of hypnotics and sedatives	
4. Maintain patent airway through suction and ventilatory support if indicated (see Chapter 21 for care of patients requiring mechanical ventilation).	4. The use of an artificial airway and ventilatory support may be necessary with respiratory depression	

Nursing Priority: Confusion
Goal: Improved thought processes

NURSING INTERVENTIONS	RATIONALE	EXPECTED OUTCOMES
1. Orient patient to time, place, date, and events around him or her.	1. Provides reality orientation to patient	• Shows improved cognitive functioning • Identifies time, place, date, and events correctly • Responds appropriately when stimulated • Responds spontaneously as treatment becomes effective • Interacts spontaneously with family and environment • Explains that change in mental and cognitive processes is a result of disease processes • Takes medications as prescribed to prevent decrease in cognitive processes
2. Provide stimulation through conversation and nonthreatening activities.	2. Provides stimulation within patient's level of tolerance for stress	
3. Explain to patient and family that change in cognitive and mental functioning is a result of disease process.	3. Reassures patient and family about the cause of the cognitive changes and that a positive outcome is possible with appropriate treatment	
4. Monitor cognitive and mental processes and response of these to medication and other therapy.	4. Permits evaluation of the effectiveness of treatment	

Collaborative Problem: Myxedema and myxedema coma
Goal: Evidence of progression to pre-coma baseline without incurring additional complications

NURSING INTERVENTIONS	RATIONALE	EXPECTED OUTCOMES
1. Monitor patient for increasing severity of signs and symptoms of hypothyroidism: a. Decreased level of consciousness b. Decreased vital signs (blood pressure, respiratory rate, temperature, pulse rate) c. Increasing difficulty in awakening or arousing patient	1. Extreme hypothyroidism may lead to myxedema, myxedema coma, and slowing of all body systems if untreated	• Exhibits reversal of myxedema and myxedema coma • Responds appropriately to questions and surroundings • Vital signs return to normal or near-normal ranges • Respiratory status improves with adequate spontaneous ventilatory effort

continued >

Plan of Nursing Care — Chart 43-4. Care of the Patient With Hypothyroidism, *Continued*

NURSING INTERVENTIONS	RATIONALE	EXPECTED OUTCOMES
2. Assist in ventilatory support if respiratory depression and failure occur.	2. Ventilatory support is necessary to maintain adequate oxygenation and maintenance of airway	• Reports no episodes of angina or other indicators of cardiac insufficiency • Experiences minimal or no complications caused by immobility
3. Administer prescribed medications (e.g., thyroxine) with extreme caution.	3. The slow metabolism and atherosclerosis of myxedema may result in angina with administration of thyroxine	
4. Turn and reposition patient at intervals.	4. Minimizes risks associated with immobility	
5. Avoid the use of hypnotic, sedative, and analgesic agents.	5. Altered metabolism of these agents greatly increases the risks of their use in myxedema	

Gerontologic Considerations

The prevalence of hypothyroidism increases with age, most often among women (Visser et al., 2013). The higher prevalence of hypothyroidism among older adults may be related to age-related alterations in immune function and complicated by multiple comorbidities.

Most patients with primary hypothyroidism present with long-standing mild to moderate hypothyroidism. Subclinical disease is common among older women and can be asymptomatic or mistaken for other medical conditions. Subtle symptoms of hypothyroidism, such as fatigue, muscle aches, and mental confusion, may be attributed to the normal aging process by patients, families, and health care providers; therefore, these symptoms require close attention (Visser et al., 2013). In addition, signs and symptoms of hypothyroidism in older adults are often atypical, and manifestations of hypothyroidism and hyperthyroidism may blur. Patients may have few or no symptoms until dysfunction is severe. Depression, apathy, and decreased mobility or activity may be the major initial symptoms and may be accompanied by significant weight loss. Constipation affects one fourth of older patients.

In older patients, treatment is recommended for those who have a TSH in excess of 10 mU/L (Visser et al., 2013). In those with mild to moderate hypothyroidism, thyroid hormone replacement is individually tailored and must be started with low dosages and increased gradually to prevent serious cardiovascular side effects (Visser et al., 2013). Angina, for example, may occur with rapid thyroid

CHART 43-5

HOME CARE CHECKLIST • The Patient With Hypothyroidism (Myxedema)

At the completion of education, the patient and/or caregiver will be able to:

- State the impact of hypothyroidism and treatment on physiologic functioning, ADLs, IADLs, roles, relationships, and spirituality.
- State precipitating factors and interventions for complications (hyperthyroidism, myxedema coma).
- Explain the purpose, dose, route, schedule, side effects, and precautions of prescribed medication (synthetic thyroid hormone).
- State that compliance with medical regimen is lifelong. Relate how to reach primary provider with questions or complications.
- State the need to avoid extreme cold temperature until condition is stable.
- State importance of regular follow-up visits with health care professional.
- Identify dietary strategies to promote weight reduction and prevent constipation (high fibre, low calorie, adequate fluid intake).
- State potential for menstrual irregularities and potential for pregnancy for women.
- State the importance of avoiding infection.
- Identify changes in personality as related to hypothyroidism.
- Identify areas of activity limitations and impact on lifestyle.

replacement in the presence of coronary artery disease secondary to the hypothyroid state. Heart failure and tachydysrhythmias may worsen during the transition from the hypothyroid state to the normal metabolic state. Dementia may become more apparent during early thyroid hormone replacement in older patients with concomitant dementia.

Older patients with severe hypothyroidism and atherosclerosis may become confused and agitated if their metabolic rate is increased too quickly. Marked clinical improvement follows the administration of hormone replacement; such medication must be continued for life, even though signs of hypothyroidism disappear within 3 to 12 weeks.

Myxedema and myxedema coma usually occur exclusively in patients older than 50 years (Ross, 2016a). The high mortality rate of myxedema coma mandates immediate IV administration of thyroid hormone and supportive management of other clinical manifestations such as hyponatremia, hypoglycemia, hypothermia, hypoventilation, and hypotension.

Older patients require periodic follow-up monitoring of serum TSH levels, because poor adherence with therapy may occur or the patient may take the medications erratically. A careful history can identify the need for further education about the importance of the medication.

Hyperthyroidism

Hyperthyroidism, a common endocrine disorder, is a form of **thyrotoxicosis** resulting from an excessive synthesis and secretion of endogenous or exogenous thyroid hormones by the thyroid (Bahn, Burch, Cooper, et al., 2011). The most common causes are Graves' disease, toxic multinodular goitre, and toxic adenoma. Other causes include thyroiditis (inflammation of the thyroid gland) and excessive ingestion of thyroid hormone.

Graves' disease, the most common cause of hyperthyroidism, is an autoimmune disorder that results from an excessive output of thyroid hormones caused by abnormal stimulation of the thyroid gland by circulating immunoglobulins (Bahn et al., 2011; Muldoon, Mai, & Burch, 2014). This disease affects women eight times more frequently than men, with onset usually between the second and fourth decades. The disorder may appear after an emotional shock, stress, or an infection, but the exact significance of these relationships is not understood.

Clinical Manifestations

Patients with hyperthyroidism exhibit a characteristic group of signs and symptoms. The presenting symptom is often nervousness. These patients are often emotionally hyperexcitable, irritable, and apprehensive; they cannot sit quietly; they suffer from palpitations; and their pulse is abnormally rapid at rest as well as on exertion. They tolerate heat poorly and perspire unusually freely. The skin is flushed continuously, with a characteristic salmon colour in Caucasians, and is likely to be warm, soft, and moist. However, patients may report dry skin and diffuse pruritus. A fine tremor of the hands may be observed. Patients may exhibit ophthalmopathy, such as exophthalmos (abnormal protrusion of one or both eyeballs), which produces a startled facial expression. Despite treatment, these ocular changes are not always reversible (Weber & Kelley, 2014).

Other manifestations include an increased appetite and dietary intake, weight loss, fatigability and weakness (difficulty in climbing stairs and rising from a chair), amenorrhea, and changes in bowel function. Atrial fibrillation occurs in 15% of older adult patients with new-onset hyperthyroidism (Muldoon et al., 2014).

Cardiac effects may include sinus tachycardia or dysrhythmias, increased pulse pressure, and palpitations; these changes may be related to increased sensitivity to catecholamines or to changes in neurotransmitter turnover. Myocardial hypertrophy and heart failure may occur if the hyperthyroidism is severe and untreated.

The course of the disease may be mild, characterized by remissions and exacerbations, and terminate with spontaneous recovery in a few months or years. Conversely, it may progress relentlessly, with the untreated person becoming emaciated, intensely nervous, delirious, and even disoriented; eventually, the heart fails.

Symptoms of hyperthyroidism may occur with the release of excessive amounts of thyroid hormone as a result of inflammation after irradiation of the thyroid or destruction of thyroid tissue by tumour. Such symptoms may also occur with excessive administration of thyroid hormone for the treatment of hypothyroidism. Long-standing use of thyroid hormone in the absence of close monitoring may be a cause of symptoms of hyperthyroidism. It is also likely to result in premature osteoporosis, particularly in women.

Assessment and Diagnostic Findings

The thyroid gland is enlarged to some extent. It is soft and may pulsate; a thrill often can be palpated, and a bruit is heard over the thyroid arteries (Weber & Kelley, 2014). These are signs of greatly increased blood flow through the thyroid gland. In advanced cases, the diagnosis is made on the basis of the symptoms, a decrease in serum TSH, increased free T_4, and an increase in radioactive iodine uptake.

Medical Management

Appropriate treatment of hyperthyroidism depends on the underlying cause and often consists of a combination of therapies, including antithyroid agents, radioactive iodine, and surgery. Treatment of hyperthyroidism is directed toward reducing thyroid hyperactivity to relieve symptoms and preventing complications. The use of radioactive iodine is the most common form of treatment for Graves' disease in Canada. Beta-adrenergic blocking agents (e.g., propranolol [Inderal], atenolol [Tenormin], metoprolol [Lopressor]) are used as adjunctive therapy for symptomatic relief, particularly in transient thyroiditis (Ross, 2016c). The three treatments (radioactive iodine therapy, antithyroid medications [e.g., thionamides], and surgery) share the same complications: relapse or recurrent hyperthyroidism and permanent hypothyroidism. The rate of relapse increases in patients who have had very severe disease, a long history of dysfunction, ocular and cardiac symptoms, large goitre, or relapse after previous treatment.

Pharmacologic Therapy

Two forms of pharmacotherapy are available for treating hyperthyroidism and controlling excessive thyroid activity: (1) use of irradiation by administration of the radioisotope iodine 131 (^{131}I) for destructive effects on the thyroid gland and (2) antithyroid medications that interfere with the synthesis of thyroid hormones and other agents that control manifestations of hyperthyroidism.

Radioactive Iodine Therapy

Radioactive iodine has been used to treat toxic adenomas, toxic multinodular goitre, and most varieties of thyrotoxicosis. Radioactive iodine is contraindicated during pregnancy because it crosses the placenta. Women of childbearing age should be given a pregnancy test 48 hours before administration of radioactive iodine and instructed to not conceive for at least 6 months following treatment. To ensure that radioactivity is no longer actively concentrated in breast tissue, radioactive iodine should not be given until at least 6 weeks after lactation stops (Bahn et al., 2011).

The goal of radioactive iodine therapy (^{131}I) is to eliminate the hyperthyroid state with the administration of sufficient radiation in a single dose (Bahn et al., 2011). Almost all of the iodine that enters and is retained in the body becomes concentrated in the thyroid gland. Therefore, the radioactive isotope of iodine is concentrated in the thyroid gland, where it destroys thyroid cells without jeopardizing other radiosensitive tissues. Over a period of several weeks, thyroid cells exposed to the radioactive iodine are destroyed, resulting in reduction of the hyperthyroid state and inevitably hypothyroidism.

Some patients at high risk for complications of hyperthyroidism (e.g., older adults, patients with cardiovascular disease) may need pretreatment with antithyroid medications. Methimazole (MMI) is given 4 to 6 weeks prior to administration of radioactive iodine. The antithyroid medications are stopped 3 days before and restarted 3 days after administering radioactive iodine and then tapered over 4 to 6 weeks (Ross, 2016g).

The use of an ablative dose of radioactive iodine initially causes an acute release of thyroid hormone from the thyroid gland and may cause increased symptoms. The patient is observed for signs of **thyroid storm** (see Chart 43-6), a life-threatening condition manifested by cardiac dysrhythmias, fever, and neurologic impairment (Davies, Laurberg, & Bahn, 2016; Ross, 2016b). Beta-blockers are used to control these symptoms.

Thyroid hormone replacement is started 4 to 18 weeks after the antithyroid medications have been stopped based on the results of thyroid function tests. TSH measurements can be misleading in the early months following treatment with radioactive iodine. Therefore, serum free T_4 is the principal test (Bahn et al., 2011; Ross, 2016e) measured at 3 to 6 weeks following administration of radioactive iodine and then every 1 to 2 months until normal thyroid function is established. If TSH and free T_4 are both persistently low, then the total T_3 must be measured to differentiate between persistent hyperthyroidism (T_3 elevated) or

CHART 43-6

Thyroid Storm (Thyrotoxic Crisis, Thyrotoxicosis)

Thyroid storm (thyrotoxic crisis) is a form of severe hyperthyroidism, usually of abrupt onset. Untreated, it is almost always fatal, but with proper treatment the mortality rate is reduced substantially. The patient with thyroid storm or crisis is critically ill and requires astute observation and aggressive and supportive nursing care during and after the acute stage of illness.

Clinical Manifestations

Thyroid storm is characterized by:

- High fever (hyperpyrexia) above 38.5°C
- Extreme tachycardia (more than 130 bpm)
- Exaggerated symptoms of hyperthyroidism with disturbances of a major system—for example, gastrointestinal (weight loss, diarrhea, abdominal pain) or cardiovascular (edema, chest pain, dyspnea, palpitations)
- Altered neurologic or mental state, which frequently appears as delirium psychosis, somnolence, or coma

Life-threatening thyroid storm is usually precipitated by stress, such as injury, infection, thyroid and nonthyroid surgery, tooth extraction, insulin reaction, diabetic ketoacidosis, pregnancy, digitalis intoxication, abrupt withdrawal of antithyroid medications, extreme emotional stress, or vigorous palpation of the thyroid. These factors can precipitate thyroid storm in the partially controlled or completely untreated patient with hyperthyroidism. Current methods of diagnosis and treatment for hyperthyroidism have greatly decreased the incidence of thyroid storm, making it uncommon today.

Management

Immediate objectives are reduction of body temperature and heart rate and prevention of vascular collapse. Measures to accomplish these objectives include:

- A hypothermia mattress or blanket, ice packs, a cool environment, hydrocortisone, and acetaminophen (Tylenol). Salicylates (e.g., aspirin) are not used because they displace thyroid hormone from binding proteins and worsen the hypermetabolism.
- Humidified oxygen is administered to improve tissue oxygenation and meet the high metabolic demands. Arterial blood gas levels or pulse oximetry may be used to monitor respiratory status.
- Intravenous fluids containing dextrose are administered to replace liver glycogen stores that have been decreased in the hyperthyroid patient.
- PTU or methimazole is administered to impede formation of thyroid hormone and block conversion of T_4 to T_3, the more active form of thyroid hormone.
- Hydrocortisone is prescribed to treat shock or adrenal insufficiency.
- Iodine is administered to decrease output of T_4 from the thyroid gland. For cardiac problems such as atrial fibrillation, dysrhythmias, and heart failure, sympatholytic agents may be administered. Propranolol, combined with digitalis, has been effective in reducing severe cardiac symptoms.

transient hypothyroidism (T_3 normal or low) (Ross, 2016e). Once a normal thyroid state has been established, TSH should be measured every 6 to 12 months for life (Ross, 2016e).

A major advantage of treatment with radioactive iodine is that it avoids many of the side effects associated with antithyroid medications. However, some patients may elect to be treated with antithyroid medications rather than radioactive iodine for a variety of reasons, including fear of radiation.

Patients who receive radioactive iodine should be informed that they can contaminate their household and other persons through saliva, urine, or radiation emitting from their body. They should avoid sexual contact, sleeping in the same bed with other persons, having close contact with children and pregnant women, and sharing utensils and cups. The patient should follow the instructions provided by the primary provider regarding the time restrictions for these cautions because they are dose related (Ross, 2016e).

Antithyroid Medications

Antithyroid medications (thionamides) are summarized in Table 43-3. The objective of pharmacotherapy is to inhibit one or more stages in thyroid hormone synthesis or hormone release. Antithyroid agents block the utilization of iodine by interfering with the iodination of tyrosine and the coupling of iodotyrosines in the synthesis of thyroid hormones. This prevents the synthesis of thyroid hormone. The most commonly used antithyroid drugs are methimazole (MMI, Tapazole) or propylthiouracil (PTU). The medications are used until the patient is euthyroid (i.e., neither hyperthyroid nor hypothyroid). These medications block extrathyroidal conversion of T_4 to T_3 (Bahn et al., 2011).

Prior to initiating therapy with these drugs, baseline blood tests are performed, including complete blood count (white blood cell [WBC] count with differential) and liver profile (transaminases and bilirubin) (Bahn et al., 2011; Ross, 2016d). The therapeutic dose is determined on the basis of clinical criteria, including changes in pulse rate, pulse pressure, body weight, size of the goitre, and results of laboratory studies. The patient should be instructed to take the medication in the morning on an empty stomach 30 minutes before eating to avoid decrease in absorption associated with some foods such as walnuts, soybean flour, cottonseed meal, and dietary fibre. Because antithyroid medications do not interfere with release or activity of previously formed thyroid hormones, it may take several weeks until symptom relief occurs. At that time, the maintenance dose is established, and the medication is gradually tapered over several months.

Toxic complications of antithyroid medications are relatively uncommon; nevertheless, the importance of periodic follow-up is emphasized, because medication sensitization, fever, rash, urticaria, or even agranulocytosis and thrombocytopenia (decrease in granulocytes and platelets) may develop (Bahn et al., 2011). With any sign of infection, especially pharyngitis and fever or the occurrence of mouth ulcers, the patient is advised to stop the medication, notify the primary provider immediately, and undergo hematologic studies (Bahn et al., 2011). PTU is recommended during the first trimester of pregnancy rather than MMI due to the teratogenic effects of MMI (Ross, 2016f). Due to risk of hepatotoxicity, PTU should be discontinued after the first trimester and the patient should be switched to MMI for the remainder of the pregnancy and when breast feeding (Ross, 2016b).

Discontinuation of antithyroid medications before therapy is complete usually results in relapse within 6 months. It is important that the possibility of relapse be discussed so that a treatment strategy will be in place if relapse occurs.

Adjunctive Therapy

Iodine or iodide is necessary for thyroid function, and deficiency or excess can lead to thyroid dysfunction. Iodine or iodide solutions were once the only therapy available for patients with hyperthyroidism but are no longer the sole method of treatment. Antithyroid medications

TABLE 43-3 Pharmacologic Agents Used to Treat Hyperthyroidism

Agent	Action	Nursing Considerations
Propylthiouracil (PTU)	Blocks synthesis of hormones (conversion of T_3 to T_4)	Monitor cardiac parameters. Observe for conversion to hypothyroidism. Must be given by mouth. Watch for rash, nausea, vomiting, agranulocytosis, SLE.
Methimazole	Blocks synthesis of thyroid hormone	More toxic than PTU. Watch for rash and other symptoms as for PTU.
Sodium iodide	Suppresses release of thyroid hormone	Given 1 hour after PTU or methimazole. Watch for edema, hemorrhage, gastrointestinal upset.
Potassium iodide	Suppresses release of thyroid hormone	Discontinue for rash. Watch for signs of toxic iodinism.
Saturated solution of potassium iodide (SSKI)	Suppresses release of thyroid hormone	Mix with juice or milk. Given by straw to prevent staining of teeth.
Beta-blocker (e.g., propranolol)	Beta-adrenergic blocking agent	Monitor cardiac status. Hold for bradycardia or decreased cardiac output. Use with caution in patients with heart failure.

T_4, thyroxine; T_3, triiodothyronine; SLE, systemic lupus erythematosus.

Adapted from Morton, P. G., & Fontaine, D. K. (2013). *Critical care nursing: A holistic approach*. Philadelphia, PA: Lippincott Williams & Wilkins.

(MMI and PTU) and radioactive iodine are not the mainstays of pharmacologic treatment for hyperthyroidism. In the short term, iodine solutions are considered effective. When treating patients with thyroid storm and those requiring surgical intervention for hyperthyroidism, iodine solutions are considered highly effective. Iodine solutions inhibit the release of T_4 and T_3 within hours of administration and inhibit thyroid hormone synthesis. The maximum inhibitory effect on serum thyroid hormone production is only 10 days (Ross, 2016g). Solutions such as potassium iodide (KI), Lugol's solution, and saturated solution of potassium iodide (SSKI) may be used in combination with antithyroid agents or beta-adrenergic blockers to prepare the patient with hyperthyroidism for surgery. Solutions of iodine and iodide compounds are more palatable in milk or fruit juice and are administered through a straw to prevent staining of the teeth. The nurse should be aware that there have been reported cases of local esophageal or duodenal mucosal injury and hemorrhage as a result of administration of Lugol's solution (960 mg/day) to manage thyroid storm (Bahn et al., 2011).

Beta-adrenergic blocking agents (e.g., propranolol, atenolol, metoprolol) are important in decreasing heart rate, systolic blood pressure, muscle weakness, nervousness, tremor, anxiety, and heat intolerance. The patient continues taking the beta-blocker until the free T_4 is within the normal range and the TSH level approaches normal.

NURSING ALERT

Patients receiving iodide medications should be observed for the development of goitre and should be cautioned against use of iodide-containing over-the-counter medications that can increase the response to iodide therapy. Cough medications, expectorants, bronchodilators, and salt substitutes may contain iodide and should be avoided.

Surgical Management

Surgery to remove thyroid tissue is reserved for special circumstances—for example, in pregnant women who are allergic to antithyroid medications, in patients with large goitres, or in patients who are unable to take antithyroid agents. Surgery for treatment of hyperthyroidism is performed soon after the thyroid function has returned to normal (4 to 6 weeks).

The surgical removal of about five sixths of the thyroid tissue (subtotal thyroidectomy) reliably results in a prolonged remission in most patients with exophthalmic goitre. Its use today is reserved for patients with obstructive symptoms, for pregnant women in the second trimester, and for patients with a need for rapid normalization of thyroid function. Before surgery, an antithyroid medication is given until signs of hyperthyroidism have disappeared. A beta-adrenergic blocking agent (e.g., propranolol) may be used to reduce the heart rate and other signs and symptoms of hyperthyroidism. Medications that may prolong clotting (e.g., aspirin) are stopped several weeks before surgery to reduce the risk of postoperative bleeding. Patients receiving iodine medication must be monitored for evidence of iodine toxicity (iodinism), which requires immediate withdrawal of the medication. Symptoms of iodinism include swelling of the buccal mucosa, excessive salivation, cold symptoms, and skin eruptions. The incidence of relapse with a total thyroidectomy is nearly 0%, whereas recurrence following a subtotal thyroidectomy is 8% at 5 years (Bahn et al., 2011).

Gerontologic Considerations

Although hyperthyroidism is much less common in older adults than hypothyroidism, patients 65 years and older need careful assessment to avoid missing subtle signs and symptoms. Subclinical hyperthyroidism has been reported in approximately 8% of this age group (Harman, 2016; Visser et al., 2013). This age group may present with atypical vague and nonspecific signs and symptoms of thyroid disease such as anorexia and weight loss with absence of ocular signs, or isolated atrial fibrillation. New or worsening heart failure or angina is more likely to occur in older patients rather than in younger patients. Symptoms such as tachycardia, fatigue, mental confusion, weight loss, change in bowel habits, and depression can be attributed to age and other illnesses that are common in older adults. The older patient may complain of difficulty climbing stairs or rising from a chair because of muscle weakness (Visser et al., 2013). Evaluation for thyroid disease with a serum TSH measurement is indicated in older patients who have unexplained physical or mental deterioration (Bahn et al., 2011). Free T_4 and T_3 should be included in the initial screening when hyperthyroidism is highly suspected. Once thyrotoxicosis is confirmed, additional tests such as radioactive iodine uptake and thyroid scan are prescribed to differentiate between causes such as Graves' disease, toxic nodular goitre, acute thyroiditis, and other disorders. Toxic nodular goitre is the most common cause of thyrotoxicosis in older patients. Patients have the option of treatment using antithyroid medications, radioactive iodine, and surgery. Radioactive iodine is generally recommended for treatment of thyrotoxicosis caused by toxic nodular goitre in older patients unless an enlarged thyroid gland is pressing on the airway. Prior to administration of radioactive iodine (Bahn et al., 2011) in this at-risk group, pretreatment with beta-blockade is indicated if the patient's resting heart rate is 90 bpm or if the patient has coexistent cardiovascular disease and symptomatic hyperthyroidism. MMI should be given prior to treatment with radioactive iodine to prevent complications due to worsening of hyperthyroidism. Patients who elect to have surgery to treat toxic nodular goitre must be pretreated with an antithyroid medication (methimazole) to achieve a euthyroid state. However, preoperative iodine should not be used to prevent exacerbating the hyperthyroidism (Bahn et al., 2011). Long-term use of certain antithyroid medications such as PTU is not recommended for treatment of toxic nodular goitre in older patients due to risk of side effects. Although rare, there is evidence that PTU can result in agranulocytosis and hepatic injury. However, the use of antithyroid medications versus radioactive iodine or surgery may be the patient's preferred choice or the option for some older patients and other ill persons with "limited longevity" who can be monitored at least every 3 months (Bahn et al., 2011).

The use of beta-adrenergic blocking agents (e.g., propranolol and atenolol) may be indicated to decrease the cardiovascular and neurologic signs and symptoms of thyrotoxicosis. These agents must be used with extreme caution in older patients to minimize adverse effects on cardiac function that may produce heart failure. The dosage of other medications used to treat other chronic illnesses in older patients may also need to be modified because of the altered rate of metabolism associated with hyperthyroidism.

Nursing Process

The Patient With Hyperthyroidism

Assessment

The health history and examination focus on symptoms related to accelerated or exaggerated metabolism. These include the patient's and family's reports of irritability and increased emotional reaction and the impact that these changes have had on the patient's interactions with family, friends, and coworkers. The history includes other stressors and the patient's ability to cope with stress.

The nurse initially and periodically assesses the patient's nutritional status and the presence of symptoms related to the hypermetabolic state. This hypermetabolic state may affect the cardiovascular system including heart rate and rhythm, blood pressure, heart sounds, and peripheral pulses. Other specific changes may also include alteration in vision and appearance of the external eye. Because emotional changes are associated with hyperthyroidism, the patient's emotional state and psychological status are evaluated, as well as such symptoms as irritability, anxiety, sleep disturbances, apathy, and lethargy, all of which may occur with hyperthyroidism (Morgan & Tsai, 2015). The family may also provide information about recent changes in the patient's emotional status.

Nursing Priorities

Based on the assessment data, major nursing priorities may include the following:

- Lack of nutrition
- Inability to cope
- Situational low self-esteem
- Imbalanced body temperature

Collaborative Problems/ Potential Complications

Based on assessment data, potential complications may include the following:

- Thyrotoxicosis or thyroid storm
- Hypothyroidism

Planning and Goals

The goals for the patient may be improved nutritional status, improved coping ability, improved self-esteem, maintenance of usual body temperature, and absence of complications.

Nursing Interventions

Improving Nutritional Status

Hyperthyroidism affects all body systems, including the GI system. The appetite is increased but may be satisfied by several well-balanced meals of small size, even up to six meals a day. Foods and fluids are selected to replace fluid lost through diarrhea and diaphoresis and to control the diarrhea that results from increased peristalsis. Rapid movement of food through the GI tract may result in nutritional imbalance and further weight loss. To reduce diarrhea, highly seasoned foods and stimulants such as coffee, tea, cola, and alcohol are discouraged. High-calorie, high-protein foods are encouraged. A quiet atmosphere during mealtime may aid digestion. Weight and dietary intake are recorded to monitor nutritional status.

Enhancing Coping Measures

The patient with hyperthyroidism needs reassurance that the emotional reactions being experienced are a result of the disorder and that with effective treatment those symptoms will be controlled. Because of the negative effect these symptoms have on family and friends, they too need reassurance that the symptoms are expected to disappear with treatment.

It is important to use a calm, unhurried approach with the patient. Stressful experiences should be minimized and a quiet, uncluttered environment should be maintained. It is important to balance periods of activity with rest.

If thyroidectomy is planned, the patient needs to know that pharmacologic therapy is necessary to prepare the thyroid gland for surgical treatment. The nurse provides education and reminds the patient to take the medications as prescribed. Because of hyperexcitability and shortened attention span, the patient may require repetition of this education and written instructions.

Improving Self-Esteem

The patient with hyperthyroidism is likely to experience changes in appearance, appetite, and weight. These factors, along with the patient's inability to cope well with family and the illness, may result in loss of self-esteem. The nurse conveys an understanding of the patient's concern about these problems and promotes the use of effective coping strategies. The patient and family should be reassured that these changes are a result of the thyroid dysfunction and are, in fact, out of the patient's control. The nurse refers the patient to professional counselling as necessary.

If the patient experiences ocular changes secondary to hyperthyroidism, eye care and protection may be necessary. The nurse educates the patient about instillation of eye drops or ointment prescribed to soothe the eyes and protect the exposed cornea. Smoking should be highly discouraged, and smoking cessation strategies are recommended. The patient may be embarrassed by the need to eat large meals. Caregivers and family should avoid commenting on the patient's large dietary intake while making sure that the patient receives sufficient nutritious food.

Maintaining Usual Body Temperature

The patient with hyperthyroidism frequently finds a normal room temperature too warm because of an exaggerated metabolic rate and increased heat production. If the patient is hospitalized, the nurse maintains the environment at a cool, comfortable temperature and changes bedding and clothing as needed. Cool baths and cool or cold fluids are encouraged, because they may provide relief.

Monitoring and Managing Potential Complications

The nurse closely monitors the patient with hyperthyroidism for signs and symptoms that may be indicative of thyroid storm. Cardiac and respiratory functions are assessed by measuring vital signs and cardiac output, electrocardiographic (ECG) monitoring, arterial blood gases, and pulse oximetry. Assessment continues after treatment is initiated because of the potential effects of treatment on cardiac function. Oxygen is administered to prevent hypoxia, to improve tissue oxygenation, and to meet the high metabolic demands. IV fluids may be necessary to maintain blood glucose levels and to replace lost fluids. Antithyroid medications (PTU or methimazole) may be prescribed to reduce thyroid hormone levels. In addition, beta-blockers and digitalis may be prescribed to treat cardiac symptoms. If shock develops, treatment strategies must be implemented (see Chapter 16).

Hypothyroidism is likely to occur with any of the treatments used for hyperthyroidism. Therefore, the nurse periodically monitors the patient. Most patients report a greatly improved sense of well-being after treatment of hyperthyroidism, and some fail to continue to take prescribed thyroid replacement therapy. Therefore, part of patient and family teaching is instruction about the importance of continuing therapy indefinitely after discharge and a discussion of the consequences of failing to take medication.

Promoting Home, Community-Based, and Transitional Care

EDUCATING PATIENTS ABOUT SELF-CARE. The nurse educates the patient with hyperthyroidism about how and when to take prescribed medication and provides instruction about the essential role of the medication in the broader therapeutic plan. Because of the hyperexcitability and decreased attention span associated with hyperthyroidism, the nurse provides a written plan for the patient to take home and use. The type and amount of information given depend on the patient's stress and anxiety levels. The patient and family members receive verbal and written education about the actions and possible side effects of the medications as well as adverse effects that should be reported if they occur (Chart 43-7).

If a total or subtotal thyroidectomy is anticipated, the patient needs information about what to expect. This information is repeated as the time of surgery approaches. The nurse also advises the patient to avoid stressful situations that may precipitate thyroid storm.

CONTINUING AND TRANSITIONAL CARE. Referral for home, community-based or transitional care, if indicated, allows the nurse to assess the home and family environment, as well as the patient's and family's understanding of the importance of adhering to the therapeutic regimen and the recommended follow-up monitoring. The nurse reinforces to the patient and family the importance of long-term follow-up because of the risk of hypothyroidism after thyroidectomy or treatment with antithyroid medications or radioactive iodine. The nurse also assesses the patient for changes indicating return to normal thyroid function and signs and symptoms of hyperthyroidism and hypothyroidism. Furthermore, the nurse reminds the patient and family about the importance of health promotion activities and recommended health screening.

Evaluation

Expected patient outcomes may include the following:

1. Improves nutritional status
   a. Reports adequate dietary intake and decreased hunger
   b. Identifies high-calorie, high-protein foods; identifies foods to be avoided
   c. Avoids use of alcohol and other stimulants
   d. Stops smoking
   e. Reports decreased episodes of diarrhea
2. Demonstrates effective coping methods in dealing with family, friends, and coworkers
   a. Explains reasons for irritability and emotional instability
   b. Avoids stressful situations, events, and people
   c. Participates in relaxing, nonstressful activities
3. Achieves increased self-esteem
   a. Verbalizes feelings about self and illness
   b. Describes feelings of frustration and loss of control
   c. Describes reasons for increased appetite
4. Maintains normal body temperature
5. Absence of complications
   a. Has serum thyroid hormone and TSH levels within expected limits
   b. Identifies signs and symptoms of thyroid storm and hypothyroidism
   c. Has vital signs and results of ECG, arterial blood gases, and pulse oximetry within expected limits
   d. States importance of regular follow-up and lifelong maintenance of prescribed therapy

CHART 43-7

HOME CARE CHECKLIST • The Patient With Hyperthyroidism

At the completion of education, the patient and/or caregiver will be able to:

- State the impact of hyperthyroidism, treatment on physiologic functioning, ADLs, IADLs, roles, relationships, and spirituality.
- State that emotional lability is part of disease process.
- Identify the potential for menstrual irregularities and pregnancy, and increased risk of osteoporosis in women.
- State that long-term treatment and follow-up is necessary.
- Describe the potential benefits and risks of surgical intervention or radioactive iodine therapy.
- State the name, dose, side effects, frequency, and schedule for all medications.
- Explain the purpose, dose, route, schedule, side effects, and precautions of treatment of hyperthyroidism (antithyroid medications, radioactive iodine).
- State the need to contact primary provider before taking over-the-counter medications.
- State changes in lifestyle (e.g., diet, activity) necessary to maintain health.
  - Identify the need for increased dietary intake until weight stabilizes.
  - Identify foods to be avoided.
  - Identify the need for planned rest periods and methods to improve sleep patterns.
  - Identify areas of stress and management techniques.
  - Identify rationale for smoking cessation and steps to stop use of any tobacco product.
- State precipitating factors and interventions for complications (hypothyroidism, thyroid storm).
- Relate how to reach primary provider with questions or complications.
- State time and date of follow-up medical appointments, therapy, and testing.
- Identify sources of support (e.g., friends, relatives, faith community, support groups, caregiver support).
- Identify the need for health promotion, disease prevention, and screening activities.

Thyroid Tumours

Tumours of the thyroid gland are classified on the basis of being benign or malignant, the presence or absence of associated thyrotoxicosis, and the diffuse or irregular quality of the glandular enlargement. If the enlargement is sufficient to cause a visible swelling in the neck, the tumour is referred to as a goitre.

All grades of goitre are encountered, from those that are barely visible to those producing disfigurement. Some are symmetric and diffuse; others are nodular. Some are accompanied by hyperthyroidism, in which case they are described as toxic; others are associated with a euthyroid state and are called nontoxic goitres.

Endemic (Iodine-Deficient) Goitre

The most common type of goitre, once encountered chiefly in geographic regions where the natural supply of iodine is deficient (e.g., the Great Lakes areas of Canada), is the so-called simple or colloid goitre. In addition to being caused by an iodine deficiency, simple goitre may be caused by an intake of large quantities of goitrogenic substances in patients with unusually susceptible glands. These substances include excessive amounts of iodine. Lithium prescribed for the treatment of bipolar disorder has also been found to also have antithyroid actions (Janicak, 2016; Shine, McKnight, Leaver, et al., 2015; Surks, 2016c).

Simple goitre represents a compensatory hypertrophy of the thyroid gland, caused by stimulation by the pituitary gland. The pituitary gland produces thyrotropin or TSH, a hormone that controls the release of thyroid hormone from the thyroid gland. Its production increases if there is subnormal thyroid activity, as when insufficient iodine is available for production of the thyroid hormone. Such goitres usually cause no symptoms, except for the swelling in the neck, which may result in tracheal compression when excessive.

Many goitres of this type recede after the iodine imbalance is corrected. Supplementary iodine, such as SSKI, is prescribed to suppress the pituitary's thyroid-stimulating activity. When surgery is recommended, the risk of postoperative complications is minimized by ensuring a preoperative euthyroid state through treatment with antithyroid medications and iodide to reduce the size and vascularity of the goitre.

Providing children in iodine-poor regions with iodine compounds can prevent simple or endemic goitre. Although the introduction of iodized salt has been the single most effective means of preventing goitre in at-risk populations, the World Health Organization (2007) is exploring alternative strategies to ensure iodine intake because of the health risks associated with excessive salt intake.

Nodular Goitre

Some thyroid glands are nodular because of areas of hyperplasia (overgrowth). No symptoms may arise as a result of this condition, but not uncommonly these nodules slowly increase in size, with some descending into the thorax, where they cause local pressure symptoms. Some nodules become malignant, and some are associated with a hyperthyroid state. Therefore, the patient with many thyroid nodules may eventually require surgery.

Thyroid Cancer

Cancer of the thyroid is much less prevalent than other forms of cancer; however, it accounts for 90% of endocrine malignancies. According to the Canadian Cancer Society's Advisory Committee on Cancer Statistics (CCSACCS, 2018), more than 7,000 new cases of thyroid cancer were diagnosed in 2017, with 1,650 (95 deaths) of the cases occurring in men and 5,400 (120 deaths) in women. There are several types of cancer of the thyroid gland; the type determines the course and prognosis (Table 43-4).

External radiation of the head, neck, or chest in infancy and childhood increases the risk of thyroid carcinoma. The incidence of thyroid cancer appears to increase 5 to 40 years after irradiation. Consequently, people who underwent radiation treatment or were otherwise exposed to radiation as children should consult a physician, request an isotope thyroid scan as part of the evaluation, follow recommended treatment of abnormalities of the gland, and continue with annual checkups (Chart 43-8).

CHART 43-8

Radiation-Induced Thyroid Damage and Cancer

The thyroid gland has a very efficient mechanism to remove iodine from the bloodstream and concentrate or "trap" it for subsequent synthesis of thyroid hormone. The effectiveness of this mechanism to concentrate iodide is reflected in a concentration of iodide 20 to 40 times the concentration of iodide in the plasma.

If milk and other food sources become contaminated with radioactivity as a result of a nuclear detonation or a nuclear power plant incident or mishap, the radioactive iodide would become concentrated in the thyroid gland at a very high concentration and would irradiate the thyroid gland, increasing the risk for thyroid gland cancer. Therefore, in communities exposed to increased radioactivity, attempts have been made to block the uptake of radioactive iodide by flooding or saturating the thyroid gland with nonradioactive iodide.

Administration of potassium iodide (KI) or other iodide preparations as soon as possible after exposure almost completely inhibits thyroid absorption of the radioactive iodide and promotes rapid excretion of any that is absorbed.

Assessment and Diagnostic Findings

Lesions that are single, hard, and fixed on palpation or associated with cervical lymphadenopathy suggest malignancy. Thyroid function tests may be helpful in evaluating thyroid nodules and masses; however, results are rarely conclusive. Needle biopsy of the thyroid gland is used as an outpatient procedure to make a diagnosis of thyroid cancer, to differentiate cancerous thyroid nodules from noncancerous nodules, and to stage the cancer if detected. The procedure is safe and usually requires only a local

TABLE 43-4 Types of Thyroid Cancers

Type of Thyroid Cancer	Characteristics
Papillary adenocarcinoma	Most common and least aggressive Asymptomatic nodule in a normal gland Starts in childhood or early adult life, remains localized Metastasizes along the lymphatics if untreated More aggressive in older adults
Follicular adenocarcinoma	Appears after 40 years of age Encapsulated; feels elastic or rubbery on palpation Spreads through the bloodstream to bone, liver, and lung Prognosis is not as favourable as for papillary adenocarcinoma
Medullary	Appears after 50 years of age Occurs as part of multiple endocrine neoplasia (MEN) Hormone-producing tumour causing endocrine dysfunction symptoms Metastasizes by lymphatics and bloodstream Moderate survival rate
Anaplastic	50% of anaplastic thyroid carcinomas occur in patients older than 60 years Hard, irregular mass that grows quickly and spreads by direct invasion to adjacent tissues May be painful and tender Survival for patients with anaplastic cancer is usually less than 6 months
Thyroid lymphoma	Appears after 40 years of age May have history of goitre, hoarseness, dyspnea, pain, and pressure Good prognosis

anesthetic agent. However, patients who undergo the procedure are monitored closely, because cancerous tissues may be missed during the procedure. A second type of aspiration or biopsy uses a large-bore needle rather than the fine needle used in standard biopsy; it may be used when the results of the standard biopsy are inconclusive or with rapidly growing tumours. Additional diagnostic studies include ultrasound, MRI, CT, thyroid scans, radioactive iodine uptake studies, and thyroid suppression tests.

Medical Management

The treatment of choice for thyroid carcinoma is surgical removal. Total or near-total thyroidectomy is performed if possible. Modified neck dissection or more extensive radical neck dissection is performed if there is lymph node involvement.

Efforts are made to spare parathyroid tissue to reduce the risk of postoperative hypocalcemia and tetany. After surgery, ablation procedures are carried out with radioactive iodine to eradicate residual microscopic disease. Radioactive iodine is also used for thyroid cancers with metastasis. The use of radioactive iodine therapy has been crucial in making thyroid one of the most curable types of cancer (Dagan & Amdur, 2013).

After surgery, thyroid hormone is given to lower the levels of TSH to a euthyroid state (Bahn et al., 2011). If the remaining thyroid tissue is inadequate to produce sufficient thyroid hormone, thyroxine is required permanently.

Several routes are available for administering radiation to the thyroid or tissues of the neck, including oral administration of radioactive iodine (Bahn et al., 2011) and external administration of radiation therapy. Short-term side effects of radioactive iodine treatment may include neck soreness, nausea, and upset stomach; salivary glands being tender and swollen; dry mouth; changes in taste; and, rarely, pain (Bahn et al., 2011). The patient who receives external sources of radiation therapy is at risk for mucositis, dryness of the mouth, dysphagia, redness of the skin, anorexia, and fatigue (see Chapter 17). Chemotherapy is infrequently used to treat thyroid cancer.

Patients whose thyroid cancer is detected early and who are appropriately treated have a good prognosis. Patients who have had papillary cancer—the most common and least aggressive tumour—have the best prognosis of all thyroid cancers (Dagan & Amdur, 2013). Long-term survival is also common in follicular cancer, which is a more aggressive form of thyroid cancer (Dagan & Amdur, 2013). However, continued thyroid hormone therapy and periodic follow-up and diagnostic testing are important to ensure the patient's well-being.

Later follow-up includes clinical assessment for recurrence of nodules or masses in the neck and signs of hoarseness, dysphagia, or dyspnea. The recommendations for long-term follow-up of patients with differentiated thyroid cancer are based on the stage of cancer and results of the follow-up examination 1 year following the initial treatment. The first-year evaluation includes clinical examination, TSH and free thyroxine, and measurement of serum thyroglobulin within 6 months following the initial treatment, and a routine neck ultrasound with the first 6 to 12 months following initial treatment. Tests used to confirm sites of metastasis if there is clinical evidence of recurrence include radioiodine imaging, CT, MRI, skeletal x-rays, and skeletal radionucleotide imaging. Fluorodeoxyglucose (FGDA) PET is useful to establish prognosis if there is evidence of distant metastases (Tuttle, 2016). Free T_4, TSH, and serum calcium and phosphorus levels are monitored to determine whether the thyroid hormone supplementation is adequate and to note whether calcium balance is maintained.

Although local and systemic reactions to radiation may occur and may include neutropenia or thrombocytopenia, these complications are rare when radioactive iodine is used. Patients who undergo surgery that is combined with radioactive iodine have a higher survival rate than those who undergo surgery alone. Patient teaching emphasizes the importance of taking prescribed medications and following recommendations for follow-up monitoring. The patient who is undergoing radiation therapy is also instructed in how to assess and manage side effects of treatment.

Nursing Management

Important preoperative goals are to prepare the patient for surgery and reduce anxiety. Often, the patient's home life has become tense because of their restlessness, irritability, and nervousness secondary to hyperthyroidism. Efforts are necessary to protect the patient from tension and stress to avoid precipitating thyroid storm. Suggestions are made to limit stressful situations. Quiet and relaxing activities are encouraged.

Providing Preoperative Care

The nurse instructs the patient about the importance of eating a diet high in carbohydrates and proteins. A high daily caloric intake is necessary because of the increased metabolic activity and rapid depletion of glycogen reserves. Supplementary vitamins, particularly thiamine and ascorbic acid, may be prescribed. The patient is reminded to avoid tea, coffee, cola, and other stimulants.

The nurse also informs the patient about the purpose of preoperative tests, if they are to be performed, and explains what preoperative preparations to expect. This information should help to reduce the patient's anxiety about the surgery. In addition, special efforts are made to ensure a good night's rest before surgery, although many patients are admitted to the hospital on the day of surgery.

Preoperative teaching includes demonstrating to the patient how to support the neck with the hands after surgery to prevent stress on the incision. This involves raising the elbows and placing the hands behind the neck to provide support and reduce strain and tension on the neck muscles and the surgical incision.

Providing Postoperative Care

The nurse periodically assesses the surgical dressings and reinforces them if necessary. When the patient is in a recumbent position, the nurse observes the sides and the back of the neck as well as the anterior dressing for bleeding. In addition to monitoring the pulse and blood pressure for any indication of internal bleeding, it is important to be alert for complaints of a sensation of pressure or fullness at the incision site. Such symptoms may indicate subcutaneous hemorrhage and hematoma formation and should be reported.

Difficulty in respiration can occur as a result of edema of the glottis, hematoma formation, or injury to the recurrent laryngeal nerve. This complication requires that an airway be inserted. Therefore, a tracheostomy set is kept at the bedside at all times, and the surgeon is summoned at the first indication of respiratory distress. If the respiratory distress is caused by hematoma, surgical evacuation is required.

The intensity of pain is assessed, and analgesic agents are administered as prescribed for pain. The nurse should anticipate apprehension in the patient and should inform the patient that oxygen will assist breathing. When moving and turning the patient, the nurse carefully supports the patient's head and avoids tension on the sutures. The most comfortable position is the semi-Fowler's position, with the head elevated and supported by pillows.

IV fluids are administered during the immediate postoperative period. Water may be given by mouth as soon as nausea subsides. Usually, there is a little difficulty in swallowing; initially, cold fluids and ice may be taken better than other fluids. Often, patients prefer a soft diet to a liquid diet in the immediate postoperative period.

The patient is advised to talk as little as possible to reduce edema to the vocal cords; however, when the patient does speak, any voice changes are noted, which might indicate injury to the recurrent laryngeal nerve, which lies just behind the thyroid next to the trachea. An overbed table is provided for access to frequently used items so the patient avoids turning his or her head. The table can also be used to support a humidifier when vapor-mist inhalations are prescribed for the relief of excessive mucus accumulation.

The patient is encouraged to be out of bed as soon as possible and to eat foods that are easily swallowed. A high-calorie diet may be prescribed to promote weight gain. The incision may be closed using absorbable sutures, nonabsorbable sutures, and adhesive strips. Absorbable sutures dissolve within the body. If nonabsorbable sutures are used, the timeline for removal may vary; however, these types of sutures are usually removed 5 to 7 days following surgery. Adhesives will peel off spontaneously. The patient is usually discharged from the hospital on the day of surgery or soon afterward if the postoperative course is uncomplicated.

Monitoring and Managing Potential Complications

Hemorrhage, hematoma formation, edema of the glottis, and injury to the laryngeal nerve are complications reviewed previously in this chapter. Occasionally in thyroid surgery, the parathyroid glands are injured or removed, producing a disturbance in calcium metabolism. As the blood calcium level falls, hyperirritability of the nerves occurs, with spasms of the hands and feet and muscle twitching (see Chapter 17). This group of symptoms is termed *tetany*, and the nurse must immediately report its appearance because laryngospasm, although rare, may occur and obstruct the airway. Tetany of this type is usually treated with IV calcium gluconate. This calcium abnormality is usually temporary after thyroidectomy unless all parathyroid tissues were removed.

> **NURSING ALERT**
>
> **Following thyroid surgery, the patient should be monitored closely for signs of tetany, including hyperirritability of the nerves, with spasms of the hands and feet and muscle twitching. Laryngospasm, although rare, may occur and obstruct the airway.**

Promoting Home, Community-Based, and Transitional Care

The patient is usually discharged within 1 or 2 days. Therefore, the patient and family need to be knowledgeable about the signs and symptoms of the complications that may occur and those that should be reported. Strategies are suggested for managing postoperative pain at home and for increasing humidification. The nurse explains to the patient and family the need for rest, relaxation, and nutrition. The patient is permitted to resume his or her former activities and responsibilities completely once recovered from surgery.

If indicated, a referral to home care is made. The home care nurse assesses the patient's recovery from surgery. The nurse also assesses the surgical incision and reinforces instruction about limiting activities that put strain on the incision and sutures. Family responsibilities and factors relating to the home environment that produce emotional tension have often been implicated as precipitating causes of thyrotoxicosis. A home visit provides an opportunity to evaluate these factors and to suggest ways to improve the home and family environment. The nurse instructs the patients about the importance of follow-up visits to the physician or the clinic for monitoring of thyroid status.

THE PARATHYROID GLANDS

Anatomic and Physiologic Overview

The parathyroid glands (normally four) are situated in the neck and embedded in the posterior aspect of the thyroid gland (see Fig. 43-5). Parathormone (parathyroid hormone)—the protein hormone produced by the parathyroid glands—regulates calcium and phosphorus metabolism. Increased secretion of parathormone results in increased calcium absorption from the kidney, intestine, and bones, which raises the serum calcium level (Grossman & Porth, 2014). Some actions of this hormone are increased by the presence of vitamin D. Parathormone also tends to lower the blood phosphorus level. The serum level of ionized calcium regulates the output of parathormone. Increased serum calcium results in decreased parathormone secretion, creating a negative feedback system.

Pathophysiology

Excess parathormone can result in markedly increased levels of serum calcium, a potentially life-threatening situation. When the product of serum calcium and serum phosphorus (calcium × phosphorus) rises, calcium phosphate may

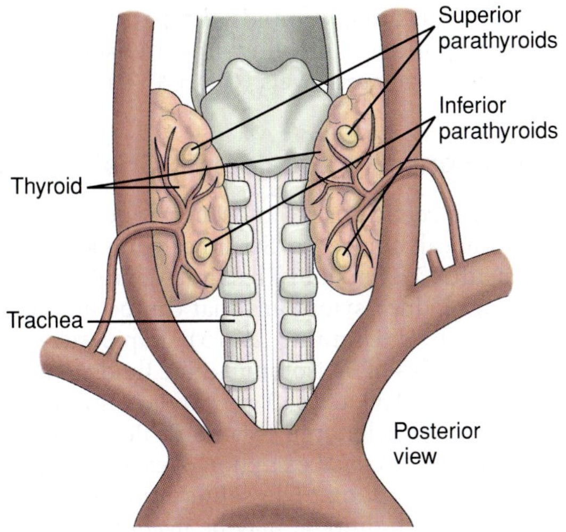

FIGURE 43-5. The parathyroid glands are located behind the thyroid gland. The parathyroids may be embedded in the thyroid tissue.

precipitate in various organs of the body (e.g., the kidneys) and cause tissue calcification.

Hyperparathyroidism

Hyperparathyroidism, which is caused by overproduction of parathormone by the parathyroid glands, is characterized by bone decalcification and the development of renal calculi (kidney stones) containing calcium. Primary hyperparathyroidism occurs two to four times more often in women than in men and is most common in people between 60 and 70 years of age. Its incidence is approximately 25 cases per 100,000 people. The disorder is rare in children younger than 15 years, but its incidence increases 10-fold between the ages of 15 and 65 years. Half of the people diagnosed with hyperparathyroidism do not have symptoms (Fuleihan & Silverberg, 2017).

Secondary hyperparathyroidism, with manifestations similar to those of primary hyperparathyroidism, occurs in patients who have chronic renal failure and the so-called renal rickets as a result of phosphorus retention, increased stimulation of the parathyroid glands, and increased parathormone secretion.

Clinical Manifestations

The patient may have no symptoms or may experience signs and symptoms resulting from involvement of several body systems. Apathy, fatigue, muscle weakness, nausea, vomiting, constipation, hypertension, and cardiac dysrhythmias may occur. All these signs and symptoms are attributable to the increased concentration of calcium in the blood. Psychological effects may vary from irritability and neurosis to psychoses caused by the direct action of calcium on the brain and nervous system. An increase in calcium produces a decrease in the excitation potential of nerve and muscle tissue.

The formation of stones in one or both kidneys (nephrolithiasis), related to the increased urinary excretion of calcium and phosphorus, is one of the major complications of hyperparathyroidism. Although the incidence is on the decline in the United States, it occurs in 15% to 20% of newly diagnosed patients (Fuleihan & Silverberg, 2017). Kidney damage can result from the precipitation of calcium phosphate in the renal pelvis and parenchyma, which causes renal calculi (kidney stones), obstruction, pyelonephritis, and kidney injury.

Musculoskeletal symptoms accompanying hyperparathyroidism may be caused by demineralization of the bones or by bone tumours composed of benign giant cells resulting from overgrowth of osteoclasts. The patient may develop skeletal pain and tenderness, especially of the back and joints; pain on weight bearing; pathologic fractures; deformities; and shortening of body stature. Bone loss attributable to hyperparathyroidism increases the risk of fracture.

The incidence of peptic ulcer and pancreatitis is increased with hyperparathyroidism and may be responsible for many of the GI symptoms that occur.

Assessment and Diagnostic Findings

Primary hyperparathyroidism is diagnosed by persistent elevation of serum calcium levels and an elevated concentration of parathormone. Radioimmunoassays for parathormone are sensitive and differentiate primary hyperparathyroidism from other causes of hypercalcemia in more than 80% of patients with elevated serum calcium levels (Fuleihan & Silverberg, 2017). An elevated serum calcium level alone is a nonspecific finding, because serum levels may be altered by diet, medications, and kidney and bone changes. Bone changes may be detected on x-ray or bone scans in advanced disease. The double-antibody parathyroid hormone test is used to distinguish between primary hyperparathyroidism and malignancy as a cause of hypercalcemia. Ultrasound, MRI, thallium scan, and fine-needle biopsy have been used to evaluate the function of the parathyroids and to localize parathyroid cysts, adenomas, or hyperplasia.

Medical Management

Surgical Management

The recommended treatment for primary hyperparathyroidism is the surgical removal of abnormal parathyroid tissue (parathyroidectomy) (Fuleihan & Silverberg, 2017). In the past, the standard parathyroidectomy involved a bilateral neck exploration under general anesthesia. Today, minimally invasive parathyroidectomy techniques allow for unilateral neck exploration using local anesthesia; these are performed on an outpatient basis. In some cases, only the removal of a single diseased gland is necessary, reducing morbidity rates associated with surgery. For asymptomatic patients who have only mildly elevated serum calcium concentrations and normal kidney function, surgery may be delayed and the patient monitored closely for worsening of hypercalcemia, bone deterioration, renal impairment, or the development of kidney stones.

Surgery is recommended for asymptomatic patients who meet one or more of the following criteria: (1) younger than 50 years, (2) any patient unable or unlikely to participate in follow-up care, (3) serum calcium level more than 1 mg/dL (0.25 mmol/L) above normal reference range, (3) GFR < 60 mL/min, (4) urinary calcium level greater than 400 mg/day (10 mmol/day, (5) bone density at hip, lumbar spine, or distal radius with T score < –2.5 or previous fracture fragility at any site, (6) nephrolithiasis or nephrocalcinosis (Fuleihan & Silverberg, 2017).

Hydration Therapy

Patients with hyperparathyroidism are at risk for renal calculi. Therefore, a daily fluid intake of 2,000 mL or more is encouraged to help prevent calculus formation. The patient is instructed to report other manifestations of renal calculi, such as abdominal pain and hematuria. Thiazide diuretics are avoided, because they decrease the renal excretion of calcium and further elevate serum calcium levels. Because of the risk of hypercalcemic crisis (see later discussion), the patient is instructed to avoid dehydration and to seek immediate health care if conditions that commonly produce dehydration (e.g., vomiting, diarrhea) occur.

Mobility

Mobility of the patient, with walking or use of a rocking chair for those with limited mobility, is encouraged as much as possible, because bones that are subjected to normal stress give up less calcium. Bed rest increases calcium excretion and the risk for renal calculi. Oral phosphates lower the serum calcium level in some patients; long-term use is not recommended because of the risk of ectopic calcium phosphate deposition in soft tissues.

Diet and Medications

Nutritional needs are met, but the patient is advised to avoid a diet with restricted or excess calcium. If the patient has a coexisting peptic ulcer, prescribed antacids and protein feedings are necessary. Because anorexia is common, efforts are made to improve the appetite. Prune juice, stool softeners, and physical activity, along with increased fluid intake, help offset constipation, which is common postoperatively.

Nursing Management

The insidious onset and chronic nature of hyperparathyroidism and its diverse and commonly vague symptoms may result in depression and frustration. The family may have considered the patient's illness to be psychosomatic. An awareness of the course of the disorder and an understanding approach by the nurse may help the patient and family deal with their reactions and feelings.

The nursing management of the patient undergoing parathyroidectomy is essentially the same as that of a patient undergoing thyroidectomy. However, the previously described precautions about airway patency, dehydration, immobility, and diet are particularly important in the patient who is awaiting or recovering from parathyroidectomy. Although not all parathyroid tissue is removed during surgery in an effort to control the calcium–phosphorus balance, the nurse closely monitors the patient to detect symptoms of tetany (which may be an early postoperative complication). Most patients quickly regain function of the remaining parathyroid tissue and experience only mild, transient postoperative hypocalcemia. In patients with significant bone disease or bone changes, a more prolonged period of hypocalcemia should be anticipated. The nurse reminds the patient and family about the importance of follow-up to ensure return to expected serum calcium levels (Chart 43-9).

Complications: Hypercalcemic Crisis

Acute hypercalcemic crisis can occur with extreme elevation of serum calcium levels. Serum calcium levels greater than 13 mg/dL (3.25 mmol/L) result in neurologic, cardiovascular, and kidney symptoms that can be life threatening (Fischbach & Dunning, 2015). Rapid rehydration with large volumes of IV isotonic saline fluids to maintain urine output of 100 to 150 mL/hr is combined with administration of calcitonin (Shane & Berenson, 2016). Calcitonin promotes renal excretion of excess calcium and reduces bone resorption. The saline infusion should be stopped and a loop diuretic may be needed if the patient develops edema. Dosage and rates of infusion depend on the patient profile. The patient should be monitored carefully for fluid overload. Loop diuretics are not recommended as initial therapy in the absence of heart failure and kidney insufficiency. Bisphosphonates are added to promote a sustained decrease in serum calcium levels by promoting calcium deposition in bone and reducing the GI absorption of calcium. Cytotoxic agents (e.g., mithramycin), calcitonin, and dialysis may be used in emergency situations to decrease serum calcium levels quickly.

NURSING ALERT

The patient in acute hypercalcemic crisis requires close monitoring for life-threatening complications and prompt treatment to reduce serum calcium levels.

A combination of calcitonin and corticosteroids has been administered in emergencies to reduce the serum calcium level by increasing calcium deposition in bone. Other agents that may be administered to decrease serum calcium levels include bisphosphonates (e.g., etidronate [Didronel], pamidronate [Aredia]) (Shane & Berenson, 2016).

Expert assessment and care are required to minimize complications and reverse the life-threatening hypercalcemia. Medications are administered with care, and attention is given to fluid balance to promote return of usual fluid and electrolyte balance. Supportive measures are necessary for the patient and family. (See Chapters 17 and 68 for further discussion of hypercalcemic crisis.)

Hypoparathyroidism

Hypoparathyroidism is caused by abnormal parathyroid development, destruction of the parathyroid glands (surgical removal or autoimmune response), and vitamin D deficiency. The most common cause is the near-total removal of the thyroid gland. The result is inadequate secretion of parathormone (Goltzman, 2016).

Deficiency of parathormone results in increased blood phosphate (hyperphosphatemia) and decreased blood calcium (hypocalcemia) levels. In the absence of parathormone, there is decreased intestinal absorption of dietary

CHART 43-9

HOME CARE CHECKLIST • The Patient's Hyperparathyroidism

At the completion of education, the patient and/or caregiver will be able to:

- State the impact of hyperparathyroidism and treatment on physiologic functioning, ADLs, IADLs, roles, relationships, and spirituality.
- Describe potential benefits and risks of parathyroidectomy.
- State the name, dose, side effects, frequency, and schedule for all medications.
- Explain the purpose, dose, route, schedule, side effects, and precautions of pharmacologic treatment (loop diuretics, phosphates, and calcitonin) of hyperparathyroidism.
- State the need to contact primary provider before taking over-the-counter medication containing calcium.
- State changes in lifestyle (e.g., diet, activity) necessary to maintain health, including:
  - Recommended intake of dietary calcium.
  - Maintenance of regular bowel habits and management of constipation (e.g., prune juice, stool softeners, increased physical activity and fluids).
  - Monitoring of fluid intake as indicated, generally 2,000 mL daily.
  - Managing pain (medication and nonpharmacologic interventions).
  - Increasing mobility as indicated
- Relate how to reach primary provider with questions or complications.
- State time and date of follow-up medical appointments, therapy, and testing.
- Identify sources of support (e.g., friends, relatives, faith community, support groups, caregiver support).
- Identify the need for health promotion, disease prevention, and screening activities.

ADL, activities of daily living; IADL, independent activities of daily living.

calcium and decreased resorption of calcium from bone and through the renal tubules. Decreased renal excretion of phosphate causes hypophosphaturia, and low serum calcium levels result in hypocalciuria.

Clinical Manifestations

Hypocalcemia causes irritability of the neuromuscular system and contributes to the chief symptom of hypoparathyroidism—tetany. Tetany is a general muscle hypertonia, with tremor and spasmodic or uncoordinated contractions occurring with or without efforts to make voluntary movements. Symptoms of latent tetany are numbness, tingling, and cramps in the extremities, and the patient reports stiffness in the hands and feet. In overt tetany, the signs include bronchospasm, laryngeal spasm, carpopedal spasm (flexion of the elbows and wrists and extension of the carpophalangeal joints and dorsiflexion of the feet), dysphagia, photophobia, cardiac dysrhythmias, and seizures. Other symptoms include anxiety, irritability, depression, and even delirium. ECG changes and hypotension also may occur.

Assessment and Diagnostic Findings

A positive **Chvostek sign** or a positive **Trousseau's sign** suggests latent tetany. Chvostek sign is positive when a sharp tapping over the facial nerve just in front of the parotid gland and anterior to the ear causes spasm or twitching of the mouth, nose, and eye (see Fig. 13-6A). Trousseau's sign is positive when carpopedal spasm is induced by occluding the blood flow to the arm for 3 minutes with a blood pressure cuff (see Fig. 13-6B). The diagnosis of hypoparathyroidism often is difficult because of the vague symptoms, such as aches and pains. Therefore, laboratory studies are especially helpful. Tetany develops at very low serum calcium levels. Serum phosphate levels are increased, and x-rays of bone show increased density. Calcification is detected on x-rays of the subcutaneous or paraspinal basal ganglia of the brain.

Medical Management

The goal of therapy is to increase the serum calcium level to 2.2 to 2.5 mmol/L and to eliminate the symptoms of hypoparathyroidism and hypocalcemia. Management is determined by the underlying cause and patient profile. Treatment may include combinations of calcitriol, calcium, magnesium, and vitamin D_2 (ergocalciferol) or vitamin D_3 (calcitriol), the latter being preferred. A thiazide diuretic (e.g., hydrochlorothiazide [HydroDIURIL]) may be given to help decrease urinary calcium excretion (Goltzman, 2016; Rosen, 2016). Recombinant parathyroid hormone

CHART 43-10

HOME CARE CHECKLIST • The Patient With Hypoparathyroidism

At the completion of education, the patient and/or caregiver will be able to:

- State the impact of hypoparathyroidism and treatment on physiologic functioning, ADLs, IADLs, roles, relationships, and spirituality.
- State purpose, dose, route, schedule, side effects, and precautions of prescribed medications (calcium, phosphate binders).
- State changes in lifestyle (e.g., diet, activity) necessary to maintain health, including:
    - Ensuring a diet high in calcium and vitamin D, low in phosphorous.
    - Alternating activity and rest periods.
- State precipitating factors and interventions for complications (seizure, cardiac dysrhythmias, cardiac arrest).
- State necessary actions for seizure activity.
- Relate how to reach primary provider with questions or complications.
- State time and date of follow-up medical appointments, therapy, and testing.
- Identify sources of support (e.g., friends, relatives, faith community, support groups, caregiver support).
- Identify the need for health promotion, disease prevention, and screening activities.

ADL, activities of daily living; IADL, independent activities of daily living.

has been approved for the treatment of osteoporosis but not for hypoparathyroidism at this time (Goltzman, 2016; Rosen, 2016).

When hypocalcemia and tetany occur after a thyroidectomy, the immediate treatment is administration of IV calcium gluconate. If this does not decrease neuromuscular irritability and seizure activity immediately, sedative agents such as pentobarbital may be given.

Because of neuromuscular irritability, the patient with hypocalcemia and tetany requires an environment that is free of noise, drafts, bright lights, or sudden movement. Tracheostomy or mechanical ventilation may become necessary, along with bronchodilating medications, if the patient develops respiratory distress.

Therapy for chronic hypoparathyroidism is determined after serum calcium levels are obtained. A diet high in calcium and low in phosphorus is prescribed. Although milk, milk products, and egg yolk are high in calcium, they are restricted because they also contain high levels of phosphorus. Spinach also is avoided because it contains oxalate, which would form insoluble calcium substances. Oral tablets of calcium salts, such as calcium gluconate, may be used to supplement the diet. Aluminum hydroxide gel or aluminum carbonate (Gelusil, Amphojel) also is given after meals to bind phosphate and promote its excretion through the GI tract.

Nursing Management

Nursing management of the patient with possible acute hypoparathyroidism includes the following:

- Care of postoperative patients who have undergone thyroidectomy, parathyroidectomy, or radical neck dissection is directed toward detecting early signs of hypocalcemia and anticipating signs of tetany, seizures, and respiratory difficulties.
- Calcium gluconate is kept at the bedside with equipment necessary for emergency IV administration. If the patient requiring administration of calcium gluconate has a cardiac disorder, is subject to dysrhythmias, or is receiving digitalis, the calcium gluconate is administered slowly and cautiously.
- Calcium and digitalis increase systolic contraction and also potentiate each other; this can produce potentially fatal dysrhythmias. Consequently, the cardiac patient requires continuous cardiac monitoring and careful assessment.

An important aspect of nursing care is teaching about medications and diet therapy. The patient needs to know the reason for high calcium and low phosphate intake and the symptoms of hypocalcemia and hypercalcemia; he or she should know to contact the physician immediately if these symptoms occur (Chart 43-10).

THE ADRENAL GLANDS

Anatomic and Physiologic Overview

Each person has two adrenal glands, one attached to the upper portion of each kidney (Porth, 2015). Each adrenal gland is, in reality, two endocrine glands with separate, independent functions. The adrenal medulla at the centre of the gland secretes catecholamines, and the outer portion of the gland, the adrenal cortex, secretes steroid hormones (see Fig. 43-6). The secretion of hormones from the adrenal cortex is regulated by the hypothalamic–pituitary–adrenal axis. The hypothalamus secretes corticotropin-releasing

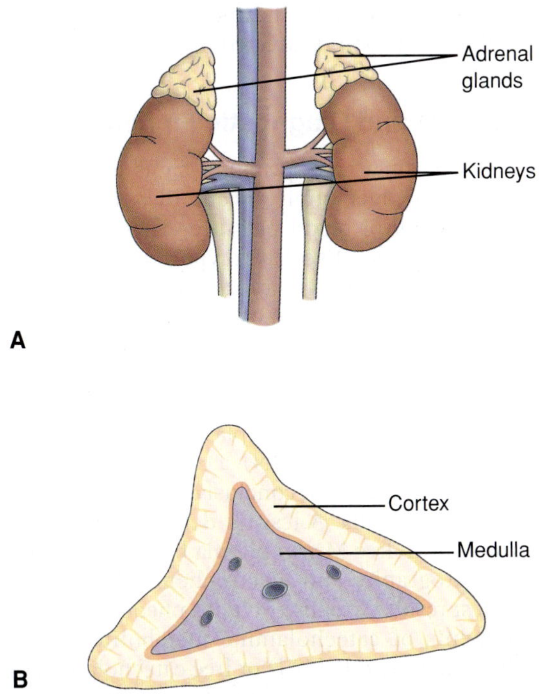

FIGURE 43-6. A. The adrenal glands sit on top of the kidneys. B. Each gland is composed of an outer cortex and an inner medulla. Each area secretes specific hormones. The adrenal medulla secretes catecholamines—epinephrine and norepinephrine; the adrenal cortex secretes glucocorticoids, mineralocorticoids, and sex hormones. (Adapted from Porth, C. M. [2006]. *Essentials of pathophysiology: Concepts of altered health states* [2nd ed.]. Philadelphia, PA: Lippincott Williams & Wilkins.)

hormone (CRH), which stimulates the pituitary gland to secrete ACTH, which in turn stimulates the adrenal cortex to secrete glucocorticoid hormone (cortisol). Increased levels of the adrenal hormone then inhibit the production or secretion of CRH and ACTH. This system is an example of a negative feedback mechanism.

Adrenal Medulla

The adrenal medulla functions as part of the autonomic nervous system. Stimulation of preganglionic sympathetic nerve fibres, which travel directly to the cells of the adrenal medulla, causes release of the catecholamine hormones epinephrine and norepinephrine. About 90% of the secretion of the human adrenal medulla is epinephrine (also called **adrenaline**). Catecholamines regulate metabolic pathways to promote catabolism of stored fuels to meet caloric needs from endogenous sources. The major effects of epinephrine release are to prepare to meet a challenge (fight-or-flight response). Secretion of epinephrine causes decreased blood flow to tissues that are not needed in emergency situations, such as the GI tract, and increased blood flow to tissues that are important for effective fight or flight, such as cardiac and skeletal muscle. Catecholamines also induce the release of free fatty acids, increase the basal metabolic rate, and elevate the blood glucose level.

Adrenal Cortex

A functioning adrenal cortex is necessary for life; adrenocortical secretions make it possible for the body to adapt to stress of all kinds. The three types of steroid hormones produced by the adrenal cortex are glucocorticoids, mainly cortisol; **mineralocorticoids**, mainly aldosterone; and sex hormones, mainly androgens (male sex hormones) (Porth, 2015). Without the adrenal cortex, severe stress would cause peripheral circulatory failure, circulatory shock, and prostration. Survival in the absence of a functioning adrenal cortex is possible only with nutritional, electrolyte, and fluid replacement and appropriate replacement with exogenous adrenocortical hormones.

Glucocorticoids

The glucocorticoids are so named because they have an important influence on glucose metabolism: Increased hydrocortisone secretion results in elevated blood glucose levels. However, the glucocorticoids have major effects on the metabolism of almost all organs of the body. Glucocorticoids are secreted from the adrenal cortex in response to the release of ACTH from the anterior lobe of the pituitary gland. This system represents an example of negative feedback. The presence of glucocorticoids in the blood inhibits the release of CRH from the hypothalamus and also inhibits ACTH secretion from the pituitary. The resultant decrease in ACTH secretion causes diminished release of glucocorticoids from the adrenal cortex.

Glucocorticoids (in the form of corticosteroids) are administered frequently to inhibit the inflammatory response to tissue injury and to suppress allergic manifestations. Their side effects include the development of diabetes mellitus, osteoporosis, peptic ulcer, increased protein breakdown resulting in muscle wasting and poor wound healing, and redistribution of body fat. Large amounts of exogenously administered glucocorticoids in the blood inhibit the release of ACTH and endogenous glucocorticoids. Because of this, the adrenal cortex can atrophy. If exogenous glucocorticoid administration is discontinued suddenly, adrenal insufficiency results because of the inability of the atrophied cortex to respond adequately.

Mineralocorticoids

Mineralocorticoids exert their major effects on electrolyte metabolism. They act principally on the renal tubular and GI epithelium to cause increased sodium ion absorption in exchange for excretion of potassium or hydrogen ions. ACTH only minimally influences aldosterone secretion. It is primarily secreted in response to the presence of angiotensin II in the bloodstream. Angiotensin II is a substance that elevates the blood pressure by constricting arterioles. Its concentration is increased when renin is released from the kidney in response to decreased perfusion pressure. The resultant increased aldosterone levels promote sodium reabsorption by the kidney and the GI tract, which tends to restore blood pressure to normal. The release of aldosterone is also increased by hyperkalemia. Aldosterone is the primary hormone for the long-term regulation of sodium balance.

Adrenal Sex Hormones (Androgens)

Androgens, the third major type of steroid hormones produced by the adrenal cortex, exert effects similar to those of male sex hormones. The adrenal gland may also secrete small amounts of some estrogens, or female sex hormones. ACTH controls the secretion of adrenal androgens. When secreted in normal amounts, the adrenal androgens probably have little effect, but when secreted in excess, as in certain inborn enzyme deficiencies, masculinization may result. This is termed the **adrenogenital syndrome**.

Pheochromocytoma

Pheochromocytoma is a tumour that is usually benign and originates from the chromaffin cells of the adrenal medulla. This tumour is the cause of high blood pressure in 0.1% of patients with hypertension and is usually fatal if undetected and untreated. Although uncommon, it is one form of hypertension that is usually cured by surgery. In 90% of patients (Porth, 2015), the tumour arises in the medulla; in the remaining patients, it occurs in the extra-adrenal chromaffin tissue located in or near the aorta, ovaries, spleen, or other organs. Pheochromocytoma may occur at any age, but its peak incidence is between 40 and 50 years of age and affects men and women equally (Young & Kaplan, 2016). Ten percent of the tumours are bilateral, and 10% are malignant. Because of the high incidence of pheochromocytoma in family members of affected people, the patient's family members should be alerted and screened for this tumour. Pheochromocytoma may occur in the familial form as part of multiple endocrine neoplasia type 2; therefore, it should be considered a possibility in patients who have medullary thyroid carcinoma and parathyroid hyperplasia or tumour.

Clinical Manifestations

The nature and severity of symptoms of functioning tumours of the adrenal medulla depend on the relative proportions of epinephrine and norepinephrine secretion. The typical triad of symptoms is headache, diaphoresis, and palpitations in the patient with hypertension. The tumour is discovered incidentally in approximately 10% of patients (Young, Kaplan, & Kebebew, 2016). Hypertension and other cardiovascular disturbances are common. The hypertension may be intermittent or persistent. If the hypertension is sustained, it may be difficult to distinguish from other causes of hypertension. Other symptoms may include tremor, headache, flushing, and anxiety. Hyperglycemia may result from conversion of liver and muscle glycogen to glucose due to epinephrine secretion; insulin may be required to maintain normal blood glucose levels.

The clinical picture in the paroxysmal form of pheochromocytoma is usually characterized by acute, unpredictable attacks lasting seconds or several hours. Symptoms usually begin abruptly and subside slowly. During these attacks, the patient is extremely anxious, tremulous, and weak. The patient may experience headache, vertigo, blurring of vision, tinnitus, air hunger, and dyspnea. Other symptoms include polyuria, nausea, vomiting, diarrhea, abdominal pain, and a feeling of impending doom. Palpitations and tachycardia are common (Porth, 2015). Blood pressures exceeding 250/150 mm Hg have been recorded. Such blood pressure elevations are life threatening and can cause severe complications, such as cardiac dysrhythmias, dissecting aneurysm, stroke, and acute kidney failure. Postural hypotension (decrease in systolic blood pressure, lightheadedness, dizziness on standing) occurs in 70% of patients with untreated pheochromocytoma.

Assessment and Diagnostic Findings

Pheochromocytoma is suspected if signs of sympathetic nervous system overactivity occur in association with marked elevation of blood pressure. These signs can be associated with the "five Hs": *h*ypertension, *h*eadache, *h*yperhidrosis (excessive sweating), *h*ypermetabolism, and *h*yperglycemia. The presence of these signs is highly predictive of pheochromocytoma. Paroxysmal symptoms of pheochromocytoma commonly develop in the fifth decade of life.

Measurements of urine and plasma levels of catecholamines and metanephrine (MN), a catecholamine metabolite, are the most direct and conclusive tests for overactivity of the adrenal medulla. A test for detecting pheochromocytoma measures free MN in plasma by high-pressure liquid chromatography and electrochemical detection. A negative test result virtually excludes pheochromocytoma. Measurements of catecholamine metabolites (MN and vanillylmandelic acid [VMA]) or free catecholamines have been extensively used in the clinical setting. In most cases, pheochromocytoma can be diagnosed or confirmed based on a properly collected 24-hour urine sample. Levels can be as high as two times the normal limit. A 24-hour urine specimen is collected to detect free catecholamines, MN, and VMA; the use of combined tests increases the diagnostic accuracy of testing. A number of medications and foods, such as coffee and tea (including decaffeinated varieties), bananas, chocolate, vanilla, and aspirin, may alter the results of these tests; therefore, careful instructions to avoid restricted items must be given to the patient. Urine collected over a 2- or 3-hour period after an attack of hypertension can be assayed for catecholamine content (Young et al., 2016).

The total plasma catecholamine (epinephrine and norepinephrine) concentration is measured with the patient supine and at rest for 30 minutes. To prevent elevation of catecholamine levels resulting from the stress of venipuncture, a butterfly needle, scalp vein needle, or venous catheter may be inserted 30 minutes before the blood specimen is obtained.

Factors that may elevate catecholamine concentrations must be controlled to obtain valid results; these factors include consumption of coffee or tea (including decaffeinated varieties), use of tobacco, emotional and physical stress, and use of many prescription and over-the-counter medications (e.g., amphetamines, nose drops or sprays, decongestant agents, bronchodilators).

Expected plasma values of epinephrine are 590 pmol/L; expected values of norepinephrine are generally less than 590 to 3,240 pmol/L. Values of epinephrine greater than 2,180 pmol/L or norepinephrine values greater than 11,800 pmol/L are considered diagnostic of pheochromocytoma. Values that fall between normal levels and those diagnostic of pheochromocytoma indicate the need for further testing.

A clonidine suppression test may be performed if the results of plasma and urine tests of catecholamines are inconclusive. Clonidine (Catapres) is a centrally acting antiadrenergic medication that suppresses the release of neurogenically mediated catecholamines. The suppression test is based on the principle that catecholamine levels are normally increased through the activity of the sympathetic nervous system. In pheochromocytoma, increased catecholamine levels result from the diffusion of excess catecholamines into the circulation, bypassing normal storage and release mechanisms. Therefore, in patients with pheochromocytoma, clonidine does not suppress the release of catecholamines (Young & Kaplan, 2016).

Imaging studies, such as CT, MRI, and ultrasonography, may also be carried out to localize the pheochromocytoma and to determine whether more than one tumour is present. The use of ^{131}I-metaiodobenzylguanidine (MIBG) scintigraphy may be required to determine the location of the pheochromocytoma and to detect metastatic sites outside the adrenal gland. MIBG is a specific isotope for catecholamine-producing tissue. It has been helpful in identifying tumours not detected by other tests or procedures. MIBG scintigraphy is a noninvasive, safe procedure that has increased the accuracy of diagnosis of adrenal tumours (Fischbach & Dunning, 2015).

Other diagnostic studies may focus on evaluating the function of other endocrine glands because of the association of pheochromocytoma in some patients with other endocrine tumours.

Medical Management

During an episode or attack of hypertension, tachycardia, anxiety, and the other symptoms of pheochromocytoma, bed rest with the head of the bed elevated is prescribed to promote an orthostatic decrease in blood pressure.

Pharmacologic Therapy

The patient may be treated preoperatively on an inpatient or outpatient basis. Regardless of the setting, monitoring of blood pressure and cardiac function is essential. The goals are to control hypertension before and during surgery and volume expansion. Although there are no randomized controlled studies that have compared the efficacy of different treatments, the use of an alpha-adrenergic blocker, sometimes in tandem with a beta-adrenergic blocker, has led to positive outcomes. In some instances, calcium channel blockers and metyrosine have been also been used successfully.

Preoperatively, the patient may begin treatment with a low dose of an alpha-adrenergic blocker (phenoxybenzamine [Dibenzyline]) 10 to 14 days or longer prior to surgery (Young et al., 2016). The patient should be informed about the potential for adverse effects of these medications, which include orthostasis, nasal stuffiness, increased fatigue, and retrograde ejaculation in men. The dosage is increased every 2 to 3 days as needed to control blood pressure, with the final dose usually ranging between 20 to 100 mg daily (Young et al., 2016). Some practitioners may prefer the use of a selective alpha$_1$-adrenergic blocker with fewer side effects, such as prazosin (Minipress), terazosin (Hytrin), or doxazosin (Cardura), when long-term therapy is indicated. Unless contraindicated, patients are encouraged to begin a high-sodium diet on the second or third day after the introduction of alpha-adrenergic blockade.

After administration of the alpha-blockers, the blood pressure should be monitored closely. In an outpatient setting, the blood pressure should be taken twice daily in a sitting and standing position. The targets are 120/80 mm Hg (seated) with a standing systolic pressure greater than 90 mm Hg. Age and comorbid disease should be taken into consideration when establishing and evaluating targets. Cautious low-dose beta-adrenergic blockade (e.g., propranolol) is only initiated once adequate alpha-adrenergic control has been achieved (Young et al., 2016). The dosage is adjusted according to the patient response and ability to tolerate the drug. The dosage may be initiated in daily divided doses and on day 2 adjusted to a single long-acting dose. On subsequent days, the dose may be increased to control tachycardia as needed with a target heart rate of 60 to 80 bpm.

Calcium channel blockers such as nifedipine (Procardia) are sometimes used as an alternative or supplement to preoperative alpha- and beta-blockers, when blood pressure control is inadequate or the patient is unable to tolerate the side effects. Nifedipine and nicardipine (Cardene) may be used safely without causing undue hypotension. For episodes of severe hypertension, nifedipine is a fast and effective treatment, because the capsules can be pierced and chewed. The patient needs to be well hydrated before, during, and after surgery to prevent hypotension. Additional medications that may be used preoperatively include catecholamine synthesis inhibitors, such as alpha-methyl-*p*-tyrosine (metyrosine [Demser]). These are occasionally used if adrenergic blocking agents (i.e., alpha- and beta-blockers) are not effective. Long-term use of metyrosine may result in many adverse effects, including sedation, depression, diarrhea, anxiety, nightmares, dysuria, impotence, elevated aspartate aminotransferase, anemia, thrombocytopenia, crystalluria, galactorrhea (breast discharge), and extrapyramidal signs (e.g., drooling, speech impairment, tremors).

Surgical Management

The definitive treatment of pheochromocytoma is surgical removal of the tumour, usually with **adrenalectomy** (removal of one or both adrenal glands). Surgery may be performed using a laparoscopic approach or an open operation. The laparoscopic approach is the preferred method for patients with solitary intra-adrenal pheochromocytomas less than 8 cm in diameter without malignancy (Young et al., 2016). Bilateral adrenalectomy may be necessary if tumours are present in both adrenal glands. Patient preparation includes control of blood pressure and blood volumes; usually, this is carried out over 10 to 14 days, as described previously. A calcium channel blocker (nicardipine [Cardene]) can be given intraoperatively exclusively or in combination with the alpha- and beta-blockers to control blood pressure.

A hypertensive crisis, however, can still arise as a result of manipulation of the tumour during surgical excision, causing a release of stored epinephrine and norepinephrine, with marked increases in blood pressure and changes in heart rate. In response to this crisis, sodium nitroprusside (Nitropress), phentolamine (OraVerse), or nicardipine can be given. Lidocaine (Xylocaine) or esmolol (Brevibloc) is used to control cardiac arrhythmias (Young et al., 2016). Exploration of other possible tumour sites is frequently undertaken to ensure removal of all tumour tissue. As a result, the patient is subject to the stress and effects of a long surgical procedure, which may increase the risk of hypertension postoperatively.

Corticosteroid replacement is required if bilateral adrenalectomy has been necessary. Corticosteroids may also be required for the first few days or weeks after removal of a single adrenal gland. IV administration of corticosteroids (methylprednisolone sodium succinate [Solu-Medrol]) may begin on the evening before surgery and continue during the early postoperative period to prevent adrenal insufficiency. Oral preparations of corticosteroids (prednisone) are prescribed after the acute stress of surgery diminishes.

Hypotension and hypoglycemia may occur in the postoperative period because of the sudden withdrawal of excessive amounts of catecholamines. Therefore, careful attention is directed toward monitoring and treating these changes. Blood pressure is expected to return to normal with treatment; however, one third of patients continue to be hypertensive after surgery. This may result if not all pheochromocytoma tissue was removed, if pheochromocytoma recurs, or if the blood vessels were damaged by severe and prolonged hypertension. Several days after surgery, urine and plasma levels of catecholamines and their metabolites are measured to determine whether the surgery was successful.

Nursing Management

The patient who has undergone surgery to treat pheochromocytoma has experienced a stressful preoperative and postoperative course and may remain fearful of repeated attacks. Although it is usually expected that all pheochromocytoma tissue has been removed, there is a possibility that other sites were undetected and that attacks may recur. The patient is monitored for several days in the intensive care unit with special attention given to ECG changes, arterial pressures, fluid and electrolyte balance, and blood glucose levels. Several IV lines are inserted for administration of fluids and medications.

Promoting Home, Community-Based, and Transitional Care

Educating Patients About Self-Care

During the pre- and postoperative phases of care, the nurse educates the patient about the importance of follow-up monitoring to ensure that pheochromocytoma does not recur undetected. After adrenalectomy, the use of corticosteroids may be needed. Therefore, the nurse educates the patient about their purpose, the medication schedule, and the risks of skipping doses or stopping their administration abruptly.

The nurse educates the patient and family about how to measure the patient's blood pressure and when to notify the primary provider about changes in blood pressure. In addition, the nurse provides verbal and written instructions about the procedure for collecting 24-hour urine specimens to monitor urine catecholamine levels.

Continuing and Transitional Care

A follow-up visit from a home care nurse may be indicated to assess the patient's postoperative recovery, surgical incision, and compliance with the medication schedule. This may help reinforce previous teaching about management and monitoring. The home care nurse also obtains blood pressure measurements and assists the patient in preventing or dealing with problems that may result from long-term use of corticosteroids.

Because of the risk of recurrence of hypertension, periodic checkups are required, especially in young patients and in those whose families have a history of pheochromocytoma. The patient is scheduled for periodic follow-up appointments to observe for return of expected blood pressure and plasma and urine levels of catecholamines.

Adrenocortical Insufficiency (Addison Disease)

Addison disease, primary adrenal insufficiency (PAI), occurs when the adrenal glands are damaged and cannot produce sufficient amounts of cortical hormones (Bornstein, Allolio, Arlt, et al., 2016). Autoimmune or idiopathic atrophy of the adrenal glands is responsible for 80% to 90% of all cases. Other causes include surgical removal of both adrenal glands and infection of the adrenal glands. Tuberculosis and histoplasmosis are the most common infections that destroy adrenal gland tissue. The use of multiple pharmacologic therapies such as anticoagulants (resulting in adrenal hemorrhage), anticonvulsants (e.g., phenytoin [Dilantin] and phenobarbital), and antibiotics (e.g., rifampicin) for chronic and severe illnesses has also resulted in manifestations of PAI (Bornstein et al., 2016). Tuberculosis should be considered in the diagnostic workup. Inadequate secretion of ACTH from the pituitary gland is a secondary cause of adrenocortical insufficiency as a result of decreased stimulation of the adrenal cortex (Bornstein et al., 2016).

Therapeutic use of corticosteroids is the most common cause of adrenocortical insufficiency (Porth, 2015). Symptoms of adrenocortical insufficiency may result from the sudden cessation of exogenous adrenocortical hormonal therapy, which suppresses the body's normal response to stress and interferes with normal feedback mechanisms. Treatment with daily administration of corticosteroids for 2 to 4 weeks may suppress function of the adrenal cortex; therefore, adrenal insufficiency should be considered in any patient who has been treated with corticosteroids.

Clinical Manifestations

Addison disease is characterized by muscle weakness; anorexia; GI symptoms; fatigue; emaciation; dark pigmentation of the mucous membranes and the skin, especially of the knuckles, knees, and elbows; hypotension; and low blood glucose, low serum sodium, and high serum potassium levels. Depression, emotional lability, apathy, and confusion are present in 20% to 40% of patients (Nieman, 2016a). In severe cases, the disturbance of sodium and potassium metabolism may be marked by depletion of sodium and water and severe, chronic dehydration.

With disease progression, **addisonian crisis** (i.e., hypotension, cyanosis, fever, nausea, vomiting, and signs of shock) develops. In addition, the patient may have pallor; complain of headache, abdominal pain, and diarrhea; and may show signs of confusion and restlessness. Even slight overexertion, exposure to cold, acute infection, or a decrease in salt intake may lead to circulatory collapse, shock, and death, if untreated. The stress of surgery or dehydration resulting from preparation for diagnostic tests or surgery may precipitate an addisonian or hypotensive crisis.

Assessment and Diagnostic Findings

Although the clinical manifestations presented appear specific, the onset of Addison disease usually occurs with nonspecific symptoms. The diagnosis is confirmed by laboratory test results. Combined measurements of early-morning serum cortisol and plasma ACTH are performed to differentiate primary adrenal insufficiency from secondary adrenal insufficiency and from normal adrenal function. Patients with primary insufficiency have a greatly increased plasma ACTH level and a serum cortisol concentration lower than the normal range or in the low-normal range (Nieman, 2016b). Other laboratory findings include decreased levels of blood glucose (hypoglycemia) and sodium (hyponatremia), an increased serum potassium concentration (hyperkalemia), and an increased white blood cell count (leukocytosis).

Medical Management

Immediate treatment is directed toward combating circulatory shock: restoring blood circulation, administering fluids and corticosteroids, monitoring vital signs, and placing the patient in a recumbent position with the legs elevated. Hydrocortisone (Solu-Cortef) is administered by IV, followed by 5% dextrose in normal saline. Vasopressor amines may be required if hypotension persists.

Antibiotics may be administered if infection has precipitated adrenal crisis in a patient with chronic adrenal insufficiency. In addition, the patient is assessed closely to identify other factors, stressors, or illnesses that led to the acute episode.

Oral intake may be initiated as soon as tolerated. IV fluids are gradually decreased after oral fluid intake is adequate to prevent hypovolemia. If the adrenal gland does not regain function, the patient needs lifelong replacement of corticosteroids and mineralocorticoids to prevent recurrence of adrenal insufficiency (Young & Kaplan, 2016). During stressful procedures or significant illnesses, additional supplementary therapy with glucocorticoids is required to prevent addisonian crisis. In addition, the patient may need to supplement dietary intake with salt during GI losses of fluids through vomiting and diarrhea.

Nursing Management

Assessing the Patient

The health history and examination focus on the presence of symptoms of fluid imbalance and on the patient's level of stress. The nurse monitors the blood pressure and pulse rate as the patient moves from a lying, sitting, and standing position to assess for inadequate fluid volume. A decrease in systolic pressure (20 mm Hg or more) may indicate depletion of fluid volume, especially if accompanied by symptoms. The skin is assessed for changes in colour and turgor, which could indicate chronic adrenal insufficiency and hypovolemia. The patient is assessed for change in weight, muscle weakness, fatigue, and any illness or stress that may have precipitated the acute crisis.

Monitoring and Managing Addisonian Crisis

The patient at risk is monitored for signs and symptoms indicative of addisonian crisis, which can include shock; hypotension; rapid, weak pulse; rapid respiratory rate; pallor; and extreme weakness (see Chapter 16). Physical and psychological stressors such as cold exposure, overexertion, infection, and emotional distress should be avoided.

The patient with addisonian crisis requires immediate treatment with IV administration of fluid, glucose, and electrolytes, especially sodium; replacement of missing steroid hormones; and vasopressors. The nurse anticipates and meets the patient's needs to promote return to a pre-crisis state.

Restoring Fluid Balance

The nurse encourages the patient to consume foods and fluids that assist in restoring and maintaining fluid and electrolyte balance. Along with the dietitian, the nurse helps the patient select foods high in sodium during GI disturbances and in very hot weather.

The nurse instructs the patient and family to administer hormone replacement as prescribed and to modify the dosage during illness and other stressful situations. Written and verbal instructions are provided about the administration of mineralocorticoid (Florinef) or corticosteroid (prednisone) as prescribed.

Improving Activity Tolerance

Until the patient's condition is stabilized, the nurse takes precautions to avoid unnecessary activity and stress that could precipitate another hypotensive episode. Efforts are made to detect signs of infection or the presence of other stressors. Explaining the rationale for minimizing stress during the acute crisis assists the patient to increase activity gradually.

Promoting Home and Community-Based, and Transitional Care

Educating Patients About Self-Care

Because of the need for lifelong replacement of adrenal cortex hormones to prevent addisonian crises, the patient and family members receive explicit education about the rationale for replacement therapy and proper dosage. In addition, the patient, family, and caregivers are educated about the signs of excessive or insufficient hormone replacement. The patient should have an emergency kit in the form of corticosteroid in prefilled syringes, 100-mg vials of hydrocortisone or 4 mg of dexamethasone and 0.9% sterile saline to reconstitute the corticosteroid and syringes (Nieman, 2016c). Specific verbal and written instructions about how and when to use the injection are also provided to the patient and family or caregivers. The entire dose of 100-mg hydrocortisone or 4 mg of dexamethasone should be given and medical attention sought immediately after administering the drug. Chart 43-11 summarizes education for patients with Addison disease and their caregivers.

CHART 43-11

HOME CARE CHECKLIST • The Patient With Adrenal Insufficiency (Addison Disease)

At the completion of education, the patient and/or caregiver will be able to:

- State the impact of adrenal insufficiency and treatment on physiologic functioning, ADLs, IADLs, roles, relationships, and spirituality.
- State the purpose, dose, route, schedule, side effects, and precautions of prescribed medications (corticosteroid replacement).
- State that compliance with medical regimen is lifelong.
- Recognize the need for dosage adjustment during times of stress.
- State changes in lifestyle (e.g., diet, activity) necessary to maintain health, including:
  - Wearing medical alert identification, and carrying medical information card.
  - Avoiding strenuous activity in hot, humid weather.
  - Identifying strategies for dealing with stress and avoiding adrenal crisis.
  - Notifying primary providers about disease before treatment or procedure.
  - Increasing fluid intake and salt with excessive perspiration.
  - Ensuring high-carbohydrate, high-protein diet with adequate sodium intake.
- State warning signs of adrenal crisis and the need for emergency care.
- Explain components of an emergency kit and indications for their use; demonstrate how to use them.
- Relate how to reach primary provider with questions or complications.
- State time and date of follow-up medical appointments, therapy, and testing.
- Identify sources of support (e.g., friends, relatives, faith community, support groups, caregiver support).
- Identify the need for health promotion, disease prevention, and screening activities.

ADL, activities of daily living; IADL, independent activities of daily living.

Continuing and Transitional Care

Although most patients can return to their job and family responsibilities soon after hospital discharge, others cannot do so because of concurrent illnesses or incomplete recovery from the episode of adrenal insufficiency. In these circumstances, a referral for home care enables the home care nurse to assess the patient's recovery, monitor hormone replacement, and evaluate stress in the home. The nurse assesses the patient's and family's knowledge about medication therapy and dietary modifications. A home visit also allows the nurse to assess the patient's plans for follow-up visits to the clinic or physician's office. The nurse reminds the patient and family about the importance of participating in health promotion activities and health screening.

Cushing Syndrome

Cushing syndrome results from excessive, rather than deficient, adrenocortical activity (Porth, 2015). Cushing syndrome is commonly caused by the use of corticosteroid medications and is infrequently the result of excessive corticosteroid production secondary to hyperplasia of the adrenal cortex. However, overproduction of endogenous corticosteroids may be caused by several mechanisms, including a tumour of the pituitary gland that produces ACTH and stimulates the adrenal cortex to increase its hormone secretion despite production of adequate amounts. Primary hyperplasia of the adrenal glands in the absence of a pituitary tumour is less common. Another less common cause of Cushing syndrome is the ectopic production of ACTH by malignancies; bronchogenic carcinoma is the most common type. Regardless of the cause, the normal feedback mechanisms that control the function of the adrenal cortex become ineffective, and the usual diurnal pattern of cortisol is lost. The signs and symptoms of Cushing syndrome are primarily a result of over secretion of glucocorticoids and androgens, although mineralocorticoid secretion may be affected as well (Porth, 2015).

NURSING ALERT

Nurses must recognize that imbalanced adrenocortical hormone secretion characterizes both Addison disease (hypoproduction) and Cushing syndrome (hyperproduction).

Clinical Manifestations

When overproduction of the adrenal cortical hormone occurs, arrest of growth, obesity, and musculoskeletal changes occur along with glucose intolerance. The classic picture of Cushing syndrome in the adult is that of central-type obesity, with a fatty "buffalo hump" in the neck and supraclavicular areas, a heavy trunk, and relatively thin extremities. The skin is thin, fragile, and easily traumatized; ecchymoses (bruises) and striae develop. The patient reports weakness and lassitude. Sleep is disturbed because of altered diurnal secretion of cortisol.

Excessive protein catabolism occurs, producing muscle wasting and osteoporosis. Kyphosis, backache, and compression fractures of the vertebrae may result. Retention of sodium and water occurs as a result of increased mineralocorticoid activity, producing hypertension and heart failure.

The patient develops a "moon-faced" appearance and may experience increased oiliness of the skin and acne. There is increased susceptibility to infection. Hyperglycemia or overt diabetes may develop. The patient may also report weight gain, slow healing of minor cuts, and bruises.

Women between the ages of 20 and 40 years are five times more likely than men to develop Cushing syndrome. In females of all ages, virilization may occur as a result of excess androgens. Virilization is characterized by the appearance of masculine traits and the recession of feminine traits. There is an excessive growth of hair on the face (hirsutism), the breasts atrophy, menses cease, the clitoris enlarges, and the voice deepens. Libido is lost in men and women.

Changes occur in mood and mental activity, and psychosis may develop. Distress and depression are common and are increased by the severity of the physical changes that occur with this syndrome. If Cushing syndrome is a consequence of pituitary tumour, visual disturbances may occur because of pressure of the growing tumour on the optic chiasm. Chart 43-12 summarizes the changes associated with Cushing syndrome.

CHART 43-12

Clinical Manifestations of Cushing Syndrome

Ophthalmic
Cataracts
Glaucoma

Cardiovascular
Hypertension
Heart failure

Endocrine/Metabolic
Altered calcium metabolism
Adrenal suppression
Buffalo hump
Hyperglycemia
Hypokalemia
Impotence
Menstrual irregularities
Metabolic alkalosis
Moon face
Negative nitrogen balance
Sodium retention
Truncal obesity

Immune Function
Decreased inflammatory responses
Impaired wound healing
Increased susceptibility to infections

Skeletal
Osteoporosis
Spontaneous fractures
Aseptic necrosis of femur
Vertebral compression fractures

Gastrointestinal
Peptic ulcer
Pancreatitis

Muscular
Myopathy
Muscle weakness

Dermatologic
Thinning of skin
Petechiae
Ecchymoses
Striae
Acne

Psychiatric
Mood alterations
Psychoses

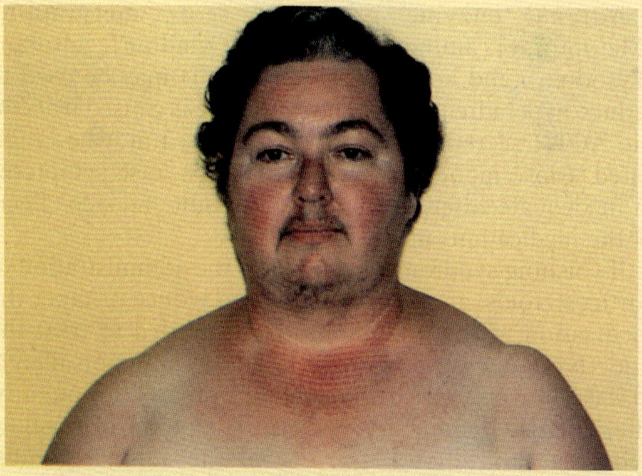

This woman with Cushing syndrome has several classic signs, including facial hair, buffalo hump, and moon face.

From Rubin, R., Strayer, D. S., & Rubin, E. (2012). *Rubin's pathology* (6th ed.). Philadelphia, PA: Lippincott Williams & Wilkins.

Assessment and Diagnostic Findings

The three tests used to diagnose Cushing syndrome are serum cortisol, urinary cortisol, and low-dose dexamethasone (Decadron) suppression tests (Nieman, 2016d). Two of these three tests need to be unequivocally abnormal to diagnose Cushing syndrome. If the results of all three tests are normal, the patient likely does not have Cushing syndrome (but may have a mild case, or the manifestations may be cyclic). For these patients, further testing is not recommended unless symptoms progress. If test results are either slightly abnormal or discordant, further testing is recommended.

Serum cortisol levels are usually higher in the early morning (6 to 8 am) and lower in the evening (4 to 6 pm). This variation is lost in patients with Cushing syndrome (Fischbach & Dunning, 2015).

A urinary cortisol test requires a 24-hour urine collection. The nurse instructs the patient how to collect and store the specimen. If the results of the urinary cortisol test are three times the upper limit of the normal range and one other test is abnormal, Cushing syndrome can be assumed.

An overnight dexamethasone suppression test is used to diagnosis pituitary and adrenal causes of Cushing syndrome. It can be performed on an outpatient basis. Dexamethasone (1 mg or 8 mg) is given orally late in the evening or at bedtime, and a plasma cortisol level is obtained at 8 am the next morning. Suppression of cortisol to less than 5 mg/dL indicates that the hypothalamic–pituitary–adrenal axis is functioning properly (Fischbach & Dunning, 2015). Stress, obesity, depression, and medications such as anticonvulsant agents, estrogen (during pregnancy or as oral medications), and rifampin (Rifadin) can falsely elevate cortisol levels.

Indicators of Cushing syndrome include an increase in serum sodium and blood glucose levels and a decrease in serum potassium, a reduction in the number of blood eosinophils, and disappearance of lymphoid tissue. Measurements of plasma and urinary cortisol levels are obtained. Several blood samples may be collected to determine whether the normal diurnal variation in plasma levels is present; this variation is frequently absent in adrenal dysfunction. If several blood samples are required, they must be collected at the times specified, and the time of collection must be noted on the requisition slip.

Medical Management

If Cushing syndrome is caused by pituitary tumours rather than tumours of the adrenal cortex, treatment is directed at the pituitary gland. Surgical removal of the tumour by transsphenoidal hypophysectomy (see Chapter 63) is the treatment of choice and has an 80% success rate. Radiation of the pituitary gland also has been successful, although it may take several months for control of symptoms. Adrenalectomy is the treatment of choice in patients with primary adrenal hypertrophy. Medical management is recommended for bilateral adrenal dysplasia.

Postoperatively, symptoms of adrenal insufficiency may begin to appear 12 to 48 hours after surgery because of reduction of the high levels of circulating adrenal hormones. Temporary replacement therapy with hydrocortisone may be necessary for several months, until the adrenal glands begin to respond normally to the body's needs. If both adrenal glands have been removed (bilateral adrenalectomy), lifetime replacement of adrenal cortex hormones is necessary.

Adrenal enzyme inhibitors (e.g., metyrapone [Metopirone], aminoglutethimide [Cytadren], mitotane [Lysodren], and ketoconazole [Nizoral]) may be used to reduce hyperadrenalism if the syndrome is caused by ectopic ACTH secretion by a tumour that cannot be eradicated. Close monitoring is necessary, because symptoms of inadequate adrenal function may result and side effects of the medications may occur.

If Cushing syndrome is a result of the administration of corticosteroids, an attempt is made to reduce or taper the medication to the minimum dosage needed to treat the underlying disease process (e.g., autoimmune or allergic disease, rejection of a transplanted organ). Frequently, alternate-day therapy decreases the symptoms of Cushing syndrome and allows recovery of the adrenal glands' responsiveness to ACTH.

Nursing Process

The Patient With Cushing Syndrome

Assessment

The health history and examination focus on the effects on the body of high concentrations of adrenal cortex hormones and on the inability of the adrenal cortex to respond to changes in cortisol and aldosterone levels. The history includes information about the patient's level of activity and ability to carry out routine and self-care activities. The skin is observed and assessed for trauma, infection, breakdown, bruising, and edema. Changes in physical appearance are noted, and the patient's responses to these changes are elicited. The nurse assesses the patient's mental function, including mood, responses to questions, awareness of environment, and level of depression. The family is often a good source of information about gradual changes in the patient's physical appearance as well as emotional status.

Nursing Priorities

Based on all the assessment data, the major nursing priorities of the patient with Cushing syndrome include the following:

- Injury due to weakness
- Infection
- Inadequate self-care
- Break in skin integrity
- Impaired body image
- Impaired thought processes

Collaborative Problems/ Potential Complications

Potential complications may include the following:

- Addisonian crisis
- Adverse effects of adrenocortical activity

Planning and Goals

The major goals for the patient include decreased risk of injury, decreased risk of infection, increased ability to carry out self-care activities, improved skin integrity, improved body image, improved mental function, and absence of complications.

Nursing Interventions

Decreasing Risk of Injury

Establishing a protective environment helps prevent falls, fractures, and other injuries to bones and soft tissues. The patient who is very weak may require assistance from the nurse in ambulating to avoid falling or bumping into sharp corners of furniture. Foods high in protein, calcium, and vitamin D are recommended to minimize muscle wasting and osteoporosis. Referral to a dietitian may assist the patient in selecting appropriate foods that are also low in sodium and calories.

Decreasing Risk of Infection

The patient should avoid unnecessary exposure to others with infections. The nurse frequently assesses the patient for subtle signs of infection, because the anti-inflammatory effects of corticosteroids may mask the common signs of inflammation and infection.

Preparing the Patient for Surgery

The patient is prepared for adrenalectomy, if indicated, and the postoperative course (see later discussion). If Cushing syndrome is a result of a pituitary tumour, a transsphenoidal hypophysectomy may be performed (see Chapter 63). Diabetes mellitus and peptic ulcer are common in patients with Cushing syndrome. Therefore, insulin therapy and medication to treat peptic ulcer are initiated if needed. Before, during, and after surgery, blood glucose monitoring and assessment of stools for blood are carried out to monitor for these complications. If the patient has other symptoms of Cushing syndrome, these are considered in the preoperative preparation. For example, if the patient has experienced weight gain, special instruction is given about postoperative breathing exercises.

Encouraging Rest and Activity

Although the patient with Cushing syndrome experiences insomnia, weakness, fatigue, and muscle wasting, the nurse should encourage moderate activity to prevent complications of immobility and promote increased self-esteem. It is important to help the patient plan and space rest periods throughout the day and promote a relaxing, quiet environment for rest and sleep.

Promoting Skin Integrity

Meticulous skin care is necessary to avoid traumatizing the patient's fragile skin. Use of adhesive tape is avoided, because it can irritate the skin and tear the fragile tissue when the tape is removed. The nurse frequently assesses the skin and bony prominences and encourages and assists the patient to change positions frequently to prevent skin breakdown.

Improving Body Image

If treated successfully, the major physical changes associated with Cushing syndrome disappear in time. The patient may benefit from discussion of the effect the changes have had on his or her self-concept and relationships with others. Weight gain and edema may be modified by a low-carbohydrate, low-sodium diet, and a high-protein intake may reduce some of the other bothersome symptoms.

Improving Thought Processes

Explanations to the patient and family members about the cause of emotional instability are important in helping them cope with the mood swings, irritability, and depression that may occur. Psychotic behaviour may occur in a few patients and should be reported. The nurse encourages the patient and family members to verbalize their feelings and concerns.

Monitoring and Managing Potential Complications

ADDISONIAN CRISIS. The patient with Cushing syndrome whose symptoms are treated by withdrawal of corticosteroids, by adrenalectomy, or by removal of a pituitary tumour is at risk for adrenal hypofunction and addisonian crisis. If high levels of circulating adrenal hormones have suppressed the function of the adrenal cortex, atrophy of the adrenal cortex is likely. If the circulating hormone level is decreased rapidly because of surgery or abrupt cessation of corticosteroid agents, manifestations of adrenal hypofunction and addisonian crisis may develop. Therefore, the patient with Cushing syndrome should be assessed for signs and symptoms of addisonian crisis as previously discussed. If addisonian crisis occurs, the patient is treated for circulatory collapse and shock (see Chapter 18).

ADVERSE EFFECTS OF ADRENOCORTICAL ACTIVITY. The nurse assesses fluid and electrolyte status by monitoring laboratory values and daily weights. Because of the increased risk of glucose intolerance and hyperglycemia, blood glucose monitoring is initiated. The nurse reports elevated blood glucose levels to the physician so that treatment can be prescribed if indicated.

Promoting Home, Community-Based, and Transitional Care

EDUCATING PATIENTS ABOUT SELF-CARE. The patient and family are informed that acute adrenal insufficiency and underlying symptoms will recur if corticosteroid therapy is stopped abruptly without medical supervision. The patient is instructed to always have an adequate supply of the corticosteroid medication to avoid running out (see Therapeutic Uses of Corticosteroids).

The nurse stresses the need for dietary modifications to ensure adequate calcium intake without increasing the risks for hypertension, hyperglycemia, and weight gain. The patient and family can be taught to monitor blood pressure, blood glucose levels, and weight. Patients are advised to wear a medical alert bracelet and to notify other health care providers (e.g., dentist) about their condition (Chart 43-13).

CONTINUING AND TRANSITIONAL CARE. The need for follow-up depends on the origin and duration of the disease and its management. The patient who has been treated by adrenalectomy or removal of a pituitary tumour requires close monitoring to ensure that adrenal function has returned to normal and to ensure adequacy of circulating adrenal hormones. The patient who requires continued corticosteroid therapy is monitored to ensure understanding of the medications and the need for a dosage that treats the underlying disorder while minimizing the side effects. Home care referral may be indicated to ensure a safe environment that minimizes stress and risk of falls and other side effects. The home care nurse assesses the patient's physical and psychological status and reports changes to the physician. The nurse also assesses the patient's understanding of the medication regimen and his or her compliance with the regimen and reinforces previous teaching about the medications and the importance of taking them as

CHART 43-13

HOME CARE CHECKLIST • The Patient With Cushing Syndrome

At the completion of education, the patient and/or caregiver will be able to:

- State the impact of Cushing syndrome and treatment on physiologic functioning, ADLs, IADLs, roles, relationships, and spirituality.
- State the relationship between adrenal hormones, emotional state, and stress.
- State the purpose, dose, route, schedule, side effects, and precautions for prescribed medications (adrenocortical inhibitors).
- State importance of compliance with medical regimen.
- State the need to contact primary provider before taking over-the-counter medications.
- State changes in lifestyle (e.g., diet, activity) necessary to maintain health, including:
  - Wearing medical alert identification and carrying medical information card.
  - Identifying methods for managing labile emotions.
  - Describing protective skin care measures and the use of protective devices and practices to decrease injury/fracture.
  - Identifying foods high in potassium and low in sodium, calories, and carbohydrates.
  - Describing measures to decrease risk of infection.
  - Balancing rest and activity.
  - Monitoring blood pressure, blood glucose levels, and weight.
- Identify signs and symptoms of excessive and insufficient adrenal hormone.
- Relate how to reach primary provider with questions or complications.
- State time and date of follow-up medical appointments, therapy, and testing.
- Identify sources of support (e.g., friends, relatives, faith community, support groups, caregiver support).
- Identify the need for health promotion, disease prevention, and screening activities.

ADL, activities of daily living; IADL, independent activities of daily living.

prescribed. The nurse emphasizes the importance of regular medical follow-up, the side effects and toxic effects of medications, and the need to wear medical identification with Addison and Cushing diseases. In addition, the nurse reminds the patient and family about the importance of health promotion activities and recommended health screening, including bone mineral density testing.

Evaluation

Expected patient outcomes may include the following:

1. Decreases risk of injury
   a. Is free of fractures or soft tissue injuries
   b. Is free of ecchymotic areas
2. Decreases risk of infection
   a. Experiences no temperature elevation, redness, pain, or other signs of infection or inflammation
   b. Avoids contact with others who have infections
3. Increases participation in self-care activities
   a. Plans activities and exercises to allow alternating periods of rest and activity
   b. Reports improved well-being
   c. Is free of complications of immobility
4. Attains/maintains skin integrity
   a. Has intact skin, without evidence of breakdown or infection
   b. Exhibits decreased edema in extremities and trunk
   c. Changes position frequently and inspects bony prominences daily
5. Achieves improved body image
   a. Verbalizes feelings about changes in appearance, sexual function, and activity level
   b. States that physical changes are a result of excessive corticosteroids
6. Exhibits improved mental functioning
7. Exhibits absence of complications
   a. Exhibits acceptable vital signs and weight and is free of symptoms of addisonian crisis
   b. Identifies signs and symptoms of adrenocortical hypofunction that should be reported and measures to take in case of severe illness and stress
   c. Identifies strategies to minimize complications of Cushing syndrome
   d. Complies with recommendations for follow-up appointments and health screening

Primary Aldosteronism

The principal action of aldosterone is to conserve body sodium. Under the influence of this hormone, the kidneys excrete less sodium and more potassium and hydrogen. Excessive production of aldosterone, which occurs in some patients with functioning tumours of the adrenal gland, causes a distinctive pattern of biochemical changes and a corresponding set of clinical manifestations that are diagnostic of this condition.

Clinical Manifestations

Hypertension is the most prominent and almost universal sign of primary aldosteronism. Patients with uncomplicated, complicated, and treatment-resistant hypertension and hypertension with hypokalemia should be considered at risk for this disorder. However, hypokalemia should no longer be considered a requisite for this diagnosis. It is now recognized that hypokalemia is not always present in primary aldosteronism. In some patients, hypokalemia only becomes evident after the introduction of a potassium-sparing diuretic (e.g., hydrochlorothiazide, furosemide) (Young, 2016; Young & Kaplan, 2016). If hypokalemia is present, it may be responsible for the variable muscle weakness or paralysis, cramping, and fatigue in patients with aldosteronism, as well as the kidneys' inability to acidify or concentrate the urine. Accordingly, the urine volume is excessive, leading to polyuria. Serum, by contrast, becomes abnormally concentrated, contributing to excessive thirst (polydipsia) and arterial hypertension. A secondary increase in blood volume and possible direct effects of aldosterone on nerve receptors, such as the carotid sinus, are other factors that result in hypertension.

Hypokalemic alkalosis may decrease the ionized serum calcium level and predispose the patient to tetany and paresthesias. Trousseau's and Chvostek signs may be used to assess neuromuscular irritability before overt paresthesia and tetany occur. Glucose intolerance may occur, because hypokalemia interferes with insulin secretion from the pancreas.

Assessment and Diagnostic Findings

Withholding antihypertensive medication before testing is not required (Young, 2016). A blood test to measure the ratio of PAC (plasma aldosterone concentration) to PRA (plasma renin activity) can be performed even while the patient is taking an antihypertensive. This should be followed by aldosterone suppression confirmatory tests and sub-type evaluation tests.

Medical Management

The recommended treatment of unilateral primary aldosteronism is total surgical removal of the adrenal tumour through laparoscopic adrenalectomy rather than open surgery. Open adrenalectomy is performed through an incision in the flank or the abdomen. In general, the postoperative care for open surgery resembles that for other abdominal surgery. However, the patient is susceptible to fluctuations in adrenocortical hormones and requires administration of corticosteroids, fluids, and other agents to maintain blood pressure and prevent acute complications. If the adrenalectomy is bilateral, replacement of corticosteroids will be lifelong. A normal serum glucose level is maintained with insulin, appropriate IV fluids, and dietary modifications.

Laparoscopic surgery is recommended over open surgery to reduce complications and hospital length of stay (Young & Kaplan, 2016). Hypokalemia should be treated with spironolactone (Aldactone) preoperatively. Hypokalemia typically resolves for all patients after surgery and hypertension is resolved in 35% to 60%. Postoperatively, spironolactone and potassium supplements should be discontinued and antihypertensives should be decreased. Potassium levels should be checked once a week for 4 weeks postoperatively (Young & Kaplan, 2016).

Medical treatment rather than surgery is recommended for patients with bilateral adrenal involvement due to poor blood pressure control and other risks.

Pharmacologic Therapy

Pharmacologic management is required for patients with bilateral adrenal hyperplasia or unilateral aldosterone hypersecretion who do not undergo surgery. Spironolactone is recommended as the first-line drug to control hypertension. Eplerenone (Inspra) a newer, more expensive drug is recommended as a second-line drug if the patient cannot tolerate side effects of spironolactone (Young & Kaplan, 2016). Serum potassium and creatinine should be monitored frequently during the first 4 to 6 weeks of taking spironolactone. Ongoing monitoring will be determined by the clinical course. The half-life of digoxin may be increased when taken with spironolactone, and its dosage may need to be adjusted. The effectiveness of spironolactone in controlling blood pressure may be affected if taken with salicylates or nonsteroidal anti-inflammatory drugs (Young & Kaplan, 2016).

Nursing Management

Nursing management in the postoperative period includes frequent assessment of vital signs to detect early signs and symptoms of adrenal insufficiency and crisis or hemorrhage. Explaining all treatments and procedures, providing comfort measures, and providing rest periods can reduce the patient's stress and anxiety level.

Corticosteroid Therapy

Corticosteroids are used extensively for adrenal insufficiency and are also widely used in suppressing inflammation and autoimmune reactions, controlling allergic reactions, and reducing the rejection process in transplantation. Commonly used corticosteroid preparations are listed in Table 43-5. Their anti-inflammatory and antiallergy actions make corticosteroids effective in treating rheumatic or connective tissue diseases, such as rheumatoid arthritis and systemic lupus erythematosus. They are also frequently used in the treatment of asthma, multiple sclerosis, and other autoimmune disorders.

High doses appear to allow patients to tolerate high degrees of stress. Such antistress action may be caused by

TABLE 43-5 Commonly Used Corticosteroid Preparations

Generic Names	Trade Names
beclomethasone	Beconase, Beclovent, Vanceril, Vancenase, Propaderm
betamethasone	Celestone, Betameth, Betnesol, Betnelan
cortisone	Cortone, Cortate, Cortogen
dexamethasone	Dexamethasone Intensol, DexPak
hydrocortisone	Cortisol, Cortef, Hydrocortone, Solu-Cortef
methylprednisolone	Medrol, Solu-Medrol, Meprolone
prednisone	Meticorten, Deltasone, Orasone, Panasol, Novo-prednisone
prednisolone	Prelone
triamcinolone	Kenalog, Triderm

Adapted from Comerford, K. C. (2015). *Nursing 2015 drug handbook*. Philadelphia, PA: Wolters Kluwer.

the ability of corticosteroids to aid circulating vasopressor substances in keeping the blood pressure elevated; other effects, such as maintenance of the serum glucose level, also may keep blood pressure elevated.

Side Effects

Although the synthetic corticosteroids are safer for some patients because of relative freedom from mineralocorticoid activity, most natural and synthetic corticosteroids produce similar kinds of side effects. The dose required for anti-inflammatory and antiallergy effects also produces metabolic effects, pituitary and adrenal gland suppression, and changes in the function of the central nervous system. Therefore, although corticosteroids are highly effective therapeutically, they may also be very dangerous. Dosages of these medications are frequently altered to allow high concentrations when necessary and then tapered in an attempt to avoid undesirable effects. This requires that patients be observed closely for side effects and that the dose be reduced when high doses are no longer required. Suppression of the adrenal cortex may persist up to 1 year after a course of corticosteroids of only 2 weeks' duration.

Therapeutic Uses of Corticosteroids

The dosage of corticosteroids is determined by the nature and chronicity of the illness as well as the patient's other medical conditions. Rheumatoid arthritis, bronchial asthma, and multiple sclerosis are chronic disorders that corticosteroids do not cure; however, these medications may be useful when other measures do not provide adequate control of symptoms. In addition, corticosteroids may be used to treat acute exacerbations of these disorders.

In such situations, the adverse effects of corticosteroids are weighed against the patient's current condition. These medications may be used for a period but then are gradually reduced or tapered as the symptoms subside. The nurse plays an important role in providing encouragement and understanding during times when the patient is experiencing (or is apprehensive about experiencing) recurrence of symptoms while taking smaller doses.

Treatment of Acute Conditions

Acute flare-ups and crises are treated with large doses of corticosteroids. Examples include emergency treatment for bronchial obstruction in status asthmaticus and for septic shock from septicemia caused by gram-negative bacteria. Other measures, such as anti-infective agents or medications, are also used with corticosteroids to treat shock and other major symptoms. At times, corticosteroids are continued past the acute flare-up stage to prevent serious complications.

Ophthalmologic Treatment

Outer eye infections can be treated by topical application of corticosteroid eye drops, because the agents do not cause systemic toxicity. However, long-term application can cause an increase in intraocular pressure, which leads to glaucoma in some patients. In addition, prolonged use of corticosteroids can sometimes lead to cataract formation.

Dermatologic Disorders

Topical administration of corticosteroids in the form of creams, ointments, lotions, and aerosols is especially effective in many dermatologic disorders. It may be more effective in some conditions to use occlusive dressings around the affected part to achieve maximum absorption of the medication. Penetration and absorption are also increased if the medication is applied when the skin is hydrated or moist (e.g., immediately after bathing).

Absorption of topical agents varies with body location. For example, absorption is greater through the layers of skin on the scalp, face, and genital area than on the forearm; as a result, use of topical agents on these sites increases the risk of side effects. The availability of over-the-counter topical corticosteroids increases the risk of side effects in patients who are unaware of their potential risks. Excessive use of these agents, especially on large surface areas of inflamed skin, can lead to decreased therapeutic effects and increased side effects.

Dosage

Attempts have been made to determine the best time to administer pharmacologic doses of steroids. If symptoms have been controlled on a 6- or 8-hour program, a once-daily or every-other-day schedule may be implemented. In keeping with the natural secretion of cortisol, the best time of day for the total corticosteroid dose is in the early morning, between 0700 and 0800 hours. Large-dose therapy at 0800 hours, when the adrenal gland is most active, produces maximal suppression of the gland. A large 0800 dose is more physiologic because it allows the body to escape effects of the steroids from 1600 hours to 0600 hours, when serum levels are usually low, hence minimizing cushingoid effects. If symptoms of the disorder being treated are suppressed, alternate-day therapy is helpful in reducing pituitary–adrenal suppression in patients requiring prolonged therapy. Some patients report discomfort associated with symptoms of their primary illness on the second day; therefore, it is important to explain to patients that this regimen is necessary to minimize side effects and suppression of adrenal function.

Tapering

Corticosteroid dosages are reduced gradually (tapered) to allow normal adrenal function to return and to prevent steroid-induced adrenal insufficiency. Up to 1 year or longer after use of corticosteroids, the patient is still at risk for adrenal insufficiency in times of stress. For example, if surgery for any reason is necessary, the patient is likely to require IV corticosteroids during and after surgery to reduce the risk of acute adrenal crisis. Patients receiving corticosteroids must have an adequate supply of medication on hand, so that they do not miss a scheduled dose and increase their risk of adrenal insufficiency.

Nursing Management

Nursing management of corticosteroid therapy includes many important interventions. Table 43-6 provides an overview of the effects of corticosteroid therapy and their nursing implications.

Promoting Home, Community-Based, and Transitional Care

Educating Patients About Self-Care

The nurse educates the patient, family, and caregivers that acute adrenal insufficiency and underlying symptoms will recur if corticosteroid therapy is stopped abruptly without medical supervision. The patient should

TABLE 43-6 Side Effects of Corticosteroid Therapy and Implications for Nursing Practice

Side Effects	Collaborative Interventions
Cardiovascular Effects	
Hypertension	Monitor for elevated blood pressure.
Thrombophlebitis	Assess for signs and symptoms of deep venous thrombosis: redness, warmth, tenderness, and edema of an extremity.
Thromboembolism	Remind patient to avoid positions and situations that restrict blood flow (e.g., crossing legs, prolonged sitting in same position).
Accelerated atherosclerosis	Encourage foot and leg exercises when recumbent. Encourage low sodium intake. Encourage limited intake of fat.
Immunologic Effects	
Increased risk of infection and masking of signs of infection	Assess for subtle signs of infection and inflammation. Encourage patient to avoid exposure to others with upper respiratory infection. Monitor patient for fungal infections. Encourage hand washing.
Ophthalmologic Changes	
Glaucoma	Encourage frequent eye examinations.
Corneal lesions	Refer patient to ophthalmologist if changes in visual acuity are detected.
Musculoskeletal Effects	
Muscle wasting	Encourage high-protein intake.
Poor wound healing	Encourage high-protein intake and vitamin C supplementation.
Osteoporosis with vertebral compression fractures, pathologic fractures of long bones, aseptic necrosis of head of the femur	Encourage diet high in calcium and vitamin D or calcium and vitamin D supplementation if indicated. Take measures to avoid falls and other trauma. Use caution in moving and turning patient. Encourage postmenopausal women on corticosteroids to consider bone mineral density testing and treatment, if indicated. Instruct patient to rise slowly from bed or chair to avoid falling due to postural hypotension.
Metabolic Effects	
Alterations in glucose metabolism	Monitor blood glucose levels at periodic intervals.
Steroid withdrawal syndrome	Instruct patient about medications, diet, and exercise prescribed to control blood glucose level. Report signs of adrenal insufficiency. Administer corticosteroids and mineralocorticoids as prescribed. Instruct patient about importance of taking corticosteroids as prescribed without abruptly stopping therapy. Encourage patient to obtain and wear a medical identification bracelet. Advise patient to notify all health care professionals (e.g., dentist) about need for corticosteroid therapy.
Changes in Appearance	
Moon face	Encourage low-calorie, low-sodium diet.
Weight gain	Assure patient that most changes in appearance are temporary and will disappear if and when corticosteroid therapy is no longer necessary.
Acne	
Fluid and Electrolyte Imbalances	Monitor intake and output and electrolytes. Administer fluids and electrolytes as prescribed.

be instructed to always have an adequate supply of the corticosteroid medication to avoid running out.

Continuing and Transitional Care

The patient who requires continued corticosteroid therapy is monitored to ensure understanding of the medications and the need for a dosage that treats the underlying disorder while minimizing the side effects. Home care referral may be indicated to ensure a safe environment that minimizes stress, risk of falls, and other side effects. The nurse assesses the patient's physical and psychological status and reports changes to the primary provider. The nurse also assesses the patient's understanding of the medication regimen and their compliance with the regimen and reinforces previous education about the medications and the importance of taking them as prescribed. The nurse emphasizes the importance of regular medical follow-up, the side effects, and effects of abruptly discontinuing corticosteroids. In addition, the nurse reminds the patient and family about the importance of health promotion activities and recommended health screening, including bone mineral density testing.

Critical Thinking Exercises

1 A 42-year-old man has been recently diagnosed with hypothyroidism. What resources would you use to identify evidence-based practices for appropriate interventions and prevention of complications for this patient? Identify the evidence, as well as the criteria used to evaluate the strength of the evidence, for the practices identified.

2 Identify the priorities, approach, and techniques you would use to perform a comprehensive assessment on a 60-year-old patient newly diagnosed with Cushing syndrome. How will your priorities, approach, and techniques differ if the patient has a visual impairment or is hard of hearing? If the patient is from a culture with very different values from your own?

3 A 75-year-old patient has a new prescription for corticosteroid therapy. Describe the assessment techniques appropriate to evaluate the patient and the use of the medication. What instructions should you provide regarding precautions to take related to corticosteroid therapy? How will your assessment and instructions differ if the patient is disoriented?

REFERENCES AND SELECTED READINGS

Books

Comerford, K. C. (2015). *Nursing 2015 drug handbook*. Philadelphia, PA: Wolters Kluwer.

Dagan, R., & Amdur, R. J. (2013). Thyroid cancer. In E. C. Halperin, D. E. Wazer, C. A. Perez, et al. (Eds.). *Perez and Brady's principles and practice of radiation oncology* (6th ed.). Philadelphia, PA: Lippincott Williams and Wilkins.

Davies, T. F., Laurberg, P., & Bahn, R. S. (2016). Thyroid disorders. In S. Melmed, K. Polonsky, P. Larsen, et al. (Eds.). *Williams textbook of endocrinology*. Philadelphia, PA: Elsevier.

Fischbach, F., & Dunning, M. B. (2015). *A manual of laboratory and diagnostic tests* (9th ed.). Philadelphia, PA: Lippincott Williams & Wilkins.

Grossman, S. C., & Porth, C. M. (2014). *Pathophysiology: Concepts of altered health states* (9th ed.). Philadelphia, PA: Lippincott Williams & Wilkins.

Kaiser, U., & Ho, K. K. Y. (2016). Pituitary physiology and diagnostic evaluation. In S. Melmed, K. Polonsky, P. Larsen, et al. (Eds.). *Williams textbook of endocrinology*. Philadelphia, PA: Elsevier.

Lazar, M. A., & Birnbaum, M. J. (2016). Principles of hormone action. In S. Melmed, K. Polonsky, P. Larsen., et al. (Eds.). *Williams textbook of endocrinology*. Philadelphia, PA: Elsevier.

Majithia, A., Altshuler, R. D., & Hirschhorn, J. N. (2016). Genetics of endocrinology. In S. Melmed, K. Polonsky, P. Larsen, et al. (Eds.). *Williams textbook of endocrinology*. Philadelphia, PA: Elsevier.

McPhee, S. J, Rabow, M. W., & Papadakis, M. (Eds.). (2016). *Current medical diagnosis and treatment*. New York: Lange Medical Books/McGraw-Hill.

Mercado, M. (2016). Endocrine and metabolic disorders. In E. T. Bope & R. D. Kellerman (Eds.). *Conn's current therapy*. Philadelphia, PA: Elsevier.

Morton, P. G., & Fontaine, D. K. (2013). *Critical care nursing: A holistic approach*. Philadelphia, PA: Lippincott Williams & Wilkins.

Porth, C. (2006). *Essentials of pathophysiology: Concepts of altered health states* (2nd ed.). Philadelphia, PA: Wolters Kluwer.

Porth, C. M. (2015). *Essentials of pathophysiology: Concepts for altered health states* (4th ed.). Philadelphia, PA: Wolters Kluwer.

Rubin, R., Strayer, D. S., & Rubin, E. (2012). *Rubin's pathology* (6th ed.). Philadelphia, PA: Lippincott Williams & Wilkins.

Salvatore, D., Davies, T. F., Sclumberger, M. J., et al. (2016). Thyroid physiology and diagnostic evaluation of patients with thyroid disorders. In S. Melmed, K. Polonsky, P. Larsen, et al. (Eds.). *Williams textbook of endocrinology*. Philadelphia, PA: Elsevier.

Sluss, P. M., & Hayes, F. J. (2016). Laboratory techniques for recognition of endocrine disorders. In S. Melmed, K. Polonsky, P. Larsen, et al. (Eds.). *Williams textbook of endocrinology*. Philadelphia, PA: Elsevier.

Weber, J. R., & Kelley, J. H. (2014). *Health assessment in nursing* (5th ed.). Philadelphia, PA: Lippincott Williams & Wilkins.

Woodworth, A., Lakhani, V., Aleryani, S. L., et al. (2014). The endocrine system. In M. Laposata (Ed.). *Laboratory medicine: The diagnosis of disease in the clinical laboratory*. New York: McGraw-Hill.

Young, W. F. (2016). Endocrine hypertension. In S. Melmed, K. Polonsky, P. Larsen, et al. (Eds.). *Williams textbook of endocrinology*. Philadelphia, PA: Elsevier.

Journals and Electronic Documents

Bahn Chair, R. S., Burch, H. B., Cooper, D. S., et al. (2011). Hyperthyroidism and other causes of thyrotoxicosis: Management guidelines of the American Thyroid Association and American Association of Clinical Endocrinologists. *Thyroid*, *21*(6), 593–646.

Bornstein, S. R., Allolio, B., Arlt, W., et al. (2016). Diagnosis and treatment of primary adrenal insufficiency: An Endocrine Society clinical practice guideline. *Journal of Clinical Endocrinology and Metabolism*, *101*(2), 364–389.

Canadian Cancer society. (2017). Thyroid cancer statistics. Retrieved from http://www.cancer.ca/en/cancer-information/cancer-type/thyroid/statistics/?region=on#ixzz5Jww3l4XB

CCSACCS. (2018). Canadian Cancer Statistics: A 2018 special report on cancer incidence by stage. Retrieved from https://www.cancer.ca/~/media/cancer.ca/CW/cancer%20information/cancer%20101/Canadian%20cancer%20statistics/Canadian-Cancer-Statistics-2018-EN.pdf?la=en

Dhyani, M., Faquin, W., Lubitz, C. C., et al. (2013). How to interpret thyroid fine-needle aspiration biopsy reports: A guide for the busy radiologist in the era of the Bethesda Classification System. *American Journal of Roentgenology*, *201*(6), 1335–1339.

Dunn, D., & Turner, C. (2016). Hypothyroidism in women. *Nursing for Women's Health*, *20*(1), 93–98.

Eugster, E. A. (2017). Pituitary gigantism. *UpToDate*. Retrieved March 31, 2017, from www.uptodate.com/contents/pituitary-gigantism

Fuleihan, G. E., & Silverberg, S. S. (2017). Primary hyperparathyroidism: Diagnosis, differential diagnosis, and evaluation. *UpToDate*. Retrieved March 31, 2017, from www.uptodate.com/contents/primary-hyperparathyroidism-diagnosis-differential-diagnosis-and-evaluation?source=search_result&search=primary+hyperparathyroidism&selectedTitle=1%7E98

Garber, J. R., Cobin, R. H., Gharib, H., et al. (2012). Clinical practice guidelines for hypothyroidism in adults: Cosponsored by the American Association of Clinical Endocrinologists and the American Thyroid Association. *Endocrine Practice*, *18*(6), 988–1028.

Goltzman, D. (2016). Hypoparathyroidism. *UpToDate*. Retrieved June 29, 2016, from www.uptodate.com/contents/hypoparathyroidism

Harman, S. M. (2016). Endocrine changes with aging. *UpToDate*. Retrieved June 22, 2016, from http://www.uptodate.com/contents/endocrine-changes-with-aging

Janicak, P. (2016). Bipolar disorder in adults and lithium: Pharmacology, administration and side effects. *UpToDate*. Retrieved June 29, 2016, from www.uptodate.com/contents/bipolar-disorder-in-adults-and-lithium-pharmacology-administration-and-side-effects/contributor-disclosure

John, C. A., & Day, M. W. (2012). Central neurogenic diabetes insipidus, syndrome of inappropriate secretion of antidiuretic hormone, and cerebral salt-wasting syndrome in traumatic brain injury. *Critical Care Nurse*, *32*(2), e1–e7.

Jonklaas, J., Bianco, A. C., Bauer, A. J., et al. (2014). Guidelines for the treatment of hypothyroidism: Prepared by the American Thyroid Association Task Force on Thyroid Hormone Replacement. *Thyroid*, *24*(12), 1670–1751.

Katznelson, L., Laws, E. R Jr., Melmed, S., et al. (2014). Acromegaly: An endocrine society clinical practice guideline. *Journal of Clinical Endocrinology and Metabolism*, *99*(11), 3933–3951.

LaFranchi, S. (2016). Congenital hypothyroidism. *UpToDate*. Retrieved June 21, 2016, from www.uptodate.com/contents/clinical-features-and-detection-of-congenital-hypothyroidism

Morgan, D., & Tsai, S. C. (2015). Sleep and the endocrine system. *Critical Care Clinics*, *31*(3), 403–418.

Muldoon, B. T., Mai, V. Q., & Burch, H. B. (2014). Management of Graves' disease: An overview and comparison of clinical practice guidelines with actual practice trends. *Endocrinology and Metabolism Clinics of North America*, *43*, 495–516.

Nieman, L. K. (2016a). Clinical manifestations of adrenal insufficiency in adults. *UpToDate*. Retrieved June 29, 2016, from www.uptodate.com/contents/clinical-manifestations-of-adrenal-insufficiency-in-aduMorganlts

Nieman, L. K. (2016b). Diagnosis of adrenal insufficiency in adults. *UpToDate*. Retrieved June 29, 2016, from www.uptodate.com/contents/diagnosis-of-adrenal-insufficiency-in-adults

Nieman, L. K. (2016c). Treatment of adrenal insufficiency in adults. *UpToDate*. Retrieved June 29, 2016, from www.uptodate.com/contents/diagnosis-of-adrenal-insufficiency-in-adults

Nieman, L. K. (2016d). Establishing the diagnosis of Cushing's syndrome. *UpToDate*. Retrieved June 29, 2016, from www.uptodate.com/contents/establishing-the-diagnosis-of-cushings-syndrome

Rosen, C. J. (2016). Parathyroid hormone therapy for osteoporosis. *UpToDate*. Retrieved June 29, 2016, from www.uptodate.com/contents/parathyroid-hormone-therapy-for-osteoporosis

Rosenthal, M. S. (2014). Ethical issues and management of thyroid disease. *Endocrinology and Metabolism Clinics of North America*, *43*(2), 545–564.

Ross, D. S. (2016a). Myxedema coma. *UpToDate*. Retrieved June 22, 2016, from www.uptodate.com/contents/myxedema-coma

Ross, D. S. (2016b). Thyroid storm. *UpToDate*. Retrieved June 22, 2016, from www.uptodate.com/contents/thyroid-storm

Ross, D. S. (2016c). Beta blockers in the treatment of hyperthyroidism. *UpToDate*. Retrieved June 22, 2016, from www.uptodate.com/contents/beta-blockers-in-the-treatment-of-hyperthyroidism

Ross, D. S. (2016d). Thionamides in the treatment of Graves' disease. *UpToDate*. Retrieved June 22, 2016, from www.uptodate.com/contents/thionamides-in-the-treatment-of-graves-disease

Ross, D. S. (2016e). Radioiodine in the treatment of hyperthyroidism. *UpToDate*. Retrieved June 29, 2016, from www.uptodate.com/contents/radioiodine-in-the-treatment-of-hyperthyroidism

Ross, D. S. (2016f). Pharmacology and toxicity of thionamides. *UpToDate*. Retrieved June 29, 2016, from www.uptodate.com/contents/pharmacology-and-toxicity-of-thionamides

Ross, D. S. (2016g). Iodine in the treatment of hyperthyroidism. *UpToDate*. Retrieved June 29, 2016, from www.uptodate.com/contents/iodine-in-the-treatment-of-hyperthyroidism?title=Hyperthyroidism

Shane, E., & Berenson, J. R. (2016). Treatment of hypercalcemia. *UpToDate*. Retrieved June 29, 2016, from www.uptodate.com/contents/treatment-of-hypercalcemia

Shine, B., McKnight, R. F., Leaver, L., et al. (2015). Long-term effects of lithium on renal, thyroid, and parathyroid function: A retrospective analysis of laboratory data. *Lancet*, *386*, 461–468.

Surks, M. I. (2016a). Manifestations of hypothyroidism. *UpToDate*. Retrieved June 21, 2016, from www.uptodate.com/contents/hypothyroidism-underactive-thyroid-beyond-the-basics

Surks, M. I. (2016b). Iodine-induced thyroid dysfunction. *UpToDate*. Retrieved June 21, 2016, from www.uptodate.com/contents/iodine-induced-thyroid-dysfunction

Surks, M. I. (2016c). Lithium and the thyroid. *UpToDate*. Retrieved June 21, 2016, from www.uptodate.com/contents/lithium-and-the-thyroid

Tuttle, R. M. (2016). Surgical treatment of differentiated thyroid cancer. *UpToDate*. Retrieved June 29, 2016, from www.uptodate.com/contents/differentiated-thyroid-cancer-surgical-treatment

U.S. Preventive Services Task Force (USPSTF). (2015). Final Update Summary: Thyroid dysfunction: Screening. Retrieved 21, 2016, from www.uspreventiveservicestaskforce.org/Page/Document/UpdateSummaryFinal/thyroid-dysfunction-screening

Visser, W. E., Visser, T. J., & Peeters R. P. (2013). Thyroid disorders in older adults. *Endocrinology and Metabolism Clinics of North America*, *42*, 287–303.

World Health Organization. (2007). Reducing Salt Intake in Populations. Retrieved from https://www.who.int/dietphysicalactivity/Salt_Report_VC_april07.pdf

Young, F., & Kaplan, N. M. (2016). Clinical presentation and diagnosis of pheochromocytoma. *UpToDate*. Retrieved 29, 2016, from www.uptodate.com/contents/pathogenesis-of-behcets-disease/abstract/130

Young, F., Kaplan, N. M., & Kebebew, E. (2016). Treatment of pheochromocytoma in adults. *UpToDate*. Retrieved June 29, 2016, from www.uptodate.com/contents/treatment-of-pheochromocytoma-in-adults

Resources

American Thyroid Association, Inc.: http://www.thyroid.org

Canadian Association of Genetic Counsellors (CAGC): http://www.cagc-accg.ca

Canadian Cancer Society/Société Canadienne du cancer, National Office: http://www.cancer.ca

Canadian Directory of Genetic Support Groups, Support Group Directory, Regional Medical Genetics Centre, Children's Hospital of Western Ontario: http://www.lhsc.on.ca/programs/medgenet

Canadian Genetic Diseases Network: http://www.cgdn.ca

Canadian Medical Association; Toward Optimized Practice (TOP) Endocrine Working Group: http://www.topalbertadoctors.org/home/

Canadian Organization for Rare Disorders (CORD): http://www.cord.ca

Cushing's Support and Research Foundation: http://csrf.net

The Endocrine Society: http://www.endo-society.org

Genetics Society of Canada: http://life.biology.mcmaster.ca/GSC

National Adrenal Disease Foundation: http://www.nadf.us

Thyroid Foundation of Canada: http://www.thyroid.ca.

The Thyroid Society for Education and Research: http://www.the-thyroid-society.org

UNIT 9

Urinary Tract Function

Case Study

DECREASING CENTRAL LINE–ASSOCIATED BLOODSTREAM INFECTIONS

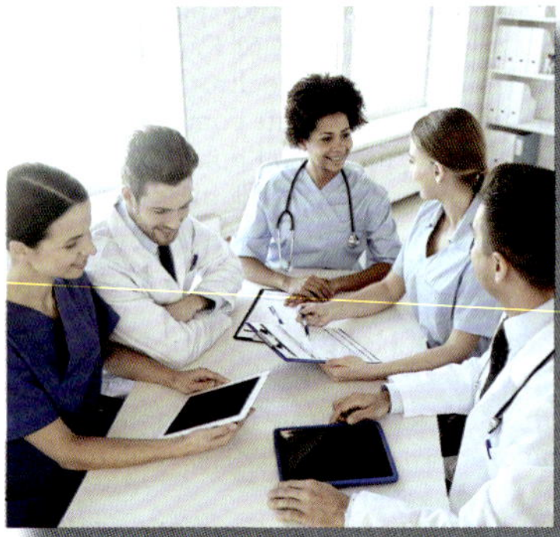

A nurse working in an acute care medical unit notes a high incidence of patients with Central line–associated bloodstream infections (CLABSIs). After accessing data about hospital admissions for CLABSI, the nurse verifies these observations. The nurse determines that many of the patients with CLABSI are receiving hemodialysis or have new kidney transplants and thus have central line access sites. The nurse sees the need for a plan that includes a unit-wide response to this problem. The plan involves arranging education programs about strategies to prevent CLABSI, including a review of hand hygiene, standard precautions/routine practices and universal precautions, and central line care.

QSEN Competency Focus: Quality Improvement

The complexities inherent in today's health care system challenge nurses to demonstrate integration of specific interdisciplinary core competencies that are aimed at ensuring the delivery of safe and quality patient care (Institute of Medicine, 2003). The Quality and Safety Education for Nurses project (QSEN, 2017; Cronenwett, Sherwood, Barnsteiner, et al., 2007) provides a framework for the knowledge, skills, and attitudes (KSAs) required for nurses to demonstrate competency in these key areas, which include ***patient-centred care***, ***interdisciplinary teamwork and collaboration***, ***evidence-based practice***, ***quality improvement***, ***safety***, and ***informatics.***

Quality Improvement Definition: Use data to monitor the outcomes of care processes and use improvement methods to design and test changes to continuously improve the quality and safety of health care systems.

SELECTED PRE-LICENSURE KSAs	APPLICATION AND REFLECTION
Knowledge	
Describe approaches for changing processes of care.	Describe how the nurse's observation of CLABSI rates in a specific population was then linked to data-derived measures that verified a need to plan a quality improvement initiative.
Skills	
Design a small test of change in daily work (using an experiential learning method such as Plan-Do-Study-Act). Practise aligning the aims, measures, and changes involved in improving care. Use measures to evaluate the effect of change.	What tools might the nurse use to gain buy-in from key constituents in his or her unit? What benchmarks of quality might he or she wish to use with these constituents?
Attitudes	
Value local change (in individual practice or team practice on a unit) and its role in creating joy in work. Appreciate the value of what individuals and teams can do to improve care.	Reflect on what you learned from this case study. Do you appreciate that variations may occur in specific populations (e.g., in this case, patients on hemodialysis and with new transplants)? If you practiced within the same setting, do you think you could have made the same observations and analyses?

Cronenwett, L., Sherwood, G., Barnsteiner, J., et al. (2007). Quality and safety education for nurses. *Nursing Outlook, 55*(3), 122–131; Institute of Medicine. (2003). *Health professions education: A bridge to quality*. Washington, DC: National Academies Press; and QSEN Institute. (2017). *QSEN competencies: Definitions and pre-licensure KSAs*. Retrieved June 12, 2019, from www.qsen.org/competencies/pre-licensure-ksas

44 Assessment of Renal and Urinary Tract Function

Adapted by Stephanie Zettel

Learning Objectives

On completion of this chapter, the learner will be able to:

1. Describe the anatomy and physiology of the renal and urinary systems.
2. Discuss the role of the kidneys in regulating fluid and electrolyte balance, acid–base balance, and blood pressure.
3. Describe the diagnostic studies used to determine upper and lower urinary tract function.
4. Identify the assessment parameters used for determining the status of upper and lower urinary tract function.
5. Initiate education and preparation for patients undergoing assessment of the urinary system.

Function of the renal and urinary systems is essential to life. The primary purpose of the renal and urinary systems is to maintain the body's state of homeostasis by carefully regulating fluid and electrolytes, removing wastes, and providing other functions (Chart 44-1). Dysfunction of the kidneys and lower urinary tract is common and may occur at any age and with varying degrees of severity. Assessment of upper and lower urinary tract function is part of every health examination and necessitates an understanding of the anatomy and physiology of the urinary system as well as the effects of changes in the system on other physiologic functions.

Anatomic and Physiologic Overview

Anatomy of the Renal and Urinary Tract Systems

The renal and urinary systems include the kidneys, ureters, bladder, and urethra. Urine is formed by the kidney and flows through the other structures to be eliminated from the body.

Kidneys

The kidneys are a pair of bean-shaped, brownish-red structures located retroperitoneally (behind and outside the peritoneal cavity) on the posterior wall of the abdomen—from the 12th thoracic vertebra to the 3rd lumbar vertebra in the adult (Fig. 44-1A). The rounded outer convex surface of each kidney is called the hilum. Each hilum is penetrated with blood vessels, nerves, and the ureter (Eaton & Pooler, 2013). The average adult kidney weighs approximately 113 to 170 g, is 10- to 12-cm long, 6-cm wide, and 2.5-cm thick (Grossman & Porth, 2014). The right kidney is slightly lower than the left due to the location of the liver.

Externally, the kidneys are well protected by the ribs and by the muscles of the abdomen and back. Internally, fat deposits surround each kidney, providing protection against jarring. The kidneys and surrounding fat are suspended from the abdominal wall by renal fascia made of connective tissue which hold the kidney in place (Skorecki, Chertow, Marsden, et al., 2015). The fibrous connective tissue, blood vessels, and lymphatics surrounding each kidney are known as the renal capsule. An adrenal gland lies on top of each kidney. The kidneys and adrenals are independent in function, blood supply, and innervation.

The renal parenchyma is divided into two parts: the cortex and the medulla (Fig. 44-1B). The medulla, which is approximately 5-cm wide, is the inner portion of the kidney. It contains the loops of Henle, the vasa recta, and the collecting ducts of the juxtamedullary nephrons. The collecting ducts from both the juxtamedullary and the cortical nephrons connect to the renal pyramids, which are triangular and are situated with the base facing the concave surface of the kidney and the point (papilla) facing the hilum, or pelvis. Each kidney contains approximately 8 to 18 pyramids. The pyramids drain into minor

CHART 44-1

Functions of the Kidney

- Urine formation
- Excretion of waste products
- Regulation of electrolytes
- Regulation of acid–base balance
- Control of water balance
- Control of blood pressure
- Renal clearance
- Regulation of red blood cell production
- Synthesis of vitamin D to active form
- Secretion of prostaglandins
- Regulates calcium and phosphorus balance

calices, which drain into major calices that open directly into the renal pelvis. The tip of each pyramid is called a papilla and projects into the minor calyx (Eaton & Pooler, 2013). The renal pelvis is the beginning of the collecting system and is composed of structures that are designed to collect and transport urine. Once the urine leaves the renal pelvis, the composition or amount of urine does not change.

The cortex, which is approximately 1-cm wide, is located farthest from the centre of the kidney and around the outermost edges. It contains the nephrons (the structural and functional units of the kidney responsible for urine formation), which are discussed below.

Blood Supply to the Kidneys

The hilum is the concave portion of the kidney through which the renal artery enters and the ureters and renal vein exit. The kidneys receive 20% to 25% of the total cardiac output, which means that all of the body's blood circulates through the kidneys approximately 12 times per hour (Grossman & Porth, 2014). The renal artery (arising from the abdominal aorta) divides into smaller and smaller vessels, eventually forming the afferent arterioles. Each afferent arteriole branches to form a glomerulus, which is the capillary bed responsible for **glomerular filtration**. Blood leaves the glomerulus through the efferent arteriole and flows back to the inferior vena cava through a network of capillaries and veins.

Nephrons

Each kidney has 1 million **nephrons** that are located within the renal parenchyma and are responsible for the formation of filtrate that will become urine (Eaton & Pooler, 2013). The large number of nephrons allows for adequate renal function even if the opposite kidney is damaged or becomes nonfunctional. If the total number of functioning nephrons is less than 20% of normal, renal replacement therapy needs to be considered.

There are two types of nephrons. The cortical nephrons, which make up 80% to 85% of the total number, are located in the outermost part of the cortex, and the juxtamedullary nephrons, which make up the remaining 15% to 20%, are located deeper in the cortex (Grossman & Porth, 2014). The juxtamedullary nephrons are distinguished by long loops of Henle and are surrounded by long capillary loops called *vasa recta* that dip into the medulla of the kidney. The length of the tubular component of the nephron is directly related to its ability to concentrate urine.

Nephrons are made up of two basic components: a filtering element composed of an enclosed capillary network (the glomerulus) and the attached tubule (Fig. 44-2). The **glomerulus** is a unique network of capillaries suspended between the afferent and efferent blood vessels, which are enclosed in an epithelial structure called *Bowman's capsule*. The glomerular membrane is composed of three filtering layers: the capillary endothelium, the basement membrane,

Glossary

aldosterone: hormone synthesized and released by the adrenal cortex; causes the kidneys to reabsorb sodium
antidiuretic hormone: hormone secreted by the posterior pituitary gland; causes the kidneys to reabsorb more water; also called vasopressin
anuria: total urine output less than 50 mL in 24 hours
bacteriuria: bacteria in the urine; bacterial count higher than 100,000 colonies/mL
creatinine: endogenous waste product of muscle energy metabolism
diuresis: increased formation and secretion of urine
dysuria: painful or difficult urination
frequency: voiding more frequently than every 3 hours
glomerular filtration: plasma filtered at the glomerulus into the kidney tubules
glomerulus: tuft of capillaries forming part of the nephron through which filtration occurs
hematuria: red blood cells in the urine
micturition: urination or voiding
nephron: structural and functional unit of the kidney responsible for urine formation
nocturia: awakening at night to urinate
oliguria: total urine output less than 500 mL in 24 hours
proteinuria: protein in the urine
pyuria: white blood cells in the urine
renal clearance: volume of plasma that the kidneys can clear of a specific solute (e.g., creatinine); expressed in millilitres per minute
renal glycosuria: recurring or persistent excretion of glucose in the urine
specific gravity: reflects the weight of particles dissolved in the urine; expression of the degree of concentration of the urine
tubular reabsorption: movement of a substance from the kidney tubule into the blood in the peritubular capillaries or vasa recta
tubular secretion: movement of a substance from the blood in the peritubular capillaries or vasa recta into the kidney tubule
urea nitrogen: nitrogenous end product of protein metabolism

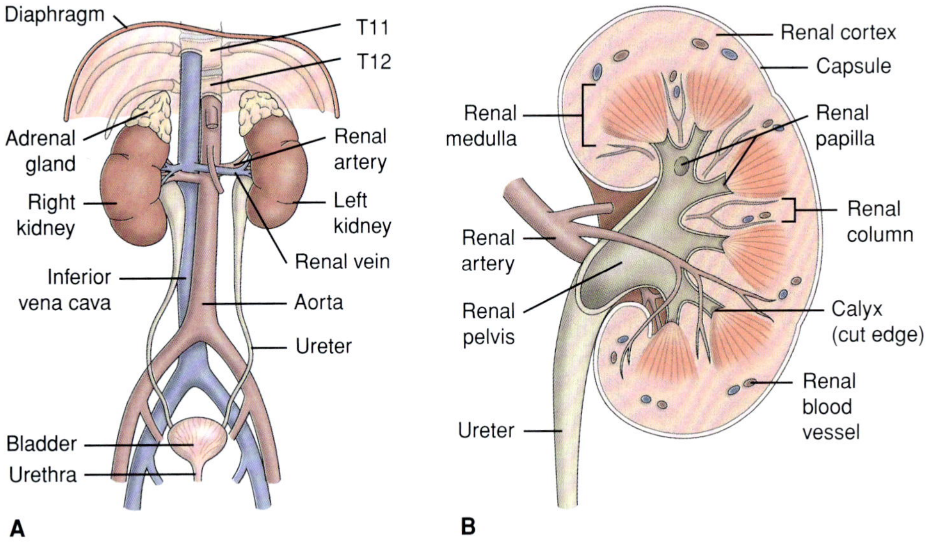

FIGURE 44-1. **A.** Kidneys, ureters, and bladder. **B.** Internal structure of the kidney. (Redrawn from Porth, C. M., & Matfin, G. (2009). *Pathophysiology: Concepts of altered health status* (8th ed.). Philadelphia, PA: Lippincott Williams & Wilkins.)

and the epithelium. This membrane normally allows filtration of fluid and small molecules, yet limits passage of larger molecules, such as blood cells and albumin. Pressure changes and the permeability of the glomerular membrane of Bowman's capsule facilitate the passage of fluids and various substances from the blood vessels, filling the space within Bowman's capsule with this filtered solution.

The tubular component of the nephron begins in the Bowman's capsule. The filtrate created in the Bowman's capsule travels first into the proximal tubule, which is made up of epithelial cells resting on the basement membrane, then the loop of Henle, the distal tubule, and either the cortical or medullary collecting ducts (Eaton & Pooler, 2013). The structural arrangement of the tubule allows the distal tubule to lie in close proximity to where the afferent and efferent arteriole respectively enter and leave the glomerulus. The distal tubular cells located in this area, known as the *macula densa*, function with the adjacent afferent arteriole and create what is known as the *juxtaglomerular apparatus*. This is the site of renin production. Renin is a hormone directly involved in the control of arterial blood pressure; it is essential for proper functioning of the glomerulus (see later discussion).

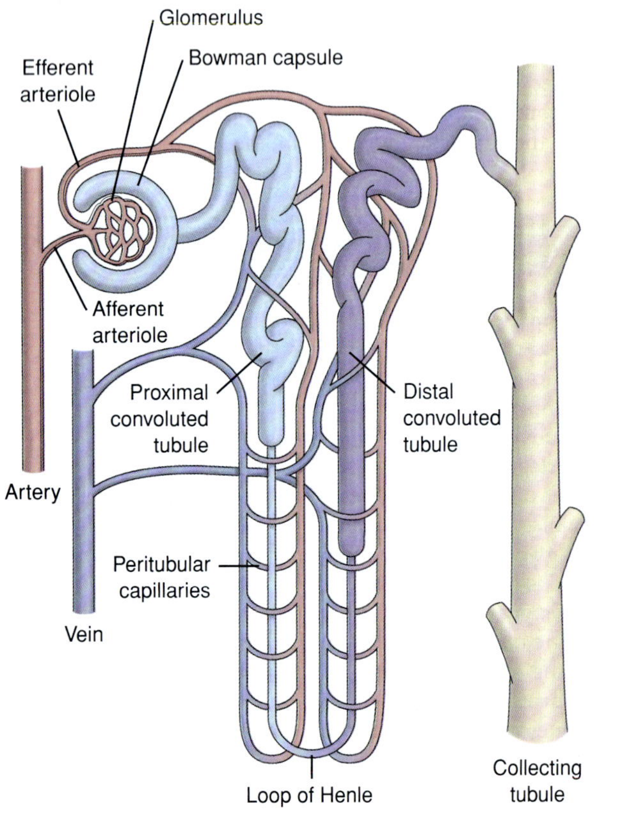

FIGURE 44-2. Representation of a nephron. Each kidney has about 1 million nephrons of two types: cortical and juxtamedullary. Cortical nephrons are located in the cortex of the kidney; juxtamedullary nephrons are adjacent to the medulla.

The tubular component consists of the Bowman's capsule, the proximal tubule, the descending and ascending limbs of the loop of Henle, and the cortical and medullary collecting ducts. This portion of the nephron is responsible for making adjustments in the filtrate, based on the body's needs. Changes are continually made as the filtrate travels through the tubules until it enters the collecting system and is expelled from the body (Fig. 44-2).

Ureters, Bladder, and Urethra

The urine formed in the nephrons flows into the renal pelvis and then into the ureters, which are long fibromuscular tubes that connect each kidney to the bladder (Hall, 2016). These narrow tubes, each 24- to 30-cm long, originate at the lower portion of the renal pelvis and terminate in the trigone (tissue between the opening of the ureters and urethra) of the bladder wall.

The left ureter is slightly shorter than the right ureter. The lining of the ureters is made up of transitional cell epithelium called *urothelium*. The urothelium prevents reabsorption of urine. The movement of urine from each renal pelvis through the ureter into the bladder is facilitated by peristaltic contraction of the smooth muscles in the ureter wall. There are three narrowed areas of each ureter: the ureteropelvic junction, the ureteral segment near the sacroiliac junction, and the ureterovesical junction. These three areas of the ureters have a propensity for obstruction by renal calculi (kidney stones) or stricture.

Obstruction of the ureteropelvic junction is the most serious because of its close proximity to the kidney and the risk of associated kidney dysfunction.

The urinary bladder is a muscular, hollow sac located just behind the pubic bone (Weber & Kelley, 2014). The capacity of the adult bladder is 400 to 500 mL but it can distend to hold a larger volume. The bladder is characterized by its central, hollow area, called the *vesicle,* which has two inlets (the ureters) and one outlet (the urethra). The area surrounding the bladder neck is called the *ureterovesical junction.* The angling of the ureterovesical junction is the primary means of providing antegrade, or downward, movement of urine, also referred to as efflux of urine. This angling prevents vesicoureteral reflux (retrograde, or backward, movement of urine) from the bladder, up the ureter, toward the kidney.

The wall of the bladder contains four layers. The outermost layer is the adventitia, which is made up of connective tissue. Immediately beneath the adventitia is a smooth muscle layer known as the *detrusor*. Beneath the detrusor is a submucosal layer of loose connective tissue that serves as an interface between the detrusor and the innermost layer, a mucosal lining. The inner layer contains specialized transitional cell epithelium, a membrane that is impermeable to water and prevents reabsorption of urine stored in the bladder. The bladder neck contains bundles of involuntary smooth muscle that form a portion of the urethral sphincter known as the internal sphincter. An important portion of the sphincteric mechanism that helps maintain continence is the external urinary sphincter at the anterior urethra, the segment most distal from the bladder (Grossman & Porth, 2014). During voiding (**micturition**), increased intravesical pressure keeps the ureterovesical junction closed and keeps urine within the ureters. As soon as micturition is completed, intravesical pressure returns to its normal low baseline value, allowing efflux of urine to resume. Therefore, the only time that the bladder is completely empty is in the last seconds of micturition, before efflux of urine resumes.

The urethra arises from the base of the bladder: In the male, it passes through the penis; in the female, it opens just anterior to the vagina. In the male, the prostate gland, which lies just below the bladder neck, surrounds the urethra posteriorly and laterally.

Function of the Renal and Urinary Tract Systems

CONCEPTS IN ACTION

Urine Formation

The healthy human body is composed of approximately 60% water. Water balance is regulated by the kidneys and results in the formation of urine. Urine is formed in the nephrons through a complex three-step process: glomerular filtration, tubular reabsorption, and tubular secretion (Fig. 44-3). Each nephron functions independently from other nephrons because each has its own blood supply (Eaton & Pooler, 2013). The various substances normally filtered by the glomerulus, reabsorbed by the tubules, and excreted in the urine include sodium, chloride, bicarbonate, potassium, glucose, urea, creatinine, and uric acid. Within the tubule, some of these substances are selectively

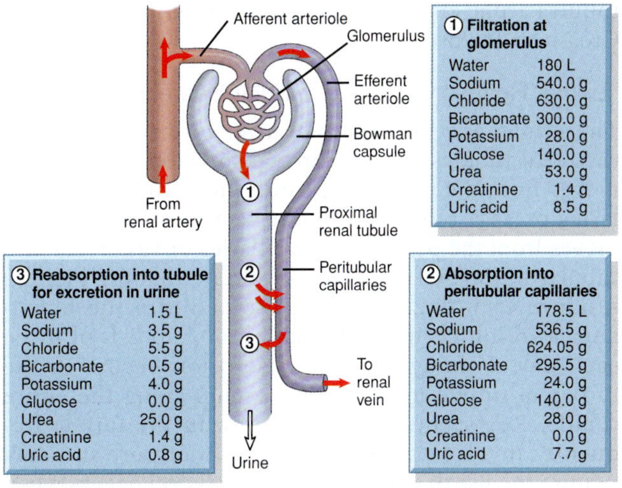

FIGURE 44-3. Urine is formed in the nephrons in a three-step process: filtration, reabsorption, and excretion. Water, electrolytes, and other substances, such as glucose and creatinine, are filtered by the glomerulus; varying amounts of these substances are reabsorbed in the renal tubule or excreted in the urine. Approximate normal volumes of these substances during the steps of urine formation are shown at the top. Wide variations may occur in these values depending on diet.

reabsorbed into the blood. Others are secreted from the blood into the filtrate as it travels down the tubule.

Amino acids and glucose are usually filtered at the level of the glomerulus and reabsorbed so that neither is excreted in the urine. Normally, glucose does not appear in the urine. However, **renal glycosuria** (recurring or persistent excretion of glucose in the urine) occurs if the amount of glucose in the blood and glomerular filtrate exceeds the amount that the tubules are able to reabsorb. Renal glycosuria can occur on its own as a benign condition (Hall, 2016). It also occurs in poorly controlled diabetes, the most common condition that causes the blood glucose level to exceed the kidney's reabsorption capacity. Renal glycosuria is also common in pregnancy.

Protein molecules also are not usually found in the urine; however, low–molecular-weight proteins (globulins and albumin) may periodically be excreted in small amounts. Protein in the urine is referred to as **proteinuria** (Eaton & Pooler, 2013).

Glomerular Filtration

The normal blood flow through the kidneys is about 1,000 and 1,300 mL/min (Grossman & Porth, 2014). As blood flows into the glomerulus from an afferent arteriole, filtration occurs. The filtered fluid, also known as filtrate or ultrafiltrate, then enters the renal tubules. Under normal conditions, about 20% of the blood passing through the glomeruli is filtered into the nephron, amounting to about 180 L/day of filtrate (Eaton & Pooler, 2013). The filtrate normally consists of water, electrolytes, and other small molecules, because water and small molecules are allowed to pass, whereas larger molecules stay in the bloodstream. Efficient filtration depends on adequate blood flow through the afferent arteriole that maintains a consistent pressure through the glomerulus (also called the hydrostatic pressure). Many factors can alter this blood flow and pressure, including hypotension, decreased oncotic pressure in the blood, and increased pressure in the renal tubules from an obstruction (Eaton & Pooler, 2013; Grossman & Porth, 2014).

Tubular Reabsorption and Tubular Secretion

The second and third steps of urine formation occur in the renal tubules. In **tubular reabsorption**, a substance moves from the filtrate back into the peritubular capillaries or vasa recta. In **tubular secretion**, a substance moves from the peritubular capillaries or vasa recta into tubular filtrate. Of the 180 L of filtrate that the kidneys produce each day, 99% is reabsorbed into the bloodstream, resulting in the formation of 1 to 2 L of urine each day. Although most reabsorption occurs in the proximal tubule, reabsorption occurs along the entire tubule. Reabsorption and secretion in the tubule frequently involve passive and active transport and may require the use of energy. Tubular secretion occurs when substances move from the peritubular capillary blood plasma (blood) into the tubular lumen (filtrate). Tubular secretion helps with the elimination of potassium, hydrogen ions, ammonia (NH_3), uric acid, some drugs, and other waste products (Headly, 2015). Filtrate becomes concentrated in the distal tubule and collecting ducts under hormonal influence and becomes urine, which then enters the renal pelvis. In the absence of tubular reabsorption, volume depletion would rapidly occur (Headly, 2015).

Antidiuretic Hormone

Antidiuretic hormone (ADH), also known as vasopressin, is a hormone that is secreted by the posterior portion of the pituitary gland in response to changes in osmolality of the blood. With decreased water intake, blood osmolality tends to increase, stimulating ADH release. ADH then acts on the kidney, increasing reabsorption of water and thereby returning the osmolality of the blood to normal. With excess water intake, the secretion of ADH by the pituitary is suppressed; therefore, less water is reabsorbed by the kidney tubule. This latter situation leads to increased urine volume (**diuresis**).

A dilute urine with a fixed specific gravity (about 1.010) or fixed osmolality (about 300 mOsm/L) indicates an inability to concentrate and dilute the urine, a common early sign of kidney disease (Skorecki et al., 2015).

Osmolarity and Osmolality

Osmolarity refers to the ratio of solute to water. The regulation of salt and water is paramount for control of the extracellular volume and both serum and urine osmolarity. Controlling either the amount of water or the amount of solute can change osmolarity. Osmolarity and ionic composition are maintained by the body within very narrow limits. As little as a 1% to 2% change in the serum osmolarity can cause a conscious desire to drink and conservation of water by the kidneys (Skorecki et al., 2015).

The degree of dilution or concentration of the urine is also measured in terms of *osmolality*, which is the number of particles (electrolytes and other molecules, referred to as osmoles) dissolved per kilogram of solution. The filtrate in the glomerular capillary normally has the same osmolality as the blood, with a value of about 280 to 300 mOsml/kg. Serum and urine osmolality and osmolarity are discussed in more detail in Chapter 17.

Regulation of Water Excretion

Regulation of the amount of water excreted is an important function of the kidney. With high fluid intake, a large volume of dilute urine is excreted. Conversely, with a low fluid intake, a small volume of concentrated urine is excreted. A person normally ingests about 1,300 mL of oral liquids and 1,000 mL of water in food per day. Of the fluid ingested, approximately 900 mL is lost through the skin and lungs (called *insensible loss*), 50 mL through sweat, and 200 mL through feces. It is important to consider all fluid gained and lost when evaluating total fluid status. Daily weight measurements are a reliable means of determining overall fluid status. One kg equals approximately 1,000 mL or 1 L, so a weight change of as little as 1 kg could suggest an overall fluid gain or loss of 1,000 mL (Grossman & Porth, 2014).

Regulation of Electrolyte Excretion

When the kidneys are functioning normally, the volume of electrolytes excreted per day is equal to the amount ingested. For example, the average Canadian daily diet contains 6 to 8 g each of sodium chloride (salt) and potassium chloride, and approximately the same amounts are excreted in the urine.

The regulation of sodium volume excreted depends on **aldosterone**, a hormone synthesized and released from the adrenal cortex. With increased aldosterone in the blood, less sodium is excreted in the urine, because aldosterone facilitates the renal reabsorption of sodium. Release of aldosterone from the adrenal cortex is largely under the control of angiotensin II. Angiotensin II levels are in turn, controlled by renin, an enzyme that is released from specialized cells in the kidneys (Fig. 44-4). This complex system is activated when pressure in the renal arterioles falls below normal levels, as occurs with shock, dehydration, or decreased sodium chloride delivery to the tubules.

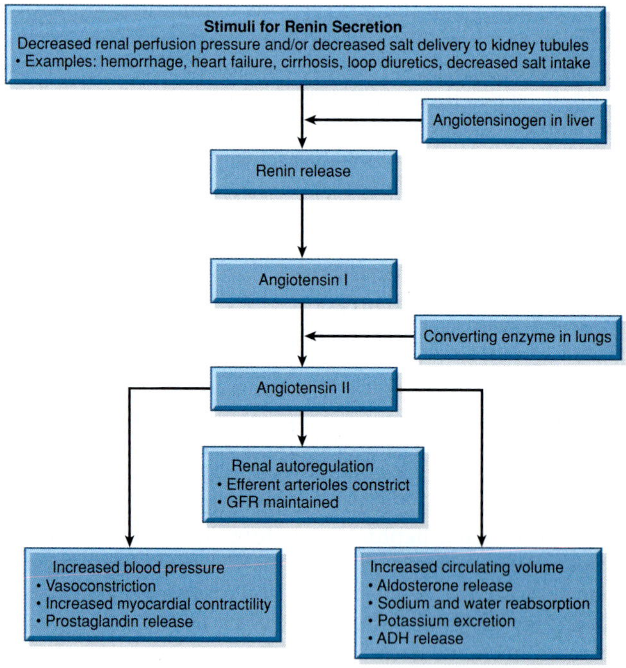

FIGURE 44-4. The renin–angiotensin system. ADH, antidiuretic hormone; GFR, glomerular filtration rate.

Activation of this system increases the retention of water and expansion of the intravascular fluid volume, thereby maintaining enough pressure within the glomerulus to ensure adequate filtration.

The regulation of serum sodium and potassium are discussed in detail in Chapter 17.

Regulation of Acid–Base Balance

The normal serum pH is about 7.35 to 7.45 and must be maintained within this narrow range for optimal physiologic function (Grossman & Porth, 2014). The kidney performs two major functions to assist in this balance. The first is to reabsorb and return to the body's circulation any bicarbonate from the urinary filtrate; the second is to excrete acid in the urine (through the synthesis of NH_3 and the excretion hydrogen ion in ammonium chloride) (Headly, 2015). Because bicarbonate is a small ion, it is freely filtered at the glomerulus. The renal tubules actively reabsorb most of the bicarbonate in the urinary filtrate. To replace any lost bicarbonate, the renal tubular cells generate new bicarbonate through a variety of chemical reactions. This newly generated bicarbonate is then reabsorbed by the tubules and returned to the body.

The body's acid production is the result of catabolism, or breakdown, of proteins, which produces acid compounds, in particular phosphoric and sulphuric acids. The normal daily diet also includes a certain amount of acid materials. Unlike carbon dioxide (CO_2), phosphoric and sulphuric acids cannot be eliminated by the lungs. Because accumulation of these acids in the blood lowers pH (making the blood more acidic) and inhibits cell function, they must be excreted in the urine. However, if the hydrogen ions are low, they will be reabsorbed. A person with normal kidney function excretes about 70 mEq of acid each day. The kidney is able to excrete some of this acid directly into the urine until the urine pH reaches 4.5, which is 1,000 times more acidic than blood (Grossman & Porth, 2014).

However, more acid usually needs to be eliminated from the body than can be secreted directly as free acid in the urine. These excess acids are bound to chemical buffers so that they can be excreted in the urine. Two important chemical buffers are phosphate ions and NH_3. When buffered with acid, NH_3 becomes ammonium (NH_4). Phosphate is present in the glomerular filtrate, and NH_3 is produced by the cells of the renal tubules and secreted into the tubular fluid. Through the buffering process, the kidney is able to excrete large quantities of acid in a bound form, without further lowering the pH of the urine.

Autoregulation of Blood Pressure

Regulation of blood pressure is an important function of the kidney. Specialized vessels of the kidney, called the *vasa recta*, constantly monitor blood pressure as blood begins its passage into the kidney. When the vasa recta detect a decrease in blood pressure, specialized juxtaglomerular cells called macula densa cells, near the afferent arteriole, distal tubule, and efferent arteriole secrete the hormone, renin. Renin converts angiotensinogen to angiotensin I, which is then converted to angiotensin II, the most powerful vasoconstrictor known; angiotensin II causes the blood pressure to increase (Hall, 2016). The adrenal cortex secretes aldosterone in response to stimulation by angiotensin II. The result is an increase in blood pressure. When the vasa recta recognize the increase in blood pressure, renin secretion stops. Failure of this feedback mechanism is one of the primary causes of hypertension (Fig. 44-4).

Renal Clearance

Renal clearance refers to the ability of the kidneys to clear solutes from the plasma. A 24-hour collection of urine is the primary test of renal clearance used to evaluate how well the kidney performs this important excretory function. Renal clearance depends on several factors: how quickly the substance is filtered across the glomerulus, how much of the substance is reabsorbed along the tubules, and how much of the substance is secreted into the tubules. It is possible to measure the renal clearance of any substance, but the one measure that is particularly useful is the *creatinine clearance.*

Creatinine is an endogenous waste product of skeletal muscle that is filtered at the glomerulus, passed through the tubules with minimal change, and excreted in the urine. Hence, creatinine clearance is a good measure of the *glomerular filtration rate* (GFR) the amount of plasma filtered through the glomeruli per unit of time. To calculate creatinine clearance, a 24-hour urine specimen is collected. Midway through the collection, the serum creatinine level is measured. The following formula is then used to calculate the creatinine clearance:

$$\frac{(\text{Volume of urine [mL/min]} \times \text{urine creatinine [mL/dL]})}{\text{Serum creatinine (mg/dL)}}$$

The adult GFR can vary from a normal of approximately 125 mL/min (1.67 to 2.0 mL/s) to a high of 200 mL/min (Grossman & Porth, 2014). Creatinine clearance is an excellent measure of renal function; as renal function declines, creatinine clearance decreases.

Regulation of Red Blood Cell Production

When the kidneys detect a decrease in the oxygen tension in renal blood flow, they release erythropoietin. *Erythropoietin* is a glycoprotein from the kidney that stimulates the bone marrow to produce red blood cells (RBCs) that carry oxygen throughout the body (Eaton & Pooler, 2013).

Vitamin D Synthesis

The kidneys are also responsible for the final conversion of inactive vitamin D to its active form, 1,25-dihydroxycholecalciferol. Vitamin D is necessary for maintaining normal calcium balance in the body and is required for intestinal absorption of calcium.

Secretion of Prostaglandins and Other Substances

The kidneys also produce prostaglandin E and prostacyclin, thromboxane and leukotrienes, which have a vasoactive effects and are important in maintaining renal blood flow. These substances contribute to autoregulation of blood flow in the kidney by causing selective vasodilation or vasoconstriction (Headly, 2015).

Excretion of Waste Products

The kidneys eliminate the body's metabolic waste products. The major waste product of protein metabolism is *urea*, of which about 25 to 30 g are produced and excreted daily (Grossman & Porth, 2014). All of this urea must be excreted in the urine; otherwise, it accumulates in body tissues. Other waste products of metabolism that must be excreted are creatinine, phosphates, and sulphates. Uric acid, formed as a waste product of purine metabolism (metabolism of DNA), is also eliminated in the urine. The kidneys also serve as the primary mechanism for excreting drug metabolites.

Urine Storage

The bladder is the reservoir for urine. Both filling and emptying of the bladder are mediated by coordinated sympathetic and parasympathetic nervous system control mechanisms involving the detrusor muscle and the bladder outlet. Conscious awareness of bladder filling occurs as a result of sympathetic neuronal pathways that travel via the spinal cord to the level of T10 through T12, where peripheral, hypogastric nerve innervation allows for continued bladder filling. As bladder filling continues, stretch receptors in the bladder wall are activated, coupled with the desire to void. This information from the detrusor muscle is relayed back to the cerebral cortex via the parasympathetic pelvic nerves at the level of S1 through S4 (Grossman & Porth, 2014). Overall bladder pressure remains low due to the bladder's compliance (ability to expand or collapse) as urine volume changes.

Bladder compliance is due in part to the smooth muscle lining of the bladder and collagen deposits within the wall of the bladder, as well as to neuronal mechanisms that inhibit the detrusor muscle from contracting (specifically, adrenergic receptors that mediate relaxation). To maintain adequate kidney filtration rates, bladder pressure during filling must remain lower than 40 cm H_2O. This low pressure allows the urine to freely leave the renal pelvis and enter the ureters. The sensation of bladder fullness is transmitted to the central nervous system when the bladder has reached about 150 to 200 mL in adults, and an initial desire to void occurs (Hall, 2016). A marked sense of fullness and discomfort with a strong desire to void usually occurs when the bladder reaches its functional capacity, 300 to 500 mL of urine. Neurologic changes to the bladder at the level of the supraspinal nerves, the spinal nerves, or the bladder wall itself can cause abnormally high volumes (up to 2,000 mL) of urine to be stored due to a decreased or absent urge to void.

Under normal circumstances with average fluid intake of approximately, 1,000 to 2,000 mL/day, the bladder should be able to store urine for periods of 2 to 4 hours at a time during the day (Hall, 2016). At night, the release of vasopressin in response to decreased fluid intake causes a decrease in the production of urine and makes urine more concentrated. This phenomenon usually allows the bladder to continue filling for periods of 6 to 8 hours in adolescents and adults, making them able to sleep for longer periods before needing to void. In older adults, decreasing bladder compliance and decreased vasopressin levels often cause ***nocturia*** (the need to wake up during the night to urinate).

Bladder Emptying

Micturition (voiding) normally occurs approximately eight times in a 24-hour period. It is activated via the micturition reflex arc within the sympathetic and parasympathetic nervous systems, which causes a coordinated sequence of events. Initiation of voiding occurs when the efferent pelvic nerve, which originates in the S1 to S4 area, stimulates the bladder to contract, resulting in complete relaxation of the striated urethral sphincter. This is followed by a decrease in urethral pressure, contraction of the detrusor muscle, opening of the vesicle neck and proximal urethra, and flow of urine. This coordinated effort by the parasympathetic system is mediated by muscarinic and, to a lesser extent, cholinergic receptors within the detrusor muscle. The pressure generated in the bladder during micturition is about 20 to 40 cm H_2O in females. This pressure is somewhat higher and more variable in males 45 years of age and older due to the normal hyperplasia of the cells of the middle lobes of the prostate gland, which surround the proximal urethra. Any obstruction of the bladder outlet, such as in advanced benign prostatic hyperplasia (BPH), results in a high voiding pressure. High voiding pressures make it more difficult to start urine flow and maintain it.

If the spinal pathways from the brain to the urinary system are destroyed (e.g., after a spinal cord injury), reflex contraction of the bladder is maintained, but voluntary control over the process is lost. In both situations, the detrusor muscle can contract and expel urine, but the contractions are generally insufficient to empty the bladder completely, so residual urine (urine left in the bladder after voiding) remains. Normally, residual urine amounts to no more than 50 mL in the middle-aged adult and less than 50 to 100 mL in the older adult.

Gerontologic Considerations

Upper and lower urinary tract function changes with age (Eliopoulos, 2018). The GFR decreases, starting between 35 and 40 years of age, and a yearly decline of about 1 mL/min continues thereafter. Older adults are more susceptible to acute and chronic kidney injury due to the structural and functional changes in the kidney. Examples include sclerosis of the glomerulus and renal vasculature, decreased blood flow, decreased GFR, altered tubular function, and acid–base imbalance. Although renal function usually remains adequate, renal reserve is decreased and may reduce the kidneys' ability to respond effectively to drastic or sudden physiologic changes. This steady decrease in glomerular filtration, combined with the use of multiple medications in which metabolites are cleared by the kidneys, puts the older adult at higher risk for adverse drug effects and drug–drug interactions (Eliopoulos, 2018).

Older adults are more prone to develop hypernatremia and fluid volume deficit, because increasing age is also associated with diminished osmotic stimulation of thirst. Thirst is defined as one's awareness of the desire to drink. The sense of thirst is so protective that hypernatremia almost never occurs in adults younger than 60 years.

Structural or functional abnormalities that occur with aging may also prevent complete emptying of the bladder. This may be due to decreased bladder wall contractility; secondary to myogenic or neurogenic factors; or related to bladder outlet obstruction, such as in BPH or after prostatectomy (Larsen & Post, 2013). Vaginal and urethral tissues atrophy (become thinner) in aging women due to decreased estrogen levels. This causes decreased blood supply to the urogenital tissues, resulting in urethral and vaginal irritation and urinary incontinence.

Urinary incontinence is present in 15% to 30% of community-dwelling older adults, 50% of older adults who are institutionalized, and 30% of older adults who are hospitalized (Eliopoulos, 2018). Many older adults and their families are unaware that urinary incontinence stems from many causes. The nurse needs to inform the patient and family that with appropriate evaluation, urinary incontinence can often be managed at home, and in many cases, it can be eliminated. Many treatments are available for urinary incontinence in the older adult, including noninvasive, behavioural interventions that the patient or caregiver can initiate (Scemons, 2013). Treatment modalities for urinary incontinence are described in further detail in Chapter 46.

Preparation of the older adult for diagnostic tests must be managed carefully to prevent dehydration, which might precipitate renal failure in a patient with marginal renal function. Limitations in mobility may affect the older adult's ability to void adequately or to consume an adequate volume of fluids. The patient may limit fluid intake to minimize the **frequency** of voiding or the risk of incontinence. Teaching the patient and family about the dangers of an inadequate fluid intake is an important role of the nurse caring for the older adult incontinent patient.

Providing education about the dangers of an inadequate fluid intake is an important role of the nurse caring for the older patient. The nurse emphasizes the need to drink throughout the day even if the patient does not feel thirsty, because the thirst stimulation is decreased.

Older women often have incomplete emptying of the bladder and urinary stasis, which may result in urinary tract infection or increasing bladder pressure, leading to overflow incontinence, hydronephrosis, pyelonephritis, or chronic kidney disease (Eliopoulos, 2018). Urologic symptoms can mimic disorders such as appendicitis, peptic ulcer disease, and cholecystitis, which can make diagnosis difficult in older adults due to decreased neurologic innervation (Eliopoulos, 2018).

CHART 44-2

Risk Factors for Selected Renal or Urologic Disorders

Risk Factor	Possible Renal or Urologic Disorder
Childhood diseases: "strep throat" impetigo, nephrotic syndrome	Chronic kidney disease
Advanced age	Incomplete emptying of bladder, leading to urinary tract infection
Instrumentation of urinary tract, cystoscopy, catheterization	Urinary tract infection, incontinence
Immobilization	Kidney stone formation
Occupational, recreational, or environmental exposure to chemicals (plastics, pitch, tar, rubber)	Acute renal failure
Diabetes	Chronic kidney disease, neurogenic bladder
Hypertension	Renal insufficiency, chronic renal failure
Multiple sclerosis	Incontinence, neurogenic bladder
Parkinson's disease	Incontinence and other complications
Systemic lupus erythematosus	Nephritis, chronic kidney disease
Gout, hyperparathyroidism, Crohn's disease, ileostomy	Kidney stone formation
Sickle cell disease, multiple myeloma	Chronic kidney disease
Benign prostatic hyperplasia	Obstruction to urine flow, leading to frequency, oliguria, anuria
Radiation therapy to pelvis	Cystitis, fibrosis of ureter, or fistula in urinary tract
Recent pelvic surgery	Inadvertent trauma to ureters or bladder
Pregnancy	Proteinuria, frequent voiding
Obstetric injury, tumours	Incontinence
Spinal cord injury	Neurogenic bladder, urinary tract infection, incontinence

Assessment of the Renal and Urinary Tract Systems

Health History

Obtaining a urologic health history requires excellent communication skills, because many patients are embarrassed or uncomfortable discussing genitourinary function or symptoms (Eliopoulos, 2018). It is important to use language the patient can understand and to avoid medical jargon. It is also important to review risk factors, particularly for those patients who are at high risk. For example, the nurse needs to be aware that multiparous women delivering their children vaginally have a high risk for stress urinary incontinence, which, if severe enough, can also lead to urge incontinence. Older women and people with neurologic disorders such as diabetic neuropathy, multiple sclerosis (MS), or Parkinson's disease often have incomplete emptying of the bladder and urinary stasis, which may result in urinary tract infection or increasing bladder pressure, leading to overflow incontinence, hydronephrosis, pyelonephritis, or chronic kidney disease.

Risk factors for specific disorders and kidney and lower urinary tract dysfunction are summarized in Chart 44-2 and discussed in Chapters 45 and 46.

When obtaining the health history, the nurse should inquire about the following:

- The patient's chief concern or reason for seeking health care, the onset of the problem, and its effect on the patient's quality of life
- The location, character, and duration of pain, if present, and its relationship to voiding; factors that precipitate pain, and those that relieve it
- History of urinary tract infections, including past treatment or hospitalization for urinary tract infection
- Fever or chills

- Previous renal or urinary diagnostic tests or use of indwelling urinary catheters
- **Dysuria** and when during voiding (i.e., at initiation or at termination of voiding) it occurs
- Hesitancy, straining, or pain during or after urination
- Urinary incontinence (stress incontinence, urge incontinence, overflow incontinence, or functional incontinence)
- **Hematuria** or change in colour or volume of urine
- Nocturia and its date of onset
- Renal calculi (kidney stones), passage of stones or gravel in urine
- Female patients: number and type (vaginal or cesarean) of deliveries; use of forceps; vaginal infection, discharge, or irritation; contraceptive practices
- History of **anuria** (decreased urine production) or other renal problem
- Presence or history of genital lesions or sexually transmitted diseases
- Use of tobacco, alcohol, or recreational drugs
- Any prescription and over-the-counter medications (including those prescribed for renal or urinary problems)

Common Symptoms

Dysfunction of the kidney can produce a complex array of symptoms throughout the body. Pain, changes in voiding, and gastrointestinal symptoms are particularly suggestive of urinary tract disease.

Pain

Genitourinary pain is usually caused by distention of some portion of the urinary tract as a result of obstructed urine flow or inflammation and swelling of tissues. Severity of pain is related to the sudden onset rather than the extent of distention.

Table 44-1 lists the various types of genitourinary pain, characteristics of the pain, associated signs and symptoms, and possible causes. However, kidney disease does not always involve pain. It tends to be diagnosed because of other symptoms that cause a patient to seek health care, such as pedal edema, shortness of breath, and changes in urine elimination (Weber & Kelley, 2014).

Changes in Voiding

Micturition is normally a painless function that occurs approximately eight times in a 24-hour period. The average person voids 1 to 2 L of urine in 24 hours, although this amount varies depending on fluid intake, sweating, environmental temperature, vomiting, or diarrhea. Common problems associated with voiding include frequency, urgency, dysuria, hesitancy, incontinence, enuresis, polyuria, **oliguria**, and hematuria. These problems and others are described in Table 44-2. Increased urinary urgency and frequency coupled with decreasing urine volumes strongly suggest urine retention. Depending on the acuity of the onset of these symptoms, immediate bladder emptying via catheterization and evaluation may be necessary to prevent kidney dysfunction.

Gastrointestinal Symptoms

Gastrointestinal signs and symptoms are often associated with urologic conditions because of shared autonomic and sensory innervation and renointestinal reflexes (Table 44-2). The proximity of the right kidney to the colon, duodenum, head of the pancreas, common bile duct, liver, and gallbladder may cause gastrointestinal disturbances. The proximity of the left kidney to the colon (splenic flexure), stomach, pancreas, and spleen may also result in intestinal symptoms. The most common signs and symptoms are nausea, vomiting, diarrhea, abdominal discomfort, and abdominal distention. Urologic symptoms can mimic such disorders as appendicitis, peptic ulcer disease, and cholecystitis; this can make diagnosis difficult, especially in the older adult, who have decreased neurologic innervation to this area.

Unexplained Anemia

Gradual kidney dysfunction can be insidious in its presentation, although fatigue is a common symptom.

TABLE 44-1 Identifying Characteristics of Genitourinary Pain

Type	Location	Character	Associated Signs and Symptoms	Possible Etiology
Kidney	Costovertebral angle, may extend to umbilicus	Dull constant ache; if sudden distention of capsule, pain is severe, sharp, stabbing, and colicky in nature	Nausea and vomiting, diaphoresis, pallor, signs of shock	Acute obstruction, kidney stone, blood clot, acute pyelonephritis, trauma
Bladder	Suprapubic area	Dull, continuous pain, may be intense with voiding, may be severe if bladder full	Urgency, pain at end of voiding, painful straining	Overdistended bladder, infection, interstitial cystitis; tumour
Ureteral	Costovertebral angle, flank, lower abdominal area, testis, or labium	Severe, sharp, stabbing pain, colicky in nature	Nausea and vomiting, paralytic ileus	Ureteral stone, edema or stricture, blood clot
Prostatic	Perineum and rectum	Vague discomfort, feeling of fullness in perineum, vague back pain	Suprapubic tenderness, obstruction to urine flow; frequency, urgency, dysuria, nocturia	Prostatic cancer, acute or chronic prostatitis
Urethral	Male: along penis to meatus; female: urethra to meatus	Pain variable, most severe during and immediately after voiding	Frequency, urgency, dysuria, nocturia, urethral discharge	Irritation of bladder neck, infection of urethra, trauma, foreign body in lower urinary tract

TABLE 44-2 Problems Associated With Changes in Voiding

Problem	Definition	Possible Etiology
Anuria	Urine output <50 mL/day	Acute or chronic kidney injury (see Chapter 45), complete obstruction
Bacteriuria	Bacterial count >100,000 colonies/mL in the urine	Infection
Dysuria	Painful or difficult voiding	Lower urinary tract infection, inflammation of bladder or urethra, acute prostatitis, stones, foreign bodies, tumours in bladder
Enuresis	Involuntary voiding during sleep	Delay in functional maturation of central nervous system (bladder control usually achieved by 5 years of age), obstructive disease of lower urinary tract, genetic factors, failure to concentrate urine, urinary tract infection, psychological stress
Frequency	Frequent voiding—more than every 3 hours	Infection, obstruction of lower urinary tract leading to residual urine and overflow, anxiety, diuretic agents, benign prostatic hyperplasia, urethral stricture, diabetic neuropathy
Hematuria	Red blood cells in the urine	Cancer of genitourinary tract, acute glomerulonephritis, renal stones, renal tuberculosis, blood dyscrasia, trauma, extreme exercise, rheumatic fever, hemophilia, leukemia, sickle cell trait or disease
Hesitancy	Delay, difficulty in initiating voiding	Benign prostatic hyperplasia, compression of urethra, outlet obstruction, neurogenic bladder
Incontinence	Involuntary loss of urine	External urinary sphincter injury, obstetric injury, lesions of bladder neck, detrusor dysfunction, infection, neurogenic bladder, medications, neurologic abnormalities
Nocturia	Awakening during the night to urinate	Decreased renal concentrating ability, heart failure, diabetes, incomplete bladder emptying, excessive fluid intake at bedtime, nephrotic syndrome, cirrhosis with ascites
Oliguria	Urine output <0.5 mL/kg/hr	Acute or chronic kidney failure (see Chapter 45), inadequate fluid intake
Polyuria	Increased volume of urine voided	Diabetes, diabetes insipidus, the use of diuretics, excess fluid intake, lithium toxicity, some forms of kidney disease (hypercalcemic and hypokalemic nephropathy)
Proteinuria	Protein in the urine	Acute and chronic kidney disease, nephrotic syndrome, vigorous exercise, heat stroke, severe heart failure, diabetic nephropathy, multiple myeloma
Urgency	Strong desire to void	Infection, chronic prostatitis, urethritis, obstruction of lower urinary tract leading to residual urine and overflow, anxiety, diuretic agents, benign prostatic hyperplasia, urethral stricture, diabetic neuropathy

Fatigue, shortness of breath, and exercise intolerance all result from the condition known as "anemia of chronic disease." Although hematocrit has historically been the blood test of choice when assessing a patient for anemia, use of the hemoglobin level rather than hematocrit is a better assessment of the oxygen transport ability of the blood.

Past Health, Family, and Social History

Data collection about previous health problems or diseases provides the health care team with useful information for evaluating the patient's current urinary status. People with diabetes who have consistent hypertension and those with primary hypertension are at risk for renal dysfunction. Older men are at risk for prostatic enlargement, which causes urethral obstruction and can result in urinary tract infections and renal failure. People with a family history of urinary tract problems are at increased risk for renal disorders. Genetics may also influence renal conditions (Chart 44-3).

It is also important to assess the patient's psychosocial status, level of anxiety, perceived threats to body image, available support systems, and sociocultural patterns.

Physical Assessment

Several body systems can affect upper and lower urinary tract dysfunction, and conversely that dysfunction can affect several end organs; therefore, a head-to-toe assessment is indicated. Areas of emphasis include the abdomen, suprapubic region, genitalia, lower back, and lower extremities.

The kidneys are not usually palpable. However, palpation of the kidneys may detect an enlargement that could prove to be very important (Weber & Kelley, 2014). The correct technique for palpation is illustrated in Figure 44-5. It may be possible to palpate the smooth, rounded lower pole of the kidney between the hands. The right kidney is easier to detect, because it is somewhat lower than the left one. In patients with obesity, palpation of the kidneys is more difficult.

Renal dysfunction may produce tenderness over the costovertebral angle, which is the angle formed by the lower border of the 12th, or bottom, rib and the spine (Fig. 44-6). The abdomen (just slightly to the right and left of the midline in both upper quadrants) is auscultated to assess for bruits (low-pitched murmurs that indicate renal artery stenosis or an aortic aneurysm). The abdomen

GENETICS IN NURSING PRACTICE

Chart 44-3. Kidney and Urinary Disorders

Various conditions that affect the renal system and urinary tract function are influenced by genetic factors. Some examples of these genetic disorders are:

Autosomal Dominant:
- Familial Wilms tumour
- Polycystic kidney disease
  - Renal cystic disease in tuberous sclerosis complex

X-Linked Recessive:
- Alport syndrome (primarily X-linked but autosomal dominant and recessive forms exist)

Congenital Kidney Disorders:
- Congenital absence of the vas deferens (caused by *CFTR* gene mutation for cystic fibrosis)
- Horseshoe kidney
  - Multicystic dysplastic kidneys

Other Genetic Disorders that Impact the Renal System:
- Alpha-1 antitrypsin deficiency
- Anderson-Fabry disease
- Diabetes
- Coronary artery disease
- Pulmonary hypertension
  - Von Hippel-Lindau syndrome

FAMILY HISTORY SPECIFIC TO KIDNEY AND URINARY DISORDERS

- Inquire about other family members with a history of renal and/or urinary tract malformations, kidney disease, or end-stage kidney disease and age of onset.
- Determine if other family members have diabetic kidney disease (clustering of this within the family could indicate genetic susceptibility).
- Identify family history of male infertility and cystic fibrosis (congenital absence of vas deferens).
- Be alert to family members with history of early-onset renal (Wilms tumour) or other cancers.

PHYSICAL ASSESSMENT SPECIFIC TO GENETIC KIDNEY AND URINARY DISORDERS

- Be alert to signs and symptoms of kidney disease at an early age.
- Ascertain for presence and frequency of kidney stones or urinary tract infections.
- Assess for the presence and frequency of:
  - Abdominal pain or presence of an abdominal mass
  - Hematuria
  - Hypertension
  - Peripheral or orbital edema
  - Proteinuria
- Assess for clinical findings suggesting that kidney disease is a component of a genetic syndrome (e.g., seizures, intellectual disability, skin involvement).
- Assess for bleeding tendencies, abnormal clotting, or history of anemia.

Genetics Resources

Alport Syndrome Foundation, www.alportsyndrome.org
The American Kidney Fund, www.kidneyfund.org

Genetics Resources for Nurses and Their Patients on the Web

Genetic Alliance—a directory of support groups for patients and families with genetic conditions, http://www.geneticalliance.org

Gene Clinics—a listing of common genetic disorders with up-to-date clinical summaries and genetic counselling and testing information, http://www.geneclinics.org

National Organization of Rare Disorders—a directory of support groups and information for patients and families with rare genetic disorders, http://www.rarediseases.org http://www.ncbi.nlm.nih.gov/projects/omim

Canadian Association of Genetic Counsellors (CAGC), http://www.cagc-accg.ca—A listing of genetic centres across Canada

Canadian Cancer Society, http://www.cancer.ca—A source of information on genetic factors/risk and genetic testing

Canadian Directory of Genetic Support Groups, http://www.lhsc.on.ca/programs/medgenet—A resource guide for families and professionals

Canadian Genetic Diseases Network, http://www.cgdn.ca—A group with the stated mission to be the primary catalyst in advancing Canada's scientific and commercial competitiveness in genetic research and the application of genetic discoveries to the prevention, diagnosis, and treatment of human disease

Canadian Organization for Rare Disorders (CORD), http://www.cord.ca—A source of information on over 6,000 rare disorders; links individuals/families with the same rare disorder

Genetics Society of Canada (GSC), http://life.biology.mcmaster.ca/GSC—A group that promotes research and communicates the results and implications of genetics to the public

GeneTests, http://www.genetests.org—A publicly funded medical genetics information resource developed for physicians, other health care providers, and researchers

OMIM Online Mendelian Inheritance in Man, http://www.ncbi.nlm.nih.gov/entrez/query.fcgi?db=OMIM—A catalogue of human genes and genetic disorders

See Chapter 11 for components of genetic counseling resources.

is also assessed for the presence of ascites (accumulation of fluid in the peritoneal cavity), which may occur with kidney as well as liver dysfunction.

To check for residual urine, the bladder should be percussed after the patient voids. Percussion of the bladder begins at the midline just above the umbilicus and proceeds downward. The sound changes from tympanic to dull when percussing over the bladder. The bladder, which can be palpated only if it is moderately distended, feels like a smooth, firm, round mass rising out of the abdomen, usually at midline (Fig. 44-7). Dullness to percussion of the bladder after voiding indicates incomplete bladder emptying (Weber & Kelley, 2014). Portable bladder ultrasonography is another method of detecting urinary

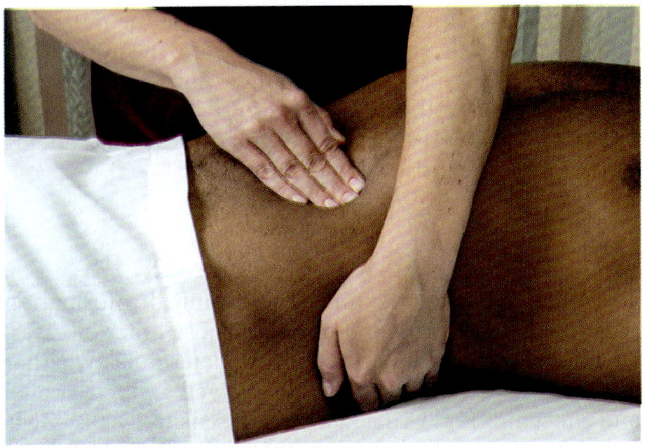

FIGURE 44-5. Technique for palpating the right kidney (*top*). Place one hand under the patient's back with the fingers under the lower rib. Place the palm of the other hand anterior to the kidney with fingers above the umbilicus. Push the hand on top forward as the patient inhales deeply. The left kidney (*bottom*) is palpated similarly by reaching over to the patient's left side and placing the right hand beneath the patient's lower left rib. (From Weber, J., & Kelley, J. (2007). *Health assessment in nursing* (3rd ed.). Philadelphia, PA: Lippincott Williams & Wilkins.)

retention. These devices provide a three-dimensional image of the bladder and should be used 10 minutes after voiding to detect urine retention (Davis, Chrisman, & Walden, 2012). See later discussion in bladder ultrasonography section.

In older men, BPH or prostatitis can cause difficulty with urination (Miller, 2012). Because the signs and symptoms of prostate cancer can mimic those of BPH, the prostate gland is palpated by digital rectal examination (DRE) as part of the yearly physical examination in men of 40 years of age and older (see Chapter 50). In addition, a blood specimen is obtained to test the prostate-specific antigen (PSA) level annually; the results of the DRE and PSA are then correlated. Blood is drawn for PSA before the DRE, because manipulation of the prostate can cause the PSA level to increase temporarily. The inguinal area is examined for enlarged nodes, an inguinal or femoral hernia, and varicocele (varicose veins of the spermatic cord).

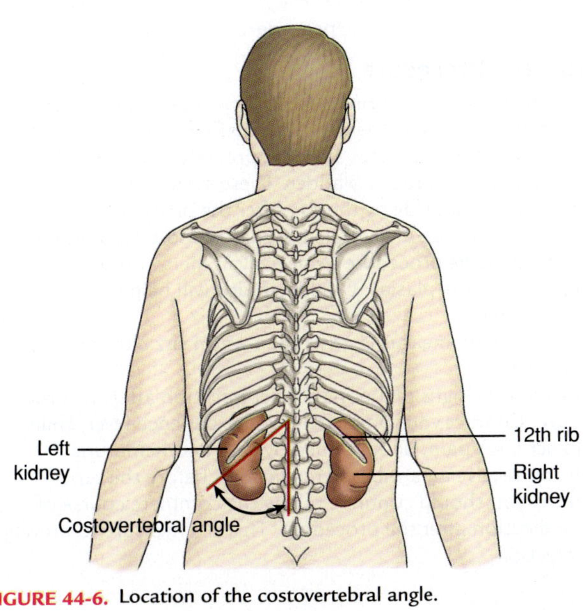

FIGURE 44-6. Location of the costovertebral angle.

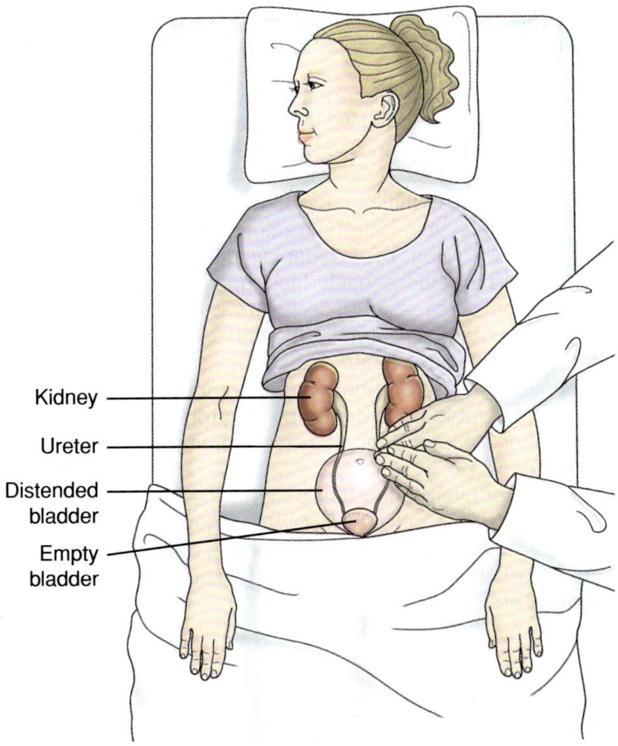

FIGURE 44-7. Palpation of the bladder.

In women, the vulva, urethral meatus, and vagina are examined (Weber & Kelley, 2014). The urethra is palpated for diverticula, and the vagina is assessed for adequate estrogen effect and any of five types of herniation: urethrocele is the bulging of the anterior vaginal wall into the urethra; cystocele is the herniation of the bladder wall into the vaginal vault; pelvic prolapse is bulging of the cervix into the vaginal vault; enterocele is herniation of the bowel into the posterior vaginal wall; and rectocele is herniation of the rectum into the vaginal wall. These prolapses are graded depending on the degree of herniation (see Chapter 48 for more information).

The woman is asked to cough and perform a Valsalva manoeuvre to assess the urethra's system of muscular and ligament support. If urine leakage occurs, the index and middle fingers of the examiner's gloved hand are used to support either side of the urethra as the woman is asked to repeat the Valsalva manoeuvre; this is called the *Marshall–Boney manoeuvre*. If this produces urinary leakage, referral is suggested.

The patient is assessed for edema and changes in body weight. Edema may be observed, particularly in the face and dependent parts of the body, such as the ankles and sacral areas, and suggests fluid retention. An increase in body weight commonly accompanies edema. A 1-kg weight gain equals approximately 1,000 mL of fluid (Hall, 2016).

The deep tendon reflexes of the knee are examined for quality and symmetry. This is an important part of testing for neurologic causes of bladder dysfunction, because the sacral area, which innervates the lower extremities, is the same peripheral nerve area responsible for urinary continence. The gait pattern of the person with bladder dysfunction is also noted, as well as the patient's ability to walk toe-to-heel. These tests evaluate possible supraspinal causes for urinary incontinence.

Unfolding Patient Story: Lloyd Bennett • Part 1

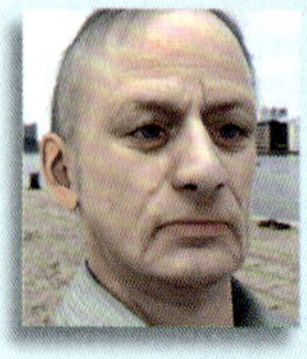

Lloyd Bennett is a 76-year-old male who fell while working outdoors. He presents to the Emergency Department with a hip fracture. What effect can significant blood loss from surgery to repair the fracture have on renal function? What clinical findings would indicate to the nurse that kidney function is impaired? What clinical assessment findings would alert the nurse of potential trauma to the urinary tract resulting from the hip fracture? What diagnostic tests may be used to identify a urinary tract complication that the nurse would consider for preparatory patient education? (Lloyd Bennett's story continues in Chapter 54.)

Care for Lloyd and other patients in a realistic virtual environment: ***vSim** for Nursing* (**thepoint.lww.com/vSimMedicalSurgical**). Practice documenting these patients' care in DocuCare (**thepoint.lww.com/DocuCareEHR**).

Diagnostic Evaluation

A comprehensive health history is used to determine the appropriate laboratory and diagnostic tests. The following sections review some of the tests that might be used.

Most patients undergoing urologic testing or imaging studies are apprehensive, even those who have had these tests in the past. Patients frequently feel discomfort and embarrassment about such a private and personal function as voiding. Voiding in the presence of others can frequently cause guarding, a natural reflex that inhibits voiding due to situational anxiety. Because the outcomes of these studies determine the plan of care, the nurse must help the patient relax by providing as much privacy and explanation about the procedure as possible (Chart 44-4). In addition, Chart 44-5 provides a plan of care for patients undergoing diagnostic testing.

Urinalysis and Urine Culture

The urinalysis provides important clinical information about kidney function and helps diagnose other diseases, such as diabetes. The urine culture determines whether bacteria are present in the urine, as well as their strains and concentration. Urine culture and sensitivity also identify the antimicrobial therapy that is best suited for the particular strains identified, taking into consideration the antibiotics that have the best rate of resolution in that particular geographic region. Appropriate evaluation of any abnormality can assist in detecting serious underlying diseases.

Components

Urine examination includes the following:

- Urine colour (Table 44-3)
- Urine clarity and odour
- Urine pH and specific gravity
- Tests to detect protein, glucose, and ketone bodies in the urine (proteinuria, renal glycosuria, and ketonuria, respectively)
- Microscopic examination of the urine sediment after centrifugation to detect RBCs (**hematuria**), white blood cells (**pyuria**), casts (cylindruria), crystals (crystalluria), and bacteria (**bacteriuria**)

CHART 44-4

Patient Education: Before and After Urodynamic Testing

The nurse instructs the patient on what to expect before, during, and after the procedure:

Preprocedure

A physician or nurse will conduct an in-depth interview. Questions related to your urologic symptoms and voiding habits will be asked.

During the Procedure

- You will be asked to describe sensations felt during the procedure
- You might be asked to change positions (e.g., from supine to sitting or standing)
- You may be asked to cough or perform the Valsalva manoeuvre (bear down) during the procedure
- You will probably need to have one or two urethral catheters inserted so that bladder pressure and bladder filling can be measured. Another catheter may be placed in the rectum or vagina to measure abdominal pressure
- You may also have electrodes (surface, wire, or needle) placed in the perianal area for electromyography (EMG). This may be uncomfortable initially during insertion and later during position changes
- Your bladder will be filled through the urethral catheter one or more times during the procedure

After the Procedure

- You may experience urinary frequency, urgency, or dysuria from the urethral catheters. Avoid caffeinated, carbonated, and alcoholic beverages after the procedure because these can further irritate the bladder. These symptoms usually decrease or subside by the day after the procedure
- You might notice a slight hematuria (blood-tinged urine) right after the procedure (especially in men with benign prostatic hyperplasia). Drinking fluids will help to clear the hematuria
- If the urinary meatus is irritated, a warm sitz bath may be helpful
- Be alert for signs of a urinary tract infection after the procedure. Contact your physician if you experience fever, chills, lower back pain, or continued dysuria and hematuria
- If you receive an antibiotic medication before the procedure, you should continue taking the complete course of medication after the procedure. This is a measure to prevent infection

Plan of Nursing Care

Chart 44-5. Care of the Patient Undergoing Diagnostic Testing of the Renal–Urologic System

Nursing Priority: Deficient knowledge

Goal: Patient demonstrates increased understanding of the procedure and tests and expected behaviours

NURSING INTERVENTIONS	RATIONALE	EXPECTED OUTCOMES
1. Assess patient's level of understanding of planned diagnostic tests	1. Provides basis for teaching and gives indication of patient's perception of tests	• States rationale for planned diagnostic tests and what tasks and behaviours are expected during the procedure
2. Provide a description of tests in language the patient can understand	2. Understanding what is expected enhances patient compliance and cooperation	• Complies with urine collection, fluid modifications, or other procedures required for diagnostic evaluation
3. Assess patient's understanding of test results after their completion.	3. Apprehension may interfere with patient's ability to understand information and results provided by health care team	• Restates in own words results of diagnostic tests • Asks for clarification of terms and procedures
4. Reinforce information provided to patient about test results and implications for follow-up care.	4. Provides opportunity for patient to clarify information and anticipate follow-up care	• Explains rationale for follow-up care • Participates in follow-up care

Nursing Priority: Acute pain

Goal: Patient reports decrease in pain and absence of discomfort

NURSING INTERVENTIONS	RATIONALE	EXPECTED OUTCOMES
1. Assess level of pain: dysuria, burning on urination, abdominal or flank pain, bladder spasm	1. Provides baseline for evaluation of pain relief strategies and progression of dysfunction	• Reports decreasing levels of pain • Reports absence of local symptoms • States ability to start and stop urinary stream without discomfort
2. Encourage fluid intake (unless contraindicated).	2. Promotes dilute urine and flushing of the lower urinary tract	• Consumes increased fluid intake if indicated
3. Encourage warm sitz baths	3. Relieves local discomfort and promotes relaxation	• Uses sitz bath as indicated
4. Report increased pain to physician	4. May indicate progression or recurrence of dysfunction, or untoward signs (e.g., bleeding, calculi)	• Identifies signs and symptoms to be reported to the health care provider • Takes medications as prescribed • Does not delay in emptying bladder
5. Administer analgesic and antispasmodic agents for pain and spasm as prescribed	5. Prescribed to relieve pain or spasm	• Uses appropriate hygienic measures, avoids use of bubble bath, uses appropriate hygiene after bowel movements
6. Assess voiding patterns and hygiene practices and provide instructions about recommended voiding patterns and hygienic practices	6. Delayed emptying of the bladder and poor hygiene may contribute to pain secondary to renal or urinary tract dysfunction	

Nursing Priority: Fear and anxiety

Goal: Patient appears relaxed and reports decreased fear and anxiety

NURSING INTERVENTIONS	RATIONALE	EXPECTED OUTCOMES
1. Assess patient's level of fear and apprehension	1. A high level of fear or apprehension can interfere with learning and cooperation	• Appears relaxed with a low level of fear or apprehension
2. Explain all procedures and tests to patient	2. Knowledge about what is expected helps reduce fear and apprehension	• States rationale for tests and procedures in a calm, relaxed manner
3. Provide privacy and respect patient's modesty by closing doors and keeping patient covered. Keep urinal and bedpan covered and out of sight	3. Communicates that you are aware of and accept patient's need for privacy and modesty	• Maintains usual privacy and modesty
4. Use correct terminology in a factual manner when questioning patient about urinary tract dysfunction	4. Conveys that you are comfortable discussing patient's urinary dysfunction and symptoms with patient	• Discusses own urinary tract dysfunction using correct terminology without overt indications of embarrassment or discomfort
5. Assess patient's fears about perceived changes associated with tests and other procedures	5. May uncover fears and misconceptions of the patient that can be alleviated by correct understanding	• Relates fears and concerns • Demonstrates correct understanding of procedures and possible outcomes
6. Instruct patient in relaxation techniques	6. Promotes relaxation and assists patient in coping with uncertainty about outcomes	• Appears relaxed with low level of fear and apprehension

TABLE 44-3 Changes in Urine Colour and Possible Causes

Urine Colour	Possible Cause
Colourless to pale yellow	Dilute urine due to diuretics, alcohol consumption, diabetes insipidus, glycosuria, excess fluid intake, renal disease
Yellow to milky white	Pyuria, infection, vaginal cream
Bright yellow	Multiple vitamin preparations
Pink to red	Hemoglobin breakdown, red blood cells, gross blood, menses, bladder or prostate surgery, beets, blackberries, medications (phenytoin [Dilantin], rifampin [Rifadin], phenothiazine [Mellaril], cascara [Sagrada], senna products)
Blue, blue green	Dyes, methylene blue, Pseudomonas species organisms, medications (amitriptyline [Amitriptyline HCL], triamterene [Dyrenium])
Orange to amber	Concentrated urine due to dehydration, fever, bile, excess bilirubin or carotene, medications (pyridium [Phenazopyridine HCL], nitrofurantoin [Furadantin])
Brown to black	Old red blood cells, urobilinogen, bilirubin, melanin, porphyrin, extremely concentrated urine due to dehydration, medications (cascara, metronidazole [Flagyl], iron preparations, quinine [Quinine Sulfate], senna products, methyldopa [Aldomet], nitrofurantoin)

Significance of Findings

Several abnormalities, such as hematuria and proteinuria, produce no symptoms but may be detected during a routine urinalysis using a dipstick. Normally, about 1 million RBCs pass into the urine daily, which is equivalent to 1 to 3 RBCs per high-power field. Hematuria (more than 3 RBCs per high-power field) can develop from an abnormality anywhere along the genitourinary tract and is more common in women than in men. Common causes include acute infection (cystitis, urethritis, or prostatitis), renal calculi, and neoplasm. Other causes include systemic disorders, such as bleeding disorders; malignant lesions; and medications, such as warfarin (Coumadin) and heparin (Heparin Sodium). Although hematuria may initially be detected using a dipstick test, further microscopic evaluation is necessary with a 24-hour collection (Fischbach & Dunning, 2015).

Proteinuria may be a benign finding, or it may signify serious disease (Israni & Kasiske, 2012). Occasional loss of up to 150 mg/day of protein in the urine, primarily albumin and Tamm–Horsfall protein (also known as *uromodulin*), is considered normal and usually does not require further evaluation. A dipstick examination, which can detect from 30 to 1,000 mg/dL of protein, should be used as a screening test only, because urine concentration, pH, hematuria, and radiocontrast materials all affect the results. Because dipstick analysis does not detect protein concentrations of less than 30 mg/dL, the test cannot be used for early detection of diabetic nephropathy. *Microalbuminuria* (excretion of 20 to 200 mg/dL of protein in the urine) is an early sign of diabetic nephropathy. Common benign causes of transient proteinuria are fever, strenuous exercise, and prolonged standing.

Causes of persistent proteinuria include glomerular diseases, malignancies, collagen diseases, diabetes mellitus, preeclampsia, hypothyroidism, heart failure, exposure to heavy metals, and use of medications, such as nonsteroidal anti-inflammatory drugs (NSAIDs) (Comerford, 2015).

Literature supports angiotensin-converting enzyme (ACE) inhibitors for hypertension in kidney disease. Many patients with proteinuria but without hypertension may also benefit from ACE inhibitors or ARBs. Medications that lower blood pressure can also significantly slow the progression of kidney disease. Two types of blood pressure–lowering medications, ACE inhibitors, and angiotensin receptor blockers (ARBs), have been shown to be effective in slowing the progression of kidney disease (National Kidney and Urologic Diseases Information Clearinghouse, 2014; Zuber, Liles, & Davies, 2013).

Specific Gravity

Specific gravity measures the density of a solution compared to the density of water, which is 1.000. Specific gravity is altered by the presence of blood, protein, and casts in the urine. The normal range of urine specific gravity is 1.010 to 1.025 (Grossman & Porth, 2014).

Methods for determination of specific gravity include the following:

- Multiple-test dipstick (most common method), with a specific reagent area for specific gravity
- Urinometer (least accurate method), in which urine is placed in a small cylinder and the urinometer is floated in the urine; a specific gravity reading is obtained at the meniscus level of the urine
- Refractometer, an instrument used in a laboratory setting, which measures differences in the speed of light passing through air and the urine sample

Urine specific gravity depends largely on hydration status. When fluid intake decreases, specific gravity normally increases. With high fluid intake, specific gravity decreases. In patients with kidney disease, urine specific gravity does not vary with fluid intake, and the patient's urine is said to have a fixed specific gravity. Disorders or conditions that cause decreased urine specific gravity include diabetes insipidus, glomerulonephritis, and severe renal damage. Those that can cause increased specific gravity include diabetes mellitus, nephritis, and fluid deficit.

Osmolality

Osmolality is the most accurate measurement of the kidney's ability to dilute and concentrate urine. It measures the number of solute particles in a kilogram of water. Serum and urine osmolality are measured simultaneously to assess the body's fluid status. The normal range of serum osmolality is about 280 to 300 mOsm/kg, and the normal range of urine osmolality is 200 to 800 mOsm/kg. For a 24-hour urine sample, the normal value is 300 to 900 mOsm/kg (Fischbach & Dunning, 2015).

TABLE 44-4 Renal Function Tests

Test	Purpose	Normal Values		
Renal Concentration				
Specific gravity	A measure of the degree of concentration of the urine	1.010–1.025		
Urine osmolality	Concentrating ability is lost early in kidney disease; hence, these test findings may disclose early defects in renal function	250–900 mOsm/kg/24 hr, 50–1,200 mOsm/kg random sample		
24-Hour Urine				
Creatinine clearance	Detects and evaluates progression of kidney disease. Test measures volume of blood cleared of endogenous creatinine in 1 minute, which provides an approximation of the glomerular filtration rate. Sensitive indicator of kidney disease used to follow progression of kidney disease	Measured in mL/min/1.73 m^2		
		Age (Years)	**Male**	**Female**
		<30	88–146	81–134
		30–40	82–140	75–128
		40–50	75–133	69–122
		50–60	68–126	64–116
		60–70	61–120	58–110
		70–80	55–113	52–105
Serum				
Creatinine level	Measures effectiveness of renal function. Creatinine is the end product of muscle energy metabolism. In normal function, the level of creatinine, which is regulated and excreted by the kidneys, remains fairly constant in the body	0.6–1.2 mg/dL (50–110 mmol/L)		
BUN	Serves as index of renal function. Urea is the nitrogenous end product of protein metabolism. Test values are affected by protein intake, tissue breakdown, and fluid volume changes	7–18 mg/dL; patients >60 years: 8–20 mg/dL		
BUN-to-creatinine ratio	Evaluates hydration status. An elevated ratio is seen in hypovolemia; a normal ratio with an elevated BUN and creatinine is seen with intrinsic kidney disease	About 10:1		

BUN, blood urea nitrogen.

Adapted from Fischbach, F., & Dunning, M. B. (2015). *A manual of laboratory and diagnostic tests* (9th ed.). Philadelphia, PA: Lippincott Williams & Wilkins.

Renal Function Tests

Renal function tests are used to evaluate the severity of kidney disease and to assess the status of the patient's kidney function. These tests also provide information about the effectiveness of the kidney in carrying out its excretory function. Renal function test results may be within normal limits until the GFR is reduced to less than 50% of normal. Renal function can be assessed most accurately if several tests are performed and their results are analyzed together. Common tests of renal function include renal concentration tests, creatinine clearance, and serum creatinine and blood **urea nitrogen** levels. Table 44-4 describes the purpose and gives the normal range for each test. Other tests for evaluating renal function that may be helpful include serum electrolyte levels and urinary biomarkers to detect acute kidney injury (Fallone & Cotton, 2015) (see Chapter 17).

Diagnostic Imaging

Kidney, Ureter, and Bladder Studies

An x-ray study of the abdomen or kidneys, ureters, and bladder (KUB) may be performed to delineate the size, shape, and position of the kidneys and to reveal urinary system abnormalities (Fischbach & Dunning, 2015).

General Ultrasonography

Ultrasonography is a noninvasive procedure that uses sound waves passed into the body through a transducer to detect abnormalities of internal tissues and organs. Abnormalities such as fluid accumulation, masses, congenital malformations, changes in organ size, and obstructions can be identified. During the test, the lower abdomen and genitalia may need to be exposed. Ultrasonography requires a full bladder; therefore, fluid intake should be encouraged before the procedure. Because of its sensitivity, ultrasonography has replaced many other tests as the initial diagnostic procedure (Boswell, Jadvar, & Palmer, 2012).

Bladder Ultrasonography

Bladder ultrasonography is a noninvasive method of measuring urine volume in the bladder. It may be indicated for urinary frequency, inability to void after removal of an indwelling urinary catheter, measurement of postvoiding residual urine volume, inability to void postoperatively, or assessment of the need for catheterization during the initial stages of an intermittent catheterization training program. Portable, battery-operated devices are available for bedside use. The scan head is placed on the patient's abdomen and directed toward the bladder. The device automatically calculates and displays urine volume.

Computed Tomography and Magnetic Resonance Imaging

Computed tomography (CT) scans and magnetic resonance imaging (MRI) are noninvasive techniques that provide excellent cross-sectional views of the kidney and urinary tract. They are used to evaluate genitourinary masses, nephrolithiasis, chronic renal infections, renal or urinary tract trauma, metastatic disease, and soft tissue abnormalities. Occasionally, an oral or intravenous radiopaque contrast material is used in CT scanning to enhance visualization (Chart 44-6).

CHART 44-6

Patient Care During Urologic Testing With Contrast Agents

For some patients, contrast agents are nephrotoxic and allergenic. Emergency equipment and medications should be available in case of an anaphylactic reaction to the contrast agent. Emergency supplies include epinephrine, corticosteroids, vasopressors, oxygen, and airway and suction equipment.

The following guidelines can help the nurse respond quickly in the event of a problem.

Nursing Actions for Patient Preparation

- Obtain the patient's allergy history with emphasis on allergy to iodine, shellfish, and other seafood, because many contrast agents contain iodine
- Notify primary provider and radiologist if the patient is allergic or suspected to be allergic to iodine
- Obtain health history. Contrast agents should be used with great caution in older patients and in patients who have multiple myeloma, renal impairment, or volume depletion
- Obtain medication history. Nephrotoxic medications such as vancomycin, amphotericin B, metformin, and nonsteroidal anti-inflammatory drugs should be discontinued before contrast media administration
- The use of both nonionic low-osmolar contrast media (LOCM, e.g., iohexol) and ionic high-osmolar contrast media (HOCM, e.g., diatrizoate), is indicated in patients with renal impairment and other risk factors to prevent contrast-induced nephropathy
- Check kidney function in at-risk patients. Patients should receive IV hydration prior to the procedure
- Inform the patient that they may experience a temporary feeling of warmth, flushing of the face, and an unusual flavour (similar to that of seafood) in the mouth when the contrast agent is infused

Nursing Actions During and Post Procedure

- Monitor patient closely for allergic reaction, and monitor urine output
- Maintain hydration status

Adapted from Andreucci, M., Solomon, R., & Tasanarong, A. (2014). *Side effects of radiographic contrast media: Pathogenesis, risk factors, and prevention.* Retrieved April 17, 2016, from www.hindawi.com/journals/bmri/2014/741018/; Rank, W. (2013). Preventing contrast media–induced nephrotoxicity. *Nursing, 43*(4), 48–51.

Nursing Interventions

Preparation includes educating the patient about relaxation techniques and explaining that they will be able to communicate with the staff by means of a microphone located inside the scanner. Many MRI suites provide headphones so that patients can listen to the music of their choice during the procedure. Nursing care guidelines for patient preparation and precautions for any imaging procedure that requires a contrast agent (contrast medium) are explained in Chart 44-6.

Before the patient enters the room where the MRI is to be performed, all metal objects and credit cards (the magnetic field can erase them) are removed. This includes medication patches (e.g., nicotine and nitroglycerin) that have a metal backing, which can cause burns if they are not removed. No metal objects (e.g., oxygen tanks, ventilators, stethoscopes) may be brought into the MRI room. The magnetic field is so strong that any metal-containing items will be pulled toward the magnet, causing severe injury and possible death. A patient history is obtained to determine the presence of any metal objects (e.g., aneurysm clips, orthopedic hardware, pacemakers, artificial heart valves, intrauterine devices). These objects could malfunction, be dislodged, or heat up as they absorb energy. Cochlear implants are inactivated by MRI; therefore, other imaging procedures are considered. A sedative agent may be prescribed, because claustrophobia is a problem for some patients.

Prior to MRI of the urinary system, the patient needs to be informed to avoid alcohol, caffeine-containing beverages, and smoking for at least 2 hours and food for at least 1 hour prior to the scan. Patients should continue taking their usual medication, except for iron supplements, which can interfere with the imaging (Fischbach & Dunning, 2015).

Nuclear Scans

Nuclear scans require injection of a radioisotope (a technetium 99m–labelled compound or iodine 123 [^{123}I] hippurate) into the circulatory system; the isotope is then monitored as it moves through the blood vessels of the kidneys. A scintillation camera is placed behind the kidney with the patient in a supine, prone, or seated position. Hypersensitivity to the radioisotope is rare. The technetium scan provides information about kidney perfusion. The ^{123}I-hippurate renal scan provides information about kidney function, such as GFR.

Nuclear scans are used to evaluate acute and chronic renal failure, renal masses, and blood flow before and after kidney transplantation. The radioisotope is injected at a specified time to achieve the proper concentration in the kidneys. After the procedure is completed, the patient is encouraged to drink fluids to promote excretion of the radioisotope by the kidneys.

Intravenous Urography

IV urography includes various tests such as excretory urography, intravenous pyelography (IVP), and infusion drip pyelography. A radiopaque contrast agent is administered by IV. An IVP shows the kidneys, ureter, and bladder via x-ray imaging as the dye moves through the upper and then the lower urinary system. A *nephrotomogram* may be carried out as part of the study to visualize different layers of the kidney and the diffuse structures within each layer and to differentiate solid masses or lesions from cysts in the kidneys or urinary tract.

IV urography may be used as the initial assessment of many suspected urologic conditions, especially lesions in the kidneys and ureters. It also provides an approximate estimate of renal function. After the contrast agent (sodium diatrizoate or meglumine diatrizoate) is administered by IV, multiple x-rays are obtained to visualize drainage structures in the upper and lower urinary systems.

Infusion drip pyelography requires IV infusion of a large volume of a dilute contrast agent to opacify the renal parenchyma and fill the urinary tract. This examination method is useful when prolonged opacification of the drainage structures is desired so that tomograms (body-section radiography) can be made. Images are obtained at specified intervals after the start of the infusion. These images show the filled and distended collecting system. The patient preparation is the same as for excretory urography, except that fluids are not restricted.

Retrograde Pyelography

In retrograde pyelography, catheters are advanced through the ureters into the renal pelvis by means of cystoscopy. A contrast agent is then injected. Retrograde pyelography is usually performed if IV urography provides inadequate visualization of the collecting systems. It may also be used before extracorporeal shock wave lithotripsy and in patients with urologic cancer who need follow-up and have an allergy to IV contrast agents. Possible complications include infection, hematuria, and perforation of the ureter. Retrograde pyelography is used infrequently because of improved techniques in excretory urography.

Cystography

Cystography aids in evaluating vesicoureteral reflux (backflow of urine from the bladder into one or both ureters) and in assessing for bladder injury. A catheter is inserted into the bladder, and a contrast agent is instilled to outline the bladder wall. The contrast agent may leak through a small bladder perforation stemming from bladder injury, but such leakage is usually harmless. Cystography can also be performed with simultaneous pressure recordings inside the bladder.

Voiding Cystourethrography

Voiding cystourethrography uses fluoroscopy to visualize the lower urinary tract and assess urine storage in the bladder. It is commonly used as a diagnostic tool to identify vesicoureteral reflux. A urethral catheter is inserted, and a contrast agent is instilled into the bladder. When the bladder is full and the patient feels the urge to void, the catheter is removed, and the patient voids.

Renal Angiography

A renal angiogram, or renal arteriogram, provides an image of the renal arteries. The femoral (or axillary) artery is pierced with a needle, and a catheter is threaded up through the femoral and iliac arteries into the aorta or renal artery. A contrast agent is injected to opacify the renal arterial supply. Angiography is used to evaluate renal blood flow in suspected renal trauma, to differentiate renal cysts from tumours, and to evaluate hypertension. It is used preoperatively for renal transplantation.

Nursing Interventions

Before the procedure, a laxative may be prescribed to evacuate the colon so that unobstructed x-rays can be obtained. Injection sites (groin for femoral approach or axilla for axillary approach) may be shaved. The peripheral pulse sites (radial, femoral, and dorsalis pedis) are marked for easy access during postprocedural assessment. The patient is informed that there may be a brief sensation of warmth along the course of the vessel when the contrast agent is injected.

After the procedure, vital signs are monitored until stable. If the axillary artery was the injection site, blood pressure measurements are taken on the opposite arm. The injection site is examined for swelling and hematoma. Peripheral pulses are palpated, and the colour and temperature of the involved extremity are noted and compared with those of the uninvolved extremity. Cold compresses may be applied to the injection site to decrease edema and pain. Possible complications include hematoma formation, arterial thrombosis or dissection, false aneurysm formation, and altered renal function.

MAG3 Renogram

This scan is used to further evaluate kidney function in some centres by permitting visualization of renal clearance (Fischbach & Dunning, 2015). The patient is given an injection containing a small amount of radioactive material, which will show how the kidneys are functioning. The patient needs to lie still for about 35 minutes while special cameras take images (Fischbach & Dunning, 2015).

Urologic Endoscopic Procedures

Endourology, or urologic endoscopic procedures, can be performed in one of two ways: using a cystoscope inserted into the urethra, or percutaneously, through a small incision.

The cystoscopic examination is used to directly visualize the urethra and bladder. The cystoscope, which is inserted through the urethra into the bladder, has an optical lens system that provides a magnified, illuminated view of the bladder (Fig. 44-8). The use of a high-intensity light and interchangeable lenses allows excellent visualization and permits still and motion pictures to be taken. The cystoscope is manipulated to allow complete visualization of the urethra and bladder as well as the ureteral orifices and prostatic urethra. Small ureteral catheters can be passed through the cystoscope for assessment of the ureters and the pelvis of each kidney.

The cystoscope also allows the urologist to obtain a urine specimen from each kidney to evaluate its function. Cup forceps can be inserted through the cystoscope for biopsy. Calculi may be removed from the urethra, bladder,

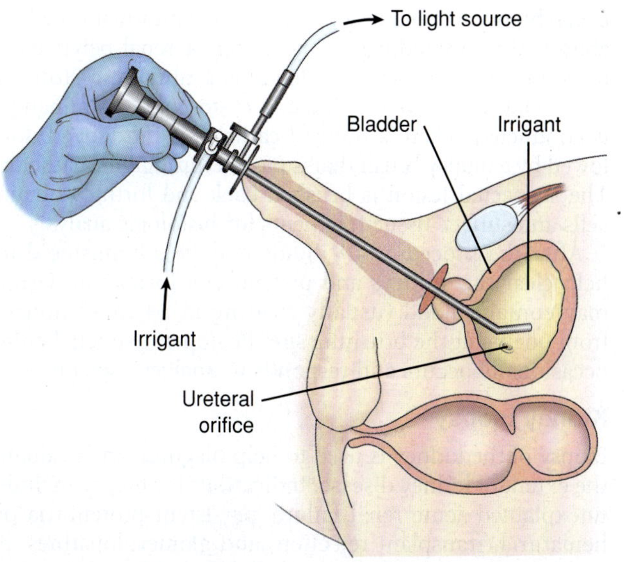

FIGURE 44-8. Cystoscopic examination. A rigid or semirigid cystoscope is introduced into the bladder. The upper cord is an electric line for the light at the distal end of the cystoscope. The lower tubing leads from a reservoir of sterile irrigant that is used to inflate the bladder.

and ureter using cystoscopy. If a lower tract cystoscopy is performed, the patient is usually conscious, and the procedure is usually no more uncomfortable than a catheterization. To minimize posttest urethral discomfort, viscous lidocaine is administered several minutes before the study. If the cystoscopy includes examination of the upper tracts, a sedative may be administered before the procedure. General anesthesia is usually administered to ensure that there are no involuntary muscle spasms when the scope is being passed through the ureters or kidney.

Nursing Interventions

The nurse describes the procedure to the patient and family to prepare them and to allay their fears. If an upper cystoscopy is to be performed, the patient is usually restricted to nothing by mouth (NPO) for several hours beforehand.

Postprocedural management is directed at relieving any discomfort resulting from the examination. Some burning on voiding, blood-tinged urine, and urinary frequency from trauma to the mucous membranes can be expected. Moist heat to the lower abdomen and warm sitz baths are helpful in relieving pain and relaxing the muscles.

After a cystoscopic examination, the patient with obstructive pathology may experience urine retention if the instruments used during the examination caused edema. The nurse carefully monitors the patient with prostatic hyperplasia for urine retention. Warm sitz baths and antispasmodic medication, such as flavoxate or flavoxate hydrochloride may be prescribed to relieve temporary urine retention caused by poor relaxation of the urinary sphincter; however, intermittent catheterization may be necessary for a few hours after the examination. The nurse monitors the patient for signs and symptoms of urinary tract infection. Because edema of the urethra secondary to local trauma may obstruct urine flow, the patient is also monitored for signs and symptoms of obstruction.

Biopsy

Renal and Ureteral Brush Biopsy

Brush biopsy techniques provide specific information when abnormal x-ray findings of the ureter or renal pelvis raise questions about whether a defect is a tumour, a stone, a blood clot, or an artefact. First, a cystoscopic examination is conducted. Then, a ureteral catheter is introduced, followed by a biopsy brush that is passed through the catheter. The suspected lesion is brushed back and forth to obtain cells and surface tissue fragments for histologic analysis.

After the procedure, IV fluids may be administered to help clear the kidneys and prevent clot formation. Urine may contain blood (usually clearing in 24 to 48 hours) from oozing at the brushing site. Postoperative renal colic occasionally occurs and responds to analgesic agents.

Kidney Biopsy

Biopsy of the kidney is used to help diagnose and evaluate the extent of kidney disease. Indications for biopsy include unexplained acute renal failure, persistent proteinuria or hematuria, transplant rejection, and glomerulopathies. A small section of renal cortex is obtained either percutaneously (needle biopsy) or by open biopsy through a small flank incision. Before the biopsy is carried out, coagulation studies are conducted to identify any risk of postbiopsy bleeding. Contraindications to kidney biopsy include bleeding tendencies, uncontrolled hypertension, a solitary kidney, and morbid obesity (Salama & Cook, 2012).

Procedure

The patient may be prescribed a fasting regimen 6 to 8 hours before the test. An IV line is established. A urine specimen is obtained and saved for comparison with the postbiopsy specimen.

If a needle biopsy is to be performed, the patient is instructed to breathe in and hold that breath (to prevent the kidney from moving) while the needle is being inserted. The sedated patient is placed in a prone position with a sandbag under the abdomen. The skin at the biopsy site is infiltrated with a local anesthetic agent. The biopsy needle is introduced just inside the renal capsule of the outer quadrant of the kidney. The location of the needle may be confirmed by fluoroscopy or by ultrasound, in which case a special probe is used.

With open biopsy, a small incision is made over the kidney, allowing direct visualization. Preparation for an open biopsy is similar to that for any major abdominal surgery.

Nursing Interventions

After a biopsy procedure, nursing care includes monitoring vital signs for the first 24 hours to detect signs and symptoms of bleeding or infection. The nurse should assess for other signs and symptoms of internal bleeding such as pallor, dizziness, and flank or back pain. IV fluids may be given to help clear the kidneys and prevent clot formation. Urine may contain blood (usually clearing in 24 to 48 hours) from oozing at the site. Bed rest should be maintained and pressure dressings applied for prescribed periods of time to control bleeding. Puncture sites should be examined for signs and symptoms of infection. Analgesic agents should be given as prescribed and needed for pain (Doss-McQuitty, 2015).

Critical Thinking Exercises

1 A patient you are caring for complains of urinary incontinence. Describe the assessment techniques appropriate to evaluate the patient. Review the possible causes and describe the actions you would take and the rationale for each action. Describe any differences in your assessments and possible action that are dependent on the gender of the patient.

2 A 30-year-old male is admitted to the emergency department for evaluation of urinary dysfunction and is scheduled for a renal angiography. The patient is now highly anxious. Describe your priorities for educating this patient about a kidney biopsy. What are your priority interventions for decreasing the patient's anxiety?

3 You make a home visit to a 70-year-old female who had a urologic examination with contrast. She complains of flu-like symptoms and reports that she thinks she notices swelling in her lower extremities. She has a history of renal impairment. Identify assessments and possible interventions that you would use to evaluate and manage the patient's symptoms. Identify the evidence for the assessments and nursing interventions you chose and the strength of that evidence.

REFERENCES AND SELECTED READINGS

Books

Boswell, W. D., Jadvar, H., & Palmer, S. L. (2012). Diagnostic kidney imaging. In M. W. Taal, G. M. Chertow, P. A. Marsden, et al. (Eds.). *Brenner & Rector's the kidney* (9th ed., pp. 930–1005). Philadelphia, PA: Elsevier.

Comerford, K. C. (2015). *Nursing 2015 drug handbook*. Philadelphia, PA: Wolters Kluwer.

Davis, C., Chrisman, J., & Walden, P. (2012). To scan or not to scan? Detecting urinary retention. *Nursing Made Incredibly Easy, 10*(4), 53–54.

Doss-McQuitty, S. J. (2015). Assessment of kidney structure and function. In C. S. Counts (Ed.). *Core curriculum for nephrology nursing* (6th ed.). Pitman, NJ: American Nephrology Nurses' Association.

Eaton, D. C., & Pooler, J. P. (2013). *Vander's renal physiology* (8th ed.). New York: McGraw-Hill Education.

Eliopoulos, C. (2018). *Gerontological nursing* (9th ed.). Philadelphia, PA: Lippincott Williams & Wilkins.

Fallone, S., & Cotton, A. B. (2015). Acute kidney injury. In C. S. Counts (Ed.). *Core curriculum for nephrology nursing* (6th ed.). Pitman, NJ: American Nephrology Nurses' Association.

Fischbach, F., & Dunning, M. B. (2015). *A manual of laboratory and diagnostic tests* (9th ed.). Philadelphia, PA: Lippincott Williams & Wilkins.

Grossman, S., & Porth, C. M. (2014). *Porth's pathophysiology: Concepts of altered health states* (9th ed.). Philadelphia, PA: Lippincott Williams & Wilkins.

Hall, J. E. (2016). *Guyton and Hall textbook of medical physiology* (13th ed.). Philadelphia, PA: Elsevier.

Headly, C. M. (2015). Anatomy and physiology. In C. S. Counts (Ed.). *Core curriculum for nephrology nursing* (6th ed.). Pitman, NJ: American Nephrology Nurses' Association.

Holcombe, D. M., & Kern Feeley, N. (2013). Renal failure. In P. G. Morton, & D. K. Fontaine (Eds.). *Critical care nursing a holistic approach* (10th ed., pp. 663–690). Philadelphia, PA: Wolters Kluwer Health/Lippincott Williams & Wilkins.

Israni, A. K., & Kasiske, B. L. (2012). Laboratory assessment of kidney disease: Glomerular filtration rate, urinalysis, and proteinuria. In M. W. Taal, G. M. Chertow, P. A. Marsden, et al. (Eds.). *Brenner & Rector's the kidney* (9th ed., pp. 868–896). Philadelphia, PA: Elsevier.

Miller, C. A. (2012). *Nursing for wellness in older adults* (6th ed.). Philadelphia, PA: Wolters Kluwer Health/Lippincott Williams & Wilkins.

Salama, A. D., & Cook, H. T. (2012). The renal biopsy. In M. W. Taal, G. M. Chertow, P. A. Marsden, et al. (Eds.). *Brenner & Rector's the kidney* (9th ed., pp. 1006–1015). Philadelphia, PA: Elsevier.

Skorecki, K., Chertow, G., Marsden P. A., et al. (2015). *Brenner and Rector's the kidney* (10th ed.). Philadelphia, PA: Elsevier Saunders.

Snyder, K. A., & Crusius, K. C. (2013). Patient assessment: Renal system. In P. G. Morton, & D. K. Fontaine (Eds.). *Critical care nursing a holistic approach* (10th ed., pp. 618–636). Philadelphia, PA: Wolters Kluwer Health/Lippincott Williams & Wilkins.

Snyder, K. A., & Haas, K. (2013). Anatomy and physiology of the renal system. In P. G. Morton, & D. K. Fontaine, (Eds.). *Critical care nursing a holistic approach* (10th ed., pp. 607–636). Philadelphia, PA: Wolters Kluwer Health/Lippincott Williams & Wilkins.

Weber, J. R., & Kelley, J. H. (2014). *Health assessment in nursing* (5th ed.). Philadelphia, PA: Lippincott Williams & Wilkins.

Journals and Electronic Documents

Alexaitis, I., & Broome, B. (2013). Implementation of a nurse-driven protocol to prevent catheter associated urinary tract infections. *Journal of Nursing Care Quality, 29*(3), 245–252.

Larsen, B., & Post, G. J. (2013). LUTS: A practical guide to alleviating lower urinary tract symptoms. *Journal of the American Academy of Physician Assistants, 26*(3), 26–30.

Mentes, J. C. (2013). The complexities of hydration issues in the elderly. *Nutrition Today, 48*(4S), S10–S12.

National Kidney and Urologic Diseases Information Clearinghouse (NKUDIC) (2014). *High blood pressure and kidney disease*. Retrieved from http://kidney.niddk.nih.gov/KUDiseases/pubs/highblood/#howcan

Robinson, J. P., Bradway, C. W., Bunting-Perry, L., et al. (2013). Lower urinary tract symptoms in men with Parkinson disease. *Journal of Neuroscience Nursing, 45*(6), 382–392.

Scemons, D. (2013). Urinary incontinence in adults. *Nursing, 43*(11), 52–60.

Shultz, J. M. (2012). Rethink urinary incontinence in older women. *Nursing, 42*(11), 32–40.

Wilde, M. H., Bliss, D. A., Booth, J., et al. (2014). Self-management of urinary & fecal incontinence. *American Journal of Nursing, 114*(1), 38–45.

Zuber, K., Liles, A. M., & Davies, J. (2013). Medication dosing in patients with chronic kidney disease. *Journal of American Academy of Physician Assistants, 26*(10), 19–25.

Resources

American Association of Kidney Patients: http://www.aakp.org
American Urological Association: http://www.auafoundation.org
Kidney Cancer Research Network of Canada: http://www.ncbi.nlm.nih.gov/entrez/query.fcgi?db=OMIM
National Institute of Diabetes and Digestive and Kidney Diseases, National Institutes of Health: http://www.niddk.nih.gov
National Kidney Foundation: http://www.kidney.org
The Kidney Foundation of Canada: http://www.kidney.ca/

45 Management of Patients With Kidney Disorders

Adapted by Lucia New

Learning Objectives

On completion of this chapter, the learner will be able to:

1. Describe the key factors associated with the development of kidney disorders.
2. Differentiate between the causes of chronic kidney disease (CKD) and acute kidney injury (AKI).
3. Compare and contrast the pathophysiology, clinical manifestations, medical management, and nursing management for patients with kidney disorders.
4. Describe the nursing management of patients with acute and chronic kidney failure.
5. Compare and contrast the kidney replacement therapies including hemodialysis, peritoneal dialysis, and kidney transplantation.
6. Describe the nursing management of the hospitalized patient on dialysis.
7. Develop a postoperative plan of nursing care and teaching plan for the patient undergoing kidney surgery and transplantation.

The kidneys and urinary system help regulate the body's internal environment and are essential for the maintenance of life. Nurses working in any clinical setting may encounter patients with various kidney disorders and thus need to be knowledgeable about these disorders. This chapter provides an overview of electrolyte imbalances that are common in patients with kidney disorders. The main causes of kidney disease are discussed, together with management strategies to prevent damage and preserve kidney function. **Chronic kidney disease** (CKD) and acute kidney injury (AKI) are discussed, as is the care of patients with other kidney conditions who require dialysis, **continuous kidney replacement therapies** (CRRTs), transplantation, and kidney surgery.

FLUID AND ELECTROLYTE IMBALANCES IN KIDNEY DISORDERS

Patients with kidney disorders commonly experience fluid and electrolyte imbalances and require careful assessment and close monitoring for signs of potential problems. The patient whose fluid intake exceeds the ability of the kidneys to excrete fluid is said to have fluid overload. If fluid intake is inadequate, the patient is said to be volume depleted and may show signs and symptoms of fluid volume deficit. The fluid intake and output (I&O) record, a key monitoring tool, is used to document important fluid parameters, including the amount of fluid taken in (orally or parenterally), the volume of urine excreted, and other fluid losses (diarrhea, vomiting, diaphoresis). Patient weight is also important, and documenting trends in weight is a key assessment strategy essential for determining the daily fluid allowance and indicating signs of fluid overload or deficit.

NURSING ALERT

The most accurate indicator of fluid loss or gain in an acutely ill patient is weight. An accurate daily weight must be obtained and recorded. A 1-kg weight gain is equal to 1,000 mL of retained fluid.

Clinical Manifestations

The signs and symptoms of common fluid and electrolyte disturbances that can occur in patients with kidney disorders and their general management strategies are listed in

Table 45-1. The nurse continually assesses, monitors, and informs appropriate members of the health care team if the patient exhibits any of these signs. Management strategies for fluid and electrolyte disturbances in kidney disease are discussed in greater depth later in this chapter (see also Chapter 17).

Gerontologic Considerations

With aging, the kidney is less able to respond to acute fluid and electrolyte changes. Older adult patients may develop atypical and nonspecific signs and symptoms of altered kidney function and fluid and electrolyte imbalances. A fluid balance deficit in older adults can lead to constipation, falls, medication toxicity, urinary tract and respiratory tract infections, delirium, seizures, electrolyte imbalances, hyperthermia, and delayed wound healing. Recognition of acute changes in fluid and electrolytes is further hampered by their association with pre-existing disorders and the misconception that they are normal changes of aging.

Changes in kidney function with normal aging increase the susceptibility of older patients to kidney dysfunction and kidney disease (Kane-Gill, Sileanu, Murugan, et al., 2015). In addition, the incidence of systemic diseases, such as atherosclerosis, hypertension, heart failure, diabetes, and cancer, increases with advancing age, predisposing older adults to kidney disease associated with these disorders. Therefore, acute problems need to be prevented if possible or recognized and treated quickly to avoid kidney damage. Thus, nurses in all settings need to be alert to signs and symptoms of kidney dysfunction in older patients.

Older patients frequently take multiple prescription and over-the-counter medications. Because alterations in kidney blood flow, glomerular filtration, and kidney clearance increase the risk of medication-associated changes in kidney function, precautions are indicated with all medications. When older patients undergo extensive diagnostic tests or when new medications (e.g., diuretic agents) are added, precautions must be taken to prevent dehydration,

Glossary

acute nephritic syndrome: type of kidney failure with glomerular inflammation

acute kidney failure: sudden rapid deterioration of kidney function that is sometimes reversible

acute tubular necrosis: type of acute kidney failure in which there is actual damage to the kidney tubules

anuria: total urine output less than 50 mL in 24 hours

arteriovenous fistula: type of vascular access for dialysis; created by surgically connecting an artery to a vein

arteriovenous graft: type of surgically created vascular access for dialysis by which a piece of biologic, semibiologic, or synthetic graft material connects the patient's artery to a vein

azotemia: abnormal concentration of nitrogenous wastes in the blood

chronic kidney disease: chronic progressive and irreversible diseases of the kidneys

continuous ambulatory peritoneal dialysis: method of peritoneal dialysis whereby a patient manually performs four or five complete exchanges or cycles throughout the day

continuous cyclic peritoneal dialysis: method of peritoneal dialysis in which a peritoneal dialysis machine (cycler) automatically performs exchanges, usually while the patient sleeps

continuous kidney replacement therapy: variety of methods used to replace normal kidney function by circulating the patient's blood through a filter and returning it to the patient

dialysate: solution that circulates through the dialyzer in hemodialysis and through the peritoneal membrane in peritoneal dialysis

dialyzer: "artificial kidney" or dialysis machine; contains a semipermeable membrane through which particles of a certain size can pass

diffusion: movement of solutes (waste products) from an area of higher concentration to an area of lower concentration

effluent: term used to describe the drained fluid from a peritoneal dialysis exchange

end-stage kidney disease: final stage of chronic kidney disease that results in retention of uremic waste products and the need for kidney replacement therapies

glomerulonephritis: inflammation of the glomerular capillaries

hemodialysis: procedure during which a patient's blood is circulated through a dialyzer to remove waste products and excess fluid

interstitial nephritis: inflammation within the kidney tissue

nephrosclerosis: hardening of the kidney arteries

nephrotic syndrome: type of kidney failure with increased glomerular permeability and massive proteinuria

nephrotoxic: any substance, medication, or action that destroys kidney tissue

osmosis: movement of water through a semipermeable membrane from an area of lower solute concentration to an area of higher solute concentration

peritoneal dialysis: procedure that uses the lining of the patient's peritoneal cavity as the semipermeable membrane for exchange of fluid and solutes

peritonitis: inflammation of the peritoneal membrane (lining of the peritoneal cavity)

pyelonephritis: inflammation of the kidney pelvis

ultrafiltration: process whereby water is removed from the blood by means of a pressure gradient between the patient's blood and the dialysate

uremia: an excess of urea and other nitrogenous wastes in the blood

urinary casts: proteins secreted by damaged kidney tubules

TABLE 45-1 Common Fluid and Electrolyte Disturbances in Kidney Disorders

Disturbance	Manifestations	General Management Strategies
Fluid volume deficit	Acute weight loss ≥5%, decreased skin turgor, dry mucous membranes, oliguria or anuria, increased hematocrit, blood urea nitrogen (BUN) level increased out of proportion to creatinine level, hypothermia	Fluid challenge, fluid replacement orally or parenterally
Fluid volume excess	Acute weight gain ≥5%, edema, crackles, shortness of breath, decreased BUN, decreased hematocrit, distended neck veins	Fluid and sodium restriction, diuretics, dialysis
Sodium deficit	Nausea, malaise, lethargy, headache, abdominal cramps, apprehension, seizures	Diet, normal saline or hypertonic saline solutions
Sodium excess	Dry, sticky mucous membranes, thirst, rough dry tongue, fever, restlessness, weakness, disorientation	Fluids, diuretics, dietary restriction
Potassium deficit	Anorexia, abdominal distention, paralytic ileus, muscle weakness, ECG changes, dysrhythmias	Diet, oral or parenteral potassium replacement therapy
Potassium excess	Diarrhea, colic, nausea, irritability, muscle weakness, ECG changes	Dietary restriction, diuretics, IV glucose, insulin and sodium bicarbonate, cation-exchange resin, calcium gluconate, dialysis
Calcium deficit	Abdominal and muscle cramps, stridor, carpopedal spasm, hyperactive reflexes, tetany, positive Chvostek's or Trousseau's sign, tingling of fingers and around mouth, ECG changes	Diet, oral or parenteral calcium salt replacement
Calcium excess	Deep bone pain, flank pain, muscle weakness, depressed deep tendon reflexes, constipation, nausea and vomiting, confusion, impaired memory, polyuria, polydipsia, ECG changes	Fluid replacement, etidronate, pamidronate, mithramycin, calcitonin, glucocorticoids, phosphate salts
Bicarbonate deficit	Headache, confusion, drowsiness, increased respiratory rate and depth, nausea and vomiting, warm flushed skin	Bicarbonate replacement, dialysis
Bicarbonate excess	Depressed respirations, muscle hypertonicity, dizziness, tingling of fingers and toes	Fluid replacement if volume depleted; ensure adequate chloride
Protein deficit	Chronic weight loss, emotional depression, pallor, fatigue, soft flabby muscles	Diet, dietary supplements, hyperalimentation, albumin
Magnesium deficit	Dysphagia, muscle cramps, hyperactive reflexes, tetany, positive Chvostek's or Trousseau's sign, tingling of fingers, dysrhythmias, vertigo	Diet, oral or parenteral magnesium replacement therapy
Magnesium excess	Facial flushing, nausea and vomiting, sensation of warmth, drowsiness, depressed deep tendon reflexes, muscle weakness, respiratory depression, cardiac arrest	Calcium gluconate, mechanical ventilation, dialysis
Phosphorus deficit	Deep bone pain, flank pain, muscle weakness and pain, paresthesia, apprehension, confusion, seizures	Diet, oral or parenteral phosphorus supplementation therapy
Phosphorus excess	Tetany, tingling of fingers and around mouth, muscle spasms, soft tissue calcification	Diet restriction, phosphate binders, normal saline solution, IV dextrose solution, and insulin

ECG, electrocardiographic; IV, intravenous.

which can compromise marginal kidney function and lead to kidney disease (Kane-Gill et al., 2015).

KIDNEY DISORDERS

Chronic Kidney Disease

Chronic kidney disease (CKD) is an abnormality of kidney structure or function for 3 months or more and is identified by the glomerular filtration rate (GFR) and other markers that indicate kidney damage. CKD is associated with decreased quality of life, increased health care expenditures, and premature death. Untreated CKD can result in **end-stage kidney disease** (ESKD) and necessitate kidney replacement therapy (dialysis or kidney transplantation). Risk factors include cardiovascular disease, diabetes, hypertension, and obesity. According to the Kidney Foundation of Canada (2018), in 2016, 1 in 10 Canadians has kidney disease and millions more are at risk. Each day an average of 15 people are told that their kidneys have failed.

Diabetes and hypertension are the highest risk factors for CKD in Canada. Other conditions include ESKD, **glomerulonephritis**, polycystic kidney disease (PKD), and systemic lupus erythematosus (Hannon & Porth, 2017).

Pathophysiology

In the early stages of CKD there can be significant damage to the kidneys without signs or symptoms. The pathophysiology of CKD is not yet clearly understood, but the damage to the kidneys is thought to be caused by prolonged acute inflammation that is not organ specific and thus has subtle systemic manifestations.

CHART 45-1

Stages of Chronic Kidney Disease

Stages are based on the glomerular filtration rate (GFR). The normal GFR is 125 mL/min/1.73 m^2

Stage 1
GFR ≥90 mL/min/1.73 m^2
Kidney damage with normal or increased GFR

Stage 2
GFR = 60–89 mL/min/1.73 m^2
Mild decrease in GFR

Stage 3
GFR = 30–59 mL/min/1.73 m^2
Moderate decrease in GFR

Stage 4
GFR = 15–29 mL/min/1.73 m^2
Severe decrease in GFR

Stage 5
GFR <15 mL/min/1.73 m^2
End-stage kidney disease or chronic kidney disease

GFR, glomerular filtration rate.
Adapted from Grossman, S. C., & Porth, C. M. (2014). *Pathophysiology: Concepts of altered health states* (9th ed.). Philadelphia, PA: Lippincott Williams & Wilkins.

Stages of Chronic Kidney Disease

CKD has been classified into five stages by the National Kidney Foundation (NKF) (see Chart 45-1). Stage 5 results when the kidneys cannot remove the body's metabolic wastes or perform their regulatory functions; thus, kidney replacement therapies are required to sustain life. Screening and early intervention are important, because not all patients progress to stage 5 CKD. Patients with CKD are at increased risk for cardiovascular disease, which is the leading cause of morbidity and mortality (Kane-Gill et al., 2015). Treatment of hypertension, anemia, and hyperglycemia and detection of proteinuria all help to slow disease progression and improve patient outcomes (Lewis, 2013).

Clinical Manifestations

Elevated serum creatinine levels indicate underlying kidney disease; as the creatinine level increases, symptoms of CKD begin. Anemia, due to decreased erythropoietin production by the kidney; metabolic acidosis; and abnormalities in calcium and phosphorus herald the development of CKD. Fluid retention, evidenced by both edema and congestive heart failure, develops. As the disease progresses, abnormalities in electrolytes occur, heart failure worsens, and hypertension becomes more difficult to control.

Assessment and Diagnostic Findings

The GFR is the amount of plasma filtered through the glomeruli per unit of time. Creatinine clearance is a measure of the amount of creatinine the kidneys are able to clear in a 24-hour period. Normal values differ in men and women. Calculation of GFR, an important assessment perimeter in CKD, is discussed in Chapter 44.

Medical Management

The management of patients with CKD includes treatment of the underlying causes. Regular clinical and laboratory assessment is important to keep the blood pressure below 130/80 mm Hg (Klein-Kauric, 2015). Medical management also includes early referral for initiation of kidney replacement therapies as indicated by the patient's kidney status. Prevention of complications is accomplished by controlling cardiovascular risk factors; treating hyperglycemia; managing anemia; smoking cessation, weight loss, and exercise programs as needed; and reduction in salt and alcohol intake.

Nephrosclerosis

Nephrosclerosis (hardening of the kidney arteries) is most often due to prolonged hypertension and diabetes. Nephrosclerosis is a major cause of CKD and ESKD secondary to many disorders.

Pathophysiology

There are two forms of nephrosclerosis: malignant (accelerated) and benign. Malignant nephrosclerosis is often associated with significant hypertension (diastolic blood pressure higher than 130 mm Hg). It usually occurs in young adults and twice as often in men compared to women (Klein-Kauric, 2015). Damage is caused by decreased blood flow to the kidney resulting in patchy necrosis of the kidney parenchyma. Over time, fibrosis occurs and glomeruli are destroyed.

The disease process progresses rapidly. Without dialysis, more than half of patients die from **uremia** (an excess of urea and other nitrogenous wastes in the blood) in a few years. Benign nephrosclerosis can be found in older adults, associated with atherosclerosis and hypertension.

Assessment and Diagnostic Findings

Symptoms are rare early in the disease, even though the urine usually contains protein and occasional casts. Kidney insufficiency and associated signs and symptoms occur late in the disease.

Medical Management

Treatment of nephrosclerosis is aggressive antihypertensive therapy. An angiotensin-converting enzyme (ACE) inhibitor, alone or in combination with other antihypertensive medications, significantly reduces its incidence. See Chapter 33 for additional information on hypertension.

Primary Glomerular Diseases

Diseases that destroy the glomerulus of the kidney are the third most common cause of stage 5 CKD. In these disorders, the glomerular capillaries are primarily involved. Antigen–antibody complexes form in the blood and become trapped in the glomerular capillaries (the filtering portion of the kidney), inducing an inflammatory response. Immunoglobulin G (IgG), the major immunoglobulin (antibody) found in the blood, can be detected in the glomerular

CHART 45-2

Terms Typically Used When Describing Glomerular Disease

Primary: Disease is mainly in glomeruli
Secondary: Glomerular diseases that are the consequence of systemic disease
Idiopathic: Cause is unknown
Acute: Occurs over days or weeks
Chronic: Occurs over months or years
Rapidly progressing: Constant loss of kidney function with minimal chance of recovery
Diffuse: Involves all glomeruli
Focal: Involves some glomeruli
Segmental: Involves portions of individual glomeruli
Membranous: Evidence of thickened glomerular capillary walls
Proliferative: Number of glomerular cells involved is increasing

Physiology/Pathophysiology

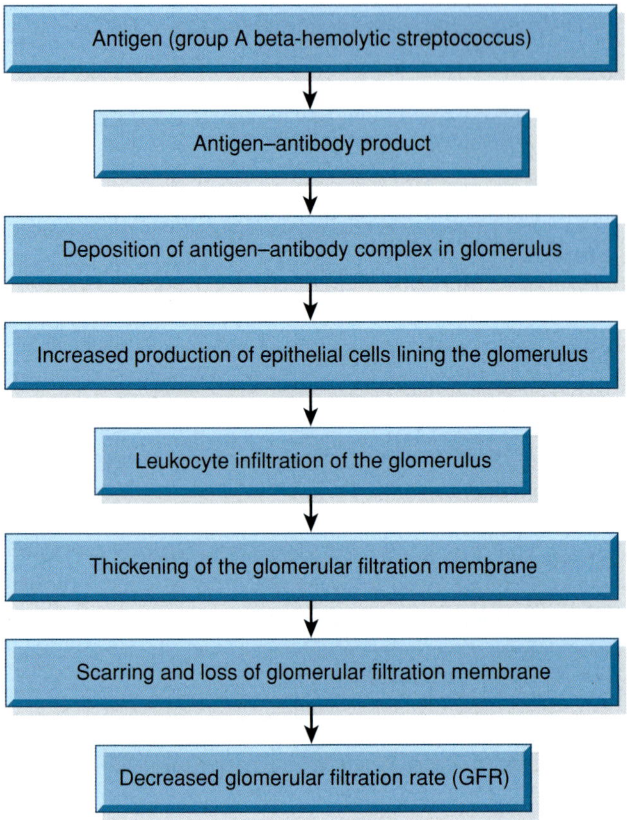

FIGURE 45-1. Sequence of events in acute nephritic syndrome.

capillary walls. The major clinical manifestations of glomerular injury include proteinuria, hematuria, decreased GFR, decreased excretion of sodium, edema, and hypertension (Chart 45-2).

Acute Nephritic Syndrome

The **acute nephritic syndrome** is the clinical manifestation of glomerular inflammation (Hannon & Porth, 2017). Glomerulonephritis is an inflammation of the glomerular capillaries that can occur in acute and chronic forms.

Pathophysiology

Primary glomerular diseases include postinfectious glomerulonephritis, rapidly progressive glomerulonephritis, membrane proliferative glomerulonephritis, membranous glomerulonephritis, IgA nephropathy, lupus nephritis, and diabetic nephropathy. Increased permeability of the glomerular filtration membrane allows for the passages of red blood cells (RBCs) and proteins (McCance & Huether, 2014). Postinfectious causes are group A beta-hemolytic streptococcal infection of the throat that precedes the onset of glomerulonephritis by 2 to 3 weeks (Fig. 45-1). It may also follow impetigo (infection of the skin) and acute viral infections (upper respiratory tract infections, mumps, varicella zoster virus, Epstein–Barr virus, hepatitis B, and human immunodeficiency virus [HIV] infection). In some patients, antigens outside the body (e.g., medications, foreign serum) initiate the process, resulting in antigen–antibody complexes being deposited in the glomeruli. In other patients, the kidney tissue itself serves as the inciting antigen.

Clinical Manifestations

The primary presenting features of an acute glomerular inflammation are hematuria, oliguria, edema, **azotemia**, an abnormal concentration of nitrogenous wastes in the blood, and proteinuria decreased GFR (Hannon & Porth, 2017). The hematuria may be microscopic (identifiable only through microscopic examination) or macroscopic (visible to the eye). The urine may appear cola-coloured because of RBCs and protein plugs or casts; RBC casts indicate glomerular injury. Glomerulonephritis may be mild and the hematuria discovered incidentally through a routine urinalysis, or the disease may be severe, with AKI and oliguria.

Some degree of edema and hypertension is present in most patients. Marked proteinuria due to the increased permeability of the glomerular membrane may also occur, with associated pitting edema, hypoalbuminemia, hyperlipidemia, and fatty casts in the urine. Blood urea nitrogen (BUN) and serum creatinine levels may increase as urine output decreases. In addition, anemia may be present.

In the more severe form of the disease, patients also complain of headache, malaise, and flank pain. Older adults may experience circulatory overload with dyspnea, engorged neck veins, cardiomegaly, and pulmonary edema. Atypical symptoms include confusion, somnolence, and seizures, which are often confused with the symptoms of a primary neurologic disorder.

Assessment and Diagnostic Findings

In acute nephritic syndrome, the kidneys become large, edematous, and congested. All kidney tissues including the glomeruli, tubules, and blood vessels are affected to varying degrees. Patients with an IgA nephropathy have an elevated serum IgA and low to normal complement levels. Electron microscopy and immunofluorescent analysis help identify the nature of the lesion; however, a kidney biopsy may be needed for definitive diagnosis. (See Chapter 44 for discussion of kidney biopsy.)

If the patient improves, the amount of urine increases and the urinary protein and sediment diminish. The percentage of adults who recover is unknown. Some patients develop severe uremia (an excess of urea and other nitrogenous wastes in the blood) within weeks and require dialysis for survival. Others, after a period of apparent recovery, insidiously develop chronic glomerulonephritis.

Complications

Complications of acute glomerulonephritis include hypertensive encephalopathy, heart failure, and pulmonary edema. Hypertensive encephalopathy is a medical emergency, and therapy is directed toward reducing the blood pressure without impairing kidney function. This can occur in acute nephritic syndrome or preeclampsia with chronic hypertension of greater than 140/90 mm Hg. Rapidly progressive glomerulonephritis is characterized by a rapid decline in kidney function. Without treatment, ESKD develops in a matter of weeks or months. Signs and symptoms are similar to those of acute glomerulonephritis (hematuria and proteinuria), but the course of the disease is more severe and rapid. Crescent-shaped cells accumulate in Bowman's space, disrupting the filtering surface. Plasma exchange (plasmapheresis) and treatment with high-dose corticosteroids and cytotoxic agents have been used to reduce the inflammatory response.

Medical Management

Management consists primarily of treating symptoms, attempting to preserve kidney function, and treating complications promptly. Treatment may include corticosteroids, antihypertensives, and controlling proteinuria. Pharmacologic therapy depends on the cause of acute glomerulonephritis. If residual streptococcal infection is suspected, penicillin is the agent of choice; however, other antibiotic agents may be prescribed. Dietary protein is restricted when kidney insufficiency and nitrogen retention (elevated BUN) develop. Sodium is restricted when the patient has hypertension, edema, and heart failure. Dialysis is initiated in acute glomerulonephritis if signs and symptoms of uremia are severe. The prognosis for patients with acute nephritic syndrome is excellent and rarely causes CKD (Hannon & Porth, 2017).

Nursing Management

Although most patients with acute uncomplicated glomerulonephritis are cared for as outpatients, nursing care is important in every setting.

Providing Care in the Hospital

In a hospital setting, carbohydrates are given liberally to provide energy and reduce the catabolism of protein. I&O are carefully measured and recorded. Fluids are given based on the patient's fluid losses and daily body weight. Insensible fluid loss through the lungs (300 mL) and skin (500 mL) is considered when estimating fluid loss (see Chapter 17). If treatment is effective, diuresis will begin, resulting in decreased edema and blood pressure. Proteinuria and microscopic hematuria may persist for many months; in fact, for acute poststreptococcal glomerulonephritis, 20% of patients have some degree of persistent proteinuria or decreased GFR 1 year after presentation (Hannon & Porth, 2017). Other nursing interventions focus on patient education about the disease process, explanations of laboratory and other diagnostic tests, and preparation for safe and effective self-care at home.

Promoting Home, Community-Based, and Transitional Care

EDUCATING PATIENTS ABOUT SELF-CARE. Patient education is directed toward symptom management and monitoring for complications. Fluid and diet restrictions must be reviewed with the patient to avoid worsening of edema and hypertension. The patient is instructed verbally and in writing to notify the physician if symptoms of kidney failure occur (e.g., fatigue, nausea, vomiting, diminishing urine output) or at the first sign of any infection.

CONTINUING AND TRANSITIONAL CARE. The importance of follow-up evaluations of blood pressure, urinalysis for protein, and BUN and serum creatinine levels to determine if the disease has progressed is stressed to the patient. A referral for home care may be indicated; a visit from a home care nurse provides an opportunity for careful assessment of the patient's progress and detection of early signs and symptoms of kidney insufficiency. If corticosteroids, immunosuppressant agents, or antibiotic medications are prescribed, the home care nurse or nurse in the outpatient setting uses the opportunity to review the dosage, desired actions, and adverse effects of medications and the precautions to be taken.

Chronic Glomerulonephritis

Chronic glomerulonephritis may be due to repeated episodes of acute nephritic syndrome, hypertensive nephrosclerosis, hyperlipidemia, chronic tubulointerstitial injury, or hemodynamically mediated glomerular sclerosis. Secondary glomerular diseases that can have systemic effects include lupus erythematosus, Goodpasture's syndrome (caused by antibodies to the glomerular basement membrane), diabetic glomerulosclerosis, and amyloidosis.

Pathophysiology

The kidneys are reduced to as little as one fifth their normal size (consisting largely of fibrous tissue). The cortex layer shrinks to 1 to 2 mm in thickness or less. Bands of scar tissue distort the remaining cortex, making the surface of the kidney rough and irregular. Numerous glomeruli and their tubules become scarred, and the branches of the kidney artery are thickened. The resulting severe glomerular damage can progress to stage 5 CKD and require kidney replacement therapies.

Clinical Manifestations

The symptoms of chronic glomerulonephritis vary. Some patients with severe disease have no symptoms at all for many years (Hannon & Porth, 2017). The condition may be discovered when hypertension or elevated BUN and serum creatinine levels are detected. Most patients report general symptoms, such as loss of weight and strength, increasing irritability, and an increased need to urinate at night (nocturia). Headaches, dizziness, and digestive disturbances are also common.

As chronic glomerulonephritis progresses, signs and symptoms of CKD may develop. The patient appears poorly nourished, with a yellow-grey pigmentation of the skin and periorbital and peripheral (dependent) edema. Blood pressure may be normal or severely elevated. Retinal findings include hemorrhage, exudate, narrowed tortuous arterioles, and papilledema. Anemia causes pale mucous membranes. Cardiomegaly, a gallop rhythm, distended neck veins, and other signs and symptoms of heart failure may be present. Crackles can be heard in the bases of the lungs.

Peripheral neuropathy with diminished deep tendon reflexes and neurosensory changes occur late in the disease. The patient becomes confused and demonstrates a limited attention span. An additional late finding includes evidence of pericarditis with a pericardial friction rub and pulsus paradoxus (difference in blood pressure during inspiration and expiration of greater than 10 mm Hg).

Assessment and Diagnostic Findings

A number of laboratory abnormalities occur. Urinalysis reveals a fixed specific gravity of about 1.010, variable proteinuria, and **urinary casts** (proteins secreted by damaged kidney tubules). As kidney failure progresses and the GFR falls below 50 mL/min, the following changes occur:

- Hyperkalemia due to decreased potassium excretion, acidosis, catabolism, and excessive potassium intake from food and medications
- Metabolic acidosis from decreased acid secretion by the kidney and inability to regenerate bicarbonate
- Anemia secondary to decreased erythropoiesis
- Hypoalbuminemia with edema secondary to protein loss through the damaged glomerular membrane
- Increased serum phosphorus level due to decreased kidney excretion of phosphorus
- Decreased serum calcium level (calcium binds to phosphorus to compensate for elevated serum phosphorus levels)
- Mental status changes
- Impaired nerve conduction due to electrolyte abnormalities and uremia

Chest x-rays may show cardiac enlargement and pulmonary edema. The electrocardiogram (ECG) may be normal or may indicate left ventricular hypertrophy associated with hypertension and signs of electrolyte disturbances, such as tall, tented (or peaked) T waves associated with hyperkalemia. Computed tomography (CT) and magnetic resonance imaging (MRI) scans show a decrease in the size of the kidney cortex.

Medical Management

Management of symptoms guides the treatment. If the patient has hypertension, efforts are made to reduce the blood pressure with sodium and water restriction, antihypertensive agents, or both. Weight is monitored daily, and diuretic medications are prescribed to treat fluid overload. Proteins of high biologic value (dairy products, eggs, meats) are provided to promote good nutritional status. Adequate calories are provided to spare protein for tissue growth and repair. Urinary tract infections (UTIs) must be treated promptly to prevent further kidney damage.

Dialysis is initiated early in the course of the disease to keep the patient in optimal physical condition, prevent fluid and electrolyte imbalances, and minimize the risk of complications of kidney failure. The course of dialysis is smoother if treatment begins before the patient develops complications.

Nursing Management

Whether the patient is hospitalized or cared for in the home, the nurse observes the patient for common fluid and electrolyte disturbances in kidney disease (Table 45-1). Changes in fluid and electrolyte status and in cardiac and neurologic status are reported promptly to the physician. Anxiety levels are often extremely high for both the patient and family. Throughout the course of the disease and treatment, the nurse gives emotional support by providing opportunities for the patient and family to verbalize their concerns, have their questions answered, and explore their options (Ahmad & Al Nazly, 2015).

Promoting Home, Community-Based, and Transitional Care

Educating Patients About Self-Care

The nurse has a major role in teaching the patient and family about the prescribed treatment plan and the risks associated with noncompliance. Instructions to the patient include explanations and scheduling for follow-up evaluations: blood pressure, urinalysis for protein and casts, and laboratory studies of BUN and serum creatinine levels. If long-term dialysis is needed, the nurse teaches the patient and family about the procedure, how to care for the access site, dietary restrictions, and other necessary lifestyle modifications. These topics are discussed later in this chapter.

Periodic hospitalization, visits to the outpatient clinic or office, and home care referrals provide the nurse in each setting with the opportunity for careful assessment of the patient's progress and continued education about changes to report to the primary health care provider (worsening signs and symptoms of kidney failure, such as nausea, vomiting, and diminished urine output). Specific teaching may include explanations about recommended diet and fluid modifications and medications (purpose, desired effects, adverse effects, dosage, and administration schedule).

Continuing and Transitional Care

Periodic laboratory evaluations of creatinine clearance and BUN and serum creatinine levels are carried out to assess residual kidney function and the need for dialysis or transplantation. If dialysis is initiated, the patient and family require considerable assistance and support in dealing with therapy and its long-term implications. The patient and family are reminded of the importance of participation in health promotion activities, including health screening. The patient is instructed to inform all health care providers about the diagnosis of glomerulonephritis so that all medical management, including pharmacologic therapy, is based on altered kidney function.

Nephrotic Syndrome

Nephrotic syndrome is a type of kidney failure characterized by increased glomerular permeability and is manifested

Physiology/Pathophysiology

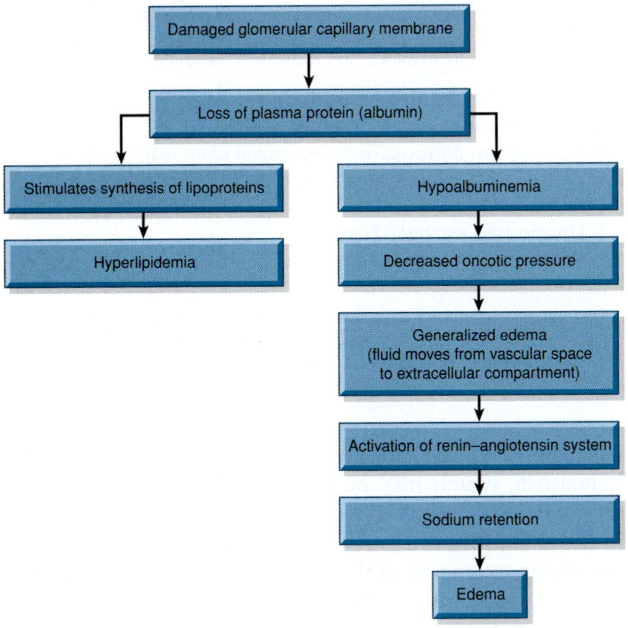

FIGURE 45-2. Sequence of events in nephrotic syndrome.

by massive proteinuria (Hannon & Porth, 2017). Clinical findings include a marked increase in protein (particularly albumin) in the urine (proteinuria), a decrease in albumin in the blood (hypoalbuminemia), diffuse edema, high serum cholesterol, and low-density lipoproteins (hyperlipidemia).

The syndrome is apparent in any condition that seriously damages the glomerular capillary membrane and results in increased glomerular permeability to plasma proteins. Although the liver is capable of increasing the production of albumin, it cannot keep up with the daily loss of albumin through the kidneys. Thus, hypoalbuminemia results (Fig. 45-2).

Pathophysiology

Nephrotic syndrome occurs with many intrinsic kidney diseases and systemic diseases that cause glomerular damage. It is not a specific glomerular disease but a constellation of clinical findings that result from the glomerular damage (Hannon & Porth, 2017).

Clinical Manifestations

The major manifestation of nephrotic syndrome is edema. It is usually soft and pitting and commonly occurs around the eyes (periorbital), in dependent areas (sacrum, ankles, and hands), and in the abdomen (ascites). Patients may also exhibit irritability, headache, and malaise.

Assessment and Diagnostic Findings

Proteinuria (predominately albumin) exceeding 3.5 g/day is the hallmark of the diagnosis of nephrotic syndrome (Hannon & Porth, 2017).

Protein electrophoresis and immunoelectrophoresis may be performed on the urine to categorize the type of proteinuria. The urine may also contain increased white blood cells (WBCs) as well as granular and epithelial casts. A needle biopsy of the kidney may be performed for histologic examination of kidney tissue to confirm the diagnosis.

Complications

Complications of nephrotic syndrome include infection (due to a deficient immune response), thromboembolism (especially of the kidney vein), pulmonary emboli, ARF (due to hypovolemia), and accelerated atherosclerosis (due to hyperlipidemia).

Medical Management

Treatment is focused on treating the underlying disease state causing proteinuria, slowing progression of CKD, and relieving symptoms. Typical treatment includes diuretics for edema, ACE inhibitors to reduce proteinuria, and lipid-lowering agents for hyperlipidemia.

Nursing Management

In the early stages of nephrotic syndrome, nursing management is similar to that of the patient with acute glomerulonephritis, but as the condition worsens, management is similar to that of the patient with ESKD (see the following section).

Patients with nephrotic syndrome need adequate instruction about the importance of following all medication and dietary regimens so that their condition can remain stable as long as possible. Patients must be made aware of the importance of communicating any health-related change to their health care providers as soon as possible so that appropriate medication and dietary changes can be made before further changes occur within the glomeruli.

Polycystic Kidney Disease

Pathophysiology

Polycystic kidney disease (PKD) is a genetic disorder characterized by the growth of numerous cysts in the kidneys. When cysts form in the kidneys, they are filled with fluid, destroying the nephrons. PKD cysts can profoundly enlarge the kidneys while replacing much of the normal structure, resulting in reduced kidney function and leading to kidney failure.

PKD can also cause cysts in the liver and problems in other organs, such as blood vessels in the brain and heart. The number of cysts as well as the complications they cause helps distinguish PKD from the usually harmless "simple" cysts that can form in the kidneys in later years of life. There are two categories of PKD: autosomal dominant (ADPKD), also known as adult polycystic disease, and autosomal recessive PKD. Of the two, ADPKD is the most common inherited form. Two major inherited forms of ADPKD exist: type I and type II. About 85% of cases are type I and 15% are type II (Hannon & Porth, 2017).

Treatment of ADPKD is largely supportive with the goal of delaying the disease progression. When ADPKD causes kidneys to fail, which usually happens after many years, the patient requires dialysis or kidney transplantation. About one half of people with the most common type of PKD progress to CKD stage 5, requiring kidney replacement.

Clinical Manifestations

Signs and symptoms of PKD result from loss of kidney function and the increasing size of the kidneys as the cysts grow. Kidney damage can result in hematuria, polyuria (large amounts of urine), hypertension, development of kidney calculi and associated UTIs, and proteinuria. The growing cysts are noted with reports of abdominal fullness and flank pain (back and lower sides).

Assessment and Diagnostic Findings

Since PKD is a genetic disease, careful evaluation of family history is necessary. Palpation of the abdomen will often reveal enlarged cystic kidneys. Diagnosis is usually made with ultrasound imaging of the kidney (Hannon & Porth, 2017).

Medical Management

PKD has no cure, and treatment is largely supportive and includes blood pressure control, pain control, and antibiotic agents to resolve infections. Once the kidneys fail, kidney replacement therapy is indicated (see later discussion in chapter). Genetic linkage studies and counselling may be indicated, particularly when screening family members for potential kidney donation (Hannon & Porth, 2017).

CHART 45-3

Risk Factors for Kidney Cancer

- Gender: Affects men more than women
- Tobacco use
- Occupational exposure to industrial chemicals, such as petroleum products, heavy metals, and asbestos
- Obesity
- Unopposed estrogen therapy
- Polycystic kidney disease

Adapted from American Cancer Society. (2015). Kidney cancer. Retrieved October 1, 2015, from www.cancer.org/cancer/kidneycancer/detailedguide/kidney-cancer-adult-key-statistics

KIDNEY CANCER

Cancer of the kidney and kidney pelvis accounts for 2 to 3% of all cancers. There were 4,200 new cases in men and 2,400 new cases in women in Canada in 2017 (Canadian Cancer Society's Advisory Committee, 2017). The incidence of all stages of kidney cancer has increased in the last two decades in Canada. Tobacco use continues to be a significant risk factor for kidney carcinoma (Chart 45-3).

The most common type of kidney carcinoma arises from the kidney epithelium and accounts for more than 80 to 90% of all kidney tumours. These tumours may metastasize early to the lungs, bone, liver, brain, and contralateral kidney. One quarter of patients have metastatic disease at the time of diagnosis. Although enhanced imaging techniques account for improved detection of early-stage kidney cancer, symptoms may not be present until the tumour reaches a considerable size (Hannon & Porth, 2017).

Clinical Manifestations

Many kidney tumours produce no symptoms and are discovered on a routine physical examination as a palpable abdominal mass. The classic signs and symptoms, which occur in only 10% of patients, include hematuria, pain, and a mass in the flank (Hannon & Porth, 2017). The usual sign that first calls attention to the tumour is painless hematuria, which may be either intermittent and microscopic or continuous and gross. There may be a dull pain in the back from the pressure produced by compression of the ureter, extension of the tumour into the perirenal area, or hemorrhage into the kidney tissue. Colicky pains occur if a clot or mass of tumour cells passes down the ureter. Symptoms from metastasis may be the first manifestations of kidney tumour and may include unexplained weight loss, increasing weakness, and anemia.

Assessment and Diagnostic Findings

Diagnosis is confirmed with ultrasonography and CT scanning. An MRI may be used to rule out the involvement of the inferior vena cava (Hannon & Porth, 2017). These tests may be exhausting for patients already debilitated by the systemic effects of a tumour as well as for older patients and those who are anxious about the diagnosis and outcome. The nurse assists the patient to prepare physically and psychologically for these procedures and monitors carefully for signs and symptoms of dehydration and exhaustion.

Treatment for kidney cancer is dependent on a host of factors, including: the stage of the cancer; the functional status of the kidneys; whether the cancer is in one or both of the kidneys; the type of cancer; and the individual's overall health. Treatment options include surgical interventions, radiation, and immunotherapy (Canadian Cancer Society, 2018).

Medical Management

The goal of management is to eradicate the tumour before metastasis occurs.

Surgical Management

Nephrectomy

A radical nephrectomy is the preferred treatment if the tumour can be removed. This includes removal of the kidney (and tumour), adrenal gland, surrounding perinephric fat and Gerota's fascia, and lymph nodes. Laparoscopic nephrectomy can be performed for removal of the kidney with a small tumour. This procedure incurs less morbidity and a shorter recovery time. Radiation therapy, hormonal therapy, or chemotherapy may be used along with surgery. Immunotherapy may also be helpful. For patients with bilateral tumour or cancer of a functional single kidney, nephron-sparing surgery (partial nephrectomy) may be considered.

Nephron-sparing surgery is increasingly being used to treat patients with solid kidney lesions. The technical success rate of nephron-sparing surgery is excellent, and operative morbidity and mortality are low.

Patients with upper tract transitional cell carcinoma may benefit from laparoscopic nephroureterectomy. Although it is a lengthier surgical procedure, it has the same efficacy and is better tolerated by patients than open nephroureterectomy.

Kidney Artery Embolization

In patients with metastatic kidney carcinoma, the kidney artery may be occluded to impede the blood supply to the tumour and thus kill the tumour cells. After angiographic studies are completed, a catheter is advanced into the kidney artery, and embolizing materials (e.g., Gelfoam, autologous blood clot, steel coils) are injected into the artery and carried with the arterial blood flow to occlude the tumour vessels mechanically. This decreases the local blood supply, making removal of the kidney (nephrectomy) easier. It also stimulates an immune response because infarction of the kidney cell carcinoma releases tumour-associated antigens that enhance the patient's response to metastatic lesions. The procedure may also reduce the number of tumour cells entering the venous circulation during surgical manipulation.

After kidney artery embolization and tumour infarction, a characteristic symptom complex called postinfarction syndrome occurs, lasting 2 to 3 days. The patient has pain localized to the flank and abdomen, elevated temperature, and gastrointestinal (GI) symptoms. Pain is treated with parenteral analgesic agents, and acetaminophen (Tylenol) is administered to control fever. Antiemetic medications, restriction of oral intake, and IV fluids are used to treat the GI symptoms.

Pharmacologic Therapy

Depending on the stage of the tumour, percutaneous partial or radical nephrectomy may be followed by treatment with chemotherapeutic agents. Treatment with biologic response modifiers such as interleukin 2 (IL-2) is effective. IL-2, a protein that regulates cell growth, is used alone or in combination with lymphokine-activated killer cells (WBCs that have been stimulated by IL-2 to increase their ability to kill cancer cells). Interferon, another biologic response modifier, appears to have a direct antiproliferative effect on kidney tumours.

Another promising experimental approach to kidney cell carcinoma is a vaccination to stimulate immune response, with autologous tumour cells with IL-2–, granulocyte-macrophage stimulating factor–, and dendritic cell–type vaccines. If patients with kidney cancer do not respond to immunotherapy, allogeneic stem cell transplantation may be indicated (see Chapter 68).

Nursing Management

The patient with a kidney tumour usually undergoes extensive diagnostic and therapeutic procedures. Treatment includes surgery, radiation therapy, and medications. After surgery, the patient usually has catheters and drains in place to maintain a patent urinary tract, to remove drainage, and to permit accurate measurement of urine output. Because of the location of the surgical incision, the patient's position during surgery, and the nature of the surgical procedure, pain and muscle soreness are common. Pharmacologic management often includes immunosuppressant agents; therefore, patients are monitored for infection.

The patient requires frequent analgesia during the postoperative period and assistance with turning, coughing, use of incentive spirometry, and deep breathing to prevent atelectasis and other pulmonary complications. The patient and family require assistance and support to cope with the diagnosis and uncertain prognosis. (See this chapter for discussion of postoperative care of the patient undergoing kidney surgery and Chapter 68 for discussion of care of the patient with cancer.)

Promoting Home, Community-Based, and Transitional Care

Educating Patients About Self-Care

The nurse teaches the patient to inspect and care for the incision and perform other general postoperative care including activity and lifting restrictions, driving, and pain management. Instructions are provided about when to notify the physician about problems (e.g., fever, breathing difficulty, wound drainage, blood in the urine, pain or swelling of the legs).

The nurse encourages the patient to eat a healthy diet and to drink adequate liquids to avoid constipation and to maintain an adequate urine volume. Education and emotional support are provided related to the diagnosis, treatment, and continuing care because many patients are concerned about the loss of the other kidney, the possible need for dialysis, or the recurrence of cancer.

Continuing and Transitional Care

Follow-up care is essential to detect signs of metastases and to reassure the patient and family about the patient's status and well-being. The patient who has had surgery for kidney carcinoma should have a yearly physical examination and chest x-ray, because late metastases are not uncommon. All subsequent symptoms should be evaluated with possible metastases in mind.

If follow-up chemotherapy is necessary, the patient and family are informed about the treatment plan or chemotherapy protocol, what to expect with each visit, and when to notify the physician. Evaluation of remaining kidney function (creatinine clearance, BUN and serum creatinine levels) may also be carried out periodically. A home care nurse may monitor the patient's physical status and psychological well-being and coordinate other indicated services and resources.

KIDNEY DISEASE

Kidney disease results when the kidneys cannot remove the body's metabolic wastes or perform their regulatory functions. The substances normally eliminated in the urine accumulate in the body fluids as a result of impaired kidney excretion, affecting endocrine and metabolic functions as well as fluid, electrolyte, and acid–base disturbances. Kidney failure is a systemic disease and is a final common pathway of many different kidney and urinary tract diseases. In 2014, 5,269 patients were newly diagnosed with ESKD. Since 2005, the number of Canadians living with ESKD has risen from 25,653 to 35,281 (Canadian Institute for Health Information [CIHI], 2016).

Acute Kidney Injury

Acute kidney injury (AKI) is a rapid loss of kidney function due to damage to the kidneys. Depending on the duration and severity of AKI, a wide range of potentially life-threatening metabolic complications can occur, including metabolic acidosis as well as fluid and electrolyte imbalances. Treatment is aimed at replacing kidney function temporarily to minimize potentially lethal complications and reduce potential causes of increased kidney injury with the goal of minimizing long-term loss of kidney function. AKI is a problem seen in hospitalized patients and those in outpatient settings.

A widely accepted criterion for AKI is a 50% or greater increase in serum creatinine above baseline (normal creatinine is less than 1 mg/dL) (Vrtis, 2013). Urine volume may be normal, or changes may occur. Possible changes include nonoliguria (greater than 800 mL/day), oliguria (less than 0.5 mL/kg/hr), or **anuria** (less than 50 mL/day) (Vrtis, 2013).

TABLE 45-2 The RIFLE Classification for Acute Kidney Injury

Class	GFR Criteria	Urinary Output Criteria
R (Risk)	Increased serum creatinine 1.5× baseline OR GFR decreased ≥25%	0.5 mL/kg/hr for 6 hours
I (Injury)	Increased serum creatinine 2× baseline OR GFR decreased ≥50%	0.5 mL/kg/hr for 12 hours
F (Failure)	Increased serum creatinine 3× baseline OR GFR decreased ≥75% OR Serum creatinine ≥354 mmol/L with an acute rise of at least 44 mmol/L	<0.3 mL/kg/hr for 24 hours OR Anuria for 12 hours
L (Loss)	Persistent acute kidney injury = complete loss of kidney function >4 weeks	
E (ESKD)	ESKD >3 months	

GFR, glomerular filtration rate; ESKD, end-stage kidney disease.

Adapted from Davies, H., & Leslie, G. (2012). Acute kidney injury and the critically ill patient. *Dimensions of Critical Care Nursing, 31*(3), 135–152.

Pathophysiology

Although the pathogenesis of AKI and oliguria is not always known, many times there is a specific underlying problem. Some of the factors may be reversible if identified and treated promptly, before kidney function is impaired. This is true of the following conditions that reduce blood flow to the kidney and impair kidney function: (1) hypovolemia; (2) hypotension; (3) reduced cardiac output and heart failure; (4) obstruction of the kidney or lower urinary tract by tumour, blood clot, or kidney stone; and (5) bilateral obstruction of the kidney arteries or veins. If these conditions are treated and corrected before the kidneys are permanently damaged, the increased BUN and creatinine levels, oliguria, and other signs may be reversed.

Although kidney stones are not a common cause of ARF, some types may increase the risk for AKI. Some hereditary stone diseases (see Chapter 46), primary struvite stones, and infection-related urolithiasis associated with anatomic and functional urinary tract anomalies and spinal cord injury may cause recurrent bouts of obstruction as well as crystal-specific damage to tubular epithelial cells and interstitial kidney cells.

Classifications of Acute Kidney Injury

The term AKI has replaced the term **acute kidney failure** because it better describes this syndrome in patients, not only simply those who require kidney replacement therapies but also those patients who experience minor changes in kidney function. Classification criteria for AKI include assessment of three grades of severity and two outcome-level classifications. This 5-point system is known as the RIFLE classification system (Davies & Leslie, 2012). RIFLE stands for risk, injury, failure, loss, and ESKD (Vrtis, 2013). Risk, injury, and failure are considered grades of AKI severity, whereas loss and ESKD are considered outcomes of loss that require some form of kidney replacement therapy, at least temporarily (Dring & Hipkiss, 2015). Table 45-2 lists the classification criteria for the RIFLE system for AKI (Vrtis, 2013). This classification system is used by health care professionals to identify kidney injury and improve patient outcomes.

Categories of Acute Kidney Injury

The major categories of AKI are prerenal (hypoperfusion of kidney), intrarenal (actual damage to kidney tissue), and postrenal (obstruction to urine flow). Prerenal AKI, which occurs in 60 to 70% of cases, is the result of impaired blood flow that leads to hypoperfusion of the kidney commonly caused by volume depletion (burns, hemorrhage, GI losses), hypotension (sepsis, shock), and kidney artery stenosis, ultimately leading to a decrease in the GFR (Vrtis, 2013). Intrarenal AKI is the result of actual parenchymal damage to the glomeruli or kidney tubules. Acute tubular necrosis (ATN), or AKI in which there is damage to the kidney tubules, is the most common type of intrinsic AKI. Characteristics of ATN are intratubular obstruction, tubular back leak (abnormal reabsorption of filtrate and decreased urine flow through the tubule), vasoconstriction, and changes in glomerular permeability. These processes result in a decrease of GFR, progressive azotemia, and fluid and electrolyte imbalances. CKD, diabetes, heart failure, hypertension, and

CHART 45-4

Causes of Acute Kidney Injury

Prerenal Failure

- Volume depletion resulting from:
  Hemorrhage
  Kidney losses (diuretics, osmotic diuresis)
  Gastrointestinal losses (vomiting, diarrhea, nasogastric suction)
- Impaired cardiac efficiency resulting from:
  Myocardial infarction
  Heart failure
  Dysrhythmias
  Cardiogenic shock
- Vasodilation resulting from:
  Sepsis
  Anaphylaxis
  Antihypertensive medications or other medications that cause vasodilation

Intrarenal Failure

- Prolonged kidney ischemia resulting from:
  Pigment nephropathy (associated with the breakdown of blood cells containing pigments that in turn occlude kidney structures)
  Myoglobinuria (trauma, crush injuries, burns)
  Hemoglobinuria (transfusion reaction, hemolytic anemia)
- Nephrotoxic agents such as:
  Aminoglycoside antibiotics (gentamicin, tobramycin)
  Radiopaque contrast agents
  Heavy metals (lead, mercury)
  Solvents and chemicals (ethylene glycol, carbon tetrachloride, arsenic)
  Nonsteroidal anti-inflammatory drugs (NSAIDs)
  Angiotensin-converting enzyme inhibitors (ACE inhibitors)
- Infectious processes such as:
  Acute **pyelonephritis**
  Acute glomerulonephritis

Postrenal Failure

- Urinary tract obstruction, including:
  Calculi (stones)
  Tumours
  Benign prostatic hyperplasia
  Strictures
  Blood clots

cirrhosis can lead to ATN. Postrenal AKI usually results from obstruction distal to the kidney by conditions such as kidney calculi, strictures, blood clots, benign prostatic hypertrophy, malignancies, and pregnancy. Pressure rises in the kidney tubules, and eventually the GFR decreases. Common causes of each type of AKI are further summarized in Chart 45-4.

Phases of Acute Kidney Injury

There are four phases of AKI: initiation, oliguria, diuresis, and recovery.

- The **initiation period** begins with the initial insult and ends when oliguria develops.
- The **oliguria period** is accompanied by an increase in the serum concentration of substances usually excreted by the kidneys (urea, creatinine, uric acid, organic acids, and the intracellular cations [potassium and magnesium]). The minimum amount of urine needed to rid the body of normal metabolic waste products is 400 mL in 24 hours or 0.5 mL/kg/hr. In this phase uremic symptoms first appear and life-threatening conditions such as hyperkalemia develop.
- The **diuresis period** is marked by a gradual increase in urine output, which signals that glomerular filtration has started to recover. Laboratory values stabilize and eventually decrease. Although the volume of urinary output may reach normal or elevated levels, kidney function may still be markedly abnormal. Because uremic symptoms may still be present, the need for expert medical and nursing management continues. The patient must be observed closely for dehydration during this phase; if dehydration occurs, the uremic symptoms are likely to increase.
- The **recovery period** signals the improvement of kidney function and may take 3 to 12 months. Laboratory values return to the patient's normal level. Although a permanent 1% to 3% reduction in the GFR is common, it is not clinically significant.

Some patients have decreased kidney function with increasing nitrogen retention, yet actually excrete normal amounts of urine (2 L/day or more). This is the nonoliguric form of kidney failure and occurs predominantly after exposure of the patient to **nephrotoxic** agents, burns, traumatic injury, and the use of halogenated anesthetic agents.

Clinical Manifestations

Almost every system of the body is affected with failure of the normal kidney regulatory mechanisms. The patient may appear critically ill and lethargic. The skin and mucous membranes are dry from dehydration. Central nervous system signs and symptoms include drowsiness, headache, muscle twitching, and seizures. Table 45-3 summarizes common clinical characteristics in all three categories of AKI.

Assessment and Diagnostic Findings

Assessment of the patient with AKI includes evaluation for changes in the urine, diagnostic tests that evaluate the kidney contour, and a variety of laboratory values. See Chapter 44 for information about the normal characteristics of urine, diagnostic findings, and laboratory values in the kidney system.

In AKI, urine output varies from scanty to a normal volume, hematuria may be present, and the urine has a low specific gravity (compared with a normal value of 1.010 to 1.025). One of the earliest manifestations of tubular damage is the inability to concentrate the urine

TABLE 45-3 Comparing Clinical Characteristics of Acute Kidney Injury

Characteristics	Categories		
	Prerenal	*Intrarenal*	*Postrenal*
Etiology	Hypoperfusion	Parenchymal damage	Obstruction
Blood urea nitrogen value	Increased (out of normal 20:1 proportion to creatinine)	Increased	Increased
Creatinine	Increased	Increased	Increased
Urine output	Decreased	Varies, often decreased	Varies, may be decreased, or sudden anuria
Urine sodium	Decreased to <20 mEq/L	Increased to >40 mEq/L	Varies, often decreased to 20 mEq/L or less
Urinary sediment	Normal, few hyaline casts	Abnormal casts and debris	Usually normal
Urine osmolality	Increased to 500 mOsm	About 350 mOsm similar to serum	Varies, increased or equal to serum
Urine specific gravity	Increased	Low normal	Varies

(Hannon & Porth, 2017). Patients with prerenal azotemia have a decreased amount of sodium in the urine (less than 20 mEq/L) and normal urinary sediment. Patients with intrarenal azotemia usually have urinary sodium levels greater than 40 mEq/L with urinary casts and other cellular debris.

Ultrasonography is a critical component of the evaluation of patients with kidney failure. A kidney sonogram or a CT or MRI scan may show evidence of anatomic changes.

The BUN level increases steadily at a rate dependent on the degree of catabolism (breakdown of protein), kidney perfusion, and protein intake. Serum creatinine levels are useful in monitoring kidney function and disease progression and increase with glomerular damage.

With a decline in the GFR, oliguria, and anuria, patients are at high risk for hyperkalemia. Protein catabolism results in the release of cellular potassium into the body fluids, causing severe hyperkalemia (high serum potassium levels). Hyperkalemia may lead to dysrhythmias, such as ventricular tachycardia and cardiac arrest. Sources of potassium include normal tissue catabolism, dietary intake, blood in the GI tract, or blood transfusion and other sources (e.g., IV infusions, potassium penicillin, and extracellular shift in response to metabolic acidosis).

Progressive metabolic acidosis occurs in kidney failure because patients cannot eliminate the daily metabolic load of acid-type substances produced by the normal metabolic processes. In addition, normal kidney buffering mechanisms fail. This is reflected by a decrease in the serum CO_2-combining power and blood pH.

Blood phosphate concentrations may increase; calcium levels may be low due to decreased absorption of calcium from the intestine and as a compensatory mechanism for the elevated blood phosphate levels. Anemia is another common laboratory finding in AKI, as a result of reduced erythropoietin production, uremic GI lesions, reduced RBC lifespan, and blood loss from the GI tract.

Prevention

AKI has a high mortality rate that ranges from 40% to 90%. Factors that influence mortality include increased age, comorbid conditions, and pre-existing kidney and vascular diseases and respiratory failure (Vrtis, 2013). Therefore, prevention of AKI is essential (see Chart 45-5).

A careful history is obtained to identify exposure to nephrotoxic agents or environmental toxins. The kidneys are susceptible to the adverse effects of medications because the kidneys are repeatedly exposed to substances in the blood. Patients taking nephrotoxic medications (e.g., aminoglycosides, gentamicin, tobramycin, colistimethate, polymyxin B, amphotericin B, vancomycin, amikacin, cyclosporine) should be monitored closely for changes in kidney function. BUN and serum creatinine levels should be obtained at baseline within 24 hours after initiation of

CHART 45-5

Preventing Acute Kidney Injury

1. Provide adequate hydration to patients at risk for dehydration including:
   Before, during, and after surgery
   Patients undergoing intensive diagnostic studies requiring fluid restriction and contrast agents (e.g., barium enema, intravenous pyelograms), especially older patients who may have marginal kidney reserve
   Patients with neoplastic disorders or disorders of metabolism (e.g., gout) and those receiving chemotherapy
2. Prevent and treat shock promptly with blood and fluid replacement.
3. Monitor central venous and arterial pressures and hourly urine output of critically ill patients to detect the onset of kidney failure as early as possible.
4. Treat hypotension promptly.
5. Continually assess kidney function (urine output, laboratory values) when appropriate.
6. Take precautions to ensure that the appropriate blood is administered to the correct patient in order to avoid severe transfusion reactions, which can precipitate kidney failure.
7. Prevent and treat infections promptly. Infections can produce progressive kidney damage.
8. Pay special attention to wounds, burns, and other precursors of sepsis.
9. To prevent infections from ascending in the urinary tract, give meticulous care to patients with indwelling catheters. Remove catheters as soon as possible.
10. To prevent toxic drug effects, closely monitor dosage, duration of use, and blood levels of all medications metabolized or excreted by the kidneys.

these medications and at least twice a week while the patient is receiving them.

Any agent that reduces kidney blood flow (e.g., long-term analgesic use) may cause kidney insufficiency. Chronic use of analgesic agents, particularly nonsteroidal anti-inflammatory drugs (NSAIDs), may cause **interstitial nephritis** (inflammation within the kidney tissue) and papillary necrosis. Patients with heart failure or cirrhosis with ascites are at particular risk for NSAID-induced kidney failure. Increased age, pre-existing kidney disease, and the simultaneous administration of several nephrotoxic agents increase the risk for kidney damage.

Contrast-induced nephropathy (CIN) is a major cause of hospital-acquired AKI. From prospective studies conducted on patients admitted with AKI, 11% to 14.5% of the cases were possibly due to intravascular contrast media. More cardiac and systemic in-hospital complications are experienced by patients with CIN, including prolonged length of stay in the hospital as well as an increased need for dialysis (Owen, Hiremath, Myers, et al., 2014). This is a potentially preventable condition. Baseline levels of creatinine greater than 2 mg/dL identify patients at high risk. Limiting the patient's exposure to contrast agents and nephrotoxic medications will reduce the risk of CIN (Jorgensen, 2013).

Administration of *N*-acetylcysteine and sodium bicarbonate before and during procedures reduces risk, but prehydration with saline is considered the most effective method to prevent RIN (Rank, 2013).

Gerontologic Considerations

About half of all patients who develop AKI during hospitalization are older than 60 years. The etiology of AKI in older adults includes prerenal causes such as dehydration, intrarenal causes such as nephrotoxic agents (e.g., medications, contrast agents), and complications of major surgery (Holcombe & Kern Feeely, 2013). Suppression of thirst, enforced bed rest, lack of access to drinking water, and confusion all contribute to the older patient's failure to consume adequate fluids and may lead to dehydration, further compromising already decreased kidney function.

AKI in older adults is also often seen in the community setting. Nurses in the ambulatory setting need to be aware of the risk. All medications need to be monitored for potential side effects that could result in damage to the kidney either through reduced circulation or nephrotoxicity. Outpatient procedures that require fasting or a bowel preparation may cause dehydration and therefore require careful monitoring.

Medical Management

The kidneys have a remarkable ability to recover from insult. The objectives of treatment of AKI are to restore normal chemical balance and prevent complications until repair of kidney tissue and restoration of kidney function can occur. Management includes eliminating the underlying cause; maintaining fluid balance; avoiding fluid excesses; and, when indicated, providing kidney replacement therapy. Prerenal azotemia is treated by optimizing kidney perfusion, whereas postrenal failure is treated by relieving the obstruction. Intrarenal azotemia is treated with supportive therapy, with removal of causative agents, aggressive management of prerenal and postrenal failure, and avoidance of associated risk factors. Shock and infection, if present, are treated promptly (see Chapter 18).

Maintenance of fluid balance is based on daily body weight, serial measurements of central venous pressure, serum and urine concentrations, fluid losses, blood pressure, and the clinical status of the patient. The parenteral and oral intake and the output of urine, gastric drainage, stools, wound drainage, and perspiration are calculated and are used as the basis for fluid replacement. The insensible fluid produced through the normal metabolic processes and lost through the skin and lungs is also considered in fluid management.

Fluid excesses can be detected by the clinical findings of dyspnea, tachycardia, and distended neck veins. The patient's lungs are auscultated for moist crackles. Because pulmonary edema may be caused by excessive administration of parenteral fluids, extreme caution must be used to prevent fluid overload. The development of generalized edema is assessed by examining the presacral and pretibial areas several times daily. Mannitol (Osmitrol), furosemide (Lasix), or ethacrynic acid (Edecrin) may be prescribed to initiate diuresis (Walton, 2015).

Adequate kidney blood flow in patients with prerenal causes of ARF may be restored by IV fluids or transfusions of blood products. If ARF is caused by hypovolemia secondary to hypoproteinemia, an infusion of albumin may be prescribed. Dialysis may be initiated to prevent complications of ARF, such as hyperkalemia, metabolic acidosis, pericarditis, and pulmonary edema. Dialysis corrects many biochemical abnormalities; allows for liberalization of fluid, protein, and sodium intake; diminishes bleeding tendencies; and promotes wound healing. **Hemodialysis** (a procedure that circulates the patient's blood through a **dialyzer** to remove waste products and excess fluid), **peritoneal dialysis** (PD) (a procedure that uses the patient's peritoneal membrane [the lining of the peritoneal cavity] as the semipermeable membrane to exchange fluid and solutes), or a variety of CRRTs (methods used to replace normal kidney function by circulating the patient's blood through a hemofilter) may be performed. These and other treatment modalities for patients with kidney dysfunction are discussed later in this chapter.

Pharmacologic Therapy

Hyperkalemia is the most life-threatening of the fluid and electrolyte changes that occur in patients with kidney disturbances. Therefore, the patient is monitored for hyperkalemia through serial serum electrolyte levels (potassium value greater than 5.5 mmol/L), ECG changes (tall, tented, or peaked T waves), and changes in clinical status (see Chapter 17). Other symptoms of hyperkalemia include irritability, abdominal cramping, diarrhea, paresthesia, and generalized muscle weakness. Muscle weakness may present as slurred speech, difficulty breathing, paresthesia, and paralysis. As the potassium level increases, both cardiac and other muscular function declines, making this a true medical emergency (Mount & Zandi-Nejad, 2012).

The elevated potassium levels may be reduced by administering cation-exchange resins (sodium polystyrene sulfonate [Kayexalate]) orally or by retention enema. Kayexalate works by exchanging sodium ions for potassium ions in the intestinal tract. Sorbitol may be administered in combination with Kayexalate to induce a diarrhea-type effect by inducing water loss in the GI tract.

If a Kayexalate retention enema is given (the colon is the major site of potassium exchange), a rectal catheter with a balloon may be used to facilitate retention if necessary. The patient should retain the Kayexalate for at least 30 to 60 minutes (preferable 6 to 10 hours) to promote potassium removal (Comerford, 2015). Afterward, a cleansing enema may be prescribed to remove remaining medication as a precaution against fecal impaction.

If the patient is hemodynamically unstable (low blood pressure, changes in mental status, dysrhythmia), IV dextrose 50%, insulin, and calcium replacement may be administered to shift potassium back into the cells. Salbutamol sulphate (Ventolin HFA) by nebulizer can lower plasma potassium concentration by 0.3 to 0.6 mmol/L within 30 minutes (Sterns, Grieff, & Bernstein, 2016). The shift of potassium into the intracellular space is temporary, so arrangements for dialysis need to be made on an emergent basis.

Since many medications are eliminated through the kidneys, dosages must be reduced when a patient has AKI. Examples of commonly used agents that require adjustment are antibiotic medications (especially aminoglycosides), digoxin, ACE inhibitors, and magnesium-containing agents.

In addition, many medications have been used in patients with AKI in an attempt to improve patient outcomes. Diuretic agents are often used to control fluid volume, but they have not been shown to improve recovery from AKI.

In patients with severe acidosis, the arterial blood gases and serum bicarbonate levels (CO_2-combining power) must be monitored because the patient may require sodium bicarbonate therapy or dialysis. If respiratory problems develop, appropriate ventilatory measures must be instituted. The elevated serum phosphate level may be controlled with phosphate-binding agents (e.g., calcium or lanthanum carbonate) that help prevent a continuing rise in serum phosphate levels by decreasing the absorption of phosphate from the intestinal tract.

Nutritional Therapy

ARF causes severe nutritional imbalances (because nausea and vomiting contribute to inadequate dietary intake), impaired glucose use and protein synthesis, and increased tissue catabolism. The patient is weighed daily and loses 0.2 to 0.5 kg daily if the nitrogen balance is negative (i.e., caloric intake falls below caloric requirements). If the patient gains or does not lose weight or develops hypertension, fluid retention should be suspected.

Nutritional support is based on the underlying cause of ARF, the catabolic response, the type and frequency of kidney replacement therapy, comorbidities, and nutritional status. Replacement of dietary proteins is individualized to provide the maximum benefit and minimize uremic symptoms. Caloric requirements are met with high-carbohydrate meals, because carbohydrates have a protein-sparing effect (i.e., in a high-carbohydrate diet, protein is not used for meeting energy requirements but is "spared" for growth and tissue healing). Foods and fluids containing potassium or phosphorus (e.g., bananas, citrus fruits and juices, coffee) are restricted.

The oliguric phase of ARF may last 10 to 20 days and is followed by the diuretic phase, at which time urine output begins to increase, signalling that kidney function is returning. Results of blood chemistry tests are used to determine the amounts of sodium, potassium, and water needed for replacement, along with assessment for overhydration or underhydration. Following the diuretic phase, the patient is placed on a high-protein, high-calorie diet and is encouraged to resume activities gradually.

Nursing Management

The nurse has an important role in caring for the patient with ARF. The nurse monitors for complications, participates in emergency treatment of fluid and electrolyte imbalances, assesses the patient's progress and response to treatment, and provides physical and emotional support. In addition, the nurse keeps family members informed about the patient's condition, helps them understand the treatments, and provides psychological support. Although the development of ARF may be the most serious problem, the nurse continues to provide nursing care indicated for the primary disorder (e.g., burns, shock, trauma, obstruction of the urinary tract).

Monitoring Fluid and Electrolyte Balance

Because of the serious fluid and electrolyte imbalances that can occur with ARF, the nurse monitors the patient's serum electrolyte levels and physical indicators of these complications during all phases of the disorder. IV solutions must be carefully selected based on the patient's fluid and electrolyte status. The patient's cardiac function and musculoskeletal status are monitored closely for signs of hyperkalemia.

! QUALITY AND SAFETY NURSING ALERT

Hyperkalemia is the most immediate life-threatening imbalance seen in AKI. Parenteral fluids, all oral intake, and all medications are screened carefully to ensure that hidden sources of potassium are not inadvertently administered or consumed.

The nurse monitors fluid status by paying careful attention to fluid intake (IV medications should be administered in the smallest volume possible), urine output, apparent edema, distention of the jugular veins, alterations in heart sounds and breath sounds, and increasing difficulty in breathing. Accurate daily weights, as well as I&O records, are essential. Indicators of deteriorating fluid and electrolyte status are reported immediately to the physician, and preparation is made for emergency treatment. Severe fluid and electrolyte disturbances may be treated with hemodialysis, PD, or CRRT.

Reducing Metabolic Rate

The nurse takes steps to reduce the patient's metabolic rate. Bed rest may be indicated to reduce exertion and the metabolic rate during the most acute stage of the disorder. Fever and infection, both of which increase the metabolic rate and catabolism, are prevented or treated promptly.

Promoting Pulmonary Function

Attention is given to pulmonary function, and the patient is assisted to turn, cough, and take deep breaths frequently to prevent atelectasis and respiratory tract infection. Drowsiness and lethargy may prevent the patient from moving and turning without encouragement and assistance.

Preventing Infection

Asepsis is essential with invasive lines and catheters to minimize the risk of infection and increased metabolism. An indwelling urinary catheter is avoided whenever possible due to the high risk of UTI associated with its use but may be required to provide ongoing data required to monitor fluid I&O.

Providing Skin Care

The skin may be dry or susceptible to breakdown as a result of edema; therefore, meticulous skin care is important. In addition, excoriation and itching of the skin may result from the deposit of irritating toxins in the patient's tissues. Bathing the patient with cool water, frequent turning, and keeping the skin clean and well moisturized and the fingernails trimmed to avoid excoriation are often comforting and prevent skin breakdown.

Providing Psychosocial Support

The patient with ARF may require treatment with hemodialysis, PD, or CRRT. The length of time that these treatments are necessary varies with the cause and extent of damage to the kidneys. The patient and family need assistance, explanation, and support during this period. The purpose of the treatment is explained to the patient and family by the physician. However, high levels of anxiety and fear may necessitate repeated explanation and clarification by the nurse. The family members may initially be afraid to touch and talk to the patient during these procedures but should be encouraged and assisted to do so.

In an intensive care setting, many of the nurse's functions are devoted to the technical aspects of patient care; however, it is essential that the psychological needs and other concerns of the patient and family be addressed. Continued assessment of the patient for complications of ARF and precipitating causes is essential.

End-Stage Kidney Disease or Chronic Kidney Disease

PRACTICE & LEARN

When a patient has sustained enough kidney damage to require kidney replacement therapy on a permanent basis, the patient has moved into the fifth or final stage of CKD, also referred to as ESKD.

Pathophysiology

As kidney function declines, the end products of protein metabolism (normally excreted in urine) accumulate in the blood. Uremia develops and adversely affects every system in the body. The greater the buildup of waste products, the more pronounced the symptoms are.

The rate of decline in kidney function and progression of ESKD is related to the underlying disorder, the urinary excretion of protein, and the presence of hypertension. The disease tends to progress more rapidly in patients who excrete significant amounts of protein or have elevated blood pressure than in those without these conditions. Cardiovascular disease is the predominant cause of death in patients with ESRD.

Clinical Manifestations

Because virtually every body system is affected in ESKD, patients exhibit a number of signs and symptoms (Hannon & Porth, 2017; McCance & Huether, 2014). The severity of these signs and symptoms depends in part on the degree of kidney impairment, other underlying conditions, and the patient's age. Cardiovascular disease is the predominant cause of death in patients with ESKD (Walton, 2015). Peripheral neuropathy, a disorder of the peripheral nervous system, is present in some patients. Patients complain of severe pain and discomfort. Restless leg syndrome and burning feet can occur in the early stage of uremic peripheral neuropathy. The precise mechanisms for many of these systemic signs and symptoms have not been identified. However, it is generally thought that the accumulation of uremic waste products is the probable cause. Chart 45-6 summarizes the systemic signs and symptoms.

Assessment and Diagnostic Findings

Glomerular Filtration Rate

As the GFR decreases (due to nonfunctioning glomeruli), the creatinine clearance decreases, while the serum creatinine and BUN levels increase. Serum creatinine is a more sensitive indicator of kidney function than BUN. The BUN is affected not only by kidney disease but also by protein intake in the diet, catabolism (tissue and RBC breakdown), parenteral nutrition, and medications such as corticosteroids.

Sodium and Water Retention

The kidney cannot concentrate or dilute the urine normally in ESKD. Appropriate responses by the kidney to changes in the daily intake of water and electrolytes, therefore, do not occur. Some patients retain sodium and water, increasing the risk for edema, heart failure, and hypertension. Hypertension may also result from activation of the renin–angiotensin–aldosterone axis and the concomitant increased aldosterone secretion. Other patients have a tendency to lose sodium and run the risk of developing hypotension and hypovolemia. Vomiting and diarrhea may cause sodium and water depletion, which worsens the uremic state.

Acidosis

Metabolic acidosis occurs in ESKD because the kidneys are unable to excrete increased loads of acid. Decreased acid secretion results from the inability of the kidney tubules to excrete ammonia (NH_3^-) and to reabsorb sodium bicarbonate (HCO_3^-). There is also decreased excretion of phosphates and other organic acids.

CHART 45-6

Assessing for End-Stage Kidney Disease

Be alert for the following signs and symptoms:

Neurologic
- Weakness and fatigue
- Confusion
- Inability to concentrate
- Disorientation
- Tremors
- Seizures
- Asterixis
- Restlessness of legs
- Burning of soles of feet
- Behaviour changes

Integumentary
- Grey-bronze skin colour
- Dry, flaky skin
- Pruritus
- Ecchymosis
- Purpura
- Thin, brittle nails
- Coarse, thinning hair

Cardiovascular
- Hypertension
- Pitting edema (feet, hands, sacrum)
- Periorbital edema
- Pericardial friction rub
- Engorged neck veins
- Pericarditis
- Pericardial effusion
- Pericardial tamponade
- Hyperkalemia
- Hyperlipidemia

Pulmonary
- Crackles
- Thick, tenacious sputum
- Depressed cough reflex
- Pleuritic pain
- Shortness of breath
- Tachypnea
- Kussmaul-type respirations
- Uremic pneumonitis

Gastrointestinal
- Ammonia odour to breath ("uremic fetor")
- Metallic taste
- Mouth ulcerations and bleeding
- Anorexia, nausea, and vomiting
- Hiccups
- Constipation or diarrhea
- Bleeding from gastrointestinal tract

Hematologic
- Anemia
- Thrombocytopenia

Reproductive
- Amenorrhea
- Testicular atrophy
- Infertility
- Decreased libido

Musculoskeletal
- Muscle cramps
- Loss of muscle strength
- Kidney osteodystrophy
- Bone pain
- Bone fractures
- Foot drop

Anemia

Anemia develops as a result of inadequate erythropoietin production, the shortened lifespan of RBCs, nutritional deficiencies, and the patient's tendency to bleed, particularly from the GI tract. Erythropoietin, a substance normally produced by the kidneys, stimulates bone marrow to produce RBCs (Muzzy & Snyder, 2013). In ESKD, erythropoietin production decreases and profound anemia results, producing fatigue, angina, and shortness of breath.

Calcium and Phosphorus Imbalance

Another abnormality seen in ESKD is a disorder in calcium and phosphorus metabolism (Hannon et al., 2010). Serum calcium and phosphate levels have a reciprocal relationship in the body: as one increases, the other decreases. With a decrease in filtration through the glomerulus of the kidney, there is an increase in the serum phosphate level and a reciprocal or corresponding decrease in the serum calcium level. The decreased serum calcium level causes increased secretion of parathormone from the parathyroid glands. However, in kidney failure, the body does not respond normally to the increased secretion of parathormone; as a result, calcium leaves the bone, often producing bone changes and bone disease as well as calcification of major blood vessels in the body. In addition, the active metabolite of vitamin D (1,25-dihydroxycholecalciferol) normally manufactured by the kidney decreases as kidney failure progresses (Hannon & Porth, 2017). Uremic bone disease, often called kidney osteodystrophy, develops from the complex changes in calcium, phosphate, and parathormone balance. There is also evidence of calcification of blood vessels.

Complications

Potential complications of ESKD that concern the nurse and necessitate a collaborative approach to care include the following:

- Hyperkalemia due to decreased excretion, metabolic acidosis, catabolism, and excessive intake (diet, medications, fluids)
- Pericarditis, pericardial effusion, and pericardial tamponade due to retention of uremic waste products and inadequate dialysis

- Hypertension due to sodium and water retention and malfunction of the renin–angiotensin–aldosterone system
- Anemia due to decreased erythropoietin production, decreased RBC lifespan, bleeding in the GI tract from irritating toxins and ulcer formation, and blood loss during hemodialysis
- Bone disease and metastatic and vascular calcifications due to retention of phosphorus, low serum calcium levels, abnormal vitamin D metabolism, and elevated aluminum levels

Medical Management

The goal of management is to maintain kidney function and homeostasis for as long as possible. All factors that contribute to ESKD and all factors that are reversible (e.g., obstruction) are identified and treated. Management is accomplished primarily with medications and diet therapy, although dialysis may also be needed to decrease the level of uremic waste products in the blood and to control electrolyte balance.

Pharmacologic Therapy

Complications can be prevented or delayed by administering prescribed phosphate-binding agents, calcium supplements, antihypertensive and cardiac medications, anticonvulsant medications, and erythropoietin Eprex.

Calcium and Phosphorus Binders

Hyperphosphatemia and hypocalcemia are treated with medications that bind dietary phosphorus in the GI tract. Binders such as calcium carbonate (Os-Cal) or calcium acetate (PhosLo) are prescribed, but there is a risk of hypercalcemia. If calcium is high or the calcium–phosphorus product exceeds 55 mg/dL, a polymeric phosphate binder such as sevelamer hydrochloride (Renagel) may be prescribed (Muzzy & Snyder, 2013). These medications bind dietary phosphorus in the intestinal tract. All binding agents must be administered with food to be effective. Magnesium-based antacids are avoided to prevent magnesium toxicity.

Antihypertensive and Cardiovascular Agents

Hypertension is managed by intravascular volume control and a variety of antihypertensive agents. Heart failure and pulmonary edema may also require treatment with fluid restriction, low-sodium diets, diuretic agents, inotropic agents such as digoxin (Lanoxin) or dobutamine (Dobutrex), and dialysis. The metabolic acidosis of ESKD usually produces no symptoms and requires no treatment; however, sodium bicarbonate supplements or dialysis may be needed to correct the acidosis if it causes symptoms (Holcombe & Kern Feeley, 2013).

Anticonvulsant Agents

Neurologic abnormalities may occur, so the patient must be observed for early evidence of slight twitching, headache, delirium, or seizure activity. If seizures occur, the onset of the seizure is recorded along with the type, duration, and general effect on the patient. The physician is notified immediately. IV diazepam (Valium) or phenytoin (Dilantin) is usually administered to control seizures. The side rails of the bed should be raised and padded to protect the patient. The nursing management of the patient with seizures is discussed in Chapter 63.

Erythropoietin

Anemia associated with ESKD is treated with recombinant human erythropoietin (Eprex). Patients with anemia (hemoglobin less than 110 g/L) present with nonspecific symptoms, such as malaise, general fatigability, and decreased activity tolerance. Erythropoietin therapy is initiated to achieve a hemoglobin level of 110 to 120 g/L.

Erythropoietin is administered intravenously or subcutaneously three times a week in ESKD. It may take 2 to 6 weeks for the hematocrit to increase; therefore, the medication is not indicated for patients who need immediate correction of severe anemia. Management involves adjustment of heparin to prevent clotting of the lines during hemodialysis treatments, frequent monitoring of hemoglobin and periodic assessment of serum iron and transferrin levels. Because adequate stores of iron are necessary for an adequate response to erythropoietin, supplementary iron may be prescribed. The patient's blood pressure and serum potassium level are monitored to detect hypertension and increasing serum potassium levels, which may occur with therapy and the increasing RBC mass. The occurrence of hypertension requires initiation or adjustment of the patient's antihypertensive therapy. Hypertension that cannot be controlled is a contraindication to recombinant erythropoietin therapy.

Patients who have received erythropoietin therapy have reported decreased levels of fatigue, increased feelings of well-being, better tolerance of dialysis, higher energy levels, and improved exercise tolerance. In addition, this therapy has decreased the need for transfusion and its associated risks, including bloodborne infectious disease, antibody formation, and iron overload.

Nutritional Therapy

Dietary intervention is necessary with deterioration of kidney function and includes careful regulation of protein intake, fluid intake to balance fluid losses, sodium intake to balance sodium losses, and some restriction of potassium. At the same time, adequate caloric intake and vitamin supplementation must be ensured. Protein is restricted because urea, uric acid, and organic acids—the breakdown products of dietary and tissue proteins—accumulate rapidly in the blood when there is impaired kidney clearance. The allowed protein must be of high biologic value (dairy products, eggs, meats). High–biologic-value proteins are those that are complete proteins and supply the essential amino acids necessary for growth and cell repair.

Usually, the fluid allowance per day is 500 to 600 mL more than the previous day's 24-hour urine output. Calories are supplied by carbohydrates and fat to prevent wasting. Vitamin supplementation is necessary because a protein-restricted diet does not provide the necessary complement of vitamins. In addition, the patient on dialysis may lose water-soluble vitamins during the dialysis treatment.

Hyperkalemia is usually prevented by ensuring adequate dialysis treatments with potassium removal and careful monitoring of diet, medications, and fluids for their potassium content. Sodium polystyrene sulfonate (Kayexalate), a cation-exchange resin, may be needed for acute hyperkalemia.

Dialysis

The patient with increasing symptoms of kidney failure is referred to a dialysis and transplantation centre early in the course of progressive kidney disease. Dialysis is usually initiated when the patient cannot maintain a reasonable lifestyle with conservative treatment. In Canada, for 2016, the number of patients receiving dialysis was 21,986 (Canadian Organ Replacement Register/Canadian Institute for Health Information, 2018).

Nursing Management

The patient with ESKD requires astute nursing care to avoid the complications of reduced kidney function and the stresses and anxieties of dealing with a life-threatening illness.

Nursing care is directed toward assessing fluid status and identifying potential sources of imbalance, implementing a dietary program to ensure proper nutritional intake within the limits of the treatment regimen, and promoting positive feelings by encouraging increased self-care and greater independence. It is extremely important to provide explanations and information to the patient and family concerning ESKD, treatment options, and potential complications. A great deal of emotional support is needed by the patient and family because of the numerous changes experienced. Specific interventions, along with rationale and evaluation criteria, are presented in more detail in the plan of nursing care for the patient with ESKD (Chart 45-7).

Promoting Home, Community-Based, and Transitional Care

Educating Patients About Self-Care

The nurse plays an important role in teaching the patient with ESKD. Because of the extensive teaching needed, the home care nurse, dialysis nurse, and nurses in the hospital and outpatient settings all provide ongoing education and reinforcement while monitoring the patient's progress and compliance with the treatment regimen.

A referral to a nutritionist is made because of the dietary changes required. The patient is taught how to check the vascular access device for patency and appropriate precautions, such as avoiding venipuncture and blood pressure measurements on the arm with the access device.

In addition, the patient and family need to know what problems to report to the health care provider. These include the following:

- Worsening signs and symptoms of kidney failure (nausea, vomiting, change in usual urine output [if any], ammonia odour on breath)
- Signs and symptoms of hyperkalemia (muscle weakness, diarrhea, abdominal cramps)
- Signs and symptoms of access problems (clotted fistula or graft, infection)

These signs and symptoms of decreasing kidney function, in addition to increasing BUN and serum creatinine levels, may indicate a need to alter the dialysis prescription. The dialysis nurses also provide ongoing education and support at each treatment visit.

Continuing and Transitional Care

The importance of follow-up examinations and treatment is stressed to the patient and family because of changing physical status, kidney function, and dialysis requirements. Referral for home care provides the home care nurse with the opportunity to assess the patient's environment and emotional status and the coping strategies used by the patient and family to deal with the changes in family roles often associated with chronic illness.

The home care nurse also assesses the patient for further deterioration of kidney function and signs and symptoms of complications resulting from the primary kidney disorder, the resulting kidney failure, and effects of treatment strategies (e.g., dialysis, medications, dietary restrictions). Patients need education and reinforcement of the dietary restrictions required, including fluid, sodium, potassium, and protein restriction. Reminders about the need for health promotion activities and health screening are an important part of nursing care for the patient with kidney failure.

Gerontologic Considerations

Diabetes, hypertension, chronic glomerulonephritis, interstitial nephritis, and urinary tract obstruction are the causes of ESKD in the older adult. The signs and symptoms of kidney disease in the older adult are often nonspecific. The occurrence of symptoms of other disorders (heart failure, dementia) can mask the symptoms of kidney disease and delay or prevent diagnosis and treatment. Patients often develop signs and symptoms of nephrotic syndrome, such as edema and proteinuria.

Hemodialysis and PD are used effectively in treating older patients. The number of older patients initiating dialysis has dramatically increased in the past decade (Terner, Redding, & Wu, 2016). Although there is no specific age limitation for kidney transplantation, concomitant disorders (e.g., coronary artery disease, peripheral vascular disease) have made it a less common treatment for the older patients. However, the outcome is comparable to that of younger patients. Some older patients elect not to undergo dialysis or transplantation. Conservative management, including nutritional therapy, fluid control, and medications such as phosphate binders, may be considered in patients who are not suitable for or elect not to have dialysis or transplantation.

KIDNEY REPLACEMENT THERAPIES

The use of kidney replacement therapies becomes necessary when the kidneys can no longer remove wastes, maintain electrolytes, and regulate fluid balance. This can occur rapidly or over a long period of time and the need for replacement therapy can be acute (short term) or chronic (long term). The main kidney replacement therapies include the various types of dialysis and kidney transplantation.

Dialysis

Types of dialysis include hemodialysis, CRRT, and PD. Acute dialysis is indicated when there is a high and

(text continued on page 1305)

Plan of Nursing Care Chart 45-7. The Patient With End-Stage Kidney Disease

NURSING INTERVENTIONS	RATIONALE	EXPECTED OUTCOMES
Nursing Priority: Excess fluid volume **Goal:** Maintenance of ideal body weight		
1. Assess fluid status: a. Daily weight b. Intake and output balance c. Skin turgor and presence of edema d. Distention of neck veins e. Blood pressure, pulse rate, and rhythm f. Respiratory rate and effort	1. Assessment provides baseline and ongoing database for monitoring changes and evaluating interventions.	• Demonstrates no rapid weight changes • Maintains dietary and fluid restrictions • Exhibits normal skin turgor without edema • Exhibits normal vital signs • Exhibits no neck vein distention • Reports no difficulty breathing or shortness of breath • Performs oral hygiene frequently • Reports decreased thirst • Reports decreased dryness of oral mucous membranes
2. Limit fluid intake to prescribed volume.	2. Fluid restriction will be determined on basis of weight, urine output, and response to therapy.	
3. Identify potential sources of fluid: a. Medications and fluids used to take or administer medications: oral and intravenous b. Foods	3. Unrecognized sources of excess fluids may be identified.	
4. Explain to patient and family rationale for fluid restriction.	4. Understanding promotes patient and family cooperation with fluid restriction.	
5. Assist patient to cope with the discomforts resulting from fluid restriction.	5. Increasing patient comfort promotes compliance with dietary restrictions.	
6. Provide or encourage frequent oral hygiene.	6. Oral hygiene minimizes dryness of oral mucous membranes.	
Nursing Priority: Nutrition **Goal:** Maintenance of adequate nutritional intake		
1. Assess nutritional status: a. Weight changes b. Laboratory values (serum electrolyte, BUN, creatinine, protein, transferrin, and iron levels)	1. Baseline data allow for monitoring of changes and evaluating effectiveness of interventions.	• Consumes protein of high biologic value • Chooses foods within dietary restrictions that are appealing • Consumes high-calorie foods within dietary restrictions • Explains in own words rationale for dietary restrictions and relationship to urea and creatinine levels • Takes medications on schedule that does not produce anorexia or feeling of fullness • Consults written lists of acceptable foods • Reports increased appetite at meals • Exhibits no rapid increases or decreases in weight • Demonstrates normal skin turgor without edema; wound healing and acceptable plasma albumin levels
2. Assess patient's nutritional dietary patterns: a. Diet history b. Food preferences c. Calorie counts	2. Past and present dietary patterns are considered in planning meals.	
3. Assess for factors contributing to altered nutritional intake: a. Anorexia, nausea, or vomiting b. Diet unpalatable to patient c. Depression d. Lack of understanding of dietary restrictions e. Stomatitis	3. Information about other factors that may be altered or eliminated to promote adequate dietary intake is provided.	
4. Provide patient's food preferences within dietary restrictions.	4. Increased dietary intake is encouraged.	
5. Promote intake of high–biologic-value protein foods: eggs, dairy products, meats.	5. Complete proteins are provided for positive nitrogen balance needed for growth and healing.	
6. Encourage high-calorie, low-protein, low-sodium, and low-potassium snacks between meals.	6. Reduces source of restricted foods and proteins and provides calories for energy, sparing protein for tissue growth and healing.	
7. Alter schedule of medications so that they are not given immediately before meals.	7. Ingestion of medications just before meals may produce anorexia and feeling of fullness.	

continued >

Plan of Nursing Care

Chart 45-7. The Patient With End-Stage Kidney Disease, *Continued*

NURSING INTERVENTIONS	RATIONALE	EXPECTED OUTCOMES
8. Explain rationale for dietary restrictions and relationship to kidney disease and increased urea and creatinine levels.	8. Promotes patient understanding of relationships between diet and urea and creatinine levels to kidney disease.	
9. Provide written lists of foods allowed and suggestions for improving their taste without use of sodium or potassium.	9. Lists provide a positive approach to dietary restrictions and a reference for patient and family to use when at home.	
10. Weigh patient daily	10. Allows monitoring of fluid and nutritional status.	
11. Assess for evidence of inadequate protein intake: a. Edema formation b. Delayed wound healing c. Decreased serum albumin levels	11. Inadequate protein intake can lead to decreased albumin and other proteins, edema formation, and delay in wound healing.	
12. Provide pleasant surroundings at meal-times.	12. Unpleasant factors that contribute to patient's anorexia are eliminated.	
Nursing Priority: Patient education **Goal:** Increased knowledge about condition and related treatment		
1. Assess understanding of cause of kidney disease, consequences of kidney disease, and its treatment: a. Cause of patient's kidney disease b. Meaning of kidney disease c. Understanding of kidney function d. Relationship of fluid and dietary restrictions to kidney disease e. Rationale for treatment (hemodialysis, peritoneal dialysis, transplantation)	1. Provides baseline for further explanations and education.	• Verbalizes relationship of cause of kidney disease to consequences • Explains fluid and dietary restrictions as they relate to failure of kidney's regulatory functions • States in own words relationship of kidney disease and need for treatment • Asks questions about treatment options, indicating readiness to learn • Verbalizes plans to continue as normal a life as possible • Uses written information and instructions to clarify questions and seek additional information
2. Provide explanation of kidney function and consequences of kidney disease at patient's level of understanding and guided by patient's readiness to learn.	2. Patient can learn about kidney disease and treatment as he or she becomes ready to understand and accept the diagnosis and consequences.	
3. Assist patient to identify ways to incorporate changes related to illness and its treatment into lifestyle	3. Patient can see that his or her life does not have to revolve around the disease.	
4. Provide oral and written information as appropriate about: a. Kidney function and failure b. Fluid and dietary restrictions c. Medications d. Reportable problems, signs, and symptoms e. Follow-up schedule f. Community resources g. Treatment options	4. Provides patient with information that can be used for further clarification at home.	
Nursing Priority: Activity/Mobility **Goal:** Participation in activity within tolerance		
1. Assess factors contributing to activity intolerance: a. Fatigue b. Anemia c. Fluid and electrolyte imbalances d. Retention of waste products e. Depression	1. Indicates factors contributing to severity of fatigue.	• Participates in increasing levels of activity and exercise • Reports increased sense of well-being • Alternates rest and activity • Participates in selected self-care activities

Plan of Nursing Care

Chart 45-7. The Patient With End-Stage Kidney Disease, *Continued*

NURSING INTERVENTIONS	RATIONALE	EXPECTED OUTCOMES
2. Promote independence in self-care activities as tolerated; assist if fatigued.	2. Promotes improved self-esteem.	
3. Encourage alternating activity with rest.	3. Promotes activity and exercise within limits and adequate rest.	
4. Encourage patient to rest after dialysis treatments.	4. Adequate rest is encouraged after dialysis treatments, which are exhausting to many patients.	

Nursing Priority: Low self-esteem and body image
Goal: Improved self-esteem

NURSING INTERVENTIONS	RATIONALE	EXPECTED OUTCOMES
1. Assess patient's and family's responses and reactions to illness and treatment.	1. Provides data about problems encountered by patient and family in coping with changes in life.	• Identifies previously used coping styles that have been effective and those no longer possible due to disease and treatment (alcohol or drug use; extreme physical exertion) • Patient and family identify and verbalize feelings and reactions to disease and necessary changes in their lives • Seeks professional counselling, if necessary, to cope with changes resulting from kidney disease • Reports satisfaction with method of sexual expression
2. Assess relationship of patient and significant family members.	2. Identifies strengths and supports of patient and family.	
3. Assess usual coping patterns of patient and family members.	3. Coping patterns that may have been effective in past may be harmful in view of restrictions imposed by disease and treatment.	
4. Encourage open discussion of concerns about changes produced by disease and treatment: a. Role changes b. Changes in lifestyle c. Changes in occupation d. Sexual changes e. Dependence on health care team	4. Encourages patient to identify concerns and steps necessary to deal with them.	
5. Explore alternate ways of sexual expression other than sexual intercourse.	5. Alternative forms of sexual expression may be acceptable.	
6. Discuss role of giving and receiving love, warmth, and affection.	6. Sexuality means different things to different people, depending on stage of maturity	

Collaborative Problems: Hyperkalemia; pericarditis, pericardial effusion, and pericardial tamponade; hypertension; anemia; bone disease and metastatic calcifications
Goal: Absence of complications

Hyperkalemia

NURSING INTERVENTIONS	RATIONALE	EXPECTED OUTCOMES
1. Monitor serum potassium levels. Notify physician if level greater than 5.5 mEq/L, and prepare to treat hyperkalemia.	1. Hyperkalemia causes potentially life-threatening changes in the body.	• Has normal potassium level • Experiences no muscle weakness or diarrhea • Exhibits normal ECG pattern • Vital signs are within normal limits
2. Assess patient for muscle weakness, diarrhea, ECG changes (tall-tented T waves and widened QRS).	2. Cardiovascular signs and symptoms are characteristic of hyperkalemia.	

Pericarditis, Pericardial Effusion, and Pericardial Tamponade

NURSING INTERVENTIONS	RATIONALE	EXPECTED OUTCOMES
1. Assess patient for fever, chest pain, and a pericardial friction rub (signs of pericarditis) and, if present, notify primary provider.	1. About 30%–50% of patients with chronic kidney disease develop pericarditis due to uremia; fever, chest pain, and a pericardial friction rub are classic signs.	• Has strong and equal peripheral pulses • Absence of a paradoxical pulse • Absence of pericardial effusion or tamponade on cardiac ultrasound • Has normal heart sounds

continued >

Plan of Nursing Care

Chart 45-7. The Patient With End-Stage Kidney Disease, *Continued*

NURSING INTERVENTIONS	RATIONALE	EXPECTED OUTCOMES
2. If patient has pericarditis, assess for the following every 4 hours: a. Paradoxical pulse >10 mm Hg b. Extreme hypotension c. Weak or absent peripheral pulses d. Altered level of consciousness e. Jugular venous distention	2. Pericardial effusion is a common fatal sequela of pericarditis. Signs of an effusion include a paradoxical pulse (>10 mm Hg drop in blood pressure during inspiration) and signs of shock due to compression of the heart by a large effusion. Cardiac tamponade exists when the patient is severely compromised hemodynamically.	
3. Prepare patient for echocardiogram to aid in diagnosis of pericardial effusion and cardiac tamponade.	3. Echocardiogram is useful in visualizing pericardial effusions and cardiac tamponade.	
4. If cardiac tamponade develops, prepare patient for emergency pericardiocentesis	4. Cardiac tamponade is a life-threatening condition, with a high mortality rate. Immediate aspiration of fluid from the pericardial space is essential.	
Hypertension		
1. Monitor and record blood pressure as indicated.	1. Provides objective data for monitoring. Elevated levels may indicate nonadherence to the treatment regimen.	• Blood pressure within normal limits • Reports no headaches, visual problems, or seizures • Edema is absent • Demonstrates compliance with dietary and fluid restrictions
2. Administer antihypertensive medications as prescribed.	2. Antihypertensive medications play a key role in treatment of hypertension associated with chronic kidney disease.	
3. Encourage adherence to dietary and fluid restriction therapy.	3. Adherence to diet and fluid restrictions and dialysis schedule prevents excess fluid and sodium accumulation	
4. Instruct patient to report signs of fluid overload, vision changes, headaches, edema, or seizures.	4. These are indications of inadequate control of hypertension and the need to alter therapy.	
Anemia		
1. Monitor RBC count, hemoglobin, and hematocrit levels as indicated.	1. Provides assessment of degree of anemia.	• Patient has a normal skin colour without pallor • Exhibits hemoglobin values within acceptable limits • Experiences no bleeding from any site
2. Administer medications as prescribed, including iron and folic acid supplements, Epogen, and multivitamins.	2. RBCs need iron, folic acid, and vitamins to be produced. Epogen stimulates the bone marrow to produce RBC.	
3. Avoid drawing unnecessary blood specimens.	3. Anemia is worsened by drawing numerous specimens.	
4. Educate patient to prevent bleeding: avoid vigorous nose blowing and contact sports, and use a soft toothbrush.	4. Bleeding from anywhere in the body worsens anemia.	
5. Administer blood component therapy as indicated.	5. Blood component therapy may be needed if the patient has symptoms.	
Bone Disease and Metastatic Calcifications		
1. Administer the following medications as prescribed: phosphate binders, calcium supplements, vitamin D supplements.	1. Chronic kidney disease causes numerous physiologic changes affecting calcium, phosphorus, and vitamin D metabolism.	• Exhibits serum calcium, phosphorus, and aluminum levels within acceptable ranges • Exhibits no symptoms of hypocalcemia • Has no bone demineralization on bone scan • Discusses importance of maintaining activity level and exercise program
2. Monitor serum lab values as indicated (calcium, phosphorus, aluminum levels) and report abnormal findings to primary provider.	2. Hyperphosphatemia, hypocalcemia, and excess aluminum accumulation are common in chronic kidney disease.	
3. Assist patient with an exercise program.	3. Bone demineralization increases with immobility.	

increasing level of serum potassium, fluid overload, or impending pulmonary edema, increasing acidosis, pericarditis, and severe confusion due to advanced uremia (Hannon & Porth, 2017). It may also be used to remove medications or toxins (poisoning or medication overdose) from the blood or for edema that does not respond to other treatment, hepatic coma, hyperkalemia, hypercalcemia, hypertension, and uremia.

Chronic or maintenance dialysis is indicated in advanced CKD and ESKD in the following instances: the presence of uremic signs and symptoms affecting all body systems (nausea and vomiting, severe anorexia, increasing lethargy, mental confusion), hyperkalemia, fluid overload not responsive to diuretics and fluid restriction, and a general lack of well-being. An urgent indication for dialysis in patients with kidney failure is pericardial friction rub.

The decision to initiate dialysis should be reached only after thoughtful discussion among the patient, family, physician, and others as appropriate. Many potentially life-threatening issues are associated with the need for dialysis. The nurse can assist the patient and family by answering their questions, clarifying the information provided, and supporting their decision.

Successful kidney transplantation eliminates the need for dialysis. Not only is the quality of life much improved in patients with ESKD who undergo transplantation, but also physiologic function is improved as well (Tonelli, Wiebe, Knoll, et al., 2011). The benefits of preemptive (prior to the initiation of dialysis) transplantation have been discussed for more than a decade. Despite the discussion, it still evades current clinical practices. Greater awareness is needed to encourage a change in practice. One strategy may be to discuss the financial incentives and disincentives for the many stakeholders involved: patients; living donors (if applicable); physicians; and health care organizations.

Hemodialysis

Hemodialysis is used for patients who are acutely ill and require short-term dialysis (days to weeks) and for patients with advanced CKD and ESKD who require long-term or permanent kidney replacement therapy. Hemodialysis prevents death but does not cure kidney disease and does not compensate for the loss of endocrine or metabolic activities of the kidneys. Most patients receive intermittent hemodialysis that involves treatments three times a week with the average treatment duration of 3 to 4 hours in an outpatient setting. Hemodialysis can also be performed at home by the patient and a caregiver. With home dialysis, treatment time and frequency can be adjusted to meet optimal patient needs.

The objectives of hemodialysis are to extract toxic nitrogenous substances from the blood and to remove excess water. A dialyzer (also referred to as an artificial kidney) serves as a synthetic semipermeable membrane, replacing the kidney glomeruli and tubules as the filter for the impaired kidneys. In hemodialysis, the blood, laden with toxins and nitrogenous wastes, is diverted from the patient to a machine, a dialyzer, where toxins are filtered out and removed and the blood is returned to the patient.

Diffusion, **osmosis**, and **ultrafiltration** are the principles on which hemodialysis is based (see Chapter 17). The toxins and wastes in the blood are removed by diffusion—that is, they move from an area of higher concentration in the blood to an area of lower concentration in the **dialysate**. The dialysate is a solution made up of all the important electrolytes in their ideal extracellular concentrations. The electrolyte level in the patient's blood can be brought under control by properly adjusting the dialysate bath. The semipermeable membrane impedes the diffusion of large molecules, such as RBCs and proteins.

Excess fluid is removed from the blood by osmosis, in which water moves from an area of low concentration potential (the blood) to an area of high concentration potential (the dialysate bath). In ultrafiltration, water moves under high pressure to an area of lower pressure. This process is much more efficient than osmosis at water removal and is accomplished by applying negative pressure or a suctioning force to the dialysis membrane. Because patients with kidney disease usually cannot excrete water, this force is necessary to remove fluid to achieve fluid balance.

The body's buffer system is maintained using a dialysate bath made up of bicarbonate (most common) or acetate, which is metabolized to form bicarbonate. The anticoagulant heparin is administered to keep blood from clotting in the dialysis circuit. Cleansed blood is returned to the body. By the end of the dialysis treatment, many waste products have been removed, the electrolyte balance has been restored to normal, and the buffer system has been replenished.

Dialyzers

Dialyzers are hollow-fibre devices containing thousands of tiny strawlike tubes that carry the blood through the dialyzer. The tubes are porous and act as a semipermeable membrane allowing toxins, fluid, and electrolytes to pass through. The constant flow of the solution maintains the concentration gradient to facilitate the exchange of wastes from the blood through the semipermeable membrane into the dialysate solution, where they are removed and discarded (Fig. 45-3).

Dialyzers have undergone many technologic changes in performance and biocompatibility. High-flux dialysis uses highly permeable membranes to increase the clearance of low- and mid-molecular-weight molecules. These special membranes are used with higher than traditional rates of flow for the blood entering and exiting the dialyzer (500 to 550 mL/min). High-flux dialysis increases the efficiency of treatments while shortening their duration and reducing the need for heparin.

Vascular Access

Access to the patient's vascular system must be established to allow blood to be removed, cleansed, and returned to the patient's vascular system at rates between 300 and 800 mL/min. Several types of access are available.

Vascular Access Devices

Immediate access to the patient's circulation for acute hemodialysis is achieved by inserting a double-lumen, noncuffed, large-bore catheter into the subclavian, internal jugular, or femoral vein by the physician (Fig. 45-4).

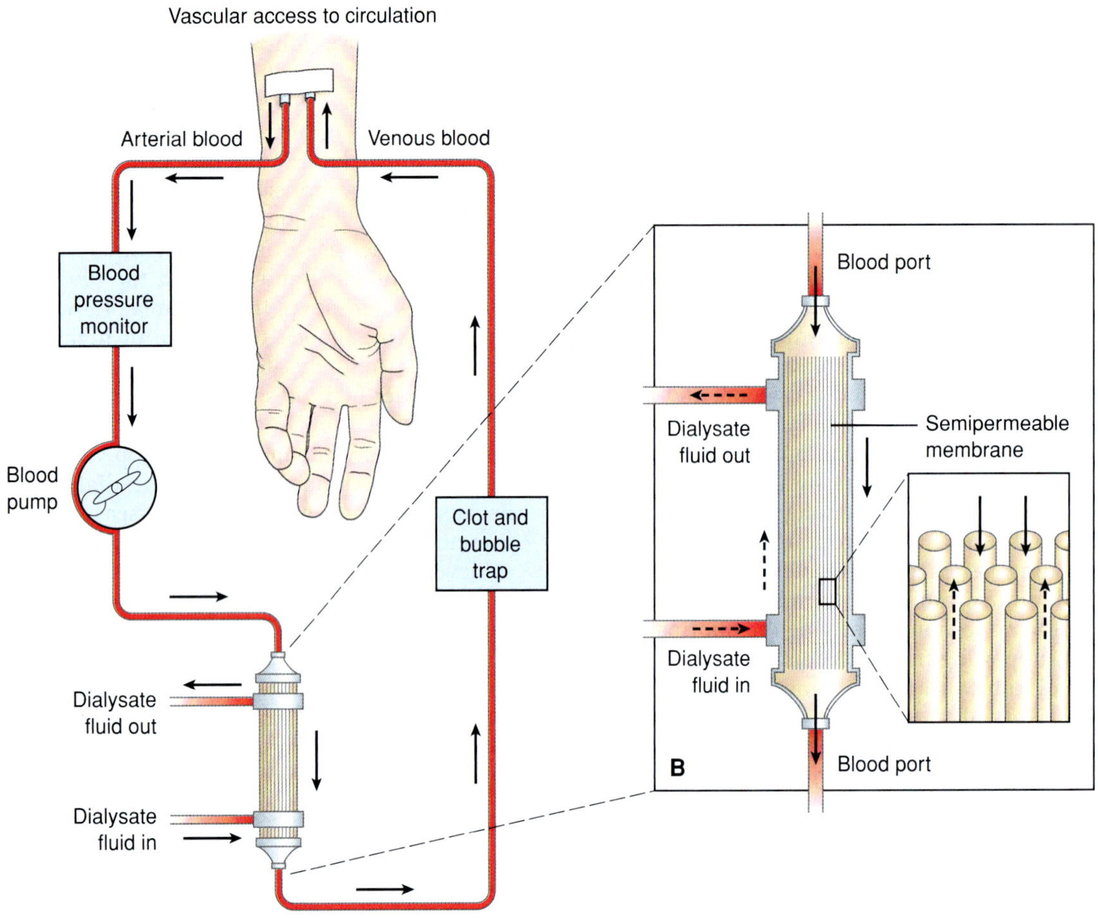

FIGURE 45-3. Hemodialysis system. Blood from an artery is pumped into (**A**) a dialyzer where it flows through the synthetic capillary tubes (**B**), which act as the semipermeable membrane (*inset*). The dialysate, which has a particular chemical composition, flows into the dialyzer around the capillary tubes that the blood flows through. The waste products in the blood diffuse across the semipermeable membrane into the dialysate solution.

This method of vascular access involves some risk (e.g., hematoma, pneumothorax, infection, thrombosis of the subclavian vein, inadequate flow). The catheter is removed when no longer needed (e.g., because the patient's condition has improved or another type of access has been established). Double-lumen, cuffed catheters may also be inserted, usually by either a surgeon or interventional radiologist, into the internal jugular vein of the patient. Since these catheters have cuffs under the skin, the insertion site heals, sealing the wound and reducing the risk for ascending infection. This feature makes these catheters safe for longer-term use. Infection rates, however, remain high and septicemia continues to be a common cause for hospital admission.

Arteriovenous Fistula

The preferred method of permanent access is an **arteriovenous fistula** (AVF) that is created surgically (usually in the forearm) by joining (anastomosing) an artery to a vein, either side to side or end to side (Fig. 45-5A). Needles are inserted into the vessel to obtain blood flow adequate to pass through the dialyzer. The arterial segment of the fistula is used for arterial flow to the dialyzer and the venous segment for reinfusion of the dialyzed blood. This access will need time (2 to 3 months) to "mature" before it can be used. As the AVF matures, the venous segment dilates due to the increased blood flow coming directly from the artery. Once sufficiently dilated it will then accommodate two large-bore (14-, 15-, or 16-gauge) needles that are inserted for each dialysis treatment. The patient is encouraged to perform hand exercises to increase the size of these vessels (i.e., squeezing a rubber ball for forearm fistulas) to accommodate the large-bore needles.

Once established, this access has the longest useful life and thus is the best option for vascular access for the patient requiring ongoing hemodialysis (MacRae, Ahmed, & Hemmelgam, 2014).

Arteriovenous Graft

An **arteriovenous graft** can be created by subcutaneously interposing a biologic, semibiologic, or synthetic graft material between an artery and vein (Fig. 45-5B). Usually a graft is created when the patient's vessels are not suitable for creation of an AVF. Patients with compromised vascular systems (e.g., from diabetes) will require a graft because their native vessels are not suitable for creation of an AVF. Grafts are usually placed in the arm but may be placed in the thigh or chest area. Stenosis, infection, and thrombosis are the most common complications that result in loss of

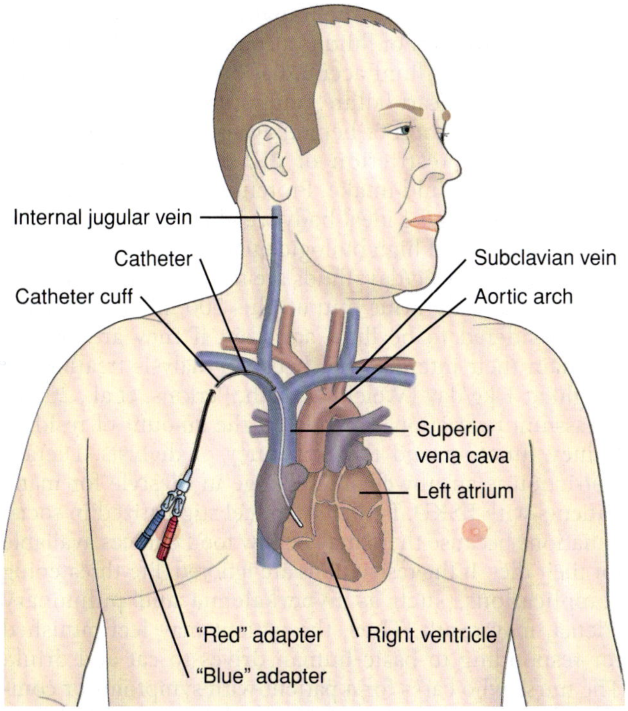

FIGURE 45-4. Double-lumen, cuffed hemodialysis catheter used in acute hemodialysis. The red lumen is attached to a blood line through which blood is pumped from the patient to the dialyzer. After the blood passes through the dialyzer (artificial kidney), it returns to the patient through the blue lumen of the catheter.

this access. It is not at all uncommon to see a dialysis patient with numerous "old" or "nonfunctioning" accesses present on their arms. The patient is asked to identify which is the current access in use and it is checked carefully for the presence of a bruit and thrill.

See the Special Considerations: Nursing Management of the Hospitalized Patient on Dialysis section later in this chapter for nursing interventions and care of the patient with an arteriovenous graft or fistula.

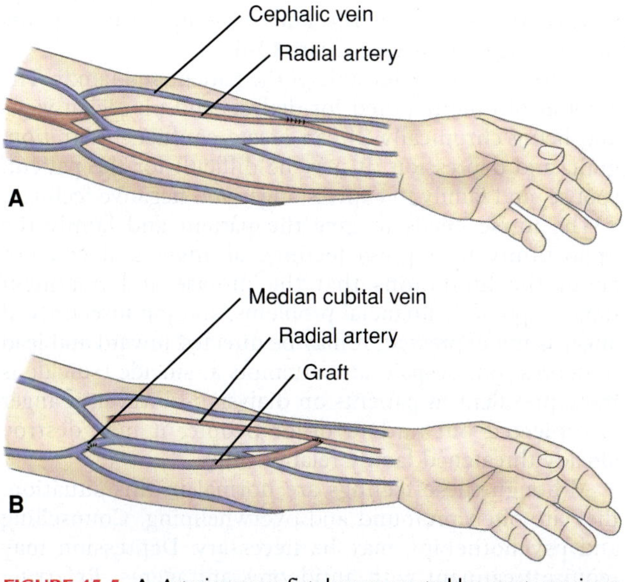

FIGURE 45-5. A. Arteriovenous fistulas are created by anastomosing a patient's vein to an artery. This illustrates a side-to-side anastomosis. **B.** Arteriovenous grafts are established by connecting the artery and vein using synthetic tubing.

> **QUALITY AND SAFETY NURSING ALERT**
>
> **Failure of the permanent dialysis access (fistula or graft) accounts for most hospital admissions of patients undergoing chronic hemodialysis. Thus, protection of the access is of high priority. The extremity with the vascular access is not to be used for measuring blood pressure or for obtaining blood specimens; tight dressings, restraints, or jewellery over the vascular access must be avoided as well.**

Complications

While hemodialysis can prolong life indefinitely, it does not alter the natural course of the underlying CKD, nor does it completely replace kidney function. The CKD complications previously discussed will continue to worsen and require more aggressive treatment. With the initiation of dialysis, disturbances of lipid metabolism (hypertriglyceridemia) are accentuated and contribute to cardiovascular complications. Heart failure, coronary heart disease, angina, stroke, and peripheral vascular insufficiency may occur and can incapacitate the patient. Cardiovascular disease remains the leading cause of death in patients receiving dialysis (Deng & Forbes, 2015; Vasundhara, Kozman, Liu, et al., 2014).

Anemia is compounded by blood lost during hemodialysis. Gastric ulcers may result from the physiologic stress of chronic illness, medication, and pre-existing medical conditions (e.g., diabetes). Patients with uremia report a metallic taste and nausea when they require dialysis. Vomiting may occur during the hemodialysis treatment when rapid fluid shifts and hypotension occur. These contribute to the malnutrition seen in patients on dialysis. Worsening calcium metabolism and kidney osteodystrophy can result in bone pain and fractures, interfering with mobility. As time on dialysis continues, calcification of major blood vessels has been reported and linked to hypertension and other vascular complications. Phosphorus deposits in the skin can occur and cause itching.

Many dialysis patients experience fatigue while undergoing hemodialysis. Up to 85% of people undergoing hemodialysis experience major sleep problems that further complicate their overall health status. Early-morning or late-afternoon dialysis may be a risk factor for developing sleep disturbances.

Other complications of dialysis treatment may include the following:

- Episodes of shortness of breath often occur as fluid accumulates between dialysis treatments.
- Hypotension may occur during the treatment as fluid is removed. Nausea and vomiting, diaphoresis, tachycardia, and dizziness are common signs of hypotension.
- Painful muscle cramping may occur, usually late in dialysis as fluid and electrolytes rapidly leave the extracellular space.

- Exsanguination may occur if blood lines separate or dialysis needles become dislodged.
- Dysrhythmias may result from electrolyte and pH changes or from removal of antiarrhythmic medications during dialysis.
- Air embolism is rare but can occur if air enters the vascular system.
- Chest pain may occur in patients with anemia or arteriosclerotic heart disease.
- Dialysis disequilibrium results from cerebral fluid shifts. Signs and symptoms include headache, nausea and vomiting, restlessness, decreased level of consciousness, and seizures. It is more likely to occur in ARF or when BUN levels are very high, exceeding 54 mmol/L.

Nursing Management

The nurse in the dialysis unit has an important role in monitoring, supporting, assessing, and educating the patient. During dialysis, the patient, the dialyzer, and the dialysate bath require constant monitoring because numerous complications are possible, including clotting of the circuit, air embolism, inadequate or excessive ultrafiltration hypotension, cramping, vomiting, blood leaks, contamination, and access complications. Nursing care of the patient and maintenance of the vascular access device are especially important and are discussed later in this chapter in the section titled Special Considerations: Nursing Management of the Hospitalized Patient on Dialysis.

Promoting Pharmacologic Therapy

Many medications are removed from the blood during hemodialysis; therefore, dosage or timing of the medication administration may require adjustment. Medications that are water soluble are readily removed during hemodialysis treatment and those that are fat soluble or adhere to other substances (like albumin) are not dialyzed out very well. This is the reason some drug overdoses are treated with emergency hemodialysis and others are not.

Patients undergoing hemodialysis who require medications (e.g., cardiac glycosides, antibiotic agents, antiarrhythmic medications, antihypertensive agents) are monitored closely to ensure that blood and tissue levels of these medications are maintained without toxic accumulation. Antihypertensive therapy, often part of the regimen of patients on dialysis, is one example when communication, teaching, and evaluation can make a difference in patient outcomes. The patient must know when and when not to take the medication. For example, if an antihypertensive agent is taken on a dialysis day, hypotension may occur during dialysis, causing dangerously low blood pressure. Many medications that are taken once daily can be held until after the dialysis treatment.

Promoting Nutritional and Fluid Therapy

Diet is important for patients on hemodialysis because of the effects of uremia. Goals of nutritional therapy are to minimize uremic symptoms and fluid and electrolyte imbalances; to maintain good nutritional status through adequate protein, calorie, vitamin, and mineral intake; and to enable the patient to eat a palatable and enjoyable diet. Restricting dietary protein decreases the accumulation of nitrogenous wastes, reduces uremic symptoms, and may even postpone the initiation of dialysis for a few months. Restriction of fluid is also part of the dietary prescription because fluid accumulation may occur, leading to weight gain, heart failure, and pulmonary edema.

With the initiation of hemodialysis, the patient usually requires some restriction of dietary protein, sodium, potassium, and fluid intake. Protein intake is restricted to about 1.2 to 1.3 g/kg ideal body weight per day; therefore, protein must be of high biologic quality. Sodium is usually restricted to 2 to 3 g/day; fluids are restricted to an amount equal to the daily urine output plus 500 mL/day. Patients are considered to be fluid adherent if they are able to maintain their interdialytic (between dialysis treatments) weight at 1 kg/day (Welch, Astroth, Perkins, et al., 2013). Potassium restriction depends on the amount of residual kidney function and the frequency of dialysis. Dietary restriction is an unwelcome change in lifestyle for many patients with ESKD. Patients can feel stigmatized in social situations because there may be few food choices available for their diet. If the restrictions are ignored, life-threatening complications, such as hyperkalemia and pulmonary edema, may result. Thus, the patient may feel punished for responding to basic human drives to eat and drink. The nurse who cares for a patient with symptoms or complications resulting from dietary indiscretion must avoid harsh, judgmental, or punitive tones when communicating with him or her. Regular education with reinforcement is needed to achieve this difficult change in lifestyle.

Meeting Psychosocial Needs

Patients requiring long-term hemodialysis are often concerned about the unpredictability of the illness and the disruption of their lives. They often have financial problems, difficulty holding a job, waning sexual desire and impotence, depression from being chronically ill, and fear of dying. Younger patients worry about marriage, having children, and the burden that they bring to their families. The regimented lifestyle that frequent dialysis treatments and restrictions in food and fluid intake impose is often demoralizing to the patient and family. Researchers have studied the quality of life and self-efficacy in patients undergoing dialysis (see Chart 45-8).

Dialysis alters the lifestyle of the patient and family. The amount of time required for dialysis and physician visits and being chronically ill can create conflict, frustration, guilt, and depression. It may be difficult for the patient, spouse, and family to express anger and negative feelings.

The nurse needs to give the patient and family the opportunity to express feelings of anger and concern about the limitations that the disease and treatment impose, possible financial problems, and job insecurity. If anger is not expressed, it may be directed inward and lead to depression, despair, and attempts at suicide (suicide is more prevalent in patients on dialysis); however, if anger is projected outward to other people, it may destroy already threatened family relationships.

Although these feelings are normal in this situation, they are often profound and overwhelming. Counselling and psychotherapy may be necessary. Depression may require treatment with antidepressant agents. Referring the patient and family to a mental health provider with expertise in the care of patients receiving dialysis may also be helpful. An interdisciplinary approach, consisting of

NURSING RESEARCH PROFILE

Chart 45-8. Quality of Life in Patients Receiving Dialysis

Wright, L. S., & Wilson, L. (2015). Quality of life and self-efficacy in three dialysis modalities: Incenter hemodialysis, home hemodialysis, and home peritoneal dialysis. *Nephrology Nursing Journal*, *42*(5), 463–476.

Purpose

Previous research has focused almost exclusively on the quality of life among patients receiving incentre hemodialysis (HD). The purpose of this study was to describe the quality of life and self-efficacy of patients receiving incentre HD compared to those receiving a home HD (HD or peritoneal dialysis [PD]).

Design

This study utilized a correlational cross-sectional design and quota sampling to achieve equal group size. Patients were recruited from outpatient dialysis facilities and included 77 community dwelling adult patients who had been on dialysis for at least 6 months. Quality of life was measured using the Kidney Disease Quality of Life (QOL) Instrument, and self-efficacy was measured using the Strategies Used by People to Promote Health instrument.

Findings

The sample included 29 participants receiving incentre HD treatments, 22 on home HD, and 26 on home PD. There were no significant differences in demographic characteristics. Participants on PD scored the highest in 6 of the 11 CKDs specific to QOL measures. Patients on PD also scored highest in 8 of the 9 generic QOL measures. The results of this study suggest a possible benefit for patients on PD with regard to QOL and self-efficacy.

Nursing Implications

This information helps nurses to understand patient needs, both medical and social, and to recognize their key role in educating patients about treatment options and other care-related issues. By knowing the differences in reported self-efficacy and QOL across dialysis modalities, nurses can help empower patients to make decisions about which mode of dialysis treatment will meet their individual needs.

clinical nurse specialists, psychologists, and social workers may be helpful in assisting the patient and family to cope with the changes brought about by kidney failure and its treatment.

The "sense of loss" that the patient experiences cannot be underestimated because every aspect of a "normal life" is disrupted. Some patients use denial to deal with the overwhelming array of medical problems (e.g., infections, hypertension, anemia, neuropathy). Staff who are tempted to label the patient as noncompliant must consider the impact of kidney failure and its treatment on the patient and family and the coping strategies that they may use.

Palliative care principles that focus on symptom control are becoming increasingly important as greater attention is focused on quality-of-life issues (Kane, Vinen, & Murtagh, 2013).

Patients and their families should be encouraged to discuss end-of-life options and have developed advanced directives or living wills.

Promoting Home, Community-Based, and Transitional Care

Educating Patients About Self-Care

Preparing a patient for hemodialysis is challenging. Often the patient does not fully comprehend the impact of dialysis, and learning needs may go unrecognized. Good communication between dialysis staff and home care nurses is essential.

Assessment helps identify the learning needs of the patient and family members. In many cases, the patient is discharged home before learning needs and readiness to learn can be thoroughly evaluated; therefore, hospital-based nurses, dialysis staff, and home care nurses must work together to provide appropriate teaching that meets the patient's and family's changing needs and readiness to learn.

The diagnosis of CRF and the need for dialysis often overwhelm the patient and family. In addition, many patients with ESRD have depressed mentation, a shortened attention span, a decreased level of concentration, and altered perception. Therefore, teaching must occur in brief, 10- to 15-minute sessions, with time added for clarification, repetition, reinforcement, and questions from the patient and family. The nurse needs to convey a nonjudgmental attitude to enable the patient and family to discuss options and their feelings about those options. Team conferences are helpful for sharing information and providing every team member the opportunity to discuss the needs of the patient and family.

Home Hemodialysis

Most patients who undergo hemodialysis do so in an outpatient setting, but home hemodialysis is an option for some. Home hemodialysis requires a highly motivated patient who is willing to take responsibility for the procedure and is able to adjust each treatment to meet the body's changing needs. It also requires the commitment and cooperation of a caregiver to assist the patient. However, many patients are not comfortable imposing on others this way and do not wish to subject family members to the feeling that their home is being turned into a clinic. The health care team never forces a patient to use home hemodialysis because this treatment requires significant changes in the home and family. Home hemodialysis must be the patient's and family's decision because full cooperation and participation are required (Peters, 2014; Wright & Wilson, 2015).

The patient undergoing home hemodialysis and the caregiver assisting that patient must be trained to prepare, operate, and disassemble the dialysis machine; maintain and clean the equipment; administer medications (e.g.,

CHART 45-9

HOME CARE CHECKLIST • The Patient Undergoing Hemodialysis

At the completion of education, the patient and/or caregiver will be able to:

- Discuss kidney disease and its effects on the body.
- State the goal and purpose of hemodialysis and its impact on physiologic functioning, ADLs, IADLs, roles, relationships, and spirituality.
- Discuss common problems that may occur during hemodialysis and their prevention and management.
- State the name, dose, side effects, frequency, and schedule for all medications on dialysis and nondialysis days.
- Describe commonly measured laboratory values, results, and implications.
- State changes in lifestyle (e.g., diet, activity) necessary to maintain health.
- Acknowledge dietary and fluid restrictions, rationale, and consequences of nonadherence.
- State dietary restrictions and changes required to provide adequate protein, calorie, vitamin, and mineral intake.
- List guidelines for prevention and detection of fluid overload, meaning of "dry" weight, and how to weigh self.
- Demonstrate vascular access care, how to check patency, signs and symptoms of infection, and prevention of complications.
- Develop strategies to manage or reduce anxiety and maintain independence.
- Discuss strategies for detection, management, and relief of pruritus, neuropathy, and other potential complications of kidney disease.
- Relate how to reach primary provider with questions or complications.
- State time and date of follow-up medical appointments, therapy, and testing.
- Coordinate financial arrangements for hemodialysis and strategies to identify and obtain resources.
- Identify sources of support (e.g., friends, relatives, faith community, support groups, caregiver support).
- Identify the need for health promotion, disease prevention, and screening activities.

ADL, activities of daily living; IADL, independent activities of daily living.

heparin) into the machine lines; and handle emergency problems (hemodialysis dialyzer rupture, electrical or mechanical problems, hypotension, shock, and seizures) (Tennankore, d'Gama, Faratro, et al., 2015). Because home hemodialysis places primary responsibility for the treatment on the patient and the family member, they must understand and be capable of performing all aspects of the hemodialysis procedure (Chart 45-9).

Before home hemodialysis is initiated, the home environment, household and community resources, and ability and willingness of the patient and family to carry out this treatment are assessed. The home is surveyed to see if electrical outlets, plumbing facilities, and storage space are adequate. Modifications may be needed to enable the patient and assistant to perform dialysis safely and to deal with emergencies.

Once home hemodialysis is initiated, the home care nurse must visit periodically to evaluate compliance with the recommended techniques, to assess the patient for complications, to reinforce previous teaching, and to provide reassurance.

Continuing and Transitional Care

The health care team's goal in treating patients with CKD is to maximize their vocational potential, functional status, and quality of life (Wright & Wilson, 2015). To facilitate kidney rehabilitation, appropriate follow-up and monitoring by members of the health care team (physicians, dialysis nurses, social worker, psychologist, home care nurses, and others as appropriate) are essential to identify and resolve problems early on. Many patients with CKD can resume relatively normal lives, doing the things that are important to them: travelling, exercising, working, or actively participating in family activities. If appropriate interventions are available early in the course of dialysis, the potential for better health improves, and the patient can remain active in family and community life. Outcome goals for kidney rehabilitation include employment for those able to work, improved physical functioning of all patients, improved understanding about adaptation and options for living well, increased control over the effects of kidney disease and dialysis, and resumption of activities enjoyed before dialysis.

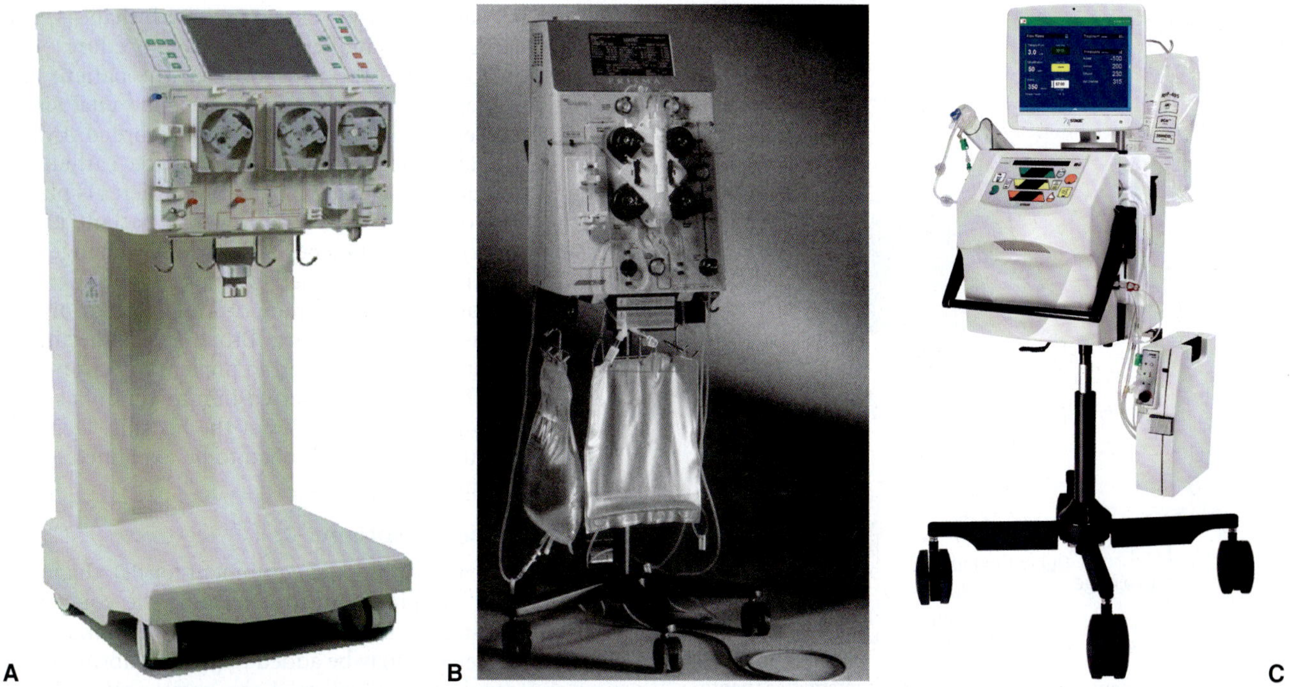

FIGURE 45-6. Devices for administering continuous kidney replacement therapy (CRRT) offer an integrated fluid warmer for the heating of infusion and dialysate fluids, a weighing system to reduce the possibility of error in assessing fluid balance, and a battery backup that allows treatments to continue when the patient is moved. (**A.** Diapact CRRT System, B-Braun Medical, Inc., Bethlehem, PA. **B.** PRISMA, Gambro Corporation, Lakewood, CO. **C.** System One, NxStage Medical Inc., Lawrence, MA.)

Continuous Kidney Replacement Therapies

CRRTs may be indicated for patients with AKI or CKD who are too clinically unstable for traditional hemodialysis, for patients with fluid overload secondary to oliguric (low urine output) kidney failure, and for patients whose kidneys cannot handle their acutely high metabolic or nutritional needs. CRRT does not produce rapid fluid shifts, does not require dialysis machines or dialysis personnel to carry out the procedures, and can be initiated quickly. Several types of CRRT are available and widely used in critical care units (Fig. 45-6). The methods are similar as they require access to the circulation and blood to pass through an artificial filter. A hemofilter (an extremely porous blood filter containing a semipermeable membrane) is used in all types.

Continuous Venovenous Hemofiltration

Continuous venovenous hemofiltration (CVVH) is used to manage ARF. Blood from a double-lumen venous catheter is pumped (using a small blood pump) through a hemofilter and then returned to the patient through the same catheter. CVVH provides continuous slow fluid removal (ultrafiltration); therefore, hemodynamic effects are mild and better tolerated by patients with unstable conditions. CVVH does not require arterial access, and critical care nurses can set up, initiate, maintain, and terminate the system.

Continuous Venovenous Hemodialysis

Continuous venovenous hemodialysis (CVVHD) is similar to CVVH. Blood is pumped from a double-lumen venous catheter through a hemofilter and returned to the patient through the same catheter. In addition to the benefits of ultrafiltration, CVVHD uses a concentration gradient to facilitate the removal of uremic toxins and fluid. No arterial access is required, hemodynamic effects are usually mild, and critical care nurses can set up, initiate, maintain, and terminate the system (Muzzy & Snyder, 2013).

Other types of CRRT include slow continuous ultrafiltration (SCUF) and continuous venovenous hemodiafiltration (CVVHDF). SCUF is indicated for patients who are fluid overloaded but without being uremic or have significant electrolyte imbalance. CVVHDF is indicated when metabolic control is not being achieved with CVVH (Richardson & Whatmore, 2014).

Peritoneal Dialysis

The goals of peritoneal dialysis (PD) are to remove toxic substances and metabolic wastes and to reestablish normal fluid and electrolyte balance. PD may be the treatment of choice for patients with kidney failure who are unable or unwilling to undergo hemodialysis or kidney transplantation. Patients who are susceptible to the rapid fluid, electrolyte, and metabolic changes that occur during hemodialysis experience fewer of these problems with the slower rate of PD. Therefore, patients with diabetes or cardiovascular disease, many older patients, and those who may be at risk for adverse effects of systemic heparin are likely candidates for PD. In addition, severe hypertension, heart failure, and pulmonary edema not responsive to usual treatment regimens have been successfully treated with PD.

In PD, the peritoneal membrane that covers the abdominal organs and lines the abdominal wall serves as the

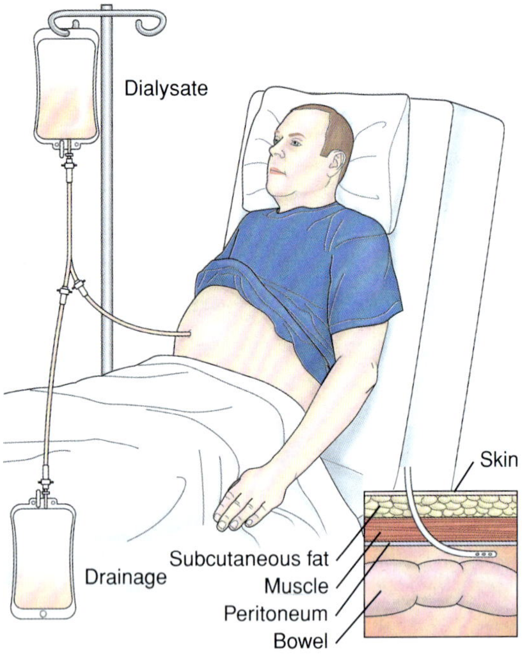

FIGURE 45-7. In peritoneal dialysis and in acute intermittent peritoneal dialysis, dialysate is infused into the peritoneal cavity by gravity, after which the clamp on the infusion line is closed. After a dwell time (when the dialysate is in the peritoneal cavity), the drainage tube is unclamped and the fluid drains from the peritoneal cavity, again by gravity. A new container of dialysate is infused as soon as drainage is complete. The duration of the dwell time depends on the type of peritoneal dialysis.

semipermeable membrane. Sterile dialysate fluid is introduced into the peritoneal cavity through an abdominal catheter at intervals (Fig. 45-7). Once the sterile solution is in the peritoneal cavity, uremic toxins such as urea and creatinine begin to be cleared from the blood. Diffusion and osmosis occur as waste products move from an area of higher concentration (the blood stream) to an area of lesser concentration (the dialysate fluid) through a semipermeable membrane (the peritoneum). This movement of solute from the blood into the dialysate fluid is called clearance. Since substances cross the peritoneal membrane at different rates, adjustments in dwell time and amount of fluid used are made to facilitate the process. Ultrafiltration (water removal) occurs in PD through an osmotic gradient created by using a dialysate fluid with a higher glucose concentration. PD usually takes 36 to 48 hours to achieve what hemodialysis accomplishes in 6 to 8 hours.

Procedure

As with other forms of treatment, the decision to begin PD is made by the patient and family in consultation with the physician. The patient may be acutely ill, thus requiring short-term treatment to correct severe disturbances in fluid and electrolyte status, or may have ESKD and need to receive ongoing treatments.

Preparing the Patient

The nurse's preparation of the patient and family for PD depends on the patient's physical and psychological status, level of alertness, previous experience with dialysis, and understanding of and familiarity with the procedure.

The nurse explains the procedure to the patient and assists in obtaining signed consent. Baseline vital signs, weight, and serum electrolyte levels are recorded. Evaluation of the abdomen for placement of the catheter is done to facilitate self-care. Typically the catheter is placed on the nondominant side to allow the patient easier access to the catheter connection site when exchanges are done. The patient is encouraged to empty the bladder and bowel to reduce the risk of puncture of internal organs during the insertion procedure. Broad-spectrum antibiotic agents may be administered to prevent infection. The peritoneal catheter can be inserted in interventional radiology, in the operating room, or at the bedside. Depending on the situation, this will need to be explained to the patient and family.

Preparing the Equipment

In addition to assembling the equipment for PD, the nurse consults with the physician to determine the concentration of dialysate to be used and the medications to be added to it. Heparin may be added to prevent fibrin formation and resultant occlusion of the peritoneal catheter. Potassium chloride may be prescribed to prevent hypokalemia. Antibiotics may be added to treat **peritonitis** (inflammation of the peritoneal membrane) caused by infection. Regular insulin may be added for patients with diabetes. Aseptic technique is imperative whenever medications are added.

Before medications are added, the dialysate is warmed to body temperature to prevent patient discomfort and abdominal pain and to dilate the vessels of the peritoneum to increase urea clearance. Solutions that are too cold cause pain, cramping, and vasoconstriction and reduce clearance. Dry heating (heating cabinet, incubator, or heating pad) is recommended. Methods not recommended include soaking the bags of solution in warm water (can introduce bacteria to the exterior of the bags of solution and increase the chance of peritonitis) and use of a microwave to heat the fluid (increases the danger of burning the peritoneum).

Immediately before initiating dialysis, using aseptic technique, the nurse assembles the administration set and tubing. The tubing is filled with the prepared dialysate to reduce the amount of air entering the catheter and peritoneal cavity, which could increase abdominal discomfort and interfere with instillation and drainage of the fluid.

Inserting the Catheter

Ideally, the peritoneal catheter is inserted in the operating room or radiology suite to maintain surgical asepsis and minimize the risk of contamination. However, in some circumstances, the physician may insert the rigid stylet catheter at the bedside using strict asepsis. Whenever a rigid catheter is used, careful securing and close observation for bowel perforation is essential to minimize complications.

Catheters for long-term use (e.g., Tenckhoff, Swan, or Cruz) are usually soft and flexible and made of silicone with a radiopaque strip to permit visualization on x-ray. These catheters have three sections: (1) an intraperitoneal section, with numerous openings and an open tip to let dialysate flow freely; (2) a subcutaneous section that

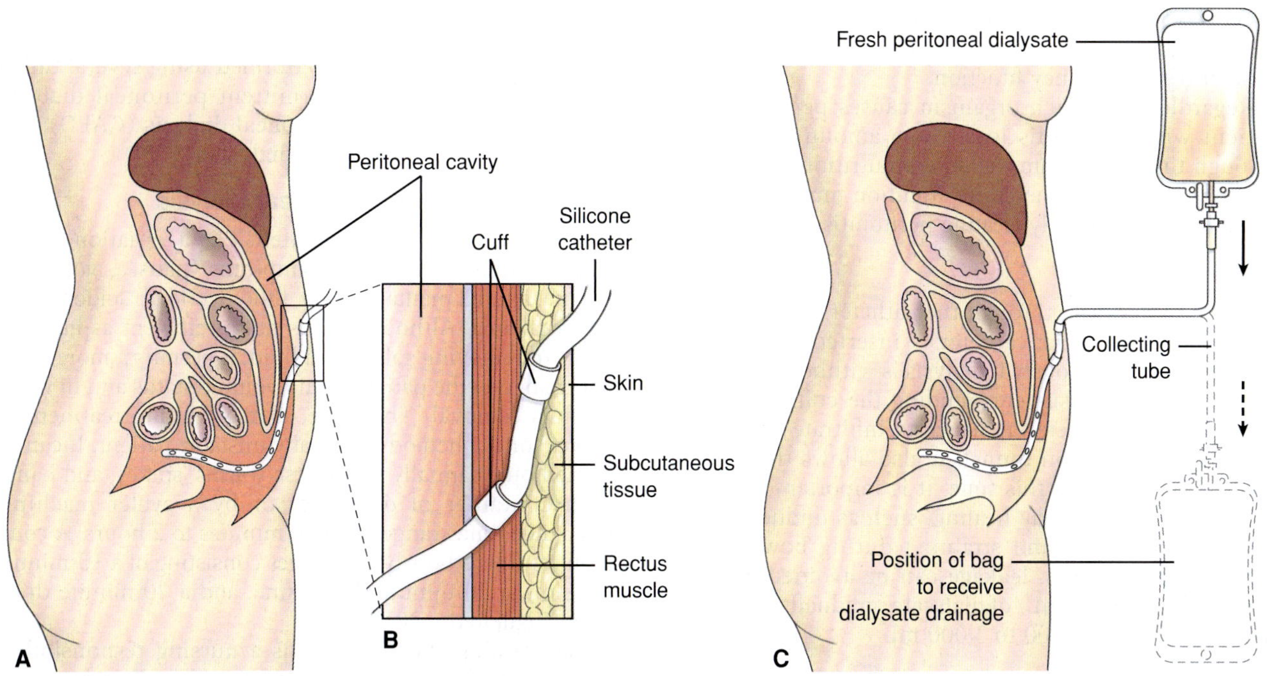

FIGURE 45-8. Continuous ambulatory peritoneal dialysis. **A.** The peritoneal catheter is implanted through the abdominal wall. **B.** Dacron cuffs and a subcutaneous tunnel provide protection against bacterial infection. **C.** Dialysate flows by gravity through the peritoneal catheter into the peritoneal cavity. After a prescribed period of time, the fluid is drained by gravity and discarded. New solution is then infused into the peritoneal cavity until the next drainage period. Dialysis thus continues on a 24-hour-a-day basis, during which the patient is free to move around and engage in his or her usual activities.

passes from the peritoneal membrane and tunnels through muscle and subcutaneous fat to the skin; and (3) an external section for connection to the dialysate system. Most of these catheters have two cuffs, which are made of Dacron polyester. The cuffs stabilize the catheter, limit movement, prevent leaks, and provide a barrier against microorganisms. One cuff is placed just distal to the peritoneum, and the other cuff is placed subcutaneously. The subcutaneous tunnel (5 to 10 cm long) further protects against bacterial infection (Fig. 45-8).

Performing the Exchange

Peritoneal dialysis involves a series of exchanges or cycles. An exchange is defined as the infusion (fill), dwell, and drainage of the dialysate. This cycle is repeated throughout the course of the dialysis. The dialysate is infused by gravity into the peritoneal cavity. A period of about 5 to 10 minutes is usually required to infuse 2 to 3 L of fluid. The prescribed dwell, or equilibration, time allows diffusion and osmosis to occur. At the end of the dwell time, the drainage portion of the exchange begins. The tube is unclamped and the solution drains from the peritoneal cavity by gravity through a closed system. Drainage is usually completed in 10 to 20 minutes. The drainage fluid is normally colourless or straw-coloured and should not be cloudy. Bloody drainage may be seen in the first few exchanges after insertion of a new catheter but should not occur after that time. The number of cycles or exchanges and their frequency are prescribed based on monthly laboratory values and presence of uremic symptoms.

The removal of excess water during PD occurs because dialysate has a high dextrose concentration, making it hypertonic. An osmotic gradient is created between the blood and the dialysate solution. Dextrose solutions of 1.5%, 2.5%, and 4.25% are available in several volumes, from 1,000 to 3,000 mL. The higher the dextrose concentration, the greater the osmotic gradient and the more water will be removed. Selection of the appropriate solution is based on the patient's fluid status.

Complications

Most complications of PD are minor, but several, if unattended, can have serious consequences.

Acute Complications

Peritonitis

Peritonitis is the most common and serious complication of PD. The first sign of peritonitis is cloudy dialysate drainage fluid. Diffuse abdominal pain and rebound tenderness occur much later. Hypotension and other signs of shock may also occur with advancing infection. The patient with peritonitis may be treated as an inpatient or outpatient (most common), depending on the severity of the infection and the patient's clinical status. Drainage fluid is examined for cell count; Gram stain and culture are used to identify the organism and guide treatment. Antibiotic agents (aminoglycosides or cephalosporins) are usually added to subsequent exchanges until Gram stain or culture results are available for appropriate antibiotic determination. Intraperitoneal administration of antibiotics is as effective as IV administration and therefore most often used. Antibiotic therapy continues for 10 to 14 days.

Careful selection and calculation of the antibiotic dosage are needed to prevent nephrotoxicity and further compromise of residual kidney function.

Regardless of which organism causes peritonitis, the patient with peritonitis loses large amounts of protein through the peritoneum. Acute malnutrition and delayed healing may result. Therefore, attention must be given to detecting and promptly treating peritonitis.

Leakage

Leakage of dialysate through the catheter site may occur immediately after the catheter is inserted. Usually, the leak stops spontaneously if dialysis is withheld for several days, giving the tissue surrounding the cuffs located on the abdominal catheter a chance to infiltrate the Dacron and seal the insertion tunnel. It also allows the exit site time to heal. During this time, it is important to reduce factors that might delay healing, such as undue abdominal muscle activity and straining during bowel movement. In many cases, leakage can be avoided by using small volumes (500 mL) of dialysate, gradually increasing the volume up to 2,000 to 3,000 mL.

Bleeding

A bloody **effluent** (drainage) may be observed occasionally, especially in young, menstruating women. The hypertonic fluid pulls blood from the uterus, through the opening in the fallopian tubes, and into the peritoneal cavity. Bleeding is also common during the first few exchanges after a new catheter insertion because some blood enters the abdominal cavity following insertion. In many cases, no cause can be found for the bleeding, although catheter displacement from the pelvis has occasionally been associated with bleeding. Some patients have had bloody effluent after an enema or from minor trauma. Invariably, bleeding stops in 1 to 2 days and requires no specific intervention. More frequent exchanges and the addition of heparin to the dialysate during this time may be necessary to prevent blood clots from obstructing the catheter.

Long-Term Complications

Hypertriglyceridemia is common in patients undergoing long-term PD, suggesting that the therapy may accelerate atherogenesis. Despite this, the use of cardioprotective medications is relatively uncommon, and many patients have suboptimal blood pressure control. Given the high burden of disease in these patients, beta-blockers and ACE inhibitors should be used to control hypertension or protect the heart, and the use of aspirin and statins should be considered (James, Oparil, Carter, et al., 2014).

Other complications that may occur with long-term PD include abdominal hernias (incisional, inguinal, diaphragmatic, and umbilical), probably resulting from continuously increased intra-abdominal pressure. The persistently elevated intra-abdominal pressure also aggravates symptoms of hiatal hernia and hemorrhoids. Low back pain and anorexia from fluid in the abdomen and a constant sweet taste related to glucose absorption may also occur.

Mechanical problems occasionally occur and may interfere with instillation or drainage of the dialysate. Formation of clots in the peritoneal catheter and constipation are factors that may contribute to these problems.

Approaches

Peritoneal dialysis can be performed using several different approaches: acute intermittent peritoneal dialysis, **continuous ambulatory peritoneal dialysis** (CAPD), and **continuous cyclic peritoneal dialysis** (CCPD).

Acute Intermittent Peritoneal Dialysis

Indications for acute intermittent PD, a variation of PD, include uremic signs and symptoms (nausea, vomiting, fatigue, altered mental status), fluid overload, acidosis, and hyperkalemia. Although PD is not as efficient as hemodialysis in removing solute and fluid, it permits a more gradual change in the patient's fluid volume status and in waste product removal. Therefore, it may be the treatment of choice for the hemodynamically unstable patient. It can be carried out manually (the nurse warms, spikes, and hangs each container of dialysate) or by a cycler machine. Exchange times range from 30 minutes to 2 hours. A common routine is hourly exchanges consisting of a 10-minute infusion, a 30-minute dwell time, and a 20-minute drain time (Figueiredo, 2014).

Maintaining the PD cycle is a nursing responsibility. Strict aseptic technique is maintained when changing solution containers and emptying drainage containers. Vital signs, weight, I&O, laboratory values, and patient status are frequently monitored. The nurse uses a flow sheet to document each exchange and records vital signs, dialysate concentration, medications added, exchange volume, dwell time, dialysate fluid balance for each exchange (fluid lost or gained), and cumulative fluid balance. The nurse also carefully assesses skin turgor and mucous membranes to evaluate fluid status and monitor the patient for edema.

> **! QUALITY AND SAFETY NURSING ALERT**
>
> **If the peritoneal fluid does not drain properly, the nurse can facilitate drainage by turning the patient from side to side or raising the head of the bed. The catheter should never be pushed further into the peritoneal cavity.**

Other measures to promote drainage include checking the patency of the catheter by inspecting for kinks, closed clamps, or an air lock. The nurse monitors for complications, including peritonitis, bleeding, respiratory difficulty, and leakage of peritoneal fluid. Abdominal girth may be measured periodically to determine if the patient is retaining large amounts of dialysis solution. In addition, the nurse must ensure that the PD catheter remains secure and that the dressing remains dry. Physical comfort measures, frequent turning, and skin care are provided. The patient and family are educated about the procedure and are kept informed about progress (fluid loss, weight loss, laboratory values). Emotional support and encouragement are given to the patient and family during this stressful and uncertain time.

Continuous Ambulatory Peritoneal Dialysis

CAPD is performed at home by the patient or a trained caregiver who is usually a family member. The procedure allows the patient reasonable freedom and control of daily

CHART 45-10

Considerations in Continuous Ambulatory Peritoneal Dialysis (CAPD)

Although CAPD is not suitable for all patients with end-stage kidney disease (ESKD), it is a viable therapy for those who can perform self-care and exchanges and who can fit therapy into their own routines. Often, patients report having more energy and feeling healthier once they begin CAPD. Nurses can be instrumental in helping patients with ESKD find the dialysis therapy that best suits their lifestyle. Those considering CAPD need to understand the advantages and disadvantages along with the indications and contraindications for this form of therapy.

Advantages

- Freedom from a dialysis machine
- Control over daily activities
- Opportunities to avoid dietary restrictions, increase fluid intake, raise serum hematocrit values, improve blood pressure control, avoid venipuncture, and gain a sense of well-being

Disadvantages

- Continuous dialysis 24 hours a day, 7 days a week

Indications

- Patient's willingness, motivation, and ability to perform dialysis at home
- Strong family or community support system (essential for success), particularly if the patient is an older adult
- Special problems with long-term hemodialysis, such as dysfunctional or failing vascular access devices, excessive thirst, severe hypertension, postdialysis headaches, and severe anemia requiring frequent transfusion
- Interim therapy while awaiting kidney transplantation
- ESKD secondary to diabetes because hypertension, uremia, and hyperglycemia are easier to manage with CAPD than with hemodialysis

Contraindications

- Adhesions from previous surgery (adhesions reduce clearance of solutes) or systemic inflammatory disease
- Chronic backache and pre-existing disk disease, which could be aggravated by the continuous pressure of dialysis fluid in the abdomen
- Risk of complications, for example, in patients receiving immunosuppressive medications, which impede healing of the catheter site, and in patients with a colostomy, ileostomy, nephrostomy, or ileal conduit because of the risk of peritonitis. The risk for complications is not an absolute contraindication for CAPD therapy.
- Diverticulitis because CAPD has been associated with rupture of the diverticulum
- Severe arthritis or poor hand strength necessitating assistance in performing the exchange. However, blind or partially blind patients and those with other physical limitations can learn to perform CAPD.

activities but requires a serious commitment to be successful. Chart 45-10 discusses suitability for CAPD.

CAPD works on the same principles as other forms of PD: diffusion and osmosis. Less extreme fluctuations in the patient's laboratory values occur with CAPD than with intermittent PD or hemodialysis because the dialysis is constantly in progress. The serum electrolyte levels usually remain in the normal range.

Procedure

The patient performs exchanges four or five times a day, 24 hours a day, 7 days a week, at intervals scheduled throughout the day. Different manufacturers supply different equipment. Most commonly used is a Y-shaped system, in which a bag containing dialysate solution comes connected to one branch of the "Y" and a sterile empty bag is connected to the second branch. This leaves the third part of the "Y" open and available for connection to the transfer set on the PD catheter. To perform an exchange, the patient (or person doing the exchange) washes his or her hands, dons a mask, and then removes the cap from the transfer set while maintaining sterility. The open end of the "Y" set is connected to the end of the transfer set and the dialysate infused where it will dwell. After the dialysate is infused, the patient clamps off the transfer set and the tubing set, disconnects the tubing set, and applies a new cap to the transfer set, making it a closed system. The patient drains the fluid (effluent) from the peritoneal cavity through the catheter (over about 20 to 30 minutes) into an empty bag. Once the effluent has been fully drained, fresh fluid is instilled into the peritoneal cavity.

The longer the dwell time, the better the clearance of uremic toxins is. If dwell time is excessive, the patient will absorb some of the effluent back into the body simply because the osmotic gradient is lost. Once equilibrium is reached, the movement of fluid and toxins stops.

Complications

To reduce the risk of peritonitis, the patient (and all caregivers) must use meticulous care to avoid contaminating the catheter, fluid, or tubing and to avoid accidentally disconnecting the catheter from the tubing. Whenever a connection/disconnection is made, hands must be washed and a mask worn by anyone within 6 ft of the area to avoid contamination with airborne bacteria. Excess manipulation should be avoided and meticulous care of the catheter entry site is provided using a standardized protocol.

Continuous Cyclic Peritoneal Dialysis

Continuous cyclic peritoneal dialysis (CCPD) uses a machine called a cycler to provide the exchanges. It is programmed as to how much fluid to use and how long and how many exchanges need to be done. Since it is programmed, it also keeps track of the total amounts removed and will sound an alarm if limits are not met. It requires that a person set up and break down the system for use, which typically takes about 15 minutes.

CCPD combines overnight intermittent PD with a prolonged dwell time during the day. The peritoneal catheter is connected to a cycler machine every evening, usually just before the patient goes to sleep for the night. Because the machine is very quiet, the patient can sleep, and the extra-long tubing allows the patient to move and turn normally during sleep.

In the morning, the patient disconnects from the cycler. Sometimes dialysate is left in the abdominal cavity for a longer day dwell cycle. This day exchange is drained during the day either by using a "Y" set or reattaching to the cycler. This process is done every day to achieve the effects of dialysis required.

CCPD has a lower infection rate than other forms of PD because there are fewer opportunities for contamination with bag changes and tubing disconnections. It also allows the patient to be free from exchanges throughout the day, making it possible to engage in work and activities of daily living more freely.

Nursing Management

Meeting Psychosocial Needs

In addition to the complications of PD previously described, patients who elect to do PD may experience altered body image because of the presence of the abdominal catheter, bag, tubing, and cycler. Waist size increases from 2.5 to 5 cm (or more) with fluid in the abdomen. This affects clothing selection and may make the patient feel "fat." Body image may be so altered that patients do not want to look at or care for the catheter for days or weeks. The nurse may arrange for the patient to talk with other patients who have adapted well to PD. Although some patients have no psychological problems with the catheter—they think of it as their lifeline and as a life-sustaining device—other patients feel they are doing exchanges all day long and have no free time, particularly in the beginning. They may experience depression because they feel overwhelmed with the responsibility of self-care.

Patients undergoing PD may also experience altered sexuality patterns and sexual dysfunction. The patient and partner may be reluctant to engage in sexual activities, partly because of the catheter being psychologically "in the way" of sexual performance. The peritoneal catheter, drainage bag, and about 2 L of dialysate may interfere with the patient's sexual function and body image as well. In patients on CCPD, the presence of the dialysis cycler in the bedroom and the continual connection during the sleeping hours can also cause interference with intimacy. Although these problems may resolve with time, some problems may warrant special counselling. Questions by the nurse about concerns related to sexuality and sexual function often provide the patient with a welcome opportunity to discuss these issues and a first step toward their resolution.

Promoting Home, Community-Based, and Transitional Care

Educating Patients About Self-Care

Patients are taught as inpatients or outpatients to perform PD once their condition is medically stable. Training usually takes 5 days to 2 weeks. Patients are taught according to their own learning ability and knowledge level and only as much at one time as they can handle without feeling uncomfortable or becoming overwhelmed. Education topics for the patient and family who will be performing PD at home are described in Chart 45-11. It is best to use individualized training methods that are based on adult-learning principles as much as possible, for the prevention of PD-related peritonitis (Zhang, Hawley, Johnson, et al., 2016).

Because of protein loss with continuous PD, the patient is instructed to eat a high-protein, well-balanced diet. The patient is also encouraged to increase his or her daily fibre intake to help prevent constipation, which can impede the flow of dialysate into or out of the peritoneal cavity. Many patients gain 1.5 to 2.5 kg within a month of initiating PD, so they may be asked to limit their carbohydrate intake to avoid excessive weight gain. Potassium, sodium, and fluid restrictions are not usually needed. Patients commonly lose about 2 to 3 L of fluid over and above the volume of dialysate infused into the abdomen during a 24-hour period, permitting a normal fluid intake even in an anephric patient (a patient without kidneys).

Continuing and Transitional Care

Follow-up care through phone calls, visits to the outpatient department, and continuing home care assist patients in the transition to home and promote their active participation in their own health care. Patients often depend on checking with the nurse to see if they are making the correct choices about dialysate or control of blood pressure, or simply to discuss a problem.

Patients may be seen by the PD team as outpatients once a month or more often if needed. The exchange procedure is evaluated at that time to see that strict aseptic technique is being used. Blood chemistry values are followed closely to make certain the therapy is adequate for the patient.

If a referral is made for home care, the home care nurse assesses the home environment and suggests modifications to accommodate the equipment and facilities needed to carry out PD. In addition, the nurse assesses the patient's and family's understanding of PD and evaluates their technique in performing PD. Assessments include checking for changes related to kidney disease, complications such as peritonitis, and treatment-related problems such as heart failure, inadequate drainage, and weight gain or loss. The nurse continues to reinforce and clarify teaching about PD and kidney disease and assesses the patient's and family's progress in coping with the procedure. This is also an opportunity to remind patients about the need to participate in appropriate health promotion activities and health screening (e.g., gynecologic examinations, colonoscopy).

Because of the projected high numbers of older adult patients who will develop ESKD, the nursing home or extended care facility is likely to become an increasingly important site for both rehabilitation and long-term management of patients with kidney failure.

Special Considerations: Nursing Management of the Hospitalized Patient on Dialysis

Whether undergoing hemodialysis or PD, the patient may be hospitalized for treatment of complications related to the dialysis treatment, the underlying kidney disorder, or health problems not related to kidney dysfunction or its treatment.

Protecting Vascular Access

When the patient undergoing hemodialysis is hospitalized for any reason, care must be taken to protect the vascular access. The nurse assesses the vascular access for patency and takes precautions to ensure that the extremity with the

CHART 45-11

HOME CARE CHECKLIST • Peritoneal Dialysis, Continuous Ambulatory Peritoneal Dialysis, or Continuous Cycling Peritoneal Dialysis

At the completion of education, the patient and/or caregiver will be able to:

- Discuss kidney disease and its effects on the body.
- State the goal and purpose of dialysis and its impact on physiologic functioning, ADLs, IADLs, roles, relationships, and spirituality.
- Describe the basic principles of peritoneal dialysis (PD) and exchange options such as continuous ambulatory peritoneal dialysis (CAPD), or continuous cycling peritoneal dialysis (CCPD).
- State what types of changes are needed (if any) to support home PD therapy and maintain a clean home environment and prevent infection.
- State how to contact the primary provider, the team of home care professionals overseeing care, and supply vendor.
- Discuss ordering, storage, and inventory of dialysis supplies.
- List emergency phone numbers.
- State the name, dose, side effects, frequency, and schedule for all medications.
- Demonstrate procedure for adding medications to the dialysis solution.
- Demonstrate catheter and exit site care.
- Demonstrate measurement of vital signs and weight measurement.
- Discuss monitoring and management of fluid balance.
- Discuss basic principles of aseptic technique.
- Demonstrate the CAPD or CCPD exchange procedure using aseptic technique (patients receiving CCPD should also demonstrate exchange procedure in case of failure or unavailability of cycling machine) and discuss cycling machine warning signals and how to address these signals.
- Demonstrate maintenance of home dialysis records.
- Demonstrate procedure for obtaining sterile peritoneal dialysis fluid samples.
- Discuss routine laboratory tests needed and implications of results.
- Discuss high protein diet and diet to avoid constipation, any other dietary restrictions as indicated.
- Discuss complications of peritoneal dialysis; prevention, recognition, and management of complications.
- Describe actions in case of emergency.
- Relate how to reach primary provider with questions or complications.
- State time and date of follow-up medical appointments, therapy, and testing.
- Coordinate financial arrangements for peritoneal dialysis and strategies to identify and obtain resources.
- Identify sources of support (e.g., friends, relatives, faith community, support groups, caregiver support).
- Identify the need for health promotion, disease prevention, and screening activities.

ADL, activities of daily living; IADL, independent activities of daily living.

vascular access is not used for measuring blood pressure or for obtaining blood specimens; tight dressings, restraints, or jewellery over the vascular access must be avoided as well.

The bruit, or "thrill," over the venous access site must be evaluated at least every 8 hours. Absence of a palpable thrill or audible bruit may indicate blockage or clotting in the vascular access. Clotting can occur if the patient has an infection anywhere in the body (serum viscosity increases) or if the blood pressure has dropped. When blood flow is reduced through the access for any reason (hypotension, application of blood pressure cuff or tourniquet), the access can clot. If a patient has a hemodialysis catheter or implanted hemodialysis access device, the nurse must observe for signs and symptoms of infection such as redness, swelling, drainage from the exit site, fever, and chills. The nurse must assess the integrity of the dressing and change it as needed. Patients with kidney disease are more prone to infection; therefore, infection control measures must be used for all procedures.

Taking Precautions During Intravenous Therapy

When the patient needs IV therapy, the rate of administration must be as slow as possible and should be strictly controlled by a volumetric infusion pump.

> **QUALITY AND SAFETY NURSING ALERT**
>
> **Because patients on dialysis cannot excrete water, rapid or excessive administration of IV fluid can result in pulmonary edema. Accurate I&O records are essential.**

Monitoring Symptoms of Uremia

As metabolic end products accumulate, symptoms of uremia worsen. Patients whose metabolic rate accelerates (those receiving corticosteroid medications or parenteral nutrition, those with infections or bleeding disorders, those undergoing surgery) accumulate waste products more quickly and may require daily dialysis. These same patients are more likely than other patients receiving dialysis to experience complications.

Detecting Cardiac and Respiratory Complications

Cardiac and respiratory assessment must be conducted frequently. As fluid builds up, fluid overload, heart failure, and pulmonary edema develop. Crackles in the bases of the lungs may indicate pulmonary edema.

Pericarditis may result from the accumulation of uremic toxins. If not detected and treated promptly, this serious complication may progress to pericardial effusion and cardiac tamponade. Pericarditis is detected by the patient's report of substernal chest pain (if the patient can communicate), low-grade fever (often overlooked), and pericardial friction rub. A pulsus paradoxus (a decrease in blood pressure of more than 10 mm Hg during inspiration) is often present. When pericarditis progresses to effusion, the friction rub disappears, heart sounds become distant and muffled, ECG waves show very low voltage, and the pulsus paradoxus worsens.

The effusion may progress to life-threatening cardiac tamponade, noted by narrowing of the pulse pressure in addition to muffled or inaudible heart sounds, crushing chest pain, dyspnea, and hypotension.

> **QUALITY AND SAFETY NURSING ALERT**
>
> **Although pericarditis, pericardial effusion, and cardiac tamponade can be detected by chest x-ray, they should also be detected through astute nursing assessment. Because of their clinical significance, assessment of the patient for these complications is a priority.**

Controlling Electrolyte Levels and Diet

Electrolyte alterations are common, and potassium changes can be life-threatening. All IV solutions and medications to be administered are evaluated for their electrolyte content. Serum laboratory values are assessed daily. If blood transfusions are required, they may be administered during hemodialysis, if possible, so that excess potassium can be removed. Dietary intake must also be monitored. The patient's frustrations related to dietary restrictions typically increase if the hospital food is unappetizing. The nurse needs to recognize that this may lead to dietary indiscretion and hyperkalemia.

Hypoalbuminemia is an indicator of malnutrition in patients undergoing long-term or maintenance dialysis. Although some patients can be treated with adequate nutrition alone, some patients remain hypoalbuminemic for reasons that are poorly understood.

Managing Discomfort and Pain

Complications such as pruritus and pain secondary to neuropathy must be managed. Antihistamine agents, such as diphenhydramine hydrochloride (Benadryl), are commonly used, and analgesic medications may be prescribed. However, because elimination of the metabolites of medications occurs through dialysis rather than through kidney excretion, medication dosages may need to be adjusted. Keeping the skin clean and well moisturized using bath oils, superfatted soap, and creams or lotions helps promote comfort and reduce itching. Teaching the patient to keep the nails trimmed to avoid scratching and excoriation also promotes comfort.

Monitoring Blood Pressure

Hypertension in kidney failure is common. It is usually the result of fluid overload and, in part, oversecretion of renin. Many patients undergoing dialysis receive some form of antihypertensive therapy and require ongoing teaching about its purpose and adverse effects. The trial-and-error approach that may be necessary to identify the most effective antihypertensive agent and dosage may confuse the patient if no explanation is provided. Antihypertensive agents must be withheld before dialysis to avoid hypotension due to the combined effect of the dialysis and the medication (Doss-McQuitty, 2014).

Typically these patients require single or multiple antihypertensive agents to achieve normal blood pressure, thus adding to the total number of medications needed on an ongoing basis.

Preventing Infection

Patients with ESKD commonly have low WBC counts (and decreased phagocytic ability), low RBC counts (anemia), and impaired platelet function. Together, these pose a high risk for infection and potential for bleeding after even minor trauma. Preventing and controlling infection are essential because the incidence of infection is high. Infection of the vascular access site and pneumonia are common.

Caring for the Catheter Site

Patients receiving CAPD usually know how to care for the catheter site; however, the hospital stay is an opportunity to assess catheter care technique and correct misperceptions or deviations from recommended technique. Recommended daily or three-or-four-times-weekly routine catheter site care is typically performed during showering or bathing. The exit site should not be submerged in bath water. The most common cleaning method is soap and water; liquid soap is recommended. During care, the nurse and patient need to make sure that the catheter remains secure to avoid tension and trauma. The patient may wear a gauze or semi-transparent dressing over the exit site.

Administering Medications

All medications and the dosage prescribed for any patient on dialysis must be closely monitored to avoid those that are toxic to the kidneys and may threaten remaining kidney function. Medications are also scrutinized for potassium and magnesium content, because medications containing potassium or magnesium must be avoided. Care must be taken to evaluate all problems and symptoms that the patient reports without automatically attributing them to kidney failure or to dialysis therapy.

Providing Psychological Support

Patients undergoing dialysis for a while may begin to reevaluate their status, the treatment modality, their satisfaction with life, and the impact of these factors on their families and support systems. Opportunities must be provided for these patients to express their feelings and reactions and to explore options. The decision to begin dialysis does not require that dialysis be continued indefinitely, and it is not uncommon for patients to consider discontinuing treatment. These feelings and reactions must be taken seriously, and the patient should have the opportunity to discuss them with the dialysis team as well as with a psychologist, psychiatrist, psychiatric nurse, trusted friend, or spiritual advisor. The patient's informed decision about discontinuing treatment, after thoughtful deliberation, should be respected.

KIDNEY SURGERY

A patient may undergo surgery to remove obstructions that affect the kidney (tumours or calculi), to insert a tube for draining the kidney (nephrostomy, ureterostomy), or to remove the kidney involved in unilateral kidney disease, kidney carcinoma, or kidney transplantation.

Management of Patients Undergoing Kidney Surgery

Preoperative Considerations

Surgery is performed only after a thorough evaluation of kidney function. Patient preparation to ensure that optimal kidney function is maintained is essential. Fluids are encouraged to promote increased excretion of waste products before surgery unless contraindicated because of preexisting kidney or cardiac dysfunction. If kidney infection is present preoperatively, broad-spectrum antimicrobial agents may be prescribed to prevent bacteremia. Antibiotic agents must be given with extreme care because many are toxic to the kidneys. Coagulation studies (prothrombin time, partial thromboplastin time, platelet count) may be indicated if the patient has a history of bruising and bleeding. The preoperative preparation is similar to that described in Chapter 19.

Because many patients facing kidney surgery are apprehensive, the nurse encourages the patient to recognize and verbalize concerns. Confidence is reinforced by establishing a relationship of trust and by providing expert care. Patients faced with the prospect of losing a kidney may think that they will be dependent on dialysis for the rest of their lives. It is important to teach the patient and family that normal function may be maintained by a single healthy kidney.

Perioperative Concerns

Kidney surgery requires various patient positions to expose the surgical site adequately. Three surgical approaches are common: flank, lumbar, and thoracoabdominal (Fig. 45-9). During surgery, plans are carried out for managing altered urinary drainage. These may include inserting a nephrostomy or other drainage tube.

Postoperative Management

Because the kidney is a highly vascular organ, hemorrhage and shock are the chief complications of kidney surgery. Fluid and blood component replacement is frequently necessary in the immediate postoperative period to treat intraoperative blood loss.

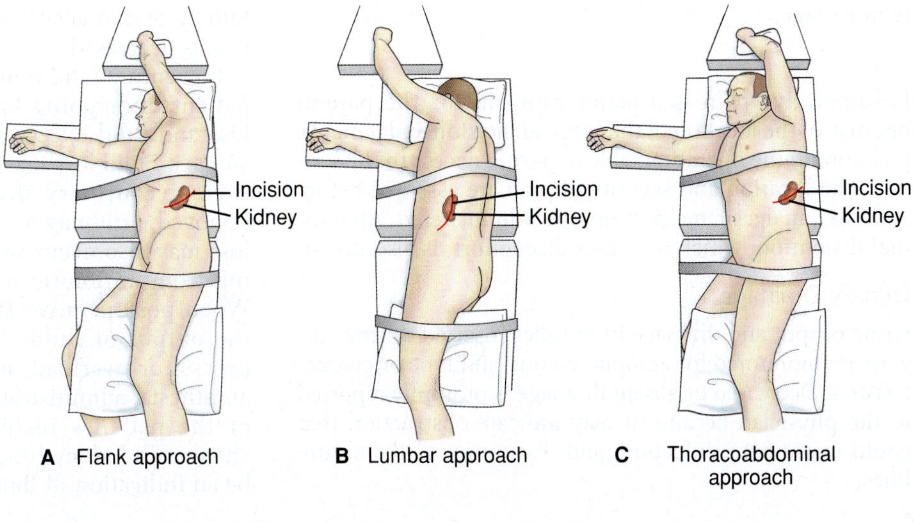

FIGURE 45-9. Patient positioning and incisional approaches (**A**, flank; **B**, lumbar; **C**, thoracoabdominal) for kidney surgery are associated with significant postoperative discomfort.

Abdominal distention and paralytic ileus are fairly common after kidney and ureteral surgery and are thought to be due to a reflex paralysis of intestinal peristalsis and manipulation of the colon or duodenum during surgery. Abdominal distention is relieved by decompression through a nasogastric tube (see Chapter 38 for treatment of paralytic ileus). Oral fluids are permitted when the passage of flatus is noted.

If infection occurs, antibiotics are prescribed after a culture reveals the causative organism. The toxic effects that antibiotic agents have on the kidneys (nephrotoxicity) must be kept in mind when assessing the patient. Low-dose heparin therapy may be initiated postoperatively to prevent thromboembolism in patients who had any type of urologic surgery.

Nursing Management

In addition to those interventions listed in this section, Chart 45-12 provides a plan of nursing care for the patient undergoing kidney surgery.

Providing Immediate Postoperative Care

Immediate postoperative care of the patient who has undergone surgery of the kidney includes assessment of all body systems. Respiratory and circulatory status, pain level, fluid and electrolyte status, and patency and adequacy of urinary drainage systems are assessed.

Respiratory Status

As with any surgery, the use of anesthesia increases the risk for respiratory complications. Noting the location of the surgical incision assists the nurse in anticipating respiratory problems and pain. Respiratory status is assessed by monitoring the rate, depth, and pattern of respirations. The location of the incision frequently causes pain on inspiration and coughing; therefore, the patient tends to splint the chest wall and take shallow respirations. Auscultation is performed to assess normal and adventitious breath sounds.

Circulatory Status and Blood Loss

The patient's vital signs and arterial or central venous pressure are monitored. Skin colour and temperature and urine output provide information about circulatory status. The surgical incision and drainage tubes are observed frequently to help detect unexpected blood loss and hemorrhage.

Pain

Postoperative pain is a major problem for the patient because of the location of the surgical incision and patient's position on the operating table to permit access to the kidney. The location and severity of pain are assessed before and after analgesic medications are administered. Abdominal distention, which increases discomfort, is also noted.

Urinary Drainage

Urine output and drainage from tubes inserted during surgery are monitored for amount, colour, and type or characteristics. Decreased or absent drainage is promptly reported to the physician because it may indicate obstruction that could cause pain, infection, and disruption of the suture lines.

Monitoring and Managing Potential Complications

Bleeding is a major complication of kidney surgery. If undetected and untreated it can result in hypovolemia and hemorrhagic shock. The nurse's role is to observe for these complications, to report their signs and symptoms, and to administer prescribed parenteral fluids and blood and blood components. Monitoring of vital signs, skin colour and temperature, the urinary drainage system, the surgical incision, and the level of consciousness is necessary to detect evidence of bleeding, decreased circulating blood, and fluid volume and cardiac output. Frequent monitoring of vital signs (initially monitored at least at hourly intervals) and urinary output is necessary for early detection of these complications.

If bleeding goes undetected or is not detected promptly, the patient may lose significant amounts of blood and may experience hypoxemia. In addition to hypovolemic shock due to hemorrhage, this type of blood loss may precipitate a myocardial infarction or transient ischemic attack. Bleeding may be suspected when the patient experiences fatigue and when urine output is less than 30 mL/hr. As bleeding persists, late signs of hypovolemia occur, such as cool skin, flat neck veins, and change in level of consciousness or responsiveness. Transfusions of blood components are indicated, along with surgical repair of the bleeding vessel.

Pneumonia may be prevented through use of an incentive spirometer, adequate pain control, and early ambulation. Early signs of pneumonia include fever, increased heart and respiratory rates, and adventitious breath sounds.

Preventing infection is the rationale for using asepsis when changing dressings and handling and preparing catheters, other drainage tubes, central venous catheters, and IV catheters for administration of fluids. Insertion sites are monitored closely for signs and symptoms of inflammation: redness, drainage, heat, and pain. Special care must be taken to prevent UTI, which is associated with the use of indwelling urinary catheters. Catheters and other invasive tubes are removed as soon as they are no longer needed.

Antibiotics are commonly administered postoperatively to prevent infection. If antibiotic agents are prescribed, serum creatinine and BUN values must be monitored closely because many antibiotic agents are toxic to the kidney or can accumulate to toxic levels if kidney function is decreased.

Preventing fluid imbalance is critical when caring for a patient undergoing kidney surgery, because both fluid loss and fluid excess are possible adverse effects of the surgery. Fluid loss may occur during surgery as a result of excessive urinary drainage when the obstruction is removed, or it may occur if diuretic agents are used. Such loss may also occur with GI losses, with diarrhea resulting from antibiotic use, or with nasogastric drainage. When postoperative IV therapy is inadequate to match the output or fluids lost, a fluid deficit results. Fluid excess, or overload, may result from cardiac effects of anesthesia, administration of excessive amounts of fluids, or the patient's inability to excrete fluid because of changes in kidney function. Decreased urine output may be an indication of fluid excess.

Plan of Nursing Care

Chart 45-12. Care of Patient Undergoing Kidney Surgery

Nursing Priority: Airway clearance
Goal: Improved airway clearance

NURSING INTERVENTIONS	RATIONALE
1. Administer analgesic agent as prescribed.	1. Enables patient to take deep breaths and cough
2. Splint incision with hands or pillow to assist patient in coughing.	2. Splints incision and promotes adequate cough and prevention of atelectasis
3. Assist patient to change positions frequently.	3. Promotes drainage and inflation of all lobes of the lungs
4. Encourage use of incentive spirometer if indicated or prescribed.	4. Encourages adequate deep breaths
5. Assist with and encourage early ambulation.	5. Mobilizes pulmonary secretions

EXPECTED OUTCOMES

- Takes deep breaths and coughs adequately when encouraged and assisted
- Exhibits respiratory rate of 12–18 breaths/min
- Exhibits normal breath sounds without adventitious sounds
- Exhibits full thoracic excursion without shallow respirations
- Uses incentive spirometer with encouragement
- Splints incision while taking deep breaths and coughing
- Reports progressively less pain and discomfort with coughing and deep breaths
- Exhibits normal blood gas levels and chest x-ray
- Exhibits normal body temperature with no signs of atelectasis or pneumonia on assessment

Nursing Priority: Acute pain and discomfort
Goal: Relief of pain and discomfort

NURSING INTERVENTIONS	RATIONALE
1. Assess level of pain.	1. Provides baseline for later evaluation of pain relief strategies
2. Administer analgesic agents as prescribed.	2. Promotes pain relief
3. Splint incision with hands or pillow during movement or deep breathing and coughing exercises.	3. Minimizes sensation of pulling or tension on incision and provides sense of support to the patient
4. Assist and encourage early ambulation.	4. Promotes resumption of muscle activity exercise

EXPECTED OUTCOMES

- Reports relief of severe pain and discomfort
- Takes analgesia as prescribed
- Exercises aching muscles within recommendations
- Uses distraction, relaxation exercises, and imagery to relieve pain
- Exhibits no behavioural manifestations of pain and discomfort (e.g., restlessness, perspiration, verbal expressions of pain)
- Participates in deep breathing and coughing exercises
- Gradually increases physical activity and exercise

Nursing Priority: Fear and anxiety
Goal: Reduction of fear and anxiety

NURSING INTERVENTIONS	RATIONALE
1. Assess patient's anxiety and fear before surgery if possible.	1. Provides a baseline for postoperative assessment
2. Assess patient's knowledge about procedure and expected surgical outcome preoperatively.	2. Provides a basis for further teaching
3. Evaluate the meaning of alterations resulting from surgical procedure for the patient and family or partner.	3. Enables understanding of patient's reactions and responses to expected and unexpected results of surgery
4. Encourage patient to verbalize reactions, feelings, and fears.	4. Affirms patient's understanding of and ultimate resolution of feelings and fears
5. Encourage patient to share feelings with spouse or partner.	5. Enables patient and partner to receive mutual support and reduces sense of isolation from each other

EXPECTED OUTCOMES

- Verbalizes reactions and feelings to staff
- Shares reactions and feelings with family or partner
- Grieves appropriately for self and for changes in role and function
- Identifies information needed to promote own adaptation and coping
- Participates in activities and events in immediate environment
- Accepts visit from ostomy group if indicated
- Identifies support person or support group

continued >

Plan of Nursing Care — Chart 45-12. Care of Patient Undergoing Kidney Surgery, *Continued*

NURSING INTERVENTIONS	RATIONALE
6. Offer and arrange for visit from member of support group (e.g., ostomy group, if indicated).	6. Provides support from another person who has encountered the same or a similar surgical procedure and an example of how others have coped with the alteration

Nursing Priority: Urinary elimination.
Goal: Maintenance of urinary elimination; infection-free urinary tract

NURSING INTERVENTIONS	RATIONALE
1. Assess urinary drainage system immediately.	1. Provides basis for further assessment and action
2. Assess adequacy of urinary output and patency of drainage system.	2. Provides baseline
3. Use asepsis and hand hygiene when providing care and manipulating drainage system.	3. Prevents or reduces risk of contamination of urinary drainage system
4. Maintain closed urinary drainage system.	4. Reduces risk of bacterial contamination and infection
5. If irrigation of the drainage system is necessary, use sterile gloves and sterile irrigating solution and a closed drainage and irrigation system.	5. Permits irrigation when necessary while maintaining closed drainage system, minimizing risk of infection
6. If irrigation is necessary and prescribed, perform it gently with sterile saline and the prescribed amount of irrigating fluid.	6. Maintains patency of the catheter or drainage system and prevents sudden increases in pressure in the urinary tract that may cause trauma, pressure on sutures or urinary tract structures, and pain
7. Assist patient in turning and moving in bed and when ambulating to prevent displacement or inadvertent removal of urinary stent or ureteral catheters if in place.	7. Prevents trauma from accidental displacement of urinary stent or ureteral catheter necessitating repeated instrumentation of the urinary tract (e.g., cystoscopy) to replace them
8. Observe urine colour, volume, odour, and components.	8. Provides information about adequacy of urine output, condition and patency of drainage system, and debris in urine
9. Minimize trauma and manipulation of catheter, drainage system, and urethra.	9. Reduces risk of contamination of drainage system and eliminates site of bacterial invasion
10. Clean catheter gently with soap during bath, avoiding any to-and-fro movement of catheter.	10. Removes debris and encrustations without causing trauma to or contamination of urethra
11. Anchor drainage tube.	11. Prevents movement or slipping of drainage tube, minimizing trauma to and contamination of urethra or catheter
12. Maintain adequate fluid intake.	12. Promotes adequate urine output and prevents urinary stasis
13. Assist with and encourage early ambulation while ensuring placement of urinary drainage system.	13. Minimizes cardiovascular and pulmonary complications while preventing loss, dislodging, or disruption of drainage system
14. If patient is to be discharged with urinary drainage system (catheter) in place or a urinary diversion, instruct patient and family member in care.	14. Knowledge and understanding of the drainage system or urinary diversion are essential to prevent infection and other complications

EXPECTED OUTCOMES

- Exhibits adequate urinary output and patent drainage system
- Exhibits urinary output consistent with fluid intake
- Demonstrates normal laboratory values: BUN, serum creatinine levels, urine specific gravity, and osmolality
- Exhibits sterile urine on urine culture
- Exhibits clear, dilute urine without debris or encrustation in the drainage system
- States rationale for avoiding manipulation of catheter, drainage, or irrigation system
- Exhibits normal placement of urinary stent or ureteral catheters until removed by physician
- Maintains closed urinary drainage system
- Exhibits normal body temperature without signs or symptoms of urinary tract infection
- Cleans catheter with soap and water
- Consumes adequate fluid intake (six to eight glasses of water or more per day, unless contraindicated)
- Urinary drainage system remains in place until physician removes or discontinues it
- Maintains urinary drainage system without infection or obstruction
- Maintains urinary diversion as instructed
- Maintains self-care so that environment is odour-free
- States rationale for close follow-up and maintains recommended schedule of appointments with health care providers

Plan of Nursing Care — Chart 45-12. Care of Patient Undergoing Kidney Surgery, *Continued*

NURSING INTERVENTIONS	RATIONALE	EXPECTED OUTCOMES
Nursing Priority: Fluid and electrolyte balance **Goal:** Normal fluid balance will be maintained		
1. Weigh patient daily.	1. Daily weight is the most sensitive indicator of fluid loss or gain	• Patient's weight will be within 2–3 lb of patient's baseline
2. Take accurate intake and output measurements.	2. Detects fluid retention due to poor cardiac or kidney output	• Intake that exceeds output will be detected early
3. Place all parenteral therapy on an infusion pump.	3. Ensures that the patient does not receive excess or insufficient intravenous fluids	• The exact amount of solution is infused with no adverse effects resulting from overinfusion or underinfusion
4. Monitor amount and characteristics of urine.	4. Assists in early detection of possible complications of surgery or tube insertion	• Urine is clear and absent of blood, pus, or any foreign substances
5. Monitor vital signs: temperature, pulse, respirations, and blood pressure.	5. When fluid volume or cardiac output is altered, vital signs are affected	• Temperature, pulse, respiration, and blood pressure are normal
6. Auscultate heart and lungs every shift.	6. When fluid volume is increased because of poor cardiac or kidney output, fluid accumulates in the lungs. Also, heart sounds change as heart failure develops; frequent auscultation ensures early detection.	• Normal heart and lung sounds are present

Astute assessment skills are needed to detect early signs of fluid excess, such as weight gain, pedal edema, urine output below 30 mL/hr, and slightly elevated pulmonary wedge pressure (if available) before they become severe. Appearance of adventitious breath sounds and shortness of breath also indicate fluid overload.

Fluid excess may be treated with fluid restriction and administration of furosemide (Lasix) or other diuretic agents. If kidney insufficiency is present, these medications may prove ineffective; therefore, dialysis may be necessary to prevent heart failure and pulmonary edema.

Deep venous thrombosis (DVT) may occur postoperatively because of surgical manipulation of the iliac vessels during surgery or prolonged immobility. Antiembolism stockings are applied, and the patient is monitored closely for signs and symptoms of thrombosis and encouraged to exercise the legs. Heparin may be administered postoperatively to reduce the risk of thrombosis.

Promoting Home, Community-Based, and Transitional Care

Educating Patients About Self-Care

If the patient has a drainage system in place, measures are taken to ensure that both the patient and family understand the importance of maintaining the system correctly at home and preventing infection. Verbal and written instructions and guidelines are provided to the patient and family at the time of hospital discharge. The patient may be asked to demonstrate management of the drainage system to ensure understanding. The importance of strategies to prevent postoperative complications (UTI and obstruction, DVT, atelectasis, and pneumonia) is stressed to the patient and family. Those signs, symptoms, problems, and questions that should be referred to the physician or other primary health care provider are reviewed by the nurse with the patient and family.

Continuing and Transitional Care

The need for postoperative assessment and care after kidney surgery continues regardless of the setting: the home, subacute care unit, outpatient clinic or office, or rehabilitation facility. Referral for home care is indicated for the patient going home with a urinary drainage system in place. During the home visit, the home care nurse reviews the instructions and guidelines given to the patient at hospital discharge. The nurse assesses the patient's ability to carry out the instructions in the home and answers questions that the patient or family has about management of the drainage system and the surgical incision.

In addition, the home care nurse obtains vital signs and assesses the patient for signs and symptoms of UTI and obstruction. The nurse also ensures that pain is adequately controlled and that the patient is complying with recommendations. The home care nurse encourages adequate fluid intake and increased levels of activity. Together the nurse, patient, and family review the signs, symptoms, problems, and questions that should be referred to the physician or other primary health care provider. If the patient has a drainage tube in place, the nurse assesses the site and the patency of the system and monitors the patient for complications, such as DVT, bleeding, or pneumonia.

Because it is easy for the patient, family, and health care team to focus on the patient's immediate disorder to the exclusion of other health issues, the nurse reminds the patient and family about the importance of participating in health promotion activities, including health screening.

Kidney Transplantation

Kidney transplantation has become the treatment of choice for most patients with ESKD. At the end of 2016, there were 37,647 Canadians (excluding Quebec) living with ESKD; also by the end of that year, 1,731 Canadians underwent kidney transplantation, including simultaneous kidney–pancreas transplants, which was an increase of 33% since 2007 (CIHI, 2018).

Patients choose kidney transplantation for various reasons, such as the desire to avoid dialysis or to improve their sense of well-being and the wish to lead a more normal life. In addition, the cost of maintaining a successful transplantation is one third the cost of dialysis treatment. Kidney transplantation is an elective procedure, not an emergency life-saving procedure. Therefore, patients should be in the best possible condition prior to transplantation.

Kidney transplantation involves transplanting a kidney from a living donor or deceased donor to a recipient who no longer has kidney function (Chart 45-13). A living donor is a person who is alive at the time of donation and may or may not be related to the recipient. A deceased or cadaveric transplant comes from someone who has died and donated his or her organs. Transplantation from well-matched living donors who are related to the patient (those with compatible ABO and human leukocyte antigens) is slightly more successful than from cadaver donors. Prior to either receiving or donating an organ, an extensive medical evaluation is performed. Not everyone is suitable for a kidney transplant. Contraindications include recent malignancy, active or chronic infection, severe irreversible extrarenal disease (e.g., inoperable cardiac disease, chronic lung disease, severe peripheral vascular disease), active autoimmune disease (e.g., HIV, hepatitis B and C), morbid obesity (body mass index greater than 35), current substance abuse, inability to give informed consent, and history of nonadherence to treatment regimens. Donors may be rejected for the same reasons or any condition that is determined to have an impact on the remaining kidney. Examples include hypertension and diabetes mellitus since both are known causes of kidney disease. It is imperative when donors are evaluated that serious consideration be given to the overall long-term health of the donor. Every precaution must be taken to ensure that the remaining kidney in the donor will remain healthy. If these conditions are met, the donor should remain healthy after donation and have a normal lifespan. Since one kidney can easily handle the body's needs, no long-term adjustments will need to be made.

The recipient's native kidneys are not usually removed. The transplanted kidney is placed in the patient's iliac fossa anterior to the iliac crest because it allows for easier access to the blood supply needed to perfuse the kidney. The ureter of the newly transplanted kidney is transplanted into the bladder or anastomosed to the ureter of the recipient (Fig. 45-10). Once the blood supply has been reestablished

CHART 45-13

Kidney Donation

An inadequate number of available kidneys remains the greatest limitation to treating patients with end-stage kidney disease successfully. For those interested in donating a kidney, the National Kidney Foundation provides written information describing the organ donation program and a card specifying the organs to be donated in the event of death.

The organ donation card is signed by the donor and two witnesses and should be carried by the donor at all times. Procurement of an adequate number of kidneys for potential recipients is still a major problem, despite national legislation that requires relatives of deceased patients or patients declared brain-dead to be asked if they would consider organ donation.

In some states in the United States, drivers can indicate their desire to be organ donors on their driver's license application on renewal.

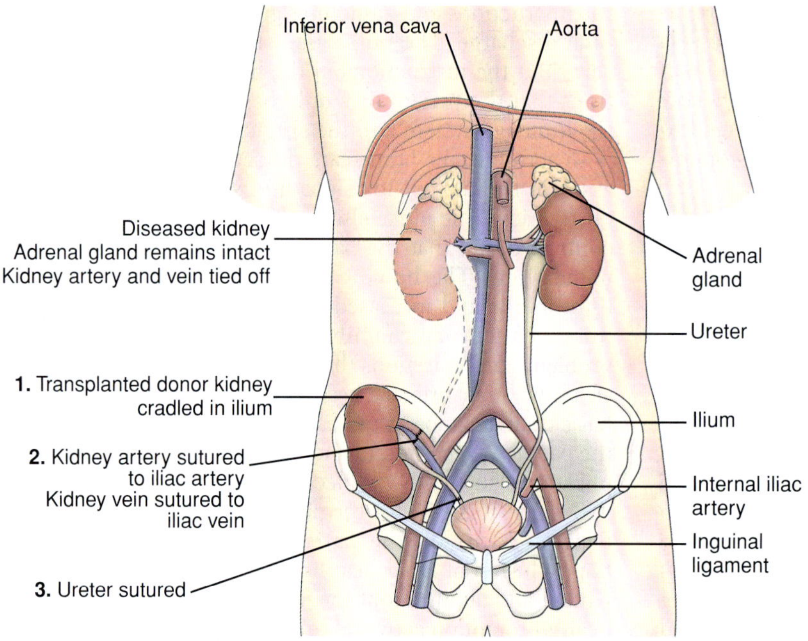

FIGURE 45-10. Kidney transplantation: **1**, The transplanted kidney is placed in the iliac fossa. **2**, The kidney artery of the donated kidney is sutured to the ileac artery, and the kidney vein is sutured to the iliac vein. **3**, The ureter of the donated kidney is sutured to the bladder or to the patient's ureter.

CHART 45-14

Kidney Transplant Rejection and Infection

Kidney graft rejection and failure may occur within 24 hours (hyperacute), within 3 to 14 days (acute), or after many years (chronic). It is not uncommon for rejection to occur during the first year after transplantation.

Detecting Rejection

Ultrasonography may be used to detect enlargement of the kidney; percutaneous kidney biopsy (most reliable) and x-ray techniques are used to evaluate transplant rejection. If the body rejects the transplanted kidney, the patient needs to return to dialysis. The rejected kidney may or may not be removed, depending on when the rejection occurs (acute vs. chronic) and the risk for infection if the kidney is left in place.

Potential Infection

About 75% of kidney transplant recipients have at least one episode of infection in the first year after transplantation because of immunosuppressant therapy. Immunosuppressants of the past made the transplant recipient more vulnerable to opportunistic infections (candidiasis, cytomegalovirus, *Pneumocystis* pneumonia) and infection with other relatively nonpathogenic viruses, fungi, and protozoa, which can be a major hazard. Cyclosporine therapy has reduced the incidence of opportunistic infections because it selectively exerts its effect, sparing T cells that protect the patient from life-threatening infections. In addition, combination immunosuppressant therapy and improved clinical care have produced 1-year patient survival rates approaching 100% and graft survival exceeding 90%. Infections, however, remain a major cause of death at all points in time for kidney transplant recipients.

Adapted from Colaneri, J. (2014). An overview of transplant immunosuppression—History, principles, and current practices in kidney transplantation. *Nephrology Nursing Journal*, *41*(6), 549–560.

to the transplanted kidney in the operating room, urine should begin to flow. The production of urine at this stage is an important indicator of the overall success of the procedure and ultimate long-term outcome.

Preoperative Management

Preoperative management goals include bringing the patient's metabolic state to a level as close to normal as possible, making sure that the patient is free of infection, and preparing the patient for surgery and the postoperative course.

Medical Management

A complete physical examination is performed on the donor and the recipient to detect and treat any conditions that could cause complications after the donor and transplantation procedure. Tissue typing, blood typing, and antibody screening are performed to determine compatibility of the tissues and cells of the donor and recipient. Other diagnostic tests must be completed to identify conditions requiring treatment before transplantation for either individual. The lower urinary tract is studied to assess bladder neck function and to detect ureteral reflux.

Both patients must be free of infection at the time of kidney transplantation. After surgery, medications to prevent transplant rejection will be prescribed to the transplant recipient. These medications suppress the immune response, leaving the patient immunosuppressed and at risk for infection. Therefore, both the donor and recipient are evaluated and treated for any infections, including gingival (gum) disease and dental caries.

A psychosocial evaluation is conducted to assess the organ recipient's ability to adjust to the transplant, coping styles, social history, social support available, and financial resources. A history of psychiatric illness is important to obtain because psychiatric conditions are often aggravated by the corticosteroids needed for immunosuppression after transplantation (Colaneri, 2014). A psychosocial evaluation is also conducted to assess the organ donor's motive for giving the organ. The donor should not be coerced to donate this organ; it should be an altruistic act (Choudhury, Jotterand, Casenave, et al., 2014; Robbins, 2014) (see Chart 45-14). If a dialysis routine has been established, hemodialysis is often performed the day before the scheduled transplantation procedure to optimize the physical status of the patient receiving the transplant.

Nursing Management

The nursing aspects of preoperative care for the patient undergoing kidney transplant are similar to those for patients undergoing other types of kidney or elective abdominal surgery. Preoperative teaching can be conducted in a variety of settings, including the outpatient preadmission area, the hospital, or the transplantation clinic during the preliminary workup phase. Patient teaching addresses postoperative pulmonary hygiene, pain management options, dietary restrictions, IV and arterial lines, tubes (indwelling catheter and possibly a nasogastric tube), and early ambulation. The patient who receives a kidney from a living related donor may be concerned about the donor and how the donor will tolerate the surgical procedure.

Most patients have been on dialysis for months or years before transplantation. Many have waited months to years for a kidney transplant and are anxious about the surgery, possible rejection, and the need to return to dialysis. Helping the patient to deal with these concerns is part of the nurse's role in preoperative management, as is teaching the patient about what to expect after surgery.

Postoperative Management

The goal of care is to maintain homeostasis until the transplanted kidney is functioning well. The patient whose kidney functions immediately has a more favourable prognosis than the patient whose kidney does not.

Medical Management

After a kidney transplantation, rejection and failure can occur within 24 hours (hyperacute), within 3 to 14 days (acute), or after many years. A hyperacute rejection is caused by an immediate antibody-mediated reaction that leads to generalized glomerular capillary thrombosis and necrosis. An acute rejection typically occurs within a few days to weeks of the transplant surgery, and the patient experiences tenderness at the transplant site, a decrease in serum creatinine values, fever, malaise, and oliguria (Colaneri, 2014). An acute rejection requires early recognition and treatment with immunosuppressant therapy, whereas a hyperacute reaction requires immediate removal of the transplanted organ (Colaneri, 2014). The long-term survival of a transplanted kidney depends on how well it matches the recipient and how well the body's immune response is controlled. The body's immune system views the transplanted kidney as "foreign"; therefore, it continually works to reject it. To overcome or minimize the body's defence mechanisms, immunosuppressive agents are given. Optimally, medications modify the immune system enough to prevent rejection, although not enough to allow infections or malignancies to occur (see Table 45-4).

Combinations of corticosteroids and medications specifically developed to affect the action of lymphocytes are used to minimize the body's reaction to the transplanted organ. Treatment with combinations of new agents has dramatically improved survival rates, and now 90% to 95% of transplanted kidneys still function after 1 year (Colaneri, 2014). Doses of immunosuppressive agents are often adjusted depending on the patient's immunologic response to the transplant. However, the patient will be required to take some form of immunosuppressive therapy for the entire time that they have the transplanted kidney.

The risks associated with taking these medications include nephrotoxicity, hypertension, hyperlipidemia, hirsutism, tremors, blood dyscrasias, cataracts, gingival hyperplasia, and several types of cancer (Colaneri, 2014).

Nursing Management

Assessing the Patient for Transplant Rejection

After kidney transplantation, the nurse assesses the patient for signs and symptoms of transplant rejection: oliguria, edema, fever, increasing blood pressure, weight gain, and swelling or tenderness over the transplanted kidney or graft. Patients receiving cyclosporine may not exhibit the usual signs and symptoms of acute rejection. In these patients, the only sign may be an asymptomatic rise in the serum creatinine level (more than a 20% rise is considered acute rejection) (Colaneri, 2014).

Preventing Infection

The results of blood chemistry tests and leukocyte and platelet counts are monitored closely because immunosuppression depresses the formation of leukocytes and platelets. The patient is closely monitored for infection because of susceptibility to impaired healing and infection related to immunosuppressive therapy and complications of kidney failure. Clinical manifestations of infection include shaking chills, fever, tachycardia, and tachypnea, as well as either an increase or a decrease in WBCs (leukocytosis or leukopenia).

Infection may be introduced through the urinary tract, the respiratory tract, the surgical site, or other sources. Urine cultures are performed frequently because of the high incidence of bacteriuria during early and late stages of transplantation. Any type of wound drainage should be viewed as a potential source of infection because drainage is an excellent culture medium for bacteria. Catheter and drain tips may be cultured when removed by cutting off the tip of the catheter or drain (using aseptic technique) and placing the tip in a sterile container to be taken to the laboratory for culture (Chart 45-14).

The nurse ensures that the patient is protected from exposure to infection by hospital staff, visitors, and other patients with active infections. Attention to hand hygiene by all who come in contact with the patient is imperative.

Monitoring Urinary Function

A kidney from a living donor related to the patient usually begins to function immediately after surgery and may produce large quantities of dilute urine. A kidney from a cadaver donor may undergo ATN and therefore may not function for 2 or 3 weeks, during which time anuria, oliguria, or polyuria may be present. During this stage, the patient may experience significant changes in fluid and electrolyte status. Therefore, careful monitoring is indicated. The output from the urinary catheter (connected to a closed drainage system) is measured every hour. IV fluids are administered on the basis of urine volume and serum electrolyte levels and as prescribed by the physician. Hemodialysis may be necessary postoperatively to maintain homeostasis until the transplanted kidney is functioning well. It may also be required if fluid overload and hyperkalemia occur. After successful kidney transplantation, the vascular access device may clot, possibly from improved coagulation with the return of kidney function. The vascular access for hemodialysis is monitored to ensure patency and to evaluate for evidence of infection.

Addressing Psychological Concerns

The rejection of a transplanted kidney is of great concern to the patient, the family, and the health care team for many months. The fear of kidney rejection and the complications of immunosuppressive therapy (Cushing's syndrome, diabetes, capillary fragility, osteoporosis, glaucoma, cataracts, acne, nephrotoxicity) place tremendous psychological stress on the patient. Anxiety and uncertainty about the future and difficult posttransplantation adjustment are often sources of stress for the patient and family.

An important nursing function is the assessment of the patient's stress and coping. The nurse uses each visit with the patient to determine if the patient and family are coping effectively and the patient is adhering to the prescribed medication regimen. If indicated or requested, the nurse refers the patient for counselling.

Monitoring and Managing Potential Complications

The patient undergoing kidney transplantation is at risk for the postoperative complications that are associated

TABLE 45-4 Immunosuppressive Agents Used Following Organ Transplant

Agent	Action	Nursing Implications
azathioprine (Azasan, Imuran)	Antagonizes purine metabolism and appears to inhibit DNA, RNA, and normal protein synthesis in rapidly growing cells; suppresses T-cell effects	Give oral drug in divided doses with food. Monitor leukocyte and platelet counts and bleeding.
belatacept (Nulojix)	Inhibition of T-lymphocyte proliferation and cytokine production	Contraindicated in patients with EBV seronegativity or unknown EBV serostatus, liver transplantation, breast-feeding. Monitor for symptoms of infection, hypertension, progressive multifocal leukoencephalopathy. Administer IV.
cyclosporine (Gengraf, Neoral, Sandimmune)	Selective and reversible inhibition of first phase of T-cell activation with T lymphocytes	Do not dilute oral solution with grapefruit juice (use orange juice, regular or chocolate milk, or apple juice and administer immediately after mixing). Observe for adverse reactions for 30 minutes after initiation of the IV infusion. Be aware that nephrotoxicity is reported in up to 1/3 of transplant recipients. Give medication with food to reduce gastrointestinal upset. Administer medication at the same time each day.
everolimus (Afinitor, Zortress)	Protein–tyrosine kinase inhibitor	Monitor for hypersensitivity reaction. Watch for changes in pulmonary status and cough. Avoid administration of live vaccines. Administer at the same time each day with food; do not crush or allow patient to chew tablet.
mycophenolate mofetil (CellCept) mycophenolic acid (Myfortic)	Inhibition of T- and B-lymphocyte responses, thus inhibiting antibody formation and generation of cytotoxic T cells	Administer on an empty stomach. Do not crush or open capsules. Avoid contact with powder in capsules; wash thoroughly with soap and water if contact occurs. Obtain baseline complete blood count with differential prior to initiating therapy. Instruct the patient to avoid over-the-counter antacids.
prednisone (Apo-Prednisone, Deltasone, Orasone, Panasol, Winpred)	Immediate-acting synthetic analog of hydrocortisone that has anti-inflammatory and immunosuppressant properties	Give with meals or a snack. Crush tablet and give with fluid if patient is unable to swallow it whole. Note that the drug should not be stopped abruptly; the dosage is reduced gradually. Monitor weight, blood pressure, blood glucose levels, and sleep patterns. Monitor for hypocalcemia. Instruct patient to avoid or minimize alcohol intake.
sirolimus (Rapamune)	Inhibits the response of helper T and B lymphocytes	Administer 4 hours after oral cyclosporine. Instruct patient to swallow tablets whole and to avoid chewing or crushing tablets. Refrigerate drug and protect from light. Instruct patient to avoid grapefruit juice within 2 hours of taking drug and to mix the drug only with orange juice or water. Instruct the patient to limit exposure to sunlight.
tacrolimus (Prograf)	Inhibits helper T lymphocytes	Monitor for neurotoxicity (tremors and changes in mental status). Assess for hypertension. Monitor tacrolimus levels.

DNA, deoxyribonucleic acid; RNA, ribonucleic acid; EBV, Epstein–Barr virus; IV, intravenous.

Adapted from Comerford, K. C. (2015). *Nursing 2015 drug handbook*. Philadelphia, PA: Wolters Kluwer.

with any surgical procedure. In addition, the patient's physical condition may be compromised because of the effects of long-standing kidney failure and its treatment. Therefore, careful assessment for the complications related to kidney failure and those associated with a major surgery are important aspects of nursing care. Breathing exercises, early ambulation, and care of the surgical incision are important aspects of postoperative care.

GI ulceration and corticosteroid-induced bleeding may occur. Fungal colonization of the GI tract (especially the mouth) and urinary bladder may occur secondary to corticosteroid and antibiotic therapy. Closely monitoring the patient and notifying the physician about the occurrence of these complications are important nursing interventions. In addition, the patient is monitored closely for signs and symptoms of adrenal insufficiency if the treatment has included use of corticosteroids.

Promoting Home, Community-Based, and Transitional Care

Educating Patients About Self-Care

The nurse works closely with the patient and family to be sure that they understand the need for continuing immunosuppressive therapy as prescribed. In addition, the patient and family are instructed to assess for and report signs and symptoms of transplant rejection, infection, or significant adverse effects of the immunosuppressive regimen. These include decreased urine output; weight gain; malaise; fever; respiratory distress; tenderness over the transplanted kidney; anxiety; depression; changes in eating, drinking, or other habits; and changes in blood pressure. The patient is instructed to inform other health care providers (e.g., dentist) about the kidney transplant and the use of immunosuppressive agents.

Continuing and Transitional Care

The patient needs to know that follow-up care after transplantation is a lifelong necessity. Individual verbal and written instructions are provided concerning diet, medication, fluids, daily weight, daily measurement of urine, management of I&O, prevention of infection, resumption of activity, and avoidance of contact sports in which the transplanted kidney may be injured. Because of the risk for other potential complications, the patient is followed closely.

Cardiovascular disease is the major cause of morbidity and mortality after transplantation, due in part to the increasing age of patients with transplants. An additional problem is possible malignancy; patients receiving long-term immunosuppressive therapy are at higher risk for cancers than the general population. So the patient is reminded of the importance of health promotion and health screening.

The Kidney Foundation of Canada and its provincial branches provide information and support to patients with kidney disease and their families.

It can provide many helpful suggestions for patients and family members learning to cope with dialysis and transplantation.

KIDNEY TRAUMA

The kidneys are protected by the rib cage and musculature of the back posteriorly and by a cushion of abdominal wall and viscera anteriorly. They are highly mobile and are fixed only at the kidney pedicle (stem of kidney blood vessels and the ureter). With traumatic injury, the kidneys can be thrust against the lower ribs, resulting in contusion and rupture. Rib fractures or fractures of the transverse process of the upper lumbar vertebrae may be associated with kidney contusion or laceration. Failure to wear seat belts contributes to the incidence of kidney trauma in motor vehicle crashes. Up to 80% of patients with kidney trauma have associated injuries of other internal organs.

Injuries may be blunt (automobile and motorcycle crashes, falls, athletic injuries, assaults) or penetrating (gunshot wounds, stabbings). Blunt kidney trauma accounts for 80% to 90% of all kidney injuries; penetrating kidney trauma accounts for the remaining 10% to 20%.

Blunt kidney trauma is classified into one of four groups, as follows:

- Contusion: bruises or hemorrhages under the kidney capsule; capsule and collecting system intact
- Minor laceration: superficial disruption of the cortex; kidney medulla and collecting system are not involved
- Major laceration: parenchymal disruption extending into cortex and medulla, possibly involving the collecting system
- Vascular injury: tears of kidney artery or vein

The most common kidney injuries are contusions, lacerations, ruptures, and kidney pedicle injuries or small internal lacerations of the kidney (Fig. 45-11). The kidneys receive half of the blood flow from the abdominal aorta; therefore, even a fairly small kidney laceration can produce massive bleeding. About 70% of patients are in shock when admitted to the hospital. In some cases, there is an isolated kidney artery thrombosis.

Clinical manifestations include pain, kidney colic (due to blood clots or fragments obstructing the collecting system), hematuria, mass or swelling in the flank, ecchymoses, and lacerations or wounds of the lateral abdomen and flank. Hematuria is the most common manifestation of kidney trauma; its presence after trauma suggests kidney injury. There is no relationship between the degree of hematuria and the degree of injury. Hematuria may not occur, or it may be detectable only on microscopic examination. Signs and symptoms of hypovolemia and shock are likely with significant hemorrhage.

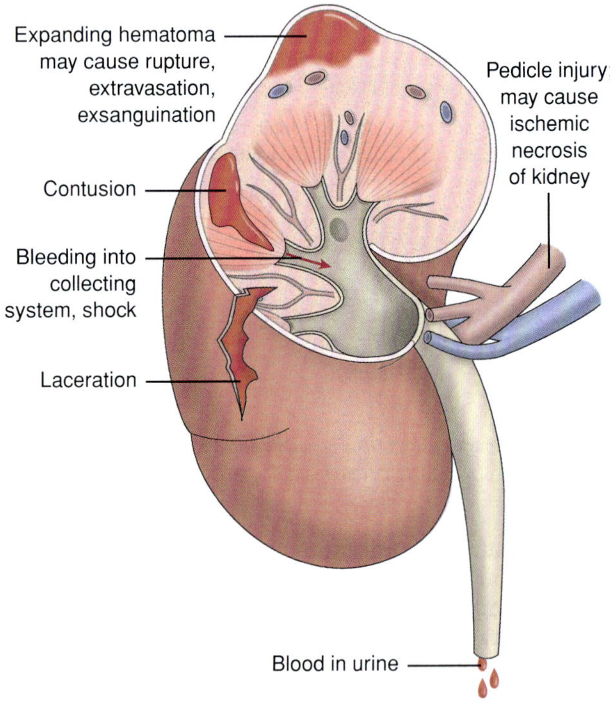

FIGURE 45-11. Types and pathophysiologic effects of kidney injuries: contusions, lacerations, rupture, and pedicle injury.

Medical Management

The goals of management in patients with kidney trauma are to control hemorrhage, pain, and infection as well as to preserve and restore kidney function. All urine is saved and sent to the laboratory for analysis to detect RBCs and to evaluate the course of bleeding. Hematocrit and hemoglobin levels are monitored closely; decreasing values indicate hemorrhage.

The patient is monitored for oliguria and signs of hemorrhagic shock, because a pedicle injury or shattered kidney can lead to rapid exsanguination. An expanding hematoma may cause rupture of the kidney capsule. To detect hematoma, the area around the lower ribs, upper lumbar vertebrae, flank, and abdomen is palpated for tenderness. A palpable flank or abdominal mass with local tenderness, swelling, and ecchymosis suggests kidney hemorrhage. The area of the original mass can be outlined with a marking pen so that the examiner can evaluate the area for change.

Kidney trauma is often associated with other injuries to the abdominal organs (liver, colon, small intestines); therefore, the patient is assessed for skin abrasions, lacerations, and entry and exit wounds of the upper abdomen and lower thorax because these may be associated with kidney injury.

With a contusion of the kidney, healing may take place with conservative measures. If the patient has microscopic hematuria and a normal IV urogram, outpatient management is possible. If gross hematuria or a minor laceration is present, the patient is hospitalized and kept on bed rest until the hematuria clears. Antimicrobial medications may be prescribed to prevent infection from perirenal hematoma or urinoma (a cyst containing urine). Patients with retroperitoneal hematomas may develop low-grade fever as absorption of the clot takes place.

Surgical Management

In kidney trauma, any sudden change in the patient's condition suggests hemorrhage and requires rapid surgical intervention. Depending on the patient's condition and the nature of the injury, major lacerations may be treated through surgical intervention or conservatively (bed rest, no surgery). Vascular injuries require immediate exploratory surgery because of the high incidence of involvement of other organ systems and the serious complications that may result if these injuries are untreated. The patient is often in shock and requires aggressive fluid resuscitation. The damaged kidney may have to be removed (nephrectomy).

Early postoperative complications (within 6 months) include rebleeding, perinephritic abscess formation, sepsis, urine extravasation, and fistula formation. Other complications include stone formation, infection, cysts, vascular aneurysms, and loss of kidney function. Hypertension can be a complication of any kidney surgery but usually is a late complication of kidney injury.

Nursing Management

The patient with kidney trauma must be assessed frequently during the first few days after injury to detect flank and abdominal pain, muscle spasm, and swelling over the flank. During this time, the patient who has undergone surgery is instructed about care of the incision and the importance of an adequate fluid intake. In addition, instructions about changes that should be reported to the physician, such as fever, hematuria, flank pain, or any signs and symptoms of decreasing kidney function, are provided. Guidelines for gradually increasing activity, lifting, and driving are also provided in accordance with the physician's prescription.

Follow-up nursing care includes monitoring the blood pressure to detect hypertension and advising the patient to restrict activities for about 1 month after trauma to minimize the incidence of delayed or secondary bleeding. The patient should be advised to schedule periodic follow-up assessments of kidney function (creatinine clearance, BUN, and serum creatinine analyses). If a nephrectomy was necessary, the patient is advised to wear medical identification.

Critical Thinking Exercises

1 You are a staff nurse in an outpatient dialysis facility. A 50-year-old woman with ESKD is scheduled to be seen in the clinic; it is anticipated that she will need dialysis in the near future. The patient lives alone and will require teaching about the dialysis options. Develop a teaching plan to explain the different types of dialysis, goals, and level of involvement on the part of the patient.

2 A 45-year-old married man visits the nephrology department to discuss options for dealing with his ESKD. His brother has begun the workup to donate one of his kidneys and the preliminary reports show that a match is possible. The patient states that he does not want his brother to go through the process of kidney donation if dialysis is possible. Identify the evidence for and the criteria used to evaluate the strength of the evidence for dialysis compared to kidney transplantation.

3 You are caring for a 35-year-old woman who has been recently diagnosed with kidney cancer. Identify possible treatment options. What nursing assessment and interventions should you make at this time? What explanations would you give the patient about kidney cancer?

4 A 55-year-old man who is blind has just had a catheter placed for PD. His wife, his primary caretaker, is deaf. Develop a teaching plan to explain peritoneal dialysis, goals, and level of involvement to the patient and family.

REFERENCES AND SELECTED READINGS

Books

Comerford, K. C. (2015). *Nursing 2015 drug handbook*. Philadelphia, PA: Wolters Kluwer.

Hannon, R. A., & Porth, C. M. (2017). *Porth pathophysiology: Concepts of altered health states* (2nd Canadian ed.). Philadelphia, PA: Wolters Kluwer Health/Lippincott Williams & Wilkins.

Holcombe, D. M., & Feeley, N. K. (2013). Acute kidney injury and chronic kidney disease. Retrieved from http://downloads.lww.com/wolterskluwer_vitalstream_com/sample-content/9781496315625_Morton11e/samples/Morton_Ch31.pdf

McCance, K. L., & Huether, S. E. (2014). *Pathophysiology: The biologic basis for disease in adults and children*. St. Louis, Missouri: Elsevier Mosby.

Mount, D. B., & Zandi-Nejad, K. (2012). Disorders of potassium balance. In M. W. Taal, G. M. Chertow, P. A. Marsden, et al. (Eds.). *Brenner & Rector's the kidney* (9th ed., pp. 640–688). Philadelphia, PA: Elsevier.

Muzzy, A. C., & Snyder, K. A. (2013). Patient management: Renal system. In P. G. Morton, & D. K. Fontaine (Eds.). *Critical care nursing: A holistic approach* (10th ed., pp. 637–662). Philadelphia, PA: Wolters Kluwer Health/Lippincott Williams & Wilkins.

Journals and Electronic Documents

General

Ahmad, M. M., & Al Nazly, E. K. (2015). Hemodialysis: Stressors and coping strategies. *Psychology Health and Medicine, 20*(4), 477–487.

Canadian Cancer Society. (2018). *Treatments for kidney cancer*. Retrieved May 20, 2018, from http://www.cancer.ca/en/cancer-information/cancer-type/kidney/treatment/?region=sk

Canadian Cancer Society's Advisory Committee on Cancer Statistics. (2017). *Canadian cancer statistics 2017*. Toronto, ON. Retrieved May 20, 2018, from http://www.cancer.ca/~/media/cancer.ca/CW/cancer%20information/cancer%20101/Canadian%20cancer%20statistics/Canadian-Cancer-Statistics-2017-EN.pdf?la=en

Canadian Institute for Health Information, & Canadian Organ Replacement Register. (2018). *Methodological notes and supplementary information, 2007 to 2016*. Ottawa, ON: Retrieved from https://www.cihi.ca/sites/default/files/document/corr_ar-meth-notes-2017-en.pdf

Choudhury, D., Jotterand, F., Casenave, G., et al. (2014). Independent donor ethical assessment: Aiming to standardize donor advocacy. *Progress in Transplantation, 24*(2), 163–168.

CIHI. (2016). *Treatment of end-stage organ failure in Canada, Canadian Organ Replacement Register, 2005–2014*. Retrieved May 20, 2018, from https://secure.cihi.ca/free_products/2016_CORR_Snapshot_EN(web).pdf

CIHI. (2017). *Annual Statistics on Organ Replacement in Canada: Dialysis, Transplantation and Donation, 2007–2016*. Retrieved May, 2018, from https://www.cihi.ca/sites/default/files/document/corr_ar-snapshot-en.pdf

CIHI. (2018). *CORR Annual Statistics, 2007 to 2016*. Retrieved from https://www.cihi.ca/en/corr-annual-statistics-2007-to-2016

Colaneri, J. (2014). An overview of transplant immunosuppression—History, principles, and current practices in kidney transplantation. *Nephrology Nursing Journal, 41*(6), 549–560.

Davies, H., & Leslie, G. (2012). Acute kidney injury and the critically ill patient. *Dimensions of Critical Care Nursing, 31*(3), 135–152.

Deng, D., & Forbes, A. (2015). Cardiovascular risk factors in patients on dialysis. *Nephrology Nursing Journal, 42*(1), 45–50.

Doss-McQuitty, S. (2014). Strategies for removing fluids during hemodialysis. *Nephrology Nursing Journal, 41*(3), 257–263.

Dring, B., & Hipkiss, V. (2015). Managing and treating chronic kidney disease. *Nursing Times, 111*(7), 16–19.

Figueiredo, A. E. (2014). The challenges in preventing infection in peritoneal dialysis: A nurse's viewpoint. *Renal Society of Australasia Journal, 10*(3), 120–125.

James, P. A., Oparil, S., Carter, B. L, et al. (2014). 2014 Evidence-based guidelines for the management of high blood pressure in adults: Report from the panel members appointed to the Eighth Joint National Committee (JNC 8). *JAMA, 311*(5), 507–520.

Jorgensen, A. L. (2013). Contrast-induced nephropathy: Pathophysiology & preventive strategies. *Critical Care Nurse, 33*(1), 37–47.

Kane, P. M., Vinen, K., & Murtagh, F. E. (2013). Palliative care for advance renal disease: A summary of the evidence and future direction. *Palliative Medicine, 27*(9), 817–821.

Kane-Gill, S. L., Sileanu, F. E., Murugan, R., et al. (2015). Risk factors for acute kidney injury in older adults with critical illness: A retrospective cohort study. *American Journal of Kidney Diseases, 65*(6), 860–869.

The Kidney Foundation of Canada (2018). *Facing the facts: Includes highlights from the Canadian Organ Replacement Register*. Retrieved from https://www.kidney.ca/file/kidney.ca_nat/news-press-releases/2016-Facing-the-Facts.docx

Klein-Kauric, Z. (2015). Understanding hypertension in patients on hemodialysis. *Nephrology Nursing Journal, 42*(1), 69–75.

Lewis, R. (2013). An overview of chronic kidney disease in older people. *Nursing Older People, 25*(10), 31–38.

MacRae, J. M., Ahmed, S. B., & Hemmelgam, B. R. (2014). Arteriovenous fistula survival and needling technique: Long-term results from a randomized buttonhole trial. *American Journal of Kidney Disease, 63*(4), 636–642.

Owen, R. J., Hiremath, S., Myers, A., et al. (2014). Canadian Association of Radiologists consensus guidelines for the prevention of contrast-induced nephropathy: Update 2012. *Canadian Association of Radiologists Journal, 65*(2), 96–105.

Rank, W. (2013). Preventing contrast media-induced nephrotoxicity. *Nursing, 43*(4), 48–51.

Richardson, A., & Whatmore, J. (2014). Nursing essential principles: Continuous renal replacement therapy. *Nursing in Critical Care, 20*(1), 8–15.

Robbins, K. C. (2014). The independent living donor advocate: An essential role for living kidney donation. *Nephrology Nursing Journal, 41*(6), 569–586.

Sterns, R. H., Grieff, M., & Bernstein, P. L. (2016). Treatment of hyperkalemia: Something old, something new. *Kidney International, 89*(3), 546–554.

Tennankore, K. K., d'Gama, C., Faratro, R., et al. (2015). Adverse technical events in home hemodialysis. *American Journal of Kidney Diseases, 65*(1), 116–121.

Terner, M., Redding, N., & Wu, J. (2016). Increasing rates of kidney failure care in Canada strains demand for kidney donors. *Health Care Quarterly, 19*(3), 10–12.

Tonelli, M., Wiebe, N., Knoll, G., et al. (2011). Systematic review: Kidney transplantation compared with dialysis in clinically relevant outcomes. *American Journal of Transplantation, 11*(10), 2093–2109.

Vasundhara, M., Kozman, H., Liu, K., et al. (2014). Cardiac troponins: Bench to bedside interpretation in cardiac disease. *The American Journal of Medical Sciences, 347*(4), 331–337.

Vrtis, M. C. (2013). Preventing and responding to acute kidney injury. *The American Journal of Nursing, 113*(4), 38–47.

Walton, B. (2015). Chronic kidney disease. *Ohio Nurse, 8*(3), 5–6

Welch, J. L., Astroth, K. S., Perkins, S. M., et al. (2013). Using a mobile application to self-monitor diet and fluid intake among adults receiving hemodialysis. *Research in Nursing & Health, 36*(3), 284–298.

Wright, L. S., & Wilson, L. (2015). Quality of life and self-efficacy in three dialysis modalities: Incenter hemodialysis, home hemodialysis, and home peritoneal dialysis. *Nephrology Nursing Journal, 42*(5), 463–476.

Zhang, L., Hawley, C. M., & Johnson, D. W. (2016). Focus on peritoneal dialysis training: Working to decrease peritonitis rates. *Nephrology Dialysis Transplantation, 31*(2), 214–222.

Renal Replacement Therapies

Peters, A. (2014). Safety issues in home dialysis. *Nephrology Nursing Journal, 41*(1), 89–92.

Resources

Canadian Cancer Society: http://www.cancer.ca
Canadian Society of Nephrology: http://www.csnscn.ca/
Canadian Society of Transplantation: http://www.cst-transplant.ca
Canadian Urological Association: http://www.uroinfo.ca/
Kidney Cancer Research Network of Canada: https://www.kcrnc.ca/
Kidney Foundation of Canada: http://www.kidney.ca/
Polycystic Kidney Disease Foundation of Canada: http://www.endpkd.ca/

46 Management of Patients With Urinary Disorders

Adapted by Lucia New

Learning Objectives

On completion of this chapter, the learner will be able to:

1. Identify factors contributing to upper and lower urinary tract infections (UTIs).
2. Use the nursing process as a framework for care of the patient with a UTI.
3. Differentiate between the various adult dysfunctional voiding patterns.
4. Develop a patient education plan for a patient who has mixed (stress and urge) urinary incontinence.
5. Identify potential causes of an obstruction of the urinary tract and management of the patient with this condition.
6. Develop a teaching plan for the patient undergoing treatment for renal calculi (kidney stones).
7. Apply the nursing process as a framework for care of the patient with kidney stones.
8. Describe the pathophysiology, clinical manifestations, medical management, and nursing management for patients with genitourinary trauma and urinary tract cancers.
9. Use the nursing process as a framework for care of the patient undergoing urinary diversion surgery.
10. Identify pre- and postoperative nursing priorities for the patient undergoing surgery for urinary diversion.

The urinary system is responsible for providing the route for drainage of urine formed by the kidneys. The field of urologic nursing requires an understanding of the anatomy, physiology, diagnostic testing, nursing care, and rehabilitation of patients with multiple processes that interfere with the urinary system. Nurses care for patients with urologic disorders in all settings. This chapter focuses on the nursing management of patients with common urinary dysfunctions, including infections, dysfunctional voiding patterns, urolithiasis, genitourinary trauma, cancer of the urinary tract, and urinary diversions.

INFECTIONS OF THE URINARY TRACT

Urinary tract infections (UTIs) are caused by pathogenic microorganisms in the urinary tract (the normal urinary tract is sterile above the urethra). UTIs are generally classified as infections involving the upper or lower urinary tract (Chart 46-1).

Lower UTIs include bacterial **cystitis** (inflammation of the urinary bladder), bacterial **prostatitis** (inflammation of the prostate gland), and bacterial **urethritis** (inflammation of the urethra). There can be acute or chronic nonbacterial causes of inflammation in any of these areas that can be misdiagnosed as bacterial infections. Upper UTIs are much less common and include acute or chronic **pyelonephritis** (inflammation of the renal pelvis), **interstitial nephritis** (inflammation of the kidney), and renal abscesses. Upper and lower UTIs are further classified as uncomplicated or complicated, depending on other patient-related conditions (e.g., whether the UTI is recurrent and the duration of the infection). Most uncomplicated UTIs are community acquired. Complicated UTIs usually occur in people with urologic abnormalities or recent catheterization and are often hospital acquired. A UTI is the second most common reason patients seek out health care (Hannon & Porth, 2017). Women are more likely to develop a UTI than men (Gupta, Grigoryan, & Trautner, 2017). Population-based research in Canada reflects an annual incidence of community-onset UTIs of 17.5 per 1,000. Women, as well as the very old and the very young, are at increased risk. The most common organisms identified were *Escherichia coli, Staphylococcus saprophyticus, Klebsiella* species, *Enterobacter* species, *and Pseudomonas aeruginosa* (Hannon & Porth, 2017; McCance & Huether, 2014). The urinary tract is also the most common site of nosocomial infection. In most of these hospital-acquired UTIs, instrumentation of the urinary tract or catheterization is the precipitating cause.

Lower Urinary Tract Infections

Several mechanisms maintain the sterility of the bladder: the physical barrier of the urethra, urine flow, ureterovesical junction competence, various antibacterial enzymes and antibodies, and antiadherent effects mediated by the mucosal cells of the bladder. Abnormalities or dysfunctions of these mechanisms are contributing factors to lower UTIs (Chart 46-2).

Pathophysiology

For infection to occur, bacteria must gain access to the bladder, attach to and colonize the epithelium of the urinary tract to avoid being washed out with voiding, evade host defence mechanisms, and initiate inflammation. Most UTIs result from fecal organisms that ascend from the perineum to the urethra and the bladder and then adhere to the mucosal surfaces.

Bacterial Invasion of the Urinary Tract

By increasing the normal slow shedding of bladder epithelial cells (resulting in bacteria removal), the bladder can clear itself of even large numbers of bacteria. Glycosaminoglycan (GAG), a hydrophilic protein, normally exerts a nonadherent protective effect against various bacteria.

Glossary

bacteriuria: bacteria in the urine

Charleston pouch: uses the ileum and ascending colon as the pouch, with the appendix and colon junction serving as the one-way valve mechanism

continent urinary diversion (Kock or Charleston pouch): transplantation of the ureters to a segment of bowel with construction of an effective continence mechanism or valve

cystectomy: removal of the urinary bladder

cystitis: inflammation of the urinary bladder

dysuria: painful or difficult urination

frequency: voiding more often than every 3 hours

functional incontinence: physical impairments make it difficult or impossible for the patient to reach the toilet in time for voiding

iatrogenic incontinence: the involuntary loss of urine due to extrinsic medical factors, predominantly medications

ileal conduit: transplantation of the ureters to an isolated section of the terminal ileum, with one end of the ureters brought to the abdominal wall

interstitial cystitis: inflammation of the bladder wall that eventually causes disintegration of the lining and loss of bladder elasticity

interstitial nephritis: inflammation of the kidney

Kock pouch: U-shaped pouch constructed of ileum, with a nipple-like one-way valve

micturition: voiding or urination

mixed incontinence: a combination of stress and urge incontinence

neurogenic bladder: bladder dysfunction that results from a disorder or dysfunction of the nervous system; may result in either urinary retention or bladder overactivity, resulting in urinary urgency and urge incontinence

nocturia: awakening at night to urinate

overflow incontinence: involuntary urine loss associated with overdistension of the bladder due to mechanical or anatomic bladder outlet obstruction

prostatitis: inflammation of the prostate gland

pyelonephritis: inflammation of the renal pelvis

pyuria: white blood cells in the urine

reflex incontinence: involuntary loss of urine due to hyperreflexia or involuntary urethral relaxation in the absence of normal sensations; usually associated with micturition (voiding)

residual urine: urine that remains in the bladder after voiding

stress incontinence: involuntary loss of urine through an intact urethra as a result of a sudden increase in intra-abdominal pressure

suprapubic catheter: a urinary catheter that is inserted through a suprapubic incision into the bladder

ureterosigmoidostomy: transplantation of the ureters into the sigmoid colon, allowing urine to flow through the colon and out the rectum

ureterovesical or vesicoureteral reflux: backward flow of urine from the bladder into one or both ureters

urethritis: inflammation of the urethra

urethrovesical reflux: backward flow of urine from the urethra into the bladder

urge incontinence: involuntary loss of urine associated with urinary urgency due to hypersensory disorders of the bladder, motor instability, or both

urinary incontinence: involuntary or uncontrolled loss of urine from the bladder sufficient to cause a social or hygienic problem

urosepsis: sepsis resulting from infected urine, most often a urinary tract infection (UTI)

wound care specialist: a nurse specially educated in appropriate skin, wound, ostomy, and continence care; often referred to as an enterostomal therapist or a wound-ostomy-continence nurse (WOCN)

CHART 46-1

Classifying Urinary Tract Infections

Urinary tract infections (UTIs) are classified by location: the lower urinary tract (which includes the bladder and structures below the bladder) or the upper urinary tract (which includes the kidneys and ureters). They can also be classified as uncomplicated or complicated UTIs.

Lower UTIs

Cystitis, prostatitis, urethritis

Upper UTIs

Acute pyelonephritis, chronic pyelonephritis, renal abscess, interstitial nephritis, perirenal abscess

Uncomplicated Lower or Upper UTIs

Community-acquired infection; common in young women and not usually recurrent

Complicated Lower or Upper UTIs

Often nosocomial (acquired in the hospital) and related to catheterization; occur in patients with urologic abnormalities, pregnancy, immunosuppression, diabetes mellitus, and obstructions and are often recurrent

The GAG molecule attracts water molecules, forming a water barrier that serves as a defensive layer between the bladder and the urine. GAG may be impaired by certain agents (cyclamate, saccharin, aspartame, and tryptophan metabolites). The normal bacterial flora of the vagina and urethral area also interfere with adherence of *E. coli* (the most common microorganism causing UTI). Urinary immunoglobulin A (IgA) in the urethra may also provide a barrier to bacteria.

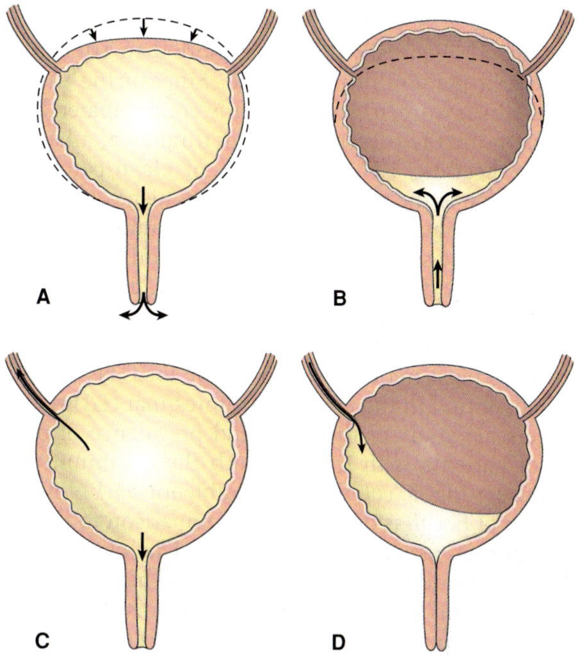

FIGURE 46-1. Mechanisms of urethrovesical and ureterovesical reflux may cause urinary tract infection. Urethrovesical reflux: With coughing and straining, bladder pressure rises, which may force urine from the bladder into the urethra. **A.** When bladder pressure returns to normal, the urine flows back to the bladder (**B**), which introduces bacteria from the urethra to the bladder. Ureterovesical reflux: With failure of the ureterovesical valve, urine moves up the ureters during voiding (**C**) and flows into the bladder when voiding stops (**D**). This prevents complete emptying of the bladder. It also leads to urinary stasis and contamination of the ureters with bacteria-laden urine.

CHART 46-2

Risk Factors: Urinary Tract Infection

- Contributing conditions such as:
  - Female gender
  - Diabetes
  - Pregnancy
  - Neurologic disorders
  - Gout
  - Altered states caused by incomplete emptying of the bladder and urinary stasis
- Decreased natural host defences or immunosuppression
- Inability or failure to empty the bladder completely
- Inflammation or abrasion of the urethral mucosa
- Instrumentation of the urinary tract (e.g., catheterization, cystoscopic procedures)
- Obstructed urinary flow caused by:
  - Congenital abnormalities
  - Urethral strictures
  - Contracture of the bladder neck
  - Bladder tumours
  - Calculi (stones) in the ureters or kidneys
  - Compression of the ureters

Adapted from Hagerty, T., Kertesz, L., Schmidt, J. M., et al. (2015). Risk factors for catheter associated urinary tract infections in critically ill patients with subarachnoid hemorrhage. *Journal of Neuroscience Nursing, 47*(1), 51–54; Hopkins, L., McCroskey, D., Reeves, G., et al. (2014). Implementing a urinary tract infection clinical practice guideline in an ambulatory urgent care practice. *The Nurse Practitioner, 39*(4), 50–54.

Reflux

An obstruction to free-flowing urine is a problem known as **urethrovesical reflux**, which is the reflux (backward flow) of urine from the urethra into the bladder (Fig. 46-1). With coughing, sneezing, or straining, the bladder pressure rises, which may force urine from the bladder into the urethra. When the pressure returns to normal, the urine flows back into the bladder, bringing into the bladder bacteria from the anterior portions of the urethra. Urethrovesical reflux is also caused by dysfunction of the bladder neck or urethra. The urethrovesical angle and urethral closure pressure may be altered with menopause, increasing the incidence of infection in postmenopausal women. Reflux is most often noted, however, in young children. Treatment is based on its severity.

Ureterovesical or **vesicoureteral reflux** refers to the backward flow of urine from the bladder into one or both ureters (see Fig. 46-1). Normally, the ureterovesical junction prevents urine from travelling back into the ureter. The ureters tunnel into the bladder wall so that the bladder musculature compresses a small portion of the ureter during normal voiding. When the ureterovesical valve is impaired by congenital causes or ureteral abnormalities, the bacteria may reach the kidneys and eventually destroy them (Hannon & Porth, 2017).

Uropathogenic Bacteria

Bacteriuria is generally defined as more than 10^5 colonies of bacteria per millilitre of urine. Since urine samples (especially in women) are commonly contaminated by the bacteria normally present in the urethral area, a bacterial count exceeding 10^5 colonies/mL of clean-catch midstream urine is the measure that distinguishes true bacteriuria from contamination. In men, contamination of the collected urine sample occurs less frequently; hence, bacteriuria can be defined as 10^4 colonies/mL urine. UTIs are the second most common type of bacterial infections seen by health care professionals (Hannon & Porth, 2017). The organisms most frequently responsible for UTIs are those normally found in the lower gastrointestinal (GI) tract. In a large-scale study of the types and prevalence of organisms of patients with UTIs in both the community and hospital setting, *E. coli* was responsible for 54.7% of UTIs. Isolation of *E. coli* is decreasing in comparison to previous observations, especially in males and in patients with indwelling bladder catheters, who instead had higher rates of *Pseudomonas* and *Enterococcus* organisms than females and noncatheterized patients (Hannon & Porth, 2017).

Routes of Infection

There are three well-recognized routes by which bacteria enter the urinary tract: up the urethra (ascending infection), through the bloodstream (hematogenous spread), or by means of a fistula from the intestine (direct extension).

The most common route of infection is transurethral, in which bacteria (often from fecal contamination) colonize the periurethral area and subsequently enter the bladder by means of the urethra. In women, the short urethra offers little resistance to the movement of uropathogenic bacteria (Hannon & Porth, 2017). Sexual intercourse or massage of the urethra forces the bacteria up into the bladder. This accounts for the increased incidence of UTIs in sexually active women. Bacteria may also enter the urinary tract by means of the blood (hematogenous spread) from a distant site of infection or through direct extension by way of a fistula from the intestinal tract.

Clinical Manifestations

Signs and symptoms of UTI depend on whether the infection involves the lower (bladder) or upper (kidney) urinary tract and whether the infection is acute or chronic. Signs and symptoms of an uncomplicated lower UTI include burning on urination, urinary **frequency** (voiding more than every 3 hours), urgency, **nocturia** (awakening at night to urinate), incontinence, and suprapubic or pelvic pain. Hematuria and back pain may also be present. In older adults, these symptoms are less common (see Gerontologic Considerations section).

In patients with complicated UTIs, manifestations can range from asymptomatic bacteriuria to gram-negative sepsis with shock. Complicated UTIs often are caused by a broader spectrum of organisms, have a lower response rate to treatment, and tend to recur. Many patients with catheter-associated UTIs are asymptomatic; however, any patient with a catheter who suddenly develops signs and symptoms of septic shock should be evaluated for **urosepsis** (the spread of infection from the urinary tract to the bloodstream that results in a systemic infection).

Gerontologic Considerations

The incidence of bacteriuria in the older adult differs from that in younger adults. Bacteriuria increases with age and disability, and women are affected more frequently than men. UTI is the most common cause of acute bacterial sepsis in patients older than 65 years of age, in whom gram-negative sepsis carries a mortality rate exceeding 50%. Urologists see many asymptomatic older patients with bacteriuria, and these individuals represent 20% of women over the age of 65 years. In the nursing home environment, older adults present with generalized symptoms initially and not all residents present with UTI symptoms (Rowe & Juthani-Mehta, 2014). UTIs occur more frequently in women than in men at younger ages but the gap between the sexes narrows in later life, which is due to reduced sexual intercourse in women and a higher incidence of bladder outlet obstruction secondary to benign prostatic hyperplasia in men (Eliopoulos, 2018).

In the older adult population at large, structural abnormalities secondary to decreased bladder tone and neurogenic bladder (dysfunctional bladder) secondary to stroke or autonomic neuropathy of diabetes may prevent complete emptying of the bladder and increase the risk for UTI (Rowe & Juthani-Mehta, 2014). When indwelling catheters are used, the risk for UTI increases dramatically. Older adult women often have incomplete emptying of the bladder and urinary stasis. In the absence of estrogen, following menopause, women are susceptible to colonization and increased adherence of bacteria to the vagina and urethra. Oral or topical estrogen has been used to restore the glycogen content of vaginal epithelial cells and an acidic pH for some of these women with recurrent cystitis.

The antibacterial activity of prostatic secretions that protects men from bacterial colonization of the urethra and bladder decreases with aging (Hannon & Porth, 2017). Although UTIs are rare in men, the prevalence of infection in men older than 50 years of age approaches that of women in the same age group. The dramatic rise in UTI in men as they age is largely due to prostatic hyperplasia or carcinoma, strictures of the urethra, and neuropathic bladder. The use of catheterization or cystoscopy in evaluation or treatment may contribute further to the higher incidence of UTI. The incidence of bacteriuria rises in men with confusion, dementia, or bowel or bladder incontinence. The most common cause of recurrent UTI in the older male patient is chronic bacterial prostatitis. Resection of the prostate gland may help to reduce its incidence (see Chapter 50).

In older patients in institutions, such as those in long-term care facilities, infecting pathogens are often resistant to many antibiotics. Factors that may contribute to UTI include high incidence of chronic illness; frequent use of antimicrobial agents; infected pressure ulcers; immobility and incomplete emptying of the bladder; and use of a bedpan rather than a commode or toilet (Chart 46-3).

Diligent hand hygiene, careful perineal care, and frequent toileting may decrease the incidence of UTIs. The organisms responsible for UTIs in the older adult in long-term care

CHART 46-3

Gerontologic Considerations

Factors That Contribute to Urinary Tract Infection in Older Adults

- Cognitive impairment
- Frequent use of antimicrobial agents
- High incidence of multiple chronic medical conditions
- Immunocompromise
- Immobility and incomplete emptying of bladder
- Obstructed flow of urine (e.g., urethral strictures, neoplasms, or a clogged indwelling catheter)

Adapted from Eliopoulos, C. (2018). *Gerontological nursing* (9th ed.). Philadelphia, PA: Lippincott Williams & Wilkins.

facilities may differ from those found in patients residing in the community; this is thought to be due in part to the frequent use of antibiotic agents by patients in these facilities. *E. coli* is the most common organism seen in older patients in the community or hospital. Patients with indwelling catheters, however, are more likely to be infected with *E. coli*, *Pseudomonas*, or *Staphylococcus* spp, and *Candida* spp. Patients who have been previously treated with antibiotics may be infected with *Enterococcus* sp. Frequent reinfections are common in older adults (Nicolle, 2014).

Controversy continues about the need for treatment of asymptomatic bacteriuria in older patients in long-term care facilities, because resulting antibiotic-resistant organisms and sepsis may be greater threats to patients. Most experts now recommend withholding antibiotics unless symptoms develop. However, treatment regimens are generally the same as those for younger adults, although age-related changes in the intestinal absorption of medications and decreased renal function and hepatic flow may necessitate alterations in the antimicrobial regimen. Renal function must be monitored, and medication dosages should be altered accordingly.

NURSING ALERT

Older adult patients often lack the typical symptoms of UTI and sepsis. Although frequency, urgency, and dysuria may occur, nonspecific symptoms, such as altered sensorium, lethargy, anorexia, new incontinence, hyperventilation, and low-grade fever, may be the only clues.

Assessment and Diagnostic Findings

Results of various tests, such as colony counts, cellular studies, and urine cultures, help to confirm the diagnosis of UTI. Pregnant women are generally screened for asymptomatic bacteriuria because the bladder may not empty as well as it usually does. In an uncomplicated UTI, the strain of bacteria will determine the antibiotic of choice.

Colony Counts

UTI is diagnosed by bacteria in the urine. A colony count of at least 10^5 colony-forming units (CFU) per millilitre of urine on a clean-catch midstream or catheterized specimen is a major criterion for infection (Hannon & Porth, 2017). However, UTI and subsequent sepsis have occurred with lower bacterial colony counts. About one third of women with symptoms of acute infections have negative midstream urine culture results and may go untreated if 10^5 CFU/mL is used as the criterion for infection. The presence of any bacteria in specimens obtained by suprapubic needle aspiration of the urinary bladder or catheterization is considered indicative of infection.

The following groups of patients should have urine cultures obtained when bacteriuria is present:

- All men (because of the likelihood of structural or functional abnormalities)
- All children
- Women with a history of compromised immune function or renal problems
- Patients with diabetes mellitus
- Patients who have undergone recent instrumentation (including catheterization) of the urinary tract
- Patients who were recently hospitalized or who live in long-term care facilities
- Patients with prolonged or persistent symptoms
- Patients with three or more UTIs in the past year
- Pregnant women
- Women following menopause
- Women who are sexually active or have new sexual partners

Cellular Studies

Microscopic hematuria (greater than four red blood cells [RBCs] per high-power field) is present in about half of patients with acute infection. **Pyuria** (greater than four white blood cells [WBCs] per high-power field) occurs in all patients with UTI; however, it is not specific for bacterial infection. Pyuria can also be seen with kidney stones, interstitial nephritis, and renal tuberculosis.

Urine Cultures

Urine cultures remain the gold standard in documenting a UTI and can identify the specific organism present. Due to the high probability that the organism in young women with their first UTI is *E. coli*, cultures are often omitted.

Other Testing Methods

Multistrip dipstick testing for WBCs, known as the leukocyte esterase test, and nitrite testing (nitrate reduction test) are common. If the leukocyte esterase test is positive, it is assumed that the patient has pyuria (WBCs in the urine) and should be treated. The nitrate reduction test is considered positive if bacteria that reduce normal urinary nitrates to nitrites are present.

Tests for sexually transmitted infections (STIs) may be performed because acute urethritis caused by sexually transmitted organisms (i.e., *Chlamydia trachomatis, Neisseria gonorrhoeae*, herpes simplex) or acute vaginitis infections (caused by *Trichomonas* or *Candida* sp.) may be responsible for symptoms similar to those of UTI. Therefore, evaluation for STIs may be performed (see Chapter 55).

Diagnostic studies such as computed tomography (CT) and ultrasonography are useful diagnostic tools. A CT scan may detect pyelonephritis or abscesses, and ultrasonography is extremely sensitive for detecting obstruction, abscesses, tumours, and cysts. Transrectal ultrasonography (to assess the prostate and bladder) is the procedure of choice for men with recurrent or complicated UTIs. A cystourethroscopy may be indicated to visualize the ureters or to detect strictures, calculi, or tumours (Hannon & Porth, 2017).

Medical Management

Management of UTIs typically involves pharmacologic therapy and patient education. The nurse is a key figure in teaching the patient about medication regimens and infection prevention measures.

Acute Pharmacologic Therapy

The ideal treatment of UTI is an antibacterial agent that eradicates bacteria from the urinary tract with minimal effects on fecal and vaginal flora, thereby minimizing the incidence of vaginal yeast infections. Yeast vaginitis occurs in as many as 25% of patients treated with antimicrobial agents that affect vaginal flora. Yeast vaginitis often causes more symptoms and is more difficult and costly to treat than the original UTI. In addition, the antibacterial agent should be affordable and should produce few adverse effects and low resistance. Since the organism in initial, uncomplicated UTIs in women is most likely *E. coli* or other fecal flora, the agent should be effective against these organisms. Various treatment regimens have been successful in treating uncomplicated lower UTIs in women: single-dose administration, short-course (3 to 4 days) medication regimens, or 7- to 10-day therapeutic courses. The trend is toward a shortened course of antibiotic therapy for uncomplicated UTIs because most are cured after 3 days of treatment.

In a complicated UTI (i.e., pyelonephritis), the general treatment of choice is usually a cephalosporin or an ampicillin/aminoglycoside combination. Patients in institutional settings may require 7 to 10 days of medication for the treatment to be effective. Other commonly used medications include trimethoprim/sulfamethoxazole (TMP-SMZ, Bactrim, Septra) and nitrofurantoin (Macrodantin, Furantoin). Occasionally, medications such as ampicillin or amoxicillin are used, but *E. coli* organisms have developed resistance to these agents.

Nitrofurantoin should not be used in patients with renal insufficiency because it is ineffective at glomerular filtration rates (GFRs) of less than 50 mL/minute and may cause peripheral neuropathy. A urinary analgesic may be prescribed to relieve the discomfort associated with the infection.

Regardless of the regimen prescribed, the patient is instructed to take all the doses prescribed, even if relief of symptoms occurs promptly. Longer medication courses are indicated for men, pregnant women, and women with pyelonephritis and other types of complicated UTIs. Hospitalization and intravenous (IV) antibiotics are occasionally needed.

Long-Term Pharmacologic Therapy

Although brief pharmacologic treatment of UTI for 3 days is usually adequate in women, infection recurs in about 20% of women treated for uncomplicated UTI. Infections that recur within 2 weeks after therapy (referred to as a relapse) do so because organisms of the original offending strain remain in the vagina. Relapses suggest that the source of bacteriuria may be the upper urinary tract or that initial treatment was inadequate or administered for too short a time. Recurrent infections in men are usually due to persistence of the same organism; further evaluation and treatment are indicated (Hopkins, McCroskey, Reeves, et al., 2014).

Reinfection of the female patient with new bacteria is the reason for more than 90% of recurrent UTIs in women. If the diagnostic evaluation reveals no structural abnormalities in the urinary tract, the woman with recurrent UTIs may be instructed to begin treatment on her own whenever symptoms occur and to contact the health care provider only when symptoms persist, fever occurs, or the number of treatment episodes exceeds four in a 6-month period. The patient may be taught to use dip-slide culture devices to detect bacteria.

If infection recurs after completing antimicrobial therapy, another short course (3 to 4 days) of full-dose antimicrobial therapy followed by a regular bedtime dose of an antimicrobial agent may be prescribed. If there is no recurrence, medication is taken every other night for 6 to 7 months. Other options include a dose of an antimicrobial agent after sexual intercourse, a dose at bedtime, or a dose every other night or three times per week. Long-term use of antimicrobial agents decreases the risk of reinfection and may be indicated in patients with recurrent infections.

If recurrence is caused by persistent bacteria from preceding infections, the cause (i.e., kidney stone, abscess), if known, must be treated. After treatment and sterilization of the urine, low-dose preventive therapy (trimethoprim with or without sulfamethoxazole) each night at bedtime is often prescribed (Hopkins et al., 2014).

Earlier studies suggested that the regular use of cranberry juice or blueberry juice reduces bacterial adherence to the epithelial lining of the urinary tract thus acting as a prevention rather than treatment of UTIs (Bass-Ware, Weed, Johnson, et al., 2014; Hannon & Porth, 2017). However, more recent studies have demonstrated that the use of cranberry juice may be effective in the prevention of UTI from *E. coli* strains mainly (Stapleton, Dziura, Hooton, et al., 2012).

Nursing Process

The Patient With a Lower Urinary Tract Infection

Nursing care of the patient with lower UTI focuses on treating the underlying infection and preventing its recurrence.

Assessment

A history of signs and symptoms related to UTI is obtained from the patient with a suspected UTI. The presence of pain, frequency, urgency, and hesitancy and changes in urine are assessed, documented, and reported. The patient's usual pattern of voiding is assessed to detect factors that may predispose him or her to UTI. Infrequent emptying of the bladder, the association of symptoms of UTI with sexual intercourse, contraceptive practices, and personal hygiene are assessed. The patient's knowledge about prescribed antimicrobial medications and preventive health care measures is also assessed. In addition, the urine is assessed for volume, colour, concentration, cloudiness, and odour, all of which are altered by bacteria in the urinary tract.

Nursing Priorities

Based on assessment data, the nursing priorities may include the following:

- Acute pain
- Deficient knowledge

Collaborative Problems/ Potential Complications

Based on assessment data, the following complications may develop:

- Sepsis
- Renal failure, which may occur as the long-term result of either an extensive infective or inflammatory process

Planning and Goals

Major goals for the patient may include relief of pain and discomfort, increased knowledge of preventive measures and treatment modalities, and absence of complications.

Nursing Interventions

Relieving Pain

The pain associated with UTI is quickly relieved once effective antimicrobial therapy is initiated. Antispasmodic agents may also be useful in relieving bladder irritability and pain. Analgesia and applying heat to the perineum help to relieve pain and spasm. The patient is encouraged to drink liberal amounts of fluids (water is the best choice) in order to promote renal blood flow and to flush the bacteria from the urinary tract. Urinary tract irritants (e.g., coffee, tea, citrus, spices, colas, alcohol) are avoided. Frequent voiding (every 2 to 3 hours) is encouraged to empty the bladder completely, as this can significantly lower urine bacterial counts, reduce urinary stasis, and prevent reinfection.

Monitoring and Managing Potential Complications

Early recognition of UTI and prompt treatment are essential to prevent recurrent infection and the possibility of complications, such as kidney disease, sepsis (urosepsis), strictures, and obstructions. The goal of treatment is to prevent infection from progressing and causing permanent kidney damage and injury. Thus, the patient must be taught to recognize early signs and symptoms, to test for bacteriuria, and to initiate treatment as prescribed. Appropriate antimicrobial therapy, liberal fluid intake, frequent voiding, and hygienic measures are commonly prescribed for managing UTI. The patient is instructed to notify the physician if fatigue, nausea, vomiting, or pruritus occurs. Periodic monitoring of renal function (creatinine clearance, blood urea nitrogen [BUN], and serum creatinine levels) and evaluation for strictures, obstructions, or stones may be indicated for patients with recurrent UTIs.

Patients with UTIs are at increased risk for gram-negative sepsis. For each day a urinary catheter is in place, the risk of developing catheter-associated urinary tract infection (CAUTI) increases. The risk of sepsis in patients with a urinary catheter is about 15% (Booker, 2015). CAUTIs should be avoided as they result in unpleasant symptoms, additional pharmacologic therapy, serious complications, and delayed discharge (Booker, 2015; Carter, Reitmeier, & Goodloe, 2014).

If an indwelling catheter is necessary, the following specific nursing interventions are initiated to prevent infection and urosepsis:

- Using strict aseptic technique during insertion of the smallest catheter possible
- Securing the catheter with tape to prevent movement
- Frequently inspecting urine colour, odour, and consistency
- Performing meticulous daily perineal care with soap and water
- Maintaining a closed system
- Following the manufacturer's instructions when using the catheter port to obtain urine specimens
- Careful assessment of vital signs and level of consciousness may alert the nurse to kidney involvement or impending sepsis. Positive blood cultures and elevated WBC counts must be reported immediately. At the same time, appropriate antibiotic therapy and increased fluid intake are prescribed (IV antibiotic therapy and fluids may be required). Aggressive early treatment is the key to reducing the mortality rate associated with CAUTI especially in older patients, those with anemia, and those with elevated blood sugar levels (Hagerty, Kertesz, Schmidt, et al., 2015). See Chart 46-4 for more information on risk factors for CAUTIs.

Promoting Home and Community-Based Care

EDUCATING PATIENTS ABOUT SELF-CARE. In helping patients learn about and prevent or manage a recurrent UTI, the nurse needs to implement teaching that meets individual patient needs. Health-related behaviours that help to prevent recurrent UTIs include practicing careful personal hygiene, increasing fluid intake to promote voiding and dilution of urine, urinating regularly and more frequently, and adhering to the therapeutic regime. For a detailed discussion of patient teaching interventions, refer to Chart 46-5.

NURSING RESEARCH PROFILE

Chart 46-4. Risk Factors for Catheter-Associated Urinary Tract Infections

Hagerty, T., Kertesz, L., Schmidt, J. M., et al. (2015). Risk factors for catheter associated urinary tract infections in critically ill patients with subarachnoid hemorrhage. *Journal of Neuroscience Nursing, 47*(1), 51–54.

Purpose

The use of indwelling urinary catheters can lead to complications, most importantly catheter-associated urinary tract infections (CAUTIs). These infections are the most common health care–associated infections in the United States. The purpose of this study was to assess the prevalence of and risk factors for CAUTIs among patients with subarachnoid hemorrhage (SAH) in one neurologic intensive care unit.

Design

This quantitative study used a retrospective design and included 242 patients with SAH admitted between 2005 and 2012 for whom data had been included in an existing data set. Logistic regression was used to identify predictors of CAUTI.

Findings

Catheterized adult patients ($n = 242$) with SAH over the 8-year period were included in the analysis. The rate of CAUTIs was 21%, or six times higher than the reported national average. Variables statistically significantly associated with CAUTI were older age (odds ratio [OR] = 1.06, 95% confidence interval [CI] [1.01, 1.11]), increased blood sugar levels (OR = 13.0, 95% CI [1.28, 107.4]), and anemia requiring transfusion (OR = 3.78, 95% CI [0.977, 14.67]).

Nursing Implications

Nurses should know that the high rates of CAUTI in this study were likely associated with prolonged catheterization. These findings indicate that nurses should carefully assess the need for catheterization and have increased vigilance regarding urinary catheter care in patients admitted with an SAH. Particular attention should be paid to patients who are older, those with anemia requiring transfusion, and those with elevated blood glucose levels due to their increased risk of CAUTI.

Evaluation

Expected patient outcomes may include the following:

1. Experiences relief of pain
   a. Reports absence of pain, urgency, dysuria, nocturia, or hesitancy on voiding
   b. Takes analgesic and antibiotic agents as prescribed
2. Explains UTIs and their treatment
   a. Demonstrates knowledge of preventive measures and prescribed treatments
   b. Drinks 8 to 10 glasses of fluids daily
   c. Voids every 2 to 3 hours
   d. Voids urine that is clear and odourless
3. Experiences no complications
   a. Reports no symptoms of infection (fever, **dysuria**, frequency) or renal failure (nausea, vomiting, fatigue, pruritus)
   b. Has normal BUN and serum creatinine levels; negative urine and blood cultures
   c. Exhibits normal vital signs and temperature; no signs or symptoms of sepsis (urosepsis)
   d. Maintains adequate urine output of more than 30 mL/hour

CHART 46-5

Patient Education: Preventing Recurrent Urinary Tract Infections

Hygiene

- Shower rather than bathe in tub because bacteria in the bathwater may enter the urethra.
- After each bowel movement, clean the perineum and urethral meatus from front to back. This will help to reduce concentrations of pathogens at the urethral opening and, in women, the vaginal opening.

Fluid Intake

- Drink liberal amounts of fluids daily to flush out bacteria.
- Avoid coffee, tea, colas, alcohol, and other fluids that are urinary tract irritants.

Voiding Habits

- Void every 2 to 3 hours during the day, and completely empty the bladder. This prevents overdistension of the bladder and compromised blood supply to the bladder wall. Both predispose the patient to urinary tract infection.

Precautions expressly for women include voiding immediately after sexual intercourse.

Interventions

- Take medication *exactly* as prescribed.
- If bacteria continue to appear in the urine, long-term antimicrobial therapy may be required to prevent colonization of the periurethral area and recurrence of infection.
- Special timing of administration may be required.
- For recurrent infection, consider acidification of the urine through ascorbic acid (vitamin C), 1,000 mg daily, or cranberry juice.
- If prescribed, test urine for presence of bacteria following manufacturer and health care provider's instructions.
- Notify the primary health care provider if fever occurs or if signs and symptoms persist.
- Consult the primary health care provider regularly for follow-up.

Upper Urinary Tract Infection

Pyelonephritis is a bacterial infection of the renal pelvis, tubules, and interstitial tissue of one or both kidneys. Causes involve either the upward spread of bacteria from the bladder or spread from systemic sources reaching the kidney via the bloodstream. It is not uncommon for bacteria that are causing a bladder infection to ascend into the kidney, causing pyelonephritis. An incompetent ureterovesical valve or obstruction occurring in the urinary tract increases the susceptibility of the kidneys to infection (see Fig. 46-1), because static urine provides a good medium for bacterial growth. Bladder tumours, strictures, benign prostatic hyperplasia, and urinary stones are some potential causes of obstruction that can lead to infections. Systemic infections (such as tuberculosis) can spread to the kidneys and result in abscesses.

Pyelonephritis may be acute or chronic. Acute pyelonephritis is an infection of the renal parenchyma and renal pelvis. It is usually manifested by enlarged kidneys with interstitial infiltrations of inflammatory cells. Abscesses may be noted on the renal capsule and at the corticomedullary junction. Eventually, atrophy and destruction of tubules and the glomeruli may result. When pyelonephritis becomes chronic, there is scarring and deformation of the renal calyces and pelvis.

Acute Pyelonephritis

Clinical Manifestations

The patient with acute pyelonephritis is acutely ill with chills, fever, leukocytosis, bacteriuria, and pyuria. Low back pain, flank pain, nausea and vomiting, headache, malaise, and painful urination are common findings. Physical examination reveals pain and tenderness in the area of the costovertebral angle (see Fig. 44-6 in Chapter 44). In addition, symptoms of lower urinary tract involvement, such as dysuria and frequency, are common.

Assessment and Diagnostic Findings

An ultrasound study or a CT scan may be performed to locate an obstruction in the urinary tract. Relief of obstruction is essential to prevent complications and eventual kidney damage. An IV pyelogram may be indicated with pyelonephritis if functional and structural renal abnormalities are suspected (Fischbach & Dunning, 2015). Radionuclide imaging with gallium citrate and indium-111 (^{111}In)–labelled WBCs may be useful to identify sites of infection that may not be visualized on CT scan or ultrasound. Urine culture and sensitivity tests are performed to determine the causative organism so that appropriate antimicrobial agents can be prescribed (Fischbach & Dunning, 2015).

Medical Management

Patients with acute uncomplicated pyelonephritis are most often treated on an outpatient basis if they are not exhibiting dehydration, nausea or vomiting, or symptoms of sepsis. In addition, they must be responsible and reliable to ensure that all medications are taken as prescribed. Other patients, including all pregnant women, may be hospitalized for at least 2 or 3 days of parenteral therapy. Oral agents may be substituted once the patient is afebrile and showing clinical improvement.

Pharmacologic Therapy

Antibiotic therapy is longer for pyelonephritis (7 to 14 days) than cystitis (1 dose—7 days) because renal parenchymal infection is more difficult to eradicate than mucosal bladder infections. Increased resistance to *E. coli*, the primary causative bacteria in pyelonephritis, has changed the treatment options and monitoring required for this infection. An oral third-generation cephalosporin drug (i.e., cefixime) is now the drug of choice for the treatment of uncomplicated pyelonephritis (Blondel-Hill & Fryters, 2012). Other agents such as TMP-SMZ, ciprofloxacin, and amoxicillin-clavulanate may be used, however, pretreatment urine cultures should be collected to detect any drug resistance (Baudry-Simner, Singh, Karlowsky, et al., 2012; Blondel-Hill & Fryters, 2012). IV third-generation cephalosporin agents (i.e., ceftriaxone) and gentamicin are used, as first-line and second-line therapies, respectively, in pregnant patients or those with severe disease. Oral antibiotic agents, tailored to urine culture and sensitivity results, may be prescribed once the patient is afebrile and showing clinical improvement.

A possible issue in acute pyelonephritis treatment is a chronic or recurring symptomless infection persisting for months or years. After the initial antibiotic regimen, the patient may need antibiotic therapy for up to 6 weeks if evidence of a relapse is seen. A follow-up urine culture is obtained 2 weeks after completion of antibiotic therapy to document clearing of the infection. Similarly, monthly urine cultures following pyelonephritis are recommended in pregnant females for the duration of their pregnancy (Blondel-Hill & Fryters, 2012).

Chronic Pyelonephritis

Repeated bouts of acute pyelonephritis may lead to chronic pyelonephritis, resulting from damage to the renal calyces and pelvis. The most common cause of chronic pyelonephritis is reflux involving either a single kidney or both, with the eventual development of chronic renal insufficiency (Hannon & Porth, 2017).

Clinical Manifestations

The patient with chronic pyelonephritis usually has no symptoms of infection unless an acute exacerbation occurs. Noticeable signs and symptoms may include fatigue, headache, poor appetite, polyuria, excessive thirst, and weight loss. Persistent and recurring infection may produce progressive scarring of the kidney resulting in chronic kidney disease (see Chapter 45).

Assessment and Diagnostic Findings

The extent of the disease is assessed by an IV urogram and measurements of creatinine clearance, blood urea nitrogen, and creatinine levels.

Complications

Complications of chronic pyelonephritis include end-stage kidney disease (from progressive loss of nephrons secondary to chronic inflammation and scarring), hypertension, and formation of kidney stones (from chronic infection with urea-splitting organisms).

Medical Management

Bacteria, if detected in the urine, are eradicated if possible. Long-term use of prophylactic antimicrobial therapy may help to limit recurrence of infections (McCance & Huether, 2014). Impaired renal function alters the excretion of antimicrobial agents and necessitates careful monitoring of renal function, especially if the medications are potentially toxic to the kidneys.

Nursing Management

The patient may require hospitalization or may be treated as an outpatient. When the patient is hospitalized, fluid intake and output are carefully measured and recorded. Unless contraindicated, fluids are encouraged (3 to 4 L/day) to dilute the urine, decrease burning on urination, and prevent dehydration. The patient's temperature is assessed every 4 hours and antipyretic and antibiotic agents are administered as prescribed. Often, the patient is more comfortable on bed rest during the acute phase of the illness.

Patient teaching focuses on prevention of UTIs by consuming adequate fluids, emptying the bladder regularly, and performing recommended perineal hygiene. The importance of taking antimicrobial medications exactly as prescribed is stressed to the patient, as is the need for keeping follow-up appointments.

ADULT VOIDING DYSFUNCTION

Both neurogenic and nonneurogenic disorders can cause adult voiding dysfunction (Table 46-1). The **micturition** (voiding or urination) process involves several highly coordinated neurologic responses that mediate bladder function. A functional urinary system allows for appropriate bladder filling and complete bladder emptying (see Chapter 44). If voiding dysfunction goes undetected and untreated, the upper urinary system may be compromised. Chronic incomplete bladder emptying from poor detrusor pressure results in recurrent bladder infection. Incomplete bladder emptying due to bladder outlet obstruction (such as benign prostatic hyperplasia), causing high-pressure detrusor contractions, can result in hydronephrosis from the high detrusor pressure that radiates up the ureters to the renal pelvis.

TABLE 46-1 Conditions Causing Adult Voiding Dysfunction

Condition	Voiding Dysfunction	Treatment
Neurogenic Disorders		
Cerebellar ataxia	Incontinence or dyssynergia	Timed voiding; anticholinergic agents
Stroke	Retention or incontinence	Anticholinergic agents; bladder retraining
Dementia	Incontinence	Prompted voiding; anticholinergic agents
Diabetes	Incontinence and/or incomplete bladder emptying	Timed voiding; EMG/biofeedback; pelvic floor nerve stimulation; anticholinergic/antispasmodic agents; well-controlled blood glucose levels
Multiple sclerosis	Incontinence or incomplete bladder emptying	Timed voiding; EMG/biofeedback to learn pelvic muscle exercises and urge inhibition; pelvic floor nerve stimulation; antispasmodic agents
Parkinson's disease	Incontinence	Anticholinergic/antispasmodic agents
Spinal Cord Dysfunction		
Acute injury	Urinary retention	Indwelling catheter
Degenerative disease	Incontinence and/or incomplete bladder emptying	EMG/biofeedback; pelvic floor nerve stimulation; anticholinergic agents
Nonneurogenic Disorder		
"Bashful bladder"	Inability to initiate voiding in public bathrooms	Relaxation therapy; EMG/biofeedback
Overactive bladder	Urgency, frequency, and/or urge incontinence	EMG/biofeedback; pelvic floor nerve stimulation; bladder drill (see Chart 46-8); anticholinergic agents
Post general surgery	Acute urine retention	Catheterization
Post prostatectomy	Incontinence	*Mild:* Biofeedback; bladder drill (see Chart 46-8); pelvic floor nerve stimulation *Moderate/severe:* Surgery—artificial sphincter
Stress incontinence	Incontinence with cough, laugh, sneeze, position change	*Mild:* Biofeedback; bladder drill (see Chart 46-8); periurethral bulking with collagen *Moderate/severe:* Surgery

EMG, electromyogram.

Adapted from Bader, M. K., Littlejohns, L. R., & Olson, D. M. (2016). *AANN core curriculum for neuroscience nursing* (6th ed.). Chicago, IL: American Association of Neuroscience Nurses.

Urinary Incontinence

It is estimated that as many as 3.3 million Canadians have **urinary incontinence** in some form (The Canadian Continence Foundation, 2014). Rather than a disease per se, it is a symptom with many causes (Hannon & Porth, 2017). Despite widespread media coverage, urinary incontinence remains underdiagnosed and underreported. Patients may be too embarrassed to seek help, causing them to ignore or conceal symptoms. Many patients resort to using absorbent pads or other devices without having their condition properly diagnosed and treated. Health care providers must be alert to subtle cues of urinary incontinence and stay informed about current management strategies.

The costs of care for patients with urinary incontinence include cost of absorbent products, medications, and surgical or nonsurgical treatment modalities as well as the psychosocial costs of urinary incontinence. These include embarrassment, loss of self-esteem, and social isolation.

Urinary incontinence affects people of all ages but is particularly common among the older adult; it can decrease their ability to maintain an independent lifestyle. This increases dependence on caregivers and may lead to institutionalization. More than half of all residents of long-term care have urinary incontinence. Although urinary incontinence is not a normal consequence of aging, age-related changes in the urinary tract predispose the older person to incontinence.

Although urinary incontinence is commonly regarded as a condition that occurs in older multiparous women, it is also common in young nulliparous women, especially during vigorous high-impact activity. Age, gender, and number of vaginal deliveries are established risk factors (Chart 46-6); they explain, in part, the increased incidence in women. Urinary incontinence is a symptom of many possible disorders.

CHART 46-6

Risk Factors: Urinary Incontinence

- Age-related changes in the urinary tract
- Caregiver or toilet unavailable
- Cognitive disturbances—dementia, Parkinson's disease
- Diabetes
- Genitourinary surgery
- High-impact exercise
- Immobility
- Incompetent urethra due to trauma or sphincter relaxation
- Medications—diuretic, sedative, hypnotic, and opioid agents
- Menopause
- Morbid obesity
- Pelvic muscle weakness
- Pregnancy—vaginal delivery, episiotomy
- Stroke

Adapted from Robinson, J. P., Bradway, C. W., Bunting-Perry, L., et al. (2013). Lower urinary tract symptoms in men with Parkinson's disease. *Journal of Neuroscience Nursing, 45*(6), 382–392.

Types of Urinary Incontinence

There are many types of urinary incontinence, including the following:

Stress incontinence is the involuntary loss of urine through an intact urethra as a result of sneezing, coughing, or changing position (Miller, 2015; Weber & Kelley, 2014). It predominantly affects women who have had vaginal deliveries and is thought to be the result of decreasing ligament and pelvic floor support of the urethra and decreasing or absent estrogen levels within the urethral walls and bladder base. In men, stress incontinence is often experienced after a radical prostatectomy for prostate cancer because of the loss of urethral compression that the prostate had supplied before the surgery, and possibly bladder wall irritability.

Urge incontinence is the involuntary loss of urine associated with a strong urge to void that cannot be suppressed (Miller, 2015; Weber & Kelley, 2014). The patient is aware of the need to void but is unable to reach a toilet in time. An uninhibited detrusor contraction is the precipitating factor. This can occur in a patient with neurologic dysfunction that impairs inhibition of bladder contraction or in a patient without overt neurologic dysfunction.

Functional incontinence refers to those instances in which lower urinary tract function is intact but other factors, such as severe cognitive impairment (e.g., Alzheimer's dementia), make it difficult for the patient to identify the need to void or physical impairments make it difficult or impossible for the patient to reach the toilet in time for voiding (Miller, 2015).

Iatrogenic incontinence refers to the involuntary loss of urine due to extrinsic medical factors, predominantly medications. One such example is the use of alpha-adrenergic agents to decrease blood pressure. In some people with an intact urinary system, these agents adversely affect the alpha receptors responsible for bladder neck closing pressure; the bladder neck relaxes to the point of incontinence with a minimal increase in intra-abdominal pressure, thus mimicking stress incontinence. As soon as the medication is discontinued, the apparent incontinence resolves.

Mixed urinary incontinence, which encompasses several types of urinary incontinence, is involuntary leakage associated with urgency and also with exertion, effort, sneezing, or coughing (Miller, 2015).

Only with appropriate recognition of the problem, assessment, and referral for diagnostic evaluation and treatment can the outcome of incontinence be determined. All people with incontinence should be considered for evaluation and treatment.

Gerontologic Considerations

If nurses and other health care providers accept incontinence as an inevitable part of illness or aging or consider it irreversible and untreatable, it cannot be treated successfully. Collaborative, interdisciplinary efforts are essential in assessing and effectively treating urinary incontinence.

Many older people experience transient episodes of incontinence that tend to be abrupt in onset. When this occurs, the nurse should question the patient, as well as the family if possible, about the onset of symptoms and any signs or symptoms of a change in other organ systems. Acute UTI, infection elsewhere in the body, constipation, decreased fluid intake, or a change in a chronic disease pattern, such as elevated blood glucose levels in patients with diabetes or decreased estrogen levels in menopausal women, can provoke the onset of urinary incontinence. If the cause is identified and modified or eliminated early at the onset of incontinence, the incontinence itself may be eliminated. Although the bladder of the older person is more vulnerable to altered detrusor activity, age alone is not a risk factor for urinary incontinence. Investigation of incontinence should include the duration, severity, and impact of the problem; the type of incontinence; the possibility of cognitive or behavioural factors; a physical examination; and a urinalysis.

Decreased bladder muscle tone is a normal age-related change found in the older adult. This leads to decreased bladder capacity, increased residual urine, and an increase in urgency. Many medications affect urinary continence in addition to causing other unwanted or unexpected effects (Miller, 2015). All medications need to be assessed for potential interactions.

Assessment and Diagnostic Findings

Once incontinence is recognized, a thorough history is necessary. This includes a detailed description of the problem and a history of medication use. The patient's voiding history, a diary of fluid intake and output, and bedside tests (e.g., residual urine, stress manoeuvres) may be used to help determine the type of urinary incontinence involved. Extensive urodynamic tests may be performed (see Chapter 44). Urinalysis and urine culture are performed to identify infection.

Urinary incontinence may be transient or reversible if the underlying cause is successfully treated and the voiding pattern reverts to normal (Chart 46-7).

Medical Management

Management depends on the type of urinary incontinence and its causes. Management of urinary incontinence may be behavioural, pharmacologic, or surgical.

CHART 46-7

Causes of Transient Incontinence

- Atrophic vaginitis, urethritis, prostatitis
- Delirium or confusion
- Excessive urine production (increased intake, diabetes, diabetic ketoacidosis)
- Limited or restricted activity
- Pharmacologic agents (anticholinergic agents, sedatives, alcohol, analgesic agents, diuretics, muscle relaxants, adrenergic agents)
- Psychological factors (depression, regression)
- Stool impaction or constipation
- Urinary tract infections (UTIs)

Behavioural Therapy

Behavioural therapies are the first choice to decrease or eliminate urinary incontinence (Chart 46-8). In using these techniques, health care professionals help patients avoid potential adverse effects of pharmacologic or surgical interventions. Pelvic floor muscle exercises (sometimes called *Kegel exercises*) represent the cornerstone of behavioural intervention for addressing symptoms of stress, urge, and mixed incontinence. Other behavioural treatments include use of a voiding diary, biofeedback, verbal instruction (prompted voiding), and physical therapy (McCooty & Latthe, 2014). Pessaries can be used as an additional conservative treatment for women with stress urinary incontinence or obstruction related to pelvic organ prolapse.

Pharmacologic Therapy

Pharmacologic therapy works best when used as an adjunct to behavioural interventions. Anticholinergic agents inhibit bladder contraction and are considered first-line medications for urge incontinence. A tricyclic antidepressant medication (e.g., amitriptyline [Elavil]) can also decrease bladder contractions as well as increase bladder neck resistance (Comerford, 2015). Pseudoephedrine sulfate (Sudafed), which acts on alpha-adrenergic receptors, causing urinary retention, may be used to treat stress incontinence; it needs to be used with caution in men with prostatic hyperplasia and patients with hypertension.

Although previously only used for the treatment of neurogenic urge incontinence (multiple sclerosis, spinal cord injury), Canadian researchers have found a clinical reduction in urinary urge incontinence by injecting botulinum toxin A injections into the detrusor muscle (Jabs & Carleton, 2013; Nitti, Dmochowski, Herschorn, et al., 2017).

Surgical Management

Surgical correction may be indicated in patients who have not achieved continence using behavioural and pharmacologic therapy. Surgical options vary according to the underlying anatomy and the physiologic problem. Most procedures involve lifting and stabilizing the bladder or urethra to restore the normal urethrovesical angle or to lengthen the urethra.

Women with stress incontinence may undergo an anterior vaginal repair, retropubic suspension, or needle suspension to reposition the urethra. Procedures to compress the urethra and increase resistance to urine flow include sling procedures and placement of periurethral bulking agents such as artificial collagen. Recent introduction of minimally invasive procedures for placement of a mesh midurethral sling has been demonstrated as effective treatment of stress incontinence in women who have failed conservative therapy such as pelvic floor muscle therapy and behaviour modification.

Periurethral bulking is a semipermanent procedure in which small amounts of artificial collagen are placed within the walls of the urethra to enhance the closing pressure of the urethra (Matsuoka, Locali, Pacetta, et al., 2016). This procedure takes only 10 to 20 minutes and may be performed under local anesthesia or moderate sedation. A cystoscope is inserted into the urethra. An instrument is inserted through the cystoscope to deliver a small amount

CHART 46-8

Health Promotion: Interventions for Urinary Incontinence

Behavioural strategies are largely carried out, coordinated, and monitored by the nurse. These interventions may or may not be augmented by the use of medications.

Fluid Management

An adequate daily fluid intake of approximately 50 to 60 oz (1,500 to 1,600 mL), taken as small increments between breakfast and the evening meal, helps to reduce urinary urgency related to concentrated urine production, decreases the risk of urinary tract infection, and maintains bowel functioning. (Constipation, resulting from inadequate daily fluid intake, can increase urinary urgency and urine retention.) The best fluid is water, although some suggest it may be helpful to include at least one glass of cranberry juice per day. Fluids containing caffeine, carbonation, alcohol, or artificial sweetener should be avoided because they irritate the bladder wall, thus resulting in urinary urgency. Some patients who have heart failure or end-stage kidney disease need to discuss their daily fluid limit with their primary provider.

Standardized Voiding Frequency

After establishing a patient's natural voiding and urinary incontinence tendencies, voiding on a schedule can be very effective in those with and without cognitive impairment, although patients with cognitive impairment may require assistance with this technique from nursing personnel or family members. The object is to purposely empty the bladder before the bladder reaches the critical volume that would cause an urge or stress incontinence episode. This approach involves the following:

- **Timed voiding** involves establishing a set voiding frequency (such as every 2 hours if incontinent episodes tend to occur 2 or more hours after voiding). The individual chooses to "void by the clock" at the given interval while awake rather than wait until a voiding urge occurs.
- **Prompted voiding** is timed voiding that is carried out by staff or family members when the individual has cognitive difficulties that make it difficult to remember to void at set intervals. The caregiver checks the patient to assess if he or she has remained dry and, if so, assists the patient to use the bathroom while providing positive reinforcement for remaining dry.
- **Habit retraining** is timed voiding at an interval that is more frequent than the individual would usually choose. This technique helps to restore the sensation of the need to void in individuals who are experiencing diminished sensation of bladder filling due to various medical conditions such as a stroke.
- **Bladder retraining**, also known as "bladder drill," incorporates a timed voiding schedule and urinary urge inhibition exercises to inhibit voiding, or leaking urine, in an attempt to remain dry for a set time. When the first timing interval is easily reached on a consistent basis without urinary urgency or incontinence, a new voiding interval, usually 10 to 15 minutes beyond the last, is established. Again, the individual practices urge inhibition exercises to delay voiding or avoid incontinence until the next preset interval arrives. When an acceptable voiding interval is reached, the patient continues that timed voiding sequence throughout the day.

Pelvic Muscle Exercise

Also known as Kegel exercises, pelvic muscle exercise (PME) aims to strengthen the voluntary muscles that assist in bladder and bowel continence in both men and women. Research shows that written or verbal instruction alone is usually inadequate to educate an individual about how to identify and strengthen the pelvic floor for sufficient bladder and bowel control. Biofeedback-assisted PME uses either electromyography or manometry to help the individual identify the pelvic muscles as they attempt to learn which muscle group is involved when performing PME. The biofeedback method also allows assessment of the strength of this muscle area.

PME involves gently tightening the same muscles used to stop flatus or the stream of urine for 5- to 10-second increments, followed by 10-second resting phases. To be effective, these exercises need to be performed two or three times a day for at least 6 weeks. Depending on the strength of the pelvic musculature when initially evaluated, anywhere from 10 to 30 repetitions of PME are prescribed at each session. Older patients may need to exercise for an even longer time to strengthen the pelvic floor muscles. PMEs are helpful for women with stress, urge, or mixed incontinence and for men who have undergone prostate surgery.

Vaginal Cone Retention Exercises

Vaginal cone retention exercises are an adjunct to the Kegel exercises. Vaginal cones of varying weight are inserted intravaginally twice a day. The patient tries to retain the cone for 15 minutes by contracting the pelvic muscles.

Transvaginal or Transrectal Electrical Stimulation

Commonly used to treat urinary incontinence, electrical stimulation is known to elicit a passive contraction of the pelvic floor musculature, thus reeducating these muscles to provide enhanced levels of continence. This modality is often used with biofeedback-assisted PME training and voiding schedules. At high frequencies, it is effective for stress incontinence. At low frequencies, electrical stimulation can also relieve symptoms of urinary urgency, frequency, and urge incontinence. Intermediate ranges are used for mixed incontinence.

Neuromodulation

Neuromodulation via transvaginal or transrectal nerve stimulation of the pelvic floor inhibits detrusor overactivity and hypersensory bladder signals and strengthens weak sphincter muscles.

Adapted from Bader, M. K., Littlejohns, L. R., & Olson, D. M. (2016). *AANN core curriculum for neuroscience nursing* (6th ed.). Chicago, IL: American Association of Neuroscience Nurses; Bass-Ware, A., Weed, D., Johnson, T., et al. (2014). Evaluation of the effect of cranberry juice on symptoms associated with a urinary tract infection. *Urologic Nursing, 34*(3), 121–127; Chisholm, A. H. (2015). Probiotics in preventing recurrent urinary tract infections in women: A literature review. *Urologic Nursing, 35*(1), 18–21, 29.

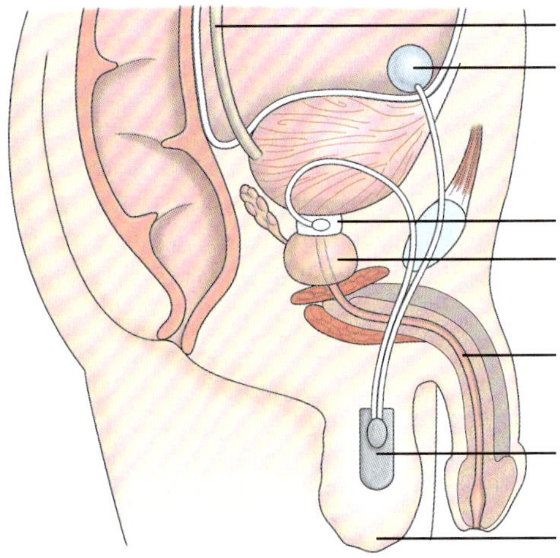

FIGURE 46-2. Male artificial urinary sphincter. An inflatable cuff is inserted surgically around the urethra or neck of the bladder. To empty the bladder, the cuff is deflated by squeezing the control pump located in the scrotum.

CHART 46-9

Patient Education: Strategies for Promoting Urinary Continence

The nurse instructs the patient to:

- Increase awareness of the amount and timing of all fluid intake.
- Avoid taking diuretics after 4 PM.
- Avoid bladder irritants, such as caffeine, alcohol, and aspartame (NutraSweet).
- Take steps to avoid constipation: Drink adequate fluids, eat a well-balanced diet high in fibre, exercise regularly, and take stool softeners if recommended.
- Void regularly, five to eight times a day (about every 2 to 3 hours):
  - First thing in the morning
  - Before each meal
  - Before retiring to bed
  - Once during night if necessary
- Perform all pelvic floor muscle exercises as prescribed, every day.
- Stop smoking (smokers usually cough frequently, which increases incontinence).

of collagen into the urethral wall at locations selected by the urologist. The patient is usually discharged home after voiding. There are no restrictions following the procedure, although occasionally more than one collagen bulking session may be necessary if the initial procedure has not halted the stress urinary incontinence. Collagen placement anywhere in the body is considered semipermanent because its durability averages between 12 and 24 months, until the body absorbs the material. Periurethral bulking with collagen offers an alternative to surgery, as in a frail, older adult person. It is also an option for people who are seeking help with stress urinary incontinence who prefer to avoid surgery and who do not have access to behavioural therapies. Studies on the efficacy of the various bulking agents are low and therefore, agents of choice for individuals are dependent on the availability of the products, physician preference, and cost.

An artificial urinary sphincter can be used to close the urethra and promote continence. Two types of artificial sphincters are a periurethral cuff and a cuff inflation pump. This type of device is available for men and women (Hannon & Porth, 2017).

Men with overflow and stress incontinence may undergo a transurethral or laser resection to relieve symptoms of prostatic enlargement. An artificial sphincter can be used after prostatic surgery for sphincter incompetence (Fig. 46-2). After surgery, periurethral bulking agents can be injected into the periurethral area to increase compression of the urethra.

Nursing Management

Nursing management is based on the premise that incontinence is not inevitable with illness or aging and that it is often reversible and treatable. The nursing interventions are determined in part by the type of treatment that is undertaken. For behavioural therapy to be effective, the nurse must provide support and encouragement because it is easy for the patient to become discouraged if therapy does not quickly improve the level of continence. Patient teaching is important and should be provided verbally and in writing (Chart 46-9). The patient should be taught to develop and use a log or diary to record timing of pelvic floor muscle exercises, frequency of voiding, any changes in bladder function, and any episodes of incontinence (Miller, 2015).

If pharmacologic treatment is used, its purpose is explained to the patient and family. It is important to educate patients who have **mixed incontinence** (both stress and urge incontinence) that anticholinergic and antispasmodic agents can help to decrease urinary urgency and frequency and urge incontinence but that they do not decrease the urinary incontinence related to stress incontinence. If surgical correction is undertaken, the procedure and its desired outcomes are described to the patient and family. Follow-up contact with the patient enables the nurse to answer the patient's questions and to provide reinforcement and encouragement.

Urinary Retention

Urinary retention is the inability to empty the bladder completely during attempts to void. Chronic urine retention often leads to **overflow incontinence** (from the pressure of the retained urine in the bladder). **Residual urine** is urine that remains in the bladder after voiding. In a healthy adult younger than 60 years, complete bladder emptying should occur with each voiding. In adults older than 60 years, 50 to 100 mL of residual urine may remain after each voiding because of the decreased contractility of the detrusor muscle.

Urinary retention can occur postoperatively in any patient, particularly if the surgery affected the perineal or anal regions and resulted in reflex spasm of the sphincters. General anesthesia reduces bladder muscle innervation and suppresses the urge to void, impeding bladder emptying.

Pathophysiology

Urinary retention may result from diabetes, prostatic enlargement, urethral pathology (infection, tumour, calculus), trauma (pelvic injuries), pregnancy, or neurologic disorders (e.g., stroke, spinal cord injury, multiple sclerosis, or Parkinson's disease). Some medications cause urinary retention either by inhibiting bladder contractility or by increasing bladder outlet resistance (Comerford, 2015).

Medications that cause retention by inhibiting bladder contractility include anticholinergic agents (atropine sulfate, dicyclomine hydrochloride [Antispas, Bentyl]); antispasmodic agents (oxybutynin chloride [Ditropan], belladonna, and opioid suppositories); and tricyclic antidepressant medications (imipramine [Tofranil], doxepin [Sinequan]). Medications that cause urine retention by increasing bladder outlet resistance include alpha-adrenergic agents (ephedrine sulfate, pseudoephedrine), beta-adrenergic blockers (propranolol), and estrogens.

Assessment and Diagnostic Findings

The assessment of a patient for urinary retention is multifaceted because the signs and symptoms may be easily overlooked. The following questions serve as a guide in assessment:

- What was the time of the last voiding, and how much urine was voided?
- Is the patient voiding small amounts of urine frequently?
- Is the patient dribbling urine?
- Does the patient complain of pain or discomfort in the lower abdomen? (Discomfort may be relatively mild if the bladder distends slowly.)
- Is the pelvic area rounded and swollen (could indicate urine retention and a distended bladder)?
- Does percussion of the suprapubic region elicit dullness (possibly indicating urine retention and a distended bladder)?
- Are other indicators of urinary retention present, such as restlessness and agitation?
- Does a postvoid bladder ultrasound test reveal residual urine?

The patient may verbalize an awareness of bladder fullness and a sensation of incomplete bladder emptying. Signs and symptoms of UTI (hematuria, urgency, frequency, nocturia, and dysuria) may be present. A series of urodynamic studies, described in Chapter 44, may be performed to identify the type of bladder dysfunction and to aid in determining appropriate treatment. The patient may complete a voiding diary to provide a written record of the amount of urine voided and the frequency of voiding. Postvoid residual urine may be assessed either using straight catheterization or an ultrasound bladder scanner and is considered diagnostic of urinary retention if there is more than 100 mL of residual urine.

Complications

Urine retention can lead to chronic infection. Infections that are unresolved predispose the patient to renal calculi (urolithiasis or nephrolithiasis), pyelonephritis, and sepsis. The kidney may also eventually deteriorate if large volumes of urine are retained, causing hydronephrosis. In addition, urine leakage can lead to perineal skin breakdown, especially if regular hygiene measures are neglected.

Nursing Management

Management strategies are instituted to prevent overdistension of the bladder and to treat infection or correct obstruction. However, many problems can be prevented with careful assessment and appropriate nursing interventions. The nurse explains why normal voiding is not occurring and monitors urine output closely. The nurse also provides reassurance about the temporary nature of retention and successful management strategies.

Promoting Urinary Elimination

Nursing measures to encourage normal voiding patterns include providing privacy, ensuring an environment and a position conducive to voiding, and assisting the patient with the use of the bathroom or bedside commode, rather than a bedpan, to provide a more natural setting for voiding. The male patient may stand beside the bed while using the urinal; most men find this position more comfortable and natural.

Additional measures include applying warmth to relax the sphincters (i.e., sitz baths, warm compresses to the perineum, showers), giving the patient hot tea, and offering encouragement and reassurance. Simple trigger techniques, such as turning on the water faucet while the patient is trying to void, may also be used. Other examples of trigger techniques are stroking the abdomen or inner thighs, tapping above the pubic area, and dipping the patient's hands in warm water. A combination of techniques may be necessary to initiate voiding.

After surgery or childbirth, prescribed analgesics should be administered because pain in the perineal area can make voiding difficult.

When the patient cannot void, catheterization is used to prevent overdistension of the bladder (see later Neurogenic Bladder and Catheterization sections). Consider using a portable ultrasound device in patients undergoing intermittent catheterization to assess urine volume and reduce unnecessary catheter insertions (Canadian Patient Safety Institute [CPSI], 2016). In the case of prostatic obstruction, attempts at catheterization (by the urologist) may not be successful, requiring insertion of a **suprapubic catheter** (catheter inserted through a small abdominal incision into the bladder). After urinary drainage is restored, bladder retraining is initiated for the patient who cannot void spontaneously.

Promoting Home, Community-Based, and Transitional Care

In addition to the strategies listed for promoting urinary continence found in Chart 46-8, modifications to the home environment can provide simple and effective ways to assist in treating urinary incontinence and retention. For example, the patient may need to remove obstacles, such as throw rugs or other objects, to provide easy, safe access to the bathroom. Other modifications that the nurse may recommend include installing support bars in the bathroom; placing a bedside commode, bedpan, or urinal within easy reach; leaving lights on in the bedroom and bathroom; and wearing clothing that is easy to remove quickly.

Neurogenic Bladder

Neurogenic bladder is a dysfunction that results from a lesion of the nervous system and leads to urinary incontinence. It may be caused by spinal cord injury, spinal tumour, herniated vertebral disk, multiple sclerosis, congenital disorders (spina bifida or myelomeningocele), infection, or diabetes mellitus (see Chapters 41, 64, and 65).

Pathophysiology

The two types of neurogenic bladder are spastic (or reflex) bladder and flaccid bladder. Spastic bladder is the more common type and is caused by any spinal cord lesion above the voiding reflex arc (upper motor neuron lesion) (Bader, Littlejohns, & Olson, 2016). The result is a loss of conscious sensation and cerebral motor control. A spastic bladder empties on reflex, with minimal or no controlling influence to regulate its activity.

Flaccid bladder is caused by a lower motor neuron lesion, commonly resulting from trauma. This form of neurogenic bladder is also increasingly being recognized in patients with diabetes mellitus. The bladder continues to fill and becomes greatly distended, and overflow incontinence occurs. The bladder muscle does not contract forcefully at any time. Because sensory loss may accompany a flaccid bladder, the patient feels no discomfort.

Assessment and Diagnostic Findings

Evaluation for neurogenic bladder involves measurement of fluid intake, urine output, and residual urine volume; urinalysis; and assessment of sensory awareness of bladder fullness and degree of motor control. Comprehensive urodynamic studies are also performed.

Complications

The most common complication of neurogenic bladder is infection resulting from urinary stasis and catheterizations. Long-term complications include urolithiasis (stones in the urinary tract), vesicoureteral reflux, and hydronephrosis, all of which can lead to destruction of the kidneys. Other complications include renal calculi, impaired skin integrity, and urinary incontinence or retention (Bader et al., 2016).

NURSING ALERT

Autonomic dysreflexia, a complication associated with spinal cord injuries, is caused by distension of the bladder. Classic symptoms include high blood pressure, bradycardia, sweating, hot flushes, and headaches. Autonomic dysreflexia is considered a medical emergency as it is a high risk factor for intracranial hemorrhage (Taweel & Seyam, 2015).

Medical Management

The problems resulting from neurogenic bladder disorders vary considerably from patient to patient and are a major challenge to the health care team. There are several long-term objectives appropriate for all types of neurogenic bladders:

- Preventing overdistension of the bladder
- Emptying the bladder regularly and completely
- Maintaining urine sterility with no stone formation
- Maintaining adequate bladder capacity with no reflux

Specific interventions include continuous, intermittent, or self-catheterization (discussed later in this chapter); use of an external condom-type catheter; a diet low in calcium (to prevent calculi); and encouragement of mobility and ambulation. A liberal fluid intake is encouraged to reduce the urinary bacterial count, reduce stasis, decrease the concentration of calcium in the urine, and minimize the precipitation of urinary crystals and subsequent stone formation.

A bladder retraining program may be effective in treating a spastic bladder or urine retention. Use of a timed, or habit, voiding schedule may be established. To further enhance emptying of a flaccid bladder, the patient may be taught to "double void." After each voiding, the patient is instructed to remain on the toilet, relax for 1 to 2 minutes, and then attempt to void again in an effort to further empty the bladder.

Pharmacologic Therapy

Parasympathomimetic medications, such as bethanechol (Urecholine), may help to increase the contraction of the detrusor muscle in acute retention not related to obstruction. These medications are not effective in chronic urinary retention.

Surgical Management

In some cases, surgery may be carried out to correct bladder neck contractures or vesicoureteral reflux or to perform some type of urinary diversion procedure.

Catheterization

WATCH & LEARN PRACTICE & LEARN

In patients with a urologic disorder or with marginal kidney function, care must be taken to ensure that urinary drainage is adequate and that kidney function is preserved. When urine cannot be eliminated naturally and must be drained artificially, catheters may be inserted directly into the bladder, the ureter, or the renal pelvis. Catheters vary in size, shape, length, material, and configuration (Carter et al., 2014). The type of catheter used depends on its purpose.

Catheterization is performed to achieve the following:

- Relieve urinary tract obstruction
- Assist with postoperative drainage in urologic and other surgeries
- Provide a means to monitor accurate urine output in critically ill patients
- Promote urinary drainage in patients with neurogenic bladder dysfunction or urine retention
- Prevent urinary leakage in patients with stage III to IV pressure injuries (see Chapter 13)

A patient should be catheterized only if necessary, as catheterization commonly leads to UTI. Catheters impede most of the natural defences of the lower urinary tract by obstructing the periurethral ducts, irritating the bladder mucosa, and providing an artificial route for organisms to enter the bladder (Hagerty et al., 2015). Organisms may be introduced from the urethra into the bladder during catheterization, or they may migrate along the epithelial surface of the urethra or external surface of the catheter. Many of the organisms can form a bacterial biofilm impenetrable to antibiotics. In addition, urinary catheters have been associated with other complications, such as bladder spasms, urethral strictures, and pressure necrosis (Bader et al., 2016).

Indwelling Catheters

When an indwelling catheter cannot be avoided, a closed drainage system is essential. This drainage system is designed to prevent any disconnections, thereby reducing the risk of contamination. Triple-lumen catheters are commonly used after transurethral prostate surgery (see Chapter 50). This system has a triple-lumen indwelling urethral catheter attached to a closed sterile drainage system. With the triple-lumen catheter, urinary drainage occurs through one channel. The retention balloon of the catheter is inflated with water or air through the second channel, and the bladder is continuously irrigated with sterile irrigating solution through the third channel.

The spout (or drainage port) of any urinary drainage bag can become contaminated when opened to drain the bag. Bacteria enter the urinary drainage bag, multiply rapidly, and then migrate to the drainage tubing, catheter, and bladder. By keeping the drainage bag lower than the patient's bladder and not allowing urine to flow back into the bladder, this risk is minimized.

Suprapubic Catheters

Suprapubic catheterization allows bladder drainage by inserting a catheter or tube into the bladder through a suprapubic (above the pubis) incision or puncture (Fig. 46-3). The catheter or suprapubic drainage tube is then threaded into the bladder and secured with sutures or tape, and the area around the catheter is covered with a sterile dressing. The catheter is connected to a sterile closed drainage system, and the tubing is secured to prevent tension on the catheter. This may be a temporary measure to divert the flow of urine from the urethra when the urethral route is impassable (because of injuries, strictures, prostatic obstruction), after gynecologic or other abdominal surgery when bladder dysfunction is likely to occur, and occasionally after pelvic fractures.

Suprapubic bladder drainage may be maintained continuously for several weeks. When the patient's ability to void is to be tested, the catheter is clamped for 4 hours, during which time the patient attempts to void. After the patient voids, the catheter is unclamped, and the residual urine is measured. If the amount of residual urine is less than 100 mL on two separate occasions (morning and evening), the catheter is usually removed. However, if the patient complains of pain or discomfort, the suprapubic catheter is usually left in place until the patient can void successfully.

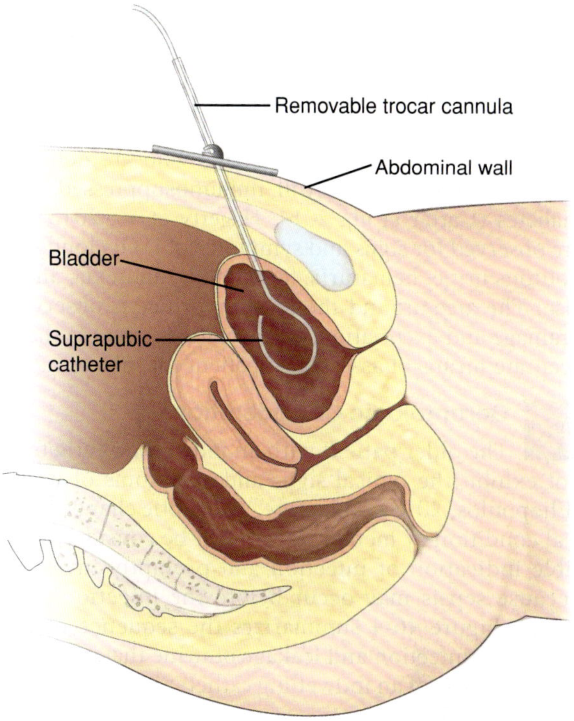

FIGURE 46-3. Suprapubic bladder drainage. A trocar cannula is used to puncture the abdominal and bladder walls. The catheter is threaded through the trocar cannula, which is then removed, leaving the catheter in place. The catheter is secured by tape or sutures to prevent unintentional removal.

Suprapubic drainage offers certain advantages. Patients can usually void sooner after surgery than those with urethral catheters, and they may be more comfortable. The catheter allows greater mobility, permits measurement of residual urine without urethral instrumentation, and presents less risk of bladder infection. The suprapubic catheter is removed when it is no longer required, and a sterile dressing is placed over the site.

The patient requires liberal amounts of fluid to prevent encrustation around the catheter. Other potential problems include the formation of bladder stones, acute and chronic infections, and problems collecting urine. A **wound care specialist**/enterostomal therapist, also referred to as a wound-ostomy-continence nurse, may be consulted to assist the patient and family in selecting the most suitable urine collection system and to teach them about its use and care.

Nursing Management

Assessing the Patient and the System

For patients with indwelling catheters, the nurse assesses the drainage system to ensure that it provides adequate urinary drainage. The colour, odour, and volume of urine are also monitored. An accurate record of fluid intake and urine output provides essential information about the adequacy of renal function and urinary drainage.

The nurse observes the catheter to make sure that it is properly anchored, to prevent pressure on the urethra at the penoscrotal junction in male patients, and to prevent tension and traction on the bladder in both male and female patients.

Patients at high risk for UTI from catheterization need to be identified and monitored carefully. These include women; older adults; and patients who are debilitated, malnourished, chronically ill, immunosuppressed, or have diabetes (Carter et al., 2014; Hagerty et al., 2015). They are observed for signs and symptoms of UTI: cloudy malodourous urine, hematuria, fever, chills, anorexia, and malaise. The area around the urethral orifice is observed for drainage and excoriation. Urine cultures provide the most accurate means of assessing a patient for infection.

Gerontologic Considerations

The older patient with an indwelling catheter may not exhibit the typical signs and symptoms of infection (Eliopoulos, 2018). Therefore, any subtle change in physical condition or mental status must be considered a possible indication of infection and promptly investigated because sepsis may occur before the infection is diagnosed. Figure 46-4 summarizes the sequence of events leading to infection and leakage of urine that often follow long-term use of an indwelling catheter in an older patient (Miller, 2015).

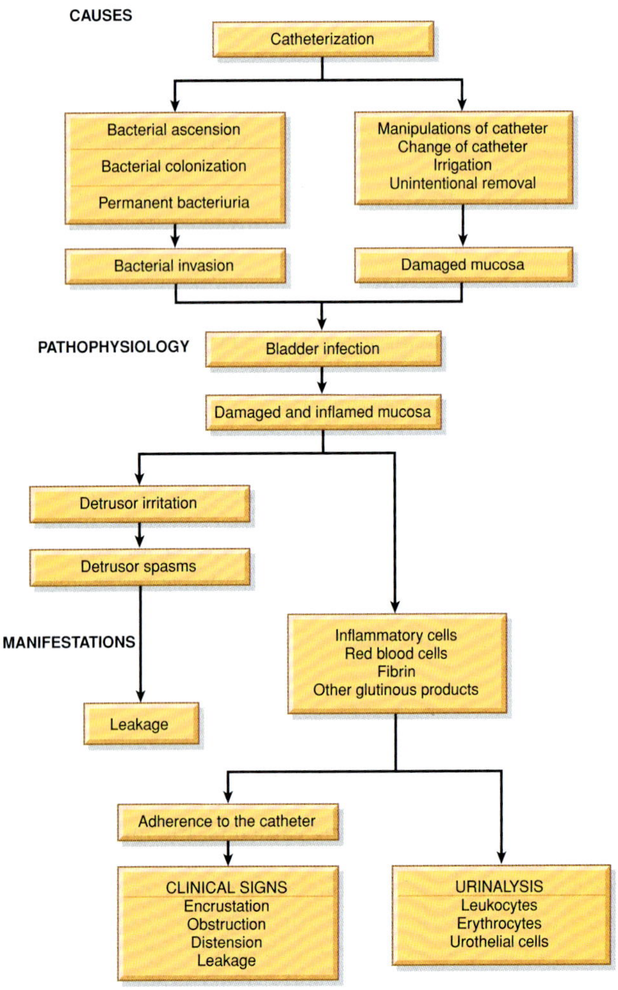

FIGURE 46-4. Pathophysiology and manifestations of bladder infection in long-term catheterized older patients.

Preventing Infection

Certain principles of care are essential to prevent infection in patients with a closed urinary drainage system (Chart 46-10). The catheter is an object foreign to the body and produces a reaction in the urethral mucosa with some urethral discharge. Vigorous cleansing of the meatus while the catheter is in place is discouraged because the cleansing action can move the catheter back and forth, increasing the risk of infection. To clean the external catheter surface, gentle washing with soap and water or wipes during the daily bath is used by some (Strouse, 2015). Others report that using 2% chlorhexidine gluconate no-rinse wipes during the daily bath helps decrease CAUTI rates (Carter et al., 2014). The catheter is anchored as securely as possible to prevent it from moving in the urethra (Carter et al., 2014; Mori, 2014).

A liberal fluid intake, within the limits of the patient's cardiac and renal reserve, and an increased urine output must be ensured to flush the catheter and to dilute urinary substances that might form encrustations (Carter et al., 2014; Hagerty et al., 2015).

Urine cultures are obtained as prescribed or indicated when monitoring the patient for infection; many catheters have an aspiration (puncture) port from which a specimen can be obtained.

Bacteriuria is considered inevitable in patients with indwelling catheters; therefore, controversy remains about the usefulness of taking cultures and treating asymptomatic bacteriuria, because overtreatment may lead to resistant strains of bacteria. Continual observation for fever, chills, and other signs and symptoms of systemic infection is necessary; these symptoms are generally treated aggressively.

Minimizing Trauma

Trauma to the urethra can be minimized by the following:

- Using an appropriate-sized catheter
- Lubricating the catheter adequately with a water-soluble lubricant during insertion
- Inserting the catheter far enough into the bladder to prevent trauma to the urethral tissues when the retention balloon of the catheter is inflated

Manipulation of the catheter is the most common cause of trauma to the bladder mucosa in the catheterized patient. Infection then inevitably occurs when urine invades the damaged mucosa.

The catheter is secured properly to prevent it from moving, causing traction on the urethra, or being unintentionally removed, and care is taken to ensure that the catheter position permits leg movement. In male patients, the drainage tube (not the catheter) is taped laterally to the thigh to prevent pressure on the urethra at the penoscrotal junction, which can eventually lead to formation of a urethrocutaneous fistula. In female patients, the drainage tubing attached to the catheter is taped to the thigh to prevent tension and traction on the bladder.

Special care should be taken to ensure that any patient who is confused does not remove the catheter with the retention balloon still inflated, as this could cause bleeding and considerable injury to the urethra.

Retraining the Bladder

When an indwelling urinary catheter is in place, the detrusor muscle does not actively contract the bladder wall to

CHART 46-10

Preventing Infection in the Patient With an Indwelling Urinary Catheter

- Avoid contamination of the drainage spout. A receptacle in which to empty the bag is provided for each patient.
- Avoid routine catheter changes. The catheter is changed only to correct problems such as leakage, blockage, or encrustations.
- Avoid unnecessary handling or manipulation of the catheter by the patient or staff.
- Carry out hand hygiene before and after handling the catheter, tubing, or drainage bag.
- Ensure a free flow of urine to prevent infection. Improper drainage occurs when the tubing is kinked or twisted, allowing pools of urine to collect in the tubing loops.
- Evaluate the benefit of placing an indwelling urinary catheter versus the risk for the patient developing a catheter-associated urinary tract infection.
- If the collection bag *must* be raised above the level of the patient's bladder, clamp the drainage tube. This prevents backflow of contaminated urine into the patient's bladder from the bag.
- Monitor the patient's voiding when the catheter is removed. The patient must void within 8 hours; if unable to void, the patient may require catheterization with a straight catheter.
- Never disconnect the tubing to obtain urine samples, to irrigate the catheter, or to ambulate or transport the patient.
- Never irrigate the catheter routinely. If the patient is prone to obstruction from clots or large amounts of sediment, use a three-way system with continuous irrigation.
- Never leave the catheter in place longer than is necessary to decrease the risk of CAUTI.
- Obtain a urine specimen for culture at the first sign of infection.
- To prevent contamination of the closed system, *never* disconnect the tubing. The drainage bag must *never* touch the floor. The bag and collecting tubing are changed if contamination occurs, if urine flow becomes obstructed, or if tubing junctions start to leak at the connections.
- To reduce the risk of bacterial proliferation, empty the collection bag at least every 8 hours through the drainage spout—more frequently if there is a large volume of urine.
- Use scrupulous aseptic technique during insertion of the catheter. Use a preassembled, sterile, closed urinary drainage system of the smallest catheter size possible to minimize trauma.
- Wash the perineal area with soap and water at least twice a day; avoid a to-and-fro motion of the catheter. Dry the area well, but avoid applying powder because it may irritate the perineum.

Adapted from Carter, N. M., Reitmeier, L., & Goodloe, L. R. (2014). An evidence-based approach to the prevention of catheter-associated urinary tract infections. *Urologic Nursing, 34*(5), 238–245.

stimulate emptying, because urine is continuously draining from the bladder. As a result, the detrusor may not immediately respond to bladder filling when the catheter is removed, resulting in either urine retention or urinary incontinence. This condition, known as postcatheterization detrusor instability, can be managed with bladder retraining (Chart 46-11).

Immediately after the indwelling catheter is removed, the patient is placed on a timed voiding schedule, usually every 2 to 3 hours. At the given time interval, the patient is instructed to void. The bladder is then scanned using a portable ultrasonic bladder scanner, and if the bladder has not emptied completely, straight catheterization may be performed (Carter et al., 2014; Mori, 2014). After a few days, as the nerve endings in the bladder wall become resensitized to the bladder filling and emptying, bladder function usually returns to normal. If the patient has had an indwelling catheter in place for an extended period (e.g., greater than 1 month), bladder retraining will take longer; in some cases, function may never return to normal, and long-term intermittent catheterization may become necessary.

Assisting With Intermittent Self-Catheterization

Intermittent self-catheterization provides periodic drainage of urine from the bladder. By promoting drainage and eliminating excessive residual urine, intermittent catheterization protects the kidneys, reduces the incidence of UTIs, and improves continence. It is the treatment of choice in patients with spinal cord injury and other neurologic disorders, such as multiple sclerosis, when the ability to empty the bladder is impaired. Self-catheterization promotes independence, results in few complications, and enhances self-esteem and quality of life.

When teaching the patient how to perform self-catheterization, the nurse must use aseptic technique to

CHART 46-11

Bladder Retraining After Indwelling Catheterization

- Instruct the patient to drink a measured amount of fluid from 8 AM to 10 PM to avoid bladder overdistension. Offer no fluids (except sips) after 10 PM.
- At specific times, ask the patient to void by applying pressure over the bladder, tapping the abdomen, or running water to trigger the bladder.
- Immediately after the voiding attempt, perform a bladder scan to determine the amount of residual urine.
- Measure the volumes of urine voided.
- Palpate the bladder at repeated intervals to assess for distension.
- Instruct the patient who has no voiding sensation to be alert to any signs that indicate a full bladder, such as perspiration, cold hands or feet, or feelings of anxiety.
- Perform straight catheterization, as prescribed, usually for residual urine of >300 mL.
- Lengthen the intervals between catheterizations as the volume of residual urine decreases. Catheterization is usually discontinued when the volume of residual urine is <100 mL.

Adapted from Carter, N. M., Reitmeier, L., & Goodloe, L. R. (2014). An evidence-based approach to the prevention of catheter-associated urinary tract infections. *Urologic Nursing, 34*(5), 238–245.

minimize the risk of cross-contamination. However, the patient may use a "clean" (nonsterile) technique at home, where the risk of cross-contamination is reduced. Either antibacterial liquid soap or povidone-iodine (Betadine) solution is recommended for cleaning urinary catheters at home. The catheter is thoroughly rinsed with tap water after soaking in the cleaning solution. It must dry before reuse. It should be kept in its own container, such as a plastic food-storage bag.

In teaching the patient, the nurse emphasizes the importance of frequent catheterization and emptying the bladder at the prescribed time. The average daytime clean intermittent catheterization schedule is every 4 to 6 hours and just before bedtime. If the patient is awakened at night with an urge to void, catheterization may be performed after an attempt is made to void normally.

The female patient assumes a Fowler's position and uses a mirror to help locate the urinary meatus. She inserts the lubricated catheter 7.5 cm (3 in) into the urethra, in a downward and backward direction. The male patient assumes a Fowler's or sitting position, lubricates the catheter, retracts the foreskin of the penis with one hand while grasping the penis and holding it at a right angle to the body. (This manoeuvre straightens the urethra and makes it easier to insert the catheter.) He inserts the catheter 15 to 25 cm until urine begins to flow. After removal, the catheter is cleaned, rinsed, and wrapped in a paper towel or placed in a plastic bag or case. Patients who follow this routine should consult a primary health care provider at regular intervals to assess urinary function and detect complications.

If the patient cannot perform intermittent self-catheterization, a family member may be taught to carry out the procedure at regular intervals during the day.

An alternative to self-catheterization that requires an extensive surgical procedure is creation of the Mitrofanoff umbilical appendicovesicostomy, which provides easy access to the bladder. In this procedure, the bladder neck is closed and the appendix is used to create access to the bladder from the skin surface through a submucosal tunnel created with the appendix. One end of the appendix is brought to the skin surface and used as a stoma, and the other end is tunnelled into the bladder. The appendix serves as an artificial urinary sphincter when an alternative is necessary to empty the bladder. A surgically prepared continent urine reservoir with a sphincter mechanism is required in cases of bladder cancer and severe **interstitial cystitis** (inflammation of the bladder wall). Various types of urologic stomas may be used when a radical **cystectomy** (surgical removal of the bladder) is necessary.

UROLITHIASIS AND NEPHROLITHIASIS

Urolithiasis and nephrolithiasis refer to stones (calculi) in the urinary tract and kidney, respectively. Urinary stones predominantly occur in the third to fifth decades of life and affect men twice as often as women (Cunningham, Noble, Al-Modhefer, et al., 2016). Stones may develop in one or both kidneys and yearly episodes are increasing (Cunningham et al., 2016).

Most stones develop in the kidneys, although they can form along any part of the urinary tract. One in 10 Canadians is affected by kidney stones, with the highest incidence in males in the fourth to sixth decades of life (Hannon & Porth, 2017). About half of patients with a single renal stone have another episode within 5 years.

Pathophysiology

Stones are formed in the urinary tract when urinary concentrations of substances such as calcium oxalate, calcium phosphate, and uric acid increase. Referred to as supersaturation, this is dependent on the amount of the substance, ionic strength, and pH of the urine. Stones may be found anywhere from the kidney to the bladder and may vary in size from minute granular deposits, called *sand* or *gravel*, to bladder stones as large as an orange. The different sites of calculi formation in the urinary tract are shown in Figure 46-5.

Stone formation is not clearly understood, and there are a number of theories about their causes. One theory is that there is a deficiency of substances that normally prevent crystallization in the urine, such as citrate, magnesium, nephrocalcin, and uropontin (Hannon & Porth, 2017). Another theory relates to fluid volume status of the patient (stones tend to occur more often in dehydrated patients). Certain factors favour the formation of stones, including infection, urinary stasis, and periods of immobility, all of which slow renal drainage and alter calcium metabolism. In addition, increased calcium concentrations in the blood and urine promote precipitation of calcium and formation of stones (about 80% of all kidney stones are calcium based) (Cunningham et al., 2016). Causes of hypercalcemia (high serum calcium) and hypercalciuria (high urine calcium) include the following:

- Hyperparathyroidism
- Renal tubular acidosis
- Cancers

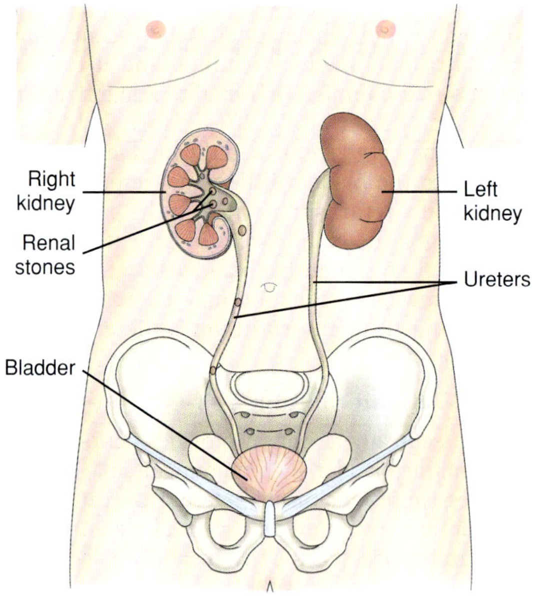

FIGURE 46-5. Examples of potential sites of calculi formation (urolithiasis) in the urinary tract.

- Granulomatous diseases (e.g., sarcoidosis, tuberculosis), which may cause increased vitamin D production by the granulomatous tissue
- Excessive intake of vitamin D
- Excessive intake of milk and alkali
- Myeloproliferative diseases (leukemia, polycythemia vera, multiple myeloma), which produce an unusual proliferation of blood cells from the bone marrow

There are four main types of stones: calcium, struvite, uric acid, and cystine. Of these four types, 70% are calcium stones. Hypercalcemia, hypercalciuria, hyperparathyroidism, diffuse bone disease, and immobilization are contributing factors to calcium stone formation. Magnesium ammonium phosphate (struvite) stones form from urea-splitting UTIs. Uric acid stones are most commonly found in individuals who have gout or consume a high-purine diet. Cystine stones are the least common type, making for less than 1% of urinary stones. Cystine stones can occur as a result of disorders of amino acid metabolism (Hannon & Porth, 2017; McCance & Huether, 2014).

Several conditions, as well as certain metabolic risk factors, predispose patients to stone formation. These include anatomic derangements such as polycystic kidney disease, horseshoe kidneys, chronic strictures, and medullary sponge disease. Urinary stone formation can occur in patients with inflammatory bowel disease and in those with an ileostomy or bowel resection because these patients absorb more oxalate. Medications known to cause stones in some patients include antacids, acetazolamide (Diamox), vitamin D, laxatives, and high doses of aspirin (Comerford, 2015). However, in many patients, no cause may be found.

Clinical Manifestations

Signs and symptoms of stones in the urinary system depend on the presence of obstruction, infection, and edema. When stones block the flow of urine, obstruction develops, producing an increase in hydrostatic pressure and distending the renal pelvis and proximal ureter. Some stones cause few, if any, symptoms while slowly destroying the functional units (nephrons) of the kidney; others cause excruciating pain and discomfort.

Stones in the renal pelvis may be associated with an intense, deep ache in the costovertebral region. Hematuria is often present; pyuria may also be noted. Pain originating in the renal area radiates anteriorly and downward toward the bladder in the female and toward the testis in the male. If the pain suddenly becomes acute, with tenderness over the costovertebral area, and nausea and vomiting appear, the patient is having an episode of renal colic. Diarrhea and abdominal discomfort may occur. These GI symptoms are due to renointestinal reflexes and the anatomic proximity of the kidneys to the stomach, pancreas, and large intestine.

Stones lodged in the ureter (ureteral obstruction) cause acute, excruciating, colicky, wave-like pain, radiating down the thigh and to the genitalia. Often, the patient has a desire to void, but little urine is passed, and it usually contains blood because of the abrasive action of the stone. This group of symptoms is called *ureteral colic*. Colic is mediated by prostaglandin E, a substance that increases ureteral contractility and renal blood flow and leads to increased intraureteral pressure and pain. In general, the patient spontaneously passes stones 0.5 to 1 cm in diameter. Stones larger than 1 cm in diameter usually must be removed or fragmented (broken up by lithotripsy) so that they can be removed or passed spontaneously.

Stones lodged in the bladder usually produce symptoms of irritation and may be associated with UTI and hematuria. If the stone obstructs the bladder neck, urinary retention occurs. If infection is associated with a stone, the condition is far more serious, with urosepsis threatening the patient's life.

Assessment and Diagnostic Findings

The diagnosis is confirmed by x-rays of the kidneys, ureters, and bladder (KUB) or by ultrasonography, IV urography, or retrograde pyelography. The noncontrast spiral CT is the optimum diagnostic test for confirming or ruling out acute renal colic (Hannon & Porth, 2017). Blood chemistries and urine tests are a part of the diagnostic workup. Dietary and medication histories and family history of renal stones are obtained to identify factors predisposing the patient to the formation of stones.

When stones are recovered (stones may be freely passed by the patient or removed through special procedures), chemical analysis is carried out to determine their composition. Stone analysis can provide a clear indication of the underlying disorder.

Medical Management

Treatment is mainly supportive with the goals of managing the acute pain, promoting passage of the stone(s), reducing the size of the stones, and preventing recurrence of stone formation (Hannon & Porth, 2017; McCance & Huether, 2014). Opioid analgesics are administered to prevent shock and syncope that may result from the excruciating pain. Nonsteroidal anti-inflammatory drugs (NSAIDs) are effective in treating kidney stone pain because they provide specific pain relief. They also inhibit the synthesis of prostaglandin E, reducing swelling and facilitating passage of the stone. Generally, once the stone has passed, the pain is relieved. Hot baths or moist heat to the flank areas may also be useful. Unless the patient is vomiting or has heart failure or any other condition requiring fluid restriction, fluids are encouraged. This increases the hydrostatic pressure behind the stone, assisting it in its downward passage. A high, around-the-clock fluid intake reduces the concentration of urinary crystalloids, dilutes the urine, and ensures a high urine output. Depending on the type of stone, changes in either dietary consumption, medications, or both may be necessary to modify the concentration of stone-forming elements in the urinary system (Hannon & Porth, 2017).

Nutritional Therapy

Nutritional therapy plays an important role in preventing kidney stones; it is safer and more economical than pharmacologic treatments (Chart 46-12) (Cunningham et al., 2016; Morgan & Pearle, 2016). Fluid intake is the mainstay of most medical therapy for kidney stones. Unless fluids are contraindicated, patients with kidney stones

CHART 46-12

Patient Education: Preventing Kidney Stones

The nurse instructs the patient to:

- Avoid protein intake; usually, protein is restricted to 60 g/day to decrease urinary excretion of calcium and uric acid.
- Limited sodium intake of 3 to 4 g/day is recommended. Table salt and high-sodium foods should be reduced, because sodium competes with calcium for reabsorption in the kidneys.
- Be aware that low-calcium diets are not generally recommended, except for true absorptive hypercalciuria. Evidence shows that limiting calcium, especially in women, can lead to osteoporosis and does not prevent stones.
- Avoid intake of oxalate-containing foods (e.g., spinach, strawberries, rhubarb, tea, peanuts, wheat bran).
- Drink fluids (ideally water and one glass of cranberry juice per day) every 1 to 2 hours during the day.
- Drink two glasses of water at bedtime and an additional glass at each nighttime awakening to prevent urine from becoming too concentrated during the night.
- Avoid activities leading to sudden increases in environmental temperatures that may cause excessive sweating and dehydration.
- Contact the primary health care provider at the first sign of a urinary tract infection.

should drink eight to ten 8-oz glasses of water daily or have IV fluids prescribed to keep the urine dilute. A urine output exceeding 2 L/day is advisable.

Interventional Procedures

If the stone does not pass spontaneously or if complications occur, common interventions include endoscopic or other procedures—for example, ureteroscopy, extracorporeal shock wave lithotripsy (ESWL), or endourologic (percutaneous) stone removal.

Ureteroscopy (Fig. 46-6A) involves first visualizing the stone and then destroying it. Access to the stone is accomplished by inserting a ureteroscope into the ureter and then inserting a laser, electrohydraulic lithotriptor, or ultrasound device through the ureteroscope to fragment and remove the stones. A stent may be inserted and left in place for 48 hours or more after the procedure to keep the ureter patent. Hospital stays are generally brief, and some patients can be treated as outpatients.

ESWL is a noninvasive procedure used to break up stones in the calyx of the kidney (Fig. 46-6B). After the stones are fragmented to the size of grains of sand, the remnants of the stones are spontaneously voided. In ESWL, a high-energy amplitude of pressure, or shock wave, is generated by the abrupt release of energy and transmitted through water and soft tissues. When the shock wave encounters a substance of different intensity (a kidney stone), a compression wave causes the surface of the stone to fragment. Repeated shock waves focused on the stone eventually reduce it to many small pieces that are excreted in the urine.

Discomfort from the multiple shocks may occur, although the shock waves usually do not cause damage to other tissue. The patient is observed for obstruction and infection resulting from blockage of the urinary tract by stone fragments. All urine is strained after the procedure; voided gravel or sand is sent to the laboratory for chemical analysis. Several treatments may be necessary to ensure disintegration of stones. Although lithotripsy is a costly treatment, its cost is offset by a decrease in the length of hospital stay and avoidance of a surgical procedure.

Endourologic methods of stone removal (Fig. 46-6C) may be used to extract renal calculi that cannot be removed by other procedures. A percutaneous nephrostomy or a percutaneous nephrolithotomy (which are similar procedures) may be performed. A nephroscope is introduced through a percutaneous route into the renal parenchyma. Depending on its size, the stone may be extracted with forceps or by a stone retrieval basket. If the stone is too large to initially be removed, an ultrasound probe inserted through a nephrostomy tube is used to pulverize the stone. Small stone fragments and stone dust are then removed from the collecting system.

Electrohydraulic lithotripsy is a similar method in which an electrical discharge is used to create a hydraulic shock wave to break up the stone. A probe is passed through the cystoscope, and the tip of the lithotriptor is placed near the stone. The strength of the discharge and pulse frequency can be varied. This procedure is performed under topical anesthesia. After the stone is extracted, the percutaneous nephrostomy tube is left in place for a time to ensure that the ureter is not obstructed by edema or blood clots. The most common complications are hemorrhage, infection, and urinary extravasation. After the tube is removed, the nephrostomy tract closes spontaneously.

Chemolysis, which is stone dissolution using infusions of chemical solutions (e.g., alkylating agents, acidifying agents) for the purpose of dissolving the stone, is an alternative treatment sometimes used in patients who are at risk of complications of other types of therapy, who refuse to undergo other methods, or who have stones (struvite) that dissolve easily. A percutaneous nephrostomy is performed, and the warm chemical solution is allowed to flow continuously onto the stone. The solution exits the renal collecting system by means of the ureter or the nephrostomy tube. The pressure inside the renal pelvis is monitored during the procedure.

Several of these treatment modalities may be used in combination to ensure removal of the stones.

Surgical Management

Surgical removal was the major mode of therapy before the advent of lithotripsy. However, today, surgery is performed in only 1% to 2% of patients. Surgical intervention is indicated if the stone does not respond to other forms of treatment. It may also be performed to correct anatomic abnormalities within the kidney to improve urinary drainage. If the stone is in the kidney, the surgery performed may be a nephrolithotomy (incision into the kidney with removal of the stone) or a nephrectomy if the kidney is nonfunctional secondary to infection or hydronephrosis. Stones in the kidney pelvis are removed by a pyelolithotomy, those in the ureter by ureterolithotomy, and those in the bladder by cystotomy. If the stone is in the bladder, an instrument may be inserted through the urethra into the bladder, and the stone is crushed in the jaws of this instrument. Such a procedure is called *cystolitholapaxy*. Nursing management following kidney surgery is discussed in Chapter 45.

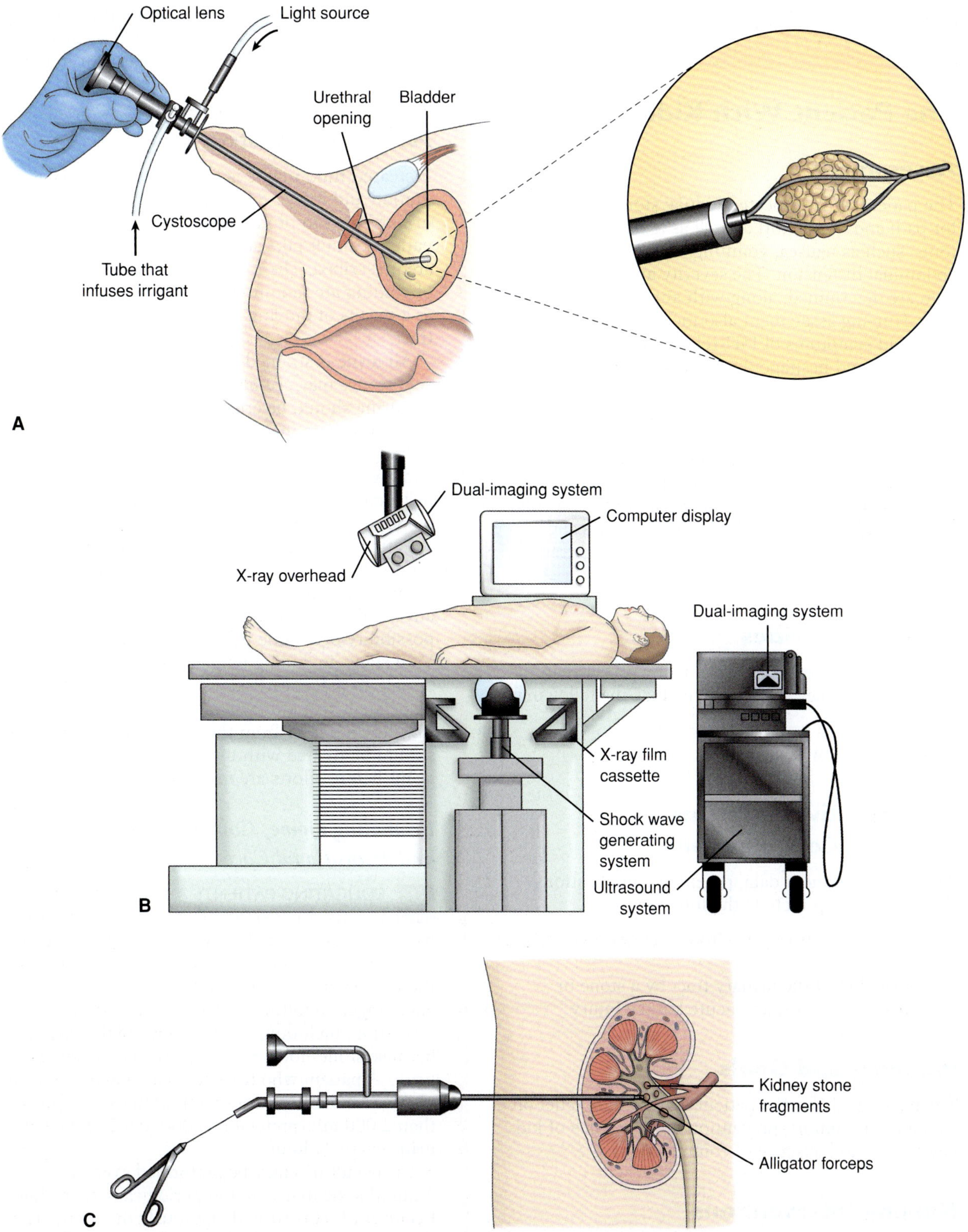

FIGURE 46-6. Methods of treating kidney stones. **A:** During a cystoscopy, which is used for removing small stones located in the ureter close to the bladder, a ureteroscope is inserted into the ureter to visualize the stone. The stone is then fragmented or captured and removed. **B:** Extracorporeal shock wave lithotripsy (ESWL) is used for most symptomatic, nonpassable upper urinary tract stones. Electromagnetically generated shock waves are focused over the area of the kidney stone. The high-energy dry shock waves pass through the skin and fragment the stone. **C:** Percutaneous nephrolithotomy is used to treat larger stones. A percutaneous tract is formed, and a nephroscope is inserted through it. Then, the stone is extracted or pulverized.

Nursing Process

The Patient With Kidney Stones

Assessment

The patient with suspected kidney stones is assessed for pain and discomfort as well as associated symptoms, such as nausea, vomiting, diarrhea, and abdominal distension. The severity and location of pain are determined, along with any radiation of the pain. Nursing assessment also includes observing for signs and symptoms of UTI (chills, fever, dysuria, frequency, and hesitancy) and obstruction (frequent urination of small amounts, oliguria, or anuria). The urine is inspected for blood and is strained for stones or gravel.

The history focuses on factors that predispose the patient to urinary tract stones or that may have precipitated the current episode of renal or ureteral colic. The patient's knowledge about kidney stones and measures to prevent their occurrence or recurrence is also assessed.

Nursing Priorities

Based on assessment data, the nursing priorities in the patient with kidney stones may include the following:

- Acute pain
- Deficient knowledge

Collaborative Problems/ Potential Complications

Based on assessment data, potential complications that may develop include the following:

- Infection and urosepsis (from UTI and pyelonephritis)
- Obstruction of the urinary tract by a stone or edema with subsequent acute kidney injury

Planning and Goals

The major goals for the patient may include relief of pain and discomfort, prevention of recurrence of kidney stones, and absence of complications.

Nursing Interventions

Relieving Pain

Severe and acute pain is often the presenting symptom of a patient with renal and urinary calculi and requires immediate attention. Opioid analgesic agents (IV or intramuscular) may be prescribed and administered to provide rapid relief along with an IV NSAID. The patient is encouraged and assisted to assume a position of comfort. If activity brings pain relief, the patient is assisted to ambulate. The pain level is monitored closely, and an increase in severity is reported promptly to the physician so that relief can be provided and additional treatment initiated.

Monitoring and Managing Potential Complications

Increased fluid intake is encouraged to prevent dehydration and increase hydrostatic pressure within the urinary tract to promote passage of the stone. If the patient cannot take adequate fluids orally, IV fluids are prescribed. The total urine output and patterns of voiding are monitored. Ambulation is encouraged as a means of moving the stone through the urinary tract.

All urine is strained through gauze because uric acid stones may crumble. Any blood clots passed in the urine should be crushed and the sides of the urinal and bedpan inspected for clinging stones. Because kidney stones increase the risk of infection, sepsis, and obstruction of the urinary tract, the patient is instructed to report decreased urine volume and bloody or cloudy urine.

Patients with calculi require frequent nursing observation to detect the spontaneous passage of a stone. The patient is instructed to immediately report any sudden increases in pain intensity because of the possibility of a stone fragment obstructing a ureter. Vital signs, including temperature, are monitored closely to detect early signs of infection. UTIs may be associated with kidney stones due to an obstruction from the stone or from the stone itself. All infections should be treated with the appropriate antibiotic agent before efforts are made to dissolve the stone.

Promoting Home, Community-Based, and Transitional Care

EDUCATING PATIENTS ABOUT SELF-CARE. Because the risk of recurring kidney stones is high, the nurse provides education about the causes of kidney stones and recommendations to prevent their recurrence (see Chart 46-12). The patient is encouraged to follow a regimen to avoid further stone formation, including maintaining a high fluid intake because stones form more readily in concentrated urine. A patient who has shown a tendency to form stones should drink enough fluid to excrete greater than 2,000 mL (preferably 3,000 to 4,000 mL) of urine every 24 hours.

Urine cultures may be performed every 1 to 2 months the first year and periodically thereafter. Recurrent UTI is treated vigorously due to the fact that prolonged immobilization slows renal drainage and alters calcium metabolism; increased mobility is encouraged whenever possible. In addition, excessive ingestion of vitamins (especially vitamin D) and minerals is discouraged.

If lithotripsy, percutaneous stone removal, ureteroscopy, or other surgical procedures for stone removal have been performed, the nurse instructs the patient about the signs and symptoms of complications that need to be reported to the physician.

The importance of follow-up to assess kidney function and to ensure the eradication or removal of all kidney stones is emphasized to the patient and family.

If ESWL has been performed, the nurse must provide instructions for home care and necessary follow-up. The patient is encouraged to increase fluid intake to assist in the passage of stone fragments, which may occur for 6 weeks to several months after the procedure. The patient and family are instructed about signs and symptoms that indicate complications, such as fever, decreasing urine output, and pain. It is also important to inform the patient to expect hematuria (it is anticipated in all patients), but it should disappear within 4 to 5 days. If the patient has a stent in the ureter, hematuria may be expected until the stent is removed. The patient is instructed to check his or her temperature daily and notify the physician if the temperature is greater than 38°C or the pain is unrelieved by the prescribed medication. The patient is also informed that a bruise may be observed on the treated side of the back.

CONTINUING AND TRANSITIONAL CARE. The patient is monitored closely in follow-up care to ensure that treatment has been effective and that no complications, such as obstruction, infection, renal hematoma, or hypertension, have developed. During the patient's visits to the clinic or physician's office, the nurse has the opportunity to assess the patient's understanding of ESWL and possible complications. In addition, the nurse has the opportunity to assess the patient's understanding of factors that increase the risk of recurrence of renal calculi and strategies to reduce those risks.

The patient's ability to monitor urinary pH and interpret the results is assessed during follow-up visits to the clinic or physician's office. Due to the high risk of recurrence, the patient with kidney stones needs to understand the signs and symptoms of stone formation, obstruction, and infection and the importance of reporting these signs promptly. If medications are prescribed for the prevention of stone formation, the actions and importance of the medications are explained to the patient.

Evaluation

Expected patient outcomes may include the following:

1. Reports relief of pain
2. States increased knowledge of health-seeking behaviours to prevent recurrence
   a. Increases fluid intake (at least eight 8-oz glasses of fluid per day)
   b. Participates in appropriate activity
   c. Consumes diet prescribed to reduce dietary factors predisposing to stone formation
   d. Recognizes symptoms (fever, chills, flank pain, hematuria) to be reported to health care provider
   e. Monitors urinary pH as directed
   f. Takes prescribed medication as directed to reduce stone formation
3. Experiences no complications
   a. Reports no signs or symptoms of infection or urosepsis
   b. Voids 200 to 400 mL per voiding of clear urine without evidence of bleeding
   c. Experiences absence of dysuria, frequency, and hesitancy
   d. Maintains normal body temperature

GENITOURINARY TRAUMA

Various types of injuries to the flank, back, or upper abdomen may result in trauma to the ureters, bladder, or urethra. Abdominal trauma is responsible for approximately 90% of all genitourinary trauma (Hallis, Amasyali, Yucak, et al., 2015). Of the 2.8 million trauma patients admitted yearly in the United States, 10% of them had sustained genitourinary injuries (McGeady & Breyer, 2013). In that same study, statistics for renal injuries were reported for Toronto and British Columbia, 3.25% and 1.4%, respectively. (Renal trauma is discussed in Chapter 45.)

Specific Injuries

Ureteral Trauma

Ureteral trauma is the least common injury of the genitourinary tract (Canadian Urological Association [CUA], 2016). Penetrating trauma and unintentional injury during surgery are the major causes of trauma to the ureters. Unintentional injury to the ureter may occur during gynecologic or urologic surgery. There are no specific signs or symptoms of ureteral injury; many traumatic injuries are discovered during exploratory surgery. If the ureteral trauma is not detected and urine leakage continues, fistulas can develop.

IV pyelogram detects 94% of ureteral injuries but direct inspection during laparotomy is the optimal diagnostic test (CUA, 2016). Surgical repair with placement of stents (to divert urine away from an anastomosis) is usually necessary.

Bladder Trauma

Injury to the bladder may occur with pelvic fractures and multiple trauma or from a blow to the lower abdomen when the bladder is full. In fact, 10% of pelvic fractures have bladder injuries (CUA, 2016). Blunt trauma may result in contusion evident as an ecchymosis—a large bruise resulting from escape of blood into the tissues and involving a segment of the bladder wall—or in rupture of the bladder extraperitoneally, intraperitoneally, or both. Complications from these injuries include hemorrhage, shock, sepsis, and extravasation of blood into the tissues, which must be treated promptly. If a bladder injury is suspected, a cystogram is the most important test (CUA, 2016).

Urethral Trauma

Urethral injuries usually occur with blunt trauma to the lower abdomen or pelvic region. Many patients also have associated pelvic fractures (5%) (CUA, 2016). The classic triad of symptoms comprises blood at the urinary meatus, inability to void, and a distended bladder.

Medical Management

The goals of management in patients with genitourinary trauma are to control hemorrhage, pain, and infection and to maintain urinary drainage. Genitourinary trauma is frequently associated with renal trauma (see Chapter 45). Hematocrit and hemoglobin levels are monitored closely; decreasing values indicate hemorrhage within the genitourinary system. The patient is also monitored for oliguria, signs of hemorrhagic shock, and signs and symptoms of acute peritonitis.

Surgical Management

In urethral trauma, unstable patients who need monitoring of urine output may need a suprapubic catheter inserted. The patient is catheterized after urethrography is performed to minimize the risk of urethral disruption and extensive, long-term complications, such as stricture, incontinence, and impotence. Surgical repair may be performed using either open or laparoscopic approaches (Hallis et al., 2015), and may be performed immediately or at a later time. Delayed surgical repair tends to be the preferred procedure because it is associated with fewer long-term complications, such as impotence, strictures, and incontinence. After surgery, an indwelling urinary catheter may remain in place for up to 1 month.

Nursing Management

The patient with genitourinary trauma should be assessed frequently during the first few days after injury to detect flank and abdominal pain, muscle spasm, and swelling over the flank.

During this time, patients can be instructed about care of the incision and the importance of an adequate fluid intake. In addition, instructions about changes that should be reported to the physician, such as fever, hematuria, flank pain, or any signs and symptoms of decreasing kidney function, are provided. The patient with a ruptured bladder may have gross bleeding for several days after repair. Guidelines for increasing activity gradually, lifting, and driving are also provided in accordance with the physician's prescription.

Follow-up nursing care includes monitoring the blood pressure to detect hypertension and advising the patient to restrict activities for about 1 month after trauma to minimize the incidence of delayed or secondary bleeding.

URINARY TRACT CANCERS

Urinary tract cancers include those of the urinary bladder; kidney and renal pelvis; ureters; and other urinary structures, such as the prostate. According to the Canadian Cancer Society's Cancer Statistics Report (2017) prostate cancer is the fourth most common type, accounting for 21% of cancers among males. The greatest number of prostate cancers is diagnosed in males in the sixth decade of life. (Renal cancer is discussed in Chapter 45, and prostate cancer is discussed in Chapter 50.) Malignant tumours of the urinary tract include transitional cell carcinomas (90%), squamous cell carcinomas (5% to 8%), adenocarcinomas (1% to 2%), sarcomas (less than 1%), and other types of cancers.

Cancer of the Bladder

Cancer of the urinary bladder affects more men than women at approximately a 4:1 ratio. Bladder cancer is the 4th most commonly diagnosed cancer in males and the 12th most commonly diagnosed cancer in females (Canadian Cancer Society's Advisory Committee, 2017). Bladder cancer has a high worldwide incidence.

Bladder cancer, combined with prostatic cancer, is among the most common urologic malignancies. Cancers arising from the prostate, colon, and rectum in males and from the lower gynecologic tract in females may metastasize to the bladder (Chart 46-13). The risk of developing bladder cancer increases with age. It usually occurs in people over the age of 65 years. Men develop bladder cancer more often than women. Bladder cancer is more common in Caucasians.

It was estimated that in 2017:

- 8,900 Canadians will be diagnosed with bladder cancer.
- 2,400 Canadians will die from bladder cancer.
- 6,700 men will be diagnosed with bladder cancer and 1,700 will die from it.
- 2,200 women will be diagnosed with bladder cancer and 680 will die from it.

Most bladder cancers are linked to smoking tobacco. Carcinogens that are found in tobacco smoke are also found in the urine of smokers. In the urine, these chemicals damage the cells that line the inside of the bladder (urothelial cells), which could lead to cancer. The carcinogens from tobacco smoke found in urine include:

- aromatic amines—alpha naphthylamine and beta naphthylamine
- some cyclic N-nitrosamines
- arsenic

CHART 46-13

Selected Risk Factors: Bladder Cancer

- Certain genetic mutations including:
  - *HRAS* mutation (Costello syndrome, Facio-cutaneous-skeletal syndrome)
  - *RB1* mutation
  - *PTEN/MMAC1* mutation (Cowden syndrome)
  - *NAT2* slow acetylator phenotype
  - *GSTM1* null phenotype
- Exposure to arsenic
- Occupational exposure to chemicals in processed paint, dye, metal, and petroleum products
- Positive family history of bladder cancer
- Pelvic radiation therapy or treatment for other cancers
- Tobacco use, cigarette smoking in particular

Adapted from National Cancer Institute (NCI). (2016). *Bladder cancer treatment (PDQ®)—Health professional version*. Retrieved December 13, 2016, from www.cancer.gov/types/bladder/hp/bladder-treatment-pdq#section/all

The risk of bladder cancer is associated with the number of cigarettes smoked per day, the number of years a person has smoked, and the age at which a person started smoking (Canadian Cancer Society [CCS], 2018).

Clinical Manifestations

Bladder tumours usually arise at the base of the bladder and involve the ureteral orifices and bladder neck. Visible, painless hematuria is the most common symptom of bladder cancer. Infection of the urinary tract is a common complication, producing frequency, urgency, and dysuria. However, any alteration in voiding or change in the urine may indicate cancer of the bladder. Pelvic or back pain may occur with metastasis.

Assessment and Diagnostic Findings

The diagnostic evaluation includes cystoscopy (the mainstay of diagnosis), excretory urography, CT, ultrasonography, and bimanual examination with the patient anaesthetized. Biopsies of the tumour and adjacent mucosa are the definitive diagnostic procedures. Transitional cell carcinomas and carcinoma in situ shed recognizable cancer cells. Cytologic examination of fresh urine and saline bladder washings provide information about the prognosis and staging, especially for patients at high risk for recurrence of primary bladder tumours.

Although the mainstay diagnostic tools such as cytology and CT have a high detection rate, they are costly. Newer diagnostic tools such as bladder tumour antigens, nuclear matrix proteins, adhesion molecules, cytoskeletal proteins, and growth factors are being studied to support the early detection and diagnosis of bladder cancer. Regular cystoscopy continues to be the standard test for finding bladder cancer (CCS, 2018).

Medical Management

Treatment of bladder cancer depends on the grade of the tumour (the degree of cellular differentiation), the stage of tumour growth (the degree of local invasion and the presence or absence of metastasis), and the multicentricity (having many centres) of the tumour. The patient's age and physical, mental, and emotional status are considered when determining treatment modalities.

Surgical Management

Transurethral resection or fulguration (cauterization) may be performed for simple papillomas (benign epithelial tumours). These procedures, described in more detail in Chapter 50, eradicate the tumours through surgical incision or electrical current with the use of instruments inserted through the urethra. After this bladder-sparing surgery, intravesical administration of bacille Calmette–Guérin (BCG) is the treatment of choice. BCG is an attenuated live strain of *Mycobacterium bovis*, the causative agent for tuberculosis. The exact action of BCG is unknown, but it is thought to have a component of direct toxicity as well as a systemic immunologic response (Hannon & Porth, 2017).

Management of superficial bladder cancers presents a challenge because there are usually widespread abnormalities in the bladder mucosa. The entire lining of the urinary tract, or urothelium, is at risk because carcinomatous changes can occur in the mucosa of the bladder, renal pelvis, ureter, and urethra. Tumour recurrence is common even after transurethral resection or fulguration (Jancke, Rosell, Jahnson, 2012). Patients with benign papillomas should undergo cytology and cystoscopy periodically for the rest of their lives because aggressive malignancies may develop from these tumours.

A simple cystectomy or a radical cystectomy is performed for invasive or multifocal bladder cancer. Radical cystectomy in men involves removal of the bladder, prostate, and seminal vesicles and immediate adjacent perivesical tissues. In women, radical cystectomy involves removal of the bladder, lower ureter, uterus, fallopian tubes, ovaries, anterior vagina, and urethra. It may include removal of pelvic lymph nodes. Removal of the bladder requires a urinary diversion procedure. This is described later in this chapter.

Although radical cystectomy remains the standard of care for invasive bladder cancer, researchers are exploring trimodality therapy—transurethral resection of the bladder tumour, radiation, and chemotherapy—in an effort to spare patients the need for cystectomy. This approach to transitional cell bladder cancer mandates lifelong surveillance with periodic cystoscopy. Although most patients respond completely and their bladders remain free from invasive relapse, one fourth develop a relapse of noninvasive disease. This may be managed with transurethral resection of the bladder tumour and intravesical therapies but carries an additional risk that a late cystectomy may be required. Outcomes are similar for patients who undergo the trimodality therapy and those who had had radical cystectomy (Kulkarni, Hermanns, Wei, et al., 2017).

Pharmacologic Therapy

Chemotherapy with a combination of methotrexate, 5-fluorouracil, vinblastine, doxorubicin (Adriamycin), and cisplatin has been effective in producing partial remission of transitional cell carcinoma of the bladder in some patients. IV chemotherapy may be accompanied by radiation therapy. Topical chemotherapy (intravesical chemotherapy or instillation of antineoplastic agents into the bladder, resulting in contact of the agent with the bladder wall) is considered when there is a high risk of recurrence, when cancer in situ is present, or when tumour resection has been incomplete. Topical chemotherapy delivers a high concentration of medication (thiotepa, doxorubicin, mitomycin, ethoglucid, and BCG) to the tumour to promote tumour destruction. Bladder cancer may also be treated by direct infusion of the cytotoxic agent through the bladder's arterial blood supply to achieve a higher concentration of the chemotherapeutic agent with fewer systemic toxic effects.

BCG is now considered the most effective intravesical agent for recurrent bladder cancer, especially superficial transitional cell carcinoma, because it is an immunotherapeutic agent that enhances the body's immune response to cancer. BCG has a 43% advantage in preventing tumour recurrence, a significantly better rate than the 16% to 21% advantage of intravesical chemotherapy. In addition, BCG is particularly effective in the treatment of carcinoma in situ, eradicating it in more than 80% of cases. In contrast to intravesical chemotherapy, BCG has also been shown to decrease the risk of tumour progression.

The optimal course of BCG appears to be a 6-week course of weekly instillations, followed by a 3-week course at 3 months for tumours that do not respond. In high-risk cancers, maintenance BCG is administered in a 3-week course at 3 and 6 months, then every 6 months up to 36 years (Kassouf, Traboulsi, Kulkarni, et al., 2015). However, the adverse effects associated with this prolonged therapy may limit its widespread applicability.

The patient is allowed to eat and drink before the instillation procedure. Once the bladder is full, the patient must retain the intravesical solution for 2 hours before voiding. At the end of the procedure, the patient is encouraged to void and to drink liberal amounts of fluid to flush the medication from the bladder.

Radiation Therapy

Radiation of the tumour may be performed preoperatively to reduce microextension of the neoplasm and viability of tumour cells, thus reducing the chances that the cancer may recur in the immediate area or spread through the circulatory or lymphatic systems. Radiation therapy is also used in combination with surgery or to control the disease in patients with inoperable tumours.

For more advanced bladder cancer or for patients with intractable hematuria (especially after radiation therapy), a large, water-filled balloon placed in the bladder produces tumour necrosis by reducing the blood supply of the bladder wall (hydrostatic therapy). The instillation of formalin, phenol, or silver nitrate relieves hematuria and strangury (slow and painful discharge of urine) in some patients.

Photodynamic Therapy

The use of photodynamic therapies (PDT) in treating superficial bladder cancer continues to be refined. PDT is based on the interaction between light, oxygen within the body tissues, and a photosensitive agent. The interaction between the three components leads to the release of a singlet oxygen and antioxidant enzymes. Death to tumour cells are caused by apoptosis or induction of necrosis. PDT can also cause destruction of the tumour vasculature producing an inflammatory response and the subsequent arrival of leukocytes (Bozzini, Colin, Betrouni, et al., 2012).

URINARY DIVERSIONS

Urinary diversion procedures are performed to divert urine from the bladder to a new exit site, usually through a surgically created opening (stoma) in the skin. These procedures are primarily performed when a bladder tumour necessitates cystectomy. Urinary diversion has also been used in managing pelvic malignancy, birth defects, strictures, trauma to the ureters and urethra, neurogenic bladder, chronic infection causing severe ureteral and renal damage, and intractable interstitial cystitis. It may also be used as a last resort in managing incontinence.

Controversy exists regarding the best method of establishing permanent diversion of the urinary tract. New techniques are frequently introduced in an effort to improve patient outcomes and quality of life. The age of the patient, condition of the bladder, body build, degree of obesity, degree of ureteral dilation, status of renal function, and the patient's learning ability and willingness to participate in postoperative care are all taken into consideration when determining the appropriate surgical procedure.

The extent to which the patient accepts urinary diversion depends to a large degree on the location or position of the stoma, whether the drainage device (pouch or bag) establishes a watertight seal to the skin, and the patient's ability to manage the pouch and drainage apparatus (Rubenwolf, Hampel, Roos, et al., 2016).

There are two types of urinary diversion. In a cutaneous urinary diversion, urine drains through an opening created in the abdominal wall and skin (Fig. 46-7). In a **continent urinary diversion**, a portion of the intestine is used to create a new reservoir for urine (Fig. 46-8). Chart 46-14 provides a plan of care for patients with urinary diversions.

Cutaneous Urinary Diversions

Ileal Conduit

The **ileal conduit** (ileal loop) is the oldest and most common of the urinary diversion procedures in use because of the low number of complications and surgeons' familiarity with the procedure. In an ileal conduit, the urine is diverted by implanting the ureter into a 12-cm loop of ileum that is led out through the abdominal wall. This loop of ileum is a simple conduit (passageway) for urine from the ureters to the surface. A loop of the sigmoid colon may also be used (Rubenwolf et al., 2016). An ileostomy bag is used to collect the urine. The resected (cut) ends of the remaining intestine are anastomosed (connected) to provide an intact bowel.

Stents, usually made of thin, pliable tubing, are placed in the ureters to prevent occlusion secondary to postsurgical edema. The bilateral ureteral stents allow urine to drain from the kidney to the stoma and provide a method for accurate measurement of urine output. They may be left in place for 10 to 21 days postoperatively. Jackson–Pratt tubes or other types of drains are inserted to prevent the accumulation of fluid in the space created by removal of the bladder.

After surgery, a skin barrier and a transparent, disposable urinary drainage bag are applied around the conduit and connected to drainage. A custom-cut appliance is used until the edema subsides and the stoma shrinks to normal size. The clear bag allows the stoma to be inspected and the patency of the stent and the urine output to be monitored. The ileal bag drains urine (not feces) continuously. The appliance (bag) usually remains in place as long as it is watertight; it is changed when necessary to prevent leakage of urine.

Complications

Complications that may follow placement of an ileal conduit include wound infection or wound dehiscence, urinary leakage, ureteral obstruction, hyperchloremic acidosis, small bowel obstruction, ileus, and gangrene of the stoma. Delayed complications include ureteral obstruction, contraction or narrowing of the stoma (stenosis), kidney deterioration due

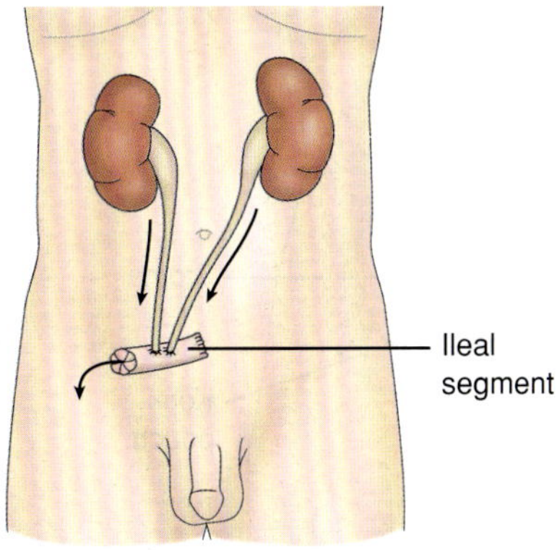

A Conventional ileal conduit.
The surgeon transplants the ureters to an isolated section of the terminal ileum (ileal conduit), bringing one end to the abdominal wall. The ureter may also be transplanted into the transverse sigmoid colon (colon conduit) or proximal jejunum (jejunal conduit).

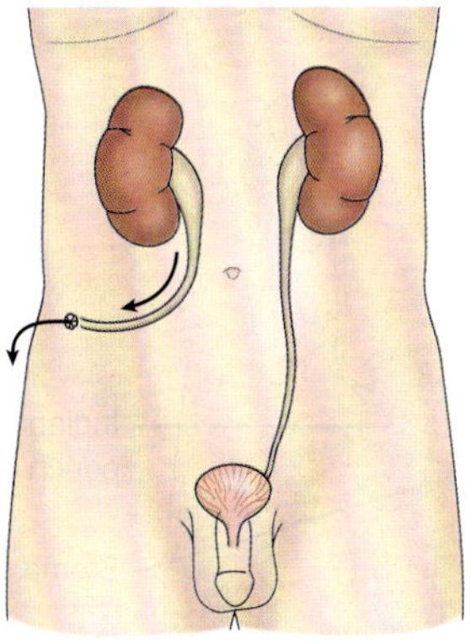

B Cutaneous ureterostomy.
The surgeon brings the detached ureter through the abdominal wall and attaches it to an opening in the skin.

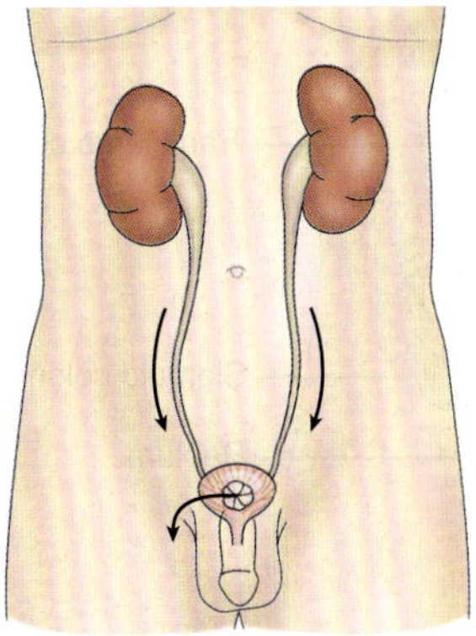

C Vesicostomy.
The surgeon sutures the bladder to the abdominal wall and creates an opening (stoma) through the abdominal and bladder walls for urinary drainage.

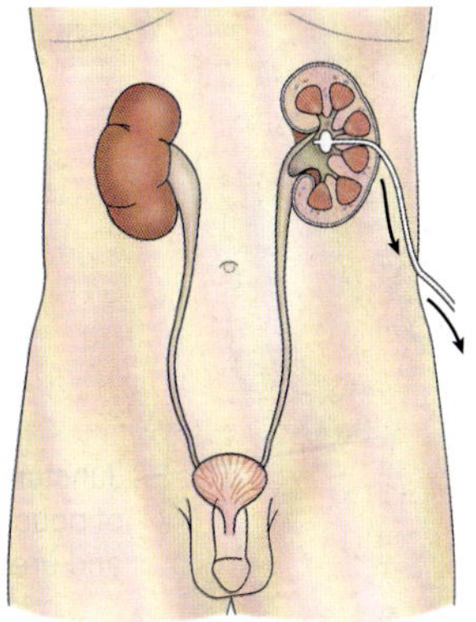

D Nephrostomy.
The surgeon inserts a catheter into the renal pelvis via an incision in the flank or by percutaneous catheter placement into the kidney.

FIGURE 46-7. Types of cutaneous diversions include the conventional ileal conduit (**A**), cutaneous ureterostomy (**B**), vesicostomy (**C**), and nephrostomy (**D**).

to chronic reflux, pyelonephritis, renal calculi, and cancer recurrence (Rubenwolf et al., 2016; Smolar, Salemi, Horst, et al., 2016).

Nursing Management

In the immediate postoperative period, urine volumes are monitored hourly. Throughout the patient's hospitalization, the nurse monitors closely for complications, reports signs and symptoms of them promptly, and intervenes quickly to prevent their progression.

A urine output below 30 mL/hour may indicate dehydration or an obstruction in the ileal conduit, with possible backflow or leakage from the ureteroileal anastomosis. After the physician's order is obtained, a catheter may be inserted through the urinary conduit to monitor the patient for possible stasis or residual urine from a constricted stoma. Urine may drain through the bilateral ureteral stents as well as around the stents. If the ureteral stents are not draining, the nurse may be instructed to carefully irrigate with 5 to 10 mL of sterile normal saline solution, being careful not to exert tension that could dislodge the stent. Hematuria may be noted in the first 48 hours after surgery but usually resolves spontaneously.

Providing Stoma and Skin Care

Because the patient requires specialized care, a consultation is initiated with a wound care specialist/enterostomal therapist. The stoma is inspected frequently for colour and viability. A healthy stoma is beefy red. A change from this normal colour to a dark purplish colour suggests that the vascular supply may be compromised. If cyanosis and a compromised blood supply persist, surgical intervention may be necessary. The stoma is not sensitive to touch, but the skin around the stoma becomes sensitive if urine or the appliance irritates it. The skin is inspected for (a) signs of irritation and bleeding of the stoma mucosa, (b) encrustation and skin irritation around the stoma (from alkaline urine coming in contact with exposed skin), and (c) wound infections.

Testing Urine and Caring for the Ostomy

Moisture in bed linens or clothing or the odour of urine around the patient should alert the nurse to the possibility

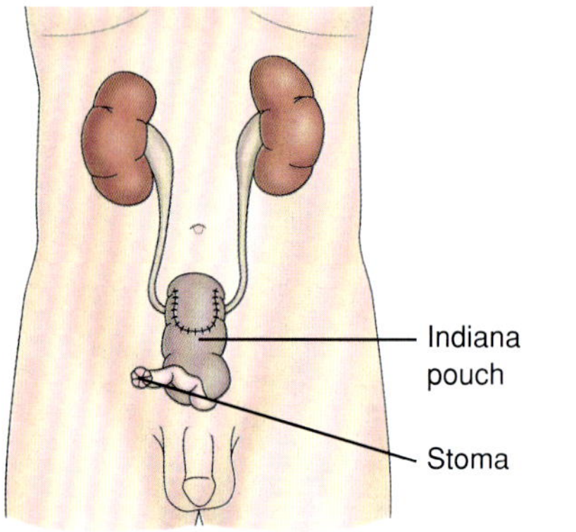

A Indiana pouch.
The surgeon introduces the ureters into a segment of ileum and cecum. Urine is drained periodically by inserting a catheter into the stoma.

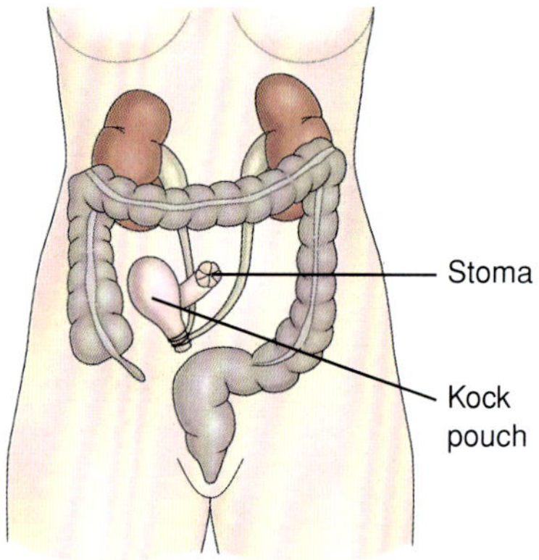

B Continent ileal urinary diversions (Kock pouch).
The surgeon transplants the ureters to an isolated segment of small bowel, ascending colon, or ileocolonic segment and develops an effective continence mechanism or valve. Urine is drained by inserting a catheter into the stoma.

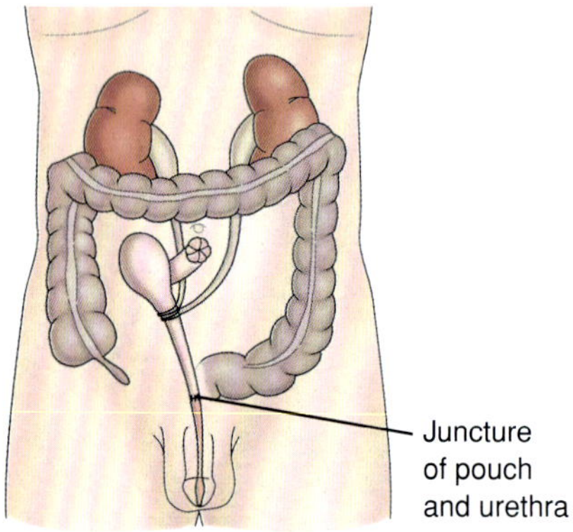

C
In male patients, the Kock pouch can be modified by attaching one end of the pouch to the urethra, allowing more normal voiding. The female urethra is too short for this modification.

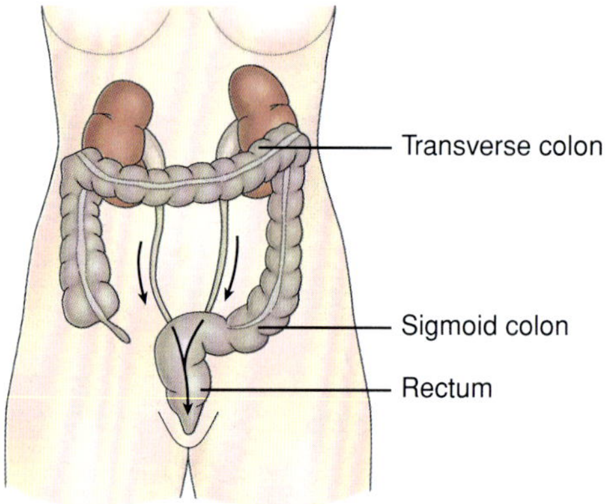

D Ureterosigmoidostomy.
The surgeon introduces the ureters into the sigmoid colon, thereby allowing urine to flow through the colon and out of the rectum.

FIGURE 46-8. Types of continent urinary diversions include the Indiana pouch (**A**), the Kock pouch (**B, C**), also called a *continent ileal diversion*, and a ureterosigmoidostomy (**D**).

of leakage from the appliance, potential infection, or a problem in hygienic management. Because severe alkaline encrustation can accumulate rapidly around the stoma, the urine pH is kept below 6.5 by administration of ascorbic acid by mouth. Urine pH can be determined by testing the urine draining from the stoma, not from the collecting appliance. A properly fitted appliance is essential to prevent exposure of the skin around the stoma to urine. The opening of the appliance should be no more than 1 to 2 mm larger than the actual stoma and the same shape (Burch, 2013). If the urine is foul smelling, the stoma is catheterized, if prescribed, to obtain a urine specimen for culture and sensitivity testing.

Encouraging Fluids and Relieving Anxiety

Because mucous membrane is used in forming the conduit, the patient may excrete a large amount of mucus mixed with urine. This causes anxiety in many patients. To help relieve this anxiety, the nurse reassures the patient that this is a normal occurrence after an ileal conduit procedure. The nurse encourages adequate fluid intake to flush the ileal conduit and decrease the accumulation of mucus.

Selecting the Ostomy Appliance

Various urine collection appliances are available, and the nurse is instrumental in selecting an appropriate one. The urinary appliance may consist of one or two pieces and may be disposable (usually used once and discarded) or reusable. The choice of appliance is determined by the location of the stoma and by the patient's normal activity, manual dexterity, visual function, body build, economic resources, and preference.

Promoting Home, Community-Based, and Transitional Care

Educating Patients About Self-Care

Patient education begins in the hospital but continues into the home setting because patients are usually discharged within days of surgery. The nurse teaches the patient how to assess and manage the urinary diversion as well as how to deal with body image changes. A wound care specialist/enterostomal therapist is invaluable in consulting with the nurse on various aspects of care and patient education.

Plan of Nursing Care

Chart 46-14. Care of the Patient With a Urinary Diversion

Nursing Priority: Disturbed body image
Goal: Healthy body image will be maintained

NURSING INTERVENTIONS	RATIONALE	EXPECTED OUTCOMES
1. Assess for patient's mood and affect with respect to urinary diversion	1. Patient's reaction to diversion will enable the nurse to assess for further psychosocial interventions as necessary	• Voices acceptance of urinary diversion, stoma, and appliance • Demonstrates increasingly independent self-care, including hygiene and grooming • Accepts support and assistance from family members, health care providers, and other ostomates
2. Encourage the patient to discuss concerns and anxiety about diversion	2. Allowing the patient to express concerns and anxious feelings can help, especially in adjusting to the changes in toileting habits	
3. Teach the patient the skills needed to be independent in managing the urinary drainage devices	3. Acquiring the skills to manage the devices can improve the patient's self-concept	
4. Provide education about ostomy care in a private setting	4. A private setting may encourage the patient to ask questions without fear of embarrassment	
5. Explain the reason for wearing gloves when assisting with ostomy care for the patient	5. Providing an explanation can prevent the patient from misinterpreting the use of gloves as a sign of aversion to the stoma	

Nursing Priority: Impaired skin integrity
Goal: Condition of skin around stoma will remain intact

NURSING INTERVENTIONS	RATIONALE	EXPECTED OUTCOMES
1. Inspect stoma and skin around stoma	1. Can give an indication of any signs of skin irritation or breakdown, allowing for the implementation of treatment measures as necessary	• Pink and moist appearance of stoma • Intact condition of skin around stoma • State actions to take if skin excoriation occurs • Demonstrates skill in managing drainage system
2. Ensure that the opening of the stoma is 1 to 2 mm larger than the actual stoma. (Initial opening may be larger due to swelling of the stoma but should be adjusted as edema decreases)	2. Prevents exposure of the skin around the stoma to urine	
3. Consult enterostomal therapist/wound care specialist if service is available	3. Patient will benefit from expert knowledge and experience on various aspects of care and education	
4. Encourage patient to maintain adequate nutritional intake	4. Poor nutrition will delay wound healing	
5. Investigate any complaints of burning or itching of the skin	5. Prompt assessment and treatment will prevent further skin breakdown	
6. Teach the patient self-management of stoma and appliance/drainage system care	6. Self-management is essential to maintaining skin integrity	

Nursing Priority: Deficient knowledge
Goal: Informed self-management of altered urinary diversion and accompanying external devices

NURSING INTERVENTIONS	RATIONALE	EXPECTED OUTCOMES
1. Assess patient's level of knowledge and understanding	1. Allows for the education to be tailored to patient's needs	• Performs self-care and proficient management of urinary diversion and appliance • Asks questions relevant to self-management and prevention of complications • Identifies signs and symptoms needing care from physician, nurse, or other health care providers
2. Teach patient and family about appearance of normal stoma	2. Assists with the self-management of the chronic condition	
3. Provide teaching with each drainage device change (refer to Chart 46-14)	3. Assists with development of competence with self-care of stoma and appliance. Involvement of patients also tailors the teaching	
4. Gradually transfer responsibility of care over to the patient and family	4. Repeated practice under guidance (if necessary) will help to develop confidence in caring for stoma and appliance	

CHART 46-15

Patient Education: Using Urinary Diversion Collection Appliances

Applying a Reusable Pouch System

The nurse instructs the patient to:

1. Gather all necessary supplies.
2. Prepare new appliance according to the manufacturer's directions:
   - Apply double-faced adhesive disc that has been properly sized to fit the reusable pouch faceplate.
   - Remove paper backing and set pouch aside, or apply thin layer of contact cement to one side of the reusable pouch faceplate.
   - Set pouch aside.
3. Remove soiled pouch gently. Lay aside to clean later.
4. Clean peristomal skin (skin around stoma) with small amount of soap and water. Rinse thoroughly and dry. If a film of soap remains on the skin and the site does not dry, the appliance will not adhere adequately.
5. Use a wick (rolled gauze pad or tampon) over the stoma to absorb urine and keep the skin dry throughout the appliance change.
6. Inspect peristomal skin for irritation.
7. Note that a skin protector wipe or barrier ring may be applied before centring the faceplate opening directly over the stoma.
8. Position appliance over stoma, and press gently into place.
9. If desired, use a pouch cover or apply cornstarch under the pouch to prevent perspiration and skin irritation.
10. Clean soiled pouch, and prepare for reuse.

Applying a Disposable Pouch System

The nurse instructs the patient to:

1. Gather all necessary supplies.
2. Measure stoma, and prepare an opening in the skin barrier about 1/8 in larger than the stoma and the same shape as the stoma.
3. Remove paper backing from skin barrier, and set aside.
4. Gently remove old appliance, and set aside.
5. Clean peristomal skin with warm water, and dry thoroughly.
6. Inspect peristomal skin (skin around stoma) for irritation.
7. Use a wick (rolled gauze pad or tampon) over the stoma to absorb urine, and keep the skin dry during the appliance change.
8. Centre opening of skin barrier over stoma, and apply with firm, gentle pressure to attain a watertight seal.
9. If using a two-piece system, snap pouch onto the flanged wafer that adheres to skin.
10. Close drainage tap or spout at bottom of pouch.
11. Note that a pouch cover can be used or cornstarch applied under pouch to prevent perspiration and skin irritation.
12. Apply hypoallergenic tape around the skin barrier in a picture-frame manner.
13. Dispose of soiled appliance.

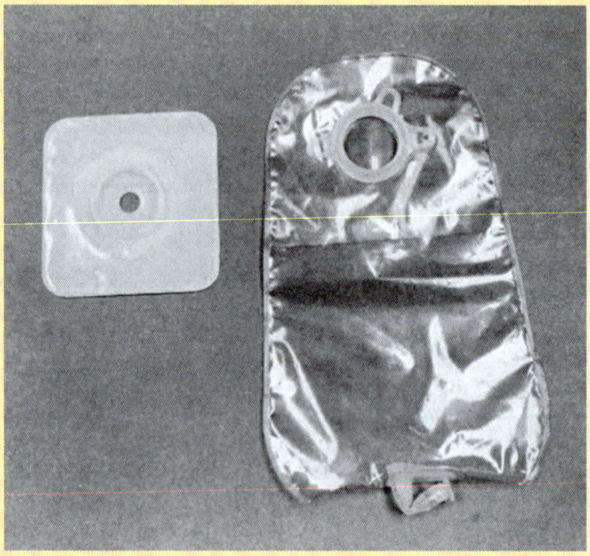

Adapted from Dukes, S., Lowther, C., Martin, T., et al. (2013). Guidelines for standardising the treatment of stoma granulomas at the mucocutaneous junction. *World Council of Enterostomal Therapists Journal*, *33*(1), 12–15.

CHANGING THE APPLIANCE. The patient and family are taught to apply and change the appliance so that they are comfortable carrying out the procedure and can do so proficiently. Ideally, the appliance system is changed before the system leaks and at a time that is convenient for the patient. Many patients find early morning most convenient because the urine output is reduced. A variety of appliances are available; an average collecting appliance lasts 3 to 7 days before leakage occurs.

Regardless of the type of appliance used, a skin barrier is essential to protect the skin from irritation and excoriation. To maintain skin integrity, a skin barrier or leaking pouch is never patched with tape to prevent accumulation of urine under the skin barrier or faceplate. The patient is instructed to avoid moisturizing soaps when cleaning the area because they interfere with the adhesion of the pouch. Because the degree to which the stoma protrudes is not the same in all patients, there are various accessories and custom-made appliances to solve individual problems. Guidelines for applying reusable and disposable systems are presented in Chart 46-15.

CONTROLLING ODOUR. The patient is instructed to avoid foods that give the urine a strong odour (e.g., asparagus, cheese, eggs). Today, most appliances contain odour barriers, but a few drops of liquid deodorizer or diluted white vinegar may be introduced through the drain spout into the bottom of the pouch with a syringe or eyedropper to reduce odours. Ascorbic acid by mouth helps to acidify the urine and suppress urine odour. Patients should be cautioned not to put aspirin tablets in the pouch to control odour, as they may ulcerate the stoma. Also, the patient is reminded that odour will develop if the pouch is worn longer than recommended and not cared for properly.

MANAGING THE OSTOMY APPLIANCE. The patient is instructed to empty the pouch by means of a drain valve when it is one third full because the weight of more urine will cause the pouch to separate from the skin. Some patients prefer wearing a leg bag attached with an adapter to the drainage apparatus. To promote uninterrupted sleep, a collecting bottle and tubing (one unit) are snapped onto an adapter that connects to the ileal appliance. A small amount of urine is left in the bag when the adapter is attached to prevent the bag from collapsing against itself. The tubing may be threaded down the pajama or pants leg to prevent kinking. The collecting bottle and tubing are rinsed daily with cool water and once a week with a 3:1 solution of water and white vinegar.

CLEANING AND DEODORIZING THE APPLIANCE. Usually, the reusable appliance is rinsed in warm water and soaked in a 3:1 solution of water and white vinegar or a commercial deodorizing solution for 30 minutes. It is rinsed with tepid water and air-dried away from direct sunlight. (Hot water and exposure to direct sunlight dry the pouch and increase the incidence of cracking.) After drying, the appliance may be powdered with cornstarch and stored. Two appliances are necessary—one to be worn while the other is air-drying.

Continuing and Transitional Care

Follow-up care is essential to determine how the patient has adapted to the body image changes as well as lifestyle changes. Referral for home care is indicated to determine how well the patient and family are coping with the changes necessitated by altered urinary drainage. The home care nurse assesses the patient's physical status and emotional response to urinary diversion. Additionally, the nurse assesses the ability of the patient and family to manage the urinary diversion and appliance, reinforces previous teaching, and provides additional information (e.g., community resources, sources of ostomy supplies, insurance coverage for supplies).

As the postoperative edema subsides, the home care nurse assists in determining the appropriate changes needed in the ostomy appliance. The size of the stoma is measured every 3 to 6 weeks for the first few months postoperatively. The correct appliance size is determined by measuring the widest part of the stoma with a ruler. The permanent appliance should be no more than 1 to 2 mm larger than the actual stoma and the same shape as the stoma to prevent contact of the skin with drainage (Burch, 2013).

The nurse teaches the patient and family about resources (see the Resources section). Local chapters of the CCS can provide resources for the patient who has undergone ostomy surgery for cancer.

The home care nurse assesses the patient for potential long-term complications such as ureteral obstruction, stenosis, hernias, or deterioration of renal function and reinforces previous teaching about these complications.

Cutaneous Ureterostomy

Cutaneous ureterostomy (see Fig. 46-7), in which the ureters are directed through the abdominal wall and attached to an opening in the skin, is used for selected patients with ureteral obstruction (i.e., advanced pelvic cancer) because it requires less extensive surgery than other urinary diversion procedures. It is also an appropriate procedure for patients who have had previous abdominal irradiation.

A urinary appliance is fitted immediately after surgery. The management of the patient with a cutaneous ureterostomy is similar to the care of the patient with an ileal conduit, although the stomas are usually flush with the skin or retracted.

Continent Urinary Diversions

Continent Ileal Urinary Reservoir (Indiana Pouch)

The most common continent urinary diversion is the Indiana pouch, created for the patient whose bladder is removed or no longer functions. The Indiana pouch uses a segment of the ileum and cecum to form the reservoir for urine (Fig. 46-8A). The ureters are tunnelled through the muscular bands of the intestinal pouch and anastomosed. The reservoir is made continent by narrowing the efferent portion of the ileum and sewing the terminal ileum to the subcutaneous tissue, forming a continent stoma flush with the skin. The pouch is sewn to the anterior abdominal wall around a cecostomy tube. Urine collects in the pouch until a catheter is inserted and the urine is drained.

The pouch must be drained at regular intervals by a catheter to prevent absorption of metabolic waste products from the urine, reflux of urine to the ureters, and UTI. Postoperative nursing care of the patient with a continent ileal urinary pouch is similar to nursing care of the patient with an ileal conduit. However, these patients usually have additional drainage tubes (cecostomy catheter from the pouch, stoma catheter exiting from the stoma, ureteral stents, and Penrose drain as well as a urethral catheter). All drainage tubes must be carefully monitored for patency and amount and type of drainage. In the immediate postoperative period, the cecostomy tube is irrigated two or three times daily to remove mucus and prevent blockage.

Other variations of continent urinary reservoirs include the **Kock pouch** (U-shaped pouch constructed of ileum, with a nipple-like one-way valve; see Fig. 46-8B,C) and the **Charleston pouch** (uses the ileum and ascending colon as the pouch, with the appendix and colon junction serving as the one-way valve mechanism). With both of these methods, the pouch must be drained at regular intervals by a catheter. For guidelines for draining a continent ileostomy (Kock pouch), see Chart 38-6.

Ureterosigmoidostomy

Ureterosigmoidostomy, another form of continent urinary diversion, is an implantation of the ureters into the sigmoid colon (see Fig. 46-8D). It is usually performed in patients who have had extensive pelvic irradiation, previous small bowel resection, or coexisting small bowel disease.

After surgery, voiding occurs from the rectum (for life), and an adjustment in lifestyle will be necessary because of urinary frequency. Drainage has a consistency equivalent to watery diarrhea, and the patient has some degree of nocturia. Patients usually need to plan activities around the frequent need to urinate, which in turn may affect the patient's social life. However, patients have the advantage of urinary control without having to wear an external appliance.

Nursing Management

In addition to the usual preoperative regimen, the patient may be placed on a liquid diet for several days preoperatively to reduce residue in the colon. Antibiotic agents (neomycin, kanamycin) are administered to disinfect the bowel. Ureterosigmoidostomy requires a competent anal sphincter, adequate renal function, and active renal peristalsis. The degree of anal sphincter control may be determined by assessing the patient's ability to retain enemas.

The postoperative regimen initially includes placing a catheter in the rectum to drain the urine and prevent reflux of urine into the ureters and kidneys. The tube is taped to the buttocks, and special skin care is given around the anus to prevent excoriation. Irrigations of the rectal tube may be prescribed, but force is never used because of the danger of introducing bacteria into the newly implanted ureters.

Monitoring Fluid and Electrolytes

In ureterosigmoidostomy, larger areas of the bowel mucosa are exposed to urine and electrolyte reabsorption. As a result, electrolyte imbalance and acidosis may occur. Potassium and magnesium in the urine may cause diarrhea. Fluid and electrolyte balance is maintained in the immediate postoperative period by closely monitoring the serum electrolyte levels and administering appropriate IV fluids. Acidosis may be prevented by placing the patient on a low-chloride diet supplemented with sodium potassium citrate.

The patient should be instructed never to wait longer than 2 to 3 hours before emptying urine from the intestine. This keeps rectal pressure low and minimizes the absorption of urinary constituents from the colon. It is essential to teach the patient about the symptoms of UTI: fever, flank pain, and dysuria.

Retraining the Anal Sphincter

After the rectal catheter is removed, the patient learns to control the anal sphincter through special sphincter exercises. At first, urination is frequent. With reassurance and encouragement and the passage of time, the patient gains greater control and learns to differentiate between the need to void and the need to defecate.

Promoting Dietary Measures

Specific dietary instructions include avoidance of gas-forming foods (flatus can cause stress incontinence and offensive odours). Other ways to avoid gas are to avoid chewing gum, smoking, and any other activity that involves swallowing air. Salt intake may be restricted to prevent hyperchloremic acidosis. Potassium intake is increased through foods and medication because potassium may be lost in acidosis.

Monitoring and Managing Potential Complications

Pyelonephritis (upper UTI) due to reflux of bacteria from the colon is fairly common. Long-term antibiotic therapy may be prescribed to prevent infection. A late complication is adenocarcinoma of the sigmoid colon, possibly from cellular changes due to exposure of the colonic mucosa to urine. Urinary carcinogens promote late malignant transformation of the colon after a ureterosigmoidostomy, warranting lifelong medical follow-up.

Orthotopic Neobladder

This procedure involves the anastomosis of a detubularized segment of bowel to the urethra; this type of diversion keeps the patient free from external devices and the preservation of anatomical voiding (Bachir & Kassouf, 2013). Such patients are advised to increase intra-abdominal pressure while relaxing the pelvic floor muscles in order to void. The maintenance of body image is a major factor in patients choosing this type of diversion. The goals of the neobladder procedure are to maintain urinary continence and to allow voluntary emptying of the neobladder without the need for self-catheterization, while preserving kidney function (Lee et al., 2014).

Nursing Process

The Patient Undergoing Urinary Diversion Surgery

Preoperative Assessment

The following are key preoperative nursing assessment concerns:

- Cardiopulmonary function assessments are performed because patients undergoing cystectomy are often older people who may be at greater risk for cardiac and respiratory complications.
- A nutritional status assessment is important because of possible poor nutritional intake related to underlying health problems.
- Learning needs are assessed to evaluate the patient's and the family's understanding of the procedure and the changes in physical structure and function that result from the surgery. The patient's self-concept and self-esteem are assessed in addition to methods for coping with stress and loss. The patient's mental status, manual dexterity and coordination, and preferred method of learning are noted because they will affect postoperative self-care.

Preoperative Priorities

Nursing Priorities

Based on the assessment data, the preoperative nursing priorities for the patient undergoing urinary diversion surgery may include the following:

- Anxiety
- Imbalanced nutrition
- Deficient knowledge

Preoperative Planning and Goals

The major goals for the patient may include relief of anxiety; improved preoperative nutritional status; and increased knowledge about the surgical procedure, expected outcomes, and postoperative care.

Preoperative Nursing Interventions

Relieving Anxiety

The threat of cancer and removal of the bladder create anxiety related to changes in body image. Patients may face problems adapting to an external appliance, a stoma, a surgical incision, and altered toileting habits. Men must also adapt to sexual impotency; a penile implant is considered if the patient is a candidate for the procedure. Women also have anxiety related to altered appearance, body image, and self-esteem. A supportive approach, both physical and psychosocial, is needed and includes assessing the patient's self-concept and manner of coping with stress and loss; helping the patient identify ways to maintain his or her lifestyle and independence with as few changes as possible; and encouraging the patient to express fears and anxieties about the ramifications of the upcoming surgery.

Ensuring Adequate Nutrition

In addition to cleansing the bowel to minimize fecal stasis, decompress the bowel, and minimize postoperative ileus; a low-residue diet is prescribed. In addition, antibiotic medications are administered to reduce pathogenic flora in the bowel and the risk of infection. Because the patient undergoing a urinary diversion procedure for cancer may be severely malnourished due to the tumour, radiation enteritis, and anorexia, enteral or parenteral nutrition may be prescribed to promote healing. Adequate preoperative hydration is imperative to ensure urine flow during surgery and to prevent hypovolemia during the prolonged surgical procedure.

Explaining Surgery and Its Effects

Participation of a wound care specialist/enterostomal therapist is invaluable for informed preoperative teaching and postoperative care planning. Explanations of the surgical procedure, the appearance of the stoma, the rationale for preoperative bowel preparation, the reasons for wearing a collection device, and the anticipated effects of the surgery on sexual functioning are part of patient teaching. The placement of the stoma site is planned preoperatively with the patient standing, sitting, and lying down to locate the stoma away from bony prominences, skin creases, and folds. The stoma should also be placed away from old scars, the umbilicus, and the belt line.

For ease of self-care, the patient must be able to see and reach the site comfortably. The site is marked with indelible ink so that it can be located easily during surgery. The patient is assessed for allergies or sensitivity to tape or adhesives. Patch testing of certain appliances may be necessary before the ostomy equipment is selected. This is particularly important if the patient is or may be allergic to latex (see Chapter 18).

Preoperative Evaluation

To measure the effectiveness of care, the nurse evaluates the patient's preoperative anxiety level and nutritional status as well as pre-existing knowledge and expectations of surgery.

Expected patient outcomes may include the following:

1. Exhibits reduced anxiety about surgery and expected losses
   a. Verbalizes fears with health care team and family
   b. Expresses positive attitude about outcome of surgery
2. Exhibits adequate nutritional status
   a. Maintains adequate intake before surgery
   b. Maintains body weight
   c. States rationale for enteral or parenteral nutrition if needed
   d. Exhibits normal skin turgor, moist mucous membranes, adequate urine output, and absence of excessive thirst
3. Demonstrates knowledge about the surgical procedure and postoperative course
   a. Identifies limitations expected after surgery
   b. Discusses expected immediate postoperative environment (tubes, equipment, nursing surveillance)
   c. Practices deep-breathing, coughing, and foot exercises

Postoperative Assessment

The role of the nurse in the immediate postoperative period is to prevent complications and to assess the patient carefully for any signs and symptoms of complications. The catheters and any drainage devices are monitored closely. Urine volume, patency of the drainage system, and colour of the drainage are assessed. A sudden decrease in urine volume or increase in drainage is reported promptly to the physician because these may indicate obstruction of the urinary tract, inadequate blood volume, or bleeding. In addition, the patient's need for pain control is assessed regularly, as with all postoperative patients.

Postoperative Priorities

Nursing Priorities

Based on assessment data, the major postoperative nursing priorities for the patient following urinary diversion surgery may include the following:

- Risk for impaired skin integrity
- Acute pain
- Disturbed body image
- Potential for sexual dysfunction
- Deficient knowledge

Collaborative Problems/ Potential Complications

Potential complications may include the following:

- Peritonitis due to disruption of anastomosis
- Stoma ischemia and necrosis due to compromised blood supply to stoma

- Stoma retraction and separation of mucocutaneous border due to tension or trauma

Postoperative Planning and Goals

The major goals for the patient may include maintaining skin integrity, relieving pain, increasing self-esteem, developing appropriate coping mechanisms to accept and deal with altered urinary function and sexuality, increasing knowledge about management of urinary function, and preventing potential complications.

Postoperative Nursing Interventions

Postoperative management focuses on monitoring urinary function, preventing postoperative complications (infection and sepsis, respiratory complications, fluid and electrolyte imbalances, fistula formation, and urine leakage), and promoting patient comfort. Catheters or drainage systems are monitored, and urine output is monitored carefully. A nasogastric tube is inserted during surgery to decompress the GI tract and to relieve pressure on the intestinal anastomosis. It is usually kept in place for several days after surgery. As soon as bowel function resumes, as indicated by bowel sounds, the passage of flatus, and a soft abdomen, oral fluids are permitted. Until that time, IV fluids and electrolytes are administered. The patient is assisted to ambulate as soon as possible to prevent complications of immobility.

Maintaining Skin Integrity

Strategies to promote skin integrity begin with reducing and controlling those factors that increase the patient's risk of poor nutrition and poor healing. As indicated previously, meticulous skin care and management of the drainage system are provided by the nurse until the patient can manage them and is comfortable doing so. Care is taken to keep the drainage system intact to protect the skin from exposure to drainage. Supplies must be readily available to manage the drainage in the immediate postoperative period. Consistency in implementing the skin care program throughout the postoperative period results in maintenance of skin integrity and patient comfort. Additionally, maintenance of skin integrity around the stoma enables the patient and family to adjust more easily to the alterations in urinary function and helps them learn skin care techniques.

Relieving Pain

Analgesic medications are administered liberally postoperatively to relieve pain and promote comfort, thereby allowing the patient to turn, cough, and perform deep-breathing exercises. Patient-controlled analgesia (PCA) and administration of analgesic agents regularly around the clock are two options that may be used to ensure adequate pain relief. A pain intensity scale is used to evaluate the adequacy of the medication and the approach to pain management.

Improving Body Image

The patient's ability to cope with the changes associated with the surgery depends to some degree on his or her body image and self-esteem before the surgery and the support and reaction of others. Allowing the patient to express concerns and anxious feelings can help, especially in adjusting to the changes in toileting habits. The nurse can also help to improve the patient's self-concept by teaching the skills needed to be independent in managing the urinary drainage devices. Education about ostomy care is conducted in a private setting to encourage the patient to ask questions without fear of embarrassment. Explaining why the nurse must wear gloves when performing ostomy care can prevent the patient from misinterpreting the use of gloves as a sign of aversion to the stoma.

Exploring Sexuality Issues

Patients who experience altered sexual function as a result of the surgical procedure may mourn this loss. Encouraging the patient and partner to share their feelings about this loss with each other and acknowledging the importance of sexual function and expression may encourage the patient and partner to seek sexual counselling and to explore alternative ways of expressing sexuality. A visit from another "ostomate" who is functioning fully in society and family life may also assist the patient and family in recognizing that full recovery is possible.

Monitoring and Managing Potential Complications

Complications are not unusual because of the complexity of the surgery, the underlying reason (cancer, trauma) for the urinary diversion procedure, and the patient's frequently less-than-optimal nutritional status. Complications may include respiratory complications (e.g., atelectasis, pneumonia), fluid and electrolyte imbalances, breakdown of any anastomosis, sepsis, fistula formation, fecal or urine leakage, and skin irritation. If these occur, the patient will remain hospitalized for an extended length of time and will probably require parenteral nutrition, GI decompression by means of nasogastric suction, and further surgery. The goals of management are to establish drainage, provide adequate nutrition for healing to occur, and prevent sepsis.

PERITONITIS. Peritonitis can occur postoperatively if urine leaks at the anastomosis. Signs and symptoms include abdominal pain and distension, muscle rigidity with guarding, nausea and vomiting, paralytic ileus (absence of bowel sounds), fever, and leukocytosis.

Urine output must be monitored closely, because a sudden decrease in output with a corresponding increase in drainage from the incision or drains may indicate urine leakage. In addition, the urine drainage device is observed for leakage. The pouch is changed if a leak is observed. Small leaks in the anastomosis may seal themselves, but surgery may be needed for larger leaks.

Vital signs (blood pressure, pulse and respiratory rates, temperature) are monitored. Changes in vital signs, as well as increasing pain, nausea and vomiting, and abdominal distension, are reported to the physician and may indicate peritonitis.

STOMA ISCHEMIA AND NECROSIS. The stoma is monitored because ischemia and necrosis of the stoma can result from tension on the mesentery blood vessels, twisting of the bowel segment (conduit) during surgery, or arterial insufficiency. The new stoma must be inspected at least every 4 hours to assess the adequacy of its blood supply. The stoma should be red or pink. If the blood supply to the stoma is compromised, the colour changes to purple, brown, or black. These changes are reported immediately to the physician. The physician or wound care specialist/enterostomal therapist may insert a small, lubricated tube into the stoma and shine a flashlight into the lumen of the tube to assess for superficial ischemia or necrosis. A necrotic stoma requires surgical intervention. If the ischemia is superficial, the dusky stoma is observed and may slough its outer layer in several days.

STOMA RETRACTION AND SEPARATION. Stoma retraction and separation of the mucocutaneous border can occur as a result of trauma or tension on the internal bowel segment used for creation of the stoma. In addition, mucocutaneous separation can occur if the stoma does not heal as a result of accumulation of urine on the stoma and mucocutaneous border. Using a collection drainage pouch with an antireflux valve is helpful because the valve prevents urine from pooling on the stoma and mucocutaneous border. Meticulous skin care to keep the area around the stoma clean and dry promotes healing. If a separation of the mucocutaneous border occurs, surgery is not usually needed. The separated area is protected by applying Karaya Powder, stoma adhesive paste, and a properly fitted skin barrier and pouch. By protecting the separation, healing is promoted. If the stoma retracts into the peritoneum, surgical intervention is mandatory.

If surgery is needed to manage these complications, the nurse provides explanations to the patient and family. The need for additional surgery is usually perceived as a setback by the patient and family. Emotional support of the patient and family is provided along with physical preparation of the patient for surgery.

Promoting Home, Community-Based, and Transitional Care

EDUCATING PATIENTS ABOUT SELF-CARE. A major postoperative objective is to assist the patient to achieve the highest level of independence and self-care possible. The nurse and wound care specialist/enterostomal therapist work closely with the patient and family to instruct and assist them in all phases of managing the ostomy. Adequate supplies and complete instruction are necessary to enable the patient and a family member to develop competence and confidence in their skills. Written and verbal instructions are provided, and the patient is encouraged to contact the nurse or physician with follow-up questions. Follow-up telephone calls from the nurse to the patient and family after discharge may provide added support as well as provide another opportunity to answer their questions. Follow-up visits and reinforcement of correct skin care and appliance management techniques also promote skin integrity. Specific techniques for managing the appliance are described in Chart 46-13.

The patient is encouraged to participate in decisions regarding the type of collecting appliance and the time of day to change the appliance. The patient is assisted and encouraged to look at and touch the stoma early to overcome any fears. The patient and family need to know the characteristics of a normal stoma:

- Pink and moist, like the inside of the mouth
- Insensitive to pain, because it has no nerve endings
- Vascular and may bleed when cleaned

Additionally, if a segment of the GI tract was used to create the urinary diversion, mucus may be visible in the urine. By learning what is normal, the patient and family become familiar with what signs and symptoms they should report to the physician or nurse and what problems they can handle themselves.

Information provided to the patient and the extent of involvement in self-care are determined by the patient's physical recovery and ability to accept and acquire the knowledge and skill needed for independence. Verbal and written instructions are provided, and the patient is given the opportunity to practice and demonstrate the knowledge and skills needed to manage urinary drainage.

CONTINUING AND TRANSITIONAL CARE. Follow-up care is essential to determine how the patient has adapted to the body image changes and lifestyle adjustments. Visits from a home care nurse are important to assess the patient's adaptation to the home setting and management of the ostomy. Teaching and reinforcement may assist the patient and family to cope with altered urinary function. It is also necessary to assess for long-term complications that may occur, such as pouch leakage or rupture, stone formation, stenosis of the stoma, deterioration in renal function, or incontinence.

Long-term monitoring for anemia is performed to identify vitamin B deficiency, which may occur when a significant portion of the terminal ileum is removed. This may take several years to develop and can be treated with vitamin B injections. The patient and family are informed of the United Ostomy Association of Canada and any local ostomy support groups to provide ongoing support, assistance, and education.

Postoperative Evaluation

In addition to the expected patient outcomes addressed in Chart 46-13, additional outcomes may include the following:

1. Reports relief of pain
2. Copes with sexuality issues
   a. Verbalizes concern about possible alterations in sexuality and sexual function

   b. Reports discussion of sexual concerns with partner and appropriate counsellor
3. Absence of complications as evidenced by the following:
   a. Reports absence of pain or tenderness in abdomen
   b. Has temperature within normal range
   c. Reports no urine leakage from incision or drains
   d. Has urine output within desired volume limits
   e. Maintains stoma that is red or pink, moist, and appropriate in size without edema
   f. Has intact and healed border of the stoma

Critical Thinking Exercises

1 As the supervisor in a long-term care facility, you are approached by the daughter of one of the residents. She requests that her mother, who can ambulate with assistance, have an indwelling urinary catheter inserted "for convenience sake." What is the evidence base that supports your response? Identify the criteria used to evaluate the strength of the evidence.

2 As one of the nurses in a busy urology practice, you are performing telephone triage. A 62-year-old man who was seen 2 days ago for increasing urinary frequency, including several awakenings at night, phones to report increasing abdominal pain. He states that he has not voided for more than 12 hours, although he has made several unsuccessful attempts. Explain the instructions you would provide. What medical and nursing interventions would you anticipate?

3 A 50-year-old woman comes for her annual pelvic checkup with complaints of occasional urinary urgency, sometimes with "near incontinences" just as she reaches the toilet. She denies the intake of any potentially bladder-irritating substances, such as beverages containing caffeine or synthetic sweeteners. She also mentions that she is having difficulty with decreased lubrication during intercourse, and her menses are irregular. On physical examination, thinning of the vaginal mucosa is noted. Identify the evidence for and the criteria used to evaluate the strength of the evidence for and against the use of estrogen in maintaining continence.

4 A 55-year-old man returns to your unit following a Camey procedure after cystectomy for bladder cancer. What immediate nursing assessment and interventions should you take at this time? Describe the nursing diagnoses and plan of care in the postoperative period. How will you modify the plan if the patient is a 75-year-old?

REFERENCES AND SELECTED READINGS

Books

Bader, M. K., Littlejohns, L. R., & Olson, D. M. (2016). *AANN core curriculum for neuroscience nursing* (6th ed.). Chicago, IL: American Association of Neuroscience Nurses.
Blondel-Hill, E., & Fryters, S. (2012). Bugs & drugs: an antimicrobial/infectious diseases reference. Alberta Health Services.
Booker, K. (2015). *Critical care nursing: Monitoring and treatment for advanced nursing practice*. Oxford: Wiley Blackwell.
Comerford, K. C. (2015). *Nursing 2015 drug handbook*. Philadelphia, PA: Wolters Kluwer.
Eliopoulos, C. (2018). *Gerontological nursing* (9th ed.). Philadelphia, PA: Lippincott Williams & Wilkins.
Fischbach, F., & Dunning, M. B. (2015). *A manual of laboratory and diagnostic tests* (9th ed.). Philadelphia, PA: Lippincott Williams & Wilkins.
Hannon, R. A., & Porth, C. M. (2017). *Porth pathophysiology: Concepts of altered health states* (2nd Canadian ed.). Philadelphia, PA: Wolters Kluwer.
McCance, K., & Huether, H. (2014). *Pathophysiology: The biologic basis for disease in adults and children* (7th ed.). St. Louis, MO: Elsevier Mosby.
Miller, C. A. (2015). *Nursing for wellness in older adults* (7th ed.). Philadelphia, PA: Lippincott Williams & Wilkins.
Weber, J., & Kelley, J. (2014). *Health assessment in nursing* (5th ed.). Philadelphia, PA: Lippincott Williams & Wilkins.

Journals and Electronic Documents

Bachir, B. G., & Kassouf, W. (2013). Urinary diversions: Advantages and disadvantages of the major types of diversions. *Current Opinion in Supportive and Palliative Care*, *7*(3), 249–253.
Bass-Ware, A., Weed, D., Johnson, T., et al. (2014). Evaluation of the effect of cranberry juice on symptoms associated with a urinary tract infection. *Urologic Nursing*, *34*(3), 121–127.
Baudry-Simner, P. J., Singh, A., Karlowsky, J. A., et al. (2012). Mechanisms of reduced susceptibility to ciprofloxacin in Escherichia coli isolates from Canadian hospitals. *Canadian Journal of Infectious Disease and Medical Microbiology*, 23(3), e60–e64.
Bozzini, G., Colin, P., Betrouni, N., et al. (2012). Photodynamic therapy in urology: What can we do now and where are we heading? *Photodiagnosis and Photodynamic Therapy*, 9(3), 261–273.
Burch, J. (2013). Care of patients with a stoma. *Nursing Standard*, 27(32), 49–56; quiz 58.
Canadian Cancer Society (CCS). (2013a). *Research and development in bladder cancer*. Retrieved from http://www.cancer.ca/en/cancer-information/cancer-type/bladder/research/?region=on
Canadian Cancer Society (CCS). (2013b). *Risk factors for bladder cancer*. Retrieved from http://www.cancer.ca/en/cancer-information/cancer-type/bladder/risks/
Canadian Cancer Society (CCS). (2013c). *Causes of bladder cancer*. Retrieved from http://www.cancer.ca/~/media/cancer.ca/CW/publications/Bladder%20cancer%20UYD/32086-1-NO.pdf
Canadian Cancer Society (CCS). (2018). *Bladder cancer statistics*. Retrieved May 20, 2018, from http://www.cancer.ca/en/cancer-information/cancer-type/bladder/statistics/?region=on
Canadian Cancer Society's Advisory Committee on Cancer Statistics. *Canadian cancer statistics 2017*. Toronto, ON: Canadian Cancer Society. Retrieved May 20, 2018, from www.cancer.ca/Canadian-Cancer-Statistics-2017-EN
Canadian Cancer Society's Cancer Statistics Report. (2017). Retrieved from https://www.cancer.ca/~/media/cancer.ca/CW/cancer%20information/cancer%20101/Canadian%20cancer%20statistics/Canadian-Cancer-Statistics-2017-EN.pdf?la=en
Canadian Patient Safety Institute (CPSI). (2016). Hospital harm improvement resource: Urinary tract infection. Retrieved from http://www.patientsafetyinstitute.ca/en/toolsResources/Hospital-Harm-Measure/Documents/Resource-Library/HHIR%20UTI.pdf
Canadian Urological Association (CUA). (2016). *Canadian undergraduate urology curriculum (CanUUC): Genitourinary trauma (PowerPoint Slides)*. Retrieved May 27, 2018, from https://www.cua.org/themes/web/assets/files/podcasts/en/trauma/canuuc_gu_trauma.pdf
Carter, N. M., Reitmeier, L., & Goodloe, L. R. (2014). An evidence-based approach to the prevention of catheter-associated urinary tract infections. *Urologic Nursing*, *34*(5), 238–245.
Crawshaw, A., Williams, J., & Woodhouse, F. (2014). The Kock pouch reconsidered: An alternative surgical technique. *British Journal of Nursing*, *23*(17), S26–S29.
Cunningham, P., Noble, H., Al-Modhefer, A., et al. (2016). Kidney stones: Pathophysiology, diagnosis and management. *British Journal of Nursing*, *25*(20), 1112–1116.
Davis, N. F., Kheradmand, F., & Creagh, T. (2013). Injectable biomaterials for the treatment of stress urinary incontinence: Their potential

and pitfalls as urethral bulking agents. *International Urogynecology Journal*, *24*(6), 913–919.
Gupta, K., Grigoryan, L., & Trautner, B. (2017). Urinary tract infection. *Annals of Internal Medicine*, *167*(7), ITC49–ITC64.
Hagerty, T., Kertesz, L., Schmidt, J. M., et al. (2015). Risk factors for catheter associated urinary tract infections in critically ill patients with subarachnoid hemorrhage. *Journal of Neuroscience Nursing*, *47*(1), 51–54.
Hallis, F., Amasyali, A. S., Yucak, A., et al. (2015). Intrathoracic kidney after blunt abdominal trauma: A case report and review of the literature. *Case Reports in Urology*, *2015*, 1–3.
Hopkins, L., McCroskey, D., Reeves, G., et al. (2014). Implementing a urinary tract infection clinical practice guideline in an ambulatory urgent care practice. *The Nurse Practitioner*, *39*(4), 50–54.
Jabs, C., & Carleton, E. (2013). Efficacy of botulinum toxin A intradetrusor injections for non-neurogenic urinary urge incontinence: A randomized double-blind controlled trial. *Journal of Obstetrical Gynecology of Canada*, *35*(1), 53–60.
Jancke, G., Rosell, J., & Jahnson, S. (2012). Residual tumour in the marginal resection after a complete transurethral resection is associated with local recurrence in Ta/T1 urinary bladder cancer. *Scandinavian Journal of Urology and Nephrology*, *46*(5), 343–347.
Kassouf, W., Traboulsi, S. L., Kulkarni, G. S., et al. (2015). *CUA guidelines on the management of non-muscle invasive bladder cancer*. Retrieved May 27, 2018, from https://www.cua.org/themes/web/assets/files/non_muscle_invasive_bladder_cancer_cuaguidelines3320.pdf
Kulkarni, G. S., Hermanns, T., Wei, Y., et al. (2017). Propensity score analysis of radical cystectomy versus bladder-sparing trimodal therapy in the setting of a multidisciplinary bladder cancer clinic. *Journal of Clinical Oncology*, *35*(20), 2299–2305.
Lee, R. K., Abol Enein, H., Artibani, W., et al. (2014). Urinary diversion after radical cystectomy for bladder cancer: Options, patient selection, and outcomes. *BJU International*, *113*(1), 11–23.
Li, J., Yang, L., Pu, C., et al. (2013). The role of duloxetine in stress urinary incontinence: A systematic review and meta-analysis. *International Urology and Nephrology*, *45*(3), 679–686.
Matsuoka, P. K., Locali, R. F., Pacetta, A. M., et al. (2016). The efficacy and safety of urethral injection therapy for urinary incontinence in women: A systematic review. *Clinics*, *71*(2), 94–100.
McCooty, S., & Latthe, P. (2014). Electronic pelvic floor assessment questionnaire: A systematic review. *British Journal of Nursing*, *23*(18), S32–S37.
McGeady, J. B., & Breyer, B. N. (2013). Current epidemiology of genitourinary trauma. *The Urologic Clinics of North America*, *40*(3), 323–334.
Morgan, M. S., & Pearle, M. S. (2016). Medical management of renal stones. *BMJ: British Medical Journal*, *352*, i52.
Mori, C. (2014). A-voiding catastrophe: Implementing a nurse-driven protocol. *Medsurg Nursing*, *23*(1), 15–21, 28.
National Cancer Institute (NCI). (2016). *Bladder cancer treatment (PDQ®)—Health professional version*. Retrieved December 13, 2016, from www.cancer.gov/types/bladder/hp/bladder-treatment-pdq#section/all
Nicolle, L. E. (2014). Catheter associated urinary tract infections. *Antimicrobial Resistance and Infection Control*, *3*(1), 23.
Nitti, V. W., Dmochowski, R., Herschorn, S., et al. (2017). OnabotulinumtoxinA for the treatment of patients with overactive bladder and urinary incontinence: Results of a phase 3, randomized, placebo controlled trial. *The Journal of Urology*, *197*(2), S216–S223.
Public Health Agency of Canada (PHAC). (2012). *The Canadian nosocomial infection surveillance program*. Retrieved from http://www.phac-aspc.gc.ca/nois-sinp/survprog-eng.php
Rowe, T. A., & Juthani-Mehta, M. (2014). Diagnosis and management of urinary tract infection in older adults. *Infectious Disease Clinics of North America*, *28*(1), 75–89.
Rubenwolf, P. C., Hampel, C., Roos, F., et al. (2016). Continent anal urinary diversion in Classic bladder exstrophy: 45-year experience. *Urology*, *100*, 249–254.
Smolar, J., Salemi, S., Horst, H., et al. (2016). Stem cells in functional bladder engineering. *Transfusion Medicine and Hemotherapy*, *43*(5), 328–335.
Stapleton, A. E., Dziura, J., Hooton, T. M., et al. (2012). Recurrent urinary tract infection and urinary Escherichia coli in women ingesting cranberry juice daily: A randomized controlled trial. *Mayo Clinic Proceedings*, *87*(2), 143–150.
Strouse, A. (2015). Appraising the literature on bathing practices and catheter-associated urinary tract infection prevention. *Urologic Nursing*, *35*(1), 11–17.
Taweel, W. A., & Seyam, R. (2015). Neurogenic bladder in spinal cord injury patients. *Research and Reports in Urology*, *7*, 85–99.
The Canadian Continence Foundation. (2014). *Incontinence: The Canadian perspective*. Retrieved from http://www.continence-fdn.ca/pdf/Research_paper_August2007.pdf

Resources

Association de la C.I. du Québec: http://www.cystiteinterstitielle.org/
Canadian Association for Enterostomal Therapy: http://www.caet.ca
Canadian Association of Nephrology Nurses and Technologists: http://www.cannt.ca
Canadian Cancer Society: http://www.cancer.ca
Canadian Continence Foundation: http://www.canadiancontinence.ca/EN/
Canadian Society of Transplantation: http://www.transplant.ca
Interstitial Cystitis Association: http://www.ichelp.com
The Kidney Foundation of Canada: http://www.kidney.ca
Ostomy Canada Society: http://www.ostomycanada.ca
Urology Nurses of Canada: http://www.unc.org/
Wound, Ostomy and Continence Nurses Society: http://www.wocn.org

UNIT 10

Reproductive Function

Case Study

INCORPORATING TECHNOLOGY IN MANAGING A PATIENT WITH NEWLY DIAGNOSED PROSTATE CANCER

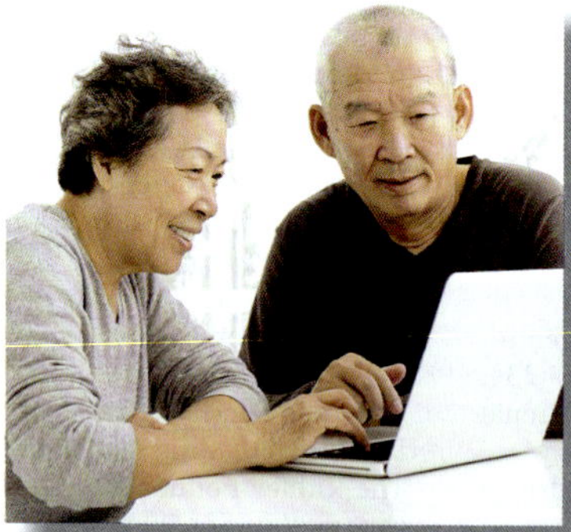

The nurse working in an infusion clinic is assigned to care for a 68-year-old patient who is retired and newly diagnosed with prostate cancer. He is accompanied by his wife and prescribed a course of chemotherapy that necessitates close monitoring of several key laboratory values. The patient and his wife live in a rural area with harsh, snowy winters. Their home is 100 km from the infusion centre. The patient and his wife are invited to enrol in a telehealth program. The program will provide education webinars about prostate cancer; it also will have access to chat rooms with other patients who have a diagnosis of prostate cancer and offer chat rooms for spouses. In addition, the patient will be able to provide periodic data to his primary provider on his laboratory values.

QSEN Competency Focus: Informatics

The complexities inherent in today's health care system challenge nurses to demonstrate integration of specific interdisciplinary core competencies that are aimed at ensuring the delivery of safe and quality patient care (Institute of Medicine, 2003). The Quality and Safety Education for Nurses project (QSEN, 2017; Cronenwett, Sherwood, Barnsteiner, et al., 2007) provides a framework for the knowledge, skills, and attitudes (KSAs) required for nurses to demonstrate competency in these key areas, which include ***patient-centred care***, ***interdisciplinary teamwork and collaboration***, ***evidence-based practice***, ***quality improvement***, ***safety***, and ***informatics.***

Informatics Definition: Use information and technology to communicate, manage knowledge, mitigate error, and support decision making.

SELECTED PRE-LICENSURE KSAs	APPLICATION AND REFLECTION
Knowledge	
Explain why information and technology skills are essential for safe patient care.	Describe the differences in this patient's ability to self-manage his therapeutic regimen with and without the telehealth system. How can telehealth improve the quality of care that he receives?
Skills	
Apply technology and information management tools to support safe processes of care.	Identify the skill set required by both the patient and his health care providers if the telehealth system is to be effective in improving his health.
Attitudes	
Appreciate the necessity for all health professionals to seek lifelong, continuous learning of information technology skills.	Reflect on your attitudes toward use of technology by older adult patients. Do you feel threatened by monitoring patients from a distance, rather than having face-to-face encounters? If so, how might this attitude create barriers to effective patient care?

Cronenwett, L., Sherwood, G., Barnsteiner, J., et al. (2007). Quality and safety education for nurses. *Nursing Outlook, 55*(3), 122–131; Institute of Medicine. (2003). *Health professions education: A bridge to quality*. Washington, DC: National Academies Press; and QSEN Institute. (2017). *QSEN competencies: Definitions and pre-licensure KSAs*. Retrieved June 12, 2019, from www.qsen.org/competencies/pre-licensure-ksas

47 Assessment and Management of Female Physiologic Processes

Adapted by Kelly Power-Kean

Learning Objectives

On completion of this chapter, the learner will be able to:

1. Describe the structures and functions of the female reproductive function.
2. Explain approaches to effective assessment of female physiologic processes.
3. Describe indicators of intimate partner violence and abuse of women and methods of identifying and treating women who are survivors of abuse.
4. Identify the diagnostic examinations and tests used to determine alteration in female reproductive function and describe the nurse's role before, during, and after these examinations and procedures.
5. Recognize common female physiologic processes and related nursing implications.
6. Describe the physiologic process and related nursing implications for women who are approaching or have completed menopause.
7. Compare the various methods of contraception and implications for care and education.
8. Describe the causes and management of infertility.
9. Use the nursing process to plan for the care of the patient with an ectopic pregnancy.

Nurses who work with women need to understand normal female anatomy and physiology and the physical, developmental, psychological, and sociocultural influences on women's health, health practices, and use of health care resources. Health assessment, maintenance, and promotion across the lifespan must consider women's growth and development, sexuality, contraception, preconception care, conception, prenatal care, effects of pregnancy on health, perimenopause, menopause, and aging. It is also necessary to consider how medications and diseases affect women. In addition, women's sexuality is complex and often affected by many factors, and related issues need careful evaluation and treatment.

ROLE OF NURSES IN WOMEN'S HEALTH

As their presence in the labour market continues to increase, women face challenges in their roles, lifestyles, and family patterns. Furthermore, they encounter environmental hazards and stress, prompting greater attention on health and health-promoting practices. As a result, many women are taking a greater interest in and responsibility for their own health and health care.

Many women delay pregnancy and childbearing until they have established careers. This is made possible because of the wide variety of contraceptive methods that are available. Advances in the treatment of infertility have enabled many women previously unable to have children to become pregnant and have allowed couples well into their 40s to have children. Women who have many roles and multiple responsibilities (e.g., workers, wives, mothers, parental caretakers) often have little time for themselves and often put the needs of others before their own health needs. Nurses must be sensitive to these needs and knowledgeable about preventive health care for women. Nurses are in an ideal position to encourage women to determine their own health goals and behaviour, teach about health promotion and illness prevention, offer intervention strategies, and provide support, counselling, and ongoing monitoring. Areas of women's health promotion include the following:

- Normal physical changes
- Strategies for detecting and preventing disease, especially sexually transmitted infections (STIs) including human immunodeficiency virus (HIV) infection and acquired immunodeficiency syndrome (AIDS)
- Issues related to sexuality and sexual function, such as contraception; preconception, prenatal, and postnatal care; sexual satisfaction; and menopause
- Diet, exercise, and health-promoting practices that maintain and enhance health
- Stress management to reduce the detrimental effects of stress on health and well-being
- Treatment for substance abuse and smoking cessation strategies

It is important that nurses promote positive practices and behaviour related to the reproductive and sexual health of all patients. Necessary strategies include the following:

- Recommending regular examinations to promote health and early detection of gynecologic and reproductive related health issues
- Providing an open, nonjudgmental environment conveying understanding and sensitivity
- Recognizing signs and symptoms of abuse and screening all patients in a private and safe environment
- Recognizing cultural differences and beliefs and respecting sexual orientation

ASSESSMENT OF THE FEMALE REPRODUCTIVE SYSTEM

Anatomic and Physiologic Overview

The female reproductive system is complex because it involves many external and internal structures that are under hormonal control.

Glossary

adnexa: the fallopian tubes and ovaries
amenorrhea: absence of menstrual flow
androgens: hormones produced by the ovaries and adrenals that affect many aspects of female health, including follicle development, libido, oiliness of hair and skin, and hair growth
cervix: bottom (inferior) part of the uterus, located in the vagina
chandelier sign: pain on gentle movement of the cervix; associated with pelvic infection
corpus luteum: site of a follicle that changes after ovulation to produce progesterone
cystocele: weakness of the anterior vaginal wall that allows the bladder to protrude into the vagina
dysmenorrhea: painful menstruation
dyspareunia: difficult or painful sexual intercourse
endometrial ablation: procedure performed through a hysteroscope in which the lining of the uterus is burned away or ablated to treat abnormal uterine bleeding
endometriosis: condition in which endometrial tissue implants in other areas of the pelvis; may produce dysmenorrhea or infertility
endometrium: lining of the uterus
estrogens: hormones that develop and maintain the female reproductive system
follicle-stimulating hormone (FSH): hormone released by the pituitary gland to stimulate estrogen production and ovulation
fornix: upper part of the vagina
fundus: body of the uterus
graafian follicle: cystic structure that develops on the ovary as ovulation begins
hymen: tissue that covers the vaginal opening partially or completely before vaginal penetration
hysteroscopy: a procedure performed using a long telescope like instrument inserted through the cervix to diagnose uterine problems
introitus: perineal opening to the vagina
luteal phase: stage in the menstrual cycle in which the endometrium becomes thicker and more vascular
luteinizing hormone (LH): hormone released by the pituitary gland that stimulates progesterone production
menarche: beginning of menstrual function
menopause: permanent cessation of menstruation resulting from the loss of ovarian follicular activity
menstruation: sloughing and discharge of the lining of the uterus if conception does not take place
ovaries: almond-shaped reproductive organs that produce eggs at ovulation and play a major role in hormone production
ovulation: discharge of a mature ovum from the ovary
perimenopause: the period immediately prior to menopause and the first year after menopause
polyp: growth of tissue on the cervix or endometrial lining; usually benign
progesterone: hormone produced by the corpus luteum
proliferative phase: stage in the menstrual cycle before ovulation when the endometrium proliferates
rectocele: weakness of the posterior vaginal wall that allows the rectal cavity to protrude into the submucosa of the vagina
secretory phase: stage of the menstrual cycle in which the endometrium becomes thickened, more vascular, and edematous
uterine prolapse: relaxation of pelvic tone that allows the cervix and uterus to descend into the lower vagina

Anatomy of the Female Reproductive System

The female reproductive system consists of external and internal pelvic structures. Other anatomic structures that affect the female reproductive system include the hypothalamus and pituitary gland of the endocrine system.

External Genitalia

The external genitalia (vulva) include two thick folds of tissue called the labia majora and two smaller lips of delicate tissue called the labia minora, which lie within the labia majora. The upper portions of the labia minora unite, forming a partial covering for the clitoris, a highly sensitive organ composed of erectile tissue. Between the labia minora, below and posterior to the clitoris, is the urinary meatus, the external opening of the female urethra, which is about 3 cm (less than 1.5 in) long. Below this orifice is a larger opening, the vaginal orifice or **introitus** (Fig. 47-1). The Skene's gland, located within the urethral meatus, produces mucous for lubrication (Ball, Dains, Flynn, et al., 2015).

On each side of the vaginal orifice is a vestibular (Bartholin's) gland, a bean-sized structure that empties its mucous secretion through a small duct. The opening of the duct lies within the labia minora, external to the hymen (membrane that encircles the introitus). The Bartholin glands can become blocked (cyst formation) or infected (abscess formation). Treatment is different for each, but pain is common with both. Pain can interfere with sitting and walking.

The hymen opening varies widely among women, and the size of the opening is an unreliable indicator of sexual experience (Ball et al., 2015). The fourchette is located in the midline below the vaginal opening where the labia majora and labia minor merge. The perineum is the area between the vagina and the rectum or anus; it is a skin-covered muscular tissue (Ball et al., 2015). The area between the vagina and rectum is called the perineum.

A number of muscles support the external genitalia. Support for the pelvic organs is from the deep muscle layer known as the levator ani. This muscle, which forms most of the pelvic diaphragm, is composed of the iliococcygeus, pubococcygeus, and the puborectalis muscles. It supports the organs of reproduction and provides elasticity of the pelvic floor. When viewed from above, it looks like joined cupped hands. Its main function is to provide support to the organs of the pelvis when increased pressure from coughing and sneezing occurs. When this muscle group is contracted, the pelvic floor is lifted upward, supporting continence (Schuiling & Likis, 2013). Muscles that contribute to the strength of the pelvic floor may be damaged during childbirth (Schuiling & Likis, 2013). The bulbocavernosus, ischiocavernosus, and transverse perineal muscles encircle and support the vagina and urethra as well as the anal sphincter.

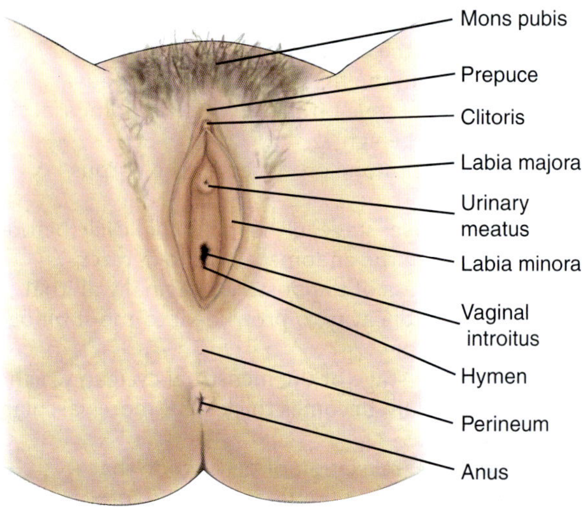

FIGURE 47-1. External female genitalia.

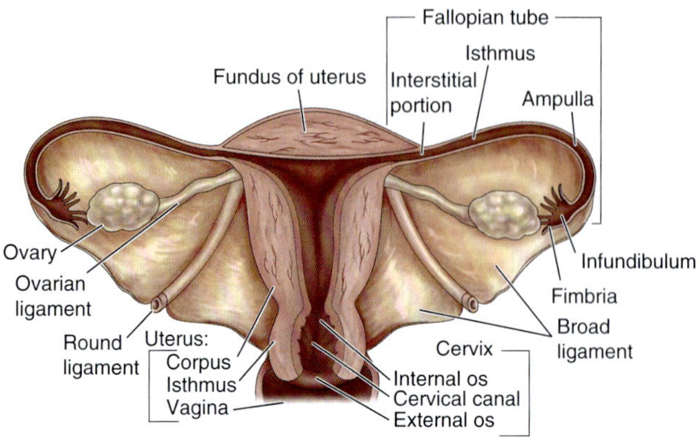

FIGURE 47-2. Internal female reproductive structures.

Internal Reproductive Structures

The internal structures consist of the vagina, uterus, ovaries, and fallopian or uterine tubes (Fig. 47-2).

Vagina

The vagina, a canal lined with a thin, glandular, highly vascular mucous membrane, is 7.5 to 10 cm (3 to 4 in) long and extends upward and backward from the vulva to the cervix. Anterior to it are the bladder and the urethra, and posterior to it lies the rectum. The anterior and posterior walls of the vagina normally touch each other. The upper part of the vagina, the **fornix**, surrounds the **cervix** (the inferior part of the uterus).

Uterus

The uterus, a pear-shaped, muscular organ, is about 7.5 cm (3 in) long and 5 cm (2 in) wide at its upper part. Its walls are about 1.25 cm (0.5 in) thick. The size of the uterus varies, depending on parity (number of pregnancies) and uterine abnormalities (e.g., fibroids, which are a type of tumour that may distort the uterus). A nulliparous woman (one who has not completed a pregnancy to the stage of fetal viability) usually has a smaller uterus than a multiparous woman (one who has completed two or more pregnancies to the stage of fetal viability). The uterus lies posterior to the bladder and is held in position by several ligaments. The round ligaments extend anteriorly and laterally to the internal inguinal ring and down the inguinal canal, where they blend with the tissues of the labia majora. The broad ligaments are folds of peritoneum extending from the lateral pelvic walls and enveloping the fallopian tubes. The uterosacral ligaments extend posteriorly to the sacrum.

The uterus has four parts: the cervix, **fundus**, corpus, and isthmus. The cervix is the opening to the uterus and projects into the vagina. A larger upper part, the fundus, is the rounded portion above the insertion of the fallopian tubes. The corpus or body is the main portion of the uterus located between the fundus and the isthmus. The isthmus is referred to as the lower uterine segment during pregnancy and joins the corpus to the cervix.

The cervix is divided into two portions. The portion above the site of attachment of the cervix to the vaginal vault is known as the supravaginal portion; the portion below the attachment site that protrudes into the vagina is known as the vaginal portion. The cervix is composed of fibrous connective tissue. The diameter varies from 2 to 5 cm depending on the childbearing history. The length is usually 2.5 to 3 cm in the woman who is not pregnant. The vaginal portion is smooth, firm, and doughnut shaped with a visible central opening referred to as the external os. The external os is round before the first birth and is often slit-like in shape after childbirth. The internal os is the opening in the cervix to the uterine cavity. In response to cyclic hormones, the cervix produces mucus, which is an important factor in fertility awareness. The vaginal surface of the cervix is covered with squamous epithelium, a rapid cellular growth site of cervical cancer and precancerous changes.

The uterine wall has three layers. The endometrium, the innermost layer, is highly vascular and responds to hormone stimulation to prepare to receive the developing ovum. It sloughs if pregnancy does not occur, resulting in menstruation; if pregnancy occurs, it sloughs after delivery. The myometrium, the middle layer, is made up of several smooth muscle layers. The outer layer of the myometrium is composed of longitudinal fibres, chiefly in the fundus, which provide the power to expel the fetus. The middle layer of the myometrium is composed of fibres interlaced with blood vessels in a figure-of-eight pattern called a *living ligature* because it contracts after childbirth to help control blood loss (Schuiling & Likis, 2013). The inner layer of the myometrium is composed of circular fibres that are concentrated around the internal cervical os to help keep the cervix closed during pregnancy. The other layer of the uterus is composed of parietal peritoneum, which covers most of the uterus.

From here the fallopian tubes extend outward, and their lumina are internally continuous with the uterine cavity (Hannon & Porth, 2016). The fallopian tubes or oviducts are the passageway for eggs from the ovary to the uterus. They curve around each ovary and are attached to the uterine fundus. Fallopian tubes are about 10 cm in length and are comprised of four parts. The infundibulum, the most distal portion, is covered in fimbriae, whose wave-like motion helps to pull the egg into the tube. The ampulla is usually the site of fertilization of the egg or ovum. The fallopian tube then narrows from its 0.6 cm diameter in the isthmus, ending in the narrowest part of the interstitial portion, which opens into the uterine cavity. The fallopian tube also secretes nutrients for growth and development of the ovum after fertilization while it passes down the tube to the uterus.

Ovaries

The **ovaries** lie behind the broad ligaments and behind and below the fallopian tubes. They are oval bodies about 3 cm (1.2 in) long. At birth, they contain thousands of tiny egg cells, or ova. The ovaries and the fallopian tubes together are referred to as the **adnexa**.

Function of the Female Reproductive System

Ovulation

At puberty (usually between 11 and 13 years of age), the ova begin to mature and menstrual cycles begin. In the follicular phase, an ovum enlarges as a type of cyst called a **graafian follicle** until it reaches the surface of the ovary, where transport occurs. The ovum (or oocyte) is discharged into the peritoneal cavity. This periodic discharge of matured ovum is referred to as **ovulation**. The ovum usually finds its way into the fallopian tube, where it is carried to the uterus. If it is penetrated by a spermatozoon, the male reproductive cell, a union occurs, and conception takes place. After the discharge of the ovum, the cells of the graafian follicle undergo a rapid change. Gradually, they become yellow (**corpus luteum**) and produce **progesterone**, a hormone that prepares the uterus for receiving the fertilized ovum. Ovulation usually occurs 2 weeks prior to the next menstrual period (Hannon & Porth, 2016).

Menstrual Cycle

The menstrual cycle is a complex process involving the reproductive and endocrine systems. The ovaries produce steroid hormones, predominantly estrogens and progesterone. Several different **estrogens** are produced by the ovarian follicle, which consists of the developing ovum and its surrounding cells. The most potent of the ovarian estrogens is estradiol. Estrogens are responsible for developing and maintaining the female reproductive organs and the secondary sex characteristics associated with the adult female. Estrogens play an important role in breast development and in monthly cyclic changes in the uterus (Schuiling & Likis, 2013).

Progesterone is also important in regulating the changes that occur in the uterus during the menstrual cycle. It is secreted by the corpus luteum, which is the ovarian follicle after the ovum has been released. Progesterone is the most important hormone for conditioning the **endometrium** (the mucous membrane lining the uterus) in preparation for implantation of a fertilized ovum. If pregnancy occurs, the progesterone secretion becomes largely a function of the placenta and is essential for maintaining a normal pregnancy. In addition, progesterone, working with estrogen, prepares the breast for producing and secreting milk. **Androgens** are also produced by the ovaries and adrenal glands, but only in small amounts. These hormones affect many aspects of female health, including follicle development, libido, oiliness of hair and skin, and hair growth (Schuiling & Likis, 2013).

Two gonadotropic hormones are released by the pituitary gland: **follicle-stimulating hormone (FSH)** and **luteinizing hormone (LH)**. FSH is primarily responsible for stimulating the ovaries to secrete estrogen. LH is primarily responsible for stimulating progesterone production. Feedback mechanisms, in part, regulate FSH and LH secretion. For example, elevated estrogen levels in the blood inhibit FSH secretion but promote LH secretion, whereas elevated progesterone levels inhibit LH secretion. In addition, gonadotropin-releasing hormone (GnRH)

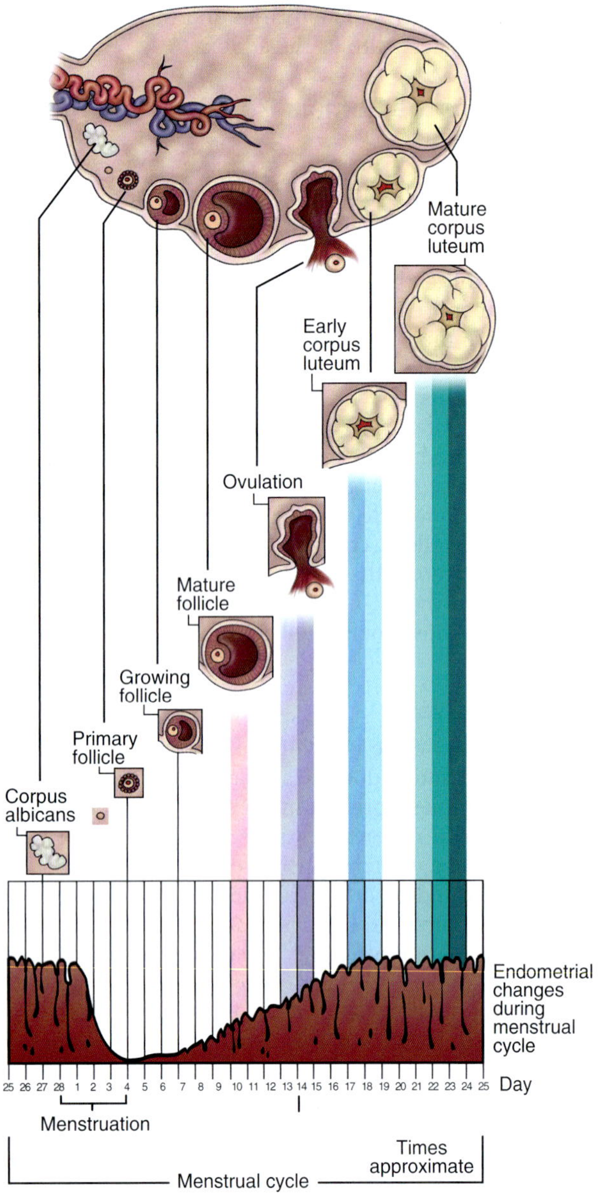

FIGURE 47-3. The menstrual cycle and the corresponding changes in the endometrium.

from the hypothalamus affects the rate of FSH and LH release (Schuiling & Likis, 2013).

The secretion of ovarian hormones follows a cyclic pattern that results in changes in the uterine endometrium and in **menstruation** (Fig. 47-3, Table 47-1). This cycle is typically 28 days in length, but there are many normal variations (from 21 to 42 days). In the **proliferative phase** at the beginning of the cycle (just after menstruation), FSH output increases, stimulating estrogen secretion. This causes the endometrium to thicken and become more vascular. In the **secretory phase** near the middle portion of the cycle (day 14 in a 28-day cycle), LH output increases, stimulating ovulation. Under the combined stimulus of estrogen and progesterone, the endometrium reaches the peak of the luteal phase, in which the endometrium is thick and highly vascular. In the **luteal phase**, which begins after ovulation, progesterone is secreted by the corpus luteum.

If the ovum is fertilized, estrogen and progesterone levels remain high, and the complex hormonal changes of pregnancy follow. If the ovum has not been fertilized, FSH and LH output diminishes, estrogen and progesterone secretion falls, the ovum disintegrates, and the endometrium, which has become thick and congested, becomes hemorrhagic. The product, menstrual flow, consisting of old blood, mucus, and endometrial tissue, is discharged through the cervix and into the vagina. After the menstrual flow stops, the cycle begins again; the endometrium proliferates and thickens from estrogenic stimulation, and ovulation recurs (Schuiling & Likis, 2013).

Menopausal Period

The menopausal period marks the end of a woman's reproductive capacity. It usually occurs between 45 and 52 years of age (Hannon & Porth, 2016). Perimenopause precedes this and can begin as early as 35 years of age. Physical, emotional, and menstrual changes may occur, and this transition offers another opportunity for health promotion and disease prevention teaching and counselling. Menopause is a normal part of aging and maturation. Menstruation ceases, and because the ovaries are no longer active, the reproductive organs become smaller. No more ova mature; therefore, no ovarian hormones are produced. (An earlier menopause may occur if the ovaries are surgically removed or are destroyed by radiation or chemotherapy or because of an unknown etiology.) Multifaceted changes also occur throughout the woman's body. These changes are neuroendocrinologic, biochemical, and metabolic and are related to normal maturation or aging (Table 47-2).

Perimenopause

Perimenopause is the period around menopause, lasting between 3 and 6 years before the last menstrual period (Eliopoulos, 2018). Women often have varied beliefs about aging, and these must be considered when caring for or educating patients who are perimenopausal.

Nursing Management

Women who are perimenopausal often benefit from information about the subtle physiologic changes they are experiencing. Perimenopause has been described as an opportune time for educating women about health promotion and disease prevention strategies. When discussing health-related concerns with women who are in midlife, nurses should consider the following issues:

- Sexuality, fertility, contraception, and STIs
- Unintended pregnancy (if contraception is not used correctly and consistently)
- Oral contraceptive use. Oral contraceptives provide women with protection against uterine cancer, ovarian cancer, anemia, pregnancy, and fibrocystic breast changes as well as relief from perimenopausal symptoms (Eliopoulos, 2018). This option should be discussed with women who are perimenopausal. Women who smoke and are 35 years or older should not take oral contraceptive agents because of an increased risk of CVD.

TABLE 47-1 Hormonal Changes During the Menstrual Cycle

(Times approximate)

Phase	Menstrual	Follicular	Ovulation	Luteal	Premenstrual
Days	1 2 3 4 5 6 7 8 9 10	11 12 13 14 15	16 17	18 19 20 21 22 23 24	25 26 27 28 1 2
Ovary					
	Degenerating corpus luteum; beginning follicular development	Growth and maturation of follicle	Ovulation	Active corpus luteum	Degenerating corpus luteum
Estrogen Production					
	Low	Increasing	High	Declining, then a secondary rise	Decreasing
Progesterone Production					
	None	Low	Low	Increasing	Decreasing
FSH Production					
	Increasing	High, then declining	Low	Low	Increasing
LH Production					
	Low	Low, then increasing	High	High	Decreasing
Endometrium					
	Degeneration and shedding of superficial layer. Coiled arteries dilate, then constrict again	Reorganization and proliferation of superficial layer	Continued growth	Active secretion and glandular dilation; highly vascular; edematous	Vasoconstriction of coiled arteries; beginning degeneration

FSH, follicle-stimulating hormone; LH, luteinizing hormone.

- Breast health. About 16% of cases of breast cancer occur in women who are perimenopausal, so breast self-examination, recommended physical examinations, and mammograms are essential.

Menopause

Menopause is the permanent physiologic cessation of menses associated with declining ovarian function (Ball et al., 2015). Most women stop menstruating between 48 and 55 years of age. Postmenopause is the period beginning from about 1 year after menses cease. Due to a decrease in estrogen levels, menopause may be associated with some atrophy of breast tissue and genital organs, loss in bone density, and vascular changes.

Menopause starts gradually and is usually signaled by changes in menstruation. The monthly flow may increase or decrease, become irregular, and finally cease. Often, the interval between periods is longer; a lapse of several months between periods is not uncommon. Ovulation occurs less frequently, estrogen levels fluctuate, and FSH levels increase in an attempt to stimulate estrogen production (Ball et al., 2015).

Postmenopausal Bleeding

Bleeding 1 year after menses cease at menopause must be investigated, and a malignant condition must be considered until proven otherwise. A transvaginal ultrasound can be used to measure the thickness of the endometrial

TABLE 47-2 Age-Related Changes in the Female Reproductive System

	Physiologic Changes	Signs and Symptoms
Cessation of ovarian function and decreased estrogen production	Decreased ovulation	Decreased/loss of ability to conceive; increased infertility
	Onset of menopause	Irregular menses with eventual cessation of menses
	Vasomotor instability and hormonal fluctuations	Hot flashes or flushing; night sweats, sleep disturbances; mood swings; fatigue
	Decreased bone formation	Bone loss and increased risk for osteoporosis and osteoporotic fractures; loss of height
	Decreased vaginal lubrication	Dyspareunia, resulting in lack of interest in sex
	Thinning of urinary and genital tracts	Increased risk for urinary tract infection
	Increased pH of vagina	Increased incidence of inflammation (atrophic vaginitis) with discharge, itching, and vulvar burning
	Thinning of pubic hair and shrinking of labia	
Relaxation of pelvic musculature	Prolapse of uterus, cystocele, rectocele	Dyspareunia, incontinence, feelings of perineal pressure

The age-related changes described above pertain to women ages 45 years and older.

lining (Fischbach & Dunning, 2015). The uterine lining in women who are postmenopausal should be thin because of low estrogen levels. A thicker lining warrants further evaluation by endometrial biopsy or a dilation and curettage (D&C).

Clinical Manifestations

Menopause has systemic effects that include an increase in body fat and intra-abdominal deposition of body fat. Also, levels of total and LDL cholesterol increase. Hot flashes occur in many women going through menopause due to alterations in thermoregulation. Because of these hormonal changes, some women notice irregular menses, breast tenderness, and mood changes long before menopause occurs (Eliopoulos, 2018). The hot or warm flashes and night sweats reported by some women are thought to be caused by hormonal changes and denote vasomotor instability. They may vary in intensity from a barely perceptible warm feeling to a sensation of extreme warmth accompanied by profuse sweating, causing discomfort, sleep disturbances, and subsequent fatigue. Other physical changes may include increased bone loss.

The entire genitourinary system is affected by the reduced estrogen level. Changes in the vulvovaginal area may include a gradual thinning of pubic hair and a gradual shrinkage of the labia. Vaginal secretions decrease, and women may report dyspareunia (discomfort during intercourse). The vaginal pH increases during menopause, predisposing women to bacterial infections and atrophic vaginitis. Discharge, itching, and vulvar burning may result.

Some women report fatigue, forgetfulness, weight gain, irritability, trouble sleeping, feeling "blue," and feelings of panic. Menopausal complaints need to be evaluated carefully because they may indicate other disorders. Most women have few problems and are relieved to be free from menstrual periods. Nurses should provide women with education and health promotion strategies appropriate for those approaching menopause (see Chart 47-1).

Psychological Considerations

Women's reactions and feelings related to loss of reproductive capacity may vary. Some women may experience role confusion, whereas others experience a sense of sexual and personal freedom. Women may be relieved that the childbearing phase of their lives is over. Each woman's personal views about menopause and circumstances affect her response and must be considered on an individual basis. Nurses need to be sensitive to all possibilities and take their cues from the patient.

Medical Management

Women approaching menopause often have many concerns about their health. Some have concerns based on a family history of heart disease, osteoporosis, or cancer. Each woman needs to be as knowledgeable as possible about her health options and should be encouraged to

CHART 47-1

Health Promotion: Strategies for Women Approaching Menopause

- An annual physical examination can help screen for problems and promote general health.
- Changes in lifestyle (e.g., diet, activity) to promote health and wellness.
  - A nutritious diet (decrease fat and calories, increase fibre and whole grains) and weight control will enhance physical and emotional well-being.
  - Exercise for at least 30 minutes 3 or 4 times a week to maintain good health.
  - Involvement in outside activities is beneficial in reducing anxiety and tension.
- Recognize the following about sexual activity:
  - Sexual functioning may be enhanced at midlife.
  - Frequent sexual activity helps to maintain the elasticity of the vagina.
  - Contraception is advised until 1 year passes without menses.
  - Safer sex is important at any age.
- Strategies and methods to prevent or manage potential problems:
  - *Hot flashes:* See primary provider to discuss hormone replacement therapy (HRT) indications (lowest dose for shortest period of time) and alternative therapy (e.g., vitamin therapy, black cohosh, and other herbal preparations). Fatigue and stress may worsen hot flashes.
  - *Itching or burning of vulvar areas:* See primary provider to rule out dermatologic abnormalities and, if appropriate, to obtain a prescription for a lubricating or hormonal cream.
  - *Dyspareunia (painful intercourse) due to vaginal dryness:* Use a water-soluble lubricant (e.g., K-Y Jelly, Astroglide, Replens), hormone cream, or contraceptive foam.
  - *Decreased perineal muscle tone and bladder control:* Practice Kegel exercises daily (contract the perineal muscles as though stopping urination; hold for 5–10 seconds and release; repeat frequently during the day).
  - *Dry skin:* Use mild emollient skin cream and lotions to prevent dry skin.
  - *Weight control:* Join a weight reduction support group such as Weight Watchers or a similar group if appropriate, or consult a registered dietitian for guidance about the tendency to gain weight, particularly around the hips, thighs, and abdomen.
  - *Osteoporosis:* Observe recommended calcium and vitamin D intake, including calcium supplements, if indicated, to slow the process of osteoporosis; avoid smoking, alcohol, and excessive caffeine, all of which increase bone loss. Perform weight-bearing exercises. Undergo bone density testing when appropriate.
  - *Risk for urinary tract infection (UTI):* Drink 6–8 glasses of water daily as a possible way to reduce the incidence of UTI related to atrophic changes of the urethra.
  - *Vaginal bleeding:* Report any bleeding after 1 year of no menses to the primary provider *immediately, no matter how minimal.*

discuss her concerns with her primary provider so that she can make an informed decision about managing menopausal symptoms and maintaining her health.

Hormone Therapy

HT or menopausal hormonal therapy (previously referred to as hormone replacement therapy [HRT]) is medication that contains estrogen or estrogen and progestin together, to replace the ones the body is no longer making. HT use is controversial, but it is prescribed to treat moderate to severe menopause-related vasomotor symptoms (hot flashes and night sweats) in women without contraindications to estrogen and progesterone whose quality of life is being affected (Eliopoulos, 2018; Fantasia & Sutherland, 2014). The current recommendation for treatment of hot flashes with HT is to use the lowest dose possible for the shortest time possible (Eliopoulos, 2018).

Methods of Administration

Both estrogen and progestin are prescribed for women who have not had a hysterectomy; progestin prevents proliferation of the uterine lining and hyperplasia. Women who no longer have a uterus because of hysterectomy can take estrogen without progestin (i.e., unopposed estrogen) because there is no longer a risk of estrogen-induced hyperplasia of the uterine lining. Although there is a slight increase of risk of stroke in women taking estrogen alone following hysterectomy, the risk of breast cancer is unchanged (Fantasia & Sutherland, 2014).

Some women take both estrogen and progestin daily; others take estrogen for 25 consecutive days each month, with progestin taken in cycles (e.g., 10 to 14 days of the month). Women who take HT for 25 days often experience bleeding after completing the progestin. Other women take estrogen and progestin every day and usually experience no bleeding. They occasionally have irregular spotting, which should be evaluated by their primary provider. Progestin administration may be oral, transdermal, vaginal, or intrauterine.

Estrogen patches, which are replaced once or twice weekly, are another option but require a progestin along with them if the woman still has a uterus. Another type of patch provides estrogen and progestin treatment (Comerford, 2015). Skin should be dry at the area of application and cleansing the site with alcohol may improve adhesiveness. Vaginal treatment with an estrogen cream, suppository, or a vaginal ring may be used for vasomotor symptoms, vaginal dryness, or atrophy (Comerford, 2015).

Risks and Benefits

HT is contraindicated in women with a history of breast cancer, vascular thrombosis, impaired liver function, uterine cancer, and undiagnosed abnormal vaginal bleeding. The risk of venous thromboembolism is increased with HT (Santen, Loprinzi, & Casper, 2016). Women who elect to take HT should be educated about the signs and symptoms of deep vein thrombosis (DVT) and pulmonary embolism (PE) and instructed to report these signs and symptoms (i.e., leg redness, tenderness, chest pain, shortness of breath) immediately. Women who take HT need to be informed about the importance of regular follow-up care, including a yearly physical examination and mammogram. An endometrial biopsy is indicated for any irregular bleeding. Because the risk of complications increases the longer HT is used, HT should be used for the shortest time possible (Eliopoulos, 2018). Estrogen alone or in combination with a progestin does not reduce the risk of dementia or cognitive impairment.

Alternative Therapy for Hot Flashes

Because women often seek information about alternatives to the use of HT, nurses must be knowledgeable about other approaches that women can use to promote their health in the peri- and postmenopausal periods. Problematic hot flashes have been treated with low-dose venlafaxine (Effexor), psychoeducational approaches, and diet and lifestyle changes (Santen et al., 2016). Similarly, vitamin B_6 and vitamin E may be effective. Some women have expressed interest in other alternative treatments (e.g., natural estrogens and progestins, black cohosh, ginseng, dongquai, soy products, and several other herbal preparations); however, limited data exist about their safety or effectiveness. A few studies have shown some improvement in vasomotor symptoms (hot flashes and night sweats) with the use of complementary therapies. These include reflexology, aromatherapy, yoga, hypnotherapy, breathing exercises, and meditation (Eliopoulos, 2018; Santen et al., 2016). When taking a medical history of a patient who is perimenopausal or menopausal, the nurse should always address their use of complementary and alternative therapies and supplements.

Maintaining Bone Health

Acceleration of bone loss resulting in osteoporosis and microarchitectural deterioration of bone tissue occurs at menopause and leads to increased bone fragility and risk of fracture (see Chapter 70).

Maintaining Cardiovascular Health

A variety of strategies can help to lower the risk of heart disease in women, including lifestyle changes and behavioural strategies.

Behavioural Strategies

As stated previously, regular physical exercise is beneficial. It may also reduce stress, enhance well-being, and improve self-image. In addition, weight-bearing exercise may prevent loss of muscle tissue and bone tissue.

Women are also encouraged to participate in other health-promoting activities. These include regular health screening recommended for women at the time of menopause: gynecologic examinations, mammograms, colonoscopy, fecal occult blood testing, and bone mineral density testing if at risk for osteoporosis.

Nutritional Therapy

Women are encouraged to decrease their fat and caloric intake and increase their intake of whole grains, fibre, fruit, and vegetables.

Nursing Management

Nurses can encourage women to view menopause as a natural change resulting in freedom from symptoms related to menses. No relationship exists between menopause and mental health problems; however, social circumstances (e.g., adolescent children, ill partners, and dependent or ill parents) that may coincide with menopause can be stressful.

Measures should be taken to promote general health (Eliopoulos, 2018). The nurse explains to the patient that cessation of menses is a normal occurrence that is rarely accompanied by nervous symptoms or illness. The current expected lifespan after menopause for the average woman is 30 to 35 years, which may encompass as many years as the childbearing phase of her life. Normal sexual urges continue, and women retain their usual response to sex long after menopause. Many women enjoy better health after menopause than before, especially those who have experienced dysmenorrhea. The individual woman's evaluation of herself and her worth, now and in the future, is likely to affect her emotional reaction to menopause. Patient education and counselling regarding healthy lifestyles, health promotion, and health screening are of paramount importance (Santen et al., 2016).

Gerontologic Considerations

Older women function at various levels across the health spectrum; some function at a high level in their jobs or families, whereas others may be very ill. Nurses need to be prepared to care for older women who may be bright, energetic, and ambitious or who are coping with multiple family crises, including their own health issues as well as for those who are experiencing a life-altering or life-threatening health problem. Older women are at risk for several conditions, including diabetes, dyslipidemia, hypertension, and thyroid disease, all of which have symptoms that may be dismissed as typical aging. Nurses can help prevent morbidity and mortality from these conditions by encouraging women to obtain regular health screenings (Eliopoulos, 2018). Knowledge related to heart disease prevention, pharmacology, diet, signs of dementia or cognitive decline, fall prevention, osteoporosis prevention, gynecologic and breast cancers, and sexuality are important for providing high-level nursing care. Health disparities, cultural competency, and end-of-life issues also need to be considered.

Assessment

A nurse who is obtaining information from a patient for the health history and performing physical assessment is in an ideal position to discuss the woman's general health issues, health promotion, and health-related concerns. Relevant topics include fitness, nutrition, cardiovascular risks, health screening, sexuality, menopause, abuse, health risk behaviours, emotional well-being, and immunizations. Recommendations for health screening are summarized in Chart 47-2.

Health History

In addition to the general health history, the nurse asks about past illnesses and experiences specific to a woman's health. Data should be collected about the following:

- Menstrual history (including menarche, length of cycles, duration and amount of flow, presence of cramps or pain, bleeding between periods or after intercourse, bleeding after menopause)
- Pregnancies (number of pregnancies, outcomes of pregnancies)
- Exposure to medications (diethylstilbestrol [DES], immunosuppressive agents, others)
- **Dysmenorrhea** (pain with menses), **dyspareunia** (pain with intercourse), pelvic pain
- Symptoms of vaginitis (i.e., odour or itching)
- Problems with urinary function, including frequency, urgency, and incontinence
- Bowel problems
- Sexual history
- STIs and methods of treatment
- Current or previous sexual abuse or physical abuse
- Past surgery or other procedures on reproductive tract structures (including female genital mutilation [FGM] or female circumcision)
- Chronic illness or disability that may affect health status, reproductive health, need for health screening, or access to health care
- Presence of or family history of a genetic disorder. Chart 47-3 presents information about genetic reproductive disorders.

In collecting data related to reproductive health, the nurse can teach the patient about normal physiologic processes, such as menstruation and menopause, and assess possible abnormalities. Many problems experienced by young or middle-aged women can be corrected easily. However, if they are not treated, they may result in anxiety and health problems. Issues related to sexuality and sexual function are typically more often brought to the attention of the gynecologic or women's health care provider than other health care providers; however, nurses caring for all women should consider these issues part of routine health assessment.

Sexual History

A sexual assessment includes both subjective and objective data and should be included in care of individuals from adolescence through advanced age. Health and sexual histories, physical examination findings, and laboratory results are all part of the database. The purpose of a sexual history is to obtain information that provides a picture of a woman's sexuality and sexual practices and to promote sexual health. It may lead to discussion about sexually transmitted illnesses, unintended pregnancies, and ways of reducing high-risk sexual behaviours (Sargant, Smallwood, Finley, et al., 2014). This information can be obtained after the gynecologic–obstetric or genitourinary history is completed. By incorporating the sexual history into the general health history, the nurse can move from areas of lesser sensitivity to areas of greater sensitivity after establishing initial rapport.

Obtaining the sexual history becomes a dynamic process reflecting an exchange of information between the patient and the nurse and provides the opportunity to clarify myths and explore areas of concern that the patient may not have felt comfortable discussing in the past. In obtaining a sexual history, the nurse must not assume the patient's sexual preference until clarified. When asking about sexual health, the nurse also cannot assume that the patient is married or unmarried. Asking a patient to label herself as single, married, widowed, or divorced may be

CHART 47-2

Summary of Health Screening and Counselling Issues for Women

Ages 19–39

SEXUALITY AND REPRODUCTIVE ISSUES

Annual pelvic examination to begin at age 25
Contraceptive options
High-risk sexual behaviours

HEALTH AND RISK BEHAVIOURS

Hygiene
Injury prevention
Nutrition
Exercise patterns
Risk for domestic abuse
Use of tobacco, drugs, and alcohol
Life stresses
Immunizations

DIAGNOSTIC TESTING[1]

Cervical cytology (Pap smear) every 3 years from ages 25 for all women who have been sexually active
Provincial or territorial screening guidelines vary STI screening as indicated

Ages 40–69

SEXUALITY AND REPRODUCTIVE ISSUES

Annual pelvic examination
Annual clinical breast exam (CBE)
Breast self-examination (BSE)
Contraceptive options
High-risk sexual behaviours
Menopausal concerns

HEALTH AND RISK BEHAVIOURS

Hygiene
Bone loss and injury prevention
Nutrition
Exercise patterns
Risk for domestic abuse
Use of tobacco, drugs, and alcohol
Life stresses
Immunizations

DIAGNOSTIC TESTING[1]

Pap smear every 3 years after three consecutive negative tests if no history of cervical abnormalities, HIV infection, or DES exposure
Mammography as per provincial guidelines
Cholesterol and lipid profile
Colorectal cancer screening
Bone mineral density testing
Thyroid-stimulating hormone testing
Hearing and eye examinations

Ages 69 and Over

Clinical breast exam (CBE) and breast self-examination (BSE) are recommended for women up to the age of 74 years

SEXUALITY AND REPRODUCTIVE ISSUES

High-risk sexual behaviours

HEALTH AND RISK BEHAVIOURS

Hygiene
Injury prevention
Nutrition
Exercise patterns
Risk for domestic abuse
Use of tobacco, drugs, and alcohol
Life stresses
Immunizations

DIAGNOSTIC TESTING[1]

Mammography as per provincial guidelines
Cholesterol and lipid profile
Colorectal cancer screening
Bone mineral density testing
Thyroid-stimulating hormone testing
Hearing and eye examinations

[1]Each individual's risks (family history, personal history) influence the need for specific assessments and their frequency.

considered by some women as inappropriate. Asking about a partner or about current meaningful relationships may be a less offensive way to initiate a sexual history.

The PLISSIT (permission, limited information, specific suggestions, intensive therapy) model of sexual assessment and intervention may be used to provide a framework for nursing interventions (Annon, 1974). The assessment begins by introducing the topic and asking the woman for permission to discuss issues related to sexuality with her.

The nurse can begin by explaining the purpose of obtaining a sexual history (e.g., "I ask all my patients about their sexual health. May I ask you some questions about this?"). History taking continues by inquiring about present sexual activity and sexual orientation (e.g., "Are you currently having sex? With a man, a woman, or both?"). Inquiries about possible sexual dysfunction may include, "Are you having any problems related to your current sexual performance?" Such problems may be related to medication, life changes, disability, or the onset of physical or emotional illness. A patient can be asked about her thoughts on what is causing the current problem (Weber & Kelley, 2014).

Information about sexual function can be introduced during the health history. By initiating an assessment about sexual concerns, the nurse communicates to the patient that issues about changes or problems in sexual functioning are valid health issues, which provides a safe environment for discussing these sensitive topics. Young women may be apprehensive about having irregular periods, may be concerned about STIs, or may require contraception. They may want information about using tampons, emergency contraception, or issues related to pregnancy. Perimenopausal women may have concerns about irregular menses. Menopausal women may be concerned about vaginal dryness and discomfort with intercourse. Women of any age may have concerns about relationships, sexual satisfaction, orgasm, or masturbation.

Risk of STIs can be assessed by asking about the number of sexual partners in the past year or in the patient's

GENETICS IN NURSING PRACTICE

Chart 47-3. Female Reproductive Processes

Various female reproductive disorders are influenced by genetic factors. Some examples include:

- Hereditary breast or ovarian cancer syndromes
- Hereditary nonpolyposis colon cancer syndrome (risk for uterine cancer)
- Kallmann syndrome
- Müllerian aplasia
- 21-Hydroxylase deficiency (female masculinization)
- Turner syndrome (45,XO)
- Klinefelter syndrome (47,XXY)

Nursing Assessments

FAMILY HISTORY ASSESSMENT SPECIFIC TO FEMALE REPRODUCTIVE PROCESSES

- Assess family history for other family members with similar reproductive problems/abnormalities. If the female is a carrier of fragile X, she may be at risk for premature ovarian failure.
- Ask about age at the start and completion of puberty. Failure to complete puberty can lead to infertility.
- The absence of the sense of smell is noted with Kallmann syndrome which, if untreated, can lead to infertility.
- Inquire about ethnic background (e.g., Ashkenazi Jewish populations and hereditary breast/ovarian cancer mutations).
- Inquire about relatives with other cancers, including early-onset ovarian, uterine, renal, prostate cancers.
- Obtain family history that includes a thorough review of reproductive history which addresses spontaneous abortions (miscarriages), infant deaths, or difficulties during pregnancy.
- If possible, obtain ages of the parents during pregnancy.

PATIENT ASSESSMENT SPECIFIC TO FEMALE REPRODUCTIVE PROCESSES

- In females with delayed puberty or primary amenorrhea, assess for clinical features of Turner syndrome (short stature, webbing of the neck, widely spaced nipples).
- Assess for other congenital anomalies in females with müllerian defect, including renal and vertebral anomalies.
- Assess for exposure to toxic chemicals, radiation, or medications during pregnancy.
- Obtain prior reproductive history.
- Inquire about use and frequency of alcohol or tobacco during pregnancy.

Genetic Resources

Genetic Alliance—a directory of support groups for patients and families with genetic conditions, http://www.geneticalliance.org

Canadian Cancer Society—offers general information about cancer and support resources for families, http://www.cancer.ca

National Organization of Rare Disorders—a directory of support groups and information for patients and families with rare genetic disorders, http://www.rarediseases.org

National Cancer Institute—current information about cancer research, treatment, resources for health care providers, individuals and families, http://www.nci.nih.gov

OMIM: Online Mendelian Inheritance in Man—a complete listing of inherited genetic conditions, https://www.omim.org/

lifetime. An open-ended question related to the patient's need for further information should be included (e.g., "Do you have any questions or concerns about your sexual health?"). Women can be advised that intercourse should never be painful; pain should be investigated by a care provider. They should also be encouraged to talk openly about their sexual feelings with their partner.

Female Genital Mutilation or Cutting

Female genital mutilation (FGM), or cutting, refers to the partial or total removal of the external female genitalia or other injury to female organs for non-medical reasons. FGM is recognized internationally as a violation of the human rights of girls and women. It reflects deep-rooted inequality between the sexes and constitutes an extreme form of discrimination against women. It is nearly always carried out on minors and is a violation of the rights of children. The practice also violates a person's rights to health, security and physical integrity, the right to be free from torture and cruel, inhuman or degrading treatment, and the right to life when the procedure results in death (World Health Organization [WHO], 2016). FGM is illegal in Canada, and many organizations (e.g., WHO, Amnesty International) consider it a health and human rights issue and are working to end it.

Complications for patients who have undergone FGM can include infertility, childbirth complications, impaired bladder function, and urinary complications. The practice is most common in the western, eastern, and northeastern regions of Africa, in some countries in Asia and the Middle East, and among migrants from these areas (WHO, 2016).

Nurses who care for patients who have undergone FGM need to be sensitive, empathetic, knowledgeable, culturally competent, and nonjudgmental. Respect for others' health beliefs, practices, and behaviour, and recognition of the complexity of issues involved is crucial. The nurse should use the woman's terminology. "Cutting" is a more acceptable term than mutilation. Speculums are not used in some developing countries; the function of this instrument should be explained, and an appropriate-sized speculum used to examine women who have experienced FGM.

Intimate Partner Violence

Intimate partner violence (IPV) is a public health problem that affects millions of Canadians each year. In Canada it is estimated that in 2013 there were over 90,300 victims of police reported IPV (Statistics Canada, 2019). IPV involves four main types of violence: Physical violence, sexual violence, stalking, and psychological aggression (CDC, 2014).

In 2016, IPV was the leading type of violence experienced by women. The most common violent offences included common assault (58%), uttering threats (11%), major assault (15%), sexual offences (8%), and criminal harassment (stalking) (4%). Spouses were responsible for 91% of the police-reported family violence (Statistics Canada, 2018). Battering involves repeated physical or sexual assault in a context of coercive control and, more broadly, emotional degradation, threats, and intimidation.

Violence is rarely a one-time occurrence in a relationship; it usually continues and escalates in severity. This is an important point to emphasize when a woman states that her partner has hurt her but has promised to change. Batterers can change their behaviour but not without extensive counselling and motivation. If a woman states that she is being hurt, sensitive care is required (Chart 47-4).

By knowing about this major public health problem, being alert to abuse-related problems, and learning how to elicit information from women about abuse, maltreatment and neglect in their lives, nurses can offer intervention for a problem that might otherwise go undetected and can save lives by making women safer through education and support. Asking each woman about violence in her life in a safe environment (i.e., a private room with the door closed) is part of a comprehensive assessment and universal screening.

No specific signs or symptoms are diagnostic of battering; however, nurses may see an injury that does not fit the account of how it happened (e.g., a bruise on the side of the upper arm after "I walked into a door"). Manifestations of abuse, maltreatment and neglect may involve suicide attempts, drug and alcohol abuse, frequent emergency department visits, vague pelvic pain, somatic complaints, and depression. However, there may be no obvious signs or symptoms. Women in abusive situations have higher levels of depression and often report that they "do not feel well," possibly due to the stress or fear and anticipation of impending abuse.

The assessment for abuse by health professionals has lagged behind community awareness and response (Hooker, Ward, & Verrinder, 2012). In addition to asking about IPV, nurses need to provide resources and referral, as

CHART 47-4

Strategies for Providing Sensitive Care Following Abuse, Maltreatment, and Neglect

Strategy	Rationale
Reassure the woman that she is not alone.	Women often believe that they are alone in experiencing abuse, maltreatment, and neglect at the hands of their partners.
Express your belief that no one should be hurt, that abuse is the fault of the batterer and is against the law.	Doing so lets the woman know that no one deserves to be abused and that she has not caused the abuse.
Assure the woman that her information is confidential, although it does become part of her medical record. *If children are suspected of being abused or are being abused, the law requires that this be reported to the authorities.* If nurses are in doubt about laws on reporting abuse, they need to check with their local or provincial domestic violence agency.	Women are often afraid that their information will be reported to the police or protective services and their children may be taken away.
Document the woman's statement of abuse and take photographs of any visible injuries if written formal consent has been obtained. (Emergency departments usually have a camera available if one is not on the nursing unit.)	Doing so provides documentation of injuries that may be needed for later legal or criminal proceedings.
Provide education that includes the following: • Inform the woman that shelters are available to ensure safety for her and her children. (Lengths of stay in shelters vary by organization but are often up to 2 months. Staff often assists with housing, jobs, and the emotional distress that accompanies the breakup of the family.) Provide list of shelters. • Inform the woman that violence gets worse, not better. • If the woman chooses to go to a shelter, let her make the call. • If the woman chooses to return to the abuser, remain nonjudgmental and provide information that will make her safer than she was before disclosing her situation. • Make sure that the woman has a 24-hour hotline telephone number that provides information and support, police number, and 911. • Assist her to setup a safety plan in case she decides to return home. (A safety plan is an organized plan for departure with packed bags and important papers hidden in a safe spot.)	Options may be lifesaving for the woman and her children.

Adapted from Centers for Disease Control and Prevention (CDC). (2019). *Preventing intimate partner violence.* Retrieved from www.cdc.gov/violenceprevention/pdf/ipv-factsheet.pdf

well as to follow written protocols of their institution or agency to ensure comprehensive care (Hooker et al., 2012).

Incest and Childhood Sexual Abuse

Nurses may encounter women who have been sexually traumatized. Female survivors of sexual abuse are reported to have more mental and physical health problems than women who were not victims of abuse (Pyra, Weber, Wilson, et al., 2014). Victims of childhood sexual abuse are reported to experience more chronic depression, posttraumatic stress disorder, morbid obesity, marital instability, gastrointestinal problems, and headaches, as well as use health care services more frequently than people who were not victims. In women, chronic pelvic pain is often associated with physical violence, emotional neglect, and sexual abuse in childhood (Schuiling & Likis, 2013). Women who have experienced rape or sexual abuse may be very anxious about pelvic examinations, labour, pelvic or breast irradiation, or any treatment or examination that involves hands-on treatment or requires removal of clothing. Nurses should be prepared to offer support and referral to psychologists, community resources, and self-help groups.

Sexual Assault

A woman is sexually assaulted about every 17 minutes in Canada (Rape Victims Support Network, 2012). Men, women, and children may be victims. Many sexual assaults occur on dates. Sexual assault nurse examiners, emergency department staff, and gynecologists perform the painstaking collection of forensic evidence that is needed for criminal prosecution. Oral, anal, and genital tissue is examined for evidence of trauma, semen, or infection. Saliva, hair, and fingernail evidence is also collected. Cultures are obtained for STIs, and prophylactic antibiotics are prescribed. The postexposure prophylaxis (PEP) recommended by the Public Health Agency of Canada (PHAC) consists of Cefixime or Ciprofloxacin, metronidazole (Flagyl), and azithromycin (Zithromax) or Doxycycline (PHAC, 2014). Hepatitis B immune globulin (HBIG) should be given up to 14 days post exposure with Hepatitis B vaccine given at 0, 1, and 6 months post exposure with an accelerated schedule if appropriate (PHAC, 2014). Recommendations for HIV PEP testing vary across the country. Decisions for treatment should be made according to provincial/territorial/regional protocols or in conjunction with an HIV specialist. HIV PEP is recommended when the assailant is known to be HIV infected and significant exposure (e.g., anal, oral, or vaginal) has occurred. PEP is also available on a case-by-case basis when other high-risk exposures occur (e.g., injection drug abuser). Emergency contraception is explained and provided if requested and appropriate. Emotional counselling is provided, and follow-up treatment visits are arranged. Rape trauma syndrome, a form of posttraumatic stress disorder (Tannura, 2014), is the emotional reaction to a sexual assault and may consist of shock, sleep disturbances, nightmares, flashbacks, anxiety, anger, mood swings, and depression. It is important and helpful for survivors to discuss the experience and to obtain professional counselling.

Screening for abuse, sexual assault, and violence should be part of routine assessment because women often do not report or seek treatment for assault. Often, the assailant is a partner, husband, or date. Nurses may encounter women with infections or pregnancies related to sexual assault who require support, understanding, and comprehensive care.

Health Issues of Women With Disabilities

Approximately 15% of women in Canada live with disabilities. Aboriginal women aged 15 or older were more than 1.5 times as likely as non-Aboriginal women to report disabilities (Statistics Canada, 2017). Women with disabilities may encounter physical, architectural, and attitudinal barriers that may limit their full participation in society (Courtney-Long, Carroll, Znang, et al., 2013). Women with disabilities may also experience stereotyping and increased risk of abuse, maltreatment, and neglect. Studies have shown that women with disabilities receive less primary health care and preventive health screening than other women, often because of access problems and health care providers who focus on the causes of disability rather than on health issues that are of concern to all women (Courtney-Long et al., 2013). To address these issues, the health history must include questions about barriers to health care encountered by women with disabilities and the effect of their disability on their health status and health care (see Chart 47-5).

Nurses assessing women with disabilities may require additional time and the assistance of others to be certain that accurate information is obtained in a sensitive and unhurried manner (Smeltzer, Avery, & Haynor, 2012). Women with disabilities may have had previous negative experiences with health care providers (Smeltzer et al., 2012), and it is important that nurses provide them with knowledgeable and sensitive care. See Chapter 12 for further discussion of health care of patients with disabilities.

Lesbians, Gay, Bisexual, Transgender, Queer/Questioning, and Others (LGBTQ$^+$)

Many health care providers are insufficiently prepared to meet the health needs of patients who identify as lesbian, gay, bisexual, transgender, queer (LGBTQ$^+$), and those who are questioning their gender (Rager Zuzelo, 2014).

Many health assessments presume a heterosexual orientation. Nursing organizations have called for recognition of LGBTQ$^+$ health disparities (Rager Zuzelo, 2014).

Those who identify themselves as LGBTQ$^+$ may have concerns about disclosure and confidentiality, discriminatory attitudes, and treatment (Bosse, Nesteby, & Randall, 2015; Johnson & Amella, 2014; Rager Zuzelo, 2014) (see Chart 47-6). Youth who identify as LGBTQ$^+$ are at higher risk of HIV and STIs (Bosse et al., 2015). Some research has reported that lesbians abuse alcohol and drugs to a greater degree than women who are heterosexual because their social venues may contribute to alcohol and drug use. In addition, youth who self-identify as lesbian, gay, or bisexual or who lack support from parents and families may experience increased physical and mental health issues (e.g., depression and substance abuse) as well as isolation (Johnson & Amella, 2014) (see Chart 47-7). Nurses need to understand the unique needs of this population and provide appropriate and sensitive care.

Physical Assessment

Periodic examinations and routine cancer screening are important for all women. A clinical breast exam (CBE)

CHART 47-5

Assessment: Assessing a Woman With a Disability

Health History

Address questions directly to the woman herself rather than to people accompanying her. Ask about:

- Self-care limitations resulting from her disability (ability to feed and dress self, the use of assistive devices, transportation requirements, other assistance needed)
- Sensory limitations (lack of sensation, low vision, deaf or hard of hearing)
- Accessibility issues (ability to get to health care provider, transfer to examination table, accessibility of office/clinic of health care provider, previous experiences with health care providers, health screening practices; her understanding of physical examination)
- Cognitive or developmental changes that affect understanding
- Limitations secondary to disability that affect general health issues and reproductive health and health care
- Sexual function and concerns (those of all women and those that may be affected by the presence of a disabling condition)
- Menstrual history and menstrual hygiene practices
- Physical, sexual, or psychological abuse (including abuse by care providers; abuse by neglect, withholding or withdrawing assistive devices or personal or health care)
- Presence of secondary disabilities (i.e., those resulting from the patient's primary disability: pressure ulcers, spasticity, osteoporosis, etc.)
- Health concerns related to aging with a disability

Physical Assessment

Provide instructions directly to the woman herself rather than to people accompanying her; provide written or audiotaped instructions.

Ask the woman what assistance she needs for the physical examination and provide assistance if needed:

- Undressing and dressing
- Providing a urine specimen
- Standing on scale to be weighed (provide alternative means of obtaining weight if she is unable to stand on scale)
- Moving on and off the examination table
- Assuming, changing, and maintaining positions

Consider the fatigue experienced by the woman during a lengthy examination and allow rest.

Provide assistive devices and other aids/methods needed to allow adequate communication with the patient (interpreters, signers, large-print written materials).

Complete examination that would be indicated for any other woman; having a disability is *never* justification for omitting parts of the physical examination, including the pelvic examination.

Adapted from Smeltzer, S. C., Mitra, M., Iezzoni, L. I., et al. (2016). Perinatal experiences of women with physical disabilities and their recommendations for Clinicians. *Journal of Obstetric, Gynecologic & Neonatal Nursing, 45*(6), 781–789.

CHART 47-6

Health Care for Those Who Identify as LGBTQ⁺

Nurses working with those who identify as LGBTQ⁺ should consider that these individuals:

- Are found in every ethnic group and socioeconomic class.
- Are seen in all age groups, including teens and seniors.
- Can be single, celibate, or divorced.
- Have often encountered insensitivity in health care encounters.
- Are typically offered contraception when asked if they are sexually active and respond affirmatively, as health care providers may assume incorrectly that they practice heterosexual intercourse.
- Have lower health screening rates than other women.
- Often feel invisible and underuse health care, similar to many other marginalized groups of women.

Nurses need to:

- Use gender-neutral questions and terms that are nonjudgmental and accepting.
- Recognize that lesbian teens are at risk for suicide and screen for those at risk.
- Recognize that many lesbians do participate in heterosexual activity but consider themselves at low risk for STIs. Because human papilloma virus, herpes infections, and other organisms implicated in STIs are transmitted by secretions and contact, lesbians may need information on STIs and contraception. If sex toys are used and not cleaned, pelvic infections can occur.

Women who identify as LGBTQ⁺ are at high risk for cancer, heart disease, depression, and alcohol abuse. They may have a higher body mass index, may bear fewer or no children, and often have fewer health preventive screenings than women who are heterosexual. These factors may increase the risk of colon, endometrial, ovarian, and breast cancer, as well as cardiovascular disease and diabetes. Adolescents are at risk for smoking and suicide/depression.

Adapted from Johnson, M. J., & Amella, E. J. (2014). Isolation of lesbian, gay, bisexual and transgender youth: A dimensional concept analysis. *Journal of Advanced Nursing, 70*(3), 523–532; Rager Zuzelo, P. (2014). Improving nursing care for lesbian, bisexual and transgender women. *Journal of Obstetric Gynecologic and Neonatal Nursing, 43*, 520–530.

NURSING RESEARCH PROFILE

Chart 47-7. Isolation in LGBTQ+ Youth

Johnson, M. J., & Amella, E. J. (2014). Isolation of lesbian, gay, bisexual and transgender youth: A dimensional concept analysis. *Journal of Advanced Nursing, 70*(3), 523–532.

Purpose

Few nursing studies have looked at isolation in youth who identify as lesbian, gay, bisexual, transgender, or queer (LGBTQ+) despite the fact that nurses have many interactions with them in hospitals, community, and school settings. Some research suggests isolation in youth who identify as LGBTQ+ is related to increased risk for mental and physical health disparities. The aim of this dimensional concept analysis was to understand isolation in the context, and from the perspective of youth identifying as LGBTQ+.

Design

Procedures for the concept analysis included describing the social construction of the concept, describing the logic of a concept from multiple perspectives and as part of multiple contexts, differentiating the relationship between perspectives and use or definition of the concept and identifying and examining assumptions. To accomplish the analysis, the two authors read each paper in its entirety and then identified the findings of each article using a table. Additional tables allowed for the identification of patterns or relationships across dimensions, discipline perspectives, and publication dates.

Results

The analysis revealed five socially constructed dimensions and four sub-dimensions. These findings indicate that there is substantial variability in the concept of isolation in LGBTQ+ youth. These differences and variations are most notably observed in the 20 articles (57%) that had more than one dimension. Although some articles were explicit about the different meanings and use of the concept, most of the papers had wide variability in the use and meaning of the concept.

Nursing Implications

It is imperative that nurses and other professionals understand the significance of isolation in youth who identify as LGBTQ+. Nurses who understand the concept have the potential, in their interactions with these youth in hospitals, community, and school settings, to intervene and suggest strategies to mitigate the isolation.

and breast self-examination (BSE) are recommended for women aged 40 to 74 without personal or family history of breast cancer, known BRCA1 or 2 mutation, or prior chest wall radiation. Cervical screening guidelines vary across the country. The CTFPHC recommends routine cervical screening, for asymptomatic patients, starting at the age of 25 years. Patients deserve understanding and support because of the emotional and physical considerations associated with gynecologic examinations. Women may be embarrassed by the usual questions asked by a gynecologist or women's health care provider. Because gynecologic conditions are of a personal and private nature to most women, such information is shared only with those directly involved in patient care.

Throughout the examination, the nurse explains the procedures to be performed. This not only encourages the woman to relax but also provides an opportunity for her to ask questions and minimizes the negative feelings that many women associate with gynecologic examinations.

The approach to the gynecologic examination needs to be systematic and thorough (Weber & Kelley, 2014). The nurse can alleviate feelings of anxiety with explanations and education (Chart 47-8). It may be helpful to emphasize that a pelvic examination should not usually be uncomfortable. Before the examination begins, the patient is asked to empty her bladder and to provide a urine specimen if urine tests are part of the total assessment. Voiding ensures patient comfort and eases the examination because a full bladder can make palpation of pelvic organs uncomfortable for the patient and difficult for the examiner.

Positioning

The supine lithotomy position is used most commonly (Weber & Kelley, 2014). If the patient chooses, alternative positions are sometimes used (Ball et al., 2015). The lithotomy position offers several advantages:

- It is more comfortable for some women.
- It allows better eye contact between patient and examiner.

CHART 47-8

Patient Education: The Pelvic Examination

A pelvic examination includes assessment of the appearance of the vulva, vagina, and cervix and the size and shape of the uterus and ovaries to ensure reproductive health and absence of illness. Providing education for the patient should make the examination proceed more smoothly.

The nurse instructs the patient to:

- Expect to have a feeling of fullness or pressure during the examination, but you should not feel pain. It is important to relax, because if you are very tense, you may feel discomfort.
- Recognize that it is normal to feel uncomfortable and apprehensive.
- Be aware that a narrow, warmed speculum will be inserted to visualize the cervix and a Papanicolaou (Pap) smear will be obtained, if indicated, and should not be uncomfortable.
- Note that you may watch the examination with a mirror if you choose; the examination usually takes no longer than 5 minutes.
- Understand that draping will be used to minimize exposure and reduce embarrassment.

Adapted from Weber, J., & Kelley, J. (2014). *Health assessment in nursing* (5th ed.). Philadelphia, PA: Lippincott Williams & Wilkins.

- It may provide an easier means for the examiner to complete the bimanual examination.
- It enables the woman to use a mirror to see her anatomy (if she chooses) to visualize any conditions that require treatment or to learn about using certain types of contraceptive methods.

Inspection

After the patient is prepared, the examiner inspects the external genitalia, noting the epidermal tissue of the labia majora; the skin fades to the pink mucous membrane of the vaginal introitus. Lesions of any type (e.g., genital warts, pigmented lesions [melanoma]) are evaluated. In the nulliparous woman, the labia minora come together at the opening of the vagina. In a woman who has delivered children vaginally, the labia minora may gape and vaginal tissue may protrude.

Trauma to the anterior vaginal wall during childbirth may have resulted in incompetency of the musculature, and a **cystocele** (a bulge caused by the bladder protruding into the submucosa of the anterior vaginal wall) may be seen. Childbirth trauma may also have affected the posterior vaginal wall, producing a **rectocele** (a bulge caused by rectal cavity protrusion). A **uterine prolapse** may also occur where the cervix descends under pressure through the vaginal canal and may be seen at the introitus. To identify such protrusions, the examiner asks the patient to "bear down."

The introitus should be free of superficial mucosal lesions. The labia minora may be separated by the fingers of the gloved hand and the lower part of the vagina palpated. In women who have not had vaginal intercourse, a **hymen** of variable thickness may be felt circumferentially within the vaginal opening. The hymenal ring usually permits the insertion of one finger. Rarely, the hymen totally occludes the vaginal entrance (imperforate hymen).

Examination

Examination techniques include the speculum examination and several palpation methods.

Speculum Examination (Fig. 47-4)

The bivalved speculum, either metal or plastic, is available in many sizes (Ball et al., 2015). Metal specula are cleaned and sterilized between patients; plastic specula are for one-time use. Water-soluble lubricant or warm water is used to lubricate the speculum (Ball et al., 2015).

The speculum is gently inserted into the posterior portion of the introitus and slowly advanced to the top of the vagina; this should not be painful or uncomfortable for the woman. The speculum is then slowly opened. In the metal types, a set-screw of the thumb rest is tightened; in

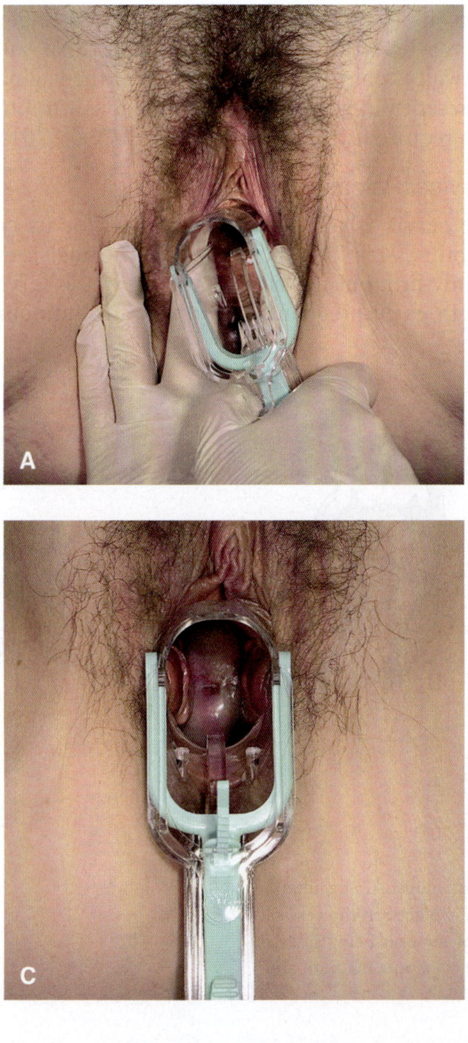

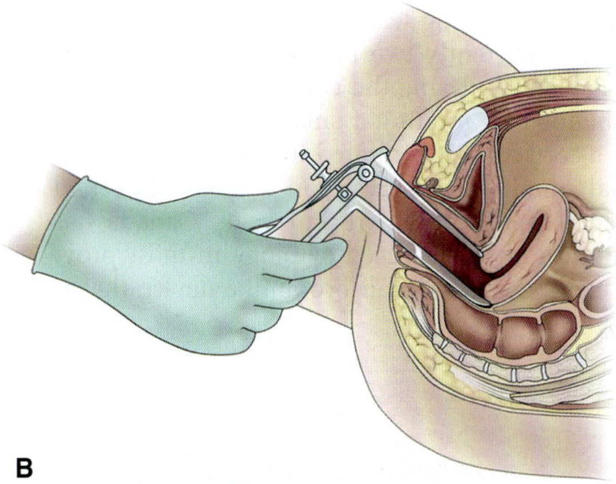

B

FIGURE 47-4. Technique for speculum examination of the vagina and cervix. **A.** The labia are spread apart with a gloved left hand, while the speculum is grasped in the right hand and turned counterclockwise before being inserted into the vagina. Once the speculum is inserted, the blades are then spread apart (**B**) to reveal the cervical os (**C**).

the plastic types, a clip is locked to hold the blades in place (Ball et al., 2015).

Inspecting the Cervix

The cervix is inspected for colour, position, size, surface characteristics, discharge, and size and shape of the cervical os (Ball et al., 2015). In nulliparous women, the cervix usually is 2 to 3 cm wide and smooth. In women who have borne children, the cervix may have a laceration, usually transverse, giving the cervical os a "fishmouth" appearance. Epithelium from the endocervical canal may have grown onto the surface of the cervix, appearing as beefy-red surface epithelium circumferentially around the os. Occasionally, the cervix of a woman whose mother took DES during pregnancy has a hooded appearance (a peaked aspect superiorly or a ridge of tissue surrounding it); this is evaluated by colposcopy when identified.

Malignant changes may not be obviously differentiated from the rest of the cervical mucosa. Small, benign cysts may appear on the cervical surface. Called *nabothian (retention) cysts,* these are usually bluish or white and are a normal finding after childbirth (Ball et al., 2015). A **polyp** of endocervical mucosa may protrude through the os and usually is dark red. Polyps can cause irregular bleeding; they are rarely malignant and usually are removed easily in an office or clinic setting. A carcinoma may appear as a cauliflowerlike growth (Ball et al., 2015). Bluish colouration of the cervix is a sign of early pregnancy (Chadwick's sign).

Obtaining Papanicolaou (Pap) Smears and Other Samples

A Pap smear is a screening test for abnormal cells of the cervix. There are currently two methods used in Canada to collect a Pap smear. Using the conventional method, a sample is obtained by rotating a small spatula at the os, followed by a cervical brush rotated in the os (Fig. 47-5). The material obtained is spread on a glass slide and sprayed/fixed immediately. In recent years Canada has seen the addition of liquid-based cytology in most provinces. This method uses a small broomlike device that is used to "sweep" the cervical os. The top of the device is then inserted into the liquid filled specimen bottle (thin "prep"). The procedural guidelines for obtaining an optimal Pap smear are presented in Chart 47-9.

A specimen of any purulent material appearing at the cervical os is obtained for culture. A sterile applicator is used to obtain the specimen, which is immediately placed in an appropriate medium for transfer to a laboratory. In a patient who has a high risk of infection, routine cultures for gonococcal and chlamydial organisms are recommended because of the high incidence of both diseases and the complications of pelvic infection, fallopian tube damage, and subsequent infertility.

Vaginal discharge, which may be normal or may result from vaginitis, may be present. Table 47-3 summarizes the characteristics of vaginal discharge found in different conditions.

Inspecting the Vagina

The vagina is inspected as the examiner withdraws the speculum. It is smooth in young girls and thickens after puberty, with many rugae (folds) and redundancy in the epithelium. In menopausal women, the vagina thins and has fewer rugae because of decreased estrogen.

Bimanual Palpation

To complete the pelvic examination, the examiner performs a bimanual examination. The examiner should inform the woman that she will be examined internally with the examiners' fingers. The gloved fingers are then advanced vertically along the vaginal canal, and the vaginal wall is palpated. Any firm part of the vaginal wall may represent old scar tissue from childbirth trauma but may also require further evaluation (Ball et al., 2015).

Cervical Palpation

The cervix is palpated and assessed for its consistency, mobility, size, and position. The normal cervix is uniformly firm but not hard. Softening of the cervix is a finding in early pregnancy. Hardness and immobility of the

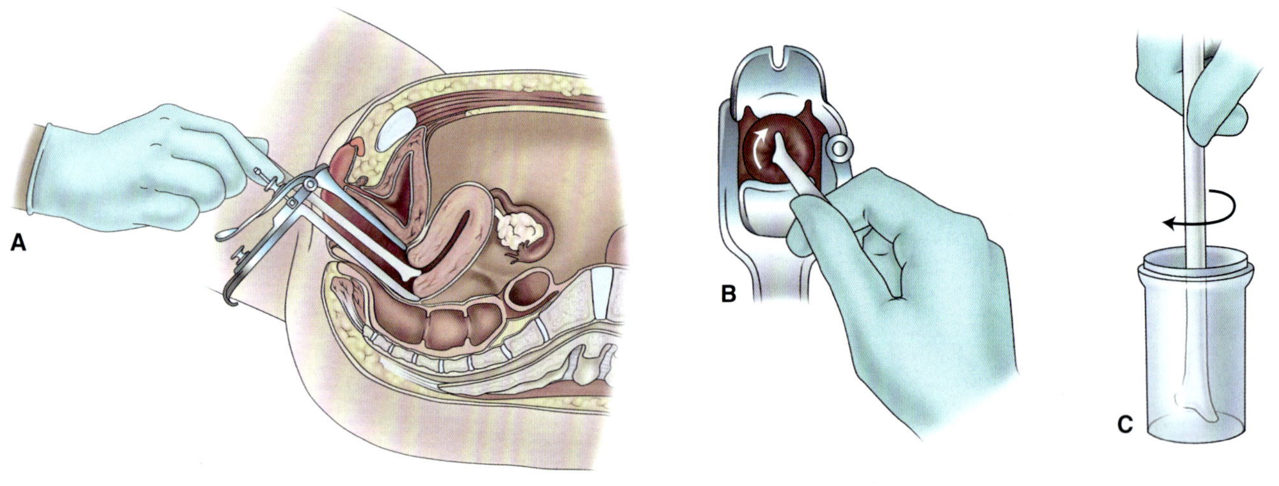

FIGURE 47-5. Method of using an Ayre spatula to obtain cervical secretions for cytology. **A.** Speculum in place and the Ayre spatula in position at the cervical os. **B.** The tip of the spatula is placed in the cervical os and the spatula rotated 360 degrees, firmly but nontraumatically. **C.** Instead of the cells being smeared on a slide, the sampling device is rinsed or twirled in the small vial containing the transport medium and sent to the laboratory.

CHART 47-9

GUIDELINES for Obtaining an Optimal Pap Smear

Equipment

- Speculum
- Gloves
- Slide, spatula, and cytobrush or thin prep kit

Implementation

NURSING ACTIONS	RATIONALE
1. Do not obtain a Papanicolaou (Pap) smear if the woman is menstruating or has other frank bleeding (*Exception:* High suspicion of neoplasia).	1. Blood obscures a proper reading of cells.
2. If performing more than one test, obtain the Pap smear first.	2. By performing the Pap smear first, the chance of a bloody smear is avoided.
3. Label the frosted end of the slide with the patient's name in pencil, or label ThinPrep Pap bottle.	3. Ink may rub off or blur. Labelling with a pencil prevents improper identification.
4. Put on gloves before gently inserting the unlubricated speculum. (Speculum may be moistened with warm water or a water-based lubricant.)	4. Gloves provide protection and warm water prevents discomfort. Non-water-based lubricants may obscure cells on Pap smear.
5. Place the longer end of the Ayre spatula in the cervical canal and rotate it in a full circle to obtain a sample from the exocervix. Spread the material obtained onto the Pap smear slide.	5. This technique obtains a sampling of the exocervix and squamocolumnar junction.
6. Insert a cytobrush 2 cm into the cervical canal and rotate 180 degrees. Roll the brush onto the Pap smear slide. (With ThinPrep Pap smears, the brushings are not spread onto a slide. The spatula and/or brush are placed in a bottle of fixative and swirled.)	6. This technique obtains a sampling of the endocervical cells and may sample cells from the squamocolumnar junction if it is high in the canal.
7. In women who have had a hysterectomy for a gynecologic cancer, use a cotton applicator moistened with normal saline solution to obtain a sampling of cells from the vaginal cuff or posterior vagina. Women who have had a hysterectomy for benign conditions do not require frequent Pap smears.	7. Normal saline solution prevents drying, which makes interpretation difficult for the cytologist and prevents absorption of cells into the cotton, increasing the yield on the slide.
8. Immediately spray the slide, or, if a ThinPrep, swirl the brush and spatula in the solution.	8. Exposure to light or air causes distortion of cells.

Adapted from Ball, J., Dains, J., Flynn, J., et al. (2015). *Seidel's guide to physical examination*. (8th ed.). St. Louis, MO: Elsevier Mosby.

cervix may reflect invasion by a neoplasm. Pain on gentle movement of the cervix is called a positive **chandelier sign** or positive cervical motion tenderness (recorded as + CMT) and usually indicates a pelvic infection.

Uterine Palpation

To palpate the uterus, the examiner places the opposite hand on the abdominal wall halfway between the umbilicus and the pubis and presses firmly toward the vagina. Movement of the abdominal wall causes the body of the uterus to descend, and the organ becomes freely movable between the hand used to examine the abdomen and the fingers of the hand used to examine the pelvis. Uterine size, mobility, and contour can be estimated through palpation. Fixation of the uterus in the pelvis may be a sign of **endometriosis** or malignancy.

The body of the uterus is normally twice the diameter and twice the length of the cervix, curving anteriorly

TABLE 47-3 Characteristics of Vaginal Discharge

Cause of Discharge	Symptoms	Odour	Consistency/Colour
Physiologic	None	None	Mucus/white
Candida species infection	Itching, irritation	Yeast odour or none	Thin to thick, curdlike/white
Bacterial vaginosis	Odour	Fishy, often noticed after intercourse	Thin/grayish or yellow
Trichomonas species infection	Irritation, odour	Malodourous	Copious, often frothy/yellow-green
Atrophic	Vulvar or vaginal dryness	Occasional mild malodour	Usually scant and mucoid/may be blood tinged

toward the abdominal wall. Some women have a retroverted or retroflexed uterus, which tips posteriorly toward the sacrum, whereas others have a uterus that is neither anterior nor posterior and is described as midline.

Adnexal Palpation

Next, the right and left adnexal areas are palpated to evaluate the fallopian tubes and ovaries. The fingers of the hand examining the pelvis are moved first to one side, then to the other, while the hand palpating the abdominal area is moved correspondingly to either side of the abdomen and downward. The adnexa (ovaries and fallopian tubes) are trapped between the two hands and palpated for an obvious mass, tenderness, and mobility. Commonly, the ovaries are slightly tender, and the patient is informed that slight discomfort on palpation is normal.

Vaginal and Rectal Palpation

Bimanual palpation of the vagina and cul-de-sac is accomplished by placing the index finger in the vagina and the middle finger in the rectum. To prevent cross-contamination between the vaginal and rectal orifices, the examiner puts on new gloves. A gentle movement of these fingers toward each other compresses the posterior vaginal wall and the anterior rectal wall and assists the examiner in identifying the integrity of these structures. During this procedure, the patient may sense an urge to defecate. The nurse assures the patient that this is unlikely to occur. Ongoing explanations are provided to reassure and educate the patient about the procedure.

Gerontologic Considerations

Annual examinations are important; they identify problems of the reproductive tract in aging women (Eliopoulos, 2018). Nurses play an important role; they can encourage all women to have regularly scheduled gynecologic examinations. The CTFPHC recommends that women aged ≥ 70 years who have been adequately screened (i.e., 3 successive negative Pap tests in the last 10 years) may cease routine screening. For women aged 70 years or over who have not been adequately screened, it is recommended that they continue screening until three negative test results have been obtained.

Perineal pruritus is abnormal in older women and should be evaluated because it may indicate a disease process (diabetes or malignancy). Vulvar dystrophy, a thickened or whitish discolouration of tissue, may be visible, and biopsy is needed to rule out abnormal cells. Topical cortisone and hormone creams may be prescribed for symptomatic relief.

With relaxing pelvic musculature, uterine prolapse and relaxation of the vaginal walls can occur (Eliopoulos, 2018). Appropriate evaluation and surgical repair can provide relief if the patient is a candidate for surgery. After surgery, the patient should know that tissue repair and healing may require more time with aging. Pessaries (latex devices that provide support) are often used if surgery is contraindicated or before surgery to see if surgery can be avoided. They are fitted by a health care provider and may reduce discomfort and pressure. Use of a pessary requires the patient to have routine gynecologic examinations to monitor for irritation or infection. The patient must be assessed for allergy prior to insertion of a latex pessary (see Chapter 48 for details about pessaries).

Diagnostic Evaluation

A wide range of diagnostic studies may be performed in the management of female physiologic processes. The nurse should educate the patient about the purpose, what to expect, and any possible side effects related to these examinations prior to testing. The nurse should be aware of contraindications, potential complications, and trends in results. Trends provide information about disease progression as well as the patient's response to therapy.

Cytologic Test for Cancer (Pap Smear)

The Pap smear is used to detect cervical cancer. Cervical secretions are gently removed from the cervical os and collected for laboratory analysis. If the Pap smear reveals atypical cells, the liquid method allows for human papillomavirus (HPV) testing. HPV DNA testing is helpful in that it can detect high-risk types that may require careful monitoring. HPV infection is often temporary, especially in healthy young women.

Terminology used to describe findings includes the following categories:

- No abnormal or atypical cells
- Atypical squamous cells of undetermined significance
- Inflammatory reactions and microbes identified
- Positive deoxyribonucleic acid (DNA) test for HPV
- Precancerous and cancerous lesions of the cervix identified

The patient may incorrectly assume that an abnormal Pap smear signifies cancer. If the Pap smear (liquid immersion method) shows atypical cells and no high-risk HPV types, the next Pap smear is performed in 1 year. If a specific infection is causing inflammation, it is treated appropriately, and the Pap smear is repeated. If the repeat Pap smear reveals atypical squamous cells with high-risk HPV types, colposcopy may be indicated. Pap smears that indicate precancerous lesions should be repeated in 4 to 6 months and colposcopy performed if the lesion has not resolved. Patients with Pap smears that indicate cancerous lesions require prompt colposcopy (Fischbach & Dunning, 2015).

If the Pap smear results are abnormal, prompt notification, evaluation, and treatment are crucial. Notification of patients is often the responsibility of nurses in a women's health care practice or clinic. Pap smear follow-up is essential because it can prevent cervical cancer. Interventions are tailored to meet the needs of the particular patient. Intensive telephone counselling, tracking systems, brochures, videos, and financial incentives have all been used to encourage follow-up. The nurse provides clear explanations and emotional support along with a carefully designed setting-specific follow-up protocol designed to meet the needs of the patient.

The Society of Obstetricians and Gynaecologists of Canada (SOGC) issued a set of guidelines for the evaluation and management of abnormal cervical cytology and histology in adolescent females (Bentley, 2012).

Colposcopy and Cervical Biopsy

If the cervical cytology result requires evaluation, a colposcopy is performed. The colposcope is an instrument with a magnifying lens that allows the examiner to visualize the cervix and obtain a sample of abnormal tissue for analysis (Fischbach & Dunning, 2015). Nurse practitioners and gynecologists require special training in this diagnostic technique.

After inserting a speculum and visualizing the cervix and vaginal walls, the examiner applies acetic acid to the cervix. Subsequent abnormal findings that indicate the need for biopsy include leukoplakia (white plaque visible before applying acetic acid), acetowhite tissue (white epithelium after applying acetic acid), punctation (dilated capillaries occurring in a dotted or stippled pattern), mosaicism (a tile-like pattern), and atypical vascular patterns. If biopsy specimens show premalignant cells, the patient usually requires cryotherapy, laser therapy, or a cone biopsy (excision of an inverted tissue cone from the cervix).

Cryotherapy and Laser Therapy

Cryotherapy (freezing cervical tissue with nitrous oxide) and laser treatment are used in the outpatient setting. Cryotherapy may result in cramping and occasional feelings of faintness (vasovagal response). A watery discharge is normal for a few weeks after the procedure as the cervix heals; however, excessive bleeding, pain, or fever should be reported to the primary provider (Fischbach & Dunning, 2015).

Cone Biopsy and Loop Electrosurgical Excision Procedure

If endocervical curettage findings indicate abnormal changes or if the lesion extends into the canal, the patient may undergo a cone biopsy. This can be performed surgically or with a procedure called loop electrosurgical excision procedure (LEEP), which uses a laser beam (Fischbach & Dunning, 2015).

Usually performed in the outpatient setting, LEEP is associated with a high success rate in removal of abnormal cervical tissue. The gynecologist excises a small amount of cervical tissue, and the pathologist examines the borders of the specimen to determine if disease is present. A patient who has received anesthesia for a surgical cone biopsy is advised to rest for 24 hours after the procedure and to leave any vaginal packing in place until it is removed (usually the next day). The patient is instructed to report any excessive bleeding.

The primary provider provides guidelines regarding postoperative sexual activity, bathing, and other activities. Because open tissue may be potentially exposed to HIV and other pathogens, the patient is cautioned to avoid intercourse until healing is complete and verified at follow-up.

Endometrial (Aspiration) Biopsy

Endometrial biopsy, a method of obtaining endometrial tissue, is performed as an outpatient procedure. This procedure is usually indicated in cases of midlife irregular bleeding, postmenopausal bleeding, and irregular bleeding while taking hormone therapy (HT) or tamoxifen. A tissue sample obtained through biopsy permits diagnosis of cellular changes in the endometrium. The only absolute contraindication to an endometrial biopsy is the presence of a viable and desired pregnancy (Del Priore, 2015).

Women who undergo endometrial biopsy may experience slight discomfort. The examiner may apply a tenaculum (a clamplike instrument that stabilizes the uterus) after the pelvic examination and then inserts a thin, hollow, flexible suction tube through the cervix into the uterus.

Findings on aspiration may include normal endometrial tissue, hyperplasia, or endometrial cancer. Simple hyperplasia is an overgrowth of the uterine lining and is usually treated with progesterone. Complex hyperplasia, which refers to overgrowth of cells with abnormal features, is a risk factor for uterine cancer and is treated with progesterone and careful follow-up. Women who are overweight, who are older than 45 years of age, who have a history of nulliparity and infertility, or who have a family history of colon cancer seem to be at higher risk for hyperplasia. Endometrial cancer is discussed in Chapter 48.

Dilation and Curettage

D&C may be diagnostic (identifies the cause of irregular bleeding) or therapeutic (often temporarily stops irregular bleeding). The cervical canal is widened with a dilator, and the uterine endometrium is scraped with a curette. The purpose of the procedure is to secure endometrial or endocervical tissue for cytologic examination, to control abnormal uterine bleeding, and as a therapeutic measure for incomplete abortion.

Because D&C is usually carried out under anesthesia and requires surgical asepsis, it is usually performed in the operating room. However, it may take place in the outpatient setting with the patient receiving a local anesthetic supplemented with diazepam (Valium) or midazolam (Versed).

The nurse explains the procedure, preparation, and expectations regarding postoperative discomfort and bleeding. The patient is instructed to void before the procedure. The patient is placed in the lithotomy position, the cervix is dilated with a dilating instrument, and endometrial scrapings are obtained by a curette. A perineal pad is placed over the perineum after the procedure, and excessive bleeding is reported. No restrictions are placed on dietary intake. If pelvic discomfort or low back pain occurs, mild analgesics usually provide relief. The primary provider indicates when sexual intercourse may be safely resumed. To reduce the risk of infection and bleeding, most providers advise no vaginal penetration or use of tampons for 2 weeks.

Endoscopic Examinations

Laparoscopy (Pelvic Peritoneoscopy)

A laparoscopy involves inserting a laparoscope (a tube about 10 mm wide and similar to a small periscope) into the peritoneal cavity through a 2-cm (0.75-in) incision below the umbilicus to allow visualization of the pelvic structures

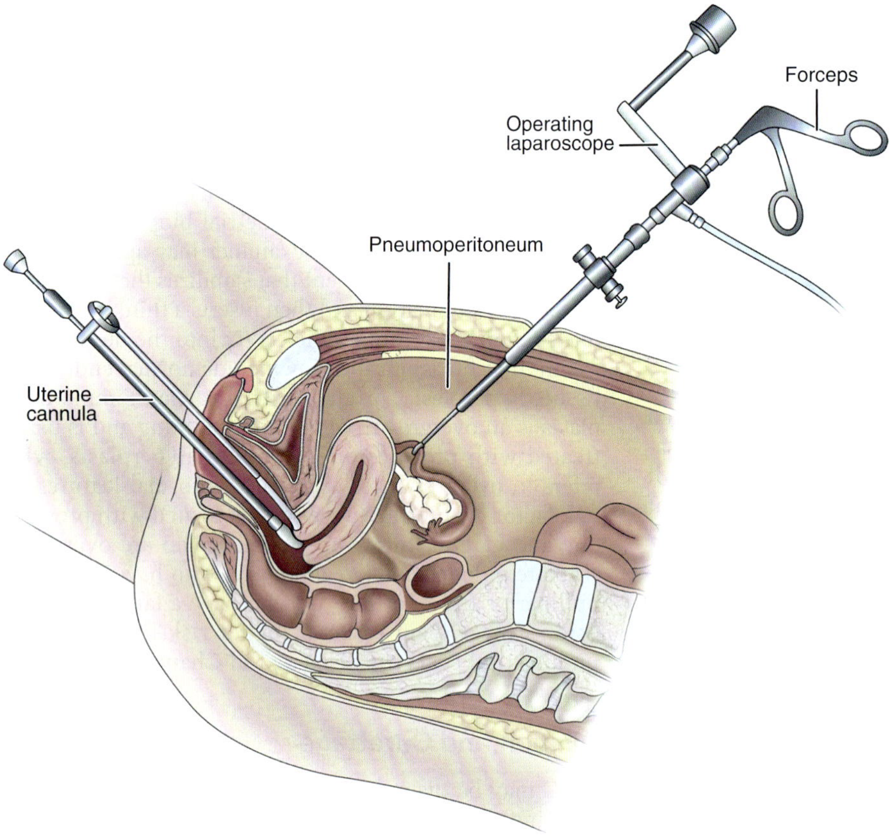

FIGURE 47-6. Laparoscopy. The laparoscope (*right*) is inserted through a small incision in the abdomen. A forceps is inserted through the scope to grasp the fallopian tube. To improve the view, a uterine cannula (*left*) is inserted into the vagina to push the uterus upward. Insufflation of gas creates an air pocket (pneumoperitoneum), and the pelvis is elevated (note the angle), which forces the intestines higher in the abdomen.

(Fig. 47-6). Laparoscopy may be used for diagnostic purposes (e.g., in cases of pelvic pain when no cause can be found) or treatment. Laparoscopy facilitates many surgical procedures, such as tubal ligation, ovarian biopsy, myomectomy, hysterectomy, and lysis of adhesions (scar tissue that can cause pelvic discomfort) (Sharp, 2016). A surgical instrument (intrauterine sound or cannula) may be positioned inside the uterus to permit manipulation or movement during laparoscopy, affording better visualization. The pelvic organs can be visualized after the injection of carbon dioxide intraperitoneally into the cavity. Called insufflation, this technique separates the intestines from the pelvic organs (Sharp, 2016). If a patient is undergoing sterilization, the fallopian tubes may be electrocoagulated, sutured, or ligated and a segment removed for histologic verification (clips are an alternative device for occluding the tubes).

After the laparoscopy is completed, the laparoscope is withdrawn, carbon dioxide is allowed to escape through the outer cannula, the small skin incision is closed with sutures or a clip, and the incision is covered with an adhesive bandage. The patient is carefully monitored for several hours to detect any untoward signs indicating bleeding (most commonly from vascular injury to the hypogastric vessels), bowel or bladder injury, or burns from the coagulator. These complications are rare, making laparoscopy a cost-effective and safe short-stay procedure. The patient may experience abdominal or shoulder pain related to the use of carbon dioxide gas.

Hysteroscopy

Hysteroscopy (transcervical intrauterine endoscopy) allows direct visualization of all parts of the uterine cavity by means of a lighted optical instrument. The procedure is best performed about 5 days after menstruation ceases, in the estrogenic phase of the menstrual cycle. The vagina and vulva are cleansed, and a paracervical anesthetic block is performed or lidocaine spray is used. The instrument used for the procedure, a hysteroscope, is passed into the cervical canal and advanced 1 or 2 cm under direct vision. Uterine-distending fluid (normal saline solution or 5% dextrose in water) is infused through the instrument to dilate the uterine cavity and enhance visibility. Hysteroscopy, which has few complications, is useful for evaluating endometrial pathology or for evaluating and treating retained products of conception (Bradley, 2016).

Hysteroscopy may be indicated as an adjunct to a D&C and laparoscopy in cases of infertility, unexplained bleeding, retained intrauterine device (IUD), and recurrent early pregnancy loss (Bradley, 2016). Treatment for some conditions (e.g., fibroid tumours) can be accomplished during this procedure, and sterilization may also be performed. Hysteroscopy is contraindicated in patients with cervical or endometrial carcinoma or acute pelvic inflammation.

An **endometrial ablation** (destruction of the uterine lining) procedure is performed with a hysteroscope and resector (cutting loop), roller ball (a barrel-shaped electrode), or laser beam in cases of severe bleeding not responsive to other therapies. Performed in an outpatient setting under general, regional, or local anesthesia, this rapid procedure is an alternative to hysterectomy for some patients. Following uterine distension with fluid infusion, the lining of the uterus is destroyed. Hemorrhage, perforation, and burns can occur.

Other Diagnostic Procedures

Many diagnostic procedures are helpful in evaluating pelvic conditions. These may include x-rays, barium enemas, gastrointestinal x-ray series, intravenous urography, and cystography studies. In addition, because the uterus, ovaries, and fallopian tubes are near the structures of the urinary tract, urologic diagnostic studies, such as x-ray study of the kidney, ureters, and bladder (KUB) and pyelography are used, as are angiography and radioisotope scanning, if needed. Other diagnostic procedures include hysterosalpingography (HSC) and computed tomography (CT) scanning.

Hysterosalpingography or Uterotubography

HSG is an x-ray study of the uterus and the fallopian tubes after injection of a contrast agent. The diagnostic procedure is performed to evaluate infertility or tubal patency and to detect any abnormal condition in the uterine cavity. Sometimes the procedure is therapeutic because the flowing contrast agent flushes debris or loosens adhesions.

Prior to HSG, laxatives and an enema may be administered to evacuate the intestinal tract so that gas shadows do not distort the x-ray findings. A mild sedative or an analgesic agent, such as ibuprofen (Advil, Motrin) may be prescribed. The patient is placed in the lithotomy position and the cervix is exposed with a bivalved speculum. A cannula is inserted into the cervix and the contrast agent is injected into the uterine cavity and the fallopian tubes. X-rays are taken to show the path and the distribution of the contrast agent.

Some patients experience nausea, vomiting, cramps, and faintness. After the test, the patient is advised to wear a perineal pad for several hours, because the radiopaque contrast agent may stain clothing.

Computed Tomography

CT scans has several advantages over ultrasonography, even though it involves radiation exposure and is more costly. It is more effective than ultrasonography for patients with obesity or for patients with a distended bowel. CT scans can also demonstrate a tumour and any extension into the retroperitoneal lymph nodes and skeletal tissue, although it has limited value in diagnosing other gynecologic abnormalities (Fischbach & Dunning, 2015).

Ultrasonography

Ultrasonography (or ultrasound) is a useful adjunct to the physical examination, particularly in patients receiving obstetrical care or in patients with abnormal pelvic examination findings. It is a simple procedure based on sound wave transmission that uses pulsed ultrasonic waves at frequencies exceeding 20,000 Hz by way of a transducer placed in contact with the abdomen (abdominal scan) or a vaginal probe (vaginal ultrasound). Mechanical energy is converted into electrical impulses, which in turn are amplified and recorded on an oscilloscope screen while a photograph or video recording of the patterns is taken. The entire procedure takes usually less than 15 to 30 minutes and involves no ionizing radiation and no discomfort other than a full bladder, which is necessary for good visualization during an abdominal scan. A vaginal ultrasound or sonogram does not require a full bladder; however, the vaginal probe can cause mild discomfort in some women.

Magnetic Resonance Imaging

Magnetic resonance imaging (MRI) produces patterns that are finer and more definitive than other imaging procedures, and it does not expose patients to radiation. However, MRI is more costly.

> **NURSING ALERT**
>
> **All metal devices, including medication skin patches with foil backing, must be removed before MRI is performed to avoid burns.**

MANAGEMENT OF FEMALE PHYSIOLOGIC PROCESSES

Many health concerns of women are related to normal changes or abnormalities of the menstrual cycle and may result from women's lack of understanding of the menstrual cycle, developmental changes, and factors that may affect the pattern of the menstrual cycle. Educating women about the menstrual cycle and changes over time is an important aspect of the nurse's role in providing quality care to women. Teaching should begin early, so that menstruation and the lifelong changes in the menstrual cycle can be anticipated and accepted as a normal part of life.

Menstruation

Menstruation, the sloughing and discharge of the lining of the uterus that takes place if conception does not occur, happens about every 28 days during the reproductive years, although normal cycles can vary from 25 to 35 days (Schuiling & Likis, 2013). The flow usually lasts 4 to 5 days, during which time 50 to 60 mL of blood are lost.

A perineal pad or tampon is generally used to absorb menstrual discharge. Tampons are used extensively. There is no significant evidence of untoward effects from their use, provided that there is no difficulty in inserting them. However, tampons should not be used for more than 4 to 6 hours, and lower absorbency tampons should be used to prevent toxic shock syndrome (Mayo Clinic, 2014). If a tampon is difficult to remove or shreds when removed, less absorbent tampons should be used. If the string breaks or retracts, the woman should squat in a comfortable position, insert one finger into the vagina, try to locate the tampon, and remove it. If she feels uncomfortable attempting this manoeuvre or cannot remove the tampon, she should consult a gynecologic health care provider promptly.

Psychosocial Considerations

Girls who are approaching **menarche** (the onset of menstruation) should be instructed about the normal process of the menstrual cycle before it occurs. Psychologically, it is much healthier and appropriate to refer to this event as a "period" rather than as "being sick." With adequate nutrition, rest, and exercise, most women feel little discomfort, although some report breast tenderness and a feeling of fullness 1 or 2 days before menstruation begins. Others report fatigue and some discomfort in the lower back, legs, and pelvis on the first day and temperament or mood changes. Slight deviations from a usual pattern of daily living are considered normal, but excessive deviation may require evaluation. Regular exercise and a healthy diet have been found to decrease discomfort for some women. Heating pads or nonsteroidal anti-inflammatory drugs (NSAIDs) may be very effective for cramps. For women with excessive cramping or dysmenorrhea, referral to a women's health care provider is appropriate; following evaluation, practitioners may prescribe oral contraceptive agents.

Cultural Considerations

Culture refers to knowledge, beliefs, customs, and values acquired as members of a racial, ethnic, religious, or social group. Canada is becoming more culturally diverse. Various aspects of culture affect many health care encounters, and these encounters can be positive if nurses understand the various cultures of their patients.

Cultural views and beliefs about menstruation differ. Some women believe that it is detrimental to change a pad or tampon too frequently; they think that allowing the discharge to accumulate increases the flow, which is considered desirable. Some women believe they are vulnerable to illness during menstruation. Others believe it is harmful to swim, shower, have their hair permed, have their teeth filled, or eat certain foods during menstruation. They may also avoid using contraception during menstruation.

In such situations, nurses are in a position to provide women with facts in an accepting and culturally sensitive manner. The objective is to be mindful of these unexpressed, deep-rooted beliefs and to provide the facts with care. Aspects of gynecologic problems cannot always be expressed easily. The nurse needs to convey confidence and openness and to offer facts to facilitate communication. Suggestions to improve care include overcoming language barriers, providing appropriate materials in the patient's language, asking about traditional beliefs and dietary practices, and asking about fears regarding care. Patience, sensitivity, and a desire to learn about other cultures and groups will enhance the nursing care of all women.

Menstrual Disorders

Menstrual disorders may include premenstrual syndrome (PMS); dysmenorrhea; amenorrhea; and excessive bleeding, irregular bleeding, or bleeding between cycles or unrelated to cycles. These disorders need to be discussed with a health care provider and managed individually.

Premenstrual Syndrome

PMS is a cluster of physical, emotional, and behavioural symptoms that are usually related to the luteal phase of the menstrual cycle. PMS is very common, affecting many women at some time in their lives (Tharpe, Farley, & Jordan, 2013) (see Chart 47-10).

CHART 47-10

Causes, Manifestations, and Treatment of Premenstrual Syndrome

Cause

- Unknown; may be related to hormonal changes combined with other factors (diet, stress, and lack of exercise)
- Many women have some symptoms related to menses, but premenstrual syndrome affects 75–95% of women at some point and is a complex of symptoms that result in dysfunction.

Physical Symptoms

- Fluid retention (e.g., bloating, breast tenderness)
- Headache
- Low back pain

Affective Symptoms

- Depression
- Anger
- Irritability
- Anxiety
- Confusion
- Withdrawal
- Symptoms begin in the 5 days preceding menses and relief occurs within 4 days of onset of menses. Dysfunction usually occurs in relationships, parenting, work, or school.

Treatment

- The use of social support and family resources.
- Nutritious diet consisting of whole grains, fruits, and vegetables; increased water intake may help.
- Selective serotonin reuptake inhibitors (SSRIs).
- Alprazolam (Xanax) has been effective but risk of physical and psychological dependence is high.
- Spironolactone, a diuretic, may be effective in treating fluid retention.
- Initiation/maintenance of exercise program.
- Stress reduction techniques.

Adapted from Hawkins, J. W., Roberto-Nichols, D. M., & Stanley-Haney, J. L. (2015). *Guidelines for nurse practitioners in gynecologic settings* (11th ed.). New York: Springer; Tharpe, N., Farley, C., & Jordan, R. (2013). *Clinical practice guidelines for midwifery & women's health*. Boston, MA: Jones & Bartlett.

Clinical Manifestations

Major symptoms of PMS include physical symptoms such as headache, fatigue, low back pain, painful breasts, and a feeling of abdominal fullness. Behavioural and emotional symptoms may include general irritability, mood swings, fear of losing control, binge eating, and crying spells. Symptoms vary widely from one woman to another and from one cycle to the next in the same woman. Great variability is found in the degree of symptoms. Many women are affected to some degree, but some are severely affected. Premenstrual dysphoric disorder (PMDD) is a severe form of PMS with significant severity of symptoms (Hawkins, Roberto-Nichols, & Stanley-Haney, 2015).

Medical Management

Because there is no single treatment or known cure for PMS, it is helpful for women to keep a record of their symptoms so they can anticipate and therefore cope with them. Regular exercise may be helpful. Although women have been advised to avoid caffeine, high-fat foods, and refined sugars, little research demonstrates the efficacy of dietary changes. Alternative therapies that have been used include vitamins B_6 (pyridoxine) and E, calcium, magnesium, and oil of evening primrose capsules (Hawkins et al., 2015).

Pharmacologic treatments include selective serotonin reuptake inhibitors (SSRIs) (e.g., fluoxetine [Prozac, Sarafem]), prostaglandin inhibitors (e.g., ibuprofen and naproxen [Anaprox, Aleve]), diuretics, antianxiety agents, and calcium supplements. Oral contraceptives containing drospirenone (a synthetic progestin) and extended regimens also may be effective (Tharpe et al., 2013).

Nursing Management

The nurse obtains a health history, noting the time when symptoms began and their nature and intensity. The nurse then determines whether symptoms occur before or shortly after the menstrual flow begins. In addition, the nurse can show the patient how to record the timing and intensity of symptoms. A nutritional history is also elicited to determine if the diet is high in salt, caffeine, or alcohol or low in essential nutrients.

The patient's goals may include reduction of anxiety, mood swings, crying, binge eating, fear of losing control, improved coping with day-to-day stressors, improved relationships with family and coworkers, and increased knowledge about PMS. Positive coping measures are promoted. This may involve encouraging the woman's partner to offer support and assistance with child care. The patient can try to plan her working time to accommodate the days she is less productive because of PMS. The nurse encourages the patient to use exercise, meditation, imagery, and creative activities to reduce stress. The nurse also encourages the patient to take medications as prescribed and provides instructions about the desired effects of the medications. Enrolling in a PMS group may help the patient learn to recognize and cope with this condition.

If the patient has severe symptoms of PMS or PMDD, the nurse assesses her for suicidal, uncontrollable, and violent behaviour. An immediate psychiatric evaluation is necessary for women with any suggestions of suicidal tendencies. In rare cases, uncontrollable behaviour may lead to violence toward family members. If abuse, maltreatment, or neglect of any member of a patient's family is suspected, it is important to implement and follow reporting protocols.

Dysmenorrhea

Primary dysmenorrhea is painful menstruation, with no identifiable pelvic pathology. It occurs at the time of menarche or shortly thereafter. It is characterized by crampy pain that begins before or shortly after the onset of menstrual flow and continues for 48 to 72 hours. Pelvic examination findings are normal. Dysmenorrhea is thought to result from excessive production of prostaglandins, which causes painful contraction of the uterus.

In secondary dysmenorrhea, pelvic pathology such as endometriosis, tumour, or pelvic inflammatory disease (PID) contributes to symptoms. Patients frequently have pain that occurs several days before menses, with ovulation, and occasionally with intercourse. It may be accompanied by nausea, diarrhea, dizziness, and backache (Hawkins et al., 2015).

Assessment and Diagnostic Findings

A pelvic examination is performed to rule out possible disorders, such as endometriosis, PID, adenomyosis, and uterine fibroids. A laparoscopy may be required to identify organic causes.

Management

In primary dysmenorrhea, the reason for the discomfort is explained, and the patient is assured that menstruation is a normal function of the reproductive system. If the patient is young and accompanied by her mother, the mother may also need reassurance. Many young women expect to have painful periods if their mothers did. The discomfort of cramps can be treated once anxiety and concern about its cause are dispelled by adequate explanation. Symptoms usually subside with appropriate medication. Useful medications include prostaglandin antagonists such as NSAIDs (e.g., ibuprofen [Motrin], naproxen [Anaprox], and mefenamic acid [Ponstel] or aspirin). If one medication does not provide relief, another may be recommended. Usually these medications are well tolerated, but some women experience gastrointestinal side effects. Contraindications include allergy, peptic ulcer history, sensitivity to aspirin-containing medications, asthma, and pregnancy. Low-dose oral contraceptives provide relief in more than 90% of patients and may be prescribed for women with dysmenorrhea who are sexually active but do not desire pregnancy (Hawkins et al., 2015).

Continuous low-level local heat may also be effective in relieving primary dysmenorrhea. Heat therapy and medication have been found to work well in combination. The patient is encouraged to continue her usual activities and to increase physical exercise if possible because this relieves discomfort for some women. Taking analgesic agents before cramps start, in anticipation of discomfort, is advised.

Management of secondary dysmenorrhea is directed at diagnosis and treatment of the underlying cause (e.g., endometriosis or PID).

Amenorrhea

Amenorrhea (absence of menstrual flow) is a symptom of a variety of disorders and dysfunctions. Primary amenorrhea (delayed menarche) refers to the situation in which a young woman who by age 15 years has not begun developing secondary sex characteristics or who by age 16 years or older has developed secondary sex characteristics but has not started menstruation (Welt & Barbieri, 2016). There are many reasons for primary amenorrhea, including genetic and anatomical disorders, Turner syndrome, anorexia, and polycystic ovarian syndrome (POS) (Welt & Barbieri, 2016).

The nurse encourages the patient to express her concerns and anxiety about this problem because the patient may feel that she is different from her peers. A complete physical examination, careful health history, and simple laboratory tests help rule out possible causes, such as metabolic or endocrine disorders and systemic diseases. Treatment is directed toward correcting any abnormalities.

Secondary amenorrhea (an absence of menses for three cycles or 6 months after a normal menarche) may be caused by functional hypothalamic amenorrhea, pituitary disease, primary ovarian failure, pregnancy, breastfeeding, menopause, too little body fat (about 22% required for menses), eating disorder, thyroid disease, or polycystic ovary syndrome (Welt & Barbieri, 2016). In adolescents, secondary amenorrhea can be caused by minor emotional upset related to being away from home, attending college, tension due to schoolwork, or interpersonal problems.

Secondary nutritional disturbances may also be factors. Obesity can result in anovulation and subsequent amenorrhea. Eating disorders, such as anorexia and bulimia, often result in lack of menses because the decrease in body fat and caloric intake affects hormonal function. Intense exercise can induce menstrual disturbances. Females who are competitive athletes often experience amenorrhea. Infrequent periods (oligomenorrhea) may be related to thyroid disorders, POS, or premature ovarian failure. Women who are HIV positive are apt to miss menstrual periods and need to be evaluated for pregnancy, thyroid disorders, hyperprolactinemia, and menopause.

Abnormal Uterine Bleeding

Dysfunctional uterine bleeding (DUB) is defined as irregular, painless bleeding of endometrial origin that may be excessive, prolonged, or without pattern. DUB can occur at any age but is most common at opposite ends of the reproductive lifespan. It is usually secondary to anovulation (lack of ovulation) and is common in adolescents and women approaching menopause.

Adolescents account for many cases of abnormal uterine bleeding; they often do not ovulate regularly as the pituitary–ovarian axis matures. Women who are perimenopausal also experience this condition because of irregular ovulation secondary to decreasing ovarian hormone production. Other causes may include fibroids, obesity, and hypothalamic dysfunction.

Abnormal or unusual vaginal bleeding that is atypical in time or amount must be evaluated because it could possibly be a manifestation of a major disorder. A physical examination is performed, and the patient is evaluated for conditions such as pregnancy, neoplasm, infection, anatomic abnormalities, endocrine disorders, trauma, blood dyscrasias, platelet dysfunction, and hypothalamic disorders.

Menorrhagia

Menorrhagia is prolonged or excessive bleeding at the time of the regular menstrual flow. In young women the cause is usually related to endocrine disturbance; in later life it usually results from inflammatory disturbances, tumours of the uterus, or hormonal imbalance.

Women with menorrhagia are urged to see a primary provider and to describe the amount of bleeding by pad count and saturation (i.e., absorbency of perineal pad or tampon and number saturated hourly). Persistent heavy bleeding can result in anemia. It can also be a sign of a bleeding disorder or a result of anticoagulant therapy. Treatment may involve endometrial ablation or hysterectomy.

Metrorrhagia

Metrorrhagia (vaginal bleeding between regular menstrual periods) is probably the most significant form of menstrual dysfunction because it may signal cancer, benign tumours of the uterus, or other gynecologic problems. This condition warrants prompt evaluation and treatment. Although bleeding between menstrual periods by women taking oral contraceptive agents is usually not serious, irregular bleeding by women taking HT should be evaluated.

Menometrorrhagia is heavy vaginal bleeding between and during periods. It, too, requires evaluation.

Postmenopausal Bleeding

Bleeding 1 year after menses cease at menopause must be investigated, and a malignant condition must be considered until proven otherwise. A vaginal ultrasound can be used to measure the thickness of the endometrial lining. The uterine lining in postmenopausal women should be thin because of low estrogen levels. A lining thicker than 5 mm usually warrants evaluation by endometrial biopsy or a D&C.

Dyspareunia

Dyspareunia (difficult or painful intercourse) can be superficial, deep, primary, or secondary and may occur at the beginning of, during, or after intercourse. Dyspareunia may be related to many factors, including injury during childbirth; lack of vaginal lubrication; a history of incest, sexual abuse, or assault; endometriosis; pelvic infection; vaginal dryness due to breastfeeding or menopause; gastrointestinal disorders; fibroids; urinary tract infection; STIs; or vulvodynia (vulvar pain that affects women of all ages without any discernible physical cause). Depending on the cause of dyspareunia, counselling, extra lubrication, or antidepressant medications may be prescribed (Schuiling & Likis, 2013). Women's health issues related to sexuality may be affected by many factors. Thus, these issues need to be taken seriously, carefully assessed, and treated.

Contraception

Each year, many pregnancies in Canada are unintended. Although unintended pregnancies occur in women of all ages, incomes, and racial and ethnic groups, the highest rates occur among adolescents and perimenopausal women. Adolescents are more likely to experience pregnancy complications and are more prone to have low–birth-weight babies. In addition, adolescent mothers are less likely to obtain a high school diploma and are more likely subsequently to live in poverty.

Women may fail to use effective methods of contraception consistently or at all. Of the women who undergo abortions, many were not using contraception when they became pregnant, and others have never used any method of contraception. Decreasing unwanted pregnancies may reduce the number of abortions, abused children, stressed families, and infant mortality and morbidity.

Nurses can assist with information and support. Women can be asked directly when they plan to have their next pregnancy and about their need for contraception. Many women who are sexually active or who are considering becoming sexually active can benefit from learning about contraception. Nurses who are involved in helping patients make contraceptive choices need to listen, take time to answer questions, and teach and assist patients in choosing the method they prefer. It is important for women to receive unbiased and nonjudgmental information, understand the benefits and risks of each method, learn about alternatives and how to use them, and receive positive reinforcement and acceptance of their choice. Some women have received misinformation (i.e., contraception causes cancer or weight gain).

Contraindications

Coexisting medical disorders may make contraception a complex issue. Contraception needs to be addressed individually in women with pre-existing conditions. With the aid of a thorough history, nurses are well positioned to aid patients in choosing the safest, most effective method of contraception to meet their individual needs. A valuable resource when counselling patients about contraceptive method choice is the SOGC Canadian Contraception Consensus (Black, Guilbert, Costescu, et al., 2015). These guidelines provide guidance on the safety of a contraceptive method for women with a wide variety of pre-existing conditions.

Abstinence

Abstinence, or celibacy, is the only completely effective means of preventing pregnancy. Abstinence may not be a desired or available option for many women because of cultural expectations and their own and their partner's values and sexual needs.

Sterilization

After abstinence, sterilization by bilateral tubal occlusion (female sterilization) or vasectomy (male sterilization) are the most effective means of contraception. Both procedures must be considered permanent because neither is easily reversible. Women and men who choose these methods should be certain that they no longer wish to have children.

Tubal Ligation

Sterilization by tubal ligation is one of the most common surgical procedures performed on women. Tubal ligation is usually performed as a same-day surgical procedure and is carried out by laparoscopy or hysteroscopy, with the patient receiving a general or local anesthetic. After the laparoscope is inserted, the fallopian tubes are visualized and may be coagulated, sutured (Pomeroy procedure), or ligated with silicone bands or a spring clip, thereby disrupting their patency.

Despite a very high rate of effectiveness, all women who have undergone tubal ligation but miss a period should be tested for pregnancy because ectopic and intrauterine pregnancies, although rare, may occur. Ovulation and menstruation are not affected by sterilization, although some women report heavier menstrual bleeding and more cramping after tubal ligation.

Before undergoing tubal ligation, the patient should be informed that an IUD, if present, will be removed. If the patient is taking oral contraceptives, she usually continues them up to the time of the procedure. If a laparoscopic procedure is performed, the patient may experience postoperative abdominal or shoulder discomfort for a few days, related to the carbon dioxide gas and the manipulation of organs. The patient is instructed to report heavy bleeding, fever, or pain that persists or increases. She should avoid intercourse, strenuous exercise, and lifting for 2 weeks. Risks associated with tubal ligation are minimal and are more often related to anesthesia than to the surgery itself. Risk is increased in women with diabetes, previous abdominal or pelvic surgery, or obesity.

Vasectomy

Vasectomy (male sterilization) and hysteroscopic/laparoscopic tubal ligation are compared in Table 47-4. See Chapter 50 for a discussion of vasectomy.

Hormonal Contraception

Various hormonal methods of birth control are approved by Health Canada. Hormonal contraceptive agents may be intrauterine, implantable, injectable, oral, transdermal, or intravaginal. These methods contain either a combination of estrogen and progestin or progestin-only. The combined methods include combination oral contraceptives, the transdermal patch, and the intravaginal ring. The progestin-only methods include the intrauterine system, the implant, the injectable, and the "mini" pill (Black et al., 2015).

NURSING ALERT

Patients need to be aware that hormonal contraceptives protect them from pregnancy but not from STIs or HIV infection. In addition, sex with multiple partners or sex without a condom may also result in chlamydial and other infections, including HIV infection.

Benefits and Risks

Benefits of combined hormonal contraceptive use include a reduction in the incidence of benign breast disease; improvement in acne; and reduced risk of uterine and ovarian cancers, anemia, and pelvic infection. In general, prolonged hormonal contraceptive use has resulted in no definite long-term undesirable effects, although there is an increased risk of gallbladder problems (e.g., cholestasis).

TABLE 47-4 Comparison of Sterilization Methods

Sterilization Method	Advantages	Disadvantages
Vasectomy	• Highly effective • Relieves female of contraceptive burden • Inexpensive in long run • Permanent • Highly acceptable procedure to most patients • Very safe • Quickly performed	• Expensive in short term • Serious long-term effects suggested (although currently unproved) • Permanent (although reversal is possible, it is expensive and requires highly technical and major surgery, and results cannot be guaranteed) • Regret in 5–10% of patients • No protection against STIs, including HIV • Not effective until sperm remaining in reproductive system are ejaculated
Hysteroscopic and laparoscopic tubal sterilization	• Low incidence of complications • Short recovery • Leaves small or no scar • Quickly performed	• Permanent • Reversal difficult and expensive • Sterilization procedures technically difficult • Requires surgeon, operating room (aseptic conditions), trained assistants, medications, surgical equipment (Essure [insertion of coil or spring in fallopian tubes] requires hysteroscopy rather than surgery) • Expensive at the time performed • If failure, high probability of ectopic pregnancy • No protection against STIs, including HIV

Resumption of normal menses is delayed 2 to 3 months or longer in about 20% of hormonal contraceptive users. Risks include venous thromboembolism, although its incidence has decreased because the estrogen concentrations used today are less than that used in early preparations. Venous thromboembolism is less than half as likely with hormonal contraceptives than with pregnancy. Fetal anomalies do not appear to be an issue, and normal reproductive tract function and fertility resume after hormonal contraceptive use is discontinued. However, most providers recommend that women who wish to become pregnant use a barrier contraceptive method for 1 to 2 months after stopping hormonal contraceptives before attempting to become pregnant to permit a normal period for accurate dating of the pregnancy.

A few patients experience adverse reactions when using hormonal contraceptives. These include nausea, depression, headache, leg cramps, and breast soreness. Usually, these symptoms subside after 3 or 4 months. Because such symptoms are sometimes related to sodium and water retention caused by estrogen, a smaller dose of the hormone or a different hormonal combination may alleviate the problem. Many patients experience spotting in the first month of use of hormonal contraceptive or if they use it irregularly, so they need to be reassured and advised to use it as prescribed. Chart 47-11 compares different oral contraceptive regimens, and Chart 47-12 describes the benefits and risks of oral contraceptive use.

Contraindications

Absolute contraindications to hormonal contraceptives include active thrombophlebitis, venous thromboembolic disorder, arterial thrombosis/ischemic heart disease migraines with focal neurologic signs, known or suspected breast cancer, known or suspected pregnancy, acute or chronic liver disease with increased liver enzyme levels or compromised liver function, smoking in women over

CHART 47-11

Patient Education: Using Contraceptives

The nurse provides education to enhance the chosen method of contraception.

The nurse instructs patients who have chosen male or female sterilization to:

- Use another contraceptive method for the first 3 months.
- Use condoms to protect against sexually transmitted infections.

The nurse instructs women who have chosen an injectable method to:

- Use condoms to protect against sexually transmitted infections.
- Obtain repeat injections on time.

The nurse instructs women who have chosen pills to:

- Use condoms to protect against sexually transmitted infections.
- Take the pill at exactly the same time every day.

The nurse instructs women who have chosen the patch to:

- Use condoms to protect against sexually transmitted infections.
- Change the patch once a week.

The nurse instructs women who have chosen a ring to:

- Use condoms to protect against sexually transmitted infections.
- Remove the vaginal ring after 3 weeks.

The nurse instructs women who have chosen a diaphragm to:

- Use correctly each time you have sex.

The nurse instructs women who have chosen condoms, a sponge, withdrawal, or spermicides to:

- Use correctly each time you have sex.

Adapted from Centers for Disease Control and Prevention (CDC). (2016). U.S. selected practice recommendations for contraceptive use, 2016. *Morbidity and Mortality Weekly Report*, *65*(4), 1–72.

CHART 47-12

Pharmacology: Benefits and Risks of Combination Hormonal Contraceptives

Benefits

- Decreased cramps and bleeding
- Regular bleeding cycle
- Decreased incidence of anemia
- Decrease in acne with some formulations
- Protection from uterine and ovarian cancer
- Decreased incidence of ectopic pregnancy
- Protection from benign breast disease
- Decreased incidence of pelvic infection

Risks

- Rare in healthy women
- Bothersome side effects (e.g., breakthrough bleeding, breast tenderness)
- Nausea, weight gain, mood changes
- Small increased risk of developing blood clots, stroke, or heart attack related more to smoking than to oral contraceptive use alone
- Possible increased incidence of benign liver tumours and gallbladder disorders
- No protection from STIs (possible increased risk with unsafe sex)

35 years; and undiagnosed genital bleeding (SexualityandU.ca, 2018).

Coexisting medical disorders may make contraception a complex issue. These disorders include chronic hypertension, lipid disorders, diabetes, migraines, fibroids, obesity, lupus, depression, seizures, and HIV infection or AIDS. Contraception needs to be addressed individually in women with these conditions.

Oral Hormonal Contraception

Oral contraceptives block ovarian stimulation by preventing the release of FSH from the anterior pituitary gland. In the absence of FSH, a follicle does not ripen, and ovulation does not occur. Progestins (synthetic forms of progesterone) suppress the LH surge, prevent ovulation, and also render the cervical mucus impenetrable to sperm.

Many women currently use oral contraceptive preparations of synthetic estrogens and progestins. A variety of formulations are available. Extended regimens of oral hormonal contraceptive agents are an option for women who have heavy or uncomfortable menstrual bleeding or who wish to have fewer periods. With the use of these regimens, women may have an increased occurrence of breakthrough bleeding; the blood may be dark brown rather than red. It may be more difficult to tell if a pregnancy occurs with this method, although pregnancy is unlikely if pills are taken as prescribed (CDC, 2016).

Transdermal Contraceptives

Ortho Evra is a thin, beige, matchbook-sized skin patch that releases an estrogen and a progestin continuously. It is changed every week for 3 weeks, and no patch is used during the fourth week, resulting in withdrawal bleeding. The effectiveness of Ortho Evra is comparable to that of oral contraceptives. Its risks are similar to those of oral contraceptives and include an increased risk of thromboembolic formation. The patch may be applied to the torso, chest, arms, or thighs; it should not be applied to the breasts. The patch is convenient and more easily remembered than a daily pill but is not as effective for women who weigh more than 90 kg (198 lb). In addition, it may also irritate skin conditions (e.g., psoriasis) in some women and results in higher blood estrogen levels than oral contraceptives. One additional side effect with the patch includes possible skin reaction such as irritation, redness, pigment changes, or rash at the site of the patch (CDC, 2016).

Vaginal Contraceptives

NuvaRing (etonogestrel/ethinyl estradiol vaginal ring) is a combination hormonal contraceptive that releases estrogen and progestin. It is inserted in the vagina for 3 weeks and then removed, resulting in withdrawal bleeding. It is as effective as oral contraceptives and results in lower hormone blood levels than oral contraceptives. NuvaRing is flexible, does not require sizing or fitting, and is effective when placed anywhere in the vagina. Patients are occasionally reluctant to consider vaginal methods of contraception unless discussed openly and as a convenient alternative to other routes of administration. Some women are uncomfortable with this method and may fear that the ring may migrate or be uncomfortable or be noticed by a partner. The patient can be informed that some women notice a slight increase in vaginal discharge (SexualityandU.ca, 2018). NuvaRing is usually more expensive than oral contraceptives.

Injectable Contraceptives

An intramuscular injection of Depo-Provera (a long-acting progestin) every 3 months inhibits ovulation and provides a reliable, private, and convenient contraceptive method (Black et al., 2015). A subcutaneous formulation is also available. It can be used by lactating women and those with hypertension, liver disease, migraine headaches, heart disease, and hemoglobinopathies. With continued use, women must be prepared for irregular bleeding episodes and spotting decrease, or amenorrhea.

Advantages of Depo-Provera include reduction of menorrhagia, dysmenorrhea, and anemia due to heavy menstrual bleeding. It may reduce the risk of pelvic infection, has been associated with improvement in hematologic status in women with sickle cell disease, and does not interfere with the efficacy of seizure agents. It decreases the risk of endometrial cancer, PID, endometriosis, and uterine fibroids (CDC, 2016).

Possible side effects of Depo-Provera include irregular menstrual bleeding, bloating, mood alteration, headaches, hair loss, decreased sex drive, bone loss, and weight loss or weight gain. The contraceptive does not protect against STIs. Fertility may be delayed when women discontinue this method; therefore, other methods of contraception may be more appropriate for the woman who wishes to conceive within a year of discontinuing contraception. Bone loss may occur while using the injection. When the injections are stopped, sometimes all of the bone loss is regained. Use of Depo-Provera should be limited to

2 years of use because of loss of bone mineral density (Comerford, 2015).

Depo-Provera is contraindicated in women who are pregnant and those who have abnormal vaginal bleeding of unknown cause, breast or pelvic cancer, or sensitivity to synthetic progestin.

Intrauterine Device

An IUD is a small plastic device, usually T-shaped, that is inserted into the uterine cavity to prevent pregnancy. A string attached to the IUD is visible and palpable at the cervical os. Two types of IUDs are the hormonal and nonhormonal. The hormonal IUD (also called an intrauterine system or IUS) releases progestin; a 3-year type and a 5-year are approved for use (Black et al., 2015). The nonhormonal IUD is effective for up to 10 years (Black et al., 2015).

Advantages include effectiveness over a long period of time, few if any systemic effects, and reduction of patient error. Almost all women are able to use an IUD. This reversible method of birth control is as effective as sterilization and more effective than barrier methods (Black et al., 2015).

Disadvantages include possible excessive bleeding, cramps, and backaches; a slight risk of tubal pregnancy; slight risk of pelvic infection on insertion; displacement of the device; and, rarely, perforation of the cervix and uterus. If a pregnancy occurs with an IUD in place, the device is removed immediately to avoid infection. Spontaneous abortion (miscarriage) may occur on removal (Black et al., 2015).

Implants

One type of single-rod subdermal implant, effective for 3 years, is approved for use in Canada and is usually placed inside the upper arm using a small incision (Black et al., 2015). It has been reported that 22% of etonogestrel implant users experienced amenorrhea and 34% experienced infrequent spotting, whereas 7% reported frequent bleeding (CDC, 2016). Women should be warned about possible discomforts that can be treated with NSAIDs. Heavy or prolonged bleeding should be evaluated for an underlying gynecologic problem, such as interactions with other medications, an STI pregnancy, or new pathologic uterine conditions (e.g., polyps or fibroids) (CDC, 2016).

Almost all women are able to use the implant, even those who are lactating. The implant is very convenient as once it is in place the patient does not have to do anything else to prevent pregnancy.

Mechanical Barriers

Diaphragm

The diaphragm is an effective contraceptive device that consists of a round, flexible spring (50 to 90 mm wide) covered with a domelike latex rubber cup. A spermicidal (contraceptive) jelly or cream is used to coat the concave side of the diaphragm before it is inserted deep into the vagina, covering the cervix completely. The spermicide inhibits spermatozoa from entering the cervical canal. The diaphragm is not felt by the user or her partner when properly fitted and inserted. Because women vary in size, the diaphragm must be sized and fitted by an experienced clinician. The woman is instructed in using and caring for the device. A return demonstration ensures that the woman can insert the diaphragm correctly and that it covers the cervix.

Each time the woman uses the diaphragm, she should examine it carefully. By holding it up to a bright light, she should ensure that it has no pinpoint holes, cracks, or tears; if any are present, the diaphragm should not be used. The woman then applies spermicidal jelly or cream and inserts the diaphragm. The diaphragm should remain in place at least 6 to 8 hours after coitus (no more than 12 hours). Additional spermicide is necessary if more than 6 hours have passed before intercourse occurs and before each act of repeated intercourse. On removal, the diaphragm should be cleansed thoroughly with mild soap and water, rinsed, and dried before being stored in its original container.

Disadvantages include allergic reactions in those who are sensitive to latex and an increased incidence of urinary tract infections. Toxic shock syndrome has been reported in some diaphragm users but is rare.

NURSING ALERT

The nurse must assess the woman for possible latex allergy because use of latex barrier methods (e.g., diaphragm, cervical cap, male condoms) may cause severe allergic reactions, including anaphylaxis, in patients with latex allergy.

Cervical Cap

The cervical cap is much smaller (22 to 35 mm) than the diaphragm and covers only the cervix. If a woman can feel her cervix, she can usually learn to use a cervical cap. The chief advantage is that the cap may be left in place for 2 days after coitus. Although convenient to use, the cervical cap may cause cervical irritation; therefore, before fitting a cap, most providers obtain a Pap smear and repeat the smear after 3 months. The cap is used with a spermicide and does not require additional spermicide for repeated intercourse.

Female Condom

The female condom was developed to give control of barrier protection to women—to provide them with protection from STIs and HIV as well as pregnancy. The female condom consists of a cylinder of polyurethane enclosed at one end by a closed ring that covers the cervix and at the other end by an open ring that covers the perineum (Fig. 47-7). Advantages include some degree of protection from STIs (HPV, herpes simplex virus, and HIV) (CDC, 2016). Disadvantages are that female condoms are more costly than male condoms and the inability to use the female condom with some positions (i.e., standing).

Spermicides

Spermicides are made from nonoxynol-9 or octoxynol and are available over the counter as foams, gels, films, and

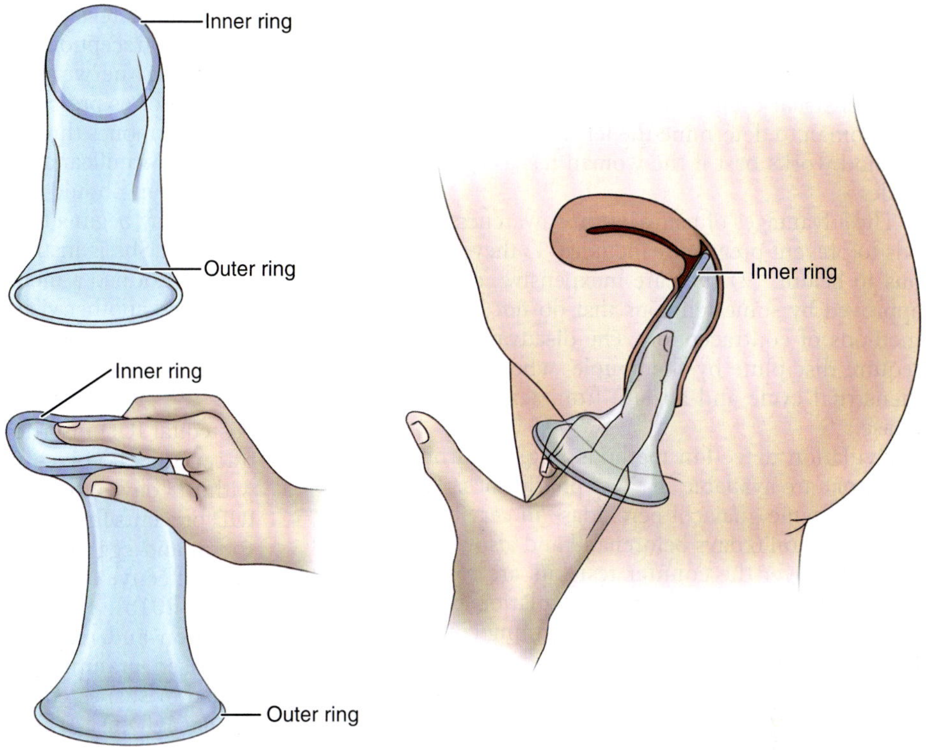

FIGURE 47-7. Female condom. To insert the female condom, hold the inner ring between the thumb and middle finger. Put the index finger on the pouch between the thumb and other fingers and squeeze the ring. Slide the condom into the vagina as far as it will go. The inner ring keeps the condom in place.

suppositories and also on condoms. Spermicides do not protect women from HIV or other STIs (Alan Guttmacher Institute, 2016; CDC, 2016). Advantages of spermicides include they are nonhormonal, are user controlled, do not cause systemic side effects, and are immediately effective (Alan Guttmacher Institute, 2016).

Male Condom

The male condom is an impermeable, snug-fitting cover applied to the erect penis before it enters the vaginal canal. The tip of the condom is pinched while being applied to leave space for ejaculate. If no space is left, ejaculation may cause a tear or hole in the condom and reduce its effectiveness. The penis, with the condom held in place, is removed from the vagina while still erect to prevent the ejaculate from leaking. Condoms are now available in large and small sizes.

The latex condom also creates a barrier against transmission of STDs (gonorrhea, chlamydial infection, and HIV) by body fluids and may reduce the risk of herpes virus transmission. However, natural condoms (those made from animal tissue) do not protect against HIV infection. Nurses need to reassure women that they have a right to insist that their male partners use condoms and a right to refuse sex without condoms, although women in abusive relationships may increase their risk of abuse by doing so. Some women carry condoms with them to be certain that one is available. Nurses should be familiar and comfortable with instructions about using condoms because many women need to know about this way of protecting themselves from HIV and other STIs. Condoms do not provide complete protection from STIs because HPV may be transmitted by skin-to-skin contact. Other STIs may be transmitted if any abraded skin is exposed to body fluids. This information should be included in patient education.

The nurse needs to consider the possibility of latex allergy. Swelling and itching can also occur. Possible warning signs of latex allergy include oral itching after blowing up a balloon or eating kiwis, bananas, pineapples, passion fruit, avocados, or chestnuts. Because many contraceptives are made of latex, patients who experience burning or itching while using latex contraceptives are instructed to see their primary provider. Alternatives to latex condoms include the female condom (Reality) and the male condom (Avanti), made of polyurethane.

Coitus Interruptus or Withdrawal

Coitus interruptus (removing the penis from the vagina before ejaculation) requires careful control by the male partner. Although it is a frequently used method of preventing pregnancy and better than no method, it is considered an unreliable method of contraception.

Fertility Awareness–Based Methods

Fertility awareness is knowing and recognizing when the fertile time occurs in the menstrual cycle. If a couple is practicing fertility awareness as a birth control method to prevent pregnancy, the couple needs to avoid having intercourse or use a barrier method during the fertile period. If the woman would like to get pregnant, the couple should have intercourse during the women's fertile days. When used to prevent pregnancy, during the first year of typical use, up to 18 women out of 100 will become pregnant (CDC, 2016).

The most common fertility awareness–based method is the Standard Days method. With this method, users must avoid unprotected sexual intercourse on days 8 to 19 of the menstrual cycle. The Standard Days method requires the woman to determine the fertile days of her cycle. This method works best if the woman has a regular menstrual cycle.

The advantages of using fertility awareness–based methods to prevent pregnancy include: (1) they are not hazardous to health, (2) they are inexpensive, and (3) they are approved by some religions that do not approve of other methods of contraception. The disadvantage is that they require discipline by the couple, who must monitor the menstrual cycle and abstain from sex during the fertile phase.

Ovulation detection methods (e.g., Clearblue Fertility Monitor) are available in most pharmacies. The presence of the enzyme guaiacol peroxidase in cervical mucus signals ovulation 6 days beforehand and also affects mucosal viscosity. Over-the-counter test kits are easy to use and reliable but can be expensive. Ovulation prediction kits and apps are more effective for planning conception than for avoiding it.

Emergency Contraception

Emergency contraception are methods that can be used by women after unprotected sexual intercourse to prevent pregnancy (Black et al., 2015). Nurses need to be aware of emergency contraception as an option for women and the indications for its use. It is clearly not suitable for long-term avoidance of pregnancy because it is not as effective as oral contraceptives or other reliable methods used regularly. However, it is valuable following intercourse when a pregnancy is not intended and in emergency situations such as sexual assault, a defective or torn condom or diaphragm, or other situations that may result in unintended conception.

Methods of Emergency Contraception

Emergency Contraceptive Pills

Three kinds of emergency contraceptive pills are available in Canada. A properly timed, adequate dose of estrogen and a progestin or progestin-only medication after intercourse without effective contraception, or when a method has failed, can prevent pregnancy by inhibiting or delaying ovulation.

Emergency contraception is considered safe and effective by the Canada Food and Drug Act and can be prescribed or purchased as Plan B (progestin only) packages of emergency contraception. It can also be prescribed as a specific number of contraceptive pills, depending on the medication and dose used.

Nausea, a common side effect, can be minimized by taking the medication with meals and with an antiemetic agent. Other side effects, such as breast soreness and irregular bleeding, may occur but are transient. Patients who use this method should be advised of the potential failure rate and also counselled about other contraceptive methods. There are no known contraindications to the use of this method, except an established pregnancy (CDC, 2016).

The nurse reviews with the patient instructions for emergency contraception based on the medication regimen prescribed. If the woman is breastfeeding, a progestin-only formulation is prescribed. To avoid exposing infants to synthetic hormones through breast milk, the patient can manually express milk and bottle feed for 24 hours after treatment. The patient should be informed that her next menstrual period may begin a few days earlier or a few days later than expected. She is instructed to return for a pregnancy test if she has not had a menstrual period in 3 weeks and should be offered another visit to provide a regular method of contraception if she does not have one currently.

Postcoital Intrauterine Device Insertion

Postcoital IUD insertion, another form of emergency contraception, involves insertion of a copper-bearing IUD within 5 days of coitus (CDC, 2016). The copper-bearing IUD prevents fertilization by causing a chemical change in sperm and egg before they can meet. This method is the most effective form of emergency contraception available (CDC, 2016). The patient may experience discomfort on insertion and may have heavier menstrual periods and increased cramping. Contraindications include a confirmed or suspected pregnancy or any contraindication to regular IUD use. The patient must be informed that there is a risk that insertion of an IUD may disrupt a pregnancy that is already present.

Nursing Management

Patients who use emergency contraception may be anxious, embarrassed, and lacking information about birth control. The nurse must be supportive and nonjudgmental and provide facts and appropriate patient teaching. If the patient repeatedly uses this method of birth control, she should be informed that the failure rate with this method is higher than with a regularly used method. Nurses can educate and inform women about emergency contraception options to reduce unwanted pregnancies and abortions. See the resources section at the end of this chapter for more information.

Abortion

Interruption of pregnancy or expulsion of the product of conception before the fetus is viable is called abortion. The fetus is generally considered to be viable any time after the 5th to 6th month of gestation.

Spontaneous Abortion

It is estimated that 1 of every 5 to 10 conceptions ends in spontaneous abortion. Most of these occur because an abnormality in the fetus makes survival impossible. Other causes may include systemic diseases, hormonal imbalance, or anatomic abnormalities. If a woman who is pregnant experiences bleeding and cramping, a threatened abortion is diagnosed because an actual abortion is usually imminent. Spontaneous abortion occurs most commonly in the 2nd or 3rd month of gestation.

There are various types of spontaneous abortion, depending on the nature of the process (threatened, inevitable, incomplete, or complete). In a threatened abortion, the cervix does not dilate. With bed rest and conservative treatment, the abortion may be prevented. If not, an abortion is imminent. If only some of the tissue is passed, the abortion is referred to as incomplete. An emptying or evacuation procedure (D&C, or dilation and evacuation [D&E]) or administration of oral misoprostol (Cytotec) is usually required to remove the remaining tissue. If the fetus and all related tissue are spontaneously evacuated, the abortion is termed complete, and no further treatment is required.

Habitual Abortion

Habitual or recurrent abortion is defined as successive, repeated, spontaneous abortions of unknown cause. As many as 60% of abortions may result from chromosomal anomalies. After two consecutive abortions, the patient is referred for genetic counselling and testing and other possible causes are explored.

If bleeding occurs in a woman who is pregnant with a past history of habitual abortion, conservative measures, such as bed rest and administration of progesterone to support the endometrium, are attempted to save the pregnancy. Supportive counselling is crucial in this stressful condition. Bed rest, sexual abstinence, a light diet, and no straining on defecation may be recommended in an effort to prevent spontaneous abortion. If infection is suspected, antibiotics may be prescribed.

In the condition known as incompetent or dysfunctional cervix, the cervix dilates painlessly in the second trimester of pregnancy, often resulting in a spontaneous abortion. In such cases, a surgical procedure called cervical cerclage may be used to prevent the cervix from dilating prematurely. It involves placing a purse-string suture around the cervix at the level of the internal os. Bed rest is usually advised to keep the weight of the uterus off the cervix. About 2 to 3 weeks before term or at the onset of labour, the suture is cut.

Medical Management

After a spontaneous abortion, all tissue passed vaginally is saved for examination. The patient and all personnel who care for her are alerted to save any discharged material. In the rare case of heavy bleeding, the patient may require blood component transfusions and fluid replacement. An estimate of the bleeding volume can be determined by recording the number of perineal pads and the degree of saturation over 24 hours. When an incomplete abortion occurs, oxytocin may be prescribed to cause uterine contractions before D&E or uterine suctioning.

Nursing Management

Because patients experience loss and anxiety, emotional support and understanding are important aspects of nursing care. Women may be grieving or relieved, depending on their feelings about the pregnancy. Providing opportunities for the patient to talk and express her emotions is helpful and also provides clues for the nurse in planning more specific care.

Induced Abortion

A voluntary-induced termination of pregnancy is performed by skilled health care providers. Decisions about abortion reside with a woman and her primary provider in the first trimester. During the second trimester, the province may regulate practice in the interest of a woman's health, and during the final weeks of pregnancy may choose to protect the life of the fetus, except when necessary to preserve the life or health of the woman.

Medical Management

Before the abortion procedure is performed (Chart 47-13), a nurse or counsellor trained in pregnancy counselling should talk with the patient and explore her fears, feelings, and options. The nurse then identifies the patient's choice (i.e., continuing pregnancy and parenthood; continuing pregnancy followed by adoption; or terminating pregnancy by abortion). If abortion is chosen, the patient has a pelvic examination to determine uterine size. A pelvic ultrasound may also be performed. Laboratory studies before an abortion must include a pregnancy test to confirm the pregnancy, hematocrit to rule out anemia, and Rh determination. Patients with anemia may need an iron supplement, and patients who are Rh-negative may require Rho(D) immune globulin (RhoGAM) to prevent isoimmunization. Before the procedure, all patients should be screened for STIs to prevent introducing pathogens upward through the cervix during the procedure.

NURSING ALERT

Women who have resorted to unskilled attempts to end a pregnancy are often critically ill because of infection, hemorrhage, or uterine rupture. If a woman has undergone such efforts to end a pregnancy, prompt medical attention, broad-spectrum antibiotics, and replacement of fluids and blood components may be required before careful attempts are made to evacuate the uterus.

Surgical terminations include D&C or vacuum aspiration of uterine contents. Medications can also be used. Mifepristone (Mifeprex), formerly known as RU-486, is used only in early pregnancy (up to 49 days from the last menstrual period). It works by blocking progesterone. Cramping and bleeding similar to a heavy menstrual period occur. After counselling and consent and often a sonogram to confirm the pregnancy, mifepristone is given. This is followed by a dose of misoprostol orally or vaginally. If the pregnancy persists, a suction aspiration is performed. Contraindications include ectopic pregnancy, adrenal failure, allergy to the medications, bleeding disorder, irritable bowel syndrome, or uncontrolled seizure disorders. Several deaths from sepsis have occurred following medical abortion; researchers and governmental agencies are closely monitoring the morbidity and mortality associated with medical abortion. Medical and surgical abortions used in the first trimester are both highly effective with low complication rates (Ireland, Geffen, & Chen, 2015).

CHART 47-13

Types of Elective Abortions

Vacuum Aspiration

- The cervix is dilated manually with instrumentation or by laminaria (small suppositories made of seaweed that swells as it absorbs water).
- A uterine aspirator is introduced.
- Suction is applied, and tissue is removed from the uterus.

This is the most common type of termination procedure and is used early in pregnancy, up to 14 weeks. Laminaria may be used to soften and dilate the cervix prior to the procedure.

Dilation and Evacuation

Cervical dilation with laminaria followed by vacuum aspiration

Labour Induction

These procedures account for less than 1% of all terminations and generally take place in an inpatient setting.

1. Installation of saline or urea results in uterine contractions
   - Although rare, serious complications can occur, including cardiovascular collapse, cerebral edema, pulmonary edema, renal failure, and disseminated intravascular coagulopathy (DIC).
2. Prostaglandins
   - Prostaglandins are introduced into the amniotic fluid or by vaginal suppository or intramuscular injection in later pregnancy.
   - Strong uterine contractions begin within 4 hours and usually result in abortion.
   - Gastrointestinal side effects (e.g., nausea, vomiting, diarrhea, and abdominal cramping) and fever can occur.
3. IV oxytocin
   Used for later abortions for genetic indications. Requires patient to go through labour.

Medical Abortion

METHOTREXATE

- Methotrexate has also been used to terminate pregnancy because it is a teratogen that is lethal to the fetus. It has been found to have minimal risk and few side effects in the woman. Its low cost may provide an alternative for some women.

MISOPROSTOL

- Misoprostol is a synthetic prostaglandin analog that produces cervical effacement and uterine contractions.
- Inserted vaginally, misoprostol is effective in terminating a pregnancy in about 75% of cases.
- When combined with methotrexate, misoprostol's effectiveness rate is high.

Nursing Management

Patient teaching is an important aspect of care for women who elect to terminate a pregnancy. A patient undergoing elective abortion is informed about what the procedure entails and the expected course after the procedure. The patient is scheduled for a follow-up appointment 2 weeks after the procedure and is instructed about signs and symptoms (i.e., fever, heavy bleeding, or pain) that should be reported.

Available contraceptive methods are reviewed with the patient at this time. Effectiveness depends on the method used and the extent to which the woman and her partner follow the instructions for use. A woman who has used any method of birth control should be assessed for her understanding of the method and its potential side effects as well as her satisfaction with the method. If the woman has not been using contraception, the nurse explains all methods and their benefits and risks and helps the patient make a contraceptive choice for use after abortion. Related teaching issues, such as the need to use barrier contraceptive devices (i.e., condoms) for protection against transmission of STIs and HIV infection and the availability of emergency contraception, are becoming increasingly important.

Psychological support is another important aspect of nursing care. The nurse needs to be aware that women terminate pregnancies for many reasons. Some women terminate pregnancies because of severe genetic defects. Women who have been raped or impregnated in incestuous relationships or by an abusive partner may elect to terminate their pregnancies. The care of a woman undergoing termination of pregnancy is stressful, and assistance needs to be provided in a safe and nonjudgmental way. Nurses have the right to refuse to participate in a procedure that is against their religious beliefs but are professionally obligated not to impose their beliefs or judgments on their patients.

Infertility

Infertility is defined as a couple's inability to achieve pregnancy after 1 year of unprotected intercourse (Tarin, Garci-Perez, Hamatani, et al., 2015). Primary infertility refers to a couple who has never had a child. Secondary infertility means that at least one conception has occurred, but currently the couple cannot achieve a pregnancy. In Canada, infertility affects 6 million couples. It is often a complex physical problem, and its causes are usually related to azoospermia, anovulation, or tubal obstruction.

Diagnostic Findings

Ovarian and Ovulation Factors

Diagnostic studies performed to determine if ovulation is regular and whether the progestational endometrium is adequate for implantation may include a serum progesterone level and an ovulation index. The ovulation index involves a urine dipstick test to determine whether the surge in LH that precedes follicular rupture has occurred.

Tubal and Uterine Factors

HSG is used to rule out uterine or tubal abnormalities. A contrast agent injected into the uterus through the cervix produces an outline of the shape of the uterine cavity and the patency of the tubes. This process sometimes removes mucus or tissue that is lodged in the tubes. Laparoscopy permits direct visualization of the tubes and other pelvic structures and can assist in identifying conditions that may interfere with fertility (e.g., endometriosis).

Fibroids, polyps, and congenital malformations are possible causative factors affecting the uterus. Their presence may be determined by pelvic examination, hysteroscopy, saline sonogram (a variation of a sonogram), and HSG. Endometriosis, even if mild, is associated with reduced fertility (Schuiling & Likis, 2013).

Male Factors

An analysis of semen provides information about the number of sperm (density), percentage of moving forms, quality of forward movement (forward progression), and morphology (shape and form). From 2 to 6 mL of watery alkaline semen is normal. A normal count has 60 to 100 million sperm/mL. However, the incidence of impregnation is lessened only when the count decreases to less than 20 million sperm/mL.

Men may also be affected by varicoceles, varicose veins around the testicle, which decrease semen quality by increasing testicular temperature. Retrograde ejaculation or ejaculation into the bladder is assessed by urinalysis after ejaculation. Blood tests for male partners may include measuring testosterone; FSH and LH (both of which are involved in maintaining testicular function); and prolactin levels.

Medical Management

The treatment of infertility is complex and often requires advanced technology. The specific type of treatment depends on the cause of the problem, if it can be identified. Many infertile couples have normal test results for ovulation, sperm production, and fallopian tube patency.

Ovulatory dysfunction is complex, but many women with ovulation disorders have polycystic ovary syndrome and may be treated with 5 days of clomiphene (Clomid) to induce ovulation (Comerford, 2015). Insulin sensitizing agents are sometimes used, and once insulin levels are normalized, ovulation often occurs. Some women have high prolactin levels, which inhibit ovulation, and they are treated with dopaminergic drugs after a pituitary adenoma is ruled out by MRI. If a woman has premature ovarian failure, oocyte donation may be considered.

Pharmacologic Therapy

Pharmacologically induced ovulation is undertaken when women do not ovulate on their own or ovulate irregularly. These couples are often treated with clomiphene to stimulate ovulation. Gonadotropin treatment may also be used if conception does not occur. Various other medications are used, depending on the primary cause of infertility (Chart 47-14).

CHART 47-14

Pharmacology: Medications That Induce Ovulation

- Clomiphene citrate (Clomid, Serophene) is an estrogen antagonist that increases gonadotropin release, resulting in follicular rupture or ovulation. Clomiphene is used when the hypothalamus is not stimulating the pituitary gland to release follicle-stimulating hormone (FSH) and luteinizing hormone (LH). This medication stimulates follicles in the ovary. It is usually taken for 5 days beginning on the 5th day of the menstrual cycle. Ovulation should occur 4–8 days after the last dose. Patients receive instructions about timing intercourse to facilitate fertilization.
- Menotropins (Repronex, Pergonal), a combination of FSH and LH, may be used to stimulate the ovaries to produce eggs. These agents are used for women with deficiencies in FSH and LH. When followed by administration of human chorionic gonadotropin, menotropins stimulates the ovaries, so monitoring by ultrasound and hormone levels is essential because overstimulation may occur.
- Follitropin-alpha (Gonal-F), follitropin-beta (Follistim), and urofollitropin (Bravelle) may be used to treat ovulation disorders or to stimulate a follicle and egg production for intrauterine insemination or in vitro fertilization or other assisted reproductive technologies.
- Gonadotropin-releasing hormone agonists (leuprolide [Lupron, Synarel]) suppress FSH, prevent premature egg release, and shrink fibroids.
- Bromocriptine (Parlodel) may be used in treatment of infertility due to elevated prolactin levels.
- Progesterone (Prometrium Crinone, progesterone in oil) vaginal suppositories help improve the uterine lining after ovulation.
- Urofollitropin (Metrodin, Bravelle), which contains FSH with a small amount of LH, is used in some disorders (e.g., polycystic ovarian syndrome) to stimulate follicle growth. Clomiphene is then used to stimulate ovulation.
- Chorionic gonadotropin (Ovidrel, Novarel, Pregnyl), which mimics LH, releases an egg after hyperstimulation and supports the corpus luteum.
- Metformin (Glucophage, Fortamet) may be used in polycystic ovarian syndrome to induce regular ovulation.
- Aspirin and heparin may be used to prevent recurrent pregnancy loss in patients with elevated antiphospholipid antibodies.

Adapted from Comerford, K. C. (2015). *Nursing2015 drug handbook*. Philadelphia, PA: Wolters Kluwer.

Blood tests and ultrasounds are used to monitor ovulation. Multiple pregnancies (i.e., twins, triplets, or more) may occur with use of these medications. Ovarian hyperstimulation syndrome (OHSS) may also occur. This condition is characterized by enlarged multicystic ovaries and is complicated by a shift of fluid from the intravascular space into the abdominal cavity. The fluid shift can result in ascites, pleural effusion, and edema; hypovolemia may also occur. Risk factors include younger age, history of POS, high serum estradiol levels, a larger number of follicles, and pregnancy.

Artificial Insemination

Artificial insemination is the deposit of semen into the female genital tract by artificial means. If the sperm cannot penetrate the cervical canal normally, artificial insemination using a partner's or husband's semen or that of a donor may be considered. When the sperm of the woman's partner is defective or absent (azoospermia) or when there is a risk of transmitting a genetic disease, donor sperm may be used. Safeguards are put in place to address legal, ethical, emotional, and religious issues. Written consent is obtained to protect all parties involved, including the woman, the donor, and the resulting child. The donor's semen is frozen, and the donor is evaluated to ensure that he is free of genetic disorders and STIs, including HIV infection (Ginsburg & Srouji, 2016).

Certain conditions must be optimal before semen is transferred to the vagina or uterus. The woman must have no abnormalities of the genital system, the fallopian tubes must be patent, and ova must be available. In the male, sperm need to be normal in shape, amount, motility, and endurance. The time of ovulation should be determined as accurately as possible so that the 2 or 3 days during which fertilization is possible each month can be targeted for treatment.

Ultrasonography and blood studies of varying hormone levels are used to pinpoint the best time for insemination and to monitor for OHSS. Fertilization seldom occurs from a single insemination. Usually, insemination is attempted between days 10 and 17 of the cycle; three different attempts may be made during one cycle. The woman may have received clomiphene or other medications to stimulate ovulation before insemination. The recipient is placed in the lithotomy position on the examination table, a speculum is inserted, and the vagina and cervix are swabbed with a cotton-tipped applicator to remove any excess secretions. The sperm are washed before insertion to remove biochemicals and to select the most active sperm. Semen is drawn into a sterile syringe, and a cannula is attached. The semen is then directed to the external os. In IUI, semen is placed into the uterine cavity.

Assisted Reproductive Technologies

Assisted reproductive technologies include in vitro fertilization (IVF) and its modifications. Currently, between 1% and 3% of all live births each year in the United States are achieved through assisted technology (Paulson, 2016).

IVF refers to a set of procedures that, if successful, results in a pregnancy. These procedures involve ovarian stimulation, egg retrieval, fertilization, and embryo transfer. The ovaries are stimulated to produce multiple eggs or ova, usually with medications, because success rates are greater with more than one embryo. Many different protocols exist for inducing ovulation with one or more agents. Patients are carefully selected and evaluated, and cycles are carefully monitored using ultrasound and monitoring hormone levels. At the appropriate time, the ova are recovered by transvaginal ultrasound retrieval. Sperm and eggs are co-incubated for up to 36 hours, and the embryos are transferred about 48 hours after retrieval. Implantation should occur in 3 to 5 days.

Gamete intrafallopian transfer (GIFT), a variation of IVF, is the treatment of choice for patients with ovarian failure. GIFT is considered in unexplained infertility and when there is religion-based discomfort with IVF. The most common indications for IVF and GIFT are irreparable tubal damage, endometriosis, unexplained infertility, inadequate sperm, and exposure to DES. Success rates for GIFT are similar to those for IVF (Paulson, 2016).

Other Assisted Reproductive Technologies

In intracytoplasmic sperm injection (ICSI), an ovum is retrieved and a single sperm is injected through the zona pellucida, through the egg membrane, and into the cytoplasm of the oocyte. The fertilized egg is then transferred back to the donor. ICSI is the treatment of choice in severe male factor infertility.

Women who cannot produce their own eggs (i.e., premature ovarian failure) have the option of using the eggs of a donor after stimulation of the donor's ovaries. The recipient also receives hormones in preparation for these procedures. Couples may also choose this modality if the female partner has a genetic disorder that may be passed on to children.

Tubal embryo transfer (TET) involves the placement of fertilized eggs or embryos into the fallopian tube. A laparoscopic procedure is needed to place the embryos in the fallopian tubes. Some women choose TET after IVF failure (Paulson, 2016).

Nursing Management

Nursing interventions when working with couples during infertility evaluations include assisting in reducing stress in the relationship, encouraging cooperation, protecting privacy, fostering understanding, and referring the couple to appropriate resources when necessary. Because infertility evaluations and treatments are expensive, time-consuming, invasive, stressful, and not always successful, couples need support in working together to deal with this process.

The Infertility Awareness Association of Canada (IAAC) a nonprofit self-help group that provides information and support for infertile patients, was founded by a group of volunteers in Ottawa. The literature on infertility that is produced by this group is an important resource for patients and professionals. Most areas of the country have local support groups. More information can be obtained by visiting the web site or contacting the Infertility Awareness Association of Canada.

Smoking cessation is strongly encouraged because smoking has an adverse effect on the success of assisted reproduction. Diet, exercise, stress reduction techniques, folic acid supplementation, health maintenance, and disease prevention are emphasized in many infertility programs. Couples may also consider adoption, child-free living, and gestational carriers (the use of a surrogate to carry the fetus for the infertile couple). Nurses can be helpful listeners and information resources in these deliberations.

Preconception/Periconception Health Care

Nurses can be instrumental in encouraging all women of childbearing age, including those with chronic illness or disabilities, to consider issues that may affect health during pregnancy (Smeltzer et al., 2016). Preconception health care is a concept that expands on the definition of prenatal care to include the time before conception (Waggoner, 2013). Women who plan their pregnancies and are healthy and well informed tend to have better outcomes. There are currently nine consensus recommendations for advancing preconception health (see Chart 47-15).

CHART 47-15

Preconception Wellness Strategies

Nurses can help advance pre- and periconception care of women by establishing the following:

- Pregnancy intention
- Access to care
- Preconception multivitamin with folic acid
- Tobacco avoidance
- Absence of uncontrolled depression
- Healthy weight
- Absence of sexually transmitted infections
- Optimal glycemic control in women with pregestational diabetes
- Teratogenic medication avoidance

Adapted from Frayne, D., Verbiest, S., Chelmow, D., et al. (2016). Health care system measures to advance preconception wellness: Consensus recommendations of the clinical workgroup of the national preconception health and health care initiative. *Obstetrics & Gynecology*, *127*(5), 863–872.

Nurses can make a difference in preconception health through education and counselling. Women who use tobacco products should be encouraged to stop smoking, and it may help to offer smoking cessation classes. Women should take folic acid supplements to prevent neural tube defects. Women with diabetes should have good glycemic control prior to conception. It is necessary to assess rubella immunity and other immunizations as well as a family history of genetic defects; genetic counselling may be appropriate. Women taking teratogenic medications and women concerned about genetic disorders should be encouraged to discuss effective contraception and childbearing plans with their primary provider (see Chart 47-3).

Ectopic Pregnancy

The incidence of ectopic pregnancy and the risk of death due to ectopic pregnancy are decreasing. However, ectopic pregnancy remains the leading cause of pregnancy-related death in the first trimester (Hannon & Porth, 2016). Ectopic pregnancy occurs when a fertilized ovum (a blastocyst) becomes implanted on any tissue other than the uterine lining. The most common site of ectopic implantation is the fallopian tube (Hannon & Porth, 2016) (Fig. 47-8).

Possible causes of ectopic pregnancy include salpingitis, peritubal adhesions (after pelvic infection, endometriosis, appendicitis), structural abnormalities of the fallopian tube, previous ectopic pregnancy, previous tubal surgery, multiple previous induced abortions and tumours that distort the tube (Hannon & Porth, 2016). Additional risk factors include smoking, IUD use, history of PID, and use of fertility drugs to induce ovulation (Hannon & Porth, 2016).

Risk factors are important, but all women need to be educated about early treatment and have a high index of suspicion in the case of a period that does not seem normal, the presence of pain, or pain with a suspected pregnancy. Women may have fatal hemorrhage with ruptured ectopic pregnancies if they delay seeking attention or if their health care providers are not alert to the possibility of this diagnosis.

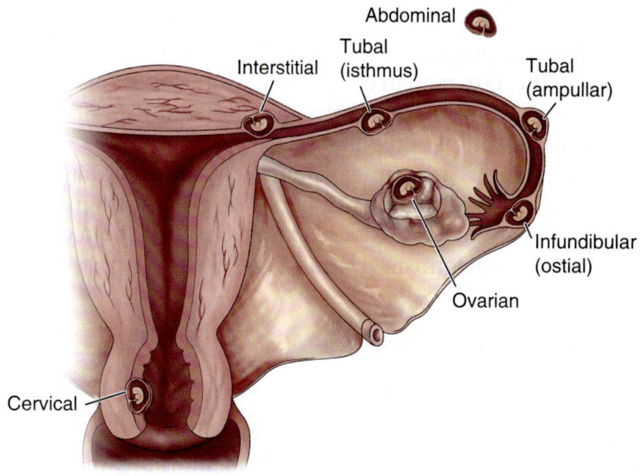

FIGURE 47-8. Sites of ectopic pregnancy.

Clinical Manifestations

Signs and symptoms vary depending on whether tubal rupture has occurred. Delay in menstruation from 1 to 2 weeks followed by slight bleeding (spotting) or a report of a slightly abnormal period suggests the possibility of an ectopic pregnancy. Symptoms may begin late, with vague soreness on the affected side (probably due to uterine contractions and distension of the tube), and may proceed to sharp, colicky pain. Most patients experience some pelvic or abdominal pain and some spotting or bleeding. Gastrointestinal symptoms, dizziness, or lightheadedness may occur. Patients may think the abnormal bleeding is a menstrual period, especially if a recent period occurred and was normal.

If implantation occurs in the fallopian tube, the tube becomes more and more distended and can rupture if the ectopic pregnancy remains undetected for 4 to 6 weeks or longer after conception. When the tube ruptures, the ovum is discharged into the abdominal cavity, and the woman experiences agonizing pain, dizziness, faintness, and nausea and vomiting due to the peritoneal reaction to blood escaping from the tube. Air hunger and symptoms of shock may occur, and the signs of hemorrhage—rapid and thready pulse, decreased blood pressure, subnormal temperature, restlessness, pallor, and sweating—are evident. Later, the pain becomes generalized in the abdomen and radiates to the shoulder and neck because of accumulating intraperitoneal blood that irritates the diaphragm.

Assessment and Diagnostic Findings

Ectopic pregnancies must be diagnosed promptly to prevent life-threatening hemorrhage, which is the major complication of rupture. During vaginal examination, a large mass of clotted blood that has collected in the pelvis behind the uterus or a tender adnexal mass may be palpable, although there are often no abnormal findings. If an ectopic pregnancy is suspected, the patient is evaluated by sonography and human chorionic gonadotropin (hCG) levels. Serial hCG tests may be needed (Hannon & Porth, 2016). The levels of hCG (the diagnostic hormone of pregnancy) double in early normal pregnancies every 3 days but are reduced in abnormal or ectopic pregnancies. A less-than-normal increase is cause for suspicion.

Transvaginal ultrasound, the usual method of diagnosis, can detect a pregnancy between 5 and 6 weeks from the time of the last menstrual period. Detectable fetal heart movement outside the uterus on ultrasound is firm evidence of an ectopic pregnancy.

Occasionally, the clinical picture makes the diagnosis relatively easy. However, when the clinical signs and symptoms are inconclusive, laparoscopy may be required for definitive diagnosis (Hannon & Porth, 2016).

Medical Management

Surgical Management

When surgery is performed early, almost all patients recover rapidly; if tubal rupture occurs, mortality increases. The type of surgery is determined by the size and extent of local tubal damage. Resection of the involved fallopian tube with end-to-end anastomosis may be effective. Some surgeons attempt to salvage the tube with a salpingotomy, which involves opening and evacuating the tube and controlling bleeding. More extensive surgery includes removing the tube alone (salpingectomy) or with the ovary (salpingo-oophorectomy).

Pharmacologic Therapy

Another option is the use of methotrexate without surgery (Hannon & Porth, 2016). Because methotrexate stops the pregnancy from progressing by interfering with DNA synthesis and the multiplication of cells, it interrupts early, small, unruptured ectopic pregnancies. The patient must be hemodynamically stable, have no active renal or hepatic disease, have no evidence of thrombocytopenia or leukopenia, and have a very small, unruptured ectopic pregnancy on ultrasound. Other indications may include no fetal cardiac activity and no active abdominal bleeding. Methotrexate is occasionally used to eliminate residual ectopic pregnancy tissue following a laparoscopy (Hannon & Porth, 2016).

Nursing Process

The Patient With an Ectopic Pregnancy

Assessment

The health history includes the menstrual pattern and any (even slight) bleeding since the last menstrual period. The nurse elicits the patient's description of pain and its location. The nurse asks the patient whether any sharp, colicky pains have occurred and whether pain radiates to the shoulder and neck (possibly caused by rupture and pressure on the diaphragm).

In addition, the nurse monitors vital signs, level of consciousness, and the nature and amount of vaginal bleeding. If possible, the nurse assesses how the patient is coping with the abnormal pregnancy and likely loss.

Nursing Priorities

Based on the assessment data, major nursing priorities may include the following:

- Acute pain
- Anticipatory grieving
- Deficient knowledge

Collaborative Problems/ Potential Complications

Potential major complications may include:

- Hemorrhage
- Hemorrhagic shock

Planning and Goals

The major goals may include relief of pain; acceptance and resolution of grief and pregnancy loss; increased knowledge about ectopic pregnancy, its treatment, and its outcome; and absence of complications.

Nursing Interventions

Relieving Pain

The abdominal pain associated with ectopic pregnancy may be described as cramping or severe continuous pain. If the patient is to have surgery, preanesthetic medications may provide pain relief. Postoperatively, analgesic agents are administered liberally; this promotes early ambulation and enables the patient to cough and take deep breaths.

Supporting the Grieving Process

Patients experience varying levels of distress. If the pregnancy was desired, loss may or may not be expressed verbally by the patient and her partner. The impact may not be fully realized until much later. The nurse should be available to listen and provide support. The patient's partner, if appropriate, should participate in this process. Even if the pregnancy was unintended, a loss has been experienced, and a grief reaction may occur.

Monitoring and Managing Potential Complications

Potential complications of ectopic pregnancy are hemorrhage and shock. Careful assessment is essential to detect the development of these complications. Continuous monitoring of vital signs, level of consciousness, amount of bleeding, and intake and output provides information about the possibility of hemorrhage and the need to prepare for IV therapy. Bed rest is indicated. Hematocrit, hemoglobin, and blood gases are monitored to assess hematologic status and adequacy of tissue perfusion. Significant deviations in these laboratory values are reported immediately, and the patient is prepared for possible surgery. Blood component therapy may be required if blood loss has been rapid and extensive. If hypovolemic shock occurs, the treatment is directed toward reestablishing tissue perfusion and adequate blood volume. See Chapter 18 for a discussion of the IV fluids and medications used in treating shock.

The nurse has an important role in prevention by being alert to patients with abnormal bleeding who may be at risk for an ectopic pregnancy and referring them immediately for care. It is necessary to keep a high index of suspicion in daily practice when a woman of childbearing age, particularly one who is not using an effective method of contraception consistently, reports abdominal discomfort or abnormal bleeding.

Promoting Home, Community-Based, and Transitional Care

EDUCATING PATIENTS ABOUT SELF-CARE. If the patient has experienced life-threatening hemorrhage and shock, these complications are addressed and treated before any in-depth teaching can begin. At this time, the patient's and the nurse's attention is focused on the crisis, not on learning. Once hemodynamically stable, the patient begins to ask questions about what happened and why certain procedures were performed. Procedures are explained in terms that are understandable to a patient who is distressed and apprehensive. The patient's partner is included in education when possible. After the patient recovers from postoperative discomfort, it may be more appropriate to address any questions and concerns that she and her partner have, including the effect of this pregnancy or its treatment on future pregnancies. The patient should be advised that ectopic pregnancies may recur. The patient is educated about possible complications and instructed to report early signs and symptoms. It is important to review signs and symptoms with the patient and instruct her to report an abnormal menstrual period promptly.

CONTINUING CARE. Because of the risk of subsequent ectopic pregnancies, the patient is advised to seek preconception counselling before considering future pregnancies and to seek early prenatal care. Follow-up contact allows the nurse to answer questions and clarify information for the patient and her partner.

Evaluation

Expected patient outcomes may include:

1. Experiences relief of pain
   a. Reports a decrease in pain and discomfort
   b. Ambulates as prescribed; performs coughing and deep breathing
2. Begins to accept loss of pregnancy and expresses grief by verbalizing feelings and reactions to loss
3. Verbalizes an understanding of the causes of ectopic pregnancy
4. Experiences no complications
   a. Exhibits no signs of bleeding, hemorrhage, or shock
   b. Has decreased amounts of discharge (on perineal pad)
   c. Has normal skin colour and turgor
   d. Exhibits stable vital signs and adequate urine output
   e. Levels of beta-hCG return to normal

Critical Thinking Exercises

1 A 20-year-old female college student comes to the student health clinic for a gynecologic examination and contraception. She asks you for advice about the most reliable method of contraception. She would like a method that is convenient. What is the evidence base for contraceptive methods for this college student? Specify the criteria used to evaluate the strength of the evidence for the practices that you identify.

2 You receive report that a 32-year-old patient will be arriving on your unit post-surgery for an ectopic pregnancy. Describe the nursing plan of care. What specific interventions and nursing management strategies are indicated? Develop a plan of patient education, and identify outcomes measures to assess the effectiveness of the education.

3 During her annual physical examination, a 55-year-old woman complains of night sweats and hot flashes. What are the immediate nursing priorities in providing care to this patient? What assessment data are needed to determine if this patient is in perimenopause or menopause?

REFERENCES AND SELECTED READINGS

Books

Annon, J. S. (1974). *The behavioral treatment of sexual problems* (1st ed.). Honolulu, HI: Enabling Systems.

Ball, J., Dains, J., Flynn, J., et al. (2015). *Seidel's guide to physical examination* (8th ed.). St. Louis, MO: Elsevier Mosby.

Comerford, K. C. (2015). *Nursing 2015 drug handbook*. Philadelphia, PA: Wolters Kluwer.

Eliopoulos, C. (2018). *Gerontological nursing* (9th ed.). Philadelphia, PA: Lippincott Williams & Wilkins.

Fischbach, F. T., & Dunning, M. B. (2015). *A manual of laboratory and diagnostic tests* (9th ed.). Philadelphia, PA: Lippincott Williams & Wilkins.

Hannon, R. A., & Porth, C. M. (2016). Porth pathophysiology: Concepts of altered health states (21st Canadian ed.). Philadelphia, PA: Wolters Kluwer Health/Lippincott Williams & Wilkins.

Hawkins, J. W., Roberto-Nichols, D. M., & Stanley-Haney, J. L. (2015). *Protocols for nurse practitioners in gynecologic settings* (11th ed.). New York: Tiresias Press.

Schuiling, K., & Likis, F. (2013). *Women's gynecologic health*. Boston, MA: Jones & Bartlett.

Statistics Canada. (2019). *Family violence in Canada: A statistical profile, 2016*. Ottawa, On: Author.

Tharpe, N., Farley, C., & Jordan, R. (2013). *Clinical practice guidelines for midwifery & women's health*. Boston, MA: Jones & Bartlett.

Weber, J., & Kelley, J. (2014). *Health assessment in nursing* (5th ed.). Philadelphia, PA: Lippincott Williams & Wilkins.

Journals and Electronic Documents

General

Alan Guttmacher Institute. (2016). *Contraceptive use in the United States*. Retrieved August 16, 2016, from www.guttmacher.org/fact-sheet/contraceptive-use-united-states

Bentley, J. (2012). Colposcopic management of abnormal cervical cytology and histology. *Journal of Obstetrics and Gynaecology Canada*, *34*(12), 1188–1203.

Black, A., Guilbert, E., Costescu, D., et al. (2015). Canadian Contraception Consensus. *Journal of Obstetrics and Gynaecology Canada*, *37*(10), S1–S4.

Bosse, J. D., Nesteby, A., & Randall, C. E. (2015). Integrating sexual minority health issues into a health assessment class. *Journal of Professional Nursing*, *31*(6) 498–507.

Bradley, L. D. (2016). *Overview of hysteroscopy*. Retrieved November 10, 2016, from www.uptodate.com/contents/overview-of-hysteroscopy?source=search_result&search=Overview+of+GynecOverview+of+Hysteroscopy%2C+ologic+Laparoscopic+Surgery+and+Non-umbilical+Entry+Sites&selectedTitle=1%7E150
Centers for Disease Control and Prevention (CDC). (2014). *Understanding intimate partner violence fact sheet*. Retrieved November 18, 2016, from https://www.cdc.gov/violenceprevention/pdf/ipv-factsheet.pdf
Centers for Disease Control and Prevention (CDC). (2016). U.S. selected practice recommendations for contraceptive use, 2016. *Morbidity and Mortality Weekly Report*, *65*(4), 1–72.
Courtney-Long, E., Carroll, D., Znang, O., et al. (2013). Prevalence of disability and disability types among adults. *Morbidity and Mortality Weekly Report*, *64*(29), 777–783.
Del Priore, G. (2015). Endometrial sampling procedure. Retrieved November 1, 2016, from www.uptodate.com/contents/endometrial-sampling-procedures
Fantasia, H. C., & Sutherland, M. A. (2014). Hormone therapy for the management of menopause symptoms. *Journal of Obstetric, Gynecologic and Neonatal Nursing*, *43*(2), 226–235.
Frayne, D., Verbiest, S., Chelmow, D., et al. (2016). Health care system measures to advance preconception wellness: Consensus recommendations of the clinical workgroup of the national preconception health and health care initiative. *Obstetrics & Gynecology*, *127*(5), 863–872.
Ginsburg, E. S., & Srouji, S. S. (2016). Donor insemination. Retrieved November 23, 2016, from www.uptodate.com/contents/donor-insemination
Hooker, L., Ward, B., & Verrinder, G. (2012). Domestic violence screening in maternal and child health nursing practice: A scoping review. *Contemporary Nurse: A Journal for the Australian Nursing Profession*, *4*(2), 198–215.
Ireland, L. D., Geffen, D., & Chen, A. Y. (2015). Medical compared with surgical abortion for effective pregnancy termination in the first trimester. *Obstetrics and Gynecology*, *126*(1), 22–28.
Johnson, M. J., & Amella, E. J. (2014). Isolation of lesbian, gay, bisexual and transgender youth: A dimensional concept analysis. *Journal of Advanced Nursing*, *70*(3), 523–532.
Mayo Clinic. (2014). *Toxic shock syndrome: Prevention*. Retrieved August 16, 2016, from www.mayoclinic.com/health/toxic-shock-syndrome/DS00221/DSECTION=prevention
Paulson, R. (2016). *In vitro fertilization*. Retrieved November 23, 2016, from www.uptodate.com/contents/in-vitro-fertilization?source=search_result&search=In+Vitro+Fertilitzation&selectedTitle=1%7E150
Public Health Agency of Canada (PHAC). (2014). *Specific populations: Sexual assault in postpubertal adolescents and adults*. Retrieved from http://www.phac-aspc.gc.ca/std-mts/sti-its/cgsti-ldcits/section-6-6-eng.php
Pyra, M., Weber, K. M., Wilson, T. E., et al. (2014). Sexual minority women and depressive symptoms throughout adulthood. *American Journal of Public Health*, *104*(12), E83–E90.
Rager Zuzelo, P. (2014). Improving nursing care for lesbian, bisexual and transgender women. *Journal of Obstetric Gynecologic and Neonatal Nursing*, *43*, 520–530.
Rape Victims Support Network. (2012). Sexual assault statistics. Retrieved from http://www.assaultcare.ca/index.php?option=com_content&view=article&id=49&Itemid=58
Santen, R. J., Loprinzi, C. L., & Casper, R. F. (2016). *Menopausal hot flashes*. Retrieved November 28, 2016, from www.uptodate.com/contents/menopausal-hot-flashes?source=search_result&search=Managing+menopausal+symptoms&selectedTitle=1%7E150
Sargant, N., Smallwood, N., Finley, F., et al. (2014). Sexual history taking: A dying skill? *Journal of Palliative Medicine*, *17*(7), 829–831.
SexualityandU.ca. (2018). *Sex & U: Your trusted resource for sexual and reproductive health*. Retrieved from https://www.sexandu.ca/
Sharp, H. T. (2016). Overview of gynecologic laparoscopic surgery and non-umbilical entry sites. *UpToDate*. Retrieved November 10, 2016, from www.uptodate.com/contents/overview-of-gynecologic-laparoscopic-surgery-and-non-umbilical-entry-sites?source=search_result&search=Overview+of+Gynecologic+Laparoscopic+Surgery+and+Non-umbilical+Entry+Sites&selectedTitle=1%7E150
Smeltzer, S. C., Avery, C., & Haynor, P. (2012). Interactions of people with disabilities and nursing staff during hospitalization. *American Journal of Nursing*, *112*(4), 30–37.
Smeltzer, S. C., Mitra, M., Iezzoni, L. I., et al. (2016). Perinatal experiences of women with physical disabilities and their recommendations for Clinicians. *Journal of Obstetric, Gynecologic & Neonatal Nursing*, *45*(6), 781–789.
Statistics Canada. (2013). *Measuring violence against women: Statistical trends*. Retrieved from http://www.statcan.gc.ca/pub/85-002-x/2013001/article/11766-eng.pdf
Statistics Canada. (2017). *Women with disabilities*. Retrieved from https://www.statcan.gc.ca/pub/89-503-x/2015001/article/14695-eng.htm
Statistics Canada. (2018). Retrieved from https://www150.statcan.gc.ca/n1/pub/85-002-x/2018001/article/54978/02-eng.htm
Tannura, T. A. (2014). Rape trauma syndrome. *American Journal of Sexuality Education*, *9*(2), 247–256.
Tarin, J. J., Garcia-Perez, M. A., Hamatani, T., et al. (2015). Infertility etiologies are genetically and clinically linked with other diseases in single meta-diseases. *Reproductive Biology and Endocrinology*, *13*, 31. doi: 10.1186/s12958-015-0029-9
Waggoner, M. (2013). Mother preconceived: The emergence of the preconception health and health care initiative. *Journal of Health Politics, Policy and Law*, *38*(2), 345–371.
Welt, C. K., & Barbieri, R. L. (2016). Evaluation and management of primary amenorrhea. Retrieved November 15, 2016, from www.uptodate.com/contents/evaluation-and-management-of-primary-amenorrhea
World Health Organization (WHO). (2013). *Female genital mutilation*. Retrieved from http://www.who.int/mediacentre/factsheets/fs241/en/
World Health Organization (WHO). (2016). *Female genital mutilation. Fact sheet number 241*. Retrieved from www.who.int/mediacentre/factsheets/fs241/en/

Resources

Amnesty International (resource for activists to end female genital mutilation): http://www.amnesty.org
Association of Reproductive Health Professionals: http://www.arhp.org
Association of Women's Health, Obstetrical and Neonatal Nurses (AWHONN): http://www.awhonn.org
Canadian Association of Perinatal and Women's Health Nursing (CAPWHN): http://www.capwhn.ca/en/capwhn/News_p2469.html
Canadian Women's Health Network: http://www.cwhn.ca/e
D.E.S. Action Canada: http://www.desaction.ca
Female Genital Mutilation Education and Networking Project (provides fact sheets, state policies, periodicals): http://www.fgmnetwork.org
Guttmacher Institute: http://www.guttmacher.org
Health Promotion for Women with Disabilities Project, Villanova University College of Nursing: http://www1.villanova.edu/villanova/nursing/community/womendisabilities.html
Infertility Awareness Association of Canada: http://www.iaac.ca/
National Association of Nurse Practitioners in Women's Health (NPWH): http://www.npwh.org
National Coalition Against Domestic Violence: http://www.ncadv.org
North American Menopause Society: http://www.menopause.org
Planned Parenthood Federation of America, http://www.plannedparenthood.org

48 Management of Patients With Female Reproductive Disorders

Adapted by Kelly Power-Kean

Learning Objectives

On completion of this chapter, the learner will be able to:

1. Compare the various types of vaginal infections and the signs, symptoms, and treatments of each.
2. Use the nursing process as a framework for care of the patient with a vulvovaginal infection.
3. Apply the nursing process as a framework for care of the patient with genital herpes.
4. Discuss the signs and symptoms, management, and nursing care of patients with inflammatory processes and structural disorders of the female reproductive tract.
5. Explain the signs and symptoms, management, and nursing care implications of benign and malignant disorders of the female reproductive tract.
6. Use the nursing process as a framework for care of the patient undergoing a hysterectomy.
7. Describe the nursing management of the patient undergoing radiation therapy for cancer of the female reproductive tract.

Disorders of the female reproductive system can be minor or serious but are often anxiety producing and distressing. Some disorders are self-limited and cause only minor inconvenience; others are life threatening and require immediate attention and long-term therapy. Many disorders are managed by the patient at home, whereas others require hospitalization and surgical intervention. Nurses not only need to be knowledgeable about these disorders but need to be sensitive to the woman's concerns and possible discomfort in discussing and dealing with these disorders.

VULVOVAGINAL INFECTIONS

Vulvovaginal infections are common, and nurses have an important role in providing information that may prevent their occurrence. To help prevent these infections, women need to understand their anatomy and vulvovaginal health.

The vagina is protected against infection by its normally low pH (3.5 to 4.5), which is maintained in part by the actions of *Lactobacillus acidophilus*, the dominant bacteria in a healthy vaginal ecosystem. These bacteria suppress the growth of anaerobes and produce lactic acid, which maintains normal pH. They also produce hydrogen peroxide, which is toxic to anaerobes (Powell & Nyirjesy, 2015). The risk of infection increases if a woman's resistance is reduced by stress or illness, if the pH is altered, or if a pathogen is introduced. Continued research into causes and treatments is needed, along with better ways to encourage growth of lactobacilli.

The epithelium of the vagina is highly responsive to estrogen, which induces glycogen formation. The subsequent breakdown of glycogen into lactic acid assists in producing a low vaginal pH. When estrogen decreases during lactation and menopause, glycogen also decreases. With reduced glycogen formation, infections may occur. In addition, as estrogen production ceases during the peri- and postmenopausal periods, the vagina and labia may atrophy (thin), making the vaginal area more susceptible to infection. When patients are treated with antibiotic agents, the normal vaginal flora is reduced. This results in altered pH and growth of fungal organisms. Other factors that may initiate or predispose to infections include contact with an infected partner and wearing tight, nonabsorbent, and heat-retaining and moisture-retaining clothing (Chart 48-1).

Vaginitis (inflammation of the vagina) is a group of conditions that cause vulvovaginal symptoms such as itching, irritation, burning, and abnormal discharge. Bacterial vaginosis is the most common cause (10% to 30% of pregnant women), followed by vulvovaginal **candidiasis** (75% of women will have at least one episode) and trichomoniasis (Table 48-1) (Public Health Agency of Canada [PHAC], 2013a). Other types include desquamative vaginitis, atrophic vaginitis, various vulvar dermatologic conditions, and **vulvodynia**. Normal vaginal discharge, which may occur in slight amounts during ovulation or just before the onset of menstruation, is clear to white, odourless, and viscous. It becomes more profuse when vaginitis occurs. Urethritis may accompany vaginitis because of the proximity of the urethra to the vagina. Discharge that occurs with vaginitis may produce itching, odour, redness, burning, or edema, which may be aggravated by voiding and defecation. After the causative organism has been identified, appropriate treatment (discussed later) is prescribed. This may include an oral medication or a local medication that is inserted into the vagina using an applicator.

CHART 48-1

Risk Factors for Vulvovaginal Infections

- Allergies
- Diabetes
- Frequent douching
- HIV infection
- Intercourse with infected partner
- Long-term or repeated use of broad-spectrum antibiotics
- Low estrogen levels
- Oral–genital contact (yeast can inhabit the mouth and intestinal tract)
- Perimenopause/menopause
- Poor personal hygiene
- Pregnancy
- Premenarche
- Synthetic clothing
- Tight undergarments
- Use of oral contraceptives

HIV, human immunodeficiency virus.
Adapted from Beckmann, C. R., Ling, F. W., Herbert, W. N., et al. (Eds.). (2014). *Obstetrics and gynecology* (7th ed.). Philadelphia, PA: Wolters Kluwer.

Glossary

abscess: a collection of purulent material
Bartholin's cyst: a cyst in a paired Bartholin or vestibular gland in the vulva
brachytherapy: delivery of radiation therapy through internal implants to a localized area of tissue
candidiasis: infection caused by *Candida* species or yeast; also referred to as monilial vaginitis or yeast infection
condylomata: warty growths indicative of the human papillomavirus (HPV)
cryotherapy: destruction of tissue by freezing (e.g., with liquid nitrogen)
cystocele: displacement of the bladder downward into the vagina
douche: rinsing the vaginal canal with fluid
dysplasia: term related to abnormal cell changes found on Pap smear and cervical biopsy reports
endocervicitis: inflammation of the mucosa and the glands of the cervix
endometriosis: endometrial tissue in abnormal locations; causes pain with menstruation, scarring, and possible infertility
enterocele: is a protrusion of the intestinal wall into the vagina
fibroid tumour: usually benign tumour arising from the muscle tissue of the uterus
fistula: abnormal opening between two organs or sites (e.g., vesicovaginal, between bladder and vagina; rectovaginal, between rectum and vagina)
hyphae: long, branching filamentous structures characteristic of fungi such as *Candida* seen under microscopic examination
hysterectomy: surgical removal of the uterus
loop electrocautery excision procedure (LEEP): procedure in which laser is used to remove a portion of cervical tissue after abnormal biopsy findings
myomectomy: surgical removal of uterine fibroids
oophorectomy: surgical removal of an ovary
pelvic exenteration: major surgical procedure in which the pelvic organs are removed
pelvic inflammatory disease (PID): inflammatory condition of the pelvic cavity, usually from a sexually transmitted infection usually from a sexually transmitted infection
polycystic ovary syndrome (PCOS): complex endocrine condition resulting in chronic anovulation, androgen excess, and multiple ovarian cysts
rectocele: bulging of the rectum into the vagina
salpingitis: inflammation of the fallopian tube
salpingo-oophorectomy: removal of the ovary and its fallopian tube (removal of the fallopian tube alone is a salpingectomy)
vaginitis: inflammation of the vagina, usually secondary to infection
vulvar dystrophy: thickening or lesions of the vulva; usually causes itching and may require biopsy to exclude malignancy
vulvectomy: removal of the tissue of the vulva
vulvitis: inflammation of the vulva, usually secondary to infection or irritation
vulvodynia: painful condition that affects the vulva

TABLE 48-1 Vaginal Infections and Vaginitis

Infection	Cause	Clinical Manifestations	Management Strategies
Candidiasis	Candida albicans, glabrata, or tropicalis	Inflammation of vaginal epithelium, producing itching, reddish irritation White, cheeselike discharge clinging to epithelium	Eradicate the fungus by administering an antifungal agent. Some more frequently used vaginal creams and suppositories are miconazole (Monistat) and clotrimazole (Gyne-Lotrimin). Review other causative factors (e.g., antibiotic therapy, nylon underwear, tight clothing, pregnancy, oral contraceptive agents). Assess for diabetes and HIV infection in patients with recurrent monilia.
Gardnerella-associated bacterial vaginosis	Gardnerella vaginalis and vaginal anaerobes	Usually no edema or erythema of vulva or vagina Grey-white to yellow-white discharge clinging to external vulva and vaginal walls	Administer metronidazole (Flagyl), with instructions about avoiding alcohol while taking this medication. If infection is recurrent, may treat partner.
Trichomonas vaginalis vaginitis	Trichomonas vaginalis	Inflammation of vaginal epithelium, producing burning and itching Frothy yellow-white or yellow-green vaginal discharge	Relieve inflammation, restore acidity, and reestablish normal bacterial flora; provide oral metronidazole for patient and partner.
Bartholinitis (infection of greater vestibular gland)	Escherichia coli T. vaginalis Staphylococcus Streptococcus Gonococcus	Erythema around vestibular gland Swelling and edema Abscessed vestibular gland	Drain the abscess; provide antibiotic therapy; excise gland of patients with chronic bartholinitis.
Cervicitis—acute and chronic	Chlamydia Gonococcus Streptococcus Many pathogenic bacteria	Profuse purulent discharge Backache Urinary frequency and urgency	Determine the cause—perform cytologic examination of cervical smear and appropriate cultures. Eradicate the gonococcal organism, if present: penicillin (as directed) or spectinomycin or tetracycline, if patient is allergic to penicillin. Tetracycline, doxycycline (Vibramycin) to eradicate chlamydia. Eradicate other causes.
Atrophic vaginitis	Lack of estrogen; glycogen deficiency	Discharge and irritation from alkaline pH of vaginal secretions	Provide topical vaginal estrogen therapy; improve nutrition if necessary; relieve dryness through the use of moisturizing medications.

Adapted from Karch, A. M. (2015). *Lippincott nursing drug guide*. Philadelphia, PA: Wolters Kluwer.

Candidiasis

Vulvovaginal candidiasis is a fungal or yeast infection caused by strains of Candida (see Table 48-1). *Candida albicans* accounts for most cases, but other strains, such as *C. glabrata*, may also be implicated. Approximately 75% of women will experience at least one episode of vulvovaginal candidiasis during their lifetime, and 5% to 10% have more than one episode (PHAC, 2013a). *C. albicans* accounts for approximately 90% of the cases, but other strains, such as *C. glabrata*, may also be implicated (Beckmann, Ling, Herbert, et al., 2014). Many women with a healthy vaginal ecosystem harbour Candida but are asymptomatic. Certain conditions favour the change from an asymptomatic state to colonization with symptoms. For example, use of antibiotic agents decreases bacteria, thereby altering the natural protective organisms usually present in the vagina. Although infections can occur at any time, they occur more commonly in pregnancy or with a systemic condition such as diabetes or human immunodeficiency virus (HIV) infection, or when patients are taking medications such as corticosteroids or oral contraceptive agents (Beckmann et al., 2014).

Clinical Manifestations

Clinical manifestations include a vaginal discharge that causes pruritus (itching) and subsequent irritation. The discharge may be watery or thick but usually has a white, cottage cheese–like appearance. Symptoms are usually more severe just before menstruation and may be less responsive to treatment during pregnancy. Diagnosis is made by microscopic identification of spores and **hyphae** (long, branching filamentous structures) on a glass slide prepared from a discharge specimen mixed with potassium hydroxide. With candidiasis, the pH is 4.5 or less (Beckmann et al., 2014). Manifestations may be uncomplicated, occurring sporadically in women who are healthy, or recurrent and complicated in women who have diabetes, are pregnant, have a compromised immune system, or have obesity.

Medical Management

The goal of management is to eliminate symptoms. Treatments include antifungal agents such as miconazole (Monistat), nystatin (Mycostatin), clotrimazole (Gyne-Lotrimin), and terconazole (Terazol) cream. These agents are inserted into the vagina with an applicator at bedtime. There are 1-, 3-, and 7-night treatment courses available (Karch, 2015). Oral medication (fluconazole [Diflucan]) is also available in a one-pill dose. Relief should be noted within 3 days.

Some vaginal creams are available without a prescription; however, patients are cautioned to use these creams only if they are certain that they have a yeast or monilial infection. Patients often use these remedies for problems other than yeast infections. If a woman is uncertain about the cause of her symptoms or if relief has not been obtained after using these creams, she should be instructed to seek health care promptly. Yeast infections can become recurrent or complicated. Women may have more than four infections in a year and severe symptoms due to pre-existing conditions such as diabetes or immunosuppression. Cell-mediated immunity may be a factor. Women with recurrent yeast infections benefit from a comprehensive gynecologic assessment.

Bacterial Vaginosis

Bacterial vaginosis is caused by an overgrowth of anaerobic bacteria and *Gardnerella vaginalis* normally found in the vagina and an absence of lactobacilli (see Table 48-1). Risk factors include douching after menses, smoking, multiple sex partners, and other sexually transmitted infections (STIs). Bacterial vaginosis is not considered an STI but is associated with sexual activity, and incidence is increased in female same-sex partners (Schuiling & Likis, 2013).

Clinical Manifestations

Bacterial vaginosis can occur throughout the menstrual cycle and does not produce local discomfort or pain. More than half of patients with bacterial vaginosis do not notice any symptoms. Discharge, if noticed, is heavier than normal and grey to yellowish white in colour. It is characterized by a fishlike odour that is particularly noticeable after sexual intercourse or during menstruation because of an increase in vaginal pH. The pH of the discharge is usually greater than 4.7 because of the amines that result from enzymes from anaerobes. The fishlike odour can be detected readily by adding a drop of potassium hydroxide to a glass slide with a sample of vaginal discharge, which releases amines; this is referred to as a positive "whiff" test. Under the microscope, vaginal cells are coated with bacteria and are described as "clue cells." Lactobacilli, which serve as a natural host defence, are usually absent. Bacterial vaginosis is not usually considered a serious condition, although it can be associated with premature labour, premature rupture of membranes, endometritis, and pelvic infection (Schuiling & Likis, 2013).

Medical Management

Metronidazole (Flagyl), given orally twice a day for 1 week, is effective; a vaginal gel is also available. Clindamycin (Cleocin) vaginal cream or ovules (oval suppositories) are also effective. Treatment of patients' partners does not seem to prevent recurrence but the use of condoms may be helpful. Bacterial vaginosis is highly persistent and tends to recur after treatment; therefore, women are encouraged to seek follow-up care if symptoms recur.

Trichomoniasis

Trichomonas vaginalis is a flagellated protozoan that causes a common STI often called *trich*. Trichomoniasis may be transmitted by an asymptomatic carrier who harbours the organism in the urogenital tract (see Table 48-1). It may increase the risk of contracting HIV from an infected partner and may play a role in the development of cervical neoplasia, postoperative infections, adverse pregnancy outcomes, pelvic inflammatory disease (PID), and infertility. Incidence is 10 times higher in African-American women, and approximately 70% to 85% of those affected are asymptomatic (CDC, 2015a). The prevalence of trichomoniasis in Canada has not been well determined; however, approximately 3.7 million cases occur each year in the United States (CDC, 2015a). Approximately 50% of those affected are asymptomatic (PHAC, 2013a).

Clinical Manifestations

Clinical manifestations include a vaginal discharge that is thin (sometimes frothy), yellow to yellow-green, malodorous, and very irritating. An accompanying **vulvitis** may result, with vulvovaginal burning and itching. Diagnosis is made most often by microscopic detection of the motile causative organisms or less frequently by culture. Inspection with a speculum often reveals vaginal and cervical erythema (redness) with multiple small petechiae ("strawberry spots") (Beckmann et al., 2014). Testing of a trichomonal discharge demonstrates a pH greater than 4.5.

Medical Management

The most effective treatment for trichomoniasis is metronidazole or tinidazole (Tindamax). Both partners receive a one-time loading dose or a smaller dose two times a day for 7 days. The one-time dose is more convenient; consequently, adherence tends to be improved. The week-long treatment has occasionally been noted to be more effective. Some patients complain of an unpleasant but transient metallic taste when taking metronidazole. Nausea and vomiting, as well as a hot, flushed feeling can occur when this medication is taken with an alcoholic beverage. Patients are strongly advised to abstain from alcohol during and for 24 hours after treatment (PHAC, 2013a). The sexual partner(s) should be treated, and abstinence is recommended during treatment to avoid reinfection (PHAC, 2013a).

Gerontologic Considerations

After menopause, the vaginal mucosa becomes thinner and may atrophy. While vulvovaginal atrophy can occur at any time in a woman's life, it is most common in women who are postmenopausal, with an incidence of nearly 50% (Lev-Sagie, 2015; Nyirjesy, 2014). This condition can be complicated by infection from phytogenic bacteria, resulting in atrophic vaginitis (see Table 48-1). Leukorrhea (vaginal discharge) may cause itching and burning. Management is similar to bacterial vaginosis. Estrogenic hormones, either taken orally or inserted into the vagina in a cream form, can also be effective in restoring the epithelium.

Desquamative inflammatory vaginitis is an uncommon but severe purulent form of vaginal infection that occurs mostly in Caucasian women who are perimenopausal. It results in vaginal inflammation, burning, discharge, and dyspareunia. Topical anti-inflammatory and antibiotic treatment is usually effective (Nyirjesy, 2014; Reichman & Sobel, 2014).

Nursing Process

The Patient With a Vulvovaginal Infection

Assessment

The woman with vulvovaginal symptoms should be examined as soon as possible after the onset of symptoms. She should be instructed not to **douche** (rinse the vaginal canal), because doing so removes the discharge needed to make the diagnosis. The area is observed for erythema, edema, excoriation, and discharge. Each of the infection-producing organisms produces its own characteristic discharge and effect (see Table 48-1). The patient is asked to describe any discharge and other symptoms, such as odour, itching, or burning. Dysuria often occurs because of local irritation of the urinary meatus. A urinary tract infection may need to be ruled out by obtaining a urine specimen for culture and sensitivity testing.

The patient is asked about the occurrence of factors that may contribute to vulvovaginal infection:

- Physical and chemical factors, such as constant moisture from tight or synthetic clothing, perfumes and powders, soaps, bubble bath, poor hygiene, and use of feminine hygiene products
- Psychogenic factors (e.g., stress, fear of STIs, abuse)
- Medical conditions or endocrine factors, such as a predisposition to *Monilia* in a patient who has diabetes
- Use of medications such as antibiotics, which may alter the vaginal flora and allow an overgrowth of monilial organisms
- New sex partner, multiple sex partners, previous vaginal infection

The patient is also asked about factors that could contribute to infection, including hygiene practices (douching), and use or nonuse of condoms.

The nurse may prepare a vaginal smear (wet mount) to assist in diagnosing the infection. A common method for preparing the smear is to collect vaginal secretions with an applicator and place the secretions on two separate glass slides. A drop of saline solution is added to one slide and a drop of 10% potassium hydroxide is added to another slide for examination under a microscope. If bacterial vaginosis is present, the slide with normal saline solution added shows epithelial cells dotted with bacteria (clue cells). If *Trichomonas* species is present, small motile cells are seen. In the presence of yeast, the potassium hydroxide slide reveals branching hyphae (Beckmann et al., 2014). Discharge associated with bacterial vaginosis produces a strong odour when mixed with potassium hydroxide. Testing the pH of the discharge with nitrazine paper assists in proper diagnosis (Beckmann et al., 2014).

Nursing Priorities

Based on the nursing assessment and other data, major nursing priorities may include the following:

- Discomfort
- Anxiety
- Infection
- Lack of knowledge about preventive measures

Planning and Goals

Major goals may include relief of discomfort, reduction of anxiety related to symptoms, prevention of reinfection or infection of sexual partner, and acquisition of knowledge about methods for preventing vulvovaginal infections and managing self-care.

Nursing Interventions

Relieving Discomfort

Treatment with the appropriate medication usually relieves discomfort. Sitz baths may be occasionally recommended and may provide temporary relief of symptoms.

Reducing Anxiety

Vulvovaginal infections are upsetting and require treatment. The patient who experiences such an infection may be very anxious about the significance of the symptoms and possible causes. Explaining the cause of symptoms may reduce anxiety related to fear of a more serious illness. Discussing ways to help prevent vulvovaginal infections may help patients adopt specific strategies to decrease infection and the related symptoms.

Preventing Reinfection or Spread of Infection

Patient education should include the fact that vulvovaginal candidiasis is not an STI and incidence can be decreased by completing treatment, avoiding unnecessary antibiotic agents, wearing cotton underwear, and not douching. Prevention strategies for vaginal infections include promotion of adequate rest, reduction of life stress, and a healthy diet low in refined sugars (Schuiling & Likis, 2013).

The patient needs to be informed about the importance of adequate treatment of herself and her partner, if indicated. Other strategies to prevent persistence or spread of infection include abstaining from sexual intercourse when infected, treatment of sexual partners, and minimizing irritation of the affected area. When medications such as antibiotic agents are prescribed for any infection, the nurse instructs the patient about the usual precautions related to using these agents. If vaginal itching occurs several days after use, the patient can be reassured that this is usually not an allergic reaction but may be a yeast or monilial infection resulting from altered vaginal bacteria. Treatment for monilial infection is prescribed if indicated.

Another goal of treatment is to reduce tissue irritation caused by scratching or wearing tight clothing. The area needs to be kept clean by daily bathing and adequate hygiene after voiding and defecation. The use of a hairdryer on a cool setting will dry the area and application of topical corticosteroids may decrease irritation.

When educating the patient about medications such as suppositories and devices such as applicators to dispense cream or ointment, the nurse may demonstrate the procedure by using a plastic model of the pelvis and vagina. The nurse should also stress the importance of handwashing before and after each administration of medication. To prevent the medication from escaping from the vagina, the patient should recline for 30 minutes after it is inserted, if possible. The patient is informed that seepage of medication may occur, and the use of a perineal pad may be helpful.

Promoting Home, Community-Based, and Transitional Care

EDUCATING PATIENTS ABOUT SELF-CARE. Vulvovaginal conditions are treated on an outpatient basis unless a patient has other medical problems. Patient teaching, tact, and reassurance are important aspects of nursing care. Women may express embarrassment, guilt, or anger and may be concerned that the infection could be serious or that it may have been acquired from a sex partner. (In some instances, treatment plans include the partner.)

The nurse assesses the patient's learning needs about the immediate problem. The patient needs to know the characteristics of normal as opposed to abnormal discharge. Questions often arise about douching. Normally, douching and use of feminine hygiene sprays are unnecessary because daily baths or showers and proper hygiene after voiding and defecating keep the perineal area clean. Douching tends to eliminate normal flora, reducing the body's ability to ward off infection. In addition, repeated douching may result in vaginal epithelial breakdown and chemical irritation and has been associated with other pelvic disorders (HealthLinkBC, 2016). In the case of recurrent yeast infections, the perineum should be kept as dry as possible. Loose-fitting cotton instead of tight-fitting synthetic, nonabsorbent, heat-retaining underwear is recommended.

Vulvar self-examination is a good health practice for all women. Becoming familiar with one's own anatomy and reporting anything that seems new or different may result in early detection and treatment of any new disorders. Nurses can also play a role in teaching women about the risks of unprotected intercourse, particularly with partners who have had sex with others.

Evaluation

Expected patient outcomes may include:

1. Experiences increased comfort
   a. Cleans the perineum as instructed
   b. Reports that itching is relieved
   c. Maintains urine output within normal limits and without dysuria
2. Experiences relief of anxiety
3. Remains free from infection
   a. Has no signs of inflammation, pruritus, odour, or dysuria
   b. Notes that vaginal discharge appears normal (thin, clear, not frothy)
4. Participates in self-care
   a. Takes medication as prescribed
   b. Wears absorbent underwear
   c. Avoids unprotected sexual intercourse
   d. Douches only as prescribed
   e. Performs vulvar self-examination regularly and reports any new findings to primary provider

Human Papillomavirus

Human papillomavirus (HPV) is the most common STI in young, sexually active people. Most adults who are sexually active will be infected with at least one type of HPV during their lifetime. In Canada, the prevalence of HPV in young women is approximately 29% (PHAC, 2015a). Studies have shown that the prevalence of HPV infections is higher in socially disadvantaged females, such as those living in low-income housing or Aboriginal communities (PHAC, 2015a). Most infections are self-limiting and without symptoms, and others can cause cervical and anogenital cancers. Infections can be latent (asymptomatic and detected only by deoxyribonucleic acid [DNA] hybridization tests for HPV), subclinical (visualized only after application of acetic acid followed by inspection under magnification), or clinical (visible **condylomata** acuminata).

Pathophysiology

HPV can be found in lesions of the skin, cervix, vagina, anus, penis, and oral cavity. Of the more than 100 genotypes of HPV that exist, about 30 genotypes affect the anogenital tract (Beckmann et al., 2014). Some are low risk in that they are unlikely to cause cancerous changes. These include types 6, 11, 42, 43, 44, 54, 61, 70, and 72. The most common strains of HPV, 6 and 11, usually cause condylomata (warty growths) that can appear on the vulva, vagina, cervix, and anus. These are often visible or may be palpable by patients. Condylomata are rarely premalignant but are an outward manifestation of the virus (Beckmann et al., 2014). High-risk oncogenic types, including 16, 18, 31, 33, 45, and 52, affect the cervix, causing abnormal cell changes or **dysplasia** (found on a Papanicolaou [Pap] smear). HPV types 16 and 18 account for 66% of cervical cancer cases, while types 31, 33, 45, and 52 account for another 15% (American College of Obstetricians and Gynecologists [ACOG], 2015a).

The incidence of HPV in young women who are sexually active is high. The infection often disappears as the result of an effective immune system response. It is thought that two proteins produced by high-risk types of HPV interfere with tumour suppression by normal cells. Risk factors include being young, being sexually active, having multiple sex partners, and having sex with a partner who has or has had multiple partners. It can be transmitted by other means, however, as it has been found in young girls who have not been sexually active.

Medical Management

Options for the treatment of external genital warts by a primary provider include topical application of trichloroacetic acid, podophyllin (Podofin, Podocon), **cryotherapy**, as well as surgical removal. Topical agents that can be applied by patients to external lesions include podofilox (Condylox) and imiquimod (Aldara). Because the safety of podophyllin, imiquimod, and podofilox during pregnancy has not been determined, these agents should not be used during pregnancy. Electrocautery and laser therapy are alternative therapies that may be indicated for patients with a large number or area of genital warts.

Treatment usually eradicates perineal warts or condylomata. However, they may resolve spontaneously without treatment and may also recur even with treatment (PHAC, 2015a). Genital warts are more resistant to treatment in patients with diabetes, those who are pregnant, who smoke, or are immunocompromised (Beckmann et al., 2014).

If the treatment includes application of a topical agent by the patient, the patient needs to be carefully instructed in the use of the agent prescribed and must be able to identify the warts and be able to apply the medication to them. The patient is instructed to anticipate mild pain or local irritation with the use of these agents.

Women with HPV should have annual Pap smears because of the potential of HPV to cause dysplasia. Much remains unknown about subclinical and latent HPV disease. Women are often exposed to HPV by partners who are unknowing carriers. Use of condoms can reduce the likelihood of transmission, but transmission can also occur during skin-to-skin contact in areas not covered by condoms.

In many cases, patients are angry about having warts or HPV and do not know who infected them because the incubation period can be long, and partners may have no symptoms. Acknowledging the emotional distress that occurs when an STI is diagnosed and providing support and facts are important nursing actions.

Prevention

The best strategy is prevention of HPV. The PHAC (2018) recommends vaccination of all females and males 9 to 26 years of age. They also recommend that vaccination be administered to individuals 27 years of age and older at ongoing risk of exposure to HPV (PHAC, 2018). Routine vaccination of boys and girls 9 to 14 years of age is offered across Canada. Currently, Gardasil and Gardasil 9 are approved for use in females aged 9 to 45 and males aged 9 to 26; Cervarix is approved for use in females aged 9 to 45 (PHAC, 2018). Gardasil provides protection against HPV 16, 18, 6, and 11; Gardasil 9 includes five additional HPV types (31, 33, 45, 52, 58). Cervarix provides protection against HPV 16 and 18 (PHAC, 2018).

The vaccination is given in three intramuscular doses, with the initial dose followed by a second dose in 2 months and a third dose 6 months after the first dose. Completion of all three doses of the vaccine is important for immunity to develop. The vaccination is contraindicated for use in women who are pregnant (PHAC, 2018).

Although this vaccine is considered an important medical breakthrough with the potential to decrease the impact of HPV-related disease in men and women, it does not replace other strategies important in prevention of HPV. Women still need cervical cancer screening (PHAC, 2018).

Herpesvirus Type 2 Infection (Herpes Genitalis, Herpes Simplex Virus)

Herpes simplex virus 2 (HSV-2) is a recurrent, lifelong viral infection that causes herpetic lesions (blisters) on the external genitalia and occasionally the vagina and cervix. It is an STI but may also be transmitted asexually from wet surfaces or by self-transmission (i.e., touching a cold sore and then touching the genital area). The initial infection is usually very painful, and blisters may take 2 to 4 weeks to heal, but it can also be asymptomatic. Over 87% of infected individuals are unaware of their infection; most HSV transmission occurs from asymptomatic viral shedding (Bechtel & Trout, 2015; CDC, 2015b). Recurrences can be associated with stress, sunburn, dental work, or inadequate rest or nutrition, or any situations that may tax the immune system.

The incidence of herpes infection in Canada is unknown (PHAC, 2013a). Transmission is possible even when a carrier does not have symptoms (subclinical shedding). Lesions increase vulnerability to HIV infection and other STIs. Vaccines for herpes genitalis are in clinical trials; however, currently, there is no commercially available vaccine (PHAC, 2013a).

Pathophysiology

There are nine types of herpesviruses belonging to three different groups that cause infections in humans (Beckmann et al., 2014). These include herpes simplex type 1

(HSV-1), usually associated with cold sores of the lips; HSV-2, usually associated with genital herpes; varicella zoster or shingles; Epstein–Barr virus; cytomegalovirus; human B-lymphotropic virus; and others.

Close human contact by the mouth, oropharynx, mucosal surface, vagina, or cervix appears necessary to acquire the infection. Other susceptible sites are skin lacerations and conjunctivae. Usually, the virus is killed at room temperature by drying. When viral replication diminishes, the virus ascends the peripheral sensory nerves and remains inactive in the nerve ganglia. Another outbreak may occur when the host is subjected to stress. In women who are pregnant and have active herpes, infants delivered vaginally may become infected with the virus. There is a risk of fetal morbidity and mortality if this occurs; therefore, a cesarean delivery may be performed if the virus recurs near the time of delivery.

Clinical Manifestations

Itching and pain occur as the infected area becomes red and edematous. Infection may begin with macules and papules and progress to vesicles and ulcers. The vesicular state often appears as a blister, which later coalesces, ulcerates, and encrusts. In women, the labia are the usual primary site, although the cervix, vagina, and perianal skin may be affected. In men, the glans penis, foreskin, or penile shaft is typically affected. Influenza-like symptoms may occur 3 or 4 days after the lesions appear. Inguinal lymphadenopathy (enlarged lymph nodes in the groin), minor temperature elevation, malaise, headache, myalgia (aching muscles), and dysuria (pain on urination) are often noted. Pain is evident during the first week and then decreases. The lesions last 2 to 12 days before crusting over (Bechtel & Trout, 2015).

Rarely, complications may arise from extragenital spread, such as to the buttocks, upper thighs, or even the eyes because of touching lesions and then touching other areas. Patients should be advised to wash their hands after contact with lesions. Other potential problems are aseptic meningitis, neonatal transmission, and severe emotional stress related to the diagnosis.

Medical Management

Currently there is no cure for genital herpes infection, but treatment is aimed at relieving the symptoms. Management goals include preventing the spread of infection, making patients comfortable, decreasing potential health risks, and initiating a counselling and education program. Three antiviral agents—acyclovir (Zovirax), valacyclovir (Valtrex), and famciclovir (Famvir)—can suppress symptoms and shorten the course of the infection (Bechtel & Trout, 2015). These agents are effective at reducing the duration of lesions and preventing recurrences. Analgesics and a saline compress can provide additional relief of symptoms. Resistance and long-term side effects do not appear to be major problems. Recurrent episodes are often milder than the initial episode. Prophylactic vaccine and topical gel development for genital herpes continues to be investigated in clinical trials (Bechtel & Trout, 2015; National Institute of Allergy and Infectious Disease [NIAID], 2015).

Nursing Process

The Patient With a Genital Herpesvirus Infection

Assessment

The health history and a physical and pelvic examination are important in establishing the nature of the infectious condition. In addition, patients are assessed for risk of STIs. The perineum is inspected for painful lesions. Inguinal nodes are assessed and are often enlarged and tender during an occurrence of genital herpes.

Nursing Priorities

Based on the assessment data, major nursing priorities may include the following:

- Pain
- Infection
- Anxiety
- Lack of knowledge

Planning and Goals

Major goals may include relief of pain and discomfort, control of infection and its spread, relief of anxiety, knowledge of and adherence to the treatment regimen and self-care, and knowledge about implications for the future.

Nursing Interventions

Relieving Pain

The lesions should be kept clean, and proper hygiene practices are advocated. Sitz baths may ease discomfort. Clothing should be clean, loose, soft, and absorbent. Aspirin and other analgesics are usually effective in controlling pain. Occlusive ointments and powders are avoided because they prevent the lesions from drying.

The patient is encouraged to increase fluid intake, to be alert for possible bladder distention, and to contact her primary provider immediately if she cannot void because of discomfort. Painful voiding may occur if urine comes in contact with the herpes lesions. Discomfort with urination can be reduced by pouring warm water over the vulva during voiding. When oral antiviral agents are prescribed, the patient is instructed about when to take the medication and what side effects to note, such as rash and headache.

Preventing Infection and Its Spread

The risk of reinfection and spread of infection to others or to other structures of the body can be reduced by proper hand hygiene, the use of barrier methods with sexual contact, and adherence to prescribed medication regimens. Avoidance of contact when obvious lesions are present does not eliminate the risk because the virus can be shed in the absence of symptoms, and lesions may not be visible.

Relieving Anxiety

Concern about the presence of herpes infection, future occurrences of lesions, and the impact of the infection on future relationships and childbearing may cause considerable patient anxiety. Nurses serve as important sources of support by listening to patients' concerns and providing information and instruction. The patient may be angry with her partner if the partner is the probable source of the infection. The patient may need assistance in discussing the infection and its implications with her current sexual partners and in future sexual relationships. The nurse can refer the patient to a support group to assist in coping with the diagnosis (see Resources at the end of the chapter).

Increasing Knowledge About the Disease and Its Treatment

Patient education is an essential part of nursing care of the patient with a genital herpes infection. This includes an adequate explanation about the infection and how it is transmitted, management and treatment strategies, strategies to minimize spread of infection, the importance of adherence to the treatment regimen, and self-care strategies. Because of the increased risk of HIV and other STIs in the presence of skin lesions, an important part of education involves informing the patient of strategies to protect herself from exposure to HIV and other STIs (Chart 48-2).

Promoting Home, Community-Based, and Transitional Care

EDUCATING PATIENTS ABOUT SELF-CARE. Health promotion strategies and self-care measures for the patient with genital herpes are described in Chart 48-2.

Evaluation

Expected patient outcomes may include:

1. Experiences a reduction in pain and discomfort
2. Keeps infection under control
   a. Demonstrates proper hygiene techniques
   b. Takes medication as prescribed
   c. Consumes adequate fluids
   d. Assesses own current lifestyle (diet, adequate fluid intake, safer sex practices, stress management)
3. Uses strategies to reduce anxiety
   a. Verbalizes issues and concerns related to genital herpes infection
   b. Discusses strategies to deal with issues and concerns with current and future sexual partners
   c. Initiates contact with support group if indicated

CHART 48-2

Health Promotion: Strategies for the Patient With Genital Herpes

Herpes is transmitted mainly by direct contact. Intercourse during a herpes outbreak not only increases the risk of transmission but also increases the likelihood of contracting HIV and other STIs. Women therefore take the following measures:

- Abstains from sexual intercourse during treatment for active disease (other options such as hand holding and kissing are acceptable).
- Avoids exposure to the sun, which can cause recurrences (and skin cancer).
- Avoids self-infection by not touching lesions during an outbreak.
- Uses barrier methods when engaging in intercourse to provide protection against viral transmission.
- Informs sexual partners of herpes diagnosis as transmission is possible even in the absence of active lesions.
- Informs obstetric care provider about the history of genital herpes. In cases of recurrence at time of delivery, cesarean section may be considered.
- Joins a support group to share solutions and experiences and hear about newer treatments (see Resources section).
- Keeps follow-up appointments with health care provider, and reports repeated recurrences (may not be as severe as the initial episode).
- Takes medication prescribed for outbreaks and avoids occlusive ointments, strong perfumed soaps, or bubble bath.
- Takes aspirin and other analgesic agents to control pain during outbreaks.
- Uses the appropriate hygiene practices including hand hygiene, perineal cleanliness, gentle washing of lesions with mild soap and running water and lightly drying lesions (i.e., lesions can become infected from germs on the hand, and the virus from the lesion can be transmitted from the hand to another area of the body or another person).
- Wears loose, comfortable clothing; eats a balanced diet; ingests adequate fluids; gets adequate rest during outbreaks.

4. Demonstrates knowledge about genital herpes and strategies to control and minimize recurrences
   a. Identifies methods of transmission of herpes infection and strategies to prevent transmission to others
   b. Discusses strategies to reduce recurrence of lesions
   c. Takes medications as prescribed
   d. Reports no recurrence of lesions

Endocervicitis and Cervicitis

Endocervicitis is an inflammation of the mucosa and the glands of the cervix that may occur when organisms gain access to the cervical glands after intercourse and, less often, after procedures such as abortion, intrauterine manipulation, or vaginal delivery. If untreated, the infection may extend into the uterus, fallopian tubes, and pelvic cavity. Inflammation can irritate the cervical tissue, resulting in spotting or bleeding and mucopurulent cervicitis (inflammation of the cervix with exudate).

Chlamydia and Gonorrhea

Chlamydia and gonorrhea are the most common causes of endocervicitis, although *Mycoplasma* may also be involved. Rates of infection have been increasing since 1997, and in 2010, 277.6/100,000 cases of chlamydia were reported (PHAC, 2013b). It is most commonly found in young, sexually active people with more than one partner and is transmitted through sexual intercourse. Untreated chlamydia infections can spread to the fallopian tubes and uterus leading to serious complications, including PID, an increased risk for ectopic pregnancy, and infertility (CDC, 2015c). At least 10% to 15% of Canadian women of reproductive age have had one occasion of PID (PHAC, 2013a). There are 100,000 reports of symptomatic PID annually, but two thirds of the cases are unrecognized and underreported. Chlamydial infections of the cervix often produce no symptoms, but cervical discharge, dyspareunia, dysuria, and bleeding may occur. Other complications include conjunctivitis and perihepatitis (Fitz-Hugh–Curtis syndrome) (CDC, 2015c).

Chlamydial infection and gonorrhea often coexist. Females who have chlamydial infections may be coinfected with gonorrhea (PHAC, 2013b). The inflamed cervix that results from infection may leave a woman more vulnerable to HIV transmission from an infected partner. Gonorrhea often is asymptomatic and is a major cause of PID, tubal infertility, ectopic pregnancy, and chronic pelvic pain (CDC, 2015d). Diagnosis can be confirmed by urine culture or other methods such as using a swab to obtain a sample of cervical or penile discharge from the patient's partner (CDC, 2015d).

Medical Management

The PHAC (2013b) recommends treating chlamydia with doxycycline (Vibramycin) for 7 days or with a single dose of azithromycin (Zithromax). Antimicrobial resistance to fluoroquinolones in the treatment of gonorrhea has left cephalosporins as the remaining recommended treatment (ACOG, 2015b; CDC, 2015d). Because of the high incidence of coinfection with chlamydia and gonorrhea, treatment for gonorrhea should include treatment for chlamydia as well (PHAC, 2013b). Partners must also be treated. Women who are pregnant are cautioned not to take tetracycline because of potential adverse effects on the fetus. In these cases, erythromycin may be prescribed. Results are usually good if treatment begins early. Possible complications from delayed or no treatment include tubal disease, ectopic pregnancy, PID, and infertility.

Cultures for chlamydia and other STIs should be obtained from all patients who have been sexually assaulted when they first seek medical attention; patients are treated prophylactically. Cultures should then be repeated in 2 weeks. Annual screening for chlamydia is recommended for all young women who are sexually active and older women with new sex partners or multiple partners (CDC, 2015c).

Nursing Management

All women who are sexually active may be at risk for chlamydia, gonorrhea, and other STIs, including HIV. Nurses can assist patients in assessing their own risk. Recognition of risk is a first step before changes in behaviour occur. Patients should be discouraged from assuming that a partner is "safe" without open, honest discussion. Nonjudgmental attitudes, educational counselling, and role playing may be helpful.

Because chlamydia, gonorrhea, and other STIs may have a serious effect on future health and fertility and because many of these disorders can be prevented using condoms and spermicides and careful choice of partners, nurses can play a major role in counselling patients about safer sex practices. Exploring options with patients, addressing knowledge deficits, and correcting misinformation may reduce morbidity and mortality.

Patients should be advised to refer partners for evaluation and treatment. All women aged 25 and younger who are sexually active should be screened annually. Those older than 25 years should be screened if risk factors are present. Repeat testing should occur 6 months after treatment (PHAC, 2013b).

Promoting Home, Community-Based, and Transitional Care

Educating Patients About Self-Care

Nurses can educate women and help them develop communication skills and initiate discussions about sex with their partners. Communicating with partners about sex, risk, postponing intercourse, and using safer sex behaviours, including the use of condoms, may be lifesaving. Some young women report having sex but not being comfortable enough to discuss sexual risk issues. Nurses can help women to advocate for their own health by discussing safety with partners prior to sexual activity.

Reinforcing the need for annual screening for chlamydia and other STIs is an important part of patient education. Instructions also include the need for the patient to abstain from sexual intercourse until all of her sex partners are treated (PHAC, 2013b).

Pelvic Infection (Pelvic Inflammatory Disease)

PID is an inflammatory condition of the pelvic cavity that may begin with cervicitis and involve the uterus (endometritis), fallopian tubes (salpingitis), ovaries (oophoritis), pelvic peritoneum, or pelvic vascular system. Infection, which may be acute, subacute, recurrent, or chronic and localized or widespread, is usually caused by bacteria but may be attributed to a virus, fungus, or parasite. Gonorrheal and chlamydial organisms are common causes but most cases of PID are polymicrobial. There are approximately 100,000 cases of symptomatic PID annually in Canada (PHAC, 2013b).

Short- and long-term consequences can occur. The fallopian tubes become narrow and scarred, which increases the risk of ectopic pregnancy (fertilized eggs trapped in the tube), infertility, recurrent pelvic pain, tubo-ovarian **abscess** (a collection of purulent material), and recurrent disease.

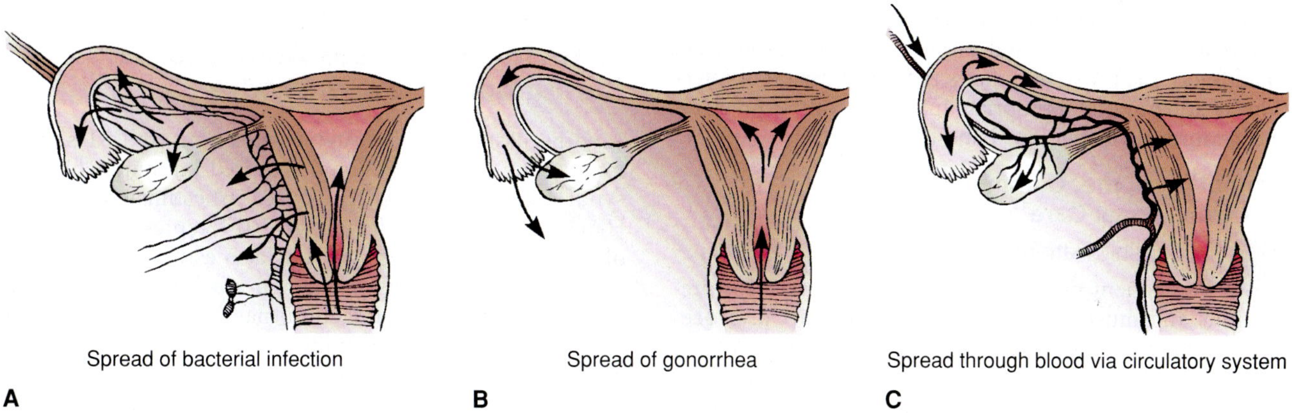

FIGURE 48-1. Pathway by which microorganisms spread in pelvic infections. **A.** Bacterial infection spreads up the vagina into the uterus and through the lymphatics. **B.** Gonorrhea spreads up the vagina into the uterus and then to the tubes and ovaries. **C.** Bacterial infection can reach the reproductive organs through the bloodstream (hematogenous spread).

Pathophysiology

The exact pathogenesis of PID has not been determined, but it is presumed that organisms usually enter the body through the vagina, pass through the cervical canal, colonize the endocervix, and move upward into the uterus. Under various conditions, the organisms may proceed to one or both fallopian tubes and ovaries and into the pelvis. In bacterial infections that occur after childbirth or abortion, pathogens are disseminated directly through the tissues that support the uterus by way of the lymphatics and blood vessels (Fig. 48-1). In pregnancy, the increased blood supply required by the placenta provides more pathways for infection. These postpartum and postabortion infections tend to be unilateral. Infections can cause perihepatic inflammation when the organism invades the peritoneum.

In gonorrheal infections, the gonococci pass through the cervical canal and into the uterus, where the environment, especially during menstruation, allows them to multiply rapidly and spread to the fallopian tubes and into the pelvis (see Fig. 48-1). The infection is usually bilateral.

In rare instances, organisms (e.g., tuberculosis) gain access to the reproductive organs by way of the bloodstream from the lungs (see Fig. 48-1). One of the most common causes of salpingitis (inflammation of the fallopian tube) is chlamydia, possibly accompanied by gonorrhea.

Pelvic infection is most often sexually transmitted but can also occur with invasive procedures such as endometrial biopsy, abortion, hysteroscopy, or insertion of an intrauterine device. Bacterial vaginosis, a vaginal infection, may predispose women to pelvic infection. Risk factors include early age at first intercourse, multiple sexual partners, frequent intercourse, intercourse without condoms, sex with a partner with an STI, and a history of STIs or previous pelvic infection.

Clinical Manifestations

Symptoms of pelvic infection usually begin with vaginal discharge, dyspareunia, dysuria, pelvic or lower abdominal pain, tenderness that occur after menses, and postcoital bleeding. Other symptoms include fever, general malaise, anorexia, nausea, headache, and possibly vomiting. On pelvic examination, intense tenderness may be noted on palpation of the uterus or movement of the cervix (cervical motion tenderness). Symptoms may be acute and severe or low grade and subtle (Brunham, Gottlieb, & Paavonen, 2015; PHAC, 2013b).

Complications

Pelvic or generalized peritonitis, abscesses, strictures, and fallopian tube obstruction may develop. Obstruction may cause an ectopic pregnancy in the future if a fertilized egg cannot pass a tubal stricture, or scar tissue may occlude the tubes, resulting in sterility. Adhesions are common and often result in chronic pelvic pain; they eventually may require removal of the uterus, fallopian tubes, and ovaries.

Medical Management

Broad-spectrum antibiotic therapy is prescribed, usually a combination of ceftriaxone (Rocephin), doxycycline, and metronidazole (Flagyl). Women are most often treated as outpatients and monitored carefully. Indications for hospitalization include surgical emergencies, pregnancy, no clinical response to oral antimicrobial therapy, inability to follow or tolerate an outpatient oral regimen, severe illness (i.e., nausea, vomiting, or high fever), and tubo-ovarian abscess (Brunham et al., 2015). Treatment of sexual partners is necessary to prevent reinfection.

Nursing Management

The nurse assesses for both the physical and emotional effects of PID. The patient may feel well one day and experience vague symptoms and discomfort the next. She may also suffer from constipation and menstrual difficulties.

If the patient is hospitalized, the nurse prepares the patient for further diagnostic evaluation and surgical intervention as prescribed. Accurate recording of vital signs, intake and output, and the characteristics and amount of vaginal discharge is necessary as a guide to therapy.

The nurse administers analgesic agents as prescribed for pain relief. Adequate rest and a healthy diet are encouraged. In addition, the nurse minimizes the transmission of infection by adhering to appropriate infection control practices and performing meticulous hand hygiene.

Promoting Home, Community-Based, and Transitional Care

Educating Patients About Self-Care

The patient must be informed of the need for precautions and must be encouraged to take part in procedures to prevent infecting others and protect herself from reinfection. The use of condoms is essential to prevent infection and sequelae. If reinfection occurs or if the infection spreads, symptoms may include abdominal pain, nausea and vomiting, fever, malaise, malodorous purulent vaginal discharge, and leukocytosis. Patient teaching consists of explaining how pelvic infections occur, how they can be controlled and avoided, and the associated signs and symptoms. Guidelines and instructions provided to the patient are summarized in Chart 48-3.

All patients who have had PID need to be informed of the signs and symptoms of ectopic pregnancy (pain, abnormal bleeding, delayed menses, faintness, dizziness, and shoulder pain) because they are prone to this complication. (See Chapter 47 for a discussion of ectopic pregnancy.)

Human Immunodeficiency Virus Infection and Acquired Immunodeficiency Syndrome

Any discussion of vulvovaginal infections and STIs must include the topic of HIV and acquired immunodeficiency syndrome (AIDS). The PHAC (2015b) estimated 595 new HIV infections among females in 2014, representing 23.2% of all new 2014 infections. They also estimate that 79.2% of new HIV infections in women are from heterosexual contact. Because HIV infection may be detected through prenatal testing and screening for STIs, nurses and other women's health care clinicians are often the first professionals to provide care for a woman with HIV infection. Thus, they need to be knowledgeable about this disorder and sensitive to women's issues and concerns (Chart 48-4).

After informed consent is obtained, women who are at risk for HIV are offered testing by a nurse or counsellor. Because patients may be reluctant to discuss risk-taking behaviour, routine screening should be offered to all women between the ages of 13 and 64 years in all health care settings (Schuiling & Likis, 2013). Early detection permits early treatment to delay progression of the disease. The nurse needs to remember that many women do not see themselves as at risk for acquiring HIV infection. See Chapter 52 for further discussion of HIV infection and AIDS.

CHART 48-3

HOME CARE CHECKLIST • The Patient With Pelvic Inflammatory Disease

At the completion of education, the patient and/or caregiver will be able to:

- State the impact of pelvic inflammatory disease on physiologic functioning, ADLs, IADLs, roles, relationships, and spirituality.
- Identify the name, dose, side effects, frequency, and schedule for all medications.
  - State the importance of completing the course of antibiotic therapy.
- Understand interventions that may prevent reoccurrence:
  - Describe proper perineal care procedures (wiping from front to back after defecation or urination).
  - Takes full course of antibiotic agents, if prescribed, after insertion of intrauterine devices.
  - Recognize that sexual partners may need treatment.
- Discuss the importance of following health practices (e.g., proper nutrition, exercise, and weight control), and safer sex practices (e.g., avoiding multiple sexual partners, consistent use of condoms before intercourse or any penile–vaginal contact if there is any chance of transmitting infection).
- State symptoms which require evaluation by a health care provider:
  - Pelvic pain or abnormal discharge, particularly after sexual exposure, childbirth, or pelvic surgery.
  - Unusual vaginal discharge or odour.
  - Pain, abnormal bleeding, delayed menses, faintness, dizziness, and shoulder pain (symptoms may indicate ectopic pregnancy).
- Relate how to reach primary provider with questions or complications.
- State time and date of follow-up medical appointments, therapy, and testing.
  - State that a gynecologic examination should be performed at least once a year.
- Identify sources of support (e.g., friends, relatives, faith community, support groups).
- Identify the need for health promotion, disease prevention, and screening activities.

ADLs, activities of daily living; IADLs, independent activities of daily living.

NURSING RESEARCH PROFILE

Chart 48-4. Life With HIV Infection

Peltzer, J., Domain, E., & Teel, C. (2015). Living in the everydayness of HIV infection: Experiences of young African-American women. *Medsurg Nursing, 24*(2), 111–118.

Purpose

The purpose of this study was to understand the lived experience of being a young African-American woman infected with HIV, and how she defines and practices both spirituality and self-care. Of US females who are HIV positive, 64% are African Americans; yet, little research has been done examining the self-care behaviours among African-American women who are infected with HIV.

Design

This study used a qualitative phenomenologic methodology. In-depth interviews were conducted with 11 African-American women, 18 to 35 years of age, who were HIV positive. The women were recruited through links provided from case managers at a safety net clinic and through an infectious disease clinic in a Midwestern, metropolitan city.

Findings

The study characterized the lived experiences of the women with HIV infection as infected lives. This predominant pattern portrays how living with HIV has impacted every aspect of their lives. The women were for the most part physically able to continue their daily routines. However, mentally and emotionally, the women were experiencing significant distress leading to chronic depression, isolation, and strained family and community relations.

Nursing Implications

Nurses should receive comprehensive HIV education that includes an overview of common, everyday experiences of women with HIV infection. Themes throughout this study clearly indicate that African-American women with HIV infection are affected in every aspect of their lives. Nurses should use the results from this study to add depression screening and assessments regarding self-care and spiritual beliefs and practices to their care of these women.

In Canada, Aboriginal people are over-represented in the HIV epidemic, with approximately 10.8% of all new infections occurring from that population (PHAC, 2015b). Women with HIV and women with partners who have HIV must be counselled about safer sex and informed about the dangers of unprotected sex. Inconsistent use of condoms results in a higher seroconversion rate. Because there is a risk of perinatal transmission, decisions to conceive or to use contraception must be based on education, accurate information, and care. Women who are pregnant are advised to have an HIV test.

The use of antiretroviral agents by women who are pregnant significantly decreases perinatal transmission of HIV infection. Therefore, the use of these agents during pregnancy is critical and must also be discussed. For women who choose to avoid conception, the use of condoms alone and with oral contraceptives are possible choices.

STRUCTURAL DISORDERS

Fistulas of the Vagina

A fistula is an abnormal opening between two internal hollow organs or between an internal hollow organ and the exterior of the body. The name of the fistula indicates the two areas that are connected abnormally: for example, a vesicovaginal fistula is an opening between the bladder and the vagina, and a rectovaginal fistula is an opening between the rectum and the vagina (Fig. 48-2). Fistulas may be congenital in origin but are most common in developing countries due to obstructed labour complications. In developed countries, they occur most often as a result of injury during pelvic surgery, vaginal delivery, radiation therapy, complications from surgical insertion of vaginal mesh, or disease processes such as carcinoma (Mellano & Tarney, 2014).

Clinical Manifestations

Symptoms depend on the specific defect. For example, in a patient with a vesicovaginal **fistula**, urine escapes continuously into the vagina. With a rectovaginal fistula, there is fecal incontinence, and flatus is discharged through the vagina. The combination of fecal discharge with leukorrhea results in malodour that is difficult to control.

Assessment and Diagnostic Findings

A history of the symptoms experienced by the patient is important to identify the structural alterations and to assess the impact of the symptoms on the patient's quality of life. Although there is no reported specificity for its use, methylene blue dye is commonly used to help delineate

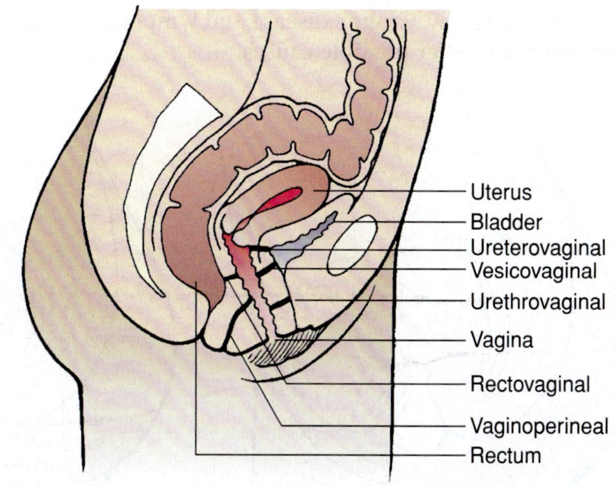

FIGURE 48-2. Common sites for vaginal fistulas: *vesicovaginal*—bladder and vagina; *urethrovaginal*—urethra and vagina; *vaginoperineal*—vagina and perineal area; *ureterovaginal*—ureter and vagina; *rectovaginal*—rectum and vagina.

the course of the fistula (Mellano & Tarney, 2014). In a vesicovaginal fistula, the dye is instilled into the bladder along with placement of vaginal packing known as the "tampon test"; stained vaginal packing can be indicative of a fistula (Mellano & Tarney, 2014). Cystourethroscopy is useful in identifying fistula while cystoscopy or IV pyelography may then be used to determine the exact location.

Medical Management

The goal is to eliminate the fistula and to treat infection and excoriation. A fistula may heal without surgical intervention, but surgery is often required. If the primary provider determines that a fistula will heal without surgical intervention, care is planned to relieve discomfort, prevent infection, and improve the patient's self-concept and self-care abilities. Measures to promote healing include proper nutrition, cleansing douches and enemas, rest, and administration of prescribed intestinal antibiotic agents. A rectovaginal fistula heals faster when the patient eats a low-residue diet and when the affected tissue drains properly. Warm perineal irrigations promote healing.

Sometimes a fistula does not heal and cannot be surgically repaired. In this situation, care must be planned and implemented on an individual basis. Cleanliness, frequent sitz baths, and deodorizing douches are required, as are perineal pads and protective undergarments. Meticulous skin care is necessary to prevent excoriation. Applying bland creams or lightly dusting with cornstarch may be soothing. In addition, attending to the patient's social and psychological needs is an essential aspect of care.

If the patient is to have a fistula repaired surgically, preoperative treatment of any existing vaginitis is important to ensure success. Usually, the vaginal approach is used to repair vesicovaginal and urethrovaginal fistulas; the abdominal approach is used to repair fistulas that are large or complex. Fistulas that are difficult to repair or very large may require surgical repair with a urinary or fecal diversion. Tissue transfer techniques (skin or tissue grafting) may be used (Mellano & Tarney, 2014).

Because fistulas usually are related to obstetric, surgical, or radiation trauma, occurrence in a patient without previous vaginal delivery or a history of surgery must be evaluated carefully. Crohn's disease and lymphogranuloma venereum are other possible causes.

Despite the best surgical intervention, fistulas may recur. After surgery, medical follow-up continues for at least 2 years to monitor for a possible recurrence.

Pelvic Organ Prolapse: Cystocele, Rectocele, Enterocele

Age and parity can put strain on the ligaments and structures that make up the female pelvis and pelvic floor. Childbirth can result in tears of the levator sling musculature, resulting in structural weakness. Hormone deficiency also may play a role. Some degree of prolapse (weakening of the vaginal walls allowing the pelvic organs to descend and protrude into the vaginal canal) may be found in many older women. Risk factors include age, parity (particularly vaginal delivery), menopause, previous pelvic surgery, and possibly a genetic predisposition (Beckmann et al., 2014).

Cystocele is a downward displacement of the bladder toward the vaginal orifice (Fig. 48-3), resulting from damage to the anterior vaginal support structures. It usually results from injury and strain during childbirth. The condition usually appears some years later when genital atrophy associated with aging occurs, but younger women who are multiparous and premenopausal may also be affected.

Rectocele is an upward pouching of the rectum that pushes the posterior wall of the vagina forward. Both rectoceles and perineal lacerations, which occur because of muscle tears below the vagina, may affect the muscles and tissues of the pelvic floor and may occur during childbirth. Sometimes the lacerations may completely sever the fibres of the anal sphincter (complete tear). An **enterocele** is a protrusion of the intestinal wall into the vagina. Prolapse results from a weakening of the support structures of the uterus itself; the cervix drops and may protrude from the vagina. If complete prolapse occurs (cervix descending beyond vulva), it may also be referred to as procidentia.

Clinical Manifestations

Because a cystocele causes the anterior vaginal wall to bulge downward, the patient may report a sense of pelvic pressure and urinary problems such as incontinence, frequency, and urgency. Back pain and pelvic pain may occur

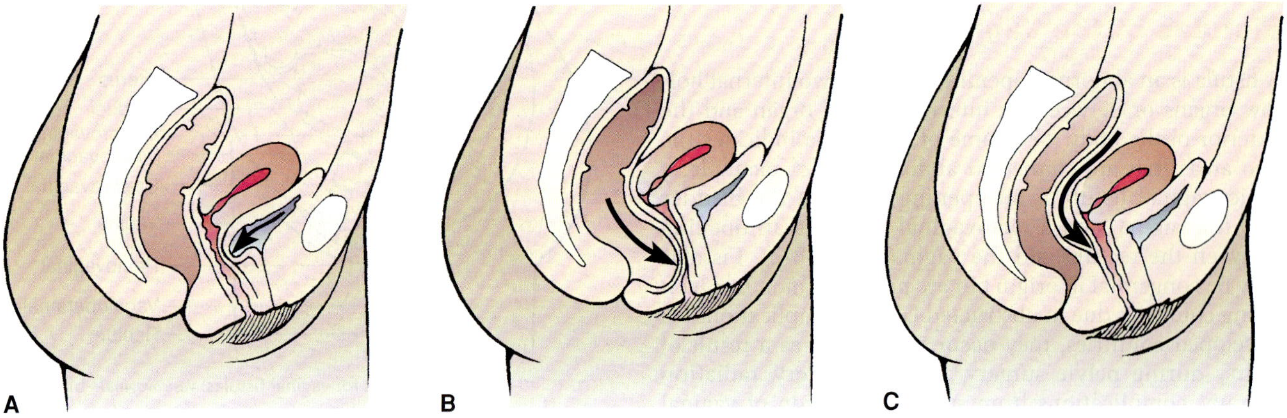

FIGURE 48-3. Diagrammatic representation of the three most common types of pelvic floor relaxation: cystocele (A), rectocele (B), and enterocele (C). *Arrows* depict sites of maximum protrusion.

as well. The symptoms of rectocele resemble those of cystocele, with one exception: instead of urinary symptoms, patients may experience rectal pressure. Constipation, uncontrollable gas, and fecal incontinence may occur in patients with complete tears. Prolapse can result in feelings of pressure and ulcerations and bleeding. Dyspareunia may occur with these disorders.

Medical Management

Kegel exercises, which involve contracting or tightening the vaginal muscles, are prescribed to help strengthen these weakened muscles (Beckmann et al., 2014). The exercises are more effective in the early stages of a cystocele. Kegel exercises are easy to perform and are recommended for all women, including those with strong pelvic floor muscles (Chart 48-5).

A pessary can be used alone or in conjunction with other treatments to avoid surgery (McIntosh, Andersen, & Reekie, 2015). This device is inserted into the vagina and positioned to keep an organ, such as the bladder, uterus, or intestine, properly aligned when a cystocele, rectocele, or prolapse has occurred. Pessaries are usually ring or doughnut shaped and are made of various materials, such as rubber or plastic (Fig. 48-4). Rubber pessaries must be avoided in women with latex allergy. The size and type of pessary are selected and fitted by a gynecologic health care provider. The patient should have the pessary removed, examined, and cleaned by her health care provider at prescribed intervals. At these checkups, vaginal walls should be examined for pressure points or signs of irritation. Normally, the patient experiences no pain, discomfort, or discharge with a pessary, but if chronic irritation, excessive discharge, or bleeding occurs, alternative measures may be needed (McIntosh et al., 2015).

A Colpexin Sphere is another nonsurgical device used to treat pelvic organ prolapse. This intravaginal device is similar to a pessary, but it supports the pelvic floor muscles and facilitates exercise of these muscles. It is removed daily for cleaning.

CHART 48-5

Patient Education: Performing Kegel (Pelvic Muscle) Exercises

Purposes: To strengthen and maintain the tone of the pubococcygeal muscle, which supports the pelvic organs; reduce or prevent stress incontinence and uterine prolapse; enhance sensation during sexual intercourse; and hasten postpartum healing.

The nurse instructs the patient to:

1. Become aware of pelvic muscle function by "drawing in" the perivaginal muscles and anal sphincter as if to control urine or defecation, but not contracting the abdominal, buttock, or inner thigh muscles.
2. Sustain contraction of the muscles for up to 10 seconds, followed by at least 10 seconds of relaxation.
3. Perform these exercises 30 to 80 times a day.

Surgical Management

In many cases, surgery helps correct structural abnormalities. The procedure to repair the anterior vaginal wall is called anterior colporrhaphy, repair of a rectocele is referred to as a posterior colporrhaphy, and repair of perineal lacerations is called a perineorrhaphy. These repairs are frequently performed laparoscopically, resulting in short hospital lengths of stay and good outcomes. A laparoscope is inserted through a small abdominal incision, the pelvis is visualized, and surgical repairs are performed. Transvaginal surgical mesh as a treatment option has been associated with the complications of vaginal erosion, pain, and infection leading to a 2014 advisory issued from Health Canada for recommendations and close monitoring of adverse outcomes (Health Canada, 2014).

Uterine Prolapse

Usually the uterus and the cervix lie at right angles to the long axis of the vagina with the body of the uterus inclined

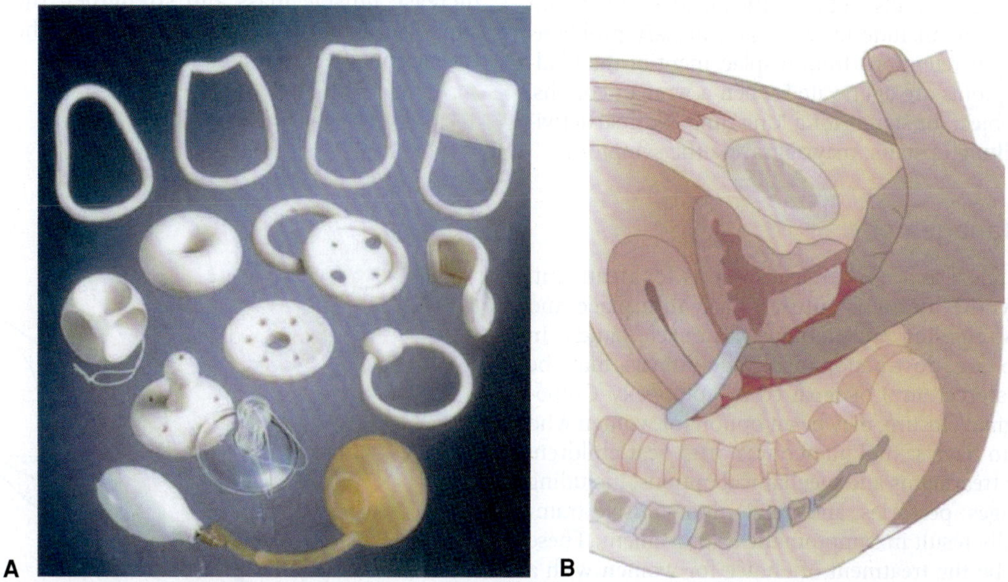

FIGURE 48-4. Examples of pessaries. **A.** Various shapes and sizes of pessaries available. **B.** Insertion of one type of pessary.

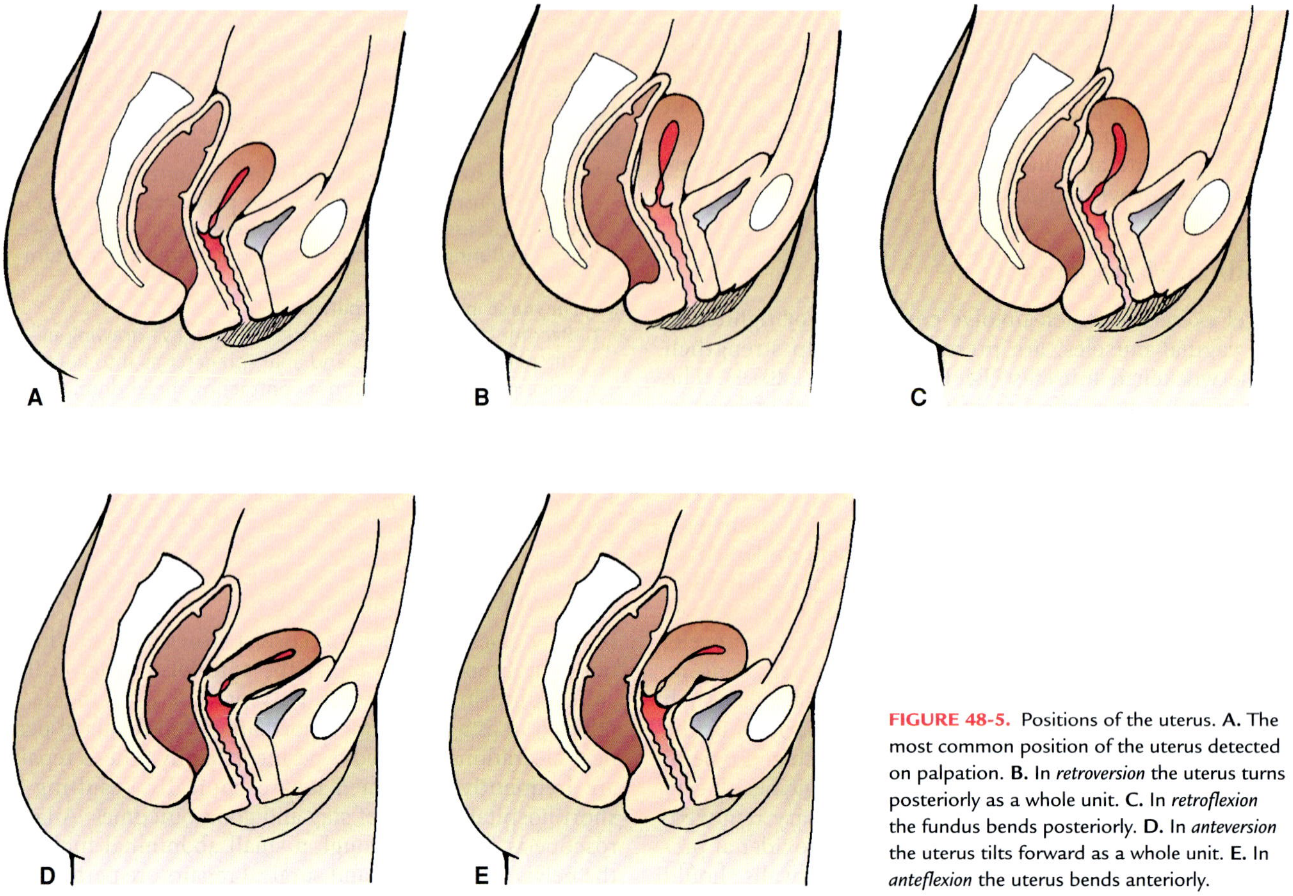

FIGURE 48-5. Positions of the uterus. **A.** The most common position of the uterus detected on palpation. **B.** In *retroversion* the uterus turns posteriorly as a whole unit. **C.** In *retroflexion* the fundus bends posteriorly. **D.** In *anteversion* the uterus tilts forward as a whole unit. **E.** In *anteflexion* the uterus bends anteriorly.

slightly forward. The uterus is normally freely movable on examination. Individual variations may result in an anterior, middle, or posterior uterine position. A backward positioning of the uterus, known as retroversion and retroflexion, is not uncommon (Fig. 48-5).

If the structures that support the uterus weaken (typically from childbirth), the uterus may work its way down the vaginal canal (prolapse) and even appear outside the vaginal orifice (procidentia) (Fig. 48-6). As the uterus descends, it may pull the vaginal walls and even the bladder and rectum with it. Symptoms include pressure and urinary problems (incontinence or retention) from displacement of the bladder. The symptoms are aggravated when a woman coughs, lifts a heavy object, or stands for a long time. Normal activities, even walking upstairs, may aggravate the symptoms.

Medical Management

There are surgical and nonsurgical options for treatment. With surgery, the uterus is sutured back into place and repaired to strengthen and tighten the muscle bands. In women who are postmenopausal, the uterus may be removed (**hysterectomy**) or repaired by colpopexy. Colpocleisis, or vaginal closure, may be an option for women who do not wish to have sexual intercourse or to bear children. Conservative treatments and mechanical options, including lifestyle changes, pessaries, and pelvic floor muscle training, can usually result in symptomatic improvement. These options may be the treatment of choice for women with a mild prolapse, who desire additional children, or who are unable to tolerate surgery (Jepson & Sung, 2014).

Nursing Management

Implementing Preventive Measures

Some disorders related to "relaxed" pelvic muscles (cystocele, rectocele, and uterine prolapse) may be prevented. During pregnancy, early visits to the primary provider permit early detection of problems. During the postpartum period, the woman can be educated to perform pelvic muscle exercises, commonly known as Kegel exercises, to increase muscle mass and strengthen the muscles that support the uterus and then to continue them as a preventive action (Beckmann et al., 2014).

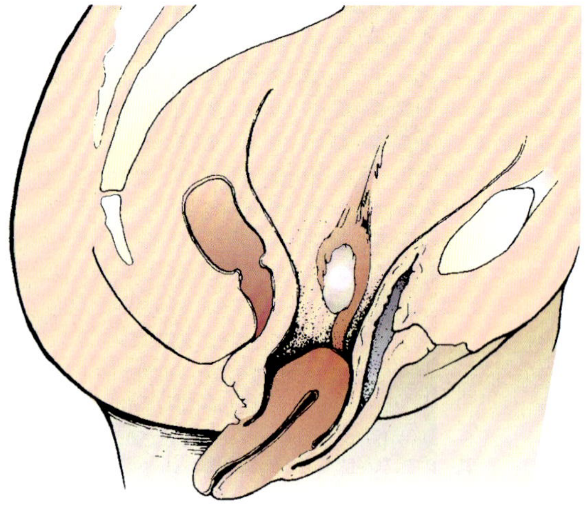

FIGURE 48-6. Complete prolapse of the uterus through the introitus.

Delays in obtaining evaluation and treatment may result in complications such as infection, cervical ulceration, cystitis, and hemorrhoids. The nurse encourages the patient to obtain prompt treatment for these structural disorders.

Implementing Preoperative Nursing Care

Before surgery, the patient needs to know the extent of the proposed surgery, the expectations for the postoperative period, and the effect of surgery on future sexual function. In addition, the patient having a rectocele repair needs to know that before surgery, a laxative and a cleansing enema may be prescribed. She may be asked to administer these at home the day before surgery. The patient is usually placed in a lithotomy position for surgery, with special attention given to moving both legs in and out of the stirrups simultaneously to prevent muscle strain and excess pressure on the legs and thighs. Other preoperative interventions are similar to those described in Chapter 19.

Initiating Postoperative Nursing Care

Immediate postoperative goals include preventing infection and pressure on any existing suture line. This may require perineal care and may preclude using dressings. The patient is encouraged to void within a few hours after surgery for cystocele and complete tear. If the patient does not void within this period and reports discomfort or pain in the bladder region after 6 hours, she needs to be catheterized. An indwelling catheter may be indicated for 2 to 4 days, so some women may return home with a catheter in place. Various other bladder care methods are described in Chapter 46. After each voiding or bowel movement, the perineum may be cleansed with warm, sterile saline solution and dried with sterile absorbent material if a perineal incision has been made.

After an external perineal repair, the perineum is kept as clean as possible. Commercially available sprays containing combined antiseptic and anesthetic solutions are soothing and effective, and an ice pack applied locally may relieve discomfort. However, the weight of the ice bag must rest on the bed, not on the patient.

Routine postoperative care is similar to that given after abdominal surgery. The patient is positioned in bed with her head and knees elevated slightly. The patient may go home the day of or the day after surgery; the length of hospital stay depends on the surgical approach used.

After surgery for a complete perineal laceration (through the rectal sphincter), special care and attention are required. The bladder is drained through the catheter to prevent strain on the sutures. Throughout recovery, stool-softening agents are given nightly after the patient begins a soft diet.

Promoting Home, Community-Based, and Transitional Care

Educating Patients About Self-Care

Prior to discharge, education is provided about cleanliness, prevention of constipation, recommended exercises, and avoiding lifting heavy objects or standing for prolonged periods. The patient is instructed to report any pelvic pain, unusual discharge, inability to carry out personal hygiene, and vaginal bleeding.

Continuing and Transitional Care

The patient is advised to continue with perineal exercises, which are recommended to improve muscle strength and tone. She is reminded to return to the gynecologist for a follow-up visit and to consult with the primary provider about when it is safe to resume sexual activity.

BENIGN DISORDERS

Vulvitis and Vulvodynia

Vulvitis (an inflammation of the vulva) may occur with other disorders, such as diabetes, dermatologic problems, or poor hygiene, or it may be secondary to irritation from a vaginal discharge related to a specific vaginitis.

Vulvodynia is a chronic vulvar pain syndrome. Symptoms may include burning, stinging, irritation, or stabbing pain. The syndrome has been described as primary, with onset at first tampon insertion or sexual experience, or secondary, beginning months or years after first tampon insertion or sexual experience. Women affected by this are usually between 18 and 25 years of age. Vulvodynia may be classified as organic if it has a known cause (infection, trauma, or irritants) or idiopathic if no cause is known. It can be chronic or unremitting, intermittent or episodic, or may occur only in response to contact (Hoffstetter & Shah, 2015). The pathophysiology is unknown. Vestibulodynia is the most frequent type of vulvodynia, producing sharp pain on pressure on the vestibule or posterior aspect of the vaginal opening.

Medical Management

Treatment methods for vulvodynia vary and depend on cause. Topical treatments, self-management care (strict vulvar care/hygiene), surgery, as well as biofeedback and dietary changes have been used. Some cases seem to be similar to peripheral neuralgia and may respond to treatment with tricyclic antidepressant agents. Patients with dyspareunia or painful intercourse may benefit from referral to a behavioural or mental health professional. Research continues on the use of hypnotherapy for symptom management (Hoffstetter & Shah, 2015).

Vulvar Cysts

Bartholin's cyst results from the obstruction of a duct in one of the paired Bartholin or vestibular mucous-secreting glands located in the posterior third of the vulva, near the vestibule. This cyst is the most common vulvar disorder. A simple cyst may be asymptomatic, but an infected cyst or abscess may cause discomfort. Infection may be due to a gonococcal organism, *Escherichia coli*, or *Staphylococcus aureus* and can cause an abscess with or without involving the inguinal lymph nodes. Skene's duct cysts may result in pressure, dyspareunia, altered urinary stream, and pain, especially if infection is present. Vestibular cysts, located inferior to the hymen, may also occur. Cysts can be treated by resection or with laser, ablation with silver nitrate, and puncture. Asymptomatic cysts do not require treatment. Malignancy can occur, usually in women older than 50 years of age; so drainage and biopsy may be considered (Maldonado, 2014).

Medical Management

The usual treatment for a Bartholin's cyst or abscess is drainage. If a cyst is asymptomatic, treatment is unnecessary. Moist heat or sitz baths may promote drainage and resolution. If drainage is necessary, several techniques are available. The simplest technique is incision and drainage. Using a Word catheter is another method. This catheter, which is a short latex stem with an inflatable bulb at the distal end, creates a tract that preserves the gland and allows for drainage. A nonopioid analgesic agent may be given before this outpatient procedure. A local anesthetic agent is injected, and the cyst is incised or lanced and irrigated with normal saline; the catheter is inserted and inflated with 2 to 3 mL of water. The catheter stem is then tucked into the vagina to allow freedom of movement. The catheter is left in place for 4 to 6 weeks (Maldonado, 2014). The patient is informed that discharge should be expected because the catheter allows drainage of the cyst. She is instructed to contact her primary provider if pain occurs, in which case the bulb may be too large for the cavity and fluid may need to be removed. Routine hygiene is encouraged. Marsupialization (creation of small pouch) and gland removal are additional treatment options (Maldonado, 2014).

Vulvar Dystrophy

Vulvar dystrophy is a condition found in older women that causes dry, thickened skin on the vulva or slightly raised, whitish papules, fissures, or macules. Symptoms usually consist of varying degrees of itching, but some patients have no symptoms. A few patients with vulvar cancer have associated dystrophy (vulvar cancer is discussed later in this chapter). Biopsy with careful follow-up is the standard intervention. Benign dystrophies include lichen planus, lichen simplex chronicus, lichen sclerosus (benign disorder of the vulva), squamous cell hyperplasia, vulvar vestibulitis (inflammation of the vulvar vestibule), and other dermatoses (Beckmann et al., 2014).

Medical Management

Topical corticosteroids (i.e., hydrocortisone creams) are the usual treatment. Petrolatum jelly may relieve pruritus. Use is decreased as symptoms resolve. Topical corticosteroids are effective in treating squamous cell hyperplasia. Treatment is often complete in 2 to 3 weeks, but ongoing assessment for vulvar atrophy should occur at least annually (Beckmann et al., 2014).

If malignant cells are detected on biopsy, local excision, laser therapy, local chemotherapy, and immunologic treatment are used. **Vulvectomy** is avoided, if possible, to spare the patient from the stress of disfigurement and possible sexual dysfunction.

Nursing Management

Key nursing responsibilities for patients with vulvar dystrophies focus on teaching. Important topics include hygiene and self-monitoring for signs and symptoms of complications.

Promoting Home, Community-Based, and Transitional Care

Educating Patients About Self-Care

Instructions for patients with benign vulvar dystrophies include the importance of maintaining good personal hygiene and keeping the vulva dry. Lanolin or hydrogenated vegetable oil is recommended for relief of dryness. Sitz baths may help but should not be overused because dryness may result or increase. The patient is instructed to notify her primary provider about any change or ulceration because biopsy may be necessary to rule out squamous cell carcinoma.

By encouraging all patients to perform genital self-examinations regularly and have any itching, lesions, or unusual symptoms assessed by a health care provider, nurses can help prevent complications and progression of vulvar lesions. Ongoing assessment should occur at least annually.

Ovarian Cysts

The ovary is a common site for cysts, which may be simple enlargements of normal ovarian constituents, the graafian follicle, or the corpus luteum, or they may arise from abnormal growth of the ovarian epithelium. Ovarian cysts are often detected on routine pelvic examination. Although these cysts are typically benign, they nevertheless should be evaluated to exclude ovarian cancer, particularly in women who are postmenopausal (ACOG, 2007, reaffirmed 2015).

The patient may or may not report acute or chronic abdominal pain. Symptoms of a ruptured cyst mimic various acute abdominal emergencies, such as appendicitis or ectopic pregnancy. Larger cysts may produce abdominal swelling and exert pressure on adjacent abdominal organs.

Postoperative nursing care after surgery to remove an ovarian cyst is similar to that after abdominal surgery, with one exception. The marked decrease in intra-abdominal pressure resulting from removal of a very large cyst usually leads to considerable abdominal distention. This may be prevented to some extent by applying a snug-fitting abdominal binder.

Some surgeons discuss the option of a hysterectomy when a woman is undergoing bilateral ovary removal because of a suspicious mass; it may increase life expectancy and avoid a later second surgery. Patient preference is a priority in determining its appropriateness.

Polycystic ovary syndrome (PCOS) is a type of hormonal imbalance or cystic disorder that affects the ovaries. This complex endocrine condition involves a disorder in the hypothalamic–pituitary and ovarian network or axis, resulting in chronic anovulation and hyperandrogenism, often along with multiple small ovarian cysts. It is common and occurs in approximately 6% to 15% of women of childbearing age (Trikudanathan, 2015). Features can include obesity, insulin resistance, impaired glucose tolerance, dyslipidemia, sleep apnea, and infertility. Symptoms are related to androgen excess. Irregular menstrual periods, resulting from lack of regular ovulation, infertility, obesity, and hirsutism, may be a presenting complaint. Cysts form in the ovaries because the hormonal milieu cannot cause ovulation on a regular basis.

Diagnosis is based on clinical criteria, including hyperandrogenism, chronic anovulation, and polycystic ovaries on ultrasound examination. Two out of three of these criteria must be present to make the diagnosis (Trikudanathan, 2015). Women with PCOS are at an increased risk for diabetes, increased blood lipids, cardiovascular disease, nonalcoholic fatty liver disease as well as anxiety and depression (Trikudanathan, 2015).

Medical Management

The treatment of large ovarian cysts is usually surgical removal. However, oral contraceptives may be used in young, healthy patients to suppress ovarian activity and resolve small cysts that appear to be fluid filled or physiologic.

Oral contraceptive agents are also usually prescribed to treat PCOS (Trikudanathan, 2015). When pregnancy is desired, medications to stimulate ovulation (clomiphene citrate [Clomid]) are often effective. Lifestyle modification is critical, and weight management is part of the treatment plan.

Weight loss as little as 5% to 10% of total body weight can help with hormone imbalance and infertility. Metformin (Glucophage) often regulates periods and can help with weight loss (Trikudanathan, 2015). Women with this diagnosis are at increased risk for endometrial cancer due to anovulation.

Benign Tumours of the Uterus: Fibroids (Leiomyomas, Myomas)

Myomatous or **fibroid tumours** of the uterus are estimated to occur in one in three women during their reproductive years. It is thought that women are genetically predisposed to develop this condition, which is almost always benign. Fibroids arise from the muscle tissue of the uterus and can be solitary or multiple, in the lining (intracavitary), muscle wall (intramural), and outside surface (serosal) of the uterus. They usually develop slowly in women between 25 and 40 years of age and may become quite large. A growth spurt with enlargement of the fibroid tumour may occur in the decade before menopause, possibly related to anovulatory cycles and high levels of unopposed estrogen. Fibroids are a common reason for hysterectomy because they often result in menorrhagia, which can be difficult to control.

Clinical Manifestations

Fibroids may cause no symptoms, or they may produce abnormal vaginal bleeding. Other symptoms result from pressure on the surrounding organs and include pain, backache, pressure, bloating, constipation, and urinary problems. Menorrhagia (excessive bleeding) and metrorrhagia (irregular bleeding) may occur because fibroids may distort the uterine lining (Fig. 48-7). Fibroids may interfere with fertility.

Medical Management

Treatment of uterine fibroids may include medical or surgical intervention and depends to a large extent on the size, symptoms, and location, as well as the woman's age and her reproductive plans. Fibroids usually shrink and disappear during menopause, when estrogen is no longer

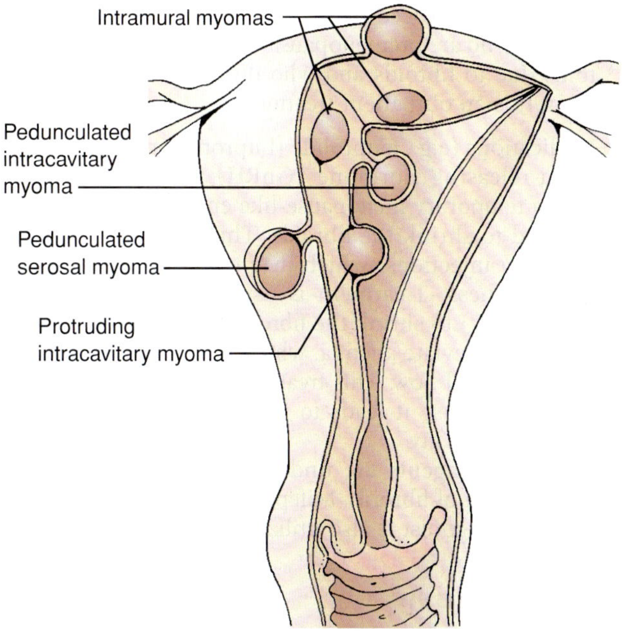

FIGURE 48-7. Myomas (fibroids). Those that impinge on the uterine cavity are called intracavitary myomas.

produced. Simple observation and follow-up may be all the management that is necessary. The patient with minor symptoms is closely monitored. If she plans to have children, treatment is as conservative as possible. As a rule, **myomectomy** (surgical removal of uterine fibroids) is performed for large tumours that produce pressure symptoms. A hysterectomy may be performed if symptoms are severe and childbearing is completed (see later discussion of nursing care for a patient having a hysterectomy).

Several alternatives to hysterectomy have been developed for the treatment of excessive bleeding due to fibroids (Canadian Women's Health Network [CWHN], 2012). These include the following:

- *Hysteroscopic resection of myomas:* A laser is used through a hysteroscope passed through the cervix; no incision or overnight stay is needed.
- *Laparoscopic myomectomy:* Removal of a fibroid through a laparoscope inserted through a small abdominal incision.
- *Laparoscopic myolysis:* The use of a laser or electrical needles to cauterize and shrink the fibroid.
- *Laparoscopic cryomyolysis:* Electric current is used to coagulate the fibroid.
- *Uterine artery embolization (UAE):* Polyvinyl alcohol or gelatin particles are injected into the blood vessels that supply the fibroid via the femoral artery, resulting in infarction and resultant shrinkage. This percutaneous image–guided therapy offers an alternative to hormone therapy or surgery. UAE may result in infrequent but serious complications such as pain, infection, amenorrhea, necrosis, and bleeding. Although rare, deaths and ovarian failure may occur. Women need to weigh the risks and benefits carefully, especially if they have not completed childbearing.
- *Magnetic resonance–guided focused ultrasound surgery (MRgFUS):* Ultrasonic energy is passed through the abdominal wall to target and destroy the fibroid. This

noninvasive procedure is approved by the FDA for women who are premenopausal with bothersome symptoms due to fibroids and who do not want more children. It is an outpatient treatment.

Medications (e.g., leuprolide [Lupron]) or other gonadotropin-releasing hormone (GnRH) analogues, which induce a temporary menopause-like environment, may be prescribed to shrink the fibroids. This treatment consists of monthly injections, which may cause hot flashes and vaginal dryness. Treatment is usually short term (i.e., before surgery) to shrink the fibroids, allowing easier surgery, and to alleviate anemia, which may occur because of heavy menstrual flow. This treatment is used on a temporary basis because it leads to vasomotor symptoms and loss of bone density.

Antifibrotic agents are under investigation for long-term treatment of fibroids. Mifepristone (Mifeprex), a progesterone antagonist is also utilized.

Endometriosis

Endometriosis is a chronic disease affecting between 7% and 10% of women of reproductive age, occurring more frequently in women who have never had children (Beckmann et al., 2014). Endometriosis consists of a benign lesion or lesions that contain endometrial tissue (similar to that lining the uterus) found in the pelvic cavity outside the uterus. Extensive endometriosis may cause few symptoms or an isolated lesion may produce severe symptoms. It is a major cause of chronic pelvic pain and infertility.

Endometriosis has been diagnosed more frequently because of the increased use of laparoscopy. There is a high incidence among patients who bear children late and among those who have fewer children. In countries where tradition favours early marriage and early childbearing, endometriosis is rare. There also appears to be a familial predisposition to endometriosis; it is more common in women whose close female relatives are affected. Other factors that may suggest increased risk include a shorter menstrual cycle (less than every 27 days), flow longer than 7 days, outflow obstruction, and younger age at menarche.

Pathophysiology

Misplaced endometrial tissue responds to and depends on ovarian hormonal stimulation. During menstruation, this ectopic tissue bleeds, mostly into areas having no outlet, which causes pain and adhesions. The lesions are typically small and puckered, with a blue/brown/grey powder-burn appearance and brown or blue-black appearance, indicating concealed bleeding.

Endometrial tissue contained within an ovarian cyst has no outlet for the bleeding; this formation is referred to as a pseudocyst or chocolate cyst. Adhesions, cysts, and scar tissue may result, causing pain and infertility (Beckmann et al., 2014). **Endometriosis** may increase the risk of ovarian cancer.

Currently the best-accepted theory regarding the origin of endometrial lesions is the transplantation theory, which suggests that a backflow of menses (retrograde menstruation) transports endometrial tissue to ectopic sites through the fallopian tubes. Why some women with retrograde menstruation develop endometriosis and others do not is unknown. Endometrial tissue can also be spread by lymphatic or venous channels.

Clinical Manifestations

Symptoms vary but include dysmenorrhea, dyspareunia, and pelvic discomfort or pain. Dyschezia (pain with bowel movements) and radiation of pain to the back or leg may occur. Depression, loss of work due to pain, and relationship difficulties may result. Infertility may occur because of fibrosis and adhesions or because of a variety of substances (prostaglandins, cytokines, other factors) produced by the implants of endometriosis and scar tissue on anatomical sites.

Assessment and Diagnostic Findings

A health history, including an account of the menstrual pattern, is necessary to elicit specific symptoms. On bimanual pelvic examination, fixed tender nodules are sometimes palpated, and uterine mobility may be limited, indicating adhesions. Laparoscopic examination confirms the diagnosis and helps stage the disease. In stage 1, patients have superficial or minimal lesions; stage 2, mild involvement; stage 3, moderate involvement; and stage 4, extensive involvement and dense adhesions, with obliteration of the cul-de-sac. Ultrasonography, magnetic resonance imaging (MRI), and CT scans may also be useful to visualize endometriosis (Beckmann et al., 2014).

Medical Management

Treatment depends on the symptoms, the patient's desire for pregnancy, and the extent of the disease. If the woman does not have symptoms, routine examination may be all that is required. Other therapies for varying degrees of symptoms may be NSAIDs, oral contraceptive agents, GnRH agonists, or surgery. Pregnancy often alleviates symptoms because neither ovulation nor menstruation occur.

Pharmacologic Therapy

Palliative measures include use of medications, such as analgesic agents and prostaglandin inhibitors, for pain. Hormonal therapy is effective in suppressing endometriosis and relieving dysmenorrhea (menstrual pain). Oral contraceptive agents provide effective pain relief and may prevent disease progression (Beckmann et al., 2014). Infrequently, side effects may occur with oral contraceptive agents, such as fluid retention, weight gain, and nausea. These can usually be managed by changing brands or formulations.

Several types of hormonal therapy are also available in addition to oral contraceptives. A synthetic androgen, danazol (Danocrine), causes atrophy of the endometrium and subsequent amenorrhea. The medication inhibits the release of gonadotropin with minimal overt sex hormone stimulation. The drawbacks of this medication are that it is expensive and may cause troublesome side effects such as fatigue, depression, weight gain, oily skin, decreased breast size, mild acne, hot flashes, and vaginal atrophy (Beckmann et al., 2014). GnRH agonists decrease estrogen production and cause subsequent amenorrhea. Side effects are related to low estrogen levels (e.g., hot flashes and vaginal dryness). Loss of bone density is often offset by concurrent use of estrogen. If side effects from GnRH develop, treatment is needed long term, or repeated treatments are necessary, additional therapy should be considered. Norethindrone acetate (Aygestin) (low-dose hormone) given along with GnRH agonist will mitigate the bone density side effects as well as not affect the drug's control of pelvic pain. Aromatase inhibitor therapy is emerging as an alternative therapy (Beckmann et al., 2014). Most women continue treatment despite side effects, and symptoms diminish for 80% to 90% of women with mild to moderate endometriosis. Hormonal medications are not used in patients with a history of abnormal vaginal bleeding or liver, heart, or kidney disease. Bone density is followed carefully because of the risk of bone loss; hormone therapy is usually short term.

Surgical Management

If conservative measures are not helpful, surgery may be necessary to relieve pain and improve the possibility of pregnancy. Surgery may be combined with the use of medical therapy. The procedure selected depends on the patient. Laparoscopy may be used to fulgurate (cut with high-frequency current) endometrial implants and to release adhesions. Laser surgery is another option made possible by laparoscopy. Laser therapy vaporizes or coagulates the endometrial implants, thereby destroying this tissue. Other surgical options include endocoagulation and electrocoagulation, laparotomy, abdominal hysterectomy, **oophorectomy** (removal of the ovary), bilateral **salpingo-oophorectomy** (removal of the ovary and its fallopian tube), and appendectomy. Many women require further intervention following conservative surgeries; therefore, total hysterectomy is the definitive procedure (Beckmann et al., 2014).

Nursing Management

The health history and physical examination focus on specific symptoms (e.g., pain), the effect of prescribed medications, and the woman's reproductive plans. This information helps in determining the treatment plan. Explaining the various diagnostic procedures may help to alleviate the patient's anxiety. Patient goals include relief of pain, dysmenorrhea, dyspareunia, and avoidance of infertility.

As the treatment progresses, the woman with endometriosis and her partner may find that pregnancy is not easily possible, and the psychosocial impact of this realization must be recognized and addressed. Alternatives, such as assisted reproductive technologies or adoption, may be discussed at an appropriate time and referrals offered.

The nurse's role in patient education is to dispel myths and encourage the patient to seek care if dysmenorrhea or dyspareunia occurs. The Endometriosis Association (Endometriosisinfo.ca) is a helpful resource for patients seeking further information and support for this condition, which can cause disabling pain and severe emotional distress.

Chronic Pelvic Pain

Chronic pelvic pain is a common disorder of women that may be related to several of the previously discussed gynecologic disorders. Chronic pelvic pain is defined as noncyclic pain concentrated in the pelvis, anterior abdominal wall, and buttock or lumbosacral region for a period greater than 6 months (Steege & Siedhoff, 2014). Causes may be of reproductive, genitourinary, or gastrointestinal origin. A history of sexual and physical abuse, PID, endometriosis, interstitial cystitis, musculoskeletal disorders, irritable bowel syndrome, and previous surgery resulting in abdominal adhesions may be associated with chronic pelvic pain. Dysmenorrhea, dyspareunia, and lower abdominal pain may also be associated with sexual and physical abuse.

Chronic pelvic pain is often difficult to treat. Treatment depends on physical and diagnostic test results and may include antidepressant, analgesic, anxiolytics, and oral contraceptive agents; GnRH agonists; exercise; diet modification; and various surgical procedures (Steege & Siedhoff, 2014).

Adenomyosis

In adenomyosis, the tissue that lines the endometrium invades the uterine wall. Symptoms include hypermenorrhea (excessive and prolonged bleeding), dysmenorrhea, polymenorrhea (abnormally frequent bleeding), and pelvic pain. Physical examination findings on palpation include a symmetrically enlarged, tender, and boggy uterus (Beckmann et al., 2014). Treatment depends on the severity of bleeding and pain. Hysterectomy may be the best option in providing relief of symptoms.

Endometrial Hyperplasia

Endometrial hyperplasia (a build-up of endometrial tissue) is the most common precursor to endometrial cancer and often results from unopposed estrogen from any source. Estrogen therapy alone without progesterone in a woman with a uterus can cause this condition. Women with anovulatory cycles, PCOS, or obesity may have high circulating levels of estrogen. Tamoxifen (Nolvadex) may also be a causative factor. Diagnosis is by biopsy or ultrasound findings of thickness of the endometrium. Hyperplasia with atypia on a pathology or biopsy report indicates risk of progression. Progestin treatment may be effective, but hysterectomy may be advised if pathology from an endometrial biopsy shows atypia. Abnormal bleeding is the most common symptom.

MALIGNANT CONDITIONS

In Canada, reproductive system cancers accounted for 12% of all new cases of cancer. The most common types of female reproductive system cancers were cancers of the uterus, ovary, and cervix, with 90% of cases developing in one of these three sites (Statistics Canada, 2015). The Canadian Cancer Society (CCS, 2017) projected the 2017 incidence and estimated mortality for female reproductive cancers in Canada as follows:

- Cervical cancer: about 1,550 new cases and 400 deaths
- Uterine cancer: about 7,300 new cases and 1,150 deaths
- Ovarian cancer: about 2,800 new cases and 1,800 deaths

Cervical cancer is the second most prevalent cancer in women worldwide and the fifth leading cause of cancer deaths. Worldwide, the incidence is declining. Pap smears in developed countries have resulted in increased detection of preinvasive lesions and decreased cancer death rates.

Death rates from all cancers are decreasing in Canada and other developed countries, while cancer in developing countries is increasing. Many of these cases affect women. Although infectious diseases and HIV are often high priorities in these countries, the toll of increasing malignancies needs to be considered.

Although some cancers are difficult to detect or prevent, annual pelvic examination with a Pap smear is a painless and relatively inexpensive method of early detection (CCS, 2018b). Primary providers can encourage women to follow this health practice by providing examinations that are educational and supportive and offer women an opportunity to ask questions and clarify misinformation.

Women diagnosed with gynecologic malignancies experience anxiety related to their prognosis. The occurrence of physical symptoms may cause more psychological distress. Intervention directed toward physical and psychological symptoms requires a multidisciplinary approach.

Nurses should be aware of ongoing clinical trials to identify options for many conditions. They are often able to answer questions about clinical trials and to encourage patients to consider participation if appropriate. Women's participation in cancer research may not occur in part because women are unaware of ongoing relevant research.

Cancer of the Cervix

Death from cervical cancer is less common due to early detection of cell changes by Pap smear (CCS, 2018b). However, in Canada, it is still the 13th most common female cancer and has an estimated incidence rate of 6.5 to 10.7 per 100,000 (CCS, 2017).

Carcinoma of the cervix is predominantly squamous cell cancer. Cervical cancer is less common than it once was because of early detection of cell changes by Pap smear. Risk factors are presented in Chart 48-6.

Preventive measures include regular pelvic examinations and Pap tests for all women, especially older women past childbearing age. Preventive counselling should encourage delaying first intercourse, avoiding HPV infection, participating only in safer sex, smoking cessation, and receiving HPV immunization.

There are several different types of cervical cancer. Most of these cancers are squamous cell carcinomas and the remainder are adenocarcinomas or mixed adenosquamous carcinomas. Adenocarcinomas begin in mucous-producing glands and are often due to HPV infection. Most cervical cancers, if not detected and treated, spread to regional pelvic lymph nodes, and local recurrence is not uncommon.

Clinical Manifestations

Early cervical cancer rarely produces symptoms. If symptoms are present, they may go unnoticed as a thin watery vaginal discharge often noticed after intercourse or douching. When symptoms such as discharge, irregular bleeding, or pain or bleeding after sexual intercourse occur, the disease may be advanced. Advanced disease should not occur if all women have access to gynecologic care and avail themselves of it. The nurse's role in access to care and its utilization is crucial.

CHART 48-6

Risk Factors: Cervical Cancer

- Chronic cervical infection
- Early childbearing
- Exposure to diethylstilbestrol in utero
- Exposure to human papillomavirus, types 16 and 18
- Family history of cervical cancer
- HIV infection and other causes of immune deficiency
- Low socioeconomic status (may be related to early marriage and early childbearing)
- Nutritional deficiencies (folate, beta-carotene, and vitamin C levels are lower in women with cervical cancer than in women without it)
- Overweight status
- Prolonged use of oral contraceptives
- Sexual activity:
  - Multiple sex partners
  - Early age (<20 years) at first coitus (exposes the vulnerable young cervix to potential viruses from a partner)
- Sexual contact with men whose partners have had cervical cancer
- Sex with uncircumcised men
- Smoking and exposure to secondhand smoke

HIV, human immunodeficiency virus.
Adapted from Canadian Cancer Society (CCS). (2018b). *Cervical cancer*. Retrieved from http://www.cancer.ca/en/cancer-information/cancer-type/cervical/screening/?region=nl; Barakat, R. R., Berchuk, A., Markman, M., et al. (Eds.). (2013). *Principles and practice of gynecologic oncology* (6th ed.). Philadelphia, PA: Lippincott Williams & Wilkins.

In advanced cervical cancer, the vaginal discharge gradually increases and becomes watery and, finally, dark and foul smelling from necrosis and infection. The bleeding, which occurs at irregular intervals between periods (metrorrhagia) or after menopause, may be slight (just enough to spot the undergarments) and occurs usually after mild trauma or pressure (e.g., intercourse, douching, or bearing down during defecation). As the disease continues, the bleeding may persist and increase. Leg pain, dysuria, rectal bleeding, and edema of the extremities signal advanced disease.

As the cancer advances, it may invade the tissues outside the cervix, including the lymph glands anterior to the sacrum. In one third of patients with invasive cervical cancer, the disease involves the fundus. The nerves in this region may be affected, producing excruciating pain in the back and the legs that is relieved only by large doses of opioid analgesic agents. If the disease progresses, it often produces extreme emaciation and anemia that is usually accompanied by fever due to secondary infection and abscesses in the ulcerating mass, and by fistula formation. Because the survival rate for in situ cancer is 100% and the rate for women with more advanced stages of cervical cancer decreases dramatically, early detection is essential.

Assessment and Diagnostic Findings

Diagnosis may be made based on abnormal Pap smear results, followed by biopsy results identifying severe dysplasia (cervical intraepithelial neoplasia type III [CIN III], high-grade squamous intraepithelial lesions [HGSIL; also referred to as HSIL], or carcinoma in situ). HPV infections are usually implicated in these conditions. Carcinoma in situ is technically classified as severe dysplasia and is defined as cancer that has extended through the full thickness of the epithelium of the cervix, but not beyond. This is often referred to as preinvasive cancer.

In its very early stages, cervical cancer is found microscopically by Pap smear. In later stages, pelvic examination may reveal a large, reddish growth or a deep, ulcerating lesion. The patient may report spotting or bloody discharge.

When the patient has been diagnosed with invasive cervical cancer, clinical staging estimates the extent of the disease so that treatment can be planned more specifically, and prognosis reasonably predicted. Staging is based on the International Federation of Gynecology and Obstetrics (FIGO) Staging Classification (Beckmann et al., 2014):

- Stage I, the carcinoma is strictly confined to the cervix.
- Stage II, the carcinoma invades beyond the uterus but not the pelvic wall or vagina.
- Stage III, the tumour spreads to the pelvic wall and/or the vagina, and/or causes hydronephrosis of the kidneys.
- Stage IV, the tumour has extended beyond the pelvis and involves the bladder or rectum.

Signs and symptoms are evaluated, and x-rays, laboratory tests, and special examinations, such as biopsy and colposcopy, are performed (Beckmann et al., 2014). Depending on the stage of the cancer, other tests and procedures may be performed to determine the extent of disease and appropriate treatment. These tests may include dilation and curettage (D&C), CT scan, MRI scan, IV urography, cystography, positron emission tomography (PET) scan, and barium x-ray studies. Treatment depends on the stage of the disease.

Medical Management

Precursor or Preinvasive Lesions

When precursor lesions, such as low-grade squamous intraepithelial lesion (LGSIL; also referred to as LSIL; CIN I and II or mild to moderate dysplasia), are found by colposcopy and biopsy, careful monitoring by frequent Pap smears or conservative treatment is possible. Conservative treatment may consist of monitoring, cryotherapy (freezing with nitrous oxide), or laser therapy. A **loop electrocautery excision procedure (LEEP)** may also be used to remove abnormal cells. In this procedure, a thin wire loop with laser is used to cut away a thin layer of cervical tissue. LEEP is an outpatient procedure that usually is performed in a gynecologist's office; it takes only a few minutes. Analgesia is given before the procedure, and a local anesthetic agent is injected into the area. This procedure allows the pathologist to examine the removed tissue sample to determine if the borders of the tissue are disease free. Another procedure called a cone biopsy or conization (removing a cone-shaped portion of the cervix) is performed when biopsy findings demonstrate CIN III or HGSIL (equivalent to severe dysplasia) and carcinoma in situ.

If preinvasive cervical cancer (carcinoma in situ) occurs when a woman has completed childbearing, a simple hysterectomy (removal of the uterus only) is usually recommended (Beckmann et al., 2014). If a woman is pregnant or wishes to have children and invasion is less than 1 mm, conization may be sufficient. Frequent follow-up examinations are necessary to monitor for recurrence (Beckmann et al., 2014).

Patients who have precursor or premalignant lesions need reassurance that they do not have invasive cancer. However, the importance of close follow-up is emphasized because the condition, if untreated for a long time, may progress to cancer. Patients with cervical cancer in situ also need to know that this is usually a slow-growing and nonaggressive type of cancer that is not expected to recur after appropriate treatment.

Invasive Cancer

Treatment of invasive cervical cancer depends on the stage of the lesion, the patient's age and general health, and the judgment and experience of the provider. Surgery and radiation treatment (intracavitary and external) are most often used. Surgical procedures that may be used to treat cervical cancer are summarized in Chart 48-7. Robot-assisted technology for the treatment of cervical cancer is a rapidly growing alternative to more invasive surgical options with decreased length of stay, recovery time, decreased blood loss, and increase in total number of retrievable lymph nodes (ACOG, 2015c). Ethical issues often arise in the treatment of invasive cancers. These issues are summarized in Chart 48-8.

Frequent follow-up after surgery is imperative because the risk of recurrence is high and usually occurs within the first 2 years. Recurrences are often in the upper quarter of the vagina, and ureteral obstruction may be a sign. Weight loss, leg edema, and pelvic pain may be signs of lymphatic obstruction and metastasis.

CHART 48-7

Surgical Procedures for Cervical Cancer

- Total hysterectomy—removal of the uterus, cervix, and ovaries
- Radical hysterectomy—removal of the uterus, ovaries, fallopian tubes, proximal vagina, and bilateral lymph nodes through an abdominal incision (*Note:* "radical" indicates that an extensive area of the paravaginal, paracervical, parametrial, and uterosacral tissues is removed with the uterus.)
- Radical vaginal hysterectomy—vaginal removal of the uterus, ovaries, fallopian tubes, and proximal vagina
- Bilateral pelvic lymphadenectomy—removal of the common iliac, external iliac, hypogastric, and obturator lymphatic vessels and nodes
- Pelvic exenteration—removal of the pelvic organs, including the bladder or rectum and pelvic lymph nodes, and construction of diversional conduit, colostomy, and vagina
- Radical trachelectomy—removal of the cervix and selected nodes to preserve childbearing capacity in a woman of reproductive age with cervical cancer

Adapted from Canadian Cancer Society (CCS). (2018b). *Cervical cancer.* Retrieved from http://www.cancer.ca/en/cancer-information/cancer-type/cervical/screening/?region=nl; Barakat, R. R., Berchuk, A., Markman, M., et al. (Eds.). (2013). *Principles and practice of gynecologic oncology* (6th ed.). Philadelphia, PA: Lippincott Williams & Wilkins.

CHART 48-8

Ethical Dilemma: What If the Patient Refuses to Autonomously Make Decisions?

Case Scenario

You work on a gynecology-oncology unit in a small rural community hospital. The patient, a 60-year-old woman, has been admitted with a diagnosis of cancer of the vulva. She has been married to her husband since she was 16 years old. Both the patient and her husband are recent immigrants to Canada from India. It has been determined that her disease is advanced and that she will need surgical removal of the vulva and radical node dissection. In addition, it is likely she will need chemotherapy and may be a candidate for enrolment in a clinical trial. After the treatment is explained using a medical translator, she asks her physician, "What would you do if it was your mother?" The physician reiterates the information about the surgery, and the patient states, "It is up to my husband to decide; he always makes our important decisions."

Discussion

Some cultures adhere to paternalistic tenets; the male "head of household" makes all major decisions, including health care decisions. The patient may be adhering to her cultural norms when she tells you that she will acquiesce to whatever decision her husband makes for her. Arguably, however, she may feel coerced or obligated to acquiesce to his decisions.

Analysis

- Describe the ethical principles that are in conflict in this case. Which principle should have pre-eminence as you proceed with your assessment of this patient?
- Describe any concerns the nurse may have regarding beneficence and autonomy.
- Discuss any concerns that the nurse may have about the patient's refusal to make a health care decision that will have a significant impact on her life. Assume that the nurse has spoken in private with the patient and have verified that she understands that failure to have this surgery may put her life in jeopardy, but she still refuses to make the decision. How can the nurse professionally reconcile her decision to put her life at greater risk so that she may adhere to her cultural norms (i.e., decision making done solely by the spouse)? Does this type of decision truly preserve her autonomy?
- What resources are available to help the nurse and his/her professional colleagues, the patient, and her husband reach consensus on the best treatment or care in this situation?

Radiation, which is often part of treatment to reduce recurrent disease, may be delivered by an external beam or by **brachytherapy** (method by which the radiation source is placed near the tumour in a sealed source) or both. The field to be irradiated as well as the dose and method of radiation are determined by stage, volume of tumour, and lymph node involvement (Beckmann et al., 2014).

A variety of chemotherapeutic approaches are used to treat advanced cervical cancer. They are often used in combination with surgery and radiation. Vaginal stenosis is a frequent side effect of radiation. Preventive therapy (i.e., vaginal dilator) can be used to avoid severe permanent vaginal stenosis.

Some patients with recurrences of cervical cancer are considered for **pelvic exenteration**, in which several pelvic organs are removed. This is a complex, extensive surgical procedure that is reserved for women with a high likelihood of cure. Unilateral leg edema, sciatica, and ureteral obstruction indicate likely disease progression. Patients with these symptoms have advanced disease and are not considered candidates for this major surgical procedure. Surgery is complex because it is performed close to the bowel, bladder, ureters, and great vessels. Possible complications include pulmonary embolism (PE), pulmonary edema, myocardial infarction, cerebrovascular accident, hemorrhage, sepsis, small bowel obstruction, fistula formation, obstruction of the ileal conduit, bladder dysfunction, and pyelonephritis, most often in the first 18 months postoperatively. Vein constriction must be avoided postoperatively. Patients with varicose veins or a history of thromboembolic disease may be treated prophylactically with heparin. Antiembolism stockings are prescribed to reduce the risk of deep vein thrombosis (DVT). Nursing care of these patients is complex and requires coordination and care by experienced health care professionals.

Cancer of the Uterus (Endometrium)

Over the last decade there has been an increase in both the incidence and death rates of cancer of the uterine endometrium (fundus or corpus), possibly because of increased life span and coexisting comorbidities. This cancer is the most frequently occurring gynecologic cancer in Canada. After breast, lung, and colorectal cancer, endometrial cancer is the fourth most common cancer in women. It is estimated that 7,300 Canadian women were diagnosed with uterine cancer in 2017 and an estimated 1,150 died from the disease (CCS, 2018c). Many women with endometrial cancer have obesity, which increases the risk of morbidity and mortality from this disease. Cumulative exposure to estrogen is considered the major risk factor (Chart 48-9). This exposure occurs with the use of estrogen therapy without the use of progestin, early menarche, late menopause, nulliparity, and anovulation. Other risk factors include obesity, infertility, and diabetes, as well as use of tamoxifen. Tamoxifen, taken for treatment or prevention of breast cancer, may cause proliferation of the uterine lining (CCS, 2018d). Women who take tamoxifen should be monitored by their oncologists and gynecologic health care providers.

Pathophysiology

Most uterine cancers are endometrioid (i.e., originating in the lining of the uterus). There are two types. Type 1, which accounts for about 90% of cases, is estrogen dependent. It is usually low grade with a favourable prognosis. Type 2, which occurs in about 10% of cases, is high grade and

CHART 48-9

Risk Factors: Uterine Cancer

- Age—usually >50 years; average age, 63 years
- Obesity that results in increased estrone levels (related to excess weight) resulting from conversion of androstenedione to estrone in body fat, which exposes the uterus to unopposed estrogen
- Unopposed estrogen therapy (estrogen used without progesterone, which offsets the risk of unopposed estrogen)
- Other: nulliparity, truncal obesity, late menopause (after 52 years of age), and the use of tamoxifen

Adapted from American College of Obstetricians and Gynecologists (ACOG). (2015d). Practice bulletin no. 149: endometrial cancer. *Obstetrics and Gynecology, 125*(4), 1006–1026.

usually serous cell or clear cell. Type 2 is estrogen independent. Older and African-American women are at higher risk for type 2 (ACOG, 2015d; Beckmann et al., 2014).

Assessment and Diagnostic Findings

All women should be encouraged to have annual checkups, including a gynecologic examination. Any woman who is experiencing irregular bleeding should be evaluated promptly. If a menopausal woman experiences bleeding, an endometrial aspiration or biopsy is performed to rule out hyperplasia, which is a possible precursor of endometrial cancer. The procedure is quick and usually not painful. Transvaginal ultrasound can also be used to measure the thickness of the endometrium (ACOG, 2015d). (Women who are postmenopausal should have a very thin endometrium due to low levels of estrogen; a thicker lining warrants further investigation.) A biopsy or aspiration for tissue pathology is diagnostic.

Medical Management

Treatment of endometrial cancer consists of surgical staging, total or radical hysterectomy (discussed later in this chapter), and bilateral salpingo-oophorectomy and lymph node sampling. Laparoscopy or a robot-assisted laparoscopic surgery is less invasive than abdominal surgery (ACOG, 2015d). Lymph node sampling and visualization of the peritoneum can be accomplished in many women in this manner. Cancer antigen 125 (CA-125) levels must be monitored, because elevated levels are a significant predictor of extrauterine disease or metastasis. Depending on the stage, the therapeutic approach is individualized and is based on stage, type, differentiation, degree of invasion, and node involvement. Radiation may be used in the form of external-beam radiation or vaginal brachytherapy (ACOG, 2015d). Whole pelvis radiotherapy may be used if there is any spread beyond the uterus. Recurrent cancer usually occurs inside the vaginal vault or in the upper vagina, and metastasis usually occurs in lymph nodes or the ovary. Recurrent lesions in the vagina are treated with surgery and radiation. Recurrent lesions beyond the vagina are treated with hormonal therapy or chemotherapy. Progestin therapy is used frequently. Patients should be prepared for such side effects as nausea, depression, rash, or mild fluid retention with progestin therapy.

Cancer of the Vulva

Primary cancer of the vulva is rare, representing 5% of all gynecologic malignancies and 1% of cancer in women (Zweizig, Korets, & Cain, 2014). It is most common in women who are postmenopausal, although its incidence in younger women is increasing. In Canada, specific numbers for vulvar cancer are not reported separately but are included in the general category of other and unspecified female genital organ cancers (CCS, 2018e). In the 2013 incidence and mortality statistics for other and unspecified female genital organ cancers, 955 Canadian women were diagnosed with other and unspecified female genital organ cancers, and 280 Canadian women died from these cancers (CCS, 2018e). Possible risk factors include smoking, HPV infection, HIV infection, and immunosuppression. Squamous cell carcinoma accounts for most primary vulvar tumours. Less common are Bartholin's gland cancer, vulvar sarcoma, and malignant melanoma. Little is known about what causes this disease; however, increased risk may be related to chronic vulvar irritation. In younger women, HPV infection may be implicated, especially types 16, 18, and 31. Prevention includes delaying onset of sexual activity to avoid early exposure to HPV and avoidance of smoking. Regular pelvic examinations, Pap smears, and vulvar self-examination are helpful in early detection. Women with persistent irritation or itching should be encouraged to seek evaluation.

Clinical Manifestations

Vulvar cancers are rarely asymptomatic (Zweizig et al., 2014). Long-standing pruritus and soreness are the most common symptoms of vulvar cancer. Itching occurs in half of all patients with vulvar malignancy. Bleeding, dysuria, foul-smelling discharge, and pain may also be present and are usually signs of advanced disease. Cancerous lesions of the vulva are visible and accessible and grow relatively slowly. Early lesions appear as a chronic dermatitis; later, patients may note a lump that continues to grow and becomes a hard, ulcerated, cauliflower-like growth. Biopsy should be performed on any vulvar lesion that persists, ulcerates, or fails to heal quickly with proper therapy. Vulvar malignancies may appear as a lump or mass, redness, or a lesion that fails to heal.

Medical Management

Vulvar intraepithelial lesions are preinvasive and are also called vulvar carcinoma in situ. They may be treated by local excision, laser ablation, application of chemotherapeutic creams, or cryosurgery.

When invasive vulvar carcinoma exists, primary treatment may include wide excision **vulvectomy** (removal of the vulva). An effort is made to individualize treatment, depending on the extent of the disease. A wide excision is performed only if lymph nodes are normal. More pervasive lesions require vulvectomy with deep pelvic node dissection. Vulvectomy is very effective at prolonging life but is frequently followed by complications (i.e., scarring, wound breakdown, leg swelling, vaginal stenosis, or rectocele). To reduce complications, only necessary tissue is removed. External beam radiation may be used, resulting in sunburn-like irritation that usually resolves in 6 to 12 months. Laser therapy and chemotherapy are other possible treatment options.

If a widespread area is involved or the disease is advanced, a radical vulvectomy with bilateral groin dissection may be performed. Antibiotic and heparin prophylaxis may be prescribed preoperatively and continued postoperatively to prevent infection, DVT, and PE. Sequential compression devices (SCDs) are applied to reduce the risk of venous thromboembolism (VTE).

Although the role of systemic chemotherapy in the treatment of vulvar cancer remains to be determined, chemotherapy may be useful when used in combination with radiation therapy in treatment of advanced disease. The combination of radiation and chemotherapy may reduce the size of the cancer, resulting in less extensive subsequent surgery (CCS, 2018a).

Clinical trials to determine the most effective treatment are difficult to conduct because there are few patients with this condition. Morbidity with recurrence of the disease is high, and patterns of recurrence vary. Reconstruction after vulvectomy is performed by plastic surgeons when appropriate and desired.

Nursing Management

Obtaining the Health History

The health history is a valuable tool for establishing rapport with the patient. The reason the patient is seeking health care is apparent. What the nurse can tactfully elicit is the reason a delay, if any, occurred, in seeking health care—for example, because of modesty, economics, denial, neglect, or fear (partners who are abusive sometimes prevent women from seeking health care). Factors involved in any delay in seeking health care and treatment may also affect recovery. The patient's health habits and lifestyle are assessed, and her receptivity to teaching is evaluated. Psychosocial factors are also assessed. Preoperative preparation and psychological support begin at this time.

Providing Preoperative Care

Relieving Anxiety

Prior to surgery, the patient must be allowed time to talk and ask questions. Fear often decreases when a woman who is to undergo wide excision of the vulva or vulvectomy learns that the possibility for subsequent sexual relations is good. The nurse reinforces the information the surgeon has given to the patient and addresses the patient's questions and concerns.

Preparing Skin for Surgery

Skin preparation may include cleansing the lower abdomen, inguinal areas, upper thighs, and vulva with chlorhexidine for several days before the surgical procedure. The patient may be instructed to do this at home.

Providing Postoperative Care

Relieving Pain

Because of the wide excision, the patient may experience severe pain and discomfort even with minimal movement. Therefore, analgesic agents are given preventively (i.e., around the clock at designated times) to relieve pain, increase the patient's comfort level, and allow mobility. Patient-controlled analgesia (see Chapter 16) may be used to relieve pain and promote patient comfort. Careful positioning using pillows usually increases comfort, as do soothing back rubs. A low Fowler's position or, occasionally, a pillow placed under the knees reduces pain by relieving tension on the incision; however, efforts must be made to avoid pressure behind the knees, which increases the risk of DVT. Positioning the patient on her side, with pillows between her legs and against the lumbar region, provides comfort and reduces tension on the surgical wound.

Improving Skin Integrity

A pressure-reducing mattress may be used to prevent pressure ulcers. Moving from one position to another requires time and effort; use of an overbed trapeze bar may help the patient move herself more easily. The extent of the surgical incision and the type of dressing are considered when choosing strategies to promote skin integrity. Intact skin needs to be protected from drainage and moisture. Dressings are changed as needed to ensure patient comfort, to perform wound care and irrigation (if prescribed), and to permit observation of the surgical site.

The wound is usually cleansed daily with warm, normal saline irrigations or other antiseptic solutions as prescribed, or a transparent dressing may be in place over the wound to minimize exposure to the air and subsequent pain. The appearance of the surgical site and the characteristics of drainage are assessed and documented. After the dressings are removed, a bed cradle may be used to keep the bed linens away from the surgical site.

Supporting Positive Sexuality and Sexual Function

The patient who undergoes vulvar surgery usually experiences concerns about body image, sexual attractiveness, and functioning. Establishing a trusting nurse–patient relationship is important for the patient to feel comfortable expressing her concerns and fears. The patient is encouraged to discuss her concerns with her sexual partner as well.

Because alterations in sexual sensation and functioning depend on the extent of surgery, the nurse needs to know about any structural and functional changes resulting from the surgery. Referral of the patient and her partner to a sex counsellor may help them address these changes and resume satisfying sexual activity.

Monitoring and Managing Potential Complications

Location, extent, and exposure of the surgical site and incision put the patient at risk for contamination of the site and infection and sepsis. The patient is monitored closely for local and systemic signs and symptoms of infection: purulent drainage, redness, increased pain, fever, and increased white blood cell count. The nurse assists in obtaining specimens for culture if infection is suspected and administers antibiotic agents as prescribed. Hand hygiene, always a crucial infection-preventing measure, is of importance along with wearing masks whenever there is an extensive area of exposed tissue. Catheters, drains, and dressings are handled carefully with gloves on to avoid cross-contamination. A low-residue diet prevents straining on defecation and wound contamination.

The patient is at risk for complications of VTE, which include DVT and PE, because of the positioning required during surgery, postoperative edema, and the immobility needed to promote healing. SCDs are applied, and other prophylactic measures may be prescribed for patients at high risk. The patient is encouraged and reminded to perform ankle exercises to minimize venous pooling, which leads to DVT. The patient is encouraged and assisted in changing positions by using the overhead trapeze bar. Pressure behind the knees is avoided when positioning the patient because this may increase venous pooling. The patient is assessed for signs and symptoms of DVT (leg pain, redness, warmth, edema) and PE (chest pain, tachycardia, dyspnea). Fluid intake is encouraged to prevent dehydration, which also increases the risk of DVT.

The extent of the surgical incision and possibly wide excision of tissue increase the risk of postoperative bleeding and hemorrhage. Pressure dressings that are applied after surgery minimize the risk.

NURSING ALERT

The patient must be monitored closely for signs of hemorrhage and resulting hypovolemic shock. These signs may include decreased blood pressure; increased pulse rate; decreased urine output; decreased mental status; and cold, clammy skin.

If hemorrhage and shock occur, interventions include fluid replacement, blood component therapy, and vasopressor medications. Laboratory results (e.g., hematocrit and hemoglobin levels) and hemodynamic monitoring are used to assess the patient's response to treatment. Depending on the specific cause of hemorrhage, the patient may be returned to the operating room. See Chapter 18 for a detailed discussion of shock.

Promoting Home, Community-Based, and Transitional Care

Educating Patients About Self-Care

Preparing the patient for hospital discharge begins before hospital admission. The patient and family are informed about what to expect during the immediate postoperative and recovery periods. Depending on the changes resulting from the surgery, the patient and her family may need instruction about wound care, urinary catheterization, and possible complications. The patient is encouraged to share her concerns and to assume increasing responsibility for her own care. She is encouraged and assisted in learning to care for the surgical site. A referral for home care is made as indicated.

Nurses are in an ideal position to educate women about performing regular vulvar self-examinations. Using a mirror, patients can see what constitutes normal female anatomy and learn about changes that should be reported (e.g., lesions, ulcers, masses, and persistent itching). Nurses must urge women to seek health care if they notice anything abnormal, because vulvar cancer is one of the most curable of all malignant conditions.

Continuing and Transitional Care

Patients may be discharged early in their postoperative recovery to home or a subacute facility. During this phase, the patient's physical status and psychological responses to the surgery are assessed. In addition, the patient is assessed for complications and healing of the surgical site. During home visits, the nurse assesses the home to determine if modifications are needed to facilitate care. The home visit is used to reinforce previous teaching and to assess the patient's and the family's understanding of and adherence to the prescribed treatment strategies. Follow-up phone calls by the nurse to the patient between home visits are usually reassuring to the patient and family, who may be responsible for performing complex care procedures. Attention to the patient's psychological responses is important because the patient may become discouraged and depressed because of alterations in body image and a slow recovery. Communication between the nurse involved in the patient's immediate postoperative care and the home care nurse is essential to ensure continuity of care.

Cancer of the Vagina

Cancer of the vagina is uncommon, representing 1% to 3% of gynecologic cancers; it is usually squamous in origin (Beckmann et al., 2014). Malignant melanoma and sarcomas can occur. Most vaginal cancers are secondary and invasive at the time of diagnosis. Risk factors include previous cervical cancer, in utero exposure to diethylstilbestrol (DES), previous vaginal or vulvar cancer, previous radiation therapy, history of HPV, or pessary use. Any patient with previous cervical cancer should be examined regularly for vaginal lesions.

Vaginal pessaries, which are used to support prolapsed tissues, can be a source of chronic irritation. As such, they have been associated with vaginal cancer, but only when the devices were not cared for properly (i.e., the device was not cleaned regularly, or the patient did not return to the health care provider regularly for vaginal examinations).

Patients often do not have symptoms but may report slight bleeding after intercourse, spontaneous bleeding, vaginal discharge, pain, and urinary or rectal symptoms (or both). Diagnosis is often by Pap smear. Encouraging close follow-up is the focus of nursing interventions with women who were exposed to DES in utero. Emotional support for mothers who received DES before its risks were discovered and their daughters who were exposed to DES in utero is essential.

Medical Management

Treatment of early lesions may include local excision, topical chemotherapy, or laser. Laser therapy is a common treatment option in early vaginal and vulvar cancer. Surgery for more advanced lesions depends on the size and the stage of the cancer. If radical vaginectomy is required, a vagina can be reconstructed with tissue from the intestine, muscle, or skin grafts. After vaginal reconstructive surgery and radiation, regular intercourse may be helpful in preventing vaginal stenosis. Water-soluble lubricants are helpful in reducing pain with intercourse (dyspareunia).

Following surgery, radiation therapy may be given by a variety of methods, including external beam radiation, which is usually an outpatient procedure, or brachytherapy, which is internal radiation therapy. Internal radiation may be given with intracavitary radioactive material contained in a seed, wire, needle, or tube, which is placed into a cavity such as the uterus or vagina. Interstitial radiation is another type of internal radiation treatment in which the radioactive material is placed in or near the cancer but not into a body cavity and is used in cervical and ovarian malignancies. These treatments may be high dose for a short period or low dose, which may take longer. Treatment during hospitalization or during outpatient therapy depends on several factors, including the status of the patient and the mode of delivery.

Cancer of the Fallopian Tubes

Malignancies of the fallopian tube are the least common type of genital cancer (American Cancer Society [ACS], 2015b). Although this type of cancer can occur at any age, it is most common in women who are postmenopausal. Symptoms are often minimal, causing diagnosis to be made at an advanced stage (Beckmann et al., 2014). Symptoms include abdominal pain, abnormal bleeding, and vaginal discharge. An enlarged fallopian tube may be found on sonogram if dilated and fluid filled, or it may appear or be palpated as a mass. Surgery followed by radiation therapy is the usual treatment.

Cancer of the Ovary

Ovarian cancer is the third most common reproductive cancer in Canada, and the fifth deadliest cancer for women following lung, breast, colorectal, and pancreatic (Beckmann et al., 2014; CCS, 2018f). Despite careful physical examination, ovarian tumours are often difficult to detect because they are usually deep in the pelvis. No early screening mechanism exists at present. Tumour-associated antigens are helpful in determining follow-up care after diagnosis and treatment and to evaluate for recurrent disease but are not useful in early general screening (Beckmann et al., 2014).

Epidemiology

One in 70 women will develop ovarian cancer in her lifetime. The incidence of this type of cancer increases with age until 70 years, with most cases diagnosed by age 60 (Beckmann et al., 2014). The frequency of ovarian cancer is highest in industrialized countries and affects women of all races and ethnic backgrounds.

Family history is the most significant risk factor. Most cases are random, but 5% to 10% of ovarian cancers are familial (Beckmann et al., 2014). In most cases, the mutations are in the *BRCA1* gene and sometimes in the *BRCA2* gene. A family history in a first-degree relative (mother, daughter, or sister), older age, early menarche, late menopause, and obesity may increase the risk of ovarian cancer. However, most women who develop ovarian cancer have no known risk factors, and no definitive causative factors have been determined.

Patients with concerns about their family history should be referred to a cancer genetics centre to obtain information and testing, if indicated. Women with inherited types of ovarian cancer tend to be younger when the diagnosis is made than the average age at the time of diagnosis. Hereditary nonpolyposis colorectal cancer (HNPCC, also known as Lynch syndrome) increases the risk of ovarian cancer 13-fold (Beckmann et al., 2014). Lifetime risk of developing ovarian cancer has been shown to be decreased by one half with long-term suppression (greater than 5 years) of ovulation through use of oral contraceptives (Beckmann et al., 2014).

Pathophysiology

Types of tumours include germ cell tumours, which arise from the cells that produce eggs and are the most common cause of ovarian cancer in women younger than 20 years (Beckmann et al., 2014); stromal cell tumours, which arise in connective tissue cells that produce hormones; and epithelial tumours, which originate from the outer surface of the ovary. Most ovarian cancers are epithelial in origin. Of the many different cell types in ovarian cancer, epithelial tumours constitute 90%. Germ cell tumours and stromal tumours make up the other 10% (Beckmann et al., 2014).

Primary peritoneal carcinoma is closely related to ovarian cancer. Extraovarian primary peritoneal carcinoma (EOPPC) resembles ovarian cancer histologically and can occur in women with and without ovaries. Symptoms and treatment are similar. Because of the possibility of EOPPC, oophorectomy lessens the chance, but does not guarantee that the patient will not develop carcinoma.

Clinical Manifestations

Symptoms of ovarian cancer are nonspecific and may include increased abdominal girth, pelvic pressure, bloating, back pain, constipation, abdominal pain, urinary urgency, indigestion, flatulence, increased waist size, leg pain, and pelvic pain. Symptoms are often vague, so many women tend to ignore them. Ovarian cancer is often silent, but enlargement of the abdomen from an accumulation of fluid is a common sign. All women with gastrointestinal symptoms without a known diagnosis must be evaluated for potential ovarian cancer. Vague, undiagnosed, persistent gastrointestinal symptoms should alert the nurse to the possibility of an early ovarian malignancy. A palpable ovary in a woman who has gone through menopause is investigated immediately because ovaries normally become smaller and less palpable after menopause.

Assessment and Diagnostic Findings

Any enlarged ovary must be investigated. Pelvic examination often does not detect early ovarian cancer, and pelvic imaging techniques are not always definitive. Ovarian tumours are classified as benign if there is no proliferation or invasion, borderline if there is proliferation but no invasion, and malignant if there is invasion. Of all new cases of ovarian tumours, 20% are classified as borderline and have low malignancy potential. However, by the time of diagnosis, most ovarian cancers are advanced (Beckmann et al., 2014; CCS, 2018a).

CHART 48-10

Main Stages of Ovarian Cancer

I. Cancer is contained within the ovary (or ovaries).
II. Cancer is in one or both ovaries and has involved other organs (i.e., uterus, fallopian tubes, bladder, the sigmoid colon, or the rectum) within the pelvis.
III. Cancer involves one or both ovaries, and one or both of the following are present: (1) cancer has spread beyond the pelvis to the lining of the abdomen; (2) cancer has spread to lymph nodes.
IV. The most advanced stage of ovarian cancer. Cancer is in one or both ovaries. There is distant metastasis to the liver, lungs, or other organs outside the peritoneal cavity; ovarian cancer cells in the pleural cavity are evidence of stage IV disease.

Adapted from Beckmann, C. R., Ling, F. W., Herbert, W. N., et al. (Eds.). (2014). *Obstetrics and gynecology* (7th ed.). Philadelphia, PA: Wolters Kluwer.

Medical Management

Surgical Management

Surgical staging, exploration, and reduction of tumour mass are the basics of treatment. Surgical removal is the treatment of choice. Staging the tumour by the FIGO staging system is performed to guide treatment (Chart 48-10). Likely treatment involves a total abdominal hysterectomy with removal of the fallopian tubes and ovaries and possibly the omentum (bilateral salpingo-oophorectomy and omentectomy); tumour debulking; para-aortic and pelvic lymph node sampling; diaphragmatic biopsies; random peritoneal biopsies; and cytologic washings. Postoperative management may include taxanes or platinum-based chemotherapy (discussed in next section).

Borderline tumours resemble ovarian cancer but have much more favourable outcomes. Women diagnosed with this type of cancer tend to be younger (early 40s). A conservative surgical approach is used. The affected ovary is removed, but the uterus and the contralateral ovary may remain in place. Adjuvant therapy may not be warranted.

Pharmacologic Therapy

Chemotherapy is usually administered IV on an outpatient basis using a combination of platinum and taxane agents. Paclitaxel (Taxol) plus carboplatin (Paraplatin) are most often used because of their excellent clinical benefits and manageable toxicity. Leukopenia, neurotoxicity, and fever may occur.

Because paclitaxel often causes leukopenia, patients may need to take granulocyte colony-stimulating factor as well. Paclitaxel is contraindicated in patients with hypersensitivity to medications formulated in polyoxyethylated castor oil and in patients with baseline neutropenia. Because of possible adverse cardiac effects, paclitaxel is not used in patients with cardiac disorders. Hypotension, dyspnea, angioedema, and urticaria indicate severe reactions that usually occur soon after the first and second doses are given. Nurses who administer chemotherapy are prepared to assist in treating anaphylaxis. Patients should be prepared for inevitable hair loss.

Carboplatin may be used in the initial treatment and in patients with recurrence. It should be used with caution in patients with renal impairment. Usually, six cycles are given. A positive clinical response is normalization of the tumour marker CA-125, negative CT results, and a normal physical and gynecologic examination.

Liposomal therapy, delivery of chemotherapy in a liposome, allows the highest possible dose of chemotherapy to the tumour target with a reduction in adverse effects. Liposomes are used as drug carriers because they are nontoxic, biodegradable, easily available, and relatively inexpensive. This encapsulated chemotherapy allows increased duration of action and better targeting. The encapsulation of doxorubicin (Doxil) lessens the incidence of nausea, vomiting, and alopecia. Patients must be monitored for bone marrow suppression and gastrointestinal and cardiac effects.

Combination IV and intraperitoneal chemotherapy is an option for some patients. However, this treatment is more toxic and side effects are more severe than regular chemotherapy (ACS, 2015b). Intraperitoneal chemotherapy is reserved for women with good kidney function (ACS, 2015b).

Genetic engineering and identification of cancer genes may make gene therapy a future possibility; gene therapy is under investigation. Emerging proteomic technologies (tissue-based protein analysis) look promising; they may allow earlier diagnosis and treatment decision making. New biomarkers need further validation, but protein signature patterns are now being tested. These technologies may result in individualized treatment strategies for epithelial ovarian cancer (ACS, 2015b).

Recurrence of ovarian cancer is common, and many patients may require treatment with multiple agents. Treatment is directed toward control of the cancer, maintenance of quality of life, and palliation. Liposomal preparations, intraperitoneal drug administration, anti-cancer vaccines, monoclonal antibodies directed against cancer antigens, gene therapy, and antiangiogenic treatments (to prevent formation of new blood vessels to halt growth of ovarian cancer) may be used in the treatment of recurrence.

Nursing Management

Nursing measures include those related to the patient's treatment plan, which may include surgery, chemotherapy, palliative care, or a combination of these. Nursing interventions after pelvic surgery to remove the tumour are similar to those after other abdominal surgeries. If ovarian cancer occurs in a young woman and the tumour is unilateral, it is removed. Childbearing, if desired, is encouraged in the near future. After childbirth, surgical reexploration may be performed, and the remaining ovary may be removed. If both ovaries are involved, bilateral oophorectomy is performed, and chemotherapy follows.

Patients with advanced ovarian cancer may develop ascites and pleural effusion. Nursing care may include administering IV fluids prescribed to alleviate fluid and electrolyte imbalances, administering parenteral nutrition to provide adequate nutrition, providing postoperative care after intestinal bypass to alleviate any obstruction, controlling pain, and managing drainage tubes. Comfort measures for women with ascites may include providing small frequent meals, decreasing fluid intake, administering diuretic agents, and providing rest. Patients with pleural effusion may experience shortness of breath, hypoxia, pleuritic chest pain, and cough. Thoracentesis is usually performed to relieve these symptoms. The patient with ovarian cancer often has complex needs and benefits from the assistance and support of an oncology clinical nurse specialist.

Hysterectomy

Hysterectomy is the surgical removal of the uterus to treat cancer, dysfunctional uterine bleeding, endometriosis, nonmalignant growths, persistent pain, pelvic relaxation and prolapse, and previous injury to the uterus. Hysterectomies have been steadily declining over the last decade as the number of other therapeutic options (i.e., laser therapy, endometrial ablation, UAE, and medications to shrink fibroid tumours) has increased (Wright, Herzog, Tsui, et al., 2013). Despite the decline in hysterectomies, it is still the most common gynecologic procedure affecting one in nine women in their lifetime; 90% of all hysterectomies are for benign causes. In Canada, approximately 346 of every 100,000 women undergo hysterectomy each year (Women's Health Data Directory, 2013). Canada has one of the highest rates in the world.

A total hysterectomy involves removal of the uterus and the cervix. Hysterectomy can be supracervical or subtotal, in which the uterus is removed but the cervix is spared. Radical hysterectomy involves removal of the uterus as well as the surrounding tissue, including the upper third of the vagina and pelvic lymph nodes. The procedure can be performed through the vagina, through an abdominal incision, or laparoscopically (in which the uterus is removed in sections through small incisions using a laparoscope). Malignant conditions usually require a total abdominal hysterectomy and bilateral salpingo-oophorectomy.

A laparoscopically assisted approach can also be used for vaginal hysterectomy. This procedure is performed as a short-stay procedure or ambulatory surgery in patients who are carefully selected. Robot-assisted hysterectomies are performed in more than 20% of cases, with similar outcomes compared to laparoscopic and vaginal methods at a higher cost (Ridgeway & Falcone, 2014).

Preoperative Management

Patients are advised to discontinue anticoagulant medications, NSAIDs such as aspirin, and vitamin E prior to surgery to reduce the risk of bleeding. Pregnancy is ruled out on the day of surgery. Prophylactic antibiotic agents may be given prior to surgery and discontinued the next day. Prevention of thromboembolic events is critical, and methods depend on the risk profile of the patient.

Postoperative Management

The principles of general postoperative care for abdominal surgery apply. Major risks are infection and hemorrhage. In addition, because the surgical site is close to the bladder, voiding problems may occur, particularly after a vaginal hysterectomy. Also, edema or nerve trauma may cause temporary loss of bladder tone (bladder atony), and an indwelling catheter may be inserted.

Nursing Process

The Patient Undergoing a Hysterectomy

Assessment

The health history and the physical and pelvic examination are completed, and laboratory tests are performed. Additional assessment data include the patient's psychosocial responses because the need for a hysterectomy may elicit strong emotional reactions. If the hysterectomy is performed to remove a malignant tumour, anxiety related to fear of cancer and its consequences adds to the stress of the patient and her family. Women who have had a hysterectomy may be at risk for psychological and physical symptoms. Alternatively, women may note improved physical and mental health after hysterectomy as troublesome symptoms may be alleviated.

Nursing Priorities

Based on the assessment data, the major nursing priorities may include the following:

- Anxiety
- Alerted body image
- Acute pain
- Lack of knowledge

Collaborative Problems/ Potential Complications

Potential complications may include the following:

- Hemorrhage
- VTE
- Bladder dysfunction
- Infection

Planning and Goals

The major goals may include relief of anxiety, acceptance of loss of the uterus, absence of pain or discomfort, increased knowledge of self-care requirements, and absence of complications.

Nursing Interventions

Relieving Anxiety

Anxiety stems from several factors: unfamiliar environment, the effects of surgery on body image and reproductive ability, fear of pain and other discomfort, and, possibly, feelings of embarrassment about exposure in the perioperative period. The nurse determines what the experience means to the patient and encourages her to verbalize her concerns. Throughout the preoperative, postoperative, and recovery periods, explanations are given about physical preparations and procedures that are performed.

Patient education addresses the outcomes of surgery, possible feelings of loss, and options for management of any symptoms that occur. Women vary in their preferences for information and participation in decision making, including choice of treatment options, accurate and useful information at the appropriate time, support from their health care providers, and access to professional and lay support systems.

Improving Body Image

The patient may have strong emotional reactions to having a hysterectomy and personal feelings related to the diagnosis, views of significant others who may be involved (family, partner), religious beliefs, and fears about prognosis. Concerns such as the inability to have children and the effect on femininity may surface, as may questions about the effects of surgery on sexual relationships, function, and satisfaction. The patient needs reassurance that she will still have a vagina and that she can experience sexual activity after temporary postoperative abstinence while tissues heal. Information that sexual satisfaction and orgasm arise from clitoral stimulation rather than from the uterus reassures many women. Most women note some change in sexual feelings after hysterectomy, but they vary in intensity. In some cases, the vagina is shortened by surgery, and this may affect sensitivity or comfort.

When hormonal balance is upset, as often occurs with reproductive system disorders, the patient may experience depressed mood and heightened emotional sensitivity to people and situations. The nurse needs to approach and evaluate each patient individually considering these factors. A nurse who exhibits interest, concern, and willingness to listen to the patient's fears will help the patient progress through the surgical experience.

Relieving Pain

Postoperative pain and discomfort are common. Therefore, the nurse assesses the intensity of the patient's pain and assists the patient with analgesia as prescribed. If the patient has abdominal distention or flatus, a rectal tube and application of heat to the abdomen may be prescribed. When abdominal auscultation reveals return of bowel sounds and peristalsis, additional fluids and a soft diet are permitted. Early ambulation facilitates the return of normal peristalsis.

Monitoring and Managing Potential Complications

HEMORRHAGE. Vaginal bleeding and hemorrhage may occur after hysterectomy. To detect these complications early, the nurse counts the perineal pads used or checks the incision site, assesses the extent of saturation with blood, and monitors vital signs. Abdominal dressings are monitored for drainage if an abdominal surgical approach has been used. In preparation for hospital discharge, the nurse gives prescribed guidelines for activity restrictions to promote healing and to prevent postoperative bleeding. Because many women may go home the day of surgery or within a day or two, they are instructed to contact the nurse or surgeon if bleeding is beyond what is expected, which should be minimal.

VENOUS THROMBOEMBOLISM. Because of positioning during surgery, postoperative edema, and decreased activity postoperatively, the patient is at risk for DVT and PE. To minimize the risk, antiembolism stockings are applied. In addition, the patient is encouraged and assisted to change positions frequently, although pressure under the knees is avoided, and to exercise her legs and feet while in bed. The nurse helps the patient ambulate early in the postoperative period. The nurse also assesses for DVT (leg pain, redness, warmth, edema) and PE (chest pain, tachycardia, dyspnea). If the patient is being discharged home soon after surgery, she is instructed to avoid prolonged sitting in a chair with pressure at the knees, sitting with crossed legs, and inactivity. Furthermore, she is instructed to contact her primary provider if symptoms of DVT or PE occur.

BLADDER DYSFUNCTION. Because of possible difficulty in voiding postoperatively, occasionally an indwelling catheter may be inserted before or during surgery and is left in place in the immediate postoperative period. If a catheter is in place, it is usually removed shortly after the patient begins to ambulate. After the catheter is removed, urinary output is monitored; additionally, the abdomen is assessed for distention. If the patient does not void within a prescribed time, measures are initiated to encourage voiding (e.g., assisting the patient to the bathroom, pouring warm water over the perineum). If the patient cannot void, catheterization may be necessary. On rare occasions, the patient may be discharged home with the catheter in place and is instructed in its management.

Promoting Home, Community-Based, and Transitional Care

EDUCATING PATIENTS ABOUT SELF-CARE. The information provided to the patient is tailored to her needs. She must know what limitations or restrictions, if any, to expect. She is instructed to check the surgical incision daily and to contact her primary provider if redness or purulent drainage or discharge occurs. She is informed that her periods are now over but that she may have a slightly bloody discharge for a few days; if bleeding recurs after this time, it should be reported immediately. The patient is instructed about the importance of an adequate oral intake and of maintaining bowel and urinary tract function. The patient is informed that she is likely to recover quickly, but that postoperative fatigue is not unusual.

The patient should resume activities gradually. This does not mean sitting for long periods, because doing so may cause blood to pool in the pelvis, increasing the risk of VTE. The nurse explains that showers are preferable to tub baths to reduce the possibility of infection and to avoid the dangers of injury that may occur when getting in and out of the bathtub. The patient is instructed to avoid straining, lifting, having sexual intercourse, or driving until permitted. Vaginal discharge, foul odour, excessive bleeding, any leg redness or pain, or an elevated temperature should be reported, and the nurse reinforces education regarding activities and restrictions.

CONTINUING AND TRANSITIONAL CARE. Follow-up telephone contact provides the nurse with the opportunity to determine whether the patient is recovering without problems and to answer any questions that may have arisen. The patient is reminded about postoperative follow-up appointments. If the patient's ovaries were removed and she finds vasomotor symptoms troublesome, hormone therapy may be considered at a low dose for a short amount of time. The patient is reminded to discuss risks and benefits of hormone therapy and alternative therapies with her primary and gynecologic care provider. Decisions about use of hormone therapy need to be made individually in consultation with the provider.

Evaluation

Expected patient outcomes may include:

1. Experiences decreased anxiety
2. Has improved body image
   a. Discusses changes resulting from surgery with her partner
   b. Verbalizes understanding of her disorder and the treatment plan
   c. Displays minimal depression or anxiety
3. Experiences minimal pain and discomfort
   a. Reports relief of abdominal pain and discomfort
   b. Ambulates without pain
4. Verbalizes knowledge and understanding of self-care
   a. Practices deep breathing, turning, and leg exercises as instructed
   b. Increases activity and ambulation daily
   c. Reports adequate fluid intake and adequate urinary output
   d. Identifies reportable symptoms
   e. Schedules and keeps follow-up appointments
5. Absence of complications
   a. Has minimal vaginal bleeding and exhibits normal vital signs
   b. Ambulates early
   c. Notes no chest or calf pain and no redness, tenderness, or swelling in the extremities
   d. Reports no urinary problems or abdominal distention

Unfolding Patient Stories: Doris Bowman • Part 1

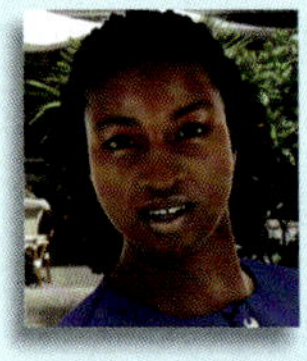

Doris Bowman, a 39-year-old diagnosed with uterine fibroids, dysmenorrhea, and menorrhagia, is considering undergoing a total abdominal hysterectomy with bilateral salpingo-oophorectomy. What are potential postoperative complications that the nurse should consider? What assessments and interventions would be done by the nurse to monitor for early detection or to prevent these complications? Describe the discharge education that would be provided by the nurse on self-care monitoring required of the patient at home and what should be reported to the health care provider. (Doris Bowman's story continues in Chapter 68.)

Care for Doris and other patients in a realistic virtual environment: ***vSim** for Nursing* **(thepoint.lww.com/vSimMedicalSurgical)**. Practice documenting these patients' care in DocuCare **(thepoint.lww.com/DocuCareEHR)**.

Radiation Therapy

Radiation may be used in the treatment of cervical, uterine, and less frequently in ovarian cancers either alone or in combination with surgery and chemotherapy. Several approaches are used to deliver radiation to the female reproductive system: external radiation, intraoperative radiation therapy (IORT), and internal (intracavitary) irradiation or brachytherapy (Halperin, Wazer, Perez, et al., 2013). The cervix and uterus can serve as a receptacle for radioactive sources for internal radiation therapy.

Methods of Radiation Therapy

External Radiation Therapy

This method of delivering radiation destroys cancerous cells at the skin surface or deeper in the body. Other methods of delivering radiation therapy are more commonly used to treat cancer of the female reproductive system than this method.

Intraoperative Radiation Therapy

IORT allows radiation to be applied directly to the affected area during surgery. An electron beam is directed at the disease site. This direct-view irradiation may be used when para-aortic nodes are involved or for unresectable (inoperable) or partially resectable neoplasms. Benefits include accurate beam direction (which precisely limits the radiation to the tumour) and the ability during treatment to block sensitive organs from radiation. IORT is usually combined with external beam irradiation preoperatively or postoperatively.

Internal (Intracavitary) Irradiation

After the patient receives an anesthetic agent and an examination, specially prepared applicators are inserted into the endometrial cavity and vagina. These devices are not loaded with radioactive material until the patient returns to her room. X-rays are obtained to verify the precise relationship of the applicator to the normal pelvic anatomy and to the tumour. When this step is completed, the radiation oncologist loads the applicators with predetermined amounts of radioactive material. This procedure, called afterloading, allows for precise control of the radiation exposure received by the patient, with minimal exposure of physicians, nurses, and other health care personnel. A patient undergoing internal radiation treatment remains isolated in a private room until the application is completed. Adjacent rooms may need to be evacuated and a lead shield placed at the doorway to the patient's room.

Of the various applicators developed for intracavitary treatment, some are inserted into the endometrial cavity and endocervical canal as multiple small irradiators (e.g., Heyman capsules). Others consist of a central tube (a tandem or intrauterine "stem") placed through the dilated endocervical canal into the uterine cavity, which remains in a fixed relationship with the irradiators placed in the upper vagina on each side of the cervix (vaginal ovoids) (Fig. 48-8).

When the applicator is inserted, an indwelling urinary catheter is also inserted. Vaginal packing is inserted to keep the applicator in place and to keep other organs, such as the bladder and rectum, as far from the radioactive source as possible. The objective of the internal treatment

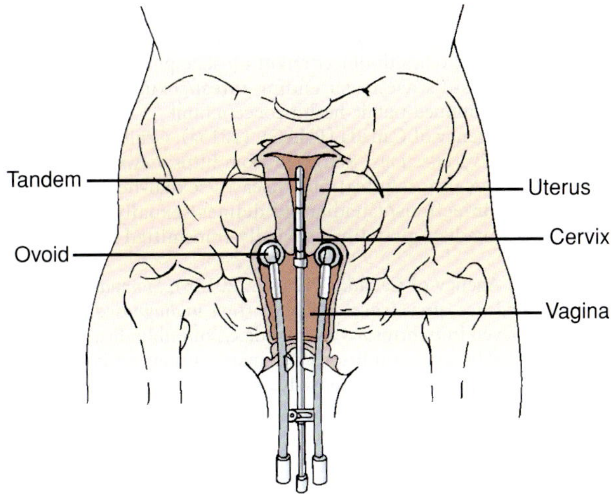

FIGURE 48-8. Placement of tandem and ovoids for internal radiation therapy.

is to maintain the distribution of internal radiation at a fixed dosage throughout the application, which may last 24 to 72 hours, depending on dose calculations made by the radiation physicist.

Automated high-dose rate intracavitary brachytherapy systems have been developed that allow outpatient radiation therapy. Treatment time is shorter, thereby decreasing patient discomfort. Staff exposure to radiation is also avoided. Isotopes of radium and cesium are used for intracavitary irradiation.

Nursing Considerations for Radiation Safety

Special precautions for the safety of the patient and the nurse are important considerations when the patient is receiving radiation therapy. The Radiation Safety Department will identify specific safety precautions to those people who will be in contact with the patient, including health care providers and family. Nursing concerns include providing the patient with emotional support and physical comfort. Further details about nursing management are provided in Chapter 68.

Critical Thinking Exercises

1 **ebp** A 60-year-old woman has been diagnosed with ovarian cancer. She reports a strong family history of cancer; her mother and a sister both died from breast cancer. She is concerned of the health status of her two daughters, both of whom are in their 30s. She has asked the nurse to discuss the risks of cancer with them. Explain what counselling and education the nurse should provide to the patient and her daughters. Identify the evidence base for the counselling and education and the strength of that evidence.

2 **pq** Identify the priorities, approach, and techniques the nurse would use to provide care for a 25-year-old woman who is being seen in an outpatient clinic for a new diagnosis of genital herpes. How will the nurse's priorities, approach, and techniques differ if the patient says she is not in a monogamous relationship? If the patient is from a culture with very different values from the nurse's background? Describe priorities, approach, and techniques to prevent reinfection or spread of the infection.

3 A 46-year-old woman has been admitted the unit for repair of a prolapsed uterus. Describe the preoperative education for her and the postoperative care that can be anticipated. What modifications in care, postoperative education, and discharge planning may be necessary if repair of a rectocele is also done?

REFERENCES AND SELECTED READINGS

Books

American Cancer Society (ACS). (2015a). *Cancer facts and figures 2015*. Atlanta, GA: Author.

Beckmann, C. R., Ling, F. W., Herbert, W. N., et al. (Eds.). (2014). *Obstetrics and gynecology* (7th ed.). Philadelphia, PA: Wolters Kluwer.

Halperin, E. C., Wazer, D. E., Perez, C. A., et al. (Eds.). (2013). *Perez and Brady's principles and practice of radiation oncology* (6th ed.). Philadelphia, PA: Lippincott Williams & Wilkins.

Karch, A. M. (2015). *Lippincott nursing drug guide*. Philadelphia, PA: Wolters Kluwer.

Schuiling, K. D., & Likis, F. E. (2013). *Women's gynecologic health* (2nd ed.). Burlington, MA: Jones & Bartlett.

Journals and Electronic Documents

American Cancer Society (ACS). (2015b). *Ovarian cancer*. Retrieved December 6, 2015, from www.cancer.org/cancer/ovariancancer/detailedguide/ovarian-cancer-new-research

American College of Obstetricians and Gynecologists (ACOG). (2007, reaffirmed 2015). Practice Bulletin No. 83: Management of adnexal masses. *Obstetrics and Gynecology*, *110*(1), 201–214.

American College of Obstetricians and Gynecologists (ACOG). (2015a). *Human papillomavirus vaccination. Committee Opinion No. 641*. Retrieved November 1, 2015, from www.acog.org/Resources-And-Publications/Committee-Opinions/Committee-on-Adolescent-Health-Care/Human-Papillomavirus-Vaccination

American College of Obstetricians and Gynecologists (ACOG). (2015b). *Dual therapy for gonococcal infections. Committee Opinion No. 645*. Retrieved November 1, 2015, from www.acog.org/Resources-And-Publications/Committee-Opinions/Committee-on-Gynecologic-Practice/Dual-Therapy-for-Gonococcal-Infections

American College of Obstetricians and Gynecologists (ACOG). (2015c). *Robotic surgery in gynecology. Committee Opinion No. 628*. Retrieved November 27, 2015, from www.acog.org/Resources-And-Publications/Committee-Opinions/Committee-on-Gynecologic-Practice/Robotic-Surgery-in-Gynecology

American College of Obstetricians and Gynecologists (ACOG). (2015d). Practice bulletin no. 149: Endometrial cancer. *Obstetrics and Gynecology*, *125*(4), 1006–1026.

Bechtel, M. A., & Trout, W. (2015). Sexually transmitted diseases. *Clinical Obstetrics and Gynecology*, *58*(1), 172–184.

Brunham, R. C., Gottlieb, S. L., & Paavonen, J. (2015). Pelvic inflammatory disease. *The New England Journal of Medicine*, *372*(21), 2039–2043.

Canadian Cancer Society (CCS). (2017). *Canadian cancer statistics 2017*. Retrieved from http://www.cancer.ca/~/media/cancer.ca/CW/cancer%20information/cancer%20101/Canadian%20cancer%20statistics/Canadian-Cancer-Statistics-2017-EN.pdf?la=en

Canadian Cancer Society (CCS). (2018a). *Cancer information*. Retrieved from http://www.cancer.ca/en/?region=nl

Canadian Cancer Society (CCS). (2018b). *Cervical cancer*. Retrieved from http://www.cancer.ca/en/cancer-information/cancer-type/cervical/screening/?region=nl

Canadian Cancer Society (CCS). (2018c). *Uterine cancer statistics*. Retrieved from http://www.cancer.ca/en/cancer-information/cancer-type/uterine/statistics/?region=nl

Canadian Cancer Society (CCS). (2018d). *Risk factors for uterine cancer*. Retrieved from http://www.cancer.ca/en/cancer-information/cancer-type/uterine/risks/?region=nl
Canadian Cancer Society (CCS). (2018e). *Vulvar cancer statistics*. Retrieved from http://www.cancer.ca/en/cancer-information/cancer-type/vulvar/statistics/?region=nl
Canadian Cancer Society (CCS). (2018f). *Ovarian cancer statistics*. Retrieved from http://www.cancer.ca/en/cancer-information/cancer-type/ovarian/statistics/?region=on
Canadian Women's Health Network (CWHN). (2012). *Fibroids*. Retrieved from http://www.cwhn.ca/en/yourhealth/faqs/fibroids
Centers for Disease Control and Prevention (CDC). (2015a). *Trichomoniasis—CDC fact sheet*. Retrieved October 29, 2015, from www.cdc.gov/std/trichomonas/STDFact-Trichomoniasis.htm
Centers for Disease Control and Prevention (CDC). (2015b). *Genital herpes—CDC fact sheet*. Retrieved November 1, 2015, from www.cdc.gov/std/herpes/stdfact-herpes-detailed.htm
Centers for Disease Control and Prevention (CDC). (2015c). *Chlamydia—CDC fact sheet*. Retrieved November 7, 2015, from www.cdc.gov/std/chlamydia/stdfact-chlamydia-detailed.htm
Centers for Disease Control and Prevention (CDC). (2015d). *Gonorrhea—CDC fact sheet*. Retrieved November 7, 2015, from www.cdc.gov/std/gonorrhea/stdfact-gonorrhea-detailed.htm
Centers for Disease Control and Prevention (CDC). (2015e). *Pelvic inflammatory disease (PID)—CDC fact sheet*. Retrieved November 7, 2015, from www.cdc.gov/std/pid/stdfact-pid-detailed.htm
Health Canada. (2014). *Surgical mesh—Complications associated with transvaginal implantation for the treatment of stress urinary incontinence and pelvic organ prolapse—Notice to hospitals*. Retrieved from http://www.healthycanadians.gc.ca/recall-alert-rappel-avis/hc-sc/2014/39475a-eng.php?_ga=2.106422467.1906023556.1527694014-189286785.1526158271
HealthLinkBC. (2016). *Vaginitis*. Retrieved from http://www.healthlinkbc.ca/kb/content/special/zx1776.html
Hoffstetter, S., & Shah, M. (2015). Vulvodynia. *Clinical Obstetrics and Gynecology*, *58*(3), 536–545.
Jepson, P. C., & Sung, V. W. (2014). Hysterectomy for pelvic organ prolapse: Indications and treatments. *Clinical Obstetrics and Gynecology*, *57*(1), 72–82.
Lev-Sagie, A. (2015). Vulvar and vaginal atrophy: Physiology, clinical presentation, and treatment considerations. *Clinical Obstetrics and Gynecology*, *58*(3), 476–491.
Maldonado, V. A. (2014). Benign vulvar tumors. *Best Practices & Research: Clinical Obstetrics & Gynecology*, *28*(7), 1088–1097.
McIntosh, L., Andersen, E., & Reekie, M. (2015). Conservative treatment of stress urinary incontinence in women: A 10-year (2004–2013) scoping review of the literature. *Urologic Nursing*, *35*(4), 179–186, 203.
Mellano, E. M., & Tarney, C. M. (2014). Management of genitourinary fistula. *Current Opinions in Obstetrics & Gynecology*, *26*(5), 415–423.
National Institute of Allergy and Infectious Diseases (NIAID). (2015). *NIAID research on genital herpes*. Retrieved November 7, 2015, from www.niaid.nih.gov/topics/genitalHerpes/research/Pages/research.aspx
Nyirjesy, P. (2014). Management of persistent vaginitis. *Obstetrics and Gynecology*, *124*(6), 1135–1146.
Petrosky, E., Bocchini, J. A., Hariri, S., et al. (2015). Use of 9-Valent human papillomavirus (HPV) vaccine: Updated HPV vaccination recommendations of the advisory committee on immunization practices. *CDC: Morbidity and Mortality Weekly Report*, *64*(11), 300–304.
Powell, A. M., & Nyirjesy, P. (2015). New perspectives on the normal vagina and noninfectious causes of discharge. *Clinical Obstetrics and Gynecology*, *58*(3), 453–463.
Public Health Agency of Canada (PHAC). (2013a). *Vaginal discharge (bacterial vaginosis, vulvovaginal candidiasis, trichomoniasis)*. Retrieved from http://www.phac-aspc.gc.ca/std-mts/sti-its/guide-lignesdir-eng.php
Public Health Agency of Canada (PHAC). (2013b). *The Chief Public Health Officer's Report on the State of Public Health in Canada 2013—Sexually transmitted infections—A continued public health concern*. Retrieved from https://www.canada.ca/en/public-health/corporate/publications/chief-public-health-officer-reports-state-public-health-canada/chief-public-health-officer-report-on-state-public-health-canada-2013-infectious-disease-never-ending-threat/sexually-transmitted-infections-a-continued-public-health-concern.html
Public Health Agency of Canada (PHAC). (2015a). *Genital human papillomavirus (HPV) infections*. Retrieved from https://www.canada.ca/en/public-health/services/infectious-diseases/sexual-health-sexually-transmitted-infections/canadian-guidelines/sexually-transmitted-infections/canadian-guidelines-sexually-transmitted-infections-33.html
Public Health Agency of Canada (PHAC). (2015b). *Summary: Estimates of HIV incidence, prevalence and proportion undiagnosed in Canada, 2014*. Retrieved from https://www.canada.ca/en/public-health/services/publications/diseases-conditions/summary-estimates-hiv-incidence-prevalence-proportion-undiagnosed-canada-2014.html#a2
Public Health Agency of Canada (PHAC). (2018). *Human papillomavirus (HPV) prevention and HPV vaccines: Questions and answers*. Retrieved from https://www.canada.ca/en/public-health/services/infectious-diseases/sexual-health-sexually-transmitted-infections/hpv-prevention-vaccines-questions-answers.html
Reichman, O., & Sobel, J. (2014). Desquamative inflammatory vaginitis. *Best Practice & Research: Clinical Obstetrics and Gynecology*, *28*(7), 1042–1050.
Ridgeway, B., & Falcone, T. (2014). Innovations in minimally invasive hysterectomies. *Clinical Obstetrics & Gynecology*, *57*(1), 83–94.
Statistics Canada. (2015). *Trends in the incidence and mortality of female reproductive system cancers*. Retrieved from http://publications.gc.ca/collections/collection_2015/statcan/82-624-x/CS82-624-x2015001-1-eng.pdf
Steege, J. F., & Siedhoff, M. T. (2014). Chronic pelvic pain. *Obstetrics and Gynecology*, *124*(3), 616–629.
Trikudanathan, S. (2015). Polycystic ovarian syndrome. *Medical Clinics of North America*, *99*(1), 221–235.
Women's Health Data Directory. (2013). *Hysterectomy rate*. Retrieved from http://www.womenshealthdata.ca/category.aspx?catid=125&rt=3
Wright, J. D., Herzog, T. J., Tsui, J., et al. (2013). Nationwide trends in the performance of inpatient hysterectomies in the United States. *Obstetrics & Gynecology*, *122*(2), 233–241.
Zweizig, S., Korets, S., & Cain, J. (2014). Key concepts in management of vulvar cancer. *Best Practices & Research: Clinical Obstetrics & Gynecology*, *28*(7), 959–966.

Resources

Association of Reproductive Health Professionals: http://www.arhp.org
Association of Women's Health, Obstetric and Neonatal Nurses (AWHONN): http://www.awhonn.org
Canadian Association of Perinatal and Women's Health Nurses: http://www.capwhn.ca/en/capwhn/index.php?page=3788
Canadian Cancer Society: http://www.cancer.ca
Canadian Federation for Sexual Health: http://www.cfsh.ca
Canadian Women's Health Network: http://www.cwhn.ca/en
Centers for Disease Control and Prevention, Office of Women's Health: http://www.cdc.gov/women/
Endometriosisinfo.ca: http://www.endometriosisinfo.ca/index_e.aspx
Endometriosis Association: http://www.endometriosisassn.org
Gay and Lesbian Medical Association: http://www.glma.org
Health Canada: http://www.hc-sc.gc.ca/index-eng.php
Infertility Awareness Association of Canada: http://www.selfhelp.on.ca/2014/10/infertility-awareness-association-of-canada/
Ovarian Cancer Canada: http://www.ovariancanada.org/
Planned Parenthood Associations in Canada: https://www.plannedparenthood.org/
Public Health Agency of Canada: http://www.phac-aspc.gc.ca/index-eng.php

49 Management of Patients With Breast Disorders

Adapted by Kelly Power-Kean

Learning Objectives

On completion of this chapter, the learner will be able to:

1. Describe the anatomy and physiology of the breast.
2. Identify the assessment and diagnostic studies used to diagnose breast disorders.
3. Compare and contrast the pathophysiology of benign and malignant breast disorders.
4. Summarize the evidence-based guidelines for the early detection of breast cancer.
5. Develop a plan for educating for patients and consumer groups about breast self-awareness.
6. Explain the different modalities used to treat breast cancer.
7. Use the nursing process as a framework for care of the patient undergoing surgery for the treatment of breast cancer.
8. Recognize the physical, psychosocial, and rehabilitative needs of the patient who has had breast surgery for the treatment of breast cancer.

Nurses care for patients with breast disorders in many settings. To care for these patients effectively, nurses require an understanding of the assessment, diagnostic testing, nursing management, and rehabilitation needs of patients with multiple processes that affect the breasts. A breast disorder, whether benign or malignant, can cause great anxiety and fear of potential disfigurement, loss of sexual attractiveness, and even death. Nurses, therefore, need the expertise in the assessment and management of not only the physical symptoms but also the psychosocial symptoms associated with breast disorders.

BREAST ASSESSMENT

Anatomic and Physiologic Overview

Male and female breasts mature comparably until puberty, when estrogen and other hormones initiate breast development. This development usually occurs from 10 to 16 years of age, although the range can vary from 9 to 18 years. Stages of breast development are described as Tanner stages 1 through 5.

- Stage 1 describes a prepubertal breast.
- Stage 2 is breast budding, the first sign of puberty in a female.
- Stage 3 involves further enlargement of breast tissue and the areola (a darker tissue ring around the nipple).
- Stage 4 occurs when the nipple and areola form a secondary mound on top of the breast tissue.
- Stage 5 is the continued development of a larger breast with a single contour.

The breasts are located between the second and sixth ribs over the pectoralis muscle from the sternum to the midaxillary line. An area of breast tissue, called the tail of Spence, extends into the axilla (Osborne & Boolbol, 2014). Fascial bands, called Cooper's ligaments, support the breast on the chest wall. The inframammary fold (or crease) is a ridge of fat at the bottom of the breast.

Each breast contains 12 to 20 cone-shaped lobes, which are made up of glandular elements (lobules and ducts) and separated by fat and fibrous tissue that binds the lobes together. Milk is produced in the lobules and then carried through the ducts to the nipple. Figure 49-1 shows the anatomy of the fully developed breast.

Assessment

Health History

When a patient presents with a breast problem, the nurse conducts a general health assessment, including history of medical disorders and previous surgery; family history of diseases, particularly cancer; gynecologic and obstetric history; present medications (including prescriptions, vitamins, and herbal); past and present use of hormonal contraceptives, hormone therapy (HT) (formerly referred to as hormone replacement therapy [HRT]), or fertility treatments; and social habits (e.g., smoking, drinking alcohol, illicit drug use). Psychosocial information, such as the patient's marital status, occupation, and availability of resources and support people, is obtained. Any recent x-rays or other diagnostic tests are noted. Focused questions pertaining to the breast disorder are asked concerning the onset of the disorder and the length of time it has been present. In addition, the patient is asked if any masses are palpable and if there is any associated pain, swelling, redness, nipple discharge, or changes in the skin. Knowledge and comfort related to breast self-awareness, which can include breast self-examination (BSE), should also be ascertained from the patient.

Glossary

adjuvant chemotherapy: use of anticancer medications in addition to other treatments to delay or prevent a recurrence of the disease

adjuvant hormonal therapy: use of synthetic hormones or other medications given after primary treatment to increase the chances of a cure by stopping or slowing the growth of certain cancers that are affected by hormone stimulation (sometimes called endocrine or antiestrogen therapy)

aromatase inhibitors: medications that block the production of estrogens by the adrenal glands

atypical hyperplasia: abnormal increase in the number of cells in a specific area within the ductal or lobular areas of the breast; this abnormal proliferation increases the risk for cancer

benign proliferative breast disease: various types of atypical, yet noncancerous, breast tissue that increase the risk for breast cancer

brachytherapy: delivery of radiation therapy through internal implants to a localized area of tissue

BRCA1 and BRCA2: genes on chromosome 17 that, when damaged or mutated, increase a woman's risk for breast and/or ovarian cancer compared with women without the mutation

Breast-conservation treatment: surgery to remove a breast tumour and a margin of tissue around the tumour without removing any other part of the breast; may or may not include lymph node removal and radiation therapy

dose-dense chemotherapy: administration of chemotherapeutic agents at standard doses with shorter time intervals between each cycle of treatment

ductal carcinoma in situ (DCIS): cancer cells starting in the ductal system of the breast but not penetrating surrounding tissue

fibrocystic breast changes: term used to describe certain benign changes in the breast, typically associated with palpable nodularity, lumpiness, swelling, or pain

fine-needle aspiration (FNA): removal of fluid for diagnostic analysis from a cyst or cells from a mass using a needle and syringe

gynecomastia: overdeveloped breast tissue typically seen in adolescent boys

HER-2/neu: a protein, when found in larger amounts, indicates an aggressive tumour

lobular carcinoma in situ (LCIS): atypical change and proliferation of the lobular cells of the breast

lymphedema: chronic swelling of an extremity due to interrupted lymphatic circulation, typically from an axillary lymph node dissection (ALND)

mammoplasty: surgery to reconstruct or change the size or shape of the breast; can be performed for reduction or augmentation

mastalgia: breast pain, usually related to hormonal fluctuations or irritation of a nerve

mastectomy: removal of the breast tissue and nipple–areola complex

mastitis: inflammation or infection of the breast

modified radical mastectomy: removal of the breast tissue, nipple–areola complex, and a portion of the axillary lymph nodes

Paget's disease: form of breast cancer that begins in the ductal system and involves scaly changes in the nipple, areola, and surrounding skin

sentinel lymph node: first lymph node(s) in the lymphatic basin that receives drainage from the primary tumour in the breast; identified by a radioisotope and/or blue dye

stereotactic core biopsy: computer-guided method of core needle biopsy that is useful when masses or calcifications in the breast cannot be felt but can be visualized using mammography

surgical biopsy: surgical removal of all or a portion of a mass for microscopic examination by a pathologist

tissue expander followed by permanent implant: series of breast-reconstructive surgeries after a mastectomy; involves stretching the skin and muscle before inserting the permanent implant

transverse rectus abdominis myocutaneous (TRAM) flap: method of breast reconstruction in which a flap of skin, fat, and muscle from the lower abdomen, with its attached blood supply, is rotated to the mastectomy site

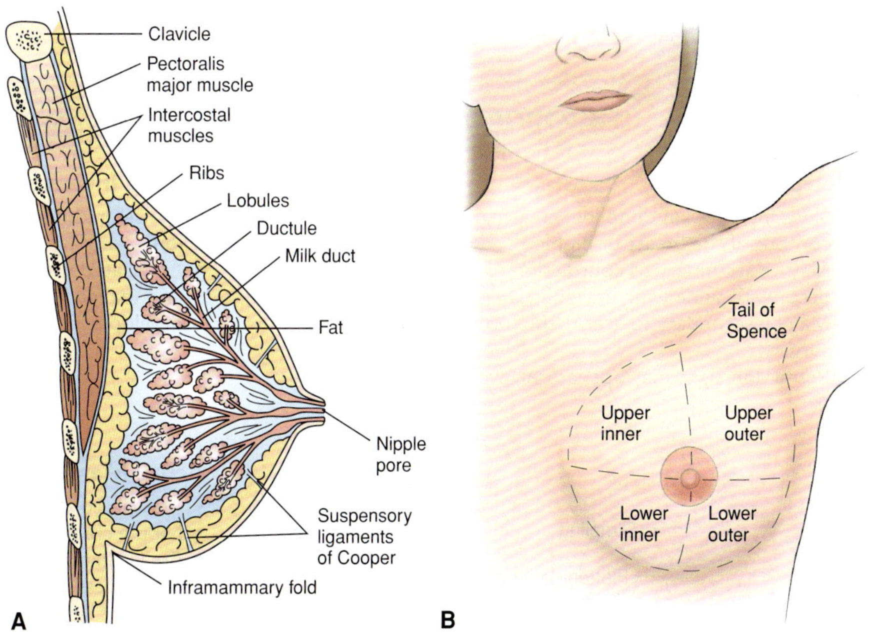

FIGURE 49-1. **A.** Anatomy of the breast. **B.** Areas of breast, including the tail of Spence.

Physical Assessment: Female Breast

A female breast examination can be conducted during any general physical or gynecologic examination or whenever the patient reports an abnormality. The Canadian Task Force for Preventative Health Care (CTFPHC) screening guidelines are for women considered average risk for breast cancer from the ages of 40 to 74 years. Both routine BSE and clinical breast examination is not recommended alone or in conjunction with mammography as no evidence has been found indicating that these practices reduce breast cancer mortality or all-cause mortality. A clinical breast examination remains appropriate when women present with, or physicians have concerns about, abnormal breast changes.

Inspection

Examination begins with inspection. The patient is asked to disrobe to the waist and sit in a comfortable position facing the examiner. The breasts are inspected for size and symmetry. A slight variation in the size of each breast is common and generally normal. The skin is inspected for colour, venous pattern, thickening, or edema. Erythema (redness) may indicate benign local inflammation or superficial lymphatic invasion by a neoplasm. A prominent venous pattern can signal increased blood supply required by a tumour. Edema and pitting of the skin may result from a neoplasm blocking lymphatic drainage, giving the skin an orange-peel appearance (peau d'orange), a classic sign of advanced breast cancer. Nipple inversion of one or both breasts is not uncommon and is significant only when of recent origin. Ulceration, rashes, or spontaneous nipple discharge requires evaluation. Examples of abnormal breast findings on inspection can be found in Chart 49-1.

To elicit skin dimpling or retraction that may otherwise go undetected, the examiner instructs the patient to raise both arms overhead. This manoeuvre usually elevates both breasts equally. The patient is then instructed to place her hands on her waist and push in. These movements, which cause contraction of the pectoral muscles, do not usually alter the breast contour or nipple direction. Any dimpling or retraction during these position changes suggests an underlying mass. The clavicular and axillary regions are inspected for swelling, discolouration, lesions, or enlarged lymph nodes (Morrow, 2014).

Palpation

The breasts are palpated with the patient sitting up (upright) and lying down (supine). In the supine position the patient's shoulder is first elevated with a small pillow to help balance the breast on the chest wall. Failure to do this allows the breast tissue to slip laterally, and a breast mass may be missed. The entire surface of the breast and the axillary tail is systematically palpated using the flat part (pads) of the second, third, and fourth fingertips, held together, making dime-sized circles. The examiner may choose to proceed in a clockwise direction, following imaginary concentric circles from the outer limits of the breast toward the nipple. Other acceptable methods are to palpate from each number on the face of the clock toward the nipple in a clockwise fashion or along imaginary vertical lines on the breast (Fig. 49-2).

Palpation of the axillary and clavicular areas is easily performed with the patient seated (Fig. 49-3). To examine the axillary lymph nodes, the examiner gently abducts the patient's arm from the thorax. With the left hand, the patient's left forearm is grasped and supported. The right hand is then free to palpate the axilla. Any lymph nodes that may be lying against the thoracic wall are noted. These lymph nodes are not normally palpable, but if they are enlarged, their location, size, mobility, and consistency are noted. During palpation, the examiner notes any patient-reported tenderness or masses. If a mass is detected, it is described by its location (e.g., right breast, 2 cm from the nipple at 2 o'clock position). Size, shape, consistency, border delineation, and mobility are included in the description (Morrow, 2014). The examiner then

CHART 49-1

Abnormal Findings During Inspection of the Breasts

Retraction Signs

- Signs include skin dimpling, creasing, or changes in the contour of the breast or nipple
- May be secondary to contraction of fibrotic tissue that can occur with underlying malignancy
- May be secondary to scar tissue formation after breast surgery
- Retraction signs may appear only with position changes

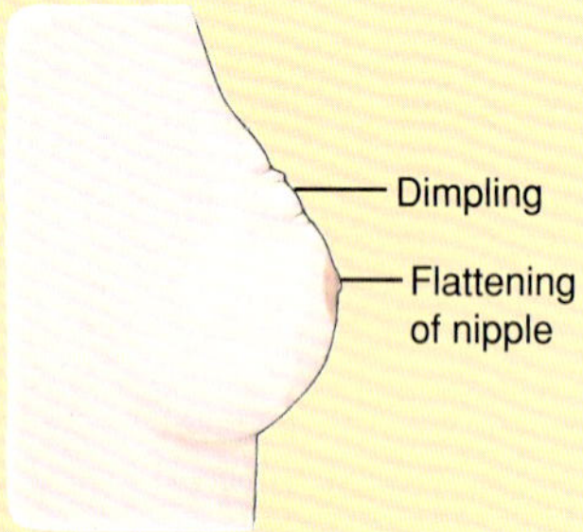

Retraction signs

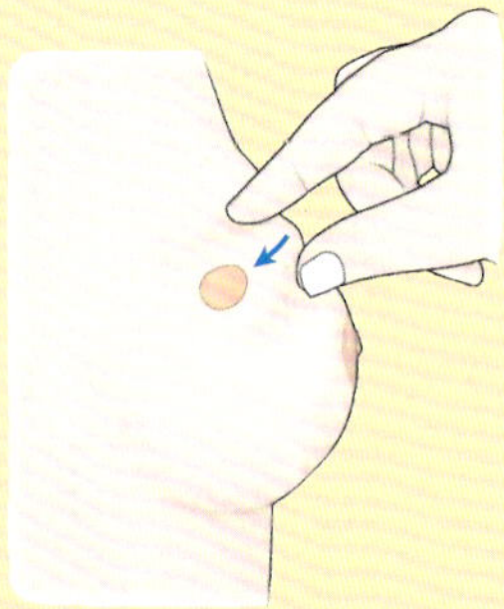

Retraction with compression

Increased Venous Prominence

- Unilateral localized increase in venous pattern associated with malignant tumours
- Normal with bilateral and symmetrical breast enlargement associated with pregnancy and lactation

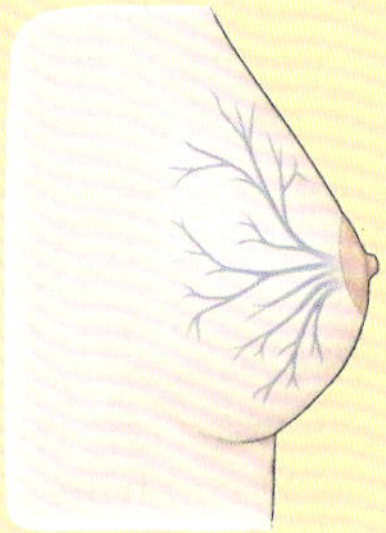

Increased venous prominence

Peau d'Orange (Edema)

- Associated with inflammatory breast cancer
- Caused by interference with lymphatic drainage
- Breast skin has orange peel appearance
- Skin pores enlarge
- May be noted on the areola
- Skin becomes thick, hard, and immobile

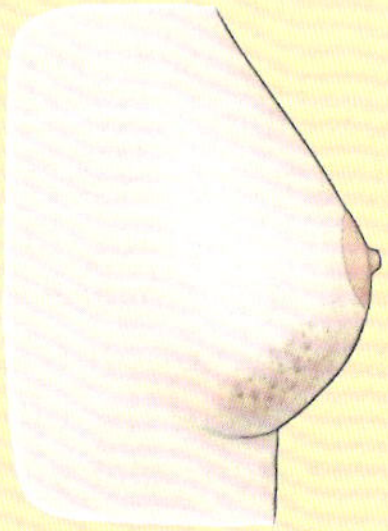

Peau d'orange

Nipple Inversion

- Considered normal if long-standing
- Associated with fibrosis and malignancy if recent development

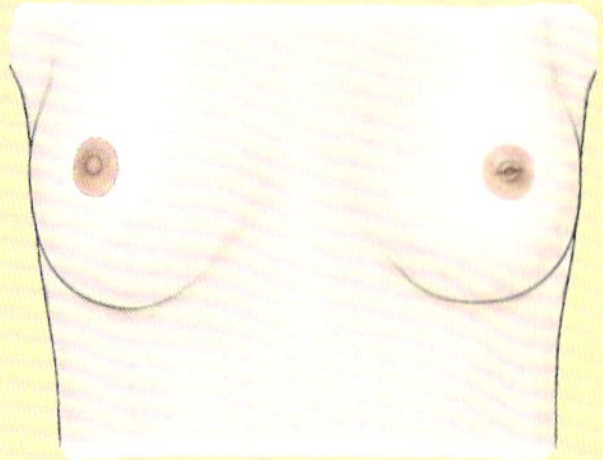

Nipple inversion

Acute Mastitis (Inflammation of the Breasts)

- Associated with lactation but may occur at any age
- Nipple cracks or abrasions noted
- Breast skin reddened and warm to touch
- Tenderness
- Systemic signs include fever and increased pulse

Paget's Disease (Malignancy of Mammary Ducts)

- Early signs: erythema of nipple and areola
- Late signs: thickening, scaling, and erosion of the nipple and areola

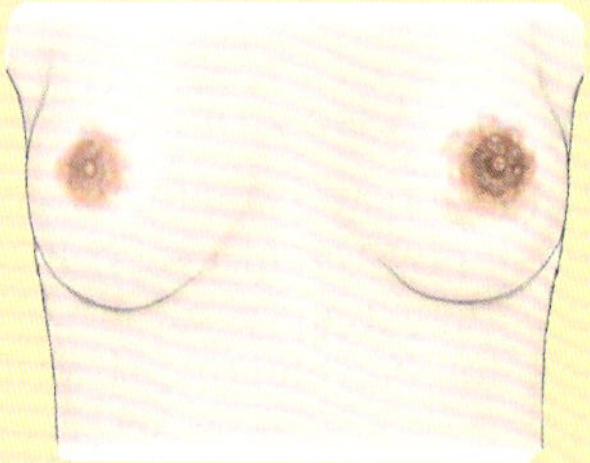

Paget's disease

modifies these steps to use the right hand to grasp the patient's left forearm, and then uses the left hand to palpate the axilla of the left breast.

The breast tissue of the adolescent is usually firm and lobular, whereas that of the postmenopausal woman is more likely to feel thinner and fattier. During pregnancy and lactation, the breasts are firmer and larger with lobules that are more distinct. Hormonal changes cause the areola to darken.

Cysts are commonly found in women who are menstruating and are usually well defined and freely movable. During the premenstrual period, cysts may be larger and more tender. Malignant tumours, on the other hand, tend to be hard, poorly defined, and nontender. The clinician should further evaluate any abnormalities detected during inspection and palpation.

Obesity may have a proinflammatory effect on the breast that can contribute to increased rates of atypia. Atypia in breast ductal lavage and C-reactive protein levels in the nipple are significantly correlated with body mass index (BMI). Excessive body weight, as reflected by a BMI of 25 kg/m^2 or higher, is associated with postmenopausal breast cancer and increases the risk of dying of this disease (Gucalp, Morris, Hudis, et al., 2014).

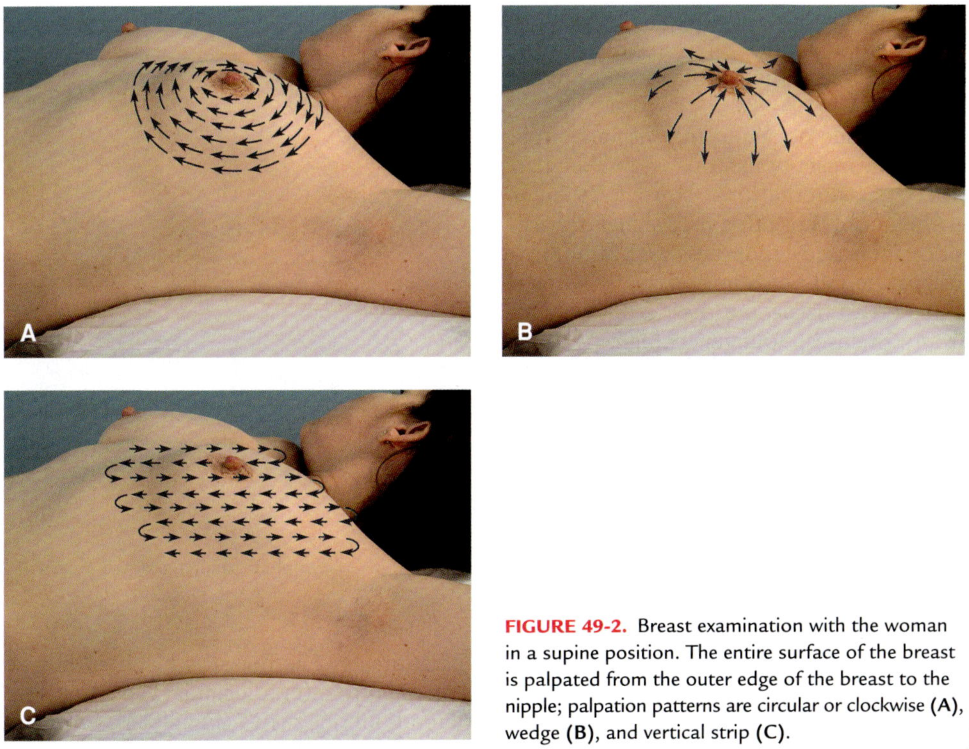

FIGURE 49-2. Breast examination with the woman in a supine position. The entire surface of the breast is palpated from the outer edge of the breast to the nipple; palpation patterns are circular or clockwise (**A**), wedge (**B**), and vertical strip (**C**).

Physical Assessment: Male Breast

Breast cancer can occur in men. Assessment of the male breast and axilla is brief but important and should be included in a physical examination. The nipple and areola are inspected for swelling, nodules, ulcerations, and nipple discharge. The flat disk of undeveloped breast tissue under the nipple is palpated. The same procedure for palpating the female axilla is used when assessing the male axilla (Weber & Kelley, 2014).

Gynecomastia is the firm enlargement of glandular tissue beneath and immediately surrounding the areola of the male. This is different from the enlargement of soft, fatty tissue, which is caused by obesity.

Diagnostic Evaluation

A wide range of diagnostic studies may be performed in patients with breast conditions (Fig. 49-4). The nurse should educate the patient about the purpose, what to expect, and any possible side effects related to these examinations prior to testing. The nurse should note trends in the patient's test results because they often provide information about disease progression as well as the patient's response to therapy.

Breast Self-Examination

The nurse plays an important role in breast awareness education, a modality used for the early detection of breast

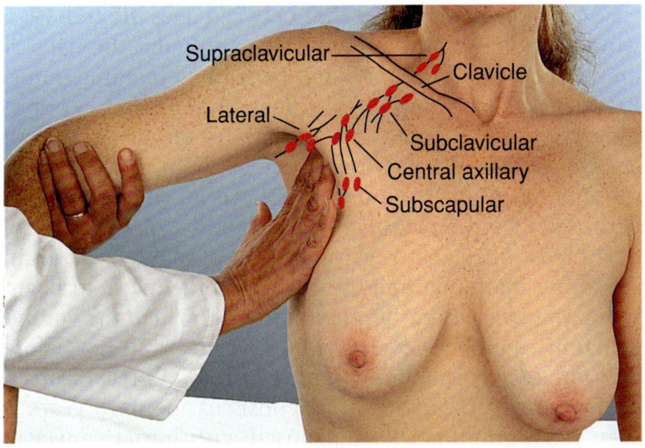

FIGURE 49-3. Palpating axillary nodes in breast examination.

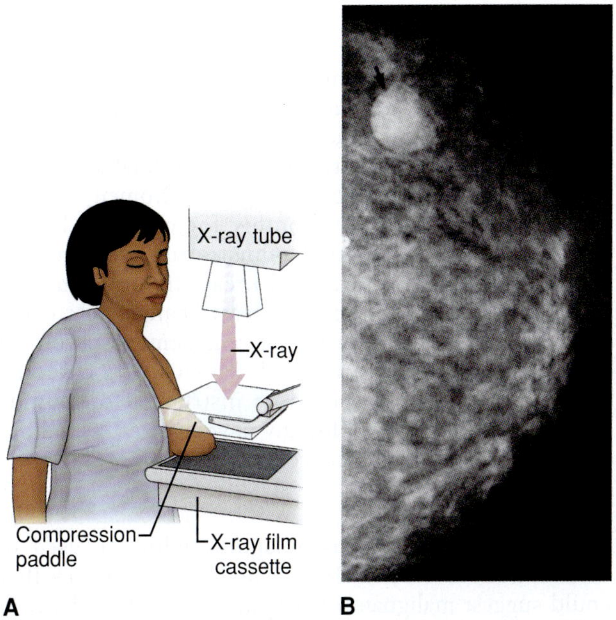

FIGURE 49-4. The mammography procedure (**A**) relies on x-ray imaging to produce the mammogram (**B**), which in this case reveals a breast lump.

cancer. The Canadian Cancer Society (CCS) (2018g) recommends that all women, regardless of age, should know what is normal for their breasts and tell their care provider if they notice any changes.

Variations in breast tissue occur during the menstrual cycle, pregnancy, and the onset of menopause. Women on HT can also experience fluctuations. Normal changes must be distinguished from those that may signal disease. Most women notice increased tenderness and lumpiness before their menstrual periods. In addition, many women have grainy-textured breast tissue, but these areas are usually less nodular after menses. Younger women may find discovering changes more difficult because of the density of their breast tissue. As women age, their breasts become fattier and may be easier to examine.

Practice has shifted from educating women about BSE to promoting breast self-awareness, which is a woman's attentiveness to the normal appearance and feel of her breasts. However, self-examination still may be appropriate for some women who are at high risk and for those who prefer it. Breast self-awareness can include self-examination. For every woman, knowing how her breasts normally feel helps detect any changes or signs of a problem. BSE may play an important role in screening, especially for women who develop cancer in the interval after a negative result on mammography or clinical breast examination or who have a false-negative imaging or clinical examination result. It can also promote detection in women who have not been screened. The goal, with or without BSE, is to report any breast changes to a primary provider.

Family history can increase the risk of breast cancer in men, particularly if other men in the family have had breast cancer. The risk is also higher if there is a breast cancer gene abnormality in the family. An abnormal *BRCA2* gene accounts for up to 40% of male breast cancers (Jain & Gradishar, 2014). Instructions about BSE should be provided to men if they have a family history of breast cancer.

Patients who elect to perform BSE should receive proper instruction on technique (Chart 49-2). They should be informed that routine monthly BSE will help them become familiar with their "normal abnormalities." If a change is detected, they should seek medical attention.

Patients should be instructed about optimal timing for BSE (5 to 7 days after menses begin for women who are premenopausal and once monthly for women who are postmenopausal). When demonstrating examination techniques, the feel of normal breast tissue should be reviewed and ways to identify breast changes discussed. Patients should then perform a BSE demonstration on themselves or on a breast model. Patients who have had breast cancer surgery should be instructed to examine their breast or chest wall for any new changes or nodules that may indicate a recurrence of the disease.

Mammography

Mammography is a breast-imaging technique used to visualize the breast to detect small abnormalities that could suggest malignant or benign disease (Fischbach & Dunning, 2015). The procedure takes about 15 minutes and can be performed in a hospital radiology department or independent imaging centre. Two views are taken of

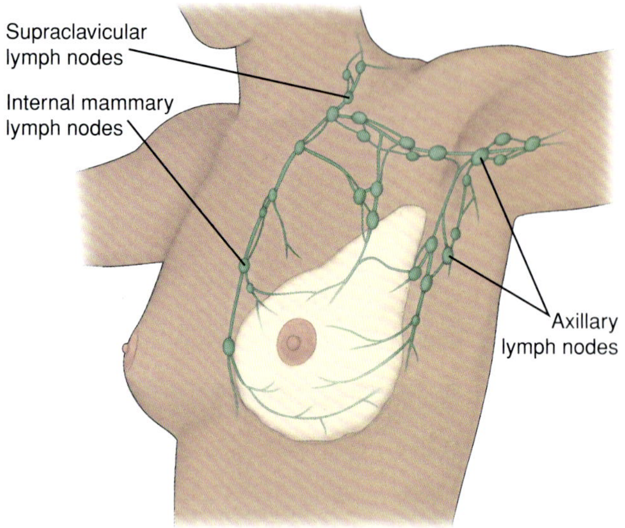

FIGURE 49-5. Lymphatic drainage of the breast.

each breast. The breast is mechanically compressed from top to bottom (craniocaudal view) and side to side (mediolateral oblique view) (Fig. 49-5). Women may experience some fleeting discomfort because maximum compression is necessary for proper visualization. The new mammogram is compared with previous mammograms, and any changes may indicate a need for further investigation. Mammography may detect a breast tumour before it is clinically palpable (i.e., smaller than 1 cm); however, it has limitations (Fischbach & Dunning, 2015). The false-negative rate ranges between 5% and 10% (Helvie & Patterson, 2014). Younger women, or those taking HT, may have dense breast tissue, making it more difficult to detect lesions with mammography.

Patients scheduled for a mammogram may voice concern about exposure to radiation. The radiation exposure is equivalent to about 1 hour of exposure to sunlight, so patients would have to have many mammograms in a year to increase their cancer risk. The benefits of this test outweigh the risks. To ensure that a mammogram is reliable, it is important to note that the responsibility for the quality of mammograms in Canada is shared among the federal, provincial, and territorial governments and is directed by the Canadian Mammogram Quality Guidelines.

Current mammographic screening guidelines of the CCS (2018a) recommend that between ages 40 and 49, a woman should discuss with her care provider the risks of breast cancer and the risks and benefits of mammograms. Between ages 50 and 69, a woman should have a mammogram every 2 years. After 70 years of age, a woman should discuss with her care provider about the frequency of mammograms. Women who are at increased risk because of a strong family history should seek the opinion of a breast specialist regarding the optimal age to begin screening mammography. A general guideline is to begin screening 10 years earlier than the age at which the youngest family member developed breast cancer but not before 25 years of age. In families with a history of breast cancer, a downward shift in age of diagnosis of about 10 years is seen (e.g., grandmother diagnosed with breast cancer at 48 years of age, mother diagnosed with breast cancer at

CHART 49-2

Patient Education: Breast Self-Examination

The nurse instructs the patient to perform the following steps:

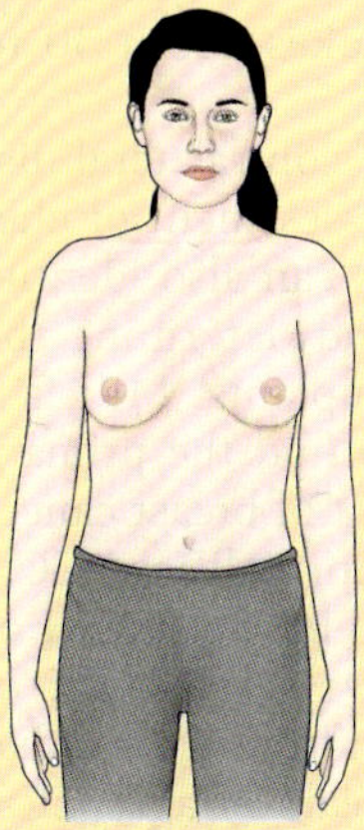

Step 1

1. Stand in front of a mirror.
2. Check both breasts for anything unusual.
3. Look for discharge from the nipple, puckering, dimpling, or scaling of the skin.

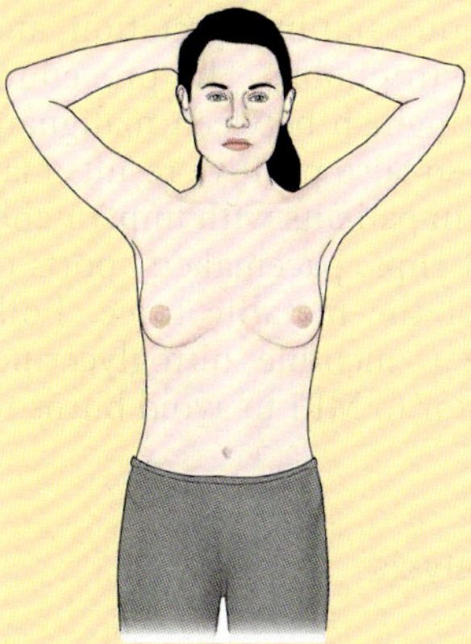

Step 2

Steps 2 and 3 are done to check for any changes in the contour of your breasts. As you do them, you should be able to feel your muscles tighten.

1. Watch closely in the mirror as you clasp your hands behind your head and press your hands forward.
2. Note any change in the contour of your breasts.

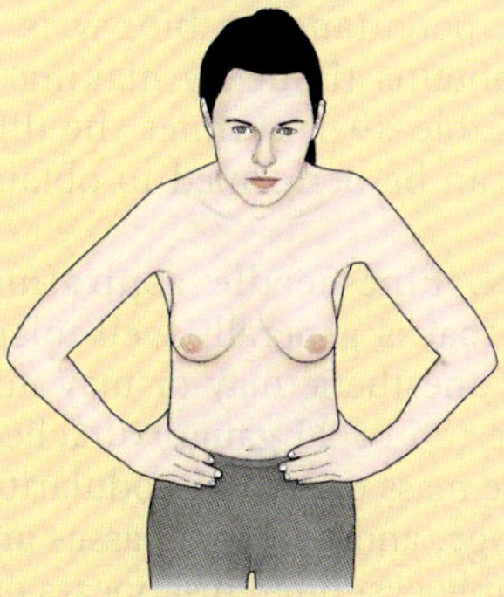

Step 3

1. Next, press your hands firmly on your hips, and bow slightly toward the mirror as you pull your shoulders and elbows forward.
2. Note any change in the contour of your breasts.

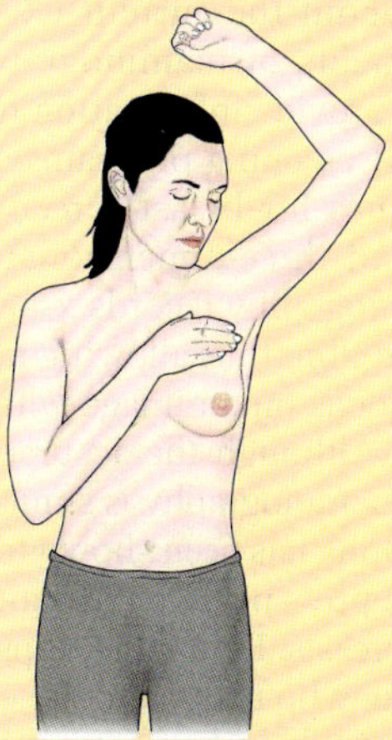

Step 4

Some women do step 4 in the shower. Your fingers will glide easily over soapy skin, so you can concentrate on feeling for changes inside the breast.

1. Raise your left arm.
2. Use three or four fingers of your right hand to feel your left breast firmly, carefully, and thoroughly.
3. Beginning at the outer edge, press the flat part of your fingers in small circles, moving the circles slowly around the breast.
4. Gradually work toward the nipple.
5. Be sure to cover the whole breast.
6. Pay special attention to the area between the breast and the underarm, including the underarm itself.
7. Feel for any unusual lumps or masses under the skin.
8. If you have any spontaneous discharge during the month, whether or not it is during your breast self-examination, see your primary provider.
9. Repeat the examination on your right breast.

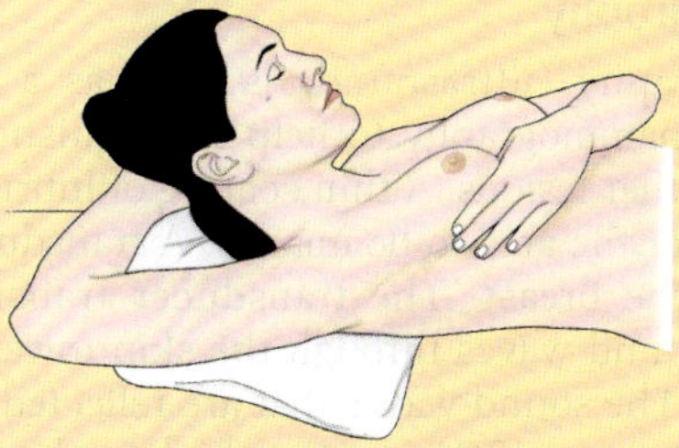

Step 5

1. Step 5 should be repeated lying down.
2. Lie flat on your back with your left arm over your head and a pillow or folded towel under your left shoulder. (This position flattens your breast and makes it easier to check.)
3. Use the same circular motion described earlier.
4. Repeat on your right breast.

Adapted from Stephen, T. C., Skillen, D. L., Day, R. A., et al. (Eds.). (2010). *Canadian Bates' guide to health assessment for nurses* (1st ed.). Philadelphia, PA: Lippincott Williams & Wilkins.

38 years of age, then daughter should begin screening at age 28 years of age).

Despite the decreased mortality rates associated with mammographic screening, many women are not undergoing this simple procedure. Nurses are in key positions to educate women about the current CCS screening guidelines and the benefits of mammography. They can also help identify and provide information to women who may benefit from such screening programs.

Newer techniques for breast screening include digital mammography and three-dimensional (3D) mammography. Digital mammography records x-ray images on a computer instead of on film, thus allowing radiologists to adjust the contrast and focus on an image without having to take additional x-rays. Although the accuracy of both film and digital screening mammography is similar for most women, digital mammography has been shown to be better at detecting estrogen receptor–negative tumours and cancer in extremely dense breasts. Both subgroups are more common in younger women, who may therefore choose digital mammography if they wish to have screening mammography. The 3D mammography obtains multiple projections of the compressed breast and results in fewer call backs for additional imaging (Jochelson, 2014). Computer-aided detection (CAD) is an option for radiologists and can be helpful in finding abnormal areas that should be checked more closely for early cancers. Refinements and improvements have been made to CAD software with a focus on increasing sensitivity for masses and reducing false-positive rates.

Contrast Mammography

A contrast-enhanced digital mammography (CEDM) is a diagnostic procedure that involves injection of less than 1 mL of radiopaque material through a cannula inserted into a ductal opening on the areola, which is followed by a mammogram (Fischbach & Dunning, 2015). It is performed to evaluate an abnormality within the duct when the patient has bloody nipple discharge on expression, spontaneous nipple discharge, or a solitary dilated duct noted on mammography.

Ultrasonography

Ultrasonography (ultrasound) is used as a diagnostic adjunct to mammography to help distinguish fluid-filled cysts from other lesions. A thin coating of lubricating jelly is spread over the area to be imaged. A transducer is then placed on the breast. The transducer transmits high-frequency sound waves through the skin toward the area of concern. The sound waves that are reflected back form a two-dimensional (2D) image, which is then displayed on a computer screen. No radiation is emitted during the procedure. Ultrasound is also used as an adjunct to mammography in women with dense breast tissue.

Ultrasonography has advantages and disadvantages. Although it can diagnose cysts with great accuracy, it cannot definitively rule out malignant lesions. Microcalcifications, which are detectable on mammography, cannot be identified on ultrasonography. Finally, examination techniques and interpretation criteria are not standardized.

Magnetic Resonance Imaging

Magnetic resonance imaging (MRI) of the breast is a highly sensitive test that has become a useful diagnostic adjunct to mammography. A magnet is linked to a computer that creates detailed images of the breast without exposure to radiation. An intravenous (IV) injection of gadolinium, a contrast dye, is given to improve visibility. The patient lies face down and the breast is placed through a depression in the table. A coil is placed around the breast, and the patient is placed inside the MRI machine. The entire procedure takes about 30 to 40 minutes.

Breast MRI is useful for evaluation of contralateral disease, invasive lobular carcinoma, and assessment of chemotherapeutic response. The procedure can also identify occult (undetectable) breast cancer and determine the integrity of saline or silicone breast implants. MRI is a highly sensitive screening tool that can find the primary tumour in the breast, examine the extent of breast cancer in the tissue, and better examine abnormalities (CCS, 2018b). Candidates include women who have a *BRCA1* or *BRCA2* mutation, a first-degree relative with either of these mutations, certain rare genetic syndromes, or radiation to the chest between 10 and 30 years of age (CCS, 2018g). MRI should be used in addition to mammography, not instead of it. Some disadvantages of MRI include high cost, variations in technique and interpretation, and the potential for patient claustrophobia. The procedure cannot always accurately distinguish between malignant and benign breast conditions, so false-positive results may occur. MRI is contraindicated in patients with implantable metal devices (e.g., aneurysm clips, pacemakers, ports of tissue expanders) because of the metallic force. Foil-backed medication patches (e.g., nicotine, nitroglycerine, fentanyl) must be removed prior to MRI to avoid burns to the skin.

Procedures for Tissue Analysis

Percutaneous Biopsy

Percutaneous biopsy is performed on an outpatient basis to sample palpable and nonpalpable lesions. Less invasive than a **surgical biopsy**, percutaneous biopsy is a needle or core biopsy that obtains tissue by making a small puncture in the skin. Table 49-1 outlines the different types of biopsies that can be performed to obtain a tissue diagnosis.

FINE-NEEDLE ASPIRATION. Fine-needle aspiration (FNA) is a biopsy technique that is generally well tolerated by most women. A local anesthetic may or may not be used. A small gauge needle (25 or 22 gauge) attached to a syringe is inserted into the mass or area of nodularity. Suction is applied to the syringe, and multiple passes are made through the mass. A simple cyst often disappears on aspiration, and the fluid is usually discarded. If no fluid is obtained, any cellular material obtained in the hub of the needle is spread on a glass slide or placed in a preservative and sent to the laboratory for analysis (CancerQuest, 2015). For nonpalpable masses, the same procedure can be performed by a radiologist using ultrasound guidance (ultrasound-guided FNA).

FNA is less expensive than other diagnostic methods and results are usually available quickly. However, false-negative or false-positive results are possible, and appropriate follow-up depends on the clinical judgment of the treating physician.

TABLE 49-1 Types of Breast Biopsies

Procedure	Palpable Mass	Health Professional Who Performs Procedure	Nature of Breast Tissue Removed
Fine-needle aspiration	Yes	Surgeon	Cellular material
Core needle biopsy	Yes	Surgeon	Tissue core
Stereotactic core biopsy	No	Radiologist	Tissue core
Ultrasound-guided core biopsy	No	Radiologist	Tissue core
MRI-guided core biopsy	No	Radiologist	Tissue core
Excisional biopsy	Yes	Surgeon	Entire mass
Incisional biopsy	Yes	Surgeon	Tissue core
Wire needle localization biopsy; may be guided by mammogram, ultrasound, or MRI	No	Radiologist inserts wire, surgeon performs biopsy	Entire mass

CORE NEEDLE BIOPSY. Core needle biopsy is similar to FNA, except a larger gauge needle is used (usually 14 gauge). A local anesthetic is applied, and tissue cores are removed via a spring-loaded device. This procedure allows for a more definitive diagnosis than FNA, because actual tissue, not just cells, is removed. It is often performed for relatively large tumours that are close to the skin surface but is also utilized for smaller, deeper lesions that are visible on ultrasound.

STEREOTACTIC CORE BIOPSY. Stereotactic core biopsy is performed on nonpalpable lesions detected by mammography. The patient lies prone on the stereotactic table. The breast is suspended through an opening in the table and compressed between two x-ray plates. Images are then obtained using digital mammography. The exact coordinates of the lesion to be sampled are located with the aid of a computer. Next, a local anesthetic is injected into the entry site on the breast. A small nick is made in the skin, a core needle is inserted, and samples of the tissue are taken for pathologic examination. Often, several passes are taken to ensure that the lesion is well sampled. Postbiopsy films are then taken to check that sampling has been adequate. A small titanium clip is almost always placed at the biopsy site so that the site can easily be located if further treatment is indicated.

Stereotactic biopsy is quite accurate and often allows the patient to avoid a surgical biopsy. However, there is a small false-negative rate. Appropriate follow-up depends on the final pathologic diagnosis and the clinical judgment of the treating physician. Use of a titanium clip does not preclude subsequent MRIs.

ULTRASOUND-GUIDED CORE BIOPSY. The principles for ultrasound-guided core biopsy are similar to those of stereotactic core biopsy, but by using ultrasound guidance, computer coordination and mammographic compression are not necessary. An ultrasound-guided core biopsy does not use radiation and is usually faster and less expensive than stereotactic core biopsy.

MAGNETIC RESONANCE IMAGING–GUIDED CORE BIOPSY. MRI-guided core biopsy can be performed by a radiologist and technologist when the abnormal area in the breast is too small to be felt but is visible on MRI.

Surgical Biopsy

Surgical biopsy is usually performed using local anesthesia and IV sedation. After an incision is made, the lesion is excised and sent to a laboratory for pathologic examination. Surgical biopsy is usually preceded by a core biopsy or stereotactic biopsy for pathologic determination.

TYPES OF SURGICAL BREAST BIOPSY

Excisional Biopsy. Excisional biopsy is the standard procedure for complete pathologic assessment of a palpable breast mass. The entire mass, plus a margin of surrounding tissue, is removed. This type of biopsy may also be referred to as a lumpectomy. Depending on the clinical situation, a frozen section analysis of the specimen may be performed at the time of the biopsy by the pathologist, who does an immediate reading intraoperatively and provides a provisional diagnosis. This can help confirm a diagnosis in a patient who had no previous tissue analysis performed.

Incisional Biopsy. Incisional biopsy surgically removes a portion of a mass. This is performed to confirm a diagnosis and to conduct special studies (e.g., ER/PR, **HER-2/neu** [also referred to as ERBB2]; see later discussion for explanation of these terms) that will aid in determining treatment, which are discussed later in this chapter. Complete excision of the area may not be possible or immediately beneficial to the patient, depending on the clinical situation. This procedure is often performed on women with locally advanced breast cancer or on women with suspected cancer recurrence, whose treatment may depend on the results of these special studies. However, pathologic information may be easily obtained from core needle biopsy, and incisional biopsy is becoming less common.

Wire Needle Localization. Wire needle localization is a technique used to locate nonpalpable masses or suspicious calcium deposits detected on a mammogram, ultrasound, or MRI that require an excisional biopsy. The radiologist inserts a long, thin wire through a needle, which is then inserted into the area of abnormality using x-ray or ultrasound guidance (whichever imaging technique originally identified the abnormality). The wire remains in place after the needle is withdrawn to ensure the precise location. The patient is then taken to the operating room, where the surgeon follows the wire to the tip and excises the area.

NURSING MANAGEMENT. During the preoperative or preprocedural visit, the nurse assesses the patient for any specific educational, physical, or psychosocial needs. This can be accomplished by reviewing the medical and psychosocial history and encouraging her to verbalize her fears, concerns, and questions. Patients are often worried not only about the procedure but also about the potential implications of the pathology results. Providing a thorough explanation about what to expect in a supportive manner can help alleviate anxiety. Patients often have difficulty absorbing all the information given to them; therefore, written materials should be provided to reinforce and clarify education.

The nurse instructs the patient to discontinue any agents that can increase the risk of bleeding, including products containing aspirin, nonsteroidal anti-inflammatory drugs, vitamin E supplements, herbal substances (such as ginkgo biloba and garlic supplements). Patients taking prescription anticoagulants must contact their health care provider (physician or NP) prior to the procedure of surgical biopsy to check whether a temporary cessation of anticoagulant is needed in order to prevent the occurrence of prolonged bleeding or development of hematomas. The patient may be instructed not to eat or drink for several hours prior to the procedure or after midnight the night before the procedure, depending on the type of biopsy and anesthesia planned. Most breast biopsy procedures today are performed with the use of moderate sedation and local anesthesia.

Immediate postoperative assessment includes monitoring the effects of the anesthesia and inspecting the surgical dressing for any signs of bleeding. Once the sedation has worn off, the nurse reviews the care of the biopsy site, pain management, and activity restrictions with the patient. Prior to discharge from the ambulatory surgical centre or the office, the patient must be able to tolerate fluids, ambulate, and void. The patient must be accompanied home. The dressing covering the incision is usually removed after 48 hours, but the Steri-Strips, which are applied directly over the incision, should remain in place for approximately 7 to 10 days or until they fall off. The use of a supportive bra following surgery is encouraged to limit movement of the breast and reduce discomfort. A follow-up telephone call from the nurse 24 to 48 hours after the procedure can provide the patient with the opportunity to ask any questions and can be a source of great comfort and reassurance.

Most women return to their usual activities the day after the procedure but are encouraged to avoid jarring or high-impact activities for 1 week to promote healing of the biopsy site. Discomfort is usually minimal, and most women find acetaminophen (Tylenol) sufficient for pain relief, although a mild opioid analgesic agent may be prescribed if needed.

Follow-up after the biopsy includes a return visit to the surgeon for discussion of the final pathology report and assessment of the healing of the biopsy site. Depending on the results of the biopsy, the nurse's role varies. If the pathology report is benign, the nurse reviews incision care and explains what the patient should expect as the biopsy site heals (i.e., changes in sensation may occur weeks or months after the biopsy due to nerve injury within the breast tissue). If a diagnosis of cancer is made, the nurse's role changes dramatically. This is discussed in depth later in this chapter.

CONDITIONS AFFECTING THE NIPPLE

Nipple Discharge

Nipple discharge in a woman who is not lactating may be related to many causes, such as carcinoma, papilloma, pituitary adenoma, cystic breasts, and various medications. Oral contraceptives, pregnancy, HT, chlorpromazine (Thorazine)-type medications, and frequent breast stimulation may be contributing factors. In some women, nipple discharge may occur during running or aerobic exercises. Nipple discharge should be evaluated by a health care provider, but it is not often a cause for alarm. One in three women has clear discharge on expression, which is usually normal. A green discharge could indicate an infection. Any discharge that is spontaneous, persistent, or unilateral is of concern. Although bloody discharge can indicate a malignancy, it is often caused by a benign wart-like growth on the lining of the duct called an intraductal papilloma.

Nipple discharge should be evaluated for the presence of occult (hidden) blood by performing a guaiac test. A negative test can be reassuring as it indicates there is no blood, but it does not prove there is no malignancy. A galactogram can also be performed to detect abnormalities within the duct that may be causing the discharge. If there is a high level of suspicion, an excisional biopsy may be indicated.

Fissure

A fissure is a longitudinal ulcer that may develop in women who are breastfeeding. If the nipple becomes irritated, a painful, raw area may form and become a site of infection. Daily washing with water, massage with breast milk or lanolin, and exposure to air are helpful. Breastfeeding can be continued with the use of a nipple shield. If the fissure is severe or extremely painful, the woman is advised to stop breastfeeding. A breast pump can be used until breastfeeding can be resumed. Persistent ulceration requires further diagnosis and therapy. Guidance from a nurse or lactation consultant may be helpful because nipple irritation can result from improper positioning (i.e., the infant has not grasped the areola fully) during breastfeeding.

BREAST INFECTIONS

Mastitis

Mastitis, an inflammation or infection of breast tissue, occurs most commonly in women who are breastfeeding, although it may also occur in women who are nonlactating. The infection may result from a transfer of microorganisms to the breast by the patient's hands or from a breastfed infant with an oral, eye, or skin infection. Mastitis may also be caused by blood-borne organisms. As inflammation progresses, the breast texture becomes tough or doughy, and the patient reports dull to severe pain in the infected region. A nipple that is discharging purulent material, serum, or blood should be promptly investigated.

Treatment consists of antibiotics and local application of cold compresses to relieve discomfort. A broad-spectrum antibiotic agent may be prescribed for 7 to 10 days. The patient should wear a snug bra and perform personal hygiene carefully. Adequate rest and hydration are important aspects of management.

Lactational Abscess

A breast abscess may develop as a consequence of acute mastitis. The area affected becomes tender and red. Purulent matter can usually be aspirated with a needle, but incision and drainage may be required. Specimens of the aspirated material are obtained for culture so that an organism-specific antibiotic agent can be prescribed.

BENIGN CONDITIONS OF THE BREAST

Breast Pain

Mastalgia (breast pain) may be cyclical or noncyclical. Cyclical pain is usually related to hormonal fluctuations usually during the menstrual cycle, and accounts for the majority of complaints. Noncyclical pain is far less common and does not vary with the menstrual cycle. Women who experience injury or trauma to the breast or those who have had a breast biopsy may experience noncyclical pain. Patients should be reassured that breast pain is rarely indicative of cancer. However, if the pain persists after menses begins, the patient should see her primary provider.

Nursing Management

The nurse may recommend that the patient wear a supportive bra both day and night for a week, decrease her salt and caffeine intake, and take ibuprofen (Advil) as needed for its anti-inflammatory actions. Vitamin E supplements may also be helpful.

Cysts

Cysts are fluid-filled sacs that develop as breast ducts dilate. Cysts occur most commonly in women 30 to 55 years of age and may be exacerbated during perimenopause. Although their cause is unknown, cysts usually disappear after menopause, suggesting that estrogen is a factor. Cystic areas often fluctuate in size and are usually larger premenstrually. They may be painless or may become very tender premenstrually. Occasionally, a patient may report an intermittent shooting sensation or a dull ache. Various breast masses are compared in Table 49-2. Cysts that are confirmed on an ultrasound and are not bothersome can often be left alone. To confirm a diagnosis or to relieve pain, FNA can be performed. Cysts do not increase the risk of breast cancer (ACS, 2015).

Fibrocystic breast changes, which are often called fibrocystic breast disease, is a nonspecific term used to describe an array of benign findings including palpable nodularity, lumpiness, swelling, or pain. The changes do not necessarily indicate a cystic or disease process.

Fibroadenomas

Fibroadenomas are firm, round, movable, benign tumours. They can occur from puberty to menopause with a peak

TABLE 49-2 Comparison of Various Breast Masses

The most common breast masses are due to cysts, fibroadenomas, or malignancy. Biopsy is usually needed for confirmation, but the following characteristics are diagnostic clues:

Characteristics	Cysts	Fibroadenomas	Malignancy
	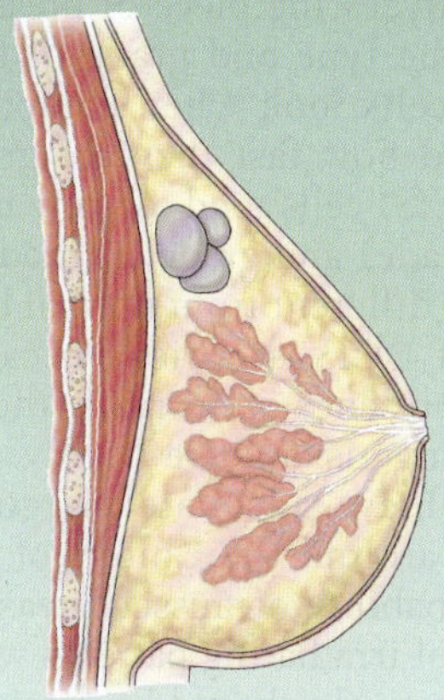	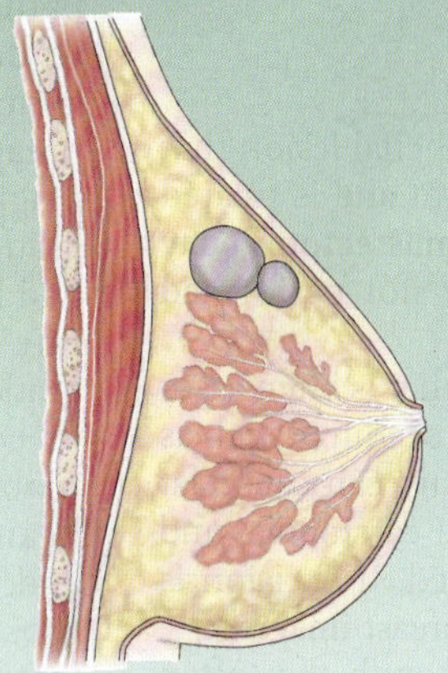	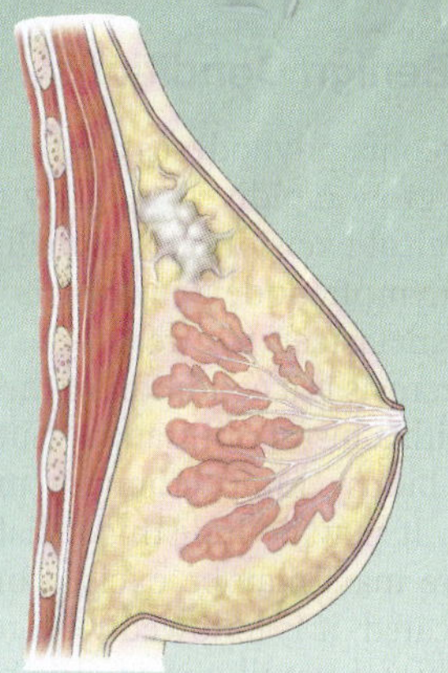
Age	30–55 yrs, regress after menopause except with use of estrogen therapy	Puberty to menopause	30–90 yrs; most common, 40–80 yrs
Number	Single or multiple	Usually single	Usually single
Shape	Round	Round, disk, or lobular	Irregular or stellate
Consistency	Soft to firm, usually elastic	Usually firm	Firm or hard
Mobility	Mobile	Mobile	May be fixed to skin or underlying tissues
Tenderness	Usually tender	Usually nontender	Usually nontender
Retraction signs	Absent	Absent	May be present

Adapted from Weber, J., & Kelley, J. (2014). *Health assessment in nursing* (5th ed.). Philadelphia, PA: Lippincott Williams & Wilkins.

incidence at 30 years of age. These masses are nontender and are sometimes biopsied or removed for definitive diagnosis.

Benign Proliferative Breast Disease

The two most common types of **benign proliferative breast disease** (atypical, yet noncancerous, breast tissue) found on biopsy are **atypical hyperplasia** and **lobular carcinoma in situ (LCIS)**. These diagnoses increase a woman's risk of breast cancer.

Atypical Hyperplasia

Atypical hyperplasia can be ductal or lobular and is a premalignant lesion of the breast. It is recognized as a precursor lesion to both noninvasive and invasive breast cancer. Imbalance in the normal regulation of cell proliferation is a defining feature. Women with atypical hyperplasia have a fourfold increased risk of breast cancer compared to women in the general population, with a cumulative incidence approaching 30% at 25 years of age (Collins & Schnitt, 2014).

Lobular Carcinoma In Situ

LCIS is an incidental microscopic finding of abnormal tissue growth in the lobules of the breast. LCIS is a risk indicator and some studies describe half of affected women will develop breast cancer within 15 to 30 years (King & Reis-Filho, 2014). Affected women should undergo rigorous breast cancer surveillance that consists of annual mammography and clinical breast examination every 6 months (National Comprehensive Cancer Network [NCCN], 2015). Patients should be offered information about chemoprevention with selective estrogen receptor modulators (SERMs), such as tamoxifen (Soltamox, Nolvadex).

Other Benign Conditions

Cystosarcoma phyllodes is a rare fibroepithelial lesion that tends to grow rapidly. It is rarely malignant and is treated with surgical excision. If it is malignant, **mastectomy** may follow. Lymph node removal is usually not performed because metastasis is rare.

Fat necrosis is a condition of the breast that is often associated with a history of trauma. Surgical procedures such as a breast biopsy, lumpectomy or mastectomy can cause fat necrosis. It may be indistinguishable from carcinoma, and the entire mass may be excised or biopsied. If excision is not indicated, it is followed with regular breast imaging.

Intraductal papilloma is a wart-like growth that often involves the large milk ducts near the nipple, causing bloody nipple discharge. Surgery usually involves removal of the papilloma and a segment of the duct where the papilloma is found.

Superficial thrombophlebitis of the breast (Mondor disease) is an uncommon condition that is usually associated with pregnancy, trauma, or breast surgery. Pain and redness occur as a result of a superficial thrombophlebitis in the vein that drains the outer part of the breast. The mass is usually linear, tender, and erythematous. Treatment consists of analgesic agents and heat.

MALIGNANT CONDITIONS OF THE BREAST

Breast cancer is the most common cancer among Canadian women, with an estimated 26,300 cases in 2017 (CCS, 2018c). Breast cancer is the second leading cause of death from cancer in Canadian women with just over 5,000 deaths in 2017.

Based on 2017 estimates, 1 in 8 Canadian women will develop breast cancer and 1 in 31 women will die from it (CCS, 2018c).

Types of Breast Cancer

Ductal Carcinoma In Situ

Ductal carcinoma in situ (DCIS) is characterized by the proliferation of malignant cells inside the milk ducts without invasion into the surrounding tissue. Unlike invasive breast cancer, DCIS does not metastasize, and a woman generally does not die of DCIS unless it develops into invasive breast cancer. DCIS can develop into invasive breast cancer if left untreated. The best estimates are that 14% to 53% of untreated DCIS progresses to invasive breast cancer over a period of 10 years or more. However, the natural history of DCIS is not well understood, and it is currently not possible to accurately predict which women with DCIS will go on to develop invasive breast cancer (ACS, 2015). DCIS is frequently manifested on a mammogram with the appearance of calcifications, and it is considered breast cancer stage 0.

Medical Management

Current management takes into account (1) assurance of an accurate diagnosis, (2) assessment of DCIS size and grade, and (3) careful margin evaluation. The pathologist analyzes the piece of breast tissue removed to determine the type and grade of the DCIS or how abnormal the cells look when compared with normal breast cells and how fast they are growing. Grade III (high-grade DCIS) cells tend to grow more quickly than grade I (low-grade) and grade II (moderate-grade) cells and look much different from normal breast cells. Accurate grading of DCIS is critical, because high nuclear grade and the presence of necrosis (the premature death of cells in living tissue) are highly predictive of the inability to achieve adequate margins or borders of healthy tissue around the cancer, of local recurrence, and of the probability of missed areas of invasion. The pros and cons of irradiating patients with DCIS who are treated conservatively should be carefully weighed on a case-by-case basis, considering recent trials have shown that radiation has a beneficial effect on distant recurrence, breast cancer–specific mortality, and overall survival. Breast conservation (treatment of a breast cancer without the loss of the breast) can be curative for well-defined subsets of women with DCIS (ACS, 2015).

Invasive Cancer

The National Comprehensive Cancer Network (NCCN), a nonprofit group of the world's 21 leading cancer centres, disseminates estimates for various types of cancer.

Infiltrating Ductal Carcinoma

Infiltrating ductal carcinoma, the most common histologic type of breast cancer, accounts for 80% of all cases. The tumours arise from the duct system and invade the surrounding tissues. They often form a solid irregular mass in the breast.

Infiltrating Lobular Carcinoma

Infiltrating lobular carcinoma accounts for 10% to 15% of breast cancers. The tumours arise from the lobular epithelium and typically occur as an area of ill-defined thickening in the breast. They are often multicentric and can be bilateral.

Medullary Carcinoma

Medullary carcinoma accounts for about 5% of breast cancers, and it tends to be diagnosed more often in women younger than 50 years. The tumours grow in a capsule inside a duct. They can become large and may be mistaken for a fibroadenoma. The prognosis is often favourable.

Mucinous Carcinoma

Mucinous carcinoma accounts for about 3% of breast cancers and often presents in women who are postmenopausal and are 75 years and older. A mucin producer, the tumour is also slow growing; thus, the prognosis is more favourable than in many other types.

Tubular Ductal Carcinoma

Tubular ductal carcinoma accounts for about 2% of breast cancers. Because axillary metastases are uncommon with this histology, prognosis is usually excellent. Micropapillary invasive ductal carcinoma is a rare type of aggressive ductal cancer characterized by a high rate of axillary node metastasis and skin involvement.

Inflammatory Carcinoma

Inflammatory carcinoma is a rare (1% to 3%) and aggressive type of breast cancer that has unique symptoms. The cancer is characterized by diffuse edema and erythema of the skin, often referred to as peau d'orange (resembling an orange peel). This is caused by malignant cells blocking the lymph channels in the skin. An associated mass may or may not be present; if there is a mass, it is often a large area of indiscrete thickening. Inflammatory carcinoma can be confused with an infection because of its presentation. The disease can spread to other parts of the body rapidly. Chemotherapy often plays an initial role in controlling disease progression, but radiation and surgery may also follow.

Paget's Disease

Paget's disease of the breast accounts for 1% of diagnosed cases of breast cancer (Grossman & Porth, 2014). Symptoms typically include a scaly, erythematous, pruritic lesion of the nipple. Paget's disease often represents DCIS of the nipple but may have an invasive component. If no lump can be felt in the breast tissue and the biopsy shows DCIS without invasion, the prognosis is very favourable.

Risk Factors

There is no single, specific cause of breast cancer. A combination of genetic, hormonal, and possibly environmental factors may increase the risk of its development (Table 49-3). More than 80% of all cases of breast cancer are sporadic, meaning that patients have no known family history of the disease. The remaining cases are either familial (there is a family history of breast cancer, but it is not passed on genetically) or genetically acquired. There is no evidence that smoking, silicone breast implants, use of antiperspirants, underwire bras, or abortion (induced or spontaneous) increases the risk of the disease. There is some evidence that long-term smoking, starting before first pregnancy, and night shift work may increase the risk for breast cancer (ACS, 2015).

As stated previously, breast cancer can be genetically inherited, resulting in significant risk. Approximately 5% to 10% of breast cancer cases have been linked to specific genetic mutations. Factors that may indicate a genetic link include multiple first-degree relatives with early-onset breast cancer, breast and ovarian cancer in the same family, male breast cancer, and Ashkenazi Jewish background. ***BRCA1* and *BRCA2*** are tumour suppressor genes that normally function to identify damaged deoxyribonucleic acid (DNA) and thereby restrain abnormal cell growth (Yarbo, Wujcik, & Gobel, 2013). Mutations in these genes on chromosome 17 are responsible for the majority of hereditary breast cancer in the United States. *BRCA* mutations in women have been associated with an overall risk of breast cancer up to 65% (ACS, 2015). Currently, women who are *BRCA* positive are counselled to start screening, typically using mammography, once a year and then MRI 6 months after the yearly mammography by 25 years of age, or 5 to 10 years earlier than their youngest affected family member. Mutations in the PALB2 gene confer similar risk. Males who carry the *BRCA2* mutation may have a lifetime risk of 6% to 7% of developing breast cancer (Jain & Gradishar, 2014).

Protective Factors

Certain factors may be protective against the development of breast cancer. Breastfeeding for at least 1 year, regular or moderate physical activity and maintaining a healthy body weight are cited as protective (ACS, 2015). Some research suggests that the use of extra virgin olive oil regularly in one's diet may be preventive (Toledo, Salas-Salvad, Donat-Vargas, et al., 2015).

Breast Cancer Prevention Strategies in the Patient Who Is at High Risk

Patients often over- or underestimate their risk of developing breast cancer. A consultation with a breast specialist is of paramount importance prior to embarking on any of the prevention strategies that follow. Once patients have an accurate assessment of their risk, along with the knowledge of the pros and cons of each prevention strategy, they can make a decision that is most appropriate for their situation.

Long-Term Surveillance

Long-term surveillance focuses on early detection. As recommended by the CCS, women with a strong family history of breast cancer, genetic mutations of BRCA1 or BRCA2, or history of breast changes may need to test earlier and more often. The frequency of clinical breast examinations and

TABLE 49-3 Risk Factors for Breast Cancer

Risk Factor	Comments
Female gender	99% of cases occur in women.
Increasing age	Increasing age is associated with an increased risk.
Personal history of breast cancer	Once treated for breast cancer, the risk of developing breast cancer in same or opposite breast is significantly increased.
Family history of breast cancer	Having first-degree relative with breast cancer (mother, sister, daughter) increases the risk twofold; having two first-degree relatives increases the risk fivefold. The risk is higher if the relative was premenopausal at the time of diagnosis. The risk is increased if a father or brother had breast cancer (exact risk is unknown).
Genetic mutation	*BRCA1* and *BRCA2* mutations account for the majority of inherited cases of breast cancer (see additional information in text).
Hormonal Factors	
• Early menarche	Before 12 yrs of age
• Late menopause	After 55 yrs of age
• Nulliparity	No full-term pregnancies
• Late age at first full-term pregnancy	After 30 yrs of age
• Hormone therapy (formerly referred to as hormone replacement therapy)	Current or recent use of combined postmenopausal hormone therapy (estrogen and progesterone) Long-term use (several years or more)
Exposure to ionizing radiation during adolescence and early adulthood	The risk is highest if breast tissue was exposed while still developing (during adolescence) such as women who received mantle radiation (to the chest area) for treatment of Hodgkin's lymphoma in their younger years.
History of benign proliferative breast disease	Having had atypical ductal or lobular hyperplasia or lobular carcinoma in situ increases the risk.
Obesity	Obesity and weight gain during adulthood increases the risk of postmenopausal breast cancer. During menopause, estrogen is primarily produced in fat tissue. More fat tissue can increase estrogen levels, thereby increasing breast cancer risk.
High-fat diet (controversial)	More research is needed.
Alcohol intake (beer, wine, or liquor)	Two to five drinks daily increases the risk about one and a half times.

Adapted from National Comprehensive Cancer Network (NCCN). (2015). Clinical practice guidelines: Breast. Retrieved on March 7, 2016 at: www.nccn.org/professionals/physician_gls/PDF/infections.pdf

mammograms may be discussed with a primary provider. In addition to yearly mammography, other screening tests, including ultrasonography, may be useful.

Chemoprevention

Chemoprevention is the main modality that aims to prevent the disease. Several national, randomized clinical trials in the past two decades have led to FDA approval of tamoxifen and raloxifene (Evista) as effective chemopreventive agents for use in women who are at high risk (Cummings, Eckert, Krueger, et al., 1999; Fisher, Constantino, Wickerham, et al., 1998; Vogel, Costantino, Wickerham, et al., 2006). In addition, anastrozole (Arimidex) and exemestane (Aromasin) are now used for chemoprevention (Comerford, 2015). Nurses can help women who are considering chemoprevention by providing them with information about the benefits, risks, and possible side effects of these medications.

Prophylactic Mastectomy

Prophylactic mastectomy is another primary prevention modality that can reduce the risk of breast cancer by 90% (National Cancer Institute [NCI], 2013) and is sometimes referred to as a "risk-reducing" mastectomy. The procedure consists of a total mastectomy (removal of breast tissue) and is usually accompanied by immediate breast reconstruction. Possible candidates include women with a strong family history of breast cancer, a diagnosis of LCIS or atypical hyperplasia, a mutation in a *BRCA* gene or previous cancer in one breast. Because of physical and psychological ramifications including anxiety, depression, and altered body image, this procedure should be undertaken only after extensive counselling related to its risks and benefits. The procedure does not confer 100% protection against the development of breast cancer (NCI, 2013).

A multidisciplinary approach should be used to help the patient arrive at a decision that is best for her. Consultation with a genetic counsellor, plastic surgeon, medical oncologist, and psychiatrist can be invaluable. The patient needs to understand that this surgery is elective and not emergent. The nurse can play a valuable role in providing the patient with information, clarification, and support during the decision-making process.

Clinical Manifestations

Breast cancers can occur anywhere in the breast but are usually found in the upper outer quadrant, where the most breast tissue is located. Generally, the lesions are nontender, fixed rather than mobile, and hard with irregular borders. Reports of diffuse breast pain and tenderness with menstruation are usually associated with benign breast disease.

With the increased use of mammography, more women are seeking treatment at earlier stages of the disease. These women often have no signs or symptoms other than a mammographic abnormality. Some women with advanced disease seek initial treatment after ignoring symptoms. Advanced signs may include skin dimpling, nipple retraction, or skin ulceration.

Assessment and Diagnostic Findings

Techniques to determine the diagnosis of breast cancer include various types of biopsy, which have been described previously. Tumour staging and analysis of additional prognostic factors are used to determine the prognosis and optimal treatment regimen (see below).

Staging

Staging involves classifying the cancer by the extent of disease. It is based on whether the cancer is invasive or noninvasive, the size of the tumour, how many lymph nodes are involved, and if it has spread to other parts of the body. The stage of a cancer is one of the most important factors in determining prognosis and treatment options. The most common system used to describe the stages of breast cancer is the TNM (tumour, nodes, metastasis) system (CCS, 2018d) (see Chapter 68). Other factors considered in staging include hormone receptors and genetic mutations.

Other diagnostic tests may be performed before or after the surgery to help in the staging of the disease. The extent of testing often depends on the clinical presentation of the disease and may include chest x-rays, computed tomography (CT) scan, MRI scan, positron emission tomography (PET) scan, bone scans, and blood work (complete blood count, comprehensive metabolic panel, tumour markers [i.e., carcinoembryonic antigen, cancer antigen 15-3]).

Prognosis

Several different factors must be taken into consideration when determining the prognosis of a patient with breast cancer. The two most important factors are tumour size and whether the tumour has spread to the lymph nodes under the arm (axilla).

In general, the smaller the tumour, the better the prognosis. A tumour starts with a genetic alteration in a single cell and takes time to divide and double in size. A carcinoma may double in size 30 times to become 1 cm or larger, at which point it becomes clinically apparent. Doubling time varies, but breast tumours are often present for several years before they become palpable. Nurses can reassure patients that once breast cancer is diagnosed, they have a safe period of several weeks to make decisions regarding treatment; however, a lengthy delay is not advisable.

CHART 49-3

Pathologic Factors Associated With Favourable Prognosis for Breast Cancer

- Noninvasive tumours or invasive tumours less than 1 cm
- Negative axillary lymph nodes
- Estrogen receptor (ER) and progesterone receptor (PR) proteins
- Well-differentiated tumours
- Low expression of HER-2/neu oncogene (also known as ERBB2)
- No vascular or lymphatic invasion
- Diploid tumours with low S-phase fraction

Adapted from U.S. Department of Health and Human Services, Public Health Service. (2012). *What you need to know about breast cancer*. Bethesda, MD: National Institutes of Health.

Prognosis also depends on the extent of spread of the breast cancer. The 5-year survival rate is approximately 100% for a stage I breast cancer and 22% for a stage IV breast cancer (CCS, 2018e). The most common route of regional spread is to the axillary lymph nodes. Other sites of lymphatic spread include the internal mammary and supraclavicular nodes (Fig. 49-5). Distant metastasis can affect any organ, but the most common sites are bone, lung, liver, chest muscle, breast skin, and brain (CCS, 2018f).

In addition to the type of breast cancer and the stage, other factors may help determine prognosis (Chart 49-3). Excessive number of copies of certain genes (amplification) or excessive amounts of their protein product (overexpression) may represent a poorer prognosis. The HER-2/neu (also known as ERBB2) oncogene is the classic example; approximately 25% of invasive breast cancers, which typically involve the more aggressive tumours, have amplification or overexpression of this gene (Press & Ma, 2014). The proliferative rate or rapidity in growth rate (S-phase fraction) and DNA content (ploidy) of a tumour are factors that are also associated with overall survival rate.

Surgical Management

The main goal of surgery is to gain local control of the disease. With breast cancer being diagnosed today at earlier stages, options for less invasive, breast-conserving surgical procedures are available. Surgical treatment options for noninvasive and invasive breast cancer are summarized in Table 49-4.

Modified Radical Mastectomy

Modified radical mastectomy is performed to treat invasive breast cancer. The procedure involves removal of breast tissue, including the nipple–areola complex. In addition, a portion of the axillary lymph nodes are also removed in axillary lymph node dissection (ALND). If immediate breast reconstruction is desired, the patient is referred to a plastic surgeon prior to the mastectomy so

TABLE 49-4 Surgical Treatment Options for Noninvasive and Invasive Breast Cancer

Noninvasive Breast Cancer	Invasive Breast Cancer
Breast conservation[a] alone	Breast conservation[a] with one of the following: Sentinel lymph node biopsy Axillary lymph node dissection
Total mastectomy alone	Total mastectomy with sentinel lymph node biopsy or Modified radical mastectomy

[a]Breast-conservation treatment includes lumpectomy, wide excision, partial or segmental mastectomy, and quadrantectomy. These are relatively synonymous terms that describe removal of varying amounts of breast tissue.

TABLE 49-5 Comparison of Sentinel Lymph Node Biopsy and Axillary Lymph Node Dissection

Sentinel Lymph Node Biopsy (SLNB)	Axillary Lymph Node Dissection (ALND)
Shorter operating room time (approximately 15–30 min)	Longer operating room time (approximately 60–90 min)
No surgical drain	Surgical drain
Local anesthesia with IV moderate sedation as outpatient surgery (unless being performed in conjunction with total mastectomy)	General anesthesia; usually overnight admission (sometimes done as outpatient surgery)
Lymphedema incidence approximately 0–7%	Lymphedema incidence approximately 0–20%
Presence of neuropathic sensations postoperatively (prevalence lower than after axillary lymph node dissection) Figure 49-3	Presence of neuropathic sensations postoperatively
Decreased range of motion in affected arm unlikely postoperatively but may occur	Decreased range of motion likely postoperatively
Seroma (collection of serous fluid in the axilla) may occur postoperatively	Seroma may occur postoperatively

that she has the opportunity to explore all available options. In modified radical mastectomy, the pectoralis major and pectoralis minor muscles are left intact, unlike in radical mastectomy, in which the muscles are removed.

Total Mastectomy

Like modified radical mastectomy, total mastectomy (i.e., simple mastectomy) also involves removal of the breast and nipple–areola complex but does not include ALND. Total mastectomy may be performed in patients with noninvasive breast cancer (e.g., DCIS), which does not have a tendency to spread to the lymph nodes. It may also be performed prophylactically in patients who are at high risk for breast cancer (e.g., LCIS, *BRCA* mutation). A total mastectomy may also be performed in conjunction with sentinel lymph node biopsy (SLNB) for patients with invasive breast cancer.

Breast-Conservation Treatment

The goal of **breast-conservation treatment** (i.e., lumpectomy, wide excision, partial or segmental mastectomy, quadrantectomy) is to excise the tumour in the breast completely and obtain clear margins while achieving an acceptable cosmetic result. If the procedure is being performed to treat a noninvasive breast cancer, lymph node removal is not necessary. For an invasive breast cancer, lymph node removal (SLNB or ALND) is indicated. The lymph nodes are removed through a separate semicircular incision in the axilla.

Sentinel Lymph Node Biopsy

The status of the lymph nodes is the most important prognostic factor in breast cancer. SLNB is a less invasive alternative to ALND and is considered a standard of care for the treatment of early-stage breast cancer. ALND is associated with potential morbidity, including **lymphedema**, cellulitis, decreased arm mobility, and sensory changes. Studies suggest that SLNB is highly accurate and is associated with a local recurrence rate similar to that of ANLD (Chung & Giuliano, 2014). Table 49-5 compares SLNB and ALND.

The sentinel lymph node, which is the first node (or nodes) in the lymphatic basin that receives drainage from the primary tumour in the breast, is identified by injecting a radioisotope and/or blue dye into the breast; the radioisotope or dye then travels via the lymphatic pathways to the node. In SLNB, the surgeon uses a hand-held probe to locate the **sentinel lymph node**, excises it, and sends it for pathologic analysis, which is often performed immediately during the surgery using frozen section analysis. If the sentinel lymph node is positive, the surgeon can proceed with an immediate ALND, thus sparing the patient a return trip to the operating room and additional anesthesia. (The patient could also return for additional surgery at a later time.) If the sentinel lymph node is negative, a standard ALND is not needed, thus sparing the patient the possible complications of the procedure. After the procedure is complete, all specimens are sent to pathology for more thorough analysis.

Nursing Management

Patients who undergo SLNB in conjunction with breast-conservation treatments are generally discharged the same day. Patients who undergo SLNB with total mastectomy usually stay in the hospital overnight, possibly longer if breast reconstruction is being performed. The patient must be informed that although frozen section analysis is highly accurate, false-negative results can occur. A negative sentinel lymph node on frozen section analysis may show metastatic disease on subsequent analysis, indicating that ALND is still necessary. The patient should also be reassured that the radioisotope and blue dye are generally safe. The patient may notice a blue-green discolouration in the urine or stool for the first 24 hours as the blue dye is excreted. The incidence of lymphedema, decreased arm mobility, and seroma formation (collection of serous fluid) in the axilla is generally low, but the patient should be prepared for these possibilities. Women who have SLNB alone have neuropathic sensations similar to those who undergo ALND, although the prevalence and severity of these sensations and the resulting distress are lower with SLNB (Chung & Giuliano, 2014).

The nurse must not overlook the psychosocial needs of the patient who has undergone SLNB. Although SLNB is a less invasive procedure than ALND and results in a shorter recovery period, a patient who has undergone SLNB also has many difficult issues surrounding her breast cancer diagnosis and treatment. The nurse must listen, provides emotional support, and refer the patient to appropriate specialists when indicated.

Nursing Process

The Patient Undergoing Surgery for Breast Cancer

Assessment

The health history is a valuable tool to assess the patient's reaction to the diagnosis and her ability to cope with it. Pertinent questions include the following:

- How is the patient responding to the diagnosis?
- What coping mechanisms does she find most helpful?
- What psychological or emotional supports does she have and use?
- Is there a partner, family member, or friend available to assist her in making treatment choices?
- What are her educational needs?
- Is she experiencing any discomfort?

Nursing Priorities

Preoperative Nursing Priorities

Based on the health history and other assessment data, major preoperative nursing priorities may include the following:

- Lack of knowledge
- Anxiety
- Fear
- Lack of coping (individual or family)
- Conflict with regard to treatment options

Postoperative Nursing Priorities

Based on the health history and other assessment data, major postoperative nursing priorities may include the following:

- Pain
- Neurovascular dysfunction and nerve irritation
- Altered body image
- Ineffective coping
- Self-care deficit
- Sexual dysfunction
- Lack of knowledge

Collaborative Problems/ Potential Complications

Potential complications may include the following:

- Lymphedema
- Hematoma/seroma formation
- Infection

Planning and Goals

The major goals may include increased knowledge about the disease and its treatment; reduction of preoperative and postoperative fear, anxiety, and emotional stress; improvement of decision-making ability; pain management; neurovascular function management; maintenance of a positive body image; improvement in coping abilities; increased self-care abilities; improvement in sexual function; and the absence of complications.

Preoperative Nursing Interventions

Providing Education and Preparation About Surgical Treatments

Patients with newly diagnosed breast cancer are expected to absorb an abundance of new information during a very emotionally difficult time, and this may lead to difficulty in making treatment decisions. The nurse plays a key role in reviewing treatment options by reinforcing information provided to the patient and answering any questions. The nurse fully prepares the patient for what to expect before, during, and after surgery. Patients undergoing breast conservation with ALND, or a total or modified radical mastectomy, generally remain in the hospital overnight (or longer if they have immediate reconstruction). Surgical drains will be inserted in the mastectomy incision and in the axilla if the patient undergoes ALND. A surgical drain is generally not needed after SLNB. The patient should be informed that she will go home with the drain(s) and that complete instructions about drain care will be provided prior to discharge. In addition, the patient should be informed that she will often have decreased arm and shoulder mobility after ALND and that she will be shown range-of-motion exercises prior to discharge. The patient should also be reassured that appropriate analgesia and comfort measures will be provided to alleviate any postoperative discomfort.

Reducing Fear and Anxiety and Improving Coping Ability

The nurse helps the patient cope with the physical and emotional effects of surgery. Many fears may emerge during the preoperative phase. These can include fear of pain, mutilation (after mastectomy), and loss of sexual attractiveness; concern about inability to care for oneself and one's family; concern about taking time off from work; and coping with an uncertain future. Providing the patient with realistic expectations about the healing process and expected recovery can help alleviate fears. Maintaining open communication and assuring the patient that she can contact the nurse at any time with questions or concerns can be a source of comfort. The patient should also be made aware of available resources at the treatment facility as well as in the breast cancer community such as social workers, psychiatrists, and support groups. Some women find it helpful and reassuring to talk to a survivor of breast cancer who has undergone similar treatments.

Promoting Decision-Making Ability

The patient may be eligible for more than one therapeutic approach; she may be presented with treatment options and then asked to make a choice. This can be very frightening for some patients, and they may prefer to have someone else make the decision for them (e.g., surgeon, family member). The nurse can be instrumental in ensuring that the patient and family members truly understand their options. The nurse can then help the patient weigh the risks and benefits of each option. The patient may be presented with the option of having breast-conservation treatment followed by radiation or a mastectomy. The nurse can explore the issues with the patient by asking questions such as the following:

- How do you think you might feel about losing your breast?
- Are you considering breast reconstruction?
- If you choose to retain your breast, would you consider undergoing radiation treatments 5 days a week for 5 to 6 weeks?

Questions such as these can help the patient focus. Once the patient's decision is made, it is very important to support it.

Postoperative Nursing Interventions

Relieving Pain and Discomfort

Many patients tolerate breast surgery quite well and have minimal pain during the postoperative period. This is particularly true of less invasive procedures such as breast-conservation treatment with SLNB. However, all patients must be carefully assessed, because individual patients can have varying degrees of pain. Patients who have had more invasive procedures such as a modified radical mastectomy with immediate reconstruction may have considerably more pain. All patients are discharged home with analgesic medication (e.g., oxycodone and acetaminophen [Percocet]) and are encouraged to take it if needed. An over-the-counter analgesic agent such as acetaminophen may provide sufficient relief. Patients sometimes report a slight increase in pain after the first few days of surgery; this may occur as patients regain sensation around the surgical site and become more active. However, patients who report more than moderate pain must be evaluated to rule out any potential complications such as infection or a hematoma. Postoperative pain may be more common in patients who have had axillary dissection and correlates with the number of nodes removed (Cherny & Truong, 2014). Alternative methods of pain management such as taking warm showers (if permitted by the surgeon) and using distraction methods (e.g., guided imagery) may also be helpful.

Managing Postoperative Sensations

Because nerves in the skin and axilla are often cut or injured during breast surgery, patients experience a variety of sensations. Common sensations include tenderness, soreness, numbness, tightness, pulling, and twinges. These sensations may occur along the chest wall, in the axilla, and along the inside aspect of the upper arm. After mastectomy, some patients experience phantom sensations and report a feeling that the breast or nipple is still present. Overall, patients do not find these sensations severe or distressing. Sensations usually persist for several months and then begin to diminish, although some may persist for as long as 5 years and possibly longer. Patients should be reassured that this is a usual part of healing and that these sensations are not indicative of a problem.

Promoting Positive Body Image

Patients who have undergone mastectomy often find it very difficult to view the surgical site for the first time. No matter how prepared the patient may think she is, the appearance of an absent breast can be very emotionally distressing. Ideally, the patient sees the incision for the first time when she is with the nurse or another health care provider who is available for support.

The nurse first assesses the patient's readiness and provides gentle encouragement. It is important to maintain the patient's privacy while assisting her as she views the incision; this allows her to express feelings safely to the nurse. Asking the patient what she perceives, acknowledging her feelings, and allowing her to express her emotions are important nursing actions. Reassuring the patient that her feelings are a usual response to breast cancer surgery may be comforting. If the patient has not had immediate reconstruction, providing her with a temporary breast form or soft padding to place in her bra on discharge can help alleviate feelings of embarrassment or self-consciousness.

Promoting Positive Adjustment and Coping

Providing ongoing assessment of how the patient is coping with her diagnosis of breast cancer and her surgical treatment is important in determining her overall adjustment. Assisting the patient in

NURSING RESEARCH PROFILE

Chart 49-4. Nurse Navigators and Breast Biopsy

Harding, M. (2015). Effect of nurse navigation on patient care satisfaction and distress associated with breast biopsy. *Clinical Journal Oncology Nursing, 19*(1), E15–E20.

Purpose

This study was conducted to evaluate the impact of nurse navigation on satisfaction with care and level of stress in patients having a breast biopsy.

Design

This study used a descriptive cross-sectional survey design. Two outpatient radiology sites were utilized including a community centre and a breast centre in Appalachia, following institutional review board (IRB) approval. The breast centre used a multidisciplinary approach coordinated by a nurse navigator; the community centre had no nurse navigator. Patients were invited to participate in the study prior to their biopsy. Study instruments included the Hospital Anxiety and Depression Scale (HADS), the State Trait Anxiety Inventory Scale (STAI-S), and the Patient Satisfaction Questionnaire (PSQ-18). Descriptive statistics were used to analyze demographic characteristics, *t* tests, chi square tests and Pearson correlations were used to examine variables.

Findings

One hundred and thirty-seven women completed the study instruments at home following a core needle biopsy. The majority (68%) of the women were older than 50 years of age. Women who received navigation services ($N = 85$) had lower scores on all three distress measures (HAD-A [anxiety subscale], HAD-D [depression subscale], & STAI-S), with significantly lower anxiety levels on the HADS-A. There were no significant differences in patient satisfaction between the two groups. Sixty-six women (48%) sought outside information regarding an aspect of the diagnostic experience. Women not receiving navigation services were significantly more likely to seek outside information ($X^2 = 7.949$; $p < 0.01$), with a majority (67%) using the internet as an information source.

Nursing Implications

This study suggests that nurse navigators providing information and support can improve decision making and help prepare women for explanatory educational sessions with radiologists and surgeons. Nurses working with women having a breast biopsy should also keep in mind that this study reported.

identifying and mobilizing her support systems can be beneficial to her well-being. The patient's spouse or partner may also need guidance, support, and education. The patient and partner may benefit from a wide network of available community resources, including the Reach to Recovery program of the CCS advocacy groups, social worker or a spiritual advisor. Encouraging the patient to discuss issues and concerns with other patients who have had breast cancer may help her to understand that her feelings are normal and that other women who have had breast cancer can provide invaluable support and understanding.

The patient may also have considerable anxiety about the treatments that will follow surgery (i.e., chemotherapy and radiation) and their implications. Providing her with information about the plan of care and referring her to the appropriate members of the health care team also promote coping during recovery. Some women require additional support to adjust to their diagnosis and the changes that it brings. If a woman displays ineffective coping, consultation with a mental health practitioner may be indicated. Research suggests that nurse navigators can help those undergoing breast biopsy to cope (Harding, 2015) (see Chart 49-4).

Improving Sexual Function

Once discharged from the hospital and feeling well, most patients are physically allowed to engage in sexual activity, if interested. However, any change in the patient's body image, self-esteem, or the response of her partner may increase her anxiety level and affect sexual function. Some partners may have difficulty looking at the incision, whereas others may be completely unaffected. Encouraging the patient to openly discuss how she feels about herself and about possible reasons for a decrease in libido (e.g., fatigue, anxiety, self-consciousness) may help clarify issues for her. Helpful suggestions for the patient may include varying the time of day for sexual activity (when the patient is less tired), assuming positions that are more comfortable, and expressing affection using alternative measures (e.g., hugging, kissing, manual stimulation).

Most patients and their partners adjust with minimal difficulty if they openly discuss their concerns. However, if issues cannot be resolved, a referral for counselling (e.g., psychologist, psychiatrist, psychiatric clinical nurse specialist, social worker, sex therapist) may be helpful. The ambulatory care nurse in the outpatient clinic or hospital should inquire whether the patient who was sexually active prior to surgery has resumed activities, because many patients are reluctant or embarrassed to bring this topic up themselves.

Monitoring and Managing Potential Complications

LYMPHEDEMA. Lymphedema is a complication characterized by a chronic swelling of an extremity due to interrupted lymphatic circulation. The swelling is due to the accumulation of protein-rich fluid in the interstitial space and is a somewhat common postoperative complication after ALND. It often affects both the breast and ipsilateral limb. It is associated with a painful swelling of the arm as well as weakness, shoulder pain, and tingling sensations in the arm and shoulder. Research results suggest that within 5 years of ALND, there is a 20% risk of lymphedema. Because sentinel lymph node dissection (SLND) involves more focused surgery and less disruption of the axilla, the risk is only up to 7% within 5 years. Risk factors for lymphedema in mixed-age groups include ALND, concomitant radiation therapy, increased age, presence of a concomitant infection, pre-existing cardiovascular conditions, and obesity (McLaughlin, 2014).

Lymphedema results if functioning lymphatic channels are inadequate to ensure a return flow of lymph fluid to the general circulation. After axillary lymph nodes are removed, collateral circulation must assume this function. Transient edema in the postoperative period occurs until collateral circulation has completely taken over this function, which generally occurs within a month. Performing prescribed exercises, elevating the arm above the heart several times a day, and gentle muscle pumping (making a fist and releasing) can help reduce the transient edema. The patient needs reassurance that this transient swelling is not lymphedema.

Once lymphedema develops, it tends to be chronic, so preventive strategies are vital. After ALND, the patient is taught hand and arm care to prevent injury or trauma to the affected extremity, thus decreasing the likelihood for lymphedema development (Chart 49-5). The patient is instructed to follow these guidelines for the rest of her life. She is also instructed to contact the physician or a nurse immediately if she suspects that she has lymphedema, because early intervention provides the best chance for control. If allowed to progress without treatment, the swelling can become more difficult to manage. Treatment may consist of a course of antibiotic agents if an infection is present. A referral to a rehabilitation specialist (e.g., occupational or physical therapist) may be necessary for a compression sleeve or glove, exercises, manual lymph drainage, and a discussion of ways to modify daily activities to avoid worsening lymphedema. Ongoing research is seeking to identify which lymph nodes drain the arm before surgery so that they can be preserved when possible, helping to prevent the development of lymphedema.

CHART 49-5

Patient Education: Hand and Arm Care After Axillary Lymph Node Dissection

The nurse instructs the patient to:

- Avoid blood pressures, injections, and blood draws in affected extremity.
- Use sunscreen (higher than 15 SPF) for extended exposure to sun.
- Apply insect repellent to avoid insect bites.
- Wear gloves for gardening.
- Use cooking mitt for removing objects from oven.
- Avoid cutting cuticles; push them back during manicures.
- Use electric razor for shaving armpit.
- Avoid lifting objects greater than 2.5–5.0 kg.
- If a trauma or break in the skin occurs, wash the area with soap and water, and apply an over-the-counter antibacterial ointment (Bacitracin or Neosporin).
- Observe the area and extremity for 24 hours; if redness, swelling, or a fever occurs, call the surgeon or nurse.

HEMATOMA OR SEROMA FORMATION. Hematoma formation (collection of blood inside a cavity) may occur after either mastectomy or breast conservation and usually develops within the first 12 hours after surgery. The nurse assesses for signs and symptoms of a hematoma at the surgical site, which may include swelling, tightness, pain, and bruising of the skin. The surgeon should be notified immediately if there is gross swelling or increased bloody output from the drain. Depending on the surgeon's assessment, a compression wrap may be applied to the incision for approximately 12 hours, or the patient may be returned to the operating room so that the incision may be reopened to identify the source of bleeding. Some hematomas are small, and the body absorbs the blood naturally. The patient may take warm showers (if permitted by the surgeon) or apply warm compresses to help increase the absorption. A hematoma usually resolves in 4 to 5 weeks.

A seroma, a collection of serous fluid, may accumulate under the breast incision after mastectomy or breast conservation or in the axilla. Signs and symptoms may include swelling, heaviness, discomfort, and a sloshing of fluid. Seromas may develop temporarily after the drain is removed or if the drain is in place and becomes obstructed. Seromas rarely pose a threat and may be treated by unclogging the drain or manually aspirating the fluid with a needle and syringe. Large, long-standing seromas that have not been aspirated could lead to infection. Small seromas that are not bothersome to the patient usually resolve on their own.

INFECTION. Although infection is rare, it is a risk after any surgical procedure. This risk may be higher in patients with conditions such as diabetes, immune disorders, and advanced age, as well as in those with poor hygiene. Patients are taught to monitor for signs and symptoms of infection (redness, warmth around incision, tenderness, foul-smelling drainage, temperature greater than 40°C, chills) and to contact the surgeon or nurse for evaluation. Treatment consists of oral or IV antibiotics (for more severe infections) for 1 or 2 weeks. Cultures are taken of any foul-smelling discharge.

Promoting Home, Community-Based and Transitional Care

EDUCATING PATIENTS ABOUT SELF-CARE. Patients who undergo breast cancer surgery receive a tremendous amount of information both pre- and postoperatively. It is often difficult for the patient to absorb all of the information, partly because of the emotional distress that often accompanies the diagnosis and treatment. Prior to discharge, the nurse must assess the patient's readiness to assume self-care responsibilities and identify any gaps in knowledge. A review of education provided in written and oral forms, with reinforcement, may be required to ensure that the patient and family are prepared to manage the necessary care at home. The nurse reiterates symptoms that the patient should report, such as infection, seroma, hematoma, or arm swelling. All instruction should be reinforced during office visits and by telephone.

Most patients are discharged 1 or 2 days after ALND or mastectomy (possibly later if they have had immediate reconstruction) with surgical drains in place. Initially, the drainage fluid appears bloody, but it gradually changes to a serosanguineous and then a serous fluid over the next several days. The patient is given instructions about drainage management at home (Chart 49-6). If the patient lives alone and drainage management is difficult, a referral for a home care nurse should be made. The drains are usually removed when the output is less than 30 mL in a 24-hour period (approximately 7 to 10 days). The home care nurse also reviews pain management and incision care.

In general, the patient may shower on the second postoperative day and wash the incision and drain site with soap and water to prevent infection. Some surgeons do not permit showers until 48 hours after drains are removed. If immediate reconstruction has been performed, showering may be contraindicated until the drain is removed. A dry dressing may be applied to the incision each day for 7 days. The patient should realize that sensation may be decreased in the operative area because the nerves were disrupted during surgery and she should be informed that gentle care is needed to avoid injury. After the incision has completely healed (usually after 4 to 6 weeks), lotions or creams may be applied to the area to increase skin elasticity. The patient can begin to use deodorant on the affected side, although many women note that they no longer perspire as much as before the surgery.

After ALND, patients are taught arm exercises on the affected side to restore range of motion (Chart 49-7). After SLNB, patients may also benefit from these exercises, although they are less likely to have decreased range of motion than those who have undergone ALND. Range-of-motion exercises are initiated on the second postoperative day; however, instruction often occurs on the first postoperative day. The goals of the exercise regimen are to increase circulation and muscle strength, prevent joint

CHART 49-6

HOME CARE CHECKLIST • Patient With a Drainage Device Following Breast Surgery

At the completion of education, the patient and/or caregiver will be able to:

- Name the procedure that was performed and identify changes in anatomic structure or function as well as changes in ADLs, IADLs, roles, relationships, and spirituality.
- Identify interventions and strategies (e.g., prosthesis) used in adapting to any permanent changes in structure or function.
- Describe ongoing postoperative therapeutic regimen, including diet and activities to perform (e.g., when to shower, arm exercises) and to limit or avoid (e.g., lifting weights, driving a car, contact sports).
- State the name, dose, side effects, frequency, and schedule for all medications.
    - Describe approaches to controlling pain (e.g., take analgesics as prescribed; use nonpharmacologic interventions).
- State how to obtain medical supplies and carry out dressing changes, wound care, and other prescribed regimens.
    - Care for the drain site and incision as per surgeon's recommendation.
    - Demonstrate how to empty and measure fluid from the drainage device.
    - Demonstrate how to milk clots through the tubing of the drainage device.
    - Identify when the drain is ready for removal (usually when draining <30 mL for a 24-hour period).
- Describe signs and symptoms of complications.
    - State observations that require contacting the physician or nurse (e.g., sudden change in color of drainage, sudden cessation of drainage, signs or symptoms of an infection).
- Relate how to reach primary provider with questions or complications.
- State time and date of follow-up appointments, therapy, and testing.
- Identify sources of support (e.g., friends, relatives, faith community, cancer support groups, caregiver support).
- Identify the need for health promotion, disease prevention, and screening activities (e.g., gynecologic examination, mammogram).

CHART 49-7

Patient Education: Exercise After Breast Surgery

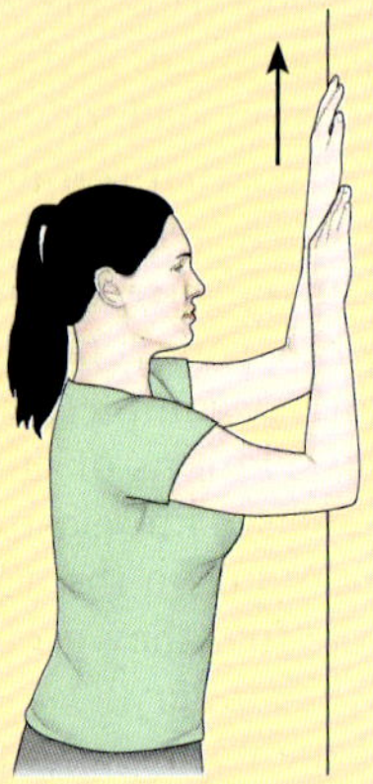

1. *Wall handclimbing.* Stand facing the wall with feet apart and toes as close to the wall as possible. With elbows slightly bent, place the palms of the hand on the wall at shoulder level. By flexing the fingers, work the hands up the wall until arms are fully extended. Then reverse the process, working the hands down to the starting point.

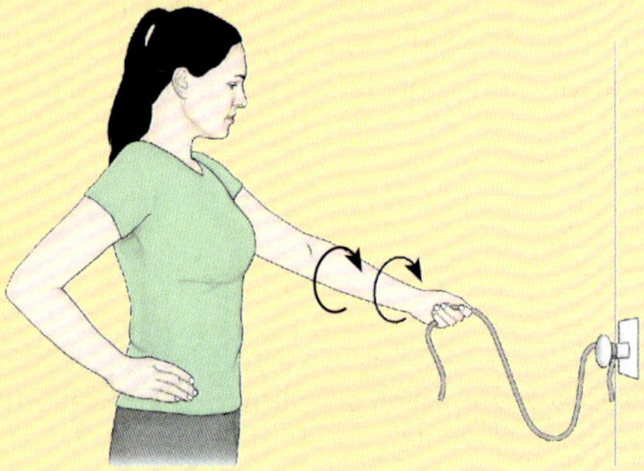

2. *Rope turning.* Tie a light rope to a doorknob. Stand facing the door. Take the free end of the rope in the hand on the side of surgery. Place the other hand on the hip. With the rope-holding arm extended and held away from the body (nearly parallel with the floor), turn the rope, making as wide swings as possible. Begin slowly at first; speed up later.

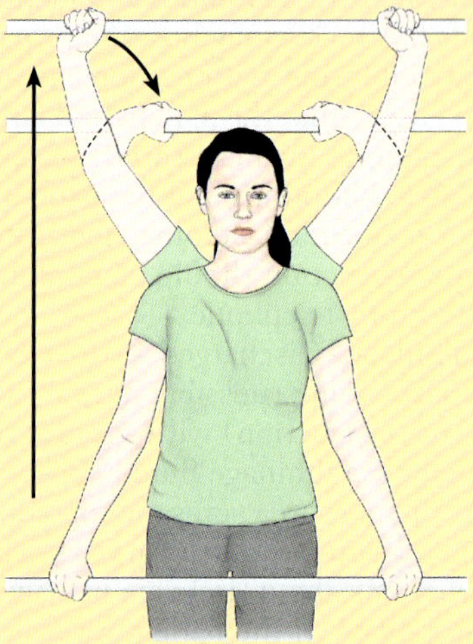

3. *Rod or broomstick lifting.* Grasp a rod with both hands, held about 2 ft apart. Keeping the arms straight, raise the rod over the head. Bend elbows to lower the rod behind the head. Reverse manoeuvre, raising the rod above the head, then return to the starting position.

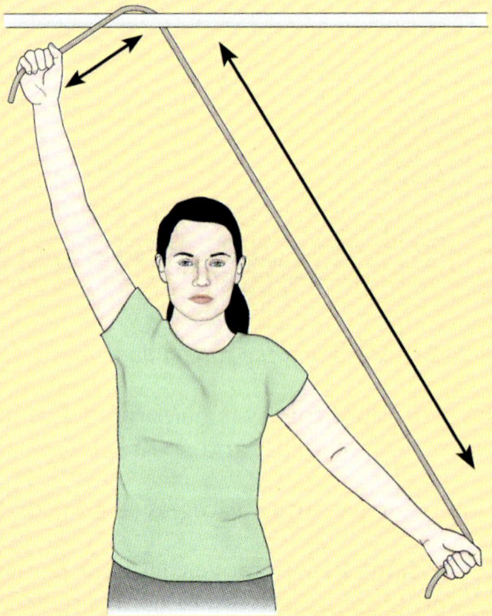

4. *Pulley tugging.* Toss a light rope over a shower curtain rod or doorway curtain rod. Stand as nearly under the rope as possible. Grasp an end in each hand. Extend the arms straight and away from the body. Pull the left arm up by tugging down with the right arm, then the right arm up and the left down in a see-sawing motion.

stiffness and contractures, and restore full range of motion. The patient is instructed to perform range-of-motion exercises at home three times a day for 20 minutes at a time until full range of motion is restored (generally 4 to 6 weeks). Most patients find that after the drain is removed, range of motion returns quickly if they have adhered to their exercise program.

If the patient is having any discomfort, taking an analgesic agent 30 minutes before beginning the exercises can be helpful. Taking a warm shower before exercising can also loosen stiff muscles and provide comfort. When exercising, the patient is encouraged to use the muscles in both arms and to maintain proper posture. Specific exercises may need to be prescribed and introduced gradually if the patient has had skin grafts; has a tense, tight surgical incision; or has had immediate reconstruction. Self-care activities, such as brushing the teeth, washing the face, and brushing the hair, are physically and emotionally therapeutic because they aid in restoring arm function and provide a sense of normalcy for the patient.

The patient is instructed about postoperative activity limitation. Generally, heavy lifting (more than 2 to 4 kg) is avoided for about 4 to 6 weeks, although normal household and work-related activities are promoted to maintain muscle tone. Brisk walking, use of stationary bikes and stepping machines, and stretching exercises may begin as soon as the patient feels comfortable. Once the drain is removed, the patient may begin to drive if she has full arm range of motion and is no longer taking opioid analgesic agents. General guidelines for activity focus on the gradual introduction of previous activities (e.g., bowling, weight training) once fully healed.

CONTINUING AND TRANSITIONAL CARE. Patients who have difficulty managing their postoperative care at home may benefit from a referral for home health, transitional, or community-based care. The nurse making a home visit assesses the patient's incision and surgical drain(s), adequacy of pain management, adherence to the exercise plan, and overall physical and psychological functioning. In addition, the home care nurse reinforces previous education and communicates important physiologic findings and psychosocial issues to the patient's primary provider, nurse, or surgeon.

The frequency of follow-up visits after surgery may vary but generally should occur every 3 to 6 months for the first several years. The patient may alternate visits with the surgeon, medical oncologist, or radiation oncologist, depending on the treatment regimen. The ambulatory care nurse can also be a great source of education for the patient and family and should encourage them to telephone if they have any questions or concerns. It is common for people to ignore routine health care when a major health issue arises, so women who have been treated for breast cancer are reminded of the importance of participating in routine health screening.

Evaluation

Expected preoperative patient outcomes may include:

1. Exhibits knowledge about diagnosis and surgical treatment options
   a. Asks relevant questions about diagnosis and available surgical treatments
   b. States rationale for surgery
   c. Describes advantages and disadvantages of treatment options
2. Verbalizes willingness to deal with anxiety and fears related to the diagnosis and the effects of surgery on self-image and sexual functioning
3. Demonstrates ability to cope with diagnosis and treatment
   a. Verbalizes feelings appropriately and recognizes normalcy of mood lability
   b. Proceeds with treatment in timely fashion
   c. Discusses impact of diagnosis and treatment on family and work
4. Makes decisions regarding treatment options in timely fashion

Expected Postoperative Patient Outcomes

Expected postoperative patient outcomes may include:

1. Reports that pain has decreased and states pain and discomfort management strategies are effective
2. Identifies postoperative sensations and recognizes that they are a normal part of healing
3. Exhibits clean, dry, and intact surgical incisions without signs of inflammation or infection
4. Lists the signs and symptoms of infection to be reported to the nurse or surgeon
5. Verbalizes feelings regarding change in body image
6. Discusses meaning of the diagnosis, surgical treatment, and fears appropriately
7. Participates actively in self-care measures
   a. Performs exercises as prescribed
   b. Participates in self-care measures as prescribed
8. Discusses issues of sexuality and resumption of sexual relations
9. Demonstrates knowledge of postdischarge recommendations and restrictions
   a. Describes follow-up care and activities
   b. Demonstrates appropriate care of incisions and drainage system
   c. Demonstrates arm exercises and describes exercise regimen and activity limitations during postoperative period
   d. Describes care of affected arm and hand and lists indications to contact the surgeon or nurse
10. Experiences no complications
    a. Identifies signs and symptoms of reportable complications (e.g., redness, heat, pain, edema)
    b. Explains how to contact appropriate care providers in case of complications

Radiation Therapy

Radiation therapy is used to decrease the chance of a local recurrence in the breast by eradicating residual microscopic cancer cells. Breast-conservation treatment followed by radiation therapy for stages I and II breast cancer results in a survival rate equal to that of a modified radical mastectomy (NCCN, 2015). If radiation therapy, which is part of breast-conservation treatment (Chart 49-8), is contraindicated, a mastectomy would then be indicated.

External-beam radiation (the most common type) typically begins about 6 weeks after breast conservation to allow the surgical site to heal. If systemic chemotherapy is indicated, radiation therapy usually begins after its completion. Before radiation begins, the patient undergoes a planning session called a simulation in which the anatomic areas to be treated are mapped out and then identified with small permanent ink markings. External-beam radiation, which delivers high-energy photons from a linear accelerator, is given to the entire breast region (whole-breast radiation). Each treatment lasts only a few minutes and is generally given 5 days a week for 5 to 6 weeks. After completion of radiation to the entire breast, many patients

CHART 49-8

Contraindications to Breast-Conservation Treatment

Note: Breast-conservation treatment includes both surgery and radiation.

Absolute Contraindications

- First or second trimester of pregnancy
- Presence of multicentric disease in the breast
- Prior radiation to the breast or chest region

Relative Contraindications

- History of collagen vascular disease
- Large tumour-to-breast ratio
- Tumour beneath nipple

Adapted from Harris, J., & Morrow, M. (2014). Breast-conserving therapy. In J. Harris, M. Lippman, M. Morrow, et al. (Eds.). *Diseases of the breast* (5th ed.). Philadelphia, PA: Wolters Kluwer.

receive a "boost," a dose of radiation to the lumpectomy site where the cancer cells were located. The boost consists of the same dose of radiation but is less penetrating and directed to a smaller area. The treatments are not painful.

Because most breast cancer recurrences appear at or near the lumpectomy site, the need for whole-breast radiation has been questioned. Partial breast radiation (radiation to the lumpectomy site alone) continues to be evaluated at some institutions in patients who have been carefully selected. One approach is **brachytherapy**, in which radiation is delivered by an internal device that is placed close to the tumour within the breast. This technique can lead to an improved quality of life because the treatments are administered over 4 to 5 days instead of 5 to 6 weeks.

After mastectomy, postoperative radiation is indicated for women at high risk for cancer recurrence (i.e., chest wall involvement, four or more positive lymph nodes, tumours larger than 5 cm, positive surgical margins).

Side Effects

In general, radiation therapy is well tolerated. Acute side effects consist of mild to moderate erythema, breast edema, and fatigue. Occasionally, skin breakdown may occur in the inframammary fold or near the axilla toward the end of treatment. Fatigue can be depressing, as can the frequent trips to the radiation oncology site for treatment. The patient needs to be reassured that the fatigue is normal and not a sign of recurrence. Side effects usually resolve within a few weeks to a few months after treatment is completed. Rare long-term effects of radiation therapy include pneumonitis, rib fracture, heart disease, necrosis, and breast fibrosis (Harris & Morrow, 2014).

Nursing Management

Nurses play a significant role in supporting patients throughout their treatment with radiation therapy.

Self-care instructions for patients receiving radiation are provided to assist in the maintenance of skin integrity during the treatments and for several weeks after completion. They pertain only to the area being treated and not to the rest of the body. Instructions include:

- Use mild soap with minimal rubbing.
- Avoid perfumed soaps or deodorants.
- Use hydrophilic lotions (Lubriderm, Eucerin, Aquaphor) for dryness.
- Use a nondrying, antipruritic soap (Aveeno) if pruritus occurs.
- Avoid tight clothes, underwire bras, excessive temperatures, and ultraviolet light.

Follow-up care includes teaching the patient to minimize sun exposure to the treated area (i.e., using sunblock with sun protection factor [SPF] 15 or above) and reassuring the patient that minor twinges and shooting pain in the breast are usual after radiation treatment.

Systemic Treatments

Chemotherapy

Adjuvant chemotherapy involves the use of anticancer agents in addition to other treatments (i.e., surgery, radiation) to delay or prevent a recurrence of breast cancer. It is recommended for patients who have positive lymph nodes or who have invasive tumours greater than 1 cm in size, regardless of nodal status. It is considered in patients with tumours that are 0.6 cm to 1 cm, are moderately to poorly differentiated, or have unfavourable features (NCCN, 2014). Table 49-6 outlines general indications for adjuvant chemotherapy. A survival benefit has been shown in both women who are pre- and postmenopausal and who have received chemotherapy, although data are limited in women older than 70 years. Chemotherapy is

TABLE 49-6 General Indications for Adjuvant Chemotherapy for Breast Cancer

Nodal Status, Tumour Size	Adjuvant Chemotherapy
Node negative, 0.5 cm or less	None
Node negative 0.6–1 cm (well differentiated)	None
Node negative, 0.6–1 cm (moderately or poorly differentiated and/or unfavourable features)	Consider chemotherapy
Node negative, greater than 1 cm	Chemotherapy
Node positive, any tumour size	Chemotherapy

- In addition to chemotherapy, patients with HER-2/neu-positive tumours will receive trastuzumab if they have node-positive disease; or node-negative disease with a tumour greater than 1 cm. Trastuzumab is a monoclonal antibody that targets and inactivates the HER-2/neu protein. HER-2/neu is overproduced in 25–30% of tumours and is associated with rapid growth and poor prognosis.
- Following chemotherapy, patients with hormone receptor–positive (ER+/PR+) tumours will receive hormonal therapy (tamoxifen or aromatase inhibitor) if they have either node-positive disease, node-negative disease with a tumour >1 cm, or node negative with a tumour 0.6–1 cm and moderately or poorly differentiated and/or unfavourable features.

Note: These are only general guidelines. Recommendations may vary depending on factors such as prognostic variables, patient age, and comorbid conditions.

Adapted from National Comprehensive Cancer Network (NCCN). (2015). Clinical practice guidelines: Breast. Retrieved on 3/7/2016 at: www.nccn.org/professionals/physician_gls/PDF/infections.pdf

most commonly initiated after breast surgery and before radiation. Patients who delay initiation of chemotherapy beyond 90 days postsurgery have an increased risk of adverse outcomes (Chavez-McGregor, Clarke, Lichtensztajn, et al., 2016). Nurses encourage and assist in facilitating timely treatment to optimize outcomes.

Chemotherapy regimens for breast cancer combine several agents (polychemotherapy), generally given over a period of 3 to 6 months. Decisions regarding the optimal regimen are based on a variety of factors, including tumour characteristics (i.e., tumour size, lymph node status, hormone receptor status, HER-2/neu status) and the patient's age, physical status, and existing comorbid conditions. A regimen that includes cyclophosphamide (Cytoxan), methotrexate (Trexall), and fluorouracil (Fluoroplex) (collectively referred to as CMF) has been the most widely used adjuvant therapy. It is usually well tolerated and may be considered for patients with a low risk of recurrence. CMF also may be considered for use in patients who have a high risk of cardiac toxicity or who have other limiting comorbidities. Anthracycline-based regimens (e.g., doxorubicin [Adriamycin], epirubicin [Ellence]) have shown longer survival in patients. However, the benefit relative to CMF is modest and is accompanied by increased toxicity (Meneses & Walker, 2014). Selection of patients most likely to benefit from anthracycline therapy would allow better use of current cytotoxic agents and reduce the risk of patients receiving toxicity with little or no effect. Identifying biomarkers that can accurately predict benefit from anthracyclines will also highlight key resistance/susceptibility pathways that can then be exploited clinically to further increase efficacy (Meneses & Walker, 2014). Selection of patients most likely to benefit from anthracycline therapy would allow better use of current cytotoxic agents and reduce the risk of patients receiving toxicity with little or no effect. Identifying biomarkers that can accurately predict benefit from anthracyclines will also highlight key resistance/susceptibility pathways that can then be exploited clinically to further increase efficacy (Meneses & Walker, 2014). Cyclophosphamide, doxorubicin, and fluorouracil (CAF) and doxorubicin and cyclophosphamide (AC) are examples of combination regimens often given to patients who are at high risk.

The taxanes (paclitaxel [Taxol], docetaxel [Taxotere]) are generally incorporated into treatment regimens for patients with larger, node-negative cancers and for those with positive axillary lymph nodes. The addition of four cycles of paclitaxel after a standard course of AC (regimen known as ACT) has been found to increase the disease-free period and improve overall survival in patients with operable breast cancer and positive lymph nodes (Meneses & Walker, 2014).

Much attention has been focused on dose-dense chemotherapy, which is the administration of chemotherapeutic agents at standard doses with shorter time intervals between each cycle of treatment. A systematic review and meta-analysis of existing data from randomized controlled trials that compared dose-dense chemotherapy with a standard chemotherapy schedule in women with nonmetastatic breast cancer demonstrated that dose-dense chemotherapy results in better overall and disease-free survival, particularly in women with hormone receptor–negative breast cancer (Bonilla, Ben-Aharon, Vidal, et al., 2010). However, additional data from randomized controlled trials are needed before **dose-dense chemotherapy** can be considered the standard of care (Bardia & Baselga, 2014).

SIDE EFFECTS. Many of the side effects of adjuvant chemotherapy can be managed well, allowing patients to maintain their daily routines and work schedules. In large part, this has been a result of the meticulous educational and psychological preparation provided to patients and their families by oncology nurses, oncologists, social workers, and other members of the health care team. In addition, strides have been made in the effectiveness of antiemetic agents used to alleviate nausea and vomiting and the use of hematopoietic growth factors to treat neutropenia and anemia.

Common physical side effects of chemotherapy for breast cancer may include nausea, vomiting, bone marrow suppression, taste changes, alopecia (hair loss), mucositis, neuropathy, skin changes, and fatigue. A weight gain of more than 4 kg occurs in about half of all patients; the cause is unknown. Women who are premenopausal may also experience temporary or permanent amenorrhea.

Specific side effects vary with the type of chemotherapeutic agent used. In general, CMF and the taxanes are better tolerated than the anthracyclines. However, the taxanes can cause peripheral neuropathy, arthralgias, and myalgias, particularly at high doses. During taxane administration, hypersensitivity reactions may occur; therefore, the patient must be premedicated. Alopecia is also common. The side effects of the anthracyclines may be severe and include cardiotoxicity in addition to nausea and vomiting, bone marrow suppression, and alopecia. Their vesicant properties can lead to tissue necrosis if infiltration of the medication infusion occurs.

NURSING MANAGEMENT. Nurses play an important role in helping patients manage the physical and psychosocial sequelae of chemotherapy. (Chapter 68 provides an in-depth discussion of side-effect management.) Educating the patient about the use of antiemetic agents and reviewing the optimal dosage schedule can help minimize nausea and vomiting. The different classes of antiemetic agents include serotonin (5-HT-3) receptor antagonists (palonosetron [Aloxi], granisetron [Kytril], ondansetron [Zofran]); neurokinin-1 receptor antagonists (aprepitant [Emend]); dopamine receptor antagonists (prochlorperazine [Compazine], metoclopramide [Reglan]); benzodiazepines (lorazepam [Ativan]); and corticosteroids (dexamethasone [Decadron]). Measures to ease the symptoms of mucositis may include rinsing with normal saline or sodium bicarbonate solution, avoiding hot and spicy foods, and using a soft toothbrush.

Some patients may require hematopoietic growth factors to minimize the effects of chemotherapy-induced neutropenia and anemia. Granulocyte colony-stimulating factors boost the white blood cell count, helping to reduce the incidence of neutropenic fever and infection. The short-acting form, filgrastim (Neupogen), is injected subcutaneously or IV for 7 to 10 days after chemotherapy administration. The long-acting form, pegfilgrastim (Neulasta), is injected once, no earlier than 24 hours after chemotherapy (Comerford, 2015). Erythropoietin growth factor increases the production of red blood cells, thus decreasing the symptoms of anemia. The short-acting

CHART 49-9

HOME CARE CHECKLIST • Self-Administration of Hematopoietic Growth Factors

At the completion of education, the patient and/or caregiver will be able to:

- State the impact of treatment on physiologic functioning, ADLs, IADLs, roles, relationships, and spirituality.
- Identify the benefits and expected outcome of hematopoietic growth factors.
- Locate list of names and telephone numbers of resource personnel involved in care (e.g., health care professionals, home care nurse, hematopoietic growth factor and supply vendor).
- Identify the equipment necessary for self-injection and how to obtain hematopoietic growth factor and supplies.
- Demonstrate how to give an injection properly, including:
  - How to draw up the solution in a syringe if indicated. (Note: Darbepoetin and pegfilgrastim come in prefilled syringes.)
  - Identify appropriate body sites for self-injection.
  - Demonstrate correct disposal of sharps.
  - Describe proper storage of supplies.
- State what types of lifestyle and environmental changes are needed (if any) to maintain a clean home environment and prevent infection.
- State the name, dose, side effects, frequency, and schedule for all medications.
- List complications of medications/therapeutic regimen necessitating a call to the nurse or primary provider (e.g., excessive pain, fever).
- List complications of medications/therapeutic regimen necessitating a visit to the emergency department.
- Explain treatment plan and importance of follow-up care to all health care providers.
- State time and date of follow-up appointments, therapy, and testing.
- Identify community resources for peer and caregiver/family support:
  - Identify sources of support (e.g., friends, relatives, faith community).
  - Identify phone numbers of support groups for people with cancer and their caregivers/families.
  - State meeting locations and times.
- Identify the need for health promotion, disease prevention, and screening activities.

form, epoetin alfa (Epogen) is usually given weekly. The long-acting form, darbepoetin alfa (Aranesp), can be given every 2 to 3 weeks. The nurse educates the patient and family on proper injection technique of hematopoietic growth factors and about symptoms that require follow-up with a primary provider (Chart 49-9).

To prevent some of the emotional trauma associated with alopecia, it often helps to have a patient obtain a wig before hair loss begins to occur. The nurse may provide a list of wig suppliers in the patient's geographic region. Familiarity with creative ways to use scarves and turbans may also help minimize the patient's distress. The patient needs reassurance that new hair will grow back when treatment is completed, although the colour and texture may be different. The CCS offers a program called Look Good, Feel Better that provides useful tips for applying cosmetics during the period a patient is receiving chemotherapy.

Chemotherapy may negatively affect the patient's self-esteem, sexuality, and sense of well-being. This, combined with the stress of a potentially life-threatening disease, can be overwhelming. Providing support and promoting open communication are important aspects of nursing care. Referring the patient to the dietitian, social worker, psychologist, or spiritual advisor can provide additional support. Numerous community support and advocacy groups are available for patients and their families. Complementary therapies, such as guided imagery, meditation, and relaxation exercises, can also be used in conjunction with conventional treatments.

Hormonal Therapy

The use of **adjuvant hormonal therapy**, with or without the addition of chemotherapy, is considered in women who have hormone receptor–positive tumours. Its use can be determined by the results of an estrogen and progesterone receptor assay (a test to determine whether the breast tumour is nourished by hormones). About two thirds of breast cancers are dependent on estrogen for growth and express a nuclear receptor that binds to the estrogen; thus, they are estrogen receptor–positive (ER+). Similarly, tumours that express the progesterone receptor are progesterone receptor–positive (PR+). Hormonal therapy involves the use of synthetic hormones or other medications that compete with estrogen by binding to the receptor sites (SERMs), or the use of **aromatase inhibitors**, which block estrogen production by the adrenal glands. In general, tumours that are ER+/PR+ have the greatest likelihood of responding to hormonal therapy and have a more favourable prognosis than those that are ER–/PR–. Women who are pre- and perimenopausal are more likely to have non–hormone-dependent lesions, whereas women who are postmenopausal women are more likely to have hormone-dependent lesions.

Traditionally, the SERM tamoxifen has been the main hormonal agent used in treatment of pre- and postmenopausal breast cancer and remains the mainstay in women who are premenopausal women. As an SERM, tamoxifen has estrogen antagonistic (estrogen-blocking) and agonistic (estrogen-like) effects on certain tissues. Its antagonistic effects in the breast prevent estrogen from binding to the receptor sites, thus preventing tumour growth. Tamoxifen has positive agonistic effects on blood lipid profiles and bone mineral density in women who are postmenopausal. It also has agonistic effects on endometrial tissue and blood coagulation processes, leading to an increased incidence of endometrial cancer and thromboembolic events (e.g., deep vein thrombosis, superficial phlebitis, pulmonary embolism). Nevertheless, the benefits of tamoxifen in most women with breast cancer outweigh the risks.

The aromatase inhibitors—anastrazole (Arimidex), letrozole (Femara), and exemestane (Aromasin)—are important components in the hormonal management of women who are postmenopausal. Most of the circulating estrogens in women who are postmenopausal are derived from the conversion of the adrenal androgen androstenedione to estrone and the conversion of testosterone to estradiol. Aromatase inhibitors work by blocking the enzyme aromatase from performing the conversion, thereby decreasing the level of circulating estrogen in peripheral tissues. Clinical trials have demonstrated that the aromatase inhibitors are superior to tamoxifen in terms of overall response rate and clinical benefit and that inhibitors appear to be effective and feasible compared with tamoxifen as first-line hormonal therapy in women who are postmenopausal with advanced breast cancer (Rimawi & Osborne, 2014). These data ensure that aromatase inhibitors will play an increasingly central role in the long-term management of breast cancer. Trials are ongoing to determine the optimal treatment regimen and the timing of the treatment. Table 49-7 outlines the adverse effects of adjuvant hormonal therapy. Chart 49-10 outlines appropriate patient education to manage the adverse effects.

Targeted Therapy

An exciting area of research in the systemic treatment of breast cancer involves the use of targeted therapies. Trastuzumab (Herceptin) is a monoclonal antibody that binds specifically to the HER-2/neu protein. This protein, which regulates cell growth, is present in small amounts on the surface of normal breast cells and in most breast cancers. Approximately 25% to 30% of tumours overexpress (overproduce) the HER-2/neu protein and are associated with rapid growth and poor prognosis. Trastuzumab targets and inactivates the HER-2/neu protein, thus slowing tumour growth.

Unlike chemotherapy, trastuzumab spares the normal cells and has limited adverse reactions, which may include fever, chills, nausea, vomiting, diarrhea, and headache.

TABLE 49-7 Adverse Reactions Associated With Adjuvant Hormonal Therapy Used to Treat Breast Cancer

Therapeutic Agent	Adverse Reactions/Side Effects
Selective Estrogen Receptor Modulator	
Tamoxifen (Nolvadex)	Hot flashes, vaginal dryness/discharge/bleeding, irregular menses, nausea, mood disturbances; increased risk for endometrial cancer; increased risk for thromboembolic events (deep vein thrombosis, pulmonary embolism, superficial phlebitis)
Aromatase Inhibitors	
Anastrozole (Arimidex)	Musculoskeletal symptoms (arthritis, arthralgia, myalgia), increased risk of osteoporosis/fractures, nausea/vomiting, hot flashes, fatigue, mood disturbances
Letrozole (Femara)	
Exemestane (Aromasin)	

Adapted from Comerford, K. C. (2015). *Nursing 2015 drug handbook*. Philadelphia, PA: Wolters Kluwer.

CHART 49-10

Patient Education: Managing Side Effects of Adjuvant Hormonal Therapy in Breast Cancer

Hot Flashes
- Wear breathable, layered clothing (e.g., cotton).
- Avoid caffeine and spicy foods.
- Perform breathing exercises (paced respirations).
- Consider medications (vitamin E, antidepressants) or acupuncture.

Vaginal Dryness
- Use vaginal moisturizers for everyday dryness (e.g., Replens, vitamin E suppository).
- Apply vaginal lubrication during intercourse (e.g., Astroglide, K-Y jelly).

Nausea and Vomiting
- Consume a bland diet.
- Try to take medication in the evening.

Musculoskeletal Symptoms
- Take nonsteroidal analgesics as recommended.
- Take warm baths.

Risk of Endometrial Cancer
- Report any irregular bleeding to a gynecologist for evaluation.

Risk for Thromboembolic Events
- Report any redness, swelling, or tenderness in the lower extremities, or any unexplained shortness of breath.

Risk for Osteoporosis or Fractures
- Undergo a baseline bone density scan.
- Perform regular weight-bearing exercises.
- Take calcium supplements with vitamin D.
- Take bisphosphonates (e.g., alendronate) or calcitonin as prescribed.

However, when trastuzumab is given to patients who have previously been treated with an anthracycline, the risk of cardiac toxicity is increased. The medication has been shown to improve survival rates in women with HER-2/neu–positive metastatic breast cancer and is now regarded as standard therapy. It may be given as a single agent or in combination with chemotherapy. More recently, trastuzumab has been shown to be effective in treating early-stage breast cancer that is HER-2/neu positive. Assessing the benefits and risks of trastuzumab is complex, and medical oncologists often use a variety of aids in their decision making (Kimmick, Hughes, & Muss, 2014).

Treatment of Recurrent and Metastatic Breast Cancer

Despite the advances made in the treatment of breast cancer, it may recur locally (on the chest wall or in the conserved breast), regionally (in the remaining lymph nodes), or systemically (in distant organs). In metastatic disease, the bone, usually the hips, spine, ribs, skull, or pelvis, is the most common site of spread. Other sites of metastasis include the lungs, liver, pleura, and brain.

The overall prognosis and optimal treatment are determined by a variety of factors such as the site and extent of recurrence, the time to recurrence from the original diagnosis, history of prior treatments, the patient's performance status, and any existing comorbid conditions. Patients with bone metastases generally have a longer overall survival compared with metastases in visceral organs.

Local recurrence in the absence of systemic disease is treated aggressively with surgery, radiation, and hormonal therapy. Chemotherapy may also be used for tumours that are not hormonally sensitive. Local recurrence may be an indicator that systemic disease will develop in the future, particularly if it occurs within 2 years of the original diagnosis (NCCN, 2015).

Metastatic breast cancer involves control of the disease rather than cure (NCCN, 2015). Treatment includes hormonal therapy, chemotherapy, and targeted therapy. Surgery or radiation may be indicated in select situations. Women who are premenopausal and who have hormonally dependent tumours may eliminate the production of estrogen by the ovaries through oophorectomy (removal of the ovaries) or suppression of estrogen production by medications such as leuprolide (Lupron) or goserelin (Zoladex).

Patients with advanced breast cancer are monitored closely for signs of disease progression. Baseline studies are obtained at the time of recurrence. These may include complete blood count; comprehensive metabolic panel; tumour markers (i.e., carcinoembryonic antigen, cancer antigen 15-3); bone scan; CT of the chest, abdomen, and pelvis; and MRI of symptomatic areas. Additional x-rays may be performed to evaluate areas of pain or abnormal areas seen on bone scan (e.g., long bones, pelvis). These studies are repeated at regular intervals to assess for effectiveness of treatment and to monitor progression of disease.

Nursing Management

Nurses play an important role in not only educating patients and managing their symptoms but also in providing emotional support. Many patients find that recurrence of the disease is more distressing than the initial cancer diagnosis. They not only have to contend with another round of treatments but are also faced with a greater uncertainty about their future and long-term survival. The nurse can help the patient identify coping strategies and set priorities to optimize quality of life. Family members and significant others should be included in the treatment plan and follow-up care. Referrals to support groups, in addition to psychiatry or psychiatric clinical nurse specialist, social work, and complementary medicine programs (e.g., guided imagery, meditation, yoga) should be made as indicated.

Nurses also play important roles in providing palliative care, if indicated. The highest priorities include alleviating pain and providing comfort measures. A frank discussion with the patient and family regarding their preferences for end-of-life care should occur before the need arises to ensure a smooth transition without disruption of care. Referrals to hospice and home health care should be initiated as necessary.

Reconstructive Procedures After Mastectomy

Breast reconstruction can provide a significant psychological benefit for women who are already struggling with the emotional distress of losing a breast. A consultation with a plastic surgeon can help the patient understand procedures for which she is a candidate and the pros and cons of each. Factors to consider include body size and shape, comorbid conditions (e.g., hypertension, diabetes, obesity), personal habits such as smoking, and patient preference. The patient must be informed that although breast reconstruction can provide a good cosmetic result, it will never precisely duplicate the natural breast. Realistic preparation can help the patient avoid unrealistic expectations. Once reconstruction is complete, the opposite breast may require augmentation, reduction, or mastopexy to achieve symmetry on both sides. The patient must also be informed that breast reconstruction neither will interfere with breast cancer treatments nor affect the risk of cancer recurrence. Reconstruction is considered an integral component in the surgical treatment of breast cancer and is usually covered by provincial and territorial health plans.

Many women elect immediate reconstruction at the time of the mastectomy operation. This can be beneficial in that it saves the woman from undergoing general anesthesia a second time and saves the cost and stress of future hospitalizations. However, it does increase the length of the surgical procedure. Delayed reconstruction is preferable in women who are having a difficult time deciding on the type of reconstruction that they desire. It may also be preferable in patients with advanced disease such as inflammatory breast cancer, where the breast cancer treatments should begin without delay. Any delays in healing after immediate reconstruction may interfere with the initiation of treatment.

Tissue Expander Followed by Permanent Implant

Breast reconstruction using a **tissue expander followed by a permanent implant** is the simplest and most common method used today (Fig. 49-6). To accommodate an implant, the skin remaining after a mastectomy and the

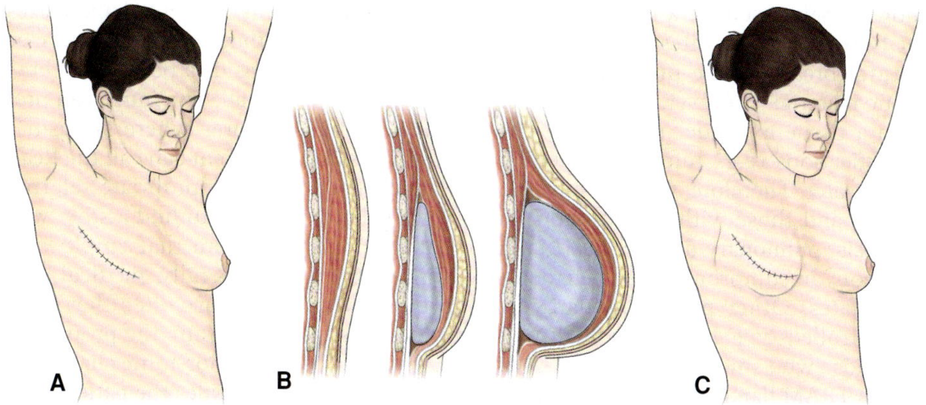

FIGURE 49-6. Breast reconstruction with tissue expander. **A.** Mastectomy incision line prior to tissue expansion. **B.** The expander is placed under the pectoralis muscle and is gradually filled with saline solution through a port to stretch the skin enough to accept a permanent implant. **C.** The breast mound is restored. Although permanent, scars will fade with time. The nipple and areola are reconstructed later. (Adapted from American Society of Plastic Surgeons.)

underlying muscle must gradually be stretched by a process called tissue expansion. The surgeon places a tissue expander (a balloon-like device) through the mastectomy incision underneath the pectoralis muscle. A small amount of saline is injected through a metal port intraoperatively to partially inflate the expander. Then, for about 6 to 8 weeks, at weekly intervals, the patient receives additional saline injections through the port until the expander is fully inflated. It remains fully expanded for about 6 weeks to allow the skin to loosen. The expander is then exchanged for a permanent implant. This is usually performed as an outpatient surgical procedure.

Advantages of this expansion procedure are a shorter operating time and a shorter recuperation period than for autologous reconstruction (see Tissue Transfer Procedures below). A disadvantage is a tendency for the implant to feel firm and round, with little natural ptosis (sag). Women with a small to medium opposite breast with little ptosis are good candidates for this procedure. Women who have had radiation or who have connective tissue disease are not good candidates because of the decreased elasticity of the skin.

NURSING ALERT

The patient must be cautioned not to have an MRI while the tissue expander is in place because the port contains metal. This is not an issue once the permanent implant is in place because it does not contain any metal.

The patient should be informed that for the rest of her life she should not engage in any exercises that will develop the pectoralis muscle because this can result in distortion of the reconstructed breast.

Tissue Transfer Procedures

Autologous reconstruction is the use of the patient's own tissue to create a breast mound. A flap of skin, fat, and muscle with its attached blood supply is rotated to the mastectomy site to create a mound that simulates the breast. Donor sites may include the **transverse rectus abdominis myocutaneous (TRAM) flap** (abdominal muscle) (Fig. 49-7), gluteal flap (buttock muscle), or the latissimus dorsi flap (back muscle) (Fig. 49-8). The results

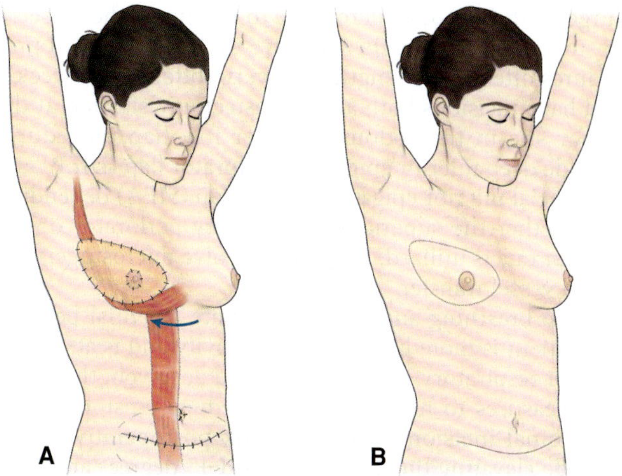

FIGURE 49-7. Breast reconstruction: Transverse rectus abdominis myocutaneous (TRAM) flap. **A.** A breast mound is created by tunnelling abdominal skin, fat, and muscle to the mastectomy site. **B.** Final location of scars. (Adapted from American Society of Plastic Surgeons.)

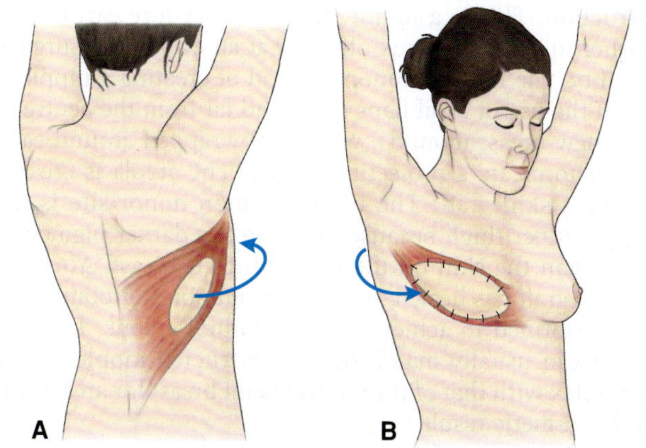

FIGURE 49-8. Breast reconstruction: Latissimus dorsi flap. **A.** The latissimus muscle with an ellipse of skin is rotated from the back to the mastectomy site. **B.** Because the flap is usually not bulky enough to provide an adequate breast mound, an implant is often also required. (Adapted from American Society of Plastic Surgeons.)

more closely resemble a real breast because the skin and fat from the donor sites are similar in consistency to a natural breast. These procedures avoid the use of synthetic material. However, they involve longer recuperation than a tissue expander procedure. The risk of potential complications (e.g., infection, bleeding, flap necrosis) is also greater. Therefore, patients must be in relatively good health, and those with medical conditions (e.g., atherosclerosis, pulmonary disease, heart failure) that affect circulation or compromise oxygen delivery are not good candidates. Other poor candidates include those with uncontrolled type 1 diabetes mellitus or morbid obesity and those who smoke.

The TRAM flap is the most commonly performed tissue transfer procedure. A free TRAM procedure may also be performed; in this case, the skin, fat, muscle, and blood supply are completely detached from the body and then transplanted to the mastectomy site using microvascular surgery (the use of a microscope to reconnect the vessels). Postoperatively, patients who have undergone TRAM procedures often face a lengthy recovery (often 6 to 8 weeks) and have incisions both at the mastectomy site and at the donor site in the abdomen. Other free flap procedures include deep inferior epigastric perforator flap (DIEP) and superficial inferior epigastric artery flap (SIEA) depending on whether the superior gluteal artery perforator or the inferior one is utilized. Free flaps involve microsurgery for blood vessel transfer.

Deep breathing and leg exercises are essential because the patient is more limited in her activity and is at greater risk for respiratory complications and deep vein thrombosis. Measures to help the patient reduce tension on the abdominal incision during the first postoperative week include elevating the head of the bed 45 degrees and flexing the patient's knees.

Once the patient is able to ambulate, she can protect the surgical incision by splinting it and will gradually achieve a more upright position. The patient is instructed to avoid high-impact activities and lifting (more than 2 to 4 kg for 6 to 8 weeks after surgery) to prevent stress on the incision.

Nipple–Areola Reconstruction

After the breast mound has been created and the site has healed, some women choose to have nipple–areola reconstruction. This is a minor surgical procedure carried out either in the physician's office or at an outpatient surgical facility. The most common method of creating a nipple is with the use of local flaps (skin and fat from the centre of the new breast mound), which are wrapped around each other to create a projecting nipple. The areola is created using a skin graft. The most common donor site is the upper inner thigh because this skin has darker pigmentation than the skin on the reconstructed breast. After the nipple graft has healed, micropigmentation (tattooing) can be performed to achieve a more natural colour. The surgeon can usually match the reconstructed nipple–areola complex with that of the contralateral breast for an acceptable cosmetic result.

Prosthetics

Not all patients desire or are candidates for reconstructive surgery. A breast prosthesis, an external form that simulates the breast, is another option. Prostheses are available in different shapes, sizes, colours, and materials, although they are most often made of silicone. They can be placed inside a pocket in a bra or can adhere directly to the chest wall. The nurse can provide the patient with the names of stores where she can be fitted for a prosthesis, or the patient can call the Reach to Recovery program of the CCS for appropriate referrals. The patient should be encouraged to find a store with a comfortable, supportive atmosphere that employs a certified prosthetics consultant. Generally, medical supply shops are not recommended because often they do not have the appropriate resources to ensure the proper fitting of a prosthesis.

Prior to discharge from the hospital, the nurse usually provides the patient with a temporary, lightweight, cotton-filled form that can be worn until the surgical incision is well healed (4 to 6 weeks). After that, the patient can be fitted for a prosthesis. Insurance companies generally cover the cost of the prosthesis and the special bras that hold it in place. A breast prosthesis can provide a psychological benefit and assist the woman in resuming proper posture because it helps balance the weight of the remaining breast.

Special Issues in Breast Cancer Management

Implications of Genetic Testing

The rapid advancement in genetics not only has brought new knowledge about inherited breast cancer, but it has also raised potential ethical and psychosocial issues. Although the actual testing for the *BRCA1* and *BRCA2* and several other genes that increase risk involves a simple blood or saliva test, ethical and psychosocial issues must first be addressed. Before undergoing genetic testing, a person should meet either with a clinician who has expertise in this area or with a certified genetics counsellor to discuss risk factors as well as the benefits, sequelae, and limitations of testing.

How people react when they receive their actual test results is not always easy to predict. A negative test in a person who comes from a family with a known mutation may lead to enormous relief. However, a negative test in a family with no known mutation may be a source of undue reassurance; the possibility of existing genes that cannot yet be detected remains. A negative test may also lead to feelings of guilt in a person whose family members did not receive favourable test results; this is known as survivor's guilt. A positive test could act as a motivator in a person to pursue appropriate screening or treatment, or it could cause tremendous anxiety, depression, and worry.

In addition, test results may be ambiguous, leading to feelings of confusion and uncertainty. People must be informed that not all gene carriers develop breast cancer (incomplete penetrance) and that not all noncarriers are protected or immune.

People must be well informed of all issues and potential implications prior to undergoing genetic testing (see Chapter 11). Nurses play a role in educating and counselling patients and their family members about the implications of genetic testing. Nurses provide support and clarification and make referrals to appropriate specialists when indicated.

Pregnancy and Breast Cancer

Breast cancer during pregnancy is defined as breast cancer diagnosed during gestation or within 1 year of childbirth and occurs in 1 in 3,000 women. Because of increased levels of hormones produced during pregnancy and subsequent lactation, the breast tissue becomes tender and swollen, making it more difficult to detect a mass. If a mass is found during pregnancy, ultrasound is the preferred diagnostic method because it involves no exposure to radiation. If indicated, mammography with appropriate shielding, FNA, and biopsy can be performed. Modified radical mastectomy remains the most common form of surgical treatment. SLNB is typically not performed because of the unknown effects of the radioisotope and the blue dye on the fetus. Breast-conservation treatment may be considered if the breast cancer is diagnosed during the third trimester. Radiation can then be delayed until after delivery because it is contraindicated during pregnancy. If a woman is close to term, a cesarean section may be performed as soon as maturation of the fetus allows and then treatment is initiated. If aggressive disease is detected early in pregnancy and chemotherapy is advised, termination of the pregnancy may be considered. If a mass is found while a woman is breastfeeding, she is urged to stop to allow the breast to involute (return to its baseline state) before any type of surgery is performed (NCCN, 2015).

Fertility issues and the future desire for children are major concerns of young women who are survivors of breast cancer. Most cancer therapies have a substantial morbidity on reproductive function, not only because they increase the risk of early menopause but also because they are associated with a decreased ovarian reserve and a loss of fertility. It is estimated that physiologic age of the ovaries in a survivor of cancer may be 10 years older than the actual chronologic age.

Chemotherapy causes a progressive dose-related depletion of ovarian follicles and granulosa cells that translates into oligomenorrhea and subsequent premature ovarian failure, ultimately leading to what is known as chemotherapy-induced amenorrhea (CIA). Regardless of the beneficial effects that hormonal changes can have as part of the adjuvant endocrine strategy, CIA is an adverse event to consider when selecting the best adjuvant treatment. Patients with cancer need to be informed about their reproductive future and options to preserve fertility before treatment (Ruddy & Ginsburg, 2014).

Quality of Life and Survivorship

With increased early detection and improved treatment modalities, women with breast cancer have become the largest group of cancer survivors. However, the treatment or simply the diagnosis of breast cancer may have long-term effects that negatively affect the patient and her family. The patient should be prepared early on for the potential long-term effects of the disease, so she has realistic expectations and can make informed decisions.

Survivors of breast cancer may experience a variety of issues as a result of their diagnosis and treatment. Estrogen withdrawal from chemotherapy-induced menopause and hormonal treatments can lead to a variety of symptoms, including hot flashes, vaginal dryness, urinary tract infections, weight gain, decreased sex drive, and increased risk of osteoporosis. HT to alleviate symptoms is contraindicated in women with breast cancer. Certain chemotherapeutic agents can cause long-term cardiac effects and neuropathy. In addition, patients may experience impaired cognitive functioning such as difficulty concentrating (often referred to as chemo-brain). Rare long-term effects of radiation can include pneumonitis, rib fractures, heart disease, and breast fibrosis or necrosis (Harris & Morrow, 2014). Long-term sequelae after breast surgery may include lymphedema (mainly after ALND), pain, and sensory disturbances. Once lymphedema develops, it tends to be a chronic problem, so prevention strategies (discussed earlier) are vital. Weight gain and infections are risk factors for lymphedema (Ahn & Port, 2016). Nurses need to encourage patients to maintain an active lifestyle and avoid weight gain.

Long-term psychosocial sequelae may include fears of recurrence, mood changes (e.g., worry, sadness, anger, frustration), an increased sense of vulnerability, uncertainty, feelings of loss (e.g., fertility), concerns about body image, self-concept, and sexuality; emotional distress related to role adjustments and family response; and concerns about finances and employment. Depression and anxiety have been documented in 20% to 30% of women with breast cancer. Interventions should be targeted to meet informational needs, manage uncertainty, control symptoms, address cultural differences, and enhance social and emotional support (Heinz & Williams, 2015; Ligabel & Denlinger, 2013).

Gerontologic Considerations

Breast reconstruction in older women with breast cancer is a feasible option that should be offered to patients. Most women tolerate the procedure well and have good cosmetic outcomes. Patients can be offered both implant-based reconstruction and autologous tissue transfer with minimal complications as long as appropriate preoperative selection criteria are used. The safety of reconstruction, together with increase in life expectancy and healthier lifestyles, makes breast reconstruction after mastectomy desirable at any age (NCCN, 2015).

A thorough assessment must be performed before any treatment is initiated, and careful monitoring must occur throughout the course of treatment to avoid complications. The physical and psychosocial assessment of the older woman should include general health, currently existing comorbidities, performance status, cognitive status, current medications, available resources, and support systems.

Breast Health of Women With Disabilities

Disparities in obtaining a mammogram at recommended screening intervals persist for many women, including those with disabilities. Prevalence of self-reported use of mammography is lower for women with a disability. It is estimated that women with a disability are less likely to have received a mammogram within the 2-year recommended period (Courtney-Long, Armour, Frammartino, et al., 2011). Many imaging facilities do not have accessible mammography equipment, and staff members may be unfamiliar with modifications in positioning needed to obtain acceptable scans (Canadian Breast Cancer Network [CBCN], 2012). Furthermore, health care providers often neglect to recommend health screening for women with disabilities, despite the fact that they have the same risks for breast cancer as other women and generally have a normal or near-normal life expectancy. The more severe the disability, the less likely that a woman will undergo mammography. For those women who cannot be adequately positioned for a mammogram, ultrasound may be used as an alternative; however, these women may need more frequent clinical breast examinations.

Efforts to reduce disparities in breast cancer screening might be more effective if all segments of the population are targeted. Possible barriers to the use of mammography in women with disabilities include physical inaccessibility of office space and medical equipment; limited transportation and parking options; and time and assistance constraints associated with undressing, transferring, and positioning for medical examinations. To promote health and wellness, health agencies, providers, and health care plans must promote cancer prevention and educational programs that are inclusive and responsive to the special needs of women with disabilities (Swaine, Parish, Luken, et al., 2014).

An essential role of the nurse is to assist all women, including those with disabilities to identify accessible health screening and to advocate for greater accessibility of imaging centres and other health care facilities. Reminding women of the need for recommended clinical breast examinations and mammograms is an important part of nursing care.

RECONSTRUCTIVE BREAST SURGERY

Breast-reconstruction surgery, called **mammoplasty**, is an elective procedure that can enhance a woman's self-image and sense of well-being. Women desire reconstruction for a variety of physical and psychological reasons. Therefore, it is important for the health care team to conduct a thorough assessment prior to reconstructive surgery to evaluate the woman's underlying desire, motivation, and expectations. Preparing a woman realistically could help her to avoid potential disappointment. A variety of reconstructive options are available today for women who desire a correction in the size or the shape of the breast, including reduction mammoplasty (breast reduction), augmentation mammoplasty (breast enlargement), and mastopexy (breast lift). Several options are also available to reconstruct the breast after a mastectomy.

Reduction Mammoplasty

Reduction mammoplasty is usually performed on women who have breast hypertrophy (excessively large breasts). The weight of the enlarged breasts can cause discomfort, fatigue, embarrassment, and poor posture.

Reduction mammoplasty is an outpatient procedure that is performed under general anesthesia. Most commonly, an anchor-shaped incision that circles the areola is made, extending downward and following the natural curve of the crease beneath the breast (inframammary fold). Depending on the size of the breast, the nipple may be moved up to a higher position while still attached to the breast tissue or it may be separated and transplanted to a new location. Drains are placed in the incision and remain for 2 to 5 days.

During the preoperative consultation, the patient should be informed that there is a possibility that sensory changes of the nipple (such as numbness) may occur. These sensations are normal and usually resolve after several months but can sometimes persist. The procedure may also make breastfeeding impossible, although some women have breastfed successfully. The patient must also be aware that if she gains weight (usually more than 4 kg), her breasts may also enlarge.

After reduction mammoplasty, many women verbalize feelings of extreme satisfaction, possibly because of the relief they experience. The patient is instructed to wear a supportive bra 24 hours a day for 2 weeks to prevent tension on the swollen breast and incision line. Vigorous exercise (e.g., jumping, jogging) should be avoided for about 6 weeks after surgery.

Augmentation Mammoplasty

Augmentation mammoplasty is requested by women who desire larger or fuller breasts. The procedure is performed by placing a breast implant either under the pectoralis muscle (subpectoral) or under the breast tissue (subglandular). The subpectoral approach is preferred because it interferes less with clinical breast examinations and mammograms. The incision line can be placed in the inframammary fold, in the axilla, or around the areola. The procedure is performed as an outpatient procedure under general anesthesia. A drain is not necessary. Postoperative instructions are the same as for reduction mammoplasty.

Saline implants are typically used for augmentation mammoplasty. At this time, both saline-filled and silicone-gel–filled breast implants are available in Canada (Government of Canada, 2017). Women with breast implants should be aware that mammograms may be more difficult to read, so they should seek experienced breast radiologists.

Mastopexy

Mastopexy is performed when the patient is happy with the size of her breasts but wishes to have the shape improved and a lift performed. This is also an outpatient surgical procedure, and postoperative instructions are the same as for reduction mammoplasty.

DISEASES OF THE MALE BREAST

Gynecomastia

Gynecomastia is the most common breast condition in the male. Adolescent boys can be affected because of hormones secreted by the testes. This type of gynecomastia is virtually always benign and resolves spontaneously in 1 to 2 years. Gynecomastia can also occur in older men and usually presents as a firm, tender mass underneath the areola. In these patients, gynecomastia may be diffuse and related to use of certain medications (e.g., digitalis, ranitidine [Zantac]). It may also be associated with certain conditions, including feminizing testicular tumours, infection in the testes, and liver disease resulting from factors such as alcohol abuse or a parasitic infection.

Patients in their late teens to late 40s presenting with idiopathic (unknown cause) gynecomastia should have a testicular examination and possibly a testicular ultrasound. Treatment of the enlarged breast tissue is based on patient preference and is usually reserved for those men who cannot tolerate the cosmetic appearance of the breast or who have severe pain associated with the condition. Mammography and ultrasound are utilized if there is a concern about malignancy. Observation is acceptable in most cases because gynecomastia may resolve on its own. Surgical removal of the tissue through a small incision around the areola is the best treatment option. Liposuction performed by a plastic surgeon is another possibility, although this does not allow for pathologic examination of the tissue.

Male Breast Cancer

Cancer of the male breast accounted for approximately 1% of all cases of breast cancer with an estimated 230 cases in 2017 (CCS, 2018c). The average age at the time of diagnosis is 67 years, but the disease may occur in younger men, especially if there is a genetic link (Mattarella, 2010). Although breast carcinoma in both genders shares certain characteristics, notable differences have emerged. Familial cases in men usually have *BRCA2* rather than *BRCA1* mutations. Klinefelter's syndrome, a chromosomal condition reflecting decreased testosterone levels, is the strongest risk factor for developing male breast carcinoma. Presentation is usually a painless lump, but is often late, with more than 40% of individuals having stage III or IV disease. When survival is adjusted for age at diagnosis and stage of disease, outcomes for male and female patients with breast cancer is similar (Jain & Gradishar, 2014).

Early detection is uncommon in male breast cancer because of the rare nature of the disease. Often neither patient nor physician suspects male breast cancer early in its development. Treatment generally consists of a total mastectomy with either SLNB or ALND. As in women with breast cancer, prognosis depends on the stage of disease at presentation. Involvement of the axillary lymph nodes is the most important prognostic indicator. Male breast cancers are very likely to be ER+, and tamoxifen, although it has several side effects, is a mainstay of treatment.

Because breast cancer is primarily a disease of women, men may feel that a certain stigma is attached to their diagnosis. Health care professionals must be sensitive to their needs and provide information and support.

Critical Thinking Exercises

1 **ebp** A 27-year-old woman has no significant medical history but has a positive family history for breast cancer. What evidence-based recommendations are indicated for the regularity of assessments and screening for this woman? Identify the criteria to evaluate the strength of the evidence for these recommendations.

2 **pq** A 64-year-old woman with a new diagnosis of breast cancer is admitted for a mastectomy. What are the priorities for care of this patient in the preoperative phase? How will your priorities change in the postoperative phase? What are the priorities for discharge instructions and education for this patient? How will your priorities change if the patient is being discharged with a drain?

3 A 54-year-old woman with breast cancer has been prescribed adjuvant hormonal therapy. What would be most important to include in patient education? Describe at least three topics that need to be addressed.

REFERENCES AND SELECTED READINGS

Books

Bardia, A., & Baselga, J. (2014). Preoperative chemotherapy for operable breast cancer. In J. Harris, M. Lippman, M. Morrow, et al. (Eds.). *Diseases of the breast* (5th ed.). Philadelphia, PA: Wolters Kluwer.

Cherny, N., & Truong, P. (2014). Brachial plexopathy in patients with breast cancer. In J. Harris, M. Lippman, M. Morrow, et al. (Eds.). *Diseases of the breast* (5th ed.). Philadelphia, PA: Wolters Kluwer.

Chung, A., & Giuliano, A. (2014). Sentinel lymph node biopsy. In J. Harris, M. Lippman, M. Morrow, et al. (Eds.). *Diseases of the breast* (5th ed.). Philadelphia, PA: Wolters Kluwer.

Collins, L., & Schnitt, S. (2014). Pathology of benign breast disorders. In J. Harris, M. Lippman, M. Morrow, et al. (Eds.). *Diseases of the breast* (5th ed.). Philadelphia, PA: Wolters Kluwer.

Comerford, K. C. (2015). *Nursing 2015 drug handbook*. Philadelphia, PA: Wolters Kluwer.

Day, R. A. (2012). Breasts and axillae assessment. In T. C. Stephen, D. L. Skillen, Day, R. A., et al. (Eds.), *Canadian Jensen's nursing health assessment: A best practice approach* (Canadian ed., revised reprint., pp. 57–60). Philadelphia, PA: Wolters Kluwer Health/Lippincott Williams & Wilkins.

Fischbach, F., & Dunning, M. B. (2015). *A manual of laboratory and diagnostic tests* (9th ed.). Philadelphia, PA: Wolters Kluwer.

Grossman, S., & Porth, C. M. (2014). *Porth's pathophysiology: Concepts of altered health states* (9th ed.). Philadelphia, PA: Lippincott Williams & Wilkins.

Gucalp, A., Morris, P., Hudis, C., et al. (2014). Implications of obesity in breast cancer. In J. Harris, M. Lippman, M. Morrow, et al. (Eds.). *Diseases of the breast* (5th ed.). Philadelphia, PA: Wolters Kluwer.

Harris, J., & Morrow, M. (2014). Breast-conserving therapy. In J. Harris, M. Lippman, M. Morrow, et al. (Eds.). *Diseases of the breast* (5th ed.). Philadelphia, PA: Wolters Kluwer.

Helvie, M., & Patterson, S. (2014). Imaging analysis: Mammography. In J. Harris, M. Lippman, M. Morrow, et al. (Eds.). *Diseases of the breast* (5th ed.). Philadelphia, PA: Wolters Kluwer.

Jain, S., & Gradishar, W. (2014). Male breast cancer. In J. Harris, M. Lippman, M. Morrow, et al. (Eds.). *Diseases of the breast* (5th ed.). Philadelphia, PA: Wolters Kluwer.

Jochelson, M. (2014). New breast imaging techniques. In J. Harris, M. Lippman, M. Morrow, et al. (Eds.). *Diseases of the breast* (5th ed.). Philadelphia, PA: Wolters Kluwer.

Kimmick, G., Hughes, K., & Muss, H. (2014). Breast cancer in older women. In J. Harris, M. Lippman, M. Morrow, et al. (Eds.). *Diseases of the breast* (5th ed.). Philadelphia, PA: Wolters Kluwer.

King, T., & Reis-Filho, J. (2014). Lobular carcinoma in situ: Biology and management. In J. Harris, M. Lippman, M. Morrow, et al. (Eds.). *Diseases of the breast* (5th ed.). Philadelphia, PA: Wolters Kluwer.

McLaughlin, S. (2014). Lymphedema. In J. Harris, M. Lippman, M. Morrow, et al. (Eds.). *Diseases of the breast* (5th ed.). Philadelphia, PA: Wolters Kluwer.

Meneses, K., & Walker, D. (2014). Nursing care in patient management and quality of life. In J. Harris, M. Lippman, M. Morrow, et al. (Eds.). *Diseases of the breast* (5th ed.). Philadelphia, PA: Wolters Kluwer.

Morrow, M. (2014). Physical examination of the breast. In J. Harris, M. Lippman, M. Morrow, et al. (Eds.). *Diseases of the breast* (5th ed.). Philadelphia, PA: Wolters Kluwer.

National Comprehensive Cancer Network (NCCN). (2014). *Breast cancer treatment guidelines in oncology. Breast Cancer. Version* 2. Atlanta, GA: American Cancer Society.

Osborne, M., & Boolbol, S. (2014). Breast anatomy and development. In J. Harris, M. Lippman, M. Morrow, et al. (Eds.). *Diseases of the breast* (5th ed.). Philadelphia, PA: Wolters Kluwer.

Press, M., & Ma, Y. (2014). HER2/ERBB2 testing: Assessment of status for targeted therapies. In J. Harris, M. Lippman, M. Morrow, et al. (Eds.). *Diseases of the breast* (5th ed.). Philadelphia, PA: Wolters Kluwer.

Rimawi, M., & Osborne, C. (2014). Adjuvant systemic therapy: Endocrine therapy. In J. Harris, M. Lippman, M. Morrow, et al. (Eds.). *Diseases of the breast* (5th ed.). Philadelphia, PA: Wolters Kluwer.

Ruddy, K., & Ginsburg, E. (2014). Reproductive issues in breast cancer survivors. In J. Harris, M. Lippman, M. Morrow, et al. (Eds.). *Diseases of the breast* (5th ed.). Philadelphia, PA: Wolters Kluwer.

Weber, J., & Kelley, J. (2014). *Health assessment in nursing* (5th ed.). Philadelphia, PA: Lippincott Williams & Wilkins.

Yarbo, C. H., Wujcik, D., & Gobel, B. H. (Eds.). (2013). *Breast Cancer*. Sudbury, MA: Jones & Bartlett.

Journals and Electronic Documents

Ahn, S., & Port, E. (2016) Lymphedema precautions: Time to abandon old practices? *Journal of Clinical Oncology*, *34*(12), 655–658.

American Cancer Society. (2015). Cancer facts and figures 2015. Retrieved on February 22, 2016, from: www.cancer.org/acs/groups/content/@editorial/documents/document/acspc-044552.pdf

Bonilla, L., Ben-Aharon, I., Vidal, L., et al. (2010). Dose-dense chemotherapy in nonmetastatic breast cancer: A systematic review and meta-analysis of randomized controlled trials. *Journal of the National Cancer Institute*, *102*(24), 1845–1854.

Canadian Breast Cancer Network. (2012). *Women with Disabilities & Breast Cancer Screening: An Environmental Scan. Identified Problems, Strategies and Recommended Next Steps*. Ottawa: Author. Retrieved from: http://www.cbcn.ca/index.php?pageaction=content.page&id=7947&lang=en

Canadian Cancer Society (CCS). (2018a). *Screening for breast cancer*. Toronto: Author. Retrieved from: http://www.cancer.ca/en/cancer-information/cancer-type/breast/screening/?region=bc

Canadian Cancer Society (CCS). (2018b). Diagnosis of breast cancer. Retrieved from: http://www.cancer.ca/en/cancer-information/cancer-type/breast/diagnosis/?region=bc

Canadian Cancer Society (CCS). (2018c). *Canadian Cancer Statistics*. Ottawa: Public Health Agency of Canada, and Statistics Canada. Retrieved from: http://www.cancer.ca/en/cancer-information/cancer-type/breast/statistics/?region=bc

Canadian Cancer Society (CCS). (2018d). Staging cancer. Retrieved from Canadian Cancer Society (CCS). (2018). Screening for breast cancer. Toronto: Author. Retrieved from: http://www.cancer.ca/en/cancer-information/cancer-type/breast/screening/?region=bc

Canadian Cancer Society (CCS). (2018e). Survival statistics for breast cancer. Retrieved from: http://www.cancer.ca/en/cancer-information/cancer-type/breast/prognosis-and-survival/survival-statistics/?region=on

Canadian Cancer Society. (CCS). (2018f). If breast cancer spreads. Retrieved from: http://www.cancer.ca/en/cancer-information/cancer-type/breast/if-cancer-spreads/?region=on

Canadian Cancer Society. (2018g). Find cancer early: When should I be screened for breast cancer? Retrieved from: http://www.cancer.ca/en/prevention-and-screening/reduce-cancer-risk/find-cancer-early/get-screened-for-breast-cancer/when-should-i-be-screened-for-breast-cancer/?region=bc

Canadian Task Force for Preventative Health Care. (2011). Recommendations on screening for breast cancer in average-risk women aged 40–74 years. *CMAJ*, *183*(17), 1991–2001.

CancerQuest. (2015). Introduction to patient information, detection and diagnosis, fine needle aspiration. Retrieved on May 22, 2016, from: www.cancerquest.org

Chavez-McGregor, M., Clarke, C. A., Lichtensztajn, D. Y., et al. (2016). Delayed initiation of adjuvant chemotherapy among patients with breast cancer. *JAMA Oncology*, 2(3), 322–329.

Courtney-Long, E., Armour, B., Frammartino, B., et al. (2011). Factors associated with self-reported mammography use for women with and women without a disability. *Journal of Women's Health 20*, 1279–1286.

Cummings, S. R., Eckert, S., Krueger, K. A., et al. (1999). The effect of raloxifene on risk of breast cancer in postmenopausal women: Results from the MORE randomized trial. *Journal of the American Medical Association*, *281*(23), 2189–2197.

Fisher, B., Costantino, J. P., Wickerham, D. L., et al. (1998). Tamoxifen for prevention of breast cancer. Report of the National Surgical Adjuvant Breast and Bowel Project P-1 study. *Journal of the National Cancer Institute*, *90*(18), 1371–1388.

Government of Canada. (2017). Breast implants. Retrieved from: https://www.canada.ca/en/health-canada/services/drugs-medical-devices/breast-implants.html

Harding, M. (2015). Effect of nurse navigation on patient care satisfaction and distress associated with breast biopsy. *Clinical Journal Oncology Nursing*, *19*(1), E15–E20.

Heinz, S., & Williams, P. (2015). Symptom alleviation and self-care among breast cancer survivors after treatment completion. *Clinical Journal of Oncology Nursing*, *19*(3), 343–349.

Kim, H.-J., Barsevick, A. M., & Tulman, L. (2009). Predictors of the intensity of cluster symptoms in patients with breast cancer. *Journal of Nursing Scholarship*, *41*(2), 158–165.

Ligabel, J., & Denlinger, C. (2013). New NCCN guidelines for survivorship care. *Journal of the National Comprehensive Care Network*, *11* (5 Suppl), 640–644.

Mattarella, A. (2010). Breast cancer in men. *Radiologic Technology*, *35*(23), 18–20.

National Cancer Institute (NCI). (2013). Surgery to reduce the risk of breast cancer. Retrieved on February 26, 2016, from: www.cancer.gov/types/breast/risk-reducing-surgery-fact-sheet

National Comprehensive Cancer Network (NCCN). (2015). Clinical practice guidelines: Breast. Retrieved on March 7, 2016, from: www.nccn.org/professionals/physician_gls/PDF/infections.pdf

Swaine, J., Parish, S., Luken, K., et al. (2014). Test of an intervention to improve knowledge of women with intellectual disability about cervical and breast cancer screening. *Journal of Intellectual Disability Research*, *58*(7), 651–663.

Toledo, E., Salas-Salvad, J., Donat-Vargas, C., et al. (2015). Mediterranean diet and invasive breast cancer risk among women at high cardiovascular risk in the PREDIMED trial: A randomized clinical trial. *JAMA Internal Medicine*, *175*(11), 1752–1760.

Vogel, V. G., Costantino, J. P., Wickerham, D. L., et al. (2006). Effects of tamoxifen vs raloxifene on the risk of developing invasive breast cancer and other disease outcomes. The NSABP study of tamoxifen and raloxifene (STAR) P-2 trial. *Journal of the American Medical Association*, *295*(23), 2727–2741.

Resources

American Cancer Society: http://www.cancer.org
Canadian Cancer Society: http://www.cancer.ca
Canadian Cancer Survivor Network: http://survivornet.ca/en/
Canadian Society of Plastic Surgeons: http://www.plasticsurgery.ca/
Cancer Care, Inc. (provides free professional support services to anyone affected by cancer): http://www.cancercare.org
Fertile Future: http://www.fertilefuture.ca
National Cancer Institute: http://www.cancer.gov/cancertopics/types/breast
National Lymphedema Network: https://www.nationallymphedemanetwork.org/
Oncology Nursing Society: http://www.ons.org
Reach to Recovery Program (Information available through local Canadian Cancer Society chapters).
Susan G. Komen for the Cure: ww5.komen.org

50 Assessment and Management of Problems Related to Male Reproductive Disorders

Adapted by Mohamed Toufic El Hussein and Joseph Osuji

Learning Objectives

On completion of this chapter, the learner will be able to:

1. Describe structures and function of the male reproductive system.
2. Discuss nursing assessment of the male reproductive system; identify diagnostic tests used and their related nursing implications.
3. Explain the causes and management of male sexual dysfunction.
4. Compare the types of prostatectomy with regard to advantages and disadvantages.
5. Use the nursing process as a framework for care of the patient with prostate cancer or undergoing prostatectomy.
6. Identify the nursing management of patients with testicular cancer.
7. Compare and contrast the various disorders of the penis, including pathophysiology, clinical manifestations, and management.

Introduction

Disorders of the male reproductive system include a wide variety of conditions that usually affect both the urinary and reproductive systems. Because these disorders focus on the genitalia and in some instances sexuality, the patient may experience anxiety and embarrassment. Nurses must recognize the patient's need for privacy as well as his need for education. This requires both an openness to discuss critical and sensitive issues with the patient and effective assessment, management, and communication on the part of the nurse. Nurses must be comfortable when examining male genitalia and must recognize their own attitudes and perceptions about male reproductive disorders. Education of the patient and partner about treatment and self-care strategies is essential (Tabloski, 2014).

ASSESSMENT OF THE MALE REPRODUCTIVE SYSTEM

Anatomic and Physiologic Overview

In the male, several organs serve as parts of both the urinary tract and the reproductive system. Disorders in the male reproductive organs may interfere with the functions of one or both of these systems. As a result, diseases of the male reproductive system are usually treated by a urologist. The structures in the male reproductive system are the testes, the vas deferens (ductus deferens) and the seminal vesicles, the **penis**, and certain accessory glands, such as the prostate gland and Cowper's gland (bulbourethral gland) (Fig. 50-1).

The **testes** are formed in the embryo within the abdominal cavity near the kidney. During the last month of fetal life, they descend posterior to the peritoneum and pierce the abdominal wall in the groin. Later, they progress along the inguinal canal into the scrotum. In this descent, they are accompanied by blood vessels, lymphatics, nerves, and ducts, which support the tissue and make up the spermatic cord. This cord extends from the internal inguinal ring through the abdominal wall and the inguinal canal to the scrotum. As the testes descend into the scrotum, a tubular extension of peritoneum accompanies them (Hall, 2015). Normally, this tissue is obliterated during fetal development, the only remaining portion being that which covers the testes, the tunica vaginalis. (When this peritoneal process is not obliterated but remains open into the abdominal cavity, a potential sac remains into which abdominal contents may enter to form an indirect inguinal hernia.)

The testes are encased in the scrotum, which keeps them at a slightly lower temperature than the rest of the body to facilitate **spermatogenesis** (production of sperm) (Hall, 2015). The testes consist of numerous seminiferous tubules in which the spermatozoa form. Collecting tubules transmit the spermatozoa into the epididymis, which is a hoodlike structure lying on the testes containing winding ducts that lead into the vas deferens. This firm, tubular structure passes upward through the inguinal canal to enter the abdominal cavity behind the peritoneum. It then extends downward toward the base of the bladder. An outpouching from this structure is the seminal vesicle, which acts as a reservoir for testicular secretions. The tract is continued as the ejaculatory duct, which passes through the prostate gland to enter the urethra. Testicular secretions take this pathway when they exit the penis during ejaculation.

The testes have a dual function: the formation of spermatozoa from the germinal cells of the seminiferous tubules and the secretion of the male sex hormone **testosterone**, which induces and preserves the male sex characteristics.

The **prostate gland** lies just below the base of the bladder. It surrounds the urethra and is traversed by the ejaculatory duct, which is a continuation of the vas deferens. This gland produces a secretion that is chemically and physiologically suitable to the needs of the spermatozoa in their passage from the testes.

The Cowper's gland lies below the prostate within the posterior aspect of the urethra. This gland empties its

Glossary

benign prostatic hyperplasia (BPH): noncancerous enlargement or hypertrophy of the prostate. BPH is the most common pathologic condition in older men and the second most common cause of surgical intervention in men older than 60 years.

Bowen disease: form of squamous cell carcinoma in situ of the penile shaft

circumcision: excision of the foreskin, or prepuce, of the glans penis

cryosurgery of the prostate: localized treatment of the prostate by application of freezing temperatures

cryptorchidism: most common congenital defect, characterized by failure of one or both of the testes to descend into the scrotum

epididymitis: infection of the epididymis that usually descends from an infected prostate or urinary tract; also may develop as a complication of gonorrhea

erectile dysfunction: also called *impotence*; the inability to either achieve or maintain an erection sufficient to accomplish sexual intercourse

hydrocele: collection of fluid, generally in the tunica vaginalis of the testis, although it also may collect within the spermatic cord

nocturia: urination during the night

orchiectomy: surgical removal of one or both of the testes

orchitis: inflammation of the testes (testicular congestion) caused by pyogenic, viral, spirochetal, parasitic, traumatic, chemical, or unknown factors

penile cancer: rare type of cancer that occurs in the skin or tissues; can involve the glans, the body of the penis, the urethra, and regional or distant lymph nodes

penis: male organ for copulation and urination; consists of glans penis, body, and root

Peyronie disease: buildup of fibrous plaques in the sheath of the corpus cavernosum, causing curvature of the penis when it is erect

phimosis: condition in which the foreskin is constricted so that it cannot be retracted over the glans; can occur congenitally or from inflammation and edema

priapism: uncontrolled, persistent erection of the penis occurring from either neural or vascular causes, including medications, sickle cell thrombosis, leukemic cell infiltration, spinal cord tumours, and tumour invasion of the penis or its vessels

prostate cancer: the most common cancer in men; risk factors include increasing age, African or Caribbean descent, and possibly a low fibre and higher-fat diet; the genetic association of prostate cancer and the increased incidence within certain families is being investigated

prostate gland: gland that lies just below the neck of the bladder, surrounds the urethra, and is traversed by the ejaculatory duct, which is a continuation of the vas deferens; produces a secretion that is chemically and physiologically suitable to the needs of the spermatozoa in their passage from the testes

prostate-specific antigen (PSA): substance that is produced by the prostate gland and measured in a blood specimen; PSA levels are increased with prostate cancer; the PSA test is used in combination with digital rectal examination to detect prostate cancer

prostatism: obstructive and irritative symptom complex that includes increased frequency and hesitancy in starting urination, a decrease in the volume and force of the urinary stream, acute urinary retention, and recurrent urinary tract infections

prostatitis: inflammation of the prostate gland caused by infectious agents (bacteria, fungi, mycoplasma) or various other conditions (e.g., urethral stricture, prostatic hyperplasia)

spermatogenesis: production of sperm in the testes

testes: the ovoid sex glands encased in the scrotum; the testes produce sperm

testicular cancer: the most common cancer in men 15 to 29 years of age and the second most common malignancy in those 35 to 39 years of age; its cause is unknown

testosterone: male sex hormone secreted by the testes; induces and preserves the male sex characteristics

transurethral resection of the prostate (TURP, or TUR): resection of the prostate through endoscopy; the surgical and optical instrument is introduced directly through the urethra to the prostate, and the gland is then removed in small chips with an electrical cutting loop

varicocele: abnormal dilation of the veins of the pampiniform venous plexus in the scrotum (the network of veins from the testis and the epididymis, which constitute part of the spermatic cord)

vasectomy: also called *male sterilization*; ligation and transection of part of the vas deferens, with or without removal of a segment of the vas to prevent the passage of the sperm from the testes

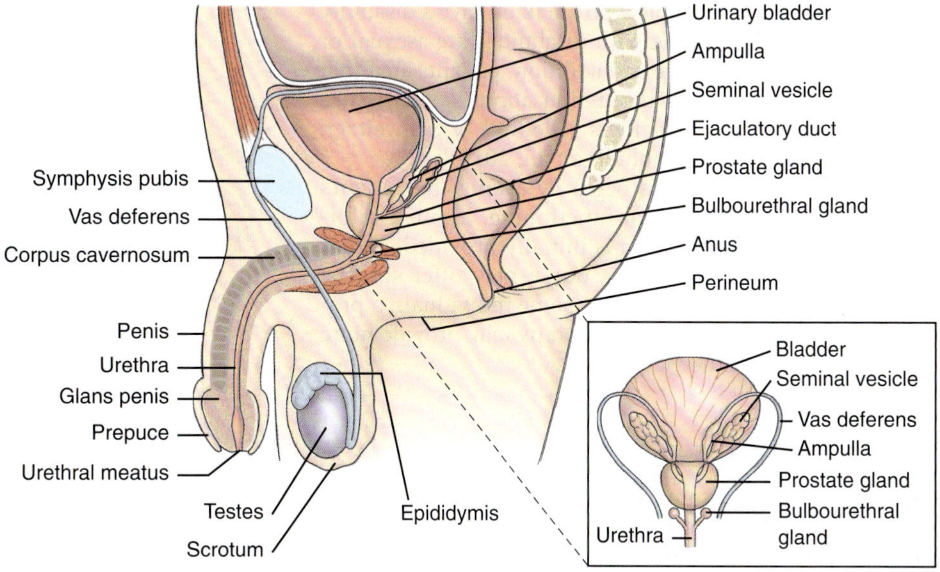

FIGURE 50-1. Structures of the male reproductive system.

secretions into the urethra during ejaculation, providing lubrication. The penis has a dual function: It is the organ for copulation and for urination. Anatomically, it consists of the glans penis, body, and root. The glans penis is the soft, rounded portion at the distal end of the penis. The urethra, a tube that carries urine, opens at the tip of the glans. The glans is naturally covered or protected by elongated penile skin—the foreskin—which may be retracted to expose the glans. However, many men have had the foreskin removed (**circumcision**) as newborns. The body of the penis is composed of erectile tissues containing numerous blood vessels that become distended, leading to an erection during sexual excitement. The urethra, which passes through the penis, extends from the bladder through the prostate to the distal end of the penis.

Assessment

Health History and Clinical Manifestations

Male sexuality is a complex phenomenon that is strongly influenced by personal, cultural, religious, and social factors. Sexuality and male reproductive function become concerns in the presence of illness and disability (Norton & Tremayne, 2015). Throughout the assessment process, the nurse must recognize the importance of sexuality to the patient.

Assessment of male reproductive function begins with an evaluation of urinary function and symptoms. This assessment also includes a focus on sexual function as well as manifestations of sexual dysfunction. The patient is asked about his usual state of health and any recent change in general physical and sexual activity. Any symptoms or changes in function are explored fully and described in detail. These symptoms may include those associated with an obstruction caused by an enlarged prostate gland (benign prostatic hyperplasia [BPH]): decreased force of urine stream, straining to start stream, hesitancy, intermittent/disrupted stream, or "double" or "triple" voiding (urinates two or three times over a period of several minutes to completely empty his bladder). Bladder symptoms may also be present: frequency (every two or fewer hours), **nocturia** more than twice a night, urgency, or urge incontinence. The patient is also assessed for dysuria, hematuria, and hematospermia (blood in the ejaculate).

Assessment of sexual function is an essential part of every health history. Discussing sexuality with patients with an illness or who have a disability can be uncomfortable for nurses and other health care providers. Health care professionals may unconsciously have stereotypes related to sexuality (e.g., ill or persons with a disability are asexual or should remain sexually inactive). Patients may be embarrassed to initiate a discussion about these issues with their health care providers, or they may feel as though the issue is not a serious medical issue and cannot be helped or is a normal part of the aging process (Quinn & Happell, 2012). Because changes in sexual functioning are a common concern of patients, it is important to address these issues. By initiating a discussion about sexual concerns, the nurse demonstrates that changes in sexual functioning are valid topics for discussion and provides a safe environment for discussing these sensitive topics. There are three models for sexual intervention which can assist health care providers to have a structured approach when addressing sexual health issues. The PLISSIT (*p*ermission, *l*imited *i*nformation, *s*pecific *s*uggestions, *i*ntensive *t*herapy), the BETTER (*b*ringing up the topic, *e*xplaining, *t*elling, *t*iming, *e*ducate about treatment-related sexual side effects, *r*ecording) model, and the ALARM (*a*ctivity, *l*ibido, *a*rousal, *r*esolution, and *m*edical information) are commonly identified in the literature. These models may be used to provide a framework for nursing interventions (Norton & Tremayne, 2015; Quinn & Happell, 2012). The BETTER model was developed more recently to assist health care professionals to include sexuality in the assessment of patients with cancer (Tannenbaum, 2015).

Patients may find it difficult to express their feelings and concerns regarding their sexuality, especially after a body image change (e.g., after major surgery such as amputation). Discussing sexuality with patients who have an illness or disability can be uncomfortable for nurses and other health care providers; this, in turn, makes discussion of these issues more difficult and uncomfortable for patients. Health care professionals may unconsciously have stereotypes about the sexuality of people who are ill or have a disability (e.g., the belief that people with disabilities are asexual or should be sexually inactive). In addition, patients are often embarrassed to initiate a discussion about sexual issues with their health care providers (Gledhill & Schweitzer, 2013; Mitchell, Mercer, Ploubidis, et al., 2013).

The nurse should always begin by asking the patient's permission to discuss sexual functioning. Limited information about sexual function is initially provided, and as the discussion progresses, the nurse may offer specific suggestions for interventions. For some individuals, a professional who specializes in sex therapy may provide more intensive therapy as needed.

Physical Assessment

In addition to the customary aspects of the physical examination, two essential components address disorders of the male genital or reproductive system: the digital rectal examination (DRE) and the testicular examination.

Digital Rectal Examination

The DRE is used to screen for prostate cancer and is recommended annually for every man older than 50 years (45 years for men at high risk [African American men and men with a family history of prostate cancer in first-degree relatives]) (American Cancer Society [ACS], 2015). The DRE enables the skilled examiner, using a lubricated, gloved finger placed in the rectum, to assess the size, symmetry, shape, and consistency of the posterior surface of the prostate gland (see Fig. 50-2). The clinician assesses for tenderness of the prostate gland on palpation and for the presence and consistency of any nodules. The DRE may be performed with the patient leaning over an examination table or positioning the man in a side-lying position with legs flexed toward the abdomen or supine with legs resting in stirrups. To minimize discomfort and relax the anal sphincter during the rectal examination, the patient is instructed to take a deep breath and exhale slowly as the practitioner inserts a finger. If possible, he should turn his feet inward so his toes are touching. Although this examination may be uncomfortable and embarrassing for the patient, it is an important screening tool.

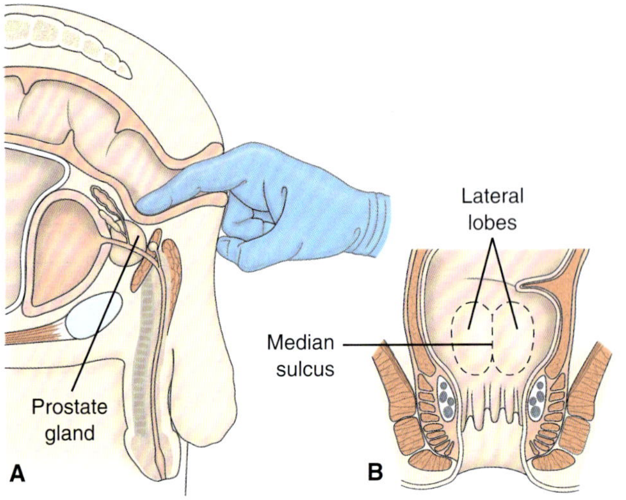

FIGURE 50-2. **A.** Palpation of the prostate gland during digital rectal examination (DRE) enables the examiner to assess the size, shape, and texture of the gland. **B.** The prostate is round, with a palpable median sulcus or groove separating the two lobes. It should feel rubbery and free of nodules and masses.

Testicular Examination

The male genitalia are inspected for abnormalities and palpated for masses. The penis is inspected and palpated for ulcerations, nodules, inflammation, and discharge. The scrotum is palpated carefully for nodules, masses, or inflammation. Examining the scrotum can reveal such disorders as hydrocele, hernia, or tumour of the testis. The testicular examination provides an excellent opportunity to instruct the patient about techniques for testicular self-examination (TSE) and its importance in early detection of testicular cancer (discussed later in this chapter). This self-examination should begin during adolescence.

Gerontologic Considerations

As men age, the prostate gland enlarges, prostate secretion decreases, the scrotum hangs lower, the testes become smaller and firmer, and pubic hair becomes sparser and stiffer. Changes in gonadal function include a decline in plasma testosterone levels and reduced production of progesterone (Table 50-1). Other changes include an increased

TABLE 50-1 Age-Related Change in Male Reproductive System

Age-related Change	Physiologic Changes	Manifestations
Decrease in sex hormone secretion, especially testosterone	Decreased muscle strength and sexual energy	Changes in sexual response: prolonged time to reach full erection, rapid penile detumescence, and prolonged refractory period Decrease in number of viable sperm
	Shrinkage and loss of firmness of testes; thickening of seminiferous tubules	Smaller testes
	Fibrotic changes of corpora cavernosa	Erectile dysfunction
	Enlargement of prostate gland	Weakening of prostatic contractions Hyperplasia of prostate gland Signs and symptoms of obstruction of lower urinary tract (urgency, frequency, nocturia)

Adapted from Tabloski, P. A. (2014). *Gerontological nursing: The essential guide to clinical practice* (3rd ed.). New York: Pearson.

incidence of genitourinary tract cancer, and risk of urinary incontinence for various reasons. Libido and potency often decrease in as many as two thirds of men older than 70 years (Tabloski, 2014). Vascular problems cause about half of the cases of impotence in men older than 50 years.

Male reproductive capability is maintained with advancing age, and many men are sexually active their entire adult lives. Although degenerative changes occur in the seminiferous tubules, spermatogenesis (production of sperm) continues allowing men to produce viable sperm throughout their lives.

Male hypogonadism (decreased function of the testes) starts gradually at approximately 50 years of age, resulting in decreased testosterone production. The older man notices that the sexual response slows, erection takes longer, full erections may not be attained, and ejaculation takes longer to occur and control or resolution may occur without orgasm. Sexual function can be affected by psychological problems, illnesses, and medications (Mulhall & Hsiao, 2014). In general, the entire sexual act takes longer. Sexual activity is closely correlated with the man's sexual activity in his earlier years; if he was more active than average as a young man, he will most likely continue to be more active than average in his later years.

Men older than 50 years are at increased risk for genitourinary tract cancers, including those of the kidney, bladder, prostate, and penis. The DRE, **prostate-specific antigen (PSA)** test, and urinalysis, which screens for hematuria, may uncover a higher percentage of malignancies at earlier stages and lead to lower treatment-associated morbidity as well as a lower mortality.

Urinary incontinence occurs in one fifth of community-dwelling older men and rises to nearly 50% in men in long-term care settings (Tabloski, 2014). Older adults admitted to acute care settings should be screened for this problem. Urinary incontinence may have many causes, including medications, neurologic disease, or benign prostatic hyperplasia (BPH). Incontinence may also be linked to erectile dysfunction when there is damage to the neural pathways that initiate an erection (Lim, 2013). Diagnostic tests are performed to exclude reversible causes. New-onset urinary incontinence is a nursing priority that requires evaluation.

Diagnostic Evaluation

Prostate-Specific Antigen Test

The cells within the prostate gland produce a protein that can be measured in the blood called the PSA. It is a sensitive but not specific test for prostate cancer. In the absence of prostate cancer, serum PSA levels vary with age, race, and prostate volume. Increased levels may indicate prostate cancer. However, a number of other conditions such as BPH, acute urinary retention, and acute prostatitis may cause high PSA levels. Values of PSA may also increase after ejaculation. PSA levels are measured in nanograms per milliliter (ng/mL). In most laboratories, values less than 4 ng/mL are generally considered normal, and values greater than 4 ng/mL are considered elevated (Barry & Hayes, 2015; Pagana & Pagana, 2013). The use of age-specific reference ranges is encouraged to help minimize unnecessary biopsies.

A serum PSA level and a DRE, which are recommended by the ACS (2015), are used to screen for prostate cancer for men with at least a 10-year life expectancy and for men at high risk, including those with a strong family history of prostate cancer and of African American ethnicity. The perceptions of some African American men and women reflect the belief that PSA screening saves lives and needs to be done despite recommendations against screening due to a number of false positives resulting in unnecessary treatment (Hunter, Vines, & Carlisle, 2015). The PSA test is also used to monitor patients for recurrence after treatment for cancer of the prostate, based on evidence-based guidelines (National Comprehensive Cancer Network [NCCN], 2016b). Neither the DRE nor PSA is 100% accurate, but when used together, their accuracy increases.

Ultrasonography

Transrectal ultrasound (TRUS) may be performed in patients with abnormalities detected by DRE and in those with elevated PSA levels. After DRE has been completed, a lubricated, condom-covered, rectal probe transducer is inserted into the rectum (Itano, Brant, Conde, et al., 2016). Water may be introduced into the condom to help transmit sound waves to the prostate. TRUS may be used in detecting nonpalpable prostate cancers and in staging localized prostate cancer. Needle biopsies of the prostate are commonly guided by TRUS.

Prostate Fluid or Tissue Analysis

Specimens of prostate fluid or tissue may be obtained for culture when disease or inflammation of the prostate gland is suspected. A biopsy of the prostate gland may be necessary to obtain tissue for histologic examination. This may be performed at the time of prostatectomy or by means of a perineal or transrectal needle biopsy. Six to 12 biopsies from all four prostate zones may be obtained during a TRUS-guided biopsy.

Tests of Male Sexual Function

If the patient cannot engage in sexual intercourse to his satisfaction, a detailed history is obtained. Nocturnal erections occur in healthy males of all ages. Nocturnal penile tumescence tests may be conducted in a sleep laboratory to monitor changes in penile circumference during sleep using various methods to determine number, duration, rigidity, and circumference of penile erections; the results help identify whether the erectile dysfunction is caused by physiologic or psychological factors. Additional tests, including psychological evaluations, are also part of the diagnostic workup and are usually conducted by a specialized team of health care providers.

DISORDERS OF MALE SEXUAL FUNCTION

Erectile Dysfunction

Erectile dysfunction (ED), also called *impotence*, is the inability to achieve or maintain an erection sufficient to accomplish intercourse (Grossman & Porth, 2014). The man may report decreased frequency of erections, inability to achieve a firm erection, or rapid detumescence (subsiding of erection). The physiology of erection and ejaculation is complex and involves parasympathetic and sympathetic components. Erection involves the release of nitric oxide into the corpus cavernosum during sexual stimulation. Its release activates cyclic guanosine monophosphate (cGMP), causing smooth muscle relaxation. This allows flow of blood into the corpus cavernosum, resulting in erection (Grossman & Porth, 2014; McDougal, Wein, Kavoussi, et al., 2016). Erective dysfunction has both psychogenic and organic causes. Psychogenic causes include anxiety, fatigue, depression, and pressure to perform sexually. Organic causes include occlusive vascular disease, endocrine disease (diabetes, pituitary tumours, hypogonadism with testosterone deficiency, hyperthyroidism, and hypothyroidism), cirrhosis, chronic renal failure, genitourinary conditions (radical pelvic surgery), hematologic conditions (Hodgkin disease, leukemia), neurologic disorders (neuropathies, parkinsonism, spinal cord injury, multiple sclerosis), trauma to the pelvic or genital area, alcohol, medications (Chart 50-1), and drug abuse.

Assessment and Diagnostic Findings

The diagnosis of ED requires a sexual and medical history; an analysis of presenting symptoms; a physical examination, including a neurologic examination; a detailed assessment of all medications, alcohol, and drugs used; and various laboratory studies. The extent of the history will depend on the patient's presenting symptoms and the presence of factors that may affect sexual function: chronic illnesses (e.g., diabetes, multiple sclerosis, stroke, cardiac disease), use of medications (e.g., many antihypertensive medications including thiazide diuretics, spironolactone, beta-blockers, methyldopa and clonidine, anticholinergic medications, psychotropic agents including selective serotonin reuptake inhibitors and tricyclics) and laboratory tests (e.g., gonadotrophins, testosterone, sex-binding globulin levels, prolactin levels, fasting lipid profile, and thyroid function tests) (Grant, Jackson, Baig, et al., 2013), stress, and alcohol use.

Nocturnal penile tumescence tests are conducted in sleep laboratories to monitor changes in penile circumference. In healthy men, nocturnal penile erections closely parallel rapid eye movement (REM) sleep in occurrence and duration. Organically impotent men show inadequate sleep-related erections that correspond to their waking performance. The nocturnal penile tumescence test can help to determine whether erectile impotence has an organic or psychological cause. Arterial blood flow to the penis is measured using a Doppler probe. In addition, nerve conduction tests and extensive psychological evaluations are carried out. Figure 50-3 describes the evaluation and treatment of men with ED.

Medical Management

Treatment, which depends on the cause, can be medical, surgical, or both (Table 50-2). Nonsurgical therapy includes treating associated conditions, such as alcoholism and diabetes, and readjusting hypertensive agents or other medications (Mola, 2015). Endocrine therapy may be instituted for ED secondary to hypothalamic–pituitary–gonadal dysfunction and may reverse the condition. Patients with ED from psychogenic causes are referred to a health care provider or therapist specializing in sexual dysfunction.

Pharmacologic Therapy

Phosphodiesterase type 5 (PDE-5) inhibitors (oral medications that are used to treat ED) are first-line therapy

CHART 50-1

Pharmacology: Classes of Medications Associated With Erectile Dysfunction

- *Antiadrenergics and antihypertensives:* guanethidine (Ismelin), clonidine (Catapres), hydralazine (Apresoline)
- *Anticholinergics and phenothiazines:* prochlorperazine (Compazine), trihexyphenidyl (Artane)
- *Antidepressants:* tricyclic antidepressants: amitriptyline (Elavil), desipramine (Norpramin); selective serotonin reuptake inhibitors: fluoxetine (Prozac), sertraline (Zoloft)
- *Antifungals:* ketoconazole (Nizoral)
- *Antihistamines:* diphenhydramine (Benadryl), dimenhydrinate (Dramamine)
- *Antihormone (prostate cancer treatment):* flutamide (Eulexin), leuprolide (Lupron)
- *Antipsychotics:* haloperidol (Haldol), chlorpromazine (Thorazine)
- *Anticonvulsant agents:* carbamazepine (Tegretol)
- *Antispasmodics:* oxybutynin (Ditropan)
- *Anxiolytics, sedative–hypnotics, tranquilizers:* lorazepam (Ativan), triazolam (Halcion)
- *Beta-blockers:* nadolol (Corgard), metoprolol (Lopressor)
- *Calcium channel blockers:* nifedipine (Adalat, Procardia)
- *Carbonic anhydrase inhibitors:* acetazolamide (Diamox)
- *Chemotherapeutic agents:* busulfan (Myleran), cyclophosphamide (Cytoxan)
- *Diuretics:* hydrochlorothiazide (HydroDIURIL), furosemide (Lasix), spironolactone (Aldactone), verapamil (Calan)
- *Histamine-2 antagonists:* nizatidine (Axid), ranitidine (Zantac)
- *Nonsteroidal anti-inflammatory drugs:* naproxen (Naprosyn), indomethacin (Indocin)
- *Other substances:* alcohol, amphetamines, barbiturates, cocaine, marijuana, methadone, nicotine, opioids
- *Parkinson disease medications:* carbidopa/levodopa (Sinemet), benztropine (Cogentin)

Adapted from Karch, A. M. (2016). *2016 Lippincott pocket drug guide for nurses* (4th ed.). Philadelphia, PA: Wolters Kluwer.

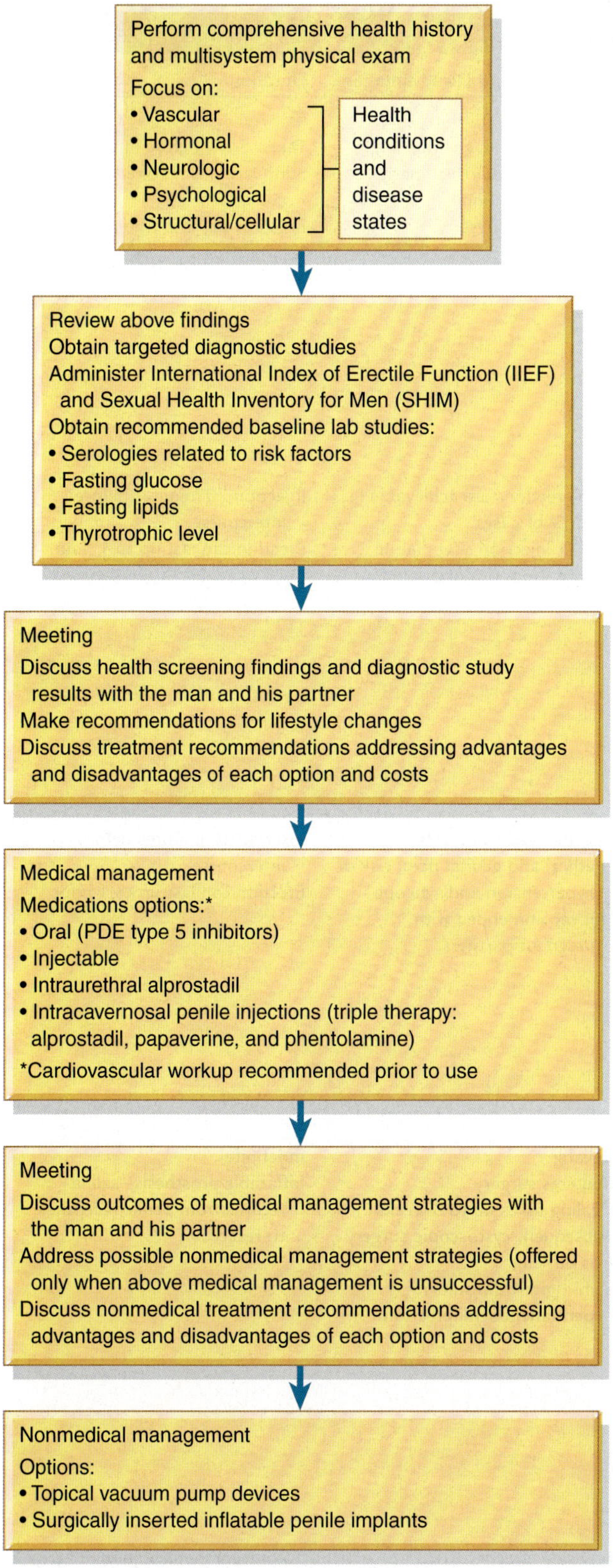

FIGURE 50-3. Evaluation and treatment of men with erectile dysfunction.

(Liu, Yen, & Wu, et al., 2014). Currently available PDE-5 inhibitors include sildenafil (Viagra), vardenafil (Levitra), and tadalafil (Cialis). Each of these agents has a similar mechanism of action but a different pharmacologic action and clinical use. Erection involves the release of nitric oxide in the vasculature of the corpus cavernosum as a result of sexual stimulation. This subsequently leads to smooth muscle relaxation in blood vessels supplying the corpus cavernosum, resulting in increased blood flow and an erection. During sexual stimulation, PDE-5 inhibitors increase blood flow to the penis (Grossman & Porth, 2014).

When PDE-5 inhibitors are taken about 1 hour before sexual activity, they are effective in producing an erection with sexual stimulation; the erection can last about 1 to 2 hours. The most common side effects of these medications include headache, flushing, dyspepsia, diarrhea, nasal congestion, and lightheadedness. These agents are contraindicated in men who take organic nitrates (e.g., isosorbide [Isordil], nitroglycerin), because taken together, these medications can cause side effects such as severe hypotension (Grossman & Porth, 2014; McDougal et al., 2016). In addition, PDE-5 inhibitors must be used with caution in patients with retinopathy, especially in those with diabetic retinopathy. Patient education about the use of these medications and their side effects is summarized in Table 50-3.

For patients in whom PDE-5 inhibitors are contraindicated or ineffective, other pharmacologic measures to induce erections include injecting vasoactive agents, such as alprostadil, papaverine, and phentolamine, directly into the penis. Complications include priapism (a persistent abnormal erection) and development of fibrotic plaques at the injection sites. Alprostadil is also formulated in a gel pellet that can be inserted into the tip of the urethra with an applicator to create an erection.

Penile Implants

Two general types of penile implants are available: the malleable, noninflatable, nonhydraulic prosthesis (also called the *semi-rigid rod*) and the inflatable, hydraulic prostheses (Keane & Graham, 2016). The semi-rigid rod (e.g., the Small-Carrion prosthesis) results in a permanent semi-erection but can be bent into an unnoticeable position when appropriate. The inflatable prosthesis simulates natural erections and natural flaccidity. Complications after implantation include infection, erosion of the prosthesis through the skin (more common with the semi-rigid rod than with the inflatable prosthesis), and persistent pain, which may require removal of the implant. Subsequent cystoscopic surgery is more difficult with a semi-rigid rod than with the inflatable prosthesis.

Factors to consider in choosing a penile prosthesis are the patient's activities of daily living, social activities, and the expectations of the patient and his partner. Ongoing counselling for the patient and his partner is usually necessary to help them adapt to the prosthesis.

Negative Pressure Devices

Negative pressure (vacuum) devices may also be used to induce an erection. A plastic cylinder is placed over the flaccid penis, and negative pressure is applied. When an erection is attained, a constriction band is placed around the base of the penis to maintain the erection. To avoid penile injury, the patient is instructed not to leave the constricting band in place for longer than 1 hour. Only devices with a vacuum limiter are recommended for use

TABLE 50-2 Treatments for Erectile Dysfunction

Method	Description	Advantages and Disadvantages	Duration
Pharmacologic Therapy			
Oral medications (sildenafil [Viagra]; vardenafil [Levitra]; tadalafil [Cialis]) 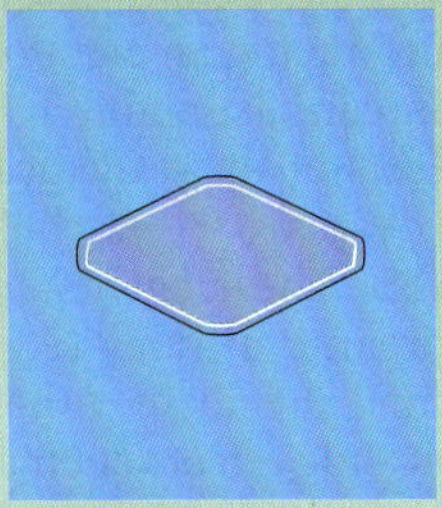 Oral medication	Smooth muscle relaxant causing blood to flow into penis	Can cause headache flushing, dyspepsia, diarrhea, nasal congestion, and lightheadedness See contraindications in Table 59-3	Taken orally before intercourse Stimulation is required to achieve erection Erection can last 1 hour
Injection (alprostadil, papaverine, phentolamine) 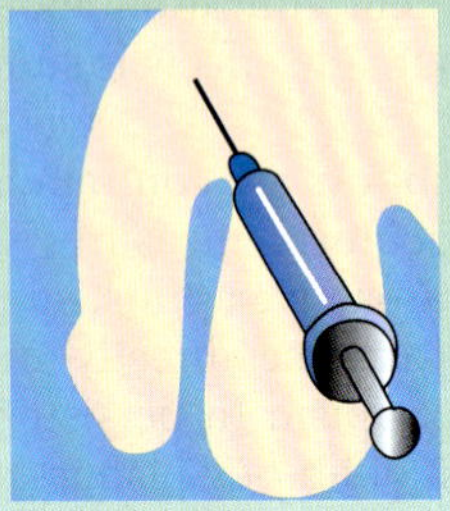 Penile injection	Smooth muscle relaxant causing blood to flow into penis	Firm erections are achievable in >50% of cases Pain at injection site; plaque formation, risk of priapism	Injection 20 minutes before intercourse Erection can last up to 1 hour
Urethral suppository (alprostadil) 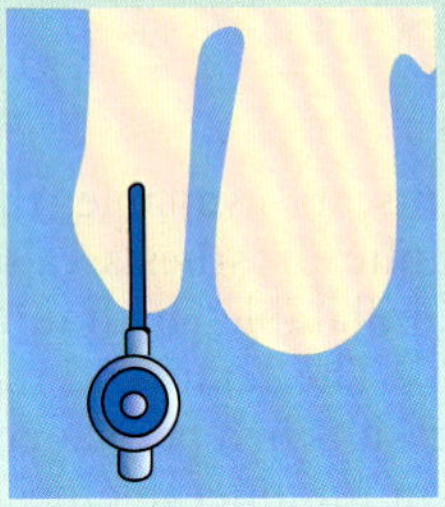 Penile suppository	Smooth muscle relaxant causing blood to flow into penis	May be used twice a day Urethral and genital pain; risk of hypertension and syncope Not recommended with pregnant partners	Inserted 10 minutes before intercourse Erection can last up to 1 hour
Penile Implants • Semi-rigid rod • Inflatable • Soft silicone 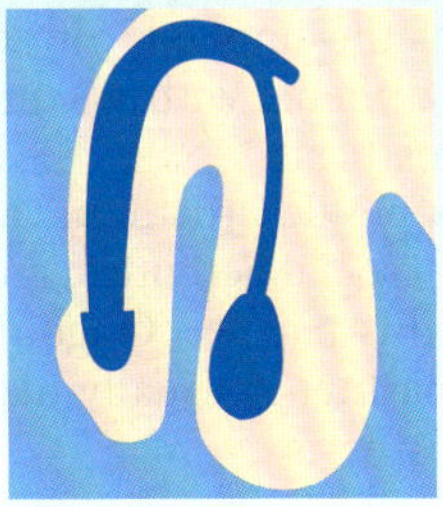 Penile implant	Surgically implanted into corpus cavernosum	Reliable Requires surgery Healing takes up to 3 weeks Subsequent cystoscopic surgery is difficult Semi-rigid rod results in permanent semi-erection	Indefinite Inflatable prosthesis—saline returns from penile receptacle to reservoir
Negative Pressure (Vacuum) Devices 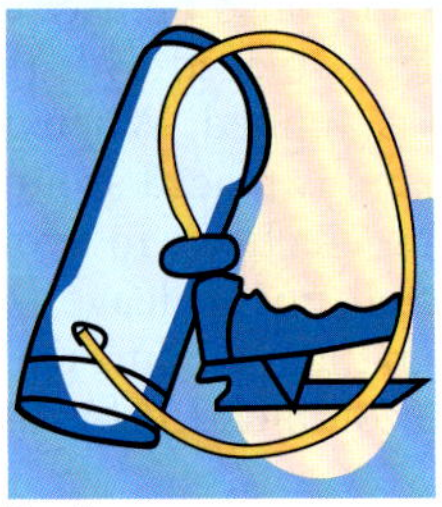 Penile vacuum pump	Induction of erection with vacuum; maintained with constriction band around base of penis	Few side effects Cumbersome to use before intercourse Vasocongestion of penis can cause pain or numbness	To prevent penile injury, constriction band must not be left in place >1 hour

TABLE 50-3 Pharmacologic Treatment of Erectile Dysfunction

	Sildenafil (Viagra)	Vardenafil (Levitra)	Tadalafil (Cialis)
When to take	Take the medication 30 minutes to 4 hours before intercourse. *There must be sexual stimulation to produce an erection*	Follow the same directions as with sildenafil; take the medication 1 hour before intercourse. The peak action occurs in 30–120 minutes. *There must be sexual stimulation to produce an erection*	Take the medication before sexual activity. Effect peaks at 30 minutes to 6 hours; effect may last up to 36 hours. *There must be sexual stimulation to produce an erection*
Frequency of use	If you take this medication more than once a day, it will not have an increased effect. You may take it 7 days per week if you wish, but only once in 24 hours. It does not build up in your bloodstream. Remember to take it only when you want to have intercourse	The recommended frequency for this medication is 10 mg in 24 hours	The effects of this medication may last up to 36 hours. This allows for increased spontaneity in the sexual experience
Side effects	Side effects include headache, flushing, indigestion, nasal congestion, abnormal vision, diarrhea, dizziness, and rash. You may also have low blood sugar and abnormal liver function tests; your primary provider can determine this	Side effects include headache, flushing, runny nose, indigestion, sinusitis, flu-like syndrome, dizziness, nausea, back pain, and joint pain. Tell your primary provider if you experience any of these effects. You may also have abnormally elevated liver enzymes; your primary provider can determine this	Side effects are similar to those of sildenafil and vardenafil. Tadalafil may also cause back pain and muscle aches. Tell your primary provider if you experience any of these side effects
Contraindications	Do not take if you are taking nitrate medications such as nitroglycerin (e.g., Nitro-Bid) or isosorbide mononitrate (e.g., Imdur) Do not take if you have high uncontrolled blood pressure, coronary artery disease, or have had a heart attack within the past 6 months Do not take if you have been diagnosed with a cardiac dysrhythmia or kidney or liver dysfunction		
Drug interactions	This medication can react with other medications that you may be taking. Provide your primary provider and pharmacist with a complete list of all prescribed and over-the-counter medications that you are using		
Use of PDE-5 inhibitors with penile injections or urethral suppositories	The use of PDE-5 inhibitors with other forms of therapy for erectile dysfunction has not been tested and should be avoided		

PDE-5, phosphodiesterase type 5.

Adapted from Hsu, J. C., Tang, D. H., & Lu, C. Y. (2015). Risk-benefit assessment of oral phosphodiesterase type 5 inhibitors for treatment of erectile dysfunction: A multiple criteria decision analysis. *International Journal of Clinical Practice*, *69*(4), 436–443.

(Mulhall & Hsiao, 2014). Although many men find this method satisfactory, others experience premature loss of penile rigidity or pain when applying suction or during intercourse.

Nursing Management

Personal satisfaction and the ability to sexually satisfy a partner are common concerns of patients. ED can have a significant impact on a man, his partner(s), and their relationship(s). There may be a reduction of self-esteem or poor quality of life in men who suffer from ED (Peate, 2012). The literature states that nurses must help men identify both the physical and psychological impact of ED (Peate, 2012; Steggall, 2012). Men with illnesses and disabilities may need the assistance of a sex therapist to find, implement, and integrate their sexual beliefs and behaviours into a healthy and satisfying lifestyle. The nurse can inform patients that support groups for men with ED and their partners have been established.

Disorders of Ejaculation

Premature ejaculation (PE) is defined as the occurrence of ejaculation sooner than desired, either before or shortly after penetration, causing distress to either one or both partners. It is one of the most common complaints of men or couples, affecting 20% to 30% of men (Keane & Graham, 2016; McDougal et al., 2016). The spectrum of responses ranges from occasional ejaculation with intercourse or self-stimulation to complete inability to ejaculate under any circumstances. Various forms of PE have been identified: (1) lifelong PE caused by neurobiologic or genetic conditions; (2) acquired PE (medical or psychological); (3) natural variable PE (normal variation); and (4) premature-like ejaculatory dysfunction (psychological). In young men aged 18 to 25 years, factors associated with PE and ED include smoking, use of illegal drugs or medications without prescriptions, poor physical and mental health, lack of physical activity and lack of sexual experience (Akre, Berchtold, Gmel, et al., 2014). Other ejaculatory problems may include inhibited (delayed or

GENETICS IN NURSING PRACTICE

Chart 50-2. Male Reproductive Disorders

Various male reproductive disorders are influenced by genetic factors. Some examples are:

- 21-Hydroxylase deficiency
- Congenital absence of the vas deferens, prostate gland, or seminal vesicles
- Kallmann syndrome
- Klinefelter syndrome (47, XXY)
- Prostate cancer
- Y chromosome deletions

Nursing Assessments

FAMILY HISTORY ASSESSMENT SPECIFIC TO MALE REPRODUCTIVE DISORDERS

- Collect a three-generation family history on both maternal and paternal sides of the family.
- Assess family history for other family members with similar reproductive problems/abnormalities.

PATIENT ASSESSMENT SPECIFIC TO MALE REPRODUCTIVE DISORDERS

- In males with delayed puberty or infertility, assess for clinical features of Klinefelter syndrome (tall stature, gynecomastia, learning disabilities).
- Assess males with delayed or absent puberty for clinical features of Kallmann syndrome (cleft lip with or without cleft palate, abnormal eye movements, hearing loss, and abnormalities of tooth development).
- Assess males for history of early growth spurt, which is a symptom of 21-hydroxylase deficiency.
- Inquire about history of prostate inflammation, genital infections, medication use (steroids), or prior history of mumps.
- Assess for physical abnormalities of the genitalia.

Genetics Resources

Association for X and Y chromosome variations: www.genetic.org

Klinefelter syndrome support group: www.klinefeltersyndrome.org

retarded) ejaculation, which is the involuntary inhibition of the ejaculatory reflex (see Chart 50-2). Retrograde ejaculation occurs when semen travels toward the bladder instead of exiting through the penis, resulting in infertility. This form of PE may occur after prior prostate or urethral surgery, with diabetes, or with the use of medications such as antihypertensive agents.

Evaluation of PE involves a thorough sexual history focusing on the duration of symptoms, time to ejaculation, degree of voluntary control over ejaculation, frequency of occurrence, and course of the problem since the first sexual encounter (Keane & Graham, 2016; McDougal et al., 2016). Treatment, which depends on the nature and severity of PE and perceived distress that it causes, includes behavioural and psychological approaches, as well as pharmacologic therapy that attempts to alter the sensory input or retard the ejaculatory response. Behavioural therapy (e.g., counselling, sex therapy, psychoeducation, and couples therapy) often involves both the man and his sexual partner. The couple is encouraged to identify their sexual needs and to communicate those needs to each other. Pharmacologic management involves selective serotonin reuptake inhibitors dapoxetine (Priligy), alpha-1 adrenoceptor antagonists, the tricyclic antidepressant clomipramine (Anafranil), and topical anesthetic agents. In some cases, a combination of pharmacologic and behavioural therapy may be effective.

Inhibited ejaculation is most often caused by psychological factors, neurologic disorders (e.g., SCI, multiple sclerosis, neuropathy secondary to diabetes), surgery (prostatectomy), and medications. Chemical, vibratory, and electrical methods of stimulation have been used with some success. Treatment usually addresses the physical and psychological factors involved in inhibited ejaculation (Wincze & Weisberg, 2015). Although outpatient therapy may involve numerous sessions (12 to 18), it often results in a success rate of 70% to 80%. The outcome depends on a previous satisfying sexual experience history, a short duration of the ejaculatory problem, feelings of sexual desire, feelings of attraction to one's sexual partner, motivation for treatment, and absence of serious psychological problems.

For men with retrograde ejaculation, the urine may be collected shortly after ejaculation, revealing a large amount of sperm in the urine. This urine may also be collected to obtain adequate viable sperm for use in artificial insemination. In men with SCI, techniques that may be used to obtain sperm for artificial insemination include self-stimulation, vibratory stimulation, or electroejaculation. Electroejaculation involves the use of a specially designed probe that is inserted into the rectum next to the prostate. The probe delivers a current that stimulates the nerves and produces contraction of the pelvic muscles and ejaculation. However, spontaneous or stimulated ejaculation may cause autonomic dysreflexia (overstimulation of the autonomic nervous system) in patients with SCI at T6 or higher, creating a life-threatening situation (see Chapter 65). If this disorder is not treated promptly, it may lead to seizures, stroke, and even death.

INFECTIONS OF THE MALE GENITOURINARY TRACT

Acute uncomplicated cystitis in adult men is uncommon but occasionally occurs in men whose sexual partners have vaginal infections with *Escherichia coli* (asymptomatic bacteriuria may also occur from genitourinary manipulation, catheterization, or instrumentation). Urinary tract infections in the male are discussed in Chapter 46.

The incidence of sexually transmitted infections (STIs) in Canada is increasing in men and women. It is unclear whether these increasing rates are a result of actual increase in the number of people with STIs or because of changes in diagnosing and reporting procedures (Public Health Agency of Canada [PHAC], 2013). The PHAC (2013) indicates that regardless, STIs remain a public health concern. In 2008, 70% of the 161,592 cases of notifiable diseases reported by the CNDSS were sexually transmitted and bloodborne infections. Several infections are classified as STIs: urethritis (gonococcal and nongonococcal), genital ulcers (genital herpes infections, primary syphilis, chancroid, granuloma inguinale, and lymphogranuloma venereum), genital warts (human papillomavirus [HPV]), scabies, pediculosis pubis, molluscum contagiosum, hepatitis and enteric infections, proctitis, genital chlamydia, and acquired immunodeficiency syndrome (AIDS). In Canada, the most commonly reported STI is *chlamydia*. In 2010, 94,690 cases of chlamydia infections were reported in Canada (PHAC, 2013). Gonorrhea is the second most commonly reported STI, with the gender ratio being reversed and males accounting for two thirds of cases. Syphilis infections have been rising dramatically since the year 2000. In 2010, 1,757 cases of infectious syphilis were reported with an overall rate of 5.2 per 100,000 people. The PHAC (2013) reports that the rates for males, particularly those of ages 30 to 39 years were higher than rates for females. A dramatic increase in syphilis incidence has been most notable among men who have sex with men (MSM) (PHAC, 2013). Trichomoniasis or STIs characterized by genital ulcers are thought to increase susceptibility to human immunodeficiency virus (HIV) infection. Trichomoniasis is associated with nonchlamydial, nongonococcal urethritis.

Prevention of STIs includes identifying individual risk behaviours. Nurses can assist patients with risk reduction strategies which can include abstinence, limiting sexual relations to long-term and monogamous partners, condom use, and sharing information on sexual history with partners (PHAC, 2013). Nurses must also encourage patients to seek and follow through with testing and treatment (where necessary) for sexually transmitted and bloodborne infections.

Treatment of STIs must be targeted at the patient as well as his or her sexual partners and sometimes the unborn child. A thorough history that includes a sexual history is crucial to identify patients at risk and to direct care and teaching. Partners of men with STIs must also be examined, treated, and counselled to prevent reinfection and complications in both partners and to limit the spread of the disease. Sexual abstinence during treatment and recovery is advised to prevent the transmission of STIs (PHAC, 2013). Using latex condoms for at least 6 months after completion of treatment is recommended to decrease transmission of HPV infections as well as other STIs. Because patients with one STI may also have another, it is important to examine and test for other STIs. The use of spermicides with nonoxynol 9 ("N-9") is discouraged, as they do not protect against HIV infection and may increase the risk for transmission of the virus. Refer to Chapters 52 and 55 for more detailed discussions of HIV infection, AIDS, and other STIs.

Immunizations can also be used to prevent and control the spread of infections, including STIs (HPV and hepatitis). Since 2008, all provinces and territories have introduced HPV vaccines for young females. In 2012, the National Advisory Committee on Immunization extended the recommended use of the HPV vaccine to include older females (up to 45 years old) and young males (9 to 26 years). Future evaluations will need to measure how the vaccine affects men, women, and various at-risk subpopulations as well as the long-term effectiveness in reducing incidence of related cancers (PHAC, 2013).

PROSTATIC DISORDERS

Prostatitis

Prostatitis is an inflammation of the prostate gland caused by infectious agents (bacteria, fungi, mycoplasma) or other conditions (e.g., urethral stricture, prostatic hyperplasia). *E. coli* is the most commonly isolated organism although *Klebsiella* and *Proteus* species are also found (Chen, Hu, Peng, et al., 2016). Microorganisms are usually carried to the prostate from the urethra. Prostatitis may be classified as acute or chronic and bacterial or abacterial, depending on the presence or absence of microorganisms in the prostatic fluid.

Clinical Manifestations

Symptoms of prostatitis may include perineal discomfort, burning, urgency, frequency, and pain with or after ejaculation. Prostatodynia (pain in the prostate) is manifested by pain on voiding or perineal pain without evidence of inflammation or bacterial growth in the prostate fluid.

Acute bacterial prostatitis may produce sudden fever and chills and perineal, rectal, or low back pain. Urinary symptoms, such as dysuria, frequency, urgency, and nocturia (urination during the night), may occur. Some patients do not have symptoms. Chronic bacterial prostatitis is a major cause of relapsing urinary tract infection in men. Symptoms are usually mild when compared with acute infections, including increased frequency, dysuria, and occasionally urethral discharge. High temperature and chills are uncommon.

Complications of prostatitis may include swelling of the prostate gland and urinary retention. Other complications include epididymitis, bacteremia, and pyelonephritis.

Assessment and Diagnostic Findings

The diagnosis of prostatitis requires a careful history, culture of prostate fluid or tissue, and occasionally a histologic examination of the tissue. To locate the source of a lower genitourinary infection (bladder neck, urethra, prostate), it is necessary to collect a divided urinary specimen for segmental urine culture. After cleaning the glans penis and retracting the foreskin (if present), the patient voids 10 to 15 mL of urine into a container. This represents urethral urine. Without interrupting the urinary stream, he then collects 50 to 75 mL of urine in a second container; this represents bladder urine.

If the patient does not have acute prostatitis, the physician immediately performs a prostatic massage and collects any prostatic fluid that is expressed into a third container. If it is not possible to collect prostatic fluid, the patient voids a small quantity of urine. The specimen may contain the bacteria present in the prostatic fluid. Urinalysis after prostate examination commonly reveals many white blood cells.

Medical Management

The goal of therapy for acute bacterial prostatitis is to avoid the complications of abscess formation and septicemia. A broad-spectrum antibiotic agent (to which the causative organism is sensitive) is administered for 10 to 14 days, typically fluoroquinolones. Intravenous administration of the antibiotic may be necessary to achieve high serum and tissue levels.

Chronic bacterial prostatitis is difficult to treat because most antibiotics diffuse poorly from the plasma into the prostatic fluid. Nevertheless, antibiotics may be prescribed, including trimethoprim–sulfamethoxazole (TMP–SMZ or Septra) or a fluoroquinolone. Continuous therapy with low-dose antibiotics to suppress the infection may also be indicated. The patient is advised that the infection may recur and is taught to recognize its symptoms. In addition, treatment for chronic prostatitis may include reducing the retention of prostatic fluid by ejaculation through sexual intercourse or self-stimulation. Research indicates that physical therapy, acupuncture, trigger point injections, and home exercise therapy may also help patients obtain relief from chronic prostatitis (Ulbricht & Rusie, 2012).

Nursing Management

Acute prostatitis (fever, severe pain and discomfort, inability to urinate, malaise) may require the patient to receive intravenous antibiotics. Nursing management includes administration of prescribed antibiotics and patient teaching about the medication and the possible side effects. As well, the nurse will describe the use of comfort measures. Comfort is promoted with analgesic agents (to relieve pain), antispasmodic medications and bladder sedatives (to relieve bladder irritability), sitz baths (to relieve pain and spasm), and stool softeners (to prevent pain from straining). The patient is encouraged to remain on bed rest to alleviate symptoms quickly.

Promoting Home, Community-Based, and Transitional Care

Educating Patients About Self-Care

The nurse instructs the patient to complete the prescribed course of antibiotics. If intravenous antibiotics are to be administered at home, the nurse instructs the patient and family about correct and safe administration. Arrangements for home care to oversee administration may be needed. Hot sitz baths (10 to 20 minutes) may be taken several times daily. Fluids are encouraged to satisfy thirst but are not "forced" because an effective medication level must be maintained in the urine. Foods and liquids that have diuretic action or that increase prostatic secretions, such as alcohol, coffee, tea, chocolate, cola, and spices, should be avoided. During periods of acute inflammation, sexual arousal and intercourse should be avoided.

To minimize discomfort, the patient should avoid sitting for long periods. Medical follow-up is often necessary for at least 6 months to 1 year because prostatitis caused by the same or different organisms can recur.

Benign Prostatic Hyperplasia (Enlarged Prostate)

Benign prostatic hyperplasia (BPH) is a condition in which the prostate gland enlarges due to the increased number of cells and then gradually extends upward into the bladder and obstructs the outflow of urine. It is one of the most common pathologic conditions in men older than 50 years, because the prostate naturally gets larger as men age. According to the Canadian Cancer Society (2014a) almost all men by the age of 70 will have some prostate enlargement. It is important to note that BPH does not increase the risk of prostate cancer. Smoking, heavy alcohol consumption, obesity, reduced activity level, hypertension, heart disease, diabetes, and a Western diet (high in animal fat and protein and refined carbohydrates, low in fibre) are risk factors for BPH (Tantamango-Bartley, Knutsen, Knutsen, et al., 2016).

Clinical Manifestations

In the literature, lower urinary tract symptoms (LUTS) are often used to describe clinical manifestations of BPH. LUTS symptoms are thought to be caused by increased muscle tone and resistance and direct mechanical obstruction of the bladder (Cohen & Parsons, 2012). The hypertrophied lobes may obstruct the vesicle neck or prostatic urethra, causing incomplete emptying of the bladder and urinary retention. As a result, a gradual dilation of the ureters (hydroureter) and kidneys (hydronephrosis) can occur. Urinary tract infections may result from urinary stasis, because some urine remains in the urinary tract and serves as a medium for infective organisms. Men with BPH often report frequent urination (nocturia, frequency, urgency), straining, feeling unable to empty bladder, urinary incontinence, dysuria, and hematuria.

Assessment and Diagnostic Findings

Examination reveals a prostate gland that is large, rubbery, and nontender. The irritative and obstructive symptom complex (referred to as **prostatism**) includes increased frequency of urination, nocturia, urgency, hesitancy in starting urination, abdominal straining with urination, a decrease in the volume and force of the urinary stream, interruption of the urinary stream, dribbling (urine dribbles out after urination), a sensation that the bladder has not been completely emptied, acute urinary retention, and recurrent urinary tract infections. Ultimately, azotemia (accumulation of nitrogenous waste products) and renal failure can occur with chronic urinary retention and large residual volumes. Generalized symptoms may also be noted, including fatigue, anorexia, nausea, vomiting, and epigastric discomfort. Other disorders producing similar obstructive symptoms include urethral stricture, prostate cancer, neurogenic bladder, and urinary bladder stones.

A physical examination with DRE and diagnostic studies may be performed to determine the degree to which the prostate is enlarged, the presence of any changes in the bladder wall, and the efficiency of renal function. These tests may include urinalysis and urodynamic studies to assess urine flow. Renal function tests, including serum creatinine levels, may be performed to determine if there is renal impairment from prostatic back pressure and to evaluate renal reserve. If surgery is planned, complete blood studies are performed. Because hemorrhage is a major complication of prostate surgery, all clotting defects must be corrected. A high percentage of patients with BPH have cardiac or respiratory complications, or both, because of their age; therefore, cardiac and respiratory function is assessed as well as medications, particularly medications affecting clotting.

Medical Management

The treatment plan depends on the cause of BPH, the severity of the obstruction, and the patient's condition. If the patient is admitted on an emergency basis because of complete urinary retention, urethral catheterization is required. In cases of severe prostatic enlargement or stricture, a urologist may be the only professional skilled enough to pass the catheter to allow urine drainage. An ordinary catheter may be too soft and pliable to advance through the urethra into the bladder. In such cases, a thin wire, called a *stylet*, is introduced (by a urologist) into the catheter. Sometimes, an incision is made into the bladder (a suprapubic cystostomy) to provide drainage.

Pharmacologic Therapy

Pharmacologic treatment for BPH includes use of alpha-adrenergic blockers and 5-alpha-reductase inhibitors, or a combination of both. PDE-5 inhibitors such as tadalafil (Cialis) may also be used, whether or not the patient has erection problems (Cohen & Parsons, 2012). Alpha-adrenergic blockers (e.g., terazosin [Hytrin], doxazosin [Cardura], tamsulosin [Flomax]) relax the smooth muscle of the bladder neck and prostate. Alfuzosin (Uroxatral) is an extended-release alpha-adrenergic antagonist that exerts its effects on the prostate, bladder neck, and posterior urethra. The smooth muscle blockade improves urine flow and relieves BPH symptoms (Cohen & Parsons, 2012).

Because a hormonal component of BPH has been identified, one method of treatment involves hormonal manipulation with antiandrogen agents (e.g., finasteride [Proscar], dutasteride [Avodart]). 5-Alpha-reductase inhibitors such as finasteride prevent the conversion of testosterone to dihydrotestosterone (DHT). Decreased levels of DHT lead to decreased glandular cell activity and prostate size. Side effects include gynecomastia (breast enlargement), ED, and flushing. There is some evidence the 5-alpha-reductase inhibitors may decrease the risk of prostate cancer (Cohen & Parsons, 2012).

Saw palmetto is a herbal product used to treat the symptoms associated with BPH. The active element comes from the fruit of the American dwarf palm tree. Research has shown that the efficacy of saw palmetto is similar to that of medications such as finasteride, and the herbal product may be better tolerated and less expensive (Cohen & Parsons, 2012). In theory, it functions by interfering with the conversion of testosterone to DHT. In addition, saw palmetto may directly block the ability of DHT to stimulate prostate cell growth. It should not be used with finasteride, dutasteride, or medications containing estrogen.

Surgical Procedures

Several approaches can be used to remove a noncancerous hypertrophied portion of the prostate gland: TURP, transurethral incision of the prostate (TUIP and suprapubic prostatectomy (Table 50-4). In these approaches, the surgeon removes all hyperplastic tissue, leaving behind only

TABLE 50-4 Surgical Approaches for Treatment of Prostate Disorders

The surgical approach of choice depends on: (1) the size of the gland; (2) the severity of the obstruction; (3) the age of the patient; (4) the condition of the patient; and (5) the presence of associated diseases.

Surgical Approach	Advantages	Disadvantages	Nursing Implications
Transurethral Resection (TURP) Removal of prostatic tissue by optical instrument introduced through urethra; used for glands of varying size. Ideal for patients who are poor surgical risks	Avoids abdominal incision Safer for surgical-risk patient Shorter length of hospital stay and recovery periods Lower morbidity rate Causes less pain Can be used as a palliative approach with history of radiation therapy	Requires highly skilled surgeon Recurrent obstruction, urethral trauma, and stricture may develop Delayed bleeding may occur	Monitor for hemorrhage Observe for symptoms of urethral stricture (dysuria, straining, weak urinary stream)
Open Surgical Removal			
Suprapubic approach Removal of prostatic tissue through abdominal incision; can be used for gland of any size	Technically simple Offers wide area of exploration Permits exploration for cancerous lymph nodes Allows more complete removal of obstructing gland Permits treatment of associated bladder lesions	Requires surgical approach through the bladder Control of hemorrhage is difficult Urine may leak around the suprapubic tube Recovery may be prolonged and uncomfortable	Monitor for indications of hemorrhage and shock Provide meticulous aseptic care to the area around suprapubic tube

continued >

TABLE 50-4 Surgical Approaches for Treatment of Prostate Disorders (Continued)

Surgical Approach	Advantages	Disadvantages	Nursing Implications
Perineal Approach Removal of gland through an incision in the perineum; preferred approach for patients with obesity	Offers direct anatomic approach Permits gravity drainage Particularly effective for radical cancer therapy Allows hemostasis under direct vision Low mortality rate Low incidence of shock Ideal for patients with large prostate who are very old, frail, and poor surgical risks	Higher postoperative incidence of impotence and urinary incontinence Possible damage to rectum and external sphincter Restricted operative field Greater potential for contamination and infection of incision	Avoid using rectal tubes or thermometers and enemas after perineal surgery Use drainage pads to absorb excess urinary drainage Provide foam rubber ring for patient comfort in sitting Anticipate urinary leakage around the wound for several days after the catheter is removed
Retropubic Approach Low abdominal incision; bladder is not entered	Avoids incision into the bladder Permits surgeon to see and control bleeding Shorter recovery period Less bladder sphincter damage Suitable for removal of large glands	Cannot treat associated bladder disease Increased incidence of hemorrhage from prostatic venous plexus; osteitis pubis	Monitor for hemorrhage Anticipate posturinary leakage for several days after removing the catheter
Transurethral Incision (TUIP) Urethral approach; 1–2 cuts are made in the prostate and prostate capsule to reduce pressure on the urethra and to reduce urethral constriction	Results comparable to TURP Low incidence of erectile dysfunction and retrograde ejaculation No bladder neck contracture	Recurrent obstruction and urethral trauma Delayed bleeding	Monitor for hemorrhage
Laparoscopic Radical Prostatectomy In this approach, 4–6 small (1 cm [0.5 inch]) incisions are made in the abdomen; laparoscopic instruments inserted through the incisions are used to dissect the prostate	Minimally invasive technique Improved patient satisfaction and quality of life Shorter length of hospital stay Short convalescence More rapid return to normal activity Short indwelling catheter duration Decreased blood loss to 400 mL Reduced infection risk Less scarring Better visualization of surgical field than other approaches	Lack of tactile sensation available with open prostatectomy Inability to palpably assess for induration and palpable nodules Inability to delineate the proximity of involvement of the neurovascular bundles due to lack of palpation Long surgical time (4–5 hours)	Observe for symptoms of urethral stricture (dysuria), straining, weak urinary stream Monitor for hemorrhage and shock Provide meticulous aseptic care to area around suprapubic tube Monitor for changes in bowel function Avoid using rectal tubes or thermometers and enemas after perineal surgery Use drainage pads to absorb excess urinary drainage Provide foam rubber ring for patient comfort in sitting Anticipate urinary leakage around the wound for several days after the catheter is removed
Robotic-Assisted Laparoscopic Radical Prostatectomy Involves using computer console and da Vinci. In this approach, 6 small (1 cm [0.5 inch]) incisions are made in the abdomen; laparoscopic instruments inserted through the incisions are used to dissect the prostate	Minimally invasive technique Improved patient satisfaction and quality of life Shorter length of hospital stay Short convalescence More rapid return to normal activity Short indwelling catheter duration Decreased blood loss to 150 mL Improved magnification of operative field, using a 3-dimensional view (includes, magnification, high resolution, and depth perception) Less postoperative pain Reduced risk of infection Less scarring Laparoscopic instruments have 6 degrees of movement with joints, allowing extensive range of motion and precision Nerve sparing with less incontinence and sexual dysfunction	Lack of tactile sensation available with open prostatectomy Inability to palpably assess for induration and palpable nodules Inability to delineate the proximity of involvement of the neurovascular bundles due to lack of palpation	Observe for symptoms of urethral stricture (dysuria), straining, weak urinary stream. Monitor for hemorrhage and shock. Provide meticulous aseptic care to the area around suprapubic tube Monitor for changes in bowel function Avoid using rectal tubes or thermometers and enemas after perineal surgery Use drainage pads to absorb excess urinary drainage Provide foam rubber ring for patient comfort in sitting Anticipate urinary leakage around the wound for several days after the catheter is removed

Adapted from Keane, T. E., & Graham, S. D. (Eds.). (2016). *Glenn's urologic surgery*. Philadelphia, PA: Wolters Kluwer; McDougal, W. S., Wein, A. J., Kavoussi, L. R., et al. (Eds.). (2016). *Campbell-Walsh urology* (11th ed.). Philadelphia, PA: Elsevier.

the capsule of the prostate. The transurethral approaches (TURP, TUIP) are closed procedures; suprapubic prostatectomy is an open procedure (i.e., a surgical incision is required). The procedure chosen depends on the underlying disorder, the patient's age and physical status, and patient preference.

Transurethral Resection of the Prostate

Transurethral resection of the prostate (TURP, or TUR), the most common procedure used in men with small- to moderate-sized prostates. In Canada, the TURP is performed on 90% of men with BPH (Ben-Zvi, Hueber, Valdivieso, et al., 2014). This procedure is carried out through endoscopy. The surgical and optical instrument is introduced directly through the urethra to the prostate, which can then be viewed directly. The gland is removed in small chips with an electrical cutting loop (Fig. 50-4A). This procedure eliminates the risk of transurethral resection syndrome (hyponatremia, hypovolemia). Transurethral resection syndrome is a potential but rare complication of TURP that occurs in approximately 2% of men who undergo the procedure (Lycken, Garmo, Adolfsson, et al., 2013; Rathkopf & Scher, 2013) (see Chart 50-3).

This approach usually requires an overnight hospital stay. Over time, repeated procedures may be necessary because the residual prostatic tissue can grow back. TURP rarely causes ED, but it may cause retrograde ejaculation because removing the prostatic tissue at the bladder neck can cause the seminal fluid to flow backward into the bladder rather than forward through the urethra during ejaculation.

Transurethral Incision of the Prostate

TUIP is another procedure used in treating BPH. An instrument is passed through the urethra (Fig. 50-4B). One or two incisions are made in the prostate and prostate capsule to reduce prostate pressure on the urethra and to reduce urethral constriction. TUIP is indicated when the

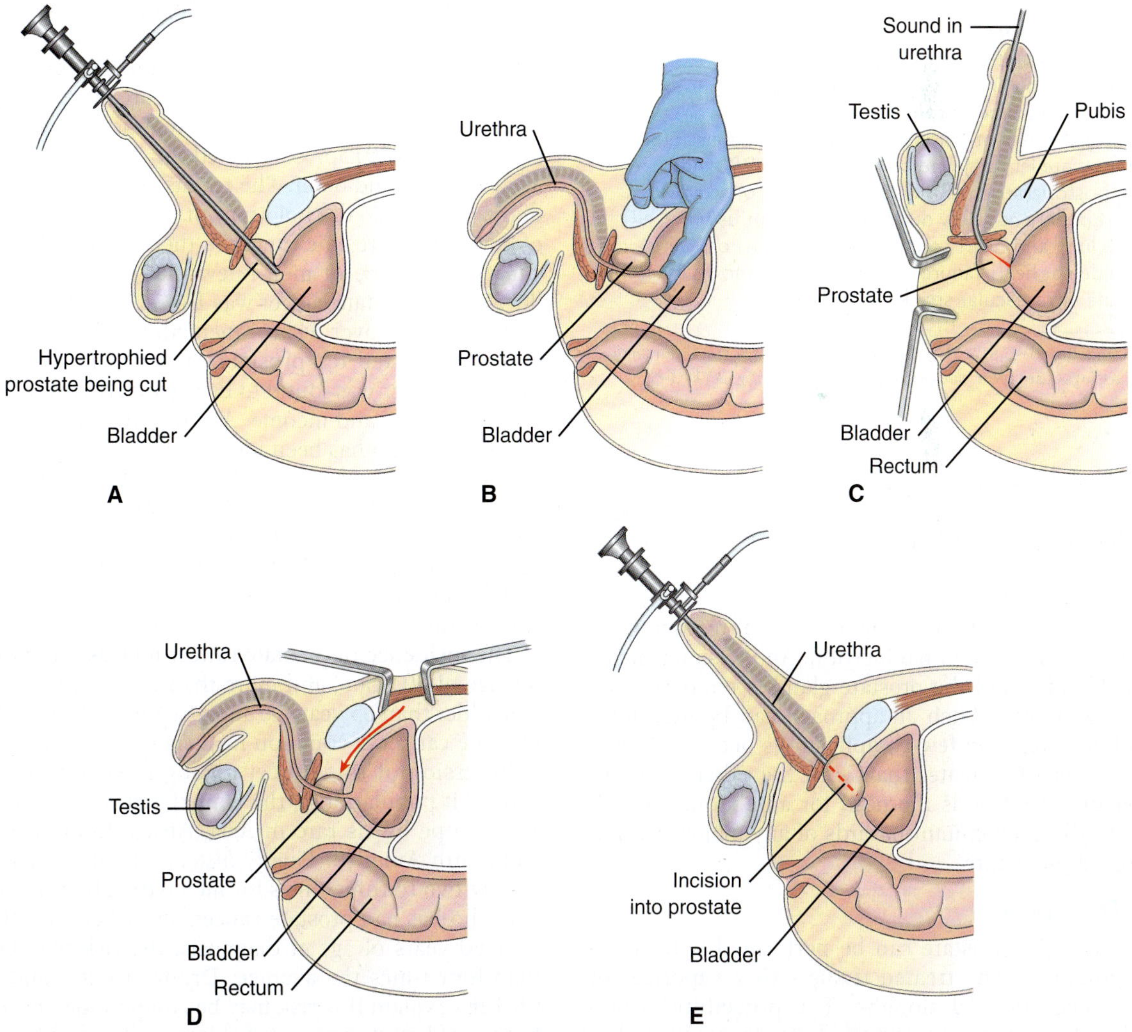

FIGURE 50-4. Prostate surgery procedures. **A.** Transurethral resection (TUR). A loop of wire connected with a cutting current is rotated in the cystoscope to remove shavings of prostate at the bladder orifice. **B.** Transurethral incision of the prostate (TUIP) involves one or two incisions into the prostate to reduce pressure on the urethra. **C.** Suprapubic prostatectomy. With an abdominal approach, the prostate is shelled out of its bed. **D.** Perineal prostatectomy. Two retractors on the left spread the perineal incision to provide a view of the prostate. **E.** Retropubic prostatectomy is performed through a low abdominal incision. Note two abdominal retractors and *arrow* pointing to the prostate gland.

CHART 50-3

Transurethral Resection Syndrome

Transurethral resection syndrome is a rare but potentially serious complication of transurethral prostatectomy (TURP). Signs and symptoms are caused by neurologic, cardiovascular, and electrolyte imbalances associated with absorption of the solution used to irrigate the surgical site during the surgical procedure. Hyponatremia, hypovolemia, and occasionally hyperammonemia may occur.

Signs and Symptoms

- Collapse
- Headache
- Hypotension
- Lethargy and confusion
- Muscle spasms
- Nausea and vomiting
- Seizures
- Tachycardia

Interventions

- Discontinue irrigation
- Administer diuretic agents as prescribed
- Replace bladder irrigation with normal saline
- Monitor intake and output
- Monitor the patient's vital signs and level of consciousness
- Differentiate lethargy and confusion of TURP syndrome from postoperative disorientation and hyponatremia
- Maintain patient safety during times of confusion
- Assess lung and heart sounds for indications of pulmonary edema, heart failure, or both as fluid moves back into the intravascular space

Adapted from Brown, C. S. (2014). Dilutional hyponatremia in a community hospital setting: Case report. *Intensive and Critical Care Nursing, 30*(1), 1–5.

prostate gland is small (30 g or less). It can be performed on an outpatient basis and has a lower complication rate than other invasive prostate procedures.

Suprapubic Prostatectomy

Suprapubic prostatectomy is one method of removing the gland through an abdominal incision. An incision is made into the bladder, and the prostate gland is removed from above (Fig. 50-4C). Such an approach can be used for a gland of any size, and few complications occur, although blood loss may be greater than with the other methods. Another disadvantage is the need for an abdominal incision, with the concomitant hazards of any major abdominal surgical procedure.

Other Therapies

Resection of the prostate can be performed with ultrasound guidance. The treated tissue either vaporizes or becomes necrotic and sloughs. The procedure is performed in the outpatient setting and usually results in less postoperative bleeding than in a traditional surgical prostatectomy.

Transurethral needle ablation uses low-level radio frequencies to produce localized heat that destroys prostate tissue while sparing the urethra, nerves, muscles, and membranes. The radio frequencies are delivered by thin needles placed in the prostate gland through use of a catheter. The body then resorbs the dead tissue.

Transurethral microwave thermotherapy (TUMT) involves the application of heat to the prostatic tissue. A transurethral probe is inserted into the urethra, and microwaves are carefully directed to the prostate tissue. A water-cooling system helps to minimize damage to the urethra and decreases the discomfort from the procedure. The tissue becomes necrotic and sloughs.

Finally, "watchful waiting," in which patients are monitored periodically for severity of symptoms, physical findings, laboratory tests, and diagnostic urologic tests, is the appropriate treatment for many patients, because the likelihood of progression of the disease or the development of complications is unknown.

Cancer of the Prostate

PRACTICE & LEARN

Prostate cancer is the most common form of cancer in Canadian men and about 25% of all new cancer cases (Prostate Cancer Canada [PCC], 2013f). PCC estimates that 23,600 will be diagnosed with prostate cancer in 2013 and that 43,900 will die of the disease. Prostate cancer rates are twice as high in Black Canadian men than in white men, and Black Canadian men are more likely to die of prostate cancer than men in any other racial or ethnic group. PCC (2013c) conducted an online poll for men aged 18 years and older. The results showed that over half of the men (55%) did not know or underestimated the risk of developing prostate cancer in their lifetime. Within the survey, only 16% of men knew that the lifetime risk of developing prostate cancer was 1 in 7. The PCC continues to explain that over 44% of men admitted to being reluctant to be tested for prostate cancer. Knowledge about prostate cancer was found to be negatively correlated with education, age, and income. A culturally sensitive promotional campaign has been identified as an important strategy to increase awareness of the racial disparities in the incidence of prostate cancer and mortality rates. Nurses are in an ideal position to use these research findings to improve the health of Black Canadian men by teaching and counselling them about prostate cancer, screening, and treatment.

The incidence of prostate cancer increases rapidly after the age of 50 years, and more than 75% of cases occur in men older than 65 year (Drudge-Coates & Turner, 2012b). Prostate cancer is common in Canada (see Chart 50-4 for a discussion of this cancer among First Nations, Metis, and Inuit populations), the United States, and northwestern Europe but is rare in Asia, Africa, Central America, and South America. *Family history* can also increase the risk by two to three times for men with a first-degree relative who has had prostate cancer, and when the relative is over 60 years of age at diagnosis, the risk may be more than four times the average. Drudge-Coates and Turner (2012b) explain this risk may be compounded by a family history of breast cancer. *A diet* low in fibre and high in fat, may lead to higher rates of prostate cancer. Research suggests that saturated fat (commonly found in processed foods, whole-milk dairy products, and fatty cuts of meat) increases the production of the hormone testosterone, which may help prostate cancer cells grow (PCC, 2013e). *Lifestyle risks* that may make prostate cancer more likely

CHART 50-4

Prostate Cancer in First Nations, Metis and Inuit Populations

One of the most common cancers diagnosed in Alberta from 1997 to 2010 include prostate cancer, but the number of prostate cancers are lower rates than those of non-First Nation men (Health Canada, 2013). According to the same report, even though First Nation males are less likely to be diagnosed with prostate cancer, they are more likely to die of the disease. Some of the barriers related to prostate cancer, include inadequate access to cancer screening. Reason include: lack of transportation, fear of cancer and diagnosis, geographic location, lack of culturally relevant services and shyness/discomfort in discussing sexual health related disorders/diseases. Recommendations to encourage First Nation males to access prostate cancer screening include aligning culturally sensitive services with various First Nation cultures.

include obesity or increased BMI, along with a sedentary lifestyle or lack of exercise.

Clinical Manifestations

Cancer of the prostate in its early stages rarely produces symptoms. The symptoms that develop from urinary obstruction occur late in the disease. This cancer tends to vary in its course. If the neoplasm is large enough to encroach on the bladder neck, signs and symptoms of urinary obstruction occur: difficulty and frequency of urination, urinary retention, and decreased size and force of the urinary stream. Other symptoms may include blood in the urine or semen and painful ejaculation. Hematuria may result if the cancer invades the urethra or bladder, or both. Prostate cancer can metastasize to bone and lymph nodes. Symptoms related to metastases include backache, hip pain, perineal and rectal discomfort, anemia, weight loss, weakness, nausea, and oliguria (decreased urine output). Unfortunately, these symptoms may be the first indications of prostate cancer.

Assessment and Diagnostic Findings

The diagnosis of prostate cancer is usually made using a triage approach which uses patient history, physical examination, and investigations such as PSA and biopsies (Drudge-Coates & Turner, 2012b). When prostate cancer is detected early, the likelihood of cure is high. Every man older than 50 years should have a DRE as part of his regular health checkup. Routine annual DRE (preferably by the same examiner) is important because early cancer may be detected as a nodule within the substance of the gland or as an extensive hardening in the posterior lobe. The more advanced lesions are "stony hard," "woody," and fixed. DRE also provides useful clinical information about the rectum, anal sphincter, and quality of stool. The combination of DRE and PSA testing appears to be a cost-effective method of detecting prostate cancer.

Prostate cancer is confirmed by a histologic examination of tissue removed by TRUS-guided needle biopsy. The most frequent scoring tool is the Gleason Score, used to grade prostate cancer and to guide the physician in determining the most appropriate treatment (Drudge-Coates & Turner, 2012b; PCC, 2013b). Men with a Gleason Score of 2 to 4 are at low risk, those with a score of 5 to 7 are at moderate risk, and a score of 8 to 10 indicates a high risk of the prostate cancer extending beyond the prostatic capsule.

Other tests include bone scans or skeletal x-rays to detect metastatic bone disease, excretory urography to detect changes caused by ureteral obstruction, renal function tests, and computed tomography (CT) scans or lymphangiography to identify metastases in the pelvic lymph nodes.

Sexual Complications

Treatment for prostate cancer increases the risk of sexual dysfunction. With nerve-sparing radical prostatectomy, the chance of recovering erections is better for men who are younger and in whom both neurovascular bundles are spared. Men who experienced some sexual dysfunction prior to surgery must be counselled that they have a high risk of ED after surgery. Hormonal therapy also affects the central nervous system mechanisms that mediate sexual desire and arousability.

The PDE-5 inhibitors have been found to be effective for treating ED in younger men after radiation therapy or after radical retropubic prostatectomy, especially if the neurovascular bundles were preserved.

Treatment Options

Watchful Waiting

Watchful waiting is one option after the diagnosis of prostate cancer. This includes monitoring the prostate cancer and using treatment only if symptoms exist. This option may be chosen in older men with comorbidities. It can also be considered as an option in men with localized prostate cancer, with a limited life-expectancy (Drudge-Coates & Turner, 2012b).

Active Surveillance

Active surveillance is another way to monitor prostate cancer, when there are aims to avoid or delay treatment. Some factors that may be used when considering active surveillance include small, slow growing cells that are composed of relatively normal-looking cells (this is determined by the pathologist from the prostate biopsy); the likelihood of the patient dying from other causes (including old age); and the possible side effects or the treatments outweigh the benefits of treatment (PCC, 2013a).

Surgical Management

Radical Prostatectomy

A radical prostatectomy (removal of the prostate and seminal vesicles) remains the standard surgical procedure for patients who have early-stage, potentially curable disease and a life expectancy of 10 years or more (Drudge-Coates & Turner, 2012b). It is done through an abdominal or perineal incision (Fig. 50-4D, E). More frequently, radical prostatectomy is performed laparoscopically or robotically. Sexual dysfunction may follow a radical prostatectomy, and some patients experience various degrees of urinary incontinence (Isbarn, Huland, & Graefen, 2013).

Robotic-Assisted Laparoscopic Radical Prostatectomy

In the last few years, the minimally invasive surgical approaches called robotic-assisted laparoscopic radical prostatectomy (RALP) have been used as a standard of treatment for prostate cancer. Some literature supports the idea that there is a decrease in morbidity with the use of RALP (Jung, Seo, Lim, et al., 2012). Laparoscopic radical prostatectomy provides better visualization of the surgical site and surrounding areas. Preliminary data suggest that patients who undergo this procedure have less bleeding and reduced need for blood transfusion, a shorter hospital stay, less postoperative pain, a shorter duration of indwelling catheterization, and more rapid return to normal activity when compared with open radical prostatectomy (Jung et al., 2012). Research is ongoing to assess long-term outcomes and cancer control.

Cryosurgery of the Prostate

Cryosurgery of the prostate is used to ablate prostate cancer in patients who may not tolerate surgery or in those with recurrent prostate cancer. Transperineal probes are inserted into the prostate under ultrasound guidance to freeze the tissue directly.

Complications

Complications depend on the type of prostatectomy performed and may include hemorrhage, clot formation, catheter obstruction, and sexual dysfunction. All prostatectomies carry a risk of impotence because of potential damage to the penile nerve supply. In most instances, sexual activity may be resumed in 6 to 8 weeks, which is the time required for the prostatic fossa to heal. According to PCC (2013d), a *nerve-sparing technique* may be used to try to preserve the nerves that control erections, rather than removing them with the prostate. However, this may not be an option for all patients because there is a risk that cancer cells may remain if the nerves are left intact. With ejaculation, the seminal fluid goes into the bladder and is excreted with the urine. (The anatomic changes in the posterior urethra lead to retrograde ejaculation.)

Medical Management

Radiation Therapy

If prostate cancer is detected in its early stage, the treatment may be curative radiation therapy. Two major forms of radiation therapy are used to treat cancer of the prostate: teletherapy (external) and brachytherapy (internal).

Teletherapy (external beam radiation therapy) involves 6 to 7 weeks of daily (5 days/week) radiation treatments. Intensity-modulated radiation therapy (IMRT) has revolutionized the delivery of external beam radiation therapy. IMRT sets a dose for the target volume and restricts the dose to adjacent structures. It is thought to be accurate within 1 to 3 mm.

Brachytherapy involves the implantation of interstitial radioactive seeds under anesthesia. This therapy can be permanent or temporary. The surgeon uses ultrasound guidance to insert needles into the prostate which will deliver the radioactive strands, and the patient returns home after the procedure. Radiation safety guidelines include straining urine for seeds and using a condom during sexual intercourse for 2 weeks after implantation, to catch any seeds that pass through the urethra.

Side effects of teletherapy and brachytherapy, which usually are transitory, include inflammation of the rectum, bowel, and bladder (proctitis, enteritis, and cystitis) due to their proximity to the prostate and the radiation doses. Irritation of the bladder and urethra from radiation therapy can cause pain with urination and during ejaculation until the irritation subsides. However, there is a greater preservation of sexual potency with radiation therapy than with surgery. For patients with clinically localized but high-risk prostate cancer, multimodal treatment may result in improved cancer control. In patients with larger tumours, combination therapy (radiation therapy followed by hormonal therapy) may improve overall survival.

Hormonal Therapy

Hormone therapy is considered a treatment option in older men with prostate cancer who are not suitable for the more radical treatments. Typically, these men still require treatments to control the cancer. The goal of hormone therapy is to shrink and control the growth of prostate cancer cells, wherever they may be in the body (Malik, 2014). Hormonal therapy for advanced prostate cancer suppresses androgenic stimuli to the prostate by decreasing the circulating plasma testosterone levels or interrupting the conversion to or binding of DHT. As a result, the prostatic epithelium atrophies (decreases). Up until the 1980s the only option available to reduce the production of testosterone was through surgical castration. This effect is accomplished either by **orchiectomy** (surgical removal of the testes). Currently pharmacologic advances have provided hormonal therapy to include the administration of medications.

Orchiectomy lowers plasma testosterone levels because about 93% of circulating testosterone is of testicular origin (7% is from the adrenal glands). As a result, the testicular stimulus required for continued prostatic growth is removed, resulting in prostatic atrophy. Although orchiectomy does not cause the side effects associated with other hormonal therapies, it carries a significant emotional impact.

Estrogen therapy, usually in the form of diethylstilbestrol (DES), has long been used to inhibit the gonadotropins responsible for testicular androgenic activity, thereby removing the androgenic hormone that promotes the growth of the malignancy. DES relieves symptoms of advanced prostate cancer, reduces tumour size, decreases pain from metastatic nodules, and promotes well-being. However, DES significantly increases the risk for thromboembolism, pulmonary embolism, myocardial infarction, and stroke. Other side effects of estrogen therapy include impotence, decreased libido, difficulty in achieving orgasm, decreased sperm production, and gynecomastia (enlargement of breasts in men).

See Chart 50-5 for the Plan of Nursing Care for a patient with prostate cancer.

Newer hormonal therapies include the luteinizing hormone–releasing hormone (LHRH) agonists (leuprolide [Lupron] and goserelin [Zoladex]) and antiandrogen agents (flutamide [Euflex]). LHRH suppresses testicular androgen, whereas flutamide causes adrenal androgen

(text continued on page 1500)

Plan of Nursing Care — Chart 50-5. The Patient With Prostate Cancer

NURSING INTERVENTIONS	RATIONALE	EXPECTED OUTCOMES
Nursing Priority: Anxiety **Goal:** Reduced stress and improved ability to cope		
1. Obtain health history to determine the following: a. Patient's concerns b. His level of understanding of his health concern c. His past experience with cancer d. Whether he knows his diagnosis of malignancy and its prognosis e. His support systems and coping methods	1. Nurse clarifies information and facilitates patient's understanding and coping.	• Appears relaxed • States that anxiety has been reduced or relieved • Demonstrates understanding of illness and treatment when questioned • Engages in open communication with others
2. Provide education about diagnosis and treatment plan a. Explain in simple terms what diagnostic tests to expect, how long they will take, and what will be experienced during each test b. Review treatment plan, and allow patient to ask questions	2. Helping the patient to understand the diagnostic tests and treatment plan will help to decrease his anxiety and promote cooperation	
3. Assess his psychological reaction to his diagnosis/prognosis and how he has coped with past stresses	3. This information provides clues in determining appropriate measures to facilitate coping	
4. Provide information about institutional and community resources for coping with prostate cancer, such as social services, support groups, and community agencies	4. Institutional and community resources can help the patient and family cope with the illness and treatment on an ongoing basis	
Nursing Priority: Urinary retention **Goal:** Improved pattern of urinary elimination		
1. Determine patient's usual pattern of urinary function	1. Provides a baseline for comparison and a goal to work toward	• Voids at normal intervals • Reports absence of frequency, urgency, or bladder fullness • Displays no palpable suprapubic distention after voiding • Maintains balanced intake and output
2. Assess for signs and symptoms of urinary retention: amount and frequency of urination, suprapubic distention, complaints of urgency, and discomfort	2. Voiding 20 to 30 mL frequently and output less than intake suggests retention	
3. Catheterize patient or do ultrasound to determine amount of residual urine	3. Determines the amount of urine remaining in the bladder after voiding	
4. Initiate measures to treat retention a. Encourage normal position for voiding b. Recommend using Valsalva manoeuvre c. Administer prescribed cholinergic agent d. Monitor effects of medication	4. Promotes voiding a. Usual position provides relaxed conditions conducive to voiding b. Valsalva manoeuvre exerts pressure to force urine out of the bladder c. Stimulates bladder contraction d. If unsuccessful, another measure may be required	
5. Consult with physician regarding intermittent or indwelling catheterization; assist with procedure as required	5. Catheterization will relieve urinary retention until the specific cause is determined; treatment with an alpha blocker may be initiated with catheter in place	
6. Monitor catheter function; maintain sterility of closed system; irrigate as required	6. Adequate functioning of catheter is to be ensured to empty the bladder and to prevent infection	

continued >

Plan of Nursing Care — Chart 50-5. The Patient With Prostate Cancer, *Continued*

NURSING INTERVENTIONS	RATIONALE	EXPECTED OUTCOMES
7. Monitor voiding if catheter removed	7. Trial without catheter will assess effectiveness of medication and whether surgery is indicated	
8. Prepare patient for surgery if indicated	8. Surgical removal of the obstruction may be necessary	
Nursing Priority: Lack of knowledge **Goal:** Understanding of the diagnosis and ability to care for self		
1. Encourage communication with patient	1. This is designed to establish rapport and trust	• Discusses his concerns and issues freely • Asks questions and shows interest in his condition • Describes activities that help or hinder recovery • Identifies ways of attaining/maintaining bladder control • Demonstrates satisfactory technique and understanding of catheter care • Lists signs and symptoms that must be reported should they occur
2. Review the anatomy of the involved area	2. Orientation to one's anatomy is basic to understanding its function	
3. Be specific in selecting information that is relevant to patient's particular treatment plan	3. This is based on the treatment plan; as it varies with each patient, individualization is desirable	
4. Identify ways to reduce pressure on the operative area after prostatectomy a. Avoid prolonged sitting (in a chair, long automobile rides), standing, or walking b. Avoid straining, such as during exercises, bowel movement, lifting, and sexual intercourse	4. This is to prevent bleeding; such precautions are in order for 6 to 8 weeks postoperatively	
5. Familiarize patient with ways of attaining/maintaining bladder control a. Encourage urination every 2 to 3 hours; discourage voiding when supine b. Avoid drinking cola and caffeine beverages; suggest an evening cut-off time for drinking fluids to minimize nocturia c. Describe pelvic floor muscle exercises to be performed two to three times a day d. Develop a schedule with the patient that will fit into his routine	5. These measures will help to control frequency and dribbling and aid in preventing retention a. By sitting or standing, the patient is more likely to empty his bladder b. Spacing the kind and amount of liquid intake will help to prevent frequency c. Exercises will assist him in starting and stopping the urinary stream d. A schedule will assist in developing a workable pattern of normal activities	
6. Demonstrate catheter care; encourage his questions; stress the importance of the position of the urinary receptacle	6. By requiring a return demonstration of care, collection, and emptying of the device, he will become more independent	
Nursing Priority: Imbalanced nutrition **Goal:** Maintain optimal nutritional status		
1. Assess amount of food eaten	1. This assessment will help to determine nutrient intake	• Responds positively to his favourite foods • Assumes responsibility for his oral hygiene • Notes increase in weight after improved appetite
2. Routinely weigh patient	2. Weighing the patient on the same scale under similar conditions can help to monitor changes in weight	
3. Elicit patient's explanation of poor appetite	3. His explanation may present easily corrected practices	
4. Cater to his individual food preferences (e.g., avoiding foods that are too spicy or too cold)	4. Food should be palatable and appealing	
5. Recognize effect of medication or radiation therapy on appetite	5. Many chemotherapeutic agents and radiation therapy promote anorexia	

Plan of Nursing Care — Chart 50-5. The Patient With Prostate Cancer, *Continued*

NURSING INTERVENTIONS	RATIONALE	EXPECTED OUTCOMES
6. Inform patient that alterations in taste can occur	6. Aging and the disease process can reduce taste sensitivity. In addition, smell and taste can be altered as a result of the body's absorption of by-products of cellular destruction (brought on by malignancy and its treatment)	
7. Use measures to control nausea and vomiting a. Administer prescribed antiemetics, around the clock if necessary b. Provide oral hygiene after vomiting episodes c. Provide rest periods after meals	7. Prevention of nausea and vomiting can stimulate appetite	
8. Provide frequent small meals and a comfortable and pleasant environment	8. Smaller portions of food are less overwhelming to the patient	
9. Assess patient's ability to obtain and prepare foods	9. Disability or lack of social support can hinder the patient's ability to obtain and prepare foods	
Nursing Priority: Sexual dysfunction **Goal:** Ability to resume/enjoy modified sexual functioning		
1. Determine from nursing history what effect patient's medical condition is having on his sexual functioning	1. Decreased libido and erectile dysfunction may be experienced	• Describes the reasons for changes in sexual functioning • Discusses with appropriate health care personnel alternative approaches and methods of sexual expression • Includes partner in discussions related to changes in sexual function
2. Inform patient of effects of prostate surgery, orchiectomy (when applicable), chemotherapy, irradiation, and hormonal therapy on sexual function	2. Treatment modalities may alter sexual function, but each is evaluated separately with regard to its effect on a particular patient	
3. Include his partner in developing understanding and in discovering alternative, satisfying close relations with each other	3. Bonds between a couple can be strengthened with new appreciation and support that had not been evident before the current illness	
Nursing Priority: Pain **Goal:** Relief of pain		
1. Evaluate nature of patient's pain, its location, and intensity using pain rating scale	1. Determining the nature and causes of pain and its intensity helps to select proper relief modality and provide a baseline for later comparison	• Reports relief of pain • Expects exacerbations, reports their quality and intensity, and obtains relief • Uses pain relief strategies appropriately and effectively • Identifies strategies to avoid complications of analgesic use
2. Avoid activities that aggravate or worsen pain	2. Bumping the bed is an example of an action that can intensify the patient's pain	
3. Because pain is usually related to bone metastasis, ensure that patient's bed has a bed board on a firm mattress. Also, protect patient from falls/injuries	3. This will provide added support and is more comfortable. Protecting the patient from injury protects him from additional pain	
4. Provide support for affected extremities	4. More support, coupled with reduced movement of the part, helps in pain control	
5. Prepare patient for radiation therapy if prescribed	5. Radiation therapy may be effective in controlling pain	
6. Administer analgesics or opioids at regularly scheduled intervals as prescribed	6. Analgesics alter the perception of pain and provide comfort. Regularly scheduled analgesics around the clock rather than as needed provide more consistent pain relief	
7. Initiate bowel program to prevent constipation	7. Opioid analgesics and inactivity contribute to constipation	

continued >

Plan of Nursing Care — Chart 50-5. The Patient With Prostate Cancer, *Continued*

Nursing Priority: Impaired physical mobility and activity intolerance
Goal: Improved physical mobility

NURSING INTERVENTIONS	RATIONALE	EXPECTED OUTCOMES
1. Assess for factors causing limited mobility (e.g., pain, hypercalcemia, limited exercise tolerance)	1. This information offers clues to the cause; if possible, the cause is treated	• Achieves improved physical mobility • Relates that short-term goals are encouraging him because they are attainable
2. Provide pain relief by administering prescribed medications	2. Analgesics/opioids allow the patient to increase his activity more comfortably	
3. Encourage use of assistive devices: cane, walker	3. Support may offer the security needed to become mobile	
4. Involve significant others in helping patient with range-of-motion exercises, positioning, and walking	4. Assistance from the partner or others encourages the patient to repeat activities and achieve goals	
5. Provide positive reinforcement for achievement of small gains	5. Encouragement stimulates improvement of performance	
6. Assess nutritional status	6. See Nursing Diagnosis: Imbalanced Nutrition (less than body requirements)	

Collaborative Problems: Hemorrhage, infection, bladder neck obstruction
Goal: Absence of complications

NURSING INTERVENTIONS	RATIONALE	EXPECTED OUTCOMES
1. Alert the patient to changes that may occur (after discharge) and that need to be reported:	1. Certain changes signal early complications, requiring nursing and medical interventions.	• Experiences no bleeding or passage of blood clots • Reports no pain around the catheter • Experiences normal frequency of urination • Reports normal urinary output • Maintains bladder control
a. Continued bloody urine; passing blood clots	a. Hematuria with or without blood clot formation may occur postoperatively	
b. Pain; burning around catheter	b. Indwelling urinary catheters may be a source of infections	
c. Frequency of urination	c. Urinary frequency may be caused by urinary tract infections or by bladder neck obstruction, resulting in incomplete voiding	
d. Diminished urinary output	d. Bladder neck obstruction decreases the amount of urine that is voided	
e. Increasing loss of bladder control	e. Urinary incontinence may be a result of urinary retention	

suppression. Cyproterone acetate (Androcur) is a synthetic progesterone derivative that provides effective, competitive inhibition of androgens at the target cells. In contrast to estrogen, the newer hormonal agents are associated with a lower incidence of cardiovascular side effects, gynecomastia, and decreased sexual function. Side effects experienced by men undergoing hormonal therapy can include hot flashes, mood swings, altered libido, fatigue, gynecomastia, osteoporosis, and loss of muscle mass (Malik, 2014).

Other Therapies

For men with advanced prostate cancer, palliative measures are indicated. Although cure is unlikely with advanced prostate cancer, many men survive for long intervals apparently free of metastatic disease. If prostate cancer metastasizes to the bones, these bone lesions can be very painful. Opioid and nonopioid medications are used to control the pain. In addition, external beam radiation therapy can be delivered to skeletal lesions to relieve pain. Radiopharmaceuticals, such as strontium 89 and samarium 153, can also be intravenously injected to treat multiple sites of bone metastases. If antiandrogen therapies are not effective, medications such as prednisone and mitoxantrone may reduce pain and improve quality of life. With advanced prostate cancer, blood transfusions are administered to maintain adequate hemoglobin levels when bone marrow is replaced by tumour.

Chemotherapy

Prior to 2004 there were no treatments available to improve the survival rate for men with metastatic prostate cancer. Chemotherapy may be used in certain cases to treat metastatic prostate cancer (Turner & Drudge-Coates, 2012). The standard of care is to use docetaxel 75 mg/m^2

plus prednisone 5 mg BID. Using this type of chemotherapy has improved quality of life, overall pain reduction, and overall survival for approximately 18 months (Drudge-Coates & Turner, 2012a). Several other medications are under development for men with advanced prostate cancer and are in trial phases.

Naturopathic or nutritional supplements are used by many patients who have been diagnosed with cancer (Braun, Gupta, Birdsall, et al., 2013). PCC (2013d) explains that alternative therapies can sometimes be used in place of conventional treatment options. At this time alternative therapies are considered scientifically unproven treatments.

Patients should be encouraged to speak with their physician if they want to choose this route (Braun et al., 2013).

Nursing Process

The Patient Undergoing Prostatectomy

Prostate surgery may be indicated for the patient with BPH or prostate cancer. The objectives before prostate surgery are to assess the patient's general health status and to establish optimal renal function. Prostate surgery should be performed before acute urinary retention develops and damages the upper urinary tract and collecting system or, in the case of prostate cancer, before cancer progresses.

Assessment

The nurse assesses how the underlying disorder (BPH or prostate cancer) has affected the patient's lifestyle. Has he been reasonably active for his age? What is his presenting urinary concern (described in his own words)? Has he experienced decreased force of urinary flow, decreased ability to initiate voiding, urgency, frequency, nocturia, dysuria, urinary retention, or hematuria? Does the patient report associated issues, such as back pain, flank pain, and lower abdominal or suprapubic discomfort? If he reports such discomfort, possible causes include infection, retention, and renal colic. Has he experienced ED or changes in frequency or enjoyment of sexual activity?

The nurse obtains further information about the patient's family history of cancer and heart or kidney disease, including hypertension. Has he lost weight? Does he appear pale? Can he raise himself out of bed and return to bed without assistance? Can he perform usual activities of daily living? This information will help in determining how soon he will return to normal activities after prostatectomy.

Preoperative Nursing Priorities

Based on assessment data, the patient's major preoperative nursing priorities may include the following:

- Anxiety about surgery and its outcome
- Acute pain related to bladder distention
- Deficient knowledge about factors related to the disorder and the treatment protocol

Postoperative Nursing Priorities

Based on assessment data, the patient's major postoperative nursing priorities may include the following:

- Acute pain related to surgical incision, catheter placement, and bladder spasms
- Deficient knowledge about postoperative care and management

Collaborative Problems/ Potential Complications

Based on assessment data, the potential complications may include the following:

- Hemorrhage and shock
- Infection
- Deep vein thrombosis (DVT)
- Catheter obstruction
- Sexual dysfunction
- Urinary incontinence

Planning and Goals

The major preoperative goals for the patient may include reduced anxiety and learning about his prostate disorder and the perioperative experience. The major postoperative goals may include maintenance of fluid volume balance, relief of pain and discomfort, ability to perform self-care activities, and absence of complications.

Preoperative Nursing Interventions

Reducing Anxiety

The patient is frequently admitted to the hospital on the morning of surgery. Because contact with the patient may be limited before surgery, the nurse must establish communication with the patient to assess his understanding of the diagnosis and the planned surgical procedure. The nurse clarifies the nature of the surgery and expected postoperative outcomes. In addition, the nurse familiarizes the patient with the pre- and postoperative routines and initiates measures to reduce anxiety. Because the patient may be sensitive and embarrassed discussing issues and concerns related to the genitalia and sexuality, the nurse provides privacy and establishes a trusting and professional relationship. He is encouraged to verbalize his feelings and concerns.

Relieving Discomfort

If discomfort is present before the day of surgery because of urinary obstruction, analgesic agents are administered and measures to relieve anxiety are initiated. If the patient is hospitalized, the nurse monitors the patient's voiding patterns, evaluates bladder distention, and assists with catheterization if indicated.

An indwelling catheter is inserted if the patient has continuing urinary retention or if laboratory test results indicate azotemia. For a few days after the bladder begins draining, the blood pressure may fluctuate and renal function may decline. If the patient cannot tolerate a urinary catheter, he is prepared for a cystostomy (see Chapters 45 and 46).

Providing Instruction

Before surgery, the nurse reviews with the patient the anatomy of the urinary and reproductive system, using diagrams and other teaching aids if indicated. This is often done either during the preadmission testing visit or in the urologist's office. The nurse explains what will take place as the patient is prepared for diagnostic tests and then for surgery (depending on the kind of prostatectomy planned). The nurse describes the type of incision, which varies with the type of surgical approach. The patient is informed about the type of urinary drainage system that is expected, the type of anesthesia, and the recovery room procedure. The amount of information given is based on the patient's needs and questions. Procedures expected during the immediate perioperative period are explained, questions are answered, and support is provided. In addition, the patient is instructed about postoperative use of medications for pain management.

Preparing the Patient

Preoperative preparation is described in Chapter 19. Elastic compression stockings are applied before surgery and are particularly important for prevention of DVT if the patient is placed in a lithotomy position during surgery. An enema is usually administered at home the evening before surgery or the morning of surgery to prevent postoperative straining, which can induce bleeding.

Postoperative Nursing Interventions

Maintaining Fluid Balance

During the postoperative period after TURP, the patient is at risk for imbalanced fluid volume because of the irrigation of the surgical site during and after surgery. With continuous bladder irrigation (CBI) of the urinary catheter to prevent its obstruction by blood clots, fluid may be absorbed through the open surgical site and retained, increasing the risk for excessive fluid retention, fluid imbalance, and water intoxication (called *TURP syndrome*). The urine output and the amount of fluid used for irrigation must be closely monitored. The patient is also monitored for electrolyte imbalances (i.e., hyponatremia), rising blood pressure, confusion, and respiratory distress. The risk for fluid and electrolyte imbalance is increased in older adult patients with pre-existing cardiovascular or respiratory disease. These signs and symptoms are documented and reported to the surgeon immediately.

Relieving Pain

After a prostatectomy, the patient is assisted to sit and dangle his legs over the side of the bed on the day of surgery. The next morning, he is assisted to ambulate. If pain occurs, the cause and location are determined. It may be related to the incision or may be the result of excoriation of the skin at the catheter site. It may be in the flank area, indicating a kidney condition, or it may be due to bladder spasms. Bladder irritability can initiate bleeding and result in clot formation, leading to urinary retention.

Patients experiencing bladder spasms may note an urgency to void, a feeling of pressure or fullness in the bladder, and bleeding from the urethra around the catheter. Anticholinergic medications, such as oxybutynin, that relax the smooth muscles can help to ease the spasms, which can be intermittent and severe. Warm compresses to the pubis may also relieve the spasms.

The nurse monitors the drainage tubing and irrigates the system as prescribed to relieve any obstruction that may cause discomfort. Usually, the catheter is irrigated with 50 mL of irrigating fluid at a time. It is important to make sure that the same amount is recovered in the drainage receptacle. Securing the catheter drainage tubing to the leg or abdomen can help to decrease tension on the catheter and prevent bladder irritation. Discomfort may be caused by dressings that are too snug, saturated with drainage, or improperly placed. Analgesic agents are administered as prescribed.

When ambulatory, the patient is encouraged to walk but not to sit for prolonged periods, as this increases intra-abdominal pressure and the possibility of discomfort and bleeding. Prune juice and stool softeners are provided to ease bowel movements and to prevent excessive straining. An enema, if prescribed, is administered with caution to avoid rectal perforation.

Monitoring and Managing Potential Complications

After prostatectomy, the patient is monitored for major complications such as hemorrhage, infection, DVT, and catheter obstruction.

HEMORRHAGE. The immediate dangers after a prostatectomy are bleeding and hemorrhagic shock. This risk is increased with BPH because a hyperplastic prostate gland is very vascular. Bleeding may occur from the prostatic bed. Bleeding may also result in the formation of clots, which then obstruct urine flow. The urine drainage normally begins as reddish-pink and then clears to a light pink within 24 hours after surgery. Bright-red bleeding with increased viscosity and numerous clots usually indicates arterial bleeding. Venous blood appears darker and less viscous. Arterial hemorrhage usually requires surgical intervention (e.g., suturing of bleeders or transurethral coagulation of bleeding vessels), whereas venous bleeding may be controlled by applying prescribed traction to the catheter so that the balloon holding the catheter in place applies pressure to the prostatic fossa. The surgeon applies traction by securely taping the catheter to the patient's thigh.

Nursing management includes strategies to stop the bleeding and to prevent or reverse hemorrhagic shock. If blood loss is extensive, fluids and blood component therapy may be administered. If hemorrhagic shock occurs, treatments described in Chapter 18 are initiated.

Nursing interventions include close monitoring of vital signs; administering medications, intravenous fluids, and blood component therapy as prescribed; maintaining an accurate record of intake and output; and careful monitoring of drainage to ensure adequate urine flow and patency of the drainage system. The patient who experiences hemorrhage and his family are often anxious and benefit from explanations and reassurance about the event and the procedures that are performed.

INFECTION. After perineal prostatectomy, the surgeon usually changes the dressing on the first postoperative day. Further dressing changes may become the nurse's responsibility. Careful aseptic technique is used because the possibility for infection is high. Dressings can be held in place by a double-tailed, T-binder bandage or a padded athletic supporter. The tails cross over the incision to give double thickness and then each tail is drawn up on either side of the scrotum to the waistline and fastened.

Rectal thermometers, rectal tubes, and enemas are avoided because of the risk for injury to and bleeding in the prostatic fossa. After the perineal sutures are removed, the perineum is cleansed as indicated. Sitz baths are also used to promote healing.

Urinary tract infections and epididymitis are possible complications after prostatectomy. The patient is assessed for their occurrence; if they occur, the nurse administers antibiotics as prescribed.

Because the risk for infection continues after discharge from the hospital, the patient and family need to be instructed on the signs and symptoms of infection (fever, chills, sweats, myalgias, dysuria, urinary frequency, and urgency). The patient and family are instructed to contact the urologist if these symptoms occur.

DEEP VEIN THROMBOSIS. Because patients undergoing prostatectomy have a high incidence of DVT and pulmonary embolism, the physician may prescribe prophylactic (preventive) low-dose heparin therapy. The nurse assesses the patient frequently after surgery for manifestations of DVT and applies elastic compression stockings to reduce the risk for DVT and pulmonary embolism. Nursing and medical management of DVT and pulmonary embolism are detailed in Chapters 32 and 24, respectively. The patient who is receiving heparin must be closely monitored for excessive bleeding.

OBSTRUCTED CATHETER. After a TURP, the catheter must drain well; an obstructed catheter produces distention of the prostatic capsule and resultant hemorrhage. Furosemide (Lasix) may be prescribed to promote urination and initiate postoperative diuresis, thereby helping to keep the catheter patent.

The nurse observes the lower abdomen to ensure that the catheter has not become blocked. An overdistended bladder presents a distinct, rounded swelling above the pubis.

The drainage bag, dressings, and incisional site are examined for bleeding. The colour of the urine is noted and documented; a change in colour from pink to amber indicates reduced bleeding. Blood pressure, pulse, and respirations are monitored and compared with baseline preoperative vital signs to detect hypotension. The nurse also observes the patient for restlessness, cold sweats, pallor, any drop in blood pressure, and an increasing pulse rate.

Drainage of the bladder may be accomplished by gravity through a closed sterile drainage system. A *three-way drainage* system is used to irrigate the bladder and prevent clot formation (Fig. 50-5). Continuous or intermittent irrigation may be used. Gentle manual irrigation of the catheter may be prescribed to remove any obstructing clots.

If the patient complains of pain, the tubing is examined. The drainage system is irrigated, if indicated and prescribed, to clear any obstruction. Usually, the catheter is irrigated with 50 mL of irrigating fluid at a time. The amount of fluid recovered in the drainage bag must equal the amount of fluid injected. Overdistention of the bladder is avoided because it can induce secondary hemorrhage by stretching the coagulated blood vessels in the prostatic capsule.

The drainage tube or catheter is taped to the shaved inner thigh to prevent traction on the bladder. If a cystostomy catheter is in place, it is taped to the abdomen. The nurse explains the purpose of the catheter to the patient and assures him that the urge

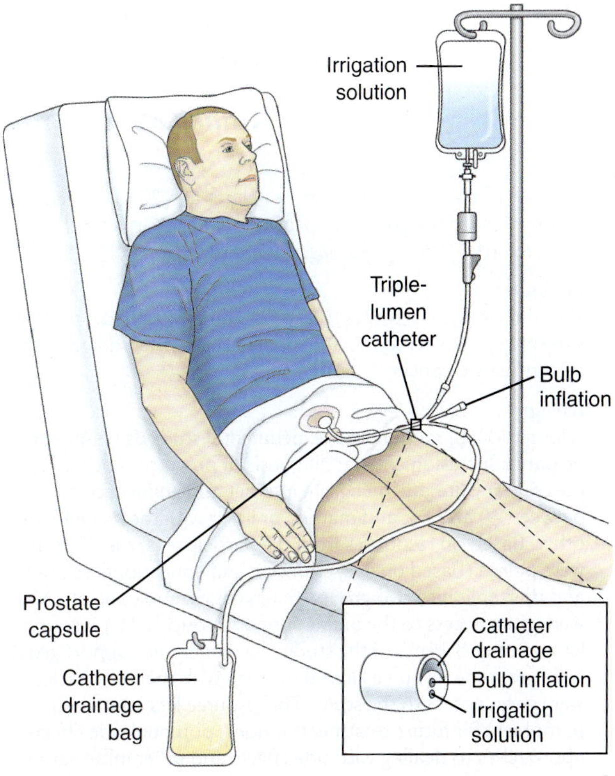

FIGURE 50-5. A three-way system for bladder irrigation.

to void results from the presence of the catheter and from bladder spasms. He is cautioned not to pull on the catheter, as this causes bleeding and subsequent catheter blockage, which leads to urinary retention.

COMPLICATIONS WITH CATHETER REMOVAL. After the catheter is removed (usually when the urine appears clear), urine may leak around the wound for several days in patients who have undergone perineal, suprapubic, and retropubic surgery. The cystostomy tube may be removed before or after the urethral catheter is removed. Some urinary incontinence may occur after catheter removal, and the patient is informed that this is likely to subside in time.

SEXUAL DYSFUNCTION. Depending on the type of surgery, the patient may experience sexual dysfunction related to ED, decreased libido, and fatigue. These issues may become a concern of the patient soon after surgery or in the weeks to months during rehabilitation. Reassurance that the usual level of libido will return following recuperation from surgery is often helpful to the patient and his partner. The patient may also experience fatigue during rehabilitation from surgery. This fatigue may also decrease his libido and alter his enjoyment of usual activities.

Nursing interventions include assessing for the presence of sexual dysfunction following surgery. Providing a private and confidential environment to discuss issues of sexuality is important. The emotional challenges of prostate surgery and its consequences need to be carefully explored with the patient and his partner. Providing the opportunity to discuss these issues can be very beneficial to the patient (Chart 50-6).

Promoting Home, Community-Based, and Transitional Care

EDUCATING PATIENTS ABOUT SELF-CARE. Men undergoing prostatectomy may be discharged within 3 to 4 days or less. The length of the hospital stay depends on the type of prostatectomy performed. Patients undergoing a perineal prostatectomy are hospitalized for 3 to 5 days. If a retropubic or suprapubic prostatectomy is performed, the hospital stay is 5 to 7 days. The patient and family require instructions about how to manage the drainage system, how to assess for complications, and how to promote recovery. Verbal and written instructions are provided about the need to maintain the drainage system and to monitor urinary output; about wound care; and about strategies to prevent complications, such as infection, bleeding, and thrombosis. They are informed about signs and symptoms that should be reported to the physician (e.g., blood in urine, decreased urine output, fever, change in wound drainage, calf tenderness).

As the patient recovers and drainage tubes are removed, he may become discouraged and depressed because he does not immediately regain bladder control. Moreover, urinary frequency and burning may occur after the catheter is removed. Teaching the following exercises, known as pelvic floor muscle exercises, may help the patient regain urinary control:

- Tighten the pelvic floor by tensing the muscles around the rectum as if trying to stop from passing gas. The buttocks, thighs, and stomach should stay relaxed. If the penis twitches and contracts inward slightly, the patient is tightening the correct muscles.

NURSING RESEARCH PROFILE

Chart 50-6. Impact of Prostate Cancer

Osei, D. K., Lee, J. W., Modest, N. N., et al. (2013). Effects of an online support group for prostate cancer survivors: A randomized trial. *Urologic Nursing, 33*(3), 123–133.

Purpose

The aim of this study was to explore the effects of an on-line support system on the quality of life among men diagnosed with prostate cancer.

Design

A longitudinal, randomized, experimental study using 40 participants. Inclusion criteria: diagnosis of prostate cancer in the past 5 years; literate in English, internet and email access; between 40 and 85; and married or living with their significant other. Based on responses from the participants, the 40 men were paired (based on age, ethnicity, and educational status) and then split into two groups (intervention and control). Men were given access to the online support group or to a resource kit and after 8 weeks of the study, the men in the support group were given the resource kit and the men with the resource kit were given access to the study. The resource kits contained pamphlets for future treatment options, potential side effects, approaches to dealing with side effects and other information.

After the baseline data was completed, Cronbach's alphas were calculated for 10 quality-of-life scales. This included SF-12 (physical health and mental health), EPIC-26 (urinary obstruction, urinary incontinence, bowels, sexual and hormonal). The Satisfaction with Life (life satisfaction and MIDUS [relationship satisfaction]).

Findings

Overall, the intervention group experienced improvement in urinary retention and obstruction health, sexual health, and hormonal health. In contrast, the control group reported quality of life had dropped on six quality-of-life measures: physical health, perceived sexual health, hormonal health, life satisfaction, and spouse negative characteristics.

Nursing Implications

Although more research is needed, online support groups do have some positive impact on perceived quality of life and recovery process. In the future, nurses could consider studying the differences between face to face groups and internet support groups. Because the internet has become such a part of our day to day lives, potential is enormous.

- Squeeze firmly for 5 to 10 seconds per contraction
- Try to perform 10 to 12 contractions two to three times a day, relaxing the muscle for 10 to 20 seconds between each contraction

Pelvic floor muscle exercises should continue until the patient gains full urinary control. The patient is instructed to urinate as soon as he feels the first urge to do so. It is important for the patient to know that regaining urinary control is a gradual process; he may continue to "dribble" after being discharged from the hospital, but the dribbling should gradually diminish (within up to 1 year). Lining underwear with absorbent pads can help to minimize embarrassing stains on clothing. The urine may be cloudy for several weeks after surgery but should clear as the prostate area heals.

While the prostatic fossa heals (6 to 8 weeks), the patient should avoid activities that produce Valsalva effects (straining at stool, heavy lifting) because this increases venous pressure and may produce hematuria. He should avoid long motor trips and strenuous exercise, which increase the tendency to bleed. He should also know that spicy foods, alcohol, and coffee may cause bladder discomfort. The patient is cautioned to drink enough fluids to avoid dehydration and thus decrease the risk for a blood clot to form and obstruct the flow of urine. Signs of complications, such as bleeding, passage of blood clots, a decrease in the urinary stream, urinary retention, or urinary tract infection symptoms, should be reported to the physician (Chart 50-7).

CONTINUING AND TRANSITIONAL CARE. Referral for home, community-based, or transitional care may be indicated if the patient is an older adult or has other health problems, if the patient and family cannot provide care in the home, or if the patient lives alone without available supports. The home care nurse assesses the patient's physical status (cardiovascular and respiratory status, fluid and nutritional status, patency of the urinary drainage system, wound and nutritional status) and provides catheter and wound care, if indicated. The nurse reinforces previous teaching and assesses the ability of the patient and family to manage required care. The home care nurse encourages the patient to ambulate and to carry out pelvic floor muscle exercises as prescribed. The patient may

CHART 50-7

HOME CARE CHECKLIST • Postprostatectomy Care

At the completion of education, the patient and/or caregiver will be able to:

- Name the procedure that was performed and identify any permanent changes in anatomic structure or function as well as changes in ADLs, IADLs, roles, relationships, and spirituality.
- Locate list of names and telephone numbers of resource personnel involved in care (e.g., health care professionals, home care nurse, urinary catheter/dressing supply vendor).
- Identify the equipment necessary and how to obtain medical supplies to carry out dressing changes, wound care, and other prescribed regimens.
- Describe ongoing postoperative therapeutic regimen, including diet and activities to perform (e.g., increased activity and ambulation, perineal exercises) and to limit or avoid (e.g., lifting weights, driving a car, contact sports).
  - Describe measures to relieve postoperative pain and discomfort (e.g., take analgesics as prescribed; use nonpharmacologic interventions).
  - Demonstrate appropriate care of urinary catheter and collection receptacle.
  - Demonstrate appropriate dressing change/wound care.
  - When appropriate, demonstrate performance of perineal muscle exercises to facilitate bladder control.
- State the name, dose, side effects, frequency, and schedule for all medications.
- Identify signs and symptoms of complications that should be reported to the surgeon (e.g., decreased output, blood or clots in urine or urine drainage system, change in wound drainage, fever or symptoms of urinary tract infections, calf tenderness).
- Explain treatment plan and importance of follow-up care to all health care providers.
  - State time and date of follow-up appointments, therapy, and testing.
- Identify community resources for peer and caregiver/family support:
  - Identify sources of support (e.g., friends, relatives, faith community).
  - Identify phone numbers of support groups for people with cancer and their caregivers/families.
- State meeting locations and times for support groups.
- Identify the need for health promotion, disease prevention, and screening activities.

ADL, activities of daily living; IADL, independent activities of daily living.

need to be reminded that return of bladder control may take time.

The patient is reminded about the importance of participating in routine health screening and other health promotion activities. If the prostatectomy was performed to treat prostate cancer, the patient and family are also instructed about the importance of follow-up and monitoring with the physician.

Evaluation

Expected preoperative patient outcomes may include the following:

1. Demonstrates reduced anxiety
2. States that pain and discomfort are decreased
3. Relates understanding of surgical procedure and postoperative course and practices pelvic floor muscle exercises and other techniques useful in facilitating bladder control

Expected postoperative patient outcomes may include the following:

1. Relates relief of discomfort
2. Exhibits fluid and electrolyte balance
    a. Irrigation fluid and urinary output within parameters determined by surgeon
    b. Experiences no signs or symptoms of fluid retention
3. Participates in self-care measures
    a. Increases activity and ambulation daily
    b. Produces urine output within normal ranges and consistent with intake
    c. Performs pelvic floor muscle exercises and interrupts urinary stream to promote bladder control
    d. Avoids straining and lifting heavy objects
4. Is free of complications
    a. Maintains vital signs within normal limits
    b. Exhibits wound healing, without signs of inflammation or hemorrhage
    c. Maintains acceptable level of urinary elimination
    d. Maintains optimal drainage of catheter and other drainage tubes
    e. Reports understanding of changes in sexual function

DISORDERS AFFECTING THE TESTES AND ADJACENT STRUCTURES

Undescended Testis (Cryptorchidism)

Cryptorchidism is a congenital condition characterized by failure of one or both of the testes to descend into the scrotum. One or both testes may be absent. The testis may be located in the abdominal cavity or inguinal canal. If the testis does not descend as the boy matures, a surgical procedure known as orchiopexy is performed to position it properly. An incision is made over the inguinal canal, and the testis is brought down and anchored in the scrotum.

Orchitis

Orchitis is an inflammation of the testes (testicular congestion) caused by pyogenic, viral, spirochetal, parasitic, traumatic, chemical, or unknown factors. Mumps is one such factor. Mumps vaccination is recommended for postpubertal men who have not been infected. When postpubertal men contract mumps, about one in five develops some form of orchitis 4 to 7 days after the jaw and neck swell. The testis may show some atrophy. In the past, sterility and impotence often resulted. Today, a man who has never had mumps and who is exposed to the disease receives gamma globulin immediately; the disease is likely to be less severe, with minimal or no complications.

Medical Management

If the cause of orchitis is bacterial, viral, or fungal, therapy is directed at the specific infecting organism. Rest, elevation of the scrotum, ice packs to reduce scrotal edema, antibiotics, analgesic agents, and anti-inflammatory medications are recommended.

Epididymitis

Epididymitis is an infection of the epididymis that usually descends from an infected prostate or urinary tract. It may also develop as a complication of gonorrhea. In men younger than 35 years, the major cause of epididymitis is *Chlamydia trachomatis*. The infection passes upward through the urethra and the ejaculatory duct and then along the vas deferens to the epididymis.

The patient complains of unilateral pain and soreness in the inguinal canal along the course of the vas deferens and then develops pain and swelling in the scrotum and the groin. The epididymis becomes swollen and extremely painful; the patient's temperature is elevated. The urine may contain pus (pyuria) and bacteria (bacteriuria), and the patient may experience chills and fever.

Medical Management

If the patient is seen within the first 24 hours after onset of pain, the spermatic cord may be infiltrated with a local anesthetic agent to relieve pain. If the epididymitis is from a chlamydial infection, the patient and his sexual partner must be treated with antibiotics. The patient is observed for abscess formation as well. If no improvement occurs within 2 weeks, an underlying testicular tumour should be considered. An epididymectomy (excision of the epididymis from the testis) may be performed for patients with recurrent, incapacitating episodes of epididymitis or for those with chronic, painful conditions. With long-term epididymitis, the passage of sperm may be obstructed. If the obstruction is bilateral, infertility may result.

Nursing Management

The patient is placed on bed rest, and the scrotum is elevated with a scrotal bridge or folded towel to prevent traction on the spermatic cord and to promote venous drainage and relieve pain. Antimicrobial agents are administered as prescribed until the acute inflammation subsides. Intermittent cold compresses to the scrotum may help to ease the pain. Later, local heat or sitz baths may help to resolve the inflammation. Analgesic medications are administered for pain relief as prescribed.

The nurse instructs the patient to avoid straining, lifting, and sexual stimulation until the infection is under control. He should continue taking analgesic agents and antibiotics as prescribed and using ice packs if necessary to relieve discomfort. He needs to know that it may take 4 weeks or longer for the epididymis to return to normal.

Testicular Cancer

Testicular cancer is the most common cancer in Canadian adolescents and men 15 to 29 years of age. In 2013, there were approximately 940 cases of testicular cancer diagnosed. Although testicular cancer occurs most often between age 15 and 40 years, it can occur in males of any age. It is one of the most curable forms of cancer in Canada. If found and treated early there is a 95% cure rate and a 96% longer-term survival rate (Movember Canada, 2014).

The testicles contain several types of cells, each of which may develop into one or more types of cancer. It typically presents as a small hard lump, which may produce swelling or a change in the consistency of the testicle (Movember Canada, 2014). The type of cancer determines the appropriate treatment and affects the prognosis. Testicular cancers are classified as germinal or nongerminal (stromal); secondary testicular cancers may also occur.

Classification of Testicular Tumours

Germinal Tumours

Over 90% of all cancers of the testicle are germinal; **germinal tumours** may be further classified as seminomas or nonseminomas. About half of all germinal tumours are seminomas, or tumours that develop from the sperm-producing cells of the testes. *Nonseminoma germinal cell tumours* tend to develop earlier in life than seminomas, usually occurring in men in their 20s. Examples of nonseminomas include teratocarcinomas, choriocarcinomas, yolk sac carcinomas, and embryonal carcinomas. *Seminomas* tend to remain localized, whereas nonseminomatous tumours grow quickly.

Nongerminal Tumours

Testicular cancer may also develop in the supportive and hormone-producing tissues, or stroma, of the testicles. These tumours account for about 4% of testicular tumours in adults and 20% of testicular tumours in children. The two main types of **stromal tumours** are *Leydig cell tumours* and *Sertoli cell tumours*. Although these tumours infrequently spread beyond the testicle, a small number of these tumours metastasize and tend to be resistant to chemotherapy and radiation therapy.

Secondary Testicular Tumours

Secondary testicular tumours are those that have **metastasized** to the testicle from other organs. *Lymphoma* is the most common cause of secondary testicular cancer. Cancers may also spread to the testicles from the prostate gland, lung, skin (melanoma), kidney, and other organs. The prognosis for these cancers is usually poor, as these cancers generally also spread to other organs. Treatment depends on the specific type of cancer.

Risk Factors

Risk factors for testicular cancer include undescended testicles (cryptorchidism), a family history of testicular cancer, and cancer of one testicle, which increases the risk in the other testicle. Race and ethnicity have been identified as risk factors. For example, white Canadian men have a five times greater risk than that of Black Canadian men and more than double the risk of Asian Canadian men. Occupational hazards, including exposure to chemicals encountered in mining, oil and gas production, and leather processing, have been suggested as possible risk factors.

Clinical Manifestations

Men with testicular cancer may experience few or no symptoms. The symptoms of testicular cancer appear gradually, with a mass or lump on the testicle and generally painless enlargement of the testis (Movember Canada, 2014). The patient may complain of heaviness in the scrotum, inguinal area, or lower abdomen. Back ache (from retroperitoneal node extension), abdominal pain, weight loss, and general weakness may result from metastasis. Enlargement of the testis without pain is a significant diagnostic finding. Testicular tumours tend to metastasize early, spreading from the testis to the lymph nodes in the retroperitoneum and to the lungs. Sexual function and fertility are quality-of-life issues that are also associated with testicular cancer (Kim, McGlynn, McCorkle, et al., 2012).

Assessment and Diagnostic Findings

Monthly TSEs are effective in detecting testicular cancer (Chart 50-8). Teaching men of all ages to perform TSE is an important health promotion intervention for early detection of testicular cancer. Since testicular cancer occurs most often in young adults, TSE should begin during adolescence.

Human chorionic gonadotropin and alpha-fetoprotein are tumour markers that may be elevated in patients with testicular cancer. (Tumour markers are substances synthesized by the tumour cells and released into the circulation in abnormal amounts.) Tumour marker levels in the blood are used for diagnosis, staging, and monitoring the response to treatment. Other diagnostic tests include intravenous urography to detect any ureteral deviation caused by a tumour mass; lymphangiography to assess the extent of tumour spread to the lymphatic system; ultrasound to determine the presence and size of the testicular mass; and CT scan of the chest, abdomen, and pelvis to determine the extent of the disease in the lungs, retroperitoneum, and pelvis. Microscopic analysis of tissue is the only definitive way to determine if cancer is present but is usually performed at the time of surgery rather than as a part of the diagnostic workup to reduce the risk of promoting spread of the cancer.

CHART 50-8

Patient Education

Testicular Self-Examination

Testicular self-examination (TSE) is to be performed once a month. The test is neither difficult nor time-consuming. A convenient time is usually after a warm bath or shower, when the scrotum is more relaxed.

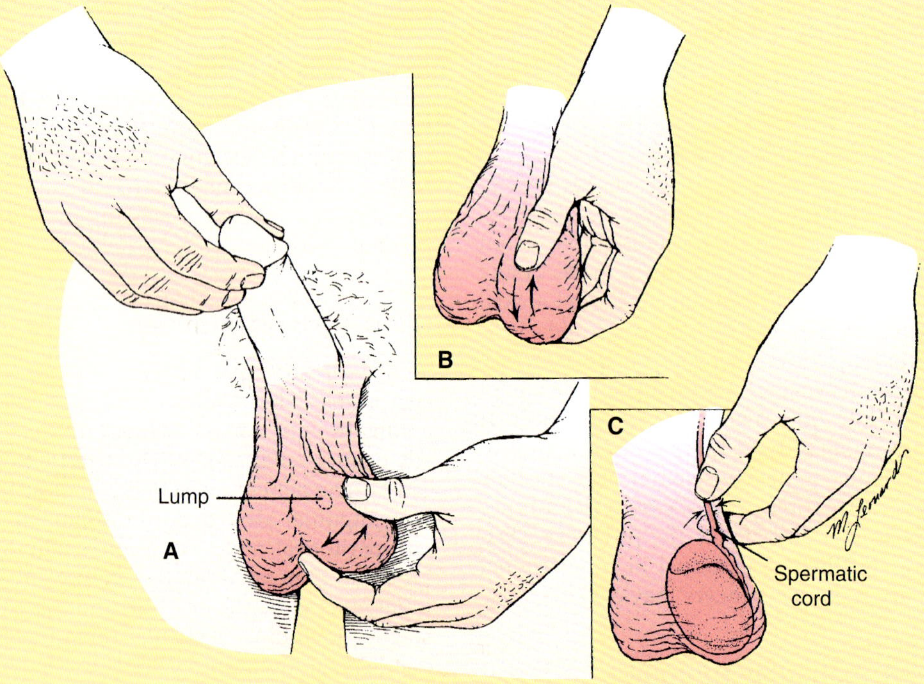

1. Use both hands to palpate the testis. The normal testicle is smooth and uniform in consistency.
2. With the index and middle fingers under the testis and the thumb on top, roll the testis gently in a horizontal plane between the thumb and fingers (**A**).
3. Feel for any evidence of a small lump or abnormality.
4. Follow the same procedure and palpate upward along the testis (**B**).
5. Locate and palpate the epididymis (**C**), a cordlike structure on the top and back of the testicle that stores and transports sperm. Also locate and palpate the spermatic cord.
6. Repeat the examination for the other testis, epididymis, and spermatic cord. It is normal to find that one testis is larger than the other.
7. If you find any evidence of a small, pea-like lump or if the testis is swollen (possibly from an infection or tumour), consult your physician.

Adapted from Weber, J. R., & Kelley, J. H. (2014). *Health assessment in nursing* (5th ed.). Philadelphia, PA: Lippincott Williams & Wilkins.

Medical Management

Testicular cancer is one of the most curable solid tumours. The goals of management are to eradicate the disease and achieve a cure. Treatment selection is based on the cell type and the anatomic extent of the disease. The testis is removed by orchiectomy through an inguinal incision with a high ligation of the spermatic cord. A gel-filled prosthesis can be implanted. After unilateral orchiectomy for testicular cancer, most patients experience no impairment of endocrine function. Some patients, however, have decreased hormonal levels, suggesting that the unaffected testis is not functioning at normal levels. Retroperitoneal lymph node dissection (RPLND) may be performed after orchiectomy to prevent lymphatic spread of the cancer. Laparoscopic RPLND (L-RPLND) has become a preferred alternative to the more invasive open RPLND for early-stage nonseminomatous germ cell testicular cancer. Patients who underwent L-RPLND had decreased morbidity, hospital stay, and time to return to normal activity. Although libido and orgasm are usually unimpaired after RPLND, the patient may develop ejaculatory dysfunction with resultant infertility.

As stated previously, testicular cancers are classified as either seminomas or nonseminomas for determining treatment; seminomatous types are more sensitive to radiation therapy. Research has demonstrated that for stage IIA/B seminomas, radiation therapy alone provides excellent results for the majority of patients. Postoperative irradiation of the lymph nodes from the diaphragm to the iliac region is used to treat seminomas. Radiation is delivered only to the affected side; the other testis is shielded from radiation to preserve fertility. Radiation is also used for patients whose disease does not respond to chemotherapy and those for whom lymph node surgery is not recommended. Lymphangiography and CT are used to determine spread of the disease to the lymph nodes.

Chemotherapy is reserved for the treatment of stage IIC testicular cancer as well as more advanced stages. The standard treatment for testicular germ cell cancer includes bleomycin, etoposide, and cisplatin (Bradford, 2012). This regimen results in a high percentage of complete remissions. Good results may be obtained by combining different types of treatment, including surgery, radiation therapy, and chemotherapy. Even with disseminated testicular cancer, the prognosis is favourable, and the disease is probably curable because of advances in diagnosis and treatment. Patients who undergo chemotherapy should discuss fertility options with their physician. Sperm cryopreservation is the only choice available at this time for conserving fertility in men with cancer (Bradford, 2012).

A patient with a history of one testicular tumour has a greater chance of developing subsequent tumours. The most common site of recurrence is the retroperitoneum. Follow-up studies include chest x-rays, excretory urography, radioimmunoassay of human chorionic gonadotropins and alpha-fetoprotein levels, and examination of lymph nodes to detect recurrent malignancy.

Long-term side effects associated with chemotherapy or radiation treatment for testicular cancer include kidney damage, hearing issues, gonadal damage, neurologic changes, and rarely secondary cancers. Chemotherapy has improved survival rates among patients with testicular cancer, giving it the highest cure rate of any solid tumour cancer.

Nursing Management

Nursing management includes assessment of the patient's physical and psychological status and monitoring the patient for response to and possible effects of surgery, chemotherapy, and radiation therapy (see Chapter 68). Pre- and postoperative care is described in Chapters 19 and 21, respectively. In addition, because the patient may have difficulty coping with his condition, issues related to body image and sexuality are addressed. He needs encouragement to maintain a positive attitude during what may be a long course of therapy. He also needs to know that radiation therapy will not necessarily prevent him from fathering children, nor does unilateral excision of a testis necessarily decrease virility. The nurse reminds the patient about the importance of performing TSE and keeping follow-up appointments with the physician. The patient is also encouraged to participate in health promotion and health screening activities.

Hydrocele

A **hydrocele** is a collection of fluid, generally in the tunica vaginalis of the testis, although it may also collect within the spermatic cord. The tunica vaginalis becomes widely distended with fluid. Hydrocele can be differentiated from a hernia by transillumination; a hydrocele transmits light, whereas a hernia does not. Hydrocele may be acute or chronic. Acute hydrocele may occur in association with acute infectious diseases of the epididymis or as a result of local injury or systemic infectious diseases, such as mumps. The cause of chronic hydrocele is unknown. Ultrasonography is recommended for large hydroceles to differentiate them from testicular tumours (Crawford, 2014).

Usually, therapy is not required. Treatment is necessary only if the hydrocele becomes tense and compromises testicular circulation or if the scrotal mass becomes large, uncomfortable, or embarrassing. In the surgical treatment of hydrocele, an incision is made through the wall of the scrotum down to the distended tunica vaginalis. The sac is resected or, after being opened, is sutured together to collapse the wall. Postoperatively, the patient wears an athletic supporter for comfort and support. The major complication is hematoma in the loose scrotal tissues.

Varicocele

A **varicocele** is an abnormal dilation of the veins of the pampiniform venous plexus in the scrotum (the network of veins from the testis and the epididymis that constitute part of the spermatic cord). Varicoceles usually occur in the veins on the upper portion of the left testicle in adults. In some men, a varicocele has been associated with infertility. Few, if any, subjective symptoms may be produced by the enlarged spermatic vein, and no treatment is required unless fertility is a concern. Symptomatic varicocele (pain, tenderness, and discomfort in the inguinal region) is corrected surgically by ligating the external spermatic vein at the inguinal area. An ice pack may be applied to the scrotum for the first few hours after surgery to relieve edema. The patient then wears a scrotal supporter.

Vasectomy

Vasectomy, or male sterilization, is the ligation and transection of part of the vas deferens, with or without removal of a segment of the vas deferens. To prevent the passage of the sperm from the testes, the vas deferens is exposed through a surgical opening in the scrotum or a puncture using a sharp, curved hemostat (Fig. 50-6). The severed

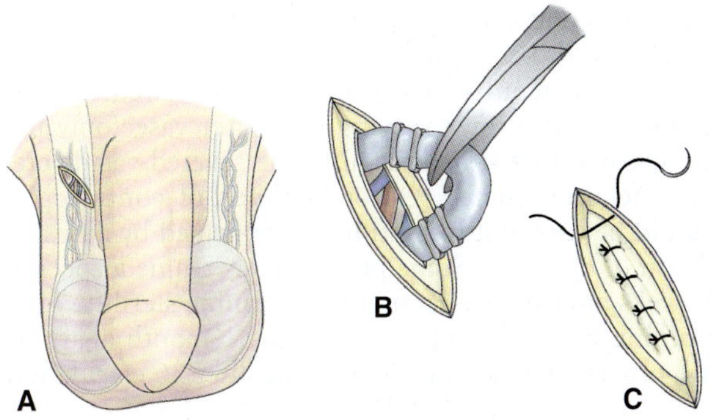

FIGURE 50-6. A vasectomy is a resection of the vas deferens to prevent passage of sperm from the testes to the urethra during ejaculation. **A.** An incision or small puncture is made to expose the vas deferens. **B.** The vas deferens is isolated and severed. **C.** The severed ends are occluded with ligatures or clips, or the lumen of each vas is sealed by electrocautery and the incision is sutured closed. (Suturing may not be required if a puncture approach has been used.)

ends are occluded with ligatures or clips, or the lumen of each vas deferens is sealed by cautery. The spermatozoa, which are manufactured in the testes, cannot travel up the vas deferens after this surgery.

Because seminal fluid is manufactured predominantly in the seminal vesicles and prostate gland, which are unaffected by vasectomy, no noticeable decrease occurs in the amount of ejaculate even though it contains no spermatozoa. Because the sperm cells have no exit, they are resorbed into the body. This procedure has no effect on sexual potency, erection, ejaculation, or production of male hormones and provides no protection against STIs.

Couples who were worried about pregnancy resulting from contraceptive failure often report a decrease in concern and an increase in spontaneous sexual arousal after vasectomy. Concise and factual preoperative explanations may minimize or relieve the patient's concerns related to masculinity. Although a relationship between vasectomy and autoimmune disorders and prostatic cancer has been suggested, there is no clinical evidence of either.

The patient is advised that he will be sterile but that potency will not be altered. As with any surgical procedure, a surgical consent form must be signed. On rare occasions, a spontaneous reanastomosis of the vas deferens occurs, making it possible to impregnate a partner.

Complications of vasectomy include scrotal ecchymoses and swelling, superficial wound infection, vasitis (inflammation of the vas deferens), epididymitis or epididymo-orchitis, hematomas, and spermatic granuloma. A spermatic granuloma is an inflammatory response to the collection of sperm leaking into the scrotum from the severed end of the proximal vas deferens. This can initiate recanalization of the vas deferens, making pregnancy possible.

Nursing Management

Ice bags are applied intermittently to the scrotum for several hours after surgery to reduce swelling and to relieve discomfort. The nurse advises the patient to wear cotton, supportive briefs for added comfort and support. He may become greatly concerned about the discolouration of the scrotal skin and superficial swelling. These are temporary conditions that occur frequently after vasectomy and may be relieved by sitz baths.

Sexual intercourse may be resumed as desired, although fertility remains for a varying time after vasectomy until the spermatozoa stored distal to the severed vas deferens have been evacuated. Other methods of contraception should be used until infertility is confirmed by an examination of ejaculate. Some physicians examine a specimen 4 weeks after the vasectomy to determine sterility; others examine two consecutive specimens 1 month apart; and still others consider a patient sterile after 36 ejaculations.

Vasovasostomy (Sterilization Reversal)

Microsurgical techniques are used to reverse a vasectomy (vasovasostomy), thus restoring patency to the vas deferens. Many men have sperm in their ejaculate after a reversal, and 40% to 75% can impregnate a partner.

Banking Sperm

Storing fertile semen in a sperm bank before a vasectomy is an option for men who face an unforeseen life event that may cause them to want to father a child at a later time. In addition, if a man is about to undergo a procedure or treatment (e.g., radiation therapy to the pelvis or chemotherapy) that may affect his fertility, sperm banking may be considered. This procedure usually requires several visits to the facility where the sperm is stored under hypothermic conditions. The semen is produced by self-stimulation and collected in a sterile container for storage.

DISORDERS AFFECTING THE PENIS

Hypospadias and Epispadias

Hypospadias and epispadias are congenital anomalies of the urethral opening. In hypospadias, the urethral opening is a groove on the underside of the penis. In epispadias, the urethral opening is on the dorsum. These anatomic abnormalities may be repaired by various types of plastic surgery, usually when the boy is very young.

Phimosis

Phimosis, a condition in which the foreskin is constricted so that it cannot be retracted over the glans, can occur congenitally or from inflammation and edema. With the trend away from routine circumcision of newborns, early instruction should be given about cleansing the prepuce. If the preputial area is not cleaned, normal secretions accumulate, causing inflammation (balanitis), which can lead to adhesions and fibrosis. The thickened secretions become encrusted with urinary salts and calcify, forming calculi in the prepuce. In older adult men, penile carcinoma may develop. Phimosis is corrected by circumcision (see later discussion).

Paraphimosis is a condition in which the foreskin is retracted behind the glans and because of narrowness and subsequent edema cannot be returned to its usual position (covering the glans). Paraphimosis is treated by firmly compressing the glans to reduce its size and then pushing the glans back while simultaneously moving the prepuce forward (manual reduction). Circumcision is usually indicated after the inflammation and edema subside.

Cancer of the Penis

Penile cancer predominantly occurs in men over 60 years of age; however, 22% of patients are younger than the age of 40 (Bullen, Edwards, Marke, et al., 2013; Turner, Drudge-Coates, & Henderson, 2013). In 2013, 220 Canadian men were diagnosed with penile cancer; 41 died from it (Canadian Cancer Society) (http://www.cancer.ca/en/cancer-information/cancer-type/penile/statistics/?region=nu#ixzz5ZyTYiibL). In some countries such as Asia, Africa, and South America, penile cancer is more prevalent. A publication by Turner, Drudge-Coates, and Henderson (2013) states that HPV appears to have a role in this type of cancer. However, the "protective" effect of circumcision is seen only in males who are circumcised in the neonatal period; circumcision that occurs at puberty or after does not confer the same benefit (Bullen et al., 2013). Cancer of the penis is a rare type of cancer that appears on the skin of the penis as a painless, wart-like growth or ulcer. Cancer of the penis can involve the glans, the coronal sulcus under the prepuce, the corporal bodies, the urethra, and regional or distant lymph nodes (Turner et al., 2013). **Bowen disease** is a form of squamous cell carcinoma in situ of the penile shaft. Typically, a man delays seeking treatment for more than a year, probably because of guilt, embarrassment, or ignorance.

Prevention

Circumcision in infancy almost eliminates the possibility of penile cancer because chronic irritation and inflammation of the glans penis predispose to penile tumours (Bullen et al., 2013; Canadian Cancer Society, 2014a; Turner et al., 2013). In uncircumcised men, personal hygiene is an important preventive measure.

Medical Management

The aim in managing penile cancer is to cure the client with minimal disfigurement. Treatment modalities include surgery (circumcision, glans resurfacing, glansectomy, or partial penectomy), chemotherapy, radiotherapy, or a combination of these approaches (Turner et al., 2013). Smaller lesions involving only the skin may be controlled by excision (Turner et al., 2013). Topical chemotherapy with 5-fluorouracil cream is an option in selected patients. Radiation therapy is used to treat small squamous cell carcinomas of the penis or for palliation in advanced tumours or lymph node metastasis. Partial penectomy (removal of the penis) is preferred to total penectomy if possible; about 40% of patients can then participate in sexual intercourse and stand for urination. The shaft of the penis can still respond to sexual arousal with an erection and has the sensory capacity for orgasm and ejaculation. Total penectomy is indicated when the tumour is not amenable to conservative treatment. After a total penectomy, the patient may still experience orgasm with stimulation of the perineum and scrotal area.

Priapism

Priapism is an uncontrolled, persistent erection of the penis that causes the penis to remain engorged and painful. It occurs from either neural or vascular causes, including sickle cell thrombosis, leukemic cell infiltration, spinal cord tumours or injury, and tumour invasion of the penis or its vessels. It may also occur with use of medications that affect the central nervous system, antihypertensive agents, antidepressant medications, and substances injected into the penis to treat ED. This condition may result in gangrene and often results in impotence, whether treated or not.

Priapism is a urologic emergency, but men often delay seeking treatment because of embarrassment. By the time they arrive in the emergency department, several hours may have passed and permanent penile damage has occurred. The goal of therapy is to improve venous drainage of the corpora cavernosa to prevent ischemia, fibrosis, and impotence. The initial treatment is directed at relieving the erection and includes bed rest and sedation. The corpora may be irrigated with an anticoagulant, which allows stagnant blood to be aspirated. Shunting procedures to divert the blood from the turgid corpora cavernosa to the venous system (corpora cavernosa–saphenous vein shunt) or into the corpus spongiosum–glans penis compartment may be attempted.

Peyronie Disease

Peyronie disease involves the buildup of fibrous plaques in the sheath of the corpus cavernosum. These plaques are not visible when the penis is relaxed. When erect, however, curvature of the penis occurs that can be painful and can make sexual intercourse difficult or impossible. Peyronie disease primarily occurs in middle-aged and older men. Although the plaques may shrink over time, surgical removal of the plaques may be necessary.

Urethral Stricture

Urethral stricture is a condition in which a section of the urethra is narrowed. It can occur congenitally or from a scar along the urethra. Traumatic injury to the urethra (e.g., from instrumentation, pelvic fractures, or STIs) can result in strictures. Treatment involves dilation of the urethra or, in severe cases, urethrotomy (surgical removal of the stricture).

Circumcision

Circumcision is the excision of the foreskin, or prepuce, of the glans penis. It is usually performed in infancy. In adults, it is part of the treatment for phimosis, paraphimosis, and recurrent infections of the glans and foreskin and may be performed at the personal desire of the patient.

Postoperatively, a petrolatum (Vaseline) gauze dressing is applied and changed as indicated. The patient is observed for bleeding. Because considerable pain may occur after circumcision, analgesic agents are administered as needed.

Critical Thinking Exercises

1 During a community health fair, you are approached by a 49-year-old Black Canadian man who asks you about his risks for prostate cancer. Develop a plan to address this issue with him at the health fair, and provide the rationale for your plan. How would your responses differ if you saw the patient during an office visit to follow-up an elevated PSA test result?

2 One of your patients, a 44-year-old man with multiple sclerosis, asks you about PDE-5 inhibitors. What information would you give him about this class of medications and what teaching approach would you use? How would your approach differ if your patient were a 56-year-old man with long-standing diabetes? If your patient were a 68-year-old man with coronary artery disease?

3 You are caring for two patients who have undergone prostatectomy. One has had surgery to treat BPH and the other a radical prostatectomy to treat malignant prostate cancer. How would your care differ for these two patients? How would the patient's underlying disorder alter your hospital care and your discharge planning?

4 A 34-year-old man is seeking treatment for an STI. When you are obtaining the health history, he reports that this is his fifth or sixth episode of STI. In addition to assisting with medical management and follow-up, what other interventions would you consider for this patient? What strategies would you suggest to him to reduce his risk for subsequent STIs and the risk of transmitting an STI to his sexual partner? How would your teaching differ if the patient revealed that he had sex with men only?

5 A college athlete who describes his health as excellent comes to the student health clinic because he noticed a walnut-size mass in his testicle when showering. Describe the specific components of the history and physical examination that would be appropriate. What would be your concerns, and what referrals would be warranted for him? What is the evidence base for the effectiveness of TSE in detection of testicular cancer? How strong is that evidence, and what criteria did you use to determine the strength of the evidence?

REFERENCES AND SELECTED READINGS

Books

American Cancer Society. (2015). *Cancer facts and figures 2015*. Atlanta, GA.

Grossman, S., & Porth, C. M. (2014). *Pathophysiology: Concepts of altered health states* (9th ed.). Philadelphia, PA: Lippincott Williams & Wilkins.

Hall, J. E. (2015). *Guyton & Hall textbook of medical physiology* (13th ed.). Philadelphia, PA: Saunders Elsevier.

Itano, J. K., Brant, J. M., Conde, F. A., et al. (2016). *Core curriculum for oncology nursing* (5th ed.). St. Louis, MO: Mosby Elsevier.

Keane, T. E., & Graham, S. D. (Eds.). (2016). *Glenn's urologic surgery*. Philadelphia, PA: Wolters Kluwer.

McCance, K. L., Huether, S. E., Brashers, V. L., et al. (Eds.). (2013). *Pathophysiology: The biologic basis for disease in adults and children* (7th ed.). St. Louis, MO: Mosby Elsevier.

McDougal, W. S., Wein, A. J., Kavoussi, L. R., et al. (Eds.). (2016). *Campbell-Walsh urology* (11th ed.). Philadelphia, PA: Elsevier.

Mulhall, J. P., & Hsiao, W. (Eds.). (2014). *Men's sexual health and fertility: A clinician's guide*. New York: Springer.

Pagana, K. D., & Pagana, T. J. (2013). *Mosby's diagnostic and laboratory test reference* (11th ed.). St. Louis, MO: Mosby Elsevier.

Tabloski, P. A. (2014). *Gerontological nursing: The essential guide to clinical practice* (3rd ed.). New York: Pearson.

Wincze, J. P., & Weisberg, R. B. (2015). *Sexual dysfunction: A guide for assessment and treatment*. New York: Guildford Press.

Journals and Electronic Documents

Akre, C., Berchtold, A., Gmel, G., et al. (2014). The evolution of sexual dysfunction in young men aged 18–25 years. *Journal of Adolescent Health, 55*(14), 736–743.

Barry, M. J., & Hayes, J. H. (2015). Evaluating an elevated screening PSA test. *Journal of the American Medical Association, 314*(19), 2073–2074.

Ben-Zvi, T., Hueber, P. A., Valdivieso, R., et al. (2014). Urological resident exposure to transurethral options for BPH management in 2012–2013: A pan-Canadian survey. *Canadian Urological Association Journal, 8*(1–2), 54–60.

Braun, D. P., Gupta, D., Birdsall, T. C., et al. (2013). Effect of naturopathic and nutritional supplement treatment on tumor response, control, and recurrence in patients with prostate cancer treated with radiation therapy. *Journal of Alternative and Complementary Medicine, 19*(3), 198–203.

Bullen, K., Edwards, S., Marke, V., et al. (2013). Looking past the obvious: Experiences of altered masculinity in penile cancer. *Psycho-Oncology, 19*, 933–940.

Canadian Cancer Society's Advisory Committee on Cancer Statistics. (2013). *Canadian Cancer Statistics 2013*. Toronto, ON: Canadian Cancer Society. Retrieved from http://www.cancer.ca/~/media/cancer.ca/CW/cancer%20information/cancer%20101/Canadian%20cancer%20statistics/canadian-cancer-statistics-2013-EN.pdf

Canadian Cancer Society. (2014a). *Early Detection of Penile Cancer*. Toronto, ON: Author. Retrieved February 18, 2014, from http://www.cancer.ca/en/cancer-information/cancer-type/penile/early-detection/?region=ab

Canadian Cancer Society. (2014b). *Penile Cancer Statistics*. Toronto, ON: Author. Retrieved from http://www.cancer.ca/en/cancer-information/cancer-type/penile/statistics/?region=ab

Chen, X., Hu, C., Peng, Y., et al. (2016). Association of diet and lifestyle with chronic prostatitis/chronic pelvic pain syndrome and pain severity: A case–control study. *Prostate Cancer and Prostatic Diseases, 19*, 92–99.

Cohen, S. A., & Parsons, J. K. (2012). Combination pharmacological therapies for the management of benign prostatic hyperplasia. *Drugs and Aging, 29*(4), 275–284.

Crawford, P. (2014). Evaluation of scrotal masses. *American Family Physician, 89*(9), 723–727

Curran, M. P. (2012). Tadalafil: In the treatment of signs and symptoms of benign prostatic hyperplasia with or without erectile dysfunction. *Drugs and Aging, 29*, 771–781.

Drudge-Coates, L., & Turner, B. (2012a). Prostate cancer overview. Part 2: Metastatic prostate disease. *British Journal of Nursing, 21*(18), S23–S28.

Drudge-Coates, L., & Turner, B. (2012b). Prostate cancer overview. Part 1: Non-metastatic prostate cancer. *British Journal of Nursing, 21*(18), S23–S28.

Gledhill, S., & Schweitzer, R. D. (2013). Sexual desire, erectile dysfunction and the biomedicalization of sex in older heterosexual men. *Journal of Advanced Nursing, 70*(4), 894–903.

Grant, P., Jackson, G., Baig, I., et al. (2013). Erectile dysfunction in general medicine. *Clinical Medicine, 13*(2), 136–140.

Health Canada. (2013). *First Nations Health Status Report: Alberta Region 2011–2012*. Ottawa, ON: Author. http://publications.gc.ca/collections/collection_2013/sc-hc/H26-4-2012-eng.pdf

Hunter, J. C., Vines, A. I., & Carlisle, V. (2015). African Americans' perceptions of prostate-specific antigen prostate cancer screening. *Health Education and Behavior, 42*(4), 539–544

Isbarn, H., Huland, H., & Graefen, M. (2013). Results of radical prostatectomy in newly diagnosed prostate cancer. *Deutsches Arzteblatt International, 110*(29–30), 497–503.

Jung, J. H., Seo, J. W., Lim, M. S., et al. (2012). Extended pelvic lymph node dissection including internal iliac packet should be performed during robot-assisted laparoscopic radical prostatectomy for high-risk prostate cancer. *Journal of Laparoendoscopic and Advanced Surgical Techniques, 22*(8), 785–790.

Kim, C., McGlynn, K. A., McCorkle, R., et al. (2012). Sexual functioning among testicular cancer survivors: A case-control study in the U.S. *Journal of Psychosomatic Research, 73*(1), 68–73.

Lim, P. H. (2013). How incontinence affects sexual health. *Australian and New Zealand Continence Journal, 19*(4), 117–121.

Liu, K. C., Yen, C. Y., Wu, R. S. C., et al. (2014). The roles of endoplasmic reticulum stress and mitochondrial apoptotic signaling pathway in quercetin-mediated cell death of human prostate cancer PC-3 cells. *Environmental Toxicology, 29*(4), 428–439.

Lycken, M., Garmo, H., Adolfsson, J., et al. (2013). Patterns of androgen deprivation therapies among men diagnosed with localized prostatic cancer: A population based study. *European Journal of Cancer, 49*(9), 1789–1798

Malik, S. (2014). Using hormone therapy for the management of prostate cancer. *Nursing and Residential Care, 16*(2), 75–77.

Mitchell, K. R., Mercer, C. H., Ploubidis, G. B., et al. (2013). Sexual function in Britain: Findings from the Third National Survey of Sexual Attitudes and Lifestyles (Natsal-3). *Lancet, 382*, 1817–1829.

Mola, J. R. (2015). Erectile dysfunction in the older adult male. *Urologic Nursing, 35*(2), 87–93.

Movember Canada. (2014). *Men's health: testicular cancer*. Retrieved from http://ca.movember.com/mens-health/testicular-cancer

National Comprehensive Cancer Network [NCCN]. (2016b). *Clinical practice guidelines in oncology: Prostate cancer*. Retrieved on March 6, 2017, from www.nccn.org/professionals/default.aspx

Norton, W., & Tremayne, P. (2015). Sex and the older man. *British Journal of Nursing*, *24*(4), 218–221.

Osei, D. K., Lee, J. W., Modest, N. N., et al. (2013). Effects of an online support group for prostate cancer survivors: A randomized trial. *Urologic Nursing*, *33*(3), 123–133.

Peate, I. (2012). Breaking the silence: Helping men with erectile dysfunction. *British Journal of Community Nursing*, *17*(7), 310, 312, 314–317.

Prostate Cancer Canada (PCC). (2013a). *Active Surveillance*. Retrieved from http://prostatecancer.ca/Prostate-Cancer/Treatment/Active-Surveillance#.UzRnu2BOW70

Prostate Cancer Canada (PCC). (2013b). *Grading*. Retrieved from http://prostatecancer.ca/Prostate-Cancer/Testing-and-Diagnosis/Grading#.UzRoGGBOW70

Prostate Cancer Canada (PCC). (2013c). *Prostate Cancer Canada releases new recommendations*. Retrieved from http://prostatecancer.ca/In-The-News/Foundation-News-Releases/Prostate-Cancer-Canada-Releases-New-Recommendation#.UzRlyGBOW70

Prostate Cancer Canada (PCC). (2013d). *Radical Prostatectomy*. Retrieved from http://prostatecancer.ca/Prostate-Cancer/Treatment/Radical-Prostatectomy#.UzRoWWBOW70

Prostate Cancer Canada (PCC). (2013e). *Risk Factors*. Retrieved. http://prostatecancer.ca/Prostate-Cancer/About-Prostate-Cancer/Risk-Factors#.UzRnO2BOW70

Prostate Cancer Canada (PCC). (2013f). *Statistics*. Retrieved from http://prostatecancer.ca/Prostate-Cancer/About-Prostate-Cancer/Statistics#.UzRl9GBOW70

Public Health Agency of Canada. (2013). *The chief public health officer's report on the state of public health in Canada, 2013 infectious disease—The never-ending threat*. Ottawa, ON: Author.

Quinn, C., & Happell, B. (2012). Getting BETTER: Breaking the ice and warming to the inclusion of sexuality in mental health nursing care. *International Journal of Mental Health Nursing*, *21*, 154–162.

Rathkopf, D., & Scher, H. I. (2013). Androgen receptor antagonists in castration-resistant cancer. *The Cancer Journal*, *19*(1), 43–49.

Robbins-Cherry, S. A., Hayter, M., Wylie, K. R., et al. (2011). The experiences of men living with inhibited ejaculation. *Sexual and Relationship Therapy*, *26*(3), 242–253.

Steggall, M. (2012). Pharmacological management of premature ejaculation. *Nurse Prescribing*, *10*(11), 545–550.

Tannenbaum, C. (2015). Associations between urinary symptoms and sexual health in older adults. *Clinics in Geriatric Medicine*, *31*(4), 581–590.

Tantamango-Bartley, Y., Knutsen, S. F., Knutsen, R., et al. (2016). Are strict vegetarians protected against cancer? *American Journal of Clinical Nutrition*, *103*, 153–160.

Turner, B., & Drudge-Coates, L. (2012). New pharmacological treatments for prostate cancer. *Nurse Prescribing*, *10*(10), 498–502.

Turner, B., Drudge-Coates, L., & Henderson, S. (2013). Penile cancer: Diagnosis, clinical features and management. *Nursing Standard*, *27*(29), 50–57.

Ulbricht, C., & Rusie, E. (2012). Clinical Roundup: Evidenced-based systematic review results. *Alternative and Complementary Therapies*, *18*(1), 51–55.

Resources and Web Sites

Canadian Cancer Society: http://www.cancer.ca.
Canadian Continence Foundation: http://www.continence-fdn.ca.
Canadian Prostate Cancer Network: http://www.cpcn.org.
Canadian Prostate Health Council: http://www.canadian-prostate.com.
Canadian Urological Association: http://www.cua.org/.
Prostate Cancer Information, Health Canada and the Department of Urology, Dalhousie University: http://www.caprostate.com.

UNIT 11

Immunologic and Hematologic Function

Case Study

SUPPORTING THE PATIENT WITH SYSTEMIC LUPUS ERYTHEMATOSUS

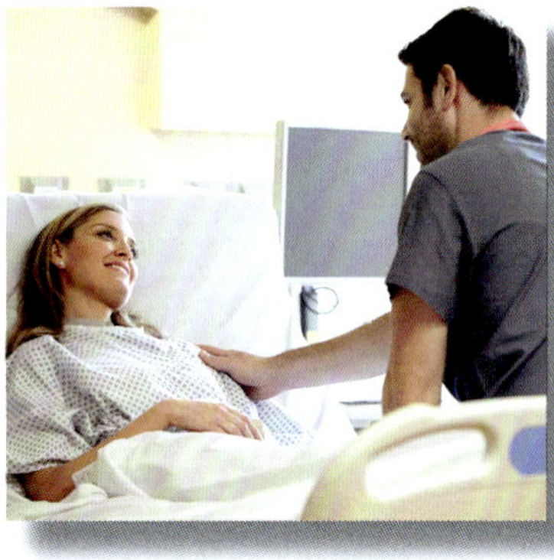

A 24-year-old female is hospitalized with an autoimmune disorder, systemic lupus erythematosus (SLE). She has a toddler at home and reports that she and her husband wish to conceive another child. She has recently stopped taking her medications prescribed to treat SLE, which include hydroxychloroquine (Plaquenil) and prednisone. As a result of stopping her medications, she is experiencing a flare-up of SLE. She is currently experiencing fatigue, acute pain in her joints, and fever. She has a WBC of 2.1/mm^3 and Hgb 7.6 mg/dL. She is reluctant to resume medical treatment, including resuming her prescribed medications, as it may have teratogenic effects.

QSEN Competency Focus: Patient-Centred Care

The complexities inherent in today's health care system challenge nurses to demonstrate integration of specific interdisciplinary core competencies that are aimed at ensuring the delivery of safe and quality patient care (Institute of Medicine, 2003). The Quality and Safety Education for Nurses project (QSEN, 2017; Cronenwett, Sherwood, Barnsteiner, et al., 2007) provides a framework for the knowledge, skills, and attitudes (KSAs) required for nurses to demonstrate competency in these key areas, which include ***patient-centred care***, ***interdisciplinary teamwork and collaboration***, ***evidence-based practice***, ***quality improvement***, ***safety***, and ***informatics.***

Patient-Centred Care Definition: Recognize the patient or designee as the source of control and full partner in providing compassionate and coordinated care based on respect for patient's preferences, values, and needs.

SELECTED PRE-LICENSURE KSAs	APPLICATION AND REFLECTION
Knowledge	
Describe strategies to empower patients or families in all aspects of the health care process.	Describe strategies you would use to ensure that this patient is fully engaged in all aspects of her care. How might this empower her?
Skills	
Engage patients or designated surrogates in active partnerships that promote health, safety, well-being, and self-care management.	Discuss how you would assess the threats to this patient's active involvement in her health, safety, well-being, and self-care management. What measures might you take to mitigate these threats?
Attitudes	
Value active partnership with patients or designated surrogates in planning, implementation, and evaluation of care.	Reflect on your attitudes toward patients with chronic illness who stop taking their medication for personal reasons, such as wanting to conceive another child. What impact does this have on the plan of care?

Cronenwett, L., Sherwood, G., Barnsteiner, J., et al. (2007). Quality and safety education for nurses. *Nursing Outlook, 55*(3), 122–131; Institute of Medicine. (2003). *Health professions education: A bridge to quality*. Washington, DC: National Academies Press; and QSEN Institute. (2017). *QSEN competencies: Definitions and pre-licensure KSAs*. Retrieved June 12, 2019, from www.qsen.org/competencies/pre-licensure-ksas

51 Assessment of Immune Function

Adapted by Kelly Power-Kean

Learning Objectives

On completion of this chapter, the learner will be able to:

1. Describe the body's general immune responses.
2. Discuss the stages of the immune response.
3. Differentiate between cellular and humoral immune responses.
4. Describe the effects of selected variables on function of the immune system.
5. Use assessment parameters for determining the status of patients' immune function.

Immunity is the body's specific protective response to a foreign agent or organism. The **immune system** functions as the body's defense mechanism against invasion and allows a rapid response to foreign substances in a specific manner. Genetic and cellular responses result. Any qualitative or quantitative change in the components of the immune system can produce profound effects on the integrity of the human organism. Immune function is affected by a variety of factors, such as central nervous system integrity, general physical and emotional status, medications, dietary patterns, and the stress of illness, trauma, or surgery. Dysfunctions involving the immune system occur across the life span. Many are genetically based; others are acquired. Immune memory is a property of the immune system that provides protection against harmful microbial agents despite the timing of reexposure to the agent. Tolerance is the mechanism by which the immune system is programmed to eliminate foreign substances such as microbes, toxins, and cellular mutations but maintains the ability to accept self-antigens. Some credence is given to the concept of surveillance, in which the immune system is in a perpetual state of vigilance, screening and rejecting any invader that is recognized as foreign to the host. The term **immunopathology** refers to the study of diseases that result from dysfunctions within the immune system. Disorders of the immune system may stem from excesses or deficiencies of immunocompetent cells, alterations in the function of these cells, immunologic attack on self-antigens, or inappropriate or exaggerated responses to specific **antigens** (Table 51-1).

Growing numbers of patients with primary immune deficiencies live to adulthood and many others acquire immune disorders during their adult years. Thus, nurses in many practice settings need to understand how the immune system functions as well as immunopathologic processes. In addition, knowledge about assessment and care of people with immunologic disorders enables nurses to make appropriate management decisions.

Anatomic and Physiologic Overview

Anatomy of the Immune System

The immune system is composed of an integrated collection of various cell types, each with a designated function in defending against infection and invasion by other organisms. Supporting this system are molecules that are responsible for the interactions, modulations, and regulation of the system. These molecules and cells participate in specific interactions with immunogenic **epitopes** (**antigenic determinants**) present on foreign materials, initiating a series of actions in a host, including the inflammatory response, the lysis of microbial agents, and the disposal of foreign toxins. The major components of the immune system include central and peripheral organs, tissues, and cells.

Bone Marrow

The white blood cells (WBCs) involved in immunity are produced in the bone marrow (Fig. 51-1). Like other blood cells, lymphocytes are generated from stem cells (undifferentiated cells). There are two types of lymphocytes—B lymphocytes (**B cells**) and T lymphocytes (**T cells**).

TABLE 51-1 Immune System Disorders

Disorder	Description
Autoimmunity	Normal protective immune response paradoxically turns against or attacks the body, leading to tissue damage
Hypersensitivity	Body produces inappropriate or exaggerated responses to specific antigens
Gammopathies	Immunoglobulins are overproduced
Immune Deficiencies	
Primary	Deficiency results from improper development of immune cells or tissues; usually congenital or inherited
Secondary	Deficiency results from some interference with an already developed immune system; usually acquired later in life

Lymphoid Tissues

The spleen, composed of red and white pulp, acts somewhat like a filter. The red pulp is the site where old and injured red blood cells (RBCs) are destroyed. The white pulp contains concentrations of lymphocytes. The lymph nodes, which are connected by lymph channels and capillaries, are distributed throughout the body. They remove foreign material from the lymph system before it enters the bloodstream. The lymph nodes also serve as centres for immune cell proliferation. The remaining lymphoid tissues contain immune cells that defend the body's mucosal surfaces against microorganisms (McComb, Thiriot, Krishnan, et al., 2013).

Function of the Immune System

CONCEPTS IN ACTION

The basic function of the immune system is to remove foreign antigens such as viruses and bacteria to maintain

Glossary

agglutination: clumping effect occurring when an antibody acts as a cross-link between two antigens

antibody: a protein substance developed by the body in response to and interacting with a specific antigen

antigen: substance that induces the production of antibodies

antigenic determinant: the specific area of an antigen that binds with an antibody combining site and determines the specificity of the antigen–antibody reaction

apoptosis: programmed cell death that results from the digestion of deoxyribonucleic acid by endonucleases

B cells: cells that are important for producing a humoral immune response

cellular immune response: the immune system's third line of defense, involving the attack of pathogens by T cells

complement: series of enzymatic proteins in the serum that, when activated, destroy bacteria and other cells

cytokines: generic term for nonantibody proteins that act as intercellular mediators, as in the generation of immune response

cytotoxic T cells: lymphocytes that lyse cells infected with virus; also play a role in graft rejection

epitope: any component of an antigen molecule that functions as an antigenetic determinant by permitting the attachment of certain antibodies

genetic engineering: emerging technology designed to enable replacement of missing or defective genes

helper T cells: lymphocytes that attack foreign invaders (antigens) directly

humoral immune response: emerging technology designed to enable replacement of missing or defective genes

immune response: the coordinated response of the components of the immune system to a foreign agent or organism

immune system: the collection of organs, cells, tissues, and molecules that mediate the immune response

immunity: the body's specific protective response to a foreign agent or organism; resistance to disease, specifically infectious diseases

immunopathology: study of diseases resulting in dysfunctions within the immune system

immunoregulation: complex system of checks and balances that regulates or controls immune responses

immunosenescence: the gradual deterioration of the immune system brought on by the aging process

interferons: proteins formed when cells are exposed to viral or foreign agents; capable of activating other components of the immune system

lymphokines: substances released by sensitized lymphocytes when they come in contact with specific antigens

memory cells: cells that are responsible for recognizing antigens from previous exposure and mounting an immune response

natural killer (NK) cells: lymphocytes that defend against microorganisms and malignant cells

null lymphocytes: lymphocytes that destroy antigens already coated with the antibody

opsonization: the coating of antigen–antibody molecules with a sticky substance to facilitate phagocytosis

phagocytic cells: cells that engulf, ingest, and destroy foreign bodies or toxins

phagocytic immune response: the immune system's first line of defense, involving white blood cells that have the ability to ingest foreign particles

stem cells: precursors of all blood cells; reside primarily in bone marrow

suppressor T cells: lymphocytes that decrease B-cell activity to a level at which the immune system is compatible with life

T cells: cells that are important for producing a cellular immune response

Physiology/Pathophysiology

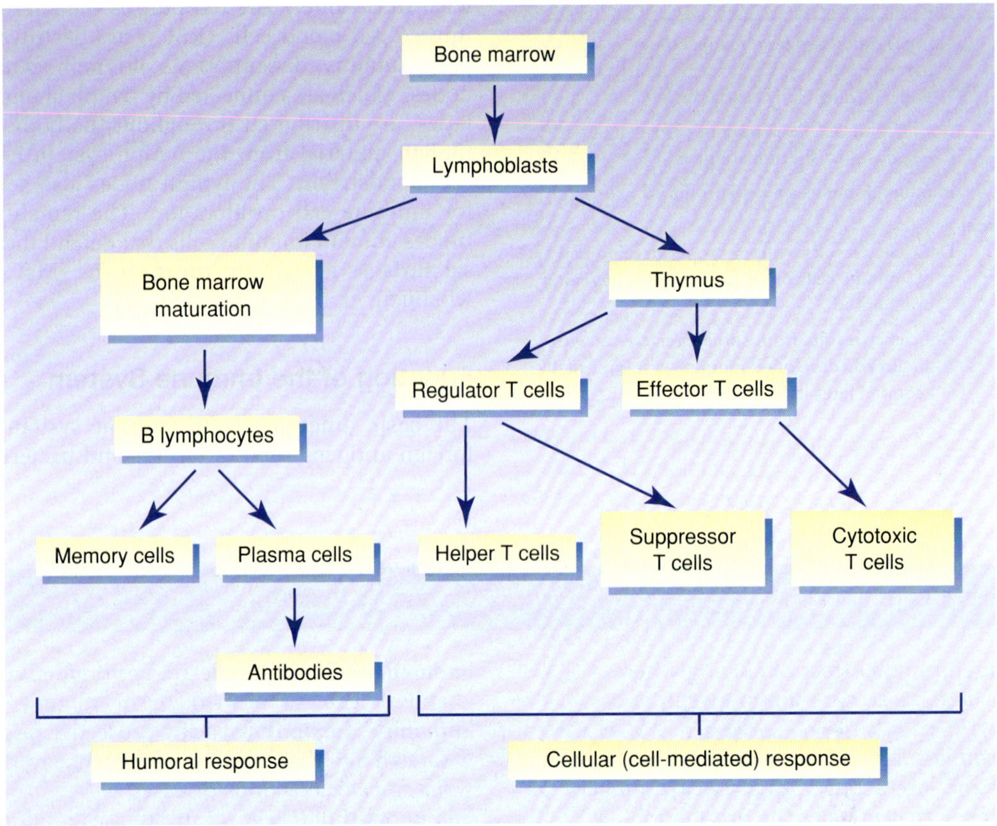

FIGURE 51-1. Development of cells of the immune system.

homeostasis. There are two general types of immunity: natural (innate) and acquired (adaptive). Natural immunity or nonspecific immunity is present at birth. Acquired or specific immunity develops after birth. Each type of immunity has a distinct role in defending the body against harmful invaders, but the various components are usually interdependent (Levinson, 2014).

Natural Immunity

Natural immunity, which is nonspecific, provides a broad spectrum of defense against and resistance to infection. It is considered the first line of host defense following antigen exposure, because it protects the host without remembering prior contact with an infectious agent (Levinson, 2014). Natural (innate) immunity co-coordinates the initial response to pathogens through the production of **cytokines** and other effector molecules, which either activate cells for control of the pathogen (by elimination) or promote the development of the acquired **immune response**. The cells involved in this response include macrophages, dendritic cells, **natural killer (NK) cells**, basophils, eosinophils, and granulocytes. The early events in this process are critical in determining the nature of the adaptive immune response. Natural immune mechanisms can be divided into two stages: immediate (generally occurring within minutes) and delayed (occurring within several days after exposure) (Levinson, 2014).

White Blood Cell Action

The cellular response is key to the effective initiation of the immune response. WBCs, or leukocytes, participate in both the natural and the acquired immune responses. Granular leukocytes, or granulocytes (so called because of granules in their cytoplasm), fight invasion by foreign bodies or toxins by releasing cell mediators, such as histamine, bradykinin, and prostaglandins, and engulfing the foreign bodies or toxins. Granulocytes include neutrophils, eosinophils, and basophils.

Neutrophils (polymorphonuclear leukocytes) are the first cells to arrive at the site where inflammation occurs. Eosinophils and basophils, other types of granulocytes, increase in number during allergic reactions and stress responses. Nongranular leukocytes include monocytes or macrophages (referred to as histiocytes when they enter tissue spaces) and lymphocytes. Monocytes are the first to arrive on the scene and function as **phagocytic cells**, engulfing, ingesting, and destroying greater numbers and quantities of foreign bodies or toxins than granulocytes do. Lymphocytes, consisting of B cells and T cells, play major roles in humoral and cell-mediated immune responses. About 60% to 70% of lymphocytes in the blood are T cells, and about 10% to 15% are B cells (Haynes, Soderberg, & Fauci, 2015).

Inflammatory Response

The inflammatory response is a major function of the natural immune system that is elicited in response to tissue injury or invading organisms. Chemical mediators assist this response by minimizing blood loss, walling off the invading organism, activating phagocytes, and promoting formation of fibrous scar tissue and regeneration of injured tissue. The inflammatory response (discussed further in Chapter 9) is facilitated by physical and chemical barriers that are part of the human organism.

Physical and Chemical Barriers

Activation of the natural immunity response is enhanced by processes inherent in physical and chemical barriers. Physical surface barriers include intact skin, mucous membranes, and cilia of the respiratory tract, which prevent pathogens from gaining access to the body. The cilia of the respiratory tract, along with coughing and sneezing responses, filter and clear pathogens from the upper respiratory tract before they can invade the body further. Chemical barriers, such as mucus, acidic gastric secretions, enzymes in tears and saliva, and substances in sebaceous and sweat secretions, act in a nonspecific way to destroy invading bacteria and fungi. Viruses are countered by other means, such as interferon.

Immune Regulation

Regulation of the immune response involves balance and counterbalance. Dysfunction of the natural immune system can occur when the immune components are inactivated or when they remain active long after their effects are beneficial. A successful immune response eliminates the responsible antigen. If an immune response fails to develop and clear an antigen sufficiently, the host is considered to be immunocompromised or immunodeficient. If the response is overly robust or misdirected, allergies, asthma, or autoimmune disease results. The immune system's recognition of one's own cells or tissues as "foreign" rather than as self is the basis of many autoimmune disorders (Grossman & Porth, 2014). Despite the fact that the immune response is critical to the prevention of disease, it must be well controlled to curtail immunopathology. Most microbial infections induce an inflammatory response mediated by T cells and cytokines, which, in excess, can cause tissue damage (Haynes et al., 2015). Therefore, regulatory mechanisms must be in place to suppress or halt the immune response. This is mainly achieved by the production of cytokines and transformation of growth factor that inhibits macrophage activation. In some cases, T-cell activation is so acute that these mechanisms fail, and pathology develops. Ongoing research on **immunoregulation** holds the promise of preventing graft rejection and aiding the body in eliminating cancerous or infected cells (Kannan, Madden, & Andrews, 2013; Lo, Lee, & Powell, 2014).

Although natural immunity can often effectively combat infections, many pathogenic microbes have evolved that resist natural immunity. Adaptive immunity is necessary to defend against these resistant agents.

Acquired Immunity

Acquired (adaptive) immunity usually develops as a result of prior exposure to an antigen through immunization (vaccination) or by contracting a disease, both of which generate a protective immune response. Weeks or months after exposure to the disease or vaccine, the body produces an immune response that is sufficient to defend against the disease on re-exposure. In contrast to the rapid but nonspecific natural immune response, this form of immunity relies on the recognition of specific foreign antigens. The adaptive immune response is broadly divided into two mechanisms: (1) the cell-mediated response, involving T-cell activation; and (2) effector mechanisms, involving B-cell maturation and production of antibodies (Haynes et al., 2015).

The two types of acquired immunity are known as active and passive and are interrelated. Active adaptive immunity refers to immunologic defenses developed by the person's own body. This immunity typically lasts many years or even a lifetime. Passive adaptive immunity is temporary immunity transmitted from a source outside the body that has developed immunity through previous disease or immunization. Examples include immunity resulting from the transfer of antibodies from the mother to an infant in utero or through breast feeding or receiving injections of immune globulin. Active and passive adaptive immunity involve humoral and cellular (cell-mediated) immunologic responses (described later in this chapter).

Response to Invasion

When the body is invaded or attacked by bacteria, viruses, or other pathogens, it has three means of defense:

- The phagocytic immune response
- The humoral or antibody immune response
- The cellular immune response

The first line of defense, the **phagocytic immune response**, primarily involves the WBCs (granulocytes and macrophages), which have the ability to ingest foreign particles and destroy the invading agent; eosinophils are only weakly phagocytic. Phagocytes also remove the body's own dying or dead cells. Cells in necrotic tissue that are dying release substances that trigger an inflammatory response. **Apoptosis**, or programmed cell death, is the body's way of destroying worn-out cells such as blood or skin cells or cells that need to be renewed (Grossman & Porth, 2014).

A second protective response, the **humoral immune response** (sometimes called the **antibody** response), begins with the B lymphocytes, which can transform themselves into plasma cells that manufacture antibodies. These antibodies are highly specific proteins that are transported in the bloodstream and attempt to disable invaders. The third mechanism of defense, the **cellular immune response**, also involves the T lymphocytes, which can turn into special cytotoxic (or killer) T cells that can attack the pathogens.

The structural part of the invading or attacking organism that is responsible for stimulating antibody production is called an antigen (or an immunogen). For example, an antigen can be a small patch of proteins on the outer surface of a microorganism. Not all antigens are naturally immunogenic; some must be coupled to other molecules to stimulate the immune response. A single bacterium or large molecule, such as a diphtheria or tetanus toxin, may have several antigens, or markers, on its surface, thus inducing the body to produce a number of different antibodies. Once produced, an antibody is released into the

Physiology/Pathophysiology

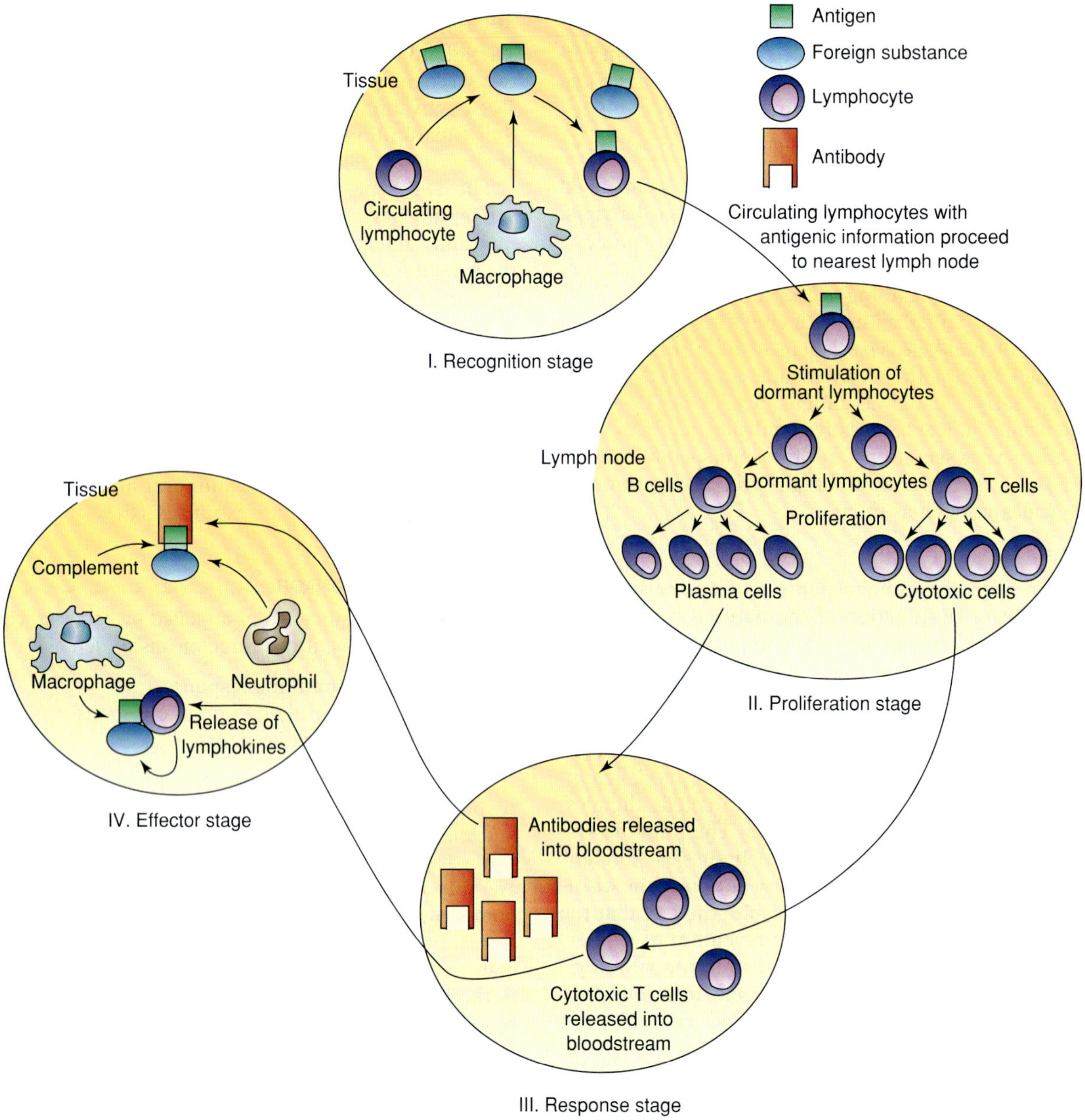

FIGURE 51-2. Stages of the immune response. **I.** In the *recognition stage*, antigens are recognized by circulating lymphocytes and macrophages. **II.** In the *proliferation stage*, the dormant lymphocytes proliferate and differentiate into cytotoxic (killer) T cells or B cells responsible for formation and release of antibodies. **III.** In the *response stage*, the cytotoxic T cells and the B cells perform cellular and humoral functions, respectively. **IV.** In the *effector stage*, antigens are destroyed or neutralized through the action of antibodies, complement, macrophages, and cytotoxic T cells.

bloodstream and carried to the attacking organism. There, it combines with the antigen, binding with it like an interlocking piece of a jigsaw puzzle. There are four well-defined stages in an immune response: recognition, proliferation, response, and effector (Fig. 51-2).

Recognition Stage

Recognition of antigens as foreign, or non-self, by the immune system is the initiating event in any immune response. Recognition involves the use of lymph nodes and lymphocytes for surveillance. Lymph nodes are widely distributed internally throughout the body and in the circulating blood as well as externally near the body's surfaces. They continuously discharge small lymphocytes into the bloodstream. These lymphocytes patrol the tissues and vessels that drain the areas served by that node. Lymphocytes recirculate from the blood to lymph nodes and from the lymph nodes back into the bloodstream in a continuous circuit. Lymphocytes and other cells have "microbial sensors" that identify molecules on microbes and other microorganisms. The interaction of these sensors with the offending agent sets off a cascade aimed at destroying the microbe (Paul, 2013). Invading organisms have pathogen-associated molecular patterns (PAMPs) contained in their cell membranes that are recognized by the immune system cells. Once the receptors on the immune cells come into contact with the PAMPs, the immune response is triggered (Grossman & Porth, 2014). Macrophages play an important role in helping the circulating lymphocytes process the antigens. Both macrophages and neutrophils have receptors for antibodies and **complement**; as a result, they coat microorganisms with antibodies, complement, or both, enhancing phagocytosis.

In a streptococcal throat infection, for example, the streptococcal organism gains access to the mucous membranes of the throat. A circulating lymphocyte moving through the tissues of the throat comes in contact with the organism. The lymphocyte recognizes the antigens on the microbe as different (non-self) and the streptococcal organism as antigenic (foreign). This triggers the second stage of the immune response—proliferation.

Proliferation Stage

The circulating lymphocytes containing the antigenic message return to the nearest lymph node. Once in the node, these sensitized lymphocytes stimulate some of the resident T and B lymphocytes to enlarge, divide, and proliferate. T lymphocytes differentiate into cytotoxic (or killer) T cells, whereas B lymphocytes produce and release antibodies. Enlargement of the lymph nodes in the neck in conjunction with a sore throat is one example of the immune response.

Response Stage

In the response stage, the differentiated lymphocytes function in either a humoral or a cellular capacity. This stage begins with the production of antibodies by the B lymphocytes in response to a specific antigen. The cellular response stimulates the resident lymphocytes to become cells that attack microbes directly rather than through the action of antibodies. These transformed lymphocytes are known as cytotoxic (killer) T cells.

Viral rather than bacterial antigens induce a cellular response. This response is manifested by the increasing number of T lymphocytes (lymphocytosis) seen in the blood tests of people with viral illnesses such as infectious mononucleosis. Cellular immunity is discussed in further detail later in this chapter. Most immune responses to antigens involve both humoral and cellular responses, although one usually predominates. For example, during transplant rejection, the cellular response involving T cells predominates, whereas in the bacterial pneumonias and sepsis, the humoral response involving B cells plays the dominant protective role (Chart 51-1).

Effector Stage

In the effector stage, either the antibody of the humoral response or the cytotoxic (killer) T cell of the cellular response reaches and connects with the antigen on the surface of the foreign invader. This initiates activities involving interplay of antibodies (humoral immunity), complement, and action by the **cytotoxic T cells** (cellular immunity).

Humoral Immune Response

The humoral response is characterized by the production of antibodies by B lymphocytes in response to a specific antigen. While B lymphocytes are responsible for the production of antibodies, both the macrophages of natural immunity and the special T lymphocytes of cellular immunity are involved in recognition.

CHART 51-1

Comparison of Cellular and Humoral Immune Responses

Humoral Responses (B Cells)

- Bacterial phagocytosis and lysis
- Anaphylaxis
- Allergic hay fever and asthma
- Immune complex disease
- Bacterial and some viral infections

Cellular Responses (T Cells)

- Transplant rejection
- Delayed hypersensitivity (tuberculin reaction)
- Graft-versus-host disease
- Tumour surveillance or destruction
- Intracellular infections
- Viral, fungal, and parasitic infections

Antigen Recognition

Several theories explain the mechanisms by which B lymphocytes recognize the invading antigen and respond by producing antibodies. It is known that B lymphocytes recognize and respond to invading antigens in more than one way.

The B lymphocytes respond to some antigens by directly triggering antibody formation; however, in response to other antigens, they need the assistance of T cells to trigger antibody formation. With the help of macrophages, the T lymphocytes are believed to recognize the antigen of a foreign invader. The T lymphocyte picks up the antigenic message, or "blueprint," of the antigen and returns to the nearest lymph node with that message. B lymphocytes stored in the lymph nodes are subdivided into thousands of clones, which are stimulated to enlarge, divide, proliferate, and differentiate into plasma cells capable of producing specific antibodies to the antigen. Other B lymphocytes differentiate into B-lymphocyte clones with a memory for the antigen. These **memory cells** are responsible for the more exaggerated and rapid immune response in a person who is repeatedly exposed to the same antigen.

Role of Antibodies

Antibodies are large proteins called *immunoglobulins* that consist of two subunits, each containing a light and a heavy peptide chain held together by a chemical link composed of disulfide bonds. Each subunit has one portion that serves as a binding site for a specific antigen and another portion that allows the antibody molecule to take part in the complement system.

Antibodies defend against foreign invaders in several ways, and the type of defense used depends on the structure and composition of both the antigen and the immunoglobulin. The antibody molecule has at least two combining sites, or Fab fragments. One antibody can act as a cross-link between two antigens, causing them to bind or clump together. This clumping effect, referred to as **agglutination**, helps to clear the body of the invading organism by facilitating phagocytosis. Some antibodies assist in removing offending organisms through **opsonization**. In this process, the antigen–antibody molecule is coated with a sticky substance that also facilitates phagocytosis.

Antibodies also promote the release of vasoactive substances, such as histamine and slow-reacting substance, two of the chemical mediators of the inflammatory response. Antibodies do not function in isolation; rather, they mobilize other components of the immune system to defend against the invader.

The body can produce five different types of immunoglobulins (Ig). Each of the five types, or classes, is identified by a specific letter of the alphabet, IgA, IgD, IgE, IgG, and IgM. Classification is based on the chemical structure and biologic role of the individual immunoglobulin. Major characteristics of the immunoglobulins are summarized in Chart 51-2.

CHART 51-2

Major Characteristics of the Immunoglobulins

IgG (75% of Total Immunoglobulin)

- Appears in serum and tissues (interstitial fluid)
- Assumes a major role in bloodborne and tissue infections
- Activates the complement system
- Enhances phagocytosis
- Crosses the placenta

IgA (15% of Total Immunoglobulin)

- Appears in body fluids (blood, saliva, tears, breast milk, as well as pulmonary, gastrointestinal, prostatic, and vaginal secretions)
- Protects against respiratory, gastrointestinal, and genitourinary infections
- Prevents absorption of antigens from food
- Passes to neonate in breast milk for protection

IgM (10% of Total Immunoglobulin)

- Appears mostly in intravascular serum
- Appears as the first immunoglobulin produced in response to bacterial and viral infections
- Activates the complement system

IgD (0.2% of Total Immunoglobulin)

- Appears in small amounts in serum
- Possibly influences B-lymphocyte differentiation, but role is unclear

IgE (0.004% of Total Immunoglobulin)

- Appears in serum
- Takes part in allergic and some hypersensitivity reactions
- Combats parasitic infections

Ig, immunoglobulin.
Adapted from Grossman, S. C., & Porth, C. M. (2014). *Porth's pathophysiology: Concepts of altered health states* (9th ed., p. 278). Philadelphia, PA: Lippincott Williams & Wilkins.

Antigen–Antibody Binding

The portion of the antigen involved in binding with the antibody is referred to as the antigenic determinant. The most efficient immunologic responses occur when the antibody and antigen fit like a lock and key. Poor fit can occur with an antibody that was produced in response to a different antigen. This phenomenon is known as cross-reactivity. For example, in acute rheumatic fever, the antibody produced against *Streptococcus pyogenes* in the upper respiratory tract may cross-react with the patient's heart tissue, leading to heart valve damage.

Cellular Immune Response

The T lymphocytes are primarily responsible for cellular immunity. Stem cells continuously migrate from the bone marrow to the thymus gland, where they develop into T cells. Despite the partial degeneration of the gland at puberty, T cells continue to develop in the thymus gland. Several types of T cells exist, each with designated roles in the defense against bacteria, viruses, fungi, parasites, and malignant cells. T cells attack foreign invaders directly rather than by producing antibodies.

Cellular reactions are initiated, with or without the assistance of macrophages, by the binding of an antigen to an antigen receptor located on the surface of a T cell. The T cells then carry the antigenic message, or blueprint, to the lymph nodes, where the production of other T cells is stimulated. Some T cells remain in the lymph nodes and retain a memory for the antigen. Other T cells migrate from the lymph nodes into the general circulatory system and ultimately to the tissues, where they remain until they either come in contact with their respective antigens or die (Grossman & Porth, 2014).

Types of T Lymphocytes

T cells include effector T cells, **suppressor T cells**, and memory T cells. The two major categories of effector T cells—**helper T cells** (also referred to as CD4+ cells) and cytotoxic T cells (also referred to as CD8+ cells)—participate in the destruction of foreign organisms. T cells interact closely with B cells, indicating that humoral and cellular immune responses are not separate, unrelated processes but rather are branches of the immune response that interact.

Helper T cells are activated on recognition of antigens and stimulate the rest of the immune system. When activated, helper T cells secrete cytokines, which attract and activate B cells, cytotoxic T cells, NK cells, macrophages, and other cells of the immune system. Cytokines are proteins produced by the cells of the immune system that determine the actions of the immune system cells. Separate subpopulations of helper T cells produce different types of cytokines and determine whether the immune response will be the production of antibodies or a cell-mediated immune response. Helper T cells also produce **lymphokines**, one category of cytokines (Table 51-2).

Cytotoxic T cells (killer T cells) attack the antigen directly by altering the cell membrane and causing cell lysis (disintegration) and releasing cytolytic enzymes and cytokines. Lymphokines can recruit, activate, and regulate other lymphocytes and WBCs. These cells then assist in destroying the invading organism. Delayed-type hypersensitivity is an example of an immune reaction that

TABLE 51-2 Cytokines and Their Biologic Activity

Cytokine[a]	Biologic Activity
Interleukin-1 (alpha and beta)	Promotes differentiation of T and B lymphocytes, natural killer (NK) cells, and null cells
Interleukin-2	Stimulates growth of T lymphocytes and special activated killer lymphocytes (known as lymphocyte-activated killer cells [LAK cells])
Interleukin-3	Stimulates growth of mast cells and other blood cells
Interleukin-4	Stimulates growth of T and B lymphocytes, mast cells, and macrophages
Interleukin-5	Stimulates antibody responses
Interleukin-6	Stimulates growth and function of B lymphocytes and antibodies
Interleukin-7	Stimulates growth of pre-B, CD4+ and CD8+ T lymphocytes and activates mature T lymphocytes
Interleukin-8	Promotes chemotaxis and activation of neutrophils
Interleukin-9	Stimulates growth and proliferation of T lymphocytes
Interleukin-10	Inhibits interferon-gamma and mononuclear cell inflammation
Interleukin-11	Promotes induction of acute phase proteins
Interleukin-12	Introduces helper T lymphocytes
Interleukin-13	Inhibits mononuclear phagocyte inflammation and promotes differentiation of B cells
Interleukin-16	Promotes chemotaxis CD4+ T lymphocytes and eosinophils
Permeability factor	Increases vascular permeability, allowing white cells into area
Interferon gamma	Activates macrophages; increases expression of class I and II MHC antigen processing and presentation
Interferon (type 1 alpha and type beta)	Exerts antiviral activity in body cells; induces class I antigen expression; activates NK cells
Migration inhibitory factor	Suppresses movement of macrophages, keeping macrophages in area of foreign cells
Skin reactive factor	Induces inflammatory response
Cytotoxic factor (lymphotoxin)	Kills certain antigenic cells
Macrophage chemotactic factor	Attracts macrophages into the area
Lymphocyte blastogenic factor	Stimulates more lymphocytes, recruiting additional lymphocytes into the area
Macrophage aggregation factor	Causes clumping of macrophages and lymphocytes
Macrophage activation factor	Allows macrophages to adhere to surfaces more readily
Proliferation inhibitor factor	Inhibits growth of certain antigenic cells
Cytophilic antibody	Binds to an Fc receptor on macrophages, thereby permitting macrophages to bind to antigens
Tumour necrosis factor alpha	Stimulates inflammation, wound healing, and tissue remodelling
Tumour necrosis factor beta	Mediates inflammation and graft rejection

[a]Cytokines are biologically active substances that are released by cells to regulate growth and function of other cells within the immune system.

Lymphocytes produce lymphokines, and monocytes and macrophages produce monokines. This table lists some of the cytokines that play a role in immune system functioning.

NK, natural killer; T_H2, T-helper type 2; IgE, immunoglobulin E; T_H1, T-helper type 1; MHC, major histocompatibility complex; CSF, colony-stimulating factor.

Adapted from Grossman, S. C., & Porth, C. M. (2014). *Porth's pathophysiology: Concepts of altered health states* (9th ed.). Philadelphia, PA: Lippincott Williams & Wilkins.

protects the body from antigens through the production and release of lymphokines (see later discussion).

Suppressor T cells have the ability to decrease B-cell production, thereby keeping the immune response at a level that is compatible with health (e.g., sufficient to fight infection adequately without attacking the body's healthy tissues). Memory cells are responsible for recognizing antigens from previous exposure and mounting an immune response (Table 51-3).

Null Lymphocytes and Natural Killer Cells

Null lymphocytes and NK cells are other lymphocytes that assist in combating organisms. These cells are distinct from B cells and T cells and lack the usual characteristics of those cells. Null lymphocytes, a subpopulation of lymphocytes, destroy antigens already coated with antibody. These cells have special receptor sites on their surface that allow them to connect with the end of antibodies; this is known as antibody-dependent, cell-mediated cytotoxicity.

NK cells are a class of lymphocytes that recognize infected and stressed cells and respond by killing these cells and by secreting macrophage-activating cytokine. The helper T cells contribute to the differentiation of null and NK cells.

Complement System

Circulating plasma proteins, known as complement, are made in the liver and activated when an antibody connects with its antigen. Complement plays an important role in the defense against microbes. Destruction of an invading or attacking organism or toxin is not achieved merely by the binding of the antibody and antigens; it also requires activation of complement, the arrival of killer T cells, or the attraction of macrophages. Complement has three major physiologic functions: defending the body against bacterial infection, bridging natural and acquired immunity, and disposing of immune complexes and the byproducts associated with inflammation (Grossman & Porth, 2014).

TABLE 51-3 Lymphocytes Involved in Immune Responses

Type of Immune Response	Cell Type	Function
Humoral	B lymphocyte	Produces antibodies or immunoglobulins (IgA, IgD, IgE, IgG, IgM)
Cellular	T lymphocyte	
	Helper T	Attacks foreign invaders (antigens) directly Initiates and augments inflammatory response
	Helper T_1	Increases activated cytotoxic T cells
	Helper T_2	Increases B cell (BG8) antibody production
	Suppressor T	Suppresses the immune response
	Memory T	Remembers contact with an antigen and on subsequent exposures mounts an immune response
	Cytotoxic T (killer T)	Lyses cells infected with virus; plays a role in graft rejection
Nonspecific	Non-T or non-B lymphocyte null cell	Destroys antigens already coated with antibody
	Natural killer (NK) cell (granular lymphocyte)	Defends against microorganisms and some types of malignant cells; produces cytokines

The proteins that comprise complement interact sequentially with one another in a cascading effect. The complement cascade is important in modifying the effector arm of the immune system. Activation of complement allows important events, such as removal of infectious agents and initiation of the inflammatory response, to take place. These events involve active parts of the pathway that enhance chemotaxis of macrophages and granulocytes, alter blood vessel permeability, change blood vessel diameters, cause cells to lyse, alter blood clotting, and cause other points of modification. These macrophages and granulocytes continue the body's defense by devouring the antibody-coated microbes and by releasing bacterial products.

The complement cascade may be activated by any of three pathways: classic, lectin, and alternative. The classic pathway is triggered after antibodies bind to microbes or other antigens and is part of the humoral type of adaptive immunity. The lectin pathway is activated when a plasma protein (mannose-binding lectin) binds to terminal mannose residue on the surface glycoproteins of microbes. The alternative pathway is triggered when complement proteins are activated on microbial surfaces. This pathway is part of innate immunity.

Complement components, prostaglandins, leukotrienes, and other inflammatory mediators all contribute to the recruitment of inflammatory cells, as do chemokines, a group of cytokines. The activated neutrophils pass through the vessel walls to accumulate at the site of infection, where they phagocytose complement-coated microbes (Abbas, Lichtman, & Pillai, 2014). This response is usually therapeutic and can be lifesaving if the cell attacked by the complement system is a true foreign invader. However, if that cell is part of the human organism, the result can be devastating disease and even death. Many autoimmune diseases and disorders characterized by chronic infection are thought to be caused in part by continued or chronic activation of complement, which in turn results in chronic inflammation. The RBCs and platelets have complement receptors and, as a result, play an important role in the clearance of immune complexes that consist of antigen, antibody, and components of the complement system (Abbas et al., 2014).

Immunomodulators

Antimicrobial agents and vaccines have yielded considerable therapeutic success and the immune system usually works effectively; however, many infectious diseases remain difficult clinical challenges. Treatment success may be compromised by defects of the immune system; in this case, enhancement of the host immune response may be therapeutically beneficial. An immunomodulator (also known as a biologic response modifier) affects the host via direct or indirect effects on one or more components of the immunoregulatory network. **Interferons**, colony-stimulating factors, and monoclonal antibodies (MoAbs) are examples of agents used to help enhance the immune system (Page & Liles, 2015).

Interferons

Interferon, one type of biologic response modifier, is a nonspecific viricidal protein that is naturally produced by the body and is capable of activating other components of the immune system. Interferons continue to be investigated to determine their roles in the immune system and their potential therapeutic effects in disorders characterized by disturbed immune responses. These substances have antiviral and antitumour properties. In addition to responding to viral infection, interferons are produced by T lymphocytes, B lymphocytes, and macrophages in response to antigens. They are thought to modify the immune response by suppressing antibody production and cellular immunity. They also facilitate the cytolytic role of macrophages and NK cells. Interferons are used to treat immune-related disorders (e.g., multiple sclerosis) and chronic inflammatory conditions (e.g., chronic hepatitis). Research continues to evaluate the effectiveness of interferons in treating cancers (Booy, Hofland, & van Eijck, 2015) and acquired immunodeficiency syndrome.

Colony-Stimulating Factors

Colony-stimulating factors are a group of naturally occurring glycoprotein cytokines that regulate production, differentiation, survival, and activation of hematopoietic cells. Erythropoietin stimulates RBC production. Thrombopoietin plays a key regulatory role in the growth and differentiation of bone marrow cells. Interleukin-5 (IL-5) stimulates the growth and survival of eosinophils and basophils. Stem cell factor and IL-3 serve as stimuli for multiple hematopoietic cell lines. Granulocyte colony–stimulating factor, granulocyte macrophage–colony-stimulating factor, and macrophage colony–stimulating factor all serve as growth factors for specific cell lines. These cytokines have attracted considerable interest for their potential role in immunomodulation (Page & Liles, 2015).

Monoclonal Antibodies

MoAbs have become available through technologic advances, enabling investigators to grow and produce targeted antibodies for specific pathologic organisms. This type of specificity allows MoAbs to destroy pathologic organisms and spare normal cells. The specificity of MoAbs depends on identifying key antigen proteins that are present on the surface of tumours, but not on normal tissues. When the MoAb attaches to the cell surface antigen, it blocks an important signal transduction pathway for communication between the malignant cells and the extracellular environment. The results may include an inability to initiate apoptosis, reproduce, or invade surrounding tissues. To date, more than 1,000 tumour antigens have been identified (Glassman & Balthasar, 2014). See Chapter 68 for a discussion on the use of MoAbs in cancer.

Advances in Immunology

Genetic Engineering

One of the more remarkable evolving technologies is **genetic engineering**, which uses recombinant deoxyribonucleic acid (DNA) technology. Two facets of this technology exist. The first permits scientists to combine genes from one type of organism with genes of a second organism. This type of technology allows cells and microorganisms to manufacture proteins, monokines, and lymphokines, which can alter and enhance immune system function. The second facet of recombinant DNA technology involves gene therapy. If a particular gene is abnormal or missing, experimental recombinant DNA technology may be capable of restoring normal gene function. For example, a recombinant gene is inserted onto a virus particle. When the virus particle splices its genes, the virus automatically inserts the missing gene and theoretically corrects the genetic anomaly. Extensive research into recombinant DNA technology and gene therapy is ongoing (Geering & Fussenegger, 2015).

Stem Cells

Stem cells are capable of self-renewal and differentiation; they continually replenish the body's entire supply of both RBCs and WBCs. Some stem cells, described as totipotent cells, have tremendous capacity to self-renew and differentiate. Embryonic stem cells, described as pluripotent, give rise to numerous cell types that are able to form tissues. Research has shown that stem cells can restore an immune system that has been destroyed (Kessler, 2015). Stem cell transplantation has been carried out in humans with certain types of immune dysfunction, such as severe combined immunodeficiency; clinical trials using stem cells are under way in patients with a variety of disorders having an autoimmune component, including systemic lupus erythematosus, rheumatoid arthritis, scleroderma, and multiple sclerosis. Research with embryonic stem cells has enabled investigators to make substantial gains in developmental biology, gene therapy, therapeutic tissue engineering, and the treatment of a variety of diseases (Kessler, 2015). However, along with these remarkable opportunities, many ethical challenges arise, which are largely based on concerns about safety, efficacy, resource allocation, and human cloning.

Cancer and Immunotherapy

It has long been understood that the immune system plays a role in fighting off malignancies. Recent advances in cancer treatment have sought to augment the body's natural antitumour activity and to shut down the pathways that allow malignancies to elude the immune system, which has led to the development of such treatments as MoAbs, cancer vaccines, immune adjuvants, immune checkpoint inhibitors, and cytokines (Kannan et al., 2013). These immunotherapeutic treatments are designed to stimulate the patient's immune system to mount its own defense against the cancer and have shown very promising results in a number of different cancer types.

Assessment of the Immune System

An assessment of immune function begins during the health history and physical examination. Areas to be assessed include nutritional status; infections and immunizations; allergies; disorders and disease states, such as autoimmune disorders, cancer, and chronic illnesses; surgeries; medications; and blood transfusions. In addition to inspection of general characteristics, palpation of the lymph nodes and examinations of the skin, mucous membranes, and respiratory, gastrointestinal, musculoskeletal, genitourinary, cardiovascular, and neurosensory systems are performed (Chart 51-3).

Health History

The history should note the patient's age along with information about past and present conditions and events that may provide clues to the status of the patient's immune system.

Gender

There are differences in the immune system functions of men and women. For example, many autoimmune diseases have a higher incidence in females than in males, a phenomenon believed to be correlated with sex hormones. Sex hormones have long been recognized for their role in reproductive function, and in the past two decades research has revealed that these hormones are integral signaling modulators of the immune system. Sex hormones play definitive roles in lymphocyte maturation, activation, and synthesis of antibodies and cytokines. In autoimmune disease, expression of sex hormones is altered, and this change contributes to immune dysregulation (Ngo, Steyn, & McCombe, 2014).

Gerontologic Considerations

Immunosenescence is a complex route in which the aging process stimulates changes in the immune system

CHART 51-3

Assessing for Immune Dysfunction

Be alert for the following signs and symptoms:

Respiratory System
- Changes in respiratory rate
- Cough (dry or productive)
- Abnormal lung sounds (wheezing, crackles, rhonchi)
- Rhinitis
- Hyperventilation
- Bronchospasm

Cardiovascular System
- Hypotension
- Tachycardia
- Dysrhythmia
- Vasculitis
- Anemia

Gastrointestinal System
- Hepatosplenomegaly
- Colitis
- Vomiting
- Diarrhea

Genitourinary System
- Frequency and burning on urination
- Hematuria
- Discharge

Musculoskeletal System
- Joint mobility, edema, and pain

Skin
- Rashes
- Lesions
- Dermatitis
- Hematomas or purpura
- Edema or urticaria
- Inflammation
- Discharge

Neurosensory System
- Cognitive dysfunction
- Hearing loss
- Visual changes
- Headaches and migraines
- Ataxia
- Tetany

(Shekarabi & Asgari, 2014). Some of the changes that occur in immunosenescence include, but are not limited to, bone marrow defects, dysfunction of the thymus gland, and impaired lymphocytes. Cellular changes occur as the result of aging and include impaired neutrophil function, decreased number of circulating macrophages, impaired dendritic cell function, and reduced T-cell activation (Müller & Pawelec, 2014). As the immune system undergoes age-associated alterations, its response to infections progressively deteriorates. The capacity for self-renewal of hematopoietic stem cells diminishes. There is a notable decline in the total number of phagocytes, coupled with an intrinsic reduction in their activity. The cytotoxicity of NK cells decreases, contributing to a decline in humoral immunity (Müller & Pawelec, 2014). Acquired immunity may be negatively affected; the efficacy of vaccines is frequently decreased in older adults (Goronzy & Weyand, 2013). Inflammatory cytokines tend to increase with age.

Older adults have increased incidence of infections, autoimmune diseases, metabolic diseases, osteoporosis, and neurologic disorders (Müller & Pawelec, 2014). The increased incidence of autoimmune diseases may be from a decreased ability of antibodies to differentiate between self and nonself. Failure of the surveillance system to recognize mutant or abnormal cells also may be responsible, in part, for the high incidence of cancer associated with increasing age.

Age-related changes in many body systems also contribute to impaired immunity (Table 51-4). For example, postmenopausal females are at a greater risk for urinary tract infections due to residual urine, urinary incontinence, and estrogen deficiency (Mody & Juthani-Mehta, 2014). Secondary changes, including malnutrition and poor circulation, as well as the breakdown of natural mechanical barriers such as the skin, place the aging immune system at even greater disadvantage against infection (Carlsson, Haglin, Rosendahl, et al., 2013).

The effects of the aging process and psychological stress interact, with the potential to negatively influence immune integrity (Epel & Lithgow, 2014). Consequently, continual assessment of the physical and emotional status of the older adult is imperative, because early recognition and management of factors influencing immune response may prevent or mitigate the high morbidity and mortality seen with illness in the older adult population (Müller & Pawelec, 2014).

Nutrition

The relationship of infection to nutritional status is a key determinant of health. Traditionally, this relationship focused on the effect of nutrients on host defenses and the effect of infection on nutritional needs. This has expanded in scope to encompass the role of specific nutrients in acquired immune function—the modulation of inflammatory processes and the virulence of the infectious agent itself. Iron and the immune system are linked in homeostasis and pathology, thus making it essential for maximum function (Cassat & Skaar, 2013). The list of nutrients affecting infection, immunity, inflammation, and cell injury has expanded from traditional proteins to several vitamins, multiple minerals, and, more recently, specific lipid components of the diet. One review looked at the role of vitamins A, C, D, E, and K in treatment of pancreatic cancer but concluded that not enough evidence based on clinical trials is available to fully support the use of these vitamins as an intervention (Davis-Yadley & Malafa, 2015). The role of micronutrients and fatty acids on the response of cells and tissues to hypoxic and toxic damage has been recognized, suggesting that there is another dimension to the relationship. Deficiencies in micronutrients have been connected to impairment in various body functions, including immunity. Zinc deficiency in particular has been linked to the development of a number of diseases. Zinc plays an important role in homeostasis, immune function, and apoptosis, among other functions (Müller & Pawelec, 2014).

TABLE 51-4 Age-Related Changes in Immunologic Function

Body System	Changes	Consequences
Immune	Impaired function of B and T lymphocytes Failure of lymphocytes to recognize mutant or abnormal cells Decreased antibody production Failure of immune system to differentiate "self" from "nonself" Suppressed phagocytic immune response	Suppressed responses to pathogenic organisms with increased risk for infection Increased incidence of cancers Anergy (lack of response to antigens applied to the skin [allergens]) Increased incidence of autoimmune diseases Absence of typical signs and symptoms of infection and inflammation Dissemination of organisms usually destroyed or suppressed by phagocytes (e.g., reactivation or spread of tuberculosis)
Gastrointestinal	Decreased gastric secretions and motility Decreased phagocytosis by the liver's Kupffer cells Altered nutritional intake with inadequate protein intake	Proliferation of intestinal organisms resulting in gastroenteritis and diarrhea Increased incidence and severity of hepatitis B; increased incidence of liver abscesses Suppressed immune response
Urinary	Decreased kidney function and changes in lower urinary tract function (enlargement of prostate gland, neurogenic bladder). Altered genitourinary tract flora	Urinary stasis and increased incidence of urinary tract infections
Pulmonary	Impaired ciliary action due to exposure to smoke and environmental toxins	Impaired clearance of pulmonary secretions; increased incidence of respiratory infections
Integumentary	Thinning of skin with less elasticity; loss of adipose tissue	Increased risk of skin injury, breakdown, and infection
Circulatory	Impaired microcirculation	Stasis and pressure ulcers
Neurologic function	Decreased sensation and slowing of reflexes	Increased risk of injury, skin ulcers, abrasions, and burns

The effects exerted by polyunsaturated fatty acids on immune system functions are under investigation. Studies show that these elements play a role in diminishing the incidence and severity of inflammatory disorders (Hardin-Fanning, Boissonneault, & Lennie, 2011). Recent studies show that diets high in olive oil are not as immunosuppressive as diets rich in fish oil. The contribution of immune modulation by lipids to the high risk of infectious complications associated with the use of parenteral nutrition is unclear; however, a recent meta-analysis revealed that the use of glutamine-supplemented parenteral nutrition decreased the incidence of infections postoperatively (Yue, Tian, Wang, et al., 2013).

Depletion of protein reserves results in atrophy of lymphoid tissues, depression of antibody response, reduction in the number of circulating T cells, and impaired phagocytic function. As a result, susceptibility to infection is greatly increased. During periods of infection or serious illness, nutritional requirements may be further altered, potentially contributing to depletion of protein, fatty acid, vitamin, and trace elements and causing even greater risk of impaired immune response and sepsis. Nutritional intake that supports a competent immune response plays an important role in reducing the incidence of infections; patients whose nutritional status is compromised have a delayed postoperative recovery and often experience more severe infections and delayed wound healing. The nurse must assess the patient's nutritional status, caloric intake, and quality of foods ingested. There is evidence that nutrition plays a role in the development of cancer and that diet and lifestyle can alter the risk of cancer development as well as other chronic diseases (Supic, Jagodic, & Magic, 2013). The nurse must assume a proactive role in ensuring the best possible nutritional intake for all patients as a vital step in preventing disease and poor outcomes (Tappenden, Quatrara, Parkhurst, et al., 2013).

Immunization

The patient is asked about childhood and adult immunizations, including vaccinations, to provide protection against influenza, pneumococcal disease (Pneumovax), pertussis, herpes simplex, and the usual childhood diseases (e.g., measles, mumps). Herpes simplex virus infections have a significant impact on health, causing a wide range of diseases (e.g., oral and genital herpes). Teaching about the importance of adhering to the recommended schedule for these vaccines should be initiated.

Infection

Known past or present exposure to tuberculosis is assessed, and the dates and results of any tuberculin tests (purified protein derivative [PPD] test) and chest x-rays are documented. Recent exposure to any infections and the exposure dates are elicited. The nurse must assess whether the patient has been exposed to any sexually transmitted infections (STIs) or bloodborne pathogens such as hepatitis B, C, and D viruses and human immunodeficiency virus (HIV). A history of STIs such as gonorrhea, syphilis, human papillomavirus infection, and chlamydia can alert the nurse that the patient may have been exposed to HIV or hepatitis. Patients who have had an ischemic stroke or transient ischemic attack (TIA) are at risk for infection following the event (Ross, Lee, & Brewer, 2014). In an effort to fight infection, patients mount a peripheral immune response (PIR) consisting of neutrophilia, lymphocytopenia, and elevated monocytes (Ross et al., 2014). Researchers are investigating the time course, trajectory, and significance of the PIR following stroke or TIA (Ross et al., 2014; Ross &

NURSING RESEARCH PROFILE

Chart 51-4. Peripheral Immune Response Trajectories

Ross, A. M., & Lee, C. (2015). Description and identification of the peripheral immune response trajectories over time in first-time and recurrent stroke/transient ischemic attack. *Journal of Neuroscience Nursing, 47*(5), 256–262.

Purpose

It is not known how the immune response changes over time in patients after a stroke or transient ischemic attack (TIA). The purpose of this study was to describe the peripheral immune response (PIR) trajectories over time following a first-time and recurrent stroke or transient ischemic attack. The two aims were first to compare changes in the PIR over time in patients with a first versus a recurrent stroke or TIA, and second to identify trajectories of change in the PIR in patients after a stroke or TIA.

Design

This was a secondary analysis of data collected during a retrospective cross-sectional study on the PIR in the acute phase of care after a stroke or TIA. Data for the parent study were collected using a detailed retrospective medical record review. Descriptive statistics and latent growth mixture modelling were used to investigate the changes in PIR over time.

Findings

Of the 192 adult men and women included in the study 84 (44%) had a first-time stroke or TIA and 108 (56%) had a recurrent event. Participants with recurrent stroke or TIA had a persistent elevation in lymphocyte percentage compared to a significant decline in lymphocyte percentage observed in patients with a first-time event. The first trajectory (80% of the sample) had persistently lower lymphocyte percentages and higher neutrophil percentages over time, while the second trajectory (20% of the sample) had higher lymphocyte percentages and lower neutrophil percentages over time.

Nursing Implications

Nurses monitoring laboratory values after stroke or TIA need to recognize that different trajectories of PIRs exist. This may have future implications for identification of patients who may benefit from novel immune therapies. Nurses caring for patients who have any signs of depressed immune function need to be more vigilant in their assessments, watching for possible signs and symptoms of infection.

Lee, 2015) (Chart 51-4). A history of past and present infections and the dates and types of treatments, along with a history of any multiple persistent infections, fevers of unknown origin, lesions or sores, or any type of drainage, as well as the response to treatment, are obtained.

Allergy

The patient is asked about any allergies, including types of allergens (e.g., pollens, dust, plants, cosmetics, food, medications, vaccines, latex), the symptoms experienced, and seasonal variations in occurrence or severity in the symptoms. A history of testing and treatments, including prescribed and over-the-counter medications that the patient has taken or is currently taking for these allergies and the effectiveness of the treatments, is obtained. All medication and food allergies are listed on an allergy alert sticker and placed on the front of the patient's health or medical record to alert others. Continued assessment for potential allergic reactions in the patient is vital.

Disorders and Diseases

Autoimmune Disorders

Autoimmune disorders affect people of both genders of all ages, ethnicities, and social classes. Autoimmune disorders are a group of disorders that can affect almost any cell or tissue in the body (Grossman & Porth, 2014). As mentioned previously, they tend to be more common in women because estrogen tends to enhance immunity. Androgen, on the other hand, tends to be immunosuppressive. Autoimmune diseases are a leading cause of death by disease in females of reproductive age.

The patient is asked about any autoimmune disorders, such as lupus erythematosus, rheumatoid arthritis, multiple sclerosis, or psoriasis. The onset, severity, remissions and exacerbations, functional limitations, treatments that the patient has received or is currently receiving, and effectiveness of the treatments are described. The occurrence of different autoimmune diseases within a family strongly suggests a genetic predisposition to more than one autoimmune disease (Brooks & Renaudineau, 2015) (see Chart 51-5).

Neoplastic Disease

If there is a history of cancer in the family, more information is obtained, including the type of cancer, age at onset, and relationship (maternal or paternal) of the patient to the affected family members. Dates and results of any cancer screening tests for the patient are documented.

A history of cancer in the patient is also obtained, along with the type of cancer, date of diagnosis, and treatment modalities used. Immunosuppression contributes to the development of cancers; however, cancer itself is immunosuppressive, as is the treatment for cancer. Large tumours can release antigens into the blood, and these antigens combine with circulating antibodies and prevent them from attacking the tumour cells. Furthermore, tumour cells may possess special blocking factors that coat tumour cells and prevent their destruction by killer T lymphocytes. During the early development of tumours, the body may fail to recognize the tumour antigens as foreign and subsequently fail to initiate destruction of the malignant cells. Hematologic cancers, such as leukemia and lymphoma, are associated with altered production and function of WBCs and lymphocytes.

All treatments that the patient has received or is currently receiving, such as radiation or chemotherapy, are

GENETICS IN NURSING PRACTICE

Chart 51-5. Immunologic Disorders

An immunologic disorder is a disorder of an individual's immune system, which is a network of cells, tissues, and organs that work together to defend the body against attacks by foreign invaders such as bacteria, parasites, and fungi that can cause infection. A number of immunologic disorders have a known inheritance pattern, while others are noted to have a genetic abnormality that is influenced by environmental exposures. Therefore, the pattern of inheritance is unclear in some immunologic disorders. Examples of immunologic disorders caused by a genetic abnormality include:

- Adenosine deaminase deficiency (autosomal recessive)
- Alopecia areata
- Alopecia totalis
- Asthma
- Ataxia telangiectasia (autosomal recessive)
- Autoimmune polyglandular syndrome
- Bruton's agammaglobulinemia (X linked)
- Burkitt lymphoma
- Crohn's disease
- Diabetes, type 1
- DiGeorge syndrome (Autosomal dominant)
- Familial Mediterranean fever
- Job syndrome (autosomal dominant and recessive)
- Purine nucleoside phosphorylase deficiency (autosomal dominant)
- Severe combined immunodeficiency (primarily X linked)
- Wiskott-Aldrich syndrome (X linked)

Nursing Assessments

FAMILY HISTORY ASSESSMENT SPECIFIC TO IMMUNOLOGIC DISORDERS

- Collect a family history for both maternal and paternal relatives for three generations.
- Assess family history for other family members with histories of immunologic disorders.
- Obtain information about family members with a history of recurrent infections or illness.
- Recognize ethnic risk (non-Ashkenazi Jewish, Armenian, Arab, and Turkish are at greater risk for Familial Mediterranean fever; Caucasians have a higher incidence of Crohn's disease).

PATIENT ASSESSMENT

- Assess for symptoms such as changes in respiratory status associated with asthma (e.g., wheezing, or airway hyperresponsiveness; mucosal edema; and mucus production).
- Gather information regarding immunizations and whether an altered response to any immunization has occurred.
- Assess for symptoms of immunodeficiency disorders, such as unexplained weight gain or loss, skin rashes, changes in hair texture or distribution, joint or muscle pain, intolerance to cold, irregular menstrual periods, abdominal discomfort, or the presence of diarrhea.
- Identify pattern of sickness with regard to frequency of colds, respiratory infections, or history of illness that tends to linger.
- Obtain history of childhood illnesses and details of the illness experience.
- Assess for medical history of frequent or recurrent infections.
- Learn about susceptibility to infections, assess for patterns (frequency, length of illness, severity of symptoms), and recognize infections that would be atypical for age.
- Inquire about environmental exposures (e.g., smoke, chloroform, metal or dust particles, paint).
- Ask about exposure to other viruses such as Epstein-Barr or influenza.

recorded in the health history. In addition, the nurse should elicit information related to complementary or alternative modalities that have been used and the response to these efforts. Radiation destroys lymphocytes and decreases the ability to mount an effective immune response. The size and extent of the irradiated area determine the extent of immunosuppression. Whole-body irradiation may leave the patient totally immunosuppressed. Chemotherapy and other cancer treatments also affect bone marrow function, destroying cells that contribute to an effective immune response and resulting in immunosuppression (Morrison, 2014).

Chronic Illness and Surgery

The health assessment includes a history of chronic illness, such as diabetes, renal disease, chronic obstructive pulmonary disease (COPD), or fibromyalgia. The onset and severity of illnesses, as well as treatment that the patient is receiving for the illness, are obtained. Chronic illness may contribute to immune system impairments in various ways. Kidney injury is associated with a deficiency in circulating lymphocytes. In addition, immune defenses may be altered by acidosis and uremic toxins. In diabetes, an increased incidence of infection has been associated with vascular insufficiency, neuropathy, and poor control of serum glucose levels. Recurrent respiratory tract infections are associated with COPD as a result of altered inspiratory and expiratory function and ineffective airway clearance. In addition, a history of organ transplantation or surgical removal of the spleen, lymph nodes, or thymus is noted, because these conditions may place the patient at risk for impaired immune function (Bronte & Pittet, 2013).

Special Problems

Conditions such as burns and other forms of injury and infection may contribute to altered immune system function. Major burns cause impaired skin integrity and compromise the body's first line of defense. Loss of large amounts of serum occurs with burn injuries and depletes the body of essential proteins, including immunoglobulins. The physiologic and psychological stressors associated with surgery or injury stimulates cortisol release from the adrenal cortex; increased serum cortisol also contributes to suppression of normal immune responses (Eng, Kokolus, Reed, et al., 2014).

TABLE 51-5 Selected Medications and Effects on the Immune System

Drug Classification (and Examples)	Effects on the Immune System
Antibiotics (in large doses)	**Bone Marrow Suppression**
ceftriaxone (Rocephin)	Eosinophilia, hemolytic anemia, hypoprothrombinemia, neutropenia, thrombocytopenia
cefuroxime sodium (Ceftin)	Eosinophilia, hemolytic anemia, hypoprothrombinemia, neutropenia, thrombocytopenia
chloramphenicol (Chloromycetin)	Leukopenia, aplastic anemia
dactinomycin (Cosmegen)	Agranulocytosis, neutropenia
fluoroquinolones (ciprofloxacin [Cipro], levofloxacin [Levaquin])	Hemolytic anemia, methemoglobinemia, eosinophilia, leukopenia, pancytopenia
gentamicin sulphate (Garamycin)	Agranulocytosis, granulocytosis
macrolides (erythromycin, azithromycin [Zithromax], clarithromycin [Biaxin])	Neutropenia, leukopenia
penicillins	Agranulocytosis
streptomycin	Leukopenia, neutropenia, pancytopenia
vancomycin (Vancocin, Vancoled)	Transient leukopenia
Antithyroid Drugs	
propylthiouracil (PTU)	Agranulocytosis, leukopenia
Nonsteroidal Anti-Inflammatory Drugs (NSAIDs) (in large doses)	**Inhibit Prostaglandin Synthesis or Release**
aspirin	Agranulocytosis
COX-2 inhibitors (celecoxib [Celebrex])	Anemia, allergy, no other major adverse effects
ibuprofen (Advil, Motrin)	Leukopenia, Neutropenia
indomethacin (Indocid, Indocin)	Agranulocytosis, leukopenia
phenylbutazone	Pancytopenia, agranulocytosis, aplastic anemia
Adrenal Corticosteroids	**Immunosuppression**
prednisone	
Antineoplastic Agents (cytotoxic agents)	**Immunosuppression**
cyclophosphamide (Cytoxan)	Leukopenia, neutropenia
mechlorethamine HCl (Mustargen)	Agranulocytosis, neutropenia
cyclosporine (Neoral)	Leukopenia, inhibits T-lymphocyte function
Antimetabolites	**Immunosuppression**
pyrimidine antagonist (Fluorouracil [5-FU])	Leukopenia, eosinophilia
folic acid antagonist (Methotrexate)	Leukopenia, aplastic bone marrow
purine antagonist (Mercaptopurine[(6-MP])	Leukopenia, pancytopenia

COX, cyclo-oxygenase.

Adapted from Comerford, K. C. (2015). *Nursing 2015 drug handbook*. Philadelphia, PA: Wolters Kluwer.

Medications and Blood Transfusions

A list of past and present medications is obtained. In large doses, antibiotics, corticosteroids, cytotoxic agents, salicylates, nonsteroidal anti-inflammatory drugs, and anesthetic agents can cause immune suppression (Table 51-5).

A history of blood transfusions is obtained, because previous exposure to foreign antigens through transfusion may be associated with abnormal immune function. In addition, although the risk of HIV transmission through blood transfusion is extremely low in patients who received a transfusion after 1985 (when testing of blood for HIV was initiated in Canada), a small risk remains.

The patient is also asked about the use of herbal agents and over-the-counter medications. Because many of these products have not been subjected to rigorous testing, their effects have not been fully identified. It is important, therefore, to ask patients about their use of these substances, to document their use, and to educate patients about untoward effects that may alter immune responsiveness.

Lifestyle Factors

Like any other body system, the functions of the immune system are interrelated with other body systems. Poor nutritional status, smoking (Sheils, Katki, Freedman, et al., 2014), excessive consumption of alcohol, illicit drug use, STIs, and occupational or residential exposure to environmental radiation and pollutants have been associated with impaired immune function and are assessed in a detailed patient history. Although factors that are not consistent with a healthy lifestyle are predominately responsible for ineffective immune function, positive lifestyle factors can also negatively affect immune function and require assessment. For example, rigorous exercise or competitive exercise—usually considered a positive lifestyle factor—can be a physiologic stressor and cause negative effects on immune response (Jin, Paik, Kwak, et al., 2015). This outcome is compounded if the person also faces stressful environmental conditions while undergoing exercise. Given the cumulative impact of various environmental stressors on the immune system, every effort should be made to minimize the person's exposure to stressors other than the exercise performed (Jin et al., 2015).

Psychoneuroimmunologic Factors

Patient assessment must also address psychoneuroimmunologic factors. The bidirectional pathway between the brain and immune system is referred to as psychoneuroimmunology (Fagundes, Lindgren, & Kiecolt-Glaser, 2013). The immune response is regulated and modulated in part by neuroendocrine influences. Lymphocytes and macrophages have receptors that can respond to neurotransmitters and endocrine hormones. Lymphocytes can produce and secrete adrenocorticotropic hormone and endorphin-like compounds. Cells in the brain, especially in the hypothalamus, can recognize prostaglandins, interferons, and interleukins as well as histamine and serotonin, all which are released during the inflammatory process. Like all other biologic systems functioning to maintain homeostasis, the immune system is integrated with other psychophysiologic processes and is regulated and modulated by the brain. These relationships may have immunologic consequences.

Conversely, the immune processes can affect neural and endocrine function, including behaviour. Growing evidence indicates that measurable immune system response can be positively influenced by biobehavioural strategies such as relaxation and imagery techniques, biofeedback, humor, hypnosis, and conditioning (Bennett, Parsons, Ben-Moshe, et al., 2014; Palsson & van Tilburg, 2015). Therefore, the assessment should address the patient's general psychological status and the patient's use of and response to these strategies.

Physical Assessment

During the physical examination (see Chart 51-3), the skin and mucous membranes are assessed for lesions, dermatitis, purpura (subcutaneous bleeding), urticaria, inflammation, or any discharge. Any signs of infection are noted. The patient's temperature is recorded, and the patient is observed for chills and sweating. The anterior and posterior cervical, supraclavicular, axillary, and inguinal lymph nodes are palpated for enlargement. If palpable nodes are detected, their location, size, consistency, and reports of tenderness on palpation are noted. Joints are assessed for tenderness, swelling, increased warmth, and limited range of motion. The patient's respiratory, cardiovascular, genitourinary, gastrointestinal, and neurosensory systems are evaluated for signs and symptoms indicative of immune dysfunction. Any functional limitations or disabilities the patient may have are also assessed.

Diagnostic Evaluation

A series of blood tests and skin tests as well as a bone marrow biopsy may be performed to evaluate the patient's immune competence. Specific laboratory and diagnostic tests are discussed in greater detail along with individual disease processes in subsequent chapters in this unit. Selected laboratory and diagnostic tests used to evaluate immune competence are summarized in Chart 51-6.

CHART 51-6

Selected Tests for Evaluating Immunologic Status

Various laboratory tests may be performed to assess immune system activity or dysfunction. The studies assess leukocytes and lymphocytes, humoral immunity, cellular immunity, phagocytic cell function; complement activity, hypersensitivity reactions, specific antigen–antibodies, or human immunodeficiency virus infection.

Humoral (Antibody-Mediated) Immunity Tests

- B-cell quantification with monoclonal antibody
- In vivo immunoglobulin synthesis with T-cell subsets
- Specific antibody response
- Total serum globulins and individual immunoglobulins (electrophoresis, immunoelectrophoresis, single radial immunodiffusion, nephelometry, and isohemagglutinin techniques)

Cellular (Cell-Mediated) Immunity Tests

- Total lymphocyte count
- T-cell and T-cell–subset quantification with monoclonal antibody
- Delayed hypersensitivity skin test
- Cytokine production
- Lymphocyte response to mitogens, antigens, and allogenic cells
- Helper and suppressor T-cell functions

Nursing Management

The nurse needs to be aware that patients undergoing evaluation for possible immune system disorders experience not only physical pain and discomfort with certain types of diagnostic procedures, but also many psychological reactions. It is the nurse's role to counsel, educate, and support patients throughout the diagnostic process. Many patients may be extremely anxious about the results of diagnostic tests and the possible implications of those results for their future health, employment, and personal relationships. This is an ideal time for the nurse to provide counselling and education, should these interventions be warranted.

Critical Thinking Exercises

1 An 80-year-old woman presents to her primary provider for evaluation of a recurrent urinary tract infection for which she has received several courses of antibiotics. What diagnostic tests would you expect to be prescribed? What is the rationale for these tests? What further assessment data would you want to obtain from this patient?

2 **ebp** A 40-year-old woman with systemic lupus erythematosus (SLE) is admitted to the hospital for a kidney transplant and is prescribed immunosuppressant medications. Describe how her altered immune system would affect the care you provide. Develop an evidence-based education plan for the patient and her family before hospital discharge. Discuss the criteria used to assess the strength of the evidence for your education plan.

3 **pq** **A 35-year-old woman with rheumatoid arthritis presents with an acute flare-up of her symptoms and is prescribed corticosteroids. What are your priority nursing observations and assessments? Identify priorities for patient education appropriate for the new prescription of steroids.**

REFERENCES AND SELECTED READINGS

Books

Abbas, A., Lichtman, A., & Pillai, S. (2014). *Basic immunology, functions and disorders of the immune system* (4th ed.). Philadelphia, PA: W. B. Saunders.

Bulechek, G. M., Butcher, H. K., & Dochterman, J. M. (2012). *Nursing interventions classification (NIC)* (6th ed.). St. Louis, MO: Mosby.

Fagundes, C. P., Lindgren, M. E., & Kiecolt-Glaser, J. K. (2013). Psychoneuroimmunology and cancer: Incidence, progression, and quality of life. In B. I. Carr, & J. Steel (Eds.). *Psychological aspects of cancer: A guide to emotional and psychological consequences of cancer, their causes and their management*. New York: Springer.

Grossman, S. C., & Porth, C. M. (2014). *Porth's pathophysiology: Concepts of altered health states* (9th ed.). Philadelphia, PA: Lippincott Williams & Wilkins.

Hannon, R. A., Pooler, C., & Porth, C. M. (2010). *Porth pathophysiology: Concepts of altered health states* (1st Canadian ed.). Philadelphia, PA: Wolters Kluwer Health/Lippincott Williams & Wilkins.

Haynes, B. F., Soderberg, K. A., & Fauci, A. S. (2015). Introduction to the immune system. In D. L. Kasper, A. S. Fauci, S. L. Hauser, et al. (Eds.). *Harrison's principles of internal medicine* (19th ed.). New York: McGraw-Hill Education.

Johnson, M., Bulechek, G., Butcher, H. K., et al. (2011). *NOC and NIC linkages to NANDA-I and clinical conditions: Supporting critical thinking and quality care* (3rd ed.). St. Louis, MO: Mosby.

Kessler, J. A. (2015). Applications of stem cell biology in clinical medicine. In D. L. Kasper, A. S. Fauci, S. L. Hauser, et al. (Eds.). *Harrison's principles of internal medicine* (19th ed.). New York: McGraw-Hill Education.

Levinson, W. (2014). *Review of medical microbiology and immunology* (13th ed.). New York: McGraw-Hill Education.

McComb, S., Thiriot, A., Krishnan, L., et al. (2013). Introduction to the immune system. In K. M. Fulton, & S. M. Twine (Eds.). *Immunoproteomics: Methods and protocols*. Totowa: Humana Press.

Page, A. V., & Liles, W. C. (2015). Immunomodulators. In J. E. Bennett, R. Dolin, & M. J. Blaser (Eds.). *Principles and practices of infectious diseases* (8th ed.). Philadelphia, PA: Elsevier Saunders.

Paul, W. E. (Ed.) (2013). *Fundamental immunology* (7th ed.). Philadelphia, PA: Lippincott Williams & Wilkins.

Shekarabi, M., & Asgari, F. (2014). Aging immunity and infection. In A. N. Massoud, & N. Rezaei (Eds.). *Immunology of aging*. New York: Springer Heidelberg.

Journals

Bennett, P. N., Parsons, T., Ben-Moshe, R., et al. (2014). Laughter and humor therapy in dialysis. *Seminars in Dialysis*, 27(5), 488–493. doi:10.1111/sdi.12194.

Booy, S., Hofland, L., & van Eijck, C. (2015). Potentials of interferon therapy in the treatment of pancreatic cancer. *Journal of Interferon and Cytokine Research*, *35*(5), 327–339.

Bronte, V., & Pittet, M. J. (2013). The spleen in local and systemic regulation of immunity. *Immunity*, *39*(5), 809–818.

Brooks, W. H., & Renaudineau, Y. (2015). Epigenetics and autoimmune diseases: The X chromosome-nucleolus nexus. *Frontiers in Genetics*, 6(22), 1–20.

Carlsson, M., Haglin, L., Rosendahl, E., et al. (2013). Poor functional status is associated with urinary tract infection among older people living in residential care facilities. *The Journal of Nutrition, Health & Aging*, *17*(2), 186–191.

Cassat, J. E., & Skaar, E. P. (2013). Iron in infection and immunity. *Cell Host & Microbe*, *13*(5), 509–519.

Davis-Yadley, A. H., & Malafa, M. P. (2015). Vitamins in pancreatic cancer: A review of underlying mechanisms and future applications. *Advances in Nutrition*, *6*, 774–802.

Eng, J. W., Kokolus, K. M., Reed, C. B., et al. (2014). A nervous tumor microenvironment: The impact of adrenergic stress on cancer cells, immunosuppression, and immunotherapeutic response. *Cancer Immunology and Immunotherapy*, *63*(11), 1115–1128.

Epel, E. S., & Lithgow, G. J. (2014). Stress biology and aging mechanisms: Toward understanding the deep connection between adaptation to stress and longevity. *The Journals of Gerontology Series A: Biological Sciences and Medical Sciences*, *69*(Suppl 1), S10–S16.

Geering, B., & Fussenegger, M. (2015). Synthetic immunology: Modulating the human immune system. *Trends in Biotechnology*, *33*(2), 65–79.

Glassman, P. M., & Balthasar, J. P. (2014). Mechanistic considerations for the use of monoclonal antibodies for cancer therapy. *Cancer Biology & Medicine*, *11*(1), 20–33.

Goronzy, J. J., & Weyand, C. M. (2013). Understanding immunosenescence to improve responses to vaccines. *Nature Immunology*, *14*, 428–436.

Hardin-Fanning, F., Boissonneault, G. A, & Lennie, T. A. (2011). Polyunsaturated fatty acids. *Journal of Gerontological Nursing*, *37*(5), 20–28.

Jin, C. H., Paik, I. Y., Kwak, Y. S., et al. (2015). Exhaustive submaximal endurance and resistance exercises induce temporary immunosuppression via physical and oxidative stress. *Journal of Exercise and Rehabilitation*, *11*(4), 198–203.

Kang, D. H., McArdle, T., Park, N. J., et al. (2011). Dose effects of relaxation practice on immune responses in women newly diagnosed with breast cancer: An exploratory study. *Oncology Nursing Forum*, *38*(3), E240–E252.

Kannan, R., Madden, K., & Andrews, S. (2013). Primer on immune-oncology and immune response. *Clinical Journal of Oncology Nursing*, *18*(3), 311–317.

Lo, Y. C., Lee, C. F., & Powell, J. D. (2014). Insight into the role of mTOR and metabolism in T cells reveals new potential approaches to preventing graft rejection. *Current Opinion in Organ Transplantation*, *19*(4), 363–371.

Mody, L., & Juthani-Mehta, M. (2014). Urinary tract infections in older women: A clinical review. *JAMA*, *311*(8), 844–854.

Morrison, V. A. (2014). Immunosuppression associated with novel chemotherapy agents and monoclonal antibodies. *Clinical Infectious Diseases*, *59*(Suppl 5), S360–S364.

Müller, L., & Pawelec, G. (2014). Aging and immunity: Impact of behavioral intervention. *Brain, Behavior, and Immunity*, *39*, 8–22.

Ngo, S. T., Steyn, F. J., & McCombe, P. A. (2014). Gender differences in autoimmune disease. *Frontiers in Neuroendocrinology*, *35*(3), 347–369.

Palsson, O. S., & van Tilburg, M. (2015). Hypnosis and guided imagery treatment for gastrointestinal disorders: Experience with scripted protocols developed at the University of North Carolina. *American Journal of Clinical Hypnosis*, *58*(1), 5–21.

Ross, A. M., & Lee, C. (2015). Description and identification of the peripheral immune response trajectories over time in first-time and recurrent stroke/transient ischemic attack. *Journal of Neuroscience Nursing*, *47*(5), 256–262.

Ross, A. M., Lee, C. S., & Brewer, M. (2014). Peripheral immune response and infection in first-time and recurrent ischemic stroke or transient ischemic attack. *Journal of Neuroscience Nursing*, *46*(4), 199–206.

Sheils, M. S., Katki, H. A., Freedman, N. D., et al. (2014). Cigarette smoking and variations in systemic immune and inflammation markers. *Journal of the National Cancer Institute*, *106*(11), 1–8.

Supic, G., Jagodic, M., & Magic, Z. (2013). Epigenetics: A new link between nutrition and cancer. *Nutrition and Cancer*, *65*(6), 781–792.

Tappenden, K. A., Quatrara, B., Parkhurst, M. L., et al. (2013). Critical role of nutrition in improving quality of care: An interdisciplinary call to action to address adult hospital malnutrition. *MEDSURG Nursing*, *22*(3), 147–165.

Yue, C., Tian, W., Wang, W., et al. (2013). The impact of perioperative glutamine-supplemented parenteral nutrition on outcomes of patients undergoing abdominal surgery: A meta-analysis of randomized clinical trials. *The American Surgeon*, *79*(5), 506–513.

Resources

Canadian Allergy, Asthma and Immunology Foundation: http://allergyfoundation.ca/

Canadian Society of Allergy and Clinical Immunology: http://www.csaci.ca/

Genetic Alliance: http://www.geneticalliance.org/

National Organization for Rare Disorders: https://www.rarediseases.org/

OMIM—Online Mendelian Inheritance in Man: https://www.omim.org/

52 Management of Patients With Immune Deficiency Disorders

Adapted by Kelly Power-Kean

Learning Objectives

On completion of this chapter, the learner will be able to:

1. Identify the pathophysiology, clinical manifestations, and nursing management of patients with primary immune deficiency disorders (PIDD).
2. Describe the modes of transmission of human immune deficiency virus (HIV) infection and prevention strategies.
3. Explain the pathophysiology associated with the clinical manifestations of HIV and acquired immune deficiency syndrome (AIDS) and the purpose of antiretroviral therapy (ART).
4. Identify resources available to patient and family that promote self-management of immune deficiency disorders.
5. Use the nursing process as a framework for care of the patient with HIV/AIDS.

The human immune system is complex and multidimensional. It works to protect against invasion by foreign substances, protect against the proliferation of neoplastic cells, and plays a key role in inflammation and healing. Immunodeficiencies may be classified as either primary or secondary and by the affected components of the immune system. Patients with primary or secondary immune system disorders require care from nurses who are knowledgeable about the pathophysiology, diagnostic procedures, and interventions that are used in the management of these disorders.

PRIMARY IMMUNE DEFICIENCIES

The majority of primary immune deficiency diseases (PIDDs) are diagnosed in infancy, with a male-to-female ratio of 5 to 1. However, some PIDDs are not diagnosed until adolescence or early adulthood, when the gender distribution equalizes. Diagnosis at this stage frequently is confounded by frequent use of antibiotics that mask symptoms. On occasion, adults present with clinical episodes of infectious diseases that are beyond the scope of normal immunocompetence. Examples include infections that are unusually persistent, recurrent, or resistant to treatment and those involving unexpected dissemination of disease or atypical pathogens.

Pathophysiology

There are more than 300 different forms of PIDDs affecting about 29,000 people in Canada (Immunodeficiency Canada, 2018). More than 270 different genes are associated with PIDDs that are recognized by the International Union of Immunological Societies (Hernandez-Trujillo, Orange, Roy, et al., 2015). These rare genetic diseases prevent the body from developing normal immune responses resulting in a complex group of disorders with a wide array of clinical presentations. Many present during the first year of life and may be chronic, debilitating, and costly (National Institute of Allergies and Infectious Diseases [NIAID], 2015).

Clinical Manifestations

Major signs and symptoms include multiple infections despite aggressive treatment, infections with unusual or opportunistic organisms, failure to thrive or poor growth, and a positive family history (Costa-Carvalho, Grumach, Franco, et al., 2014). Table 52-1 contains selected PIDDs along with some of their clinical manifestations.

Assessment and Diagnostic Findings

There is often a considerable delay between the onset of symptoms and time of diagnosis of PIDD (Lehman,

Hernandez-Trujillo, & Ballow, 2015). Because of the genetic origins of PIDD, family history should be carefully assessed but epidemiologic data about specific infectious agents should be considered as well (Costa-Carvalho et al., 2014).

Laboratory tests are used to identify antibody deficiencies, cellular (T-cell) defects, neutrophil disorders, and complement deficiencies (Blaese, Stiehm, Bonilla, et al., 2013). A complete blood cell count with manual differential should always be analyzed first. Lymphopenia may indicate an immunologic abnormality; serum Ig levels (IgG, IgM, and IgA), and antibody responses to vaccines should be assessed to detect a humoral immune defect. Age-matched normal ranges need to be used since antibody levels change as the person ages (Younger, Epland, Zampelli, et al., 2015).

Prevention

Live vaccines are contraindicated in patients with antibody deficiency disorders (Younger et al., 2015). The patient is incapable of generating antibodies and the live substance in the vaccine can cause disease. Family planning should be addressed in terms of future pregnancies; in some situations, prenatal in utero testing of a fetus can determine whether the infant will be affected (Blaese et al., 2013).

Medical Management

A pattern of unusually frequent, opportunistic, or severe infections generates the possibility of a PIDD and initial testing or referral to an immunologist (Younger et al., 2015). Patients with neutropenia are at increased risk for developing severe infections despite substantial advances in supportive care. Epidemiologic shifts occur periodically and must be detected early because they influence prophylactic, empiric, and specific strategies for medical management. Attention to infection control practices is important, especially with the emergence of multidrug-resistant organisms.

Hematopoietic stem cell transplantation (HSCT) is a curative modality. The stem cells may be from embryos or adults. Toxicity and reduced efficacy are frequent limitations of HSCT.

Another therapy involves the use of cells as vehicles for the delivery of genes or gene products. Gene therapy has many adverse effects; the first studies in human participants

Glossary

candidiasis: fungal infection, usually of skin or mucous membranes, caused by *Candida* species

enzyme immunoassay (EIA): a blood test that can determine the presence of antibodies to HIV in the blood or saliva; also referred to as **enzyme-linked immunosorbent assay (ELISA)**. Positive results must be validated, usually with Western blot test or the Geenius HIV-1/2 confirmatory assay

HIV-1: retrovirus isolated and recognized as the etiologic agent of AIDS

HIV encephalopathy: clinical syndrome characterized by a progressive decline in cognitive, behavioural, and motor functions

immune reconstitution inflammatory syndrome (IRIS): a syndrome that results from rapid restoration of pathogen-specific immune responses to opportunistic infections

Kaposi's sarcoma: malignancy that involves the epithelial layer of blood and lymphatic vessels

latent reservoir: the integrated HIV provirus within the CD4+ T cell during the resting memory state; does not express viral proteins and is invisible to the immune system and antiviral medications.

***Mycobacterium avium* complex (MAC):** opportunistic infection caused by mycobacterial organisms that commonly causes a respiratory illness but can also infect other body systems

opportunistic infection: illness caused by various organisms, some of which usually do not cause disease in people with normal immune systems

peripheral neuropathy: disorder characterized by sensory loss, pain, muscle weakness, and wasting of muscles in the hands or legs and feet

***Pneumocystis* pneumonia (PCP):** common opportunistic lung infection; pathogen implicated is most commonly a fungus

polymerase chain reaction: a sensitive laboratory technique that can detect and quantify HIV in a person's blood or lymph nodes

postexposure prophylaxis (PEP): taking antiretroviral medicines as soon as possible, but no more than 72 hours (3 days) after possible HIV exposure; two to three drugs are usually prescribed which must be taken for 28 days.

pre-exposure prophylaxis (PrEP): prevention method for HIV-negative people who are at high risk of HIV infection; involves taking a specific combination of HIV medicines daily; use with condoms and other prevention tools.

progressive multifocal leukoencephalopathy: opportunistic infection that infects brain tissue and causes damage to the brain and spinal cord

retrovirus: a virus that carries genetic material in ribonucleic acid (RNA) instead of DNA and contains reverse transcriptase

reverse transcriptase: enzyme that transforms single-stranded RNA into a double-stranded DNA

viral load test: measures the quantity of HIV RNA or DNA in the blood

viral set point: amount of virus present in the blood after the initial burst of viremia and the immune response that follows

wasting syndrome: involuntary weight loss consisting of both lean and fat body mass

Wiskott–Aldrich syndrome: immunodeficiency characterized by thrombocytopenia and the absence of T and B cells

TABLE 52-1 Selected Primary Immune Deficiency Disorders (PIDDs)

Disorder	Characteristics
Autoimmune lymphoproliferative syndrome (ALPS)	Unusually high numbers of lymphocytes accumulate in the lymph nodes, liver, and spleen leading to enlargement of those organs. Causes numerous autoimmune problems including low levels of red blood cells, platelets, and neutrophils
Autoimmune polyglandular syndrome type 1 (APS-1) (also called autoimmune polyendocrinopathy-candidiasis-ectodermal dystrophy [APECED])	Causes a diverse range of symptoms, including autoimmunity against different types of organs and candidiasis, a fungal infection caused by *Candida* yeast
CARD9 deficiency and other syndromes of susceptibility to candidiasis	Results in susceptibility to fungal infections such as candidiasis; fungi are usually present on the skin; does not cause severe problems in healthy people
Chronic granulomatous disease (CGD)	May be caused by mutations in one of five different genes. Phagocytes are unable to kill certain bacteria and fungi resulting in increased susceptibility to infections
Common variable immunodeficiency (CVID)	Caused by a variety of genetic abnormalities resulting in defective ability of immune cells to produce normal amounts of antibodies, resulting in frequent bacterial or viral infections of the upper airway, sinuses, and lungs
Congenital neutropenia syndromes	Characterized by low levels of neutrophils from birth
CTLA4 deficiency	Autoimmunity, low levels of antibodies, and excessive numbers of lymphocytes which infiltrate the gut, lungs, bone marrow, central nervous system, kidneys resulting in recurrent infections
DOCK8 deficiency	Genetic defect named after mutated gene responsible for the disease which causes decreased numbers and defective function of immune cells and recurrent infections
GATA2 deficiency	Can manifest as five different syndromes with a wide variety of symptoms including severe infections, respiratory problems, hearing loss, leg swelling, and cancer. These symptoms can appear early in childhood but also later on in life
Glycosylation disorders with immune deficiency	Defects in glycosylation, which refers to the attachment of sugars to proteins; can disrupt the immune system resulting in immune deficiency
Hyperimmunoglobulin E syndrome (HIES). Also called Job syndrome	Results from mutations in a gene that encodes a signaling module called STAT3 resulting in recurrent bacterial infections of skin and lungs
Hyperimmunoglobulin M (hyper-IgM) syndromes	Immune system fails to produce normal IgA, IgG, and IgE antibodies but can produce normal or elevated IgM. Infants usually develop severe respiratory infections
Interferon gamma, interleukin 12, interleukin 23 deficiencies	Interferon gamma, interleukin 12, and interleukin 23 are key signals that raise alert against bacteria and other infectious microbes; deficiencies result in susceptibility to infections caused by bacteria and viruses
Leukocyte adhesion deficiency (LAD)	Phagocytes are unable to move to the site of an infection resulting in an inability to fight pathogens resulting in recurrent, life-threatening infections and poor wound healing
NF-kB Essential modifier (NEMO) mutations	Mutations in the NEMO gene cannot "turn on" other genes especially those involved in inflammation and the immune response and are, therefore, highly susceptible to infections with mycobacteria
PI3 Kinase disease	Genetic mutations overactivate an important immune signaling pathway causing a change reaction that disrupts the infection-fighting B and T cells resulting in a weakened immune system and frequent bacterial and viral infections
PLCG2-associated antibody deficiency and immune dysregulation (PLAID)	Rare disorder with allergic response to cold (cold urticaria) as the most distinct symptom
Severe combined immune deficiency (SCID)	Group of rare, life-threatening disorders caused by mutations in different genes involved in development and function of T and B cells; infants appear healthy at birth but are highly susceptible to severe infections
Warts, hypogammaglobulinemia, infections, and myelokathexis syndrome (WHIMS)	Low levels of white blood cells, especially neutrophils, which predispose to frequent infections and persistent warts
Wiskott–Aldrich syndrome (WAS)	Problems with B and T cells and platelets resulting in prolonged episodes of bleeding, recurrent bacterial and fungal infections, and increased risk of cancers and autoimmune diseases

Adapted from National Institute of Allergies and Infectious Diseases. (2015). *Types of primary immune deficiency disorders*. Retrieved May 10, 2016, from www.niaid.nih.gov/topics/immuneDeficiency/Pages/majorPIDDs.aspx.

revealed numerous toxicities with this therapy. Knowledge of these toxicities is being used in planning further studies to increase tolerability (Blaese et al., 2013).

Pharmacologic Therapy

Pharmacologic treatment depends upon the type and severity of presenting infection and the particular PIDD diagnosis (see Table 52-1). Prophylactic drug treatment prevents some bacterial and fungal infections, but it must be used with caution because it has been implicated in the emergence of resistant organisms. The choices for empiric therapy include combination regimens and monotherapy. Specific choices depend on local factors (epidemiology, susceptibility/resistance patterns, availability, cost). Patients with antibody deficiencies receive regular Ig replacement therapy including both IV immunoglobulin (IVIG) and subcutaneous immunoglobulin (SCIG) to provide functional antibodies (Cherin, Marie, Michallet, et al., 2016). Chart 52-1 provides guidelines for management of IVIG.

CHART 52-1

GUIDELINES for Managing Immunoglobulin Therapy

Immunoglobulin therapy is an important treatment for a variety of disease states that are characterized by deficient production of antibodies. Immunoglobulin can be administered for replacement therapy as an IV infusion or subcutaneous (SQ) injection. It can safely be administered in outpatient as well as inpatient settings.

Equipment (as Needed)

- Single-use tourniquet
- Single-use scissors or clippers for hair removal
- IVIG solution, tubing, connector, catheter, or syringe
- Chlorhexidine gluconate, povidone-iodine, or alcohol swabs
- Nonlatex gloves
- Transparent dressing, bandage, or sterile gauze
- Padded, appropriate-length arm board
- Tape
- Topical analgesics
- Preservative-free 0.9% NaCl flush solution
- Padded, appropriate-length arm board or finger splint
- Electronic infusion pump

Implementation

NURSING ACTIONS	RATIONALE
1. Verify prescription for IVIG therapy and identify patient	1. Serious errors can be avoided by careful checking. Immunoglobulin is supplied in a 5% solution or a lyophilized powder with a reconstituting diluent prepared from Cohn fraction II obtained from pools of 1,000 to 20,000 donors. Currently, several different IV preparations are approved for use and have been shown to be effective and safe by the U.S. Food and Drug Administration. Immunoglobulin can also be administered via SQ injection
2. Check for allergies (i.e., latex, iodine)	2. Checking for allergies reduces risk of allergic reaction
3. Explain procedure to patient	3. Knowledge increases patient comfort and cooperation
4. Perform hand hygiene and put on disposable nonlatex gloves	4. Asepsis is essential to prevent infection. The use of nonlatex gloves prevents exposure of nurse to patient's blood and of patient and nurse to latex
5. Obtain Ht. and Wt. of patient before treatment	5. Obtaining Ht. and Wt. helps verify accurate dosing
6. Assess baseline vital signs before, during, and after treatment	6. An elevated temperature at the beginning of treatment may be an indication to delay the therapy to avoid misinterpreting this as an adverse reaction
7. Premedicate with acetaminophen (Tylenol) and diphenhydramine (Benadryl) as prescribed 30 minutes before the start of infusion therapy. Corticosteroids may be prescribed as well	7. Premedicating may help avert adverse reactions. Corticosteroids may be used to prevent possible severe reactions in patients who are perceived to be at risk
8. Verify the route and dose of IVIG therapy	8. IVIG can be administered via the IV or SQ routes. The optimal dose is determined by the patient's response. In most instances, an IV dose of 200 to 800 mg/kg of body weight is administered every 3 to 4 weeks to ensure adequate serum levels of immunoglobulin G (IgG)
9. Insert IV cannula or catheter according to Guidelines for Starting a Peripheral Intravenous Infusion, as needed	9. Patient may need IV access, may have a port or long-term catheter for an IV infusion
10. Administer the IV infusion at a slow rate, not to exceed 3 mL/minute, usually at 100 to 200 mL/hour	10. Administer according to manufacturer's instructions. Beginning at a slow rate helps minimize adverse reactions
11. Continually assess the patient for adverse reactions	11. Be aware of complaints of a tickle or lump in the throat as the precursor to laryngospasm that precedes bronchoconstriction. Caution should be exercised when changing IVIG products, because they are not biologically equivalent. Understand that long-term tolerance of an older IVIG product does not necessarily imply tolerance to a newer product, even if it is technically superior
12. Stop IV infusion at the first sign of reaction	12. Initiate the institutional protocol to be followed in an emergent situation. Patients who have an IgA deficiency have IgE antibodies to IgA, which requires administration of plasma or immunoglobulin replacement from IgA-deficient patients. Because all IV immunoglobulin preparations contain some IgA, they may cause an anaphylactic reaction in patients with IgE anti-IgA antibodies
13. Administer SQ immunoglobulin as orders	13. The pharmacokinetics of IgG differ when smaller doses are given more frequently, as is commonly done with SQ regimens

Ht., height; Wt., weight.

Adapted from Cherin, P., Marie, I., Michallet, M., et al. (2016). Management of adverse events in the treatment of patients with immunoglobulin therapy: A review of evidence. *Autoimmunity Reviews*, *15*, 71–81.

CHART 52-2

HOME CARE CHECKLIST • Home Administration of Ig Replacement Therapy

At the completion of education, the patient and/or caregiver will be able to:

- State the impact of immune deficiency on physiologic functioning, ADLs, IADLs, roles, relationships, and spirituality
- State what types of changes are needed (if any) to maintain a clean home environment and prevent infection
- State how to contact the primary provider, the team of home care professionals overseeing care, and intravenous supply vendor
- State how to obtain medical supplies and carry out dressing changes, IV access site care, and other prescribed regimens
- Identify the benefits and expected outcome of regular Ig replacement therapy
- State rationale for prophylactic use of acetaminophen (Tylenol) and diphenhydramine (Benadryl) before treatment begins
- State the rationale for prehydration on the day before infusion
- Demonstrate how to prepare regular Ig replacement therapy
- Demonstrate how to administer regular Ig replacement therapy
- Demonstrate how to clean and maintain IV equipment, as applicable
- Identify side effects and adverse effects of regular Ig replacement therapy
- Demonstrate how to monitor for adverse effects of regular Ig replacement therapy
- Describe to whom, how, and when to report adverse effects of regular Ig replacement therapy
- Describe appropriate actions to take for adverse effects
- Verbalize understanding of emergency measures for anaphylactic shock

ADL, activities of daily living; IADL, independent activities of daily living.

Nursing Management

Many patients with PIDDs have comorbid autoimmune disorders, such as thyroid disease, rheumatoid arthritis, cytopenias, and inflammatory bowel disease (Younger et al., 2015). Many patients require immunosuppression to ensure engraftment of depleted bone marrow during transplantation procedures. For this reason, nursing care must be meticulous. Appropriate hand hygiene and infection prevention precautions are essential. Institutional policies and procedures related to infection prevention care must be followed scrupulously until definitive evidence demonstrates that precautions are unnecessary. Continual monitoring of the patient's condition is critical, so early signs of impending infection may be detected and treated before they seriously compromise the patient's status.

Patients and caregivers in the home are taught how to administer medications, including regular Ig replacement therapy, if prescribed. Instruction is provided to the patient and family about how to administer the therapy at home (see Chart 52-2). Nurses provide ongoing education and support for the patient and family.

ACQUIRED IMMUNE DEFICIENCY

Immune deficiency can be acquired due to medical treatment such as chemotherapy or infection from agents such as human immune deficiency virus (HIV). Advances have been made in treating HIV infection and acquired immune deficiency syndrome (AIDS); however, AIDS remains a critical public health issue in communities across the country and around the world. Prevention, early detection, and ongoing treatment remain important aspects of care for persons living with HIV infection or AIDS, sometimes referred to as PLWHA.

HIV Infection and AIDS

Since the disease now known as AIDS was first identified more than 35 years ago, remarkable progress has been made in improving the length and quality of life for people living with HIV disease. During the first decade, progress was associated with the recognition and treatment of opportunistic diseases and introduction of prophylaxis against **opportunistic infections** (illnesses caused by various organisms, some of which usually do not cause disease in people with normal immune systems). The second decade witnessed progress in the development of highly active antiretroviral drug therapies (HAARTs) as well as continuing progress in the treatment of opportunistic infections. The third decade has focused on issues of preventing new infections, adherence to antiretroviral therapy (ART), development of second-generation combination medications that affect different stages of the viral life cycle, and continued need for an effective vaccine. The

HIV antibody test, an **enzyme immunoassay** (EIA; or a variant of this test called enzyme-linked immunosorbent assay [ELISA]), became available in 1984, allowing early diagnosis of the infection before the onset of symptoms. Since then, HIV infection has been best managed as a chronic disease, most appropriately in an outpatient care setting, whereas AIDS may involve acute conditions that require hospitalization.

Epidemiology

After the first case of AIDS was reported in Canada in 1982, the Centers for Disease Control and Prevention (CDC) issued a case definition of AIDS. Since 1982, many different definitions have been used for national and international reporting. The CDC has revised the case definition several times with the last update occurring in 2014. In May 2003, HIV disease became legally notifiable in all Canadian provinces and territories (CATIE, 2017). All jurisdictions voluntarily report positive HIV tests to the Centre for Infectious Disease Prevention and Control (CIDPC).

Criteria for a confirmed case of HIV infection can be met by either laboratory evidence or clinical evidence but laboratory evidence, usually obtained through blood tests, is preferred over clinical evidence (e.g., patient signs and symptoms). A case of HIV infection can be classified in one of five HIV infection stages (0, 1, 2, 3, or unknown). Stage 0 indicates early HIV infection, inferred from laboratory testing; stages 1, 2, and 3 are based on the $CD4^+$ T-lymphocyte count; while cases with no information on $CD4^+$ T-lymphocyte count or percentage are classified as stage unknown (Selik, Mokotoff, Branson, et al., 2014).

Three types of HIV tests may be available in Canada, depending on the province or territory where testing occurs: nominal, nonnominal, and anonymous (CATIE, 2017). Nominal, or name-based testing, means that the test is ordered using the name of the person being tested. A nonnominal, or nonidentifying test, is requested using a code or the initials of the person being tested. An anonymous test uses a code known only to the person being tested. This process offers the highest degree of confidentiality and may encourage more people to come forward for testing (Jürgens, 2006). However, anonymous HIV testing is available in some, but not all, provinces (CATIE, 2014).

The CATIE (2018) estimated that at the end of 2016, there were 63,110 people living with HIV in Canada. This represents a 5% increase since 2014. The increase in the number of people living with HIV is attributed to mainly to new infections continuing to occur each year and fewer HIV-related deaths among people living with HIV because antiretroviral (ARV) treatment has improved survival. The estimated all-age HIV prevalence rate in Canada in 2016 was 173 per 100,000 population (CATIE, 2018).

Unprotected sex and sharing of injection drug use equipment are the major means of transmission of HIV. Among reported cases of AIDS in adult males in 2010, 34.7% were in the exposure category of men who have sex with men (MSM); 35.3% from injection drug use; and 26.7% from heterosexual contact. Aboriginal women, women from countries where HIV is endemic, women who use injection drugs, and women in prison continue to be overrepresented and disproportionately affected by HIV infection (Public Health Agency of Canada [PHAC], 2019). Aboriginal Canadians made up 4.9% of the total Canadian population in 2016 but represented 11.3% of new HIV infections in 2016 (CATIE, 2019). Approximately 6,055 Aboriginal people in Canada were living with HIV at the end of 2016, representing 9.6% of all prevalent HIV infections in 2016. In 2016, 245 new HIV infections (11.3%) occurred in aboriginal people compared to 217 new infections in 2014. Aboriginal populations have incidence rates 2.7 times higher than people of other ethnicities (CATIE, 2018).

The all-age HIV incidence rate for people in Canada from HIV-endemic countries is 6.4 times higher than people of other ethnicities. In addition, people from countries where HIV is endemic made up 2.5% of the Canadian population in 2011 but represent 13.6% of new infections in 2016. The all-age HIV incidence rate for males was 3.4 times greater than that of females (CATIE, 2018).

Considering intensive efforts globally, the HIV pandemic has been addressed but the burden remains significant. According to the World Health Organization (WHO) (2015), there were approximately 36.9 million people living with HIV at the end of 2014 with 2 million people becoming newly infected with HIV in 2014 globally. Sub-Saharan Africa is the most affected region, with 25.8 million people living with HIV in 2014 and almost 70% of the global total of new HIV infections. About 51% of people with HIV know that they are infected; 40% of those needing ART are accessing treatment globally. Forty-seven percent of adults living with HIV/AIDS are female (17.4 million) (WHO, 2015), many of whom are in their childbearing years. The diagnosis and treatment of HIV infection remain highly dependent upon the geographic location of where the person is living.

HIV Transmission

Inflammation and breaks in the skin or mucosa result in the increased probability that an HIV exposure will lead to infection. Human immune deficiency virus type 1 (**HIV-1**) is transmitted in body fluids (blood, seminal fluid, vaginal secretions, amniotic fluid, and breast milk) that contain infected cells. Higher amounts of HIV and infected cells in the body fluid are associated with the probability that the exposure will result in infection. Mother-to-child transmission of HIV-1 may occur in utero, at the time of delivery, or through breast-feeding, but most perinatal infections are thought to occur after exposure during delivery. HIV is not transmitted through casual contact (see Chart 52-3).

Blood and blood products can transmit HIV to recipients. However, the risk associated with transfusions has been virtually eliminated as a result of voluntary self-deferral, completion of a detailed health history, extensive testing, heat treatment of clotting factor concentrates, and more effective virus inactivation methods. Donated blood is tested for antibodies to HIV-1, human immunodeficiency virus type 2 (**retrovirus** identified in 1986 in patients with AIDS in Western Africa), and the p24 antigen; since 1999, additional testing has been performed.

CHART 52-3

Risk Factors: Risks Associated With HIV Infection

- Sharing infected injection drug use equipment
- Having sexual relations with infected individuals (both male and female)
- Infants born to mothers with HIV infection and/or who are breast-fed by HIV-infected mothers
- People who received organ transplants, HIV-infected blood, or blood products (especially between 1978 and 1985)

Gerontologic Considerations

A growing number of adults aged 50 and older have HIV/AIDS (National Institute on Aging [NIA], 2015). Many were diagnosed with HIV in their younger years and are benefitting from effective treatment. However, thousands of older adults unknowingly become infected with HIV every year. Older adults are less likely than younger people to get tested. Signs of HIV/AIDS can be mistaken for the aches and pains of normal aging. Older adults might be coping with other diseases common to aging that can mask the signs of HIV/AIDS.

Tillman and Mark (2015) examined published research on the frequency of HIV and sexually transmitted infection (STI) testing among older adults (aged 50 and older), factors related to HIV and STI testing among older adults, and the perspectives and practices of older adults and health care providers related to patient-provider communication regarding sexual health. They found that low rates of HIV and STI testing were influenced by low perceived risk of infection by older adults and their health care providers. Providers bring societal age and gender biases to their perceptions of patient sexuality, which influence their communication about sexual health with older adult patients. Providers' assumptions that discussions about sexual health will offend their patients, as well as their own discomfort with talking to older adults about sex, inhibit them from assessing risk factors that may indicate a need for HIV and STI testing. Older adults living with HIV/AIDS also experience the development of other comorbidities such as cardiovascular disease and diabetes occurring within that specific demographic population, and HIV/AIDS becomes a contributing, but not necessarily primary, cause of mortality.

Prevention of HIV Infection

Nurses need to help in efforts to prevent HIV infection by educating how to eliminate or reduce risks associated with HIV infection and AIDS. HIV is transmitted through the exchange of some infected body fluids. While behavioural interventions such as encouraging the use of condoms are highly effective in reducing the transmission of HIV, the HIV-negative person must be motivated and have the freedom to choose to use the method. In some situations, however, that freedom is absent. For example, a lack of freedom exists in a discordant couple (those in which only one partner has HIV) if the husband refuses to use condoms and the wife's cultural and religious beliefs require intercourse with her husband. In this context, **pre-exposure prophylaxis** (PrEP) might be appropriate. PrEP involves taking one pill containing two HIV medications (tenofovir disoproxil fumarate 300 mg and emtricitabine 200 mg [Truvada]) daily in order to avoid the risk of sexual HIV acquisition in adults and adolescents age 12 and older (Comerford, 2015). HIV status should be checked every 3 months to be sure that the person has not become infected. The ultimate goal of PrEP is to reduce the acquisition of HIV infection with its resulting morbidity, mortality, and cost to individuals and society (US Public Health Service, 2014).

Preventive Education

Prevention of HIV infection is achieved through: (a) behavioural interventions have been effective in reducing the risk of acquiring or transmitting HIV by ensuring that people have the information, motivation, and skills necessary to reduce their risk; (b) HIV testing, because most people change behaviours to protect their partners if they know they are infected with HIV; and (c) linkage to treatment and care, which enables individuals with HIV to live longer, healthier lives, and reduce their risk of transmitting HIV (CDC, 2015a). Other than abstinence, consistent and correct use of condoms (Chart 52-4) is the only effective method of decreasing the risk of sexual transmission of HIV infection. When latex male condoms are used consistently during vaginal or anal intercourse they are highly effective in preventing the sexual transmission of HIV. Non-latex condoms made of natural materials such as lambskin are available for people with latex allergy but will not protect against HIV infection. A male condom should be used for oral contact with the penis, and a dental dam (a flat piece of latex used by dentists to isolate a tooth for treatment) or an altered condom can be used for oral contact with the vagina or rectum. Medical male circumcision, when safely provided by well-trained health professionals, reduces the risk of heterosexually acquired HIV infection in men by approximately 60%. This is a key intervention in generalized epidemic settings with high HIV prevalence and a low male circumcision rate (WHO, 2015).

The polyurethane female condom, which is an effective contraceptive, provides a physical barrier that prevents exposure to genital secretions containing HIV such as semen and vaginal fluid. The female condom is the only barrier method that can be controlled by the woman. Other safe and effective woman-controlled methods such as microbicides remain elusive although clinical trials continue globally.

Microbicides are gels, creams, films, or suppositories that can kill or neutralize viruses and bacteria; *vaginal* and *rectal* microbicides are being researched to see if they can prevent sexual transmission of HIV.

Total abstinence from addictive drugs might not be a realistic short-term goal. Using a harm reduction framework, the nurse works with people who inject drugs to assist them to increase their healthy behaviours. Harm reduction frameworks use practical strategies and ideas aimed at reducing negative consequences associated with drug use and a movement for social justice built on a belief in, and respect for, the rights of people who use drugs. Therefore, under this framework, needle exchange

CHART 52-4

Patient Education: The Right Way to Use a Male Condom

1. Put on a new condom before any kind of sex
2. Hold the condom by the tip to squeeze out the air

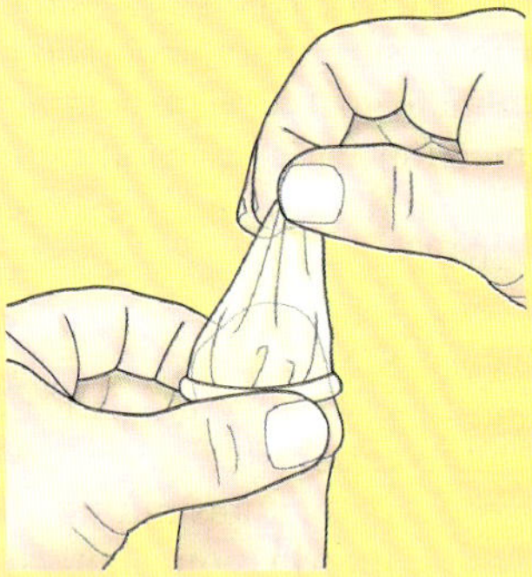

3. Unroll the condom all the way over the erect penis

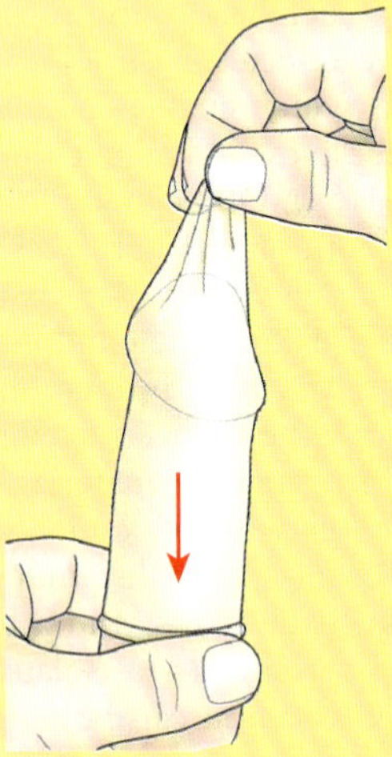

4. Have sex
5. Hold the condom so it cannot come off the penis
6. Pull out
7. Use a new condom if you want to have sex again or if you want to have sex in a different place (e.g., in the anus and then in the vagina)

Keep condoms cool and dry. Never use skin lotions, baby oil, petroleum jelly, or cold cream with condoms. The oil in these products will cause the condom to break. Products made with water or silicone (such as K-Y jelly) are safer to use.

programs are usually free and do not promote increased drug use; on the contrary, they have been found to decrease the incidence of blood-borne infections in people who inject drugs. Nurses should refer clients to needle exchange programs in their neighborhood whenever available. If new needles and syringes are not available, cleaning used needles and syringes with bleach may reduce the risk of HIV (CDC, 2015b). Sharing of drug-use equipment is a high-risk behaviour for a number of blood-borne infections and should be avoided.

Related Reproductive Education

Because HIV infection in women often occurs during the childbearing years, family planning issues need to be addressed. Attempts to achieve pregnancy by couples in which only one partner has HIV (known as discordant couples) expose the unaffected partner to the virus. Efforts at artificial insemination using processed semen from an HIV-infected partner continue. Studies are needed, because HIV has been found in the spermatozoa of patients with HIV infection, and it is possible that HIV can replicate in the male germ cell. Women considering pregnancy need to have accurate information about the risks of transmitting HIV infection to themselves, their partner, and their future children, and about the benefits of taking ART to reduce perinatal HIV transmission. Women in resource-rich settings who are HIV positive should be instructed not to breast-feed their infants, because HIV is transmitted through breast milk.

An increased risk of HIV infection in women is associated with hormonal contraceptive use, but a cause-and-effect relationship has not been established (Sharma & Walmsley, 2015). Women who are HIV negative and who use hormonal contraceptives to prevent pregnancy should be encouraged to use methods to block HIV infection including PrEP; providers should explore drug–drug interactions between hormonal contraceptives and ART in women infected with HIV (Sharma & Walmsley, 2015).

Prevention in Lesbian, Gay, Bisexual, Transsexual and Queer

Many health care providers are insufficiently prepared to meet the unique health needs of those who identify as lesbian, gay, bisexual, transgender and queer (LGBTQ). LGBTQ youth, in particular, are at higher risk for contracting HIV (Bosse, Nesteby, & Randall, 2015; Johnson & Amella, 2013). At the same time, this population experiences significant challenges due to family rejection, lack of social support, stigma, isolation, minority stress, as well as abuse and harassment (Bosse et al., 2015; Johnson & Amella, 2013). Nurses need to be nonjudgmental in order to be effective in educating this population about prevention methods.

Reducing the Risk of Transmission to Health Care Providers

Standard Precautions

Implementation of appropriate hand hygiene measures remains the most effective measure to prevent transmission of organisms. To reduce the risk of exposure of health care workers to HIV, the CDC developed standard precautions (see Chart 52-5) which are designed to reduce the risk of transmission of pathogens. Standard precautions are used when working with all patients in all health care settings, regardless of their diagnosis or presumed infectious status.

Postexposure Prophylaxis for Health Care Providers

The occupational transmission of HIV to health care providers is extremely rare. As of 2013, 58 confirmed occupational exposures to HIV and 150 possible transmissions had been reported in the United States and only one confirmed case has been reported since 1999. **Postexposure prophylaxis (PEP)** includes taking ARV medicines as soon as possible, but no more than 72 hours (3 days) after

CHART 52-5

Recommendations for Standard Precautions

1. **Hand hygiene:** Use after touching blood, body fluids, secretions, excretions, or contaminated items; immediately after removing gloves; and between patient contacts
2. **Personal protective equipment:**
   - *Gloves:* Use for touching blood, body fluids, secretions, excretions, and contaminated items, and for touching mucous membranes and nonintact skin
   - *Gown:* Use during procedures and patient care activities when contact of clothing/exposed skin with blood or body fluids, secretions, and excretions is anticipated
   - *Mask, eye protection (goggles), face shield*[a]: Use during procedures and patient care activities likely to generate splashes or sprays of blood, body fluids, and secretions, especially suctioning or endotracheal intubation
3. **Soiled patient care equipment:** Handle in a manner that prevents transfer of microorganisms to others and to the environment; wear gloves if visibly contaminated; and perform hand hygiene
4. **Environmental control:** Develop procedures for routine care, cleaning, and disinfection of environmental surfaces, especially frequently touched surfaces in patient care areas
5. **Textiles and laundry:** Handle in a manner that prevents transfer of microorganisms to others and to the environment
6. **Needles and other sharps:** Do not recap, bend, break, or hand manipulate used needles; if recapping is required, use a one-handed scoop technique only; use safety features when available; and place used sharps in a puncture-resistant container
7. **Patient resuscitation:** Use mouthpiece, resuscitation bag, and other ventilation devices to prevent contact with mouth and oral secretions
8. **Patient placement:** Prioritize for single-patient room if patient is at increased risk for transmission, is likely to contaminate the environment, does not maintain appropriate hygiene, or is at increased risk for acquiring infection or developing adverse outcome following infection
9. **Respiratory hygiene/cough etiquette** (source containment of infectious respiratory secretions in symptomatic patients, beginning at initial point of encounter, such as triage and reception areas in emergency departments and physician offices): Instruct symptomatic people to cover mouth and nose when sneezing or coughing, use tissues and dispose in no-touch receptacle, observe hand hygiene after soiling of hands with respiratory secretions, and wear surgical mask if tolerated

[a]During aerosol-generating procedures on patients with suspected or proven infections transmitted by respiratory aerosols (e.g., severe acute respiratory syndrome), wear a fit-tested N95 or higher respirator in addition to gloves, gown, and face/eye protection.

From Centers for Disease Control and Prevention (CDC). (2007). *2007 Guideline for Isolation Precautions: Preventing Transmission of Infectious Agents in Healthcare Settings.* Retrieved May 13, 2016, from www.cdc.gov/hicpac/2007ip/2007ip_part1.html

possible HIV exposure; two to three drugs are usually prescribed which must be taken for 28 days. Health care providers who are exposed to a needle stick involving HIV-infected blood in a health care setting have a 0.23% risk of becoming HIV infected; the risk of infection due to occupational exposure is very low (CDC, 2019).

Occupational exposure is considered an urgent medical concern and should be managed immediately after possible exposure—the sooner the better; every hour counts (CDC, 2019). The CDC is suggesting that these postexposure guidelines be followed after occupational and other exposures such as sexual assault. Chart 52-6 provides the strategies and emphasizes the need for quick action.

Vaccination

In the face of a global pandemic, the search for an effective vaccine against the HIV remains an urgent priority (Fauci & Marston, 2015). In 2010 the Government of Canada and the Bill and Melinda Gates Foundation joined together to support the establishment of a new Canadian HIV Vaccine Initiative (CHVI) Research and Development Alliance which will enable Canada to be a leading contributor to global efforts in developing a safe effective, affordable, and globally accessible HIV vaccine (Health Canada, 2015).

Pathophysiology

Because HIV is an infectious disease, it is important to understand how HIV-1 integrates itself into a person's immune system and how the immune response plays a pivotal role in the course of HIV disease. This knowledge is also essential for understanding medication therapy and vaccine development. Viruses are intracellular parasites. HIV is in the subfamily of lentiviruses and is a retrovirus because it carries its genetic material in the form of ribonucleic acid (RNA) rather than deoxyribonucleic acid (DNA) (Grossman & Porth, 2014).

Two genetically different but closely related forms of HIV (HIV-1 and HIV-2) have been identified. The course of illness is slower when infection is caused by HIV-2, which seems to be more common in Western Africa compared to HIV-1, which is more common in other regions of the globe. Blood tests may be used to screen for both forms of HIV. As shown in Figure 52-1A, HIV consists of a viral core containing viral RNA, surrounded by an envelope consisting of protruding glycoproteins.

All viruses target specific cells. HIV targets cells with CD4 receptors, which are expressed on the surface of T lymphocytes, monocytes, dendritic cells, and brain microglia. Mature T cells (T lymphocytes) are composed of two major subpopulations that are defined by cell surface receptors of CD4 or CD8. Approximately two thirds of peripheral blood T cells are CD4+, and approximately one third are CD8+. Most people have about 700 to 1,000 CD4+ cells/mm^3, but a level as low as 500 cells/mm^3 can be considered within normal limits. During stage 0, which is also known as acute/recent infection, most varieties of HIV-1 use the chemokine receptor molecule CCR5 (R5 virus) for entry to T cells in addition to the CD4+ receptor, which suggests that the R5 variant is preferred to a

CHART 52-6

Post-HIV Exposure Prophylaxis for Health Care Providers

If you sustain an occupational exposure to HIV, take the following actions immediately:

- Alert your supervisor and initiate the occupational exposure reporting system used in the setting
- Determine the HIV status of the exposure source (i.e., patient) when possible to guide appropriate use of HIV postexposure prophylaxis (PEP). Use rapid-testing if the HIV status of the patient is unknown. Check laws in your state as you proceed to determine HIV status of the source patient
- Get counseling at the time of exposure and at follow-up appointments
- Exposed health care providers (HCP) are advised to use precautions (e.g., use of barrier contraception and avoidance of blood or tissue donations, pregnancy, and, if possible, breast feeding) to prevent secondary transmission, especially during the first 6 to 12 weeks after exposure
- For exposures for which three drug PEP is prescribed, HCPs are informed regarding the following:
  - Possible drug toxicities (e.g., rash and hypersensitivity reactions that could imitate acute HIV seroconversion and the need for monitoring)
  - Possible drug interactions
  - The need for adherence to PEP regimens

Undergo early reevaluation after exposure:

- Regardless of whether an HCP is taking PEP, reevaluation of exposed HCP within 72 hours after exposure is strongly recommended, as additional information about the exposure or the source patient may be available

Follow-up with HIV testing and appointments. At a minimum, this follow-up should include:

- HIV testing at baseline and at 6 weeks, 12 weeks, and 6 months after exposure; alternatively, if the HCP is certain that a fourth-generation combination HIV p24 antigen–HIV antibody test is being utilized, then HIV testing could be performed at baseline, 6 weeks after exposure, and 4 months after exposure
  - Complete blood counts and renal and hepatic function tests (at baseline and 2 weeks after exposure; further testing may be indicated if abnormalities are detected)

Note: All HIV testing results should preferably be given to the exposed HCP during face-to-face appointments.

Adapted from Kuhar, D., Henderson, D., Struble, K., et al. (2013). Updated US Public Health Service guidelines for the management of occupational exposures to human immunodeficiency virus and recommendations for post-exposure prophylaxis. *Infection Control and Hospital Epidemiology*, *34*(9), 875–892.

different variant (CXCR4) but the preferred coreceptor can shift over the course of infection.

The HIV life cycle is complex (Fig. 52-1B) and consists of the following steps (Grossman & Porth, 2014):

1. Attachment/Binding. In this first step, the GP120 and GP41 glycoproteins of HIV bind with the host's uninfected CD4+ receptor and chemokine coreceptors, usually CCR5, which results in fusion of HIV with the CD4+ T-cell membrane

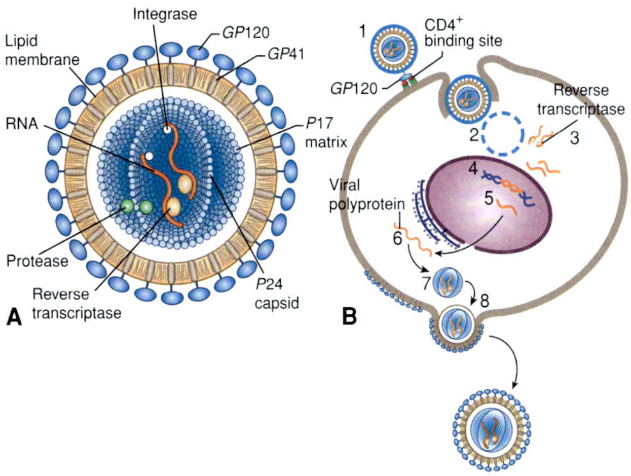

FIGURE 52-1. **A.** Structure of HIV-1 virus. The virus surrounded by a lipid envelope. **B.** Life cycle of HIV-1. (Reprinted with permission from Grossman, S., & Porth, C. (2014). *Porth's pathophysiology: Concepts of altered health states* (9th ed.). Philadelphia, PA: Lippincott Williams & Wilkins.)

2. Uncoating/Fusion. The contents of HIV's viral core (two single strands of viral RNA and three viral enzymes: **reverse transcriptase**, integrase, and protease) are emptied into the CD4+ T cell
3. DNA synthesis. HIV changes its genetic material from RNA to DNA through action of reverse transcriptase, resulting in double-stranded DNA that carries instruction for viral replication
4. Integration. New viral DNA enters the nucleus of the CD4+ T cell and through action of integrase is blended with the DNA of the CD4+ T cell, resulting in permanent, lifelong infection. Prior to this step, the uninfected person has been only exposed to, not infected with, HIV. With this step, HIV infection is permanent
5. Transcription. When the CD4+ T cell is activated, the double-stranded DNA forms single-stranded messenger RNA (mRNA), which builds new viruses
6. Translation. The mRNA creates chains of new proteins and enzymes (polyproteins) that contain the components needed in the construction of new viruses
7. Cleavage. The HIV enzyme protease cuts the polyprotein chain into the individual proteins that make up the new virus
8. Budding. New proteins and viral RNA migrate to the membrane of the infected CD4+ T cell, exit from the cell, and start the process all over

In resting (nondividing) CD4+ cells, HIV survives in a latent state as an integrated provirus that produces few or no viral particles. These resting CD4+ T cells can be stimulated to produce new particles if something activates them, such as another infection. When a resting T cell that harbours this integrated DNA (also known as provirus) becomes activated against HIV or other microbes, the cell begins to produce new copies of both RNA and viral proteins. Consequently whenever the infected $CD4^+$ cell is activated, HIV replication and budding occur, which can destroy the host cell. Newly formed HIV released into the blood can infect other CD4+ cells.

A mutation of CCR5 that is common in Caucasians, but not other ethnic groups, has been identified. About 1% of Caucasians lack functional CCR5 and are highly protected against HIV infection even if exposed (although protection is not absolute); about 18% are not markedly protected against infection but, if infected, demonstrate significantly slower rates of disease progression. CCR5 levels on T cells influence HIV acquisition, disease progression rates, viral load, and immune recovery during ART (Gornalusse, Mummidi, Gaitan, et al., 2015).

HIV-1 mutates quickly, at a relatively constant rate, with about 1% of the virus's genetic material changing annually. HIV-1 exhibits substantial genetic diversity and several different genotypes of HIV-1 exist throughout the world. There is a major group (group M), which consists of subtypes A through L, and a more diverse collection of outliers, which has been referred to as groups N and O. Subtype B HIV-1 viruses predominate in the Western world; this genetic variation is one of the major reasons why effective vaccine development has been such a challenge.

Stages of HIV Infection

There are five stages of HIV infection based on clinical history, physical examination, laboratory evidence of immune dysfunction, signs and symptoms, and infections and malignancies. See Table 52-2.

The period from infection with HIV to the development of HIV-specific antibodies is known as primary infection **or acute HIV infection** (previously known as the window period) and is part of stage 0 (Selik et al., 2014). Acute HIV infection is the interval between the appearance of detectable HIV RNA and the first detection of antibodies. Its duration also depends on the design of the antibody immunoassay and the sensitivity of the immunoassay during seroconversion (CDC, 2014). Initially, there is a period during which those who are HIV positive test negative on the HIV antibody blood test, although they are infected and highly infectious, because their viral loads are very high. About 40% to 80% of patients develop clinical symptoms of a nonspecific viral illness (e.g., fever, fatigue, or rash) lasting 1 to 2 weeks. After 2 to 3 weeks, antibodies

TABLE 52-2 HIV Infection Stages 1, 2, and 3 Based on Age-Specific Laboratory Data

	Age on Date of $CD4^+$ T-lymphocyte Test					
	<1 Year		1–5 Years		≥6 Years	
Stage	Cells/IL	%	Cells/IL	%	Cells/IL	%
1	≥1,500	≥34	≥1,000	≥30	≥500	≥26
2	750–1,499	26–33	500–999	22–29	200–499	14–25
3	<750	<26	<500	<22	<200	<14

If a stage-3-defining opportunistic illness has been diagnosed, then the stage is 3 regardless of $CD4^+$ T-lymphocyte test.

Stage-3-Defining Opportunistic Illnesses in HIV Infection

Bacterial infections, multiple or recurrent (only among children aged less than 6 years)
Candidiasis of bronchi, trachea, or lungs
Candidiasis of esophagus
Cervical cancer, invasive (only in persons aged 6 years or older)
Coccidioidomycosis, disseminated or extrapulmonary
Cryptococcosis, extrapulmonary
Cryptosporidiosis, chronic intestinal (>1 month's duration)
Cytomegalovirus disease (other than liver, spleen, or nodes), onset at age >1 month
Cytomegalovirus retinitis (with loss of vision)
Encephalopathy attributed to HIV
Herpes simplex: chronic ulcers (>1 month's duration) or bronchitis, pneumonitis, or esophagitis (onset at age >1 month)
Histoplasmosis, disseminated or extrapulmonary isosporiasis, chronic intestinal (>1 month's duration)
Kaposi sarcoma
Lymphoma, Burkitt (or equivalent term)
Lymphoma, immunoblastic (or equivalent term)
Lymphoma, primary, of brain
Mycobacterium avium complex or *Mycobacterium kansasii,* disseminated or extrapulmonary
Mycobacterium tuberculosis of any site, pulmonary (only in persons aged 6 years or older) disseminated, or extrapulmonary
Mycobacterium, other species or unidentified species, disseminated or extrapulmonary
Pneumocystis jirovecii (previously known as "*Pneumocystis carinii*") pneumonia (PCP)
Pneumonia, recurrent (only in persons aged 6 years or older)
Progressive multifocal leukoencephalopathy
Salmonella septicemia (recurrent)
Toxoplasmosis of brain, onset at age >1 month
Wasting syndrome attributed to HIV

Adapted from Selik, R., Mokotoff, E., Branson, B., et al. (2014). Revised surveillance case definition for HIV infection—United States, 2014. *Morbidity and Mortality Weekly Report, 63*(RR03), 1–10.

to the glycoproteins of the HIV envelope can be detected in the sera of HIV-infected people, but most of these antibodies lack the ability to totally control the virus. By the time neutralizing antibodies can be detected, HIV-1 is firmly established in the host.

Primary or acute infection is characterized by high levels of viral replication, widespread dissemination of HIV throughout the body, and destruction of CD4+ T cells. This leads to dramatic drops in CD4+ T-cell counts (normally 500 to 1,500 cells/mm^3 of blood). The host responds to the HIV infection through a CD4+ T-cell response that causes other immune cells, such as CD8+ lymphocytes, to increase their killing of infected, virus-producing cells. The body produces antibody molecules in an effort to contain the free HIV particles (outside cells) and assist in their removal. During this stage, the virus is widely disseminated in lymphoid tissue, and a **latent reservoir** within resting memory CD4$^+$ T cells is created.

The amount of virus in the body after the initial immune response subsides is referred to as the **viral set point**, which results in an equilibrium between HIV levels and the immune response that may be elicited. This can last for years and is inversely correlated with disease prognosis. The higher the viral set point, the poorer the prognosis. After the viral set point is reached, a chronic stage persists in which the immune system cannot eliminate the virus despite its best efforts. This set point varies greatly from patient to patient and dictates the subsequent rate of disease progression; on an average, 8 to 10 years pass before a major HIV-related complication develops. In this prolonged, chronic stage, patients feel well and have few, if any, symptoms. Apparent good health continues because CD4+ T-cell levels remain high enough to preserve immune defensive responses but over time, the number of CD4$^+$ T cells continues to decrease.

Stage 2 occurs when CD4$^+$ T-lymphocyte cells are between 200 and 499, stage 3 when the count drops below 200 cells/mm^3 of blood and at this point, the person is considered to have AIDS for surveillance purposes. HIV disease progression is classified from less to more severe; once a case is classified into a surveillance severity stage, it cannot be reclassified into a less severe stage even if the CD4$^+$ T-lymphocytes increase, which often occurs when a person receives ART. A stage 3 diagnosis has implications for services (e.g., disability benefits, housing, and income support).

Assessment and Diagnostic Findings in HIV Infection

During the first stage of HIV infection, the patient may be asymptomatic or may exhibit various signs and symptoms such as fatigue or skin rash. Patients who are in later stages of HIV infection may have a variety of symptoms related to their immunosuppressed state. The staging system requires laboratory evidence of HIV infection in order to diagnose HIV or AIDS (see Table 52-2).

HIV Tests

Screening Tests

Several screening tests are used to diagnose HIV infection, and others are used to determine the stage and severity of the infection. There are three types of HIV diagnostic tests: antibody tests, antigen/antibody tests, and nucleic acid (RNA) tests. Antibody tests detect antibodies, not HIV itself, while antigen and RNA tests directly detect HIV.

The newest HIV tests, fourth-generation tests, screen for HIV antibodies and the virus itself. This test detects the HIV protein called the p24 antigen (p24 antigen test) (CATIE, 2018). All laboratories in Canada use fourth-generation HIV testing technologies for screening blood samples. These antigen-antibody combination tests are more sensitive and have reduced the window period.

Rapid point of care (POC) testing, another technology, can improve access to testing because the entire testing process. This test only detects anti-HIV antibodies and is known as the INSTI test. POC testing is not available in all provinces or territories (CATIE, 2018).

Another test, called the HIV nucleic acid amplification test (NAAT or NAT), detects HIV RNA as early as 7 to 14 days after infection.

To overcome barriers that currently impede efforts to reduce the number of undiagnosed cases of HIV in Canada, PHAC (2014b) recommends the following:

1. Normalize HIV testing; make it part of routine medical care
2. Simplify risk assessments
3. Accept verbal consent for voluntary testing
4. Emphasize that HIV is a chronic manageable condition

Before an HIV antibody test is performed, the meaning of the test and possible test results are explained, and informed consent for the test is obtained from the patient. When the result of the HIV antibody test is received, it is carefully explained to the patient in private (Chart 52-7). All test results are kept confidential. Education and counselling about the test result and about preventing transmission are essential. The patient's psychological response to a positive test result may include feelings of panic, depression, and hopelessness. The social and interpersonal consequences of a positive test result can be devastating. The patient may lose his or her sexual partner, housing, and health insurance because of disclosure. He or she may experience discrimination in employment and housing, as well as social ostracism. For these reasons and others, patients who test positive may need ongoing counselling as well as referrals for social, financial, medical, and psychological support services. Patients whose test results are seronegative may develop a false sense of security, possibly resulting in continued high-risk behaviours or feelings that they are immune to the virus. These patients may need ongoing counselling to help modify high-risk behaviours and to encourage returns for repeated testing. Other patients may experience anxiety regarding the uncertainty of their status.

Confirmation Tests

When a person is infected with HIV, the immune system responds by producing antibodies against the virus, usually within 3 to 12 weeks after infection. Various tests are used to determine the presence of antibodies to HIV.

The Geenius HIV-1/2 Confirmatory Assay has replaced the Western blot as the confirmatory diagnostic test

CHART 52-7

HIV Test Results: Implications for Patients

Interpretation of Positive Test Results

- Antibodies to HIV are present in the blood (the patient has been infected with the virus, and the body has produced antibodies)
- HIV is active in the body, and the patient can transmit the virus to others
- Despite HIV infection, the patient does not necessarily have AIDS
- The patient is not immune to HIV (the antibodies do not indicate immunity)

Interpretation of Negative Test Results

- Antibodies to HIV are not present in the blood at this time, which can mean that the patient has not been infected with HIV or, if infected, the body has not yet produced antibodies (stage 0)
- The patient should continue taking precautions. The test result does not mean that the patient is immune to the virus, nor does it mean the patient is not infected; it just means that the body may not have produced antibodies yet. If viral test used, a negative result is more consistent with the conclusion that the patient is uninfected

HIV, human immune deficiency virus; AIDS, acquired immune deficiency syndrome.

following a positive HIV screening test. This test is used by all Public Health laboratories in Canada that conduct HIV confirmatory tests.

According to CATIE (2018), the nucleic acid amplification tests (NAATs) have the shortest window period of all HIV tests and can detect HIV infection as early as 14 days postinfection. NAATs are used as confirmatory tests in some laboratories in Canada. They may also be used when the HIV confirmation is indeterminate or differs from the screening test. Some provinces/territories are considering using NAATs as screening tests because of their very short window period however the high cost of the test is prohibitive.

The p24 antigen test is used as confirmatory tests in some laboratories in Canada. They may also be used when the confirmatory test for HIV is indeterminate or has a different result from the screening test (CATIE, 2018).

In 2012 the FDA in the United States approved the first over-the-counter rapid oral home HIV test. However, use of home testing kits raises concerns because of the lack of counselling and possible inaccurate results, including both false-positive and false-negative results. Currently, there are no approved home-based testing kits licensed by Health Canada, although there are rapid-testing kits available for use in clinical settings supported by a laboratory that performs HIV testing.

Staging

Two surrogate markers are used routinely to assess immune function and level of HIV viremia: CD4⁺ T-cell count (CD4⁺ count) and plasma HIV RNA (viral load). CD4⁺ count should be measured in all patients at entry into care. **Viral load tests** use target amplification methods to quantify HIV RNA or DNA levels in the plasma. Target amplification methods include reverse transcriptase–**polymerase chain reaction** (RT-PCR) and NAAT. A widely used viral load test measures plasma HIV RNA levels. Currently, these tests are used to track viral load and response to treatment of HIV infection. RT-PCR is also used to detect HIV in high-risk seronegative people before antibodies are measurable, to confirm a positive EIA result, and to screen neonates. HIV culture or quantitative plasma culture and plasma viremia are additional tests that measure viral burden, but they are used infrequently. Viral load is a better predictor of the risk of HIV disease progression than the CD4+ count. The lower the viral load, the longer the time to AIDS diagnosis and the longer the survival time. The key goal of ART is to achieve and maintain durable viral suppression.

Treatment of HIV Illness

The U.S. Department of Health and Human Services Panel on Antiretroviral Guidelines for Adults and Adolescents (Panel) (2016) is composed of HIV specialists from across the country who regularly meet to review the latest scientific evidence. These recommendations are generally used by Canadian health care providers to guide treatment protocols. The CD4⁺ count serves as the major laboratory indicator of immune function and prophylaxis for opportunistic infections and is the strongest predictor of subsequent disease progression and survival (Panel, 2016). New drugs that offer new mechanisms of action, improvements in potency and activity even against multidrug-resistant viruses, dosing convenience, and tolerability have been approved. The overarching goal of ART is to suppress HIV replication to a level below which drug-resistant mutations do not emerge; related goals are to: (a) reduce HIV-associated morbidity and prolong the duration and quality of survival; (b) restore and preserve immunologic function; (c) maximally and durably suppress plasma HIV viral load; and (d) prevent HIV transmission (Panel, 2016). In Canada, ART is now recommended for all HIV-infected patients regardless of their viral load or CD4⁺ count (Panel, 2016). Optimal viral suppression is defined generally as a viral load persistently below the level of detection (HIV RNA less than 20 to 75 copies/mL, depending on the assay used). Clinicians, in partnership with patients, make treatment decisions based on a number of factors, including whether the patient has already taken ART or is ART-naive and the willingness of the patient to adhere to the lifelong treatment regimen.

Achieving viral suppression requires the use of ART with at least two, and preferably three, active drugs from two or more drug classes and should occur within the first 12 to 24 weeks of therapy especially if the patient is new to ART (Panel, 2016). More than 30 ARV drugs, in 6 classes are Food and Drug Administration (FDA) approved for the treatment of HIV infection. The different drug classes of ART target some of the steps in the HIV/host cycle (see Fig. 52-1). These seven classes include the nucleoside/nucleotide reverse transcriptase inhibitors (NRTIs), non-nucleoside reverse transcriptase inhibitors (NNRTIs), protease inhibitors (PIs), integrase strand transfer inhibitors (INSTIs), a fusion inhibitor, a CCR5 antagonist, and a CD4 postattachment inhibitor (Table 52-3). In addition, two

TABLE 52-3 Antiretroviral Agents

Generic Name (Abbreviation) and Trade Names (Italic)	Food Interactions	Adverse Effects
Nucleoside Reverse Transcriptase Inhibitors (NRTIs)		
Abacavir (ABC) *Ziagen* *Trizivir* (ABC/ZDV/3TC) *Epzicom* (ABC/3TC) *Triumeq* (ABC/3TC/DTG)	Take without regard to meals	Hypersensitivity reaction, which can be fatal; symptoms may include fever, rash, nausea, vomiting, diarrhea, abdominal pain, malaise or fatigue, loss of appetite, and respiratory symptoms such as sore throat, cough, shortness of breath
Didanosine (ddI) *Videx* *Videx EC*	Take half hour before or 2 hours after meals	Pancreatitis, peripheral neuropathy, retinal changes, nausea, diarrhea, lactic acidosis with fatty degeneration of the liver, insulin resistance/diabetes
Emtricitabine (FTC) *Emtriva*	Take without regard to meals	Minimal toxicity, hyperpigmentation/skin discolouration. Severe acute exacerbation of hepatitis
Atripla (FTC/EFV/TDF)	Take on empty stomach to reduce side effects	Minimal toxicity, lactic acidosis with hepatic steatosis.
Complera (FTC/RPV/TDF)	Take with a snack	Peripheral neuropathy, lipodystrophy, pancreatitis, lactic acidosis with hepatic steatosis (higher incidence with d4 T than with other NRTIs), hyperlipidemia, rapidly progressive ascending neuromuscular weakness (rare)
Stribild (FTC/EVG/c/TDF)	Take with a snack	
Truvada (FTC/TDF)	Take without regard to meals	
lamivudine (3TC) *Epivir* *Combivir* (3TC/ZDV) Epzicom (3TC/ABC) *Trizivir* (ABC/3TC/ZDV) stavudine (d4 T) *Zerit*	Take without regard to meals	
Tenofovir disoproxil fumarate (TDF) *Viread*	Take without regard to meals	Asthenia, headache, diarrhea, nausea, vomiting, and flatulence; kidney insufficiency; lactic acidosis with hepatic steatosis
Zidovudine (AZT or ZDV) *Retrovir* *Combivir* (3TC/AZT) *Trizivir* (ABC/3TC/AZT)	Take without regard to meals	Bone marrow suppression; macrocytic anemia or neutropenia; nail pigmentation, GI intolerance, headache, insomnia, asthenia; lactic acidosis with hepatic steatosis
Nonnucleoside Reverse Transcriptase Inhibitors		
Efavirenz (EFV) *Sustiva* *Atripla (EFV/TDF/FTC)*	Take on empty stomach	Rash (rare cases of Stevens–Johnson syndrome have been reported), central nervous system symptoms (dizziness, somnolence, insomnia, abnormal dreams, confusion, abnormal thinking, impaired concentration, amnesia, agitation, depersonalization, hallucinations, and euphoria), increased transaminase levels, false-positive cannabinoid test, teratogenic in monkeys and potentially teratogenic in humans during first trimester of pregnancy
Etravirine (ETR) *Intelence*	Take following a meal	Rash, including Stevens–Johnsons syndrome, hypersensitivity reaction, nausea
Nevirapine (NVP) *Viramune* *Viramune XR*	Take without regard to meals	Rash including Stevens–Johnson syndrome, symptomatic hepatitis including fatal hepatic necrosis has been reported. Single dose has been used in developing countries to prevent vertical transmission
Rilpivirine (RPV) *Edurant* *Complera (RPV/TDF/FTC)*	Take with a meal of between 400 and 600 calories	Rash, depression, insomnia, headache, hepatotoxicity
Protease Inhibitors		
Atazanavir (ATV) *Reyataz* *Evotaz (ATV/c)*	Take with a snack	Indirect hyperbilirubinemia; prolonged PR interval (some patients experience asymptomatic first-degree AV block); EKG changes; hyperglycemia; fat maldistribution; possible increased bleeding episodes in patients with hemophilia. Check creatinine clearance
Darunavir (DRV) *Prezista* *Prezcobix (DRV/c)*	Take with a snack	Skin rash (10%), Stevens–Johnson syndrome, diarrhea, nausea, headache, cold-like symptoms (including runny nose or sore throat), inflammation of the liver, abnormal liver function tests, fever, and abnormally high cholesterol and triglyceride levels have been reported
Fosamprenavir (FPV) *Lexiva*	Tablets may be taken with or without food	Skin rash (19%), diarrhea, nausea, vomiting, headache, hyperlipidemia, transaminase elevation, hyperglycemia, fat maldistribution, possible increased bleeding episodes in patients with hemophilia
Indinavir (IDV) *Crixivan*	For unboosted IDV: Should be taken 1 hour before or 2 hours after meals; may take with skim milk or low-fat meal For RTV-boosted IDV: Can be taken with or without food	Nephrolithiasis, GI intolerance, nausea, indirect hyperbilirubinemia, hyperlipidemia, headache, asthenia, blurred vision, dizziness, rash, metallic taste, thrombocytopenia, alopecia, hemolytic anemia, hyperglycemia, fat maldistribution, possible increased bleeding episodes in patients with hemophilia

TABLE 52-3 Antiretroviral Agents (Continued)

Generic Name (Abbreviation) and Trade Names (Italic)	Food Interactions	Adverse Effects
Lopinavir + ritonavir (LPV/r) *Kaletra*	Liquid forms are taken with a snack; no restrictions for tablet	GI intolerance, nausea, vomiting, diarrhea, asthenia, hyperlipidemia (especially hypertriglyceridemia), elevated serum transaminase, hyperglycemia, fat maldistribution, possible increased bleeding episodes in patients with hemophilia, EKG changes
Nelfinavir (NFV) *Viracept*	Take with a snack	Diarrhea, hyperlipidemia, hyperglycemia, fat maldistribution, possible increased bleeding episodes in patients with hemophilia, serum transaminase elevation
Ritonavir (RTV) *Norvir*	Take with a snack	GI intolerance, nausea, vomiting, diarrhea, paresthesias (circumoral and extremities), hyperlipidemia (especially hypertriglyceridemia), hepatitis, asthenia, taste perversion, hyperglycemia, fat maldistribution, possible increased bleeding in patients with hemophilia. Lower doses used as a booster
Saquinavir (SQV) *Invirase*	Take with meals or within 2 hours after meal	GI intolerance, nausea, diarrhea, abdominal pain and dyspepsia, headache, hyperlipidemia, elevated transaminase enzymes, hyperglycemia, fat maldistribution, possible increased bleeding episodes in patients with hemophilia, EKG changes
Tipranavir (TPV) *Aptivus*	Take with a snack	Serious liver problems, bleeding on the brain, skin rash (21%), increased cholesterol and triglyceride levels, and changes in body fat; women taking birth control pills that contain estrogen may be more likely to develop a rash. Individuals with hemophilia may have increased bleeding. Take with RTV, if prescribed
Fusion Inhibitor		
Enfuvirtide (T-20) *Fuzeon*	Injected subcutaneously, so meals are not an issue	Local injection site reactions—almost 100% of patients (pain, erythema, induration, nodules and cysts, pruritus, ecchymosis); increased rate of bacterial pneumonia; hypersensitivity reaction—symptoms may include rash, fever, nausea, vomiting, chills, rigors, hypotension, or elevated serum transaminases
Integrase Inhibitor (INSTIs)		
Dolutegravir (DTG) *Tivicay*	Take without regard to meals	Hypersensitivity reaction including rash, constitutional symptoms, and organ dysfunction, insomnia, headache
Elvitegravir (EVG)	Take with a snack	Nausea, diarrhea
Vitekta *Stribild (EVG/c/FTC/TDF)*	Take with a snack	Nausea, diarrhea, renal impairment, decrease in bone density, acute exacerbation of hepatitis, lactic acidosis
Raltegravir (RAL) *Isentress*	Take without regard to meals	Rash including Stevens-Johnson syndrome, diarrhea, nausea, headache, fever, insomnia
CCR5 Antagonist		
Maraviroc (MVC) *Selzentry*	Take without regard to meals; requires CCR5 tropism blood test before starting	Cough, fever, dizziness, headache, orthostatic hypotension, nausea, bladder irritation; possible liver problems and cardiac events; an increased risk for some infections; a slight increase in cholesterol levels

[a]This information changes often. Check the panel and also the U.S. Food and Drug Administration website, http://www.fda.gov/forpatients/illness/hivaids/ucm118915.htm) for current information when using ART.

GI, gastrointestinal; AV, atrioventricular; EKG, electrocardiogram.

Adapted from Panel on Antiretroviral Guidelines for Adults and Adolescents (Panel). (2016). *Guidelines for the use of antiretroviral agents in HIV-1-infected adults and adolescents*. Department of Health and Human Services. Retrieved May 12, 2016, from www.aidsinfo.nih.gov/ContentFiles/AdultandAdolescentGL.pdf. Appendix B, Tables 1 through 6.

drugs (cobicistat and ritonavir) are used to improve the pharmacokinetic profiles of some of the other ART drugs. Some pharmaceutical companies have combined two to three agents into one tablet or capsule. The Panel (2016) provides clear directions regarding which medications should be prescribed for both ART-naive and experienced patients. CATIE (2018) provides a comprehensive guide to medications that are available in Canada for the treatment of HIV.

The PHAC (2017) estimates that 76% of persons diagnosed with HIV were on treatment, and 89% of persons on treatment had suppressed viral loads. Viral loads are often not suppressed because the patient is not adhering to the treatment plan. Psychosocial barriers such as depression and other mental illnesses, neurocognitive impairment, low health literacy, low levels of social support, stressful life events, high levels of alcohol consumption and active substance use, homelessness, poverty, nondisclosure of HIV serostatus, denial, stigma, and inconsistent access to medications affect adherence to ART. Failure to adopt practices that facilitate adherence, such as linking medication taking to daily activities or using a medication reminder system or a pill organizer, is also associated with treatment failure (Panel, 2016). Simplifying treatment regimens and decreasing the number of medications that must be taken each day may increase patients' adherence to therapy. It is difficult to predict which patients will adhere to medication regimens but a positive relationship between the patient and health care provider is associated with better adherence. Individualized plans of care that take into consideration housing and social support issues, in addition to health indicators, are essential.

Adherence to the ARV treatment plan involves very complex behaviour that can change over the duration of the medication regimen. Self-reported adherence measures can distinguish clinically meaningful patterns of medication-taking behaviours; therefore, nurses should assess if patients can describe how they are taking their ART (see Chart 52-8 for strategies for adhering to medication therapy for HIV).

Laboratory tests evaluate whether ART is effective for a specific patient. An adequate $CD4^+$ response for most patients on ART is an increase in $CD4^+$ count in the range of 50 to 150 mm^3 per year, generally with an accelerated response in the first 3 months (Panel, 2016). Viral load should be measured at baseline and on a regular basis thereafter because viral load is the most important indicator of response to ART.

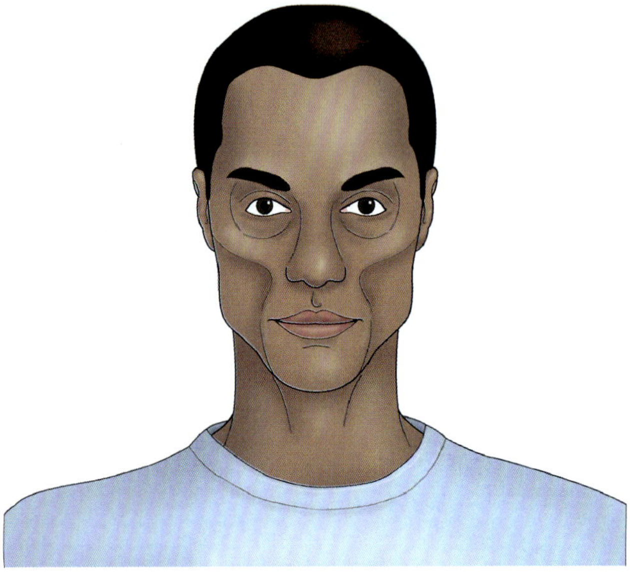

FIGURE 52-2. Facial lipoatrophy.

NURSING ALERT

Nurses must recognize the differences among common laboratory tests used to diagnose and assess HIV infection and guide therapy. For example, the EIA is a diagnostic screening test that determines the presence of antibodies to HIV. The RT-PCR test, which measures viral load, is used along with the $CD4^+$ count, which indicates the level of immune dysfunction, to assess the stage and severity of HIV infection. It is important to assess the extent of damage to the immune system before initiation of ART and/or prophylactic treatment for opportunistic infections.

Adverse effects associated with all HIV treatment regimens include hepatotoxicity, nephrotoxicity, and osteopenia, along with increased risk of cardiovascular disease and myocardial infarction (Table 52-3). Many of the ARV agents may cause fat redistribution syndrome (lipodystrophy) which consists of lipoatrophy (localized subcutaneous fat loss in the face, arms, legs, and buttocks) and lipohypertrophy (central visceral fat [lipomata] accumulation in the abdomen, although possibly in the breasts, dorsocervical region [buffalo hump], and within the muscle and liver). Facial wasting, characterized as a sinking of the cheeks, eyes, and temples caused by the loss of fat tissue under the skin, may be treated by injectable fillers such as poly-L-lactic acid (Sculptra) (see Fig. 52-2). These changes can disturb the body image of people living with HIV/AIDS and may be a reason they decline or stop ART. Nurses could use an instrument such as the assessment of body change distress (ABCD) questionnaire that assesses subjective report of bodily changes and body dissatisfaction and the impact of bodily changes on psychosocial variables, quality of life, and HIV self-care behaviours (Blashill, Wilson, Baker, et al., 2014).

Drug Resistance

Drug resistance is the ability of pathogens to withstand the effects of medications that should be toxic to them. There are two major components of ART resistance: (a) transmission of drug-resistant HIV at the time of initial infection;

CHART 52-8

Promoting Adherence to ART

Strategies	Examples
Use a multidisciplinary team approach. Provide an accessible, trustworthy health care team	• Nonjudgmental providers, nurses, social workers, pharmacists, and medication managers
Strengthen early linkage to care and retention in care	• Encourage health care team participation in linkage to and retention in care
Assess patient readiness to start ART	
Evaluate patient's knowledge about HIV disease, prevention and treatment and, on the basis of the assessment, provide HIV-related information	• Consider the patient's current knowledge base, provide information about HIV, including the natural history of the disease, HIV viral load and $CD4^+$ count and expected clinical outcomes according to these parameters, and therapeutic and prevention consequences of nonadherence

CHART 52-8 Promoting Adherence to ART (Continued)

Strategies	Examples
Identify facilitators, potential barriers to adherence, and necessary medication management skills before starting ART medication	• Assess patient's cognitive competence and any impairment • Assess behavioural and psychosocial challenges including depression, mental illnesses, levels of social support, high levels of alcohol consumption and active substance use, nondisclosure of HIV serostatus and stigma • Identify and address language and literacy barriers • Assess beliefs, perceptions, and expectations about taking ART (e.g., impact on health, side effects, disclosure issues, consequences of nonadherence) • Ask about medication taking skills and foreseeable challenges with adherence (e.g., past difficulty keeping appointments, adverse effects from previous medications, issues managing other chronic medications, need for medication reminders and organizers) • Assess structural issues including unstable housing, lack of income, unpredictable daily schedule, lack of prescription drug coverage, lack of continuous access to medications
Provide needed resources	• Provide or refer for mental health and/or substance abuse treatment • Provide resources to obtain prescription drug coverage, stable housing, social support, and income and food security
Involve the patient in ARV regimen selection	• Review regimen potency, potential side effects, dosing frequency, pill burden, storage requirements, food requirements, and consequences of nonadherence • Assess daily activities and tailor regimen to predictable and routine daily events • Consider use of fixed-dose combination formulation • Assess if cost/copayment for drugs can affect access to medications and adherence
Assess adherence at every clinic visit	• Monitor viral load as a strong biologic measure of adherence • Use a simple behavioural rating scale • Employ a structured format that normalizes or assumes less-than-perfect adherence and minimizes socially desirable or "white coat adherence" responses • Ensure that other members of the health care team also assess adherence
Use positive reinforcement to foster adherence success	• Inform patients of low or nondetectable levels of HIV viral load and increases in $CD4^+$ cell counts • When needed, consider providing incentives and rewards for achieving high levels of adherence and treatment success
Identify the type of and reasons for nonadherence	• Failure to fill the prescription(s) • Failure to understand dosing instructions • Complexity of regimen (e.g., pill burden, size, dosing schedule, food requirements) • Pill aversion • Pill fatigue • Adverse effects • Inadequate understanding of drug resistance and its relationship to adherence • Cost-related issues • Depression, drug and alcohol use, homelessness, poverty • Stigma • Nondisclosure • Other potential barriers
Select from among available effective treatment adherence interventions	• Use evidence-based interventions to promote adherence • Use adherence-related tools to complement education and counseling interventions (e.g., pill boxes, dose planners, reminder devices) • Use community resources to support adherence (e.g., visiting nurses, community workers, family, peer advocates) • Use patient prescription assistance programs • Use motivational interviews
Systematically monitor retention in care	• Record and follow-up on missed visits
On the basis of any problems identified through systematic monitoring, consider options to enhance retention in care given resources available	• Provide outreach for those patients who drop out of care • Use peer or paraprofessional treatment navigators • Employ incentives to encourage clinic attendance or recognize positive clinical outcomes resulting from good adherence • Arrange for directly observed therapy (if feasible)

Adapted from Panel on Antiretroviral Guidelines for Adults and Adolescents (Panel). (2016). *Guidelines for the use of antiretroviral agents in HIV-1-infected adults and adolescents.* Department of Health and Human Services. Retrieved May 12, 2016, from www.aidsinfo.nih.gov/ContentFiles/AdultandAdolescentGL.pdf. Table 13. Strategies to Improve Adherence to Antiretroviral Therapy and Retention in Care.

and (b) selective drug resistance in patients who are receiving nonsuppressive regimens. Genotypic and phenotypic resistance assays are used to assess viral strains and inform selection of treatment strategies. Genotypic assays detect drug-resistant mutations present in relevant viral genes while phenotypic assays measure the ability of a virus to grow in different concentrations of ART drugs. Resistance testing in persons who are chronically infected is recommended at the time of entry into HIV care. Although no definitive prospective data exist to support the choice of one type of resistance testing over another, genotypic testing is generally preferred because of lower cost, more rapid turnaround time, the assay's ability to detect mixtures of wild-type and resistant virus, and the relative ease of interpreting test results. If therapy is deferred, repeat testing soon before initiation of ART should be considered because the patient may have acquired drug-resistant virus (i.e., superinfection) (Panel, 2016).

Immune Reconstitution Inflammatory Syndrome

Immune reconstitution inflammatory syndrome (IRIS) results from rapid restoration of pathogen-specific immune responses to opportunistic infections that cause either the deterioration of a treated infection or new presentation of a subclinical infection. This syndrome typically occurs during the initial months after beginning ART and is associated with a wide spectrum of organisms, most commonly mycobacteria, herpes viruses, and deep fungal infections. IRIS is characterized by fever, respiratory and/or abdominal symptoms, and worsening of the clinical manifestations of an opportunistic infection or the appearance of new manifestations. IRIS is treated with anti-inflammatory medications such as cortisone. The nurse should be alert to the possibility of IRIS, especially in the 3-month period after treatment with ART is initiated, because this syndrome is associated with significant morbidity and patients often require hospital admission.

Paradoxical tuberculosis-associated–immune reconstitution inflammatory syndrome (TB-IRIS) is a serious complication that arises during successful ART in patients with HIV–TB coinfection who are receiving TB treatment. In most patients, TB-IRIS occurs within the first few weeks of ART but can occur much later. Patients with HIV–TB coinfection with low $CD4^+$ counts who start ART are at high risk of developing TB-IRIS. Although the immunopathogenesis of TB-IRIS is still not completely understood, the explosive restoration of T-cell function is believed to play a distinct role.

Clinical Manifestations

Respiratory Manifestations

Shortness of breath, dyspnea (laboured breathing), cough, chest pain, and fever are associated with various opportunistic infections such as those caused by *Pneumocystis jiroveci*, *Mycobacterium avium-intracellulare*, cytomegalovirus (CMV), and *Legionella* species.

Pneumocystis Pneumonia

***Pneumocystis* pneumonia (PCP)** is caused by *P. jirovecii* (formerly *P. carinii*) (Panel on Opportunistic Infections in HIV-Infected Adults and Adolescents [OI-Panel], 2015) and the incidence has declined substantially with widespread use of PCP prophylaxis, which is used to prevent PCP, and ART. The most common manifestations of PCP are subacute onset of progressive dyspnea, fever, nonproductive cough, and chest discomfort that worsens within days to weeks. In mild cases, pulmonary examination usually is normal at rest. With exertion, tachypnea, tachycardia, and diffuse dry (cellophane) rales may be auscultated. Oral thrush is a common coinfection. Fever is apparent in most cases and may be the predominant symptom. Hypoxemia is the most characteristic laboratory abnormality, along with elevated lactate dehydrogenase levels. Because clinical presentation, blood tests, and chest radiographs are not pathognomonic for PCP, and because the organism cannot be cultivated routinely, histopathologic or cytopathologic demonstration of organisms in tissue, bronchoalveolar lavage fluid, or induced sputum samples is required for a definitive diagnosis (OI-Panel, 2015).

Mycobacterium avium Complex

***Mycobacterium avium* complex (MAC)** disease is a common opportunistic infection that typically occurs in patients with $CD4^+$ T-lymphocyte ($CD4^+$) cell counts less than 50 cells/mm^3. MAC is caused by infection with different types of mycobacterium: *Mycobacterium avium, Mycobacterium intracellulare,* or *Mycobacterium kansasii.* Early symptoms may be minimal and can precede detectable mycobacteremia by several weeks and include fever, night sweats, weight loss, fatigue, diarrhea, and abdominal pain. A confirmed diagnosis of disseminated MAC disease is based on compatible clinical signs and symptoms coupled with the isolation of MAC from cultures of blood, lymph node, bone marrow, or other normally sterile tissue or body fluids (OI-Panel, 2015).

Tuberculosis

The estimated annual risk of reactivation with TB among those with untreated HIV infection and latent TB infection is 3% to 16% and approximates the lifetime risk for individuals without HIV infection who have latent TB infection. TB disease can occur at any $CD4^+$ T-lymphocyte ($CD4^+$ cell) count, although the risk increases with progressive immune deficiency. Testing for latent TB at the time of HIV diagnosis should be routine, regardless of an individual's risk of TB exposure. Individuals with negative diagnostic tests for latent TB who have stage 3 HIV infection should be retested once their $CD4^+$ count increases due to ART. Screening for symptoms (asking for cough of *any* duration) coupled with chest radiography is recommended to exclude TB disease in a patient with a positive skin test or interferon-gamma release assays. Latent TB in a person with HIV infection is treated with isoniazid (INH), supplemented with pyridoxine (Aminoxin) to prevent peripheral neuropathy, for 9 months since it has proven efficacy, good tolerability, and infrequent severe toxicity.

TB disease can develop in the lungs as well as in extrapulmonary sites such as the central nervous system (CNS), bone, pericardium, stomach, peritoneum, and scrotum and initial diagnostic testing is directed at the anatomic site of symptoms or signs, such as the lungs, lymph nodes, and cerebrospinal fluid (CSF). TB in individuals with advanced immune deficiency can be rapidly progressive and fatal if treatment is delayed and such patients often have smear-negative sputum specimens. Therefore, after collection of available specimens for culture and molecular diagnostic tests, empiric treatment for TB is warranted in patients with clinical and radiographic presentation suggestive of HIV-related TB. Treatment of suspected TB in individuals with HIV infection is the same as for those who are HIV uninfected and should include an initial four-drug combination of isoniazid, rifampin (Rifadin), pyrazinamide, and ethambutol (Etibi) (OI-Panel, 2015).

Gastrointestinal Manifestations

The gastrointestinal manifestations of HIV infection and AIDS include loss of appetite, nausea, vomiting, oral and esophageal candidiasis, and chronic diarrhea. Gastrointestinal symptoms may be related to the direct inflammatory effect of HIV on the cells lining the intestines. Some of the enteric pathogens that occur most frequently, identified by stool cultures or intestinal biopsy, are *Cryptosporidium muris, Salmonella* species, *Isospora belli, Giardia lamblia*, CMV, *Clostridium difficile*, and *M. avium-intracellulare*. In patients with AIDS, the effects of diarrhea can be devastating in terms of profound weight loss (more than 10% of body weight), fluid and electrolyte imbalances, perianal skin excoriation, weakness, and inability to perform the usual activities of daily living.

Candidiasis

Oropharyngeal and esophageal **candidiasis** (fungal infections) are common in patients with HIV infection. Oropharyngeal candidiasis is characterized by painless, creamy-white, plaque-like lesions that can occur on the buccal surface, hard or soft palate, oropharyngeal mucosa, or tongue surface. Lesions can be easily scraped off with a tongue depressor or other instrument which is in contrast to lesions associated with oral hairy leukoplakia. In women with early-stage HIV infection, *Candida* vulvovaginitis usually presents the same as in women without HIV infection, with white adherent vaginal discharge associated with mucosal burning and itching of mild-to-moderate severity and sporadic recurrences (OI-Panel, 2015).

Wasting Syndrome

Wasting syndrome is defined as the involuntary loss of more than 10% of one's body weight while having experienced diarrhea or weakness and fever for more than 30 days. Wasting refers to the loss of muscle mass, although part of the weight loss may also be due to loss of fat.

Oncologic Manifestations

Those with HIV/AIDS are at greater risk of developing certain cancers. These include **Kaposi's sarcoma** (KS), lymphoma, and invasive cervical cancer. KS and lymphoma are discussed below. Cervical carcinoma is described later in Gynecologic Manifestations section.

Kaposi's Sarcoma

KS is caused by human t (HHV-8); affects eight times more men than women; and may spread through sexual contact. It involves the epithelial layer of blood and lymphatic vessels. AIDS-related KS exhibits a variable and aggressive course, ranging from localized cutaneous lesions to disseminated disease involving multiple organ systems. Cutaneous signs may be the first manifestation of HIV; they can appear anywhere on the body and are usually brownish pink to deep purple. They may be flat or raised and surrounded by ecchymosis (hemorrhagic patches) and edema (Fig. 52-3). Rapid development of lesions involving large areas of skin is associated with extensive disfigurement and significant body image issues. The location and size of some lesions can lead to venous stasis, lymphedema, and pain. Ulcerative lesions disrupt skin integrity and increase discomfort and susceptibility to infection. The most common sites of visceral involvement are the lymph nodes, gastrointestinal tract, and lungs. Involvement of internal organs may eventually lead to organ failure, hemorrhage, infection, and death.

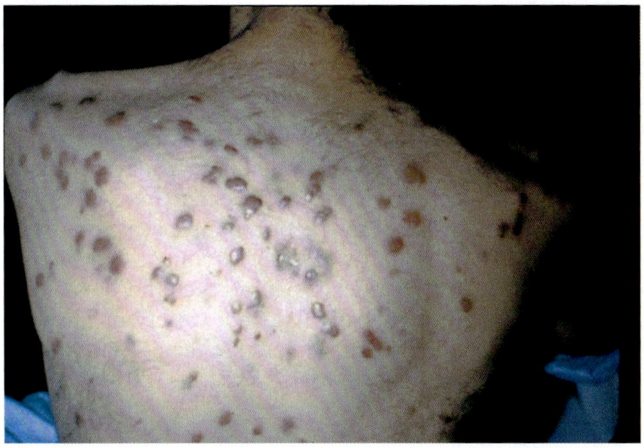

FIGURE 52-3. Lesions of the AIDS-related Kaposi's sarcoma. Whereas some patients may have lesions that remain flat, others experience extensively disseminated, raised lesions with edema. (Reprinted with permission from DeVita Jr., V. T., Hellman, S., & Rosenberg, S. (Eds.) (1993). *AIDS: Etiology, diagnosis, treatment, and prevention* (4th ed.). Philadelphia, PA: Lippincott Williams & Wilkins.)

Diagnosis of KS is confirmed by biopsy of suspected lesions. Prognosis depends on the extent of the tumour, the presence of other symptoms of HIV infection, and the CD4+ count. Death may result from tumour progression. More often, however, it results from other complications of HIV infection.

AIDS-Related Lymphomas

AIDS-related lymphomas include both Hodgkin lymphoma and non-Hodgkin lymphoma. Non-Hodgkin lymphoma is more common. AIDS-related lymphoma is usually aggressive; there are three main types: diffuse large B-cell; B-cell immunoblastic; and small noncleaved cell lymphoma. Symptoms include weight loss, night sweats, and fever. The complete blood count might be abnormal and a biopsy will confirm the diagnosis (National Cancer Institute [NCI], 2015).

Neurologic Manifestations

HIV-related brain changes have profound effects on cognition, including motor function, executive function, attention, visual memory, and visuospatial function. Neurologic dysfunction results from direct effects of HIV on nervous system tissue, opportunistic infections, primary or metastatic neoplasms, cerebrovascular changes, metabolic encephalopathies, or complications secondary to therapy. Immune system response to HIV infection in the CNS includes inflammation, atrophy, demyelination, degeneration, and necrosis.

Peripheral Neuropathy

Peripheral neuropathy is the most common neurologic symptom at any stage of HIV infection. It may be a side effect of some ART drugs, and may occur in a variety of patterns, with distal sensory polyneuropathy or distal symmetric polyneuropathy the most frequently occurring type. It can lead to significant pain of feet and hands and functional impairment. Patients use a variety of physical and psychological self-management strategies to minimize this symptom (Nicholas, Corless, & Evans, 2014).

HIV Encephalopathy

HIV encephalopathy was formerly referred to as AIDS dementia complex (see Chart 52-9). It is a clinical syndrome is characterized by a progressive decline in cognitive, behavioural, and motor functions as a direct result of HIV infection. HIV has been found in the brain and CSF of patients with HIV encephalopathy. The brain cells infected by HIV are predominantly the $CD4^+$ cells of monocyte–macrophage lineage. HIV infection is thought to trigger the release of toxins or lymphokines that result in cellular dysfunction inflammation, or interference with neurotransmitter function rather than cellular damage.

Signs and symptoms may be subtle and difficult to distinguish from fatigue, depression, or the adverse effects of treatment for infections and malignancies. Early manifestations include memory deficits, headache, difficulty concentrating, progressive confusion, psychomotor slowing, apathy, and ataxia. Later stages include global cognitive impairments, delay in verbal responses, a vacant stare, spastic paraparesis, hyperreflexia, psychosis, hallucinations, tremor, incontinence, seizures, mutism, and death.

Confirming the diagnosis of HIV encephalopathy can be difficult. Extensive neurologic evaluation includes a computed tomography scan which may indicate diffuse cerebral atrophy and ventricular enlargement. Other tests that may detect abnormalities include magnetic resonance imaging, analysis of CSF through lumbar puncture, and brain biopsy.

Cryptococcus Neoformans

A fungal infection, *Cryptococcus neoformans*, is another common opportunistic infection among patients with AIDS, and it causes neurologic disease. Cryptococcal meningitis is characterized by symptoms such as fever, headache, malaise, stiff neck, nausea, vomiting, mental status changes, and seizures. Diagnosis is confirmed by CSF analysis.

Progressive Multifocal Leukoencephalopathy

Progressive multifocal leukoencephalopathy (PML) is a demyelinating CNS disorder that affects the oligodendroglia. Clinical manifestations often begin with mental confusion and rapidly progress to include blindness, aphasia, muscle weakness, paresis (partial or complete paralysis), and death. ART has greatly reduced the threat of mortality associated with this disorder.

CHART 52-9

Care of the Patient With HIV Encephalopathy

Chronic Confusion

- Assess mental status and neurologic functioning
- Monitor for medication interactions, infections, electrolyte imbalance, and depression
- Frequently orient the patient to time, place, person, reality, and the environment
- Use simple explanations
- Instruct the patient to perform tasks in incremental steps
- Provide memory aids (clocks and calendars)
- Provide memory aids for medication administration
- Postactivity schedule
- Give positive feedback for appropriate behaviour.
- Educate caretakers about orienting patient to time, place, person, reality, and the environment
- Encourage the patient to designate a responsible person to assume power of attorney

Disturbed Sensation

- Assess sensory impairment
- Decrease amount of stimuli in the patient's environment
- Correct inaccurate perceptions
- Provide reassurance and safety if the patient displays fear
- Provide a secure and stable environment
- Educate caregivers about recognizing inaccurate sensory perceptions
- Provide caregivers techniques to correct inaccurate perceptions
- Instruct the patient and caregivers to report any changes in the patient's vision to the patient's health care provider

Risk for Injury

- Assess the patient's level of anxiety, confusion, or disorientation
- Assess the patient for delusions or hallucinations
- Remove potentially dangerous objects from the patient's environment
- Structure the environment for safety (ensure adequate lighting, avoid clutter, provide bed rails if needed)
- Supervise smoking
- Do not let the patient drive a car if confusion is present
- Instruct the patient and caregiver in home safety
- Provide assistance as needed for ambulation and in getting in and out of bed
- Pad headboard and side rails if the patient has seizures

Self-Care Deficits

- Encourage activities of daily living within the patient's level of ability
- Encourage independence, but assist if the patient cannot perform an activity
- Demonstrate any activity that the patient is having difficulty accomplishing
- Monitor food and fluid intake
- Weigh patient weekly
- Encourage the patient to eat, and offer nutritious meals, snacks, and adequate fluids
- If patient is incontinent, establish a routine toileting schedule
- Educate caregivers about meeting the patient's self-care needs

Other Neurologic Disorders

Other infections involving the nervous system include *Toxoplasma gondii*, CMV, and *Mycobacterium tuberculosis* infections.

Depressive Manifestations

Depression and apathy are neuropsychiatric complications of HIV infection. Estimates suggest that the prevalence of current depression is between 30% and 40% in persons with HIV/AIDS. Similarly, apathy, which refers to reduced, self-initiated, cognitive, emotional, and behavioural activity, is also commonly reported among those living with a diagnosis of HIV with rates as high as 65% (Bryant, Whitehead, Burrell, et al., 2015). Alcohol and cocaine use—both current and former—have been associated with depression and apathy in this population, and depression has been associated with less adherence with ART.

Integumentary Manifestations

Cutaneous manifestations are associated with HIV infection and the accompanying opportunistic infections and malignancies. KS (described earlier) and opportunistic infections such as herpes zoster and herpes simplex are associated with painful vesicles that disrupt skin integrity. Molluscum contagiosum is a viral infection characterized by deforming plaque formation. Seborrheic dermatitis is associated with an indurated, diffuse, scaly rash involving the scalp and face. Patients with AIDS may also exhibit a generalized folliculitis associated with dry, flaking skin or atopic dermatitis, such as eczema or psoriasis. Up to 60% of patients treated with the antibacterial agent trimethoprim–sulfamethoxazole (TMP–SMZ) develop a drug-related rash that is pruritic with pinkish-red macules and papules (Comerford, 2015). Patients with any of these rashes experience discomfort, have body image changes, and are at increased risk for infection from disrupted skin integrity.

Gynecologic Manifestations

Persistent, recurrent vaginal candidiasis may be the first sign of HIV illness in women. Past or present genital ulcers are a risk factor for the transmission of HIV infection. Women with HIV infection are more susceptible to genital ulcers and venereal warts and have increased rates of incidence and recurrence of these conditions. Ulcerative STIs such as chancroid, syphilis, and herpes are more severe in women with HIV infection. Human papillomavirus (HPV) causes venereal warts and is a risk factor for cervical intraepithelial neoplasia, a cellular change that is frequently a precursor to cervical cancer. Women who are HIV-seropositive and have cervical carcinoma present at a more advanced stage of disease and have more persistent and recurrent disease and a shorter interval to recurrence and death than women without HIV infection.

Women with HIV are at increased risk for **pelvic inflammatory disease (PID)**, and the associated inflammation may potentiate the transmission of HIV infection. Moreover, women with HIV infection appear to have a higher incidence of menstrual abnormalities, including amenorrhea or bleeding between periods, than do women without HIV infection. The failure of health care providers to consider HIV infection in women may lead to a later diagnosis, thereby denying these patients appropriate and timely treatment.

Medical Management

Treatment of Opportunistic Infections

Guidelines for the treatment of opportunistic infections should be consulted for the most current recommendations (OI-Panel, 2015). Although ART is highly effective in keeping the $CD4^+$ cell count high, opportunistic infections continue to cause considerable morbidity and mortality for three main reasons: (a) many patients are unaware of their HIV infection and present with an opportunistic infection as the initial indicator of their disease; (b) some patients are aware of their HIV infection but do not take ARV agents because of psychosocial or economic factors; and (c) others receive prescriptions for ARV medications but fail to attain adequate virologic and immunologic response as a result of issues related to adherence, pharmacokinetics, or unexplained biologic factors.

Pneumocystis Pneumonia

Persons in stage 3 HIV infection should receive chemoprophylaxis to prevent PCP with trimethoprim–sulfamethoxazole (TMP–SMX) if they have $CD4^+$ counts less than 200 cells/mm^3 or a history of oropharyngeal candidiasis (OI-Panel, 2015). Once the $CD4^+$ count improves, prophylaxis can be discontinued. When a person is diagnosed with PCP, TMP–SMX is the treatment of choice, lowering the dose if there is abnormal renal function. Adjunctive corticosteroids (Prednisone) are indicated as early as possible, preferentially within 72 hours after starting specific PCP therapy. Treatment duration is usually 21 days; rates of adverse reaction to TMP–SMX are high including rash (30% to 55%) (including Stevens–Johnson syndrome), fever (30% to 40%), leukopenia (30% to 40%), hepatitis (20%), thrombocytopenia (15%), azotemia (1% to 5%), and hyperkalemia. Because long-term survival is possible for patients in whom ART is effective, individuals with AIDS and severe PCP should be given the option to choose mechanical ventilation and critical care management if their functional status is such that it would be appropriate, just as with patients without HIV infection. Paradoxical IRIS has been reported following PCP and starting ART (OI-Panel, 2015).

Mycobacterium Avium Complex

Initial treatment of MAC disease should consist of two or more antimycobacterial drugs to prevent or delay the emergence of resistance. Clarithromycin (Biaxin) is the preferred first agent; however, azithromycin (Zithromax) can be substituted for clarithromycin when drug interactions or intolerance to clarithromycin preclude its use. Ethambutol is the recommended second drug (OI-Panel, 2015).

Cryptococcal Meningitis

Cryptococcosis among patients with HIV infection most commonly occurs as a subacute meningitis or meningoencephalitis with fever, malaise, and headache. Treating cryptococcosis consists of three phases: induction, consolidation, and maintenance therapy. The preferred induction treatment for cryptococcal meningitis and other forms of extrapulmonary cryptococcosis is the IV lipid formulation of amphotericin B in combination with fluconazole (Diflucan). Serious potential adverse effects of amphotericin B include anaphylaxis, kidney and hepatic impairment, electrolyte imbalances, anemia, fever, and severe chills. After at least 2 weeks of successful induction therapy—defined as substantial clinical improvement and a negative CSF culture after a repeat lumbar puncture—amphotericin B and flucytosine can be discontinued. Follow-up or consolidation therapy is then initiated with oral fluconazole daily which should continue for at least 8 weeks (OI-Panel, 2015).

Cytomegalovirus Retinitis

Retinitis caused by CMV is a leading cause of blindness in patients with AIDS. Oral valganciclovir (Valcyte), IV ganciclovir (Cytovene), IV ganciclovir followed by oral valganciclovir, IV foscarnet (Foscavir), IV cidofovir (Vistide), and a ganciclovir intraocular implant coupled with valganciclovir are all effective treatments for CMV retinitis (OI-Panel, 2015). All of these drugs have significant toxicities (bone marrow suppression, neutropenia, hepatitis, renal toxicity, seizures, etc.) and are used with caution (Comerford, 2015).

Antidiarrheal Therapy

Although many forms of diarrhea respond to treatment, it is not unusual for this condition to recur and become a chronic problem for the patient with HIV infection. Therapy with octreotide acetate (Sandostatin), a synthetic analogue of somatostatin, has been shown to effectively manage chronic severe diarrhea. High concentrations of somatostatin receptors have been found in the gastrointestinal tract and in other tissues. Somatostatin inhibits many physiologic functions, including gastrointestinal motility and intestinal secretion of water and electrolytes.

Chemotherapy

Kaposi's Sarcoma

KS can be treated with local therapy, radiation therapy, chemotherapy, and biologic therapy depending upon the location of the lesions.

Lymphoma

There is no standard treatment for AIDS-related peripheral or systemic lymphoma. The treatment plan is adjusted for each patient and usually includes one or more of combination chemotherapy, high-dose chemotherapy and stem cell transplant. There are many ongoing clinical trials (using monoclonal antibodies; different treatment combinations) that patients with AIDS-related lymphoma may be eligible to enter (NCI, 2015).

Antidepressant Therapy

Treatment for depression in people with HIV infection involves cognitive behavioural therapy integrated with pharmacotherapy. If depressive symptoms are severe and of sufficient duration, treatment with antidepressants may be initiated. Antidepressants such as imipramine (Tofranil), desipramine (Norpramin), and fluoxetine (Prozac) may be used because these medications also alleviate the fatigue and lethargy that are associated with depression. A psychostimulant such as methylphenidate (Ritalin) may be used in low doses in patients with neuropsychiatric impairment. Electroconvulsive therapy may be an option for patients with severe depression who do not respond to pharmacologic interventions.

Nutrition Therapy

Alterations in lipid metabolism are associated with HIV infection and ART. Malnutrition increases the risk of infection and the incidence of opportunistic infections. Nutrition therapy should be part of the overall management plan and should be tailored to meet the nutritional needs of the patient, whether by oral diet, enteral tube feedings, or parenteral nutritional support, if needed. As with all patients, a healthy diet is essential for the patient with HIV infection. For all patients with AIDS who experience unexplained weight loss, calorie counts and weight monitoring should be obtained to evaluate nutritional status and initiate appropriate therapy. The goal is to maintain the ideal weight and, when necessary, to increase weight.

Appetite stimulants have been successfully used in patients with AIDS-related anorexia. Megestrol acetate (Megace), a synthetic oral progesterone preparation, promotes significant weight gain and inhibits cytokine IL-1 synthesis. In patients with HIV infection, it increases body weight primarily by increasing body fat stores. Dronabinol (Marinol), which is a synthetic tetrahydrocannabinol (THC), the active ingredient in marijuana, has been used to relieve nausea and vomiting associated with cancer chemotherapy. After beginning dronabinol therapy, almost all patients with HIV infection experience a modest weight gain. The effects on body composition are unknown.

Oral supplements may be used when the diet is deficient in calories and protein. Ideally, oral supplements should be lactose-free (people with HIV infection may be intolerant to lactose), high in calories and easily digestible protein, low in fat with the fat easily digestible, palatable, inexpensive, and tolerated without causing diarrhea. Nutritional supplements have been developed specifically for people with HIV infection and AIDS. Parenteral nutrition is the final option because of its prohibitive cost and associated risks, including possible infection.

Complementary, Alternative and Integrative Modalities

Complementary and alternative medicine (or CAM) refers to medical practices that are "outside the standard Western medical model" (CATIE 2017) and is also known as holistic or integrative medicine. Combined with traditional therapies, these may improve the patient's overall well-being. However, there can be adverse drug–drug interactions between certain therapies (e.g., St. John wort) and some ART.

Although there is insufficient research on the effects of complementary, alternative, and integrative therapies, a growing body of literature reports benefits for modalities involving nutrition, exercise, psychosocial treatment, and Chinese medicine (NCCIH, 2019). PHAC (2015) found that since Aboriginal women's views about the etiology and treatment for their HIV illness were different from the conventional biomedical view of HIV disease, the women used a combination of biomedical, traditional, and alternative treatments for their illness. At other times fear of judgment, discrimination, and stigma have made it less likely for Aboriginal women to access Western health care (McCall & Pauly, 2012) (Chart 52-10).

NURSING RESEARCH PROFILE

Chart 52-10. Aboriginal Women's View of HIV Care

McCall, J., & Pauly, B. (2012). Providing a safe place: Adopting a culturally safe perspective in the care of Aboriginal women living with HIV/AIDS. *Canadian Journal of Nursing Research*, *44*(2), 130–145.

Purpose

Aboriginal women living HIV/AIDS are more likely to die of AIDS-related illnesses and less likely to access treatment for their HIV infection than the general population infected with HIV. The study examines the lives and experiences of Aboriginal women facing significant social-economic barriers and living with HIV illness in relation to accessing care.

Study Sample and Design

A qualitative research design was selected for the study, and in-depth semi-structured interviews were the primary data collection methods. The sample consisted of eight Aboriginal women who self-identified as HIV positive. Participants were recruited through one inpatient HIV unit and one outpatient HIV clinic. The interviews were audio recorded and transcribed verbatim. The transcripts were read repeatedly to identify recurring, converting, and contradictory patterns of interaction; key concept; emerging themes; symbolic examples; and possible connections to the underlying theory. The transcripts were coded, and emerging themes and categories were identified and reviewed with participants.

Findings

A number of themes were uncovered related to Aboriginal women's experiences with health care, including fear of rejection. The participants were reluctant to access health services because they felt unsafe. The participants in this study faced barriers to forming therapeutic relationships with the providers with whom they came in contact, due to a lack of communication and a sense of powerlessness and fearfulness about how they would be treated. The women's experiences of judgment and stigma compounded their discomforts with the care that was provided.

Nursing Implications

The authors examine how cultural safety principles might be applied in therapeutic relationships with Aboriginal women as part of the process of facilitating access to care that is acceptable and timely. It is clear from the findings that it is critical for nurses and other health care workers to understand the positioning of Aboriginal women in the health care system and the need for safer environments. Through the use of a cultural safety framework, nurses are able to develop therapeutic and safe relationships with their patients. When nurses practice in a culturally safe manner, they not only help improve the lives of their patients, but they also stand to achieve a heightened state of self-awareness and professional growth.

Clinical trials are in progress to examine the effect of Chinese herbal treatments of HIV-associated symptoms related to inadequate nutrition, such as fatigue, nausea, vomiting, painful or difficulty swallowing, altered taste sensation, and diarrhea. At present, there are no definitive study results indicating that these treatments are effective, but some appear promising. In a recent randomized trial at Mount Sinai Hospital in Toronto researchers explore mindfulness-based stress reduction for HIV positive men. While the results are mixed they seem to indicate that enhanced psychological function is supported by mindfulness-based stress reduction therapy (Vollestad, Sivertsen, & Nielsen, 2011).

Many patients who use these therapies do not report their use to their health care providers. To obtain a complete health history, the nurse should ask about the patient's use of complementary, alternative, and integrative therapies. Patients may need to be encouraged to report their use of these therapies to their primary provider. Problems may arise, for example, when patients are using complementary, alternative, and integrative therapies while participating in clinical drug trials; alternative therapies can have significant adverse side effects, making it difficult to assess the effects of the medications in the clinical trial. The nurse who suspects that complementary, alternative, and integrative therapies is causing a side effect needs to discuss this with the patient, the alternative therapy provider, and the primary provider. The nurse needs to view complementary, alternative, and integrative therapies with an open mind and try to understand the importance of this treatment to the patient. This approach will improve communication with the patient and reduce conflict.

Supportive Care

Patients who are weak and debilitated as a result of chronic illness associated with HIV infection and AIDS typically require many kinds of supportive care. Nutritional support may be as simple as providing assistance in obtaining or preparing meals. For patients with more advanced nutritional impairment resulting from decreased intake, wasting syndrome, or gastrointestinal malabsorption associated with diarrhea, parenteral feedings may be required. Imbalances that result from nausea, vomiting, and profuse diarrhea often necessitate IV fluid and electrolyte replacement.

Management of skin breakdown associated with KS, perianal skin excoriation, or immobility entails thorough and meticulous skin care that involves regular turning, cleansing, and applications of medicated ointments and dressings. To combat pain associated with skin breakdown, abdominal cramping, peripheral neuropathy, or KS, the nurse administers analgesic agents at regular intervals around the clock. Patients with a history of drug abuse will need to have tailored approaches for pain management. Relaxation and guided imagery may be helpful in reducing pain and anxiety.

Pulmonary symptoms, such as dyspnea and shortness of breath, may be related to opportunistic infection, KS, or fatigue. For patients with these symptoms, oxygen therapy, relaxation training, and energy conservation techniques may be effective. Patients with severe respiratory dysfunction may require mechanical ventilation. Before mechanical ventilation is instituted, the procedure is explained to the patient and the caregiver.

As noted previously, with the advent of ART, there are generally more positive outcomes than could be achieved a few years ago, and a patient mechanically ventilated has a reasonable likelihood of survival. However, if the patient decides to forgo mechanical ventilation, their wishes should be followed. Ideally, the patient has prepared an advance directive identifying preferences for treatments and end-of-life care, including hospice care. If the patient has not identified preferences in advance, treatment options are described so that the patient can make informed decisions and have those wishes respected.

Nurses should anticipate that patients as well as family and friends will need support and time to share concerns. In some family systems, more than one person might be living with HIV/AIDS.

Nursing Process

The Patient With HIV/AIDS Illness

The nursing care of patients with HIV/AIDS is challenging because of the potential for any organ system to be involved due to infections or cancer. In addition, this disease is complicated by many emotional, social, and ethical issues. The plan of care for the patient with AIDS (Chart 52-11) is individualized to meet the needs of the patient. The best practice guidelines of HIV/AIDS nursing developed by the Canadian Association of Nurses in AIDS Care (2012)

(text continued on page 1561)

Plan of Nursing Care — Chart 52-11. Care of the Patient With AIDS

NURSING INTERVENTIONS	RATIONALE	EXPECTED OUTCOMES
Nursing Priority: Diarrhea **Goal:** Resumption of usual bowel habits		
1. Assess patient's normal bowel habits	1. Provides baseline for evaluation	• Exhibits return to normal bowel patterns • Reports decreasing episodes of diarrhea and abdominal cramping • Identifies and avoids foods that irritate the gastrointestinal tract • Takes appropriate therapy as prescribed • Exhibits normal stool cultures • Maintains adequate fluid intake • Maintains body weight and reports no additional weight loss • States rationale for avoiding smoking • Enrolls in program to stop smoking • Uses medication as prescribed • Maintains adequate fluid status • Exhibits normal skin turgor, moist mucous membranes, adequate urine output, and absence of excessive thirst
2. Assess for diarrhea: frequent, loose stools; abdominal pain or cramping, volume of liquid stools, and exacerbating and alleviating factors	2. Detects changes in status, quantifies loss of fluid, and provides basis for nursing measures	
3. Obtain stool cultures, and administer antimicrobial therapy as prescribed	3. Identifies pathogenic organism; therapy targets specific organism	
4. Initiate measures to reduce hyperactivity of bowel	4. Promotes bowel rest, which may decrease acute episodes	
a. Maintain food and fluid restrictions as prescribed. Suggest BRAT diet (*b*ananas, *r*ice, *a*pplesauce, *t*ea, and *t*oast)	a. Reduces stimulation of bowel	
b. Discourage smoking	b. Eliminates nicotine, which acts as bowel stimulant	
c. Avoid bowel irritants such as fatty or fried foods, raw vegetables, and nuts. Offer small, frequent meals	c. Prevents stimulation of bowel and abdominal distention and promotes adequate nutrition	
5. Administer anticholinergic antispasmodics and opioids or other medications as prescribed	5. Decreases intestinal spasms and motility	
6. Maintain fluid intake of at least 3 L/day unless contraindicated	6. Prevents hypovolemia	
Nursing Priority: Risk for infection **Goal:** Absence of infection		
1. Monitor for infection: fever, chills, and diaphoresis; cough; shortness of breath; oral pain or painful swallowing; creamy-white patches in oral cavity; urinary frequency, urgency, or dysuria; redness, swelling, or drainage from wounds; vesicular lesions on face, lips, or perianal area	1. Allows for early detection of infection, essential for prompt initiation of treatment. Repeated and prolonged infections contribute to patient's debilitation	• Identifies reportable signs and symptoms of infection • Reports signs and symptoms of infection if present • Exhibits and reports absence of fever, chills, and diaphoresis • Exhibits normal (clear) breath sounds without adventitious breath sounds

Plan of Nursing Care

Chart 52-11. Care of the Patient With AIDS, *Continued*

NURSING INTERVENTIONS

2. Educate patient or caregiver about need to report possible infection
3. Monitor white blood cell (WBC) count and differential
4. Obtain cultures of wound drainage, skin lesions, urine, stool, sputum, mouth, and blood as prescribed. Administer antimicrobial therapy as prescribed
5. Instruct patient in ways to prevent infection
6. Clean kitchen and bathroom surfaces with disinfectants
   a. Clean hands thoroughly after exposure to body fluids
   b. Avoid exposure to others' body fluids or sharing eating utensils
   c. Turn, cough, and deep breathe, especially when activity is decreased
   d. Maintain cleanliness of perianal area
   e. Avoid handling pet excreta or cleaning litter boxes, birdcages, or aquariums
   f. Cook meat and eggs thoroughly
7. Maintain aseptic technique when performing invasive procedures such as venipunctures, bladder catheterizations, and injections

RATIONALE

2. Allows early detection of infection
3. Elevated WBC count possibly associated with infection
4. Assists in determining offending organism to initiate appropriate treatment
5. Minimizes exposure to infection and transmission of HIV infection to others
6. Prevents hospital-acquired infections

EXPECTED OUTCOMES

- Maintains weight
- Reports adequate energy level without excessive fatigue
- Reports absence of shortness of breath and cough
- Exhibits pink, moist oral mucous membranes without fissures or lesions
- Takes appropriate therapy as prescribed
- Experiences no infection
- States rationale for strategies to avoid infection
- Modifies activities to reduce exposure to infection or infectious persons
- Practices "safer sex"
- Avoids sharing eating utensils and toothbrush
- Exhibits normal body temperature
- Uses recommended techniques to maintain cleanliness of skin, skin lesions, and perianal area
- Has others handle pet excreta and cleanup
- Uses recommended cooking techniques

Nursing Priority: Ineffective airway clearance
Goal: Improved airway clearance

NURSING INTERVENTIONS

1. Assess and report signs and symptoms of altered respiratory status, tachypnea, the use of accessory muscles, cough, colour and amount of sputum, abnormal breath sounds, dusky or cyanotic skin colour, restlessness, confusion, or somnolence
2. Obtain sputum sample for culture as prescribed. Administer antimicrobial therapy as prescribed
3. Provide pulmonary care (cough, deep breathing, postural drainage, and vibration) every 2 to 4 hours
4. Assist patient in attaining semi- or high Fowler's position
5. Encourage adequate rest periods
6. Initiate measures to decrease viscosity of secretions
   a. Maintain fluid intake of at least 3 L/day unless contraindicated
   b. Humidify inspired air as prescribed
   c. Consult with primary provider concerning the use of mucolytic agents delivered through nebulizer or intermittent positive pressure breathing treatment

RATIONALE

1. Indicates abnormal respiratory function
2. Aids in identification of pathogenic organisms
3. Prevents stasis of secretions and promotes airway clearance
4. Facilitates breathing and airway clearance
5. Maximizes energy expenditure and prevents excessive fatigue
6. Facilitates expectoration of secretions; prevents stasis of secretions

EXPECTED OUTCOMES

- Maintains normal airway clearance:
  - Respiratory rate <20 breaths/minute
  - Unlaboured breathing without the use of accessory muscles and flaring nares (nostrils)
  - Skin colour pink (without cyanosis)
  - Alert and aware of surroundings
  - Arterial blood gas values normal
  - Normal breath sounds without adventitious breath sounds
- Begins appropriate therapy
- Takes medication as prescribed
- Reports improved breathing
- Maintains clear airway
- Coughs and takes deep breaths every 2 to 4 hours as recommended
- Demonstrates appropriate positions and practices postural drainage every 2 to 4 hours
- Reports reduced breathing difficulty when in semi- or high-Fowler's position
- Practices energy-conserving strategies and alternates rest with activity
- Demonstrates reduction in thickness (viscosity) of pulmonary secretions
- Reports increased ease in coughing up sputum

continued >

Plan of Nursing Care — Chart 52-11. Care of the Patient With AIDS, *Continued*

NURSING INTERVENTIONS	RATIONALE	EXPECTED OUTCOMES
7. Perform tracheal suctioning as needed	7. Removes secretions if patient is unable to do so	• Uses humidified air or oxygen as prescribed and indicated • Indicates need for assistance with removal of pulmonary secretions • Understands need for and cooperates with endotracheal intubation and the use of a mechanical ventilator • Verbalizes concerns about respiratory difficulty, intubation, and mechanical ventilation
8. Administer oxygen therapy as prescribed	8. Increases availability of oxygen	
9. Assist with endotracheal intubation; maintain ventilator settings as prescribed	9. Maintains ventilation	

Nursing Priority: Imbalanced nutrition
Goal: Intake of nutrients sufficient to meet metabolic needs

NURSING INTERVENTIONS	RATIONALE	EXPECTED OUTCOMES
1. Assess nutritional status with height, weight, age; blood urea nitrogen, serum protein, albumin, transferrin, hemoglobin, and hematocrit levels; and cutaneous anergy	1. Provides objective measurement of nutritional status	• Identifies factors limiting oral intake, and uses resources to promote adequate dietary intake • Reports increased appetite • States understanding of nutritional needs • Identifies ways to reduce factors that limit oral intake • Rests before meals • Eats in pleasant, odor-free environment • Arranges meals to coincide with visitors' visits • Reports increased dietary intake • Uses oral hygiene before meals • Takes analgesic agents before meals as prescribed • Identifies ways to increase protein and caloric intake • Identifies foods high in protein and calories • Consumes foods high in protein and calories • Reports decreased rate of weight loss • Maintains adequate caloric intake • States rationale for enteral or parenteral nutrition if needed • Demonstrates skill in preparing alternate sources of nutrition
2. Obtain dietary history, including likes and dislikes and food intolerances	2. Defines need for nutritional education; helps individualize interventions	
3. Assess factors that interfere with oral intake	3. Provides basis and directions for interventions	
4. Consult with dietitian to determine patient's nutritional needs	4. Facilitates meal planning	
5. Reduce factors limiting oral intake	5. Addresses factors limiting intake	
a. Encourage patient to rest before meals	a. Minimizes fatigue, which can decrease appetite	
b. Plan meals so that they do not occur immediately after painful or unpleasant procedures	b. Decreases noxious stimuli	
c. Encourage patient to eat meals with visitors or others when possible	c. Limits social isolation	
d. Encourage patient to prepare simple meals or to obtain assistance with meal preparation if possible	d. Limits energy expenditure	
e. Serve small, frequent meals: 6/day.	e. Prevents overwhelming patient	
f. Limit fluids 1 hour before meals and with meals	f. Reduces satiety	
6. Instruct patient in ways to supplement nutrition: consume protein-rich foods (meat, poultry, fish) and carbohydrates (pasta, fruit, breads)	6. Provides additional proteins and calories	
7. Consult with primary provider and dietitian about alternative feeding (enteral or parenteral nutrition)	7. Provides nutritional support if patient is unable to take sufficient amounts by mouth	
8. Consult with social worker or community liaison about financial assistance if patient cannot afford food	8. Increases availability of resources and nutrition	

Nursing Priority: Deficient knowledge
Goal: Increased knowledge concerning means of preventing disease transmission

NURSING INTERVENTIONS	RATIONALE	EXPECTED OUTCOMES
1. Instruct patient, family, and friends about routes of transmission of HIV	1. Knowledge about disease transmission can help prevent spread of disease; may also alleviate fears	• Patient, family, and friends state means of transmission

Plan of Nursing Care

Chart 52-11. Care of the Patient With AIDS, *Continued*

NURSING INTERVENTIONS	RATIONALE	EXPECTED OUTCOMES
2. Instruct patient, family, and friends about means of preventing transmission of HIV	2. Reduces transmission risk	• Reports and demonstrates practices to reduce exposure of others to HIV • Demonstrates knowledge of safer sexual practices • Identifies means of preventing disease transmission • States that sexual partners are informed about patient's positive HIV status in blood • Avoids IV/injection drug use and sharing of drug equipment with others • Understands risks and benefits associated with PrEP
a. Avoid sexual contact with multiple partners, and use precautions if sexual partner's HIV status is not certain	a. The risk of infection increases with the number of sexual partners, male or female, and sexual contact with those who engage in high-risk behaviours	
b. Use condoms during sexual intercourse (vaginal, anal, oral–genital); avoid mouth contact with the penis, vagina, or rectum; avoid sexual practices that can cause cuts or tears in the lining of the rectum, vagina, or penis	b. Risk of HIV transmission is reduced	
c. Avoid sex with sex workers and others at high risk	c. Many sex workers are infected with HIV through sexual contact with multiple partners or IV/injection drug use	
d. Do not use IV/injection drugs; if addicted and unable or unwilling to change behaviour, use clean needles and syringes	d. Clean needles and syringes are the only way to prevent HIV transmission for those who continue to use drugs. Taking precautions is important for those who are antibody positive to prevent transmitting HIV	
e. Women who may have been exposed to HIV through sexual or drug practices should consult with a physician before becoming pregnant; consider the use of antiretroviral agents if pregnant	e. HIV can be transmitted from mother to child in utero; the use of antiretroviral agents during pregnancy significantly reduces perinatal transmission of HIV	
f. Consider using PrEP	f. Taking ART before engaging in high-risk activity seems to protect against infection	
Nursing Priority: Social isolation **Goal:** Decreased sense of social isolation		
1. Assess patient's usual patterns of social interaction	1. Establishes basis for individualized interventions	• Shares with others the need for valued social interaction • Demonstrates interest in events, activities, and communication • Verbalizes feelings and reactions to diagnosis, prognosis, and life changes • Identifies modes of transmission of HIV • States ways of preventing transmission of HIV to others while maintaining contact with valued friends and relatives • Reveals HIV/AIDS diagnosis to others when appropriate • Identifies resources (i.e., family, friends, and support groups) • Uses resources when appropriate • Accepts offers of assistance and support • Reports decreased sense of isolation • Maintains contacts with those of importance to him or her • Develops or continues hobbies that effectively serve as diversion or distraction
2. Observe for behaviours indicative of social isolation, such as decreased interaction with others, hostility, noncompliance, sad affect, and stated feelings of rejection or loneliness	2. Promotes early detection of social isolation, which may be manifested in several ways	
3. Provide instruction concerning modes of transmission of HIV	3. Provides accurate information, corrects misconceptions, and alleviates anxiety	
4. Assist patient to identify and explore resources for support and positive mechanisms for coping (e.g., contact with family, friends, AIDS task force)	4. Enables mobilization of resources and supports	
5. Allow time to be with patient other than for medications and procedures	5. Promotes feelings of self-worth and provides social interaction	
6. Encourage participation in diversional activities such as reading, television, or handcrafts	6. Provides distraction	

continued >

Plan of Nursing Care

Chart 52-11. Care of the Patient With AIDS, *Continued*

NURSING INTERVENTIONS	RATIONALE	EXPECTED OUTCOMES
Collaborative Problems: Opportunistic infections; impaired breathing; wasting syndrome and fluid and electrolyte imbalances; adverse reaction to medications		
Goal: Absence of complications		
Opportunistic Infections		
1. Monitor vital signs including temperature	1. Changes in vital signs such as increases in pulse rate, respirations, blood pressure, and temperature may indicate infection	• Exhibits stable vital signs • Experiences control of infection • Identifies signs and symptoms correctly and experiences no complications • Identifies signs and symptoms that are reportable to the primary provider • Takes medications as prescribed
2. Obtain laboratory specimens, and monitor test results	2. Smears and cultures can identify causative agents such as bacteria, fungi, and protozoa, and sensitivity studies can identify antibiotics or other medications effective against the causative agent	
3. Instruct the patient and caregiver about signs and symptoms of infection and the need to report them early	3. Early recognition of symptoms facilitates prompt treatment and avoids extra complications	
Impaired Breathing		
1. Monitor respiratory rate and pattern	1. Rapid shallow breathing, diminished breath sounds, and shortness of breath may indicate respiratory failure resulting in hypoxia	• Maintains stable respiratory rate and pattern within the normal limits • Exhibits no adventitious lung sounds; normal breath sounds • Has stable pulse rate and blood pressure within normal limits, and exhibits no evidence of hypoxia • Oxygen saturation levels within acceptable range
2. Auscultate the chest for breath sounds and abnormal lung sounds	2. Crackles and wheezes may indicate fluid in the lungs, which disrupts respiratory function and alters the blood's oxygen-carrying capacity	
3. Monitor pulse rate, blood pressure, and oxygen saturation levels	3. Changes in pulse rate, blood pressure, and oxygen levels may indicate the development of respiratory or cardiac failure	
Wasting Syndrome and Fluid and Electrolyte Disturbances		
1. Monitor weight and laboratory values for nutritional status	1. Weight loss, malnutrition, and anemia are common in HIV infection and increase risk of superinfection	• Maintains stable weight • Eats a nutritious diet • Attains and maintains hemoglobin, hematocrit, and ferritin levels within normal limits • Sustains fluid and electrolyte balance within normal limits • Exhibits no signs and symptoms of dehydration
2. Monitor intake and output and laboratory values for fluid and electrolyte imbalance (potassium, sodium, calcium, phosphorus, magnesium, and zinc)	2. Chronic diarrhea, inadequate oral intake, vomiting, and profuse sweating deplete electrolytes. Small intestine inflammation may impair the absorption of fluids and electrolytes	
3. Monitor for and report signs and symptoms of dehydration	3. Fluid loss results in decreased circulating volume leading to tachycardia, dry skin and mucous membranes, poor skin turgor, elevated urine specific gravity, and thirst. Early detection allows early treatment	
Reactions to Medications		
1. Monitor for medication interactions	1. People with HIV infection receive many medications for HIV and for disease complications. Early detection of medication interactions is necessary to prevent complications	• Experiences no serious side effects or complications from medications • Correctly describes medication regimen and complies with therapy, including adaptations in eating routines and type of food used with prescribed medications

Plan of Nursing Care

Chart 52-11. Care of the Patient With AIDS, *Continued*

NURSING INTERVENTIONS	RATIONALE	EXPECTED OUTCOMES
2. Monitor for and promptly report side effects from antiretroviral agents	2. Side effects from antiretroviral agents can be life-threatening. Serious side effects include anemia, pancreatitis, peripheral neuropathy, mental confusion, and persistent nausea and vomiting. Corrective measures need to be instituted	
3. Instruct the patient and caregiver in the medication regimen	3. Knowledge of the medication purpose, correct administration, side effects, and strategies to manage or prevent side effects promotes safety and greater compliance with treatment	

direct nursing practice. Care includes many of the interventions and concerns mentioned in the section on supportive care.

Assessment

Nursing assessment includes identification of potential risk factors, including a history of risky sexual practices or IV/injection drug use. The patient's physical status and psychological status are assessed. All factors affecting immune system functioning are thoroughly explored. A number of instruments can be used to assess symptoms and self-management strategies (Fierz, Nicca, & Spirig, 2013).

Nutritional Status

Nutritional status is assessed by obtaining a dietary history and identifying factors that may interfere with oral intake, such as anorexia, nausea, vomiting, oral pain, or difficulty swallowing. In addition, the patient's ability to purchase, prepare, and safely store food is assessed. Weight history (i.e., changes over time); anthropometric measurements; and blood urea nitrogen (BUN), serum protein, albumin, and transferrin levels provide objective measurements of nutritional status.

Skin Integrity

The skin and mucous membranes are inspected daily for evidence of breakdown, ulceration, or infection. The oral cavity is monitored for redness, ulcerations, and the presence of creamy-white patches indicative of candidiasis. Assessment of the perianal area for excoriation and infection in patients with profuse diarrhea is important. Wounds are cultured to identify infectious organisms.

Respiratory Status

Respiratory status is assessed by monitoring the patient for cough, sputum production (i.e., amount and colour), shortness of breath, orthopnea, tachypnea, and chest pain. The presence and quality of breath sounds are investigated. Other measures of pulmonary function include chest x-ray results, arterial blood gas values, pulse oximetry, and pulmonary function test results.

Neurologic Status

Neurologic status is determined by assessing level of consciousness; orientation to person, place, and time; and memory lapses. Mental status is assessed as early as possible to provide a baseline. The patient is also assessed for sensory deficits (visual changes, headache, or numbness and tingling in the extremities), motor involvement (altered gait, paresis, or paralysis), and seizure activity.

Fluid and Electrolyte Balance

Fluid and electrolyte status is assessed by examining the skin and mucous membranes for turgor and dryness. Dehydration may be indicated by increased thirst, decreased urine output, postural hypotension, weak and rapid pulse, and urine specific gravity of 1.025 or more. Electrolyte imbalances, such as decreased serum sodium, potassium, calcium, magnesium, and chloride, typically result from profuse diarrhea. The patient is assessed for signs and symptoms of electrolyte deficits, including decreased mental status, muscle twitching, muscle cramps, irregular pulse, nausea and vomiting, and shallow respirations.

Knowledge Level

The patient's level of knowledge about the disease, modes of disease transmission, and adherence to ART are evaluated. In addition, the level of knowledge of family (biologic and family of choice) and friends is assessed. The patient's psychological reaction to the diagnosis of HIV infection or AIDS is important to explore. Reactions vary among patients and may include denial, anger, fear, shame, withdrawal from social interactions, and depressive symptoms. It is often helpful to gain an understanding of how the patient has dealt with illness and major life stresses in the past. The patient's resources for support are also identified.

Nursing Priorities

The list of potential nursing priorities is extensive because of the complex nature of HIV/AIDS. However, based on assessment data, major nursing priorities may include the following:

- Impaired skin integrity
- Diarrhea
- Risk for infection
- Activity intolerance
- Chronic confusion related to cognitive changes associated with HIV encephalopathy
- Ineffective airway clearance
- Acute and chronic pain
- Imbalanced nutrition
- Social isolation
- Grieving
- Deficient knowledge

Collaborative Problems/ Potential Complications

Possible complications may include the following:

- Opportunistic infections
- Impaired breathing or respiratory failure
- Wasting syndrome and fluid and electrolyte imbalance
- Adverse reaction to medications
- Body image changes

Planning and Goals

Goals for the patient may include achievement and maintenance of skin integrity, resumption of usual bowel patterns, absence of infection, improved activity tolerance, improved thought processes, improved airway clearance, increased comfort, improved nutritional status, increased socialization, expression of grief, increased knowledge regarding disease prevention and self-care, and absence of complications.

Nursing Interventions

Promoting Skin Integrity

The skin and oral mucosa are assessed routinely for changes in appearance, location and size of lesions, and evidence of infection and breakdown. The patient is encouraged to maintain a balance between rest and mobility whenever possible. Patients who are immobile are assisted to change position at least every 2 hours and more often as needed. Devices such as alternating-pressure mattresses and low–air-loss beds are used to prevent skin breakdown. Patients are encouraged to avoid scratching; to use nonabrasive, nondrying soaps; and to apply unscented skin moisturizers to dry skin. Regular oral care is also encouraged.

Medicated lotions, ointments, and dressings are applied to affected skin surfaces as prescribed. Adhesive tape is avoided. Skin surfaces are protected from friction and rubbing by keeping bed linens free of wrinkles and avoiding tight or restrictive clothing. Patients with foot lesions are advised to wear cotton socks and shoes that do not cause the feet to perspire. Antipruritic, antibiotic, and analgesic agents are administered as prescribed.

The perianal region is assessed frequently for infection and impairment of skin integrity. The patient is instructed to keep the area as clean as possible. The perianal area is cleaned after each bowel movement with nonabrasive soap and water to prevent further excoriation and breakdown of the skin and infection. If the area is very painful, soft cloths or cotton sponges may be less irritating than washcloths. In addition, sitz baths or gentle irrigation may facilitate cleaning and promote comfort. The area is dried thoroughly after cleaning. Topical lotions or ointments may be prescribed to promote healing. Wounds are cultured if infection is suspected, so that the appropriate antimicrobial treatment can be initiated. Debilitated patients may require assistance in maintaining hygienic practices.

Promoting Usual Bowel Patterns

Bowel patterns are assessed for diarrhea. The nurse monitors the frequency and consistency of stools and the patient's reports of abdominal pain or cramping associated with bowel movements. Factors that exacerbate frequent diarrhea are also assessed. The quantity and volume of liquid stools are measured to document fluid volume losses. Stool cultures are obtained to identify pathogenic organisms.

The patient is counselled about ways to decrease diarrhea. The physician may recommend restriction of oral intake to rest the bowel during periods of acute inflammation associated with severe enteric infections. As the patient's dietary intake is increased, foods that act as bowel irritants, such as raw fruits and vegetables, popcorn, carbonated beverages, spicy foods, and foods of extreme temperatures, should be avoided. Small, frequent meals help to prevent abdominal distention. Medications, such as anticholinergic agents, antispasmodic, agents, or opioids, can be prescribed to decrease diarrhea by decreasing intestinal spasms and motility. Administering antidiarrheal agents on a regular schedule may be more beneficial than administering them on an as-needed basis. Antibiotics and antifungal agents may also be prescribed to combat pathogens identified by stool cultures. Assessment of self-care strategies being used is essential.

Preventing Infection

The patient and caregivers are instructed to monitor for signs and symptoms of infection: fever; chills; night sweats; cough with or without sputum production; shortness of breath; difficulty breathing; oral

HIV illness may be overwhelmed with emotions such as anxiety, guilt, shame, and fear. They also may be faced with multiple losses, including financial security; normal roles and functions; self-esteem; privacy; ability to control bodily functions; ability to interact meaningfully with the environment; and sexual functioning, as well as rejection by sexual partners, family, and friends. Some patients may harbour feelings of guilt because of their lifestyle or because they may have infected others in current or previous relationships. Other patients may feel anger toward sexual partners who transmitted the virus to them. Infection control measures used in the hospital or at home may further contribute to the patient's emotional isolation. Any or all of these stressors may cause the patient with AIDS to withdraw both physically and emotionally from social contact

Nurses are in a key position to provide an atmosphere of acceptance and understanding for people with HIV and their families and partners. The patient's usual level of social interaction is assessed as early as possible to provide a baseline for monitoring changes in behaviours that suggest social isolation (e.g., decreased interaction with staff or family, hostility, nonadherence). Patients are encouraged to express feelings of isolation and loneliness, with the assurance that these feelings are not unique or abnormal.

Providing information about how to protect themselves and others may help patients avoid social isolation. Patients, family, and friends must be reassured that HIV is not spread through casual contact. Education of ancillary personnel, nurses, and physicians helps reduce factors that might contribute to patients' feelings of isolation. Patient care conferences that address the psychosocial issues associated with HIV infection may help sensitize the health care team to patients' needs.

Coping With Grief

The nurse can help the patient verbalize feelings and explore and identify resources for support and mechanisms for coping, especially when the patient is grieving anticipated losses. The patient is encouraged to maintain contact with family, friends, and coworkers and to use local or national HIV support groups and hotlines. If possible, losses are identified and addressed. The patient is encouraged to continue usual activities whenever possible. Consultations with mental health counsellors are useful for many patients and their families.

Improving Knowledge of HIV

The patient and family are educated about HIV infection, means of preventing HIV transmission, ART, and appropriate self-care measures. Information about the purpose of the medications, their correct administration, side effects, and strategies to manage or prevent side effects is provided. The patient is instructed to avoid others with active infections, such as upper respiratory infections.

Monitoring and Managing Potential Complications

OPPORTUNISTIC INFECTIONS. Patients who are severely immunosuppressed are at risk for opportunistic infections. Therefore, anti-infective agents may be prescribed, and laboratory tests obtained to monitor their effect. Signs and symptoms of opportunistic infections, including fever, malaise, difficulty breathing, nausea or vomiting, diarrhea, difficulty swallowing, and any occurrences of swelling or discharge, should be reported as treated as indicated.

RESPIRATORY FAILURE. Impaired breathing is a major complication that increases the patient's discomfort and anxiety and may lead to respiratory and cardiac failure. The respiratory rate and pattern are monitored, and the lungs are auscultated for abnormal breath sounds. The patient is instructed to report shortness of breath and increasing difficulty in carrying out usual activities. Pulse rate and rhythm, blood pressure, and oxygen saturation are monitored. Suctioning and oxygen therapy may be prescribed to ensure an adequate airway and to prevent hypoxia. Mechanical ventilation may be necessary for the patient who cannot maintain adequate ventilation as a result of pulmonary infection, fluid and electrolyte imbalance, or respiratory muscle weakness. Arterial blood gas values are used to guide ventilator settings. If the patient is intubated, methods must be established to allow communication with the nurse and others. The patient receiving mechanical ventilation will require support to cope with the stress associated with intubation and ventilator assistance. The use of mechanical ventilation should be consistent with the patient's decisions about end-of-life treatment. (Further discussion of end-of-life care can be found in Chapter 15.)

WASTING SYNDROME. Wasting syndrome and fluid and electrolyte disturbances, including dehydration, are common complications of stage 3 of infection. The patient's nutritional and electrolyte status is evaluated by monitoring weight gains or losses, skin turgor, ferritin levels, hemoglobin and hematocrit values, and electrolyte levels. Fluid and electrolyte status is monitored on an ongoing basis; fluid intake and output and urine-specific gravity may be monitored daily if the patient is hospitalized with complications. The skin is assessed for dryness and adequate turgor. Vital signs are monitored for decreased systolic blood pressure or increased pulse rate on sitting or standing. Signs and symptoms of electrolyte disturbances, such as muscle cramping, weakness, irregular pulse, decreased mental status, nausea, and vomiting, are documented and reported to the physician. Serum electrolyte values are monitored, and abnormalities are reported.

The nurse helps the patient select foods that will replenish electrolytes, such as oranges and bananas (potassium) and cheese and soups (sodium). A fluid intake of 3 L or more per day, unless contraindicated, is encouraged to replace fluid lost with diarrhea, and measures to control diarrhea are initiated. If fluid and electrolyte imbalances persist, the nurse administers

CHART 52-13

Health Promotion: Protecting Against HIV Infection

All patients should be advised to:

- Abstain from exchanging sexual fluids (semen and vaginal fluid)
- Reduce the number of sexual partners to one
- Always use latex condoms. If the patient is allergic to latex, nonlatex condoms should be used; however, they will not protect against HIV infection
- Not reuse condoms
- Avoid using cervical caps or diaphragms without using a condom as well
- Always use dental dams for oral–genital or anal stimulation
- Avoid anal intercourse, because this practice may injure tissues; if not possible, use lubricant—there are water and silicone-based products designed for anal sex
- Avoid manual–anal intercourse ("fisting")
- Avoid sharing needles, razors, toothbrushes, sex toys, or blood-contaminated articles
- Consider PrEP if regularly engage in high-risk behaviours

Patients who are HIV seropositive should also be advised to:

- Take ART regularly to achieve viral suppression
- Inform previous, present, and prospective sexual and drug-using partners of their HIV-positive status. If the patient is concerned for their safety, advise the patient that many states have established mechanisms through the public health department in which professionals are available to notify exposed contacts
- Avoid having unprotected sex with another HIV-seropositive person. Cross-infection with that person's HIV can increase the severity of infection
- Not donate blood, plasma, body organs, or sperm.

ART, antiretroviral therapy; PrEP, pre-exposure prophylaxis.

IV fluids and electrolytes as prescribed. Effects of parenteral therapy are monitored.

SIDE EFFECTS OF MEDICATIONS. Adverse effects are of concern in patients who receive many medications to treat HIV infection or its complications. Many medications can cause severe toxic effects. Patients and their caregivers need to know which signs and symptoms of side effects should be reported immediately to their primary provider (Chart 52-13).

In addition to medications used to treat HIV infection, other medications that may be required include opioids, tricyclic antidepressants, and NSAIDs for pain relief; medications for treatment of opportunistic infections; antihistamines (diphenhydramine [Benadryl]) for relief of pruritus; acetaminophen (Tylenol) or aspirin for management of fever; and antiemetic agents for control of nausea and vomiting. Concurrent use of these medications can cause many drug interactions, resulting in hepatic and hematologic abnormalities. Therefore, careful monitoring of laboratory test results is essential.

During each contact with the patient, the nurse not only asks about side effects but also about how well the patient is managing the medication regimen. To promote adherence, the nurse should assist the patient to organize and plan the medication regimen.

Body Image Changes

Body image changes often occur in patients with HIV and are an important collaborative problem. The nurse helps the patient verbalize feelings and explore and identify resources for support and mechanisms for coping with body image changes. Consultations with mental health counselors may be indicated for patients adjusting to body image changes.

Promoting Home, Community-Based, and Transitional Care

EDUCATING PATIENTS ABOUT SELF-CARE. Patients, families, and friends are educated about the routes of transmission of HIV. As discussed earlier, the nurse discusses precautions the patient can use to avoid transmitting HIV sexually or through sharing of body fluids, especially blood. Patients and their families or caregivers must receive instructions about how to prevent disease transmission, including handwashing techniques and methods for safely handling and disposing of items soiled with body fluids. Clear guidelines about avoiding and controlling infection, keeping regular health care appointments, symptom management, nutrition, rest, and exercise are necessary (see Chart 52-14). The importance of personal and environmental hygiene is emphasized. Kitchen and bathroom surfaces should be cleaned regularly with disinfectants to prevent growth of fungi and bacteria. Patients with pets are encouraged to have another person clean areas soiled by animals, such as bird cages and litter boxes. If this is not possible, patients should use gloves and should wash their hands after they clean the area. Patients are advised to avoid exposure to others who are sick or who have been recently vaccinated, especially with live vaccine. The importance of avoiding smoking, excessive alcohol, and over-the-counter and street drugs is emphasized. Patients who are HIV positive or who inject drugs are instructed not to donate blood. IV/injection drug users who are unwilling to stop using drugs are advised to avoid sharing drug equipment with others.

Caregivers in the home are taught how to administer medications, including IV preparations. The medication regimens used for patients with HIV illness and AIDS are often complex and expensive. Patients receiving combination therapies for the treatment of HIV infection and its complications require careful education about the importance of taking medications as prescribed and explanations and assistance in fitting the medication regimen into their lives (see Chart 52-8). If the patient requires enteral or parenteral nutrition, instruction is provided to the patient and family about how to administer nutritional therapies at home. Nurses provide ongoing education and support for the patient and family.

CONTINUING AND TRANSITIONAL CARE. Home, community-based, transitional, and hospice nurses are in an excellent position to provide the support

CHART 52-14

HOME CARE CHECKLIST • Infection Prevention for the Patient With Immune Deficiency

At the completion of education, the patient and/or caregiver will be able to:

- State the impact of immune deficiency on physiologic functioning, ADLs, IADLs, roles, relationships, and spirituality
- State changes in lifestyle (e.g., hygiene, activity) necessary to decrease risk for infection
  - Maintain good hand hygiene technique before eating, after using the bathroom, and before and after performing health care procedures
  - Maintain total body hygiene and foot care to prevent bacterial and fungal diseases
  - Maintain skin integrity, using cream and emollients to prevent or manage dry, chafed, or cracked skin
  - Maintain good oral hygiene and dental checkups
  - Avoid people with infections, recent vaccinations, and crowds
  - Perform deep breathing; use incentive spirometer every 4 hours while awake if mobility is restricted
  - Provide adequate lubrication with gentle vaginal manipulation during sexual intercourse; avoid anal intercourse
- State changes in home environment necessary to decrease risk for infection
  - Avoid cleaning birdcages and litter boxes; consider avoiding garden work (soil) and fresh flowers in stagnant water
  - Identify the rationale for frequent cleaning of kitchen and bathroom surfaces with disinfectant
- Verbalize understanding of ways to maintain a nutritious diet and adequate calories and necessary changes to decrease risk of infection
- State the reason for avoiding the eating of raw fruits and vegetables, cooking all foods thoroughly, and immediately refrigerating all leftover food
- Identify rationale and benefits of avoiding alcohol, tobacco, and unprescribed medications
- State the name, dose, side effects, frequency, and schedule for all medications
- Verbalize ways to cope with stress successfully, plans for regular exercise, and rationale for obtaining adequate rest
- Identify signs and symptoms of infection to report to the primary provider, such as fever; chills; wet or dry cough; breathing problems; white patches in the mouth; swollen glands; nausea; vomiting; persistent abdominal pain; persistent diarrhea; problems with urination or changes in the character of the urine; red, swollen, or draining wounds; sores or lesions on the body; persistent vaginal discharge with or without itching; and severe fatigue
- Demonstrate how to monitor for signs of infection
- Describe to whom, how, and when to report signs of infection
- Describe appropriate actions to take should infection occur

ADL, activities of daily living; IADL, independent activities of daily living.

and guidance that is so often needed in the home setting. Home care nurses are key to the safe and effective administration of parenteral antibiotics, chemotherapy, and nutrition in the home.

Many people with HIV/AIDS remain in their community and continue their usual daily activities, whereas others can no longer work or maintain their independence. Families or caregivers may need assistance in providing supportive care. Many community-based organizations that provide a variety of services for people living with HIV illness and AIDS; nurses can help identify these services.

During home visits, the nurse evaluates the patient's physical and emotional status and home environment. The patient's adherence to the therapeutic regimen is assessed, and strategies are suggested to assist with adherence. The patient is assessed for progression of disease and for adverse side effects of medications. Previous teaching is reinforced, and the importance of keeping follow-up appointments is stressed.

Complex wound care or respiratory care may be required in the home. Patients and families are often unable to meet these skilled care needs without assistance. Nurses may refer patients to community programs that offer a range of services for patients, friends, and families, including help with housekeeping, hygiene, and meals; transportation and shopping; individual and group therapy; support for caregivers; telephone networks for the homebound; and legal and financial assistance. These services are typically provided by both professionals and nonprofessional volunteers. A social worker may be consulted to identify sources of financial support, if needed.

Home care and hospice nurses are increasingly called on to provide physical and emotional support to patients and families as patients with AIDS enter the terminal stages of disease. This support takes on special meaning when people with AIDS lose friends and when family members fear the disease or feel anger concerning the patient's lifestyle. The nurse encourages the patient and family to discuss end-of-life decisions and to ensure that care is consistent with those decisions, all comfort measures are employed, and the patient is treated with dignity at all times.

Evaluation

Expected patient outcomes may include:

1. Maintains skin integrity
2. Resumes usual bowel habits
3. Experiences no infections
4. Maintains adequate level of activity tolerance
5. Maintains usual level of thought processes
6. Maintains effective airway clearance
7. Experiences increased sense of comfort and less pain
8. Maintains adequate nutritional status
9. Experiences decreased sense of social isolation
10. Progresses through grieving process
11. Reports increased understanding of AIDS, prevention of HIV transmission and ART, and participates in self-care activities as possible
12. Remains free of complications

Detailed outcomes are included in the plan of nursing care for a patient with AIDS (see Chart 52-11).

Emotional and Ethical Concerns

Nurses in all settings are called on to provide care for patients with HIV illness. In doing so, they encounter not only the physical challenges of this epidemic but also emotional and ethical concerns. The concerns raised by health care professionals involve issues such as fear of infection, responsibility for giving care, values clarification, confidentiality, developmental stages of patients and caregivers, and poor prognostic outcomes.

Many patients with HIV illness have engaged in "stigmatized" behaviours. Because these behaviours challenge some traditional religious and moral values, some nurses may feel reluctant to care for these patients. In addition, health care providers may still have fear and anxiety about disease transmission despite education concerning infection control and the low incidence of transmission to health care providers. Nurses are encouraged to examine their personal beliefs and to use the process of values clarification to approach controversial issues. The Canadian Nurses Association Code of Ethics for Registered Nurses (2017) can also be used to help resolve ethical dilemmas that might affect the quality of care given to patients with HIV infection and AIDS.

Nurses are responsible for protecting the patient's right to privacy by safeguarding confidential information. Inadvertent disclosure of confidential patient information may result in personal, financial, and emotional hardships for the patient. The controversy surrounding confidentiality concerns the circumstances in which information may be disclosed to others. Health care team members need accurate patient information to conduct assessment, planning, implementation, and evaluation of patient care. Failure to disclose HIV status could compromise the quality of patient care. Sexual partners of patients infected with HIV should know about the potential for infection and the need to engage in safer sex practices, as well as the possible need for testing and health care. Nurses are advised to discuss concerns about confidentiality with nurse administrators and to consult professional nursing organizations such as the Canadian Association of Nurses in AIDS Care and legal experts in their province to identify the most appropriate course of action.

Chart 52-15 explores issues related to revealing one's HIV status. Nurses also must ensure that HIV-infected clients are aware of the legal obligations to report their HIV status to their sexual partners. This legislation is controversial, and nurses should be aware of the issues (see Canadian HIV/AIDS Legal Network web site and resources).

During the early years of the AIDS epidemic, the mortality rate was high. But medication advances have controlled the disease progression, resulting in what is called "functional cure" or HIV remission, which is characterized by

CHART 52-15

Ethics and Related Issues: Revealing One's HIV Status

Should all People who are Infected With HIV Be Required to Reveal This Status to all Their Sexual and Drug-Sharing Contacts?

Situation

The human immunodeficiency virus (HIV) causes infection, which may progress to AIDS. Because sexual contacts and needle-sharing partners are at risk for developing the disease, would a policy that requires notification of contacts infringe on the liberty and privacy of the known HIV-infected person?

Dilemma

The person's right to privacy conflicts with notifying all people who are contacts either through sexual or needle-sharing behaviour (autonomy vs. justice). The person's right to privacy conflicts with society's need to contain the deadly virus and stem a deadly epidemic (autonomy vs. justice).

Discussion

1. What arguments would you offer in favour of notifying all the person's contacts?
2. What arguments would you offer against notifying all or some of the person's contacts?
3. Each state has various laws that pertain to whether contacts can be notified and who is responsible for notifying contacts. Is there a law for contact notification in the state in which you live? If there is such a law in your state, who is responsible for contact notification?
4. What would you do if the person responsible for contact notification refuses to do so based on his or her own beliefs for confidentiality of HIV infection status? How would you respond if the HIV-positive person said that he or she is afraid to notify his or her contact because of fear of a violent response?

viral loads at low or undetectable levels (Vanham, Buvé, Florence, et al., 2014). Many strategies have been used by nurses to cope with the stress associated with caring for HIV-infected patients. Education and provision of up-to-date information help to alleviate apprehension and prepare nurses to deliver safe, high-quality patient care. Interdisciplinary meetings allow participants to support one another and provide comprehensive patient care. Staff support groups give nurses an opportunity to solve problems and explore values and feelings about caring for patients with AIDS and their families; they also provide a forum for grieving. Other sources of support include nursing administrators, peers, and spiritual advisors.

Critical Thinking Exercises

1 A 43-year-old man who is an IV drug user and in a committed relationship wants to reduce the risk of HIV infection. What is the evidence base on strategies to reduce risk from use of IV/injection drugs? What is the evidence about the effectiveness of needle exchange programs? What is the evidence for the effectiveness of PrEP? How would the nurse determine the strength of the evidence and how would the nurse present information to him?

2 A 20-year-old female college student comes to the student health clinic stating she had unprotected sex with a partner she suspects is HIV positive. What further questions does the nurse ask the patient? What is the nurse's priority focus for the physical examination? What diagnostic tests and treatments may the nurse anticipate?

3 The nurse is making a home visit to a patient with AIDS who lives alone and has become weak and debilitated. Describe the aspects of the home environment that the nurse would assess to ensure safety and adequate care. Describe the nursing plan of care to promote adherence with ART and other medications since the patient is taking multiple different medications many times during the day. Identify the resources the nurse could use to help support this patient to remain at home.

REFERENCES AND SELECTED READINGS

Books

Blaese, R., Stiehm, E., Bonilla, F., et al. (2013). *Patient & family handbook for primary immunodeficiency diseases* (5th ed.). Towson, MD: Immune Deficiency Foundation.

Canadian Association of Nurses in AIDS Care. (2012). *Caring for clients who are at risk for and living with HIV/AIDS: Best practice guidelines.* Vancouver, BC: Author. Retrieved from http://www.catie.ca/sites/default/files/Best%20Practice%20Guidelines%20Final%20April%202012.pdf

Comerford, K. C. (2015). *Nursing 2015 drug handbook.* Philadelphia, PA: Wolters Kluwer.

Grossman, S., & Porth, C. (2014). *Porth's pathophysiology: Concepts of altered health states* (9th ed.). Philadelphia, PA: Lippincott Williams & Wilkins.

Haynes, B. F., Soderberg, K. A., & Fauci, A. S. (2015). Introduction to the immune system. In D. L. Kasper, A. S. Fauci, S. L. Hauser, et al. (Eds.). *Harrison's principles of internal medicine* (19th ed.). New York: McGraw-Hill Education.

Jurgens R. (2006). HIV Testing and Confidentiality: Final Report. Montréal: Canadian HIV/AIDS Legal Network and Canadian AIDS Society. ISBN 1-896735-16-9.

Page, A. V., & Liles, W. C. (2015). Immunomodulators. In J. E. Bennett, R. Dolin, & M. J. Blaser (Eds.). *Principles and practices of infectious diseases* (8th ed.). Philadelphia, PA: Elsevier Saunders.

Public Health Agency of Canada (PHAC). (2012). *Routine practices and additional precautions assessment and educational tools.* Ottawa, ON: Author. Retrieved from http://publications.gc.ca/site/archivee-archived.html?url=http://publications.gc.ca/collections/collection_2013/aspc-phac/HP40-65-2012-eng.pdf

Journals and Electronic Documents

Blashill, A., Wilson, J. M., Baker, J. S., et al. (2014). Assessing appearance-related disturbances in HIV-infected men who have sex with men (MSM): Psychometrics of the body change and distress questionnaire—Short Form (ABCD-SF). *AIDS Behavior, 18*(6), 1075–1084.

Bosse, J. D., Nesteby, A., & Randall, C. E. (2015). Integrating sexual minority health issues into a health assessment class. *Journal of Professional Nursing, 31*(6) 498–507.

Bryant, V., Whitehead, N., Burrell, L., et al. (2015). Depression and apathy among people living with HIV: Implications for treatment of HIV. Associated Neurocognitive Disorders. *AIDS and Behavior, 19*(8), 1430–1437.

Canadian AIDS Treatment Information Exchange (CATIE). (2014). *Anonymous HIV Testing Program.* Retrieved from https://www.catie.ca/en/pc/program/anon

Canadian AIDS Treatment Information Exchange (CATIE). (2017). *HIV testing process.* Retrieved from http://www.catie.ca/en/fact-sheets/testing/hiv-testing-process

Canadian AIDS Treatment Information Exchange (CATIE). (2018). *HIV testing technologies.* Retrieved from http://www.catie.ca/en/fact-sheets/testing/hiv-testing-technologies

Canadian Nurses Association (CNS). (2017). *2017 code of ethic for registered nurses.* Retrieved from https://cna-aiic.ca/en/nursing-practice/the-practice-of-nursing/nursing-ethics

CATIE (2017). *HIV testing process.* Retrieved from: https://www.catie.ca/en/fact-sheets/testing/hiv-testing-process

CATIE (2018). *The epidemiology of HIV in Canada.* https://www.catie.ca/en/fact-sheets/epidemiology/epidemiology-hiv-canada

Ceballos, K., Waterman, K., Hulett, T., et al. (2013). Nurse-driven quality improvement interventions to reduce hospital-acquired infection in the NICU. *Advances in Neonatal Care (Elsevier Science), 13*(3), 154–165.

Centers for Disease Control and Prevention (CDC). (2014). *Laboratory testing for the diagnosis of HIV infection: Updated recommendations.* Retrieved May 13, 2016, from stacks.cdc.gov/view/cdc/23447

Centers for Disease Control and Prevention (CDC). (2015a). *CDC's HIV prevention progress in the United States.* Retrieved May 13, 2016, from www.cdc.gov/hiv/dhap/progress/index.html

Centers for Disease Control and Prevention (CDC). (2015b). *HIV and injection drug use in the United States.* Retrieved May 31, 2016, from: www.cdc.gov/hiv/riskbehaviors/idu.html

Centers for Disease Control and Prevention (CDC). (2019). *Occupational HIV Transmission and Prevention among Health Care Workers.* Retrieved from https://www.cdc.gov/hiv/workplace/healthcareworkers.html

Cherin, P., Marie, I., Michallet, M., et al. (2016). Management of adverse events in the treatment of patients with immunoglobulin therapy: A review of evidence. *Autoimmunity Reviews, 15*, 71–81.

Costa-Carvalho, B. T., Grumach, A. S., Franco, J. L., et al. (2014). Attending to warning signs of primary immunodeficiency diseases across the range of clinical practice. *Journal of Clinical Immunology, 34*(1), 10–22.

Fauci, A., & Marston, H. (2015). Toward an HIV vaccine: A scientific journey. *Science, 349*(6246), 386–387.

Fierz, K., Nicca, D., & Spirig, R. (2013). Perceived HIV symptom manageability: Synthesis of a new use for a known concept. *Journal of Advanced Nursing, 69*(1), 229–241.

Gornalusse, G., Mummidi, S., Gaitan, A., et al. (2015). Epigenetic mechanisms, T-cell activation, and CCR5 genetics interact to regulate T-cell expression of CCR5, the major HIV-1 coreceptor. *Proceedings of the National Academy of Sciences of the United States of America, 112*(34), E4762–E4771.

Health Canada. (2015). *Canadian HIV vaccine initiative.* Retrieved from https://www.canada.ca/en/public-health/programs/canadian-hiv-vaccine-initiative/frequently-asked-questions.html

Hernandez-Trujillo, H., Orange, J., Roy, J., et al. (2015). Validity of primary immunodeficiency disease diagnoses in United States Medicaid data. *Journal of Clinical Immunology*, *35*(6), 566–572.
Immunodeficiency Canada. (2018). *Primary immunodeficiency*. Retrieved from http://immunodeficiency.ca/primary-immunodeficiency/primary-immunodeficiency-pi/
Johnson, M. J., & Amella, E. J. (2013). Isolation of lesbian, gay, bisexual and transgender youth: A dimensional concept analysis. *Journal of Advanced Nursing*, *70*(3), 523–532.
Lehman, H., Hernandez-Trujillo, V., & Ballow, M. (2015). Brief review: Diagnosing primary immunodeficiency: A practical approach for the non-immunologist. *Current Medical Research & Opinion*, *31*(4), 697–706.
McCall, J., & Pauly, B. (2012). Providing a safe place: Adopting a culturally safe perspective in the care of Aboriginal women living with HIV/AIDS. *Canadian Journal of Nursing Research*, *44*(2), 130–145.
National Cancer Institute (NCI). (2015). *AIDS-related lymphoma treatment*. Retrieved May 31, 2016, from www.cancer.gov/types/lymphoma/patient/aids-related-treatment-pdq
National Center for Complementary and Integrative Health (NCCIH). (2019). *Terms Related to Complementary and Integrative Health*. Retrieved from https://nccih.nih.gov/health/providers/camterms.htm
National Institute of Allergies and Infectious Diseases (NIAID). (2015). *Types of primary immune deficiency disorders*. Retrieved May 10, 2016, from www.niaid.nih.gov/topics/immuneDeficiency/Pages/majorPIDDs.aspx.
National Institute on Aging (NIA). (2015). *HIV, AIDS, and older people*. Retrieved May 11, 2016, from www.nia.nih.gov/health/publication/hiv-aids-and-older-people
Nicholas, P., Corless, I., & Evans, L. (2014). Peripheral neuropathy in HIV: An analysis of evidence-based approaches. *Journal of the Association of Nurses in AIDS Care*, *25*(4), 318–329.
Panel on Antiretroviral Guidelines for Adults and Adolescents (Panel). (2016). *Guidelines for the use of antiretroviral agents in HIV-1-infected adults and adolescents*. Department of Health and Human Services. Retrieved May 12, 2016, from www.aidsinfo.nih.gov/ContentFiles/AdultandAdolescentGL.pdf
Panel on Opportunistic Infections in HIV-Infected Adults and Adolescents (OI-Panel). (2015). *Guidelines for the prevention and treatment of opportunistic infections in HIV-infected adults and adolescents: recommendations from the Centers for Disease Control and Prevention, the National Institutes of Health, and the HIV Medicine Association of the Infectious Diseases Society of America (OI-Panel)*. Retrieved May 12, 2016, from aidsinfo.nih.gov/contentfiles/lvguidelines/adult_oi.pdf
Public Health Agency of Canada (PHAC). (2014a). *HIV/AIDS Epi updates, October 2014—National HIV Prevalence and Incidence Estimates for 2011*. Retrieved from https://www.canada.ca/en/public-health/services/hiv-aids/publications/epi-updates/chapter-1-national-hiv-prevalence-incidence-estimates-2011.html
Public Health Agency of Canada (PHAC). (2014b). *Human immunodeficiency virus—HIV screening and testing guide*. Retrieved from https://www.canada.ca/en/public-health/services/hiv-aids/hiv-screening-testing-guide.html
Public Health Agency of Canada (PHAC). (2015). *Chapter 8: HIV/AIDS Epi updates, July 2010—HIV/AIDS among Aboriginal people in Canada*. Retrieved from https://www.canada.ca/en/public-health/services/hiv-aids/publications/epi-updates/chapter-8-hiv-aids-among-aboriginal-people-canada.html#a33
Public Health Agency of Canada (PHAC). (2017). *PHAC (2017). Summary: Measuring Canada's progress on the 90-90-90 HIV targets*. Retrieved from https://www.canada.ca/en/public-health/services/publications/diseases-conditions/summary-measuring-canada-progress-90-90-90-hiv-targets.html
Public Health Agency of Canada (PHAC). (2019). *Summary: Estimates of HIV incidence, prevalence and Canada's progress on meeting the 90-90-90 HIV targets, 2016*. Retrieved from: https://www.canada.ca/en/public-health/services/publications/diseases-conditions/summary-estimates-hiv-incidence-prevalence-canadas-progress-90-90-90.html
Schnall, R., Wantland, D., Velez, O., et al. (2014). Feasibility testing of a web-based symptom self-management system for persons living with HIV. *Journal of the Association of Nurses in AIDS Care*, *25*(4), 364–371.
Selik, R., Mokotoff, E., Branson, B., et al. (2014). Revised surveillance case definition for HIV infection—United States, 2014. *Morbidity and Mortality Weekly Report*, *63*(RR03),1–10.
Sharma, M., & Walmsley, S. (2015) Contraceptive options for HIV-positive women: Making evidence-based patient centered decisions. *HIV Medicine*, *16*(6), 329–336.
Tillman, J. L., & Mark, H. D. (2015). HIV and STI testing in older adults: An integrative review. *Journal of Clinical Nursing*, *24*(15–18), 2074–2095. doi: 10.1111/jocn.12797
US Public Health Service. (2014). *Preexposure prophylaxis for the prevention of HIV infection in the United States: Clinical practice guideline*. Retrieved May 11, 2016, from www.cdc.gov/hiv/pdf/prepguidelines2014.pdf
Vanham, G., Buvé, A., Florence, E., et al. (2014). What is the significance of post treatment control of HIV infection vis-à-vis functional cure? *AIDS*, *28*(4), 603–605.
Vollestad, J., Sivertsen, B., & Nielsen, G. H. (2011). Mindfulness-based stress reduction for patients with anxiety disorders: Evaluation in a randomized controlled trial. *Behaviour Research and Therapy*, *49*(4), 281–288.
World Health Organization (WHO). (2015). *HIV/AIDS: Fact sheet N°360*. Retrieved August 8, 2016, from www.who.int/mediacentre/factsheets/fs360/en/
Younger, E., Epland, K., Zampelli, A., et al. (2015). Primary immunodeficiency diseases: A primer for PCPs. *The Nurse Practitioner*, *40*(2), 1–7.

Resources

AIDS Action: http://www.aac.org/
AIDS Education and Training Centers (ETCs) Program (regional, national, and international training opportunities): http://www.aidsetc.org
Antiretroviral medication information Web sites: www.AIDSmeds.com: www.projectinform.org; www.sfaf.org; http://hivinsite.ucsf.edu; http://www.amfAR.org; http://www.natap.org; http://www.thebody.com (many of these sites are coordinated by people living with HIV/AIDS
British Columbia Centre for Excellence in HIV/AIDS: http://www.cfenet.ubc.ca/index.php#
Canadian Aboriginal AIDS Network: http://www.caan.ca/
Canadian AIDS Society: http://www.cdnaids.ca/
Canadian AIDS Treatment Information Exchange: http://www.catie.ca/
Canadian Allergy, Asthma and Immunology Foundation, 774 Echo Drive, Ottawa, ON K1S 5N8, (613) 730–6272: http://allergyfoundation.ca/
Canadian Association for HIV Research: http://www.cahr-acrv.ca
Canadian Association of Nurses in AIDS Care: http://www.canac.org
Canadian Blood Services: http://www.blood.ca/
Canadian Harm Reduction Network: http://www.canadianharmreduction.com/
Canadian HIV/AIDS Information Centre: http://www.aidssida.cpha.ca/
Canadian HIV/AIDS Legal Network: http://www.aidslaw.ca/
Canadian HIV Trials Network: http://www.hivnet.ubc.ca/e/home/
Canadian Hospice Palliative Care Association: http://www.chpca.net/
Canadian Immunodeficiencies Patient Organization, 362 Concession 12 East, RR #2, Hastings, Ontario, K0L 1Y0, (877) 262-CIPO: http://www.cipo.ca.
Canadian Institute for Health Information, 495 Richmond Road, Suite 600, Ottawa, ON K2A 4H6, (613) 241–7860: https://www.cihi.ca/en
Canadian Institutes of Health Research: http://www.cihr-irsc.gc.ca/
Canadian International Development Agency: https://www.tbs-sct.gc.ca/cla/idevi01-eng.asp
Canadian Nurses Association: https://www.cna-aiic.ca/en
Canadian Public Health Association: http://www.cpha.ca/
Canadian Society of Allergy and Clinical Immunology, 774 Echo Drive, Ottawa, ON K1S 5N8, (613) 730–6272: http://www.csaci.org.
Centers for Disease Control and Prevention: http://www.cdc.gov
Gay Men's Health Crisis Network: http://www.gmhc.org
Genetic Alliance, 4301 Connecticut Avenue NW, Suite 404, Washington, DC 20008–2369, (202) 966–5557: http://www.geneticalliance.org.
Hemophilia and AIDS/HIV Network for the Dissemination of Information: http://www.hemophilia.org
Immunodeficiency Canada, 3299 Bayview Avenue, Toronto, ON M2K 2Y5, (416) 964–3434: http://immunodeficiency.ca
International AIDS Vaccine Initiative: http://www.iavi.org
International Council of Nurses: http://www.icn.ch/
International Development Research Centre: http://www.idrc.ca/
International Partnership for Microbicides: https://www.ipmglobal.org/
Joint United Nations Programme on HIV/AIDS: http://www.unaids.org/en/default.asp
Public Health Agency of Canada, Centre for Infectious Disease Prevention and Control: https://stephenlewisfoundation.org/
United Nations Association in Canada: http://www.unac.org/en/index.asp
U.S. Department of Health and Human Services AIDS Info Drug Database: https://aidsinfo.nih.gov/
World Health Organization: http://www.who.int/en/

53 Assessment and Management of Patients With Allergic Disorders

Adapted by Kelly Power-Kean

Learning Objectives

On completion of this chapter, the learner will be able to:

1. Explain the physiologic events involved with allergic reactions.
2. Describe the types of hypersensitivity.
3. Use appropriate parameters for assessment of the status of patients with allergic disorders.
4. Describe the pathophysiologic changes, clinical manifestations, and management of patients with allergic disorders.
5. Describe measures to prevent and manage anaphylaxis.
6. Use the nursing process as a framework for care of the patient with allergic rhinitis.
7. Discuss the different allergic disorders according to type.

The human body is menaced by a host of potential invaders—**allergens** as well as microbial organisms—that constantly threaten its defences. After penetrating those defences, these allergens and organisms, if allowed to continue unimpeded, disrupt the body's enzyme systems and destroy its vital tissues. To protect against these agents, the body is equipped with an elaborate defence system.

The epithelial cells coating the skin and making up the lining of the respiratory, gastrointestinal, and genitourinary tracts provide the first line of defence against microbial invaders. The structure and continuity of these surfaces and their resistance to penetration are initial deterrents to invaders.

One of the most effective defence mechanisms is the body's capacity to equip itself rapidly with weapons (antibodies) individually designed to meet each new invader, namely specific **antigens**. Antibodies react with antigens in a variety of ways: (a) by coating the antigens' surfaces if they are particular substances, (b) by neutralizing the antigens if they are toxins, and (c) by precipitating the antigens out of solution if they are dissolved. The antibodies prepare the antigens so that the phagocytic cells of the blood and the tissues can dispose of them. However, despite being usually protective, in some cases the immune system produces inappropriate or exaggerated responses to specific antigens, and the result is an allergic or **hypersensitivity** disorder.

ALLERGIC ASSESSMENT

Physiologic Overview

An allergic reaction is a manifestation of tissue injury resulting from interaction between an antigen and an **antibody**. **Allergy** is an inappropriate and often harmful response of the immune system to normally harmless substances, called allergens (e.g., dust, weeds, pollen, dander). Chemical mediators released in allergic reactions may produce symptoms that range from mild to life threatening.

In allergic reactions, the body encounters allergens that are types of antigens, usually proteins that the body's defences recognize as foreign, and a series of events occurs in an attempt to render the invaders harmless, destroy them, and remove them from the body. When lymphocytes respond to the antigens, antibodies (protein substances that protect against antigens) are produced.

Antibodies combine with antigens in a special way, which has been likened as keys fitting into a lock. Antigens (the keys) fit only certain antibodies (the locks). Hence, the term *specificity* refers to the specific reaction of an antibody to an antigen. There are many variations and complexities in these patterns.

Function of Immunoglobulins

Antibodies that are formed by lymphocytes and plasma cells in response to an immunogenic stimulus constitute a group of serum proteins called **immunoglobulins**. Grouped into five classes (IgE, IgD, IgG, IgM, and IgA), immunoglobulins can be found in the lymph nodes, tonsils, appendix, and Peyer's patches of the intestinal tract, or circulating in the blood and lymph. These antibodies are capable of binding with a wide variety of antigens. Immunoglobulins of the IgE class are involved in allergic disorders and some parasitic infections. IgE-producing cells are located in the respiratory and intestinal mucosa. Two or more IgE molecules bind together to an allergen and trigger mast cells or basophils to release chemical mediators, such as **histamine**; **serotonin**; kinins; slow-reacting substance of **anaphylaxis**; and the neutrophil factor, which produces allergic skin reactions, asthma, and hay fever. **Atopy** refers to IgE-mediated diseases such as allergic rhinitis that have a genetic component.

Role of B Cells

B cells, or B lymphocytes, are programmed to produce one specific antibody. On encountering a specific antigen, B cells stimulate production of plasma cells, the site of antibody production. The result is the outpouring of antibodies for the purpose of destroying and removing the antigens.

Role of T Cells

T cells, or T lymphocytes, assist the B cells. T cells secrete substances that direct the flow of cell activity, destroy target cells, and stimulate the macrophages. The macrophages present the antigens to the **T cells** and initiate the immune response. They also digest antigens and assist in removing cells and other debris. Unlike a specific antibody, a T cell does not bind free antigens.

Function of Antigens

Antigens are divided into two groups: complete protein antigens and low–molecular-weight substances. Complete protein antigens, such as animal dander, pollen, and horse serum, stimulate a complete humoural response. (Refer to Chapter 51 for a discussion of humoural immunity.) Low–molecular-weight substances, such as medications, function as **haptens** (incomplete antigens), binding to tissue or serum proteins to produce a carrier complex that initiates an antibody response. In an allergic reaction, the production of antibodies requires active communication between cells. When the allergen is absorbed through the respiratory tract, gastrointestinal tract, or skin, allergen sensitization occurs. Macrophages process the antigen and present it to the appropriate cells. These cells mature into allergen-specific secreting plasma cells that synthesize and secrete antigen-specific antibodies.

Function of Chemical Mediators

Mast cells, which are located in the skin and mucous membranes, play a major role in IgE-mediated immediate hypersensitivity. When mast cells are stimulated by antigens, powerful chemical mediators are released causing a sequence of physiologic events that results in symptoms of immediate hypersensitivity (Fig. 53-1). There are two types of chemical mediators: primary and secondary. Primary mediators are preformed and are found in mast cells or basophils. Secondary mediators are inactive precursors that are formed or released in response to primary

Glossary

allergen: substance that causes manifestations of allergy
allergy: inappropriate and often harmful immune system response to substances that are usually harmless
anaphylaxis: rapid clinical response to an immediate immunologic reaction between a specific antigen and antibody
angioneurotic edema: condition characterized by urticaria and diffuse swelling of the deeper layers of the skin (i.e., angioedema)
antibody: protein substance developed by the body in response to and interacting with a specific antigen
antigen: substance that induces the production of antibodies
antihistamine: medication that opposes the action of histamine
atopic dermatitis: type I hypersensitivity involving inflammation of the skin evidenced by itching, redness, and a variety of skin lesions
atopy: term often used to describe immunoglobulin E–mediated diseases (i.e., atopic dermatitis, asthma, and allergic rhinitis) with a genetic component
B cells: lymphocytic cells that are important in producing circulating antibodies
bradykinin: a substance that stimulates nerve fibres and causes pain
eosinophil: granular leukocyte
erythema: diffuse redness of the skin
hapten: incomplete antigen
histamine: substance in the body that causes increased gastric secretion, dilation of capillaries, and constriction of the bronchial smooth muscle
hypersensitivity: abnormal heightened reaction to a stimulus of any kind
immunoglobulins: a family of closely related proteins capable of acting as antibodies
leukotrienes: a group of chemical mediators that initiate the inflammatory response
mast cells: connective tissue cells that contain heparin and histamine in their granules
prostaglandins: unsaturated fatty acids that have a wide assortment of biologic activity
serotonin: chemical mediator that acts as a potent vasoconstrictor and bronchoconstrictor
T cells: cells that can cause graft rejection, kill foreign cells, or suppress production of antibodies
urticaria: hives

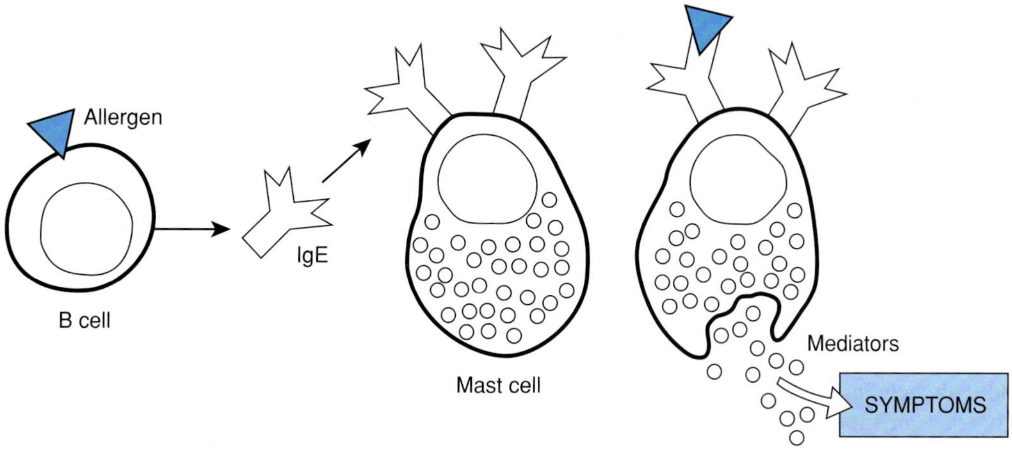

FIGURE 53-1. Allergen triggers the B cell to make immunoglobulin E (IgE) antibody, which attaches to the mast cell. When that allergen reappears, it binds to the IgE and triggers the mast cell to release its chemicals. (Courtesy of U.S. Department of Health and Human Services, National Institutes of Health.)

mediators. Table 53-1 summarizes the actions of primary and secondary chemical mediators.

Primary Mediators

Histamine

Histamine, which is released by mast cells, plays an important role in the immune response. It is the first chemical mediator to be released in immune and inflammatory responses. It is synthesized and stored in high concentrations in body tissues exposed to environmental substances (Frandsen & Pennington, 2014). Histamine's effects peak 5 to 10 minutes after antigen contact and include the following: **erythema**; localized edema in the form of wheals; pruritus; contraction of bronchial smooth muscle, resulting in wheezing and bronchospasm; dilation of small venules and constriction of larger vessels; and increased secretion of gastric and mucosal cells, resulting in diarrhea (Abbas, Lichtman, & Pillai, 2014; Rich, Fleisher, Shearer, et al., 2013). Histamine action results from stimulation of histamine-1 (H_1) and histamine-2 (H_2) receptors. H_1 receptors are found predominantly on bronchiolar and vascular smooth muscle cells. H_2 receptors are found on gastric parietal cells.

Certain medications are categorized by their action at these receptors. Diphenhydramine (Benadryl) is an example

TABLE 53-1 Chemical Mediators of Hypersensitivity

Mediators	Action
Primary Mediators (Preformed and found in mast cells or basophils)	
Histamine (preformed in mast cells) Smooth muscle contraction, increased vascular permeability, increased mucus secretions	Vasodilation
Eosinophil chemotactic factor of anaphylaxis (preformed in mast cells)	Attracts eosinophils
Platelet-activating factor (requires synthesis by mast cells, neutrophils, and macrophages)	Smooth muscle contraction Incites platelets to aggregate and release serotonin and histamine
Prostaglandins (chemically derived from arachidonic acid; require synthesis by cells)	D and F series → bronchoconstriction E series → bronchodilation D, E, and F series → vasodilation
Basophil kallikrein (preformed in mast cells)	Frees bradykinin, which causes bronchoconstriction, vasodilation, and nerve stimulation
Secondary Mediators (Inactive precursors formed or released in response to primary mediators)	
Bradykinin (derived from precursor kininogen)	Smooth muscle contraction, increased vascular permeability, stimulates pain receptors, increased mucus production
Serotonin (preformed in platelets)	Smooth muscle contraction, increased vascular permeability
Heparin (preformed in mast cells)	Anticoagulant
Leukotrienes (derived from arachidonic acid and activated by mast cell degranulation) C, D, and E or slow-reacting substance of anaphylaxis (SRS-A)	Smooth muscle contraction, increased vascular permeability

Adapted from Grossman, S. C., & Porth, C. M. (2014). *Porth's pathophysiology: Concepts of altered health states* (9th ed.). Philadelphia, PA: Lippincott Williams & Wilkins.

of an **antihistamine**, a medication that displays an affinity for H_1 receptors. Cimetidine (Tagamet) and ranitidine (Zantac) target H_2 receptors to inhibit gastric secretions in peptic ulcer disease.

Eosinophil Chemotactic Factor of Anaphylaxis

Eosinophil chemotactic factor of anaphylaxis affects movement of eosinophils (granular leukocytes) to the site of allergens. It is performed in the mast cells and is released from disrupted mast cells.

Platelet-activating Factor

Platelet-activating factor is responsible for initiating platelet aggregation and leukocyte infiltration at sites of immediate hypersensitivity reactions. It also causes bronchoconstriction and increased vascular permeability (Frandsen & Pennington, 2014).

Prostaglandins

Prostaglandins produce smooth muscle contraction as well as vasodilation and increased capillary permeability. They sensitize pain receptors and increase the pain associated with inflammation. In addition, prostaglandins induce inflammation and enhance the effects of mediators of inflammatory response. Local manifestations include erythema, heat, and edema (Frandsen & Pennington, 2014).

Secondary Mediators

Leukotrienes

Leukotrienes are chemical mediators that initiate the inflammatory response. Many manifestations of inflammation can be attributed in part to leukotrienes. In addition, leukotrienes cause smooth muscle contraction, bronchial constriction, mucus secretion in the airways, and the typical wheal-and-flare reactions of the skin. Compared with histamine, leukotrienes are 100 to 1,000 times more potent in causing bronchospasm.

Bradykinin

Bradykinin is a substance that has the ability to cause increased vascular permeability, vasodilation, hypotension, and contraction of many types of smooth muscle, such as the bronchi. Increased permeability of the capillaries results in edema. Bradykinin stimulates nerve cell fibres and produces pain.

Serotonin

Serotonin acts as a potent vasoconstrictor, causing contraction of bronchial smooth muscle.

Hypersensitivity

Although the immune system defends the host against infections and foreign antigens, immune responses can themselves cause tissue injury and disease. Hypersensitivity is an excessive or aberrant immune response to any type of stimulus (Abbas et al., 2014). It usually does not occur with the first exposure to an allergen. Rather, the reaction follows a re-exposure after sensitization, or buildup of antibodies, in a predisposed individual. Injurious or pathologic immune reactions are classed as hypersensitivity reactions. To promote understanding of the immunopathogenesis of disease, hypersensitivity reactions have been classified into four specific types of reactions (Fig. 53-2). Most allergic reactions are either type I or type IV hypersensitivity reactions.

Anaphylactic (Type I) Hypersensitivity

The most severe hypersensitivity reaction is anaphylaxis. An unanticipated severe allergic reaction that is rapid in onset, anaphylaxis is characterized by edema in many tissues, including the larynx, and is often accompanied by hypotension, bronchospasm, and cardiovascular collapse in severe cases. Type I or anaphylactic hypersensitivity is an immediate reaction beginning within minutes of exposure to an antigen. Primary chemical mediators are responsible for the symptoms of type I hypersensitivity because of their effects on the skin, lungs, and gastrointestinal tract. If chemical mediators continue to be released, a delayed reaction may occur and may last for up to 24 hours.

Clinical symptoms are determined by the amount of the allergen, the amount of mediator released, the sensitivity of the target organ, and the route of allergen entry. Type I hypersensitivity reactions may include both local and systemic anaphylaxis.

Cytotoxic (Type II) Hypersensitivity

Type II, or cytotoxic, hypersensitivity occurs when the immune system mistakenly identifies a normal constituent of the body as foreign. This reaction may be a result of a cross-reacting antibody, possibly leading to cell and tissue damage.

Type II hypersensitivity reactions are associated with several disorders. For example, in myasthenia gravis, the body mistakenly generates antibodies against normal nerve-ending receptors. In Goodpasture's syndrome, it generates antibodies against lung and renal tissue, producing lung damage and kidney injury (Grossman & Porth, 2014).

Immune Complex (Type III) Hypersensitivity

Type III, or immune complex, hypersensitivity involves immune complexes that are formed when antigens bind to antibodies. These complexes are cleared from the circulation by phagocytic action. If these type III complexes are deposited in tissues or vascular endothelium, two factors contribute to injury: the increased amount of circulating complexes and the presence of vasoactive amines. As a result, there is an increase in vascular permeability and tissue injury.

Type III, or immune complex, hypersensitivity involves immune complexes that are formed when antigens bind to antibodies. These complexes are then cleared from the circulation by phagocytic action. If these type III complexes are deposited in tissues or vascular endothelium, two factors contribute to injury: the increased amount of circulating complexes and the presence of vasoactive amines. As a result, there is an increase in vascular permeability and tissue injury.

Delayed-Type (Type IV) Hypersensitivity

Type IV, or delayed-type hypersensitivity (DTH), is an immune reaction in which T-cell–dependent macrophage activation and inflammation cause tissue injury. This type of reaction to the subcutaneous injection of antigen is often used as an assay for cell-mediated immunity (e.g., the purified protein derivative skin test for immunity to *Mycobacterium tuberculosis*) (Abbas et al., 2014).

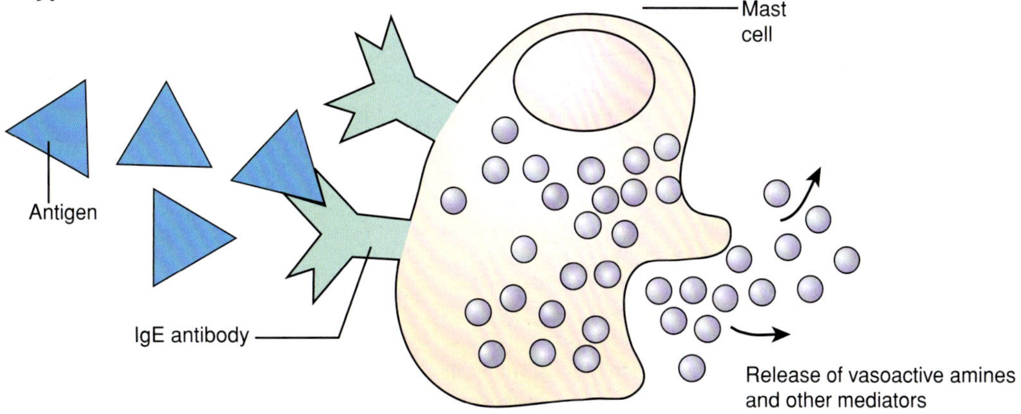

Type I. An anaphylactic reaction is characterized by vasodilation, increased capillary permeability, smooth muscle contraction, and eosinophilia. Systemic reactions may involve laryngeal stridor, angioedema, hypotension, and bronchial, GI, or uterine spasm; local reactions are characterized by hives. Examples of type I reactions include extrinsic asthma, allergic rhinitis, systemic anaphylaxis, and reactions to insect stings.

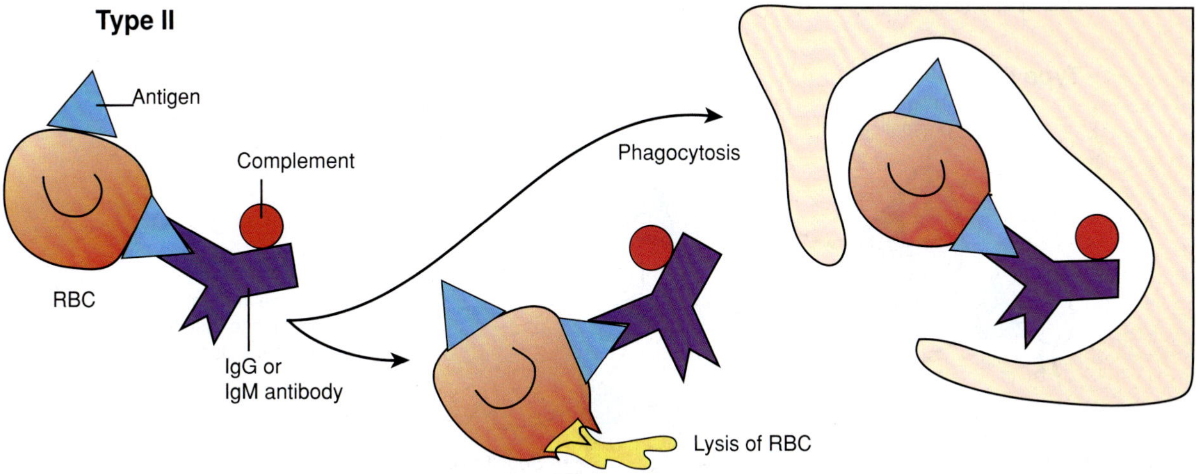

Type II. A cytotoxic reaction, which involves the binding of either the IgG or IgM antibody to a cell-bound antigen, may lead to eventual cell and tissue damage. The reaction is the result of mistaken identity when the system identifies a normal constituent of the body as foreign and activates the complement cascade. Examples of type II reactions are myasthenia gravis, Goodpasture syndrome, pernicious anemia, hemolytic disease of the newborn, transfusion reaction, and thrombocytopenia.

FIGURE 53-2. Four types of hypersensitivity reactions. (GI, gastrointestinal; Ig, immunoglobulin; PMN, polymorphonuclear; RBC, red blood cell.) (*continued*)

Assessment

A comprehensive allergy history and a thorough physical examination provide useful data for the diagnosis and management of allergic disorders. An allergy assessment form is useful for obtaining and organizing pertinent information (Chart 53-1).

The degree of difficulty and discomfort experienced by the patient because of allergic symptoms and the degree of improvement in those symptoms with and without treatment are assessed and documented. The relationship of symptoms to exposure to possible allergens is noted.

Diagnostic Evaluation

Diagnostic evaluation of the patient with allergic disorders commonly includes blood tests, smears of body secretions, skin tests, and the serum-specific IgE test (formerly known as radioallergosorbent test [RAST]). Results of laboratory blood studies provide supportive data for various diagnostic possibilities; however, they are not the major criteria for the diagnosis of allergic disease.

Complete Blood Count With Differential

The white blood cell (WBC) count is usually normal except with infection and inflammation (Pagana & Pagana, 2013). Eosinophils, which are granular leukocytes, normally make up 2% to 5% of the total number of WBCs. They can be found in blood, sputum, and nasal secretions. A level greater than 5% to 10% is considered abnormal and may be found in patients with allergic disorders (Rich et al., 2013).

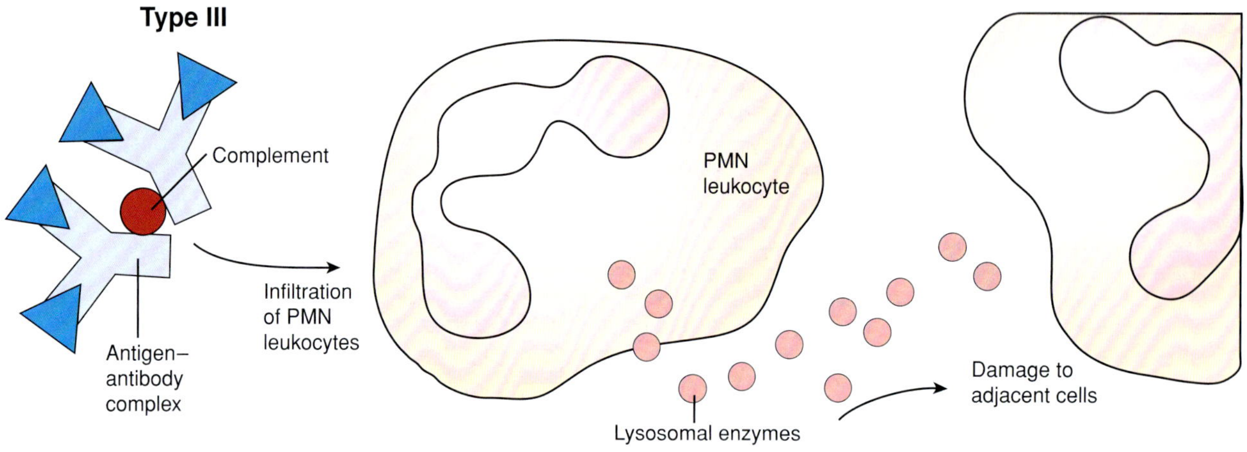

Type III. An immune complex reaction is marked by acute inflammation resulting from formation and deposition of immune complexes. The joints and kidneys are particularly susceptible to this kind of reaction, which is associated with systemic lupus erythematosus, serum sickness, nephritis, and rheumatoid arthritis. Some signs and symptoms include urticaria, joint pain, fever, rash, and adenopathy (swollen glands).

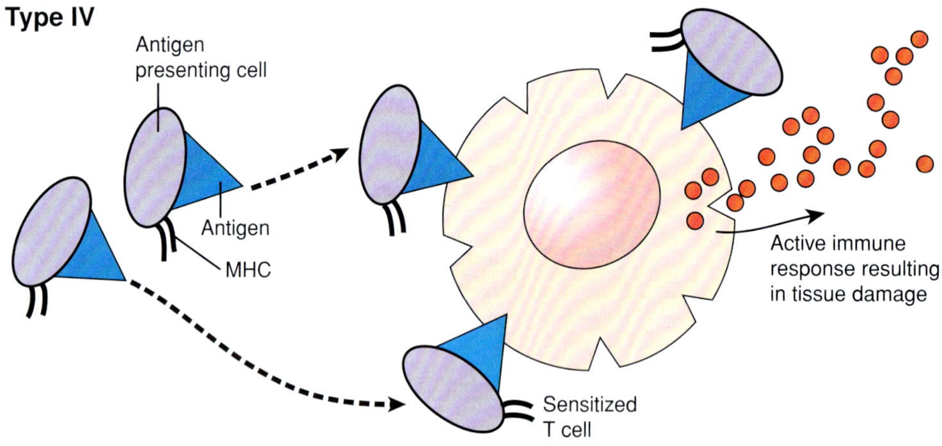

Type IV. A delayed, or cellular, reaction occurs 1 to 3 days after exposure to an antigen. The reaction, which results in tissue damage, involves activity by lymphokines, macrophages, and lysozymes. Erythema and itching are common; a few examples include contact dermatitis, graft-versus-host disease, Hashimoto's thyroiditis, and sarcoidosis.

FIGURE 53-2. (*Continued*)

Eosinophil Count

An actual count of eosinophils can be obtained from blood samples or smears of secretions. During symptomatic episodes, smears obtained from nasal secretions and sputum of patients with allergies usually reveal an increase in eosinophils, indicating an active allergic response (Rich et al., 2013).

Total Serum Immunoglobulin E Levels

High total serum IgE levels support the diagnosis of allergic disease. In the majority of cases, the antibody typically responsible for an allergic reaction belongs to the IgE isotype. Patients with this disorder are said to have an IgE-mediated allergic disease (Portnoy, 2015).

Skin Tests

Skin testing entails the intradermal injection or superficial application (epicutaneous) of solutions at several sites. Depending on the suspected cause of allergic signs and symptoms, several different solutions may be applied at separate sites. These solutions contain individual antigens representing an assortment of allergens most likely to be implicated in the patient's disease. Positive (wheal-and-flare) reactions are clinically significant when correlated with the history, physical findings, and results of other laboratory tests. Skin testing is considered the most accurate confirmation of allergy (Oppenheimer, Durham, Nelson, et al., 2014).

The results of skin tests complement the data obtained from the history. They indicate which of several antigens are most likely to provoke symptoms and indicate the

CHART 53-1

Allergy Assessment Form

Name ____ Age ____ Sex ____ Date ____

I. Chief concern:

II. Present illness:

III. Collateral allergic symptoms:

Eyes: Pruritus ____ Burning ____ Lacrimation ____
Swelling ____ Injection ____ Discharge ____

Ears: Pruritus ____ Fullness ____ Popping ____
Frequent infections

Nose: Sneezing ____ Rhinorrhea ____ Obstruction ____
Pruritus ____ Mouth ____ breathing
Purulent discharge ____

Throat: Soreness ____ Postnasal discharge ____
Palatal pruritus ____ Mucus in the morning ____

Chest: Cough ____ Pain ____ Wheezing ____
Sputum ____ Dyspnea ____
Colour ____ Rest ____
Amount ____ Exertion ____

Skin: Dermatitis ____ Eczema ____ Urticaria ____

IV. Family allergies: ____

V. Previous allergic treatment or testing: ____

Prior skin testing: ____

Medications:

Antihistamines	Improved ____	Unimproved ____
Bronchodilators	Improved ____	Unimproved ____
Nose drops	Improved ____	Unimproved ____
Hyposensitization	Improved ____	Unimproved ____
Duration ____		
Antigens ____		
Reactions ____		
Antibiotics	Improved ____	Unimproved ____
Corticosteroids	Improved ____	Unimproved ____

VI. Physical agents and habits: ____

Bothered by:

Tobacco for ____ years	Alcohol ____	Air conditioning ____
Cigarettes ____ packs/day	Heat ____	Muggy weather ____
Cigars ____ per day	Cold ____	Weather changes ____
Pipes ____ per day	Perfumes ____	Chemicals ____
Never smoked ____	Paints ____	Hair spray ____
Bothered by smoke ____	Insecticides ____	Newspapers ____
	Cosmetics ____	Latex ____

VII. When symptoms occur: ____

Time and circumstances of 1st episode: ____

Prior health: ____

Course of illness over decades: progressing ____ regressing ____

Time of year: ____ Exact dates: ____

Perennial ____

Seasonal ____

Seasonally exacerbated ____

Monthly variations (menses, occupation): ____

Time of week (weekends vs. weekdays): ____

Time of day or night: ____

After insect stings: ____

VIII. Where symptoms occur: ____

Living where at onset: ____

Living where since onset: ____

Effect of vacation or major geographic change: ____

Symptoms better indoors? Or outdoors?: ____

Effect of school/work: ____

Effect of staying elsewhere nearby: ____

Effect of hospitalization: ____

Effect of specific environments: ____

continued >

CHART 53-1 Allergy Assessment Form (Continued)

Do symptoms occur around: ____
old leaves ____ hay ____ lakeside ____ barns ____
summer homes ____ damp basement ____ dry attic ____
lawn mowing ____ animals ____ other ____
Do symptoms occur after eating:
cheese ____ mushrooms ____ beer ____ melons ____
bananas ____ fish ____ nuts ____ citrus fruits ____
other foods (list)
Home: city ____ rural ____
house ____ age ____
apartment ____ basement ____ damp ____ dry ____
heating system ____
pets (how long) ____ dog ____ cat ____ other ____

Bedroom:	Type	Age	*Living room:*	Type	Age
Pillow	____	____	Rug	____	____
Mattress	____	____	Matting	____	____
Blankets	____	____	Furniture	____	____
Quilts	____	____			
Furniture	____	____			

Anywhere in home symptoms are worse: ____
IX. What does patient think makes symptoms worse? ____
X. Under what circumstances is patient free of symptoms? ____
XI. Summary and additional comments: ____

intensity of the patient's sensitization. The dosage of the antigen (allergen) injected is also important. Most patients are hypersensitive to more than one allergen. Under testing conditions, they may not react (although they usually do) to the specific allergens that induce their attacks.

In cases of doubt about the validity of the skin tests, a serum-specific IgE test or a provocative challenge test may be performed. If a skin test is indicated, there is a reasonable suspicion that a specific allergen is producing symptoms in a patient with allergies. However, several precautionary steps must be observed before skin testing with allergens is performed:

- Testing is not performed during periods of bronchospasm.
- Epicutaneous tests (scratch or prick tests) are performed before other testing methods in an effort to minimize the risk of systemic reaction.
- Emergency equipment must be readily available to treat anaphylaxis.

Types of Skin Tests

The methods of skin testing include prick skin tests, scratch tests, and intradermal skin testing. After negative prick or scratch tests, intradermal skin testing is performed with allergens that are suggested by the patient's history to be problematic. The back is the most suitable area of the body for skin testing because it permits the performance of many tests. A multitest applicator with multiple test heads is commercially available for simultaneous administration of antigens by multiple punctures at different sites. A negative response on a skin test cannot be interpreted as an absence of sensitivity to an allergen. Such a response may occur with insufficient sensitivity of the test or with use of an inappropriate allergen in testing. Therefore, it is essential to observe the patient undergoing skin testing for an allergic reaction even if the previous response was negative.

Interpretation of Skin Test Results

Familiarity with and consistent use of a grading system are essential. The grading system used should be identified on a skin test record for later interpretation. A positive reaction, evidenced by the appearance of a **urticarial** wheal (round, reddened skin elevation) (Fig. 53-3), localized erythema (diffuse redness) in the area of inoculation or contact, or pseudopodia (irregular projection at the end of a wheal) with associated erythema is considered indicative of sensitivity to the corresponding antigen. False-positive results may occur because of improper preparation or administration of allergen solutions.

NURSING ALERT

Corticosteroids and antihistamines, including over-the-counter allergy medications, suppress skin test reactivity and are usually withheld 48 to 96 hours before testing, depending on the duration of their activity. False-positive skin tests may result from improper preparation or administration of allergen solutions.

Positive or negative skin tests are interpreted in the context of the patient's history, clinical signs, and exposure to allergens (Australasian Society of Clinical Immunology and Allergy [ASCIA], 2015). The following guidelines are used for the interpretation of skin test results:

- Skin tests are used most frequently with the diagnosis of allergic rhinitis (Baran, Ozcan, Selcuk, et al., 2014).

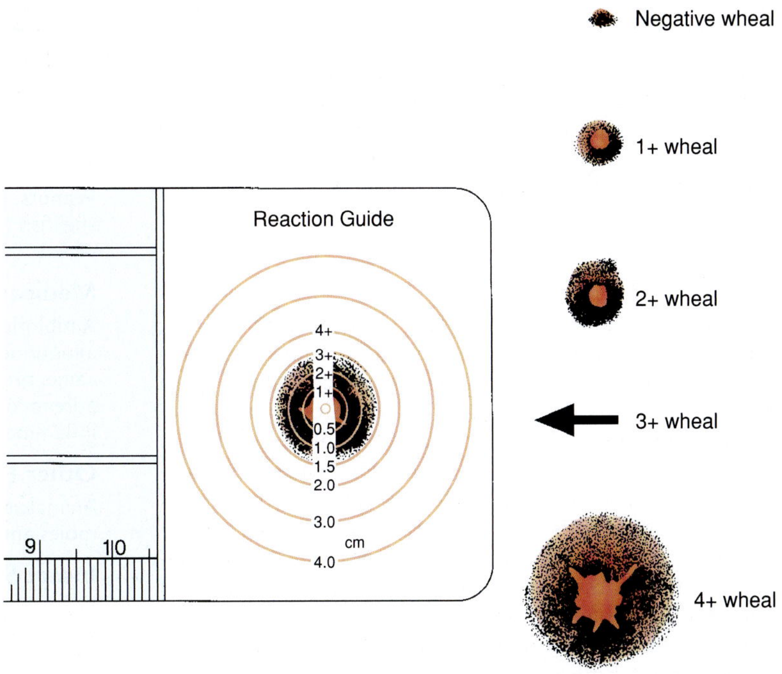

FIGURE 53-3. Interpretation of reactions: Negative, wheal soft with minimal erythema; 1+, wheal present (5 to 8 mm) with associated erythema; 2+, wheal (7 to 10 mm) with associated erythema; 3+, wheal (9 to 15 mm), slight pseudopodia possible with associated erythema; 4+, wheal (12 mm+) with pseudopodia and diffuse erythema.

- Negative test results are helpful in ruling out food allergy.
- Positive skin tests correlate highly with food allergy (ASCIA, 2015).

The use of skin tests to diagnose immediate hypersensitivity to medications is limited, because metabolites of medications, not the medications themselves, are usually responsible for causing hypersensitivity.

Provocative Testing

Provocative testing involves the direct administration of the suspected allergen to the sensitive tissue, such as the conjunctiva, nasal or bronchial mucosa, or gastrointestinal tract (by ingestion of the allergen), with observation of target organ response. This type of testing is helpful in identifying clinically significant allergens in patients who have a large number of positive tests. Major disadvantages of this type of testing are the limitation of one antigen per session and the risk of producing severe symptoms, particularly bronchospasm, in patients with asthma.

Serum-Specific IgE Test

The serum-specific IgE test, formerly known as RAST, is an automated test performed on blood samples by a pathology laboratory. As the name suggests, it detects free antigen-specific IgE in serum as opposed to antigen-specific IgE bound to mast cells in the skin (ASCIA, 2015; Portnoy, 2015). The advantages of this test over other tests include decreased risk of systemic reaction, stability of antigens, and lack of dependence on skin reactivity modified by medications. The major disadvantages include limited allergen selection and reduced sensitivity compared with intradermal skin tests, lack of immediate results, and higher cost (ASCIA, 2015).

ALLERGIC DISORDERS

There are two types of IgE-mediated allergic reactions: atopic and nonatopic disorders. Although the underlying immunologic reactions of the two types of disorders are the same, the predisposing factors and manifestations are different. Atopy is defined as the genetic predisposition to mount an IgE response to inhaled or ingested innocuous proteins (Rich et al., 2013). Atopic diseases consist of allergic rhinitis, asthma, and **atopic dermatitis**. All share a common pathogenesis, mediated by IgE, and are frequently present together in the same individual and in families. The nonatopic disorders lack the genetic component and organ specificity of the atopic disorders (Rich et al., 2013). Latex allergy (see later discussion) can present as an IgE-mediated anaphylaxis, type I reaction or a type IV hypersensitivity referred to as contact dermatitis (American Academy of Allergy, Asthma, & Immunology [AAAAI], 2015; Habif, 2016; Rich et al., 2013).

Unfolding Patient Stories: Jennifer Hoffman • Part 2

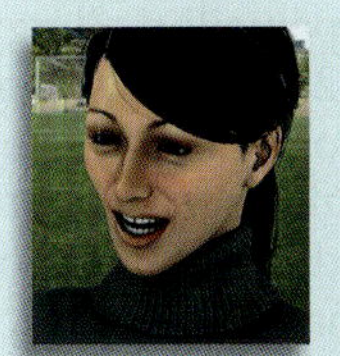

Recall from Chapter 25 Jennifer Hoffman, who came to the clinic with continued symptoms of asthma. The nurse confirmed that she was following the asthma action plan; however, Jennifer now returns to the clinic with worsening symptoms. What assessment findings would indicate to the nurse that Jennifer is having a hypersensitivity reaction to an allergen(s)? What questions can assist the nurse in identifying the causative agent(s)? What interventions should be implemented when allergen(s) are identified?

Care for Jennifer and other patients in a realistic virtual environment: ***vSim** for Nursing* (**thepoint.lww.com/vSimMedicalSurgical**). Practice documenting these patients' care in DocuCare (**thepoint.lww.com/DocuCareEHR**).

Anaphylaxis

Anaphylaxis is a clinical response to an immediate (type I hypersensitivity) immunologic reaction between a specific antigen and an antibody. The reaction results from a rapid release of IgE-mediated chemicals, which can induce a severe, life-threatening reaction (Abbas et al., 2014).

Pathophysiology

Anaphylaxis is a type I IgE allergic reaction to an antigen, a foreign substance that has entered the body (Frandsen & Pennington, 2014). It is caused by the cross-links of an allergen with allergen-specific IgE antibodies found on the surface membrane of mast cells and basophils, leading to cellular degranulation. The subsequent release of histamine and other bioactive mediators causes activation of platelets, eosinophils, and neutrophils. Histamine, prostaglandins, and inflammatory leukotrienes are potent vasoactive mediators that are implicated in the vascular permeability changes, flushing, urticaria, angioedema, hypotension, and bronchoconstriction that characterize anaphylaxis. Smooth muscle spasm, bronchospasm, mucosal edema and inflammation, and increased capillary permeability result. Symptoms of anaphylaxis are sudden in onset and progress in severity over minutes to hours (Campbell, Li, Nicklas, et al., 2014).

Closely resembling anaphylaxis is an anaphylactoid, reaction, which is caused by the release of mast cell and basophil mediators triggered by non–immunoglobulin E (IgE)-mediated events.

This nonallergenic anaphylaxis reaction may occur with medications, food, exercise, or cytotoxic antibody transfusions. The reaction may be local or systemic. Local reactions usually involve urticaria and angioedema at the site of the antigen exposure. Although possibly severe, nonallergenic anaphylaxis reactions are rarely fatal. Systemic reactions occur within about 30 minutes after exposure and involve cardiovascular, respiratory, gastrointestinal, and integumentary organ systems. For the most part, the treatment of nonallergenic anaphylaxis reaction is identical to that of anaphylaxis.

Common causes of anaphylaxis are listed in Chart 53-2. Antibiotics and radiocontrast agents cause the most serious anaphylactic reactions. Penicillin is the most common medication to cause anaphylaxis. In a study of an outpatient adult population, the prevalence of penicillin allergy was found to be 12% (Albin & Agarwal, 2014). However, only 6% of these patients were referred to an allergist for testing. Patients with reported penicillin allergy who were evaluated with skin testing experienced decreased use of broad spectrum antibiotics and fewer anaphylactic reactions (Albin & Agarwal, 2014).

CHART 53-2

Common Causes of Anaphylaxis

Foods

Peanuts, tree nuts (e.g., walnuts, pecans, cashews, almonds), shellfish (e.g., shrimp, lobster, crab), fish, milk, eggs, soy, wheat

Medications

Antibiotics, especially penicillin and sulfa antibiotics, allopurinol, radiocontrast agents, anesthetic agents (lidocaine, procaine), vaccines, hormones (insulin, vasopressin, adrenocorticotropic hormone), aspirin, nonsteroidal anti-inflammatory drugs

Other Pharmaceutical/Biologic Agents

Animal serums (tetanus antitoxin, snake venom antitoxin, rabies antitoxin), antigens used in skin testing

Insect Stings

Bees, wasps, hornets, yellow jackets, ants (including fire ants)

Latex

Medical and nonmedical products containing latex

Clinical Manifestations

Anaphylactic reactions produce a clinical syndrome that affects multiple organ systems. Reactions may be categorized as mild, moderate, or severe. The time from the exposure to the antigen to the onset of symptoms is a good indicator of the severity of the reaction: the faster the onset, the more severe the reaction. The severity of previous reactions does not determine the severity of subsequent reactions, which could be the same or more or less severe. The severity depends on the degree of allergy and the dose of allergen exposure (Campbell et al., 2014).

Mild systemic reactions consist of peripheral tingling and a sensation of warmth, possibly accompanied by a sensation of fullness in the mouth and throat. Nasal congestion, periorbital swelling, pruritus, sneezing, and tearing of the eyes can also be expected. The onset of symptoms begins within the first 2 hours after the exposure.

Moderate systemic reactions may include flushing, warmth, anxiety, and itching in addition to any of the milder symptoms. More serious reactions include bronchospasm and edema of the airways or larynx with dyspnea, cough, and wheezing. The onset of symptoms is the same as for a mild reaction.

Severe systemic reactions have an abrupt onset with the same signs and symptoms described previously. These symptoms progress rapidly to bronchospasm, laryngeal edema, severe dyspnea, cyanosis, and hypotension. Dysphagia (difficulty swallowing), abdominal cramping, vomiting, diarrhea, and seizures can also occur. Cardiac arrest and coma may follow. Severe reactions are also referred to as anaphylactic shock.

Prevention

Strict avoidance of potential allergens is an important preventive measure for the patient at risk for anaphylaxis. Those at risk for anaphylaxis from insect stings should avoid areas populated by insects and should use appropriate clothing, insect repellent, and caution to avoid further stings.

If avoidance of exposure to allergens is impossible, an autoinjector system for epinephrine will be prescribed. The patient should be instructed to carry and administer epinephrine to prevent an anaphylactic reaction in the event of exposure to the allergen. People who are sensitive to insect bites and stings, those who have experienced food or medication reactions, and those who have experienced idiopathic or exercise-induced anaphylactic reactions should always carry an emergency kit that contains epinephrine. The EpiPen is an autoinjection device that is commercially available for first aid that delivers premeasured doses of epinephrine (Food Allergy Canada, 2018). The autoinjection system requires no preparation, and the self-administration technique is uncomplicated. The patients must be given an opportunity to demonstrate the correct technique for use; an EpiPen training device can be used for educating about the correct technique. Verbal and written information about the emergency kit, as well as strategies to avoid exposure to threatening allergens, must also be provided.

Screening for allergies before a medication is prescribed or first given is an important preventive measure. A careful history of any sensitivity to suspected antigens must be obtained before administering any medication, particularly in parenteral form, because this route is associated with the most severe anaphylaxis. Nurses caring for patients in any setting (hospital, home, outpatient diagnostic testing sites, long-term care facilities) must assess patients' risks for anaphylactic reactions. Patients are asked about previous exposure to contrast agents used for diagnostic tests and any allergic reactions as well as reactions to any medications, foods, insect stings, and latex. People who are predisposed to anaphylaxis should wear medical identification, such as a bracelet or necklace, which names allergies to medications, food, and other substances.

People who are allergic to insect venom may require venom immunotherapy, which is used as a control measure and not a cure. The most common serious allergic reactions to insect stings are from the Hymenoptera family, which includes bees, ants, wasps, and yellow jackets (Perez-Riverol, Justo-Jacomini, de Lima Zollner, et al., 2015). Venom is an effective treatment for people with systemic reactions to an insect sting. It reduces the systemic reaction, reduces the risk of future large local reactions, and improves quality of life (Ludman & Boyle, 2015).

Insulin-allergic patients with diabetes and those who are allergic to penicillin may require desensitization. Desensitization is based on controlled anaphylaxis, with a gradual release of mediators. Patients who undergo desensitization are cautioned to avoid lapses in therapy, because this may lead to the reappearance of the allergic reaction when the use of the medication is resumed.

Medical Management

Management depends on the severity of the reaction. Initially, respiratory and cardiovascular functions are evaluated. If the patient is in cardiac arrest, cardiopulmonary resuscitation (CPR) is instituted (Link, Berkow, Kudenchuk, et al., 2015). Supplemental oxygen is provided during CPR or if the patient is cyanotic, dyspneic, or wheezing. Epinephrine, in a 1:1,000 dilution, is given subcutaneously in the upper extremity or thigh and may be followed by a continuous intravenous infusion. Most adverse events associated with administration of epinephrine (i.e., Adrenaline) occur when the dose is excessive, or it is given intravenously. Patients at risk for adverse effects include older patients and those with hypertension, arteriopathies, or known ischemic heart disease.

Antihistamines and corticosteroids should not be given in place of epinephrine. However, they may also be given as adjunct therapy (Campbell et al., 2014).

Intravenous fluids (e.g., normal saline solution), volume expanders, and vasopressor agents are given to maintain blood pressure and normal hemodynamic status. In patients with episodes of bronchospasm or a history of bronchial asthma or chronic obstructive pulmonary disease, aminophylline and corticosteroids may also be given to improve airway patency and function.

Patients who have experienced anaphylactic reactions and received epinephrine should be transported to the local emergency department (ED) for observation and monitoring because of the risk for a "rebound" or delayed reaction 4 to 8 hours after the initial allergic reaction. However, the observation time should be individualized based on the severity of the anaphylaxis. Longer periods of observation should be considered for patients who ingested the allergen, required more than one dose of epinephrine, had hypotension or pharyngeal edema, or have a history of asthma (Campbell et al., 2014).

Nursing Management

If a patient is experiencing an allergic response, the nurse assesses the patient for signs and symptoms of anaphylaxis. Airway, breathing pattern, and vital signs are assessed. The patient is observed for signs of increasing edema and respiratory distress. Prompt notification of the rapid response team, the provider, or both is required. Rapid initiation of emergency measures (e.g., intubation, administration of emergency medications, insertion of intravenous lines, fluid administration, and oxygen administration) is important to reduce the severity of the reaction and to restore cardiovascular function. The nurse documents the interventions used and the patient's vital signs and response to treatment.

The patient who has recovered from anaphylaxis needs an explanation of what occurred, instruction about avoiding future exposure to antigens, and how to administer emergency medications to treat anaphylaxis. The patient must be instructed about antigens that should be avoided and about other strategies to prevent recurrence of anaphylaxis. All patients who have experienced an anaphylactic reaction should receive a prescription for autoinjectable epinephrine devices. The nurse instructs the patient and family in their use and has the patient and family demonstrate correct administration (Chart 53-3).

Allergic Rhinitis

Allergic rhinitis (hay fever, seasonal allergic rhinitis) is the most common form of respiratory allergy, which is presumed to be mediated by an immediate (type I hypersensitivity) immunologic reaction, and it is among the top 10 reasons for visits to primary care physicians (Braido,

CHART 53-3

Patient Education: Self-Administration of Epinephrine

The nurse instructs the patient to:

1. After removing the EpiPen autoinjector from its carrying tube, grasp the unit with the orange tip (injecting end) pointing downward. Form fist around the unit with the orange tip down; with your other hand, remove the blue safety release cap.

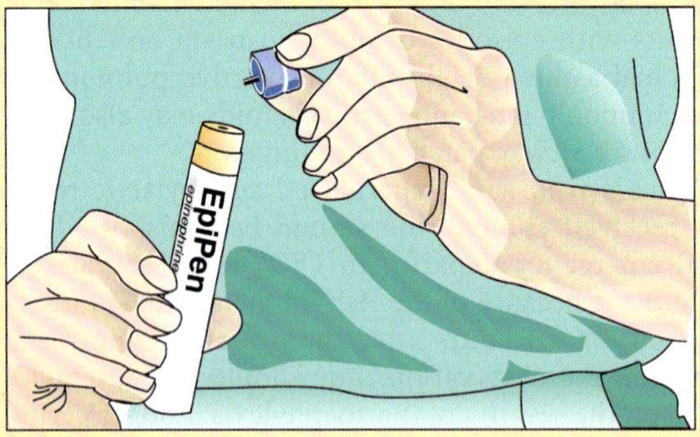

2. Hold black tip near outer thigh. Swing and **jab firmly** into outer thigh until a click is heard with the device perpendicular (90-degree angle) to the thigh. Do NOT inject into buttocks.

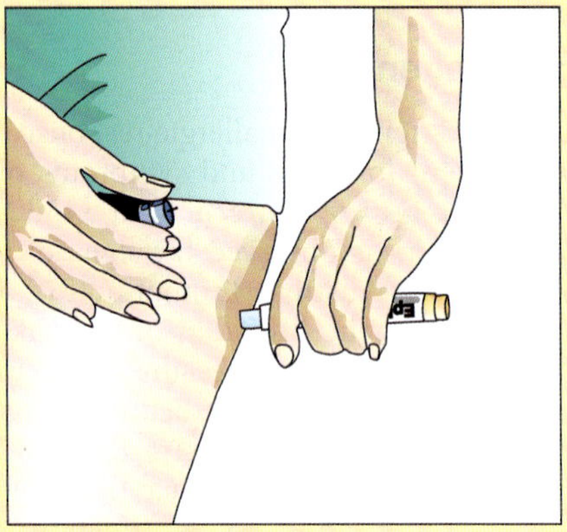

3. Hold firmly against the thigh for approximately 10 seconds. Remove the unit from the thigh and gently massage the injection area for 10 seconds. Call 911 and seek immediate medical attention. Carefully place the used autoinjector unit, needle-end first, into the device storage tube without bending the needle. Screw on the storage tube completely and take it with you to the hospital emergency room.

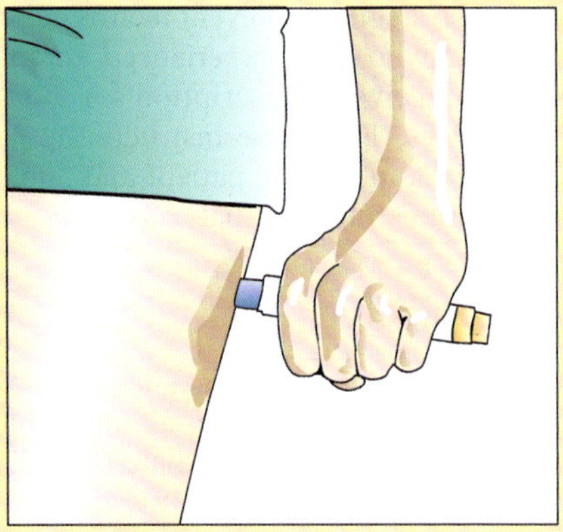

Sclifò, & Ferrando, 2014). It affects about 20% to 25% of the Canadian population (Keith, Desrosiers, Laister, et al., 2012). Symptoms are similar to those of viral rhinitis but are usually more persistent and demonstrate seasonal variation; rhinitis is considered to be the allergic form if the symptoms are caused by an allergen-specific IgE-mediated immunologic response. However, approximately one third of patients with rhinitis have associated conjunctivitis, sinusitis, and asthma (Baran et al., 2014; Lehrer, Mullol, Agredo, et al., 2014). The proportion of patients with the allergic form of rhinitis increases with age. It often occurs with other conditions, such as asthma, and cystic fibrosis (Rosenfeld, Piccirillo, Chandrasekhar, et al., 2015). If symptoms are severe, allergic rhinitis may interfere with sleep, leisure, school, and overall quality of life (Sheikh, 2015). Chronic rhinitis accounts for an average of 1 to 2 missed work days per patient per year. These patients experience a 36% reduction in on-the-job effectiveness and 38% loss of productivity (Sheikh, 2015).

Early diagnosis and adequate treatment are essential to reduce complications and relieve symptoms.

Because allergic rhinitis is induced by airborne pollens or moulds, it is characterized by the following seasonal occurrences (Sheikh, 2015):

- *Early spring:* Tree pollen (oak, elm, poplar)
- *Early summer:* Grass pollen (Timothy, Red-top)
- *Early fall:* Weed pollen (ragweed)

Each year attacks begin and end at about the same time. Airborne mould spores require warm, damp weather. Although there is no rigid seasonal pattern, these spores appear in early spring, are rampant during the summer and taper off and disappear by the first frost in areas that experience dramatic seasonal temperature variation. In temperate areas that do not experience freezing temperatures, these allergens, especially mould, can persist throughout the year.

Pathophysiology

Sensitization begins by ingestion or inhalation of an antigen. On re-exposure, the nasal mucosa reacts by the slowing of ciliary action, edema formation, and leukocyte (primarily eosinophil) infiltration. Histamine is the major mediator of allergic reactions in the nasal mucosa. Tissue edema results from vasodilation and increased capillary permeability.

Clinical Manifestations

The four major signs and symptoms of allergic rhinitis include copious amounts of serous nasal discharge, nasal congestion, sneezing, as well as nose and throat itching. Patients may experience postnasal drip, itching, watery eyes, headache, and hyposomnia (Baran et al., 2014). Bronchial asthma is more persistent in patients with chronic rhinitis than in those with allergic rhinitis (Lehrer et al., 2014). The symptoms of this chronic condition depend on environmental exposure and intrinsic host responsiveness. Allergic rhinitis can affect quality of life by also producing sleep disturbance, impairment of daily activities, and missed school and work (Rich et al., 2013).

Assessment and Diagnostic Findings

Diagnosis of seasonal allergic rhinitis is based on history, physical examination, and diagnostic test results. Diagnostic tests include nasal smears, peripheral blood counts, total serum IgE, epicutaneous and intradermal testing, serum-specific IgE, and nasal provocation tests. Results indicative of allergy as the cause of rhinitis include increased IgE and eosinophil levels and positive reactions on allergen testing. False-positive and false-negative responses to these tests, particularly skin testing, may occur (Rich et al., 2013).

Medical Management

The goal of therapy is to provide relief from symptoms. Therapy may include one or all of the following interventions: avoidance therapy, pharmacologic therapy, and immunotherapy. Verbal instructions must be reinforced by written information. Knowledge of general concepts regarding assessment and therapy in allergic diseases is important so that patients can learn to manage certain conditions as well as prevent severe reactions and illnesses.

Avoidance Therapy

In avoidance therapy, every attempt is made to remove the allergens that act as precipitating factors. Simple measures and environmental controls are often effective in decreasing symptoms. Examples include the use of air conditioners, air cleaners, humidifiers and dehumidifiers; removal of dust-catching furnishings, carpets, and window coverings; removal of pets from the home or bedroom; the use of pillow and mattress covers that are impermeable to dust mites; and a smoke-free environment (Sheikh, 2015). Additional measures include changing clothing when coming in from outside, showering to wash allergens from hair and skin, and using an over-the-counter nasal irrigation device or saline nasal spray to reduce allergens in the nasal passages. Because multiple allergens are often implicated, multiple measures to avoid exposure to allergens are often necessary (Bleier, 2015; Sheikh, 2015). High-efficiency particulate air (HEPA) purifiers and vacuum cleaner filters may also be used to reduce allergens in the environment. Research has shown that multiple avoidance strategies tailored to a person's risk factors can reduce the severity of symptoms, the number of work or school days missed because of symptoms, and the number of unscheduled health care visits for treatment (Sheikh, 2015). In many cases, it is impossible to avoid exposure to all environmental allergens, so pharmacologic therapy or immunotherapy is needed.

Pharmacologic Therapy

Antihistamines

Antihistamines, classified as H_1-receptor antagonists (or H_1 blockers), are used in the management of mild allergic disorders. H_1 blockers bind selectively to H_1 receptors, preventing the actions of histamines at these sites. They do not prevent the release of histamine from mast cells or basophils. The H_1 antagonists have no effect on H_2 receptors, but they do have the ability to bind to nonhistaminic receptors. The ability of certain antihistamines to bind to and block muscarinic receptors underlines several of the prominent anticholinergic side effects of these medications.

Oral antihistamines, which are readily absorbed, are most effective when given at the first occurrence of symptoms because they prevent the development of new symptoms. The effectiveness of these medications is limited to certain patients with hay fever, vasomotor rhinitis, urticaria (hives), and mild asthma. They are rarely effective in other conditions or in any severe conditions (Frandsen & Pennington, 2014; Hodgson & Kizior, 2014).

Antihistamines are frequently prescribed for the symptomatic relief of allergic rhinitis. The major side effects are drowsiness and dry mouth (Hwang & Patel, 2015; Rosenfeld et al., 2015). Additional side effects include anxiety, agitation, urinary retention, blurred vision, anorexia, nausea, and vomiting (Frandsen & Pennington, 2014; Hodgson & Kizior, 2014).

Antihistamines are contraindicated during pregnancy, in nursing mothers and newborns, in children and older adults, and in patients with hypersensitivity to the drugs whose conditions may be aggravated by muscarinic blockade (e.g., asthma, urinary retention, open-angle glaucoma, hypertension, and prostatic hyperplasia) (Frandsen & Pennington, 2014; Hodgson & Kizior, 2014; Katzung & Trevor, 2015).

Second-generation or nonsedating H_1-receptor antagonists are newer types of antihistamines. Unlike first-generation H_1-receptor antagonists, they do not readily enter the brain from the blood (Frandsen & Pennington, 2014; Rich et al., 2013). They bind to peripheral rather than central nervous system H_1 receptors, causing less sedation. Examples of these medications are loratadine (Claritin), fexofenadine (Allegra), and cetirizine (Zyrtec). Selected H_1 antihistamines are shown in Table 53-2.

Antihistamines may also be combined with decongestants to reduce the nasal congestion associated with allergies. Most combination products are available as over-the-counter (nonprescription) medications; examples are desloratadine/pseudoephedrine (Claritin-D) and cetirizine/pseudoephedrine (Zyrtec-D). Decongestants can cause an increase in blood pressure; therefore, patients with a history of hypertension should be cautioned about long-term use of any medication containing decongestants (Bleier, 2015; Hodgson & Kizior, 2014).

Adrenergic Agents

Adrenergic agents, which are vasoconstrictors of mucosal vessels, are used topically in nasal (Afrin) and ophthalmic (Alphagan P) formulations in addition to the oral route (pseudoephedrine [Sudafed]) (Frandsen & Pennington, 2014; Hodgson & Kizior, 2014). The topical route (drops and sprays) causes fewer side effects than oral administration; however, the use of drops and sprays should be limited to a few days to avoid rebound congestion. Adrenergic nasal decongestants are applied topically to the nasal mucosa for the relief of nasal congestion. They activate the alpha-adrenergic receptor sites on the smooth muscle of the nasal mucosal blood vessels, reducing local blood flow, fluid exudation, and mucosal edema. Topical ophthalmic drops are used for symptomatic relief of eye irritations caused by allergies. Potential side effects include hypertension, dysrhythmias, palpitations, central nervous system stimulation, irritability, tremor, and tachyphylaxis (acceleration of hemodynamic status).

TABLE 53-2 Selected H_1 Antihistamines

H_1 Antihistamine	Contraindications	Major Side Effects	Nursing Implications and Patient Education
First-Generation H_1 Antihistamines (Sedating)			
Diphenhydramine (Benadryl)	Allergy to any antihistamines Third trimester of pregnancy Lactation Use cautiously with narrow-angle glaucoma, asthma, stenosing peptic ulcer, benign prostatic hyperplasia (BPH) or bladder neck obstruction, first and second trimester of pregnancy, older patients, hypertension	Drowsiness, confusion, dizziness, dry mouth, nausea, vomiting, photosensitivity, urinary retention	Administer with food if gastrointestinal (GI) upset occurs. Caution patients to avoid alcohol, driving, or engaging in any hazardous activities until central nervous system (CNS) response to medication is stabilized. Suggest sucking on sugarless lozenges or ice chips for relief of dry mouth. Encourage use of sunscreen and hat while outdoors. Assess for urinary retention; monitor urinary output.
Chlorpheniramine (Chlor-Trimeton)	Allergy to any antihistamines Third trimester of pregnancy Lactation Use cautiously with narrow-angle glaucoma, asthma, stenosing peptic ulcer, BPH or bladder neck obstruction, first and second trimester of pregnancy, older patients, hypertension	Drowsiness, sedation, and dizziness, although less than other sedating agents; confusion, dry mouth, nausea, vomiting, urinary retention, epigastric distress, thickening of bronchial secretions	Caution patients to avoid alcohol, driving, or engaging in any hazardous activities until CNS response to medication is stabilized. Suggest sucking on sugarless lozenges or ice chips for relief of dry mouth. Recommend use of humidifier.
Hydroxyzine (Atarax)	Allergy to hydroxyzine or cetirizine (Zyrtec), pregnancy, lactation, hypertension	Drowsiness, dry mouth, involuntary motor activity, including tremor and seizures	Caution patients to avoid alcohol, driving, or engaging in any hazardous activities until CNS response to medication is stabilized. Suggest sucking on sugarless lozenges or ice chips for relief of dry mouth. Instruct patients to report tremors.
Second-Generation H_1 Antihistamines (Nonsedating)			
Cetirizine (Zyrtec)	Allergy to any antihistamines Narrow-angle glaucoma Asthma Stenosing peptic ulcer BPH or bladder neck obstruction Lactation Hypertension	Dry nasal mucosa, thickening of bronchial secretions	Can be taken without regard to meals. Instruct patients to use caution if driving or performing tasks that require alertness. Recommend use of humidifier.
Desloratadine (Clarinex)	Allergy to loratadine (Alavert, Claritin) Lactation Use cautiously with renal or hepatic impairment pregnancy, hypertension	Somnolence, nervousness, dizziness, fatigue, dry mouth	Can be taken without regard to meals. Suggest sucking on sugarless lozenges or ice chips for relief of dry mouth. Recommend use of humidifier.
Loratadine (Alavert, Claritin)	Allergy to any antihistamines Narrow-angle glaucoma Asthma Stenosing peptic ulcer BPH or bladder neck obstruction, hypertension	Headache, nervousness, dizziness, depression, edema, increased appetite	Instruct patients to take on empty stomach (1 hour before or 2 hours after meals or food). Instruct patients to avoid alcohol and to use caution if driving or performing tasks that require alertness. Suggest sucking on sugarless lozenges or ice chips for relief of dry mouth. Recommend use of humidifier.
Fexofenadine (Allegra)	Allergy to any antihistamines Pregnancy Lactation Use cautiously with hepatic or renal impairment, older patients, hypertension	Fatigue, drowsiness, GI upset	Should not be administered within 15 minutes of ingestion of antacids. Instruct patients to use caution if driving or performing tasks that require alertness. Recommend use of humidifier.
Levocetirizine (Xyzal)	Hypersensitivity to any antihistamines End-stage renal disease Hemodialysis Use cautiously with pregnancy, lactation, older patients.	Drowsiness, GI disturbance, headache	Can be taken without regard to meals. Instruct patients to use caution if driving or performing tasks that require alertness. Recommend the use of a humidifier.

Adapted from Comerford, K. C. (2015). *Nursing 2015 drug handbook*. Philadelphia, PA: Wolters Kluwer.

Mast Cell Stabilizers

Intranasal cromolyn sodium (NasalCrom) is a spray that acts by stabilizing the mast cell membrane, thus reducing the release of histamine and other mediators of the allergic response. In addition, it inhibits macrophages, eosinophils, monocytes, and platelets involved in the immune response (Arcangelo & Peterson, 2013). Cromolyn interrupts the physiologic response to nasal antigens and is used prophylactically (before exposure to allergens) to prevent the onset of symptoms and to treat symptoms once they occur. It is also used therapeutically in chronic allergic rhinitis. This spray is as effective as antihistamines but is less effective than intranasal corticosteroids in the treatment of seasonal allergic rhinitis. The patient must be informed that the beneficial effects of the medication may take a week or so to manifest. The medication is of no benefit in the treatment of nonallergic rhinitis. Adverse effects (e.g., sneezing, local stinging, and burning sensations) are usually mild.

Corticosteroids

Intranasal corticosteroids are indicated in more severe cases of allergic and perennial rhinitis that cannot be controlled by more conventional medications such as decongestants, antihistamines, and intranasal cromolyn. Examples of these medications include beclomethasone (Beconase, Qnasl), budesonide (Rhinocort), flunisolide (AeroSpan), and triamcinolone (Nasacort) (Comerford, 2015).

Because of their anti-inflammatory actions, corticosteroids are equally effective in preventing or suppressing the major symptoms of allergic rhinitis. These medications are given by metered-spray devices. If the nasal passages are blocked, a topical decongestant may be used to clear the passages before the administration of the intranasal corticosteroid. Patients must be aware that full benefit may not be achieved for several days to 2 weeks. Adverse effects of intranasal corticosteroids are mild and include drying of the nasal mucosa and burning and itching sensations caused by the vehicle used to administer the medication. Recommended use of this medication is limited to 30 days. Beclomethasone, budesonide, flunisolide, and triamcinolone are deactivated rapidly after absorption, so they do not achieve significant blood levels. Because corticosteroids suppress host defences, they must be used with caution in patients with tuberculosis or untreated bacterial infections of the lungs. Patients taking corticosteroids are at risk for infection and for suppression of typical manifestations of inflammation because host defences are compromised. Inhaled corticosteroids do not affect the immune system to the same degree as systemic corticosteroids (i.e., oral corticosteroids). Because corticosteroids are inhaled into the upper respiratory tract, tuberculosis or untreated bacterial infections of the lungs may become apparent and progress. Whenever possible, patients with tuberculosis or other bacterial infections of the lungs should avoid inhaled corticosteroids.

Oral and parenteral corticosteroids are used when conventional therapy has failed, and symptoms are severe and of short duration (Frandsen & Pennington, 2014; Hodgson & Kizior, 2014). They can control symptoms of allergic reactions such as hay fever, medication-induced allergies, and allergic reactions to insect stings. Because the response to corticosteroids is delayed, these agents have little or no value in acute therapy for severe reactions such as anaphylaxis. The patient is also instructed about side effects, which include fluid retention, weight gain, hypertension, gastric irritation, glucose intolerance, and adrenal suppression.

NURSING ALERT

Patients who receive high-dose or long-term corticosteroid therapy must be cautioned not to stop taking the medication suddenly. Doses are tapered when discontinuing this medication to avoid adrenal insufficiency.

Leukotriene Modifiers

Leukotrienes have many effects on the inflammatory cycle. Leukotriene modifiers, such as zafirlukast (Accolate) and montelukast (Singulair), block the synthesis or action of leukotrienes and prevent the signs and symptoms associated with asthma (Table 53-3).

Leukotriene modifiers are for long-term use, and patients should be advised to take their medication daily. Patients take appropriate "rescue" medications for symptom exacerbation but continue to take the leukotriene modifier on a daily basis. The National Asthma Education and Prevention Program (NAEPP) suggests using a leukotriene modifier in conjunction with an inhaled corticosteroid for mild persistent asthma (National Institute of Allergy and Infectious Disease [NIAID], 2013).

Immunotherapy

Allergen desensitization (allergen immunotherapy, hyposensitization) is primarily used to treat IgE-mediated diseases by injections of allergen extracts. Immunotherapy, also referred to as allergy vaccine therapy, involves the administration of gradually increasing quantities of specific allergens to the patient until a dose is reached that is effective in reducing disease severity from natural exposure. This is an effective treatment for 80% to 90% of certain allergens such as grass and pollen (ASCIA, 2015; Senti,

TABLE 53-3 Leukotriene Modifiers

Leukotriene Modifier	Available Formulations	Frequency of Dosing
Leukotriene-Receptor Antagonists (LTRAs)		
Zafirlukast (Accolate)	Tablets: 10 mg; 20 mg	Taken twice a day
Montelukast (Singulair)	Tablets: 10 mg Chewable tablets: 4 mg; 5 mg Granules: 4 mg/packet	Taken once a day in PM
Leukotriene-Receptor Inhibitors (LTRIs)		
Zileuton (Zyflo CR)	Tables: 600 mg extended release	Taken twice a day within 1 hour after morning and evening meals

CHART 53-4

Immunotherapy: Indications and Contraindications

Indications

- Allergic rhinitis, conjunctivitis, or allergic asthma
- History of a systemic reaction to Hymenoptera and specific immunoglobulin E antibodies to Hymenoptera venom
- Desire to avoid the long-term use, potential adverse effects, or costs of medications
- Lack of control of symptoms by avoidance measures or use of medications

Contraindications

- The use of beta-blocker or angiotensin-converting enzyme inhibitor therapy, which may mask early signs of anaphylaxis
- Presence of significant pulmonary or cardiac disease or organ failure
- Inability of the patient to recognize or report signs and symptoms of a systemic reaction
- Nonadherence of the patient to other therapeutic regimens and no likelihood that patient will adhere to the immunization schedule (often weekly for an indefinite period)
- Inability to monitor the patient for at least 30 minutes after administration of immunotherapy
- Absence of equipment or adequate personnel to respond to allergic reaction if one occurs

von Moos, Graf, et al., 2015; Sheikh, 2015). This type of therapy provides an adjunct to symptomatic pharmacologic therapy and can be used when allergen avoidance is not possible. Specific immunotherapy has been used in the treatment of allergic disorders for many years. Goals of immunotherapy include reducing the level of circulating IgE, increasing the level of blocking antibody IgG, and reducing mediator cell sensitivity. Immunotherapy has been most effective for ragweed pollen; however, treatment for grass, tree pollen, cat dander, and house dust mite allergens has also been effective. Indications and contraindications for immunotherapy are presented in Chart 53-4.

Correlation of a positive skin test with a positive allergy history is an indication for immunotherapy if the allergen cannot be avoided. The benefit of immunotherapy has been fairly well established in instances of allergic rhinitis and bronchial asthma that are clearly due to sensitivity to one of the common pollens, moulds, or household dust. Unlike antiallergy medication, allergen immunotherapy has the potential to alter the allergic disease course after 3 to 5 years of therapy. Because it may prevent the progression or development of asthma or multiple or additional allergies, it is also considered to be a potential preventive measure (Sheikh, 2015). The patient needs to understand what to expect and the importance of continuing therapy for several years before immunotherapy is accomplished. When skin tests are performed, the results are correlated with symptoms; treatment is based on the patient's needs rather than just on the results of skin tests.

There are three methods of immunotherapy: subcutaneous immunotherapy (SIT), sublingual immunotherapy (SLIT), and epicutaneous immunotherapy (EPIT).

Subcutaneous Immunotherapy

The most common method of treatment is SIT, which consists of the serial injection of one or more antigens that are selected in each particular case on the basis of skin testing. This method provides a simple and efficient technique for identifying IgE antibodies to specific antigens. Specific treatment consists of injecting extracts of the allergens that cause symptoms in a particular patient. Injections begin with very small amounts and are gradually increased, usually at weekly intervals, until a maximum tolerated dose is attained. Maintenance booster injections are given at 2- to 4-week intervals, frequently for a period of several years, before maximum benefit is achieved, although some patients will note early improvement in their symptoms, which tends to occur most frequently at the induction or "up-dosing" phase. Therefore, the patient must be monitored after administration of immunotherapy.

NURSING ALERT

Because the injection of an allergen may induce systemic reactions, such injections are given only in a setting where epinephrine is immediately available (i.e., primary provider's office, clinic).

Because of the risk for anaphylaxis, injections should not be given by a lay person or by the patient. The patient must remain in the office or clinic for at least 30 minutes after the injection and is observed for possible systemic symptoms. If a large, local swelling develops at the injection site, the next dose should not be increased, because this may be a warning sign of a possible systemic reaction (ASCIA, 2015; Sheikh, 2015).

Maintenance booster injections are given at 2- to 4-week intervals, frequently for a period of several years, before the maximum benefit is achieved, although some patients will note early improvement in their symptoms. Long-term benefit seems to be related to the cumulative dose of vaccine given over time (ASCIA, 2015; Sheikh, 2015).

Sublingual Immunotherapy

In 2001 Health Canada approved the use of a SLIT. SLIT has been reported to have a 30% to 40% reduction in reactions and rescue medication usage in seasonal allergic rhinitis. Administration of SLIT includes a buildup phase that is followed by a treatment plan of three times per week with a rapid dissolving tablet or liquid containing allergen extracts. Recent studies show comparable efficacy of SLIT with SIT (Senti et al., 2015). Systemic side effects are rare but have been reported in patients who also report systemic reactions with SIT. Side effects include irritation, minor swelling or itching inside the mouth, and stomach upset and nausea.

Epicutaneous Immunotherapy

EPIT represents an alternative allergen immunotherapy with delivery of the allergen to the epidermis. Because the epidermis is less vascular, there is reduced risk of systemic allergic side effects due to inadvertent intravascular allergen delivery. Reports from the completed trials of EPIT may find potential application in the management of IgE-mediated allergies, but more research is needed to define an optimal regimen that balances clinical efficacy and safety (Senti et al., 2015).

Immunotherapy should not be initiated during pregnancy; for patients who have been receiving immunotherapy before pregnancy, the dosage should not be increased during pregnancy.

Therapeutic failure is evident when a patient does not experience a decrease of symptoms within 12 to 24 months, fails to develop increased tolerance to known allergens, and cannot decrease the use of medications to reduce symptoms. Potential causes of treatment failure include misdiagnosis of allergies, inadequate doses of allergen, newly developed allergies, and inadequate environmental controls.

Nursing Process

The Patient With Allergic Rhinitis

Assessment

The examination and history of the patient reveal sneezing, often in paroxysms; thin and watery nasal discharge; itching eyes and nose; lacrimation; and occasionally headache. The health history includes a personal and family history of allergy. The allergy assessment identifies the nature of antigens, seasonal changes in symptoms, and medication history. The nurse also obtains subjective data about how the patient feels just before symptoms become obvious, such as the occurrence of pruritus, breathing issues, and tingling sensations. In addition to these symptoms, hoarseness, wheezing, hives, rash, erythema, and edema are noted. Any relationship between emotional concerns or stress and the triggering of allergy symptoms is assessed.

Nursing Priorities

Based on the assessment data, the major nursing priorities may include:

- Problematic breathing pattern
- Lack of knowledge about allergy and self-care practices
- Lack of coping with condition

Collaborative Problems/ Potential Complications

Potential complications may include the following:

- Anaphylaxis
- Impaired breathing
- Nonadherence to the therapeutic regimen

Planning and Goals

The goals for the patient may include restoration of a breathing pattern that provides adequate ventilation, increased knowledge about the causes and control of allergic symptoms, improved coping with alterations and modifications, and absence of complications.

Nursing Interventions

Improving Breathing Pattern

The patient is instructed and assisted to modify the environment to reduce the severity of allergic symptoms or to prevent their occurrence. The patient is also instructed to reduce exposure to people with upper respiratory tract infections. Adherence to medication schedules and other treatment regimens is encouraged and reinforced.

Promoting Understanding of Allergy and Allergy Control

Instruction includes strategies to minimize exposure to allergens, and explanations about desensitization procedures, and correct use of medications. The nurse informs and reminds the patient of the importance of keeping appointments for desensitization procedures, because dosages are usually adjusted on a weekly basis and missed appointments may interfere with the dosage adjustment.

Patients need to understand the difference between rescue medications for allergy exacerbation and seasonal flares (e.g., antihistamines) and medications used for allergy control throughout the year (e.g., inhaled corticosteroids, leukotriene modifiers). Patients also need to understand that medications for allergy exacerbation and seasonal flares should be used only when the allergy is apparent. Continued use of these medications when not required can result in tolerance; consequently, the medication will not be effective when needed.

Coping With a Chronic Disorder

Although allergic reactions are infrequently life-threatening, they require vigilance to avoid allergens and modification of the lifestyle or environment to prevent recurrence of symptoms. Allergic symptoms are often present year-round and create discomfort and inconvenience for the patient. Although patients may not feel ill during allergy seasons, they often do not feel well either. The need to be alert for possible allergens in the environment may be tiresome, placing a burden on the patient's ability to lead a normal life. Stress related to these difficulties may in turn increase the frequency or severity of symptoms. To assist the patient in adjusting to these modifications, the nurse must have an appreciation of the difficulties encountered by the patient. The patient is encouraged to verbalize feelings and concerns in a supportive environment and to identify strategies to deal with them effectively.

Monitoring and Managing Potential Complications

ANAPHYLAXIS AND IMPAIRED BREATHING. Respiratory and cardiovascular functioning can be significantly altered during allergic reactions by the reaction itself or by the medications used to treat reactions. The respiratory status is evaluated by monitoring the respiratory rate and pattern and by assessing for breathing difficulties or unexpected lung sounds. The pulse rate and rhythm and blood pressure are monitored to assess cardiovascular status regularly or any time the patient reports symptoms such as itching or difficulty breathing. In the event of signs and symptoms suggestive of anaphylaxis, emergency medications and equipment must be available for immediate use.

NONADHERENCE TO THERAPEUTIC REGIMEN. Knowledge about the treatment regimen does not ensure adherence. Having the patient identify potential barriers and explore acceptable solutions for effective management of the condition (e.g., installing tile floors rather than carpet, not gardening in the spring) can increase adherence to the treatment regimen.

Promoting Home, Community-based and Transitional Care

EDUCATING PATIENTS ABOUT SELF-CARE. The patient is instructed about strategies to minimize exposure to allergens, the actions and adverse effects of medications, and the correct use of medications. The patient should know the name, dose, frequency, actions, and side effects of all medications taken.

Instruction about strategies to control allergic symptoms is based on the needs of the patient as determined by the results of tests, the severity of symptoms, and the motivation of the patient and family to deal with the condition. Suggestions for patients who are sensitive to dust and mould in the home are given in Chart 53-5.

If the patient is to undergo SIT immunotherapy, the nurse reinforces the primary provider's explanation regarding the purpose and procedure. Instructions are given regarding the series of injections, which are usually given initially every week and then at 2- to 4-week intervals. These instructions include remaining in the primary provider's office or the clinic for at least 30 minutes after the injection so that emergency treatment can be given if the patient has a reaction, avoiding rubbing or scratching the injection site, and continuing with the series for the period of time required. In addition, the patient and family are informed about emergency treatment of severe allergic symptoms.

Because antihistamines may produce drowsiness, the patient is cautioned about this and other side effects of the particular medication. Operating machinery, driving a car, and performing activities that require intense concentration should be postponed. The patient is also informed about the dangers of drinking alcohol when taking antihistamines, because they tend to exaggerate the effects of alcohol.

The patient must be aware of the effects caused by overuse of the sympathomimetic agents in nose drops or sprays, because a condition referred to as rhinitis medicamentosa may result. After topical application of the medication, a rebound period occurs in which the nasal mucous membranes become more edematous and congested than they were before the medication was used. Such a reaction encourages the use of more medication, and a cyclic pattern results. The topical agent must be discontinued immediately and completely to correct this problem.

CONTINUING AND TRANSITIONAL CARE. Follow-up telephone calls to the patient are often reassuring to the patient and family and provide an opportunity for the nurse to answer any questions. The patient is reminded to keep follow-up appointments and informed about the importance of continuing with treatment. The importance of participating in health promotion activities and health screening is also emphasized.

Evaluation

Expected patient outcomes may include:

1. Exhibits a breathing pattern that provides adequate ventilation
   a. Demonstrates lungs clear on auscultation
   b. Exhibits absence of adventitious breath sounds (crackles, rhonchi, wheezing)
   c. Has an acceptable respiratory rate and pattern
   d. Reports no complaints of respiratory distress (shortness of breath, difficulty on inspiration or expiration)
2. Demonstrates knowledge about allergy and strategies to control symptoms
   a. Identifies causative allergens, if known
   b. States methods of avoiding allergens and controlling indoor and outdoor precipitating factors
   c. Removes from environment items that retain dust
   d. Wears a dampened mask if dust or mould may be a problem
   e. Avoids smoke-filled rooms and dust-filled or freshly sprayed areas
   f. Uses air conditioning for a major part of the day when allergens are high
   g. Takes antihistamines as prescribed; participates in hyposensitization program, if applicable
   h. Describes name, purpose, side effects, and method of administration of prescribed medications
   i. Identifies when to seek immediate medical attention for severe allergic responses
   j. Describes activities that are possible, including ways to participate in activities without activating the allergies
3. Adapts to the inconveniences of an allergy
   a. Relates the emotional aspects of the allergic response

CHART 53-5

HOME CARE CHECKLIST • Allergy Management

At the completion of education, the patient, caregiver, or both will be able to:

- State the impact of environmental allergens (e.g., dust, moulds, perfumes, foods) on physiologic functioning, ADLs, IADLs, roles, relationships, and spirituality.
- State changes in home environment necessary to minimize exposure to allergens.
  - Removing drapes, curtains, and venetian blinds and replacing them with pull shades; covering the mattress with a hypoallergenic cover that can be zipped; and removing rugs and replacing them with wood flooring or linoleum.
  - Reducing dust in the house as a whole by using steam or hot water for heating and using high-efficiency particulate air (HEPA) purifiers or air conditioning.
  - Washing the floor and dusting and vacuuming daily, using clean filters, wearing a mask whenever cleaning is being done.
  - Replacing stuffed furniture with wood pieces that can easily be dusted.
  - Avoiding the use of tufted bedspreads, stuffed toys, and feather pillows and replacing them with washable cotton material.
  - Avoiding the use of any clothing that causes itching.
- Verbalize ways to reduce exposure to pollens or moulds by identifying seasons of the year when pollen counts are high; wearing a mask at times of increased exposure (windy days and when grass is being cut); and avoiding contact with weeds, dry leaves, and freshly cut grass.
- State rationale for seeking air-conditioned areas at the height of the allergy season.
- State rationale for avoiding sprays and perfumes.
- State rationale for the use of hypoallergenic cosmetics.
- State rationale for taking prescribed medications as ordered.
- Identify specific foods that may cause allergic symptoms and develop a list of foods to avoid (e.g., fish, nuts, eggs, chocolate).
- Verbalize ways to cope with stress successfully, plans for regular exercise, and rationale for obtaining adequate rest.
- State how to reach primary provider with questions or complications.
- State time and date of follow-up appointments, testing.
- Identify the need for health promotion, disease prevention, and screening activities.

ADLs, activities of daily living; IADLs, independent activities of daily living.

b. Demonstrates use of measures to cope positively with allergy
c. Demonstrates absence of complications
d. Exhibits vital signs within appropriate limits
e. Reports no symptoms or episodes of anaphylaxis (urticaria, itching, peripheral tingling, fullness in the mouth and throat, flushing, difficulty swallowing, coughing, wheezing, or difficulty breathing)
f. Demonstrates correct procedure to self-administer emergency medications to treat severe allergic reaction
g. Correctly states medication names, dose and frequency of administration, and medication actions
h. Correctly identifies side effects and untoward signs and symptoms to report to primary provider
i. Discusses acceptable lifestyle changes and solutions for identified potential barriers to adherence to treatment and medication regimen

Contact Dermatitis

Contact dermatitis, a type IV delayed hypersensitivity reaction, is an acute or chronic skin condition caused by contact with an exogenous substance that elicits an allergic response. There are four basic types: allergic, irritant, phototoxic, and photo allergic (Table 53-4). Eighty percent of cases are caused by excessive exposure to or additive effects of irritants (e.g., soaps, detergents, organic solvents). Skin sensitivity may develop after brief or prolonged periods of exposure, and the clinical picture may appear hours or weeks after the sensitized skin has been exposed.

Clinical Manifestations

Symptoms include itching, burning, erythema, skin lesions (vesicles and papules), and edema, followed by skin thickening, hardening, and scaling (Fonacier, Bernstein, Pacheco, et al., 2015). In severe responses, hemorrhagic bullae may develop. Repeated reactions may be accompanied by

TABLE 53-4 Types, Testing, and Treatment of Contact Dermatitis

Type	Etiology	Clinical Presentation	Diagnostic Testing	Treatment
Allergic	Results from contact of skin and allergenic substance. Has a sensitization period of 10 to 14 days.	Vasodilation and perivascular infiltrates on the dermis Intracellular edema Usually seen on dorsal aspects of hand	Patch testing (contraindicated in acute, widespread dermatitis)	Avoidance of offending material Burow's solution or cool water compress Systemic corticosteroids (prednisone) for 7 to 10 days Topical corticosteroids for mild cases Oral antihistamines to relieve pruritus
Irritant	Results from contact with a substance that chemically or physically damages the skin on a nonimmunologic basis. Occurs after first exposure to irritant or repeated exposures to milder irritants over an extended time.	Dryness lasting days to months Vesiculation, fissures, cracks Hands and lower arms most common areas	Clinical picture Appropriate negative patch tests	Identification and removal of source of irritation Application of hydrophilic cream or petrolatum to soothe and protect Topical corticosteroids and compresses for weeping lesions Antibiotics for infection and oral antihistamines for pruritus
Phototoxic	Resembles the irritant type but requires sun and a chemical in combination to damage the epidermis	Similar to irritant dermatitis	Photopatch test	Same as for allergic and irritant dermatitis
Photoallergic	Resembles allergic dermatitis but requires light exposure in addition to allergen contact to produce immunologic reactivity.	Similar to allergic dermatitis	Photopatch test	Same as for allergic and irritant dermatitis

Adapted from Comerford, K. C. (2015). *Nursing 2015 drug handbook*. Philadelphia, PA: Wolters Kluwer.

thickening of the skin and pigmentary changes. Secondary invasion by bacteria may develop in skin that is abraded by rubbing or scratching. Usually, there are no systemic symptoms unless the eruption is widespread (Habif, 2016).

Assessment and Diagnostic Findings

Determining allergens responsible requires a history, physical examination, and patch testing.

Assessment should include the date of onset, and any identifiable relationship to work environment and skin care products (Habif, 2016). The location of the lesions, distribution of the dermatitis, absence of other etiologies, and the history of exposure aid in determining the condition (Fonacier et al., 2015). Patch testing and environmental history of exposure to contact allergens are required to verify the diagnosis. Patch testing is indicated in cases in which inflammation persists despite avoidance therapy. The patch test most commonly used is the Thin-layer Rapid Use Epicutaneous (TRUE) test (Habif, 2016).

Atopic Dermatitis

Atopic dermatitis is a type I immediate hypersensitivity disorder characterized by inflammation and hyper reactivity of the skin. The term is used synonymously with atopic eczema (AAAAI, 2015). Other terms used to describe this kind of disorder include atopic eczema, atopic dermatitis, and atopic dermatitis/eczema syndrome (AEDS). In a revised classification system developed to clarify terminology, AEDS includes both allergic and nonallergic disorders (Habif, 2016). Currently *atopic dermatitis* is the most commonly used of these terms and is used for the purpose of this discussion.

Atopic dermatitis is a chronic pruritis inflammatory skin disease. Increased serum IgE levels have been indicated in 80% of the patients with a family history of type I allergies, allergic rhinitis, and asthma. This disorder affects 15% to 30% of children and 2% to 10% of adults in developed countries (AAAAI, 2015). Most patients have significant elevations of serum IgE and peripheral eosinophilia. The eosinophil count may be increased depending on concomitant respiratory allergies (Habif, 2016).

Pruritus and hyperirritability of the skin are the most consistent features of atopic dermatitis and are related to large amounts of histamine in the skin. Excessive dryness of the skin with resultant itching is related to changes in lipid content, sebaceous gland activity, and sweating. In response to stroking of the skin, immediate redness appears on the skin. Pallor follows in 15 to 30 seconds and persists for 1 to 3 minutes. Patterns of inflammation result from scratching of erythematous papules. Lesions develop secondary to the trauma of scratching and appear in areas of increased sweating and hypervascularity. Atopic dermatitis is chronic, with remissions and exacerbations. This condition has a tendency to recur, with remission from adolescence to 20 years of age (Habif, 2016).

Nurses should be aware that atopic dermatitis is often linked in a process called the atopic march that often leads to asthma, allergic rhinitis, or food allergy (Fonacier et al., 2015). It is the result of interactions between susceptibility genes, the environment, defective function of the skin barrier, and immunologic responses.

Medical Management

Treatment of patients with atopic dermatitis must be individualized. Guidelines for treatment include identification and avoidance of contact with the offending agents; elimination of inflammatory disorders and infections; prescription of topical corticosteroids and nonsteroidal anti-inflammatory agents; preservation and restoration of the stratum corneum layer; and prescription of antipruritic agents, oral antibiotics, and oral immunosuppressants for severely affected patients (Fonacier et al., 2015; Habif, 2016).

Itching can be decreased by wearing cotton fabrics; washing with a mild detergent; humidifying dry heat in winter; maintaining room temperature at 20° to 22.2°C (68° to 72°F); using antihistamines such as diphenhydramine; and avoiding animals, dust, sprays, and perfumes. Keeping the skin moisturized with daily baths to hydrate the skin and the use of topical skin moisturizers is encouraged. Topical corticosteroids are used to prevent inflammation, and any infection is treated with antibiotics to eliminate *Staphylococcus aureus* when indicated (Fonacier et al., 2015; Habif, 2016).

The use of immunosuppressive agents, such as cyclosporine (Neoral, Sandimmune), tacrolimus (Prograf, Protopic), and pimecrolimus (Elidel), may be effective in inhibiting T cells and mast cells involved in atopic dermatitis (Fonacier et al., 2015; Habif, 2016).

Research is needed to assess the effectiveness and the adverse side effects of medications used to treat atopic dermatitis.

Nursing Management

Patients who experience atopic dermatitis and their families require assistance and support from the nurse to cope with the disorder. The symptoms are often disturbing to the patient and disruptive to the family. The appearance of the skin may affect the patient's self-esteem and their willingness to interact with others. Instructions and counselling about strategies to incorporate preventive measures and treatments into the lifestyle of the family may be helpful.

The patient and family need to be aware of signs of secondary infection and of the need to seek treatment if infection occurs. The nurse also educates the patient and family about the side effects of medications used in treatment.

Dermatitis Medicamentosa (Drug Reactions)

Dermatitis medicamentosa, a type I hypersensitivity disorder, is the term applied to skin rashes associated with certain medications. Although people react differently to each medication, certain medications tend to induce eruptions of similar types. This disorder is the leading cause of fatal anaphylaxis, comprising 43% of deaths from anaphylaxis. All routes of administration are potentially fatal, but drugs given parenterally incur the greatest risk. Cutaneous rashes are among the most common adverse reactions to medications and occur in approximately 2% to 3% of hospitalized patients (Habif, 2016; Rich et al., 2013).

In general, drug reactions appear suddenly with characteristics that are more intense than the somewhat similar eruptions of infectious origin, and, with the exception of bromide and the iodide rashes, disappear rapidly after the medication is withdrawn (Comerford, 2015). Rashes may be accompanied by systemic or generalized symptoms. On discovery of a medication allergy, patients are warned that they have a hypersensitivity to a particular medication and are advised not to take it again. Penicillin, cephalosporin, and sulfonamide antibiotics are most commonly implicated (Habif, 2016). Patients should carry information identifying the hypersensitivity with them at all times.

Skin eruptions related to medication therapy suggest more serious hypersensitivities. Frequent assessment and prompt reporting of the appearance of any eruptions are important so that early treatment can be initiated. Some cutaneous drug reactions may indicate involvement of other organs and are known as complex drug reactions. Patients who suspect that a new rash may be caused by a drug allergy (newly prescribed medications, especially antibiotics such as penicillin or sulfa medications) should stop taking the medication immediately and contact their prescribing clinician, who will determine whether the medication and the rash are related.

Urticaria and Angioneurotic Edema

Urticaria (hives) is a type I hypersensitive allergic reaction of the skin that is characterized by the sudden appearance of edematous, pink or red wheals of variable size from 2 to 4 mm, and general pruritus. They may involve any part of the body, including the mucous membranes (especially those of the mouth), the larynx (occasionally with serious respiratory complications), and the gastrointestinal tract. This is a common condition with approximately 10% to 20% of people having one episode during their lifetime. Urticaria is most commonly instigated by infections, allergic reaction to food, insect stings, and medications (American Osteopathic College of Dermatology, 2015).

Each hive remains for a few minutes to several hours before disappearing. They usually fade within 24 to 48 hours, but new lesions may be developing simultaneously at other skin sites (Bernstein, Lang, Khan, et al., 2014). The condition usually resolves in 3 weeks. However, if this sequence continues for longer than 6 weeks, the condition is called *chronic urticaria*.

Management of the condition includes eliminating the causative drug or food; avoiding the use of nonsteroidal anti-inflammatory drugs (NSAIDs); minimizing potential aggravators, including heat, stress, alcohol, and tight clothes; administering antihistamines, and possibly a short course of corticosteroids (Prednisone) (AAAAI, 2015; American Osteopathic College of Dermatology, 2015; Habif, 2016; Rich et al., 2013).

Angioneurotic edema (i.e., angioedema) involves the deeper layers of the skin, resulting in more diffuse swelling rather than the discrete lesions characteristic of hives. It is manifested by nonpruritis, brawny, nonpitting edema with well-defined margins and erythema similar to urticaria (Bernstein et al., 2014). Urticaria and angioedema often occur together (Habif, 2016).

The regions most often involved in angioedema are the lips, eyelids, cheeks, hands, feet, genitalia, and tongue; the mucous membranes of the larynx, bronchi, and gastrointestinal canal may also be affected, particularly in the hereditary type (see discussion in the following section). On occasion, this reaction covers the entire back. Swellings may appear suddenly, in a few seconds or minutes, or slowly in 1 or 2 hours. In the latter case, their appearance is often preceded by itching or burning sensations. Seldom does more than a single swelling appear at one time, although one may develop while another is disappearing. Infrequently, swelling recurs in the same region. Individual lesions usually resolve in 24 hours (AAAAI, 2015; Rich et al., 2013). On rare occasions, swelling may recur with remarkable regularity at intervals of 3 to 4 weeks.

Several frequently prescribed medications, such as angiotensin-converting enzyme inhibitors (captopril [Capoten]) and penicillin, may cause angioedema. The nurse needs to be aware of all medications the patient is taking and be alert to the potential of angioedema as a side effect.

Hereditary Angioedema

Hereditary angioedema is a rare, potentially life-threatening, autosomal dominant disorder (Cicardi & Zuraw, 2015). Although not an immunologic disorder in the usual sense, this condition is included because of its resemblance to allergic angioedema and because of the potential seriousness of the condition. Symptoms are due to edema of the skin, the respiratory tract, or the digestive tract. Attacks may be precipitated by trauma or may seem to occur spontaneously.

Clinical Manifestations

When skin is involved, the swelling is usually diffuse, does not itch, and is usually not accompanied by urticaria. Gastrointestinal edema may cause abdominal pain severe enough to be incapacitating. Typically, attacks last 2 to 4 days and resolve without intervention; however, attacks can occasionally affect the subcutaneous and submucosal tissues in the region of the upper airway and can be associated with respiratory obstruction and asphyxiation (Cicardi & Zuraw, 2015).

Medical Management

Attacks usually subside within 3 to 4 days, but during this time the patient should be observed carefully for signs of laryngeal obstruction, which may necessitate tracheostomy as a life-saving measure. Epinephrine, antihistamines, and corticosteroids are usually used in treatment, although their success is limited (Cicardi & Zuraw, 2015; Habif, 2016; Rich et al., 2013).

Cold Urticaria

Familial atypical cold urticaria (FACU) and acquired cold urticaria (ACU) are additional diseases within the spectrum of urticaria induced by temperature exposure. FACU is an autosomal dominant condition, inherited from one affected parent, and symptoms usually begin at birth within the first 6 months of life (Rich et al., 2013). ACU most frequently affects children and young adults (Habif, 2016; Rich et al., 2013).

Clinical Manifestations

Patients with FACU break out in hives (i.e., urticaria) when exposed to cold. The urticaria may be prompted by exposure to cold weather or cold water or after coming in contact with cold objects. Lesions occur within a few hours and usually subside in 2 days (Rich et al., 2013). Symptoms include fever, chills, conjunctiva infection, sweating, headache, and arthralgia. During the attack, the patient may develop leukocytosis, an increase in the erythrocyte sedimentation rate (ESR) and raised C-reactive protein levels (Ciccarelli, De Martinis, & Ginaldi, 2014).

Cold urticaria is diagnosed by physical testing. Ice cube provocation testing involves applying an ice cube to the skin of the forearm for 1 to 5 minutes. A positive test results in development of urticaria at the site in a patient with ACU. Clinical manifestations of FACU can be precipitated by the patient merely entering a 4°C (39°F) room.

Medical Management

Prevention involves avoidance of cold stimuli. Treatment involves bed rest, warmth, and corticosteroids to treat an acute attack (Ciccarelli et al., 2014).

All patients with any form of cold urticaria should carry an autoinjectable epinephrine device for emergency use because hives can progress to anaphylaxis.

Food Allergy

IgE-mediated food allergy, a type I hypersensitivity reaction, occurs in about 2% of the adult population; it is thought to occur in people who have a genetic predisposition combined with exposure to allergens early in life through the gastrointestinal or respiratory tract or nasal mucosa. More than 170 foods have been reported to cause IgE-mediated reactions (Sampson, Aceves, Brock, et al., 2014).

Almost any food can cause allergic symptoms. Any food can contain an allergen that results in anaphylaxis. The most common offenders are seafood (lobster, shrimp, crab, clams, fish), peanuts, tree nuts, berries, eggs, wheat, milk, and chocolate (Sampson et al., 2014). Peanut and tree nut (e.g., cashew, walnut) allergies are responsible for the most severe food allergy reactions. There is insufficient evidence that maternal diet during pregnancy or lactation affects the development of food allergies later in life (AAAAI, 2015; NIAID, 2013; Sampson et al., 2014).

One of the dangers of food allergens is that they may be hidden in other foods and not apparent to people who are susceptible to the allergen. For example, peanuts and peanut butter are often used in salad dressings and in Asian, African, and Mexican cooking and may result in severe allergic reactions, including anaphylaxis. Previous contamination of equipment with allergens (e.g., peanuts) during preparation of another food product (e.g., chocolate cake) is enough to produce anaphylaxis in people with severe allergy (Fleischer, Sicherer, Greenhawt, et al., 2015).

Clinical Manifestations

Food allergy is the most common trigger for anaphylaxis. Symptoms occur in a few minutes to hours from exposure. The clinical symptoms are classic allergic symptoms (urticaria, dermatitis, wheezing, cough, laryngeal edema, angioedema) and gastrointestinal symptoms (itching; swelling of lips, tongue, and palate; abdominal pain; nausea; cramps; vomiting; and diarrhea) (NIAID, 2013; Sampson et al., 2015).

Assessment and Diagnostic Findings

A careful diagnostic workup is required in any patient with a suspected food hypersensitivity. Included are a detailed allergy history, a physical examination, and pertinent diagnostic tests. Skin prick testing is used to identify the source of symptoms and assists in identifying specific foods as causative agents.

Medical Management

Therapy for food hypersensitivity includes elimination of the food responsible for the hypersensitivity (see Chart 53-6). Pharmacologic therapy is necessary for patients who cannot avoid exposure to offending foods and for patients with multiple food sensitivities not responsive to avoidance measures. Medication therapy involves the use of H_1 blockers, antihistamines, adrenergic agents, corticosteroids, and cromolyn sodium. All patients with food allergies, especially seafood and nuts, should have an autoinjectable epinephrine (e.g., EpiPen or Auvi-Q) device prescribed. Another essential aspect of management is educating patients and family members about how to recognize and manage the early stages of an acute anaphylactic reaction (AAAAI, 2015; Campbell et al., 2014). Many food allergies disappear with time, particularly in children.

Nursing Management

In addition to participating in management of the allergic reaction, the nurse focuses on preventing future exposure of the patient to the food allergen. If a severe allergic or anaphylactic reaction to food allergens has occurred, the nurse must instruct the patient and family about strategies to prevent its recurrence. Patients' food allergies should be noted on their medical records, because there may be risk of allergic reactions not only to food but also to some medications containing similar substances (Sampson et al., 2014).

Latex Allergy

Latex allergy, the allergic reaction to natural rubber proteins, has been implicated in rhinitis, conjunctivitis, contact dermatitis, urticaria, asthma, and anaphylaxis. The prevalence has been steadily declining, possibly because of the use of nonpowdered latex and latex-free gloves (Mayo Foundation for Medical Education and Research, 2015).

CHART 53-6

HOME CARE CHECKLIST • Managing Food Allergies

At the completion of education, the patient, caregiver, or both will be able to:

- State the impact of food allergies on physiologic functioning, ADLs, IADLs, roles, relationships, and spirituality.
- Verbalize understanding of the need to maintain an allergen-free diet.
- Demonstrate reading of food labels to identify hidden allergens in food.
- Identify ways to manage an allergen-free diet when eating away from home.
- State the need to wear medical identification bracelet or necklace.
- List symptoms of food allergy.
- Demonstrate emergency administration of epinephrine.
- State the importance of replacing epinephrine when outdated.
- State the importance of prompt treatment of allergic reactions and health care follow-up.
- State how to reach primary provider with questions or complications.
- State time and date of follow-up appointments, testing.
- Verbalize ways to cope with stress successfully, plans for regular exercise, and rationale for obtaining adequate rest.
- Identify the need for health promotion, disease prevention, and screening activities.

ADLs, activities of daily living; IADLs, independent activities of daily living.

Natural rubber latex is derived from the sap of the rubber tree (*Hevea brasiliensis*). The conversion of the liquid rubber latex into a finished product entails the addition of more than 200 chemicals. The proteins in the natural rubber latex (Hevea proteins) or the various chemicals that are used in the manufacturing process are thought to be the source of the allergic reactions. Not all objects composed of latex have the same ability to stimulate an allergic response. For example, the antigenicity of latex gloves can vary widely depending on the manufacturing method used (AAAAI, 2015; Mayo Foundation for Medical Education and Research, 2015).

Those at risk include 8% to 17% of health care workers, patients with atopic allergies or multiple surgeries, people working in factories that manufacture latex products, females, and 67% of patients with spina bifida (Rich et al., 2013). Because more food handlers, hair dressers, automobile mechanics, and police wear latex gloves, they are at risk for latex allergy. Patients are at risk for anaphylactic reactions due to contact with latex during medical treatments, especially surgical procedures. Food that has been handled by people wearing latex gloves may stimulate an allergic response. Cross-reactions have been reported in people who are allergic to certain food products, such as kiwis, bananas, pineapples, mangos, passion fruits, avocados, and chestnuts (AAAAI, 2015; Mayo Foundation for Medical Education and Research, 2015).

Routes of exposure to latex products can be cutaneous, percutaneous, mucosal, parenteral, and aerosol. Allergic reactions are more likely with parenteral or mucous membrane exposure but can also occur with cutaneous contact or inhalation. The most frequent source of exposure is cutaneous, which usually involves the wearing of natural latex gloves. The powder used to facilitate putting on latex gloves can become a carrier of latex proteins from the gloves; when the gloves are put on or removed, the particles become airborne and can be inhaled or settle on skin, mucous membranes, or clothing. Mucosal exposure can occur from the use of latex condoms, catheters, airways, and nipples. Parenteral exposure can occur from intravenous lines or

TABLE 53-5 Selected Products Containing Natural Rubber Latex and Latex-free Alternatives

Products Containing Latex	Examples of Latex-safe Alternatives[a]
Hospital Environment	
Ace bandage (brown)	Ace bandage, white, all cotton
Adhesive bandages, Band-Aid dressing, Telfa	Cotton pads and plastic or silk tape, Active Strip (3M), Duoderm
Anesthesia equipment	Neoprene anesthesia kit (King)
Blood pressure cuff, tubing, and bladder	Clean Cuff, single-use nylon or vinyl blood pressure cuffs or wrap with stockinette or apply over clothing
Catheters	All-silicone or vinyl catheters
Catheter leg bag straps	Velcro straps
Crutch axillary pads and hand grips, tips	Cover with cloth, tape
ECG pads	Baxter, Red Dot 3M ECG pads
Elastic compression stockings	Kendall SCD stockings with stockinette
Gloves	Derma Prene, neoprene, polymer, or vinyl gloves
IV catheters	Jelko, Deseret IV catheters
IV rubber injection ports	Cover Y sites and ports; do not puncture. Use three-way stopcocks on plastic tubing.
Levin tube	Salem sump tube
Medication vials	Remove rubber stopper
Penrose drains	Jackson-Pratt, Zimmer Hemovac drains
Prepackaged enema kits	Theravac, Fleet Ready-to-Use
Pulse oximeters	Noninoximeters
Resuscitation bags	Laerdal, Puritan Bennett, *certain* Ambu
Stethoscope tubing	PVC tubing; cover with latex-free stockinette
Suction tubing	PVC (Davol, Laerdal)
Syringes—single use (Monoject, BD)	Terumo syringes, Abbott PCA Abboject
Tapes	Dermicel, Micropore
Theraband	New Thera-band Exercisers, plastic tubing
Thermometer probes	Diatec probe covers
Tourniquets	X-Tourn straps (Avcor)
Home Environment	
Balloons	Mylar balloons
Condoms, diaphragms	Polyurethane products, Durex Avanti and Reality products (female condom)
Diapers, incontinence pads	Huggies, Always, *some* Attends
Feminine hygiene pad	Kimberly-Clark products
Wheelchair cushions	ROHO cushions, Sof Care bed/chair cushions

[a]Confirmation is essential to verify that all items are latex-free before using, especially if risk of latex allergy is present.

ECG, electrocardiogram; IV, intravenous; PVC, polyvinyl chloride.

Adapted from American Academy of Allergy, Asthma, and Immunology (AAAAI). (2015). *Anaphylaxis overview*. Retrieved November 11, 2015, from www.aaaai.org; Australasian Society of Clinical Immunology and Allergy (ASCIA). (2015). *Immunotherapy for treatment of allergy*. Retrieved November 15, 2015, from allergy.org.au; Campbell, R. L., Li, J., Nicklas, R. A., et al. (2014). Emergency department diagnosis and treatment of anaphylaxis: A practice parameter. Annals of Allergy Asthma & Immunology, *113*, 599–608; Centers for Disease Control and Prevention (CDC). (2014). *Latex allergy: A prevention guide*. Retrieved November 20, 2015, from www.cdc.gov/niosh/docs/98-113/default.html; Mayo Foundation for Medical Education and Research. (2015). *Diseases and conditions: Latex allergy*. Retrieved November 20, 2015, from www.mayoclinic.org/diseases-conditions/latex-allergy/basics/definition/CON-20024233 hemodialysis equipment. In addition to latex-derived medical devices, many household items also contain latex. Examples of medical and household items containing latex and a list of alternative products are found in Table 53-5. It is estimated that more than 40,000 medical devices and nonmedical products contain latex. Chemical additives used in the manufacture of nonlatex gloves and other items have been associated with allergic symptoms, although these otherwise have a low potential to stimulate an allergic response (AAAAI, 2015; Mayo Foundation for Medical Education and Research, 2015).

Clinical Manifestations

Many different types of reactions to latex are possible (see Table 53-6). Irritant contact dermatitis, a nonimmunologic response, may be caused by mechanical skin irritation or an alkaline pH associated with latex gloves. Common symptoms of irritant dermatitis include erythema and pruritus. These symptoms can be eliminated by changing the brand of gloves or by using powder-free gloves. The use of hand lotion before donning latex gloves can worsen the symptoms, because lotions may leach latex proteins from the gloves, thus increasing skin exposure and the risk of developing true allergic reactions (Mayo Foundation for Medical Education and Research, 2015).

Delayed hypersensitivity to latex, a type IV reaction mediated by T cells in the immune system, is localized to the area of exposure and is characterized by symptoms of contact dermatitis, including vesicular skin lesions, papules, pruritus, edema, erythema, and crusting and thickening of the skin. These symptoms usually appear on the

TABLE 53-6 Types of Reactions to Latex

Type of Reaction	Cause	Signs/Symptoms	Treatment
Irritant contact dermatitis	Damage to skin because of irritation and loss of epidermoid skin layer; not an allergic reaction. Can be caused by excessive use of soaps and cleansers, repeated handwashing, inadequate hand drying, mechanical irritation (e.g., sweating, rubbing inside powdered gloves), exposure to chemicals added during the manufacturing of gloves, and alkaline pH of powdered gloves. Reaction may occur with first exposure, is usually benign, and is not life-threatening.	Acute: Redness, edema, burning, discomfort, itching Chronic: Dry, thickened, cracked skin	Referral for diagnostic testing Avoidance of exposure to irritant Thorough washing and drying of hands Use of powder-free gloves with more frequent changes of gloves Changing glove types Use of water- or silicone-based moisturizing creams, lotions, or topical barrier agents Avoidance of oil- or petroleum-based skin agents with latex products, because they cause breakdown of the latex product
Allergic contact dermatitis	Delayed hypersensitivity (type IV) reaction. Usually affects only area in contact with latex; reaction is usually to chemical additives used in the manufacturing process rather than to latex itself. Cause of reaction is T cell–mediated sensitization to additives of latex. Reaction is not life-threatening and is far more common than a type I reaction. Slow onset; occurs 18–24 hours after exposure. Resolves within 3–4 days after exposure. More severe reactions may occur with subsequent exposures.	Pruritus, erythema, swelling, crusty thickened skin, blisters, other skin lesions	Referral for diagnosis (patch tests) and treatment Thorough washing and drying of hands Use of water- or silicone-based moisturizing creams, lotions, or topical barrier agents Avoidance of oil- or petroleum-based products unless they are latex compatible Avoidance of identified causative agent, because continued exposure to latex products in presence of breaks in skin may contribute to latex protein sensitization
Latex allergy	Type I IgE-mediated immediate hypersensitivity to plant proteins in natural rubber latex. In sensitized people, antilatex IgE antibody stimulates mast cell proliferation and basophil histamine release. Exposure can be through contact with the skin, mucous membranes, or internal tissues, or through inhalation of traces of powder from latex gloves. Severe reactions usually occur shortly after parenteral or mucous membrane exposure. People with any type I reaction to latex are at high risk for anaphylaxis. Local swelling, redness, edema, itching, and systemic reactions, including anaphylaxis, occur within minutes after exposure.	Rhinitis, flushing, conjunctivitis, urticaria, laryngeal edema, bronchospasm, asthma, severe vasodilation angioedema, anaphylaxis, cardiovascular collapse, death	Immediate treatment of reaction with epinephrine, fluids, vasopressors, and corticosteroids, and airway and ventilator support, with close monitoring for recurrence for the next 12–14 hours Prompt referral for diagnostic evaluation Treatment and diagnostic evaluation in latex-free environment Assessment of all patients for symptoms of latex allergy Teaching of patients and family members about the disorder and about the importance of preventing future reactions by avoiding latex (e.g., wearing medical alert bracelet, carrying EpiPen)

back of the hands. This reaction is thought to be caused by chemicals that are used in the manufacturing of latex products. It is the most common allergic reaction to latex. Although usually not life threatening, delayed hypersensitivity reactions often require major changes in the patient's home and work environment to avoid further exposure. People who are sensitized to latex are at increased risk for development of type I allergic reactions (AAAAI, 2015; Mayo Foundation for Medical Education and Research, 2015).

Immediate hypersensitivity, a type I allergic reaction, is mediated by the IgE mast cell system (Abbas et al., 2014). Symptoms can include rhinitis, conjunctivitis, asthma, and anaphylaxis. Clinical manifestations have a rapid onset and can include urticaria, wheezing, dyspnea, laryngeal edema, bronchospasm, tachycardia, angioedema, hypotension, and cardiac arrest.

Localized itching, erythema, or local urticaria within minutes after exposure to latex are often the initial symptoms. Symptoms of subsequent reactions can include generalized urticaria, angioedema, rhinitis, conjunctivitis, asthma, and anaphylactic shock minutes after dermal or mucosal exposure to latex. An increasing number of patients who are allergic to latex experience severe reactions characterized by generalized urticaria, bronchospasm, and hypotension.

Assessment and Diagnostic Findings

The diagnosis of latex allergy is based on the history and diagnostic test results (Mayo Foundation for Medical Education and Research, 2015). Sensitization is detected by skin testing, serum-specific IgE, EIA, or ELISA or the level of Hevea latex-specific IgE antibody in the serum. Testing for the chemicals found in the rubber production that makes latex is performed using the patch test. Skin patch testing is the preferred method for patients with contact allergies. The TRUE test and other skin tests should be performed only by clinicians who have expertise in their administration and interpretation and who have the necessary equipment available to treat local or systemic allergic reactions to the reagent (Habif, 2016).

Medical Management

The best treatment available for latex allergy is the avoidance of latex-based products, although avoidance is often difficult because of the widespread use of such products. Patients who have experienced an anaphylactic reaction to latex should be instructed to wear medical identification. Antihistamines and an emergency kit containing epinephrine should be provided to these patients, along with instructions about emergency management of latex allergy symptoms. Patients must be counselled to notify all health care workers as well as local paramedic and ambulance companies about their allergy. Warning labels can be attached to car windows to alert police and paramedics about the driver's or passenger's latex allergy in case of a motor vehicle crash. People with latex allergy should be provided with a list of alternative products and referred to local support groups; they are also urged to carry their own supply of nonlatex gloves.

People with type I latex sensitivity may be unable to continue to work if a latex-free work environment is not possible. This may occur with surgeons, dentists, operating room personnel, or intensive care nurses. Occupational implications for employees with type IV latex sensitivity are usually easier to manage by changing to nonlatex gloves and avoiding direct contact with latex-based medical equipment. Although latex-specific immunotherapy has been attempted, this method of treatment remains experimental.

Nursing Management

The nurse can assume a pivotal role in the management of latex allergies in both patients and staff. All patients should be asked about latex allergy, although special attention should be given to those at particularly high risk (e.g., patients with spina bifida, patients who have undergone multiple surgical procedures). Every time an invasive procedure must be performed, the nurse should consider the possibility of latex allergies. Nurses working in operating rooms, intensive care units, endoscopy units, and EDs need to pay particular attention to latex allergy. Refer to Chart 53-1 for an allergy assessment form.

Although the type I reaction is the most significant of the reactions to latex, care must be taken in the presence of irritant contact dermatitis and delayed hypersensitivity reaction to avoid further exposure of the person to latex. Patients with latex allergy are advised to notify their health care providers and to wear a medical identification. Patients must be knowledgeable about what products contain latex and what products are safe, nonlatex alternatives. They must also become knowledgeable about signs and symptoms of latex allergy and emergency treatment and self-injection of epinephrine in case of an allergic reaction.

Nurses can be instrumental in establishing and participating in multidisciplinary committees to address latex allergy and to promote a latex-free environment. Latex allergy protocols and education of staff about latex allergy and precautions are important strategies to reduce this growing problem and to ensure assessment and prompt treatment of those affected by allergy to latex.

Critical Thinking Exercises

1 **pq** You are the nurse working in a preoperative holding area. A 38-year-old patient tells you that she has had a reaction to latex in the past. What are the immediate nursing priorities in providing care to this patient? What assessment data are needed to determine if this patient has a latex allergy?

2 **ebp** A 47-year-old mail carrier presents to the ED complaining of difficulty breathing after being stung by a bee. He states that this has happened two other times in his recent past and seems to be worse each time. What are the priority interventions? What medication is the drug of choice for severe allergic reactions, and how is it given? Describe the strength of the evidence and criteria used to assess its strength.

REFERENCES AND SELECTED READINGS

Books

Abbas, A. K., Lichtman, A. H., & Pillai, S. (2014). *Basic immunology: Functions and disorders of the immune system* (4th ed.). Philadelphia, PA: Elsevier Health Sciences.

Arcangelo, V. P., & Peterson, A. (Eds.). (2013). *Pharmacotherapeutics for advanced practice: A practical approach* (3rd ed.). Philadelphia, PA: Lippincott Williams & Wilkins.

Comerford, K. C. (2015). *Nursing 2015 drug handbook*. Philadelphia, PA: Wolters Kluwer.

Frandsen, G., & Pennington, S. (2014). *Abrams's clinical drug therapy* (10th ed.). Philadelphia, PA: Wolters Kluwer Health/Lippincott Williams & Wilkins.

Grossman, S. C., & Porth, C. M. (2014). *Porth's pathophysiology: Concepts of altered health states* (9th ed.). Philadelphia, PA: Lippincott Williams & Wilkins.

Habif, T. (2016). *Clinical dermatology: A color guide to diagnosis and therapy* (6th ed.). St Louis, MO: Elsevier.

Hodgson, B., & Kizior, R. (2014). *Saunders nursing drug book*. St Louis, MO: Elsevier.

Katzung, B., & Trevor, A. (2015). *Basic & clinical pharmacology* (13th ed.). New York: McGraw-Hill Education.

Pagana, K., & Pagana, T. (2013). *Mosby's diagnostic & laboratory test reference* (11th ed.). St Louis, MO: Elsevier.

Rich, R. R., Fleisher, T., Shearer, W., et al. (2013). *Clinical immunology* (4th ed.). St Louis, MO: Elsevier.

Journals and Electronic Documents

Albin, S., & Agarwal, S. (2014). Prevalence and characteristics of reported penicillin allergy in an urban outpatient population. *Allergy and Asthma Proceedings*, *35*(6), 489–494.

American Academy of Allergy, Asthma, and Immunology (AAAAI). (2015). Anaphylaxis overview. Retrieved November 15, 2015, from www.aaaai.org

American Osteopathic College of Dermatology. (2015). Urticaria. Retrieved November 15, 2015, from www.aocd.org

Australasian Society of Clinical Immunology and Allergy (ASCIA). (2015). Immunotherapy for treatment of allergy. Retrieved November 15, 2015, from allergy.org.au

Baran, H., Ozcan, K., Selcuk, A., et al. (2014). Allergic rhinitis and its impact on asthma classification correlations. *The Journal of Laryngology & Otology*, *128*, 431–437.

Bernstein, J., Lang, D., Khan, D., et al. (2014). The diagnosis and management of acute and chronic urticaria: 2014 update. *Journal of Allergy and Clinical Immunology in Practice*, *133*(5), 1270–1277.

Bleier, B. (2015). Nasal/sinus irrigation. Retrieved November 15, 2015, from care.american-rhinologic.org

Braido, F., Sclifò, F., Ferrando, M., et al. (2014). New therapies for allergic rhinitis. *Current Allergy and Asthma Reports*, *14*(4), 1–8.

Burks, A. (2008). Peanut allergy. *Lancet*, *371*(3), 1538–1546.

Campbell, R. L., Li, J., Nicklas, R. A., et al. (2014). Emergency department diagnosis and treatment of anaphylaxis: A practice parameter. *Annals of Allergy Asthma & Immunology*, *113*, 599–608.

Cicardi, M., & Zuraw, B. (2015). Hereditary angioedema: Treatment of acute attacks. Retrieved November 15, 2015, from www.uptodate.com/contents/hereditary-angioedema-treatment-of-acute-attacks

Ciccarelli, F., De Martinis, M., & Ginaldi, L. (2014). An update on autoinflammatory diseases. *Current Medical Chemistry*, *21*(3), 261–269.

Fleischer, D., Sicherer, S., Greenhawt, M., et al. (2015). Consensus communication on early peanut introduction and the prevention of peanut allergy in high-risk infants. *Journal of Allergy and Immunology*, *136*(2), 258–261.

Fonacier, L., Bernstein, D., Pacheco, K., et al. (2015). Contact dermatitis: A practice parameter-update 2015. *Journal of Allergy and Clinical Immunology in Practice*, *3*, S1–S39.

Food Allergy Canada. (2018). *Anaphylaxis*. Retrieved from http://foodallergycanada.ca/about-allergies/anaphylaxis/

Hwang, P., & Patel, Z. (2015). Acute sinusitis and rhinosinusitis in adults: Treatment. Retrieved November 2015, from www.uptodate.co

Keith, P., Desrosiers, M., Laister, T., et al. (2012). The burden of allergic rhinitis (AR) in Canada: perspectives of physicians and patients. *Allergy, Asthma & Clinical Immunology*, *8*(7), https://doi.org/10.1186/1710-1492-8-7

Lehrer, E., Mullol, J., Agredo, F., et al. (2014). Management of chronic rhinitis in asthma patients: Is there still a debate. *Current Allergy and Asthma Report*, *14*(6), 1–6.

Link, M. S., Berkow, L. C., Kudenchuk, P. J., et al. (2015). Part 7: Adult advanced cardiovascular life support: 2015 American Heart Association Guidelines update for cardiopulmonary resuscitation and emergency cardiovascular care. *Circulation*, *132*(Suppl 2), S444–S464.

Ludman, S., & Boyle, R. (2015). Stinging insect allergy: Current perspectives on venom immunotherapy. *Journal of Allergy and Asthma*, *2015*(8), 75–86.

Mayo Foundation for Medical Education and Research. (2015). Diseases and conditions: Latex allergy. Retrieved November 20, 2015, from www.mayoclinic.org/diseases-conditions/latex-allergy/basics/definition/CON-20024233

National Institute of Allergy and Infectious Disease (NIAID). (2013). The national asthma education and prevention program. Retrieved November 20, 2015, from www.nhlbi.nih.gov/about/org/naepp/

Oppenheimer, J., Durham, S., Nelson, H., et al. (2014). *Allergy diagnostic testing*. Retrieved November 20, 2015, from www.worldallergy.org

Perez-Riverol, A., Justo-Jacomini, D., de Lima Zollner, R., et al. (2015). Facing hymenoptera venom allergy: From natural to recombinant allergens. *Toxins*, *7*(7), 2551–2570.

Portnoy, J. (2015). World allergy. Retrieved November 20, 2015, from www.worldallergy.org

Rosenfeld, R., Piccirillo, J. F., Chandrasekhar, S., et al. (2015). Clinical practice guideline (Update): Adult sinusitis. *Otolaryngology-Head and Neck Surgery*, *152*(2S), S1–S39.

Sampson, H., Aceves, S., Brock, S., et al. (2014). Food allergy: A practice parameter update—2014. *Journal of Allergy and Clinical Immunology*, *134*(5), 1025.e1–e43.

Senti, G., von Moos, S., Graf, N., et al. (2015). Determinants of efficacy and safety in epicutaneous allergen immunotherapy: Summary of three clinical trials. *European Journal of Allergy and Clinical Immunology*, *70*(6), 707–710.

Sheikh, J. (2015). Allergic rhinitis treatment and management. Retrieved November 15, 2015, from emedicine.medscape.com/article/134825-treatment

Resources

Asthma Society of Canada: http://www.asthma.ca.

Canadian Allergy, Asthma and Immunology Foundation: http://www.allergyfoundation.ca.

Canadian Society of Allergy and Clinical Immunology: http://csaci.ca.

Food Allergy Canada: http://foodallergycanada.ca/

54 Assessment and Management of Patients With Hematologic Disorders

Adapted by Stephanie Zettel

Learning Objectives

On completion of this chapter, the learner will be able to:

1. Describe the process of hematopoiesis.
2. Specify the proper techniques utilized to perform a comprehensive physical assessment of hematologic function.
3. Describe the processes involved in maintaining hemostasis.
4. Differentiate between the hypoproliferative and the hemolytic anemias and compare and contrast the physiologic mechanisms, clinical manifestations, medical management, and nursing interventions for each.
5. Discuss the diverse etiologies and management of secondary polycythemias.
6. Use the nursing process as a framework for care of patients with anemia.
7. Compare the leukemias in terms of their incidence, physiologic alterations, clinical manifestations, management, and prognosis.
8. Use the nursing process as a framework for care of patients with acute leukemia.
9. Use the nursing process as a framework for care of patients with lymphoma and multiple myeloma.
10. Describe the processes involved in neutropenia and lymphopenia and the general principles of medical and nursing management of patients with these disorders.
11. Use the nursing process as a framework for care of patients with bleeding and thrombotic disorders.
12. Identify therapies for blood disorders, including the nursing implications for the administration of blood components.

Unlike many other body systems, the hematologic system involves the entire human body. Patients with hematologic disorders often have significant abnormalities in blood tests but few or no symptoms. Therefore, the nurse must have a good understanding of the pathophysiology of the patient's condition and the ability to make a thorough assessment that relies heavily on the interpretation of laboratory tests. It is equally important for the nurse to anticipate potential patient needs and to target nursing interventions accordingly. Because it is so important to the understanding of most hematologic diseases, a basic appreciation of blood cells and bone marrow function is necessary.

HEMATOLOGIC ASSESSMENT

Anatomic and Physiologic Overview

The hematologic system consists of the blood and the sites where blood is produced, including the bone marrow and the **reticuloendothelial system** (RES). Blood is a specialized organ that differs from other organs in that it exists in a fluid state. Blood is composed of **plasma** and various types of cells. Plasma is the fluid portion of blood; it contains various proteins, such as albumin, globulin, **fibrinogen**, and other factors necessary for clotting, as well as electrolytes, waste

Glossary

absolute neutrophil count: a calculation of the number of circulating neutrophils, derived from the total white blood cells (WBCs) and the percentage of neutrophils counted in a microscope's visual field

anemia: decreased red blood cell (RBC) count

anergy: diminished reactivity to antigens (transient or complete)

angiogenesis: formation of new blood vessels

angular cheilosis: cracking sore at corner of mouth

aplasia: lack of cellular development (e.g., of cells within the bone marrow)

band cell: slightly immature neutrophil

blast cell: primitive WBC

cytokines: hormones produced by leukocytes that are vital to regulation of hematopoiesis, apoptosis, and immune responses

D-dimer: test to measure fibrin breakdown; considered more specific than fibrin degradation products in the diagnosis of disseminated intravascular coagulation

differentiation: development of functions and characteristics that are different from those of the parent stem cell

erythrocyte: see red blood cell

erythrocyte sedimentation rate: laboratory test that measures the rate of settling of RBCs; elevation is indicative of inflammation; also called the "sed rate"

erythroid cells: any cell that is or will become a mature RBC

erythropoiesis: process of formation of RBCs

erythropoietin: hormone produced primarily by the kidney; necessary for erythropoiesis

fibrin: filamentous protein; basis of thrombus and blood clot

fibrinogen: protein converted into fibrin to form thrombus and clot

fibrinolysis: process of breakdown of fibrin clot

granulocyte: granulated WBC (neutrophil, eosinophil, basophil); sometimes used synonymously with neutrophil

haptoglobin: blood protein synthesized by liver; binds free hemoglobin released from erythrocytes, which is then removed by the reticuloendothelial system

hematocrit: percentage of total blood volume consisting of RBCs

hematopoiesis: complex process of the formation and maturation of blood cells

hemoglobin: iron-containing protein of RBCs; delivers oxygen to tissues

hemolysis: destruction of RBCs; can occur within or outside of the vasculature

hemosiderin: iron-containing pigment derived from breakdown of hemoglobin

hemostasis: intricate balance between clot formation and clot dissolution

histiocytes: cells present in all loose connective tissue, capable of phagocytosis

hypochromia: pallor within the RBC caused by decreased hemoglobin content

left shift, or shift to the left: increased release of immature forms of WBCs from the bone marrow in response to need

leukemia: uncontrolled proliferation of WBCs, often immature

leukocyte: see white blood cell

leukopenia: less-than-normal amount of WBCs in circulation

lymphocyte: form of WBC involved in immune functions

lymphoid: pertaining to lymphocytes

lysis: destruction of cells

macrophage: reticuloendothelial cells capable of phagocytosis

microcytosis: smaller-than-normal RBCs

monocyte: large WBC that becomes a macrophage when it leaves the circulation and moves into body tissues

myeloid: pertaining to nonlymphoid blood cells that differentiate into RBCs, platelets, macrophages, mast cells, and various WBCs

myelopoiesis: formation and maturation of cells derived from myeloid stem cell

neutropenia: lower-than-normal number of neutrophils

neutrophil: fully mature WBC capable of phagocytosis; primary defense against bacterial infection

normochromic: normal RBC colour, indicating normal amount of hemoglobin

normocytic: normal size of RBC

nucleated RBC: immature form of RBC; portion of nucleus remains within the RBC

oxyhemoglobin: combined form of oxygen and hemoglobin; found in arterial blood

pancytopenia: abnormal decrease in WBCs, RBCs, and platelets

petechiae: tiny capillary hemorrhages

phagocytosis: process of cellular ingestion and digestion of foreign bodies

plasma: liquid portion of blood

plasminogen: protein converted to plasmin to dissolve thrombi and clots

platelet: thrombocyte; a cellular component of blood involved in blood coagulation

polycythemia: excess RBCs

red blood cell (RBC): erythrocyte; a cellular component of blood involved in the transport of oxygen and carbon dioxide

reticulocytes: slightly immature RBCs, usually only 1% of total circulating RBCs

reticuloendothelial system (RES): complex system of cells throughout body capable of phagocytosis

serum: portion of blood remaining after coagulation occurs

stem cell: primitive cell, capable of self-replication and differentiation into myeloid or lymphoid stem cell

thrombin: enzyme necessary to convert fibrinogen into fibrin clot

thrombocyte: see platelet

thrombocytopenia: lower-than-normal platelet count

thrombocytosis: higher-than-normal platelet count

white blood cell (WBC): leukocyte; one of several cellular components of blood involved in defense of the body; subtypes include neutrophils, eosinophils, basophils, monocytes, and lymphocytes

TABLE 54-1 Blood Cells

Cell Type	Major Function
WBC (Leukocyte)	Fights infection
Neutrophil	Essential in preventing or limiting bacterial infection via phagocytosis
Monocyte	Enters tissue as macrophage; highly phagocytic, especially against fungus; immune surveillance
Eosinophil	Involved in allergic reactions (neutralizes histamine); digests foreign proteins
Basophil	Contains histamine; integral part of hypersensitivity reactions
Lymphocyte	Integral component of immune system
T lymphocyte	Responsible for cell-mediated immunity; recognizes material as "foreign" (surveillance system)
B lymphocyte	Responsible for humoral immunity; many mature into plasma cells to form antibodies
Plasma cell	Secretes immunoglobulin (antibody); most mature form of B lymphocyte
RBC (Erythrocyte)	Carries hemoglobin to provide oxygen to tissues; average lifespan is 120 days
Platelet (Thrombocyte)	Fragment of megakaryocyte; provides basis for coagulation to occur; maintains hemostasis; average lifespan is 10 days

WBC, white blood cell; RBC, red blood cell.

products, and nutrients. About 55% of blood volume is plasma.

Blood

The cellular component of blood consists of three primary cell types (Table 54-1): **erythrocytes** (red blood cells [RBCs], red cells), **leukocytes** (**white blood cells [WBCs]**), and **thrombocytes** (**platelets**). These cellular components of blood normally make up 40% to 45% of the blood volume. Because most blood cells have a short lifespan, the need for the body to replenish its supply of cells is continuous; this process is termed **hematopoiesis**. The primary site for hematopoiesis is the bone marrow. During embryonic development and in other conditions, the liver and spleen may also be involved.

Under normal conditions, the adult bone marrow produces about 175 billion erythrocytes, 70 billion **neutrophils** (a mature type of WBC), and 175 billion platelets each day. When the body needs more blood cells, as in infection (when neutrophils are needed to fight the invading pathogen) or in bleeding (when more RBCs are required), the marrow increases its production of the cells required. Thus, under normal conditions, the marrow responds to increased demand and releases adequate numbers of cells into the circulation.

Blood makes up approximately 7% to 10% of the normal body weight and amounts to 5 to 6 L of volume. Circulating through the vascular system and serving as a link between body organs, blood carries oxygen absorbed from the lungs and nutrients absorbed from the gastrointestinal (GI) tract to the body cells for cellular metabolism. Blood also carries hormones, antibodies, and other substances to their sites of action or use. In addition, blood carries waste products produced by cellular metabolism to the lungs, skin, liver, and kidneys, where they are transformed and eliminated from the body.

The body has developed an elaborate mechanism through the hematologic system by which it protects itself from trauma. An intricate clotting mechanism is activated when necessary to seal any leak in the blood vessels. Excessive clotting is equally dangerous, because thrombi can obstruct blood flow to vital tissues. Similarly, the body has a fibrinolytic mechanism that eventually dissolves clots (thrombi) formed within blood vessels. The balance between these two systems, clot (thrombus) formation and clot dissolution or **fibrinolysis**, is called **hemostasis**.

Bone Marrow

The bone marrow is the site of hematopoiesis, or blood cell formation (Fig. 54-1). In adults, blood cell formation is usually limited to the pelvis, ribs, vertebrae, and sternum. Marrow is one of the largest organs of the body, making up 4% to 5% of total body weight. It consists of islands of cellular components (red marrow) separated by fat (yellow marrow). As people age, the proportion of active marrow is gradually replaced by fat; however, in healthy adults, the fat can again be replaced by active marrow when more blood cell production is required. In adults with disease that causes marrow destruction, fibrosis, or scarring, the liver and spleen can also resume production of blood cells by a process known as extramedullary hematopoiesis.

The marrow is highly vascular. Primitive cells called **stem cells** exist within marrow and have the ability to self-replicate, thereby ensuring a continuous supply of stem cells throughout the life cycle. Stem cells can also begin a process of **differentiation** into either **myeloid** or **lymphoid** stem cells with appropriate stimulation. These stem cells are further committed to produce specific types of blood cells; lymphoid stem cells produce either T or B **lymphocytes**, and myeloid stem cells differentiate into three broad cell types: erythrocytes, leukocytes, and platelets. Thus, with the exception of lymphocytes, all blood cells are derived from myeloid stem cells. A defect in a myeloid stem cell can cause problems with erythrocyte, leukocyte, and platelet production.

Blood Cells

Erythrocytes (Red Blood Cells)

The normal erythrocyte is a biconcave disk that resembles a soft ball compressed between two fingers (Fig. 54-2). It has a diameter of about 8 μm and is so flexible that it can pass easily through capillaries that may be as small as 2.8 μm in diameter. The membrane of the red cell is very thin so that gases, such as oxygen and carbon dioxide, can easily diffuse across it; the disk shape provides a large surface area that facilitates the absorption and release of oxygen molecules.

Mature erythrocytes consist primarily of **hemoglobin**, which contains iron and makes up 95% of the cell mass. Mature erythrocytes have no nuclei, and they have many fewer metabolic enzymes than do most other cells. The presence of a large amount of hemoglobin enables the red cell to perform its principal function; the transport of oxygen between the lungs and tissues. Occasionally the marrow releases slightly immature forms of erythrocytes,

Physiology/Pathophysiology

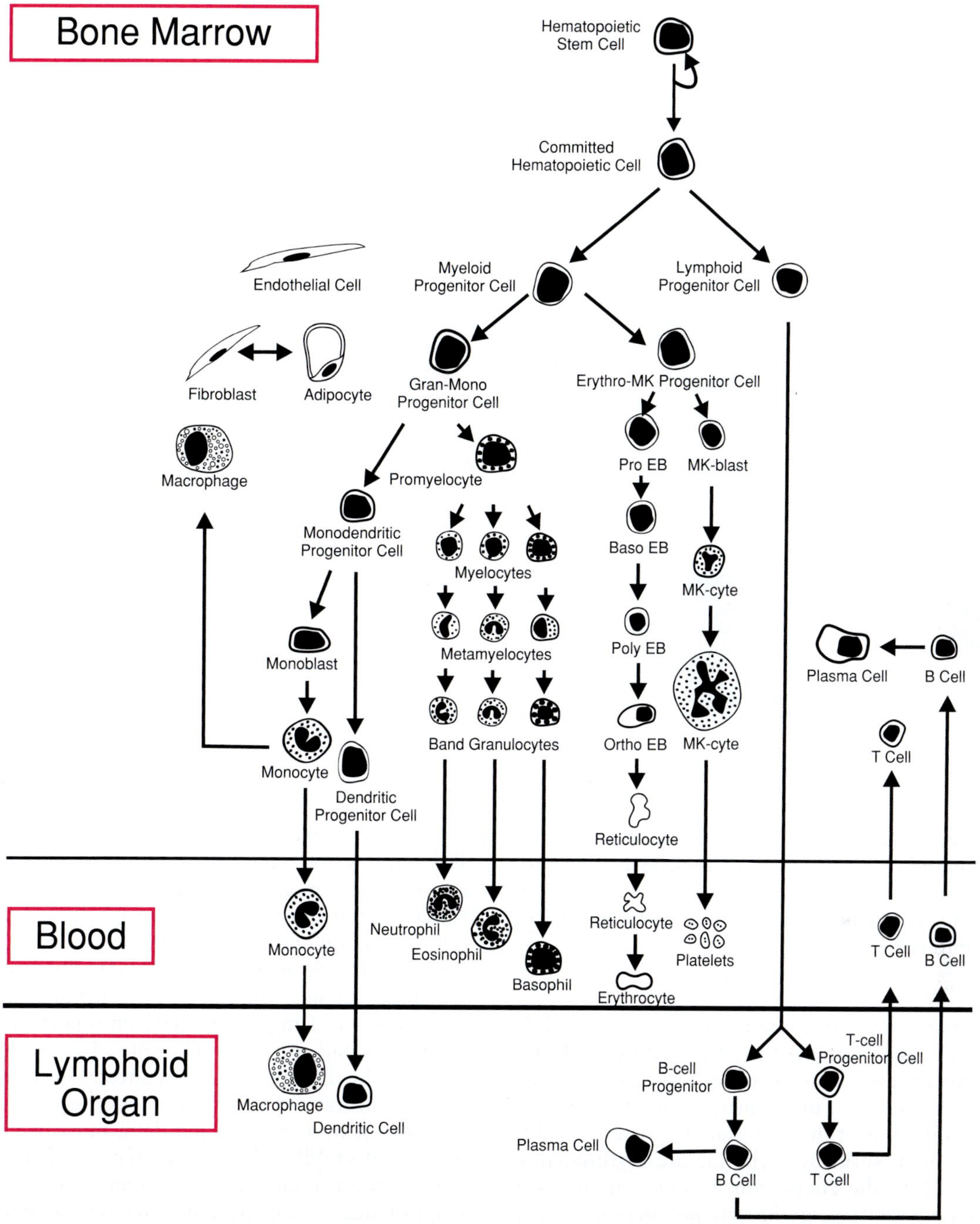

FIGURE 54-1. Hematopoiesis. Uncommitted (pluripotent) stem cells can differentiate into myeloid or lymphoid stem cells. These stem cells then undergo a complex process of differentiation and maturation into normal cells that are released into the circulation. The myeloid stem cell is responsible not only for all non-lymphoid white blood cells but also for the production of red blood cells (RBCs) and platelets. Each step of the differentiation process depends in part on the presence of specific growth factors for each cell type. When the stem cells are dysfunctional, they may respond inadequately to the need for more cells, or they may respond excessively, sometimes uncontrollably, as in leukemia.

called **reticulocytes**, into the circulation. This occurs as a normal response to an increased demand for erythrocytes (as in bleeding) or in some disease states.

The oxygen-carrying hemoglobin molecule is made up of four subunits, each containing a heme portion attached to a globin chain. Iron is present in the heme component of the molecule. An important property of heme is its ability to bind to oxygen loosely and reversibly. Oxygen readily binds to hemoglobin in the lungs and is carried as **oxyhemoglobin** in arterial blood. Oxyhemoglobin is a brighter red than hemoglobin that does not contain oxygen (reduced hemoglobin); thus, arterial blood is a brighter red than venous blood. The oxygen readily dissociates (detaches) from hemoglobin in the tissues, where

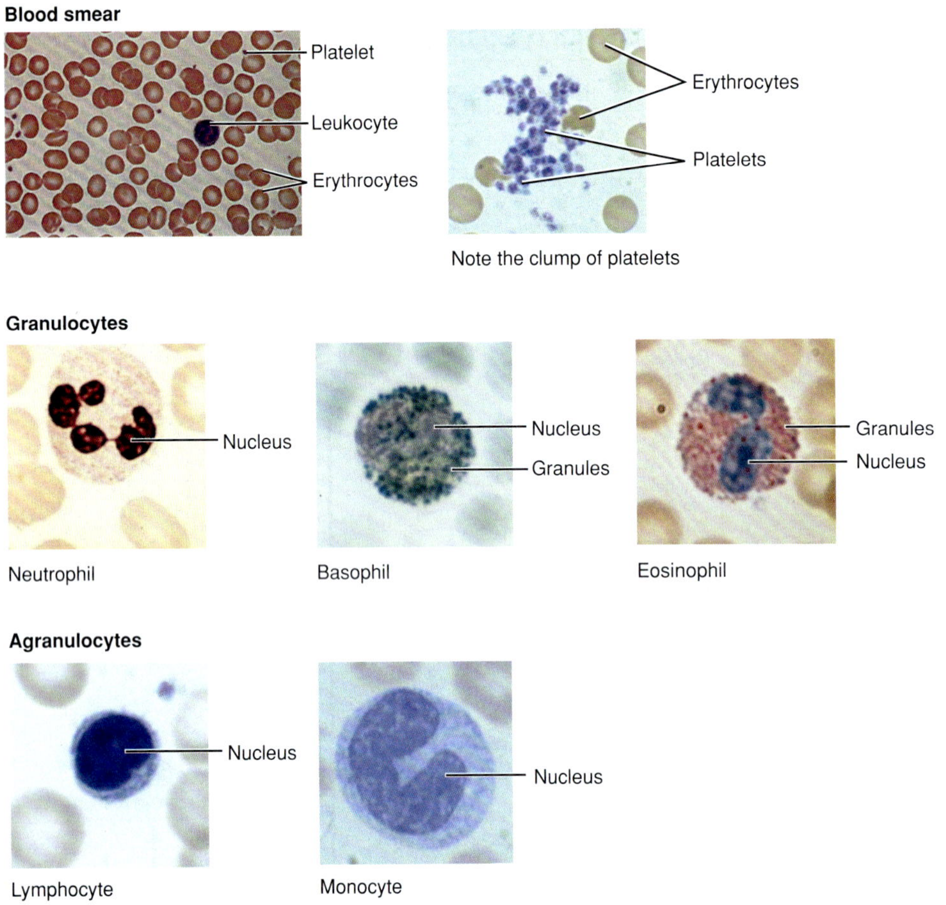

FIGURE 54-2. Normal types of blood cells. (From Cohen, B. J. (2005). *Memmler's the human body in health and disease* (10th ed.). Philadelphia, PA: Lippincott Williams & Wilkins.)

the oxygen is needed for cellular metabolism. In venous blood, hemoglobin combines with hydrogen ions produced by cellular metabolism and also acts as a buffer for excessive acid. Whole blood normally contains about 15 g of hemoglobin per 100 mL of blood.

Erythropoiesis

Erythroblasts arise from the primitive myeloid stem cells in bone marrow. The erythroblast is an immature nucleated cell that gradually loses its nucleus. At this stage, the cell is known as a reticulocyte. Further maturation into an erythrocyte entails the loss of the dark-staining material within the cell and slight shrinkage. The mature erythrocyte is then released into the circulation. Under conditions of rapid **erythropoiesis** (i.e., erythrocyte production), reticulocytes and other immature cells (e.g., **nucleated RBCs**) may be released prematurely into the circulation. This is often seen when the liver or spleen takes over as the site of erythropoiesis and more nucleated red cells appear within the circulation.

Differentiation of the primitive myeloid stem cell into an erythroblast is stimulated by **erythropoietin**, a hormone produced primarily by the kidney. If the kidney detects low levels of oxygen, as occurs when fewer red cells are available to bind oxygen (i.e., **anemia**), or with people living at high altitudes with lower atmospheric oxygen concentrations, erythropoietin levels increase. The increased erythropoietin then stimulates the marrow to increase production of erythrocytes. The entire process of erythropoiesis typically takes 5 days.

For normal erythrocyte production, the bone marrow also requires iron, vitamin B_{12}, folic acid, pyridoxine (vitamin B_6), protein, and other factors. A deficiency of these factors during erythropoiesis can result in decreased red cell production and anemia.

IRON STORES AND METABOLISM. The average daily diet in the Canada contains 10 to 15 mg of elemental iron, but only 0.5 to 1 mg of ingested iron is normally absorbed from the small intestine. The rate of iron absorption is regulated by the amount of iron already stored in the body and by the rate of erythrocyte production. Additional amounts of iron, up to 2 mg daily, must be absorbed by women of childbearing age to replace that lost during menstruation. Total body iron content in the average adult is approximately 3 g, most of which is present in hemoglobin or in one of its breakdown products. Iron is stored as **ferritin** and when required, the iron is released into the plasma, binds to transferrin, and is transported into the membranes of the normoblasts (erythrocyte precursor cells) within the marrow, where it is incorporated into hemoglobin. Iron is lost in the feces, either in bile, blood, or mucosal cells from the intestine.

The concentration of iron in blood is normally about 13 to 31 μmol/L for men and 11 to 29 μmol/L for women. With iron deficiency, bone marrow iron stores are rapidly depleted; hemoglobin synthesis is depressed, and the erythrocytes produced by the marrow are small and low in hemoglobin. Iron deficiency in the adult generally indicates blood loss (e.g., from bleeding in the GI tract or heavy menstrual flow). Lack of dietary iron is rarely the sole cause of iron deficiency anemia in adults. The source of iron deficiency should be investigated promptly because iron deficiency in an adult may be a sign of bleeding in the GI tract or colon cancer.

VITAMIN B_{12} AND FOLIC ACID METABOLISM. Vitamin B_{12} and folic acid are required for the synthesis of deoxyribonucleic acid (DNA) in RBCs. Both vitamin B_{12} and folic acid are derived from the diet. Folic acid is absorbed in the proximal small intestine, but only small amounts are stored within the body. If the diet is deficient in folic acid, stores within the body quickly become depleted. Because vitamin B_{12} is found only in foods of animal origin, strict vegetarians may ingest little vitamin B_{12}. Vitamin B_{12} combines with intrinsic factor produced in the stomach in order to be absorbed. The vitamin B_{12}–intrinsic factor complex is then absorbed in the distal ileum. People who have had a partial or total gastrectomy may have limited amounts of intrinsic factor; and therefore, the absorption of vitamin B_{12} may be diminished. The effects of either decreased absorption or decreased intake of vitamin B_{12} are not apparent for 2 to 4 years.

Vitamin B_{12} and folic acid deficiencies are characterized by the production of abnormally large erythrocytes called megaloblasts. Because these cells are abnormal, many are sequestered (trapped) while still in the bone marrow, and their rate of release is decreased. Some of these cells actually die in the marrow before they can be released into the circulation. This results in megaloblastic anemia.

Red Blood Cell Destruction

The average lifespan of a normal circulating erythrocyte is 120 days. Aged erythrocytes lose their elasticity and become trapped in small blood vessels and the spleen. They are removed from the blood by the reticuloendothelial cells, particularly in the liver and the spleen. As the erythrocytes are destroyed, most of their hemoglobin is recycled. Some hemoglobin also breaks down to form bilirubin and is secreted in the bile. Most of the iron is recycled to form new hemoglobin molecules within the bone marrow; small amounts are lost daily in the feces and urine and monthly in menstrual flow.

Leukocytes (White Blood Cells)

Leukocytes are divided into two general categories: **granulocytes** and **lymphocytes**. In normal blood, the total leukocyte count is 4,000 to 11,000 cells/mm^3. Of these, approximately 60% to 80% are granulocytes and 20% to 40% are lymphocytes. Both of these types of leukocytes primarily protect the body against infection and tissue injury.

Granulocytes

Granulocytes are defined by the presence of granules in the cytoplasm of the cell. Granulocytes are divided into three main subgroups, which are characterized by the staining properties of these granules (see Fig. 54-2). Eosinophils have bright-red granules in their cytoplasm, whereas the granules in basophils stain deep blue. The third and most numerous cell in this class is the neutrophil, with granules that stain a pink to violet hue. Neutrophils are also called polymorphonuclear neutrophils (PMNs, or polys) or segmented neutrophils (segs).

The nucleus of the mature neutrophil has multiple lobes (usually two to five) that are connected by thin filaments of nuclear material, or a "segmented" nucleus; it is usually twice the size of an erythrocyte. The somewhat less mature granulocyte has a single-lobed, elongated nucleus and is called a **band cell**. Ordinarily, band cells account for only a small percentage of circulating granulocytes, although their percentage can increase greatly under conditions in which neutrophil production increases, such as infection. An increased number of band cells are sometimes called a **left shift or shift to the left**. (Traditionally, the diagram of neutrophil maturation showed the myeloid stem cell on the left with progressive maturation stages toward the right, ending with a fully mature neutrophil on the far right side. A shift to the left indicates that more immature cells are present in the blood than normal.)

Fully mature neutrophils result from the gradual differentiation of myeloid stem cells, specifically myeloid **blast cells**. The process, called **myelopoiesis**, is highly complex and depends on many factors. These factors, including specific **cytokines** such as growth factors, are normally present within the marrow itself. As the blast cell matures, the cytoplasm of the cell changes in colour (from blue to violet) and granules begin to form with the cytoplasm. The shape of the nucleus also changes. The entire process of maturation and differentiation takes about 10 days (see Fig. 54-1). Once the neutrophil is released into the circulation from the marrow, it stays there for only about 6 hours before it migrates into the body tissues to perform its function of **phagocytosis** (ingestion and digestion of bacteria and particles). Neutrophils die here within 1 to 2 days. The number of circulating granulocytes found in the healthy person is relatively constant, but in infection large numbers of these cells are rapidly released into the circulation.

Agranulocytes

MONOCYTES. Monocytes (also called mononuclear leukocytes) are leukocytes with a single-lobed nucleus and a granule-free cytoplasm—hence the term *agranulocyte* (see Fig. 54-2). In normal adult blood, monocytes account for approximately 5% of the total leukocytes. Monocytes are the largest of the leukocytes. Produced by the bone marrow, they remain in the circulation for a short time before entering the tissues and transforming into **macrophages**. Macrophages are particularly active in the spleen, liver, peritoneum, and alveoli; they remove debris from these areas and phagocytize bacteria within the tissues.

LYMPHOCYTES. Mature lymphocytes are small cells with scanty cytoplasm (see Fig. 54-2). Immature lymphocytes are produced in the marrow from the lymphoid stem cells. A second major source of production is the thymus. Cells derived from the thymus are known as T lymphocytes (or T cells); those derived from the marrow can also be T cells but are more commonly B lymphocytes (or B cells). Lymphocytes complete their differentiation and maturation primarily in the lymph nodes and in the lymphoid tissue of the intestine and spleen after exposure to a specific antigen. Mature lymphocytes are the principal cells of the immune system, producing antibodies and identifying other cells and organisms as "foreign."

Function of Leukocytes

Leukocytes protect the body from invasion by bacteria and other foreign entities. The major function of neutrophils is phagocytosis. Neutrophils arrive at a given site within 1 hour after the onset of an inflammatory reaction and initiate phagocytosis, but they are short-lived. An influx of monocytes follows; these cells continue their phagocytic activities for long periods as macrophages. This process constitutes a second line of defense for the body against inflammation and infection. Although neutrophils can often work adequately against bacteria without the help of macrophages, macrophages are particularly effective against fungi and viruses. Macrophages also digest senescent (aging or aged) blood cells, primarily within the spleen.

The primary function of lymphocytes is to attack foreign material. One group of lymphocytes (T lymphocytes) kills foreign cells directly or releases lymphokines, substances that enhance the activity of phagocytic cells. T lymphocytes are responsible for delayed allergic reactions, rejection of foreign tissue (e.g., transplanted organs), and destruction of tumour cells. This process is known as *cellular immunity*. The other group of lymphocytes (B lymphocytes) is capable of differentiating into plasma cells. Plasma cells, in turn, produce antibodies called immunoglobulins (Ig), which are protein molecules that destroy foreign material by several mechanisms. This process is known as *humoral immunity*.

Eosinophils and basophils function in hypersensitivity reactions. Eosinophils are important in the phagocytosis of parasites. The increase in eosinophil levels in allergic states indicates that these cells are involved in the hypersensitivity reaction; they neutralize histamine. Basophils produce and store histamine as well as other substances involved in hypersensitivity reactions. The release of these substances provokes allergic reactions.

Platelets (Thrombocytes)

Platelets, or thrombocytes, are not technically cells; rather, they are granular fragments of giant cells in the bone marrow called megakaryocytes (see Fig. 54-2). Platelet production in the marrow is regulated in part by the hormone **thrombopoietin**, which stimulates the production and differentiation of megakaryocytes from the myeloid stem cell. Thrombopoietin is synthesized by the liver, the kidney, and in small amounts by skeletal muscles cells.

Platelets play an essential role in the control of bleeding. They circulate freely in the blood in an inactive state, where they nurture the endothelium of the blood vessels, maintaining the integrity of the vessel. When vascular injury occurs, platelets collect at the site and are activated. They adhere to the site of injury and to each other, forming a platelet plug that temporarily stops bleeding. Substances released from platelet granules activate coagulation factors in the blood plasma and initiate the formation of a stable clot composed of **fibrin**, a filamentous protein. Platelets have a normal lifespan of 7 to 10 days.

Plasma and Plasma Proteins

After cellular elements are removed from blood, the remaining liquid portion is called **plasma**. More than 90% of plasma is water. The remainder consists primarily of plasma proteins, clotting factors (particularly fibrinogen), and small amounts of other substances such as nutrients, enzymes, waste products, and gases. If plasma is allowed to clot, the remaining fluid is called **serum**. Serum has essentially the same composition as plasma, except that fibrinogen and several clotting factors have been removed during the clotting process.

Plasma proteins consist primarily of albumin and the globulins. The globulins can be separated into three main fractions (alpha, beta, and gamma), each of which consists of distinct proteins that have different functions. Important proteins in the alpha and beta fractions are the transport globulins and the clotting factors that are made in the liver. The transport globulins carry various substances in bound form in the circulation. For example, thyroid-binding globulin carries thyroxin, and transferrin carries iron. The clotting factors, including fibrinogen, remain in an inactive form in the blood plasma until activated by the clotting cascade. The gamma-globulin fraction refers to the immunoglobulins, or antibodies. These proteins are produced by well-differentiated B lymphocytes and plasma cells. The actual fractionation of the globulins can be seen on a specific laboratory test (serum protein electrophoresis).

Albumin is particularly important for the maintenance of fluid balance within the vascular system. Capillary walls are impermeable to albumin, so its presence in the plasma creates an osmotic force that keeps fluid within the vascular space. Albumin, which is produced by the liver, has the capacity to bind to several substances that are transported in plasma (e.g., certain medications, bilirubin, and some hormones). People with impaired hepatic function may have low concentrations of albumin, with a resultant decrease in osmotic pressure and the development of edema.

Reticuloendothelial System (RES)

The RES is composed of special tissue macrophages. When released from the marrow, monocytes spend a short time in the circulation (about 24 hours) and then enter the body tissues. Within the tissues, the monocytes continue to differentiate into macrophages, which can survive for months or years. Macrophages have a variety of important functions. They defend the body against foreign invaders (i.e., bacteria and other pathogens) via phagocytosis. They remove old or damaged cells from the circulation. They stimulate the inflammatory process and present antigens to the immune system (see Chapter 51). Macrophages give rise to tissue **histiocytes**, including Kupffer cells of the liver, peritoneal macrophages, alveolar macrophages, and other components of the RES. Thus, the RES is a component of many other organs within the body, particularly the spleen, lymph nodes, lungs, and liver.

The spleen is the site of activity for most macrophages. Most of the spleen (75%) is made of red pulp; here the blood enters the venous sinuses through capillaries that are surrounded by macrophages. Within the red pulp are tiny aggregates of white pulp, consisting of B and T lymphocytes. The spleen sequesters newly released reticulocytes from the marrow, removing nuclear fragments and other materials (e.g., denatured hemoglobin, iron) before the now fully mature erythrocyte returns to the circulation. Essentially, the spleen filters the blood to ensure its optimal function in circulation. Although a minority of erythrocytes (less than 5%) pool in the spleen, a significant proportion of platelets (20% to 40%) pool here. If the spleen is enlarged, a greater proportion of red cells and platelets can be sequestered. The spleen is a major source of hematopoiesis in fetal life. It can resume hematopoiesis later in adulthood if necessary, particularly when marrow function is compromised (e.g., in bone marrow fibrosis). The spleen has important immunologic functions as well. It forms substances called opsonins that promote the phagocytosis of neutrophils; it also forms the antibody immunoglobulin M (IgM), the antibody formed after first exposure to an antigen.

Hemostasis

Hemostasis is the process of preventing blood loss from intact vessels and of stopping bleeding from a severed vessel, which requires adequate numbers of functional platelets. Platelets nurture the endothelium and thereby maintain the structural integrity of the vessel wall. Two processes are involved in arresting bleeding: primary and secondary hemostases.

In **primary hemostasis**, the severed blood vessel constricts. Circulating platelets aggregate at the site and adhere to the vessel and to one another. An unstable hemostatic plug is formed. For the coagulation process to be correctly activated, circulating inactive coagulation factors must be converted to active forms. This process occurs on the surface of the aggregated platelets at the site of vessel injury. The end result is the formation of fibrin, which reinforces the platelet plug and anchors it to the injury site. This process is termed **secondary hemostasis**. The process of blood coagulation is highly complex. It can be activated by the *intrinsic* or the *extrinsic* pathway. Both pathways are needed for maintenance of normal hemostasis.

Many factors are involved in the reaction cascade that forms fibrin. When tissue is injured, the extrinsic pathway is activated by the release of thromboplastin from the tissue. As the result of a series of reactions, prothrombin is converted to **thrombin**, which in turn, catalyzes the conversion of fibrinogen to fibrin. Clotting by the intrinsic pathway is activated when the collagen that lines blood vessels is exposed. Clotting factors are activated sequentially until, as with the extrinsic pathway, fibrin is ultimately formed. Although the intrinsic pathway is slower, this sequence is probably most often responsible for clotting in vivo.

As the injured vessel is repaired and again covered with endothelial cells, the fibrin clot is no longer needed. The fibrin is digested via two systems: the *plasma fibrinolytic system* and the *cellular fibrinolytic system*. The substance **plasminogen** is required to lyse (break down) the fibrin. Plasminogen, which is present in all body fluids, circulates with fibrinogen and is actually incorporated into the fibrin clot as it forms. When the clot is no longer needed (e.g., after an injured blood vessel has healed), the plasminogen is activated to form plasmin. Plasmin digests the fibrinogen and fibrin. The breakdown particles of the clot, called fibrin degradation products, are released into the circulation. Through this system, clots are dissolved as tissue is repaired, and the vascular system returns to its normal baseline state.

Gerontologic Considerations

In older adults, the bone marrow's ability to respond to the body's need for blood cells (erythrocytes, leukocytes, and platelets) may be decreased. This decreased ability is a result of many factors, including diminished production of the growth factors necessary for hematopoiesis by stromal cells within the marrow or a diminished response to the growth factors (in the case of erythropoietin). In addition, in older adults, the bone marrow may be more susceptible to the myelosuppressive effects of medications. As a result of these factors, when an older adult needs more blood cells, the bone marrow may not be able to adequately increase production of these cells. **Leukopenia** (a decreased number of circulating leukocytes) or anemia can result.

Assessment

Health History

A careful health history and physical assessment can provide important information related to a patient's known or potential hematologic diagnosis. Because many hematologic disorders are more prevalent in certain ethnic groups, assessments of ethnicity and family history are useful (see Chart 54-1). Similarly, obtaining a nutritional history and assessing the use of prescription and over-the-counter medications, as well as herbal supplements, are important to note, because several conditions can result from nutritional deficiencies, or from the use of certain herbs or medications. Careful attention to the onset of a symptom or finding (e.g., rapid vs. gradual; persistent vs. intermittent), its severity, and any contributing factors can further differentiate potential causes. Of equal importance is assessing the impact of these findings on the patient's functional ability, manifestations of distress, and coping mechanisms.

Physical Assessment

The physical assessment should be comprehensive and include careful attention to the skin, oral cavity, lymph nodes, and spleen (see Fig. 54-3). Table 54-2 highlights a general approach to the physical assessment findings in hematologic disorders.

Diagnostic Evaluation

Most hematologic diseases reflect a defect in the hematopoietic, hemostatic, or reticuloendothelial system. The defect can be *quantitative* (e.g., increased or decreased production of cells), *qualitative* (e.g., the cells that are produced are defective in their normal functional capacity), or both. Initially, many hematologic conditions cause few symptoms. Therefore, extensive laboratory tests are often required to diagnose a hematologic disorder. For most hematologic conditions, continued monitoring via

GENETICS IN NURSING PRACTICE

Chart 54-1. Hematologic Disorders

Hematologic disorders are marked by aberrations in the structure or function of the blood cells or the blood clotting mechanism. Some examples of genetic hematologic disorders are:

Autosomal dominant:
- Factor V Leiden
- Familial hypercholesterolemia
- Hereditary angioedema
- Hereditary spherocytosis
- von Willebrand's disease

Autosomal recessive:
- Hemochromatosis
- Sickle cell disease
- Thalassemia

X-linked:
- Hemophilia

Nursing Assessments

Refer to Chart 5-2: Genetics in Nursing Practice: Genetic Aspects of Health Assessment

FAMILY HISTORY ASSESSMENT SPECIFIC TO HEMATOLOGIC DISORDERS
- Collect family history information on maternal and paternal relatives from three generations of the family.
- Assess family history for other family members with histories of blood disorders or episodes of abnormal bleeding.
- If a family history or personal risk is suspected, the person should be carefully screened for bleeding disorders prior to surgical procedures.

PATIENT ASSESSMENT SPECIFIC TO HEMATOLOGIC DISORDERS
- Assess for specific symptoms of hematologic diseases:
  - Extreme fatigue (the most common symptom of hematologic disorders)
  - Delayed clotting of blood
  - Easy or deep bruising
  - Abnormal bleeding (e.g., frequent nosebleeds)
  - Abdominal pain (hemochromatosis) or joint pain (sickle cell disease)
- Review blood cell counts for abnormalities
- Assess for presence of illness despite low risk for the illness (e.g., a young adult with a blood clot)

Resources

Sickle Cell Association of Ontario (SCAO): https://sicklecellontario.ca/

Canadian Hemophilia Society: https://www.hemophilia.ca/

Hemophilia Federation of America: www.hemophiliafed.org

Iron Disorders Institute: Hemochromatosis: www.hemochromatosis.org

Sickle Cell Association of America: www.sicklecelldisease.org

See Chapter 11, for components of genetic counselling.

specific blood tests is required because it is very important to assess for changes in test results over time. In general, it is important to assess trends in test results because these trends help the clinician decide whether the patient is responding appropriately to interventions.

Hematologic Studies

The most common tests used are the complete blood count (CBC) and the peripheral blood smear. The CBC identifies the total number of blood cells (leukocytes, erythrocytes, and platelets), as well as the hemoglobin, **hematocrit** (percentage of blood volume consisting of erythrocytes), and RBC indices. Because cellular morphology (shape and appearance of the cells) is particularly important in accurately diagnosing most hematologic disorders, the blood cells involved must be examined. This process is referred to as the manual examination of the peripheral smear, which may be part of the CBC. In this test, a drop of blood is spread on a glass slide, stained, and examined under a microscope. The shape and size of the erythrocytes and platelets, as well as the actual appearance of the leukocytes, provide useful information in identifying hematologic conditions. Blood for the CBC is typically obtained by venipuncture (Fischbach & Dunning, 2015).

Other common tests of coagulation are the prothrombin time (PT), typically replaced by the standardized test, international normalized ratio (INR), and the activated partial thromboplastin time (aPTT). The INR and aPTT serve as useful screening tools for evaluating a patient's clotting ability and monitoring the therapeutic effectiveness of anticoagulant medications. In both tests, specific reagents are mixed into the plasma sample, and the time taken to form a clot is measured. For these tests to be accurate, the test tube must be filled with the correct amount of the patient's blood; either excess or inadequate blood volume within the tube can render the results inaccurate.

Bone Marrow Aspiration and Biopsy

The bone marrow aspiration and biopsy are crucial when additional information is needed to assess how a person's blood cells are being formed and to assess the quantity and quality of each type of cell produced within the marrow. These tests are also used to document infection or tumour within the marrow.

Normal bone marrow is in a semifluid state and can be aspirated through a special large needle. In adults, bone marrow is usually aspirated from the iliac crest and occasionally from the sternum. The aspirate provides only a sample of cells. Aspirate alone may be adequate for evaluating certain conditions, such as anemia. However, when more information is required, a biopsy is also performed. Biopsy samples are taken from the posterior iliac crest;

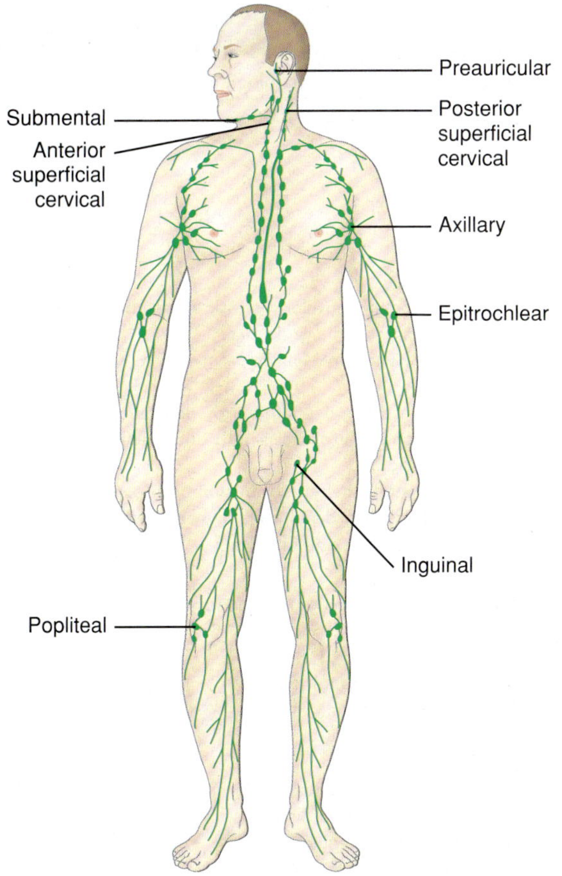

FIGURE 54-3. Lymphatic system. *Arrows* indicate sites of lymph nodes accessible for palpation. (Developed by Thomas, M., & Morrow, K. (2011). Veterans Administration Palo Alto Health Care System.)

occasionally, an anterior approach is required. A marrow biopsy shows the architecture of the bone marrow as well as its degree of cellularity.

Most patients need no more preparation than a careful explanation of the procedure, but for some very anxious patients, an antianxiety agent such as lorazepam (Ativan) may be useful. It is always important for the physician or nurse to describe and explain the procedure and any anticipated sensations to the patient. The risks, benefits, and alternatives are also discussed. A signed informed consent is needed before the procedure is performed.

Before aspiration, the skin is cleansed using aseptic technique. A small area is then anesthetized with a local anesthetic agent extending through the skin and subcutaneous tissue to the periosteum of the bone. It is not possible to anesthetize the bone itself. The bone marrow needle is introduced with a stylet in place. When the needle is felt to go through the outer cortex of bone and enter the marrow cavity, the stylet is removed, a syringe is attached, and a small volume (5 mL) of blood and marrow is aspirated. Patients typically feel a pressure sensation as the needle is advanced into position. The actual aspiration always causes sharp but brief pain, resulting from the suction exerted as the marrow is aspirated into the syringe; the patient should be warned about this. Taking deep breaths or using relaxation techniques often helps ease the discomfort (see Fig. 54-4).

If a bone marrow biopsy is necessary, it is best performed after the aspiration and in a slightly different location, because the marrow structure may be altered after aspiration. A special biopsy needle is used. Because these needles are large, the skin may be punctured first with a surgical blade to make a 3- or 4-mm incision. The biopsy needle is advanced well into the marrow cavity. When the needle is properly positioned, a portion of marrow is cored out. The patient feels a pressure sensation but should not feel actual pain. The nurse should instruct the patient to inform the physician if pain occurs so that an additional anesthetic agent can be administered.

Complications of either bone marrow aspiration or biopsy include bleeding and infection. The risk of bleeding is somewhat increased if the patient's platelet count is low or if the patient has been taking a medication (e.g., aspirin) that alters platelet function. After the marrow sample is obtained, pressure is applied to the site for several minutes. The site is then covered with a sterile dressing. Most patients have no discomfort after a bone marrow aspiration, but the site of a biopsy may ache for 1 or 2 days. Warm tub baths and a mild analgesic agent (e.g., acetaminophen [Tylenol]) may be useful. Aspirin-containing analgesic agents should be avoided because they can aggravate or potentiate bleeding.

Unfolding Patient Stories: Lloyd Bennett • Part 2

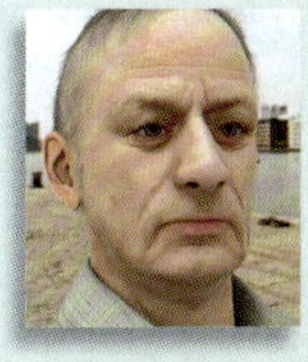

Recall from Chapter 44 Lloyd Bennett, who presented to the emergency department with a hip fracture. What physical assessment and laboratory data can assist the nurse in evaluation for possible internal blood loss from the fracture or indications that the patient is at higher risk of bleeding?

Care for Lloyd and other patients in a realistic virtual environment: ***vSim** for Nursing* **(thepoint.lww.com/vSimMedicalSurgical).** Practice documenting these patients' care in DocuCare **(thepoint.lww.com/DocuCareEHR).**

Anemia

Anemia is a condition in which the hemoglobin concentration is lower than normal and reflects the presence of fewer than the normal number of erythrocytes within the circulation. As a result, the amount of oxygen delivered to body tissues is also diminished. Anemia is not a specific disease state but a sign of an underlying disorder. ***It is by far the most common hematologic condition.***

Classification of Anemias

Anemia may be classified in several ways (Table 54-3). A physiologic approach classifies anemia according to whether the deficiency in erythrocytes is caused by a defect in their production (hypoproliferative anemia), by their destruction (hemolytic anemia), or by their loss (bleeding).

In *hypoproliferative* anemias, the marrow cannot produce adequate numbers of erythrocytes. Decreased erythrocyte production is reflected by an inappropriately normal or low reticulocyte count. Inadequate production of

TABLE 54-2 Health History and Physical Assessment in Hematologic Disorders[a]

	Findings	Potential Indications of Hematologic Disorder
Health History	Prior episodes of bleeding (epistaxis, tooth, gum, hematuria, menorrhagia, hematochezia, gastrointestinal bleeding, and/or ulcers)	Thrombocytopenia, coagulopathy, anemia
	Prior blood clots, pulmonary emboli, miscarriages	Thrombotic disorder
	Fatigue and weakness	Anemia, infection, malignancy, clonal disorders
	Dyspnea, particularly dyspnea on exertion, orthopnea, shortness of breath	Anemia, infection
	Prior radiation therapy (especially pelvic irradiation)	Anemia, pancytopenia, myelodysplastic syndrome, leukemia
	Prior chemotherapy	Myelodysplastic syndrome, leukemia
	Hobbies/occupational/military exposure history (especially benzene, Agent Orange)	Myelodysplastic syndrome, leukemia, myeloma, lymphoma
	Diet history	Anemia (due to vitamin B_{12}, folate, iron deficiency)
	Alcohol consumption	Anemia (effect on hematopoiesis, nutritional deficiency)
	Use of herbal supplements	Platelet dysfunction
	Concurrent medications	Neutropenia, anemia, hemolysis, thrombocytopenia
	Family history/ethnicity	Some hematologic disorders have a higher prevalence in certain ethnic groups and families
Physical Assessment		
Skin	Gray-tan or bronze skin colour (especially genitalia, scars, exposed areas)	Hemochromatosis (primary or secondary)
	Ruddy complexion (face, conjunctiva, hands, feet)	Polycythemia
	Ecchymoses (i.e., bruises)	Thrombocytopenia, coagulopathy
	Petechiae (i.e., pinpoint hemorrhagic lesions, usually more prominent on trunk or anterior aspects of lower extremities)	Severe thrombocytopenia
	Rash	Variable; if pruritic, may indicate polycythemia, other nonhematologic-related disorders
	Bleeding (including around vascular lines, tubes)	Thrombocytopenia, coagulopathy
	Conjunctival hemorrhage	Severe thrombocytopenia, coagulopathy
	Pallor, especially in mucous membranes (including conjunctiva), nail beds	Anemia
	Jaundice in mucous membranes (including conjunctiva), nail beds, palate	Hemolysis
Oral cavity	Petechiae in the buccal mucosa, gingiva, hard palate	Severe thrombocytopenia
	Ulceration of oral mucosa	Infection, leukemia
	Tongue: Smooth	Pernicious anemia
	Beefy red	Vitamin B_{12}/folate deficiency
	Enlarged	Amyloidosis
	Angular cheilosis (ulceration at corners of mouth)	Anemia
	Enlarged gums: hyperplasia	Leukemia
Lymph nodes	Enlarged size, firm and fixed vs. mobile and tender	Leukemia, lymphoma
Respiratory	Increased rate and depth of respirations; adventitious breath sounds	Anemia; infection
Cardiovascular	Distended neck veins, edema, chest pain on exertion, murmurs, gallops	Severe anemia
	Hypotension (below baseline)	Polycythemia
	Hypertension (above baseline)	
Genitourinary	Hematuria	Hemolysis, thrombocytopenia
	Proteinuria	Myeloma
Musculoskeletal	Rib/sternal tenderness to palpation	Leukemia, myeloma
	Back pain; tenderness to palpation over spine, loss of height, kyphosis	Myeloma
	Pain/swelling in knees, wrists, hands	Hemophilia, sickle cell disease
Abdominal	Enlarged spleen	Leukemia, myelofibrosis
	Enlarged liver	Myelofibrosis
	Stool positive for occult blood	Anemia, thrombocytopenia
Central nervous system	Cranial nerve dysfunction	Vitamin B_{12} deficiency
	Peripheral nerve dysfunction (especially sensory)	Vitamin B_{12} deficiency, amyloidosis, myeloma
	Visual changes, headache, alteration in mental status	Severe thrombocytopenia
Gynecologic	Menorrhagia	Thrombocytopenia, coagulopathy
Constitutional	Fever, chills, sweats, asthenia	Leukemia, lymphoma; infection

[a]Common findings (obtained via health history and physical assessment) that occur in patients with hematologic disorders. Note that signs and symptoms are not disease specific but are useful in guiding the nurse to establishing an etiology for the findings noted.

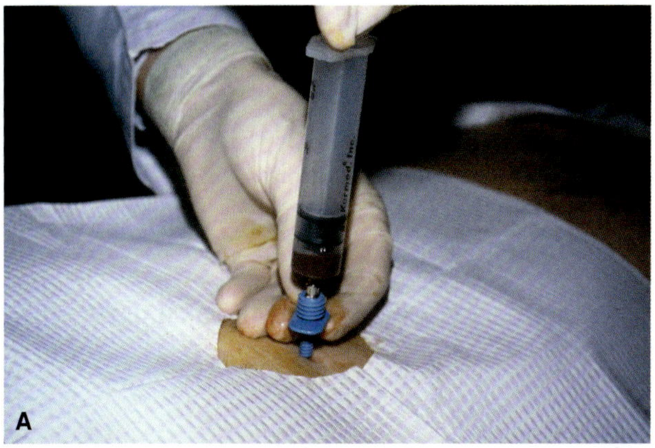

A

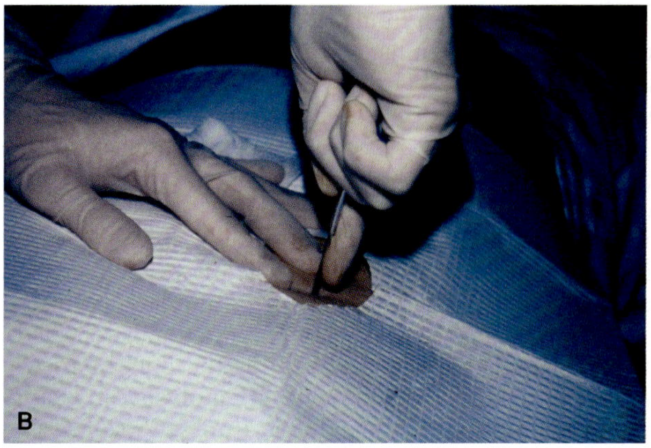

B

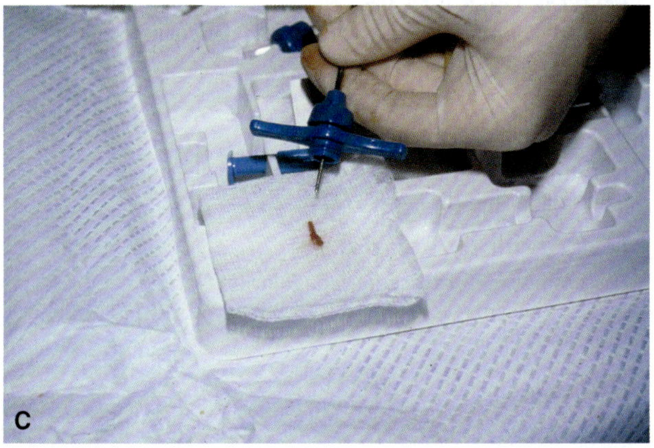

C

FIGURE 54-4. Bone marrow aspiration procedure. The posterior superior iliac crest is the preferred site for bone marrow aspiration and biopsy because no vital organs or vessels are nearby. The patient is placed either in the lateral position with one leg flexed or in the prone position. The anterior iliac crest or sternum may also be used. Note that the sternum cannot be used for a marrow biopsy. **A.** Bone marrow aspiration. **B.** Inserting a Jamshidi biopsy needle. **C.** Dispensing the bone marrow core. (From Farhi, D. C. (2009). *Pathology of bone marrow and blood cells* (2nd ed.). Philadelphia, PA: Lippincott Williams & Wilkins.)

TABLE 54-3 Classification of Anemias

	Laboratory Findings	
Type of Anemia	**CBC**	**Other**
Hypoproliferative (Resulting from Defective RBC Production)		
Iron deficiency	↓ MCV, ↓ reticulocytes	↓ Iron, % saturation, ferritin ↑ TIBC
Vitamin B_{12} deficiency (megaloblastic)	↑ MCV	↓ Vitamin B_{12}
Folate deficiency (megaloblastic)	↑ MCV	↓ Folate
Decreased erythropoietin production (e.g., from renal dysfunction)	Normal MCV	↓ Erythropoietin level ↑ Creatinine
Cancer/inflammation	Normal MCV	↑ Ferritin, % saturation ↓ Iron, TIBC ↓ Erythropoietin level (usually)
Bleeding (Resulting from RBC Loss)		
Bleeding from gastrointestinal tract, epistaxis (nosebleed), trauma, bleeding from genitourinary tract (e.g., menorrhagia)	↓ Hgb and Hct (*Note:* Hgb and Hct may be normal if measured soon after bleeding starts) ↓ MCV (normal MCV initially) ↑ Reticulocytes	↓ Iron, % saturation, ferritin (later)
Hemolytic (Resulting from RBC Destruction)		
Altered erythropoiesis (sickle cell disease, thalassemia, other hemoglobinopathies)	↓ MCV ↑ Reticulocytes Fragmented RBCs (various shapes)	
Hypersplenism (hemolysis)	↑ MCV	
Drug-induced anemia	↑ Presence of spherocytes	
Autoimmune anemia	↑ Presence of spherocytes	
Mechanical heart valve–related anemia	Fragmented red cells	

CBC, complete blood count; RBC, red blood cell; ↓, decreased; MCV, mean corpuscular volume; %, percent; ↑, increased; TIBC, total iron-binding capacity; Hgb, hemoglobin; Hct, hematocrit.

Adapted from Prchal, J. T. (2016a). Clinical manifestations and classification of erythrocyte disorders. In K. Kaushansky, M. A. Lichtman, J. T. Prchal, et al. (Eds.). *Williams hematology* (9th ed.). New York: McGraw-Hill Medical.

erythrocytes may result from marrow damage due to medications (e.g., chloramphenicol) or chemicals (e.g., benzene) or from a lack of factors (e.g., iron, vitamin B_{12}, folic acid, erythropoietin) necessary for erythrocyte formation.

In hemolytic anemias, premature destruction of erythrocytes results in the liberation of hemoglobin from the erythrocytes into the plasma; the released hemoglobin is converted into bilirubin, thus causing the bilirubin concentration to rise. The *increased erythrocyte destruction* leads to tissue hypoxia, which in turn, stimulates erythropoietin production. This increased production is reflected in an increased reticulocyte count as the bone marrow responds to the loss of erythrocytes. **Hemolysis** can result from an abnormality within the erythrocyte itself (e.g., sickle cell disease, glucose-6-phosphate dehydrogenase [G-6-PD] deficiency) or within the plasma (e.g., immune hemolytic anemias), or from direct injury to the erythrocyte within the circulation (e.g., hemolysis caused by mechanical heart valve). Chart 54-2 identifies causes of hemolytic anemia.

It is usually possible to determine whether the presence of anemia in a given patient is caused by destruction or by inadequate production of erythrocytes on the basis of the following factors:

- The marrow's ability to respond to decreased erythrocytes (as evidenced by an increased reticulocyte count in the circulating blood)
- The degree to which young erythrocytes proliferate in the bone marrow and the manner in which they mature (as observed on bone marrow biopsy)
- The presence or absence of end products of erythrocyte destruction within the circulation (e.g., increased bilirubin level; decreased haptoglobin level, as the **haptoglobin** binds the free hemoglobin released from erythrocytes)

CHART 54-2

Causes of Hemolytic Anemias

Inherited Hemolytic Anemia

ABNORMAL HEMOGLOBIN

Sickle cell disease[a]
Thalassemia[b]

RED BLOOD CELL MEMBRANE ABNORMALITY

Acanthocytosis
Hereditary elliptocytosis
Hereditary spherocytosis
Stomatocytosis

ENZYME DEFICIENCIES

Glucose-6-phosphate dehydrogenase deficiency[c]

Acquired Hemolytic Anemia

ANTIBODY RELATED

Autoimmune hemolytic anemia[d]
Iso-antibody/transfusion reaction[e]
Cold agglutinin disease

Not Antibody Related

Disseminated intravascular coagulation[f]
Hypersplenism[g]
Infection
  Bacterial
  Parasitic
Liver disease
Mechanical heart valve
Microangiopathic hemolytic anemia
Paroxysmal nocturnal hemoglobinuria
Toxins
Trauma
Uremia

[a]Discussed in text.
[b]Discussed in text.
[c]Discussed in text.
[d]Discussed in text.
[e]Discussed in text.
[f]Discussed in text.
[g]Discussed in text.

Clinical Manifestations

Aside from the severity of the anemia itself, several factors influence the development of anemia-associated symptoms: the rapidity with which the anemia has developed, the duration of the anemia (i.e., its chronicity), the metabolic requirements of the patient, other concurrent disorders or disabilities (e.g., cardiac or pulmonary disease), and complications or concomitant features of the condition that produced the anemia.

In general, a rapidly developing anemia has more severe symptoms. An otherwise healthy person can often tolerate as much as a 50% gradual reduction in hemoglobin without pronounced symptoms or significant incapacity, whereas the rapid loss of as little as 30% may precipitate profound vascular collapse in the same person. A person who has become gradually anemic, with hemoglobin levels at generally 120 g/L or less (Van Leeuwen & Bladh, 2017) usually has few or no symptoms other than slight tachycardia on exertion and fatigue.

People who customarily are very active or who have significant demands on their lives (e.g., a single, working mother of small children) are more likely to have symptoms, and those symptoms are more likely to be pronounced than in more sedentary people. Patients with hypothyroidism with decreased oxygen needs may be completely asymptomatic, without tachycardia or increased cardiac output, at an even lower hemoglobin level. Similarly, patients with coexistent cardiac, vascular, or pulmonary disease may develop more pronounced symptoms of anemia (e.g., dyspnea, chest pain, muscle pain, or cramping) at a higher hemoglobin level than those without these concurrent health problems.

Finally, some anemias are complicated by various other abnormalities that do not result from the anemia but are inherently associated with these particular diseases. These abnormalities may give rise to symptoms that completely overshadow those of the anemia, as in the painful crises of sickle cell anemia.

Assessment and Diagnostic Findings

A variety of hematologic studies are performed to determine the type and cause of the anemia. In an initial evaluation, the hemoglobin, hematocrit, reticulocyte count, and RBC indices (the mean corpuscular volume [MCV] and red cell distribution width [RDW], are particularly useful). Iron studies (serum iron level, total iron-binding capacity [TIBC], percent saturation, and ferritin), as well as serum vitamin B_{12} and folate levels are also frequently obtained. Other tests include haptoglobin (the protein that binds free hemoglobin from erythrocytes and transports this to the spleen for further processing) and erythropoietin levels. The remaining CBC values are useful in determining whether the anemia is an isolated problem or part of another hematologic condition, such as **leukemia** or myelodysplastic syndrome (MDS). Bone marrow aspiration may be performed. In addition, other diagnostic studies may be performed to determine the presence of underlying chronic illness, such as malignancy, or the source of any blood loss, such as polyps or ulcers within the GI tract.

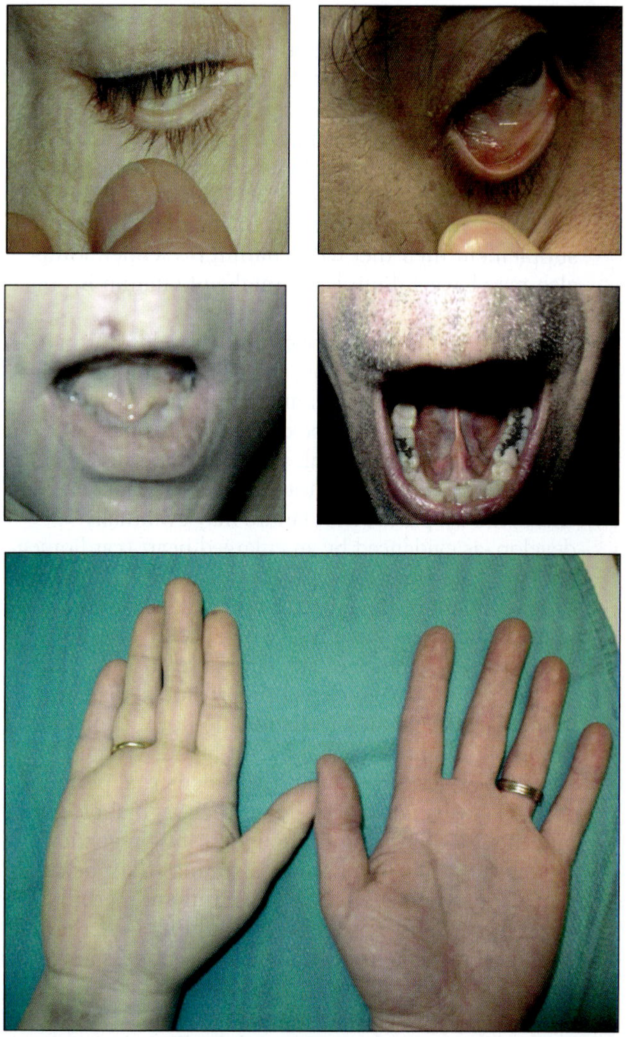

FIGURE 54-5. Pallor seen in the patient with anemia. (From Tkachuk, D. C., & Hirschman, J. V. (2007). *Wintrobe's atlas of clinical hematology* (Fig. 1.1, p. 9). Philadelphia, PA: Lippincott Williams & Wilkins.)

Complications

General complications of severe anemia include heart failure, paresthesias, and delirium. Patients with underlying heart disease are far more likely to have angina or symptoms of heart failure than those without heart disease. Complications associated with specific types of anemia are included in the description of each type.

Medical Management

Management of anemia is directed toward correcting or controlling the cause of the anemia; if the anemia is severe, the erythrocytes that are lost or destroyed may be replaced with a transfusion of packed red blood cells (PRBCs). Similarly, too few erythrocytes from deficient production can also be treated with a blood transfusion. The management of the various types of anemia is covered in the discussions that follow.

Gerontologic Considerations

A recent study indicates that approximately 3% of Canadians have anemia. Anemia was found to be more prevalent in households that have lower income, and in adults who were 65- to 79-year-old. In this group, deficiency in vitamin B_{12} is a significant contributing factor (Cooper, Greene-Finestone, Lowell, et al., 2012). The impact of anemia on function is significant. A review among the older adult has noted that increased fragility, decreased mobility and exercise performance, increased risk of falling, diminished cognitive function, increased risk of developing dementia (Hong, Falvey, Harris, et al., 2013) and major depression, and lower skeletal muscle and bone density are associated with anemia (Valderrabano et al., 2017).

Nursing Process

The Patient With Anemia

Assessment

The health history and physical examination provide important data about the type of anemia involved, the extent and type of symptoms it produces, and the impact of those symptoms on the patient's life. Weakness, fatigue, and general malaise are common, as are pallor of the skin and mucous membranes (conjunctivae, oral mucosa) (see Fig. 54-5).

Jaundice may be present in patients with megaloblastic anemia or hemolytic anemia but is much more common with hemolytic anemia. The tongue may be smooth and red (in iron deficiency anemia) or beefy red and sore (in megaloblastic anemia); the corners of the mouth may be ulcerated (**angular cheilosis**) in both iron deficiency and megaloblastic anemia. People with iron deficiency anemia may additionally crave ice, starch, or dirt; this craving is known as *pica*. The nails may be brittle, ridged, and concave.

The health history should include a medication history, because some medications can depress bone marrow activity, induce hemolysis, or interfere with folate metabolism (e.g., ethyl alcohol). An accurate history of alcohol intake, including the amount and duration, should be obtained. Family history is important, because certain anemias are inherited. It is necessary to ask about athletic endeavours because extreme exercise can decrease erythropoiesis and erythrocyte survival.

A nutritional assessment is important because this may indicate deficiencies in essential nutrients such as iron, vitamin B_{12}, and folic acid. Strict vegetarians are at risk for megaloblastic types of anemia if they do not supplement their diet with vitamin B_{12}. Older adults also may have a diminished intake of vitamin B_{12} or folate.

Cardiac status should be carefully assessed. When the hemoglobin level is low, the heart attempts to compensate by pumping faster and harder in an effort to deliver more blood to hypoxic tissue. This increased cardiac workload can result in such symptoms as tachycardia, palpitations, dyspnea, dizziness, orthopnea, and exertional dyspnea. Heart failure may eventually develop, as evidenced by an enlarged heart (cardiomegaly) and liver (hepatomegaly) and by peripheral edema.

Assessment of the GI system may disclose complaints of nausea, vomiting (with specific questions about the appearance of any emesis [e.g., looks like "coffee grounds"]), melena or dark stools, diarrhea, anorexia, and glossitis (inflammation of the tongue). Stools should be tested for occult blood. Women should be questioned about their menstrual periods (e.g., excessive menstrual flow, other vaginal bleeding) and the use of iron supplements during pregnancy.

Neurologic examination is also important because pernicious anemia affects the central and peripheral nervous systems. Assessment should include the presence and extent of peripheral numbness and paresthesias, ataxia, poor coordination, and confusion. Delirium can sometimes result from other types of anemia, particularly in older adults. Finally, it is important to monitor relevant laboratory test results and to note any changes over time.

Nursing Priorities

Based on the assessment data, major nursing priorities for the patient with anemia may include:

- Fatigue
- Altered nutrition
- Altered tissue perfusion
- Nonadherence with prescribed therapy

Collaborative Problems/ Potential Complications

Based on the assessment data, potential complications that may develop include:

- Heart failure
- Angina
- Paresthesias
- Confusion

Planning and Goals

The major goals for the patient may include decreased fatigue, attainment or maintenance of adequate nutrition, maintenance of adequate tissue perfusion, compliance with prescribed therapy, and absence of complications.

Nursing Interventions

Managing Fatigue

The most common symptom and complication of anemia is fatigue. Fatigue is often the symptom that has the greatest negative impact on a patient's level of functioning and consequent quality of life. Therefore, it should not be minimized. Patients often describe the fatigue from anemia as oppressive. Fatigue can be significant, yet the anemia may not be severe enough to warrant transfusion. Fatigue can interfere with a person's ability to work and to participate in activities with family and friends. Patients often lose interest in hobbies and activities, including sexual activity. The distress from fatigue is often related to a person's responsibilities and life demands, as well as the amount of assistance and support received from others.

Nursing interventions can focus on assisting the patient to prioritize activities and to establish a balance between activities and rest that is acceptable to the patient. Patients with chronic anemia need to maintain some physical activity and exercise to prevent the deconditioning that results from inactivity.

Maintaining Adequate Nutrition

Inadequate intake of essential nutrients, such as iron, vitamin B_{12}, folic acid, and protein, can cause some anemias. The symptoms associated with anemia (e.g., fatigue, anorexia) can in turn interfere with maintaining adequate nutrition. A healthy diet should be encouraged. The nurse should inform the patient that alcohol interferes with the utilization of essential nutrients and should advise the patient to avoid or limit his or her intake of alcoholic beverages. Dietary teaching sessions should be individualized, involve family members, and include cultural aspects related to food preferences and food preparation. Dietary supplements (e.g., vitamins, iron, folate, protein) may be prescribed.

Equally important, the patient and family must understand the role of nutritional supplements in the proper context, because many forms of anemia are not the result of a nutritional deficiency. In such cases, even an excessive intake of nutritional supplements will not improve the anemia. A potential problem in patients with chronic transfusion requirements occurs with the indiscriminate use of iron supplements. Unless an aggressive program of chelation therapy is implemented, these people are at risk for iron overload from their transfusions. The addition of an iron supplement only exacerbates the situation.

Maintaining Adequate Perfusion

Patients with acute blood loss or severe hemolysis may have decreased tissue perfusion from decreased blood volume or reduced circulating erythrocytes (decreased hematocrit). Lost volume is replaced with transfusions or intravenous (IV) fluids, based on symptoms and laboratory test results. Supplemental oxygen may be necessary, but it is rarely needed on a long-term basis unless there is underlying severe cardiac or pulmonary disease. The nurse monitors the patient's vital signs and pulse oximeter readings closely; other medications, such as antihypertensive agents, may need to be adjusted or withheld.

Promoting Adherence With Prescribed Therapy

For patients with anemia, medications or nutritional supplements are often prescribed to treat the condition. These patients need to understand the purpose of the medication, how to take the medication and over what time period, and how to manage any side effects of therapy. To enhance compliance, the nurse assists the patient to develop ways to incorporate the therapeutic plan into everyday activities, rather than merely giving the patient a list of instructions. For example, many patients have difficulty taking iron supplements because of related GI effects. Rather than seeking assistance from a health care provider in managing the problem, some patients simply stop taking the iron.

Abruptly stopping some medications can have serious consequences, as in the case of high-dose corticosteroids to manage hemolytic anemias. Some medications, such as growth factors, are extremely expensive. Patients receiving these medications may need assistance to obtain needed insurance coverage or to explore alternative ways to obtain these medications.

Monitoring and Managing Potential Complications

A significant complication of anemia is heart failure from chronic diminished blood volume and the heart's compensatory effort to increase cardiac output. Patients with anemia should be assessed for signs and symptoms of heart failure (see Chapter 31).

In megaloblastic forms of anemia, the significant potential complications are neurologic. A neurologic assessment should be performed for patients with known or suspected megaloblastic anemia. Patients may initially complain of paresthesias in their lower extremities. These paresthesias are usually manifested as numbness and tingling on the bottom of the foot, and they gradually progress. As the anemia progresses, other signs become apparent. Position and vibration sense may be diminished; difficulty maintaining balance is not uncommon, and some patients have gait disturbances as well. Initially mild confusion may develop and may become severe.

Evaluation

Expected patient outcomes may include:

1. Reports less fatigue
   a. Follows a progressive plan of rest, activity, and exercise
   b. Prioritizes activities
   c. Paces activities according to energy level
2. Attains and maintains adequate nutrition
   a. Eats a healthy diet
   b. Develops a meal plan that promotes optimal nutrition
   c. Maintains adequate amounts of iron, vitamins, and protein from diet or supplements
   d. Adheres to nutritional supplement therapy when prescribed
   e. Verbalizes understanding of rationale for using recommended nutritional supplements
   f. Verbalizes understanding of rationale for avoiding nonrecommended nutritional supplements
3. Maintains adequate perfusion
   a. Has vital signs within baseline for patient
   b. Has pulse oximetry (arterial oxygenation) value within normal limits
4. Absence of complications
   a. Avoids or limits activities that cause dyspnea, palpitations, dizziness, or tachycardia
   b. Uses rest and comfort measures to alleviate dyspnea
   c. Has vital signs within baseline for patient
   d. Has no signs of increasing fluid retention (e.g., peripheral edema, decreased urine output, neck vein distention)
   e. Remains oriented to time, place, and situation
   f. Ambulates safely, using assistive devices as necessary
   g. Remains free of injury
   h. Verbalizes understanding of importance of serial CBC measurements
   i. Maintains safe home environment; obtains assistance as necessary

Hypoproliferative Anemias

Iron Deficiency Anemia

Iron deficiency anemia typically results when the intake of dietary iron is inadequate for hemoglobin synthesis. The body can store about one fourth to one third of its iron, and iron deficiency anemia does not actually develop until these stores are depleted. Iron deficiency anemia is the most common type of anemia in all age groups, and it is the most common anemia in the world. It is particularly prevalent in developing countries, where inadequate iron stores can result from inadequate intake of iron (seen with vegetarian diets) or from blood loss (e.g., from intestinal hookworm). Iron deficiency in Canada is most often related to blood loss. In fact, the cause of iron deficiency anemia should be considered to be bleeding until proven otherwise.

The most common cause of iron deficiency anemia in men and postmenopausal women is bleeding from ulcers, gastritis, inflammatory bowel disease, or GI tumours. The most common causes of iron deficiency anemia in premenopausal women are menorrhagia (i.e., excessive menstrual bleeding) and pregnancy with inadequate iron supplementation. Patients with chronic alcoholism often have chronic blood loss from the GI tract, which causes iron loss and eventual anemia. Other causes include iron malabsorption, as is seen after gastrectomy or with celiac disease.

Clinical Manifestations

Patients with iron deficiency primarily have symptoms of anemia. If the deficiency is severe or prolonged, they may also have a smooth, sore tongue; brittle and ridged nails; and angular cheilosis. These signs subside after iron replacement therapy. The health history may be significant for multiple pregnancies, GI bleeding, and pica.

Assessment and Diagnostic Findings

The definitive method of establishing the diagnosis of iron deficiency anemia is bone marrow aspiration. The aspirate is stained to detect iron, which is at a low level or even absent. However, few patients with suspected iron deficiency anemia undergo bone marrow aspiration. In many patients, the diagnosis can be established with other tests, particularly in patients with a history of conditions that predispose them to this type of anemia.

There is a strong correlation between laboratory values that measure iron stores and hemoglobin levels. After iron stores are depleted (as reflected by low serum ferritin levels), the hemoglobin level falls. The diminished iron stores cause small erythrocytes to be produced by the marrow. Therefore, as the anemia progresses, the MCV, which is a measure of the size of the erythrocytes, also decreases. Hematocrit and RBC levels are also low in relation to the hemoglobin level. Other laboratory tests that measure iron stores are useful but are not as consistent indicators as a low ferritin level, which reflects low iron stores. Typically, patients with iron deficiency anemia have a low serum iron level and an elevated TIBC, which measures the transport protein supplying the marrow with iron as needed (also referred to as **transferrin**). However, other disease states, such as infection and inflammatory conditions, can also cause a low serum iron level and TIBC, as well as an elevated ferritin level. Currently, the most reliable and clinically useful laboratory findings in evaluating iron deficiency anemia are the ferritin and hemoglobin values.

Medical Management

Except in the case of pregnancy, the cause of iron deficiency should be investigated. Anemia may be a sign of a curable GI cancer or of uterine fibroid tumours. Stool specimens should be tested for occult blood. People 50 years of age or older should have periodic colonoscopy, endoscopy, or x-ray examination of the GI tract to detect ulcerations, gastritis, polyps, or cancer. Several oral iron preparations—ferrous sulphate, ferrous gluconate, and ferrous fumarate—are available for treating iron deficiency anemia. The hemoglobin level may increase in only a few weeks, and the anemia can be corrected in a few months. Iron store replenishment takes much longer, so it is important that the patient continue taking the iron for as long as 6 to 12 months.

CHART 54-3

Parenteral Iron Formulations

- Older formulations of parenteral iron had a high molecular weight, and the risk of hypersensitivity reactions, including anaphylaxis, was significant. Newer formulations have a low molecular weight, and the risk of anaphylaxis is markedly reduced.
- Ferric gluconate (Ferrlecit): Each 5 mL contains 62.5-mg elemental iron; 125 mg is diluted in 100 mL normal saline and infused over 1 hour, or 5 mL undiluted is given as a slow IV push injection over 5 minutes. Although the likelihood of an allergic reaction is extremely low, a test dose is often given prior to the first infusion.
- Iron sucrose (Venofer): Each 5 mL contains 100-mg elemental iron; 100 to 200 mg can be given undiluted as a slow IV push injection over 2 to 5 minutes. This procedure can be repeated as often as every 3 days for a total cumulative dose of 1,000 mg within a 2-week period.

In some cases, oral iron is poorly absorbed or poorly tolerated, or iron supplementation is needed in large amounts. In these situations, IV or, infrequently, intramuscular (IM) administration of iron may be needed. Before parenteral administration of a full dose, a small test dose should be administered parenterally to avoid the risk of anaphylaxis. Emergency medications (e.g., epinephrine) should be close at hand. If no signs of allergic reaction have occurred after 30 minutes, the remaining dose of iron may be administered. Newer formulations of iron are associated with a lower incidence of anaphylaxis and test doses may not be necessary. Several doses are required to replenish the patient's iron stores (see Chart 54-3).

Nursing Management

Preventive education is important, because iron deficiency anemia is common in menstruating and pregnant women. Food sources high in iron include organ meats (e.g., beef or calf's liver, chicken liver), other meats, beans (e.g., black, pinto, and garbanzo), leafy green vegetables, raisins, and molasses. Taking iron-rich foods with a source of vitamin C (e.g., orange juice) enhances the absorption of iron.

The nurse helps the patient select a healthy diet. Nutritional counselling can be provided for those whose usual diet is inadequate. Patients with a history of eating fad diets or strict vegetarian diets are counselled that such diets often contain inadequate amounts of absorbable iron. The nurse encourages the patient to continue iron therapy as long as it is prescribed, although the patient may no longer feel fatigued.

Because iron is best absorbed on an empty stomach, the patient is instructed to take the supplement an hour before meals. Iron supplements are usually given in the oral form, typically as ferrous sulphate. Most patients can use the less expensive, more standard forms of ferrous sulphate. Tablets with enteric coating may be poorly absorbed and should be avoided. Many patients have difficulty tolerating iron supplements because of GI side effects (primarily constipation, but also cramping, nausea, and

CHART 54-4

Patient Education: Taking Oral Iron Supplements

The nurse instructs the patient to:

- Take iron on an empty stomach (1 hour before or 2 hours after a meal), preferably with orange juice or other forms of vitamin C. Iron absorption is reduced with food, especially dairy products.
- Prevent gastrointestinal distress by using the following schedule if more than one tablet a day is prescribed: Start with only one tablet per day for a few days, then increase to two tablets per day, then three tablets per day. This method permits the body to adjust gradually to the iron. If unable to tolerate oral iron supplements due to gastrointestinal distress and these interventions are inadequate, take at least one tablet daily rather than stop completely. However, reduced dosage will necessitate longer treatment duration to adequately replete iron stores.
- Increase the intake of vitamin C (citrus fruits and juices, strawberries, tomatoes, broccoli) to enhance iron absorption.
- Eat foods high in fibre to minimize problems with constipation; add stool softener if needed.
- Remember that stools will become dark in colour.
- Prevent staining the teeth with a liquid preparation by using a straw or placing a spoon at the back of the mouth to take the supplement. Rinse the mouth thoroughly afterward.

vomiting). Some iron formulations are designed to limit GI side effects by the addition of a stool softener or use of sustained-release formulations to limit nausea or gastritis. Specific patient teaching aids (Chart 54-4) can assist patients with the use of iron supplements.

If taking iron on an empty stomach causes gastric distress, the patient may need to take it with meals. However, doing so diminishes iron absorption by as much as 50%, thus prolonging the time required to replenish iron stores. Antacids or dairy products should not be taken with iron, because they greatly diminish its absorption. Polysaccharide iron complex forms are also available; they have less GI toxicity but are more expensive.

Liquid forms of iron that cause less GI distress are available. However, they can stain the teeth; the patient should be instructed to take this medication through a straw, to rinse the mouth with water, and to practice good oral hygiene after taking this medication. Finally, the patient should be informed that iron salts may colour the stool dark green or black. However, iron replacement therapy does not cause a false-positive result on stool analyses for occult blood.

IV supplementation may be used when the patient's iron stores are completely depleted, the patient cannot tolerate oral forms of iron supplementation (see Medical Management), or both. The volume of iron required when IM administration is used may be excessive, causing some local pain and possibly staining the skin. These side effects are minimized by using the Z-track technique for administering iron dextran deep into the gluteus maximus muscle (buttock). The nurse avoids vigorously rubbing the injection site after the injection. Because of the problems with IM administration, the IV route is preferred when oral administration is not possible.

Anemias in Renal Disease

The degree of anemia in patients with end-stage renal disease varies greatly, but in general patients do not become significantly anemic until the serum creatinine level exceeds 265 umol/L. The symptoms of anemia are often the most disturbing of the patient's symptoms. If untreated, the hematocrit usually falls to between 20% and 30%, although in rare cases it may fall to less than 15%. The erythrocytes are normal in appearance.

This anemia is caused by both a mild shortening of erythrocyte lifespan and a deficiency of erythropoietin (necessary for erythropoiesis). As renal function decreases, erythropoietin, which is produced by the kidney, also decreases. Because erythropoietin is also produced outside the kidney, some erythropoiesis continues, even in patients whose kidneys have been removed. However, the number of RBCs produced is small, and the degree of erythropoiesis is inadequate for normal function.

Patients undergoing long-term hemodialysis lose blood into the dialyzer and therefore may become iron deficient. Folic acid deficiency develops because this vitamin passes into the dialysate. Therefore, patients who receive hemodialysis and who have anemia should be evaluated for iron and folate deficiency and treated appropriately.

The availability of recombinant erythropoietin (epoetin alfa [Epogen, Procrit], darbepoetin alfa [Aranesp]) has dramatically altered the management of anemia in end-stage renal disease by decreasing the need for RBC transfusion, with its associated risks. Erythropoietin, in combination with oral iron supplements, can raise and maintain hematocrit levels significantly, and this can increase the risk for heart failure, heart attack, and stroke. Therefore, the hemoglobin should be checked frequently and the dose of erythropoietin titrated to maintain an appropriate hemoglobin level.

Anemia of Chronic Disease

The term *anemia of chronic disease* is a misnomer in that only the chronic diseases of inflammation, infection, and malignancy cause this type of anemia. Many chronic inflammatory diseases are associated with a **normochromic, normocytic** anemia (i.e., the erythrocytes are normal in colour and size). These disorders include rheumatoid arthritis; severe, chronic infections; and many cancers. It is therefore imperative that the specific "chronic disease" be accurately diagnosed when this form of anemia is identified so that the anemia can be appropriately managed.

The anemia is usually mild to moderate and nonprogressive. It develops gradually over 6 to 8 weeks and then stabilizes at a hematocrit seldom less than 25%. The hemoglobin level rarely falls below 100 g/L, and the bone marrow has normal cellularity with increased stores of iron as the iron is diverted from the serum. Erythropoiesis is impaired because of decreased levels of erythropoietin, as well as decreased responsiveness of the marrow to erythropoietin. Iron use is also blocked by **erythroid cells** because of increased levels of hepcidin, which inhibits iron absorption and recycling. A moderate shortening of erythrocyte survival also occurs in response to inflammatory cytokines produced in patients with cancer or chronic granulomatous infections.

Most of these patients have few symptoms and do not require treatment for the anemia. With successful treatment of the underlying disorder, the bone marrow iron is used to make erythrocytes and the hemoglobin level rises. These patients do not benefit from additional iron supplementation.

Gerontologic Considerations

Increasing evidence suggests that inflammation may have a significant role in the development of anemia in older adults (Goodnough & Schrier, 2014). Higher-than-normal levels of inflammatory cytokines (proteins) are found in the older adult population, which may also be associated with anemia (Fairweather-Tait, Wawer, Gilings, et al., 2014). This pro-inflammatory state may predispose older adults to frailty and chronic disease, manifested by weight loss, decreased mobility, generalized weakness, and poor balance; frailty is strongly associated with the anemia of chronic disease (Chang, Weis, Xue, et al., 2013). Erythropoietin levels may not rise appropriately in response to decreased hemoglobin.

Aplastic Anemia

Aplastic anemia is a rare disease caused by a decrease in or damage to marrow stem cells, damage to the microenvironment within the marrow, and replacement of the marrow with fat. The primary cause consists of an autoimmune disorder in which the body's T cells mediate an inappropriate attack against the bone marrow (Peslak, Olson, & Babushok, 2017), resulting in bone marrow **aplasia** (i.e., markedly reduced hematopoiesis). Therefore, in addition to severe anemia, significant **neutropenia** and **thrombocytopenia** (i.e., a deficiency of platelets) also occur. Other causal factors include exposure to toxins such as benzene and chloramphenicol. Some viral infections such as hepatitis and Epstein–Barr virus are also considered to be associated with aplastic anemia (Jain, Kumar, Tyagi, et al., 2012).

Pathophysiology

Aplastic anemia can be congenital or acquired, but most cases are idiopathic (i.e., without apparent cause). Infections and pregnancy can trigger this disorder; it also may be caused by certain medications, chemicals, or radiation damage. Agents that may produce marrow aplasia include benzene and benzene derivatives (e.g., airplane glue, paint remover, dry-cleaning solutions). Certain toxic materials, such as inorganic arsenic, glycol ethers, plutonium, and radon, have also been implicated as potential causes.

Clinical Manifestations

The manifestations of aplastic anemia are often insidious. Complications resulting from bone marrow failure may occur before the diagnosis is established. Typical complications are infection and the symptoms of anemia (e.g., fatigue, pallor, dyspnea). Purpura (bruising) may develop later and should trigger a CBC and hematologic evaluation if these were not performed initially. If the patient has had repeated throat infections, cervical lymphadenopathy may be seen. Other lymphadenopathies and splenomegaly sometimes occur. Retinal hemorrhages are common.

Assessment and Diagnostic Findings

In many situations, aplastic anemia occurs when a medication or chemical is ingested in toxic amounts. However, in a few people, it develops after a medication has been taken at the recommended dosage. This may be considered an idiosyncratic reaction in those who are highly susceptible, possibly caused by a genetic defect in the medication biotransformation or elimination process. A CBC reveals **pancytopenia** (a decrease in all myeloid stem cell–derived cells) with an absolute neutrophil count (ANC) less than 1,500/μL, hemoglobin less than 100 g/L, and platelets less than 50,000/μL (Segel & Lichtman, 2016). A bone marrow aspirate shows an extremely hypoplastic or even aplastic (very few to no cells) marrow replaced with fat.

Medical Management

The lymphocytes of patients with aplastic anemia destroy the stem cells and consequently impair the production of erythrocytes, leukocytes, and platelets. Despite its severity, aplastic anemia can be treated in most people. Those who are younger than 60 years, who are otherwise healthy, and who have a compatible donor can be cured of the disease by a bone marrow transplant (BMT) or hematopoietic stem cell transplant (HSCT) (Maury & Aljurf, 2013). In others, the disease can be managed with immunosuppressive therapy, commonly using a combination of antithymocyte globulin (ATG) and cyclosporine or androgens. ATG, a purified gamma-globulin solution, is obtained from horses or rabbits immunized with human T lymphocytes. Side effects during the infusion are common and may include fever and chills. The sudden onset of a rash or bronchospasm may herald anaphylaxis and requires prompt management (see Chapters 53 and 73). Serum sickness, as evidenced by fever, rash, arthralgias, and pruritus, may develop in some patients; it may take weeks to resolve.

Immunosuppressants prevent the patient's lymphocytes from destroying the stem cells. If relapse occurs (i.e., the patient becomes pancytopenic again), reinstitution of the same immunologic agents may induce another remission. Corticosteroids are not very useful as immunosuppressive agents, because patients with aplastic anemia are particularly susceptible to the development of bone complications from corticosteroids (e.g., aseptic necrosis of the head of the femur).

Supportive therapy plays a major role in the management of aplastic anemia. Any offending agent is discontinued. The patient is supported with transfusions of PRBCs and platelets as necessary. Death usually is caused by hemorrhage or infection.

Nursing Management

Patients with aplastic anemia are vulnerable to problems related to erythrocyte, leukocyte, and platelet deficiencies.

They should be assessed carefully for signs of infection and bleeding. Specific interventions are delineated in the sections on neutropenia and thrombocytopenia. Nurses must also monitor for side effects of therapy, particularly for hypersensitivity reactions while administering ATG. If patients require long-term cyclosporine therapy, they should be monitored for long-term effects, including renal or liver dysfunction, hypertension, pruritus, visual impairment, tremor, and skin cancer. Patients should also be informed that the metabolism of ATG is altered by many other medications; thus, each new prescription needs careful assessment for drug–drug interactions. Patients also need to understand the importance of not abruptly stopping their immunosuppressive therapy.

Megaloblastic Anemias

Identical bone marrow and peripheral blood changes occur with both vitamin B_{12} and folic acid deficiency because both vitamins are essential for normal DNA synthesis. With either anemia, the erythrocytes that are produced are abnormally large and are called **megaloblastic** red cells. Other cells derived from the myeloid stem cell (nonlymphoid leukocytes, platelets) are also abnormal. A bone marrow analysis reveals hyperplasia (abnormal increase in the number of cells), and the precursor erythroid and myeloid cells are large and bizarre in appearance. However, many of these abnormal erythroid and myeloid cells are destroyed within the marrow, and the mature cells that do leave the marrow are actually fewer in number. Thus, pancytopenia (a decrease in all myeloid-derived cells) can develop. In advanced stages of disease, the hemoglobin value may be as low as 44 to 55 g/L, the leukocyte count 2,000 to 3,000/mm^3, and the platelet count less than 50,000/mm^3. Those cells that are released into the circulation are often abnormally shaped. The neutrophils are also hypersegmented. The platelets may be abnormally large. The erythrocytes are abnormally shaped, and the shapes may vary widely. Because the erythrocytes are very large, the MCV is very high, usually exceeding 110 μm^3.

Pathophysiology

Folic Acid Deficiency

Folic acid is stored as compounds referred to as folates. The folate stores in the body are much smaller than those of vitamin B_{12}, and they are quickly depleted when the dietary intake of folate is deficient (within 4 months). Folate is found in green vegetables and liver. Folate deficiency occurs in people who rarely eat uncooked vegetables. Alcohol increases folic acid requirements, and at the same time, patients with alcoholism usually have a diet that is deficient in the vitamin. Folic acid requirements are also increased in patients with chronic hemolytic anemias and in women who are pregnant, because the need for erythrocyte production is increased in these conditions. Some patients with malabsorptive diseases of the small bowel, such as sprue, may not absorb folic acid normally.

Vitamin B_{12} Deficiency

A deficiency of vitamin B_{12} can occur in several ways. Inadequate dietary intake is rare but can develop in strict vegetarians who consume no meat or dairy products. Faulty absorption from the GI tract is more common. This occurs in conditions such as Crohn's disease, or after ileal resection bariatric surgery, or gastrectomy. Chronic use of histamine blockers, antacids, or proton pump inhibitors to reduce gastric acid production can also inhibit B_{12} absorption, as can the use of the drug metformin (Glucophage) in managing diabetes (Goroll & Mulley, 2014a; Singh, Kumar, Karmakar, et al., 2013). Another cause is the absence of intrinsic factor, as in *pernicious anemia*. Intrinsic factor is normally secreted by cells within the gastric mucosa; it binds with dietary vitamin B_{12} and travels with it to the ileum, where the vitamin is absorbed. Without intrinsic factor, orally consumed vitamin B_{12} cannot be absorbed, and erythrocyte production is eventually diminished. Even if adequate vitamin B_{12} and intrinsic factor are present, a deficiency may occur if a condition involving the ileum or pancreas impairs absorption. Pernicious anemia, which tends to run in families, is primarily a disorder of adults, particularly the elderly.

The body normally has large stores of vitamin B_{12}, so years may pass before the deficiency results in anemia. Because the body compensates so well, the anemia can be severe before the patient becomes symptomatic. Patients with pernicious anemia have a higher incidence of gastric cancer than the general population; these patients may benefit from having endoscopies at regular intervals to screen for early gastric cancer (Vannella, Lahner, Osborn, et al., 2013).

Clinical Manifestations

Symptoms of folic acid and vitamin B_{12} deficiencies are similar, and the two anemias may coexist. However, the neurologic manifestations of vitamin B_{12} deficiency do not occur with folic acid deficiency, and they persist if vitamin B_{12} is not replaced. Therefore, careful distinction between the two anemias must be made. Serum levels of both vitamins can be measured. In the case of folic acid deficiency, even small amounts of folate increase the serum folate level, sometimes to normal. Measuring the amount of folate within the red cell itself (red cell folate) is therefore a more sensitive test in determining true folate deficiency.

After the body stores of vitamin B_{12} are depleted, the patient may begin to show signs and symptoms of the anemia. However, because the onset and progression of the anemia are so gradual, the body can compensate very well until the anemia is severe, so that the typical manifestations of anemia (weakness, listlessness, fatigue) may not be apparent initially. The hematologic effects of deficiency are accompanied by effects on other organ systems, particularly the GI tract and nervous system. Patients with pernicious anemia develop a smooth, sore, red tongue and mild diarrhea. They are extremely pale, particularly in the mucous membranes. They may become confused; more often they have paresthesias in the extremities (particularly numbness and tingling in the feet and lower legs). They may have difficulty maintaining their balance because of damage to the spinal cord, and they also lose position sense (proprioception). These symptoms are progressive, although the course of illness may be marked by spontaneous partial remissions and exacerbations. Without treatment, patients can die after several years, usually from heart failure secondary to anemia.

Assessment and Diagnostic Findings

The classic method of determining the cause of vitamin B_{12} deficiency is the Schilling test, in which the patient receives a small oral dose of radioactive vitamin B_{12}, followed in a few hours by a large, nonradioactive parenteral dose of vitamin B_{12} (this aids in renal excretion of the radioactive dose). If the oral vitamin is absorbed, more than 8% is excreted in the urine within 24 hours; therefore, if no radioactivity is present in the urine (i.e., the radioactive vitamin B_{12} stays within the GI tract), the cause is GI malabsorption of the vitamin B_{12}. Conversely, if radioactivity is detected in the urine, the cause of the deficiency is not ileal disease or pernicious anemia. Later, the same procedure is repeated, but this time intrinsic factor is added to the oral radioactive vitamin B_{12}. If radioactivity is now detected in the urine (i.e., the vitamin B_{12} was absorbed from the GI tract in the presence of intrinsic factor), the diagnosis of pernicious anemia can be made. The Schilling test is useful only if the urine collections are complete; therefore, the nurse must promote the patient's understanding and compliance with this collection.

Other methods of establishing the diagnosis may be used. Although it is possible to measure levels of methylmalonic acid (one of the substrates for the Kreb's cycle that relies on vitamin B_{12} as a cofactor for its conversion to succinyl-CoA) in vitamin B_{12} deficiency, these levels also increase in the setting of renal insufficiency. Furthermore, it is expensive to measure these levels, which also limits the utility of the test. A more useful, easier test is the intrinsic factor antibody test. A positive test indicates the presence of antibodies that bind the vitamin B_{12}–intrinsic factor complex and prevent it from binding to receptors in the ileum, thus preventing its absorption. Although this test is not specific for pernicious anemia alone, it can aid in the diagnosis.

Medical Management

Folate deficiency is treated by increasing the amount of folic acid in the diet and administering 1 mg of folic acid daily. Folic acid is administered intramuscularly only to people with malabsorption problems. Although many multivitamin preparations now contain folic acid, additional supplements may be necessary because the amount may be inadequate to fully replace deficient body stores. Patients with alcoholism should receive folic acid as long as they continue to consume alcohol.

Vitamin B_{12} deficiency is treated by vitamin B_{12} replacement. Vegetarians can prevent or treat deficiency with oral supplements with vitamins or fortified soy milk. When the deficiency is due to the more common defect in absorption or the absence of intrinsic factor, replacement is by monthly IM injections of vitamin B_{12}. A small amount of an oral dose of vitamin B_{12} can be absorbed by passive diffusion, even in the absence of intrinsic factor, but large doses (2 mg/day) are required if vitamin B_{12} is to be replaced orally.

As vitamin B_{12} is replaced, the reticulocyte count rises within 1 week, and in several weeks the blood counts are all normal. The tongue feels better and appears less red in several days. However, the neurologic manifestations require more time for recovery; if there is severe neuropathy, the patient may never recover fully. To prevent recurrence of pernicious anemia, vitamin B_{12} therapy must be continued for life.

Nursing Management

Assessment of patients who have or are at risk for megaloblastic anemia includes inspection of the skin, mucous membranes, and tongue. Mild jaundice may be apparent and is best seen in the sclera without using fluorescent lights. Vitiligo (patchy loss of skin pigmentation) and premature greying of the hair are often seen in patients with pernicious anemia. Because of the neurologic complications associated with vitamin B_{12} deficiency anemia, a careful neurologic assessment is important, including tests of position and vibration sense.

The nurse needs to pay particular attention to ambulation and should assess the patient's gait and stability as well as the need for assistive devices (e.g., canes, walkers) and for assistance in managing daily activities. Of particular concern is ensuring safety when position sense, coordination, and gait are affected. Physical and occupational therapy referrals may be needed. If sensation is altered, the patient needs to be instructed to avoid excessive heat and cold.

Because mouth and tongue soreness may limit nutritional intake, the nurse advises the patient to eat small amounts of bland, soft foods frequently. The nurse also may explain that other nutritional deficiencies, such as alcohol-induced anemia, can induce neurologic problems.

Promoting Home, Community-Based, and Transitional Care

The patient must be taught about the chronicity of the disorder and the need for monthly vitamin B_{12} injections or daily oral vitamin B_{12}, even in the absence of symptoms. If parenteral replacement is used, many patients can be taught to self-administer their injections. The gastric atrophy associated with pernicious anemia increases the risk for gastric carcinoma, so the patient needs to understand that ongoing medical follow-up and screening are important.

Myelodysplastic Syndrome

MDS is a group of disorders of the myeloid stem cell that causes dysplasia (abnormal development) in one or more types of cell lines. The most common feature of MDS—dysplasia of the erythrocytes—is manifested as a macrocytic anemia; however, the leukocytes (myeloid cells, particularly neutrophils) and platelets can also be affected. Although the bone marrow is actually hypercellular, many of the cells within it die before being released into the circulation. Therefore, the actual number of cells in the circulation is typically lower than normal. In addition to the quantitative defect (i.e., fewer cells than normal), there is also a qualitative defect: the cells do not function normally. The neutrophils have diminished ability to destroy bacteria by phagocytosis; platelets are less able to aggregate and are less adhesive than usual. The result of these qualitative defects is an increased risk of infection and bleeding, even when the actual number of circulating cells may not be excessively low.

Primary MDS tends to be a disease of people older than 60 years of age. Because the initial findings are so subtle, the disease may not be diagnosed until later in the illness trajectory, if at all. Thus, the actual incidence of MDS is not known.

Secondary MDS can occur at any age and result from prior toxic exposure to chemicals, including chemotherapeutic medications (particularly alkylating agents). Secondary MDS tends to have a poorer prognosis than does primary MDS. Thirty percent of MDS cases evolve into acute myeloid leukemia (AML); this type of leukemia tends to be resistant to standard therapy.

Clinical Manifestations

The manifestations of MDS can vary widely. Many patients are asymptomatic, and the illness is often discovered incidentally when a CBC is performed for other purposes. Similarly other patients have profound symptoms and complications from the illness. Fatigue is often present, at varying levels. Neutrophil dysfunction puts the person at risk for recurrent pneumonias and other infections. Because platelet function can also be altered, bleeding can occur. These problems may persist in a fairly steady state for months or even years. They may also progress over time; as the dysplasia evolves into a leukemic state, the complications increase in severity.

Assessment and Diagnostic Findings

The CBC typically reveals a macrocytic anemia; leukocyte and platelet counts may be diminished as well. Serum erythropoietin levels and the reticulocyte count may be inappropriately low. If the disease evolves into AML, more immature blast cells are noted on the CBC.

The official diagnosis of MDS is based on the results of a bone marrow aspiration and biopsy. Cytogenetic analysis of the bone marrow is important in determining the overall prognosis, risk of evolution into AML, and method of treatment.

Medical Management

Allogeneic BMT or stem cell transplant (SCT) is the only cure for MDS. Medical management strategies are based on the stage of disease and prognosis. The goal for treating patients with low-risk disease is to improve cytopenias, decrease blood transfusion requirements, and improve quality of life. The goal for treating patients with high-risk disease is to decrease the likelihood that the disease transforms into AML and to extend survival (Adès, Itzykson, & Fenaux, 2014; Pandita & Mukherjee, 2014).

Patients frequently need repeated transfusions (**red blood cells [RBCs]**, platelets, or both) throughout the illness trajectory to maintain adequate hemoglobin and platelet levels (termed *transfusion dependence*). Attempts to improve anemia and decrease RBC transfusion are often successful with the use of erythroid-stimulating agents (epoetin alfa [Procrit] or darbopoetin alfa [Aranesp]). Higher-than-normal doses may be required to achieve an adequate improvement in hemoglobin. Adding myeloid growth factors such as G-CSF (filgrastim [Neupogen]) or GM-CSF (sargramostim [Leukine]) can boost responsiveness to these agents (Pandita & Mukherjee, 2014). The median duration of response to this therapy is 2 years; transfusion requirements typically increase by this point.

Thrombocytopenia is a difficult challenge to manage in the MDS patient population. It develops in 40% to 80% of patients over the course of the disease (Santini & Fenaux, 2015) and is seen in 30% of those with lower-risk MDS (Pandita & Mukherjee, 2014). Severe thrombocytopenia is difficult to manage because patients can quickly develop refractoriness to platelet transfusions due to alloimmunization (Pandita & Mukherjee, 2014). Moreover, bleeding can develop even when the platelet level is not excessively low, due to poor platelet function. The cause of thrombocytopenia appears to be increased apoptosis (programmed cell death) and premature marrow destruction of the platelets prior to their release into the circulation (Santini & Fenaux, 2015). The recombinant thrombopoietin receptor agonists romiplastim (Nplate) and eltrombopag (Promacta) have been developed to stimulate the proliferation and differentiation of megakaryocytes into platelets within the bone marrow. These agents are now being evaluated for efficacy in the context of managing thrombocytopenia in MDS. Both drugs have demonstrated the ability to significantly raise platelet counts in this population, but their duration of action may not be long. Increased rates of marrow fibrosis and AML evolution seem to be ameliorated by discontinuing the drug, but additional study is needed.

Unique findings in subsets of MDS can be used to guide special approaches to therapy. Lenalidomide (Revlimid) is extremely effective in treating patients who have a specific cytogenetic/chromosomal abnormality, such as the deletion of 5q. Patients with hypocellular marrows may respond well to immunosuppressive therapy using ATG (Garcia-Manero, 2015).

Patients with intermediate-risk disease are typically treated with either of two available hypomethylating agents—azacitidine or decitabine (Dacogen). These drugs work by inhibiting the abnormal genes regulating methylation, promoting tumour suppression genes, and permitting myeloid differentiation within the bone marrow. Neither drug has been shown to modify the natural trajectory of lower-risk MDS; therefore, hypomethylating agents are not typically used until erythroid-stimulating agents are no longer effective in controlling transfusion dependence (Garcia-Manero, 2015). Response to azacitidine can result in improved cytopenias, reduced transfusion requirements, reduced transformation to AML, and improved overall survival. A recent meta-analysis suggests a higher rate of partial and overall response and overall hematologic improvement with azacitidine compared with decitabine (Xie, Jiang, & Xie, 2015). Azacitidine also may be more effective when used in those of older age or who have higher-risk disease. However, as each drug has a slightly different mechanism of action, changing to the alternate drug may still be effective if the disease becomes resistant.

Traditionally, intensive chemotherapy has been used in patients with more aggressive forms of the illness. Results are disappointing, particularly in the context of unfavourable cytogenetic abnormalities (Adès et al., 2014). Secondary MDS and MDS that evolves into AML tend to be refractory to conventional therapy for leukemia.

Infection rates are high in the MDS population. In a retrospective review, infections were identified in 21% of MDS patients; infections requiring hospitalization occurred in 15% of these patients within the first year from the time of diagnosis (Sullivan, Sekeres, Shrestha, et al., 2013). In this study, rates of infection were similar between those patients with low-risk disease and those with high-risk disease. Severe neutropenia, coexisting chronic obstructive pulmonary disease (COPD) or autoimmune disease, and history of other malignancy were associated with higher risk for developing infection, whereas the extent of thrombocytopenia, age, MDS therapy, or diabetes were not. Pneumonia was the most common type of infection in this study; bacteria (gram negative and gram positive) were the predominant pathogens.

The administration of myeloid growth factors alone may be useful in some patients with infections and severe neutropenia, but they are not typically used to prevent infection. Studies have not found them useful in improving overall survival (Pandita & Mukherjee, 2014). Prophylactic antibiotics are not routinely used so that resistant organisms do not develop, but prompt initiation of antimicrobial therapy is crucial at the onset of infection to diminish the risk of increased mortality.

Iron overload is another significant problem for patients with MDS. Data suggest that ineffective erythropoiesis in MDS results in increased iron absorption from the intestinal tract, thereby resulting in elevated ferritin levels even in the absence of repeated red cell transfusions (Nolte, Angelucci, Breccia, et al., 2015; Steensma & Gatterman, 2013). However, red cell transfusion dependence is the primary cause for iron overload in this patient population. Here, surplus iron is deposited in cells within the RES, and later in parenchymal organs (e.g., liver). While a true cause-and-effect has not yet been established, there is significant concern that patients with transfusion-dependent MDS are at high risk for developing cardiac events, particularly heart failure. Excess iron, and the resultant increased oxidative stress, is also associated with hepatic and pancreatic dysfunction, the development of diabetes, increased rates of infection, and decreased hematopoiesis. Studies are ongoing to further investigate if iron overload actually causes these complications.

In patients with MDS, iron overload is typically managed by chelation therapy. Iron is bound to the chelating agent and then excreted in the urine. Because chelation therapy removes only a small amount of iron with each treatment, patients with chronic iron overload from RBC transfusions need to continue chelation therapy as long as the iron overload exists. Oral iron chelation with deferasirox (Exjade) has replaced the need for long subcutaneous infusions of deferoxamine (Desferal). However, adherence remains a challenge, largely due to toxicity associated with the drug.

Because MDS tends to occur in older adults, other concurrent chronic conditions may limit treatment options.

Nursing Management

Caring for patients with MDS can be challenging because the illness is unpredictable. As with other hematologic conditions, some patients (especially those with no symptoms) have difficulty perceiving that they have a serious illness that can place them at risk of life-threatening complications. At the other extreme, many patients have tremendous difficulty coping with the uncertain trajectory of the illness and fear that the illness will evolve into AML. Thus, it is important for patients to understand their unique risk of the disease transforming to AML and to recognize that MDS is a chronic illness.

Patients with MDS need extensive instruction about infection risk, measures to avoid such risk, signs and symptoms of developing infection, and appropriate actions to take should such symptoms occur. Instruction should also be given regarding the risk of bleeding. Patients with MDS who are hospitalized may require neutropenic precautions.

Laboratory values need to be monitored closely to anticipate the need for transfusion and to determine response to treatment with growth factors. Patients with chronic transfusion requirements often benefit from the insertion of a vascular access device for this purpose. Patients receiving growth factors or chelation therapy need instruction about these medications, their side effects, and administration techniques, if self-administered.

Chelation therapy is a process that is used to remove excess iron acquired from chronic transfusions. Iron is bound to a substance, the chelating agent, and then excreted in the urine. Because chelation therapy removes only a small amount of iron with each treatment, patients with chronic transfusion requirements (and iron overload) need to continue chelation therapy as long as the iron overload exists, potentially for the rest of their lives. Renal and liver dysfunction are possible, so serum creatinine and liver function tests should be monitored and the medication held until the laboratory results return to baseline; the medication is typically resumed at a reduced dose. Patients should also have baseline and annual auditory and eye examinations, because hearing loss and visual changes can occur with chelation treatment.

Hemolytic Anemias

In hemolytic anemias, the erythrocytes have a shortened lifespan; thus, their number in the circulation is reduced. Fewer erythrocytes result in decreased available oxygen, causing hypoxia, which in turn stimulates an increase in erythropoietin release from the kidney. The erythropoietin stimulates the bone marrow to compensate by producing new erythrocytes and releasing some of them into the circulation somewhat prematurely as reticulocytes. If the red cell destruction persists, the hemoglobin is broken down excessively; about 80% of the heme is converted to bilirubin, conjugated in the liver, and excreted in the bile.

The mechanism of erythrocyte destruction varies, but all types of hemolytic anemia share certain laboratory features. The reticulocyte count is elevated, the fraction of indirect (unconjugated) bilirubin is increased, and the supply of haptoglobin (a binding protein for free hemoglobin) is depleted as more hemoglobin is released. As a result, the plasma haptoglobin level is low. If the marrow cannot compensate to replace the erythrocytes (indicated by a decreased reticulocyte count), the anemia will progress.

Hemolytic anemia has various forms. Inherited forms include sickle cell anemia, thalassemia and thalassemia major, G-6-PD deficiency, and hereditary spherocytosis (erythrocytes are sphere shaped rather than in the form of a biconcave disk). Acquired forms include autoimmune hemolytic anemia, non–immune-mediated paroxysmal nocturnal hemoglobinuria, microangiopathic hemolytic anemia, and heart valve hemolysis, as well as anemias associated with hypersplenism.

Sickle Cell Disease

Sickle cell anemia is a severe hemolytic anemia that results from inheritance of the sickle hemoglobin gene. This gene causes the hemoglobin molecule to be defective. The sickle hemoglobin (HbS) acquires a crystal-like formation when exposed to low oxygen tension. The oxygen level in venous blood can be low enough to cause this change; consequently, the erythrocyte containing HbS loses its round, pliable, biconcave disk shape and becomes deformed, rigid, and sickle shaped (Fig. 54-6). These long, rigid erythrocytes can adhere to the endothelium of small vessels; when they adhere to each other, blood flow to a region or an organ may be reduced. If ischemia or infarction results, the patient may have pain, swelling, and fever. The sickling process takes time; if the erythrocyte is again exposed to adequate amounts of oxygen (e.g., when it travels through the pulmonary circulation) before the membrane becomes too rigid, it can revert to a normal shape. For this reason, the "sickling crises" are intermittent. Cold can aggravate the sickling process, because vasoconstriction slows the blood flow. Oxygen delivery can also be impaired by an increased blood viscosity, with or without occlusion due to adhesion of sickled cells; in this situation, the effects are seen in larger vessels, such as arterioles.

The *HbS* gene is inherited in people of African descent and to a lesser extent in people from the Middle East, the Mediterranean area, and aboriginal tribes in India. Sickle cell anemia is the most severe form of sickle cell disease. Less severe forms include sickle cell hemoglobin C (SC) disease, sickle cell hemoglobin D (SD) disease, and sickle cell beta-thalassemia. The clinical manifestations and management are the same as for sickle cell anemia. The term *sickle cell trait* refers to the carrier state for SC diseases; it is the most benign type of SC disease, in that less than 50% of the hemoglobin within an erythrocyte is HbS. However, if two people with sickle cell trait have children, the children may inherit two abnormal genes and will have sickle cell anemia. (Refer to Chapter 11 for additional discussion of genetic diseases.)

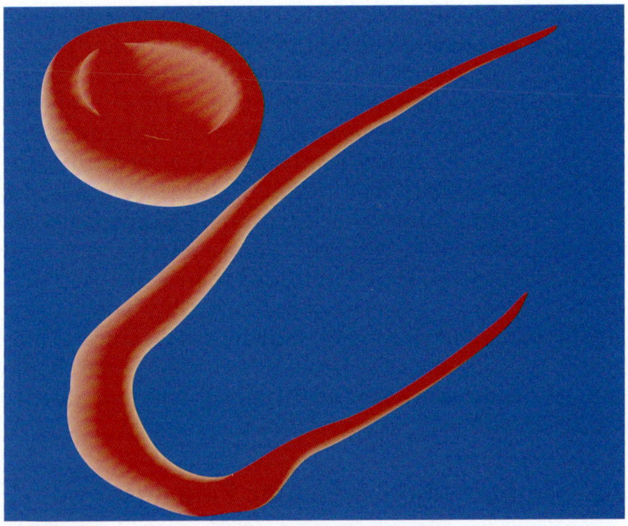

FIGURE 54-6. A normal red blood cell (**upper left**) and a sickled red blood cell.

Clinical Manifestations

Symptoms of sickle cell disease vary and are only somewhat based on the amount of HbS. Symptoms and complications result from chronic hemolysis or thrombosis. Sickled cells are rapidly hemolyzed and thus have a very short lifespan (10 to 12 days). Anemia is always present; usually hemoglobin values are 75 to 100 g/L. Jaundice is characteristic and is usually obvious in the sclerae. The bone marrow expands in childhood in a compensatory effort to offset the anemia, sometimes leading to enlargement of the bones of the face and skull. The chronic anemia is associated with tachycardia, cardiac murmurs, and often an enlarged heart (cardiomegaly). Dysrhythmias and heart failure may occur in adults.

Virtually any organ may be affected by thrombosis, but the primary sites for sickle cell crises involve those areas with slower circulation, such as the spleen, lungs, and central nervous system. All the tissues and organs are vulnerable to microcirculatory interruptions by the sickling process and therefore are susceptible to hypoxic damage or ischemic necrosis. Patients with sickle cell anemia are unusually susceptible to infection, particularly pneumonia and osteomyelitis. Complications of sickle cell anemia include infection, stroke, renal failure, impotence, heart failure, and pulmonary hypertension (Table 54-4).

Sickle Cell Crisis

There are three types of sickle cell crisis in the adult population. The most common is the very painful *sickle crisis*, which results from tissue hypoxia and necrosis due to inadequate blood flow to a specific region of tissue or organ. *Aplastic crisis* results from infection with the human parvovirus. The hemoglobin level falls rapidly and the marrow cannot compensate, as evidenced by an absence of reticulocytes. *Sequestration crisis* results when other organs pool the sickled cells. Although the spleen is the most common organ responsible for sequestration in children, most children with sickle cell anemia have had a splenic infarction by 10 years of age, and the spleen is then no longer functional (autosplenectomy). In adults, the common organs involved in sequestration are the liver and, more seriously, the lungs.

Acute Chest Syndrome

Acute chest syndrome is a complication of the pulmonary vasculature where blood flow is occluded; it is commonly seen with people who have sickle cell disease and is manifested by fever, cough, tachycardia, and new infiltrates seen on the chest x-ray. These signs often mimic infection, which is often the cause. However, the infectious etiology appears to be atypical bacteria such as *Chlamydia pneumoniae* and *Mycoplasma pneumoniae,* as well as viruses such as respiratory syncytial virus (RSV) and parvovirus.

TABLE 54-4 Complications in Sickle Cell Disease[a]

Organ Involved	Mechanisms[a]	Diagnostic Findings	Signs and Symptoms
Spleen	Primary site of sickling → infarctions → ↓ phagocytic function of macrophages	Autosplenectomy; ↑ infection (especially pneumonia, osteomyelitis)	Abdominal pain; fever, signs of infection
Lungs	Infection	Pulmonary infiltrate	Chest pain; dyspnea
	Infarction → ↑ pulmonary pressure → pulmonary hypertension	↑ $sPLA_2$[b]	Chest pain; dyspnea
Central nervous system	Infarction	Stroke	Weakness (if severe); learning difficulties (if mild)
Kidney	Sickling → damage to renal medulla	Hematuria; inability to concentrate urine; kidney injury	Dehydration
Heart	Anemia	Tachycardia; cardiomegaly → heart failure	Weakness, fatigue, dyspnea
Bone	↑ Erythroid production	Widening of medullary spaces and cortical thinning	Ache, arthralgias
	Infarction of bone	Osteosclerosis → avascular necrosis	Bone pain, especially hips
Liver	Hemolysis	Jaundice and gallstone formation; hepatomegaly	Abdominal pain
Skin and peripheral vasculature	↑ Viscosity/stasis → infarction → skin ulcers	Skin ulcers; ↓ wound healing	Pain
Eye	Infarction	Scarring, hemorrhage, retinal detachment	↓ Vision; blindness
Penis	Sickling → vascular thrombosis	Priapism → impotence	Pain, impotence

[a]Problems encountered in sickle cell disease vary and are the result of a variety of mechanisms, as depicted in this table. Common physical findings and symptoms are also variable.

[b]Elevated $sPLA_2$ levels can predict impending acute chest syndrome (see text).

→, leading to; ↓, decreased; ↑, increased; $sPLA_2$, secretory phospholipase A_2.

Other causes include pulmonary fat embolism, pulmonary infarction, and pulmonary thromboembolism. Increased secretory phospholipase A_2 concentration has been identified as a predictor of impending acute chest syndrome; the increased amounts of free fatty acids can cause increased permeability of the pulmonary endothelium and leakage of the pulmonary capillaries). Although this syndrome can progress to acute respiratory distress syndrome and death, prompt and aggressive intervention can result in a favourable outcome; some people benefit from taking hydroxycarbamide (or hydroxyurea and Hydrea) as a preventative measure. This medication helps to increase the production of both fetal and normal hemoglobin.

Pulmonary Hypertension

Pulmonary hypertension is a common sequela of sickle cell disease, and often the cause of death (Howard et al., 2015). Diagnosing pulmonary hypertension is difficult because clinical symptoms rarely occur until damage is irreversible. Pulse oximetry measurements are typically normal, and breath sounds are clear to auscultation until the disease has progressed to later stages. Although changes are not evident on chest x-ray, computed tomography (CT) of the chest often demonstrates microvascular pulmonary occlusion and diminished perfusion of the lung. The diagnosis of pulmonary hypertension is elusive, but screening patients with sickle cell disease with Doppler echocardiography is useful in identifying patients with elevated pulmonary artery pressures (Howard et al., 2015).

Stroke

Stroke is a devastating complication of SCD that affects 11% of patients under 20 years of age (Natrajan & Kutlar, 2016). While ischemic strokes are most common, particularly in young children and older adults, hemorrhagic stroke is more common in younger adults. The mechanisms are varied, but often result from decreased cerebral blood flow due to anemia, hemolysis, and increased hypoxic stress. Silent cerebral infarction is more common, with a prevalence of 40% (Quinn, 2014). Even without abnormal brain imaging, asymptomatic adults may have evidence of decline in neurocognitive function. These individuals are at risk for developing overt stroke (Quinn, 2014). Medical management of stroke includes red cell transfusions to reduce the level of hemoglobin S to less than 30%, thereby preventing cerebral edema (Chou, 2013).

Reproductive Problems

As patients live longer with SCD, the adverse impact on sexual function is now better appreciated. Almost 25% of men with SCD develop hypogonadism (Smith-Whitley, 2014). Low testosterone levels, low libido, erectile dysfunction, and infertility can occur. Frequent episodes of priapism (prolonged erection of the penis, typically without sexual stimulation) can also contribute to significant pain, decreased libido, and impotence. These problems can be a source of extreme embarrassment and depression. Menarche may be delayed in females, but menstrual patterns appear normal (Smith-Whitley, 2014). Pain episodes may be increased during menstruation. Fertility issues are not well assessed in women. Contraception is important when hydroxyurea (Hydrea) is used to treat SCD as it may be teratogenic. Concerns about infertility when using hydroxyurea may adversely influence adherence to this therapy among men (DeBaun, 2014). The nurse should initiate open discussions about sexual and reproductive concerns with patients prescribed this therapy.

Assessment and Diagnostic Findings

The patient with sickle cell trait usually has a normal hemoglobin level, a normal hematocrit, and a normal blood smear. In contrast, the patient with sickle cell anemia has a low hematocrit and sickled cells on the smear. The diagnosis is confirmed by hemoglobin electrophoresis.

Prognosis

Patients with sickle cell disease are usually diagnosed in childhood because they become anemic in infancy and begin to have sickle cell crises at 1 or 2 years of age. Some children die in the first years of life, typically of infection, but antibiotic use and parent teaching strategies have greatly improved the outcomes for these children. However, with current management strategies, the average life expectancy is still suboptimal: 42 to 48 years. Young adults are often forced to live with multiple, often severe, complications from their disease. In some patients, the symptoms and complications diminish by 30 years of age; these patients live into the sixth decade or longer. Currently, there is no way to predict which patients will fall into this subgroup.

Medical Management

Treatment for sickle cell disease is the focus of continued research. However, aside from the equally important aggressive management of symptoms and complications, there are currently few primary treatment modalities for sickle cell diseases.

Hematopoietic Stem Cell Transplant (HSCT)

HSCT may cure sickle cell disease. However, this treatment modality is available to only a small subset of affected patients because of either the lack of a compatible donor or because severe organ damage (e.g., renal, liver, lung) that may be already present in the patient is a contraindication for HSCT.

Pharmacologic Therapy

Hydroxyurea is a chemotherapy agent that is effective in increasing fetal hemoglobin (i.e., hemoglobin F) levels in patients with SCD, thereby decreasing the formation of sickled cells; it currently is the only FDA-approved drug for this disease in the United States (Ataga & Stocker, 2015). In a landmark study, patients who received hydroxyurea had fewer painful episodes of sickle cell crisis, a lower incidence of acute chest syndrome, and less need for transfusions (Charache, Terrin, Moore, et al., 1995); subsequent studies revealed a 40% decrease in mortality in those individuals who received the drug (Natrajan & Kutlar, 2016). However, whether hydroxyurea can prevent or reverse actual organ damage needs to be investigated further. Side effects of hydroxyurea include chronic suppression of leukocyte formation, teratogenesis, and potential for later development of a malignancy. Patient response to this agent varies significantly. The incidence and severity of side effects are also highly variable within a dose range. Adherence to taking this medication as prescribed is a common problem.

Patients with sickle cell disease require daily folic acid replacements to maintain the supply required for increased erythropoiesis from hemolysis. Infections must be treated promptly with appropriate antibiotics; infection, particularly pneumococcal infection, remains a major cause of death. These patients should receive pneumococcal and annual influenza vaccinations (Howard et al., 2015).

Acute chest syndrome, a vaso-occlusive crisis of the pulmonary vasculature commonly seen in people with sickle cell disease, is managed by prompt initiation of antibiotic therapy. Incentive spirometry has been shown to decrease the incidence of pulmonary complications significantly. In severe cases, bronchoscopy may be required to identify the source of pulmonary disease. Hydration is important but must be carefully monitored. Corticosteroids may also be useful. Transfusions reverse the hypoxia and decrease the level of secretory phospholipase A_2. Pulmonary function should be monitored regularly to detect pulmonary hypertension early, when therapy (hydroxyurea, arginine, transfusions, or BMT) may have a positive impact.

Transfusion Therapy

RBC transfusions have been shown to be highly effective in several situations: in an acute exacerbation of anemia (e.g., aplastic crisis), in the prevention of severe complications from anesthesia and surgery, in improving the response to infection (when the infection results in exacerbated anemia), and in severe cases of acute chest syndrome (Chou, 2013). Transfusions are also effective in diminishing episodes of sickle cell crisis in pregnant women, but this does not improve fetal survival. Chronic transfusion therapy may be effective in preventing or managing complications from sickle cell disease, including stroke, acute chest syndrome, and acute exacerbation of anemia (Chou, 2013).

The risk of complications from transfusion is important to consider. These risks include iron overload, which necessitates chelation therapy (see Myelodysplastic Syndrome, Nursing Management); poor venous access, which necessitates a vascular access device (and its attendant risk of infection or thrombosis); infections (hepatitis, human immunodeficiency virus [HIV]); and especially alloimmunization (an immune response to antigens from donor cells) from repeated transfusions. Another complication from transfusion is increased blood viscosity without reduction in the concentration of hemoglobin S. Exchange transfusion (in which the patient's own blood is removed and replaced via transfusion) may be performed to diminish the risk of increasing the viscosity excessively; the objective is to reduce the hematocrit to less than 30%, with transfusions supplying more than 80% of the patient's blood volume. Finally, it is important to consider the significant financial cost of an aggressive transfusion and chelation program.

Chelation therapy is a process that is used to remove excess iron acquired from chronic transfusions. Side effects from oral chelators commonly include diarrhea and abdominal cramping. Instructing the patient to take the medication in the evening prior to dinner and gradually increasing the dosage over time may diminish these side effects (Nolte et al., 2015; Steensma & Gatterman, 2013). Skin rash is usually mild and rarely warrants temporarily stopping the drug. Monitoring renal function is important as a rise in serum creatinine is common. The dosage should be reduced if the serum creatinine rises by more than one third of baseline. Patients with pre-existing liver disease, including cirrhosis, should not receive oral iron chelators.

Because repeated blood transfusions are necessary, patients may develop multiple autoantibodies, making cross-matching difficult. In this patient population, a hemolytic transfusion reaction (see later discussion) may mimic the signs and symptoms of a sickle cell crisis. The classic distinguishing factor is that with a hemolytic transfusion reaction, the patient becomes *more* anemic after being transfused. These patients need very close observation. Further transfusion is avoided if possible until the hemolytic process abates. If possible, the patient is supported with corticosteroids (prednisone), IV immunoglobulin (IVIG), and erythropoietin (Epogen).

Supportive Therapy

Supportive care is equally important. Pain management is a significant issue. The incidence of painful sickle cell crises is highly variable; many patients have pain on a daily basis. The severity of the pain may not be enough to cause the patient to seek assistance from health care providers but severe enough to interfere with the ability to work and function within the family unit. Acute pain episodes tend to be self-limited, lasting hours to days. If the patient cannot manage the pain at home, intervention is frequently sought in an urgent care facility or emergency department. Adequate hydration is important during a painful sickling episode. Oral hydration is acceptable if the patient can maintain adequate fluid intake; IV hydration with dextrose 5% in water (D_5W) or dextrose 5% in 0.25 normal saline solution (3 $L/m^2/24$ hours) is usually required for sickle crisis. Supplemental oxygen may also be needed.

The use of medication to relieve pain is important (see Chapter 16 for a discussion of pain management). Aspirin is very useful in diminishing mild to moderate pain; it also diminishes inflammation and potential thrombosis (due to its ability to decrease platelet adhesion). Nonsteroidal anti-inflammatory drugs (NSAIDs) are useful for moderate pain or in combination with opioid analgesics. Although no tolerance develops with NSAIDs, a "ceiling effect" does develop whereby an increase in dosage does not increase analgesia. NSAID use must be carefully monitored, because these medications can precipitate renal dysfunction. When opioid analgesic agents are used, morphine is the medication of choice for acute pain. Patient-controlled analgesia (PCA) is frequently used. Patients using PCA morphine tend to have less sedation side effects.

Chronic pain increases in incidence as the patient ages and is caused by continued complications (e.g., avascular necrosis of the hip) from the sickling. With chronic pain management, the principal goal is to maximize functioning; pain may not be completely eliminated without sacrificing function. This concept may be difficult for patients to accept; they may need repeated explanations and support from nonjudgmental health care providers. Nonpharmacologic approaches to pain management are crucial in this setting. Examples include physical and occupational therapy, physiotherapy (including the use of heat, massage, and exercise), cognitive and behavioural intervention (including distraction, relaxation, and motivational therapy), and support groups.

Working with patients who have multiple episodes of severe pain can be challenging. It is important for health care providers to realize that patients with sickle cell disease must face a lifelong experience with severe and unpredictable pain. Such pain is disruptive to the patient's level of functioning, including social functioning, and may result in a feeling of helplessness. Patients with inadequate social support systems may have more difficulty coping with chronic pain.

Nursing Process

The Patient With Sickle Cell Crisis

Assessment

The patient is asked to identify factors that precipitated previous crises and measures he or she uses to prevent and manage crises. Pain levels should always be monitored using a pain intensity scale, such as a 0-to-10 scale. The quality of the pain (e.g., sharp, dull, burning), the frequency of the pain (constant vs. intermittent), and factors that aggravate or alleviate the pain are included in this assessment. If a sickle cell crisis is suspected, the nurse needs to determine whether the pain currently experienced is the same as or different from the pain typically encountered in crisis.

Because the sickling process can interrupt circulation in any tissue or organ, with resultant hypoxia and ischemia, a careful assessment of all body systems is necessary. Particular emphasis is placed on pain, swelling, and fever. All joint areas are carefully examined for pain and swelling. The abdomen is assessed for pain and tenderness because of the possibility of splenic infarction.

The cardiopulmonary systems must be assessed carefully, including auscultation of breath sounds, measurement of oxygen saturation levels, and signs of cardiac failure, such as the presence and extent of dependent edema, an increased point of maximal impulse (PMI), and cardiomegaly (as seen on a chest x-ray). The patient is assessed for signs of dehydration by a history of fluid intake and careful examination of mucous membranes, skin turgor, urine output, and serum creatinine and blood urea nitrogen (BUN) values.

A careful neurologic examination is important to elicit symptoms of cerebral hypoxia. However, ischemic findings on magnetic resonance imaging (MRI) or Doppler studies may precede findings on the physical examination. MRI and Doppler studies are used for early diagnosis and may result in improved patient outcome because therapy can be initiated promptly.

Because patients with sickle cell anemia are susceptible to infections, they are assessed for the presence of any infectious process. Particular attention is given to examination of the chest, long bones, and femoral head, because pneumonia and osteomyelitis are especially common. Leg ulcers, which may be infected and slow to heal, are common (see Fig. 54-7).

The extent of anemia and the ability of the marrow to replenish erythrocytes are assessed by the hemoglobin level, hematocrit, and reticulocyte counts, and they are compared with the patient's baseline values. The patient's current and past history of medical management is also obtained, particularly chronic transfusion therapy, hydroxyurea use, and prior treatment for infection.

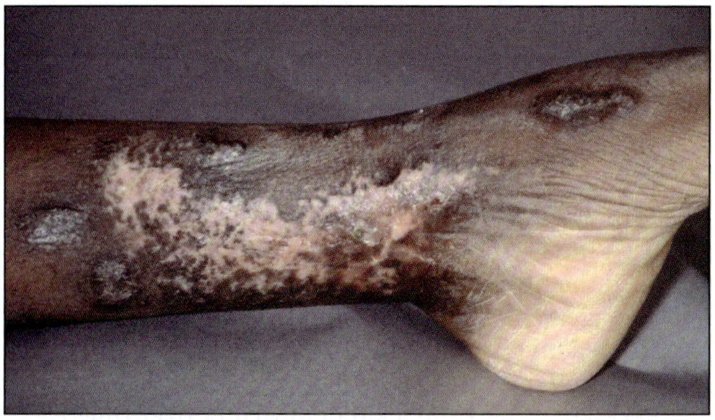

FIGURE 54-7. Chronic skin ulcers seen in a patient with sickle cell anemia. (From Tkachuk, D. C., & Hirschman, J. V. (2007). *Wintrobe's atlas of clinical hematology* (Fig. 1.71, p. 36). Philadelphia, PA: Lippincott Williams & Wilkins.)

Nursing Priorities

Based on the assessment data, major nursing priorities for the patient with sickle cell crisis may include:

- Acute pain and fatigue
- Risk for infection
- Risk for powerlessness and helplessness
- Deficient knowledge

Collaborative Problems/ Potential Complications

Based on the assessment data, potential complications may include:

- Hypoxia, ischemia, infection, and poor wound healing leading to skin breakdown and ulcers
- Dehydration
- Cerebrovascular accident (CVA, brain attack, stroke)
- Anemia
- Acute and chronic renal failure
- Heart failure, pulmonary hypertension, and acute chest syndrome
- Impotence
- Poor compliance
- Substance abuse related to poorly managed chronic pain

Planning and Goals

The major goals for the patient are relief of pain, decreased incidence of crisis, enhanced sense of self-esteem and power, and absence of complications.

Nursing Interventions

Managing Pain

Acute pain during a sickle cell crisis can be severe and unpredictable. The patient's subjective description and rating of pain on a pain scale must guide the use of analgesic agents. Any joint that is acutely swollen should be supported and elevated until the swelling diminishes. Relaxation techniques, breathing exercises, and distraction are helpful for some patients. After the acute painful episode has diminished, aggressive measures should be implemented to preserve function. Physical therapy, whirlpool baths, and transcutaneous electrical nerve stimulation (TENS) are examples of such modalities.

Managing Fatigue

The fatigue experienced can be acute or chronic in nature. Assisting the patient to find an appropriate balance between exercise and rest can be a useful strategy. Patients will need to develop strategies to cope with daily life demands in the setting of chronic fatigue. Maximizing nutrition, hydration, healthy sleep cycles, and diminishing tissue hypoxia can all serve to minimize fatigue. Research is needed to better understand fatigue in this patient population as well as to delineate the most effective ways to ameliorate it.

Preventing and Managing Infection

Nursing care focuses on monitoring patients for signs and symptoms of infection. Prescribed antibiotics should be initiated promptly, and patients should be assessed for signs of dehydration. If patients are to take prescribed oral antibiotics at home, they must understand the importance of completing the entire course of antibiotic therapy.

Promoting Coping Skills

This illness frequently leaves the patient feeling powerless and with decreased self-esteem because its acute exacerbations often result in chronic health problems. These feelings can be exacerbated by inadequate pain management, and enhancing pain management can be extremely useful in establishing a therapeutic relationship based on mutual trust. Nursing care that focuses on the patient's strengths rather than deficits can enhance effective coping skills. Providing the patient with opportunities to make decisions about daily care may increase the patient's feelings of control. The patient needs to understand the rationale for and importance of compliance with a therapeutic medication regimen.

Minimizing Deficient Knowledge

Patients with sickle cell anemia benefit from understanding what situations can precipitate a sickle cell crisis and the steps they can take to prevent or diminish such crises. Keeping warm and maintaining adequate hydration can be effective in diminishing the occurrence and severity of attacks.

If hydroxyurea is prescribed for a woman of childbearing age, she should be told that the drug can cause congenital harm to unborn children and advised about pregnancy prevention.

Monitoring and Managing Potential Complications

Management measures for many of the potential complications have been described in previous sections. Other measures follow.

LEG ULCERS. Leg ulcers require careful management and protection from trauma and contamination. Referral to a wound–ostomy–continence nurse (WOCN) may facilitate healing and assist with prevention. If leg ulcers fail to heal, skin grafting may be necessary. Scrupulous aseptic technique is warranted to prevent nosocomial infections.

PRIAPISM LEADING TO IMPOTENCE. Male patients may develop sudden, painful episodes of priapism (persistent penile erection). The patient is taught to empty his bladder at the onset of the attack, exercise, and take a warm bath. If an episode persists longer than 3 hours, medical attention, which consists of IV hydration, administration of analgesic agents, and possible penile intracavernosal aspiration, is recommended. Repeated episodes may lead to extensive vascular thrombosis, resulting in impotence.

CHRONIC AND ACUTE PAIN. Many patients have considerable difficulty coping with chronic pain and repeated episodes of sickle cell crisis and may find it difficult to adhere to a prescribed treatment plan. Some patients with SCD develop problems with substance abuse, although the rate of abuse in this patient population is similar to populations of patients with other diseases (Natrajan & Kutlar, 2016). This results from inadequate management of acute pain during episodes of crisis, which then promotes mistrust of the health care system and (from the patient's perspective) the need to seek care from other sources. In a qualitative study of health care system engagement and opioid pain use, patients with SCD who viewed themselves as "allies" and used interpersonal and symptom-specific strategies used the hospital setting less frequently for pain management than those who had a more defensive and reactive approach with their health care providers (Brown, Weisberg, Balf-Soran, et al., 2014). Receiving care from a single provider over time is much more beneficial than receiving care from rotating physicians and staff in an ED. Prior negative ED experiences often result in the patient delaying appropriate care during a subsequent painful episode (Jenerette, Brewer, & Ataga, 2014). When crises occur, the staff in the ED should be in contact with the patient's primary provider so that optimal management can be achieved. Frank, open discussion can be instrumental in promoting trust and improved outcomes. Health care providers' attitudes toward patients with SCD are also important if improved outcomes are to be achieved (Freiermuth, Haywood, Silva, et al., 2014) (see Chart 54-5).

NURSING RESEARCH PROFILE

Chart 54-5. Attitudes Toward Patients With Sickle Cell Disease in a Multicentre Sample of Emergency Department Providers

Freiermuth, C. E., Haywood, C., Silva, S., et al. (2014). Attitudes toward patients with sickle cell disease in a multicenter sample of emergency department providers. *Advanced Emergency Nursing Journal*, *36*(4), 335–347.

Purpose

Pain management for vaso-occlusive crisis is a common reason patients with sickle cell disease (SCD) seek care in the emergency department (ED). An earlier systematic literature review noted strong evidence that negative attitudes from health care providers can be a barrier to adequate pain management in this patient population. Being able to accurately measure health care provider attitudes toward patients with SCD is important for assessing the efficacy of interventions to address these barriers. The purpose of this study was threefold: (1) to validate an assessment scale to assess attitudes of health care providers toward patients with SCD, (2) to measure the attitudes of health care providers working in the ED setting toward patients with SCD, and (3) to explore differences in attitudes between types of health care professionals working in the ED.

Design

A convenience sample of 214 providers (120 registered nurses [RNs], 50 resident physicians, 33 attending physicians, 11 nurse practitioners and physician assistants) from two Level 1 trauma centres in North Carolina consented to participate in this study by completing the General Perceptions about SCD Patients Scale and the Medical Condition Regard Scale (used to test the validity of the General Perceptions scale). Demographic data from the participants were also gathered, including age, gender, ethnicity, years of experience in the role, and average number of patients with SCD cared for during an average week.

Findings

The majority of all providers were white; only 6.5% were black. When compared with physicians, nurses reported higher negative attitude scores and lower uneasiness scores; there was no significant difference in positive attitude scores between these two groups of professionals. Nurses also reported higher mean levels of frustration in caring for adults with SCD than the physicians. When compared with physicians, more nurses reported feeling that opioid addiction was prevalent in the general population of adults with SCD and in those with SCD treated in the ED. Scores related to beliefs about addiction were markedly higher in the RN group than the physician group. Given the small numbers of non-white participants, it was not possible to analyze difference in scores between ethnic groups.

Nursing Implications

Data from this study suggest that the General Perceptions about SCD Patients Scale is reliable and valid for use in health care professional staff. The data also support the need to improve attitudes of those health care professionals caring for individuals with SCD, particularly RNs, in the context of pain and pain management. Developing appropriate education, peer support, and multidisciplinary quality improvement team tracking can improve the ED care experience of patients with SCD.

Promoting Home, Community-Based, and Transitional Care

EDUCATING PATIENTS ABOUT SELF-CARE. Because patients with sickle cell disease are typically diagnosed as children, parents participate in the initial education. As the child ages, educational interventions prepare the child to assume more responsibility for self-care. Most families can learn about vascular access device management and chelation therapy. Nurses in outpatient facilities or home care nurses may need to provide follow-up care for patients with vascular access devices.

CONTINUING AND TRANSITIONAL CARE. The illness trajectory of sickle cell disease is highly varied, with unpredictable episodes of complications and crises. Care is often provided on an emergency basis, especially for some patients with pain management problems (see previous section). All health care providers who provide services to patients with sickle cell disease and their families need to communicate regularly with each other. Patients need to learn which parameters are important for them to monitor and how to monitor them. Guidelines should also be given regarding when it is appropriate to seek urgent care.

Evaluation

Expected patient outcomes may include:

1. Control of pain
   a. Uses analgesic agents to control acute pain
   b. Uses relaxation techniques, breathing exercises, and distraction to help relieve pain
2. Is free of infection
   a. Has normal temperature
   b. Has leukocyte count within normal range ($4{,}500/mm^3$ to $11{,}000/mm^3$)
   c. Identifies importance of continuing antibiotics at home (if applicable)
3. Expresses improved sense of control
   a. Participates in goal setting and in planning and implementing daily activities
   b. Participates in decisions about care
4. Increases knowledge about disease process
   a. Identifies situations and factors that can precipitate sickle cell crisis
   b. Describes lifestyle changes needed to prevent crisis
   c. Describes the importance of warmth, adequate hydration, and prevention of infection in preventing crisis
5. Absence of complications

Thalassemia

The thalassemias are a group of hereditary anemias characterized by **hypochromia** (an abnormal decrease in the hemoglobin content of erythrocytes), extreme **microcytosis** (smaller-than-normal erythrocytes), destruction of blood elements (hemolysis), and variable degrees of anemia. The thalassemias occur worldwide, but the highest prevalence is found in people of Mediterranean, African, and Southeast Asian ancestry.

Thalassemias are associated with defective synthesis of hemoglobin; the production of one or more globulin chains within the hemoglobin molecule is reduced. When this occurs, the imbalance in the configuration of the hemoglobin causes it to precipitate in the erythroid precursors or the erythrocytes themselves. This increases the rigidity of the erythrocytes and thus, the premature destruction of these cells.

Thalassemias are classified into two major groups according to which hemoglobin chain is diminished: alpha or beta. The alpha-thalassemias occur mainly in people from Asia and the Middle East, and the beta-thalassemias are most prevalent in people from Mediterranean regions but also occur in those from the Middle East or Asia. The alpha-thalassemias are milder than the beta forms and often occur without symptoms; the erythrocytes are extremely microcytic, but the anemia, if present, is mild.

The severity of beta-thalassemia varies depending on the extent to which the hemoglobin chains are affected. Patients with mild forms have microcytosis (erythrocytes with reduced MCV) and mild anemia. If left untreated, severe beta-thalassemia (i.e., thalassemia major or Cooley's anemia) can be fatal within the first few years of life. BMT offers a chance of cure, but when this is not possible, the disease is usually treated with transfusion of PRBCs. Patients may survive into their 50s. Patient teaching during the reproductive years should include preconception counselling about the risk of thalassemia major in offspring.

Thalassemia Major

Thalassemia major is characterized by severe anemia, marked hemolysis, and ineffective erythropoiesis. With early regular transfusion therapy, growth and development through childhood are facilitated. Organ dysfunction due to iron overload results from the excessive amounts of iron in multiple PRBC transfusions. Regular chelation therapy can reduce the complications of iron overload and prolong the life of these patients. This disease is potentially curable by HSCT if the procedure can be performed before liver damage occurs (i.e., during childhood).

Glucose-6-Phosphate Dehydrogenase Deficiency

The G-6-PD gene is the source of the abnormality in this disorder; this gene produces an enzyme within the erythrocyte that is essential for membrane stability. A few patients have inherited an enzyme that is so defective that they have a chronic hemolytic anemia; however, the most common type of defect results in hemolysis only when the erythrocytes are stressed by certain situations, such as fever or the use of certain medications. African Americans and people of Greek or Italian origin are those primarily affected by this disorder. The type of deficiency found in the Mediterranean population is more severe than that in the African American population, resulting in greater hemolysis and sometimes in life-threatening anemia. All types of G-6-PD deficiency are inherited as X-linked defects; therefore, many more men are at risk than women. In the United States, about 12% of African American males are affected. The deficiency is also common in those of Asian ancestry and in certain Jewish populations.

Oxidant drugs (drugs that induce an oxidative stress on the body) have hemolytic effects for people with G-6-PD deficiency. These medications include antimalarial agents (e.g., chloroquine [Aralen]), sulfonamides (e.g., trimethoprim–sulfamethoxazole [Bactrim, Septra]), nitrofurantoin (e.g., Macrodantin), common coal tar analgesics (including Aspirin in high doses), thiazide diuretics (e.g., hydrochlorothiazide [HydroDIURIL], chlorothiazide [Diuril]), oral hypoglycemic agents (e.g., glyburide [Micronase], metformin [Glucophage]), dapsone, primaquine, phenazopyridine, chloramphenicol (Chloromycetin), the street drug amyl nitrite ("poppers"), and vitamin K (phytonadione [AquaMEPHYTON]). In affected people, a severe hemolytic episode can also result from ingestion of fava beans.

Clinical Manifestations

Patients are asymptomatic and have normal hemoglobin levels and reticulocyte counts most of the time. However, several days after exposure to an offending medication, they may develop pallor, jaundice, and hemoglobinuria (hemoglobin in the urine). The reticulocyte count increases, and symptoms of hemolysis develop. Special stains of the peripheral blood may then disclose Heinz bodies (degraded hemoglobin) within the erythrocytes. Hemolysis is often mild and self-limited. However, in the more severe Mediterranean type of G-6-PD deficiency, spontaneous recovery may not occur.

Assessment and Diagnostic Findings

The diagnosis is made by a screening test or by a quantitative assay of G-6-PD.

Medical Management

The treatment is to arrest the source and stop the offending medication. Transfusion is necessary only in the severe hemolytic state, which is more commonly seen in the Mediterranean variety of G-6-PD deficiency.

Nursing Management

Patients are educated about the disease and given a list of medications to avoid. If hemolysis develops, nursing interventions are the same as for hemolysis from other causes. Patients should be instructed to wear MedicAlert bracelets that identify that they have G-6-PD deficiency. Genetic counselling may be indicated.

Immune Hemolytic Anemia

Hemolytic anemias can result from exposure of the erythrocyte to antibodies. Alloantibodies (i.e., antibodies against the host, or "self") result from the immunization of a person with foreign antigens (e.g., the immunization of an Rh-negative person with Rh-positive blood). *Alloantibodies* tend to be large (IgM type) and cause immediate destruction of the sensitized erythrocytes, either within the blood vessel (intravascular hemolysis) or within the liver. An example of alloimmune hemolytic anemia in adults is anemia that results from a hemolytic transfusion reaction.

Autoantibodies may develop for many reasons. In many instances, the person's immune system is dysfunctional, so that it falsely recognizes its own erythrocytes as foreign and produces antibodies against them. This mechanism is seen in people with chronic lymphocytic leukemia (CLL). Another mechanism is a deficiency in suppressor lymphocytes which normally prevent antibody formation against a person's own antigens. *Autoantibodies* tend to be of the IgG type. The erythrocytes are sequestered in the spleen and destroyed by the macrophages outside the blood vessel (extravascular hemolysis).

Autoimmune hemolytic anemias can be classified based on the body temperature involved when the antibodies react with the red blood cell antigen. Warm-body antibodies bind to erythrocytes most actively in warm conditions (37°C); cold-body antibodies react in cold conditions (0°C). Most autoimmune hemolytic anemias are the warm-body type. Autoimmune hemolytic anemia is associated with other disorders in most cases (e.g., medication exposure, lymphoma, CLL, other malignancy, collagen vascular disease, autoimmune disease, infection). In idiopathic autoimmune hemolytic states, the reason why the immune system produces the antibodies is not known. This primary form affects patients of all ages and both genders equally, whereas the incidence of secondary forms is greater in people older than 45 years of age and in females.

Clinical Manifestations

Clinical manifestations can vary, and they usually reflect the degree of anemia. The hemolysis may be very mild, so that the patient's marrow compensates adequately and the patient is asymptomatic. At the other extreme, the hemolysis can be so severe that the resultant anemia is life-threatening. Most patients complain of fatigue and dizziness. Splenomegaly is the most common physical finding, occurring in more than 80% of patients; hepatomegaly, lymphadenopathy, and jaundice are also common.

Assessment and Diagnostic Findings

Laboratory tests show a low hemoglobin level and hematocrit, most often with an accompanying increase in the reticulocyte count. Erythrocytes appear abnormal; spherocytes are common. The serum bilirubin level is elevated, and if the hemolysis is severe, the haptoglobin level is low or absent. The Coombs test (also referred to as the direct antiglobulin test [DAT]), which detects antibodies on the surface of erythrocytes, shows a positive result.

Medical Management

Any possible offending medication should be immediately discontinued. The treatment consists of high doses of corticosteroids until hemolysis decreases. Corticosteroids decrease the macrophage's ability to clear the antibody-coated erythrocytes. If the hemoglobin level returns toward normal, usually after several weeks, the corticosteroid dose can be lowered or, in some cases, tapered and discontinued. However, corticosteroids rarely produce a lasting remission. In severe cases, blood transfusions may be required. Because the antibody may react with all possible donor cells, careful blood typing is necessary, and the transfusion should be administered slowly and cautiously.

Splenectomy (i.e., removal of the spleen) may be performed if corticosteroids do not produce a remission, because this procedure removes the major site of erythrocyte destruction. If neither corticosteroid therapy nor splenectomy is successful, immunosuppressive agents may be administered. The two immunosuppressive agents most frequently used are cyclophosphamide (Cytoxan) and azathioprine (Imuran). Cyclophosphamide has a more rapid effect but more toxicity, and azathioprine has a less rapid effect but less toxicity. The synthetic androgen danazol (Danocrine) can be useful in some patients, particularly in combination with corticosteroids. If corticosteroids or immunosuppressive agents are used, the taper must be gradual to prevent a rebound "hyperimmune" response and exacerbation of the hemolysis. Monoclonal antibodies (e.g., rituximab [Rituxan]) can also be effective for some patients. Immunoglobulin administration is effective in about one third of patients, but the effect is transient, and the medication is expensive. Transfusions may be necessary if the anemia is severe; it may be extremely difficult to cross-match samples of available units of PRBCs with that of the patient.

For patients with cold-antibody hemolytic anemia, no treatment may be required other than to advise the patient to keep warm; relocation to a warm climate may be advisable. However, in other situations, the hemolysis may warrant more aggressive interventions as described previously.

Nursing Management

Patients may have great difficulty understanding the pathologic mechanisms underlying the disease and may need repeated explanations in terms they can understand. Patients who have had a splenectomy should be vaccinated against pneumococcal infections (e.g., with Pneumovax) and informed that they are permanently at greater risk for infection. Patients receiving long-term corticosteroid therapy, particularly those with concurrent diabetes or hypertension, need careful monitoring. They must understand the need for the medication and the importance of never abruptly discontinuing it. A written explanation and a tapering schedule should be provided, and adjustments based on hemoglobin levels should be emphasized. Similar teaching should be provided when immunosuppressive agents are used. Corticosteroid therapy is not without significant risk, and patients need to be monitored closely for complications. The short- and long-term complications of corticosteroid therapy are presented in Chapter 43.

NURSING ALERT

It can be difficult to cross-match blood when antibodies are present. If imperfectly cross-matched RBCs must be transfused, the nurse should begin the infusion very slowly (10 to 15 mL over 20 to 30 minutes) and monitor the patient very closely for signs and symptoms of a hemolytic transfusion reaction.

Hereditary Hemochromatosis

Hemochromatosis is a genetic condition in which excess iron is absorbed from the GI tract. Normally, the GI tract absorbs 1 to 2 mg of iron daily, but in those with hereditary hemochromatosis, this rate increases significantly. The excess iron is deposited in various organs, particularly the liver, myocardium, testes, thyroid, and pancreas. Eventually, the affected organs become dysfunctional. This condition is found in approximately 1 in 327 Canadians (Canadian Liver Foundation, 2012). The genetic defect associated with hemochromatosis is most commonly seen as a specific mutation (C282Y homozygosity) of the *HFE* gene whose protein is responsible for regulating iron uptake by transferrin (the iron transporter). Women are less often affected than men because women lose iron through menses.

Clinical Manifestations

There is generally no evidence of tissue damage until middle age, because the accumulation of iron in body organs occurs gradually. Symptoms of weakness, lethargy, arthralgia, weight loss, and loss of libido are common and occur earlier in the illness trajectory. The skin may appear hyperpigmented from melanin deposits (and occasionally **hemosiderin**, an iron-containing pigment) or appear bronze in colour. Cardiac dysrhythmias and cardiomyopathy can occur, with resulting dyspnea and edema. Endocrine dysfunction is manifested as hypothyroidism, diabetes mellitus, and hypogonadism (testicular atrophy, diminished libido, and impotence). Cirrhosis is common in later stages of the disease, as well as a shortened life expectancy. Hemochromatosis is also a risk factor for hepatocellular carcinoma (Canadian Liver Foundation, 2012).

Assessment and Diagnostic Findings

Diagnostic laboratory findings include an elevated serum iron level and high transferrin saturation (more than 60% in men, more than 50% in women). CBC values are typically normal. The definitive diagnostic test for hemochromatosis was formerly the liver biopsy, but testing for the associated genetic mutation is now more commonly used.

Medical Management

Therapy involves the removal of excess iron via therapeutic phlebotomy (removal of whole blood from a vein). Each unit of blood removed results in a decrease of 200 to 250 mg of iron. The objective is to reduce the hemoglobin level to between 105 and 110 g/L and the transferrin saturation to 30% or less (Canadian Hemochromatosis Society, 2014). To achieve this, frequent phlebotomy is required (1 to 2 units weekly). Phlebotomy is then necessary only every 1 to 4 months until the hemoglobin levels are maintained at 130 to 180 g/L for men and 120 to 160 g/L for women with transferrin saturation between 30% and 40%. After 1 to 3 years, the frequency of phlebotomy can often be further reduced to prevent reaccumulation of iron deposits. Aggressive removal of excess iron can prevent end-organ dysfunction, particularly liver cirrhosis and its complications (ascites, hemorrhage, hepatocellular carcinoma).

Nursing Management

Patients with hemochromatosis often limit their dietary intake of iron, although this is not effective. However, it is important for these patients to avoid any additional insults to the liver, such as alcohol abuse. Serial screening tests for hepatoma (e.g., through monitoring alpha-fetoprotein) are important. Other body systems should be monitored for signs of organ dysfunction, particularly the endocrine and cardiac systems to ensure that appropriate management can be implemented quickly. Because patients with hemochromatosis require frequent phlebotomies, problems with venous access are common. Children of patients who are homozygous for the *HFE* gene mutation should be screened for the mutation as well. Patients who are heterozygous for the *HFE* gene do not develop the disease but need to be advised that they can transmit the gene to their children.

Polycythemia

Polycythemia refers to an increased volume of erythrocytes. The term is used when the hematocrit is elevated (more than 55% in males, more than 50% in females). Dehydration (decreased volume of plasma) can cause an elevated hematocrit but not typically to the level to be considered polycythemia. Polycythemia is classified as either primary or secondary.

Polycythemia Vera

Polycythemia vera ("P vera"), or primary polycythemia, is a proliferative disorder of the myeloid stem cells. The bone marrow is hypercellular, and the erythrocyte, leukocyte, and platelet counts in the peripheral blood are elevated. However, erythrocyte elevation predominates; the hematocrit can exceed 60%. This increase in production can last for an extended period of 10 years or more. Over time, the spleen resumes its embryonic function of hematopoiesis and enlarges. Eventually, the bone marrow may become fibrotic, with a resultant inability to produce as many cells. The disease then evolves into myeloid metaplasia with myelofibrosis, MDS, or AML in a significant proportion of patients; this form of AML is usually refractory to standard treatment. The incidence of PV in North American varies from a low of 22 to a high of 57 per 100,000 people. This means that there are between 8,000 and 21,000 people living with PV in Canada with about 180 to 600 new cases being diagnosed each year. The average age at which PV is diagnosed is about 60 to 65 years old, and only 10% of patients are under the age 40 (Leukemia and Lymphoma Society of Canada, 2016).

Clinical Manifestations

Patients typically have a ruddy complexion and splenomegaly. Symptoms result from increased blood volumes and may include headache, dizziness, tinnitus, fatigue, paresthesias, and blurred vision, or from increased blood viscosity and may include angina, claudication, dyspnea, and thrombophlebitis, particularly if the patient has atherosclerotic blood vessels. For this reason, blood pressure is often elevated. Uric acid may be elevated, resulting in gout and renal stone formation. Another common and bothersome problem is generalized pruritus, which may be caused by histamine release due to an increased number of basophils. Erythromelalgia, a burning sensation in the fingers and toes, may be reported and is only partially relieved by cooling.

Assessment and Diagnostic Findings

Diagnosis is based on an elevated erythrocyte mass, a normal oxygen saturation level, and often an enlarged spleen. Other factors useful in establishing the diagnosis include elevated leukocyte and platelet counts. The erythropoietin level is not as low as would be expected with an elevated hematocrit; it is normal or only slightly low. Causes of secondary erythrocytosis should not be present (see later discussion).

The mutation of the enzyme JAK2 causes an erythrocyte hypersensitivity to the effects of erythropoietin, and the protein encoded by this mutated gene can be measured to determine if there are problems with overproduction of cells in the bone marrow. Although a mutation in JAK2 is found in the majority of people with polycythemia vera, it is not specific for the disease.

Complications

Patients with polycythemia vera are at increased risk for thromboses that may result in CVAs (strokes, brain attacks) or myocardial infarctions (MIs); thrombotic complications are the most common cause of death. Bleeding is also a complication, possibly because the platelets are often very large and somewhat dysfunctional. The bleeding can be significant and can occur in the form of nosebleeds, ulcers, frank GI bleeding, hematuria, and intracranial hemorrhage.

Medical Management

The objective of management is to reduce the high blood cell mass. Phlebotomy is an important part of therapy (see Fig. 54-8). It involves removing enough blood (initially 500 mL once or twice weekly) to reduce blood viscosity and to deplete the patient's iron stores, thereby rendering the patient iron deficient and consequently unable to continue to manufacture erythrocytes excessively. Many patients are managed by routine phlebotomy on an intermittent basis, with the target of maintaining the hematocrit less than 45%.

Chemotherapeutic agents (e.g., hydroxyurea) can be used to suppress marrow function, but this may increase the risk of leukemia. Patients receiving hydroxyurea appear to have a lower incidence of thrombotic complications than those treated by phlebotomy alone; this may result with a normal platelet count. Anagrelide (Agrylin), which inhibits platelet aggregation, can also be useful in

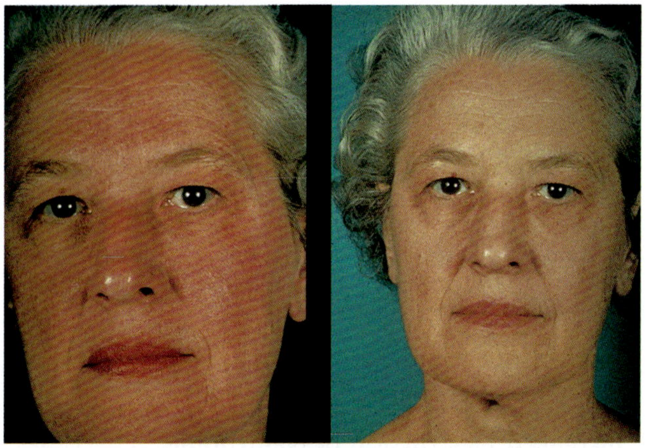

FIGURE 54-8. Phlebotomy can markedly reduce the plethora seen in polycythemia vera. This is evidenced here by a marked reduction in facial rubor in a patient with polycythemia vera. (From Turgeon, M. L. (2012). *Clinical hematology: Theory & procedures* (5th ed., Fig. 21.10, p. 373). Philadelphia, PA: Lippincott Williams & Wilkins.)

TABLE 54-5 Common Symptoms Associated With Myeloproliferative Neoplasms

Symptoms vary between the three myeloproliferative neoplasms, both in frequency and severity. Nurses should assess these patients frequently for the presence of these symptoms and initiate appropriate measures to ameliorate them.

Symptom	P Vera (%)	ET (%)	Myelofibrosis (%)
Fatigue	85	84	94
Concentration	62	58	68
Early satiety	60	56	74
Night sweats	52	47	63
Pruritus	62	46	52
Abdominal discomfort	48	48	65
Bone pain	48	45	53
Weight loss	33	28	47
Fever	19	17	24

P vera, polycythemia vera; ET, essential thrombocythemia.

Adapted from Geyer, H. L., & Mesa, R. A. (2014). Therapy for myeloproliferative neoplasms: When, which agent, and how? *Hematology American Society of Hematology Education Program*, *2014*(1), 277–286.

controlling the **thrombocytosis** associated with polycythemia vera. However, many patients have difficulty tolerating the medication; it can cause significant side effects, including headache, fluid retention, cardiac dysrhythmias, and heart failure. Interferon alfa-2b (Intron-A) is the most effective treatment for managing the pruritus associated with polycythemia vera but may be difficult for patients to tolerate because of its frequent side effects (e.g., flu-like syndrome, depression). Antihistamines, including histamine-2 blockers, are not particularly effective in controlling itching. Allopurinol (Zyloprim) is used to prevent gouty attacks in patients with elevated uric acid concentrations.

The use of aspirin to prevent thrombotic complications is controversial. High-dose aspirin may be associated with an increased risk of bleeding and no decreased risk of thrombosis. In contrast, low-dose aspirin decreases the risk of significant thrombotic complications (deep vein thrombosis [DVT], pulmonary embolism, MI, stroke) but does not increase the risk of significant bleeding; therefore, aspirin (ASA) is now recommended as an antithrombotic prophylaxis. Aspirin is also useful in reducing the pain associated with erythromelalgia.

Nursing Management

Patients with polycythemia vera can exhibit a variety of symptoms that have an adverse impact on quality of life (Abelsson, Andréasson, Samuelsson, et al., 2013; Stein, Moliterno, & Tiu, 2014). As symptoms vary and are not related to extent of disease (Scherber, Geyer, & Mesa, 2014), it is important to assess for symptoms carefully and regularly throughout the illness trajectory. Table 54-5 identifies common symptoms associated with polycythemia vera.

The nurse focuses on symptom management. Fatigue is the most common symptom, and can occur in 85% of patients (Radia & Geyer, 2015; Scherber, Kosiorek, Senyak, et al., 2016). Concurrent comorbidities (e.g., hypothyroidism, depression) and medications (e.g., antihypertensives, antihistamines) can exacerbate the fatigue (Scherber et al., 2016). Fatigue is not always correlated with the level of disease risk; patients with low-risk disease are as troubled with fatigue as are those with high-risk disease (Radia & Geyer, 2015).

Pruritus is also a common and frustrating symptom, occurring in up to 65% of patients with polycythemia vera (Radia & Geyer, 2015). It is described as strong itching, stinging, or burning. Pruritus is frequently triggered by contact with water (Siegel, Tauscher, & Petrides, 2013), alcohol consumption, diaphoresis, or change in body temperature. Antihistamines, including histamine-2 blockers, are not particularly effective in controlling itching, nor are emollient lotions. Interferon alfa-2b, selective serotonin uptake inhibitors (e.g., paroxetine), and ultraviolet therapy have marginal effectiveness in diminishing the pruritus (Stein et al., 2014). As the efficacy of pharmacologic strategies may not be optimal, it is important to individualize therapy and monitor its effectiveness (Siegel et al., 2013). The nurse may recommend bathing in tepid or cool water and avoiding vigorous toweling off after bathing. Cocoa butter or oatmeal-based lotions and bath products or baking soda dissolved in bathwater may also be helpful.

Potentially life-threatening complications from the disease are thrombosis or hemorrhage. Risk factors for thrombotic complications, particularly a prior history of thrombosis, smoking, obesity, and poorly controlled hypertension and diabetes, should be assessed, and patients should be encouraged to modify the cardiovascular risk factors within their control (e.g., smoking, obesity). Adopting or maintaining a healthy lifestyle should be encouraged. Patients should be instructed about the signs and symptoms of thrombosis. To reduce the likelihood of DVT, sedentary behaviour, crossing the legs, and wearing tight or restrictive clothing (particularly stockings) should be discouraged. Patients with a history of significant bleeding are usually advised to avoid high-dose aspirin and aspirin-containing medications, because these medications alter platelet function. Minimizing alcohol intake should also be emphasized to further diminish the risk of bleeding. Patients should be counselled about the signs of bleeding. The patient needs to be instructed to avoid iron supplements, including those in over-the-counter multivitamin supplements, because the iron can further stimulate RBC production.

Secondary Polycythemia

Secondary polycythemia is caused by excessive production of erythropoietin. This may occur in response to a reduced amount of oxygen, which acts as a hypoxic stimulus, as in heavy cigarette smoking, chronic obstructive pulmonary disease, or cyanotic heart disease, or in nonpathologic conditions such as living at a high altitude. It can also result from certain hemoglobinopathies (e.g., hemoglobin Chesapeake), in which the hemoglobin has an abnormally high affinity for oxygen. Secondary polycythemia can also occur from neoplasms (e.g., renal cell carcinoma) that stimulate erythropoietin production.

Medical Management

When secondary polycythemia is mild, treatment may not be necessary; when treatment is necessary, it involves treating the primary conditions. If the cause cannot be corrected (e.g., by treating the renal cell carcinoma or improving pulmonary function with smoking cessation), therapeutic phlebotomy may be necessary in symptomatic patients to reduce blood viscosity and volume as well as when the hematocrit is significantly elevated.

Leukopenia

Leukopenia, a condition in which there are fewer leukocytes than normal, results from neutropenia (diminished neutrophils) or lymphopenia (diminished lymphocytes). Even if other types of leukocytes (e.g., monocytes, basophils) are diminished, their numbers are too few to reduce the total leukocyte count significantly.

Neutropenia

Neutropenia (a neutrophil count of less than 2,000/mm^3) results from decreased production of neutrophils or increased destruction of these cells (Chart 54-6). Neutrophils are essential in preventing and limiting bacterial infection. A patient with neutropenia is at increased risk for infection from both exogenous and endogenous sources. (The GI tract and skin are common endogenous sources.) The risk of infection is based not only on the severity of the neutropenia but also on its duration. The actual number of neutrophils, known as the **absolute neutrophil count** (ANC), is determined by a simple mathematical calculation using data obtained from the CBC and differential. The risk of infection increases proportionately with the decrease in neutrophil count. The risk is significant when the ANC is less than 1,000/mm^3, is high when it is less than 500/mm^3, and is almost certain when it is less than 100/mm^3. The risk of developing infection also increases with the length of time during which neutropenia persists, even when the ANC is not dangerously low.

CHART 54-6

Causes of Neutropenia

Decreased Production of Neutrophils

- Aplastic anemia, due to medications or toxins
- Chemotherapy
- Metastatic cancer, lymphoma, leukemia
- Myelodysplastic syndromes
- Radiation therapy

Ineffective Granulocytopoiesis

- Megaloblastic anemia

Increased Destruction of Neutrophils

- Bacterial infections
- Hypersplenism
- Immunologic disorders (e.g., systemic lupus erythematosus)
- Medication induced[a]
- Viral disease (e.g., infectious hepatitis, mononucleosis)

[a]Formation of antibody to medication, leading to a rapid decrease in neutrophils.

Conversely, even a severe neutropenia may not result in infection if the duration of the neutropenia is brief, as is often seen after chemotherapy (Chart 54-7).

Clinical Manifestations

There are no definite symptoms of neutropenia until the patient becomes infected. A routine CBC with differential, as obtained after chemotherapy treatment, can reveal neutropenia before the onset of infection.

NURSING ALERT

Patients with neutropenia often do not exhibit classic signs of infection. Fever is the most common indicator of infection, yet fever is not always present, particularly if the patient is taking corticosteroids.

Medical Management

Treatment of the neutropenia varies, depending on its cause. If the neutropenia is medication induced, the offending agent is stopped immediately, if possible. Treatment of an underlying neoplasm can temporarily make the neutropenia worse, but with bone marrow recovery, treatment may actually improve it. Corticosteroids may be used if the cause is an immunologic disorder. The use of growth factors such as G-CSF or granulocyte-macrophage colony-stimulating factor (GM-CSF) can be effective in increasing neutrophil production when the cause of the neutropenia is decreased production. Withholding or reducing the dose of chemotherapy or radiation therapy may be required when the neutropenia is caused by these

CHART 54-7

Risk Factors: Development of Infection and Bleeding in Patients With Hematologic Disorders

Risk of Infection

- *Severity of neutropenia:* Risk of infection is proportional to severity of neutropenia.
- *Duration of neutropenia:* Increased duration leads to increased risk of infection.
- *Nutritional status:* Decreased protein stores lead to decreased immune response and anergy.
- *Deconditioning:* Decreased mobility leads to decreased respiratory effort, leading to increased pooling of secretions.
- *Lymphocytopenia; disorders of lymphoid system (chronic lymphocytic leukemia, lymphoma, myeloma):* Decreased cell-mediated and humoral immunity.
- *Invasive procedures:* Break in skin integrity leads to increased opportunity for organisms to enter blood system.
- *Hypogammaglobulinemia:* Decreased antibody formation.
- *Poor hygiene:* Increased organisms on skin and mucous membranes, including perineum.
- *Poor dentition; mucositis:* Decreased endothelial integrity leads to increased opportunity for organisms to enter blood system.
- *Antibiotic therapy:* Increased risk for superinfection, often fungal.
- *Certain medications:* See text.

Risk of Bleeding

- *Severity of thrombocytopenia:* Risk increases when platelet count decreases; usually not a significant risk until platelet count is less than 10,000/mm^3, or less than 50,000/mm^3 when invasive procedure is performed.
- *Duration of thrombocytopenia:* Risk increases when duration increases (e.g., risk is less when duration is transient after chemotherapy than when duration is permanent with poor marrow production).
- *Sepsis:* Mechanism unknown; appears to cause increased platelet consumption.
- *Increased intracranial pressure:* Increased blood pressure leads to rupture of blood vessels.
- *Liver dysfunction:* Decreased synthesis of clotting factors.
- *Renal dysfunction:* Decreased platelet function.
- *Dysproteinemia:* Protein coats surface of platelet, leading to decreased platelet function; protein causes increased viscosity, which leads to increased stretching of capillaries and thus increased bleeding.
- *Alcohol abuse:* Suppressive effect on marrow leads to decreased platelet production and decreased ability to function; decreased liver function results in decreased production of clotting factors.
- *Splenomegaly:* Increased platelet destruction; spleen traps circulating platelets.
- *Concurrent medications:* See text.

treatments; however, in the case of potentially curative therapy, administration of growth factor is considered to be preferable to ensure that the maximum antitumour effect can be achieved by maintaining the chemotherapy regimen as originally planned.

If the neutropenia is accompanied by fever, the patient is considered to have an infection and is usually admitted to the hospital. Cultures of blood, urine, and sputum, as well as a chest x-ray, are obtained. To ensure adequate therapy against the infectious organisms, broad-spectrum antibiotics are initiated as soon as the cultures are obtained, although the antibiotics may be changed after culture and sensitivity results are available.

Nursing Management

Nurses in all settings have a crucial role in assessing the severity of neutropenia and in preventing and managing complications, which most often include infections. Patient teaching is equally important, particularly in the outpatient setting, so that the patient can implement appropriate self-care measures and know when and how to seek medical care (Chart 54-8). Patients at risk of neutropenia should have blood drawn for a CBC with differential; the frequency is based on the suspected severity and duration of the neutropenia. Nurses need to be able to calculate the ANC to assess the severity of neutropenia and the risk of infection. Chart 54-9 identifies nursing interventions related to neutropenia.

Lymphopenia

Lymphopenia (a lymphocyte count less than 1,500/mm^3) can result from ionizing radiation, long-term use of corticosteroids, uremia, some neoplasms (e.g., breast and lung cancers, advanced Hodgkin's disease), and some protein-losing enteropathies (in which the lymphocytes within the intestines are lost). Although when lymphopenia is mild, it is often without sequelae; when severe, it can result in bacterial infections (due to low B lymphocytes) or in opportunistic infections (due to low T lymphocytes).

Clonal Stem Cell Disorders

When some hematologic neoplasms develop, hematopoietic control mechanisms may be in place to continue to produce adequate numbers of normal blood cells. These are commonly referred to as **indolent neoplasms**, where the increased numbers of cells produced from a culprit clone all have the same genotype (see Chapter 11 for further discussion of genotypes). However, at some time, the control mechanisms may fail and the "indolent" clone may then evolve into a more aggressive clone.

Not all malignancies arise from an indolent neoplasm, however. Rather, they may evolve directly from changes in the stem cell. Similarly, not all indolent neoplasms will eventually evolve into a malignancy. Nonetheless, such evolution is possible for virtually any clonal disorder. Figure 54-9 illustrates this concept for myeloid stem cell disorders. Similar neoplastic conditions are derived from

CHART 54-8

HOME CARE CHECKLIST • The Patient at Risk for Infection

At the completion of education, the patient and/or caregiver will be able to:

- State the impact of alterations in neutrophils, lymphocytes, immunoglobulins on physiologic functioning, ADLs, IADLs, roles, relationships, and spirituality.
- State changes in lifestyle (e.g., diet, activity) or home environment necessary to decrease risk for infection.
  - Maintain good hand hygiene technique, oral hygiene, total body hygiene, and skin integrity.
  - Avoid cleaning birdcages and litter boxes; consider avoiding garden work (soil) and fresh flowers in stagnant water.
  - Maintain a high-calorie, high-protein diet, with fluid intake of 3,000 mL daily (unless fluids are restricted).
  - Avoid people with infections and crowds.
  - Perform deep breathing; use incentive spirometer every 4 hours while awake if mobility is restricted.
  - Provide adequate lubrication with gentle vaginal manipulation during sexual intercourse; avoid anal intercourse.
- Identify signs and symptoms of infection to report to the primary provider, such as fever; chills; wet or dry cough; breathing problems; white patches in the mouth; swollen glands; nausea; vomiting; persistent abdominal pain; persistent diarrhea; problems with urination or changes in the character of the urine; red, swollen, or draining wounds; sores or lesions on the body; persistent vaginal discharge with or without itching; and severe fatigue.
- Demonstrate how to monitor for signs of infection.
- Describe to whom, how, and when to report signs of infection.
- Describe appropriate actions to take should infection occur.

ADLs, activities of daily living; IADLs, independent activities of daily living.

disorders within the lymphoid stem cell disorder (Shlush & Minden, 2015). Refer to later discussions about specific diseases noted in Figure 54-9.

LEUKEMIA

The term *leukocytosis* refers to an increased level of leukocytes in the circulation. Typically, only one specific cell type is increased. Because the proportions of several types of leukocytes (e.g., eosinophils, basophils, monocytes) are small, only an increase in neutrophils or lymphocytes can be great enough to elevate the total leukocyte count. Although leukocytosis can be a normal response to increased need (e.g., in acute infection), the elevation in leukocytes should decrease as the physiologic need decreases. A prolonged or progressively increasing elevation in leukocytes is abnormal and should be evaluated. A significant cause of persistent leukocytosis is hematologic malignancy.

Hematopoiesis is characterized by a rapid, continuous turnover of cells. Normally, production of specific blood cells from their stem cell precursors is carefully regulated according to the body's needs. If the mechanisms that control the production of these cells are disrupted, the cells can proliferate excessively. Hematopoietic malignancies are often classified by the cells involved. Leukemia is a neoplastic proliferation of one particular cell type (granulocytes, monocytes, lymphocytes, or infrequently erythrocytes or megakaryocytes). The defect originates in the hematopoietic stem cell, the myeloid, or the lymphoid stem cell. The lymphomas are neoplasms of lymphoid tissue, usually derived from B lymphocytes. Multiple myeloma is a malignancy of the most mature form of B lymphocyte, the plasma cell.

The common feature of the leukemias is an *unregulated proliferation of leukocytes in the bone marrow*. In acute

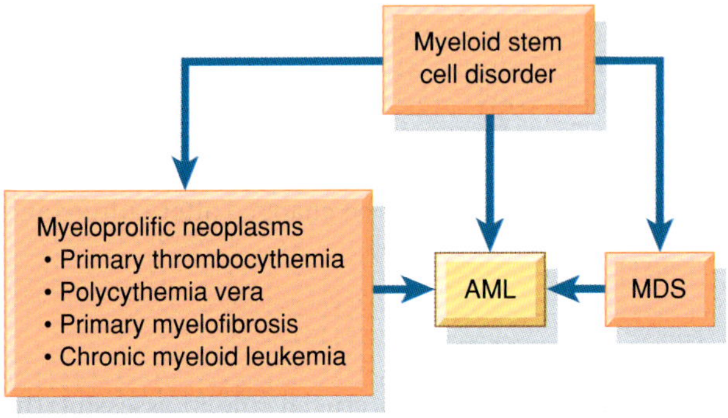

FIGURE 54-9. The development of myeloid neoplasms. Changes within the myeloid stem cell can cause the development of neoplasms that are either proliferative or, in the case of myelodysplastic syndrome, dysplastic. Although any indolent myeloid neoplasm can evolve into a malignant condition (e.g., acute myeloid leukemia [AML]), in most instances this will not occur. For example, the incidence of evolution from primary thrombocythemia is very low, yet it is much higher when from primary myelofibrosis. The actual incidence of evolution continues to change as therapy before more effective, as in the case of chronic myeloid leukemia. Note that AML can arise directly from the altered myeloid stem cell; it need not evolve from an existing indolent neoplasm. Similar events occur with lymphoid malignancy development.

CHART 54-9

Neutropenia Precautions

Nursing Priorities

Risk for infection secondary to impaired immunocompetence due to:

- Diminished neutrophil count (see below) or hypocellularity due to disease or treatment
- Dysfunctional neutrophils (e.g., secondary to myelodysplastic syndrome [MDS])
- Dysfunctional or diminished lymphocytes
- Hypogammaglobulinemia
- Diminished immune response or anergy
- Malnutrition
- Surgery or invasive procedures
- Antibiotic therapy (increased risk of superimposed infection)

Assessment

PATIENT

Assess the following areas thoroughly every shift or visit (with spot checks throughout shift if the patient is hospitalized) and notify physician of any signs of infection or worsening of status:

- *Skin:* Check for tenderness, edema, breaks in skin integrity, moisture, drainage, lesions (especially under breasts, axillae, groin, skin folds, bony prominences, perineum); check all puncture sites (e.g., intravenous sites) for signs and symptoms of inflammation/infection.
  - Skin and mucous membranes are the body's first line of defense against infection; loss of endothelial cell integrity allows organisms to enter the blood and lymph systems.
- *Oral mucosa:* Check for moisture, lesions, colour (check palate, tongue, buccal mucosa, gums, lips, oropharynx).
- *Respiratory:* Check for presence of sinus pressure or tenderness, cough, sore throat; auscultate breath sounds; assess rate and depth of respiration, use of accessory muscles.
- *Gastrointestinal:* Check for abdominal discomfort/distention, nausea, change in bowel pattern; auscultate bowel sounds.
- *Genitourinary:* Check for dysuria, urgency, frequency; check urine for colour, clarity, odour.
- *Neurologic:* Check for complaints of headache, neck stiffness, visual disturbances; assess level of consciousness, orientation, behaviour.
- *Temperature:* Check every 4 hours or every visit; call primary health care provider if temperature is >38°C (>101°F), fever is unresponsive to acetaminophen, or patient shows a decline in hemodynamic status.
  - Neutropenic, infected patients often do not exhibit the classic signs of inflammation/infection (i.e., redness, cloudiness of any drainage); the only initial sign may be fever (and it often occurs later in the infectious process with neutropenia).

DIAGNOSTIC STUDIES

- Monitor complete blood count (CBC) and differential daily (especially absolute neutrophil count [ANC], lymphocyte count).
- Call physician if ANC is <1,000/mm^3 or is significantly different from previous count, or whenever patient becomes symptomatic (e.g., febrile).
- Monitor globulin, albumin, total protein levels.
- Monitor all culture and sensitivity reports.
- Monitor x-ray reports.

Nursing Interventions

ENVIRONMENT AND STAFF

- Thorough hand hygiene must be performed by everyone before entering patient's room each and every time.
- Allow no one with a cold or sore throat to care for the patient or to enter room, or come in contact with patient at home.
- Care for neutropenic patients before caring for other patients (as much as possible).
- Use private room for patient if ANC is <1,000/mm^3.
- Allow no fresh flowers or plants (stagnant water, risk of *Aspergillus* infection).
- Change water in containers every shift (include O_2 humidification systems every 24 hours).
- Ensure room is cleaned daily.

DIETARY

- Provide low-microbial diet.[a]
- Encourage adequate hydration.

PATIENT

- Avoid suppositories, enemas, rectal temperatures.
- Practice deep breathing (with incentive spirometer) every 4 hours while awake.
- Ambulate; wear high-efficiency particulate air (HEPA) filter mask if neutropenia is severe.
- Prevent skin dryness with water-soluble lubricants, especially in high-risk areas (e.g., lips, corners of mouth, elbows, feet, bony prominences).

HYGIENE

- Provide meticulous total body hygiene daily (preferably with antimicrobial solution), including perineal care after every bowel movement.
- Provide thorough oral hygiene after meals and every 4 hours while awake; warm saline, or salt and soda solution, is effective; avoid use of lemon-glycerine swabs, commercial mouthwashes, and hydrogen peroxide.

INTRAVENOUS (IV) THERAPY

- Avoid plastic cannulas for peripheral IVs when ANC is <500/mm^3 if possible; a central vascular access device is preferred for long-term or intensive IV therapy.
- Inspect IV sites every shift; monitor closely for any discomfort; erythema may not be present.
- Maintain meticulous IV site care.
- Cleanse skin with antimicrobial solution before venipuncture (unless patient is allergic).
- Moisture-vapour-permeable dressings are permissible with strict adherence to institutional protocol.
- Change IV tubing per institution policy, using aseptic technique.
- Administer antimicrobial agents on time.

Expected Patient Outcomes

- Patient demonstrates an absence of infection as evidenced by an absence of fever, chills, inflammation, drainage, cough, dyspnea, sore throat, dysuria, or urinary frequency.
- Patient demonstrates an absence of infection as evidenced by the presence of vital signs within normal limits, including intact neurologic status and intact skin.

Duration of Evaluation

Until patient is no longer neutropenic and any infection is resolved.

[a]Note that although it is certainly prudent to avoid uncooked eggs, seafood, and meats as well as unwashed fruits and vegetables, there is little evidence to support this guideline.

forms (or late stages of chronic forms), the proliferation of leukemic cells leaves little room for normal cell production. There can also be a proliferation of cells in the liver and spleen (extramedullary hematopoiesis). With acute forms, there can be infiltration of leukemic cells in other organs, such as the meninges, lymph nodes, gums, and skin. The cause of leukemia is not fully known, but there is some evidence that genetic influences and viral pathogenesis may be involved. Bone marrow damage from radiation exposure or from chemicals such as benzene and alkylating agents (e.g., melphalan [Alkeran]) can cause leukemia.

The leukemias are commonly classified according to the stem cell line involved, either lymphoid or myeloid. They are also classified as either acute or chronic, based on the time it takes for symptoms to evolve and the phase of cell development that is halted (i.e., with few leukocytes differentiating beyond that phase).

In acute leukemia, the onset of symptoms is abrupt, often occurring within a few weeks. Leukocyte development is halted at the blast phase, so that most leukocytes are undifferentiated cells or are blasts. Acute leukemia progresses very rapidly; death occurs within weeks to months without aggressive treatment.

In chronic leukemia, symptoms evolve over a period of months to years, and the majority of leukocytes produced are mature. Chronic leukemia progresses more slowly; the disease trajectory can extend for years.

Acute Myeloid Leukemia

AML results from a defect in the hematopoietic stem cell that differentiates into all myeloid cells: monocytes, granulocytes (e.g., neutrophils, basophils, eosinophils), erythrocytes, and platelets. All age groups are affected, although it infrequently occurs before age 40 and the incidence rises with age, with a peak incidence at age 67. Slightly more men than women are affected (Canadian Cancer Society, 2016). AML is the most common nonlymphocytic leukemia.

The prognosis is highly variable. Patient age is a significant factor; patients who are younger may survive for 5 years or more after diagnosis of AML. However, patients who are older or have a more undifferentiated form of AML tend to have a worse prognosis.

The prognosis is highly variable. Patient age may be a factor; patients who are younger may survive for 5 years or more after diagnosis of AML. The development of AML in people with pre-existing MDS or in those who previously received alkylating agents for cancer (secondary AML) is also associated with a much worse prognosis; the leukemia tends to be more resistant to treatment, resulting in a much shorter duration of remission. With treatment, patients with secondary AML survive an average of less than 1 year, with death usually a result of infection or hemorrhage. Patients receiving supportive care also usually survive less than 1 year, dying of infection or bleeding.

Clinical Manifestations

AML develops without warning, with symptoms typically occurring over a period of weeks. Signs and symptoms result from insufficient production of normal blood cells.

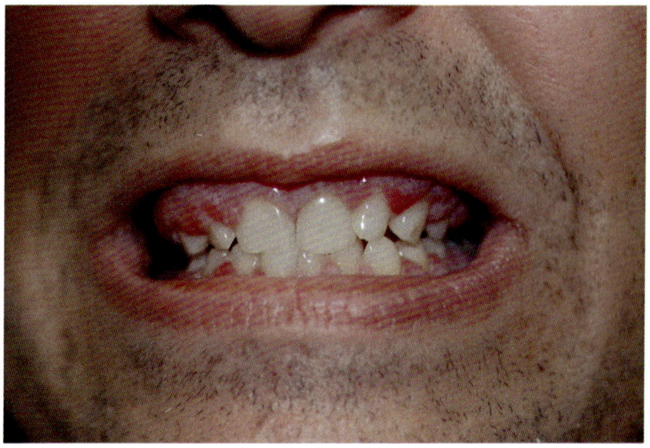

FIGURE 54-10. Gingival infiltration of leukemic cells in a patient with acute myeloid leukemia. (From Greer, J. P., Foerster, J., Rodgers, G. M., et al. (2009). *Wintrobe's clinical hematology* (12th ed., Fig. 72.8, p. 1680). Philadelphia, PA: Lippincott Williams & Wilkins.)

Fever and infection result from neutropenia (low neutrophil count); weakness and fatigue, dyspnea on exertion, and pallor from anemia; and **petechiae**, ecchymoses, and bleeding tendencies from thrombocytopenia. The proliferation of leukemic cells within organs leads to a variety of additional symptoms: pain from an enlarged liver or spleen, hyperplasia of the gums, and bone pain from expansion of marrow (see Fig. 54-10). Petechiae (pinpoint red or purple hemorrhagic spots on the skin) or ecchymoses (bruises) are common on the skin occasionally, leukemic infiltrates are also seen (see Fig. 54-11). Leukemic cells can also infiltrate the gingiva or synovial spaces of joints. Lymphadenopathy (enlargement of lymph nodes) or splenomegaly (enlargement of the spleen) is rare. Fevers may occur and are not always due to infection.

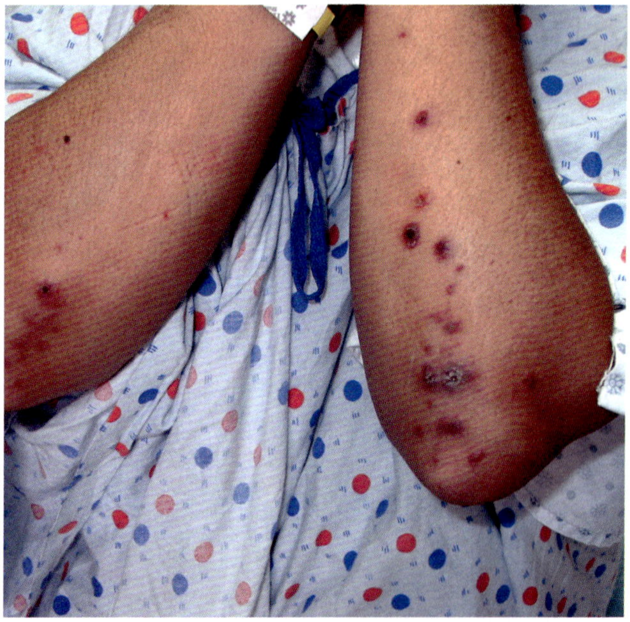

FIGURE 54-11. Leukemia cutis. Infiltration of leukemic cells in skin on extensor surface of forearms. (Reproduced with permission from Stedman's Medical Dictionary. Copyright 2008 Lippincott Williams & Wilkins.)

Assessment and Diagnostic Findings

AML develops without warning, with symptoms occurring over a period of weeks to months. The CBC shows a decrease in both erythrocytes and platelets. Although the total leukocyte count can be low, normal, or high, the percentage of normal cells is usually vastly decreased. A bone marrow analysis shows an excess of immature blast cells (more than 30%). AML can be further classified into seven different subgroups, based on cytogenetics, histology, and morphology of the blasts. The actual prognosis varies somewhat between subgroups and with the extent of cytogenetic abnormalities and genetic mutations. The clinical course and treatment differ substantially with only one subtype. Patients with acute promyelocytic leukemia (APL or AML-M3) often have significantly more problems with bleeding, in that they have underlying coagulopathy and a higher incidence of disseminated intravascular coagulation (DIC).

Complications

Complications of AML include bleeding and infection, which are the major causes of death. The risk of bleeding correlates with the level and duration of platelet deficiency (thrombocytopenia). The low platelet count can cause ecchymoses and petechiae. Major hemorrhages also may develop when the platelet count drops to less than 10,000/mm^3. The most common bleeding sources include GI, pulmonary, vaginal, and intracranial. For undetermined reasons, fever and infection also increase the likelihood of bleeding. DIC is common, particularly in patients with APL (Coombs, Tavakkoli, & Tallman, 2015). A very high WBC count (greater than 100,000 × 10^9/L) can cause stasis within the cerebral or pulmonary circulation.

Because of the lack of mature and normal granulocytes that help fight infection, patients with leukemia are prone to infection. The likelihood of infection increases with the degree and duration of neutropenia; neutrophil counts that persist at less than 100/mm^3 dramatically increase the risk of systemic infections. As the duration of severe neutropenia increases, the patient's risk of developing fungal infections also increases. Fungal infections remain difficult to treat despite the development of new antifungal agents, particularly if the patient has persistent neutropenia (Perfect, Hachem, & Wingard, 2014). However, improvement in reducing the incidence of fungal disease was noted in a study evaluating the efficacy of the drug posaconazole (Noxafil) as antifungal prophylaxis (Pagano, Verga, Busca, et al., 2014).

Massive leukemic cell destruction from chemotherapy results in the release of intracellular electrolytes and fluids into the systemic circulation. Increases in uric acid levels, potassium, and phosphate are seen; this process is referred to as tumour **lysis** (cell destruction) syndrome (see Chapter 68). The increased uric acid and phosphorus levels make the patient vulnerable to renal stone formation and renal colic, which can progress to acute kidney injury. Hyperkalemia and hypocalcemia can lead to cardiac dysrhythmias; hypotension; neuromuscular effects such as muscle cramps, weakness, and spasm/tetany; and confusion; and seizures may also develop. Patients require a high fluid intake, and prophylaxis with allopurinol (Zyloprim) to prevent crystallization of uric acid and subsequent stone formation. If necessary, uric acid degradation can be promoted by the administration of the enzyme rasburicase (Elitek) (Röllig & Ehninger, 2015).

GI problems may result from the infiltration of abnormal leukocytes into the abdominal organs and from the toxicity of the chemotherapeutic agents. Anorexia, nausea, vomiting, diarrhea, and severe mucositis are common. Because of the profound myelosuppressive effects of chemotherapy, significant neutropenia and thrombocytopenia typically result in serious infection and increased risk of bleeding.

Medical Management

Despite advances in understanding the biology of the AML, substantive advances in treatment response rates and survival rates have not occurred for decades, with the exception of advances made in treating APL (see later discussion). Even for those subtypes that have not benefited from advances in treatment, cure is still possible. The overall objective of treatment is to achieve complete remission, in which there is no evidence of residual leukemia in the bone marrow. Attempts are made to achieve remission by the aggressive administration of chemotherapy, called *induction therapy*, which usually requires hospitalization for several weeks. Induction therapy typically involves high doses of cytarabine (Cytosar, Ara-C) and daunorubicin (Cerubidine) or mitoxantrone (Novantrone) or idarubicin (Idamycin); sometimes etoposide (VP-16, VePesid) is added to the regimen. The choice of agents is based on the patient's physical status and history of prior antineoplastic treatment.

Treatment of APL revolves around induction therapy using the differentiating agent all-trans retinoic acid (ATRA), which induces the promyelocytic blast cells to differentiate, thereby deterring the cells from proliferating. ATRA is typically combined with a conventional chemotherapeutic agent, usually an anthracycline drug. This regimen yields a very high response rate, and cure is possible.

The aim of induction therapy is to eradicate the leukemic cells, but this is also accompanied by the eradication of normal types of myeloid cells. Thus, the patient becomes severely neutropenic (an ANC of 0 is not uncommon), anemic, and thrombocytopenic (a platelet count of less than 10,000/mm^3 is common). During this time, the patient is typically very ill, with bacterial, fungal, and occasionally viral infections; bleeding; and severe mucositis, which cause diarrhea and an inability to maintain adequate nutrition. Supportive care consists of administering blood products (PRBCs and platelets) and promptly treating infections. The use of granulocytic growth factors, either G-CSF (filgrastim [Neupogen]) or GM-CSF (sargramostim [Leukine]), can shorten the period of significant neutropenia by stimulating the bone marrow to produce leukocytes more quickly; these agents do not appear to increase the risk of producing more leukemic cells.

When the patient has recovered from the induction therapy (i.e., the neutrophil and platelet counts have returned to normal and any infection has resolved), *consolidation therapy* (postremission therapy) is administered to eliminate any residual leukemia cells that are not clinically detectable and reduce the chance for recurrence. Multiple treatment cycles of various agents are used, usually containing some form of cytarabine. Frequently, the patient receives one cycle of treatment that is almost the same, if not identical, to the induction treatment but at lower dosages, thereby resulting in less toxicity.

Another aggressive treatment option is BMT or HSCT. When a suitable tissue match can be obtained, the patient embarks on an even more aggressive regimen of chemotherapy (sometimes in combination with radiation therapy), with the treatment goal of destroying the hematopoietic function of the patient's bone marrow. The patient is then "rescued" with the infusion of the donor stem cells to reinitiate blood cell production. Patients who undergo HSCT have a significant risk for infection, graft-versus-host disease (GVHD, in which the donor's lymphocytes [graft] recognize the patient's body as "foreign" and set up reactions to attack the "foreign" host), and other complications. The most appropriate use and timing of HSCT remain unclear. Patients with a poorer prognosis may benefit from early HSCT; those with a good prognosis may not need transplant at all.

Another important option for the patient to consider is supportive care alone. In fact, supportive care may be the only option if the patient has significant comorbidity, such as extremely poor cardiac, pulmonary, renal, or hepatic function, and/or is extremely old. In such cases, aggressive antileukemia therapy is not used; occasionally, hydroxyurea (Hydrea) may be used briefly to control the increase of blast cells. Patients are more commonly supported with antimicrobial therapy and transfusions as needed. This treatment approach provides the patient with some additional time outside the hospital (e.g., at home); however, death frequently occurs within months, typically from infection or bleeding. (Refer to Chapter 15 for a discussion of end-of-life care.)

Nursing Management

Nursing management of the patient with acute leukemia is presented at the end of the discussion of leukemia in this chapter.

Chronic Myeloid Leukemia

Chronic myeloid leukemia (CML) arises from a mutation in the myeloid stem cell. Normal myeloid cells continue to be produced, but there is a pathologic increase in the production of forms of blast cells. Therefore, a wide spectrum of cell types exists within the blood, from blast forms through mature neutrophils. Because there is an uncontrolled proliferation of cells, the marrow expands into the cavities of long bones (e.g., the femur), and cells are also formed in the liver and spleen (extramedullary hematopoiesis), resulting in enlargement of these organs that is sometimes painful. In 90% to 95% of patients with CML, a section of DNA is missing from chromosome 22 (the Philadelphia chromosome); it is translocated onto chromosome 9. The specific location of these changes is on the *BCR* gene of chromosome 22 and the *ABL* gene on chromosome 9. When these two genes fuse (*BCR-ABL* gene), they produce an abnormal protein (a tyrosine kinase protein) that causes leukocytes to divide rapidly. This *BCR-ABL* gene is present in virtually all patients with this disease.

CML is uncommon in people younger than 20 years of age; the incidence increases with age (mean age is 67 years) (Canadian Cancer Society, 2016). Patients diagnosed with CML in the chronic phase have an overall median life expectancy exceeding 5 years. During that time, they have few symptoms and complications from the disease itself. Problems with infections and bleeding are rare. However, once the disease transforms to the acute phase (blast crisis), the overall survival rarely exceeds several months.

Clinical Manifestations

The clinical picture of CML varies. Many patients are asymptomatic, and leukocytosis is detected by a CBC performed for some other reason. The leukocyte count commonly exceeds 100,000/mm^3. Patients with extremely high leukocyte counts may be somewhat short of breath or slightly confused because of decreased capillary perfusion to the lungs and brain from leukostasis (the excessive volume of leukocytes inhibits blood flow through the capillaries). The patient may have an enlarged, tender spleen. The liver may also be enlarged. Some patients have insidious symptoms, such as malaise, anorexia, and weight loss. Lymphadenopathy is rare. There are three stages in CML: chronic, transformation, and accelerated or blast crisis. Patients develop more symptoms and complications as the disease progresses.

Medical Management

Advances in understanding of the pathology of CML at a molecular level have led to dramatic changes in its treatment. An oral formulation of a tyrosine kinase inhibitor, imatinib mesylate (Gleevec), works by blocking signals within the leukemia cells that express the *BCR-ABL* protein, thus preventing a series of chemical reactions that cause the cell to grow and divide. Imatinib therapy appears to be most useful in the chronic phase of the illness. It can induce complete remission at the cellular and even the molecular level. Imatinib is metabolized by the cytochrome P450 pathway, which means that drug–drug interactions are common. Also, antacids and grapefruit juice may limit drug absorption, and large doses of acetaminophen can cause hepatotoxicity.

In those instances where imatinib (at conventional doses) does not elicit a molecular remission, or when that remission is not maintained, other treatment options may be considered. The dosage of imatinib can be increased (with increased toxicity), another inhibitor of *BCR-ABL* can be used (e.g., dasatinib [Sprycel]), or an allogeneic transplant can be used. CML is a disease that can potentially be cured with BMT or HSCT in otherwise healthy patients who are younger than 65 years of age. However, with the development of tyrosine kinase inhibitors such as imatinib and dasatinib, the timing of transplant has come into question. Patients who receive such transplants while still in the chronic phase of the illness tend to have a greater chance for cure than those who receive them in the acute phase. The use of imatinib therapy may decrease the need for transplantation in CML; however, the long-term efficacy of imatinib as well as its effects on transplant morbidity, mortality, and risk of relapse remains unknown.

The *transformation phase* can be insidious or rapid; it marks the process of evolution (or transformation) to the acute form of leukemia (blast crisis). In the transformation phase, the patient may complain of bone pain and may report fevers (without any obvious sign of infection) and weight loss. Even with chemotherapy, the spleen may continue to enlarge. The patient may become more anemic and thrombocytopenic; an increased basophil level is detected by the CBC.

In the acute form of CML (blast crisis), treatment may resemble induction therapy for acute leukemia, using the same medications as for AML or acute lymphocytic leukemia. Patients whose disease evolves into a "lymphoid" blast crisis are more likely to be able to re-enter a chronic phase after induction therapy. For those whose disease evolves into AML, therapy has been largely ineffective in achieving a second chronic phase. However, an increased dose of imatinib or dasatinib can be effective in the later stages of CML. Nonetheless, life-threatening infections and bleeding occur frequently in this phase.

In rare instances, when a purely palliative approach is desired, the therapeutic approach focuses on reducing the leukocyte count to a more normal level but does not alter cytogenetic changes. This goal can be achieved by using oral chemotherapeutic agents, typically hydroxyurea or busulfan (Myleran). In the case of an extreme leukocytosis at diagnosis (e.g., leukocyte count greater than 300,000/mm^3), a more emergent treatment may be required. In this instance, leukapheresis (in which the patient's blood is removed and separated, with the leukocytes withdrawn and the remaining blood returned to the patient) can temporarily reduce the number of leukocytes. An anthracycline chemotherapeutic agent (e.g., daunomycin [Cerubidine]) may also be used to bring the leukocyte count down quickly to a safer level, where more conservative therapy can be instituted.

Nursing Management

Advances in treatment of CML have changed the trajectory of the disease, from life-threatening and likely fatal to being a chronic illness. However, nurses must understand that the effectiveness of the drugs used to treat CML is based on the patient's ability to adhere to the prescribed medication regimen and on appropriate monitoring of the therapeutic response.

Drugs used to treat CML may cause side effects for the patient that may be difficult to manage. Fatigue, asthenia, pruritus, headache, skin rash, and oropharyngeal pain are common side effects that often can be effectively managed with nursing intervention (Coleman, 2014).

Blood testing, using a specific polymerase chain reaction (PCR) to detect the level of *BCR-ABL*, is performed at regular intervals to assess for a major molecular response. Major molecular response is the benchmark for determining the efficacy of therapy and the need to change to a different drug (Deninger, 2015). Yet studies have documented the lack of adherence to this assessment with rates of adherence from less than 40% (Goldberg, 2015) to only 21% within the initial 3 months of therapy (Di Bella, Bhowmik, Bhor, et al., 2015).

Patient adherence to therapy is critical for optimal outcomes to be achieved. Several studies have documented suboptimal adherence rates to taking tyrosine kinase inhibitors as prescribed. A large study conducted in Italy discovered a self-reported rate of complete adherence to be only 60% (Breccia, Efficace, Sica, et al., 2015). In that study, forgetting to take the drug was the most common reported reason for decreased adherence. A review of 34 studies was conducted to better determine adherence rates to therapy and issues related to poor adherence in patients receiving tyrosine kinase inhibitor therapy (Hall, Paul, Bryant, et al., 2016). In this review, 100% adherence rates ranged from 20% to 53%. The investigators explored factors associated with reduced adherence, many of which have significant relevance for nursing and are depicted in Table 54-6.

TABLE 54-6 Risk Factors Associated With Lower Adherence to Oral Therapy for Chronic Myeloid Leukemia (CML)

Risk Factor Category	Risk Factor	Nursing Intervention
Patient Characteristics	Lower education level (below high school)	
	Higher self-report of functional status	
	Low self-efficacy regarding medication administration[a]	Explore with patient perceived barriers related to medication administration
	Taking medication independent of meals[a]	Develop medication administration schedule with patient; use timer/watch alarm to alert patient when to take medication
	Lack of knowledge regarding disease and treatment[a]	Provide relevant information in format understandable to patient
Social Characteristics	Living alone[a]	Evaluate need for phone follow-up, initiation of home care
	Low levels of social support	
	Low socioeconomic status	
Disease and Treatment Characteristics	Farther time from diagnosis	
	Higher rates of treatment-related side effects[a]	Monitor patient closely for side effects
	Higher number of cancer-related complications[a]	Monitor patient closely for complications
	Not participating in a clinical trial[a]	Provide patient with information on enrolment eligibility as advisable

[a]indicates risk factor amenable to nursing intervention.

Adapted from Hall, A. E., Paul, C., Bryant, J., et al. (2016). To adhere or not to adhere: Rates and reasons of medication adherence in hematological cancer patients. *Critical Reviews in Oncology/Hematology*, *97*(1), 247–262.

These data highlight the importance of nurses educating patients and assisting them to identify methods that help them remember to take their medication, to manage side effects, and to obtain prescription renewals on time. Furthermore, nurses must encourage patients to raise issues of concern that interfere with their adherence to their prescribed therapy. As adherence may decrease over time, it is important that nurses continue to assess patients for risk factors that may diminish adherence and proactively address them. To facilitate this process, acknowledging that the patient is ultimately responsible for their own care and targeting educational interventions to enhance the patient's ability to think critically are crucial (Coleman, 2014).

Acute Lymphocytic Leukemia

Acute lymphocytic leukemia (ALL) results from an uncontrolled proliferation of immature cells (lymphoblasts) derived from the lymphoid stem cell. The cell of origin is the precursor to the B lymphocyte in approximately 75% of ALL cases; T-lymphocyte ALL occurs in approximately 25% of cases. The *BCR-ABL* translocation (see earlier discussion) is found in 20% of ALL blast cells. ALL is most common in young children, with boys affected more often than girls; the peak incidence is 4 years of age. After 15 years of age, it is relatively uncommon. Increasing age appears to be associated with diminished survival; the 5-year event-free survival rate is almost 73% for children with ALL (Canadian Cancer Society, 2016) but drops to 58% to 59% for adults (Leukemia and Lymphoma Society of Canada, 2016). Yet even if relapse occurs, resumption of induction therapy can often achieve a second complete remission. Moreover, BMT may be successful even after a second relapse, particularly in certain subsets of patients (e.g., those with Philadelphia chromosome–positive ALL [Ph+ ALL]) (Chen, Campbell, & Chen, 2014).

Clinical Manifestations

Immature lymphocytes proliferate in the marrow and impede the development of normal myeloid cells. As a result, normal hematopoiesis is inhibited, resulting in reduced numbers of leukocytes, erythrocytes, and platelets. Leukocyte counts may be either low or high, but there is always a high proportion of immature cells. Manifestations of leukemic cell infiltration into other organs are more common with ALL than with other forms of leukemia and include pain from an enlarged liver or spleen and bone pain. The central nervous system is frequently a site for leukemic cells; thus, patients may exhibit headache and vomiting because of meningeal involvement. Other extranodal sites include the testes and breasts.

Medical Management

The goal of treatment is to obtain remission without excess toxicity and with a rapid hematologic recovery so that additional therapy can be given if needed. Because of the heterogeneity of the disease, treatment plans are based on genetic markers of the disease as well as risk factors of the patient, primarily age. Because ALL frequently invades the CNS, preventive intrathecal chemotherapy or, less frequently, cranial irradiation is also a key part of the treatment plan.

Treatment protocols for ALL tend to be complex, using a wide variety of chemotherapeutic agents and complicated administration schedules. The expected outcome of treatment is complete remission. Lymphoid blast cells are typically very sensitive to corticosteroids and to vinca alkaloids; therefore, these medications are an integral part of the initial induction therapy. The corticosteroid dexamethasone is preferred to prednisone, as it is more toxic to lymphoid cells and has better CNS penetration. Typically, an anthracycline is included, sometimes with asparaginase (Elspar). Once a patient is in remission, special testing (immunophenotyping, immunoglobulin gene rearrangements, T-cell receptor genes, molecular testing) is done to look for residual leukemia cells; these tests can detect as fewer as 1 ALL cell among 10,000 to 100,000 normal cells. This minimal residual disease testing is useful as a prognostic indicator. Based on these results and the rapidity in which remission is achieved, a consolidation regimen ensues, using different combinations and dosages of the drugs used in induction therapy; the goal of consolidation is to improve outcomes in those patients at high risk for relapse. HSCT may be considered during initial remission if disease features and testing suggest the risk of relapse is high (Mathisen, Kantarjian, Thomas, et al., 2013). In the context of average-risk disease, HSCT may be postponed until the time of relapse, should it occur. The therapeutic goal at the time of relapse is to reinitiate treatment to obtain a remission and then move quickly to HSCT (Mathisen et al., 2013). HSCT can improve long-term disease-free survival; however, this potential benefit must be weighed with the risks associated with the procedure, including death and long-term morbid complications (see Chapter 68).

Despite its complexity, treatment can be provided in the outpatient setting in some circumstances until severe complications develop. Tyrosine kinase inhibitors (e.g., imatinib) appear effective in patients with Ph+ ALL; these drugs can be used alone or in combination with conventional chemotherapy (Chiaretti & Foà, 2015). Commercially available monoclonal antibodies (MoAbs), in which the antibody specific to the antigen expressed on the ALL blast cell is selected for treatment, are being utilized in the context of salvage therapy; new MoAbs are under investigation (DeAngelo, 2015).

Patients with ALL can experience some unique adverse effects from treatment. The use of corticosteroids to treat ALL increases the patient's susceptibility to infection; viral infections are common. Avascular necrosis can occur in patients treated with corticosteroid-based chemotherapy, as well as with transplantation. Patients treated with asparaginase are at increased risk for thrombosis. Hepatic toxicity is also common and may necessitate cessation of supportive drugs, such as proton pump inhibitors and certain antibacterial and antifungal drugs.

Nursing Management

Nursing management of the patient with acute leukemia is presented at the end of the leukemia section in this chapter.

Chronic Lymphocytic Leukemia

CLL is a common malignancy of older adults; the median age at diagnosis is 71 years (Canadian Cancer Society, 2016). CLL is the most common form of leukemia in the United States and Europe, affecting more than 120,000 people. It is rarely seen in persons of Asian descent. On average, patients with CLL survive up to 12.5 years (early-stage CLL); this period may be as low as 1.5 years (late-stage CLL).

Pathophysiology

CLL is typically derived from a malignant clone of B lymphocytes. What was formerly called T-lymphocyte CLL is rare and is now reclassified as T-cell prolymphocytic leukemia (Hallek, 2015). In contrast to the acute forms of leukemia, most leukemia cells in CLL are fully mature. One possible mechanism that explains this oncogenesis is that these cells can escape apoptosis (programmed cell death), resulting in an excessive accumulation of the cells in the marrow and circulation. The disease is historically classified into three or four stages, based on the two classification systems that are used. In the early stage, an elevated lymphocyte count is seen; it can exceed 100,000/mm^3.

Because the lymphocytes are small, they can easily travel through the small capillaries within the circulation, and the pulmonary and cerebral complications of leukocytosis (as seen with myeloid leukemias) are not typically found in CLL. However, these cells often accumulate within the lymph nodes and spleen. When it takes less than 12 months for the absolute number of lymphocytes to double (lymphocyte doubling time), a more aggressive disease course may ensue.

Immunophenotyping of the circulating B cells is critical to establish the diagnosis by identifying the presence of a malignant clone of these cells; it is also used to gauge the prognosis (Hallek, 2015). Other special cytogenetic and molecular analyses (e.g., fluorescence in situ hybridization [FISH]) are also used to guide prognosis and therapy. Beta-2 microglobulin, a protein found on the surface of lymphocytes, can be measured in the serum; an elevated level correlates with more advanced clinical stage and poorer prognosis.

Autoimmune complications can occur at any stage, as either autoimmune hemolytic anemia or idiopathic thrombocytopenic purpura. In the autoimmune process, the RES destroys the body's own erythrocytes or platelets. Patients with CLL also have a greater risk for developing other cancers; the risk is 2.2 times higher than the expected incidence per the SEER database (Randhawa & Ferrajoli, 2016). Second cancers typically involve the skin, colon, lung, breast, prostate, and kidney. Roughly 10% of patients will experience a gradual transformation of their disease to one that becomes refractory to chemotherapy (prolymphocytic leukemia transformation) (Awan & Byrd, 2016). Slightly fewer patients will experience a sudden transformation to a very aggressive lymphoma, known as Richter's transformation; this transformation results in markedly increased lymphadenopathy, splenomegaly, worsening B symptoms (see later discussion), and survival of only a few months despite treatment.

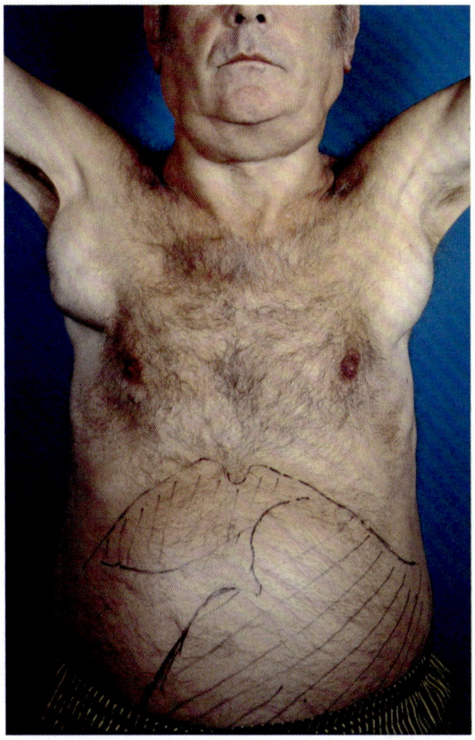

FIGURE 54-12. Massive lymphadenopathy in a patient with chronic lymphocytic leukemia. Note the enlarged liver and spleen as well. (From Tkachuk, D. C., & Hirschman, J. V. (2007). *Wintrobe's atlas of clinical hematology* (Fig. 5.1, p. 154). Philadelphia, PA: Lippincott Williams & Wilkins.)

Clinical Manifestations

Many patients are asymptomatic and are diagnosed incidentally during routine physical examinations or during treatment for another disease. An increased lymphocyte count (lymphocytosis) is always present. The erythrocyte and platelet counts may be normal or, in later stages of the illness, decreased. Enlargement of lymph nodes (lymphadenopathy) is common; this can be severe and sometimes painful (see Fig. 54-12). The spleen can also be enlarged (splenomegaly).

Patients with CLL can develop "B symptoms," a constellation of symptoms including fevers, drenching sweats (especially at night), and unintentional weight loss. Patients with CLL have defects in their humoral and cell-mediated immune systems; therefore, infections are common. The defect in cellular immunity is evidenced by an absent or decreased reaction to skin sensitivity tests (e.g., *Candida*, mumps), which is known as **anergy**. Life-threatening infections are common, particularly with advanced disease. Viral infections, such as herpes zoster, can become widely disseminated. Defects in the complement system are also seen, which result in increased risk of developing infection with encapsulated organisms (e.g., *Haemophilus influenzae*).

Medical Management

For patients with no symptoms at the time of diagnosis, the traditional "watch and wait" approach is still used, even in the face of genetic markers associated with poor prognosis (Stilgenbauer, 2015). However, with the advent of newer treatment modalities and of more sensitive means of determining prognosis, achieving a complete remission and eradicating even minimal residual disease in patients in the early stages of CLL result in improved survival (Hallek, 2015). As a result, treatment may be initiated sooner in the illness trajectory; clinical trials are ongoing to assess for an advantage in survival with this approach. Various parameters are considered when treatment is selected, including the clinical stage of the disease, disease-associated symptoms, the functional status of the patient, genetic risk for poor prognosis, and the extent of any prior therapy and efficacy of that therapy (Hallek, 2015). Functional status is a complex consideration; in this context, it incorporates the individual's life expectancy independent of CLL (due to other health problems), the ability to tolerate aggressive therapy (where creatinine clearance is particularly important), and the ability to perform activities of daily living (Shanafelt, 2013). Individuals with good functional status can typically tolerate aggressive therapy and often achieve a lasting complete remission. Whereas, the objective of treatment in those with more impaired physical status focuses on controlling bothersome symptoms (e.g., drenching night sweats, painful lymphadenopathy).

The use of combination therapy, using an immunotherapeutic antibody against CD20 (e.g., rituximab [Rituxan], ofatumumab [Arzerra], or obinutuzumab [Gazyva]) with chemotherapy agents (e.g., fludarabine [Fludara], cyclophosphamide [Cytoxan], bendamustine [Treanda] and/or chlorambucil [Leukeran]) is typically given as initial therapy; the patient's functional status (as described above) guides the specific treatment selection. When the disease is accompanied by a deletion of the TP53 gene or a mutation of this gene, the combination of chemo-immunotherapy is largely ineffective. However, two kinase inhibitors, ibrutinib (Imbruvica) and idelalisib (Zydelig), are now available that are efficacious in this context (Hallek, 2015).

The effectiveness of conventional treatment must be balanced by the risk of toxicity. For example, the chemotherapy drugs fludarabine and cyclophosphamide are often given in combination with the MoAb rituximab. This regimen can result in remissions that last 5 years, but has a high associated rate of toxicity (76%) (Shanafelt, 2013). In contrast, chlorambucil has a remission time of 12 months, but the associated toxicity is negligible. These data emphasize the importance of determining the goals of treatment with the patient *a priori*.

The major side effect of fludarabine is prolonged bone marrow suppression, manifested by prolonged periods of neutropenia, lymphopenia, and thrombocytopenia, which puts patients at risk for such infections as *Pneumocystis jiroveci, Listeria,* mycobacteria, herpes viruses, and cytomegalovirus (CMV). The MoAb alemtuzumab (Campath) is often used in combination with other chemotherapeutic agents when the disease is refractory to fludarabine, the patient has very poor prognostic markers, or it is necessary to eradicate residual disease after initial treatment. Alemtuzumab targets the CD52 antigen commonly found on CLL cells, and it is effective in clearing the marrow and circulation of these cells without affecting the stem cells. Because CD52 is present on both B and T lymphocytes, patients receiving alemtuzumab are at significant risk for infection; prophylactic use of antiviral agents and antibiotics (e.g., trimethoprim–sulfamethoxazole [Bactrim, Septra]) is important and needs to continue for several months after treatment ends. CMV infection is also common with alemtuzumab and prophylaxis is important; among commonly prescribed antiviral agents, Valacuclovir (Valtrex) is more effective than acyclovir (Zovirax) for treating CMV (Randhawa & Ferrajoli, 2016).

Virtually all patients with CLL have reduced levels of immunoglobulins, and bacterial infections are common, independent of treatment. Intravenous treatment with immunoglobulin (IVIG) may be given to selected patients with recurrent infection. While studies have not demonstrated improved survival, the rate of developing major infections is reduced (Randhawa & Ferrajoli, 2016). Patients with CLL should receive both pneumonia and flu vaccinations as indicated (see Chapter 23). Live vaccines should be avoided.

Because of the older age of most patients with CLL, transplantation may not be an option, particularly if significant comorbidities exist. Yet, allogeneic HSCT can be effective in patients with P53 deletions or mutations who otherwise have a poor prognosis. Morbidity and mortality rates remain high (20%); thus, this treatment modality may be reserved for those patients with high-risk disease, younger age, and high degree of match from the donor (Stilgenbauer, 2015).

Nursing Process

The Patient With Acute Leukemia

Assessment

Although the clinical picture varies with the type of leukemia as well as the treatment, the health history may reveal a range of subtle symptoms reported by the patient before the problem is detectable on physical examination. Weakness and fatigue are common manifestations, not only of the leukemia, but also of the resulting complications of anemia and infection. If the patient is hospitalized, the assessments should be performed daily, or more frequently as warranted. Because the physical findings may be subtle initially, a thorough, systematic assessment incorporating all body systems is essential. For example, a dry cough, mild dyspnea, and diminished breath sounds may indicate a pulmonary infection. However, the infection may not be seen initially on the chest x-ray; the absence of neutrophils delays the inflammatory response against the pulmonary infection, thus delaying the changes seen on x-ray. The platelet count can become dangerously low, leaving the patient at risk for significant bleeding. When serial assessments are performed, current findings are compared with previous findings to evaluate improvement or worsening.

The nurse also must closely monitor the results of laboratory studies. Flow sheets and spreadsheets are particularly useful in tracking the leukocyte count,

ANC, hematocrit, platelet, creatinine and electrolyte levels, and hepatic function tests. Culture results need to be reported immediately so that appropriate antimicrobial therapy can begin or be modified.

Nursing Priorities

Based on the assessment data, major nursing priorities for the patient with acute leukemia may include:

- Risk for infection
- Risk for impaired skin integrity
- Impaired gas exchange
- Impaired mucous membranes
- Imbalanced nutrition
- Acute pain and discomfort
- Hyperthermia
- Fatigue and activity intolerance
- Impaired physical mobility
- Risk for excess fluid volume
- Diarrhea
- Risk for deficient fluid volume
- Self-care deficit
- Anxiety
- Disturbed body image
- Grieving
- Potential for spiritual distress
- Deficient knowledge

Collaborative Problems/ Potential Complications

Based on the assessment data, potential complications that may develop include:

- Infection
- Bleeding/DIC
- Renal dysfunction
- Tumour lysis syndrome
- Nutritional depletion
- Mucositis
- Depression and anxiety

Planning and Goals

The major goals for the patient may include absence of complications and pain, attainment and maintenance of adequate nutrition, activity tolerance, ability to provide self-care and to cope with the diagnosis and prognosis, positive body image, and an understanding of the disease process and its treatment.

Nursing Interventions

Preventing or Managing Infection and Bleeding

The nursing interventions related to diminishing the risk of infection and bleeding are delineated in Chart 54-8.

Managing Mucositis

Although emphasis is placed on the oral mucosa, the entire GI mucosa can be altered, not only by the effects of chemotherapy but also from prolonged administration of antibiotics.

Improving Nutritional Intake

The disease process can increase the patient's metabolic rate and nutritional requirements. (Sepsis further increases them.) Nutritional intake is often reduced because of pain and discomfort associated with stomatitis. Encouraging or providing mouth care before and after meals and the administration of analgesic agents before eating can help increase intake. If oral anesthetic agents are used, the patient must be warned to chew with extreme care to avoid inadvertently biting the tongue or buccal mucosa.

Nausea should not deter nutritional intake, because antiemetic therapy is highly effective. However, nausea can result from antimicrobial therapy, so some antiemetic therapy may still be required after the chemotherapy has been completed.

Small, frequent feedings of foods that are soft in texture and moderate in temperature may be better tolerated. Nutritional supplements are frequently used. Daily body weight (as well as intake and output measurements) is useful in monitoring fluid status. Both calorie counts and more formal nutritional assessments are useful. Parenteral nutrition is often required to maintain adequate nutrition.

Easing Pain and Discomfort

Recurrent fevers are common in acute leukemia; at times, they are accompanied by shaking chills (rigours), which can be severe. Myalgias and arthralgias can result. Acetaminophen is typically given to decrease fever, but it does so by increasing diaphoresis. Sponging with cool water may be useful, but cold water or ice packs should be avoided because the heat cannot dissipate from constricted blood vessels. Bedclothes need frequent changing as well. Gentle back and shoulder massage may provide comfort.

Mucositis can also cause significant discomfort. In addition to oral hygiene practices, PCA can be effective in controlling the pain (see Chapter 16). With the exception of severe mucositis, less pain is associated with acute leukemia than with many other forms of cancer. However, the amount of psychological suffering that the patient must endure can be immense. Patients often benefit from active listening.

Because patients with acute leukemia require hospitalization for extensive nursing care (either during induction or consolidation therapy or during resultant complications), sleep deprivation frequently results. Nurses need to implement creative strategies that permit uninterrupted sleep for at least a few hours while still administering necessary medications on time.

Decreasing Fatigue and Activity Intolerance

Fatigue is a common and oppressive symptom. Nursing interventions should focus on assisting the patient to establish a balance between activity and rest. Patients with acute leukemia need to maintain some physical activity and exercise to prevent the deconditioning that results from inactivity. The use of a high-efficiency particulate air (HEPA) filter mask can permit the patient to ambulate outside the room despite severe neutropenia. Stationary bicycles may also be set up in the room; however, many patients lack the motivation or stamina to use them. At a minimum, patients should be encouraged to sit up in a chair while awake rather than staying in bed; even this simple activity can improve the patient's tidal volume and enhance circulation. Physical therapy can also be beneficial. Patients with acute leukemia may require hospitalization for extensive nursing care (either during induction or consolidation therapy or during resultant complications); sleep deprivation frequently results. Nurses need to implement creative strategies that permit uninterrupted sleep for at least a few hours while still administering necessary medications on schedule (see Chart 54-10).

Maintaining Fluid and Electrolyte Balance

Febrile episodes, bleeding, and inadequate or overly aggressive fluid replacement can alter the patient's fluid status. Similarly, persistent diarrhea, vomiting, and long-term use of certain antimicrobial agents can cause significant deficits in electrolytes. Intake and output need to be measured accurately, and daily weights should also be monitored. The patient should be assessed for signs of dehydration as well as fluid overload, with particular attention to pulmonary status and the development of dependent edema. Laboratory test results, particularly electrolytes, blood urea nitrogen, creatinine, and hematocrit, should be monitored and compared with previous results. Replacement of electrolytes, particularly potassium and magnesium, is commonly required. Patients receiving amphotericin or certain antibiotics are at increased risk for electrolyte depletion.

Improving Self-Care

Because hygiene measures are so important in this patient population, they must be performed by the nurse when the patient cannot do so. However, the patient should be encouraged to do as much as possible to preserve mobility and function as well as self-esteem. Patients may have negative feelings

NURSING RESEARCH PROFILE

Chart 54-10. Sleep Disturbances Among Patients Post-HSCT

Hacker, E. D., Patel, P., & Stainthorpe, M. (2013). Sleep interrupted: Nocturnal care disturbances following hematopoietic stem cell transplantation. *Clinical Journal of Oncology Nursing, 17*(5), 517–523.

Purpose

Sleep is a physiologic process essential for health and well-being. Patients admitted to the hospital for hematopoietic stem cell transplantation (HCST) are at risk for sleep-wake disturbance due to the acuity of their illness, the need for continuous nursing care, environmental issues, and individual patient factors. The purpose of this exploratory retrospective study was to examine reports of sleep disturbance and nocturnal disturbances in patients receiving HSCT.

Design

Forty adults who were hospitalized for HSCT comprised the convenience sample for this study. Patients were receiving HSCT for a malignancy (not specified) on a single bone marrow transplantation unit in an academic medical centre. Twenty-four of the participants were male, and 16 were female. Data were obtained from the patients' electronic medical records to complete the hourly nocturnal care interactions checklist, a standardized checklist designed to record interactions between the patient and all health care team members between the hours of 9 PM and 7 AM. Standardization of data abstraction was achieved by performing separate reviews of the record and identifying any inconsistencies in coding the data. The investigators also recorded any documentation of sleep disturbance within the progress notes of the medical record.

Results

Data were obtained from 160 unique nights; 1,642 care interactions were identified. The mean number of interactions over a 4-day time period was 41 per patient (range 20 to 58), approximately 10 interactions per patient per night. Five categories accounted for 88% of the nocturnal interactions: medication administration (40%), vital sign measurement (21%), obtaining blood samples (11%), intravenous catheter maintenance (10%), and patient assessment (6%). Nursing documentation of sleep disturbance was noted 145 times for 29 patients, and 17 times for 11 patients by physicians. Sleep aid medication was prescribed *(pro re nata* [PRN]) for 25 of the 40 patients. The peak time of nocturnal interaction occurred between 12 AM and 1 AM and between 4 AM and 5 AM, coinciding with obtaining routine vital sign measurements.

Nursing Implications

This study highlights that patients who have had HSCT have their sleep frequently interrupted while hospitalized. While the frequency is less than that reported in other studies documenting sleep interruption in the ICU setting, this study suggests that care (and thus sleep interruptions) is more clustered in the transplant unit setting. Nonetheless, clustering interventions is only partially responsible for disturbing sleep in that 50% of the interactions occur outside the two peak periods identified (i.e., 12 AM and 4 AM). Of note, toileting activities were not documented. As diarrhea is common in this patient population, the amount of sleep interruption may be greater than the data from this study suggest.

Given that a normal sleep cycle (REM sleep) is 90 to 120 minutes in length, most patients do not obtain the amount and quality of sleep needed to maximize—or regain—health. Nurses need to work collaboratively to cluster activities and interventions as much as possible. The timing of routine care practices may need to be modified so that the opportunity for patients to obtain needed sleep without interruption is realized.

because they can no longer care for themselves. Empathetic listening is helpful, as is realistic reassurance that these deficits are temporary. As the patient recovers, it is important to assist him or her to resume more self-care. Patients are usually discharged from the hospital with a vascular access device (e.g., Hickman catheter, peripherally inserted central catheter [PICC]), and most patients can care for the catheter with adequate instruction and practice under observation.

Managing Anxiety and Grief

Being diagnosed with acute leukemia can be extremely frightening. In many instances, the need to begin treatment is emergent, and the patient has little time to process the fact that he or she has the illness before making decisions about therapy. Providing emotional support and discussing the uncertain future are crucial. The nurse also needs to assess how much information the patient wants to have regarding the illness, its treatment, and potential complications. This desire should be reassessed at intervals, because needs and interest in information change throughout the course of the disease and treatment. Priorities must be identified so that procedures, assessments, and self-care expectations are adequately explained even to those who do not wish extensive information.

Many patients become depressed and begin to grieve for the losses they feel, such as normal family functioning, professional roles and responsibilities, and social roles, as well as physical functioning. The nurse can assist the patient to identify the source of the grief and encourage him or her to allow time to adjust to the major life changes produced by the illness. Role restructuring, in both family and professional life, may be required. Again, when possible, encouraging the patient to identify options and to take time making important decisions is helpful.

Discharge from the hospital can also provoke anxiety. Although most patients are eager to go home, they may lack confidence in their ability to manage potential complications and to resume their normal activity. Close communication between nurses across care settings can reassure patients that they will not be abandoned.

Encouraging Spiritual Well-Being

Because acute leukemia is a serious, potentially life-threatening illness, the nurse may offer support to enhance the patient's spiritual well-being. The patient's spiritual and religious practices should be assessed and pastoral services offered. Throughout the patient's illness, it is important that the nurse assist the patient to maintain hope. However, that hope should be realistic and will certainly change over the course of the illness. For example, the patient may initially hope to be cured, but with repeated relapses and a change to hospice or palliative care the same patient may hope for a quiet, dignified death (see Chart 54-11). (Refer to Chapter 15 for a discussion of end-of-life care.)

Promoting Home, Community-Based, and Transitional Care

EDUCATING PATIENTS ABOUT SELF-CARE. Most patients cope better when they have an understanding of what is happening to them. Based on their education, literacy level, and interest, teaching of the patient and family should focus on the disease (including some pathophysiology), its treatment, and certainly the resulting significant risk of infection and bleeding (see Chart 54-8).

Management of a vascular access device can be taught to most patients or family members. Nurses in outpatient facilities or home care nurses may need to provide follow-up care for patients with vascular access devices.

CONTINUING AND TRANSITIONAL CARE. Shortened hospital stays and outpatient care have significantly altered care for patients with acute leukemia. In many instances, when the patient is clinically stable but still requires parenteral antibiotics or blood products, these procedures can be performed in an outpatient setting. Nurses in these various settings must communicate regularly. They need to tell the patient which parameters are important to monitor and how to monitor them, and give the patient specific instructions about when to seek care from the physician or other health care provider. The primary care provider is responsible for monitoring the patient who is cured or in sustained remission.

The patient and family need to have a clear understanding of the disease, the prognosis, and how to monitor for complications or recurrence. The nurse ensures that this information is provided. Should the patient no longer respond to therapy, it is important to respect the patient's choices about treatment, including measures to prolong life and other end-of-life measures. Advance directives, including living wills, provide patients with some measure of control during terminal illness.

Most patients in this stage choose to be cared for at home, and families often need support when considering this option. Coordination of home care services and instruction can help alleviate anxiety about managing the patient's care in the home. As the patient becomes weaker, the caregivers must assume more of the patient's care. In addition, caregivers often need to be encouraged to take care of themselves, allowing time for rest and accepting emotional support. Hospice staff can assist in providing respite for family members as well as care for the patient. Patients and families also need assistance to cope with changes in their roles and responsibilities. Anticipatory grieving is an essential task during this time (see Chapter 15).

In patients with acute leukemia, death typically occurs from infection or bleeding. Family members need to have information about these complications and the measures to take should either occur. Many family members cannot cope with the care required when a patient begins to bleed actively. It is important to delineate alternatives to keeping the

CHART 54-11

Ethical Dilemma: Can Comfort Care at End of Life Equate to Assisted Suicide or Active Euthanasia?

Case Scenario

A 34-year-old patient, wife and mother of two young children, has been on the oncology unit with a terminal diagnosis of acute myeloid leukemia (AML). She has recently decided to stop all treatments and begin palliative care. Over the course of the past few weeks, she has developed intractable bone pain, nausea, and episodes of severe bleeding. The patient, who is of sound mental capacity, discusses further treatment options with the oncologist and her family and wants to die peacefully. The patient is placed on a midazolam (Versed) and morphine intravenous drip that you titrate to achieve relief of symptoms. The patient dies peacefully within 72 hours of you starting this new medication regimen with her family at her bedside.

Discussion

There is a great deal of discomfort among both clinicians and laymen around what constitutes comfort care (i.e., palliative care) at end of life and what may constitute either assisted suicide or euthanasia. The premise is that palliative care should ameliorate pain and physical suffering in the patient who is terminally ill, but it should not significantly shorten the patient's life. There is never the intent to deliberately kill the patient. Although the American Nurses Association (ANA) clearly does not advocate that nurses participate in either assisted suicide or euthanasia, and avows that nurses should not participate in acts that intentionally cause patient death (ANA, 2015), the ANA does advocate that nurses provide competent palliative care at end of life that preserves each individual patient's dignity and autonomy (ANA, 2015).

Analysis

- Would you describe your role in this case as complicit in assisted suicide, active euthanasia, or providing palliation? What distinction, if any, might there be among these three acts?
- Describe how the ethical principles of autonomy, beneficence, and nonmaleficence may intersect or be at odds with each other in this case (see Chart 3-3 in Chapter 3).
- Discuss how palliative sedation meets the moral justification of the four principles of the doctrine of double effect (Chapter 15).
- Note that the ANA (2015) *Code of Ethics* clearly states that nurses should not *intentionally* cause a patient's death. What were your "intentions" in this case? How might intentionality be instrumental in making this act of titrating medications that provided palliation morally defensible?

REFERENCES

American Nurses Association (ANA). (2015). *Code of ethics for nurses with interpretive statements*. Washington, DC: Nursesbooks.org.

Broeckaert, B. (2011). Palliative sedation, physician assisted suicide, and euthanasia: "Same, same but different?" *American Journal of Bioethics, 11*(6), 62–64.

Carvalho, T. B., Radt, M. Y., Verheijde, J. L., et al. (2011). Continuous deep sedation in end-of-life care: Disentangling palliation from physician-assisted death. *American Journal of Bioethics, 11*(6), 60–62.

Wilson, O., Avalos, G., & Dowling, M. (2016). Knowledge of palliative care and attitudes towards nursing the dying patient. *British Journal of Nursing, 25*(11), 600–605.

Resource

See Chapter 3, Chart 3-3 for ethics resources.

patient at home, such as inpatient hospice units. Should another option be sought, family members who may feel guilty that they could not keep the patient at home will require support from the nurse.

Evaluation

Expected patient outcomes may include:

1. Shows no evidence of infection
2. Experiences no bleeding
3. Has intact oral mucous membranes
   a. Participates in oral hygiene regimen
   b. Reports no discomfort in mouth
4. Attains optimal level of nutrition
   a. Maintains weight with increased food and fluid intake
   b. Maintains adequate protein stores (e.g., albumin, prealbumin)
5. Reports satisfaction with pain and comfort levels
6. Has less fatigue and increased activity
7. Maintains fluid and electrolyte balance
8. Participates in self-care
9. Copes with anxiety and grief
   a. Discusses concerns and fears
   b. Uses stress management strategies appropriately
   c. Participates in decisions regarding end-of-life care
   d. Discusses hope for peaceful death
10. Absence of complications

Primary Myelofibrosis

Primary myelofibrosis, also known as agnogenic myeloid metaplasia or myelofibrosis with myeloid metaplasia, is a chronic myeloproliferative disorder that arises from neoplastic transformation of an early hematopoietic stem cell. The disease is characterized by marrow fibrosis or scarring, extramedullary hematopoiesis (typically involving the spleen and the liver), leukocytosis, thrombocytosis, and anemia. Some patients have diminished leukocyte, platelet, and erythrocyte counts (i.e., pancytopenia). Patients with myelofibrosis have increased **angiogenesis** (formation of new blood vessels) within the marrow. Early forms of blood cells (including nucleated RBCs [immature

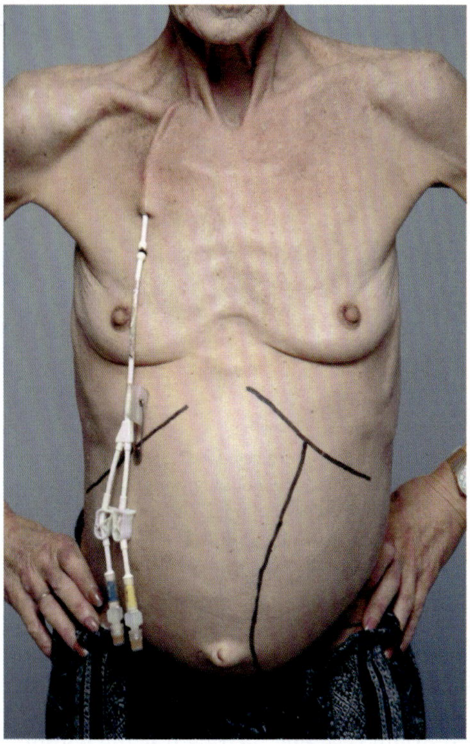

FIGURE 54-13. Cachexia, severe wasting, and massively enlarged liver and spleen (hepatosplenomegaly) are seen in advanced myeloproliferative disorders, particularly myelofibrosis. (Note also the lack of adequate dressing over the patient's vascular access device.) (From Tkachuk, D. C., & Hirschman, J. V. (2007). *Wintrobe's atlas of clinical hematology* (Fig. 4.1, p. 111). Philadelphia, PA: Lippincott Williams & Wilkins.)

RBCs] and megakaryocyte fragments) are frequently found in the circulation. The cause is unknown. Secondary myelofibrosis evolves from polycythemia vera or, much less frequently, from ET. As with ET and polycythemia vera, mutations of the JAK2 gene or calreticulin are frequently seen; prognosis is worse in those without genetic mutations (Lichtman & Prchal, 2016).

Myelofibrosis is the rarest of the classic myeloproliferative neoplasms that do not involve the *BCR-ABL* gene (i.e., CML). It is a disease of the older adult, with a median age at diagnosis of 65 to 70 years, and is more common in males. Symptoms may result from an often massively enlarged spleen, causing discomfort and early satiety. Other signs and symptoms include profound fatigue, pruritus, bone pain, weight loss, infection and bleeding (from pancytopenia), and cachexia (see Fig. 54-13). Arterial or venous thrombosis can occur but is less frequent than that found in polycythemia vera or ET. Average survival ranges from 2 to 10 years based on the occurrence of such adverse prognostic indicators as increased age; anemia; leukocytosis; presence of blast cells in the circulation; and the presence of fever, diaphoresis, or weight loss at the time of diagnosis (Lichtman & Prchal, 2016). Common causes of death are heart or liver failure, complications of marrow failure (e.g., infection, bleeding), and transformation to AML. AML is especially difficult to treat successfully in these situations.

Medical Management

Goals of therapy are based on reducing the burden of the disease (by decreasing symptoms and splenomegaly) and improving blood counts (Geyer & Mesa, 2014). Risk is determined based on several factors, including age (over 65 years of age), elevated WBC count (above 25,000/mm^3), severe anemia (hemoglobin less than 10 g/dL), the presence of constitutional symptoms (e.g., weight loss), the presence of blast cells in the peripheral blood, RBC transfusion requirement, and unfavourable cytogenetic profile. Patients assessed to have low-risk disease may not require therapy initially, reserving it when more symptoms develop (see Table 54-5).

Anemia is most commonly managed with RBC transfusions. Erythroid-stimulating agents may improve anemia to the extent that transfusion requirement is reduced but the effect is not durable (Manea, 2014). Androgens have been used in the past, but they are largely ineffective. Other pharmacologic agents are used to diminish splenomegaly and improve cytopenias. Hydroxyurea is often used to control high leukocyte and platelet counts and to reduce the size of the spleen. Thalidomide (Thalomid) or pomalidomide (Pomalyst) may be useful in improving anemia and reducing an enlarged spleen, but the effect is transient, lasting an average of 8 months (Odenike, 2013).

Ruxolitinib (Jakafi) is an inhibitor of the JAK2 kinase. It can be highly effective in decreasing splenomegaly, improves fatigue and weight gain, and decreases night sweats and pruritus and the need for RBC transfusions. Thrombocytopenia can be significant, as well as anemia. However, the anemia may improve after several months of therapy.

HSCT is a useful treatment modality in younger, otherwise healthy people, and is the only current therapy that can reverse the fibrosis within the marrow (Odenike, 2013). Patients with high risk of disease should be promptly evaluated to determine candidacy (Geyer & Mesa, 2014).

Splenectomy may be used to control the complications that result from a massively enlarged spleen. The mortality rate associated with this procedure is 10%, and the morbidity associated with the procedure (e.g., infection, bleeding, thrombosis) is 47% (Geyer & Mesa, 2014; Lichtman & Prchal, 2016). Furthermore, a reactive thrombocytosis and leukocytosis can develop because the cells are no longer sequestered out of the circulation. The decision to undergo splenectomy warrants careful consideration of the advantages and disadvantages.

Nursing Management

Splenomegaly can be profound in patients with myelofibrosis, with enlargement of the spleen that may extend to the pelvic rim. This condition is extremely uncomfortable and can severely limit nutritional intake. Analgesic agents are usually ineffective. Splenomegaly, coupled with a hypermetabolic state, results in significant weight loss and muscle wasting. Patients benefit from small, frequent meals of foods that are high in calories and protein. Weakness, fatigue, and altered body image are other significant problems. Energy conservation methods and active listening are important nursing interventions. The patient needs to be educated about signs and symptoms of infection, bleeding, and thrombosis, as well as appropriate interventions if these occur. Ensuring that the patient takes steps to decrease risks associated with developing thrombosis (e.g., smoking; obesity; poorly controlled hyperlipidemia,

TABLE 54-7 Fatigue in Patients With Myeloproliferative Neoplasms

Self-reported strategies used to ameliorate fatigue by patients with myeloproliferative neoplasms. Data obtained from online surveys (*N* = 1,788) gathered via myeloproliferative neoplasm web sites.

Strategy	Patients Reported Use (%)
Setting priorities	75
Postponing nonessential activities	74
Exercise	73
Naps	70
Walking	66
Socializing	65
Nutrition	64
Reading	62
Scheduling activity during peak energy periods	62
Pacing activities	58
Structured daily routine	54
Delegation	52

Adapted from Scherber, R. M., Kosiorek, H. E., Senyak, Z., et al. (2016). Comprehensively understanding fatigue in patients with myeloproliferative neoplasms. *Cancer*, *122*(3), 477–485.

hypertension, or diabetes) is also important. Table 54-7 identifies useful strategies aimed at managing fatigue.

LYMPHOMA

The lymphomas are neoplasms of cells of lymphoid origin. These tumours usually start in lymph nodes but can involve lymphoid tissue in the spleen, GI tract (e.g., the wall of the stomach), liver, or bone marrow. They are often classified according to the degree of cell differentiation and the origin of the predominant malignant cell. Lymphomas can be broadly classified into two categories: Hodgkin's lymphoma and non-Hodgkin's lymphoma (NHL).

Hodgkin's Lymphoma

Hodgkin's lymphoma is a relatively rare malignancy that has an impressive cure rate. It is somewhat more common in men than women and has two peaks of incidence: one in the early 20s and the other after 50 years of age. Disease occurrence has a familial pattern: First-degree relatives have a higher-than-normal frequency of disease, but the actual incidence of this pattern is low. No increased incidence for nonblood relatives (e.g., spouses) has been documented. Hodgkin's lymphoma is seen more commonly in patients receiving chronic immunosuppressive therapy (e.g., for renal transplant) and also in veterans of the military who were exposed to the herbicide Agent Orange.

Pathophysiology

Unlike other lymphomas, Hodgkin's lymphoma is unicentric in origin in that it initiates in a single node. The disease spreads by contiguous extension along the lymphatic system. The malignant cell of Hodgkin's lymphoma is the Reed–Sternberg cell, a gigantic tumour cell that is morphologically unique and is thought to be of immature lymphoid origin (see Fig. 54-14). It is the pathologic hallmark and essential diagnostic criterion. However, the tumour is very heterogeneous and may actually contain few Reed–Sternberg cells. Repeated biopsies may be required to establish the diagnosis.

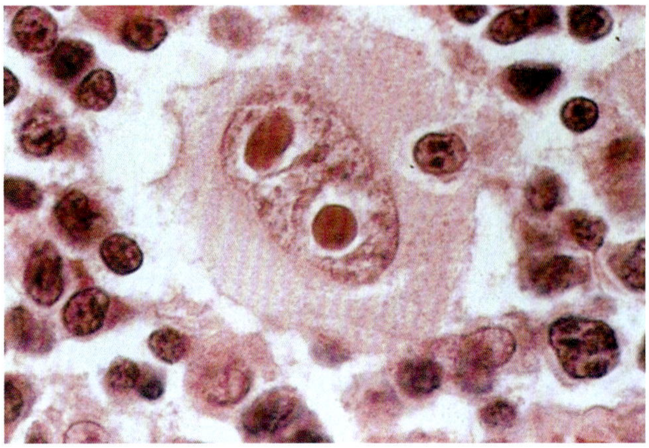

FIGURE 54-14. Reed–Sternberg cell. Reed–Sternberg cells are large, abnormal lymphocytes that may contain more than one nucleus. These cells are found in Hodgkin's lymphoma. (Adapted with permission from Rubin, R., Strayer, D. S., & Rubin, E. (2011). *Rubin's pathology* (6th ed.). Philadelphia, PA: Lippincott Williams & Wilkins.)

The cause of Hodgkin's lymphoma is unknown, but a viral etiology is suspected. Although fragments of the Epstein–Barr virus have been found in some Reed–Sternberg cells, the precise role of this virus in the development of Hodgkin's lymphoma remains unknown.

Hodgkin's lymphoma is customarily classified into five subgroups based on pathologic analyses that reflect the natural history of the malignancy and suggest the prognosis. For example, when lymphocytes predominate, with few Reed–Sternberg cells and minimal involvement of the lymph nodes, the prognosis is much more favourable than when the lymphocyte count is low and the lymph nodes are virtually replaced by tumour cells of the most primitive type. Most patients with Hodgkin's lymphoma have the types currently designated "nodular sclerosis" or "mixed cellularity." The nodular sclerosis type tends to occur more often in young women, at an earlier stage but with a worse prognosis than the mixed cellularity subgroup, which occurs more commonly in men and causes more constitutional symptoms but has a better prognosis.

Clinical Manifestations

Hodgkin's lymphoma usually begins as a painless enlargement of one or more lymph nodes on one side of the neck. The individual nodes are painless and firm but not hard. The most common sites for lymphadenopathy are the cervical, supraclavicular, and mediastinal nodes; involvement of the iliac or inguinal nodes or spleen is much less common. A mediastinal mass may be seen on chest x-ray; occasionally, the mass is large enough to compress the trachea and cause dyspnea. Pruritus is common; it can be extremely distressing, and the cause is unknown. Some

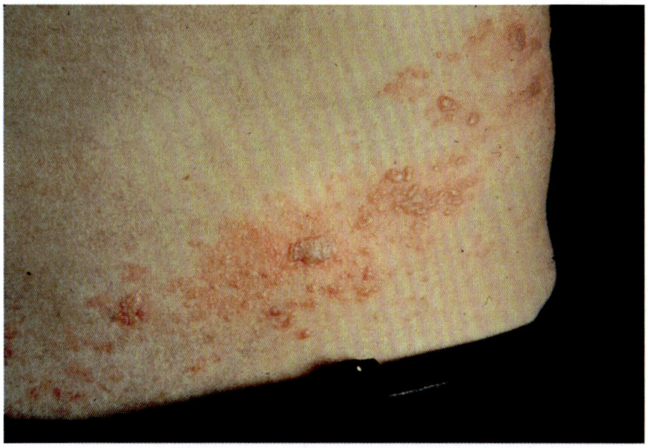

FIGURE 54-15. Herpes zoster is a common complication in patients with lymphoproliferative disease, such as Hodgkin's lymphoma here. Zoster infections are also common in patients on chronic steroid use for hematologic conditions and some chemotherapy regimens. (From Tkachuk, D. C., & Hirschman, J. V. (2007). *Wintrobe's atlas of clinical hematology* (Fig. 5.152, p. 207). Philadelphia, PA: Lippincott Williams & Wilkins.)

patients experience brief but severe pain after drinking alcohol, usually at the site of the tumour. Again, the cause of this is unknown.

All organs are vulnerable to invasion by tumour cells. The symptoms result from compression of organs by the tumour, such as cough and pulmonary effusion (from pulmonary infiltrates), jaundice (from hepatic involvement or bile duct obstruction), abdominal pain (from splenomegaly or retroperitoneal adenopathy), or bone pain (from skeletal involvement). Herpes zoster infections are common. A cluster of constitutional symptoms has important prognostic implications. Referred to as "B symptoms," they include fever (without chills), drenching sweats (particularly at night), and unintentional weight loss of more than 10% of body weight. B symptoms are found in 40% of patients and are more common in advanced disease.

A mild anemia is the most common hematologic finding. The leukocyte count may be elevated or decreased. The platelet count is typically normal, unless the tumour has invaded the bone marrow, suppressing hematopoiesis. The **erythrocyte sedimentation rate (ESR)** and the serum copper level are used by some clinicians to assess disease activity. Patients with Hodgkin's lymphoma have impaired cellular immunity, as evidenced by an absent or decreased reaction to skin sensitivity tests (e.g., *Candida*, mumps). Infections, including viral infections, are common (see Fig. 54-15).

Assessment and Diagnostic Findings

Because many manifestations are similar to those occurring with infection, diagnostic studies are performed to rule out an infectious origin for the disease. The diagnosis is made by means of an excisional lymph node biopsy and the finding of the Reed–Sternberg cell. Once the diagnosis is confirmed and the histologic type is established, it is necessary to assess the extent of the disease, a process referred to as staging.

During the health history, the patient is assessed for any B symptoms. Physical examination requires a careful, systematic evaluation of the lymph node chains, as well as the size of the spleen and liver. A chest x-ray and a CT scan of the chest, abdomen, and pelvis are crucial to identify the extent of lymphadenopathy within these regions. A positron emission tomography (PET) scan may be the most sensitive imaging test in identifying residual disease. Laboratory tests include CBC, platelet count, ESR, and liver and renal function studies. A bone marrow biopsy is performed if there are signs of marrow involvement, and some physicians routinely perform bilateral biopsies. Bone scans may be performed.

Medical Management

The goal in the treatment of Hodgkin's lymphoma is cure. Cure rates are 85% to 90% for patients with early-stage disease and 65% to 85% for those with advanced-stage disease (Matasar, Ford, Riedel, et al., 2015). Treatment is determined primarily by the stage of the disease, not by the histologic type; however, extensive research is ongoing to target treatment regimens more to the histologic subtypes or prognostic features. Because of long-term survival and potential for cure from the disease, consideration must be made of potential long-term morbidity associated with treatment, particularly cardiac disease and second malignancies. Treatment choice must be balanced between using high-intensity therapy, where the likelihood of cure or long-lasting remission is high but has a risk of late toxicity and potential mortality, and less-intensive therapy that may have less toxicity but greater likelihood of relapsed disease. This dilemma is particularly relevant when treating young patients with early-stage disease (Johnson, 2013).

Treatment of limited-stage Hodgkin's lymphoma commonly involves a short course (2 to 4 months) of chemotherapy followed by radiation therapy to the specific involved area. This strategy has reduced the radiation dosage, with subsequent decrease in long-term side effects (particularly second malignancies and late cardiovascular events) and without decreasing the likelihood of controlling the disease. However, with the effectiveness of second-line therapies, even this amount of radiation is being questioned (Johnson, 2013). Combination chemotherapy with doxorubicin (Adriamycin), bleomycin (Blenoxane), vinblastine (Velban), and dacarbazine (DTIC), referred to as ABVD, is considered the standard treatment for more advanced disease (stages III and IV and all stages with B symptoms). Chemotherapy is often successful in obtaining remission even when relapse occurs. Other combinations of chemotherapy are used, which may have more toxicity. The MoAb brentuximab vedotin (Adcetris) has approval for use in refractory relapsed Hodgkin's lymphoma. This drug targets a receptor that is expressed on the surface of activated T and B lymphocytes, but also on Reed–Sternberg cells. Current studies are ongoing to determine the best time to use this therapy: prior to transplant (HSCT), as maintenance therapy post-transplant, or when transplant is not an option (Graf & Gopal, 2014).

HSCT is used for advanced or refractory disease. Most patients diagnosed with Hodgkin's lymphoma are either cured or experience prolonged remissions, and thus live for many years post diagnosis. As a result, much is now known about the long-term effects of chemotherapy and radiation therapy. Second malignancies are the leading cause of death in long-term survivors of Hodgkin's lymphoma (Ng, 2014). There is a latency period of 5 years, after which time the risk progressively increases and remains greater than would be expected in the general population, at least 25 years after diagnosis (Ng, 2014). In a study of 465 adults previously treated for Hodgkin's lymphoma, the risk of developing a nonfatal second malignancy was 3.41 times higher (Matasar et al., 2015). The most common to develop are breast, lung, GI, and skin cancers. Prior radiation therapy is more closely associated with the development of secondary cancers, but chemotherapy that used alkylator drugs is associated with lung and GI cancer development (Ng, 2014). Leukemia more commonly developed in patients who received the chemotherapy regimen MOPP (i.e., nitrogen mustard, vincristine, procarbazine, and prednisone).

Cardiovascular disease is also frequently seen in the Hodgkin's lymphoma survivor population. The risk develops after a latency of 10 years after diagnosis and is directly related to doses of radiation to the anterior chest region. Coronary artery disease, dysrhythmias, valvular disease, and cardiomyopathy are noted after radiation; congestive heart failure, decreased systolic function, and dilated cardiomyopathy are more commonly associated with prior anthracycline therapy (Ng, 2014).

Other organ dysfunction is also well documented, including that of the endocrine system. A high incidence of anxiety and depression that also persist over time was reported in several studies (Matasar et al., 2015; Oerlemans, Mols, Nijziel, et al., 2014). Persistent fatigue is common in survivors and can be exacerbated by depression and other treatment-related comorbidities (Daniëls, Oerlemans, Krol, et al., 2013; Daniëls, Oerlemans, Krol, et al., 2014; Soares, Biasoli, Scheliga, et al., 2013). See Chapter 68 for long-term potential complications associated with chemotherapy or radiation therapy.

Late effects of treatment can have an adverse effect on a survivor's quality of life (Oerlemans et al., 2014; Khimani, Chen, Mauch, et al., 2013). A study of 40 young adult survivors found improvements in quality of life as soon as 1 month after completing therapy, and this improvement was still noted 6 months after therapy (Roper, Cooley, McDermott, et al., 2013). These data need to be replicated in larger studies and for longer periods of time; it may be that early improvements in quality of life do not persist long term, particularly as late complications arise. Adequate social support and social network are associated with better quality of life (Soares et al., 2013).

Nursing Management

The potential development of a second malignancy should be addressed with the patient when treatment decisions are made. However, it is also important to tell patients that Hodgkin's lymphoma is often curable. The nurse should encourage patients to reduce other factors that increase the risk of developing second cancers, such as use of tobacco and alcohol and exposure to environmental carcinogens and excessive sunlight. Screening for late effects of treatment (see Chapter 68, Chart 68-5) is necessary. In addition, the nurse should provide education about relevant self-care strategies and disease management.

Non-Hodgkin's Lymphomas

The non-Hodgkin's lymphomas (NHLs) are a heterogeneous group of cancers that originate from the neoplastic growth of lymphoid tissue. As in CLL, the neoplastic cells are thought to arise from a single clone of lymphocytes; however, in NHL, the cells may vary morphologically. Most NHLs involve malignant B lymphocytes; only 5% involve T lymphocytes. In contrast to Hodgkin's lymphoma, the lymphoid tissues involved are largely infiltrated with malignant cells. The spread of these malignant lymphoid cells occurs unpredictably, and true localized disease is uncommon. Lymph nodes from multiple sites may be infiltrated, as may sites outside the lymphoid system (extranodal tissue; see Fig. 54-16).

NHL is now the fifth most common type of cancer diagnosed in Canada. The incidence increases with each decade of life; the median age at diagnosis is 66 years (Canadian Cancer Society, 2016). Although no common etiologic factor has been identified, the incidence of NHL has increased in people with immunodeficiencies or autoimmune disorders; prior treatment for cancer; prior organ transplant; viral infections (including Epstein–Barr virus and HIV); and exposure to pesticides, solvents, dyes, or defoliating agents, including Agent Orange. The prognosis varies greatly among the more than 30 subtypes of NHL. Diffuse large B-cell lymphoma is the most common form and accounts for about 30% of all newly diagnosed lymphomas (80% of all aggressive types) with a great variety in 5-year

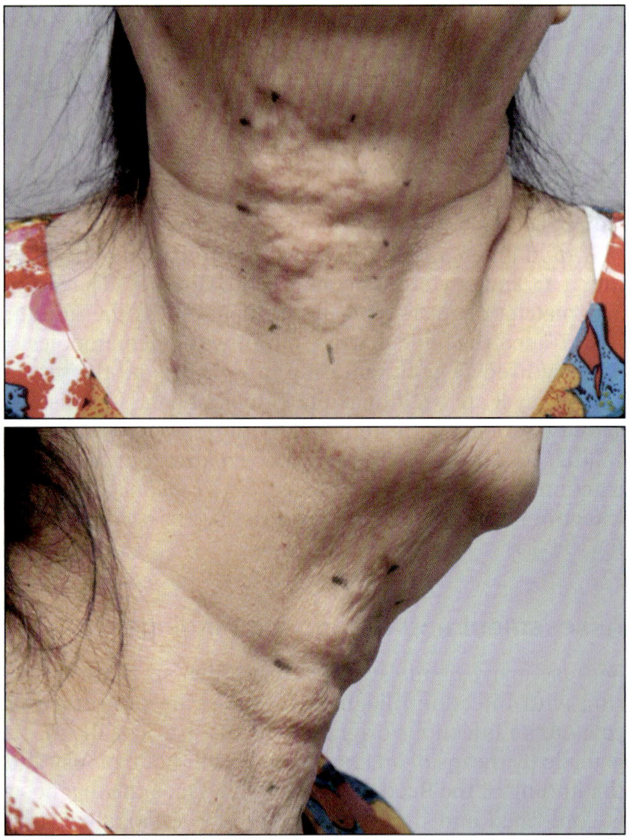

FIGURE 54-16. Any extranodal location can be a site for diffuse B-cell lymphoma, such as the thyroid, as shown here. (From Tkachuk, D. C., & Hirschman, J. V. (2007). *Wintrobe's atlas of clinical hematology* (Fig. 5.87, p. 183). Philadelphia, PA: Lippincott Williams & Wilkins.)

survival rates. Follicular lymphoma is the second most common form and accounts for 22% of all new cases (70% of all indolent [less aggressive] types) with a larger median survival rate (Canadian Cancer Society, 2016).

Clinical Manifestations

Symptoms are highly variable, reflecting the diverse nature of the NHLs. Lymphadenopathy is most common (66%); however, in indolent (or relatively benign) types of lymphomas, the lymphadenopathy can wax and wane. With early-stage disease, or with the types that are considered indolent, symptoms may be virtually absent or very minor, and the illness typically is not diagnosed until it progresses to a later stage, when the patient is symptomatic. At these stages (III or IV), lymphadenopathy is distinctly noticeable. One third of patients with NHLs have B symptoms (fever, drenching night sweats, and unintentional weight loss). Lymphomatous masses can compromise organ function. For example, a mass in the mediastinum can cause respiratory distress; abdominal masses can compromise the ureters, leading to renal dysfunction; and splenomegaly can cause abdominal discomfort, nausea, early satiety, anorexia, and weight loss. Involvement of the central nervous system with lymphoma is becoming increasingly common.

Assessment and Diagnostic Findings

The actual diagnosis of NHL is categorized into a highly complex classification system based on histopathology, immunophenotyping, and cytogenetic analyses of the malignant cells (see Table 54-8). The specific histopathologic type of the disease has important prognostic implications. Treatment also varies and is based on these features. Indolent types tend to have small cells that are distributed in a follicular pattern. Aggressive types tend to have large or immature cells distributed through the nodes in a diffuse pattern. Staging is typically based on data obtained from CT and PET scans, bone marrow biopsies, and occasionally cerebrospinal fluid analysis. The stage is based on the site of disease and its spread to other sites. For example, in stage I disease, only one area of involvement is detected; thus, stage I disease is highly localized and may respond well to localized therapy (e.g., radiation therapy).

TABLE 54-8 Types of Lymphomas[a]

Indolent	Aggressive	Highly Aggressive
Follicular	Diffuse large cell	Burkitt
Small lymphocytic	Mantle cell	Lymphoblastic
Marginal zone: MALT		AIDS-related B cell
Splenic		
Nodal		
Lymphoplasmacytic: Waldenstrom's macroglobulinemia		

[a]Major types of lymphomas, many of which are indolent in nature. Table does not present an all-inclusive list.

MALT, mucosa-associated lymphoidal tissue; AIDS, acquired immunodeficiency syndrome.

In contrast, in stage IV disease at least one extranodal site is detected.

Although stage of disease is important, it is often not an accurate predictor of prognosis. Two prognostic classification systems have been developed that are particularly useful in the elderly patient population, the International Prognostic Index (IPI) and, for follicular lymphomas, the Follicular Lymphoma International Prognostic Index (FLIPI). Age, performance status, lactate dehydrogenase levels, and extent of disease are scored to determine risk of failure or death from disease. Based on the IPI, 5-year overall survival rates are 71% overall but vary greatly, depending on the particular type of lymphoma.

Medical Management

Treatment is determined by the classification of disease, the stage of disease, prior treatment (if any), and the patient's ability to tolerate therapy. Tolerance to therapy is largely dictated by renal, hepatic, and cardiac function; the presence of concurrent diseases; functional status; and age. If the disease is not aggressive and is localized, radiation alone may be the treatment of choice. With aggressive types of NHL, aggressive combinations of chemotherapeutic agents are used; the combination of the monoclonal antibody rituximab with conventional chemotherapy (Cytoxan, doxorubicin, vincristine, and prednisone [R-CHOP]) is now considered standard treatment for common lymphomas. Central nervous system involvement is common with some aggressive forms of NHL; in this situation, cranial radiation or intrathecal chemotherapy is used in addition to systemic chemotherapy.

There is no standard therapy for follicular lymphoma. "Watchful waiting" is often used in those with indolent disease. Rituximab or radiopharmaceutical agents (e.g., tositumomab/iodine-131 [Bexxar] or ibritumomab tiuxetan [Zevalin]) are also used, although the latter agents cause technical difficulties with administration due to the radioactivity of the agent. More aggressive treatment (often R-CHOP) may provide a longer duration of remission in which additional treatment is not needed. Unfortunately, in most situations, relapse is commonly seen in patients with low-grade lymphomas. Treatment after relapse is controversial. BMT or HSCT may be considered for patients younger than 60 years of age (see Chapter 68).

Nursing Management

Lymphoma is a highly complex constellation of diseases. When caring for patients with lymphoma, it is extremely important for the nurse to know the specific disease type, stage of disease, treatment history, and current treatment plan. Most of the care for patients with Hodgkin's lymphoma or NHL takes place in the outpatient setting, unless complications occur (e.g., infection, respiratory compromise due to mediastinal mass). The most commonly used treatment methods are chemotherapy (often combined with an MoAb) and radiation therapy. Chemotherapy causes systemic side effects (e.g., myelosuppression, nausea, hair loss, risk of infection), whereas radiation therapy causes specific side effects that are limited to the area being irradiated. For example, patients receiving abdominal radiation therapy may experience nausea and diarrhea but not hair loss. Regardless of the type of treatment, all patients may experience fatigue.

The risk of infection is significant for these patients, not only from treatment-related myelosuppression but also from the defective immune response that results from the disease itself. Patients need to be educated to minimize the risks of infection, to recognize signs of possible infection, and to contact their primary provider if such signs develop.

Additional complications depend on the location of the lymphoma. Therefore, the nurse must know the tumour location so that assessments can be targeted appropriately. For example, patients with lymphomatous masses in the upper chest should be assessed for superior vena cava obstruction or airway obstruction, if the mass is near the bronchus or trachea.

Patient education is an integral component of nursing care. A longitudinal study of more than 1,000 patients with various types of lymphoma confirmed that informational needs vary over the course of the survival trajectory (Husson, Oerlemans, Mols, et al., 2014). Those patients diagnosed with lymphoma within the past 2 years voiced the need for disease and medical information; whereas, those diagnosed beyond 2 years voiced the need for information related to long-term effects of therapy. These results lend credence to the importance of tailoring information provided to the unique learning needs of the patient, as well as the coping styles that patient uses in living with lymphoma.

Many lymphomas can be cured with current treatments. However, as survival rates increase, the incidence of second malignancies, particularly AML or MDS, also increases. Therefore, survivors should be screened regularly for the development of second malignancies. As is true with long-term survivors of Hodgkin's lymphoma, survivors of NHL may be faced with managing persistent fatigue, depression, anxiety, cardiac, and pulmonary toxicity (Spector, Noonan, Mayer, et al., 2015). A study of quality of life among survivors of diffuse large B cell lymphoma found that younger-aged survivors (18 to 59 years of age) reported worse cognitive and social function and more financial problems and dyspnea compared to age-matched controls (van der Poel, Oerlemans, Schouten, et al., 2014). In contrast, the reported quality of life of older-aged survivors was similar to those of the control group, albeit lower than those of the younger-aged survivor group.

The Canadian Cancer Society developed health behaviour recommendations for cancer survivors, which include avoiding smoking, maintaining a normal body mass index (BMI), improving nutrition (i.e., consuming fruits and vegetables), and engaging in at least 150 minutes of aerobic physical activity per week.

MULTIPLE MYELOMA

Multiple myeloma is a malignant disease of the most mature form of B lymphocyte, the plasma cell. Plasma cells secrete immunoglobulins, proteins necessary for antibody production to fight infection. In 2016, 2,700 people in Canada were diagnosed with the disease (Canadian Cancer Society, 2016). There is a slightly higher incidence in men than women. The 5-year standardized survival rate for patients is a little over 42% (Canadian Cancer Society, 2016). Currently, prognosis is based on two simple markers: serum albumin (presumed to be a negative acute-phase reactant), and serum beta-2 microglobulin (presumed to be an indirect measure of tumour burden, defined as an approximation of the amount of cancer or the number of cancer cells in the body) (Landgren & Morgan, 2014). Research is currently directed at identifying specific types of chromosomal abnormalities that will further determine prognosis and treatment.

Pathophysiology

In multiple myeloma, the malignant plasma cells produce an increased amount of a specific immunoglobulin that is nonfunctional. Functional types of immunoglobulin are still produced by nonmalignant plasma cells, although in lower-than-normal quantity. The specific immunoglobulin secreted by the myeloma cells is detectable in the blood or urine and is referred to as the monoclonal protein, or M protein. This protein serves as a useful marker to monitor the extent of disease and the patient's response to therapy. It is commonly measured by serum or urine protein electrophoresis, or free light chain assay (see Fig. 54-17). The patient's total protein level is also typically elevated because of the production of M protein. Malignant plasma cells also secrete certain substances to stimulate angiogenesis to enhance the growth of these clusters of plasma cell. Occasionally, the plasma cells infiltrate other tissue, in which case they are referred to as plasmacytomas. Plasmacytomas can occur in the sinuses, spinal cord, and soft tissues.

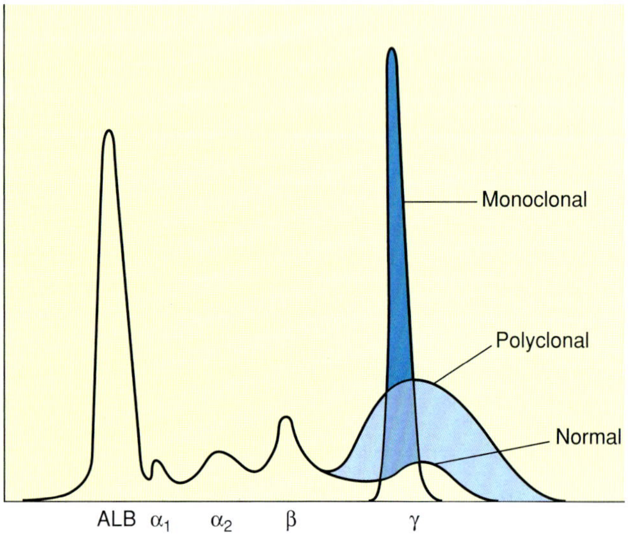

FIGURE 54-17. Abnormal serum protein electrophoresis patterns contrasted with a normal pattern. Polyclonal peaks are characterized by a broad-based increase in immunoglobulin (Ig) by myriad reactive plasma cells and indicate a benign reactive process. In contrast, a narrow spike indicates homogeneity of the Ig secreted by a single clone of plasma cells. M spikes are seen in monoclonal gammopathies of undetermined significance or in plasma malignancies (myeloma, Waldenstrom's macroglobulinemia). (From Turgeon, M. (2012). *Clinical hematology theory & procedures* (5th ed., Fig. 20.7, p. 347). Philadelphia, PA: Lippincott Williams & Wilkins.)

Myeloma may evolve from a premalignant stage, known as monoclonal gammopathy of undetermined significance, or MGUS (Rajkumar, Dimopoulos, Palumbo, et al., 2014). At this point in the disease, there is no evidence of end-organ dysfunction that is seen in multiple myeloma: hypercalcemia, renal insufficiency, anemia, or bone lesions. This constellation of organ damage is referred to by the acronym *CRAB* (elevated *c*alcium, *r*enal insufficiency, *a*nemia, and/or *b*one lesions). In MGUS, while there is no evidence of CRAB features, there is a mild elevation in the M protein. The rate of progression from the MGUS state to multiple myeloma is 0.5% to 1% per year.

Clinical Manifestations

The classic presenting symptom of multiple myeloma is bone pain, usually in the back or ribs. Bone pain is reported by two thirds of all patients at diagnosis. The bone pain associated with myeloma increases with movement and decreases with rest; patients may report that they have less pain on awakening but more during the day. In myeloma, a substance secreted by the plasma cells, osteoclast activating factor, and other substances (e.g., interleukin-6 [IL-6]) are involved in stimulating osteoclasts. Both mechanisms appear to be involved in the process of bone breakdown. Thus, lytic lesions as well as osteoporosis may be seen on bone x-rays but do not visualize on bone scans. The bone destruction can be severe enough to cause vertebral collapse and fractures, including spinal fractures, which can impinge on the spinal cord and result in spinal cord compression (see Fig. 54-18).

If the bone destruction is fairly extensive, excessive ionized calcium is lost from the bone and enters the serum; hypercalcemia may therefore develop (frequently manifested by excessive thirst, dehydration, constipation, altered mental status, confusion, and perhaps coma). Renal failure may also occur; the configuration of the circulating immunoglobulin molecule (particularly the shape of lambda light chains) can damage the renal tubules.

NURSING ALERT

Any older adult patient whose chief complaint is back pain and who has an elevated total protein level should be evaluated for possible myeloma.

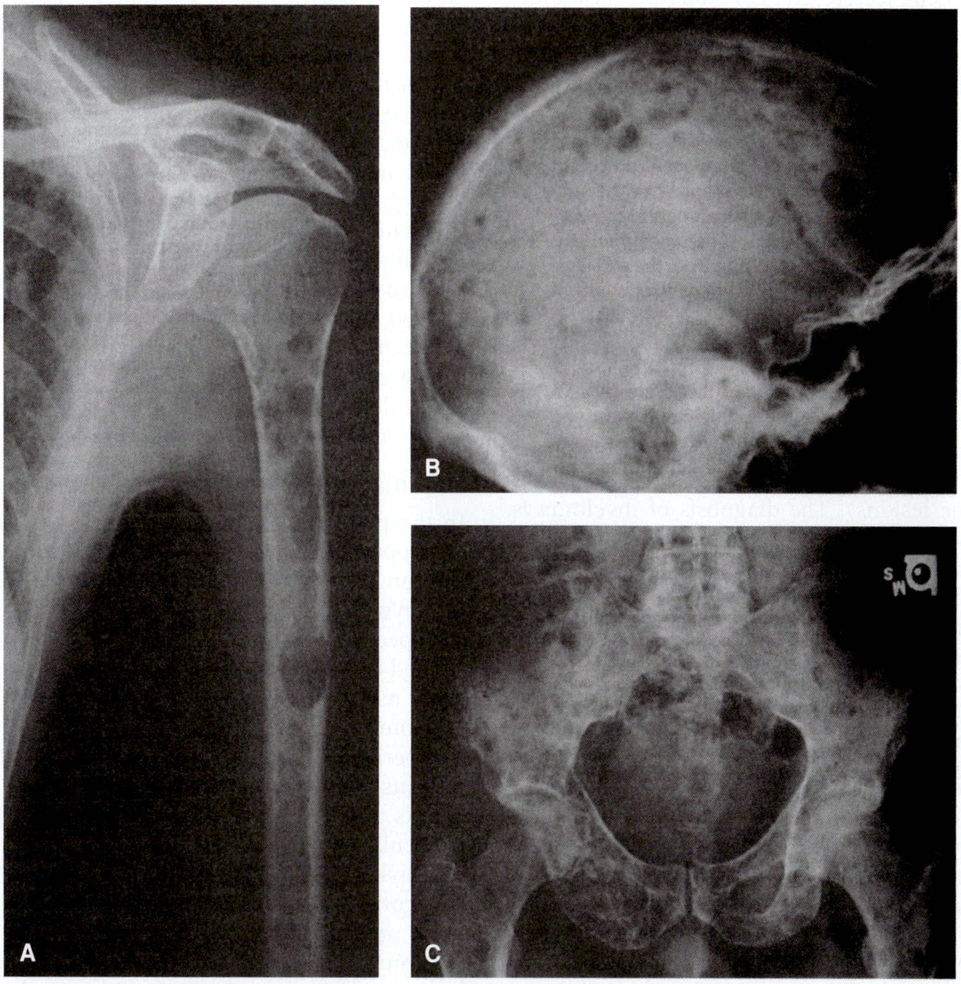

FIGURE 54-18. Lytic lesions seen in the humerus and skull in patients with multiple myeloma. These lesions typically occur in the long bones, vertebrae, and skull. Long bones are susceptible to fracture when the lesion occurs near the surface of the bone; vertebrae are susceptible to collapse, resulting in loss of height and potential for spinal cord compression. (From Foerster, J., & Greer, J. P. (1999). *Wintrobe's clinical hematology* (10th ed., p. 2640). Philadelphia, PA: Lippincott Williams & Wilkins.)

As more and more malignant plasma cells are produced, the marrow has less space for erythrocyte production, and anemia may develop. This anemia is also caused to a great extent by a diminished production of erythropoietin by the kidney. In the late stage of the disease, a reduced number of leukocytes and platelets may also be seen because the bone marrow is infiltrated by malignant plasma cells.

Infection is a concern. Infections occur most commonly within the first 2 months of beginning therapy and in the setting of advanced, refractory disease. In multiple myeloma, in contrast to other hematologic malignancies, the incidence of infection does not appear to be related to the extent of neutropenia. Infections occurring at the beginning of treatment are often caused by *S. pneumoniae*; those that occur when the disease is advanced or in the setting of renal failure are most often caused by gram-negative bacilli or *Staphylococcus aureus*. Infection is frequently the cause of death from multiple myeloma.

Neurologic manifestations can also occur. Spinal cord compression is the most common, and other neurologic symptoms may be present. When the M protein is IgM, peripheral neuropathy is more likely. Nerve root compression, the presence of intracranial neoplastic cells, and meningeal involvement are quite rare.

When plasma cells secrete excessive amounts of immunoglobulin, the serum viscosity can increase. Hyperviscosity may be manifested by bleeding from the nose or mouth, headache, blurred vision, paresthesias, or heart failure. Thromboembolic events (blood clots) may occur in patients with myeloma; the incidence is thought to be 3% to 10% (Alves et al., 2017).

Assessment and Diagnostic Findings

An elevated monoclonal protein spike in the serum (via serum protein electrophoresis), urine (via urine protein electrophoresis), or light chain (via serum free light chain analysis) is considered to be a major criterion in the diagnosis of multiple myeloma. Evidence of end-organ damage is necessary to establish the diagnosis, using the acronym CRAB (elevated calcium, renal insufficiency, anemia, and/or bone lesions). The diagnosis of myeloma is confirmed by bone marrow biopsy; the presence of more than 10% plasma cells is the hallmark diagnostic criterion. Because the infiltration of the marrow by these malignant plasma cells is not uniform, the plasma cells may not be increased in a given sample (a false-negative result).

Medical Management

There is no cure for multiple myeloma. Even autologous HSCT is considered to extend remission rather than provide a cure. However, for many patients, it is possible to control the illness and maintain their level of functioning quite well for several years or longer. For those who are not candidates for HSCT, chemotherapy is the primary treatment. A significant improvement in response rates is largely due to the marked increase in new types of drugs used to treat this disease. The decision when to treat and with which regimen is highly complex. The time interval between treatment and relapse, development of drug resistance, adverse features of the disease (such as certain cytogenetic abnormalities), patient factors (especially comorbidities), and goals of treatment must all be considered.

Early Treatment Options

Because treatment has vastly improved, some experts advocate initiating therapy prior to the development of CRAB features, when the myeloma is considered "smoldering" (Rajkumar, Landgren, & Mateos, 2015). Corticosteroids, particularly dexamethasone, often form the backbone in myeloma therapy. They are typically combined with an immunomodulatory drug (lenalidomide, pomalidomide, or thalidomide) or a proteasome inhibitor (bortezomib [Velcade], carfilzomib [Kyprolis]). These drugs all target the disease via different mechanisms than do conventional chemotherapeutic agents. Combinations of two or three drugs are commonly used with the goal of reducing the tumour burden as much as possible.

Autologous Stem Cell Transplantation

Therapy has changed substantively for multiple myeloma, and has resulted in impressive increases in duration of survival. Importantly, patients not only live longer, the new treatment modalities provide the opportunity for enhanced quality of life. Therapeutic options are based on the determination of eligibility for receiving an autologous HSCT. Patient's age, functional status, and comorbidities are used to determine eligibility for transplant. For those deemed eligible, initial treatment is focused on reducing the amount of tumour burden (decrease the number of myeloma cells and reducing monoclonal protein) without damaging the patient's stem cells, which are harvested and then later used in the transplant process. Patients who are not eligible for autologous HSCT typically receive lower-intensity therapy with the objective of reducing tumour burden as much as possible. In both situations, maintenance therapy may be used to enhance the duration of remission. Therapeutic goals for patients who are frail when diagnosed focus on improving disease-associated symptoms and quality of life.

Pharmacologic Therapy

In the past decade, two new classes of drugs have been developed that have significant impact in treating multiple myeloma. Immunomodulatory drugs (IMiDs) have broad antimyeloma effects by inhibiting angiogenesis and affecting specific cytokines, Il-6, tumour necrosis factor, both needed to support myeloma cell growth. Thalidomide, initially used as an antiemetic, was the first IMiD used in myeloma therapy. Fatigue, dizziness, constipation, rash, and peripheral neuropathy are commonly encountered in patients treated with thalidomide, whereas myelosuppression is not. There is also an increased incidence of DVT, particularly when the drug is used with corticosteroids; prophylactic anticoagulation should be used to prevent this complication. The thalidomide analogues lenalidomide and pomalidomide are also effective in treating myeloma. Side effects are quite different from those of thalidomide—myelosuppression, skin rash, and VTE are common, whereas sedation, neuropathy (including peripheral neuropathy), and constipation are not. Muscle cramps are more commonly associated with lenalidomide. These drugs are excreted by the kidneys, so careful monitoring of renal function is required, and dose reduction may be necessary. Because of teratogenic effects of all of these drugs, the female patient of child bearing age must be counselled and agree to use approved methods of birth control prior to taking any of them. While thalidomide is not used as frequently in treating multiple myeloma, the lack of associated myelosuppression makes it a viable option for select patients.

Proteasome inhibitors are a class of drugs that have significant antimyeloma effects. Myeloma cells produce large amounts of immunoglobulin protein, and proteasomes are needed to process and clear the excess mis/unfolded protein that accumulates within the cell. Inhibiting this process causes an excess accumulation of these proteins that results in apoptosis of the myeloma cell (Merin & Kelly, 2015). Bortezomib (Velcade) was the first proteasome inhibitor used in treating multiple myeloma. A recent systematic review reported that the inclusion of bortezomib in various treatment regimens resulted in improved response to treatment and in some studies, in overall survival (Kouroukis, Baldassarre, Haynes, et al., 2014).

Side effects of bortezomib include transient thrombocytopenia, orthostatic hypotension, nausea and vomiting, skin rash, neuropathy, and asthenia (i.e., weakness, malaise, fatigue). Because neuropathy is potentially serious, the dosage needs to be decreased as soon as the neuropathy begins to interfere with function; however, administering the drug subcutaneously rather than intravenously markedly reduces this problem, as does changing the dosing schedule (weekly administration rather than twice weekly). Bortezomib is metabolized by the cytochrome P450 pathway, which means that a careful review of concurrent medications for drug–drug interaction is crucial. An oral formulation of the drug, ixazomib (Ninlaro) has been approved by Health Canada.

Carfilzomib has greater proteasome selectivity than bortezomib and causes irreversible proteasome inhibition (Colson, 2015). It has a different side effect profile from bortezomib. Whereas peripheral neuropathy is not a side effect, pulmonary and cardiac toxicity are side effects, including dyspnea, which is more common early in treatment, as well as congestive heart failure, dysrhythmia formation, and ischemic heart disease (Wang & Cheng, 2013). Patients should be screened for cardiac disease prior to starting carfilzomib-based therapy, including obtaining baseline electrocardiograms (ECGs) and pulmonary function tests. Patients with pre-existing heart disease should be carefully monitored throughout their treatment and hypertension well controlled.

Corticosteroids induce apoptosis in myeloma cells and markedly decrease bone pain (Colson, 2015). As a result, corticosteroids, particularly dexamethasone, have been used in combination with other myeloma therapy for decades. Reduced dosage (40-mg dexamethasone weekly as opposed to 160 mg weekly) has been associated with decreased adverse events, particularly VTE. Nonetheless, long-term use of corticosteroids can cause significant morbidity, including infection, VTE, proximal muscle weakness, osteoporosis, cataract formation, mood and behaviour changes, and dental caries.

In additional to conventional chemotherapy, new drugs are now available for treating multiple myeloma (Lonial & Nooka, 2015). MoAbs have been targeted against specific antigens found on the surface of myeloma cells; daratumumab (Darzalex) is the first MoAb approved for myeloma therapy. Deacetylase inhibitors work to prevent the accumulation of mis/unfolded proteins that are not cleared by proteasomes; panobinostat (Farydak) is the first histone deacetylase inhibitor approved for use in multiple myeloma (Colson, 2015; Lonial & Nooka, 2015). Additional MoAbs, deacetylase inhibitors, and drugs with yet different mechanisms of action are under development. For all these new therapies, additional research is needed to guide clinicians and patients in determining how best—and when—to incorporate them in the multiple myeloma treatment armamentarium.

Managing Complications

Radiation therapy is useful in strengthening the bone at a specific lesion, particularly a bone at risk for fracture or spinal cord compression. It is also extremely useful in relieving bone pain and reducing the size of plasma cell tumours that occur outside the skeletal system as in plasmacytomas (Walker, Lawson, Buckle, et al., 2014). However, because it is a nonsystemic form of treatment, it does not diminish the source of the bone conditions (i.e., the production of malignant plasma cells). Therefore, radiation therapy is typically used in combination with systemic treatment such as chemotherapy.

When lytic lesions result in vertebral compression fractures, vertebroplasty may be performed (Jurczyszyn, Czepko, Banach, et al., 2015). This procedure may be enhanced by concomitant kyphoplasty (see Chapter 71 for further discussion of both vertebroplasty and kyphoplasty).

Some bisphosphonates, such as pamidronate (Aredia) and zoledronic acid (Zometa), have been shown to strengthen bone in multiple myeloma by diminishing survival of osteoclasts, thus controlling bone pain and potentially preventing bone fracture. These agents are also effective in managing and preventing hypercalcemia. Some evidence suggests that bisphosphonates may activate an antimyeloma immune response, inducing myeloma cell death, acting synergistically with antineoplastic drugs, and enhancing immune surveillance (van Acker, Anguille, Willemen, et al., 2015) (see Chapter 71 for further discussion of bisphosphonates).

When patients have significant signs and symptoms of hyperviscosity, plasmapheresis may be used to lower the immunoglobulin level. Symptoms may be more useful than serum viscosity levels in determining the need for this intervention.

Gerontologic Considerations

Historically, aggressive myeloma therapy, particularly HSCT, was limited to patients younger than age 65, but recently this approach has been challenged. Patients older than age 65 who have excellent organ function (i.e., renal, hepatic, cardiopulmonary) and who have fewer comorbidities may tolerate more intense treatment, including reduced-dose autologous HSCT (Cerrato, Mina, & Palumbo, 2014). Determining an older adult patient's ability to tolerate therapy *a priori* is important. In addition to chronologic age, organ function, and comorbidity, the ability to independently perform activities of daily living is another important factor. A comprehensive assessment of all these factors is useful to better determine the level of "fitness" in a given patient. Data suggest that patients categorized as frail develop more severe toxicity associated with therapy and consequently are more likely to discontinue that treatment (Wildes, Rosko, & Tuchman, 2014).

The older adult patient may have different goals of care from that of younger patients. Effective symptom control, preserving cognitive function, and maintaining independence are often viewed as higher priority than survival in the older adult (Wildes et al., 2014). Discussing these goals of care as well as the patient's physical and social needs can provide a more personalized approach to treating the older adult with multiple myeloma. Using lower doses and focusing on side effect management are important treatment strategies (Cerrato et al., 2014; Wildes et al., 2014). Side effects should be managed without additional medications to reduce the burden of "polypharmacy." Incorporating the expertise of a palliative care clinician may be extremely beneficial, not only in devising an appropriate treatment plan, but also in more effective symptom and side effect management.

Nursing Management

Pain management is very important in patients with multiple myeloma. NSAIDs can be very useful for mild pain or can be given in combination with opioid analgesics. Because NSAIDs can cause gastritis and renal dysfunction, renal function must be carefully monitored and patients assessed for gastritis; many patients are unable to use NSAIDs due to concurrent or newly developed renal insufficiency. Long-acting opioids are often prescribed to afford adequate pain relief.

Promoting Home, Community-Based, and Transitional Care

Educating Patients About Self-Care

The patient needs to be educated about activity restrictions (e.g., lifting no more than 10 lb, the use of proper body mechanics). Braces are occasionally needed to support the spinal column, but may be uncomfortable and hamper adherence. Bisphosphonate therapy has markedly reduced the severity and extent of bone pain. Patients need to understand the importance of comprehensive oral hygiene and good dental care to diminish the likelihood of developing osteonecrosis of the jaw that may arise from bisphosphonate therapy.

Renal function must be monitored closely. Kidney injury can become severe, and dialysis may be needed. Maintaining high urine output (3 L/day) can be very useful in preventing or limiting this complication, as is treating the underlying disease. The patient also needs to be instructed about the signs and symptoms of hypercalcemia. While hypercalcemia usually occurs at the onset of the disease, it can also develop at the time of disease progression or when multiple myeloma becomes refractory to therapy. Maintaining mobility and hydration are important to diminish exacerbations of this complication.

Because antibody production is impaired, infections, particularly bacterial infections, are common and can be life-threatening. The patient needs to be instructed in appropriate infection prevention measures and should be advised to contact the primary provider immediately if fever or other signs and symptoms of infection develop. The patient should receive pneumococcal and influenza vaccines. Prophylactic antibiotics, such as trimethoprim–sulfamethoxazole, are often used, particularly when patients are treated with corticosteroid-containing regimens to prevent *Pneumocystis jirovecii* pneumonia (Raje, Yee, & Roodman, 2014). The antiviral agent acyclovir is recommended when patients are treated with bortezomib-based regimens to diminish the potential development of viral infection, such as herpes zoster.

Continuing and Transitional Care

Many newer medications, particularly the IMiDs, are associated with higher risks of thromboembolism formation, particularly when used concurrently with high doses of corticosteroids or erythropoietin (Raje et al., 2014). Other risk factors include decreased mobility, obesity, prior thromboembolic events, diabetes, cardiac or renal disease, and the presence of a vascular access device (e.g., PICC). It is important to maintain mobility and to use strategies that enhance venous return (e.g., antiembolism stockings, avoid crossing the legs). For patients without additional risk factors, VTE can be prevented by taking low-dose aspirin. Those patients with additional risk factors for developing VTE should receive anticoagulation therapy.

Peripheral neuropathy is a frequent issue for patients with multiple myeloma, affecting over 50% at the time of diagnosis (Koeppen, 2014). That incidence has increased with the use of thalidomide or bortezomib. The neuropathy is primarily sensory, but motor or autonomic nervous system neuropathy is also seen (Jongen, Broijl, & Sonneveld, 2015) (see Table 54-9).

Painful neuropathy can be quite disabling and may interfere with the patient's ability to perform normal activities of daily living. The nurse needs to carefully assess for symptoms related to peripheral neuropathy and make assessments of the home for safety. Sensation (touch, temperature, pain, vibration, proprioception), ankle reflexes, distal muscle strength, and blood pressure should be evaluated. Other risk factors for peripheral neuropathy (e.g., diabetes, vitamin deficiencies, viral infection, or excessive alcohol consumption) should be aggressively managed. Patients should be educated to report any symptoms of peripheral neuropathy and to not minimize such symptoms, because prompt cessation of therapy or reducing the dose can prevent the neuropathy from progressing. Resuming treatment with a lower dosage and at a longer interval between dosing may diminish the worsening of peripheral nerve damage. Recovery can occur over time, although it may be incomplete. There is inadequate evidence to support the use of neuroprotective substances (e.g., l-carnitine) or additional nutritional supplements in treating this form of peripheral neuropathy (Jongen et al., 2015; Koeppen, 2014). Gabapentinoids (e.g., gabapentin [Neurontin], pregabalin [Lyrica]), tricyclic antidepressants (e.g., amitriptyline [Elavil], nortriptyline [Aventyl]), and selective serotonin reuptake inhibitors (e.g., duloxetine [Cymbalta]) can be used to diminish pain; opioids are fairly ineffective in this context.

As many drugs used in treating multiple myeloma are given orally, the nurse must ensure that the patient fully understands how to take the medication, manage side

TABLE 54-9 Peripheral Neuropathy

Type of Neuropathy	Manifestations	Nursing Intervention/Patient Education
Sensory	Hypoesthesia	Warn patient to avoid extreme temperatures (e.g., bathwater). Inspect feet for trauma, potential infection. Use loose-fitting stockings.
	Paresthesia (tingling)	Gentle massage Gentle ROM exercises
	Hyperalgesia (pain) Toes and fingers Soles of feet/palms	Gentle massage (cocoa butter or menthol-based cream/lotion) Apply lidocaine 5% patch to affected area every 12 hours. Consider gabapentin (Neurontin), tricyclic antidepressants (e.g., amitriptyline [Elavil]).
Motor	Muscle cramps Tremor ↓ Strength in distal muscles	Maximize hydration, ambulation (Quinine is not recommended).
	Gait disturbance ↓ Fine motor function (e.g., handwriting, buttoning clothes)	Encourage the use of appropriate footwear. Consider ambulatory aides (e.g., walker). Remove scatter rugs; perform a home safety evaluation. PT referral OT referral (if severe limitations)
Autonomic Nervous System	Orthostatic hypotension	Warn patient to avoid abrupt position change. Maximize hydration. Consider adjusting antihypertensive medications, diuretics.
	Bradycardia	Assess/warn patient for impact (fatigue, impairment in function). Consider adjusting drugs that cause bradycardia (e.g., calcium channel blockers, beta-blockers, alpha-/beta-adrenergic blockers, digoxin). Explore the use of activity to increase heart rate.
	Sexual dysfunction	Explore alternative means of sexual activity beyond intercourse. Consider the use of erectile dysfunction medication.
	Constipation	Maximize fluid intake, fibre. Use stool softeners, laxatives.

ROM, range of motion; ↓, decreased; PT, physical therapy; OT, occupational therapy.

Note: Peripheral neuropathy can be classified into three main categories. Within each category, specific manifestations are delineated as well as relevant nursing interventions. If the neuropathy is related to myeloma therapy, it is crucial to promptly stop the potentially offending medication. It is also important to reduce the impact from other predisposing factors. For example, diabetes should be well controlled and alcohol consumption reduced.

effects, and know what steps can be taken to diminish or mitigate toxicity. For example, cigarette smoking may decrease the efficacy of pomalidomide as it impacts its metabolism via the cytochrome P450 pathway. Therefore, patients need to be strongly encouraged to cease smoking and be provided assistance to do so.

BLEEDING DISORDERS

Failure of normal hemostatic mechanisms can result in bleeding, which may be severe. This bleeding is commonly provoked by trauma, but in certain circumstances it can occur spontaneously. When the source is platelet or coagulation factor abnormalities, the site of bleeding can be anywhere in the body. When the source is vascular abnormalities, the site of bleeding may be more localized. Some patients have simultaneous defects in more than one hemostatic mechanism.

The bone marrow may be stimulated to increase platelet production (thrombopoiesis). This may be a reactive response, as in a compensatory response to significant bleeding, or a more general response to increased hematopoiesis, as in iron deficiency anemia. Sometimes, the increase in platelets does not result from increased production but from a loss in platelet pooling within the spleen. The spleen typically holds about one third of the circulating platelets at any time. If the spleen is absent (e.g., splenectomy), the platelet reservoir is also lost, and an abnormally high number of platelets enters the circulation. In time, the rate of thrombopoiesis slows to re-establish a more normal platelet level.

Clinical Manifestations

Signs and symptoms of bleeding disorders vary depending on the type of defect. A careful history and physical examination can be useful in determining the source of the hemostatic defect. Abnormalities of the vascular system give rise to local bleeding, usually into the skin. Because platelets are primarily responsible for stopping bleeding from small vessels, patients with platelet defects develop petechiae, often in clusters; these are seen on the skin and mucous membranes but also occur throughout the body (Fig. 54-19). Bleeding from platelet disorders can be severe. Unless the platelet disorder is severe, bleeding can often be stopped promptly when local pressure is applied; it does not typically recur when the pressure is released.

In contrast, coagulation factor defects do not tend to cause superficial bleeding, because the primary hemostatic mechanisms are still intact. Instead, bleeding occurs deeper within the body (e.g., subcutaneous or IM hematomas, hemorrhage into joint spaces). External bleeding diminishes very slowly when local pressure is applied; it

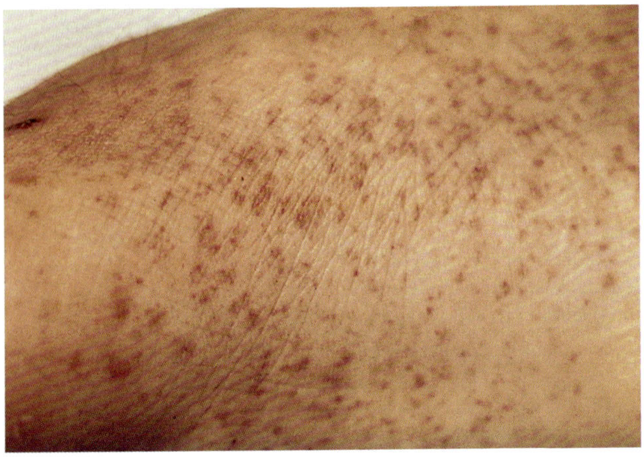

FIGURE 54-19. Petechiae. (From Foerster, J., & Greer, J. P. (1999a). *Wintrobe's clinical hematology* (10th ed.). Color plate 62.4. Philadelphia, PA: Lippincott Williams & Wilkins.)

often recurs several hours after pressure is removed. For example, severe bleeding may start several hours after a tooth extraction. Risk factors for bleeding are listed in Chart 54-7.

Medical Management

Management varies based on the underlying cause of the bleeding disorder. If bleeding is significant, transfusions of blood products are indicated. The specific blood product used is determined by the underlying defect and the extent of the blood loss. If fibrinolysis is excessive, hemostatic agents such as aminocaproic acid (Amicar) can be used to inhibit this process. This agent must be used with caution, because excessive inhibition of fibrinolysis can result in thrombosis. A patient scheduled for an invasive procedure, including a dental extraction, may need a transfusion prior to the procedure to minimize the risk of excessive bleeding.

Nursing Management

Patients who have bleeding disorders or who have the potential for development of such disorders as a result of disease or therapeutic agents must be taught to observe themselves carefully and frequently for bleeding (Chart 54-12). They need to understand the importance of avoiding activities that increase the risk of bleeding, such as contact sports. It is necessary to examine the skin for petechiae and ecchymoses (bruises) and the nose and gums for bleeding. Hospitalized patients are monitored for bleeding by testing all drainage and excreta (feces, urine, emesis, and gastric drainage) for occult as well as obvious blood. Outpatients are often given fecal occult blood screening cards to detect occult blood in stools.

Essential Thrombocythemia

Essential thrombocythemia (ET), also called *primary thrombocythemia*, is a stem cell disorder within the bone marrow. A mutation of the JAK2 gene promotes cell proliferation and resistance to cell death and a hypersensitivity to erythropoietin and thrombopoietin; it is found in 55% of patients with ET (Geyer & Mesa, 2014). A marked increase in platelet production occurs, with the platelet

CHART 54-12

HOME CARE CHECKLIST • The Patient at Risk for Bleeding

At the completion of education, the patient and/or caregiver will be able to:

- Describe the source and function of platelets and clotting factors.
- State the impact of an alteration in platelets on physiologic functioning, ADLs, IADLs, roles, relationships, and spirituality.
- State changes in lifestyle (e.g., diet, activity) or home environment necessary to decrease risk of bleeding.
  - Avoid the use of suppositories, enemas, and tampons
  - Avoid constipation
  - Avoid vigorous sexual intercourse and anal sex
  - Avoid contact sports
  - Avoid or limit aggressive manual labor
  - Use an electric razor for shaving and a soft-bristled toothbrush for teeth brushing
  - Notify health care professional before having dental work or other invasive procedures
- Identify medications and other substances to avoid (e.g., aspirin-containing medications, alcohol).
- Identify signs and symptoms of bleeding.
- Demonstrate how to monitor for signs of bleeding.
- Describe to whom, how, and when to report signs of bleeding.
- Demonstrate appropriate actions to take should bleeding occur.

ADLs, activities of daily living; IADLs, independent activities of daily living.

count consistently greater than 450,000/mm^3. The platelet count can exceed 1 to 2 million/mm^3. Occasionally, the increase in platelets (i.e., thrombocythemia) is accompanied by an increase in erythrocytes, leukocytes, or both; however, these cells are not increased to the extent that they are in polycythemia vera, CML, or myelofibrosis. Platelet size may be abnormal; these circulate throughout the vascular system in an activated state. Extremely high levels of platelets (exceeding 1 million/mm^3) are associated with acquired von Willebrand's disease; therefore, these patients are at higher risk for bleeding complications.

The exact cause of ET is unknown. This disease affects women twice as often as men and tends to occur later in life (median age at diagnosis is 65 to 70 years). Overall, survival does not differ from the general population. However, survival rates vary based on the type of mutations seen in this disease. For example, 25% of patients with ET have a mutation in the calreticulin gene; the presence of this mutation appears to be associated with fewer thrombotic events and higher survival rates (Radia & Geyer, 2015). Patients without mutations may have a lower survival rate. The evolution to AML is very low (0.8%) (Birgegård, 2013). Death is typically due to thrombosis (arterial or venous) or hemorrhage.

Clinical Manifestations

Many patients with ET are asymptomatic; the illness is diagnosed as the result of finding an elevated platelet count on a CBC. Symptoms occur most often when the platelet count exceeds 1 million/mm^3; however, they do not always correlate with the extent to which the platelet count is elevated. When symptoms do occur, they primarily result from vascular occlusion. This occlusion can occur in large arterial vessels (cerebrovascular, coronary, or peripheral arteries) and deep veins, as well as in the microcirculation. The interactive effects of platelet substances within the surface of the vascular endothelium can cause microthrombi in the arterioles and inflammation within the endothelium; these interactions result in erythromelalgia, the development of painful burning, warmth, and redness in a localized distal area of the extremities. More common forms of venous thromboembolism (VTE) include DVT and pulmonary embolism (PE).

Headaches are the most common neurologic manifestations; other manifestations include transient ischemic attacks and diplopia. Tinnitus, paresthesias, or atypical chest pain may also occur (Tefferi & Barbui, 2015).

Because the platelets can be dysfunctional, minor or major hemorrhage may occur. Bleeding is commonly limited to recurrent skin manifestations (ecchymoses, hematomas, epistaxis, gum bleeding), although significant GI bleeding and intracranial hemorrhage are both possible. Bleeding typically does not occur unless the platelet count exceeds 1.5 million/mm^3. It results from a deficiency in von Willebrand factor (vWF) as the platelet count increases (Alvarez-Larrán & Besses, 2014; Tefferi & Barbui, 2015).

Assessment and Diagnostic Findings

The diagnosis of ET is made by ruling out other potential disorders—either other myeloproliferative disorders or underlying illnesses that cause a reactive or secondary thrombocytosis (see later discussion). Iron deficiency should be excluded, because a reactive increase in the platelet count often accompanies this deficiency. Occult malignancy should be excluded. The CBC shows markedly large and abnormal platelets; the platelet count is persistently elevated (greater than 450,000/mm^3). An analysis of the JAK2 mutation or calreticulin is very useful, whereas an analysis of the bone marrow (by aspiration and biopsy) can aid in distinguishing between true ET and early myelofibrosis.

Complications

Complications include inappropriate formation of thrombi and hemorrhage. Patients with cardiovascular risk factors (such as poorly controlled hypertension, diabetes, obesity, hyperlipidemia, and smoking) are at higher risk for thrombotic complications (Barbui, Finazzi, & Falanga, 2013; Lekovic, Gotic, Sefer, et al., 2015). Patients older than 60 years and those with a history of prior thrombosis are also at higher risk for complications. Major bleeding tends to occur when the platelet count is very high (greater than 1.5 million/mm^3) and there is a prior history of major bleeding. In contrast, patients who are younger than 60 years, have no previous history of a thrombotic or hemorrhagic event, and have a normal WBC count and platelet counts less than 1 million/mm^3 are considered to be at low risk for developing thrombotic or hemorrhagic complications (Geyer & Mesa, 2014).

Medical Management

The management of ET is based on risk for developing thrombosis or hemorrhage, and the presence of symptoms (see Table 54-5). A careful assessment of risk factors, history of peripheral vascular disease, tobacco use, atherosclerosis, diabetes, and prior thrombotic or bleeding events are all considered in developing the treatment plan.

In younger patients with no risk factors, patients may receive no therapy and be closely observed. Low-dose aspirin therapy is commonly recommended as it is felt to be sufficient to prevent thrombotic complications (Alvarez-Larrán & Besses, 2014; Barbui et al., 2013; Tefferi & Barbui, 2015). However, the use of aspirin can increase the risk of hemorrhagic complications, particularly when the platelet count exceeds 1 million/mm^3. Determining the presence of acquired von Willebrand's disease is important prior to initiating aspirin therapy in these patients. Aspirin use in this context is associated with a much higher risk of hemorrhage. Aspirin therapy is also contraindicated in patients with a history of GI bleeding. Aspirin can relieve the neurologic symptoms (e.g., headache), erythromelalgias, and visual symptoms of ET, and is considered safe and effective in preventing complications during pregnancy (Tefferi & Barbui, 2015).

In older patients and in those with a history of prior thrombosis, more aggressive measures are necessary to prevent thrombosis or bleeding. Hydroxyurea is effective in lowering the platelet count to a level below 400,000/mm^3 and is effective in reducing the risk for developing arterial thrombosis and hemorrhage (Tefferi & Barbui, 2015). This agent is taken orally and causes minimal side effects other than dose-related leukopenia. With long-term use, some patients develop painful leg ulcers or actinic keratosis (Cozzani, Iurlo, Merlo, et al., 2015). Resistance develops in up to 25% of patients over time, necessitating changing pharmacologic management (Sever, Newberry, & Verstovsek, 2014).

Anagrelide is more specific in lowering the platelet count than hydroxyurea but has more side effects and may not be as effective. Severe headaches cause many patients to stop taking the medication. Tachycardia and chest pain may also occur, and anagrelide is contraindicated in patients with concurrent cardiac problems. Anagrelide is also associated with disease progression; for these reasons, it is infrequently used (Tefferi & Barbui, 2015).

Interferon alfa-2b has been shown to effectively lower platelet counts due to its antiproliferative effects on hematopoietic precursor cells and its ability to reduce the extent of molecular changes (Birgegård, 2013; Sever et al., 2014). Significant side effects such as fatigue, fever, depression, and flu-like symptoms are common. Subclinical depression may not be recognized until the drug is discontinued (Birgegård, 2013). A pegylated formulation of interferon alpha-2b is more commonly used, which may have improved tolerance and longer duration of use. Interferon is also safe for use in pregnancy.

Rarely, the occlusive symptoms require emergent reduction in the platelet count. When necessary, platelet apheresis reduces the amount of circulating platelets, but only transiently. The extent to which symptoms and complications (e.g., thromboses) are reduced by apheresis is unclear.

Patients who develop arterial or venous thrombosis may require additional therapy beyond reducing the platelet count (e.g., with hydroxyurea). Data suggest that those who develop cerebrovascular disease are more effectively managed with antiplatelet therapy (e.g., aspirin), whereas those who develop VTE may be more effectively managed with anticoagulation than antiplatelet therapy (Alvarez-Larrán & Besses, 2014).

Nursing Management

Symptoms associated with ET are now used as one criterion for initiating and selecting therapy (see Table 54-5). Because thrombosis and hemorrhage are the primary cause of morbidity or mortality, it is important to assess patients for a history of prior thrombotic or hemorrhagic events. Risk factors for thrombosis are assessed, such as obesity, hypertension, hyperlipidemia, diabetes, and smoking; measures to diminish these risk factors are strongly encouraged. Patients with ET need to be educated about the risks of hemorrhage and thrombosis. The patient is informed about signs and symptoms of thrombosis, particularly the neurologic manifestations, such as visual changes, numbness, tingling, and weakness. Patients taking aspirin should be informed about the importance of taking this medication as well as the increased risk of bleeding. Patients who are at risk for bleeding should be instructed about medications (e.g., aspirin, nonsteroidal anti-inflammatory agents [NSAIDs]) and other substances (e.g., alcohol, certain herbal therapies) that can alter platelet function. Patients taking interferon may be taught to self-administer the medication and how to manage side effects. Patients taking hydroxyurea should have CBCs monitored regularly; the dosage is adjusted based on the platelet and WBC count.

Secondary Thrombocytosis

Increased platelet production is the primary mechanism of secondary, or reactive, thrombocytosis. The platelet count is above normal, but, in contrast to primary thrombocythemia, an increase of more than 1 million/mm^3 is rare. Platelet function is normal; the platelet survival time is normal or decreased. Consequently, symptoms associated with hemorrhage or thrombosis are rare. Many disorders or conditions can cause a reactive increase in platelets, including infection, chronic inflammatory disorders, iron deficiency, malignant disease, acute hemorrhage, and splenectomy (see previous discussion of primary thrombocythemia). Treatment is aimed at the underlying disorder. With successful management, the platelet count usually returns to normal.

Thrombocytopenia

Thrombocytopenia (low platelet level) can result from various factors: decreased production of platelets within the bone marrow, increased destruction of platelets, or increased consumption of platelets. Causes and treatments are summarized in Table 54-10.

Clinical Manifestations

Bleeding and petechiae usually do not occur with platelet counts greater than 50,000/mm^3, although excessive bleeding can follow surgery or other trauma. When the platelet count drops to less than 20,000/mm^3, petechiae can appear, along with nasal and gingival bleeding, excessive menstrual bleeding, and excessive bleeding after surgery or dental extractions. When the platelet count is less than 5,000/mm^3, spontaneous, potentially fatal central nervous system or GI hemorrhage can occur. If the platelets are dysfunctional as a result of disease (e.g., MDS) or medications (e.g., aspirin), the risk of bleeding may be much greater even when the actual platelet count is not significantly reduced, because the function of the platelets is altered.

Assessment and Diagnostic Findings

A platelet deficiency that results from decreased production (e.g., leukemia, MDS) can usually be diagnosed by examining the bone marrow via aspiration and biopsy. Numerous genetic causes of thrombocytopenia have been discovered, including autosomal dominant, autosomal recessive, and X-linked mutations. If platelet destruction is the cause of thrombocytopenia, the marrow shows increased megakaryocytes and normal or even increased platelet production as the body attempts to compensate for the decreased platelets in circulation.

An important cause to exclude is "pseudothrombocytopenia." Here, platelets aggregate and clump in the presence of ethylenediamine tetra-acetic acid (EDTA), the anticoagulant present in the tube used for CBC collection.

TABLE 54-10 Causes and Management of Thrombocytopenia

Cause	Management
Decreased Platelet Production	
Hematologic malignancy, especially acute leukemias	Treat leukemia; platelet transfusion
MDS	Treat MDS; platelet transfusion
Metastatic involvement of bone marrow from solid tumours	Treat solid tumour
Aplastic anemia	Treat underlying condition
Megaloblastic anemia	Treat underlying anemia
Toxins	Remove toxin
Medications (e.g., sulfa drugs, methotrexate)	Stop medication
Infection (especially septicemia, viral infection, tuberculosis, chronic hepatitis C)	Treat infection
Chronic alcohol abuse	Refrain from alcohol consumption
Chemotherapy	Delay or decrease dose; platelet transfusion
Chronic liver disease	Treat underlying disease
Radiation (e.g., pelvic irradiation)	Platelet transfusion
Delayed engraftment after stem cell transplantation	Platelet transfusion
Increased Platelet Destruction	
Due to antibodies:	Treat condition
ITP	
Lupus erythematosus	
Malignant lymphoma	
CLL	Treat CLL and/or treat as ITP
Medications	Stop medication
Due to infection:	Treat infection
Bacteremia/sepsis	
Postviral infection	
Sequestration of platelets in an enlarged spleen	If thrombocytopenia is severe, splenectomy may be needed
Increased Platelet Consumption	
DIC	Treat underlying condition triggering DIC; administer heparin, aminocaproic acid (Amicar), blood products
Major bleeding	Transfusion support, surgery if appropriate
Severe pulmonary embolism/ severe thrombosis	Treat clot
Intravascular devices (intra-aortic balloon pump, cardiac assist devices)	Transfusion support as needed
Extracorporeal circulation (hemofiltration, extracorporeal lung assist)	Transfusion support as needed

MDS, myelodysplastic syndrome; ITP, idiopathic thrombocytopenic purpura; CLL, chronic lymphocytic leukemia; DIC, disseminated intravascular coagulation.

A manual examination of the peripheral smear can easily determine platelet clumping as the cause of thrombocytopenia; newer cell counter machines can also detect this.

Medical Management

The management of secondary thrombocytopenia is usually treatment of the underlying disease. If platelet production is impaired, platelet transfusions may increase the platelet count and stop bleeding or prevent spontaneous hemorrhage. If excessive platelet destruction occurs, transfused platelets are also destroyed, and the platelet count does not increase. The most common cause of excessive platelet destruction is ITP (see the following discussion). In some instances splenectomy can be a useful therapeutic intervention, but often it is not an option; for example, in patients in whom the enlarged spleen is due to portal hypertension related to cirrhosis, splenectomy may cause more bleeding disorders.

Nursing Management

When selecting nursing interventions, the nurse considers the cause of the thrombocytopenia, the likely duration, and the overall condition of the patient. Education is important, as are interventions to promote patient safety, particularly fall prevention in the older adult or patient who is frail. The interventions for a patient with thrombocytopenia are the same as those for a patient with cancer who is at risk for bleeding (see Chapter 68).

Immune Thrombocytopenic Purpura

ITP is a disease that affects people of all ages, but it is more common among children and young women. Other names for the disorder are idiopathic thrombocytopenic purpura and immune thrombocytopenia. Primary ITP occurs in isolation; secondary ITP often results from autoimmune diseases (e.g., antiphospholipid antibody syndrome), viral infections (e.g., hepatitis C, HIV), and various drugs (e.g., sulfa drugs). Primary ITP is defined as a platelet count less than 100×10^9/L with an inexplicable absence of a cause for thrombocytopenia (Neunert, 2013).

Pathophysiology

ITP is an autoimmune disorder characterized by a destruction of normal platelets by an unknown stimulus. Antiplatelet antibodies develop in the blood and bind to the patient's platelets. These antibody-bound platelets are then ingested and destroyed by the RES or tissue macrophages. The body attempts to compensate for this destruction by increasing platelet production within the marrow. However, platelet production may also be impaired as the antibodies may also induce cell death (via apoptosis) of the megakaryocytes and thus inhibit platelet production within the bone marrow (Neunert, 2013).

Clinical Manifestations

Many patients have no symptoms, and the low platelet count is an incidental finding (often less than 30,000/mm^3; less than 5000/mm^3 is not uncommon). Common physical manifestations are easy bruising, heavy menses, and petechiae on the extremities or trunk (see Fig. 54-19). Patients with simple bruising or petechiae ("dry purpura") tend to have fewer complications from bleeding than those with bleeding from mucosal surfaces, such as the GI tract (including the mouth) and pulmonary system (e.g., hemoptysis), which is termed *wet purpura.* Patients with wet purpura have a greater risk of life-threatening bleeding than do those with dry purpura; aggressive treatment should be promptly initiated (Diz-Küçükkaya & López, 2016). Severe thrombocytopenia (platelet count less than 20,000/mm^3), a history of prior minor bleeding episodes, and advanced age also are predictive of severe bleeding (Arnold, 2015). Despite low platelet counts, the platelets are young and very functional. They adhere to endothelial surfaces and to one another, so spontaneous bleeding does not always occur. Thus, treatment may not be initiated unless bleeding becomes severe or life-threatening, or the platelet count is extremely low (less than 30,000/mm^3) (Diz-Küçükkaya & López, 2016).

Assessment and Diagnostic Findings

A careful history and physical assessment must be obtained to exclude causes of the thrombocytopenia and identify evidence of bleeding. Patients should be tested for hepatitis C and HIV, if not previously done to rule out these potential causes. If a bone marrow aspirate is performed, an increase in megakaryocytes may be seen. The severity of the thrombocytopenia is highly variable, but a platelet count that is less than 20,000/mm^3 is a common finding.

Some patients are found to be infected with *Helicobacter pylori*, and eradicating the infection may improve platelet counts (Neunert, Lim, Crowther, et al., 2011). It is unclear why *H. pylori* and ITP are correlated, but possible causes are that *H. pylori* may trigger an autoimmune reaction or that it binds to vWF, both of which may result in accelerated platelet demise.

Medical Management

The primary goal of treatment is a "safe" platelet count (i.e., platelets adequate to maintain hemostasis). Because the risk of bleeding typically does not increase until the platelet count is less than 30,000/mm^3, a patient whose count exceeds 30,000/mm^3 to 50,000/mm^3 may be carefully observed without additional intervention. However, if the count is less than 30,000/mm^3 or if bleeding occurs, the goal is to improve the patient's platelet count rather than to cure the disease. The decision to treat should not be made merely on the basis of the patient's platelet count but, more importantly, on the severity of bleeding (if any); likely treatment-related side effects; and the patient's lifestyle, activity level, concurrent use of medications, and overall preference. A person with a sedentary lifestyle can tolerate a low platelet count more safely than one with a more active lifestyle; however, increasing age is also associated with increased bleeding risk and mortality (Diz-Küçükkaya & López, 2016).

Treatment for ITP usually involves several approaches. If the patient is taking a medication known to be associated with ITP (e.g., quinine, sulfa-containing medications), then that medication must be stopped immediately. Transfusions tend to be ineffective because the patient's antiplatelet antibodies bind with the transfused platelets, causing them to be destroyed. Platelet counts can actually drop further after platelet transfusion. Thus, despite extremely low platelet counts, platelet transfusions are not indicated. Occasionally, transfusion of platelets may protect against catastrophic bleeding in patients with severe wet purpura. Aminocaproic acid—a fibrinolytic enzyme inhibitor that slows the dissolution of clots—may be useful for patients with significant mucosal bleeding refractory to other treatments.

The mainstay of short-term therapy is the use of immunosuppressive agents. These agents block the binding receptors on macrophages so that the platelets are not destroyed. The American Society of Hematology recommends administering the corticosteroid prednisone at a dose of 1 mg per kilogram of body weight for 21 days and then tapering the dose until the patient is off the medication (Neunert et al., 2011). Because of the associated side effects, patients cannot take high doses of corticosteroids indefinitely. Platelet counts typically begin to rise within a few days after institution of corticosteroid therapy. The platelet count tends to drop once the corticosteroid dose is tapered, but it often can remain at an adequate level.

IVIG is also commonly used to treat ITP. It is effective in binding the receptors on the macrophages; however, high doses are required, the drug is very expensive, and the effect is transient. Another approach to the management of chronic ITP involves the use of anti-D (WinRho) in patients who are Rh (D) positive. The actual mechanism of action is unknown. One theory is that the anti-D binds to the patient's erythrocytes, which are in turn destroyed by the body's macrophages. The receptors in the RES may become saturated with the sensitized erythrocytes, diminishing removal of antibody-coated platelets. Anti-D produces a transient decreased hematocrit and increased platelet count in many, but not all, patients with ITP.

At some point, the platelet count will usually decline; at that time, additional therapy is required. Second-line therapy options should consider the patient's specific needs and potential treatment-related side effects.

Splenectomy is an alternative treatment and results in a sustained normal platelet count approximately 50% of the time, although many patients can maintain a "safe" platelet count of more than 30,000/mm^3 after the removal of the spleen (Rodeghiero & Ruggeri, 2015). Even those who do respond to splenectomy may have recurrences of severe thrombocytopenia months or years later. Patients who have undergone splenectomy are permanently at risk for sepsis and should receive pneumococcal, *Haemophilus influenzae* type B, and meningococcal vaccines, preferably 2 to 3 weeks before the splenectomy is performed (see Chapter 24 for information on pneumonia vaccine).

Other management options include certain monoclonal antibodies (e.g., rituximab). This agent may increase platelet counts for up to 1 year in 20% to 35% of those treated, but when that response is lost, the platelet count may not fall so low as to warrant additional therapy (Rodeghiero & Ruggeri, 2015).

In addition, two thrombopoietin receptor agonists have been approved for use in steroid-refractory ITP. Romiplostim (Nplate) is given weekly as a subcutaneous injection; eltrombopag (Promacta) is given orally. The timing of taking eltrombopag is somewhat complex, as the drug metabolism is altered with food and many medications. Side effects include headache, blistering of the oral mucosa, and ecchymoses. Platelet counts can fluctuate widely and treatment needs to be continued indefinitely (Rodeghiero & Ruggeri, 2015). However, in some situations, the platelet count can remain at a safe level after the drug is stopped.

Nursing Management

Nursing care includes an assessment of the patient's lifestyle to determine the risk of bleeding from activity. A careful medication history is also obtained, including use of over-the-counter (OTC) medications, herbs, and nutritional supplements. The nurse must be alert for sulfa-containing medications and others that alter platelet function (e.g., aspirin-based or other NSAIDs). The nurse assesses for any history of recent viral illness and reports of headache or visual disturbances, which could be initial symptoms of intracranial bleeding. Patients who are admitted to the hospital with wet purpura and low platelet counts should have a neurologic assessment incorporated into their routine vital sign measurements. All injections or rectal medications should be avoided, and rectal temperature measurements should not be performed, because they can stimulate bleeding.

Studies of patients with ITP have demonstrated a significant increase in fatigue compared to those without the disease that was not associated with the duration of the disease, corticosteroid use, bleeding episodes, and low platelet count (Diz-Küçükkaya & López, 2016). Nurses should explore the extent the patient experiences fatigue and offer strategies to ameliorate this problem.

Patient education addresses signs of exacerbation of disease (e.g., petechiae, ecchymoses), how to contact appropriate health care personnel, the name and type of medication inducing ITP (if appropriate), current medical treatment (medications, side effects, tapering schedule if relevant), and the frequency of monitoring the platelet count. The patient is instructed to avoid all agents that interfere with platelet function, including herbal therapies and OTC medications. The patient should avoid constipation, the Valsalva manoeuvre (e.g., straining at stool), and vigorous flossing of the teeth. Electric razors should be used for shaving, and soft-bristled toothbrushes should replace stiff-bristled ones. The patient may also be counselled to refrain from vigorous sexual intercourse when the platelet count is less than 10,000/mm^3. Patients who are receiving corticosteroids long term are at risk for complications including osteoporosis, proximal muscle wasting, cataract formation, and dental caries. Bone mineral density should be monitored, and these patients may benefit from calcium and vitamin D supplementation and bisphosphonate therapy to prevent significant bone disease.

Platelet Defects

Quantitative platelet defects are relatively common (thrombocytopenia), but qualitative defects can also occur. With qualitative defects, the number of platelets may be normal, but the platelets do not function normally. In the past, the bleeding time was most commonly used to evaluate platelet function. Now a platelet function analyzer is often used; this method is particularly valuable for rapid and simple screening.

Aspirin may induce a functional platelet disorder. Even small amounts of aspirin reduce normal platelet aggregation, and the prolonged bleeding time lasts for several days after aspirin ingestion. Although this does not cause bleeding in most people, patients with a coagulation disorder (e.g., hemophilia) or thrombocytopenia can have significant bleeding after taking aspirin, particularly if invasive procedures or trauma has occurred.

NSAIDs can also inhibit platelet function, but the effect is not as prolonged as with aspirin (about 5 days vs. 7 to 10 days). Other causes of platelet dysfunction include end-stage renal disease, possibly from metabolic products affecting platelet function; MDS; multiple myeloma (due to abnormal protein interfering with platelet function); cardiopulmonary bypass; and herbs and other medications (Chart 54-13).

Clinical Manifestations

Bleeding may be mild or severe. Its extent is not necessarily correlated with the platelet count or with tests that measure coagulation (PT, aPTT). Ecchymoses are common, particularly on the extremities. Patients with platelet dysfunction may be at risk for significant bleeding after trauma or invasive procedures (e.g., biopsy, dental extraction).

Medical Management

If the platelet dysfunction is caused by medication, its use should be stopped, if possible, particularly when bleeding occurs. If platelet dysfunction is marked, bleeding can often be prevented by transfusion of normal platelets before invasive procedures. Aminocaproic acid may be required to prevent significant bleeding after such procedures.

Nursing Management

Patients with significant platelet dysfunction need to be instructed to avoid substances that can diminish platelet function, such as certain over-the-counter medications, herbs, nutritional supplements, and alcohol. They also need to inform their health care providers (including dentists) of the underlying condition before any invasive procedure is performed, so that appropriate steps can be initiated to diminish the risk of bleeding. Bleeding precautions should be initiated as appropriate (see Chart 54-12).

Hemophilia

Two inherited bleeding disorders—hemophilia A and hemophilia B—are clinically indistinguishable, although they can be distinguished by laboratory tests. Hemophilia A is caused by a genetic defect that results in deficient or defective factor VIII. Hemophilia B (also called *Christmas disease*) stems from a genetic defect that causes deficient or defective factor IX. Hemophilia is a relatively common disease; hemophilia A occurs in 1 of every 5,000 to 7,000 births and is five times more common than hemophilia B (Escobar & Key, 2016). Both types of hemophilia are inherited as X-linked traits, so most affected people are males; females can be carriers but are almost always asymptomatic. However, it is estimated that one third of cases result from spontaneous mutations, rather than through familial transmission (Dunn, 2015). The disease occurs in all ethnic groups (Escobar & Key, 2016).

CHART 54-13

Pharmacology: Medications and Substances That Impair Platelet Function

Anesthetic Agents
- Halothane (Fluothane)
- Local anesthetic agents

Antibiotics
- Aminoglycosides
- Beta-lactam antibiotics
  - Penicillins
  - Cephalosporins
- Nitrofurantoin
- Sulfonamides

Anticoagulation and Antiplatelet Agents
- Abciximab (ReoPro)
- Antithrombin agents
- Clopidogrel (Plavix)
- Dipyridamole (Persantine)
- Fibrinolytic agents
- Heparin
  - Unfractionated heparin
  - Low-molecular-weight heparins
- Ticlopidine (Ticlid)
- Tirofiban (Aggrastat)

Anti-Inflammatory Agents (Nonsteroidal)
- Aspirin
- Colchicine (Colcrys)
- Ibuprofen (Advil, Motrin)
- Indomethacin (Indocin)
- Naproxen (Aleve)

Antineoplastic Agents
- Carmustine (BCNU)
- Daunorubicin (Cerubidine)
- Mithramycin (Mithracin)
- Vinblastine (Velban)
- Vincristine (Oncovin)

Cardiovascular/Respiratory Drugs
- Angiotensin-converting enzyme inhibitors
- Angiotensin receptor blockers
- Beta-blockers
- Calcium channel blockers
- Cilostazol (Pletal)
- Clofibrate (Atromid-S)
- Diuretics
  - Ethacrynic acid (Edecrin)
  - Furosemide (Lasix)
- Hydralazine (Apresoline)
- Methylxanthines
  - Aminophylline
  - Theophylline (Theo-Dur)
- Nitrates
  - Isosorbide (Isordil)
- Phentolamine (Regitine)
- Prasugel (Effient)
- Prostacyclin
- Quinidine

Food and Food Additives
- Caffeine
- Chinese black tree fungus
- Clove
- Cumin
- Ethanol (i.e., alcohol)
- Fish oils
- Garlic
- Ginger
- Onion extract
- Turmeric

Plasma Expanders
- Dextrans
- Hydroxyethyl starch (HES)

Psychotropic Agents
- Phenothiazines
- Serotonin reuptake inhibitors
  - Fluoxetine (Prozac)
  - Fluvoxamine (Luvox)
  - Paroxetine (Plaxil)
  - Sertraline (Zoloft)
- Tricyclic antidepressants
  - Doxepin (Sinequan)
  - Imipramine (Tofranil)
- Valproic acid (Dapacon)

Miscellaneous
- Antihistamines
- Contrast agents
- Glyceryl guaiacolate (cough syrup base)
- Hepatitis B vaccine
- Heroin
- Hydroxychloroquine (Plaquenil; Quineprox)
- Phenytoin (Dilantin)
- Vitamin E

Herbal Supplements
- Feverfew
- Gingko
- Ginseng
- Kava kava

The tendency for developing bleeding serves as the basis for hemophilia classification (Escobar & Key, 2016):

- Severe disease is defined as a plasma factor activity level of less than 1 IU/dL, or less than 1% normal factor VIII levels
- Moderate disease reflects a level of 1 to 5 IU/dL or factor VIII level between 1% and 5% of normal
- Mild disease reflects a level above 5 IU/dL or factor VIII level above 5%

Hemophilia is recognized in early childhood, usually in the toddler age group. However, patients with mild hemophilia may not be diagnosed until they experience severe trauma (e.g., a high school football injury) or surgery.

Clinical Manifestations

Hemophilia is manifested by hemorrhages into various parts of the body; these hemorrhages can be severe and can occur even after minimal trauma. The frequency and severity of the bleeding depend on the degree of factor deficiency as well as the intensity of the precipitating trauma. For example, patients with a mild factor VIII deficiency rarely develop hemorrhage spontaneously; hemorrhage tends to occur secondary to trauma. In contrast, spontaneous hemorrhages, particularly hemarthroses and hematomas, can frequently occur in patients with severe factor VIII deficiency (Escobar & Key, 2016).

About 75% of all bleeding in patients with hemophilia occurs into joints. The most commonly affected joints are the knees, elbows, ankles, shoulders, wrists, and hips. Patients often note pain in a joint before they are aware of swelling and limitation of motion. Recurrent joint hemorrhages can result in damage so severe that chronic pain, ankylosis (fixation), or arthropathy of the joint occurs (see Fig. 54-20). Patients with severe factor deficiency can become disabled by the joint damage before they become adults. Bleeding can be superficial as hematomas or as deep hemorrhages into muscle or subcutaneous tissue. With severe factor VIII deficiency, hematomas can occur without known trauma and progressively extend in all directions. When the hematomas occur within muscle, particularly in the extremities, peripheral nerves can be compressed. Over time, this compression results in decreased sensation, weakness, and atrophy of the area involved.

Bleeding is not limited to the joints and muscles. Bleeding is commonly associated with dental extraction. Spontaneous hematuria and GI bleeding can also occur. Bleeding is also common in other mucous membranes, such as the nasal passages, and in soft tissues. The most dangerous site of hemorrhage is in the head (intracranial or extracranial). Any head trauma requires prompt evaluation and treatment. Surgical procedures typically result in excessive bleeding at the surgical site. Because clot formation is poor, wound healing may also be poor.

Falls carry significant risk for morbidity in adults. A retrospective study of 74 adults over age 40 with severe or moderate hemophilia and independent in their mobility was evaluated for risk factors for falling (Sammels, Vandesande, Vlaeyen, et al., 2014). Falling was not uncommon in this sample; 32.4% fell in the previous year, and 42% of those who fell did so repeatedly (i.e., average 4 falls yearly). Most falls occurred outdoors and among those adults more physically active. This finding differs from other research that suggests physical activity decreased fall risk and may be due to higher confidence and thus less care when ambulating. Arthropathy and urinary incontinence were also associated with increased fall risk.

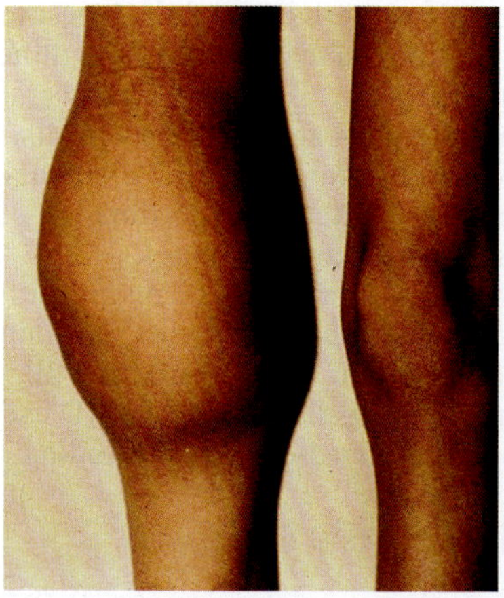

FIGURE 54-20. Hemophilic arthropathy: Sequelae of recurrent joint bleeding. (From Foerster, J., & Greer, J. P. (1999b). *Wintrobe's clinical hematology* (10th ed.). Color plate 68. Philadelphia, PA: Lippincott Williams & Wilkins.)

Medical Management

Recombinant forms of factor VIII and X concentrates are available and decrease the need for using factor concentrates, or, more infrequently, fresh-frozen plasma. Patients are given concentrates when they are actively bleeding; it is crucial to initiate treatment as soon as possible so that bleeding complications can be avoided. Prophylactic use of these factors as a preventive measure before traumatic procedures (e.g., lumbar puncture, dental extraction, surgery) is an important strategy in preventing bleeding (Escobar & Key, 2016). Children typically receive factor administration prophylactically, three to four times each week; this approach has markedly reduced the incidence and severity of joint complications (Josephson, 2013). However, cost and adherence can limit the effectiveness of this approach. Studies suggest that initiating a prophylactic program later in life (adolescents or young adults) can still afford a positive outcome on joint complications, pain, physical function, and quality of life (Josephson, 2013).

Developing neutralizing antibodies (inhibitors) to factor concentrates is the most significant complication of factor replacement therapy. Between 13% and 33% of patients with hemophilia A and up to 3% of patients with hemophilia B develop antibodies (inhibitors) to factor concentrates (Kempton & Meeks, 2014). Although one third of such inhibitors are transient, their effects can be significant and induce partial or complete refractoriness to factor replacement, thus resulting in a markedly increased risk of bleeding. Treatment success is optimal when antibody titers remain low; thus, it is important to identify rising titers and act promptly. The mainstay of inhibitor management is inducing immune tolerance. Special formulations of factor replacement products are given on a daily basis. Some form of immunosuppression therapy (e.g., cyclophosphamide, IVIG, prednisone) may be used to facilitate eradicating the inhibitor. Patients with severe factor deficiency should be screened for antibodies, particularly before major surgery so that appropriate therapy can be initiated and major bleeding complications from surgery averted.

Other therapeutic options include administering recombinant factor VIIa (Novoseven, Novo Nordisk) or activated prothrombin complex concentrates (IaPCC, FEIBA) (Kempton & Meeks, 2014). An efficacy of 80% has been reported for both agents (Kempton & Meeks, 2014).

Aminocaproic acid inhibits fibrinolysis and therefore stabilizes the clot; it is very effective as an adjunctive measure after oral surgery and in treating mucosal bleeding. Another agent—desmopressin—induces a significant but transient rise in factor VIII levels; the mechanism for this response is unknown. In patients with mild forms of hemophilia A, desmopressin is extremely useful, significantly reducing the amount of blood products required. However, desmopressin is not effective in patients with severe factor VIII deficiency (Collins, Chalmers, Hart, et al., 2013).

Nursing Management

Most patients with hemophilia are diagnosed as children. They often require assistance in coping with the condition because it is chronic, places restrictions on their lives, and is an inherited disorder that can be passed to future generations. From childhood, patients are helped to cope with the disease and to identify the positive aspects of their lives. They are encouraged to be self-sufficient and to maintain independence by preventing unnecessary trauma that can cause acute bleeding episodes and temporarily interfere with normal activities. As they work through their feelings about the condition and progress to accepting it, they can assume more and more responsibility for maintaining optimal health.

Patients with mild factor deficiency may not be diagnosed until adulthood if they do not experience significant trauma or surgery as children. These patients need extensive education about activity restrictions and self-care measures to diminish the chance of hemorrhage and complications of bleeding. The nurse should emphasize safety at home and in the workplace.

Patients and family members are instructed how to administer the factor concentrate at home at the first sign of bleeding so that bleeding is minimized and complications avoided. The use of prophylactic factor replacement can be very effective in diminishing the morbidity associated with repeated bleeding. However, this method requires administration of these factors as often as two to three times each week. Adherence to prophylactic infusions can problematic. A recent study reported the adherence rate to be only 76%; those who had used prophylactic therapy for longer periods of time had higher adherence rates (Ho, Gue, McIntosh, et al., 2014). Nurses can assist patients to consider that the potential benefits of prophylactic therapy outweigh the disadvantages (i.e., time-consuming), particularly early in prophylaxis therapy. Patients with hemophilia are instructed to avoid agents that interfere with platelet aggregation, such as aspirin, NSAIDs, some herbal and nutritional supplements (e.g., chamomile, nettle, alfalfa), and alcohol. This restriction applies to OTC medications such as cold remedies. Oral hygiene is very important as a preventive measure because dental extractions are hazardous. Applying pressure to a minor wound may be sufficient to control bleeding if the factor deficiency is not severe. Nasal packing should be avoided, because bleeding frequently resumes when the packing is removed. Splints and other orthopedic devices may be useful in patients with joint or muscle hemorrhages. All injections should be avoided; invasive procedures (e.g., endoscopy, lumbar puncture) should be minimized or performed after administration of appropriate factor replacement. Patients with hemophilia should carry or wear medical identification (e.g., Medic-Alert bracelets). In addition, patients or families should have a written emergency plan that includes what to do in specific situations as well as names and phone numbers of emergency contacts.

During hemorrhagic episodes, the extent of bleeding must be assessed carefully. Patients who are at risk for significant compromise (e.g., bleeding into the respiratory tract or brain) warrant close observation and systematic assessment for emergent complications (e.g., respiratory distress, altered level of consciousness). If the patient has had recent surgery, the nurse frequently and carefully assesses the surgical site for bleeding. Frequent monitoring of vital signs is needed until the nurse is certain that there is no excessive postoperative bleeding.

Analgesic agents are commonly required to alleviate the pain associated with hematomas and hemorrhage into joints. Many patients report that warm baths promote relaxation, improve mobility, and lessen pain. However, during bleeding episodes, heat is avoided because it can accentuate bleeding; applications of cold are used instead.

Although the formulation of heat-solvent or detergent-treated factor concentrates has rendered factor VIII and IX preparations free of viruses such as HIV and hepatitis C, many patients treated prior to 1985 have already been exposed to these viruses through previous transfusions (Escobar & Key, 2016). These patients and their families may need assistance in coping with the diagnosis and the consequences of these infections.

Genetic testing and counselling should be provided to female carriers so that they can make informed decisions regarding having children and managing pregnancy (see Chapter 11).

Gerontologic Considerations

With improved therapy, the average lifespan of the patient with hemophilia continues to rise. Several unique challenges are seen in this patient population. The older adult patient with hemophilia was likely managed with blood component transfusion, at least early in life. Thus, hepatitis B and C infections are very common in this population, particularly hepatitis C (Canaro, Goranova-Marinova, & Berntorp, 2014); patients with HIV or hepatitis C are at increased risk for liver disease, which can be fatal. Intracranial hemorrhage is the third most common cause of death after HIV and hepatitis and may not result from trauma. The likelihood of acquiring inhibitors, especially hemophilia A inhibitors, also increases with age.

Although patients with hemophilia less commonly have concomitant cardiovascular disease, it is difficult to manage when it is present. Coronary bypass graft surgery is extremely high risk, as are stent placements. Antiplatelet therapy (including aspirin) can be challenging in those with severe hemophilia. Close coordination of care with a hematologist can improve outcomes.

Arthropathy is a major cause of morbidity in older patients with hemophilia and results in diminished range of motion, and chronic pain (Canaro et al., 2014). Pain management can be challenging as NSAID use is contraindicated due to the increased risk of bleeding.

Von Willebrand's Disease

Usually inherited as a dominant trait, vWD is a common bleeding disorder that affects males and females equally. The prevalence of this disease is estimated to be 1% of the world population (Canadian Hemophilia Society, 2019).

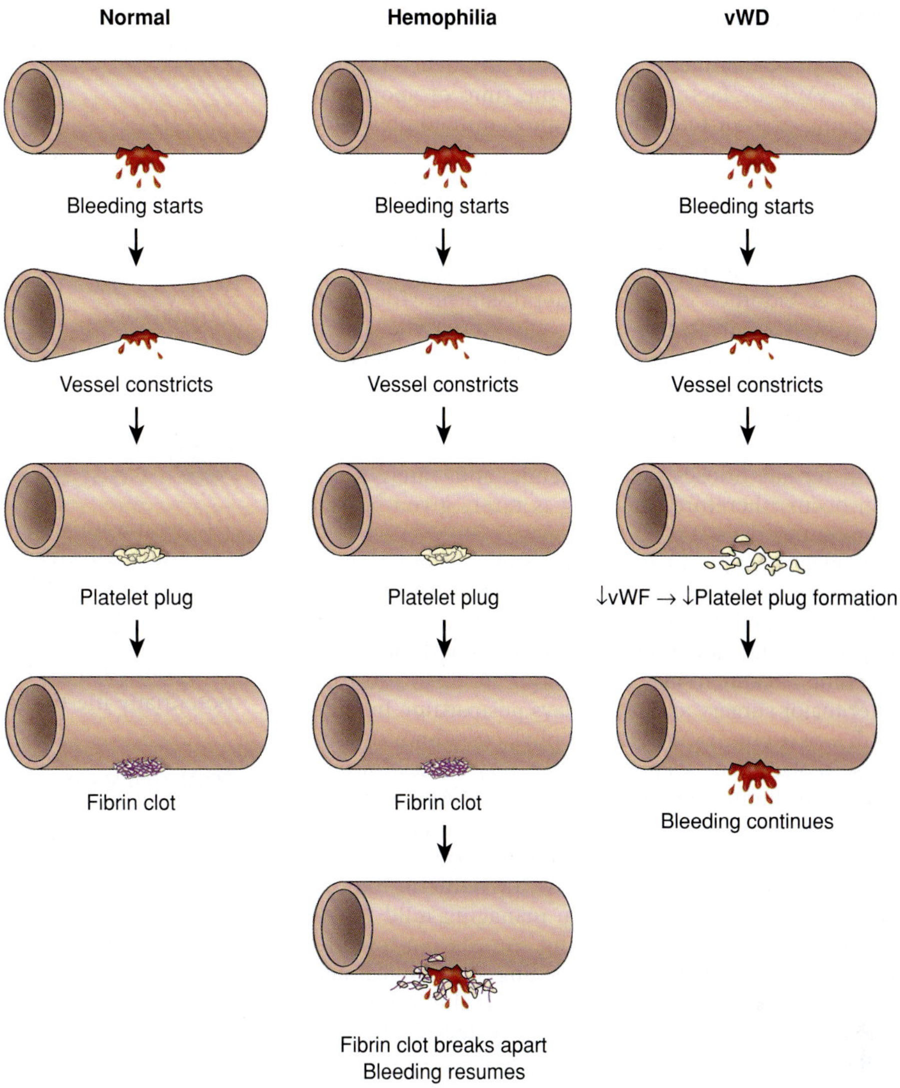

FIGURE 54-21. Differences in bleeding. Normal, hemophilia, and von Willebrand's disease (vWD). (From Thomas, M., & Morrow, K. Veterans Administration Palo Alto Health Care System. Palo Alto: CA.)

The disease is caused by a deficiency of vWF, which is necessary for factor VIII activity. vWF is also necessary for platelet adhesion at the site of vascular injury. Although synthesis of factor VIII is normal, its half-life is shortened; therefore, factor VIII levels commonly are mildly low (15% to 50% of normal).

There are three types of vWD. Type 1, the most common, is characterized by decreases in structurally normal vWF. Type 2 shows variable qualitative defects based on the specific vWF subtype involved. Type 3 is very rare (less than 5% of cases) and is characterized by a severe vWF deficiency as well as significant deficiency of factor VIII. Figure 54-21 depicts the abnormal differences in clotting found in hemophilia and vWD.

Clinical Manifestations

Bleeding tends to be mucosal. Patients commonly have recurrent nosebleeds, easy bruising, heavy menses, prolonged bleeding from cuts, and postoperative bleeding. Massive soft tissue or joint hemorrhages are not often seen, unless the patient has severe type 3 vWD. As the laboratory values fluctuate (see the following Assessment and Diagnostic Findings section), so does the bleeding. For example, a careful history of prior bleeding may show little problem with postoperative bleeding on one occasion but significant bleeding from a dental extraction at another time.

Assessment and Diagnostic Findings

The diagnosis is established by the patient meeting all of these criteria: a history of bleeding since childhood, reduced vWF activity in plasma, and a history of bleeding within the family (Federici, 2014). Laboratory test results show a normal platelet count but a prolonged bleeding time and a slightly prolonged aPTT. These defects are not static, and laboratory test results can vary widely within the same patient over time. Thus, it is crucial to review these values over time rather than rely on a single measurement. More important tests include the ristocetin cofactor, or vWF collagen binding assay, which measures vWF activity. While these tests are specific for vWF abnormalities, they are not very sensitive. Thus, other tests are often needed to establish the diagnosis, such as the vWF antigen, factor VIII, and, for patients with suspected type 2 defects, vWF multimers, which measure specific subtypes of vWF.

Medical Management

The goal of treatment is to replace the deficient protein (e.g., vWF or factor VIII) at the time of spontaneous bleeding or prior to an invasive procedure to prevent subsequent bleeding. Desmopressin, a synthetic vasopressin analogue, can be used to prevent bleeding associated with dental or surgical procedures or to manage mild bleeding after surgery in those individuals with mild vWD, although it is often ineffective in treating those with type 3 vWD (Neff & Sidonio, 2014). Desmopressin provides a transient increase in factor VIII coagulant activity and may also correct the bleeding time. Desmopressin can be given as an IV infusion or intranasally. With major surgery or invasive procedures, IV administration is preferable. Side effects include headache, facial flushing, and tachycardia. With repeated doses, hyponatremia, and, rarely, seizures can occur; therefore, the drug is rarely given beyond 3 consecutive days.

Replacement products include Humate-P and Alphanate, which are commercial concentrates of vWF and factor VIII. The dosage and frequency of administration of these agents depend on the patient's factor VIII levels and the extent of bleeding. Treatment may be necessary for up to 7 to 10 days after major surgery and 3 to 4 days postpartum. In patients with severe type 3 vWD, the prophylactic administration of these replacement agents has been very successful in preventing or limiting spontaneous bleeding. Antibody formation to these products usually occurs only in patients with type 3 vWD, after administration of high doses.

Other agents may be effective in reducing bleeding. Aminocaproic acid is useful in managing mild forms of mucosal bleeding by inhibiting the dissolution of the thrombus that forms at the bleeding site. Topical agents that enhance thrombin formation at the site of application are useful to achieve hemostasis in dental procedures (Neff & Sidonio, 2014). Estrogen–progesterone compounds may diminish the extent of menses. Platelet transfusions are useful when there is significant bleeding. While rich in vWF and factor VIII, cryoprecipitate is typically used only in emergent situations due to the associated risk of iatrogenic transmission of viruses (e.g., hepatitis). Herbs and medications that interfere with platelet function (e.g., aspirin) should be avoided.

ACQUIRED COAGULATION DISORDERS

Liver Disease

With the exception of factor VIII, most blood coagulation factors are synthesized in the liver. Therefore, hepatic dysfunction (due to cirrhosis, tumour, or hepatitis; see Chapter 39) can result in diminished amounts of the factors needed to maintain coagulation and hemostasis. Prolongation of the PT, unless it is caused by vitamin K deficiency, may indicate severe hepatic dysfunction. Although bleeding is usually minor (e.g., ecchymoses), these patients are also at risk for significant bleeding, related especially to trauma or surgery. Transfusion of fresh-frozen plasma may be required to replace clotting factors and to prevent or stop bleeding. Patients may also have life-threatening hemorrhage from peptic ulcers or esophageal varices. In these cases, replacement with fresh-frozen plasma, PRBCs, and platelets is usually required.

Vitamin K Deficiency

The synthesis of many coagulation factors depends on vitamin K. Vitamin K deficiency is common in malnourished patients. Prolonged use of some antibiotics decreases the intestinal flora that produces vitamin K, depleting vitamin K stores. Administration of vitamin K (phytonadione [Mephyton]), either orally or as a subcutaneous injection, can correct the deficiency quickly; adequate synthesis of coagulation factors is reflected by normalization of the PT.

Disseminated Intravascular Coagulation

DIC is not an actual disease but a sign of an underlying condition. DIC may be triggered by sepsis, trauma, cancer, shock, abruptio placentae, toxins, allergic reactions, and other conditions; the vast majority (two thirds) of cases of DIC are initiated by an infection or a malignancy (Levi & Seligsohn, 2016). The severity of DIC is variable, but it is potentially life-threatening.

Pathophysiology

In DIC, normal hemostatic mechanisms are altered. The inflammatory response generated by the underlying disease initiates the process of inflammation and coagulation within the vasculature. The natural anticoagulant pathways within the body are simultaneously impaired, and the fibrinolytic system is suppressed so that a massive amount of tiny clots forms in the microcirculation. Initially, the coagulation time is normal. However, as the platelets and clotting factors form microthrombi, coagulation fails. Thus, the paradoxical result includes excessive clotting and bleeding (see Fig. 54-22).

The clinical manifestations of DIC are primarily reflected in compromised organ function or failure. Decline in organ function is usually a result of excessive clot formation (with resultant ischemia to all or part of the organ) or, less often, of bleeding. The excessive clotting triggers the fibrinolytic system to release fibrin degradation products, which are potent anticoagulants, furthering the bleeding. The bleeding is characterized by low platelet and fibrinogen levels; prolonged PT, aPTT, and thrombin time; and elevated fibrin degradation products and **D-dimers**.

The mortality rate can exceed 80% in patients who develop severe DIC with ischemic thrombosis, frank hemorrhage, and multiple organ dysfunction syndrome (MODS). Identification of patients who are at risk for DIC and recognition of the early clinical manifestations of this syndrome can result in prompt medical intervention, which may improve the prognosis. However, the primary prognostic factor is the ability to treat the underlying condition that precipitated DIC.

Clinical Manifestations

Patients with frank DIC may bleed from mucous membranes, venipuncture sites, and the GI and urinary tracts.

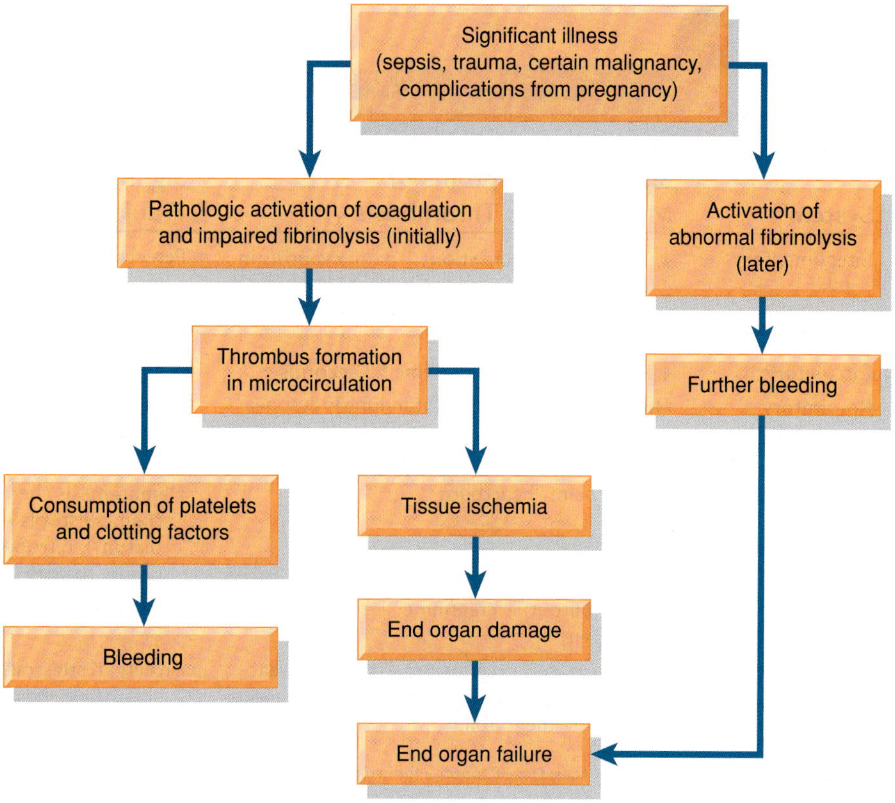

FIGURE 54-22. Pathophysiology of disseminated intravascular coagulation.

The bleeding can range from minimal occult internal bleeding to profuse hemorrhage from all orifices. Patients typically develop MODS, and they may exhibit acute kidney injury as well as pulmonary and multifocal central nervous system infarctions as a result of microthromboses, macrothromboses, or hemorrhages.

During the initial process of DIC, the patient may have no new symptoms—the only manifestation being a progressive decrease in the platelet count. As the thrombosis becomes more extensive, the patient exhibits signs and symptoms of thrombosis in the organs involved. Then, as the clotting factors and platelets are consumed to form these thrombi, bleeding occurs. Initially, the bleeding is subtle, but it can develop into frank hemorrhage. Signs and symptoms depend on the organs involved and are listed in Chart 54-14.

Assessment and Diagnostic Findings

Clinically, the diagnosis of DIC is often established by laboratory tests that reflect consumption of platelets and clotting factors (i.e., drop in platelet count, an elevation in fibrin degradation products and D-dimer, an increase in PT and aPTT, and a low fibrinogen level) (see Table 54-11). Although each of these tests is useful in establishing the diagnosis of DIC, the specificity of each individual parameter is lacking, although D-dimer levels are more accurate than fibrin degradation products. The International Society on Thrombosis and Haemostasis has developed a highly sensitive and specific scoring system using the platelet count, fibrin degradation products, PT, and fibrinogen level to diagnose DIC (Levi & Seligsohn, 2016) (see Table 54-12). This system is also useful in predicting the

TABLE 54-11 Laboratory Values Commonly Found in Disseminated Intravascular Coagulation[a]

Test	Function Evaluated	Normal Range	Changes in DIC
Platelet count	Platelet number	150,000–450,000/mm^3	↓
Prothrombin time (PT)	Extrinsic pathway	11–12.5 seconds	↑
Partial thromboplastin time (activated) (aPTT)	Intrinsic pathway	23–35 seconds	↑
Thrombin time (TT)	Clot formation	8–11 seconds	↑
Fibrinogen	Amount available for coagulation	170–340 mg/dL	↓
D-dimer	Local fibrinolysis	0–250 ng/mL	↑
Fibrin degradation products (FDPs)	Fibrinolysis	0–5 mcg/mL	↑
Euglobulin clot lysis	Fibrinolytic activity	≥2 hours	≤1 hour

[a]Because DIC is a dynamic condition, the laboratory values measured will change over time. Therefore, a progressive increase or decrease in a given laboratory value is likely to be more important than the actual value of a test at a single point in time.

DIC, disseminated intravascular coagulation; ↓, decreased; ↑, increased.

CHART 54-14

Assessment: Assessing for Thrombosis and Bleeding in Disseminated Intravascular Coagulation

System	Signs and Symptoms of Microvascular Thrombosis	Signs and Symptoms of Microvascular and Frank Bleeding
Integumentary (skin)	↓ Temperature, sensation; ↑ pain; cyanosis in extremities, nose, earlobes; focal ischemia, superficial gangrene	Petechiae, including periorbital and oral mucosa; bleeding: gums, oozing from wounds, previous injection sites, around catheters (IVs, tracheostomies); epistaxis; diffuse ecchymoses; subcutaneous hemorrhage; joint pain
Circulatory	↓ Pulses; capillary filling time >3 seconds	Tachycardia
Respiratory	Hypoxia (secondary to clot in lung); dyspnea; chest pain with deep inspiration; ↓ breath sounds over areas of large embolism	High-pitched bronchial breath sounds; tachypnea; ↑ consolidation; signs and symptoms of acute respiratory distress syndrome
Gastrointestinal	Gastric pain; "heartburn"	Hematemesis (heme⊕ nasogastric output); melena (heme⊕ stools → tarry stools → bright-red blood from rectum); retroperitoneal bleeding (abdomen firm and tender to palpation; distended; ↑ abdominal girth)
Renal	↓ Urine output; ↑ creatinine, ↑ blood urea nitrogen	Hematuria
Neurologic	↓ Alertness and orientation; ↓ pupillary reaction; ↓ response to commands; ↓ strength and movement ability	Anxiety; restlessness; ↓ mentation, altered level of consciousness; headache; visual disturbances; conjunctival hemorrhage

↓, decreased; ↑, increased; IV, intravenous; heme⊕, positive for hemoglobin.

Note: Signs of microvascular thrombosis are the result of an inappropriate activation of the coagulation system, causing thrombotic occlusion of small vessels within all body organs. As the clotting factors and platelets are consumed, signs of microvascular bleeding appear. This bleeding can quickly extend into frank hemorrhage. Treatment must be aimed at the disorder underlying the disseminated intravascular coagulation; otherwise, the stimulus for the syndrome will persist.

severity of the disease over time and subsequent mortality. Other tests, such as thromboelastography, can be performed at the bedside and can better assess platelet function as well as fibrinolytic activity; studies suggest it is more useful to assess the status of the coagulation system in critically ill patients at the bedside than use more conventional laboratory tests (Haase, Ostrowski, Wettersley, et al., 2015; Mishra, Thekkudan, Sahajanadan, et al., 2015).

Medical Management

The most important factor in managing DIC is aggressively treating the underlying cause; until the cause is controlled, DIC will persist. Correcting the secondary effects of tissue ischemia by improving oxygenation, replacing fluids, correcting electrolyte imbalances, and administering vasopressor medications is also important. If serious hemorrhage occurs, the depleted coagulation factors and platelets may be replaced to reestablish the potential for normal hemostasis and thereby diminish bleeding. However, decisions to provide transfusion support should not be solely based on the laboratory results, but on the extent of hemorrhage or need to initiate an invasive procedure. Cryoprecipitate is given to replace fibrinogen and factors V and VII. Administering fresh frozen plasma replaces coagulation factors, but can exacerbate capillary leak, further compromising pulmonary function. Platelets are transfused to correct severely low platelet levels, control bleeding (with factor replacement), or prior to an invasive procedure (Levi & Seligsohn, 2016).

A controversial treatment strategy is to interrupt the thrombosis process through the use of heparin infusion. Heparin may inhibit the formation of microthrombi and thus permit perfusion of the organs (skin, kidneys, or brain) to resume. Heparin use was traditionally reserved for patients in whom thrombotic manifestations predominated or in whom extensive blood component

TABLE 54-12 Scoring System for Disseminated Intravascular Coagulation

Laboratory Test	0	1	2	3
Platelet count	>100,000/mm^3	>50,000/mm^3, <100,000/mm^3	<50,000/mm^3	
Fibrin degradation products	No increase		Moderate increase	Strong increase
Prothrombin time (upper limit of normal)	<3 seconds	>3 seconds, <6 seconds	>6 seconds	
Fibrinogen	>100 mg/dL	<100 mg/dL		

Note: 5 or more is compatible with overt disseminated intravascular coagulation.

Adapted from Taylor, F. B., Toh, C. H., Hoots, W. K., et al. (2007). Towards a definition, clinical and laboratory criteria, and a scoring system for DIC. *Journal of Thrombosis and Haemostasis*, *5*(3), 445–659.

replacement failed to halt the hemorrhage or increased fibrinogen and other clotting levels. In the absence of bleeding, prophylactic doses of unfractionated heparin or low–molecular-weight heparin (LMWH) may be used to prevent VTE, whereas therapeutic doses of unfractionated heparin may be used when severe thrombosis predominates. The effectiveness of heparin can be determined by observing for normalization of the plasma fibrinogen concentration and diminishing signs of bleeding. However, there is little evidence to suggest that heparin reverses organ dysfunction, whereas there is stronger evidence that LMWH may be associated with this benefit (Toh & Alhamdi, 2013). Fibrinolytic inhibitors, such as aminocaproic acid, are not routinely advised; they block the lysis of fibrin needed to preserve tissue perfusion. However, if the bleeding is profuse and there is evidence of excessive fibrinolysis, fibrinolytic inhibitors are used concomitantly with a continuous infusion of IV heparin (Levi & Seligsohn, 2016).

Recent studies suggest that recombinant forms of thrombomodulin can effectively bind to thrombin and inactivate thrombin's coagulant activity (Hoppensteadt, Tsuruta, Cunanan, et al., 2014; Matsushita, Watanabe, Honda, et al., 2014). This treatment may be a useful means to control profound bleeding associated with DIC. All management strategies must be individualized to the specific patient, underlying cause of DIC, and response to interventions.

Nursing Management

Nurses need to be aware of which patients are at risk for DIC (see previous discussion on "triggers"). Patients need to be assessed thoroughly and frequently for signs and symptoms of thrombi and bleeding and monitored for any progression of these signs (see Chart 54-14). Lab values must be monitored frequently, not only for the actual result but to note trends over time as well as the rate of change in values.

Chart 54-15 describes care of the patient with DIC. Assessment and interventions should target potential sites of end-organ damage. As organs become ischemic from microthrombi, organ function diminishes; the kidneys, lungs, brain, and skin are particularly vulnerable. Lack of renal perfusion may result in acute tubular necrosis and kidney injury, sometimes requiring dialysis. Placement of a large-bore dialysis catheter is extremely hazardous for this patient population and should be accompanied by adequate platelet and plasma transfusions. Hepatic dysfunction is also relatively common, reflected in altered liver function tests, depleted albumin stores, and diminished synthesis of clotting factors. Respiratory function warrants careful monitoring and aggressive measures to diminish alveolar compromise. Suctioning should be performed as gently as possible to diminish the risk of additional bleeding. Central nervous system involvement can be manifested as headache, visual changes, and alteration in level of consciousness.

Thrombotic Disorders

Several conditions can alter balance within the normal hemostasis process, causing excessive thrombosis that may be arterial (due to platelet aggregation) or venous (composed of platelets, red cells, and thrombin). Abnormalities that predispose a person to thrombotic events include decreased clotting inhibitors within the circulation (which enhances coagulation), altered hepatic function (which may decrease the production of clotting factors or clearance of activated coagulation factors), lack of fibrinolytic enzymes, and tortuous or atherosclerotic vessels (which promote platelet aggregation). Thrombosis may occur as an initial manifestation of an occult malignancy or as a complication from a pre-existing cancer. It can also be caused by more than one predisposing factor. Several inherited or acquired deficiency conditions, including hyperhomocysteinemia, antithrombin (AT) deficiency, protein C deficiency, protein S deficiency, activated protein C (APC) resistance, and factor V Leiden deficiency, can predispose a patient to repeated episodes of thrombosis; they are referred to as hypercoagulable states or thrombophilia. Those disorders that are inherited should trigger the need for familial genetic testing for the disorder (see Chapter 11); acquired disorders do not warrant familial testing.

Conditions that may result from thrombosis include acute coronary syndrome (ACS) (see Chapter 29), ischemic stroke (see Chapter 64), and peripheral arterial occlusive disease (see Chapter 32). Anticoagulation therapy is necessary. The duration of therapy varies with the location and extent of the thrombosis, precipitating events (e.g., trauma, immobilization), and concurrent risk factors (e.g., the use of oral contraceptives or cigarettes, obesity, tortuous blood vessels, history of thrombotic events; see Table 54-13). A recent study found that taking aspirin after completing standard anticoagulation therapy for treating VTE reduced the risk of recurrent thrombosis (Simes, Becattini, Agnellis, et al., 2014). With some conditions, or with repeated thrombosis, lifelong anticoagulant therapy is necessary.

Hyperhomocysteinemia

Homocysteine can promote platelet aggregation. Increased plasma levels of homocysteine are a significant risk factor for VTE (e.g., DVT, pulmonary embolism [PE]), recurrent VTE, and arterial thrombosis (e.g., ischemic stroke, ACS) (Reitter-Pfoertner, Waldhoer, Mayerhofer, et al., 2013). Hyperhomocysteinemia can be hereditary, or it can result from a nutritional deficiency of folate and, to a lesser extent, of vitamins B_{12} and B_6, because these vitamins are cofactors in homocysteine metabolism. For unknown reasons, people who are older and those with kidney injury may also have elevated levels of homocysteine in the absence of nutritional deficiencies of these vitamins (Middeldorp & Coppens, 2016). Although a simple fasting measurement of plasma homocysteine can serve as a useful screening test, people with genetically inherited hyperhomocysteinemia and those who are vitamin B_6 deficient may have normal or minimally elevated levels. A more sensitive method involves obtaining a second measurement 4 hours after the patient consumes methionine; hyperhomocysteinemia is found twice as often when this method is used. In hyperhomocysteinemia, the endothelial lining of the vessel walls is denuded,

(text continued on page 1674)

Plan of Nursing Care — Chart 54-15. The Patient With Disseminated Intravascular Coagulation

Nursing Priority: Bleeding
Goals: Hemodynamic status maintained; urine output ≥0.5 mL/kg/hr

NURSING INTERVENTIONS	RATIONALE	EXPECTED OUTCOMES
1. Avoid procedures/activities that can increase intracranial pressure (e.g., coughing, straining to have a bowel movement).	1. Prevents intracranial bleeding	• Level of consciousness (LOC) stable • Central venous pressure 5–12 cm H_2O, systolic blood pressure ≥70 mm Hg • Urine output ≥0.5 mL/kg/hr • Decreased bleeding • Decreased oozing • Decreased ecchymoses • Amenorrhea • Absence of oral and bronchial bleeding • Oral mucosa clean, moist, intact
2. Monitor vital signs closely, including neurologic checks: a. Monitor hemodynamics. b. Monitor abdominal girth. c. Monitor urine output.	2. Identifies signs of hemorrhage/shock quickly	
3. Avoid medications that interfere with platelet function if possible (e.g., aspirin, nonsteroidal anti-inflammatory drugs, beta-lactam antibiotics).	3. Decreases problems with platelet aggregation and adhesion	
4. Avoid rectal probes, rectal medications.	4. Decreases risk of rectal bleeding	
5. Avoid intramuscular injections.	5. Decreases risk of intramuscular bleeding a. Provides accurate, objective assessment of extent of bleeding b. Identifies presence of or quantifies extent of bleeding c. Quantifies extent of bleeding d. Decreases chance for gynecologic source of hemorrhage	
6. Monitor amount of external bleeding carefully: a. Monitor number of dressings, percentage of dressing saturated; time to saturate a dressing is more objective than "dressing saturated a moderate amount." b. Assess suction output, all excreta for frank or occult blood. c. Monitor pad counts in women with vaginal bleeding. d. Females may receive progesterone to prevent menses.	6. Prevents excessive trauma that could cause bleeding	
7. Use low pressure with any suctioning.	7. Prevents excessive trauma that could cause bleeding. Glycerin and alcohol (in commercial mouthwashes) will dry mucosa, increasing risk for bleeding.	
8. Administer oral hygiene carefully. a. Avoid lemon-glycerin swabs, hydrogen peroxide, commercial mouthwashes. b. Use sponge-tipped swabs, salt/baking soda (bicarbonate of soda) mouth rinses.	8. Prevents excessive bleeding at sites	
9. Avoid dislodging any clots, including those around IV sites and injection sites.		

Nursing Priority: Impaired skin integrity
Goals: Skin integrity remains intact; oral mucosa remains intact

NURSING INTERVENTIONS	RATIONALE	EXPECTED OUTCOMES
1. Assess skin, with particular attention to bony prominences, skin folds.	1. Prompt identification of any area at risk for skin breakdown or showing early signs of breakdown can facilitate prompt intervention and thus prevent complications.	• Skin integrity remains intact; skin is warm, and of normal colour. • Oral mucosa is intact, pink, moist, without bleeding.

Plan of Nursing Care — Chart 54-15. The Patient With Disseminated Intravascular Coagulation, *Continued*

NURSING INTERVENTIONS	RATIONALE	EXPECTED OUTCOMES
2. Reposition carefully; use pressure-reducing mattress. 3. Perform careful skin care every 2 hours, emphasizing dependent areas, all bony prominences, perineum. 4. Use lamb's wool between digits, around ears, as needed.	2–4. Meticulous skin care and the use of measures to prevent pressure on bony prominences decrease the risk of skin trauma.	
5. Use prolonged pressure after injection or procedure when such measures must be performed (at least 5 minutes).	5. Initial platelet plug is very unstable and easily dislodged, which can lead to increased bleeding.	
6. Perform oral hygiene carefully (see earlier discussion).	6. Meticulous care is needed to decrease trauma, bleeding, and risk of infection.	

Nursing Priority: Imbalanced fluid volume
Goals: Absence of edema; absence of crackles; intake not greater than output

NURSING INTERVENTIONS	RATIONALE	EXPECTED OUTCOMES
1. Auscultate breath sounds every 2–4 hours.	1. Crackles can develop quickly.	• Breath sounds clear • Absence of edema • Intake does not exceed output • Weight stable
2. Monitor extent of edema.	2. Fluid may extend beyond intravascular system.	
3. Monitor volume of IVs, blood products; decrease volume of IV medications if indicated.	3. Helps prevent fluid overload	
4. Administer diuretics as prescribed.	4. Decreases fluid volume	

Nursing Priority: Microthrombi/clotting
Goals: Neurologic status remains intact; absence of hypoxemia; peripheral pulses remain intact; skin integrity remains intact; urine output remains ≥0.5 mL/kg/hr

NURSING INTERVENTIONS	RATIONALE	EXPECTED OUTCOMES
1. Assess neurologic, pulmonary, integumentary systems.	1. Initial signs of thrombosis can be subtle.	• Arterial blood gases, O_2 saturation, pulse oximetry, LOC within normal limits • Breath sounds clear • Absence of edema • Intake does not exceed output • Weight stable
2. Monitor response to heparin therapy.	2. Assure anticoagulation effectiveness that may prevent formation of additional thromboses.	
3. Assess extent of bleeding.	3. Objective measurements of all sites of bleeding are crucial to accurately assess extent of blood loss.	
4. Monitor fibrinogen levels.	4. Response to heparin is most accurately reflected in fibrinogen level.	
5. Stop aminocaproic acid, if prescribed, if symptoms of thrombosis occur.	5. Aminocaproic acid should be used only in setting of extensive hemorrhage not responding to replacement therapy.	

Nursing Priority: Anxiety
Goals: Feelings verbalized/identified; realistic hope maintained

NURSING INTERVENTIONS	RATIONALE	EXPECTED OUTCOMES
1. Identify previous coping mechanisms, if possible; encourage patient to use them as appropriate.	1. Identifying previous stressful situations can aid in recall of successful coping mechanisms.	• Previously used coping strategies identified and tried, to extent patient is able to do so • Patient indicates understanding of procedures and situation as condition permits.
2. Explain all procedures and their rationale in terms that patient and family can understand.	2. Decreased knowledge and uncertainty can increase anxiety.	
3. Assist family in supporting patient.	3. Family can be useful in assisting patient to use coping strategies and to maintain hope.	
4. Use services from behavioural medicine, chaplain as needed.	4. Additional professional intervention may be necessary, particularly if previous coping mechanisms are maladaptive or ineffective. Spiritual dimension should be supported.	

LOC, level of consciousness.

TABLE 54-13 Risk Factors for Thrombosis

Acquired	Inherited	Mixed/Unknown
Advanced age	Antithrombin deficiency	Activated protein C resistance
Antiphospholipid antibody syndrome	Factor V Leiden	↑ Factor VII
Atrial fibrillation	Factor XII deficiency	↑ Factor VIII
Diabetes	Protein C deficiency	↑ Factor IX
Drugs (e.g., cocaine, ergot)	Protein S deficiency	↑ Factor XI
Estrogen use	Prothrombin 20210a	↓ Fibrinolytic activity
Hypertension		↑ Homocysteine
Inflammatory bowel disease		
Immobility		
Lupus anticoagulant		
Major surgery		
Myeloproliferative disease		
Nephrotic syndrome		
Obesity		
Paralysis		
Pregnancy/postpartum period		
Prior stroke		
Prior superficial vein thrombosis		
Smoking		
Trauma/fracture		
Vascular access catheters		

↑, increased; ↓, decreased.

Note: Risk factors for first, unprovoked venous thromboembolism. Note that the factor levels that are increased are procoagulant proteins.

Adapted from Heit, J. A. (2015). Epidemiology of venous thromboembolism. *Nature Reviews. Cardiology, 2015*(8), 464–474; Kreidy, R. (2014). Influence of acquired and genetic risk factors on the prevention, management, and treatment of thromboembolic disease. *International Journal of Vascular Medicine, 2014*: 859726; Martinelli I., Passamonti, S. M., & Bucciarelli, P. (2014). Thrombophilic states. *Handbook of Clinical Neurology, 120*, 1061–1071.

which can precipitate thrombus formation. Research findings do not support that taking folic acid, vitamin B_6, and vitamin B_{12} supplements is effective in decreasing the risk of recurrent venous or arterial thromboembolism (Middeldorp & Coppens, 2016). Smoking causes low levels of vitamins B_6 and B_{12} and folate; thus, homocysteine levels rise. Patients need to be encouraged to refrain from smoking.

Antithrombin Deficiency

AT is a protein that inhibits thrombin and certain coagulation factors, and it may also play a role in diminishing inflammation within the endothelium of blood vessels. AT deficiency is a hereditary condition that can cause venous thrombosis, particularly when the AT level is less than 60% of normal. Patients with AT deficiency rarely develop thrombosis before puberty. By 50 years of age, two thirds of patients with AT deficiency have venous thrombosis. The most common sites for thrombosis are the deep veins of the leg and the mesentery. Recurrent thrombosis often occurs, particularly as the patient ages. Patients tend to exhibit heparin resistance; thus, they may require greater amounts of heparin to achieve adequate anticoagulation. Patients with AT deficiency should be encouraged to have their family members tested for the deficiency.

AT deficiency can also be acquired by four mechanisms: accelerated consumption of AT (as in DIC), reduced synthesis of AT (as in hepatic dysfunction), increased excretion of AT (as in nephrotic syndrome), and medication induced (e.g., estrogens, L-asparaginase).

Protein C Deficiency

Protein C is an enzyme that, when activated, inhibits coagulation. When levels of protein C are deficient, the risk of thrombosis increases, and thrombosis can often occur spontaneously. People who are deficient in protein C are often without symptoms until their 20s; the risk of having a thrombotic event then increases, with a median age at first thrombosis ranging from 30 to 45 years. A rare but significant complication of anticoagulation management in patients with protein C deficiency is warfarin-induced skin necrosis. This complication appears to result from progressive thrombosis in the capillaries within the skin. The extent of the necrosis can be extreme. Prompt cessation of warfarin, treatment with vitamin K, and infusions of heparin and fresh-frozen plasma are crucial to arrest the pathophysiologic process and reverse the effects of the warfarin. Treatment with purified protein C concentrate is sometimes indicated.

Protein S Deficiency

Protein S is another natural anticoagulant normally produced by the liver. APC requires protein S to inactivate certain clotting factors. When the level of protein S is deficient, this inactivation process is diminished, and the risk of thrombosis can be increased. Like patients with protein C deficiency, those with protein S deficiency have a greater risk of recurrent venous thrombosis early in life, as early as 15 years of age. More than 50% of these thromboses are spontaneous. Thromboses most commonly occur in the axillary, mesenteric, and cerebral veins. Warfarin-induced skin necrosis is possible. Acquired protein S deficiency can also occur. Pregnancy, DIC, liver disease, nephritic syndrome, HIV infection, and the use of L-asparaginase have all been associated with reduced protein S levels.

Activated Protein C Resistance and Factor V Leiden Mutation

APC resistance is a common condition that can occur with other hypercoagulable states. APC is an anticoagulant, and resistance to APC increases the risk of venous thrombosis. A molecular defect in the factor V gene has been identified in most (90%) patients with APC resistance. This factor V Leiden mutation is the most common cause of inherited hypercoagulability in Caucasians, but its incidence appears to be much lower in other ethnic groups. Factor V Leiden mutation synergistically increases the risk of thrombosis in patients with other risk factors (e.g., use of oral contraceptives, hyperhomocysteinemia, increased age). People who are homozygous for the factor V Leiden mutation are at extremely high risk of thrombosis and need anticoagulation for life, whereas those who are heterozygous for the mutation may need anticoagulation for only several months after a thrombotic event.

Acquired Thrombophilias

Acquired thrombophilias are types of clotting disorders that do not have inherited/genetic causes.

Etiology

Acquired thrombophilias result in inappropriate clot formation, typically caused by either an excess in antibodies that cause clotting or an increase in clotting factors.

Antiphospholipid Syndrome

Antibodies to phospholipids are common acquired causes of thrombophilia (i.e., hypercoagulable states); up to 5% of the general population may have this disorder. These antibodies reduce levels of annexin V, a protein that binds phospholipids and has anticoagulant activity (Chaturvedi & McCrae, 2015). The most common of these phospholipid antibodies are either lupus or anticardiolipin antibodies, or an antibody to B_2-glycoprotein (Rand & Wolgast, 2016). Antiphospholipid syndrome is classified as primary or secondary, with a reaction secondary to a pre-existing autoimmune disease—with systemic lupus erythematosus being the most common disease implicated. Primary antiphospholipid syndrome is associated with certain infections (hepatitis C, HIV, syphilis, malaria) or certain medications (e.g., antibiotics, quinine [Qualaquin], hydralazine [Apresoline], procainamide [Pronestyl]); a genetic predisposition to this syndrome has been postulated but not yet proven. Antiphospholipid antibodies are associated with repeated miscarriages and felt to be a significant cause of stroke. Most thrombotic events are venous, but arterial thrombosis can occur in up to one third of the cases. Recurrent thromboses tend to be of the same type—that is, venous thrombosis after an initial venous thrombosis, arterial thrombosis after an initial arterial thrombosis. Thrombi typically occur in large vessels. Therapy varies, based on the type of syndrome (e.g., secondary forms may be treated with immunosuppressive therapy), history of prior thrombosis, and location of thrombosis (venous versus arterial); arterial thrombosis often necessitates adding low-dose aspirin to some form of heparin (see later discussion).

Malignancy

Another common acquired cause of thrombophilia is cancer, particularly stomach, pancreatic, lung, and ovarian cancers. The type of thrombosis that results is unusual. Rather than DVT or PE, the thrombosis occurs in unusual sites, such as the portal, hepatic, or renal vein or the inferior vena cava. Migratory superficial thrombophlebitis or nonbacterial thrombotic endocarditis can also occur. In these patients, anticoagulation can be difficult to manage, and the thrombosis can progress despite standard doses of anticoagulants. LMWH appears to be a more effective anticoagulant than warfarin in treating this patient population (Connolly & Francis, 2013).

Medical Management

The primary method of treating thrombotic disorders is anticoagulation. However, in thrombophilic conditions, when to treat (prophylaxis or not) and how long to treat (lifelong or not) can be controversial. Anticoagulation therapy is not without risks; the most significant risk is bleeding. The most common anticoagulant medications are identified in the following section.

Pharmacologic Therapy

Anticoagulant agents are used in the treatment or prevention of thrombosis. These agents, particularly warfarin or unfractionated heparin (see later discussion), can cause bleeding, particularly if their use is not carefully monitored. Along with administering anticoagulant agents, any modifiable risk factors that predispose a patient to thrombosis should be identified and modified, as appropriate. When risk factors (e.g., immobility after surgery, pregnancy) are nonmodifiable, prophylactic anticoagulation may be necessary.

Heparin

UNFRACTIONATED HEPARIN. Heparin is a naturally occurring anticoagulant agent that enhances AT III and inhibits platelet function. To prevent thrombosis, heparin is typically given as a subcutaneous injection two or three times daily. A recent systematic review found that administering heparin slowly (over 30 seconds) resulted in less pain and smaller ecchymoses at the infection site than when the injection was given more rapidly (over 10 seconds) (Akbari, Janani, Mohammady, et al., 2014; Visvanathan, 2015).

To treat thrombosis, heparin is usually administered IV. The therapeutic effect of heparin is monitored by serial measurements of the aPTT; the dose is adjusted to maintain the range at 1.5 to 2.5 times the laboratory control. Protamine sulphate is rarely needed for heparin toxicity (to prevent or treat bleeding complications), because the half-life of heparin is very short (Sartori & Prandoni, 2016).

LOW-MOLECULAR-WEIGHT HEPARIN. LMWHs (e.g., dalteparin [Fragmin], enoxaparin [Lovenox]) are special forms of heparin that have more selective effects on coagulation. Based on their biochemical properties, LMWHs have a longer half-life and a less variable anticoagulant response than unfractionated heparin. These differences permit LMWHs to be safely given only once or twice daily, without the need for laboratory monitoring for dose adjustments. The incidence of heparin-induced thrombocytopenia (HIT) (see later discussion) is much lower when an LMWH is used; however, LMWH is 100% cross-reactive with HIT antibodies and therefore contraindicated in HIT. In certain conditions, the use of an LMWH has allowed anticoagulation therapy to be moved entirely to the outpatient setting. Many cases of uncomplicated DVT are being managed outside the hospital. LMWHs are also used as "bridge therapy" when patients receiving anticoagulation therapy (warfarin) require a major invasive procedure such as surgery. In this situation, warfarin is stopped 2 to 3 days preoperatively, and an LMWH is used in its place until the procedure is performed. After the procedure, warfarin therapy is resumed. If the LMWH is resumed after the procedure, it is discontinued when a therapeutic level of warfarin is achieved.

HEPARIN-INDUCED THROMBOCYTOPENIA. HIT is a significant complication of heparin-based therapy. HIT involves the formation of antibodies against the heparin–platelet complex. HIT may occur in as many as 5% of patients receiving heparin (Lee & Arepally, 2013). The type of heparin used, duration of heparin therapy (beyond 4 days), and surgery (especially if it requires use of cardiopulmonary bypass) appear to be risk factors for developing HIT. Bovine preparations are more likely to lead to HIT than porcine preparations, and LMWH formulations carry a lower risk. Neither the dose nor the route of administration (IV vs. subcutaneous) is a risk. Women appear to be at a higher risk and young adults are at a very low risk for developing the disorder for reasons that are not clear. A decline in platelet count is a hallmark sign that typically occurs after 5 to 10 days of heparin therapy; therefore, the platelet count should be monitored in any patient beginning heparin therapy. The platelet count can drop significantly, usually by 50% of baseline over a period of 1 to 3 days (Greinacher, 2015). The antibodies typically disappear in 2 to 3 months.

Affected patients are at increased risk for thrombosis, either venous, arterial, or both, and the thrombosis can range from DVT to ACS or stroke, or to ischemic damage to an extremity, necessitating amputation. VTE is the most common, typically DVT or PE (Lee & Arepally, 2013).

Treatment for HIT includes prompt cessation of heparin (including any heparin-coated catheters) and initiation of an alternative means of anticoagulation. If the heparin is stopped without providing additional anticoagulation, the patient is at increased risk for developing new thrombi. Argatroban is an inhibitor of thrombin and an FDA-approved anticoagulant for the treatment of HIT. Oral anticoagulation with warfarin is contraindicated because it initially promotes thrombosis in the microvasculature by depleting protein C, which can lead to ischemia and gangrenous limbs (Greinacher, 2015). Once the platelet count has recovered, transitioning to treatment with warfarin is possible. Individuals who develop thrombosis in the setting of HIT should receive anticoagulation for 3 to 6 months; the duration of anticoagulation in the absence of thrombosis is shorter (Lee & Arepally, 2013). Patients need to be aware of their risk for reactivation of the disorder should they be exposed to any amount of heparin within 3 to 4 months after diagnosis. This time frame is thought to be sufficient to remove anti–heparin-platelet antibodies from the circulation by the RES.

Warfarin (Coumadin)

Warfarin (Coumadin) is a vitamin K antagonist; therefore, it interferes with the synthesis of vitamin K–dependent clotting factors. Warfarin binds to albumin, is metabolized in the liver, and has an extremely long half-life. Typically, a patient with VTE is initially treated with both heparin (either unfractionated or an LMWH) and warfarin. When the INR reaches the desired therapeutic range, the heparin is stopped. The dosage required to maintain the therapeutic range (typically an INR of 2.0 to 3.0) varies widely among patients and even within the same patient, depending on the diagnosis and the rationale for anticoagulation. Frequent monitoring of the INR is extremely important so that the dosage of warfarin can be adjusted as needed.

Some patients can monitor their own INR testing and adjust their warfarin dosage based on pre-established algorithms (Michaels & Regan, 2013). Nurses play a critical role in evaluating which patients may be candidates for this self-management approach. Patient education is critical; eligible patients must demonstrate the ability to accurately calibrate and use the INR diagnostic machine, obtain a blood sample correctly, interpret the results, and adjust the warfarin dosage correctly.

Warfarin is affected by many medications; consultation with a pharmacist is important to assess the extent to which concurrently given medications, herbs, and nutritional supplements may interact with warfarin. It is also affected by many foods, so patients need dietary instruction and may benefit from consultation with a dietitian. In particular, foods with high vitamin K content antagonize the effects of warfarin. Some of these foods include spinach, broccoli, and lettuce. Patients need not avoid such foods but do need to maintain consistent intake; for example, eating a salad daily as opposed to weekly will diminish the antagonistic effect (although will likely necessitate a higher dose of warfarin). Chart 54-16 lists agents that interact with warfarin. A significant complication of warfarin therapy is bleeding. The antidote for warfarin is vitamin K, which will rapidly reverse its anticoagulant effects (i.e., within 30 minutes when given IV) (Garcia, 2014). With significant bleeding, transfusions of fresh-frozen plasma are indicated to replace the vitamin K-dependent coagulation factors.

Thrombin and Factor Xa Inhibitors

Several oral anticoagulant agents have been approved for use that are not vitamin K antagonists (such as warfarin). Dabigatran (Pradaxa) is a direct thrombin inhibitor, whereas rivaroxaban (Xarelto), apixaban (Eliquis), and edoxaban (Savaysa) are factor Xa inhibitors. These drugs are indicated for prevention of DVT, PE, or stroke in patients with atrial fibrillation. With the exception of edoxaban, these drugs are also indicated as prophylaxis to prevent DVT in patients having knee or hip replacement surgery. These drugs appear to be as efficacious as warfarin but have the advantage of not requiring frequent INR monitoring and dose adjustment. All of these drugs are metabolized by the cytochrome P450 pathway; therefore, it is important to assess for potential drug–drug interactions.

Studies show that each of these new oral anticoagulant agents is associated with less risk of bleeding than warfarin. However, this benefit may not be seen in adults over 75 years of age; studies show similar rates of hemorrhage independent of oral anticoagulant used (Levine & Goldstein, 2014). Each of these agents still carries some risk of bleeding in all age groups. Dabigatran can be cleared if necessary via hemodialysis, and its absorption can be reduced with oral activated charcoal. Prothrombin complex concentrate, activated prothrombin concentrate, or recombinant factor VIIa can be used to reverse the effect of these oral anticoagulant agents; more specific antidotes are under development.

A challenge associated with the use of these oral agents is that it is not possible to easily measure their anticoagulant

CHART 54-16

Pharmacology: Agents That Interact With Warfarin (Coumadin)

Although warfarin (Coumadin), an anticoagulant medication, is commonly used to treat and prevent thrombosis, many drug-drug and drug-food interactions are associated with its use. A careful medication history (including OTC medications, herbs, and other substances, such as vitamins and minerals) is important when oral anticoagulation therapy is prescribed. Consultation with a pharmacist is recommended to assess the extent to which concurrent medications may affect the anticoagulant and for appropriate dosage adjustments. The following list contains a few examples of agents that interact with warfarin.

Agents That Inhibit Warfarin Function

Azathioprine (Imuran)
Barbiturates
Carbamazepine (Tegretol)
Cholestyramine (Questran)
Corticosteroids
Cyclosporine (Sandimmune)
Dicloxacillin (Dynapen)
Digitalis
Estrogens
Ethanol (Alcohol)
Glutethimide (Doriden)
Griseofulvin (Grisovin)
Haloperidol (Haldol)
Herbal medicines: coenzyme Q, ginseng, St. John's wort, Cat's claw, green tea
Nafcillin
Oral contraceptives
Phenytoin (Dilantin) (long term)
Primidone (Mysoline)
Ribavirin (Copegus)
Rifampin (Rifadin)
Secobarbital (Seconal)
Spironolactone (Aldactone)
Sucralfate (Carafate)
Trazodone (Desyrel)
Vitamin K

Agents That Potentiate Warfarin Function

Acetaminophen (Tylenol)
Allopurinol (Zyloprim)
Amiodarone
Anabolic steroids
Anti-inflammatory agents, including nonsteroidal anti-inflammatory drugs
Antimalarial agents
Argatroban
Aspirin
Broad-spectrum antibiotics
Chloral hydrate
Chloramphenicol
Cimetidine (Tagamet)
Colchicine (Colcrys)
Clofibrate (Atromid-S)
Chlorpromazine (Thorazine)
Danazol (Danocrine)
Diltiazem (Cardizem)
Disulfiram (Antabuse)
Erythromycin (E-Mycin)
Ethacrynic acid (Edecrin)
Feprazone (Prenazone)
Fluconazole (Diflucan)
Gemfibrozil (Lopid)
Herbal medicines: anise, danshen, devil's claw, dong quai, feverfew, fish oil, garlic, ginkgo, ginseng, green tea, licorice root, papain, turmeric, willow bark
Influenza vaccine
Isoniazid (INH)
Lovastatin (Mevacor)
Mefenamic acid (Ponstel)
Methotrexate (MTX)
Metronidazole (Flagyl)
Miconazole (Monistat)
Omeprazole (Prilosec)
Oral hypoglycemic agents
Oxyphenbutazone (Tandearil)
Phenytoin (Dilantin) (short term)
Piroxicam (Feldene)
Probenecid (Benemid)
Propranolol (Inderal)
Propylthiouracil (PTU)
Quinidine (Quinaglute)
Quinine (Qualiquin)
Salicylates
Simvastatin (Zocor)
Sulfinpyrazone (Anturane)
Sulfonamides (long acting)
Tamoxifen (Nolvadex)
Testosterone
Thyroxine
Triclofos
Tricyclic antidepressants
Vitamin C (in very large doses)
Vitamin E (in very large doses)
Voriconazole (Vfend)

effect. Values obtained from standard tests of coagulation (e.g., PT, PTT) yield inconsistent results when measured during administration of these drugs. Measuring anti-Xa activity can be more reliable; however, this test is not available in many laboratories and the time required to obtain results limits its clinical utility (Garcia, 2014). Nevertheless, these drugs are rapidly cleared from the circulation, so long as the patient's renal function is normal. Therefore, their anticoagulant effect may be stopped simply by withdrawing drug administration.

When choosing an oral anticoagulant agent, bleeding risk (lower with thrombin or factor Xa inhibitors) and ability to reverse the anticoagulant effect (easier to manage and control with warfarin) are important considerations. As noted previously, patients with poor renal function exhibit reduced drug clearance. Therefore, the risks of bleeding are higher when anticoagulant agents are prescribed for these patients and those risks need to be carefully weighed against the benefit of decreasing risk of thrombosis. There are additional factors that support the selection of warfarin over the newer agents. Concerns about adherence, the presence of a prosthetic heart valve, and extremes in body weight are factors that support the prescription of warfarin (Garcia, 2014). Drug cost is another important consideration; warfarin is inexpensive, the new drugs are not.

Aspirin

Patients with VTE (e.g., DVT, PE) remain at risk for recurrent thrombosis upon completion of anticoagulant therapy (10% risk within the first year, 5% risk with each subsequent year). An analysis of two large studies (1,224 patients with VTE) revealed a 42% reduction in risk of recurrent VTE in patients who took 100-mg enteric-coated aspirin daily compared with those who took a placebo. Importantly, the risk of bleeding was not increased in those who took aspirin (Simes et al., 2014). The results of this study may increase the recommended use of aspirin after the conclusion of anticoagulation therapy in patients diagnosed with VTE.

Nursing Management

Patients with thrombotic disorders should avoid activities that lead to circulatory stasis (e.g., immobility, crossing the legs). Exercise, especially ambulation, should be performed frequently throughout the day, particularly during long trips by car or plane. Antiembolism stockings are often prescribed, and patients usually need assistance in learning how to use them properly. Surgery further increases the risk of thrombosis. Medications that alter platelet aggregation, such as low-dose aspirin or clopidogrel (Plavix), may be prescribed. Some patients require lifelong therapy with anticoagulants such as warfarin. No evidence supports the use of bed rest as a therapeutic intervention in people with DVT or PE (Partsch, 2014; Pillai & Raval, 2015).

Patients with thrombotic disorders, particularly those with thrombophilia, should be assessed for concurrent risk factors for thrombosis and should avoid them if possible. For example, the use of tobacco and nicotine products should be avoided, blood pressure controlled, and alcohol consumption moderated (Levine & Goldstein, 2014). In many instances, younger patients with thrombophilia may not require prophylactic anticoagulation; however, with concomitant risk factors (e.g., pregnancy), increasing age, or subsequent thrombotic events, prophylactic or long-term anticoagulation therapy may be required. Being able to provide the health care provider with an accurate health history can be extremely useful and can help guide the selection of appropriate therapeutic interventions. Patients need to understand risk factors for thrombosis and what they can do to diminish or reduce them, such as avoiding smoking, using alternative forms of contraception, increasing mobility, and maintaining a healthy weight. Patients with hereditary disorders should encourage their siblings and children to be tested for the disorder.

When a patient with a thrombotic disorder is hospitalized, frequent assessments should be performed for signs and symptoms of beginning thrombus formation, particularly in the legs (DVT) and lungs (PE). Ambulation or range-of-motion exercises as well as the use of antiembolism stockings should be initiated promptly to decrease stasis. Properly fitted graduated compression stockings may reduce pain and edema associated with the acute stage of DVT; however, studies evaluating their efficacy have yielded conflicting results and adherence to wearing them is often poor (Raskob, Hull, Buller, et al., 2016; Sachdeva, Dalton, Amaragiri, et al., 2014).

Therapies for Blood Disorders

Splenectomy

The surgical removal of the spleen (splenectomy) is sometimes necessary. Splenectomy may be required after trauma to the abdomen. Severe hemorrhage can occur if the spleen is ruptured because the spleen is very vascular. Splenectomy is also a possible treatment for hematologic disorders. For example, an enlarged spleen may be the site of excessive destruction of blood cells. If either of these conditions occurs, splenectomy is performed as an emergency procedure. In addition, some patients with grossly enlarged spleens develop severe thrombocytopenia as a result of platelets being sequestered in the spleen. Splenectomy removes the "trap," and platelet counts may normalize over time.

In general, the mortality rate after splenectomy is low. Laparoscopic splenectomy can be performed in selected patients, with a resultant decrease in postoperative morbidity. Complications that may result from surgery are atelectasis, pneumonia, abdominal distention, and abscess formation. Although young children are at the highest risk after splenectomy, all age groups are vulnerable to overwhelming lethal infections and should receive the pneumococcal vaccine (Pneumovax) before undergoing splenectomy, if possible.

The patient is instructed to seek prompt medical attention if even relatively minor symptoms of infection occur. Often, patients with high platelet counts have even higher counts after splenectomy (more than 1 million/mm^3), which can predispose them to serious thrombotic or hemorrhagic problems. However, this increase is transient and usually does not warrant additional treatment.

Therapeutic Apheresis

Apheresis is a Greek word meaning separation. In therapeutic apheresis (or pheresis), blood is taken from the patient and passed through a centrifuge, where a specific component is separated from the blood and removed (Table 54-14). The remaining blood is then returned to the patient. The entire system is closed, so the risk of bacterial contamination is low. When platelets or leukocytes are removed, the decrease in these cells within the circulation is temporary. However, the temporary decrease provides a window of time until suppressive medications (e.g., chemotherapy) can have therapeutic effects. Sometimes plasma is removed rather than blood cells—typically so that specific, abnormal proteins within the plasma are transiently lowered until a long-term therapy can be initiated.

Apheresis is also used to obtain larger amounts of platelets from a donor than can be provided from a single unit of whole blood. A unit of platelets obtained in this way is equivalent to 6 to 8 units of platelets obtained from six to eight separate donors via standard blood donation methods. Platelet donors can have their platelets apheresed as

TABLE 54-14 Types of Apheresis[a]

Procedure	Purpose	Examples of Clinical Use
Plateletpheresis	Remove platelets	Extreme thrombocytosis, essential thrombocythemia (temporary measure); single-donor platelet transfusion
Leukapheresis	Remove WBCs (can be specific to neutrophils or lymphocytes)	Extreme leukocytosis (e.g., AML, CML) (very temporary measure); harvest WBCs for transfusion
Erythrocytapheresis (RBC exchange)	Remove RBCs	RBC dyscrasias (e.g., sickle cell disease); RBCs replaced via transfusion
Plasmapheresis (plasma exchange)	Remove plasma proteins	Hyperviscosity syndromes; treatment for some renal and neurologic diseases (e.g., Goodpasture syndrome, TTP, Guillain–Barré, myasthenia gravis)
Stem cell harvest	Remove circulating stem cells	Transplantation (donor harvest or autologous)

[a]Therapeutic apheresis can be used to treat a wide variety of conditions. When it is used to treat a disease that causes an increase in a specific cell type with a short life in circulation (i.e., WBCs, platelets), the reduction in those cells is temporary. However, this temporary reduction permits a margin of safety while waiting for a longer-lasting treatment modality (e.g., chemotherapy) to take effect. Apheresis can also be used to obtain stem cells for transplantation, either from a matched donor (allogeneic) or from the patient (autologous).

WBC, white blood cell; AML, acute myeloid leukemia; CML, chronic myeloid leukemia; RBC, red blood cell; TTP, thrombotic thrombocytopenic purpura.

Adapted from Stowell, C. P., & Hass, J. J. (2014). Transfusion medicine. In M. Laposata (Ed.). *Laboratory medicine: The diagnosis of disease in the clinical lab*. New York: McGraw-Hill.

often as every 14 days. Leukocytes can be obtained similarly, typically after the donor has received growth factors (G-CSF, GM-CSF) to stimulate the formation of additional leukocytes and thereby increase the leukocyte count. The use of these growth factors also stimulates the release of stem cells within the circulation. Apheresis is used to harvest these stem cells (typically over a period of several days) for use in HSCT.

Hematopoietic Stem Cell Transplantation

HSCT is a therapeutic modality that offers the possibility of cure for some patients with hematologic disorders such as severe aplastic anemia, some forms of leukemia, and thalassemia. It can also provide longer remission from disease even when cure is not possible, such as in multiple myeloma. Hematopoietic stem cells may be transplanted from either allogeneic or autologous donors. For most hematologic diseases, allogeneic transplant is more effective (Fakih, Shah, & Nieto, 2016); here, stem cells are obtained from a donor whose cells match those of the patient. In contrast, the patient's own stem cells are harvested and then used in autologous transplant. (See Chapter 68 for a detailed discussion of HSCT.)

Therapeutic Phlebotomy

Therapeutic phlebotomy is the removal of a certain amount of blood under controlled conditions. Patients with elevated hematocrits (e.g., those with polycythemia vera) or excessive iron absorption (e.g., hemochromatosis) can usually be managed by periodically removing 1 unit (about 500 mL) of whole blood. Eventually this process can produce iron deficiency, leaving the patient unable to produce as many erythrocytes. The actual procedure for therapeutic phlebotomy is similar to that for blood donation (see later discussion).

Blood Component Therapy

A single unit of whole blood contains 450 mL of blood and 50 mL of an anticoagulant, which can be processed and dispensed for administration. However, it is more appropriate, economical, and practical to separate that unit of whole blood into its primary components: erythrocytes, platelets, and plasma (leukocytes are rarely used; see later discussion). Because the plasma is removed, a unit of PRBCs is very concentrated (hematocrit approximately 70%).

Each component must be processed and stored differently to maximize the longevity of the viable cells and factors within it; each individual blood component has a different storage life. PRBCs are stored at 4°C. With special preservatives, they can be stored safely for up to 42 days before they must be discarded. In contrast, platelets must be stored at room temperature because they cannot withstand cold temperatures, and they last for only 5 days before they must be discarded. To prevent clumping, platelets are gently agitated while stored. Plasma is immediately frozen to maintain the activity of the clotting factors within; it lasts for 1 year if it remains frozen. Alternatively, plasma can be further pooled and processed into blood derivatives, such as albumin, immune globulin, factor VIII, and factor IX. Table 54-15 describes each blood component and how it is commonly used.

Special Preparations

Factor VIII concentrate (antihemophilic factor) is a lyophilized, freeze-dried concentrate of pooled fractionated human plasma. It is used in treating hemophilia A. Factor IX concentrate (prothrombin complex) is similarly prepared and contains factors II, VII, IX, and X. It is used primarily for treatment of factor IX deficiency (hemophilia B). Factor IX concentrate is also useful in treating congenital factor VII and factor X deficiencies. Recombinant forms of factor VIII, such as Humate-P or Alphanate, are also useful. Because they contain vWF, these agents are used in vWD as well as in hemophilia A, particularly when patients develop factor VIII inhibitors.

Plasma albumin is a large protein molecule that usually stays within vessels and is a major contributor to plasma oncotic pressure. This protein is used to expand the blood volume of patients in hypovolemic shock and, rarely, to increase the concentration of circulating albumin in patients with hypoalbuminemia.

TABLE 54-15 Blood and Blood Components Commonly Used in Transfusion Therapy[a]

Component	Composition	Indications and Considerations
Whole blood	Cells and plasma, hematocrit about 40%	Volume replacement and oxygen-carrying capacity; usually used only in significant bleeding (>25% blood volume lost)
PRBCs	RBCs with little plasma (hematocrit about 75%); some platelets and WBCs remain	↑ RBC mass; symptomatic anemia: • Platelets within the unit are not functional • WBCs within the unit may cause reaction and are not functional
Platelets—random	Platelets (5.5×10^{10} platelets/unit), plasma; some RBCs, WBCs	Bleeding due to severe ↓ platelets Prevent bleeding when platelets <5,000–10,000/mm^3 Survival ↓ in presence of fever, chills, infection Repeated treatment leads to ↓ survival due to alloimmunization.
Platelets—single donor	Platelets (3×10^{11} platelets/unit) 1 unit is equivalent to 6–8 units of random platelets.	Used for repeated treatment: ↓ alloimmunization risk by limiting exposure to multiple donors
Plasma	Plasma; all coagulation factors Complement	Bleeding in patients with coagulation factor deficiencies; plasmapheresis
Granulocytes	Neutrophils ($>1 \times 10^{10}$/unit); some lymphocytes, RBCs, and platelets will remain within the unit.	Severe neutropenia in selected patients; controversial
Lymphocytes	Lymphocytes (number varies)	Stimulate graft-vs.-host disease effect
Cryoprecipitate	Fibrinogen ≥150 mg/bag, AHF (VIII:C) 80–110 units/bag, von Willebrand factor; fibronectin	von Willebrand's disease Hypofibrinogenemia Hemophilia A
AHF	Factor VIII	Hemophilia A
Factor IX concentrate	Factor IX	Hemophilia B (Christmas disease)
Factor IX complex	Factors II, VII, IX, X	Hereditary factor VII, IX, X deficiency; hemophilia A with factor VII inhibitors
Albumin	Albumin 5%, 25%	Hypoproteinemia; burns; volume expansion by 5% to ↑ blood volume; 25% leads to ↓ hematocrit
IV gamma-globulin	Immunoglobulin G antibodies	Hypogammaglobulinemia (in CLL, recurrent infections); ITP; primary immunodeficiency states
Antithrombin III concentrate (AT III)	AT III (trace amounts of other plasma proteins)	AT III deficiency with or at risk for thrombosis

[a]The composition of each type of blood component is described as well as the most common indications for using a given blood component. RBCs, platelets, and fresh-frozen plasma are the blood products most commonly used. When transfusing these blood products, it is important to realize that the individual product is always "contaminated" with very small amounts of other blood products (e.g., WBCs mixed in a unit of platelets). This contamination can cause some difficulties, particularly isosensitization, in certain patients.

PRBC, packed red blood cell; RBC, red blood cell; WBC, white blood cell; ↑, increased; ↓, decreased; AHF, antihemophilic factor; IV, intravenous; CLL, chronic lymphocytic leukemia; ITP, idiopathic thrombocytopenic purpura.

Adapted from American Red Cross. (2015a). *Blood components*. Retrieved September 14, 2015, from www.redcrossblood.org/learn-about-blood/bloodcomponents; Dzieczkowski, J. S., & Anderson, K.C. (2015). Transfusion biology and therapy. In D. Kasper, A. Fauci, S. Hauser, et al. (Eds.). *Harrison's principles of internal medicine* (19th ed.). Retrieved May 25, 2016, from accessmedicine.mhmedical.com.laneproxy.stanford.edu/content.aspx?bookid=1130&Sectionid=79732248

Immune globulin is a concentrated solution of the antibody IgG; it contains very little IgA or IgM. It is prepared from large pools of plasma. The IV form (IVIG) is used in various clinical situations to replace inadequate amounts of IgG in patients who are at risk for recurrent bacterial infection (e.g., those with CLL, those receiving BMT or HSCT). It is also used in certain autoimmune disorders, such as ITP. Both albumin and IVIG, in contrast to all other fractions of human blood, cells, or plasma, can survive being subjected to heating at 60°C for 10 hours to free them of the viral contaminants that may be present (Chart 54-17).

Procuring Blood and Blood Products

Blood Donation

To protect both the donor and the recipients, all prospective donors are examined and interviewed before they are allowed to donate their blood. The intent of the interview is to assess the general health status of the donor and to identify risk factors that might harm a recipient of the donor's blood. Donors should be in good health and without any of the following:

- A history of viral hepatitis at any time in the past, or a history of close contact with a patient who had hepatitis or was undergoing dialysis within 6 months
- A history of receiving a blood transfusion or an infusion of any blood derivative (other than serum albumin) within 12 months
- Previous transfusion in the United Kingdom, Gibraltar, or Falkland Islands. People who received these transfusions are not allowed to donate blood in the United States because they may have an increased likelihood of transmitting Creutzfeldt–Jakob disease.
- A cumulative total stay since 1980 in the United Kingdom of more than 3 months or in any other European country exceeding 6 months, because the likelihood

CHART 54-17

Diseases Potentially Transmitted by Blood Transfusion

Hepatitis (Viral Hepatitis B, C)

- There is greater risk from pooled blood products and blood of paid donors than from volunteer donors.
- A screening test detects most hepatitis B and C.
- Transmittal risk for hepatitis B is estimated at 1:350,000 donated units.

AIDS (HIV and HTLV)

- Donated blood is screened for antibodies to HIV.
- Transmittal risk is estimated at 1:1.5 million donated units.
- People with high-risk behaviours (multiple sex partners, anal sex, IV/injection drug use) and people with signs and symptoms that suggest AIDS should not donate blood.

Cytomegalovirus (CMV)

- Transmittal risk is greater for premature newborns with CMV antibody–negative mothers and for immunocompromised recipients who are CMV negative (e.g., those with acute leukemia, organ or tissue transplant recipients).
- Blood products rendered "leukocyte reduced" help reduce transmission of virus.

Graft-Versus-Host Disease (GVHD)

- GVHD occurs only in severely immunocompromised recipients (e.g., Hodgkin's disease, bone marrow transplantation).
- Transfused lymphocytes engraft in recipient and attack host lymphocytes or body tissues; signs and symptoms are fever, diffuse reddened skin rash, nausea, vomiting, and diarrhea.
- Preventive measures include irradiating blood products to inactivate donor lymphocytes (no known radiation risks to transfusion recipient) and processing donor blood with leukocyte reduction filters.

Creutzfeldt–Jakob Disease (CJD)

- CJD is a rare, fatal disease that causes irreversible brain damage.
- There is no evidence of transmittal by transfusion.
- All blood donors must be screened for positive family history of CJD.
- Potential donors who spent a cumulative time of 5 years or more (January 1980 to present) in certain areas of Europe cannot donate blood; blood products from a donor who develops CJD are recalled.

AIDS, acquired immunodeficiency syndrome; HIV, human immunodeficiency virus; HTLV, human T-lymphotropic virus.

Adapted from Katz, L. M., & Dodd, R. Y. (2013). Transfusion-transmitted diseases. In B. A. Shaz, C. D. Hillyer, M. Roshal, et al. (Eds.). *Transfusion medicine and hemostasis: Clinical and laboratory aspects* (2nd ed.). Waltham, MA: Elsevier.

of transmitting Creutzfeldt–Jakob disease may be increased

- A history of untreated syphilis or malaria, because these diseases can be transmitted by transfusion even years later. A person who has been free of symptoms and off therapy for 3 years after malaria may be a donor.
- A history or evidence of drug abuse in which illicit drugs were self-injected, because many IV/injection drug users are carriers of hepatitis and because the risk of HIV is high in this group
- A history of possible exposure to HIV. The population at risk includes people who engage in anal sex, people with multiple sexual partners, IV/injection drug users, sexual partners of people at risk for HIV, and people with hemophilia.
- A skin infection, because of the possibility of contaminating the phlebotomy needle, and subsequently the blood itself
- A recent history of asthma, urticaria, or allergy to medications, because hypersensitivity can be transferred passively to the recipient
- Pregnancy, because of the nutritional demands of pregnancy on the mother
- A history of tooth extraction or oral surgery within 72 hours, because such procedures are frequently associated with transient bacteremia
- A history of untreated exposure to infectious disease within the past 3 weeks, because of the risk of transmission to the recipient
- Recent immunizations, because of the risk of transmitting live organisms (2-week waiting period for live, attenuated organisms; 1 month for rubella, mumps, varicella; 1 year for rabies)
- A history of recent tattoo, because of the risk of blood-borne infections (e.g., hepatitis, HIV)
- Cancer, because of the uncertainty about transmission of the disease. People who have a history of a nonhematologic cancer treated with surgery or radiation and who are without evidence of recurrence for at least 5 years are eligible to donate.
- A diagnosis of hemochromatosis (although this exclusion varies among blood centres)
- A history of whole blood donation within the past 56 days

Potential donors should be asked whether they have consumed any aspirin or aspirin-containing medications within the past 3 days. Although aspirin use does not render the donor ineligible, the platelets obtained may be dysfunctional and therefore not useful; aspirin use within 48 to 72 hours contraindicates platelet donation. Aspirin does not affect the erythrocytes or plasma obtained from the donor.

All donors are expected to meet the following minimal requirements:

- Body weight should exceed 50 kg for a standard 450-mL donation. Donors weighing less than 50 kg donate proportionately less blood. People younger than 17 years of age are disqualified from donation.
- The oral temperature should not exceed 37.5°C.
- The pulse rate should be regular and between 50 and 100 bpm.
- The systolic arterial blood pressure should be 90 to 180 mm Hg, and the diastolic pressure should be 50 to 100 mm Hg.
- The hemoglobin level should be at least 125 g/L for women and 130 for men.

Directed Donation

At times, friends and family of a patient wish to donate blood for that person. These blood donations are termed directed donations. These donations are not any safer than those provided by random donors, because directed donors may not be as willing to identify themselves as having a history of any of the risk factors that disqualify a person from donating blood.

Standard Donation

Phlebotomy consists of venipuncture and blood withdrawal. Standard precautions are used. Donors are placed in a semirecumbent position. The skin over the antecubital fossa is carefully cleansed with an antiseptic preparation, a tourniquet is applied, and venipuncture is performed. Withdrawal of 450 mL of blood usually takes less than 15 minutes. After the needle is removed, donors are asked to hold the involved arm straight up, and firm pressure is applied with sterile gauze for 2 to 3 minutes or until bleeding stops. A firm bandage is then applied. The donor remains recumbent until he or she feels able to sit up, usually within a few minutes. Donors who experience weakness or faintness should rest for a longer period. The donor then receives food and fluids and is asked to remain another 15 minutes.

The donor is instructed to leave the dressing on and to avoid heavy lifting for several hours, to avoid smoking for 1 hour, to avoid drinking alcoholic beverages for 3 hours, to increase fluid intake for 2 days, and to eat healthy meals for at least 2 weeks. Specimens from this donated blood are tested to detect infections and to identify the specific blood type (see later discussion).

Autologous Donation

A patient's own blood may be collected for future transfusion; this method is useful for many elective surgeries where the potential need for transfusion is high (e.g., orthopedic surgery). Preoperative donations are ideally collected 4 to 6 weeks before surgery. Iron supplements are prescribed during this period to prevent depletion of iron stores. Typically, 1 unit of blood is drawn each week; the number of units obtained varies with the type of surgical procedure to be performed (i.e., the amount of blood anticipated to be transfused). Phlebotomies are not performed within 72 hours of surgery. Individual blood components can also be collected.

The primary advantage of autologous transfusions is the prevention of viral infections from another person's blood. Other advantages include safe transfusion for patients with a history of transfusion reactions, prevention of alloimmunization, and avoidance of complications in patients with alloantibodies. Autologous donations are regulated by provincial and territorial policies.

Needless autologous donation (i.e., performed when the likelihood of transfusion is small) is discouraged because it is expensive, takes time, and uses resources inappropriately. Moreover, in an emergency situation, the autologous units available may be inadequate, and the patient may still require additional units from the general donor supply. Furthermore, although autologous transfusion can eliminate the risk of viral contamination, the risk of bacterial contamination is the same as that in transfusion from random donors.

Contraindications to donation of blood for autologous transfusion are acute infection, severely debilitating chronic disease, hemoglobin level less than 1.94 mmol/L, hematocrit less than 38%, unstable angina, and acute cardiovascular or cerebrovascular disease. A history of poorly controlled epilepsy may be considered a contraindication in some centres.

Intraoperative Blood Salvage

This transfusion method provides replacement for patients who cannot donate blood before surgery and for those undergoing vascular, orthopedic, or thoracic surgery. During a surgical procedure, blood lost into a sterile cavity (e.g., hip joint) is suctioned into a cell-saver machine. The whole blood or PRBCs are washed, often with saline solution; filtered; and then returned to the patient as an IV infusion. Salvaged blood cannot be stored, because bacteria cannot be completely removed from the blood and it cannot be used when it is contaminated with bacteria. The use of intraoperative blood salvage has decreased the need for autologous blood donation.

Hemodilution

This transfusion method may be initiated before or after induction of anesthesia. About 1 to 2 units of blood are removed from the patient through a venous or arterial line and simultaneously replaced with a colloid or crystalloid solution. The blood obtained is then reinfused after surgery. The advantage of this method is that the patient loses fewer erythrocytes during surgery, because the added IV solutions dilute the concentration of erythrocytes and lower the hematocrit. However, patients who are at risk for myocardial injury should not be further stressed by hemodilution.

Complications of Blood Donation

Excessive bleeding at the donor's venipuncture site is sometimes caused by a bleeding disorder but more often results from a technique error: laceration of the vein, excessive tourniquet pressure, or failure to apply enough pressure after the needle is withdrawn.

Fainting is common after blood donation and may be related to emotional factors, a vasovagal reaction, or prolonged fasting before donation. Because of the loss of blood volume, hypotension and syncope may occur when the donor assumes an erect position. A donor who appears pale or complains of faintness should immediately lie down or sit with the head lowered below the knees. He or she should be observed for another 30 minutes.

Anginal chest pain may be precipitated in patients with unsuspected coronary artery disease. Seizures can occur in donors with epilepsy, although the incidence is very low. Both angina and seizures require further medical evaluation and treatment.

Blood Processing

Samples of the unit of blood are always taken immediately after donation so that the blood can be typed and tested.

Each donation is tested for antibodies to HIV 1 and 2, hepatitis B core antibody (anti-HBc), hepatitis C virus (HCV), human T-cell lymphotropic virus type I (anti-HTLV-I/II), hepatitis B surface antigen (HbsAG), and syphilis. Negative reactions are required for the blood to be used, and each unit of blood is labelled to certify the results. Nucleic acid amplification testing has increased the ability to detect the presence of HCV, HIV, and West Nile virus infections, because it directly tests for genomic nucleic acids of the viruses rather than for the presence of antibodies to the viruses. This testing significantly shortens the "window" of inability to detect HIV and HCV from a donated unit, further ensuring the safety of the blood; the risk of transmission of HIV or HCV is now very low. Blood is also screened for CMV; if it tests positive for CMV, it can still be used, except in recipients who are negative for CMV and who are immunocompromised (e.g., BMT or HSCT recipients).

Equally important to viral testing is accurate determination of the blood type. More than 200 antigens have been identified on the surface of RBC membranes. Of these, the most important for safe transfusion are the ABO and Rh systems. The ABO system identifies which sugars are present on the membrane of a person's erythrocytes: A, B, both A and B, or neither A nor B (type O). To prevent a significant reaction, the same type of PRBCs should be transfused. Previously, it was thought that in an emergency situation in which the patient's blood type was not known, type O blood could be safely transfused. This practice is no longer recommended.

The Rh antigen (also called D) is present on the surface of erythrocytes in 85% of the population (Rh positive). Those who lack the D antigen are called Rh negative. PRBCs are routinely tested for the D antigen as well as ABO. Patients should receive PRBCs with a compatible Rh type.

The majority of transfusion reactions (other than those due to procedural error) are due to the presence of donor leukocytes within the blood component unit (PRBCs or platelets); the recipient may form antibodies to the antigens present on these leukocytes. PRBC components typically have 1 to 3×10^9 leukocytes remaining in each unit. Leukocytes from the blood product are frequently filtered to diminish the likelihood of developing reactions and refractoriness to transfusions, particularly in patients who have chronic transfusion needs. The process of leukocyte filtration renders the blood component "leukocyte poor" (i.e., leukopoor). Filtration can occur at the time the unit is collected from the donor and processed, which achieves better results but is more expensive, or at the time the blood component is transfused by attaching a leukocyte filter to the blood administration tubing. Many centres advocate routinely using leukopoor filtered blood components for people who have or are likely to develop chronic transfusion requirements.

When a patient is immunocompromised, as in the case of bone or stem cell transplant, any donor lymphocytes must be removed from the blood components. In this situation, the blood component is exposed to low amounts of radiation (25 Gy) that kill any lymphocytes within the blood component. Irradiated blood products are highly effective in preventing transfusion-associated GVHD, which is fatal in most cases. Irradiated blood products have a shorter shelf life.

Transfusion

Administration of blood and blood components requires knowledge of correct administration techniques and possible complications. It is very important to be familiar with the agency's policies and procedures for transfusion therapy. Methods for transfusing blood components are presented in Charts 54-18 and 54-19.

Setting

Most blood transfusions are performed in the acute care setting, and sometimes must be done emergently. However, the processes utilized to ensure safe transfusion of blood cannot be abridged for the sake of rapidity; all procedural details outlined in Chart 54-18 must be followed, including obtaining informed consent (see Chart 54-20).

Patients with chronic transfusion requirements often can receive transfusions in other settings. Freestanding infusion centres, ambulatory care clinics, physicians' offices, and even patients' homes may be appropriate settings for transfusion. Typically, patients who need chronic transfusions but are otherwise stable physically are appropriate candidates for outpatient therapy. Verification and administration of the blood product are performed as in a hospital setting. Although most blood products can be transfused in the outpatient setting, the home is typically limited to transfusions of PRBCs and factor components (e.g., factor VIII for patients with hemophilia).

Pretransfusion Assessment

Patient History

Patient history is an important component of the pretransfusion assessment to determine the history of previous transfusions as well as previous reactions to transfusion. The history should include the type of reaction, its manifestations, the interventions required, and whether any preventive interventions were used in subsequent transfusions. It is important to assess the number of pregnancies a woman has had, because a high number can increase her risk of reaction due to antibodies developed from exposure to fetal circulation. Other concurrent health problems should be noted, with careful attention to cardiac, pulmonary, and vascular disease.

> **NURSING ALERT**
>
> **The nurse should establish a baseline by taking vital signs before the transfusion. Also, written consent to perform the procedure is required.**

Physical Assessment

A systematic physical assessment and measurement of baseline vital signs are important before transfusing any blood product. The respiratory system should be assessed, including careful auscultation of the lungs and the patient's use of accessory muscles. Cardiac system assessment should include careful inspection for any edema as well as other signs of cardiac failure (e.g., jugular venous distention).

CHART 54-18

Transfusion of Packed Red Blood Cells

Preprocedure

1. Confirm that the transfusion has been prescribed.
2. Check that patient's blood has been typed and cross-matched.
3. Verify that patient has signed a written consent form per institution or agency policy and agrees to procedure.
4. Explain procedure to patient. Instruct patient in signs and symptoms of transfusion reaction (itching, hives, swelling, shortness of breath, fever, chills).
5. Take patient's temperature, pulse, respiration, blood pressure and assess fluid volume status (e.g., auscultate lungs, assess for jugular venous distention) to serve as a baseline for comparison during transfusion.
6. Note if signs of increased fluid overload present (e.g., heart failure, see Chapter 31), contact primary provider to discuss potential need for a prescription for diuretic, as warranted.
7. Use hand hygiene and wear gloves in accordance with standard precautions.
8. Use appropriately sized needle for insertion in a peripheral vein.[a] Use special tubing that contains a blood filter to screen out fibrin clots and other particulate matter. Do not vent blood container.

Procedure

1. Obtain packed red blood cells (PRBCs) from the blood bank *after* the IV line is started. (Institution policy may limit release to only 1 unit at a time.)
2. Double-check labels with another nurse or physician to ensure that the ABO group and Rh type agree with the compatibility record. Check to see that number and type on donor blood label and on patient's medical record are correct. Confirm patient's identification by asking the patient's name and checking the identification wristband.
3. Check blood for gas bubbles and any unusual colour or cloudiness. (Gas bubbles may indicate bacterial growth. Abnormal colour or cloudiness may be a sign of hemolysis.)
4. Make sure that PRBC transfusion is initiated within 30 minutes after removal of PRBCs from blood bank refrigerator.
5. For the first 15 minutes, run the transfusion slowly—no faster than 5 mL/min. Observe patient carefully for adverse effects. If no adverse effects occur during the first 15 minutes, increase the flow rate unless patient is at high risk for circulatory overload.
6. Monitor closely for 15–30 minutes to detect signs of reaction. Monitor vital signs at regular intervals per institution or agency policy; compare results with baseline measurements. Increase frequency of measurements based on patient's condition. Observe patient frequently throughout the transfusion for any signs of adverse reaction, including restlessness, hives, nausea, vomiting, torso or back pain, shortness of breath, flushing, hematuria, fever, or chills. Should any adverse reaction occur, stop infusion immediately, notify primary provider, and follow the agency's transfusion reaction standard.
7. Note that administration time does not exceed 4 hours because of increased risk of bacterial proliferation.
8. Be alert for signs of adverse reactions: circulatory overload, sepsis, febrile reaction, allergic reaction, and acute hemolytic reaction.
9. Change blood tubing after every 2 units transfused to decrease chance of bacterial contamination.

Postprocedure

1. Obtain vital signs and breath sounds; compare with baseline measurements. If signs of increased fluid overload present (e.g., heart failure, see Chapter 31), consider obtaining prescription for diuretic as warranted.
2. Dispose of used materials properly.
3. Document procedure in patient's medical record, including patient assessment findings and tolerance to procedure.
4. Monitor patient for response to and effectiveness of procedure. If patient is at risk, monitor for at least 6 hours for signs of transfusion-associated circulatory overload (TACO); also monitor for signs of delayed hemolytic reaction.

Note: Never add medications to blood or blood products; if blood is too thick to run freely, normal saline may be added to the unit. If blood must be warmed, use an in-line blood warmer with a monitoring system. Adapted from Gorski, L., Hadaway, L., Hagle, M., et al. (2016). Infusion therapy: Standards of practice. *Journal of Infusion Nursing, 39*(1S), S135–S137; Stupnyckyj, C., Smolarek, S., Reeves, C., et al. (2014). Changing blood transfusion policy and practice. *The American Journal of Nursing, 114*(12), 50–59.

[a]Most policies stipulate using an IV with a minimum of 20 gauge. A recent evidence-based synthesis did not find increased hemolysis when packed red cells are infused through a small-gauge needle (Stupnyckyj, Smolarek, Reeves, et al., 2014).

The skin should be observed for rashes, petechiae, and ecchymoses. The sclera should be examined for icterus. In the event of a transfusion reaction, a comparison of findings can help differentiate between types of reactions.

Patient Education

Reviewing the signs and symptoms of a transfusion reaction is crucial for patients who have not received a previous transfusion. Even for patients who have received prior transfusions, a brief review of the signs and symptoms of transfusion reactions is advised. Signs and symptoms of a reaction include fever, chills, respiratory distress, low back pain, nausea, pain at the IV site, or anything "unusual." Although a thorough review is very important, it is also important to reassure the patient that the blood is carefully tested against the patient's own blood (cross-matched) to diminish the likelihood of any untoward reaction. Similarly, the patient can be reassured about the very low possibility of contracting HIV from the transfusion; this fear persists among many people.

Complications

Any patient who receives a blood transfusion may develop complications from that transfusion. When explaining the reasons for the transfusion, it is important to include the risks and benefits and what to expect during and after the transfusion. Patients must be informed that, although it has been tested carefully, the supply of blood is not

CHART 54-19

Transfusion of Platelets or Fresh-Frozen Plasma

Preprocedure

1. Confirm that the transfusion has been prescribed.
2. Verify that patient has signed a written consent form per institution or agency policy and agrees to procedure.
3. Explain procedure to patient. Instruct patient in signs and symptoms of transfusion reaction (itching, hives, swelling, shortness of breath, fever, chills).
4. Take patient's temperature, pulse, respiration, blood pressure, and assess fluid status, and auscultate breath sounds to establish a baseline for comparison during transfusion.
5. Note if signs of increased fluid overload present (e.g., heart failure, see Chapter 31), contact primary provider to discuss potential need for a prescription for diuretic, as warranted; this is particularly important when plasma is also infused.
6. Use hand hygiene and wear gloves in accordance with standard precautions.
7. Use a 22-gauge or larger needle for placement in a large vein, if possible. Use appropriate tubing per institution policy (platelets often require different tubing from that used for other blood products).

Procedure

1. Obtain platelets or fresh-frozen plasma (FFP) from the blood bank (only *after* the IV line is started).
2. Double-check labels with another nurse or physician to ensure that the ABO group matches the compatibility record (not usually necessary for platelets; here only if compatible platelets are ordered). Check to see that the number and type on donor blood label and on patient's medical record are correct. Confirm patient's identification by asking the patient's name and checking the identification wristband.
3. Check blood product for any unusual colour or clumps (excessive redness indicates contamination with larger amounts of red blood cells).
4. Make sure that platelets or FFP units are given immediately after they are obtained.
5. Infuse each unit of FFP over 30–60 minutes per patient tolerance; be prepared to infuse at a significantly lower rate in the context of fluid overload. Infuse each unit of platelets as fast as patient can tolerate to diminish platelet clumping during administration. Observe patient carefully for adverse effects, especially circulatory overload. Decrease rate of infusion if necessary.
6. Observe patient closely throughout transfusion for any signs of adverse reaction, including restlessness, hives, nausea, vomiting, torso or back pain, shortness of breath, flushing, hematuria, fever, or chills. Should any adverse reaction occur, stop infusion immediately, notify primary provider, and follow the agency's transfusion reaction standard.
7. Monitor vital signs at the end of transfusion per institution policy; compare results with baseline measurements.
8. Flush line with saline after transfusion to remove blood component from tubing.

Postprocedure

1. Obtain vital signs and auscultate breath sounds; compare with baseline measurements. If signs of increased fluid overload present, consider obtaining prescription for diuretic, as warranted.
2. Dispose of used materials properly.
3. Document procedure in patient's medical record, including patient assessment findings and tolerance to procedure.
4. Monitor patient for response to and effectiveness of procedure. A platelet count may be ordered 1 hour after platelet transfusion to facilitate this evaluation.
5. If patient is at risk for transfusion-associated circulatory overload (TACO), monitor closely for 6 hours after transfusion if possible.

Note: FFP requires ABO but not Rh compatibility. Platelets are not typically cross-matched for ABO compatibility. Never add medications to blood or blood products.

completely risk-free. Nursing management is directed toward preventing complications, promptly recognizing complications if they develop, and promptly initiating measures to control complications. The following sections describe the most common or potentially severe transfusion-related complications.

Febrile Nonhemolytic Reaction

A febrile nonhemolytic reaction is caused by antibodies to donor leukocytes that remain in the unit of blood or blood component; it is the most common type of transfusion reaction, accounting for more than 90% of reactions. It occurs more frequently in patients who have had previous transfusions (exposure to multiple antigens from previous blood products) and in Rh-negative women who have borne Rh-positive children (exposure to an Rh-positive fetus raises antibody levels in the untreated mother). These reactions occur in 3% of PRBC transfusions and 20% of platelet transfusions. More than 10% of patients with chronic transfusion requirements develop this type of reaction.

The diagnosis of a febrile nonhemolytic reaction is made by excluding other potential causes, such as a hemolytic reaction or bacterial contamination of the blood product. The signs and symptoms of a febrile nonhemolytic transfusion reaction are chills (minimal to severe) followed by fever (more than 1°C elevation). The fever typically begins within 2 hours after the transfusion is begun. Although the reaction is not life-threatening, the fever, and particularly the chills and muscle stiffness, can be frightening to the patient.

This reaction can be diminished, even prevented, by further depleting the blood component of donor leukocytes; this is accomplished by a leukocyte reduction filter. Antipyretics can be given to prevent fever, but routine premedication is not advised because it can mask the beginning of a more serious transfusion reaction.

Acute Hemolytic Reaction

The most dangerous, and potentially life-threatening, type of transfusion reaction occurs when the donor blood is incompatible with that of the recipient. Antibodies already present in the recipient's plasma rapidly combine with antigens on donor erythrocytes, and the erythrocytes are destroyed in the circulation (i.e., intravascular hemolysis).

CHART 54-20

Ethical Dilemma: What If the Patient Does Not Consent to Blood Transfusions?

Case Scenario

An 18-year-old male is admitted with severe bleeding due to a stab wound. The surgeon states that the patient will need to receive several units of blood products to stabilize him. When he is presented with the informed consent, he refuses to sign because of his religious convictions. The surgeon states, "If you were my son, I would insist that you sign." His mother is adamant that he receives the blood, because the surgeon has told her that her son will likely die of his injuries without the transfusions. The patient acknowledges that he fully understands the consequences of his failure to consent and refuses. The patient dies as a result of hypovolemic shock.

Discussion

A patient's religious and cultural beliefs may significantly impact their decision whether to consent to a procedure such as a blood transfusion. Differences in moral perspectives can complicate the provision of quality nursing care. The patient who has mental capacity, is fully informed of the benefits and risks of a procedure, and is at least 18 years of age has the right to sign or refuse to sign an informed consent. In this particular case scenario, although his mother and the surgeon know his decision to refuse blood products will likely end in his death, only the patient has the autonomy to make this decision, regardless of his young age. The nurse should support the autonomous decision that the patient makes, even when his decision to refuse blood transfusions may cause the nurse to experience moral distress.

Analysis

- Describe the ethical principles that are in conflict in this case (see Chart 3-3). Which principle should have preeminence when you obtain informed consent from patients?
- Discuss the surgeon's response to the patient's decision as it relates to coercion and paternalism.
- How might the nurse respond to this patient and his family in an ethically sensitive and responsive manner?
- What resources would you utilize in this situation that would meet the needs of the patient and his family?

Resources

See Chapter 3, Chart 3-3 for ethics resources.

Adapted from Pavlish, C., Brown-Saltzman, K., Jakel, P., et al. (2014). The nature of ethical conflicts and the meaning of moral community in oncology practice. *Oncology Nursing Forum*, *41*(2), 130–140.

The most rapid hemolysis occurs in ABO incompatibility. This reaction can occur after transfusion of as little as 10 mL of PRBCs. Rh incompatibility often causes a less severe reaction. The most common causes of acute hemolytic reaction are errors in blood component labelling and patient identification that result in the administration of an ABO-incompatible transfusion.

Symptoms consist of fever, chills, low back pain, nausea, chest tightness, dyspnea, and anxiety. As the erythrocytes are destroyed, the hemoglobin is released from the cells and excreted by the kidneys; therefore, hemoglobin appears in the urine (hemoglobinuria). Hypotension, bronchospasm, and vascular collapse may result. Diminished renal perfusion results in acute renal failure, and DIC may also occur.

The reaction must be recognized promptly and the transfusion discontinued immediately. Blood and urine specimens must be obtained and analyzed for evidence of hemolysis. Treatment goals include maintaining blood volume and renal perfusion and preventing and managing DIC.

Acute hemolytic transfusion reactions are preventable. Meticulous attention to detail in labelling blood samples and blood components and accurately identifying the recipient cannot be overemphasized.

Allergic Reaction

Some patients develop urticaria (hives) or generalized itching during a transfusion. The cause of these reactions is thought to be a sensitivity reaction to a plasma protein within the blood component being transfused. Symptoms of an allergic reaction are urticaria, itching, and flushing. The reactions are usually mild and respond to antihistamines. If the symptoms resolve after administration of an antihistamine (e.g., diphenhydramine [Benadryl]), the transfusion may be resumed. Rarely, the allergic reaction is severe, with bronchospasm, laryngeal edema, and shock. These reactions are managed with epinephrine, corticosteroids, and vasopressor support, if necessary.

Giving the patient antihistamines before the transfusion may prevent future reactions. For severe reactions, future blood components are washed to remove any remaining plasma proteins. Leukocyte filters are not useful to prevent such reactions, because the offending plasma proteins can pass through the filter.

Transfusion-Associated Circulatory Overload (TACO)

If too much blood is infused too quickly, hypervolemia can occur. This condition can be aggravated in patients who already have increased circulatory volume (e.g., those with heart failure, renal dysfunction, advanced age, acute myocardial infarction) (Alam, Lin, Lima, et al., 2013). A careful assessment for signs of circulatory overload or positive fluid status prior to initiating the transfusion is required, particularly in those individuals at risk for developing transfusion-related acute lung injury (TRALI). PRBCs are safer to use than whole blood. If the administration rate is sufficiently slow, circulatory overload may be prevented. For patients who are at risk for, or already in, circulatory overload, diuretics are given prior to the transfusion or between units of PRBCs. Patients receiving fresh-frozen plasma or even platelets may also develop circulatory overload. The infusion rate of these blood components must also be titrated to the patient's tolerance. Rates of transfusion may need to decrease to less than 100 to 120 mL/hr (Alam et al., 2013).

Signs of circulatory overload include dyspnea, orthopnea, tachycardia, an increase in blood pressure, and sudden anxiety. Jugular vein distention, crackles at the base of the lungs, and hypoxemia will also develop. Pulmonary edema can quickly develop, as manifested by severe dyspnea and coughing of pink, frothy sputum.

If fluid overload is mild, the transfusion can often be continued after slowing the rate of infusion and administering diuretics. However, if the overload is severe, the patient is placed upright with the feet in a dependent position, the transfusion is discontinued, and the primary provider is notified. The IV line is kept patent with a very slow infusion of normal saline solution or a saline lock device to maintain access to the vein in case IV medications are necessary. Oxygen and morphine may be needed to treat severe dyspnea (see Chapter 31).

TACO can develop as late as 6 hours after transfusion (Alam et al., 2013). Therefore, patients need close monitoring after the transfusion is completed, particularly those who are at higher risk for developing this complication (e.g., older adults, those with a positive fluid balance prior to transfusion, patients with renal dysfunction, patients with left ventricular dysfunction). Monitoring vital signs, auscultating breath sounds, and assessing for jugular venous distention should be included in patient monitoring.

Bacterial Contamination

The incidence of bacterial contamination of blood components is very low; however, administration of contaminated products puts the patient at great risk. Contamination can occur at any point during procurement or processing but often results from organisms on the donor's skin. Many bacteria cannot survive in the cold temperatures used to store PRBCs, but some organisms can do so. Platelets are at greater risk of contamination because they are stored at room temperature. Recently, blood centres have developed rapid methods of culturing platelet units, thereby diminishing the risk of using a contaminated platelet unit for transfusion.

Preventive measures include meticulous care in the procurement and processing of blood components. When PRBCs or whole blood is transfused, it should be administered within a 4-hour period, because warm room temperatures promote bacterial growth. A contaminated unit of blood product may appear normal, or it may have an abnormal colour.

The signs of bacterial contamination are fever, chills, and hypotension. These signs may not occur until the transfusion is complete, occasionally not until several hours after the transfusion. If the condition is not treated immediately with fluids and broad-spectrum antibiotics, septic shock can occur. Even with aggressive management, including vasopressor support, the mortality rate is high.

As soon as the reaction is recognized, any remaining transfusion is discontinued, and the IV line is kept open with normal saline solution. The physician and the blood bank are notified, and the blood container is returned to the blood bank for testing and culture. Sepsis is treated with IV fluids and antibiotics; corticosteroids and vasopressors are often also necessary (see Chapter 18).

Transfusion-Related Acute Lung Injury (TRALI)

TRALI is a potentially fatal, idiosyncratic reaction that is defined as the development of acute lung injury occurring within 6 hours after the blood transfusion. All blood components have been implicated in TRALI, including IVIG, cryoprecipitate, and stem cells. TRALI is the most common cause of transfusion-related death (Alam et al., 2013).

The underlying pathophysiologic mechanism for TRALI is unknown but is thought to involve specific human leukocyte antigen (HLA) or human neutrophil antigen (HNA) antibodies in the donor's plasma that react to the leukocytes in the recipient's blood. Occasionally, the reverse occurs, and antibodies present in the recipient's plasma agglutinate the antigens on the few remaining leukocytes in the blood component being transfused. Another theory suggests that an initial insult to the patient's vascular endothelium can predispose the neutrophils to aggregate at the injured endothelium. Various substances within the transfused blood component (lipids, cytokines) then activate these neutrophils. Each of these pathophysiologic mechanisms can contribute to the process. The end result of this process is interstitial and intra-alveolar edema, as well as extensive sequestration of WBCs within the pulmonary capillaries (Bockhold & Crumpler, 2015).

Onset is abrupt (usually within 6 hours of transfusion, often within 2 hours). Signs and symptoms include acute shortness of breath, hypoxia (arterial oxygen saturation [SaO_2] less than 90%; partial pressure of arterial oxygen [PaO_2] to fraction of inspired oxygen [FIO_2] ratio of less than 300), hypotension, fever, and eventual pulmonary edema. Diagnostic criteria include hypoxemia, bilateral pulmonary infiltrates (seen on chest x-ray), no evidence of cardiac cause for the pulmonary edema, and no other plausible alternative cause within 6 hours of completing transfusion. Aggressive supportive therapy (e.g., oxygen, intubation, fluid support) may prevent death. Immunologic therapy (e.g., corticosteroids) has not been shown to be effective in this setting; diuretics can worsen the situation (Bockhold & Crumpler, 2015; Kenz & van der Linden, 2014).

Although TRALI can occur with the transfusion of any blood component, it is more likely to occur when plasma and, to a lesser extent, platelets are transfused. One commonly used preventive strategy involves limiting the frequency and amount of blood products transfused. Another entails obtaining plasma and possibly platelets only from men because women who have been pregnant may have developed offending antibodies. A third strategy involves screening donors for the presence of these antibodies and discarding any plasma-containing blood products from those donors who screen positive. The efficacy of these approaches in preventing TRALI remains unclear (Alam et al., 2013).

Delayed Hemolytic Reaction

Delayed hemolytic reactions usually occur within 14 days after transfusion, when the level of antibody has been increased to the extent that a reaction can occur. The hemolysis of the erythrocytes is extravascular via the RES and occurs gradually.

Signs and symptoms of delayed hemolytic reactions are fever, anemia, increased bilirubin level, decreased or absent haptoglobin, and possibly jaundice. Rarely, there is hemoglobinuria. Generally, these reactions are not dangerous, but it is important to recognize them, because subsequent transfusions with blood products containing these antibodies may cause a more severe hemolytic reaction. However, recognition is also difficult, because the patient may not be in a health care setting to be tested for this reaction, and even if the patient is hospitalized, the reaction may be too mild to be recognized clinically. Because the amount of antibody present can be too low to detect, it is difficult to prevent delayed hemolytic reactions. Fortunately, the reaction is usually mild and requires no intervention.

Disease Acquisition

Despite advances in donor screening and blood testing, certain diseases can still be transmitted by transfusion of blood components (see Chart 54-17).

Complications of Long-Term Transfusion Therapy

The complications that have been described represent a real risk to any patient any time a blood component is administered. However, patients with long-term transfusion requirements (e.g., those with MDS, thalassemia, aplastic anemia, sickle cell anemia) are at greater risk for infection transmission and for becoming more sensitized to donor antigens, simply because they are exposed to more units of blood and, consequently, more donors. A summary of complications associated with long-term transfusion therapy is given in Table 54-16.

Iron overload is a complication unique to people who have had long-term PRBC transfusions. One unit of PRBCs contains 250 mg of iron. Patients with chronic transfusion requirements can quickly acquire more iron than they can use, leading to iron overload. Over time, the excess iron deposits in body tissues and can cause organ damage, particularly in the liver, heart, testes, and pancreas. Promptly initiating a program of iron chelation therapy can prevent end-organ damage from iron toxicity (see Myelodysplastic Syndrome, Nursing Management, and Hereditary Hemochromatosis, Nursing Management).

Nursing Management for Transfusion Reactions

If a transfusion reaction is suspected, the transfusion must be immediately stopped and the physician notified. A thorough patient assessment is crucial, because many complications have similar signs and symptoms. The following steps are taken to determine the type and severity of the reaction:

- Stop the transfusion. Maintain the IV line with normal saline solution through new IV tubing, administered at a slow rate.
- Assess the patient carefully. Compare the vital signs with baseline, including oxygen saturation. Assess the patient's respiratory status carefully. Note the presence of adventitious breath sounds, use of accessory muscles, extent of dyspnea, and changes in mental status, including anxiety and confusion. Note any chills, diaphoresis, jugular vein distention, and reports of back pain or urticaria.
- Notify the physician of the assessment findings, and implement any treatments prescribed. Continue to monitor the patient's vital signs and respiratory, cardiovascular, and renal status.
- Notify the blood bank that a suspected transfusion reaction has occurred.
- Send the blood container and tubing to the blood bank for repeat typing and culture. The identifying tags and numbers are verified.

If a hemolytic transfusion reaction or bacterial infection is suspected, the nurse does the following:

- Obtains appropriate blood specimens from the patient
- Collects a urine sample as soon as possible to detect hemoglobin in the urine
- Documents the reaction according to the institution's policy

TABLE 54-16 Common Complications Resulting From Long-Term Packed Red Blood Cell Transfusion Therapy[a]

Complication	Manifestation	Management
Infection	Hepatitis (B, C)	May immunize against hepatitis B; treat hepatitis C; monitor hepatic function
	CMV	WBC filters to protect against CMV
Iron overload	Heart failure	Prevent by chelation therapy
	Endocrine failure (diabetes, hypothyroidism, hypoparathyroidism, hypogonadism)	
Transfusion reaction	Sensitization	Diminish by RBC phenotyping, using WBC-filtered products
	Febrile reactions	Diminish by using WBC-filtered products

[a]Patients with long-term transfusion therapy requirements are at risk not only for the transfusion reactions discussed in the text but also for the complications noted in the table. In many cases, the use of WBC-filtered (i.e., leukocyte-poor) blood products is standard for patients who receive long-term packed RBC transfusion therapy. An aggressive chelation program initiated early in the course of therapy can prevent problems with iron overload.

CMV, cytomegalovirus; WBC, white blood cell; RBC, red blood cell.

Adapted from McCullough, J., Refaai, M. A., & Cohn, C. S. (2015). Blood procurement and red cell transfusion. In K. Kaushansky, M. Lichtman, J. Prchal, et al. (Eds.). *Williams hematology* (9th ed.). New York: McGraw-Hill.

CHART 54-21

Pharmacology: Pharmacologic Alternatives to Blood Transfusions

Growth Factors

Recombinant technology has provided a means to produce hematopoietic growth factors necessary for the production of blood cells within the bone marrow. By increasing the body's production of blood cells, transfusions and complications resulting from diminished blood cells (e.g., infection from neutropenia) may be avoided. However, the successful use of growth factors requires functional bone marrow. Moreover, the safety of these products has been questioned, and the U.S. Food and Drug Administration is limiting their use in some patient populations.

Erythropoietin

Erythropoietin (epoetin alfa [Epogen, Procrit]; darbopoietin [Aranesp]) is an effective alternative treatment for patients with chronic anemia secondary to diminished levels of erythropoietin, as in chronic renal disease. This medication stimulates erythropoiesis. It also has been used for patients who are anemic from chemotherapy or zidovudine (AZT) therapy and for those who have diseases involving bone marrow suppression, such as myelodysplastic syndrome (MDS). The use of erythropoietin can also enable a patient to donate several units of blood for future use (e.g., preoperative autologous donation). The medication can be administered IV or subcutaneously, although plasma levels are better sustained with the subcutaneous route. Side effects are rare, but erythropoietin can cause or exacerbate hypertension. If the anemia is corrected too quickly or is overcorrected, the elevated hematocrit can cause headache and, potentially, seizures. Thrombosis has been noted in some patients whose hemoglobins were raised to a high level; thus, it is recommended that a target hemoglobin level of less than 12 g/dL be used. These adverse effects are rare except for patients with renal failure. Serial complete blood counts (CBCs) must be performed to evaluate the response to the medication. The dose and frequency of administration are titrated to the hemoglobin level.

Granulocyte Colony-Stimulating Factor (G-CSF)

G-CSF (filgrastim [Neupogen, Zarxio, Granix]) is a cytokine that stimulates the proliferation and differentiation of myeloid stem cells; a rapid increase in neutrophils is seen within the circulation. G-CSF is effective in improving transient but severe neutropenia after chemotherapy or in some forms of MDS. It is particularly useful in preventing bacterial infections that would be likely to occur with neutropenia. G-CSF is given subcutaneously on a daily basis. The primary side effect is bone pain; this probably reflects the increase in hematopoiesis within the marrow. Serial CBCs should be performed to evaluate the response to the medication and to ensure that the rise in white blood cells is not excessive. The effect of G-CSF on myelopoiesis is short; the neutrophil count drops once the medication is stopped.

Granulocyte-Macrophage Colony-Stimulating Factor (GM-CSF)

GM-CSF (sargramostim [Leukine]) is a cytokine that is naturally produced by a variety of cells, including monocytes and endothelial cells. It works either directly or synergistically with other growth factors to stimulate myelopoiesis. GM-CSF is not as specific to neutrophils as is G-CSF; thus, an increase in erythroid (red blood cell) and megakaryocytic (platelet) production may also be seen. GM-CSF serves the same purpose as G-CSF. However, it may have a greater effect on macrophage function and therefore may be more useful against fungal infections, whereas G-CSF may be better used to fight bacterial infections. GM-CSF is also given subcutaneously. Side effects include bone pain, fevers, and myalgias.

Thrombopoietin

Thrombopoietin (TPO) is a cytokine that is necessary for the proliferation of megakaryocytes and subsequent platelet formation. Nonimmunogenic second-generation thrombopoietic growth factors (romiplostim [Nplate]; eltrombopag [Promacta]) are used for the treatment of idiopathic thrombocytopenic purpura. Eltrombopag is also approved for use in certain situations for patients with aplastic anemia and in patients requiring hepatitis C treatment that can cause significant thrombocytopenia.

Adapted from Seeber, P., & Shander, A. (2012a). Anemia therapy I: Erythropoiesis-stimulating agents. In P. Seeber & A. Shander (Eds.). *Basics of blood management* (2nd ed.). Oxford, UK: Wiley-Blackwell; Seeber, P., & Shander, A. (2012b). Growth factors. In P. Seeber & A. Shander (Eds.). *Basics of blood management* (2nd ed.). Oxford, UK: Wiley-Blackwell.

Pharmacologic Alternatives to Blood Transfusions

Pharmacologic agents that stimulate the production of one or more types of blood cells by the marrow are commonly used (see Chart 54-21). Researchers continue to seek a blood substitute that is practical and safe. Manufacturing artificial blood is problematic, given the myriad functions of blood components. Currently, there are two types of products in development: hemoglobin-based oxygen carriers and perfluorocarbons (which have great ability to dissolve gases and thus carry oxygen indirectly) (Goodnough & Shander, 2013; van Veen & Hunt, 2015). None of these products are available for use in the United States (Tao & Ghoroghchian, 2014).

Hematopoietic Stem Cell Transplantation and Bone Marrow Transplantation

HSCT and BMT are therapeutic modalities that offer the possibility of cure for some patients with hematologic disorders such as severe aplastic anemia, some forms of leukemia, and thalassemia.

Critical Thinking Exercises

1 You are working in a hematology-oncology clinic. The laboratory reports a critical laboratory result for one of your patients with possible MDS: The leukocyte count is 1,800/mm^3 with 40% neutrophils. What other laboratory results would be important to review or consider? The patient is also anemic (hemoglobin 8.2 mg/dL) and platelets are 65,000/mm^3. What observations will you include in your assessment of this patient? Determine the extent to which this patient is neutropenic. What medical treatments would you anticipate? How would you educate the patient about neutropenia precautions? What evidence exists to support your educational interventions? What is the strength of that evidence?

2 You are caring for a 32-year-old woman who has had repeated hospitalizations for sickle cell crisis. What is the evidence base that indicates which factors should be assessed to determine the patient's educational, coping, and pain management needs? What is the strength of that evidence? Identify the evidence base that supports concepts that you will incorporate into the patient's discharge plan.

3 A 63-year-old man presents to the emergency department with unilateral swelling and pain of the left lower extremity. He reports this is the third time he has had a blood clot (DVT). How would you determine if he is at risk for having a hypercoagulable disorder? What would you include in your history to help you? How would you respond if he asks you if he will "ever get off Coumadin"? What would you include in your patient education to aid him in adhering to lifelong anticoagulation? What would your interventions be to decrease the risk of postphlebitic syndrome?

4 You are caring for a patient who is septic and is now receiving a transfusion of 2 units of PRBCs. The patient's temperature spikes to 38.5°C (101.3°F) after half of the second unit has been transfused. What are the possible causes of the fever? How would you differentiate the cause as sepsis versus a transfusion reaction? What are the appropriate nursing interventions? What are the potential causes of transfusion reaction? How are they manifested?

REFERENCES AND SELECTED READINGS

Books

Adamson, J. W. (2015). Iron deficiency and other hypoproliferative anemias. In D. Kasper, A. Fauci, S. Hauser, et al. (Eds.). *Harrison's principles of internal medicine* (19th ed.). Retrieved September 13, 2015, from accessmedicine.mhmedical.com.laneproxy.stanford.edu/content.aspx?bookid=1130&Sectionid=79731112

Adamson, J. W., & Longo, D. L. (2015). Anemia and polycythemia. In D. Kasper, A. Fauci, S. Hauser, et al. (Eds.). *Harrison's principles of internal medicine* (19th ed.). Retrieved September 22, 2015, from accessmedicine.mhmedical.com.laneproxy.stanford.edu/content.aspx?bookid=1130&Sectionid=79727787

American Nurses Association (ANA). (2015). *Code of ethics for nurses with interpretive statements*. Washington, DC: Nursesbooks.org.

Awan, F. T., & Byrd, J. C. (2016). Chronic lymphocytic leukemia. In K. Kaushansky, M. A. Lichtman, J. T. Prchal, et al. (Eds.). *Williams hematology* (9th ed.). New York: McGraw-Hill.

Bunn, H. (2017). Overview of the anemias. In J. C. Aster, & H. Bunn (Eds.). *Pathophysiology of blood disorders* (2nd ed.). New York: McGraw-Hill. Retrieved October 25, 2016, from accessmedicine.mhmedical.com.laneproxy.stanford.edu/content.aspx?bookid=1900&Sectionid=137394689

Butterworth, J. F., Mackey, D. C., & Wasnick, J. D. (2013). Fluid management & blood component therapy. In J. F. Butterworth IV, D. C. Mackey, & J. D. Wasnick (Eds.). *Morgan & Mikhail's clinical anesthesiology* (5th ed.). Retrieved September 15, 2015, from accessmedicine.mhmedical.com.laneproxy.stanford.edu/content.aspx?bookid=564&Sectionid=42800585

Canadian Cancer Society's Advisory Committee on Cancer Statistics. *Canadian Cancer Statistics 2013*. Toronto, ON: Author. Retrieved from http://www.cancer.ca/~/media/cancer.ca/CW/cancer%20information/cancer%20101/Canadian%20cancer%20statistics/canadian-cancer-statistics-2013-EN.pdf

Dale, D.C., & Welte, K. (2016). Neutropenia and neutrophilia. In K. Kaushansky, M. A. Lichtman, J. T. Prchal, et al. (Eds.). *Williams hematology* (9th ed.). New York: McGraw-Hill Medical.

Davoren, J. B., & Wang, S. (2013). Blood disorders. In G. D. Hammer & S. J. McPhee (Eds.). *Pathophysiology of disease: An introduction to clinical medicine* (7th ed.). Retrieved September 13, 2015, from accessmedicine.mhmedical.com.laneproxy.stanford.edu/content.aspx?bookid=961&Sectionid=53555687

Diz-Küçükkaya, R., & López, J. (2016). Thrombocytopenia. In K. Kaushansky, M. A. Lichtman, J. T. Prchal, et al. (Eds.). *Williams hematology* (9th ed.). New York: McGraw-Hill Medical.

Doherty, G. M. (Ed.) (2015). *Spleen. Current diagnosis & treatment: Surgery* (14th ed.). Retrieved September 13, 2015, from accessmedicine.mhmedical.com.laneproxy.stanford.edu/content.aspx?bookid=1202&Sectionid=71521945

Dzieczkowski, J. S., & Anderson, K. C. (2015). Transfusion biology and therapy. In D. Kasper, A. Fauci, S. Hauser, et al. (Eds.). *Harrison's principles of internal medicine* (19th ed.). Retrieved May 25, 2016, from accessmedicine.mhmedical.com.laneproxy.stanford.edu/content.aspx?bookid=1130&Sectionid=79732248

Escobar, M. A., & Key, N. S. (2016). Hemophilia A and hemophilia B. In K. Kaushansky, M. A. Lichtman, J. T. Prchal, et al. (Eds.). *Williams hematology* (9th ed.). New York: McGraw-Hill Medical.

Fakih, R., Shah, N., & Nieto, Y. (2016). Autologous hematopoietic progenitor cell transplantation. In H. M. Kantarjian & R. A. Wolff (Eds.). *The MD Anderson manual of medical oncology* (3rd ed.). Retrieved May 25, 2016, from accessmedicine.mhmedical.com.laneproxy.stanford.edu/content.aspx?bookid=1772&Sectionid=121897865.

Ferri, F. F. (2014). *Ferri's clinical advisor*. Philadelphia, PA: Mosby.

Fischbach, F. T., & Dunning, M. B. (2009). *A manual of laboratory and diagnostic tests* (8th ed.). Philadelphia, PA: Lippincott Williams & Wilkins.

Fischbach, F., & Dunning, M. (2015). *A manual of laboratory and diagnostic tests*. (9th ed.). Philadelphia, PA: Lippincott Williams & Wilkins.

Ganz, T. (2016a). Anemia of chronic disease. In K. Kaushansky, M. A. Lichtman, J. T. Prchal, et al. (Eds.). *Williams hematology* (9th ed.). New York: McGraw-Hill Medical.

Ganz, T. (2016b). Iron deficiency and overload. In K. Kaushansky, M. A. Lichtman, J. T. Prchal, et al. (Eds.). *Williams hematology* (9th ed.). New York: McGraw-Hill Medical.

Goroll, A. H., & Mulley, A. G. (Eds.). (2014a). Approach to the patient with heartburn and reflux (gastroesophageal disease). In *Primary care medicine: Office evaluation and management of the adult patient*. Philadelphia, PA: Lippincott Williams & Wilkins.

Goroll, A. H., & Mulley, A. G. (Eds.) (2014b). Evaluation of anemia. In *Primary care medicine: Office evaluation and management of the adult patient*. Philadelphia, PA: Lippincott Williams & Wilkins.

Green, R. (2016). Folate, cobalamin, and megaloblastic anemias. In K. Kaushansky, M. A. Lichtman, J. T. Prchal, et al. (Eds.). *Williams hematology* (9th ed.). New York: McGraw-Hill Medical.

Henry, P. H., & Longo, D. L. (2015). Enlargement of lymph nodes and spleen. In D. Kasper, A. Fauci, S. Hauser, et al. (Eds.). *Harrison's principles of internal medicine* (19th ed.) Retrieved May 5, 25, 2016, from accessmedicine.mhmedical.com.laneproxy.stanford.edu/content.aspx?bookid=1130&Sectionid=7973242

Hoffbrand, A. V., & Pettit, J. E. (2009). *Color atlas of clinical hematology* (4th ed.). Philadelphia, PA: Mosby.

Hoffman, R. (2008). *Hematology: Basic principles and practice* (5th ed.). Philadelphia, PA: Churchill Livingstone/Elsevier.

Katz, L. M., & Dodd, R. Y. (2013). Transfusion-transmitted diseases. In B. A. Shaz, C. D. Hillyer, M. Roshal, et al. (Eds.). *Transfusion medicine and hemostasis: Clinical and laboratory aspects* (2nd ed.). Waltham, MA: Elsevier.

Kaushansky, K. (2016). Reactive thrombocytosis. In K. Kaushansky, M. A. Lichtman, J. T. Prchal, et al. (Eds.). *Williams hematology* (9th ed.). New York: McGraw-Hill Medical.

Konkle, B. A. (2015). Disorders of platelets and vessel wall. In D. Kasper, A. Fauci, S. Hauser, et al. (Eds.). *Harrison's principles of internal medicine* (19th ed.). Retrieved September 13, 2015, from accessmedicine.mhmedical.com.laneproxy.stanford.edu/content.aspx?bookid=1130&Sectionid=7973242

Larson, R. A., & Richard, L. M. (2016). Acute lymphoblastic leukemia. In K. Kaushansky, M. A. Lichtman, J. T. Prchal, et al. (Eds.). *Williams hematology* (9th ed.). New York: McGraw-Hill.

Levi, M., & Seligsohn, U. (2016). Disseminated intravascular coagulation. In K. Kaushansky, M. A. Lichtman, J. T. Prchal, et al. (Eds.). *Williams hematology* (9th ed.). New York: McGraw-Hill Medical.

Levi, M., Seligsohn, U., & Kaushansky, K. (2016). Classification, clinical manifestations, and evaluation of disorders of hemostasis. In K. Kaushansky, M. A. Lichtman, J. T. Prchal, et al. (Eds.). *Williams hematology* (9th ed.). New York: McGraw-Hill Medical.

Lichtman, M. A., & Prchal, J. T. (2016). Primary myelofibrosis. In K. Kaushansky, M. A. Lichtman, J. T. Prchal, et al. (Eds.). *Williams hematology* (9th ed.). New York: McGraw-Hill.

Liesveld, J. L., & Lichtman, M. A. (2016). Acute myelogenous leukemia. In K. Kaushansky, M. A. Lichtman, J. T. Prchal, et al. (Eds.). *Williams hematology* (9th ed.). New York: McGraw-Hill.

McCullough, J., Refaai, M. A., & Cohn, C. S. (2015). Blood procurement and red cell transfusion. In K. Kaushansky, M. Lichtman, J. Prchal, et al. (Eds.). *Williams hematology* (9th ed.). New York: McGraw-Hill.

Mescher, A. L. (2013). *Blood. Junqueira's basic histology: Text & atlas* (13th ed.). Retrieved September 13, 2015, from accessmedicine.mhmedical.com.laneproxy.stanford.edu/content.aspx?bookid=574&Sectionid=42524598

Middeldorp, S., & Coppens, M. (2016). Hereditary thrombophilia. In K. Kaushansky, M. A. Lichtman, J. T. Prchal, et al. (Eds.). *Williams hematology* (9th ed.). New York: McGraw-Hill Medical.

Natrajan, K., & Kutlar, A. (2016). Disorders of hemoglobin structure: Sickle cell anemia and related abnormalities. In K. Kaushansky, M. A. Lichtman, J. T. Prchal, et al. (Eds.). *Williams hematology* (9th ed.). New York: McGraw-Hill Medical.

O'Donnell, E., Cottini, F., Raje, N., et al. (2016). *Myeloma*. In K. Kaushansky, M. A. Lichtman, J. T. Prchal, et al. (Eds.). *Williams hematology* (9th ed.). New York: McGraw-Hill.

Packman, C. H. (2016). Hemolytic anemia resulting from immune injury. In K. Kaushansky, M. A. Lichtman, J. T. Prchal, et al. (Eds.). *Williams hematology* (9th ed.). New York: McGraw-Hill Medical.

Papayannopoulou, T., & Migliaccio, A. (2013). Biology of erythropoiesis, erythroid differentiation, and maturation. In R. Hoffman, E. J. Benz, L. Silberstein, et al. (Eds.). *Hematology: Basic principles and practice* (6th ed.). Waltham, MA: Elsevier.

Prchal, J. T. (2016a). Clinical manifestations and classification of erythrocyte disorders. In K. Kaushansky, M. A. Lichtman, J. T. Prchal, et al. (Eds.). *Williams hematology* (9th ed.). New York: McGraw-Hill Medical.

Prchal, J. T. (2016b). Primary and secondary erythrocytoses. In K. Kaushansky, M. A. Lichtman, J. T. Prchal, et al. (Eds.). *Williams hematology* (9th ed.). New York: McGraw-Hill Medical.

Prchal, J. F., & Prchal, J. T. (2016). Polycythemia vera. In K. Kaushansky, M. A. Lichtman, J. T. Prchal, et al. (Eds.). *Williams hematology* (9th ed.). New York: McGraw-Hill.

Press, O. (2016). Hodgkin lymphoma. In K. Kaushansky, M. A. Lichtman, J. T. Prchal, et al. (Eds.). *Williams hematology* (9th ed.). New York: McGraw-Hill.

Rand, J. H., & Wolgast, L. (2016). The antiphospholipid syndrome. In K. Kaushansky, M. A. Lichtman, J. T. Prchal, et al. (Eds.). *Williams hematology* (9th ed.). New York: McGraw-Hill Medical.

Raskob, G. E., Hull, R. D., Buller, H. R., et al. (2016). Venous thrombosis. In K. Kaushansky, M. A. Lichtman, J. T. Prchal, et al. (Eds.). *Williams hematology* (9th ed.). New York: McGraw-Hill Medical.

Ryan, D. H. (2015). Examination of the marrow. In K. Kaushansky, M. Lichtman, J. Prchal, et al. (Eds.). *Williams hematology* (9th ed.). New York: McGraw-Hill.

Schneider, K. I. (2008). *Transfusion medicine: A clinical guide*. Austin, TX: Landes Bioscience.

Seeber, P., & Shander, A. (2012a). Anemia therapy I: Erythropoiesis-stimulating agents. In P. Seeber & A. Shander (Eds.). *Basics of blood management* (2nd ed.). Oxford, UK: Wiley-Blackwell.

Seeber, P., & Shander, A. (2012b). Growth factors. In P. Seeber & A. Shander (Eds.). *Basics of blood management* (2nd ed.). Oxford, UK: Wiley-Blackwell.

Segel, G. B., & Lichtman, M. A. (2016). Aplastic anemia: Acquired and inherited. In K. Kaushansky, M. A. Lichtman, J. T. Prchal, et al. (Eds.). *Williams hematology* (9th ed.). New York: McGraw-Hill Medical.

Stowell, C. P., & Hass, J. J. (2014). Transfusion medicine. In M. Laposata (Ed.). *Laboratory medicine: The diagnosis of disease in the clinical lab*. New York: McGraw-Hill

Tkachuk, D. C., & Hirschman, J. V. (2007). *Wintrobe's atlas of clinical hematology (Fig. 1.1, p. 9)*. Philadelphia, PA: Lippincott Williams & Wilkins.

Van Leeuwen, A. M., & Bladh, M. L. (2017). *Davis's comprehensive handbook of laboratory & diagnostic tests*, 7th edition. Philadelphia, PA: F.A. Davis.

van Solinge, W. W., & van Wijk, R. (2016). Erythrocyte enzyme disorders. In K. Kaushansky, M. A. Lichtman, J. T. Prchal, et al. (Eds.). *Williams hematology* (9th ed.). New York: McGraw-Hill Medical.

Vasu, S., & Caligiuri, M. A. (2016). Lymphocytosis and lymphocytopenia. In K. Kaushansky, M. A. Lichtman, J. T. Prchal, et al. (Eds.). *Williams hematology* (9th ed.). New York: McGraw-Hill Medical.

Weatherall, D. J. (2016). The thalassemias: Disorders of globin synthesis. In K. Kaushansky, M. A. Lichtman, J. T. Prchal, et al. (Eds.). *Williams hematology* (9th ed.). New York: McGraw-Hill Medical.

Journals and Electronic Documents

Abelsson, J., Andréasson, B., Samuelsson, J., et al. (2013). Patients with polycythemia have worst impairment of quality of life among patients with newly diagnosed acute myeloid leukemia. *Journal of Clinical Oncology*, *30*(21), 2670–2677.

Adams, P. C. (2015). Epidemiology and diagnostic testing for hemochromatosis and iron overload. *International Journal of Laboratory Hematology*, *37*(Suppl 1), 25–30.

Adès, L., Itzykson, R., & Fenaux, P. (2014). Myelodysplastic syndromes. *Lancet*, *383*(9936), 2239–2252.

Akbari, S., Janani, L., Mohammady, M., et al. (2014). Slow versus fast subcutaneous heparin injections for prevention of bruising and site-pain intensity. *The Cochrane Database of Systematic Reviews*, *7*:CD008077.

Alam, A., Lin, Y., Lima, A., et al. (2013). The prevention of transfusion-associated circulatory overload. *Transfusion Medicine Reviews*, *27*(2), 105–112.

Alvarez-Larrán, A., & Besses, C. (2014). Antiplatelet therapy in the management of myeloproliferative neoplasms. *Current Hematologic Malignancy Reports*, *9*(4), 319–323.

Alves, C., Ramalheira, S., Tavares, M., et al. (2017). Thromboembolic events in multiple myeloma patients—Incidence in 235 Patients. *Ann Hematol Oncol*, *4*(2), 1134.

American Cancer Society. (2013). *Possible risks of blood transfusions*. Retrieved September 14, 2015, from www.cancer.org/treatment/treatmentsandsideeffects/treatmenttypes/bloodproductdonationandtransfusion/blood-product-donation-and-transfusion-possible-transfusion-risks

American Cancer Society (ACS). (2014a). *Leukemia—Acute myeloid (myelogenous)*. Retrieved December 10, 2015, from www.cancer.org/cancer/leukemia-acutemyeloidaml/detailedguide/leukemia-acute-myeloid-myelogenous-key-statistics

American Cancer Society (ACS). (2014b). *Survival rates for myelodysplastic syndrome*. Retrieved December 20, 2015, from www.cancer.org/cancer/myelodysplasticsyndrome/overviewguide/myelodysplastic-syndromes-overview-survival

American Cancer Society. (2015). *Colorectal cancer screening tests*. Retrieved October 31, 2015, from www.cancer.org/cancer/colonandrectumcancer/moreinformation/colonandrectumcancerearlydetection/colorectal-cancer-early-detection-screening-tests-used?gclid=CLfqt5mU7cgCFVGCfgodMG0E_Q

American Cancer Society (ACS). (2015a). *Do we know what causes chronic myeloid leukemia?* Retrieved December 16, 2015, from http://www.cancer.org/cancer/leukemia-chronicmyeloidcml/detailedguide/leukemia-chronic-myeloid-myelogenous-diagnosis

American Cancer Society (ACS). (2015b). *Survival rates and factors that affect prognosis (outlook) for non-Hodgkin lymphoma*. Retrieved January

10, 2016, from www.cancer.org/cancer/non-hodgkinlymphoma/detailedguide/non-hodgkin-lymphoma-factors-prognosis
American Cancer Society (ACS). (2015c). *Survival rates for Hodgkin disease by stage*. Retrieved January 2, 2016, from www.cancer.org/cancer/hodgkindisease/detailedguide/hodgkin-disease-survival-rates
American Cancer Society (ACS). (2015d). *Types of non-Hodgkin lymphoma*. Retrieved January 10, 2016, from www.cancer.org/cancer/non-hodgkinlymphoma/detailedguide/non-hodgkin-lymphoma-types-of-non-hodgkin-lymphoma
American Cancer Society (ACS). (2015e). *What are the key statistics about non-Hodgkin lymphoma?* Retrieved January 10, 2016, from www.cancer.org/cancer/non-hodgkinlymphoma/detailedguide/non-hodgkin-lymphoma-key-statistics
American Red Cross. (2015a). *Blood components*. Retrieved September 14, 2015, from www.redcrossblood.org/learn-about-blood/bloodcomponents.
American Red Cross. (2015b). *Eligibility requirements*. Retrieved September 19, 2015, from www.redcrossblood.org/donating-blood/eligibility-requirements.
Ameringer, S., Elswick, R. K., & Smith, W. (2014). Fatigue in adolescents and young adults with sickle cell disease: Biological and behavioral correlates and health-related quality of life. *Journal of Pediatric Oncology Nursing*, *31*(1), 6–17.
Andro, M., Le Squere, P., Estivin, S., et al. (2013). Anaemia and cognitive performances in the elderly: A systematic review. *European Journal of Neurology*, *20*(9), 1234–1240.
Arnold, D. M. (2015). Bleeding complications in immune thrombocytopenia. *Hematology American Society of Hematology Education Program*, *2015*(1), 237–242.
Ataga, K. I., & Klings, E. S. (2014). Pulmonary hypertension in sickle cell disease: Diagnosis and management. *Hematology American Society of Hematology Education Program*, *2014*(1), 425–431.
Ataga, K. I., & Stocker, J. (2015). The trials and hopes for drug development in sickle cell disease. *British Journal of Haematology*, *170*(6), 768–780.
Barbui, T., Finazzi, G., & Falanga, A. (2013). Myeloproliferative neoplasms and thrombosis. *Blood*, *122*(13), 2176–2184.
Batlevi, C. L., & Younes, A. (2013). Novel therapy for Hodgkin lymphomas. *Hematology American Society of Hematology Education Program*, *2013*(1), 394–399.
Berliner, N. (2013). Anemia in the elderly. *Transactions of the American Clinical and Climatological Association*, *124*, 230–237.
Birgegård, G. (2013). Pharmacological management of essential thrombocythemia. *Expert Opinion on Pharmacotherapy*, *14*(10), 1295–1306.
Bockhold, C., & Crumpler, S. (2015). Responding to pulmonary-related blood transfusion reactions. *Nursing*, *45*(9), 36–41.
Boehringer Ingelheim Pharmaceuticals. (2015). *Pradaxa product information*. Retrieved March 18, 2016, from http://docs.boehringer-ingelheim.com/Prescribing%20Information/PIs/Pradaxa/Pradaxa.pdf
Bowen, D. T. (2013). Occupational and environmental etiology of MDS. *Best Practice and Research in Clinical Haematology*, *26*(4), 319–326.
Breccia, M., Efficace, F., Sica, S., et al. (2015). Adherence and future discontinuation of tyrosine kinase inhibitors in chronic phase chronic myeloid leukemia. A patient-based survey on 1133 patients. *Leukemia Research*, *39*(10), 1055–1059.
Broadway-Duren, J. B., & Klaassen, H. (2013). Anemias. *Critical Care Nursing Clinics of North America*, *25*(4), 411–426.
Broeckaert, B. (2011). Palliative sedation, physician assisted suicide, and euthanasia: "Same, same but different?" *American Journal of Bioethics*, *11*(6), 62–64.
Brown, S. E., Weisberg, D. F., Balf-Soran, G., et al. (2014). Sickle cell disease patients with and without extremely high hospital use: Pain, opioids, and coping. *Journal of Pain and Symptom Management*, *49*(3), 539–547.
Camaschella, C. (2015). Iron deficiency: New insights into diagnosis and treatment. *Hematology American Society of Hematology Education Program*, *2015*(1), 8–13.
Camp, M. A. (2014). Hemostatic agents: A guide to safe practice for perioperative nurses. *AORN Journal*, *100*(2), 131–147.
Canadian Hemochromatosis Society. (2014). *Therapeutic phlebotomy techniques-A patients view*. Retrieved from https://www.toomuchiron.ca/2014/04/therapeutic-phlebotomy-techniques-a-patients-view/
Canadian Hemophilia Society. (2019). *All about Von Willibrands Disease*. Retrieved from https://www.hemophilia.ca/files/All%20About%20VWD%202011%20-%20FINAL.pdf
Canadian Liver Foundation. (2012). *Hemochromatosis*. Retrieved from http://www.liver.ca/liver-disease/types/hemochromatosis.aspx?gclid=CNn41Kr40b0CFURlfgodEQcAWw
Canaro, M., Goranova-Marinova, V., & Berntorp, E. (2014). The ageing patient with haemophilia. *European Journal of Haematology*, *94*(Suppl 77), 17–22.
Carvalho, T. B., Radt, M. Y., Verheijde, J. L., et al. (2011). Continuous deep sedation in end-of-life care: disentangling palliation from physician-assisted death. *American Journal of Bioethics*, *11*(6), 60–62.
Caughey, M. C., Poole, C., Ataga, K. I., et al. (2015). Estimated pulmonary artery systolic pressure and sickle cell disease: A meta-analysis and systematic review. *British Journal of Haematology*, *170*(3), 416–424.
Centers for Disease Control and Prevention. (2013). Bacterial contamination of platelets. Retrieved September 20, 2015, from www.cdc.gov/bloodsafety/bbp/bacterial-contamination-of-platelets.html
Cerrato, C., Mina, R., & Palumbo, A. (2014). Optimal management of elderly patients with myeloma. *Expert Review of Anticancer Therapy*, *14*(2), 217–228.
Chang, E. T., Boffetta, P., Adami, H. O., et al. (2015). A critical review of the epidemiology of Agent Orange or 2,3,7,8-tetrachlorodibenzo-p-dioxin and lymphoid malignancies. *Annals of Epidemiology*, *25*(4), 275–292.
Chang, S., Weis, C., Xue, Q., et al. (2013). Association between inflammatory-related disease burden and frailty: Results from the Women's Health and Aging Studies (WHAS) I and II. *Archives of Gerontology and Geriatrics*, *54*(1), 9–15.
Charache, S., Terrin, M. L., Moore, R. D., et al. (1995). Effect of hydroxyurea on the frequency of painful crises in sickle cell anemia. Investigators of the Multicenter Study of Hydroxyurea in Sickle Cell Anemia. *New England Journal of Medicine*, *332*(20), 1317–1322.
Chaturvedi, S., & McCrae, K. R. (2015). The antiphospholipid syndrome: Still an enigma. *Hematology American Society of Hematology Education Program*, *2015*(1), 53–60.
Chen, R., Campbell, J. Chen, B. (2014). Prophylaxis and treatment of acute lymphoblastic leukemia relapse after allogenic hematopoetic stem cell transplantation. *OncoTargets and Therapy, 2015*(8), 405–412. doi: https://doi.org/10.2147/OTT.S78567
Cheson, B. D., Fisher, R. I., Barrington, S. F., et al. (2014). Recommendations for initial evaluation, staging, and response assessment of Hodgkin and non-Hodgkin lymphoma: The Lugano classification. *Journal of Clinical Oncology*, *32*(27), 3059–3067.
Chiaretti, S., & Foà, R. (2015). Management of adult Ph-positive acute lymphoblastic leukemia. *Hematology American Society of Hematology Education Program*, *2015*(1), 406–413.
Chou, S. T. (2013). Transfusion therapy for sickle cell disease: A balancing act. *Hematology. The American Society of Hematology Education Program*, *2013*(1), 439–446.
Coleman, M. (2014). Patient empowerment in the management of chronic myeloid leukemia. *Clinical Journal of Oncology Nursing*, *18*(2), E12–E18.
Collins, W., Chalmers, E., Hart, D., et al. (2013). Diagnosis and management of acquired coagulation inhibitors: A guideline from UKHCDO. *British Journal of Haematology*, *162*(6), 758–773.
Colson, K. (2015). Treatment-related symptom management in patients with multiple myeloma: A review. *Supportive Care in Cancer*, *23*(5), 1431–1445.
Connolly, G. C., & Francis, C. W. (2013). Cancer-associated thrombosis. *Hematology American Society of Hematology*, *2013*(1), 684–691.
Coombs, C. C., Tavakkoli, M., & Tallman, M. S. (2015). Acute promyelocytic leukemia: Where did we start, where are we not, and the future. *Blood Cancer Journal*, *5*, e304.
Cooper, M., Greene-Finestone, L., Lowell, H., et al. (2012). *Iron insufficiency in Canadians. Component of Statistics Canada Catalogue no. 82-003-X Health Reports*. Retrieved from http://www.statcan.gc.ca/pub/82-003-x/2012004/article/11742-eng.htm
Cozzani, E., Iurlo, A., Merlo, G., et al. (2015). Essential thrombocythemia: The dermatologic point of view. *Clinical Lymphoma Myeloma and Leukemia*, *15*(12), 739–747.
Cylwik, B., Naklicki, N., Gruszewska, E., et al. (2013). The distribution of serum folate concentration and red blood cell indices in alcoholics. *Journal of Nutritional Science and Vitaminology*, *59*(1), 1–8.
Daniëls, L. A., Oerlemans, S., Krol, A. D., et al. (2013). Persisting fatigue in Hodgkin lymphoma survivors: A systematic review. *Annals of Hematology*, *9*(8), 1023–1032.
Daniëls, L. A., Oerlemans, S., Krol, A. D., et al. (2014). Chronic fatigue in Hodgkin lymphoma survivors and associations with anxiety, depression and comorbidity. *British Journal of Cancer*, *110*(4), 868–874.
Darbari, D., Ballas, S. K., & Clauw, D. J. (2014). Thinking beyond sickling to better understand pain in sickle cell disease. *European Journal of Haematology*, *93*(2), 89–95.

DeAngelo, D. J. (2015). The use of novel monoclonal antibodies in the treatment of acute lymphoblastic leukemia. *Hematology American Society of Hematology Education Program, 2015*(1), 400–405.
DeBaun, M. R. (2014). Hydroxyurea therapy contributes to infertility in adult men with sickle cell disease: A review. *Expert Review of Hematology*, *7*(6), 767–773.
de Prost, N., Sasanelli, M., Deux, J. F., et al. (2015). Positron emission tomography with 18F-fluorodeoxyglucose in patients with sickle cell acute chest syndrome. *Medicine*, *94*(18), e821.
Deninger, M. W. (2015). Molecular monitoring in CML and the prospects for treatment-free remissions. *Hematology American Society of Hematology Education Program*, *2015*(1), 257–263.
Di Bella, N. J., Bhowmik, D., Bhor, M., et al. (2015). The effectiveness of tyrosine kinase inhibitors and molecular monitoring patterns in newly diagnosed patients with chronic myeloid leukemia in the community setting. *Clinical Lymphoma, Myeloma and Leukemia*, *15*(10), 599–605.
Diericix, D., Kentos, A., & Delannoy, A. (2015). The role of rituximab in adults with warm antibody autoimmune hemolytic anemia. *Blood*, *125*(21), 3223–3229.
Dmitrieva, O., de Lusignan, S., Macdougnall, I., et al. (2013). Association of anaemia in primary care patients with chronic kidney disease: Cross-sectional study of quality improvement in chronic kidney disease (QICKD) trial data. *BMC Nephrology*, *14*(1), 24.
Donovan, A. K., Smith, K. J., & Ragni, M. V. (2013). Anticoagulation duration in heterozygous factor V Leiden: A decision analysis. *Thrombosis Research*, *132*(6), 724–728.
Dunn, A. (2015). The long and short of it: Using the new factor products. *Hematology American Society of Hematology Education Program*, *2015*(1), 26–32.
Elmariah, H., Garrett, M. E., De Castro, L. M., et al. (2014). Factors associated with survival in a contemporary adult sickle cell disease cohort. *American Journal of Hematology*, *89*(5), 530–535.
Erba, H. P. (2015). Finding the optimal combination therapy for the treatment of newly diagnosed AML in older patients unfit for intensive therapy. *Leukemia Research*, *39*(2), 183–191.
Evens, A. M., & Kostakoglu, L. (2014). The role of FDG-PET in defining prognosis of Hodgkin lymphoma for early stage disease. *Hematology. American Society of Hematology Education Program*, *2014*(1), 135–143.
Fairweather-Tait, S., Wawer, A., Gilings, R., et al. (2014). Iron status in the elderly. *Mechanisms of Ageing and Development*, *136–137*(100), 22–28.
Federici, A. B. (2014). Clinical and laboratory diagnosis of vWD. *Hematology American Society of Hematology*, *2014*(1), 524–530.
Food and Drug Administration (2015). *Ixazomib*. Retrieved January 13, 2016, from www.fda.gov/Drugs/InformationOnDrugs/ApprovedDrugs/ucm473804.htm
Foster, M. (2014). Reevaluating the neutropenic diet: Time to change. *Clinical Journal of Oncology Nursing*, *18*(2), 239–241.
Freiermuth, C. E., Haywood, C., Silva, S., et al. (2014). Attitudes toward patients with sickle cell disease in a multicenter sample of emergency department providers. *Advanced Emergency Nursing Journal*, *36*(4), 335–347.
Furukawa, Y., & Kikuchi, J. (2015). Molecular pathogenesis of multiple myeloma. *International Journal of Clinical Oncology*, *20*(3), 413–422.
G6PD Deficiency Association. (2015). Drugs to avoid list. Retrieved November 22, 2015, from g6pddeficiency.org/wp/living-with-g6pd-deficiency/drugs-to-avoid-list/#.VlfncHarRhE
Garcia, D. A. (2014). The target-specific oral anticoagulants: Practical considerations. *Hematology American Society of Hematology*, *2014*(1), 510–513.
Garcia-Manero, G. (2015). Myelodysplastic syndromes: 2015 update on diagnosis, risk-stratification and management. *American Journal of Hematology*, *90*(9), 832–841.
Geyer, H. L., & Mesa, R. A. (2014). Therapy for myeloproliferative neoplasms: When, which agent, and how? *Hematology American Society of Hematology Education Program*, *2014*(1), 277–286.
Goldberg, S. L. (2015). Monitoring chronic myeloid leukemia in the real world: Gaps and opportunities. *Clinical Lymphoma Myeloma and Leukemia*, *15*(12), 711–714.
Goodnough, L. T., & Schrier, S. L. (2014). Evaluation and management of anemia in the elderly. *American Journal of Hematology*, *89*(1), 88–96.
Goodnough, L. T., & Shander, A. (2013). Current status of pharmacologic therapies in patient blood management. *Anesthesia & Analgesia*, *116*(1), 15–34.
Gorski, L., Hadaway, L., Hagle, M., et al. (2016). Infusion therapy: Standards of practice. *Journal of Infusion Nursing*, *39*(1S), S135–S137.
Graf, S. A., & Gopal, A. K. (2014). Treatment of relapsed classical Hodgkin lymphoma in the brentuximab vedotin era. *Hematology American Society of Hematology Education Program*, *2014*(1), 151–157.
Greinacher, A. (2015). Heparin-induced thrombocytopenia. *New England Journal of Medicine*, *373*(3), 252–261.
Haase, N., Ostrowski, S. R., Wettersley, J., et al. (2015). Thromboelastography in patients with severe sepsis: A prospective cohort study. *Intensive Care Medicine*, *41*(1), 77–85.
Hacker, E. D., Patel, P., & Stainthorpe, M. (2013). Sleep interrupted: Nocturnal care disturbances following hematopoietic stem cell transplantation. *Clinical Journal of Oncology Nursing*, *17*(5), 517–523.
Hall, A. E., Paul, C., Bryant, J., et al. (2016). To adhere or not to adhere: Rates and reasons of medication adherence in hematological cancer patients. *Critical Reviews in Oncology/Hematology*, *97*(1), 247–262.
Hallek, M. (2015). Chronic lymphocytic leukemia: 2015 update on diagnosis, risk stratification, and treatment. *American Journal of Hematology*, *90*(5), 446–460.
Hamideh, D., & Alvarez, O. (2013). Sickle cell disease related mortality in the United States (1999–2009). *Pediatric Blood & Cancer*, *60*(9), 1482–1486.
Heeney, M. M. (2014). Iron clad: Iron hemostasis and the diagnosis of hereditary iron overload. *Hematology American Society of Hematology*, *2014*(1), 202–209.
Heit, J. A. (2015). Epidemiology of venous thromboembolism. *Nature Reviews. Cardiology*, *2015*(8), 464–474.
Hiddemann, W., & Cheson, B. D. (2014). How we manage follicular lymphoma. *Leukemia*, *28*(7), 1388–1395.
Ho, S., Gue, D., McIntosh, K., et al. (2014). An objective method for assessing adherence to prophylaxis in adults with severe haemophilia. *Haemophilia*, *20*(1), 39–43.
Hong, C. H., Falvey, C., Harris, T. B., et al. (2013). Anemia and risk of dementia in older adults: Findings from the Health ABC study. *Neurology*, *81*(6), 528–533.
Hoppensteadt, D., Tsuruta, K., Cunanan, J., et al. (2014). Thrombin generation mediators and markers in sepsis-associated coagulopathy and their modulation by recombinant thrombomodulin. *Clinical and Applied Thrombosis/Hemostasis*, *20*(2), 129–135.
Howard, J., Hart, N., Roberts-Harewood, M., et al; BCSH Committee. (2015). Guideline on the management of acute syndrome in sickle cell disease. *British Journal of Haematology* *166*(4), 492–505. doi: 10.1111/bjh.13348
Hughes, T., & White, D. (2013). Which TKI? An embarrassment of riches for chronic myeloid leukemia patients. *Hematology American Society of Hematology Education Program*, *2013*(1), 168–175.
Hurrell, K. (2014). Safe administration of blood components. *Nursing Times*, *110*(38), 16–19.
Husson, O., Oerlemans, S., Mols, F., et al. (2014). Satisfaction with information provision is associated with baseline but not with follow-up quality of life among lymphoma patients: Results from the PROFILES registry. *Acta Ongologica*, *53*(7), 917–926.
Izutsu, K. (2014). Treatment of follicular lymphoma. *Journal of Clinical and Experimental Hematopathology*, *54*(1), 31–37.
Jain, D., Kumar, R., Tyagi, N., et al. (2012). Etiology and survival of aplastic anemia: A study based on clinical investigation. *Journal of Clinical Laboratory Analysis*, *26*(6), 452–458.
Jenerette, C. M., Brewer, C. A., & Ataga, K. I. (2014). Care seeking for pain in young adults with sickle cell disease. *Pain Management Nursing*, *15*(1), 324–330.
Johnson, P. W. (2013). Management of early stage Hodgkin lymphoma: Is there still a role for radiation? *Hematology American Society of Hematology Education Program*, *2013*(1), 400–405.
Jongen, J. L., Broijl, A., & Sonneveld, P. (2015). Chemotherapy-induced peripheral neuropathies in hematological malignancies. *Journal of Neuro-Oncology*, *121*(2), 229–237.
Jordan, L., Adams-Graves, P., Kanter-Washko, J., et al. (2015). Multicenter COMPACT study of complications in patients with sickle cell disease and utilization of iron chelation therapy. *Current Medical Research and Opinion*, *31*(3), 513–523.
Josephson, N. (2013). The hemophilias and their clinical management. *Hematology American Society of Hematology Education Program*, *2013*(1), 261–267.
Jurczyszyn, A., Czepko, R., Banach, M., et al. (2015). Percutaneous vertebroplasty for pathological vertebral compression fractures secondary to multiple myeloma—medium-term and long-term assessment of pain relief and quality of life. *Advances in Clinical and Experimental Medicine*, *24*(4), 651–656.

Kam, G., Yiu, R., Loh, Y., et al. (2015). Impact of pegylated filgrastim in comparison to filgrastim for patients with acute myeloid leukaemia (AML) on high-dose cytarabine (HIDAC) consolidation therapy. *Supportive Care in Cancer, 23*(3), 643–649.

Kanwar, P., & Kowdley, K. D. (2014). Metal storage disorders. *Medical Clinics of North America, 98*(1), 87–102.

Kempton, C., & Meeks, S. L. (2014). Toward optimal therapy for inhibitors in hemophilia. *Hematology American Society of Hematology Education Program, 2014*(1), 364–371.

Kenz, H. E., & Van der Linden, P. (2014). Transfusion-related acute lung injury. *The European Journal of Anaesthesiology, 31*(7), 345–350.

Khimani, N., Chen, Y. H., Mauch, P. M., et al. (2013). Influence of new late effects on quality of life over time in Hodgkin lymphoma survivors: A longitudinal study. *Annals of Oncology, 24*(1), 226–230.

Kim, H. C. (2014). Red cell exchange: Special focus on sickle cell disease. *Hematology American Society of Hematology Education Program, 2014*(1), 450–456.

Koeppen, S. (2014). Treatment of multiple myeloma: Thalidomide, bortezomib, and lenalidomide-induced peripheral neuropathy. *Oncology Research and Treatment, 37*(9), 506–513.

Kouroukis, T. C., Baldassarre, F. G., Haynes, A. E., et al. (2014). Bortezomib in multiple myeloma: Systematic review and clinical considerations. *Current Oncology, 21*(4), e573–e603.

Kreidy, R. (2014). Influence of acquired and genetic risk factors on the prevention, management, and treatment of thromboembolic disease. *International Journal of Vascular Medicine, 2014*, 859726.

Landgren, O., & Morgan, G. J. (2014). Biologic frontiers in multiple myeloma: From biomarker identification to clinical practice. *Clinical Cancer Research 20*(4), 804–813.

Lee, G. M., & Arepally, G. M. (2013). Heparin-induced thrombocytopenia. *Hematology American Society of Hematology, 2013*(1), 668–674.

Lekovic, D., Gotic, M., Sefer, D., et al. (2015). Predictors of survival and cause of death in patients with essential thrombocythemia. *European Journal of Haematology, 95*(5), 461–466.

Leukemia & Lymphoma Society. (2013). *Hodgkin lymphoma*. Retrieved June 2, 2016, from www.lls.org/sites/default/files/file_assets/PS57_Hogkin_Lymphoma%20FINAL_with%20insert%20May2016.pdf

Leukemia & Lymphoma Society. (2015a). *Acute myeloid leukemia*. Retrieved June 2, 2015, from www.lls.org/sites/default/files/file_assets/PS32_AML_Booklet_FINAL6.15.pdf

Leukemia & Lymphoma Society. (2015b). Somewhere is today. Facts 2014–2015. Retrieved December 10, 2015, from www.lls.org/sites/default/files/file_assets/facts.pdf

Levine, M., & Goldstein, J. N. (2014). Bleeding complications of targeted oral anticoagulants: What is the risk? *Hematology American Society of Hematology, 2014*(1), 504–509.

Lonial, S., & Nooka, A. K. (2015). Novel combination approaches for myeloma. *Hematology American Society of Hematology Education Program, 2015*(1), 286–293.

Lopez, A., Cacoub, P., Macdougall, I., et al. (2015). Iron-deficiency anaemia. *Lancet, 387*(10021), 907–916.

Maggio, A., Vitrano, A., Calvaruso, G., et al. (2013). Serial echocardiographic left ventricular ejection fraction measurements: A tool for detecting thalassemia major patients at risk for cardiac death. *Blood Cells, Molecules, & Diseases, 50*(4), 241–246.

Manea, P. J. (2014). Optimizing the management of patients with myelofibrosis. *Clinical Journal of Oncology Nursing, 18*(3), 330–337.

Marsh, J., & Kulasekararaj, A. (2013). Management of the refractory aplastic anemia patient: What are the options? *American Society of Hematology Educational Program, 2013*(1), 87–94.

Martelli, M., Ferreria, A., Agostinelli, C., et al. (2013). Diffuse B-cell lymphoma. *Critical Reviews in Oncology/Hematology, 87*(2), 146–171.

Martinelli, I., Passamonti, S. M., & Bucciarelli, P. (2014). Thrombophilic states. *Handbook of Clinical Neurology, 120*, 1061–1071.

Matasar, M. J., Ford, J. S., Riedel, E. R., et al. (2015). Late morbidity and mortality in patients with Hodgkin's lymphoma treated during adulthood. *Journal of the National Cancer Institute, 107*(4), djv018.

Mathisen, M. S., Kantarjian, H., Thomas, D., et al. (2013). Acute lymphoblastic leukemia in adults: Encouraging developments on the way to higher cure rates. *Leukemia & Lymphoma, 54*(12), 2592–2600.

Matsushita, T., Watanabe, J., Honda, G., et al. (2014). Thrombomodulin alpha treatment in patients with acute promyelocytic leukemia and disseminated intravascular coagulation: A retrospective analysis of an open-label, multicenter, post-marketing surveillance study cohort. *Thrombosis Research, 133*(5), 772–781.

Maury, S., & Aljurf, M. (2013). Management of adult patients older than 40 years refractory to at least one immunosuppressive course: HLA-identical sibling HSCT using fludarabine-based conditioning. *Bone Marrow Transplantation, 48*(2), 196–197.

McClish, D. K., Smith, W. R., Dahman, B. A., et al. (2009). Pain site frequency and location in sickle cell disease: The PISCES project. *Pain, 145*(1–2), 246–251.

Mehta, R. H., Castelvecchio, S., Ballotta, A., et al. (2013). Association of gender and lowest hematocrit on cardiopulmonary bypass with acute kidney injury and operative mortality in patients undergoing cardiac surgery. *The Annals of Thoracic Surgery, 96*(1), 133–140.

Merin, N. M., & Kelly, K. R. (2015). Clinical use of proteosome inhibitors in treatment of multiple myeloma. *Pharmaceuticals, 8*(1), 1–20.

Michaels, K., & Regan, E. N. (2013). Teaching patients INR self-management. *Nursing, 43*(5), 67–69.

Michel, M. (2014). Warm autoimmune hemolytic anemia: Advances in pathophysiology and treatment. *Presse médicale, 43*(4 Pt 2), e97–e104.

Mihailovic, J., & Goldsmith, S. J. (2015). Multiple myeloma: 18F-FDG-PET/CT and diagnostic imaging. *Seminars in Nuclear Medicine, 45*(1), 16–31.

Mishra, P. K., Thekkudan, J., Sahajanadan, R., et al. (2015). The role of point-of-care assessment of platelet function in predicting postoperative bleeding and transfusion requirements after coronary artery bypass grafting. *Annals of Cardiac Anaesthesia, 18*(1), 45–51.

National Cancer Institute. (2013). *SEER Stat Fact Sheets: Myeloma*. Retrieved January 13, 2016, from seer.cancer.gov/statfacts/html/mulmy.html

National Clinical Guideline Centre (UK). (2015). *Anaemia management in chronic kidney disease: Partial update 2015 [Internet]*. London: Royal College of Physicians (UK). Retrieved October 24, 2016, from ww-ncbi-nlm-nih-gov.laneproxy.stanford.edu/books/NBK299242/ PubMed PMID: 26065064.

National Heart, Lung, and Blood Institute. (2015). *Who is at risk for sickle cell anemia?* Retrieved March 14, 2016, from www.nhlbi.nih.gov/health/health-topics/topics/sca/atrisk.html.

National Hemophilia Foundation. (2014). *What is von Willebrand disease?* Retrieved November 19, 2015, from www.hemophilia.org

Neff, A. T., & Sidonio, R. F. (2014). Management of vWD. *Hematology American Society of Hematology, 2014*(1), 536–541.

Nemtsas, P., Arnaoutoglou, M., Perifanis, V., et al. (2015). Neurological complications of beta-thalassemia. *Annals of Hematology, 94*(8), 1261–1265.

Neunert, C. E. (2013). Current management of immune thrombocytopenia. *Hematology American Society of Hematology Education Program, 2013*(1), 276–282.

Neunert, C., Lim, W., Crowther, M., et al. (2011). The American Society of Hematology 2011 evidence-based practice guideline for immune thrombocytopenia. *Blood, 117*(16), 4190–4207.

Ng, A. K. (2014). Current survivorship recommendations for patients with Hodgkin lymphoma: Focus on late effects. *Hematology American Society of Hematology Education Program, 2014*(1), 488–494.

Nielson, O., Ainsworth, M., Coskun, M., et al. (2015). Management of iron-deficiency anemia in inflammatory bowel disease: A systematic review. *Medicine, 94*(23), 1–14.

Nolte, F., Angelucci, E., Breccia, M., et al. (2015). Updated recommendations on the management of gastrointestinal disturbances during iron chelation therapy with deferasirox in transfusion dependent patients with myelodysplastic syndrome: Emphasis on optimized dosing schedules and new formulations. *Leukemia Research, 39*(10), 1028–1033.

O'Brien, C., Dempsey, O., & Kennedy, M. J. (2014). Febrile neutropenia risk assessment tool: Improving clinical outcomes for oncology patients. *European Journal of Oncology Nursing, 18*(2), 167–174.

Odenike, O. (2013). Beyond JAK inhibitor therapy in myelofibrosis. *Hematology American Society of Hematology Education Program, 2015*(1), 545–552.

Oerlemans, S., Mols, F., Nijziel, M. R., et al. (2014). The course of anxiety and depression for patients with Hodgkin's lymphoma or diffuse large B cell lymphoma: A longitudinal study of the PROFILES registry. *Journal of Cancer Survivorship, 8*(4), 555–564.

Pagano, L., Verga, L., Busca, A., et al. (2014). Systemic antifungal treatment after posaconazole prophylaxis: Results from the SEIFEM 2010-C survey. *Journal of Antimicrobial Chemotherapy, 69*(11), 3142–3147.

Palumbo, A., Avet-Loiseau, H., Oliva, S., et al. (2015). Revised International Staging System for multiple myeloma: A report from International Myeloma Working Group. *Journal of Clinical Oncology, 33*(26), 2863–2869.

Pandita, A., & Mukherjee, S. (2014). Resuscitating a dying marrow: The role of hematopoietic growth factors. *Current Hematologic Malignancy Reports, 9*(4), 412–420.

Papamerkouriou, Y. M., Kenanaidis, E., Gamie, Z., et al. (2015). Treatment of multiple myeloma bone disease: Experimental and clinical data. *Expert Opinion on Biological Therapy, 15*(2), 213–230.

Partsch, H. (2014). The role of leg compression in the treatment of deep vein thrombosis. *Phlebology/Venous Forum of the Royal Society of Medicine, 29*(Suppl 1), 66–70.

Pavlish, C., Brown-Saltzman, K., Jakel, P., et al. (2014). The nature of ethical conflicts and the meaning of moral community in oncology practice. *Oncology Nursing Forum, 41*(2), 130–140.

Perfect, J. R., Hachem, R., & Wingard, J. R. (2014). Update on epidemiology of and preventive strategies for invasive fungal infections in cancer patients. *Clinical Infectious Diseases, 59*(Suppl 5), S352–S355.

Peslak, S., Olson, T., & Babushok, D. (2017). Diagnosis and treatment of aplastic anemia. *Current Treatment Options in Oncology, 18*(12), 1–20.

Piel, F. B., & Weatherall, D. J. (2014). The α-Thalassemias. *The New England Journal of Medicine, 371*(20), 1908–1916.

Pillai, A. R., & Raval, J. S. (2015). Does early ambulation increase the risk of pulmonary embolism in deep vein thrombosis? A review of the literature. *Home Healthcare Nurse, 32*(6), 336–342.

Porter, J., & Garbowski, M. (2013). Consequences and management of iron overload in sickle cell disease. *Hematology American Society of Hematology Education Program, 2013*(1), 447–456.

Quinn, C. T. (2014). Breakthrough: New guidelines for silent cerebral ischemia and infarction in sickle cell disease. *Hematology American Society of Hematology Education Program, 2014*(1), 438–443.

Radia, D., & Geyer, H. L. (2015). Management of symptoms in polycythemia vera and essential thrombocythemia patients. *Hematology American Society of Hematology Education Program, 2015*(1), 340–348.

Raje, N. S., Yee, A. J., & Roodman, G. D. (2014). Advances in supportive care for multiple myeloma. *Journal of the National Comprehensive Cancer Network, 12*(4), 502–511.

Rajkumar, S. V., Dimopoulos, M. A., Palumbo, A., et al. (2014). International Myeloma Working Group updated criteria for the diagnosis of multiple myeloma. *Lancet Oncology, 15*(12), e538–e548.

Rajkumar, S. V., Landgren, O., & Mateos, M. V. (2015). Smoldering multiple myeloma. *Blood, 125*(20), 3069–3075.

Randhawa, J. K., & Ferrajoli, A. (2016). A review of supportive care and recommendations to preventive approaches for patients with chronic lymphocytic leukemia. *Expert Review of Hematology, 9*(3), 235–244.

Raphael, J. L., & Oyeku, S. O. (2013). Sickle cell disease pain management and the medical home. *Hematology American Society of Hematology Education Program, 2014*(1), 433–438.

Reitter-Pfoertner, S., Waldhoer, T., Mayerhofer, M., et al. (2013). The influence of thrombophilia on the long-term survival of patients with a history of venous thromboembolism. *Thrombosis and Haemostasis, 109*(1), 79–84.

Reyes, M., Blank, H. M., & Grossniklaus, D. (2015). *Hemochromatosis*. National Center on Birth Defects and Developmental Disabilities, Centers for Disease Control and Prevention. Retrieved November 26, 2015, from www.cdc.gov/ncbddd/hemochromatosis/training/epidemiology/prevalence.html

Rodeghiero, R., & Ruggeri, M. (2015). Treatment of immune thrombocytopenia in adults: The role of thrombopoietin-receptor agonists. *Seminars in Hematology, 52*(1), 16–24.

Röllig, C., & Ehninger, G. (2015). How I treat hyperleukocytosis in acute myeloid leukemia. *Blood, 125*(21), 3246–3252.

Roper, K., Cooley, M. E., McDermott, K., et al. (2013). Health-related quality of life after treatment of Hodgkin lymphoma in young adults. *Oncology Nursing Forum, 40*(4), 349–360.

Ryblom, H., Hast, R., Hellström-Lindberg, E., et al. (2015). Self-perception of symptoms of anemia and fatigue before and after blood transfusions in patients with myelodysplastic syndromes. *European Journal of Oncology Nursing, 19*(2), 99–106.

Sachdeva, A., Dalton, M., Amaragiri, S. V., et al. (2014). Graduated compression stockings for prevention of deep vein thrombosis. *The Cochrane Database of Systematic Reviews, 12*, CD001484.

Sammels, M., Vandesande, J., Vlaeyen, E., et al. (2014). Falling and fall risk factors in adults with haemophilia: An exploratory study. *Haemophilia, 20*(6), 836–845.

Santini, V., & Fenaux, P. (2015). Treatment of myelodysplastic syndrome with thrombomimetic drugs. *Seminars in Hematology, 52*(1), 38–45.

Sartori, M. T., & Prandoni, P. (2016). How to effectively manage the event of bleeding complications when using anticoagulants. *Expert Review of Hematology, 9*(1), 37–50.

Scherber, R. A., Geyer, H. L., & Mesa, R. A. (2014). Quality of life in MPN comes of age as a therapeutic target. *Current Hematologic Malignancy Reports, 9*(4), 324–330.

Scherber, R. M., Kosiorek, H. E., Senyak, Z., et al. (2016). Comprehensively understanding fatigue in patients with myeloproliferative neoplasms. *Cancer, 122*(3), 477–485.

Schiffer, C. A. (2014). Optimal dose and schedule of consolidation in AML: Is there a standard? Best Practice & Research. *Clinical Haematology, 27*(3–4), 259–264.

Schuff-Werner, P., Steiner, M., Fenger, S., et al. (2013). Effective estimation of correct platelet counts in pseudothrombocytopenia using an alternative anticoagulant based on magnesium salt. *British Journal of Haematology, 162*(5), 684–692.

Sever, M., Newberry, K. J., & Verstovsek, S. (2014). Therapeutic options for patients with polycythemia vera and essential thrombocythemia refractory/resistant to hydroxyurea. *Leukemia & Lymphoma, 55*(12), 2685–2690.

Shanafelt, T. (2013). Treatment of older patients with chronic lymphocytic leukemia: Key questions and current answers. *Hematology American Society of Hematology Education Program, 2013*(1), 158–167.

Shipton, M. J., & Thachil, J. (2015). Vitamin B12 deficiency: A 21st century perspective. *Clinical Medicine, 15*(2), 145–150.

Shlush, L. I., & Minden, M. D. (2015). Preleukemia: The normal side of cancer. *Current Opinion in Hematology, 22*(2), 77–84.

Siegel, F. P., Tauscher, J., & Petrides, P. E. (2013). Aquagenic pruritus in polycythemia vera: Characteristics and influence on quality of life in 441 patients. *American Journal of Hematology, 88*(8), 665–669.

Simes, J., Becattini, C., Agnellis, G., et al. (2014). Aspirin for the prevention of recurrent venous thromboembolism: The INSPIRE Collaboration. *Circulation, 130*(13), 1062–1071.

Singh, A. K., Kumar, A., Karmakar, D., et al. (2013). Association of B12 deficiency and clinical neuropathy with metformin use in type 2 diabetes patients. *Journal of Postgraduate Medicine, 60*(4), 253–257.

Smith-Whitley, K. (2014). Reproductive issues in sickle cell disease. *Hematology. American Society Hematology Education Program, 2014*(1), 418–424.

Snoeck, H. W. (2013). Aging of the hematopoietic system. *Current Opinion In Hematology, 20*(4), 355–361.

Soares, A., Biasoli, I., Scheliga, A., et al. (2013). Association of social network and social support with health-related quality of life and fatigue in long-term survivors of Hodgkin lymphoma. *Supportive Care in Cancer, 21*(8), 2153–2159.

Spector, D. J., Noonan, D., Mayer, D. K., et al. (2015). Are lifestyle behavioral factors associated with health-related quality of life in long-term survivors of non-Hodgkin lymphoma? *Cancer, 121*(18), 3343–4451.

Squizzato, A., Romualdi, E., Passamonti, F., et al. (2013). Antiplatelet drugs for polycythemia vera and essential thrombocythemia. *Cochrane Database of Systematic Reviews, 4*, CD006503.

Stabler, S. (2013). Vitamin B12 deficiency. *The New England Journal of Medicine, 368*(2), 149–160.

Steensma, D. P., & Gatterman, N. (2013). When is iron overload deleterious, and when and how should iron chelation therapy be administered in myelodysplastic syndromes? *Best Practice & Research. Clinical Hematology, 26*(4), 431–444.

Stein, B. L., Moliterno, A. R., & Tiu, R. V. (2014). Polycythemia vera disease burden: Contributing factors, impact on quality of life, and emerging treatment options. *Annals of Hematology, 93*(12), 1965–1976.

Stilgenbauer, S. (2015). Prognostic markers and standard management of chronic lymphocytic leukemia. *Hematology American Society of Hematology Education Program, 2015*(1), 368–377.

Stupnyckyj, C., Smolarek, S., Reeves, C., et al. (2014). Changing blood transfusion policy and practice. *The American Journal of Nursing, 114*(12), 50–59.

Sullivan, L. R., Sekeres M. A., Shrestha, N. K., et al. (2013). Epidemiology and risk factors for infections in myelodysplastic syndromes. *Transplant Infectious Disease, 15*(6), 652–657.

Tao, Z., & Ghoroghchian, P. P. (2014). Microparticle, nanoparticle, and stem cell-based oxygen carriers as advanced blood substitutes. *Trends in Biotechnology, 32*(9), 466–473.

Taylor, F. B., Toh, C. H., Hoots, W. K., et al. (2007). Towards a definition, clinical and laboratory criteria, and a scoring system for DIC. *Journal of Thrombosis and Haemostasis, 5*(3), 445–659.

Tefferi, A., & Barbui, T. (2015). Polycythemia vera and essential thrombocythemia: 2015 update on diagnosis, risk-stratification and management. *American Journal of Hematology*, *90*(2), 162–173.

Telen, M. J., Afenyi-Annan, A., Garrett, M. E., et al. (2015). Alloimmunization in sickle cell disease: Changing antibody specificities and association with chronic pain and decreased survival. *Transfusion*, *55*(6 Pt 2), 1378–1387.

Thompson, P. A., Kantarjian, H. M., & Cortes, J. E. (2015). Diagnosis and treatment of chronic myeloid leukemia in 2015. *Mayo Clinic Proceedings*, *90*(10), 1440–1454.

Toh, C. H., & Alhamdi, Y. (2013). Current consideration and management of disseminated intravascular coagulation. *Hematology American Society of Hematology Education Program*, *2013*(1), 286–291.

Troy, J. D., Atallah, E., Geyer, J. T., et al. (2014). Myelodysplastic syndromes in the United States: An update for clinicians. *Annals of Medicine*, *46*(5), 283–289.

Truelove, E., Fielding, A. K., & Hunt, B. J. (2013). The coagulopathy and thrombotic risk associated with L-asparaginase treatment in adults with acute lymphoblastic leukemia. *Leukemia*, *27*(3), 553–559.

Turan, O., Ündar, B., Güany, T., et al. (2013). Investigation of inherited thrombophilias in patients with pulmonary embolism. *Blood Coagulation & Fibrinolysis*, *24*(2), 140–149.

U.S. Food and Drug Administration. (2015). *Information on erythropoiesis-stimulating agents (ESA) epoetin alfa (marketed as Procrit, Epogen), darbepoetin alfa (marketed as Aranesp)*. Retrieved March 12, 2016, from www.fda.gov/drugs/drugsafety/postmarketdrugsafetyinformationforpatientsandproviders/ucm109375.htm

Valderrabano, R. J., Lee, J., Lui, L., et al. (2017). Older men with anemia have increased fracture risk independent of bone mineral density. *The Journal of Endocrinology and Metabolism 102*(7), 2199–2206. Retrieved from https://doi.org/10.1210/jc.2017-00266

van Acker, H. H., Anguille, S., Willemen, Y., et al. (2015). Bisphosphonates for cancer treatment: Mechanisms of action and lessons from clinical trials. *Pharmacology & Therapeutics*, *158*(2016), 24–40.

van der Poel, M. W., Oerlemans, S., Schouten, H. C., et al. (2014). Quality of life more impaired in younger than in older diffuse large B cell lymphoma survivors compared to a normative population: A study from the population-based PROFILES registry. *Annals of Hematology*, *93*(5), 811–819.

van Meer, S., de Man, R. A., Siersema, P. D., et al. (2013). Surveillance for hepatocellular carcinoma in chronic liver disease: Evidence and controversies. *World Journal of Gastroenterology*, *19*(40), 6744–6756.

Vannella, L., Lahner, E., Osborn, J., et al. (2013). Systematic review: Gastric cancer incidence in pernicious anaemia. *Alimentary Pharmacology & Therapeutics*, *37*(4), 375–382.

Vannucchi, A. M. (2014). How I treat polycythemia vera. *Blood*, *124*(22), 3212–3220.

van Veen, T., & Hunt, J. A. (2015). Tissue engineering red blood cells: A therapeutic. *Journal of Tissue Engineering and Regenerative Medicine*, *9*(7), 760–770.

Visvanathan, V. (2015). Slow vs. fast subcutaneous heparin injections for prevention of pain and bruising. *American Journal of Nursing*, *115*(12), 27.

Vonk, A. B., Meesters, M. I., Garnier, R. P., et al. (2013). Intraoperative cell salvage is associated with reduced postoperative blood loss and transfusion requirements in cardiac surgery: A cohort study. *Transfusion*, *53*(11), 2782–2789.

Walker, R. E., Lawson, M. A., Buckle, C. H., et al. (2014). Myeloma bone disease: Pathogenesis, current treatments and future targets. *British Medical Bulletin*, *111*(1), 117–138.

Wallen, G. R., Minnitti, C. P., Krumlauf, M., et al. (2014). Sleep disturbance, depression and pain in adults with sickle cell disease. *BMC Psychiatry*, *14*, 207.

Wang, M., & Cheng, J. (2013). Overview and management of cardiac and pulmonary adverse events in patients with relapsed and/or refractory multiple myeloma treated with single-agent carfilzomib. *Oncology*, *27*(Suppl 3), 24–30.

Weyrich, A. S. (2014). Platelets: More than a sack of glue. *Hematology. American Society of Hematology. Education Program*, *2014*(1), 400–403.

Wildes, T. M., Rosko, A., & Tuchman, S. A. (2014). Multiple myeloma in the older adult: Better prospects, more challenges. *Journal of Clinical Oncology*, *32*(24), 2531–2540.

Wilson, O., Avalos, G., & Dowling, M. (2016). Knowledge of palliative care and attitudes towards nursing the dying patient. *British Journal of Nursing*, *25*(11), 600–605.

Xie, M., Jiang, Q., & Xie, Y. (2015). Comparison between decitabine and azacitidine for the treatment of myelodysplastic syndrome: A meta-analysis with 1392 participants. *Clinical Lymphoma, Myeloma & Leukemia*, *15*(1), 22–28.

Yawn, B. P., Buchanan, G. R., Afenyi-Annan, A. N., et al. (2014). Management of sickle cell disease: Summary of the 2014 evidence-based report by expert panel members. *Clinical Review & Education*, *312*(10), 1033–1048.

Zanella A., & Barcellini, W. (2014). Treatment of autoimmune hemolytic anemias. *Haematologica*, *99*(10), 1547–1554.

Resources

Aplastic Anemia and Myelodysplasia Association of Canada: http://www.aamac.ca/research.html

Aplastic Anemia and MDS International Foundation: http://www.aamds.org/aplastic

Blood and Marrow Transplant InfoNet: http://www.bmtinfonet.org

Canadian Blood Services: http://www.blood.ca/

Canadian Cancer Society: http://www.cancer.ca

Canadian Hemochromatosis Society: http://www.toomuchiron.ca/

Canadian Hemophilia Society: https://www.facebook.com/CanadianHemophiliaSociety

Canadian Hemophilia Society: https://www.hemophilia.ca/what-is-von-willebrand-disease/

International Myeloma Foundation: http://www.myeloma.org

Leukemia and Lymphoma Society: http://www.leukemia-lymphoma.org

Myelodysplastic Syndromes Foundation: http://www.mds-foundation.org

Sickle Cell Disease Association of Canada: http://www.sicklecelldisease.ca/fr/

55 Management of Patients With Infectious Diseases

Adapted by Bernice Heinrichs and Lisa Acorn

Learning Objectives

On completion of this chapter, the learner will be able to:

1. Differentiate between the concepts of colonization, infection, and disease.
2. Identify federal and local resources available when seeking information about infectious diseases and infection prevention and control.
3. Identify and describe Routine Practices and Additional Precautions (RPAP) and how to apply these into nursing practice.
4. Identify the benefits of adherence with an immunization schedule of recommended vaccines.
5. Describe emerging infectious diseases and factors that lead to their development.
6. Use the nursing process as a framework for care of patients with infectious diseases and sexually transmitted infections.

An **infectious disease** is any disease caused by the growth of pathogenic microbes in the body. It may or may not be communicable (i.e., contagious). Modern science has controlled, eradicated, or decreased the incidence of many infectious diseases. However, increases in other **infections**, such as those caused by antibiotic-resistant organisms and emerging infectious diseases, are a major concern.

This chapter explains/describes the infectious process, chain of infection, IPC measures including Routine Practices and Additional Precautions, specific organisms with potential to cause health care–associated infection (HAI), immunization, and emerging diseases. Other infectious diseases are discussed in the appropriate chapters, for example, refer to Chapter 24 for information on tuberculosis TB. It is important to understand infectious causes and the treatment of contagious, serious, and common infections. Table 55-1 presents selected infectious diseases, their causative organisms, routes of transmission, and usual **incubation periods** (time between contact and development of the first signs and symptoms).

Infection Prevention and Control

Health Canada and the Public Health Agency of Canada (PHAC) are the main federal departments in Canada involved in preventing and controlling infections in humans. The World Health Organization (WHO) and the Centers for Disease Control and Prevention (CDC) are principal international agencies with similar goals. In recent years, attention to **HAIs** has grown. Health Canada and the PHAC routinely publish recommendations, guidelines, and summaries through their Internet sites (http://www.hc-sc.gc.ca and http://www.phac-aspc.gc.ca, respectively) and the weekly journal, the Canada Communicable Disease Report (CCDR), in which significant cases, outbreaks, environmental hazards, or other public health problems are reported. Examples of important PHAC Guidelines include *Routine Practices and Additional Precautions for Preventing the Transmission of Infection in Health Care Settings* (PHAC, 2016); *Hand Hygiene Practices in Health care Settings* (PHAC, 2012); and *Clostridium Difficile Infection: Infection Prevention and Control Guidance for Management in Acute Care Settings* (PHAC, 2013a).

This chapter summarizes several aspects of infectious diseases. However, the field of infection prevention and control (IPC) is changing very rapidly. Health care workers should seek the most current information when they address patient care concerns or develop IPC policies.

The Infectious Process

The Chain of Infection

There are six links in the chain of infection; causative organism, reservoir, portal of exit, route of transmission,

susceptible host, and portal of entry. All of these elements are required for an infection to occur.

Figure 55-1 illustrates the elements of the chain and identifies points where health care workers can intervene to interrupt the chain

Understanding the chain of infection can help with both the prevention and treatment of infectious diseases.

Causative Organism

The types of microorganisms that cause infections are bacteria, rickettsiae, viruses, protozoa, fungi, and helminths.

Reservoir

Reservoir means any person, plant, animal, substance, or location that provides nourishment for microorganisms and enables further dispersal of the organism. Infections may be prevented by eliminating the causative organisms from the reservoir. For example, performing hand hygiene before and after contact with patients and their environment, and cleaning the environment to reduce the number of microorganisms help to break this link in the chain of infection.

Portal of Exit

The portal of exit means the route by which an infectious agent (microorganism) leaves the reservoir. For example, blood, body fluids, excretions, secretions exit the host from the respiratory, gastrointestinal, or skin/mucous membranes. Covering portals of exit, for example, dressing wounds, or wearing masks to control respiratory secretions help break this link in the chain of infection.

Glossary

Additional Precautions (AP): Extra measures used in addition to Routine Practices, to interrupt transmission of an infectious agent. AP are initiated based on a point-of-care risk assessment of the patient's condition or clinical symptoms or on a specific diagnosis.

alcohol-based hand rub (ABHR): A liquid, gel, or foam formulation of 60% to 90% alcohol (e.g., ethanol, isopropanol) used to reduce the number of microorganisms on hands. ABHRs contain emollients to reduce skin irritation and are less time-consuming to use than washing with soap and water.

bacteremia: laboratory proven presence of bacteria in the bloodstream

colonization: microorganisms present in or on a host, without host interference or interaction and without eliciting symptoms in the host

community-associated methicillin-resistant *Staphylococcus aureus (CA-MRSA)*: MRSA colonization or infection in a person who has not been treated in a health care setting

emerging infectious diseases: human infectious diseases with incidence increased within the past two decades or potential increase in the near future

fungemia: a bloodstream infection caused by a fungal organism

health care–associated infection (HAI): an infection not present or incubating at the time of admission to the health care setting

host: an organism that provides living conditions to support a microorganism

immune: person who has protection from a previous infection or immunization who resists reinfection when exposed to the same agent

incubation period: time between contact and onset of signs and symptoms

infection: condition in which the host interacts physiologically and immunologically with a microorganism

infectious disease: the consequences that result from invasion of the body by microorganisms that can produce harm and/or potential death

latency: time interval after primary infection when a microorganism lives within the host without producing clinical evidence of infection

methicillin-resistant *Staphylococcus aureus* (MRSA): *Staphylococcus aureus* bacterium that is not susceptible to extended penicillin antibiotic formulas, such as methicillin, oxacillin, or nafcillin; MRSA may be acquired in a health care facility or community setting.

normal flora: persistent nonpathogenic organisms colonizing a host

point-of-care risk assessment: before each patient interaction, the assessment of the risk of exposure to blood, body fluids, and nonintact skin prior to patient care; and the implementation of actions (e.g., performing hand hygiene and using the appropriate personal protective equipment [PPE]) to decrease exposure and prevent transmission of microorganisms

reservoir: any person, plant, animal, substance, or location that provides living conditions for microorganisms and enables further dispersal of the organism

Routine Practices (RP): A comprehensive set of infection prevention and control (IPC) measures that have been developed for use in the care of all patients at all times in all health care settings. Routine Practices aim to minimize or prevent health care–associated infections in all individuals in the health care setting, including patients, health care workers, other staff, visitors, and contractors. Routine Practices is synonymous with CDC standard precautions.

susceptible: not possessing immunity to a particular pathogen

transient flora: organisms that have been recently acquired and are likely to be shed in a relatively short period

vancomycin-resistant *Enterococcus (VRE)*: Enterococcus bacterium that is resistant to the antibiotic vancomycin

virulence: degree of pathogenicity of an organism

TABLE 55-1 Infectious Diseases, Causative Organisms, Routes of Transmission, and Usual Incubation Periods

Disease or Condition	Organism	Usual Mode of Transmission	Usual Incubation Period (Infection to First Symptom)
Acquired immunodeficiency syndrome	Human immunodeficiency virus	Sexual; percutaneous; perinatal	Median of 10 years
Anthrax	*Bacillus anthracis*	Airborne, contact, or ingestion	1–6 days
Chancroid	*Haemophilus ducreyi*	Sexual	3–5 days
Chickenpox	Varicella zoster	Airborne or contact	~10–21 days
Cytomegalovirus infection	Cytomegalovirus	Transfusion and transplantation; sexual; perinatal	Highly variable: 3–8 weeks after transfusion, 3–12 weeks after delivery of newborn
Diarrheal disease (common causes)	*Campylobacter* species	Ingestion of contaminated food	3–5 days
	Clostridium difficile	Fecal–oral	Variable; in part related to the influence of antibiotic agents
	Salmonella species	Ingestion of contaminated food or drink	12–36 hours
	Shigella species	Ingestion of contaminated food or drink; direct contact with carrier	1–3 days
	Yersinia species	Ingestion of contaminated food or drink; direct contact with carrier	1–3 days
Ebola	Ebola virus	Contact with blood or body fluids	2–21 days
Gonorrhea	*Neisseria gonorrhoeae*	Sexual; perinatal	2–7 days
Hand, foot, and mouth disease	Coxsackievirus	Direct contact with nose and throat secretions and with feces of people who are infected	3–5 days
Hantavirus pulmonary syndrome	Sin Nombre virus	Contact (direct or indirect) with rodents	Unclear
Hepatitis, foodborne	Hepatitis A virus	Ingestion of contaminated food or drink; direct contact with carrier	15–50 days
	Hepatitis E virus	Ingestion of contaminated food or drink; direct contact with carrier	15–65 days
Hepatitis, bloodborne	Hepatitis B virus	Sexual; perinatal; percutaneous	45–160 days
	Hepatitis C virus	Sexual; perinatal; percutaneous	15–160 days
	Hepatitis D	Sexual; perinatal; percutaneous	30–150 days
	Hepatitis G	Percutaneous	14–145 days
Herpes simplex	Human herpes viruses 1 and 2	Contact with mucous membrane secretions	2–12 days
Histoplasmosis	*Histoplasma capsulatum*	Inhalation of airborne spores	5–18 days
Hookworm disease	*Necator americanus; Ancylostoma duodenale*	Contact with soil contaminated with human feces	A few weeks to many months
Impetigo	*Staphylococcus aureus, Streptococcus pyogenes*	Contact with *S. aureus* carrier or with patient's soiled towels or combs	4–10 days
Influenza	Influenza virus A, B, or C	Droplet spread	24–72 hours
Legionnaires disease	*Legionella pneumophila*	Airborne from water source	2–10 days
Lyme disease	*Borrelia burgdorferi*	Tick bite	14–23 days
Lymphogranuloma venereum	*Chlamydia trachomatis*	Sexual	Weeks to years
Malaria	*Plasmodium vivax; Plasmodium malariae; Plasmodium falciparum; Plasmodium ovale*	Bite from *Anopheles* species mosquito	12–30 days
Marburg hemorrhagic fever	Marburg virus	Unknown route of transmission from animals to humans; person-to-person by droplets and direct contact	5–10 days
Meningococcal meningitis or bacteremia	*Neisseria meningitidis*	Contact with pharyngeal secretions; perhaps airborne	2–10 days
Mononucleosis	Epstein–Barr virus	Contact with pharyngeal secretions	4–6 weeks
Mycobacterial diseases (nontuberculosis *Mycobacterium* species)	*Mycobacterium avium; Mycobacterium kansasii; Mycobacterium fortuitum; Mycobacterium gordonae;* other *Mycobacterium* species	Variable; probably contact with soil, water, or other environmental source; none is person-to-person transmissible	Variable
Mycoplasmal pneumonia	*Mycoplasma pneumoniae*	Droplet inhalation	14–21 days

continued >

TABLE 55-1 Infectious Diseases, Causative Organisms, Routes of Transmission, and Usual Incubation Periods (Continued)

Disease or Condition	Organism	Usual Mode of Transmission	Usual Incubation Period (Infection to First Symptom)
Norovirus	*Norovirus*	Fecal–oral by food or water or by person-to-person spread	24–48 hours
Pediculosis	*Pediculus humanus capitis* (head louse); *Pediculosis pubis* (crab louse)	Direct contact	1–2 weeks
Pertussis (whooping cough)	*Bordetella pertussis*	Contact with respiratory droplets	7–10 days
Pinworm disease	*Enterobius vermicularis*	Direct contact with egg-contaminated articles	4- to 6-week life cycle; often takes months of infection before recognition
Pneumocystis jiroveci pneumonia	*Pneumocystis jiroveci*	Unknown; not transmitted person to person	Infants: 1–2 months; adults: unclear
Pneumococcal pneumonia	*Streptococcus pneumoniae*	Droplet spread	Probably 1–3 days
Rabies	Rabies virus	Bite from rabid animal	2–8 weeks
Respiratory syncytial disease	Respiratory syncytial virus	Self-inoculation by mouth or nose after contact with infectious respiratory secretions	3–7 days
Ringworm	*Microsporum* species; *Trichophyton* species	Direct and indirect contact with lesions	4–10 days
Rocky Mountain spotted fever	*Rickettsia rickettsii*	Bite from infected tick	3–14 days
Roseola infantum	Human herpes virus 6	Saliva	10–15 days
Rotavirus gastroenteritis	*Rotavirus*	Fecal–oral route	~48 hours
Rubella	Rubella virus	Droplet spread; direct contact	14–21 days
Scabies	*Sarcoptes scabei*	Direct skin contact	2–6 weeks
Smallpox	*Variola major and minor*	Airborne and contact	7–14 days
Syphilis	*Treponema pallidum*	Sexual; perinatal	10 days to 10 weeks
Tetanus	*Clostridium tetani*	Puncture wound	4–21 days
Trichinosis	*Trichinella spiralis*	Ingestion of insufficiently cooked foods, especially pork and beef	10–14 days
Tuberculosis	*Mycobacterium tuberculosis*	Airborne	4–12 weeks to the formation of primary lesion
West Nile virus	West Nile virus	Bite of infected mosquitoes; from transfusions and transplants; perinatal	3–14 days
Zika virus	Zika virus	Bite of infected *Aedes* mosquitoes	Unclear

Route of Transmission

A route of transmission is necessary to connect the infectious source with a new host.

Contact, droplet, airborne, ingestion, common vehicle, and vectorborne are potential routes of infectious disease transmission. Transmission routes vary by microorganism and some microorganisms have more than one route of transmission. Refer to Table 55-1 for examples.

Use of barriers such as personal protective equipment (PPE) and hand hygiene help break this link in the chain of infection.

Susceptible Host

For infection to occur, the host must be susceptible to a particular organism. Previous infection or immunization may render the host **immune**, and not susceptible, to an infection from that organism. Although exposure to potentially infectious microorganisms occurs on a continual basis, healthy immune systems generally prevent infection.

Maximizing host defenses through activities such as immunization, improved nutrition, and diabetes control help break this link in the chain of infection (PHAC, 2016).

Portal of Entry

A portal of entry is needed for an organism to enter the host, for example, mucous membranes, respiratory tract, broken skin, and devices such as intravenous (IV) lines. Specific organisms require different portals of entry for infection to occur (see Fig. 55-1).

Measures to protect the portal of entry include covering wounds, wearing PPE, use of aseptic technique, and performing hand hygiene (PHAC, 2016).

Measures to Minimize the Risk of Infection

The PHAC recommends use of Routine Practices in the care of all patients to minimize or prevent HAIs in the health care setting. Routine Practices address the infectious agent, infected source control, susceptible host protection, and environmental hygiene through use of engineering measures, administrative measures, and PPE (PHAC, 2016).

Engineering Measures

Engineering controls are built into facility and include single-patient rooms, traffic flow, negative pressure

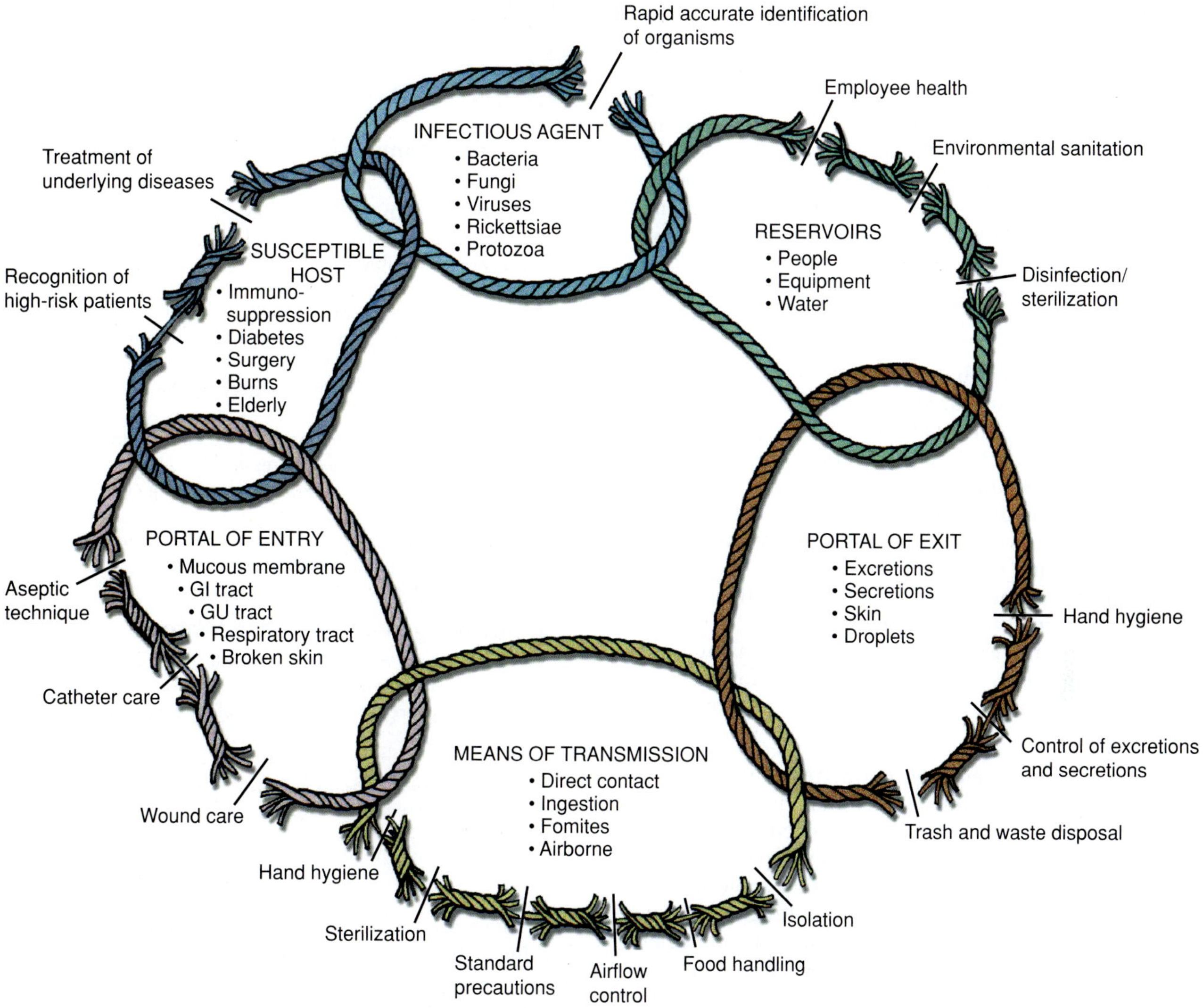

FIGURE 55-1. Health care workers' interventions used to break the chain of infection transmission. GI, gastrointestinal; GU, genitourinary.

ventilation, hand hygiene facilities, and temperature and humidity controls.

Administrative Measures

Administrative controls include development of policies, procedures and practices that support patient and staff safety such as education and training, immunization, staffing ratios, environmental cleaning, monitoring of hand hygiene compliance and outbreak management.

Routine Practices

Routine Practices include point-of-care risk assessment, source control, hand hygiene, aseptic care of IV catheters and other invasive equipment, safe handling and use of sharps, selection and use of PPE, and cleaning and disinfection of the environment and equipment. Nurses also provide education to patients, families, and visitors regarding disease transmission including preventative measures such as respiratory hygiene, and if applicable, the reason for Additional Precautions necessary for care. The following are recommendations for routine practices:

1. **Hand hygiene:** Use after touching blood, body fluids, secretions, excretions, or contaminated items; immediately after removing gloves; and between patient contacts
2. **PPE:**
   - *Gloves:* Use for touching blood, body fluids, secretions, excretions, and contaminated items, and for touching mucous membranes and nonintact skin
   - *Gown:* Use during procedures and patient care activities when contact of clothing/exposed skin with blood or body fluids, secretions, and excretions is anticipated
   - *Mask, eye protection (goggles), face shield*[1]: Use during procedures and patient care activities likely to generate splashes or sprays of blood, body fluids,

[1]During aerosol-generating procedures on patients with suspected or proven infections transmitted by respiratory aerosols (e.g., severe acute respiratory syndrome), wear a fit-tested N95 or higher respirator in addition to gloves, gown, and face/eye protection.

and secretions, especially suctioning or endotracheal intubation
3. **Soiled patient care equipment:** Handle in a manner that prevents transfer of microorganisms to others and to the environment; wear gloves if visibly contaminated; and perform hand hygiene
4. **Environmental control:** Develop procedures for routine care, cleaning, and disinfection of environmental surfaces, especially frequently touched surfaces in patient care areas
5. **Textiles and laundry:** Handle in a manner that prevents transfer of microorganisms to others and to the environment
6. **Needles and other sharps:** Do not recap, bend, break, or hand manipulate used needles; if recapping is required, use a one-handed scoop technique only; use safety features when available; and place used sharps in a puncture-resistant container
7. **Patient resuscitation:** Use mouthpiece, resuscitation bag, and other ventilation devices to prevent contact with mouth and oral secretions
8. **Patient placement:** Prioritize for single-patient room if patient is at increased risk for transmission, is likely to contaminate the environment, does not maintain appropriate hygiene, or is at increased risk for acquiring infection or developing adverse outcome following infection.

Respiratory hygiene/cough etiquette (source containment of infectious respiratory secretions in symptomatic patients, beginning at initial point of encounter, such as triage and reception areas in emergency departments and physician offices): Instruct symptomatic people to cover mouth and nose when sneezing or coughing, use tissues and dispose in no-touch receptacle, observe hand hygiene after soiling of hands with respiratory secretions, and wear surgical mask if tolerated (CDC, 2007).

Point-of-Care Risk Assessment

A **point-of-care risk assessment** (PCRA) is performed before each patient contact to evaluate the likelihood of exposure to an infectious agent and to guide control measures.

Source Control

Early identification and source control (e.g., triage, spatial separation of patients with potentially infectious disease) is facilitated by prompt assessment of patients for signs and symptoms of acute infection. Visual reminders can be used to cue patients who are potentially infectious to perform hand hygiene and wear a mask if necessary. Physical barriers at triage and reception areas may be used to protect staff.

Hand Hygiene

Hand hygiene is the most effective way to prevent transmission of microorganisms that cause HAIs in health care settings (PHAC, 2012). Chart 55-1 describes hand hygiene methods. Hand hygiene reduces the bacterial load and decreases the risk of transfer to other patients. All health care settings should evaluate compliance with hand hygiene by all personnel who care for patients.

Health care workers should not wear artificial fingernails, fingernail enhancements, nail extenders or jewellery, other than a simple ring, when providing patient care, working with sterile linen/supplies, medical device reprocessing, or in the clinical laboratory, as they may impede effective hand hygiene (PHAC, 2012). Natural nails should be kept less than 0.6-cm long and clear nail polish, if worn, should not be chipped as it can support increased bacterial growth (PHAC, 2012).

Alcohol-based hand rubs (ABHRs) are the preferred method of hand hygiene in health care settings. ABHRs provide a rapid kill of most transient microorganisms, are less time consuming than washing with soap and water, and are easier on skin (PHAC, 2012).

Hands should be washed with soap and water if visibly soiled, or if exposure to norovirus or *C. difficile* is suspected.

CHART 55-1

Hand Hygiene Methods

Hand Decontamination With Alcohol-Based Product

- After contact with body fluids, excretions, mucous membranes, nonintact skin, or wound dressings as long as hands are not visibly soiled
- After contact with a patient's intact skin (e.g., after taking pulse or blood pressure or lifting a patient)
- In patient care, when moving from a contaminated body site to a clean body site
- After contact with inanimate objects in the patient's immediate vicinity
- Before caring for patients with severe neutropenia or other forms of severe immune suppression
- Before donning sterile gloves when inserting central catheters
- Before inserting urinary catheters or other devices that do not require a surgical procedure
- After removing gloves

Handwashing With Soap and Water

- When hands are visibly dirty or contaminated with biologic material from patient care
- When health care workers do not tolerate waterless alcohol product

Adapted from Centers for Disease Control and Prevention. (2002). Guideline for hand hygiene in health care settings. *MMWR: Morbidity and Mortality Weekly Report, 51*(RR 16), 1–56.

Aseptic Technique

Aseptic technique is used to prevent transfer of microorganisms from the patient's body surface to a normally sterile body site or from one person to another by keeping patient's skin, supplies, and surfaces free from microorganisms.

Safe injection practices include considering a syringe or needle contaminated after it has been used to enter or connect to a patient's IV catheter, infusion bag, or administration set; never entering a vial or bag/bottle with a used syringe or needle; never administering medications from the same syringe to more than one patient; using single-use vials for only one patient; using IV solution for only one patient and dedicating multidose vials to a single patient whenever possible (PHAC, 2016).

Sharps Safety

The risk of bloodborne infection is reduced by handling needles, scalpels, and other sharp objects with care to avoid percutaneous injury. Used needles should not be recapped. Instead, they are placed directly into puncture-resistant containers immediately after use. Safety engineered sharps, for example, needleless devices, should be used when possible (PHAC, 2016a).

If there is a blood or body fluids exposure, the nurse immediately: (1) performs first aid, for example, rinses thoroughly with warm water; (2) reports the exposure to the employer; and (3) seeks medical attention.

Use of Personal Protective Equipment

PPE such as gloves, gowns, facial protection and respirators, are used to prevent exposure to infectious disease.

Glove use is determined by the point of care risk assessment. Gloves are worn if contact with blood, body fluids, secretions and excretions, mucous membranes, draining wounds or nonintact skin is anticipated or during direct care if the health care worker has an open cut or abrasions on hands. Gloves are single use and discarded after patient care contact. Gloves do not completely eliminate hand contamination, as hands can become soiled through glove defects and during glove removal. Hand hygiene is performed after gloves are removed. Gloves are not required for routine patient care activities in which contact is limited to patient's intact skin (PHAC, 2016a).

As patient advocates, nurses have an important role in promoting hand hygiene and glove use by other health care workers, such as laboratory personnel, technicians, and others who have contact with patients.

Latex gloves are preferred over vinyl gloves because of comfort and fit; they also may offer greater protection from exposures. However, use of latex gloves can lead to reactions ranging from local skin irritation to more severe reactions. If reactions occur, vinyl, nitrile, powder-free gloves or "low-protein" latex gloves may be used. The nurse who experiences irritation or an allergic reaction associated with glove use should report symptoms to occupational health or a physician.

Gowns are worn to protect skin and clothing during patient care activities that may produce soiling or generate splashes or sprays of blood, body fluids, secretions, or excretions.

Facial protection is worn during activities or procedures that may result in splashes or sprays of blood, body fluids, secretions or excretions. Facial protection requires both mask and eye protection, for example, use of mask with visor attachment or face shields that cover the mucous membranes of the eyes, nose, and mouth.

N95 respirators are disposable particulate filtering face pieces that fit closely over the mouth, nose and chin worn to protect the wearer from diseases spread through the air, for example, pulmonary tuberculosis. Occupational Health requires fit-testing for health care workers to determine appropriate respirator use for Airborne Precautions.

Cleaning and Disinfection of Patient Care Equipment

Reusable equipment that has been in direct contact with a patient or in that patient's environment should be cleaned and disinfected or sterilized before use on another patient.

Handling of Linen and Waste

Handle linens in a manner that reduces the potential risk of cross contamination, for example, use of laundry hampers close to the point of care.

Follow local protocols for proper handling and disposal for the types of waste created, for example, biomedical.

Patient Placement and Accommodation

Patient placement is used to reduce the risk of exposure to a patient who is infectious, for example, single or multi-patient room is determined by the point-of-care risk assessment for presence of known or suspected infection.

Patient Flow

Transfer of patients within and between facilities should be limited unless medically required.

Additional Precautions

Additional Precautions are used in addition to Routine Practices to prevent the transmission of specific infectious agents that are highly contagious, epidemiologically significant, or infectious syndromes spread via airborne, droplet, or contact routes (PHAC, 2016).

Airborne Precautions are required for patients with suspect or confirmed pulmonary tuberculosis, chickenpox, or other airborne pathogens. When hospitalized, patients should be in airborne infection isolation rooms (AIIR), engineered to provide negative air pressure, rapid turnover of air, and air either highly filtered or exhausted directly to the outside. Health care professionals are required to wear a fit-tested N95 respirator at all times while in the patient's room.

Droplet Precautions are used for organisms such as influenza or meningococcus transmitted by close, face-to-face, within 2 metres, exposure to respiratory secretions. While taking care of a patient requiring Droplet Precautions, the nurse wears a face mask and eye protection, but because the risk of transmission is limited to close proximity, the door may remain open (PHAC, 2016).

Contact Precautions are used to prevent the transmission of organisms such as antibiotic-resistant organisms or *C. difficile* that are spread by direct contact (skin-to-skin), or by indirect contact with the patient's environment. Contact precautions are also used when the presence of body fluids, or secretions such as uncontained wound drainage or fecal incontinence, pose a higher risk of transmission. When possible, the patient requiring Contact Precautions is placed in a private room to facilitate hand hygiene and decrease environmental contamination. Masks are not needed, and doors do not need to be closed (see Chart 55-2).

Home-Based Care of the Patient With an Infectious Disease

The nurse who cares for the patient with an infectious disease in the home provides information about infection risk prevention to the patient, the family, and the caregiver. Refer to Chart 55-3. As in other health care settings the nurse implements Routine Practices to reduce the risk of infection.

CHART 55-2

Summary of Types of Precautions and Patients Requiring the Precautions

Routine Practices

Use Routine Practices for the care of all patients.
Add Additional Precautions which include:

Airborne Precautions

In addition to Routine Practices, use Airborne Precautions for patients known or suspected to have serious illnesses transmitted by airborne droplet nuclei. Examples of such illnesses include the following:

- Measles
- Varicella (including disseminated zoster)[2]
- Tuberculosis

Droplet Precautions

In addition to Routine Practices, use Droplet Precautions for patients known or suspected to have serious illnesses transmitted by large particle droplets. Examples of such illnesses include:

- Invasive *Haemophilus influenzae* type b disease, including meningitis, pneumonia, epiglottitis, and sepsis
- Invasive *Neisseria meningitidis* disease, including meningitis, pneumonia, and sepsis
- Other serious bacterial respiratory infections spread by droplet transmission, including:
  - Diphtheria (pharyngeal)
  - Primary atypical pneumonia (*Mycoplasma pneumoniae*)
  - Pertussis
  - Pneumonic plague
  - Streptococcal (group A) pharyngitis, pneumonia, or scarlet fever in infants and young children
- Serious viral infections spread by droplet transmission, including:
  - Adenovirus[3]
  - Influenza
  - Mumps
  - Parvovirus B19
  - Rubella

Contact Precautions

In addition to Routine Practices, use Contact Precautions for patients known or suspected to have serious illnesses easily transmitted by direct patient contact or by contact with items in the patient's environment. Examples of such illnesses include:

- Gastrointestinal, respiratory, skin, or wound infections or colonization with multidrug-resistant bacteria judged by the infection control program, based on current provincial, regional, or national recommendations, to be of special clinical and epidemiologic significance
- Enteric infections with a low infectious dose or prolonged environmental survival, including:
  - *Clostridium difficile*
  - For diapered or incontinent patients: enterohemorrhagic *Escherichia coli* O157:H7, *Shigella* species, hepatitis A, or rotavirus
- Respiratory syncytial virus, parainfluenza virus, or enteroviral infections in infants and young children
- Skin infections that are highly contagious or that may occur on dry skin, including:
  - Diphtheria (cutaneous)
  - Herpes simplex virus (neonatal or mucocutaneous)
  - Major (noncontained) abscesses, cellulitis, or pressure ulcers
  - Scabies
  - Staphylococcal furunculosis in infants and young children
  - Zoster (disseminated or in the immunocompromised host)[4]
- Viral and hemorrhagic conjunctivitis
- Viral hemorrhagic infections (Ebola, Lassa, or Marburg)

[2]Certain infections require more than one type of precaution. From PHAC Routine Practices and Additional Precautions for Preventing the Transmission of Infection in Health care (2016a).
[3]Certain infections require more than one type of precaution. From PHAC Routine Practices and Additional Precautions for Preventing the Transmission of Infection in Health care (2016a).

Patient Education

When assessing the risk for infection of the patient in the home environment who is immunosuppressed, it is important to realize that intrinsic colonizing bacteria and latent viral infections present a greater risk than do extrinsic environmental contaminants. The nurse reassures the patient and family that their home needs to be clean but not sterile. For patients with neutropenia or T-cell dysfunction (e.g., patients with acquired immunodeficiency syndrome [AIDS]), it is wise to restrict visits of people with potentially contagious illnesses. The immunosuppressed patient is vulnerable to acquiring bacterial infection with enteric pathogens from food; therefore, family members should be reminded about the need to follow recommendations for hygiene and safe cooking times and temperatures.

Reducing Risk to Household Members

Establishing reasonable barriers to infection transmission in the household is an important part of home care. The nurse can teach household members strategies to reduce their risk of becoming infected based on the route of transmission of the disease-causing organism. The family should be reassured that frequent hand washing and use of common household disinfectants are effective measures to prevent the spread of infection.

Family members assisting in the care of a patient with a bloodborne infection such as HIV or hepatitis C can prevent transmission by carefully handling any sharp objects that are contaminated with blood. Family teaching may include discussion about the importance of avoiding sharing items like razors and toothbrushes and measures to avoid exposure to blood when shaving the patient; performing dressing changes; or administering any IV, intramuscular, or subcutaneous medication. Used needles, syringes, and vascular access equipment should be discarded into containers designed for sharps disposal. With the exception of TB, the opportunistic infections associated with AIDS do not usually pose a risk to healthy family members. Dishes are safe to use after being washed

CHART 55-3

HOME CARE CHECKLIST • Prevention of Infection in the Home Care Setting

At the completion of education, the patient and/or caregiver will be able to:

- State the impact of infectious disease and treatment on physiologic functioning, ADLs, IADLs, roles, relationships, and spirituality
- State the need for infection risk prevention for the patient (preventing recurrence or new infections) caregivers, and family in the home
  - Verbalize the route of transmission for agent of infection
- State the purpose, dose, route, schedule, side effects, and precautions for prescribed medications
  - Adhere to antibiotic regimen (patient) or completion of vaccination series (patient and caregiver)
- State how to contact all members of the treatment team (e.g., health care providers, home care professionals, and durable medical equipment and supply vendor)
- State changes in lifestyle (e.g., diet, activity) or home environment necessary to decrease risk for infection
  - Perform satisfactory hand hygiene technique, oral hygiene, total body hygiene, and maintain skin integrity (patient)
  - Ensure thorough hand hygiene (alcohol-based disinfectant or handwashing) after care (family/caregiver)
  - Avoid contact with someone who has a known infectious disease
  - Cook all foods thoroughly and store meat products separate from other food groups
  - Use separate eating utensils and towels
  - Demonstrate aseptic technique in the care of technical equipment such as IV catheter and indwelling urinary catheter
- Identify signs and symptoms of infection to report to the primary provider, such as fever, chills, wet or dry cough; breathing problems; white patches in the mouth; swollen glands; nausea; vomiting; persistent abdominal pain; persistent diarrhea; problems with urination or changes in the character of the urine; red, swollen, or draining wounds; sores or lesions on the body; persistent vaginal discharge with or without itching; and severe fatigue
- Demonstrate how to monitor for signs of infection
- Describe to whom, how, and when to report signs of infection
- Describe appropriate actions to take should infection occur
- Relate how to reach primary provider with questions or complications
- State time and date of follow-up medical appointments, therapy, and testing
- Identify sources of support (e.g., friends, relatives, faith community, support groups, caregiver support)
- Identify the need for health-promotion, disease prevention, and screening activities

with hot water, and bedding, towels, and clothing are safe to use after being washed in a hot water cycle.

Colonization, Infection, and Infectious Disease

Relatively few anatomic sites (e.g., brain, blood, bone, heart, vascular system) are sterile. Bacteria found throughout the body usually provide beneficial **normal flora** to compete with potential pathogens, to facilitate digestion, or to work in sync with the host.

Colonization

The term **colonization** is used to describe microorganisms present without host interference or interaction. Organisms reported in microbiology test results may reflect colonization rather than infection. Colonization can be present without causing harm or infection and may not require treatment.

Infection

Infection indicates a host interaction with an organism. A patient colonized with *S. aureus* may have staphylococci on the skin without any skin interruption or irritation. However, if the patient has an incision, *S. aureus* could enter the wound, resulting in an immune system reaction of local inflammation and migration of white cells to the site. Clinical evidence of redness, heat, and pain and laboratory evidence of white blood cells on the wound specimen smear suggest infection. In this situation, the host identifies the staphylococci as *foreign*. Infection is recognized by the host reaction (manifested by signs and symptoms) and by laboratory-based evidence of white blood cell reaction and microbiologic organism identification.

Infectious Disease

It is important to recognize the difference between infection and infectious disease. Infectious disease is the state

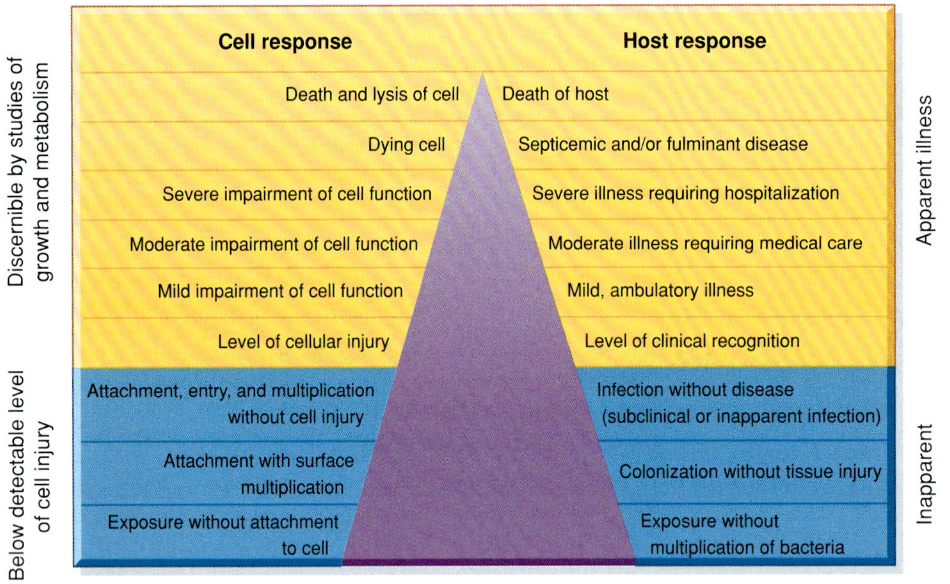

FIGURE 55-2. Biologic spectrum of response to bacterial infection at the cellular level (*left*) and of the intact host (*right*). (Redrawn from Evans, A. S., & Brachman, P. S. (1998). *Bacterial infections in humans*. New York: Plenum.)

in which the infected host displays a decline in wellness due to the infection. When the host interacts immunologically with an organism but remains symptom free, the definition of infectious disease has not been met. For example, when a person is first infected with *M. tuberculosis*, infection can be detected by a positive tuberculin skin test (TST), which demonstrates immunologic recognition. Most people who are infected with *M. tuberculosis* have latent infection, but few people (approximately 10%) actually become ill and demonstrate symptoms of TB (fever, weight loss, and advancing pneumonia). Figure 55-2 depicts the range of response to bacterial infection at the cellular and host level.

The primary source of information about most bacterial infections is the microbiology laboratory report, which is a tool used along with clinical indicators to determine if a patient is colonized, infected, or diseased. Microbiology reports from clinical specimens usually show three components: the smear and stain, the culture and organism identification, and the antimicrobial susceptibility, that is, sensitivity. As a marker of infection, the smear and stain generally provide the most helpful information because they describe the mix of cells present at the anatomic site at the time of specimen collection. Culture and sensitivity results specify which organisms are recognized and which antibiotics actively affect the bacteria.

Nurses serve important roles in preventing the transfer of organisms as they have many opportunities for spreading organisms, given their frequent encounters with patients and families. It is essential for the nurse to model appropriate and effective hand hygiene practices in all aspects of patient care. Nurses can also help reduce hand-to-hand spread of organisms by serving as patient advocates. The nurse should observe the hand hygiene activities of other professionals and alert them to lapses in technique that are observed. Nurses need to educate patients and their families to feel comfortable in reminding health care workers to perform hand hygiene before patient contact.

The following sections summarizes several aspects of infectious diseases. However, the field of infection control and prevention changes rapidly. Nurses should seek the most current information when they address patient care concerns or develop infection control policies (see the Resources section).

Specific Organisms With Health Care–Associated Infection Potential

Antimicrobial-Resistant Organisms

Antimicrobial-resistant organisms (AROs) are microorganisms that have developed resistance to one or more antimicrobial agents and are of clinical or epidemiologic significance. In Canada, **methicillin-resistant *Staphylococcus aureus*** (MRSA), vancomycin-resistant enterococci (VRE), *C. difficile* infection (CDI), extended spectrum β-lactamase (ESBL), and carbapenemase-producing Enterobacteriaceae (CPE) are considered AROs.

Transmission of AROs occurs directly by a health care worker's hand contact with infected or colonized patients and indirectly by hand contact with contaminated equipment or environments (PHAC, 2016a).

Elements of ARO control may also include careful selection and use of antibiotics, clinical microbiology support and identification, differentiation of resistant strains, and active surveillance cultures for ARO colonization (PHAC, 2016b).

MRSA (Methicillin-Resistant Staphylococcus aureus)

MRSA, a common human pathogen, refers to *S. aureus* that is resistant to beta lactam antibiotics such as methicillin, oxacillin, penicillin, and amoxicillin. Soon after penicillin was discovered in the 1940s, *S. aureus* became almost universally penicillin resistant. Alternative therapies in the form of cephalosporins and synthetic penicillin solutions such as methicillin were introduced.

MRSA can colonize the skin and mucosal surfaces of healthy people or cause infections such as wound, urine, skin and soft tissue infections, osteomyelitis, endocarditis, and bacteremia, especially in people who are immunocompromised.

Health care–associated MRSA (HA-MRSA) infections are associated with increased morbidity and mortality and costs.

MRSA is transmitted by direct contact or indirectly through contact with contaminated items or surfaces.

COMMUNITY-ASSOCIATED MRSA (CA-MRSA). **Community-associated MRSA (CA-MRSA)** has rapidly emerged over the past decade, causing infection in young, healthy people (e.g., skin, soft tissue, and pneumonia). CA-MRSA is linked to increased illness severity and deaths. Risk factors include overcrowding, frequent skin-to-skin contact, abraded or compromised skin surfaces, sharing of potentially contaminated personal items, challenges in maintaining personal cleanliness and hygiene, and limited access to health care (Irvine, 2017).

CA-MRSA strains introduced into Canadian hospitals are transmitted in the same manner as health care strains and may become indistinguishable from HA-MRSA strains.

A 2016 laboratory analysis of MRSA strain types found the overall proportion of CA-MRSA continues to surpass the overall proportion of HA-MRSA (45% vs. 32%) (Canadian Antimicrobial Resistance Surveillance System, 2018). CA-MRSA can usually be treated with trimethoprim–sulfamethoxazole, clindamycin, and tetracyclines. Invasive, severe, and complicated infections are often treated with parental vancomycin.

Vancomycin-resistant MRSA strains have emerged in the United States and Europe but are rare in Canada (Canadian Antimicrobial Resistance Surveillance System, 2018).

VRE (Vancomycin-Resistant Enterococcus)

Enterococci are gram-positive bacteria that live in the gastrointestinal tract. They are commonly found in the environment and rarely cause infection. A person is infected with **vancomycin-resistant *Enterococcus* (VRE)** when they become symptomatic, for example, urinary tract or blood stream infection. People are at higher risk for VRE infection if they are immunocompromised; were previously treated with vancomycin or other antibiotics; or if they had surgery or have medical devices such as urinary catheters (PHAC, 2017c).

VRE is usually spread by person-to-person contact or by contact with contaminated surfaces (PHAC, 2017c).

Many VRE strains are resistant to all other antimicrobial therapies so there may be few effective therapy options. VRE colonization and infection can also serve as a reservoir of vancomycin-resistant coded genes that may be transferred to the more virulent *S. aureus* (Canadian Antimicrobial Resistance Surveillance System, 2018).

Clostridium difficile

C. difficile, a spore-forming bacterium, is the most frequent cause of health care–associated infectious diarrhea resulting in increased morbidity and mortality, length of stay, and cost. In Canada, NAP1, a hypervirulent strain, accounted for approximately 24% of isolates from hospitalized patients in 2015 (Loo et al., 2018). It is estimated 37,900 cases of *C. difficile* infection (CDI), of which 27% are recurrent infection, occur annually in Canada, costing about $281 million (Loo et al., 2018).

After previous increases in the health care–associated rate of CDI, the Canadian Nosocomial Infection Surveillance Program reported a decreased incidence in participating hospitals from 7.9/10,000 patient-days in 2011 to 4.3/10,000 patient-days in 2015. Implementation of effective antimicrobial stewardship programs and IPC measures may have impacted this rate (Loo et al., 2018).

Antibiotic use often precedes CDI as antibiotics disrupt the intestinal flora and cause pathologic conditions by releasing toxins into the lumen of the bowel. In pseudomembranous colitis, the most extreme form of CDI, debris from the injured lumen and from white blood cells accumulates in the form of pseudomembranes or studded areas of the colon. The destruction of such a large anatomic area can produce profound sepsis and can be fatal.

C. difficile can be transmitted within health care facilities by person-to-person contact or environmental contamination. Contact Precautions should be implemented for patients with acute diarrhea, and suspected or confirmed CDI. *C. difficile* spores are resistant to alcohol and some disinfectants. Hand hygiene should be performed with soap and water. Sporicidal disinfectants such as bleach (hypochlorites) may be recommended for environmental cleaning (PHAC, 2013a).

Treatment of CDI usually involves discontinuation of antibiotics prescribed for other indications and treatment with Vancomycin. Fecal microbiota transplantation may be used as an alternative therapy for recurrent CDI (Loo et al., 2018). Fecal donors must be healthy and free of infectious diseases, including HIV, hepatitis, and intestinal pathogens that could be harmful to the recipient (Health Canada, 2016).

Multidrug-Resistant Gram-Negative Organisms

During the past several decades, the incidence of infections caused by multidrug-resistant gram-negative organisms has increased dramatically.

Resistance to the carbapenem antibiotics, especially in Enterobacteriaceae, is particularly concerning. Enterobacteriaceae are gram-negative organisms including *E. coli*, *Klebsiella* spp., and *Enterobacter* spp. Limited available treatment options for infections caused by carbapenemase-producing Enterobacteriaceae result in poorer health outcomes (CARSS, 2018; Bonomo, Burd, Conly, et al., 2018).

Amidst rapid intercontinental spread of CPE, rates in sentinel Canadian hospitals remain relatively low; however, the number of CPE isolates reported to provincial laboratories is rising, for example, 4 in 2009 and 779 in 2016, with the largest increase (1.8-fold) between 2015 and 2016 (CARRS, 2018).

Once introduced into health care environments, these organisms can spread easily during contact with contaminated equipment and on health care workers' hands. Routine Practices and implementation of Contact Precautions diminishes the risk of patient-to-patient transmission.

Preventing Health Care–Associated Bloodstream Infections (Bacteremia and Fungemia)

Bacteremia is defined as the laboratory-confirmed presence of bacteria in the bloodstream. **Fungemia** is a bloodstream infection caused by a fungal organism. Most health care–associated blood stream infections (BSIs) are associated with the use of a central venous catheter (CVC)

CHART 55-4

Conditions That Suggest the Presence of Health Care–Associated Vascular Access Device-Related Bacteremia or Fungemia

- The patient has catheter in place, appears septic, but has no obvious reason to suggest predisposition to sepsis
- There is no infection at another body site to indicate probable source of sepsis
- The site of vascular line insertion is red, swollen, or draining (especially purulent drainage)
- The patient has a central vascular line in place at the onset of sepsis
- The bloodstream infection is caused by *Candida* species or by common skin organisms such as coagulase-negative staphylococci, *Bacillus* species, or *Corynebacterium* species
- The patient remains septic after appropriate therapy without removal of the vascular access device

(PHAC, 2014). Microorganisms can migrate along the catheter from the insertion site or may be introduced into the catheter lumen at junction sites, especially when these are disconnected.

In the United States, approximately 16,000 CVC-BSIs occur in ICUs, and 500 to 4,000 patients die annually from the infection. CVC-BSIs are also associated with increased length of hospital stay and medical costs. Cost of a CVC-BSI are estimated to range from $34,000 to $56,000 US with an estimated annual cost of $60 to $460 million. There are no equivalent Canadian figures (PHAC, 2014).

The most common causative microorganisms for CVC-BSI are coagulase-negative staphylococci, *Staphylococcus aureus*, enterococci, *Candida* spp. and gram-negative bacilli. Antibiotic-resistant strains are frequently encountered (PHAC, 2014).

The Canadian Patient Safety Institute recommends a bundle approach for catheter insertion and care to prevent CVC-BSI:

> During catheter insertion the recommended bundle includes: (1) hand hygiene (see Chart 55-5); (2) maximal barrier precautions; (3) chlorhexidine skin antisepsis; (4) optimal catheter site selection, with avoidance of the femoral vein for central venous access in adult patients; and (5) daily review of line necessity with prompt removal of unnecessary lines.

- For central line care the bundle of actions includes:
  - Daily review and prompt removal of unnecessary lines
  - Aseptic access to lumens
- Catheter site and tubing care (Canadian Patient Safety Institute, 2016).

Refer to Chart 55-5 for Nursing Research Profile: Does Washing the Hands of Patients Decrease HAIs?

Changing Infusion Sets, Caps, and Solutions

Infusion sets and stopcock caps should be changed no more frequently than every 4 days, but at least every 7 days, unless an infusion set is used for the delivery of blood or lipid solutions. Infusion sets and tubing for blood, blood products, or lipid emulsions should be changed within 24 hours of initiating the infusion. Blood infusions should finish within 4 hours of hanging the blood; lipid solutions should be completed within 24 hours of hanging. Needleless system components should be changed at the same frequency as tubing. Injection ports should be scrubbed with chlorhexidine, povidone-iodine, an iodophor, or 70% alcohol before accessing the system with a sterile device (Gorski et al., 2016; SHN, 2012).

NURSING RESEARCH PROFILE

Chart 55-5. Does Washing the Hands of Patients Decrease HAIs?

Fox, C., Wavra, T., Drake, D. A., et al. (2015). Use of a patient hand hygiene protocol to reduce hospital acquired infections and improve nurses' hand washing. *American Journal of Critical Care*, *24*(3), 216–224.

Purpose

Patients who are critically ill are at increased risk of health care-associated infections (HAIs) and associated increases in morbidity and mortality. The purpose of this study was to investigate whether a new patient hand hygiene protocol would reduce HAIs in an intensive care unit (ICU).

Design

A posttest with a retrospective comparison group design was used. Data were collected from a single ICU over approximately 2 and a half years. There were three consecutive phases: (1) a comparison 12-month period before protocol implementation; (2) a 10-week protocol training period; and (3) a 12-month period during the protocol implementation. The two HAIs tracked were central line-associated bloodstream infection (CLABSI) and catheter-associated urinary tract infection (CAUTI). The protocol consisted of the use of 2% chlorhexidine gluconate (CHG) wipes used to wash the hands of patients three times a day.

Findings

There were reductions in 12-month CLABSI and CAUTI rates overall, but the differences were not statistically significant. The rates of nurses washing the hands of the patients with CHG wipes also increased, but the increase was not statistically significant.

Nursing Implications

This study used a unique protocol whereby nurses washed the hands of patient in an ICU with CHG wipes three times each day. While statistically significant results were not found, this protocol deserves further study with a stronger research design. There are no known disadvantages to washing the hands of patients and instructing family members to use CHG wipes on their own hands unless there are breaks in the skin on the hands.

Preventing Infection in the Community

Health Canada, the PHAC, provincial/territorial governments, and local public health departments share responsibility for prevention and control of infection in the community. Methods of infection prevention include sanitation techniques (e.g., water purification, disposal of sewage and other potentially infectious materials), regulated health practices (e.g., the handling, storage, packaging, and preparation of food by institutions), and immunization programs. In Canada, immunization programs have markedly decreased the incidence of infectious diseases.

Immunization Programs

Immunization is an effective public health strategy for the elimination, containment and control of diseases that previously caused serious illness, hospitalization and death, for example, diphtheria, pertussis, measles and polio (PHAC, 2016a). While now rare in Canada, the diseases would reappear if current vaccination programs were reduced or stopped. Immunization protects the people receiving vaccines and enhances group immunity.

More than 25 vaccines are currently licensed in Canada. Vaccines are suspensions of antigen preparations, intended to produce a human immune response to protect the host from future encounters with the organism. Vaccine manufacturer's instructions must be followed, for example, the package insert includes contraindications; details about studied experiences with allergy and other complications; and information about refrigeration, storage, dosage, and administration. The most common adverse effects are allergic reaction to the antigen or carrier solution and the occurrence of the actual disease, often in modified form, when live vaccine is used.

The PHAC outlines immunization competencies for nurses and other health care workers that support safe and competent immunization practices and higher vaccine coverage rates. The Canadian Immunization Guide publishes and updates recommended immunization schedules for infants, children, youth, and adults (PHAC, 2017a). The Guide also describes common concerns and information to respond, for example, contraindications or precautions. People may have concerns about vaccination even when there is no increased risk. Vaccine providers must distinguish among these different reasons for hesitancy to be immunized and respond accordingly. Information about vaccines and vaccine-preventable diseases can be found on the PHAC website.

The recommended vaccines for adults are designed to protect those with underlying diseases with increased infection risk; those with potential for occupational exposure; or those who may be exposed to infectious agents during travel. Adults who are immunosuppressed, including those who have had a splenectomy, should be vaccinated for pneumococcus (*Streptococcus pneumoniae*) and meningococcus (*Neisseria meningitidis*). Health care workers should be immune to measles, mumps, rubella, pertussis, tetanus, hepatitis B, and varicella.

The incidence of vaccine-preventable diseases, such as measles, mumps, rubella, and diphtheria, is affected by immigration from developing countries. Vaccine campaigns in developing countries are often financially and logistically constrained, and immigrants from such areas may be more likely than Canadian residents to be unprotected. Individual risk and epidemic risk are reduced when vaccination campaigns reach all communities, including those with a high proportion of immigrants.

Common Vaccines

MEASLES, MUMPS, AND RUBELLA VACCINE. Since the measles, mumps, and rubella (MMR) vaccines are included in routine infant and child immunization, these diseases have decreased substantially but imported cases and occasional measles outbreaks still occur. To maintain this effective public health strategy, routine MMR vaccination should be administered to children at 12 to 15 months of age, with repeat dosing at 4 to 6 years of age. Measles-containing vaccine is recommended for susceptible adults born in or after 1970. MMR vaccine or human immune globulin (Ig) may be used for measles postexposure immunization in susceptible persons (PHAC, 2017a).

Patients should be advised that fever, transient lymphadenopathy, or hypersensitivity reaction might occur following an MMR vaccination. The risk of side effects is greater in vaccine recipients who have not previously received the vaccine than in those who have received repeat doses. Antipyretics may be used to decrease the risk of fever, but aspirin must be avoided in infants and children because of the risk of Reye's syndrome.

VARICELLA (CHICKENPOX) VACCINE AND ZOSTER (SHINGLES) VACCINE. Varicella zoster is the virus that causes chickenpox and reactivated infection results in herpes zoster. Adolescents, adults, and individuals who are immunocompromised are most likely to have complications such as severe varicella or death (Government of Canada, 2018a).

Transmission occurs by airborne and contact routes. With rare exception, varicella infects a person only once. The incubation period is about 2 weeks, with a range of 10 to 21 days. During a prodrome of general malaise often noticed about 2 days before the rash develops. The newly infected host is capable of transmitting the virus to other susceptible contacts. Typically, the vesicular, pustular rash spreads rapidly from a few to many lesions in a matter of hours. New lesions continue to form for 2 to 3 days and appear at different stages throughout this time. By the fourth symptomatic day the lesions begin to dry and new lesions usually do not develop. Fever is common during the 4 to 6 days of rash progression. When the lesions are dry and crusted the patient is no longer contagious.

Herpes zoster, also known as shingles, is a painful, localized rash caused by recurrent varicella. Vesicles are restricted to areas supplied by single-associated nerve groups. Varicella may be transmitted from those with shingles to people who are susceptible to varicella; the new varicella infections are manifested as chickenpox. Varicella-containing vaccine is available as univalent varicella vaccine or combined multivalent measles-mumps-rubella-varicella (MMRV) vaccine. The efficacy of varicella vaccines in children is estimated to be 94.4% following a single dose and 98.3% following a second dose (Government of Canada, 2018a).

The vaccine should not be given to those who are pregnant, or have demonstrated allergy to varicella vaccine. Patients who are immunocompromised should be assessed on a case-by-case basis. Refer to the Canadian Immunization Guide for specific recommendations for blood products, human Ig, and timing of immunization (Government of Canada, 2018a).

INFLUENZA VACCINE. Influenza is an acute viral respiratory disease that predictably and periodically causes worldwide epidemics known as pandemics. Epidemics occur every 2 to 3 years, with a variable degree of severity. Influenza and pneumonia are ranked among the top 10 leading causes of death in Canada. Each year, there are approximately 23,000 laboratory-confirmed cases of influenza, which are related to about 12,200 hospitalizations and 3,500 deaths (PHAC, 2017d).

Two types of influenza vaccines are available in Canada: inactivated influenza vaccines for intramuscular injection and a live attenuated influenza vaccine for intranasal administration (LAIV) (Moore, 2018).

The inactivated influenza vaccine is available as a trivalent vaccine, composed of three strains, two type A influenza and one type B influenza, or a quadrivalent vaccine composed of four strains, two of type A and two of type B (Moore, 2018). Health Canada authorizes trivalent influenza vaccine for use in persons ≥3 years of age (PHAC, 2017d).

An annual influenza vaccine is recommended for all those over 6 months of age without contraindications, especially people at increased risk of influenza-related complications or hospitalization, for example, pregnant women, people over 65, continuing care residents, Indigenous people, and anyone caring for high-risk individuals (PHAC, 2017d).

Reporting Problems With Vaccines

Nurses ask parents or adult vaccine recipients to provide information about any issues encountered after vaccination. An Adverse Events Following Immunization form must be completed with the following information: type of vaccine received, timing of vaccination, onset of the adverse event, current illnesses or medication, history of adverse events after vaccination, and demographic information about the recipient. Forms are available on the PHAC website.

Contraindications to Vaccines

In general, all vaccines may be given at the same visit. If doses must be given on separate visits, it is then wise to separate by at least 4 weeks so that there is no immune reaction interfering with the response to the second vaccine (CDC, 2016a). The nurse assesses each patient to identify contraindications to vaccinations, for example, anaphylaxis after a previous dose; encephalopathy within 7 days of a previous pertussis vaccine; or persons severely immunocompromised or pregnant. Some live vaccines, for example, varicella, MMR, yellow fever, are contraindicated for patients who are severely immunosuppressed or pregnant. All decisions about vaccination should be made by the patient's primary provider after careful review of vaccine-specific contraindication.

Planning for an Influenza Pandemic

A pandemic is a global outbreak of a disease. Influenza has caused three pandemics in the 20th century: "Spanish flu" during 1918–1919, "Asian flu" during 1957–1958, and "Hong Kong flu" during 1968–1969. The worst pandemic, in 1918–1919, killed between 30,000 and 50,000 people in Canada and 20 to 50 million people worldwide.

The 2009 influenza A (H1N1) pandemic tested Canada's pandemic preparedness and required unprecedented collaboration among all levels of government and stakeholders. Antiviral stockpiles were deployed and pandemic vaccine was administered to millions of Canadians (Government of Canada, 2018b).

Subtypes of influenza viruses have pandemic potential because they continually change within animals and secondarily within humans. As a result of these changes, new viruses may emerge and expose entire populations who are immunologically unprotected (Government of Canada, 2018b).

Influenza pandemics are likely to be more catastrophic than other anticipated public health problems because they last longer than other emergency events, often occur in waves, deplete the available health care workforce, and reduce the supply of medical equipment because of their widespread nature. The Canadian Pandemic Influenza Plan assumes 70% of the population may become infected; many will be asymptomatic; 15% to 35% of the population will become ill; and of those about 50% will seek outpatient care, 1% will require hospitalization, and about 0.4% will die. The PHAC encourages all health care institutions to have a pandemic plan and to test the components of the plan regularly (Government of Canada, 2018b).

Avian Influenza Pandemic

Avian influenza (bird flu) is an infection caused by influenza viruses that chiefly infect birds and poultry. While there are four types of influenza virus (A, B, C and D), only influenza A and B viruses cause seasonal outbreaks in humans, and only influenza A viruses have been known to cause pandemics. Aquatic birds are natural hosts for influenza A viruses, but a wide range of species can be infected, for example, poultry, pigs. Most animal influenza virus strains do not cause human disease but infections can occur by close contact with infected poultry or animals (Government of Canada, 2018b).

Novel influenza A viruses may arise through mixing of animal and human influenza genes or by genetic mutation allowing the virus to infect humans. Novel influenza viruses do not usually evolve into pandemic viruses, but once the virus becomes transmissible between humans community outbreaks or pandemics can occur. For example, avian A, H5N1 viruses, have caused sporadic human cases since 1997 but don't spread easily in humans. The case fatality rate for A (H5N1) infections has been over 50%, so if this virus becomes able to spread easily between people the resulting pandemic could have serious implications (Government of Canada, 2018b).

Nursing Process

The Patient With an Infectious Disease

Assessment

The health history, physical examination, and the use of diagnostic tests are important for determining the presence of infection and infectious diseases. Symptoms of infectious diseases vary significantly between and within diseases. For some infections, visible symptoms such as rash, redness, or swelling provide early warnings of infection. In other infections, such as TB and HIV, asymptomatic latency is prolonged, and infection must be determined through diagnostic procedures.

The history is obtained to establish the likelihood and probable source of infection as well as the degree of associated pathology and symptoms. The patient's previous medical record is reviewed when possible. In obtaining a health history, the following questions may be asked:

- Does the patient have a history of previous or recurrent infections?
- Has the patient had a fever? How high has the patient's temperature been? Is the temperature constant? Or does it rise and fall? Has fever been associated with chills? Has the patient taken any medication to relieve fever?
- Is there cough? Is the cough chronic? Or acute? Is it associated with shortness of breath? Does the cough produce sputum? What colour is the sputum? Is the sputum bloody? Has the patient had a tuberculin skin test (TST) recently? If so, what were the results? Has the patient been given isoniazid (INH) prophylaxis for TB infection? Has the patient been treated for TB in the past?
- Is there pain? Where is the pain? What is the nature of the pain? Does the patient have a sore throat? Headache? Myalgias?, or Arthralgias? Is there pain on urination? Or pain with other activity?
- Is there edema? Is there drainage associated with the edema? Is the edematous area warm to touch?
- Is there a draining lesion? Is the drainage associated with trauma? Or a previous procedure? Is the drainage purulent? Or clear?
- Does the patient have diarrhea? Vomiting? Or abdominal pain?
- Is there a rash? What is the nature of the rash—is it flat? Raised? Red? Crusted? Or lacelike? Is drainage purulent? Has the patient taken medications that could induce rash? Has there been exposure to another person who has an identified infectious disease or rash?
- What is the patient's immunization history?
- Has there been an insect bite? Or animal bite? Has there been an animal scratch? Other exposure to pets? Farm animals? Or experimental animals?
- What medications are used? Have antibiotics been taken recently? Or long term? Is the patient being treated with corticosteroids? Immunosuppressive agents? Or chemotherapy?
- Is there a history of substance abuse?
- Has the patient been treated in the past for other infectious diseases? Has the patient been hospitalized for infectious diseases?
- If sexual history is pertinent, has there been sexual exposure to another person with a known sexually transmitted infection (STI)? Has the patient been treated for STIs in the past? Is the patient pregnant? Or has she recently been pregnant? Has the patient been tested for HIV?
- Has the patient travelled abroad, including developing countries? What was the immunization or antimicrobial prophylaxis used for protection while travelling?
- What is the patient's occupation? What are the patient's recreational activities? Hobbies?

Because infection may occur in any body system, physical examination may reveal signs of infection at any body site. Generalized signs of chronic infection may include significant weight loss or pallor associated with anemia of chronic diseases. Acute infection may manifest with fever, chills, lymphadenopathy, or rash. Localized signs vary by source of infection. Purulent drainage, pain, edema, and redness are strongly associated with localized infection. Cough and shortness of breath may be caused by influenza, pneumonia, or TB, as well as many noninfectious causes.

Nursing Priorities

Based on assessment data, the patient's major nursing priorities related specifically to infection may include the following:

- Risk for infection transmission
- Deficient knowledge about disease
- Risk for (fever)

Infection may interrupt the usual function of any affected body system. These system alterations can be found in the appropriate chapters.

Collaborative Issues/ Potential Complications

Based on assessment data, potential complications that may develop include the following:

- Septicemia, bacteremia, or sepsis
- Septic shock
- Dehydration
- Abscess formation
- Endocarditis
- Infectious disease–related cancers
- Infertility
- Congenital abnormalities

Planning and Goals

Major goals for the patient may include prevention of spread of infection, increased knowledge about the infection and its treatment, control of fever and related discomforts, and absence of complications.

Nursing Interventions

Preventing Infection Transmission

Consistent use of Routine Practices and implementation of Additional Precautions when indicated reduces the risk of infection transmission.

Teaching About the Infectious Process

Interruption of transmission requires diagnosis and patient adherence with the treatment regimen. The nurse's role is to educate the patient and, in some situations, to report the case to public health officials for contact tracing and verification of follow-up.

The nurse stresses the importance of immunization to parents of young children and to others for whom vaccines are recommended, such as patients who are older, are immunosuppressed, or have chronic illnesses or disabilities. Nurses have a personal responsibility to keep their immunizations up-to-date, for example, hepatitis B, and receive an annual influenza vaccine to reduce potential transmission to themselves and vulnerable patient groups.

Infectious diseases may seem mysterious and are frequently socially stigmatizing. Patient teaching efforts require empathy and sensitivity. For example, in the past, TB was a stigmatizing disease. The nurse may need to provide basic information to the patient who needs INH prophylaxis to promote understanding and allay anxiety that the patient may feel.

Controlling Fever and Accompanying Discomforts

Fever must always be investigated to determine whether infection is the source. Evidence indicates that fever, mediated by the hypothalamus, may potentiate beneficial functions in the syndrome of reactions known as *acute-phase reaction*. These reactions include changes in liver protein synthesis; alterations in serum metals, such as iron; and increased production of certain classes of white blood cells and other cells of the immune system. Most fevers are physiologically controlled so that the temperature remains below 41°C. However, severe fever, as occurs with meningococcal meningitis, may cause heat stroke and other complications. Even milder fevers accompanied by fatigue, chills, and diaphoresis are often uncomfortable for the patient. Whether fever is treated or untreated, adequate fluid intake is important during febrile episodes.

NURSING ALERT

Because fever offers clues about infection severity and the success of antibiotic therapy, outpatients with fever are taught to obtain accurate temperature readings. Frequently, family caregivers know that a patient has warm skin but do not disturb the patient by taking a temperature reading. Body temperature information can be very helpful in adjusting therapy or in reevaluating a preliminary diagnosis.

Evaluation

Expected patient outcomes may include the following:

1. Uses appropriate methods to prevent the spread of infection
2. Acquires knowledge about the infectious process
3. Exhibits absence of elevated body temperature

Monitoring and Managing Potential Complications

The patient with a rapidly progressive infectious disease needs vital signs and level of consciousness closely monitored. X-ray findings and microbiologic, immunologic, hematologic, cytologic, and parasitologic laboratory values must be interpreted in the context of other clinical findings to assess the course of the infectious disease.

Antibiotic therapy is frequently complex, and modifications are necessary because of sensitivity test results and disease progression. To ensure therapeutic blood levels rise rapidly, antibiotic therapy should be initiated as soon as it is prescribed rather than waiting until routine medication scheduling times. The Plan of Nursing Care in Chart 55-6 describes nursing interventions for specific complications of infection.

Diarrheal Diseases

Diarrheal diseases are especially prevalent in the developing world and cause significant morbidity and mortality. It is estimated that diarrheal diseases kill more than 6,000 children per day in Asia, Africa, and Latin America. The most important cause of death associated with these diseases is dehydration, and the most important treatment that decreases death rates is oral rehydration therapy (ORT) (Porth, 2017).

In Canada, the epidemiology of diarrheal diseases is changing constantly. Water disinfection, pasteurization, and appropriate food packaging have decreased the incidence of diseases such as typhoid and cholera. However, importation of foreign foods, environmental and ecologic changes, and changes in diagnostic test modalities have contributed to important new trends and outbreaks.

Transmission

The portal of entry of all diarrheal pathogens is oral ingestion. About 4 million Canadians get sick annually from contaminated food, leading to over 11,500 hospitalizations and 240 deaths (Government of Canada, 2016c).

Infection can occur when the infectious dose is high enough or if the food neutralizes the acidic environment of the stomach. Decreased gastric acidity with disruption of usual bowel flora, as occurs after surgery; use of antimicrobial agents; and the immune dysfunction of AIDS all decrease intestinal defenses.

Causes

There are many bacterial, viral, and parasitic causes of diarrheal diseases. Common causes of bacterial infection include *Campylobacter*, *Salmonella*, *Shigella*, *E. coli*, and *Yersinia* species. The most significant viral causes of diarrhea are *Rotavirus*, which commonly results in diarrhea in young children, and *Calicivirus*, often called *Norovirus*, a virus associated with outbreaks in continuing care facilities and cruise ships. Parasitic infections of importance include *Giardia* and *Cryptosporidium* species and *Entamoeba histolytica*.

(text continued on page 1718)

Plan of Nursing Care

Chart 55-6. Care of the Patient With an Infectious Disease

Nursing Priority: Infection
Goal: Prevention of transmission of infectious agents

NURSING INTERVENTIONS	RATIONALE	EXPECTED OUTCOMES
1. Prevent patient-to-patient infection spread	1. Organisms can be spread through direct or indirect contact and/or via airborne or droplet routes	• No evidence of patient-to patient transmission of infection • Absence of health care-associated infections including central line related bacteremia and sepsis; urinary tract infection; and pneumonia. • Patient actively participates in treatment • Patient complies with infection control measures
a. Follow Public Health Agency of Canada (PHAC, 2016a) Routine Practices and Additional Precautions (RPAP) such as placement in single patient room)	a. Routine Practices are used to reduce the likelihood of transmission from patient to patient	
b. Ensure that patients with airborne infections remain in single-patient rooms during the hospital stay. If they must leave their rooms, arrangements should be made to decrease the likelihood of contact with other patients. Rooms should be ventilated according to PHAC criteria. Personal protective equipment in the form of fit-tested N95 respirators should be worn as indicated The N95 respirator is the minimal level of personal protection for tuberculosis control. The "N" indicates the filter is not oil resistant; and the "95" indicates that the respirator has 95% effectiveness in filtering particles at 0.3 microns; the most penetrating particle size (PHAC, 2016a) Health care providers, and anyone at high risk of getting influenza, for example, adults and children with chronic health conditions, people in continuing care facilities; people >65 years of age should get an annual influenza vaccination	b. Additional Precautions are implemented in addition to Routine Practices to prevent the transmission of specific infectious agents that are highly contagious, epidemiologically significant or infectious syndromes spread via airborne, droplet, or contact routes	
	c. Engineering controls are important in the prevention of airborne diseases Influenza vaccine safely reduces risk of respiratory infection associated with this highly communicable virus	
2. Prevent health care workers' transfer of organisms from patient to patient. Perform hand hygiene before and after each patient contact; before clean or aseptic procedures; and after exposure or risk of exposure to blood or body fluids	2. Transfer of organisms on the contaminated hands of health care workers is a common route of transmission. Disease causing organisms may colonize the hands of health care workers.	• Health care workers adhere to PHAC hand hygiene recommendations • No evidence of transmission via health care workers
a. Alcohol-based hand rubs (ABHR) are the preferred method of hand hygiene in health care settings. Hand washing with soap and water is required when hands are visibly soiled; or if exposure to infectious diarrhea	a. Hand hygiene reduces **transient flora** on outer epidermal layers of skin. Alcohol-based hand rubs (ABHR) are usually effective to reduce transient flora. Handwashing with soap and water is more effective than ABHR when hands are visibly soiled and for diarrhea especially when caused by CDI	

continued >

Plan of Nursing Care — Chart 55-6. Care of the Patient With an Infectious Disease, *Continued*

NURSING INTERVENTIONS	RATIONALE	EXPECTED OUTCOMES
b. Use gloves when handling any body fluid from any patient. Change gloves between patient care activities, and perform hand hygiene after gloves are removed	b. Gloves provide a barrier from blood or body fluid exposure. Gloves quickly become contaminated and then become a potential vehicle for the transfer of organisms between patients. Microflora on the hands are likely to proliferate while gloves are worn	
c. Avoid wearing artificial fingernails or extenders when providing patient care. Keep natural nails less than 0.6 cm long and remove nail polish when chipped	c. Artificial fingernails, nail extenders and chipped fingernails harbour microorganisms	
d. Model hand hygiene compliance and correct glove use for other health care professionals	d. Role models help promote and sustain hand hygiene compliance among other health care professionals. (Dombecki, Shah, Eke-Usim, et al., 2015)	
3. Prevent patient-to-health care worker transmission of infection.	3. Health care workers may acquire occupational infections due to close contact with patients	• No occupationally acquired infections in nurses and other health care workers
a. Avoid risk of infection with tuberculosis	a. The most important element in the reduction of tuberculosis is early identification. Many of the symptoms of tuberculosis are subtle and may be first observed by the nurse who had prolonged contact with the patient	• Health care workers follow Routine Practices, Additional Precautions and immunization recommendations
(1) Participate in the early identification of patients with active disease. Patients will be asked about risk factors, symptoms, previous exposure, and tuberculin skin test (TST) status	(1) Identification of patients at risk can help to prevent exposure	
(2) Expedite diagnostic workup with chest x-ray, sputum analysis for organisms, and TST administration as appropriate	(2) Confirmation of diagnosis facilitates development of an appropriate treatment plan, including prevention of spread of infection	
(3) Maintain engineering controls. Keep the patient in a private room with a closed door	(3) Confining airflow to the immediate vicinity of the patient and exhausting air to the outside reduce the likelihood of transmission to health care workers in areas outside of the patient room	
(4) Use respiratory protection in the isolation room or when participating in procedures that are likely to generate cough, such as suctioning, intubation, or administering nebulized medications	(4) N95 respirators are designed to reduce health care workers' risk	

Plan of Nursing Care

Chart 55-6. Care of the Patient With an Infectious Disease, *Continued*

NURSING INTERVENTIONS	RATIONALE	EXPECTED OUTCOMES
b. Avoid risk of transmission of bloodborne diseases such as hepatitis B, hepatitis C, and HIV	b. Health care workers can contract bloodborne diseases via percutaneous injury such as needlestick or by contact with blood or body fluids to mucous membranes, such as eyes and mouth	
(1) Get the hepatitis B vaccination	(1) Hepatitis B vaccine should be administered to reduce risk from this contagious bloodborne virus	
(2) Use Routine Practices as defined by (PHAC, 2016a) (e.g., puncture-resistant sharps container at point of use and proper handling and disposal of sharps)	(2) Routine Practices are based on the recognition that most patients are not identified as infected by physical assessment or history taking. Health care workers must assume that all patients may be infected with bloodborne or other infection and must use barrier precautions appropriately for all patients	
(3) Use "needleless" syringes and other injury-preventing devices	(3) Use of safety-engineered sharp devices decreases the risk of transmission of bloodborne diseases.	
c. Avoid the risk of influenza transmission	c. Up-to-date immunizations of health care workers reduce their risk of infection.	
(1) Get an influenza vaccination annually		
(2) Get vaccinated or produce proof of immunity to measles, mumps, rubella, and varicella		
4. Prevent patient exposure to contaminated medical equipment	4. Contaminated equipment is a reservoir for harboring organisms. Equipment must be cleaned, disinfected, or sterilized between patients to prevent the transmission of infection	• Equipment is cleaned, disinfected or sterilized between patients as required for patient safety • No evidence of transmission due to contaminated equipment
a. Ensure equipment inserted through intact skin is sterile	a. Sterile equipment is free of all microorganisms including spores	
b. Ensure equipment that contacts mucous membranes, for example, respiratory equipment is, at minimum, high level disinfected or sterilized between patients	b. Equipment contacting mucous membranes requires high-level disinfection rendering it free of all microorganisms, with the exception of spores	
c. Ensure equipment which touches intact skin is thoroughly cleaned and is low-level disinfected between patients	c. Low-level disinfection reduces microorganisms to a safe level for the patient with intact skin	
5. Follow established guidelines for the routine removal and replacement of intravenous devices	5. Indwelling intravenous devices can serve as a conduit for organisms to migrate into the bloodstream	• Reduced risk of health care associated bloodstream infection related to intravenous devices
6. Remove urinary catheters at the earliest time possible	6. The risk of urinary tract infections is directly related to the length of time that a urinary catheter remains in place	• Reduced risk of health care–associated urinary tract infection related to urinary catheter use

continued >

Plan of Nursing Care

Chart 55-6. Care of the Patient With an Infectious Disease, *Continued*

NURSING INTERVENTIONS	RATIONALE	EXPECTED OUTCOMES
7. Remove endotracheal and nasogastric tubes as soon as possible	7. The risk for pneumonia is increased with the use and duration of indwelling devices	• Reduced risk of health care–associated pneumonia related to indwelling devices

Nursing Priority: Deficient knowledge
Goal: Acquisition of knowledge about the infectious process

NURSING INTERVENTIONS	RATIONALE	EXPECTED OUTCOMES
1. Listen carefully to what the patient says about symptoms, illness and previous treatment 2. Provide pertinent explanations about: a. Organism and route of transmission b. Treatment goals c. Follow-up schedule d. Prevention of transmission to others	1. Listening detects any misunderstanding or misinformation and provides an opportunity for education 2. Knowledge about specific diagnoses and treatments may increase adherence	• Patient actively participates in treatment • Patient adheres to infection control measures • Patient demonstrates knowledge about their diagnosis and adheres to treatment
3. Allow opportunities for questions and discussions 4. Teach the patient and family about: a. Prophylaxis or immunization, if recommended b. Community resources, if necessary c. Means of preventing transmission within the home	3. The patient's questions indicate issues that need clarification 4. Understanding of the risks and precautions associated with an infectious disease may reduce the opportunity for transmission	• Patient asks for clarification as needed • Patient and family perform actions to protect themselves and others from infectious disease

Nursing Priority: Imbalanced body temperature (fever)
Goal: Patient comfort and return of normal temperature

NURSING INTERVENTIONS	RATIONALE	EXPECTED OUTCOMES
1. Monitor temperature, pulse, and respirations at regular intervals	1. Graph fever curve to help evaluate when fever occurs, how long it lasts, and whether it responds to therapy	• Body temperature within expected limits • Maintenance of fluid and electrolyte balance • Patient comfortable

Collaborative Problems: Among potential complications are septicemia, bacteremia, or sepsis; septic shock; dehydration; abscess formation; endocarditis; infectious disease–related cancers; and infertility
Goal: Absence of complications

Septicemia, Bacteremia, Sepsis

NURSING INTERVENTIONS	RATIONALE	EXPECTED OUTCOMES
1. Monitor patient for evidence of infection 2. Assess treatment effectiveness 3. Administer antibiotics as prescribed, with the first dose given at the earliest time possible	1. Early recognition and treatment of infection reduces the likelihood of secondary infections 2. Some infections progress rapidly unless antibiotics are administered promptly 3. Prompt treatment will improve outcomes	• Identification and effective treatment of infection prevents progression to more severe infection, for example, bloodstream infection

Septic Illness

NURSING INTERVENTIONS	RATIONALE	EXPECTED OUTCOMES
1. Monitor vital signs for patients with recognized infections, that is, pneumonia, intra-abdominal, and urinary tract infections, and severely immunosuppressed patients at risk for septic illness, for example, premature infants, older adults, those with implanted medical devices (Safer Healthcare Now, 2015)	1. Early recognition of the signs of septic illness and prompt treatment of impending shock may reduce the severity or mortality	• Infections are identified and treated promptly reducing risk of septic illness • Hemodynamic and respiratory status are within expected range

Plan of Nursing Care

Chart 55-6. Care of the Patient With an Infectious Disease, *Continued*

NURSING INTERVENTIONS	RATIONALE	EXPECTED OUTCOMES
2. Monitor for signs of: a. Fever b. Chills and shaking, arthralgias and myalgias, nausea and vomiting, light-headedness etc. (Safer Healthcare Now, 2015) c. Hypotension d. Tachycardia >90 beats/minute e. Tachypnea >20 breaths/minute f. Evidence of decreased perfusion or dysfunction of vital organs in the form of: (1) Altered mental status (2) Decreased capillary refill or mottling (3) Elevated lactate levels (4) Urine output <0.5 mL/kg/hour for at least 2 hours	2. Therapeutic maintenance of hemodynamic and respiratory status is necessary until infection is effectively treated	
3. Administer antibiotics, fluid replacement, vasopressors, and oxygen as prescribed.		
Dehydration		
1. Assess for dehydration (thirst, dryness of mucous membranes, loss of skin turgor, reduced peripheral pulses, urine output <0.5 mL/kg/hour)	1. Signs of dehydration provide a basis for fluid replacement and suggest possible further complications of circulatory collapse	• Attains fluid balance (output approximates intake: body weight unchanged) • Mucous membranes appear moist; expected skin turgor • Serum electrolytes are within expected limits
2. Monitor weight	2. Rapid changes in weight indicate fluid volume changes	
3. Monitor intake and output and serum electrolyte levels	3. Dehydration produces a deficit in some electrolytes. Decreased urine production may indicate hypovolemia and decreased renal perfusion	
4. Replace fluids as needed. If the patient can tolerate oral fluids, offer fluids every 2 to 4 hours. Administer intravenous fluids as prescribed	4. When possible, oral hydration is preferable because the patient can select the beverage, control the rate and interval of replacement, and care for self at home. In addition, the risks associated with vascular devices are avoided. If intravenous fluid is required, intravenous solutions are selected to facilitate intestinal reabsorption of fluid and electrolytes	
Abscess Formation		
1. Assess vascular access sites, wound sites, pressure ulcers, and other appropriate sites for apparent collections of purulent material	1. Collections of purulent material often require drainage before antimicrobial therapy is effective	• Absence of abscess • Takes antibiotics as prescribed
2. Assess the patient who has had abdominal surgery or trauma to abdominal area for localized signs of intra-abdominal abscess. These signs include:	2. Intra-abdominal abscess formation is most common following traumatic or surgical disruption of the GI tract. Signs are often initially subtle	
3. Assess the patient who has had percutaneous abscess drainage to determine whether drainage has been successful. Be alert for all of the above signs and symptoms.	3. After percutaneous drainage, recurrent or persistent signs of abscess may indicate the need for surgical treatment	
4. Administer antibiotics as prescribed.	4. Antibiotics, along with drainage, are the most important elements of intra-abdominal abscess management	

continued >

Plan of Nursing Care — Chart 55-6. Care of the Patient With an Infectious Disease, *Continued*

NURSING INTERVENTIONS	RATIONALE	EXPECTED OUTCOMES
Endocarditis		
Prevention		
1. Teach patients with the following conditions about the importance of antibiotic prophylaxis for events and procedures that may introduce the risk of endocarditis: a. Valvular disease b. Congenital heart disease c. Intracardiac prosthesis d. Previous endocarditis	1. Patients with underlying valvular disease and other cardiac abnormalities are at increased risk for "seeding" of the cardiac valves during procedures that can cause bacteremia	• Informs health care professionals of cardiac conditions that require antibiotic prophylaxis before invasive procedures • Takes prophylactic antibiotics as prescribed
Management		
1. Obtain blood cultures as prescribed; carefully record results. Note persistent bloodstream infections with a particular organism	1. A definitive diagnosis of endocarditis requires blood culture confirmation	• Endocarditis is diagnosed, treated, and cured
2. Obtain a detailed history about the duration of fever in the absence of a well-recognized cause	2. Endocarditis should be suspected in patients who report an unexplained fever of more than 1 week's duration	
3. Administer intravenous antibiotic therapy at the prescribed time schedule	3. Intravenous therapy is usually required for cure. The goal of therapy is complete eradication of all organisms. Careful adherence to following the scheduled administration is therefore essential	

• Infectious Disease–Related Cancers and Infertility
These potential complications of infectious diseases are prevented by primary avoidance of infection. Management is directed toward treating each of them as a noninfectious

Food safety measures such as hand hygiene; cleaning kitchen surfaces and utensils with warm, soapy water; separating raw foods from cooked foods; cooking to a safe temperature; and refrigerating food and leftovers are key to preventing transmission of bacteria and viruses during food handling (Government of Canada, 2016c).

Campylobacter Infections

Campylobacter species are the most frequent cause of diarrheal disease worldwide. The bacterium, which is abundant in animal foods, is especially common in poultry but can also be found in beef and pork. Direct person-to-person transmission appears to be less common than it is for other enteric pathogens, such as *Shigella*. Guillain–Barré syndrome, a serious neurologic disorder characterized by temporary paralysis, is a complication of approximately 1 of 1,000 cases of *Campylobacter* infection.

After a person is infected, the bacterium directly attacks the lumen of the intestine and may cause disease through enterotoxin release. Symptoms range from mild abdominal cramping and minimal diarrhea to severe disease with profuse watery bloody diarrhea and debilitating abdominal cramping. Antimicrobial therapy is recommended only for patients who are seriously ill.

Salmonella Infection

Salmonella is a gram-negative bacillus with many species, including the very pathogenic *Salmonella typhi*, that is, typhoid fever. Of the nontyphi species, most organisms are prevalent in animal food sources. In Canada, approximately 6,500 cases of confirmed *Salmonella* are reported annually, with Enteriditis isolates the most frequently reported (Government of Canada, 2016b). Salmonella contributes to 1 in 4 hospitalizations of all food-borne illnesses, totaling 88,000 illnesses, 925 hospitalizations, and 17 deaths annually (Government of Canada, 2016c).

Salmonella species may cause gastroenteritis, and systemic infection, or an asymptomatic colonized state. Diarrhea with gastroenteritis is common. Disseminated disease and bacteremia, sometimes accompanied by diarrhea, occur less often.

The person with *Salmonella*-caused diarrhea is occasionally a source for transmission to others. The importance of good hygiene should be emphasized, and health care workers use Routine Practices including hand hygiene, PPE (e.g., gloves), and environmental cleaning principles when handling bedpans, stool specimens, or other objects that may be contaminated with feces. Although patients with systemic salmonellosis require antimicrobial therapy, those with gastroenteritis only are not usually treated, because antibiotics may increase the period of time that the patient carries the bacteria while not improving the clinical outcome.

Shigella Infection

The *Shigella* species is a gram-negative organism that invades the lumen of the intestine and causes disease and severe watery, possibly bloody, diarrhea. *Shigella* species are spread through the fecal–oral route, with easy transmission from one person to another. *Shigella* exhibits high levels of **virulence**, the degree of pathogenicity of an organism; infection with a very small number of organisms can cause disease. Because transmission occurs easily with improper hygiene, it is not surprising that *Shigella* organisms disproportionately affect pediatric populations. Disease in the very young may infrequently be complicated by pulmonary or neurologic symptoms.

Antimicrobial therapy should be instituted early. Frequently, initial therapy choices must be altered when final microbiologic testing reveals the organism's sensitivity.

Escherichia coli

E. coli is the most common aerobic organism colonizing the large bowel. When *E. coli* bacteria are cultured from fecal specimens, the results generally reflect normal flora. However, certain strains of *E. coli* with increased virulence have been responsible for significant outbreaks of diarrheal disease in recent years. These stronger pathogenic strains are subgrouped as enterotoxigenic *E. coli* (ETEC) because of their production of enterotoxins. ETEC strains often cause cholera-like disease, with rapid, severe dehydration and an increased risk of death.

Several outbreaks of an *E. coli* species, 0157:H7, have been linked to the ingestion of undercooked beef and to vegetables that have been contaminated by animal waste water. This bacterium lives in the intestines of cattle and can be introduced into meat at the time of slaughter.

Calicivirus (Norwalk-Like Virus; Norovirus)

Calicivirus, which is often referred to as the Norwalk-like virus or the *Norovirus*, is a very common cause of foodborne illness. Onset of illness is usually acute, with vomiting and watery diarrhea that generally last for approximately 2 days. Dehydration is the most common complication. Provinces and territories are required to report cases of norovirus to the PHAC (PHAC, 2014).

Calicivirus is transmitted easily from person to person by direct contact and by ingesting contaminated food. Water-borne outbreaks have been associated with sewage-contaminated wells and contaminated swimming pools. Although people with *Calicivirus* infection typically recover within 2 to 3 days, they may continue to transmit the virus to others for approximately 2 more weeks.

Caliciviruses can withstand environmental extremes of heat or cold and are resistant to chemical disinfection; characteristics which contribute to their epidemic potential. Control of *Calicivirus* in health care facilities requires a coordinated program including patient placement, environmental disinfection, diagnosis, and coordination with public health officials. Contact Precautions should be used when caring for patients with incontinence and during outbreaks of the virus. Health care workers should wear masks if they are cleaning heavily soiled areas or caring for a patient who is actively vomiting. Special attention to cleaning is needed during health care facility outbreaks, and hypochlorite solutions may be used if there is ongoing transmission (PHAC, 2014). More information on norovirus can be found on the PHAC website.

Giardia and Cryptosporidium

Transmission of enteric protozoa *Giardia* and *Cryptosporidium* occurs when food or water is contaminated by human or animal feces with viable cysts of the organism. People often become infected while travelling to endemic areas or by drinking contaminated water from mountain streams. The organism can also be transmitted by person-to-person contact, such as occurs in day care settings (Government of Canada, 2018e). Transmission by sexual contact has also been documented.

Frequently, the infection goes unnoticed. Infection is often recognized more easily in children than in adults. In extreme cases, the patient may experience abdominal pain and chronic diarrhea, usually described as containing mucous and fat but not blood. Microscopic examination of stool specimens reveals the trophozoite or cyst stages of the parasitic life cycle.

Giardiasis can be treated using a number of drugs, including metronidazole, quinacrine, furazolidone, tinidazole, ornidazole, nitazoxanide, and nimorazole, while nitazoxanide is the only drug approved for treatment of cryptosporidiosis. Patients should be advised regarding the ease of transmission and preventative measures such as hand hygiene and environmental cleaning. Drinking water in areas where water is not treated or filtered should be avoided unless it has been boiled, disinfected or is in a commercially sealed bottle (Government of Canada, 2018d).

Vibrio cholerae

Although reported cases of cholera are rare in Canada, no discussion of infectious diarrhea is complete without mention of this very serious infectious disease. Historically, epidemics of cholera have influenced all aspects of life—from medical to political—and infection rates have been significant enough to destroy governments and armies. Cholera is always a concern when wars or natural disasters result in inadequately processed waste water. *Vibrio cholerae* also may be found naturally in brackish rivers and coastal waters.

V. cholerae is a gram-negative organism with several different serotypes. The type usually associated with epidemics is toxigenic *V. cholerae* 01. The organism is transmitted by contaminated food or water.

Cholera causes disease with a very rapid onset of copious diarrhea in which up to 1 L of fluid per hour can be lost. Dehydration, with subsequent cardiopulmonary collapse, may cause rapid progression from onset of signs and symptoms to death. The principal therapy is rehydration. Rehydration efforts should be vigorous and sustained. If oral rehydration is not effective, the patient needs IV therapy.

Although most travellers to countries affected by cholera are at low risk, those at higher risk include humanitarian relief workers, and travellers visiting areas of high risk with limited access to safe water and food (Government of Canada, 2018d). Confirmation of the causative organism can be made by stool culture. All cases must be reported to local and provincial/territorial public health authorities. People travelling to areas where cholera occurs regularly should remember the simple rule of thumb: "boil it, cook it, peel it, or forget it."

Nursing Process

The Patient With Infectious Diarrhea

Assessment

The patient with diarrhea is assessed to determine their hydration status and is rehydrated if found to be dehydrated. Assessment includes evaluation for thirst, dryness of oral mucous membranes, sunken eyes, a weakened pulse, and loss of skin turgor. Careful observation for these signs is especially important in cases of rapidly dehydrating diseases, most notably cholera, and in younger children.

Intake and output measurements are crucial in determining fluid balance. Liquid stool should be measured and recorded, along with the frequency of stools. Consistency and appearance of stool are key indicators of the type and severity of the diarrheal disease. The presence of mucous or blood should also be documented.

When conducting a health history, the nurse asks if the patient has recently travelled, if the patient is being treated with antibiotics, if the patient has been in contact with anyone who has recently had diarrheal disease, and what the patient has recently eaten. Frequently, patients attribute the most recent meal eaten as the cause of symptoms. However, the incubation period for most diarrheal conditions is longer than the time interval between meals and the nurse needs to get detailed information about the meal preceding the illness and about all food intake in the previous 3 to 4 days. When eliciting this kind of history, it is helpful to ask the patient to list every food tasted. The nurse also asks the patient if he or she is employed in a food preparation service, because the local public health departments should be notified about any person with infectious diarrhea who works in the food industry.

Nursing Priorities

Based on the assessment data, the patient's major nursing priorities may include the following:

- Water and electrolyte balance
- Deficient knowledge regarding prevention of infection

Collaborative Problems/ Potential Complications

Based on the assessment data, potential complications that may develop include the following:

- Bacteremia
- Hypovolemic shock

Planning and Goals

The most important goals are maintenance of fluid and electrolyte balance, increased knowledge about the disease and risk of transmission, and absence of complications.

Nursing Interventions

Correcting Dehydration Associated With Diarrhea

The patient is assessed to determine the degree of dehydration and the amount and route of rehydration needed. Oral rehydration therapy is a strategy used to reduce the severe complications of diarrheal disease regardless of causative agent. It is inexpensive and effective for most patients, but it is often underused because of cultural beliefs discouraging oral intake during episodes of diarrhea. The World Health Organization (WHO) and the United Nations International Children's Emergency Fund (UNICEF) recommend an oral rehydration solution (ORS) for the treatment of children and adults with dehydration and electrolyte imbalance associated with cholera and other forms of diarrheal disease. It contains, in millimoles per litre: sodium, 90; potassium, 20; chloride, 80; citrate, 10; and glucose, 111.

MILD DEHYDRATION. The patient exhibits dry oral mucous membranes of the mouth and increased thirst. The rehydration goal at this level of dehydration is to deliver about 50 mL of ORS per 1 kg of weight over a 4-hour interval.

MODERATE DEHYDRATION. Common findings are sunken eyes, loss of skin turgor, increased thirst, and dry oral mucous membranes. The rehydration goal at this level of dehydration is to deliver about 100 mL/kg of ORS over 4 hours.

SEVERE DEHYDRATION. The patient with severe dehydration shows signs of shock, that is, rapid thready pulse, cyanosis, cold extremities, rapid breathing, lethargy, or coma, and should receive IV replacement until hemodynamic and mental status return to expected state. When improvement is evident, the patient can be treated with ORS.

Administering Rehydration Therapy

In Canada, commercially available preparations such as Pedialyte have been effective fluid and electrolyte replacements for children with common viral diarrheal disorders. However, when diarrheal losses are very high, greater than 10 mL/kg/hour, the lower sodium concentrations of these formulas make them less appropriate than the WHO formula.

NURSING ALERT

Sports drinks do not replace fluid losses correctly and should not be used.

For the hospitalized child, diarrheal fluid loss is weighed, and ORS should be administered at a rate of 1 mL for each gram of diarrheal stool. Stool losses can be estimated so that the patient receives about 10 mL/kg of ORS for each diarrheal stool.

It is important for children and adults with acute diarrheal symptoms to maintain caloric intake. Recommended foods include starches, cereals, yogurt, fruits, and vegetables. Foods that are high in simple sugars, such as undiluted apple juice or gelatin, should be avoided. Because diarrheal episodes are often accompanied by vomiting, rehydration and refeeding can be difficult. Oral rehydration therapy is best delivered frequently in small amounts. When patients are persistently vomiting, they often require frequent fluid administration by spoonfuls. IV therapy is necessary for the patient who is severely dehydrated or in shock.

Increasing Knowledge and Preventing Spread of Infection

Public health nurses, school nurses, and others involved in patient teaching emphasize principles of safe food preparation, with special attention to meat preparation and cooking. Bacteria can grow in temperatures between 4° and 60°C. Keep cold foods cold at or below 4°C, and keep hot foods hot at or above 60°C (PHAC, 2013a). Ground beef should be cooked until no longer pink. In planning events for groups of people, adequate provision for storage and reheating to temperature thresholds is necessary. When preparing food, it is important to use separate surfaces, knives, and other equipment for meat and nonmeat items.

Diarrheal diseases discussed in this section must be reported to local or provincial/territorial health departments. The goal of reporting is to provide information for determining incidence trends and promptly identifying any restaurants or other food preparation establishments that have served contaminated food.

The need for rehydration and refeeding is taught to parents of children with diarrheal disease. Beliefs about illness and food patterns may have a traditional or cultural basis, and any teaching of health facts requires cultural sensitivity.

In both homes and health care delivery settings, good hygiene, and principles of Routine Practices should be emphasized.

Monitoring and Managing Potential Complications

BACTEREMIA. *E. coli, Salmonella*, and *Shigella* are organisms that can enter the bloodstream and disseminate to other organs. Blood cultures are necessary in the acutely febrile patient with diarrhea. If initial smear results reveal gram-negative organisms, antibiotic therapy is instituted.

HYPOVOLEMIC SHOCK. Shock associated with diarrheal diseases requires accurate intake and output assessment and vigorous fluid replacement. In rare instances, patients with severe fluid imbalance require intensive care nursing support with aggressive hemodynamic monitoring. Refer to Chapters 17 and 18 for further information.

Evaluation

Expected patient outcomes may include the following:

1. Attains fluid balance
   a. Output approximates intake
   b. Mucous membranes appear moist
   c. Skin turgor is as expected
   d. Adequate amounts of fluids and calories ingested
   e. Absence of vomiting
   f. Stools are of usual colour and consistency
2. Acquires knowledge and understanding about infectious diarrhea and transmission potential
   a. Takes proper precautions to prevent spread of infection to others
   b. Describes principles and techniques of safe food storage, preparation, and cooking
3. Absence of complications
   a. Temperature is within expected range
   b. Blood culture reports are negative
   c. Fluid balance is achieved

Sexually Transmitted Infections

Sexually transmitted infection (STI) is the term now commonly used instead of *sexually transmitted disease* as it is a broader term that encompasses asymptomatic infections. An STI is a disease acquired through sexual contact with an infected person. Table 55-2 identifies diseases that can be classified as STIs. Infections caused by organisms not generally considered STIs can also be transmitted during sexual contact; for example, *Giardia*, can be transmitted through sexual exposure to feces.

TABLE 55-2 Sexually Transmitted Infections and Their Routes of Transmission

Sexually Transmitted Infection (STI)	Route(s) of Transmission
Chancroid, *Lymphogranuloma venereum*, and *Granuloma inguinale*	Sexual
Chlamydia	Sexual
Cytomegalovirus	Sexual, less intimate contact
Gonorrhea	Sexual, perinatal
Hepatitis B	Sexual, percutaneous, perinatal
Hepatitis C	Percutaneous, probably sexual, probably perinatal
Herpes simplex	Sexual
HIV infection/AIDS	Sexual, percutaneous, perinatal
Human papillomavirus	Sexual
Syphilis	Sexual, perinatal

HIV, human immunodeficiency virus; AIDS, acquired immunodeficiency virus.

Adapted from Centers for Disease Control and Prevention (CDC). (2015b). *CDC fact sheet: Reported STDs in the United States*. Retrieved on October, 24, 2016, from www.cdc.gov/std/stats14/std-trends-508.pdf

STIs are a significant public health concern in Canada. Rates of *Chlamydia* infection, gonorrhea, and infectious syphilis are steadily increasing and new sexually transmitted pathogens are emerging with limited treatment options, for example, *Mycoplasma genitalium* can cause nongonococcal urethritis in men and cervicitis and pelvic inflammatory disease (PID) in women (Government of Canada, 2018f).

Portals of entry and sites of infection include the skin and mucosal linings of the urethra, cervix, vagina, rectum, and oropharynx. Many STIs have few or no noticeable symptoms and individuals may not be aware they are infected. If left untreated, these infections can lead to serious health implications (PHAC, 2018a).

STI prevention activities include safer-sex awareness campaigns, screening, case finding, and partner notification (PHAC, 2018b).

Condoms provide a protective barrier from transmission of STI-related organisms. At first referred to as a method to ensure *safe sex*, the use of condoms has been shown to reduce but not eliminate the risk of transmission of HIV and other STIs. Thus, the term *safer sex* more appropriately connotes the public health message to be used when promoting the use of condoms.

STIs provide a unique set of challenges for nurses, physicians, and public health officials. Because of perceived stigma and possible threat to emotional relationships, people with symptoms of STIs are often reluctant to seek health care in a timely fashion. STIs may progress without symptoms. A delay in diagnosis and treatment is potentially harmful because the risk of complications for the infected person and the risk of transmission to others increase over time.

Infection with one STI suggests the possibility of infection with other diseases as well. After one STI is identified, diagnostic evaluation for others should be conducted. The possibility of HIV infection should be pursued when any STI is diagnosed.

Human Immunodeficiency Virus

HIV is the causative agent of AIDS. HIV is transmitted through sexual contact or percutaneous injection of contaminated blood or from infected mother to fetus. Most people infected by the percutaneous route are IV or injecting drug users who share contaminated needles, but transmission is also remotely possible through contaminated blood transfusion. Since 1985, all blood transfusions have been screened, and transfusion-related transmission of HIV is now extremely unlikely.

Human Immunodeficiency Virus–Related Complications

HIV infection, if untreated, leads to the profound immunosuppression that is characteristic of AIDS. Complications of HIV infection include many opportunistic infections, including those due to *Pneumocystis jiroveci*, *Cryptococcus neoformans*, cytomegalovirus, and *Mycobacterium avium*.

Syphilis

Syphilis is an acute and chronic infectious disease caused by the spirochete *Treponema pallidum*. It is acquired through sexual contact or may be congenital in origin. Syphilis rates are rising in Canada for both sexes but especially in men who have sex with men. The increased number of women with syphilis often corresponds with rising congenital syphilis rates. Infants can be infected in utero or by contact with an active genital lesion at the time of delivery. Screening pregnant women is crucial to prevention (PHAC, 2018b).

Stages of Syphilis

In the untreated person, the course of syphilis can be divided into three stages: primary, secondary, and tertiary (PHAC, 2018b). These stages reflect the time from infection and the clinical manifestations observed in that period, and are the basis for treatment decisions.

Primary syphilis occurs 2 to 3 weeks after initial inoculation with the organism. Symptoms can include formation of a painless chancre or wart-like lesion at the site of infection and lymphadenopathy. Untreated, these lesions usually resolve spontaneously within about 2 months.

Secondary syphilis occurs when the hematogenous spread of organisms from the original chancre leads to generalized infection. The rash of secondary syphilis occurs about 2 to 8 weeks after the chancre and involves the trunk and the extremities, including the palms of the hands and the soles of the feet. Transmission of the organism can occur through contact with these lesions. Generalized signs of infection may include lymphadenopathy, arthritis, meningitis, hair loss, fever, malaise, and weight loss.

After the secondary stage, there is a period of **latency**, when the infected person has no signs or symptoms of syphilis. Latency can be interrupted by a recurrence of secondary syphilis symptoms.

Tertiary syphilis is the final stage in the natural history of the disease. While many do not exhibit symptoms in the final stage, tertiary syphilis presents as a slowly progressive inflammatory disease with the potential to affect multiple organs. The most common manifestations at this level are aortitis and neurosyphilis, as evidenced by dementia, psychosis, paresis, stroke, or meningitis.

Assessment and Diagnostic Findings

Because syphilis shares symptoms with many diseases, clinical history and laboratory evaluation are important. The conclusive diagnosis of syphilis can be made by direct identification of the spirochete obtained from the chancre lesions of primary syphilis. Serologic tests used in the diagnosis of secondary and tertiary syphilis require clinical correlation in interpretation.

Screening for syphilis usually involves the use of nontreponemal tests (NTT) such as rapid plasma reagin (RPR) or venereal disease research laboratory (VDRL), followed by confirmatory treponemal tests if the NTT is reactive. The NTT may be nonreactive in patients with suspected primary syphilis or late latent syphilis and it is then appropriate to add a treponemal test to the initial screen or, in the case of primary syphilis, to repeat the NTT after 2 to 4 weeks (PHAC, 2018b).

After adequate therapy, the test result is expected to decrease quantitatively until it is read as negative, usually about 2 years after therapy is completed.

Treponemal tests, such as the fluorescent treponemal antibody absorption test (FTA-ABS) and the microhemagglutination test (MHA-TP), are used to verify that the screening test did not represent a false-positive result. Positive results usually are positive for life and therefore are not appropriate to determine therapeutic effectiveness (PHAC, 2018b).

Treponemal enzyme immunoassays (EIA) are now commercially available in Canada and may provide a more sensitive screening test for syphilis. Syphilis testing algorithms vary across Canada and local laboratory testing protocols should be followed (PHAC, 2018b).

Medical Management

Antibiotics are administered to treat of all stages of syphilis. Penicillin G benzathine is the medication of choice for early syphilis or early latent syphilis of less than 1 year's duration. This long-acting benzathine penicillin achieves detectable serum levels of penicillin for 2 to 4 weeks in nonpregnant adults and is required to adequately treat infectious syphilis; short-acting penicillin agents are not adequate for achieving cure (PHAC, 2018a).

Consult the PHAC website for the most recent treatment guidelines. Recommendations provide special guidelines for treatment in the setting of pregnancy, allergy, HIV infection, pediatric infection, congenital infection, and neurosyphilis.

Nursing Management

Syphilis is a reportable communicable disease. In any health care facility, a mechanism must be in place to ensure that all diagnosed patients are reported to the provincial/territorial or local public health department to ensure community follow-up. The public health department is responsible for identification of sexual contacts, contact notification, and contact screening.

Lesions of primary and secondary syphilis may be highly infective. Gloves are worn when direct contact with lesions is likely, and hand hygiene is performed after gloves are removed. Isolation in a private room is not required.

Chlamydia trachomatis and Neisseria gonorrhoeae

Chlamydia trachomatis and *Neisseria gonorrhoeae* are the most commonly reported STIs. Coinfection with *C. trachomatis* often occurs in patients infected with *N. gonorrhoeae*. Young adults 15 to 24 years of age account for about two thirds of reported Chlamydia cases in Canada (Government of Canada, 2018e).

Clinical Manifestations

Women

Both *C. trachomatis* and *N. gonorrhoeae* infections frequently do not cause symptoms in women. When symptoms are present, mucopurulent cervicitis with exudates in the endocervical canal is the most frequent finding. Women with gonorrhea can also present with symptoms of urinary tract infection or vaginitis.

Men

Although men are more likely than women to have symptoms when infected, infection with *N. gonorrhoeae* or *C. trachomatis* can be asymptomatic. When symptoms are present, they may include burning during urination and penile discharge. Patients with *N. gonorrhoeae* infection may also report painful, swollen testicles.

Complications

In women, PID, ectopic pregnancy, endometritis, and infertility are possible complications of either *N. gonorrhoeae* or *C. trachomatis* infection. In men, epididymitis, a painful disease that may lead to infertility, may result from infection with either bacterium. In both males and females, arthritis or bloodstream infection may be caused by *N. gonorrhoeae*.

Assessment and Diagnostic Findings

The patient is assessed for fever, discharge (urethral, vaginal, or rectal), and signs of arthritis. Diagnostic methods used in *N. gonorrhoeae* infection include Gram stain (appropriate only for male urethral samples), culture, and nucleic acid amplification tests (NAATs). Gram stain and the direct fluorescent antibody test can be used in chlamydia. NAATs are also available for *C. trachomatis* but demand strict attention to laboratory procedures to ensure test reliability. In the female patient, samples are obtained from the endocervix, anal canal, and pharynx. In the male patient, specimens are obtained from the urethra, anal canal, and pharynx. Because *N. gonorrhoeae* organisms are susceptible to environmental changes, specimens for culture must be delivered to the laboratory immediately after they are obtained.

Medical Management

Because patients are often coinfected with both gonorrhea and chlamydia, the PHAC recommends dual therapy even if only gonorrhea has been laboratory proven. Due to a rapid increase in quinolone-resistant *Neisseria* gonorrhea treatment with combination gonorrhea infection therapy is recommended. Quinolones such as ciprofloxacin and ofloxacin are no longer routinely recommended, but may be considered as an alternative treatment option for treating gonococcal infections (PHAC, 2013b).

Test of cure by way of a gonococcal culture is recommended for pharyngeal infections, persistent symptoms, cases treated with other than the preferred treatment and cases linked to a drug-resistant failure case treated with the same antibiotic (PHAC, 2013b). Serologic testing for syphilis and HIV should be offered to patients with gonorrhea or chlamydia, because any STI increases the risk of other STIs.

Nursing Management

Gonorrhea and chlamydia are reportable communicable diseases. In any health care facility, a mechanism should be in place to ensure that all diagnosed patients are reported to the local public health department to ensure follow-up of the patient. The public health department also is responsible for interviewing the patient to identify sexual contacts, so that contact notification and screening can be initiated.

The adolescent and young adult population is a target group for preventive patient teaching about gonorrhea and chlamydia. Along with reinforcing the importance of abstinence, when appropriate, education should address postponing the age of initial sexual exposure, limiting the number of sexual partners, and using condoms for barrier protection. Young women and women who are pregnant should also be instructed about the importance of routine screening for chlamydia.

Nursing Process

The Patient With a Sexually Transmitted Infection

Assessment

Confidentiality is important when discussing sexual issues. When a detailed sexual history is necessary, it is important to respect the patient's right to privacy. The patient is asked to describe the onset and progression of symptoms and to characterize any lesions by location and by describing drainage, if present. Brief explanations of why the information is needed are often helpful. Clarification of terms may be necessary if either the patient or nurse uses words that are unfamiliar to the other.

When obtaining a sexual history, the CDC recommends the following systematic interview of key areas, the five Ps: *p*artners, *p*revention of pregnancy, *p*rotection from STIs, *p*ractices, and *p*ast history of STIs (CDC, 2015).

Asking specific information about sexual contacts is usually done only when the nurse is part of a team that will conduct partner notification. The nurse describes to the patient the public health notification process and resources that are available to assist sexual partners or infants and children.

During the physical examination, the examiner assesses the patient for rashes, lesions, drainage, discharge, or swelling and palpates inguinal nodes to elicit tenderness. Women are examined for abdominal or uterine tenderness. The mouth and throat are examined for signs of inflammation or exudate.

Nursing Priorities

Based on assessment data, the patient's major nursing priorities may include the following:

- Deficient knowledge
- Anxiety related to anticipated stigmatization
- Nonadherence with treatment

Collaborative Problems/ Potential Complications

Based on assessment data, potential complications that may develop include the following:

- Increased risk for ectopic pregnancy
- Infertility
- Transmission of infection to fetus, resulting in congenital abnormalities and other outcomes
- Neurosyphilis
- Gonococcal meningitis
- Gonococcal arthritis
- Syphilitic aortitis
- HIV-related complications

Planning and Goals

Major goals are increased patient understanding of the natural history and treatment of the infection, reduction in anxiety, increased adherence with therapeutic and preventive goals, and absence of complications.

Nursing Interventions

Increasing Knowledge and Preventing Spread of Disease

Education about STIs and prevention of the spread to others is often accomplished simultaneously. The infected patient is told what the causative organism is and should receive an explanation of the usual course of the infection, including the interval of potential communicability to others, and possible complications. The nurse stresses the importance of following therapy as prescribed and the need to report any side effects or symptom progression.

Discussion emphasizes that the same behaviours that led to infection with one STI increases the risk for any other STI, including HIV. Methods used to contact sexual partners are discussed. The patient needs to understand that until the partner has been treated, continued sexual exposure to the same person may lead to reinfection. The relative value of condoms in reducing the risk for infection with STIs should be addressed. When appropriate, the patient is encouraged to discuss any reasons for resistance to condom use to promote thoughtful decision making about this preventive method.

Reducing Anxiety

When appropriate, the patient is encouraged to discuss anxieties and fear associated with the diagnosis, treatment, or prognosis. By individualizing teaching efforts, factual information applied to specific needs may offer reassurance. Patients may need help in planning a discussion with partners. If the patient is especially apprehensive about this aspect, referral to a social worker or other specialist may be appropriate. For example, such support is especially important when the patient has newly diagnosed HIV infection. Patients with HIV may benefit from programs that combine support, education, counselling, and therapeutic goals. Such programs are designed to offer coordinated care throughout the course of disease progression.

Increasing Adherence

In group settings, for example, an outpatient obstetric setting, or in a one-to-one setting, open discussion about STI information facilitates patient teaching. Discomfort can be reduced by factual explanation of causes, consequences, treatments, prevention, and responsibilities. Because most communities have expanded STI prevention resources, referrals to appropriate agencies can complement individual educational efforts and ensure that later questions or uncertainties can be addressed by experts.

Monitoring and Managing Potential Complications

INFERTILITY AND INCREASED RISK OF ECTOPIC PREGNANCY. STIs may lead to pelvic inflammatory disease (PID) and, with it, increased risk of ectopic pregnancy and infertility. Refer to Chapters 47 and 48 for additional information.

CONGENITAL INFECTIONS. All STIs can be transmitted to infants in utero or at the time of birth. Complications of congenital infection can range from localized infection (e.g., throat infection with *N. gonorrhoeae*), to congenital abnormalities (e.g., stunting of growth or deafness from congenital syphilis), to life-threatening disease (e.g., congenital herpes simplex virus).

NEUROSYPHILIS, GONOCOCCAL MENINGITIS, GONOCOCCAL ARTHRITIS, AND SYPHILITIC AORTITIS. STIs can cause disseminated infection. The central nervous system may be infected, as seen in cases of neurosyphilis or gonococcal meningitis. Gonorrhea that infects the skeletal system may result in gonococcal arthritis. Syphilis can infect the cardiovascular system by forming vegetative lesions on the mitral or aortic valves.

HIV-RELATED COMPLICATIONS. HIV infection leads to the profound immunosuppression characteristic of AIDS. Complications of HIV infection include many opportunistic infections, including those due to *Pneumocystis jiroveci*, *Cryptococcus neoformans*, cytomegalovirus, and *Mycobacterium avium*. Refer to Chapter 52.

Evaluation

Expected patient outcomes may include the following:

1. Exhibits knowledge about STIs and their transmission
2. Demonstrates a less anxious demeanor
   a. Discusses anxieties and goals for treatment
   b. Inspects self for lesions, rashes, and discharge
   c. Accepts support, education, and counselling when indicated
   d. Assists with sharing information about infection with sexual partners
   e. Discusses risk-reduction behaviours and safer sex practices
3. Complies with treatment
4. Achieves effective treatment
5. Reports for follow-up examinations if necessary
6. Absence of complications

Emerging Infectious Diseases

As defined by the CDC, **emerging infectious diseases** are human diseases of infectious origin that have increased within the past two decades or that are likely to increase in the near future. Examples of emerging infectious diseases presented here include Zika virus, West Nile virus, Ebola Virus Disease, Legionnaires' disease, and pertussis. Table 55-1 provides an overview of infectious diseases, including emerging infectious diseases.

Many factors contribute to newly emerging or reemerging infectious diseases. These include travel, globalization of food supply and central processing of food, population growth, increased urban crowding, population movements (e.g., those that result from war, famine, or manmade or natural disasters), ecologic changes, human behaviour (e.g., risky sexual behaviour, IV/injection drug use), antimicrobial resistance, and breakdown in public health measures.

These diseases are important from an epidemiologic standpoint because their incidence has not yet stabilized. When the pattern of disease in a community is not well understood in the medical-scientific community, patients, families, and others in the community often become alarmed about these diseases. During times of increased concern about bioterrorism, whether triggered by actual events or by hoaxes, nurses have responsibility to rationally separate facts from fears. In discussions with patients and other caregivers, it is important to keep the focus on what is known and to clarify the plan for diagnosis, treatment, and containment.

Zika Virus

The Zika virus was first discovered as a pathogen in monkeys in the Zika Forest of Uganda in the 1940s; it was found to cause human disease in the 1950s. The epidemiologic pattern changed as the first large outbreak in humans did not occur until 2007 in Micronesia. The disease was not seen in the Western Hemisphere until July 2015, when a large outbreak began in Brazil. Within the next year, infections were noted in countries throughout the Americas and Pacific Islands (WHO, 2016a).

The incubation period for Zika virus disease appears to be just a few days. There is a wide variation in clinical presentations in those infected. Among patients who are symptomatic, most have self-limiting illness of 2 to 7 days duration with mild fever, rash, headache, conjunctivitis, or joint and muscle pain. The most troubling effect is that Zika has been associated with microcephaly and other congenital abnormalities in infants of some women infected with Zika during pregnancy. The virus can also cause Guillain–Barré syndrome, a condition with nerve and muscle weakness that often quickly progresses to a paralysis (WHO, 2016a).

Zika is primarily transmitted through bites of infected mosquitos from the *Aedes* genus. Sustained outbreaks have been more common in tropical areas where these mosquitos thrive. The *Aedes* mosquito is also the carrier of other mosquito-borne viruses such as dengue, chikungunya, and yellow fever. Unlike these other mosquito-borne diseases, Zika can also be transmitted through sexual transmission. This combination of transmission routes makes prevention efforts especially challenging. People can travel to epidemic areas, and later, as asymptomatic infected carriers, transmit the virus to their sexual partners. Because of the concern about congenital infection, women who are pregnant are advised to avoid travel to endemic areas and to use abstinence or safer sex methods if their sexual partners have traveled to such regions. Similarly, couples with exposure to areas where there is ongoing transmission are counseled in contraceptive options (CDC, 2016c; Morgan, 2017).

West Nile Virus

The West Nile virus was first recognized in the 1930s in Africa and was first seen in humans in North America in 1999. Although most human infections are mild or asymptomatic, a range of presentations is possible.

Approximately 20% of people who are infected have a mild disease called *West Nile fever.* These patients usually experience headache, fever, and a persistent fatigue that may continue for several months. In these patients, fewer than 1 in 150 infections develop into more serious disease, which is characterized by severe neuroinvasive illness, meningitis, encephalitis, and paralysis or poliomyelitis. The mortality rate for people with the milder West Nile fever and meningitis is less than 1%, but this rate increases to approximately 20% for those with encephalitis. Although age-related factors do not appear to affect a person's chances of acquiring West Nile virus, the risk of neuroinvasive disease is greater in those older than 50 years (CDC, 2016c).

The incubation period, that is, from mosquito bite to onset of symptoms, is between 3 and 14 days. Currently there is no treatment for West Nile virus infection. Medical and nursing management consists of fluid replacement, airway management, and supportive nursing care when meningitis or symptoms are present.

Birds are the natural reservoir for the virus, and since 1999, the population of infected birds in Canada has increased steadily. Mosquitoes become infected when feeding on birds and can transmit the virus to animals and humans. Although human-to-human transmission of West Nile virus is very rare, transmission has occurred as the result of occupational exposure in laboratory workers, infant exposure transplacentally and from breastfeeding, and blood transfusion or organ transplant from infected donors (PHAC, 2015).

Ebola Virus Disease

The first human outbreak of Ebola virus disease occurred in 1976. For decades the virus maintained a pattern of sporadic outbreaks in remote African villages, followed by intervening periods without any recognized cases worldwide. In 2014, the virus broke through this usual pattern and rampaged through the West African countries Liberia, Guinea, and Sierra Leone, with secondary cases in other countries in Africa, Europe, and the United States (Chertow, Kleine, Edwards, et al., 2014).

Pathophysiology

Ebola is spread through direct contact with blood or body fluids (urine, vomit, feces, saliva, sweat, semen, and breast milk) from the person who is ill from the virus and possibly from contact with semen of a man who has recovered from Ebola. It is not spread through air, water, or insect bite. In Africa, it may occasionally be spread by handling infected bats or infected wild animals that are sometimes hunted for food. Ebola virus is only detected in blood after the patient becomes symptomatic and viral levels rise significantly as the disease progresses (Chertow et al., 2014).

The incubation period from exposure to first symptoms ranges from 2 to 21 days. If there are no symptoms by 21 days after exposure, there is essentially no risk of developing Ebola. Patients are not contagious to others before symptoms occur. Thorough identification of Ebola contacts and careful symptom monitoring can prevent subsequent waves of transmission.

Clinical Manifestations

The initial clinical manifestations include high fever, muscle aches, and fatigue. Between the third and fifth symptomatic day, the patient often develops severe diarrhea, abdominal pain, and vomiting. Patients are at great risk of severe dehydration at this point as many produce over 5 L of liquid stool per day. This stage can persist for a week or more, and many patients develop hemodynamic shock. Refer to Chapter 18. Patients may also show increasing neurologic symptoms during that period, such as confusion, agitation, delirium, or encephalitis. Approximately 5% will develop bleeding or hemorrhage, a very poor prognostic indicator. Patients who do not die during the first 2 weeks of the disease are most likely to survive the illness (Chertow et al., 2014).

Medical Management

Treatment is largely supportive maintenance of the circulatory system and respiratory systems. It is likely that the patient who is infected will need ventilator and dialysis support during the acute phase of illness.

Nursing Management

Nursing management mirrors that of medical management and is largely supportive. Supportive care for a patient with such a devastating disease requires psychological support for the patient and family.

Health care workers are at increased risk for acquiring Ebola because they may have contact with body fluids or equipment contaminated from exposure to body fluids. Because so much virus is present, especially in vomit and diarrhea, the patient should be isolated in a private room, away from other patients. Patients must be promptly isolated and health care workers should wear complete PPE. Systems must be set up so that an observer guides each worker to meticulously don PPE before direct contact with a patient who is infected to ensure that all equipment is worn correctly. After a worker has direct contact with a patient who is infected, an observer should direct careful doffing (removal) of PPE to ensure that no exposure occurs in the process. Equipment used for the patient with Ebola virus should be used solely for that patient and should be disposed after use. If equipment must be reused, it should be sterilized or scrupulously cleaned with a bleach-based solution before reuse. Care for the patient with Ebola requires hospitals and transport systems to develop plans to coordinate staffing, supply maintenance, handling of waste, and communication with the public (WHO, 2016b).

Legionnaires' Disease

Legionnaires' disease is a multisystem illness that usually includes pneumonia and is caused by the gram-negative bacterium *Legionella pneumophila*. Named after an outbreak among people attending a convention of the American Legion in 1976, its potential to cause outbreaks has been demonstrated repeatedly in hospitals and other settings. It continues to be considered an emerging infectious disease because there are new presentations in recent years. In Canada, fewer than 100 cases of Legionnaires' disease are reported per year; however, the actual number of cases is probably much higher, as not all people with pneumonia are tested for *Legionella* infection (Government of Canada, 2015b).

Legionella organisms are found in many man-made and naturally occurring water sources. Although the organisms may initially be introduced to the plumbing system in low numbers, growth is enhanced by water storage, sediment, temperatures ranging from 25° to 42°C, and certain amoebae frequently present in water that can support intracellular growth of legionellae. Because incidence appears to increase in the summer and autumn months, vacation-related exposure to hotel or cruise ship plumbing and air-conditioning systems, whirlpool spas, and decorative fountains may be a causative risk.

Pathophysiology

L. pneumophila is transmitted by the aerosolized route from an environmental source to a person's respiratory tract. In hospitals, patients may be exposed to aerosols created by cooling towers, water exposure from in-room plumbing, and respiratory therapy equipment. Person-to-person transmission, if it occurs at all, is extremely rare. Because underlying medical conditions can increase host susceptibility and subsequent severity of disease and because hospital plumbing systems are often very complex, outbreaks occur in hospitals more frequently than at other centres within the community. The mortality rate for Legionnaires' disease may be as high as 10% in some populations (Cooley, 2016).

Risk Factors

Risk factors for *Legionella* infection include diseases that lead to severe immunosuppression, such as AIDS, hematologic malignancy, end-stage renal disease, or use of immunosuppressive agents. Other factors associated with increased risk include advanced age, diabetes, alcohol abuse, smoking, and other pulmonary diseases (Cooley, 2016).

Clinical Manifestations

The lungs are the principal organs of infection; however, other organs may also be involved. The incubation period ranges from 2 to 10 days. Early symptoms may include malaise, myalgias, headache, and dry cough. The patient develops increasing pulmonary symptoms, including productive cough, dyspnea, and chest pain. Patients are usually febrile, and body temperatures may reach or exceed 39.4°C. Diarrhea and other gastrointestinal symptoms are common. In severe cases, multiorgan involvement and failure may follow.

Assessment and Diagnostic Findings

The diagnostic approach generally involves accumulation of information obtained from the history, physical examination, x-rays, laboratory findings, and assessment of therapeutic effectiveness. Chest x-ray abnormalities may vary in severity and in location within the lungs. Laboratory tests available for the diagnosis of *Legionella* include culture or tests that detect either antigen or antibody. The most frequently used test is the urinary antigen. The greatest limitation of the test is that it detects only one subgroup of one of the several species of *Legionella*. The CDC recommends using multiple tests when Legionnaires' disease is suspected because none of the tests are completely accurate (CDC, 2016b).

Medical Management

The antibiotic agents of choice are azithromycin (Zithromax) or a fluoroquinolone such as moxifloxacin (Avelox) (CDC, 2016c). The antibiotic doxycycline may also be used.

Nursing Management

The nursing management described for the patient with any pneumonia (see Chapter 24) should form the basis of care for the patient with *Legionella* pneumonia. Isolation is not required because *Legionella* is not transmitted between humans. When the patient has acquired the infection in a health care facility, water cultures should be performed to determine if the water supply is contaminated.

Pertussis

Pertussis, also known as whooping cough, is the second most reported vaccine preventable disease in Canada (Wierzbowski, 2017).

Pertussis is caused by the bacterium *Bordetella pertussis*. It is highly contagious, and patients usually present to health care professionals with a sudden (paroxysmal) cough that is accompanied by a characteristic whoop—a high-pitched noise heard when inhaling.

Pathophysiology

B. pertussis is primarily transmitted by droplets but transmission from direct contact with a contaminated item also occurs. People who are infected spread the illness when coughing, sneezing, or sharing breathing space and are most infectious within the 2 weeks after coughing starts. The usual incubation period is 7 to 10 days. *B. pertussis* attaches to the cilia lining the upper respiratory tract and releases toxins that cause the airway to swell (Wierzbowski, 2017).

Clinical Manifestations

Pertussis causes a range of respiratory symptoms, with cough being the most frequent. It is generally most severe for infants who have not yet been vaccinated. Pneumonia is the most common consequence of infection, but the disease can also lead to seizures, encephalopathy, and, rarely, death. People who have been vaccinated seldom have severe disease.

Assessment and Diagnostic Findings

Most diagnoses of pertussis are made, at least initially, without laboratory confirmation. The clinical case definition, unless there is a pre-existing condition to explain the symptoms, is a new cough lasting at least 2 weeks with inspiratory whoop or vomiting after cough. Laboratory confirmation can be made by clinical culture or by polymerase chain reaction assay for *B. pertussis*. Serologic testing may be used in later stages of the disease to confirm diagnosis. Nasopharyngeal specimens obtained by swab or aspirate are the best source for a culture (Wierzbowski, 2017).

Medical Management

Early treatment for pertussis is important to prevent complications. The antibiotic agents of choice are azithromycin, erythromycin (Erythrocin), or clarithromycin (Biaxin). The antibiotic trimethoprim–sulfamethaxazole (TMP–SMZ) (Bactrim) may also be used. Close contacts of a patient with proven or suspected pertussis may receive antibiotic prophylaxis to reduce the risk of disease. Patients receiving appropriate antibiotic treatment for 5 days are no longer considered infectious (Government of Canada, 2014).

Nursing Management

Patients who are hospitalized with pertussis should be isolated in droplet precautions until they have received 5 days of appropriate therapy. Household members should receive antimicrobial prophylaxis and should be advised to report any symptoms of an upper respiratory infection.

Because pertussis is most severe for infants, it is important to ensure that all women who are pregnant are vaccinated with Tdap (tetanus, diphtheria, acellular pertussis vaccine). The best time for Tdap for women who have not been vaccinated before becoming pregnant is late in the second trimester or in the third trimester. If a woman has not been vaccinated prior to delivery of the infant, Tdap should be given immediately postpartum. Fathers, siblings, grandparents, and others who are around infants under 12 months should also be vaccinated to reduce the risk of transmitting pertussis.

For the protection of both worker and patient, all health care workers should receive a single dose of Tdap vaccine. Workers who are unsure if they have ever had Tdap should receive the vaccine regardless of the possible interval since the previous vaccination.

Booster doses are recommended at ages of 12 to 23 months, 4 to 6 years, and 14 to 16 years. Immunity to pertussis wanes with time so adolescents and adults may require a booster vaccination to reduce the risk of infection and its consequent transmission of the bacteria to others (Government of Canada, 2014).

Travel and Immigration

Travel, trade, migration, and wars have led to many epidemics throughout history. The potential for epidemics is greatest when travellers and immigrants introduce microorganisms to which the host population has little or no immunity. Examples of important epidemics in the Western Hemisphere have included yellow fever, malaria, hookworm, leprosy, smallpox, measles, mumps, and syphilis. The HIV epidemic demonstrates the way that travel and immigration allow a disease to spread undetected worldwide.

The 2014 Ebola outbreak demonstrates how global travel contributes to a rapidly occurring epidemic involving an unrecognized pathogen.

In Canada, an infrastructure with enforced vaccination, clean water, and insect and rodent control decreases the risk that epidemics will progress even when travel may introduce exotic microorganisms. However, the recent experience with Zika virus has reinforced knowledge that insect transmission can lead to significant human outbreaks. Thus, the concern grows that vector-borne diseases such as dengue and malaria may increase in Canada as mosquitoes can transmit disease locally when a reservoir of infected humans is established. The PHAC maintains an active surveillance system to monitor and halt the incidence of many diseases prospectively.

Immigration and Acquired Immunodeficiency Disease Syndrome

The fact that AIDS reached pandemic proportions less than a decade after its recognition attests to the efficiency of world travel in spreading disease. Such rapid transmission rates are especially dramatic because HIV essentially requires intimate contact between two people through sexual activity or sharing blood through needles. Refer to Chapter 52 for more information.

Immigration and Tuberculosis

Immigration has always been an important influence in the dynamic epidemiology of TB in Canada. In 2007, the incidence of TB among foreign-born people accounted for 66% of all cases reported in Canada (Government of Canada, 2018g).

The association between immigration and transmission risk is greatest in urban areas because these locations are frequently heavily populated and frequently visited by foreign-born people. These locales are also often the epicentre of the HIV epidemic. Because HIV infection depletes T cells, which are necessary for TB protection, the geographic closeness of these two microorganisms potentiates increased rates of both infections.

A positive TST establishes that TB infection has occurred at some time in a person's life but does not provide information about current infectivity. The reliability of TST interpretation is decreased among foreign-born people because the Bacille Calmette–Guérin (BCG) vaccine is used in many countries. After receiving BCG, people often have some degree of TST reactivity for a prolonged time. New rapid tests are now available for the detection of TB that are not affected by prior BCG vaccination including the QuantiFERON-TB test. Refer to Chapter 24 for more detailed discussion.

Immigration and Vector-Borne Diseases

Malaria and dengue are diseases that cause significant morbidity and mortality throughout the developing world. These diseases may be "imported" to Canada via travel, immigration, or commerce. They are caused by microorganisms that can be spread to humans by mosquitoes that thrive in tropical zones and breed in stagnant water sources. Although malaria is uncommon in Canada about 488 cases are reported per year, and these patients require immediate hospitalization and treatment (Government of Canada, 2015a). Similarly dengue fever can cause severe disease and can be fatal. Medical care can help with recovery (Government of Canada, 2014a).

Critical Thinking Exercises

1 Your unit has had an increase in HAIs in the past 6 months. Identify how HAIs occur. What nursing interventions should be used to reduce the risk of new HAIs? What evidence-based strategies are used to decrease the incidence of HAIs? Identify the criteria used to evaluate the strength of the evidence for the practices you identify.

2 You are a home care nurse caring for a 75-year-old patient with multiple medical conditions. What information should be provided about infection risk prevention to the patient, the family, and the caregiver?

3 Identify the priorities, approach, and techniques you would use for a 21-year-old woman who presents to student health with symptoms of Zika after traveling to Brazil for spring break. How would your priorities, approach, and techniques differ if the patient is a 21-year-old man? If the female patient is pregnant?

REFERENCES AND SELECTED READINGS

Books

Centers for Disease Control and Prevention. (2015). *Epidemiology and Prevention of Vaccine-Preventable Diseases*. Hamborsky J, Kroger A, Wolfe S. (Eds.). 13th ed. Washington D. C: Public Health Foundation.

Guerrant, R. L., & Steiner, T. S. (2015). Principles and syndromes of enteric infection. In G. L. Mandell, R. D. Bennett, R. Dolin (Eds.). *Mandell, Douglas and Bennett's principles and practice of infectious diseases* (8th ed.). Philadelphia, PA: Elsevier.

Mandell, G. L., Bennett, R. D., & Dolin, R. (Eds.) (2014). *Principles and practice of infectious diseases* (8th ed.). Philadelphia, PA: Elsevier.

Porth, C. M. (2017). Disorders of gastrointestinal function (pp. 879–910). In R. A. Hannon, C. Pooler, & C. M. Porth (Eds.). *Porth pathophysiology: Concepts of altered health states* (Second Canadian edition). Philadelphia, PA: Wolters Kluwer Health/Lippincott Williams & Wilkins.

Journals and Electronic Documents

Bonomo, R. A., Burd, E. M., Conly, J., et al. (2018). Carbapenemase-producing organisms: A global scourge. Review article. *Clinical Infectious Diseases*, *66*(8):1290–1297.

Canadian Patient Safety Institute. (2016). *Central Line Infections*. Retrieved from http://www.patientsafetyinstitute.ca/en/Topic/Pages/Central-Line-Infections-(CLI).aspx.

Centers for Disease Control and Prevention (CDC). (2007). *2007 Guideline for Isolation Precautions: Preventing Transmission of Infectious Agents in Healthcare Settings*. Retrieved on May 13, 2016, from: www.cdc.gov/hicpac/2007ip/2007ip_part1.html

Centers for Disease Control and Prevention. (2015). *Sexually transmitted diseases treatment guidelines*. Retrieved from https://www.cdc.gov/std/tg2015/clinical.htm.

Centers for Disease Control and Prevention (CDC). (2016a). *Immunization schedules*. Retrieved from www.cdc.gov/vaccines/schedules.

Centers for Disease Control and Prevention (CDC). (2016b). *Legionnaire's disease*. Retrieved from https://www.cdc.gov/legionella/about/history.html.

Centers for Disease Control and Prevention (CDC). (2016c). *Zika virus*. Retrieved from www.cdc.gov/zika.

Chertow, D. S., Kleine, C., Edwards, J. K., et al. (2014). Ebola virus disease in West Africa—Clinical manifestations and management. *New England Journal of Medicine*, *371*(22), 2054–2057.

Cooley, L. (2016). Legionnaires disease on rise in US—2016 Update. *Medscape*. Retrieved from www.medscape.com/viewarticle/864189 Dantes.

Dombecki, C., Shah, M. M., Eke-Usim, A., et al. (2015). The impact of role models on hand hygiene compliance. *Infect Control Hosp Epidemiol*, *36*(5), 610–612.

Gilmartin, H., Sousa, K. H., & Battaglia, C. (2016). Capturing the central line bundle infection prevention interventions: Comparison of Reflective and Composite Modeling Methods. *Nursing Research*, *65*(5), 397–407.

Government of Canada. (2012). *Enteric Protozoa: Giardia and Cryptosporidium*. Retrieved from https://www.canada.ca/en/health-canada/services/environmental-workplace-health/reports-publications/water-quality/enteric-protozoa-giardia-cryptosporidium.html#a23

Government of Canada. (2014a). *Dengue fever*. Retrieved from https://www.canada.ca/en/public-health/services/infectious-diseases/viral-haemorrhagic-fevers/dengue-fever.html.

Government of Canada. (2014b). *Pertussis (whooping cough)*. Retrieved from https://www.canada.ca/en/public-health/services/immunization/vaccine-preventable-diseases/pertussis-whooping-cough/health-professionals.html.

Government of Canada. (2015a). *For health professionals: West Nile virus*. Retrieved from https://www.canada.ca/en/public-health/services/diseases/west-nile-virus/health-professionals-treating-west-nile-virus.html.

Government of Canada. (2015b). *Legionella. What is Legionella?*. Retrieved from https://www.canada.ca/en/public-health/services/infectious-diseases/legionella.html.

Government of Canada. (2016a). *For health professionals: Malaria*. Retrieved from https://www.canada.ca/en/public-health/services/diseases/malaria/health-professionals-malaria.html.

Government of Canada. (2016b). *For health professionals: Salmonellosis (salmonella)*. Retrieved from https://www.canada.ca/en/public-health/services/diseases/salmonellosis-salmonella/health-professionals.html.

Government of Canada. (2016c). *Infographic: Food-related illnesses, hospitalizations and deaths in Canada*. Retrieved from https://www.canada.ca/en/public-health/services/publications/food-nutrition/infographic-food-related-illnesses-hospitalizations-deaths-in-canada.html?_ga=2.123183307.1726313276.1538588111-1599574183.1488986256.

Government of Canada. (2018). *Canadian antimicrobial resistance surveillance system-update 2018: Executive summary*. Retrieved from https://www.canada.ca/en/public-health/services/publications/drugs-health-products/canadian-antimicrobial-resistance-surveillance-system-2018-report-executive-summary.html

Government of Canada. (2018a). *Canadian immunization guide*. Retrieved from https://www.canada.ca/en/public-health/services/canadian-immunization-guide.html.
Government of Canada. (2018b). *Canadian pandemic influenza preparedness: Planning guidance for the health sector*. Retrieved from https://www.canada.ca/en/public-health/services/flu-influenza/canadian-pandemic-influenza-preparedness-planning-guidance-health-sector.html.
Government of Canada. (2018c). *Cholera*. Retrieved from https://travel.gc.ca/travelling/health-safety/diseases/cholera.
Government of Canada. (2018d). *Eat and drink safely abroad*. Retrieved from https://travel.gc.ca/travelling/health-safety/food-water.
Government of Canada. (2018e). *Section 5-1: Canadian Guidelines on Sexually Transmitted Infections—Management and treatment of specific infections—Mycoplasma Genitalium Infections*. Retrieved from https://www.canada.ca/en/public-health/services/infectious-diseases/sexual-health-sexually-transmitted-infections/canadian-guidelines/sexually-transmitted-infections/canadian-guidelines-sexually-transmitted-infections-49.html.
Government of Canada. (2018f). *Section 5–10: Canadian Guidelines on Sexually Transmitted Infections—Management and treatment of specific infections—Syphilis*. Retrieved from https://www.canada.ca/en/public-health/services/infectious-diseases/sexual-health-sexually-transmitted-infections/canadian-guidelines/sexually-transmitted-infections/canadian-guidelines-sexually-transmitted-infections-27.html.
Government of Canada. (2018g). *Surveillance of tuberculosis (TB)*. Retrieved from https://www.canada.ca/en/public-health/services/diseases/tuberculosis-tb/surveillance-tuberculosis-tb.html.
Irvine, J. (2017). *Community-associated methicillin-resistant Staphylococcus aureus in indigenous communities in Canada. Position statement. Canadian Pediatric Society*. Retrieved from https://www.cps.ca/en/documents/position/community-associated-MRSA-in-Indigenous-communities.
Loewen, K., Schreiber, Y., Kirlew, M., et al. (2017). Community-associated methicillin-resistant staphylococcus aureus infection. Clinical review. *Canadian Family Physician, 63*(7), 512–520. Retrieved from http://www.cfp.ca/content/cfp/63/7/512.full.pdf.
Marschall, J., Mermel, L. A., Fakih, M., et al. (2014). Strategies to prevent central-line associated blood stream infections in acute care hospitals: 2014 update. *Infection Control and Hospital Epidemiology, 35*(7), 753–771.
Moore, D. L. (2018). Vaccine recommendations for children and youth for the 2017/2018 influenza season. *Paediatrics and Child Health 23*(1), e10–e13.
Morgan, S. A. (2017). Spring break? Think Zika. *American Nurse Today, 12*(3), 15.
Public Health Agency of Canada (PHAC). (2012). *Hand hygiene practices in healthcare settings*. Retrieved from http://publications.gc.ca/collections/collection_2012/aspc-phac/HP40-74-2012-eng.pdf
Public Health Agency of Canada (PHAC). (2013a). *Clostridium difficile infection: Infection prevention and control guidance for management in acute care settings*. Retrieved from https://www.canada.ca/en/public-health/services/infectious-diseases/nosocomial-occupational-infections/clostridium-difficile-infection-prevention-control-guidance-management-acute-care-settings.html
Public Health Agency of Canada (PHAC). (2013b). *Canadian guidelines on sexually transmitted infections. Gonococcal infections chapter*. Retrieved from https://www.canada.ca/content/dam/phac-aspc/migration/phac-aspc/std-mts/sti-its/cgsti-ldcits/assets/pdf/section-5-6-eng.pdf.
Public Health Agency of Canada (PHAC). (2014). *Norovirus fact sheet*. Retrieved from http://www.phac-aspc.gc.ca/fs-sa/fs-fi/norovirus-eng.php.
Public Health Agency of Canada (PHAC). (2015). *Canadian pandemic influenza preparedness: Planning guidance for the health sector. Emergency preparedness and response*. Retrieved from https://www.canada.ca/en/public-health/services/flu-influenza/canadian-pandemic-influenza-preparedness-planning-guidance-health-sector/table-of-contents.html#a1.
Public Health Agency of Canada (PHAC). (2016a). *Canadian guidelines on sexually transmitted infections*. Retrieved from https://www.canada.ca/en/public-health/services/infectious-diseases/sexual-health-sexually-transmitted-infections/canadian-guidelines/sexually-transmitted-infections/canadian-guidelines-sexually-transmitted-infections-16.html
Public Health Agency of Canada (PHAC). (2016b). *Summary report on ARO surveillance data from January 1, 2011 to December 31, 2015. Canadian Nosocomial Infection Surveillance Program (CNISP). Centre for Communicable Diseases and Infection Control*.
Public Health Agency of Canada (PHAC). (2017a). *Canadian Immunization Guide Chapter on Influenza and Statement on Seasonal Influenza Vaccine for 2017–2018. An Advisory Committee Statement (ACS). National Advisory Committee on Immunization (NACI). Minister of Health*.
Public Health Agency of Canada (PHAC). (2017b). *Central Venous Catheter-Associated Blood Stream Infections in Intensive Care Units in Canadian Acute-Care Hospitals Surveillance Report January 1, 2006 to December 31, 2006 and January 1, 2009 to December 31, 2011. Centre for Communicable Diseases and Infection Control. Minister of the Public Health Agency of Canada*.
Public Health Agency of Canada (PHAC). (2017c). *Surveillance Protocol for Vancomycin Resistant Enterococci (VRE) in CNISP Healthcare Facilities. Canadian Nosocomial Infection Surveillance Program (CNISP)* Retrieved from https://www.ammi.ca/Content/CNISP%202017%20VRE%20protocol%20FINAL__EN.pdf.
Public Health Agency of Canada (PHAC). (2017d). *Canadian immunization guide chapter on influenza and statement on seasonal influenza vaccine for 2017–2018*. Retrieved from https://www.canada.ca/en/public-health/services/publications/healthy-living/canadian-immunization-guide-statement-seasonal-influenza-vaccine-2017-2018.html
Public Health Agency of Canada (PHAC). (2018a). *Canadian Antimicrobial Resistance Surveillance System 2017 Report*. Retrieved from https://www.canada.ca/en/public-health/services/publications/drugs-health-products/canadian-antimicrobial-resistance-surveillance-system-2017-report-executive-summary.html.
Public Health Agency of Canada (PHAC). (2018b). *Sexually Transmitted Infections. Canada Communicable Disease Report*. Retrieved from https://www.canada.ca/content/dam/phac-aspc/documents/services/reports-publications/canada-communicable-disease-report-ccdr/monthly-issue/2018-44/issue-2-february-1-2018/issue-2-eng.pdf.
Safer Healthcare Now. (2012). *Prevent central line infections getting started kit*. Retrieved from http://www.patientsafetyinstitute.ca/en/toolsResources/Documents/Interventions/Central%20Line-Associated%20Bloodstream%20Infection/CLI%20Getting%20Started%20Kit.pdf.
Safer Healthcare Now. (2015). *Sepsis: Getting started kit. Section 1: Prevention, early identification and response to sepsis*. Retrieved from http://www.patientsafetyinstitute.ca/en/toolsResources/Sepsis-GSK/Documents/Sepsis%20Getting%20Started%20Kit%20-%20Section%201%20-%20Sepsis%20Prevention%20Identification%20and%20Response.pdf.
Wierzbowski, A. K. (2017). *Disease debrief: Pertussis. National Collaborating Centre for Infectious Diseases*. Retrieved from https://nccid.ca/debrief/pertussis/.
Workowski, K. A., Bolan GA., (2015). Sexually transmitted diseases treatment guidelines Centers for Disease Control and Prevention (CDC). *MMWR: Morbidity and Mortality Weekly Report, 55*(RR11), 1–94.
World Health Organization (WHO). (2016a). *Zika virus*. Retrieved on October, 24, 2016, from www.who.int/topics/zika/en/
World Health Organization (WHO). (2016b). *Ebola virus disease*. Retrieved from https://www.who.int/ebola/en/

Resources

Association of Medical Microbiology and Infectious Disease Canada: http://www.ammi.ca
Association for Professionals in Infection Control and Epidemiology (APIC), Inc.: http://www.apic.org
Canadian Centre for Occupational Health and Safety: http://www.ccohs.ca
Canadian Lung Association: http://www.lung.ca
Health Canada: http://www.hc-sc.gc.ca
Infectious Diseases Society of America (IDSA): http://www.idsociety.org
National Advisory Committee on Immunization: http://www.phac-aspc.gc.ca/naci-ccni/index-eng.php
National Foundation for Infectious Diseases (NFID): http://www.nfid.org
National Institute of Allergy and Infectious Diseases (NIAID), National Institutes of Health: http://www.niaid.nih.gov/default.htm
Occupational Safety and Health Administration (OSHA): http://www.osha.gov
Public Health Agency of Canada: http://www.phac-aspc.gc.ca
Safer Healthcare Now: http://www.saferhealthcarenow.ca
Travel Health Information: http://www.TravelHealth.gc.ca
U.S. Centers for Disease Control and Prevention (CDC): http://www.cdc.gov
World Health Organization (WHO): http://www.who.int/home-page

56 Assessment and Management of Patients With Rheumatic Disorders

Adapted by Jennifer Densmore

Learning Objectives

On completion of this chapter, the learner will be able to:

1. Explain the pathophysiology of rheumatic diseases.
2. Describe the assessment and diagnostic findings seen in patients with a suspected diagnosis of rheumatic disease or disorder.
3. Discuss appropriate nursing interventions based on nursing priorities and collaborative problems that commonly occur with rheumatic disorders.
4. Apply the nursing process as a framework for the care of the patient with a rheumatic disease, such as connective tissue disease or osteoarthritis.
5. Describe the systemic effects of a connective tissue disease.
6. Devise a teaching plan for the patient with newly diagnosed rheumatic disease.
7. Identify modifications in interventions to accommodate changes in patients' functional ability that may occur with disease progression.

Rheumatic diseases include common disorders such as **osteoarthritis** (OA) and less common conditions such as systemic lupus erythematosus (SLE) and scleroderma. These conditions can be life-threatening, or they can be minor illnesses. The problems caused by the rheumatic diseases include not only the obvious limitations in mobility and activities of daily living but also the more subtle systemic effects that can lead to organ failure and death or result in problems such as pain, fatigue, altered self-image, and sleep disturbances. The rheumatic disease may be the patient's primary health problem or a secondary diagnosis. An understanding of rheumatic diseases and their effects on a patient's function and well-being is essential to developing an appropriate plan of nursing care.

Rheumatic Diseases

Commonly called **arthritis** (inflammation of a joint) and thought of as one condition, the rheumatic diseases include more than 100 different types of disorders that primarily affect skeletal muscles, bones, cartilage, ligaments, tendons, and joints in males and females of all ages (Grossman & Porth, 2014). Some disorders are more likely to occur at a particular time of life or to affect one gender more than the other. The onset of these conditions may be acute or insidious, with a course possibly marked by periods of remission (a period when disease symptoms are reduced or absent) and exacerbation (a period when symptoms occur or increase). Treatment can be simple, aimed at localized relief, or it can be complex, directed toward relief of systemic effects. Permanent changes and disability may result from these disorders.

Rheumatologic disease processes affect males and females of all ages and ethnic groups. Some disorders are more likely to occur at a particular time of life or to affect one gender more often than the other. In general, women are two to nine times more commonly affected by rheumatologic diseases than men (Barbour, Helmick, Theis, et al., 2013). The onset of these conditions may be acute or insidious, with a course possibly marked by periods of remission (a period when disease symptoms are reduced or absent) and exacerbation (a period when symptoms occur or increase). Treatment can be simple, aimed at localized relief, or it can be complex, directed toward relief of systemic effects. Permanent changes and disability may result from these disorders.

Nurses need to understand the classification of rheumatic diseases. One basic system is to classify disease as either monoarticular (affecting a single joint) or polyarticular (affecting multiple joints), and then to further classify it as either inflammatory or noninflammatory. Conditions that may secondarily affect the musculoskeletal structure

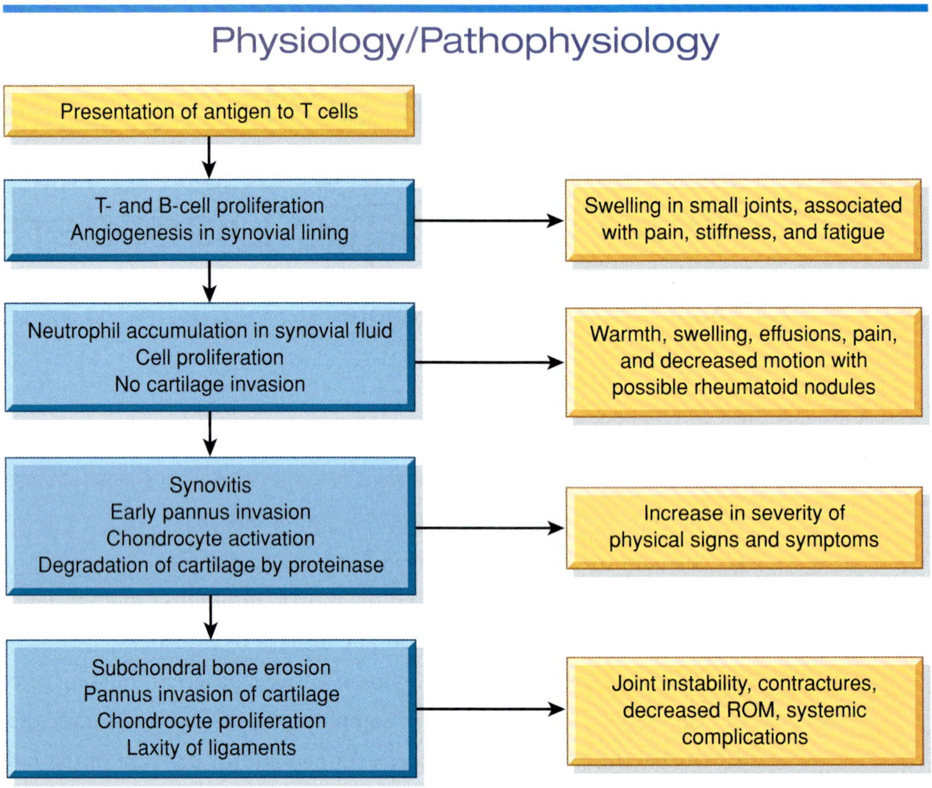

FIGURE 56-1. Pathophysiology and associated physical signs of rheumatoid arthritis. ROM, range of motion.

are also included, illustrating the diversity of the rheumatic diseases.

Pathophysiology

The joint is the area most commonly affected in rheumatic diseases. Despite the diversity of rheumatic diseases, from localized involvement of one joint to systemic, multisystem disorders, they all involve some degree of inflammation and degeneration, which may occur simultaneously. Inflammation is manifested in the joints as synovitis. In inflammatory rheumatic diseases, the primary process is inflammation caused by the immune response. Degeneration occurs as a secondary process, resulting from the effect of **pannus** (proliferation of newly formed synovial tissue infiltrated with inflammatory cells). Conversely, in degenerative rheumatic diseases, inflammation occurs as a secondary process. This synovitis is usually milder, is more likely to be seen in advanced disease, and represents a reactive process.

Inflammation

Inflammation is a series of related steps. In response to the triggering event (e.g., trauma, increased stress), the antigen stimulus activates monocytes and T lymphocytes (also called T cells). Next, the immunoglobulin antibodies form immune complexes with antigens. Phagocytosis of the immune complexes is initiated, generating an inflammatory reaction (joint effusion, pain, and edema) (Fig. 56-1).

During the next step, the immune response deviates from normal. Phagocytosis produces chemicals such as leukotrienes and prostaglandins. Leukotrienes contribute to the inflammatory process by attracting other white blood cells to the area. Prostaglandins act as modifiers to inflammation. In some cases, they increase inflammation; in other cases, they decrease it. Leukotrienes and prostaglandins produce enzymes such as collagenase that break down collagen, a vital part of a normal joint. The release of these enzymes in the joint causes edema, proliferation of the synovial membrane and pannus formation, destruction of cartilage, and erosion of bone.

Glossary

ankylosis: fixation or immobility of a joint
arthritis: inflammation of a joint
arthroplasty: replacement of a joint
osteoarthritis: degenerative joint disease
osteophyte: a bony outgrowth or protuberance; bone spur
pannus: proliferation of newly formed synovial tissue infiltrated with inflammatory cells
rheumatic diseases: numerous disorders affecting skeletal muscles, bones, cartilage, ligaments, tendons, and joints
rheumatoid arthritis: autoimmune disease of unknown origin
subchondral bone: bony plate that supports the articular cartilage
tophi: accumulation of crystalline deposits in articular surfaces, bones, soft tissue, and cartilage

The immunologic inflammatory process begins when antigens are presented to T lymphocytes, leading to a proliferation of T and B cells. B cells are a source of antibody-forming cells, or plasma cells. In response to specific antigens, plasma cells produce and release antibodies. Antibodies combine with corresponding antigens to form pairs, or immune complexes. The immune complexes build up and are deposited in the synovial tissue or other organs in the body, triggering the inflammatory reaction that can ultimately damage the involved tissue.

The systemic nature of the rheumatic diseases is reflected in the resultant widespread inflammatory process. Although focused in the joints, inflammation also involves other areas. The blood vessels (vasculitis and arteritis), lungs, heart, and kidneys may also be affected by the inflammation. In the joints, this inflammatory response is manifested as pannus extending throughout the joint space and, if persistent, eroding the articular cartilage, causing secondary degenerative changes to the joint.

Autoimmunity

A hallmark of rheumatologic diseases is autoimmunity, where the body mistakenly recognizes its own tissue as a foreign antigen. Autoimmunity leads to destruction of tissue via the same inflammatory process as discussed earlier, along with chronic and long-standing pain. Although focused in the joints, inflammation and autoimmunity also involve other areas. The blood vessels (vasculitis and arteritis), lungs, heart, and kidneys may be affected by the autoimmunity and inflammation. See Chapter 51 for more information on autoimmune disease. A large group of genes, called *human leukocyte antigen* (HLA) genes, has been linked to the immune response and the development of multiple rheumatologic diseases (Di Lorenzo, 2015).

Degeneration

Although the cause of degeneration of the articular cartilage is poorly understood, the process is known to be metabolically active and therefore is more accurately called "degradation." One theory of degradation is that genetic or hormonal influences, mechanical factors, and prior joint damage cause cartilage failure. Degradation of cartilage ensues, and increased mechanical stress on bone ends, causes stiffening of bone tissue. Another theory is that bone stiffening occurs and results in increased mechanical stress on cartilage, which in turn initiates the processes of degradation. (See Chapter 69 for more information on the structure and function of the articular system.)

Clinical Manifestations

The most common symptom of the rheumatic diseases that causes a person to seek medical attention is pain. Other common symptoms include joint swelling, limited movement, stiffness, weakness, and fatigue.

Assessment and Diagnostic Findings

Assessment begins with a general health history, which includes the onset of symptoms and how they evolved, family history, past health history, and any other contributing factors. Because many of the rheumatic diseases are chronic conditions, the health history should also include information about the patient's perception of the problem, previous treatments and their effectiveness, the patient's support systems, and the patient's current knowledge base and the source of that information. A complete health history is followed by a complete physical assessment (see Chapter 5).

Assessment for rheumatic diseases combines the physical examination with a functional assessment. Inspection of the patient's general appearance occurs during initial contact. Gait, posture, and general musculoskeletal size and structure are observed. Gross deformities and abnormalities in movement are noted. The symmetry, size, and contour of other connective tissues, such as the skin and adipose tissue, are also noted and recorded. Chart 56-1 outlines the important areas for consideration during the physical assessment. The functional assessment is a combination of history (what the patient reports that he or she can and cannot do) and examination (observation of activities: the patient demonstrates what he or she can and cannot do, such as dressing and getting in and out of a chair). Observation also includes the adaptations and adjustments the patient may have made (sometimes without awareness); for example, with shoulder or elbow involvement, the person may bend over to reach a fork, rather than raising the fork to the mouth.

The history and physical assessment data are supplemented by supportive or confirming diagnostic test findings. In some instances, tests are used to monitor the course of the disease. For example, the erythrocyte sedimentation rate (ESR) reflects inflammatory activity and, indirectly, the progression or remission of disease.

Laboratory Studies

Some of the most common laboratory studies are listed with their corresponding normal ranges and primary indications in Table 56-1. Many of the tests require special laboratory techniques and may not be performed in every health care facility. The primary health care provider determines which tests are necessary based on symptoms, stage of disease, cost, and likely benefit.

Other Diagnostic Studies

Imaging studies commonly used for patients with rheumatic diseases include x-ray studies, computed tomography (CT) scans, and magnetic resonance imaging (MRI) scans, and arthrography. See Chapter 69 for further information about these and other diagnostic studies.

Medical Management

The chronic nature of rheumatic conditions requires cooperation between the patient and the provider. The patient needs to understand the disease process and to be active in making good decisions for their care. Patient education regarding the disease process and treatment options is imperative to enable the patient to make informed decisions regarding their care. Management of rheumatologic diseases is based on the patient's self-assessment of

CHART 56-1

Assessment: Assessing for Rheumatic Disorders

In addition to the head-to-toe assessment or systems review, the following are important areas of consideration to be noted when performing the complete physical assessment of a patient with a known or suspected rheumatic disorder.

Manifestation	Significance
Skin (inquire and inspect)	
Rash, lesions	Associated with systemic lupus erythematosus (SLE) vasculitis, adverse effect of medication
Increased bruising	Associated with several rheumatic diseases and adverse effect of medication
Erythema	Sign of inflammation
Thinning	Adverse effect of medication
Warmth	Sign of inflammation
Photosensitivity	Associated with SLE, dermatomyositis, adverse effect of medication
Hair (inquire and inspect)	
Alopecia or thinning	Associated with rheumatic diseases or adverse effect of medication
Eye (inquire and inspect)	
Dryness, grittiness	Associated with Sjögren's syndrome (commonly occurring with rheumatoid arthritis [RA] and SLE)
Decreased acuity or blindness	Associated with temporal arteritis, medication complications
Cataracts	Adverse effect of medication
Decreased peripheral vision	Adverse effect of medication
Conjunctivitis, uveitis	Associated with ankylosing spondylitis and Reiter's syndrome
Ear (inquire)	
Tinnitus	Adverse effect of medication
Decreased acuity	Adverse effect of medication
Mouth (inquire and inspect)	
Buccal, sublingual lesions	Associated with vasculitis, dermatomyositis, adverse effect of medication
Altered sense of taste	Adverse effect of medication
Dryness	Associated with Sjögren's syndrome
Dysphagia	Associated with myositis
Difficulty chewing	Associated with decreased range of motion of jaw
Chest (inspect and inquire)	
Pleuritic pain	Associated with RA and SLE
Decreased chest expansion	Associated with ankylosing spondylitis
Activity intolerance (dyspnea)	Associated with pulmonary hypertension in scleroderma
Cardiovascular system (inquire, inspect, palpate)	
Blanching of fingers on exposure to cold	Associated with Raynaud's phenomenon
Peripheral pulses	Deficit may indicate vascular involvement or edema associated with medication effect or rheumatic diseases, especially SLE or scleroderma
Abdomen (inquire and palpate)	
Altered bowel habits	Associated with scleroderma, spondylosis, ulcerative colitis, decreased physical mobility, medication effect
Nausea, vomiting, bloating, and pain	Adverse effect of medication
Weight change (measure)	Associated with RA (decreased), adverse effect of medication (increased or decreased)
Genitalia (inquire and inspect)	
Dryness, itching	Associated with Sjögren's syndrome
Abnormal menses	Adverse effect of medication
Altered sexual performance	Fear of pain (or of pain caused by partner) and limitation of motion may affect sexual mobility
Hygiene	Poor hygiene may be related to limitations in activities of daily living
Urethritis, dysuria	Associated with ankylosing spondylitis and Reiter's syndrome
Lesions	Associated with vasculitis
Neurologic (inquire and inspect)	
Paresthesias of extremities; abnormal reflex pattern	Nerve compressions (e.g., carpal tunnel syndrome, spinal stenosis)
Headaches	Associated with temporal arteritis, adverse effect of medication
Musculoskeletal (inspect and palpate)	
Joint redness, warmth, swelling, tenderness, deformity—location of first joint involved, pattern of progression, symmetry, acute vs. chronic nature	Signs of inflammation
Joint range of motion	Decreased range of motion may indicate severity or progression of disease
Surrounding tissue findings	
Muscle atrophy, subcutaneous nodules, popliteal cyst	Extra-articular manifestations
Muscle strength (grip)	Muscle strength decreases with increased disease activity

TABLE 56-1 Common Blood Studies for Rheumatic Diseases

Test	Normal Value	Significance
Serum		
Creatinine		
Metabolic waste excreted through the kidneys	0.7–1.4 mg/dL (62–124 μmol/L)	Increase may indicate kidney damage in SLE, scleroderma, and polyarteritis
Erythrocyte Count		
Measures circulating erythrocytes	*Men:* 4,600,000–6,200,000/mm^3 (4.6–6.2 × 10^{12}/L) *Women:* 4,200,000–5,400,000/mm^3 (4.2–5.4 × 10^{12}/L)	Decrease can be seen in RA, SLE
Erythrocyte Sedimentation Rate (ESR)		
Measures the rate at which RBCs settle out of unclotted blood in 1 hour	Westergren: Men under 50 years: <15 mm/hr Men over 50 years: <20 mm/hr Women under 50 years: <25 mm/hr Women over 50 years: <30 mm/hr	Increase is usually seen in inflammatory connective tissue diseases. An increase indicates rising inflammation, resulting in clustering of RBCs, which makes them heavier than normal. The higher the ESR, the greater the inflammatory activity
Hematocrit		
Measures the size, capacity, and number of cells present in blood	*Men:* 42–52% *Women:* 35–47%	Decrease can be seen in chronic inflammation (anemia of chronic disease); also, blood loss through GI bleed
White Blood Cell Count		
Measures circulating leukocytes	4,500–11,000 cells/mm^3	Decrease may be seen in SLE
VDRL (Venereal Disease Research Laboratory)		
Measures antibody to syphilis	Nonreactive	False-positive results are sometimes found with SLE
Uric Acid		
Measures level of uric acid in serum	2.5–8 mg/dL (0.15–0.5 mmol/L)	Increase is seen with gout. During acute flare, levels may be normal. After flare has subsided, levels will be elevated in gout
Serum Immunology		
Antinuclear Antibody (ANA)		
Measures antibodies that react with a variety of nuclear antigens If antibodies are present, further testing determines the type of ANA circulating in the blood (anti-DNA, anti-RNP)	Negative Healthy adults may also have a positive ANA	Positive test may be associated with SLE, RA, scleroderma, Raynaud's disease, Sjögren's syndrome, necrotizing arteritis. The higher the titer, the greater the inflammation The pattern of immunofluorescence (speckled, homogeneous, or nucleolar) helps determine the diagnosis
Anti-DNA, DNA Binding		
Titer measurement of antibody to double-stranded DNA	Negative	High titer is seen in SLE; increases in titer may indicate an increase in disease activity
Complement Levels—C3, C4		
Complement is a protein substance that binds with antigen–antibody complexes for the purpose of lysis. When the number of complexes increases markedly, complement is used for lysis, thus depleting the amount available in the blood.	*C3:* 80–170 mg/dL (0.8–1.7 g/L) *C4:* 18–51 mg/dL (180–510 mg/L)	Decrease may be seen in RA and SLE Decrease indicates autoimmune and inflammatory activity
C-Reactive Protein (CRP)		
Shows presence of abnormal glycoprotein due to inflammatory process	<1 mg/dL (<10 mg/L)	A positive reading indicates active inflammation
Immunoglobulin Electrophoresis		
Measures the values of immunoglobulins	*IgA:* 80–400 mg/dL (0.8–4 g/L) *IgG:* 600–1,800 mg/dL (6–18 g/L) *IgM:* 55–250 mg/dL (0.55–2.5 g/L)	Increased levels are found in people who have autoimmune disorders
Rheumatoid Factor (RF)		
Determines the presence of abnormal antibodies seen in connective tissue disease	Negative	Positive titer >1:80 Present in 80% of those with RA Positive RF may also suggest SLE, Sjögren's syndrome, or mixed connective tissue disease. The higher the titer (number at right of colon), the greater the inflammation
Tissue Typing		
HLA-B27 Antigen		
Measures presence of HLA antigens, which are used for tissue recognition	Negative	Found in 80–90% of those with ankylosing spondylitis and Reiter's syndrome

SLE, system lupus erythematosus; RBCs, red blood cells; GI, gastrointestinal; RA, rheumatoid arthritis; DNA, deoxyribonucleic acid; RNP, ribonucleoprotein; IgA, immunoglobulin A; IgG, immunoglobulin G; IgM, immunoglobulin M; HLA, human leukocyte antigen.

Adapted from Fischbach, F., & Dunning, M. B. (2015). *A manual of laboratory and diagnostic tests* (9th ed.). Philadelphia, PA: Lippincott Williams & Wilkins.

TABLE 56-2 Management Goals and Strategies for Rheumatic Diseases

Goals	Management Strategies
Suppress inflammation and the autoimmune response	Optimize pharmacologic therapy (anti-inflammatory and disease-modifying agents)
Control pain	Protect joints; ease pain with splints, thermal modalities, relaxation techniques
Maintain or improve joint mobility	Implement exercise programs for joint motion, muscle strengthening, weight loss as appropriate, and overall health
Maintain or improve functional status	Make use of adaptive devices and techniques
Increase patient's knowledge of disease process	Provide and reinforce patient education
Promote self-management by patient adherence with the therapeutic regimen	Emphasize compatibility of therapeutic regimen and lifestyle

symptom, quality of life, and objective assessment by the provider (Schur & Moreland, 2016). Table 56-2 outlines goals and strategies for care of the patient with rheumatic diseases.

Pharmacologic Therapy

Medications are used with the rheumatic diseases to manage symptoms, to control inflammation, and, in some instances, to modify the disease. Useful medications include the salicylates, nonsteroidal anti-inflammatory drugs (NSAIDs), and both biologic and nonbiologic disease-modifying antirheumatic drugs (DMARDs). As their name suggests, DMARDs have the ability to suppress the autoimmune response; alter disease progression; and stop or decrease further tissue damage on the joints, cartilage, and organs. DMARDs have been found to halt the progression of bone loss and destruction and can induce remission (Carter, Patty-Resk, Ruffing, et al., 2015). Nonbiologic DMARDs are thought to reduce proinflammatory cytokines (cell-signaling proteins) and increase anti-inflammatory cytokines. Biologic DMARDs, in contrast, have been specifically engineered to target a certain cell or molecule within the immune system to treat the specific rheumatologic condition. Specific biologic DMARDs target tumour necrosis factor alpha (TNF-α), B cells, T cells, interleukin 1 (IL-1), and interleukin 6 (IL-6). Table 56-3 reviews commonly used medications.

Controlling the inflammation related to the disease process helps manage pain, but this is often a delayed response. Nonopioid medications are often used for pain management, especially early in the treatment program, until other measures can be instituted. Short-term use of low-dose antidepressant medications, such as amitriptyline (Elavil), may be prescribed to reestablish adequate sleep patterns and improve pain management (Karch, 2014).

Nonpharmacologic Pain Management

Nonpharmacologic methods of pain management are important. Heat applications are helpful in relieving pain, stiffness, and muscle spasm. Superficial heat may be applied in the form of warm tub baths or showers and warm moist compresses. Paraffin baths (dips), which offer concentrated heat, are helpful to patients with wrist and small-joint involvement. Maximum benefit is achieved within 20 minutes after application. More frequent use for shorter lengths of time is most beneficial. Therapeutic exercises can be carried out more comfortably and effectively after heat has been applied.

Devices such as braces, splints, and assistive devices for ambulation (e.g., canes, crutches, walkers) ease pain by limiting movement or stress from putting weight on painful joints. Acutely inflamed joints can be rested by applying splints to limit motion. Splints also support the joint to relieve spasm. Canes and crutches can relieve stress from inflamed and painful weight-bearing joints while promoting safe ambulation. Cervical collars may be used to support the weight of the head and limit cervical motion. A metatarsal bar or special pads may be put into the patient's shoes if foot pain or deformity is present. A combination of methods may be required, because different methods often work better at different times.

Exercise and Activity

The ongoing nature of most rheumatic diseases makes it important to maintain and, when possible, improve joint mobility and overall functional status. Appropriate programs of exercise have been shown to decrease pain and improve function (Miller, 2015). Changes in gait as well as joint limitations commonly require referral for rehabilitation therapy. An individualized exercise program is crucial to improve movement. Table 56-4 summarizes the exercises appropriate for patients with rheumatic diseases. Physical and occupational therapy programs and interventions are beneficial in improving physical activity and maintaining range of motion. Such interventions may include stretching exercises, muscle conditioning, aerobic exercise, massage, acupuncture, chiropractic and osteopathic manipulation. Other strategies for decreasing pain include muscle relaxation techniques, imagery, self-hypnosis, and distraction. The use of transcutaneous electrical nerve stimulation (TENS) unit has also been found to improve pain and enhance physical activity (Carter et al., 2015). A mild analgesic agent may be suggested before exercise to improve pain during exercise. A weight reduction program may be recommended to relieve stress on painful joints for some patients. Any patient who experiences acute or prolonged pain associated with exercise should report the symptoms to their primary provider for evaluation.

The major challenge for the patient and the health care provider is the need to adjust all aspects of treatment according to the activity of the disease. Especially for the patient with an active diffuse connective tissue disease, such as **rheumatoid arthritis** (RA) or systemic lupus erythematous (SLE), activity levels may vary from day to day and even within a single day.

Sleep

Short-term use of low-dose antidepressant medications, such as amitriptyline (Elavil), may be prescribed to reestablish adequate sleep patterns and improve pain management (Papadakis, McPhee, & Rabow, 2015). Patients need restful sleep so that they can cope with pain,

TABLE 56-3 Selected Medications Used in Rheumatic Diseases

Medication	Action, Use, and Indication	Nursing Considerations
Salicylates		
Acetylated: aspirin *Nonacetylated:* choline trisalicylate (Arthropan, Trilisate), salsalate (Disalcid), sodium salicylate	*Action:* Anti-inflammatory, analgesic, antipyretic Acetylated salicylates are platelet aggregation inhibitors Anti-inflammatory doses will produce blood salicylate levels of 20–30 mg/dL	Administer with meals to prevent gastric irritation. Assess for tinnitus, gastric intolerance, GI bleeding, and purpura Monitor for possible confusion in the older adult
Nonsteroidal Anti-Inflammatory Drugs (NSAIDs)		
Diclofenac (Voltaren), diflunisal (Dolobid), etodolac (Lodine), flurbiprofen (Ansaid), ibuprofen (Motrin), ketoprofen (Orudis, Oruvail), meclofenamate (Meclomen), meloxicam (Mobic), nabumetone (Relafen), naproxen (Naprosyn), oxaprozin (Daypro), piroxicam (Feldene), sulindac (Clinoril), tolmetin sodium (Tolectin)	*Action:* Anti-inflammatory, analgesic, antipyretic, platelet aggregation inhibitor Anti-inflammatory effect occurs 2–4 weeks after initiation All NSAIDs are useful for short-term treatment of acute gout attack NSAIDs are an alternative to salicylates for first-line therapy in several rheumatic diseases	Administer NSAIDs with food Monitor for GI, CNS, cardiovascular, renal, hematologic, and dermatologic adverse effects Avoid salicylates; use acetaminophen for additional analgesia Watch for possible confusion in older adults
COX-2 enzyme blockers: celecoxib (Celebrex)	*Action:* Inhibit only COX-2 enzymes, which are produced during inflammation, and spare COX-1 enzymes, which can be protective to the stomach	Monitoring is the same as for other NSAIDs Increased risk of cardiovascular events, including myocardial infarction and stroke Appropriate for older adults and patients who are at high risk for gastric ulcers
Disease-Modifying Antirheumatic Drugs (DMARDs)		
Antimalarials: hydroxychloroquine (Plaquenil), chloroquine (Aralen)	*Action:* Anti-inflammatory, inhibit lysosomal enzymes Slow acting; onset may take 2–4 months. May be used in conjunction with other DMARD therapy. Useful in RA and SLE	Administer concurrently with NSAIDs Assess for visual changes, GI upset, skin rash, headaches, photosensitivity, bleaching of hair Emphasize need for ophthalmologic examinations (every 6–12 months).
Janus Kinase (JAK) inhibitors (Xeljanz)	*Action*: Enters the cell and binds to the active JAK site, inhibits autophosphorylation and JAK activation that inhibits cytokine production. May be used in combination with methotrexate or other nonbiologic DMARDs. May also be used as monotherapy	Administer twice a day. Do not administer with biologic DMARDs or potent immunosuppressants. Monitor lipids 4–8 weeks following initiation of therapy. Monitor liver enzymes routinely
sulfasalazine (Azulfidine)	*Action:* Anti-inflammatory, reduces lymphocyte response, inhibits angiogenesis Useful in RA, seronegative spondyloarthropathies	Administer concurrently with NSAIDs. Do not use in patients with allergy to sulfa medications or salicylates Emphasize adequate fluid intake Assess for GI upset, skin rash, headache, liver abnormalities, anemia
Immunosuppressives: methotrexate (Rheumatrex), azathioprine (Imuran), cyclophosphamide (Cytoxan)	*Action:* Nonbiologic immune suppression, affect DNA synthesis and other cellular effects Have teratogenic potential; azathioprine and cyclophosphamide reserved for more aggressive or unresponsive disease Methotrexate is generally the first-line agent for RA treatment; also useful in SLE. Methotrexate may be given orally or by intramuscular or subcutaneous injection	Assess for bone marrow suppression, GI ulcerations, skin rashes, alopecia, bladder toxicity, increased infections Monitor CBC, liver enzymes, creatinine at 6 weeks after initiation, then every 2–3 months or accordingly Advise patient of contraceptive measures because of teratogenicity
cyclosporine (Neoral)	*Action:* Nonbiologic immune suppression by inhibiting T lymphocytes Used for severe, progressive RA, unresponsive to other DMARDs Used in combination with methotrexate	Assess slow dose titration upward until response noted or toxicity occurs Assess for toxic effects, such as bleeding gums, fluid retention, hair growth, tremors. Monitor blood pressure and renal function (creatinine) every 2 weeks until stable
Immunomodulators		
Pyrimidine synthesis inhibitor: leflunomide (Arava)	*Action:* Nonbiologic with antiproliferative and anti-inflammatory effects; used in moderate to severe RA May be used alone or in combination with other DMARDs	Long half-life; requires loading dose followed by daily administration. Assess for diarrhea, hair loss, skin rash, mouth sores Monitor liver function tests Contraindicated in pregnancy and breast-feeding Given orally

continued >

TABLE 56-3 Selected Medications Used in Rheumatic Diseases (Continued)

Medication	Action, Use, and Indication	Nursing Considerations
TNF blocking agents: adalimumab (Humira), certolizumab pegol (Cimzia), etanercept (Enbrel), infliximab (Remicade), golimumab (Simponi)	*Action:* Biologic response modifier that binds to TNF, a cytokine involved in inflammatory and immune responses. Used in moderate to severe RA. Can be used alone or with methotrexate or other nonbiologic DMARDs. Adalimumab is given by subcutaneous injection every 2 weeks, but may be used every week if efficacy not reached. Certolizumab pegol is given by subcutaneous injection every 2 weeks. Etanercept is given by subcutaneous injection weekly. Infliximab is given intravenously over 2 hours or more. Medication must be refrigerated Golimumab is given by subcutaneous injection once a month. Golimumab SQ is a second alternative that is administered intravenously every 8 weeks after initial 2 loading doses	Patient should be tested for tuberculosis before beginning this medication. Educate patient about subcutaneous self-injection. Monitor for injection site reactions. Educate patient about increased risk for infection and to withhold medication if fever occurs. Notify provider if any illness or infection occurs and medication is held
T-cell costimulation modulator: abatacept (Orencia)	*Action:* Blocks one of the pathways needed to fully activate T cells, decreasing inflammatory and immunologic responses. Used in moderate to severe RA unresponsive to TNF inhibitors. Used with methotrexate or DMARDs other than TNF inhibitors or anakinra	Administered IV initially, then transitions to subcutaneous dosage once weekly. Educate patient about subcutaneous self-injections given daily. Monitor for injection site reactions. Educate patient about increased risk of infection and to withhold medication if fever occurs. IV infusions are given every 4 weeks over 30-minute infusion
B-cell production blocker: rituximab (Rituxan)	*Action:* Binds to B-lymphocyte CD20 surface antigens. Used in refractory RA in patients with inadequate response to TNF antagonist. Given with methotrexate	Rituximab is given as two 1,000-mg doses via IV infusion separated by 2 weeks. Given on weeks 0 and 2, and then subsequent doses are infused 24 weeks later or based on clinical diagnosis (commonly given every 6 months). Premedicate with acetaminophen, antihistamine, and methylprednisolone (Solumedrol) 30 minutes prior to infusion of rituximab. Educate patient about increased risk of infection
Human IL-1 receptor antagonist: anakinra (Kineret)	*Action:* Blocks IL-1 receptors, decreasing inflammatory and immunologic responses. Used in moderate to severe RA. Can be used alone or with methotrexate or DMARDs other than TNF-blocking agents	Given daily by subcutaneous injection. Educate patient about subcutaneous self-injections given daily. Medication must be refrigerated. Monitor for injection site reactions. Educate patient about increased risk of infection and to withhold medication if fever occurs
Human IL-6 receptor antagonist: tocilizumab (Actemra)	*Action:* Binds to and inhibits IL-6 receptors, decreasing inflammatory and immunologic responses. Can be used alone or with methotrexate or in combination with other nonbiologic DMARDs	Administered IV every 4 weeks. Educate patient about increased risk of infection.
Corticosteroids		
Prednisone, prednisolone, hydrocortisone	*Action:* Anti-inflammatory. Used for shortest duration and at lowest dose possible to minimize adverse effects Useful for unremitting RA, SLE, polymyalgia rheumatica, myositis, arteritis Fast acting; onset in days Intra-articular injections useful for joints unresponsive to NSAIDs	Assess for toxicity: Cataracts, GI irritation, hyperglycemia, hypertension, fractures, avascular necrosis, hirsutism, psychosis Joints most amenable to injections include ankles, knees, hips, shoulders, and hands Repeated injections can cause joint damage. Use caution in patients diagnosed with diabetes, due to effects causing elevation in blood sugar
Topical Analgesics		
Capsaicin (Zostrix)	*Action:* Analgesic	Instruct patient to apply sparingly, avoid areas of open skin, and avoid contact with eyes and mucous membranes. Wash hands carefully after application Assess for local skin irritation

GI, gastrointestinal; CNS, central nervous system; COX, cyclo-oxygenase; RA, rheumatoid arthritis; SLE, systemic lupus erythematosus; IM, intramuscular; WBCs, white blood cells; CBC, complete blood count; TNF, tumour necrosis factor; IV, intravenous; IL-1, interleukin 1; IL-6, interleukin 6.

Adapted from Karch, A. (2014). *Lippincott's nursing drug guide*. Philadelphia, PA: Lippincott Williams & Wilkins.

TABLE 56-4 Exercise to Promote Mobility

Type of Exercise	Purpose	Recommended Performance	Precautions
Range of motion	Maintain flexibility and joint motion	Active or active/self-assisted at least daily	Reduce the number of repetitions when inflammation is present
Isometric exercise	Improve muscle tone, static endurance, and strength; prepare for dynamic and weight-bearing exercises	Perform at 70% of maximal voluntary contraction daily	Monitor blood pressure; isometric exercises may increase blood pressure and decrease blood flow to muscles
Dynamic exercise	Maintain or increase dynamic strength and endurance; increase muscle power; enhance synovial blood flow; promote strength of bone and cartilage	Start with repetitions against gravity and add progressive resistance; perform 2–3 days per week	May increase biomechanical stress on unstable or misaligned joints
Aerobic exercise	Improve cardiovascular fitness and endurance	Perform 3–5 days per week for 20–30 minutes of moderate-intensity exercise	Progress slowly as activity tolerance and fitness improve
Pool exercise	Water supports or resists movement; warm water may provide muscle relaxation	Provide buoyant medium for performance of dynamic or aerobic exercise	Heated swimming pool; deep water to minimize joint compression; nonslip footwear for safety and comfort. Receive appropriate instruction in a program designed for people with arthritis

Adapted from Carter S. C., Patty-Resk, C., Ruffing, V., et al. (2015). *Core curriculum for rheumatology nursing* (1st ed.). Greenville, SC: Lyons Den Solutions, LLC.

minimize physical fatigue, and deal with the changes related to having a chronic disease. In patients with acute disease, sleep time is frequently reduced and fragmented by prolonged awakenings. Stiffness, depression, and medications may also compromise the quality of sleep and increase daytime fatigue. A sleep-inducing routine, medication, and comfort measures may help improve the quality of sleep.

Education about sleep hygiene strategies may help promote restorative sleep. These strategies include establishing a set time to sleep and a regular wake-up time, creating a quiet sleep environment with a comfortable room temperature, avoiding factors that interfere with sleep (e.g., the use of alcohol and caffeine), using relaxation exercises, and getting out of bed and engaging in another activity (e.g., reading) if unable to sleep.

Nursing Management

The plan of nursing care in Chart 56-2 details the nursing priorities, interventions, and expected outcomes for the patient older with a rheumatic disorder.

Gerontologic Considerations

The various rheumatologic disease conditions in the older adult pose unique challenges. These challenges relate to disability, cognitive changes, comorbid conditions, and diagnosis. Musculoskeletal problems are the most frequently reported conditions in older adults (Miller, 2015) and will be seen more frequently by health professionals in the coming years along with associated disability, especially among frail older adults.

Comorbid conditions pose a unique challenge in diagnosing rheumatologic disease in older adults because they have the potential to mask or alter presenting symptoms (Papadakis et al., 2015). The frequency, pattern of onset, clinical features, severity, and effects on function of the rheumatic disease in older patients may be different in very old patients. In addition, other medical conditions may take precedence over the rheumatic disease, which commonly becomes a secondary diagnosis and concern. Decreased vision and altered balance, often present in older adults, may be problematic if rheumatic disease in the lower extremities affects locomotion. The combination of decreased hearing and visual acuity, memory loss, and depression contributes to failure to follow the treatment regimen in older adult patients as well (Miller, 2015). Special techniques for promoting patient safety, self-management, and strategies such as memory aids for medications may be necessary.

Behavioural clues such as gait patterns, guarding, and joint flexion may aid the nurse in assessing the patient's pain when cognitive impairment is present. Older adults, especially men, may also neglect to communicate their pain unless elicited by the provider. Pain, in general, in this population that is not treated or undertreated may impact the quality of life for these patients, which can exacerbate all other medical conditions (Carter et al., 2015).

Older adults have an increased risk of osteoporosis. Pain, loss of mobility, diminished self-image, and increasing morbidity can result from progressive osteoporosis. Therefore, diagnosis and treatment of osteoporosis should not be overlooked in this population. Pharmacologic therapy (including analgesic agents), exercise, postural assistance, modification of activities of daily living, and psychological support are useful components of the treatment program for the older adult.

Identifying the effects of the rheumatic disease on the patient's lifestyle, independence, and psychological status is important and can improve the quality of life for older adults. Depressed mood is routinely found in those suffering from chronic joint disease. The body image and

(text continued on page 1742)

Plan of Nursing Care

Chart 56-2. Care of the Patient With a Rheumatic Disorder

Nursing Priority: Acute and chronic pain

Goal: Improvement in comfort level; incorporation of pain management techniques into daily life

NURSING INTERVENTIONS	RATIONALE
1. Provide variety of comfort measures a. Application of heat or cold b. Massage, position changes, rest c. Foam mattress, supportive pillow, splints d. Relaxation techniques, diversional activities	1. Pain may respond to nonpharmacologic interventions such as joint protection, exercise, relaxation, and thermal modalities
2. Administer anti-inflammatory, analgesic, and slow-acting antirheumatic medications as prescribed	2. Pain of rheumatic disease responds to individual or combination medication regimens
3. Individualize medication schedule to meet patient's need for pain management	3. Previous pain experiences and management strategies may be different from those needed for persistent pain
4. Encourage verbalization of feelings about pain and chronicity of disease	4. Verbalization promotes coping
5. Teach pathophysiology of pain and rheumatic disease, and assist patient to recognize that pain often leads to unproven treatment methods	5. Knowledge of rheumatic pain and appropriate treatment may help patient avoid unsafe, ineffective therapies
6. Assist in identification of pain that leads to use of unproven methods of treatment	6. The impact of pain on an individual's life often leads to misconceptions about pain and pain management techniques
7. Assess for subjective changes in pain	7. The individual's description of pain is a more reliable indicator than objective measurements such as change in vital signs, body movement, and facial expression

EXPECTED OUTCOMES

- Identifies factors that exacerbate or influence pain response
- Identifies and uses pain management strategies
- Verbalizes decrease in pain
- Reports signs and symptoms of side effects in timely manner to prevent additional problems
- Verbalizes that pain is characteristic of rheumatic disease
- Establishes realistic pain relief goals
- Verbalizes that pain often leads to the use of nontraditional and unproven self-treatment methods
- Identifies changes in quality or intensity of pain

Nursing Priority: Fatigue

Goal: Incorporates as part of daily activity strategies necessary to modify fatigue

NURSING INTERVENTIONS	RATIONALE
1. Provide instruction about fatigue.	1. The patient's understanding of fatigue will affect his or her actions.
a. Describe relationship of disease activity to fatigue	a. The amount of fatigue is directly related to the activity of the disease
b. Describe comfort measures while providing them	b. Relief of discomfort can relieve fatigue
c. Develop and encourage a sleep routine (warm bath and relaxation techniques that promote sleep)	c. Effective bedtime routine promotes restorative sleep
d. Explain importance of rest for relieving systematic, articular, and emotional stress	d. Different kinds of rest are needed to relieve fatigue and are based on patient need and response
e. Explain how to use energy conservation techniques (pacing, delegating, setting priorities)	e. A variety of measures can be used to conserve energy
f. Identify physical and emotional factors that can cause fatigue	f. Awareness of the various causes of fatigue provides the basis for measures to modify the fatigue
2. Facilitate development of appropriate activity/rest schedule	2. Alternating rest and activity conserves energy while allowing most productivity
3. Encourage adherence to the treatment program	3. Overall control of disease activity can decrease the amount of fatigue
4. Refer to and encourage a conditioning program	4. Deconditioning resulting from lack of mobility, understanding, and disease activity contributes to fatigue
5. Encourage adequate nutrition, including source of iron from food and supplements	5. A nutritious diet can help counteract fatigue

EXPECTED OUTCOMES

- Self-evaluates and monitors fatigue pattern
- Verbalizes the relationship of fatigue to disease activity
- Uses comfort measures as appropriate
- Practices effective sleep hygiene and routine
- Makes use of various assistive devices (splints, canes) and strategies (bed rest, relaxation techniques) to ease different kinds of fatigue
- Incorporates time management strategies in daily activities
- Uses appropriate measures to prevent physical and emotional fatigue
- Has an established plan to ensure well-paced, therapeutic activity schedule
- Adheres to therapeutic program
- Follows a planned conditioning program
- Consumes a nutritious diet consisting of appropriate food groups and recommended daily allowance of vitamins and minerals

Plan of Nursing Care

Chart 56-2. Care of the Patient With a Rheumatic Disorder, *Continued*

Nursing Priority: Impaired physical mobility
Goal: Attains and maintains optimal functional mobility

NURSING INTERVENTIONS	RATIONALE	EXPECTED OUTCOMES
1. Encourage verbalization regarding limitations in mobility.	1. Mobility is not necessarily related to deformity. Pain, stiffness, and fatigue may temporarily limit mobility. The degree of mobility is not synonymous with the degree of independence. Decreased mobility may influence a person's self-concept and lead to social isolation	• Identifies factors that interfere with mobility • Describes and uses measures to prevent loss of motion • Identifies environmental (home, school, work, community) barriers to optimal mobility • Uses appropriate techniques and/or assistive equipment to aid mobility • Identifies community resources available to assist in managing decreased mobility
2. Assess need for occupational or physical therapy consultation: a. Emphasize range of motion of affected joints b. Promote use of assistive ambulatory devices c. Explain use of safe footwear d. Use individual appropriate positioning/posture	2. Therapeutic exercises, proper footwear, and/or assistive equipment may improve mobility. Correct posture and positioning are necessary for maintaining optimal mobility	
3. Assist to identify environmental barriers	3. Furniture and architectural adaptations may enhance mobility	
4. Encourage independence in mobility and assist as needed a. Allow ample time for activity b. Provide rest period after activity c. Reinforce principles of joint protection and work simplification	4. Changes in mobility may lead to a decrease in personal safety	
5. Initiate referral to community health agency	5. The degree of mobility may be slow to improve or may not improve with intervention	

Nursing Priority: Self-care deficits
Goal: Achieves self-care independently or with the use of resources

NURSING INTERVENTIONS	RATIONALE	EXPECTED OUTCOMES
1. Assist patient to identify self-care deficits and factors that interfere with ability to perform self-care activities	1. The ability to perform self-care activities is influenced by the disease activity and the accompanying pain, stiffness, fatigue, muscle weakness, loss of motion, and depression	• Identifies factors that interfere with the ability to perform self-care activities • Identifies alternative methods for meeting self-care needs • Uses alternative methods for meeting self-care needs • Identifies and uses other health care resources for meeting self-care needs
2. Develop a plan based on the patient's perceptions and priorities on how to establish and achieve goals to meet self-care needs, incorporating joint protection, energy conservation, and work simplification concepts a. Provide appropriate assistive devices b. Reinforce correct and safe use of assistive devices c. Allow patient to control timing of self-care activities d. Explore with the patient different ways to perform difficult tasks or ways to enlist the help of someone else	2. Assistive devices may enhance self-care abilities. Effective planning for changes must include the patient, who must accept and adopt the plan	
3. Consult with community health care agencies when individuals have attained a maximum level of self-care yet still have some deficits, especially regarding safety	3. Individuals differ in ability and willingness to perform self-care activities. Changes in ability to care for self may lead to a decrease in personal safety	

continued >

Plan of Nursing Care — Chart 56-2. Care of the Patient With a Rheumatic Disorder, *Continued*

NURSING INTERVENTIONS	RATIONALE	EXPECTED OUTCOMES
Nursing Priority: Disturbed body image **Goal:** Adapts to physical and psychological changes imposed by the rheumatic disease		
1. Help patient identify elements of control over disease symptoms and treatment 2. Encourage patient's verbalization of feelings, perceptions, and fears a. Help to assess present situation and identify problems b. Assist to identify past coping mechanisms c. Assist to identify effective coping mechanisms	1. The individual's self-concept may be altered by the disease or its treatment 2. The individual's coping strategies reflect the strength of his or her self-concept	• Verbalizes an awareness that changes taking place in self-concept are normal responses to rheumatic disease and other chronic illnesses • Identifies strategies to cope with altered self-concept
Nursing Priority: Ineffective coping **Goal:** Use of effective coping behaviours for dealing with actual or perceived limitations and role changes		
1. Identify areas of life affected by disease. Answer questions and dispel possible myths 2. Develop plan for managing symptoms and enlisting support of family and friends to promote daily function	1. The effects of disease may be more or less manageable once identified and explored reasonably 2. By taking action and involving others appropriately, patient develops or draws on coping skills and community support	• Names functions and roles affected and not affected by disease process • Describes therapeutic regimen and states actions to take to improve, change, or accept a particular situation, function, or role
Collaborative Problems: Complications secondary to effects of medications **Goal:** Absence or resolution of complications		
1. Perform periodic clinical assessment and laboratory evaluation 2. Instruct in correct self-administration, potential side effects, and importance of monitoring 3. Counsel regarding methods to reduce side effects and manage symptoms 4. Administer medications in modified doses as prescribed if complications occur	1. Skillful assessment helps detect early symptoms of side effects of medications 2. The patient needs accurate information about medications and potential side effects to avoid or manage them 3. Appropriate identification and early intervention may minimize complications 4. Modifications may help minimize side effects or other complications	• Complies with monitoring procedures and experiences minimal side effects • Takes medication as prescribed and lists potential side effects • Identifies strategies to reduce or manage side effects • Reports that side effects or complications have subsided

self-esteem of the older adult with rheumatic disease, combined with underlying depression, may interfere with the use of assistive devices such as canes. The use of adaptive equipment such as long-handled reachers or tongs may be viewed by the older adult as evidence of aging rather than as a means of increasing independence.

Because most rheumatologic diseases involve pain, especially with joints, some older adults may consider their symptoms as inevitable consequences of aging. In fact, many older adults expect and accept the immobility and self-care problems related to the rheumatic diseases and do not seek help, thinking that nothing can be done.

The older adult usually has a lifelong pattern of dealing with the stresses of daily life. Depending on the success of that pattern, the older adult can often maintain a positive attitude and self-esteem when faced with a rheumatic disease, especially if support is available. Previous stress management strategies are assessed. If these strategies have been effective, the patient is encouraged and supported in their use. If they were ineffective, the nurse assists the patient in identifying alternative strategies, encourages the use of new strategies, and assesses their effectiveness.

Pharmacologic treatment of rheumatic disease in older patients is more difficult than in younger patients. If therapeutic medications have an effect on the senses (hearing, cognition), this effect is intensified in the older adult. The cumulative effect of medications, in general, is accentuated because of the physiologic changes of aging. For example, decreased renal function in the older adult alters the metabolism of certain medications, such as NSAIDs.

Older adults are more prone to side effects associated with the use of multiple-drug therapy.

Partly because of the more frequent contact of older adults with health care providers for a variety of health issues, overtreatment or inappropriate treatment is possible. Complaints of pain may be met with a prescription for an opioid analgesic agent rather than instructions for rest, the use of an assistive device, and local comfort measures such as heat or cold. Acetaminophen (Tylenol) may be appropriate and worth trying before other medications that pose a greater chance of side effects. NSAIDs can be used; however, studies report that long-term use of NSAIDs can increase the risks of peptic ulcers, hemorrhage, and cardiovascular toxicity. New guidelines recommend NSAIDs should be used in conjunction with a proton pump inhibitor (i.e., omeprazole [Prilosec]) to decrease the likelihood of gastric ulcers forming, hemorrhage, and cardiovascular toxicity (Fujita, Kutsumi, Sanuki, et al., 2013).

Intra-articular corticosteroid injections, with their usually rapid relief of symptoms, may be requested by the patient who is unaware of the consequences of too-frequent use of this treatment. In addition, exercise programs may not be instituted or may be ineffective because the patient expects results to occur quickly or fails to appreciate the effectiveness of a program of exercise. In fact, strength training is encouraged in the older adult with chronic diseases.

Diffuse Connective Tissue Diseases

Diffuse connective tissue disease refers to a group of systematic disorders that are chronic in nature and are characterized by diffuse inflammation and degeneration in the connective tissues. These disorders share similar clinical features and may affect some of the same organs. The characteristic clinical course is one of exacerbations and remissions. Although the diffuse connective tissue diseases have unknown causes, they are thought to be the result of immunologic abnormalities. They include RA, SLE, scleroderma, polymyositis, and polymyalgia rheumatica.

Rheumatoid Arthritis

RA is an autoimmune disease of unknown origin that affects 1% of the population worldwide, with females having a 2.5 times greater incidence than males. It may occur at any age but the onset commonly occurs between the third and sixth decade of life. The incidence of RA increases after the sixth decade of life (Carter et al., 2015). Risk factors for the development of RA include environmental factors such as pollution and smoking, family history of first-degree relatives, and illnesses such as bacterial and viral illnesses. Cigarette smoking is one modifiable risk factor that has been shown to be highly related to RA (Carter et al., 2015).

Pathophysiology

The exact mechanism of action for the etiology of RA is unknown. Research has, however, identified that the autoimmune reaction (see Fig. 56-1) originates in the synovial tissue. It is hypothesized that both environmental factors, such as cigarette smoking, and genetic factors coalesce to produce inflammatory and destructive synovial fluid, starting in the more distal joints. This RA synovium breaks down collagen, causing edema, proliferation of the synovial membrane, and ultimately pannus formation. Pannus destroys cartilage and erodes the bone. The consequence is the loss of articular surfaces and joint motion. Muscle fibres undergo degenerative changes. Tendon and ligament elasticity and contractile power are lost.

The RA inflammatory process has also been implicated in other disease processes (i.e., arteriosclerosis). It is hypothesized that the RA disease process somehow interferes with the production of high-density lipoprotein cholesterol, which is the form of cholesterol responsible for decreasing cellular lipids and, therefore, is considered antiatherosclerotic.

The nervous system is also affected by the RA inflammatory process. The synovial inflammation can compress the adjacent nerve, causing neuropathies and paresthesias. Axonal degeneration and neuronal demyelination are also possible due to the infiltration of polymorphonuclear leukocytes, eosinophils, and mononuclear cells, causing necrotizing or occlusive vasculitis (Ramos-Remus, Duran-Barragan, & Castillo-Ortiz, 2012).

Clinical Manifestations

The American College of Rheumatology and the European League Against Rheumatism have collaborated and established new criteria for classifying RA. These criteria are based on a point system where a total score of 6 or greater is required for the diagnosis of RA. The scoring system is based on joint involvement (number of joints affected), serology (low-positive or high-positive rheumatoid factor [RF] or anti-citrullinated peptide antibody [ACPA]), abnormal results of the acute phase reactants (ESR or C- reactive protein [CRP]), and duration of symptoms greater than 6 weeks. Patients diagnosed with RA who are excluded from these diagnostic criteria include: (1) patients who have one joint with synovitis that is not related to any other clinical disease and who also score at least 6 to 10 points on the scale; and (2) patients diagnosed with bony erosions on x-ray (Aletaha, Neogi, Silman, et al., 2010).

The initial clinical manifestations of RA include symmetric joint pain and morning joint stiffness lasting longer than 1 hour. Over the course of the disease, clinical manifestations of RA vary, usually reflecting the stage and severity of the disease. Symmetric joint pain, swelling, warmth, erythema, and lack of function are classic symptoms. Palpation of the joints reveals spongy or boggy tissue. Often, fluid can be aspirated from the inflamed joint. Characteristically, the pattern of joint involvement begins in the small joints of the hands, wrists, and feet (Papadakis et al., 2015). As the disease progresses, the knees, shoulders, hips, elbows, ankles, cervical spine, and temporomandibular joints are affected. The onset of symptoms is usually acute. Symptoms are usually bilateral and symmetric.

In the early stages of disease, even before the presentation of bony changes, limitation in function can occur when there is active inflammation in the joints. Joints that are hot, swollen, and painful are not easily moved. The patient tends to guard or protect these joints by immobilizing them.

Immobilization for extended periods can lead to contractures, creating soft tissue deformity.

Deformities of the hands (e.g., ulnar deviation and swan neck deformity) and feet are common in RA (see Chapter 69). The deformity may be caused by misalignment resulting from swelling, progressive joint destruction, or the subluxation (partial dislocation) that occurs when one bone slips over another and eliminates the joint space. Deformities of RA differ from those seen with OA, such as Heberden's and Bouchard's nodes.

RA is a systemic disease with multiple extra-articular features. Most common are fever, weight loss, fatigue, anemia, lymph node enlargement, and Raynaud's phenomenon (cold- and stress-induced vasospasm causing episodes of digital blanching or cyanosis). Rheumatoid nodules may be noted in patients with more advanced RA, and they develop at some time in the course of the disease in about 20% of patients (Papadakis et al., 2015). These nodules are usually nontender and movable in the subcutaneous tissue. They usually appear over bony prominences such as the elbow, are varied in size, and can disappear spontaneously. Nodules occur only in people who have RF. The nodules often are associated with rapidly progressive and destructive disease. Other extra-articular features include arteritis, neuropathy, pericarditis, splenomegaly, and Sjögren's syndrome (dry eyes and dry mucous membranes).

Assessment and Diagnostic Findings

Several assessment findings are associated with RA: rheumatoid nodules, joint inflammation detected on palpation, and laboratory findings. The history and physical examination focus on manifestations, such as bilateral and symmetric stiffness, tenderness, swelling, and temperature changes in the joints. The patient is also assessed for extra-articular changes; these often include weight loss, sensory changes, lymph node enlargement, and fatigue. Symptoms and examination findings are often recorded using a Disease Activity Score-28 (DAS28) form to evaluate disease activity and help guide treatment decisions.

RA inflammatory processes have also been implicated in arterial wall stiffness and endothelial dysfunction. It is now believed that cardiovascular risks are similar to the risks of patients with diabetes. Therefore, cardiovascular risk assessment should be included in the patient's physical assessment (Palmer & El Miedany, 2014).

RF is present in about 70% to 80% of patients with RA, but its presence alone is not diagnostic of RA, and its absence does not rule out the diagnosis. Antibodies to cyclic citrullinated peptide (anti-CCP) have a specificity of approximately 95% at detecting RA (Papadakis et al., 2015). The ESR and CRP tend to be significantly elevated in the acute phases of RA and are therefore useful in monitoring active disease and disease progression. The complete blood count (CBC) should be assessed to establish a baseline count especially prior to starting medications. Patients may exhibit anemia, and platelets may be elevated due to the inflammatory process. A tuberculin (TB) skin test should be done prior to the initiation of certain medications to rule out tuberculosis. In the event the patient has latent TB and has never been treated, the infection can be reactivated. Hepatitis B and Hepatitis C should also be assessed for diagnosis, which could impact treatment strategies if positive. If the client tests positive for hepatitis, the infection should be treated prior to starting medication. Liver and kidney monitoring is recommended for most DMARD therapy because it can cause elevation of the liver enzymes and can also affect kidney function.

X-ray, ultrasound, or both of the hands, wrists, and feet can be useful in establishing a baseline for joint evaluation, and assessing the joints for erosions and synovitis. Joint damage may occur within the first 6 to 12 months of diagnosis and should be followed as indicated. MRI can also be useful to detect small erosions that may not be visible on x-ray or ultrasound.

Arthrocentesis may also be performed on any affected joint. Results of the arthrocentesis may show synovial fluid that is cloudy, milky, or dark yellow and may contain numerous inflammatory components. Recommended tests to perform on synovial fluid include WBC with differential, cultures, Gram stain and crystals (Sholter & Russell, 2016).

Medical Management

The goal of treatment at all phases of the RA disease process is to decrease joint pain and swelling, achieve clinical remission, decrease the likelihood of joint deformity, and minimize disability. Initial treatment delays have been implicated in greater long-term joint deformity. Aggressive and early treatment regimens are warranted.

Early Rheumatoid Arthritis

Once the diagnosis of RA is made, treatment should begin with either a nonbiologic or biologic DMARD. The goal of using DMARD therapy is preventing inflammation and joint damage. Recommended treatment guidelines include beginning with the nonbiologic DMARDs (methotrexate [Rheumatrex], leflunomide [Arava], sulfasalazine [Azulfidine]), or hydroxychloroquine (Plaquenil) within 3 months of disease onset. Care should be used with each of these medications, by performing routine blood testing for liver and kidney function, along with monitoring the CBC for anemia. Dosage may need to be modified for patients with renal impairment. Annual eye examinations are also recommended with the use of sulfasalazine and hydroxychloroquine (Carter et al., 2015).

After initiating treatment with a DMARD, patients generally report a beneficial effect within 6 weeks and tolerate the medication relatively well (Papadakis et al., 2015). However, some patients may take longer to see improvement. Research suggests that methotrexate combined with low-dose prednisone improves patient outcome compared to the use of methotrexate alone for early RA.

Another treatment approach for RA is the use of biologic DMARDs. These agents have been specifically engineered to target the most prominent proinflammatory mediators in RA—TNF-α, B cells, T cells, IL-1, and IL-6 (Klippel, Stone, Crofford, et al., 2008) (see Table 56-3). Biologic DMARDs are the first-targeted therapy for RA. Clinical evidence suggests that biologic DMARDs work more quickly and show a greater delay in radiologic disease progression when compared to nonbiologic DMARDs (Klippel et al., 2008). The biologic DMARDs are more expensive and have fewer years of usage with the RA population. Therefore, they tend to be reserved for patients with persistent moderate-to-severe RA who have not responded adequately to synthetic DMARDs (Papadakis et al., 2015).

NSAIDs and specifically the cyclo-oxygenase 2 (COX-2) enzyme blockers are used for pain and inflammation relief. NSAIDs, such as ibuprofen (Motrin) and naproxen (Naprosyn), are commonly prescribed because of their low cost and analgesic properties. They must be used, however, with caution in long-term chronic diseases because of the possibility of gastric ulcers. Several COX-2 enzyme blockers have been approved for treatment of RA. Cyclo-oxygenase is an enzyme that is involved in the inflammatory process. COX-2 medications block the enzyme involved in inflammation (COX-2) while leaving intact the enzyme involved in protecting the stomach lining (COX-1). As a result, COX-2 enzyme blockers are less likely to cause gastric irritation and ulceration than other NSAIDs; however, they are associated with increased risk of cardiovascular disease and must be used with caution (Karch, 2014). The nurse should be aware that no NSAIDs, not even the COX-2 inhibitors, prevent erosions or alter disease progression and, consequently, are medications useful only for symptom relief.

Additional analgesia may be prescribed for periods of extreme pain. Opioid analgesic agents are avoided because of the potential for continuing need for pain relief. Nonpharmacologic pain management techniques (e.g., relaxation techniques, heat and cold applications) are taught (Carter et al., 2015).

Moderate, Erosive Rheumatoid Arthritis

For moderate, erosive RA, a formal program with occupational and physical therapy is prescribed to educate the patient about principles of pacing activities, work simplification, range of motion, and muscle-strengthening exercises. The patient is encouraged to participate actively in the management program. The medication program is reevaluated periodically, and appropriate changes are made if indicated. Cyclosporine, an immunosuppressant, may be added to enhance the disease-modifying effect of methotrexate (Klippel et al., 2008). Combination therapy using one nonbiologic DMARD and one biologic DMARD is common.

Persistent, Erosive Rheumatoid Arthritis

For persistent, erosive RA, reconstructive surgery and corticosteroids are often used. Reconstructive surgery is indicated when pain cannot be relieved by conservative measures and the threat of loss of independence is eminent. Surgical procedures include synovectomy (excision of the synovial membrane), tenorrhaphy (suturing of a tendon), arthrodesis (surgical fusion of the joint), surgical repair, and replacement of the joint. Surgery is not performed during exacerbations.

Systemic corticosteroids are used when the patient has unremitting inflammation and pain or needs a "bridging" medication while waiting for the slower DMARDs (e.g., methotrexate) to begin taking effect. Low-dose corticosteroid therapy is prescribed for the shortest time necessary to minimize side effects (Papadakis et al., 2015). Single large joints that are severely inflamed and fail to respond promptly to the measures outlined previously may be treated by local injection of a corticosteroid.

Advanced, Unremitting Rheumatoid Arthritis

For advanced, unremitting RA, immunosuppressive agents are prescribed because of their ability to affect the production of antibodies at the cellular level. These include high-dose methotrexate, cyclophosphamide (Cytoxan), and azathioprine (Imuran). However, these medications are highly toxic and can produce bone marrow suppression, anemia, gastrointestinal disturbances, severe birth defects, and rashes (Karch, 2014).

For most patients with RA, the emotional and possible financial burden of the disease can lead to depressive symptoms and sleep deprivation. The patient may require the short-term use of low-dose antidepressant medications, such as amitriptyline (Elavil), paroxetine (Paxil), or sertraline (Zoloft), to reestablish an adequate sleep pattern and manage depressive symptoms. Patients may benefit from referrals for talk therapy or group support.

Nutrition Therapy

Patients with RA frequently experience anorexia, weight loss, and anemia. A dietary history identifies usual eating habits and food preferences. Two common problems seen in these patients are weight loss and rheumatoid cachexia (loss of skeletal muscle). Increased metabolism and decreased intake contribute to these losses. Increased and prolonged flares contribute to the increased expenditure as well. The dietician will counsel the patient about better food choices. Food selection should include the five major groups (grains, vegetables, fruits, dairy, and protein), with emphasis on foods high in vitamins, protein, and iron for tissue building and repair. For the patient who is extremely anorexic, small, frequent feedings with increased protein supplements may be prescribed. Supplemental vitamins and minerals may also be prescribed as needed. Boswellia, ginger, green tea, and turmeric have been studied for helping with inflammation and pain. However, the American College of Rheumatology does not recommend herbal supplements to treat RA as the U.S. Food and Drug Administration (FDA) does not regulate the safety and effectiveness of herbal supplements (Afshar, 2015).

Certain medications (i.e., oral corticosteroids) used in RA treatment stimulate the appetite and, when combined with decreased activity, may lead to weight gain. Therefore, patients may need to be counseled about eating a healthy, calorie-restricted diet.

Nursing Management

Nursing care of the patient with RA follows the basic plan of care presented earlier (see Chart 56-2). The most common issues for the patient with RA include pain, sleep disturbance, fatigue, altered mood, and limited mobility. The patient with newly diagnosed RA needs information about the disease to make daily self-management decisions and cope with having a chronic disease. Consultation with a dietician for assessment and assistance with appropriate food choices may be helpful.

Monitoring and Managing Potential Complications

Patients commonly have comorbid conditions such as cardiovascular disease that can lead to complications. It has been estimated that the primary cause of death for up to 40% of patients diagnosed with RA is cardiovascular disease. The cause of cardiovascular disease in these patients is thought to be due to elevated lipid values, chronic inflammation, dysfunction of the endothelium, and/or abnormal homocysteine levels (Palmer & El Miedany, 2014).

Medications used for treating RA may cause serious and adverse effects. The primary provider bases the prescribed medication regimen on clinical findings and past medical history, and then, with the help of the nurse, monitors for side effects using periodic clinical assessments and laboratory testing. The nurse, who can be available for consultation between visits with the primary provider, works to help the patient recognize and deal with these side effects (see Table 56-3). Medication may need to be stopped or the dose reduced. If the patient experiences an increase in symptoms while the complication is being resolved or a new medication is being initiated, the nurse's counseling regarding symptom management may relieve potential anxiety and distress.

Promoting Home, Community-Based, and Transitional Care

Educating Patients About Self-Care

Patient education is an essential aspect in nursing care of the patient with RA to enable the patient to maintain as much independence as possible, to take medications accurately and safely, and to use adaptive devices correctly (Cottrell, Jonas, Bergsten, et al., 2013). Patient education focuses on the disorder itself, the possible changes related to the disorder, the therapeutic regimen prescribed to treat it, and the potential side effects of medications (see Nursing Research Profile in Chart 56-3). Patients undergoing surgery need education as well. The nurse works with the patient and family on strategies to maintain independence, function, and safety in the home (see Chart 56-4).

The patient and family are encouraged to verbalize their concerns and ask questions. Because RA commonly affects young women, major concerns may be related to the effects of the disease on childbearing potential, caring for family, or work responsibilities. The patient with a chronic illness may seek a "cure" or have questions about alternative therapies. There is not enough evidence of the effectiveness of complementary, alternative, and integrative health therapies, and more rigorous research is needed (Marcus, 2015).

Pain, fatigue, and depressive symptoms can interfere with the patient's ability to learn and should be addressed before the instruction is initiated. Various educational strategies may then be used, depending on the patient's previous knowledge base, interest level, degree of comfort, social or cultural influences, and readiness to learn. The nurse educates the patient about basic disease management and necessary adaptations in lifestyle. Some types of aerobic exercise and strength training should be discussed. Because suppression of inflammation and autoimmune responses requires the use of anti-inflammatory, disease-modifying antirheumatic, and immunosuppressive agents, the patient is taught about prescribed medications, including type, dosage, rationale, potential side effects, self-administration, and required monitoring procedures. If hospitalized, the patient is encouraged to practice new self-management skills with support from caregivers and significant others. The nurse then reinforces disease management skills during each patient contact. Barriers are assessed, and measures are taken to promote adherence to medications and the treatment program.

Continuing and Transitional Care

Depending on the severity of the disorder and the patient's resources and supports, referral for home care may be warranted. Patients who are older or frail, with RA that limits function significantly, may need referral for home care.

The impact of RA on everyday life is not always evident when the patient is seen in the hospital or in an ambulatory

NURSING RESEARCH PROFILE

Chart 56-3. Addressing Unmet Needs of Patients With Rheumatoid Arthritis

Cottrell, J. D., Jonas, M., Bergsten, U., et al. (2013). The nurse's role in addressing unmet treatment and management needs of patients with rheumatoid arthritis: Delphi-based recommendations. *International Journal of Nursing Knowledge, 24*(2), 66–76.

Purpose

Nurses spend a lot of time with patients with rheumatoid arthritis (RA). The purpose of this research was to evaluate the nurse's role in management of patients with RA.

Design

The modified Delphi methodology was the design for this study. Three rheumatology nurses developed a survey questionnaire. An additional group of 12 international rheumatology nurses, with extensive patient management experience, served as an expert panel. The survey was given to the panel of 12 rheumatology nurses in two online rounds and then in a third round during an in-person meeting.

Findings

The nurse has many roles in the management of patients with RA. In this study, the nurse's reported roles involved providing care, educating about treatment, performing a disease assessment, giving the patient treatment feedback, helping patients with unmet physical and emotional needs, and explaining complex treatments.

Nursing Implications

Rheumatology nurses are in a position to be able to expand the nursing role for patients diagnosed with RA. These nurses already perform the roles of caregiver and educator, and provide disease assessment. It is important for nurses to also address unmet patient needs, provide improved patient care, and perform additional functions for the patients to meet unmet physical and emotional needs.

CHART 56-4

HOME CARE CHECKLIST • The Patient With Rheumatoid Arthritis

At the completion of education, the patient and/or caregiver will be able to:

- State the impact of rheumatoid arthritis on physiologic functioning, ADLs, IADLs, roles, relationships, and spirituality.
- State changes in lifestyle (e.g., diet, activity, rest) necessary to maintain health
- State the name, dose, side effects, frequency, and schedule for all medications
- Demonstrate accurate and safe self-administration of medications
- Describe and demonstrate the use of pain management techniques
- Demonstrate ability to perform ADLs independently or with assistive devices/adaptive equipment
- Verbalize ways to cope with stress successfully, plans for regular, safe exercise, and rationale for obtaining adequate rest
- Demonstrate a relaxation technique
- Verbalize a dietary plan that includes increased vitamins, protein, and iron for tissue building and repair
- State how to reach primary provider with questions or complications
- State time and date of follow-up appointments, testing
- Identify the need for health promotion, disease prevention, and screening activities
- Identify community resources for peer and caregiver/family information and support
- Identify sources of support (e.g., friends, relatives, faith community)
- Identify phone numbers of support groups for people with chronic illness/disabilities and their caregivers/families
- State meeting locations and times

ADLs, activities of daily living; IADLs, independent activities of daily living.

care setting. The increased frequency with which nurses see patients in the home provides opportunities for problem identification and implementation of interventions aimed at improving the quality of life of patients with RA.

During home visits, the nurse has the opportunity to assess the home environment and its adequacy for patient safety and management of the disorder. Adherence to the treatment program can be more easily monitored in the home setting, where physical and social barriers to adherence are more readily identified. For example, a patient who also has diabetes and requires insulin may be unable to fill the syringe accurately or unable to administer the insulin because of impaired joint mobility. Appropriate adaptive equipment needed for increased independence is often identified more readily when the nurse observes how the patient functions in the home. Any barriers to adherence are identified, and appropriate referrals are made.

For patients at risk for impaired skin integrity, the home care nurse can closely monitor skin status and also instruct, provide, or supervise the patient and family in preventive skin care measures. The nurse also assesses the patient's need for assistance in the home and supervises those who may meet many of the needs of the patient with RA. Referrals to physical and occupational therapists may be made as problems are identified and limitations increase. A home care nurse may visit the home to make sure the patient can function as independently as possible despite mobility problems and can safely manage treatments, including pharmacotherapy. The patient and family should be informed about support services such as Meals on Wheels and local chapters of the Arthritis Foundation.

Because many of the medications used to suppress inflammation are injectable, the nurse may administer the medication to the patient or teach self-injection. These frequent contacts allow the nurse to reinforce other disease management techniques.

The nurse also assesses the patient's physical and psychological status, adequacy of symptom management, and adherence to the management plan. Patients should know which type of rheumatic disease they have, not just that they have "arthritis" or "arthritis of the knee." The importance of attending follow-up appointments is emphasized to the patient and family, and they should be reminded about the importance of participating in other health promotion activities and health screening. Patients with chronic disorders such as RA often focus on the chronic disease and neglect general health issues.

Systemic Lupus Erythematosus

SLE is an inflammatory, autoimmune disorder that affects nearly every organ in the body. The overall prevalence of SLE is estimated to be 1 per 1,000 Canadians and it occurs ten times more frequently in women than in men. SLE usually develops in individuals in their 20s or 30s. It occurs 6 to10 times more frequently in women than in men and occurs 3 times more in African American populations than among Caucasians (CDC, 2015a; Lim, Bayakly, Helmick, et al., 2014). In addition to SLE, many other forms of adult lupus exist, including discoid lupus erythematosus (which primarily affects the skin on the face), subacute cutaneous lupus erythematous (sun exposed areas affected with sores), and drug-induced lupus (rarely includes brain or kidney effects and is usually temporary).

Pathophysiology

SLE starts with the body's immune system inaccurately recognizing one or more components of the cell's nucleus as foreign, seeing it as an antigen. The immune system starts to develop antibodies to the nuclear antigen. In particular, B cells begin to overproduce antibodies with the help of multiple cytokines such as B-lymphocyte stimulator (BLyS), which is overexpressed in SLE. The antibodies and antigens form antigen–antibody complexes and have the propensity to get trapped in the capillaries of visceral structures. The antibodies also act to destroy host cells. It is thought that those two mechanisms are responsible for the majority of the clinical manifestations of this disease process. It is hypothesized that the immunoregulatory disturbance is brought about by some combination of four distinct factors: genetic, immunologic, hormonal, and environmental (Carter et al., 2015).

Research into the genetic origins of SLE has thus far revealed that multiple genes are likely implicated in the development of SLE. In support of this theory, research with homozygous twins has shown a higher incidence of SLE, especially considering that the prevalence of SLE was low in other family members (Bartels, 2015). The large majority of SLE cases, however, remain sporadic and unrelated to family medical history.

Given the acute number of women with SLE compared with men, it is hypothesized that female sex hormones (estrogen) play a role in the predisposition to SLE. Estrogen may contribute to the body's response of overreacting to the body's own tissues.

Although genetics and hormones likely play a role in the predisposition of SLE, it is hypothesized that an exogenous or environmental trigger is implicated in the onset of the disease process. These triggers may include cigarette smoke, ultraviolet rays exposure from sunlight and fluorescent light bulbs, medications (sulfa drugs, penicillin, or antibiotic drugs), viral, infections, emotional stress, stress on the body (e.g., surgery, pregnancy), and silica dust exposure in the occupational setting (Carter et al., 2015).

Clinical Manifestations

SLE is an autoimmune, systemic disease that can affect any body system. The disease process involves chronic states where symptoms are minimal or absent and acute flares where symptoms and lab results are elevated. Systemic symptoms include fever, malaise, weight loss, and anorexia. The mucocutaneous, musculoskeletal, renal, nervous, cardiovascular, and respiratory systems are most commonly involved. Less commonly affected are the gastrointestinal tract and liver as well as the ocular system.

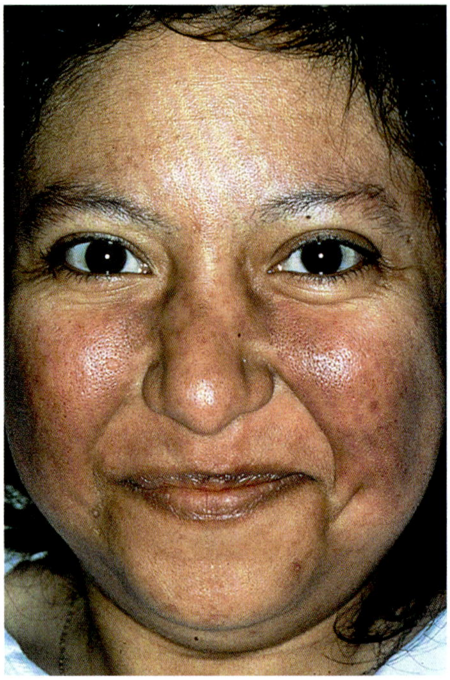

FIGURE 56-2. The characteristic butterfly rash of systemic lupus erythematosus.

Some type of cutaneous system manifestation is experienced in 80% to 90% of patients with SLE (Bartels, 2015; Klippel et al., 2008). Four of the 11 criteria used for diagnosing SLE by the American College of Rheumatology involve the cutaneous system. The most familiar skin manifestation (occurring in less than 50% of patients with SLE) is an acute cutaneous lesion consisting of a butterfly-shaped erythematous rash across the bridge of the nose and cheeks (see Fig. 56-2). Several other skin manifestations may occur in patients with SLE, including subacute cutaneous lupus erythematosus, which involves papulosquamous or annular polycyclic lesions, and a discoid rash, which is a chronic rash with erythematous papules or plaques and scaling and can cause scarring and pigmentation changes. In some cases, the only skin involvement may be a discoid rash. In some patients with SLE, the initial skin involvement is the precursor to more systemic involvement. The lesions often worsen during **exacerbations** (flares) of the systemic disease and possibly are provoked by sunlight or artificial ultraviolet light (Bartels, 2015). Oral ulcers, which may accompany skin lesions, may involve the buccal mucosa or the hard palate, occur in crops, and are often associated with exacerbations. Other cutaneous manifestations include splinter hemorrhages, alopecia, and Raynaud's phenomenon.

Joint symptoms, with arthralgias, arthritis (synovitis), or both, occur in more than 90% of patients with SLE and are commonly the earliest manifestation of the disease process (Papadakis et al., 2015). Joint swelling, tenderness, and pain on movement are also common. Frequently, these are accompanied by morning stiffness.

The cardiac system is also commonly affected in SLE. Pericarditis is the most common cardiac manifestation (Bartels, 2015). Patients may present with substernal chest pain that is aggravated by movement or inspiration. Symptoms can be acute and severe or last for weeks at a time. Other cardiac symptoms may involve myocarditis, hypertension, cardiac dysrhythmias, and valvular incompetence. Women who have SLE are also at risk for early-onset atherosclerosis, making them much more likely to suffer myocardial infarction or stroke. These events, which are believed to be secondary to the accelerated atherosclerosis, may contribute to higher rates of death for women with SLE. Inflammation is believed to be the key factor in the development and progression of atherosclerosis (Bartels, 2015).

Nephritis as a result of SLE, also referred to as lupus nephritis, occurs due to a buildup of antibodies and immune complexes that cause damage to the nephrons. Serum creatinine levels and urinalysis are used in screening for renal involvement. Early detection allows for prompt treatment so that renal damage can be prevented. Renal involvement may lead to hypertension, which also requires careful monitoring and management (see Chapter 33).

Central nervous system involvement is widespread, encompassing the entire range of neurologic disease. The varied and frequent neuropsychiatric presentations of SLE are now widely recognized and include psychosis, cognitive impairment, seizures, peripheral and cranial neuropathies, transverse myelitis, and strokes. These are generally demonstrated by subtle changes in behaviour patterns or cognitive ability.

Assessment and Diagnostic Findings

Diagnosis of SLE is based on a complete history, physical examination, and blood tests. Typically, assessment reveals classic symptoms, including fever, fatigue, weight loss, and possibly arthritis, pleurisy, and pericarditis. Interactions with the patient and family may provide further evidence of systemic involvement.

In addition to the general assessment performed for any patient with a rheumatic disease, assessment for known or suspected SLE has special features. The skin is inspected for erythematous rashes. Cutaneous erythematous plaques with an adherent scale may be observed on the scalp, face, or neck. Areas of hyperpigmentation or depigmentation may be noted, depending on the phase and type of the disease. The patient should be questioned about skin changes (because these may be transitory) and specifically about sensitivity to sunlight or artificial ultraviolet light. The scalp should be inspected for alopecia and the mouth and throat for ulcerations reflecting gastrointestinal involvement.

Cardiovascular assessment includes auscultation for pericardial friction rub, possibly associated with myocarditis and accompanying pleural effusions. The pleural effusions and infiltrations, which reflect respiratory insufficiency, are demonstrated by abnormal lung sounds. Papular, erythematous, and purpuric lesions developing on the fingertips, elbows, toes, and extensor surfaces of the forearms or lateral sides of the hand that may become necrotic suggest vascular involvement.

Joint swelling, tenderness, warmth, pain on movement, stiffness, and edema may be detected on physical examination. The joint involvement is often symmetric and similar to that found in RA.

The neurologic assessment is directed at identifying and describing any central nervous system changes. The patient and family members are asked about any behavioural changes, including manifestations of neuroses or psychosis. Signs of depression are noted, as are reports of seizures, chorea, or other central nervous system manifestations.

No single laboratory test confirms SLE; rather, blood testing reveals moderate to severe anemia, thrombocytopenia, leukocytosis, or leukopenia and positive ANAs. Other diagnostic immunologic tests support but do not confirm the diagnosis.

Medical Management

Treatment of SLE includes management of acute and chronic disease. Although SLE can be life-threatening, advances in its treatment have led to improved survival and reduced morbidity. Acute disease requires interventions directed at controlling increased disease activity or exacerbations that can involve any organ system. Disease activity is a composite of clinical and laboratory features that reflect active inflammation secondary to SLE. Management of the more chronic condition involves periodic monitoring and recognition of meaningful clinical changes requiring adjustments in therapy.

The goals of treatment include preventing progressive loss of organ function, reducing the likelihood of acute disease, minimizing disease-related disabilities, and preventing complications from therapy. Management of SLE involves regular monitoring to assess disease activity and therapeutic effectiveness.

Pharmacologic Therapy

Medication therapy for SLE is based on the concept that local tissue inflammation is mediated by exaggerated or heightened immune responses, which can vary widely in intensity and require different therapies at different times. Corticosteroids are the single most important medication available for treatment. They are used topically for cutaneous manifestations, in low oral doses for minor disease activity, and in high doses for major disease activity. Intravenous (IV) administration of corticosteroids is an alternative to traditional high-dose oral use. Antimalarial medications are effective for managing cutaneous, musculoskeletal, and mild systemic features of SLE. The NSAIDs used for minor clinical manifestations are often used along with corticosteroids in an effort to minimize corticosteroid requirements.

Immunosuppressive agents (alkylating agents and purine analogues) are used because of their effect on immune function. These medications are generally reserved for patients who have serious forms of SLE that have not responded to conservative therapies. B-cell depleting therapies are the newest treatment for SLE. Monoclonal antibodies, rituximab (Rituxan), and epratuzumab (humanized anit-CD22 antibody) have shown good therapeutic results in clinical trials (Ding & Gordon, 2013).

Nursing Management

Nursing care of the patient with SLE is based on the fundamental plan presented earlier in the chapter (see Chart 56-2). The most common nursing priorities include fatigue, impaired skin integrity, body image disturbance, and lack of knowledge regarding self-management decisions. The disease or its treatment may produce dramatic changes in appearance and considerable distress for the patient. The changes and the unpredictable course of SLE necessitate expert assessment skills and nursing care with sensitivity to the psychological reactions of the patient. The patient may benefit from participation in support groups, which can provide disease information, daily management tips, and social support. Because sun and ultraviolet light exposure can increase disease activity or cause an exacerbation, patients should be taught to avoid exposure or to protect themselves with sunscreen and clothing.

Because of the increased risk of involvement of multiple organ systems, patients should understand the need for routine periodic screenings as well as health promotion activities. A dietary consultation may be indicated to ensure that the patient is knowledgeable about dietary recommendations, given the increased risk of cardiovascular disease, including hypertension and atherosclerosis. Smoking tobacco accelerates complications in patients with SLE (Chasset, Frances, Barete, et al., 2015). In the healthy population, smoking increases the incidence of respiratory infections, lung cancer, risk of coronary artery disease; increases blood pressure, which can worsen kidney function; inhibits liver function (which can also inhibit treatment medications from working appropriately, such as hydroxychloroquine); increases the risk for skin diseases; and increases the risk for osteoporosis. Patients diagnosed with SLE are at even higher risk of developing lung cancer and other rare cancers. Therefore, smoking cessation programs should be offered to all patients who report smoking habits (Montes, Mocarzel, Lanzieri, et al., 2016).

The nurse educates the patient about the importance of continuing prescribed medications and addresses the changes and potential side effects that are likely to occur with their use. The patient is reminded of the importance of monitoring because of the increased risk of systemic involvement, including renal and cardiovascular effects.

Because of the immunosuppression associated with systemic corticosteroid usage, the nurse must watch for signs and symptoms of infection, especially with acutely ill patients.

The nurse should also screen the patient for osteoporosis, because long-term use of corticosteroids increases the incidence of osteoporosis. Patients should have a bone mineral density test performed at diagnosis and prior to beginning steroid use to determine a baseline status and then every 2 years thereafter. Educating the patient regarding calcium and Vitamin D supplementation daily is encouraged, along with the benefits of weight-bearing activities to support bone health (Cash & Glass, 2015).

Sjögren's Syndrome

Sjögren's syndrome is a systemic autoimmune disease that progressively affects the lacrimal and salivary glands of the body. More than 90% of patients affected are women, and the onset tends to begin between 35 and 50 years of age (Carter et al., 2015).

It is one of the most common autoimmune disorders, and very commonly manifests in conjunction with other autoimmune diseases such as RA or SLE.

Pathophysiology

B-cell–mediated antibodies infiltrate the exocrine glands, leading to gland dysfunction and gland destruction. This phenomenon seems to be somewhat regulated by genetics (HLA subtype). There also appears to be environmental triggers such as viruses. Given the clinical makeup and antibodies present, it may also be that Sjögren's disease is a subtype of SLE (Klippel et al., 2008).

Clinical Manifestations

The most common symptoms involve dry eyes (keratoconjunctivitis sicca) and dry mouth (xerostomia). Some patients will complain that their eyes feel "gritty," as if there is sand present. The patient's eyes will exhibit increased redness and lack of tearing. These ocular symptoms can also lead to increased levels of anxiety and depression. The mouth will have dry and sticky mucous membranes. The reduced saliva production may lead to difficulty swallowing.

Sjögren's syndrome can also exhibit symptoms in many other organ systems. Vasculitis (5% to 10%) can manifest with palpable purpura on the skin (Quemeneur, Mouthon, Cacoub, et al., 2013). Lesions may ulcerate and can be painful. Optic neuritis, trigeminal neuralgia, and sensory neuropathy may be present, with symptoms such as burning pain in the extremities, numbness, vertigo, arthralgia, and/or myalgia. Raynaud's phenomenon, which involves blood vessel spasms leading to decreased circulation to the toes, fingers, nose and ears, is noted in 13% to 62% of patients (Klippel et al., 2008). Symptoms such as cough, dyspnea, and abdominal pain may also occur.

Assessment and Diagnostic Findings

The classification criteria for diagnosis of Sjögren's syndrome identify six distinct indices (Klippel et al., 2008):

- Ocular symptoms such as chronic dry eye (keratoconjunctivitis sicca).
- Positive ocular tests (evaluating tear production, corneal, and conjunctival damage). Ocular testing may include Schemer tear test or Rose Bengal tests.
- Oral symptoms, dry mouth.
- Histopathology evaluation (of salivary glands). This will help differentiate the cause of dry mouth from other causes, such as infection, malignancy, stones, and sarcoidosis.
- Salivary gland involvement.

Laboratory tests include autoantibodies to ribonucleoprotein particles (Ro[SS-A] and/or La[SS-B]), which act as antigens in this disease process. Other laboratory indices are also useful in diagnosing Sjögren's syndrome. RF is present in 50% to 70% of patients. ANA, circulating DNA (cDNA), anti-CCP, and anticentromere antibody (ACA) are all potentially present in Sjögren's syndrome and in some cases may act as markers for disease activity (Moerman, Bootsma, Kroese, et al., 2013).

For vasculitis manifestations, a skin biopsy can yield useful information such as leukocytoclastic vasculitis found on histologic examination. If neurologic symptoms are present, nerve conduction studies, MRI, electroencephalograms, and cerebrospinal fluid testing may be used to aid in diagnosis and treatment planning.

Medical Management

There is no cure for Sjögren's syndrome, and treatment is aimed at symptom management. Artificial tears, drops such as pilocarpine (Piloptic), and ocular ointments such as topical cyclosporine are used for dry eyes. Tears normally drain through the lacrimal puncta to the nose, which can render artificial tears ineffective. Therefore, punctum plugs have become very important management tools. For dry mouth, systemic cholinergic agents such as are used regularly. Biotene oral rinse may also be useful for some patients. Additional suggestions include eating small frequent meals; omitting spicy, salty, and irritating food; and avoiding smoking, excessive alcohol use, and drugs with anticholinergic side effects. For severe cases, biologic DMARDs such as rituximab and belimumab and nonbiologic DMARDs such as hydroxychloroquine are sometimes used, but evidence regarding their effectiveness is limited (Carter et al., 2015).

Nursing Management

Nursing care is based on the fundamental plan of nursing care presented earlier (see Chart 56-2). The most frequent nursing priorities for the patient with Sjögren's syndrome are altered skin integrity, self-care deficit, and deficient knowledge of self-management techniques.

The nurse is in the unique position to reinforce the treatment regimen with the patient, especially involving the ocular treatments to avoid sequelae-like eye infections secondary to the dry eyes.

Scleroderma

Scleroderma is a compilation of autoimmune diseases affecting the connective tissue of the skin, blood vessel walls, and internal organs. There are two general types: localized (affecting only the cutaneous system) and systemic (routinely referred to as systemic sclerosis and affecting multiple organ systems). Scleroderma is a rare disease affecting 250 patients per million population (Klippel et al., 2008). Similar to other autoimmune diseases, women are affected three to five times more than men, and the onset occurs typically between the ages of 30 and 50 years. African American patients are affected much younger and have more diffuse symptoms with more severe lung disease. Scleroderma has a variable course with remissions and exacerbations (Varga, 2014).

Pathophysiology

Scleroderma commonly begins with skin involvement. Mononuclear cells cluster on the skin and stimulate lymphokines to stimulate procollagen. Insoluble collagen is formed and accumulates excessively in the tissues. Initially, the inflammatory response causes edema formation, with a resulting taut, smooth, and shiny skin appearance. The skin then undergoes fibrotic changes, leading to loss of elasticity and movement. Eventually, the tissue degenerates and becomes nonfunctional. This chain of events, from inflammation to degeneration, also occurs in blood vessels, major organs, and body systems (Varga, 2014). Both genetics and environmental factors can influence the disease process.

Clinical Manifestations

Scleroderma starts insidiously with Raynaud's phenomenon and swelling in the hands. The skin and the subcutaneous tissues become increasingly hard and rigid and cannot be pinched up from the underlying structures. Wrinkles and lines are obliterated and the skin is dry because sweat secretion over the involved region is suppressed. The extremities stiffen and lose mobility. The condition spreads slowly; for years, these changes may remain localized in the hands and the feet. The face appears mask-like, immobile, and expressionless, and the mouth becomes rigid.

The changes within the body, although not visible directly, are more important than the visible changes. The left ventricle of the heart is involved, resulting in heart failure. The esophagus hardens, interfering with swallowing. The lungs become scarred, impeding respiration. Digestive disturbances occur because of hardening (sclerosing) of the intestinal mucosa, and progressive renal failure may occur.

The patient may manifest a variety of symptoms referred to as the CREST syndrome. CREST stands for *c*alcinosis (calcium deposits in the tissues), *R*aynaud's phenomenon, *e*sophageal hardening and dysfunction, *s*clerodactyly (scleroderma of the digits), and *t*elangiectasia (capillary dilation that forms a vascular lesion) (Papadakis et al., 2015).

Assessment and Diagnostic Findings

Assessment focuses on the sclerotic changes in the skin, contractures in the fingers, and colour changes or lesions in the fingertips. Assessment of systemic involvement requires a systems review with special attention to gastrointestinal, pulmonary, renal, and cardiac symptoms. Limitations in mobility and self-care activities should be assessed, along with the impact the disease has had (or may have) on body image.

There is no one conclusive test to diagnose scleroderma. A skin biopsy is performed to identify cellular changes specific to scleroderma. Pulmonary studies show ventilation–perfusion abnormalities. Echocardiography identifies pericardial effusion (often present with cardiac involvement). Esophageal studies demonstrate decreased motility in most patients with scleroderma. Blood tests may detect ANAs, indicating a connective tissue disorder and possibly distinguishing the subgroup (diffuse or limited) of scleroderma. A positive ANA test result is common in patients with scleroderma (Varga, 2014).

Medical Management

Treatment of scleroderma is dependent on the clinical manifestations. All patients require counselling, during which realistic individual goals may be determined. Support measures include strategies to decrease pain and limit disability. A moderate exercise program is encouraged to prevent joint contractures. Patients are advised to avoid extreme temperatures and to use moisturizing lotion to minimize skin dryness.

Pharmacologic Therapy

No medication regimen is effective in modifying the disease process in scleroderma, but various medications are used to treat organ system involvement. Calcium channel blockers and other antihypertensive agents may provide improvement in symptoms of Raynaud's phenomenon. Anti-inflammatory medications can be used to control arthralgia, stiffness, and general musculoskeletal discomfort. Proton pump inhibitors are used for symptoms of gastric reflux. Aspirin and HMG-CoA (3-hydroxy-3-methylglutaryl coenzyme A) reductase inhibitors (statins) are used to help reduce cardiovascular risk factors. Given the propensity toward digital ulcers due to Raynaud's phenomenon and the potential for pulmonary hypertension, vasoactive medications such as epoprostenol (Flolan), bosentan (Tracleer), and sildenafil (Viagra) are used. Immunosuppressive agents such as cyclophosphamide and methotrexate have been used to improve skin and lung function. The antifibrotic agent imatinib mesylate is used to decrease fibrosis in various organs. Ultraviolet A irradiation is sometimes used to decrease the synthesis of collagen in dermal fibrosis and improve skin symptoms (Carter et al., 2015).

Nursing Management

The nursing care of the patient with scleroderma is based on the fundamental plan of nursing care presented earlier (see Chart 56-2). The most common nursing care priorities for the patient with scleroderma include impaired skin integrity; self-care deficits; imbalanced nutrition, less than body requirements; and disturbed body image. The patient with advanced disease may also have impaired gas exchange, decreased cardiac output, impaired swallowing, and constipation.

Providing meticulous skin care and preventing the effects of Raynaud's phenomenon are major nursing challenges. Patient teaching must include the importance of avoiding cold and protecting the fingers in cold weather and when shopping in the frozen-food section of the grocery store. Warm socks and properly fitting shoes are helpful in preventing ulcers. Careful, frequent inspection for early ulcers is important. Smoking cessation is critical.

Polymyositis

Polymyositis is a group of diseases that are termed *idiopathic inflammatory myopathies* (Klippel et al., 2008). They are rare conditions, with an incidence estimated at 2 cases per 10,000 adults per year. Polymyositis is most commonly seen in women versus men (2:1) and usually seen between 40 and 50 years of age (Miller & Viegels, 2016).

Pathophysiology

Polymyositis is classified as autoimmune because autoantibodies are present. However, these antibodies do not cause damage to muscle cells, indicating only an indirect role in tissue damage. The pathogenesis is multifactorial, and a genetic predisposition is likely. Drug-induced disease is rare. Some evidence suggests a viral link.

Clinical Manifestations

The onset may be very slow and insidious, with symptoms gradually worsening over weeks to months. Proximal muscle weakness is typically the first symptom. Muscle weakness is usually symmetric and diffuse. Common complaints include having difficulty rising from a chair, climbing steps, or holding up the head. Myalgia and muscle tenderness occur in 25% to 50% of patients. Dermatomyositis, a related condition, is most commonly identified by an erythematous smooth or scaly lesion found over the joint surface, which often occurs prior to symptoms of weakness in 50% to 60% of patients (Miller & Viegels, 2016).

Assessment and Diagnostic Findings

A complete history and physical examination assist in excluding other muscle-related disorders. As with other diffuse connective tissue disorders, no single test confirms polymyositis. An electromyogram is performed to rule out degenerative muscle disease. A muscle biopsy may reveal inflammatory infiltrate in the tissue. Serum studies indicate increased muscle enzyme activity.

Medical Management

Management involves high-dose corticosteroid therapy initially, followed by a gradual dosage reduction over several months as muscle enzyme activity decreases. Patients who do not respond to corticosteroids require the addition of an immunosuppressive agent, such as azathioprine, methotrexate, cyclosporine, or cyclophosphamide. The IV immune globulin given in combination with corticosteroids or another immunosuppressive agent has been noted to be beneficial (Carter et al., 2015). Plasmapheresis, lymphapheresis, and total body irradiation have been used if there is no response to corticosteroids and immunosuppressive medications. The antimalarial agent hydroxychloroquine may be effective for skin rashes. Physical therapy is initiated slowly, with range-of-motion exercises to maintain joint mobility, followed by gradual strengthening exercises (Klippel et al., 2008).

Nursing Management

Nursing care is based on the fundamental plan of nursing care presented earlier (see Chart 56-2). The most frequent nursing priorities for the patient with polymyositis include impaired physical mobility, fatigue, self-care deficit, and insufficient knowledge of self-management techniques.

Patients with polymyositis may have symptoms similar to those of other inflammatory diseases. However, proximal muscle weakness is characteristic, making activities such as combing the hair, reaching overhead, and using stairs difficult. Therefore, use of assistive devices may be recommended, and referral to occupational or physical therapy may be warranted.

Polymyalgia Rheumatica and Giant Cell Arteritis

PMR involves stiffness of muscles and pain in the neck, shoulder, and pelvic girdle. GCA is a form of vasculitis affecting the medium-sized and large arteries of the body (Klippel et al., 2008). GCA is also sometimes referred to as temporal arteritis because the majority of arteries affected are extracranial branches of the carotid artery. It is widely agreed, however, that both PMR and GCA represent a spectrum of one disease (Papadakis et al., 2015). Both primarily affect individuals older than 50 years and are associated with the same HLA haplotype genetic markers. PMR and GCA occur predominately in Caucasians and often in first-degree relatives. PMR has an annual incidence rate of 52 cases per 100,000 people older than 50 years. GCA varies by geographic location and has the highest incidence in Scandinavian countries. PMR is two to three times more common than GCA (Klippel et al., 2008).

Pathophysiology

The underlying mechanism of action involved with PMR and GCA is unknown. It is clear, however, that the immune system is abnormally activated in both disease processes with increases in circulating monocytes that produce IL-1 and IL-6. These circulating monocytes make the endothelial linings of blood vessels more vulnerable to vasculitis (Klippel et al., 2008). Immunoglobulin deposits in the walls of inflamed temporal arteries suggest that an autoimmune process is at work.

Clinical Manifestations

Polymyalgia rheumatica is characterized by severe proximal muscle discomfort with mild joint swelling. Severe aching in the neck, shoulder, and pelvic muscles is common. Stiffness is noticeable most often in the morning and after periods of inactivity. Systemic features include low-grade fever, weight loss, malaise, anorexia, and depression. Because polymyalgia rheumatica usually occurs in people 50 years of age and older, it may be confused with, or dismissed as, an inevitable consequence of aging.

Giant cell arteritis, sometimes associated with polymyalgia rheumatica, may cause headaches, changes in vision, and jaw claudication. These symptoms should be evaluated immediately because of the potential for a sudden and permanent loss of vision if the condition is left untreated. Polymyalgia rheumatica and giant cell arteritis typically have a self-limited course, lasting several months to several years (Klippel et al., 2008).

Assessment and Diagnostic Findings

Assessment focuses on musculoskeletal tenderness, weakness, and decreased function. Careful attention should be directed toward assessing the head (for changes in vision, headaches, and jaw claudication). An MRI scan may be used in the assessment of extra-articular synovitis in patients with PMR, regardless of symptoms.

Often, diagnosis is difficult because of the lack of specificity of tests. A markedly high ESR is a screening test but is not definitive. The CRP level and platelet count also provide valuable data. In fact, simultaneous elevation in the ESR and CRP has a sensitivity of 98.6% and a specificity of 75.7% in making the diagnosis of GCA when coupled with clinical findings (Seetharaman, 2015). Diagnosis of both GCA and PMR is more likely to be made by eliminating other potential diagnoses. The dramatic and immediate response to treatment with corticosteroids is considered by some to be diagnostic.

In the case of GCA, biopsy of the temporal artery is the definitive diagnostic tool (Seetharaman, 2015). High-resolution MRI is an alternative or adjunct to the traditional temporal artery biopsy.

Medical Management

The treatment for patients with PMR (without GCA) is moderate doses of corticosteroids. Longer durations of corticosteroid treatment are required with patients who have higher baseline inflammatory markers. Gradual tapering of the corticosteroid treatment should be monitored. NSAIDs are sometimes given in mild disease. The treatment for patients with GCA is rapid initiation of and strict adherence to a regimen of corticosteroids. This is essential to avoid the complication of blindness. Aspirin is a useful adjunctive treatment that also helps reduce the risk of visual loss (Yurdakul, Bodur, Sivas, et al., 2015).

Nursing Management

Nursing care of the patient with polymyalgia rheumatica is based on the fundamental plan of nursing care presented earlier (see Chart 56-2). The most common nursing priorities include pain and insufficient knowledge of the medication regimen.

A management concern is that the patient will take the prescribed medication, frequently corticosteroids, until symptoms improve and then discontinue the medication. The decision to discontinue the medication should be based on clinical and laboratory findings and the physician's assessment. Nursing implications include assisting the patient to prevent and monitor side effects of medications (e.g., infections, diabetes, gastrointestinal problems, and depression) and to adjust to side effects that cannot be prevented (e.g., increased appetite and altered body image).

NURSING ALERT

The nurse must emphasize to the patient the need for continued adherence to the prescribed medication regimen to avoid complications of giant cell arteritis, such as blindness.

The loss of bone mass with corticosteroid use increases the risk of osteoporosis in this already at-risk population. Interventions to promote bone health, such as adequate dietary calcium and vitamin D, measurement of bone mineral density, weight-bearing exercise, smoking cessation, and reduction of alcohol consumption if indicated, should be emphasized.

Osteoarthritis (Degenerative Joint Disease)

OA is a noninflammatory degenerative disorder of the joints. It is the most common form of joint disease and is routinely referred to as degenerative joint disease. OA is classified as either primary (idiopathic), with no prior event or disease related to the OA, or secondary, resulting from previous joint injury or inflammatory disease, similar to RA (Papadakis et al., 2015). Unlike most of the disease processes discussed in this chapter, the pathophysiology of primary OA does not involve autoimmunity or inflammation. It can occur as an end result of an autoimmune disorder where joint destruction occurs. Another distinguishing characteristic of OA is that it is limited to the affected joints; there are no systemic symptoms associated with it.

OA often begins in the third decade of life and peaks between the fifth and sixth decades. By 40 years of age, 90% of the population have degenerative joint changes in their weight-bearing joints, even though clinical symptoms are usually absent (Papadakis et al., 2015). Women, especially those who are Hispanic or African American, are more commonly affected. The incidence of OA increases with age. It is estimated that over 85% of the general population over 65 years of age has radiographic changes indicating OA (Cash & Glass, 2015). Although OA is usually thought of as a disease of aging, it also affects younger patients and results in significant losses in work-related productivity and higher costs (CDC, 2015).

Pathophysiology

All joints consist of bone, particularly **subchondral bone** or the bony plate to which the articular cartilage is attached. This articular cartilage is a lubricated, smooth tissue that protects the bone from damage with physical activity. Between the articular cartilage of the bones forming the joint is a space (called the *joint space*) that allows for movement. To aid in fluidity, each joint contains synovial fluid to help lubricate and protect the joint's movement. With OA, the articular cartilage breaks down, leading to progressive damage to the underlying bone and eventual formation of **osteophytes** (bone spurs) that protrude into the joint space. The result is that the joint space is narrowed, leading to decreased joint movement and the potential for more damage. Consequently, the joint can progressively degenerate (see Fig. 56-3). Understanding of OA pathophysiology has been greatly expanded beyond what was previously thought of as simply "wear and tear" related to aging. The basic degenerative process in the joint exemplified in OA is presented in Figure 56-4. In addition to the degeneration, an infectious arteritis can occur. See Chapter 71 for discussion of septic (infectious) arthritis.

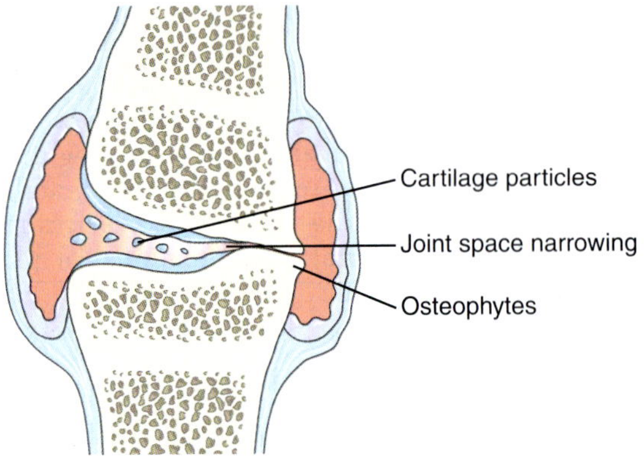

FIGURE 56-3. Joint space narrowing and osteophytes (bone spurs) are characteristic of degenerative changes in joints.

Risk factors for the disease and its progression include older age, female gender, and obesity. In addition, certain occupations (e.g., those requiring laborious tasks); engaging in sport activities; and a history of previous injuries, muscle weakness, genetic predisposition, and certain diseases can also place patients at risk for joint destruction. The most prominent modifiable risk factor for OA is obesity. In fact, both quality and quantity of life are reduced with OA, especially when obesity and OA are combined. A program of diet and exercise can help minimize symptoms of OA in patients with obesity (CDC, 2015).

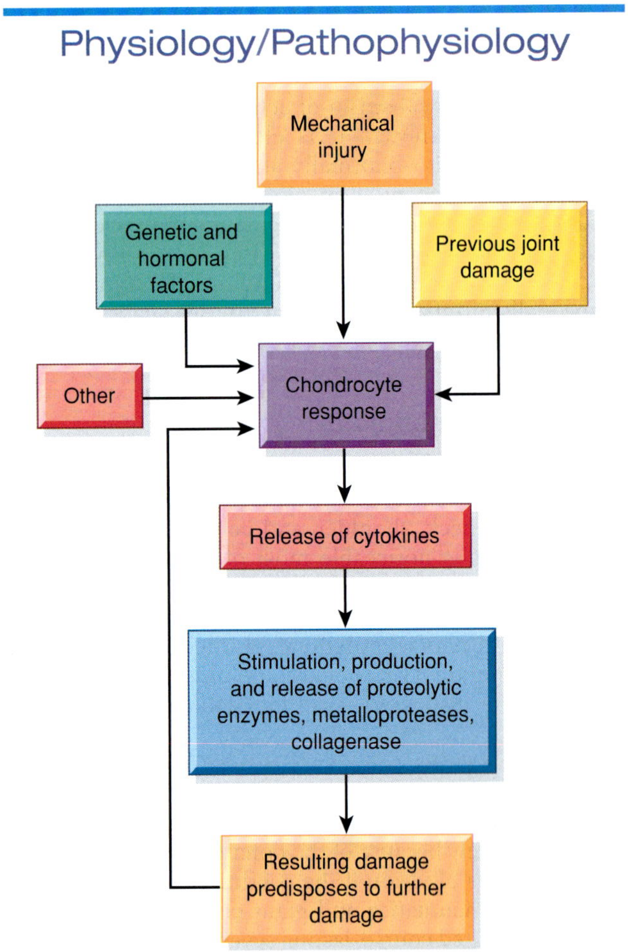

FIGURE 56-4. Pathophysiology of osteoarthritis.

Clinical Manifestations

The primary clinical manifestations of OA are pain, stiffness, and functional impairment. The pain is caused by an inflamed synovium, stretching of the joint capsule or ligaments, irritation of nerve endings in the periosteum over osteophytes (bone spurs), trabecular microfracture, intraosseous hypertension, bursitis, tendinitis, and muscle spasm. Stiffness, which is most commonly experienced in the morning or after awakening, usually lasts less than 30 minutes and decreases with movement. Functional impairment results from pain on movement and limited motion caused by structural changes in the joints.

On physical examination, the affected joint may be enlarged with a decreased range of motion. Although OA occurs most often in weight-bearing joints (hips, knees, cervical and lumbar spine), the proximal interphalangeal (PIP) and distal interphalangeal (DIP) joints are also often involved causing bony enlargements of the DIP (Heberden's nodes) and PIP (Bouchard's nodes) joints. Crepitus may be palpated, especially over the knee. Joint effusion, a sign of inflammation, is usually mild. No systemic manifestations are found.

Assessment and Diagnostic Findings

Diagnosis of OA is complicated because only 30% of patients with changes seen on x-ray report symptoms. Physical assessment of the musculoskeletal system reveals tender and enlarged joints. Inflammation, when present, is not the destructive type as seen in the connective tissue diseases such as RA. OA is characterized by a progressive loss of the joint cartilage, which appears on x-ray as a narrowing of the joint space. In addition, reactive changes occur at the joint margins and on the subchondral bone in the form of osteophytes as the cartilage attempts to regenerate(Papadakis et al., 2015). Neither the presence of osteophytes nor joint space narrowing alone is specific for OA; however, when combined, these are sensitive and specific findings. In early or mild OA, there is only a weak correlation between joint pain and synovitis. Blood tests are not useful in the diagnosis of OA.

Medical Management

The goals of management are to decrease pain and stiffness and to maintain or, when possible, improve joint mobility. Exercise, especially in the form of cardiovascular aerobic exercise and lower extremity strength training, has been found to prevent OA progression and decrease symptoms of OA. Along with exercise, weight loss, which in turn decreases excess load on the joint, can also be extremely beneficial. Occupational and physical therapy can help the patient adopt self-management strategies (Kalunian, 2015a).

Wedged insoles, knee braces, and other modalities are being evaluated as possible therapies aimed at treating the abnormalities in biomechanics found in OA. The use of orthotic devices (e.g., splints, braces) and walking aids (e.g., canes) can improve pain and function by decreasing force on the affected joint (Kalunian, 2015a).

Patients with arthritis often use complementary, alternative, and integrative health therapies, such as massage, yoga, pulsed electromagnetic fields, TENS, and music therapy. These may also include herbal and dietary supplements, other special diets, acupuncture, acupressure, wearing copper bracelets or magnets, and participation in T'ai chi. Research is under way to determine the effectiveness of many of these treatments. To date, no definitive evidence has been found regarding their efficacy (Kalunian, 2015a).

Pharmacologic Therapy

Pharmacologic management of OA is directed toward symptom management and pain control. Selection of medication is based on the patient's needs, the stage of disease, and the risk of side effects. Medications are used in conjunction with nonpharmacologic strategies. In most patients with OA, the initial analgesic therapy is acetaminophen. Some patients respond to the nonselective NSAIDs, and patients who are at increased risk for gastrointestinal complications, especially gastrointestinal bleeding, have been managed effectively with COX-2 enzyme blockers. However, COX-2 enzyme blockers must be used with caution because of the associated risk of cardiovascular disease. Other medications that may be considered are the opioids and intra-articular corticosteroids. Topical analgesic agents such as capsaicin (Capsin, Zostrix) and methylsalicylate are also used (Carter et al., 2015). Topical diclofenac sodium gel (Voltaren gel) has been FDA approved for the use of osteoarthritic joint pain in the hands and knees.

Other therapeutic approaches include glucosamine and chondroitin. Although it has been suggested that these substances modify cartilage structure, studies have not shown them to be effective (Martin, Van Sell, & Danter, 2012). Viscosupplementation, the injection of gel-like substances (hyaluronates) into a joint (intra-articular), is thought to supplement the viscous properties of synovial fluid. These viscosupplements aim to prevent the loss of cartilage and repair chondral defects (Kalunian, 2015b).

Surgical Management

In moderate to severe OA, when pain is severe or because of loss of function, surgical intervention may be used. The procedures most commonly used are osteotomy (to alter the distribution of weight within the joint) and arthroplasty. In **arthroplasty**, diseased joint components are replaced (see Chapter 70). Rehabilitation with physical therapy that is initiated within the first 24 hours is associated with decreased hospital length of stay and improved balance and gait function (Martin, Thornhill, & Katz, 2015).

Nursing Management

Pain management and optimal functional ability are major goals of nursing intervention. With those goals in mind, nursing management of the patient with OA includes pharmacologic and nonpharmacologic approaches as well as education. The patient's understanding of the disease process and symptom pattern is critical to the plan of care. Because patients with OA usually are older, they may have other health problems. Commonly they are overweight, and they may have a sedentary lifestyle. Weight loss and exercise are important approaches to lessen pain and disability. Canes or other assistive devices for ambulation should be considered, and any stigma about the use of these devices should be explored. Exercises such as walking should be begun in moderation and increased gradually. Patients should plan their daily exercise for a time when the pain is least severe or plan to use an analgesic agent, if appropriate, before exercising. Adequate pain management is important for the success of an exercise program. Open discussion regarding the use of complementary, alternative, and integrative health therapies is important to maintain safe and effective practices for patients looking for relief.

Spondyloarthropathies

The spondyloarthropathies are another category of systemic inflammatory disorders of the skeleton. The spondyloarthropathies include ankylosing spondylitis (AS), reactive arthritis (formerly known as Reiter's syndrome), and psoriatic arthritis. Spondyloarthritis is also associated with inflammatory bowel diseases such as Crohn's disease (regional enteritis) and ulcerative colitis (Grossman & Porth, 2014).

These rheumatic diseases share several clinical features. The inflammation tends to occur peripherally at the sites of attachment—at tendons, joint capsules, and ligaments. Periosteal inflammation may be present. Many patients have arthritis of the sacroiliac joints. The onset tends to occur during young adulthood, with the disease affecting men more often than women. There is a strong tendency for these conditions to occur in families. Frequently, the HLA-B27 genetic marker is found. In addition, more than one of these conditions can be found simultaneously in the same person or another family member (Carter et al., 2015).

As with other inflammatory conditions, patients with spondyloarthropathies have an increased risk for cardiovascular disease. These findings may be related to a state of chronic systemic inflammation and an increase in traditional cardiac risk factors, such as lack of exercise due to increased pain (Carter et al., 2015).

Ankylosing Spondylitis

AS is a chronic and inflammatory disease of the spine. It is more prevalent in males than in females and is usually diagnosed in the second or third decade of life. The disease is also more severe in males, and significant systemic involvement is likely.

AS affects the cartilaginous joints of the spine and surrounding tissues, making them rigid, decreasing mobility, and leading to kyphosis (a stooped position). This kyphosis can, in turn, lead to decreased stability and balance. Back pain is the characteristic feature. The back pain can be so severe that it may mask symptoms of a cervical fracture, which can lead to neurologic problems if left untreated. Occasionally, the large synovial joints, such as the hips, knees, or shoulders, may be involved (Carter et al., 2015).

AS also exhibits systemic effects. Uveitis occurs in 20% to 25% of patients with AS and may be a presenting feature (Smith, 2013). Another potential complication of AS is the risk of osteoporosis, which appears to be related to the inflammatory process as well as bone turnover and low vitamin D levels. Other complications involve atrioventricular conduction defects, aortic insufficiency, and pulmonary fibrosis (Papadakis et al., 2015). As the disease progresses, **ankylosis** of the entire spine may occur, leading to respiratory compromise and further complications.

Reactive Arthritis (Reiter's Syndrome)

The disease process involved in Reiter's syndrome is called reactive because the arthritis occurs after an infection. It mostly affects young adult males and is characterized primarily by urethritis, arthritis, and conjunctivitis. Dermatitis and ulcerations of the mouth and penis may also be present. Low back pain is common.

Psoriatic Arthritis

Psoriatic arthritis is an inflammatory arthritis associated with the skin disease psoriasis. In fact, research has suggested that between 10% and 20% of people with psoriasis will eventually develop psoriatic arthritis (Carter et al., 2015; Dewing, 2015). Psoriasis is the most common autoimmune disease in the United States, affecting 2% to 3% of the population. Psoriatic arthritis onset occurs between 30 and 50 years of age and affects equal numbers of men and women (Dewing, 2015).

Pathogenesis of the disease process is hypothesized to start in the skin with an exaggerated immune response to environmental factors and then spreads to the joints in genetically susceptible individuals. Genetics is found to be a strong predictor. Many men and women diagnosed with psoriatic arthritis usually have a first-degree relative with psoriasis. Research shows that the HLAs are also present in up to 50% of patients diagnosed with psoriatic arthritis testing positive for the HLA-B27 antigen (Dewing, 2015). Although these patients test negative for RF, levels of TNF-α and other cytokines are elevated (Dewing, 2015). The body is triggered to activate the T cells of the immune system, producing inflammatory cytokines and mediators that cause changes and inflammation in the body, which also may result in erosions and joint destruction. In addition to joint damage, this cascade may also damage the ligaments, tendons, skin, and nails. Nail psoriasis occurs in approximately 90% of patients (Dewing, 2015).

Psoriatic arthritis is characterized by synovitis, polyarthritis, and spondylitis. Inflammatory back pain is a common symptom, which is differentiated from other back pain by symptoms of back pain presenting at a young age, pain improving with activity, and pain occurring at night. Radiographic evidence of asymmetrical sacroiliitis or spondylitis may also assist with diagnosing psoriatic arthritis (Dewing, 2015). Other sites of pain commonly seen in these patients are the Achilles tendon, plantar fascia, or tibial tuberosity areas. Pain in these areas is common from the inflammation that occurs at the entheses, where tendons and ligaments attach to the bone.

In addition to pain, infections can also occur since this is a systemic disease. Uveitis occurs in approximately 1.5% to 25% of patients diagnosed with psoriatic arthritis. Uveitis should be quickly diagnosed and treated by the ophthalmologist to prevent vision loss (Dewing, 2015).

Medical Management

Medical management of spondyloarthropathies focuses on treating pain and maintaining mobility by suppressing inflammation. For the patient with AS, good body positioning and posture are essential so that if ankylosis (fixation) does occur, the patient is in the most functional position. Maintaining range of motion with regular exercise and a muscle-strengthening program is especially important and has been linked with higher quality of life for the patient (Carter et al., 2015).

Pharmacologic Management

The European League Against Rheumatism guidelines recommend NSAIDs as the first-line therapy for treating all spondylarthropathies. All chronic conditions (cardiac, renal, and gastrointestinal) should be taken into consideration when prescribing long-term NSAIDs. Methotrexate, sulfasalazine, and leflunomide may also be used; these drugs may help with skin and peripheral joint disease but may not prevent spinal changes. Corticosteroid injections may be used for periodic flares; however, oral and long-term use of steroids is not recommended due to the possibility of psoriatic skin flare when discontinuing use. More recently, anti-TNF therapy has been approved by the FDA for psoriatic arthritis. Anti-TNF medications that have been used effectively include etanercept (Enbrel), infliximab (Remicade), adalimumab (Humira), golimumab (Simponi), and certolizumabpegol (Cimzia). Two additional agents include apremilast (Otezla), which is a PDE4 inhibitor, and ustekinumab (Stelara), an anti-IL12/anti-IL23 agent (Carter et al., 2015; Dewing, 2015).

Surgical Management

With advanced AS and subsequent debilitating kyphosis, an osteotomy of the spine can be done. One study showed that an average correction of 45 degrees in the cervical spine was obtained and that quality of life also improved. Surgical management may also include total joint replacement (see Chapter 70) (Carter et al., 2015).

Nursing Management

Major nursing interventions in the spondyloarthropathies are related to symptom management and maintenance of optimal functioning. Affected patients are primarily young men. Their major concerns are often related to prognosis and job modification, especially among those who perform physical work. Patients may also express concerns about leisure and recreational activities. Focusing on physical activity and staying active and maintaining good posture will help to prevent chronic changes that may lead to deformities. It is important to address psychological changes, such as depression and emotional stress, that can occur with the diagnosis and chronicity of the disease (Carter et al., 2015). If symptoms are present, the primary provider should assess for emotional stress and treat as appropriate.

Metabolic and Endocrine Diseases Associated With Rheumatic Disorders

Metabolic and endocrine diseases may be associated with rheumatic disorders. These include biochemical abnormalities (amyloidosis and scurvy), endocrine diseases (diabetes mellitus and acromegaly), immunodeficiency diseases (human immunodeficiency virus [HIV] infection, acquired immunodeficiency syndrome [AIDS]), and some inherited disorders (hypermobility syndromes). However, the most common conditions are the crystal-induced arthropathies, in which crystals such as monosodium urate (gout) or calcium pyrophosphate (calcium pyrophosphate dihydrate disease [CPPD] or pseudogout) are deposited within joints and other tissues (Papadakis et al., 2015).

Gout

Gout is the most common form of inflammatory arthritis. The prevalence is reported to be about 3.9% and appears to be on the rise. Men are three to four times more likely to be diagnosed with gout than women. The incidence of gout increases with age, body mass index, alcohol consumption, hypertension, and diuretic use (CDC, 2015b). Evidence links the consumption of fructose-rich beverages with the risk of gout for both men and women (CDC, 2015b). Patients with gout have an increased risk of cardiovascular disease. Comorbid conditions such as hypertension, dyslipidemia, diabetes, OA, and kidney disease may be present in patients with gout (Papadakis et al., 2015).

Given that the incidence of gout increases with age, its management can be complicated by other medical conditions, medications, and age-related changes (Carter et al., 2015).

Pathophysiology

Gout is caused by hyperuricemia (increased serum uric acid). Uric acid is a by-product of purine metabolism; purines are basic chemical compounds found in high concentrations in meat products. Urate levels are affected by diet, medications, overproduction in the body, and inadequate excretion by the kidneys. Hyperuricemia (serum concentration greater than 6.8 mg/dL) can, but does not always, cause urate crystal deposition. However, as uric acid levels increase, the risk becomes greater. The initial cause for the gout attack occurs when macrophages in the joint space phagocytize urate crystals. Through a series of immunologic steps, interleukin-1 beta is secreted, increasing the inflammation. This process is exacerbated by the presence of free fatty acids. Both alcohol and consumption of a large meal, especially with red meat, can lead to increases in free fatty acid concentrations; they also are implicated as triggers to acute gout attacks (Carter et al., 2015).

With repeated attacks, accumulations of sodium urate crystals, called **tophi**, are deposited in peripheral areas of the body, such as the great toe, the hands, and the ear. Renal Urolithiasis (kidney stones), with chronic kidney disease secondary to urate deposition, may develop.

Primary hyperuricemia may be caused by severe dieting or starvation, excessive intake of foods that are high in purines (shellfish, organ meats), or heredity. In secondary hyperuricemia, gout is a clinical feature secondary to any of a number of genetic or acquired processes, including conditions in which there is an increase in cell turnover (leukemia, multiple myeloma, some types of anemias, psoriasis) and an increase in cell breakdown. Altered renal tubular function, either as a major action or as an unintended side effect of certain pharmacologic agents (e.g., diuretics such as thiazides and furosemide), low-dose salicylates, or ethanol can contribute to uric acid underexcretion (Klippel et al., 2008). The finding of urate crystals in the synovial fluid of asymptomatic joints suggests that factors other than crystals may be related to the inflammatory reaction. Recovered monosodium urate crystals are coated with immunoglobulins that are mainly IgG. IgG enhances crystal phagocytosis, thereby demonstrating immunologic activity (Klippel et al., 2008).

Clinical Manifestations

Manifestations of the gout syndrome include acute gouty arthritis (recurrent attacks of severe articular and periarticular inflammation), tophi (crystalline deposits accumulating in articular tissue, osseous tissue, soft tissue, and cartilage), gouty nephropathy (renal impairment), and uric acid urinary calculi. Four stages of gout can be identified: asymptomatic hyperuricemia, acute gouty arthritis, intercritical gout, and chronic tophaceous gout (Neoai, Jansen, Dalbeth, et al., 2015). The subsequent development of gout is directly related to the duration and magnitude of the hyperuricemia. Therefore, the commitment to lifelong pharmacologic treatment of hyperuricemia is deferred until there is an initial attack of gout.

For hyperuricemic people who are going to develop gout, acute arthritis is the most common early clinical manifestation. The metatarsophalangeal joint of the big toe is a commonly affected joint. The tarsal area, ankle, or knee may also be affected. Less commonly, the wrists, fingers, and elbows may be affected. Trauma, alcohol ingestion, dieting, medications, surgical stress, or illness may trigger the acute attack. The abrupt onset often occurs at night, awakening the patient with severe pain, redness, swelling, and warmth of the affected joint. Early attacks tend to subside spontaneously over 3 to 10 days even without treatment. The attack is followed by a symptom-free period (the intercritical stage) until the next attack, which may not come for months or years. However, with time, attacks tend to occur more frequently, involve more joints, and last longer (Becker, 2015).

Tophi (seen in chronic tophaceous gout) are generally associated with more frequent and severe inflammatory episodes. Higher serum concentrations of uric acid are also associated with more extensive tophus formation. Tophi most commonly occur in the synovium, olecranon bursa, subchondral bone, infrapatellar and Achilles tendons, and subcutaneous tissue on the extensor surface of the forearms and overlying joints. They have also been found in the aortic walls, heart valves, nasal and ear cartilage, eyelids, cornea, and sclera. Joint enlargement may cause a loss of joint motion. Uric acid deposits may cause renal stones and kidney damage.

Medical Management

A definitive diagnosis of gouty arthritis is established by polarized light microscopy of the synovial fluid of the involved joint. Uric acid crystals are seen within the polymorphonuclear leukocytes in the fluid.

Acute attacks are managed with colchicine (Colcrys) (oral or parenteral), an NSAID such as indomethacin (Indocin), or a corticosteroid. Management of hyperuricemia, tophi, joint destruction, and renal disorders is usually initiated after the acute inflammatory process has subsided. Once the acute attack has subsided, uric acid–lowering therapy should be considered. Xanthine oxidase inhibitors, such as allopurinol (Zyloprim) and febuxostat (Uloric), are the agents of choice. Given the role of IL-1 in the pathogenesis of gout, some experts suggest that there may be a role for anakinra (Kineret), an IL-1 receptor antagonist in the management of acute gout (Papadakis et al., 2015).

Management between gout attacks needs to include lifestyle changes such as avoiding purine-rich foods, weight loss, decreasing alcohol consumption, and avoiding certain medications. Uricosuric agents, such as probenecid (Benemid), may be indicated in patients with frequent acute attacks. Uricosuric medications correct hyperuricemia and dissolve deposited urate. Corticosteroids may also be used in patients who have no response to other therapy. In patients with refractory chronic gout who are not controlled with the regimens mentioned earlier, pegloticase (Krystexxa), a newer agent, has been shown to be effective in lowering uric acid levels (Becker, 2016). Specific treatment is based on the serum uric acid level, 24-hour urinary uric acid excretion, and renal function (see Table 56-5) (Carter et al., 2015).

TABLE 56-5 Common Medications Used to Treat Gout

Medication	Actions and Use	Nursing Implications
Colchicine (Colcrys)	Lowers the deposition of uric acid and interferes with leukocyte infiltration, thus reducing inflammation; does not alter serum or urine levels of uric acid; used in acute and chronic management	*Acute management:* Administer when attack begins; dosage increased until pain is relieved or diarrhea develops, then stop medication *Chronic management:* Causes gastrointestinal upset in most patients.
Probenecid (Benemid)	Uricosuric agent; inhibits renal reabsorption of urates and increases the urinary excretion of uric acid; prevents tophi formation	Be alert for nausea and rash
Allopurinol (Zyloprim), febuxostat (Uloric)	Xanthine oxidase inhibitors; interrupt the breakdown of purines before uric acid is formed; inhibit xanthinoxidase because uric acid formation is blocked	Monitor for side effects, including bone marrow depression, vomiting, and abdominal pain. Avoid starting medication or increasing dose if active flare present

Adapted from Karch, A. (2014). *Lippincott's nursing drug guide*. Philadelphia, PA: Lippincott Williams & Wilkins.

Nursing Management

Historically, gouty arthritis was thought to be a condition among royalty and the very rich, with the disease attributed to "high living." This has not been shown to be entirely true. Although severe dietary restriction is not necessary, the nurse should encourage the patient to restrict consumption of foods high in purines, especially organ meats, and to limit alcohol intake. Maintenance of normal body weight should be encouraged. In an acute episode of gouty arthritis, pain management with prescribed medications is essential, along with avoidance of factors that increase pain and inflammation, such as trauma, stress, and alcohol. Between acute episodes, the patient feels well and may abandon preventive behaviours, which may result in an acute attack. Acute attacks are most effectively treated if therapy is begun early in the course (Carter et al., 2015).

Fibromyalgia

Fibromyalgia is a chronic pain syndrome that involves chronic fatigue, generalized muscle aching, stiffness, sleep disturbances, and functional impairment. It is estimated to affect more than 5 million Americans, representing 2% to 5% of the general population, with women affected more than men. Between 25% and 65% of patients with fibromyalgia have other rheumatologic conditions such as RA, SLE, and AS (CDC, 2015c).

Pathophysiology

The amplified pain experienced by patients with fibromyalgia is neurogenic in origin (Carter et al., 2015). Specifically, the central nervous system's ascending and descending pathways (that regulate and moderate pain processing) function abnormally, causing amplification of pain signals. Some scientists describe this as if the "volume control setting" for pain were abnormally high (Carter et al., 2015). Therefore, stimulation that may not normally elicit pain, such as touch, may do so. In addition, there are a number of predisposing factors to pain, including anxiety, depression, physical trauma, emotional stress, sleep disorder, and viral infection (Carter et al., 2015).

Assessment and Diagnostic Findings

The American College of Rheumatology established preliminary diagnostic criteria and symptom severity indices for fibromyalgia (Carter et al., 2015). These criteria emphasize the regions of pain, rather than specific points, and take into account the fatigue, cognitive symptoms, and unrefreshed sleep that patients with fibromyalgia also tend to experience (Carter et al., 2015).

Medical Management

Treatment consists of attention to the specific symptoms reported by the patient. NSAIDs may be used to treat the diffuse muscle aching and stiffness. Tricyclic antidepressants such as amitriptyline (Elavil) and nortriptyline (Pamelor) as well as sleep hygiene measures are used to improve or restore normal sleep patterns (Cash & Glass, 2015). Muscle relaxants such as cyclobenzaprine (Amrix) may also be used to help with relaxation and pain. Cognitive behavioural therapy is also useful in improving sleep and attentional dysfunction. In addition, serotonin norepinephrine reuptake inhibitors, such as duloxetine (Cymbalta), venlafaxine (Effexor), and milnacipran (Savella); selective serotonin reuptake inhibitors, including fluoxetine (Prozac), paroxetine (Paxil), and sertraline (Zoloft); as well as anticonvulsants such as gabapentin (Neurontin) and pregabalin (Lyrica) have been reported to be effective (Carter et al., 2015). Individualized programs of exercise are used to decrease muscle weakness and discomfort and to improve the general deconditioning that occurs in affected patients. There has also been some promising research in complementary, alternative, and integrative health therapies, such as acupuncture, massage, homeopathy, hydrotherapy, craniosacral therapy, and myofascial therapy (Carter et al., 2015).

Nursing Management

Typically, patients with fibromyalgia have endured their symptoms for a long period of time. They may feel as if their symptoms have not been taken seriously. Nurses need to pay special attention to supporting these patients and providing encouragement as they begin their program of therapy. Patient support groups may be helpful. Careful listening to patients' descriptions of their concerns and symptoms is essential to help them make the changes that are necessary to improve their quality of life (Carter et al., 2015).

Arthritis Associated With Infectious Organisms

Arthritis, tenosynovitis, and bursitis can be associated with infectious organisms. Some inflammation of joints, tendons, and bursae is directly related to infection caused by bacterial, viral, fungal, or parasitic agents. Bacterial arthritis is the most rapidly destructive form of infectious arthritis. There are two major classes of bacterial arthritis: those caused by *Neisseria gonorrhoeae* and those caused by a nongonococcal bacterium. The most prevalent of the nongonococcal organisms include *Staphylococcus aureus* and the various streptococcal variants. Less common pathogens are related to syphilis, tuberculosis, leprosy, fungi (particularly coccidioidomycosis), mycoplasmas, and viral agents such as rubella, parvovirus, and hepatitis B.

Clinical Manifestations

The characteristic symptom is acute onset of a warm, swollen joint. Culture of the bacterium from the synovial fluid confirms the diagnosis. The patient often immobilizes the joint and elevates the affected extremity because of pain and swelling. Fever may be high, or it may be absent. Signs of systemic infection may be absent in older patients, in those with diabetes, and in those with suppressed immune systems. Diagnosis and treatment may be delayed for patients with pre-existing arthritic conditions if they attribute the symptoms to a flare-up of arthritis.

Management

This condition is a medical emergency necessitating early diagnosis and appropriate treatment to eliminate the causative organism; otherwise, the joint may be destroyed relatively quickly. Treatment consists of parenteral antibiotics and drainage of the joint. The results of cultures are used to determine the appropriate antibiotic therapy. Immobilization of the joint and repeated joint aspirations may be necessary in addition to IV antibiotics. Nursing management focuses on providing pain relief, administering antibiotics, and assisting the patient with self-care activities. If the patient is discharged home on IV antibiotic therapy, the nurse arranges home care and provides the patient and care providers with education in safe administration of the drug and changes that should be reported to a health care provider.

Neoplasms and Neurovascular, Bone, and Extra-Articular Disorders

Primary neoplasms of joints, tendon sheaths, and bursae are rare. Most neoplasms are benign, arising from the synovium. These benign tumours include lipoma, hemangioma, fibroma, and tumour-like lesions such as ganglion, bursitis, and synovial cyst. Malignant tumours include primary tumours, such as synovial and bone sarcomas, and secondary involvement as manifestations of joint invasion by leukemia, lymphoma, myeloma, or metastasis. Neoplasms may manifest as back or neck pain.

Neurovascular disorders include the compression syndromes, such as those with peripheral entrapment (e.g., carpal tunnel syndrome), radiculopathy, and spinal stenosis. Raynaud's phenomenon and erythromelalgia (throbbing and burning pain often affecting the hands and feet) are also included in this category.

Bone and cartilage disorders include osteoporosis, osteomalacia, hypertrophic osteoarthropathy, diffuse idiopathic skeletal hyperostosis, Paget's disease, osteonecrosis, avascular necrosis, costochondritis, osteolysis or chondrolysis, and biomechanical or anatomic abnormalities. Notably, these conditions involve resorption, destruction, infection, or remodeling of bone.

Extra-articular rheumatism is a descriptive term for a group of conditions that affect structures other than the joints. Included are general and regional pain syndromes, low back pain and intervertebral disk disorders, tendonitis and bursitis, and ganglion cysts.

Miscellaneous Disorders

The last category in the classification of the rheumatic diseases is aptly labelled miscellaneous disorders because it contains a mix of disorders that are frequently associated with arthritis and other conditions. These include the direct consequences of trauma (including internal derangement and loose bodies of joints), pancreatic disease (related to avascular necrosis or osteonecrosis), sarcoidosis (a multisystem disorder particularly of the lymph nodes and lungs), and palindromic rheumatism (an uncommon variety of recurring and acute arthritis and periarthritis that in some may progress to RA but is characterized by symptom-free periods of days to months). Other conditions include villonodular synovitis, chronic active hepatitis, and drug-related rheumatic syndromes. The nursing interventions related to these varied conditions are specific to the multisystemic problems experienced by the patient. However, the musculoskeletal components should not be neglected or overlooked. Further information about these rare disorders can be found in specialty references.

Critical Thinking Exercises

1 A 62-year-old patient who was recently diagnosed with OA comes in for her follow-up appointment. She wants to know why she is not being prescribed "stronger medications" for her arthritis like her friend is taking. Her friend has RA and her pain improved significantly after starting adalimumab injections. Describe your teaching plan to explain the physiologic differences between OA and RA, medications commonly used for OA and the difference between treatment regimens for OA and RA.

2 Your patient is a 52-year-old male patient with a history of hypertension, stage 3 kidney disease, diabetes, and hyperlipidemia. He smokes 1 pack of cigarettes a day and drinks alcohol on occasion. He is 189 cm tall and weighs 110 kg. Today he presents with complaints of severe pain in his right great toe that started Sunday morning. He spent a long weekend with friends, drank a lot of alcohol, and ate a lot of rich food. He woke Sunday morning with pain in his foot that has progressively gotten worse. He has been diagnosed with gout. Identify the priorities, approach, and techniques you would use to provide nursing care to this patient. How would you prioritize the physical examination and techniques performed since his pain scale is 8/10? What lifestyle modifications are a priority for this patient?

3 You are the nurse taking care of a woman with Sjögren's syndrome. What is the evidence for symptom management for this patient? What criteria would you use to assess the strength of the evidence? What is the evidence for treatment options to improve her symptoms?

REFERENCES AND SELECTED READINGS

Books

Carter S. C., Patty-Resk, C., Ruffing, V., et al. (2015). *Core curriculum for rheumatology nursing* (1st ed.). Greenville, SC: Lyons Den Solutions, LLC.

Cash, J. C., & Glass, C. A. (2015). *Adult-gerontology practice guidelines*. New York: Springer Publishing Company.

Fischbach, F., & Dunning, M. B. (2015). *A manual of laboratory and diagnostic tests* (9th ed.). Philadelphia, PA: Lippincott Williams & Wilkins.

Grossman, S. C., & Porth, C. M. (2014). *Porth's pathophysiology: Concepts of altered health states* (9th ed.). Philadelphia, PA: Lippincott Williams & Wilkins.

Karch, A. (2014). *Lippincott's nursing drug guide*. Philadelphia, PA: Lippincott Williams & Wilkins.

Klippel, J. H., Stone, J. H., Crofford, L. J., et al. (Eds.). (2008). *Primer on the rheumatic diseases* (13th ed.). New York: Springer.

Miller, C. A. (2015). *Nursing for wellness in older adults* (7th ed.). Philadelphia, PA: Lippincott Williams & Wilkins.

Papadakis, M. A., McPhee, S. J., & Rabow, M. W. (2015). *Current medical diagnosis and treatment 2016* (55th ed.). New York: McGraw-Hill.

Journals and Electronic Documents

Afshar, B. (2015). *RA: Best and worse supplements and herbs*. Retrieved on 5/14/2016 at: www.webmd.com/rheumatoid-arthritis/guide/rheumatoid-arthritis-best-wrose-supplements-herbs.

Aletaha, D., Neogi, T., Silman, A. J., et al. (2010). 2010 Rheumatoid arthritis classification criteria: An American College of Rheumatology/European League Against Rheumatism collaborative initiative. *Arthritis and Rheumatism*, *62*(9), 2569–2581.

American College of Rheumatology. (1997). *ACR-endorsed criteria for Rheumatic diseases*. Retrieved on 1/13/2016 at: www.rheumatology.org/Portals/0/Files/1997%20Update%20of%201982%20Revised.pdf

Barbour, K. E., Helmick, C. G., Theis, K. A., et al. (2013). Prevalence of doctor-diagnosed arthritis and arthritis-attributable activity limitation—United States, 2010–2012. *MMWR: Morbidity and Mortality Weekly Report*, *62*(44), 869–873.

Bartels, C. (2015). *Systemic Lupus Erythematosus*. Retrieved on May 14, 2016, from www.emedicine.medscape.com/article/332244-overview.

Becker, M. A. (2015). Clinical manifestations and diagnosis of gout. Retrieved on May 14, 2016, from www.uptodate.com/contents/search?search=Clinical+manifestations+and+diagnosis+of+gout&x=4&y=8

Becker, M. A. (2016). Prevention of recurrent gout: Pharmacologic urate-lowering therapy and treatment of tophi. Retrieved on May 14, 2016, from www.uptodate.com/contents/search?search=Prevention+of+recurrent+gout%3A+Pharmacologic+urate-lowering+therapy+and+%09treatment+of+tophi&x=4&y=9

Bultink, I. E. (2012). Osteoporosis and fractures in systemic lupus erythematosus. *Arthritis Care and Research*, *64*(1), 2–8.

Centers for Disease Control and Prevention (CDC). (2015). Osteoarthritis (OA). Retrieved on May 14, 2016, from www.cdc.gov.

Centers for Disease Control and Prevention (CDC). (2015a). *Systemic lupus erythematous (SLE or lupus): Prevalence and incidence*. Retrieved from: www.cdc.gov/arthritis/basics/lupus.htm

Centers for Disease Control and Prevention (CDC). (2015b). *Gout*. Retrieved on May 14, 2016, from www.cdc.gov/arthritis/basics/gout.htm.

Centers for Disease Control and Prevention (CDC). (2015c). *Fibromyalgia*. Retrieved from www.cdc.gov/arthritis/basics/fibromyalgia.htm

Chasset, F., Frances, C., Barete, S., et al. (2015). Influence of smoking on the efficacy of antimalarials in cutaneous lupus: A meta-analysis of the literature. *Journal of the American Academy of Dermatology*, *72*(4), 634–639.

Cottrell, J. D., Jonas, M., Bergsten, U., et al. (2013). The nurse's role in addressing unmet treatment and management needs of patients with rheumatoid arthritis: Delphi-based recommendations. *International Journal of Nursing Knowledge*, *24*(2), 66–76.

Dewing, K. A. (2015). Management of patients with psoriatic arthritis. *The Nurse Practitioner*, *40*(4), 40–46.

Di Lorenzo, A. L. (2015). HLA-B27 syndromes. Retrieved on May 14, 2016, from www.emedicine.medscape.come/article/1201027-overview

Ding, H. J., & Gordon, C. (2013). New biologic therapy for systemic lupus erythematosus. *Current opinion in pharmacology, 13*(3), 405-412.

Fonseca, R., Bernardes, M., Terroso, G., et al. (2014). Silent burdens in disease: Fatigue and depression in SLE. *Autoimmune Diseases*, *2014*, 790724.

Fujita, T., Kutsumi, H., Sanuki, T., et al. (2013). Adherence to the preventive strategies for nonsteroidal anti-inflammatory drug- or low–dose aspirin-induced gastrointestinal injuries. *Journal of Gastroenterology*, *48*(5), 559–573.

Hochberg, C. (1997). Updating the American College of Rheumatology revised criteria for the classification of systemic lupus erythematosus. *Arthritis and Rheumatism*, *40*(9), 1725

Jordan, S., Maurer, B., Toniolo, M., et al. (2015). Performance of the new ACR/EULAR classification criteria for systemic sclerosis in clinical practice. *Rheumatology*, *54*(8), 1454–1458.

Kalunian, K. C. (2015a). Nonpharmacologic therapy of osteoarthritis. Retrieved from www.uptodate.com/contents/search?search=Nonpharmacologic+therapy+of+osteoarthritis+&x=13&y=8

Kalunian, K. C. (2015b). Treatment of osteoarthritis resistant to initial pharmacologic therapy. Retrieved from www.uptodate.com/contents/search?search=Treatment+of+osteoarthritis+resistant+to+initial+pharmacologic+therapy&x=8&y=16

Lim, S., Bayakly, A. R., Helmick, C. G., et al. (2014). The incidence and prevalence of systemic lupus erythematosus, 2002–2004. *Arthritis & Rheumatology*, *66*(2), 357–368.

Marcus, D. M. (2015). Herbal remedies, supplements & acupuncture for arthritis. *The American College of Rheumatology*. Retrieved from www.rheumatology.org/i-am-a/patient-caregiver/treatments/herbal-remedies-supplements-acupuncture-for-arthritis.

Martin, G. M., Thornhill, T. S., & Katz, J. M. (2015). Total knee arthroplasty. Retrieved from www.uptodate.com/contents/search?search=Total+knee+arthroplastypolimiosite&x=16&y=10

Martin, M. S., Van Sell, S., & Danter, J. (2012). Glucosamine and chondroitin: An appropriate adjunct treatment of symptomatic osteoarthritis of the knee. *Orthopaedic Nursing*, *31*(3), 160–166.

Miller, M. L., & Viegels, R. A. (2016). Clinical manifestations of dermatomyositis and polymyositis in adults. Retrieved from www.uptodate.com/contents/clinical-manifestations-of-dermatomyositis-and-polymyositis-in-adults?source=machineLearning&search=polimiosite&selectedTitle=2%7E150&sectionRank=1&anchor=H17269403

Moerman, R., Bootsma, H., Kroese, R., et al. (2013). Sjogren's syndrome in older patients: Aetiology, diagnosis and management. *Drugs and Aging*, *30*(3), 137–153.

Montes, R. A., Mocarzel, L. O., Lanzieri, P. G., et al. (2016). Smoking and its association with morbidity in systemic lupus erythematosus. *Arthritis and Rheumatology*, *68*(2), 441–448.

Neoai, T., Jansen, T. A., Dalbeth, N., et al. (2015). 2105 Gout classification criteria: An American College of Rheumatology collaborative project. Retrieved from www.rheumatology.org/Practice-Quality/Clinical-Support/Criteria.

Palmer, D., & El Miedany, Y. (2014). Rheumatoid arthritis: Recommendations for treat to target. *British Journal of Nursing*, *23*(6), 310–315.

Quemeneur, T., Mouthon, L., Cacoub, P., et al. (2013). Systemic vasculitis during the course of systemic sclerosis: Report of 12 cases and review of the literature. *Medicine*, *92*(1), 1–9.

Ramos-Remus, C., Duran-Barragan, S., &Castillo-Ortiz, J. (2012). Beyond the joints: Neurological involvement in rheumatoid arthritis. *Clinical Rheumatology*, *31*(1), 1–12.

Schur, P. H., & Moreland, L. W. (2016). General principles of management of rheumatoid arthritis in adults. Retrieved from www.uptodate.com/contents/general-principles-of-management-of-rheumatoid-arthritis-in-adults?source=search_result&search=rheumatoid+arthritis&selectedTitle=3~150

Seetharaman, M. (2015). Giant Cell Arteritis (Temporal Arteritis) workup. Retrieved on May 15, 2016, from emedicine.medscape.com/article/332483-workup

Sholter, D. E., & Russell, A. S. (2016). Synovial fluid analysis. Retrieved on May 14, 2016, from www.uptodate.com/contents/synovial-fluid-analysis.

Smith, W. M. (2013). Gender and spondyloarthropathy-associated uveitis. *Journal of Ophthalmology*, *2013*, 928264.

Tan, E. M., Cohen, A. S., Fries, J. F., et al. (1982). The 1982 revised criteria for the classification of systemic lupus erythematosus. *Arthritis and Rheumatism*, *25*(11), 1271–1277.

Varga, J. (2014). Diagnosis and differential diagnosis of systemic sclerosis (scleroderma) in adults. Retrieved from www.uptodate.com/contents/search?search=Diagnosis+and+differential+diagnosis+of+systemic+sclerosis+%28scleroderma%29+in+%09adults&x=14&y=9

Varga, J., & Steen, V. (2015). Pulmonary arterial hypertension in systemic sclerosis (scleroderma): Definition, classification, risk factors, screening and prognosis. Retrieved on May 14, 2016, from www.uptodate.com/contents/table-of-contents/rheumatology/scleroderma.

Yurdakul, F. G., Bodur, H., Sivas, F., et al. (2015). Clinical features, treatment and monitoring in patients with olymyalgiarheumatica. *Archives of Rheumatology*, *30*(1), 28–33.

Resources

American College of Rheumatology and Association of Rheumatology Health Professionals: http://www.rheumatology.org

American Fibromyalgia Syndrome Association, Inc.: http://www.afsafund.org

Arthritis Society (National Office): http://www.arthritis.ca.

Canadian Arthritis Network/Le réseau Canadien de l'arthrite: http://www.arthritisnetwork.ca.

Canadian Spondylitis Association: http://www.spondylitis.ca/en/.

Lupus Canada: http://www.lupuscanada.org.

National Institute of Arthritis and Musculoskeletal and Skin Diseases, National Institutes of Health: http://www.niams.nih.gov

Scleroderma Society of Canada: http://www.scleroderma.ca.

Sjögren's Society of Canada: http://www.sjogrenscanada.org.

Spondylitis Association of America: http://www.spondylitis.org

UNIT 12

Integumentary Function

Case Study MANAGING A PATIENT WITH A PRESSURE ULCER

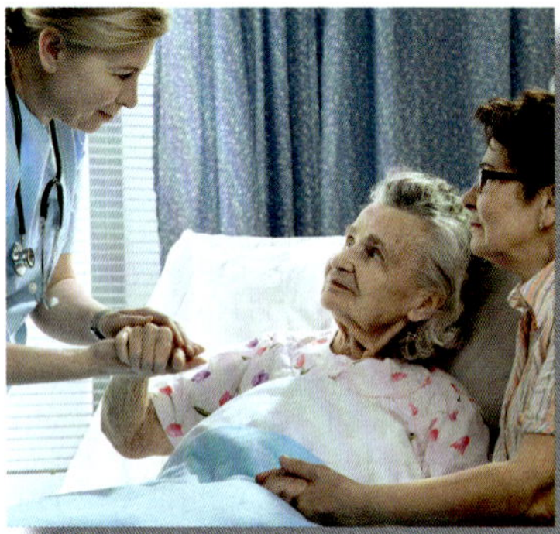

The nurse is caring for an 85-year-old female who was living with her husband at home. The patient was admitted to a medical unit for smoke inhalation after a house fire. While doing a morning assessment, the nurse notes and documents that the patient has a stage II pressure ulcer on her sacral area. No pressure ulcer was documented during the patient's admission assessment. Upon further investigation, the nurse notes that three other patients on this unit in the last 6 months also had stage II and III pressure ulcers that were not documented as present upon hospital admission.

QSEN Competency Focus: Evidence-Based Practice

The complexities inherent in today's health care system challenge nurses to demonstrate integration of specific interdisciplinary core competencies that are aimed at ensuring the delivery of safe and quality patient care (Institute of Medicine, 2003). The Quality and Safety Education for Nurses project (QSEN, 2017; Cronenwett, Sherwood, Barnsteiner, et al., 2007) provides a framework for the knowledge, skills, and attitudes (KSAs) required for nurses to demonstrate competency in these key areas, which include ***patient-centred care***, ***interdisciplinary teamwork and collaboration***, ***evidence-based practice***, ***quality improvement***, ***safety***, and ***informatics.***

The College of Nurses of Ontario (CNO) outlines entry-level practice expectations of the registered nurse. These competencies include self-regulation, professional responsibility and accountability, knowledge-based practice, service to the public, and ethical practice. According to CNO (2014), these competencies are not tasks, but behavioural outcomes "that require the registered nurse to utilize a depth and breadth of knowledge, skill and judgement that allow them safely practice and competently adapt to changes in the health care environment" (CNO, 2014).

Evidence-Based Practice Definition: Integrate best current evidence with clinical expertise and patient/family preferences and values for delivery of optimal health care.

SELECTED PRE-LICENSURE KSAs	APPLICATION AND REFLECTION
Knowledge	
Describe reliable sources for locating evidence reports and clinical practice guidelines.	Identify the sources you would use to find evidence-based reports and clinical guidelines for managing stage II pressure ulcers in this patient as well as others admitted to the medical unit.
Skills	
Read original research and evidence reports related to area of practice. Locate evidence reports related to clinical practice topics and guidelines.	Access the source or sources you have identified, and find research and evidence reports that describe how to best manage this patient's skin breakdown. What is the strength of the evidence for these management strategies? What criteria will you use to judge the strength of the evidence you have identified?
Attitudes	
Appreciate the importance of regularly reading relevant professional journals.	Reflect upon what you learned by engaging in this exercise. Think about how the best evidence you found may change in time. If you were treating a patient with a stage II pressure ulcer in 10 years' time, do you think you would likely be using these same evidence-based guidelines or reports to guide your practice? Why is the nature of clinical practice ever changing?

College of Nurses of Ontario (CNO). (2014). *Entry to practice competencies for Registered Nurses*. Retrieved June 13, 2019, from https://www.cno.org/globalassets/docs/reg/41037_entrytopracitic_final.pdf; Cronenwett, L., Sherwood, G., Barnsteiner, J., et al. (2007). Quality and safety education for nurses. *Nursing Outlook, 55*(3), 122–131; Institute of Medicine. (2003). *Health professions education: A bridge to quality*. Washington, DC: National Academies Press; and QSEN Institute. (2017). *QSEN competencies: Definitions and pre-licensure KSAs*. Retrieved June 12, 2019, from www.qsen.org/competencies/pre-licensure-ksas

57 Assessment of Integumentary Function

Adapted by Carla Wells

Learning Objectives

On completion of this chapter, the learner will be able to:

1. Identify the anatomy and physiology of the integument (skin, hair, nails).
2. Differentiate the composition and function of each skin layer: epidermis, dermis, and subcutaneous tissue.
3. Identify and describe primary and secondary skin lesions by colour, distribution, and configuration (pattern).
4. Recognize common integumentary changes associated with systemic disease.
5. Describe the aging process of the integument and common changes in older adults.
6. List appropriate questions to elicit information during an assessment of the integument.
7. Describe the focus and techniques of physical examination most useful when examining the skin, hair, and nails.
8. Discuss common skin tests and procedures used for diagnosing skin and related disorders.

Introduction

The integument is the largest organ system of the body. In addition to the skin, hair, and nails, it is composed of four types of glands: sweat, oil, ceruminous, and mammary (larger, complex apocrine sweat glands). Because the skin, hair, and nails mirror the general health of the patient, many systemic conditions may be accompanied by dermatologic manifestations. The skin also provides hints of a patient's emotional state (e.g., flushing with nervousness or humiliation) (Amerman, 2016; Martini, Timmons, & Tallitsch, 2012).

Skin disorders are encountered frequently in nursing practice. The psychological stress of illness, incapacitation, or personal and family life challenges are commonly exhibited outwardly as dermatologic conditions. A hospitalized patient may suddenly develop itching and a rash from the treatment regimen. In certain systemic conditions, such as hepatitis, thyroid alterations, and some cancers, dermatologic manifestations may be the first sign of the disorder.

Anatomic and Physiologic Overview

The skin is indispensable for human life. The skin of the integument forms a barrier between internal organs and the external environment, and participates in many vital body functions (e.g., regulation of body temperature). Skin is contiguous with the mucous membrane at the external openings of the digestive, respiratory, and urogenital systems. Because skin disorders are readily visible, dermatologic concerns are commonly the primary reason for a patient to seek health care.

Anatomy of the Skin, Hair, Nails, and Glands of the Skin

The skin is composed of three layers: epidermis, dermis, and subcutaneous tissue (Fig. 57-1).

The epidermis is the outermost layer of stratified epithelial cells and composed predominantly of **keratinocytes**. It ranges in thickness from about 0.1 mm on the eyelids to

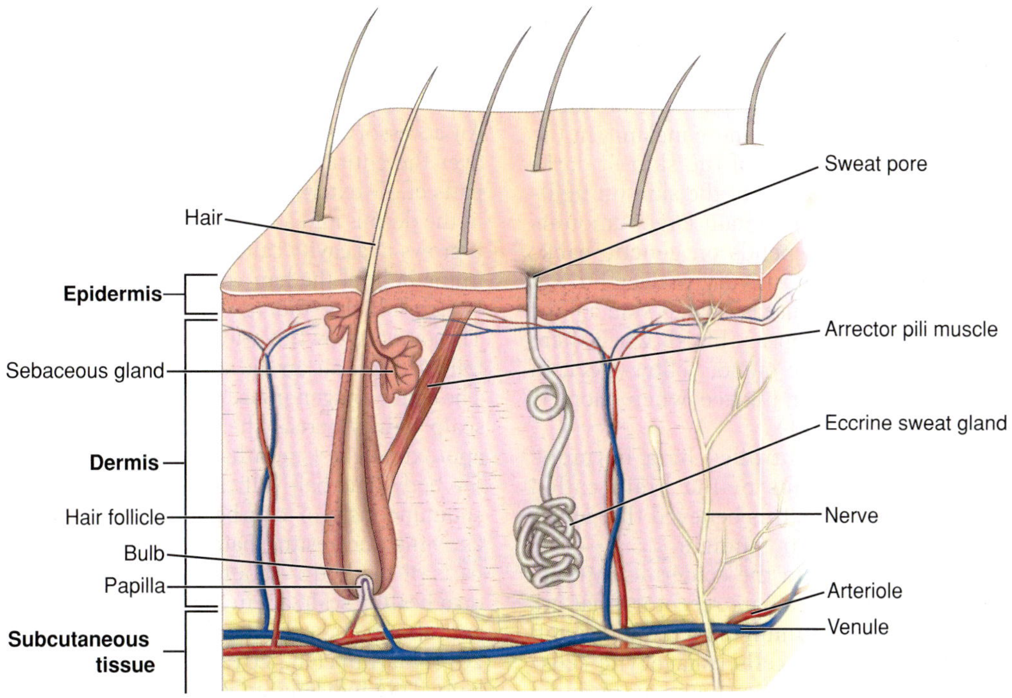

FIGURE 57-1. Anatomic structures of the skin.

about 1.0 mm on the palms of the hands and soles of the feet. Four distinct layers compose the epidermis in thin skin, from innermost to outermost: stratum germinativum, stratum spinosum, stratum granulosum, and stratum corneum. In thick skin (e.g., palms, soles), the stratum lucidum is layered over the stratum granulosum. Every layer becomes more differentiated (i.e., mature and with more specific functions) as it rises from the basal stratum germinativum layer to the outermost stratum corneum layer (Amerman, 2016; Martini et al., 2012).

Epidermis

The epidermis, which is contiguous with mucous membranes, consists of live, continuously dividing cells covered on the surface by dead cells that were originally deeper in the dermis but were pushed upward by the newly developing, more differentiated cells underneath. This external layer is almost completely replaced every 3 to 4 weeks. The dead cells contain large amounts of **keratin**, an insoluble, fibrous protein that forms the outer barrier of the skin and has the capacity to repel pathogens and

Glossary

alopecia: loss of hair from any cause
anagen phase: active phase of hair growth
dermatosis: any skin condition
erythema: redness of the skin caused by congestion of the capillaries
hirsutism: the condition of having excessive hair growth
hyperpigmentation: increase in the melanin of the skin, resulting in increased pigmentation
hypopigmentation: decrease in the melanin of the skin, resulting in diminished pigmentation
keratin: insoluble, fibrous protein the epidermis, hair, nails
keratinocytes: arising from the innermost layer of the epidermis, synthesize the insoluble protein, keratin
Langerhans cells: dendritic clear cells in the epidermis that carry surface receptors for immunoglobulin and complement; active participants in delayed hypersensitivity of the skin
melanin: the substance responsible for colouration of the skin
melanocytes: dendritic clear cells of the epidermis that produce melanin
Merkel cells: tactile cells of the epidermis; transmit sensory messages
petechiae: pinpoint, round, nonelevated red spots that appear on the skin as a result of blood leakage into the skin
rete ridges: undulations and furrows at the dermis–epidermis junction and responsible for cementing together the two layers
sebaceous glands: oil glands in the dermis that secrete sebum to lubricate and keep the skin soft and inhibit bacterial growth; accessory structures of the skin
sebum: fatty secretion of the sebaceous glands; contains epithelial debris
telangiectasia: dilatations of small blood vessels on the skin; spidery or linear
vitiligo: localized or widespread condition characterized by destruction of the melanocytes in circumscribed areas of the skin, resulting in depigmented (white) patches
Wood's light: blue light used for diagnosing skin conditions (e.g., fungus infections)

prevent excessive fluid loss from the body. Keratin is the principal hardening ingredient of the hair and nails.

Melanocytes are special cells of the epidermis that are primarily involved in producing the pigment **melanin**, which colours the skin and hair. The more melanin in the tissue, the darker the colour. Most of the skin of dark-skinned people and the darker areas of the skin on light-skinned people (e.g., the nipple) contain larger amounts of this pigment. Skin colour depends on genetic background and varies from pale, almost ivory, to deep brown, and almost pure black. Systemic disease affects skin colour as well. For example, the skin appears bluish when there is insufficient oxygenation of the blood, yellow-green in people with jaundice, or red or flushed when there is inflammation or fever (Table 57-1).

Production of melanin is controlled by a hormone secreted from the hypothalamus of the brain called *melanocyte-stimulating hormone*. It is believed that melanin can absorb ultraviolet light in sunlight.

Two other cells are common to the epidermis: Merkel and Langerhans cells. **Merkel cells** are receptors that are sensitive to touch and transmit stimuli to the axon through a chemical synapse. **Langerhans cells** (phagocytic cells) are believed to play a significant role in cutaneous immune system reactions. These cells of the afferent immune system both process invading antigens and transport the antigens to the lymph system to activate the T lymphocytes (Amerman, 2016; Martini et al., 2012).

Characteristics of the epidermis vary in different areas of the body. It is thickest over the palms of the hands and soles of the feet and contains increased amounts of keratin. Thickness of the epidermis can increase with use and may result in calluses forming on the hands or corns forming on the feet.

The junction of the epidermis and dermis is an area of many undulations and furrows called **rete** (epidermal) **ridges** that anchor the epidermis to the dermis and permit the free exchange of essential nutrients between the two layers. This interlocking produces contours on the surface of the skin; on the fingertips, they are called *fingerprints* which are an individual's most unique characteristic that does not change (Amerman, 2016; Martini et al., 2012).

Dermis

The dermis is the largest portion of the skin, providing strength and structure. It is composed of two layers: papillary and reticular. The papillary layer lies directly beneath the epidermis and is composed primarily of fibroblast cells capable of producing one form of collagen, a component of connective tissue. The reticular layer lies beneath the papillary layer and also produces collagen and elastic bundles. The dermis contains blood and lymph vessels, nerves, sweat and sebaceous glands, and hair follicles.

Subcutaneous Tissue

The subcutaneous tissue (hypodermis) is the innermost layer of the skin. It is primarily adipose tissue, which provides a cushion between the skin layers, muscles, and bones. It promotes skin mobility, moulds body contours, and insulates the body. Fat is deposited and distributed according to the individual's gender and in part accounts for the difference in body shape between men and women. Overeating results in increased deposition of fat beneath the skin. The subcutaneous tissues and amount of fat deposited are important factors in body temperature regulation.

Hair

An accessory structure of the integument, hair is present over the entire body except for the palms, soles, lips, and parts of the external genitalia. Hair consists of a root formed in the dermis and a hair shaft that projects beyond the skin. It grows in a cavity called a *hair follicle*. Proliferation of cells in the bulb of the hair causes the hair to form (Fig. 57-1).

Hair follicles undergo cycles of active and resting cycles. The rate of growth varies; beard growth is the most rapid, followed by hair on the scalp, axillae, thighs, and eyebrows. The active **anagen phase** (growth) may last up to 6 years for scalp hair, whereas the telogen (resting) phase lasts for approximately 4 months. During telogen, hair sheds from the body. The hair follicle recycles into the growing phase spontaneously or can be induced by plucking out hairs. Growing and resting hair can be found side by side on all parts of the body. About 90% of the 100,000 hair follicles on a healthy scalp are in the growing phase at any one time, and about 50 scalp hairs are shed each day (Amerman, 2016; Martini et al., 2012). Sustained loss of more than 100 hairs daily indicates an unhealthy situation.

A small bulge on the side of the hair follicle houses the stem cells that migrate down to the follicle root and begin the cycle of reproducing the hair shaft. These bulges also contain the stem cells that migrate upward to reproduce skin (Amerman, 2016; Martini et al., 2012). The location of these cells on the side of the hair shaft rather than at the base is a factor in hair loss. In conditions in which inflammation causes damage to the root of the hair, regrowth is possible; if inflammation damages the bulge on the side, stem cells are destroyed and hair does not grow.

In certain locations on the body, hair growth is controlled by sex hormones. The most vivid example is the growth of hair on the face (i.e., beard and moustache), chest, and back, which is controlled by the male hormones (androgens). Some women with higher levels of testosterone have hair in areas generally considered to be masculine (e.g., face, chest, and lower abdomen). Often a genetic variation, if it appears along with irregular menses and weight changes, it may indicate a hormonal imbalance.

Hirsutism (excessive hair growth) is distressing for women who often consider it to be a taboo subject (Weber & Kelley, 2018). Most often associated with polycystic ovary syndrome, up to 15% of women with the condition have no identifiable cause, yet the effects are negative self-worth, relationship difficulties, and emotional stress (Weber & Kelley, 2018).

Hair in different parts of the body serves different functions. The terminal hairs of the eyes (i.e., eyebrows and eye lashes), nose, and ears filter out dust, microorganisms, and airborne debris. The hair of the skin provides thermal insulation in furry mammals; during cold or fright piloerection occurs (i.e., hairs stand on end), caused by contraction of tiny erector muscles attached to hair follicles. The piloerector response that occurs in humans ("goose bumps") is not comparably insulating (Amerman, 2016; Martini et al., 2012).

Hair colour is genetically determined. Grey or white hair reflects the loss of pigment. Hair quantity and distribution can be affected by endocrine conditions. For

TABLE 57-1 Select Cutaneous Manifestations of Systemic Diseases

Common cutaneous manifestations of systemic diseases include *pruritus* (itching), which may result from chronic renal disease, scabies, pediculosis (lice), obstructive biliary disease with jaundice, Hodgkin's or non-Hodgkin's lymphoma, or medication reactions; *pallor*, which suggests anemia or a cardiopulmonary disorder; and *skin thickening and hardening*, such as that which occurs with scleroderma and dermatomyositis.

	Manifestation	Systemic Disease
Scale 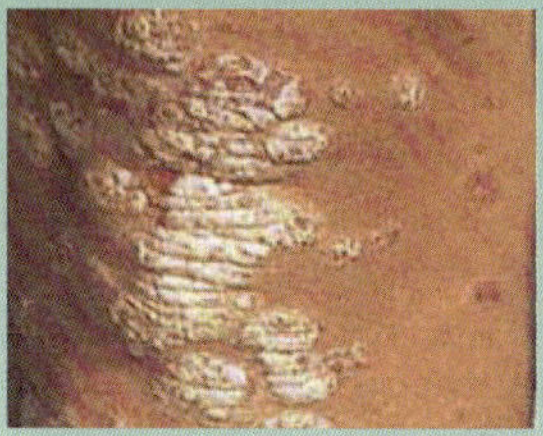	Plaques with scales (on the anterior knee, posterior elbow)	Psoriasis
Ecchymosis 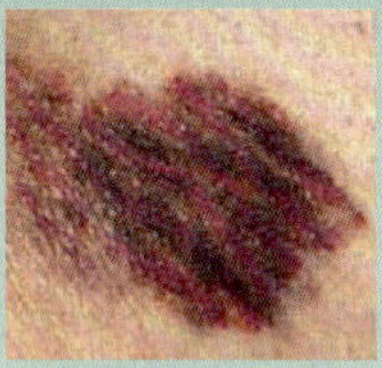 **Purpura** 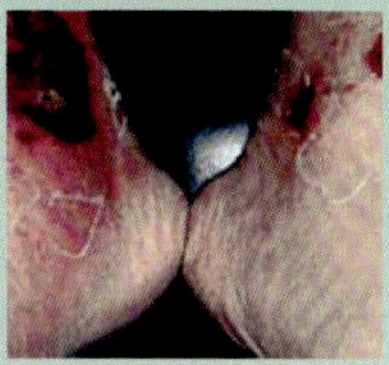	Ecchymosis (bruise) and purpura (bleeding into the skin)	Platelet disorder, vessel fragility
Urticaria 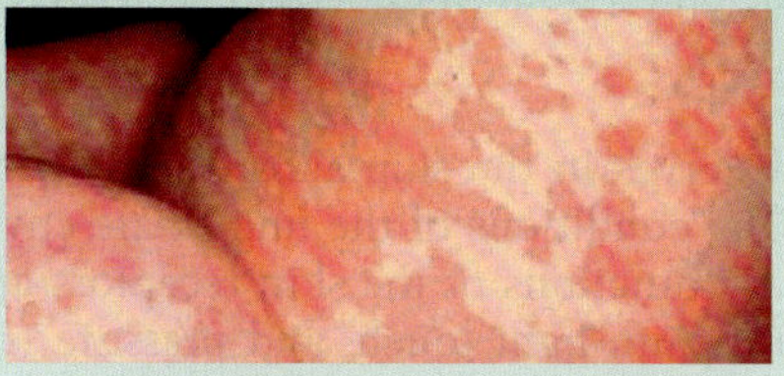	Urticaria (wheals or hives)	Infections, allergic reactions
Plaque 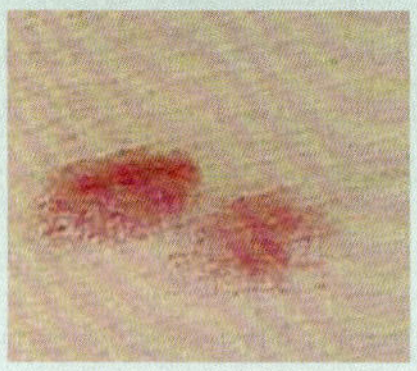 **Nodule** 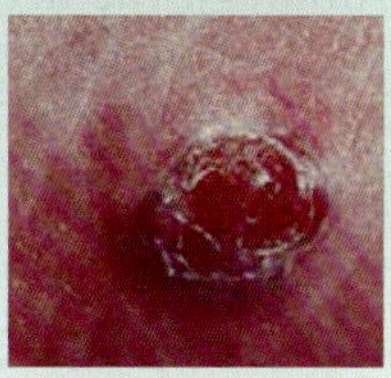	Cutaneous lesions: blue-red or dark brown plaques and nodules	Kaposi's sarcoma
Café-au-lait spot 	Macular, tan café-au-lait spots	Neurocutaneous disorders, such as neurofibromatosis type 1 (von Recklinghausen's disease)
Ulcerated lesion 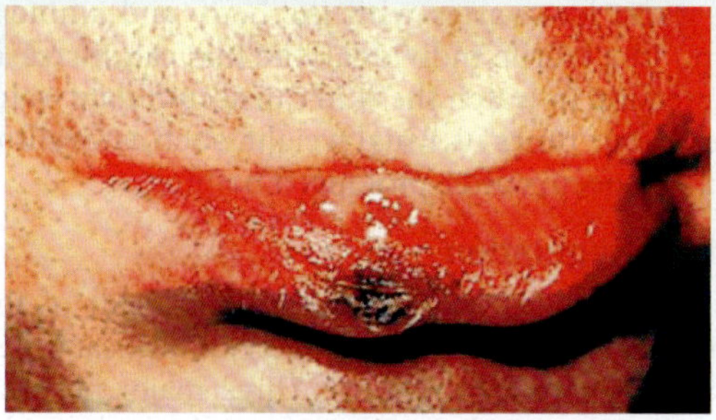	Painless chancre or ulcerated lesion	Syphilis

example, Cushing's syndrome causes hirsutism (excessive hair growth, especially in women), and hypothyroidism (underactive thyroid) causes changes in hair texture. In many cases, chemotherapy and radiation therapy cause hair thinning or weakening of the hair shaft, resulting in partial or complete **alopecia** (hair loss) from the scalp and other parts of the body.

Nails

On dorsal surfaces of fingers and toes, a hard, transparent plate of keratin, called the *nail*, overlies the skin. The nail grows from its root, an epithelial fold called the *cuticle*. The nail preserves the highly developed sensory functions of fingers and toes, such as picking up small objects.

Nail growth is continuous throughout life. Growth is faster in fingernails than toenails, with an average growth of 0.5 mm weekly and slows with aging (Amerman, 2016). Complete renewal of a fingernail takes about 170 days, whereas toenail renewal takes 12 to 18 months (Weber & Kelley, 2018).

Glands of the Skin

Two types of skin glands exist: sebaceous glands and sweat glands (Fig. 57-1). **Sebaceous glands** are associated with hair follicles. Ducts of the sebaceous glands empty **sebum** (oily secretion) into the space between the hair follicle and the hair shaft. For each hair, there is a sebaceous gland whose secretions lubricate the hair and render the skin soft and pliable.

Sweat glands are located in the skin over most of the body surface, and are heavily concentrated in the palms of the hands and soles of the feet. Only the glans penis, the margins of the lips, external ear, and nail bed are devoid of sweat glands. Sweat glands are subclassified into two categories: eccrine and apocrine.

Eccrine sweat glands are found in all areas of the skin. Their ducts open directly onto the skin surface. The thin, watery secretion called *sweat* is produced in the basal coiled portion of the eccrine gland and released into its narrow duct. Sweat is composed of predominantly water and contains about one half of the salt content of the blood plasma. Sweat is released from eccrine glands in response to elevated ambient temperature and elevated body temperature. The rate of sweat secretion is controlled by the sympathetic nervous system. Excessive sweating of the palms and soles, axillae, forehead, and other areas may occur in response to pain and stress.

Apocrine sweat glands are larger, and unlike eccrine glands, secrete odoriferous sweat. Located in the axillae, anal region, scrotum, and labia majora, their ducts generally open onto hair follicles. Apocrine glands become active at puberty. In women, they enlarge and recede with each menstrual cycle. Apocrine glands produce a milky sweat that is sometimes broken down by bacteria to produce the characteristic underarm odour. Specialized apocrine glands called *ceruminous glands* are found in the external ear, where they produce cerumen (wax).

Functions of the Skin

Protection

The skin covering most of the body is no more than 1 mm thick, but it provides very effective protection against invasion by bacteria and other foreign matter. Thickened skin of the palms and soles protects against the effects of the constant trauma that occurs in these areas.

The epidermis is the outermost layer of skin and is composed of several layers of keratinocytes that change character as they migrate to the surface. The stratum corneum, the outer layer of the epidermis, provides the most effective barrier to epidermal water loss and penetration of environmental factors such as chemicals, microbes, and insect bites.

Various lipids are synthesized in the stratum corneum and are the basis for the barrier function of this layer. These long-chain lipids are better suited than phospholipids for water resistance. The presence of these lipids in the stratum corneum creates a relatively impermeable barrier for water egress and for the entry of toxins, microbes, and other substances that come in contact with the surface of the skin.

Some substances do penetrate the skin but meet resistance in trying to move through the channels between the cell layers of the stratum corneum. Microbes and fungi, which are part of the body's usual flora, cannot penetrate unless there is a break in the skin barrier.

The dermis–epidermis junction is the basal layer composed of collagen. The basal layer serves four functions: acts as a scaffold for tissue organization and a template for regeneration; provides selective permeability for filtration of serum; creates a physical barrier between different types of cells; and binds the epithelium to underlying cell layers.

Sensation

Receptor endings of nerves in the skin allow the body to constantly monitor the conditions of the immediate environment. The primary functions of the skin receptors are to sense temperature, pain, light touch, and pressure (or heavy touch). Different nerve endings respond to each different stimulus. Although the nerve endings are distributed over the entire body, they are more concentrated in some areas than in others. For example, fingertips are more densely innervated than skin on the back.

Fluid Balance

The stratum corneum (outermost layer of the epidermis) has the capacity to absorb water, preventing excessive loss of water and electrolytes from the internal body and retaining moisture in the subcutaneous tissues. When skin is damaged, as occurs with a severe burn, large quantities of fluids and electrolytes may be lost rapidly, possibly leading to circulatory collapse, shock, and death.

Skin is not completely impermeable to water. Small amounts of water continuously evaporate from the skin surface. This evaporation, called *insensible perspiration*, amounts to approximately 600 mL daily in a healthy adult. Insensible water loss varies with the body and ambient temperature. In a febrile individual, the loss can increase. During immersion in water, the skin can accumulate water up to three or four times its usual weight, such as swelling of the skin that occurs after prolonged bathing.

Temperature Regulation

The body continuously produces heat as a result of the metabolism of food, which produces energy. This heat is dissipated primarily through the skin. Three major physical processes are involved in loss of heat from the body to the environment. First, radiation transfers heat to another object of lower temperature situated at a distance. Second, conduction transfers heat from the body to a cooler object in contact with it. Heat transferred by conduction to the air surrounding the body is removed by the third process, convection, which moves warm air molecules away from the body.

Evaporation from the skin aids heat loss by conduction. Heat is conducted through the skin into water molecules on its surface, causing the water to evaporate. The water on the skin surface may be from insensible perspiration, sweat, or the environment.

All mechanisms for heat loss are used, but when the ambient temperature is very high, radiation and convection are ineffective, and evaporation becomes the only means for heat loss.

Under usual conditions, metabolic heat production is balanced by heat loss. The internal temperature of the body is maintained constant at approximately 37°C. The rate of heat loss depends primarily on the surface temperature of the skin, which is a function of the skin blood flow. Under usual conditions, the total blood circulated through the skin is approximately 450 mL/min, or 10 to 20 times the amount of blood required to provide necessary metabolites and oxygen. The sympathetic nervous system primarily controls blood flow through skin vessels. Increased blood flow to the skin results in more heat delivered to the skin and a greater rate of heat loss from the body. In contrast, decreased skin blood flow reduces the skin temperature and helps to conserve heat for the body. When the temperature of the body begins to fall, as occurs on a cold day, the blood vessels of the skin constrict, reducing body heat.

Sweating is another process by which the body regulates the rate of heat loss. Sweating does not occur until the core body temperature exceeds 37°C, regardless of skin temperature. In extremely hot environments, the rate of sweat production may be as high as 1 L/hr. Under some circumstances (e.g., emotional stress) sweating may occur as a reflex and is unrelated to a need to lose body heat.

Vitamin Production

Skin exposed to ultraviolet light can convert substances necessary for synthesizing vitamin D_3 (cholecalciferol). Vitamin D is essential for preventing osteoporosis and rickets, which are conditions that cause bone deformities and result from deficiency of vitamin D, calcium, and phosphorus. In Canada, the only natural sources of vitamin D in the food supply are egg yolks and fatty fish (Health Canada, 2014). Vitamin D is required for healthy muscles and may prevent some types of cancers such as colorectal and breast (Canadian Cancer Society, 2014). Canada's northern geographic location does affect population exposure to ultraviolet light, resulting in inadequate ultraviolet exposure during the year. Osteoporosis Canada (2014) recommends year-round dietary supplements of vitamin D. Infants living in northern Canada require dietary supplements of 400 IU of vitamin D daily (Health Canada, 2014). The recommended daily intake for children and adults 9 to 50 years is 600 IU (Health Canada, 2014). For adults >50 years, Health Canada (2014) recommends 400 IU of vitamin D per day, and 600 IU daily for women who are pregnant or lactating. The Canadian Cancer Society recommends that adult Canadians take 1,000 IU of vitamin D_3 daily (2014). An upper limit of vitamin D_3 allows room for obtaining vitamin D from food sources such as milk, multivitamins, and the sun but varies between 2,000 and 4,000 IU, depending on the authoritative source (Canadian Cancer Society, 2014; Health Canada, 2014).

Immune Response Function

The skin functions not only as a barrier defence against environmental hazards, but also produces immune responses. The skin has the capacity to generate innate and adaptive immune responses (Bolognia, Jorizzo, & Schaffer, 2012). Innate immune functions of the skin include the closely packed layers of the stratum corneum, the nonspecific inflammatory response of pattern recognition receptors, and a chemical environment that inhibits microbial colonization (Grossman & Porth, 2014). The Langerhans cells of the skin are part of adaptive immunity. They function as antigen-presenting cells, with the ability to transport foreign substances to nearby lymph nodes for cell-mediated immune reaction (Grossman & Porth, 2014).

Gerontologic Considerations

The skin undergoes many physiologic changes associated with aging. A lifetime of excessive sun exposure, systemic diseases, and inadequate nutrition can increase the range of skin conditions and the rapidity with which they appear. In addition, certain medications (e.g., antihistamines, antibiotics, diuretics, antidepressants, antipsychotics, and antidiabetic preparations) are photosensitizing and increase the damage that results from sun exposure (Canadian Dermatology Association, 2014a). An increasing vulnerability to injury and certain diseases is the outcome. Skin conditions are common among older adults (Stephen, 2012), but signs of older adult abuse need to be differentiated (e.g., welts on palms or soles, knuckle-shaped bruises, multiple scars) (Yaffe & Tazkarji, 2012).

Significant changes occur with aging. Major changes in the skin of older adults include dryness, wrinkling, uneven pigmentation, and various proliferative lesions. Cellular changes associated with aging include a thinning at the junction of the dermis and epidermis which results in fewer anchoring sites between the two skin layers; even minor injury or stress to the epidermis can cause it to shear away from the dermis, a phenomenon that may account for the increased vulnerability of aged skin to trauma. With increasing age, the epidermis and dermis thin and flatten, causing wrinkles, sagging, and overlapping skin folds (Fig. 57-2) (Grossman & Porth, 2014; Martini et al., 2012).

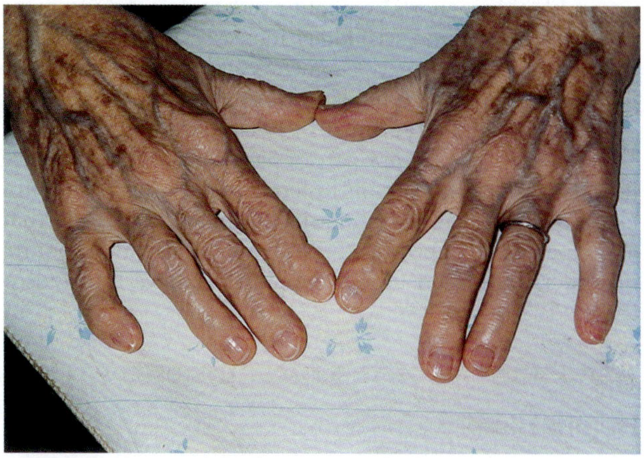

FIGURE 57-2. Hands with wrinkling and overlapping folds common to aging skin.

CHART 57-1

Benign Changes in Skin of Older Adults

- Cherry angiomas (bright red "moles")
- Diminished hair, especially on scalp and pubic area
- Dyschromias (colour variations)
  Solar lentigo (liver spots)
  Melasma (dark discolouration of the skin)
  Lentigines (freckles)
- Neurodermatitis (itchy spots)
- Seborrheic keratoses (crusty brown "stuck-on" greasy patches)
- Spider angiomas
- Telangiectasias (spidery or linear red marks on skin caused by stretching of the superficial blood vessels)
- Wrinkles
- Xerosis (dryness)
- Xanthelasma (yellowish waxy deposits on upper and lower eyelids)

Loss of the subcutaneous tissue substances of elastin, collagen, and subcutaneous fat diminishes the protection and cushioning of underlying tissues and organs, decreases muscle tone, and results in the loss of the insulating properties of fat.

Cellular replacement slows as a result of aging. As dermal layers thin, skin becomes fragile and transparent. The blood supply to the skin also changes with age. Vessels, especially the capillary loops, decrease in number and size. These vascular changes contribute to delayed wound healing, commonly seen in older adults. Sweat and sebaceous glands decrease in number and functional capacity, leading to dry and scaly skin. Reduced hormonal levels of androgens are thought to contribute to declining sebaceous gland function (Bolognia et al., 2012).

Hair growth gradually diminishes, especially over the lower legs and dorsum of the feet. Thinning is common in the scalp, axillae, and pubic areas. Other functions affected by normal aging include the barrier function of skin, sensory perception, and thermoregulation.

Photoaging (damage from excessive sun exposure), has detrimental effects on the aging of skin. A lifetime of outdoor work or outdoor activities (e.g., construction work, lifeguarding, sunbathing, sports) without prudent use of sunscreens can lead to profound wrinkling; increased loss of elasticity; mottled, pigmented areas; cutaneous atrophy; and benign or malignant lesions (Canadian Dermatology Association, 2014b; Grossman & Porth, 2014; Weber & Kelley, 2018).

Many skin lesions are part of aging. Recognizing these lesions enables the patient to feel less anxious about skin changes. Chart 57-1 summarizes some skin lesions that are expected to appear as the skin ages and which require no special attention unless the skin becomes infected or irritated.

Assessment of the Integument

Health History

Initiate the health history interview by collecting identifying data and acquiring a general impression of the overall health of the patient. Inquire about any family and personal history of medications, or chemicals; previous skin disorders, skin cancer, skin allergies, and allergic reactions to food (Mansen & Gabiola, 2015). Ongoing research is considering the success of developing tolerance from infancy based on the timing of introducing solid food (Abrams & Becker, 2013). Obtain the names of cosmetics, soaps, shampoos, and other personal hygiene products if there have been any recent skin conditions noticed with the use of these products. Perform a symptom/sign analysis of the patient's presenting integumentary concern. Determine the location and spread of the condition, the nature of any discomfort (e.g., pain, itching), the intensity or severity of discomfort, and the onset, frequency, and timing. Ask about aggravating and alleviating factors as well as associated symptoms. Determine if environmental factors are involved and explore the significance of the condition for the patient. Finally, ask what the patient thinks is the cause. Chart 57-2 lists selected questions useful in obtaining appropriate information. Chart 57-3 provides genetic factors influencing skin conditions.

CHART 57-2

Assessment: Assessing for Skin Disorders

Patient history relevant to skin disorders may be obtained by asking the following questions:

- When did you first notice this skin problem? (In addition, investigate duration and intensity.)
- Has it occurred previously?
- Are there any other symptoms?
- What site was first affected?
- What did the rash or lesion look like when it first appeared?
- Where and how fast did it spread?
- Do you have any itching, burning, tingling, or crawling sensations?
- Is there any loss of sensation?
- Is the problem worse at a particular time or season?
- How do you think it started?
- Do you have a history of hay fever, asthma, hives, eczema, or allergies?
- Who in your family has skin problems or rashes?
- Did the eruptions appear after certain foods were eaten? Which foods?
- When the problem occurred, had you recently consumed alcohol?
- What relation do you think there may be between a specific event and the outbreak of the rash or lesion?
- What medications are you taking?
- What topical medication (ointment, cream, salve) have you put on the lesion (including over-the-counter medications)?
- What skin products or cosmetics do you use?
- What is your occupation?
- What in your immediate environment (plants, animals, chemicals, infections) might be precipitating this disorder? Is there anything new, or are there any changes in the environment?
- Does anything touching your skin cause a rash?
- How has this affected you (or your life)?
- Is there anything else you wish to talk about in regard to this disorder?

GENETICS IN NURSING PRACTICE

Chart 57-3. Integumentary Conditions

Examples of integumentary conditions influenced by genetic factors include the following:

Autosomal Dominant:
- Ehlers–Danlos
- Legius syndrome
- Loeys–Dietz syndrome
- Neurofibromatosis type 1
- Tuberous sclerosis

Autosomal Recessive:
- Albinism
- Congenital ichthyosis

X-Linked Dominant:
- Incontinentia pigmenti

X-Linked Recessive:
- Hypohidrotic ectodermal dysplasia
- Pseudoxanthoma elasticum

Inheritance pattern is not distinct; however, there is a genetic predisposition for the disease:
- Ectodermal dysplasias
- Eczema
- Port wine stain
- Psoriasis

Nursing Assessments

FAMILY HISTORY ASSESSMENT
- Assess for other closely related family members with integumentary impairment or alterations.
- Inquire about the nature and type of skin lesions and age at onset (e.g., skin involvement with incontinentia pigmenti occurs in the first few weeks of life with blistering of the skin, whereas lesions of neurofibromatosis type 1 may appear in early childhood through adulthood).
- Note gender of affected individuals (e.g., mostly females with incontinentia pigmenti, mostly males with hypohidrotic ectodermal dysplasia).
- Inquire about the presence of other clinical features, such as unusual hair, teeth, or nails; thrombocytopenia; recurrent infections.

PHYSICAL EXAMINATION
- Assess for related clinical features, such as sparse eyebrows and eyelashes, unusually shaped teeth, alopecia, nail changes (e.g., hypohidrotic ectodermal dysplasia).
- Assess for related alterations in vision, such as nystagmus, strabismus; albinism; retinal changes (e.g., pseudoxanthoma elasticum); Lisch nodules and/or optic glioma (neurofibromatosis type 1).

MANAGEMENT ISSUES SPECIFIC TO GENETICS
- Inquire whether DNA mutation or other genetic testing has been performed on affected family members.
- If indicated, refer for further genetic counselling and evaluation so that family members can discuss heredity, risk to other family members, availability of genetic testing, and gene-based interventions.
- Offer appropriate genetic information and resources.
- Assess patient's understanding of genetic information.
- Provide support to families with newly diagnosed genetic-related integumentary conditions.
- Participate in management and coordination of care for patients with genetic conditions and for individuals predisposed to develop or pass on a genetic condition.

GENETIC RESOURCES FOR NURSES AND THEIR PATIENTS ON THE WEB
Canadian Association of Genetic Counsellors (CAGC): http://www.cagc-accg.ca—A listing of genetic centres across Canada

Canadian Cancer Society: http://www.cancer.ca—Information on the genetic factors/risks and genetic testing

Canadian Directory of Genetic Support Groups: http://www.lhsc.on.ca/programs/medgenet—Resource guide for families and professionals

Canadian Genetic Diseases Network: http://www.cgdn.ca—Its stated mission is to be the primary catalyst in advancing Canada's scientific and commercial competitiveness in genetic research and the application of genetic discoveries to the prevention, diagnosis, and treatment of human disease

Canadian Organization for Rare Disorders (CORD): http://www.cord.ca—Information on over 6,000 rare disorders and links individuals/families together with the same rare disorder

GeneTests: http://www.genetests.org—Publicly funded medical genetic information resource developed for physicians, other health care providers, and researchers

Genetic Alliance: http://www.geneticalliance.org—Increases the capacity of genetic advocacy groups to achieve their missions and leverages the voices of millions of individuals and families living with genetic conditions

Genetics Society of Canada (GSC): http://life.biology.mcmaster.ca/GSC/—Promotes research and communicates the results and implications of genetics to the public

OMIM Online Mendelian Inheritance in Man: http://www.ncbi.nlm.nih.gov/entrez/query.fcgi?db=OMIM—Catalogue of human genes and genetic disorders

Unfolding Patient Stories: Vincent Brody • Part 2

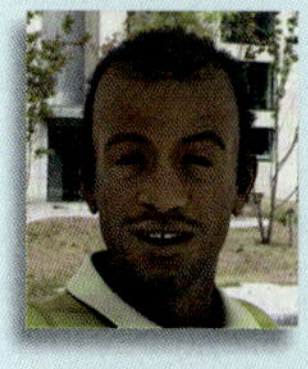

Recall from Chapter 4 Vincent Brody, with chronic obstructive pulmonary disease (COPD), who spends most of the day in a recliner chair smoking and has a poor nutritional intake due to shortness of breath. He is admitted to the hospital with COPD exacerbation. What are the factors related to his diagnosis? What background information can influence skin breakdown? Describe the skin assessment performed by the nurse.

Care for Vincent and other patients in a realistic virtual environment: ***vSim** for Nursing* **(thepoint.lww.com/vSimMedicalSurgical)**. Practice documenting these patients' care in DocuCare **(thepoint.lww.com/DocuCareEHR)**.

Physical Examination

Assessment of the integument involves the entire skin area, mucous membranes, scalp, hair, and nails. The skin reflects an individual's overall health, and alterations commonly correspond to disease in other organ systems. Use inspection and palpation to examine the integument. Find a well-lit and warm environment. Take advantage of a penlight to study lesions. Instruct the patient to disrobe and ensure adequate draping. If you anticipate palpating a rash or skin lesions, wear disposable gloves when initiating the examination. Explain that this is routine practice; it is important to avoid making the patient feel as if he or she cannot be touched. Touching skin lesions indicates a level of acceptance of the patient.

Inspection and Palpation

Inspect and palpate the skin, hair, and nails. Pay attention to colour and vascularity; palpate for temperature, mobility, turgor, moisture, texture, and edema. Inspect and palpate the condition of the hair and nails. Use gloves for inspecting the hair, not only to be protected if lice or mites are discovered, but also to avoid contact with skin lesions. Lice are the most common parasitic infestation in children and lice resistance to topical treatment is increasingly common (Smith & Goldman, 2012). Focus on the colour, distribution, and configuration (pattern) of any skin lesions.

Skin colour varies from person to person, ranging from ivory to deep brown to almost pure black. The skin of exposed portions of the body, especially in sunny, warm climates, tends to be more pigmented than the rest of the body. The vasodilation that occurs with fever, sunburn, and inflammation produces a pink or reddish hue to the skin. Pallor is absent or diminished skin colour and vascularity, and is best observed in the conjunctivae, around the mouth, on the hard palate, or the ear lobes.

The bluish hue of cyanosis indicates cellular hypoxia and is easily observed in the extremities, nail beds, lips, and mucous membranes. Jaundice, a yellowing of the skin, is directly related to an elevation in serum bilirubin and is often first observed in the sclerae and mucous membranes (Fig. 57-3).

Erythema

Erythema is redness of the skin caused by the congestion of capillaries. In light-skinned people, it is easily observed wherever it appears. Always inspect for colour changes before palpating, otherwise changes may be missed. To determine possible inflammation, palpate the skin for increased warmth, edema, or hardness (intracellular infiltration). Because dark skin tends to assume a purple-grey cast when an inflammatory process is present, it may be difficult to detect erythema; inspect the palms and soles in a dark-skinned individual.

Rash

When the patient reports itching (pruritus), ask the patient to indicate which areas of the body are involved. Stretch the skin gently to decrease the reddish tone and make the rash more visible. Pointing a penlight laterally across the skin may highlight the rash, making it easier to observe. Palpate for differences in skin texture by running the tips of the fingers lightly over the skin. The borders of a rash may be palpable. Include the patient's mouth and ears in the examination. (Sometimes, rubeola [measles] causes a red cast to appear on the tip of the ears.) Measure the patient's temperature and palpate the lymph nodes.

Cyanosis

Cyanosis is the bluish discolouration that results from a lack of oxygen in the blood. It appears with shock, or with respiratory or circulatory compromise. In people with light skin, cyanosis manifests as a bluish hue to the lips, fingertips, and nail beds (Fig. 57-3). Other indications of decreased tissue perfusion include cold, clammy skin; a rapid, thready pulse; and rapid, shallow respirations. Examine the conjunctivae of the eyelids for pallor and **petechiae** (pinpoint red spots that appear on the skin as a result of blood leakage into the skin). In a person with dark skin, the skin usually assumes a greyish cast. To detect cyanosis, observe the areas around the mouth, lips, hard palate, over the cheekbones, palms, soles, and earlobes.

Colour Changes

Almost every process that occurs in the skin causes some colour change. For example, **hypopigmentation** (decrease in the melanin of the skin, resulting in a loss of pigmentation) may be caused by a fungal infection, eczema, or **vitiligo** (a condition characterized by nonfunctional melanocytes in circumscribed areas of the skin, resulting in white patches) (Grossman & Porth, 2014). **Hyperpigmentation** (increase in the melanin of the skin, resulting in increased pigmentation) may occur as a result of aging, disease or injury to the skin (postinflammatory), or sun injury.

Changes in skin colour in individuals with dark skin are more noticeable and may cause more concern because the discolouration is more readily visible. Some variation in skin pigment levels is expected. Examples include the pigmented crease across the bridge of the nose, pigmented streaks in the nails, and pigmented spots on the sclera of the eye. Many variations of colour are genetically determined (Grossman & Porth, 2014; Weber & Kelley, 2018).

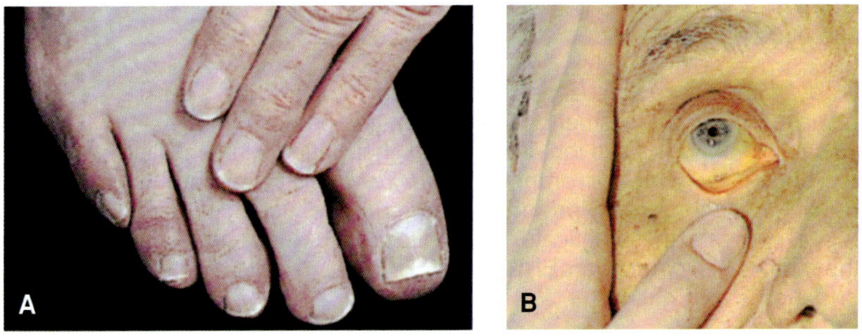

FIGURE 57-3. Examples of skin colour changes: (**A**) the bluish tint of cyanosis and (**B**) the yellow hue of jaundice. (From Weber, J. W., & Kelley, J. (2014). *Health assessment in nursing* (5th ed.). Philadelphia, PA: Lippincott Williams & Wilkins.)

Assessing Patients With Dark Skin

Colour gradations that occur in dark skin are largely determined by genetics; they may be described as light, medium, or dark. In individuals with dark skin, melanin is produced at a faster rate and in larger quantities than in people with light skin. Healthy dark skin has a reddish base or undertone. Inspect for it. The buccal mucosa, tongue, lips, and nails are pink. The degree of pigmentation of the patient's skin may affect the appearance of a lesion. Lesions may be black, purple, or grey instead of the tan or red seen in patients with light skin. Dark pigment responds with discolouration after injury or inflammation, and patients with dark skin more often experience postinflammatory hyperpigmentation than those with lighter skin. The hyperpigmentation eventually fades but may require months or a year.

In general, people with dark skin suffer the same skin conditions as those with light skin. They are less likely to have skin cancer but more likely to have keloid or scar formation, and disorders resulting from occlusion or blockage of hair follicles.

Table 57-2 provides an overview of colour changes in light-skinned and dark-skinned people, and the following section provides specific guidelines for assessing dark and light skin.

TABLE 57-2 Colour Changes in Light and Dark Skin

Etiology	Light Skin	Dark Skin
Pallor		
Anemia—decreased hematocrit		
Shock—decreased perfusion, vasoconstriction	Generalized pallor	Brown skin appears yellow-brown, dull; black skin appears ashen grey, dull. (Observe areas with least pigmentation: conjunctivae, mucous membranes.)
Local arterial insufficiency	Marked localized pallor (lower extremities, especially when elevated)	Ashen grey, dull; cool to palpation
Albinism—total absence of pigment melanin	Whitish pink	Tan, cream, white
Vitiligo—a condition characterized by destruction of the melanocytes in circumscribed areas of the skin (may be localized or widespread)	Patchy, milky white spots, often symmetric bilaterally	Same
Cyanosis		
Increased amount of unoxygenated hemoglobin:	Dusky blue	Dark but dull, lifeless; only severe cyanosis is apparent in skin, and may appear greyish. (Observe conjunctivae, oral mucosa, nail beds.)
Central—chronic heart and lung diseases cause arterial desaturation	Nail beds dusky	
Peripheral—exposure to cold, anxiety		
Erythema		
Hyperemia—increased blood flow through engorged arterial vessels, as in inflammation, fever, alcohol intake, blushing	Red, bright pink	Purplish-grey tinge, but difficult to see. (Palpate for increased warmth with inflammation, taut skin, and hardening of deep tissues.)
Polycythemia—increased red blood cells, capillary stasis	Ruddy blue in face, oral mucosa, conjunctivae, hands and feet	Well concealed by pigment. (Observe for redness in lips.)
Carbon monoxide poisoning	Bright, cherry red in face and upper torso	Cherry red nail beds, lips, and oral mucosa
Venous stasis—decreased blood flow from area, engorged venules	Dusky rubor of dependent extremities (a prelude to necrosis with pressure ulcer)	Easily masked. (Use palpation to identify warmth or edema.)
Jaundice		
Increased serum bilirubin concentration (>2 mg/dL) due to liver dysfunction or hemolysis, as after severe burns or some infections	Yellow first in sclerae, hard palate, and mucous membranes; then over skin	Check sclerae for yellow near limbus; do not mistake normal yellowish fatty deposits in the periphery under eyelids for jaundice. (Jaundice is best noted at junction of hard and soft palate, on palms.)
Carotenemia—increased level of serum carotene from ingestion of large amounts of carotene-rich foods	Yellow-orange tinge in forehead, palms and soles, and nasolabial folds, but no yellowing in sclerae or mucous membranes	Yellow-orange tinge in palms and soles
Uremia—kidney injury causes retained urochrome pigments in the blood	Orange-green or grey overlying pallor of anemia; may also have ecchymoses and purpura	Easily masked. (Rely on laboratory and clinical findings.)
Brown-Tan		
Addison disease—cortisol deficiency stimulates increased melanin production	Bronzed appearance, an "external tan"; most apparent around nipples, perineum, genitalia, and pressure points (inner thighs, buttocks, elbows, axillae)	Easily masked. (Rely on laboratory and clinical findings.)
Café-au-lait spots—caused by increased melanin pigment in basal cell layer	Tan to light brown, irregularly shaped, oval patch with well-defined borders	Often not visible in the very dark-skinned person

Adapted from Taylor, S. C., Kelly, A. P., Lim, H., et al. (2014). *Dermatology for skin of color* (2nd ed.). New York: McGraw-Hill Medical.

Assessing Skin Lesions

Skin lesions are the most prominent characteristics of dermatologic conditions. They vary in size, shape, and cause and are classified according to their appearance and origin. Skin lesions can be described as primary or secondary. Primary lesions are the initial lesions and are characteristic of the disease itself. Secondary lesions result from changes in primary lesions resulting from external causes, such as scratching, trauma, infections, or changes caused by wound healing. Depending on the stage of development, skin lesions are further categorized by type and appearance (Table 57-3).

TABLE 57-3 Primary and Secondary Skin Lesions

Lesion	Description	Examples
Primary Lesions		
MACULE, PATCH 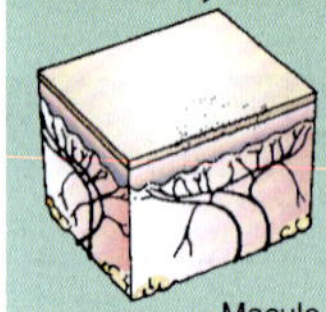 Macule 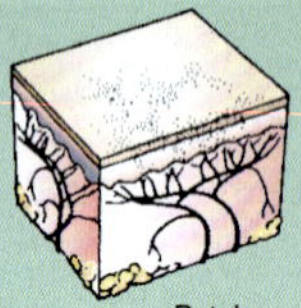 Patch	Flat, nonpalpable skin colour change (colour may be brown, white, tan, purple, red) • *Macule:* <1 cm; circumscribed border • *Patch:* >1 cm; may have irregular border	Freckles, flat moles, petechia, rubella, vitiligo, port wine stains, ecchymosis
PAPULE, PLAQUE 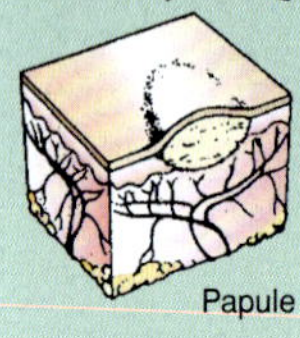 Papule 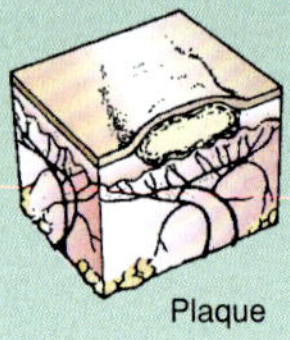 Plaque	Elevated, palpable, solid mass with a circumscribed border Plaque may be coalesced papules with flat top • *Papule:* <0.5 cm • *Plaque:* >0.5 cm	*Papules:* Elevated nevi, warts, lichen planus *Plaques:* Psoriasis, actinic keratosis
NODULE, TUMOUR 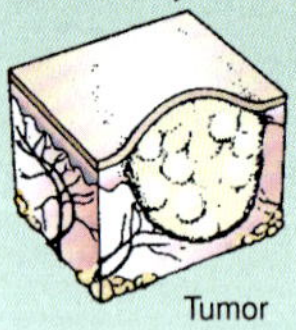 Tumor	Elevated, palpable, solid mass that extends deeper into the dermis than a papule • *Nodule:* 0.5–2 cm; circumscribed • *Tumour:* >1–2 cm; tumours do not always have sharp borders	*Nodules:* Lipoma, squamous cell carcinoma, poorly absorbed injection, dermatofibroma *Tumours:* Larger lipoma, carcinoma
VESICLE, BULLA 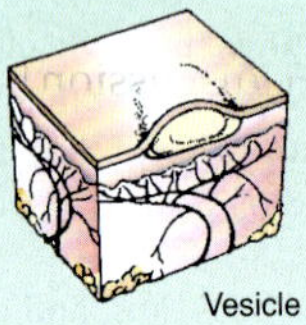 Vesicle 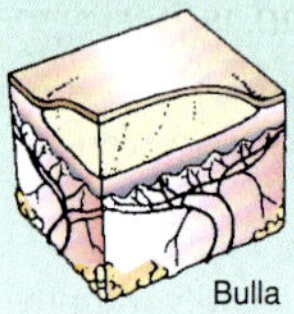 Bulla	Circumscribed, elevated, palpable mass containing serous fluid • *Vesicle:* <0.5 cm • *Bulla:* >0.5 cm	*Vesicles:* Herpes simplex/zoster, varicella, poison ivy, second-degree burn (blister) *Bulla:* Pemphigus, contact dermatitis, large burn blisters, poison ivy, bullous impetigo
WHEAL 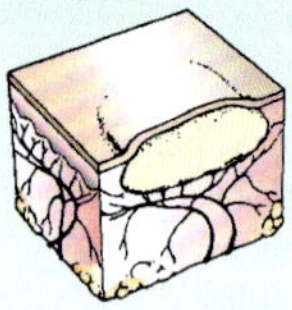	Elevated mass with transient borders; often irregular; size and colour vary Caused by movement of serous fluid into the dermis; does not contain free fluid in a cavity (e.g., as a vesicle does)	Urticaria (hives), insect bites
PUSTULE 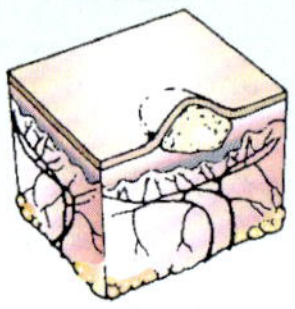	Pus-filled vesicle or bulla	Acne, impetigo, furuncles, carbuncles
CYST 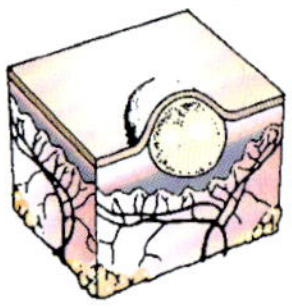	Encapsulated fluid-filled or semisolid mass in the subcutaneous tissue or dermis	Sebaceous cyst, epidermoid cysts

TABLE 57-3 Primary and Secondary Skin Lesions (Continued)

Lesion	Description	Examples
Secondary Lesions		
EROSION 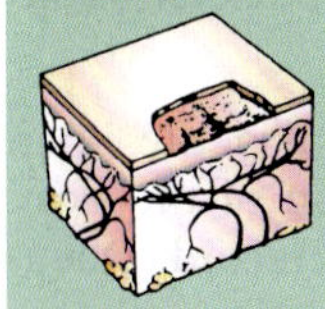	Loss of superficial epidermis that does not extend to dermis; depressed, moist area	Ruptured vesicles, scratch marks
ULCER 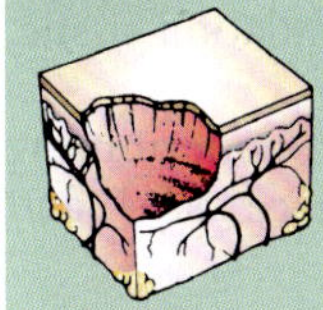	Skin loss extending past epidermis; necrotic tissue loss; bleeding and scarring possible	Stasis ulcer of venous insufficiency, pressure ulcer
FISSURE 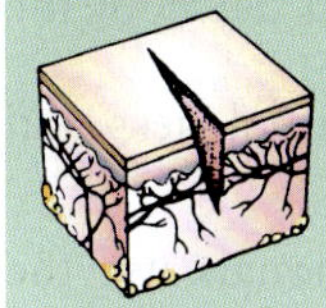	Linear crack in the skin that may extend to dermis	Chapped lips or hands, tinea pedis
SCALES 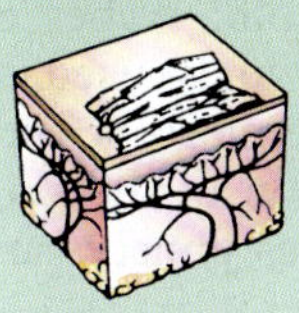	Flakes secondary to desquamated, dead epithelium that may adhere to skin surface; colour varies (silvery, white); texture varies (thick, fine)	Dandruff, psoriasis, dry skin, pityriasis rosea
CRUST 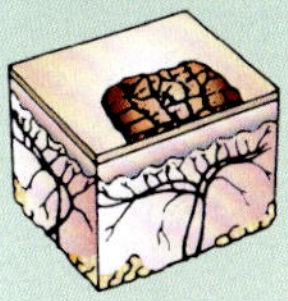	Dried residue of serum, blood, or pus on skin surface Large, adherent crust is a scab	Residue left after vesicle rupture: impetigo, herpes, eczema
SCAR (CICATRIX) 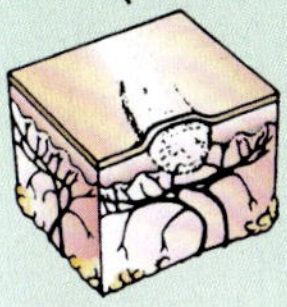	Skin mark left after healing of a wound or lesion; represents replacement by connective tissue of the injured tissue • *Young scars:* Red or purple • *Mature scars:* White or glistening	Healed wound or surgical incision
KELOID 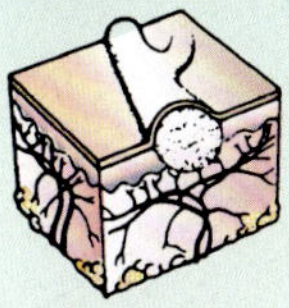	Hypertrophied scar tissue secondary to excessive collagen formation during healing; elevated, irregular, red Greater incidence among African Americans	Keloid of ear piercing or surgical incision
ATROPHY 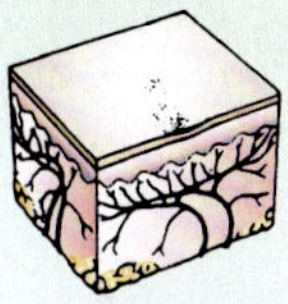	Thin, dry, transparent appearance of epidermis; loss of surface markings; secondary to loss of collagen and elastin; underlying vessels may be visible	Aged skin, arterial insufficiency
LICHENIFICATION 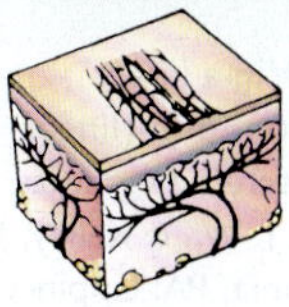	Thickening and roughening of the skin or accentuated skin markings that may be secondary to repeated rubbing, irritation, scratching	Contact dermatitis

Adapted from Bickley, L. S. (2013). *Bates' guide to physical examination and history taking* (11th ed.). Philadelphia, PA: Lippincott Williams & Wilkins; Weber, J. W., & Kelley, J. (2014). *Health assessment in nursing* (5th ed.). Philadelphia, PA: Lippincott Williams & Wilkins.

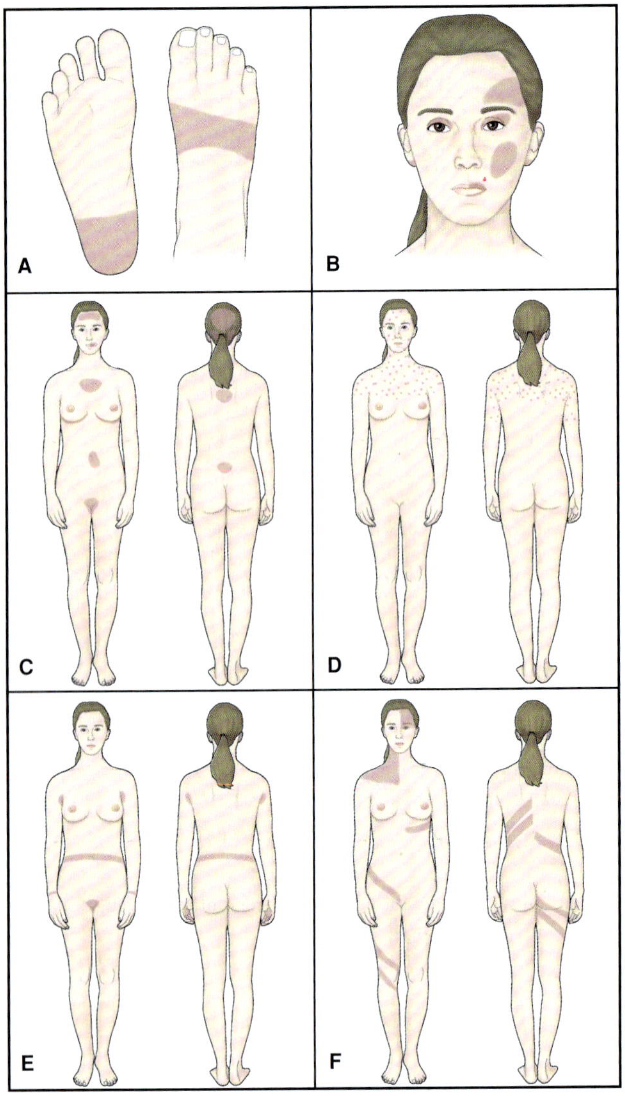

FIGURE 57-4. Anatomic distribution of common skin disorders. A. Contact dermatitis (shoes). B. Contact dermatitis (cosmetics, perfumes, earrings). C. Seborrheic dermatitis. D. Acne. E. Scabies. F. Herpes zoster (shingles).

A preliminary assessment of the eruption or lesion helps to identify the type of **dermatosis** and to detect whether the lesion is primary or secondary. Observe the anatomic distribution of the eruption because certain diseases affect known sites of the body and are distributed in characteristic patterns and shapes (Figs. 57-4 and 57-5). To determine the extent of the regional distribution, compare the left and right sides of the body while assessing the colour and shape (configuration) of the lesions. After inspection, palpate the lesions to determine their texture, shape, and border, and to detect if they are soft, filled with fluid, or hard and fixed to the surrounding tissue.

Use a metric ruler to measure the size of the lesions for future comparisons. Document the dermatosis on the patient's health record; describe the distribution, configuration, and type clearly, using precise terminology.

Determine the characteristic distribution of the lesions (e.g., bilateral, symmetric, truncal, extremities), and obtain the remaining details:

- Type of lesion (primary or secondary) (e.g., macule, papule, pustule, vesicle, bulla)
- Colour of lesion
- Any associated redness, heat, pain, or swelling
- Size and location of involved area
- Configuration (pattern) of eruption (e.g., discrete, confluent, linear, dermatomal, annular)

Perform a comprehensive assessment if acute open wounds or lesions are found on inspection of the skin. Document the description in the patient's record. Documentation includes the following characteristics:

- *Wound bed:* Inspect for necrotic and granulation tissue, epithelium, exudate, colour, and odour.
- *Wound edges and margins:* Observe for undermining (extension of the wound under the surface skin), and evaluate for condition.
- *Wound size:* Measure in millimetres or centimetres, as appropriate, to determine diameter and depth of the wound and surrounding erythema.
- *Surrounding skin:* Assess for colour, suppleness and moisture, irritation, and scaling.

Both patients and health care professionals use the ABCDE method for screening moles for possible melanoma (Canadian Dermatology Association, 2014b; Weber & Kelley, 2018). The ABCDE method is widely used in Canadian family practice, but the use of a dermoscope with a handheld light magnifier for examination of the skin increases the accuracy of diagnosis, reduces unnecessary

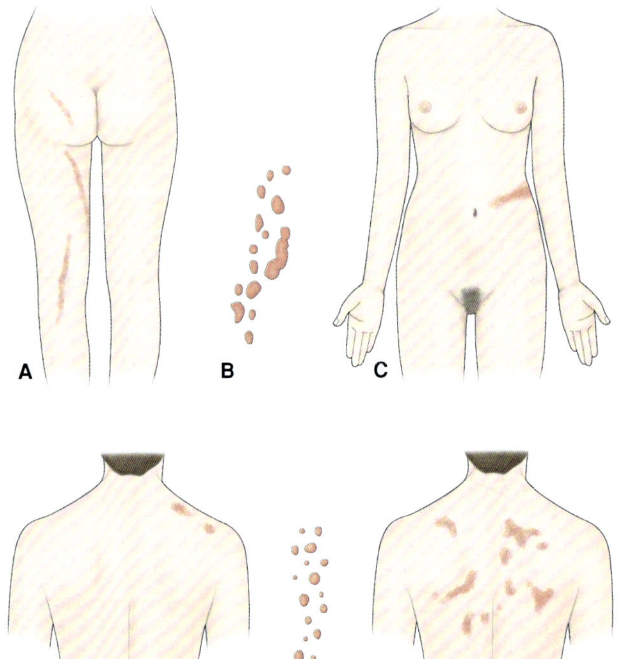

FIGURE 57-5. Skin lesion configurations. A. Linear (in a line). B. Annular and arciform (circular or arcing). C. Zosteriform (linear along a nerve route). D. Grouped (clustered). E. Discrete (separate and distinct). F. Confluent (merged). (From Weber, J. W., & Kelley, J. (2007). *Health assessment in nursing* (3rd ed.). Philadelphia, PA: Lippincott Williams & Wilkins.)

referrals, and limits the biopsy rates for benign lesions (Herschorn, 2012; Mansen & Gabiola, 2015). The letters ABCDE stand for the following:

- A for asymmetry; one half is not like the other half
- B for borders; look for irregular edges, ragged, notched, and not well-defined borders
- C for colour; look for variation or change in colour with tan, brown, black, red, blue, grey, or white areas
- D for diameter; look for growth in size of the lesion larger than a pencil eraser (6 mm)
- E for evolution; look for change in size, shape, symptoms (itchiness, tenderness), surface elevation, bleeding, or colour

Assessing Vascularity and Hydration

After the colour of the skin has been evaluated and lesions have been inspected, an assessment of vascular changes in the skin is performed. A description of vascular changes includes location, distribution, colour, size, and the presence of pulsations. Common vascular changes include petechiae, ecchymoses, **telangiectasias** (venous stars), and angiomas (see Table 57-4).

Skin moisture, temperature, and texture are assessed primarily by palpation. The turgor (i.e., elasticity) of the skin, which decreases with normal aging, may be a factor in assessing the hydration status of a patient. To assess skin turgor, the skin should be gently pinched between the thumb and forefinger. The skin is observed to see how long it takes to return to baseline. People who are dehydrated or those with dry skin will display decreased skin turgor, where the skin remains tented after being pinched rather than returning to normal almost immediately. Edema is indicated when the skin appears tense and shiny, when a finger gently pressed into the skin leaves an indentation or "pit." Assessing the depth of the pit and length of time to resolution indicates the extent of edema (LeBlond, Brown, Suneja, et al., 2014).

Assessing the Nails and Hair

Many alterations in the nail or nail bed reflect local or systemic alterations in progress or resulting from past events (Fig. 57-6). Transverse depressions known as Beau's lines in the nails may reflect retarded growth of the nail matrix because of severe illness or, more commonly, local trauma. Ridging, hypertrophy, and other changes may also be visible with local trauma. Paronychia, an inflammation of the skin around the nail, is usually accompanied by tenderness and erythema. The angle between the healthy nail and its base is 160 degrees. When palpated, the nail base is usually firm. Clubbing of the nails is manifested by a straightening of the angle (180 degrees or greater) and softening of the nail base. The softened area feels sponge like when palpated (Bickley, 2013). Clubbing can be a normal variant, but it is most often associated with pulmonary disease and can be a sign of chronic hypoxia (Habif, 2016).

Inspect and palpate the hair. Wear disposable gloves as lesions on the scalp may not be initially visible. Ensure that the examination room is well lit. Separate the hair so that you can inspect the condition of the scalp easily seen. Assess the colour, texture, moisture, and distribution of the hair. Inspect for any lesions, evidence of itching,

TABLE 57-4 Vascular Lesions

PETECHIA (*PL.* PETECHIAE) 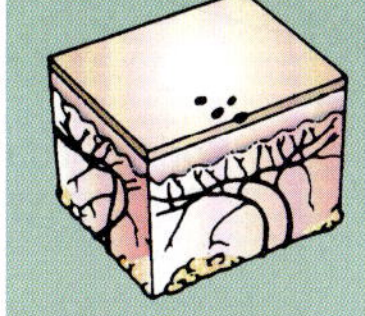	Round red or purple macule Small (1–2 mm) Secondary to blood extravasation Associated with bleeding tendencies or emboli to skin
ECCHYMOSIS (*PL.* ECCHYMOSES) 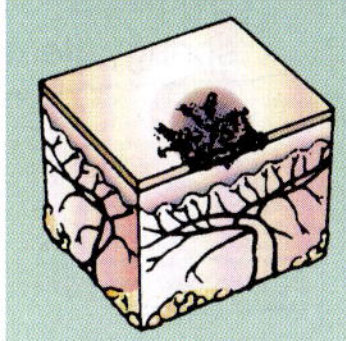	Round or irregular macular lesion Larger than petechia Colour varies and changes—black, yellow, and green hues Secondary to blood extravasation Associated with trauma, bleeding tendencies
CHERRY ANGIOMA 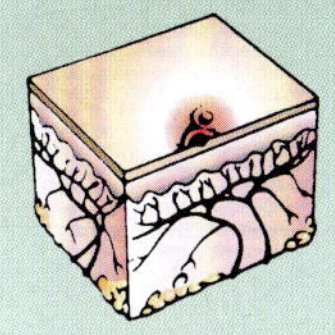	Papular and round Red or purple Noted on trunk, extremities May blanch with pressure Normal age-related skin alteration Usually not clinically significant
SPIDER ANGIOMA 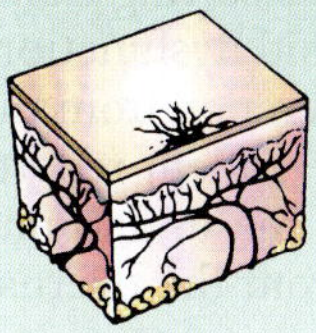	Red, arteriole lesion Central body with radiating branches Noted on face, neck, arms, trunk Rare below the waist May blanch with pressure Associated with liver disease, pregnancy, vitamin B deficiency
TELANGIECTASIA (VENOUS STAR) 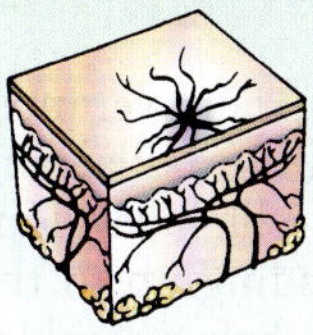	Shape varies—spider like or linear Colour bluish or red Does not blanch when pressure is applied Noted on legs, anterior chest Secondary to superficial dilation of venous vessels and capillaries Associated with increased venous pressure states (varicosities)

Adapted from Bickley, L. S. (2013). *Bates' guide to physical examination and history taking* (11th ed.). Philadelphia, PA: Lippincott Williams & Wilkins; Weber, J. W., & Kelley, J. (2014). *Health assessment in nursing* (5th ed.). Philadelphia, PA: Lippincott Williams & Wilkins.

inflammation, scaling, or signs of infestation (e.g., lice or mites) and document findings.

Colour and Texture

Natural hair colour ranges from white to black. Hair colour begins to grey with age, initially appearing during the third decade of life when the loss of melanin begins to become apparent. It is not unusual for the hair of younger people to turn grey as a result of hereditary traits. Individuals with albinism (partial or complete absence of pigmentation) have a genetic predisposition to white hair from birth. The natural state of the hair can be altered by using hair dyes, bleaches, and curling or relaxing products. Establish what types of products are used during the assessment.

The texture of scalp hair ranges from fine to coarse, silky to brittle, oily to dry, and shiny to dull; hair can be straight, curly, wavy, or kinky. Dry, brittle hair may result

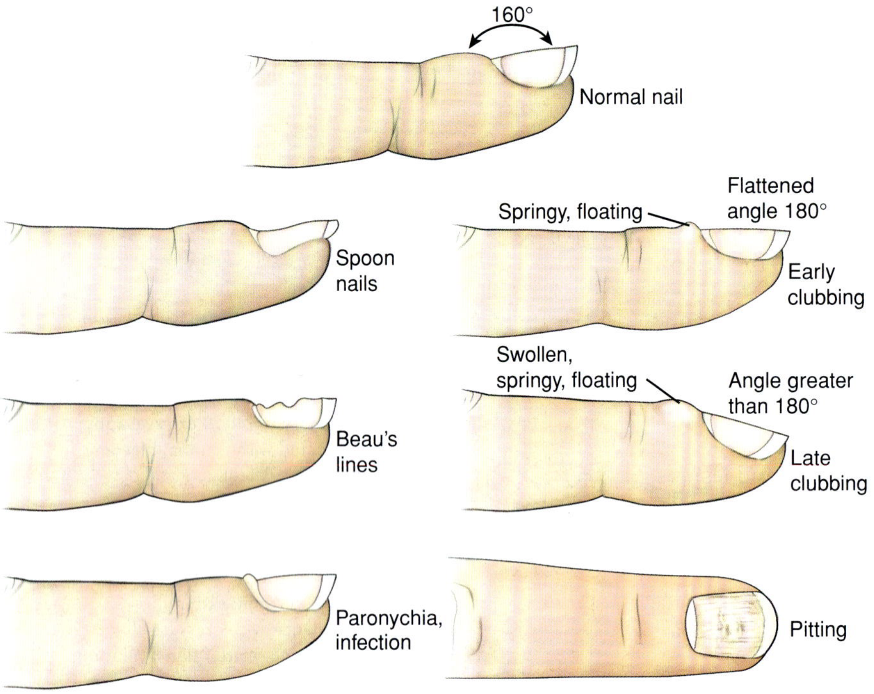

FIGURE 57-6. Common nail disorders. (From Weber, J. R., & Kelley, J. H. (2018). *Health assessment in nursing* (6th ed.). Philadelphia, PA: Wolters Kluwer.)

from overuse of hair dyes, hair dryers, and curling irons, or from endocrine disorders, such as thyroid dysfunction. Oily hair is usually caused by increased secretion from the sebaceous glands close to the scalp. If the patient reports a recent change in hair texture, explore the underlying reason; the alteration may arise simply from the overuse of commercial hair products or from changing to a new shampoo.

Distribution

Body hair distribution varies with location. Hair over most of the body is fine (vellus hair), except in the axillae and pubic areas, where it is coarse. Pubic hair, which develops at puberty, forms a diamond shape extending up to the umbilicus in boys and men. Female pubic hair resembles an inverted triangle. If a pattern found is more characteristic of the opposite gender, it may indicate an endocrine disorder that requires further investigation. Expect genetic differences in hair, such as straight hair in Asians and curly, coarser hair in people of African descent.

Men tend to have more body and facial hair than women. Loss of hair (alopecia) can occur over the entire body or be confined to a specific area. Scalp hair loss may be localized to patchy areas or may range from generalized thinning to total baldness. When assessing scalp hair loss, it is important to investigate the underlying cause with the patient. Patchy hair loss may be from habitual hair pulling or twisting; from excessive traction on the hair (e.g., braiding too tightly); excessive use of dyes, straighteners, and oils; chemotherapeutic agents (e.g., doxorubicin, cyclophosphamide); fungal infection; or moles or lesions on the scalp. Regrowth may be erratic, and distribution may never attain the previous thickness.

Hair Loss

The most common cause of hair loss is male pattern baldness, which affects more than one half of the male population and is believed to be related to heredity, aging, and androgen (male hormone) levels. Androgen is necessary for male pattern baldness to develop. The pattern of hair loss begins with receding of the hairline in the frontal–temporal area and progresses to gradual thinning and complete loss of hair over the top of the scalp and crown. Figure 57-7 illustrates the progression of typical male pattern baldness. Though androgenic alopecia is considered a male disorder, millions of women also experience it. Women tend to retain some of the hair on the crown of the scalp and never go completely bald.

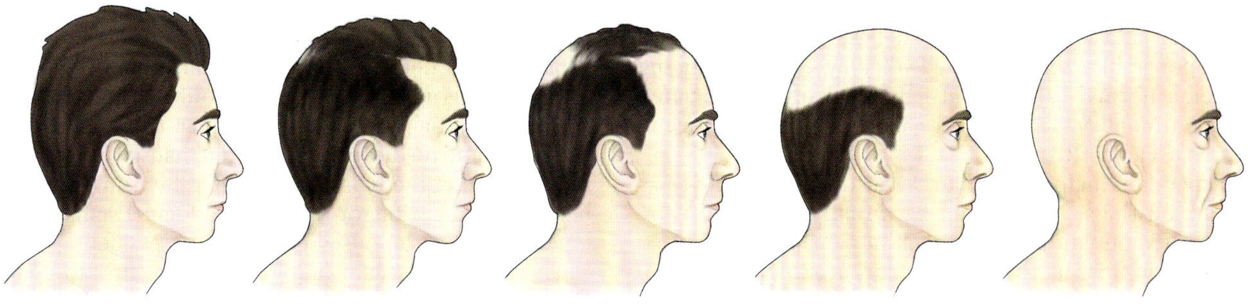

FIGURE 57-7. The progression of male pattern baldness.

Other Changes

Male pattern hair distribution may be seen in some women at the time of menopause, when the hormone estrogen is no longer produced by the ovaries. In women with hirsutism, excessive hair may grow on the face, chest, shoulders, and pubic area. For some, it is a taboo subject (e.g., having to shave). Sensitive questioning about how it affects daily life and relationships may provide nursing opportunities to support and advise (Mansen & Gabiola, 2015). When menopause is ruled out as the underlying cause, hormonal disorders related to pituitary or adrenal dysfunction are investigated.

Because patients with skin conditions may be viewed negatively by others, these patients may become distraught and avoid interaction with people. Skin conditions can lead to disfigurement, isolation, job loss, and economic hardship.

Some conditions may subject the patient to a protracted illness, leading to feelings of depression, frustration, self-consciousness, poor self-image, and rejection. Itching and skin irritation, features of many skin diseases, may be a constant annoyance. The results of these discomforts may be loss of sleep, anxiety, and depression, all of which reinforce the general distress and fatigue that frequently accompany skin disorders.

Provide understanding, explanations of the condition, and appropriate instructions related to treatment to patients suffering such physical and psychological discomforts. They benefit from nursing support, patience, and encouragement. It takes time to help patients gain insight into their challenges and resolve their difficulties. It is imperative to overcome any aversion that you may feel when caring for patients with unattractive skin disorders. Avoid demonstrating any hesitancy when approaching such patients as hesitancy only reinforces the psychological trauma of the disorder.

Skin Consequences of Selected Systemic Diseases

Skin Disorders in Diabetes

Diabetes causes changes in circulation and cell nutrition that can have a great impact on skin status. Some of the more common skin conditions encountered in diabetes are discussed in this section.

Diabetic Dermopathy

Diabetic dermopathy (shin spots) occurs in about 50% of patients with diabetes. These lesions are found on the lower anterior legs, forearms, thighs, and other bony prominences. Caused by breakdown of the small vessels that supply the skin, each shin spot starts as a dull red bump, smaller than a pencil eraser. It slowly spreads to about the size of a quarter, becomes more scaly, and eventually leaves a brownish scar on the skin. The lesions are usually bilateral and occur in linear clusters. No treatment is required (American Diabetes Association, 2014).

Stasis Dermatitis

Stasis dermatitis is not unique to diabetes, but because of the blood vessel damage that results from diabetes, it is very common in patients with this disease. Large vessels are damaged, compromising circulation to the lower arms and legs. A lack of nutrients results in the skin becoming very dry and fragile. Minor injuries heal more slowly, and ulcers form easily. The skin takes on a thick leathery texture and a yellowish, waxy hue.

Skin Infections

The skin of patients with diabetes is prone to bacterial and fungal infections. Bacterial infections appear as small pimples around hair follicles and the most frequently affected sites include the lower legs, lower abdomen, and buttocks. Sometimes, the lesions enlarge to become furuncles or carbuncles. If the blood glucose level is not well controlled, these infections may be very slow to heal.

Fungal infections are quite common in areas that remain moist all the time (under breasts, upper thighs, in axilla). *Candida* (yeast) infections appear beefy red and have small pustules around the border of the area, with the skin appearing moist and raw.

Dermatophyte infections are dry and only minimally red, with more scales. Common sites are the toenails and feet.

Be alert to the signs of these common infections. Report them to the attention of the physician and help the patient or family learn basic skin maintenance techniques.

Leg and Foot Ulcers

Because of peripheral neuropathy, patients with diabetes do not always sense irritation or minor injuries to the lower legs and feet. Any injury to the lower legs or feet can become infected. If left untreated, injured tissue may lead to ulceration. Ulcerations often go unnoticed and become quite large before being treated. Ulcerations unresponsive to treatment are a leading cause of diabetic foot and leg amputations.

Cutaneous Signs of Human Immunodeficiency Virus Disease

Cutaneous signs may be the first manifestation of human immunodeficiency virus (HIV), appearing in more than 90% of people infected with HIV as their immune function deteriorates. These skin signs correlate with helper T-cells that have low counts of CD4 molecules on the surface (Carter & Hughson, 2014). Some disorders such as Kaposi's sarcoma, oral hairy leukoplakia, facial molluscum contagiosum, and oral candidiasis suggest that CD4 counts are less than 200 to 300 mm^3 (instead of between 500 and 1,500 cells). Skin infections, both bacterial and viral, are common and will appear more severe than expected. Acute flare of chronic conditions such as seborrhea or acne may indicate a new infection. Being sensitive to these changes can alert the nurse so that early interventions can be initiated (Schwartz, 2015).

Be sensitive to these changes so that early intervention can be initiated.

Diagnostic Evaluation

A wide range of diagnostic studies may be performed in patients with altered integumentary function. The nurse educates the patient about the purpose, what to expect, and any possible side effects related to these examinations prior to testing. The nurse also notes trends in results because they provide information about whether lesions are primary or secondary, disease progression, and the patient's response to therapy.

Skin Biopsy

Performed to obtain tissue for microscopic examination, a skin biopsy may be obtained by shave, excision, or by a skin punch instrument that removes a small core of tissue. Biopsies are performed on skin nodules, plaques, blisters, and other lesions to rule out malignancy, to aid in diagnosis, and to perform additional testing such as Gram stain for bacteria or periodic acid-Schiff (PAS) for fungal elements.

Immunofluorescence

Designed to identify the site of an immunologic reaction, immunofluorescence testing combines an antigen or antibody with a fluorochrome dye. Antibodies can be made fluorescent by attaching them to a dye. Direct immunofluorescence tests on skin are techniques to detect autoantibodies directed against portions of the skin. The indirect immunofluorescence test detects specific antibodies in the patient's serum and may be used to detect bullous pemphigoid, systemic lupus erythematosus, and dermatitis herpetiformis.

Patch Testing

Performed to identify substances to which the patient has developed an allergy, patch testing involves applying the suspected allergens, such as nickel or fragrances, to normal skin under occlusive patches. Patients wear these occluded strips on their backs for 48 hours, and the area is assessed after 72 hours. The development of redness, fine elevations, or itching is considered a weak positive reaction; fine blisters, papules, and severe itching indicate a moderately positive reaction; and blisters, pain, and ulceration indicate a strong positive reaction. The nurse educates the patient with a positive reaction to avoid the allergen, which is often quite difficult, due to the prevalence of many allergens.

Skin Scrapings

Tissue samples are scraped from suspected fungal (dermatophyte) lesions with a scalpel blade moistened with oil so that the scraped skin adheres to the blade. Scrapings may also be mixed with potassium hydroxide (Binamer, 2013). The scraped material is transferred to a glass slide, covered with a coverslip, and examined microscopically. The spores and hyphae of dermatophyte infections, as well as infestations such as scabies, can be visualized. Scrapings are a quick method for identifying dermatophytes, but culturing a scraping on a medium such as agar is the criterion standard test (Binamer, 2013).

Tzanck Smear

The Tzanck smear is an age-old test used to examine cells from blistering, bullous, and pustular skin conditions, such as herpes zoster, varicella, herpes simplex, and all forms of pemphigus. The secretions from a suspected lesion are applied to a glass slide, stained, and examined. The test cannot distinguish between herpes simplex and herpes zoster infections, but is highly sensitive and specific and useful in diagnosis otherwise.

Wood's Light Examination

Wood's light is a special lamp that produces long-wave ultraviolet rays, which result in a characteristic dark purple fluorescence. The colour of the fluorescent light is best seen in a darkened room, where it is possible to differentiate epidermal from dermal lesions and hypopigmented and hyperpigmented lesions from healthy skin (which does not shine under the light). The patient is reassured that the light is not harmful to the skin or eyes, and should not wash the skin before the test. Lesions that still contain melanin almost disappear under ultraviolet light, whereas lesions that are devoid of melanin increase in whiteness with ultraviolet light.

Clinical Photographs

Photographs are taken to document the nature and extent of the skin condition and to determine progress or improvement resulting from treatment. They are sometimes used to track the status of moles to document if the characteristics of the mole are changing.

Nursing Implications

The nurse may be responsible to ensure that consent forms are completed for surgical procedures and for clinical photography, that all specimens collected are managed according to protocol, that a log is maintained tracking specimens to and from the laboratory, and that results are received in a timely manner. The nurse educates the patient regarding appropriate care of surgical sites and implication of test results.

Critical Thinking Exercise

1 A neighbour of yours tells you that her 8-year-old twin daughters have joined the swim team that is affiliated with the local pool in your community. She is looking forward to enjoying time at the pool with her daughters, but is worried that she will get sunburned. She tells you that she is thinking about getting a tan at a tanning salon before she begins to take her daughters to the pool. Is this an advisable practice that might diminish her risk of getting sunburned or from getting skin cancer? Describe evidence-based measures she might take that can reduce her risk of getting sunburned and reduce her future risk of skin cancer.

REFERENCES AND SELECTED READINGS

Books and Documents

Amerman, E. C. (2016). *Human anatomy and physiology*. United States: Pearson Education, Inc.

Bickley, L. S. (2013). *Bates' guide to physical examination and history taking* (11th ed.). Philadelphia, PA: Lippincott Williams & Wilkins.

Bobonich, M. A., & Nolen, M. E. (2014). *Dermatology for advanced practice clinicians*. Philadelphia, PA: Wolters Kluwer.

Bolognia, J., Jorizzo, J., & Schaffer, J. (2012). *Dermatology* (3rd ed.). Philadelphia, PA: Elsevier Saunders.

Grossman, S. C., & Porth, C. M. (2014). *Porth's pathophysiology: Concepts of altered health states* (9th ed.). Philadelphia, PA: Kluwer Health/Lippincott Williams & Wilkins.

Habif, T. P. (2016). *Clinical dermatology* (6th ed.). St. Louis, MO: Elsevier Health Sciences.

LeBlond, R. F., Brown, D. D., Suneja, M., et al. (2014). *DeGowin's diagnostic examination* (10th ed.). New York: McGraw-Hill.

Mansen, T. J., & Gabiola, J. (2015). *Patient-focused assessment: The art and science of clinical data gathering*. Boston, MA: Pearson.

Martini, F. H., Timmons, M. J., & Tallitsch, R. B. (2012). *Human anatomy* (7th ed.). Toronto, ON: Pearson Benjamin Cummings.

Skillen, D. L. (2012). Older adults. In T. C. Stephen, D. L. Skillen, R. A. Day, et al. (Eds.). *Canadian Jensen's nursing health assessment: A best practice approach* (1st ed., pp. 925–956). Philadelphia, PA: Wolters Kluwer Health/Lippincott Williams & Wilkins.

Stephen, T. C. (2012). Skin, hair, and nails assessment. In T. C. Stephen, D. L. Skillen, R. A. Day, et al. (Eds.). *Canadian Jensen's nursing health assessment: A best practice approach* (1st ed., pp. 267–325). Philadelphia, PA: Wolters Kluwer Health/Lippincott Williams & Wilkins.

Taylor, S. C., Kelly, A. P., Lim, H., et al. (2016). *Dermatology for skin of color* (2nd ed.). New York: McGraw-Hill Medical.

Weber, J. R., & Kelley, J. H. (2018). *Health assessment in nursing* (6th ed.). Philadelphia, PA: Wolters Kluwer.

Journals and Electronic Documents

Abrams, E. M., & Becker, A. B. (2013). Introducing solid food: Age of introduction and its effect on risk of food allergy and other atopic diseases. *Canadian Family Physician*, *59*, 721–722.

Aldeen, T., & Basra, M. (2011). Management of psoriasis and its comorbidities in primary care. *British Journal of Nursing*, *20*, 1186–1192.

American Diabetes Association. (2014). *Skin complications: General skin conditions*. Retrieved from http://www.diabetes.org/living-with-diabetes/complications/skin-complications.html

Binamer, Y. (2013). Dermacase. Can you identify this condition? Kerion (inflammatory tinea capitis). *Canadian Family Physician*, *59*, 271–272.

Canadian Cancer Society. (2014). *Vitamin D*. Retrieved from http://www.cancer.ca/en/prevention-and-screening/live-well/vitamin-d/?region=on

Canadian Dermatology Association. (2014a). *Photoaging*. Retrieved from http://www.dermatology.ca/skin-hair-nails/skin/photoaging

Canadian Dermatology Association. (2014b). *Malignant melanoma*. Retrieved from http://www.dermatology.ca/skin-hair-nails/skin/skin-cancer/malignant-melanoma

Carter, M., & Hughson, G. (2014). *CD4 cell counts*. Retrieved from http://www.aidsmap.com/CD4-cell-counts/page/1044596

Health Canada. (2012). *Vitamin D and calcium: Updated dietary reference intakes*. Retrieved from https://www.canada.ca/en/health-canada/services/food-nutrition/healthy-eating/vitamins-minerals/vitamin-calcium-updated-dietary-reference-intakes-nutrition.html#a17

Herschorn, A. (2012). Dermoscopy for melanoma detection in family practice. *Canadian Family Physician*, *58*, 740–745.

Onselen, J. V. (2011). Hirsutism: Causes and treatment for women. *British Journal of Nursing*, *20*, 985–990.

Osteoporosis Canada. (2014). *Vitamin D: An important nutrient that protects you against falls and fractures*. Retrieved from http://www.osteoporosis.ca/osteoporosis-and-you/nutrition/vitamind-d

Polasik, K., Placek, W., & Romanska-Gocka, K. (2010). The role of Langerhans cells in etiopathogenesis of atopic dermatitis. *Przegl Dermatologiczny/Dermatology Review*, *97*, 303–312.

Schwartz, R. A. (2015). Cutaneous manifestations of HIV. *Medscape*. Retrieved from emedicine.medscape.com/article/1133746-overview

Smith, C. H., & Goldman, R. D. (2012). An incurable itch: Head lice. *Canadian Family Physician*, *58*, 839–841.

Yaffe, M. J., & Tazkarji, B. (2012). Understanding elder abuse in family practice. *Canadian Family Physician*, *58*, 1336–1340.

Resources and Web Sites

Canadian Alopecia Areata Association: http://canaaf.org/
Canadian Association of Genetic Counsellors (CAGC): http://www.cagc-accg.ca
Canadian Association of Wound Care: http://www.cawc.net
Canadian Cancer Society/Société canadienne du cancer: http://www.cancer.ca
Canadian Dermatology Association: http://www.dermatology.ca
Canadian Dermatology Nurses Association: http://www.cdermnurse.org/home.htm
Canadian Directory of Genetic Support Groups, Support Group Directory, Regional Medical Genetics Centre: http://www.lhsc.on.ca/programs/medgenet
Canadian Organization for Rare Disorders (CORD): http://www.cord.ca
Dermatology Information System (DermIS): http://www.dermis.net
Eczema Canada: http://www.eczemacanada.ca
Lupus Canada: http://www.lupuscanada.org
Psoriasis Society of Canada: http://www.psoriasissociety.org
Rosacea Awareness Program: http://www.about-rosacea.com

58 Management of Patients With Dermatologic Conditions

Adapted by Carla Wells

Learning Objectives

On completion of this chapter, the learner will be able to:

1. Describe the general management of the patient with an unexpected skin condition.
2. Use the nursing process as a framework for care of the patient with psoriasis.
3. Describe the health education needs of the patient with infections of the skin and parasitic skin diseases.
4. Use the nursing process as a framework for care of patients with noninfectious, inflammatory dermatoses.
5. Describe the management and nursing care of the patient with skin cancer.
6. Use the nursing process as a framework for care of the patient with malignant melanoma.
7. Describe characteristics of the various types of Kaposi's sarcoma.
8. Compare the various types of dermatologic and plastic reconstructive surgeries.
9. Use the nursing process as a framework for care of the patient undergoing facial reconstructive surgery.

Dermatologic disorders are encountered frequently by nurses across many practice settings. Nursing management of patients with dermatologic problems includes administering topical and systemic medications and managing dressings. The nurse can also be instrumental in educating patients how to care for their skin. The objectives of nursing interventions are to prevent additional skin damage, prevent secondary infection, reverse the inflammatory process, and relieve the symptoms.

SKIN CARE FOR PATIENTS WITH SKIN CONDITIONS

Some skin problems are markedly aggravated by soap and water; therefore, bathing routines are modified according to the condition. Denuded skin, whether the area of desquamation is large or small, is excessively prone to damage by chemicals, trauma, and even bathing. The friction of a towel, if applied with vigour, is often sufficient to produce a brisk inflammatory response that can cause a lesion to flare (Inamadar & Palit, 2013).

Protecting the Skin

The essence of skin care and protection in bathing a patient with skin concerns is as follows:

- A mild, lipid-free soap or soap substitute is used.
- The area is rinsed completely and blotted dry with a soft cloth.
- Deodorant soaps are avoided.
- Laundry detergents and fabric softener free of fragrance are used.

Special care is necessary when changing dressings. The use of pledgets saturated with oil, sterile saline, or another prescribed solution helps loosen crusts, remove exudates, or free an adherent dry dressing (Dabiri, Damstetter, & Phillips, 2016).

Preventing Secondary Infection

Potentially infectious skin lesions are regarded strictly as such, and proper precautions are observed until the diagnosis is established. Most lesions with purulent drainage contain infectious material. Nurses and physicians must adhere to Routine Practices and Additional Precautions (Public Health Agency of Canada [PHAC], 2012) and wear gloves when inspecting the skin or changing the dressing. Proper disposal of any contaminated dressing is carried out according to the Canadian Centre for Occupational Health and Safety (CCOHS) regulations.

Reversing the Inflammatory Process

The type of skin lesion (e.g., oozing, infected, or dry) usually determines the type of local medication or treatment that is prescribed. As a rule, if the skin is acutely inflamed (i.e., hot, red, and swollen) and oozing, it is best to apply wet dressings and soothing lotions. For chronic conditions in which the skin surface is dry and scaly, water-soluble emulsions, creams, ointments, and pastes are used. The therapy is modified as the responses of the skin indicate. The patient and the nurse should note whether the medication or dressings seem to irritate the skin. The success or failure of therapy usually depends on adequate instruction and motivation of the patient and family as well as the support of health care personnel.

Wound Care for Skin Conditions

There are three types of wound dressings: passive, interactive, and active. Passive dressings have only a protective function and maintain a moist environment for natural healing. They include those that just cover the area (e.g., DuoDERM, Tegaderm) and may remain in place for several days. Interactive dressings are capable of absorbing wound exudate while (a) maintaining a moist environment in the area of the wound and (b) allowing the surrounding skin to remain dry. They include hydrocolloids, hydrofibers, alginates, and hydrogels. It is thought that interactive dressings are able to modify the physiology of the wound environment by modulating and stimulating cellular activity and by releasing growth factor. Active dressings improve the healing process and decrease healing time. They include skin grafts and biologic skin substitutes. Both interactive and active dressings create a moist environment at the interface of the wound with the dressing.

Because so many wound care products are available, it is often difficult to select the most appropriate product for a specific wound (Chart 58-1). Selection of products should be made carefully because of their expense. Both clinical efficacy and health-related outcomes (e.g., decreased pain, increased mobility) should be used to measure the success of a product for a wound. Even with the availability of a large variety of dressings, an appropriate selection can be made if certain principles are maintained. These principles are referred to as the five rules of wound care (Dabiri et al., 2014).

Rule 1: Categorization

The nurse learns about dressings by generic category and compares new products with those that already make up the category. As hundreds of choices become available, the nurse becomes familiar with indications, contraindications, and side effects. The best dressing may be created by combining products in different categories to achieve several goals at the same time. These categories are discussed in subsequent sections.

Rule 2: Selection

The nurse selects the safest and most effective, user-friendly, and cost-effective dressing possible. In some cases, nurses carry out the physician's prescriptions for dressings, but they should be prepared to give the physician feedback about the dressing's effect on the wound,

Glossary

acantholysis: separation of epidermal cells from each other due to damage or abnormality of the intracellular substance
balneotherapy: bath with therapeutic additives
bullae: large, fluid-filled blisters
carbuncle: localized skin infection involving several hair follicles
cheilitis: inflammation of the lip; dry, cracking, inflamed skin at the corners of the mouth is called *angular cheilitis*; when caused by sun exposure, it is called *solar cheilitis*
comedones: the primary lesions of acne, caused by sebum blockage in the hair follicle
cytotoxic: destructive of cells
debridement: removal of necrotic or dead tissue by mechanical, surgical, or autolytic means
dermatitis: any inflammation of the skin
dermatosis: any abnormal skin lesion
epidermopoiesis: development of epidermal cells
fibrinolytic: substance that acts to break up fibrin, the fine filaments of blood clots
furuncle: localized skin infection of a single hair follicle
hydrophilic: material that absorbs moisture
hydrophobic: material that repels moisture
hygroscopic: material that absorbs moisture from the air
lichenification: thickening of the horny layer of the skin
liniments: lotions with added oil for increased softening of the skin
mitogenic: substance that stimulates mitosis or cell division and reproduction
plasmapheresis: removal of whole blood from the body, separation of its cellular elements by centrifugation, and reinfusion of them suspended in saline or some other plasma substitute, thereby depleting the body's own plasma without depleting its cells
pyodermas: bacterial skin infections
striae: bandlike streaks on the skin distinguished by colour, texture, depression, or elevation from the tissue in which they are found; usually purplish or white
suspensions: liquid preparations in which powder is suspended, requiring shaking before use
tinea: superficial fungal infection on the skin or scalp
xerosis: overly dry skin

CHART 58-1

Wound Care Products

adhesives	foam dressings
adhesive removers	gauze dressings
adhesive skin closures	growth factors
adhesive tapes	hydrocolloid dressings
alginate dressings	hydrogel dressings
antibiotics	leg ulcer wraps, compression bandages or wraps
antimicrobials	lubricating, stimulating sprays
antiseptics	moisturizers
bandages	moisture barrier ointments
biosynthetic dressings	ointments
cleansers	perineal cleansers
collagen dressings	skin sealants
composite dressings	transparent film dressings
contact layers	wound fillers: pastes, powders, beads, etc.
creams or skin protectant pastes	wound pouches
dressing covers	
enzyme debriding agents	

ease of use for the patient, and other considerations when applicable.

Rule 3: Change

The nurse changes dressings based on patient, wound, and dressing assessments, not on standardized routines. Traditional nursing care plans recommended changing dressings on a routine schedule, often three or four times each day; however, with current dressings, such frequent dressing change practices are obsolete and unnecessary.

NURSING ALERT

It is believed that the natural wound-healing process should not be disrupted. Unless the wound is infected or has a heavy discharge, it is common to leave chronic wounds covered for 48 to 72 hours and acute wounds for 24 hours.

Rule 4: Evolution

As the wound progresses through the phases of wound healing, the dressing protocol is altered to optimize wound healing. It is rare, especially in cases of chronic wounds, that the same dressing material is appropriate throughout the healing process. The rule assumes that the nurse and the patient or family have access to a wide variety of products and are knowledgeable about their use. The nurse teaches the patient or family caregiver about wound care and ensures that the family has access to appropriate dressing choices.

Rule 5: Practice

Practice with dressing material is required for the nurse to learn the performance parameters of the particular dressing. Refining the skills of applying appropriate dressings correctly and learning about new dressing products are essential nursing responsibilities. Dressing changes should only be delegated to assistive personnel who possess the required skills and abilities for such procedures; wound assessments require the knowledge base and assessment skills of professional nurses.

Autolytic Debridement

Autolytic **debridement** is a process that uses the body's own digestive enzymes to break down necrotic tissue. The wound is kept moist with occlusive dressings. Eschar and necrotic debris are softened, liquefied, and separated from the bed of the wound.

Several commercially available products contain the same enzymes that the body produces naturally. These are called *enzymatic debriding agents*; examples include Accuzyme, Granulex, and Zymase. Application of these products speeds the rate at which necrotic tissue is removed. This method is still slower and no more effective than surgical debridement. When enzymatic debridement is being used under an occlusive dressing, a foul odour is produced by the breakdown of cellular debris. This odour does not indicate that the wound is infected. The nurse should expect this reaction and help the patient and family understand the reason for the odour.

Categories of Dressings

Table 58-1 is a guide to wound dressing functions and categories.

Occlusive Dressings

Occlusive dressings may be commercially produced or made inexpensively from sterile or nonsterile gauze squares or wrap. Occlusive dressings cover topical medication that is applied to a skin lesion. The area is kept airtight by using plastic film (e.g., plastic wrap). Plastic film is thin and readily adapts to all sizes, body shapes, and skin surfaces. Plastic surgical tape containing a corticosteroid in the adhesive layer can be cut to size and applied to individual lesions. Generally, plastic wrap should be used for no more than 12 hours each day.

Wet Dressings

Wet dressings (i.e., wet compresses applied to the skin) were traditionally used for acute, weeping, inflammatory lesions. They have become almost obsolete in light of the many newer products available for wound care.

Moisture-Retentive Dressings

Newer, commercially produced moisture-retentive dressings can perform the same functions as wet compresses but are more efficient at removing exudate because of their higher moisture–vapour transmission rate; some have reservoirs that can hold excessive exudate. A number of moisture-retentive dressings are already impregnated with saline solution, petrolatum, zinc-saline solution, hydrogel, or antimicrobial agents, thereby eliminating the need to coat the skin to avoid maceration. The main advantages of moisture-retentive dressings over wet compresses are improved fibrinolysis, accelerated epidermal resurfacing, reduced pain, fewer infections, less scar tissue, gentle autolytic debridement, and decreased frequency of dressing changes. Depending on the product

TABLE 58-1 Quick Guide to Function and Action of Wound Dressings

Function	Action	Example
Absorption	Absorbs exudates	Alginates, composite dressings, foams, gauze, hydrocolloids, hydrogels
Cleansing	Removes purulent drainage, foreign debris, and devitalized tissue	Wound cleansers
Debridement	*Autolytic*—covers a wound and allows enzymes to self-digest sloughed skin	Absorption beads, pastes, powders; alginates; composite dressings; foams; hydrate gauze; hydrogels; hydrocolloids; transparent films; wound care systems
	Chemical or enzymatic—applied topically to break down devitalized tissue	Enzymatic debridement agents
	Mechanical—removes devitalized tissue with mechanical force	Wound cleansers, gauze (wet to dry), whirlpool
Diathermy	Produces electrical current to promote warmth and new tissue growth	
Hydration	Adds moisture to a wound	Gauze (saturated with saline solution), hydrogels, wound care systems
Maintain moist environment	Manages moisture levels in a wound and maintains a moist environment	Composites, contact layers, foams, gauze (impregnated or saturated), hydrogels, hydrocolloids, transparent films, wound care systems
Manage high-output wounds	Manages excessive quantities of exudates	Pouching systems
Pack or fill dead space	Prevents premature wound closure or fills shallow areas and provides absorption	Absorbent beads, powders, pastes; alginates; composites, foams; gauze (impregnated and nonimpregnated)
Protect and cover wound	Provides protection from the external environment	Composites, compression bandages/wraps, foams, gauze dressings, hydrogels, hydrocolloids, transparent film dressings
Protect periwound skin	Prevents moisture and mechanical trauma from damaging delicate tissue around wound	Composites, foams, hydrocolloids, pouching systems, skin sealants, transparent film dressings
Provide therapeutic compression	Provides appropriate levels of support to the lower extremities in venous stasis disease	Compression bandages, wraps, graduated compression stockings

Adapted from Krasner, D., Rodeheaver, G., Sibbald, G., et al. (2012). *Chronic wound care: A clinical source book for healthcare professionals* (5th ed.). Malvern, PA: HMP Communications.

used and the type of dermatologic problem encountered, most moisture-retentive dressings may remain in place from 12 to 24 hours; some can remain in place as long as a week (Landriscina, Rosen, & Friedman, 2015).

Hydrogels

Hydrogels are polymers with a 90% to 95% water content. They are available in impregnated sheets or as gel in a tube. Their high moisture content makes them ideal for autolytic debridement of wounds. They are semitransparent, allowing for wound inspection without dressing removal. They are comfortable and soothing for the painful wound. They have no inherent adhesive and require a secondary dressing to keep them in place. Hydrogels are appropriate for superficial wounds with high serous output, such as abrasions, skin graft sites, and draining venous ulcers (Landriscina et al., 2015).

Hydrocolloids

Hydrocolloids are composed of a water-impermeable, polyurethane outer covering separated from the wound by a hydrocolloid material. They are adherent and nonpermeable to water vapour and oxygen. As water evaporates over the wound, water is absorbed into the dressing, which softens and discolours with the increased water content. The dressing can be removed without damage to the wound. As the dressing absorbs water, it produces a foul-smelling, yellowish covering over the wound. This is a normal chemical interaction between the dressing and wound exudate and should not be confused with purulent drainage from the wound. Unfortunately, most of the hydrocolloid dressings are opaque, limiting inspection of the wound without removal of the dressing.

Available in sheets and in gels, hydrocolloids are a good choice for both exudative and acute wounds. Easy to use and comfortable, hydrocolloid dressings promote debridement and formation of granulation tissue. Most can be left in place for as long as 7 days and can be submerged in water for bathing or showering. Hydrocolloid dressings are more effective than saline gauze or paraffin gauze dressings in completely healing chronic wounds (Landriscina et al., 2015).

Hydrofiber™ Technology Dressings

Hydrofiber™ Technology is a specially engineered soft and absorbent dressing material that transforms into a gel when it comes in contact with exudates from a wound. This gelling action is said to create the best optimum environment for wound healing. It is available in sheets and with or without composite cover dressings, Hydrofiber™ Technology dressings are a good choice for moderate to heavily exudative wounds. They fill dead space, trap bacteria, and maintain a moist wound environment. Also available with ionic silver, these dressings reduce the bioburden in wounds and provide rapid and sustained antimicrobial activity on demand. The amount of dressing can be adjusted to increase wear time. Dressings can be left in place for up to 7 days.

Foam Dressings

Foam dressings consist of microporous polyurethane with an absorptive **hydrophilic** (water-absorbing) surface that covers the wound and a **hydrophobic** (water-resistant) backing to block leakage of exudate. While some are nonadherent and require a secondary dressing to keep them in place, others contain layers of hydrofiber and act as a secondary dressing combined. Moisture is absorbed into the foam layer, decreasing maceration of surrounding tissue. A moist environment is maintained, and removal of the dressing does not damage the wound. The foams are opaque and must be removed for wound inspection. Foams are a good choice for exudative wounds. They are especially helpful over bony prominences because they provide contoured cushioning (Landriscina et al., 2015).

Calcium Alginates

Calcium alginates are derived from seaweed and consist of tremendously absorbent calcium alginate fibres. They are hemostatic and bioabsorbable and can be used as sheets, mats, or ropes of absorbent material. As the exudate is absorbed, the fibres turn into a viscous hydrogel. They are quite useful in areas where the tissue is more irritated or macerated. The alginate dressing forms a moist pocket over the wound while the surrounding skin stays dry. The dressing also reacts with wound fluid to form a foul-smelling coating. Alginates work well when packed into a deep cavity, wound, or sinus tract with heavy drainage. They are nonadherent and require a secondary dressing. Wound experts suggest that alginates are superior to other modern dressings for debriding necrotic wounds (Landriscina et al., 2015).

Advances in Wound Treatment

Increasing understanding of how skin and wounds heal has led to several advances in therapy. Growth factors are cytokines or proteins that have potent **mitogenic** activity. Low levels of cytokines circulate in the blood continuously, but activated platelets release increased amounts of preformed growth factors into a wound. This increase in cytokines in the wound stimulates cellular growth and granulation of skin. REGRANEX Gel contains becaplermin, a platelet-derived growth factor, which is applied to the wound to stimulate healing. REGRANEX Gel is used in the treatment of lower extremity diabetic neuropathic ulcers that may still have adequate blood supply. Apligraf is a skin construct (i.e., bioengineered skin substitute) imbedded in a dressing that also contains cytokines and fibroblasts. When applied to wounds, these agents stimulate platelet activity and potentially decrease wound-healing time.

Bioengineered skin substitutes have emerged in the past 20 years as the most effective method for management of chronic wounds. Most of these skin substitutes are cultures of keratinocytes delivered on a petrolatum gauze. They work by maintaining wound moisture, providing a structure for regeneration of cells, and supplying beneficial cytokines. A partial list of these substitutes includes AlloDerm, Apligraf, Dermagraft, Epicel, and Laserskin.

Some oral medications are being investigated for their benefits in healing chronic venous ulcers of the lower legs. Pentoxifylline (Trental) increases peripheral blood flow by decreasing the viscosity of blood. It has some **fibrinolytic** action and decreases leukocyte adhesion to the wall of the blood vessels. Enteric-coated aspirin has also been shown to be of value, although its exact mechanism is still not clear.

Medical Management

Medical management of skin disorders includes a host of prescribed and over-the-counter therapies.

Therapeutic Baths (Balneotherapy) and Medications

Baths or soaks, known as **balneotherapy**, are useful when large areas of skin are affected. The baths remove crusts, scales, and old medications and relieve the inflammation and itching that accompany acute dermatoses. Additional information about therapeutic baths is given in Table 58-2.

TABLE 58-2 Types of Therapeutic Baths

Bath Solution	Effects and Uses	Nursing Interventions
Water	Same effect as wet dressings	• Fill the tub half full.
Saline	Used for widely disseminated lesions	• Keep the water at a comfortable temperature.
Colloidal (Aveeno, oatmeal)	Antipruritic, soothing	• Do not allow the water to cool excessively.
Sodium bicarbonate (baking soda)	Cooling	• Use a bath mat—*medications added to the bath can cause the tub to be slippery.*
Starch	Soothing	• Apply an emollient cream to damp skin after the bath if lubrication is desired.
Medicated tars	Psoriasis and chronic eczema	• Because tars are volatile, the bath area should be well ventilated.
Bath oils	Antipruritic and emollient action; acute and subacute generalized eczematous eruptions	• Dry by gently blotting with a towel.
		• Keep room warm to minimize temperature fluctuations.
		• Encourage the patient to wear light, loose clothing after the bath.

TABLE 58-3 Common Topical Preparations and Medications

Preparation	Product Name
Moisturizer creams	AcidMantle cream, Curel cream, Dermasil, Eucerin, Lubriderm, Noxzema skin cream
Moisturizer ointments	Aquaphor Healing Ointment, Eutra Swiss SkinCream, Vaseline ointment
Topical anesthetic agents	Lidocaine (Xylocaine) of various strengths in the form of spray, ointment, gel; lidocaine 2.5% and prilocaine 2.5% (EMLA cream)
Topical antibiotic agents	Bacitracin, bacitracin and polymyxin B (Polysporin), mupirocin 2% (Bactroban ointment or cream), erythromycin 2% (Emgel, Eryderm solution), clindamycin phosphate 1% (Cleocin cream, gel, solution), gentamicin sulfate 1% (Garamycin cream or ointment), 1% silver sulfadiazine cream (Silvadene)

Adapted from Goldsmith, L., Katz, S. I., Gilchrest, B. A., et al. (2012). *Fitzpatrick's dermatology in general medicine* (8th ed.). New York: McGraw-Hill.

Pharmacologic Therapy

Because skin is easily accessible and therefore easy to treat, topical medications are often used. High concentrations of some medications can be applied directly to the affected site with little systemic absorption and therefore with few systemic side effects. However, some medications are readily absorbed through the skin and can produce systemic effects. Because topical preparations may induce allergic contact **dermatitis** (inflammation of the skin) in sensitive patients, any untoward response should be reported immediately and the medication discontinued.

Medicated lotions, creams, ointments, and powders are frequently used to treat skin lesions. In general, moisture-retentive dressings, with or without medication, are used in the acute stage; lotions and creams are reserved for the subacute stage; and ointments are used when inflammation has become chronic and the skin is dry with scaling or **lichenification** (leathery thickening).

With all types of topical medication, the patient is taught to apply the medication gently but thoroughly and, when necessary, to cover the medication with a dressing to protect clothing. Table 58-3 lists some commonly used topical preparations.

Lotions

Lotions are frequently used to replenish lost skin oils or to relieve pruritus. They are usually applied directly to the skin, but a dressing soaked in the lotion can be placed on the affected area. Lotions must be applied every 3 or 4 hours for sustained therapeutic effect. If left in place for a longer period, they may crust and cake on the skin.

Lotions are of two types: **suspensions** and **liniments**. Suspensions consist of a powder in water, requiring shaking before application, and clear solutions, containing completely dissolved active ingredients. Lotions are usually applied directly to the skin, but a dressing soaked in the lotion can be placed on the affected area. A suspension such as calamine lotion provides a rapid cooling and drying effect as it evaporates, leaving a thin, medicinal layer of powder on the affected skin. Liniments are lotions with oil added to prevent crusting. Because lotions are easy to use, therapeutic compliance is generally high.

Powders

Powders usually have a talc, zinc oxide, bentonite, or cornstarch base and are dusted on the skin with a shaker or with cotton sponges. Although their therapeutic action is brief, powders act as **hygroscopic** agents that absorb and retain moisture from the air and reduce friction between skin surfaces and clothing or bedding.

Creams

Creams may be suspensions of oil in water or emulsions of water in oil, with additional ingredients to prevent bacterial and fungal growth. Both may cause an allergic reaction such as contact dermatitis. Oil-in-water creams are easily applied and usually are the most cosmetically acceptable to the patient. Although they can be used on the face, they tend to have a drying effect. Water-in-oil emulsions are greasier and are preferred for drying and flaking dermatoses. Creams usually are rubbed into the skin by hand. They are used for their moisturizing and emollient effects.

Gels

Gels are semisolid emulsions that become liquid when applied to the skin or scalp. They are cosmetically acceptable to the patient because they are not visible after application, and they are greaseless and nonstaining. The newer water-based gels appear to penetrate the skin more effectively and cause less stinging on application. They are especially useful for acute dermatitis in which there is weeping exudate (e.g., poison ivy).

Pastes

Pastes are mixtures of powders and ointments and are used in inflammatory blistering conditions. They adhere to the skin and may be difficult to remove without using an oil (e.g., olive oil, mineral oil). Pastes are applied with a wooden tongue depressor or gloved hand.

Ointments

Ointments retard water loss and lubricate and protect the skin. They are the preferred vehicle for delivering medication to chronic or localized dry skin conditions, such as eczema or psoriasis. Ointments are applied with a wooden tongue depressor or gloved hand.

Sprays and Aerosols

Spray and aerosol preparations may be used on any widespread dermatologic condition. They evaporate on contact and are used infrequently.

Topical Corticosteroids

Corticosteroids are widely used in treating dermatologic conditions to provide anti-inflammatory, antipruritic, and vasoconstrictive effects. The patient is taught to apply this medication according to strict guidelines, using it sparingly but rubbing it into the prescribed area thoroughly. Absorption of topical corticosteroid is enhanced when the skin is hydrated or the affected area is covered by an occlusive or moisture-retentive dressing (Karch, 2015). Inappropriate use of topical corticosteroids can result in local and systemic side effects, especially when the medication is absorbed through inflamed and excoriated skin, under occlusive dressings, or when used for long periods on sensitive areas. Local side effects may include skin atrophy and thinning, **striae** (bandlike streaks), and telangiectasia. Thinning of the skin results from the ability of corticosteroids to inhibit skin collagen synthesis. The thinning process can be reversed by discontinuing the medication, but striae and telangiectasia are permanent. Systemic side effects may include hyperglycemia and symptoms of Cushing's syndrome. Caution is required when applying corticosteroids around the eyes because long-term use may cause glaucoma or cataracts, and the anti-inflammatory effect of corticosteroids may mask existing viral or fungal infections.

Concentrated (fluorinated) corticosteroids are never applied on the face or intertriginous areas (i.e., axilla and groin), because these areas have a thinner stratum corneum and absorb the medication much more quickly than areas such as the forearm or legs. Persistent use of concentrated topical corticosteroids in any location may produce acnelike dermatitis, known as steroid-induced acne, and hypertrichosis (excessive hair growth). Because some topical corticosteroid preparations are available without prescription, patients are cautioned about prolonged and inappropriate use. Table 58-4 lists topical corticosteroid preparations according to potency.

TABLE 58-4 Potency: Topical Corticosteroids

Potency	Topical Corticosteroid	Preparations
OTC	0.5–1.0% hydrocortisone	cr, lot, oint
Lowest	dexamethasone 0.1% (Decaderm)	cr, oint, aerosol, gel
	alclometasone 0.05% (Aclovate)	cr, oint
	hydrocortisone 2.5% (Hytone)	cr, lot, oint
Low–medium	desonide 0.05% (DesOwen, Tridesilon)	cr, lot, oint
	fluocinolone acetonide 0.025% (Synalar)	cr, solution
	hydrocortisone valerate 0.2% (Westcort)	cr, solution
	betamethasone valerate 0.1% (Valisone)	cr, oint
	fluticasone propionate 0.05% (Cutivate)	cr, oint
Medium–high	triamcinolone acetonide 0.1–0.5% (Aristocort)	cr, oint, lot
	fluocinonide 0.05% (Lidex)	cr, oint, gel
	desoximetasone 0.05–0.25% (Topicort)	cr, oint, gel
	fluocinolone 0.2% (Synalar)	cr, oint
	diflorasone diacetate 0.05% (Psorcon)	cr, oint
Very high	clobetasol propionate 0.05% (Temovate)	cr, oint, gel
	betamethasone dipropionate 0.05% (Diprolene)	cr, oint, gel
	halobetasol propionate 0.05% (Ultravate)	cr, oint

OTC, over the counter; cr, cream; lot, lotion; oint, ointment.

Adapted from Karch, A. M. (2015). *Lippincott's nursing drug guide* (2015th ed.). Philadelphia, PA: Lippincott Williams & Wilkins.

Intralesional Therapy

Intralesional therapy consists of injecting a sterile suspension of medication (usually a corticosteroid) into or just below a lesion. Although this treatment may have an anti-inflammatory effect, local atrophy may result if the medication is injected into subcutaneous fat. Skin lesions treated with intralesional therapy include psoriasis, keloids, and cystic acne. Occasionally, immunotherapeutic and antifungal agents are administered as intralesional therapy.

Systemic Medications

Systemic medications are also prescribed for skin conditions. These include corticosteroids for short-term therapy for contact dermatitis or for long-term treatment of a chronic **dermatosis**, such as pemphigus vulgaris. Other frequently used systemic medications include antibiotics, antifungals, antihistamines, sedatives, tranquilizers, analgesics, and **cytotoxic** agents.

Nursing Management

Management begins with a health history, direct observation, and a complete physical examination. Chapter 56 provides a description of integumentary assessment. Because of its visibility, a skin condition is usually difficult to ignore or conceal from others and may therefore cause the patient some emotional distress. The major goals for the patient may include maintenance of skin integrity, relief of discomfort, promotion of restful sleep, self-acceptance, knowledge about skin care, and avoidance of complications.

Nursing management for patients who must perform self-care for skin disorders, such as applying medications and dressings, focuses mainly on teaching the patient how to wash the affected area and pat it dry; apply medication to the lesion while the skin is moist; cover the area with plastic (e.g., Telfa pads, plastic wrap, vinyl gloves, plastic bag) if recommended; and cover it with an elastic bandage, dressing, or paper tape to seal the edges. Dressings that contain or cover a topical corticosteroid should be removed for 12 of every 24 hours to prevent skin thinning (atrophy), striae, and telangiectasia (small, red lesions caused by dilation of blood vessels).

Other forms of dressings, such as those used to cover topical medications, include soft cotton cloth and stretchable cotton dressings (e.g., Surgitube, Tubegauz) that can be used for fingers, toes, hands, and feet. The hands can be covered with disposable polyethylene or vinyl gloves sealed at the wrists; the feet can be wrapped in plastic bags covered by cotton socks. Gloves and socks that are already impregnated with emollients, making application to the hands and feet more convenient, are also available. When large areas of the body must be covered, cotton cloth topped by an expandable stockinette can be used. Disposable diapers or cloths folded in diaper fashion are useful for dressing the groin and the perineal areas. Axillary dressings can be made of cotton cloth, or a commercially prepared dressing may be used and taped in place or held by dress shields. A turban or plastic shower cap is useful for holding dressings on the scalp. A face mask, made from gauze with holes cut out for the eyes, nose, and mouth, may be held in place with gauze ties looped through holes cut in the four corners of the mask. Refer to the Chart 58-4 for more information.

PRURITUS

General Itching

Pruritus (itching) is the most common symptom of patients with dermatologic disorders (Carr, Veledar, & Chen, 2014; Tarikci, Kocatürk, Güngör, et al., 2015). Itch receptors are unmyelinated, penicillate (brushlike) nerve endings that are found exclusively in the skin, mucous membranes, and cornea. Although pruritus is usually caused by primary skin disease with resultant rash or lesions, it may occur without a rash or lesion. This is referred to as essential pruritus, which generally has a rapid onset, may be severe, and interferes with normal daily activities.

Pruritus may be the first indication of a systemic internal disease such as diabetes, blood disorder, or cancer (occult malignancy of the breast or colon, lymphoma). It may also accompany kidney, hepatic, and thyroid diseases (see Chart 58-2). Some common oral medications such as aspirin, antibiotics, hormones (e.g., estrogens, testosterone, or oral contraceptives), and opioids (e.g., morphine) may cause pruritus directly or by increasing sensitivity to ultraviolet (UV) light. Certain soaps and chemicals, radiation therapy, prickly heat (miliaria), and contact with woolen garments are associated with pruritus as well. Pruritus may also be caused by psychological factors, such as excessive stress in family or work situations, and is called *psychodermatosis* (Tarikci et al., 2015).

CHART 58-2

Systemic Disorders Associated With Generalized Pruritus

- Chronic kidney disease
- Endocrine disease (thyrotoxicosis, hypothyroidism, diabetes)
- Folliculitis (bacterial, candidiasis, dermatophyte)
- Hematologic disorders (iron deficiency anemia)
- Infestations (scabies, lice, other insects)
- Malignancies (polycythemia vera, Hodgkin's lymphoma, lymphoma, leukemia, multiple myeloma, mycosis fungoides, and cancers of the lung, breast, central nervous system, and gastrointestinal tract)
- Neurologic disorders (multiple sclerosis, brain abscess, brain tumour)
- Obstructive biliary disease (primary biliary cirrhosis, extrahepatic biliary obstruction, drug-induced cholestasis)
- Pruritus of pregnancy (pruritic urticarial papules of pregnancy, cholestasis of pregnancy, pemphigoid of pregnancy)
- Psychiatric disorders (emotional stress, anxiety, neurosis, phobias)
- Skin conditions (seborrheic dermatitis, folliculitis, atopic dermatitis)

Adapted from Tarikci, N., Kocatürk, E., Güngör, S., et al. (2015). Pruritus in systemic diseases: A review of etiological factors and new treatment modalities. *The Scientific World Journal, 2015*, 803752.

Pathophysiology

Scratching the itchy area causes the inflamed cells and nerve endings to release histamine, which produces more pruritus, generating a vicious itch–scratch cycle. If the patient responds to an itch by scratching, the integrity of the skin may be altered, and excoriation, redness, raised areas (wheals), infection, or changes in pigmentation may result. Pruritus usually is more severe at night and is less frequently reported during waking hours, probably because the person is distracted by daily activities. At night, when there are few distractions, the slightest pruritus cannot be easily ignored. Severe itching is debilitating (Bolier, Elferink, & Beuers, 2016).

Gerontologic Considerations

Pruritus occurs frequently in older adults as a result of dry skin. Older adults are also more likely to have a systemic illness that triggers pruritus, are at higher risk for occult malignancy, and are more likely to be on multiple medications than is the younger population. All of these factors increase the incidence of pruritus in the older adult (Eliopoulos, 2018).

Medical Management

A thorough history and physical examination usually provide clues to the underlying cause of the pruritus, such as hay fever, allergy, recent administration of a new medication, or a change of cosmetics or soaps. After the cause has been identified, treatment of the condition should relieve the pruritus. Signs of infection and environmental clues, such as warm, dry air or irritating bed linens, are identified. In general, washing with soap and hot water is avoided. Bath oils (e.g., Lubath, Alpha-Keri) containing a surfactant that makes the oil mix with bath water may be sufficient for cleaning. However, an older adult or a patient with unsteady balance should avoid adding oil because it increases the danger of slipping in the bathtub. A warm bath with a mild soap followed by application of a bland emollient to moist skin can control **xerosis** (dry skin). Applying a cold compress, ice cube, or cool agents that contain menthol and camphor (which constrict blood vessels) may also help to relieve pruritus (Tarikci et al., 2015).

Pharmacologic Therapy

Topical antipruritic agents (e.g., lidocaine, prilocaine) or capsaicin cream (Capzasin) may be useful in providing relief from localized pruritus. Topical corticosteroids are effective when used to diminish pruritus that occurs secondary to inflammatory conditions because of their anti-inflammatory effects. Oral antihistamines are frequently prescribed and may be effective when the pruritus is nocturnal, particularly agents such as diphenhydramine (Benadryl) or hydroxyzine (Atarax), which also cause somnolence, resulting in a restful and comfortable sleep. Other nonsedating antihistamines such as fexofenadine (Allegra) are used to relieve daytime pruritus. Selective serotonin reuptake inhibitor antidepressants (e.g., fluoxetine [Prozac], sertraline [Zoloft]) may be effective, particularly in patients with pruritus that is secondary to

NURSING RESEARCH PROFILE

Chart 58-3. Quality of Life Among Women With Acne

Gorelick, J., Daniels, S. R., Kawata, A. K., et al. (2015). Acne-related quality of life among female adults of different races/ethnicities. *Journal of the Dermatology Nurses Association*, 7(3), 154–162.

Purpose

Acne vulgaris is a common chronic dermatosis that is traditionally considered a disorder of adolescence. However, it frequently persists into adulthood, with an estimated prevalence of 43% among adults in their third decade of life. Women are more commonly affected than men, and women of colour are affected more commonly than Caucasian women. Acne is also associated with depression, distress, and lower quality of life (QOL). However, little is known about the effects of acne on QOL among women of different racial groups. The purpose of this study was to describe the QOL of women with facial acne and find whether or not there existed differences in QOL among participants based on their racial background.

Design

This was a descriptive cross-sectional web-based study that solicited participants who were part of a preregistered YouGov pool of panelists in the United States. The study was approved by a centralized institutional review board before prospective participants were invited to join the study. Eligibility criteria included women between 25 and 45 years of age with an active email address who could read and understand English and who self-reported having at least 25 visible facial acne lesions. After screening, eligible participants were invited to complete an online survey with items that provided information on demographics, comorbid health conditions, clinical characteristics of the acne, and self-assessed reports of work or school productivity. The Acne-Specific QOL Questionnaire (Acne-QOL) was a component of the survey, as were psychological symptoms measured by items included from the Patient Health Questionnaire-4 (PHQ-4).

Findings

Participants ($N = 312$) reflected a diverse racial mix including Caucasian (34.3%), African American (30.8%), Hispanic (17.6%), and Asian American (17.3%). The mean age of the sample was 35.3 years of age (SD 5.9). Caucasian participants reported more concern with lesions (i.e., "pimples," "bumps") whereas African American, Hispanic, and Asian American participants reported greater concern with postinflammatory hyperpigmentation, in addition to lesions ($p < 0.0001$). More Caucasian participants reported anxiety ($p < 0.0001$), depression ($p < 0.001$), and migraines ($p < 0.05$) than participants from other racial groups. Participants from all racial groups reported that acne hampered their QOL, and more than one third reported moderate to severe symptoms of anxiety and depression. Acne also negatively affected the ability of participants from all racial groups to concentrate on work or school.

Nursing Implications

Results from this study indicate that having acne can adversely affect QOL in women. In particular, women with acne may have different concerns, based on their racial background/skin type. African American, Hispanic, and Asian American women are more prone to the adverse consequence of hyperpigmentation from acne lesions. Results from this study confirm that this is a top concern among these women who have acne, whereas Caucasian women are primarily concerned about the appearance of lesions. Conversely, Caucasian women express more symptoms consistent with depression and anxiety related to having acne than women from other racial groups. Nurses can use information gleaned from this study to tailor individualized care toward women with acne.

cholestasis or the uremia of chronic kidney disease (Bolier et al., 2016; Chan, Li, Wong, et al., 2013; Hong, Buddenkotte, Berger, et al., 2013).

Nursing Management

The nurse reinforces the reasons for the prescribed therapeutic regimen and counsels the patient on specific points of care (Chart 58-3). If baths have been prescribed, the patient is reminded to use tepid (not hot) water and to shake off the excess water and blot between intertriginous areas (body folds) with a towel. Rubbing vigorously with the towel is avoided because this overstimulates the skin and causes more itching. It also removes water from the stratum corneum. Immediately after bathing, the skin should be lubricated with an emollient to trap moisture.

The patient is instructed to avoid situations that cause vasodilation (i.e., expansion of the blood vessels). Examples include exposure to an overly warm environment and ingestion of alcohol or hot foods and liquids. All can induce or intensify itching. Using a humidifier is helpful if environmental air is dry. Activities that result in perspiration should be limited because perspiration may irritate and promote pruritus. If the patient is troubled at night with itching that interferes with sleep, the nurse can advise wearing cotton clothing next to the skin rather than synthetic materials. The room should be kept cool and humidified. Vigorous scratching should be avoided, and nails should be kept trimmed to prevent skin damage and infection. When the underlying cause of pruritus is unknown and further testing is required, the nurse explains each test and the expected outcome.

Perineal and Perianal Itching

Pruritus of the genital and anal regions may be caused by small particles of fecal material lodged in the perianal crevices or attached to anal hairs. Alternatively, it may result from perianal skin damage caused by scratching, moisture, and decreased skin resistance as a result of corticosteroid or antibiotic therapy. Other possible causes of perianal itching include local irritants such as scabies and lice, local lesions such as hemorrhoids, fungal or yeast infections, and pinworm infestation. Conditions such as diabetes mellitus, anemia, hyperthyroidism, and pregnancy may also result in pruritus. Occasionally, no cause can be identified.

Nursing Management

The patient is instructed to follow proper hygiene measures and to discontinue home and over-the-counter remedies. The perineal or anal area should be rinsed with lukewarm water and blotted dry with cotton balls. Premoistened tissues may be used after defecation. Use a powder such as Zeasorb (Stiefel) to absorb perspiration and prevent yeast infection. Never use cornstarch as it increases yeast.

As part of health teaching, the nurse instructs the patient to avoid bathing in water that is too hot and to avoid using bubble baths, sodium bicarbonate, and detergent soaps, all of which aggravate dryness. To keep the perineal or perianal skin area as dry as possible, patients should avoid wearing underwear made of synthetic fabrics. Local anesthetic agents should not be used, as these may have allergic effects. The patient should also avoid vasodilating agents or stimulants (e.g., alcohol, caffeine) and mechanical irritants such as rough or woolen clothing. A diet that includes adequate fibre may help maintain soft stools and prevent minor trauma to the anal mucosa.

SECRETORY DISORDERS

The main secretory function of the skin is performed by the sweat glands, which help to regulate body temperature. These glands excrete perspiration that evaporates, thereby cooling the body. The sweat glands are located in various parts of the body and respond to different stimuli. Those on the trunk generally respond to thermal stimulation, those on the palms and soles respond to nervous stimulation, and those in the axillae and on the forehead respond to both kinds of stimulation. Usual perspiration has no odour. Body odour is produced by the increase in bacteria on the skin and the interaction of bacterial waste products with the chemicals of perspiration. As a rule, moist skin is warm, and dry skin is cool, but this is not always true. It is not unusual to observe warm, dry skin in a dehydrated patient and very hot, dry skin in some febrile states.

Usually, underarm sweat can be controlled with the use of antiperspirants and deodorants. Most antiperspirants are aluminum salts that block the opening to the sweat duct. Pure deodorants inhibit bacterial growth and block the metabolism of sweat; they have no antiperspirant effect. Fragrance-free deodorants are available for those with sensitive skin. Open weave products such as J-cloths can be placed under the breasts or abdomen to absorb perspiration.

Hidradenitis Suppurativa

Hidradenitis suppurativa (HS) is a chronic suppurative folliculitis of the perianal, axillary, and genital areas or under the breasts. It can produce abscesses or sinuses with scarring. It develops after puberty and diminishes in incidence after 50 years of age. African Americans are at greater risk for HS. In addition, men are at greater risk for anogenital HS, whereas women are at greater risk for axillary HS. The cause is unknown, but it appears to have a genetic basis (Wollina, Koch, Heinig, et al., 2013).

Pathophysiology

It had been assumed for many years that HS was caused by an abnormal blockage and infection of the sweat glands. However, recent evidence suggests that it is a primary disorder of follicular occlusion that causes eventual hypertrophic formation of scar tissue in the area of the sweat glands (Wollina et al., 2013).

Clinical Manifestations

HS occurs more frequently in the axillae but also appears in inguinal folds, on the mons pubis, around the buttocks, areolae of the breasts, submammary fold, nape of the neck, and shoulders. The patient may present with a firm, pea-sized nodule that causes discomfort, or with a history of this type of nodule that then ruptures and discharges purulent drainage. The nodule then propagates, and multiple similar nodules will form adjacent to the initial nodule. These nodules become deep seated and, as they rupture, form scars. The nodules may coalesce or form “bridges,” become infected, and result in abscesses. As they coalesce, the patient will present with complaints of persistent pain (Wollina et al., 2013).

Medical Management

The patient is educated to use warm compresses and wear loose-fitting clothes over the nodules or lesions. Oral antibiotic agents such as erythromycin, tetracycline, minocycline, and doxycycline are frequently prescribed. Nonsteroidal anti-inflammatory drugs (NSAIDs) may be indicated to relieve the pain. Silver-impregnated alginate dressings may be useful with some lesions. Incision and drainage of large suppurating areas with gauze packs inserted to facilitate drainage are often necessary. Rarely, the entire area is excised, removing the scar tissue and any infection. This surgery is drastic in that it may require the use of skin grafts (see later discussion) and is performed only as a last resort. CO_2 laser surgery (see later discussion) may be more effective than this type of excisional surgery (Wollina et al., 2013).

Seborrheic Dermatitis

Seborrhea is excessive production of sebum (i.e., secretion of sebaceous glands) in areas where sebaceous glands are usually found in large numbers, such as the face, scalp, eyebrows, eyelids, sides of the nose and upper lip, malar regions (cheeks), ears, axillae, under the breasts, groin, and gluteal crease of the buttocks. Seborrheic dermatitis is a chronic inflammatory disease of the skin with a predilection for areas that are well supplied with sebaceous glands or lie between skin folds, where the bacteria count is high (Borda & Wikramanayake, 2015).

Clinical Manifestations

Two forms of Seborrheic Dermatitis can occur, an oily form and a dry form. Either form may start in childhood and continue throughout life. The oily form appears moist or greasy. There may be patches of sallow, greasy skin, with or without scaling, and slight erythema (redness), predominantly on the forehead, nasolabial fold, beard area, and scalp and between adjacent skin surfaces in the regions of the axillae, groin, and breasts. Small pustules or papulopustules resembling acne may appear on the trunk. The dry form, consisting of flaky desquamation of the scalp with a profuse amount of fine, powdery scales, is commonly called *dandruff*. The mild forms of the disease are asymptomatic. When scaling occurs, it is often accompanied by pruritus, which may lead to scratching and secondary infections and excoriation.

Seborrheic dermatitis has a genetic predisposition. Hormones, nutritional status, infection, and emotional stress influence its course. The remissions and exacerbations of this condition are explained to the patient. If a person has not previously been diagnosed with this condition and suddenly appears with a severe outbreak, a complete history and physical examination are considered.

Medical Management

Because there is no known cure for seborrhea, the objectives of therapy are to control the disorder and allow the skin to repair itself. Seborrheic dermatitis of the body and face may respond to a topically applied corticosteroid cream, which allays the secondary inflammatory response. However, this medication should be used with caution near the eyelids because it can lead to glaucoma and cataracts. As an alternative treatment, patients can wash the eyelids using baby shampoo and cotton swabs (Handler, 2017).

Patients with seborrheic dermatitis may develop a secondary candidal (yeast) infection in body creases or folds. To avoid this, patients should be advised to ensure maximum aeration of the skin and to clean carefully areas where there are creases or folds in the skin (Borda & Wikramanayake, 2015). Patients with persistent candidiasis should be evaluated for diabetes.

The mainstay of dandruff treatment is proper, frequent shampooing (at least three times weekly) with medicated shampoos. Two or three different types of shampoo should be used in rotation to prevent the seborrhea from becoming resistant to a particular shampoo. The shampoo is left on at least 5 to 10 minutes. As the condition of the scalp improves, the treatment can be less frequent. Antiseborrheic shampoos include those containing selenium sulfide suspension, zinc pyrithione, salicylic acid, or sulphur compounds, and tar shampoo that contains sulphur or salicylic acid (Borda & Wikramanayake, 2015; Handler, 2017).

Nursing Management

A person with seborrheic dermatitis is advised to avoid external irritants, excessive heat, and perspiration; rubbing and scratching prolong the disorder. To avoid secondary infection, the patient should air the skin and keep skin folds clean and dry.

Instructions for using medicated shampoos are reinforced for those with dandruff that requires treatment. Frequent shampooing is contrary to some cultural practices; the nurse is sensitive to these differences when teaching the patient about home care.

The patient is cautioned that seborrheic dermatitis is a chronic problem that tends to reappear. The goal is to keep it under control. Patients need to be encouraged to adhere to the treatment program. Those who become discouraged and disheartened by the effect on body image need to be treated with sensitivity and an awareness of their need to express their feelings.

Acne Vulgaris

Acne vulgaris is a common disorder affecting susceptible hair follicles, most commonly on the face, back, chest, and upper arms (Well, 2013). It is a chronic dermatosis characterized by **comedones** (primary acne lesions), both closed and open, and by papules, pustules, nodules, and cysts (Zaenglein, Pathy, Schlosser, et al., 2016).

Acne is the most commonly encountered skin condition that affects up to 80% of Canadian young adults. Acne is most prevalent during adolescence among males but is more prevalent in adulthood among females. Acne is traditionally considered a skin disorder of adolescence; however, by age 45 years, up to 5% of adults report having acne (Rao & Chen, 2016; Well, 2013). Acne appears to stem from an interplay of genetic, hormonal, and bacterial factors (Al-Hammadi, Al-Ismaily, Al-Ali, et al., 2016).

Pathophysiology

During childhood, the sebaceous glands are small and virtually nonfunctioning. These glands are under endocrine control, especially by the androgens. During puberty, androgens stimulate the sebaceous glands, causing them to enlarge and secrete a natural oil (sebum) that rises to the top of the hair follicle and flows out onto the skin surface. In adolescents who develop acne, androgenic stimulation produces a heightened response in the sebaceous glands so that acne occurs when accumulated sebum plugs the pilosebaceous ducts. Sebaceous plugging then causes a localized inflammatory response (Al-Hammadi et al., 2016).

Clinical Manifestations

The primary lesions of acne are comedones. Closed comedones (whiteheads) are obstructive lesions formed from impacted lipids or oils and keratin that plug the dilated follicle. They are small, whitish papules with minute follicular openings that generally cannot be seen. Closed comedones may evolve into open comedones, in which the contents of the ducts are in open communication with the external environment. The colour of open comedones (blackheads) results not from dirt but from an accumulation of lipid, bacterial, and epithelial debris.

Although the exact cause is unknown, some closed comedones may rupture, resulting in an inflammatory reaction caused by leakage of follicular contents (e.g., sebum, keratin, bacteria) into the dermis. This inflammatory response may result from the action of certain skin bacteria, such as *Propionibacterium acnes*, that live in the hair follicles and break down the triglycerides of the sebum into free fatty acids and glycerin. The resultant inflammation is seen clinically as erythematous papules, inflammatory pustules, and inflammatory cysts. Mild papules and cysts drain and heal on their own without treatment. Deeper papules and cysts may result in scarring of the skin. Acne is usually graded as mild, moderate, or severe based on the number and type of lesions (e.g., comedones, papules, pustules, cysts).

Assessment and Diagnostic Findings

The diagnosis of acne is based on the history and physical examination, evidence of lesions characteristic of acne, and age. Women may report a history of flare-ups a few days before menses. The presence of the typical comedones along with oily skin is characteristic (Rao & Chen, 2016; Well, 2013). Oiliness is more prominent in the midfacial area; other parts of the face may appear dry.

There is at present no consensus on manifestations that constitute mild, moderate, and severe acne (Zaenglein et al., 2016). Generally speaking, mild acne is characterized by the presence of comedones and a few papulopustules; moderate acne is characterized by a greater number of papulopustules and comedones along with the presence of inflammatory pustules; and, severe acne is characterized by the presence of cysts (also called nodules or nodulocysts) that are greater than 5 mm in diameter (Rao & Chen, 2016).

Medical Management

The goals of management are to reduce bacterial colonies, decrease sebaceous gland activity, prevent the follicles from becoming plugged, reduce inflammation, combat secondary infection, minimize scarring, and eliminate factors that predispose the person to acne. The therapeutic regimen depends on the type of lesion (e.g., comedonal, papular, pustular, cystic).

There is no predictable cure for the disease, but combinations of therapies are available that can effectively control its activity. Topical treatment may be all that is needed to treat mild to moderate lesions and superficial inflammatory lesions (i.e., papular or pustular).

Nutrition and Hygiene Therapy

Although food restrictions have been recommended from time to time in treating acne, diet is not believed to play a major role in therapy. However, the elimination of a specific food or food product associated with a flare-up of acne, such as chocolate, cola, fried foods, or milk products, should be promoted. Maintenance of good nutrition equips the immune system for effective action against bacteria and infection.

For mild cases of acne, washing twice each day with a cleansing soap may be all that is required. These soaps can remove the excessive skin oil and the comedones in most cases. Over-the-counter acne medications contain salicylic acid and benzoyl peroxide, both of which are very effective at removing the sebaceous follicular plugs. However, the skin of some people is sensitive to these products, which can cause irritation or excessive dryness, especially when used with some prescribed topical medications. The patient is instructed to discontinue their use if severe irritation occurs. Oil-free cosmetics and creams should be chosen. These products are usually designated as useful for acne-prone skin. The duration of treatment depends on the extent and severity of the acne. In severe cases, treatment may extend over years.

Pharmacologic Therapy

Pharmacologic treatments for acne are based on the severity of the acne (Zaenglein et al., 2016). Table 58-5 summarizes the first-line treatment modalities for acne vulgaris based on severity.

Topical Pharmacologic Therapy

BENZOYL PEROXIDE. Benzoyl peroxide preparations are widely used because they produce a rapid and sustained reduction of inflammatory lesions. They depress sebum production and promote breakdown of comedo plugs (Zaenglein et al., 2016). They also produce an antibacterial effect by suppressing *P. acnes*. Initially, benzoyl peroxide causes redness and scaling, but the skin usually adjusts

TABLE 58-5 First-Line Medications Indicated for Treatment of Acne Vulgaris

Classification	Recommended Medications
Mild acne	Benzoyl peroxide
	-or-
	Topical retinoid
	-or-
	Combination[a] topical antibiotic and benzoyl peroxide
	-or-
	Combination[a] topical retinoid and benzoyl peroxide
	-or-
	Combination[a] topical retinoid and benzoyl peroxide and topical antibiotic
Moderate acne	Combination[a] topical antibiotic and benzoyl peroxide
	-or-
	Combination[a] topical retinoid and benzoyl peroxide
	-or-
	Combination[a] topical retinoid and benzoyl peroxide and topical antibiotic
	-or-
	Oral antibiotic and combination[a] topical retinoid and benzoyl peroxide
	-or-
	Oral antibiotic and combination[a] topical retinoid and benzoyl peroxide and topical antibiotic
Severe acne	Oral antibiotic and combination[a] topical retinoid and benzoyl peroxide
	-or-
	Oral antibiotic and combination[a] topical antibiotic and benzoyl peroxide
	-or-
	Oral antibiotic and combination[a] topical retinoid and benzoyl peroxide and topical antibiotic
	-or-
	Oral antibiotic and oral isotretinoin

[a]May be prescribed as combination products or as singular products.

Adapted from Zaenglein, A. L., Pathy, A. L., Schlosser, B. J., et al. (2016). Guidelines of care for the management of acne vulgaris. *Journal of the American Academy of Dermatology*, *74*(5), 945–973.

quickly to its use. Typically, the patient applies a gel of benzoyl peroxide once daily. In many instances, this is the only treatment needed. Benzoyl peroxide, benzoyl erythromycin, and benzoyl sulphur combinations are available over the counter and by prescription. Vitamin A acid (tretinoin) applied topically is used to clear the keratin plugs from the pilosebaceous ducts. Vitamin A acid speeds the cellular turnover, forces out the comedones, and prevents new comedones.

The patient is informed that symptoms may worsen during early weeks of therapy because inflammation may occur during the process. Erythema and peeling also frequently occur. Improvement may take 8 to 12 weeks. Some patients cannot tolerate this therapy. The patient is cautioned against sun exposure while using this topical medication, as it may cause an exaggerated sunburn. Package insert directions should be followed carefully.

SALICYLIC ACID PREPARATIONS. Over-the-counter salicylic acid preparations are also available for use by patients with mild acne. The effects of these agents are similar to those of benzoyl peroxide products. Although salicylic acid products have long been used by patients with acne, their efficacy has not been demonstrated in clinical trials (Zaenglein et al., 2016). Prescription topical agents used for years that have also not demonstrated efficacy in clinical trials include zinc, sulphur, and resorcinol, and are therefore not recommended for treatment (Zaenglein et al., 2016).

TOPICAL ANTIBIOTICS. Topical antibiotic treatment for acne is common. Topical antibiotic agents suppress bacterial growth; reduce superficial free fatty acid levels; decrease comedones, papules, and pustules; and produce no systemic side effects (Karch, 2015). The most commonly prescribed agents include clindamycin and erythromycin (Well, 2013). Topical combination gels that include both benzoyl peroxide and an antibiotic (e.g., benzoyl erythromycin) are commonly prescribed and can be very effective treatment (Zaenglein et al., 2016).

Systemic Pharmacologic Therapy

ANTIBIOTICS. Oral antibiotics, such as tetracycline, doxycycline, and minocycline, administered in small doses over a long period are very effective in treating moderate and severe acne, especially when the acne is inflammatory and results in pustules, abscesses, and scarring. Therapy may continue for months to years. The tetracycline family of antibiotics is contraindicated in children younger than 12 years and in pregnant women. Although these medications are considered safe for long-term use in most cases, administration during pregnancy can affect the development of teeth, causing enamel hypoplasia and permanent discolouration of teeth in infants. Side effects of tetracyclines include photosensitivity, nausea, diarrhea, cutaneous infection in either gender, and vaginitis in women. In some women, broad-spectrum antibiotics may suppress usual vaginal bacteria and predispose the patient to candidiasis, which is a fungal infection.

ORAL RETINOIDS. Synthetic vitamin A compounds (i.e., retinoids) are used with dramatic results in patients with nodular cystic acne unresponsive to conventional therapy. One compound is isotretinoin (Accutane). Isotretinoin is also used for active inflammatory papular pustular acne that has a tendency to scar. Isotretinoin reduces sebaceous gland size and inhibits sebum production. It also causes the epidermis to shed (epidermal desquamation), thereby unseating and expelling existing comedones.

The most common side effect, experienced by almost all patients, is **cheilitis** (inflammation or cracks of the lips/corners of the mouth). Dry and chafed skin and mucous membranes are frequent side effects. These changes are reversible with the withdrawal of the medication. Most important, isotretinoin, like other vitamin A metabolites, is teratogenic in humans, meaning that it can have an adverse effect on a fetus, causing central nervous system and cardiovascular defects and structural abnormalities of the face.

To avoid additive toxic effects, patients are cautioned not to take vitamin A supplements while taking isotretinoin.

NURSING ALERT

Two negative pregnancy tests are required before taking Accutane and are continued monthly until the medication is stopped. All women of childbearing age are required to abstain from sexual activity or use at least two forms of birth control from 1 month before, during treatment, and up to 8 weeks after treatment (Stephen, 2012).

HORMONE THERAPY. Estrogen therapy (including progesterone–estrogen preparations) suppresses sebum production and reduces skin oiliness. It is usually reserved for young women when the acne begins somewhat later than usual and tends to flare up at certain times in the menstrual cycle. Estrogen in the form of estrogen-dominant oral contraceptive compounds may be administered on a prescribed cyclic regimen. Estrogen is not administered to male patients because of undesirable side effects such as enlargement of the breasts and decrease in body hair (Al-Hammadi et al., 2016).

Surgical Management

Surgical treatment of acne consists of comedo extraction; injections of corticosteroids into the inflamed lesions; and incision and drainage of large, fluctuant (moving in palpable waves), nodular cystic lesions. Cryosurgery (freezing with liquid nitrogen) may be used for nodular and cystic forms of acne. Patients with deep scars may be treated with deep abrasive therapy (dermabrasion), in which the epidermis and some superficial dermis are removed down to the level of the scars.

Comedones may be removed with a comedo extractor. The site is first cleaned with alcohol. The opening of the extractor is then placed over the lesion, and direct pressure is applied to cause extrusion of the plug through the extractor. Removal of comedones leaves erythema, which may take several weeks to subside. Recurrence of comedones after extraction is common because of the continuing activity of the pilosebaceous glands.

Nursing Management

Nursing care of patients with acne consists largely of monitoring and managing potential complications of skin treatments. Major nursing activities include patient education, particularly in proper skin care techniques, and managing potential concerns related to the skin disorder or therapy. Providing positive reassurance, listening attentively, and being sensitive to the feelings of the patient with acne are essential contributors to the patient's psychological well-being and understanding of the disease and treatment plan. In particular, women with acne frequently report diminished quality of life, more anxiety, and depression (Gorelick, Daniels, Kawata, et al., 2015; Zaenglein et al., 2016) (Chart 58-3).

Preventing Scarring

Prevention of scarring is the ultimate goal of therapy. The chance of scarring increases as the grade of acne increases. Grades III and IV (25 to more than 50 comedones, papules, or pustules) usually require longer-term therapy with systemic antibiotics or isotretinoin. Patients are warned that discontinuing these medications can exacerbate acne, lead to more flare-ups, and increase the chance of deep scarring. Furthermore, manipulation of the comedones, papules, and pustules increases the potential for scarring.

When acne surgery is prescribed to extract deep-seated comedones or inflamed lesions or to incise and drain cystic lesions, the intervention itself may result in further scarring. Dermabrasion, which levels existing scar tissue, can also increase scar formation. Hyperpigmentation or hypopigmentation also may affect the tissue involved. The patient is informed of these potential outcomes before choosing surgical intervention for acne.

Preventing Infection

Female patients receiving long-term antibiotic therapy with tetracycline should be advised to watch for and report signs and symptoms of oral or vaginal candidiasis, which is a yeastlike fungal infection.

Promoting Home, Community-Based, and Transitional Care

Educating Patients About Self-Care

In addition to receiving instructions for taking prescribed medications, patients are instructed to wash the face and other affected areas with mild soap and water twice each day to remove surface oils and prevent obstruction of the oil glands. They are cautioned to avoid scrubbing the face; acne is not caused by dirt and cannot be washed away.

Mild abrasive soaps and drying agents are prescribed to eliminate the oily feeling that troubles many patients. At the same time, patients are cautioned to avoid excessive abrasion, as it makes acne worse. Excessive abrasion causes minute scratches on the skin surface and increases possible bacterial contamination. Soap itself can irritate the skin.

All forms of friction and trauma are avoided, including propping the hands against the face, rubbing the face, and wearing tight collars and helmets. **Patients are instructed to avoid manipulation of pimples or blackheads**. Squeezing merely worsens the problem, because a portion of the blackhead is pushed down into the skin, which may cause the follicle to rupture. Because cosmetics, shaving creams, and lotions can aggravate acne, these substances are best avoided unless the patient is advised otherwise. There is no evidence that a particular food can cause or aggravate acne. In general, eating a nutritious diet helps the body maintain a strong immune system.

INFECTIOUS DERMATOSES

Bacterial Skin Infections

Also called **pyodermas**, pus-forming bacterial infections of the skin may be primary or secondary. Primary skin infections originate in previously usual-appearing skin and are often caused by a single organism. Secondary skin infections arise from a pre-existing skin disorder or from disruption of the skin integrity from injury or surgery. In either case, several microorganisms may be implicated (e.g., *Staphylococcus aureus*, group A streptococci). The most common primary bacterial skin infections are impetigo and folliculitis. Folliculitis may lead to **furuncles** or **carbuncles**.

Impetigo

Impetigo is a superficial infection of the skin caused by staphylococci, streptococci, or multiple bacteria. Bullous impetigo, a more deep-seated infection of the skin caused by *S. aureus*, is characterized by the formation of **bullae** (i.e., large, fluid-filled blisters) from original vesicles. The bullae rupture, leaving raw, red areas.

The exposed areas of the body, face, hands, neck, and extremities are most frequently involved. Impetigo is contagious and may spread to other parts of the patient's skin or to other members of the family who touch the patient or use towels or combs that are soiled with the exudate of the lesions.

Although impetigo is seen at all ages, it is particularly common among children living in poor hygienic conditions. It often follows pediculosis capitis (head lice), scabies (itch mites), herpes simplex, insect bites, poison ivy, or eczema. Chronic health issues, poor hygiene, and malnutrition may predispose an adult to impetigo. Some people have been identified as asymptomatic carriers of *S. aureus*, usually in the nasal passages.

Clinical Manifestations

The lesions begin as small, red macules, which quickly become discrete, thin-walled vesicles (filled with serum, pus, or blood) (Mansen & Gabiola, 2015) that soon rupture and become covered with a loosely adherent honey-yellow crust (Fig. 58-1). These crusts are easily removed to reveal smooth, red, moist surfaces on which new crusts soon develop. If the scalp is involved, the hair is matted, which distinguishes the condition from ringworm.

Medical Management

Systemic antibiotic therapy is the usual treatment. It reduces contagious spread, treats deep infection, and prevents acute glomerulonephritis (kidney infection), which may occur as an aftermath of streptococcal skin diseases. In nonbullous impetigo, benzathine penicillin or oral penicillin may be prescribed. Bullous impetigo is treated with a penicillinase-resistant penicillin (e.g., cloxacillin,

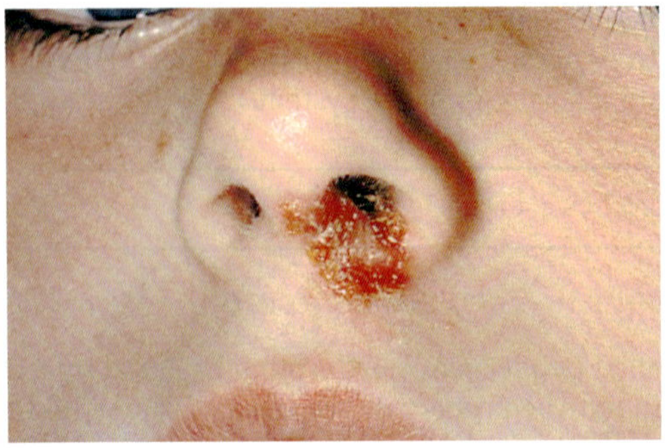

FIGURE 58-1. Impetigo of the nostril.

dicloxacillin). In penicillin-allergic patients, erythromycin is an effective alternative.

Topical antibacterial therapy (e.g., mupirocin) may be prescribed when the disease is limited to a small area. However, topical therapy requires that the medication be applied to the lesions several times daily for a week. The treatment regimen may be impossible for some patients or their caregivers to follow. Topical antibiotics generally are not as effective as systemic therapy in eradicating or preventing the spread of streptococci from the respiratory tract, thereby increasing the risk for developing glomerulonephritis.

When topical therapy is prescribed, lesions are soaked or washed with soap solution to remove the central site of bacterial growth, giving the topical antibiotic an opportunity to reach the infected site. After the crusts are removed, a topical medication (e.g., bacitracin/polymyxin [Polysporin], bacitracin) may be applied. Gloves are worn when providing patient care. An antiseptic solution, such as povidone-iodine (Betadine) may be used to clean the skin, reduce bacterial content in the infected area, and prevent spread.

Nursing Management

The nurse instructs the patient and family members to bathe at least once daily with bactericidal soap. Cleanliness and good hygiene practices help to prevent the spread of the lesions from one skin area to another and from one person to another. Each person should have a separate towel and washcloth. Because impetigo is a contagious disorder, infected people should avoid contact with other people until the lesions heal (Lewis, 2016).

Folliculitis, Furuncles, and Carbuncles

Folliculitis is an infection of bacterial or fungal origin that arises within the hair follicles. Lesions may be superficial or deep. Single or multiple papules or pustules appear close to the hair follicles. Folliculitis commonly affects the beard area of men who shave and women's legs. Other areas include the axillae, trunk, and buttocks (Van Bijnen, Paget, den Heijer, et al., 2014).

Pseudofolliculitis barbae (shaving bumps) are an inflammatory reaction that occurs predominantly on the faces of black Canadian and other curly haired men as a result of shaving. The sharp ingrowing hairs have a curved root that grows at a more acute angle and pierces the skin, provoking an irritative reaction. The only entirely effective treatment is to avoid shaving. Other treatments include using special lotions or antibiotics or using a hand brush to dislodge the hairs mechanically. If the patient must remove facial hair, a depilatory cream or electric razor may be used.

A furuncle (boil) is an acute inflammation arising deep in one or more hair follicles and spreading into the surrounding dermis. It is a deeper form of folliculitis. Furunculosis refers to multiple or recurrent lesions. Furuncles may occur anywhere on the body but are more prevalent in areas subjected to irritation, pressure, friction, and excessive perspiration, such as the back of the neck, the axillae, and the buttocks.

A furuncle may start as a small, red, raised, painful pimple. Frequently, the infection progresses and involves the skin and subcutaneous fatty tissue, causing tenderness, pain, and surrounding cellulitis. The area of redness and induration represents an effort of the body to keep the infection localized. The bacteria (usually staphylococci) produce necrosis of the invaded tissue. The characteristic pointing of a boil follows in a few days. When this occurs, the centre becomes yellow or black, and the boil is said to have "come to a head."

A carbuncle is an abscess of the skin and subcutaneous tissue that represents an extension of a furuncle that has invaded several follicles and is large and deep seated. It is usually caused by a staphylococcal infection. Carbuncles appear most commonly in areas where the skin is thick and inelastic. The back of the neck and the buttocks are common sites. In carbuncles, the extensive inflammation frequently prevents a complete walling off of the infection; absorption may occur, resulting in high fever, pain, leukocytosis, and even extension of the infection to the bloodstream.

Furuncles and carbuncles are more likely to occur in patients with underlying systemic diseases, such as diabetes or hematologic malignancies, and in those receiving immunosuppressive therapy for other diseases. Both are more prevalent in hot climates, especially on skin beneath occlusive clothing.

Medical Management

In treating staphylococcal infections, it is important not to rupture or destroy the protective wall of induration that localizes the infection. The boil or pimple should never be squeezed.

Follicular disorders, including folliculitis, furuncles, and carbuncles, are usually caused by staphylococci; although if the immune system is impaired, the causative organisms may be gram-negative bacilli. Systemic antibiotic therapy, selected by sensitivity study, is generally indicated. Oral cloxacillin, dicloxacillin, and flucloxacillin are first-line medications. Cephalosporins and erythromycin are also effective. Bed rest is advised for patients who have boils on the perineum or in the anal region, and a course of systemic antibiotic therapy is indicated to prevent the spread of the infection. If MRSA is suspected, antibiotic agents selected may include clindamycin, trimethoprim–sulfamethoxazole, or minocycline (Peebles, Morris, & Chafe, 2014).

When the pus has localized and is fluctuant, a small incision with a scalpel can speed resolution by relieving the tension and ensuring direct evacuation of the pus and slough. The patient is instructed to keep the draining lesion covered with a dressing.

Nursing Management

Intravenous fluids, fever reduction, and other supportive treatments are indicated for patients who are acutely ill from infection. Warm, moist compresses increase vascularization and hasten resolution of the furuncle or carbuncle. The surrounding skin may be cleaned gently with antibacterial soap, and an antibacterial ointment may be applied. Soiled dressings are handled according to Routine Practices and Additional Precautions (PHAC, 2012). Nursing personnel carefully follow isolation precautions to avoid becoming carriers of staphylococci. Disposable gloves are worn when caring for these patients.

NURSING ALERT

Nurses must take special precautions in caring for boils on the face, because the skin area drains directly into the cranial venous sinuses. Sinus thrombosis with fatal pyemia can develop after manipulating a boil in this location. The infection can travel through the sinus tract and penetrate the brain cavity, causing brain abscess.

Promoting Home, Community-Based, and Transitional Care

Educating Patients About Self-Care

To prevent and control staphylococcal skin infections such as boils and carbuncles, the staphylococcal pathogen must be eliminated from the skin and environment. Efforts must be made to increase the patient's resistance and provide a hygienic environment. If lesions are actively draining, the mattress and pillow are covered with plastic material and wiped off with disinfectant daily; the bedsheets, towels, and clothing are laundered after each use; and the patient should use an antibacterial soap and shampoo for an indefinite period, often for several months.

Recurrent infection is prevented with the use of prescribed antibiotic therapy (longer than about 3 months). The patient must take the full dose for the time prescribed. The purulent exudate (pus) is a source of reinfection or transmission of infection to caregivers. When the patient has a history of recurrent infections, a carrier state may exist, which should be investigated and treated with an antibacterial cream such as mupirocin.

Viral Skin Infections

Herpes Zoster

Herpes zoster, also called *shingles*, is an infection caused by the varicella-zoster virus, a member of a group of DNA viruses. The viruses causing chickenpox and herpes zoster are indistinguishable, hence the name *varicella-zoster virus*. The disease is characterized by a painful vesicular eruption along the area of distribution of the sensory nerves from one or more posterior ganglia. It is assumed that herpes zoster represents a reactivation of latent varicella virus infection and reflects lowered immunity. After a case of chickenpox runs its course, it is thought that the varicella-zoster viruses responsible for the outbreak lie dormant inside nerve cells near the brain and spinal cord. Later, when these latent viruses are reactivated, they travel by way of the peripheral nerves to the skin, where the viruses multiply and create a red rash of small, fluid-filled blisters. About 10% of adults get shingles during their lifetimes, usually after age 50 years. There is an increased frequency of herpes zoster infections in patients with weakened immune systems, including those with human immunodeficiency virus (HIV) infection and in those with cancer. In these patients, the infection can become widespread and cause significant complications (Janniger, Eastern, Hospenthal, et al., 2016).

Clinical Manifestations

The eruption is usually accompanied or preceded by pain, which may radiate over the entire region supplied by the affected nerves. The pain may be burning, lancinating (tearing or sharply cutting), stabbing, or aching. Some patients have no pain, but itching and tenderness may occur over the area. Sometimes, malaise and gastrointestinal disturbances precede the eruption. The patches of grouped vesicles appear on the red and swollen skin. The early vesicles, which contain serum, later may become purulent, rupture, and form crusts. The inflammation is usually unilateral, involving the thoracic, cervical, or cranial nerves in a bandlike configuration. The blisters are usually confined to a narrow region of the face or trunk (Fig. 58-2). The clinical course varies from 1 to 3 weeks. If an ophthalmic nerve is involved, the patient may have eye pain. Inflammation and a rash on the trunk may cause pain with the slightest touch. The healing time varies from 7 to 26 days.

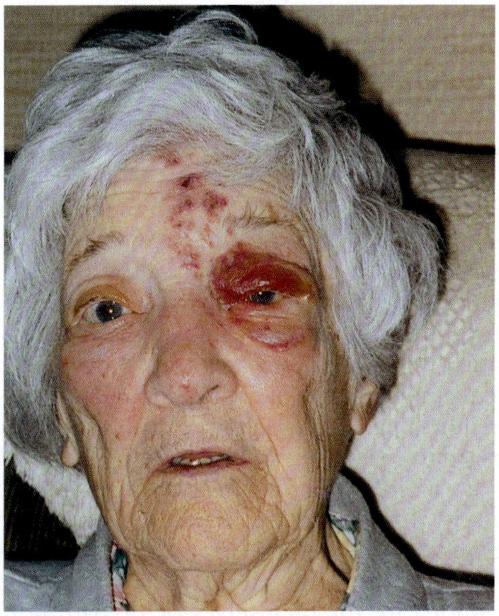

FIGURE 58-2. Herpes zoster (shingles).

Herpes zoster in healthy adults is usually localized and benign. However, in immunosuppressed patients, the disease may be severe and the clinical course acutely disabling.

Herpes zoster ophthalmicus (HZO) is a rare subtype of herpes zoster that causes severe consequences. Typically in HZO, a branch of the trigeminal nerve is affected that innervates the ocular and periocular structures. This may cause significant pain and morbid ocular complications, including blindness (Janniger et al., 2016).

Medical Management

There is evidence that infection is arrested if oral antiviral agents such as acyclovir (Avirax), valacyclovir (Valtrex), or famciclovir (Famvir) are administered within 24 hours of the initial eruption. Intravenous acyclovir, if started early, is effective in significantly reducing the pain and halting the progression of the disease. In older adults, the pain from herpes zoster may persist as postherpetic neuralgia for months after the skin lesions disappear.

The goals of herpes zoster management are to relieve the pain and to reduce or avoid complications, which include infection, scarring, and postherpetic neuralgia and eye complications. Pain is controlled with analgesics, because adequate pain control during the acute phase helps to prevent persistent pain patterns. Systemic corticosteroids may be prescribed for patients older than 50 years to reduce the incidence and duration of postherpetic neuralgia (persistent pain of the affected nerve after healing). Healing usually occurs sooner in those who have been treated with corticosteroids. Triamcinolone (Aristocort, Kenacort, Kenalog) injected subcutaneously under painful areas is effective as an anti-inflammatory agent.

Ophthalmic herpes zoster occurs when an eye is involved. This is considered an ophthalmic emergency, and the patient should be referred to an ophthalmologist immediately to prevent the possible sequelae of keratitis, uveitis, ulceration, and blindness.

People who have been exposed to varicella (chickenpox) by primary infection or by vaccination are not at risk for infection after exposure to patients with herpes zoster.

Nursing Management

The patient and family members are instructed about the importance of taking antiviral agents as prescribed and in keeping follow-up appointments with the health care professional. The nurse assesses the patient's discomfort and response to medication and collaborates with the physician to make necessary adjustments to the treatment regimen. The patient is taught how to apply wet dressings or medication to the lesions and to follow proper hand hygiene techniques to avoid spreading the virus.

Diversionary activities and relaxation techniques are encouraged to ensure restful sleep and to alleviate discomfort. A caregiver may be required to assist with dressings, particularly if the patient is older and unable to apply them. Significant others or a home care nurse may need to help with dressing changes. Food preparation for patients who cannot care for themselves or prepare nourishing meals must be arranged.

Herpes Simplex

Herpes simplex is a common skin infection. There are two types of the causative virus, which are identified by viral typing. Generally, herpes simplex type 1 occurs on the mouth and type 2 in the genital area, but both viral types can be found in both locations. About 85% of adults worldwide are seropositive for herpes type 1. The prevalence of type 2 is lower; type 2 usually appears at the onset of sexual activity. Serologic testing shows that many more people are infected than have a history of clinical disease.

Herpes simplex is classified as a true primary infection, a nonprimary initial episode, or a recurrent episode. True primary infection is the initial exposure to the virus. A nonprimary initial episode is the initial episode of type 1 or type 2 in a person previously infected with the other type. Recurrent episodes are subsequent episodes of the same viral type.

Types of Herpes Simplex

Orolabial Herpes

Orolabial herpes, also called *fever blisters* or *cold sores*, consists of erythematous-based clusters of grouped vesicles on the lips. A prodrome of tingling or burning with pain may precede the appearance of the vesicles by up to 24 hours. Certain triggers, such as sunlight exposure or increased stress, may cause recurrent episodes. Fewer than 1% of people with primary orolabial herpes infections develop herpetic gingivostomatitis. This complication occurs more in children and young adults. The onset is often accompanied by high fever, regional lymphadenopathy, and generalized malaise. Another complication of orolabial herpes is the development of erythema multiforme, an acute inflammation of the skin and mucous membranes with characteristic lesions that have the appearance of targets (i.e., concentric red rings with white bands between the red rings).

Genital Herpes

Genital herpes, or type 2 herpes simplex, manifests with a broad spectrum of clinical signs. Minor infections may produce no symptoms at all; severe primary infections with type 1 can cause systemic flulike illness. Lesions appear as grouped vesicles on an erythematous base initially involving the vagina, rectum, or penis. New lesions can continue to appear for 7 to 14 days. Lesions are symmetric and usually cause regional lymphadenopathy. Fever and flulike symptoms are common. Typical recurrences begin with a prodrome of burning, tingling, or itching about 24 hours before the vesicles appear. As the vesicles rupture, erosions and ulcerations begin to appear. Severe infections can cause extensive erosions of the vaginal or anal canal. For further information, refer to Chapter 47.

Assessment and Diagnostic Findings

Herpes simplex infections are confirmed in several ways. Generally, the appearance of the skin eruption is strongly suggestive. Viral cultures and rapid assays are available, and the type of test used depends on lesion morphology.

Acute vesicular lesions are more likely to react positively to the rapid assay, whereas older, crusted patches are better diagnosed with viral culture. In all cases, it is imperative to obtain enough viral cells for testing, and careful collection methods are therefore important. All crusts are gently removed or vesicles gently unroofed. A sterile cotton swab premoistened in viral culture preservative is used to swab the base of the vesicle to obtain a specimen for analysis.

Complications

Eczema herpeticum is a condition in which patients with eczema contract herpes that spreads throughout the eczematous areas. The same type of spread of herpes can occur in severe seborrhea, scabies, and other chronic skin conditions. Eczema herpeticum is managed with oral or intravenous acyclovir. Herpes whitlow is an infection of the pulp of a fingertip with herpes type 1 or 2. There is tenderness and erythema of the lateral fold of the cuticle. Deep-seated vesicles appear within 24 hours.

Most cases of neonatal infection with herpes occur during delivery by contact of the infant with the mother's active ulcerations. Rarely, in mothers who have primary infections during pregnancy, intrauterine neonatal infections occur. Fetal anomalies include skin lesions, microcephaly, encephalitis, and intracerebral calcifications.

Medical Management

In many patients, recurrent orolabial herpes represents more of a nuisance than a disease. Because sun exposure is a common trigger, those with recurrent orolabial herpes should use a sunscreen liberally on the lips and face. Topical treatment with drying agents may accelerate healing. In more severe outbreaks or in patients who have identified triggers, intermittent treatment with 200 mg of acyclovir administered five times each day for 5 days is often started as soon as the earliest symptoms occur.

Treatment of genital herpes depends on the severity, the frequency, and the psychological impact of recurrences and on the infectious status of the sexual partner. For people who have mild or rare outbreaks, no treatment may be required. For those who have more severe outbreaks, but for whom outbreaks are still infrequent, intermittent treatment as described for oral lesions can be used. Because intermittent treatment reduces the duration of the infection by only 24 to 36 hours, it should be initiated as early as possible.

Patients who have more than six recurrences per year may benefit from suppressive therapy. Use of acyclovir, valacyclovir, or famciclovir suppresses 85% of recurrences, and 20% of patients are free of recurrences during suppressive therapy. Suppressive therapy also reduces viral shedding by almost 95%, making the person less contagious. Treatment with suppressive doses of oral antiviral medications prevents recurrent erythema multiforme (acute eruption of macules, papules, and vesicles with a multiforme appearance).

Management of genital herpes in pregnancy is controversial. Routine prenatal cultures do not predict shedding at the time of delivery. The use of scalp electrodes during delivery should be avoided because they increase the risk for infection in the newborn. Because the risk for neonatal herpes is greater in women with their initial episode during pregnancy, suppression therapy should be started in these women to reduce outbreaks during the third trimester. All women with active lesions at the time of delivery undergo cesarean section.

In immunocompromised patients, suppression therapy should be considered. In severe infections of the hospitalized patient, intravenous acyclovir is prescribed.

Fungal (Mycotic) Skin Infections

Fungi, tiny members of a subdivision of the plant kingdom that thrive on organic matter, cause various common skin infections. In some cases, they affect only the skin and its appendages (hair and nails). In other cases, internal organs are involved, and the diseases may be life threatening. However, superficial infections rarely cause even temporary disability and respond readily to treatment. Secondary infection with bacteria, *Candida*, or both organisms may occur.

The most common fungal skin infection is **tinea**, which is also called *ringworm* because of its characteristic appearance of a ring or rounded tunnel under the skin. Tinea infections affect the head, body, groin, feet, and nails (Sahoo & Mahajan, 2016). Table 58-6 summarizes the tinea infections and treatments.

To obtain a specimen for diagnosis, the lesion is cleaned and a scalpel or glass slide is used to remove scales from the margin of the lesion. The scales are dropped onto a slide to which potassium hydroxide has been added. The diagnosis is made by examination of the infected scales microscopically for spores and hyphae or by isolating the organism in culture. Under Wood's light, a specimen of infected hair appears fluorescent; this may be helpful in diagnosing some cases of tinea capitis (Sahoo & Mahajan, 2016).

Parasitic Skin Infestation

Pediculosis: Lice Infestation

Lice infestation affects people of all ages. Three varieties of lice infest humans: *Pediculus humanus capitis* (i.e., head louse), *Pediculus humanus corporis* (i.e., body louse), and *Phthirus pubis* (i.e., pubic louse or crab louse). Lice are called *ectoparasites* because they live on the outside of the host's body. They depend on the host for their nourishment, feeding on human blood approximately five times each day. They inject their digestive juices and excrement into the skin, which causes severe itching (Dunphy, Winland-Brown, Porter, et al., 2015).

Pediculosis Capitis

Pediculosis capitis is an infestation of the scalp by the head louse. The female louse lays her eggs (i.e., nits) close to the scalp. The nits become firmly attached to the hair shafts with a tenacious substance. The young lice hatch in about 10 days and reach maturity in 2 weeks. Head lice may be transmitted directly by physical contact or indirectly by infested combs, brushes, wigs, hats, helmets, and bedding (Dunphy et al., 2015).

TABLE 58-6 Tinea (Ringworm) Infections

Type and Location	Clinical Manifestations	Treatment
Tinea capitis (scalp; contagious fungal infection of the hair shaft)	• Oval, scaling, erythematous patches • Small papules or pustules on the scalp • Brittle hair that breaks easily; patchy alopecia	• Griseofulvin for 4–6 weeks or terbinafine (Lamisil) for 2–4 weeks • Shampoo hair twice weekly with selenium sulfide shampoo for 2 weeks
Tinea corporis (body)	• Begins with red macule, which spreads to a ring of papules or vesicles with central clearing • Lesions found in clusters; many spread to the hair, scalp, or nails • Pruritis is a common complaint	• Local infections—topical antifungal creams once or twice daily (e.g., clotrimazole [Lotrimin], econazole [Spectazole], ketoconazole [Nizoral]) • Extensive infections or concomitant tinea capitis or immunosuppressive conditions (e.g., active neoplasms)—oral antifungal medications (e.g., fluconazole [Diflucan] for 2–4 weeks, itraconazole for 1 week, terbinafine for 2 weeks)
Tinea cruris (groin area; "jock itch")	• Begins with small, red scaling patches, which spread to form circular elevated plaques • Very pruritic • Clusters of pustules may be seen around borders	• Local infections—see treatment for tinea corporis • Extensive infections or concomitant tinea pedis or immunosuppressive conditions (e.g., active neoplasms)—see treatment for tinea corporis • Educate patients to avoid wearing clothing that is tight over the groin; patients should pat dry skin folds thoroughly (avoid rubbing) after bathing and use separate towels for groin and other body parts

Tinea pedis (foot; "athlete's foot")	• Soles of one or both feet have scaling and mild redness with maceration in the toe webs
	• More acute infections may have clusters of clear vesicles on dusky base
		• Local infections—see treatment for tinea corporis
		• Extensive infections or concomitant tinea pedis or immunosuppressive conditions (e.g., active neoplasms)—see treatment for tinea corporis
		• Educate patients:
		  • to put on socks before underwear to avoid cross-contamination to groin
		  • to either dispose of old shoes or treat them with antifungal powder to prevent reinfection
		  • to wear protective footwear at communal pools and tubs

Tinea unguium (toenails; onychomycosis)	• Nails thicken, crumble easily, and lack lustre • Whole nail may be destroyed • If untreated, can result in pain, loss of balance, and candida infection	• Oral antifungal medications for 12 weeks (e.g., itraconazole, terbinafine) with or without concomitant topical ciclopirox olamine nail lacquer (Penlac) • Nail avulsion may be indicated, either surgically or chemically using a 40–50% urea compound

Adapted from Handler, M. Z., Stephany, M. P., & Schwarts, R. A. (2016). Tinea capitis. *Medscape*. Retrieved February 11, 2017, from emedicine.medscape.com/article/1091351-overview; Lesher, J. L. (2016). Tinea corporis. *Medscape*. Retrieved February 11, 2017, from emedicine.medscape.com/article/1091473-overview; Robbins, C. M., & Elewski, B. E. (2016). Tinea pedis. *Medscape*. Retrieved February 11, 2017, from emedicine.medscape.com/article/1091684-overview; Tosti, A. (2016). Onychomycosis. *Medscape*. Retrieved February 11, 2017, from emedicine.medscape.com/article/1105828-overview; and Weiderkehr, M., & Schwartz, R. A. (2016). Tinea cruris. *Medscape*. Retrieved February 11, 2017, from emedicine.medscape.com/article/1091806-overview.

Clinical Manifestations

Head lice are found most commonly along the back of the head and behind the ears. The eggs are visible to the naked eye as silvery, glistening oval bodies that are difficult to remove from the hair. The bite of the insect causes intense itching, and the resultant scratching often leads to secondary bacterial infection, such as impetigo or furunculosis. The infestation is more common in children and in people with long hair. Head lice may be transmitted directly by physical contact or indirectly by infested combs, brushes, wigs, hats, and bedding.

Medical Management

Treatment involves washing the hair with a shampoo containing lindane (Kwell) or pyrethrin compounds with piperonyl butoxide (RID or R&C shampoo). The patient is instructed to shampoo the scalp and hair according to the product directions. After the hair is rinsed thoroughly, it is combed with a fine-toothed comb dipped in vinegar to remove any remaining nits or nit shells freed from the hair shafts. They are extremely difficult to remove and may have to be picked off one by one with the fingernails.

All articles, clothing, towels, and bedding that may have lice or nits should be washed in hot water—at least 54°C—or dry-cleaned to prevent reinfestation. Upholstered furniture, rugs, and floors should be vacuumed frequently. Combs and brushes are also disinfected with the shampoo. All family members and close contacts are treated. Complications such as severe pruritus, pyoderma, and dermatitis are treated with antipruritics, systemic antibiotics, and topical corticosteroids.

Nursing Management

The nurse informs the patient that head lice may infest anyone and are not a sign of uncleanliness. Because the condition spreads rapidly, treatment must be started immediately. School epidemics may be managed by having all of the students shampoo their hair on the same night. Students are warned not to share combs, brushes, and hats. Each family member should be inspected for head lice daily for at least 2 weeks. The patient is instructed that lindane may be toxic to the central nervous system when used more frequently or for longer periods of time than specified in the package insert.

Pediculosis Corporis and Pubis

Pediculosis corporis is an infestation of the body by the body louse. This is a disease of unwashed people or those who live in close quarters and do not change their clothing (e.g., survivors of natural disasters who must live with others in temporary housing without access to running water and clean clothes). Pediculosis pubis is extremely common. The infestation is generally localized in the genital region and is transmitted chiefly by sexual contact (Guenther & Maguiness, 2016).

Clinical Manifestations

Head lice are found most commonly along the back of the head and behind the ears. To the naked eye, the eggs look like silvery, glistening oval bodies. The bite of the insect causes intense pruritus, and the resultant scratching often leads to secondary bacterial infection, such as impetigo or furunculosis. The infestation is more common in children and people with long hair (Bonilla, Durden, Eremeeva, et al., 2013; Dunphy et al., 2015).

With body lice, the areas of the skin that come in closest contact with the underclothing (i.e., neck, trunk, and thighs) are chiefly involved. The body louse lives primarily in the seams of underwear and clothing, to which it clings as it pierces the skin with its proboscis. Its bites cause characteristic minute hemorrhagic points. Widespread excoriation may appear as a result of intense pruritus and scratching, especially on the trunk and neck. Among the secondary lesions produced are parallel linear scratches and a slight degree of eczema. In long-standing cases, the skin may become thick, dry, and scaly, with dark pigmented areas (Bonilla et al., 2013).

Pruritus is the most common symptom of pediculosis pubis, particularly at night. Reddish-brown dust (i.e., excretions of the insects) may be found in the patient's underclothing. The pubic area should be examined with a magnifying glass for lice crawling down a hair shaft or nits cemented to the hair or at the junction with the skin. Infestation by pubic lice may coexist with sexually transmitted infections such as gonorrhea, herpes, or syphilis. There may also be infestation of the hairs of the chest, armpit, beard, and eyelashes. Grey-blue macules may sometimes be seen on the trunk, thighs, and axillae as a result of either the reaction of the insects' saliva with bilirubin (converting it to biliverdin) or an excretion produced by the salivary glands of the louse (Bonilla et al., 2013; Dunphy et al., 2015).

Medical Management

Treatment of head and pubic lice involves washing the hair with a shampoo containing pyrethrin compounds with piperonyl butoxide (RID or R&C shampoo) or rinsing with permethrin (Nix). Although it had been first-line treatment for many years, lindane (Kwell) is no longer recommended because of its neurotoxic adverse effects (Dunphy et al., 2015). The patient is instructed to shampoo the scalp and hair according to the product directions. After the hair is rinsed thoroughly, it is combed with a fine-toothed comb dipped in vinegar to remove any remaining nits or nit shells freed from the hair shafts. They are extremely difficult to remove and may have to be picked off one by one (Dunphy et al., 2015; Gellatly, Krim, Palenchar, et al., 2016).

The patient with body lice is instructed to bathe with soap and water. Typically, no medications are indicated because the lice live on the patient's clothing. Topical medications used to treat head and pubic lice may be applied to the clothing, however, particularly in the seams of garments (see following discussion about general hygiene measures). If the eyelashes are involved, petrolatum may be thickly applied twice daily for 8 days, followed by mechanical removal of any remaining nits (Bonilla et al., 2013).

Upholstered furniture, rugs, and floors should be vacuumed frequently. Combs, brushes, and helmets are disinfected or discarded. All family members and close contacts are treated (Bonilla et al., 2013; Dunphy et al., 2015).

Complications, such as severe pruritus, pyoderma, and dermatitis, are treated with antipruritics, systemic antibiotics, and topical corticosteroids. Body lice can transmit epidemic rickettsial disease (e.g., epidemic typhus, relapsing fever, and trench fever) to humans. The causative organism may be in the gastrointestinal tract of the insect and may be excreted on the skin surface of the infested person (Bonilla et al., 2013).

Nursing Management

All family members and sexual contacts must be treated and educated in personal hygiene and methods to prevent or control infestation. The patient and partner must also be scheduled for a diagnostic workup for coexisting sexually transmitted infection. All clothing and bedding should be machine washed in hot water or dry-cleaned.

Scabies

Scabies is an infestation of the skin by the itch mite *Sarcoptes scabiei*. The disease may be found in people living in substandard hygienic conditions, but it can occur in anyone. Infestations may or may not be associated with sexual activity. The mites frequently involve the fingers, and hand contact may produce infection (Mounsey, Murray, Bielefeldt-Ohmann, et al., 2015).

In children, overnight stays with friends or the exchange of clothes may be a source of infection. Health care personnel who have prolonged hands-on physical contact with an infected patient may likewise become infected.

Clinical Manifestations

It takes approximately 4 weeks from the time of contact for a patient's symptoms to appear. The patient complains of severe itching caused by a delayed type of immunologic reaction to the mite or its fecal pellets. During examination, the patient is asked where the itch is most severe. A magnifying glass and a penlight are held at an oblique angle to the skin while a search is made for the small, raised burrows. The burrows may be multiple, straight or wavy, brown or black, threadlike lesions, most commonly observed between the fingers and on the wrists. Other sites are the extensor surfaces of the elbows; the knees; the edges of the feet; the points of the elbows; around the nipples; in the axillary folds; under pendulous breasts; and in or near the groin or gluteal fold, penis, or scrotum. Red, pruritic eruptions usually appear between adjacent skin areas. However, the burrow is not always visible (Dunphy et al., 2015; Mounsey et al., 2015).

Any patient with a rash may have scabies. One classic sign of scabies is the increased itching that occurs at night, perhaps because the increased warmth of the skin has a stimulating effect on the parasite. Hypersensitivity to the organism and its products of excretion also may contribute to the itching. If the infection has spread, other members of the family and close friends also complain of itching about a month later.

Secondary lesions are quite common and include vesicles, papules, excoriations, and crusts. Bacterial superinfection may result from constant excoriation of the burrows and papules.

Gerontologic Considerations

Older adult patients living in long-term care facilities are susceptible to outbreaks of scabies because of close living quarters, poor hygiene due to limited physical ability, and the potential for incidental spread of the organisms by staff members. The vivid inflammatory reaction seen in younger people seldom occurs; rather, the older adult may have peripheral sensory deficits and be less prone to scratch or may be physically unable to scratch. Scratching is an effective mechanism that partially eradicates mite infestation; thus, this results in a more severe subtype. The lesions crust over (causing "crusted scabies") and, in time, may become hyperkeratotic (Dunphy et al., 2015).

Health care personnel in extended-care facilities should wear gloves when providing hands-on care to a patient suspected of having scabies until the diagnosis is confirmed and treatment completed. It is advisable to treat all residents, staff, and families of patients at the same time to prevent reinfection. The scales that are present with crusted scabies must be removed so that the antiscabicidal medication may be effective. Crusts may be removed with warm water soaks followed by application of 5% salicylic acid in petrolatum cream (Thomas, Peterson, Walton, et al., 2015).

Assessment and Diagnostic Findings

The diagnosis is confirmed by recovering *S. scabiei* or the mites' by-products from the skin. A sample of superficial epidermis is scraped off the top of the burrows or papules with a small scalpel blade. The scrapings are placed on a microscope slide and examined through a low-powered microscope to demonstrate evidence of the mite at any stage (e.g., egg, egg casing, larva, nymph, adult).

Medical Management

The patient is instructed to take a warm, soapy bath or shower to remove the scaling debris from the crusts and then to dry thoroughly and allow the skin to cool. A prescription scabicide, such as lindane (Kwell), crotamiton (Eurax), or 5% permethrin (Elimite), is applied thinly to the entire skin from the neck down, sparing only the face and scalp (which are not affected in scabies). The medication is left on for 12 to 24 hours, after which the patient is instructed to wash thoroughly. One application may be curative, but it is advisable to repeat the treatment in 1 week.

NURSING ALERT

The patient must understand medication instructions, because application of a scabicide immediately after bathing and before the skin dries and cools increases percutaneous absorption of the scabicide and the potential for central nervous system abnormalities such as seizures.

Nursing Management

The patient should wear clean clothing and sleep between freshly laundered bedsheets. All bedding and clothing must be washed in hot water and dried on the hot dryer cycle because the mites can survive up to 36 hours in sheets. If bedsheets or clothing cannot be washed in hot water, dry-cleaning is advised.

After treatment is completed, the patient should apply an ointment, such as a topical corticosteroid, to skin lesions because the scabicide may irritate the skin. The patient's hypersensitivity does not cease on destruction of the mites. Pruritus may continue for several weeks as a manifestation of hypersensitivity, particularly in atopic (allergic) people. This is not a sign that the treatment has failed. The patient is instructed not to apply more scabicide, as it will cause more irritation and increased itching. As well, the patient is advised not to take frequent hot showers, as they can dry the skin and produce pruritus. Oral antihistamines such as diphenhydramine (Benadryl) or hydroxyzine (Atarax) can help to control the itching.

All family members and close contacts should be treated simultaneously to eliminate the mites. Some scabicides are approved for use in infants and pregnant women. If scabies is sexually transmitted, the patient may require treatment for coexisting sexually transmitted infection. Scabies may also coexist with pediculosis.

NONINFECTIOUS INFLAMMATORY DERMATOSES

Irritant Contact Dermatitis

Contact dermatitis (also called eczema) is an inflammatory reaction of the skin to physical, chemical, or biologic agents. The epidermis is damaged by repeated physical and chemical irritations. Contact dermatitis may be of the primary irritant type, in which a nonallergic reaction results from exposure to an irritating substance, or it may be allergic (i.e., allergic contact dermatitis), resulting from exposure of sensitized people to contact allergens. Common causes of irritant dermatitis are soaps, detergents, scouring compounds, and industrial chemicals. Predisposing factors include extremes of heat and cold, frequent contact with soap and water, and a pre-existing skin disease (Chart 58-4).

(text continued on page 1806)

Plan of Nursing Care

Chart 58-4. Patients With Dermatoses (Abnormal Skin Conditions)

NURSING INTERVENTIONS	RATIONALE	EXPECTED OUTCOMES
Nursing Priority: Skin care **Goal:** Maintenance of skin integrity		
1. Protect healthy skin from maceration (excessive hydration of stratum corneum) when applying wet dressings.	1. Maceration of healthy skin can cause skin breakdown and extension of the primary condition.	• Maintains skin integrity • Absence of maceration • No signs of thermal injury • Absence of infection • Applies prescribed topical medication • Takes prescribed medication on schedule
2. Remove moisture from skin by blotting gently and avoiding friction.	2. Friction and maceration play a major role in some skin diseases.	
3. Guard carefully against risks of thermal injuries from excessively hot wet dressings and from subtle heat injuries (heating pads, radiators).	3. Patients with dermatoses may have decreased sensitivity to heat.	
4. Advise patient to use sunscreening agents.	4. Many cosmetic issues and virtually all cutaneous malignancies can be attributed to chronic skin damage.	
Nursing Priority: Acute pain **Goal:** Relief of discomfort		
1. Examine area of involvement.	1. Understanding the extent and characteristics of the skin involved helps in planning interventions.	• Achieves relief of discomfort • Verbalizes that itching has been relieved • Demonstrates absence of skin excoriation from scratching • Complies with prescribed treatment • Keeps skin hydrated and lubricated • Demonstrates intact skin; skin regaining healthy appearance
a. Attempt to discover cause of discomfort.	a. Helps to identify appropriate comfort measures.	
b. Record observations in detail, using descriptive terminology.	b. An accurate description of a cutaneous lesion is necessary for diagnosis and treatment. Many skin conditions appear similar but have different etiologies. Cutaneous inflammatory response may be muted in older adults.	
c. Anticipate possible allergic reaction; obtain a medication history.	c. A generalized rash, particularly of sudden onset, may indicate a medication allergy.	
2. Control environmental and physical factors.	2. Itching is aggravated by heat, chemicals, and physical irritants.	
a. Keep humidity about 60%; use a humidifier.	a. At low humidity, the skin loses water.	
b. Maintain a cool environment.	b. Coolness deters itching.	
c. Use mild soap for sensitive skin (Dove, Cetaphil, Aveeno).	c. These contain no detergents, dyes, fragrances, or hardening agents.	
d. Remove excess clothing or bedding.	d. Promotes cool environment.	
e. Wash bedsheets and clothing with mild, fragrance-free soap.	e. Strong soaps and laundry additives can cause skin irritation.	
f. Stop repeated exposures to detergents, cleansers, and solvents.	f. Any substance that removes water, lipids, or protein from the epidermis alters the skin's barrier function.	
3. Use skin care measures to maintain skin integrity and promote comfort.	3. The skin is an important barrier that must be maintained intact to function properly.	
a. Provide tepid cooling baths or cool dressings for itching.	a. Gradual evaporation of water from dressings cools the skin and relieves pruritus.	
b. Treat dryness (xerosis) as prescribed.	b. Dry skin can produce areas of dermatitis with redness, itching, scaling, and, in more severe forms, swelling, blistering, cracking, and weeping.	

continued >

Plan of Nursing Care — Chart 58-4. Patients With Dermatoses (Abnormal Skin Conditions), *Continued*

NURSING INTERVENTIONS	RATIONALE	EXPECTED OUTCOMES
c. Apply skin lotion or cream immediately after bathing.	c. Effective hydration of the stratum corneum prevents compromise of the barrier layer of the skin.	
d. Keep nails trimmed.	d. Trimming decreases skin damage from scratching.	
e. Apply prescribed topical therapy.	e. This helps to relieve symptoms.	
f. Help patient accept possibly prolonged treatment.	f. Effective coping measures usually promote comfort.	
g. Advise patient refrain from using salves or lotions that are commercially available.	g. The patient's skin condition may be aggravated by self-medication.	
Nursing Priority: Restful sleep **Goal:** Achievement of restful sleep		
1. Prevent and treat dry skin.	1. Nocturnal pruritus interferes with sleep.	• Achieves restful sleep • Reports relief of itching • Maintains appropriate environmental conditions • Avoids caffeine in the late afternoon and evening • Identifies measures to promote sleep • Experiences satisfactory rest/sleep pattern
a. Advise patient to keep bedroom well ventilated and humidified.	a. Dry air will make skin feel itchy. A comfortable environment promotes relaxation.	
b. Keep skin moisturized.	b. This prevents water loss. Dry, itchy skin can usually be controlled but not cured.	
c. Bathe/shower only as necessary if skin is excessively dry. Use no soap or only mild soap. Apply skin lotion/cream immediately after bathing while skin is damp.	c. These measures preserve skin moisture.	
2. Advise patient of the following measures that may be helpful in promoting sleep:		
a. Keep a regular schedule for sleeping. Go to bed at the same time; get up at the same time.	a. Regularity of sleep schedule is important in maintaining sleep.	
b. Avoid caffeinated drinks in the evening.	b. Caffeine has peak effect 2 to 4 hours after being consumed.	
c. Exercise regularly, particularly in the late afternoon.	c. Exercise at this time appears to have beneficial sleep effect.	
d. Use a bedtime routine or ritual.	d. This eases transition from wakefulness to sleep.	
e. Use an antihistamine at bedtime if prescribed.	e. Antihistamines decrease itching and promote sleep.	
Nursing Priority: Body Image **Goal:** Development of increasing self-acceptance		
1. Assess patient for disturbance of self-image (avoidance of eye contact, self-negating verbalizations, expression of disgust about skin condition).	1. Disturbance of body image may accompany any disease or condition that is apparent to the patient. An impression of one's own body has an effect on self-concept.	• Develops increasing acceptance of own body • Follows through and participates in self-care measures • Reports feeling in control of situation • Gives self-positive reinforcement • Verbalizes a more healthful self-regard • Appears less self-conscious; is not afraid to socialize and be seen by others • Uses concealing and highlighting techniques to enhance appearance
2. Identify psychosocial stage of development.	2. There is a relationship between development stage, self-image, and the patient's reaction to and understanding of skin condition.	
3. Provide opportunity for expression. Listen (in an open, nonjudgmental way) to expressions of grief/anxiety about changes in body image.	3. The patient needs the experience of being heard and understood.	

Plan of Nursing Care

Chart 58-4. Patients With Dermatoses (Abnormal Skin Conditions), *Continued*

NURSING INTERVENTIONS	RATIONALE	EXPECTED OUTCOMES
4. Assess patient's concerns and fears. Assist anxious patient to develop insight and identify and cope with problems.	4. This gives health care personnel an opportunity to neutralize undue anxiety and restore reality to the situation. Fear is destructive to adaptation.	
5. Support patient's efforts to improve body image (participation in skin treatments; grooming), develop self-acceptance, socialize with others, and use cosmetics to conceal disfigurement.	5. A positive approach and suggestions about cosmetic techniques are often helpful in promoting self-acceptance and socialization.	

Nursing Priority: Patient teaching
Goal: Understanding of skin care

NURSING INTERVENTIONS	RATIONALE	EXPECTED OUTCOMES
1. Determine what patient knows (understands and misunderstands) about condition.	1. Provides baseline data for developing the teaching plan.	• Acquires understanding of skin care • Follows treatment as prescribed and can verbalize rationale for measures taken • Carries out prescribed baths, soaks, wet dressings • Uses topical medication appropriately • Understands importance of nutrition to skin health
2. Keep patient informed; correct misconceptions/misinformation.	2. Patients need to have a sense that there is something they can do. Most patients benefit from explanations and reassurance.	
3. Demonstrate application of prescribed therapy (wet compresses; topical medication).	3. Allows patient the opportunity to observe the correct way to perform therapies.	
4. Advise patient to keep skin moist and flexible with hydration and application of skin cream and lotion.	4. The stratum corneum needs water to stay flexible. Application of skin cream or lotion to damp skin prevents dry, rough, cracked, and scaly skin.	
5. Encourage patient to attain a healthy nutritional status.	5. The appearance of the skin reflects a person's general health. Changes may signal abnormal nutrition.	

Collaborative Problems: Infection
Goal: Absence of complications

NURSING INTERVENTIONS	RATIONALE	EXPECTED OUTCOMES
1. Have a high index of suspicion for an infection in patients with compromised immune systems.	1. Any condition that compromises the immune status increases the risk of cutaneous infection.	• Remains free of infection • Describes skin care measures that promote cleanliness and prevent skin breakdown • Identifies signs and symptoms of infection to report • Identifies adverse effects of medications that should be reported to health care personnel • Participates in skin care measures (e.g., dressing changes, soaks)
2. Instruct patient clearly and in detail about therapeutic regimen.	2. Effective patient education is dependent on the interpersonal skills of the health professionals and on giving clear instructions reinforced through written instructions.	
3. Apply intermittent wet dressings as prescribed to reduce intensity of inflammation.	3. A wet dressing produces evaporative cooling, causing constriction of superficial cutaneous vessels and thereby decreasing erythema and serum production. Wet dressings help in debridement of vesicles and crusts and control inflammatory processes.	
4. Provide tub baths and soaks as prescribed.	4. Loosens exudate and scales.	
5. Administer prescribed antimicrobial agents.	5. Kills or prevents the growth of the infectious organism.	

continued >

Plan of Nursing Care

Chart 58-4. Patients With Dermatoses (Abnormal Skin Conditions), *Continued*

NURSING INTERVENTIONS	RATIONALE	EXPECTED OUTCOMES
6. Use topical medications containing corticosteroids as prescribed and as indicated. a. Observe lesion periodically for changes in response to therapy. b. Instruct patient about possible adverse effects of long-term use of fluorinated topical corticosteroids.	6. Corticosteroids have an anti-inflammatory action, resulting in part from their ability to induce vasoconstriction of the small vessels in the upper dermis. Extensive prolonged use of topical corticosteroids can lead to antiproliferative effects on epidermal cells (loss of hair in area used; thinning of the skin).	
7. Advise patient to stop using any skin agent that makes condition worse.	7. A contact dermatitis or allergic reaction may develop from any ingredient in the medication.	

Clinical Manifestations

The eruptions begin when the causative agent contacts the skin. The first reactions include pruritus, burning, and erythema, followed closely by edema, papules, vesicles, and oozing or weeping. In the subacute phase, these vesicular changes are less marked, and they alternate with crusting, drying, fissuring, and peeling. If repeated reactions occur or if the patient continually scratches the skin, lichenification and pigmentation occur. Secondary bacterial invasion may follow (Cohen, 2014).

Medical Management

The objectives of management are to soothe and heal the involved skin and protect it from further damage. The distribution pattern of the reaction is identified to differentiate between allergic and irritant contact dermatitis. A detailed history is obtained. If possible, the offending irritant is removed. Local irritation should be avoided, and soap is not generally used until healing occurs.

Many preparations are advocated for relieving dermatitis. In general, a barrier cream that contains ceramide (e.g., Impruv, CeraVe) or dimethicone (e.g., Cetaphil) is used for small patches of erythema. A thin layer of cream or ointment containing a corticosteroid is commonly used, although the efficacy of corticosteroids has not been demonstrated in research (Cohen, 2014). The patient is educated about how to treat and prevent future bouts of irritant dermatitis (see Chart 58-5).

Psoriasis

Psoriasis is a chronic noninfectious inflammatory disease of the skin in which epidermal cells are produced at a rate that is about six to nine times faster than usual. The cells in the basal layer of the skin divide too quickly, and the newly formed cells move so rapidly to the skin surface that they become evident as profuse scales or plaques of epidermal tissue. The psoriatic epidermal cell may travel from the basal cell layer of the epidermis to the stratum corneum (i.e., skin surface) and be cast off in 3 to 4 days, which is in sharp contrast to the usual 26 to 28 days. As a result of the increased number of basal cells and rapid cell passage, the usual events of cell maturation and growth cannot take place. This abnormal process does not allow the normal protective layers of the skin to form. It is thought that the condition stems from a hereditary defect that causes overproduction of keratin. Current evidence supports an immunologic basis for the disease. Although the primary manifestation of this noncommunicable disease tends to involve the skin, psoriasis may

CHART 58-5

Patient Education: Strategies for Avoiding Contact Dermatitis

The precautions listed below may help prevent repeated cases of contact dermatitis and should be followed for at least 4 months after skin appears to be completely healed.

The nurse instructs the patient to:

- Study the pattern and location of your dermatitis and think about which things have touched your skin and which things may have caused the problem; try to avoid contact with these materials.
- Avoid heat, soap, and rubbing, all of which are external irritants.
- Choose bath soaps, laundry detergents, and cosmetics that do not contain fragrance.
- Avoid using a fabric softener dryer sheet (Bounce, ClingFree). Fabric softeners that are added to the washer may be used.
- Avoid topical medications, lotions, or ointments, except those specifically prescribed for your condition.
- Wash your skin thoroughly immediately after exposure to possible irritants.
- Ensure that when wearing gloves (such as for washing dishes or general cleaning), they are cotton lined. Do not wear them more than 15 or 20 minutes at a time.

Adapted from Hogan, D. J. (2016). Irritant contact dermatitis. *Medscape*. Retrieved February 11, 2017, from emedicine.medscape.com/article/1049352-overview involve the oral cavity, eyes (including the lids, conjunctivae, and corneas), and joints. Psoriasis is typically characterized by the appearance of silvery plaques that most commonly appear on the skin over the elbows, knees, scalp, lower back, and buttocks (Meffert, 2016). Onset may occur at any age, with a median onset at 28 years. It is more prevalent among women and Caucasians. It is thought that most patients with psoriasis have a genetic predisposition to develop the disease. Psoriasis is characterized by periods of remission and exacerbation throughout life (Meffert, 2016).

Pathophysiology

Current evidence supports an autoimmune basis for psoriasis. Periods of emotional stress and anxiety aggravate the condition, and trauma, infections, and seasonal and hormonal changes may also serve as triggers (Meffert, 2016).

In this disease, the epidermis becomes infiltrated by activated T cells and cytokines, resulting in both vascular engorgement and proliferation of keratinocytes. Epidermal hyperplasia results. These epidermal cells tend to improperly retain their nuclei, crippling their ability to release lipids that encourage cellular adhesion. This results in rapid turnover of poorly matured cells that do not adhere well to each other, resulting in the classic presentation of plaquelike lesions that have a silvery, scaly, flaky appearance (Meffert, 2016).

Clinical Manifestations

Lesions appear as red, raised patches of skin covered with silvery scales. The scaly patches are formed by the buildup of living and dead skin resulting from the vast increase in the rate of skin cell growth and turnover (Fig. 58-3). If the scales are scraped away, the dark red base of the lesion is exposed, producing multiple bleeding points. These patches are not moist and may be pruritic. One variation of this condition is called *guttate psoriasis* because the lesions remain about 1 cm wide and are scattered like raindrops over the body. This variation is believed to be associated with a recent streptococcal throat infection. Psoriasis may range in severity from a cosmetic source of annoyance to a physically disabling and disfiguring disorder.

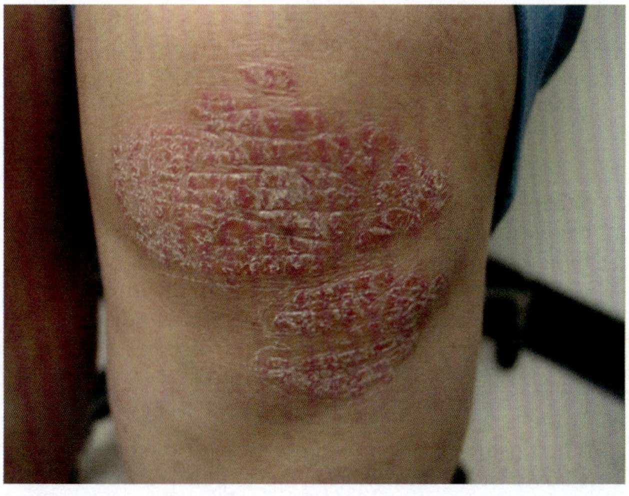

FIGURE 58-3. Psoriasis.

Particular sites of the body tend to be affected most by this condition; they include the scalp, the extensor surface of the elbows and knees, the lower part of the back, and the genitalia. Bilateral symmetry is a feature of psoriasis. In approximately one fourth to one half of patients, the nails are involved, with pitting, discolouration, crumbling beneath the free edges, and separation of the nail plate. When psoriasis occurs on the palms and soles, it can cause pustular lesions called *palmar pustular psoriasis*.

Complications

Asymmetric rheumatoid factor–negative arthritis of multiple joints occurs in up to 42% of people with psoriasis, most typically after the skin lesions appear (Nicpon, 2017). The most typical joints affected include those in the hands or feet, although sometimes larger joints such as the elbows, knees, or hips may be affected (Meffert, 2016). A rheumatologist should be consulted to assist in the diagnosis and long-term treatment of this disorder. Psoriatic arthritis is discussed in more detail later in this chapter.

Erythrodermic psoriasis, an exfoliative psoriatic state, involves disease progression that involves the total body surface. The patient is acutely ill, with fever, chills, and an electrolyte imbalance. Erythrodermic psoriasis often appears in people with chronic psoriasis after infections or after exposure to certain medications, including withdrawal of systemic corticosteroids.

Assessment and Diagnostic Findings

The presence of the classic plaque-type lesions generally confirms the diagnosis of psoriasis. Because the lesions tend to change histologically as they progress from early to chronic plaques, biopsy of the skin is of little diagnostic value. There are no specific blood tests helpful in diagnosing the condition. When in doubt, the health professional should assess for signs of nail and scalp involvement and for a positive family history.

Medical Management

The goals of management are to slow the rapid turnover of epidermis, to promote resolution of the psoriatic lesions, and to control the natural cycles of the disease. There is no known cure.

The therapeutic approach should be one that the patient understands; it should be cosmetically acceptable and minimally disruptive of lifestyle. Treatment involves the commitment of time and effort by the patient and possibly the family. Any precipitating or aggravating factors are addressed. An assessment is made of lifestyle because psoriasis is significantly affected by stress. Management of emotional factors should be addressed as part of the overall treatment of psoriasis. The patient is informed that treatment of severe psoriasis can be time consuming, expensive, and aesthetically unappealing at times. Many patients report difficulty adhering to treatment plans, either for time reasons or lack of response to the treatment (Mease & Armstrong, 2014).

TABLE 58-7 Current Treatments for Psoriasis

Topical Agents	Use	Selected Agents
Biologicals	Moderate to severe lesions	cyclosporine (Neoral), alefacept (Amevive), etanercept (Enbrel), infliximab (Remicade)
Topical corticosteroids	Mild to moderate lesions Moderate to severe lesions Severe lesions Lesions on face and groin	Aristocort, Kenalog, Valisone Lidex, Psorcon, Cutivate Temovate, Diprolene, Ultravate Aclovate, DesOwen, Hytone 2.5%
Topical nonsteroidals	Mild to severe	Retinoids such as tazarotene (Tazorac) Vitamin D_2 derivative calcipotriene (Dovonex)
Coal tar products	Mild to moderate lesions	Coal tar and salicylic acid ointment (Aquatar, Estar gel, Fototar, Zetar); anthralin (Anthra-Derm, Dritho-Creme); Neutrogena T-Derm, Psorigel
Medicated shampoos	Scalp lesions	Neutrogena T-Gel, T-Sal, Zetar, Head & Shoulders, Desenex, Selsun Blue, Bakers P&S (emulsifying agent with phenol, saline solution, and mineral oil)
Intralesional therapy	Thick plaques and nails	Kenalog, Cordran-impregnated tape, Fluoroplex
Systemic therapy	Extensive lesions and nails	methotrexate (Folex, Mexate); hydroxyurea (Hydrea); retinoic acid (Tegison) (not to be used in women of childbearing age)
	Psoriatic arthritis	Oral gold (auranofin), etretinate, methotrexate
Photochemotherapy	Moderate to severe lesions	UVA or UVB light with or without topical medications PUVA (combines UVA light with oral psoralens, or topical trisoralen)

Gentle removal of scales is an important principle of psoriasis treatment. This can be accomplished by taking baths with added oils (e.g., olive oil, mineral oil), colloidal oatmeal preparations, or coal tar preparations. A soft brush may be used to gently scrub the psoriatic plaques. After bathing, the application of emollient creams containing alpha hydroxy acids (e.g., Lac-Hydrin, Penederm) or salicylic acid can soften thick scales. The patient and family should be encouraged to establish a regular skin care routine that can be maintained even when the psoriasis is not in an acute stage (Mease & Armstrong, 2014).

Pharmacologic Therapy

Three types of therapy are commonly indicated: topical, phototherapy, and systemic. Topical agents, possibly in tandem with phototherapy, are recommended for mild disease. Patients with moderate or severe disease should receive topical agents, phototherapy, and systemic treatment (Nicpon, 2017) (Table 58-7).

Topical Agents

Topically applied agents are used to slow the overactive epidermis without affecting other tissues. These topical formulations include lotions, ointments, pastes, creams, and shampoos. Two topical treatments introduced within the last few years are a vitamin D preparation, calcipotriene (Dovonex), and a retinoid compound, tazarotene (Tazorac). Treatment with these agents tends to suppress **epidermopoiesis** (i.e., development of epidermal cells) and cause sloughing of the rapidly growing epidermal cells. Older treatments, including tar baths and application of tar preparations on involved skin, are rarely used. Tar and anthralin cause irritation of the skin at the sites of application, are malodorous and difficult to apply, and do not give reliable results. Newer preparations that cause less irritation and have more consistent results are becoming more widely used.

Topical corticosteroids may be applied for their anti-inflammatory effect. Choosing the correct strength of corticosteroid for the involved site and choosing the most effective vehicle base are important aspects of topical treatment. In general, high-potency topical corticosteroids are not used on the face and intertriginous areas, and their use on other areas should be limited to a 4-week course of twice-daily applications. A 2-week break is taken before repeating treatment with the high-potency corticosteroids. For long-term therapy, moderate-potency corticosteroids are used. On the face and intertriginous areas, only low-potency corticosteroids are appropriate for long-term use (see Table 58-4).

Occlusive dressings may be applied to increase the effectiveness of the corticosteroid. Large plastic bags may be used—one for the upper body with openings cut for the head and arms and one for the lower body with openings for the legs. Large rolls of tubular plastic can be used to cover the arms and legs. Another option is a vinyl jogging suit. The medication is applied, and the suit is put on over it. The hands can be wrapped in gloves, the feet in plastic bags, and the head in a shower cap. Occlusive dressings should not remain in place longer than 8 hours. The nurse should very carefully inspect the skin for the appearance of atrophy, hypopigmentation, striae, and telangiectasias, which are side effects of corticosteroids.

NURSING ALERT

When plastic substances are used, the nurse needs to check for flammability. Some thin plastic films burn slowly (if touched by a lighted cigarette), whereas others burst rapidly into flame. The patient should be cautioned not to smoke while wrapped in plastic dressing.

When psoriasis involves large areas of the body, topical corticosteroid treatment can be expensive and involve some systemic risk. The more potent corticosteroids, when applied to large areas of the body, have the potential to cause adrenal suppression through percutaneous absorption of the medication. In this event, other treatment modalities (e.g., nonsteroidal topical medications, UV light) may be used instead or in combination to decrease the need for corticosteroids (Bronckers, Paller, van Geel, et al., 2015; Mease & Armstrong, 2014).

Tazarotene (Tazorac), a newer nonsteroidal topical preparation, is available and effective for many patients. Treatment with this agent tends to suppress epidermopoiesis (i.e., development of epidermal cells) and causes sloughing of the scales covering psoriatic plaques. As with other retinoids, it causes increased sensitivity to sunlight, so patients are cautioned to use an effective sunscreen and avoid other photosensitizers (e.g., tetracycline, antihistamines). Tazarotene is listed as a category X drug in pregnancy; reports indicate evidence of fetal risk, and the risk of use in pregnant women clearly outweighs any possible benefits. A negative result on a pregnancy test should be obtained before initiating this medication, and an effective contraceptive should be continued during treatment. Side effects of tazarotene include burning, erythema, or irritation at the site of application and worsening of psoriasis.

Intralesional Agents

Intralesional injections of triamcinolone acetonide (Aristocort, Kenalog-10, Trymex) can be administered directly into highly visible or isolated patches of psoriasis that are resistant to other forms of therapy. Care must be taken to ensure that the medication is not injected into healthy skin.

Phototherapy

For patients who do not respond well to topical treatments, phototherapy using narrow-band ultraviolet-B (UVB) therapy may be effective as a single-therapy modality. However, phototherapy is generally more effective when it is given as ultraviolet-A (UVA) in conjunction with a photosensitizing oral medication (a combination referred to as PUVA). Here, the patient takes a photosensitizing medication (i.e., psoralen) in a standard dose and is subsequently exposed to long-wave UV light as the medication plasma levels peak. It is thought that when psoralen-treated skin is exposed to UVA light, the psoralen binds with DNA and decreases epidermal cellular proliferation. PUVA has been associated with long-term risks of skin cancer, cataracts, and premature aging of the skin (Bronckers et al., 2015; Meffert, 2016).

The patient is usually treated two or three times each week until the psoriasis clears. An interim period of 48 hours between treatments is necessary to allow any burns resulting from PUVA therapy to become evident. After the psoriasis clears, the patient begins a maintenance program. Once little or no disease is active, less potent therapies are used to keep minor flare-ups under control (Meffert, 2016).

If access to a light treatment unit is not feasible, the patient can expose himself or herself to sunlight. The risks of all light treatments are similar and include acute sunburn reaction; exacerbation of photosensitive disorders such as lupus, rosacea, and polymorphic light eruption; and other skin changes such as increased wrinkles, thickening, and an increased risk for skin cancer.

Excimer lasers have come into use in treating psoriasis. These lasers function at 308 nm. A laser can be more effective on the scalp or on other hard-to-treat areas, because the laser can be aimed very specifically on the plaque. Table 58-7 summarizes the treatment plans.

Systemic Agents

Although systemic corticosteroids may cause rapid improvement of psoriasis, their usual risks and the possibility of triggering a severe flare-up on withdrawal limit their use. Systemic cytotoxic preparations, such as methotrexate, have been used in treating extensive psoriasis that fails to respond to other forms of therapy. Other systemic medications in current use include hydroxyurea (Hydrea) and cyclosporine A (CyA).

Methotrexate appears to inhibit DNA synthesis in epidermal cells, thereby reducing the turnover time of the psoriatic epidermis. However, the medication can be toxic, especially to the liver, which can suffer irreversible damage. The kidneys and the bone marrow are other organs that may be damaged by the medication. Laboratory studies must be monitored to ensure that the hepatic, hematopoietic, and renal systems are functioning adequately. The patient should avoid drinking alcohol while taking methotrexate, because alcohol ingestion increases the possibility of liver damage. The medication is teratogenic (producing physical defects in the fetus) and is not be administered to pregnant women.

Hydroxyurea also inhibits cell replication by affecting DNA synthesis. The patient is monitored for signs and symptoms of bone marrow depression.

Cyclosporine A, a cyclic peptide used to prevent rejection of transplanted organs, has shown some success in treating severe, therapy-resistant cases of psoriasis. Its use, however, is limited by side effects such as hypertension and nephrotoxicity.

Oral retinoids (i.e., synthetic derivatives of vitamin A and its metabolite, vitamin A acid) modulate the growth and differentiation of epithelial tissue. Etretinate is especially useful for severe pustular or erythrodermic psoriasis. Etretinate is a teratogen with a very long half-life; it cannot be used in women with childbearing potential.

Nursing Management

Psoriasis may cause despair and frustration for the patient; observers may stare, comment, ask embarrassing questions, or even avoid the person. The disease can eventually exhaust the patient's resources, interfere with their job, and negatively affect many aspects of life.

The nurse assesses the impact of the disease on the patient and the coping strategies used for conducting normal activities and interactions with family and friends (Bronckers et al., 2015). Many patients need reassurance that the condition is not infectious, not a reflection of poor personal hygiene, and not skin cancer. The nurse can create an environment in which the patient feels comfortable discussing important quality-of-life issues related to their psychosocial and physical response to this chronic illness.

The nurse explains with sensitivity that although there is no cure for psoriasis and lifetime management is necessary, the condition can usually be controlled. The pathophysiology of psoriasis is reviewed, as are the factors that provoke it—irritation or injury to the skin (e.g., cut, abrasion, sunburn), current illness (e.g., pharyngeal streptococcal infection), and emotional stress. It is emphasized that repeated trauma to the skin and an unfavourable environment (e.g., cold) may exacerbate psoriasis. The patient is cautioned about taking any nonprescription medications because some may aggravate mild psoriasis. As well, the patient is advised to seek treatment from the same primary provider for any acute illnesses or chronic conditions to minimize chances of receiving prescriptions that may interfere with each other (Meffert, 2016; Nicpon, 2017).

Reviewing and explaining the treatment regimen are essential to ensure adherence to the therapeutic regimen. For example, if the patient has a mild condition confined to localized areas, such as the elbows or knees, application of an emollient to maintain softness and minimize scaling may be all that is required. Most patients need a comprehensive care plan that ranges from using topical medications and shampoos to more complex and lengthy treatment with systemic medications and photochemotherapy, such as PUVA therapy. Patient education materials that include a description of the therapy and specific guidelines are helpful but cannot replace face-to-face discussions of the treatment plan.

To avoid injuring the skin, the patient is advised not to pick at or scratch the affected areas. Measures to prevent dry skin are encouraged because dry skin worsens psoriasis. Too-frequent washing produces more soreness and scaling. Water should be warm, not hot, and the skin should be dried by patting with a towel rather than by rubbing. Emollients have a moisturizing effect, providing an occlusive film on the skin surface so that normal water loss through the skin is halted and allowing the trapped water to hydrate the stratum corneum. A bath oil or emollient cleansing agent can comfort sore and scaling skin. Softening the skin can prevent fissures.

A therapeutic relationship between health care professionals and the patient with psoriasis includes education and support. Introducing the patient to successful coping strategies used by others with psoriasis and making suggestions for reducing or coping with stressful situations at home, school, and work can facilitate a more positive outlook and acceptance of the chronicity of the disease (Bronckers et al., 2015).

Nursing Process

Care of the Patient With Psoriasis

Assessment

The nursing assessment focuses on how the patient is coping with the psoriatic skin condition, appearance of the skin, and appearance of the skin lesions. The notable manifestations are red, scaling papules that coalesce to form oval, well-defined plaques. Silver-white scales may also be present. Adjacent skin areas show red, smooth plaques with a macerated surface. It is important to examine the areas especially prone to psoriasis: elbows, knees, scalp, gluteal cleft, fingers, and toenails (for small pits).

Psoriasis may cause despair and frustration for the patient; observers may stare, comment, ask embarrassing questions, or even avoid the person. The disease can eventually exhaust the patient's resources, interfere with his or her job, and make life miserable in general. Teenagers are especially vulnerable to the psychological effects of this disorder. The family is affected as well, because time-consuming treatments, messy salves, and constant shedding of scales may disrupt home life and cause resentment. The patient's frustrations may be expressed through hostility directed at health care personnel and others.

Nursing Priorities

Based on nursing assessment data, the patient's major nursing priorities may include the following:

- Patient teaching
- Impaired skin integrity
- Disturbed body image

Collaborative Problems/ Potential Complications

Based on assessment data, potential complications include the following:

- Infection
- Psoriatic arthritis

Planning and Goals

Major goals for the patient may include increased understanding of psoriasis and the treatment regimen, achievement of smoother skin with control of lesions, development of self-acceptance, and absence of complications.

Nursing Interventions

Promoting Understanding

The nurse explains with sensitivity that although there is no cure for psoriasis, and lifetime management is necessary, the condition can usually be controlled. The pathophysiology of psoriasis is reviewed, as are the factors that provoke it—irritation or injury to the skin (e.g., cut, abrasion, sunburn), current illness (e.g., pharyngeal streptococcal infection), and emotional stress. It is emphasized that repeated trauma to the skin and an unfavourable environment (e.g., cold) or a specific medication (e.g., lithium, beta-blockers, indomethacin) may exacerbate psoriasis. The patient is cautioned about taking any nonprescription medications because some may aggravate mild psoriasis.

Reviewing and explaining the treatment regimen are essential to ensure compliance. For example, if the patient has a mild condition confined to localized areas, such as the elbows or knees, application of an emollient to maintain softness and minimize scaling may be all that is required. Most patients need a comprehensive plan of care that ranges from using topical medications and shampoos to more complex and lengthy treatment with systemic medications and photochemotherapy, such as PUVA therapy. Patient education materials that include a description of the therapy and specific guidelines are helpful but cannot replace face-to-face discussions of the treatment plan.

Increasing Skin Integrity

To avoid injuring the skin, the patient is advised not to pick at or scratch the affected areas. Measures to prevent dry skin are encouraged because dry skin worsens psoriasis. Too-frequent washing produces more soreness and scaling. Water should be warm, not hot, and the skin should be dried by patting with a towel rather than by rubbing. Emollients have a moisturizing effect, providing an occlusive film on the skin surface so that usual water loss through the skin is halted and allowing the trapped water to hydrate the stratum corneum. A bath oil or emollient cleansing agent can comfort sore and scaling skin. Softening the skin can prevent fissures (see Chart 58-4).

Improving Self-Concept and Body Image

A therapeutic relationship between health care professionals and the patient with psoriasis is one that includes education and support. After the treatment regimen is established, the patient should begin to feel more confident and empowered in carrying it out and in using coping strategies that help deal with the altered self-concept and body image brought about by the disease. Introducing the patient to successful coping strategies used by others with psoriasis and making suggestions for reducing or coping with stressful situations at home, school, and work can facilitate a more positive outlook and acceptance of the chronicity of the disease.

Monitoring and Managing Potential Complications

PSORIATIC ARTHRITIS. The diagnosis of psoriasis, especially when it is accompanied by the complication of arthritis, is usually difficult to make. Psoriatic arthritis involving the sacroiliac and distal joints of the fingers may be overlooked, especially if the patient has the typical psoriatic lesions. However, patients who report mild joint discomfort and some pitting of the fingernails may not be diagnosed with psoriasis until the more obvious cutaneous lesions appear.

The report of joint discomfort in the patient with psoriasis is noted and evaluated. The symptoms of psoriatic arthritis can mimic the symptoms of Reiter's disease and ankylosing spondylitis, and a definitive diagnosis must be made. Treatment of the condition usually involves joint rest, application of heat, and salicylates.

The patient requires education about the care and treatment of the involved joints and the need for compliance with therapy. The incidence of psoriatic arthropathy is unknown because the symptoms are so variable. It is believed, however, that when the psoriasis is extensive and a family history of inflammatory arthritis is elicited, the chance that the patient will develop psoriatic arthritis increases substantially. It is recommended that a rheumatologist be consulted to assist in the diagnosis and treatment of the arthropathy.

Promoting Home, Community-Based, and Transitional Care

EDUCATING PATIENTS ABOUT SELF-CARE. Printed patient education materials may be provided to reinforce face-to-face discussions about treatment guidelines and other considerations. Patients using topical corticosteroid preparations repeatedly on the face and around the eyes should be aware that cataract development is possible. Strict guidelines for applying these medications should be emphasized, because overuse can result in skin atrophy, striae, and medication resistance.

PUVA, which is reserved for moderate to severe psoriasis, produces photosensitization. If exposure to the sun is unavoidable, the skin must be protected with sunscreen and clothing. Gray- or green-tinted wraparound sunglasses should be worn to protect the eyes during and after treatment, and ophthalmologic examinations should be performed on a regular basis (Meffert, 2016; Nicpon, 2017).

If indicated, referral may be made to a mental health professional who can help to ease emotional strain and give support. Belonging to a support group may also help patients acknowledge that they are not alone in experiencing life adjustments in response to a visible, chronic disease. The Canadian Dermatology Association (http://www.dermatology.ca/patients_public/info_patients/psoriasis/index.html) and the Psoriasis Society of Canada (http://www.psoriasissociety.org) publish periodic bulletins and reports about new and relevant developments in this condition. Chart 58-6 is a Home Care Checklist for the patient with psoriasis.

Evaluation

Expected patient outcomes may include the following:

1. Demonstrates knowledge and understanding of disease process and its treatment
   a. Describes psoriasis and prescribed therapy
   b. Verbalizes that trauma, infection, and emotional stress may be trigger factors
   c. Maintains control with appropriate therapy
   d. Demonstrates proper application of topical therapy

CHART 58-6

HOME CARE CHECKLIST • The Patient With Psoriasis

At the completion of education, the patient and/or caregiver will be able to:

- Describe the etiology of psoriasis.
- Describe optimal skin maintenance practices to maintain moisture of skin and prevent infection.
- Demonstrate proper application of prescribed topical medications.
- Describe common side effects of oral medication, if prescribed.
- Demonstrate appropriate therapeutic bath technique, if prescribed.
- Verbalize optimism about condition.
- Identify a support person with whom to discuss feelings and concerns.

2. Achieves smoother skin and control of lesions
   a. Exhibits no new lesions
   b. Keeps skin lubricated and soft
3. Develops self-acceptance
   a. Identifies someone with whom to discuss feelings and concerns
   b. Expresses optimism about outcomes of treatment
4. Absence of complications
   a. Has no joint discomfort
   b. Reports control of cutaneous lesions with no extension of disease

Generalized Exfoliative Dermatitis

Generalized exfoliative dermatitis, also called *erythroderma,* is characterized by a scaling erythematous dermatitis that may involve more than 90% of the skin (César, Cruz, Mota, et al., 2016). Generalized exfoliative dermatitis has a variety of causes. It may occur as a result of a reactive process (e.g., drug allergy) or may be secondary to an underlying skin disease (e.g., psoriasis, contact dermatitis, atopic dermatitis) or a systemic disease (e.g., lymphoma, leukemia). The cause is idiopathic (i.e., unknown) in approximately 16% of cases (Kellen & Berlin, 2016); idiopathic generalized exfoliative dermatitis is also called *red man syndrome* (Umar & Kelly, 2016). Although generalized exfoliative dermatitis may occur at any age, it more commonly appears in those between the ages of 41 and 61 years. It occurs two to four times more commonly in men than in women (Kellen & Berlin, 2016).

Clinical Manifestations

Exfoliative dermatitis starts acutely as a patchy or a generalized erythematous eruption accompanied by fever, malaise, and occasionally gastrointestinal symptoms. The skin colour changes from pink to dark red. After a week, the characteristic exfoliation (i.e., scaling) begins, usually in the form of thin flakes that leave the underlying skin smooth and red, with new scales forming as the older ones come off. Hair loss may accompany this disorder. Relapses are common. The systemic effects include high-output heart failure, intestinal disturbances, breast enlargement, elevated levels of uric acid in the blood (i.e., hyperuricemia), and temperature disturbances.

Assessment and Diagnostic Findings

The presence of scaling erythematous dermatitis, particularly when it occurs in tandem with a known skin disease or a new prescription medication, increases the suspicion that generalized exfoliative dermatitis may be diagnosed. The patient frequently also presents with hypoalbuminemia and a negative nitrogen balance, as described previously, as well as an increased erythrocyte sedimentation rate that is consistent with an underlying acute inflammatory process. A skin biopsy is indicated, because it may confirm the underlying cause and diagnosis (Umar & Kelly, 2016).

Medical Management

The objectives of management are to discern and treat any underlying disorder, to maintain fluid and electrolyte balance, and to prevent infection. The treatment is individualized and supportive and should be initiated as soon as the condition is diagnosed.

The patient may be hospitalized. All medications that may be implicated are discontinued. A comfortable room temperature should be maintained because the patient does not have normal thermoregulatory control as a result of temperature fluctuations caused by vasodilation and evaporative water loss. Fluid and electrolyte balance must be maintained because there is considerable water and protein loss from the skin surface. Administration of plasma volume expanders may be indicated. Patients in a negative nitrogen balance may be prescribed enteral or parenteral therapy (Umar & Kelly, 2016).

Nursing Management

Continual nursing assessment is carried out to prevent sepsis. The disrupted, erythematous, moist skin is susceptible to infection and becomes colonized with pathogenic organisms, which produce more inflammation. Antibiotic agents, which are prescribed if infection is present, are selected on the basis of culture and sensitivity.

Hypothermia may occur because increased blood flow in the skin, coupled with increased water loss through the skin, leads to heat loss by radiation, conduction, and evaporation. Changes in vital signs are closely monitored and reported.

Topical therapy is used to provide symptomatic relief. Soothing baths, compresses, and lubrication with emollients are used to treat the extensive dermatitis. Topical corticosteroids are the mainstay of treatment. The patient is likely to be extremely irritable because of the severe pruritus; sedating antihistamines to be given before bedtime may be prescribed to relieve the itching and promote sleep (e.g., hydroxyzine [Atarax, Vistaril]) (Umar & Kelly, 2016).

The use of oral or parenteral corticosteroids may be prescribed; however, their use is controversial. They are contraindicated when the cause of the condition is either not known or is suspected to be secondary to an underlying skin disease, such as psoriasis. When generalized exfoliative dermatitis occurs as a complication of psoriasis, systemic corticosteroids can exacerbate the condition (Umar & Kelly, 2016). When a specific cause is known, more specific therapy may be used. The patient is advised to avoid all irritants in the future, particularly medications that are known to cause the condition (Kellen & Berlin, 2016).

NURSING ALERT

The nurse observes the patient for signs and symptoms of heart failure because hyperemia and increased cutaneous blood flow can produce high-output cardiac failure.

BLISTERING DISEASES

Blisters of the skin have many origins, including bacterial, fungal, or viral infections; allergic contact reactions; burns; metabolic disorders; and immunologically mediated reactions. Some of these have been discussed previously (e.g., herpes simplex and zoster infections, contact dermatitis). Immunologically mediated diseases are autoimmune reactions and represent a defect of immunoglobulin M (IgM), immunoglobulin E (IgE), immunoglobulin G (IgG), and protein complement 3 (C3). Some of these conditions are life threatening; others become chronic.

The diagnosis is always made by histologic examination of a biopsy specimen by a dermatopathologist. A specimen from the blister and surrounding skin demonstrates **acantholysis** (i.e., separation of epidermal cells from each other because of damage to or an abnormality of the intracellular substance). Circulating antibodies may be detected by immunofluorescent studies of the patient's serum.

Pemphigus Vulgaris

Pemphigus is a group of serious diseases of the skin characterized by the appearance of bullae (blisters) of various sizes on apparently "normal" skin and mucous membranes. Available evidence indicates that pemphigus is an autoimmune disease involving IgG. It is thought that the pemphigus antibody is directed against a specific cell-surface antigen in epidermal cells. A blister forms from the antigen–antibody reaction. The level of serum antibody is predictive of disease severity. Genetic factors may also play a role in its development, with the highest incidence among those of Jewish or Mediterranean descent. This disorder usually occurs in men and women in middle and late adulthood. The condition may be associated with penicillins and captopril and with myasthenia gravis (Santoro, Stoopler, & Werth, 2013).

Clinical Manifestations

Most patients present with oral lesions appearing as irregularly shaped erosions that are painful, bleed easily, and heal slowly. The skin bullae enlarge, rupture, and leave large, painful eroded areas that are accompanied by crusting and oozing. A characteristic offensive odour emanates from the bullae and the exuding serum. There is blistering or sloughing of uninvolved skin when minimal pressure is applied (i.e., Nikolsky's sign). The eroded skin heals slowly, and huge areas of the body eventually are involved. Bacterial superinfection is common.

Complications

The most common complications of pemphigus vulgaris arise when the disease process is widespread. Before the advent of corticosteroid and immunosuppressive therapy, patients were very susceptible to secondary bacterial infection. Skin bacteria have relatively easy access to the bullae as they ooze, rupture, and leave denuded areas that are open to the environment. Fluid and electrolyte imbalance results from the loss of both fluid and protein as the bullae rupture. Hypoalbuminemia is common when the disease process includes extensive areas of the body skin surface and mucous membranes.

Management

The goals of therapy are to bring the disease under control as rapidly as possible, to prevent loss of serum and the development of secondary infection, and to promote re-epithelization (i.e., renewal of epithelial tissue).

Corticosteroids are administered in high doses to control the disease and keep the skin free of blisters. The high dosage level is maintained until remission is apparent. In some cases, corticosteroid therapy must be maintained for life.

Corticosteroids are administered with or immediately after a meal and may be accompanied by an antacid as prophylaxis against gastric complications. Essential to therapeutic management are daily evaluations of body weight, blood pressure, blood glucose levels, and fluid balance. High-dose corticosteroid therapy has its own serious toxic effects (see Chapter 42).

Immunosuppressive agents (e.g., azathioprine, cyclophosphamide, gold) may be prescribed to help control the disease and reduce the corticosteroid dose. **Plasmapheresis** (i.e., plasma exchange) temporarily decreases the serum antibody level and has been used with variable success, although it is generally reserved for life-threatening cases.

Bullous Pemphigoid

Bullous pemphigoid is an acquired disease of flaccid blisters appearing on normal or erythematous skin. It appears more often on the flexor surfaces of the arms, legs, axilla, and groin. Oral lesions, if present, are usually transient and minimal. When the blisters break, the skin has shallow erosions that heal fairly quickly. Pruritus can be intense, even before the appearance of the blisters. Bullous pemphigoid is common in older adults, with a peak incidence at about 60 years of age. There is no gender or genetic predilection, and the disease can be found throughout the world.

Management

Medical treatment includes topical corticosteroids for localized eruptions and systemic corticosteroids for widespread involvement. Systemic corticosteroids (e.g., prednisone) may be continued for months, in alternate-day doses. The patient needs to understand the implications of long-term corticosteroid therapy, including loss of bone mass, osteoporosis, cataracts, peptic ulcers, psychotic reactions, increased risk for infection, weight gain from fluid retention, and the potential for adrenal suppression (see Chapter 43).

Dermatitis Herpetiformis

Dermatitis herpetiformis is an intensely pruritic, chronic disease that manifests with small, tense blisters that are distributed symmetrically over the elbows, knees, buttocks, and nape of the neck. It is most common between age 20 and 40 years but can appear at any age. Most patients with dermatitis herpetiformis have a subclinical defect in gluten metabolism.

Management

Most patients respond to dapsone (a combination of tetracycline and nicotinamide) and to a gluten-free diet. All patients should be screened for glucose-6-phosphate dehydrogenase deficiency, because dapsone can induce severe hemolysis in those with this deficiency. Patients benefit from dietary consultation because the dietary restrictions are lifelong, and a gluten-free diet is often difficult to follow. They need emotional support as they deal with the process of learning new habits and accepting major changes in their life.

Nursing Process

Care of the Patient With Blistering Diseases

Assessment

Patients with blistering disorders may experience significant disability. There is constant itching and possible pain in the denuded areas of skin. There may be drainage from the denuded areas, which may be malodorous. Effective assessment and nursing management become a challenge.

Disease activity is monitored clinically by examining the skin for the appearance of new blisters. Areas where healing has occurred may show signs of hyperpigmentation. Particular attention is given to assessing for signs and symptoms of infection.

Nursing Priorities

Based on nursing assessment data, the patient's major nursing priorities may include the following:

- Skin and oral cavity pain
- Impaired skin integrity
- Anxiety and ineffective coping
- Deficient knowledge

Collaborative Problems/ Potential Complications

Based on assessment data, potential complications include the following:

- Infection and sepsis related to loss of protective barrier of skin and mucous membranes
- Fluid volume deficit and electrolyte imbalance related to loss of tissue fluids

Planning and Goals

The major goals for the patient may include relief of discomfort from lesions, skin healing, reduced anxiety and improved coping capacity, and absence of complications.

Nursing Interventions

Oral Health Restoration

The patient's entire oral cavity may be affected with erosions and denuded surfaces (Scardina, Pisano, & Messina, 2010). Necrotic tissue may develop over these areas, adding to the patient's discomfort and interfering with food intake. Weight loss and hypoproteinemia may result. Meticulous oral hygiene is important to keep the oral mucosa clean and allow the epithelium to regenerate. Frequent rinsing of the mouth is prescribed to rid the mouth of debris and to soothe ulcerated areas. Commercial mouthwashes are avoided. The lips are kept moist with lanolin, petrolatum, or lip balm. Cool mist therapy helps to humidify environmental air.

Enhancing Skin Integrity and Relieving Discomfort

Cool, wet dressings or baths are protective and soothing. The patient with painful and extensive lesions should be premedicated with analgesics before skin care is initiated. Patients with large areas of blistering have a characteristic odour that decreases when secondary infection is controlled. After the patient's skin is bathed, it is dried carefully and dusted liberally with nonirritating powder, which enables the patient to move freely in bed. Fairly large amounts are necessary to keep the patient's skin from sticking to the sheets. Tape should never be used on the skin, as it may produce more blisters. Hypothermia is common, and measures to keep the patient warm and comfortable are priority nursing activities. The nursing management of patients with bullous skin conditions is similar to that for patients with extensive burns (see Chapter 58).

Anxiety Reduction

Attention to the psychological needs of the patient requires listening to the patient, being available, giving expert nursing care, and educating the patient and the family. The patient is encouraged to freely express anxieties, discomfort, and feelings of hopelessness. Arranging for a family member or a close friend to spend more time with the patient can be supportive. When patients receive information about the disease and its treatment, uncertainty and anxiety are reduced, and the patient's capacity to act on his or her own behalf is enhanced. Referral for psychological counselling may assist the patient in dealing with fears, anxiety, and depression.

Monitoring and Managing Potential Complications

INFECTION PROTECTION. The patient is susceptible to infection because the barrier function of the skin is compromised. Bullae are also susceptible to infection, and sepsis may follow. The skin is cleaned to remove debris and dead skin and to prevent infection.

Secondary infection may be accompanied by an offensive odour from skin or oral lesions. *Candida albicans* of the mouth (i.e., thrush) commonly affects patients receiving high-dose corticosteroid therapy. The oral cavity is inspected daily, and any changes are reported. Oral lesions are slow to heal.

Infection is the leading cause of death in patients with blistering diseases. Particular attention is given to assessment for signs and symptoms of local and systemic infection. Seemingly trivial concerns or minimal changes are investigated because corticosteroids can mask or alter typical signs and symptoms of infection. The patient's vital signs are taken, and temperature fluctuations are monitored. The patient is observed for chills, and all secretions and excretions are monitored for changes suggesting infection. Results of culture and sensitivity tests are monitored. Antimicrobial agents are administered as prescribed, and response to treatment is assessed. Health care personnel must perform effective hand hygiene and wear gloves.

In hospitalized patients, environmental contamination is reduced as much as possible. Protective isolation measures and standard precautions are warranted.

FLUID AND ELECTROLYTE MANAGEMENT. Extensive denudation of the skin leads to fluid and electrolyte imbalance because of significant loss of fluids and sodium chloride from the skin (Tang & Lee, 2010). This sodium chloride loss is responsible for many of the systemic symptoms associated with the disease and is treated by intravenous administration of saline solution.

A large amount of protein and blood is lost from the denuded skin areas. Blood component therapy may be prescribed to maintain the blood volume, hemoglobin level, and plasma protein concentration. Serum albumin, protein, hemoglobin, and hematocrit values are monitored.

The patient is encouraged to maintain adequate oral fluid intake. Cool, nonirritating fluids are encouraged to maintain hydration. Small, frequent meals or snacks of high-protein, high-calorie foods (e.g., Ensure, Sustacal, eggnog, milkshakes) help to maintain nutritional status. Parenteral nutrition is considered if the patient cannot eat an adequate diet.

Evaluation

Expected patient outcomes may include the following:

1. Achieves relief from pain of oral lesions
   a. Identifies therapies that reduce pain
   b. Uses mouthwashes and anesthetic or antiseptic aerosol mouth spray
   c. Drinks chilled fluids at 2-hour intervals
2. Achieves skin healing
   a. States purpose of therapeutic regimen
   b. Cooperates with soaks and bath regimen
   c. Reminds caregivers to use liberal amounts of nonirritating powder on bed linens
3. Reports that anxiety and ability to cope with condition have improved
   a. Verbalizes concerns about condition, self, and relationships with others
   b. Participates in self-care
4. Experiences no complications
   a. Has cultures from bullae, skin, and orifices that are negative for pathogenic organisms
   b. Has no purulent drainage
   c. Shows signs that skin is clearing
   d. Body temperature within expected range
   e. Keeps intake record to ensure adequate fluid intake and normal fluid and electrolyte balance
   f. Verbalizes rationale for intravenous infusion therapy
   g. Has urine output within expected limits
   h. Has serum chemistry and hemoglobin and hematocrit values within expected limits

Toxic Epidermal Necrolysis and Stevens–Johnson Syndrome

Toxic epidermal necrolysis (TEN) and Stevens–Johnson syndrome (SJS) are potentially fatal skin disorders and the most severe form of erythema multiforme. These diseases are mucocutaneous reactions that constitute a spectrum of reactions, with TEN being the most severe. The mortality rate from TEN approaches 30%. Both conditions are triggered by a reaction to medications or result from a viral infection. Antibiotics, anticonvulsant agents, NSAIDs, and sulfonamides are the most frequent medications implicated in TEN and SJS (Grossman & Porth, 2014).

Clinical Manifestations

TEN and SJS are characterized initially by conjunctival burning or itching, cutaneous tenderness, fever, cough, sore throat, headache, extreme malaise, and myalgias (aches and pains). These signs are followed by a rapid onset of erythema involving much of the skin surface and mucous membranes, including the oral mucosa, conjunctiva, and genitalia. In severe cases of mucosal involvement, there may be danger of damage to the larynx, bronchi, and esophagus from ulcerations. Large, flaccid bullae develop in some areas; in other areas, large sheets of epidermis are shed, exposing the underlying dermis. Fingernails, toenails, eyebrows, and eyelashes may be shed along with the surrounding epidermis. The skin is excruciatingly tender, and the loss of skin leaves a weeping surface similar to that of a total body, partial-thickness burn; hence, the condition is also referred to as "scalded skin syndrome."

These conditions occur in all ages and both genders. The incidence is increased in older adults because of their use of many medications. People who are immunosuppressed, including those with HIV infection and acquired immunodeficiency syndrome (AIDS), have a high risk of TEN and SJS. Although the incidence of TEN and SJS in the general population is about 2 to 3 cases per 1 million person-years, the risk associated with sulfonamides in HIV-positive individuals may approach 1 case per 1,000. Most patients with TEN have an abnormal metabolism of the culprit medication, and the mechanism leading to TEN seems to be a cell-mediated cytotoxic reaction.

Complications

Sepsis and keratoconjunctivitis are complications of TEN and SJS. Unrecognized and untreated sepsis can be life threatening. Keratoconjunctivitis can impair vision and result in conjunctival retraction, scarring, and corneal lesions.

Assessment and Diagnostic Findings

Histologic studies of frozen skin cells from a fresh lesion and cytodiagnosis of collections of cellular material from a freshly denuded area are performed. A history of ingestion of medications known to precipitate TEN or SJS may confirm medication reaction as the underlying cause.

Immunofluorescent studies may be performed to detect atypical epidermal autoantibodies. A genetic predisposition to erythema multiforme has been suggested but is not confirmed for all cases.

Medical Management

The goals of treatment include control of fluid and electrolyte balance, prevention of sepsis, and prevention of ophthalmic complications. Supportive care is the mainstay of treatment.

All nonessential medications are discontinued immediately. If possible, the patient is treated in a regional burn centre, because aggressive treatment similar to that for severe burns is required. Skin loss may approach 100% of the total body surface area. Surgical debridement or hydrotherapy in a Hubbard tank (i.e., large, steel tub) may be performed to remove involved skin.

Tissue samples from the nasopharynx, eyes, ears, blood, urine, skin, and unruptured blisters are obtained for culture to identify pathogenic organisms. Intravenous fluids are prescribed to maintain fluid and electrolyte balance, especially in the patient who has severe mucosal involvement and who cannot easily take oral nourishment. Because an indwelling intravenous catheter may be a site of infection, fluid replacement is carried out by nasogastric tube and then orally as soon as possible.

Initial treatment with systemic corticosteroids is controversial. Some experts argue for early high-dose corticosteroid treatment. However, in most cases, the risk for infection, the complication of fluid and electrolyte imbalance, the delay in the healing process, and the difficulty in initiating oral corticosteroids early in the course of the disease outweigh the perceived benefits. In patients with TEN thought to result from a medication reaction, corticosteroids may be administered; however, the patients are closely monitored for the previously stated adverse effects.

One report stated that administration of intravenous immunoglobulin (IVIG) to 10 patients led to improvement within 48 hours and skin healing within 1 week. This response is dramatically better than that obtained with immunosuppressives, and IVIG may soon become the treatment of choice.

Protecting the skin with topical agents is crucial. Various topical antibacterial and anesthetic agents are used to prevent wound sepsis and to assist with pain management. Systemic antibiotic therapy is used with extreme caution. Temporary biologic dressings (e.g., pigskin, amniotic membrane) or plastic semipermeable dressings (e.g., Vigilon) may be used to reduce pain, decrease evaporation, and prevent secondary infection until the epithelium regenerates. Meticulous oropharyngeal and eye care is essential when there is severe involvement of the mucous membranes and the eyes.

Nursing Process

Care of the Patient With Toxic Epidermal Necrolysis or Stevens–Johnson Syndrome

Assessment

For patients with toxic epidermal necrolysis, a careful inspection of the skin is made, including its appearance and the extent of involvement. The "normal" skin is closely observed to determine if new areas of blisters are developing. Seepage from blisters is monitored for amount, colour, and odour. Inspection of the oral cavity for blistering and erosive lesions is performed daily; the patient is assessed daily for itching, burning, and dryness of the eyes. The patient's ability to swallow and drink fluids, as well as speak normally, is determined.

The patient's vital signs are monitored, and special attention is given to the presence and character of fever and the respiratory rate, depth, rhythm, and cough. The characteristics and amount of respiratory secretions are reviewed. Assessment for high fever, tachycardia, and extreme weakness and fatigue is essential, because these factors indicate the process of epidermal necrosis, increased metabolic needs, and possible gastrointestinal and respiratory mucosal sloughing. Urine volume, specific gravity, and colour are monitored. The insertion sites of intravenous lines are inspected for signs of local infection. Daily body weight is recorded.

The patient is asked to describe fatigue and pain levels. An attempt is made to evaluate the patient's level of anxiety. The patient's basic coping mechanisms are assessed, and effective coping strategies are identified.

Nursing Priorities

Based on assessment data, the patient's major nursing priorities may include the following:

- Impaired tissue integrity
- Deficient fluid volume and electrolytes
- Temperature control
- Acute pain
- Anxiety

Collaborative Problems/ Potential Complications

Based on assessment data, potential complications include the following:

- Sepsis
- Conjunctival retraction, scars, and corneal lesions

Planning and Goals

The major goals for the patient may include skin and oral tissue healing, fluid balance, prevention of heat loss, relief of pain, reduced anxiety, and absence of complications.

Nursing Interventions

Maintaining Skin and Mucous Membrane Integrity

The local care of the skin is an important area of nursing management. The skin denudes easily, even when the patient is lifted and turned; it may be necessary to place the patient on a circular turning frame. The nurse applies the prescribed topical agents that reduce the bacterial population of the wound surface. Warm compresses, if prescribed, are applied gently to denuded areas. The topical antibacterial agent may be used in conjunction with hydrotherapy in a tank, bathtub, or shower. The nurse monitors the patient's condition during the treatment and encourages the patient to exercise the extremities during hydrotherapy.

The painful oral lesions make oral hygiene difficult. Careful oral hygiene is performed to keep the oral mucosa clean. Prescribed mouthwashes, anesthetics, or coating agents are used frequently to rid the mouth of debris, soothe ulcerative areas, and control foul mouth odour. The oral cavity is inspected several times each day, and any changes are documented and reported. Petrolatum or a prescribed ointment is applied to the lips.

Attaining Fluid Balance

The vital signs, urine output, and sensorium are observed for indications of hypovolemia. Mental changes from fluid and electrolyte imbalance, sensory overload, or sensory deprivation may occur. Laboratory test results are evaluated, and unexpected results are reported. The patient is weighed daily (with a bed scale if necessary).

Oral lesions may result in dysphagia, making tube feeding or parenteral nutrition necessary. Prescribed enteral nourishment or enteral supplements can be administered by tube feeding until oral ingestion can be tolerated. A daily calorie count and accurate recording of all intake and output are essential. The nurse regulates intravenous fluids at prescribed infusion rates and assesses for systemic (i.e., overinfusion or underinfusion) and local (e.g., infection) complications.

Preventing Hypothermia

The patient with TEN is prone to chilling. Dehydration may be made worse by exposing the denuded skin to a continuous current of warm air. The patient is usually sensitive to room temperature changes. Measures implemented for a burn patient, such as cotton blankets, ceiling-mounted heat lamps, and heat shields, are useful in maintaining body temperature. To minimize shivering and heat loss, the nurse works rapidly and efficiently when large wounds are exposed for wound care. The patient's temperature is monitored frequently.

Relieving Pain

The nurse assesses the patient's pain, its characteristics, any factors that influence the pain, and the patient's behavioural responses. Prescribed analgesics are administered, and the nurse documents pain relief and any side effects. Analgesics are administered before painful treatments are performed. Providing thorough explanations and speaking calmly to the patient during treatments can allay the anxiety that may intensify pain. Offering emotional support and reassurance and implementing measures that promote rest and sleep are basic in achieving pain control. As the pain diminishes and the patient has more physical and emotional energy, self-management techniques for pain relief, such as progressive muscle relaxation and imagery, may be taught.

Reducing Anxiety

Because the lifestyle of patients with TEN has been abruptly changed to one of complete dependence, an assessment of their emotional state may reveal anxiety, depression, and fear of dying. Patients can be reassured that these reactions are expected. They also need nursing support, honest communication, and hope that their situation can improve. They are encouraged to express their feelings to someone they trust. Listening to their concerns and being readily available with skilful and compassionate care are important anxiety-relieving interventions. Emotional support by a psychiatric nurse, chaplain, psychologist, or psychiatrist may be helpful to promote coping during the long recovery period.

Monitoring and Managing Potential Complications

SEPSIS. The major cause of death from TEN is infection, and the most common sites of infection are the skin and mucosal surfaces, lungs, and blood. The organisms most often involved are *S. aureus*, *Pseudomonas*, *Klebsiella*, *Escherichia coli*, *Serratia*, and *Candida*. Monitoring vital signs closely and noticing changes in respiratory, renal, and gastrointestinal function may quickly detect the beginning of an infection. Strict asepsis is always maintained during routine skin care measures. Hand hygiene and wearing sterile gloves when carrying out procedures are necessary. When the condition involves a large portion of the body, the patient should be in a private room to prevent possible cross-infection from other patients. Visitors must wear protective garments and wash their hands before and after coming into contact with the patient. People with any infectious disease should not visit the patient.

CONJUNCTIVAL RETRACTION, SCARS, AND CORNEAL LESIONS. The eyes are inspected daily for signs of itching, burning, and dryness, which may indicate progression often to keratoconjunctivitis, which is the principal eye complication. Applying a cool, damp cloth over the eyes may relieve burning sensations. The eyes are kept clean and observed for signs of discharge or discomfort, and the progression of symptoms is documented and reported. Administering an eye lubricant, when prescribed, may alleviate dryness and prevent corneal abrasion. Using eye patches or reminding the patient to blink periodically may also counteract dryness. The patient is instructed to avoid rubbing the eyes or putting any medication into the eyes that has not been prescribed or approved by the physician.

Promoting Home, Community-Based, and Transitional Care

EDUCATING PATIENTS ABOUT SELF-CARE. Patients with TEN or SJS with involvement of large areas of the skin require care that is similar to that of patients with thermal burns. As the patient completes the acute inpatient stage of illness, the focus is directed toward rehabilitation and outpatient care or care in a rehabilitation centre. Throughout this care, the patient and family members are involved in the care and are instructed in the procedures, such as wound care and dressing changes, that will need to be continued at home. The patient and family members are assisted in acquiring dressing supplies that will be needed at home.

The patient and family members are also provided with instructions about pain management, nutrition, measures to increase mobility, and prevention of complications, including prevention of infection. They are taught the signs and symptoms of complications and are instructed when to notify the health care professional. Instructions are provided in writing to the patient and family so that they can refer to these instructions when necessary at later times.

CONTINUING AND TRANSITIONAL CARE. Interdisciplinary follow-up care is imperative to ensure that the patient's progress continues. Some patients will require care in a rehabilitation centre before returning home. Others will require outpatient physical and occupational therapy for an extended period. When the patient returns home, the home care nurse coordinates the care provided by the various members of the health care team (e.g., physician, physical therapist, occupational therapist, dietician). The nurse also monitors the patient's progress, provides ongoing assessment to identify complications, and monitors the patient's adherence to the plan of care. The patient's adaptation to the home care environment and the patient and family's needs for support and assistance are also assessed. Referrals to community agencies are made as appropriate.

Evaluation

Expected patient outcomes may include the following:

1. Achieves increasing skin and oral tissue healing
   a. Demonstrates areas of healing skin
   b. Swallows fluids and speaks clearly
2. Attains fluid balance
   a. Demonstrates laboratory values within expected ranges
   b. Maintains urine volume and specific gravity within acceptable range
   c. Shows stable vital signs
   d. Increases intake of oral fluids without discomfort
   e. Gains weight, if appropriate
3. Attains thermoregulation
   a. Registers body temperature within expected range
   b. Reports no chills
4. Achieves pain relief
   a. Uses analgesics as prescribed
   b. Uses self-management techniques for relief of pain

5. Appears less anxious
   a. Discusses concerns freely
   b. Sleeps for progressively longer periods
6. Absence of complications, such as sepsis and impaired vision
   a. Body temperature within expected range
   b. Laboratory values within expected ranges
   c. Has no unexpected discharges or signs of infection
   d. Continues to see objects at baseline acuity level
   e. Shows no signs of keratoconjunctivitis

Ulcerations

Superficial loss of surface tissue as a result of death of the cells is called *ulceration*. A simple ulcer, such as the kind found in a small, superficial, partial-thickness burn, tends to heal by granulation (i.e., new tissue granules) if kept clean and protected from injury. If it is exposed to the air, the serum that escapes will dry and form a scab, under which the epithelial cells will grow and cover the surface completely. Certain diseases cause characteristic ulcers; tuberculous ulcers and syphilitic ulcers are examples.

Ulcers related to problems with arterial circulation are seen in patients with peripheral vascular disease, arteriosclerosis, Raynaud's disease, and frostbite. In these patients, treatment of the ulcers is concurrent with treatment of the arterial disease (see Chapter 32). Nursing management includes the use of the dressings discussed at the beginning of this chapter. If nursing interventions are instituted early in the progression of an ulcer, the condition can often be effectively improved. Surgical amputation of an affected limb is a last resort.

Pressure ulcers involve breakdown of the skin due to prolonged pressure, friction and shear forces, and insufficient blood supply, usually at bony prominences. Information about these ulcers is presented in Chapter 12.

TUMOURS OF THE SKIN

Tumours of the skin are common and occur along a spectrum from those that are benign to those that are highly malignant.

Benign Tumours of the Skin

Cysts

Cysts of the skin are epithelium-lined cavities that contain fluid or solid material. Epidermal cysts (i.e., epidermoid cysts) occur frequently and may be described as slow-growing, firm, elevated tumours found most frequently on the face, neck, upper chest, and back. Removal of the cysts provides a cure.

Pilar cysts (i.e., trichilemmal cysts), formerly called *sebaceous cysts*, are most frequently found on the scalp. They originate from the middle portion of the hair follicle and from the cells of the outer hair root sheath. The treatment is surgical removal.

Actinic and Seborrheic Keratoses

Seborrheic keratoses are benign, wartlike lesions of various sizes and colours, ranging from light tan to black. They are usually located on the face, shoulders, chest, and back and are the most common skin tumours seen in middle-aged and older adults. They may be cosmetically unacceptable to the patient. A black keratosis may be erroneously diagnosed as malignant melanoma. The treatment is removal of the tumour tissue by excision, electrodesiccation and curettage, or application of CO_2 or liquid nitrogen. However, there is no harm in allowing these growths to remain, as there is no medical significance to their presence.

Actinic keratoses are premalignant skin lesions that develop in chronically sun-exposed areas of the body. They appear as rough, scaly patches with underlying erythema. A small percentage of these lesions gradually transform into cutaneous squamous cell carcinoma (SCC); they are usually removed by cryotherapy or shave excision.

Verrucae: Warts

Warts are common, benign skin tumours caused by infection with the human papillomavirus, which belongs to the DNA virus group. All age groups may be affected, but the condition occurs most frequently between age 12 and 16 years. There are many types of warts.

As a rule, warts are asymptomatic, except when they occur on weight-bearing areas, such as the soles of the feet. They may be treated with locally applied laser therapy, liquid nitrogen, salicylic acid plasters, or electrodesiccation (i.e., destruction of skin lesions by monopolar high-frequency electric current).

Warts occurring on the genitalia and perianal areas are known as condylomata acuminata. They may be transmitted sexually and are treated with liquid nitrogen, cryosurgery, electrosurgery, topically applied trichloroacetic acid, and curettage. Condylomata (see Chapter 47) that affect the uterine cervix predispose the patient to cervical cancer.

Angiomas

Angiomas are benign vascular tumours that involve the skin and the subcutaneous tissues. They are present at birth and may occur as flat, violet-red patches (i.e., port-wine angiomas) or as raised, bright-red, nodular lesions (i.e., strawberry angiomas). The latter tend to involute spontaneously within the first few years of life, but port-wine angiomas usually persist indefinitely. Most patients use masking cosmetics (e.g., Covermark or Dermablend) to camouflage the lesion. The argon laser is currently being used on various angiomas with success. Treatment of strawberry angiomas is more successful if undertaken as soon after birth as possible.

Pigmented Nevi: Moles

Moles are common skin tumours of various sizes and shades, ranging from yellowish brown to black. They may be flat, macular lesions or elevated papules or nodules that occasionally contain hair. Most pigmented nevi are harmless lesions. However, in rare cases, malignant changes occur, and a melanoma develops at the site of the nevus. Some authorities believe that all congenital moles should be removed, because they may have a higher incidence of malignant change. However, depending on the quantity and location, this may be impractical. Nevi that show a change in colour or size or become symptomatic (e.g., itch) or develop irregular borders should be removed to determine if malignant changes have occurred. Moles that occur in unusual places should be examined carefully for any irregularity and for notching of the border and variation in colour. Early melanomas may display some redness and irritation and areas of bluish pigmentation where the pigment-containing cells have spread deeper into the skin. Late melanomas have areas of paler colour, where pigment cells have stopped producing melanin. Nevi larger than 1 cm should be examined carefully. Excised nevi should be examined histologically.

Keloids

Keloids are benign overgrowths of fibrous tissue at the site of a scar or trauma. They appear to be more common among dark-skinned people. Keloids are asymptomatic but may cause disfigurement and cosmetic concern. The treatment, which is not always satisfactory, consists of surgical excision, intralesional corticosteroid therapy, and radiation.

Dermatofibroma

A dermatofibroma is a common, benign tumour of connective tissue that occurs predominantly on the extremities. It is a firm, dome-shaped papule or nodule that may be skin coloured or pinkish brown. Excisional biopsy is the recommended method of treatment.

Neurofibromatosis: Von Recklinghausen's Disease

Neurofibromatosis is a hereditary condition manifested by pigmented patches (i.e., café-au-lait macules), axillary freckling, and cutaneous neurofibromas that vary in size. Developmental changes may occur in the nervous system, muscles, and bone. Malignant degeneration of the neurofibromas occurs in some patients.

Malignant Tumours of the Skin: Skin Cancer

Skin cancer, especially basal cell carcinoma (BCC) and SCC, are the most common cancers in Canada, accounting for approximately over 80,000 cases of skin cancer diagnosed in Canada every year. There are more cases of skin cancer each year than the number of breast, prostate, lung, and colon cancers combined (Canadian Skin Cancer Foundation, 2019). Because the skin is easily inspected, skin cancer is readily seen and detected and is the most successfully treated type of cancer.

Exposure to UV radiation, including the sun and artificial UV rays (e.g., tanning booths) is the leading preventable cause of skin cancer; incidence is related to the total amount of exposure to the sun. Sun damage is cumulative, and harmful effects may be severe by age 20 years. The increase in skin cancer probably reflects changing lifestyles and the emphasis on sunbathing, tanning beds, and related activities in light of changes in the environment, such as holes in the Earth's ozone layer. Protective measures should be used throughout life, and nurses need to inform patients about risk factors associated with skin cancer (Chart 58-7).

CHART 58-7

Risk Factors: Skin Cancer

- Adults <30 years[a] and >50 years of age
- Chronic ultraviolet light/sun exposure
- Family history of skin cancer
- Having a large number of nevi[b] (i.e., moles)
- History of indoor tanning
- History of sunburns
- Immunosuppression
- People who are light skinned, have blond or red hair, or have blue or green eyes

[a]These are risks that are specific to melanoma.
[b]These are risks that are specific to melanoma.
Adapted from American Cancer Society (ACS). (2016). *Risk factors for melanoma skin cancer*. Retrieved November 29, 2016, from www.cancer.org/cancer/melanoma-skin-cancer/causes-risks-prevention/risk-factors.html

Basal Cell and Squamous Cell Carcinomas

The most common types of skin cancer are BCC and squamous cell (epidermoid) carcinoma (SCC). The third most common type, malignant melanoma, is discussed separately. Skin cancer is diagnosed by biopsy and histologic evaluation.

Clinical Manifestations

BCC is the most common type of skin cancer. It generally appears on sun-exposed areas of the body and is more prevalent in regions where the population is subjected to intense and extensive exposure to the sun. The incidence is proportional to the age of the patient (average age of 60 years) and the total amount of sun exposure, and it is inversely proportional to the amount of melanin in the skin.

BCC usually begins as a small, waxy nodule with rolled, translucent, pearly borders; telangiectatic vessels may be present. As it grows, it undergoes central ulceration and sometimes crusting (Fig. 58-4). The tumours appear most frequently on the face. BCC is characterized by invasion and erosion of contiguous (adjoining) tissues. It rarely metastasizes, but recurrence is common. However, a neglected lesion can result in the loss of a nose, an ear, or a lip. Other variants of BCC may appear as shiny, flat, grey or yellowish plaques.

SCC is a malignant proliferation arising from the epidermis. Although it usually appears on sun-damaged skin, it may arise from normal skin or from pre-existing skin lesions. It is of greater concern than BCC because it is a truly invasive carcinoma, metastasizing by the blood or lymphatic system (Najjar, 2016).

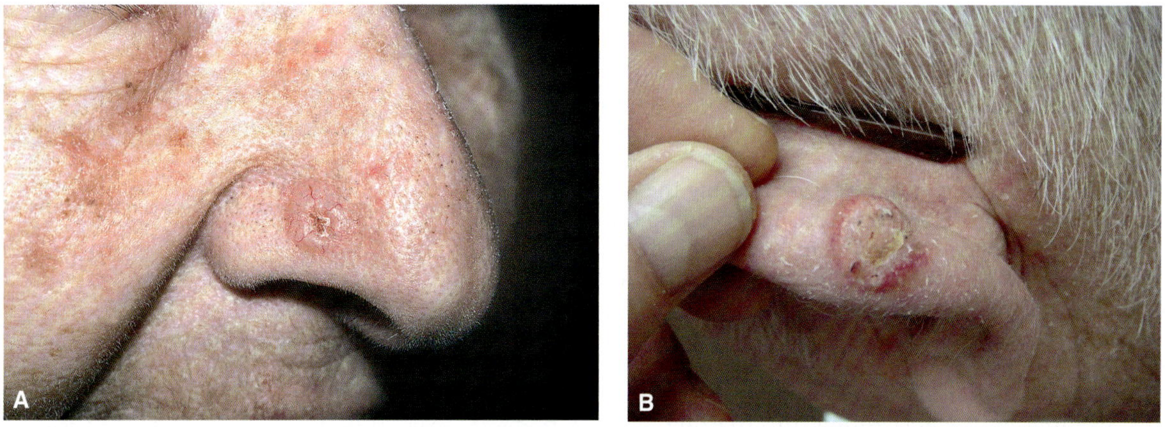

FIGURE 58-4. Basal cell carcinoma (A) and squamous cell carcinoma (B). (From Goodheart, H. P. [2011]. *Goodheart's same-site differential diagnosis: A rapid method of diagnosing and treating common skin disorders*. Philadelphia, PA: Lippincott Williams & Wilkins.)

Metastases account for 75% of deaths from SCC. The lesions may be primary, arising on the skin and mucous membranes, or they may develop from a precancerous condition, such as actinic keratosis (i.e., lesions occurring in sun-exposed areas), leukoplakia (i.e., premalignant lesion of the mucous membrane), or scarred or ulcerated lesions. SCC appears as a rough, thickened, scaly tumour that may be asymptomatic or may involve bleeding (see Fig. 58-4). The border of an SCC lesion may be wider, more infiltrated, and more inflammatory than that of a BCC lesion. Secondary infection can occur. Exposed areas, especially of the upper extremities and of the face, lower lip, ears, nose, and forehead, are common sites.

Prognosis

The prognosis for BCC is usually good. Tumours remain localized, and although some require wide excision with resultant disfigurement, the risk for death from BCC is low. The prognosis for SCC depends on the incidence of metastases, which is related to the histologic type and the level or depth of invasion. Usually, tumours arising in sun-damaged areas are less invasive and rarely cause death, whereas SCC that arises without a history of sun or arsenic exposure or scar formation appears to have a greater chance for spread.

Medical Management

The goal of treatment is to eradicate the tumour. The treatment method depends on the tumour location; the cell type, location, and depth; the cosmetic desires of the patient; the history of previous treatment; whether the tumour is invasive and whether metastatic nodes are present. The management of BCC and SCC includes surgical excision, Mohs' micrographic surgery, electrosurgery, cryosurgery, and radiation therapy.

Surgical Management

The primary goal is to remove the tumour entirely. The best way to maintain cosmetic appearance is to place the incision properly along natural skin tension lines and natural anatomic body lines (Langer's lines). In this way, scars are less noticeable. The size of the incision depends on the tumour size and location but usually involves a length to width ratio of 3:1.

The adequacy of the surgical excision is verified by microscopic evaluation of sections of the specimen. When the tumour is large, reconstructive surgery with use of a skin flap or skin grafting may be required. The incision is closed in layers to enhance cosmetic effect. A pressure dressing applied over the wound provides support. Infection after a simple excision is uncommon if proper surgical asepsis is maintained.

Mohs' Micrographic Surgery

This technique is the most accurate surgical technique and best conserves normal tissue. The procedure removes the tumour layer by layer. The first layer excised includes all evident tumour and a small margin of normal-appearing tissue. The specimen is frozen and analyzed by section to determine if all of the tumour has been removed. If not, additional layers of tissue are shaved and examined until all tissue margins are tumour free. In this manner, only the tumour and a safe, normal tissue margin are removed. Mohs' surgery is the recommended tissue-sparing procedure, with extremely high cure rates for BCC and SCC. It is the treatment of choice and the most effective for tumours around the eyes, nose, upper lip, and auricular and periauricular areas (Najjar, 2016).

The Mohs' procedure occurs in ambulatory care settings and is performed under local anesthetic. The length of the procedure depends on how many layers of tissue need to be removed and if a skin graft is required. It may take 5 to 6 hours.

Electrosurgery

Electrosurgery is the destruction or removal of tissue by electrical energy. The current is converted to heat, which then passes to the tissue from a cold electrode. Electrosurgery may be preceded by curettage (i.e., excising the skin tumour by scraping its surface with a curette). Electrodesiccation is then implemented to achieve hemostasis and to destroy any viable malignant cells at the base of the wound or along its edges. Electrodesiccation is useful for lesions smaller than 1 to 2 cm in diameter.

This method takes advantage of the fact that the tumour in each instance is softer than surrounding skin and therefore can be outlined by a curette, which "feels" the extent of the tumour. The tumour is removed, and the base is cauterized. The process is repeated twice. Usually, healing occurs within a month (Bader, Kennedy, Santacroce, et al., 2016).

Cryosurgery

Cryosurgery destroys the tumour by deep freezing the tissue. A thermocouple needle apparatus is inserted into the skin, and liquid nitrogen is directed to the centre of the tumour until the tumour base is −40° to −60°C. Liquid nitrogen has the lowest boiling point of all cryogens tried, is inexpensive, and is easy to obtain. The tumour tissue is frozen, allowed to thaw, and then refrozen. The site thaws naturally and then becomes gelatinous and heals spontaneously. Swelling and edema follow the freezing. The appearance of the lesion varies. Healing, which may take 4 to 6 weeks, occurs faster in areas with a good blood supply.

Nonsurgical Alternative Therapies

Some older adult patients may defer surgical treatment options. Furthermore, in some cases, lesions may be extensive or are located on sites where wide surgical excision is not practical to achieve (e.g., cancer of the eyelid, tip of the nose). In these cases, local radiation therapy (see Chapter 15) or Photodynamic therapy may prove reasonable alternatives. PDT involves application of 5-aminolevulinic acid (ALA-PDT) to the lesion, which is then followed by photoactivation with directed blue light for approximately 1 hour. This has the effect of locally destroying the neoplastic cells, with good cosmetic results. Topical application of 5-fluorouracil cream (a chemotherapeutic agent) may be tried as another alternative to managing superficial BCC (Bader et al., 2016).

The patient should be informed that the skin may become red and blistered after any of these therapies. A bland skin ointment prescribed by the primary provider may be applied to relieve discomfort. The patient should also be cautioned to avoid exposure to the sun.

Nursing Management

Because many skin cancers are removed by excision, patients are usually treated in outpatient surgical units. The role of the nurse is to teach the patient about prevention of skin cancer and about self-care after treatment (Chart 58-8).

Promoting Home, Community-Based, and Transitional Care

Educating Patients About Self-Care

The wound is usually covered with a dressing to protect the site from physical trauma, external irritants, and contaminants. The patient is advised when to report for a dressing change or is given written and verbal information on how to change dressings, including the type of dressing to purchase, how to remove dressings and apply fresh ones, and the importance of handwashing before and after the procedure.

The patient is advised to watch for excessive bleeding and tight dressings that compromise circulation. If the lesion is in the perioral area, the patient is instructed to drink liquids through a straw and limit talking and facial movement. Dental work should be avoided until the area is completely healed.

After the sutures are removed, an emollient cream may be used to help reduce dryness. Applying a sunscreen over the wound is advised to prevent postoperative hyperpigmentation if the patient spends time outdoors.

Follow-up examinations are at regular intervals, usually every 3 months for a year, and should include palpation of the adjacent lymph nodes. The patient is instructed to seek treatment for any moles that are subject to repeated friction and irritation and to watch for indications of potential malignancy in moles as described previously. The importance of lifelong follow-up evaluations should be emphasized.

CHART 58-8

Health Promotion: Preventing Skin Cancer

Minimize sun exposure:

- To the extent possible, avoid sun between the hours of 10 AM and 4 PM.
- Wear protective clothing (e.g., long-sleeved clothing, broad-brimmed hats).
- Seek shady areas when outdoors.
- Use caution around snow and water because of reflective sun rays.

Use sunscreen:

- Use a sunscreen with a sun protection factor (SPF) of 15 or higher that protects against both ultraviolet-A (UVA) and ultraviolet-B (UVB) rays.
- Apply generously 20 minutes prior to sun exposure (e.g., going outdoors).
- Reapply every 2 hours, or immediately after swimming.
- Use lip balm with SPF of 15 or higher.
- Do not use artificial ultraviolet sources (e.g., tanning beds and booths).

Check your skin regularly:

- Perform self-examination monthly.
- Schedule an examination by primary provider yearly, if over the age of 50 years.

Adapted from the Centers for Disease Control and Prevention (CDC). (2016b). *What can I do to reduce my risk of skin cancer?* Retrieved November 13, 2017, from www.cdc.gov/cancer/skin/basic_info/prevention.htm

Malignant Melanoma

A malignant melanoma is a cancerous neoplasm in which atypical melanocytes (i.e., pigment cells) are present in the epidermis and the dermis (and sometimes the subcutaneous cells). It is the most lethal of all the skin cancers.

It can occur in one of several forms: superficial spreading melanoma, lentigo maligna melanoma, nodular melanoma, and acral lentiginous melanoma. These types have specific clinical and histologic features as well as different biologic behaviours. Melanomas occasionally appear simultaneously with cancer of other organs.

Risk Factors

The cause of malignant melanoma is unknown, but UV rays are strongly suspected, based on indirect evidence

CHART 58-9

Risk Factors for Malignant Melanoma

- Fair-skinned or freckled, blue-eyed, light-haired people of Celtic or Scandinavian origin
- People who burn and do not tan or who have a significant history of severe sunburn
- Environmental exposure to intense sunlight
- History of melanoma (personal or family)
- Skin with giant congenital nevi

such as the increased incidence of melanoma in countries near the equator and in people younger than age 30 years who have used a tanning bed more than 10 times per year. In general, 1 in 100 whites will get melanoma every year. Up to 10% of melanoma patients are members of melanoma-prone families who have multiple changing moles (i.e., dysplastic nevi) that are susceptible to malignant transformation. Patients with dysplastic nevus syndrome have been found to have unusual moles, larger and more numerous moles, lesions with irregular outlines, and pigmentation located all over the skin. Microscopic examination of dysplastic moles shows disordered, faulty growth. Chart 58-9 lists risk factors for malignant melanoma.

Clinical Manifestations

Superficial spreading melanoma occurs anywhere on the body and is the most common form of melanoma. It usually affects middle-aged people and occurs most frequently on the trunk and lower extremities. The lesion tends to be circular, with irregular outer portions. The margins of the lesion may be flat or elevated and palpable (Fig. 58-5). This type of melanoma may appear in a combination of colours, with hues of tan, brown, and black mixed with grey, blue-black, or white. Sometimes, a dull pink rose colour can be seen in a small area within the lesion.

Lentigo Maligna Melanomas

Lentigo maligna melanomas are slowly evolving, pigmented lesions that occur on exposed skin areas, especially the dorsum of the hand, the head, and the neck in older adults. Often, the lesions are present for many years before they are examined by a physician. They first appear as tan, flat lesions, but in time they undergo changes in size and colour.

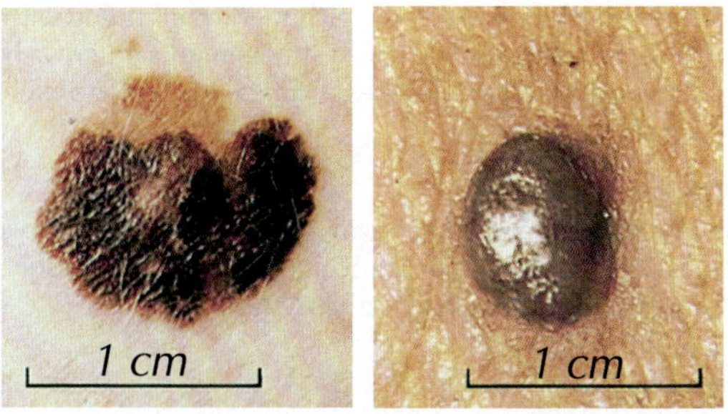

FIGURE 58-5. Two forms of malignant melanoma: superficial spreading (**left**) and nodular (**right**).

Nodular Melanoma

Nodular melanoma is a spherical, blueberrylike nodule with a relatively smooth surface and a relatively uniform, blue-black colour (see Fig. 58-5). It may be dome shaped with a smooth surface. It may have other shadings of red, grey, or purple. Sometimes, nodular melanomas appear as irregularly shaped plaques. The patient may describe this as a blood blister that fails to resolve. A nodular melanoma invades directly into adjacent dermis (i.e., vertical growth) and therefore has a poorer prognosis.

Acral Lentiginous Melanoma

Acral lentiginous melanoma occurs in areas not excessively exposed to sunlight and where hair follicles are absent. It is found on the palms of the hands, on the soles of the feet, in the nail beds, and in the mucous membranes in dark-skinned people. These melanomas appear as irregular, pigmented macules that develop nodules. They may become invasive early.

Assessment and Diagnostic Findings

Biopsy results confirm the diagnosis of melanoma. An excisional biopsy specimen provides histologic information on the type, level of invasion, and thickness of the lesion. An excisional biopsy specimen that includes a 1-cm margin of normal tissue and a portion of underlying subcutaneous fatty tissue is sufficient for staging a melanoma in situ or an early, noninvasive melanoma. Incisional biopsy should be performed when the suspicious lesion is too large to be removed safely without extensive scarring. Biopsy specimens obtained by shaving, curettage, or needle aspiration are not considered reliable histologic proof of disease (Tan, Talavera, Schulman, et al., 2016).

A thorough history and physical examination should include a meticulous skin examination and palpation of regional lymph nodes that drain the lesional area. Because melanoma occurs in families, a positive family history of melanoma is investigated so that first-degree relatives, who may be at high risk for melanoma, can be evaluated for atypical lesions. After the diagnosis of melanoma has been confirmed, a chest x-ray, CBC, complete chemistry panel with creatinine, liver function tests, and lactate dehydrogenase (LDH) are usually performed. The LDH may be elevated in the presence of metastatic disease. Depending on the results of these tests, magnetic resonance imaging of the brain, computed tomography scans of the chest, abdomen, or pelvis, and positron emission tomography scans of the lymphatics may be indicated to further stage the extent of disease (Tan et al., 2016).

Staging of the tumours follows the tumour, nodes, metastasis (TNM) classification system (see Chapter 15) and is used to determine appropriate treatment and prognosis. Patients with stage I disease (i.e., tumour less than 2 mm thick and without lymph node involvement or metastases) have a better than 92% survival 5 years post diagnosis, whereas those with stage II disease (i.e., tumour less than 4 mm thick and without lymph node involvement or metastases) and stage III disease (i.e., tumour of any thickness with lymph node involvement but no metastasis) have a likelihood of surviving 5 years post diagnosis between 53% and 81% and between 40% and 78%, respectively. The prognosis is grim for patients who present with stage IV disease (i.e., tumours with associated distant metastases), with less than 20% survival after 5 years (American Cancer Society [ACS], 2016).

Medical Management

Treatment depends on the stage of the tumour and the tumour type. Surgical excision is the treatment of choice for small, superficial lesions. Deeper lesions require wide local excision, after which skin grafting may be necessary. Sentinel lymph node biopsy is commonly performed to examine the nodes nearest the tumour and to spare the patient the long-term sequelae of extensive removal of lymph nodes if the sample nodes are negative. If these are positive, lymph node dissection may be indicated (Tan et al., 2016).

Recently, greater understanding of the stem cells of melanoma indicates that effective therapies should be individualized for each patient. The observation that 60% of all patients with melanoma have a *BRAF* genetic mutation is useful in guiding targeted therapy. Clinical observations suggest that very few single-agent therapies provide significant clinical benefits because of the complex molecular nature of melanoma and the need to further define individual cell variations (Nguyen, Couts, Luo, et al., 2015).

Patients with a stage II or stage III tumour considered at risk for relapse are typically prescribed high-dose interferon alpha-2 intravenously for 4 weeks, followed by subcutaneous dosing for an additional 48 weeks. This adjuvant immunotherapeutic agent is associated with decreased rates of relapse and overall improved survival (National Cancer Institute [NCI], 2016). Some patients with stage III tumour may also benefit from receiving the monoclonal antibody, ipilimumab (Yervoy). This agent primes the patient's T cells so that they are more adept at identifying and killing tumour cells.

Monoclonal antibodies that could be indicated for later stage tumours (i.e., late stage III and stage IV) include pembrolizumab (Keytruda) and nivolumab (Opdivo); these agents are associated with tumour regression (Tan et al., 2016). Other treatments may include traditional chemotherapeutic agents, such as dacarbazine (DTIC-Dome), or therapies that are demonstrating promise in some patients with advanced disease, including IL-2, and granulocyte-macrophage colony-stimulating factor (Tan et al., 2016).

Nursing Process

Care of the Patient With Malignant Melanoma

Assessment

Assessment of the patient with malignant melanoma is based on the patient's history and symptoms. The patient is asked specifically about pruritus, tenderness, and pain, which are not features of a benign nevus. The patient is also questioned about changes in pre-existing moles or the development of new, pigmented lesions. People at risk are assessed very carefully.

A magnifying lens and good lighting are needed for inspecting the skin for irregularity and changes in the mole. Signs that suggest malignant changes are referred to as the ABCDEs of moles (Chart 58-10).

Common sites of melanomas are the skin of the back; the legs (especially in women); between the toes; and on the feet, face, scalp, fingernails, and backs of hands. In dark-skinned people, melanomas are most likely to occur in less pigmented sites: palms, soles, subungual areas, and mucous membranes. Satellite lesions (i.e., those situated near the mole) are inspected.

CHART 58-10

Assessment: Assessing the ABCDEs of Moles

Melanomas may be distinguished from benign nevi, using the following characteristics:

A FOR ASYMMETRY
- The lesion does not appear balanced on both sides. If an imaginary line was drawn down the middle, the two halves would not look alike.
- The lesion has an irregular surface with uneven elevations (irregular topography) either palpable or visible. A change in the surface may be noted from smooth to scaly.

B FOR IRREGULAR BORDER
- Angular indentations or multiple notches appear in the border.
- The border is fuzzy or indistinct, as if rubbed with an eraser.

C FOR VARIEGATED COLOUR
- Benign moles are usually a uniform light to medium brown. Darker colouration indicates that the melanocytes have penetrated to a deeper layer of the dermis.
- Colours that may indicate malignancy if found together within a single lesion are shades of red, white, and blue; shades of blue are ominous.
- White areas within a pigmented lesion are suspicious.
- Some melanomas, however, are not variegated but are uniformly coloured (bluish-black, bluish-grey, bluish-red).

D FOR DIAMETER
- A diameter >6 mm (about the size of a pencil eraser) is considered more suspicious, although this finding without other signs is not significant. Many benign skin growths are larger than 6 mm, whereas some early melanomas may be smaller.

E FOR EVOLVING
- Benign moles appear the same over time; when a mole starts to change in appearance, in size, shape, colour, or elevation, it may suggest malignancy.

Adapted from Skin Cancer Foundation. (2016). *Warning signs: The ABCDEs of melanoma*. Retrieved February 13, 2017, from www.skincancer.org/skin-cancer-information/melanoma

Nursing Priorities

Based on nursing assessment data, the patient's major nursing priorities may include the following:

- Acute pain related to surgery
- Anxiety and depression
- Deficient knowledge

Collaborative Problems/ Potential Complications

Based on assessment data, potential complications include the following:

- Metastasis
- Infection of the surgical site

Planning and Goals

The major goals for the patient may include relief of pain and discomfort, reduced anxiety and depression, knowledge of early signs of melanoma, and absence of complications.

Nursing Interventions

Relieving Pain and Discomfort

Surgical removal of melanoma in different locations (e.g., head, neck, eye, trunk, abdomen, extremities, central nervous system) presents different challenges, taking into consideration the removal of the primary melanoma, the intervening lymphatic vessels, and the lymph nodes to which metastases may spread. Nursing management of the patient having surgery in these regions is discussed in the appropriate chapters.

Nursing intervention after surgery for a malignant melanoma centres on promoting comfort, because wide excision surgery may be necessary. A split-thickness or full-thickness skin graft may be necessary when large defects are created by surgical removal of a melanoma. Anticipating the need for and administering appropriate analgesic medications are important.

Reducing Anxiety and Depression

Psychological support is essential when disfiguring surgery is performed. Support includes allowing patients to express feelings about the seriousness of this cutaneous neoplasm, understanding their anger and depression, and conveying understanding of these feelings. During the diagnostic workup and staging of the depth, type, and extent of the tumour, the nurse answers questions, clarifies information, and helps to clarify misconceptions. Learning that they have a melanoma can cause patients considerable fear and anguish. Pointing out patients' resources, past effective coping mechanisms, and social support systems helps them cope with the challenges associated with diagnosis, treatment, and continuing follow-up. The patient's family is included in all discussions to clarify the information presented, ask questions that the patient might be reluctant to ask, and provide emotional support to the patient.

Monitoring and Managing Potential Complications

METASTASIS. The prognosis for malignant melanoma is related to metastasis: the deeper and thicker (more than 4 mm) the melanoma, the greater is the likelihood of metastasis. If the melanoma is growing radially (i.e., horizontally) and is characterized by peripheral growth with minimal or no dermal invasion, the prognosis is favourable. When the melanoma progresses to the vertical growth phase (i.e., dermal invasion), the prognosis is poor. Lesions with ulceration have a poor prognosis. Melanomas of the trunk appear to have a poorer prognosis than those of other sites, perhaps because the network of lymphatics in the trunk permits metastasis to regional lymph nodes.

The role of the nurse in caring for the patient with metastatic disease is to provide holistic care. The nurse must be knowledgeable about the most effective current therapies and deliver supportive care, provide and clarify information about the therapy and the rationale for its use, identify potential side effects of therapy and ways to manage them, and instruct the patient and family about the expected outcomes of treatment. The nurse monitors and documents symptoms that may indicate metastasis: lung (e.g., difficulty breathing, shortness of breath, increasing cough), bone (e.g., pain, decreased mobility and function, pathologic fractures), and liver (e.g., change in liver enzyme levels, pain, jaundice). Nursing care is based on the patient's symptoms and emotional needs.

Although the chance of a cure for malignant melanoma that has metastasized is poor, the nurse encourages the patient to have hope in the therapy employed while maintaining a realistic perspective about the disease and ultimate outcome. Moreover, the nurse provides time for the patient to express fears and concerns regarding future activities and relationships, offers information about support groups and contact people, and arranges palliative and hospice care if appropriate (see Chapter 15).

Promoting Home, Community-Based, and Transitional Care

EDUCATING PATIENTS ABOUT SELF-CARE. The best hope of decreasing the incidence of skin cancer lies in educating patients about the early signs. Patients at risk are educated to examine their skin and scalp monthly in a systematic manner and to seek prompt medical attention if changes are detected. The nurse also points out that a key factor in the development of melanoma is exposure to sunlight. Because melanoma is thought to be genetically linked, the family and the patient should be educated about sun-avoiding measures and the importance of annual assessment by a primary provider.

Evaluation

Expected patient outcomes may include the following:

1. Experiences relief of pain and discomfort
   a. States pain is diminishing
   b. Exhibits healing of surgical scar without heat, redness, or swelling
2. Reports feeling less anxious
   a. Expresses fears and fantasies
   b. Asks questions about medical condition
   c. Requests repetition of facts about melanoma
   d. Identifies support and comfort provided by family member or significant other
3. Demonstrates understanding of means for detecting and preventing melanoma
   a. Demonstrates how to conduct self-examination of skin on a monthly basis
   b. Verbalizes the following danger signals of melanoma: change in size, colour, shape or outline of mole, mole surface, or skin around mole
   c. Identifies measures to protect self from exposure to sunlight
4. Experiences absence of complications
   a. Recognizes abnormal signs and symptoms that should be reported to physician
   b. Complies with recommended follow-up procedures and prevention strategies

Metastatic Skin Tumours

The skin is an important, although not a common, site of metastatic cancer. All types of cancer may metastasize to the skin, but carcinoma of the breast is the primary source of cutaneous metastases in women. Other sources include cancer of the large intestine, ovaries, and lungs. In men, the most common primary sites are the lungs, large intestine, oral cavity, kidneys, or stomach. Skin metastases from melanomas are found in both genders. The clinical appearance of metastatic skin lesions is not distinctive, except perhaps in some cases of breast cancer in which diffuse, brawny hardening of the skin of the involved breast is seen. In most instances, metastatic lesions occur as multiple cutaneous or subcutaneous nodules of various sizes that may be skin coloured or different shades of red (Cho, Park, Lee, et al., 2014).

Other Malignancies of the Skin

Kaposi's Sarcoma

First described by Moritz Kaposi in 1872, Kaposi's sarcoma (KS) has received renewed attention since its association with HIV and AIDS. Its occurrence with AIDS involves a more varied and aggressive form of KS than was seen previously. Before the AIDS epidemic, KS was considered a rare malignancy. KS is a malignancy of endothelial cells that line the small blood vessels. KS is manifested clinically by lesions of the skin, oral cavity, gastrointestinal tract, and lungs. The skin lesions consist of reddish-purple to dark-blue macules, plaques, or nodules. KS is subdivided into three categories:

- *Classic KS* occurs predominantly in men of Mediterranean or Jewish ancestry between 40 and 70 years of age. Most patients have nodules or plaques on the lower extremities that rarely metastasize beyond this area. Classic KS is chronic, relatively benign, and rarely fatal.
- *Endemic (African) KS* affects people predominantly in the eastern half of Africa near the equator. Men are affected more often than women, and children can be affected as well. The disease may resemble classic KS, or it may infiltrate and progress to lymphadenopathic forms.
- *Immunosuppression-associated KS* occurs in transplant recipients and people with AIDS. This form of KS is characterized by local skin lesions and disseminated visceral and mucocutaneous diseases. The greater the degree of immunosuppression, the higher the incidence of KS. Immunosuppression-related KS that results from AIDS is an aggressive tumour that involves multiple body organs. Its presentation resembles that of KS associated with immunosuppressive therapy. Most patients are between age 20 and 40 years. More information on AIDS-related KS can be found in Chapter 52.

Basal and Squamous Cell Carcinomas in the Immunocompromised Population

The incidence of BCC and SCC is increased in all immunocompromised individuals, including those infected with HIV. Clinically, the tumours have the same appearance as in non–HIV-infected people; however, in HIV patients, the tumours may grow more rapidly and recur more frequently. These tumours are managed the same as for the general population. Frequent follow-up (every 4 to 6 months) is recommended to monitor for recurrence.

Dermatologic and Plastic, Reconstructive, and Cosmetic Procedures

The word *plastic* comes from a Greek word meaning "to form." Plastic or reconstructive surgery is performed to reconstruct or alter congenital or acquired defects to restore or improve the body's form and function. Often, the terms *plastic* and *reconstructive* are used interchangeably. This type of surgery includes closure of wounds, removal of skin tumours, repair of soft tissue injuries or burns, correction of deformities, and repair of cosmetic defects. Plastic surgery can be used to repair many parts of the body and numerous structures, such as bone, cartilage, fat, fascia, mucous membrane, muscle, nerve, and cutaneous structures. Bone inlays and transplants for deformities and nonunion can be performed, muscle can be transferred, nerves can be reconstructed and spliced, and cartilage can be replaced. As important as any of these measures is the reconstruction of the cutaneous tissues around the neck and the face; this is usually referred to as aesthetic or cosmetic surgery.

Cosmetic procedures (Table 58-8) are generally considered to be ones that correct defects that are not life threatening or caused by disease. An example would be removal of a benign mole or sebaceous cyst from the face. Most health insurance plans do not cover procedures deemed to

TABLE 58-8 Nursing Considerations in Cosmetic Procedures

Nursing Consideration	Interventions and Patient Education
Maintaining airway and pulmonary function	Cosmetic surgeries involving the face and neck can cause considerable swelling; bandages can restrict breathing or eating. Check dressings frequently, and ensure that no constriction occurs as swelling develops.
Relieving pain and achieving comfort	Procedures that involve a large surface area will cause considerable pain. Cool compresses or ice packs will relieve the burning of dermabrasion or chemical peels. Oral analgesic agents should be given regularly to control pain.
Maintaining adequate nutrition	When the face is involved, the patient may be unable to fully open the mouth, and chewing may be painful. Provide soft or liquid diet that is high in protein to assist with healing.
Enhancing communication	Depending on the type of cosmetic procedure, a nonverbal method of communication might be necessary until pain and swelling have subsided.
Improving self-concept	Recovery time from cosmetic procedures is slow. Expected results will take weeks to become apparent. Persons of colour will experience increased pigmentation long after the initial wounds have healed. Helping patients to understand postoperative expectations will allow them to feel more comfortable with the healing process.
Promoting family coping	Most cosmetic procedures are performed in an outpatient facility; therefore, family members are integral to postoperative care. They should understand what to expect as the patient emerges from the procedure room: the type of dressings that will be in place, the skin care plan that is prescribed, and how to cope with the patient's pain.
Monitoring and managing potential complications	Infection is the most common complication, but excessive pain, nerve damage, and emotional distress about appearance are also common. If opioid analgesic agents are used, there may be gastrointestinal upset, mental status changes, or allergic reaction to the medication. Alert the caregiver to signs of these complications and how and when to report changes in status.

be cosmetic, and these procedures can be expensive. Procedures that are performed to correct a surgical defect, such as removal of a skin cancer or correction of a significant congenital defect such as a cleft lip, are generally covered by insurance.

Wound Coverage: Grafts and Flaps

Various surgical techniques, including skin grafts and flaps, are used to cover skin wounds.

Skin Grafts

Skin grafting is a technique in which a section of skin is detached from its own blood supply and transferred as free tissue to a distant (recipient) site. Skin grafting can be used to repair almost any type of wound and is the most common form of reconstructive surgery.

Skin grafts are commonly used to repair defects that result from excision of skin tumours, to cover areas denuded of skin (e.g., burns), and to cover wounds in which insufficient skin is available to permit wound closure. They are also used when primary closure of the wound increases the risk for complications or when primary wound closure would interfere with function.

Skin grafts may be classified as autografts, allografts, or xenografts. An autograft is tissue obtained from the patient's own skin. An allograft is tissue obtained from a donor of the same species. These grafts are also called *allogeneic* or *homograft*. A xenograft or heterograft is tissue from another species.

Grafts are also referred to by their thickness. A skin graft may be a split-thickness (i.e., thin, intermediate, or thick) or full-thickness graft, depending on the amount of dermis included in the specimen. A split-thickness graft can be cut at various thicknesses and is commonly used to cover large wounds or defects for which a full-thickness graft or flap is impractical (Fig. 58-6). A full-thickness graft consists of epidermis and the entire dermis without the underlying fat. It is used to cover wounds that are too large to be closed directly.

Donor Site

The donor site is selected with several criteria in mind:

- Achieving the closest possible colour match
- Matching the texture and hair-bearing qualities
- Obtaining the thickest possible skin graft without jeopardizing the healing of the donor site (Fig. 58-7)
- Considering the cosmetic effects of the donor site after healing so that it is in an inconspicuous location

Donor Site Care

Detailed attention to the donor site is just as important as the care of the recipient area. The donor site heals by re-epithelization of the raw, exposed dermis. Usually, a single layer of nonadherent, fine-mesh gauze is placed directly over the donor site. Absorbent gauze dressings are then placed on top to absorb blood or serum from the wound. A membrane dressing (e.g., Opsite) may be used and provides certain advantages. It is transparent and allows the wound to be observed without disturbing the dressing, and it permits the patient to shower without fear of saturating the dressing with water.

After healing, the patient is instructed to keep the donor site soft and pliable with cream (e.g., lanolin, olive oil). Extremes in temperature, external trauma, and sunlight are to be avoided for donor sites and grafted areas because these areas are sensitive, especially to thermal injuries.

Graft Application

A graft is obtained by a variety of instruments: razor blades, skin-grafting knives, electric- or air-powered dermatomes, or drum dermatomes. The skin graft is taken from the donor or host site and applied to the desired site, called the *recipient site* or *graft bed*.

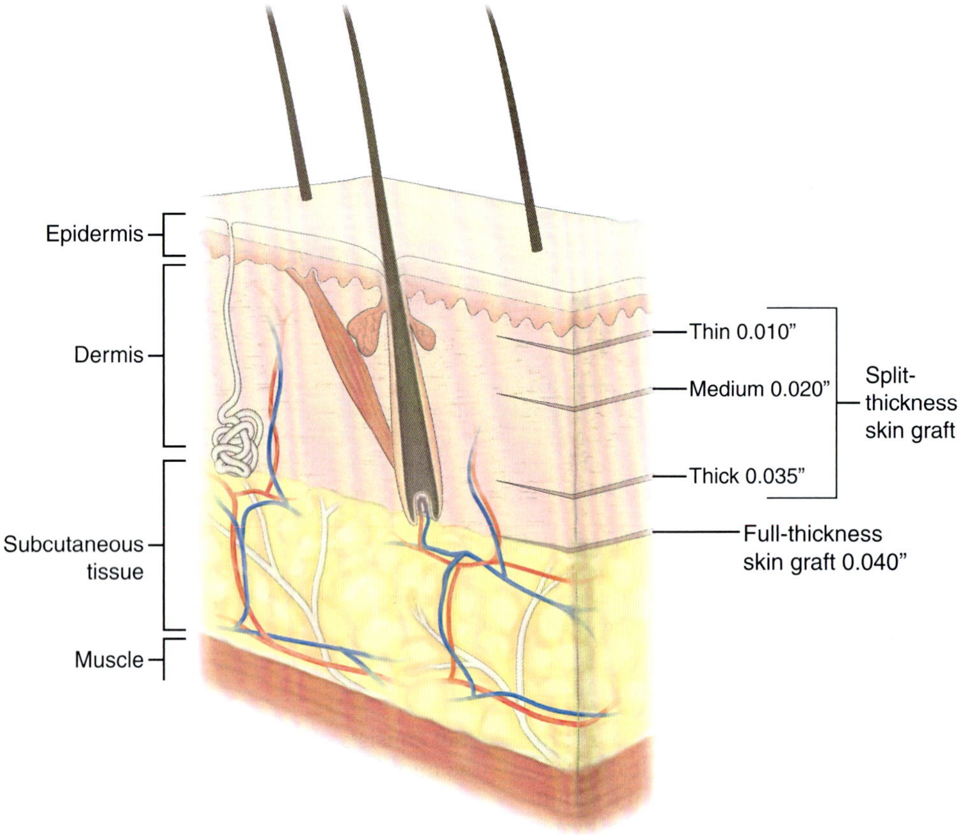

FIGURE 58-6. Layers of skin appropriate for split-thickness and full-thickness grafts.

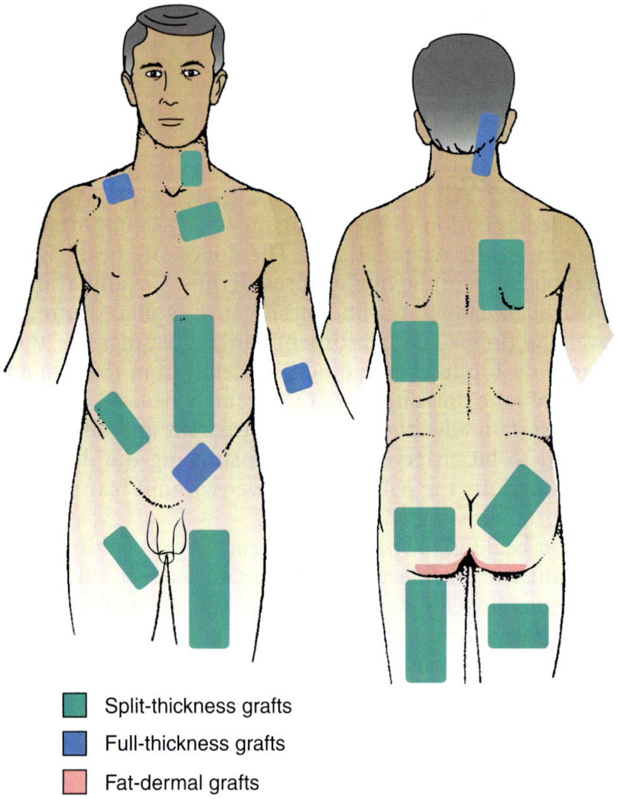

FIGURE 58-7. Common donor skin graft sites. Blue skin areas are appropriate for full-thickness grafts; green areas are used for split-thickness grafts; rose sites are used for fat-dermal grafts.

For a graft to survive and be effective, certain conditions must be met:

- The recipient site must have an adequate blood supply so that usual physiologic function can resume.
- The graft must be in close contact with its bed to avoid accumulation of blood or fluid.
- The graft must be fixed firmly (immobilized) so that it remains in place on the recipient site.
- The area must be free of infection.

The graft, when applied to the recipient site, may be sutured in place. It may be slit and spread apart to cover a greater area. The process of revascularization (i.e., establishing the blood supply) and reattachment of a skin graft to a recipient bed is referred to as a "take." After a skin graft is put in place, it may be left exposed (in areas that are impossible to immobilize) or covered with a light dressing or a pressure dressing, depending on the area (Urden, Stacy, & Lough, 2014).

Nursing Management

The nurse instructs the patient to keep the affected part immobilized as much as possible. For a facial graft, strenuous activity must be avoided. A graft on the hand or arm may be immobilized with a splint. When a graft is placed on a lower extremity, the part is kept elevated because the new capillary connections are fragile and excess venous pressure may cause rupture. When ambulation is permitted, the patient wears an elastic stocking to counterbalance venous pressure.

The nurse instructs the patient, family member, or other caregiver to inspect the dressing daily. Unusual drainage or an inflammatory reaction around the wound margin suggests infection and should be reported immediately to the physician. Any fluid, purulent drainage, blood, or serum that has collected is gently evacuated by the surgeon, because accumulation of any of these materials would cause the graft to separate from its bed.

When the graft appears pink, it is vascularized. After 2 to 3 weeks, mineral oil or a lanolin cream is massaged into the wound to moisten the graft. Because there may be loss of feeling or sensation in the grafted area for a prolonged period, the application of heating pads and exposure to sun are avoided to prevent burns and further skin trauma.

NURSING ALERT

Both the donor site and the grafted area must be protected from exposure to extremes in temperature, external trauma, and sunlight because these areas are sensitive, especially to thermal injuries.

Flaps

Another form of wound coverage is provided by flaps. A flap is a segment of tissue that remains attached at one end (i.e., a base or pedicle) while the other end is moved to a recipient area. Its survival depends on functioning arterial and venous blood supplies and lymphatic drainage in its pedicle or base. A flap differs from a graft in that a portion of the tissue is attached to its original site and retains its blood supply. An exception is the free flap, which is described later.

Flaps may consist of skin, mucosa, muscle, adipose tissue, omentum, and bone. They are used for wound coverage and provide bulk, especially when bone, tendon, blood vessels, or nerve tissue is exposed. Flaps are used to repair defects caused by congenital deformity, trauma, or tumour ablation (i.e., removal, usually by excision) in an adjacent part of the body.

Flaps offer an aesthetic solution because a flap retains the colour and texture of the donor area; is more likely to survive than a graft; and can be used to cover nerves, tendons, and blood vessels. However, several surgical procedures are usually required to advance a flap. The major complication is necrosis of the pedicle or base as a result of failure of the blood supply.

Free Flaps

A striking advance in reconstructive surgery is the use of free flaps or free-tissue transfer achieved by microvascular techniques. A free flap is completely severed from the body and transferred to another site. A free flap receives early vascular supply from microvascular anastomosis (i.e., attachment) with vessels at the recipient site. The procedure usually is completed in one step, eliminating the need for a series of surgical procedures to move the flap. Microvascular surgery allows surgeons to use a variety of donor sites for tissue reconstruction.

Cosmetic Procedures

Chemical Face Peeling

Chemical face peeling, a technique that involves applying a chemical mixture to the face for superficial destruction of the epidermis and the upper layers of the dermis, treats fine wrinkles, keratoses, and pigment issues. It is especially useful for wrinkles at the upper and lower lips, forehead, and periorbital areas.

Pretreatment may consist of cleansing the face and hair for several days before the procedure with a hexachlorophene detergent. Pretreatment medication (i.e., analgesic and tranquilizer for moderate sedation) may be prescribed to alleviate apprehension and control pain. This permits the patient to be sedated but conscious during the procedure, although some patients request general anesthesia.

The type of chemical used depends on the planned depth of the peel. A phenol-based chemical in an oil–water emulsion is commonly used because it produces a controlled, predictable chemical burn. The chemical is applied systematically to the face with cotton-tipped applicators. The conscious patient feels a burning sensation at this time. A mask of waterproof adhesive may then be applied directly to the skin and moulded closely to the contours of the face, thereby acting as an occlusive dressing that increases the chemical penetration and action. Some surgeons believe that equally good results can be obtained with occlusive tape. After the tape mask is applied, the burning sensation continues, and the tape mask remains in place for 12 to 24 hours. Frequent small doses of analgesics and tranquilizers are prescribed to keep the patient comfortable.

Complications

Complications may arise when control of the chemically induced burn cannot be sustained. Complications include pigment changes, infection, milia (i.e., small inclusion cysts that disappear after several months), scarring, atrophy, sensitivity changes, and long-term (4 to 5 months) erythema or pruritus.

Management

Because chemical face peeling is performed in the physician's office or in an outpatient surgical department, most care takes place in the home. After 6 to 8 hours, the face becomes edematous and the eyelids usually swell shut. The patient should be reassured that this reaction is expected and is usual. The patient is cautioned to move the mouth as little as possible so that the tape continues to adhere to the skin. The head of the bed is elevated, and liquids are administered through a straw. Most of the burning sensation and discomfort subside after the first 12 to 24 hours.

By the second day, the patient may feel moisture under the dressings as serous exudate seeps from the chemically exfoliated skin. Dressings are usually removed 24 to 48 hours after treatment, exposing skin resembling a second-degree burn. The patient may be alarmed by the appearance of the skin and should be reassured. After the tape mask is removed, some surgeons dust the treated skin surface with thymol iodide powder for its drying and bacteriostatic effects. Application of triple-antibiotic ointment may be substituted in some cases. The skin surface is left uncovered to dry. The patient may be permitted to wash the face with lukewarm water or advised to shower several times daily to help remove any remaining facial crusting. An ointment is prescribed to cover the face and soften and loosen the crust between washings.

The nurse reinforces the physician's explanation that the redness of the skin will gradually subside over the next 4 to 12 weeks. Although a line between treated and untreated skin may be seen, makeup is usually permitted after the first few weeks. The patient is cautioned to avoid exposure to direct or reflected sunlight, because the treatment reduces the natural protection of the skin from the sun. The skin will probably never tan evenly again. Blotchy pigmentation can occur with exposure to the sun.

Dermabrasion

Dermabrasion is a form of skin abrasion used to correct acne scarring, aging, and sun-damaged skin. A special instrument (i.e., motor-driven wire brush, diamond-impregnated disk, or serrated wheel) is used in the procedure. The epidermis and some superficial dermis are removed, while enough of the dermis is preserved to allow re-epithelization of the treated areas. Results are best in the face because it is rich in intradermal epithelial elements.

Preparation and Procedure

The primary reason for undergoing dermabrasion is to improve appearance. The surgeon explains to the patient what can be expected from the procedure. The patient should also be informed about the nature of the postoperative dressing, what discomfort may be experienced, and how long it will be before the tissues look normal.

Dermabrasion may be performed in the physician's office, the operating room, or an outpatient setting. It is performed under local or general anesthesia. During the procedure, some surgeons use refrigerant anesthetics to turn the skin into a numb, solid mass of rigid tissue and to provide a momentarily bloodless surgical field. During and after planing, the area is irrigated with copious amounts of saline solution to remove debris and allow the surgeon to see the area. A dressing impregnated with ointment is usually applied to the abraded surface.

Management

The nurse instructs the patient about postoperative effects. Edema occurs during the first 48 hours and may cause the eyelids to close. The head of the bed is elevated to hasten fluid drainage. Erythema occurs and can last for weeks or months. After 24 hours, the dressing may be removed if the physician approves. When the serum oozing from the skin begins to gel, the patient applies the prescribed ointment to the face several times each day to prevent hard crusting and to keep the abraded areas soft and flexible. With the physician's approval, clear-water cleansing or soaking of the face is started to remove crusts from the healing skin.

The patient is advised to avoid extreme cold and heat and excessive straining or lifting, which may bruise delicate new capillaries. Direct or reflected sunlight should be avoided for 3 to 6 months and a sunscreen used.

Facial Reconstructive Surgery

Reconstructive procedures on the face are individualized to the patient's needs and desired outcomes. They are performed to repair deformities or restore normal function as much as possible. They may vary from closure of small defects to complicated procedures involving implantation of prosthetic devices to conceal a large defect or reconstruct a lost part of the face (e.g., nose, ear, jaw). Each surgical procedure is customized and involves a variety of incisions, flaps, and grafts.

In correcting a primary defect, the surgeon may have to create a secondary defect. Although the procedure may restore some function, such as eating or talking, the cosmetic or aesthetic results may be limited. The original appearance of a patient who has severe damage to soft tissue and bone structure can seldom be restored. Multiple surgical procedures may be required. The process of facial reconstruction is usually slow and tedious.

Face-Lift

Rhytidectomy (face-lift) is a surgical procedure that removes soft tissue folds and minimizes cutaneous wrinkles on the face. It is performed to create a more youthful appearance. Psychological preparation requires that the patient recognize the limitations of surgery and the fact that miraculous rejuvenation will not occur. The patient is informed that the face may appear bruised and swollen after the dressings are removed and that several weeks may pass before the edema subsides. Corticosteroids (e.g., methylprednisolone) and vitamin C are prescribed postoperatively to minimize edema. Prophylactic antibiotic agents such as cephalexin (Keflex) may also be prescribed postoperatively (Warren & Neligan, 2013).

Management

The nurse encourages the patient to rest quietly for the first 2 postoperative days until the dressings are removed. The head of the bed is elevated, and neck flexion is discouraged to avoid compromising the circulation and the suture line. The patient may feel some tightness of the face and neck from pressure created by the newly tightened muscles, fascia, and skin. Analgesics may be prescribed to relieve discomfort. A liquid diet may be given by means of straws, and a soft diet is permitted if chewing is not too uncomfortable.

When the dressings are removed, the skin is gently cleaned of crusting and oozing and coated with the prescribed topical ointment. Any hair matted with drainage may be combed with warm water and a wide-toothed comb.

The patient is advised not to lift or bend for 7 to 10 days because this activity may increase edema and provoke bleeding. Activities are gradually resumed. When all sutures are removed, the hair may be shampooed and blown dry with warm, not hot, air to avoid burning the ears, which may be numb for a while.

The patient needs to know that a face-lift will not stop the aging process and that with time the tissues will resume the downward drift. Some patients have two or more face-lifts.

Sudden pain indicates that blood is accumulating underneath the skin flaps; it should be reported to the surgeon immediately. Complications include sloughing of the skin, deformities of the face and neck, and partial facial paralysis. Cigarette smoking has been implicated as a cause of skin slough in some patients.

Laser Treatment of Cutaneous Lesions

Lasers are devices that amplify or generate highly specialized light energy. They can mobilize immense heat and power when focused at close range and are valuable tools in providing dermatologic abrasion therapy. The laser modalities used for this purpose today include scanned CO_2 laser, pulsed CO_2 laser, pulsed erbium/yttrium-aluminum-garnet (Er:YAG) laser, fractional Er:YAG laser resurfacing, combination CO_2 and Er:YAG lasers, and fractionated photothermolysis (Husain & Alster, 2016).

Each of these lasers is a precise surgical instrument that vaporizes and excises water-containing tissues with minimal damage. Because the beams used can seal blood and lymphatic vessels, they create a dry surgical field that makes many procedures easier and quicker. Therefore, these lasers are generally safe to use on patients with bleeding disorders or those receiving anticoagulant therapy. They are primarily used to improve the appearance of facial wrinkles, although they are also useful in removing epidermal nevi, tattoos, certain warts, skin cancer, ingrown toenails, and keloids. Incisions made with the laser beam heal and scar much like those made by a scalpel. Patients with a history of herpes simplex viral infection typically receive preprocedural antiviral prophylaxis (Husain & Alster, 2016).

Argon Laser

The argon laser produces a visible blue-green light that is absorbed by vascular tissue and is therefore useful in treating vascular lesions: port-wine stains, telangiectasias, vascular tumours, and pigmented lesions. The argon beam can penetrate approximately 1 mm of skin and reach the pigmented layer, causing protein coagulation in this area. An immediate effect is that tiny blood vessels under the skin coagulate, causing the area to turn a much lighter colour. A crust forms within a few days.

During the procedure, the patient may require local anesthesia (lidocaine) but only if the lesion, such as a port-wine stain, is wider than 0.5 cm. Laser beams, regardless of type, are reflected and scattered in all directions during the treatment. Laser radiation is hazardous to the eye, and the eyes of the patient and all personnel involved in the surgical procedure and those who are within the immediate surgical environment must be protected with orange, argon light–absorbing safety goggles.

Management

Cold compresses are usually applied over the treatment area for approximately 6 hours to minimize edema, exudate, and loss of capillary permeability. The nurse advises the patient that swelling will subside in 1 to 2 days and will be followed by a crust that will last 7 to 10 days. The nurse instructs the patient to avoid picking at the crust, to apply an antibacterial ointment sparingly until the crust separates, to avoid applying makeup until the wound heals, and to avoid exposure to the sun. Sunscreen is to be used when exposure is unavoidable.

CO_2 Laser

The CO_2 laser emits invisible light in the infrared spectrum that is absorbed at the skin surface because of the high water content of the skin and the long wavelength of the CO_2 light. As the laser beam strikes tissue, it is absorbed by the intracellular and extracellular water, which vaporizes, destroying the tissue. The CO_2 laser is a precise surgical instrument that vaporizes and excises tissue with minimal damage. Because the beam can seal blood and lymphatic vessels, it creates a dry surgical field that makes many procedures easier and quicker. It is therefore safe to use on patients with bleeding disorders or those receiving anticoagulant therapy. It is useful for removing epidermal nevi, tattoos, certain warts, skin cancer, ingrown toenails, and keloids. Incisions made with the laser beam heal and scar much like those made by a scalpel.

In addition to wearing safety goggles, the patient and personnel wear laser-grade surgical masks to avoid inhaling the by-product smoke, referred to as a plume.

Management

Immediately after undergoing CO_2 laser surgery, the treated area turns a charcoal colour. The wound is covered with antibacterial ointment and a nonadhesive dressing. The patient is instructed to keep the wound dry except for gentle cleansing with mild soap several times each day. After the skin is cleaned, a prescribed ointment and light dressing are applied.

Because nerve endings and lymphatic vessels are sealed by the laser, less edema and pain follow the laser procedure than conventional surgery. A mild analgesic is sufficient to maintain patient comfort. Wound healing occurs by secondary intention, with granulation tissue appearing within a week; complete healing occurs in several weeks. Sun exposure to the area should be avoided for approximately 6 months. Application of a sunscreen with an SPF value of at least 15 is recommended. People at high risk for skin cancer from sun exposure are advised to use a sunscreen with an SPF greater than 15 to block UVB and UVA light.

Pulse-Dye Laser

The tunable pulse-dye laser with various wavelengths is the latest laser available for dermatologic surgery. It is especially useful in treating cutaneous vascular lesions such as port-wine stains and telangiectasia. Eye protection used for the argon and CO_2 lasers is insufficient when the pulse-dye laser is in use. Special eyeglasses, such as those made of didymium glass, are required for the patient and all personnel. The procedure is generally painless. For procedures requiring anesthesia, lidocaine without epinephrine is sufficient because local vasoconstriction (which epinephrine induces) is unnecessary.

Management

The patient is informed that there may be stinging in the treated area for several hours. Applying ice to the area and a light antibacterial ointment followed by a nonstick dressing (e.g., Telfa) usually eases discomfort.

NURSING ALERT

Telfa pads contain latex and should not be used on patients who are latex sensitive. Other dressings such as petrolatum-impregnated gauze should be used to prevent the dressing from adhering to the wound.

If crusting occurs, the patient is advised to wash the area gently with soap and water and reapply the antibacterial cream twice daily until the crust disappears. The nurse also advises the patient to avoid wearing makeup until all crust is removed. Sun exposure should be avoided as well; sunscreens with an SPF value of 15 or greater should be used for 3 to 4 months after the treatment. Complete removal of the lesion at one session, especially a port-wine stain, is rare. The patient should be informed that several treatments may be necessary.

Critical Thinking Exercises

1 You are caring for an 18-year-old female university student with chronic, cystic acne. She has been prescribed oral isotretinoin. What side effects should you review with this patient? What type of screening should be done before she is started on the isotretinoin? What are some self-care strategies you could recommend?

2 You work in a dermatology clinic. A 46-year-old woman presents to the clinic with a new onset of silvery plaques and is diagnosed with moderate psoriasis. The dermatologist has prescribed methotrexate therapy. The patient says to you "My daughter takes that drug for her Crohn's disease. How can this also work for treating what I have?" How would you answer the patient? What is the strength of the evidence that methotrexate is effective in treating moderate to severe psoriasis? Describe components of your plan to educate this woman on how to best self-manage her disease.

3 A 44-year-old construction worker presenting to the family practice clinic where you work states that his father had melanoma and that now he is concerned about several pigmented lesions on his arms and neck. He also has red, scaly, nonhealing lesions on his scalp and face. Describe your focused priority assessments and interventions. What are the priorities for education that you should provide to this patient about preventing melanoma and performing self-examination of the skin?

REFERENCES AND SELECTED READINGS

Books

Dunphy, L., Winland-Brown, J., Porter, B., et al. (2015). *Primary care: Art and science of advanced practice nursing* (4th ed.). Philadelphia, PA: FA Davis.

Eliopoulos, C. (2018). *Gerontological nursing* (9th ed.). Philadelphia, PA: Lippincott Williams & Wilkins.

Goldsmith, L., Katz, S. I., Gilchrest, B. A., et al. (2012). *Fitzpatrick's dermatology in general medicine* (8th ed.). New York: McGraw-Hill.

Grossman, S. C., & Porth, C. M. (2014). *Porth's pathophysiology: Concepts of altered health states* (9th ed.). Philadelphia, PA: Kluwer Health/Lippincott Williams & Wilkins.

Krasner, D., Rodeheaver, G., Sibbald, G., et al. (2012). *Chronic wound care: A clinical source book for healthcare professionals* (5th ed.). Malvern, PA: HMP Communications.

Mansen, T. J., & Gabiola, J. (2015). *Patient-focused assessment: The art and science of clinical data gathering*. Boston, MA: Pearson.

Stephen, T. C. (2012). Skin, hair, and nails assessment. In T. C. Stephen, D. L. Skillen, R. A. Day, et al. (Eds.). *Canadian Jensen's nursing health assessment: A best practice approach* (1st ed., pp. 267–325). Philadelphia, PA: Wolters Kluwer Health/Lippincott Williams & Wilkins.

Urden, L. D., Stacy, K. M., & Lough, M. E. (2014). *Critical care nursing: Diagnosis and management* (7th ed.). St. Louis, MO: Elsevier Mosby.

Warren, R. J., & Neligan, P. C. (2013). *Plastic surgery* (3rd ed.). St. Louis, MO: Elsevier Mosby.

Wong, B., Arnold, M., & Boeckmann, J. (2016). *Facial plastic and reconstructive surgery*. New York: Springer.

Journals and Electronic Documents

Akram, S., & Zaman, H. (2015). Warts and verrucas: Assessment and treatment. *The Pharmaceutical Journal, 294*, 7867.

Al-Hammadi, A., Al-Ismaily, A., Al-Ali, S., et al. (2016). Topical, biological and clinical challenges in the management of patients with acne vulgaris. *Sultan Qaboos University Medical Journal, 16*(2), e152–e160.

Alves, J. V., Matos, D. M., Barreiros, H. F., et al. (2014). Variants of dermatofibroma—A histopathological study. *Anais Brasileiros de Dermatologia, 89*(3), 472–477.

American Cancer Society (ACS). (2016). *Risk factors for melanoma skin cancer*. Retrieved November 29, 2016, from www.cancer.org/cancer/melanoma-skin-cancer/causes-risks-prevention/risk-factors.html

Antiga, E., & Caproni, M. (2015). The diagnosis and treatment of dermatitis herpetiformis. *Clinical, Cosmetic and Investigational Dermatology, 8*, 257–265.

Arif, T. (2015). Salicylic acid as a peeling agent: A comprehensive review. *Clinical, Cosmetic and Investigational Dermatology, 8*, 455–461.

Bader, R. S., Kennedy, A. S., Santacroce, L., et al. (2016). Basal cell carcinoma. *Medscape*. Retrieved January 15, 2019, from emedicine.medscape.com/article/276624-overview

Bolier, R., Elferink, R. P., & Beuers, U. (2016). Advances in pathogenesis and treatment of pruritus. *Clinics in Liver Disease, 17*(2), 319–329.

Bonilla, D. L., Durden, L. A., Eremeeva, M. E., et al. (2013). The biology and taxonomy of head and body lice—Implications for louse-borne disease prevention. *PLoS Pathogens, 9*(11), e1003724.

Borda, L. J., & Wikramanayake, T. C. (2015). Seborrheic dermatitis and dandruff: A comprehensive review. *Journal of Clinical and Investigative Dermatology, 3*(2). doi: 10.13188/2373-1044.1000019.

Bronckers, I. M., Paller, A. S., van Geel, M. J., et al. (2015). Psoriasis in children and adolescents: Diagnosis, management and comorbidities. *Paediatric Drugs, 17*, 373–384.

Canadian Cancer Society's Advisory Committee on Cancer Statistics. (2013). *Canadian Cancer Statistics 2013*. Toronto, ON: Canadian Cancer Society.

Canadian Cancer Society's Advisory Committee on Cancer Statistics. (2015). *Canadian Cancer Statistics 2015*. Toronto, ON: Canadian Cancer Society. Retrieved from https://www.cancer.ca/~/media/cancer.ca/CW/cancer%20information/cancer%20101/Canadian%20cancer%20statistics/Canadian-Cancer-Statistics-2015-EN.pdf

Canadian Dermatology Association. (2014a). *Skin cancer self-examination poster*. Ottawa, ON: Author. Retrieved from http://www.dermatology.ca/wp-content/uploads/2012/01/MMPoster-2009EN.gif

Canadian Dermatology Association. (2014b). *Basal cell skin cancer*. Retrieved from http://www.dermatology.ca/skin-hair-nails/skin/skin-cancer/#!/skin-hair-nails/skin/skin-cancer/basal-cell-skin-cancer

Canadian Dermatology Association. (2014c). *Melanoma*. Ottawa, ON: Author. Retrieved from http://www.dermatology.ca/wp-content/uploads/2012/01/Melanoma-handout-EN.pdf

Canadian Skin Cancer Foundation. (2019). https://www.canadianskincancerfoundation.com/

Carr, C., Veledar, E., & Chen, S. (2014). Factors mediating the impact of chronic pruritus on quality of life. *JAMA Dermatology, 150*(6), 613–620.

Centers for Disease Control and Prevention (CDC). (2016a). *What are the risk factors for skin cancer?* Retrieved November 29, 2016, from www.cdc.gov/cancer/skin/basic_info/risk_factors.htm

Centers for Disease Control and Prevention (CDC). (2016b). *What can I do to reduce my risk of skin cancer?* Retrieved November 13, 2017, from www.cdc.gov/cancer/skin/basic_info/prevention.htm

César, A., Cruz, M., Mota, A., et al. (2016). Erythroderma. A clinical and etiological study of 103 patients. *Journal of Dermatological Case Reports*, *10*(1), 1–9.

Chan, L. S. (2016). Bullous pemphigoid. *Medscape*. Retrieved November 4, 2016, from emedicine.medscape.com/article/1062391-overview

Chan, K. Y., Li, C. W., Wong, H., et al. (2013). Use of sertraline for antihistamine-refractory uremic pruritus in renal palliative care patients. *Journal of Palliative Medicine*, *16*(8), 966–970.

Cho, J., Park, Y., Lee, J. C., et al. (2014). Case series of different onset of skin metastasis according to the breast cancer subtypes. *Cancer Research and Treatment: Official Journal of Korean Cancer Association*, *46*(2), 194–199.

Clark, J. M., Wang, T. D., & Terris, D. J. (2015). Skin flap design. *Medscape*. Retrieved February 3, 2017, from emedicine.medscape.com/article/875968-overview

Cohen, P. R. (2014). Follicular contact dermatitis revisited: A review emphasizing neomycin-associated follicular contact dermatitis. *World Journal of Clinical Cases*, *2*(12), 815–821.

Cohen, V., Jellinek, S. P., & Schwartz, R. A. (2016). Toxic epidermal necrolysis. *Medscape*. Retrieved February 12, 2017, from emedicine.medscape.com/article/229698-overview

Dabiri, G., Damstetter, E., & Phillips, T. (2014). Choosing a wound dressing based on common wound characteristics. *WHS Wound Healing Society*, *5*(1), 32–40.

Dabiri, G., Elizabeth Damstetter, E., & Phillips, T. (2016). Choosing a wound dressing based on common wound characteristics. *Advances in Wound Care*, *5*(1), 32–41.

Friedman, J. M. (2014). Neurofibromatosis. *GeneReviews*. Retrieved October 14, 2016, from www.ncbi.nlm.nih.gov/books/NBK1109/

Gellatly, K. J., Krim, S., Palenchar, D. J., et al. (2016). Expansion of the knockdown resistance frequency map for human head lice (Phthiraptera: Pediculidae) in the United States using quantitative sequencing. *Journal of Medical Entomology*, *53*(3), 653–659.

Gorelick, J., Daniels, S. R., Kawata, A. K., et al. (2015). Acne-related quality of life among female adults of different races/ethnicities. *Journal of the Dermatology Nurses Association*, *7*(3), 154–162.

Guenther, L., & Maguiness, S. (2016). Pediculosis (lice). *Medscape*. Retrieved November 4, 2016, from emedicine.medscape.com/article/225013-overview

Handler, M. Z. (2017). Seborrheic dermatitis treatment and management. *Medscape*. Retrieved February 4, 2017, from emedicine.medscape.com/article/1108312-treatment

Handler, M. Z., Stephany, M. P., & Schwarts, R. A. (2016). Tinea capitis. *Medscape*. Retrieved February 11, 2017, from emedicine.medscape.com/article/1091351-overview

Hession, M. T., & Graber, E. M. (2015). Atrophic acne scarring: A review of treatment options. *The Journal of Clinical and Aesthetic Dermatology*, *8*(1), 50–58.

Hochman, B., Isoldi, F. C., Furtado, F., et al. (2015). New approach to the understanding of keloid: Psychoneuroimmune–endocrine aspects. *Clinical, Cosmetic and Investigational Dermatology*, *8*, 67–73.

Hogan, D. J. (2016). Irritant contact dermatitis. *Medscape*. Retrieved February 11, 2017, from emedicine.medscape.com/article/1049352-overview

Hong, J., Buddenkotte, J., Berger, T. G., et al. (2013). Management of itch in atopic dermatitis. *Seminars in Cutaneous Medicine and Surgery*, *30*(2), 71–86.

Husain, Z., & Alster, T. S. (2016). The role of lasers and intense pulsed light technology in dermatology. *Clinical, Cosmetic and Investigational Dermatology*, *9*, 29–40.

Inamadar, A. C., & Palit, A. (2013). Sensitive skin: An overview. *Indian Journal of Dermatology, Venereology, and Leprology*, *79*(1), 9–16.

Janniger, C. K., Eastern, J. S., Hospenthal, D. R., et al. (2016). Herpes zoster. *Medscape*. Retrieved November 4, 2016, from emedicine.medscape.com/article/1132465-overview

Karch, A. M. (2015). 2015 Lippincott's nursing drug guide. Philadelphia, PA: Lippincott Williams & Wilkins.

Kellen, R., & Berlin, J. M. (2016). Dermatology emergencies. *Journal of the Dermatology Nurses Association*, *8*(3), 193–202.

Landriscina, A., Rosen, J., & Friedman, A. (2015). Systemic approach to wound dressings. *Journal of Drugs in Dermatology*, *14*(7), 740–744.

Lesher, J. L. (2016). Tinea corporis. *Medscape*. Retrieved February 11, 2017, from emedicine.medscape.com/article/1091473-overview

Lewis, L. S. (2016). Impetigo. *Medscape*. Retrieved February 11, 2017, from emedicine.medscape.com/article/965254-overview

McCallon, S., Weir, D., & Lantis, J. (2015). Optimizing wound bed preparation with collagenase enzymatic debridement. *Journal of the American College of Clinical Wound Specialists*, *6*(1–2), 14–23.

Mease, P. J., & Armstrong, A. W. (2014). Managing patients with psoriatic disease: The diagnosis and pharmacologic treatment of psoriatic arthritis in patients with psoriasis. *Drugs*, *74*(4), 423–441.

Meffert, J. (2016). Psoriasis. *Medscape*. Retrieved November 4, 2016, from emedicine.medscape.com/article/1943419-overview

Mounsey, K. E., Murray, H. C., Bielefeldt-Ohmann, H., et al. (2015). Prospective study in a porcine model of Sarcoptes scabiei indicates the association of Th2 and Th17 pathways with the clinical severity of scabies. *PLoS Neglected Tropical Diseases*, *9*(3), e0003498.

Najjar, T. (2016). Cutaneous squamous cell carcinoma. *Medscape*. Retrieved February 13, 2017, from emedicine.medscape.com/article/1965430-overview

National Cancer Institute (NCI). (2016). *Melanoma treatment—Health professional version*. Retrieved February 13, 2017, from www.cancer.gov/types/skin/hp/melanoma-treatment-pdq

Nguyen, N., Couts, K. L., Luo, Y., et al. (2015). Understanding melanoma stem cells. *Melanoma Management*, *2*(2), 179–188.

Nicpon, J. (2017). Psoriasis management: Quality, cost, and coordination. *Journal of the Dermatology Nurses Association*, *9*(1), 21–25.

Occupational Safety and Health Administration (OSHA). (2012). *Toxic and hazardous substances: Bloodborne pathogens*. Retrieved October 11, 2016, from www.osha.gov/pls/oshaweb/owadisp.show_document?p_table = STANDARDS&p_id = 10051

Orsted, H. L., Keast, D. H., Forest-Lalande, L., et al. (2017). *Foundations of best practice for skin and wound management: Best practice recommendations for the prevention and management of wounds*. Retrieved from https://www.woundscanada.ca/docman/public/health-care-professional/bpr-workshop/165-wc-bpr-prevention-and-management-of-wounds/file

Peebles, E., Morris, R., & Chafe, R. (2014). Community-associated methicillin-resistant Staphylococcus aureus in a pediatric emergency department in Newfoundland and Labrador. *The Canadian Journal of Infectious Diseases & Medical Microbiology*, *25*(1), 13–16.

Public Health Agency of Canada (PHAC). (2012). *Routine practices and additional precautions for preventing the transmission of infection in health care settings*. Retrieved from http://www.ipac-canada.org/pdf/2013_PHAC_RPAP-EN.pdf

Radu, O., & Pantanowitz, L. (2013). Kaposi sarcoma. *Archives of Pathology & Laboratory Medicine*, *137*(2), 289–294.

Rao, J., & Chen, J. (2016). Acne vulgaris. *Medscape*. Retrieved November 4, 2016, from emedicine.medscape.com/articles/1069804-overview/showall

Robbins, C. M., & Elewski, B. E. (2016). Tinea pedis. *Medscape*. Retrieved February 11, 2017, from emedicine.medscape.com/article/1091684-overview

Rosso, J., Kircik, L., Goldenberg, G., et al. (2014). Comprehensive management of actinic keratoses. *The Journal of Clinical and Aesthetic Dermatology*, *7*(9 Suppl), S2–S12.

Sahoo, A. K., & Mahajan, R. (2016). Management of tinea corporis, tinea cruris, and tinea pedis: A comprehensive review. *Indian Dermatology Online Journal*, *7*(2), 77–86.

Santoro, F., Stoopler, E., & Werth, V. (2013). Pemphigus. *Dental Clinics of North America*, *57*(4), 597–610.

Sardana, K., Chakravarty, P., & Goel, K. (2014). Optimal management of common acquired melanocytic nevi (moles): Current perspectives. *Clinical, Cosmetic and Investigational Dermatology*, *7*, 89–103.

Scardina, G. A., Pisano, T., & Messina, P. (2010). Oral mucositis. Review of literature. *The New York State Dental Journal*, *76*(1), 34–38.

Skin Cancer Foundation. (2016). *Warning signs: The ABCDEs of melanoma*. Retrieved February 13, 2017, from www.skincancer.org/skin-cancer-information/melanoma

Smith & Nephew. (n.d.). *Regranex (becaplermin) gel 0.01%: A front-line solution to a serious problem*. Retrieved June 15, 2018, from https://regranex.com

Song, S. W., Burm, J. S., Yang, W. Y., et al. (2014). Minimally invasive excision of epidermal cysts through a small hole made by a CO2 laser. *Archives of Plastic Surgery*, *41*(1), 85–88.

Tan, W. W., Talavera, F., Schulman, P., et al. (2016). Malignant melanoma. *Medscape*. Retrieved February 13, 2017, from emedicine.medscape.com/article/280245-overview

Tang, V. C., & Lee, E. W. (2010). Fluid balance chart: do we understand it?. *Clinical Risk*, *16*(1), 10–13.

Tarikci, N., Kocatürk, E., Güngör, Ş., et al. (2015). Pruritus in systemic diseases: A review of etiological factors and new treatment modalities. *The Scientific World Journal*, *2015*, 803752.

Thomas, J., Peterson, G. M., Walton, S. F., et al. (2015). Scabies: An ancient global disease with a need for new therapies. *BMC Infectious Diseases*, *15*, 250.
Tosti, A. (2016). Onychomycosis. *Medscape*. Retrieved February 11, 2017, from emedicine.medscape.com/article/1105828-overview
Umar, S. H., & Kelly, A. P. (2016). Erythroderma (generalized exfoliative dermatitis). *Medscape*. Retrieved November 4, 2016, from emedicine.medscape.com/article/1106906-overview
Van Bijnen, E. M., Paget, W. J., den Heijer, C. D., et al. (2014). Primary care treatment guidelines for skin infections in Europe: Congruence with antimicrobial resistance found in commensal Staphylococcus aureus in the community. *BMC Family Practice*, *15*, 175.
Weiderkehr, M., & Schwartz, R. A. (2016). Tinea cruris. *Medscape*. Retrieved February 11, 2017, from emedicine.medscape.com/article/1091806-overview
Well, D. (2013). Acne vulgaris: A review of causes and treatment options. *The Nurse Practitioner*, *38*(10), 22–31.
Wernli, K. J., Henrikson, N. B., Morrison, C. C., et al. (2016). Screening for skin cancer in adults: Updated evidence report and systematic review for the US preventive services task force. *JAMA*, *316*(4), 436–447.
Wollina, U., Koch, A., Heinig, B., et al. (2013). Acne inversa (Hidradenitis suppurativa): A review with a focus on pathogenesis and treatment. *Indian Dermatology Online Journal*, *4*(1), 2–11.
Zaenglein, A. L., Pathy, A. L., Schlosser, B. J., et al. (2016). Guidelines of care for the management of acne vulgaris. *Journal of the American Academy of Dermatology*, *74*(5), 945–973.
Zeina, B., Mansoor, S., & Sakka, N. (2016). Pemphigus vulgaris. *Medscape*. Retrieved February 12, 2017, from emedicine.medscape.com/article/1064187-overview

Resources

Canadian Alopecia Areata Foundation (CANAAF): http://canaaf.org
Canadian Association of Wound Care: http://www.cawc.net
Canadian Cancer Society/Société canadienne du cancer: http://www.cancer.ca
Canadian Dermatology Association: http://www.dermatology.ca
Canadian Directory of Genetic Support Groups, Support Group Directory: http://www.lhsc.on.ca/programs/medgenet
Canadian Organization for Rare Disorders (CORD): http://www.cord.ca
Canadian Society for Molecular Biosciences (CSMB): http://www.csmb-scbm.ca/index.aspx
Center for Genetic Health Tips: http://www.cgdn.ca
Dermatology Information System, a cooperation between the Department of Clinical Social Medicine (University of Heidelberg) and the Department of Dermatology (University of Erlangen): http://www.dermis.net
Eczema Canada: http://www.eczemacanada.ca
GeneTests: http://www.genetests.org
Health Canada: http://www.hc-sc.gc.ca
Lupus Canada: http://www.lupuscanada.org
Melanoma Education Foundation: http://www.skincheck.org
Psoriasis Society of Canada: http://www.psoriasissociety.org
Rosacea Awareness Program: http://www.about-rosacea.com

59 Management of Patients With Burn Injury

Adapted by Lindsay Burnett

Learning Objectives

On completion of this chapter, the learner will be able to:

1. Discuss the classification system used for burn injuries.
2. Describe the local and systemic effects of a major burn injury.
3. Describe the three phases of burn care and the priorities of care for each phase.
4. Compare and contrast the potential fluid and electrolyte alterations of the emergent/resuscitative and acute phases of burn management.
5. Describe the goals of the following aspects of burn wound care and the nurse's role in each: wound cleaning, topical antibacterial therapy, wound dressing, dressing changes, wound débridement, and wound grafting.
6. Describe the nurse's role in the following areas of management: pain management, restrictions of activity and joint motion, psychological support of the patient and family, nutritional support, pulmonary care, and patient and family education.
7. Use the nursing process as a framework for care of the patient during the three phases of burn care.

The nurse who cares for a patient with a burn injury requires a high level of knowledge about the physiologic changes that occur after a burn as well as astute assessment skills to detect subtle changes in the patient's condition. In addition, the nurse must be able to provide sensitive, compassionate care to patients who are critically ill and must initiate rehabilitation early in the course of care. The nurse must also be able to communicate effectively with patients with burns, distraught family members, and members of the entire interdisciplinary burn management team. This will ensure quality care, which increases the likelihood of the patient's survival and promotes optimal quality of life.

Incidence of Burn Injury

According to the government of Canada (2017), 1,682 cases of burn injuries were identified and reported in 2013. Half were scalds, and 30% were contact burns from hot objects. The two leading direct causes of scalds were hot beverages and hot water (not from the tap). The two leading direct causes of contact burns were stoves/ovens and fireplaces/accessories. Overall, 13.0% of cases (218/1,682) were serious enough to require hospital admission; the highest proportion of hospitalizations was among those exposed to fire/flame/smoke.

Burns continue pose a strain on health care resources, with 177 million dollars spent on treating burns. The indirect costs are also significant, estimated at 188 million dollars attributed to decreased productivity and disability related to the burn injury. Burns are the fifth leading cause of work injury in Canada (Parachute Canada, 2015).

According to the electronic Canadian Hospital Injury Reporting and Prevention Program database for emergency department visits, the most common cause of burns in 2013 was scalds (52.3%), followed by contact burns (29.9%). Burn injury prevention through local, national, and international efforts is important to raise awareness and decrease risk of suffering from a burn injury.

Young children and older people are at particularly high risk for burn injury. Their skin is thin and fragile;

therefore, even a limited period of contact with a source of heat can create a full-thickness burn.

Prevention

Burns are preventable. An important goal of nurses in community and home settings is to provide education about the prevention of burn injury (see Chart 59-1). Nurses should capitalize on the teachable moment, an opportunity using a recent injury event, as a prime time people "are likely to be more receptive to accept guidance on how to change their behaviour to avoid future injury" (Klas, Smith, Matherly, et al., 2015, p. 434). High-risk behaviours such as alcohol consumption and alcohol abuse often precipitate many burn injuries (Sen et al., 2015). Smoking materials, particularly cigarettes, are a leading cause of fire death in the United States (ABA, 2011). The World Health Organization (WHO) recommends heightened awareness of the burden of burn injury and risk factors as imperatives to develop an effective burn prevention program (WHO, 2014).

Burns can also occur from work-related injuries. Education to prevent burn injuries in the workplace should include safe handling of chemicals and chemical products and increasing awareness of the potential for injuries caused by hot objects and substances. Patients with burns secondary to the illegal manufacturing of the drug methamphetamine are appearing with increasing frequency in burn centres. These patients are often admitted with both severe burns and inhalation injury.

Many burns can be prevented. Nurses can play an active role in preventing fires and burns by teaching prevention concepts and promoting legislation related to fire safety (see Chart 59-1). Promoting the use of smoke alarms and

CHART 59-1

Health Promotion: Burn Prevention

- Advise that matches and lighters be kept out of the reach of children.
- Emphasize the importance of never leaving children unattended around fire or in bathroom/bathtub.
- Educate about the installation and maintenance of smoke and carbon monoxide detectors on every level of the home and changing batteries annually on birthday.
- Recommend the development and practice of a home exit fire drill with all members of the household.
- Advocate setting the water heater temperature no higher than 48.9°C (120°F).
- Educate about the perils of smoking in bed, smoking while using home oxygen, or falling asleep while smoking.
- Caution against using flammable liquids to start fires and/or throwing flammable liquids onto an already burning fire.
- Warn of the danger of removing the radiator cap from a hot car engine.
- Recommend avoidance of overhead electrical wires and underground wires when working outside.
- Advise that hot irons and curling irons be kept out of the reach of children.
- Discourage running electric cords under carpets or rugs.
- Recommend storage of flammable liquids well away from a fire source, such as a pilot light.
- Educate about the importance of being aware of loose clothing when cooking over a stovetop or flame.
- Recommend having a working fire extinguisher in the home and knowing how to use it.

Glossary

Alloderm: processed dermis from human cadaver skin; can be used as dermal layer for skin grafts

allograft: graft transferred from one human (living or cadaveric) to another human; also called allograft

autograft: graft derived from one part of a patient's body and used on another part of that same patient's body

Biobrane: synthetic dressing composed of a nylon, Silastic membrane combined with a collagen derivative

carboxyhemoglobin: compound of carbon monoxide and hemoglobin, formed in the blood with exposure to carbon monoxide

collagen: protein present in skin, tendon, bone, cartilage, and connective tissue

contracture: shrinkage of burn scar through collagen maturation

cultured epithelial autografts (CEA): autologous epidermal cells that proliferate in culture and then are grafted onto the patient

débridement: removal of foreign material and devitalized tissue until surrounding healthy tissue is exposed

dermis: the second layer of skin containing sweat glands, hair follicles, and nerves

donor site: the area from which skin is taken to provide a skin graft for another part of the body

epidermis: the outermost layer of skin

eschar: devitalized tissue resulting from a burn

escharotomy: linear excision made through eschar to release constriction of underlying tissue

excision: surgical removal of tissue

fasciotomy: incision made through the fascia to release constriction of underlying muscle

hydrotherapy: cleansing of wounds through use of bath, shower, shower cart table, or immersion

hypertrophic scar: excessive scar formation that rises above the level of the skin

Integra: a synthetic dermal regeneration template that provides immediate closure and permanent regeneration of the dermis

rule of nines: method for calculating body surface area burned by dividing the body into multiples of nine

xenograft: graft obtained from an animal of a species (i.e., pigskin) other than that of the recipient; also called a xenograft carbon monoxide detectors has had the greatest impact on decreasing fire deaths in Canada.

There are four major goals relating to burns:

1. Prevention
2. Institution of lifesaving measures for the severely burned person
3. Prevention of disability and disfigurement through early, specialized, individualized treatment
4. Rehabilitation through reconstructive surgery and rehabilitative programs

Outlook for Survival and Recovery

Great strides in research have helped to increase the survival rate of patients with burn injuries. Mortality has fallen to levels never thought possible. Research in areas such as fluid resuscitation, emergent burn treatment, inhalation injury treatment, and changes in wound care practice with early **débridement** and **excision** have contributed greatly to the decrease in burn deaths. Additionally, a better understanding of the importance of adequate nutritional support has contributed to increased survival rates. Nonetheless, even in specialized burn centres, adults with greater than 40% TBSA burned remain at high risk of morbidity and mortality (Jeschke et al., 2015). Very young and very old people have a high risk of death after burn injuries due to immature and stressed immunologic systems and pre-existing medical conditions, respectively. Chances of survival are greater in children older than 5 years and in adults younger than 40 years. Outcome depends on the depth and extent of the burn as well as on the preinjury health status and age of the patient. Acute care of patients with burn injuries has improved to the point at which survival is expected for most patients, and the burn team has shifted its focus to long-term outcomes for these patients.

Gerontologic Considerations

Age-related changes such as thinning skin, decreased sensation, altered mental status, and pre-existing comorbidities place older people at higher risk for burn injury. These changes also place older people at risk for suffering a severe burn because they have difficulty in extinguishing the fire and removing themselves from the burn source.

Morbidity and mortality rates associated with burns are usually greater in older patients than in younger patients. For example, the lethal dose in 50% of the population (LD50) is 30% to 50% TBSA for older adults, which has not changed much over time (Jeschke & Peck, 2017). Thinning and loss of elasticity of the skin in the older predisposes them to a deep injury from a thermal insult that might cause a less severe burn in a younger person. Moreover, chronic illnesses decrease the older person's ability to withstand the multisystem stresses imposed by burn injury (Jeschke & Peck, 2017).

An important goal of nurses in community and home settings is preventing burn injury, especially among the older population. Nurses need to assess an older patient's ability to perform activities of daily living safely, assist older patients and families to modify the environment to ensure safety, and make referrals as needed.

Pathophysiology of Burns

Burns are caused by a transfer of energy from a heat source to the body. Heat may be transferred through conduction or electromagnetic radiation. Burns are categorized as thermal, electrical (which can include thermal), chemical, and radiation. Tissue destruction results from coagulation, protein denaturation, or ionization of cellular contents. The skin and the mucosa of the upper airways are the sites of tissue destruction. Deep tissues, including the viscera, can be damaged by electrical burns or through prolonged contact with a heat source. Disruption of the skin can lead to increased fluid loss, infection, hypothermia, scarring, compromised immunity, and changes in function, appearance, and body image.

The severity of the burn injury depends on the temperature of the burning agent and the duration of contact with the agent. Hot beverages (i.e., coffee, tea, hot chocolate) are usually served at 71° to 82°C, resulting in almost instantaneous burns that will require surgery. One second of contact with hot tap water at 68°C may result in a burn that destroys both the **epidermis** and the **dermis**, causing a full-thickness (third-degree) injury. Fifteen seconds of exposure to hot water at 56.1°C results in a similar full-thickness injury. Splash and spill burns may not be as deep as burns suffered in a bathtub if the source of the hot liquid is removed immediately from the skin, therefore lessening the severity of the burn. Temperatures less than 43°C are tolerated for long periods without injury.

Classification of Burns

Burn injuries are described according to the depth of the injury and the extent of body surface area injured.

Burn Depth

Burns are classified according to the depth of tissue destruction as superficial injuries, superficial partial-thickness injuries, deep partial-thickness injuries, or full-thickness injuries. Burn depth determines whether reepithelialization will occur. Determining burn depth can be difficult even for the experienced burn care provider (see Table 59-1). (The categories of superficial, superficial partial-thickness, deep partial-thickness, and full-thickness burns are similar to, but not the same as, first-, second-, and third-degree burns.)

In a superficial burn injury the epidermal layer of the skin is injured. The damaged skin may be painful and appear dark pink, dry, and tender, as in a sunburn. It usually heals quickly within 7 days.

In a superficial partial-thickness burn, the epidermis is destroyed and the upper layers of the dermis are injured. It is characteristically dark pink or red in colour, with blisters present. There is some mild edema and it is very painful. Capillary blanching is still present. It takes longer to heal, usually 10 to 14 days.

A deep partial-thickness burn involves destruction of the epidermis and injury to deeper portions of the dermis. The wound is painful, appears red, and exudes fluid. It has decreased sensation and has delayed capillary blanching. Hair follicles and other dermal appendages remain intact. Deep partial-thickness burns take longer to heal and are more likely to result in hypertrophic scars; skin grafting

TABLE 59-1 Characteristics of Burns According to Depth

Causes	Skin Involvement	Clinical Manifestations	Wound Appearance	Recuperative Course and Treatment
First Degree (Superficial)				
Sunburn Low-intensity flash Superficial scald	Epidermis	Tingling Hyperesthesia (hypersensitivity) Pain that is soothed by cooling Peeling Itching	Reddened; blanches with pressure; dry Minimal or no edema Possible blisters	Complete recovery within a few days Oral pain medications, cool compresses, skin lubricants (e.g., ointments, emollients); topical antimicrobial agents not indicated
Second Degree (Partial Thickness)				
Scalds Flash flame Contact	Epidermis, portion of dermis	Pain Hyperesthesia Sensitive to air currents	Blistered, mottled red base; disrupted epidermis; weeping surface Edema	Recovery in 2–3 weeks Some scarring and depigmentation possible; may require grafting
Third Degree (Full Thickness)				
Flame Prolonged exposure to hot liquids Electric current Chemical Contact	Epidermis, dermis, and sometimes subcutaneous tissue; may involve connective tissue, and muscle	Insensate Shock Myoglobinuria (red pigment in urine) and possible hemolysis (blood cell destruction) Possible contact points (entrance or exit wounds in electrical burns)	Dry; pale white, red brown, leathery, or charred Coagulated vessels may be visible Edema	Eschar may slough Grafting necessary Scarring and loss of contour and function
Fourth Degree (Full Thickness That Includes Fat, Fascia, Muscle, and/or Bone)				
Prolonged exposure or high-voltage electrical injury	Deep tissue, muscle and bone	Shock Myoglobinuria (red pigment in urine) and possible hemolysis (blood cell destruction)	Charred	Amputations likely Grafting of no benefit, given depth and severity of wound(s)

Adapted from American Burn Association. (2011). *Advanced burn life support (ABLS) course provider manual 2011*. Chicago, IL: Author; Kearns, R. D., Cairns, C. B., Holmes, J. H., et al. (2013). Thermal burns: A review of best practice. *EMS World, 42*(1), 43–51.

may be necessary. See Table 59-2 for pathophysiologic changes in severe burns.

A full-thickness burn involves total destruction of epidermis and dermis and, in some cases, may involve the subcutaneous and fascia layers as well. Wound colour ranges widely from white to red, brown, or black. The burned area is painless because nerve fibres are destroyed, and it does not blanch. The wound appears leathery; hair follicles and sweat glands are destroyed (Fig. 59-1). Excision of the burn wound and skin grafting is necessary.

The following factors are considered in determining the depth of the burn:

- How the injury occurred
- Causative agent, such as flame or scalding liquid
- Temperature of the burning agent
- Duration of contact with the agent
- Thickness of the skin

TABLE 59-2 Pathophysiologic Changes With Severe Burns

Body System	Physiologic Changes
Cardiovascular	Cardiac depression, edema, hypovolemia
Pulmonary	Vasoconstriction, edema
Gastrointestinal	Impaired motility and absorption, vasoconstriction, loss of mucosal barrier function with bacterial translocation, increased pH
Kidney	Vasoconstriction
Other	Altered thermoregulation, immunodepression, hypermetabolism

Adapted from Abdullahi, A., & Jeschke, M. G. (2014). Nutrition and anabolic pharmacotherapies in the care of burn patients. *Nutrition in Clinical Practice, 29*(5), 621–630; Snell, J. A., Loh, N. W., Mahambrey, T., et al. (2013). Clinical review: The critical care management of the burn patient. *Critical Care, 17*(5), 241.

Extent of Body Surface Area Injured

Various methods are used to estimate the TBSA affected by burns; among them are the **rule of nines**, the Lund and Browder method, and the palm method.

Rule of Nines

An estimation of the TBSA involved in a burn is simplified by using the rule of nines (Fig. 59-2). The rule of nines is a quick way to calculate the extent of burns. The system assigns percentages in multiples of nine to major body surfaces.

Lund and Browder Method

A more precise method of estimating the extent of a burn is the Lund and Browder method, which recognizes that the percentage of TBSA of various anatomic parts,

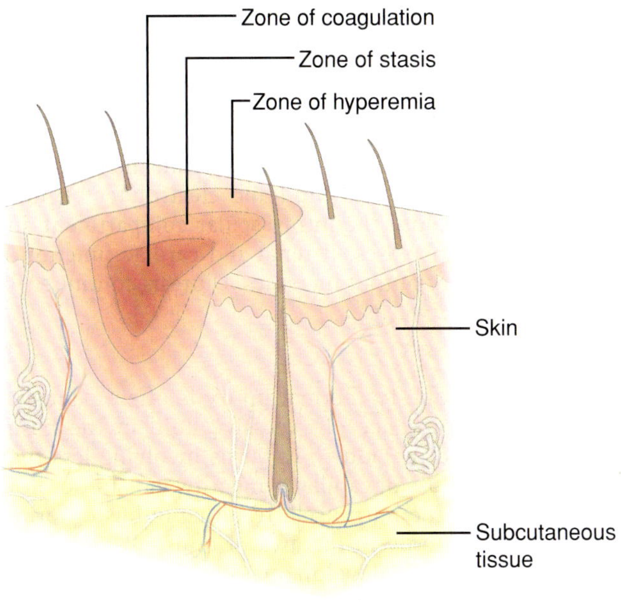

FIGURE 59-1. Zones of burn injury. Each burned area has three zones of injury. The inner zone (known as the area of coagulation, where cellular death occurs) sustains the most damage. The middle area, or zone of stasis, has a compromised blood supply, inflammation, and tissue injury. The outer zone—the zone of hyperemia—sustains the least damage.

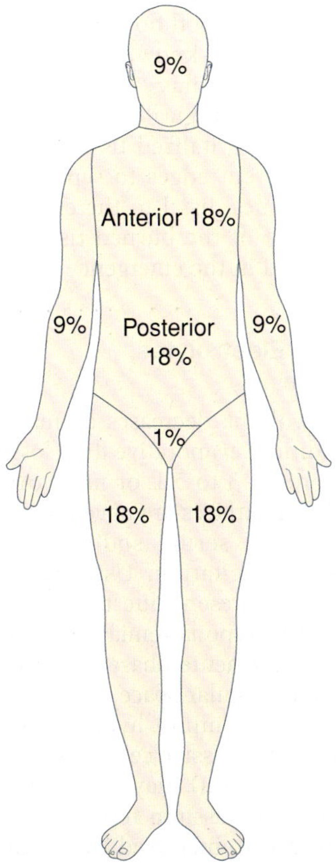

FIGURE 59-2. The rule of nines: Estimated percentage of total body surface area (TBSA) in the adult is arrived at by sectioning the body surface into areas with a numeric value related to nine. (*Note:* The anterior and posterior head total 9% of TBSA.) In patients with burns, the total estimated percentage of TBSA injured is used to calculate the patient's fluid replacement needs.

especially the head and legs, changes with growth. Because of changes in body proportion with growth, the calculated TBSA changes with age as well. By dividing the body into very small areas and providing an estimate of the proportion of TBSA accounted for by such body parts, one can obtain a reliable estimate of the TBSA burned. The initial evaluation is made on the patient's arrival at the hospital and is revised on the second and third postburn days because the demarcation usually is not clear until then.

Palmer Method

In patients with scattered burns, a method to estimate the percentage of burn is the palm method. The size of the patient's palm is approximately 1% of TBSA.

Electrical Burns

Electrical injury accounts for a small percentage of burn unit admissions each year, yet it is one of the worst types of burn injuries that can be sustained. The devastating effects of an electrical injury can cause lifelong neurovascular problems. High-voltage (more than 1,000 volts) injury can cause tissue and bone destruction resulting in amputations and may lead to cardiac and respiratory abnormalities resulting in the possible loss of life. An electrical injury results when a current of electricity travels through the body and exits to the ground itself. With an electrical injury, there is contact with the electrical source, resulting in contact points, previously referred to as entrance and exit wounds. An arc injury is the result of the electricity's travelling on the outside of the body or arcing around it. Often, the clothes catch fire because of the high energy. The patient ends up with a thermal burn and often small, spiderlike markings that make a path on the skin. The cutaneous injury from electrical sources is usually small compared with the damage under the surface of the skin. Electricity travels through areas of least resistance and destroys everything in its path—nerves and blood vessels first; bones are destroyed last, as they are most resistant. The stronger the current and the longer the duration of contact are, the more severe the injury is.

For a patient with an electrical burn, once the patient is out of the path of the electricity, emergency care can safely be provided. The ABCs of emergency care are always followed. An electrical current immediately contracts muscles as it travels through the body, and cardiac arrhythmias and spinal injuries often result from the muscular contraction. A 12-lead ECG should be performed. Continuous monitoring is only required if dysrhythmias or ectopy is evident (ABLS, 2018). Until it is known that the patient has no fractures, it is imperative that a neck collar remains in place and that the patient be logrolled to eliminate the chance of further spinal cord injury. With high-voltage electrical injuries, cervical spine immobilization is a priority until cervical spine injury is ruled out.

For a patient with an electrical burn, prompt administration of intravenous (IV) fluids using fluid resuscitation formulas and monitoring of urine output are critical components of care. Patients with electrical burns are prone to acute renal failure because of the release of myoglobin from the destruction of muscle and tissue. Myoglobin can constrict renal arteries and renal tubules blocking the flow of urine through the kidneys. Patients can have gross hematuria on admission to the hospital. Administration of high amounts of IV fluids helps to maintain the flow of urine. It is difficult to assess the amount of fluid a patient will require because the electrical injury creates so much damage inside the body. The nurse should expect 75 to 100 mL/hr of urine output for an adult patient who is receiving fluid resuscitation.

In patients with electrical injuries, neurovascular checks of affected extremities are very important. A person can have neurovascular complications for as long as 2 years after the incident occurred. Decreased blood flow may indicate the development of compartment syndrome, which requires an emergent fasciotomy. Baseline neurologic and functional status must be assessed as soon as possible to rule out any abnormalities that might appear at a later date.

Local and Systemic Responses to Burns

Burns that do not exceed 20% TBSA produce a primarily local response. Burns that exceed 20% TBSA may produce both a local and a systemic response and are considered major burn injuries. This systemic response is due to the release of cytokines and other mediators into the systemic circulation. The release of local mediators and changes in blood flow, tissue edema, and infection can cause progression of the burn injury.

Pathophysiologic changes resulting from major burns during the initial burn-shock period include tissue hypoperfusion and organ hypofunction secondary to decreased cardiac output, followed by a hyperdynamic and hypermetabolic phase. The incidence, magnitude, and duration of pathophysiologic changes in burns are proportional to the extent of burn injury, with a maximal response seen in burns covering 60% or more TBSA.

The initial systemic event after a major burn injury is hemodynamic instability, resulting from loss of capillary integrity and a subsequent shift of fluid, sodium, and protein from the intravascular space into the interstitial spaces. Figure 59-3 illustrates the pathophysiologic processes in acute major burns. Hemodynamic instability involves cardiovascular, fluid and electrolyte, blood volume, pulmonary, and other mechanisms.

Cardiovascular Response

Hypovolemia is the immediate consequence of fluid loss resulting in decreased perfusion and oxygen delivery. Cardiac output decreases before any significant change in blood volume is evident. As fluid loss continues and vascular volume decreases, cardiac output continues to fall and blood pressure drops. This is the onset of burn shock. In response, the sympathetic nervous system releases catecholamines, resulting in an increase in peripheral resistance (vasoconstriction) and an increase in pulse rate. Peripheral vasoconstriction further decreases cardiac output. Myocardial contractility may be suppressed by the release of inflammatory cytokine necrosis factor (Wurzer, Culnan, Cancio, et al., 2018).

Prompt fluid resuscitation maintains the blood pressure in the low-normal range and improves cardiac output. Despite adequate fluid resuscitation, cardiac filling pressures (central venous pressure, pulmonary artery pressure, and pulmonary artery wedge pressure) remain low during the burn-shock period. If inadequate fluid resuscitation occurs, distributive shock will occur (see Chapter 18).

In general, the greatest volume of fluid leak occurs in the first 24 to 36 hours after the burn, peaking by 6 to 8 hours. As the capillaries begin to regain their integrity, burn shock resolves and fluid and electrolytes begin to remobilize back into the intravascular compartment and blood volume increases. If renal and cardiac function is adequate, urinary output increases. Diuresis continues for several days to 2 weeks.

Burn Edema

Local swelling due to thermal injury is often extensive. Edema is the presence of excessive fluid in the tissue spaces. As noted previously, in burns involving less than 20% TBSA, the loss of capillary integrity and shift of fluid are localized to the burn itself, resulting in blister formation and edema only in the area of injury. Patients with more severe burns develop massive systemic edema. Edema is the greatest 18 to 24 hours after injury. It begins to resolve 1 to 2 days post burn and usually is completely resolved in 7 to 10 days post injury. Edema in burn wounds can be reduced by avoiding excessive fluid during the early postburn period. Unnecessary overresuscitation will increase edema formation in both burn tissue and nonburn tissue.

As edema increases in circumferential burns, pressure on small blood vessels and nerves in the distal extremities causes an obstruction of blood flow and consequent ischemia. This complication is known as compartment syndrome. The physician may need to perform an **escharotomy**, which is a surgical incision into the **eschar** and superficial fascia (devitalized tissue resulting from a burn), permitting the cut edges to separate and restore blood flow to the tissues distal to the eschar and relieve the constricting effect of the burned tissue. This procedure can be performed in the emergency department or at the bedside.

Effects on Fluids, Electrolytes, and Blood Volume

Circulating blood volume decreases dramatically during burn shock. In addition, evaporative fluid loss through the burn wound may reach 3 to 5 L or more over a 24-hour period until the burn surfaces are covered.

During burn shock, serum sodium levels vary in response to fluid resuscitation. Usually, hyponatremia (sodium depletion) is present due to sodium and water shifting into the cells. Hyponatremia is also common during the first week of the acute phase, as water shifts from the interstitial to the vascular space.

Immediately after burn injury, hyperkalemia (excessive potassium) results from massive cell destruction. Hypokalemia (potassium depletion) may occur later with fluid shifts and inadequate potassium replacement. Anaerobic metabolism begins due to increased lactic acid levels, and metabolic acidosis occurs.

At the time of burn injury, some red blood cells may be destroyed and others damaged, resulting in anemia. Despite this, the hematocrit may be elevated due to plasma loss. Blood loss during surgical procedures, wound care, and diagnostic studies and ongoing

Physiology/Pathophysiology

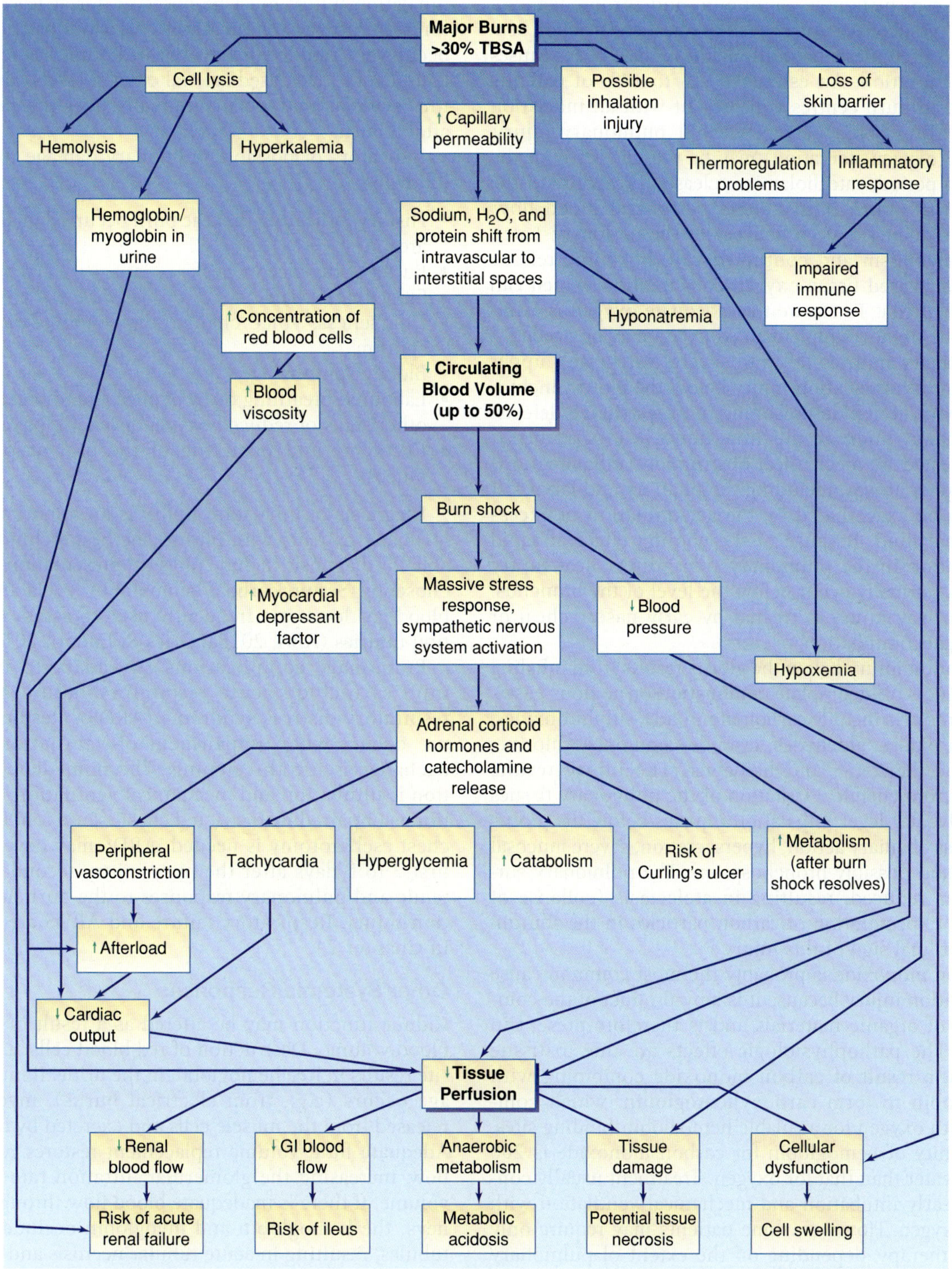

FIGURE 59-3. Overview of physiologic changes that occur after major burn. TBSA, total body surface area; H_2O, water; GI, gastrointestinal.

hemolysis further contribute to anemia. Blood transfusions are required periodically to maintain adequate hemoglobin levels for oxygen delivery. Abnormalities in coagulation, including a decrease in platelets (thrombocytopenia) and prolonged clotting and prothrombin times also occur with burn injury.

Pulmonary Response

Inhalation injury has a significant impact on survivability of a patient with burns. Inhalation injuries in combination with cutaneous burns are an important comorbid factor in burn injury that increases morbidity and mortality significantly (Dries & Endorf, 2013). Deterioration in patients who are severely burned can occur even without evidence of a smoke inhalation injury. Bronchoconstriction caused by release of histamine, serotonin, and thromboxane, a powerful vasoconstrictor, as well as chest constriction secondary to circumferential full-thickness chest burns causes this deterioration. An estimated 2% to 14% of patients admitted to burn centres will present with an inhalation injury (ABA, 2018a). Even without pulmonary injury, hypoxia (oxygen starvation) may be present. Early in the postburn period, catecholamine release in response to the stress of the burn injury alters peripheral blood flow, thereby reducing oxygen delivery to the periphery. Later, hypermetabolism and continued catecholamine release lead to increased tissue oxygen consumption, which can lead to hypoxia. To ensure that adequate oxygen is available to the tissues, supplemental oxygen may be needed.

Pulmonary injuries fall into several categories: upper airway injury; inhalation injury below the glottis, including carbon monoxide poisoning; and restrictive defects. Upper airway injury results from direct heat or edema. It is manifested by mechanical obstruction (inflammation) of the upper airway, including the pharynx and larynx. It can also be exacerbated by the accumulation of excess interstitial fluid. Because of the cooling effect of rapid vaporization in the pulmonary tract, direct heat injury does not normally occur below the level of the bronchus. Upper airway injury is treated by early nasotracheal or endotracheal intubation.

Inhalation injury below the glottis results from inhaling the products of incomplete combustion or noxious gases. These products include carbon monoxide, sulphur oxides, nitrogen oxides, aldehydes, cyanide, ammonia, chlorine, phosgene, benzene, and halogens. The injury results directly from chemical irritation of the pulmonary tissues at the alveolar level. Inhalation injuries below the glottis cause loss of ciliary action, hypersecretion, severe mucosal edema, and possibly bronchospasm. The pulmonary surfactant is reduced, resulting in atelectasis (collapse of alveoli). Expectoration of carbon particles in the sputum is the cardinal sign of this injury.

Carbon monoxide is probably the most common cause of inhalation injury because it is a by-product of the combustion of organic materials and is therefore present in smoke. The pathophysiologic effects are due to tissue hypoxia, a result of carbon monoxide combining with hemoglobin to form **carboxyhemoglobin**, which competes with oxygen for available hemoglobin-binding sites. The affinity of hemoglobin for carbon monoxide is 200 times greater than that for oxygen. Treatment usually consists of early intubation and mechanical ventilation with 100% oxygen. However, some patients may require only oxygen therapy, depending on the extent of pulmonary injury and edema. Administering 100% oxygen is essential to accelerate the removal of carbon monoxide from the hemoglobin molecule (it will reduce the half-life of carbon monoxide from 4 hours to 40 minutes).

Restrictive defects arise when edema develops under full-thickness burns encircling the neck and thorax. Chest excursion may be greatly restricted, resulting in decreased tidal volume. In such situations, escharotomy is necessary to help improve ventilation and oxygenation.

Pulmonary abnormalities are not always immediately apparent. More than half of all patients with burns with pulmonary involvement do not initially demonstrate pulmonary signs and symptoms. Any patient with possible inhalation injury must be observed for at least 48 hours for respiratory complications. Airway obstruction may occur very rapidly or develop in hours. Decreased lung compliance, decreased arterial oxygen levels, and respiratory acidosis may occur gradually over the first 5 days after a burn.

Indicators of possible pulmonary damage include the following:

- History indicating that the burn occurred in an enclosed area
- Burns of the face or neck
- Singed nasal hair
- Hoarseness, voice change, dry cough, stridor, sooty sputum
- Bloody sputum
- Laboured breathing or tachypnea (rapid breathing) and other signs of reduced oxygen levels (hypoxemia)
- Erythema and blistering of the oral or pharyngeal mucosa

Diagnosis of inhalation injury is an important priority for many patients with burns. The best techniques available for diagnosis include physical presentation and bronchoscopy. Serum carboxyhemoglobin levels and arterial blood gas levels are frequently used to assess for inhalation injuries (ABA, 2018a; Dries & Endorf, 2013).

Pulmonary complications secondary to inhalation injuries include acute respiratory failure and acute respiratory distress syndrome (ARDS). Respiratory failure occurs when impairment of ventilation and gas exchange is life threatening. The immediate intervention is intubation and mechanical ventilation. If ventilation is impaired by restricted chest excursion, immediate chest escharotomy is needed. ARDS may develop in the first 2 to 5 days after the burn injury secondary to systemic and pulmonary responses to the burn and inhalation injury. Respiratory failure and ARDS are discussed in Chapter 24.

Other Systemic Responses

Kidney function may be altered as a result of decreased blood volume. Destruction of red blood cells at the injury site results in free hemoglobin in the urine. If muscle damage occurs (e.g., from electrical burns), myoglobin is released from the muscle cells and excreted by the kidney. Adequate fluid volume replacement restores renal blood flow, increasing the glomerular filtration rate and urine volume. If there is inadequate blood flow through the kidneys, the hemoglobin and myoglobin occlude the renal tubules, resulting in acute tubular necrosis and acute kidney injury (AKI).

The immunologic defenses of the body are greatly altered by burn injury. Serious burn injury diminishes resistance to infection as alternations in the immune cells affect their ability to function. As a result, sepsis continues to be the leading cause of morbidity and mortality in patients with thermal injuries (Greenhalgh, 2017). The loss of skin integrity is compounded by the release of abnormal inflammatory factors, altered levels of immunoglobulins and serum complement, impaired neutrophil function, and a reduction in lymphocytes (lymphocytopenia). The resulting immunosuppression places the patient with burns at high risk for sepsis.

Loss of skin also results in an inability to regulate body temperature. Patients with burns may therefore exhibit low body temperatures in the early hours after injury. Then, as hypermetabolism resets core temperatures, patients with burns become hyperthermic for much of the postburn period, even in the absence of infection.

Two potential gastrointestinal complications may occur: paralytic ileus (absence of intestinal peristalsis) and Curling's ulcer. Decreased peristalsis and bowel sounds are manifestations of paralytic ileus resulting from burn trauma. Narcotics for pain management may also slow peristalsis. Gastric distention and nausea may lead to vomiting unless gastric decompression is initiated. Gastric bleeding secondary to massive physiologic stress may be signaled by occult blood in the stool, regurgitation of "coffee ground" material from the stomach, or bloody vomitus. These signs suggest gastric or duodenal erosion (Curling's ulcer).

Patients with large burn wounds are at risk for abdominal compartment syndrome, especially if fluid resuscitation is delayed and results in over resuscitation (Kollias, Stampolidis, Kourakos, et al., 2015). Fluid shifts into the abdominal cavity cause increased abdominal distention, decreasing urine output and resulting in hypotension and difficulty with ventilation. Bladder pressures greater than 25 to 30 mm Hg over time are an indicator of increasing abdominal pressure. Emergent laparotomy aids in reducing abdominal pressure.

Three components of the gastrointestinal tract are altered after burn injury: first, the mucosal barrier becomes permeable; second, the permeability allows for overgrowth of gastrointestinal bacteria; and third, the bacteria translocate to other organs, causing infection. Patients are unable to defend against their own bacteria due to immunosuppression in burn injury.

Management of Burn Injury

PRACTICE & LEARN

Burn care must be planned according to the burn depth and local response, the extent of the injury, and the presence of a systemic response. Burn care then proceeds through three phases: emergent/resuscitative phase, acute/intermediate phase, and rehabilitation phase. Although priorities exist for each of the phases, the phases overlap, and assessment and management of specific problems and complications are not limited to these phases but take place throughout burn care. The three phases and the priorities for care are summarized in Table 59-3.

Emergent/Resuscitative Phase of Burn Care

On-the-Scene Care

Anyone who encounters a person with burns for the first time may feel overwhelmed. The person's appearance can be frightening at first. It can be difficult not to get caught up with the appearance of the person and instead to concentrate on the burn wounds. However, the burn wound is not the first priority at the scene: The first priority of on-the-scene care for a person with burns is to prevent injury to the rescuer. If needed, fire and emergency medical services should be requested at the first opportunity. Additional emergency procedures are highlighted in Chart 59-2.

Primary Survey

Although the local effects of a burn are the most evident, the systemic effects pose a greater threat to life. Therefore, it is important to remember "ABCDE" of burn trauma care during the early postburn period (ABLS, 2018):

- Airway and cervical spine protection
- Breathing; assess rate and depth or breathing, chest auscultation
- Circulation and cardiac status; blood pressure, heart rate, and skin colour. Cardiac monitoring for patients with all electrical injuries for at least 24 hours after cessation of dysrhythmia. Insert two large bore IVs and initiate fluids; a starting point for adults is Ringer's lactate at 500 mL/hr.
- Disability, Neurologic Deficit, and Gross Deformity
- Exposure; undress the patient and examine for associated injuries while maintaining a warm environment

TABLE 59-3 Phases of Burn Care

Phase	Duration	Priorities
Emergent or immediate resuscitative	From onset of injury to completion of fluid resuscitation	• Primary survey: A, B, C, D, E • Prevention of shock • Prevention of respiratory distress • Detection and treatment of concomitant injuries • Wound assessment and initial care
Acute	From beginning of diuresis to near completion of wound closure	• Wound care and closure • Prevention or treatment of complications, including infection • Nutritional support
Rehabilitation	From major wound closure to return to individual's optimal level of physical and psychosocial adjustment	• Prevention of scars and contractures • Physical, occupational, and vocational rehabilitation • Functional and cosmetic reconstruction • Psychosocial counselling

Adapted from American Burn Association. (2018). Advanced burn life support (ABLS) course provider manual 2018. Chicago, IL; Serghiou, M. A., Ott, S., Cowan, A., et al. (2018). Burn rehabilitation along the continuum of care. In D. Herndon (Ed.). *Total Burn Care* (5th ed.). Edinburgh, UK: Saunders Elsevier.

CHART 59-2

Emergency Procedures at the Burn Scene

- **Extinguish the flames.** When clothes catch fire, the flames can be extinguished if the victim falls to the floor or ground and rolls **until the flames go out** ("stop, drop and roll"); anything available to smother the flames, such as a blanket, rug, or coat, may be used. Standing still forces the victim to breathe flames and smoke, and running fans the flames. If the burn source is electrical, the electrical source must be disconnected.
- **Cool the burn.** After the flames are extinguished, the burned area and adherent clothing are soaked with *cool* water, briefly, to cool the wound and halt the burning process. Once a burn has been sustained, the application of cool water is the best first aid measure. Soaking the burn area intermittently in cool water or applying cool towels gives immediate and striking relief from pain and limits local tissue edema and damage. However, *never apply ice directly to the burn, never wrap patients with burns in ice, and never use cold soaks or dressings for longer than several minutes; such procedures may worsen the tissue damage and lead to hypothermia in patients with large burns.*
- Remove restrictive objects. If possible, remove clothing immediately. Adherent clothing may be left in place once cooled. Other clothing and all jewelry should be removed to allow for assessment and to prevent constriction secondary to rapidly developing edema.
- **Cover the wound.** The burn should be covered as quickly as possible with a clean, dry sheet to minimize bacterial contamination and decrease pain by preventing air from coming into contact with the injured surface. *Ointments and salves should not be used. Other than the dressing, no medication or material should be applied to the burn wound.*
- **Irrigate chemical burns.** Chemical burns resulting from contact with a corrosive material are irrigated immediately. Most chemical laboratories have a high-pressure shower for such emergencies. If such an injury occurs at home, brush off the chemical agent, remove clothes immediately, and rinse all areas of the body that have come in contact with the chemical. Rinsing can occur in the shower or any other source of continuous running water. Flushing/rinsing should be done for *at least* 20 minutes. If a chemical gets in or near the eyes, the eyes should be flushed with cool, clean water immediately. Outcomes for the patient with chemical burns are significantly improved by rapid, sustained flushing of the injury at the scene. *Never attempt to neutralize the chemical, as this could cause further burns.*

NURSING ALERT

Breathing must be assessed and a patent airway established immediately during the initial minutes of emergency care. Immediate therapy is directed toward establishing an airway and administering humidified 100% oxygen. If such a high concentration of oxygen is not available under emergency conditions, oxygen by mask or nasal cannula is given initially. If qualified personnel and equipment are available and if the patient has severe respiratory distress or airway edema, the rescuers can insert an endotracheal tube and initiate manual ventilation.

The circulatory system must also be assessed quickly. Apical pulse and blood pressure are monitored frequently. Tachycardia (abnormally rapid heart rate) and slight hypotension are expected soon after the burn. The neurologic status is assessed quickly in the patient with extensive burns. Often, the patient with burns is awake and alert initially, and vital information can be obtained at that time. A secondary head-to-toe survey of the patient is carried out to identify other potentially life-threatening injuries. Preventing shock in a patient with burns is imperative.

NURSING ALERT

No food or fluid is given by mouth, and the patient is placed in a position (HOB elevated) that will prevent aspiration of vomitus because nausea and vomiting typically occur due to paralytic ileus resulting from the stress of injury.

The burn wound, once it has been cooled, should be wrapped in a clean, dry sheet/cloth. A pillow case is suitable for upper and lower limb injuries. Polyvinyl chloride film (cling film/Saran wrap) is a good alternative to cover the burned areas as it forms an impermeable, nonadherent barrier that minimizes contamination by shielding the burn wound from secondary infection, reduces pain produced by the exposure of the damaged nerve endings (in partial-thickness burns) to the air currents, and provides protection during transport. Being transparent, it also allows the wound to be viewed for assessment without having to be removed, it does not shed fibres into the wound, and it is easily removed without causing further trauma. It is important to lay the film on the patient, not wrap the area, as swelling may lead to constriction. It is advisable to avoid using wet dressings as heat loss during transfer can be considerable. Topical creams should not be applied as this may interfere with subsequent assessments, unless the Burn Centre has specifically requested it (ABA, 2018b). As previously mentioned, once the rescue workers have covered the burn wounds, they should keep the patient warm, have an established airway, supply oxygen, and insert at least two large-bore IV lines.

Medical Management

The patient is transported to the nearest emergency department. The hospital and physician are alerted that the patient is en route to the emergency department so that lifesaving measures can be initiated immediately by a trained team.

Initial priorities in the emergency department remain airway, breathing, and circulation. For mild pulmonary injury, inspired air is humidified and the patient is encouraged to cough so that secretions can be removed by suctioning. For more severe situations, it is necessary to remove secretions by bronchial suctioning and to administer bronchodilators and mucolytic agents. If edema of the airway develops, endotracheal intubation may be necessary. Continuous positive airway pressure and mechanical ventilation may also be required to achieve adequate oxygenation.

After adequate respiratory status and circulatory status have been established, the patient is assessed for cervical spinal injuries or head injury if the patient was involved in an explosion, a fall, a jump, or an electrical injury. Once the patient's condition is stable, attention is directed to the burn wound itself. All clothing and jewelry are removed. For chemical burns, flushing of the exposed areas is continued. The patient is checked for contact lenses. These are removed immediately if chemicals have contacted the eyes or if facial burns have occurred.

It is important to validate an account of the burn scenario provided by the patient, witnesses at the scene, and paramedics. Information needs to include time of the burn injury, source of the burn, TBSA involved, depth of the burn, the place where the burn occurred, how the burn was treated at the scene, and any history of falling with the injury. A history of pre-existing diseases, allergies, and medications and the use of drugs, alcohol, and tobacco is obtained at this point to plan care. Two large-bore (16- or 18-gauge) IV catheters should be inserted in a nonburned area (if not inserted earlier). If the burn exceeds 20% TBSA, a nasogastric tube should be inserted and connected to low intermittent suction. Often, patients with large burns become nauseated as a result of the gastrointestinal effects of the burn injury, such as paralytic ileus (absence of peristalsis), and the effects of medication such as opioids. All patients who are intubated should have a nasogastric tube inserted to decompress the abdomen and prevent vomiting. For burns greater than 20% TBSA, an indwelling urinary catheter is inserted to permit more accurate monitoring of urine output and renal function during fluid resuscitation.

The physician evaluates the patient's general condition, assesses the burn, determines the priorities of care, and directs the individualized plan of treatment, which is divided into systemic management and local care of the burned area. Nonsterile gloves, caps, masks, and gowns are worn by personnel while assessing the exposed burned areas. Clean technique is maintained while assessing burn wounds.

Assessment of both the TBSA burned and the depth of the burn is completed after soot and debris have been gently cleansed from the burn wound. Careful attention is paid to keeping the patient with burns warm during wound assessment and cleansing. Assessment is repeated frequently throughout burn wound care. Photographs may be taken of the burn areas initially and periodically throughout treatment; in this way, the initial injury and burn wound can be documented. Clean sheets are placed under and over the patient to protect the area from contamination, maintain body temperature, and reduce pain caused by air currents passing over exposed nerve endings.

Baseline height, weight, arterial blood gases, hemoglobin, hematocrit, electrolyte values, blood alcohol level, drug panel, urinalysis, and chest x-rays are obtained. If the patient is older or has an electrical burn, a baseline 12-lead electrocardiogram is obtained. Because burns are contaminated wounds, tetanus prophylaxis is administered if the patient's immunization status is not current or is unknown.

Although the major focus of care during the emergent phase is physical stabilization, the nurse must also attend to the patient's and family's psychological needs. Burn injury is a crisis, causing variable emotional responses. The patient's and family's coping abilities and available supports are assessed. Circumstances surrounding the burn injury should be considered when providing care (see Chart 59-3). Individualized psychosocial support must be given to the patient and family. Because the patient with burns is usually anxious and in pain, those in attendance should provide reassurance and support, explanations of procedures, and adequate pain relief. As poor tissue perfusion often accompanies burn injuries, only IV pain medication (usually morphine or fentanyl) is given, titrated for the patient. If the patient wishes to see a spiritual advisor, one is notified.

Transfer to a Burn Centre

The depth and extent of the burn are considered in determining whether the patient should be transferred to a burn centre. Patients with major burns, those who are at the extremes of the age continuum, those with coexisting health problems that may affect recovery, and those with circumstances that increase their risk for acute and long-term complications are transferred to a burn centre. Chart 59-4 lists the ABA's criteria for burn centre referral after initial assessment and management.

If the patient is to be transported to a burn centre, the following measures are instituted before transfer:

- A secure IV catheter is inserted with lactated Ringer's solution infusing at the rate required to maintain a urine output of 0.5 to 1.0 mL/kg/hr
- A patent airway is ensured.
- Adequate pain relief is attained.
- Adequate peripheral circulation is established in any burned extremity.
- Wounds are covered with a clean, dry sheet, and the patient is kept comfortably warm.
- An indwelling urinary catheter is inserted for burns greater than 20% TBSA.

All assessments and treatments are documented, and this information is provided to the burn centre personnel. The transferring facility must relay accurate intake and output totals to burn centre personnel so that adequate fluid resuscitation measures continue.

Management of Fluid Loss and Shock

Next to handling respiratory difficulties, the most urgent need is preventing hypovolemic shock by replacing lost fluids and electrolytes. As mentioned previously, survival of patients with burns depends on adequate fluid resuscitation. Table 59-4 summarizes the fluid and electrolyte changes in the emergent phase of burn care. IV lines and an indwelling urinary catheter must be in place before implementing fluid resuscitation. Baseline weight and laboratory test results are obtained as well. These parameters must be monitored closely in the immediate postburn (resuscitation) period.

Fluid Replacement Therapy

The total volume and rate of IV fluid replacement are gauged by the patient's response. The adequacy of fluid

CHART 59-3

Ethical Dilemma: How Much Is Enough and What Is Comfort Care?

Case Scenario

A 66-year-old man was transported to the nearest burn centre, where you work as a staff nurse. He was drinking beer and cooking steaks on top of a propane grill. He inexplicably threw lighter fluid on the grill and it engulfed his upper torso and face in flames. He sustained a full-thickness burn to 42% of his body (face, neck, both arms, and chest). He was awake at the scene of injury when paramedics arrived and indicated a past medical history of hypertension, hypercholesterolemia, and gout. He was in little pain at the time due to the depth of the burn injury; however, he was asking the team questions related to the survivability of his injury, "Am I going to die?"

Given the extensiveness of his facial burns, he was intubated upon admission to the burn centre. Family arrived, and the burn surgeon explained the extent of injury. A decision was made to proceed with care and assess his progress post resuscitation. They were prepared for a future decision regarding withdrawal of care if survival becomes futile.

Initial resuscitation has occurred, and approximately 4 days post burn, the patient begins to show signs of acute kidney injury. He has had one surgical procedure for débridement and grafting to his chest, and although grafts are intact, they do not look healthy. He is showing increased signs of discomfort and pain due to the operative procedure and the addition of another wound (the new donor site). In a team meeting, the family decides that they do not want to initiate hemodialysis and therefore place the patient on comfort measures. Approximately 3 days later, he remains on comfort care and has increased signs of restlessness and pain. You are caring for the patient and request that the physician prescribe an increase in pain medication from 5-mg morphine to 8 mg IV. Within 2 hours after administration, the patient expired without discomfort. Six months later, the facility is contacted by an attorney and informed that the family is taking legal action against you and the physician for performing euthanasia on the patient.

Discussion

Clinicians on burn teams commonly face these types of ethical dilemmas. Whenever possible, the team should attempt to elicit the patient's wishes as early as possible, including any advance directives. It is important to collaborate and communicate with the family regarding end-of-life care. Although the family agreed to "comfort care," there may have been ambiguity regarding what this entails. The problem in this case is that due to absence of pain, it is often difficult for a patient to understand the severity of their burn injury. The patient begins to experience increased pain as care progresses, and increased medication is expected. As the medication is increased to relieve pain and suffering but death ensued, the *Doctrine of Double Effect* comes into play. The medication given relieved the pain and suffering but the "bad" effect or death occurred. In such cases, the outcome may be predicted but it is not the intention of the intervention.

Analysis

- Describe the ethical principles that are in conflict in this case (see Chapter 3). Which principle should have preeminence as you proceeded to work with this family?
- Would you describe your role in this case as complicit with assisted suicide, active euthanasia, or providing palliation? What distinction, if any, might there be among these three acts? Do you believe that this was a survivable injury?
- Describe how the ethical principles of autonomy, beneficence, and nonmaleficence may intersect or be at odds with each other in this case (see Chapter 3). As a member of the burn team when the patient arrived at your facility, what could you have done differently to ensure that the patient's autonomy was preserved before he was intubated?
- What were the "intentions" in this case? How might intentionality be instrumental in making this act of titrating medications that provided palliation morally defensible? Is this nursing intervention morally defensible according to the principle of double effect (see Chapter 3).
- Note that the American Nurses Association (2015) *Code of Ethics* clearly states that nurses should not *intentionally* cause a patient's death.

REFERENCES

American Nurses Association. (2015). Code of ethics for nurses with interpretive statements. Washington, DC: American Nurses Publishing, American Nurses Foundation/ American Nurses Association.

Beauchamp, T. L., & Childress, J. F. (2012). *Principles of biomedical ethics* (7th ed.). New York: Oxford University Press.

resuscitation is determined by following urine output totals, an index of renal perfusion. Output totals of 0.5 to 1.0 mL/kg/hr (30 to 60 mL/hr) have been used as goals. Other indicators of adequate fluid replacement are vital signs, cognitive status, and extremity temperature.

NURSING ALERT

Clinical parameters are far more important in resuscitation than any formula. Indeed, the patient's individual response is the key to assessing the adequacy of fluid resuscitation.

Additional gauges of fluid requirements and response to fluid resuscitation include hematocrit, hemoglobin, and serum sodium levels. If the hematocrit and the hemoglobin levels decrease or if the urinary output exceeds 1 mL/kg/hr (60 mL/hr), the rate of IV fluid administration should be decreased. The exception is electrical injuries where urine output goals are higher, usually 1.0 to 1.5 mL/kg/hr (75 to 100 mL/hr) until myoglobin clears. The goal is to maintain serum sodium levels in the normal range during fluid replacement.

The goal of optimal fluid resuscitation is adequate organ perfusion while administering the least amount of fluid to avoid complications of overresuscitation. Factors that are associated with the increased fluid requirements include

CHART 59-4

American Burn Association Criteria for Referral to a Burn Centre

- Partial-thickness burns covering 10% of total body surface area or greater
- Burns involving the face, hands, feet, genitalia, perineum, or major joints
- Third-degree burns
- Electrical burns, including lightning injury
- Chemical burns
- Inhalation injury
- Burn injury in patients with pre-existing medical disorders
- Any patients with burns and concomitant trauma
- Children with burn injuries in facilities that do not specialize in pediatric care
- Patients who will require special social, emotional, or long-term rehabilitation

Adapted from American Burn Association. (2011). *Advanced burn life support (ABLS) course provider manual 2011*. Chicago, IL: Author.

delayed resuscitation, scald burn injuries, inhalation injuries, high-voltage electrical injuries, hyperglycemia, alcohol intoxication, and chronic diuretic therapy. Second 24-hour postburn fluid infusion rates incorporate both the maintenance amount of fluid and any additional fluid needs secondary to evaporative water loss through the burn wound. Underresuscitation can also be detrimental to the patient and lead to organ failure, with AKI being the most common consequence of hypovolemia. It is important to reassess the patient's mental status frequently; anxiety and restlessness are also early signs of hypovolemia (ABA, 2018c; Cartotto, Greenhalgh, & Cancio, 2017).

Fluid Requirements

The projected fluid requirements for the first 24 hours are calculated by the clinician based on the extent of the burn injury. Superficial burns are not included in TBSA for fluid resuscitation determination and increase the risk of overresuscitation (ABLS, 2018). Some combination of fluid categories may be used: colloids (whole blood, plasma, and plasma expanders) and crystalloids/electrolytes (lactated Ringer's solution or physiologic sodium chloride). Adequate fluid resuscitation results in slightly decreased blood volume levels during the first 24 postburn hours and restores plasma levels to normal by the end of 48 hours. Oral resuscitation can be successful in adults with less than 20% TBSA and children with less than 10% TBSA (ABA, 2018c).

Formulas have been developed for estimating fluid loss based on the estimated percentage of burned TBSA and the weight of the patient. The length of time since the burn injury occurred is also very important in calculating estimated fluid needs. Formulas must be adjusted so that initiation of fluid replacement reflects the time of injury. Resuscitation formulas are approximations only and are individualized to meet the requirements of each patient. The various formulas are discussed below and summarized in Chart 59-5.

As early as 1978, the National Institutes of Health Consensus Development Conference on Supportive Therapy in Burn Care established that salt and water are required in patients with burns but that colloid may or may not be useful during the first 24 to 48 postburn hours. In 2008, the ABA recommended a guideline as research suggests fluid resuscitation based on 4 mL/kg/hr often results in overresuscitation and excessive edema (ABA, 2018c). The American Burn Association Consensus formula, also termed the "adjusted fluid rate," provides for the volume of IV solution required in the first 24 hours after burn injury. In general, 2 mL/kg per percent second- and third-degree burns of lactated Ringer's solution may be used initially for adults as it most closely resembles extracellular (normal body) fluids. Starting from the time of injury, half of the calculated fluid total is to be given over the first 8 postburn hours. The rate and volume of the infusion must be regulated according to the patient's response by changing the hourly infusion rates. Fluid boluses are recommended only

TABLE 59-4 Fluid and Electrolyte Changes in the Emergent/Resuscitative Phase

Fluid accumulation phase (shock phase)
Plasma → interstitial fluid (edema at burn site)

Observation	Explanation
Generalized dehydration	Plasma leaks through damaged capillaries
Reduction of blood volume	Secondary to plasma loss, fall of blood pressure, and diminished cardiac output
Decreased urinary output	Secondary to: Fluid loss Decreased renal blood flow Sodium and water retention caused by increased adrenocortical activity (hemolysis of red blood cells, causing hemoglobinuria and myonecrosis or myoglobinuria)
Potassium (K^+) excess	Massive cellular trauma causes release of K^+ into extracellular fluid (ordinarily, most K^+ is intracellular)
Sodium (Na^+) deficit	Large amount of Na^+ is lost in trapped edema fluid and exudate and by shift into cells as K^+ is released from cells (ordinarily most Na^+ is extracellular)
Metabolic acidosis (base-bicarbonate deficit)	Loss of bicarbonate ions accompanies sodium loss
Hemoconcentration (elevated hematocrit)	Liquid blood component is lost into extravascular space

CHART 59-5

Guidelines and Formulas for Fluid Replacement in Burn Patients

American Burn Association Consensus Formula

Lactated Ringer's solution: 2 mL × kg body weight × % total body surface area (TBSA) burned. Half to be given in first 8 hours. Continued assessment and adjustment of fluid based on the individual patient's response.

Evans Formula

1. Colloids: 1 mL × kg body weight × % TBSA burned
2. Electrolytes (saline): 1 mL × kg body weight × % TBSA burned
3. Glucose (5% in water): 2,000 mL for insensible loss

Day 1: Half to be given in first 8 hours; remaining half over next 16 hours

Day 2: Half of previous day's colloids and electrolytes; all of insensible fluid replacement

Maximum of 10,000 mL over 24 hours. Second- and third-degree (partial- and full-thickness) burns exceeding 50% TBSA are calculated on the basis of 50% TBSA.

Brooke Army Formula

1. Colloids: 0.5 mL × kg body weight × % TBSA burned
2. Electrolytes (lactated Ringer's solution): 1.5 mL × kg body weight × % TBSA burned
3. Glucose (5% in water): 2,000 mL for insensible loss

Day 1: Half to be given in first 8 hours; remaining half over next 16 hours

Day 2: Half of colloids; half of electrolytes; all of insensible fluid replacement

Second- and third-degree (partial- and full-thickness) burns exceeding 50% TBSA are calculated on the basis of 50% TBSA.

Parkland/Baxter Formula

Lactated Ringer's solution: 4 mL × kg body weight × % TBSA burned

Day 1: Half to be given in first 8 hours; half to be given over next 16 hours

Day 2: Varies. Colloid is added

Hypertonic Saline Solution

Concentrated solutions of sodium chloride (NaCl) and lactate with concentration of 250–300 mEq of sodium per litre, administered at a rate sufficient to maintain a desired volume of urinary output. Do not increase the infusion rate during the first 8 postburn hours. The risk of hypernatremia and the risk of renal failure must be monitored closely. Goal: Increase serum sodium level and osmolality to reduce edema and prevent pulmonary complications.

in the presence of marked hypotension, not low urine output. For adult patients with an electrical injury the starting point is suggested at 4 mL/kg per percent second- and third-degree burns. For pediatric patients, the ABA suggests 3 mL/kg per percent second- and third-degree burns, again giving half in the first 8 hours. In infants and young children less than 30 kg, lactated Ringer's with 5% dextrose should be added at a maintenance rate (ABA, 2018c). There is still not complete agreement about which fluid resuscitation formula is best for burn injury. Again, practitioners should take note that the resuscitation formulas serve only as guidelines, and the patient's response to fluid therapy is the best parameter to use (ABA, 2018c).

Studies demonstrate that with large burns, there is a failure of the sodium-potassium pump (a physiologic mechanism involved in fluid–electrolyte balance) at the cellular level. Thus, patients with very large burns may need proportionately more millilitres of fluid per percent of burn than those with smaller burns. Also, patients with electrical injury, pulmonary injury, and delayed fluid resuscitation and those who were burned while intoxicated may need additional fluids.

The following example illustrates use of the Consensus formula in a 70-kg patient with a 50% TBSA burn:

1. American Burn Association Consensus formula: 2 mL/kg/% TBSA
2. 2 × 70 × 50 = 7,000 mL/24 hr
3. Plan to administer: First 8 hours = 3,500 mL, or 473 mL/hr

Most fluid replacement formulas use isotonic electrolyte solutions. Regardless of which standard replacement formula is used, the patient receives approximately the same fluid volume and sodium replacement during the first 48 hours.

Another fluid replacement method requires hypertonic electrolyte solutions. This method uses concentrated solutions of sodium chloride and lactate (a balanced salt solution) so that the resulting fluid has a concentration of 250 to 300 mEq of sodium. The rationale for this replacement method is that by increasing serum osmolality, fluid will be pulled back into the vascular space from the interstitial space. Reduced systemic and pulmonary edema has been reported after administering hypertonic solutions. There is a need for close monitoring for risk of hypernatremia and renal failure (Cartotto et al., 2017).

NURSING ALERT

Formulas are only a guide. The patient's response, evidenced by heart rate, blood pressure, and urine output, is the primary determinant of actual fluid therapy and must be assessed at least hourly. Patient outcomes are improved by optimal fluid resuscitation.

Gerontologic Considerations

Decreased function of the cardiovascular, renal, and pulmonary systems increases the need for close observation of older patients with even relatively minor burns during the emergent and acute phases. Acute renal failure is much more common in older patients than in those younger than 40 years. The margin of difference between hypovolemia and fluid overload is very small. Suppressed immunologic response, a high incidence of malnutrition, and an inability to withstand metabolic stressors (e.g., a cold environment) further compromise the older person's ability to heal. As a result of these issues in older patients who sustain burn injury, close monitoring and prompt treatment of complications are mandatory.

Nursing Management

Assessment data obtained by prehospital providers (rescuers such as emergency medical technicians) are shared with the physician and nurse in the emergency department. Nursing assessment in the emergent phase of burn injury focuses on the major priorities for any trauma patient; the burn wound is a secondary consideration. Aseptic management of the burn wounds and invasive lines continues.

The nurse monitors vital signs frequently. Respiratory status is monitored closely, and apical, carotid, and femoral pulses are evaluated. Cardiac monitoring is indicated if the patient has a history of cardiac disease, electrical injury, or respiratory problems or if the pulse is dysrhythmic or the rate is abnormally slow or rapid.

If all extremities are burned, determining blood pressure may be difficult. A sterile dressing applied under the blood pressure cuff will protect the wound from contamination. Because increasing edema makes blood pressure difficult to auscultate, a Doppler (ultrasound) device or a noninvasive electronic blood pressure device may be helpful. In severe burns, an arterial catheter is used for blood pressure measurement and for collecting blood specimens. Peripheral pulses of burned extremities are monitored hourly; the Doppler device is useful for this. Elevation of burned extremities is crucial to decrease edema. Elevation of the upper and lower extremities on pillows may be helpful.

Large-bore IV catheters and an indwelling urinary catheter are inserted, if not already in place, and the nurse's assessment includes monitoring fluid intake and output. Urine output, an indicator of renal perfusion, is monitored carefully and measured hourly. The amount of urine first obtained when the urinary catheter was inserted is recorded. This may assist in determining the extent of preburn renal function and fluid status. Urine specific gravity, pH, and glucose, acetone, protein, and hemoglobin levels are assessed frequently.

Red-tinged urine suggests the presence of hemochromogen and myoglobin resulting from muscle damage. This is associated with deep burns caused by electrical injury or prolonged contact with flames. Glucosuria, a common finding in the early postburn hours, results from the release of stored glucose from the liver in response to stress.

Although not responsible for calculating the patient's fluid requirements, the nurse needs to know the maximum volume of fluid the patient should receive. Infusion pumps and rate controllers are used to deliver a complex regimen of prescribed IV fluids. Administering and monitoring IV therapy are major nursing responsibilities.

Body temperature, body weight, preburn weight, and history of allergies, tetanus immunization, past medical and surgical problems, current illnesses, and use of medications are assessed. A head-to-toe assessment is performed, focusing on signs and symptoms of concomitant illness, injury, or developing complications. Patients with facial burns should have their eyes examined for potential injury to the corneas. An ophthalmologist is consulted for complete assessment via fluorescent staining.

Assessing the extent of the burn wound continues and is facilitated with anatomic diagrams (described previously). In addition, the nurse works with the physician to assess the depth of the wound and areas of full- and partial-thickness injury. Assessment of the circumstances surrounding the injury is important. Obtaining a history of the burn injury can help to plan the care for the patient. Assessment should include the time of injury, mechanism of burn, whether the burn occurred in a closed space, the possibility of inhalation of noxious chemicals, and any related trauma.

The neurologic assessment focuses on the patient's level of consciousness, psychological status, pain and anxiety levels, and behaviour. The patient's and family's understanding of the injury and treatment is assessed as well.

Nursing care of the patient during the emergent/resuscitative phase of burn injury is detailed in the Plan of Nursing Care (Chart 59-6).

Acute or Intermediate Phase

The acute or intermediate phase of burn care follows the emergent/resuscitative phase and begins 48 to 72 hours after the burn injury. During this phase, attention is directed toward continued assessment and maintenance of respiratory and circulatory status, fluid and electrolyte balance, and gastrointestinal function. Infection prevention, burn wound care (i.e., wound cleaning, wound débridement, topical antibacterial therapy, wound dressing, dressing changes, and skin grafting), pain management, and nutritional support are priorities at this stage and will be discussed in detail.

Medical Management

Airway obstruction caused by upper airway edema can take as long as 48 hours to develop. Changes detected by x-ray and arterial blood gases may occur as the effects of resuscitative fluid and the chemical reaction of smoke components with lung tissues become apparent. Pulmonary complications are not unusual in burn injury. Those with ventilator-associated pneumonia (VAP) have an increased mortality rate. Ideally, the best practice is to remove the endotracheal tube as soon as possible so that a route for pathogens is not accessible to the lungs. The arterial blood gas values and other parameters determine the need for intubation or mechanical ventilation.

As capillaries regain integrity, at 48 or more postburn hours, fluid moves from the interstitial to the intravascular compartment and diuresis begins (Table 59-5). If cardiac or renal function is inadequate, for instance in the older patient or in the patient with pre-existing cardiac disease, fluid overload occurs and symptoms of congestive heart failure may result (see Chapter 31). Early detection allows for early intervention and carefully calculated fluid intake. Vasoactive medications, diuretics, and fluid

(text continued on page 1854)

Plan of Nursing Care

Chart 59-6. Care of the Patient During the Emergent/Resuscitative Phase of Burn Injury

Nursing Priority: Impaired gas exchange
Goal: Maintenance of adequate tissue oxygenation

NURSING INTERVENTIONS	RATIONALE	EXPECTED OUTCOMES
1. Provide humidified oxygen.	1. Humidified oxygen provides moisture to injured tissues; supplemental oxygen increases alveolar oxygenation.	• Absence of dyspnea • Respiratory rate between 12 and 20 breaths/min • Breaths sounds clear on auscultation • Arterial oxygen saturation >94% by pulse oximetry • Arterial blood gas levels within normal limits
2. Assess breath sounds, and respiratory rate, rhythm, depth, and symmetry. Monitor patient for signs of hypoxia.	2. These factors provide baseline data for further assessment and evidence of increasing respiratory compromise.	
3. Observe for the following: a. Erythema or blistering of lips or buccal mucosa b. Singed nostrils c. Burns of face, neck, or chest d. Increasing hoarseness e. Soot in sputum or tracheal tissue in respiratory secretions	3. These signs indicate possible inhalation injury and risk of respiratory dysfunction.	
4. Monitor arterial blood gas values, pulse oximetry readings, and carboxyhemoglobin levels.	4. Increasing PCO_2 and decreasing PO_2 and O_2 saturation may indicate need for mechanical ventilation.	
5. Report laboured respirations, decreased depth of respirations, or signs of hypoxia to physician immediately.	5. Immediate intervention is indicated for respiratory difficulty.	
6. Prepare to assist with intubation and escharotomies.	6. Intubation allows airway patency and mechanical ventilation. Escharotomy enables chest excursion in circumferential chest burns.	
7. Monitor mechanically ventilated patient closely.	7. Monitoring allows early detection of decreasing respiratory status or complications of mechanical ventilation.	
8. Assist with bronchoscopy	8. Gold standard for assessment of inhalation injury. Allows for direct visualization of upper and lower airways, direct evidence of charring, soot deposition, and/or mucosal ulceration.	

Nursing Priority: Ineffective airway clearance
Goal: Maintain patent airway and adequate airway clearance

NURSING INTERVENTIONS	RATIONALE	EXPECTED OUTCOMES
1. Maintain patent airway through proper patient positioning, removal of secretions, and artificial airway if needed.	1. A patent airway is crucial to respiration.	• Patent airway • Respiratory secretions are minimal, colourless, and thin • Respiratory rate, pattern, and breath sounds normal
2. Provide humidified oxygen.	2. Humidity liquefies secretions and facilitates expectoration.	
3. Encourage patient to mobilize, turn, cough, and deep breathe. Encourage patient to use incentive spirometry. Suction as needed.	3. These activities promote mobilization and removal of secretions.	

Plan of Nursing Care

Chart 59-6. Care of the Patient During the Emergent/Resuscitative Phase of Burn Injury, *Continued*

Nursing Priority: Fluid volume deficit
Goal: Restoration of optimal fluid and electrolyte balance and perfusion of vital organs

NURSING INTERVENTIONS	RATIONALE	EXPECTED OUTCOMES
1. Observe vital signs (including central venous pressure or pulmonary artery pressure, if indicated) and urine output, and be alert for signs of hypovolemia or fluid overload.	1. Hypovolemia is a major risk immediately after the burn injury. Over resuscitation might cause fluid overload.	• Serum electrolytes within normal limits • Urine output between 30–60 mL/hr • Blood pressure higher than 90/60 mm Hg • Heart rate less than 120 beats/min • Exhibits clear sensorium • Voids clear yellow urine with specific gravity within normal limits
2. Monitor urine output at least hourly, and weigh patient daily.	2. Output and weight provide information about renal perfusion, adequacy of fluid replacement, and fluid requirement and fluid status.	
3. Maintain intravenous (IV) lines and regulate fluids at appropriate rates, as prescribed.	3. Adequate fluids are necessary to maintain fluid and electrolyte balance and perfusion of vital organs.	
4. Observe for symptoms of deficiency or excess of serum sodium, potassium, calcium, phosphorus, and bicarbonate.	4. Rapid shifts in fluid and electrolyte status are possible in the postburn period.	
5. Elevate head of patient's bed, and elevate burned extremities.	5. Elevation promotes venous return, decreases the cardiac workload of the heart, assists in the prevention of aspiration and facilitates ventilation, and reduces edema in the head, neck, and hands.	
6. Notify physician immediately of decreased urine output, blood pressure, central venous, pulmonary artery, or pulmonary artery wedge pressures, or increased pulse rate.	6. Because of the rapid fluid shifts in burn shock, fluid deficit must be detected early so that distributive shock does not occur.	

Nursing Priority: Hypothermia
Goal: Maintenance of adequate body temperature

NURSING INTERVENTIONS	RATIONALE	EXPECTED OUTCOMES
1. Provide a warm environment through use of warm blankets, heat lamps, and forced-air warming blankets (i.e., Bair huggers).	1. A stable environment minimizes evaporative heat loss.	• Body temperature remains 36.1–38.3°C • Absence of chills or shivering
2. Work quickly when wounds must be exposed.	2. Minimal exposure minimizes heat loss from wound.	
3. Assess core body temperature frequently.	3. Frequent temperature assessments help to detect developing hypothermia.	

Nursing Priority: Pain
Goal: Control of pain

NURSING INTERVENTIONS	RATIONALE	EXPECTED OUTCOMES
1. Use a pain intensity scale to assess pain level (i.e., 0–10). Differentiate from hypoxia.	1. Pain level provides baseline for evaluating effectiveness of pain relief measures. Hypoxia can cause similar signs and must be ruled out before analgesic medication is administered.	• States pain level is decreased • Absence of nonverbal cues of pain
2. Administer IV opioid analgesics as prescribed. Observe for respiratory depression in the patient who is not mechanically ventilated. Assess response to analgesic.	2. IV administration is necessary because of altered tissue perfusion from burn injury.	
3. Provide emotional support and reassurance.	3. Emotional support is essential to reduce fear and anxiety resulting from burn injury. Fear and anxiety increase the perception of pain.	

continued >

Plan of Nursing Care — Chart 59-6. Care of the Patient During the Emergent/Resuscitative Phase of Burn Injury, *Continued*

NURSING INTERVENTIONS	RATIONALE	EXPECTED OUTCOMES
Nursing Priority: Anxiety **Goal:** Minimization of patient and family's anxiety		
1. Assess patient and family's understanding of burn injury, coping skills, and family dynamics.	1. Previous successful coping strategies can be encouraged for use in the present crisis. Assessment allows planning of individualized interventions.	• Patient and family verbalize understanding of emergent burn care • Able to answer simple questions • The patient will develop effective coping strategies
2. Individualize responses to the patient and family's coping level.	2. Reactions to burn injury are extremely variable. Interventions must be appropriate to the patient and family's present level of coping.	
3. Explain all procedures to the patient and the family in clear, simple terms.	3. Increased understanding alleviates fear of the unknown. High levels of anxiety may interfere with understanding of complex explanations.	
4. Maintain adequate pain relief.	4. Pain increases anxiety.	
5. Consider administering prescribed anti-anxiety medications if the patient remains extremely anxious despite nonpharmacologic interventions.	5. Anxiety levels during the emergent phase may exceed the patient's coping abilities. Medication decreases physiologic and psychological anxiety responses.	
6. Consider consulting psychology.	6. Depression, regression, and manipulative behaviour are common responses of patients who have burn injuries.	
Collaborative Problems: Acute respiratory failure, distributive shock, acute renal failure, compartment syndrome, paralytic ileus, Curling's ulcer **Goal:** Absence of complications		
Acute Respiratory Failure		
1. Assess for increasing dyspnea, stridor, changes in respiratory patterns.	1. Such signs reflect deteriorating respiratory status.	• Arterial blood gas values within acceptable limits: • PO_2 >80 mm Hg • PCO_2 <50 mm Hg • Breathes spontaneously with adequate tidal volume • Chest x-ray findings normal • Absence of cerebral signs of hypoxia
2. Monitor pulse oximetry, arterial blood gas values for decreasing PO_2 and oxygen saturation, and increasing PCO_2.	2. Such signs reflect decreased oxygenation status.	
3. Monitor chest x-ray results.	3. X-ray may disclose pulmonary injury.	
4. Assess for restlessness, confusion, difficulty attending to questions, or decreasing level of consciousness.	4. Such manifestations may indicate cerebral hypoxia. May also indicate sepsis.	
5. Report deteriorating respiratory status immediately to physician.	5. Acute respiratory failure is life threatening, and immediate intervention is required.	
6. Prepare to assist with intubation or escharotomies as indicated.	6. Intubation allows mechanical ventilation. Escharotomies allow improved chest excursion with respirations.	
Distributive Shock		
1. Assess for decreasing urine output, central venous pressures, pulmonary artery and pulmonary artery wedge pressures, blood pressure, and cardiac output, or increasing pulse.	1. Such signs and symptoms may indicate distributive shock and inadequate intravascular volume.	• Urine output between 30–60 mL/hr • Blood pressure within patient's expected range (usually >90/60 mm Hg)

Plan of Nursing Care

Chart 59-6. Care of the Patient During the Emergent/Resuscitative Phase of Burn Injury, *Continued*

NURSING INTERVENTIONS	RATIONALE	EXPECTED OUTCOMES
2. Assess for progressive edema as fluid shifts occur.	2. As fluid shifts into the interstitial spaces in burn shock, edema occurs and may compromise tissue perfusion. A pulse rate <110 beats/min in adults usually indicates adequate volume; with rates >120 beats/min usually indicative of hypovolemia. Narrowed pulse pressure provides an earlier indication of shock than systolic blood pressure alone.	• Heart rate within patient's expected range (usually <110/min). • Pressures and cardiac output remain within normal limits
3. Adjust fluid resuscitation in collaboration with the physician in response to physiologic findings.	3. Optimal fluid resuscitation prevents distributive shock and improves patient outcomes.	
Acute Kidney Injury		
1. Monitor urine output and blood urea nitrogen (BUN) and creatinine levels.	1. These values reflect renal function.	• Adequate urine output • BUN and creatinine values remain normal
2. Report decreased urine output or increased BUN and creatinine values to physician.	2. These laboratory values indicate possible renal failure.	
3. Assess urine for hemoglobin or myoglobin.	3. Hemoglobin or myoglobin in the urine points to an increased risk of renal failure.	
4. Administer increased fluids as prescribed.	4. Fluids help to flush out hemoglobin and myoglobin from renal tubules, decreasing the potential for renal failure.	
Compartment Syndrome		
1. Assess peripheral pulses hourly with Doppler ultrasound device.	1. Assessment with Doppler device substitutes for auscultation and indicates characteristics of arterial blood flow.	• Absence of paresthesias or symptoms of ischemia of nerves and muscles • Peripheral pulses detectable by Doppler
2. Assess warmth, capillary refill, sensation, and movement of extremity hourly. Compare affected with unaffected extremity.	2. These assessments indicate characteristics of peripheral perfusion.	
3. Remove blood pressure cuff after each reading.	3. Cuff may act as a tourniquet as extremities become edematous.	
4. Elevate burned extremities.	4. Elevation reduces edema formation.	
5. Report loss of pulse or sensation or presence of pain to physician immediately.	5. These signs and symptoms may indicate inadequate tissue perfusion.	
6. Prepare to assist with escharotomies.	6. Escharotomies relieve the constriction caused by edema under circumferential burns and improve tissue perfusion.	
Paralytic Ileus		
1. For burns greater than 25%—maintain nasogastric tube on low intermittent suction until bowel sounds resume.	1. This measure relieves gastric and abdominal distention, also prevents vomiting.	• Absence of abdominal distention • Normal bowel sounds within 48 hours
2. Auscultate for bowel sounds, abdominal distention.	2. As bowel sounds resume, feeding may be slowly initiated. Abdominal distention reflects inadequate decompression.	
Curling's Ulcer		
1. Assess gastric aspirate for pH and blood.	1. Acidic pH indicates need for antacids or histamine blockers. Blood indicates possible gastric bleeding.	• Absence of abdominal distention • Normal bowel sounds within 48 hours • Gastric aspirate and stools do not contain blood
2. Assess stools for occult blood.	2. Blood in stools may indicate gastric or duodenal ulcer.	
3. Administer histamine blockers and antacids as prescribed.	3. Such medications reduce gastric acidity and risk of ulceration.	

TABLE 59-5 Fluid and Electrolyte Changes in the Acute Phase

Fluid remobilization phase (state of diuresis)
Interstitial fluid → plasma

Observation	Explanation
Hemodilution (decreased hematocrit)	Blood cell concentration is diluted as fluid enters the intravascular compartment; loss of red blood cells destroyed at burn site.
Increased urinary output	Fluid shift into intravascular compartment increases renal blood flow and causes increased urine formation.
Sodium (Na^+) deficit	With diuresis, sodium is lost with water; existing serum sodium is diluted by water influx.
Potassium (K^+) deficit (occurs occasionally in this phase)	Beginning on the fourth or fifth postburn day, K^+ shifts from extracellular fluid into cells.
Metabolic acidosis	Loss of sodium depletes fixed base; relative carbon dioxide content increases.

restriction may be used to support circulatory function and prevent congestive heart failure and pulmonary edema.

Cautious administration of fluids and electrolytes continues during this phase of burn care because of the shifts in fluid from the interstitial to intravascular compartments, losses of fluid from large burn wounds, and the patient's physiologic responses to the burn injury. Blood components are administered as needed to treat blood loss and anemia.

Fever is common in patients with burns after burn shock resolves. A resetting of the core body temperature in severely burned patients results in a body temperature a few degrees higher than normal for several weeks after the burn. Bacteremia and septicemia also cause fever in many patients. Acetaminophen and hypothermia blankets may be required to maintain body temperature in a range of 37.2° to 38.3°C to reduce metabolic stress and tissue oxygen demand.

Infection Prevention

Prevention is the best way to minimize infection. Despite aseptic precautions and the use of topical antimicrobial agents, the burn wound is an excellent medium for bacterial growth and proliferation. The burn eschar is a nonviable crust with no blood supply; therefore, neither polymorphonuclear leukocytes or antibodies nor systemic antibiotics can reach the area. The typical burn wound is initially colonized predominantly with gram-positive organisms, which are fairly quickly replaced by antibiotic-susceptible gram-negative organisms, usually within a week of the burn injury (Cambiaso-Daniel et al., 2018). Methicillin-susceptible *Staphylococcus aureus*, methicillin-resistant *Staphylococcus aureus* (MRSA), enterococci, including vancomycin-resistant enterococci (VRE), gram-negative bacteria, and *Candida* are prevalent pathogens in burn infections. If the patient becomes infected due to delays in wound closure and requires treatment with broad-spectrum antibiotics, the normal bacterial flora may be replaced by yeasts, fungi, and antibiotic-resistant bacteria.

The primary source of bacterial infection appears to be the patient's intestinal tract, which is the source of most microbes. The intestinal mucosa normally serves as a barrier to keep the internal environment free from a variety of pathogens. After a severe burn injury, the intestinal mucosal barrier becomes markedly permeable. Because of this impaired intestinal mucosal barrier, the disturbed microbial flora and endotoxins found in the intestinal lumen pass freely into the systemic circulation, finally causing infection. If the intestinal mucosa receives some type of protection against permeability change, infection could be avoided. Early enteral feeding is one step to help avoid this increased intestinal permeability and prevent early endotoxin translocation. Infection impedes burn wound healing by promoting excessive inflammation and damaging tissue. A major secondary source of pathogenic microbes is the environment. Infection control is a major role of the burn team in providing appropriate burn wound care. Personal protective equipment is worn while caring for the patient with open burn wounds. Strict aseptic technique with frequent hand washing is used when caring directly for burn wounds.

Wound bacterial swabs may obtained regularly to monitor colonization of the burn wound. Antibiotics are seldom prescribed prophylactically because of the risk of promoting resistant strains of bacteria. Systemic antibiotics are administered when there is documentation of burn wound sepsis or other positive cultures such as urine, sputum, or blood. Sensitivity of the organisms to the prescribed antibiotics should be determined before administration. Several parenteral antimicrobial agents may be given together to treat the infection. Careful attention is paid to antibiotic use in the burn unit because inappropriate use of antibiotics significantly affects the microbial flora present in the unit and increases the risk of drug resistance.

Wound Cleansing

The goal of wound cleansing is to remove bacteria and debris with as little chemical and mechanical force as possible to prevent trauma to the healthy tissue but with enough force to remove loose bacteria and debris. Always cleanse a wound before applying a new dressing (Jeschke & Peck, 2017). Individuals with small open burns (less than 10%) may shower using mild soap and running water.

Hydrotherapy equipment is an important environmental reservoir of gram-negative organisms. Its use for burn care is discouraged based on demonstrated associations between use of contaminated hydrotherapy equipment and infections. Burn wound infections and colonization as well as bloodstream infections caused by multidrug-resistant *Pseudomonas aeruginosa, Acinetobacter baumannii,* and MRSA have been associated with hydrotherapy.

Patients have their wounds cleansed at the bedside using sterile normal saline or sterile water by means of sequential cleansing to decrease the risks of cross contamination. Unburned areas, including the hair, must be washed regularly as well. At the time of wound cleaning, all skin is inspected for any hints of redness, breakdown, or local infection. Hair that is in and 5 cm around the burn area, except the eyebrows, should be shaved.

Small intact blisters, unless interfering with range of motion, may be left intact. Blisters larger than 1 cm in diameter should be deroofed and debrided 1 to 2 days postburn. All blisters that are a result of a chemical burn should be deroofed (Jeschke & Peck, 2017). There are high levels of inflammatory mediators in blister fluid, which can lead to increases in ischemia in the burn wound (Micak & Buffalo, 2007).

Conscientious management of the burn wound is essential. When nonviable loose skin is removed, aseptic conditions must be established. Wound cleaning is usually performed at least daily in wound areas that are not undergoing surgical intervention. When the eschar begins to separate from the viable tissue beneath (approximately 1.5 to 2.0 weeks after the burn), more frequent cleaning and débridement may be in order.

After the burn wounds are cleaned, the prescribed method of dressing care is performed. Physician preferences, the availability of skilled nursing staff, and resources in terms of number of personnel, supplies, and time must be considered in choosing the best method for a given patient. Whatever the method, the goal is to protect the wound from overwhelming proliferation of pathogenic organisms and invasion of deeper tissues until either spontaneous healing or skin grafting can be achieved.

Patient comfort and ability to participate in the prescribed treatment are also important considerations. Wound care procedures are metabolically stressful. Therefore, the patient is assessed for signs of chilling, fatigue, changes in hemodynamic status, and pain unrelieved by analgesic medications or relaxation techniques.

Topical Antibacterial Therapy

There is general agreement that some form of antimicrobial therapy applied to the burn wound is the best method of local care in extensive burn injury. Topical antibacterial therapy does not sterilize the burn wound; it simply reduces the number of bacteria so that the overall microbial population can be controlled by the body's host defense mechanisms. Topical therapy promotes conversion of the open, dirty wound to a closed, clean one.

Criteria for choosing a topical agent include the following:

- It is effective against gram-negative organisms, *P. aeruginosa*, *Staphylococcus aureus*, and even fungi.
- It is clinically effective.
- It penetrates the eschar but is not systemically toxic.
- It does not lose its effectiveness, allowing another infection to develop.
- It is cost-effective, available, and acceptable to the patient.
- It is easy to apply, minimizing nursing care time.

The most commonly used topical agents are Bacitracin or Polysporin, silver nitrate, mafenide acetate (Sulfamylon), and silver sulfadiazine (Flamazine). These agents are described in Table 59-6. Many other topical agents are available, including povidone–iodine

TABLE 59-6 Overview of Topical Antibacterial Agents Used for Burn Wounds

Agent	Indication/Comment	Application	Nursing Implications
General			
Antimicrobial ointment	Antibacterial coverage and promotion of a moist wound environment	Apply 1/16-in layer of ointment with a clean glove daily.	Ensure removal of old ointment at the time of wound cleaning prior to applying a new layer. Monitor closely for signs and symptoms of local infection.
Specific Agents			
Silver sulfadiazine 1% (Silvadene) water-soluble cream	Bactericidal agent for many gram-positive and gram-negative organisms, as well as yeast and *Candida albicans* Minimal penetration of eschar	Apply 1/16-in layer of cream with a clean glove 1–3 times daily.	Anticipate formation of pseudoeschar (proteinaceous gel), which can be removed.
Mafenide acetate 5–10% (Sulfamylon) hydrophilic-based solution or cream	Antimicrobial agent for gram-positive and gram-negative organisms Diffuses through eschar and avascular tissue (e.g., cartilage)	Apply twice a day with a clean glove as prescribed.	Is a strong carbonic anhydrase inhibitor and may cause metabolic acidosis. Application may cause considerable pain initially.
Silver nitrate 0.5% aqueous solution	Effective against most strains of *Staphylococcus* and *Pseudomonas* and many gram-negative organisms. Does not penetrate eschar.	Apply solution to gauze dressing and place over wound. Keep the dressing wet but covered with dry gauze and dry blankets to decrease vaporization.	Monitor serum sodium (Na^+) and potassium (K^+) levels, and replace as prescribed. Silver nitrate solution is hypotonic and acts as a wick for sodium and potassium. Protect bed linens and clothing from contact with silver nitrate, which stains everything it touches.
Silver-impregnated dressings (sheets or mesh)	Broad antimicrobial effects (product specific) Delivers a uniform, antimicrobial concentration of silver ions to the burn wound.	Apply directly to wound. Cover with absorbent secondary dressing if needed.	May produce a pseudoeschar from silver after application. Can be left in place for several days (product specific).

Adapted from Micromedex 2.0. (2015). *Formulary Advisor*, University of Texas–Medical Branch Galveston. Retrieved on July 10, 2015 (pass-protected), from www.micromedicsolutions.com/micromedex2/librarian

ointment 10% (Betadine), gentamicin sulphate, nitrofurazone (Furacin), Dakin's solution, acetic acid, miconazole, and clotrimazole.

No single topical medication is universally effective. Using different agents at different times in the postburn period may be necessary. Bacteriologic cultures are required to monitor the effect of topical medications.

NURSING ALERT

Prudent use and alternation of antimicrobial agents result in less resistant strains of bacteria, greater effectiveness of the agents, and a decreased risk of sepsis.

Before a topical agent is reapplied, the previously applied topical agent must be thoroughly removed. The number of times the dressings are changed and moistened with antimicrobial solutions is planned to promote optimal therapeutic use of the topical agent.

Wound Dressing

When the wound is clean, the prescribed topical agent is applied; the wound is then covered with layers of gauze. A light dressing is used over joint areas to allow for motion (unless the particular area has a graft and motion is contraindicated). A light dressing is also applied over areas for which a splint has been designed to conform to the body contour for proper positioning. Circumferential dressings should be applied distally to proximally. If the hand or foot is burned, the fingers and toes should be wrapped individually to promote adequate healing and prevent webbing.

Superficial burns to the face may be left open to air once they have been cleaned and the topical agent has been applied. Care must be given to ensure that the topical agent does not interfere with the eyes or mouth. A light dressing can be applied to the face to absorb excess exudates that might run into the eyes, causing irritation. Attention must be given to burns left exposed to ensure that they do not dry out and convert to a deeper burn.

Close communication and cooperation among the patient, surgeon, nurse, and other health care team members are essential for optimal burn wound care. Different wound areas on a given patient may require a variety of wound care techniques. Diagrams or photographs taken with consent posted in the patient's chart and at the bedside are useful to inform staff of the current prescription for wound care, splints to be applied over dressings, and the exercise regimen to be followed before dressings are reapplied.

NURSING ALERT

Dressings can impede circulation if they are wrapped too tightly. The peripheral pulses must be checked frequently and burned extremities elevated. If the patient's pulse is diminished, this is a critical situation and must be addressed immediately.

Dressings that adhere to the wound bed may be removed more comfortably and with less damage to healing tissue by moistening the dressing with water. The patient may participate in removing the dressings, providing some degree of control over this painful procedure. The wounds are then cleaned and débrided to remove any remaining topical agent, exudate, and nonviable tissue. Sterile scissors and forceps may be used to trim loose eschar and encourage separation of devitalized tissue. During this procedure, the wound and surrounding skin are carefully inspected. Documentation should include color, odour, size, exudate, signs of reepithelialization, any changes from the previous dressing change, and other key characteristics.

Occlusive Method

There is a role for occlusive dressings in treating specific wounds. An occlusive dressing is a thin gauze that is impregnated with a topical antimicrobial agent or that is applied after topical antimicrobial application. Occlusive dressings are most often used over areas with new skin grafts. Their purpose is to protect the graft, promoting an optimal condition for its adherence to the recipient site. Ideally, these dressings remain in place for 3 to 5 days, at which time they are removed for examination of the graft.

When these dressings are applied, precautions are taken to prevent two body surfaces from touching, such as fingers or toes, ear and scalp, the areas under the breasts, any point of flexion, or between the genital folds. Functional body alignment positions are maintained by using splints or by careful positioning of the patient.

Dressing Changes

Dressings are changed in the patient's room or treatment area approximately 20 minutes after an analgesic agent is administered. They may also be changed in the operating room after the patient is anesthetized. A mask, face shield/eye protection, water proof gown (i.e., Gortex), and gloves are worn by health care personnel when removing the dressings. The outer dressings are cut with blunt scissors, and the soiled dressings are removed and disposed of in accordance with established procedures for contaminated materials.

Dressings that adhere to the wound can be removed more comfortably if they are premoistened with sterile normal saline or sterile water. The remaining dressings are carefully and gently removed. The patient may participate in removing the dressings, providing some degree of control over this painful procedure. The wounds are then cleaned and débrided to remove debris, any remaining topical agent, exudate, and dead skin. Sterile scissors and forceps are used to trim loose eschar and encourage separation of devitalized skin. Débridement of wounds and tissues is becoming a restricted activity that requires advanced training and skills to be performed safely. The clinician must ensure that there is an institutional or agency policy in place to support them, they have the necessary skills to perform the procedure, and the skill is within their scope of practice. During this procedure, the wound and surrounding skin are carefully inspected. The colour, odour, size, exudate, signs of reepithelialization, and other characteristics of the wound and the eschar and any changes from the previous dressing change are noted.

Wound Débridement

As debris accumulates on the wound surface, it can impede keratinocyte migration, thus delaying the epithelialization process. Débridement, another facet of burn wound care, has two goals:

- To remove tissue contaminated by bacteria and foreign bodies, thereby protecting the patient from invasion of bacteria
- To remove devitalized tissue or burn eschar in preparation for wound healing or skin grafting

There are four types of débridement—natural, mechanical, chemical, and surgical.

Natural Débridement

With natural débridement, the dead tissue separates from the underlying viable tissue spontaneously. After partial- and full-thickness burns, bacteria that are present at the interface of the burned tissue and the viable tissue underneath gradually liquefy the fibrils of **collagen** that hold the eschar in place for the first or second postburn week. Proteolytic and other natural enzymes cause this phenomenon. Using antibacterial topical agents, however, tends to slow this natural process of eschar separation. It is advantageous to the patient to speed this process through other means, such as mechanical or surgical débridement, thereby reducing the time during which bacterial invasion and other iatrogenic problems may arise.

Mechanical Débridement

Mechanical débridement involves using surgical scissors and forceps to separate and remove the eschar. This technique can be performed by skilled physicians, nurses, or physical therapists and is usually done with daily dressing changes and wound cleaning procedures. Débridement by these means is carried out to the point of pain and bleeding. Hemostatic agents or pressure can be used to stop bleeding from small vessels. Wet-to-dry dressings are not advocated in burn care because of the chance of removing viable cells along with necrotic tissue. Dressing changes alone aid in the removal of wound debris.

Topical enzymatic débridement agents are available to promote débridement of the burn wounds. Because such agents do not have antimicrobial properties, they should be used with topical antibacterial therapy to protect the patient from bacterial invasion.

Chemical Débridement

Topical enzymatic agents are available to promote débridement of burn wounds. Because such agents usually do not have antimicrobial properties, they may be used together with topical antibacterial therapy to protect the patient from bacterial invasion. Heavy metals such as silver can deactivate débriding agents; therefore, caution is necessary to ensure that the topical antimicrobial agent does not interfere with the chemical débridement. Alternating topical medications with dressing changes may also be considered.

Surgical Débridement

Overall, the incidence of burn wound infection has declined in recent years with the change to early excision and wound closure (Puri, Khare, Chandramouli, et al., 2016). Early surgical excision to remove devitalized tissue along with early burn wound closure is now being recognized as one of the most important factors contributing to survival in a patient with a major burn injury. Aggressive surgical wound closure has reduced the incidence of burn wound sepsis, thus improving survival rates (Puri et al., 2016). Early excision is carried out before the natural separation of eschar is allowed to occur.

Surgical débridement is an operative procedure involving either primary excision (surgical removal of tissue) of the full thickness of the skin down to the fascia (tangential excision) or shaving the burned skin layers gradually down to freely bleeding, viable tissue. Surgical excision is initiated early in burn wound management. This may be performed a few days after the burn or as soon as the patient is hemodynamically stable and edema has decreased. Ideally, the wound is then covered immediately with a skin graft, if needed, and an occlusive dressing. If the wound bed is not ready for a skin graft at the time of excision, a temporary biologic dressing may be used until a skin graft can be applied during subsequent surgery.

The use of surgical excision carries with it risks and complications, especially with large burns. The procedure creates a high risk of extensive blood loss (Mosley, Muniz Castro, Joe, et al., 2018) and lengthy operating and anesthesia time. However, when conducted in a timely and efficient manner, surgical excision results in shorter hospital stays and possibly a decreased risk of complications from invasive burn wound sepsis.

Gerontologic Considerations

Eschar separation in full-thickness burns is typically delayed in older patients, and older patients are frequently poor risks for surgical excision. Therefore, prolonged hospitalization, immobilization, and associated problems may be common. If the older patient can tolerate surgery, early excision with skin grafting is the treatment of choice because it decreases the mortality rate in this population. Prevention of complications of prolonged hospitalization, including preventing delirium and immobility, are essential in the care of the older patient with burns.

Grafting the Burn Wound

If wounds are deep partial thickness or full thickness, or the TBSA of the burn is extensive, spontaneous reepithelialization is not possible. Therefore, coverage of the burn wound is necessary until coverage with a graft of the patient's own skin (**autograft**) is possible. The purposes of wound coverage are to decrease the risk for infection; prevent further loss of protein, fluid, and electrolytes through the wound; and minimize heat loss through evaporation. Several methods of wound coverage are available; some are temporary until grafting with permanent coverage is possible. Wound coverage may consist of biologic, biosynthetic, synthetic, and autologous methods or a combination of these approaches, as described in Table 59-7.

The main areas for skin grafting include the face (for aesthetic and psychological reasons); functional areas, such as the hands and feet; and areas that involve joints. Grafting permits earlier functional ability and reduces **contractures** (the shrinkage of burn scar through collagen maturation). When burns are very extensive, the chest and abdomen may be grafted first to reduce the burn surface.

TABLE 59-7 Temporary and Permanent Burn Wound Coverings

Name	Source	Type of Covering	Advantages	Disadvantages
Biobrane	Biosynthetic nylon on Silastic membrane Collagen derivative	Temporary	Protects wound from fluid and protein loss Reduces pain Monitor daily initially, can remain in place for weeks Multiple uses over wide-meshed grafts, donor sites, and partial-thickness burns Extended shelf life	Wound surface must be free of infection. Use on partial-thickness wounds only
Aquacel Ag	Sodium carboxymethylcellulose and ionic silver	Temporary	Ionic silver immediately kills pathogens Reduces pain Must be monitored daily initially, can remain in place up to 14 days Highly absorbent, creating moist wound environment	Difficult to cover joints Painful to remove if it needs to be removed prematurely Use on partial-thickness wounds only.
BCG Matrix	Biosynthetic beta-glucan enmeshed with collagen	Temporary	Covers partial-thickness wounds and donor sites Can be left in place until wound heals	High cost Requires the wound be clean and free of infection
Allograft (homograft)	Human fresh or cryopreserved	Temporary	Covers large areas Used until wound is ready for autografting Aids in revascularization of wound Protects granulation tissue Decreases evaporation of water and protein from wound	Eventual rejection
Xenograft (heterograft)	Pig, rabbit, dog, lizard; fresh, frozen, or freeze dried	Temporary	Readily available Long shelf life Decreases pain of wound Protects granulation tissue Covers large areas Aids in wound débridement when removed	Eventual rejection Can be used only with noninfected partial-thickness wounds
Integra	Dermal replacement; dermal matrix covered by autograft	Permanent	Cryopreserved—easy to transport Multiple uses: burns, dermal ulcers Donor site smaller with less scarring Used for burn wound covering and reconstruction	Wound surface must be free of infection for "take." High cost Rigorous postoperative care Need to stage procedures
Alloderm	Nonimmunogenic dermal replacement Freeze-dried acellular allogenic dermis engrafted with a thick epithelial autograft	Permanent	Supports autograft Less scarring and contracture formation Multiple uses in dental, abdominal, burn, and reconstructive surgery High percentage of "take"	Wound surface must be free of infection for "take." High cost
Cultured epithelial autograft (CEA)	Patient's own cells (autologous cultured epithelium)	Permanent	Lifesaving for very large full-thickness burns Covers large areas of wound from cells obtained from small biopsy of skin	Length of time to grow skin Tedious postoperative care with immobility Easily infected, fragile and affected by shear Difficult to handle graft High cost of grafts and process Increased scarring and contractures
Apligraf CE	Cultured keratinocytes with allodermis cultured fibroblast matrix	—	Bioengineered Better growth potential than CEA Good graft "take" with less chance of rejection Less scarring	High cost New in wound care market; limited experience with use
Autograft	Patient's own skin	Permanent	Multiple uses in different wounds Ideal and safest wound covering Reduced healing time and scarring Sheet or meshed grafts possible No rejection by patient's immune system	Need to stage procedures Limited amount of skin available with large burns Creates donor site wound Healing of recipient areas with irregular pattern

Granulation tissue fills the space created by the wound, creates a barrier to bacteria, and serves as a bed for epithelial cell growth. Richly vascular granulation tissue is pink, firm, shiny, and free of exudate and debris. It should have a bacterial count of less than 100,000 per gram of tissue to optimize graft take. If the wound is not ready for skin grafting, the burn wound is excised and allowed to granulate. Once the wound is excised, a wound covering is applied to keep the wound bed moist and promote the granulation process.

Biologic Dressings (Allograft and Heterografts)

Biologic dressings have several uses. In extensive burns, they save lives by providing temporary wound closure and protecting the granulation tissue until autografting is possible. Biologic dressings are commonly used in patients with large areas of burn and little remaining normal skin donor sites. Biologic dressings may also be used to débride wounds after eschar separation. With each biologic dressing change, débridement occurs. Once the biologic dressing appears to be "taking," or adhering to the granulating surface with minimal underlying exudation, the patient is ready for an autograft.

Biologic dressings also provide temporary immediate coverage for partial- to full-thickness burns and decrease the wound's evaporative water and protein loss. They decrease pain by protecting nerve endings and are an effective barrier against water loss and entry of bacteria. When applied to superficial partial-thickness wounds, they seem to speed healing. Biologic materials can be left open or covered. They stay in place for varying lengths of time but are removed in instances of infection or rejection.

Biologic dressings consist of **allografts** (or homografts) and **xenografts** (or heterografts). Allografts are skin obtained from living or recently deceased humans. The amniotic membrane (amnion) from the human placenta may also be used as a biologic dressing. Xenografts consist of skin taken from animals (usually pigs). Most biologic dressings are used as temporary coverings of burn wounds and are eventually rejected because of the body's immune reaction to them as foreign.

Cadaver allografts are available from skin banks in fresh and cryopreserved (frozen) forms, and have been the choice for resurfacing large debrided areas. Cadaver skin serves as temporary wound cover, reduces pain and fever, restores function, increases appetite, controls fluid loss, and promotes wound healing. As the grafts revascularize, they form a barrier against bacterial invasion and prevent further loss of water, electrolytes, and protein from the wound. Allografts decrease bacterial counts of underlying tissues and facilitate future grafting by promoting a sterile wound bed (Voigt, Williamson, Kagan, et al., 2018). Allografts can last 7 to 10 days before the body rejects them. They are then replaced with an autograft.

Amnion is less expensive and is available in some hospitals with burn centres and specialized tissue banks, which obtain and process it in cooperation with obstetric services. However, amnion grafts do not become vascularized by the patient's vessels and can be left in place only for short periods. Also, screening for viral disease is difficult.

Pigskin is available from commercial suppliers. It is available fresh, frozen, or lyophilized (freeze-dried) for longer shelf life. Pigskin impregnated with a topical antibacterial agent such as silver nitrate is also available. Pigskin is widely used for temporary covering of clean wounds such as superficial partial-thickness wounds and donor sites. Although pigskin does not vascularize, it will adhere to clean superficial wounds and provides excellent pain control while the underlying wound epithelializes (Kagan et al., 2013).

Biosynthetic and Synthetic Dressings

Problems with availability, sterility, and cost have prompted the search for biosynthetic and synthetic skin substitutes, which may eventually replace biologic dressings as temporary wound coverings. Currently, the most widely used synthetic dressing is **Biobrane**, which is composed of a nylon, Silastic membrane combined with a collagen derivative. The material is semitransparent and sterile. It has an extended shelf life and is less costly than xenograft or pigskin. Like biologic dressings, Biobrane protects the wound from fluid loss and bacterial invasion.

Biobrane adheres to the wound fibrin, which binds to the nylon–collagen material. Within 5 days, cells migrate into the nylon mesh. In general, adherence to the wound surface correlates directly with low bacterial counts. When the Biobrane dressing adheres to the wound, the wound remains stable and the Biobrane can remain in place for 3 to 4 weeks. Biobrane dressings (Fig 59-4) readily adhere to donor sites and meticulously clean débrided partial-thickness wounds; they will remain until spontaneous epithelialization and wound healing occur. Biobrane can be laid on top of a wide-meshed autograft to protect the wound until the autograft epithelium grows out to close the interstices. As the Biobrane gradually separates, it is trimmed, leaving a healed wound.

Biobrane is also useful for intermediate- or long-term closure of a surgically excised wound until an autograft becomes available. Like biologic dressings, Biobrane should not be used over full-thickness, grossly contaminated, or necrotic wounds. Removal of Biobrane after several weeks is similar to but easier than removal of a vascularized allograft and leaves a bleeding granulation bed that readily accepts an autograft.

Another fairly new temporary wound covering is BCG Matrix. This dressing combines beta-glucan, a complex carbohydrate, with collagen in a meshed reinforced wound

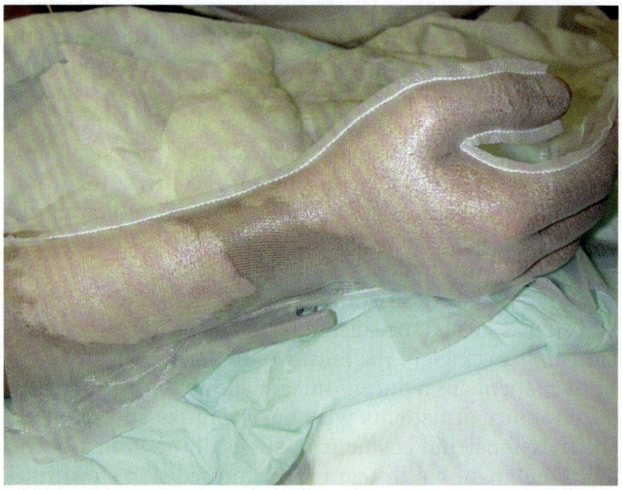

FIGURE 59-4. Biobrane applied to hand and forearm. (Used with permission from University of Texas Medical Branch, Galveston, TX.)

dressing. Beta-glucan is known to stimulate macrophages, which are vital in the inflammatory process of healing. BCG Matrix is a temporary wound covering intended for use with partial-thickness burns and donor sites. It is applied immediately after cleaning and débridement. If the burn wound surface remains free of infection, BCG Matrix can be left in place until healing is complete.

Several other synthetic dressings are available for burn wound care. Op-Site, a thin, transparent, polyurethane elastic film, can be used to cover clean small partial-thickness wounds and donor sites. This dressing is occlusive and waterproof but permeable to water vapor and air; this permeability not only provides protection from microbial contamination but also allows for the exchange of gases, which occurs much more quickly in a moist environment. Other synthetic dressings used for burn wounds include Tegaderm, N-Terface, and DuoDerm.

Burns that are between superficial and deep partial thickness in depth can be treated with a promising new temporary biologic covering, TransCyte, a material composed of human newborn fibroblasts that are cultured on the nylon mesh of Biobrane. The thin silicone membrane bonded to the mesh provides a moisture vapor barrier for the wound. TransCyte is used to treat burns in which the depth is indeterminate. TransCyte delivers a variety of biologically active proteins, which may benefit the wound healing process. Research has shown that wounds treated with TransCyte heal more quickly and with less hypertrophic scarring than do burns treated with the traditional silver sulfadiazine protocols.

Dermal Substitutes

In an attempt to develop the ideal burn wound covering product, dermal substitutes have been created. It is believed skin substitutes enhance the healing process of an open wound when autologous skin is unavailable or limited for use (Middlekoop & Sheridan, 2018). Two such products are Integra Artificial Skin and Alloderm.

A dermal analogue, **Integra** is composed of two main layers. The epidermal layer, consisting of silicone, acts as a bacterial barrier and prevents water loss from the dermis. The dermal layer is composed of animal collagen. It interfaces with the open wound surface and allows migration of fibroblasts and capillaries into the material. This "neodermis" becomes a permanent structure. The artificial dermis is biodegraded and reabsorbed. The outer silicone membrane is removed 2 to 3 weeks after application and is replaced with the patient's own skin in the form of a thin epidermal skin graft. When a thinner autologous donor graft is used, donor site healing is quicker. Long-term effects of Integra include minimal contracture formation. The graft site is very pliable, almost eliminating the need for repeated cosmetic surgery. Most importantly, Integra has resulted in less hypertrophic scarring, thus reducing the need for compression devices once the burn wound has healed. Because Integra allows for earlier excision and coverage of the burn wound, metabolic demands of the patient are reduced. Integra allows for the increased survivability of patients with burn injuries and improves the functional and cosmetic qualities of the healed burns. The combination of Integra with cultured skin substitutes has demonstrated promise in burn management (Matsumura, Matsushima, Ueyama, et al., 2016).

Another promising dermal substitute is **Alloderm**. It is processed dermis from human cadaver skin, which can be used as the dermal layer for skin grafts. When a **donor site** (the area from which skin is taken to provide a skin graft for another part of the body) is harvested for an autologous skin graft, both the epidermal and dermal layers of skin are removed from the donor site. Alloderm provides a permanent dermal layer replacement. Its use allows the burn surgeon to harvest a thinner skin graft consisting of the epidermal layer only. The patient's epidermal layer is placed directly over the dermal base (Alloderm). The new graft is then treated according to the burn unit's protocol. The use of Alloderm has also resulted in less scarring and contractures with healed grafts; donor sites heal much more quickly than conventional donor sites because only the epidermal layer has been harvested. This is important when donor sites are limited because of extensive burns.

Autografts

Autografts remain the preferred material for definitive burn wound closure following excision. Autografts are the ideal means of covering burn wounds because the grafts are the patient's own skin and thus are not rejected by the patient's immune system. They can be split-thickness, full-thickness, pedicle flaps, or epithelial grafts. Full-thickness and pedicle flaps are commonly used for reconstructive surgery months or years after the initial injury.

Split-thickness autografts can be applied in sheets, or they can be expanded by meshing so that they can cover 1.5 to 9.0 times more than a given donor site area. Skin meshers enable the surgeon to cut tiny slits into a sheet of donor skin, making it possible to cover large areas with smaller amounts of donor skin. These expanded grafts adhere to the recipient site more easily than sheet grafts and prevent the accumulation of blood, serum, air, or purulent material under the graft. However, any kind of graft other than a sheet graft will contribute to scar formation as it heals. Using expanded grafts may be necessary in large wounds but should be viewed as a compromise in terms of aesthetics.

If blood, serum, air, fat, or necrotic tissue lies between the recipient site and the graft, there may be partial or total loss of the graft. Infection and mishandling of the graft, as well as trauma during dressing changes, account for most other instances of graft loss. Using split-thickness grafts allows the remaining donor site to retain sweat glands and hair follicles and minimizes donor site healing time.

A **cultured epithelial autograft (CEA)** provides permanent coverage of large wounds when harvesting of skin for autografting is not an option. This involves a biopsy of the patient's skin in an unburned area. Keratinocytes are then isolated and epithelial cells are cultured in a laboratory. The original epithelial cell sample can multiply to 10,000 times its original size over 30 days. These cells are then attached to the burn wound, and extreme care is taken until they have adhered to the wound surface. Varying degrees of success have been reported, and results are encouraging. However, the disadvantages of CEA are that the grafts are thin and fragile and can shear easily. Current literature has shown better success with CEA graft take and can be lifesaving in burns with TBSA greater than 50% (Allen, Recht, & Litt, 2018). The area of skin substitutes continues to be a large focus of burn research today.

CARE OF THE PATIENT WITH AN AUTOGRAFT. The first dressing change is usually performed 3 to 5 days after surgery, or earlier in the case of purulent drainage or a foul odour.

The patient is positioned and turned carefully to avoid disturbing the graft or putting pressure on the graft site. If an extremity has been grafted, it is elevated to minimize edema. The patient begins exercising the grafted area 5 to 7 days after grafting.

CARE OF DONOR SITE. A moist gauze dressing is applied at the time of surgery to maintain pressure and to stop any oozing. A thrombostatic agent such as thrombin or epinephrine may be applied directly to the site as well. The donor site may be treated in several ways, from single-layer gauze impregnated with petrolatum and bismuth (i.e., Xeroform), to new biosynthetic dressings such as Biobrane. Many burn centres are also using foam, hydrofibre (i.e., Aquacel AG + extra), or hydrocolloid dressings on donor sites. Despite the type of donor site covering, donor sites must remain clean, dry, and free from pressure. Because a donor site is usually a partial-thickness wound, it will heal spontaneously within 10 to 14 days with proper care. Donor sites are painful, and additional pain management must be a part of the patient's care.

Pain Management

Pain is inevitable during recovery from any burn injury. Burn pain is thought to have both nociceptive and neuropathic pain components. Management of the often severe pain is one of the most difficult challenges facing the burn team. Many factors contribute to the patient's pain experience. These factors include but are not limited to the severity of the pain, the adequacy of the health care provider's assessment of the pain, the appropriateness and adequacy of pharmacologic treatment of pain, the multiple procedures involved in burn care (i.e., wound care, rehabilitative exercises), and appropriate evaluation of the effectiveness of pain relief measures. The outstanding features of burn pain are its intensity and long duration. Further, necessary wound care carries with it the anticipation of pain and anxiety.

In partial-thickness burns, the nerve endings are exposed, resulting in excruciating pain with exposure to air currents. Although nerve endings are destroyed in full-thickness burns, the margins of the burn wound are hypersensitive to pain, and there is pain in adjacent structures. Healing of full-thickness burns creates significant discomfort as regenerating nerve endings become entrapped in scar formation. Most severe burns are a combination of partial-thickness and full-thickness burns.

Patients with burns have been described as having many types of pain: background or resting pain, procedural pain, breakthrough pain, postoperative pain, neuropathic pain, and chronic pain. Background pain is pain that exists on a 24-hour basis. Procedural pain is pain caused by procedures such as burn wound care or range-of-motion exercises. Breakthrough pain occurs when blood levels of analgesic agents fall below the level required to control background pain. The patient's pain level must be assessed throughout the day because each type of pain is different and various pain management strategies may be needed to address different types of pain (Rerouvey & Shahrokhi, 2015).

The primary pain from the burn itself is intense in the initial acute postburn phase. In the next few weeks thereafter, until the skin heals or skin grafts are applied and heal, the pain intensity remains high because of treatment-induced pain. Wound cleaning, débridement, dressing changes, and physical therapy can all cause intense pain. Donor sites may be intensely painful for several days. Discomfort related to tissue healing, such as itching, tingling, and tightness of contracting skin and joints, adds to the duration, if not the intensity, of pain over weeks or months. Because pain cannot be eliminated short of complete anesthesia, the goal is to minimize the pain with analgesic agents to an acceptable goal set by the patient.

Opioid administration via the IV route, particularly in the emergent and acute phases of burn management, remains the mainstay for pharmacologic management of burn pain. The use of opioids is complicated by the fluctuation in the bioavailability of drugs, protein binding of the drug, and the drug clearance related to the hemodynamic and fluid volume shifts that occur with a burn injury. Absorption of the opioid also may be affected. The titrating of analgesic agents to obtain pain relief while minimizing side effects is crucial. The patient's requirements for analgesia are often high, but fear of addiction on the part of the patient and health care provider hamper adequate opioid administration.

Morphine sulphate remains the analgesic of choice for treatment of acute burn pain. It is titrated to obtain pain relief based on the patient's self-report of pain using a standardized pain rating scale.

Fentanyl is another useful opioid for burn pain, particularly procedural burn pain. It has been shown to be effective for management of intense pain of short duration. Fentanyl has a rapid onset, high potency, and short duration, all of which make it effective for use with burn wound procedures. Appropriate cardiac and respiratory monitoring must be carried out during its administration.

For patients using patient-controlled analgesia (PCA), a pump is used to self-administer a dose of an opioid at set intervals. If the patient presses the PCA button sooner than the pump allows, the patient will not receive a dose of the opioid. It is important for caregivers to monitor patients for the first 2 to 24 hours to ensure they are using the device properly.

Sustained-release opioids, such as MS Contin or oxycodone (OxyContin), have also been used successfully in the treatment of burn pain. These medications can effectively treat the resting pain that is often associated with burn injury. Additional medications must be prescribed with these medications to cover breakthrough pain.

Some burn units use self-administered nitrous oxide during burn wound procedures. Proper ventilation and monitoring equipment and availability of qualified personnel to administer nitrous oxide limit its use.

Short-acting anesthetic agents (i.e., propofol), which cause procedural sedation or general anesthesia, are being used for the management of procedural pain associated with major dressing changes and initial surgical dressing removal. Anesthetic agents are given in combination with narcotic analgesics by a qualified anesthetist or intensivist. Continuous patient cardiac monitoring is required, with emergency resuscitation equipment readily at hand.

Anxiety and pain go hand in hand for patients with burns. The entire burn experience can produce severe anxiety, which can, in turn, exacerbate pain. Therefore, the ideal pain management regimen must incorporate the treatment of pain and anxiety and must be individualized for each patient. Sedation with anxiolytic medications such as lorazepam (Ativan) and midazolam (Versed) may be indicated in addition to the administration of opioids.

Research has shown that sleep deprivation leads to increased reports of pain, and vice versa, in patients with burns. The problem arises with administration of opioids, which affect various sleep stages by decreasing rapid eye movement (REM) sleep, leading to hyper arousal (Faraklas et al., 2013). Many other agents used to treat burn injury, such as bronchodilators and antipruritics, interfere with sleep, which in turn can interfere with pain management.

The use of nonpharmacologic measures aids in the management of burn pain. These measures include relaxation techniques, deep-breathing exercises, distraction, guided imagery, hypnosis, therapeutic touch, humour, and information giving as well as music therapy. Researchers have found that music affects both physiologic and psychological aspects of the pain experience. It diverts the patient's attention from the painful stimulus; provides reality orientation, distraction, and sensory stimulation; and allows for patient self-expression.

Modulation of Hypermetabolism

Burn injuries produce profound metabolic abnormalities fueled by the exaggerated stress response to the injury. Metabolic responses are mediated by the stimulation of the sympathetic nervous system to release catecholamines, cortisol, glucagon, and insulin. The body's response has been classified as hyperdynamic, hypermetabolic, and hypercatabolic. Hypermetabolism can affect morbidity and mortality by increasing the risk of infection and slowing the healing rate. Patients' metabolic demands vary with the extent of the burn injury and age (Jeschke, 2016).

Metabolic measures using indirect calorimetry provide more accurate assessments of energy expenditure and caloric demand. Therefore, it is essential to control the stress response by increasing the anabolic process through adequate nutrition and increased muscle activity, decreasing heat loss from wounds, and maintaining a warm environment. Controlling secondary stress, such as pain and anxiety, also helps to control the stress response.

The most important of these interventions is to provide adequate nutrition and calories to decrease catabolism (Abdullahi & Jeschke, 2014). Healing of the burn wound consumes large quantities of energy. Effective nutrition management depends on how well the energy expenditure due to the burn injury can be estimated and matched with appropriate amounts of micronutrients, carbohydrates, lipids, and protein. The goal of nutritional support is to promote a state of positive nitrogen balance by optimizing nutrition to match nutrient utilization (Carson, Khosrozadeh, Norbury, et al., 2018). The nutritional support required is based on the patient's preburn status and the TBSA burned. Dietary consultations are essential in helping patients meet their nutritional needs. Daily calorie counts aid in assessing the adequacy of nutritional intake. Overfeeding must be avoided, because it increases metabolism, oxygen consumption, and carbon dioxide production.

Several formulas exist for estimating the daily metabolic expenditure and caloric requirements of patients with burn injuries. The most commonly used formulas include the Curreiri formula, which uses body weight and percent burn, and a variation of the Harris–Bennedict equation, which determines basal energy requirements based on stress and burn size (Carson et al., 2018). Nutritional targets have remained static in recent years, with most programs striving for protein goals of 2 to 3 g/kg/d and caloric targets of 1.5 times a calculated basal metabolic rate or 1.2 times the resting energy expenditure measured using indirect calorimetry. Glucose is ideally not the only fuel because high levels are not oxidized in this hormonal milieu. Additionally, adequate amounts of micronutrients and vitamins are beneficial (Nordlund, Pham, & Gibran, 2014).

The enteral route of feeding is far superior to the parenteral route, and most patients tolerate gastric feedings without difficulty. Enteral feedings preserve the intestinal barrier function and absorption of peptides and amino acids, which leads to higher nitrogen retention. Feedings are started as soon as possible. The placement of feeding tubes into the stomach is preferred as it maintains gastric peristalsis, the secretion of digestive enzymes from the stomach, and it is easier to obtain access for gastric feeds. Placement of feeding tubes into the duodenum helps prevent aspiration and allows for continuous, uninterrupted feedings during surgical procedures.

If the oral route is used, high-protein, high-calorie meals and supplements are given. Inhalation injury and prolonged intubation lead to dysphagia in patients with burn injuries. Speech therapists work closely with the burn team to help the patient preserve swallowing function.

Patients lose a great deal of weight during recovery from severe burns. Reserve fat deposits are catabolized, fluids are lost, and caloric intake may be limited. Because a burn injury lowers the patient's resistance to infection and disease, the nutritional status must be improved and maintained although the patient has a poor appetite and is weak. One goal of nutrition management is to decrease or stop the catabolic process and promote protein anabolism. Beta-blockers, such as propranolol, that alter the catabolic state are often used in patients with burns. Supplemental vitamins and minerals, including the nonessential amino acid glutamine, are given to provide support when the patient is in the hypermetabolic, infection-prone state of acute burn injury. In addition, research is focused on aggressive alteration of the hyperglycemic response and administration of insulin therapy to promote wound healing. Other treatment modalities include early excision and skin grafting of the burn wound, aggressive prevention or treatment of infections, and adequate exercise with physical therapy to lessen muscle wasting and increase strength. Additional pharmacologic modalities used to alter the hypermetabolic state of burn injury include the use of oxandrolone (Oxandrin), an anabolic steroid; an adrenergic antagonist (propranolol [Indural]); and an anabolic protein, recombinant human growth hormone (Jeschke, 2016).

Disorders of Wound Healing

Disorders of wound healing in the patient with burns result from excessive abnormal healing or inadequate new tissue formation. Hypertrophic scarring and keloid formation result from excessive abnormal healing.

Scars

One of the most devastating sequelae of a burn injury is the formation of **hypertrophic scars**. Clinicians cannot reliably predict or prevent the formation of hypertrophic scars. Hypertrophic scars are more common in children, in people with dark skin, and in areas of stretch or motion. The pathophysiology behind these scars is not completely understood, but they are characterized by an overabundant matrix formation, especially collagen.

Hypertrophic scars and wound contractures are more likely to occur if the initial burn injury extends below the level of the deep dermis. Healing of such deep wounds results in the replacement of normal integument with highly metabolically active tissues that lack the normal architecture of the skin. In the collagen layer beneath the epithelium, many fibroblasts proliferate gradually. Myofibroblasts, cells that have the ability to contract, are also present in immature wounds. As the myofibroblasts contract, the collagen fibres, which normally lie in flat bundles, tend to form a wavy pattern. Eventually, the collagen bundles take on a super-coiled appearance, and collagen nodules develop. The scar becomes red (because of its hypervascular nature), raised, and hard.

Burn personnel must be proactive in the prevention and management of scar formation. Compression measures are instituted early in burn wound treatment. Elastic bandages (ACE, Tensor) are used initially to help promote adequate circulation, but they can also be used as the first form of compression. Scar management occurs mainly in the rehabilitative phase, after the wounds are closed. Hypertrophic scarring may cause severe contracture across involved joints. Therefore, prevention and management of this type of scarring is essential (see Prevention of Hypertrophic Scarring section in the rehabilitation phase discussion). However, these scars are limited to the area of injury and gradually regress over time.

Keloids

Keloids are the result of an overgrowth of granulation tissue that may develop and extend beyond the wound surface, unlike hypertrophic scar tissue, which stays within the wound edges. Keloids tend to be found in people with darkly pigmented skin, tend to grow outside of wound margins, and are likely to recur after surgical excision.

Failure to Heal

Failure of the wound to heal may result from many factors, including infection, an underlying disease process, shearing, pressure, or inadequate nutrition. A serum albumin level of less than 2 g/dL is usually a factor in impaired healing in the patient with burns.

Contractures

Contractures are another concern as wounds heal. The burn wound tissue shortens because of the force exerted by the fibroblasts and the flexion of muscles in natural wound healing. An opposing force provided by splints, traction, and purposeful movement and positioning must be used to counteract deformity in burns affecting joints.

Nursing Process

Care of the Patient During the Acute Phase

Assessment

Continued assessment of the patient during the early weeks after the burn injury focuses on hemodynamic alterations, wound healing, pain and psychosocial responses, and early detection of complications. Assessment of respiratory and fluid status remains the highest priority for detection of potential complications.

The nurse assesses vital signs frequently. Continued assessment of peripheral pulses is essential for the first few postburn days while edema continues to increase, potentially damaging peripheral nerves and restricting blood flow. Observation of the electrocardiogram may give clues to cardiac dysrhythmias resulting from potassium imbalance, pre-existing cardiac disease, or the effects of electrical injury or burn shock.

Assessment of residual gastric volumes and pH in the patient with a nasogastric tube is also important. Blood in the gastric fluid or the stools must also be noted and reported.

Assessment of the burn wound requires an experienced eye, hand, and sense of smell. Important wound assessment features include size, colour, odour, eschar, exudate, abscess formation under the eschar, epithelial buds (small pearl-like clusters of cells on the wound surface), bleeding, granulation tissue appearance, status of grafts and donor sites, and quality of surrounding skin. Any significant changes in the wound are reported to the physician, because they usually indicate burn wound or systemic sepsis and require immediate intervention.

Other significant and ongoing assessments focus on pain and psychosocial responses; daily body weights; caloric intake; general hydration; and serum electrolyte, hemoglobin, and hematocrit levels. Assessment for excessive bleeding from blood vessels adjacent to areas of surgical exploration and débridement is necessary as well. The Plan of Nursing Care provides an outline of nursing activities in the acute phase of burn care.

Nursing Priorities

Based on assessment data, nursing priorities in the acute phase of burn care may include the following:

- Excessive fluid volume
- Infection
- Imbalanced nutrition
- Impaired skin integrity
- Acute pain
- Impaired physical mobility
- Ineffective coping
- Interrupted family processes
- Lack of knowledge

Collaborative Problems/ Potential Complications

Based on assessment data, potential complications that may develop in the acute phase of burn care may include the following:

- Heart failure and pulmonary edema
- Sepsis
- Acute respiratory failure
- ARDS
- Visceral damage (electrical burns)

Planning and Goals

The major goals for the patient may include restoration of normal fluid balance, absence of infection, attainment of anabolic state and normal weight, improved skin integrity, reduction of pain and discomfort, optimal physical mobility, adequate patient and family coping, adequate patient and family knowledge of burn treatment, and absence of complications. Achieving these goals requires a collaborative, interdisciplinary approach to patient management (Chart 59-7).

Nursing Interventions

Restoring Normal Fluid Balance

To reduce the risk of fluid overload and consequent congestive heart failure, the nurse closely monitors IV and oral fluid intake, using IV infusion pumps to minimize the risk of rapid fluid infusion. To monitor changes in fluid status, careful intake and output and daily weights are obtained. Changes, including those of blood pressure and pulse rate, are reported to the physician (invasive hemodynamic monitoring is avoided because of the high risk of infection). Low-dose dopamine to increase renal perfusion and diuretics may be prescribed to promote increased urine output. The nurse's role is to administer these medications as prescribed and to monitor the patient's response.

Preventing Infection

A major part of the nurse's role during the acute phase of burn care is detecting and preventing infection. The nurse is responsible for providing a clean and safe environment and for closely scrutinizing the burn wound to detect early signs of infection. Culture results and white blood cell counts are monitored.

Strict aseptic technique is used for wound care procedures. Aseptic technique is also used for any invasive procedures, such as insertion of IV lines and urinary catheters or tracheal suctioning. Meticulous hand hygiene before and after each patient contact or any object or furniture in the patient's environment is also an essential component of preventing infection, even though gloves are worn to provide care. Gloves are not a substitution for hand hygiene.

The nurse protects the patient from sources of contamination, including other patients, staff members, visitors, and equipment. Invasive lines and tubing must be routinely changed according to recommendations of the CDC (2014). Tube feeding reservoirs, ventilator circuits, and drainage containers are replaced regularly. Fresh flowers, plants, or fresh fruit baskets are not permitted in the patient's room because of the risk of microorganism growth. Visitors are screened to avoid exposing the immunocompromised patient to pathogens.

Patients can inadvertently promote migration of microorganisms from one burned area to another by touching their wounds or dressings. Bed linens also can spread infection through either colonization with wound microorganisms or fecal contamination. Regularly bathing unburned areas and changing linens can help to prevent infection.

Maintaining Adequate Nutrition

Oral fluids should be initiated slowly when bowel sounds resume. The patient's tolerance is noted. If vomiting and distention do not occur, fluids may be increased gradually and the patient may advance to a normal diet or to tube feedings.

The nurse collaborates with the dietitian or nutrition support team to plan a protein- and calorie-rich diet that is acceptable to the patient. Family members may be encouraged to bring nutritious and favourite foods to the hospital. Milkshakes and sandwiches made with meat, peanut butter, and cheese may be offered as snacks between meals and late in the evening. Nutritional supplements such as Ensure and Resource may be provided. Caloric intake must be documented. Vitamin and mineral supplements may be prescribed.

If caloric goals cannot be met by oral feeding, a feeding tube is inserted and used for continuous or bolus feedings of specific formulas. The volume of residual gastric secretions should be checked to ensure absorption. Parenteral nutrition may also be required but should be used only if gastrointestinal function is compromised (see Chapter 36).

Patients should be weighed each day and their weights graphed. Patients can use this information to set goals for their own nutritional intake and to monitor weight loss and gain. Ideally, the patient will lose no more than 5% of preburn weight if aggressive nutritional management is implemented.

The patient with anorexia requires encouragement and support from the nurse to increase food intake. The patient's surroundings should be as pleasant as possible at mealtime. Catering to food preferences and offering high-protein, high-vitamin snacks are ways of encouraging the patient to increase intake.

Promoting Skin Integrity

Wound care is usually the most time-consuming element of burn care after the emergent phase. The physician will prescribe the desired topical antibacterial agents and specific biologic, biosynthetic, or synthetic wound coverings and will plan for surgical excision and grafting. The nurse needs to make astute assessments of wound status, to use creative approaches to wound dressing, and to support the patient during the emotionally distressing and very painful experience of wound care.

(text continued on page 1869)

Plan of Nursing Care

Chart 59-7. Care of the Patient During the Acute Phase of Burn Injury

Nursing Priority: Fluid volume excess
Goal: Maintenance of optimal fluid balance

NURSING INTERVENTIONS	RATIONALE	EXPECTED OUTCOMES
1. Monitor vital signs, intake and output, weight. Assess for edema, jugular venous distention (JVD), crackles, and increased arterial pressures.	1. These signs reflect fluid status.	• Intake, output, and body weight correlate with expected pattern • Vital signs and arterial pressures remain within designated limits • Urine output increases in response to diuretic and vasoactive medications
2. Notify physician of urine output <30 mL/hr, weight gain, JVD, crackles, increased arterial pressures.	2. These indicate increased fluid volume.	
3. Maintain intravenous fluids on pumps or rate controllers.	3. Regulation prevents unintentional fluid bolus.	
4. Administer dopamine or diuretics as prescribed. Assess response.	4. Low-dose dopamine increases renal perfusion, which increases urine output. Diuretics promote increased urine formation and urine output and decrease intravascular volume.	

Nursing Priority: Risk for infection
Goal: Absence of localized or systemic infection

NURSING INTERVENTIONS	RATIONALE	EXPECTED OUTCOMES
1. Use asepsis in all aspects of patient care. a. Adherence to the essential 4 Moments of effective hand hygiene. b. Use clean or sterile gloves for wound care. c. Wear isolation gown or protective plastic apron for patient care. d. Wear mask and hair cover when wounds are exposed and during sterile procedures. e. Change invasive lines and tubings as recommended by the Centers for Disease Control and Prevention (CDC).	1. Aseptic techniques minimize risk of cross-contamination and spread of bacterial contamination. a. Hand hygiene remains the single most important infection control measure and reduces the incidence of health care–associated infections (HAI).	• Wound cultures show minimal bacteria • Negative blood, urine, and sputum cultures • Urine output and vital signs within acceptable range • Absence of signs and symptoms of infection and sepsis
2. Screen visitors for respiratory, gastrointestinal, or integumentary infections. Provide isolation gowns for visitors without active infection, and instruct in hand hygiene.	2. Avoiding known infecting agents prevents introduction of additional microorganisms.	
3. Exclude plants and flowers in water from patient's room.	3. Stagnant water is a potential source of bacterial growth; soil may contain insects.	
4. Inspect wound for signs of infection, purulent drainage, or discolouration.	4. Such signs indicate localized infection.	
5. Monitor white blood cell (WBC) count, culture, and sensitivity results.	5. Increased WBC count indicates infection. Culture and sensitivity indicate microorganisms present and appropriate antibiotics to be used.	
6. Administer antibiotics as prescribed.	6. Antibiotics reduce bacteria.	
7. Provide regular linen changes, and assist patient with personal hygiene.	7. These measures reduce potential bacterial colonization of burn wound.	
8. Report to physician decreased bowel sounds, tachycardia, decreased blood pressure, decreased urine output, fever, and flushing, confusion or sudden disorientation.	8. These signs may indicate sepsis.	
9. Administer fluids and vasoactive medications as prescribed. Assess response.	9. These agents are used to maintain tissue perfusion in sepsis.	

continued >

Plan of Nursing Care

Chart 59-7. Care of the Patient During the Acute Phase of Burn Injury, *Continued*

Nursing Priority: Altered nutrition
Goal: Attainment of anabolic nutritional status

NURSING INTERVENTIONS	RATIONALE	EXPECTED OUTCOMES
1. Provide high-calorie, high-protein diet; include patient preferences and homemade food. Provide nutritional supplements as prescribed.	1. The patient needs sufficient nutrients for wound healing and increased metabolic requirements.	• Gains weight daily after initial loss • Exhibits no signs of protein, vitamin, or mineral deficiencies • Meets required nutritional needs entirely by oral intake • Participates in selection of diet with prescribed nutrients • Serum protein levels within acceptable range
2. Monitor patient's daily weight and calorie count.	2. These measures assist in determining whether dietary needs are being met.	
3. Administer supplemental vitamins and minerals as prescribed.	3. These help to meet additional nutritional needs; adequate vitamins and minerals are necessary for wound healing and cellular function.	
4. Administer enteral or parenteral nutrition per protocol if dietary needs are not met through oral intake.	4. Nutritional techniques ensure that nutritional needs are met.	
5. Report abdominal distention, large gastric residual volumes, or diarrhea to physician.	5. These signs may indicate intolerance of route or type of feeding.	

Nursing Priority: Impaired skin integrity
Goal: Demonstration of improved skin integrity

NURSING INTERVENTIONS	RATIONALE	EXPECTED OUTCOMES
1. Clean wounds, body, and hair daily.	1. Daily cleaning reduces potential bacterial colonization.	• Skin is generally intact and free of signs of infection, pressure, and trauma • Open wounds are pink, reepithelializing, and free of infection • Donor sites are clean and reepithelializing • Healed wounds are soft and smooth • Skin is lubricated and elastic; soft and supple
2. Provide wound care as prescribed.	2. Care promotes wound healing.	
3. Apply topical antibacterial agents and dressing as prescribed.	3. Wound care regimen reduces bacterial colonization and promotes healing.	
4. Prevent pressure, infection, and mobilization of skin grafts.	4. These measures promote graft take and healing.	
5. Provide donor site care.	5. Care promotes healing of donor site.	
6. Provide adequate nutritional support.	6. Adequate nutrition is essential for normal granulation and healing.	
7. Assess wound and graft sites. Report signs of poor healing, poor graft take, or trauma to physician.	7. Early intervention for poor wound healing or graft take is essential. Grafted or healed burn wounds are susceptible to trauma.	

Nursing Priority: Pain
Goal: Reduction or control of pain

NURSING INTERVENTIONS	RATIONALE	EXPECTED OUTCOMES
1. Assess pain level using pain intensity scale. Observe for nonverbal indicators of pain: grimacing, tachycardia, clenched fists.	1. Pain assessment data provide baseline for assessing response to interventions.	• Requests analgesics for specific wound care procedures or physical therapy activities • States pain is minimal • Gives no physiologic or nonverbal cues of moderate or severe pain • Uses pain control measures such as nitrous oxide, relaxation, imagery, and distraction techniques to assist with coping with pain • Can sleep without being disturbed by pain • Reports skin is comfortable with no itching or tightness
2. Educate the patient about the usual pain trajectory in burn recovery and options for pain control. Allow patient as much control as possible regarding pain management.	2. Knowledge reduces fear of the unknown and provides some measure of control to the patient.	
3. Offer analgesics approximately 20 minutes before painful procedures.	3. Premedication allows time for therapeutic response.	
4. Provide analgesia before pain becomes severe.	4. Pain is more easily controlled before it becomes severe.	
5. Instruct and assist patient in relaxation, imagery, and distraction techniques.	5. Nonpharmacologic pain measures provide multiple interventions to decrease pain sensation.	

Plan of Nursing Care

Chart 59-7. Care of the Patient During the Acute Phase of Burn Injury, *Continued*

NURSING INTERVENTIONS	RATIONALE	EXPECTED OUTCOMES
6. Assess and document the patient's response to interventions.	6. Patient's responses assist in ascertaining best pain control techniques for the patient.	
7. Administer antianxiety and antipruritic agents as indicated.	7. These medications help to increase patient's comfort.	
8. Lubricate healing burn wounds with water- or silica-based lotion (nonperfumed).	8. These preparations decrease sensation of skin tightness.	

Nursing Priority: Impaired physical mobility
Goal: Achievement of optimal physical mobility

NURSING INTERVENTIONS	RATIONALE	EXPECTED OUTCOMES
1. Position patient carefully to prevent flexed position in burned areas.	1. Proper positioning reduces risk of flexion contractures.	• Improves ROM of joints daily • Demonstrates preinjury ROM of all joints • Absence of signs of periarticular calcification or HO (heterotopic ossification: abnormal formation of bone in response to soft tissue trauma) • Participates in activities of daily living
2. Implement range-of-motion (ROM) exercises several times daily.	2. ROM exercises minimize muscle atrophy.	
3. Assist with early sitting and ambulation.	3. Early mobility encourages increased use of muscles.	
4. Use splints and exercise devices recommended by occupational and physical therapists.	4. Such devices encourage activity while maintaining proper position of joints.	
5. Encourage self-care to the extent of the patient's ability.	5. Self-care promotes both independence and increased activity.	

Nursing Priority: Ineffective individual coping
Goal: Use of appropriate coping strategies to deal with postburn problems

NURSING INTERVENTIONS	RATIONALE	EXPECTED OUTCOMES
1. Assess patient for coping abilities and previous successful coping strategies.	1. Psychosocial data provide baseline for planning care.	• Verbalizes reactions to burns, therapeutic procedures, and losses • Identifies effective coping strategies used previously in stressful situations • Accepts dependency on health care providers during acute illness • Resolves grief over losses resulting from burn injury • Participates in decision making regarding care • Has hopeful attitude toward future
2. Demonstrate acceptance of patient. Provide positive feedback and support.	2. Acceptance encourages self-esteem and continued progress toward independence.	
3. Assist patient to set achievable short-term goals for increased independence in activities of daily living.	3. Short-term goal setting leads to pattern of success for patient. Long-term goals may seem unrealistic or unattainable to patient.	
4. Use multidisciplinary approach to promote mobility and independence.	4. Communication among disciplines provides consistent approach.	
5. Consult with health care team members for assistance with regressive or maladaptive behaviours.	5. Collaboration uses the expertise of others.	

Nursing Priority: Altered family processes
Goal: Achievement of appropriate patient/family processes

NURSING INTERVENTIONS	RATIONALE	EXPECTED OUTCOMES
1. Assess patient and family's perception of impact of burn injury on family functioning.	1. Assessment data provide baseline from which to plan care.	• Patient verbalizes feelings regarding alteration in family interactions • Family can emotionally support the patient during hospitalization • Family states that needs are met
2. Demonstrate willingness to listen. Provide realistic support.	2. Empathetic attitude promotes verbalizing of concerns.	
3. Refer family to social services and other resources as needed.	3. Collaboration assists to address concerns comprehensively.	
4. Explain the burn patient's coping patterns to family. Discuss ways that they can support the patient.	4. Explanations help to decrease anxiety about the unknown and promote appropriate support of patient by family.	

continued >

Plan of Nursing Care — Chart 59-7. Care of the Patient During the Acute Phase of Burn Injury, *Continued*

Nursing Priority: Lack of knowledge
Goal: Verbalization of understanding of course of burn treatment by patient and family

NURSING INTERVENTIONS	RATIONALE	EXPECTED OUTCOMES
1. Assess readiness of patient and family to learn.	1. Limit education to patient and family's ability to process information.	• States rationale for different aspects of treatment • States realistic time period for recovery • Patient and family participate in management plans as appropriate
2. Explore patient and family's previous experience with hospitalization and illness.	2. This information provides a baseline for explanations and indication of patient and family's expectations.	
3. Review general course of burn treatment with patient and family.	3. Knowing what to expect prepares patient and family for upcoming events.	
4. Explain importance of patient participation in care for optimal results.	4. This information provides specific direction to patient.	
5. Realistically explain length of time involved in burn recovery.	5. Honesty promotes realistic expectations.	

Collaborative Problems: Congestive heart failure, pulmonary edema, sepsis, acute respiratory failure, acute respiratory distress syndrome, visceral damage (electrical burns)
Goal: Absence of complications

Congestive Heart Failure (CHF) and Pulmonary Edema

NURSING INTERVENTIONS	RATIONALE	EXPECTED OUTCOMES
1. Assess for decreased urine output, JVD, or an S_3 or S_4 heart sound.	1. These signs may indicate decreased cardiac output and the onset of CHF.	• Breath sounds clear upon auscultation • Absence of dyspnea, orthopnea, JVD, and S_3 or S_4 heart sounds • Urine output, arterial pressures, and cardiac output within normal limits
2. Monitor for increases in arterial pressures or decrease in cardiac output.	2. Increased pressures indicate increased preload and intravascular volumes. Decreasing cardiac output reflects less oxygen and nutrients available to the tissues and may indicate the onset of CHF.	
3. Assess for crackles on lung auscultation, dyspnea, orthopnea, or decreased oxygenation detected by pulse oximetry or arterial blood gas values.	3. Such signs may indicate progression of CHF to pulmonary edema.	
4. Report the above mentioned signs and symptoms to the physician.	4. Prompt medical intervention is needed.	
5. Position patient with the head of bed up 45 degrees to 90 degrees as tolerated.	5. Elevation facilitates gas exchange.	
6. Administer diuretics as prescribed. Assess patient's response.	6. Diuretics increase urine output and decrease cardiac preload and intravascular volumes.	

Sepsis

NURSING INTERVENTIONS	RATIONALE	EXPECTED OUTCOMES
1. Assess for fever, increased pulse, widened pulse pressure, and flushed, dry skin in unburned areas. Watch trends and notify physician if noted.	1. Such signs may indicate impending sepsis.	• Negative blood, sputum, and urine cultures • Absence of tachycardia, widening pulse pressure, and flushed, dry skin in unburned areas
2. Monitor wound, blood, sputum, and urine cultures, and notify physician of positive cultures.	2. Positive cultures indicate infection and possible sepsis.	
3. Administer fluids, vasoactive medications, and antibiotics as prescribed. Monitor for therapeutic response. Check that infecting organisms are sensitive to prescribed antibiotics.	3. Antibiotics kill susceptible bacteria. Intravenous fluids and vasoactive medications maintain intravascular volume and blood pressure.	
4. Monitor for therapeutic serum antibiotic levels.	4. Antibiotics are most effective at therapeutic levels. Excessive levels can cause organ damage.	

Plan of Nursing Care

Chart 59-7. Care of the Patient During the Acute Phase of Burn Injury, *Continued*

NURSING INTERVENTIONS	RATIONALE	EXPECTED OUTCOMES
Acute Respiratory Failure/Acute Respiratory Distress Syndrome (ARDS)		
1. Assess for respiratory distress, changes in respiratory patterns, or onset of adventitious breath sounds. Report to physician.	1. Such problems indicate possible acute respiratory failure. Pulmonary complications may not appear for 24–48 hours after the burn injury.	• Arterial blood gases within normal limits • Normal lung compliance • Absence of respiratory distress • Improved PO_2 level
2. Monitor pulse oximetry and arterial blood gas levels for decreasing oxygen saturation and PO_2. Report to physician.	2. Decreasing oxygenation indicates deteriorating respiratory status. Medical intervention is needed.	
3. Monitor the mechanically ventilated patient for decreased spontaneous tidal volumes and lung compliance.	3. Respiratory problems reflect increased difficulty with ventilation and may indicate the onset of ARDS.	
4. In collaboration with the physician and respiratory therapist, administer positive end-expiratory pressure and pressure support. Assess patient's response.	4. These measures optimize diffusion of oxygen across the alveolar–capillary membrane.	
Visceral Damage (Electrical Burns)		
1. Assess patient for signs of deep pain. Focus on areas between the contact point with the electrical source and contact point with the grounding site.	1. Pain may reflect visceral damage.	• Absence of visceral organ damage • Stable cardiac rhythm
2. Monitor electrocardiogram (ECG) rhythm.	2. The patient with electrical burns is at risk for arrhythmias.	
3. Report to physician any complaints of deep pain or dysrhythmias.	3. Visceral damage requires immediate intervention.	
4. Monitor electrolytes, enzymes, clotting factors (CK and troponin).	4. CK-MB and troponin levels are often elevated with electrical injuries, especially if the current pathway involves the chest/thorax	

The nurse serves as the coordinator of the complex aspects of wound care and dressing changes for the patient. The nurse must be aware of the rationale and nursing implications for the various wound management approaches. Nursing functions include assessing and recording any changes or progress in wound healing and keeping all members of the health care team informed of changes in the wound or treatment. A diagram, updated daily by the nurse responsible for the patient's care, helps to inform all of those concerned about the latest wound care procedures in use for the patient.

The nurse also assists the patient and family by providing instruction, support, and encouragement to take an active part in dressing changes and wound care when appropriate. Discharge planning needs for wound care are anticipated early in the course of burn management, and the strengths of the patient and family are assessed and used in preparing for eventual discharge and home care.

Relieving Pain and Discomfort

Pain measures discussed earlier are continued during the acute phase of burn recovery. Analgesic agents and anxiolytic medications are administered as prescribed. Frequent assessment of pain and discomfort is essential. To increase its effectiveness, analgesic medication is provided before the pain becomes severe. Nursing interventions such as teaching the patient relaxation techniques, giving the patient some control over wound care and analgesia, and providing frequent reassurance are helpful. Guided imagery may be effective in altering the patient's perceptions of and responses to pain. Other pain-relieving approaches include distraction through video programs or video games, hypnosis, biofeedback, and behavioural modification.

The nurse assesses the patient's sleep patterns daily. Lack of sleep and rest interferes with healing, comfort, and restoration of energy. If necessary, sedatives are prescribed on a regular basis in addition to analgesics and anxiolytics.

The nurse works quickly to complete treatments and dressing changes to reduce pain and discomfort. The patient is encouraged to take analgesic medications before painful procedures. The patient's response to the medication and other interventions is assessed and documented.

Healing burn wounds are typically described by patients as itchy and tight. Oral antipruritic agents, a cool environment, frequent lubrication of the skin with water or a silica-based lotion, exercise and splinting to prevent skin contracture, and diversional activities help to promote comfort in this phase.

Promoting Physical Mobility

An early priority is to prevent complications resulting from immobility. Deep breathing, turning, and proper repositioning are essential nursing practices that prevent atelectasis and pneumonia, control edema, and prevent pressure ulcers and contractures. These interventions are modified to meet the patient's needs. Low–air-loss and rotation beds may be useful, and early sitting and ambulation are encouraged. Whenever the lower extremities are burned, elastic pressure bandages (ACE, Tensor) should be applied before the patient is placed in an upright position. These bandages promote venous return and minimize swelling.

The burn wound is in a dynamic state for a year or more after wound closure. During this time, aggressive efforts must be made to prevent contracture and hypertrophic scarring. Both passive and active range-of-motion exercises are initiated from the day of admission and are continued after grafting, within prescribed limitations. Splints or functional devices may be applied to extremities for contracture control. The nurse monitors the splinted areas for signs of vascular insufficiency, nerve compression, and areas of pressure.

Strengthening Coping Strategies

In the acute phase of burn care, the patient is facing the reality of the burn trauma and is grieving over obvious losses. Depression, regression, and manipulative behaviour are common responses of patients who have burn injuries. Withdrawal from participation in required treatments and regression must be viewed with an understanding that such behaviour helps the patient cope with an enormously stressful event. Although most patients recover emotionally from a burn injury, some have more difficult psychological reactions to the injury and its outcomes (Fauerbach, Wiechman, & Mason, et al., 2016).

Much of the patient's energy goes into maintaining vital physical functions and wound healing in the early postburn weeks, leaving little emotional energy for coping in a more effective manner. Nurses can assist patients to develop effective coping strategies by setting specific expectations for behaviour, promoting truthful communication to build trust, helping patients practice appropriate strategies, and giving positive reinforcement when appropriate. Most importantly, the nurse and all members of the health care team must demonstrate acceptance of the patient.

Patients with burns are very dependent on health care team members during the long period of acute illness. However, even when physically unable to contribute much to self-care, they can be included in decisions regarding care and encouraged to assert their individuality in terms of preferences and recognition of their unique identities. As patients improve in mobility and strength, the nurse works with them to set realistic expectations for self-care, including self-feeding, assistance with wound care procedures, exercise, and planning for the future. Many patients respond positively to the use of contractual agreements and other strategies (i.e., a daily schedule) that recognizes their independence and their specific role as part of the health care team moving toward the goal of self-care. Consultation with psychiatric/mental health care providers may be helpful to assist the patient in developing effective coping strategies.

Supporting Patient and Family Processes

Family functioning is disrupted with burn injury. One of the nurse's responsibilities is to support the patient and family and to address their spoken and unspoken concerns. Family members need to be instructed about ways that they can support the patient as adaptation to burn trauma occurs. The family also needs support by the health care team. The burn injury has tremendous psychological, economic, and practical impact on the patient and family. Referrals for social services or psychological counselling should be made as appropriate. The nurse should direct the patient and family to online resources, such as the Phoenix Society, and to local burn support groups if available. This support continues into the rehabilitation phase.

Patients with burns are commonly sent to burn centres far from home. Because burn injuries are not anticipated, family roles are disrupted. Therefore, both the patient and the family need thorough information about the patient's burn care and expected course of treatment. Patient and family education begins at the initiation of burn management. Barriers to learning are assessed and considered in teaching. The preferred learning styles of both the patient and family are assessed. This information is used to tailor teaching activities. The nurse assesses the ability of the patient and family to grasp and cope with the information. Verbal information is supplemented by videos, models, or printed materials, if available. Patient and family education is a priority in the acute and rehabilitation phase. Again, there are many online education resources available through the Phoenix Society and the Model System Knowledge Translation Center websites that both burn staff and patients/families can access for free.

Nurses must remain sensitive to the possibility of changing family dynamics. It is not unusual for the provider in the family to be the one who is injured. Roles begin to change, which adds more stress to the family. In addition, families are often relocated due to loss of property from a fire. Social services play an integral part in providing support at this time.

Monitoring and Managing Potential Complications

HEART FAILURE AND PULMONARY EDEMA. The patient is assessed for fluid overload, which may occur as fluid is mobilized from the interstitial compartment back into the intravascular compartment. If the cardiac and renal systems cannot compensate for the excess vascular volume, congestive heart failure and pulmonary edema may result. The patient is assessed for signs of heart failure, including decreased cardiac output, oliguria, jugular vein distention, edema, and the onset of an S_3 or S_4 heart sound. If invasive hemodynamic monitoring is used, increasing central venous, pulmonary artery, and wedge pressures indicate increased fluid volume.

Crackles in the lungs and increased difficulty with respiration may indicate a fluid buildup in the lungs, which is reported promptly to the physician. In the meantime, the patient is positioned comfortably, with the head of the bed raised (if not contraindicated because of other treatments or injuries) to promote lung expansion and gas exchange. Management of this complication includes providing supplemental oxygen, administering IV diuretic agents, carefully assessing the patient's response, and providing vasoactive medications, if indicated.

SEPSIS. The signs of early systemic sepsis are subtle and require a high index of suspicion and very close monitoring of changes in the patient's status. Early signs of sepsis may include confusion, increased temperature, increased pulse rate, widened pulse pressure, and flushed dry skin in unburned areas. As with many observations of the patient with burns, one needs to look for patterns or trends in the data. (Refer to Chapter 18 for a more detailed discussion of septic shock.)

Wound and blood cultures are performed as prescribed, and results are reported to the physician immediately. The nurse also observes for and reports early signs of sepsis and promptly intervenes, administering prescribed IV fluids and antibiotics to prevent septic shock, which is a complication with a high mortality rate. Antibiotics must be given as scheduled to maintain proper blood concentrations. Serum antibiotic levels are monitored for evidence of maximal effectiveness, and the patient is monitored for toxic side effects.

ACUTE RESPIRATORY FAILURE AND ACUTE RESPIRATORY DISTRESS SYNDROME. The patient's respiratory status is monitored closely for increased difficulty breathing, change in respiratory pattern, and onset of adventitious (abnormal) sounds. Typically, at this stage, signs and symptoms of injury to the respiratory tract become apparent. Respiratory failure may follow. As described previously, signs of hypoxia (decreased oxygen to the tissues), decreased breath sounds, wheezing, tachypnea, stridor, and sputum tinged with soot (or in some cases containing sloughed tracheal tissue) are among the many possible findings. Patients receiving mechanical ventilation must be assessed for a decrease in tidal volume and lung compliance. The key sign of the onset of ARDS is hypoxemia while receiving 100% oxygen, decreased lung compliance, and significant shunting. The physician should be notified immediately of deteriorating respiratory status.

Medical management of the patient with acute respiratory failure requires intubation and mechanical ventilation (if not already in use). If ARDS has developed, higher oxygen levels, positive end-expiratory pressure, and pressure support are used with mechanical ventilation to promote gas exchange across the alveolar–capillary membrane.

VISCERAL DAMAGE. The nurse must be alert to signs of necrosis of visceral organs due to electrical injury. Tissues affected are usually between the contact point with the electrical source and contact point with the grounding site of the electrical burn. All patients with electrical burns should undergo electrocardiographic monitoring, with arrhythmias being reported to the physician. Monitoring of electrolytes, enzymes, and clotting factors (CK and troponin) should also be done. Careful attention must also be paid to signs or reports of pain related to deep muscle ischemia. To minimize the severity of complications, visceral ischemia must be detected as early as possible. The physician can perform a **fasciotomy** to relieve the swelling and ischemia in the muscles and fascia and to promote oxygenation of the injured tissues. Because of the deep incisions involved with fasciotomy, the patient must be monitored carefully for signs of excessive blood loss and hypovolemia.

Evaluation

Expected patient outcomes may include the following:

1. Achieves optimal fluid balance
   a. Maintains intake and output and body weight that correlate with expected pattern
   b. Exhibits vital signs and central venous, pulmonary artery, and pulmonary artery wedge pressures within designated limits
   c. Demonstrates increased urine output in response to diuretic and vasoactive medications
   d. Has heart rate less than 110 beats/min
2. Has no localized or systemic infection
   a. Has wound culture results showing minimal bacteria
   b. Has normal urine and sputum culture results
3. Demonstrates anabolic nutritional status
   a. Gains weight daily after initial loss secondary to fluid diuresis and no oral intake of food or fluid
   b. Shows no signs of protein, vitamin, or mineral deficiencies
   c. Meets required nutritional needs entirely by oral intake
   d. Participates in selecting diet containing prescribed nutrients
   e. Exhibits normal serum protein levels
4. Demonstrates improved skin integrity
   a. Sustains generally intact skin that remains free of infection, pressure, and injury
   b. Demonstrates remaining open wound areas that are pink, reepithelializing, and free of infection
   c. Demonstrates donor graft sites that are clean and healing
   d. Has healed wounds that are soft and smooth
   e. Demonstrates skin that is lubricated and elastic; soft and supple
5. Has minimal pain
   a. Requests analgesic agents for specific wound care procedures or physical therapy activities
   b. Reports minimal or tolerable pain
   c. Gives no physiologic, verbal, or nonverbal cues that pain is moderate or severe

d. Uses pain control measures such as nitrous oxide, relaxation, imagery, and distraction techniques to cope with and alleviate pain and discomfort
e. Can sleep without being disturbed by pain
f. Reports skin is comfortable, with no itching or tightness
6. Demonstrates optimal physical mobility
a. Improves range of motion of joints daily
b. Demonstrates preinjury range of motion of all joints
c. Has no signs of calcification around the joints
d. Participates in activities of daily living
7. Uses appropriate coping strategies to deal with postburn problems
a. Verbalizes reactions to burns, therapeutic procedures, and losses
b. Identifies coping strategies used effectively in previous stressful situations
c. Accepts dependency on health care providers during acute phase
d. Verbalizes realistic view of problems resulting from burn injury and plans for future
e. Cooperates with health care providers in required therapy
f. Participates in decision making regarding care
g. Resolves grief over losses resulting from burn injury and circumstances surrounding injury (e.g., death of others, damage to home or other property, loss of income)
h. States realistic objectives for plastic surgery, further medical intervention, and results
i. Verbalizes realistic abilities and goals
j. Displays hopeful attitude toward future
8. Relates appropriately in patient/family processes
a. Patient and family verbalize feelings regarding change in family interactions
b. Family emotionally supports patient during hospitalization
c. Family states that own needs are met
9. Patient and family verbalize understanding of treatment course
a. States rationale for different aspects of treatment
b. States realistic time period for recovery
10. Absence of complications
a. Breath sounds clear on auscultation
b. Exhibits no dyspnea or orthopnea and can breathe easily when standing, sitting, and lying down
c. Exhibits no S_3 or S_4 heart sounds or jugular venous distention
d. Exhibits urine output; central venous, pulmonary artery, and pulmonary artery wedge pressures; and cardiac output within normal or acceptable limits
e. Exhibits normal blood, sputum, and urine culture results
f. Maintains arterial blood gas values within normal or acceptable limits
g. Has normal lung compliance
h. Has no visceral organ damage
i. Has stable cardiac rhythm

Rehabilitation Phase of Burn Care

Although long-term aspects of burn care are discussed last in this chapter, rehabilitation begins immediately after the burn has occurred—as early as the emergent period—and often extends for years after injury. In the aftermath of the acute stages of injury, the patient increasingly focuses on the alterations in self-image and lifestyle that may occur. Wound healing, psychosocial support, and restoring maximal functional activity remain priorities. The focus on maintaining fluid and electrolyte balance and improving nutritional status continues. Reconstructive surgery to improve body appearance and function may be needed. One important focus of the burn team is to evaluate the patient carefully for late complications related to burn injuries as described in Table 59-8.

Burn injuries can have a major impact on quality of life. Changes in physical activity and social, psychological, and employment status may occur. Therefore, psychological and vocational counselling and referral to support groups may be helpful to promote recovery and quality of life. Family members also need support and guidance in assisting the patient to return to optimal health.

Burn rehabilitation is comprehensive, complex, and requires a multidisciplinary approach to optimize the patient's physical and psychosocial recovery related to the injury. As patients begin to recover, they become more aware of the injuries and the challenges they face. Individualized plans of care that are specific to the severity and location of injury are developed and reevaluated frequently. The increased survival of patients with significant burn injuries has translated into the need for additional and comprehensive burn rehabilitation programs worldwide. The ultimate goal is to return patients to the highest level of function possible within the context of their injuries. Occupational and physical therapists are essential to optimize patient goals and outcomes.

Prevention of Hypertrophic Scarring

The wound is in a dynamic state for 1.5 to 2.0 years after the burn occurs. If appropriate measures are instituted during this active period, the scar tissue loses its redness and softens. Healed areas that are prone to hypertrophic scarring require the patient to wear a pressure garment. These devices are especially useful for partial-thickness wounds that require more than 2 weeks to heal and for the edges of grafted skin. Applying elastic pressure garments loosens collagen bundles and encourages parallel orientation of the collagen to the skin surface, with the disappearance of the dermal nodules. As pressure continues over time, there is a restructuring of the collagen and a decrease in vascularity and cellularity. However, pressure needs to be continuous. Many areas of the body are difficult to compress due to the contours or the presence of cartilage. Gel or gel sheets inserts are used under the pressure garments to enhance scar compression in immature scars (Nedelec et al., 2015).

The physical therapist, occupational therapist, or a representative of the manufacturer of elastic pressure garments measures the patient for correct fit. While awaiting the arrival of the garment, soft, tubular, knitted elastic pressure bandages can be used to help desensitize the patient's skin, protect healing areas, apply pressure, and

TABLE 59-8 Complications in Rehabilitation Phase of Burn Care

Complications	Contributing Factors	Interventions
Neuropathies and nerve entrapment	Electrical injury, large deep burns, improper positioning, edema, scar tissue	Assess peripheral pulses and sensation (neurovascular checks). Prevent edema and pressure by elevation, positioning, and prevention of constricting dressings. Assess splints for proper fit and application. Consult OT and PT departments for positioning.
Wound breakdown and/or pressure ulcer formation	Shearing, pressure, inadequate nutrition	Protect wound from pressure and shearing forces. Educate patient about importance of good nutrition.
Hypertrophic scarring	Partial- and full-thickness burns	Keep skin pliable and soft by using emollients. Apply pressure garments as prescribed. Massage.
Contractures	Partial- and full-thickness burns	Maintain position of joints in alignment. Perform gentle range-of-motion exercises. Consult OT and PT departments for exercises and positioning recommendations.
Joint instability	Burn wound, burn scar, and contractures	Maintain appropriate joint positioning through appropriate application of splints. Monitor joint pinning if indicated.
Complex pain	Trauma and burns	Provide adequate pain management. Consult OT and PT departments for exercises and desensitization. Promote gentle motion of affected extremities.

promote venous return. Patients must be instructed about the need for lubrication and protection of the healing skin and the need for pressure garments for at least a year after the injury. A program including elastic pressure garments, splints, and exercise under the supervision of an experienced physical and occupational therapy team is recommended for optimal functional and aesthetic results.

Nursing Process

Care of the Patient During the Rehabilitation Phase

Assessment

Information about the patient's educational level, occupation, leisure activities, cultural background, religion, and family interactions is obtained early. The patient's self-concept, mental status, emotional response to the injury and hospitalization, level of intellectual functioning, previous hospitalizations, response to pain and pain relief measures, and sleep pattern are also essential components of a comprehensive assessment. Information about the patient's general self-concept, self-esteem, and coping strategies in the past will be valuable in addressing emotional needs.

Ongoing physical assessments related to rehabilitation goals include range of motion of affected joints, functional abilities in activities of daily living, early signs of skin breakdown from splints or positioning devices, evidence of neuropathies (neurologic damage), activity tolerance, and quality or condition of healing skin. The patient's participation in care and ability to demonstrate self-care in such areas as ambulation, eating, wound cleaning, and applying pressure wraps are documented on a regular basis. In addition to these assessment parameters, specific complications and treatments require additional specific assessments; for example, the patient undergoing primary excision requires postoperative assessment.

Recovery from burn injury involves every system of the body. Therefore, assessment of the patient must be comprehensive and continuous. Priorities will vary at different points during the rehabilitation phase. Understanding the pathophysiologic responses to burn injury forms the framework for detecting early progress or signs and symptoms of complications. Early detection leads to early intervention and enhances the potential for successful rehabilitation.

Nursing Priorities

Based on assessment data, nursing priorities in the long-term rehabilitation phase of burn care may include the following:

- Activity intolerance
- Disturbed body image
- Lack of knowledge

Collaborative Problems/ Potential Complications

Based on assessment data, potential complications that may develop in the rehabilitation phase include the following:

- Contractures
- Inadequate psychological adaptation to burn injury

Planning and Goals

The major goals for the patient include increased participation in activities of daily living; increased understanding of the injury, treatment, and planned follow-up care; adaptation and adjustment to alterations in body image, self-concept, and lifestyle; and absence of complications.

Nursing Interventions

Promoting Activity Tolerance

Nursing interventions that must be carried out according to a strict regimen and the pain that accompanies movement take their toll on a patient with burns. The patient may become confused and disoriented and lack the energy to participate optimally in care. The nurse must schedule care in such a way that the patient has periods of uninterrupted rest and sleep. A good time for planned patient rest is after the stress of dressing changes and exercise, while pain interventions and sedatives may still be effective. This plan must be communicated to family members and other care providers.

Patients with burns may have insomnia related to frequent nightmares about the burn injury or to other fears and anxieties about the outcome of the injury. The nurse listens to and reassures the patient while promoting a normal sleep-wake cycle. Nonpharmacologic methods such as relaxation methods are encouraged. Hypnotic agents are administered, as prescribed, to promote sleep.

Reducing metabolic stress by relieving pain, preventing chilling or fever, and promoting the physical integrity of all body systems will help the patient conserve energy for therapeutic activities and wound healing.

The nurse incorporates physical therapy exercises in the patient's care to prevent muscle atrophy and to maintain the mobility required for daily activities. The patient's activity tolerance, strength, and endurance will gradually increase if activity occurs over increasingly longer periods. Fatigue, fever, and pain tolerance are monitored and used to determine the amount of activity to be encouraged on a daily basis. Activities such as family visits and recreational or play therapy (e.g., video games, radio, television) can provide diversion, improve the patient's outlook, and increase tolerance for physical activity.

Improving Body Image and Self-Concept

Patients with burns frequently suffer profound losses. These include not only a loss of body image due to disfigurement but also losses of personal property, homes, loved ones, and ability to work. They lack the benefit of anticipatory grief often seen in a patient approaching surgery or a person dealing with the terminal illness of a loved one.

As care progresses, the patient who is recovering from burns becomes aware of daily improvement and begins to exhibit basic concerns: Will I be disfigured? How long will I be in the hospital? What about my job and family? Will I ever be independent again? Was my burn the result of my carelessness? As the patient expresses such concerns, the nurse must take time to listen and to provide realistic support. The nurse can refer patients to a support group, such as those usually available at local burn centres. Through participation in such groups, patients will meet others with similar experiences and learn coping strategies to help them deal with their losses. Interaction with other burn survivors allows the patient to see that adaptation to the burn injury is possible. If a support group is not available, visits from burn survivors can be helpful to the patient coping with such a traumatic injury.

A major responsibility of the nurse is to assess constantly the patient's psychosocial needs. What are the patient's fears and concerns? Does the patient fear loss of control of care, independence, or sanity itself? Is the patient afraid of rejection by family and loved ones? Does he or she fear being unable to cope with pain or physical appearance? Does the patient have concerns about sexuality, including sexual function? Being aware of these anxieties and understanding the basis of the patient's fears enable the nurse to provide support and to cooperate with other members of the health care team in developing a plan to help the patient deal with these feelings.

When caring for patients with burns, the nurse needs to be aware that there are prejudices and misunderstandings in society about those who are viewed as different. Opportunities and accommodations available to others are often denied to those who are disfigured. Such amenities include social participation, employment, prestige, various roles, and status. The health care team must actively promote a healthy body image and self-concept in burn survivors so that they can accept or challenge others' perceptions of those who are disfigured. Survivors themselves must show others who they are, how they function, and how they want to be treated.

The nurse can help patients practice their responses to people who may stare or inquire about their injury once they are discharged from the hospital. The nurse can help patients build self-esteem by recognizing their uniqueness—for example, with small gestures such as providing a birthday cake, combing the patient's hair before visiting hours, giving information about the availability of a cosmetician to enhance appearance, and teaching the patient ways to direct attention away from a disfigured body to the self within. Consultants such as psychologists, social workers, vocational counsellor, and teachers are valuable participants in assisting patients with burns to regain their self-esteem.

Monitoring and Managing Potential Complications

CONTRACTURES. With early and intensive physical and occupational therapy, contractures are rarely a long-term complication. However, surgical intervention is indicated if a full range of motion in the patient with burns is not achieved. (Refer to Chapter 12 for a discussion of prevention of contractures.)

IMPAIRED PSYCHOLOGICAL ADAPTATION TO THE BURN INJURY. Some patients, particularly those with limited coping skills or psychological function or a history of psychiatric problems before the burn injury, may not achieve adequate psychological adaptation to the burn injury. Psychological counselling or psychiatric referral may be made to assess the patient's emotional status, to help the patient develop coping skills, and to intervene if major psychological issues or ineffective coping is identified.

Promoting Home, Community-Based, and Transitional Care

EDUCATING PATIENTS ABOUT SELF-CARE. As the inpatient phase of recovery becomes shorter, the focus of rehabilitative interventions is directed toward outpatient care or care in a rehabilitation centre. In the long term, much of the care of healing burns will be performed by the patient and others at home. Throughout the phases of burn care, efforts are made to prepare the patient and family for the care that will continue at home. Thus, they are instructed about the measures and procedures that they will need to perform. For example, patients commonly have small areas of clean, open wounds that are healing slowly. They are instructed to wash these areas daily with mild soap and water, and to apply the prescribed topical agent or dressing.

In addition to instructions about wound care, patients and families require careful written and verbal instructions about prevention of complications, pain management, and nutrition. Information about specific exercises and use of pressure garments and splints is reviewed with both the patient and family; written instructions are provided for reference. They are taught to recognize abnormal signs and instructed to report them to the physician. All of this information will enable patients to progress successfully through the rehabilitative phase of burn management. The patient and family are assisted in planning for the patient's continued care by identifying and acquiring supplies and equipment that are needed at home.

CONTINUING AND TRANSITIONAL CARE. Follow-up care by an interprofessional burn care team will be necessary. Preparations should begin during the early stages of care. Patients who receive care in a burn centre usually return to the burn clinic or centre periodically for evaluation by the burn team, modification of home care instructions, and planning for reconstructive surgery. Other patients receive ongoing care from the general or plastic surgeon who cared for them during the acute phase of their management. Still other patients require the services of a rehabilitation centre and may be transferred to such a centre for aggressive rehabilitation before going home. Many patients require outpatient physical or occupational therapy, often several times weekly. It is often the nurse who is responsible for coordinating all aspects of care and ensuring that the patient's needs are met. Such coordination is an important aspect in assisting a patient with burns to achieve independence.

Patients who return home after a severe burn injury, those who cannot manage their own burn care, and those with inadequate support systems will need referral for home care. During visits to the patient at home, the home care nurse assesses the patient's physical and psychological status as well as the adequacy of the home setting for safe and adequate care. The nurse monitors the patient's progress and adherence to the plan of care and notes any problems that interfere with the patient's ability to carry out the care. During the visit, the nurse assists the patient and family with wound care and exercises. Patients with severe or persistent depression or difficulty adjusting to changes in their social and/or occupational roles are identified and referred to the burn team for possible referral to a psychologist, psychiatrist, or vocational counsellor.

The burn team or home care nurse identifies community resources that may be helpful for the patient and family. Several support groups and other organizations offer services for patients with burns. They provide caring people (often those recovered from burn injuries) who can visit a patient in the hospital or home or telephone the patient and family periodically to provide support and counselling about skin care, cosmetics, and problems related to psychosocial adjustment. Such organizations sponsor group meetings and social functions at which outpatients are welcome. Some also provide school reentry programs and are active in burn prevention activities. If more information is needed regarding burn prevention, the American Burn Association can help to locate the nearest burn centre (including locations in Canada) and offer current burn prevention tips (see Chart 59-1).

Because so much attention is given to the burn wound and the treatments that are necessary to treat the burn wound and to prevent complications, the patient, family, and health care providers may inadvertently ignore the patient's ongoing needs for health promotion and screening. Thus, the patient and family are reminded of the importance of periodic health screening and preventive care (e.g., gynecologic examinations, dental care).

Evaluation

Expected patient outcomes may include the following:

1. Demonstrates activity tolerance required for desired daily activities
   a. Obtains sufficient sleep daily
   b. Reports absence of nightmares or sleep disturbances
   c. Shows gradually increasing tolerance and endurance in physical activities
   d. Can concentrate during conversations
   e. Has energy available to sustain desired daily activities
2. Adapts to altered body image
   a. Verbalizes accurate description of alterations in body image and accepts physical appearance
   b. Demonstrates interest in resources that may improve body appearance and function
   c. Uses cosmetics, wigs, and prostheses as desired to achieve acceptable appearance
   d. Socializes with significant others, peers, and usual social group
   e. Seeks and achieves return to role in family, school, and community as a contributing member

3. Demonstrates knowledge of required self-care and follow-up care
   a. Describes surgical procedures and treatments accurately
   b. Verbalizes detailed plan for follow-up care
   c. Demonstrates ability to perform wound care and prescribed exercises
   d. Returns for follow-up appointments as scheduled
   e. Identifies resource people and agencies to contact for specific problems
4. Exhibits no complications
   a. Demonstrates full range of motion
   b. Shows no signs of withdrawal or depression
   c. Displays no psychotic behaviours

Outpatient Burn Care

More and more burns are being treated exclusively in outpatient settings, including wound clinics, physicians' offices, and emergency department clinics. The outpatient setting is appropriate for the care of minor burns. However, a number of factors must be considered in determining the appropriate site of care. These factors include the age of the patient, the extent and depth of the burn, the availability of family support systems and community resources to assist the patient, the patient's adherence to the prescribed plan of care, and the distance from home to the outpatient setting.

Initially, looking at and touching the burn wound may be difficult and even frightening to some family members and patients. However, with encouragement and support, most can handle burn wound care with little need for daily professional care. Instructions, both verbal and written, are given to the patient about burn wound care, pain management strategies, the need for adequate nutrition, and the importance of exercise and rest. Instruction is also given about signs and symptoms of infection that should be reported to the physician. The importance of notifying the physician about complications early and of keeping follow-up appointments is emphasized to the patient and family.

Gerontologic Considerations

Nursing assessment of the older patient with burns should include particular attention to pulmonary function, response to fluid resuscitation, and signs of mental confusion or disorientation. A careful history of preburn medications, pre-existing illnesses, cognitive and mental assessments are essential. Delirium is a medical emergency and every effort to prevent it from occurring is of utmost importance.

Nursing care promotes early mobilization, aggressive pulmonary care, and attention to preventing complications. Because of lowered resistance, burn wound sepsis and lethal systemic septicemias are more likely in older patients. Moreover, fever may not be present in the older to signal such events. Therefore, surveillance for other signs of infection becomes even more important.

Rehabilitation must take into account pre-existing functional abilities and limitations, such as arthritis and low activity tolerance. Older patients commonly lack family members who can provide home care, so social services and community nursing services must be contacted to provide optimal care and supervision after hospital discharge.

Critical Thinking Exercises

1 A 45-year-old man sustains a steam burn while working on an offshore oil platform in the Gulf of Mexico. He sustains third-degree burns over 65% of his body. Inclement weather has delayed transportation to the nearest burn centre. What should be the priorities of the first responders on the scene? On arrival to the treating facility, the patient's temperature is 35.2°C (95.3°F), and his weight is 62 kg (137 lb). How should the treatment team at the burn treating facility prioritize this patient's care?

2 A 34-year-old woman is roasting a turkey for Thanksgiving. In the process of removing the turkey from the oven, grease spills from the roasting pan onto her right hand and forearm, and both lower legs and feet. She is transported by EMS to the hospital for care. Using the rule of nines, what is her estimated TBSA? Based on the best evidence, what type of fluid should be used for resuscitation and why? What other information would you need to calculate her fluid requirements in the emergent/resuscitative phase?

3 A 69-year-old man was found down in the hallway of his apartment by firefighters, who extracted him from the smoke-filled building after being called to the scene by neighbours. He does not sustain obvious cutaneous burns. Upon interview and examination, he is tachypneic and exhibits hoarseness when speaking. You note singed nasal hair and lips. What is your immediate concern? What treatment should you expect the physician to prescribe first? Based on the current best evidence, what tests or procedures would most likely be prescribed to assist in the diagnosis and management of this patient?

REFERENCES AND SELECTED READINGS

Books

American Burn Association (ABA). (2018a). *Advanced burn life support (ABLS) course provider manual 2011*. Chicago, IL: Author.

American Burn Association. (2018b). *Burn center referral criteria*. Retrieved March 25, 2019, from http://ameriburn.org/wp-content/uploads/2017/05/burncenterreferralcriteria.pdf

American Burn Association. (2018c). *Scalds: A Burning Issue*. A Campaign Kit for Burn Awareness Week. Retrieved March 25, 2019, from http://ameriburn.org/wp-content/uploads/2017/04/scaldinjuryeducatorsguide.pdf

Cabiaso-Daniel, J., Gallagher, J., Norbury, W., et al. (2018). Treatment of infection in burn patients. In D. N. Herndon (Ed.). *Total burn care* (5th ed.). Philadelphia, PA: Saunders Elsevier.

Carson, J. S., Khosrozadeh, H., Norbury, W. B., et al. (2018). Nutritional needs and support for the burned patient. In D. N. Herndon (Ed.). *Total burn care* (5th ed.). Philadelphia, PA: Saunders Elsevier.

Centers for Disease Control and Prevention. (2014). Guidelines for the prevention of intravascular catheter-related infections. 1–83.

Herndon, D. N. (2018). *Total burn care*. Philadelphia, PA: WB Saunders.

Lee, J. O., Dibildox, M., Jimenez, C. J., et al. (2012). Operative wound management. In D. Herndon (Ed.). *Total burn care* (4th ed.). Edinburgh, UK: Saunders Elsevier.

Mayhall, C. G. (2012). Healthcare-associated burn wound infections. In C. G. Mayhall (Ed.). *Hospital epidemiology and infection control* (4th ed.). Philadelphia, PA: Lippincott Williams & Wilkins.

Micak, R., & Buffalo, M. (2007). Pre-hospital management, transportation, and emergency care. In D. N. Herndon (Ed.). *Total burn care* (2nd ed.). Philadelphia, PA: Saunders Elsevier.

Middlekoop, E., & Sheridan, R. L. (2018). Skin substitutes and 'the next level'. In D. N. Herndon (Ed.). *Total burn care* (5th ed.). Philadelphia, PA: Saunders Elsevier.

Serghiou, M. A., Ott, S., Whitehead, C., et al. (2012). Comprehensive rehabilitation of the burn patient. In D. Herndon (Ed.). *Total burn care* (4th ed.). Edinburgh, UK: Saunders Elsevier.

Voigt, C., Williamson, S., Kagan, R., et al. (2018). The skin bank. In D. N. Herndon (Ed.). *Total burn care* (5th ed.). Philadelphia, PA: Saunders Elsevier.

Wurzer, P., Culnan, D., Cancio, L. C., et al. (2018). Pathophysiology of burn shock and burn edema. In D. N. Herndon (Ed.). *Total burn care* (5th ed.). Philadelphia, PA: Saunders Elsevier.

Journals and Electronic Documents

Abdullahi, A., & Jeschke, M. G. (2014). Nutrition and anabolic pharmacotherapies in the care of burn patients. *Nutrition in Clinical Practice, 29*(5), 621–630.

Advanced Burn Life Support (ABLS). (2018). *ABLS live course (American Burn Association)*. Retrieved from http://ameriburn.org/education/abls-program/abls-live-course/#1493046921889-efac1085-f963

Allen, A., Recht, K., & Litt, J. S. (2018). Successful posterior cultured epidermal autograft placement to a major burn victim: a university burn center experience and review of the literature. *Journal of Burn Care & Research, 39*(1), 231.

Cahill, K. C., Tiong, W. H., & Conroy, F. J. (2013). Trineural injury to the right hand after domestic electrocution. *Journal of Burn Care and Research, 35*(5), e353–e356.

Cartotto, R., Greenhalgh, D., & Cancio, C. (2017). Burn State of the Science: Fluid Resuscitation. *Journal of Burn Care & Research, 38*(3), e596–e604.

Davis, J. S., Rodriquez, L. I., Quintana, O. D., et al. (2013). Use of a warming catheter to achieve normothermia in large burns. *Journal of Burn Care and Research, 34*(1), 191–195.

Dries, D., & Endorf, F. (2013). Inhalation injury: epidemiology, pathology, treatment strategies. *Scandinavian Journal of Trauma, Resuscitation and Emergency Medicine*, 21–31. Retrieved from https://doi.org/10.1186/1757-7241-21-31

Emergency department surveillance of burns and scalds, electronic Canadian Hospitals Injury Reporting and Prevention Program, 2013—HPCDP: Volume 37-1, January 2017. Retrieved from https://www.canada.ca/en/public-health/services/reports-publications/health-promotion-chronic-disease-prevention-canada-research-policy-practice/vol-37-no-1-2017/glance-emergency-department-surveillance-thermal-burns-scalds-electronic-canadian-hospitals-injury-reporting-prevention-program-2013.html

Fahlstrom, K., Boyle, C., & Makic, M. B. (2013). Implementation of a nurse-driven burn resuscitation protocol: A quality improvement project. *Critical Care Nurse, 33*(1), 25–35.

Faraklas, I., Holt, B., Tran, S., et al. (2013). Impact of a nursing-driven sleep hygiene protocol on sleep quality. *Journal of Burn Care & Research, 34*(2), 249–254.

Fauerbach, J., Wiechman, S. A., & Mason, S. (2016). Psychological distress after burn injury. Retrieved on April 2, 2019, from https://msktc.org/burn/factsheets/Psychological-Distress

Flores, O., Stockton, K., Roberts, J. A., et al. (2015). The efficacy and safety of adrenergic blockade after burn injury: A systematic review and meta-analysis. *Journal of Trauma and Acute Care Surgery, 80*(1), 146–155.

Gabriel, V. (2011). Hypertrophic scar. *Physical Medicine and Rehabilitation Clinics of North America*, 22, 301–310.

Greenhalgh, D. (2017). Sepsis in the burn patient: A different problem than sepsis in the general population. *Burns & Trauma*, 5, 23.

Hermans, M. E. (2014). Porcine xenografts vs. (cryopreserved) allografts in the management of partial thickness burns: Is there a clinical difference? *Burns, 40*(3), 408–415.

Hobbs, K. (2014). Which factors influence the development of post-traumatic stress disorder in patients with burn injuries? A systematic review of the literature. *Burns, 41*(3), 421–430.

Hostler, D., Weaver, M. D., Ziembicki, J. A., et al. (2013). Admission temperature and survival in patients admitted to burn centers. *Journal of Burn Care and Research, 34*(5), 498–506.

Jeschke, M. G. (2016). Postburn hypermetabolism: Past, present, and future. *Journal of Burn Care & Research, 37*(2), 86–96.

Jeschke, M. G., Finnerty, C. C., Shahrokhi, S., et al. (2013). Wound coverage technologies in burn care: Novel techniques. *Journal of Burn Care and Research, 34*(6), 612–620.

Jeschke, M. G., & Peck, P. (2017). Burn Care of the Elderly. *Journal of Burn Care & Research, 38*(3), e625–e628.

Jeschke, M. G., Pinto, R., Kraft, R., et al. (2015). Morbidity and survival probability in burn patients in modern burn care. *Critical Care Medicine, 43*(4), 808–815.

Justiniano, C. F., Coffey, R. A., Evans, D. C., et al. (2015). Comorbidity-polypharmacy score predicts in-hospital complications and the need for discharge to extended care facility in older burn patients. *Journal of Burn Care and Research, 36*(1), 193–196.

Kagan, R. J., Peck, M. D., Ahrenholz, D. H., et al. (2013). Surgical management of the burn wound and use of skin substitutes: An expert panel white paper. *Journal of Burn Care & Research, 34*(2), e60–e79.

Kearns, R. D., Cairns, C. B., Holmes, J. H., et al. (2013). Thermal burns: A review of best practice. *EMS World, 42*(1), 43–51.

Klas, K. S., Smith, S. J., Matherly, A. F., et al. (2015). Multicenter assessment of burn team injury prevention knowledge. *Journal of Burn Care and Research, 36*(3), 434–439.

Kollias, S., Stampolidis, N., Kourakos, P., et al. (2015). Abdominal compartment syndrome (ACS) in a severely burned patient. *Annals of Burns and Fire Disasters, 28*(1), 5–8.

Kwon, K. H., Kim, S. H., & Minn Y. K. (2014). Electrodiagnostic study of peripheral nerves in high-voltage electrical injury. *Journal of Burn Care and Research, 35*(4), e230–e233.

Kym, D., Yim, H., Yoon, J., et al. (2015). The application of cultured epithelial autografts improves survival in burns. *Wound Repair and Regeneration, 23*, 340–344.

Mann-Salinas, E. A., Baun, M. M., Meininger, J. C., et al. (2013). Novel predictors of sepsis outperform the American Burn Association sepsis criteria in the burn intensive care unit patient. *Journal of Burn Care and Research, 34*(1), 31–43.

Matsumura, H., Matsushima, A., Ueyama, M., et al. (2016). Application of the cultured epidermal autograft "JACE®" for treatment of severe burns: Results of a 6-year multicenter surveillance in Japan. *Burns, 42*(4), 769–776.

Meyerson, J. M., Coffey, R., Jones, L. M., et al. (2015). Burn center barrier protocols during dressing change: A national survey. *Journal of Burn Care and Research, 36*(4), 238–234.

Micromedex 2.0. (2015). Formulary advisor, University of Texas–Medical Branch Galveston. Retrieved on July 10, 2015 (pass-protected), from www.micromedicsolutions.com/micromedex2/librarian

Mosley, M., Muniz Castro, J., Joe, V., et al. (2018). Time from burn injury to initial excision and its association with surgical blood loss. *Journal of Burn Care & Research, 39*(1), S69.

Nedelec, B., Carter, A., Forbes, L., et al. (2015). Practice guidelines for the application of nonsilicone or silicone gels and gel sheets after burn injury. *Journal of Burn Care & Research, 36*(3), 345–374.

Nordlund, M. J., Pham, T. N., & Gibran, N. S. (2014). Micronutrients after burn injury: a review. *Journal of Burn Care & Research, 35*(2), 121–133.

Parachutte Canada. (2015). *The Cost of Injury in Canada.* Toronto: Parachute, in collaboration with The Conference Board of Canada; 2015. Retrieved from www.parachutecanada.org/downloads/research/Cost_of_Injury-2015.pdf.

Puri, V., Khare, N. A., Chandramouli, M. V., et al. (2016). Comparative analysis of early excision and grafting vs delayed grafting in burn patients in a developing country. *Journal of Burn Care & Research, 37*(5), 278–282.

Rerouvey, H., & Shahrokhi, S. (2015). Pain and the thermally injured patient—a review of current therapies. *Journal of Burn Care and Research, 36*(2), 315–323.

Sen, S., Palmieri, T., & Greenhalgh, D. (2015). Review of burn research for year 2014. *Journal of Burn Care and Research, 36*(6), 587–594.

Trexler, S. T., Lundy, J. B., Chung, K. K., et al. (2014). Prevalence and impact of late defecation in the critically ill, thermally injured adult patient. *Journal of Burn Care and Research, 35*(4), e224–e229.

Wiechman, S. A., & Brych, S. (2019). Employment after burn injury. Retrieved on April 2, 2019, from https://msktc.org/burn/factsheets/Employment-After-Burn-Injury

World Health Organization (WHO). (2014). *Fact sheet No. 365. Burns*. Retrieved on June 12, 2016, from www.who.int/mediacentre/factsheets/fs365/en/

Resources

American Burn Association: http://www.ameriburn.org
Burn Institute: http://www.burninstitute.org
Burn Prevention Foundation: http://www.burnprevention.org
Canadian Patient Safety Institute: http://www.patientsafetyinstitute.ca/English/Pages/default.aspx#
Chemical Educational Foundation: http://www.chemed.org
Firefighters Burn Institute: http://www.ffburn.org
Integra Life Sciences Corporation: http://www.integralife.com/
International Association of Fire Fighters Burn Foundation: http://www.iaff.org
International Society for Burn Injuries: http://www.worldburn.org
LifeCell Corporation: http://www.lifecell.com
Model Systems Knowledge Translation Center: https://msktc.org/burn
Phoenix Society for Burn Survivors: http://www.phoenix-society.org
The Cost of Injury in Canada. Toronto: Parachute, in collaboration with The Conference Board of Canada; 2015. Retrieved from www.parachutecanada.org/downloads/research/Cost_of_Injury-2015.pdf

UNIT 13

Sensorineural Function

Case Study: SUPPORTING A PATIENT WHO VALUES INDEPENDENCE

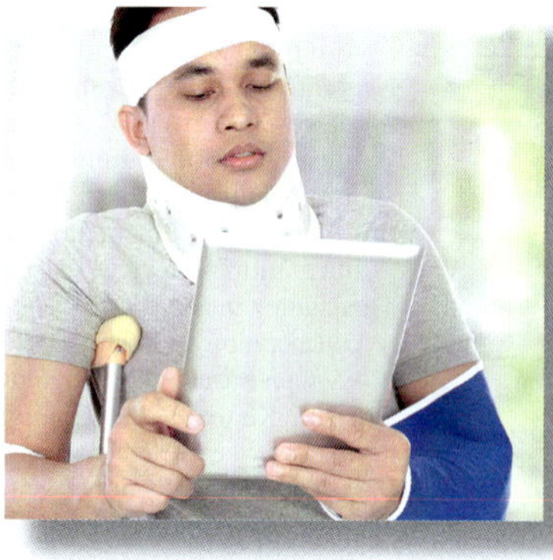

A 33-year-old patient was admitted to a surgical unit after being hit by a car crossing the street. The patient has been deaf since birth and did not hear the oncoming traffic. He lives alone with his hearing service dog and is used to being very independent. He is awaiting surgery to repair his shoulder fracture. He either does not understand or did not hear the instructions to call for help to get out of bed and got himself up to the bathroom to urinate despite the fact that he was instructed to use a bedside urinal. The nurse is concerned that he may fall while getting up alone and tried to communicate to him the importance of calling for assistance to get out of bed.

QSEN Competency Focus: Patient-Centred Care

The complexities inherent in today's health care system challenge nurses to demonstrate integration of specific interdisciplinary core competencies that are aimed at ensuring the delivery of safe and quality patient care (Institute of Medicine, 2003). The Quality and Safety Education for Nurses project (QSEN, 2017; Cronenwett, Sherwood, Barnsteiner, et al., 2007) provides a framework for the knowledge, skills, and attitudes (KSAs) required for nurses to demonstrate competency in these key areas, which include ***patient-centred care***, ***interdisciplinary teamwork and collaboration***, ***evidence-based practice***, ***quality improvement***, ***safety***, and ***informatics.***

Patient-Centred Care Definition: Recognize the patient or designee as the source of control and full partner in providing compassionate and coordinated care based on respect for patient's preferences, values, and needs.

SELECTED PRE-LICENSURE KSAs	APPLICATION AND REFLECTION
Knowledge	
Integrate understanding of multiple dimensions of patient-centred care: • Patient/family/community preferences, values • Coordination and integration of care • Information, communication, and education • Physical comfort and emotional support • Involvement of family and friends	Describe the factors that are impacting the patient's decision to get out of bed on his own. Identify the factors that should be incorporated into his care to best support him so that he is empowered to make the decision that is best for him.
Skills	
Communicate patient values, preferences, and expressed needs to other members of the health care team.	Discuss how you would advocate for this patient so that he receives the care that is best for him. How would you coordinate his care with other members of the health care team so that it reflects his wishes and desires?
Attitudes	
Value seeing health care situations "through patient's eyes." Respect and encourage individual expression of patient values, preferences, and expressed needs.	Reflect on a time you felt a loss of control. How did that fear affect your decision making? Think about how individual preferences and values affect how health care decisions are made. Can you respect decisions that others make that are different from decisions you would make in a similar situation? Why is it important for nurses to demonstrate respect for patients' autonomous decision making?

Cronenwett, L., Sherwood, G., Barnsteiner, J., et al. (2007). Quality and safety education for nurses. *Nursing Outlook, 55*(3), 122–131; Institute of Medicine. (2003). *Health professions education: A bridge to quality.* Washington, DC: National Academies Press; and QSEN Institute. (2017). *QSEN Competencies: Definitions and pre-licensure KSAs*. Retrieved June 3, 2019, from www.qsen.org/competencies/pre-licensure-ksas

60 Assessment and Management of Patients With Eye and Vision Disorders

Adapted by Mohamed Toufic El Hussein and Joseph Osuji

Learning Objectives

On completion of this chapter, the learner will be able to:

1. Identify the major structures and function of the eye.
2. Specify assessment and diagnostic findings used in the evaluation of ocular disorders.
3. Describe assessment and management strategies for patients with low vision and blindness.
4. List the pharmacologic actions and nursing management of common ophthalmic medications.
5. Recognize the clinical features, assessment and diagnostic findings, and medical or surgical management of glaucoma, cataracts, and other ocular disorders.
6. Explain the nursing management of patients with glaucoma, cataracts, and ocular trauma.
7. Discuss general discharge education for patients after ocular surgery.

The World Health Organization (WHO, 2017) estimated that 253 million people live with vision impairment: 36 million are blind and 217 million have moderate to severe vision impairment. Moreover 81% of people who are blind or have moderate or severe vision impairment are aged 50 years and above. Chronic eye diseases are the main cause of vision loss where uncorrected refractive errors and untreated cataract are the top two causes of vision impairment. Untreated cataract remains the leading cause of blindness in low- and middle-income countries. Globally over 80% of all vision impairment can be prevented or cured.

The eye is a sensitive, highly specialized sense organ subject to various disorders, many of which lead to impaired vision. Impaired vision affects an individual's independence in self-care, work and lifestyle choices, sense of self-esteem, safety, ability to interact with society and the environment, and overall quality of life. Many of the leading causes of visual impairment are associated with aging (e.g., cataracts, glaucoma, macular degeneration). Everyday 700 Canadians sustain eye injuries at work (Canadian National Institute for the Blind [CNIB], 2014e). The rapidly changing technologic advances of ophthalmic surgery affect all age groups. These include refractive procedures as well as implantation of intraocular lenses (IOLs) and telescopic devices.

Although most people with eye disorders are treated in an ambulatory care setting, many patients receiving health care have an eye disease as a comorbid condition. In addition to understanding the prevention, treatment, and consequences of eye disorders, nurses in all settings should assess visual acuity (VA) in those at risk (e.g., patients who are older, those with diabetes or acquired immunodeficiency syndrome [AIDS]), refer patients to eye care specialists as appropriate, implement health promotion measures such as wearing sunglasses to prevent further visual loss, and help patients adapt to impaired vision.

ASSESSMENT OF THE EYE

Anatomic and Physiologic Overview

Unlike most organs of the body, the eye is available for external examination, and its anatomy is more easily assessed than many other body parts (Fig. 60-1). The

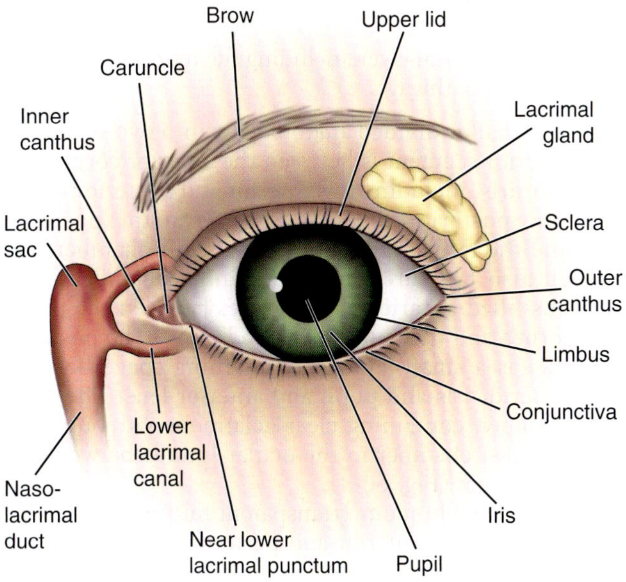

FIGURE 60-1. External structures of the eye and position of the lacrimal structures.

eyeball, or globe, sits in a protective bony structure known as the orbit. Lined with muscle and connective and adipose tissues, the orbit is about 4 cm high, wide, and deep, and it is shaped roughly like a four-sided pyramid, surrounded on three sides by the sinuses: ethmoid (medially), frontal (superiorly), and maxillary (inferiorly). The optic nerve and the ophthalmic artery enter the orbit at its apex through the optic foramen. The eyeball is moved though all fields of gaze by the extraocular muscles. The four rectus muscles and two oblique muscles (Fig. 60-2) are innervated by cranial nerves (CNs) III, IV, and VI. Usually, the movements of the two eyes are coordinated, and the brain perceives a single image.

The eyelids, composed of thin elastic skin that covers striated and smooth muscles, protect the anterior portion of the eye. The eyelids contain multiple glands, including sebaceous, sweat, and accessory lacrimal glands, and they are lined with conjunctival material. The upper lid usually covers the uppermost portion of the iris and is innervated by the oculomotor nerve (CN III). The lid margins contain meibomian glands, the inferior and superior puncta, and the eyelashes. The triangular spaces formed by the junction of the eyelids are known as the inner or medial canthus and the outer or lateral canthus. With every blink

Glossary

anterior chamber: aqueous-containing space in the eye between the posterior (endothelial) cornea and the anterior iris and pupil

aqueous humour: transparent nutrient-containing fluid that fills the anterior and posterior chambers of the eye

astigmatism: refractive error due to an irregularity in the curvature of the cornea

binocular vision: normal ability of both eyes to focus on one object and fuse the two images into one

blindness: inability to see, defined as corrected visual acuity (VA) of 20/400 or less, or a visual field of no more than 20 degrees in the better eye

cataract: progressive opacity of the lens of the eye

chemosis: edema of the conjunctiva

diplopia: seeing one object as two; double vision

emmetropia: normal refractive condition resulting in clear focus on retina; no optical defects

endophthalmitis: intraocular infection

entropion: turning in of the lower eyelid

enucleation: removal of the eyeball and part of the optic nerve

evisceration: removal of the intraocular contents through a corneal or scleral incision; the optic nerve, sclera, extraocular muscles, and sometimes the cornea are left intact

exenteration: surgical removal of the entire contents of the orbit, surrounding soft tissue, and most or all of the eyelids

glaucoma: group of conditions characterized by increased intraocular pressure (IOP)

hyperemia: red eyes resulting from dilation of the vasculature of the conjunctiva

hyperopia: farsightedness; light rays focus behind the retina

hyphema: blood in the anterior chamber

hypopyon: collection of inflammatory cells in the anterior chamber of the eye

injection: congestion of blood vessels

keratoconus: cone-shaped deformity of the cornea

myopia: nearsightedness; light rays focus in front of the retina

neovascularization: growth of abnormal new blood vessels

nystagmus: involuntary oscillation of the eyeball

papilledema: swelling of the optic disc usually due to increased intracranial pressure

photophobia: ocular pain on exposure to light

presbyopia: the loss of accommodative power in the lens due to age

proptosis or exophthalmos: abnormal protrusion of the eyeball

ptosis: drooping eyelid

refraction: determination of the refractive errors of the eye for the purpose of vision correction

scotomas: blind or partially blind areas in the visual field

sympathetic ophthalmia: an inflammatory condition created in the fellow eye by the affected eye

trachoma: an infectious disease caused by the bacterium *Chlamydia trachomatis*—the leading cause of preventable blindness in the world

trichiasis: turning in of the eyelashes

vitreous humour: transparent, colourless gelatinous material that fills the vitreous chamber behind the lens

Note: Common abbreviations related to vision and eye health are OD (oculus dexter, right eye), OS (oculus sinister, left eye), and OU (oculus uterque, both eyes).

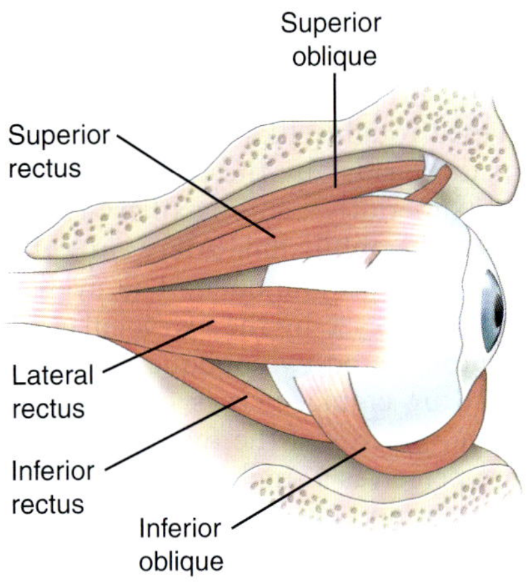

FIGURE 60-2. The extraocular muscles responsible for eye movement. The medial rectus muscle (not shown) is responsible for opposing the movement of the lateral rectus muscle.

of the eyes, the lids wash the cornea and conjunctiva with tears.

Tears are vitally important to eye health. They are formed by the lacrimal gland and the accessory lacrimal glands. A healthy tear is composed of three layers: lipoid, aqueous, and mucoid. If there is a defect in the composition of any of these layers, the integrity of the cornea may be compromised. Tears are secreted in response to reflex or emotional stimuli.

The conjunctiva, a thin transparent mucous membrane, provides a barrier to the external environment extending under the eyelids (palpebral conjunctiva) and over the sclera (bulbar conjunctiva). The junction of the two portions is known as the fornix. The conjunctiva meets the cornea at the limbus on the outermost edge of the iris.

The eyeball is composed of the following three layers:

- The outer dense fibrous layer, including the sclera and transparent cornea
- The middle vascular layer, containing the iris, ciliary body, and choroid
- The inner neural layer, including the retina, optic nerve, and visual pathway

The eyeball is divided anatomically into two segments. The anterior segment is between the anterior cornea and posterior iris, including the anterior and posterior chamber. The posterior segment is between the posterior lens and the retina, including the vitreous chamber. The eyeball also has three fluid-containing chambers. The aqueous-filled **anterior chamber** lies between the posterior cornea and the anterior iris and pupil. The posterior chamber is a small aqueous-containing space between the posterior iris and pupil and anterior lens. The vitreous chamber, containing clear gelatinous vitreous fluid, is the largest chamber in the ocular fundus between the lens and retina (Fig. 60-3).

The **aqueous humour** (transparent nutrient-containing fluid that fills the anterior and posterior chambers of the eye) is produced in the posterior chamber by the ciliary body (Grossman & Porth, 2014). It flows through the pupil into the anterior chamber and drains through the trabecular meshwork into the canal of Schlemm. Production of aqueous humour is related to the intraocular pressure (IOP). Normal IOP is less than 21 mm Hg (Eldaly, Bunce, El Sheikha, et al., 2014). **Vitreous humour,** which is composed mostly of water and encapsulated by a hyaloid membrane, helps maintain the shape of the eye. The vitreous is attached to the retina by scattered collagenous filaments. The vitreous shrinks and shifts with age. Through this degenerative process, the gel-like characteristics liquefy, causing stringy debris known as floaters.

The sclera, commonly known as the white of the eye, is a dense, fibrous structure that comprises the posterior five sixths of the eye. The sclera helps to maintain the shape of the eyeball and protects the intraocular contents from trauma. The sclera may have a slightly bluish tinge in young children, a dull white colour in adults, and a slightly

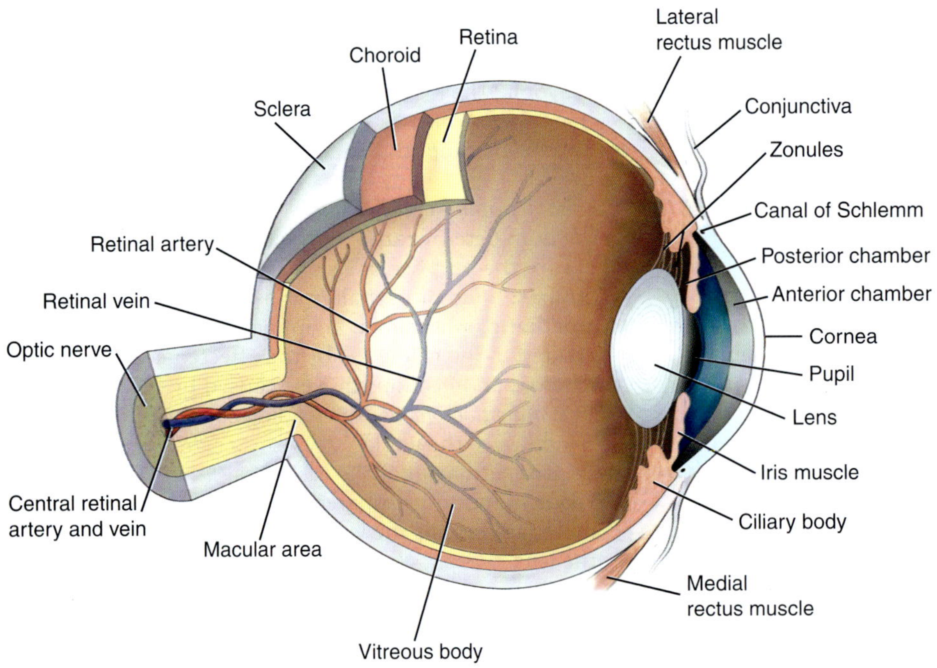

FIGURE 60-3. Three-dimensional cross-section of the eye.

yellowish colour in older adults. Externally, it is overlaid with conjunctiva, which is a thin, transparent, mucous membrane that contains fine blood vessels. The conjunctiva meets the cornea at the limbus on the outermost edge of the iris.

The cornea, a vulnerable transparent avascular domelike structure, forms the most anterior portion of the eyeball and is the main refracting surface of the eye. It is composed of five layers: the epithelium, Bowman membrane, stroma, Descemet's membrane, and endothelium. It contains high concentrations of nerve fibres and is extremely sensitive to pain. The epithelium, the outermost protective layer, absorbs oxygen and nutrients from the tear film nourishing the cornea. The epithelial cells readily regenerate, unlike the innermost endothelial cells, which do not regenerate and result in corneal edema when injured.

The uveal tract is the vascular middle layer of the eye consisting of the iris, ciliary body, and the choroid.

The iris surrounding the pupil is a highly vascularized pigmented collection of fibres that gives the eye colour. The dilator and sphincter muscles of the iris control pupil size. The dilator muscles are controlled by the sympathetic nervous system. The sphincter muscles are controlled by the parasympathetic nervous system.

The ciliary body consists of ciliary processes, ciliary muscles, and zonular fibres (ligaments) that work together to form aqueous fluid and control focusing through the zonular fibres that suspend the crystalline lens.

The choroid lies between the retina and the sclera, supplying blood and oxygen to the outer retina. Pigmented cells containing melanocytes in the choroid assist to absorb scattered light.

Directly behind the pupil and iris lies the lens, an avascular and almost completely transparent biconvex structure held in position by zonular fibres in the ciliary body. The lens enables focusing for near and distance vision through accommodation, the process by which the lens of the eye adjusts the focal length to focus a clear image on the retina. With aging and certain conditions (e.g., diabetes or trauma), the lens loses its transparency and ability to focus due to formation of a cataract (see later discussion).

The retina—the innermost surface of the fundus composed of neural tissue—is an extension of the optic nerve. Viewed through the pupil, the landmarks of the retina are the optic disc, the retinal vessels, and the macula. The point of entrance of the optic nerve into the retina is the optic disc. The optic disc is pink, either oval or circular in shape, and has sharp margins. In the disc, a physiologic depression or cup is present centrally, with the retinal blood vessels emerging from it. The retinal tissues arise from the optic disc and line the inner surface of the vitreous chamber. The retinal vessels enter the eye through the optic disc, branching out through the retina and forming superior and inferior branches. The macula is the area of the retina responsible for central vision. The rest of the retina is responsible for peripheral vision. In the centre of the macula is the most sensitive area—the fovea—which is avascular and surrounded by the superior and inferior vascular arcades. Two important layers of the retina are the retinal pigment epithelium (RPE) and the sensory retina. A single layer of cells constitutes the RPE. These cells have numerous functions, including the absorption of light. The sensory retina contains the photoreceptor cells: rods and cones. The rods are responsible for night or low-light vision. The cones are retinal photoreceptor cells essential for VA, colour discrimination, and fine detail. Cones are distributed throughout the retina, with their greatest concentration in the fovea. Rods are absent in the fovea.

VA depends on a healthy functioning eye and an intact visual pathway. This pathway is made up of the retina, optic nerve, optic chiasm, optic tracks, lateral geniculate bodies, optic radiations, and the visual cortex area of the brain. The visual pathway is part of the central nervous system.

The optic nerve (CN II) transmits impulses from the retina to the occipital lobe of the brain. The optic nerve head, or optic disc, is the physiologic blind spot in each eye. The optic nerve leaves the eye and then meets the optic nerve from the other eye at the optic chiasm. The chiasm is the anatomic point at which the nasal fibres from the nasal retina of each eye cross to the opposite side of the brain. The nerve fibres from the temporal retina of each eye remain uncrossed. Fibres from the right half of each eye, which would be the left visual field, carry impulses to the right occipital lobe. Fibres from the left half of each eye, or the right visual field, carry impulses to the left occipital lobe. Beyond the chiasm, these fibres are known as the optic tract. The optic tract continues on to the lateral geniculate body. The lateral geniculate body is connected by the optic radiations to the cortex of the occipital lobe of the brain.

Assessment

Ocular History

The eye care professional, through careful questioning, elicits the necessary information that can lead to the diagnosis of an ophthalmic condition. Pertinent questions to ask during the interview can be found in Chart 60-1. Genetics plays a role in many eye and vision disorders (Chart 60-2) (Lee & Garg, 2015).

Visual Acuity

After the patient's chief concern has been identified and the history has been obtained, VA is assessed. This is an essential part of the eye examination and a measure against which all therapeutic outcomes are based.

Most people are familiar with the standard Snellen chart. This chart is composed of a series of rows of progressively smaller letters and is used to test distance vision. The fraction 20/20 is considered the standard of "normal" vision. Most people can see the letters on the line designated as 20/20 from a distance of 6.1 m (20 ft). A person whose vision is 20/200 can see an object from 20 ft away (6.1 m) that a person whose vision is 20/20 can see from 200 ft (61 m) away (Stephen, 2012).

The patient is positioned at the prescribed distance, usually 6.1 m (20 ft), from the chart and is asked to read the smallest line that he or she can see. The patient should wear distance correction (eyeglasses or contact lenses) if required, and each eye is tested separately. The right eye is commonly tested first. The patient is asked to cover the left eye with an opaque card while the right eye is being tested. Patients are encouraged to read every letter

CHART 60-1

Assessment: Taking a History of Patients With Eye and Vision Disorders

- What does the patient perceive to be the problem?
- Is visual acuity diminished?
- Does the patient experience blurred, double, or distorted vision?
- Is there pain? Is it sharp or dull? Is it worse when blinking?
- Is the discomfort an itching sensation or more of a foreign body sensation?
- Are both eyes affected?
- Is there a history of discharge? If so, inquire about colour, consistency, and odour.
- Describe the onset of the problem (sudden, gradual). Is it worsening?
- What is the duration of the problem?
- Is this a recurrence of a previous condition?
- How has the patient self-treated?
- What makes the symptoms improve or worsen?
- Has the condition affected performance of activities of daily living?
- Are there any systemic diseases? What medications are used in their treatment?
- What other eye conditions does the patient have?
- Is there a history of eye surgery?
- Have other family members had the same symptoms or condition?

Adapted from Weber, J., & Kelley, J. (2014). *Health assessment in nursing* (5th ed.). Philadelphia, PA: Lippincott Williams & Wilkins.

possible and to guess, if necessary. If the patient successfully reads the line, the examiner encourages the patient to attempt the next line of smaller letters. The smallest line in which the patient can successfully identify more than half the letters is recorded as the VA for the eye being tested. This procedure is then repeated for the left eye, with the right eye covered, and then both eyes are tested together. If a patient is unable to read the English alphabet, a Snellen E Chart is available.

The VA is recorded in the following way. If the patient reads all five letters from the 20/20 line with the right eye and three of the five letters on the 20/15 line with the left eye, the examiner writes right eye 20/20, left eye 20/15-2, or VA 20/20, 20/15-2 (Weber & Kelley, 2014).

If the patient is unable to read the largest letter on the chart (the 20/200 line), the patient should be moved toward the chart or the chart moved toward the patient, until the patient is able to identify the largest letter on the chart. If the patient can recognize only the letter E on the top line at a distance of 10 ft (3 m), the VA would be recorded as 10 to read the largest letter on the chart (the 20/200 line), the patient should be moved toward the chart or the chart moved toward the patientexaminer holds up a random number of fingers and asks the patient to count the number he or she sees. If the patient correctly identifies the number of fingers at 3 ft (1 m), the examiner would record CF/3′.

If the patient is unable to CF, the examiner raises one hand up and down or moves it side to side and asks in which direction the hand is moving. This level of vision is known as hand motions (HM). A patient who can perceive only light is described as having light perception (LP). The vision of a patient who is unable to perceive light is described as no light perception (NLP).

External Eye Examination

After the VA has been recorded, an external eye examination is performed. The position of the eyelids is noted. Commonly, the upper 2 mm of the iris is covered by the upper lid. The patient is examined for **ptosis** (i.e., drooping eyelid) and for lid retraction (i.e., too much of the eye is exposed). Sometimes, the upper or lower lid turns out, affecting closure. The lid margins and lashes should have no edema, erythema, or lesions. The examiner looks for scaling or crusting, and the sclera is inspected. The sclera is opaque and white. Lesions on the conjunctiva, discharge, and tearing or blinking are noted.

The room is darkened so that the pupils can be examined. Examine the pupils directly. Observe the size and shape of each pupil. Next, shine a penlight on right pupil; watch for right pupil to constrict. Repeat for the other eye. Check for consensual response by shining light on the right eye and watching for the *left* pupil to constrict. Repeat by shining light on the left eye and watching for the *right* pupil to constrict. Check accommodation by having the patient stare with both eyes at a distant object (an object on the opposite wall) and then at an object up close (a pen held about 30 cm from the eyes). Pupils should dilate with distance and constrict with closeness. Record that the pupils are equal, round, and react to light and accommodation, abbreviated as PERRLA (Stephen, 2012). A pupil is usually black. An irregular pupil may result from trauma, previous surgery, or a disease process.

The patient's eyes are observed in primary or direct gaze, and any head tilt is noted. A tilt may indicate cranial nerve palsy. The patient is asked to stare at a target; each eye is covered and uncovered quickly while the examiner looks for any shift in gaze. The examiner observes for **nystagmus** (i.e., oscillating movement of the eyeball).

Using the patient's shoulders as outer edges, the extraocular movements of the eyes are tested by having the patient follow the examiner's finger through the six cardinal directions of gaze (right, right upward, right downward, left, left upward, and left downward) (Fig. 60-4). This is especially important when screening patients for ocular trauma or for neurologic disorders such as stroke or myasthenia gravis (Hickey, 2014).

Diagnostic Evaluation

Direct Ophthalmoscopy

An ophthalmoscope is a handheld instrument with various plus and minus lenses (Weber & Kelley, 2014). The lenses can be rotated into place, enabling the examiner to

GENETICS IN NURSING PRACTICE

Chart 60-2. Eye and Vision Disorders

Several eye and vision disorders are associated with genetic abnormalities. Some examples include:

Autosomal dominant:
- Aniridia
- Vitelliform macular dystrophy

Autosomal recessive:
- Achromatopsia
- Homocystinuria
- Leber congenital amaurosis

X linked:
- Choroideremia
- Colour blindness

Mitochondrial inheritance:
- Leber hereditary optic neuropathy

Multiple inheritance patterns identified:
- Glaucoma
- Macular degeneration
- Retinitis pigmentosa

Other genetic illness that will impact vision:
- Albinism
- Isolated familial congenital cataracts
- Marfan syndrome
- Stickler syndrome
- Tay-Sachs disease
- Usher syndrome

Nursing Assessments

FAMILY HISTORY ASSESSMENT
- Assess history of family members with glaucoma, cataracts, night blindness (retinitis pigmentosa), colour blindness, or other vision impairment.
- Inquire about the age of onset of symptoms (the onset of Leber hereditary optic neuropathy is in young adulthood).
- Inquire about family members with other disorders that may include visual impairment, such as cutaneous, metabolic, connective tissue disorders, and hearing loss.

PHYSICAL ASSESSMENT
- Assess for other systemic and/or clinical features such as cutaneous or skeletal conditions, or hearing loss.

Management Issues Specific to Genetics
- Inquire whether DNA gene mutation or other genetic testing has been performed on any affected family members.
- If indicated, refer for further genetic counselling and evaluation so that family members can discuss inheritance, risk to other family members, availability of genetic testing, and gene-based interventions.
- Offer appropriate genetics information and resources.
- Assess patient's understanding of genetics information.
- Provide support to families with newly diagnosed genetic-related sensorineural disorders.
- Participate in management and coordination of care of patients with genetic conditions and individuals predisposed to develop or pass on a genetic condition.

Genetics Resources

Canadian Association of Genetic Counsellors (CAGC)—a listing of genetic centres across Canada; http://www.cagc-accg.ca

Canadian Cancer Society—information on the genetic factors/risk and genetic testing; http://www.cancer.ca

Canadian Directory of Genetic Support Groups—a resource guide for families and professionals; http://www.lhsc.on.ca/programs/medgenet

Canadian Genetic Disease Network—its stated mission is to be the primary catalyst in advancing Canada's scientific and commercial competitiveness in genetic research and the application of genetic discoveries to the prevention, diagnosis, and treatment of human disease; https://www.lhsc.on.ca/canadian-directory-of-genetic-support-groups/introduction-to-the-directory

Canadian Organization for Rare Disorders (CORD)—information on over 6,000 rare disorders and links individuals/families together with the same rare disorder; http://www.cord.ca

Genetic Alliance—increases the capacity of genetic advocacy groups to achieve their missions and leverages the voices of millions of individuals and families living with genetic conditions; http://www.geneticalliance.org

Genetics Society of Canada (GSC)—promotes research and communicates the results and implications of genetics to the public; http://life.biology.mcmaster.ca/GSC

GeneTests—a publicly funded medical genetics information resource developed for physicians, other health care providers, and researchers; http://www.genetests.org

OMIM Online Mendelian Inheritance in Man—a catalogue of human genes and genetic disorders; http://www.ncbi.nlm.nih.gov/omim

bring the cornea, lens, and retina into focus sequentially. The examiner holds the ophthalmoscope in the right hand and uses the right eye to examine the patient's right eye. The examiner switches to the left hand and left eye when examining the patient's left eye. During this examination, the room is darkened, and the patient's eye is on the same level as the examiner's eye. The patient and the examiner should be comfortable, and both should breathe quietly. The patient is given a target to gaze on and is encouraged to keep both eyes open and steady.

When the fundus is examined, the vasculature comes into focus first. The veins are larger in diameter than the arteries. The examiner focuses on a large vessel and then follows it toward the midline of the body, which leads to the optic nerve. The central depression in the disc is known as the cup which is about one third of the disc. The size of the physiologic optic cup is estimated and the disc margins described as sharp or blurred. A silvery or coppery appearance, which indicates arteriolosclerosis, is noted. The periphery of the retina can be examined by having the patient shift his or her gaze. The last area of the fundus to be examined is the macula, because this area is the most sensitive to light.

The healthy fundus is free of any lesions. The examiner looks for intraretinal hemorrhages, which may appear as red smudges or, if the patient has hypertension, may look

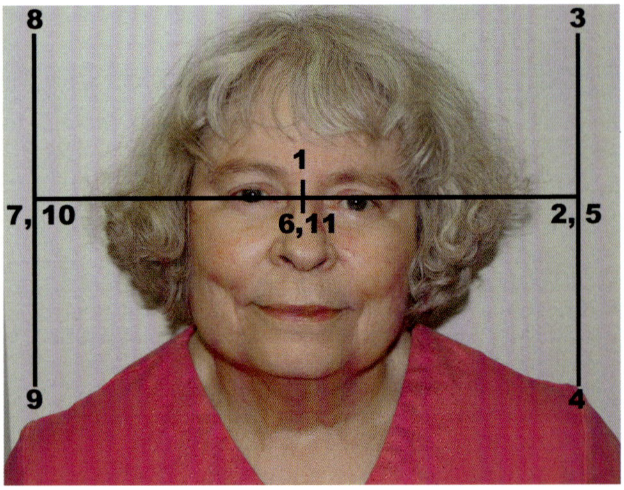

FIGURE 60-4. Testing extraocular movements.

somewhat flame shaped. Lipid may be present in the retina of patients with hypercholesterolemia or diabetes. This lipid has a yellowish appearance. Soft exudates that have a fuzzy, white appearance (i.e., cotton-wool spots) are noted. The examiner looks for microaneurysms, which look like little red dots, and nevi. Drusen (small, hyaline, globular growths), commonly found in macular degeneration, appear to be yellowish areas with indistinct edges. Small drusen have a more distinct edge. The examiner sketches the fundus and documents any abnormalities.

Indirect Ophthalmoscopy

The indirect ophthalmoscope is an instrument commonly used by eye care professionals (ophthalmologists or optometrists) to see larger areas of the retina, although in an unmagnified state. It produces a bright and intense light. The light source is affixed with a pair of binocular lenses, which are mounted on the examiner's head. The ophthalmoscope is used with a handheld, 20-diopter lens.

Slit-Lamp Examination

The slit lamp is a binocular microscope mounted on a table. This instrument enables the user to examine the eye with magnification of 10 to 40 times the real image. The illumination can be varied from a broad to a narrow beam of light for different parts of the eye. For example, by varying the width and intensity of the light, the anterior chamber can be examined for signs of inflammation. Cataracts may be evaluated by changing the angle of the light. When a handheld contact lens, such as a three-mirror lens, is used with the slit lamp, the angle of the anterior chamber may be examined, as may the ocular fundus.

Tonometry

Tonometry is an essential part of a diagnostic evaluation; it measures IOP to screen for and manage glaucoma. The device used for measuring IOP is an accurately calibrated applanation tonometer, which measures the pressure needed to flatten the cornea. Because the probe or prism touches the highly sensitive cornea, a topical anesthetic is given prior to measurement (Hogan, 2014).

Nursing Interventions

Providing patient education prior to tonometry helps avoid possible errors in IOP measurement. Patients are cautioned to avoid squeezing the eyelids, holding their breath, or performing a Valsalva manoeuvre, because these may result in abnormally increased IOP.

Colour Vision Testing

The ability to differentiate colours has a dramatic effect on the activities of daily living (ADLs). For example, the inability to differentiate between red and green can compromise traffic safety. Some careers (e.g., commercial art, colour photography, airline pilot, electrician) may be closed to people with significant colour deficiencies. The photoreceptor cells responsible for colour vision are the cones, and the greatest area of colour sensitivity is in the macula, the area of densest cone concentration.

A screening test, such as the polychromatic plates discussed in the next paragraph, can be used to establish whether a person's colour vision is within expected range. Colour vision deficits can be inherited. For example, red/green colour deficiencies are inherited in an X-linked manner, affecting approximately 8% of men and 0.5% of women (Colour Blind Awareness, 2016). Acquired colour vision losses may be caused by medications (e.g., digitalis toxicity) or pathology such as cataracts. A simple test, such as asking a patient if the red top on a bottle of eye drops appears redder to one eye than the other, can be an effective tool. A difference in the perception of the intensity of the colour red between the two eyes can be a symptom of a neurologic issue and may provide information about the location of the lesion.

Because alteration in colour vision is sometimes indicative of conditions of the optic nerve, colour vision testing is often performed in a neuro-ophthalmologic workup. The most common colour vision test is performed using Ishihara polychromatic plates. These plates are bound together in a book. On each plate of this booklet are dots of primary colours that are integrated into a background of secondary colours. The dots are arranged in simple patterns, such as numbers or geometric shapes. Patients with diminished colour vision may be unable to identify the hidden shapes. Patients with central vision conditions (e.g., macular degeneration) have more difficulty identifying colours than those with peripheral vision conditions (e.g., glaucoma) because central vision identifies colour.

Amsler Grid

The Amsler grid is a test often used for patients with macular concerns, such as macular degeneration. It consists of a geometric grid of identical squares with a central fixation point. The grid should be viewed by the patient wearing usual reading glasses. Each eye is tested separately. The patient is instructed to stare at the central fixation spot on the grid and report any distortion in the squares of the grid itself. For patients with macular concerns, some of the squares may look faded, or the lines may be wavy. Patients with age-related macular degeneration (AMD) are commonly given these Amsler grids to take home. The patient is encouraged to check them frequently, as often as daily, to detect any early signs of distortion that may indicate the development of a neovascular choroidal membrane, an advanced stage of macular degeneration characterized by the growth of abnormal choroidal vessels (Gerstenblith & Rabinowitz, 2017; Weber & Kelley, 2014).

Ultrasonography

Lesions in the globe or the orbit may not be directly visible and are evaluated by ultrasonography. Ultrasonography is a very valuable diagnostic technique, especially when the view of the retina is obscured by opaque media such as cataract or hemorrhage. An ultrasonography B-scan identifies pathology such as orbital tumours, retinal detachment, and vitreous hemorrhage. Ultrasonography A-scans are used to measure the axial length for implants prior to cataract surgery (Gerstenblith & Rabinowitz, 2017).

Optical Coherence Tomography

Optical coherence tomography is a technology that involves low-coherence interferometry (Boyd, 2016; Gerstenblith & Rabinowitz, 2017). Light is used to evaluate retinal and macular diseases as well as anterior segment conditions. This method is noninvasive and involves no physical contact with the eye.

Colour Fundus Photography

Fundus photography is a technique used to detect and document retinal lesions. The patient's pupils are widely dilated during the procedure, and VA is diminished for about 30 minutes due to retinal "bleaching" by the intense flashing lights. The resulting fundus photographs can be viewed stereoscopically so that elevations such as macular edema can be identified.

Laser Scanning

Various scanning techniques use laser light in the diagnostic evaluation of eye disorders. Confocal laser scanning ophthalmoscopy provides a three-dimensional image of the optic nerve topography and is used alone or in conjunction with fundus photography to provide comparative data for suspected optic nerve diseases such as glaucoma and **papilledema** (swelling of the optic disc due to increased intracranial pressure) (Gerstenblith & Rabinowitz, 2017). Laser scanning polarimetry is used to measure nerve fibre layer thickness and is an important indicator of glaucoma progression.

Angiography

Fluorescein angiography evaluates clinically significant macular edema, documents macular capillary nonperfusion, and identifies retinal and choroidal **neovascularization** (CNV) (i.e., growth of abnormal new blood vessels) in AMD. It is an invasive procedure in which fluorescein dye is injected, usually into an antecubital area vein. Within 10 to 15 seconds, this dye can be seen coursing through the retinal vessels. Over a 10-minute period, serial black-and-white photographs are taken of the retinal vasculature. The dye may impart a gold tone to the skin of some patients, and urine may turn deep yellow or orange. This discolouration usually disappears in 24 hours.

Indocyanine green angiography is used to evaluate abnormalities in the choroidal vasculature, conditions often seen in macular degeneration. Indocyanine green dye is injected intravenously (IV), and multiple images are captured using digital videoangiography over a period of 30 seconds to 20 minutes. The dye is generally well tolerated, but some patients experience nausea and vomiting. Allergic reactions are rare; however, indocyanine green angiography is contraindicated in patients with a history of iodide reactions.

Nursing Interventions

Prior to the angiography, the patient's blood urea nitrogen and creatinine should be checked to ensure that the kidneys will excrete the contrast agent (Fischbach & Dunning, 2015). The patient should be well hydrated, and clear liquids are usually permitted up to the time of the test. The patient is instructed to remain immobile during the angiogram process and is told to expect a brief feeling of warmth in the face, behind the eyes, or in the jaw, teeth, tongue, and lips, and a metallic taste when the contrast agent is injected.

Nursing care after angiography includes observation of the injection site (usually the antecubital vein) for bleeding or hematoma formation (a localized collection of blood). Fluorescein may impart a gold tone to the skin in some patients, and urine may turn deep yellow or orange. This discolouration usually disappears in 24 hours. Allergic reactions are rare; however, indocyanine green angiography is contraindicated in patients with a history of iodide reactions. Fluids are encouraged following the procedure to facilitate excretion of the contrast agent (Fischbach & Dunning, 2015).

Perimetry Testing

Perimetry testing evaluates the field of vision. A visual field is the area or extent of physical space visible to an eye in a given position. Its average extent is 65 degrees upward, 75 degrees downward, 60 degrees inward, and 95 degrees outward when the eye is in the primary gaze (i.e., looking directly forward). It is a three-dimensional contour representing areas of relative retinal sensitivity. VA is sharpest at the very top of the field and declines progressively toward the periphery. Visual field testing (i.e., perimetry) helps to identify which parts of the patient's central and peripheral visual fields have useful vision. It is most helpful in detecting central **scotomas** (i.e., blind areas in the visual field) in macular degeneration and the peripheral field defects in glaucoma and retinitis pigmentosa.

The two methods of perimetric testing are manual and automated perimetry. Manual perimetry involves the use of moving (kinetic) or stationary (static) stimuli or targets. An example of kinetic manual perimetry is the tangent screen. A tangent screen is a black felt material mounted on a wall that has a series of concentric circles dissected by straight lines emanating from the centre. It tests the central 30 degrees of the visual field. Automated perimetry uses stationary targets, which are harder to detect than moving targets. In this test, a computer projects light randomly in different areas of a hollow dome while the patient looks through a telescopic opening and depresses a button whenever he or she detects the light stimulus. Automated perimetry is more accurate than manual perimetry.

IMPAIRED VISION

Refractive Errors

In refractive errors, vision is impaired because a shortened or elongated eyeball prevents light rays from focusing sharply on the retina. Blurred vision from refractive error can be corrected with eyeglasses or contact lenses. The appropriate eyeglass or contact lens is determined by **refraction**. Refraction ophthalmology consists of placing various types of lenses in front of the patient's eyes to determine which lens best improves the patient's vision.

The depth of the eyeball is important in determining refractive error (Fig. 60-5). Patients for whom the visual image focuses precisely on the macula and who do not need eyeglasses or contact lenses are said to have **emmetropia** (normal vision). People who have **myopia** are said to be nearsighted. They have deeper eyeballs; the distant visual image focuses in front of, or short of, the retina. People with myopia experience blurred distance vision. When people have a shorter depth to their eyes, the visual image focuses beyond the retina; the eyes are shallower and are called hyperopic. People with **hyperopia** are farsighted. These patients experience near-vision blurriness, whereas their distance vision is excellent.

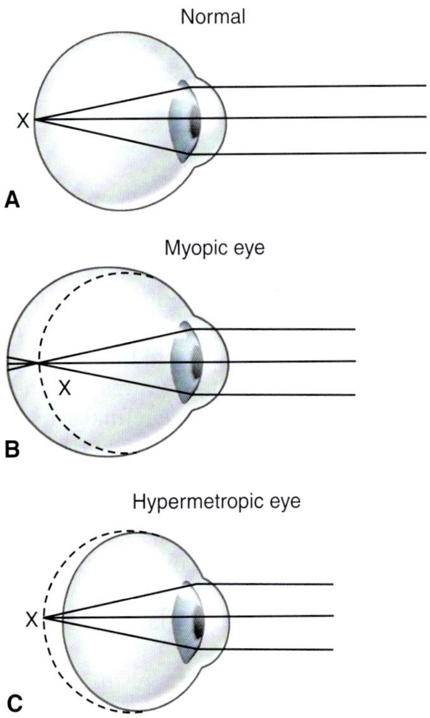

FIGURE 60-5. Eyeball shape determines visual acuity in refractive errors. **A.** Normal eye. **B.** Myopic eye. **C.** Hypermetropic eye.

Another important cause of refractive error is **astigmatism**, an irregularity in the curve of the cornea. Because astigmatism causes a distortion of the visual image, acuity of distance and near vision can be decreased. Eyeglasses with a cylinder correction may be used for correction. Hard contact lenses, which by means of their tear film correct astigmatic errors, or soft toric contact lenses with a cylinder correction may be used in place of eyeglasses for patients with astigmatism.

Ophthalmology has entered the era of customized vision correction in its desire to achieve "super-normal vision." A new method of measuring refractive error that includes sphere, cylinder, and higher-order aberrations is called wavefront technology. The most promising application for this technology is wavefront-guided refractive surgery. A customized laser ablation pattern is generated to reshape the cornea.

Low Vision and Blindness

Vision impairment is defined as having best corrected VA of 20/40 or worse in the better-seeing eye. *Low vision* describes visual impairment that requires the use of devices and strategies to perform visual tasks.

Blindness is defined as a BCVA of 20/400 to NLP. The clinical definition of absolute blindness is the absence of LP. Legal blindness is a condition of impaired vision in which an individual has a BCVA that does not exceed 20/200 in the better eye or whose widest visual field diameter is 20 degrees or less (Prevent Blindness America, 2012). This definition does not equate with functional ability, nor does it classify the degrees of visual impairment. Legal blindness ranges from an inability to perceive light to having some vision remaining. An individual who meets the criteria for legal blindness may obtain government financial assistance. There are approximately 1 million Canadians who are blind, with the largest portion of this group being over 65 years of age. Someone in Canada begins to lose his or her vision every 12 minutes (CNIB, 2014g).

Impaired vision is often accompanied by difficulty in performing functional activities. People with VA of 20/80 to 20/100 with a visual field restriction of 60 degrees to greater than 20 degrees can read at a nearly usual level with optical aids. Their visual orientation is near normal but requires increased scanning of the environment (i.e., systematic use of head and eye movements). In a VA range of 20/200 to 20/400 with a 20-degree to greater than 10-degree visual field restriction, the person can read slowly with optical aids. His or her visual orientation is slow, with constant scanning of the environment. People in this category may have the ability to negotiate their environment without auxiliary aids. This ability is termed "travel vision." People with HM vision or no vision may benefit from the use of mobility devices (e.g., cane, guide dog) and should be encouraged to learn Braille and to use computer aids.

The most common causes of blindness and visual impairment among adults 40 years of age or older are diabetic retinopathy, macular degeneration, glaucoma, and

TABLE 60-1 Age-Related Changes in the Eye

The External Eye	Structural Change	Functional Change	History and Physical Findings
Eyelids and lacrimal structures	Loss of skin elasticity and orbital fat, decreased muscle tone; wrinkles develop	Lid margins turn in causing lashes to irritate cornea and conjunctiva (entropion); or lid margins may turn out, resulting in increased corneal exposure (ectropion)	Reports of burning, foreign body sensation, increased tearing (epiphora); injection, inflammation, and ulceration may occur
Refractive changes; presbyopia	Loss of accommodative power in the lens with age	Reading materials must be held at increasing distance in order to focus	Patient reports, "Arms are too short!"; need for increased light; reading glasses or bifocals needed
Cataract	Opacities in the normally crystalline lens	Interference with the focus of a sharp image on the retina	Patients report increased glare, decreased vision, changes in colour values (blue and yellow especially affected)
Posterior vitreous detachment	Liquefaction and shrinkage of vitreous body	May lead to retinal tears and detachment	Reports light flashes, cobwebs, floaters
Age-related macular degeneration (AMD)	Drusen (yellowish aging spots in the retina) appear and coalesce in the macula. Abnormal choroidal blood vessels may lead to formation of fibrotic disciform scars in the macula	Central vision is affected; onset is more gradual in dry AMD, more rapid in wet AMD; distortion and loss of central vision may occur	Reading vision is affected; words may be missing letters, faded areas appear on the page, straight lines may appear wavy; drusen, pigmentary changes in retina; abnormal submacular choroidal vessels

Adapted from Eliopoulos, C. (2018). *Gerontological nursing* (9th ed.). Philadelphia, PA: Lippincott Williams & Wilkins.

cataracts (CNIB, 2014b). Macular degeneration is more prevalent among Caucasians, whereas glaucoma is more prevalent among African Canadians. Age-related changes in the eye are discussed below and described in Table 60-1.

Assessment and Diagnostic Testing

The assessment of low vision includes a thorough history and the examination of distance and near visual acuity, visual field, contrast sensitivity, glare, colour perception, and refraction. Specially designed, low-vision VA charts are used to evaluate patients.

Patient Interview

During history taking, the cause and duration of the patient's visual impairment are identified. Patients with retinitis pigmentosa, for example, have a genetic abnormality (see Chart 60-2). Patients with diabetic macular edema typically have fluctuating VA. Patients with macular degeneration have central acuity issues. Central acuity concerns cause difficulty in performing activities that require finer vision, such as reading. People with peripheral field defects have more difficulties with mobility. The patient's customary ADLs, medication regimen, habits (e.g., smoking), acceptance of the physical limitations brought about by the visual impairment, and realistic expectations of low-vision aids must also be identified and included in the plan of care, including provision of guidelines for safety and referrals to social services.

Contrast-Sensitivity Testing and Glare Testing

Contrast-sensitivity testing measures VA in different degrees of contrast. The initial test may take the form of simply turning on the lights while testing the distance acuity. If the patient can read better with the lights on, the patient can benefit from magnification. Glare testing enables the examiner to obtain a more realistic evaluation of the patient's ability to function in his or her environment. Glare can reduce a person's ability to see, especially in patients with cataracts. Devices that test glare, such as the Brightness Acuity Tester, produce three degrees of bright light to create a dazzle effect while the patient is viewing a target, such as Snellen letters on the wall. The lights have been calibrated to imitate certain objects that create glare, such as the brightness of a car's headlights at night.

Gerontologic Considerations

Approximately half of all individuals who are identified as legally blind each year are 65 years of age or older (Eliopoulos, 2018). With aging, structural and functional changes occur in the eye. **Presbyopia**, the loss of accommodative power in the lens, interferes with the ability to adequately focus and is the factor responsible for most older adults requiring some form of corrective lenses (Eliopoulos, 2018). Age-related changes in the eye are summarized in Table 60-1.

The most common causes of blindness and visual impairment among adults 40 years and older are diabetic retinopathy, macular degeneration, glaucoma, and cataracts (Prevent Blindness America, 2012).

Medical Management

Managing low vision involves magnification and image enhancement through the use of low-vision aids and strategies and through referrals to social services and community agencies serving those with visual impairment. The goals

TABLE 60-2 Activities Affected by Visual Impairment and Suggestions for Low-Vision Aids

Activity	Optical Aids	Nonoptical Aids
Shopping	Hand magnifier	Lighting, colour cues
Fixing a snack	Bifocals	Colour cues, consistent food storage plan
Eating out	Hand magnifier	Flashlight, portable lamp
Identifying money	Bifocals, hand magnifier	Arrange paper money in wallet compartments
Reading print	High-power spectacle, bifocals, hand magnifier, stand magnifier, closed-circuit television	Lighting, high-contrast print, large print, reading slit
Writing	Hand magnifier	Lighting, bold-tip pen, black ink
Using a telephone	Hand magnifier	Large-print buttons, hand-printed directory Braille phones, picture/photo phones, and talking phones
Crossing streets	Lightweight handheld monoscopes/telescopes	Cane, ask directions
Finding taxis and bus signs	Lightweight handheld monoscopes/telescopes	Ask for assistance
Reading medication labels	Hand magnifier	Colour codes, large print
Reading stove dials	Hand magnifier	Colour codes, raised dots
Adjusting the thermostat	Hand magnifier	Enlarged-print model
Using a computer	Spectacles	High-contrast colour, large-print program. Screen-reader programs convert text on the computer screen to synthesized speech
Reading signs	Spectacles	Move closer
Watching sporting event	Lightweight handheld monoscopes/telescopes	Sit in front rows

Adapted from Pagliuca, L. M., Macedo-Costa, K. N., Reboucas, G. B., et al. (2014). Validation of the general guidelines of communication between the nurse and the blind. *Reviews Bras Enferm*, *67*(5), 715–725.

are to enhance visual function and assist patients with low vision to perform customary activities. Low-vision aids include optical and nonoptical devices (Table 60-2). The optical devices include convex lens aids, such as magnifiers and glasses; telescopic devices; antireflective lenses that diminish glare; and electronic reading systems, such as closed-circuit television and computers with large print. Continuing advances in computer software provide very useful products for patients with low vision. Scanners with the appropriate software enable the user to scan printed data into the computer and have it read by computer voice or to enlarge the print for reading. Magnifiers can be handheld or attached to a stand with or without illumination. Telescopic devices can be spectacle telescopes or clip-on or handheld loupes.

Nonoptical aids include large-print publications and a variety of writing aids. The Internet continues to expand, and a telephone system has been developed that allows access to the Internet and e-mail using voice commands.

Strategies that enhance the performance of visual tasks include modification of body movements and illumination and training for independent living skills. Head movements and positions can be modified to place images in functional areas of the visual field. Illumination is an added feature in magnifiers. Adjusting the lighting helps with reading and other activities. Simple optical and nonoptical aids are available in low-vision clinics.

Referrals to community agencies may be necessary for patients with low vision living alone who are unable to self-administer their medications. Community agencies offer services to patients with low vision that include training in independent living skills and the provision of occupational and recreational activities and a wide variety of assistive devices for vision enhancement and orientation and mobility. Lam and Leat (2013) examined patients' perspectives of accessing a low-vision care program. Their reasons for not accessing low-vision programs included: "didn't know what it was," "vision is not bad enough," "wanted to appear independent," stigma attached to using aids, admitting they have a disability, other health issues, transportation, and education level. The irony is that low-vision care programs help people with low vision to be more independent.

Vision Restoration for the Blind

Ophthalmologists have worked for years toward visual restoration for people who are blind, and computer technology now provides opportunities for restoring sight. Research is ongoing all over the world. Retinal implants for those whose optic nerves are functional as well as cortical implants for those whose optic nerves are diseased are being developed. For example, an experimental artificial silicon retina microchip is being developed for the treatment of patients with retinitis pigmentosa (Chow, Chow, Packo, et al., 2004). The rapid changes in technology and miniaturization of computer chips may enable dramatic advances in synthetic vision in the future.

Nursing Management

Coping with blindness involves three types of adaptation: emotional, physical, and social. The emotional adjustment to blindness or severe visual impairment determines the success of the physical and social adjustments of the patient. Successful emotional adjustment means acceptance of blindness or severe visual impairment.

Promoting Coping Efforts

Effective coping may not occur until the patient recognizes the permanence of the blindness. Clinging to false hopes of regaining vision hampers effective adaptation to blindness. A patient who is newly blind and his or her family members (especially those who live with the patient) undergo the various steps of grieving: denial and shock, anger and protest, restitution, loss resolution, and acceptance. The ability to accept the changes that must come with visual loss and willingness to adapt to those changes influence the successful rehabilitation of the patient who is blind. Additional aspects to consider are value changes, independence–dependence conflicts, coping with stigma, and learning to function in social settings without visual cues and landmarks.

Promoting Spatial Orientation and Mobility

A person who is blind or severely visually impaired requires strategies for adapting to the environment. ADLs, such as walking to a chair from a bed, require spatial concepts. The person needs to know where he or she is in relation to the rest of the room, to understand the changes that may occur, and to know how to approach the desired location safely. This requires a collaborative effort between the patient and the responsible adult who serves as the sighted guide.

A patient whose visual impairment results from a chronic progressive eye disorder, such as glaucoma, has better cognitive mapping skills than the patient who becomes blind suddenly. Patients with progressive eye disorders develop the use of spatial and topographic concepts early and gradually; hence, remembering a room layout is easier for them. Patients who become blind suddenly have more difficulty in adjusting, and emotional and behavioural issues of coping with blindness may hinder their learning. These patients require intensive emotional support. The nurse assesses the degree of physical assistance the person with vision loss requires and communicates this to other health care personnel.

In the hospital, the bedside table and the call button must always be within reach. The parts of the call button are explained, and the patient is taught to touch and press the buttons or dials until the activity is mastered. The patient is familiarized with the location of the telephone, water pitcher, and other objects on the bedside table. The food tray's composition is likened to the face of a clock; for example, the main plate may be described as being at 12 o'clock or the coffee cup at 3 o'clock. All articles and furniture must remain in the same positions throughout the patient's hospitalization. Nurses should always introduce themselves upon entering a patient's room and alert the patient to their departure. Such habits are always polite and help in the care of a patient with vision loss.

The nurse should be aware of the importance of techniques in providing physical assistance, encouraging independence, and ensuring safety. Specific guidelines for interacting with the patient with vision loss are presented in Chart 60-3. The readiness of the patient and his or her family to learn is assessed before initiating orientation and mobility training. Research supports the use of a validated protocol to educate staff to perform therapeutic communication, deliver services, and minimize communication

CHART 60-3

Strategies for Interacting With People Who Are Blind or Have Low Vision

- Remember that the only difference between you and people who are blind or have low vision is that they are not able to see through their eyes what you are able to see through yours.
- Do not be uncomfortable when in the company of a person who is blind or has low vision. Talk with the person as you would talk with any other individual, honestly and without pity; do not be concerned about using words like "see" and "look." There is no need to raise your voice unless the person asks you to do so.
- Identify yourself as you approach the person and before you make physical contact. Tell the person your name and your role. If another person approaches, introduce him or her. When you leave the room, be sure to tell the person that you are leaving and if anyone else remains in the room.
- It is often appropriate to touch the person's hand or arm lightly to indicate that you are about to speak.
- When talking, face the person and speak directly to him or her using a normal tone of voice.
- Be specific when communicating direction. Mention a specific distance or use clock cues when possible (e.g., walk left about 2 m; walk about 6 m to the right; the telephone is at 2 o'clock). Avoid using phrases such as "over there."
- When you offer to assist someone, allow the person to hold onto your arm just above the elbow and to walk a half-step behind you.
- When offering the person a seat, place the person's hand on the back or the arm of the seat.
- When you are about to go up or down a flight of stairs, tell the person and place his or her hand on the banister.
- Make sure that the environment is free of obstacles; close doors and cabinets so they are not in the path.
- Offer to read written information, such as a menu.
- If you serve food to the person, use clock cues to specify where everything is on the plate.
- When the person who is blind or who has low vision is a patient in a health care facility:
  - Make sure all objects the person will need are close at hand.
  - Identify the location of objects that the person may need (e.g., "The call light is near your right hand"; "The telephone is on the table on the left side of your bed").
  - Remove obstacles that may be in the person's pathway and could cause a fall.
  - Place all assistive devices the person uses close at hand; let the person feel the devices so that he or she knows their location.
- Do not distract the service animal unless the owner has given permission.
- Ask the person, "How can I help you?" At some times the person needs help, but at other times help may not be needed.

Adapted from Pagliuca, L. M., Macedo-Costa, K. N., Reboucas, G. B., et al. (2014). Validation of the general guidelines of communication between the nurse and the blind. *Reviews Bras Enferm*, *67*(5), 715–725.

barriers with patients who are blind (Pagliuca, Macedo-Costa, Reboucas, et al., 2014).

Promoting Home, Community-Based, and Transitional Care

The nurse, social workers, family, and others collaborate to assess the patient's home condition and support system. If available, a low-vision specialist should be consulted before discharge, particularly for patients for whom identifying and administering medications pose a challenge.

The level of VA and patient preference help to determine appropriate interventions. For example, a plastic pill container with dividers that has been prefilled with a week's supply of medication can make medication administration easier for some patients, whereas others may prefer to have medication bottles marked with textured paints. Many patients require referral to social services. Patients with habits that may jeopardize safety, such as smoking, need to be cautioned and assisted to make their environment safe.

Other interventions that are appropriate for some people with low vision or blindness include Braille and guide dogs. Recent rapid advances in technology have led to the erroneous conclusion by some that Braille is an outmoded communication tool. There has been an ever-increasing reliance on print magnification technology as well as computer-assisted speech output. However, although the use of Braille may be less important for adults who have already learned language and grammar skills, educators and low-vision specialists have continued to advocate that children who are legally blind be given the opportunity to learn Braille.

Guide dogs, also known as seeing-eye dogs, are dogs that are specially bred, raised, and rigourously trained to assist people who are blind. The guide dog is a constant companion to the person who is blind (also referred to as the animal's handler) and is allowed on airplanes and in restaurants, stores, hotels, and other public places. With the assistance of the guide dog, the person who is blind can be extremely mobile and accomplish usual activities both within and outside of the home and workplace. A dog in harness is a working dog, not a pet. The dog should not be distracted from his job by well-intentioned strangers who want to pet, feed, or play with him. The dog's handler should always be consulted before approaching the working guide dog. Most health care facilities have a service animal policy that outlines the responsibilities of the handler with regard to the care of the animal.

In Canada, laws such as the Canadian Charter of Human Rights and Freedoms, Access to Information Act, and Canadian Human Rights Act support assistance of people who are blind. Governmental services include income assistance and health insurance through Family and Community Services, support services through programs such as the CNIB and the Alliance for Equality of Blind Canadians, tax exemptions and tax deductions, educational services through programs such as the Canadian Association Disability Service Providers in Post Secondary Education and National Educational Association of Disabled Students, reduced or free postage for Braille materials through the Canada Post Corporation Act, and assistance for veterans through Veteran Affairs Canada. Other resources and services are identified in "Resources" at the end of this chapter.

Unfolding Patient Stories: Vernon Watkins • Part 2

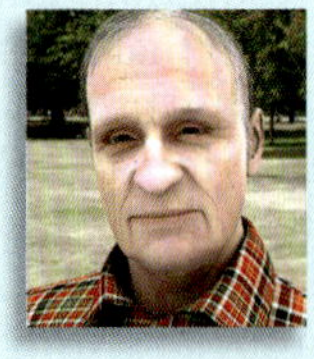

Recall from Chapter 19 Vernon Watkins, who came to the emergency department with severe abdominal pain and underwent a hemicolectomy for a bowel perforation. During postoperative care the nurse determines that he has poor vision. What measures can the nurse take to maintain a safe environment for a patient with visual impairment? How will the discovery of impaired vision impact the nursing plan of care, discharge planning, and delivery of patient education?

Care for Vernon and other patients in a realistic virtual environment: ***vSim** for Nursing* **(thepoint.lww.com/vSimMedicalSurgical).** Practice documenting these patients' care in DocuCare **(thepoint.lww.com/DocuCareEHR).**

OCULAR MEDICATION ADMINISTRATION

Because medications are often prescribed to treat ocular disorders, nurses must understand the actions of the commonly used medications and effective administration. The main objective of ocular medication delivery is to maximize the amount of medication that reaches the ocular site of action in sufficient concentration to produce a beneficial therapeutic effect. This is determined by the dynamics of ocular pharmacokinetics: absorption, distribution, metabolism, and excretion.

Ocular absorption involves the entry of a medication into the aqueous humour through the different routes of ocular medication administration. The rate and extent of aqueous humour absorption are determined by the characteristics of the medication and the anatomy and physiology of the eye. Natural barriers of absorption that diminish the efficacy of ocular medications include the following:

- *Limited size of the conjunctival sac.* The conjunctival sac can hold only 50 mcL, and any excess is wasted. The volume of one eye drop from commercial topical ocular solutions typically ranges from 20 to 35 mcL.
- *Corneal membrane barriers.* The epithelial, stromal, and endothelial layers are barriers to absorption.
- *Blood–ocular barriers.* Blood–ocular barriers prevent high ocular tissue concentration of most ophthalmic medications because they separate the bloodstream from the ocular tissues and keep foreign substances from entering the eye, thereby limiting a medication's efficacy.
- *Tearing, blinking, and drainage.* Increased tear production and drainage due to ocular irritation or an ocular condition may dilute or wash out an instilled eye drop; blinking expels an instilled eye drop from the conjunctival sac.

Distribution of an ocular medication into the various ocular tissues varies by tissue type—the conjunctiva, cornea, lens, iris, ciliary body, and choroids absorb medications to varying degrees. Medications penetrate the corneal epithelium by diffusion by passing through the cells (intracellular) or by passing between the cells (intercellular). Water-soluble (hydrophilic) medications diffuse through the intracellular route, and fat-soluble (lipophilic) medications diffuse through the intercellular route. Topical administration usually does not reach the retina in significant concentrations. Because the space between the ciliary process and the lens is small, medication diffusion in the vitreous is slow. When high concentrations of medication in the vitreous are required, intraocular injection is often chosen to bypass the natural ocular anatomic and physiologic barriers (American Society of Ophthalmic Registered Nurses [ASORN], 2013).

Aqueous solutions are most commonly used for the eye. They are the least expensive medications and interfere the least with vision. However, corneal contact time is brief because tears dilute the medication. Ophthalmic ointments have extended retention time in the conjunctival sac and provide a higher concentration than eye drops. The major disadvantage of ointments is the blurred vision that results after application. In general, eyelids and eyelid margins are best treated with ointments. The conjunctiva, limbus, cornea, and anterior chamber are treated most effectively with instilled solutions or suspensions. Subconjunctival injection may be necessary for better absorption in the anterior chamber. If high medication concentrations are required in the posterior chamber, intravitreal injections or systemically absorbed medications are considered. Contact lenses and collagen shields soaked in antibiotic agents are alternative delivery methods for treating corneal infections.

Of all these delivery methods, the topical route of administration—instilled eye drops and applied ointments—remains the most common (ASORN, 2013). Topical instillation, which is the least invasive method, permits self-administration of medication and produces fewer side effects.

Preservatives are commonly used in ocular medications. Benzalkonium chloride, for example, prevents the growth of organisms and enhances the corneal permeability of most medications; however, some patients are allergic to this preservative. This may be suspected even if the patient had never before experienced an allergic reaction to systemic use of the medication in question. Eye drops without preservatives can be prepared by pharmacists.

Common Ocular Medications

Common ocular medications include topical anesthetic, mydriatic, and cycloplegic agents that reduce IOP; anti-infective medications; corticosteroids; nonsteroidal anti-inflammatory drugs (NSAIDs); antiallergy medications; eye irrigants; and lubricants.

Topical Anesthetic Agents

One or two drops of proparacaine hydrochloride (Ophthaine 0.5%) and tetracaine hydrochloride (Pontocaine 0.5%) are instilled before diagnostic procedures such as tonometry and minor ocular procedures such as removal of sutures or conjunctival or corneal scrapings. Topical anesthetic agents are also used for severe eye pain to allow the patient to open their eyes for examination or treatment (e.g., eye irrigation for chemical burns). Anesthesia occurs within 20 seconds to 1 minute and lasts 10 to 20 minutes. The nurse must educate the patient not to rub the eyes while anesthetized because this may result in corneal damage.

Mydriatic and Cycloplegic Agents

Mydriasis, or pupil dilation, is the main objective of the administration of mydriatics and cycloplegics (Table 60-3). These two types of medications function differently and are used in combination to achieve the maximal dilation

TABLE 60-3 Mydriatics and Cycloplegics

Medication	Available Preparation/ Concentration	Indication/Dosage	Peak: Mydriasis (Minutes)	Peak: Cycloplegia (Minutes)	Recovery Time: Mydriasis	Recovery Time: Cycloplegia
phenylephrine (Neo-Synephrine)	Solutions (2.5%, 10%)	Given with cycloplegics in pupillary dilation for ophthalmoscopy and surgical procedures every 5–10 minutes × 3 or until the pupils are fully dilated	10–60	–	3–6 hours	–
atropine (Isopto Ophthalmic)	Ointment (0.5–2%) Solutions (0.5–3%)	In uveitis, or after surgery, 2–4 × daily	30–40	60–180	7–10 days	6–12 days
scopolamine (Isopto Hyoscine Ophthalmic)	Solution (0.25%)	Same as atropine	20–30	30–60	3–7 days	3–7 days
homatropine (Homatropine HBr)	Solution (5–2.5%)	Same as atropine and scopolamine	40–60	30–60	1–3 days	1–3 days
cyclopentolate (AK-Pentolate)	Solution (0.5–2%)	Given with mydriatics every 5–10 minutes × 3 or until the pupils are fully dilated for ophthalmoscopy and surgical procedures	30–60	25–75	1 day	6–24 hours
tropicamide (Myrdal)	Solution (0.25–1%)	–	20–40	20–35	6 hours	6 hours

Adapted from Comerford, K. C. (2015). *Nursing 2015 drug handbook*. Philadelphia, PA: Wolters Kluwer.

that is needed during surgery and fundus examinations to give the ophthalmologist a better view of the internal eye structures. Mydriatics potentiate alpha-adrenergic sympathetic effects that result in the relaxation of the ciliary muscle. This causes the pupil to dilate. However, this sympathetic action alone is not enough to sustain mydriasis because of its short duration of action. The strong light used during an eye examination also stimulates miosis (i.e., pupillary contraction). Cycloplegic medications are given to paralyze the iris sphincter.

The patient is educated about the temporary effects of mydriasis on vision, such as glare and the inability to focus properly. The patient may have difficulty reading. The effects of the various mydriatics and cycloplegics can last 3 hours to several days. The patient is advised to wear sunglasses (most eye clinics provide protective sunglasses). The ability to drive depends on the person's age, vision, and comfort level. Some patients can drive safely with the use of sunglasses, whereas others may need to be driven home.

Mydriatic and cycloplegic agents affect the central nervous system. Their effects are most prominent in younger and older adult patients; these patients must be assessed closely for symptoms, such as increased blood pressure, tachycardia, dizziness, ataxia, confusion, disorientation, incoherent speech, and hallucination. These medications are contraindicated in patients with narrow angles or shallow anterior chambers and in patients taking monoamine oxidase inhibitors or tricyclic antidepressants.

Medications Used to Treat Glaucoma

Therapeutic medications for glaucoma are used to lower IOP by decreasing aqueous production or increasing aqueous outflow. Because glaucoma calls for lifetime therapy, the patient must be educated with regard to both the ocular and systemic side effects of the medications. See section on glaucoma later in this chapter.

Anti-Infective Medications

Anti-infective medications include antibiotic, antifungal, and antiviral agents. Most are available as drops, ointments, or subconjunctival or intravitreal injections. Antibiotics include penicillin, cephalosporins, aminoglycosides, and fluoroquinolones. The main antifungal agent is amphotericin B. Side effects of amphotericin are serious and include severe pain, conjunctival necrosis, iritis, and retinal toxicity. Antiviral medications include acyclovir (Zovirax) and ganciclovir (Cytovene). They are used to treat ocular infections associated with herpes virus and cytomegalovirus (CMV). Patients receiving ocular anti-infective agents are subject to the same side effects and adverse reactions as those receiving oral or parenteral medications.

Corticosteroids and Nonsteroidal Anti-Inflammatory Drugs

Topical preparations of corticosteroids are commonly used in inflammatory conditions of the eyelids, conjunctiva, cornea, anterior chamber, lens, and uvea. In posterior segment diseases that involve the posterior sclera, retina, and optic nerve, topical agents are less effective and parenteral and oral routes are preferred. When a suspension is prescribed, the patient is instructed to shake the bottle several times to promote mixture of the medication and maximize its therapeutic effect. The most common ocular side effects of long-term topical corticosteroid administration are glaucoma, cataracts, susceptibility to infection, impaired wound healing, mydriasis, and ptosis. High IOP may develop, which is reversible after corticosteroid use is discontinued. To avoid the side effects of corticosteroids, NSAIDs are used as an alternative in controlling inflammatory eye conditions and postoperatively to reduce inflammation.

Antiallergy Medications

Ocular hypersensitivity reactions, such as allergic conjunctivitis, are extremely common. These conditions result primarily from responses to environmental allergens. Most allergens are airborne or carried to the eye by the hand or by other means, although allergic reactions may also be drug induced. Corticosteroids are commonly used as anti-inflammatory and immunosuppressive agents to control ocular hypersensitivity reactions.

Ocular Irrigants and Lubricants

Most irrigating solutions are used to cleanse the external lids to maintain lid hygiene, to irrigate the external corneal surface to regain normal pH (e.g., in chemical burns), to irrigate the corneal surface to eliminate debris, or to inflate the globe intraoperatively. These solutions have various compositions that include sodium, potassium, magnesium, calcium, bicarbonate, glucose, and glutathione (i.e., substance found in the aqueous humour). Sterile irrigating solutions, such as Dacriose, for lid hygiene are available. Irrigating solutions are safe to use with an intact corneal surface; however, the corneal surface should not be irrigated in cases of threatened corneal perforation. For patients with severe corneal ulcer, specific instructions from the ophthalmologist must be obtained regarding whether it is safe to irrigate the corneal surface or just to cleanse the external lids. Although it is good practice to promote hygiene, prevention of complications must be the primary concern. Normal saline solutions are commonly used to irrigate the corneal surface when chemical burns occur.

Lubricants, such as artificial tears, help alleviate corneal irritation, such as dry eye syndrome. Artificial tears are topical preparations of carboxymethylcellulose or hydroxypropyl methylcellulose that are prepared as eye drop solutions, ointments, or ocular inserts (inserted at the lower conjunctival cul-de-sac once each day). The eye drops can be instilled as often as every hour, depending on the severity of symptoms.

Nursing Management

The objectives in administering ocular medications are to ensure proper administration to maximize the therapeutic effects and to ensure the safety of the patient by monitoring for systemic and local side effects (ASORN, 2013). Absorption of eye drops by the nasolacrimal duct is undesirable because of the potential systemic side effects of ocular medications. To diminish systemic absorption and minimize the side effects, it is important to occlude the puncta (Chart 60-4). This is especially important for patients who are most vulnerable to

CHART 60-4

Patient Education: Instilling Eye Medications

The nurse instructs the patient to:

- Never use eye solutions that have changed colours.
- Perform hand hygiene before and after the procedure.
- Ensure adequate lighting.
- Read the label of the eye medication to verify that it is the correct medication.
- Remove contact lens as needed.
- Assume a comfortable position.
- Avoid touching the tip of the medication container to any part of the eye or face.
- Hold the lower lid down; do not press on the eyeball. Apply gentle pressure to the cheekbone to anchor the finger holding the lid.

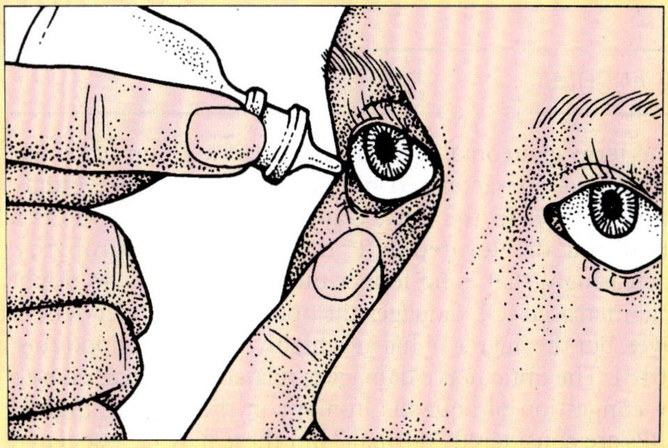

- Instill eye drops before applying ointments.
- Apply a 0.25- to 0.5-in ribbon of ointment to the lower conjunctival sac.

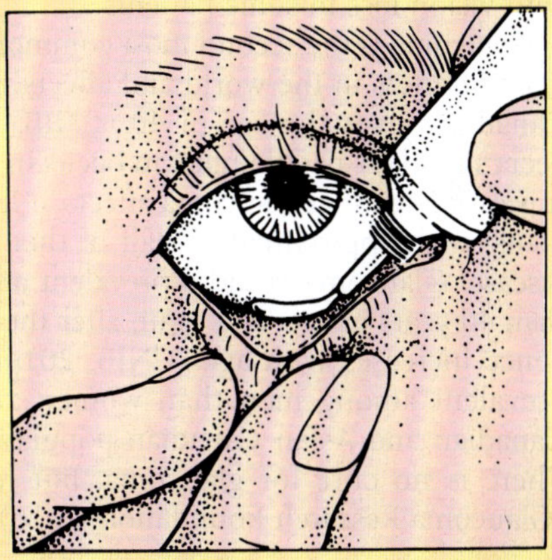

- Keep the eyelids closed, and apply gentle pressure on the inner canthus (punctal occlusion) near the bridge of the nose for 1 or 2 minutes immediately after instilling eye drops.
- Use a clean tissue to gently pat skin to absorb excess eye drops that run onto the cheeks.
- Wait 5 minutes before instilling another eye drop and 10 minutes before instilling another ointment.
- Reinsert contact lens if applicable.

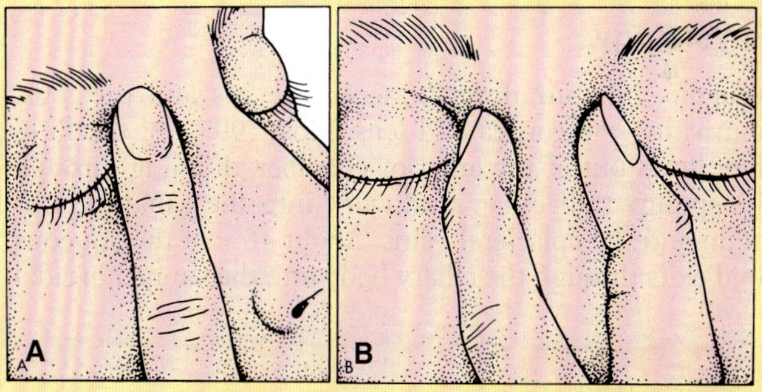

Adapted from American Society of Ophthalmic Registered Nurses (ASORN). (2013). *Recommended practice for registered nurses: Use of multi-dose medications*. San Francisco, CA: Author; Comerford, K. C. (2015). *Nursing 2015 drug handbook*. Philadelphia, PA: Wolters Kluwer.

medication overdose, including older adults; women who are pregnant or lactating; and patients with cardiac, pulmonary, hepatic, or kidney disease. A 5-minute interval between instillation of different types of ocular drops is recommended.

Before the administration of ocular medications, the nurse warns the patient that blurred vision, stinging, and a burning sensation are symptoms that ordinarily occur after instillation and are temporary. Risk for interactions of the ocular medication with other ocular and systemic medications must be emphasized; therefore, a careful patient interview regarding the medications being taken must be obtained.

NURSING ALERT

To prevent infection, meticulous hand hygiene before and after medication instillation is crucial. In addition, the tip of the eye drop bottle or the ointment tube must never touch any part of the eye, and the medication must be recapped immediately after each use.

If a patient who instills their own medications cannot feel the eye drops when they are instilled, the eye medication may be refrigerated, because a cold drop is easier to detect. A 5-minute interval between successive administrations allows adequate drug retention and absorption. The patient or the caregiver at home should be asked to demonstrate actual eye drop or ointment instillation and punctal occlusion.

GLAUCOMA

The term **glaucoma** is used to refer to a group of ocular conditions characterized by optic nerve damage (Eldaly et al., 2014). In the past, glaucoma was seen more as a condition of elevated IOP than of optic neuropathy. Increasingly, that is no longer the case. There is no doubt that increased IOP damages the optic nerve and nerve fibre layer, but the degree of harm is highly variable (Eliopoulos, 2018). The optic nerve damage is related to the IOP caused by congestion of aqueous humour in the eye. A range of IOPs are considered "normal," but these may be associated with vision loss in some patients.

Glaucoma is the second most common cause of irreversible blindness in the world and affects more than 250,000 Canadians over the age of 40 (CNIB, 2014f). It usually occurs in older people but can occur in people of any age. It is estimated that glaucoma affects at least 300,000 Canadians, with approximately half of them unaware of their disease. Glaucoma is more prevalent among people older than 40 years of age, and again after the age of 60 the incidence increases with age (CNIB, 2014f). It is also more prevalent among men than women and in the African Canadian and Asian Canadian populations (Chart 60-5). There is no cure for glaucoma, but research continues (Glaucoma Research Foundation, 2016).

Physiology

Aqueous humour flows between the iris and the lens, nourishing the cornea and lens. Most (90%) of the fluid then flows out of the anterior chamber, draining through the spongy trabecular meshwork into the canal of Schlemm and the episcleral veins. About 10% of the aqueous fluid exits through the ciliary body into the suprachoroidal space and then drains into the venous circulation of the ciliary body, choroid, and sclera. Unimpeded outflow of aqueous fluid depends on an intact drainage system and an open angle (about 45 degrees) between the iris and the cornea. A narrower angle places the iris closer to the trabecular meshwork, diminishing the angle. The amount of aqueous humour produced tends to decrease with age, in systemic diseases such as diabetes, and in ocular inflammatory conditions.

IOP is determined by the rate of aqueous production, the resistance encountered by the aqueous humour as it flows out of the passages, and the venous pressure of the episcleral veins that drain into the anterior ciliary vein. When aqueous fluid production and drainage are in balance, the IOP is between 10 and 21 mm Hg. When aqueous fluid is inhibited from flowing out, pressure builds up within the eye. Fluctuations in IOP occur with time of day, exertion, diet, and medications. It tends to increase with blinking, tight lid squeezing, and upward gazing. Systemic conditions such as hypertension and intraocular conditions such as uveitis and retinal detachment have been associated with elevated IOP. Exposure to cold weather, alcohol, a fat-free diet, heroin, and marijuana have been found to lower IOP.

Pathophysiology

There are two accepted theories regarding how increased IOP damages the optic nerve in glaucoma. The direct mechanical theory suggests that high IOP damages the retinal layer as it passes through the optic nerve head. The indirect ischemic theory suggests that high IOP compresses the microcirculation in the optic nerve head, resulting in cell injury and death. Some glaucomas appear as exclusively mechanical, and some are exclusively ischemic types. Typically, most cases are a combination of both. Regardless of the cause of damage, glaucomatous changes typically evolve through clearly discernible stages (Chart 60-6).

CHART 60-5

Risk Factors for Glaucoma

- African American race
- Cardiovascular disease
- Diabetes
- Family history of glaucoma
- Migraine syndromes
- Nearsightedness (myopia)
- Older age
- Previous eye trauma
- Prolonged use of topical or systemic corticosteroids
- Thin cornea

Adapted from Grossman, S. C., & Porth, C. M. (2014). *Porth's Pathophysiology: Concepts of altered health states* (9th ed.). Philadelphia, PA: Lippincott Williams & Wilkins.

CHART 60-6

Stages of Glaucoma

1. **Initiating events.** Precipitating factors include illness, emotional stress, congenital narrow angles, long-term use of corticosteroids, and use of mydriatics (i.e., medications causing pupillary dilation). These events lead to the second stage.
2. **Structural alterations in the aqueous outflow system.** Tissue and cellular changes caused by factors that affect aqueous humour dynamics lead to structural alterations and to the third stage.
3. **Functional alterations.** Conditions such as increased intraocular pressure or impaired blood flow create functional changes that lead to the fourth stage.
4. **Optic nerve damage.** Atrophy of the optic nerve is characterized by loss of nerve fibres and blood supply. This fourth stage inevitably progresses to the fifth stage.
5. **Visual loss.** Progressive loss of vision is characterized by visual field defects.

TABLE 60-4 Selected Glaucoma Types, Clinical Manifestation, and Treatment

Types of Glaucoma	Clinical Manifestations	Treatment
Wide Angle		
Usually bilateral, but one eye may be more severely affected than the other. In wide-angle glaucoma, the anterior chamber angle is open and appears normal.		
Normal tension glaucoma	IOP ≤21 mm Hg. Optic nerve damage, visual field defects.	If medical treatment is unsuccessful, LT can decrease IOP by 20%. Glaucoma filtering surgery if continued optic nerve damage despite medication therapy and LT.
Ocular hypertension	Elevated IOP. Possible ocular pain or headache.	The best management for normal tension glaucoma is yet to be established. Goal is to lower the IOP by at least 30%.
Narrow Angle		
Obstruction in aqueous humour outflow due to the complete or partial closure of the angle from the forward shift of the peripheral iris to the trabecula. The obstruction results in an increased IOP.		
Acute angle-closure glaucoma	Rapidly progressive visual impairment, periocular pain, conjunctival hyperemia, and congestion. Pain may be associated with nausea, vomiting, bradycardia, and profuse sweating. Reduced central visual acuity, severely elevated IOP, corneal edema. Pupil is vertically oval, fixed in a semidilated position, and unreactive to light and accommodation.	Ocular emergency; administration of hyperosmotics, acetazolamide, and topical ocular hypotensive agents, such as pilocarpine and beta-blockers (betaxolol). Possible laser incision in the iris (iridotomy) to release blocked aqueous and reduce IOP. Other eye is also treated with pilocarpine eye drops and/or surgical management to avoid a similar spontaneous attack.
Subacute angle-closure glaucoma	Transient blurring of vision, halos around lights; temporal headaches and/or ocular pain; pupil may be semidilated.	Prophylactic peripheral laser iridotomy. Can lead to acute or chronic angle-closure glaucoma if untreated.
Chronic angle-closure glaucoma	Progression of glaucomatous cupping and significant visual field loss; IOP may be normal or elevated; ocular pain and headache.	Management includes laser iridotomy and medications.

IOP, intraocular pressure.

Adapted from Eldaly, M. A., Bunce, C., El Sheikha, O. Z., et al. (2014). Non-penetrating filtration surgery versus trabeculectomy for open-angle glaucoma. *Cochrane Database of Systematic Reviews*, *(2)*, CD007059; Grossman, S. C., & Porth, C. M. (2014). *Porth's Pathophysiology: Concepts of altered health states* (9th ed.). Philadelphia, PA: Lippincott Williams & Wilkins.

Classification of Glaucoma

There are several types of glaucoma. Although glaucoma classification is changing as knowledge increases, current clinical forms of glaucoma are identified as open-angle glaucoma (accounting for 90% of all cases in Canada [CNIB, 2014f]), angle-closure glaucoma (also called pupillary block), congenital glaucoma, and glaucoma associated with other conditions, such as developmental anomalies or corticosteroid use. Glaucoma can be primary or secondary, depending on whether associated factors contribute to the rise in IOP. The two common clinical forms of glaucoma encountered in adults are open-angle and angle-closure glaucoma, which are differentiated by the mechanisms that cause impaired aqueous outflow (Grossman & Porth, 2014). Table 60-4 summarizes the characteristics of the different types of open-angle and angle-closure glaucoma.

Clinical Manifestations

Glaucoma is often called the silent thief of sight because most patients are unaware that they have the disease until they have experienced visual changes and vision loss. The patient may not seek health care until he or she experiences blurred vision or "halos" around lights, difficulty focusing, difficulty adjusting eyes in low lighting, loss of peripheral vision, aching or discomfort around the eyes, and headache.

Assessment and Diagnostic Findings

Access to ophthalmologists is limited, especially in Northern Canada. Eye examinations via a University of Alberta teleglaucoma program in northern Alberta found that only 27% of patients needed an in-person assessment by an ophthalmologist while the remainder could be managed by their referral optometrist (Verma, Arora, Kassam, et al., 2014). The purpose of a glaucoma workup is to establish the diagnostic category, assess the optic nerve damage, and formulate a treatment plan. The patient's ocular and medical history are detailed to investigate the history of predisposing factors. There are four major types of examinations used in glaucoma evaluation, diagnosis, and management: tonometry to measure the IOP, ophthalmoscopy to inspect the optic nerve, gonioscopy to examine the filtration angle of the anterior chamber, and perimetry to assess the visual fields (Glaucoma Research Foundation, 2016; Grossman & Porth, 2014).

The changes in the optic nerve significant for the diagnosis of glaucoma are pallor and cupping of the optic nerve disc. The pallor of the optic nerve is caused by a lack of blood supply that results from cellular destruction. Cupping is characterized by exaggerated bending of the blood vessels as they cross the optic disc, resulting in an enlarged optic cup that appears more basinlike compared with a normal cup. The progression of cupping in glaucoma is caused by the gradual loss of retinal nerve fibres accompanied by the loss of blood supply, resulting in increased pallor of the optic disc.

As the optic nerve damage increases, visual perception in the area is lost. The localized areas of visual loss (i.e., scotomas) represent loss of retinal sensitivity and are measured and mapped by perimetry. The results are mapped on a graph. In patients with glaucoma, the graph has a distinct pattern that is different from other ocular diseases and is useful in establishing the diagnosis.

Medical Management

The aim of all glaucoma treatment is prevention of optic nerve damage through pharmacologic therapy, laser procedures, surgery, or a combination of these approaches. Lifelong therapy is almost always necessary because glaucoma cannot be cured. Although treatment cannot reverse optic nerve damage, further damage can be controlled. The treatment goal is to maintain an IOP within a range unlikely to cause further damage (Eldaly et al., 2014).

The initial target for IOP among patients with elevated IOP and those with low-tension glaucoma with progressive visual field loss is typically set at 30% lower than the current pressure. The patient is monitored for the stability of the optic nerve. If there is evidence of progressive damage, the target IOP is again lowered until the optic nerve shows stability.

Treatment focuses on achieving the greatest benefit at the least risk, cost, and inconvenience to the patient. All treatment options have potential complications, especially surgery, which yields the best success rates. In Canada, medical management is utilized in conjunction with surgical treatment, depending on the severity and type of glaucoma.

Pharmacologic Therapy

Medical management of glaucoma relies on systemic and topical ocular medications that lower IOP. Periodic follow-up examinations are essential to monitor IOP, appearance of the optic nerve, visual fields, and side effects of medications. For patients who react to the preservative in their eye drops, preservative-free dorzolamide HCl/timolol maleate is now available in Canada. In considering a therapeutic regimen, the ophthalmologist/optometrist aims for the greatest effectiveness with the least side effects, inconvenience, and cost. Therapy takes into account the patient's health and stage of glaucoma. Comfort, affordability, convenience, lifestyle, and personality are factors to consider in the patient's compliance with the medical regimen (Eliopoulos, 2018).

The patient is usually started on the lowest dose of topical medication and then advanced to increased concentrations until the desired IOP level is reached and maintained. Because of their efficacy, minimal dosing (can be used once each day), and low-cost, beta-blockers are the preferred initial topical medications. One eye is treated first, with the other eye used as a control in determining the efficacy of the medication; once efficacy has been established, treatment of the fellow eye is started. If the IOP is elevated in both eyes, both are treated. When results are not satisfactory, a new medication is substituted. The main markers of the efficacy of the medication in glaucoma control are lowering of the IOP to the target pressure, appearance of the optic nerve head, and the visual field.

Several types of ocular medications are used to treat glaucoma (Table 60-5), including miotics (i.e., cause pupillary constriction), adrenergic agonists (i.e., sympathomimetic agents), beta-blockers, alpha$_2$-agonists (i.e., adrenergic agents), carbonic anhydrase inhibitors, and prostaglandins. Cholinergics (i.e., miotics) increase the outflow of the aqueous humour by affecting ciliary muscle contraction and pupil constriction, allowing flow through a larger opening between the iris and the trabecular meshwork. Adrenergic agonists increase aqueous outflow but primarily decrease aqueous production with an action similar to beta-blockers and carbonic anhydrase inhibitors (Comerford, 2015; Grossman & Porth, 2014).

Surgical Management

Surgery is reserved for patients in whom pharmacologic treatment has not controlled the IOP. This minimally invasive procedure is specifically designed to improve fluid drainage from the eye to balance IOP. By restoring the eye's natural fluid balance, trabeculectomy surgery stabilizes the optic nerve and minimizes further visual field damage (Eldaly et al., 2014). The surgery is performed through a small incision and does not require creation of a permanent hole in the eye wall or an external filtering bleb or an implant.

In *laser trabeculoplasty* for glaucoma, laser burns are applied to the inner surface of the trabecular meshwork to open the intratrabecular spaces and widen the canal of Schlemm, thereby promoting outflow of aqueous humour and decreasing IOP. The procedure is indicated when IOP is inadequately controlled by medications; it is contraindicated when the trabecular meshwork cannot be fully visualized because of narrow angles. A serious complication of this procedure is a transient rise in IOP (usually 2 hours after surgery) that may become persistent. IOP assessment in the immediate postoperative period is essential.

In *laser iridotomy* for pupillary block glaucoma, an opening is made in the iris to eliminate the pupillary block. Laser iridotomy is contraindicated in patients with corneal edema, which interferes with laser targeting and strength. Potential complications are burns to the cornea, lens, or retina; transient elevated IOP; closure of the iridotomy; uveitis; and blurring. Pilocarpine is usually prescribed to prevent closure of the iridotomy.

Filtering procedures for chronic glaucoma are used to create an opening or fistula in the trabecular meshwork to drain aqueous humour from the anterior chamber to the subconjunctival space into a bleb, thereby bypassing the usual drainage structures. This allows the aqueous humour to flow and exit by different routes (i.e., absorption by the conjunctival vessels or mixing with tears). *Trabeculectomy* is the standard filtering technique used to remove part of the trabecular meshwork (Eldaly et al., 2014). Complications include hemorrhage, an extremely low (hypotony) or elevated IOP, uveitis, cataracts, bleb failure, bleb leak, and **endophthalmitis**. Unlike other surgical procedures, the filtering procedure's goal in glaucoma treatment is to achieve incomplete healing of the surgical wound. The outflow of aqueous humour in a newly created drainage fistula is circumvented by the granulation of fibrovascular tissue or scar tissue formation on the surgical site. Scarring is inhibited by using antifibrosis agents such as the antimetabolites fluorouracil (Efudex) and mitomycin

TABLE 60-5 Medications Used in the Management of Glaucoma

Medication	Action	Side Effects	Nursing Implications
Cholinergics (miotics) (pilocarpine, carbachol)	Increase aqueous fluid outflow by contracting the ciliary muscle and causing miosis (constriction of the pupil) and opening of trabecular meshwork	Periorbital pain, blurry vision, difficulty seeing in the dark	Caution patients about diminished vision in dimly lit areas. Pilocarpine can be stored at room temperature for up to 8 weeks and then should be discarded.
Beta-blockers (timolol maleate)	Decrease aqueous humour production	Can have systemic effects, including bradycardia, exacerbation of pulmonary disease, and hypotension	Contraindicated in patients with asthma, chronic obstructive pulmonary disease, 2nd- or 3rd-degree heart block, bradycardia, or cardiac failure; educate patients about punctal occlusion to limit systemic effects.
Alpha-adrenergic agonists (apraclonidine, brimonidine)	Decrease aqueous humour production	Eye redness, dry mouth and nasal passages	Educate patients about punctal occlusion to limit systemic effects.
Carbonic anhydrase inhibitors (acetazolamide, dorzolamide)	Decrease aqueous humour production	Oral medications (acetazolamide) are associated with serious side effects, including anaphylactic reactions, electrolyte loss, depression, lethargy, gastrointestinal upset, impotence, and weight loss; side effects of topical form (dorzolamide) include topical allergy	Do not administer to patients with sulfa allergies; monitor electrolyte levels.
Prostaglandin analogues (latanoprost, bimatoprost)	Increase uveoscleral outflow	Darkening of the iris, conjunctival redness, possible rash	Instruct patients to report any side effects.

Adapted from Comerford, K. C. (2015). *Nursing 2015 drug handbook*. Philadelphia, PA: Wolters Kluwer.

(Mutamycin). Like all antineoplastic agents, they require special handling procedures before, during, and after the procedure. Fluorouracil can be administered intraoperatively and by subconjunctival injection during follow-up; mitomycin is much more potent and is administered only intraoperatively.

Drainage implants or shunts are open tubes implanted in the anterior chamber to shunt aqueous humour to an attached plate in the conjunctival space. A fibrous capsule develops around the episcleral plate and filters the aqueous humour, thereby regulating the outflow and controlling IOP.

Nursing Management

Nurses in all settings encounter patients with glaucoma. Even patients with long-standing disease and those with glaucoma as a secondary diagnosis should be assessed for knowledge level and adherence to their prescribed therapeutic regimen.

Promoting Home, Community-Based, and Transitional Care

Educating Patients About Self-Care

The medical and surgical management of glaucoma slows the progression of glaucoma but does not cure it. The lifelong therapeutic regimen mandates patient education. The nature of the disease and the importance of strict adherence to the medication regimen are explained to help ensure compliance. A thorough patient interview is essential to determine systemic conditions, current systemic and ocular medications, family history, and problems with compliance to glaucoma medications. Then the medication program can be discussed, particularly the interactions of glaucoma-control medications with other medications. For example, the diuretic effect of acetazolamide has an additive effect on the diuretic effects of other antihypertensive medications (Comerford, 2015). The effects of glaucoma-control medications on vision must also be explained. Miotics and sympathomimetics result in altered focus; therefore, patients need to be cautious in navigating their surroundings. Chart 60-7 contains points to review with patients with glaucoma.

Information about instilling ocular medication and preventing systemic absorption with punctal occlusion is described in the section on ocular medication administration.

Continuing and Transitional Care

Patients with severe glaucoma and impaired function may need referral to home, community-based, or transitional services that provide assistance in the home. The loss of peripheral vision impairs mobility the most. These patients need to be referred to low-vision and rehabilitation services. Patients who meet the criteria for legal blindness should be offered referrals to agencies that assist in obtaining federal/territorial assistance.

CHART 60-7

Patient Education: Managing Glaucoma

The nurse instructs the patient to:

- Know your intraocular pressure (IOP) measurement and the desired range.
- Be informed about the extent of your vision loss and optic nerve damage.
- Keep a record of your eye pressure measurements and visual field test results to monitor your own progress.
- Review all your medications (including over-the-counter and herbal medications) with your ophthalmologist, and mention any side effects each time you visit.
- Ask about potential side effects and drug interactions of your eye medications.
- Ask whether generic or less costly forms of your eye medications are available.
- Review the dosing schedule with your ophthalmologist and inform him or her if you have trouble complying with the schedule.
- Participate in the decision-making process. Let your doctor know what dosing schedule works for you and other preferences regarding your eye care.
- Have the nurse observe you instilling eye medication to determine whether you are administering it properly.
- Be aware that glaucoma medications can cause adverse effects if used inappropriately. Eye drops are to be administered as prescribed, not when eyes feel irritated.
- Ask your ophthalmologist/optometrist to send a report to your physician after each appointment.
- Keep all follow-up appointments.

Reassurance and emotional support are important aspects of care. A lifelong disease involving a possible loss of sight has psychological, physical, social, and vocational ramifications. The family is integrated into the plan of care, and because the disease has a familial tendency, family members is encouraged to undergo examinations at least once every 2 years to detect glaucoma early.

CATARACTS

A **cataract** is a lens opacity or cloudiness (Fig. 60-6). Cataracts rank only behind arthritis and heart disease as a leading cause of disability in older adults. More than 2.5 million Canadians have cataracts (CNIB, 2014a). In Canada, cataract surgery is the most commonly performed surgical procedure (CNIB, 2014a). Cataracts are a leading cause of blindness in the world (Prevent Blindness America, 2012).

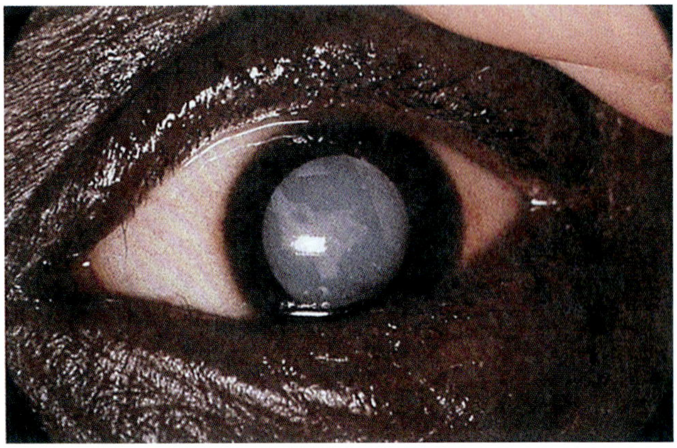

FIGURE 60-6. A cataract is a cloudy or opaque lens. On visual inspection, the lens appears grey or milky. (Rubin, R., Strayer, D. S., & Rubin, E. [2012]. *Rubin's pathology: Clinicopathologic foundations of medicine* [6th ed.]. Philadelphia, PA: Lippincott Williams & Wilkins.)

Pathophysiology

Cataracts can develop in one or both eyes at any age for a variety of causes (Chart 60-8). Cataract risk is related to lower income and educational levels, smoking history for 35 or more pack-years, diabetes, excessive sun exposure, medications, and high triglyceride levels in men (CNIB, 2014a). Visual impairment normally progresses at the same rate in both eyes over many years or in a matter of months. The three most common types of senile (age-related) cataracts are defined by their location in the lens: nuclear, cortical, and posterior subcapsular. The extent of visual impairment depends on the size, density, and location in the lens. More than one type can be present in one eye.

A nuclear cataract is associated with myopia (i.e., nearsightedness), which worsens when the cataract progresses. If dense, the cataract severely blurs vision. Periodic changes in prescription eyeglasses help manage this condition.

A cortical cataract involves the anterior, posterior, or equatorial cortex of the lens. A cataract in the equator or periphery of the cortex does not interfere with the passage of light through the centre of the lens and has little effect on vision. Cortical cataracts progress at a highly variable rate. Vision is worse in very bright light. People with the highest levels of sunlight exposure have twice the risk of developing cortical cataracts than those with low-level sunlight exposure. Occupational sun exposure in people between 20 and 29 years of age is associated with nuclear cataract formation.

Posterior subcapsular cataracts occur in front of the posterior capsule. This type typically develops in younger people and, in some cases, is associated with prolonged corticosteroid use, inflammation, or trauma. Near vision is diminished, and the eye is increasingly sensitive to glare from bright light (e.g., sunlight, headlights).

Clinical Manifestations

Painless, blurry vision is characteristic of cataracts. The patient perceives that surroundings are dimmer, as if glasses need cleaning. Light scattering is common, and the individual experiences reduced contrast sensitivity, sensitivity to glare, and reduced VA. Other effects include myopic shift (return of ability to do close work [e.g., reading fine print] without eyeglasses), astigmatism (refractive error due to an irregularity in the curvature of the cornea), monocular **diplopia** (i.e., double vision), colour shift (i.e., the aging lens becomes progressively more absorbent at the blue end of the spectrum), brunescens (i.e., colour values shift to yellow-brown), and reduced light transmission (Cash & Glass, 2016; Eliopoulos, 2018).

CHART 60-8

Risk Factors for Cataract Formation

Aging
- Loss of lens transparency
- Clumping or aggregation of lens protein (which leads to light scattering)
- Accumulation of a yellow-brown pigment due to the breakdown of lens protein
- Decreased oxygen uptake
- Increase in sodium and calcium
- Decrease in levels of vitamin C, protein, and glutathione (an antioxidant)

Associated Ocular Conditions
- Retinitis pigmentosa
- Myopia
- Retinal detachment and retinal surgery
- Infection (e.g., herpes zoster, uveitis)

Toxic Factors
- Corticosteroids, especially at high doses and in long-term use
- Alkaline chemical eye burns, poisoning
- Cigarette smoking
- Calcium, copper, iron, gold, silver, and mercury, which tend to deposit in the pupillary area of the lens

Nutritional Factors
- Reduced levels of antioxidants
- Poor nutrition
- Obesity

Physical Factors
- Dehydration associated with chronic diarrhea, use of purgatives in anorexia nervosa, and use of hyperbaric oxygenation
- Blunt trauma, perforation of the lens with a sharp object or foreign body, electric shock
- Ultraviolet radiation in sunlight and x-ray

Systemic Diseases and Syndromes
- Diabetes
- Down syndrome
- Disorders related to lipid metabolism
- Renal disorders
- Musculoskeletal disorders

Adapted from Grossman, S. C., & Porth, C. M. (2014). *Porth's Pathophysiology: Concepts of altered health states* (9th ed.). Philadelphia, PA: Lippincott Williams & Wilkins; Kumar, C. M., Seet, E., Eke, T., et al. (2016). Glycaemic control during cataract surgery under loco-regional anesthesia: A growing problem and we are none the wiser. *British Journal of Anesthesia, 117*(6), 687–691.

Assessment and Diagnostic Findings

Decreased VA is directly proportionate to cataract density. The Snellen VA test, ophthalmoscopy, and slit-lamp biomicroscopic examination are used to establish the degree of cataract formation. The degree of lens opacity does not always correlate with the patient's functional status. Some patients can perform usual activities despite clinically significant cataracts. Others with less lens opacification have a disproportionate decrease in VA; hence, VA is an imperfect measure of visual impairment.

Medical Management

No nonsurgical (medications, eye drops, eyeglasses) treatment cures cataracts or prevents age-related cataracts. However, cigarette smoking; long-term use of corticosteroids, especially at high doses; sunlight and ionizing radiation; diabetes; obesity; and eye injuries can increase the risk for cataracts. In the early stages of cataract development, glasses, contact lenses, strong bifocals, or magnifying lenses may improve vision (Cash & Glass, 2016).

Surgical Management

In general, if reduced vision from cataract does not interfere with usual activities (e.g., able to drive legally), surgery may be delayed. In deciding when cataract surgery is to be performed, the patient's functional and visual status should be a primary consideration (Eliopoulos, 2018). Surgery is performed on an outpatient basis and usually takes less than 1 hour, with the patient being discharged in 30 minutes or less afterward. Although complications from cataract surgery are uncommon, they can have significant effects on vision (Table 60-6). Restoration of visual function through a safe and minimally invasive procedure is the surgical goal, which is achieved with advances in topical anesthesia, smaller wound incision (i.e., clear cornea incision), and lens design (i.e., foldable and more accurate IOL measurements).

Injection-free topical and intraocular anesthesia, such as 1% lidocaine gel applied to the surface of the eye, eliminates the hazards of regional (retrobulbar and peribulbar) anesthesia, such as ocular perforation, retrobulbar hemorrhage, optic injuries, diplopia, and ptosis, and is ideal for patients receiving anticoagulants. Furthermore, patients can communicate and cooperate during surgery. IV moderate sedation may be used to minimize anxiety and discomfort.

When both eyes have cataracts, one eye is treated first, with at least several weeks, preferably months, separating the two operations. Because cataract surgery is performed to improve visual functioning, the delay for the other eye gives time for the patient and the surgeon to evaluate whether the results from the first surgery are adequate enough to preclude the need for a second operation. The delay also provides time for the first eye to recover; if there are any complications, the surgeon may decide to perform the second procedure differently.

Phacoemulsification

In this method of extracapsular cataract surgery, a portion of the anterior capsule is removed, allowing extraction of the lens nucleus and cortex while the posterior capsule and zonular support are left intact. An ultrasonic device is used to liquefy the nucleus and cortex, which are then suctioned out through a tube. An intact zonular–capsular diaphragm provides the needed safe anchor for the posterior chamber IOL. The pupil is dilated to 7 mm or greater (Peng, Fong, Phaik, et al., 2012). The surgeon makes a small incision on the upper edge of the cornea and a viscoelastic substance (clear gel) is injected into the space between the cornea and the lens. This prevents the space from collapsing and facilitates insertion of the IOL. Because the incision is smaller than the manual extracapsular cataract extraction, the wound heals more rapidly,

TABLE 60-6 Potential Complications of Cataract Surgery

Complication	Effects	Management and Outcome
Immediate Preoperative		
Retrobulbar hemorrhage: can result from retrobulbar infiltration of anesthetic agents if the short ciliary artery is located by the injectia	Increased IOP, proptosis, lid tightness, and subconjunctival hemorrhage with or without edema	Emergent lateral canthotomy (slitting of the canthus) is performed to stop central retinal perfusion when the IOP is dangerously elevated. If this procedure fails to reduce IOP, a puncture of the anterior chamber with removal of fluid is considered. The patient must be closely monitored for at least a few hours. Postponement of cataract surgery for 2 to 4 weeks is advised. Complications such as iris prolapse, vitreous loss, and choroidal hemorrhage could result in a catastrophic visual outcome.
Intraoperative Complications		
Rupture of the posterior capsule	May result in loss of vitreous	Anterior vitrectomy is required if vitreous loss occurs.
Suprachoroidal (expulsive) hemorrhage: profuse bleeding into the suprachoroidal space	Extrusion of intraocular contents from the eye or opposition of retinal surfaces	Closure of the incision and administration of a hyperosmotic agent to reduce IOP or corticosteroids to reduce intraocular inflammation. Vitrectomy is performed 1 to 2 weeks later. Visual prognosis is poor; some useful vision may be salvaged on rare occasions.
Early Postoperative Complications		
Acute bacterial endophthalmitis: devastating complication that occurs in about 1 in 1,000 cases; the most common causative organisms are *Staphylococcus epidermidis, S. aureus, Pseudomonas,* and *Proteus* species	Characterized by marked visual loss, pain, lid edema, hypopyon, corneal haze, and chemosis	Managed by aggressive antibiotic therapy. Broad-spectrum antibiotics are administered while awaiting culture and sensitivity results. Once results are obtained, the appropriate antibiotics are administered via intravitreal injection. Corticosteroid therapy is also administered.
Toxic anterior segment syndrome—noninfectious inflammation that is a complication of anterior chamber surgery; caused by a toxic agent such as an agent used to sterilize surgical instruments	Corneal edema occurs <24 hours after surgery; symptoms include reduced visual acuity and pain	If there is no growth of microorganisms, the treatment is topical steroids alone.
Late Postoperative Complications		
Suture-related problems	Toxic reactions or mechanical injury from broken or loose sutures	Suture removal relieves the symptoms. Topical corticosteroids are used when the incision is not healed and sutures cannot be removed.
Malposition of the IOL	Results in astigmatism, sensitivity to glare, or appearance of halos	Miotics are used for mild cases, whereas IOL removal and replacement are necessary for severe cases.
Chronic endophthalmitis	Persistent, low-grade inflammation and granuloma	Corticosteroids and antibiotics are administered systematically. If the condition persists, removal of the IOL and capsular bag, vitrectomy, and intravitreal injection of antibiotics are required.
Opacification of the posterior capsule (most common late complication of extracapsular cataract extraction)	Visual acuity is diminished.	Nd:YAG laser is used to create a hole in the posterior capsule. Blurred vision is cleared immediately.

IOP, intraocular pressure; IOL, intraocular lens; Nd:YAG, neodymium:yttrium aluminum garnet.

and there is early stabilization of refractive error and less astigmatism.

Lens Replacement

After removal of the crystalline lens, the patient is referred to as *aphakic* (i.e., without lens). The lens, which focuses light on the retina, must be replaced for the patient to see clearly. There are three lens replacement options: aphakic eyeglasses, contact lenses, and IOL implants.

Aphakic glasses are effective but heavy. Objects are magnified by 25%, making them appear closer than they actually are. Objects are magnified unequally, creating distortion. Peripheral vision is also limited, and **binocular vision** (i.e., ability of both eyes to focus on one object and fuse the two images into one) is impossible if the other eye is phakic (normal).

Contact lenses provide patients with almost normal vision, but because contact lenses need to be removed occasionally, the patient also needs a pair of aphakic glasses. Contact lenses are not advised for patients who have difficulty inserting, removing, and cleaning them. Frequent handling and improper disinfection increase the risk for infection.

Insertion of IOLs during cataract surgery is the usual approach to lens replacement (Eliopoulos, 2018). After ICCE, the surgeon implants an anterior chamber IOL in front of the iris. Posterior chamber lenses, generally used in ECCE, are implanted behind the iris. ECCE and posterior chamber IOLs are associated with a relatively low incidence of complications (e.g., hyphema, macular edema, secondary glaucoma, damage to the corneal endothelium) (Eliopoulos, 2018). IOL implantation is contraindicated in patients with recurrent uveitis, proliferative diabetic retinopathy, neovascular glaucoma, or rubeosis iridis. Like any device, IOLs can malfunction and cause complications.

The most common IOL is the single-focus lens. Eyeglasses are still needed for distant or close vision, because the single-focus lens, unlike the natural lens of the eye, cannot alter its shape to bring objects at different distances into focus. Multifocal IOLs reduce the need for eyeglasses but patients can experience halos and glare. In the future, older patients may benefit from a combined surgical approach using customized IOLs and refractive surgery for a customized vision correction.

Also known as toxic endothelial cell destruction or sterile endophthalmitis, toxic anterior segment syndrome is a noninfectious inflammation caused by a toxic agent after an uncomplicated and uneventful surgery. This relatively newly recognized disorder is a complication of anterior chamber surgery. Investigations have shown that it may be caused by toxins from improperly rinsed surgical instruments soaked in enzymatic detergents, residue from instruments sterilized with plasma gas, abnormalities in the pH or ionic composition of irrigation solutions, ophthalmic viscoelastic devices, intraocular medications, or even the finish of the IOL.

Toxic anterior segment syndrome is characterized by corneal edema less than 24 hours after surgery, compared to the classic endophthalmitis, which appears 48 to 72 hours after surgery and is bacterial in nature. Like the classic endophthalmitis, the symptoms include reduction in VA and pain. In the absence of microorganism growth, improvement has occurred with topical steroid treatment alone.

Nursing Management

The patient with cataracts should receive the usual preoperative care for ambulatory surgical patients undergoing eye surgery. The standard battery of preoperative tests (complete blood count, ECG, and urinalysis) should be prescribed only when they would have been indicated by the patient's medical history.

Providing Preoperative Care

Alpha-antagonists (particularly tamsulosin [Flomax], which is used for treatment of enlarged prostate) are known to cause a condition called *intraoperative floppy iris syndrome*. Alpha-antagonists can interfere with pupil dilation during the surgical procedure, resulting in miosis and iris prolapse and leading to complications. Intraoperative floppy iris syndrome can occur even though a patient has stopped taking the drug. The nurse needs to ask patients about a history of taking alpha-antagonists. Surgical team members are then alerted to the risk of this complication (Comerford, 2015).

Dilating drops are given prior to surgery. Nurses in the ambulatory surgery setting begin patient education about eye medications (antibiotic, corticosteroid, and anti-inflammatory drops) that will need to be self-administered to prevent postoperative infection and inflammation.

Providing Postoperative Care

Before discharge, the patient receives verbal and written education regarding eye protection, administration of medications, recognition of complications, activities to avoid, and obtaining emergency care (Chart 60-9). An eye shield is usually worn at night for the first week to avoid injury. The nurse also explains that there should be minimal discomfort after surgery and educates the patient about taking a mild analgesic agent, such as acetaminophen, as needed. Antibiotic, anti-inflammatory, and corticosteroid eye drops or ointments are prescribed postoperatively. Patients prescribed anti-inflammatory or corticosteroid eye drops are monitored for possible increases in IOP (Kusne, Kang, & Fintelmann, 2016).

Promoting Home, Community-Based, and Transitional Care

Educating Patients About Self-Care

To prevent accidental rubbing or poking of the eye, the patient wears a protective eye patch for 24 hours after surgery, followed by eyeglasses worn during the day and a metal shield worn at night for 1 to 4 weeks. The nurse instructs the patient and family in applying and caring for the eye shield. Sunglasses should be worn while outdoors during the day because the eye is sensitive to light.

Slight morning discharge, some redness, and a scratchy feeling may be expected for a few days. A clean, damp washcloth may be used to remove slight morning eye discharge. Because cataract surgery increases the risk for retinal detachment, the patient must know to notify the surgeon if new floaters (i.e., dots) in vision, flashing lights, decrease in vision, pain, or increase in redness occurs.

Continuing and Transitional Care

The eye patch is removed after the first follow-up appointment. Patients may experience blurring of vision for several days to weeks. Sutures left in the eye alter the curvature of the cornea, resulting in temporary blurring and some astigmatism. Vision gradually improves as the eye heals. Patients with IOL implants have visual improvement faster than those waiting for aphakic glasses or contact lenses. Vision is stabilized when the eye is completely healed, usually within 6 to 12 weeks, when final corrective prescription is completed. Visual correction is needed for any remaining near- or farsightedness (even in patients with IOL implants). Patients who choose multifocal IOLs should be aware that there may be increased night glare and contrast sensitivity.

CORNEAL DISORDERS

Corneal Dystrophies

Corneal dystrophies are inherited as autosomal dominant traits and manifest when the person is about 20 years of age. They are characterized by deposits in the corneal layers. Decreased vision is caused by the irregular corneal surface and corneal deposits. Corneal endothelial decompensation leads to corneal edema and blurring of vision. Persistent edema leads to **bullous keratopathy**, which is formation of blisters that cause pain and discomfort on rupturing. The two main types are keratoconus and Fuchs endothelial dystrophy.

CHART 60-9

HOME CARE CHECKLIST • Intraocular Lens Implant

At the completion of education, the patient and/or caregiver will be able to:

- Name the procedure that was performed and identify any permanent changes in anatomic structure or function as well as changes in ADLs, IADLs, roles, relationships, and spirituality.
- State the name, dose, side effects, frequency, and schedule for all medications.
- Describe ongoing postoperative therapeutic regimen and activities to limit or avoid (e.g., lifting weights, driving a car, contact sports).
    - Wear glasses or eye shield following surgery as instructed.
    - Always wash hands before touching or cleaning the postoperative eye.
    - Clean postoperative eye with a clean tissue; wipe the closed eye with a single gesture from the inner canthus outward.
    - When bathing or showering, shampoo hair cautiously or seek assistance.
    - Avoid lying on the side of the affected eye the night after surgery.
    - Keep activity light (e.g., walking, reading, watching television). Resume the following activities only as directed by the ophthalmologist: driving, sexual activity, unusually strenuous activity.
    - Avoid lifting, pushing, or pulling objects heavier than 15 lb.
    - Avoid bending or stooping for an extended period.
    - Be careful when climbing or descending stairs.
- Describe signs and symptoms of complications (e.g., vision change, continuous flashing lights appear to the affected eye, redness, swelling or increased pain near the eye, change in amount or type of eye drainage, any eye injury, significant pain not relieved by prescribed analgesia).
- Relate how to reach ophthalmologist with questions or complications.
- State time and date of follow-up appointments.
- Identify sources of assistance (e.g., meals, transportation) and support (e.g., friends, relatives, faith community).
- Identify the need for health promotion, disease prevention, and screening activities.

Keratoconus

Keratoconus is a condition characterized by a conical protuberance of the cornea with progressive thinning on protrusion and irregular astigmatism. This hereditary condition has a higher incidence among women. Onset occurs at puberty; the condition may progress for more than 20 years and is bilateral. Corneal scarring occurs in severe cases. Blurred vision is a prominent symptom. Rigid, gas-permeable contact lenses correct irregular astigmatism and improve vision. Advances in contact lens design have reduced the need for surgery. Penetrating keratoplasty is indicated when contact lens correction is no longer effective.

Fuchs Endothelial Dystrophy

Fuchs (pronounced *Fooks*) dystrophy is manifested by a slow death of cells in the endothelial cornea. It affects women more than men and is usually not noted until 50 years of age. Corneal endothelial cell death leads to corneal edema and blurring of vision. Persistent edema leads to bullous keratopathy. A bandage contact lens is used to flatten the bullae, protect the exposed corneal nerve endings, and relieve discomfort. Symptomatic treatments, such as hypertonic drops or ointment (5% sodium chloride), may reduce epithelial edema. Currently, the only cure is a corneal transplant (Dickman, Peeters, Van Den Biggelaar, et al., 2016).

Corneal Surgeries

Among the surgical procedures used to treat diseased corneal tissue are phototherapeutic keratectomy (PTK) and keratoplasty. The success rate of ocular surface transplantation using autologous oral mucosal epithelium or amniotic membrane recipient–derived bone stem cells is now reasonable. Tissue rejection remains a major cause of failure.

Phototherapeutic Keratectomy

PTK is a laser procedure that is used to treat diseased corneal tissue by removing or reducing corneal opacities and smoothening the anterior corneal surface to improve functional vision. PTK is a safer, more effective (when indicated) alternative than penetrating or lamellar keratoplasty. PTK is contraindicated in patients with active herpetic keratitis because the ultraviolet rays may reactivate latent virus. Common side effects are induced hyperopia and stromal haze. Complications are delayed reepithelialization (particularly in patients with diabetes) and bacterial keratitis. Postoperative management consists of oral analgesic agents for eye pain. Reepithelialization is promoted with a pressure patch or therapeutic soft contact lens. Antibiotic and corticosteroid ointment and NSAIDs are prescribed postoperatively. Follow-up examinations are required for up to 2 years.

Penetrating Keratoplasty

PKP (corneal transplantation or corneal grafting) involves replacing abnormal host tissue with healthy donor (cadaver) corneal tissue. Common indications are keratoconus, corneal scarring from herpes simplex, keratitis, and chemical burns.

Several factors affect the success of the graft: the condition of the ocular structures (e.g., lids, conjunctiva), quality of the tears, adequacy of blinking, and viability of the donor endothelium. Contraindications for the use of donor tissue are outlined in Chart 60-10.

In PKP, the surgeon determines the graft size before the procedure, and the appropriate size is marked on the surface of the cornea. The surgeon prepares the donor cornea and the recipient bed, removes the diseased cornea, places the donor cornea on the recipient bed, and sutures it in place. Sutures remain in place for 12 to 18 months and are then removed. Potential complications include early graft failure due to poor quality of donor tissue, surgical trauma, acute infection, and persistently increased IOP and late graft failure due to rejection.

Postoperatively, the patient receives mydriatics for 2 weeks and topical corticosteroids for 12 months (daily doses for 6 months and tapered doses thereafter). These mydriatics and corticosteroid drops should be preservative free to prevent a reactive inflammation. Patients typically describe a sensation of postoperative eye discomfort rather than acute pain.

CHART 60-10

Contraindications to the Use of Donor Tissue for Corneal Transplantation: Donor Characteristics

Systemic Disorders

- Death from unknown cause
- Creutzfeldt–Jakob disease
- AIDS or high risk for HIV infection
- Hepatitis
- Eye infection, systemic infection

Intrinsic Eye Disease

- Retinoblastoma
- Ocular inflammation
- Malignant tumours of anterior segment
- Disorders of the conjunctiva or corneal surface involving the optical zone of the cornea

Other

- History of eye trauma
- Corneal scars
- Previous surgical procedure
- Corneal graft
- LASIK eye surgery

Additional Keratoplasty Surgeries

For many years, PKP was the standard of care for patients with corneal endothelial failure but with poor refractive results. Subsequently, other techniques have been developed. Anterior lamellar keratoplasty (ALK) involves a partial-thickness graft for disorders such as anterior corneal dystrophies or scarring not involving the endothelial portion of the cornea. Deep anterior lamellar keratoplasty (DALK) involves replacement of only anterior corneal layers and not Descemet's membrane or endothelial layers for disorders such as keratoconus. Posterior lamellar keratoplasty (PLK or EK) and Descemet's stripping endothelial keratoplasty (DSEK) (which replaces only the endothelial layer of the cornea) are procedures indicated for conditions such as Fuchs endothelial dystrophy or bullous keratopathy (Dickman et al., 2016). In DSEK, layers of the cornea are dissected and selectively replaced by donor cornea tissue. DSEK offers several advantages, such as less postoperative astigmatism, faster visual recovery, and stronger wound integrity. Theoretically, the risk of rejection is less because less of the patient's tissue is replaced.

Keratoprosthesis

An additional therapeutic option for patients with multiple graft failures or severe corneal disease is keratoprosthesis (artificial cornea; e.g., U.S. Food and Drug Administration [FDA]-approved Boston Keratoprosthesis [KPro] and AlphaCor). The design of the keratoprosthesis consists of a central optic core and an outer rim that secures the prosthesis. This procedure has serious potential complications (e.g., glaucoma, endophthalmitis) and requires close follow-up and monitoring (Patel, Moster, Kishfy, et al., 2016).

Nursing Management

The nurse reinforces the surgeon's recommendations and instructions regarding visual rehabilitation and visual improvement by explaining why a technically successful graft may initially produce disappointing results because the procedure has produced a new optical surface and only after several months do patients start seeing the natural and true colours of their environment. Correction of a resultant refractive error with eyeglasses or contact lenses determines the final visual outcome. The nurse assesses the patient's support system and his or her ability to comply with long-term follow-up, which includes frequent clinic visits for several months for tapering of topical corticosteroid therapy, selective suture removal, and ongoing evaluation of the graft site and VA. The nurse also initiates appropriate referral to community services when indicated.

Because graft failure is an ophthalmic emergency that can occur at any time, the primary goal of nursing care is to teach the patient to identify signs and symptoms of graft failure. The early symptoms are blurred vision, discomfort, tearing, or redness of the eye. Decreased vision results after graft destruction. Patients must contact the ophthalmologist as soon as symptoms occur. Treatment of graft rejection is prompt administration of hourly topical corticosteroids and periocular corticosteroid injections. Systemic immunosuppressive agents may be necessary for severe, resistant cases.

Refractive Surgeries

Refractive surgeries are elective procedures performed to correct refractive errors (myopia or hyperopia) and astigmatism by reshaping the cornea (Li, Zhan, Li, et al., 2016). Laser vision correction alters the major optical function of the eye and carries risks. Refractive surgery does not alter the normal aging process of the eye. If the reason for the procedure is to meet vision requirements for the patient's occupation, the results must satisfy both the patient and the employer. Precise visual outcome cannot be guaranteed.

The corneal structure must be normal and the refractive error must be stable. The patient is required to discontinue using contact lenses for a period before the procedure (2 to 3 weeks for soft lenses and 4 weeks for hard lenses). Patients with conditions that are likely to adversely affect corneal wound healing (e.g., corticosteroid use, immunosuppression, elevated IOP) are not good candidates for the procedure. Any superficial eye disease must be diagnosed and fully treated before a refractive procedure.

Patient satisfaction is the ultimate goal; therefore, patient education and counselling about potential risks, complications, and postoperative follow-up are critical. Minimal postoperative care includes topical corticosteroid or NSAID and antibiotic drops.

Laser Vision Correction

Photorefractive Keratectomy

Photorefractive keratectomy (PRK) is used to treat myopia and hyperopia with or without astigmatism (Li et al., 2016). The excimer laser is applied directly to the cornea according to carefully calculated measurements. For myopia, the relative curvature is decreased; for hyperopia, the relative curvature is increased. A bandage contact lens is placed over the cornea to promote epithelial healing and reduce pain, which is similar to that of a severe corneal abrasion.

Laser-Assisted In Situ Keratomileusis

LASIK involves flattening the anterior curvature of the cornea by removing a stromal lamella or layer. The surgeon creates a corneal flap with a microkeratome, which is an automatic corneal shaper. The surgeon retracts a flap of corneal tissue less than one third the thickness of a human hair to access the corneal stroma and then uses the excimer laser on the stromal bed to reshape the cornea according to calculated measurements. Data are insufficient to determine whether LASIK or PRK is better at correcting nearsightedness (Li et al., 2016). There are few adverse outcomes of either procedure.

Perioperative Complications

Surgically Induced Abnormalities

Corneal surface irregularities can occur after LASIK treatment. These include central islands (central areas of stiffness or elevation), decentred ablations resulting from misalignment of the laser treatment or from involuntary eye movement during laser treatment, and forms of irregular astigmatism. Symptoms of central islands and decentred ablations include monocular diplopia or ghost images, halos, glare, and decreased VA.

Phakic Intraocular Lenses

Increasingly, phakic IOL implantation has been used for patients with moderate to severe myopia (Barsam & Allan, 2014). Phakic IOLs may be used in either the anterior or posterior chamber. The implantation of such devices is reversible because the natural lens is left in place and the normal architecture of the cornea is preserved. This procedure provides more predictable refractive results than procedures that alter the corneal curvature, is safer, and has higher patient satisfaction scores (Barsam & Allan, 2014). Potential complications include cataract, iritis or uveitis, endothelial cell loss, and increased IOP.

Conductive Keratoplasty

A recent innovation in refractive surgery for the correction of low to mild hyperopia uses the principles of thermal keratoplasty by applying radiofrequency current to the peripheral cornea using a thin, handheld probe. It does not involve the removal of cornea tissue. Clinical trials have shown that postprocedure VA, predictability, and stability are as good as, if not better than, with other refractive procedures.

Nursing Management

The length of postoperative follow-up depends on the refractive procedure, with PRK requiring a longer course, followed by RK and then LASIK.

RETINAL DISORDERS

Although the retina is composed of multiple microscopic layers, the two innermost layers, the sensory retina and the RPE, are the most relevant to common retinal disorders (Grossman & Porth, 2014). Just as the film in a camera captures an image, so does the retina, the neural tissue of the eye. The rods and cones, the photoreceptor cells, are found in the sensory layer of the retina. Beneath the sensory layer lies the RPE, the pigmented layer. When the rods and cones are stimulated by light, an electrical impulse is generated, and the image is transmitted to the brain.

Retinal Detachment

Retinal detachment refers to the separation of the RPE from the sensory layer. The four types of retinal detachment are rhegmatogenous, traction, a combination of rhegmatogenous and traction, and exudative. *Rhegmatogenous detachment* is the most common form. In this condition, a hole or tear develops in the sensory retina, allowing some of the liquid vitreous to seep through the sensory retina and

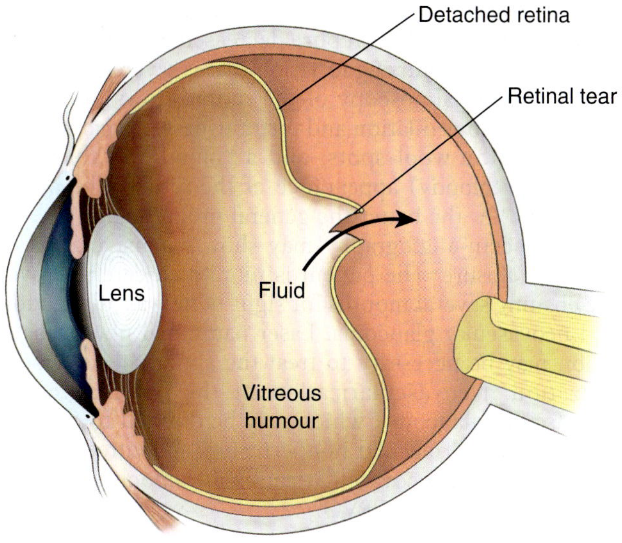

FIGURE 60-7. Retinal detachment.

detach it from the RPE (Fig. 60-7). People at risk for this type of detachment include those with high myopia or aphakia after cataract surgery. Trauma may also play a role in rhegmatogenous retinal detachment. Between 5% and 10% of all rhegmatogenous retinal detachments are associated with proliferative retinopathy, a retinopathy associated with diabetic neovascularization (see Chapter 41).

Tension, or a pulling force, is responsible for *traction retinal detachment*. An ophthalmologist must ascertain all of the areas of retinal break and identify and release the scars or bands of fibrous material providing traction on the retina. Generally, patients with this condition have developed fibrous scar tissue from conditions such as diabetic retinopathy, vitreous hemorrhage, or the retinopathy of prematurity. The hemorrhages and fibrous proliferation associated with these conditions exert a pulling force on the delicate retina.

Patients can have both rhegmatogenous and traction retinal detachment. *Exudative retinal detachments* are the result of the production of a serous fluid under the retina from the choroid. Conditions such as uveitis and macular degeneration may cause the production of this serous fluid.

Clinical Manifestations

Patients may report the sensation of a shade or curtain coming across the vision of one eye, cobwebs, bright flashing lights, or the sudden onset of a great number of floaters. Patients do not report pain.

Assessment and Diagnostic Findings

After VA is determined, the patient must have a dilated fundus examination using an indirect ophthalmoscope as well as slit-lamp biomicroscopy. Stereo fundus photography and fluorescein angiography are commonly used during the evaluation.

Increasingly, optical coherence tomography and ultrasound are used for the complete retinal assessment, especially if the view is obscured by a dense cataract or vitreous hemorrhage. All retinal breaks, all fibrous bands that may be causing traction on the retina, and all degenerative changes must be identified.

Surgical Management

In rhegmatogenous detachment, an attempt is made to surgically reattach the sensory retina to the RPE. In traction detachment, the source of traction must be removed and the sensory retina reattached. New surgical techniques as well as advances in instrumentation have led to an increased rate of success of surgical reattachment and better visual outcomes. The most commonly used surgical interventions are the scleral buckle, the pars plana vitrectomy, and pneumatic retinopexy.

Scleral Buckle

The retinal surgeon compresses the sclera (often with a scleral buckle or a silicone band; Fig. 60-8) to indent the scleral wall from the outside of the eye and bring the two retinal layers in contact with each other (Boyd, 2016). This type of surgery has a high success rate in the hands of experienced retinal surgeons. It causes less damage to the lens of the eye in phakic patients, and there is a low risk of endophthalmitis. However, there is an increased incidence of diplopia and other complications, such as induced myopia and increased postoperative pain.

Vitrectomy

A vitrectomy is an intraocular procedure in which 1- to 4-mm incisions are made at the pars plana. One incision allows the introduction of a light source, and another incision serves as the portal for the vitrectomy instrument. The surgeon dissects preretinal membranes under direct visualization while the retina is stabilized by an intraoperative vitreous substitute.

This surgical technique was originally introduced as a treatment for eyes with conditions that were previously inoperable (e.g., vitreous hemorrhage, proliferative diabetic retinopathy). Technologic improvements, including

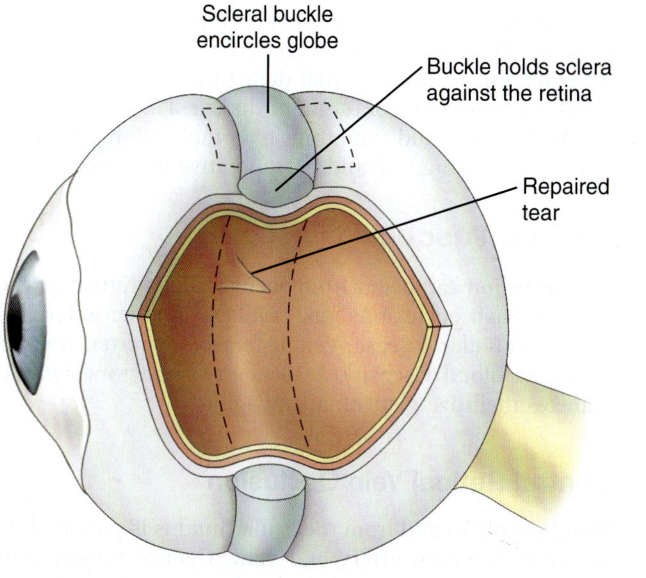

FIGURE 60-8. Scleral buckle.

the use of operating microscopes, microinstrumentation, and instruments that combine vitreous cutting, aspiration, and illumination capabilities in one device, have advanced vitreoretinal surgery. The techniques of vitreoretinal surgery can be used in various procedures, including the removal of foreign bodies, vitreous opacities such as blood, and dislocated lenses. Traction on the retina may be relieved through vitrectomy and may be combined with scleral buckling to repair retinal breaks. Treatment of macular holes includes vitrectomy, laser photocoagulation, air–fluid–gas exchanges, and the use of growth factor.

Pneumatic Retinopexy

This technique is used for the repair of a rhegmatogenous retinal detachment. It is the least invasive of the three procedures described. A gas bubble, silicone oil, or perfluorocarbon and liquids may be injected into the vitreous cavity to help push the sensory retina up against the RPE. Postoperative positioning of the patient is critical, because the injected bubble must float into a position overlying the area of detachment, providing consistent pressure to reattach the sensory retina. Argon laser photocoagulation or cryotherapy is also used to "spot-weld" small holes (Boyd, 2016).

Nursing Management

For the most part, nursing interventions consist of educating the patient and providing supportive care.

Promoting Comfort

If gas tamponade is used to flatten the retina, the patient may have to be specially positioned to make the gas bubble float into the best position. Some patients must lie face down or on their side for days. Patients and family members are made aware of these special needs beforehand, so that the patient can be made as comfortable as possible.

Teaching About Complications

In many cases, vitreoretinal procedures are performed on an outpatient basis, and the patient is seen the next day for a follow-up examination and closely monitored thereafter as required. Postoperative complications in these patients may include increased IOP, endophthalmitis, development of other retinal detachments, development of cataracts, and loss of turgor of the eye. Patients must be taught the signs and symptoms of complications, particularly of increasing IOP and postoperative infection.

Retinal Vascular Disorders

Loss of vision can occur from occlusion of a retinal artery or vein. Such occlusions may result from atherosclerosis, cardiac valvular disease, venous stasis, hypertension, or increased blood viscosity. Associated risk factors include diabetes mellitus, glaucoma, and aging.

Central Retinal Vein Occlusion

Blood supply to and from the ocular fundus is provided by the central retinal artery and vein. Central retinal vein occlusions (CRVOs) are relatively common and found most often in people older than 50 years of age. Patients who have suffered a CRVO report decreased VA, which may range from mild blurring to vision that is severely limited.

Direct ophthalmoscopy of the retina shows optic disc swelling, venous dilation and tortuousness, retinal hemorrhages, cotton-wool spots, and a "blood and thunder" (extremely bloody) appearance of the retina. The better the initial VA, the better the general prognosis is.

Fluorescein angiography may show extensive areas of capillary closure. The patient is monitored carefully over the ensuing several months for signs of neovascularization and neovascular glaucoma. Laser panretinal photocoagulation may be necessary to treat the abnormal neovascularization. Neovascularization of the iris may cause neovascular glaucoma, which may be difficult to control. Macular edema, macular nonperfusion, and vitreous hemorrhage from the neovascularization are among the potential complications of CRVO.

Branch Retinal Vein Occlusion

Some patients with branch retinal vein occlusions are symptom free, whereas others report a sudden loss of vision if the macular area is involved. A more gradual loss of vision may occur if macular edema associated with the branch retinal vein occlusion develops.

On examination, the ocular fundus appears similar to that found with CRVO; however, only those portions of the retina affected by the obstructive veins have what is known as a "blood and thunder" appearance. The diagnostic evaluation and follow-up assessments are the same as for CRVO. Potential complications are similar. Potential associated conditions include glaucoma, systemic hypertension, diabetes mellitus, hyperlipidemia, and hyperviscosity syndrome.

Central Retinal Artery Occlusion

The patient with central retinal artery occlusion, a relatively rare disorder, presents with a sudden loss of vision. VA is reduced to counting the examiner's fingers, or the field of vision is tremendously restricted. A relative afferent pupillary defect is present. Examination of the ocular fundus reveals a pale retina with a cherry-red spot at the fovea. The retinal arteries are thin, and emboli are occasionally seen in the central retinal artery or its branches. Central retinal artery occlusion is a true ocular emergency. Various treatments are used, including ocular massage, anterior chamber paracentesis, IV administration of hyperosmotic agents such as acetazolamide, and high concentrations of oxygen. Most visual loss associated with central retinal artery occlusion is severe and permanent.

Age-Related Macular Degeneration

Macular degeneration is the leading cause of severe vision loss in Canadians, especially among older adults, and is responsible for one in three cases of reported vision loss (CNIB, 2014c). Commonly called AMD, it is characterized by tiny, yellowish spots called drusen (Fig. 60-9) beneath the retina. Most people older than 60 years of age have at least a few small drusen. There is a wide range of

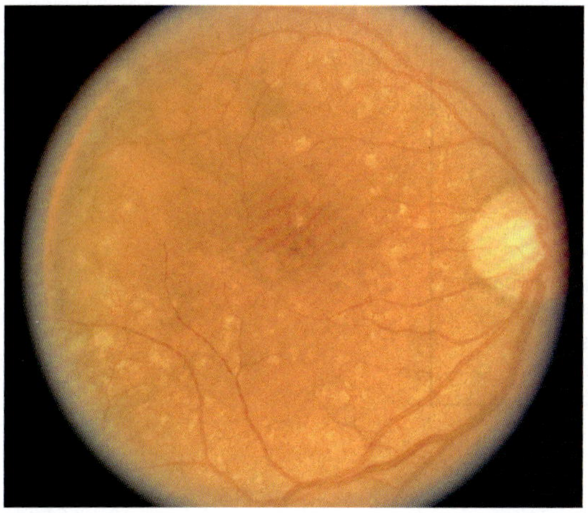

FIGURE 60-9. Retina showing drusen and age-related macular degeneration (AMD).

visual loss in patients with macular degeneration, but most patients do not experience total blindness. At present, more than one million Canadians have AMD (CNIB, 2014c). Of those, about 100,000 have blindness or partial sight. Central vision is mainly affected, with most patients retaining peripheral vision (Fig. 60-10). There are two types of AMD, commonly known as the dry type and wet type.

Between 85% and 90% of people with AMD have the dry or nonexudative type, in which the outer layers of the retina slowly break down (Fig. 60-11). With this breakdown comes the appearance of drusen. When the drusen occur outside of the macular area, patients generally have no symptoms. When the drusen occur within the macula, there is a gradual blurring of vision that patients may notice when they try to read. There is no known treatment that can cure this type of AMD. The results from a recent meta-analysis indicated a "small but statistically significant association between aspirin use and early ARMD" (Kahawita & Casson, 2014, p. 35).

The second type of AMD, the wet or exudative type, may have an abrupt onset and is more damaging to the vision. Patients report that straight lines appear crooked and distorted or that letters in words appear broken up.

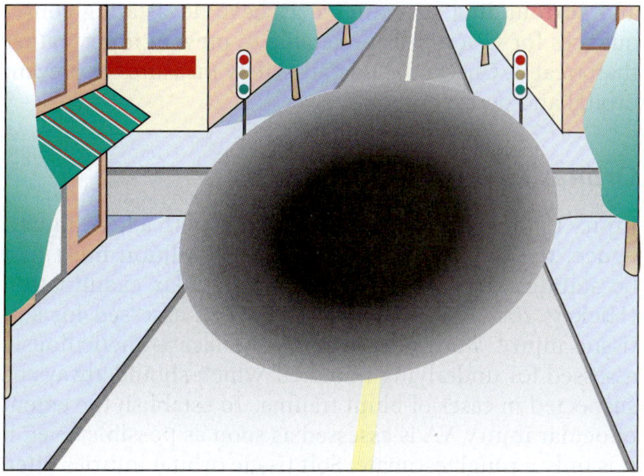

FIGURE 60-10. Visual loss associated with macular degeneration.

This effect results from proliferation of abnormal blood vessels growing under the retina, within the choroid layer of the eye, a condition known as choroidal neovascularization (CNV). The affected vessels can leak fluid and blood, elevating the retina. Some patients can be treated with the laser to stop the leakage from these vessels. This treatment is not ideal because vision may be affected by the laser treatment and abnormal vessels often grow back after treatment.

Medical Management

There is no known effective therapy for the dry (nonneovascular, nonexudative) type of AMD (Grossman & Porth, 2014).

An important component of treatment of wet (neovascular, exudative) AMD targets development and progression of angiogenesis (abnormal blood vessel formation). Vasoproliferation in wet AMD is believed to be caused by an underlying angiogenic stimulus known as vascular endothelial growth factor (VEGF) (Grossman & Porth, 2014). Examples of VEGF inhibitors given by intravitreal injection include ranibizumab (Lucentis) and bevacizumab (Avastin) (Comerford, 2015; Grossman & Porth, 2014).

Nursing Management

Nursing management is primarily educational. Most patients benefit from the use of bright lighting and magnification devices and from referral to a low-vision centre. Some low-vision centres send representatives to the patient's home or place of employment to evaluate the living and working conditions and make recommendations to improve lighting, thereby improving vision and promoting safety. The home care nurse can make the same assessment and recommendations.

Amsler grids are given to patients to use in their home to monitor for a sudden onset or distortion of vision. These may provide the earliest sign that macular degeneration is getting worse. Patients are encouraged to use these grids and to look at them, one eye at a time, several times each week with glasses on. If there is a change in the grid (e.g., if the lines or squares appear distorted or faded), the patient should notify the ophthalmologist immediately and should arrange to be seen promptly.

Ongoing Research

Angiogenesis

An important component of the effort against neovascular AMD is research into the development and progression of angiogenesis (abnormal blood vessel formation). Studies continue toward identification of agents that can be used to inhibit angiogenesis. This has implications for ocular neovascularization and the treatment of other disorders, such as solid tumours.

Vasoproliferation in exudative AMD is believed to be caused by an underlying angiogenic stimulus known as vascular endothelial growth factor (VEGF). Research is ongoing in phase III trials on two intravitreal agents designed to inhibit angiogenesis. Macugen (pegaptanib

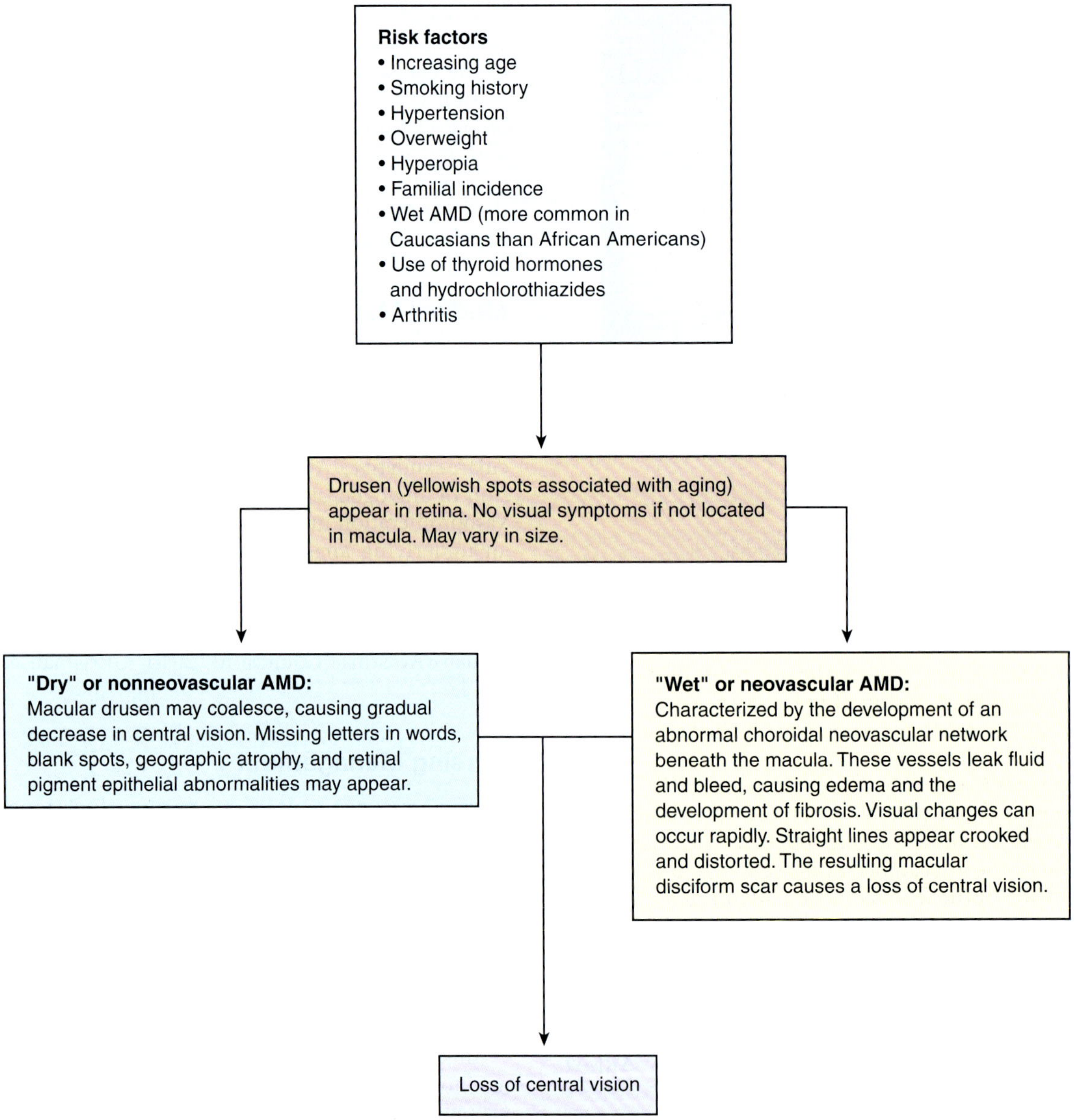

FIGURE 60-11. Progression of age-related macular degeneration (AMD): pathways to vision loss.

sodium) is designed to inhibit the ability of VEGF to bind to cellular receptors. Thus far Macugen has been shown to be safe and more effective than a placebo. Lucentis (ranibizumab) is designed to bind and inactivate all isoforms of VEGF. The results of animal studies and a small study of 64 patients have been promising. A larger phase III trial is under way.

Macular Translocation

Wet macular degeneration is characterized by the development of an abnormal CNV membrane to the detriment of central vision. One approach to this condition is the surgical procedure known as macular translocation, in which a 360-degree retinal detachment is surgically created and the retina is gently lifted and resettled, placing the macular area a slight distance away from the area of CNV. Laser treatment can then be applied to the abnormal neovascular network with minimal damage occurring to the macula. This surgical technique is being refined.

Orbital and Ocular Trauma

Whether affecting the eye or the orbit, trauma to the eye and surrounding structures may have devastating consequences for vision. It is preferable to prevent injury rather than treat it. Chart 60-11 details safety measures to prevent orbital and ocular trauma.

Orbital Trauma

Injury to the orbit is usually associated with a head injury; hence, the patient's general medical condition must first be stabilized before conducting an ocular examination (Hickey, 2014). Only then is the globe assessed for soft tissue injury. During inspection, the face is meticulously assessed for underlying fractures, which should always be suspected in cases of blunt trauma. To establish the extent of ocular injury, VA is assessed as soon as possible, even if it is only a rough estimate. Soft tissue orbital injuries often result in damage to the optic nerve. Major ocular injuries

CHART 60-11

Patient Education: Education for Patients About Preventing Eye Injuries

In and Around the House

- Make sure that all spray nozzles are directed away from you before you press down on the handle.
- Read instructions carefully before using cleaning fluids, detergents, ammonia, or harsh chemicals. Wash hands thoroughly after use.
- Use grease shields on frying pans to decrease spattering.
- Wear special goggles to shield your eyes from fumes and splashes when using powerful chemicals.
- Use opaque goggles to avoid burns from sunlamps.

In the Workshop

- Protect your eyes from flying fragments, fumes, dust particles, sparks, and splashed chemicals by wearing safety glasses.
- Read instructions thoroughly before using tools and chemicals, and follow precautions for their use.

Around Children

- Pay attention to age and maturity level of a child when selecting toys and games. Avoid projectile toys, such as darts and pellet guns.
- Supervise children when they are playing with toys or games that can be dangerous.
- Teach children the correct way to handle potentially dangerous items, such as scissors and pencils.

In the Garden/Yard

- Wear safety glasses when mowing grass or trimming hedges, shrubs, trees, etc.
- Do not let anyone stand at the side of or in front of a moving lawn mower.
- Pick up rocks and stones before going over them with the lawn mower. These stones can be hurled out of the rotary blades and rebound off curbs or walls, causing severe injury to the eye.
- Make sure that pesticide spray can nozzles are directed away from your face.
- Avoid low-hanging branches.

Around the Car

- Before opening the hood of the car, put out all smoking materials and matches. Use a flashlight, not a match or lighter, to look at the battery at night.
- Wear goggles when grinding metal or striking metal against metal while performing auto body repair.
- When using jumper cables to start the car, wear goggles; make sure the cars are not touching one another; make sure the jumper cable clamps never touch each other; never lean over the battery when attaching cables. Never attach a cable to the negative terminal of the dead battery.

In Sports

- Wear protective safety glasses, especially for sports such as racquetball, squash, tennis, baseball, and basketball.
- Wear protective caps, helmets, or face protectors when appropriate, especially for sports such as ice hockey.

Around Fireworks

- Wear eye glasses or safety goggles.
- Do not use explosive fireworks.
- Never allow children to ignite fireworks.
- Do not stand near others when lighting fireworks.
- Do not try to relight duds. Douse them in water.

indicated by a soft globe, prolapsing tissue, ruptured globe, hemorrhage, and loss of red reflex require immediate surgical attention.

Soft Tissue Injury and Hemorrhage

The signs and symptoms of soft tissue injury from blunt or penetrating trauma include tenderness, ecchymosis, lid swelling, **proptosis** (i.e., downward displacement of the eyeball), and hemorrhage. Closed injuries lead to contusions with subconjunctival hemorrhage, commonly known as a *black eye*. Blood accumulates in the tissues of the conjunctiva. Hemorrhage may be caused by a soft tissue injury to the eyelid or by an underlying fracture.

Management of soft tissue hemorrhage that does not threaten vision is usually conservative and consists of thorough inspection, cleansing, and repair of wounds. Cold compresses are used in the early phase, followed by warm compresses. Hematomas that appear as swollen, fluctuating areas may be surgically drained or aspirated; if they are causing significant orbital pressure, they may be surgically evacuated.

Penetrating injuries or severe blow to the head can result in severe optic nerve damage. Visual loss can be sudden or delayed and progressive. Immediate loss of vision after an ocular injury is usually irreversible. Delayed visual loss has a better prognosis. Corticosteroid therapy is indicated to reduce optic nerve swelling. Surgery, such as optic nerve decompression, may be performed.

Orbital Fractures

Orbital fractures are detected by facial x-rays. Depending on the orbital structures involved, orbital fractures can be classified as blow-out, zygomatic or tripod, maxillary, midfacial, orbital apex, and orbital roof fractures. Blow-out fractures result from compression of soft tissue and sudden increase in orbital pressure when the force is transmitted to the orbital floor, the area of least resistance.

The inferior rectus and inferior oblique muscles, with their fat and fascial attachments, or the nerve that courses along the inferior oblique muscle may become entrapped, and the globe may be displaced inward (i.e., enophthalmos). Computed tomography (CT) can clearly identify the muscle and its auxiliary structures that are entrapped. These fractures are usually caused by blunt small objects, such as a fist, knee, elbow, or tennis or golf ball (Hickey, 2014).

Orbital roof fractures are dangerous because of potential complications to the brain. Surgical management of these fractures requires a neurosurgeon and an ophthalmologist. The most common indications for surgical intervention are displacement of bone fragments disfiguring the usual facial contours, interference with binocular vision caused by extraocular muscle entrapment, interference with mastication in zygomatic fracture, and obstruction of the nasolacrimal duct. Surgery is usually nonemergent, and a period of 10 to 14 days gives the ophthalmologist time to assess ocular function, especially the extraocular muscles and the nasolacrimal duct. Emergency surgical repair is usually not performed unless the globe is displaced to the maxillary sinus. Surgical repair is primarily directed at freeing the entrapped ocular structures and restoring the integrity of the orbital floor.

Foreign Bodies

Foreign bodies that enter the orbit are usually tolerated, except for copper, iron, and vegetable materials such as those from plants or trees, which may cause purulent infection. X-rays and CT scans are used to identify the foreign body. Careful history taking is important, especially if the foreign body has been in the orbit for a period of time and the incident forgotten. It is important to identify metallic foreign bodies because they prohibit the use of magnetic resonance imaging (MRI) as a diagnostic tool.

After the extent of the orbital damage is assessed, the decision is made between conservative treatment and surgical removal. In general, orbital foreign bodies are usually removed if they are superficial and anterior in location, have sharp edges that may affect adjacent orbital structures, or are composed of copper, iron, or vegetable material. The surgical intervention is directed at prevention of further ocular injury and maintaining the integrity of the affected areas. Cultures are usually obtained, and the patient is placed on prophylactic IV antibiotics that are later changed to oral antibiotics.

Ocular Trauma

Ocular trauma is the leading cause of blindness among children and young adults, especially male trauma victims. The most common circumstances of ocular trauma are occupational injuries (e.g., construction industry), sports (e.g., baseball, basketball, hockey, racket sports, boxing), weapons (e.g., air guns, BB guns), assault, motor vehicle crashes (e.g., broken windshields), and war (e.g., blast fragments).

There are two types of ocular trauma in which the first response is critical: chemical burn and foreign object in the eye. With a chemical burn, the eye must be immediately irrigated with copious amounts of tap water or normal saline. With a foreign body, no attempt should be made to remove the foreign object. The object is protected from jarring or movement to prevent further ocular damage. No pressure or patch is applied to the affected eye. All traumatic eye injuries should be protected using a metal shield if available or a stiff paper cup until medical treatment can be obtained (Fig. 60-12).

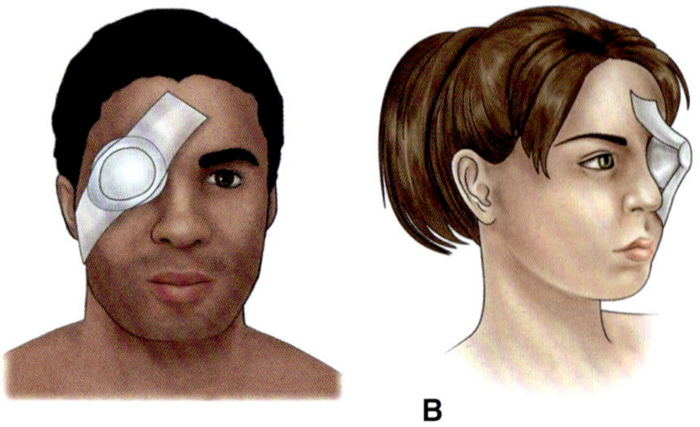

FIGURE 60-12. Two kinds of eye patches. **A.** Aluminum shield. **B.** Stiff paper cup shield (innovative substitute when aluminum shield is unavailable).

Assessment and Diagnostic Findings

A thorough history is obtained, particularly assessing the patient's ocular history, such as preinjury vision in the affected eye or past ocular surgery. Details related to the injury that help in the diagnosis and assessment of need for further tests include the nature of the ocular injury (i.e., blunt or penetrating trauma), the type of activity causing the injury to determine the nature of the force striking the eye, and whether onset of vision loss was sudden, slow, or progressive. For chemical eye burns, the chemical agent must be identified and tested for pH if a sample is available. The corneal surface is examined for foreign bodies, wounds, and abrasions, after which the other external structures of the eye are examined. Pupillary size, shape, and light reaction of the pupil of the affected eye are compared with the other eye. Ocular motility, which is the ability of the eyes to move synchronously up, down, right, and left, is also assessed.

Medical Management

Splash Injuries

Splash injuries are irrigated with normal saline solution before further evaluation. In cases of ruptured globe, cycloplegic agents (i.e., agents that paralyze the ciliary muscle) or topical antibiotics must be deferred because of potential toxicity to exposed intraocular tissues. Further manipulation of the eye must be avoided until the patient is under general anesthesia. Parenteral, broad-spectrum antibiotics are initiated. Tetanus antitoxin is administered, if indicated, as well as analgesic agents. (Tetanus prophylaxis is recommended for full-thickness ocular and skin wounds.) Any topical medication (e.g., anesthetic agents, dyes) must be sterile.

Foreign Bodies and Corneal Abrasions

After removal of a foreign body from the surface of the eye, an antibiotic ointment is applied, and the eye is patched. The eye is examined daily for evidence of infection until the wound is completely healed.

Contact lens wear is a common cause of corneal abrasion. The patient experiences severe pain and **photophobia** (i.e., ocular pain on exposure to light). Corneal epithelial defects are treated with antibiotic ointment and a pressure patch to immobilize the eyelids. It is of utmost importance that topical anesthetic eye drops are not given to a patient for repeated use after corneal injury because their effects mask further damage, delay healing, and can lead to permanent corneal scarring. Corticosteroids are avoided while the epithelial defect exists.

Penetrating Injuries and Contusions of the Eyeball

Sharp penetrating injury or blunt contusion force can rupture the eyeball. When the eyeball, cornea, and sclera rupture, rapid decompression or herniation of the orbital contents into adjacent sinuses can occur. In general, blunt traumatic injuries (with an increased incidence of retinal detachment, intraocular tissue avulsion, and herniation) have a worse prognosis than penetrating injuries. Most penetrating injuries result in marked loss of vision with the following signs: hemorrhagic **chemosis** (i.e., edema of the conjunctiva), conjunctival laceration, shallow anterior chamber with or without an eccentrically placed pupil, **hyphema** (i.e., hemorrhage within the chamber), or vitreous hemorrhage.

Hyphema is caused by contusion forces that tear the vessels of the iris and damage the anterior chamber angle. Preventing rebleeding and prolonged increased IOP are the goals of treatment for hyphema. In severe cases in which patient compliance is questionable, the patient is hospitalized with moderate activity restriction. An eye shield is applied. Topical corticosteroids are prescribed to reduce inflammation. An antifibrinolytic agent, aminocaproic acid (Amicar), stabilizes clot formation at the site of hemorrhage. Aspirin is contraindicated.

A ruptured globe and severe injuries with intraocular hemorrhage require surgical intervention. Vitrectomy is performed for traumatic retinal detachments (Boyd, 2016). Primary **enucleation** (i.e., complete removal of the eyeball and part of the optic nerve) is considered only if the globe is irreparable and has NLP. It is a general rule that enucleation is performed within 2 weeks of the initial injury (in an eye that has no useful vision after sustaining penetrating injury) to prevent the risk of **sympathetic ophthalmia**, an inflammation created in the uninjured eye by the affected eye that can result in blindness of the uninjured eye.

Intraocular Foreign Bodies

A patient who reports blurred vision and discomfort is questioned carefully about recent injuries and exposures. Patients may be injured in a number of different situations and suffer an intraocular foreign body (IOFB). Precipitating circumstances can include working in construction, striking metal against metal, being involved in motor vehicle crashes with facial injury, gunshot wounds, grinding-wheel work, and an explosion.

IOFB is diagnosed and localized by slit-lamp biomicroscopy and indirect ophthalmoscopy, as well as CT or ultrasonography. MRI is contraindicated because most foreign bodies are metallic and magnetic. It is important to determine the composition, size, and location of the IOFB and affected eye structures. Every effort should be made to identify the type of IOFB and whether it is magnetic. Iron, steel, copper, and vegetable matter cause intense inflammatory reactions. The incidence of endophthalmitis is also high. If the cornea is perforated, tetanus prophylaxis and IV antibiotics are administered. The extraction route (i.e., surgical incision) of the foreign body depends on its location and composition and associated ocular injuries. Specially designed IOFB forceps and magnets are used to grasp and remove the foreign body. Any damaged area of the retina is treated to prevent retinal detachment.

Ocular Burns

Alkali, acid, and other chemically active organic substances, such as mace and tear gas, cause chemical burns. Alkali burns (e.g., lye, ammonia) result in the most injury because they penetrate the ocular tissues rapidly and continue to cause damage long after the initial injury is sustained. They also cause an immediate rise in IOP. Acids (e.g., bleach, car batteries, refrigerant) generally cause less damage because the precipitated necrotic tissue proteins form a barrier to further penetration and damage. Chemical burns may appear as superficial punctate keratopathy (i.e., spotty damage to the cornea), subconjunctival hemorrhage, or complete marbleizing of the cornea.

In treating chemical burns, every minute counts. Immediate tap water irrigation should be started on site before transport of the patient to an emergency department. Only a brief history and examination are performed. The corneal surfaces and conjunctival fornices are immediately and copiously irrigated with normal saline or any neutral solution. A local anesthetic agent is instilled, and a lid speculum is applied to overcome blepharospasm (i.e., spasms of the eyelid muscles that result in closure of the lids). Particulate matter must be removed from the fornices using moistened, cotton-tip applicators and minimal pressure on the globe. Irrigation continues until the conjunctival pH normalizes (between 7.3 and 7.6). The pH of the corneal surface is checked by placing a pH paper strip in the fornix. Antibiotics are instilled, and the eye is patched.

The goal of intermediate treatment is to prevent tissue ulceration and promote reepithelialization. Intense lubrication using nonpreserved (i.e., without preservatives to avoid allergic reactions) tears is essential. Reepithelialization is promoted with patching or therapeutic soft lenses. The patient is usually monitored daily for several days. Prognosis depends on the type of injury and adequacy of the irrigation immediately after exposure. Long-term treatment consists of two phases: restoration of the ocular surface through grafting procedures and surgical restoration of corneal integrity and optical clarity.

Thermal injury is caused by exposure to a hot object (e.g., curling iron, tobacco, ash), whereas photochemical injury results from ultraviolet irradiation or infrared exposure (e.g., exposure to the reflections from snow, sun gazing, viewing an eclipse of the sun without an adequate filter). These injuries can cause corneal epithelial defect, corneal opacity, conjunctival chemosis and **injection** (i.e., congestion of blood vessels), and burns of the eyelids and periocular region. Antibiotics and a pressure patch for 24 hours constitute the treatment of mild injuries. Scarring of the eyelids may require oculoplastic surgery, whereas corneal scarring may require corneal surgery.

INFECTIOUS AND INFLAMMATORY CONDITIONS

Inflammation and infection of eye structures are common. Eye infection is a leading cause of blindness worldwide. Table 60-7 describes selected common infections and their treatment.

TABLE 60-7 Common Infections and Inflammatory Disorders of Eye Structures

Disorder	Description	Management
Hordeolum (stye) **Chalazion**	Acute suppurative infection of the glands of the eyelids caused by *Staphylococcus aureus*. The lid is red and edematous with a small collection of pus in the form of an abscess. There is considerable discomfort.	Warm compresses are applied directly to the affected lid area three to four times a day for 10 to 15 minutes. If the condition is not improved after 48 hours, incision and drainage may be indicated. Application of topical antibiotics may be prescribed thereafter.
Blepharitis	Sterile inflammatory process involving chronic granulomatous inflammation of the meibomian glands; can appear as a single granuloma or multiple granulomas in the upper or lower eyelids.	Warm compresses applied three to four times a day for 10 to 15 minutes may resolve the inflammation in the early stages. Most often, however, surgical excision is indicated. Corticosteroid injection to the chalazion lesion may be used for smaller lesions.
Bacterial keratitis	Chronic bilateral inflammation of the eyelid margins. There are two types: staphylococcal and seborrheic. Staphylococcal blepharitis is usually ulcerative and is more serious due to the involvement of the base of hair follicles. Permanent scarring can result.	The seborrheic type is chronic and is usually resistant to treatment, but the milder cases may respond to lid hygiene. Staphylococcal blepharitis requires topical antibiotic treatment. Instructions on lid hygiene (to keep the lid margins clean and free of exudates) are given to the patient.
Herpes simplex keratitis	Infection of the cornea by *Staphylococcus aureus, Streptococcus pneumoniae,* and *Pseudomonas aeruginosa.*	Fortified (high-concentration) antibiotic eye drops are administered every 30 minutes around the clock for the first few days, then every 1–2 hours. Systemic antibiotics may be administered. Cycloplegics are administered to reduce pain caused by ciliary spasm. Corticosteroid therapy and subconjunctival injections of antibiotics are controversial.
	Leading cause of corneal blindness. Symptoms are severe pain, tearing, and photophobia. The dendritic ulcer has a branching, linear pattern with feathery edges and terminal bulbs at its ends. Herpes simplex keratitis can lead to recurrent stromal keratitis and persist to 12 months with residual corneal scarring.	Many lesions heal without treatment and residual effects. The treatment goal is to minimize the damaging effect of the inflammatory response and eliminate viral replication within the cornea. Penetrating keratoplasty is indicated for corneal scarring and must be performed when the herpetic disease has been inactive for many months.

Dry Eye Syndrome

Dry eyes can be caused by decreased tear production or increased tear evaporation, which can be episodic or chronic (Grossman & Porth, 2014). Decreased tear production (aqueous deficiency) can be caused by systemic disease (Sjögren's, connective tissue disease), lacrimal gland obstruction, and systemic drugs (e.g., diuretics, antihistamines, psychotropic drugs). Increased tear evaporation (evaporative dry eye) can be caused by meibomian gland deficiency, lid aperture disorder, vitamin A deficiency, reduced lid blinking rate, preservatives from topical drugs, ocular surface disease (allergy), and contact lens wear. Risk factors include increasing age, smoking, recent refractive surgery, and postmenopausal status (in women). An increase in the intake of omega-3 fatty acids may be beneficial in reducing the risk (Grossman & Porth, 2014).

Clinical Manifestations

The most common concern in dry eye syndrome is a scratchy or foreign body sensation. Other symptoms include itching, excessive mucous secretion, inability to produce tears, a burning sensation, redness, pain, and difficulty moving the lids.

Assessment and Diagnostic Findings

Slit-lamp examination shows an absent or interrupted tear meniscus at the lower lid margin, and the conjunctiva is thickened, edematous, and hyperemic and has lost its lustre. A tear meniscus is the crescent-shaped edge of the tear film in the lower lid margin. Chronic dry eyes may result in chronic conjunctival and corneal irritation that can lead to corneal erosion, scarring, ulceration, thinning, or perforation that can seriously threaten vision. Secondary bacterial infection can occur.

Management

Management of dry eye syndrome requires the complete cooperation of the patient with a regimen that needs to be followed at home for a long period, or complete relief of symptoms is unlikely. Instillation of artificial tears during the day and an ointment at night has been the usual regimen to hydrate and lubricate the eye through stimulating tears and preserving a moist ocular surface. Anti-inflammatory medications have also been used, along with moisture chambers (e.g., moisture chamber spectacles, swim goggles) to provide additional relief. Restasis (cyclosporine ophthalmic emulsion, 0.05% w/v with no preservative) is now available in Canada. These eye drops are used every 12 hours. These drops are different from other treatments in that they promote actual healing of the ocular surface, with improvement continuing for a number of months.

Patients may become hypersensitive to chemical preservatives such as benzalkonium chloride and thimerosal. For these patients, preservative-free ophthalmic solutions are used. Management of the dry eye syndrome also includes the concurrent treatment of infections, such as chronic blepharitis and acne rosacea, and treating the underlying systemic disease, such as Sjögren's syndrome (an autoimmune disease).

In advanced cases of dry eye syndrome, surgical treatment that includes punctal occlusion, grafting procedures, and lateral tarsorrhaphy (i.e., uniting the edges of the lids) are options. Punctal plugs are made of silicone material for the temporary or permanent occlusion of the puncta. This helps preserve the natural tears and prolongs the effects of artificial tears. Short-term occlusion is performed by inserting punctal or silicone rods in all four puncta. If tearing is induced, the upper plugs are removed, and the remaining lower plugs are removed in another week. Permanent occlusion is performed only in severe cases among adults who do not develop tearing after partial occlusion and who have results on a repeated Schirmer's test of 2 mm or less (filter paper is used to measure tear production).

Conjunctivitis

Conjunctivitis (i.e., inflammation of the conjunctiva) is the most common ocular disease worldwide. It is characterized by a pink appearance (hence the common term *pink eye*) because of subconjunctival blood vessel hemorrhages.

Clinical Manifestations

General symptoms include foreign body sensation, scratching or burning sensation, itching, and photophobia. Conjunctivitis may be uni- or bilateral, but the infection usually starts in one eye and then spreads to the other eye by hand contact.

Assessment and Diagnostic Findings

The four main clinical features important to evaluate are the type of discharge (i.e., watery, mucoid, purulent, or mucopurulent), type of conjunctival reaction (i.e., follicular or papillary), presence of pseudomembranes or true membranes, and presence or absence of lymphadenopathy (i.e., enlargement of the preauricular and submandibular lymph nodes where the eyelids drain). Pseudomembranes consist of coagulated exudate that adheres to the surface of the inflamed conjunctiva. True membranes form when the exudate adheres to the superficial layer of the conjunctiva, and removal results in bleeding. Follicles are multiple, slightly elevated lesions encircled by tiny blood vessels; they look like grains of rice. Papillae are hyperplastic conjunctival epithelium in numerous projections that are usually seen as a fine mosaic pattern under slit-lamp examination. Diagnosis is based on the distinctive characteristics of ocular signs, acute or chronic presentation, and identification of any precipitating events. Positive results of swab smear preparations and cultures confirm the diagnosis.

Types of Conjunctivitis

Conjunctivitis is classified according to its cause. The major causes are microbial infection, allergy, and irritating toxic stimuli. A wide spectrum of exogenous microbes can cause conjunctivitis, including bacteria (e.g., *Chlamydia*), viruses, fungus, and parasites. Conjunctivitis can also result from infection of an existing ocular infection or can be a manifestation of a systemic disease.

Microbial Conjunctivitis

Bacterial Conjunctivitis

Bacterial conjunctivitis can be acute or chronic. The acute type can develop into a chronic condition. Signs and symptoms can vary from mild to severe. Chronic bacterial conjunctivitis is usually seen in patients with lacrimal duct obstruction, chronic dacryocystitis, and chronic blepharitis. The most common causative microorganisms are *Streptococcus pneumoniae, Haemophilus influenzae*, and *Staphylococcus aureus*.

Bacterial conjunctivitis manifests with an acute onset of redness, burning, and discharge. There is papillary formation, conjunctival irritation, and injection in the fornices. The exudates are variable but are usually present on waking in the morning. The eyes may be difficult to open because of adhesions caused by the exudate. Purulent discharge occurs in severe acute bacterial infections, whereas mucopurulent discharge appears in mild cases. In gonococcal conjunctivitis, the symptoms are more acute. The exudate is profuse and purulent, and there is lymphadenopathy. Pseudomembranes may be present.

Chlamydial conjunctivitis includes **trachoma** (a bilateral chronic follicular conjunctivitis of childhood that leads to blindness during adulthood if left untreated) and inclusion conjunctivitis. Trachoma is an ancient disease and is the leading cause of preventable blindness in the world. It is prevalent in areas with hot, dry, and dusty climates and in areas with poor living conditions. It is spread by direct contact with fomites, and the vectors can be insects such as flies and gnats. The onset of trachoma in children is usually insidious, but it can be acute or subacute in adults. The initial symptoms include red inflamed eyes, tearing, photophobia, ocular pain, purulent exudates, preauricular lymphadenopathy, and lid edema. Initial ocular signs include follicular and papillary formations. At the middle stage of the disease, there is an acute inflammation with papillary hypertrophy and follicular necrosis, after which **trichiasis** (turning inward of hair follicles) and **entropion** begin to develop. The lashes that are turned in rub against the cornea and, after prolonged irritation, cause corneal erosion and ulceration. The late stage of the disease is characterized by scarred conjunctiva, subepithelial keratitis, abnormal vascularization of the cornea (pannus), and residual scars from the follicles that look like depressions in the conjunctiva (Herbert's pits). Severe corneal ulceration can lead to perforation and blindness.

Inclusion conjunctivitis affects sexually active young people who have genital chlamydial infection. Transmission is by oral–genital sex or hand-to-eye transmission. It has been reported that indirect transmission has been acquired from inadequately chlorinated swimming pools. The eye lesions usually appear a week after exposure and may be associated with a nonspecific urethritis or cervicitis. The discharge is mucopurulent, follicles are present, and there is lymphadenopathy.

Viral Conjunctivitis

Viral conjunctivitis (Fig. 60-13) can also be acute and chronic. The discharge is watery, and follicles are prominent.

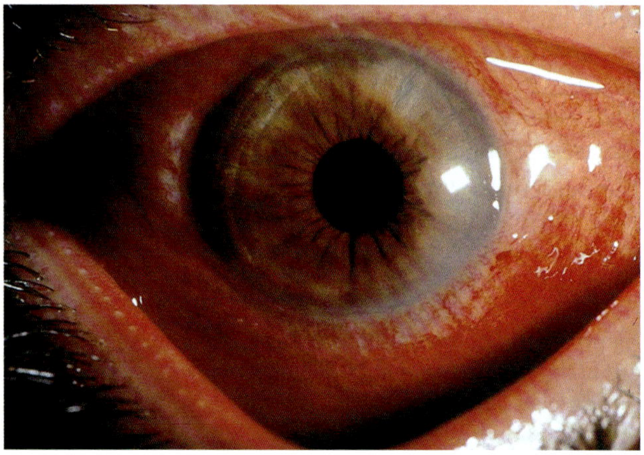

FIGURE 60-13. Conjunctival hyperemia in viral conjunctivitis.

Severe cases include pseudomembranes. The common causative organisms are adenovirus and herpes simplex virus. Conjunctivitis caused by adenovirus is highly contagious. The symptoms include extreme tearing, redness, and foreign body sensation that can involve one or both eyes. The condition is usually preceded by symptoms of upper respiratory infection. Corneal involvement causes extreme photophobia. There is lid edema, ptosis, conjunctival **hyperemia** (i.e., dilation of the conjunctival blood vessels), watery discharge, follicles, and papillae. These signs and symptoms vary from mild to severe and may last for 2 weeks. Viral conjunctivitis, although self-limited, tends to last longer than bacterial conjunctivitis.

Epidemic keratoconjunctivitis (EKC) is most often accompanied by preauricular lymphadenopathy and occasionally periorbital pain. There are marked follicular and papillary formations. EKC can lead to keratopathy. EKC is a highly contagious viral conjunctivitis that is easily transmitted from one person to another among household members, school children, and health care workers. The outbreak of epidemics is seasonal, especially during the summer when people frequent swimming pools.

Allergic Conjunctivitis

Immunologic or allergic conjunctivitis is a hypersensitivity reaction as a part of allergic rhinitis (hay fever), or it can be an independent allergic reaction. The patient usually has a history of an allergy to pollens and other environmental allergens. There is extreme itching, epiphora (i.e., excessive secretion of tears), injection, and usually severe photophobia. The stringlike mucoid discharge is usually associated with rubbing the eyes because of severe itching. Vernal conjunctivitis is also known as seasonal conjunctivitis because it appears mostly during warm weather. There may be large formations of papillae that have a cobblestone appearance. It is more common in children and young adults. Most affected individuals have a history of asthma or eczema.

Toxic Conjunctivitis

Chemical conjunctivitis can be the result of medications, chlorine from swimming pools (more common during the summer), exposure to toxic fumes among industrial workers, or exposure to other irritants such as smoke, hair sprays, acids, and alkalis.

Management

The management of conjunctivitis depends on the type. Most types of mild and viral conjunctivitis are self-limiting, benign conditions that may not require treatment and laboratory procedures. For more severe cases, topical antibiotics, eye drops, or ointment is prescribed. Patients with gonococcal conjunctivitis require urgent antibiotic therapy. If left untreated, this ocular disease can lead to corneal perforation and blindness. The systemic complications can include meningitis and generalized septicemia.

Bacterial Conjunctivitis

Acute bacterial conjunctivitis is almost always self-limiting, lasting 2 weeks if left untreated. If treated with antibiotics, it may last a few days, except for gonococcal and staphylococcal conjunctivitis.

For trachoma, usually broad-spectrum antibiotics are administered topically and systemically. Surgical management includes the correction of trichiasis (eyelashes growing inward toward the conjunctiva and cornea) to prevent conjunctival scarring.

Adult inclusion conjunctivitis requires 1 week of antibiotics. Prevention of reinfection is important, and affected individuals and their sexual partners must seek treatment for sexually transmitted disease, if indicated.

Viral Conjunctivitis

Viral conjunctivitis is not responsive to any treatment. Cold compresses may alleviate some symptoms. It is extremely important to remember that viral conjunctivitis, especially EKC, is highly transmissible. Patients must be made aware of the contagious nature of the disease, and adequate instructions must be given. These instructions should include an emphasis on handwashing and avoiding sharing hand towels, face cloths, and eye drops. Tissues should be directly discarded into the garbage.

Proper steps must be taken to avoid nosocomial infections. Frequent hand hygiene, procedures for environmental cleaning, and disinfection of equipment used for eye examination must be strictly followed at all times (Chart 60-12). During outbreaks of conjunctivitis caused by adenovirus, it is necessary that health care facilities assign specified areas for treating patients with or suspected of having conjunctivitis caused by adenovirus to prevent spread. All forms of tonometry must be avoided unless medically indicated. All multidose medications must be discarded at the end of each day or when contaminated. Infected employees and others must not be allowed to work or attend school until symptoms have resolved, which can take 3 to 7 days.

Allergic Conjunctivitis

Patients with allergic conjunctivitis, especially recurrent vernal or seasonal conjunctivitis, are usually given corticosteroids in ophthalmic preparations. Depending on the severity of the disease, they may be given oral preparations. Use of vasoconstrictors, such as topical epinephrine solution; cold compresses; ice packs; and cool ventilation usually provide comfort by decreasing swelling.

Toxic Conjunctivitis

For conjunctivitis caused by chemical irritants, the eye must be irrigated immediately and profusely with saline or sterile water.

CHART 60-12

Patient Education: Education for Patients With Viral Conjunctivitis

Viral conjunctivitis is a highly contagious eye infection that can easily spread from one person to another. The symptoms can be alarming but are not serious.

The nurse instructs the patient about this eye condition and the following self-care strategies:

- Be aware that your eyes will look red and will have watery discharge, and your lids will be swollen for about a week.
- Expect to experience eye pain, a sandy sensation in your eye, and sensitivity to light.
- Keep in mind that symptoms will resolve after about 1 week.
- Use lightweight cold compresses over your eyes for about 10 minutes four to five times a day to soothe the pain.
- Use artificial tears for the sandy sensation in your eye and mild pain medications such as acetaminophen (Tylenol).
- Stay at home and not go outside. You may return to work or school after 7 days, when the redness and discharge have cleared. Obtain a note from your primary provider to return to work or school.
- Do not share towels, linens, makeup, or any items that have come in contact with your eyes.
- Wash your hands thoroughly with soap and water frequently, including before and after you apply artificial tears or cold compresses.
- Use a new tissue every time you wipe the discharge from your eye. Dampen the tissue with clean water to clean the outside of the eye.
- Wash your face and take a shower as you normally do.
- Discard all of your makeup articles and do not apply makeup until the infection has resolved.
- Wear dark glasses if bright lights bother you.
- Note if the discharge from your eye turns yellowish and purulent or if your vision changes and return to the primary provider for an examination.

Uveitis

Inflammation of the uveal tract is called uveitis and can affect the iris, the ciliary body, or the choroid. There are two types of uveitis: nongranulomatous and granulomatous.

The most common type of uveitis is the nongranulomatous type, which manifests as an acute condition with pain, photophobia, and a pattern of conjunctival injection, especially around the cornea. The pupil is small or irregular, and vision is blurred. There may be small, fine precipitates on the posterior corneal surface and cells in the aqueous humour (i.e., cell and flare). If severe, a **hypopyon** (i.e., accumulation of pus in the anterior chamber) may occur. The condition may be uni- or bilateral and may be recurrent. Repeated attacks of nongranulomatous anterior uveitis can cause anterior synechia (i.e., peripheral iris adheres to the cornea and impedes outflow of aqueous humour). The development of posterior synechia (i.e., adherence of the iris and lens) blocks aqueous outflow from the posterior chamber. Secondary glaucoma can result from either anterior or posterior synechia. Cataracts may also occur as a sequela to uveitis.

Granulomatous uveitis can have a more insidious onset and can involve any portion of the uveal tract. It tends to be chronic. Symptoms such as photophobia and pain may be minimal. The keratic precipitate may be large and greyish. Vision is markedly and adversely affected. Conjunctival injection is diffuse, and there may be vitreous clouding. In a severe posterior uveitis, such as chorioretinitis, there may be retinal and choroidal hemorrhages.

In Manitoba, Roy (2014) completed a retrospective chart review of uveitis in 43 First Nations (FN) patients and a control group of 45 non-FN patients in Manitoba. Significant differences were found in the age of onset (FN 30.4 years vs. non-FN 40.2 years); bilateral uveitis (FN 86% vs. non-FN 51%); granulomatous uveitis (FN 53% vs. non-FN 11%); panuveitis (FN 67% vs. non-FN 16%); and anterior uveitis (FN 26% vs. non-FN 73%). The result was that FN patients needed more aggressive therapies but had an increased complication rate, and ended up with poorer vision. There is a need across Canada to "improve uveitis management and visual outcomes in this rapidly growing Canadian population" (Hooper, 2014, p. 119).

Medical Management

Because photophobia is a common symptom, patients should wear dark glasses outdoors. Ciliary spasm and synechia are best avoided through mydriasis; cyclopentolate (Cyclogyl) and atropine are commonly used. Local corticosteroid drops, such as Pred Forte 1% and Flarex 0.1%, instilled four to six times a day are also used to decrease inflammation. In very severe cases, systemic corticosteroids, as well as intravitreal corticosteroids, may be used.

If the uveitis is recurrent, a medical workup is initiated to discover any underlying cause. This evaluation should include a physical examination, complete systems review, and diagnostic tests, including a complete blood cell count, erythrocyte sedimentation rate, antinuclear antibodies (ANAs), Venereal Disease Research Laboratories (VDRL), and Lyme disease titre. Underlying causes include toxoplasmosis, herpes zoster virus, ocular candidiasis, histoplasmosis, herpes simplex virus, tuberculosis, and syphilis.

Orbital Cellulitis

Orbital cellulitis is inflammation of the tissues surrounding the eye and may result from bacterial, fungal, or viral inflammatory conditions of contiguous structures, such as the face, oropharynx, dental structures, or intracranial structures. It can also result from foreign bodies and from a pre-existing ocular infection, such as dacryocystitis and panophthalmitis, or from generalized septicemia. Infection of the sinuses is the most frequent cause. Infection originating in the sinuses can spread easily to the orbit through the thin bony walls and foramina or by means of the interconnecting venous system of the orbit and sinuses. The most common causative organisms are staphylococci and streptococci in adults and *H. influenzae* in children. The symptoms include pain, lid swelling, conjunctival edema, proptosis, and decreased ocular motility. With such edema, optic nerve compression can occur and IOP may increase.

The severe intraorbital tension caused by abscess formation and the impairment of optic nerve function in orbital cellulitis can result in permanent visual loss. Because of the orbit's proximity to the brain, orbital cellulitis can lead to life-threatening complications, such as intracranial abscess and cavernous sinus thrombosis.

Medical Management

Immediate administration of high-dose, broad-spectrum, systemic antibiotics is indicated. Cultures and Gram-stained smears are obtained. Monitoring changes in VA, degree of proptosis, central nervous system function (e.g., nausea, vomiting, fever, level of consciousness), displacement of the globe, extraocular movements, pupillary signs, and the fundus is extremely important. Consultation with an otolaryngologist is necessary, especially when sinusitis is suspected. In the event of abscess formation or progressive loss of vision, surgical drainage of the abscess or sinus is performed. Sinusotomy and antibiotic irrigation are also performed.

ORBITAL AND OCULAR TUMOURS

Benign Tumours of the Orbit

Benign tumours can develop from infancy and grow rapidly or slowly and present themselves in later life. Some benign tumours are superficial and are easily identifiable by external presentation, palpation, and x-rays, but some are deep and may require a CT scan for a more thorough and precise diagnosis. There can be a significant proptosis, and visual function may be jeopardized. Benign tumours are masses characterized by the lack of infiltration in the surrounding tissues. Examples are cystic dermoid cysts and mucocele, hemangiomas, lymphangiomas, lacrimal tumours, and neurofibromas.

To prevent recurrence, benign masses are excised completely when possible. Sometimes, excision is difficult because of the involvement of some portions of the orbital bones, such as deep dermoid cysts, in which dissection of the bone is required. Subtotal resection may be indicated in deep benign tumours that intertwine with other orbital structures, such as optic nerve meningiomas. Complete removal of the tumour may endanger visual function.

Benign Tumours of the Eyelid

Benign tumours include a wide variety of neoplasms and increase in frequency with age. Nevi may be unpigmented at birth and may enlarge and darken in adolescence or may never acquire any pigment at all. Hemangiomas are vascular capillary tumours that may be bright, superficial, strawberry-red lesions (i.e., strawberry nevus) or bluish and purplish deeper lesions. Milia are small, white, slightly elevated cysts of the eyelid that, when in multiples, create a blemish. Xanthelasma are yellowish, lipoid deposits on both lids near the inner angle of the eye that commonly appear as a result of the aging of the skin or a lipid disorder. Molluscum contagiosum lesions are flat, symmetric growths along the lid margin caused by a virus that can result in conjunctivitis and keratitis after debris gets into the conjunctival sac.

Treatment of benign congenital lid lesions is rarely indicated, except when visual function is affected. Corticosteroid injection to the hemangioma lesion is usually effective, but surgical excision may be performed. Benign lid lesions usually present aesthetic concerns rather than visual function problems. Surgical excision, or electrocautery, is primarily performed for cosmetic reasons, except for cases of molluscum contagiosum, for which surgical intervention is performed to prevent an infectious process that may ensue.

Benign Tumours of the Conjunctiva

Conjunctival nevus, a congenital, benign neoplasm, is a flat, slightly elevated, brown spot that becomes pigmented during late childhood or adolescence. This should be differentiated from the pigmented lesion melanosis acquired at middle age, which tends to wax and wane and become malignant melanoma. Keratin- and sebum-containing dermoid cysts are congenital and can be found in the conjunctiva. Dermolipoma is a congenital tumour that manifests as a smooth, rounded growth in the conjunctiva near the lateral canthus. Papillomas are usually soft with irregular surfaces and appear on the lid margins. Treatment consists of surgical excision.

Malignant Tumours of the Orbit

Rhabdomyosarcoma is the most common malignant primary orbital tumour in childhood, but it can also develop in older persons. The symptoms of rhabdomyosarcoma include sudden painless proptosis of one eye followed by lid swelling, conjunctival chemosis, and impairment of ocular motility. Imaging of these tumours establishes the size, configuration, location, and stage of the disease; delineates the degree of bone destruction; and is useful in estimating the field for radiation therapy, if needed. The most common site of metastasis is the lung.

Management of these primary malignant orbital tumours involves three major therapeutic modalities: surgery, radiation therapy, and adjuvant chemotherapy. The degree of orbital destruction is important in planning the surgical approach. In the orbit, resection often involves removal of the globe. The psychological needs of the patient and family, especially the parents of a pediatric patient, are paramount in planning the management approach.

Malignant Tumours of the Eyelid

Basal cell carcinoma is the most common malignant tumour of the eyelid. Squamous cell carcinoma occurs less frequently but is considered the second most common malignant tumour. Malignant melanoma is rare. Malignant eyelid tumours occur more frequently among people with fair complexion who have a history of chronic exposure to the sun.

Basal cell carcinoma appears as a painless nodule that may ulcerate. The lesion is invasive, spreads to the surrounding tissues, and grows slowly but does not metastasize. It usually appears on the lower lid margin near the inner canthus with a pearly white margin. Squamous cell carcinoma of the eyelids may resemble basal cell carcinoma initially because it also grows slowly and painlessly. It tends to ulcerate and invade the surrounding tissues, but it can metastasize to the regional lymph nodes. Malignant melanoma may not be pigmented and can arise from nevi. It spreads to the surrounding tissues and metastasizes to other organs.

Complete excision of these carcinomas is followed by reconstruction with skin grafting if the surgical excision is extensive. The ocular postoperative site and the graft donor site are monitored for bleeding. Donor graft sites may include the buccal mucosa, the thigh, or the abdomen. The patient is referred to an oncologist for evaluation for the need for radiation therapy treatment and monitoring for metastasis. Early diagnosis and surgical management are the basis of a good prognosis. These conditions have life-threatening consequences, and surgical excisions may result in facial disfigurement. Emotional support and reassurance are important aspects of nursing management.

Malignant Tumours of the Conjunctiva

Conjunctival carcinoma most often grows in the exposed areas of the conjunctiva. The typical lesions are usually gelatinous and whitish due to keratin formation. They grow gradually, and deep invasion and metastasis are rare. Malignant melanoma is rare but may arise from a preexisting nevus or acquired melanosis during middle age. Squamous cell carcinoma is also rare but invasive.

The management is surgical incision. Some benign tumours and most malignant tumours recur. To avoid recurrences, patients usually undergo radiation therapy and cryotherapy after the excision of malignant tumours. Cosmetic disfigurement may result from extensive excision when deep invasion by the malignant tumour is involved.

Malignant Tumour of the Globe: Ocular Melanoma

Ocular melanoma is a rare malignant choroidal tumour sometimes discovered on a retinal examination. In its early stages, it could be mistaken for a nevus. In addition to a complete physical examination to discover any evidence of metastasis (to the liver, lung, and breast), retinal fundus photography, fluorescein angiography, and ultrasonography are performed. The diagnosis is confirmed at biopsy after enucleation.

Tumours are classified according to boundary lines (apical height and basal diameter) as small, medium, or large. Small tumours are generally monitored, whereas medium and large tumours require treatment. Treatment consists of radiation, enucleation, or both. Radiation therapy may be achieved by external beam performed in repeated episodes over several days or through the implantation of a small plaque that contains radioactive iodine (I-125) pellets over the tumour.

SURGICAL PROCEDURES AND ENUCLEATION

Orbital Surgeries

Orbital surgeries may be performed to repair fractures, remove a foreign body, or remove benign or malignant growths. Surgical procedures involving the orbit and lids affect facial appearance (i.e., cosmesis). The goals are to recover and preserve visual function and to maintain the anatomic relationship of the ocular structures to achieve cosmesis. During the repair of orbital fractures, the orbital bones are realigned to follow the anatomic positions of facial structures.

Orbital surgical procedures involve working around delicate structures of the eye, such as the optic nerve, retinal blood vessels, and ocular muscles. Complications of orbital surgical procedures may include blindness as a result of damage to the optic nerve and its blood supply. Sudden pain and loss of vision may indicate intraorbital hemorrhage or compression of the optic nerve. Ptosis and diplopia may result from trauma to the extraocular muscles during the surgical procedure, but these conditions typically resolve after a few weeks.

Prophylaxis with IV antibiotics is the usual postoperative regimen after orbital surgery, especially with repair of orbital fractures and intraorbital foreign body removal. IV corticosteroids are used if there is a concern about optic nerve swelling. Topical ocular antibiotics are typically instilled, and antibiotic ointments are applied externally to the skin suture sites.

For the first 24 to 48 hours postoperatively, ice compresses are applied over the periocular area to decrease periorbital swelling, facial swelling, and hematoma. The head of the patient's bed is elevated to a comfortable position (30 to 45 degrees).

Discharge teaching includes medication instructions for oral antibiotics, instillation of ophthalmic medications, and application of ocular compresses.

Enucleation

Enucleation is the removal of the entire eye and part of the optic nerve. It may be performed for the following conditions:

- Severe injury resulting in prolapse of uveal tissue or loss of light projection or perception
- An irritated, blind, painful, deformed, or disfigured eye, usually caused by glaucoma, retinal detachment, or chronic inflammation
- An eye without useful vision that is producing or has produced sympathetic ophthalmia in the other eye
- Intraocular tumours that are untreatable by other means

The procedure for enucleation involves the separation and cutting of each of the ocular muscles, dissection of the Tenon's capsule (i.e., fibrous membrane covering the sclera), and the cutting of the optic nerve from the eyeball. The insertion of an orbital implant typically follows, and the conjunctiva is closed. A large pressure dressing is applied over the area.

Evisceration involves the surgical removal of the intraocular contents through an incision or opening in the cornea or sclera. The optic nerve, sclera, extraocular muscles, and sometimes the cornea are left intact. The main advantage of evisceration over enucleation is that the final cosmetic result and motility after fitting the ocular prosthesis are enhanced. This procedure would be more acceptable to a patient whose concept of the alteration of body image is severely threatened. The main disadvantage is the high risk of sympathetic ophthalmia.

Exenteration is the removal of the eyelids, the eye, and various amounts of orbital contents. It is indicated in malignancies in the orbit that are life threatening or when more conservative modalities of treatment have failed or are inappropriate. An example is squamous cell carcinoma of the paranasal sinuses, skin, and conjunctiva with deep orbital involvement. In its most extensive form, exenteration may include the removal of all orbital tissues and resection of the orbital bones.

Ocular Prostheses

Orbital implants and conformers (i.e., ocular prostheses usually made of silicone rubber) maintain the shape of the eye after enucleation or evisceration to prevent a contracted sunken appearance. The temporary conformer is placed over the conjunctival closure after the implantation of an orbital implant. A conformer is placed after the enucleation or evisceration procedure to protect the suture line, maintain the fornices, prevent contracture of the socket in preparation for the ocular prosthesis, and promote the integrity of the eyelids.

All ocular prosthetics have limitations in their motility. There are two designs of eye prostheses. The anophthalmic ocular prostheses are used in the absence of the globe. Scleral shells look just like the anophthalmic prosthesis (Fig. 60-14) but are thinner and fit over a globe with intact corneal sensation. An eye prosthesis usually lasts about 6 years, depending on the quality of fit, comfort, and cosmetic appearance. When the anophthalmic socket is completely healed, conformers are replaced with prosthetic eyes.

An ocularist is a specially trained and skilled professional who makes prosthetic eyes. After the ophthalmologist is satisfied that the anophthalmic socket is completely healed and is ready for prosthetic fitting, the patient is referred to an ocularist. The healing period is usually 6 to 8 weeks. It is advisable for the patient to have a consultation with the ocularist before the fitting. Obtaining accurate information and verbalizing concerns can lessen anxiety about wearing an ocular prosthesis.

Medical Management

Removal of an eye has physical, social, and psychological ramifications for any person. The significance of loss of the eye and vision must be addressed in the plan of care. The patient's preparation includes information about the surgical procedure and placement of orbital implants and conformers and the availability of ocular prosthetics to enhance cosmetic appearance. In some cases, patients may choose to see an ocularist before the surgery to discuss ocular prosthetics.

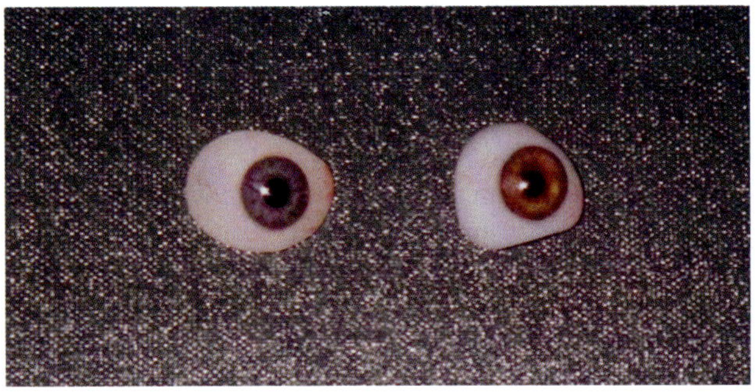

FIGURE 60-14. Eye prostheses. (**Left**) Anophthalmic ocular prosthesis. (**Right**) Scleral shell.

Nursing Management

Providing Education About Postsurgical and Prosthetic Care

Patients who undergo eye removal need to know that they will usually have a large ocular pressure dressing, which is typically removed after a week. Then an ophthalmic topical antibiotic ointment is applied in the socket three times daily.

After the removal of an eye, there is a loss of depth perception. Patients are advised to take extra caution in their ambulation and movement to avoid miscalculations that may result in injury. It may take some time to adjust to monocular vision.

The patient is advised that conformers may accidentally fall out of the socket. If this happens, the conformer is washed, wiped dry, and placed back in the socket. When surgical eye removal is unexpected, such as in severe ocular trauma, leaving no time for the patient and family to prepare for the loss, the nurse's role in providing reassurance and emotional support is crucial.

Promoting Home, Community-Based, and Transitional Care

Educating Patients About Self-Care

Patients are taught how to insert, remove, and care for the prosthetic eye. Thorough handwashing must be observed before inserting and removing an ocular prosthesis. A suction cup may be used if there are issues with manual dexterity. Precautions, such as draping a towel over the sink and closing the sink drain, are taken to avoid loss of the prosthesis. When instructing patients or family members, a return demonstration is important to assess the level of understanding and ability to perform the procedure.

Before insertion, the inner punctal or outer lateral aspects and the superior and inferior aspects of the prosthesis are identified by locating the identifying marks, such as a reddish colour in the inner punctal area. For people with low vision, other forms of identifying markers, such as dots or notches, are used. The upper lid is raised high enough to create a space; then the patient learns to slide the prosthesis up, underneath, and behind the upper eyelid. Meanwhile, the patient pulls the lower eyelid down to help put the prosthesis in place and to have its inferior edge fall back gradually to the lower eyelid. The lower eyelid is checked for correct positioning.

To remove the prosthesis, the patient cups one hand on the cheek to catch the prosthesis, places the forefinger of the free hand against the midportion of the lower eyelid, and gazes upward. Gazing upward brings the inferior edge of the prosthesis nearer the inferior eyelid margin. With the finger pushing inward, downward, and laterally against the lower eyelid, the prosthesis slides out, and the cupped hand acts as the receptacle.

CONTINUING AND TRANSITIONAL CARE. An eye prosthesis can be worn and left in place for several months. Hygiene and comfort are usually maintained with daily irrigation of the prosthesis in place with the use of a balanced salt solution, hard contact lens solution, or artificial tears. In the case of dry eye symptoms, the use of ophthalmic ointment lubricants or oil-based drops, such as vitamin E and mineral oil, can be helpful. Removing crusting and mucous discharge that accumulates overnight is performed with the prosthesis in place. Malpositions may occur when wiping or rubbing the prosthesis in the socket. The prosthesis can be turned back in place with the use of clean fingers. Proper wiping of the prosthesis is a gentle temporal-to-nasal motion to avoid malpositions.

The prosthesis needs to be removed and cleaned when it becomes uncomfortable and when there is increased mucous discharge. The socket should also be rendered free of mucus and inspected for any signs of infection. Any unusual discomfort, irritation, or redness of the globe or eyelids may indicate excessive wear, debris under the shell, or lack of proper hygiene. Any infection or irritation that does not subside needs medical attention.

OCULAR CONSEQUENCES OF SYSTEMIC DISEASE

Diabetic Retinopathy

Of all of the medical disorders that the nurse encounters, diabetes is one of the most common and one that can have devastating effects on the patient. Diabetes affects every system of the body in a deleterious way and consequently affects the patient's family and society in general. Diabetes is the leading cause of new cases of blindness in Canada in people younger than 50 years of age (CNIB, 2014d). The condition is called diabetic retinopathy, and it affects 500,000 Canadians. Regular eye examinations by optometrists and ophthalmologists can detect the condition early and treatment may prevent further loss of vision. Chapter 41 provides a detailed discussion of diabetic retinopathy.

Cytomegalovirus Retinitis

Many ophthalmic complications are associated with AIDS. On autopsy, up to 90% of patients have ocular lesions directly related to AIDS. CMV is the most common cause of retinal inflammation in patients with AIDS. About 40% of patients who have CMV retinitis lose their central vision in both eyes by the time of death.

Early symptoms of CMV retinitis vary from patient to patient. Some patients report floaters or a decrease in peripheral vision. Some patients have a paracentral or central scotoma, whereas others have a fluctuation in vision from macular edema. The retina often becomes thin and atrophic and susceptible to retinal tears and breaks.

CMV retinitis generally takes one of three forms: hemorrhagic, brushfire, or granular. In the hemorrhagic type, large areas of white, necrotic retina may be associated retinal hemorrhage. The brushfire form appears to have a yellow-white margin, which begins at the edge of burned-out atrophic retina. This retinitis expands and, if untreated, involves the entire retina. The granular form of CMV retinitis consists of white, granular lesions in the periphery of the retina that gradually expand. The white, feathery infiltration of the retina destroys sensory retina and leads to necrosis, optic atrophy, and retinal detachment.

Medical Management

Pharmacologic agents available for treatment of CMV retinitis include ganciclovir (Cytovene), foscarnet (Foscavir), and cidofovir (Vistide).

Ganciclovir is administered IV, orally, or intravitreously in the acute stage of CMV retinitis. A surgically implanted intraocular device has provided a new mode of effective ganciclovir administration. This enables a higher, more effective dose of medication to be administered and is well tolerated by patients. This constant intraocular concentration of ganciclovir lasts for about 6 to 10 months before the inserts must be replaced. Once begun, ganciclovir must be given continuously. A study that combined the use of the intravitreous implant with oral ganciclovir demonstrated a reduction in the risk of new CMV disease as well as a delay in the progression of the retinitis. This very potent medication, when administered systemically, can cause neutropenia, thrombocytopenia, anemia, and elevated serum creatinine levels. Although the surgically implanted sustained-release device enables higher concentrations of ganciclovir to reach the CMV retinitis, there are risks and complications associated with the devices, including endophthalmitis, retinal detachment, and hypotony.

Foscarnet inhibits viral deoxyribonucleic acid (DNA) replication. It may be the medication of choice when ganciclovir is ineffective. It may be administered IV or locally by intravitreal injections. The combination of foscarnet and ganciclovir has been more effective than either medication alone. Nephrotoxicity may occur with systemic foscarnet, and renal function is monitored carefully.

Cidofovir impedes CMV replication. This medication is administered IV. Cidofovir has been shown to delay the progression of CMV retinitis significantly. Nephrotoxicity, proteinuria, and increased serum creatinine levels are significant side effects of its administration.

The routine management of patients with AIDS, including those with CMV retinitis, changed with the introduction of highly active antiretroviral therapy (HAART). HAART is a combination of two or three medications of different categories. For example, a nucleoside analogue such as zidovudine administered in combination with one or more protease inhibitors such as ritonavir has led to a suppression of human immunodeficiency virus (HIV) replication for sustained periods. The immune system can then recover to a functional level. Several patients who had been treated for CMV retinitis have been able to discontinue treatment for CMV retinitis as their immune systems rebounded. However, some patients develop immune recovery uveitis, characterized by intraocular inflammation, cystoid macular edema, and the formation of epiretinal membranes. Immune recovery uveitis is managed by corticosteroids or by injection of corticosteroids into the sub-Tenon's area of the eye.

Hypertension-Related Eye Changes

Hypertension, known as the silent killer, can shorten the life span by as many as 20 years. An estimated 7.4 million Canadians have hypertension (Hypertension Canada, 2014), and more than 9 in 10 Canadians will develop hypertension unless they follow a healthy lifestyle. End-organ damage affects the heart, brain, kidney, and eye. Hypertension may be manifested in one of two forms: chronic or acute. This differentiation is determined by the rapidity in rise of the blood pressure as well as the degree of elevation. The retinal changes observed with each form are different and have different consequences for the eye.

Chronic hypertension and atherosclerosis go hand in hand, and the associated retinal changes are evidenced by the development of retinal arteriolar changes, such as tortuousness, narrowing, and a change in light reflex. Funduscopic examination reveals a copper or silver colouration of the arterioles and venous compression (arteriovenous nicking) at the arteriolar and venous crossings. Intraretinal hemorrhages from hypertension appear flame shaped because they occur in the nerve fibre layer of the retina.

Acute hypertension can result from pheochromocytoma, acute renal failure, pregnancy-induced hypertension, and malignant essential hypertension. The retinopathy associated with these crisis states is extensive, and the manifestations include cotton-wool spots, retinal hemorrhages, retinal edema, and retinal exudates, often clustered around the macula.

The choroid is also affected by the profound and abrupt rise in blood pressure and resulting vasoconstriction, and ischemia may result in serous retinal detachments and infarction of the RPE. Ischemic optic neuropathy and papilledema (i.e., swelling of the optic disc due to increased IOP) may also result. Blood pressure in these more severe stages should be lowered in a controlled gradual fashion to avoid ischemia of the optic nerve and brain secondary to a too-rapid fall in blood pressure. For further information about hypertension, see Chapter 33.

Issues in Ophthalmology

Issues that arise in any area of health care usually pose more questions than answers. In ophthalmology, the well-being of the patient physically, emotionally, financially, socially, and spiritually can be at risk when vision is threatened. Patients with a deteriorating eye condition often worry about the impact that visual loss will have on their lives. As they experience visual distortions, scotomas, or gradual visual loss, what was a vague worry can become a consuming preoccupation. The patient may equate a decrease in VA with a loss of independence. The loss of a driver's licence may force a patient to relocate his or her home or give up or change careers.

Major goals should include the preservation of vision and the prevention of further visual loss in patients who have already experienced some degree of loss. Effective communication is essential to promote rehabilitation of the distressed patient. The nurse together with the patient should establish goals. The nurse listens to the patient, tries to determine his or her level of health care need, and makes suggestions and recommendations. Lines of communication are kept open so that the patient is comfortable exploring all treatment options. Genetic counselling may also be a necessary component of the communication (see Chart 60-2).

Patient Safety

Nurses must be aware of patient safety practices unique to ophthalmology and must be an active participant in the development of a culture of safety. High-volume, efficient, fast-paced procedures characterize ophthalmic practice. This means that patient identification is critical. Active identification (asking the patient his or her name vs. asking, "Are you Ms. Smith?") and a second identifier (birth date, history, hospital number) must be verified before any procedure. As with other organs involving laterality, the correct eye must be verified before medication administration and surgery. Verification of the correct eye before surgery with the involvement of the patient or caregiver (for pediatric patients and adults with cognitive impairment) must be done before initiating any procedure or transferring the patient to another unit. Marking of the operative eye by the surgeon and a final verification of the correct eye by the surgeon, anesthesiologist, and nurse immediately before incision must be performed in all cases.

Cataract surgery with an IOL implant is one of the most frequently performed surgeries. Each facility must have a policy for multiple checks and verification of the IOL type, power, and diopter, as well as the operative eye. The surgeon, scrub nurse or technician, and circulating nurse should each verify the correct IOL measurements, the correct patient, and the patient's chart.

Critical Thinking Exercises

1 You are making a home visit to a 75-year-old male who has a long history of diabetes and complains that recently he is having trouble with his vision. Describe what priority assessment data you would focus on obtaining during your initial visit. What are your priorities of care of this patient with low vision? How would your priorities change if the man were blind?

2 A 45-year-old woman presents to the emergency department with family members, complaining she has had progressive loss of vision of her right eye since this morning. What are your priority assessments for this patient? What focused questions would you ask her? How would you focus your physical assessment? What surgical interventions could be appropriate to treat her? How would you prepare the patient and her family members for possible surgery?

3 A 56-year-old patient reports to you that he has been diagnosed with glaucoma but it is "no big deal" since his vision is fine. Although prescribed ophthalmic medications to treat glaucoma, he has not been self-administering them. What is the strength of the evidence that prescriptive medications are useful in preventing glaucoma-related complications? Identify the risk he is taking by not adhering to his prescribed medication regimen. Describe how you would educate him to gain his adherence to his prescribed regimen.

REFERENCES AND SELECTED READINGS

Books

American Society of Ophthalmic Registered Nurses (ASORN). (2013). *Recommended practice for registered nurses: Use of multi-dose medications*. San Francisco, CA: Author.

Bowling, B. (2015). *Kanski's clinical ophthalmology e-book: A systematic approach*. Elsevier Health Sciences.

Cash, J., & Glass, C. (2016). *Adult-gerontology practice guidelines*. New York: Springer Publishing Company.

Comerford, K. C. (2015). *Nursing 2015 drug handbook*. Philadelphia, PA: Wolters Kluwer.

Eliopoulos, C. (2018). *Gerontological nursing* (9th ed.). Philadelphia, PA: Lippincott Williams & Wilkins.

Fischbach, F. T., & Dunning, M. B. (2015). *A manual of laboratory and diagnostic tests* (9th ed.). Philadelphia, PA: Lippincott Williams & Wilkins.

Gerstenblith, A. T., & Rabinowitz, M. P. (2017). *The Wills eye manual: Office and emergency room diagnosis and treatment of eye disease* (7th ed.). Philadelphia, PA: Lippincott Williams & Wilkins.

Grossman, S. C., & Porth, C. M. (2014). *Porth's Pathophysiology: Concepts of altered health states* (9th ed.). Philadelphia, PA: Lippincott Williams & Wilkins.

Hickey, J. V. (2014). *The clinical practice of neurological and neurosurgical nursing* (7th ed.). Philadelphia, PA: Wolters Kluwer Health/Lippincott Williams & Wilkins.

Hogan, M. (2014). *Pearson's review & rationales: Pathophysiology with nursing reviews & rationales* (3rd ed.). Avenel, NJ: Prentice Hall, Inc.

Lewis, S. L., Bucher, L., Heitkemper, M. M., et al. (2016). *Medical-surgical nursing-e-book: Assessment and management of clinical problems, single volume*. Elsevier Health Sciences.

Oliveira, R. F., Stonecipher, K. G., Ignacio, T. S., et al. (2018). Complications related to femtosecond laser-assisted LASIK. In J. L. Alio, & D. T. Azar. *Management of complications in refractive surgery* (pp. 227–241). Cham: Springer.

Prevent Blindness America. (2012). *Vision problems in the U.S.: Update to the fifth edition*. Schaumberg, IL: Prevent Blindness America/National Eye Institute.

Stephen, T. C. (2012). Eyes assessment. In T. C. Stephen, D. L. Skillen, R. A. Day, et al. (Eds.). *Canadian Jensen's nursing health assessment: A best practice approach* (1st ed., pp. 267–325). Philadelphia, PA: Wolters Kluwer Health/Lippincott Williams & Wilkins.

Weber, J., & Kelley, J. (2014). *Health assessment in nursing* (5th ed.). Philadelphia, PA: Lippincott Williams & Wilkins.

Journals and Electronic Documents

Aref, A. A. (2016). Current management of glaucoma and vascular occlusive disease. *Current Opinion in Ophthalmology*, *27*(2), 140–145.

Barsam, A., & Allan, B. D. (2014). Excimer laser refractive surgery versus phakic intraocular lenses for the correction of moderate to high myopia. *Cochrane Database of Systematic Reviews*, *6*, CD007679.

Boyd, K. (2016). *Retinal detachment: Torn or detached retina treatment*. Retrieved March 1, 2017, from www.aao.org/eye-health/diseases/detached-torn-retina-treatment

Canadian National Institute for the Blind (CNIB). (2014a). *Cataracts*. Retrieved from http://www.cnib.ca/en/your-eyes/eye-conditions/Cataracts/Pages/default.aspx

Canadian National Institute for the Blind (CNIB). (2014b). *Eye conditions, understanding the facts of vision loss*. Retrieved from http://www.cnib.ca/en/Pages/default.aspx

Canadian National Institute for the Blind (CNIB). (2014c). *Age-related macular degeneration*. Retrieved from http://www.cnib.ca/en/your-eyes/eye-conditions/eye-connect/amd/Pages/default.aspx

Canadian National Institute for the Blind (CNIB). (2014d). *Diabetic retinopathy*. Retrieved from http://www.cnib.ca/en/your-eyes/eye-conditions/eye-connect/DR/Pages/default.aspx

Canadian National Institute for the Blind (CNIB). (2014e). *Eye safety at work*. Toronto: Author. Retrieved from http://www.cnib.ca/en/your-eyes/safety/at-work/Pages/default.aspx

Canadian National Institute for the Blind (CNIB). (2014f). *Glaucoma*. Retrieved from http://www.cnib.ca/en/your-eyes/eye-conditions/Glaucoma/Pages/default.aspx

Canadian National Institute for the Blind (CNIB). (2014g). *Seeing beyond vision loss*. Retrieved from http://www.cnib.ca/en/your-eyes/Pages/default.aspx

Centers for Disease Control and Prevention (CDC). (2016). *Learn about age-related macular degeneration*. Retrieved December 27, 2016, from www.cdc.gov/features/healthyvisionmonth/index.html

Chow, A. Y., Chow, V. Y., Packo, K. H., et al. (2004). The artificial silicon retina microchip for the treatment of visionloss from retinitis pigmentosa. *Archives of Ophthalmology*, *122*(4), 460–469.

Colour Blind Awareness. (2016). *Inherited colour vision deficiency*. Retrieved October 10, 2016, from www.colourblindawareness.org/colour-blindness/inherited

Dickman, M. M., Peeters, J. M., Van Den Biggelaar, F., et al. (2016). Changing practice patterns and long-term outcomes of endothelial versus penetrating keratoplasty: A prospective Dutch registry study. *American Journal of Ophthalmology*, *170*, 133–142.

Durand, M. L. (2017). Bacterial and fungal endophthalmitis. *Clinical Microbiology Reviews*, *30*(3), 597–613.

Eldaly, M. A., Bunce, C., & ElSheikha, O. Z., et al. (2014). Non-penetrating filtration surgery versus trabeculectomy for open-angle glaucoma. *Cochrane Database of Systematic Reviews*, (2).

Glaucoma Research Foundation. (2016). *Five common glaucoma tests*. Retrieved October 11, 2016, from www.glaucoma.org/glaucoma/diagnostic-tests.php

Grand, M. G., & Walia, H. S. (2016). Hemorrhagic risk of vitreoretinal surgery in patients maintained on novel oral anticoagulant therapy. *Retina*, *36*(2), 299–304.

Hooper, P. (2014). Ocular inflammatory disease in Canadian First Nations communities. *Canadian Journal of Ophthalmology*, *49*(2), 119.

Hypertension Canada. (2014). *Welcome to Hypertension Canada*. Retrieved from http://www.hypertension.ca/en/

Ing, E., & Doukeris, J. (2014). New oral anticoagulants and oculoplastic surgery. *Canadian Journal of Ophthalmology*, *49*(2), 123–127.

Kahawita, S. K., & Casson, R. J. (2014). Aspirin use and early age-related macular degeneration: A meta-analysis. *Canadian Journal of Ophthalmology*, *49*(1), 35–39.

Kara-Junior, N., Koch, C. R., Santhiago, M. R. D., et al. (2018). Anticoagulants and antiplatelet drugs during cataract surgery. *Arquivos Brasileiros de Oftalmologia*, *81*(4), 348–353.

Kusne, Y., Kang, P., & Fintelmann, R. E. (2016). A retrospective analysis of intraocular pressure changes after cataract surgery with the use of prednisolone acetate 1% versus difluprednate 0.05%. *Clinical Ophthalmology*, *10*, 2326–2336.

Lam, N., & Leat, S. J. (2013). Barriers to accessing low-vision care: The patient's perspective. *Canadian Journal of Ophthalmology*, *48*(6), 458–462.

Leat, S. J., Zecevic, A. A., Keeling, A., et al. (2018). Prevalence of vision loss among hospital in patients; a risk factor for falls? *Ophthalmic and Physiological Optics*, *38*(1), 106–114.

Lee, K., & Garg, S. (2015). Navigating the current landscape of clinical genetic testing for inherited retinal dystrophies. *Genetics in Medicine*, *17*(4), 245–252.

Li, S., Li, D., Zhang, Y., et al. (2018). Association between serum lipids concentration and patients with age-related cataract in China: A cross-sectional, case–control study. *BMJ Open*, *8*(4), e021496.

Li, S. M., Zhan, S., Li, S. Y., et al. (2016). Laser-assisted subepithelial keratectomy (LASEK) versus photorefractive keratectomy (PRK) for correction of myopia. *Cochrane Database of Systematic Reviews*, *2*, CD009799.

Lusthaus, J. A., & Goldberg, I. (2016). Investigational and experimental drugs for intraocular pressure reduction in ocular hypertension and glaucoma. *Expert Opinion on Investigational Drugs*, *25*(10), 1201–1208.

Mamalis, N. (2016). Phacoemulsification technology update. *Journal of Cataract & Refractive Surgery*, *42*(5), 651–652.

Markowitz, S. N. (2016). State-of-the-art: Low vision rehabilitation. *Canadian Journal of Ophthalmology*, *51*(2), 59–66.

Pagliuca, L. M., Macedo-Costa, K. N., Reboucas, G. B., et al. (2014). Validation of the general guidelines of communication between the nurse and the blind. *Reviews Bras Enferm*, *67*(5), 715–725.

Patel, V., Moster, M., Kishfy, L., et al. (2016). Sequential versus concomitant surgery of glaucoma drainage implant and Boston keratoprosthesis type 1. *European Journal of Ophthalmology*, *26*(6), 556–563.

Peng, L. H., Fong, A., Phaik, C. S., et al. (2012). Improving presurgical pupil dilation for cataract surgery patients. *Joint Commission Journal on Quality and Patient Safety*, *38*(9), 420–425.

Roy, M. (2014). Analysis of uveitis in a Canadian aboriginal population. *Canadian Journal of Ophthalmology*, *49*(2), 128–134.

The World Health Organization (WHO). (2017). *Blindness and vision impairment*. Retrieved from http://www.who.int/en/news-room/fact-sheets/detail/blindness-and-visual-impairment

Tripathy, K., Mittal, K., Venkatesh, P., et al. (2017). Treatment of unilateral zone I cytomegalovirus retinitis in acute lymphoblastic leukemia with oral valganciclovir and intravitreal ganciclovir. *Oman Journal of Ophthalmology*, *10*(3), 250.

Varma, R., Vajaranant, T. S., Burkemper, B., et al. (2016). Visual impairment and blindness in adults in the United States: Demographic and geographic variations from 2015 to 2050. *JAMA Ophthalmology*, *134*(7), 802–809.

Veritti, D., Sarao, V., & Lanzetta, P. (2017). Optimal keratoplasty for the correction of presbyopia and hypermetropia. *Journal of Ophthalmology*, *2017*, 6.

Verma, S., Arora, S., Kassam, F., et al. (2014). Northern Alberta remote teleglaucoma program: Clinical outcomes and patient disposition. *Canadian Journal of Ophthalmology*, *49*(1), 135–140.

Weinreb, R. N., Leung, C. K., Crowston, J. G., et al. (2016). Primary open-angle glaucoma. *Nature Reviews Disease Primers*, *2*, 16067.

Resources

Adaptive Technology Resource Centre: http://www.atrc.utoronto.ca/
Alliance for Equality of Blind Canadians: http://www.blindcanadians.ca/
American Macular Degeneration Foundation: http://www.macular.org/
Canadian Association Disability Service Providers in Post-Secondary Education: https://www.cacuss.ca/en/divisions/CADSPPE.
Canadian Association of Genetic Counsellors (CAGC): http://www.cagc-accg.ca/
Canadian Braille Authority: http://www.canadianbrailleauthority.ca/index.php
Canadian Cancer Society/Société canadienne du cancer, National Office: http://www.cancer.ca
Canadian Council of the Blind, CCB National Office: http://ccbnational.net/
Canadian Council on Social Development: http://www.ccsd.ca/
Canadian Deaf-Blind Council: http://www.cdbc-csac.ca/
Canadian Glaucoma Society: http://www.eyesite.ca/cgs/
Canadian Library Association: http://www.cla.ca/AM/Template.cfm?Section=Home
Canadian National Institute for the Blind, National Office: https://cnib.ca/en?region=ab
Canadian National Society for the Deaf Blind: http://www.blindcanadians.ca/publications/cbm/14/canadian-national-society-deaf-blind-cnsdb
Canadian Ophthalmological Society: http://www.eyesite.ca/
Canadian Organization for Rare Disorders (CORD): http://www.cord.ca/
Council of Canadians with Disabilities: http://www.ccdonline.ca/
Council on Access to Information for Print-Disabled Canadians, Library and Archives Canada: http://www.collectionscanada.gc.ca/accessinfo/
Glaucoma Research Foundation: http://www.glaucoma.org/index.php
Head Cancer Informatics, Ontario Cancer Institute/Princess Margaret Hospital, University Health Network: http://www.retinoblastoma.ca/
Help the Aged Canada, HTAC Head Office: http://www.helptheaged.ca/
Independent Living Canada: http://www.cailc.ca/
National Educational Association of Disabled Students: https://mssociety.ca/support-services/programs-and-services/1082/national-educational-association-of-disabled-students-neads
Prevent Blindness America: https://www.preventblindness.org/
Public Health Agency of Canada: http://www.phac-aspc.gc.ca/index-eng.php
Research to Prevent Blindness: http://www.rpbusa.org
The Canadian Association of Optometrists: http://www.opto.ca/
The Learning Disabilities Association of Canada, National Office: https://www.ldac-acta.ca/
Veterans Affairs Canada: https://www.veterans.gc.ca/eng

61 Assessment and Management of Patients With Hearing and Balance Disorders

Adapted by Mohamed Toufic El Hussein and Joseph Osuji

Learning Objectives

On completion of this chapter, the learner will be able to:

1. Describe the anatomy and physiology of the ear.
2. Explain methods used to assess hearing and balance disorders.
3. List the manifestations that may be exhibited by a person with hearing and balance disorders.
4. Identify ways to communicate effectively with a person with a hearing disorder.
5. Differentiate problems of the external ear from those of the middle ear and inner ear.
6. Compare the various types of surgical procedures used for managing middle ear disorders and appropriate nursing care.
7. Use the nursing process as a framework of care for patients undergoing mastoid surgery.
8. Apply the nursing process as a framework of care for patients with vertigo.
9. Recognize the different types of inner ear disorders, including the clinical manifestations, diagnosis, and management.

The ear is a sensory organ with dual functions—hearing and balance. The sense of hearing is critical for human development, maintenance of speech, and the ability to communicate with others. Balance (equilibrium) is essential for maintaining body movement, position, and coordination.

The delicate structure and function of the ear make early detection and accurate diagnosis of disorders necessary for preservation of hearing and balance. Among the professionals involved in the diagnosis and treatment of these disorders are otolaryngologists, pediatricians, internists, audiologists, and nurses, including occupational health nurses.

This chapter addresses the assessment and management of hearing and balance disorders common to the adult population. The pediatric otolaryngology literature provides information on otologic disorders pertaining to that population.

Anatomy and Physiology Overview

The cranium encloses and protects the brain and surrounding structures, providing attachment for various muscles that control head, facial, neck, and jaw movements. Eight bones form the cranium: the occipital bone, frontal bone, two parietal bones, two temporal bones, sphenoid bone, and ethmoid bone. Some of these bones contain sinuses, which are cavities lined with mucous membranes and connected to the nasal cavity. The ears are located on either side of the cranium at approximately eye level.

Anatomy of the External Ear

The external ear, located in the temporal bone, includes the auricle (pinna) and the external auditory canal (Fig. 61-1). The external ear is separated from the middle ear by a disk-like structure called the *tympanic membrane* (eardrum).

Auricle

The auricle is composed mainly of skin and flexible cartilage, except for the fat and subcutaneous tissue in the earlobe. The auricle collects the sound waves and directs vibrations into the external auditory canal.

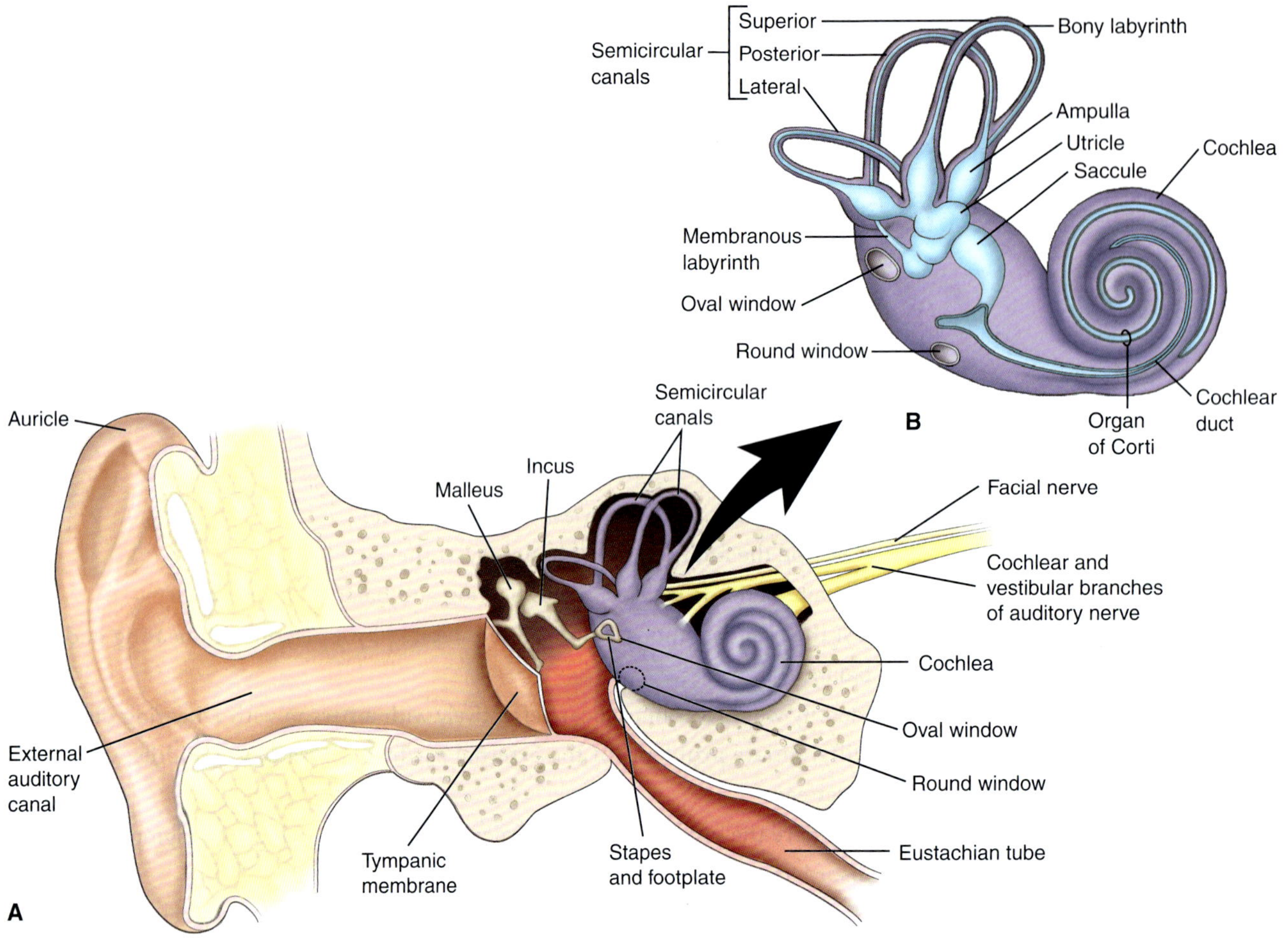

FIGURE 61-1. **A.** Anatomy of the ear. **B.** The inner ear.

Glossary

acute otitis media: inflammation in the middle ear lasting less than 6 weeks
cholesteatoma: tumour of the middle ear or mastoid, or both, that can destroy structures of the temporal bone
chronic otitis media: repeated episodes of acute otitis media causing irreversible tissue damage
conductive hearing loss: loss of hearing in which efficient sound transmission to the inner ear is interrupted by some obstruction or disease process
deafness: partial or complete loss of the ability to hear
dizziness: altered sensation of orientation in space
endolymphatic hydrops: dilation of the endolymphatic space of the inner ear; the pathologic correlate of Ménière's disease
exostoses: small, hard, bony protrusions in the lower posterior bony portion of the ear canal
external otitis (i.e., otitis externa): inflammation of the external auditory canal
labyrinthitis: inflammation of the labyrinth of the inner ear
Ménière's disease: condition of the inner ear characterized by a triad of symptoms: episodic vertigo, tinnitus, and fluctuating sensorineural hearing loss
middle ear effusion: fluid in the middle ear without evidence of infection
myringotomy (i.e., tympanotomy): incision in the tympanic membrane
nystagmus: involuntary rhythmic eye movement
ossiculoplasty: surgical reconstruction of the middle ear bones to restore hearing
otalgia: sensation of fullness or pain in the ear
otorrhea: drainage from the ear
otosclerosis: a condition characterized by abnormal spongy bone formation around the stapes
presbycusis: progressive hearing loss associated with aging
rhinorrhea: drainage from the nose
sensorineural hearing loss: loss of hearing related to damage to the end organ for hearing or cranial nerve VIII, or both
tinnitus: subjective perception of sound with internal origin; unwanted noises in the head or ear
tympanoplasty: surgical repair of the tympanic membrane
vertigo: illusion of movement in which the individual or the surroundings are sensed as moving

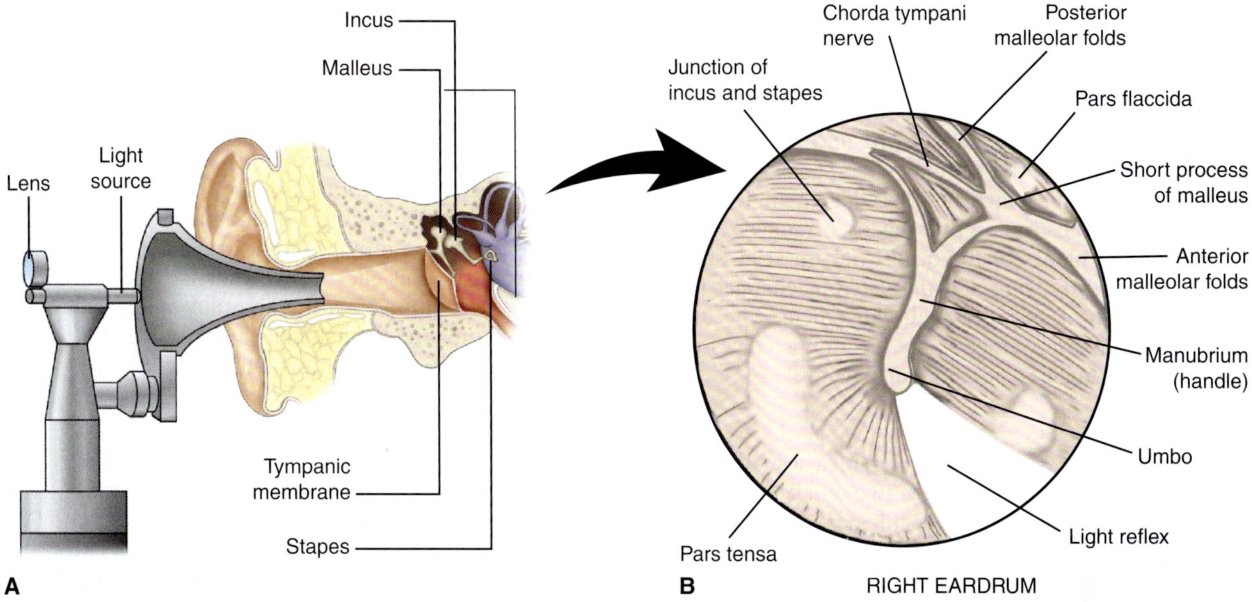

FIGURE 61-2. **A.** Technique for using the otoscope to see **(B)** the tympanic membrane.

External Auditory Canal

The external auditory canal is approximately 2.5 cm long. The lateral third is an elastic cartilaginous and dense fibrous framework covered by thin skin. The medial two thirds are bone lined with thin skin. The external auditory canal ends at the tympanic membrane.

The skin of the auditory canal contains hair, sebaceous glands, and ceruminous glands, which secrete a brown, waxy substance called *cerumen* (ear wax). The ear's self-cleaning mechanism moves old skin cells and cerumen to the outer part of the ear canal.

Just anterior to the external auditory canal is the temporomandibular joint. The head of the mandible can be felt by placing a fingertip in the joint space while the patient opens and closes the mouth.

Anatomy of the Middle Ear

The middle ear, an air-filled cavity, lies between the tympanic membrane laterally and the oval window of the cochlea medially. The middle ear is continuous with air-filled cells in the adjacent mastoid portion of the temporal bone and is connected to the nasopharynx by the eustachian tube, which is approximately 1 mm wide and 35 mm long.

Usually, the eustachian tube is closed, but it opens by action of the tensor veli palatini muscle during a Valsalva manoeuvre, yawning, or swallowing. The tube serves as a drainage channel for secretions of the middle ear and equalizes pressure in the middle ear with that of the atmosphere (Martini, Timmons, & Tallitsch, 2012).

Tympanic Membrane

The tympanic membrane (eardrum), about 1 cm in diameter and very thin, is pearly grey and translucent. It consists of three layers of tissue: an outer layer continuous with the skin of the ear canal; a fibrous middle layer; and an inner mucosal layer continuous with the lining of the middle ear cavity. Approximately 80% of the tympanic membrane is composed of all three layers stretched tightly and is called the *pars tensa*. The other 20% of the tympanic membrane lacks the middle layer, is more relaxed, and is called the *pars flaccida*. Absence of this fibrous middle layer makes the pars flaccida more vulnerable to pathologic disorders. Distinguishing landmarks of the tympanic membrane include the annulus, a fibrous border that attaches the eardrum to the temporal bone; the short process of the malleus; the long process of the malleus; the umbo of the malleus, which attaches to the tympanic membrane in the centre; the pars flaccida; and the pars tensa (Fig. 61-2).

The tympanic membrane protects the middle ear and conducts sound vibrations from the external canal to the bony ossicles. The sound pressure is magnified 22 times as a result of transmission from a larger area to a smaller one (Martini et al., 2012).

Ossicles

The middle ear contains the three smallest bones (ossicles) of the body: malleus, incus, and stapes. The ossicles, which are held in place by joints, muscles, and ligaments, and assist in sound transmission. Two small fenestrae (oval and round windows), located in the medial wall of the middle ear, separate the middle ear from the inner ear. The footplate of the stapes sits in the oval window, secured by the fibrous annulus (ring-shaped structure). The footplate transmits sound to the inner ear. The round window, covered by a thin membrane, provides an exit for sound vibrations (see Fig. 61-1).

Anatomy of the Inner Ear

The inner ear is located deep within the temporal bone. The organs for hearing (cochlea) and balance (semicircular canals), as well as cranial nerves VII (facial nerve) and VIII (vestibulocochlear nerve), are all part of this complex anatomy (see Fig. 61-1). The cochlea and semicircular canals are sheltered in the bony labyrinth. The bony labyrinth surrounds and protects the membranous labyrinth, which is bathed in a fluid called *perilymph*.

Membranous Labyrinth

Rotation, acceleration, and gravity are detected by the vestibular complex in the inner ear. The membranous labyrinth is composed of the utricle, saccule, cochlear duct, semicircular canals, and organ of Corti, and contains a fluid called *endolymph*. The three semicircular canals—posterior, superior, and lateral, which lie at 90-degree angles to one another contain sensory receptor organs, arranged to detect three rotational planes of the head (Martini et al., 2012). These receptor end organs are stimulated by changes in the rate or direction of an individual's movement. The utricle detects horizontal movements; the saccule perceives vertical acceleration such as riding in an elevator.

Organ of Corti

The organ of Corti is located in the cochlea, a snail-shaped, bony tube about 3.5 cm long with two and one half spiral turns. Membranes separate the cochlear duct (scala media) from the scala vestibuli, and the scala tympani from the basilar membrane. The organ of Corti is located on the basilar membrane stretching from the base to the apex of the cochlea. As sound vibrations enter the perilymph at the oval window and travel along the scala vestibuli, they pass through the scala tympani, enter the cochlear duct, and cause movement of the basilar membrane. The organ of Corti, also called the *end organ for hearing*, transforms mechanical energy into neural activity and separates sounds into different frequencies. This electrochemical impulse travels through the vestibulocochlear nerve to the temporal cortex of the brain for interpretation as meaningful sound. In the internal auditory canal, the cochlear branch, arising from the cochlea, joins the vestibular branch, arising from the semicircular canals, utricle, and saccule, to become the vestibulocochlear nerve (cranial nerve VIII). This canal also contains the facial nerve and the blood supply from the ear to the brain.

Function of the Ears

Hearing

Hearing is conducted along two pathways: air and bone. Sound waves transmitted by air conduction travel through the air-filled external and middle ear causing vibration of the tympanic membrane and ossicles. Sounds transmitted by bone conduction travel directly through the bony skull to the inner ear, bypassing the tympanic membrane and ossicles. Usually, air conduction is the more efficient pathway. If defects in the tympanic membrane or the ossicular chain disrupt air conduction, this results in a loss of the sound: pressure ratio and produces a **conductive hearing loss**.

Sound Conduction and Transmission

Sound waves enter the ear through the external auditory canal and cause the tympanic membrane (TM) to vibrate. Stimulated by impulses to the TM from the incus and malleus, the footplate of the stapes starts to rock (lever action) and transmits sound to the oval window as mechanical energy. This mechanical energy is then transmitted as waves to the inner ear fluids to the cochlea lodged in the labyrinth of the inner ear, stimulating the hair cells of the organ of Corti via the basilar membrane, and being converted to electrical energy. The electrical energy travels through the vestibulocochlear nerve to the auditory cortex where it is analyzed and interpreted in its final form as sound.

If the TM is intact, sound waves stimulate the oval window first, and a lag occurs before the terminal effect of the stimulus reaches the round window which opens on the opposite side of the cochlear duct. When the TM is perforated, sound waves impinge on the oval and round windows simultaneously. This effect cancels the lag and prevents the maximal effect of inner ear fluid motility and its subsequent effect in stimulating the hair cells in the organ of Corti. The result is a reduction in hearing ability (Fig. 61-3).

Balance and Equilibrium

Body balance is maintained by the coordination of muscles and joints of the body (proprioceptive system), eyes (visual system), and labyrinth (vestibular system) (Vestibular Disorders Association [VEDA], 2014). These areas send their information about equilibrium (balance) to the brain (cerebellar system) for perception and interpretation in the cerebral cortex. As the brain obtains its blood supply from the heart and arterial system, an alteration in any of these areas (e.g., arteriosclerosis, impaired vision) can cause a balance disturbance.

Assessment of Hearing and Balance

Assessment of hearing and balance requires a health history and physical examination of the external, middle, and inner ear functions. Hearing and balance are complex, coordinated systems. Nursing assessment of the effects of multifaceted interactions requires a thorough knowledge of the functional components, systematic exploration of patients' altered health issues, appropriate methods of examination, and determination of patients' responses to any alterations. In an emergency situation (e.g., trauma, clear yellow or bloody discharge from ear, sudden loss of balance or hearing) nurses perform very focused assessments (Weber & Kelley, 2014). In nonurgent interactions, nurses focus on the presenting concern or perform a comprehensive assessment to obtain baseline data for health promotion, risk assessment, and identification of change over time.

Health History

The health history is essential for capturing previous, current, and future threats to hearing and balance. Obtain an overall impression of the patient's current health status while initiating the health history. After collecting identifying data, focus on any presenting concern and complete a symptom/sign analysis. Inquire about the location (and radiation), the nature and intensity, and the timing (including onset, frequency, and duration). Determine what factors aggravate or alleviate the symptom and inquire about associated symptoms. Ask about environmental factors (at home, school, work, or leisure) that may have a role to play. Discover the effects on daily life and lastly ask what the patient thinks is the cause (Stephen, 2012).

Document the patient's medications (name, dosage, frequency, purpose, and response) and inquire about allergies.

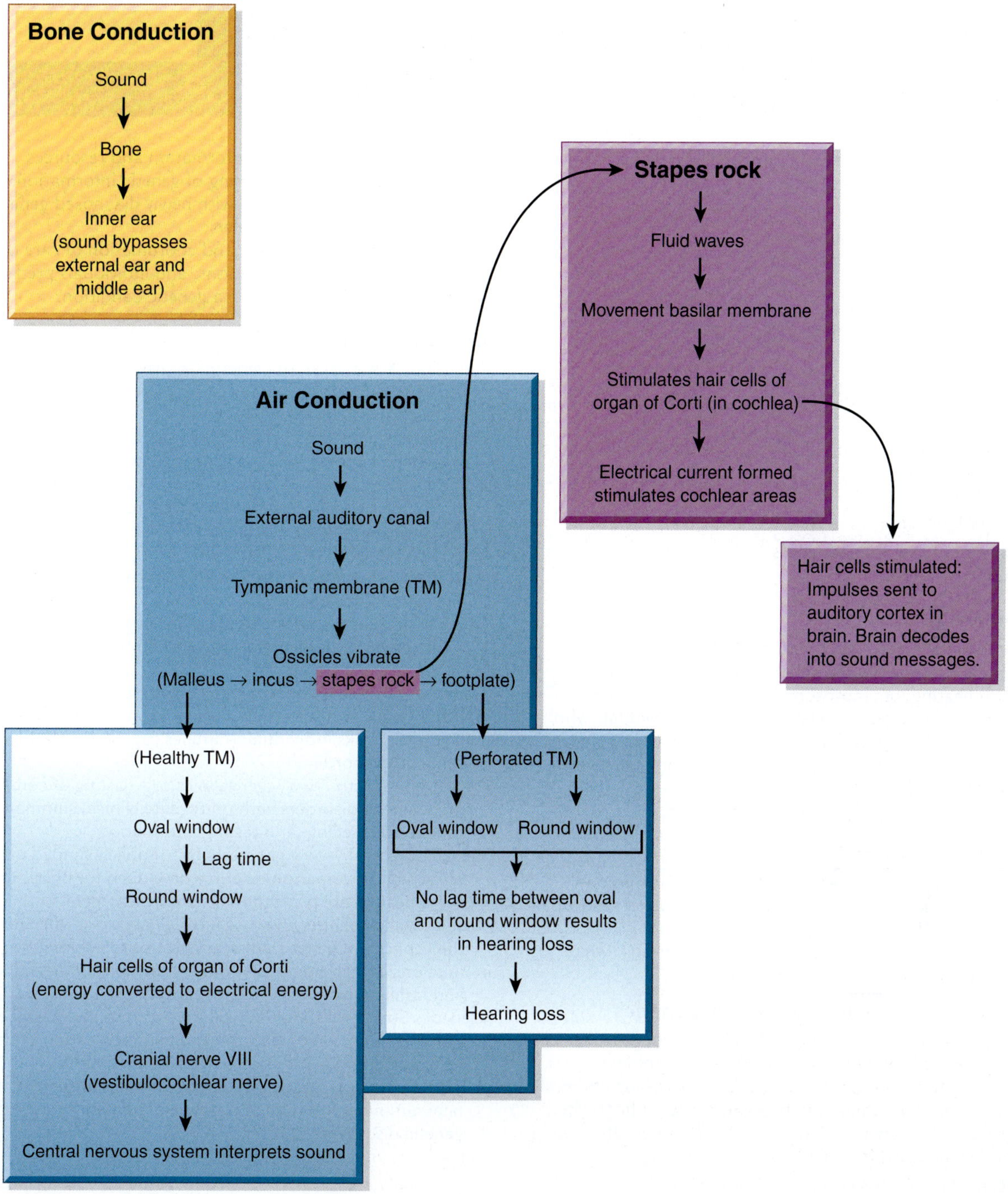

FIGURE 61-3. Bone conduction compared with air conduction.

Medications that can affect hearing or balance include salicylates, aminoglycoside antibiotics, anti-inflammatories, anti-malarials, and diuretics. Document concurrent health conditions (e.g., atrial fibrillation, blackouts, carotid artery disease, diabetes mellitus, dizziness, headaches, hypertension, sensory losses, involuntary movements) (Stephen, 2012). Inquire about past surgeries, disorders (e.g., Ménière's disease), history of mumps or prenatal rubella, and familial **deafness**. Because of progress made in recent years in genomics and genetics research, health care professionals will have a better understanding of the genetic basis for hearing impairment and the implications for clinical practice (Stanton & Griffin, 2013) (Chart 61-1).

Explore the patient's expectations for health and focus on lifestyle behaviours that can be detrimental to hearing or balance (e.g., physical risk-taking, alcohol or drug consumption, exposure to occupational or recreational noise [e.g., rock concert], dietary habits, and exposure to smoke).

Common Symptoms/Signs

Hearing loss is a significant chronic disability in Canada. In 2012/2013, an estimated 4.6 million Canadians aged 20 to 79 (19%) had hearing loss that affected their ability to hear normal speech. In Canada, the prevalence of hearing loss has often been based on self-reported data. Self-reports tend

GENETICS IN NURSING PRACTICE

Chart 61-1. Hearing Disorders

Several hearing disorders are associated with genetic abnormalities and have various patterns of inheritance.

Autosomal dominant:

- Branchiootorenal syndrome
- Neurofibromatosis type 2
- Otosclerosis
- Stickler syndrome
- Waardenburg syndrome

Autosomal recessive:

- Connexin 26 gene hearing loss (the majority of cases are recessive; however, there is an autosomal dominant form that occurs less commonly)
- Jervell and Lange-Nielsen syndrome
- Pendred syndrome
- Refsum disease
- Usher syndrome

X-Linked syndromic hearing loss:

- Alport syndrome

Nursing Assessments

FAMILY HISTORY ASSESSMENT

- Assess for other family members in several generations with hearing loss (autosomal dominant hearing loss)
- Inquire about genetic relatedness (e.g., individuals who are related, such as first cousins, have a higher chance to share the same recessive genes—autosomal recessive hearing loss)
- Inquire about age at onset of hearing loss

Physical Assessment

- Assess for related genetic conditions, such as vision impairment (e.g., retinitis pigmentosa in Usher syndrome; thyroid disorder in Pendred syndrome)
- Assess for iris, pigmentary, and hair alterations (white forelock) seen in Waardenburg syndrome

Management Issues Specific to Genetics

- Inquire whether DNA gene mutation or other genetic testing has been performed on affected family members.
- If indicated, refer for further genetic counselling and evaluation so that family members can discuss inheritance, risk to other family members, availability of genetic testing, and gene-based interventions.
- Offer appropriate genetic information and resources.
- Assess patient's understanding of genetic information.
- Provide support to families with newly diagnosed genetic-related sensorineural disorders.
- Participate in management and coordination of care of patients with genetic conditions, and individuals predisposed to develop or pass on a genetic condition.

Genetic Resources

Canadian Association of Genetic Counsellors (CAGC), http://www.cagc-accg.ca—Listing of genetic centres across Canada

Canadian Cancer Society, http://www.cancer.ca—Information on genetic factors/risks and genetic testing

Canadian Directory of Genetic Support Groups, http://www.lhsc.on.ca/programs/medgenet—Resource guide for families and professionals

Canadian Genetic Disease Network, http://www.cgdn.ca—Its stated mission is to be the primary catalyst in advancing Canada's scientific and commercial competitiveness in genetic research and the application of genetic discoveries to the prevention, diagnosis, and treatment of human disease

Canadian Organization for Rare Disorders (CORD), http://www.cord.ca—Information on over 6,000 rare disorders; links individuals/families together with the same rare disorder

Gene Clinics, http://www.geneclinics.org—Listing of common genetic disorders with up-to-date clinical summaries, genetic counselling, and testing information

GeneTests, http://www.genetests.org—Publicly funded medical genetic information resource developed for physicians, other health care professionals, and researchers

Genetic Alliance, http://www.geneticalliance.org—Increases the capacity of genetic advocacy groups to achieve their missions and leverages the voices of millions of individuals and families living with genetic conditions

Genetics Society of Canada (GSC), http://erol.mcmaster.ca/GSC/—Promotion of research and communication of the results and implications of genetics to the public

OMIM: Online Mendelian Inheritance in Man, http://www.ncbi.nlm.nih.gov/omim/Catalogue of human genes and genetic disorders

to underestimate the prevalence of hearing impairment in older adults and in people with mild- or high-frequency hearing loss.

The Hearing Foundation of Canada identifies at least 12 causes of hearing loss, including ototoxicity, tumours, trauma, repeated ear infections, prenatal conditions, and heredity. During the health history, be alert to the manifestations of hearing loss in your patient: slowness to respond, turning one ear toward you, straining to hear, misunderstanding you, asking you to repeat words, and speaking louder than necessary (Canadian Hearing Society, 2013). Although often associated with aging as *presbycusis* and the loss of upper tones of words, only about 25% of hearing loss is attributed to aging. A highly preventable cause of frequent hearing loss is precipitated by occupational exposure to loud noise or recreational exposure to noise at sports or musical events. Patients may report distress from the loss of hearing that affects socialization, relationships with family and friends, safety, and educational and recreational activities (Antonio, 2016).

According to the Canadian Tinnitus Foundation (2012), another concerning symptom is **tinnitus** which is troubling to more than 360,000 Canadians who describe up to 50 different sounds heard internally; sizzling, buzzing, chirping, clicking, pulsing, ringing, and rushing are just a few of them. Tinnitus affects all ages and may be continuous or intermittent.

Vestibular dysfunction resulting from Ménière's disease, ototoxic medications, or changes with aging poses the risk of serious injury from loss of balance. Falls are the most common cause of injuries in Canadian seniors (Seniors' Falls in Canada, 2014).

Physical Examination of the Ear

Inspection, palpation, **and screening tests** are used to examine the ears, and **to** assess hearing and balance. **Always perform inspection first, using your olfactory, visual, and auditory senses**.

External Ear

Inspection of the external ear is a simple procedure, but it is often overlooked. The external ear is examined by inspection and direct palpation; the auricle and surrounding tissues should be inspected for deformities, lesions, and discharge, as well as size, symmetry, and angle of attachment to the head. Manipulation of the auricle does not normally elicit pain. If this manoeuvre is painful, acute external otitis is suspected (Cash & Glass, 2014). Tenderness on palpation in the area of the mastoid may indicate acute mastoiditis or inflammation of the posterior auricular node. Occasionally, sebaceous cysts and tophi (subcutaneous mineral deposits) are present on the pinna. A flaky scaliness on or behind the auricle usually indicates seborrheic dermatitis and can be present on the scalp and facial structures as well.

Otoscopic Examination

Inspect the tympanic membrane with a braced otoscope and palpate indirectly using a pneumatic otoscope. Hold the otoscope in your dominant hand in a "pencil hold" position, bracing a part of your hand on the skull or face (Fig. 61-4).

Inspect the auditory canal and TM after gently straightening the canal in the adult patient by pulling up and back on the pinna. If the canal does not straighten with this technique, the TM is harder to visualize, so adjust your technique. Select the largest speculum that the canal can accommodate (usually 5 mm in adults). Gently insert the speculum downward and forward into the ear canal with your eye close to the magnifying lens. Because the distal portion of the canal is bony, sensitive, and covered with thin skin, stay central in the canal to avoid causing pain or a cough. Inspect for any discharge, inflammation, or foreign body.

The healthy TM is pearly grey and positioned obliquely. Observe for the light reflex (5 o'clock [R] ear, 7 o'clock [L] ear). Identify the visible landmarks (see Fig. 61-2): the pars tensa, umbo, manubrium of the malleus, and short process. Using a slow, circular movement of the speculum, visualize the malleolar folds and periphery. Note the presence of a perforated or scarred TM, or fluid, air bubbles, blood, or masses in the middle ear. Document the position and colour of the TM and any unusual markings or deviations. Successful otoscopic examination of the external auditory canal and TM requires that the canal be free of large amounts of cerumen. Cerumen is usually present in the external canal, and small amounts should not interfere with otoscopic examination. If the TM cannot be visualized because of cerumen, remove the cerumen by gently irrigating the external canal with warm water (if there are no contraindications to this, e.g., known perforation). If adherent cerumen is present, instill a small amount of mineral oil or over-the-counter cerumen softener in the ear canal and instruct the patient to return for subsequent removal of the cerumen and inspection of the ear. Only otolaryngologists, audiologists, and nurses with specialized training may use instruments such as a cerumen curette for cerumen removal because of the risk of perforating the TM or excoriating the external auditory canal. Cerumen buildup is a common cause of hearing loss and local irritation (Grossman & Porth, 2014).

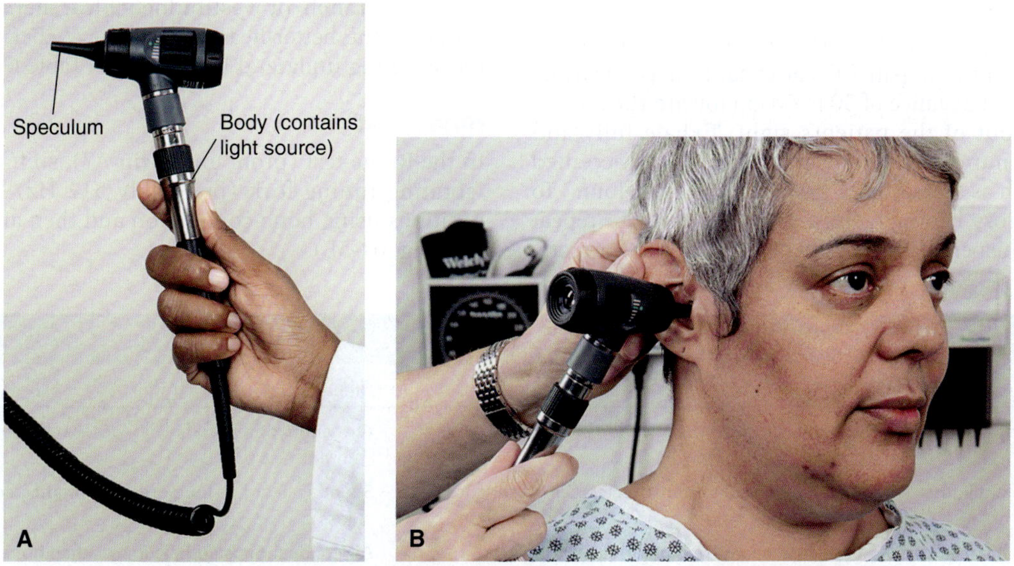

FIGURE 61-4. **A.** The otoscope. **B.** Proper technique for examining the ear. Hold the otoscope in the right or left hand, in a "pencil-hold" position. (From Weber, J., & Kelley, J. (2014). *Health assessment in nursing* (5th ed.). Philadelphia, PA: Lippincott Williams & Wilkins.)

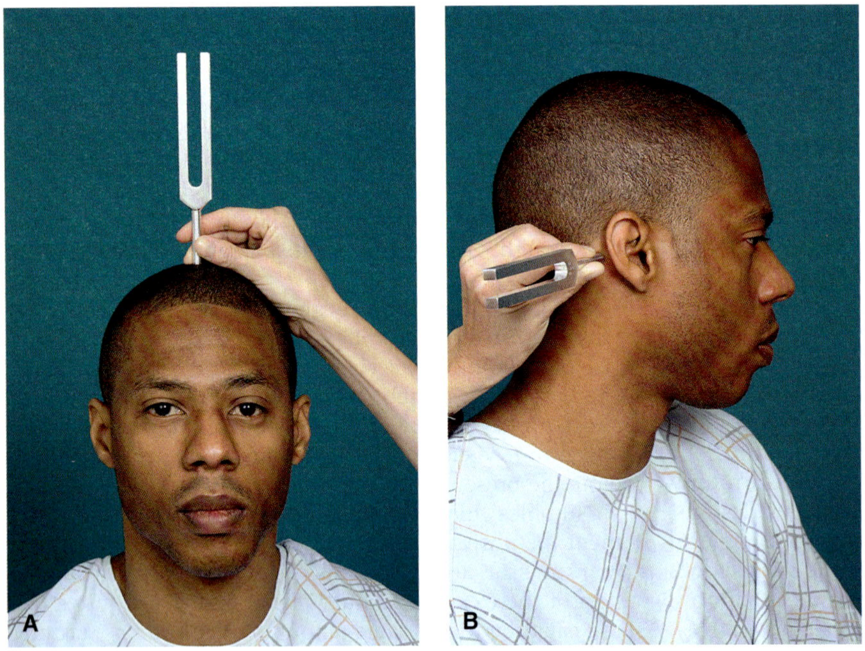

FIGURE 61-5. **A.** The Weber test assesses bone conduction of sound. **B.** The Rinne test assesses both air and bone conduction of sound.

Evaluation of Gross Auditory Acuity

Hearing assessment is a lifespan consideration. According to Speech-Language and Audiology Canada (SAC), screening for hearing loss begins with newborns and children. Auditory deprivation affects brain development, use of language, cognition, and social and emotional development (SAC, 2014). In adults, make a general estimation of hearing by assessing the patient's ability to hear a low whispered phrase or a ticking watch, testing one ear at a time. Use the Weber and Rinne tests to distinguish conductive loss from sensorineural loss when hearing is impaired (Weber & Kelley, 2014). These tests are part of the usual screening physical examination and are useful if a more specific assessment is needed, hearing loss is detected, or audiometric confirmation is desired.

Whisper Test

Occlude the ear not being tested by moving a finger or piece of cotton in the patient's ear canal to mask hearing. Whisper from a distance of 30 to 60 cm toward the nonoccluded ear, out of the patient's sight. Exhale fully and whisper two numbers or words that have equally accented syllables such as "sandbox," "baseball," or "nine-four." To determine gross hearing acuity, ask the patient to repeat what was whispered. If the patient is unable to correctly repeat the whispered words or numbers on the first attempt, try again with a slightly louder whisper.

Weber Test

The Weber test uses bone conduction to test lateralization of sound. Set a tuning fork (ideally, 512 Hz) in motion by grasping it firmly by its stem and tapping it on your hand or knee or pinching the ends of the tines between your fingers and thumb and place it midline on the patient's head or forehead (see Fig. 61-5A).

An individual with intact hearing will hear the sound equally in both ears or describe the sound as centred in the middle of the head. A person with conductive hearing loss, such as from otosclerosis or otitis media, hears the sound better in the affected ear. A person with **sensorineural hearing loss** that results from damage to the cochlear branch or vestibulocochlear nerve, hears the sound in the better-hearing ear. The Weber test is useful for detecting unilateral hearing loss (Table 61-1).

Rinne Test

In the Rinne test (pronounced rin-AY), shift the stem of a vibrating tuning fork (preferably 512 Hz) between two positions using bone conduction and then air conduction (see Fig. 61-5B).

TABLE 61-1 Comparison of Weber and Rinne Tests

Hearing Status	Weber	Rinne
Normal hearing	Sound is heard equally in both ears.	Air conduction is audible longer than bone conduction in both ears.
Conductive hearing loss	Sound is heard best in affected ear (hearing loss).	Sound is heard as long or longer in affected ear (hearing loss).
Sensorineural hearing loss	Sound is heard best in normal hearing ear.	Air conduction is audible longer than bone conduction in affected ear.

Adapted from Weber, J., & Kelley, J. (2014). *Health assessment in nursing* (5th ed.). Philadelphia, PA: Lippincott Williams & Wilkins.

Place the vibrating tuning fork on the mastoid bone behind the tested ear and ask the patient to indicate when the tone is no longer heard. Then shift the tuning fork to the opening of the ear canal and ask the patient if the tone is audible. When hearing is intact, air-conducted sound is audible longer than bone-conducted sound (e.g., AC > BC). The Rinne test distinguishes between conductive and sensorineural hearing losses. With a conductive hearing loss, bone-conducted sound is heard as long as or longer than air-conducted sound; with a sensorineural hearing loss, air-conducted sound is audible longer than bone-conducted sound.

Vestibular Dysfunction Testing to Assess Balance

Vestibular dysfunction is only one condition that contributes to impaired balance. For example, a positive Romberg test would indicate proprioceptive difficulty. (See Chapter 69 for assessment of muscle weakness, Chapter 62 for cerebellar assessment, and Chapter 60 for visual alterations.) A thorough assessment of the inner ear function will likely require several diagnostic tests guided by the history obtained (e.g., vertigo, dizziness, impaired spatial orientation, visual difficulties, response to sudden loud noises) and assessment of the various integrated systems in the vestibular system (VEDA, n.d.).

Diagnostic Evaluation of Hearing and Balance

Many diagnostic procedures are available to measure the auditory and vestibular systems indirectly. These tests are usually performed by an audiologist or speech-language pathologist who is recognized by SAC.

Audiometry

In detecting hearing loss, audiometry is the most important diagnostic instrument. Audiometric testing is of two kinds: pure-tone audiometry, in which the sound stimulus consists of a pure or musical tone (the louder the tone before the patient perceives it, the greater the hearing loss), and speech audiometry, in which the spoken word is used to determine the ability to hear and discriminate sounds and words.

When evaluating hearing, three characteristics of sound pressure waves are important: pitch (frequency), duration, and intensity. A fourth characteristic of audible sound, *timbre*, (musical quality) is not assessed. *Pitch* refers to the frequency of sound pressure waves emanating from a source per second, measured as wave cycles per second (cps) commonly expressed in Hertz (Hz). The human ear perceives sounds ranging in frequency from 20 to 20,000 Hz. The frequencies from 500 to 2,000 Hz are important for understanding everyday speech and are referred to as the speech range (speech frequencies). *Pitch* is the term used to describe frequency; a tone with 100 Hz is considered to be a low pitch and a tone of 10,000 Hz is considered to be a high pitch.

The *duration* of sound is the unit of time in seconds, minutes, or hours that a sound is heard. The unit for measuring *intensity* (loudness of sound) is the decibel (dB), the pressure exerted by sound. The physiologic perception of sound is detected by an instrument that is calibrated for the human hearing curve: the "A" scale. Hearing loss as measured in decibels is a logarithmic function of intensity that is not easily converted into a percentage. The *critical* level of loudness is approximately 30 dB(A). The shuffling of papers in quiet surroundings is about 15 dB; a low conversation, 40 dB; and a jet plane 30 m away, about 150 dB. Sound louder than 80 dB is perceived by the human ear to be harsh and can be damaging to the inner ear. Table 61-2 classifies hearing loss based on decibel level. In surgical treatment of patients with hearing loss, the aim is to improve the hearing level to 30 dB or better within the speech frequencies.

TABLE 61-2 Severity of Hearing Loss

Loss in Decibels	Interpretation
0–15	Expected (intact) hearing
>15–25	Slight hearing loss
>25–40	Mild hearing loss
>40–55	Moderate hearing loss
>55–70	Moderate to severe hearing loss
>70–90	Severe hearing loss
>90	Profound hearing loss

During audiometry, the patient wears earphones and signals to the audiologist or occupational health nurse when a tone is heard. When the tone is applied directly over the external auditory canal, air conduction is measured. When the stimulus is applied to the mastoid bone, bypassing the conductive mechanism (i.e., ossicles), nerve conduction is tested. For accuracy, audiometric evaluations are computerized and performed in a soundproof room. Responses are plotted on a graph known as an audiogram, which differentiates conductive from sensorineural hearing loss. Speech discrimination is also measured.

Tympanogram

A tympanogram, or impedance audiometry, measures middle ear muscle reflex to sound stimulation and compliance of the tympanic membrane by changing the air pressure in a sealed ear canal. Compliance is impaired with middle ear disease.

Auditory Brain Stem Response

The auditory brain stem response is a detectable electrical potential from cranial nerve VIII and the ascending auditory pathways of the brain stem in response to sound stimulation. Electrodes are placed on the patient's scalp and on each earlobe (Fischbach & Dunning, 2015). Acoustic stimuli (e.g., clicks) are made in the ear. The resulting electrophysiologic measurements can determine at which decibel level a patient hears and whether there are any impairments along the nerve pathways (e.g., tumour on cranial nerve VIII). Patients are instructed to wash and rinse their hair prior to this study but to avoid applying any other hair product. Auditory brain stem response assessment should be used in conjunction with audiometry for the most accurate results (Bhattacharyya & Meyers, 2015).

Electronystagmography

Electronystagmography is the measurement and graphic recording of the changes in electrical potentials created by eye movements during spontaneous, positional, or calorically evoked nystagmus. It identifies degree, velocity, and direction of nystagmus. It is also used to assess the oculomotor and vestibular systems and their corresponding interaction. Electronystagmography differentiates peripheral from central pathologic conditions. It helps in diagnosing conditions such as Ménière's disease and tumours of the internal auditory canal or posterior fossa. Any vestibular suppressants, such as sedatives, tranquilizers, antihistamines, and alcohol, are withheld for 24 hours before testing. No solid food is eaten prior to the test in case of vomiting. The test is contraindicated in the presence of perforations or an implanted pacemaker (Fischbach & Dunning, 2015).

Platform Posturography

Platform posturography is used to investigate postural control capabilities, such as **vertigo**. The integration of visual, vestibular, and proprioceptive cues (i.e., sensory integration) with motor response output and coordination of the lower limbs is tested. The patient stands on a platform, surrounded by a screen, and different conditions such as a moving platform with a moving screen or a stationary platform with a moving screen are presented. The responses from the patient on six different conditions are measured and indicate which of the anatomic systems may be impaired. Preparation for the testing is the same as for electronystagmography.

Sinusoidal Harmonic Acceleration

Sinusoidal harmonic acceleration, or a rotary chair, is used to assess the vestibulo-ocular system by analyzing compensatory eye movements in response to the clockwise and counterclockwise rotation of the chair.

Although such testing cannot identify the side of the lesion in unilateral disease, it helps to identify disease (e.g., Ménière's disease and tumours of the auditory canal) and evaluate the course of recovery. The same patient preparation is required as that for electronystagmography.

Middle Ear Endoscopy

Using endoscopes with very small diameters and acute angles, the ear can be examined endoscopically by an endoscopist specializing in otolaryngology. Middle ear endoscopy is performed safely and effectively as an office procedure to evaluate suspected perilymphatic fistula and new-onset conductive hearing loss, the anatomy of the round window before transtympanic treatment of Ménière's disease, and the tympanic cavity before ear surgery to treat chronic middle ear and mastoid infections.

The tympanic membrane is anesthetized topically for about 10 minutes. Then, the external auditory canal is irrigated with sterile normal saline solution. With the aid of a microscope, a tympanotomy is created with a laser beam or a myringotomy knife so that the endoscope can be inserted into the middle ear cavity. Video and photo documentation can be accomplished through the scope.

Hearing Loss

More than 3 million Canadians have some form of hearing impairment. The Canadian Association of the Deaf (CAD) (2012) estimates that there are 350,000 Canadians who are culturally deaf and 3.15 million Canadians who are hard of hearing. Culturally deaf refers to Canadians who do not consider themselves disabled because of the absence of hearing (CAD). Many hearing impaired individuals can be helped with medical or surgical therapies, or with a hearing aid. By the year 2026, Canada's population is expected to be approximately 35 million people, with 20% of the population being 65 years or older (Government of Canada, 2014). The cost of hearing loss to the Canadian economy is estimated at $18 billion per year. Of concern internationally is the evidence for early hearing loss in young people.

Conductive hearing loss usually results from an external ear disorder, such as impacted cerumen, or a middle ear disorder, such as otitis media or otosclerosis. In such instances, the efficient transmission of sound by air to the inner ear is interrupted. A sensorineural loss involves damage to the cochlea or vestibulocochlear nerve.

Mixed hearing loss and functional hearing loss also may occur. The patient with mixed hearing loss has conductive *and* sensorineural loss, resulting from dysfunction of air and bone conduction. A functional (or psychogenic) hearing loss is nonorganic and unrelated to detectable structural changes in the hearing mechanisms; it is usually a manifestation of an emotional disturbance.

Clinical Manifestations

Early manifestations of hearing impairment and loss may include tinnitus, increasing inability to hear in groups, and a need to turn up the volume of the television. Hearing impairment can also trigger changes in attitude, the ability to communicate, the awareness of surroundings, and even the ability to protect oneself, thus affecting the person's quality of life. In a classroom, a student with impaired hearing may be disinterested, inattentive, and have failing grades. A person at home may feel isolated because of an inability to hear the clock chime, doorbell ring, refrigerator hum, birds sing, or traffic pass. A pedestrian with a hearing impairment may attempt to cross the street and fail to hear an approaching car. People with hearing impairments may miss parts of a conversation. Many people are unaware of their gradual hearing impairment. Often, it is the people with whom the individual communicates who recognize the impairment first (Chart 61-2).

For various reasons, some people with hearing loss refuse to seek medical attention or wear a hearing aid. Others feel self-conscious wearing a hearing aid. Insightful people generally ask those with whom they are trying to communicate to let them know whether difficulties in communication exist. These attitudes and behaviours are

CHART 61-2

Assessment: Symptoms & Signs of Hearing Loss

Speech deterioration: The person who slurs words or drops word endings, or produces flat-sounding speech, may not be hearing correctly. The ears guide the voice, both in loudness and in pronunciation.

Fatigue: If a person tires easily when listening to conversation or to a speech, fatigue may be the result of straining to hear. Under these circumstances, the person may become irritable very easily.

Indifference: It is easy for the person who cannot hear what others say to become depressed and disinterested in life in general.

Social withdrawal: Not being able to hear what is going on causes the person who is hearing-impaired to withdraw from situations that might prove embarrassing.

Insecurity: Lack of self-confidence and fear of mistakes create a feeling of insecurity in many people who are hearing-impaired. No one likes to say the wrong thing or do anything that might appear foolish.

Indecision and procrastination: Loss of self-confidence makes it increasingly difficult for a person who is hearing-impaired to make decisions.

Suspiciousness: The person who is hearing-impaired, who often hears only part of what is being said, may suspect that others are talking about him or her or that portions of the conversation are deliberately spoken softly so that he or she will not hear them.

False pride: The person who is hearing-impaired wants to conceal the hearing loss and thus often pretends to be hearing when he or she actually is not.

Loneliness and unhappiness: Although everyone wishes for quiet now and then, enforced silence can be boring and even somewhat frightening. People with a hearing loss often feel isolated.

Tendency to dominate the conversation: Many people who are hearing-impaired tend to dominate the conversation, knowing that as long as it is centred on them and they can control it, they are not so likely to be embarrassed by some mistake.

be taken into account when counselling patients who need hearing assistance. The decision to wear a hearing aid is a personal one that is affected by attitudes and behaviours.

Prevention

Many environmental factors have an adverse effect on the auditory system and over time result in permanent sensorineural hearing loss. The World Health Organization (WHO, 2014) estimates that there are 360 million people with disabling hearing impairment and that worldwide, about a third of all people who are over 65 years of age are affected negatively by hearing impairment. Half of hearing loss and deafness is preventable. Noise exposure is the major preventable cause of hearing impairment.

Noise (unwanted, unavoidable sound) has been identified as one of the environmental hazards of the 21st century. The sheer volume of noise that surrounds us daily has increased from a simple annoyance into a potentially dangerous source of physical and psychological damage.

CHART 61-3

Risk Factors: Hearing Loss

- Family history of sensorineural impairment
- Congenital malformations of the cranial structure (ear)
- Low birth weight (<1,500 g)
- Use of ototoxic medications (e.g., gentamicin, loop diuretics)
- Recurrent ear infections
- Bacterial meningitis
- Chronic exposure to loud noises, commonly occupational and recreational
- Perforation of the tympanic membrane

Noise-induced hearing loss (NIHL) is increasing in Canadians, especially in younger persons.

In terms of physical impact, loud, persistent noise has been found to cause constriction of peripheral blood vessels, increased blood pressure and heart rate (because of increased secretion of adrenalin), and increased gastrointestinal activity. Additional research is needed to address the overall effects of noise on the human body. It seems unequivocal that a quiet environment would be more conducive to peace of mind. A person who is ill feels more at ease when noise is kept to a minimum. Numerous factors contribute to hearing loss (Chart 61-3).

The term *noise-induced hearing loss* is used to describe hearing loss that results from excessive exposure to loud sounds (both intensity and length of time exposed), such as heavy machinery, engines, and artillery. *Acoustic trauma* refers to the hearing loss caused by a single exposure to an extremely intense noise, such as an explosion. Usually, NIHL occurs at a high frequency (around 4,000 Hz). With continued noise exposure, hearing loss can become more severe and include adjacent frequencies. The minimum noise level known to cause NIHL regardless of duration, is about 85 to 90 dB.

In Canadian jurisdictions, the exposure limit to noise for 8 hours/day for 5 days/wk is 85 dB in all jurisdictions except two which permit somewhat higher levels (Canadian Centre for Occupational Health and Safety [CCOHS], 2014). Several industries (e.g., carpentry, plumbing, printing, and mining) and workplaces (e.g., shipyards, airports, breweries, and paper mills) have exposures close to or higher than these levels. Musicians and hunters are also at risk. Some equipment, such as power tools, woodworking saws, engines, and compressors, exceeds the exposure limit. For example, the sound levels from cutting machines in sawmills can reach 105 dB. The CCOHS requires that workers wear ear protection to prevent NIHL when exposed to noise above the legal limits. No medications protect against NIHL; hearing loss is permanent because the hair cells in the organ of Corti are destroyed. Ear protection against noise is the most effective preventive measure available.

Gerontologic Considerations

About 30% of people 65 years and older, and 50% of people 75 years and older have hearing difficulties. With aging, changes occur in the ear that may eventually lead to hearing deficits. Although few changes occur in the external ear, cerumen tends to become harder and drier, posing a greater chance of impaction. In the middle ear, the tympanic membrane may atrophy or become sclerotic. In the inner ear, cells at the base of the cochlea degenerate. A familial predisposition to sensorineural hearing loss is also seen, manifested by a loss in the ability to hear high-frequency sounds, followed in time by the loss of middle and lower frequencies. The term **presbycusis** describes this progressive hearing loss (Eliopoulos, 2018).

As Canadians become older, a major and serious concern relates to driving ability. Researchers at the National Centre for Audiology in Ontario studied communication difficulties when older adults are driving. They identified four themes related to driving: communication and focus, the importance of hearing conversation, the impact of missing the conversation, and responses to breakdowns in communication.

In addition to age-related changes, other factors can affect hearing in the older population, such as lifelong exposure to loud noises (e.g., jets, guns, heavy machinery, circular saws). Certain medications, such as aminoglycoside antibiotics and salicylates, have ototoxic effects when renal changes (e.g., in the older person) result in delayed medication excretion and increased levels of the medications in the blood. Some older people take quinine for treatment of leg cramps which can cause a hearing loss. Psychogenic factors and other disease processes (e.g., diabetes) also may be partially responsible for sensorineural hearing loss.

When a hearing loss occurs, an evaluation is warranted. Even with the best medical care, the individual must learn to adjust to various degrees of hearing impairment. Care of older patients includes recognizing emotional reactions related to hearing loss, such as suspicion of others because of an inability to hear adequately; frustration and anger, with repeated statements such as, "I didn't hear what you said"; and feelings of insecurity because of the inability to hear the telephone, doorbell, or alarms.

Medical Management

If a hearing loss is permanent, untreatable with medical or surgical intervention, or the patient elects not to have surgery, aural rehabilitation (discussed at the end of the chapter) may be beneficial.

Nursing Management

If you understand the different types of hearing loss, you will be more successful in adopting a communication style to fit the patient's needs. Trying to speak in a loud voice to an individual who cannot hear high-frequency sounds only makes understanding more difficult. In contrast, strategies such as talking into the less-impaired ear and using gestures and facial expressions can help (Chart 61-4).

A major issue for many deaf and hearing-impaired people is that they have other health problems that often do not receive attention, in large part because of communication problems with their health care practitioners. To effectively meet the health care needs of these patients, practitioners are legally obligated to make accommodations for the patient's inability to hear. Providing interpreters for those who can communicate through sign language is essential in many situations so that the practitioner can effectively communicate with the patient.

During health care and screening procedures, the practitioner (e.g., dentist, physician, nurse) must be aware that patients who are deaf or hearing impaired are unable to read lips, see a signer, or read written materials in the dark rooms required during some diagnostic tests. The same situation exists if the practitioner is wearing a mask or is not in sight (e.g., x-ray studies, magnetic resonance imaging [MRI], colonoscopy).

It is essential to work with patients who are deaf or hearing impaired and their families, to identify workable and effective means of communication. Equally important is to serve as catalyst and advocate throughout the health care system to ensure that accommodations are made to meet the communication needs of these patients.

CHART 61-4

Guidelines for Communicating With People Who Are Hearing Impaired

For the person who is hearingimpaired whose speech is difficult to understand:

- Devote full attention to what the person is saying. Look and listen—do not try to attend to another task while listening.
- Engage the speaker in conversation when it is possible for you to anticipate the replies. This enables you to become accustomed to any peculiarities in speech patterns.
- Try to determine the essential context of what is being said; you can often fill in the details from context.
- Do not try to appear as if you understand if you do not.
- If you cannot understand at all or have serious doubt about your ability to understand what is being said, have the person write the message rather than risk misunderstanding. Having the person repeat the message in speech, after you know its content, also aids you in becoming accustomed to the person's pattern of speech.

For the person who is hearingimpaired who speech reads:

- When speaking, always face the person as directly as possible.
- Make sure your face is as clearly visible as possible. Locate yourself so that your face is well lighted; avoid being silhouetted against strong light. Do not obscure the person's view of your mouth in any way; avoid talking with any object held in your mouth.
- Be sure that the patient knows the topic or subject before going ahead with what you plan to say. This enables the person to use contextual clues in speech reading.
- Speak slowly and distinctly, pausing more frequently than you would usually.
- If you question whether some important direction or instruction has been understood, check to be certain that the patient has the full meaning of your message.
- If for any reason your mouth must be covered (as with a mask) and you must direct or instruct the patient, write the message.

Conditions of the External Ear

Cerumen Impaction

Cerumen regularly accumulates in the external canal in various amounts and colours. Although wax does not usually need to be removed, impaction occasionally occurs, causing **otalgia** (a sensation of fullness or pain in the ear), with or without a hearing loss. Accumulation of cerumen is especially significant in the geriatric population as a cause of hearing deficit (Eliopoulos, 2018). Attempts to clear the external auditory canal with matches, hairpins, cotton-tipped applicators, and other implements are dangerous because trauma to the skin, infection, and damage to the tympanic membrane can occur.

Management

Cerumen can be removed by irrigation, suction, or instrumentation. Unless the patient has a perforated eardrum or an inflamed external ear (otitis externa), gentle irrigation usually helps to remove impacted cerumen, particularly if it is not tightly packed in the external auditory canal. For successful removal, the water stream must flow behind the obstructing cerumen to move it first laterally and then out of the canal. To prevent injury, the lowest effective pressure should be used. If the eardrum behind the impaction is perforated, water can enter the middle ear, producing acute vertigo and infection. If irrigation is unsuccessful, direct visual, mechanical removal can be performed on a cooperative patient by a trained health care professional.

> **NURSING ALERT**
>
> **Warm water (never cold or hot) and gentle (not forceful) irrigation should be used to remove cerumen. Irrigation that is too forceful can cause perforation of the tympanic membrane, and ice water causes vomiting.**

Instilling a few drops of warmed glycerin, mineral oil, or half-strength hydrogen peroxide into the ear canal for 30 minutes can soften cerumen before its removal. Ceruminolytic agents, such as carbamide peroxide (Debrox), are available; irrigation following use is necessary, as these compounds may cause an allergic dermatitis reaction. The use of any softening solution two or three times a day for several days is generally sufficient. If the cerumen cannot be dislodged by these methods, a cerumen curette, aural suction, and a binocular microscope for magnification can be used by trained professionals.

Foreign Bodies

Some objects are inserted intentionally into the ear by adults who may have been trying to clean the external canal or relieve itching or by children who introduce the objects. Other objects, such as insects, peas, beans, pebbles, toys, and beads, may enter or be introduced into the ear canal. In either case, the effects may range from no symptoms to profound pain and decreased hearing.

Management

Removing a foreign body from the external auditory canal can be quite challenging. The three standard methods for removing foreign bodies are the same as those for removing cerumen: irrigation, suction, and instrumentation. The contraindications for irrigation are also the same. Foreign vegetable bodies and insects tend to swell, precluding irrigation. Usually, an insect can be dislodged by instilling mineral oil, which will kill the insect and allow it to be removed.

Attempts to remove any foreign body from the external canal may be dangerous in unskilled hands. The object may be pushed completely into the bony portion of the canal, lacerating the skin and perforating the tympanic membrane. In difficult cases, the foreign body may have to be extracted in the operating room with the patient under general anesthesia.

External Otitis (Otitis Externa)

External otitis (otitis externa) refers to an inflammation of the external auditory canal. Causes include water in the ear canal (e.g., swimmer's ear); trauma to the skin of the ear canal, permitting entrance of organisms into the tissues; and systemic conditions, such as vitamin deficiency and endocrine disorders. Bacterial or fungal infections are most frequently encountered. The most common bacterial pathogens associated with external otitis are *Staphylococcus aureus* and *Pseudomonas* sp. The most common fungus isolated in both healthy and infected ears is *Aspergillus* (Grossman & Porth, 2014). External otitis is often caused by a dermatosis such as psoriasis, eczema, or seborrheic dermatitis. Even allergic reactions to hair spray, hair dye, and permanent wave lotions can cause dermatitis, which clears when the offending agent is removed.

Clinical Manifestations

Patients usually report pain; discharge from the external auditory canal; aural tenderness (usually not present in middle ear infections); and occasionally fever, cellulitis, and lymphadenopathy. Other symptoms may include pruritus and hearing loss or a feeling of fullness. On otoscopic examination, the ear canal is erythematous (reddened) and edematous (swollen). Discharge may be yellow or green and foul smelling. In fungal infections, the hairlike black spores may even be visible.

Medical Management

The principles of therapy are aimed at relieving the discomfort, reducing the swelling of the ear canal, and eradicating the infection. Patients may require analgesics for the first 48 to 96 hours. If the tissues of the external canal are edematous, a wick is inserted to keep the canal open so that liquid medications (e.g., Burow's solution, antibiotic otic preparations) can be introduced (Grossman & Porth, 2014). These medications may be administered by dropper at room temperature and usually are a combination of antibiotic and corticosteroid agents to soothe the inflamed tissues (Grossman & Porth, 2014). For cellulitis or fever, systemic antibiotics may be prescribed; for fungal disorders, antifungal agents are prescribed.

CHART 61-5

Patient Education: Prevention of Otitis Externa

The nurse instructs the patient to:

- Protect the external canal when swimming, showering, or washing hair. Use ear plugs or place a cotton ball covered in petrolatum jelly in the ear, and wear a swim cap. The external canal may be dried afterward with a hair dryer on low heat.
- Place alcohol drops in the external canal to act as an astringent to help prevent infection after water exposure.
- Prevent trauma to the external canal. Procedures, foreign objects (e.g., bobby pin), scratching, or any other trauma to the canal that breaks the skin integrity may cause infection.
- Be aware that if otitis externa is diagnosed, refrain from any water sport activity for approximately 7 to 10 days to allow the canal to heal completely. Recurrence is highly likely unless you allow the external canal to heal completely.

Nursing Management

Teach patients not to clean the external auditory canal with cotton-tipped applicators, to avoid swimming, and not to allow water to enter the ear when shampooing or showering. They can place a cotton ball covered in a water-insoluble gel such as petroleum jelly in the ear as a barrier to water contamination. Patients can prevent infection by using antiseptic otic preparations after swimming (e.g., Swim Ear, Ear Dry), unless there is a history of tympanic membrane perforation or a current ear infection (see Chart 61-5).

Malignant External Otitis

Malignant external otitis (temporal bone osteomyelitis) is a serious, although rare, external ear infection. This is a progressive, debilitating, and occasionally fatal infection of the external auditory canal, the surrounding tissue, and the base of the skull. *Pseudomonas aeruginosa* is usually the infecting organism in patients with low resistance to infection (e.g., patients with diabetes). Successful treatment includes control of the diabetes, administration of antibiotics (usually intravenously), and aggressive local wound care. Standard parenteral antibiotic treatment includes the combination of an antipseudomonal agent and an aminoglycoside antibiotic, both of which have potentially serious side effects. Because aminoglycosides are nephrotoxic and ototoxic, serum aminoglycoside levels and renal and auditory function must be monitored during therapy. Local wound care includes limited debridement of the infected tissue, including bone and cartilage, depending on the extent of the infection.

Masses of the External Ear

Exostoses are small, hard, bony protrusions found in the lower posterior bony portion of the ear canal and which usually occur bilaterally. The skin covering the exostosis is healthy. Exostoses are commonly considered to result from exposure to cold, wet, and windy conditions, as in scuba diving or surfing. The usual treatment, if any, is surgical excision.

Malignant tumours also may be found in the external ear. Most common are basal cell carcinomas on the pinna and squamous cell carcinomas in the ear canal. If untreated, squamous cell carcinoma may spread through the temporal bone, causing facial nerve paralysis and hearing loss. Carcinomas must be treated surgically.

Gaping Earring Puncture

Gaping earring puncture results from wearing heavy pierced earrings for a long time, an infection, or a reaction from impurities in the earring. One or more gaping punctures may result from wearing more than one earring. Whatever the cause, this deformity can only be corrected surgically. The edges of the perforations are excised on the lateral and medial surfaces of the earlobe. Next, the entire tract is removed, joining the above two incisions and resulting in a much larger defect that is closed separately on each surface.

CONDITIONS OF THE MIDDLE EAR

Tympanic Membrane Perforation

Perforation of the tympanic membrane is usually caused by infection or trauma. Sources of trauma include skull fracture, explosive injury, or a severe blow to the ear. Less frequently, perforation is caused by foreign objects (e.g., cotton-tipped applicators, bobby pins, keys) that have been pushed too far into the external auditory canal. In addition to tympanic membrane perforation, injury to the ossicles and even the inner ear may result from this type of action. Attempts by patients to clear the external auditory canal should be discouraged. During infection, the tympanic membrane can rupture if the pressure in the middle ear exceeds the atmospheric pressure in the external auditory canal.

Medical Management

Although most tympanic membrane perforations heal spontaneously within weeks after rupture, some may take several months to heal. Some perforations persist because scar tissue grows over the edges of the perforation, preventing extension of the epithelial cells across the margins and final healing. In the case of a head injury or temporal bone fracture, a patient is observed for evidence of cerebrospinal fluid **otorrhea** or **rhinorrhea**—a clear, watery drainage from the ear or nose, respectively. While healing, the ear must be protected from water.

Surgical Management

Perforations that do not heal on their own may require surgery. The decision to perform a **tympanoplasty** (surgical repair of the tympanic membrane) is usually based on the need to prevent potential infection from water entering the ear or the desire to improve the patient's hearing. Performed on an outpatient basis, tympanoplasty may involve a variety of surgical techniques. In all techniques, tissue is placed across the perforation to allow healing. Surgery is usually successful in closing the perforation permanently and improving hearing.

Acute Otitis Media

Acute otitis media is an acute infection of the middle ear, usually lasting less than 6 weeks. The pathogens that cause acute otitis media are usually *Streptococcus pneumoniae*, *Haemophilus influenzae*, and *Moraxella catarrhalis*. These enter the middle ear after eustachian tube dysfunction caused by obstruction related to upper respiratory infections, inflammation of surrounding structures (e.g., sinusitis, adenoid hypertrophy), or allergic reactions (e.g., allergic rhinitis) (Grossman & Porth, 2014). Bacteria can enter the eustachian tube from contaminated secretions in the nasopharynx, and the middle ear from a tympanic membrane perforation. Purulent exudate is usually present in the middle ear, resulting in a conductive hearing loss.

Clinical Manifestations

The symptoms of otitis media vary with the severity of the infection. The condition, usually unilateral in adults, may be accompanied by otalgia. The pain is relieved after spontaneous perforation or therapeutic incision of the tympanic membrane. Other symptoms may include drainage from the ear, fever, and hearing loss. On otoscopic examination, the external auditory canal appears healthy. The patient reports no pain with movement of the auricle. The tympanic membrane is erythematous and often bulging. Table 61-3 differentiates acute external otitis from acute otitis media.

Risk factors for acute otitis media include age (less than 12 months), chronic upper respiratory infections, medical conditions that predispose to ear infections (Down syndrome, cystic fibrosis, cleft palate), and chronic exposure to secondhand cigarette smoke.

Medical Management

The outcome of acute otitis media depends on the efficacy of therapy (the prescribed dose of an oral antibiotic and the duration of therapy), the virulence of the bacteria, and the physical status of the patient. With early and appropriate broad-spectrum antibiotic therapy, otitis media may resolve with no serious sequelae. If drainage occurs, an antibiotic otic preparation is usually prescribed. The condition may become subacute (lasting 3 weeks to 3 months), with persistent purulent discharge from the ear. Rarely does permanent hearing loss occur (Grossman & Porth, 2014). Secondary complications involving the mastoid and other serious intracranial complications, such as meningitis or brain abscess, although rare, can occur.

Surgical Management

An incision in the tympanic membrane is known as **myringotomy or tympanotomy**. The tympanic membrane is numbed with a local anesthetic such as phenol or by iontophoresis (electrical current flows through a lidocaine/epinephrine solution to numb the ear canal and tympanic membrane). The procedure is painless and takes less than 15 minutes. Under microscopic guidance, an incision is made through the tympanic membrane to relieve pressure and drain serous or purulent fluid from the middle ear.

Usually, this procedure is unnecessary for treating acute otitis media, but it may be performed if pain persists. Myringotomy also allows the drainage to be analyzed (by culture and sensitivity testing) so that the infecting organism can be identified and appropriate antibiotic therapy prescribed. The incision heals within 24 to 72 hours.

If episodes of acute otitis media recur and there is no contraindication, a ventilating, or pressure-equalizing, tube may be inserted. The ventilating tube, which temporarily takes the place of the eustachian tube in equalizing pressure, is retained for 6 to 18 months. The ventilating tube is then extruded with skin migration of the tympanic membrane, and the hole heals in nearly every case. Ventilating tubes are more commonly used to treat recurrent episodes of acute otitis media in children than in adults.

Serous Otitis Media

Serous otitis media (**middle ear effusion**) implies fluid, without evidence of active infection, in the middle ear. In theory, this fluid results from a negative pressure in the middle ear caused by eustachian tube obstruction, a condition found primarily in children. When it occurs in adults, an underlying cause for the eustachian tube dysfunction must be sought. Middle ear effusion is frequently seen in patients after radiation therapy or barotrauma, and in patients with eustachian tube dysfunction from a concurrent upper respiratory infection or allergy. Barotrauma results from sudden pressure changes in the middle ear

TABLE 61-3 Clinical Features of Otitis

Feature	Acute Otitis Externa	Acute Otitis Media
Otorrhea	May or may not be present	Present if tympanic membrane perforates; discharge is profuse
Otalgia	Persistent, may awaken patient at night	Relieved if tympanic membrane ruptures
Aural tenderness	Present on palpation of auricle or tragus	Usually absent
Systemic symptoms	Absent	Fever, upper respiratory infection, rhinitis
Edema of external auditory canal	Present	Absent
Tympanic membrane	May appear healthy	Erythema, bulging, may be perforated
Hearing loss	Conductive type	Conductive type

caused by changes in barometric pressure, as in scuba diving or airplane descent. A carcinoma (e.g., nasopharyngeal cancer) obstructing the eustachian tube should be ruled out in an adult with persistent unilateral serous otitis media.

Clinical Manifestations

Patients may report hearing loss, fullness in the ear or a sensation of congestion and perhaps even popping and crackling noises which occur as the eustachian tube attempts to open. The tympanic membrane appears dull on otoscopy and air bubbles may be visualized in the middle ear. Usually, the audiogram shows a conductive hearing loss.

Management

Serous otitis media does not need to be treated medically unless infection occurs (acute otitis media). If the hearing loss associated with middle ear effusion is problematic for the patient, a myringotomy can be performed, and a tube may be placed to keep the middle ear ventilated. Corticosteroids in small doses sometimes decrease the edema of the eustachian tube in cases of barotrauma. Decongestants have not proved effective. A Valsalva manoeuvre which forcibly opens the eustachian tube by increasing nasopharyngeal pressure may be cautiously performed. Performing the Valsalva manoeuvre may cause worsening pain or perforation of the tympanic membrane.

Chronic Otitis Media

Chronic otitis media is the result of repeated episodes of acute otitis media causing irreversible tissue pathology and persistent perforation of the tympanic membrane. Chronic infections of the middle ear damage the tympanic membrane, destroy the ossicles, and involve the mastoid. Before the discovery of antibiotics, infections of the mastoid were life threatening. The use of medications in acute otitis media has made acute mastoiditis a rare condition in developed countries.

Clinical Manifestations

Symptoms may be minimal, with varying degrees of hearing loss and the presence of a persistent or intermittent, foul-smelling otorrhea. Pain is not usually experienced, except in cases of acute mastoiditis, when the postauricular area is tender to the touch and may be erythematous and edematous. Otoscopic evaluation of the tympanic membrane may show a perforation, and cholesteatoma can be identified as a white mass behind the tympanic membrane or coming through to the external canal from a perforation.

Cholesteatoma is an ingrowth of the skin of the external layer of the eardrum into the middle ear. It is generally caused by a chronic retraction pocket of the tympanic membrane, creating a persistently high negative pressure of the middle ear. The skin forms a sac that fills with degenerated skin and sebaceous materials. The sac can attach to the structures of the middle ear or mastoid, or both.

Chronic otitis media can cause chronic mastoiditis and lead to the formation of cholesteatoma. It can occur in the middle ear, mastoid cavity, or both, often dictating the type of surgery to be performed. If untreated, cholesteatoma will continue to enlarge, possibly causing damage to the facial nerve and horizontal canal, and destruction of other surrounding structures.

Cholesteatoma alone usually does not cause pain; if treatment or surgery is delayed, the cholesteatoma may destroy structures of the temporal bone. These fast-growing tumours may cause severe sequelae such as hearing loss or neurologic disorders. Congenital cholesteatomas are usually found in children and may cause severe bone loss of the incus. Cholesteatomas found in older patients generally develop in the external canal.

Cholesteatomas may be asymptomatic or may cause hearing loss, facial pain and paralysis, tinnitus, or vertigo. Audiometric tests often show a conductive or mixed hearing loss. Based on presenting symptoms, diagnosis may be made by visual examination or by computed tomography (CT) or MRI. Therapy includes treatment of the acute infection and surgical removal of the mass to restore hearing.

Medical Management

Local treatment of chronic otitis media consists of careful suctioning of the ear under microscopic guidance. Instillation of antibiotic drops or application of antibiotic powder is used to treat a purulent discharge. Systemic antibiotics are usually not prescribed except in cases of acute infection.

Surgical Management

Surgical procedures, including tympanoplasty, ossiculoplasty, and mastoidectomy, are used after medical treatments are determined to be ineffective.

Tympanoplasty

The most common surgical procedure for chronic otitis media is tympanoplasty (surgical reconstruction of the tympanic membrane). Reconstruction of the ossicles may also be required. The purposes of a tympanoplasty are to re-establish middle ear function, close the perforation, prevent recurrent infection, and improve hearing.

There are five types of tympanoplasty. The simplest surgical procedure, type I (myringoplasty), is designed to close a perforation in the tympanic membrane. The other procedures, types II through V, involve more extensive repair of middle ear structures. The structures and the degree of involvement can differ, but all tympanoplasty procedures include restoring the continuity of the sound conduction mechanism.

Tympanoplasty is performed through the external auditory canal with a transcanal approach or postauricular incision. Contents of the middle ear are carefully inspected, and the ossicular chain is evaluated. Ossicular interruption is most frequent in chronic otitis media, but problems of reconstruction can also occur with malformations of the middle ear and ossicular dislocations due to head injuries. Dramatic improvement in hearing can result from closure of a perforation and re-establishment of the ossicles. Surgery is usually performed in an outpatient environment under moderate sedation or general anesthesia.

Ossiculoplasty

Many people use the term *tympanoplasty* to include **ossiculoplasty**, or surgical reconstruction of the middle ear bones to restore hearing. Prostheses made of materials such as Teflon, stainless steel, and hydroxyapatite are used to reconnect the ossicles, thereby re-establishing the sound conduction mechanism. Extensive damage lowers the success rate for restoring hearing.

Mastoidectomy

The objectives of mastoid surgery are to remove the cholesteatoma, gain access to diseased structures, and create a dry and healthy ear. If possible, the ossicles are reconstructed during the initial surgical procedure. Occasionally, advanced disease dictates that this be performed as part of a planned second-stage operation.

A mastoidectomy is usually performed through a postauricular incision. Infection is eliminated by removing the mastoid air cells. A second mastoidectomy may be necessary to check for recurrent or residual cholesteatoma and the hearing mechanism may be reconstructed at this time. The success rate for correcting this conductive hearing loss is approximately 75%. Surgery is usually performed in an outpatient setting. Although infrequently injured, the facial nerve, which runs through the middle ear and mastoid, is at some risk for injury during mastoid surgery. As the patient awakens from anesthesia, report any evidence of facial paresis to the physician. The patient has a mastoid pressure dressing, which can be removed 24 to 48 hours after surgery.

Nursing Process

The Patient Undergoing Mastoid Surgery

Although several otologic surgical procedures are performed under moderate sedation, mastoid surgery is performed using general anesthesia.

Assessment

The health history includes a complete description of the ear condition, including infection, otalgia, otorrhea, hearing loss, and vertigo. Collect data about the duration and intensity of the condition, its causes, and previous treatments. Obtain information about other health concerns, all medications that the patient is taking, allergies, and family history of ear disease.

Physical assessment includes observation for erythema, edema, otorrhea, lesions, and characteristics such as odour and colour of discharge. Review the results of the audiogram.

Nursing Priorities

Based on assessment data, the patient's major nursing priorities may include the following:

- Anxiety due to surgical procedure and the potential related complications
- Pain due to surgery
- Increase odds of infection after mastoidectomy and placement of grafts, prostheses, electrodes
- Decreased auditory sensory perception due to ear disorder, surgery, or packing
- Increase odds of trauma due to balance difficulties or vertigo during immediate postoperative period
- Distorted sensory perception related to potential damage to facial nerve (cranial nerve VII) and chorda tympani nerve
- Breakdown in skin integrity due to ear surgery, incisions, and graft sites
- Lack of knowledge about mastoid disease, surgical procedure, and postoperative care and expectations

Planning and Goals

The major goals of caring for a patient undergoing mastoidectomy include reduction of anxiety; freedom from pain and discomfort; prevention of infection; stable or improved hearing and communication; absence of injury from vertigo; absence of or adjustment to sensory or perceptual alterations; return of skin integrity; and increased knowledge regarding the disease, surgical procedure, and postoperative care.

Nursing Interventions

Reducing Anxiety

Reinforce the information that the otologic surgeon has discussed with the patient, including anesthesia, the location of the incision (postauricular), and expected surgical results (e.g., hearing, balance, taste, facial movement). Encourage the patient to discuss any anxieties and concerns about the surgery.

Relieving Pain

Although most patients report very little incisional pain after mastoid surgery, they do have some ear discomfort. Aural fullness or pressure after surgery is caused by residual blood or fluid in the middle ear. The prescribed analgesic may be taken for the first 24 hours after surgery and then only as needed. Instruct the patient in the use of and side effects of the medication.

A tympanoplasty may also be performed at the time of the mastoidectomy. A wick or external auditory canal packing is used after a tympanoplasty to stabilize the tympanic membrane. Inform patients that they may experience intermittent sharp, shooting pains in the ear for 2 to 3 weeks after surgery as the eustachian tube opens and allows air to enter the middle ear. Advise them to report constant, throbbing pain accompanied by fever which may indicate infection to the physician.

Preventing Infection

Measures are initiated to prevent infection in the operated ear. The external auditory canal wick, or packing, may be impregnated with an antibiotic solution before instillation. Administer prophylactic antibiotics as prescribed, and instruct the patient to prevent water from entering the external auditory canal for 6 weeks. A cotton ball or lamb's wool covered with a water-insoluble substance (e.g., petroleum jelly) and placed loosely in the ear canal usually prevents water contamination and is used when the patient showers or washes his or her hair or in any situations in which water may enter the ear. Keep the postauricular incision dry for 2 days. Report signs of infection such as an elevated temperature and purulent drainage. Some serosanguineous drainage from the external auditory canal is expected after surgery.

Improving Hearing and Communication

Hearing in the operated ear may be reduced for several weeks because of edema, accumulation of blood and tissue fluid in the middle ear, and dressings or packing. Initiate measures to improve hearing and communication, such as reducing environmental noise, facing the patient when speaking, speaking clearly and distinctly without shouting, providing good lighting if the patient relies on speech reading, and using nonverbal clues (e.g., facial expression, pointing, gestures) and other forms of communication. Instruct family members or significant others about effective ways to communicate with the patient. If the patient uses assistive hearing devices, one can be used in the unaffected ear.

Preventing Injury

Vertigo may occur after mastoid surgery if the semicircular canals or other areas of the inner ear are traumatized. This symptom is relatively uncommon after this type of ear surgery and usually is temporary. Antiemetics or antivertiginous medications (e.g., antihistamines) can be prescribed if a balance disturbance or vertigo occurs. Instruct the patient about the expected effects and potential side effects. Implement safety measures such as assisted ambulation to prevent falls. Instruct about safety measures being implemented at home to prevent falls and injury.

Preventing Altered Sensory Perception

Facial nerve injury is a potential, although rare, complication of mastoid surgery. Instruct the patient to report immediately any evidence of facial nerve (cranial nerve VII) weakness, such as drooping of the mouth on the operated side, slurred speech, decreased sensation, and difficulty swallowing. A more frequent occurrence is a temporary disturbance in the chorda tympani nerve, which is a small branch of the facial nerve that runs through the middle ear. Patients experience a taste disturbance and dry mouth on the side of surgery for several months until the nerve regenerates.

Promoting Wound Healing

Instruct the patient to avoid heavy lifting, straining, exertion, and nose blowing for 2 to 3 weeks after surgery to prevent dislodging the tympanic membrane graft or ossicular prosthesis.

CHART 61-6

Patient Education: Self-Care After Middle Ear or Mastoid Surgery

Postoperative instructions for patients who have had middle ear and mastoid surgery may vary among otolaryngologists. The nurse instructs the patient in the following general guidelines:

- Take antibiotics and other medications as prescribed.
- Avoid nose blowing for 2 to 3 weeks after surgery.
- Sneeze and cough with the mouth open for a few weeks after surgery.
- Avoid heavy lifting (>10 lb), straining, and bending over for a few weeks after surgery.
- Be aware that popping and crackling sensations in the operative ear are normal for approximately 3 to 5 weeks after surgery.
- Note that temporary hearing loss is normal in the operative ear due to fluid, blood, or packing in the ear.
- Report excessive or purulent ear drainage to the physician.
- Avoid getting water in the operative ear for 2 weeks after surgery. You may shampoo the hair 2 to 3 days postoperatively if the ear is protected from water by saturating a cotton ball with petrolatum jelly (or some other water-insoluble substance) and loosely placing it in the ear. If the postauricular suture line becomes wet, pat (not rub) the area and cover it with a thin layer of antibiotic ointment.

Promoting Home, Community-Based, and Transitional Care

EDUCATING PATIENTS ABOUT SELF-CARE. Instruct patients about prescribed medication therapy, such as analgesics, antivertiginous agents, and antihistamines for balance disturbance. Include information about the expected effects and potential side effects of the medication. Instruct patients about any activity restrictions. Advise regarding possible complications such as infection, facial nerve weakness, or taste disturbances, including the signs and symptoms to report immediately (Chart 61-6).

CONTINUING AND TRANSITIONAL CARE. Some patients, particularly older patients, who have had mastoid surgery may require the services of a home care nurse for a few days after returning home. In most cases, people find that assistance from a family member or a friend is sufficient. Caution the caregiver and patient that the patient may experience some vertigo and will therefore require help with ambulation to avoid falling. Advise them to report any symptoms of complications promptly to the surgeon. Stress the importance of scheduling and keeping follow-up appointments.

Evaluation

Expected patient outcomes may include the following:

1. Demonstrates reduced anxiety about surgical procedure
   a. Verbalizes and exhibits less stress, tension, and irritability
   b. Verbalizes acceptance of the results of surgery and adjustment to possible hearing impairment

2. Remains free of discomfort or pain
   a. Exhibits no facial grimacing, moaning, or crying, and reports absence of pain
   b. Uses analgesics appropriately
3. Demonstrates no signs or symptoms of infection
   a. Has expected vital signs, including temperature
   b. Demonstrates absence of purulent drainage from external auditory canal
   c. Describes method for preventing water from contaminating packing
4. Exhibits signs that hearing has stabilized or improved
   a. Describes surgical goal for hearing and judges whether goal has been met
   b. Verbalizes that hearing has improved
5. Remains free of injury and trauma because of vertigo
   a. Reports absence of vertigo or balance disturbance
   b. Experiences no injury or fall
   c. Modifies environment to avoid falls (e.g., night-light, no clutter on stairs)
6. Adjusts to or remains free from altered sensory perception
   a. Reports no taste disturbance, mouth dryness, or facial weakness
7. Demonstrates no skin breakdown
   a. Lists ways to prevent dislodging graft or prosthesis
   b. Is aware of limitations in activities (e.g., bathing, lifting, air travel) and for how long
8. Verbalizes the reasons for and methods of care and treatment
   a. Shares knowledge with family about treatment protocol
   b. Describes treatment and time frame for recovery phase
   c. Discusses discharge plan formulated with nurse with regard to rest periods, medication, and activities permitted and restricted
   d. Lists symptoms that should be reported to health care personnel
   e. Keeps follow-up appointments

Otosclerosis

Otosclerosis involves the stapes and is thought to result from the formation of unwanted spongy bone, especially around the oval window, with resulting fixation of the stapes (Grossman & Porth, 2014). The efficient transmission of sound is prevented because the stapes cannot vibrate and carry the sound as conducted from the malleus and incus to the inner ear. Otosclerosis is more common in women, frequently hereditary, and may be worsened by pregnancy (Eliopoulos, 2018; Grossman & Porth, 2014).

Clinical Manifestations

The condition can involve one or both ears and manifests as a progressive conductive or mixed hearing loss. The patient may or may not report tinnitus. Otoscopic examination usually reveals a healthy tympanic membrane. Bone conduction is longer than air conduction on Rinne testing. The audiogram confirms conductive hearing loss or mixed loss, especially in the low frequencies.

Medical Management

There is no known nonsurgical treatment for otosclerosis. Some physicians believe the use of Florical (a fluoride supplement) can mature the undesirable spongy bone growth. Amplification with a hearing aid also may help (Grossman & Porth, 2014).

Surgical Management

One of two surgical procedures may be performed: either stapedectomy or stapedotomy. A stapedectomy, performed through the canal, involves removing the stapes superstructure and part of the footplate and inserting a tissue graft and a suitable prosthesis (Fig. 61-6).

The surgeon drills a small hole into the footplate to hold a prosthesis. Some surgeons elect to remove only a small part of the stapes footplate (stapedotomy). Regardless of the method used, the prosthesis bridges the gap between the incus and the inner ear, providing better sound conduction. Stapes surgery is very successful; in one study, approximately 87% of patients experienced resolution of conductive hearing loss (Lachance, Bussieres, & Cote, 2012). Balance disturbance or true vertigo, which rarely occurs in other middle ear surgical procedures, may occur during the postoperative period for several days; long-term balance disorders are rare.

Middle Ear Masses

Other than cholesteatoma, masses in the middle ear are rare. Glomus jugulare is a tumour that arises from the jugular bulb. A histologically identical tumour that arises from Jacobson's nerve and remains limited to the middle ear is known as a glomus tympanicum. On otoscopy, a red blemish on or behind the tympanic membrane is indicative of a glomus tumour. The treatment for glomus tumours is surgical excision, except in poor surgical candidates, in whom radiation therapy is used.

A facial nerve neuroma is a tumour on cranial nerve VII. This type of tumour usually is not visible on otoscopic examination but is suspected when a patient presents with a facial nerve paresis. X-ray evaluation is necessary to determine the site of the tumour along the facial nerve. The treatment is surgical removal.

Other less common conditions of the middle ear include (cholesterol) granuloma and tympanosclerosis. Cholesterol granuloma is an immune system reaction to the by-products of blood (cholesterol crystals) within the middle ear. Tympanosclerosis is a deposit of collagen and minerals within the middle ear that can harden around the ossicles as a result of repeated infections. It can also be found as plaque on the tympanic membrane which can decrease hearing.

CONDITIONS OF THE INNER EAR

Disorders of balance are common (NIDCD, 2015a), and dizziness may increase the risk of falls. The term **dizziness**

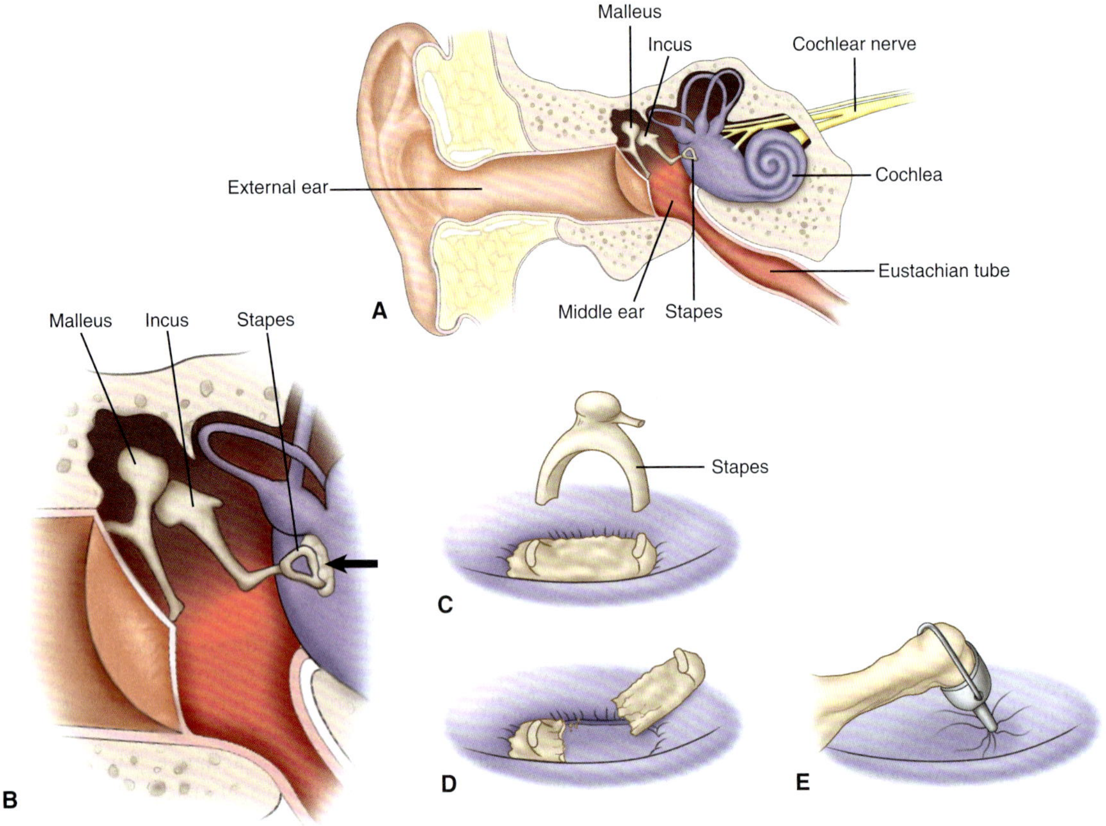

FIGURE 61-6. Stapedectomy for otosclerosis. **A.** Healthy anatomy. **B.** *Arrow* points to sclerotic process at the foot of the stapes. **C.** Stapes broken away surgically from its diseased base. The hole in the footplate provides an area where an instrument can grasp the plate. **D.** The footplate is removed from its base. Some otosclerotic tissue may remain, and tissue is placed over it. **E.** Robinson stainless steel prosthesis in position.

is used frequently by patients and health care providers to describe any altered sensation of orientation in space and is more commonly referred to as lightheadedness (Weber & Kelley, 2014).

Vertigo is defined as the misperception or illusion of motion of the person or the surroundings. Most people with vertigo describe a spinning sensation or say they feel as though objects are moving around them. Ataxia is a failure of muscular coordination and may be present in patients with vestibular disease. Syncope, fainting, and loss of consciousness are not forms of vertigo, nor are they characteristic of an ear problem; they usually indicate disease in the cardiovascular system.

Nystagmus is an involuntary rhythmic movement of the eyes that occurs when a person watches a rapidly moving object (e.g., through the side window of a moving car or train). When pathologic, it is an ocular disorder associated with vestibular dysfunction. Nystagmus can be horizontal, vertical, or rotary and can be caused by a disorder in the central or peripheral nervous system (Grossman & Porth, 2014).

Motion Sickness

Motion sickness is a disturbance of equilibrium caused by constant motion. For example, it can occur aboard a ship, on a bus, while riding on a merry-go-round or swing, or in the back seat of a car (Brainard & Gresham, 2014).

Clinical Manifestations

Motion sickness manifests itself in sweating, pallor, nausea, and vomiting caused by vestibular overstimulation. These manifestations may persist for several hours after the stimulation stops.

Management

Over-the-counter antihistamines, such as dimenhydrinate (Dramamine) or meclizine hydrochloride (Antivert), provide some relief of nausea and vomiting by blocking the conduction of the vestibular pathway of the inner ear. Anticholinergic medications, such as scopolamine patches, may also be effective because they antagonize the histamine response. These must be applied several hours before exposure to motion and replaced every 3 days (Brainard & Gresham, 2014). Side effects such as dry mouth and drowsiness occur with these medications, which may prove to be more troublesome than helpful. Potentially hazardous activities such as driving a car or operating heavy machinery should be avoided if the patient experiences drowsiness.

Ménière's Disease

PRACTICE & LEARN

Ménière's disease is an increased inner ear fluid balance caused by a malabsorption in the endolymphatic sac. Evidence indicates that many people with Ménière's disease may have a blockage in the endolymphatic duct. Regardless of the cause, **endolymphatic hydrops**, a dilation in the endolymphatic space, develops. Either increased pressure in the system or rupture of the inner ear membranes occurs, producing symptoms of Ménière's disease (Hansson & Brattmo, 2013).

Ménière's disease affects approximately 2 to 6 out of every 1,000 Canadians (MediResource, 2014). The disease has been reported in children as young as 4 years of age and in adults up to the 90s, but it is more common in adults and has an average age of onset between 40 and 60 years (Canadian Academy of Audiology, 2014). Ménière's disease appears to be equally common in both genders. Usually, one ear alone is affected, but 10% to 15% of affected individuals develop it in both ears (MediResource, 2014). Some patients report a positive family history for the disease.

Clinical Manifestations

Ménière's disease involves the following symptoms: fluctuating, progressive sensorineural hearing loss; tinnitus or a roaring sound; a feeling of pressure or fullness in the ear; and episodic, incapacitating vertigo, often accompanied by nausea and vomiting (Hansson & Brattmo, 2013). The effects of these symptoms range from a minor nuisance to extreme disability, especially if the attacks of vertigo are severe. At the onset of the disease, perhaps only one or two of the symptoms are manifested.

Some clinicians believe that there are two subsets of the disease, known as atypical Ménière's disease: cochlear and vestibular. Cochlear Ménière's disease is recognized as a fluctuating, progressive sensorineural hearing loss associated with tinnitus and aural pressure in the absence of vestibular symptoms or findings. Vestibular Ménière's disease is characterized as the occurrence of episodic vertigo associated with aural pressure but no cochlear symptoms. Patients may experience either cochlear or vestibular disease symptoms, but eventually all of these symptoms develop.

Assessment and Diagnostic Findings

Vertigo is usually the most troublesome symptom related to Ménière's disease. A careful history is taken to determine the frequency, duration, severity, and character of the vertigo attacks. Vertigo may last minutes to hours, possibly accompanied by nausea or vomiting. Patients also report diaphoresis and a persistent feeling of imbalance or disequilibrium, which may last for days. Patients may report that the attacks awaken them at night. Between attacks, they usually feel well. The hearing loss may fluctuate, with tinnitus and aural pressure waxing and waning with changes in hearing. The tinnitus and feeling of aural pressure may occur only during or before attacks, or they may be constant.

Findings of the physical examination are usually unremarkable with the exception of the evaluation of cranial nerve VIII. Sounds from a tuning fork (Weber test) may lateralize to the ear opposite the hearing loss, the one affected with Ménière's disease. An audiogram typically reveals a sensorineural hearing loss in the affected ear. This can be in the form of a "Pike's Peak" pattern, which looks like a hill or mountain, or it may show a sensorineural loss in the low frequencies. As the disease progresses, the hearing loss increases. The electronystagmogram may be negative or may show reduced vestibular response. No absolute diagnostic test exists.

Medical Management

Most patients with Ménière's disease can be successfully treated with diet and medication therapy. Many patients can control their symptoms by adhering to a low-sodium (1,000 to 1,500 mg/day or less) diet. Chart 61-7 describes dietary guidelines that may be useful in Ménière's disease. The amount of sodium is one of many factors that regulate the balance of fluid within the body. Sodium and fluid retention disrupts the delicate balance between endolymph and perilymph in the inner ear.

Psychological evaluation may be indicated if the patient is anxious, uncertain, fearful, or depressed (NIDCD, 2015b).

Pharmacologic Therapy

Pharmacologic therapy for Ménière's disease consists of antihistamines such as meclizine (Antivert), which suppress the vestibular system (NIDCD, 2015b). Tranquilizers such as diazepam (Valium) may be used in acute instances

CHART 61-7

Patient Education: Dietary Guidelines for Patients With Ménière's Disease

The nurse instructs the patient to:

- Limit foods high in salt or sugar. Be aware of foods with hidden salts and sugars.
- Eat meals and snacks at regular intervals to stay hydrated. Missing meals or snacks may alter the fluid level in the inner ear.
- Eat fresh fruits, vegetables, and whole grains. Limit the amount of canned, frozen, or processed foods with high sodium content.
- Drink plenty of fluids daily. Water, milk, and low-sugar fruit juices are recommended. Limit intake of coffee, tea, and soft drinks. Avoid caffeine because of its diuretic effect.
- Limit alcohol intake. Alcohol may change the volume and concentration of the inner ear fluid and may worsen symptoms.
- Avoid monosodium glutamate (MSG), which may increase symptoms.
- Pay attention to the intake of foods containing potassium (e.g., bananas, tomatoes, oranges) if taking a diuretic that causes potassium loss.
- Avoid aspirin and aspirin-containing medications. Aspirin may increase tinnitus and dizziness.

Adapted from National Institute on Deafness and Other Communication Disorders (NIDCD). (2015b). Ménière's disease. Retrieved June 12, 2012, from www.nidcd.nih.gov//health/balance/meniere.html

to help control vertigo. Antiemetics such as promethazine (Phenergan) suppositories help to control the nausea and vomiting and the vertigo because of their antihistamine effect. Diuretic therapy (e.g., hydrochlorothiazide) sometimes relieves symptoms by lowering the pressure in the endolymphatic system. Intratympanic injection of gentamicin (Garamycin) is used to cause ablation of the vestibular hair cells; however, the risk of significant hearing loss is high (NIDCD, 2015b).

Intake of foods containing potassium (e.g., bananas, tomatoes, oranges) is necessary if the patient takes a diuretic that causes potassium loss. No scientific basis exists for the use of vasodilators, such as nicotinic acid, papaverine hydrochloride (Pavabid), and methantheline bromide (Banthine), but they are often used in conjunction with other therapies.

Surgical Management

Although most patients respond well to conservative therapy, some continue to have disabling attacks of vertigo. If these attacks reduce their quality of life, patients may elect to undergo surgery for relief. Despite surgery, hearing loss, tinnitus, and aural fullness may continue because the surgical treatment of Ménière's disease is aimed at eliminating the attacks of vertigo.

Endolymphatic Sac Decompression

Endolymphatic sac decompression, or shunting, theoretically equalizes the pressure in the endolymphatic space. A shunt or drain is inserted in the endolymphatic sac through a postauricular incision. This procedure is favoured by many otolaryngologists as a first-line surgical approach to treat the vertigo of Ménière's disease because it is relatively simple and safe and can be performed on an outpatient basis.

Middle and Inner Ear Perfusion

Ototoxic medications, such as streptomycin or gentamicin, can be given to patients by infusion into the middle and inner ear to decrease vestibular function and vertigo. The success rate for eliminating vertigo is high, about 85%, but the risk of significant hearing loss is also high. This procedure of inner ear perfusion usually requires an overnight stay in the hospital. After the procedure, many patients have a period of imbalance lasting several weeks.

Intraotologic Catheters

In an attempt to deliver medication directly to the inner ear, catheters are being developed to provide a conduit from the outer ear to the inner ear. The route of the catheter is from the external ear canal through or around the tympanic membrane and to the round window niche or membrane. Medicinal fluids can be placed against the round window for a direct route to the inner ear fluids.

Potential uses of these catheters include treatment for sudden hearing loss and various disorders causing intractable vertigo. Future applications may include tinnitus and slowly progressing sensorineural hearing loss. Intratympanic injections of ototoxic medications for round window membrane diffusion can be used to decrease vestibular function. Established surgical techniques can be used for the patient with vertigo who has not responded to medical or physical therapeutic modalities.

Vestibular Nerve Sectioning

Vestibular nerve section provides the greatest success rate (approximately 98%) in eliminating the attacks of vertigo. It can be performed by a translabyrinthine approach (through the hearing mechanism) or in a manner that can conserve hearing (suboccipital or middle cranial fossa), depending on the degree of hearing loss. Most patients with incapacitating Ménière's disease have little or no effective hearing. Cutting the nerve prevents the brain from receiving input from the semicircular canals. This procedure requires a brief hospital stay. Nursing care for the patient with vertigo is presented in Chart 60-8, Plan of Nursing Care.

Labyrinthitis

Labyrinthitis, an inflammation of the inner ear, can be bacterial or viral in origin. Bacterial labyrinthitis is rare because of antibiotic therapy, but it sometimes occurs as a complication of otitis media. The infection can spread to the inner ear by penetrating the membranes of the oval or round windows. Viral labyrinthitis is a common diagnosis, but little is known about this disorder, which affects hearing and balance. The most commonly identified viral causes are mumps, rubella, rubeola, and influenza. Viral illnesses of the upper respiratory tract and herpetiform disorders of the facial nerve (Ramsay Hunt syndrome) also cause labyrinthitis.

Clinical Manifestations

Labyrinthitis is characterized by a sudden onset of incapacitating vertigo, usually with nausea and vomiting, various degrees of hearing loss, and possibly tinnitus. The first episode is usually the worst; subsequent attacks, which usually occur over a period of several weeks to months, are less severe.

Management

Treatment of bacterial labyrinthitis includes intravenous antibiotic therapy; fluid replacement; and administration of a vestibular suppressant, such as meclizine, and antiemetic medications. Treatment of viral labyrinthitis is based on the patient's symptoms.

Benign Paroxysmal Positional Vertigo

Benign paroxysmal positional vertigo (BPPV) is a brief period of incapacitating vertigo that occurs when the position of the patient's head is changed with respect to gravity, typically by placing the head back with the affected ear turned down. The onset is sudden and followed by a predisposition for positional vertigo, usually for hours to weeks but occasionally for months or years.

It is speculated to be caused by the disruption of debris within the semicircular canal. This debris is formed from small crystals of calcium carbonate from the inner ear structure, the utricle. This is frequently stimulated by head trauma, infection, or other events. In severe cases, vertigo may easily be induced by any head movement. The vertigo is usually accompanied by nausea and vomiting, but not hearing impairment.

Bed rest is recommended for patients with acute symptoms. There are repositioning techniques that can be used to treat vertigo. The canalith repositioning procedure is commonly used. This noninvasive procedure, which involves quick movements of the body, rearranges the debris in the canal. The procedure is performed by placing the patient in a sitting position, turning the head to a 45-degree angle on the affected side, and then quickly moving the patient to the supine position. The procedure is safe, inexpensive, and easy to perform. The Dix-Hallpike test is used to assess for BPPV. When the Dix-Hallpike test results are positive on the right side, a left-sided canalith repositioning procedure is used.

Patients with acute vertigo may be medicated with meclizine for 1 to 2 weeks. After this time, the meclizine is stopped and the patient is reassessed. Patients who continue to have severe positional vertigo may be premedicated with prochlorperazine 1 hour before the canalith repositioning procedure is performed.

Vestibular rehabilitation can be used in the management of vestibular disorders. This strategy promotes active use of the vestibular system through a multidisciplinary team approach, including medical and nursing care, stress management, biofeedback, vocational rehabilitation, and physical therapy. A physical therapist prescribes balance exercises that help the brain compensate for the impairment to the balance system. The plan of nursing care for a patient with vertigo is given in Chart 61-8.

(text continued on page 1950)

Plan of Nursing Care — Chart 61-8. Care of the Patient With Vertigo

Nursing Priority: Increased odds for injury due to altered mobility (gait disturbance and vertigo)
Goal: Remains free of any injuries associated with imbalance and/or falls

NURSING INTERVENTIONS	RATIONALE	EXPECTED PATIENT OUTCOMES
1. Assess for vertigo, including history, onset, description of attacks, duration, frequency, and any associated ear symptoms (hearing loss, tinnitus, aural fullness).	1. History provides basis for interventions.	• Takes prescribed medications appropriately • Fear and anxiety are reduced • Assumes safe position when vertigo is present • Performs exercises as prescribed • Experiences no falls due to balance disturbance • Keeps head still when vertigo is present • Reports measures that help to reduce vertigo • Describes aura and takes action to reduce severity of attack • Identifies a characteristic fullness or sense of pressure in the ear as occurring before a full-blown attack • Successfully decreases the sensation of dizziness by keeping eyes in fixed position
2. Assess extent of disability in relation to activities of daily living.	2. Extent of disability indicates risk of falling.	
3. Teach or reinforce vestibular/balance therapy as prescribed.	3. Exercises hasten labyrinthine compensation, which may decrease vertigo and gait disturbance.	
4. Administer, or teach administration of, antivertiginous medications and/or vestibular sedation medication; instruct patient about side effects.	4. Alleviates acute symptoms of vertigo	
5. Encourage patient to sit down when dizzy.	5. Decreases possibility of falling and injury	
6. Place pillow on each side of head to restrict movement.	6. Movement aggravates vertigo.	
7. Assist patient in identifying aura that suggests an impending attack.	7. Recognition of aura may trigger the need to take medication before an attack occurs, thereby minimizing the severity of effects.	
8. Recommend that the patient keep eyes open and stare straight ahead when lying down and experiencing vertigo.	8. Sensation of vertigo decreases and motion decelerates if eyes are kept in a fixed position.	

Nursing Priority: Lack of adjustment related to disability requiring change in lifestyle due to unpredictability of vertigo
Goal: Modifies lifestyle to decrease disability and exert maximum control and independence within limits posed by chronic vertigo

NURSING INTERVENTIONS	RATIONALE	EXPECTED PATIENT OUTCOMES
1. Encourage patient to identify personal strengths and roles that can still be fulfilled.	1. Maximizes sense of regaining control and independence	• Exerts maximum control of environment and independence within limits imposed by vertigo
2. Provide information about vertigo and what to expect.	2. Reduces fear and anxiety	• Demonstrates understanding Is informed about condition
3. Include family and significant others in rehabilitative process.	3. Perceived beliefs of significant others are important for patient's adherence to medical regimen.	• Family and significant others participate are included in rehabilitation process
4. Encourage patient to maintain sense of control by making decisions and assuming more responsibility for care.	4. Reinforces positive psychological and social outcomes	• Uses strengths and potentials to engage in the most independent and constructive lifestyle

continued >

Plan of Nursing Care

Chart 61-8. Care of the Patient With Vertigo, *Continued*

NURSING INTERVENTIONS	RATIONALE	EXPECTED PATIENT OUTCOMES
Nursing Priority: Altered fluid volume related to increased fluid output, altered intake, and medications **Goal:** Maintains acceptable normal fluid-electrolyte balance		
1. Assess, or have patient assess, intake and output (including emesis, liquid stools, urine, and diaphoresis). Monitor laboratory values.	1. Accurate records provide basis for fluid replacement.	• Laboratory values within expected normal limits • Alert and oriented; vital signs within accepted range normal limits, skin turgor present normal; electrolytes within range normal • Mucous membranes are moist • Vomiting or diarrhea has stopped; usual oral intake resumed
2. Assess indicators of dehydration, including blood pressure (orthostasis), pulse, skin turgor, mucous membranes, and level of consciousness.	2. Prompt recognition of dehydration allows early intervention.	
3. Encourage oral fluids as tolerated; discourage beverages containing caffeine (a vestibular stimulant).	3. Increased hydration. Oral replacement is begun as soon as possible to replace fluid losses. Caffeine may increase diarrhea.	
4. Administer, or teach administration of, antiemetics and antidiarrheal medication as prescribed and needed. Instruct patient in side effects.	4. Antiemetics reduce nausea and vomiting, reducing fluid losses and improving oral intake. Antidiarrheal medication reduces intestinal motility and fluid losses.	
Nursing Priority: Anxiety due to the disabling effects of vertigo **Goal:** Experiences less or no anxiety		
1. Assess level of anxiety. Help patient identify coping skills used successfully in the past.	1. Guides therapeutic interventions and participation in self-care. Past coping skills can relieve anxiety.	• Fear and anxiety about attacks of vertigo reduced or eliminated • Acquires knowledge and skills to deal with vertigo • Feels less tension, apprehension, and uncertainty • Uses stress management techniques when needed • Avoids upsetting encounters • Repeats instructions given and verbalizes understanding of treatments
2. Provide information about vertigo and its treatment.	2. Increased knowledge helps to decrease anxiety.	
3. Encourage patient to discuss anxieties and explore concerns about vertigo attacks.	3. Promotes awareness and understanding of relationship between anxiety level and behaviour	
4. Teach patient stress management techniques or make appropriate referral.	4. Improved stress management can reduce the frequency and severity of some vertiginous attacks.	
5. Provide comfort measures, and avoid stress-producing activities.	5. Stressful situations may exacerbate symptoms of the condition.	
6. Instruct patient in aspects of treatment regimen.	6. Patient knowledge helps to decrease anxiety.	
Nursing Priority: Increased odds for trauma related to impaired balance **Goal:** Reduces the risk of trauma by adapting the home environment and by using rehabilitative devices as necessary		
1. Assess for balance disturbance and/or vertigo by taking history and by examination for nystagmus, positive Romberg, and inability to perform tandem Romberg.	1. Peripheral vestibular disorders cause these signs and symptoms.	• Has adapted home environment or uses rehabilitative devices to reduce risk of falling • Ambulates with needed assistance • Ambulates with needed assistance • Activity level increased • Visual and proprioceptive risks identified • Visual and proprioceptive risks identified • Home environment free of hazards • Home environment free of hazards
2. Assist with ambulation when indicated.	2. Abnormal gait can predispose patient to unsteadiness and falls.	
3. Assess for visual acuity and proprioceptive deficits.	3. Balance depends on visual, vestibular, and proprioceptive systems.	
4. Encourage increased activity level with or without use of assistive devices.	4. Increased activity may help to retrain balance system.	
5. Help to identify hazards in home environment.	5. Adaptation of home environment can reduce risk of falls during rehabilitative process.	

Plan of Nursing Care

Chart 61-8. Care of the Patient With Vertigo, *Continued*

Nursing Priority: Lack of coping due to personal vulnerability and disabling effects of vertigo
Goal: Develops coping skills necessary to decrease vulnerability and unmet needs and demonstrates effective coping

NURSING INTERVENTIONS	RATIONALE	EXPECTED PATIENT OUTCOMES
1. Assess cognitive appraisal of illness and factors that may be contributing to inability to cope.	1. Improves patient's self-image and to enhances coping process	• Copes effectively with vertigo • Has acquired knowledge and skills to cope with vertigo • Verbalizes less threatening appraisal of situation • Is involved in outside activities • Identifies specific strategies for coping • Uses support groups or counselling as appropriate
2. Provide factual information about treatment and future health status.	2. Clarifies any misinformation or confusion	
3. Encourage and help patient participate in decision making about adjustments in lifestyle.	3. Helps patient regain sense of power and control in self-care with activities of daily living	
4. Encourage patient to maintain diversional or recreational activities, exercise, and social events.	4. Social isolation and avoidance of pleasant activities intensifies isolation and reduces ability to cope with vertigo.	
5. Help patient identify personal strengths and develop coping strategies based on previous positive experiences in dealing with stress and situational supports.	5. Enhances patient's strengths that help to maintain hope	
6. Refer patient to support groups or counselling as indicated.	6. May help patient feel less alone and isolated	

Nursing Priority: Lack of diversional activity related to environmental lack of such activity
Goal: Engages in diversional activities

NURSING INTERVENTIONS	RATIONALE	EXPECTED PATIENT OUTCOMES
Assess level and type of diversional activity to plan appropriate activities.	Boredom may be present as well as depression; helps to determine tolerances as well as preferences.	Verbalizes decreased feelings of boredom and appears alert and animated
Discuss usual pattern of diversional activities with patient. Suggest opportunities to continue meaningful diversional activities.	provides information about perceived and actual stressors that influence activity level; supports patient's sense of self-worth and productivity	Seeks realistic opportunities for involvement in diversional activities

Nursing Priority: Lack of ability to provide self-care: feeding, bathing/hygiene, dressing/grooming, toileting, related to labyrinth dysfunction and episodes of vertigo
Goal: Able to care for self

NURSING INTERVENTIONS	RATIONALE	EXPECTED PATIENT OUTCOMES
Administer, or teach administration of, antiemetics and other prescribed medications to relieve nausea and vomiting associated with vertigo.	Antiemetics and sedative-type medications depress stimuli in the cerebellum.	Carries out necessary functions during symptom free periods. Takes medications to relieve nausea or vomiting.
Encourage patient to perform self-care when free of vertigo.	Spacing activities is important because episodes of vertigo vary in occurrence.	Carries out daily activities
Review diet with patient and caregivers. Offer fluids as necessary.	Sodium restriction helps to improve an inner ear fluid imbalance in some patients, thereby decreasing vertigo. Fluids help to prevent dehydration.	Accepts dietary plan and reports its effectiveness Drinks fluids in sufficient amounts

Nursing Priority: Powerlessness due to illness and helplessness in certain situations due to vertigo/balance disturbance
Goal: Experiences increased sense of control over life and activities despite vertigo/balance disturbance

NURSING INTERVENTIONS	RATIONALE	EXPECTED PATIENT OUTCOMES
Assess patient's needs, values, attitudes, and readiness to initiate activities.	Involving patient in planning activities and care enhances potential for mastery.	Does not restrict activities unnecessarily due to vertigo
Provide opportunities for patient to express feelings about self and illness.	Expressing feelings increases understanding of individual coping styles and defense mechanisms.	Verbalizes positive feelings about own ability to achieve a sense of power and control
Help patient identify previous coping behaviours that were successful.	Awareness increases understanding of stressors that trigger feeling of powerlessness. Awareness of past successes enhances self-confidence.	Identifies previous successful coping behaviours

CHART 61-9

Selected Ototoxic Substances

- **Aminoglycoside antibiotic agents:** amikacin, gentamicin, kanamycin, netilmicin, neomycin, streptomycin, tobramycin
- **Anti-inflammatory agents:** salicylates (aspirin), indomethacin
- **Antimalarial agents:** quinine, chloroquine
- **Chemicals**: alcohol, arsenic
- **Chemotherapeutic (antineoplastic) agents:** cisplatin, nitrogen mustard, carboplatin
- **Loop diuretic agents:** ethacrynic acid, furosemide, acetazolamide
- **Metals:** gold, mercury, lead
- **Other antibiotic agents:** erythromycin, minocycline, polymyxin B, vancomycin

Adapted from Mudd, P. (2016). Ototoxicity. *Medscape*. Retrieved September 12, 2016, from emedicine.medscape.com/article/857679-overview.

Ototoxicity

A variety of medications may have adverse effects on the cochlea, vestibular apparatus, or cranial nerve VIII. All but a few, such as aspirin (salicylate) and quinine, cause irreversible hearing loss. At high doses, aspirin toxicity also can produce tinnitus. Intravenous medications, especially the aminoglycosides, are the most common cause of ototoxicity, and they destroy the hair cells in the organ of Corti (Chart 61-9). Antineoplastic agents also cause hair cell death in the cochlea, which can lead to hearing loss (Mudd, 2016).

Patients receiving potentially ototoxic medications are informed about the side effects of these medications (Chart 61-10). They are used with caution in patients who are at high risk for complications, such as children, older adults, women who are pregnant, patients with kidney or liver problems, and patients with current hearing disorders. Blood levels of the medications are monitored, and patients receiving long-term intravenous antibiotics are monitored with an audiogram twice each week during therapy.

Acoustic Neuroma

An acoustic neuroma is a slow-growing, benign tumour of cranial nerve VIII, usually arising from the Schwann cells of the vestibular portion of the nerve. Most acoustic tumours arise within the internal auditory canal and extend into the cerebellopontine angle to press on the brain stem, possibly destroying the vestibular nerve (Bader, Littlejohns, & Olson, 2016). Acoustic neuromas account for 5% to 10% of all intracranial tumours and seem to occur with equal frequency in men and women at any age, although most occur during middle age. Most acoustic neuromas are unilateral, except in von Recklinghausen's disease (i.e., neurofibromatosis type 1), in which bilateral tumours occur (Ghalayani, Saberi, & Sardari, 2012).

Assessment and Diagnostic Findings

The most common findings of assessment of patients with an acoustic neuroma are unilateral tinnitus and hearing loss with or without vertigo or balance disturbance. It is important to identify asymmetry in audiovestibular test results so that further workup can be performed to rule out an acoustic neuroma. Although conflicting data exist, the only known risk factor for acoustic neuroma is cell phone usage (Park, Vernick, & Ramakrishna, 2015). An MRI with a paramagnetic contrast agent (gadopentetate dimeglumine

NURSING RESEARCH PROFILE

Chart 61-10. Does Interferon Beta-1a Contribute to Hearing Loss in Patients With Multiple Sclerosis (MS)?

Lewis, M. S., McMillan, G. P., Hutter, M., et al. (2014). Does Interferon Beta-1a impact pure-tone hearing sensitivity among individuals with multiple sclerosis?. *Journal of Neuroscience Nursing*, *46*(6), 352–359.

Purpose

Previous studies reported that interferon medications, commonly used to treat multiple sclerosis (MS), might contribute to hearing loss. The purpose of this study was to assess participants with MS taking intramuscular interferon beta-1a and who have significantly poorer hearing compared to those not currently using any disease-modifying therapies.

Design

The design of this study was a secondary analysis of data that had been collected during two other large studies that evaluated hearing in those with MS. A linear mixed model was fit to the hearing thresholds of participants. The model included interferon use, MS subtype, gender, age, test frequency, MS duration in years, and a disability score.

Findings

With all participants included ($N = 52$), there was insufficient evidence to infer that intramuscular interferon-beta 1a was not ototoxic compared to nonuse of a disease-modifying therapy at all frequencies at which participants had their hearing tested. After removing two participants who were outliers, the results indicated that there was support for no ototoxic effect of intramuscular interferon beta-1a at test frequencies from 250 to 6,000 Hz. There was insufficient evidence, however, to rule out an ototoxic effect at 8,000 Hz.

Nursing Implications

More research is needed to evaluate the ototoxic effects of interferon on hearing in patients with MS. Nurses should be aware of the potential for ototoxicity with interferon use and remind patients with MS to have their hearing evaluated on a regular basis throughout the course of treatment.

[Magnevist]) is the imaging study of choice. If the patient is claustrophobic, cannot tolerate an MRI, or the scan is unavailable, CT scan with contrast dye is performed. The MRI is more sensitive than CT in delineating a small tumour.

Management

Surgical removal of acoustic tumours is the treatment of choice, because these tumours do not respond well to irradiation or chemotherapy. Because treatment of acoustic tumours crosses several specialties, the interdisciplinary treatment approach involves a neurotologist and a neurosurgeon. The objective of the surgery is to remove the tumour while preserving facial nerve function. Most acoustic tumours have damaged the cochlear branch of cranial nerve VIII, and no serviceable hearing exists before surgery. In these patients, the surgery is performed using a translabyrinthine approach, and the hearing mechanism is destroyed. If hearing is still good before surgery, a suboccipital or middle cranial fossa approach to removing the tumour may be used, and intraoperative monitoring of cranial nerve VIII is performed to save the hearing.

Complications of surgery for acoustic neuroma include facial nerve paralysis, cerebrospinal fluid leak, meningitis, and cerebral edema. Death from acoustic neuroma surgery is rare (Park et al., 2015).

AURAL REHABILITATION

If hearing loss is permanent, cannot be treated by medical or surgical means, or the patient elects not to undergo surgery, aural rehabilitation may be beneficial. The purpose of aural rehabilitation is to maximize the communication skills of the person with hearing impairment. Aural rehabilitation includes auditory training, speech reading, speech training, and the use of hearing aids and hearing guide dogs.

Auditory training emphasizes listening skills, so the person who is hearing impaired concentrates on the speaker. Speech reading (formerly known as lip reading) can help to fill the gaps left by missed or misheard words. The goals of speech training are to conserve, develop, and prevent deterioration of current communication skills.

It is important to identify the type of hearing impairment a person has so that rehabilitative efforts can be directed according to need. Surgical correction may be all that is necessary to treat and improve a conductive hearing loss. With advances in hearing aid technology, amplification for patients with sensorineural hearing loss is more helpful than ever before.

Hearing Aids

A hearing aid is a device through which speech and environmental sounds are received by a microphone, converted to electrical signals, amplified, and reconverted to acoustic signals. Many aids available for sensorineural hearing loss depress the low frequencies, or tones, and enhance hearing for the high frequencies. A general guideline for assessing the patient's need for a hearing aid is a hearing loss exceeding 30 dB in the range of 500 to 2,000 Hz in the better-hearing ear.

CHART 61-11

Options and Features of Hearing Aids to Consider

- *T-Coil:* May improve hearing on the telephone by switching the settings from normal to telephone setting. This feature also assists in amplifying voices when the patient is in larger areas, such as theatres, auditoriums, and gymnasiums. Background noise may be toned down to adequately hear close conversation.
- *Directional Microphone:* Useful in environments with a lot of background noise and activity. The microphone may be directed toward the speaker and amplifies conversation while diminishing background noise.
- *Direct Audio Input:* Directly plugs into another device, such as a computer, television, or stereo, that is attached with an extension cord.
- *Feedback Suppression:* Suppresses whistling feedback noise.

Adapted from U.S. Food and Drug Administration. (2014). Medical devices: Types of hearing aids. Retrieved August 19, 2016, from www.fda.gov/MedicalDevices/ProductsandMedicalProcedures/HomeHealthandConsumer/ConsumerProducts/HearingAids/ucm181470.htm

The evolution in technology has led to the availability of many smaller and more effective hearing aids (Chart 61-11). It is estimated that 98% of all hearing aids sold today are behind-the-ear, in-the-ear, or in-the-canal types (Table 61-4).

A hearing aid should be fitted according to the patient's needs (e.g., type of hearing loss, manual dexterity, and preferences) by a certified audiologist licensed to dispense hearing aids. Consumer protection laws allow the hearing aid to be returned after a trial use if the patient is not completely satisfied.

A hearing aid makes sounds louder, but it does not improve a patient's ability to discriminate words or understand speech. People who have low discrimination scores (i.e., 20%) on audiograms may derive little benefit from a hearing aid. Hearing aids amplify all sounds, including background noise, which may be disturbing to the wearer. Chart 61-12 identifies additional challenges associated with hearing aid use.

Computerized hearing aids are available that compensate for background noise or allow amplification at certain programmed frequencies rather than at all frequencies. Occasionally, depending on the type of hearing loss, binaural aids (i.e., one for each ear) may be indicated. Chart 61-13 provides tips for hearing aid care.

In Canada, it is not necessary to consult a physician before purchasing a hearing aid. Some provinces require a letter from a physician in order for people 65 years and older to be eligible for financial assistance for a hearing aid. The physician indicates that "there is no reason not to have a hearing aid." Children must be evaluated by a physician. Health care professionals who dispense hearing aids are required to refer prospective users to a physician if any of the following otologic conditions are evident:

- Visible congenital or traumatic deformity of the ear
- Active drainage from the ear within the previous 90 days

TABLE 61-4 Hearing Aids

Site (and Range of Hearing Loss)	Advantages	Disadvantages
Body (mild–profound)	Separation of receiver and microphone prevents acoustic feedback, allowing high amplification. Generally used in a school setting.	Bulky; requires long wire, which may be cosmetically displeasing; some loss of high-frequency response
Behind the ear (mild–profound)	Economical; powerful, with no long wires; easily used by children—adapts easily as the child grows, with only the ear mold needing replacement	Large size
In the ear (mild–moderately severe)	One-piece custom fit to contour of ear; no tubes or cords; miniature microphone is located in the ear, which is a more natural placement; more cosmetically appealing due to easy concealment	Smaller size limits output; patients who have arthritis or cannot perform tasks requiring competent manual dexterity may have difficulty with the small size of aid and/or battery; can require more repair than the behind-the-ear aid
In the canal (mild–moderately severe)	Same as in-the-ear aids; less visible, so more cosmetically pleasing	Even smaller than in-the-ear aids; requires competent manual dexterity

- Sudden or rapidly progressive hearing loss within the previous 90 days
- Report of dizziness or tinnitus
- Unilateral hearing loss that occurred suddenly or within the previous 90 days
- Audiometric air–bone gap of 15 dB or more at 500, 1,000, and 2,000 Hz
- Significant accumulation of cerumen or a foreign body in the external auditory canal
- Pain or discomfort in the ear

CHART 61-12

Hearing Aid Concerns

Whistling Noise

Loose ear mould
Improperly made
Improperly worn
Worn out

Improper Aid Selection

Too much power required in aid, with inadequate separation between microphone and receiver
Open mold used inappropriately

Inadequate Amplification

Dead batteries
Wax in ear
Wax or other material in mold
Wires or tubing disconnected from aid
Aid turned off or volume too low
Improper mold
Improper aid for degree of loss

Pain from Mold

Improperly fitted mold
Ear skin or cartilage infection
Middle ear infection
Ear tumour
Unrelated conditions of the temporomandibular joint, throat, or larynx

CHART 61-13

Patient Education: Tips for Hearing Aid Care

The nurse instructs the patient how to clean a hearing aid, check for malfunctions, and recognize complications:

Cleaning

- Keep in mind that the ear mold is the only part of the hearing aid that may be washed frequently.
- Wash the ear mold daily with soap and water.
- Allow the ear mold to dry completely before it is snapped into the receiver.
- Clean the cannula with a small pipe cleaner-like device.
- Note that properly caring for the ear device and keeping the ear canal clean and dry can prevent complications.

Checking for Malfunctions

- Be aware that inadequate amplification, a whistling noise, or pain from the mold can occur when a hearing aid is not functioning properly.
- Check for malfunctions:
  - Is the switch on properly?
  - Are the batteries charged and positioned correctly?
  - Is the ear mold clogged with cerumen? Ear wax can be easily removed with pin, pipe cleaner, or wax loop.
- Notify the hearing aid dealer if the hearing aid is still not working properly.
- Keep in mind that if the unit requires extended time for repair, the dealer may lend you a hearing aid until the repair can be accomplished.

Recognizing Complications

- Understand that common medical complications include external otitis media and pressure ulcers in the external auditory canal. Signs and symptoms of these infections include painful ear, especially when the external ear is touched; canal swelling; redness; difficulty hearing; pain radiating to the jaw area; and fever.
- Notify your health care provider for evaluation if any of these symptoms are present. You may need medication to treat infection, pain, or both.

A user instruction brochure is to accompany every hearing aid device. In this brochure, the following information is presented:

- Notification that any of the eight otologic conditions previously listed should be investigated by a physician before purchase of a hearing aid
- Instructions for proper use, maintenance, and care of the hearing aid as well as instructions for replacing or recharging the batteries
- Repair service information
- Description of avoidable conditions that could damage the hearing aid (e.g., wearing the hearing aid in the shower)
- List of any known side effects that may warrant physician consultation (e.g., skin irritation, accelerated cerumen accumulation)

Implanted Hearing Devices

Three types of implanted hearing devices are commercially available or in the investigational stage: the cochlear implant, the bone conduction device, and the semi-implantable hearing device. Cochlear implants are for patients with little or no hearing (see discussion below). Bone conduction devices, which transmit sound through the skull to the inner ear, are used in patients with a conductive hearing loss if a hearing aid is contraindicated (e.g., those with chronic infection). The device is implanted postauricularly under the skin into the skull, and an external device—worn above the ear, not in the canal—transmits the sound through the skin. Several types of implantable hearing aids exist. The bone-anchored hearing aid (BAHA) is implanted behind the ear in the mastoid area for conductive or mixed hearing loss. The middle ear implantation (MEI) is implanted in the middle ear cavity for sensorineural hearing loss in patients over 18 years of age (FDA, 2015).

The auditory brain stem implants (ABIs) are used for those with neurofibromatosis type 2 and external ear implants are used in patients with moderate high-frequency hearing loss (McNeill, 2011).

Cochlear Implant

A cochlear implant is an auditory prosthesis used for people with profound sensorineural hearing loss bilaterally who do not benefit from conventional hearing aids. The hearing loss may be congenital or acquired. An implant does not restore hearing, but it helps the person detect medium to loud environmental sounds and conversation. The implant provides stimulation directly to the auditory nerve, bypassing the nonfunctioning hair cells of the inner ear (NIDCD, 2016). The microphone and signal processor, worn outside the body, transmit electrical stimuli inside the body to the implanted electrodes. The electrical signals stimulate the auditory nerve fibres and then the brain, where they are interpreted.

Candidates for a cochlear implant, who are usually at least 1 year old, are selected after careful screening by otologic history, physical examination, audiologic testing, x-rays, and psychological testing. Several criteria apply for choosing adults who may benefit from a cochlear implant:

- Profound sensorineural hearing loss in both ears
- Inability to hear and recognize speech well with hearing aids
- No medical contraindication to a cochlear implant or general anesthesia
- Indications that being able to hear would enhance the patient's life

The surgery involves implanting a small receiver in the temporal bone through a postauricular incision and placing electrodes into the inner ear (Fig. 61-7).

The microphone and transmitter are worn on an external unit. The patient undergoes extensive cochlear rehabilitation with the interdisciplinary team, which includes an audiologist and speech pathologist. Several months may be needed to learn to interpret the sounds heard. Children and adults who lost their hearing before they learned to

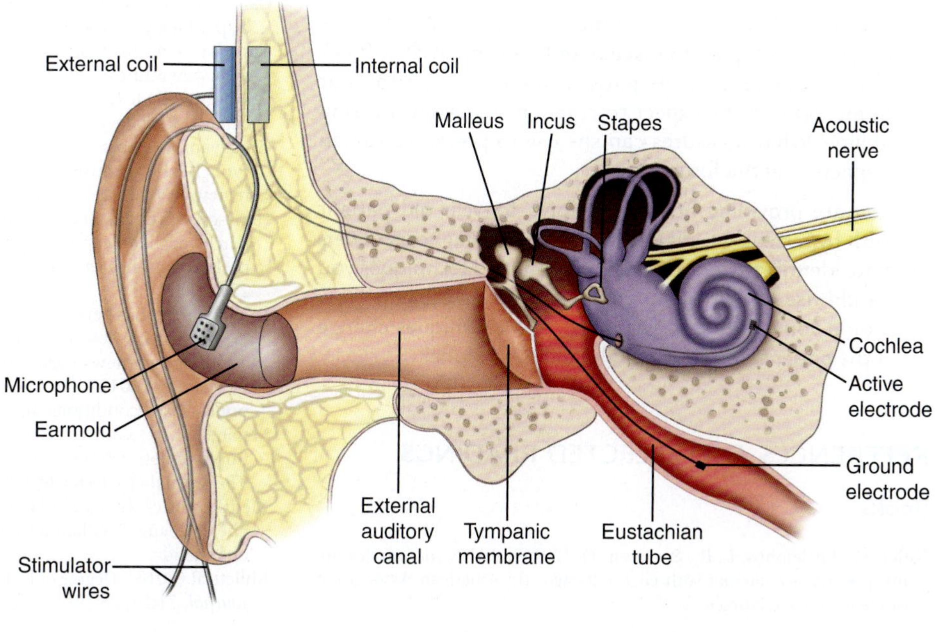

FIGURE 61-7. The cochlear implant. The internal coil has a stranded electrode lead. The electrode is inserted through the round window into the scala tympani of the cochlea. The external coil (the transmitter) is held in alignment with the internal coil (the receiver) by a magnet. The microphone receives the sound. The stimulator wire receives the signal after it has been filtered, adjusted, and modified so that the sound is at a comfortable level for the patient. Sound is passed by the external transmitter to the inner coil receiver by magnetic conduction and is then carried by the electrode to the cochlea.

speak take much longer to acquire speech. The success of cochlear implants varies widely and controversy exists about their use, especially among the Deaf community. Patients who have had a cochlear implant are cautioned that an MRI will cause the implant to become inactivated; MRI is to be used only when unavoidable.

Hearing Guide Dogs

Specially trained dogs are available to assist the person with a hearing loss. People who live alone are eligible to apply for a rescued dog, trained by International Hearing Dog, Inc. At home, the dog reacts to the sound of a telephone, a doorbell, an alarm clock, a baby's cry, a knock at the door, a smoke alarm, or an intruder. The dog does not bark but alerts its master by physical contact; the dog then runs to the source of the noise. In public, the dog positions itself between the person with hearing impairment and any potential hazard that the person cannot hear, such as an oncoming vehicle or a loud, hostile person. A person with a certified hearing guide dog is legally permitted access to public transportation, public eating places, and stores, including food markets.

Critical Thinking Exercises

1 A 45-year-old patient who has been swimming frequently in the local pool has recently been diagnosed with otitis externa. Devise an evidence-based education plan for this patient, with consideration to the diagnosis, possible medical management and treatment options, and home care instructions. Identify evidence-based techniques that the patient should perform to prevent future infections.

2 A 91-year-old female has complained of hearing loss that has gradually worsened over the past few months. She has difficulty with hearing when carrying on a conversation with others, difficulty hearing the television, and having a telephone conversation. She has seen the primary provider today and has been diagnosed with cerumen impaction. Discuss how you will educate the patient about the diagnosis of cerumen impaction. What treatments will you plan to discuss and perform in the office? List treatments that the patient will need to perform at home. Should she expect to regain her previous hearing ability? What measures can she use to prevent cerumen impaction in the future?

3 You are providing home care for a 55-year-old patient with hypertension, diabetes, and a new diagnosis of vertigo. Identify the priorities, approach, and techniques you would use to provide nursing care to this patient. How would your priorities, approach, and techniques change if the patient was 85 years old and lived alone?

REFERENCES AND SELECTED READINGS

Books

Bader, M., Littlejohns, L. R., & Olson, D. (2016). *AANN core curriculum for neuroscience nursing* (6th ed.). Chicago, IL: American Association of Neuroscience Nurses.

Brauer, R. L. (2016). *Safety and health for engineers*. John Wiley & Sons.

Cash, J. C., & Glass, C. A. (2014). *Family practice guidelines*. New York: Springer Publishing.

Dillon, P. M. (2015). *Nursing health assessment: The foundation of clinical practice: Nursing's role in health-care delivery* (3rd ed.). FA Davis.

Doenges, M. E., Moorhouse, M. F., & Murr, A. C. (2016). *Nursing diagnosis manual: Planning, individualizing, and documenting client care*. FA Davis.

Eliopoulos, C. (2018). *Gerontological nursing* (9th ed.). Philadelphia, PA: Lippincott Williams & Wilkins.

Fischbach, F., & Dunning, M. B. (2015). *A manual of laboratory and diagnostic tests* (9th ed.). Philadelphia, PA: Lippincott Williams & Wilkins.

Goolsby, M. J., & Grubbs, L. (2018). *Advanced assessment interpreting findings and formulating differential diagnoses*. FA Davis.

Grossman, S. C., & Porth, C. M. (2014). *Pathophysiology: Concepts of altered health states* (9th ed.). Philadelphia, PA: Lippincott Williams & Wilkins.

Jensen, S. (2018). *Nursing health assessment: A best practice approach*. Philadelphia, PA: Lippincott Williams & Wilkins.

Kuriger, M., Lesimple, C., Hockley, N., et al. (2018). *U.S. Patent No. 9,980,053*. Washington, DC: U.S. Patent and Trademark Office.

Martini, F. H., Timmons, M. J., & Tallitsch, R. B. (2012). *Human anatomy* (7th ed.). Boston, MA: Pearson Benjamin Cummings.

Mason, P. (2018). *Health behavior change: A guide for practitioners*. Elsevier Health Sciences.

Pagana, K. D., & Pagana, T. J. (2017). *Mosby's Manual of diagnostic and laboratory tests—eBook*. Elsevier Health Sciences.

Stephen, T. C. (2012). Ears assessment. In T. C. Stephen, D. L. Skillen, R. A. Day, et al. (Eds.). *Canadian Jensen's nursing health assessment: A best practice approach* (pp. 387–413). Philadelphia, PA: Wolters Kluwer Health/Lippincott Williams & Wilkins.

Weber, J., & Kelley, J. (2014). *Health assessment in nursing* (5th ed.). Philadelphia, PA: Lippincott Williams & Wilkins.

Journals and Electronic Documents

Antonio, S. (2016). Genetic sensorineural hearing loss clinical presentation. Retrieved August 19, 2016, from emedicine.medscape.com/article/855875-clinical#b5.

Bhattacharyya, N., & Meyers, A. D. (2015). Auditory brainstem response auditometry. Retrieved August 19, 2016, from emedicine.medscape.com/article/836277-overview#a6.

Brainard, A., & Gresham, C. (2014). Prevention and treatment of motion sickness. *American family physician*, *90*(1).

Canadian Academy of Audiology. (2014). Meniere's disease. Retrieved from http://.canadianaudiology.ca/consumer/menieres-disease.html

Canadian Association of the Deaf. (2012). Statistics on deaf Canadians. Retrieved from http://www.cad.ca/statistics on deaf canadians.php

Canadian Centre for Occupational Health and Safety. (2014). Noise—Occupational exposure limits in Canada. Retrieved from http://www.ccohs.ca/oshanswers/phys agents/exposurecan.html

Canadian Hearing Society. (2013). Signs of hearing loss. Retrieved from http://www.chs.ca/signs-hearing-loss

Canadian Tinnitus Foundation. (2012). What is tinnitus? Retrieved from http://www.findthecurenow.org

Connor, S. E. J. (2018). Contemporary imaging of auditory implants. *Clinical Radiology*, *73*(1), 19–34.

Ghalayani, P., Saberi, Z., & Sardari, F. (2012). Neurofibromatosis type 1 (von Recklinghausen's disease): A family case report and literature review. *Dental Research Journal*, *9*(4), 483–488.

Hansson, E. E., & Brattmo, M. (2013). Balance performance and self-perceived handicap among patients with Meniere's disease— A comparison with healthy controls. *European Journal of Physiotherapy*, *15*(4), 221–224.

Lachance, S., Bussieres, R., & Cote, M. (2012). Stapes surgery in profound hearing loss due to otosclerosis. Retrieved from http://www.audiology.org/news/Pages/20120829.aspex?PF=1

Mayo Clinic. (2012). Dizziness. Retrieved from http://www.mayoclinic.org/diseases-conditions/dizziness/basics/causes/con-20023004

McNeil, M. L., Gulliver, M., Morris, D. P., et al. (2011). Quality of life improvement for bone-anchored hearing aid users and their partners. *The Journal of Laryngology & Otology*, *125*(6), 554–560.

MediResource Inc. (2014). Ménière's disease. Retrieved from http://chealth.canoe.ca/channel condition info details.asp?diseaseid=180&channelid=

Millett, P. (2018). Degree of hearing loss versus hearing access. *The Hearing Journal*, *71*(9), 38–39.

Mudd, P. (2016). Ototoxicity. *Medscape*. Retrieved on September 12, 2016, from emedicine.medscape.com/article/857679-overview

National Institute on Deafness and Other Communication Disorders (NIDCD). (2015b). Ménière's disease. Retrieved June 12, 2012, from www.nidcd.nih.gov//health/balance/meniere.html

National Institute on Deafness and Other Communication Disorders (NIDCD). (2016). Strategic plan: FY 2012–2016. Retrieved September 12, 2016, from www.nidcd.nih.gov/staticresources/about/plans/strategic/FY2009–2011NIDCDStrategicPlan.pdf

Park, J. K., Vernick, D. M., & Ramakrishna, N. (2015). Vestibular schwannoma (acoustic neuroma). *UpToDate*. Retrieved August 25, 2016, from www.uptodate.com/contents/search?search=Vestibular+schwannoma+%28acoustic+neuroma%29.+&x=16&y=8

Santos, T. G., Venosa, A. R., & Sampaio, A. L. L. (2015). Association between hearing loss and vestibular disorders: A review of the interference of hearing in the balance. *International Journal of Otolaryngology and Head & Neck Surgery*, *4*(03), 173.

Shohet, J. A., & Heyers, A. D. (2012). Implantable hearing devices. Retrieved from http://emedicine.medscape.com/article/860444-overview

Speech-Language and Audiology Canada. (2014). Over half of Canadian provinces and territories lacking when it comes to newborn hearing screening. Retrieved from http://www.sac-oac.ca

Stanton, S. G., & Griffin, A. (2013). The genomics of hearing loss: A new era for clinical practice. *Canadian Journal of Speech-Language Pathology and Audiology*, 37(3), 188–205.

Strupp, M., Mandalà, M., & López-Escámez, J. A. (2019). Peripheral vestibular disorders: An update. *Current Opinion in Neurology*, *32*(1), 165–173.

The Hearing Foundation of Canada. (2014). Causes of hearing loss. Retrieved from http://www.hearingfoundation.ca/causes-of-hearing-loss/

U.S. Food and Drug Administration. (2015). Medical devices: Other products and devices to improve hearing. Retrieved August 19, 2016, from www.fda.gov/MedicalDevices/ProductsandMedicalProcedures/HomeHealthandConsumer/ConsumerProducts/HearingAids/ucm181482.htm

Vestibular Disorders Association (VEDA). (n.d.). Diagnostic tests for vestibular problems. Retrieved from http://www.vestibular.org

Vestibular Disorders Association (VEDA). (2014). What is a vestibular disorder? Retrieved from http://vestibular.org/understanding-vestibular-disorder

World Health Organization. (2014). Deafness and hearing loss. Retrieved from http://www.who.int/mediacentre/factsheets/fs300/en

Resources

Health Reports, Vol. 26, no. 7, pp. 18–25, July 2015 • Statistics Canada, Catalogue no. 82-003-X Prevalence of hearing loss among Canadians aged 20 to 79: Audiometric results from the 2012/2013 Canadian Health Measures Survey • Research Article

https://www150.statcan.gc.ca/n1/en/pub/82-003-x/2015007/article/14206-eng.pdf?st=o5Zkk1rj

https://www.canada.ca/content/dam/phac-aspc/migration/phac-aspc/seniors-aines/publications/public/injury-blessure/seniors_falls-chutes_aines/assets/pdf/seniors_falls-chutes_aines-eng.pdf

https://www.canada.ca/en/public-health/corporate/publications/chief-public-health-officer-reports-state-public-health-canada/chief-public-health-officer-report-on-state-public-health-canada-2014-public-health-future/changing-demographics.html

Acoustic Neuroma Association of Canada (ANAC): http://www.anac.ca/.

BADD—Balance and Dizziness Disorders Society: http://www.balanceanddizziness.org.

Canadian Association of the Deaf: http://www.cad.ca.

Canadian Cancer Society/Société canadienne du cancer: http://www.cancer.ca.

Canadian Centre for Occupational Health and Safety (CCOHS): http://www.ccohs.ca.

Canadian Hard of Hearing Association (CHHA): http://www.chha.ca.

Canadian Hearing Society: http://www.chs.ca.

Canadian Tinnitus and Hyperacusis Centre: http://www.canadiantinn.com.

Hearing Foundation of Canada: http://www.thfc.ca.

International Hearing Dog, Inc.: http://www.ihdi.org.

Learning Disabilities Association of Canada: http://www.ldac-taac.ca.

National Educational Association of Disabled Students: http://www.neads.ca.

National Institute on Deafness and Other Communication Disorders, National Institutes of Health: http://www.nidcd.nih.gov.

Public Health Agency of Canada: http://www.phac-aspc.gc.ca.

Seniors' Falls in Canada. 2014. http://www.phac-aspc.gc.ca/seniors-aines/publications/public/injury-blessure/seniors_falls-chutes_aines/assets/pdf/seniors_falls-chutes_aines-eng.pdf

Speech-Language & Audiology Canada: publicaffairs@sac-oac.ca

The Chief Public Health Officer's Report on the State of Public Health in Canada 2014—Changing demographics, aging and health (2014): https://www.canada.ca/en/public-health/corporate/publications/chief-public-health-officer-reports-state-public-health-canada/chief-public-health-officer-report-on-state-public-health-canada-2014-public-health-future/changing-demographics.html

Veteran Affairs Canada: http://www.vac-acc.gc.ca.

UNIT 14

Neurologic Function

Case Study EVALUATING INCREASED HYPERTENSION IN A NEUROLOGY CLINIC

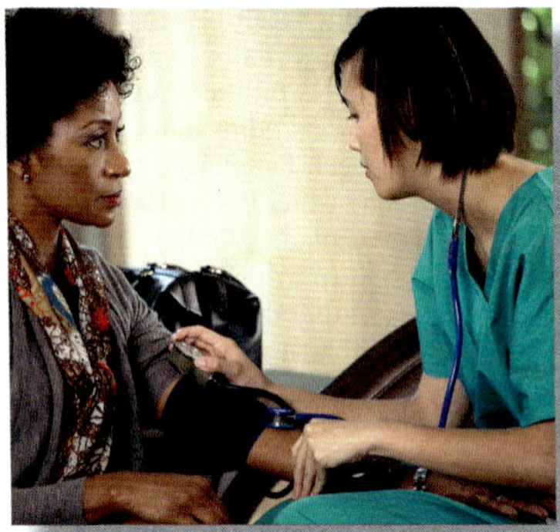

A nurse who works in a neurology clinic notes that most of the patients who are returning for care after having a stroke also have hypertension, and thus are at increased risk for another stroke. Although these patients received education while in acute care about strategies to control their hypertension, the nurse notes that this education does not seem to have been effective. The nurse wonders if a different type of intervention aimed at decreasing hypertension and the risk for another stroke should be considered.

QSEN Competency Focus: Quality Improvement

The complexities inherent in today's health care system challenge nurses to demonstrate integration of specific interdisciplinary core competencies that are aimed at ensuring the delivery of safe and quality patient care (Institute of Medicine, 2003). The Quality and Safety Education for Nurses project (QSEN, 2017; Cronenwett, Sherwood, Barnsteiner, et al., 2007) provides a framework for the knowledge, skills, and attitudes (KSAs) required for nurses to demonstrate competency in these key areas, which include ***patient-centred care***, ***interdisciplinary teamwork and collaboration***, ***evidence-based practice***, ***quality improvement***, ***safety***, and ***informatics.***

Quality Improvement Definition: Use data to monitor the outcomes of care processes and use improvement methods to design and test changes to continuously improve the quality and safety of health care systems.

SELECTED PRE-LICENSURE KSAs	APPLICATION AND REFLECTION
Knowledge	
Explain the importance of variation and measurement in assessing quality of care.	How can the nurse verify the observations made about increased hypertension rates among patients poststroke? Identify the sources of data that could be accessed to demonstrate the need for a change in the processes of care.
Skills	
Use quality measures to understand performance.	Specify the main objective that the nurse in the neurology clinic hopes to achieve with this population of patients who have had strokes. Specify measurable, time-oriented expected outcomes. Might there be an opportunity for the nurse to do a pilot test of change in this clinic? If so, how would the nurse go about designing this type of project? Who else from the neurology clinic team might need to be involved in this type of project?
Attitudes	
Value measurement and its role in good patient care.	Reflect upon the process you might follow if you were the nurse in this clinic. How would you analyze the rates of hypertension and recurrent stroke? How would you approach the patients? Would you mobilize other members of the clinic team to find a root cause for this phenomenon? Think about how mobilizing other team members could result in measurable improvements in quality of life for this population of patients.

Cronenwett, L., Sherwood, G., Barnsteiner, J., et al. (2007). Quality and safety education for nurses. *Nursing Outlook, 55*(3), 122–131; Institute of Medicine. (2003). *Health professions education: A bridge to quality*. Washington, DC: National Academies Press; and QSEN Institute. (2017). *QSEN competencies: Definitions and pre-licensure KSAs*. Retrieved June 12, 2019, from www.qsen.org/competencies/pre-licensure-ksas

62 Assessment of Neurologic Function

Adapted by Alice S.W. Khin

Learning Objectives

On completion of this chapter, the learner will be able to:

1. Describe the anatomy and physiology of the central and peripheral nervous systems.
2. Differentiate among pathologic changes that affect cranial nerves, motor and sensory pathways, and reflexes.
3. Compare the functioning of the sympathetic and parasympathetic nervous systems.
4. Relate the significance of health assessment (subjective and objective data) to the diagnosis of neurologic dysfunction.
5. Describe age-related changes in neurologic function and their impact on neurologic assessment findings.
6. Demonstrate knowledge of the diagnostic tests used for assessment of neurologic function and the related nursing implications.

Nurses in many practice settings encounter patients with altered neurologic function because the complex nervous system controls the mind, body, and spirit. Every nursing assessment is an examination of some feature of the system: cranial nerves, **mental status**, motor pathways, sensory pathways, reflexes, or speech. Alterations may occur at any time during the lifespan. They vary from mild, self-limiting symptoms to devastating, life-threatening disorders. Assessment requires knowledge of the anatomy and physiology of the nervous system, skilled history taking and physical examination, and comprehension of the array of tests and procedures used to diagnose neurologic disorders. Understanding the nursing implications and interventions related to assessment and diagnostic testing is essential.

Anatomy and Physiology Overview

The nervous system consists of two major subdivisions: the central nervous system (CNS) composed of the brain and spinal cord, and the peripheral nervous system formed by the shorter cranial and spinal nerves, and the long peripheral nerves. The brain contains more than 100 billion cells that link motor and sensory pathways, monitor body processes, respond to the internal and external environment, maintain homeostasis, and direct all psychological, biologic, and physical activity through complex chemical and electrical messages (Martini, Timmons, & Tallitsch, 2012).

Cells of the Nervous System

The basic functional unit of the brain is the neuron (Fig. 62-1). It is composed of dendrites, a cell body, and an axon. The **dendrites** are branching structures that conduct electrochemical messages to the cell body. The **axon** is a long, slender process that carries electrical impulses away from the cell body. Some neurons have a myelinated sheath that increases speed of conduction.

Nerve cell bodies occurring in clusters are called ganglia or nuclei. A cluster of cell bodies with the same function is called a centre (e.g., the respiratory centre). Neuroglial cells, five times greater in number than neurons, support, protect, and nourish neurons (Hickey, 2014; Martini et al., 2012).

Neurotransmitters

Neurotransmitters (chemical messengers) communicate messages from one neuron to another or from one neuron

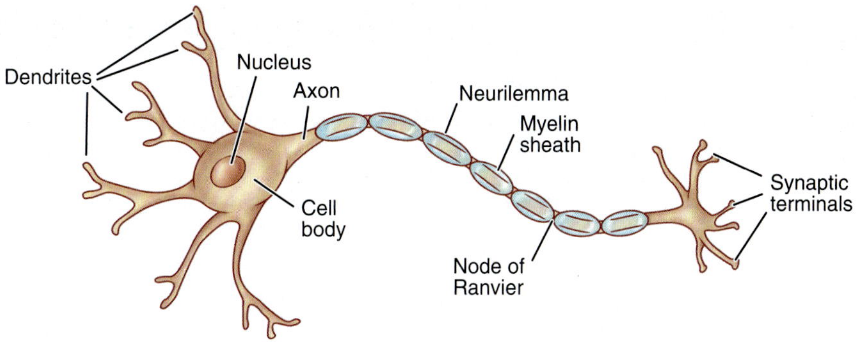

FIGURE 62-1. Neuron.

to a specific target tissue. A neurotransmitter potentiates, terminates, or modulates a specific action, and can either excite or inhibit activity of a target cell. The name of the chemical messenger, its origin, and action(s) are described in Table 62-1.

Neurotransmitters are manufactured and stored in synaptic vesicles. As an action potential (nerve impulse) is propagated along the axon and reaches the nerve terminal, neurotransmitters are released into the synapse. The neurotransmitter diffuses or is transported across the synapse, binding to receptors in the postsynaptic cell membrane. Usually, multiple neurotransmitters are at work in the neural synapse. Once released, enzymes either destroy the neurotransmitter or reabsorb it into the cell for future use.

Many neurologic disorders are associated with an imbalance in neurotransmitters. For example, Parkinson's disease develops from decreased availability of dopamine;

Glossary

agnosia: loss of ability to recognize either objects, persons, colours, images, sounds, or smells using a particular sensory system (e.g., visual, auditory, olfactory, or tactile)

ataxia: inability to coordinate muscle movements, resulting in a wide stance, and difficulty in walking, talking, and performing self-care activities

autonomic nervous system: division of the nervous system that regulates involuntary body functions (cardiac muscle, smooth muscle, and glandular activity); composed of sympathetic and parasympathetic subdivisions

axon: elongated process of the neuron that conducts impulses away from the cell body

Babinski reflex (sign): dorsiflexion (upgoing) of the great toe and spreading out of other toes when plantar superficial reflex is tested; indicative of alterations in the corticospinal tract; an expected response only in infants under 6 months of age

clonus: rapid, rhythmic muscular contractions associated with a significant hyperactive deep tendon reflex

delirium: acute, reversible, state of confusion; commonly associated with infection, medication side effects, drug or alcohol withdrawal, or dehydration

dendrite: branching cytoplasmic sensory process of the neuron that conducts impulses toward the cell body

dermatome: specific area of body surface innervated by a spinal nerve

flaccidity: decreased muscle tone (i.e., diminished residual tension); limpness, floppiness

Glasgow Coma Scale: a test of level of arousal in patients with a brain injury; assesses eye opening, motor, and verbal responses to examiner

Mental status: assessment of the workings of the patient's mind, considering the interplay of mind and body; includes orientation, alertness, memory, attention, mood, insight, judgement, and recurring thoughts

parasympathetic nervous system: craniosacral division of the autonomic nervous system; active primarily during nonstressful conditions; controls mostly visceral functions

photophobia: inability to tolerate exposure to light

position (postural) sense: awareness of position of parts of the body without using vision; also referred to as proprioception; involves position (static component) and movement (kinesthetic component) of skeletal muscles and joints, and tension in tendons and ligaments

reflex: an involuntary, automatic response to a stimulus; requires an intact neural pathway (reflex arc); may be monosynaptic or polysynaptic

rigidity: increase in muscle tone at rest; characterized by increased resistance to passive stretch

Romberg test: test for cerebellar dysfunction requiring the patient to stand with feet together, eyes closed and arms at sides; inability to maintain the position, with either significant stagger or sway, is a positive test; a test of position sense with eyes open first then closed; one test among others for static vestibular function

spasticity: sustained increase in muscle tension when it is passively lengthened or stretched, or moved voluntarily; associated with upper motor neuron lesions (i.e., found in brain or spinal cord)

sympathetic nervous system: the thoracolumbar division of the autonomic nervous system; active during stressful situations; provides predominantly excitatory responses; the "fight-or-flight" system

vertigo: illusion of an individual's movement in space, usually rotation (subjective vertigo); illusion of objects in movement around an individual (objective vertigo)

TABLE 62-1 Major Neurotransmitters

Neurotransmitter	Source	Action
Acetylcholine (major transmitter of the parasympathetic nervous system)	Many areas of the brain; autonomic nervous system	Usually excitatory; parasympathetic effects sometimes inhibitory (stimulation of heart by vagal nerve)
Serotonin	Brain stem, hypothalamus, dorsal horn of the spinal cord	Inhibitory; helps control mood and sleep, inhibits pain pathways
Dopamine	Substantia nigra and basal ganglia	Usually inhibitory; affects behaviour (attention, emotions) and fine movement
Norepinephrine (major transmitter of the sympathetic nervous system)	Brain stem, hypothalamus, postganglionic neurons of the sympathetic nervous system	Usually excitatory; affects mood and overall activity
Gamma-aminobutyric acid	Spinal cord, cerebellum, basal ganglia, some cortical areas	Inhibitory
Enkephalin, endorphin	Nerve terminals in the spine, brain stem, thalamus and hypothalamus, pituitary gland	Excitatory; pleasurable sensation, inhibits pain transmission

Adapted from Porth, C. M. (2014). *Essentials of pathophysiology* (4th ed.). Philadelphia, PA: Lippincott Williams & Wilkins.

binding of acetylcholine to muscle cells is impaired in myasthenia gravis (Porth, 2014). All brain functions are modulated through neurotransmitter receptor site activity, including memory and other cognitive processes (Hickey, 2014; Martini et al., 2012).

Ongoing research is evaluating diagnostic tests that can detect abnormal levels of neurotransmitters in the brain. Positron emission tomography (PET), for example, can detect dopamine, serotonin, and acetylcholine. Single-photon emission computed tomography (SPECT), similar to PET, can detect changes in some neurotransmitters, such as dopamine in Parkinson's disease (Fischbach & Dunning, 2015). Both PET and SPECT are discussed in more detail later in this chapter.

The Central Nervous System

The Brain

The brain accounts for approximately 2% of the total body weight; in an average young adult, the brain weighs approximately 1,400 g in an average older person, the brain weighs approximately 1,200 g (Hickey, 2014). The brain is divided into three major areas: cerebrum, brain stem, and cerebellum. The cerebrum is composed of the right and left hemispheres, thalamus, hypothalamus, and basal ganglia. The brain stem contains the midbrain, pons, and medulla. The cerebellum consists of two cerebellar hemispheres and the singular vermis (Fig. 62-2).

Cerebrum

The outside surface of the hemispheres has a wrinkled appearance that is the result of many folded layers or ridges called gyri, which increase the surface area of the brain, accounting for the high level of activity carried out by such a small-appearing organ. Between each gyrus is a sulcus or furrow that serves as an anatomic division. In between the cerebral hemispheres is the great longitudinal fissure that separates the cerebrum into the right and left hemispheres. The two hemispheres are joined at the lower portion of the fissure by the corpus callosum. The external or outer portion of the hemispheres (the cerebral cortex) is made up of grey matter approximately 2 to 5 mm in depth; it contains billions of neuron cell bodies, giving it a grey appearance. White matter makes up the innermost layer and is composed of myelinated nerve fibres and neuroglia cells that form tracts or pathways connecting various parts of the brain with one another. These pathways also connect the cortex with lower portions of the brain and spinal cord. The cerebral hemispheres are divided into pairs of lobes (Martini et al., 2018) (see Fig. 62-2):

- *Frontal*—the largest lobe, located in the front of the brain. The major functions of this lobe are concentration, abstract thought, information storage or memory, and motor function. It contains Broca's area, which is located in the left hemisphere and is critical for motor control of speech. The frontal lobe is also mostly responsible for a person's affect, judgment, personality, and inhibitions (Hickey, 2014).
- *Parietal*—a predominantly sensory lobe posterior to the frontal lobe. This lobe analyzes sensory information (e.g., taste, touch, temperature, pain, vibration, pressure) and relays its interpretation to other cortical areas; is essential to a person's awareness of body position in

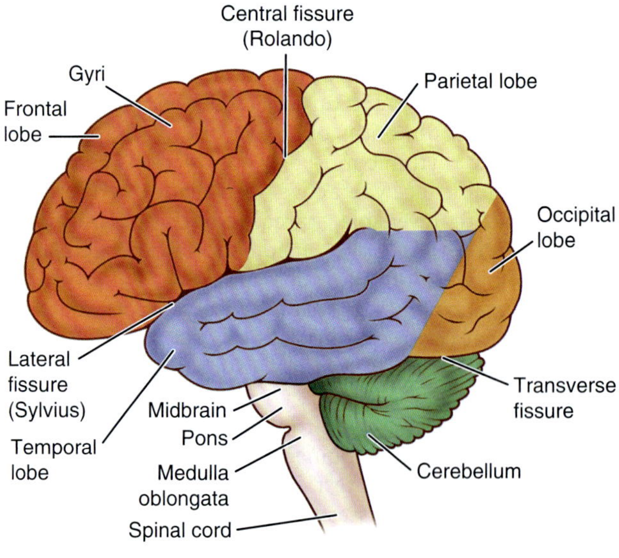

FIGURE 62-2. View of the external surface of the brain showing lobes, cerebellum, and brain stem.

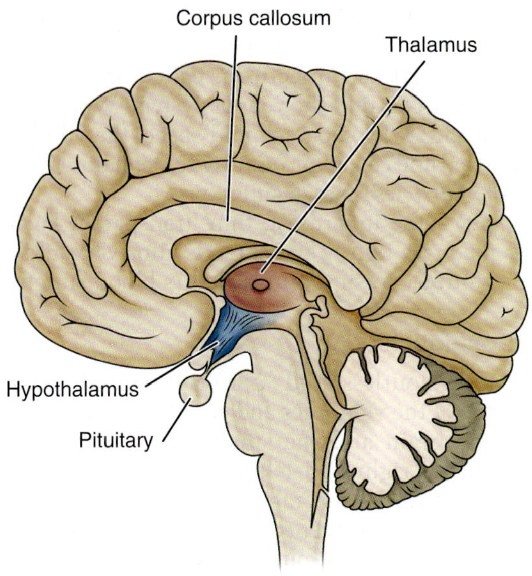

FIGURE 62-3. Medial view of the brain.

space, size, and shape discrimination, and right–left orientation (Hickey, 2014).

- *Temporal*—located inferior to the frontal and parietal lobes; contains the auditory and olfactory receptive areas and plays a role in memory of sound and understanding of language and music.
- *Occipital*—located posterior to the temporal and parietal lobes; is responsible for visual interpretation and memory.

The corpus callosum (Fig. 62-3), a thick collection of nerve fibres that connects the two cerebral hemispheres of the brain, is responsible for the transmission of information from one side of the brain to the other. Information transferred includes sensation, memory, and learned discrimination. Right-handed people and some left-handed people have cerebral dominance on the left side of the brain for verbal, linguistic, arithmetic, calculation, and analytic functions. The nondominant hemisphere is responsible for geometric, spatial, visual, pattern, and musical functions. Nuclei for cranial nerves I and II are also located in the cerebrum.

The basal ganglia are masses of nuclei located deep in the cerebral hemispheres that are responsible for control of fine motor movements, including those of the hands and lower extremities.

The thalamus (see Fig. 62-3) lies on either side of the third ventricle and acts primarily as a relay station for all sensation except smell which travels directly to the cerebral cortex. All memory, emotion, sensation, and pain impulses pass through this section of the brain.

The hypothalamus (see Fig. 62-3) is located anterior and inferior to the thalamus, and inferior and lateral to the third ventricle. The infundibulum of the hypothalamus connects it to the posterior pituitary gland. The hypothalamus plays an important role in the endocrine system by regulating the pituitary secretion of hormones that influence metabolism, reproduction, stress response, and urine production. It works with the pituitary to maintain fluid balance through hormonal release and maintains temperature regulation by promoting vasoconstriction or vasodilatation. In addition, the hypothalamus is the site of the hunger centre and is involved in appetite control. It contains centres that regulate the sleep–wake cycle, blood pressure, aggressive and sexual behaviour, and emotional responses (e.g., blushing, pleasure, rage, depression, panic, and fear). The hypothalamus also controls and regulates the autonomic nervous system. The optic chiasm (the point at which the two optic tracts cross) and the mamillary bodies (involved in olfactory reflexes, emotional response to odours, and reflex movements during eating) are also found in this area.

Brain Stem

The brain stem consists of the midbrain, pons, and medulla oblongata (see Fig. 62-2). The midbrain connects the pons and the cerebellum with the cerebral hemispheres; it contains sensory and motor pathways and serves as the centre for auditory and visual reflexes. Cranial nerves III and IV originate in the midbrain. The pons is situated anterior to the cerebellum between the midbrain and the medulla, and is a bridge between the two halves of the cerebellum, and between the medulla and the midbrain. Cranial nerves V through VII originate in the pons that contains motor and sensory pathways. Portions of the pons help regulate respiration.

Motor fibres from the brain to the spinal cord and sensory fibres from the spinal cord to the brain are located in the medulla. Most of these fibres cross, at this level. Cranial nerves VIII through XII originate in the medulla. Reflex centres for respiration, blood pressure, heart rate, coughing, vomiting, swallowing, and sneezing are located in the medulla. The reticular formation, responsible for arousal and the sleep–wake cycle, begins in the medulla and connects with numerous higher structures (Martini et al., 2018).

Cerebellum

The cerebellum is posterior to the midbrain and pons, and inferior to the occipital lobe (see Fig. 62-2). The cerebellum integrates sensory information to provide smooth coordinated voluntary and involuntary movement. It controls fine movement, balance, and **position (postural) sense** or proprioception (awareness of where each part of the body is).

Structures Protecting the Brain

The rigid skull protects the brain from injury. The major bones of the skull are the frontal, temporal, parietal, occipital, and sphenoid bones which join at the suture lines (Fig. 62-4) and form the base of the skull. Indentations in the skull base are known as fossae. The anterior fossa contains the frontal lobe; the middle fossa contains the temporal lobe; and the posterior fossa contains the cerebellum and brain stem.

The meninges (fibrous connective tissues) provide protection, support, and nourishment for the brain and spinal cord. The layers of the meninges are the dura mater, arachnoid, and pia mater (Fig. 62-5).

- *Dura mater*—the outermost layer; covers the brain and the spinal cord. It is tough, thick, inelastic, fibrous, and grey. Three major extensions of the dura permit movement of the brain: the falx cerebri, which folds between the two hemispheres; the tentorium cerebelli, which

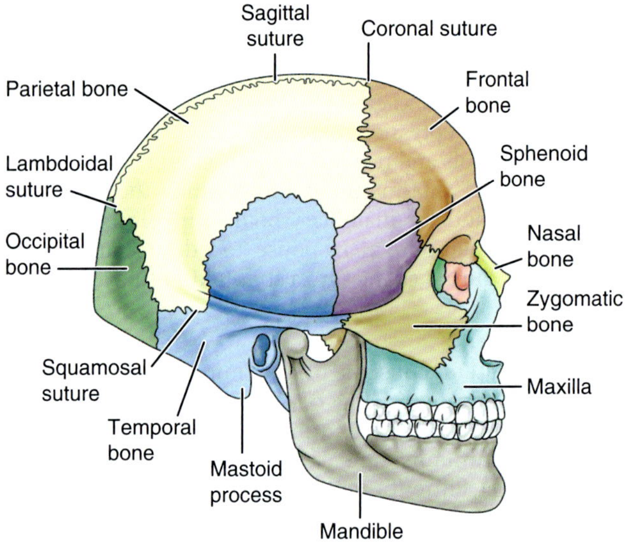

FIGURE 62-4. Bones and sutures of the skull.

folds between the occipital lobes and cerebellar hemispheres to form a tough, membranous shelf; and the falx cerebelli, which is located between the right and left cerebellar hemispheres. When excess pressure occurs in the cranial cavity, brain tissue may be compressed against these dural folds, or displaced around them or downward, a process called herniation. A potential space (the epidural space) exists between the dura and the skull, and between the periosteum and the dura in the vertebral column. Another potential space, the subdural space, exists below the dura. Blood or an abscess can accumulate in these potential spaces.

- *Arachnoid*—the middle membrane; an extremely thin, delicate membrane that closely resembles a spider web (hence the name arachnoid). The arachnoid membrane has cerebrospinal fluid (CSF) in the space below it, called the subarachnoid space. This membrane has unique fingerlike projections, called arachnoid villi, that absorb CSF into the venous system. When blood or bacteria enter the subarachnoid space, the villi become obstructed and *communicating* hydrocephalus (increased size of ventricles) may result.
- *Pia mater*—the innermost, thin, transparent layer that hugs the brain tightly and extends into every fold of the brain's surface to support the brain's blood supply.

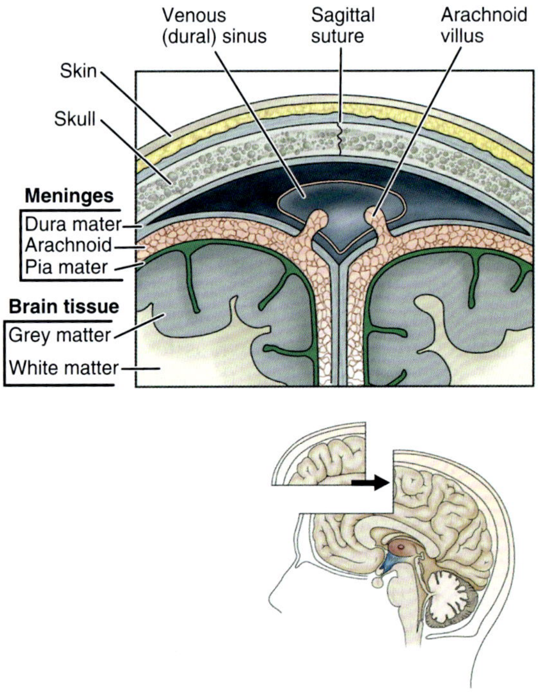

FIGURE 62-5. Meninges and related structures.

Cerebrospinal Fluid

A clear and colourless fluid (CSF) is produced in the choroid plexus of the ventricles and circulates around the surface of the brain and the spinal cord. There are four ventricles: the right and left lateral, and the third and fourth ventricles. The lateral ventricles open into the third ventricle at the interventricular foramen (foramen of Monro). The third and fourth ventricles connect via the aqueduct of Sylvius. The fourth ventricle drains CSF into the subarachnoid space on the surface of the brain and spinal cord, where it is absorbed by the arachnoid villi. Blockage of CSF flow anywhere in the ventricular system produces *obstructive* hydrocephalus.

The CSF is important in immune and metabolic functions in the brain. It is produced at a rate of about 500 mL/day; the ventricles and subarachnoid space contain approximately 150 mL of fluid (Hickey, 2014). The composition of CSF is similar to other extracellular fluids (such as blood plasma), but the concentrations of the various constituents differ. A laboratory analysis of CSF indicates colour (clear), specific gravity (1.007), protein count, white blood cell count, glucose, and other electrolyte levels (see *Understanding Clinical Pathways* on). The CSF may also be tested for immunoglobulins or presence of bacteria. The CSF may contain a few lymphocytes, but should contain no red blood cells. A CSF sample may be obtained through a lumbar puncture or intraventricular catheter (Hickey, 2014).

Cerebral Circulation

The brain does not store nutrients and requires a constant supply of oxygen. The brain receives approximately 15% of the cardiac output, or 750 mL/min blood flow. Brain circulation is unique. First, arterial and venous circulation are not parallel as in other organs in the body, partly due to the role the venous system plays in CSF absorption. Second, the brain has collateral circulation through the circle of Willis, allowing blood flow to be redirected on demand. Third, blood vessels in the brain have two rather than three layers, which may make them more prone to rupture when weakened or under pressure.

Arteries

Arterial blood supply to the brain originates from the common carotid artery, the first bifurcation off the aorta. The internal carotid arteries arise at the bifurcation of the common carotid and supply much of the anterior circulation of the brain. Branches of the internal carotid arteries, anterior and middle cerebral arteries, along with their connections, anterior and posterior communicating arteries, form the circle of Willis (Fig. 62-6).

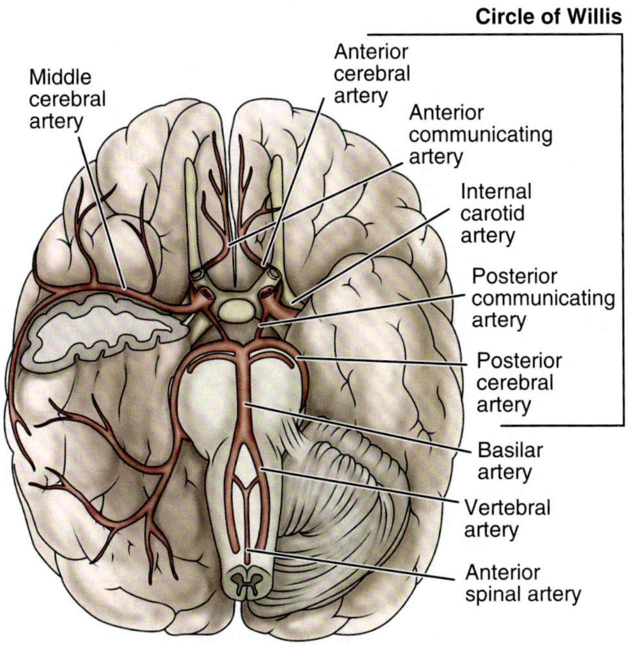

FIGURE 62-6. Arterial blood supply of the brain, including the circle of Willis, as viewed from the ventral surface.

The vertebral arteries branch from the subclavian arteries to supply most of the posterior circulation of the brain. At the level of the brain stem, the vertebral arteries join to form the basilar artery. The basilar artery divides to form the two branches of the posterior cerebral arteries. Functionally, the posterior portion of the circulation and the anterior or carotid circulation usually remain separate; the circle of Willis can provide collateral circulation if one of the vessels supplying it becomes occluded or is ligated.

The bifurcations along the circle of Willis are frequent sites of aneurysm formation. Aneurysms are outpouchings of the blood vessel due to vessel wall weakness. Aneurysms can rupture and cause a hemorrhagic stroke. (See detailed discussion in Chapter 64.)

Veins

Venous drainage for the brain does not follow the arterial circulation. Veins reach the brain's surface, join larger veins, then cross the subarachnoid space and empty into the dural sinuses which are the vascular channels lying within the dura (see Fig. 62-5). The network of the sinuses carries venous outflow from the brain and empties into the internal jugular veins, returning the blood to the heart. Cerebral veins are unique because they do not have valves to prevent blood from flowing backward and depend on both gravity and blood pressure for flow.

Blood–Brain Barrier

The blood–brain barrier isolates the CNS from many substances that circulate in the blood plasma (e.g., dyes, medications, and antibiotics). This barrier is formed by the endothelial cells of the brain's capillaries, which form continuous tight junctions, creating a barrier to macromolecules and many compounds. All substances entering the CSF must filter through the capillary endothelial cells and astrocytes. The blood–brain barrier has a protective function, but can be altered by trauma, cerebral edema, and cerebral hypoxemia. This has implications for treatment and selection of medication for CNS disorders (Hickey, 2014).

The Spinal Cord

The spinal cord is continuous with the medulla, extending from the cerebral hemispheres and serving as the connection between the brain and the periphery. Approximately 45 cm (18 in) long and about the thickness of a finger, it extends from the foramen magnum at the base of the skull to the lower border of the first lumbar vertebra, where it tapers to a fibrous band called the *conus medullaris*. Continuing below the second lumbar space are the nerve roots that extend beyond the conus, which are called the *cauda equina* because they resemble a horse's tail. Meninges surround the spinal cord (Martini et al., 2018).

In a cross-sectional view, the spinal cord has an H-shaped central core of nerve cell bodies (grey matter) surrounded by ascending and descending tracts (white matter) (Fig. 62-7).

The lower portion of the H is broader than the upper portion and corresponds to the anterior horns. The anterior horns contain cells with fibres that form the anterior (motor) root and are essential for the voluntary and reflex activity of the muscles they innervate. The thinner posterior (upper horns) portion contains cells with fibres that enter over the posterior (sensory) root and thus serve as a relay station in the sensory/reflex pathway.

The thoracic region of the spinal cord has a projection from each side at the crossbar of the H-shaped structure of grey matter called the lateral horn. It contains the cells that give rise to the autonomic fibres of the sympathetic division. The fibres leave the spinal cord through the anterior roots in the thoracic and upper lumbar segments.

The Spinal Tracts

The white matter of the spinal cord is composed of myelinated and unmyelinated nerve fibres. The fast-conducting myelinated fibres form bundles that also contain glial cells. Fibre bundles with a common function are called tracts.

There are six ascending (sensory) tracts. Two tracts, known as the fasciculus cuneatus and fasciculus gracilis or the posterior columns, conduct sensations of fine touch, pressure, vibration, position, and passive motion from the same side of the body. Before reaching the cerebral cortex, these fibres cross to the opposite side in the medulla. The

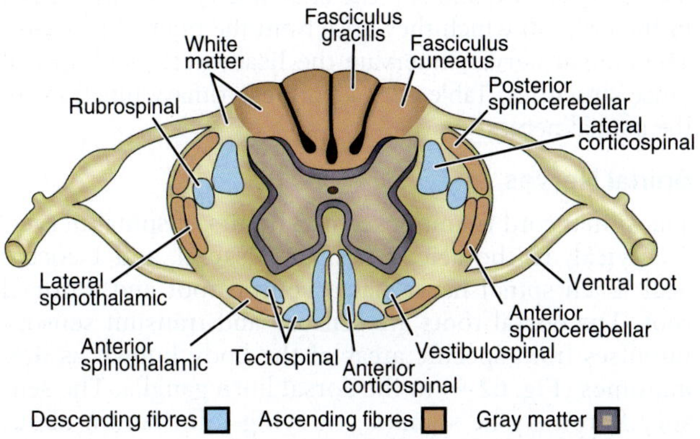

FIGURE 62-7. Cross-sectional diagram of the spinal cord showing major spinal tracts.

anterior and posterior spinocerebellar tracts conduct sensory impulses from muscle spindles, providing necessary input for coordinated muscle contraction and proprioception. They ascend essentially uncrossed and terminate in the cerebellum. The anterior and lateral spinothalamic tracts are responsible for conduction of pain, temperature, proprioception, crude touch, and pressure sensations from the upper body to the brain. They cross to the opposite side of the cord, and then ascend to the brain, terminating in the thalamus (Martini et al., 2018). There are eight descending (motor) tracts. The anterior and lateral corticospinal tracts conduct motor impulses to the anterior horn cells from the opposite side of the brain, cross in the medulla, and control voluntary muscle activity. The three vestibulospinal tracts descend uncrossed and are involved in some autonomic functions (sweating, pupil dilation, and circulation) and involuntary muscle control. The corticobulbar tract conducts impulses responsible for voluntary head and facial muscle movement and crosses at the level of the brain stem. The rubrospinal and reticulospinal tracts conduct impulses involved with involuntary muscle movement and reflex activity.

Vertebral Column

The bones of the vertebral column surround and protect the spinal cord and consist of 7 cervical, 12 thoracic, 5 lumbar vertebrae, sacrum (a fused mass of 5 vertebrae), and coccyx. Nerve roots exit from the vertebral column through the intervertebral foramina (openings). The vertebrae are separated by disks, except for the first and second cervical, the sacral, and the coccygeal vertebrae. Each vertebra has a ventral solid body and a dorsal segment or arch, which is posterior to the body. The arch is composed of two pedicles and two laminae supporting seven processes. The vertebral body, arch, pedicles, and laminae all encase and protect the spinal cord.

The Peripheral Nervous System

The peripheral nervous system includes the cranial and spinal nerves, and the autonomic nervous system.

Cranial Nerves

Twelve pairs of cranial nerves emerge from the lower surface of the brain and pass through openings in the base of the skull. Three are entirely sensory (I, II, VIII), five are motor (III, IV, VI, XI, and XII), and four are mixed sensory and motor (V, VII, IX, and X). The cranial nerves are numbered in the order in which they arise from the brain (Fig. 62-8). The cranial nerves innervate the head, neck, and special sense structures. Table 62-2 identifies primary functions of the cranial nerves.

Spinal Nerves

The spinal cord is composed of 31 pairs of spinal nerves: 8 cervical, 12 thoracic, 5 lumbar, 5 sacral, and 1 coccygeal. Each spinal nerve has a ventral root and a dorsal root. The dorsal roots are sensory and transmit sensory impulses from specific areas of the body known as **dermatomes** (Fig. 62-9) to the dorsal horn ganglia. The sensory fibre may be somatic, carrying information about pain, temperature, touch, and position sense (proprioception) from the tendons, joints, and body surfaces; or visceral, carrying information from the internal organs (Martini et al., 2018).

The ventral roots are motor, and transmit impulses from the spinal cord to the body, and these fibres are also either somatic or visceral. The visceral fibres include autonomic

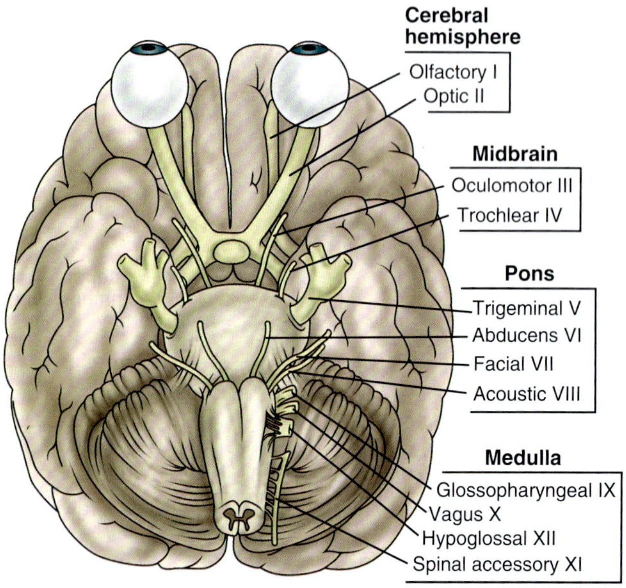

FIGURE 62-8. Diagram of the base of the brain showing entrance or exit of the cranial nerves. The right column shows the anatomic location of the connection of each cranial nerve to the central nervous system.

TABLE 62-2 Cranial Nerves

Cranial Nerve	Type	Function
I (olfactory)	Sensory	Sense of smell
II (optic)	Sensory	Visual acuity and visual fields
III (oculomotor)	Motor	Muscles that move the eye and lid, pupillary constriction, lens accommodation
IV (trochlear)	Motor	Muscles that move the eye
V (trigeminal)	Mixed	Facial sensation, corneal reflex, mastication
VI (abducens)	Motor	Muscles that move the eye
VII (facial)	Mixed	Symmetry of facial expression and muscle movement in upper and lower face, salivation and tearing, taste, sensation in the ear
VIII (acoustic)	Sensory	Hearing and equilibrium
IX (glossopharyngeal)	Mixed	Taste, sensation in pharynx and tongue, pharyngeal muscles, swallowing
X (vagus)	Mixed	Muscles of pharynx, larynx, and soft palate; sensation in external ear, pharynx, larynx, thoracic and abdominal viscera; parasympathetic innervation of thoracic and abdominal organs
XI (spinal accessory)	Motor	Sternocleidomastoid and trapezius muscles
XII (hypoglossal)	Motor	Movement of the tongue

Adapted from Bader, M., Littlejohns, L. R., & Olson, D. (2016). *AANN core curriculum for neuroscience nursing* (6th ed.). Chicago, IL: American Association of Neuroscience Nurses.

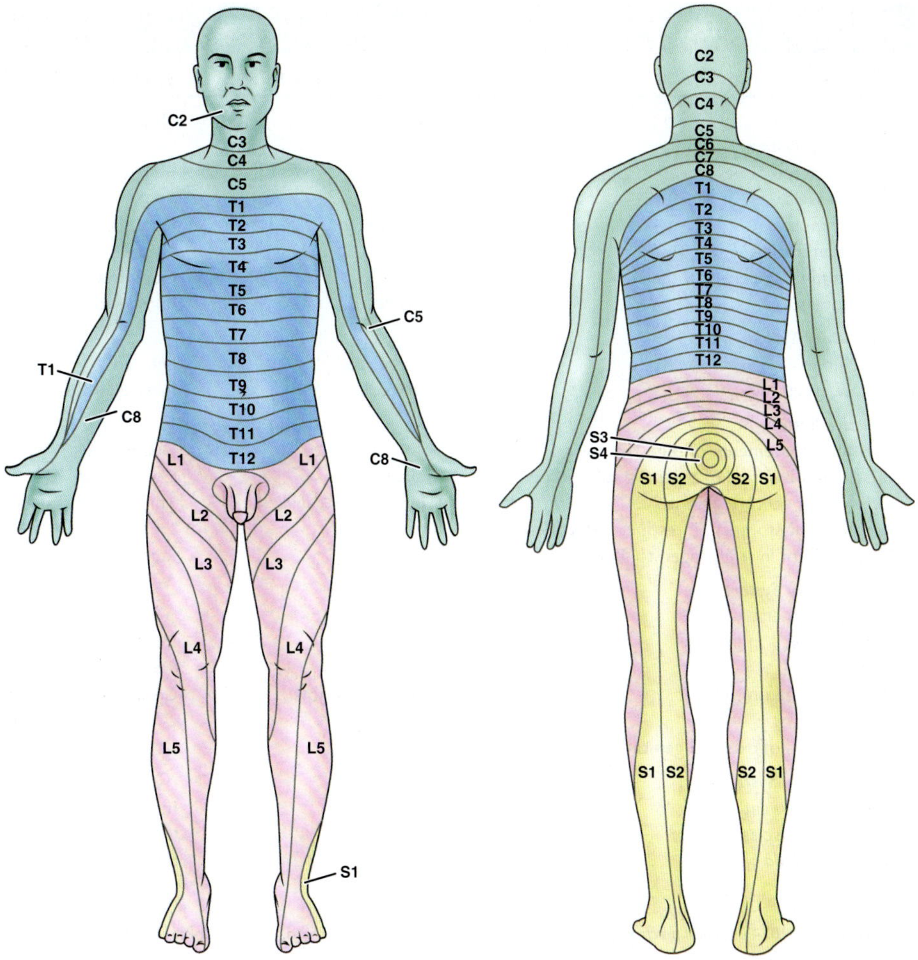

FIGURE 62-9. Dermatome distribution.

fibres that control the cardiac muscles and glandular secretions.

Autonomic Nervous System

The **autonomic nervous system** regulates the activities of internal organs such as the heart, lungs, blood vessels, digestive organs, and glands. Maintenance and restoration of internal homeostasis is largely the responsibility of the autonomic nervous system. There are two major subdivisions: the **sympathetic nervous system** (thoracolumbar division), with predominantly excitatory responses, most notably the "fight-or-flight" response, and the parasympathetic nervous system (craniosacral division), which controls mostly visceral functions and inhibition—the "rest-and-digest" response.

The autonomic nervous system innervates most body organs. Although usually considered part of the peripheral nervous system, this system is regulated by centres in the spinal cord, brain stem, and hypothalamus. The autonomic nervous system has two neurons in a series extending between the centres in the CNS and the organs innervated. The first neuron, the preganglionic neuron, is located in the brain or spinal cord, and its axon extends to the autonomic ganglia. There, it synapses with the second neuron, the postganglionic neuron, located in the autonomic ganglia, and its axon synapses with the target tissue and innervates the effector organ. Its regulatory effects are exerted not on individual cells but on large expanses of tissue and on entire organs. The responses elicited do not occur instantaneously but after a lag period. These responses are sustained far longer than other neurogenic responses to ensure maximal functional efficiency on the part of receptor organs, such as blood vessels.

The hypothalamus is the major subcortical centre for the regulation of visceral and somatic activities, serving an inhibitory–excitatory role in the autonomic nervous system. The hypothalamus has connections that link the autonomic system with the thalamus, the cortex, the olfactory apparatus, and the pituitary gland. Located here are the mechanisms for the control of visceral and somatic reactions that were originally important for defense or attack and are associated with emotional states (e.g., fear, anger, anxiety); for the control of metabolic processes, including fat, carbohydrate, and water metabolism; for the regulation of body temperature, arterial pressure, and all muscular and glandular activities of the gastrointestinal tract; for control of genital functions; and for the sleep cycle.

Most tissues and organs under autonomic control are innervated by the two divisions. For example, the parasympathetic division causes contraction (stimulation) of the urinary bladder muscles and a decrease (inhibition) in heart rate, whereas the sympathetic division produces relaxation (inhibition) of the urinary bladder and an increase (stimulation) in the rate and force of the heartbeat. Table 62-3 compares the sympathetic and the parasympathetic effects on the different systems of the body.

TABLE 62-3 Effects of the Autonomic Nervous System

Structure or Activity	Parasympathetic Effects	Sympathetic Effects
Pupil of the Eye	Constricted	Dilated
Circulatory System		
Rate and force of heartbeat	Decreased	Increased
Blood vessels		
In heart muscle	Constricted	Dilated
In skeletal muscle	[a]	Dilated
In abdominal viscera and the skin	[a]	Constricted
Blood pressure	Decreased	Increased
Respiratory System		
Bronchioles	Constricted	Dilated
Rate of breathing	Decreased	Increased
Digestive System		
Peristaltic movements of digestive tube	Increased	Decreased
Muscular sphincters of digestive tube	Relaxed	Contracted
Secretion of salivary glands	Thin, watery saliva	Thick, viscid saliva
Secretions of stomach, intestine, and pancreas	Increased	[a]
Conversion of liver glycogen to glucose	[a]	Increased
Genitourinary System		
Urinary bladder		
Muscle walls	Contracted	Relaxed
Sphincters	Relaxed	Contracted
Muscles of the uterus	Relaxed; variable	Contracted under some conditions; varies with menstrual cycle and pregnancy
Blood vessels of external genitalia	Dilated	[a]
Integumentary System		
Secretion of sweat	[a]	Increased
Pilomotor muscles	[a]	Contracted (goose-flesh)
Adrenal Medulla	[a]	Secretion of epinephrine and norepinephrine

[a]No direct effect.

From Hickey, J. (2014). *Clinical practice of neurological and neurosurgical nursing* (7th ed.). Philadelphia, PA: Wolters Kluwer Health/Lippincott Williams & Wilkins.

Sympathetic Nervous System

Under stress from either physical or emotional causes, sympathetic impulses increase greatly. As a result, the bronchioles dilate for easier gas exchange; the heart's contractions are stronger and faster; the arteries to the heart and voluntary muscles dilate, carrying more blood to these organs; peripheral blood vessels constrict, making the skin feel cool but shunting blood to essential organs; the pupils dilate; the liver releases glucose for quick energy; peristalsis slows; hair stands on end; and perspiration increases. The main sympathetic neurotransmitter is norepinephrine (noradrenaline). A sympathetic discharge is the same as if the body has been given an injection of adrenalin—hence, the term *adrenergic* is often used to refer to this division.

Sympathetic neurons are located primarily in the thoracic and the lumbar segments of the spinal cord, and their axons, or the preganglionic fibres, emerge by way of anterior nerve roots from the eighth cervical or first thoracic segment to the second or third lumbar segment. A short distance from the cord, these fibres diverge to join a chain, composed of 22 linked ganglia, that extends the entire length of the spinal column, adjacent to the vertebral bodies on both sides. Some form multiple synapses with nerve cells within the chain. Others traverse the chain without making connections or losing continuity to join large "prevertebral" ganglia in the thorax, the abdomen, or the pelvis or one of the "terminal" ganglia in the vicinity of an organ, such as the bladder or the rectum (Fig. 62-10).

Postganglionic nerve fibres originating in the sympathetic chain rejoin the spinal nerves that supply the extremities and are distributed to blood vessels, sweat glands, and smooth muscle tissue in the skin. Postganglionic fibres from the prevertebral plexuses (e.g., the cardiac, pulmonary, splanchnic, and pelvic plexuses) supply structures in the head and neck, thorax, abdomen, and pelvis, respectively, having been joined in these plexuses by fibres from the parasympathetic division.

The adrenal glands, kidneys, liver, spleen, stomach, and duodenum are under the control of the giant celiac plexus, commonly known as the solar plexus. This receives its sympathetic nerve components by way of the three splanchnic nerves, composed of preganglionic fibres from nine segments of the spinal cord (T4 to L1), and is joined by the vagus nerve, representing the parasympathetic division. From the celiac plexus, fibres of both divisions travel along the course of blood vessels to their target organs.

SYMPATHETIC SYNDROMES. Certain syndromes are distinctive to diseases of the sympathetic nerve trunks. For example, sympathetic storm is a syndrome associated with changes in level of consciousness, altered vital signs, diaphoresis, and agitation that may result from hypothalamic stimulation of the sympathetic nervous system following traumatic brain injury (Fischbach & Dunning, 2015).

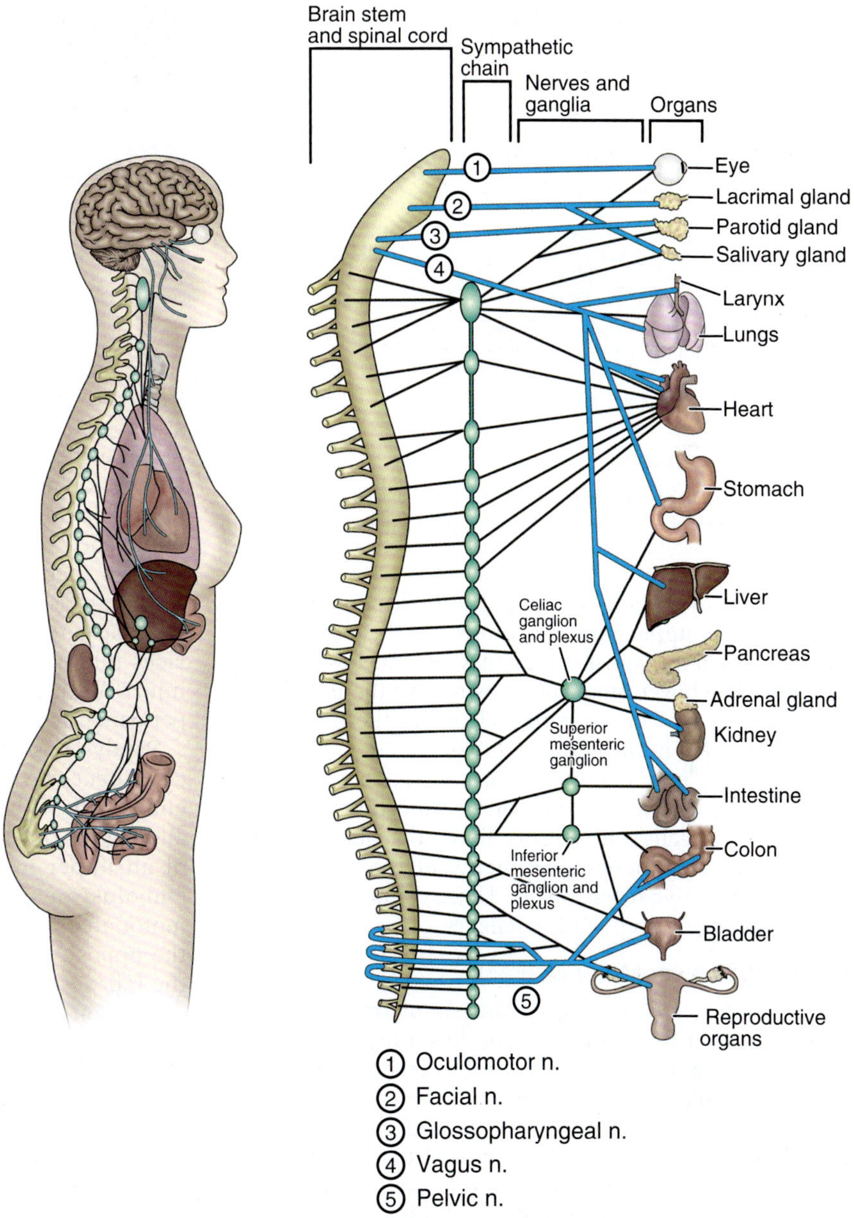

FIGURE 62-10. Anatomy of the autonomic nervous system.

Parasympathetic Nervous System

The **parasympathetic nervous system** functions as the dominant controller for most visceral effectors; the primary neurotransmitter is acetylcholine. During quiet, nonstressful conditions, impulses from parasympathetic fibres (cholinergic) predominate. The fibres of the parasympathetic system are located in two sections, one in the brain stem and the other from spinal segments below L2. Because of the location of these fibres, the parasympathetic system is referred to as the craniosacral division, as distinct from the thoracolumbar (sympathetic) division of the autonomic nervous system.

The parasympathetic nerves arise from the midbrain and the medulla oblongata. Fibres from cells in the midbrain travel with the third oculomotor nerve to the ciliary ganglia, where postganglionic fibres of this division are joined by those of the sympathetic system, creating controlled opposition, with a delicate balance maintained between the two at all times.

Motor and Sensory Pathways of the Nervous System

Motor Pathways

The corticospinal tract begins in the motor cortex, a vertical band within each frontal lobe, and controls voluntary movements of the body. The exact locations within the brain at which the voluntary movements of the muscles of the face, thumb, hand, arm, trunk, and leg originate are known (Fig. 62-11).

To initiate movement, these particular cells must send the stimulus along their fibres. Stimulation of these cells with an electric current also results in muscle contraction. En route to the pons, the motor fibres converge into a tight bundle known as the internal capsule. A comparatively small injury to the internal capsule results in a more severe paralysis than does a larger injury to the cortex itself.

At the medulla, the corticospinal tracts cross to the opposite side, continuing to the anterior horn of the spinal cord,

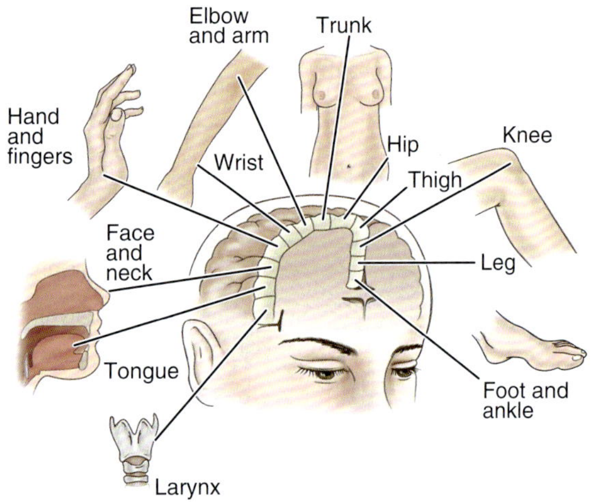

FIGURE 62-11. Diagrammatic representation of the cerebrum showing locations for control of motor movement of various parts of the body.

in proximity to a motor nerve cell. Until this point, neurons are known as **upper motor neurons**. As they connect to motor fibres of the spinal nerves, they become **lower motor neurons**. The lower motor neurons receive the impulse in the posterior part of the cord and run to the myoneural junction located in the peripheral muscle.

Involuntary motor activity is also possible and is mediated through reflex arcs. Synaptic connections between anterior horn cells and sensory fibres that have entered adjacent or neighbouring segments of the spinal cord serve as protective mechanisms. These connections occur during testing of deep tendon reflexes.

Upper and Lower Motor Neurons

The voluntary motor system consists of two groups of neurons: upper motor neurons and lower motor neurons. Upper motor neurons originate in the cerebral cortex, the cerebellum, and the brain stem. Their fibres make up the descending motor pathways, are located entirely within the CNS, and modulate the activity of the lower motor neurons. Lower motor neurons are located either in the anterior horn of the spinal cord grey matter or within cranial nerve nuclei in the brain stem. Axons of lower motor neurons in both sites extend through peripheral nerves and terminate in skeletal muscle. Lower motor neurons are located in both the CNS and the peripheral nervous system (Martini et al., 2018).

The motor pathways from the brain to the spinal cord, as well as from the cerebrum to the brain stem, are formed by upper motor neurons. They begin in the cortex of one side of the brain, descend through the internal capsule, cross to the opposite side in the brain stem, descend through the corticospinal tract, and synapse with the lower motor neurons in the cord. The lower motor neurons receive the impulse in the posterior part of the cord and run to the myoneural junction located in the peripheral muscle. The clinical features of lesions of upper and lower motor neurons are discussed in the following sections and in Table 62-4.

UPPER MOTOR NEURON LESIONS. Upper motor neuron lesions can involve the motor cortex, the internal capsule, the spinal cord grey matter, and other structures of the brain through which the corticospinal tract descends.

TABLE 62-4 Comparison of Upper Motor Neuron and Lower Motor Neuron Lesions

Upper Motor Neuron Lesions	Lower Motor Neuron Lesions
Loss of voluntary control	Loss of voluntary control
Increased muscle tone	Decreased muscle tone
Muscle spasticity	Flaccid muscle paralysis
No muscle atrophy	Muscle atrophy
Hyperactive and altered reflexes	Absent or decreased reflexes

If the upper motor neurons are damaged or destroyed, as frequently occurs with stroke or spinal cord injury, paralysis (loss of voluntary movement) results. In contrast, because the inhibitory influences of intact upper motor neurons are impaired, reflex (involuntary) movements are uninhibited resulting in hyperactive deep tendon reflexes, diminished or absent superficial reflexes, and pathologic reflexes such as a Babinski response. Severe leg spasms can occur as the result of an upper motor neuron lesion; the spasms result from the preserved reflex arc, which lacks inhibition along the spinal cord below the level of injury. With little or no muscle atrophy, muscles remain permanently tense, exhibiting spastic paralysis.

Paralysis associated with upper motor neuron lesions can affect a whole extremity, both extremities, or an entire half of the body. Hemiplegia (paralysis of an arm and leg on the same side of the body) can be the result of an upper motor neuron lesion. If hemorrhage, an embolus, or a thrombus destroys the fibres from the motor area in the internal capsule, the arm and the leg of the opposite side become stiff, weak, or paralyzed, and the reflexes are hyperactive. (See Chapter 62 for further discussion of hemiplegia.) If both legs are paralyzed, the condition is called paraplegia. If all four extremities are paralyzed, the condition is called tetraplegia (quadriplegia). (See Chapter 63 for additional discussion of these disorders.)

LOWER MOTOR NEURON LESIONS. If a motor nerve is damaged between the spinal cord and muscle, it is lower motor neuron damage which results in muscle paralysis. Reflexes are lost, and the muscle becomes flaccid (limp) and atrophied from disuse. If a patient has injured the spinal trunk and it can heal, use of the muscles connected to that section of the spinal cord may be regained, but if the anterior horn motor cells are destroyed, the nerves cannot regenerate and the muscles are never useful again.

The principal signs of lower motor neuron disease are flaccid paralysis and atrophy of the affected muscles. Lower motor neuron lesions can result from trauma, infection (e.g., poliomyelitis), toxins, vascular disorders, congenital malformations, degenerative processes, and neoplasms. Compression of nerve roots by herniated intervertebral disks is a common cause of lower motor neuron dysfunction.

Coordination of Movement

The motor system is complex, and motor function depends not only on the integrity of the corticospinal tracts but also on other pathways from the basal ganglia and cerebellum that control and coordinate voluntary motor function. The smoothness, accuracy, and strength that characterize the muscular movements of a healthy person are attributable to the influence of the cerebellum and the basal ganglia.

Through the action of the cerebellum, the contractions of opposing muscle groups are adjusted in relation to each other to maximal mechanical advantage; muscle contractions can be sustained evenly at the desired tension and without significant fluctuation, and reciprocal movements can be reproduced at high and constant speed, in stereotyped fashion and with relatively little effort.

The basal ganglia play an important role in planning and coordinating motor movements and posture. Complex neural connections link the basal ganglia with the cerebral cortex. The major effect of these structures is to inhibit unwanted muscular activity.

Impaired cerebellar function, which may occur as a result of an intracranial injury or some type of an expanding mass (e.g., hemorrhage, abscess, or tumour), results in loss of muscle tone, weakness, and fatigue. Depending on the area of the brain affected, the patient has different motor symptoms or responses. The patient may demonstrate unexpected flexion or extension, or flaccid posturing. Flaccidity (lack of muscle tone) preceded by unusual posturing in a patient with cerebral injury indicates severe neurologic impairment, which may herald brain death (see Chapter 63, Fig. 63-1 for further explanation).

Destruction or dysfunction of the basal ganglia leads to muscle **rigidity**, disturbances of posture, and difficulty initiating or changing movement. The patient tends to have involuntary movements. These may take the form of coarse tremors, most often in the upper extremities, particularly in the distal portions; athetosis, movement of a slow, squirming, writhing, twisting type; or chorea, marked by spasmodic, purposeless, irregular, uncoordinated motions of the trunk and the extremities, and facial grimacing. Disorders affecting basal ganglia activity include Parkinson's and Huntington's diseases (see Chapter 67).

Sensory System Function

Receiving Sensory Impulses

Afferent impulses travel from their points of origin to their destinations in the cerebral cortex via the ascending pathways directly, or they may cross at the level of the spinal cord or in the medulla, depending on the type of sensation carried. Knowledge of these pathways is important for neurologic assessment and for understanding symptoms and their relationship to various lesions.

Sensory impulses convey sensations of heat, cold, pain, position, and vibration sense. The axons enter the spinal cord by way of the posterior root, specifically in the posterior grey columns of the spinal cord, where they connect with the cells of secondary neurons. Pain and temperature fibres (located in the spinothalamic tract) cross immediately to the opposite side of the cord and course upward to the thalamus. Fibres carrying sensations of crude touch, light pressure, and localization do not connect immediately with the second neuron but ascend the cord for a variable distance before entering the grey matter and completing this connection. The axon of the secondary neuron traverses the cord, crosses in the medulla, and proceeds upward to the thalamus.

Position and vibratory sensations are produced by stimuli arising from muscles, joints, and bones. These stimuli are conveyed, uncrossed, all the way to the brain stem, along with fine touch, by the axon of the primary neuron. In the medulla, synaptic connections are made with cells of the secondary neurons, whose axons cross to the opposite side and then proceed to the thalamus.

Integrating Sensory Impulses

In addition to integration of all sensory impulses except olfaction, the thalamus plays a role in the conscious awareness of pain, and variation in temperature and touch. The thalamus is responsible for the sense of movement and position, and the ability to recognize the size, shape, and quality of objects. Sensory information is relayed from the thalamus to the parietal lobe for interpretation.

Sensory Losses

Destruction of a sensory nerve results in total loss of sensation in its area of distribution (see Fig. 62-9). Lesions affecting the posterior spinal nerve roots may cause impairment of tactile sensation, including intermittent severe pain that is referred to their areas of distribution.

Destruction of the spinal cord yields complete anesthesia below the level of injury. Selective destruction or degeneration of the posterior columns of the spinal cord is responsible for a loss of position and vibratory sense in segments distal to the lesion, without loss of touch, pain, or temperature perception. A cyst in the centre of the spinal cord causes dissociation of sensation—loss of pain at the level of the lesion. This occurs because the fibres carrying pain and temperature cross within the cord immediately on entering; thus, any lesion that divides the cord longitudinally divides these fibres. Other sensory fibres ascend the cord for variable distances, some even to the medulla, before crossing, thereby bypassing the lesion and avoiding destruction. Lesions in the thalamus or parietal lobe result in impaired touch, pain, temperature, and proprioceptive sensations.

Assessment of the Nervous System

The nervous system controls complex interactions in patients' internal and external environments. Nursing assessment of the effects of those interactions requires a thorough knowledge of the functioning of the neurologic system, systematic exploration of patients' potential and actual health issues related to neurologic alterations, application of appropriate methods of inquiry and physical examination techniques, and determination of patients' responses to any known alterations in health. In a potentially life-threatening situation, nurses perform very focused (emergency) assessments; in nonurgent interactions, nurses focus on a presenting concern or perform comprehensive assessments to obtain baseline data for health promotion, risk assessment, and identification of change over time. Taking into account the patient's occupation, economic status, and learning ability, they formulate an individualized plan of nursing care to assist patients to enjoy the best possible level of health.

Health History

Neurologic diseases or conditions may be stable or progressive, characterized by symptom-free periods as well as fluctuations in symptoms. Symptoms and signs may present as subtle or intense, fluctuating or permanent, inconvenient or devastating. The health history is essential for capturing previous, current, and future threats to health of the neurologic system.

Obtain an overall impression of the current health status of the patient while initiating the health history. After collecting identifying data, focus on any presenting concern and complete a symptom/sign analysis. Inquire about the location (and radiation), the nature and intensity, and the timing (including onset, frequency, and duration). Determine what factors aggravate or alleviate the symptom and inquire about associated symptoms. Ask about environmental factors (at home, school, work, or leisure) that may have a role to play. Discover the effects on daily life (significance to the patient) and only then, ask what the patient thinks is the cause (patient perspective) (Stephen, 2012). Over time, the health history will identify disorder progression, remission, or exacerbation.

Document the patient's medications (name, dosage, frequency, purpose, and response) and inquire about allergies. Document concurrent health conditions (e.g., atrial fibrillation, blackouts, carotid artery disease, diabetes mellitus, dizziness, headaches, hypertension, sensory losses, involuntary movements, weakness), and note the patient's speech, mood, attention, memory, and orientation (Stephen, 2012). Inquire about past surgeries and any history of genetic or familial disorders (Chart 62-1).

Explore the patient's expectations for health and focus on lifestyle behaviours that can be detrimental to nervous system health (e.g., physical risk-taking, alcohol or drug

GENETICS IN NURSING PRACTICE

Chart 62-1. Neurologic Disorders

Diseases and Conditions Influenced by Genetic Factors

- Alzheimer's disease
- Amyotrophic lateral sclerosis (ALS)
- Duchenne muscular dystrophy
- Epilepsy
- Friedrich's ataxia
- Huntington's disease
- Myotonic dystrophy
- Neurofibromatosis type I
- Parkinson's disease
- Spina bifida
- Tourette's syndrome

Nursing Assessments

FAMILY HISTORY ASSESSMENT

- Assess for other similarly affected relatives with neurologic impairment.
- Inquire about age of onset (e.g., present at birth—spina bifida; developed in childhood—Duchenne muscular dystrophy; developed in adulthood—Huntington's disease, Alzheimer's disease, amyotrophic lateral sclerosis).
- Inquire about the presence of related conditions such as mental retardation and/or learning disabilities (neurofibromatosis type I).

Patient Assessment

- Assess for the presence of other physical features suggestive of an underlying genetic condition, such as skin lesions seen in neurofibromatosis type 1 (café-au-lait spots).
- Assess for other congenital conditions (e.g., cardiac, ocular).

Management Specific to Genetics

- Inquire whether DNA mutation or other genetic testing has been performed on affected family members.
- If indicated, refer for further genetic counselling and evaluation so that family members can discuss inheritance, risk to other family members, availability of genetic testing, and gene-based interventions.
- Offer appropriate genetic information and resources.
- Assess patient's understanding of genetic information.
- Provide support to families with newly diagnosed genetic-related neurologic disorders.
- Participate in management and coordination of care of patients with genetic conditions and individuals predisposed to develop or pass on a genetic condition.

Genetics Resources for Nurses and Their Patients on the Web

Canadian Association of Genetic Counsellors (CAGC), http://cagc-accg.ca/-Listing of genetic centres across Canada

Canadian Directory of Genetic Support Groups, http://www.lhsc.onca/programs/medgenet-Resource guide for families and professionals

Canadian Genetic Diseases Network, http://www.cgdc.ca/-Its stated mission is to be the primary catalyst in advancing Canada's scientific and commercial competitiveness in genetic research and the application of genetic discoveries to the prevention, diagnosis, and treatment of human disease

Canadian Organization for Rare Disorders (CORD), http://www.cord.ca/-Information on over 6,000 rare disorders and links individuals/families together with the same rare disorder

Genetics Society of Canada (GSC), http://life.biology.mcmaster.ca/GSC/-Promotion of research and communication of the results and implications of genetics to the public

Genetic Alliance—a directory of support groups for patients and families with genetic conditions, http://www.geneticalliance.org

Gene Clinics—a listing of common genetic disorders with up-to-date clinical summaries, genetic counselling, and testing information, http://www.geneclinics.org

National Organization of Rare Disorders—a directory of support groups and information for patients and families with rare genetic disorders, http://www.rarediseases.org

OMIM: Online Mendelian Inheritance in Man—a complete listing of inherited genetic conditions, http://www.nchi.nlm.nih.gov/omim/stats/html

consumption, exposure to other neurotoxins [e.g., lead], dietary habits, obesity, and tobacco use).

Common Symptoms

The symptoms and signs of neurologic disorders are as varied as the disease processes. One way to organize thinking about neurologic conditions is to focus on mental status (e.g., memory, affect), speech, sensory concerns (e.g., pain, numbness, tingling), and/or motor concerns (e.g., tremor, weakness, gait). Later chapters in this unit present the relationship of specific signs and symptoms to particular disorders.

Pain

Pain is an unpleasant sensory and emotional experience associated with actual or potential tissue damage. It is multidimensional and mainly subjective, but can be observed in restlessness, irritability, facial expressions of distress, for example. Pain can be acute or chronic. In general, acute pain lasts for a relatively short period of time and remits as the pathology resolves. In neurologic disease, acute pain may be associated with meningeal irritation/infection, brain hemorrhage (e.g., subdural hematoma), spinal disk disease (e.g., sciatica with pain shooting down posterior leg) or trigeminal neuralgia (severe, jabbing facial pain) (Jarvis, 2015). In contrast, chronic or persistent pain extends for long periods of time and may represent a broader pathology. Many degenerative and chronic neurologic conditions (e.g., multiple sclerosis) present with chronic pain. (See Chapter 16 for a more detailed discussion of pain, and other chapters in this unit.)

Seizures

Seizures are the result of paroxysmal electrical discharges in the cerebral cortex, which then manifest as an alteration in sensation, behaviour, movement, perception, or consciousness. The alteration may be short, such as in a blank stare that lasts only a second, or of longer duration, such as a tonic–clonic grand mal seizure that can last several minutes. The seizure activity reflects the area of the brain affected. Seizures can occur as isolated events, such as when induced by a high fever, alcohol or drug withdrawal, or hypoglycemia. A seizure may also be the first obvious sign of a brain lesion (Hickey, 2014).

Dizziness and Vertigo

Dizziness may be a patient's term for lightheadedness, ataxia, or **vertigo**. One difficulty confronting health care providers when assessing dizziness is the vague and varied terms patients use to describe the sensation. Careful questioning clarifies the intent. Dizziness is fairly common in older adults and one of the most common concerns encountered by health professionals. Dizziness can have many causes, including viral syndromes, hot weather, roller coaster rides, and middle ear infections.

About 50% of all patients with dizziness have vertigo, which is defined as an illusion of movement, usually rotation. Vertigo is often a manifestation of vestibular dysfunction. It can be so severe as to result in spatial disorientation, lightheadedness, loss of equilibrium (staggering), nausea, vomiting, and perspiration (Hannon, 2017).

Visual Disturbances

Visual defects that cause people to seek health care can range from the decreased visual acuity associated with cataracts, double vision, or sudden blindness caused by glaucoma. Patients' concerns may or may not be associated with pain. Vision depends on functioning visual pathways through the retina and optic chiasm, and the radiations into the visual cortex in the occipital lobes. Lesions of the eye itself (e.g., cataract), lesions along the pathway (e.g., tumour), or lesions in the visual cortex (e.g., stroke) interfere with visual acuity. Unexpected eye movement (e.g., nystagmus associated with multiple sclerosis) can also compromise vision by causing diplopia (double vision). (See Chapter 60 for a more detailed discussion of disorders that affect vision.)

Muscle Weakness

Muscle weakness is a common manifestation of neurologic disease, especially distal weakness (e.g., handgrip, frequent tripping). It frequently coexists with other symptoms of disease (e.g., atrophy, fasiculations) and can affect a variety of muscles, causing a wide range of disability. Weakness can be sudden and permanent, as in stroke, or progressive, as in neuromuscular diseases such as amyotrophic lateral sclerosis. Any muscle group can be affected.

Sensory Alterations

Alterations in sensation are a neurologic manifestation of both central and peripheral nervous system disease and can affect small or large areas of the body. Frequently associated with weakness or pain, they are potentially disabling. Lack of sensation places a person at risk for falls and injury.

Past Health, Family, and Social History

Inquire about any family history of genetic diseases (see Chart 62-1).

Review of the medical history, including a system-by-system evaluation, is part of the health history. Inquire about any history of trauma or falls that may have involved the head or spinal cord and include questions regarding the use of alcohol, medications, and illicit drugs. The health history is critical in neurologic assessment and contributes to an accurate diagnosis.

Physical Examination

The neurologic examination is systematic and includes a variety of clinical tests and observations designed to evaluate a complex system. Many neurologic rating scales exist and some of the more common ones are discussed in this chapter. A complete neurologic examination includes mental status and speech, motor and sensory functions, cranial nerves, reflexes, and cerebellar function. Use the examination modes of inspection, palpation, and percussion (Bickley & Szilagyi, 2012).

The brain and spinal cord cannot be examined as directly as other systems of the body. Much of the neurologic examination is an indirect evaluation that assesses the function of the specific body part or parts controlled by the nervous system. One way to organize a neurologic assessment is to divide it into five components: consciousness and cognition, cranial nerves, motor system, sensory system, and reflexes. Depending on the patient's condition, one or more components may become the priority assessment. For example, motor, sensory, and reflex assessments are the priority in patients with spinal injury; in a comatose patient, the cranial nerves and level of consciousness become the priority; in ambulatory patients, subjective data guide the examination focus.

Assessing Consciousness and Cognition

Cerebral alterations may cause disturbances in mental status, intellectual functioning, thought content, and emotional status. There may also be alterations in language abilities. Be aware of the patient's overall level of consciousness and any changes over time.

The nurse records and reports specific observations regarding mental status, intellectual function, thought content, speech, and emotional status, all of which permit comparison by others over time. Alterations are described in specific and nonjudgmental terms. Avoid use of terms such as "inappropriate" or "demented" as they often mean different things to different people and are not useful when describing behaviour. Analysis and the conclusions that may be drawn from these findings depend on your knowledge of neuroanatomy, neurophysiology, and neuropathology.

Mental Status

Observe the patient's appearance and behaviour, noting dress, grooming, and personal hygiene. Posture, gestures, movements, and facial expressions provide useful information. Does the patient appear to be aware of and interact with the surroundings?

Assess orientation to time, place, and person. Does the patient know what day it is, what year it is, and the name of the prime minister of Canada? Is the patient aware of where he or she is? Is the patient aware of who you are or your reason for being in the room? Assess immediate and remote memory. Is the capacity for immediate memory intact?

Intellectual Function

An individual with an average IQ can repeat seven digits without faltering and can recite five digits backward. Ask the patient to count backward from 100 or to subtract 7 from 100, then 7 from that, and so forth (called serial 7s). The capacity to interpret well-known proverbs tests abstract reasoning which is a higher intellectual function. For example, does the patient know what "a stitch in time saves nine" means? The intellectual function of patients with damage to the frontal cortex may appear intact until one or more tests of intellectual capacity are performed. Questions to assess this capacity include the ability to recognize similarities. For example, how are a mouse and dog alike? A pen and pencil alike? Can the patient make judgments about situations? For example, if the patient arrived home without a house key, what options does the patient have?

Thought Content

During the health history interview, assess the patient's thought content. Are the patient's thoughts spontaneous, natural, clear, relevant, and coherent? Does the patient have any fixed ideas, illusions, or preoccupations? What are his or her insights into these thoughts? Preoccupation with death or morbid events, hallucinations, and paranoid ideation are examples of unusual thoughts or perceptions that require further evaluation.

Emotional Status

Assessment of consciousness and cognition also includes the patient's emotional status. Is the patient's affect (external manifestation of mood) natural and even, or irritable and angry, anxious, apathetic or flat, or euphoric? Does his or her mood fluctuate as you would expect, or does the patient unpredictably swing from joy to sadness during the interview? Is affect appropriate to words and thought content? Are verbal communications consistent with nonverbal cues?

Language Ability

Individuals with intact neurologic function can understand and communicate in spoken and written language. Does the patient answer questions appropriately? Can he or she read a sentence from a newspaper and explain its meaning? Can the patient write his or her name or copy a simple figure that you have drawn? Deficiency in language function is called aphasia (e.g., receptive aphasia, expressive aphasia). Different types of aphasia result from injury to different parts of the brain (Table 62-5). (See a detailed discussion in Chapter 64.)

Impact on Lifestyle

Assess the impact any impairment has on the patient's lifestyle and relationships. Consider issues such as the limitations imposed on the patient by any cognitive deficit and the patient's role in society, including family and community roles. Your plan of care needs to address adaptation to the neurologic deficit and continued function to the extent possible within the patient's support system.

Level of Consciousness

Consciousness is the patient's wakefulness and ability to respond to the environment. Level of consciousness is the most sensitive indicator of neurologic function. Observe for alertness and ability to follow commands.

If the patient is not alert or able to follow commands, observe for eye opening; verbal response and motor response to stimuli, if any; and the type of stimuli needed to obtain a response using the **Glasgow Coma Scale** (see Chapter 65). Use noxious stimuli first, then painful stimuli if no response is observed. In the patient with decreased level of consciousness, motor and cranial nerve function become the priority assessments, as the findings can indicate the area of involvement in the absence of responsiveness. (See further discussion about changes in level of consciousness in Chapter 63.)

TABLE 62-5 Types of Aphasia and Region of Brain Involved

Type of Aphasia	Brain Area Involved
Auditory-receptive	Temporal lobe
Visual-receptive	Parietal-occipital area
Expressive speaking	Inferior posterior frontal areas
Expressive writing	Posterior frontal area

Unfolding Patient Stories: Marilyn Hughes • Part 1

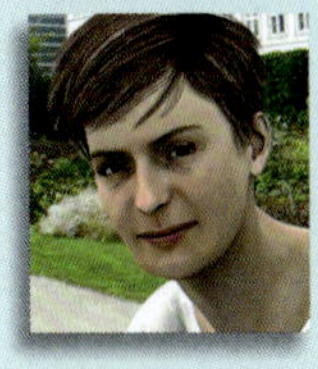

Marilyn Hughes, a 45-year-old female, was brought to the emergency department by her husband after a fall down icy stairs. She sustained a left midshaft tibia–fibula fracture, which requires surgery. Her husband informs the nurse that she also hit her head and did not respond to him for a short time after the fall. Describe the neurologic assessment performed by the nurse. Why should the nurse report this information promptly to the health care team? (Marilyn Hughes' story continues in Chapter 72.)

Care for Marilyn and other patients in a realistic virtual environment: ***vSim** for Nursing* (**thepoint.lww.com/vSimMedicalSurgical**). Practice documenting these patients' care in DocuCare (**thepoint.lww.com/DocuCareEHR**).

Examining the Cranial Nerves

Assess cranial nerves when level of consciousness is decreased, brain stem pathology exists, or peripheral nervous system disease is present. Chart 62-2 contains assessment techniques for the cranial nerves and significant findings. Compare right and left cranial nerve functions throughout the examination.

Examining the Motor System

Motor Ability

A thorough examination of the motor system includes an assessment of muscle size and tone as well as strength, coordination, and balance. Instruct the patient to walk across the room, if possible, while observing posture and gait. Inspect the muscles and palpate if necessary, for size and symmetry. Note any evidence of atrophy or involuntary movements (e.g., tremors, tics). Evaluate muscle tone (residual tension) by palpating various muscle groups at

CHART 62-2

GUIDELINES for Assessing Cranial Nerve Function

Equipment

- Tongue depressor
- Flashlight
- Sugar and salt samples
- Watch
- Cotton-tipped swab
- Cotton swabs
- Snellen chart
- Ophthalmoscope
- Samples of familiar odours
- Tuning fork
- Tubes of hot and cold water

Implementation

NURSING ACTIONS	RATIONALE
1. Explain procedure to patient.	1. Knowledge increases patient comfort and cooperation.
2. Perform hand hygiene.	2. Asepsis is essential to prevent infection.
3. Assess cranial nerve (CN) I (olfactory). With eyes closed, patient is asked to identify familiar odours (coffee, tobacco). Each nostril is tested separately.	3. The significant finding is anosmia (loss of sense of smell).
4. Assess CN II (optic). Assess vision using a Snellen eye chart. Assess visual fields. Perform ophthalmoscopic examination.	4. Significant findings include hemianopias (visual field defects) and decreased visual acuity or blindness.
5. Assess CN III (oculomotor). Test for eye movement toward the nose; inspect for conjugate movements and nystagmus. Evaluate papillary size, and test for pupillary reactivity to light; inspect ability to open eyelids.	5. Significant findings include dysconjugate gaze; gaze weakness or paralysis; double vision; dilated pupil, with or without impaired pupillary reaction to light; and inability to open the affected eyelid.
6. Assess CN IV (trochlear). Test for upward eye movement; inspect for conjugate movements and nystagmus.	6. Significant findings include dysconjugate gaze, gaze weakness or paralysis, and double vision.
7. Assess CN V (trigeminal). Have patient close the eyes. Touch cotton to forehead, cheeks, and jaw. Sensitivity to superficial pain is tested in these same three areas by using the sharp and dull ends of a broken tongue blade. Alternate between the sharp point and the dull end. Patient reports "sharp" or "dull" with each movement. If responses are incorrect, test for temperature sensation. Test tubes of cold and hot water are used alternately. While patient looks up, *lightly* touch a wisp of cotton against the temporal surface of each cornea. A blink and tearing are normal responses. Have patient clench and move the jaw from side to side. Palpate the masseter and temporal muscles, noting strength and equality.	7. Significant findings include impaired or absent corneal reflex, facial numbness, and jaw weakness.
8. Assess CN VI (abducens). Test for lateral eye movement; inspect for conjugate movement.	8. Significant findings include dysconjugate gaze, gaze weakness or paralysis, and double vision.

continued >

GUIDELINES for Assessing Cranial Nerve Function (Continued)

NURSING ACTIONS	RATIONALE
9. Assess CN VII (facial). Observe for symmetry while patient performs facial movements: smiles, whistles, elevates eyebrows, frowns, tightly closes eyelids against resistance (examiner attempts to open them). Observe face for flaccid paralysis (shallow nasolabial folds). Have patient extend tongue. Test ability to discriminate between sugar and salt.	9. Significant findings include facial weakness, inability to completely close the eyelid, and impaired taste.
10. Assess CN VIII (acoustic). Perform whisper or watch-tick test. Test for lateralization (Weber test). Test for air and bone conduction (Rinne test). Assess balance with eyes open and then closed for 20 seconds (Romberg test).	10. Significant findings include decreased hearing or deafness and impaired balance.
11. Assess CN IX (glossopharyngeal). Assess patient's ability to swallow and discriminate between sugar and salt on posterior third of the tongue.	11. Significant findings include dysphagia (difficulty swallowing) and impaired taste.
12. Assess CN X (vagus). Depress a tongue blade on posterior tongue, or stimulate posterior pharynx to elicit gag reflex. Note any hoarseness in voice. Check ability to swallow. Have patient say "ah." Observe for symmetric rise of uvula and soft palate.	12. Significant findings include weak or absent gag reflex, dysphagia, aspiration, hoarseness, and dysarthria (slurred speech).
13. Assess CN XI (spinal accessory). While patient shrugs shoulders against resistance, palpate and note strength of trapezius muscles. As patient turns head against opposing pressure of the examiner's hand, palpate and note strength of each sternocleidomastoid muscle.	13. Significant findings include weak or absent shoulder shrug and inability to turn the head to the side.
14. Assess CN XII (hypoglossal). While patient protrudes the tongue, note any deviation or tremors. Test the strength of the tongue by having patient move the protruded tongue from side to side against a tongue depressor.	14. Significant findings include dysphagia and dysarthria

Adapted from Bader, M., Littlejohns, L. R., & Olson, D. (2016). *AANN core curriculum for neuroscience nursing* (6th ed.). Chicago, IL: American Association of Neuroscience Nurses; Weber, J., & Kelley, J. (2014). *Health assessment in nursing* (5th ed.). Philadelphia, PA: Lippincott Williams & Wilkins.

rest and during passive range of motion, documenting any resistance. Unexpected muscle tone includes **spasticity** (increased muscle tension), rigidity (resistance to passive stretch), or **flaccidity** (limpness).

Muscle Strength

After assessing muscle tone, assess the patient's ability to flex or extend the extremities against resistance to test muscle strength. The function of an individual muscle or group of muscles is evaluated by placing the muscle at a disadvantage. The quadriceps, for example, is a powerful muscle responsible for straightening the leg. After the patient's leg is straightened, it is exceedingly difficult for the nurse to flex the knee. With the knee flexed, ask the patient to straighten the leg against resistance, to detect weakness. Always compare sides of the body when testing muscle strength. For example, compare the right upper extremity to the left upper extremity. Evaluate for subtle differences in strength by testing for drift. For example, when both arms are held out in front of the patient with palms up, look for drift, indicating a subtle weakness that may not have been detected during the resistance examination.

Use a 5-point scale to rate muscle strength. A 5 indicates active movement against gravity and resistance; 4 indicates active movement against gravity and some resistance; 3 indicates active movement against gravity; 2 indicates active movement with gravity eliminated; 1 indicates barely detectable contractile power; and 0 indicates no contraction, no movement. A stick figure may be used to document muscle strength in a concise format. Use the 5-point scale to record distal and proximal strength in both upper and lower extremities (Chart 62-3) (Jarvis, 2015).

When recording muscle strength, a stick figure is used as a precise form to document findings. The five-point scale is used to rate and record distal and proximal strength in both upper and lower extremities. Figure 62-12 provides further details.

Assessment of muscle strength may be as detailed as necessary. Quickly test the strength of the proximal muscles of the upper and lower extremities, comparing both

CHART 62-3

Scale for Grading Muscle Strength

Muscle strength is graded on a 0–5 scale:

0—No muscular contraction detected
1—A barely detectable flicker or trace of contraction
2—Active movement of the body part with gravity eliminated
3—Active movement against gravity
4—Active movement against gravity and some resistance
5—Active movement against full resistance without evident fatigue. This is expected muscle strength.

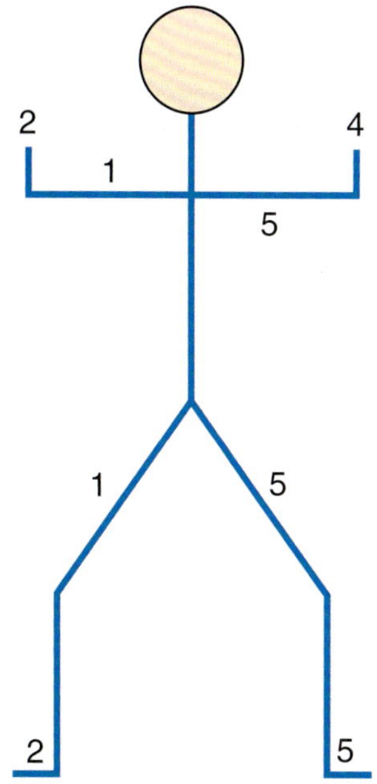

FIGURE 62-12. A stick figure may be used to record muscle strength.

sides. Then assess the strength of the finer muscles that control the function of the hand (hand grasp) and the foot (dorsiflexion and plantar flexion).

Balance and Coordination

Cerebellar and basal ganglia influence on the motor system is reflected in balance control and coordination. Test coordination in the hands and upper extremities by having the patient perform rapid, alternating movements and point-to-point testing. Instruct the patient to alternately pronate and supinate one hand at a time on his or her thigh as rapidly as possible. Ask the patient to touch each of the fingers with the thumb in a consecutive motion, one hand at a time. Note the speed, symmetry, and degree of difficulty. Carry out point-to-point testing by having the patient touch your extended finger and then his or her own nose as you move your finger in front several times. Hold your finger still and ask the patient to close eyes and touch the stationary finger. Repeat with the other arm.

Coordination in the lower extremities is tested by having the patient run the heel down the anterior surface of the tibia of the other leg and off the great toe (Stephen, Skillen, & Day, 2013–2014). Test each leg in turn. **Ataxia** is defined as incoordination of voluntary muscle action, particularly of the muscle groups used in activities such as walking or reaching for objects. Tremors (rhythmic, involuntary movements) noted at rest or during movement suggest a disorder in the anatomic areas responsible for balance and coordination.

The **Romberg test** is a screening test for balance. The patient stands with feet together and arms at the side, first with eyes open and then with both eyes closed for 20 to 30 seconds. Stand close to support the patient if he or she begins to fall. Slight swaying is expected, but a loss of balance is not and is considered to be a positive Romberg test. Additional cerebellar tests for balance in the ambulatory patient include hopping in place, alternating knee bends, and heel-to-toe walking (both forward and backward) (Stephen et al., 2013–2014).

Examining the Sensory System

The sensory system is even more complex than the motor system, because sensory modalities are more widespread throughout the central and peripheral nervous systems. The sensory examination is largely subjective and requires the cooperation of the patient. Be familiar with dermatomes that represent the distribution of the spinal nerves that arise from the spinal cord (see Fig. 62-9) (Bickley & Szilagyi, 2012). Assessment of the sensory system involves tests for tactile sensation, superficial pain, temperature, vibration, and position sense (proprioception). Instruct the patient to keep the eyes closed and demonstrate what light touch and superficial pain feel like on the patient's hand. Simple directions and demonstration of the sensation encourage the cooperation of the patient.

Assess tactile sensation by lightly touching a cotton wisp to corresponding areas on each side of the body. Compare the sensitivity of proximal areas of the extremities to that of distal areas, and of the right and left sides.

Pain and temperature sensations are transmitted together in the spinothalamic tract of the spinal cord, so it is generally unnecessary to test for temperature sense. Determine the patient's sensitivity to a sharp object assesses superficial pain perception. Pain sensation is usually tested on patients who do not respond to or cannot discriminate touch stimulation. Ask the patient to differentiate between the sharp end of a broken wooden tongue blade or cotton swab; using a safety pin is not advisable because it breaks the integrity of the skin. Occasionally, test with the dull end to check for patient reliability. Compare sides.

Vibration and proprioception are transmitted together in the posterior column of the cord. Vibration is evaluated using a low-frequency (128 Hz or 256 Hz) tuning fork. Place the handle of the vibrating fork against the distal joint of the great toes or the distal thumb joint and ask the patient what he or she feels. Stop the vibration and ask what the patient feels. If the patient does not perceive the vibrations at the distal bony prominences, progress to ankle, patella, and hip with the tuning fork until the patient perceives the vibrations. Compare side to side (Stephen et al., 2013–2014).

Position sense (proprioception) may be determined by asking the patient to close both eyes and indicate if you have moved the great toe or index finger up and down. Vibration and position sense are often lost together, frequently in circumstances in which all other sensation remains intact.

Evaluate integration of sensation in the brain by testing two-point discrimination. Touch the patient (eyes closed) with two sharp objects simultaneously. Are they perceived as two or as one? If touched simultaneously on opposite sides of the body, the patient should report being touched in two places. If only one site is reported, the one not being recognized demonstrates extinction. Another test of higher cortical sensory ability is tactile discrimination. Instruct the patient to close both eyes and identify an object (e.g., key, coin) that the nurse places in one hand; inability to identify an object by touch is known as tactile agnosia or astereognosis. **Agnosia** is the general loss of ability to recognize objects through a particular sensory

TABLE 62-6 Types of Agnosia and Corresponding Sites of Lesions

Type of Agnosia	Affected Cerebral Area
Visual	Occipital lobe
Auditory	Temporal lobe (lateral and superior portions)
Tactile	Parietal lobe
Body parts and relationships	Parietal lobe (posteroinferior regions)

system. Show the patient a familiar object and ask to identify it by name; inability to identify a visualized object is known as visual agnosia. Each of these dysfunctions implicates a different part of the brain (Table 62-6).

Decreased or absent sensations occur with conditions anywhere along the sensory pathway. Sensory deficits resulting from peripheral neuropathy or spinal cord injury follow anatomic dermatomes. Destructive lesions of the brain may affect sensation on an entire side of the body. Stroke affecting a portion of the sensory cortex will produce altered sensory discrimination.

Examining the Reflexes

Reflexes are involuntary contractions of muscles or muscle groups in response to a stimulus. Reflexes are classified as deep tendon, superficial, or pathologic. Testing reflexes enables the examiner to assess involuntary reflex arcs that depend on the presence of afferent stretch receptors, spinal or brain stem synapses, efferent motor fibres, and a variety of modifying influences from higher levels.

Deep Tendon Reflexes

Use a reflex hammer to elicit a deep tendon reflex. Hold the handle of the hammer loosely between the thumb and index finger, allowing a full swinging motion. The wrist motion is similar to that used during percussion. Position the extremity so that the tendon is slightly stretched. This requires a sound knowledge of the location of muscles and their tendon attachments. Strike the tendon briskly (Table 62-7), and compare the response with that on the opposite side of the body. Deep tendon reflex responses are often graded on a scale of 0 to 4+ (Chart 62-4).

A wide variation in reflex response may be accepted; it is more important that the reflexes be symmetrically equivalent than a certain number or designation. To compare, make sure both sides are equally relaxed and strike each tendon with equal force.

Valid findings depend on several factors: proper use of the reflex hammer, proper positioning of the extremity, and a relaxed patient (Jarvis, 2015). If the reflexes are symmetrically diminished or absent, use isometric contraction of other muscle groups to increase reflex activity. For example, if lower extremity reflexes are diminished or absent, instruct the patient to lock the fingers together and pull in opposite directions as you strike the tendon. Having the patient clench the jaw may similarly elicit more reliable biceps, triceps, and brachioradialis reflexes.

The absence of reflexes is significant, although ankle jerks (Achilles reflex) may be absent in older adults. As stated previously, scale ratings are highly subjective. Findings may be recorded as a fraction, indicating the scale range (e.g., 2/4). Some examiners prefer to use the terms

CHART 62-4

Documenting Reflexes

Deep tendon reflexes are graded on a scale of 0–4:

0—No response
1+—Diminished (hypoactive)
2+—Normal
3+—Increased (may be interpreted as normal)
4+—Hyperactive (hyperreflexia)

The deep tendon responses and plantar reflexes are commonly recorded on stick figures. The arrow points downward if the plantar response is normal and upward if the response is abnormal.

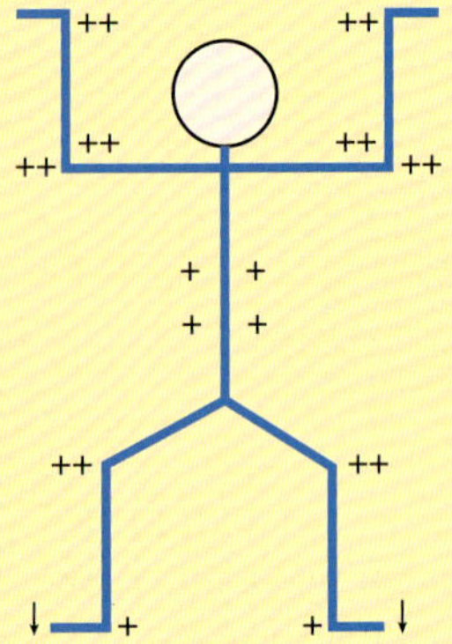

absent, diminished, present, or hyperactive when describing reflexes. As with muscle strength recording, a stick figure may be used to document numerical findings.

BICEPS REFLEX. Elicit the biceps reflex by striking the biceps tendon over a slightly flexed elbow. Support the forearm with one arm while placing the thumb against the tendon and striking the thumb with the reflex hammer. The expected response is flexion at the elbow and contraction of the biceps.

TRICEPS REFLEX. To elicit a triceps reflex, flex the patient's arm at the elbow and position it in front of the chest (bedridden patient) or at the side. Support the patient's arm and identify the triceps tendon by palpating 2.5 to 5 cm above the elbow. A direct blow on the tendon produces contraction of the triceps muscle and extension of the elbow.

BRACHIORADIALIS REFLEX. With the patient's forearm resting on the lap or across the abdomen, assess the brachioradialis reflex. Gently strike the hammer 2.5 to 5 cm above the wrist to obtain flexion and supination of the forearm (Jarvis, 2015).

PATELLAR REFLEX. Elicit the patellar reflex by striking the patellar tendon just below the patella. The patient may be in a sitting or a lying position. If the patient is supine, support the legs to facilitate relaxation of the muscles. Contractions of the quadriceps and knee extension are expected responses.

ACHILLES REFLEX. To elicit an Achilles reflex, dorsiflex the foot at the ankle and strike the stretched Achilles tendon. This reflex usually produces plantar flexion. If unable to elicit the ankle reflex and suspect that the patient cannot relax, instruct the patient to kneel on a chair or similar elevated, flat surface. This position places the ankles in

TABLE 62-7 Deep Tendon Reflexes

Level Tested	Technique
Biceps: C5 and C6 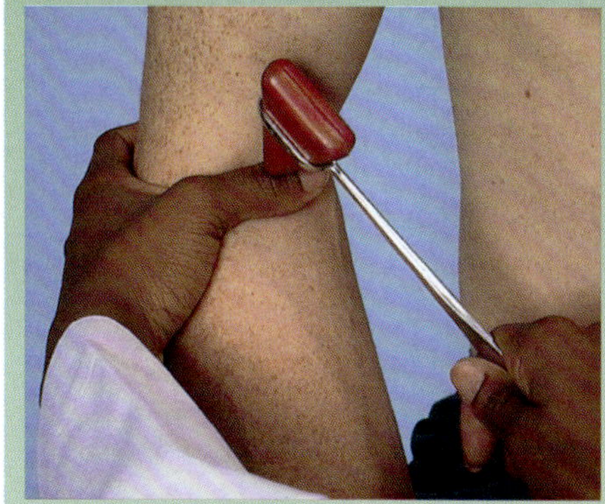	Ask the patient to partially flex the elbow and place the palm down. To assist with relaxation, the patient may rest the arm against the nurse's. Place on finger or thumb on the biceps tendon. Strike the finger or thumb with the reflex hammer briskly so that the impact is delivered through the digit to the biceps tendon. Observe for flexion at the elbow and contraction of the biceps muscle. If that patient's reflexes are symmetrically diminished or absent, ask the patient to clench the teeth or squeeze one hand tight with the opposite hand as the tendon is struck (reinforcement). This action may enhance the resulting reflex. In recording, note that reinforcement was used.
Triceps: C6 and C7 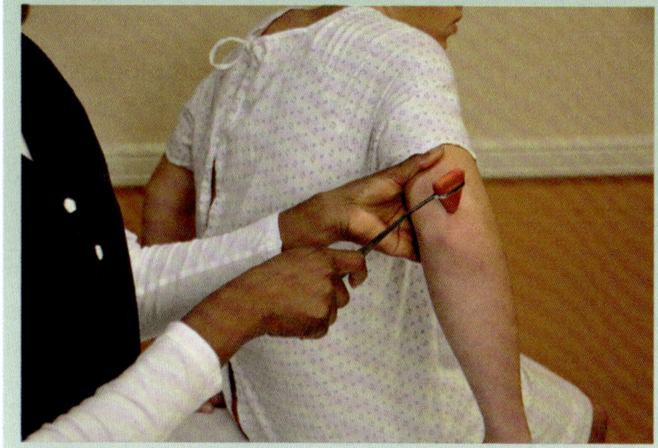	Have the patient flex the arm at the elbow and the palm toward the body if sitting or supine. If the patient is seated, it may be easiest for the nurse to hold the patient's arm in a relaxed dangling position. Palpate the triceps muscle and strike it directly just about the elbow. Observe for extension of the elbow and contraction of the triceps muscle.
Brachioradialis: C5 and C6 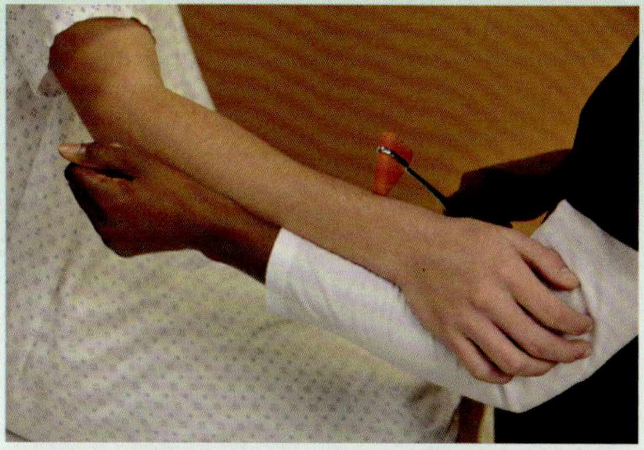	Have the patient flex the arm (up to 45 degrees) and rest the forearm on the nurse's arm with the hands slightly pronated. Palpate the brachioradial tendon approximately 2.5–5.0 cm above the wrist and strike it directly with the reflex hammer. Observe for supination of the forearm, flexion of the elbow, and contraction of the muscle.
Patellar: L2–L4 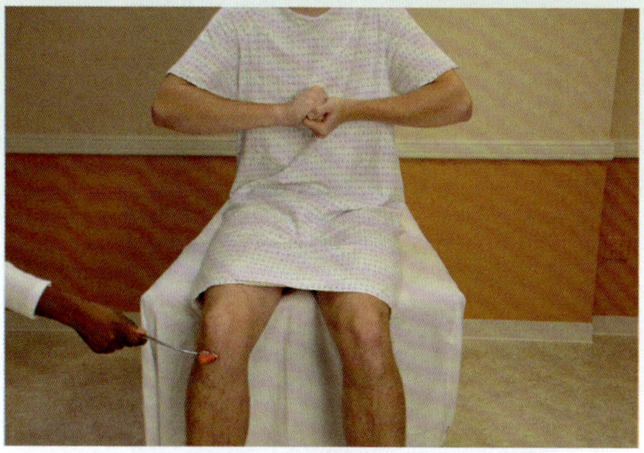	If supine, have the patient flex the knee at 90 degrees and support the upper leg with the hand. If sitting, allow the lower leg to dangle over the edge of the examining table. Palpate the patellar tendon directly below the patella and then strike it directly. Observe for extension of the lower leg and contraction of the quadriceps muscle. If the patient's reflexes are symmetrically diminished or absent, ask the patient to lock the fingers in front of the chest and pull one hand against the other (reinforcement).

continued >

TABLE 62-7 Deep Tendon Reflexes (Continued)

Level Tested	Technique
Achilles: S1 and S2 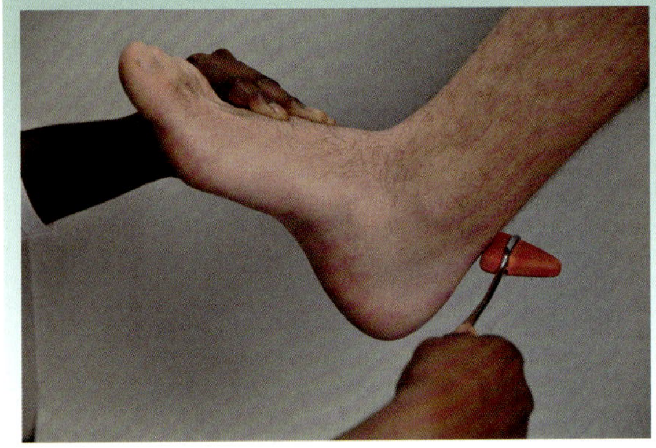	With the patient sitting and legs dangling, support the patient's foot. (The patient may also kneel on a stool with the feet dangling.) Palpate the Achilles tendon; strike the tendon directly near the ankle maleolus. Observe for plantar flexion of the foot and contraction of the gastrocnemius muscle.

dorsiflexion and reduces any muscle tension in the gastrocnemius. Strike the Achilles tendons in turn; plantar flexion is usually the result (Skillen, 2012).

CLONUS. When reflexes are very hyperactive, a phenomenon called **clonus** may be elicited. If the foot is abruptly dorsiflexed, it may continue to "beat" two or three times before it settles into a position of rest. With CNS disease this activity occasionally persists repeatedly; that is, the foot does not come to rest while the tendon is being stretched. The unsustained clonus associated with hyperactive reflexes is not considered pathologic. Sustained clonus always indicates the presence of CNS disease and requires further evaluation.

Superficial Reflexes

The major superficial reflexes include corneal, palpebral, gag, upper/lower abdominal, cremasteric (men only), plantar, and perianal. These reflexes are graded differently than the motor reflexes and are noted to be present (+) or absent (–). Of these, only the corneal, gag, and plantar reflexes are tested commonly.

Test the corneal reflex carefully using a clean wisp of cotton and lightly touching the outer corner of each eye on the cornea. The reflex is present if the action elicits a bilateral blink. A stroke or brain injury might result in loss of this reflex, either unilaterally or bilaterally. Loss of this reflex indicates the need for eye protection and possible lubrication to prevent corneal damage.

Elicit the gag reflex by gently touching the back of the pharynx with a cotton-tipped applicator, first on one side and then the other. Positive response is midline elevation of the uvula and "gag" with stimulation. Absent response on one or both sides can be seen following a stroke and requires careful evaluation and management of the resultant swallowing dysfunction to prevent aspiration of food and fluids.

Elicit the plantar reflex by stroking the sole of the foot with a tongue blade or the handle of a reflex hammer along the lateral edge and moving across the ball of the foot. Stimulation causes toe flexion.

PATHOLOGIC REFLEXES. Expect pathologic reflexes in the presence of neurologic disease. They often represent emergence of earlier reflexes that disappeared with maturity of the nervous system. A well-known pathologic reflex indicative of CNS disease affecting the corticospinal tract is the **Babinski reflex**. In a person with an intact CNS the toes contract and draw together when the plantar reflex is tested (Fig. 62-13).

If a person has CNS disease of the motor system, the toes fan out and the great toe dorsiflexes (up-toeing) (Skillen, 2012). This is expected in infants under 6 months of age, but represent a serious finding in adults. Several other pathologic reflexes convey similar information.

Gerontologic Considerations

During the aging process, the nervous system undergoes many changes, and is more vulnerable to illness. Age-related changes vary in degree throughout the nervous system. Nervous system changes due to aging must be

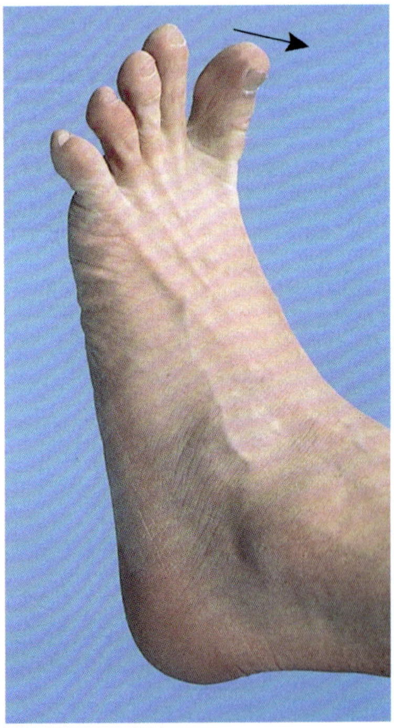

FIGURE 62-13. Babinski sign.

distinguished from those due to disease with the appropriate investigation. For example, while diminished strength and agility are an expected part of aging, localized weakness can only be attributed to disease.

Structural and Physiologic Changes

A number of alterations occur with increasing age. With a loss of neurons, the number of synapses and neurotransmitters decreases. This results in slowed nerve conduction and response time. Brain weight is decreased and the ventricle size increases to maintain cranial volume. Cerebral blood flow and metabolism are reduced, leading to slower mental functions. Temperature regulation becomes less efficient. In the peripheral nervous system, myelin is lost, resulting in a decrease in conduction velocity in some nerves. Visual and auditory nerves degenerate, leading to loss of visual acuity and hearing. Taste buds atrophy and nerve cell fibres in the olfactory bulb degenerate (Jarvis, 2015). Nerve cells in the vestibular system of the inner ear, cerebellum, and proprioceptive pathways degenerate, leading to balance difficulties. Deep tendon reflexes can be decreased or in some cases absent. Hypothalamic function is modified such that stage IV sleep is reduced. An overall slowing of autonomic nervous system responses occurs. Pupillary responses are reduced or may not appear at all in the presence of cataracts.

Motor Alterations

Reduced nerve input into muscle contributes to an overall reduction in muscle bulk, with atrophy most easily noted in the hands. Changes in motor function often result in decreased strength and agility, with increased reaction time. Gait is often slowed and wide based. These changes can create difficulties in maintaining balance, predisposing the older person to falls.

Sensory Alterations

Tactile sensation is dulled in older individuals due to a decrease in the number of sensory receptors. They may have difficulty identifying objects by touch, because fewer tactile cues are received from the bottom of the feet creating confusion about body position and location.

Sensitivity to glare, decreased peripheral vision, and a constricted visual field occur due to degeneration of visual pathways, resulting in disorientation, especially at night when there is little or no light in the room. Because older individuals take longer to recover visual sensitivity when moving from a light to dark area, nightlights and a safe and familiar arrangement of furniture are essential.

Loss of hearing can contribute to confusion, anxiety, disorientation, misinterpretation of the environment, feelings of inadequacy, and social isolation. A decreased sense of taste and smell may contribute to weight loss and disinterest in food. A decreased sense of smell may present a safety hazard, because older adults living alone may be unable to detect household gas leaks or fires. Smoke and carbon monoxide detectors, important for all, are critical for senior populations.

Temperature Regulation and Pain Perception

The older patient may feel cold more readily than heat and require extra covering in bed; a room temperature somewhat higher than usual is often desirable. Reaction to painful stimuli may decrease with age. Because pain is an important warning signal, use caution when applying hot or cold packs. The older patient may be burned or suffer frostbite before being aware of any discomfort. Reports of pain, such as abdominal discomfort or chest pain, may be more serious than the patient's perception might indicate; they require careful evaluation. Two common pain syndromes in the neurologic system in older adults are diabetic neuropathies and postherpetic neuropathies.

Mental Status

Mental processing time decreases with age, but memory, language, and judgment capacities remain intact. Change in mental status should never be assumed to be an expected process of aging. **Delirium** (mental confusion, usually with delusions and hallucinations) is seen in older patients who have underlying CNS damage or are experiencing an acute condition such as infection, adverse medication reaction, or dehydration. Drug toxicity and depression may produce impairment of attention and memory, and require evaluation as a possible cause of mental status change. Delirium must be differentiated from dementia, which is a chronic and irreversible deterioration of cognitive status. (See Chapter 14 for further discussion of delirium and dementia.)

Nursing Implications

Include the previously described modifications to your nursing care for patients with age-related changes to the nervous system, and for patients with long-term neurologic disability who are aging. Consider the consequences of any neurologic deficit and its impact on overall function such as activities of daily living, use of assistive devices, and individual coping when planning patient care. Evaluate for risk of falls, and initiate falls prevention measures for the hospitalized and home-based patient.

Understand the altered responses and changing needs of the older patient before providing education. Visual and hearing deficits require adaptations in activities such as preoperative teaching, diet therapy, and instruction about new medications. When taking advantage of visual materials for teaching or menu selection, use adequate lighting without glare, contrasting colours, and large print to offset visual difficulties caused by rigidity and opacity of the lens in the eye and slower pupillary reaction. Explain procedures and preparations needed for diagnostic tests, taking into account the possibility of impaired hearing and slowed responses in older adults. Even with hearing loss, the patient often hears adequately if you use a low-pitched, clear voice; shouting only makes it harder for the patient to understand. Providing auditory and visual cues aids understanding; if the patient has a significant hearing or visual loss, assistive devices, a signer, interpreter, or translator may be needed.

Teach at an unrushed pace and use reinforcement to enhance learning and retention. Keep material short, concise, and concrete. Match vocabulary to the patient's ability, and clearly define terms. The older patient requires adequate time to receive and respond to stimuli, to learn, and to react. These measures allow comprehension, memory, and formation of association and concepts.

Diagnostic Evaluation

Computed Tomography Scanning

Computed tomography (CT) scanning uses a narrow x-ray beam to scan body parts in successive layers. The images provide cross-sectional views of the brain, distinguishing differences in tissue densities of the skull, cortex, subcortical structures, and ventricles. An intravenous (IV) contrast agent may be used to highlight differences further. The brightness of each slice of the brain in the final image is proportional to the degree to which it absorbs x-rays. The image is displayed on an oscilloscope or TV monitor and is photographed and stored digitally. Scanning with CT is usually performed first without contrast material and then with IV contrast, if needed. The patient lies on an adjustable table with the head in a head rest while the scanning system rotates around the head and produces cross-sectional images. The patient must lie with the head held perfectly still without talking or moving the face, because head motion distorts the image. Scanning by CT is quick and painless and uses a small amount of radiation to produce images; it has a high degree of sensitivity for detecting lesions.

Spiral (helical) CT scanning can be used to avoid misinterpretations because of movement by children or adults who are unable to remain still. Spiral CT is quick.

Brain lesions have a different tissue density from the surrounding healthy brain tissue. Alterations detected on brain CT include tumour or other masses, infarction, hemorrhage, displacement of the ventricles, and cortical atrophy. Angiography by CT allows visualization of blood vessels; in some situations this eliminates the need for formal angiography. Whole-body CT scanners allow cross-sections of the spinal cord to be visualized. The injection of a water-soluble iodinated contrast agent into the subarachnoid space through lumbar puncture improves the visualization of the spinal and intracranial contents on these images. The CT scan, along with magnetic resonance imaging (MRI), has largely replaced myelography as a diagnostic procedure for the diagnosis of herniated lumbar disks.

Nursing Interventions

Essential nursing interventions include preparation for the procedure and patient monitoring. Teach the patient about the need to lie quietly throughout the procedure. Review relaxation techniques with patients who experience claustrophobia. Administer sedation if agitation, restlessness, or confusion will interfere with a successful study. Monitor the sedated patient closely. If a contrast agent is to be used, assess the patient in advance for an iodine/shellfish allergy, because the contrast agent used may be iodine based. Evaluate renal function because the contrast material is cleared through the kidneys. Prepare a suitable IV line for contrast injection and ensure fasting (usually 4 hours) prior to the study. Monitor patients who receive an IV contrast agent during and after the procedure for allergic reactions and changes in kidney function (Fischbach & Dunning, 2015).

Magnetic Resonance Imaging

Imaging using MR applies a powerful magnetic field to obtain images of different areas of the body without using ionizing radiation. Serial studies can be performed without risk. The magnetic field causes the hydrogen nuclei (protons) within the body to align like small magnets in a magnetic field. In combination with radiofrequency pulses, the protons emit signals, which are converted to images. An MRI scan can be performed with or without a contrast agent and can identify a cerebral condition earlier and more clearly than other diagnostic tests. It can provide information about the chemical changes within cells, allowing the clinician to monitor a tumour's response to treatment. It is particularly useful in the diagnosis of brain tumour, stroke, and multiple sclerosis. A complete MRI scan may take an hour or longer to complete, so use in emergency situations is limited.

Newer MRI applications allow imaging of brain blood flow and metabolism via special imaging techniques added to the MRI. Such techniques include diffusion-weighted imaging (DWI), perfusion-weighted imaging (PWI), magnetic resonance spectroscopy, and fluid attenuation inversion recovery (FLAIR). Magnetic resonance angiography (MRA) allows separate visualization of the cerebral vasculature without the administration of an arterial contrast agent. Both MRI and CT images are used as tools to plan and direct surgical intervention.

Nursing Interventions

Patient preparation includes teaching and obtaining an adequate history. Ferromagnetic substances in the body may become dislodged by the magnet, so history of working with metal fragments must be reviewed. Inquire if the patient has any implants of metal objects (e.g., aneurysm clips, orthopedic hardware, pacemakers, artificial heart valves, intrauterine devices). Understand that these objects could malfunction, be dislodged, or heat up as they absorb energy. Cochlear implants will be inactivated by MRI; therefore, other imaging procedures are considered. A complete list of metal compatibility may be found on MRI manufacturers' web sites contained in the resource section at the end of the chapter.

Before the patient enters the room where the MRI is to be performed, all metal objects and credit cards (the magnetic field can erase them) must be removed. This includes medication patches that have a metal backing and metallic lead wires; these can cause burns if not removed (Fischbach & Dunning, 2015). No metal objects may be brought into the room where the MRI is located; this includes oxygen tanks, IV poles, ventilators, or even stethoscopes. The magnetic field generated by the unit is so strong that any metal-containing items will be strongly attracted and literally can be pulled away with such force that they fly like projectiles toward the magnet. There is a risk of severe injury and death. Further, damage to expensive equipment may occur.

NURSING ALERT

For patient safety, the nurse must make sure that no patient care equipment (e.g., portable oxygen tanks) that contains metal or metal parts enters the room where the MRI is located. The patient must be assessed for the presence of medication patches with foil backing (such as nicotine) that may cause a burn.

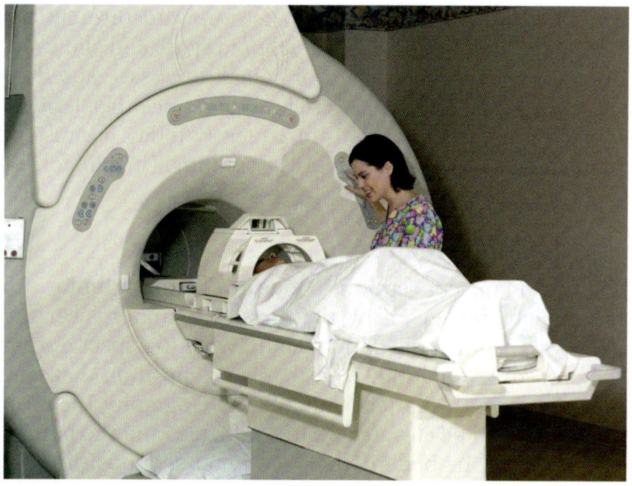

FIGURE 62-14. Technician explains what to expect during a magnetic resonance imaging procedure.

For the MRI, the patient lies with the head in a frame on a flat platform that is moved into a tube housing the magnet (Fig. 62-14).

The tube is narrow; persons with a wide girth may not fit into the scanner. Patients who are unable to lie flat will not be able to tolerate an MRI. The scanning process is painless, but the patient hears loud thumping of the magnetic coils as the magnetic field is being pulsed. Patients may experience claustrophobia while inside the narrow tube; sedation may be prescribed in these circumstances. Newer versions of MRI machines (open MRI) are less claustrophobic than the earlier devices and are available in some locations. However, the images produced on these machines are often not as detailed, and traditional devices are preferable for accurate diagnosis. The patient may be taught to use relaxation techniques while in the scanner. The patient is informed that he or she will be able to talk to the staff during the scan through a microphone inside the scanner (Fischbach & Dunning, 2015).

Positron Emission Tomography

Tomography by PE is a computer-based nuclear imaging technique that produces images of actual organ functioning. The patient either inhales a radioactive gas or is injected with a radioactive substance that emits positively charged particles. When these positrons combine with negatively charged electrons (typically found in the body's cells), the resultant gamma rays can be detected by a scanning device that produces a series of two-dimensional views at various levels of the brain. This information is integrated by a computer and gives a composite picture of the brain at work.

The PET permits the measurement of blood flow, tissue composition, and brain metabolism and thus indirectly evaluates brain function. The brain is one of the most metabolically active organs, consuming 80% of the glucose the body uses. The PET measures this activity in specific areas of the brain and can detect changes in glucose use.

This tomography is useful in showing metabolic changes in the brain (Alzheimer's disease), locating lesions (brain tumour, epileptogenic lesions), identifying blood flow and oxygen metabolism in patients with strokes, distinguishing tumour from areas of necrosis, and revealing biochemical irregularities associated with mental illness. The isotopes used have a very short half-life and are expensive to produce, requiring specialized equipment for production. This type of scanning has been useful in research settings for the last 20 years and is becoming more available in clinical settings. Improvement in the scanning procedure and production of isotopes, as well as the advent of reimbursement by third-party payers, has increased the availability of PET studies.

Nursing Interventions

Prepare the patient by explaining the test, and teaching the patient about inhalation techniques and the sensations (e.g., dizziness, lightheadedness, and headache) that may occur. Explain that the IV injection of the radioactive substance produces similar side effects. Ensure that no caffeine, alcohol, or tobacco have been used recently. Review relaxation exercises that may reduce patient anxiety during the test. Encourage the patient to drink plenty of fluids following the test to help remove radioisotopes from the body.

Single-Photon Emission Computed Tomography

Tomography by SPEC is a three-dimensional imaging technique that uses radionuclides and instruments to detect single-photons. This perfusion study captures a moment of cerebral blood flow at the time of injection of a radionuclide. Gamma photons are emitted from a radiopharmaceutical agent administered to the patient and are detected by a rotating gamma camera or cameras; the image is sent to a minicomputer. This approach allows areas behind overlying structures or background to be viewed, greatly increasing the contrast between healthy and altered tissue. It is relatively inexpensive, and the duration is similar to that of a CT scan.

The quality of brain scanning has improved significantly with SPECT which is useful in detecting the extent and location of unusually perfused areas of the brain, thus allowing detection, localization, and sizing of stroke (before it is visible by CT scan); the localization of seizure foci in epilepsy; the detection of tumour progression (and the evaluation of perfusion before and after neurosurgical procedures. Pregnancy and breast-feeding are contraindications to SPECT.

Nursing Interventions

The nursing interventions for SPECT primarily include patient preparation and patient monitoring. Teach the patient what to expect before the test to allay anxiety and ensure patient cooperation during the test. Advise premenopausal women to practise effective contraception before and for several days after testing; instruct the woman who is breast-feeding to stop nursing for the time period recommended by the nuclear medicine department.

Be prepared to accompany and monitor the patient during transport to the nuclear medicine department for the scan. Monitor patients during and after the procedure for allergic reactions to the radiopharmaceutical agent.

Cerebral Angiography

Cerebral angiography is an x-ray study of the cerebral circulation with a contrast agent injected into a selected artery. A valuable tool for investigating vascular disease or anomalies, it is used to determine vessel patency, identify presence of collateral circulation, and provides detail on vascular anomalies that can be used in planning interventions. With the advent of additional imaging techniques, formal cerebral angiography is less frequently performed.

Cerebral angiograms are performed by threading a catheter through the femoral artery in the groin and up to the desired vessel. Alternatively, direct puncture of the carotid artery or retrograde injection of a contrast agent (e.g., iodinated substance, carbon dioxide gas) into the brachial artery may be performed. X-ray images are obtained as the contrast agent flows through the vessels; the carotid and vertebral arterial systems are visualized, as well as venous drainage. Arterial access may also be used for interventional procedures, such as placing coils in an aneurysm or arteriovenous malformation.

After the groin is shaved a local anesthetic agent is administered to minimize pain at the insertion site and to reduce arterial spasm. A catheter is introduced into the femoral artery, flushed with heparinized saline, and filled with contrast agent. Fluoroscopy is used to guide the catheter to the appropriate vessels. Neurologic assessment is conducted during and immediately following cerebral angiography to observe for embolism or arterial dissection that may occur during the test. Signs of these complications include new onset of alterations in the level of consciousness, weakness on one side of the body, motor or sensory deficits, and speech disturbances.

Nursing Interventions

Ensure that the patient's blood urea nitrogen and creatinine are checked prior to the angiography to confirm that the kidneys will be able to clear the contrast agent. Usually, permit clear liquids up to the time of the test so that the patient remains well hydrated. Assess the patient's peripheral pulses as baseline data for monitoring afterwards; mark locations of the appropriate pulses with a felt-tip pen. Instruct the patient to void immediately before the test. Explain that the patient is to remain immobile during the angiogram process and to expect a brief feeling of warmth in the face, behind the eyes, or in the jaw, teeth, tongue, and lips, as well as a metallic taste when the contrast agent is injected.

Monitor vital signs frequently. Conduct neurologic assessment before and after cerebral angiography. Observe the injection site for bleeding or hematoma formation (a localized collection of blood). Monitor peripheral pulses frequently because of the risk of a hematoma at the puncture site or embolization to a distal artery. Assess the colour and temperature of the involved extremity for early detection of possible embolism. Observe for delayed allergic reaction.

Myelography

A myelogram is an x-ray of the spinal subarachnoid space taken after the injection of a contrast agent into the spinal subarachnoid space through a lumbar puncture. The water-based contrast agent disperses upward through the CSF to outline the spinal subarachnoid space and show any distortion of the spinal cord or spinal dural sac caused by tumours, cysts, herniated vertebral disks, or other lesions. Myelography is performed infrequently today because of the sensitivity of CT and MRI scanning (Fischbach & Dunning, 2015).

Nursing Interventions

Clarify any misconceptions about myelography, follow up the explanation given by the physician, and answer the questions. Inform the patient about what to expect during the procedure, including the changes in position that may occur. Inform the patient that after myelography, the head of the bed will be elevated 30 to 45 degrees and the patient is to remain in bed in the recommended position for 3 hours or as prescribed. Instruct the patient to drink liberal amounts of fluid for rehydration and replacement of CSF to decrease the incidence of post–lumbar puncture headache. Monitor the blood pressure, pulse, respiratory rate, and temperature as well as the patient's ability to void. Observe for untoward signs such as headache, fever, stiff neck, **photophobia** (sensitivity to light), seizures, and signs of chemical or bacterial meningitis (Hickey, 2014).

Noninvasive Carotid Flow Studies

Noninvasive carotid flow studies use ultrasound imagery and Doppler measurements of arterial blood flow to evaluate carotid and deep orbital circulation. The graph produced indicates blood velocity. Increased blood velocity can indicate stenosis or partial obstruction. These tests are often obtained before more invasive tests such as arteriography, or are used as screening tools. Carotid Doppler, carotid ultrasonography, oculoplethysmography, and ophthalmodynamometry are four common noninvasive vascular techniques that permit evaluation of arterial blood flow and detection of arterial stenosis, occlusion, and plaques. These vascular studies allow noninvasive imaging of extracranial and intracranial circulation (Diepenbrock, 2012).

Transcranial Doppler

Transcranial Doppler uses the same noninvasive techniques as carotid flow studies except that it records the blood flow velocities of the intracranial vessels. Arterial flow velocities can be measured through thin areas of the temporal and occipital bones of the skull. A handheld Doppler probe emits a pulsed beam; the signal is reflected by the moving red blood cells within the blood vessels. Transcranial Doppler is a noninvasive technique that is helpful in assessing vasospasm (a complication following subarachnoid hemorrhage), altered cerebral blood flow found in occlusive vascular disease, other cerebral pathology, and brain death.

Nursing Interventions

When a carotid flow study or transcranial Doppler is scheduled, describe the procedure to the patient. Inform the patient that this is a noninvasive test, that a handheld transducer will be placed over the neck and the orbits of the eyes, and that a water-soluble jelly is used on the transducer. Either one of these low-risk tests can be performed at the patient's bedside.

Electroencephalography

An electroencephalogram (EEG) represents a record of the electrical activity generated in the brain (Hickey, 2014). It is obtained using electrodes applied on the scalp or microelectrodes placed within the brain tissue. It provides an assessment of cerebral electrical activity. It is useful for diagnosing and evaluating seizure disorders, coma, or organic brain syndrome. Tumours, brain abscesses, blood clots, and infection may cause altered patterns in electrical activity. The EEG is also used in making a determination of brain death.

Electrodes are applied to the scalp to record the electrical activity in various regions of the brain. The amplified activity of the neurons between any two of these electrodes is recorded on continuously moving paper; this record is called the encephalogram.

For a baseline recording, the patient lies quietly with both eyes closed. The patient may be asked to hyperventilate for 3 to 4 minutes or to look at a bright, flashing light for photic stimulation. These activation procedures are performed to evoke unexpected electrical discharges, such as seizure potentials. A sleep EEG may be recorded after sedation because some atypical brain waves are seen only when the patient is asleep. If the epileptogenic area is inaccessible to conventional scalp electrodes, nasopharyngeal electrodes may be used.

Depth recording of EEG is performed by introducing electrodes stereotactically (radiologically placed using instrumentation) into a target area of the brain, as indicated by the patient's seizure pattern and scalp EEG. It is used to identify patients who may benefit from surgical excision of epileptogenic foci. Special transsphenoidal, mandibular, and nasopharyngeal electrodes can be used, and video recording combined with EEG monitoring and telemetry is used in hospital settings to capture epileptiform conditions and their sequelae. Some epilepsy centres provide long-term ambulatory EEG monitoring with portable recording devices (Bader et al., 2016).

Nursing Interventions

To increase the chances of recording seizure activity, it is sometimes recommended that the patient be deprived of sleep on the night before the EEG. Withold anticonvulsant agents, tranquilizers, stimulants, and depressants 24 to 48 hours before an EEG because these medications can alter the EEG wave patterns or mask the unusual wave patterns of seizure disorders (Pagana & Pagana, 2017). Ensure that coffee, tea, chocolate, and cola drinks are not served in the meal before the test because of their stimulating effect. At the same time, ensure that the patient is not fasting, because an altered (diminished) blood glucose level can cause changes in brain wave patterns.

Inform the patient that the standard EEG takes 45 to 60 minutes; a sleep EEG requires 12 hours. Assure the patient that the procedure does not cause an electric shock (the flow of electrical activity is from the patient's body) and that the EEG is a diagnostic test, not a form of treatment. Alert the patient to lie quietly during the test. Inform that sedation is not advisable, because it may lower the seizure threshold in patients with a seizure disorder and it alters brain wave activity in all patients. Check the physician's prescription regarding the administration of anticonvulsant medication prior to testing (Pagana & Pagana, 2013).

Understand that routine EEGs use a water-soluble lubricant for electrode contact, which can be wiped off and removed by shampooing later; sleep EEGs involve the use of collodion glue for electrode contact, which requires acetone for removal.

Electromyography

An electromyogram (EMG) is obtained by inserting needle electrodes into the skeletal muscles to measure changes in the electrical potential of the muscles (Pagana & Pagana, 2013). The electrical potentials are shown on an oscilloscope and amplified so that both the sound and appearance of the waves can be analyzed and compared simultaneously.

An EMG is useful in determining the presence of neuromuscular disorders and myopathies. It helps distinguish weakness due to neuropathy (functional or pathologic changes in the peripheral nervous system) from weakness resulting from other causes.

Nursing Interventions

Explain the procedure and alert the patient to expect a sensation similar to that of an intramuscular injection as the needle is inserted into the muscle. Inform the patient that the muscles examined may ache for a short time after the procedure.

Nerve Conduction Studies

Nerve conduction studies are performed by stimulating a peripheral nerve at several points along its course and recording the muscle action potential or the sensory action potential that results. Surface or needle electrodes are placed on the skin over the nerve to stimulate the nerve fibres. This test is useful in the study of peripheral neuropathies and is often included as part of the EMG.

Evoked Potential Studies

Evoked potential studies involve application of an external stimulus to specific peripheral sensory receptors with subsequent measurement of the electrical potential generated. Electrical changes are detected with the aid of computerized devices that extract the signal, display it on an oscilloscope, and store the data on magnetic tape or disk. In neurologic diagnosis, they reflect nerve conduction times in the peripheral nervous system. In clinical practice, the visual, auditory, and somatosensory systems are most often tested. These studies are used with patients who are unable to indicate recognition of a stimulus (Pagana & Pagana, 2013).

In visual evoked responses, the patient looks at a visual stimulus (flashing lights, a checkerboard pattern on a screen). The average of several hundred stimuli is recorded by EEG leads placed over the occipital lobe. The transit time from the retina to the occipital area is measured using computer-averaging methods.

Brain stem auditory evoked responses (BAERs) are measured by applying an auditory stimulus (repetitive auditory click) and measuring the transit time via the brain stem into the cortex. Specific lesions in the auditory pathway modify or delay the response. BAERs may be used in the diagnosis of brain stem alterations and in determination of brain death.

In somatosensory evoked responses (SERs), the peripheral nerves are stimulated (electrical stimulation through skin electrodes) and the transit time along the spinal cord to the cortex is measured and recorded from scalp electrodes. SERs are used to detect deficits in spinal cord or peripheral nerve conduction and to monitor spinal cord function during surgical procedures. It is also useful in the diagnosis of demyelinating diseases, such as multiple sclerosis and polyneuropathies, where nerve conduction is slowed.

Nursing Interventions

Explain the procedure to reassure the patient and encourage relaxation. Advise the patient to remain perfectly still throughout the recording to prevent artefact (signals not generated by the brain) that interfere with the recording and interpretation of the test.

Lumbar Puncture and Examination of Cerebrospinal Fluid

A lumbar puncture (spinal tap) is carried out by inserting a needle into the lumbar subarachnoid space to withdraw CSF. The test may be performed to obtain CSF for examination, to measure and reduce CSF pressure, to determine the presence or absence of blood in the CSF, and to administer medications intrathecally (into the spinal canal).

The needle is usually inserted into the subarachnoid space between the third and fourth or fourth and fifth lumbar vertebrae. Because the spinal cord ends at the first lumbar vertebra, insertion of the needle below the level of the third lumbar vertebra prevents puncture of the spinal cord.

A successful lumbar puncture requires that the patient be relaxed; an anxious patient is tense, and this may increase the pressure reading. The CSF pressure may be measured by attaching a sterile manometer to the LP needle. If the CSF pressure is equal to or greater than 20 cm H_2O, it is considered to indicate increased pressure (Pagana & Pagana, 2013). A lumbar puncture may be risky in the presence of an intracranial mass lesion because intraspinal pressure is decreased by removal of CSF, and the brain may herniate downward through the foramen magnum (Chart 62-5).

Cerebrospinal Fluid Analysis

The CSF is clear and colourless. A yellow tinge could indicate elevated protein levels, melanoma, or excess carotene or bilirubin in the blood. Pink, blood-tinged, or grossly bloody CSF may indicate a subarachnoid hemorrhage (blood does not clot). The CSF may be bloody initially because of local trauma (but it will clot), and becomes clearer as more fluid is drained. Specimens are obtained for cell count, culture, glucose, protein, and other tests as indicated. The specimens are sent to the laboratory immediately because changes will take place and alter the result if the specimens are allowed to stand. (See for CSF values.)

Post–Lumbar Puncture Headache

A post–lumbar puncture headache, ranging from mild to severe, may occur a few hours to several days after the procedure. This complication occurs in 15% to 30% of patients. It is a throbbing bifrontal or occipital headache, dull and deep in character, and particularly severe on sitting or standing, but lessens or disappears when the patient lies down.

The headache is caused by CSF leakage at the puncture site. The fluid continues to escape into the tissues by way of the needle track from the spinal canal. As a result of the leak, the supply of CSF in the cranium is depleted to a point at which it is insufficient to maintain proper mechanical stabilization of the brain. When the patient assumes an upright position, tension and stretching of the venous sinuses and pain-sensitive structures occur.

Post–lumbar puncture headache may be avoided if a small-gauge needle is used and if the patient remains prone after the procedure. When more than 20 mL of CSF are removed, position the patient supine for several hours. Keeping the patient flat overnight may reduce the incidence of headaches.

Usually, a postpuncture headache is managed by bed rest, analgesic agents, and hydration. Occasionally, if the headache persists, an epidural blood patch technique may be used. Blood is withdrawn from the antecubital vein and injected into the epidural space, usually at the site of the previous spinal puncture, with the rationale that the blood acts as a gelatinous plug to seal a hole in the dura, preventing further loss of CSF.

Other Complications of Lumbar Puncture

Herniation of the intracranial contents, spinal epidural abscess, spinal epidural hematoma, and meningitis are rare but serious complications of lumbar puncture. Other complications include temporary voiding difficulties, slight elevation of temperature, backache or spasms, and neck stiffness.

Promoting Home and Community-Based Care

Educating Patients About Self-Care

Many diagnostic tests that were once performed in a hospital stay are now carried out in short-procedure units or outpatient settings. As a result, family members often provide the postprocedure care. The patient and family must receive clear verbal and written instructions about precautions to take after the procedure, complications to avoid, and steps to take if complications occur. Because many patients undergoing neurologic diagnostic studies are older or have neurologic deficits, ensure provisions are made for transportation, postprocedure care, and appropriate monitoring.

Continuing and Transitional Care

Contact the patient and family after diagnostic testing to determine if there are any questions about the procedure or if the patient had any untoward results. Reinforce

CHART 62-5

Assisting With a Lumbar Puncture

A needle is inserted into the subarachnoid space through the third and fourth or fourth and fifth lumbar interface to withdraw spinal fluid.

Preprocedure

1. Determine whether written consent for the procedure has been obtained.
2. Explain the procedure to the patient and describe sensations that are likely during the procedure (i.e., a sensation of cold as the site is cleansed with solution, a needle prick when local anesthetic agent is injected).
3. Determine whether the patient has any questions or misconceptions about the procedure; the needle is inserted into a space outside of the spinal cord.
4. Instruct the patient to void before the procedure.

Procedure

1. The patient is positioned on one side at the edge of the bed or examining table with back toward the physician; the thighs and legs are flexed as much as possible to increase the space between the spinous processes of the vertebrae, for easier entry into the subarachnoid space.

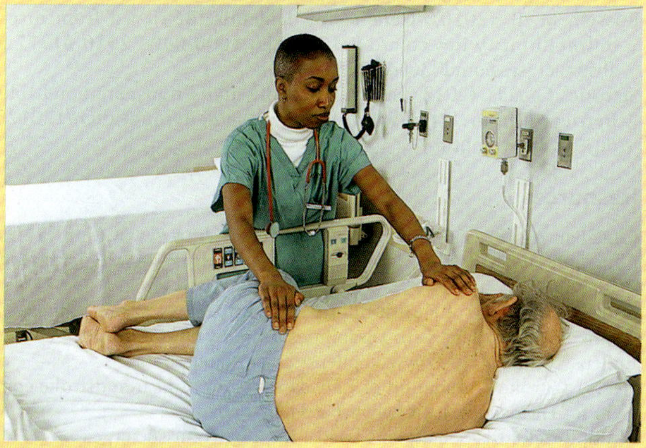

2. A small pillow may be placed under the patient's head to maintain the spine in a horizontal position; a pillow may be placed between the legs to prevent the upper leg from rolling forward.
3. The nurse assists the patient to maintain the position to avoid sudden movement, which can produce a traumatic (bloody) tap.
4. The patient is encouraged to relax and is instructed to breathe quietly and relaxed, because hyperventilation may lower an elevated pressure.
5. The nurse describes the procedure step by step to the patient as it proceeds.
6. The physician cleanses the puncture site with an antiseptic agent solution and drapes the site.
7. The physician injects local anesthetic agent to numb the puncture site, and then inserts a spinal needle into the subarachnoid space through the third and fourth or fourth and fifth lumbar interspace. A pressure reading may be obtained.
8. A specimen of CSF is removed and usually collected in three test tubes, labelled in order of collection. The needle is withdrawn.
9. The physician applies a small dressing to the puncture site.
10. The tubes of CSF are sent to the laboratory immediately.

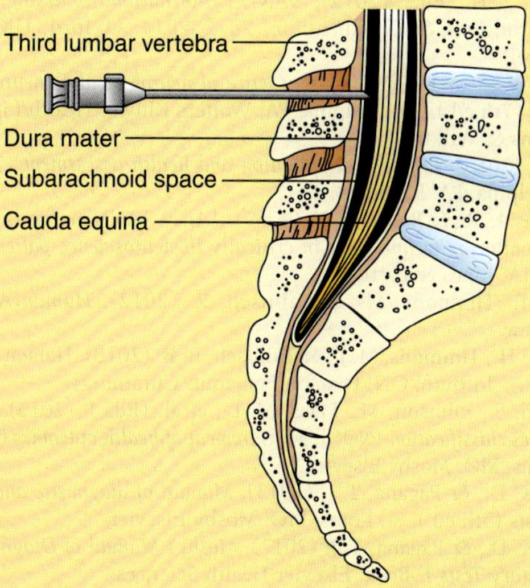

Postprocedure

1. Instruct the patient to lie prone for 4 to 6 hours to separate the alignment of the dural and arachnoid needle punctures in the meninges, to reduce leakage of CSF.
2. Monitor the patient for complications of lumbar puncture; notify physician if complications occur.
3. Encourage increased fluid intake to reduce the risk of post-procedure headache.

teaching and remind the patient and family to make and keep follow-up appointments. With patients, family members, and other health care providers, focus on the immediate needs, issues, or deficits that necessitated the diagnostic testing.

Critical Thinking Exercises

1 Identify the priorities, approach, and techniques you would use to perform a neurologic assessment on an 82-year-old patient with confusion. How will your priorities, approach, and techniques differ if the patient has a visual impairment, is hard of hearing, or has lower extremity weakness?

2 A 40-year-old patient is scheduled for an electroencephalogram (EEG). What resources would you use to identify the current guidelines for EEG ? What is the evidence base for these practices? Identify the criteria used to evaluate the strength of the evidence for these practices.

3 A 35-year-old female patient is having a lumbar puncture at the bedside. Identify the nursing interventions indicated before, during, and after the procedure. What patient education is indicated? How will your nursing interventions and patient education change if the patient is pregnant or lactating?

REFERENCES AND SELECTED READINGS

Books

Bader, M., Littlejohns, L. R., & Olson, D. (2016). *AANN core curriculum for neuroscience nursing* (6th ed.). Chicago, IL: American Association of Neuroscience Nurses.

Bickley, L., & Szilagyi, P. G. (2012). *Bates' guide to physical examination and history-taking*. Lippincott Williams & Wilkins.

Bulechek, G. M., Buthcher, H. K., Dochterman, J. M., et al. (Eds.). (2013). *Nursing interventions classification (NIC)* (6th ed.). St. Louis, MO: Mosby Elsevier.

Diepenbrock, N. H. (2012). *Quick reference to critical care* (4th ed.). Philadelphia, PA: Wolters Kluwer Health/Lippincott Williams & Wilkins.

Fischbach, F. T., & Dunning, M. B. (2015). *Nurse's quick reference to common laboratory and diagnostic tests* (6th ed.). Philadelphia, PA: Lippincott Williams & Wilkins.

Fontana, S. A., & Porth, C. M. (2017). Disorders of hearing and vestibular function. In R. A. Hannon, C. Pooler, & C. M. Porth (Eds.). *Porth Pathophysiology: Concepts of altered health states* (2nd Canadian ed.). Philadelphia, PA: Wolters Kluwer Health/Lippincott Williams & Wilkins.

Hannon, R. A. (2017). *Porth pathophysiology: concepts of altered health states*. Philadelphia, PA: Wolters Kluwer.

Herdman, T. H. (Ed.). (2012). *NANDA International Nursing Diagnoses: Definitions & Classification, 2012–2014*. Oxford, UK: Wiley Blackwell.

Hickey, J. V. (2014). *The clinical practice of neurological & neurosurgical nursing* (7th ed.). Philadelphia, PA: Wolters Kluwer Health/Lippincott Williams & Wilkins.

Jarvis, C. (2015). *Physical examination and health assessment* (7th ed.). Philadelphia, PA: Saunders.

Littlejohns, L. R., & Bader, M. K. (2009). *AACN-AANN protocols for practice: Monitoring technologies in critically ill neuroscience patients*. Sudbury, MA: Jones & Bartlett.

Martini, F., Timmons, M., & Tallitsch, R. (2012). *Human Anatomy*. Glenview.

Martini, F. H., Timmons, M. J., & Tallitsch, R. B. (2018). *Human anatomy* (9th ed.). Toronto, ON: Pearson Benjamin Cummings.

Moorhead, S., Johnson, M., Maas, M. L., et al. (Eds.). (2013). *Nursing outcomes classification (NOC). Measurement of health outcomes* (5th ed.). St. Louis, MO: Mosby Elsevier.

Pagana, K. D., & Pagana, T. J. (2013). *Manual of diagnostic and laboratory tests* (5th ed.). St. Louis, MO: Mosby Elsevier.

Pagana, K. D., & Pagana, T. J. (2017). *Mosby's Manual of Diagnostic and Laboratory Tests-E-Book*. Elsevier Health Sciences.

Porth, C. M. (2014). *Essentials of pathophysiology* (4th ed.). Philadelphia, PA: Lippincott Williams & Wilkins.

Skillen, D. L. (2012). Neurological assessment. In T. C. Stephen, D. L. Skillen, R. A. Day, et al. (Eds.). *Canadian Jensen's nursing health assessment: A best practice approach* (1st ed., pp. 697–754). Philadelphia, PA: Wolters Kluwer Health/Lippincott Williams & Wilkins.

Stephen, T. C. (2012). The health history. In T. C. Stephen, D. L. Skillen, R. A. Day, et al. (Eds.). *Canadian Jensen's nursing health assessment: A best practice approach* (1st ed., pp. 37–51). Philadelphia, PA: Wolters Kluwer Health/Lippincott Williams & Wilkins.

Stephen, T. C., Skillen, D. L., & Day, R. A. (2013–2014). *A syllabus for adult health assessment*. Edmonton, AB: University of Alberta, Faculty of Nursing.

Journals and Electronic Documents

Canadian Institute for Health Information. (2010). Seniors and falls: Fall-related hospitalizations. Retrieved from http://www.cihi.ca.

Holland, C. (2013). "Be creative and clear to learn the language of aphasia." Retrieved from http://www.nursingtimes.net/nursing-practice/clinical-zones/neurology/be-creative-and-clear-to-learn-the-language-of-aphasia/5066450.article

Krueger, H., Noonan, V. K., Trenaman, L. M., et al. (2013). The economic burden of traumatic spinal cord injury in Canada. Retrieved from http://www.ncbi.nlm.nih.gov/pubmet/23725450

Monden, K. R., Trost, Z., Catalano, D., et al. (2014). Resilience following spinal cord injury: A phenomenological view. Retrieved from http://www.nature.com/sc/journal/v52/n3/full/sc2013159a.html

Noonan, V. K., Fingas, M., Farry A., et al. (2012). Incidence and prevalence of spinal cord injury in Canada: A national perspective. Retrieved from http://www.ncbi.nlm.nih.gov/pubmet/22555590

Parkinson Society Canada. (2010). Ottawa scientists zero in on causes and treatment of Parkinson's through study of proteins, gene mutations and potential drug treatments. Retrieved from http://www.parkinson.ca/site/c.kgLNIWODKpF/b.6391465/k.D5A0/Ottawa_scientists_zero_in_on_causes_and_treatment_of_Parkinson8217s_through_study_of_proteins_gene_mutations_and_potential_drug_treatments.htm

Russell, M. B. (2010). Genetics of dementia. Retrieved from http://onlinelibrary.wiley.com/doi/10.1111/j.1600-0404.2010.01377.x/abstraact;jsessionid=366AA2C5C29

Statistics Canada. (2012). Study: Profile of seniors' transportation habits. Retrieved from http://www.statcan.gc.ca/daily-quotidien/120123/dq120123c-eng.htm

Resources

Canadian Association of Neuroscience Nurses: http://www.cann.ca
Canadian Hypertension Education Program: http://www.hypertension.ca/chep
Canadian Institute of Health Information: http://www.secure.cihi.ca
Council of Canadians with Disabilities: http://www.ccdonline.ca
Epilepsy Canada: http://www.epilepsy.ca
Heart & Stroke Foundation of Canada: http://www.heartandstroke.com
Help for Headaches: http://www.headache-help.org
Multiple Sclerosis Society of Canada: http://www.mssociety.ca
Neurological Health Charities Canada: http://www.mybrainmatters.ca
Parkinson Society of Canada: http://www.parkinson.ca
Public Health Agency of Canada: http://www.phac-aspc.gc.ca
Think First Foundation of Canada: http://www.thinkfirst.ca

63 Management of Patients With Neurologic Dysfunction

Adapted by Ron Prince

Learning Objectives

On completion of this chapter, the learner will be able to:

1. Describe the nursing needs of patients with various neurologic dysfunctions.
2. Describe the multiple needs of the patient with altered level of consciousness.
3. Use the nursing process as a framework for care of the patient with altered level of consciousness.
4. Identify the early and late clinical manifestations of increased intracranial pressure.
5. Use the nursing process as a framework for care of the patient with increased intracranial pressure.
6. Describe the needs of the patient undergoing intracranial or transsphenoidal surgery.
7. Use the nursing process as a framework for care of the patient undergoing intracranial or transsphenoidal surgery.
8. Identify the various types and causes of seizures.
9. Use the nursing process to develop a plan of care for the patient experiencing seizures.
10. Identify the needs of the patient experiencing headaches.

This chapter presents the care of the patient with an altered level of consciousness (LOC), the patient with increased **intracranial pressure** (ICP), the patient undergoing neurosurgical procedures, experiencing seizures, or experiencing headaches. Some of the topics in this chapter, such as headaches and seizures, may be symptoms of dysfunction in other body systems. Conversely, headaches and seizures can be symptoms of a severe disruption of the neurologic system. These disorders can also be diagnosed as "idiopathic," which means without an identifiable cause. The commonality in these disorders is not in the diagnosis or the medical treatment; it is in the behaviours and needs of the patient and the manner in which nurses can best support the patient through these episodes.

The central nervous system (CNS) contains a vast network of neurons controlling the body's vital functions. Yet this system is vulnerable, and its optimal function depends on several key factors. First, the neurologic system relies on its structural integrity for support and homeostasis, but this integrity may be disrupted. Examples of structural disruption can include head injury, brain tumour, intracranial hemorrhage, infection, and stroke. Due to this disruption brain tissue expands in the inflexible cranium, ICP rises, and cerebral perfusion/blood flow is impaired. Further expansion places pressure on vital centres, which can cause permanent neurologic deficits or lead to brain death.

Second, the neurologic system relies on the body's ability to maintain a homeostatic environment. It requires the body to deliver the essential elements of oxygen and glucose, and to filter out substrates toxic to the neurons. Sepsis, hypovolemia, myocardial infarction, respiratory arrest, hypoglycemia, electrolyte imbalance, drug and/or alcohol overdose, encephalopathy, and ketoacidosis are all examples of circumstances in which the neurologic system is depressed due to a toxic metabolic effect or due to the body's mechanical inability to provide essential substrates. Some conditions can be treated and neurologic impairments can be reversed; others result in permanent deficits.

Although neuroscience nursing is a specialty which requires an understanding of neuroanatomy, neurophysiology, neurodiagnostic testing, critical care nursing, and rehabilitation nursing, nurses in all settings care for patients with neurologic disorders. Ongoing assessment of the patient's neurologic function and health needs, identification of issues, mutual goal setting, development and implementation of care plans (including teaching, counselling, and coordinating activities), and evaluation of the outcomes of care are nursing actions integral to the recovery of the patient. The nurse also collaborates with other members of the health care team to provide essential care, offer a variety of solutions to issues, help the patient and family gain control of their lives, and explore the educational and supportive resources available in the community. The goals are to achieve as high a level of function as possible and to enhance the quality of life for the patient and their family with neurologic impairment and his or her family.

ALTERED LEVEL OF CONSCIOUSNESS

An **altered LOC** is apparent in the patient who is not oriented, does not follow commands, or needs persistent stimuli to achieve a state of alertness. LOC is gauged on a continuum, with a state of alertness and full cognition (consciousness) on one end and coma on the other end. **Coma** is a clinical state of unarousable unresponsiveness in which there are no purposeful responses to internal or external stimuli, although nonpurposeful responses to painful stimuli and brain stem reflexes may be present (Lee, Savage, McKee, et al., 2013). **Akinetic mutism** is a state of unresponsiveness to the environment in which the patient makes no voluntary movement or sound but sometimes opens the eyes. **Persistent vegetative state** is a condition in which the patient is described as wakeful after coma but is devoid of cognitive or affective mental function. **Locked-in syndrome** results from a lesion

Glossary

akinetic mutism: unresponsiveness to the environment; the patient makes no movement or sound but sometimes opens the eyes

altered level of consciousness: condition of being less responsive to and aware of environmental stimuli to achieve state of alertness

autoregulation: ability of cerebral blood vessels to dilate or constrict to maintain stable cerebral blood flow despite changes in systemic arterial blood pressure

brain death: irreversible loss of all functions of the entire brain, including the brain stem

coma: prolonged state of unconsciousness

craniectomy: a surgical procedure that involves removal of a portion of the skull

craniotomy: a surgical procedure that involves entry into the cranial vault

Cushing's reflex: the brain's attempt to increase blood flow by increasing arterial blood pressure to overcome the increased intracranial pressure

Cushing's triad: three classic signs—bradycardia, hypertension, and bradypnea—seen with pressure on the medulla as a result of brain stem herniation

decerebration: an abnormal body posture associated with a severe brain injury, characterized by extreme extension of the upper and lower extremities

decortication: an abnormal posture associated with severe brain injury, characterized by abnormal flexion of the upper extremities and extension of the lower extremities

epilepsy: a group of syndromes characterized by paroxysmal transient disturbances of brain function

herniation: abnormal protrusion of brain tissue through a defect or natural opening

intracranial pressure: pressure exerted by the volume of the intracranial contents within the cranial vault

locked-in syndrome: condition resulting from a lesion in the pons in which the patient lacks all distal motor activity (paralysis) but cognition is intact

microdialysis: procedure in which an intracranial catheter is inserted near an injured area of the brain to measure lactate, pyruvate, glutamate, and glucose levels

migraine headache: a severe, unrelenting headache often accompanied by symptoms such as nausea, vomiting, and visual disturbances

minimally conscious state: a state in which the patient demonstrates awareness but cannot communicate thoughts or feelings

Monro–Kellie hypothesis: theory that states that due to limited space for expansion within the skull, an increase in any one of the cranial contents—brain tissue, blood, or cerebrospinal fluid—causes a change in the volume of the others

persistent vegetative state: condition in which the patient is wakeful but devoid of conscious content, without cognitive or affective mental function

primary headache: a headache for which no specific organic cause can be found

secondary headache: headache identified as a symptom of another organic disorder (e.g., brain tumour, hypertension, hemorrhage)

seizures: paroxysmal transient disturbance of the brain resulting from a discharge of abnormal electrical activity

status epilepticus: episode in which the patient experiences multiple seizure bursts with no recovery time in between

subarachnoid screw or bolt: device placed into the subarachnoid space to measure intracranial pressure

transsphenoidal: surgical approach to the pituitary via the sphenoid sinuses through the nasal cavity

ventriculostomy: an opening into the skull in which a catheter is placed in one of the lateral ventricles of the brain to measure intracranial pressure and allow for drainage of CSF affecting the pons and results in tetraplegia (formerly called *quadriplegia*) and inability to speak, but vertical eye movements and lid elevation remain intact and are used to indicate responsiveness (Hickey, 2014). The level of responsiveness and consciousness is the most important indicator of the patient's condition.

Pathophysiology

Altered LOC is not a disorder itself; rather, it is a function and symptom of multiple pathophysiologic phenomena. The cause may be neurologic (head injury, stroke), toxicologic (drug overdose, alcohol intoxication), or metabolic (hepatic or renal failure, diabetic ketoacidosis).

The underlying causes of neurologic dysfunction are disruption in the cells of the nervous system, neurotransmitters, or brain anatomy (see Chapter 62). A disruption of the basic functional units (neurons) or neurotransmitters results in faulty impulse transmission, impeding communication within the brain or from the brain to other parts of the body. These disruptions are caused by cellular edema and other mechanisms such as antibodies disrupting chemical transmission at receptor sites.

Intact anatomic structures of the brain are needed for proper function. The two hemispheres of the cerebrum must communicate, via an intact corpus callosum, and the lobes of the brain (frontal, parietal, temporal, and occipital) must communicate and coordinate their specific functions (see Chapter 62). Additional anatomic structures of importance are the cerebellum and the brain stem. The cerebellum has both excitatory and inhibitory functions and is largely responsible for coordination of movement, balance, and fine motor skills. The brain stem contains areas that control the heart, respiration, and blood pressure. Disruptions in the anatomic structures are caused by trauma, edema, pressure from tumours, and other mechanisms such as an increase or decrease in blood or cerebrospinal fluid (CSF) circulation.

Clinical Manifestations

Alterations in LOC occur along a continuum, and the clinical manifestations depend on where the patient is on this continuum. As the patient's state of alertness and consciousness decreases, initial changes in LOC may be reflected by subtle behavioural changes such as confusion, restlessness or increased anxiety; there will be changes in the eye opening response, verbal response, motor response, and eventually the pupillary response. The pupillary response becomes sluggish (response is slower); as the patient becomes comatose, the pupils become fixed (no response to light). The patient in a coma is unable to follow commands and does not open the eyes, respond verbally, or move the extremities in response to a request to do so.

Assessment and Diagnostic Findings

The patient with an altered LOC is at risk for alterations in every body system. A complete assessment is performed, with particular attention to the neurologic system. The neurologic examination should be as complete as the patient's LOC allows (Arbour, 2013). It includes an evaluation of mental status, cranial nerve function, cerebellar function (balance and coordination), reflexes, and motor and sensory functions. LOC, the most sensitive indicator of neurologic function, is assessed based on the criteria in the Glasgow Coma Scale: eye opening, verbal response, and motor response (Morton & Fontaine, 2013). The patient's responses are rated on a scale from 3 to 15. A score of 3 indicates severe impairment of neurologic function, brain death, or pharmacologic inhibition of the neurologic response. A score of 15 indicates that the patient is fully responsive (see Chapter 65).

If the patient is comatose and has localizing signs such as abnormal pupillary and motor responses, it is assumed that neurologic disease is present until proven otherwise. Common diagnostic procedures used to identify the cause of unconsciousness include computed tomography (CT) scanning, magnetic resonance imaging (MRI), and electroencephalography (EEG). Less common procedures include positron emission tomography (PET) and single photon emission computed tomography (SPECT; see Chapter 62). Laboratory tests include analysis of blood glucose, electrolytes, serum ammonia, and liver function tests; blood urea nitrogen (BUN) levels; serum osmolality; calcium level; and partial thromboplastin and prothrombin times; and the International Normalized Ratio (INR). Other studies may be used to evaluate serum ketones, alcohol and drug levels, and arterial blood gases.

Complications

Potential complications for the patient with altered LOC include respiratory failure, pneumonia, pressure injuries, limb contracture, gastrointestinal ulcer disease and subsequent hemorrhage, and aspiration. Respiratory failure may develop shortly after the patient becomes unconscious. If the patient cannot maintain the airway or has ineffective respirations, supportive care is initiated to provide adequate ventilation. Pneumonia is common in patients receiving mechanical ventilation or in those who cannot maintain and clear their airways. The patient with altered LOC is subject to all the complications associated with immobility, such as pressure injuries, venous stasis, musculoskeletal deterioration, and disturbed gastrointestinal functioning. Pressure injuries may become infected and act as a source of sepsis. Aspiration of gastric contents or feedings may occur, precipitating the development of pneumonia or airway occlusion. Limb contractures develop due to long periods of immobility and lack of range of motion in the joints.

Medical Management

The first priority of intervention for the patient with altered LOC is to obtain and maintain a patent airway. The patient may be orally or nasally intubated, or a tracheostomy may be performed if oral intubation is contraindicated. Until the ability of the patient to breathe on their own is determined, a mechanical ventilator is used to maintain adequate oxygenation. The circulatory status (blood pressure, heart rate) is monitored to ensure adequate perfusion to the body and brain. An intravenous (IV) catheter is inserted to provide access for IV fluids and medications. Neurologic care focuses on the specific neurologic pathology, if known. Nutritional support, via a feeding tube or a gastrostomy tube, is initiated as soon as possible. In addition to measures designed to determine and treat the underlying causes of altered LOC, other medical interventions are aimed at pharmacologic management and prevention of complications.

Nursing Process

The Patient With an Altered Level of Consciousness

Assessment

Assessment of the patient with an altered LOC often starts with assessing the alertness of the patient. Alertness is measured by the patient's ability to open the eyes spontaneously or in response to a vocal or noxious stimulus (pressure or pain) to the nail bed or squeezing the trapezius muscle (Hickey, 2014). Patients with severe neurologic dysfunction cannot do this. The nurse assesses for periorbital edema (swelling around the eyes) or trauma, which may prevent the patient from opening the eyes, and documents any such condition that interferes with eye opening.

Verbal response is then assessed through determining the patient's orientation to time, person, and place. Patients are asked to identify the day, date, or season of the year and to identify where they are or to identify the clinicians, family members, or visitors present. Other questions such as, "Who is the prime minister?" or "What is the next holiday?" may be helpful in determining the patient's processing of information. (Verbal response cannot be evaluated if the patient is intubated or has a tracheostomy, and may be difficult in those patients with a language barrier, and this should be clearly documented.)

Motor response includes spontaneous, purposeful movement (e.g., the awake patient can move all four extremities with equal strength on command), movement only in response to noxious stimuli (e.g., pressure/pain), or abnormal posturing (Hickey, 2014; Morton & Fontaine, 2013). If the patient is not responding to commands, the motor response is tested by applying a noxious stimulus (firm but gentle pressure) to the nail bed or by squeezing the trapezius muscle. If the patient attempts to push away or withdraw, the response is recorded as purposeful or appropriate ("patient withdraws to painful stimulus"). Localization is a more organized response where rather than simply push away, the patient can cross the midline from one side of the body to the other in response to a painful stimulus. An inappropriate or nonpurposeful response is random and aimless. Posturing may be decorticate or decerebrate (Fig. 63-1; see also Chapter 62). The nurse always identifies and records the *best* motor response, keeping in mind that the patient may be hemiplegic. The most severe neurologic impairment results in flaccidity. The motor response cannot be elicited or assessed when the patient has been administered pharmacologic paralyzing agents.

In addition to LOC, the nurse monitors parameters such as respiratory status, vital signs, eye signs, focal signs, motor strength and sensation, and reflexes on an ongoing basis. Table 63-1 summarizes the assessment and the clinical significance of the findings. Body functions (circulation, respiration, elimination, fluid, and electrolyte balance) are examined in a systematic and ongoing manner.

Nursing Priorities

Based on the assessment data, the major nursing priorities may include the following:

- Airway clearance
- Risk of injury
- Fluid and electrolyte deficit
- Nutrition
- Impaired oral mucous membrane
- Risk for impaired skin integrity

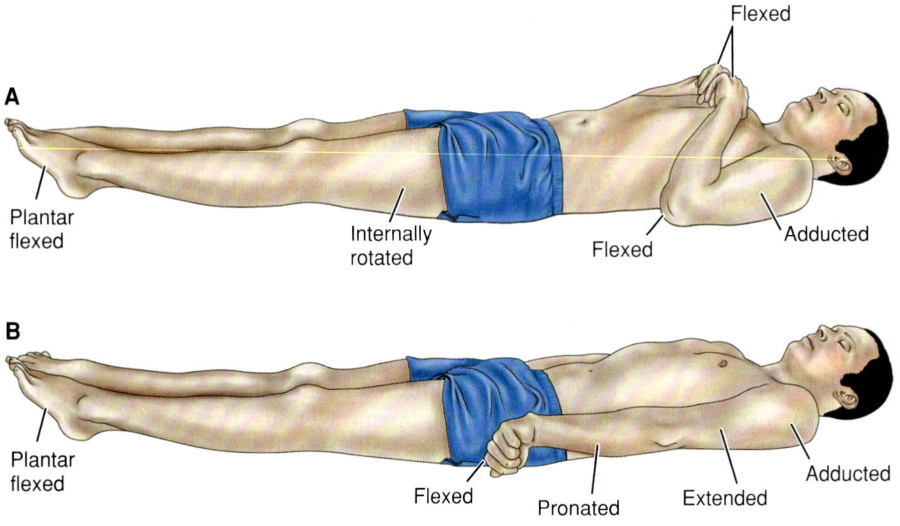

FIGURE 63-1. Abnormal posture response to stimuli. **A.** Decorticate posturing and flexion of the upper extremities, internal rotation of the lower extremities, and plantar flexion of the feet. **B.** Decerebrate posturing, involving extension and outward rotation of upper extremities and plantar flexion of the feet. (Adapted from Posner, J. B., Saper, C. B., Schiff, N. D., et al. (2007). *Plum and Posner's diagnosis of stupor and coma* (4th ed.). Oxford, UK: Oxford University Press.)

TABLE 63-1 Nursing Assessment of the Patient Who Is Unconscious

Examination	Clinical Assessment	Clinical Significance
Level of responsiveness or consciousness	Eye opening; verbal and motor responses; pupils (size, equality, reaction to light)	Obeying commands is a favourable response and demonstrates a return to consciousness
Pattern of respiration	Respiratory pattern	Disturbances of respiratory centre of brain may result in various respiratory patterns
	Cheyne–Stokes respiration	Suggests lesions deep in both hemispheres; area of basal ganglia and upper brain stem
	Hyperventilation	Suggests onset of metabolic problem or brain stem damage
	Ataxic respiration with irregularity in depth/rate	Ominous sign of damage to medullary centre
Eyes Pupils (size, equality, reaction to light) 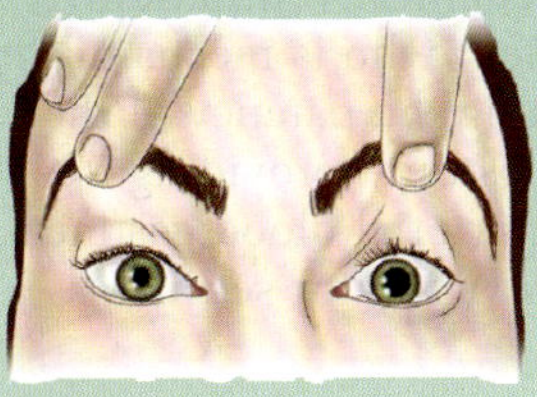	Equal, normally reactive pupils Equal or unequal diameter Progressive dilation Fixed dilated pupils	Suggests that coma is toxic or metabolic in origin Helps determine location of lesion Indicates increasing intracranial pressure Indicates injury at level of midbrain
Eye movements	Normally, eyes should move from side to side	Functional and structural integrity of brain stem is assessed by inspection of extraocular movements; usually absent in deep coma
Corneal reflex 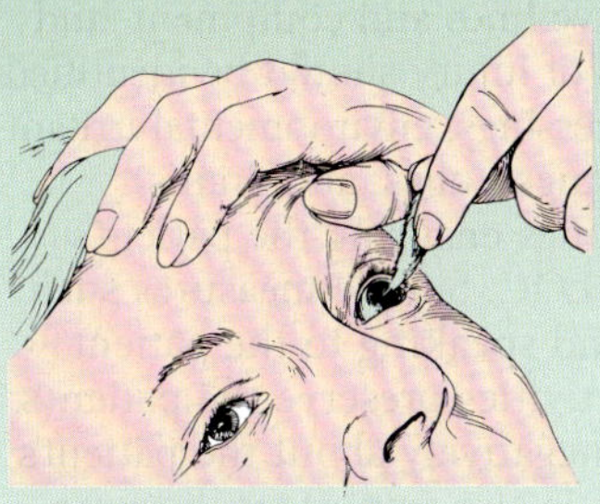	When cornea is touched with a wisp of clean cotton, blink response is normal	Tests cranial nerves V and VII; helps determine location of lesion if unilateral; absent in deep coma
Facial symmetry	Asymmetry (sagging, decrease in wrinkles)	Sign of paralysis
Swallowing reflex	Drooling vs. spontaneous swallowing	Absent in coma Paralysis of cranial nerves X and XII
Neck	Stiff neck Absence of spontaneous neck movement	Subarachnoid hemorrhage, meningitis Fracture or dislocation of cervical spine
Response of extremity to noxious stimuli	Firm pressure on a joint of the upper and lower extremities Observe spontaneous movements	Asymmetric response in paralysis Absent in deep coma
Deep tendon reflexes	Tap patellar and biceps tendons	Brisk response may have localizing value Asymmetric response in paralysis Absent in deep coma
Pathologic reflexes 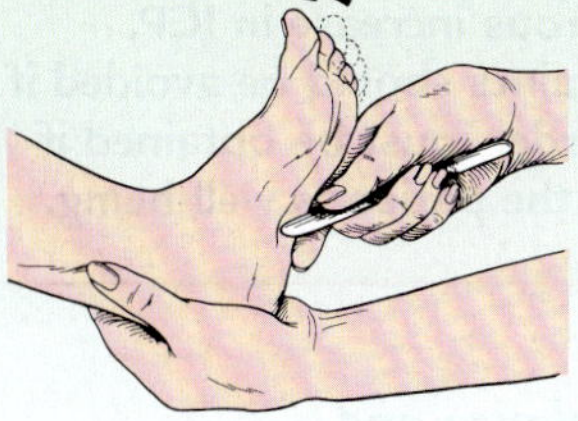	Firm pressure with blunt object on sole of foot, moving along lateral margin and crossing to the ball of foot	Flexion of the toes, especially the great toe, is normal except in newborn Dorsiflexion of toes (especially great toe) indicates contralateral pathology of corticospinal tract (Babinski reflex) Helps determine location of lesion in brain
Abnormal posture	Observation for posturing (spontaneous or in response to noxious stimuli) Flaccidity with absence of motor response Decorticate posture (flexion and internal rotation of forearms and hands) Decerebrate posture (extension and external rotation)	Deep extensive brain lesion Seen with cerebral hemisphere pathology and in metabolic depression of brain function Decerebrate posturing indicates deeper and more severe dysfunction than does decorticate posturing; implies brain pathology; poor prognostic sign

- Impaired tissue integrity
- Ineffective thermoregulation
- Impaired urinary elimination
- Bowel incontinence
- Disturbed sensory perception
- Interrupted family processes

Collaborative Problems/ Potential Complications

Based on the assessment data, potential complications may include:

- Respiratory distress or failure
- Atelectasis and pneumonia
- Aspiration
- Cardiac deconditioning and alterations in blood pressure and pulse
- Gastric ulcer
- Pressure injury
- Venous thromboembolism (VTE)
- Contractures

Planning and Goals of Care

The goals of care for the patient with altered LOC include maintenance of a clear airway, protection from injury, attainment of fluid volume balance, achievement of intact oral mucous membranes, maintenance of normal skin integrity, absence of corneal irritation, attainment of effective thermoregulation, and effective urinary elimination. Additional goals include bowel continence, accurate perception of environmental stimuli, maintenance of intact family or support system, and absence of complications (Stewart-Amidei & Klein, 2013).

Because the unconscious patient's protective reflexes are impaired, the quality of nursing care provided may mean the difference between life and death. The nurse must assume responsibility for the patient until the basic reflexes (coughing, blinking, and swallowing) return and the patient becomes conscious and oriented. Therefore, the major nursing goal is to compensate for the absence of these protective reflexes.

Nursing Interventions

Maintaining the Airway

The most important consideration in managing the patient with altered LOC is to establish an adequate airway and ensure ventilation. Obstruction of the airway is a risk because the epiglottis and tongue may relax, occluding the oropharynx, or the patient may aspirate oral and nasopharyngeal secretions and vomitus.

The accumulation of secretions in the pharynx presents a serious concern. Because the patient cannot swallow and lacks pharyngeal reflexes, these secretions must be removed to eliminate the danger of aspiration. Elevating the head of the bed to 30 degrees helps prevent aspiration. Positioning the patient in a lateral position also helps, as it permits the jaw and tongue to fall forward, thus promoting drainage of secretions.

Positioning alone is not always adequate, however. Suctioning and oral hygiene may be required. Suctioning is performed to remove secretions from the posterior pharynx and upper trachea. Before and after suctioning, the patient is adequately ventilated to prevent hypoxia (Hickey, 2014). Chest physiotherapy and postural drainage may be initiated to promote pulmonary hygiene, unless contraindicated by the patient's underlying condition. The chest should be auscultated at least every 8 hours to detect adventitious breath sounds or absence of breath sounds.

Despite these measures, or because of the severity of impairment, the patient with altered LOC often requires intubation and mechanical ventilation. Nursing actions for the patient who is mechanically ventilated include maintaining the patency of the endotracheal tube or tracheostomy, providing frequent oral care, monitoring arterial blood gas measurements, and maintaining ventilator settings (see Chapter 26).

Protecting the Patient

For the protection of the patient, padded side rails are provided and raised at all times. Care is taken to prevent injury from invasive lines and equipment, and other potential sources of injury should be identified (e.g., restraints, tight dressings, environmental irritants, damp bedding or dressings, tubes, and drains).

Protection also includes ensuring the patient's dignity during altered LOC. Simple measures such as providing privacy and speaking to the patient during nursing care activities preserve the patient's dignity. Not speaking negatively about the patient's condition or prognosis is also important, because patients in a light coma may be able to hear. The comatose patient has an increased need for advocacy, and the nurse is responsible for seeing that these advocacy needs are met.

NURSING ALERT

If the patient begins to emerge from unconsciousness, every measure that is available and appropriate for calming and quieting the patient should be used. Any form of restraint is likely to be countered with resistance, leading to self-injury or to a dangerous increase in ICP. Therefore, physical restraints should be avoided if possible; a physician's order must be obtained if their use is essential for the patient's well-being.

Maintaining Fluid Balance and Managing Nutritional Needs

Hydration status is assessed by examining tissue turgor and mucous membranes, assessing intake and output trends, and analyzing laboratory data. Fluid needs are met initially by administering the required

IV fluids. However, IV solutions (and blood component therapy) for patients with intracranial conditions must be given slowly. If they are given too rapidly, they can increase ICP. The quantity of fluids given may be restricted to minimize the possibility of cerebral edema.

If the patient does not recover quickly and sufficiently enough to take adequate fluids and calories by mouth, a feeding or gastrostomy tube will be inserted for the administration of fluids and enteral feedings. Research suggests that patients fed within 48 hours of injury have improved outcomes over those in whom nutrition is delayed (Wang, Dong, Han, et al., 2013).

Providing Oral Care

The mouth is inspected for dryness, inflammation, and crusting. The patient who is unconscious requires careful oral care, because there is a risk of parotitis if the mouth is not kept scrupulously clean. The mouth is cleansed and rinsed carefully to remove secretions and crusts and to keep the mucous membranes moist. A thin coating of petrolatum on the lips prevents drying, cracking, and encrustations. If the patient has an endotracheal tube, the tube should be moved to the opposite side of the mouth daily to prevent ulceration of the mouth and lips. If the patient is intubated and mechanically ventilated, good oral care is also necessary. Research suggests that comprehensive mouth care with antiseptic such as chlorhexidine and head of bed elevation decreases ventilator-associated pneumonia and improves the oral health in patients who are intubated (Munro & Ruggiero, 2014). Oral care should be provided every 4 hours at minimum.

Maintaining Skin and Joint Integrity

Preventing skin breakdown requires continuing nursing assessment and intervention. Special attention is given to patients who are unconscious, because they cannot respond to external stimuli and reposition themselves. Assessment includes a regular schedule of turning to avoid pressure, which can cause breakdown and necrosis of the skin. Turning also provides kinesthetic (sensation of movement), proprioceptive (awareness of position), and vestibular (equilibrium) stimulation. After turning, the patient is carefully repositioned to prevent ischemic necrosis over pressure areas; this is usually achieved by the use of pillows or other positioning aids. Dragging or pulling the patient up in bed must be avoided, because this creates a shearing force and friction on the skin surface (see Chapter 13) and will contribute to skin breakdown. Nurses must also insure they use proper body mechanics when turning the neuroscience patient in order to prevent injuries to themselves.

Maintaining correct body position is important; equally important is passive exercise of the extremities to prevent contractures. The use of splints or foam boots aids in the prevention of foot drop and eliminates the pressure of bedding on the toes. The use of trochanter rolls to support the hip joints keeps the legs in proper alignment. The arms are in abduction, the fingers lightly flexed, and the hands in slight supination. The heels of the feet are assessed for pressure areas. Specialty beds, such as fluidized or low-air-loss beds, may be used to decrease pressure on bony prominences (Hickey, 2014).

Preserving Corneal Integrity

Some unconscious patients have their eyes open and have inadequate or absent corneal reflexes. The cornea may become irritated, dried out, or scratched, leading to ulceration. If artificial tears are prescribed, they may be instilled every 2 hours. Periorbital edema (swelling around the eyes) often occurs after cranial surgery. If cold compresses are prescribed, care must be exerted to avoid contact with the cornea. Eye patches should be used cautiously because of the potential for corneal abrasion from contact with the patch.

Maintaining Body Temperature

High fever in the patient who is unconscious may be caused by infection of the respiratory or urinary tract, drug reactions, or damage to the hypothalamic temperature-regulating centre. A slight elevation of temperature may be caused by dehydration. The environment can be adjusted, depending on the patient's condition, to promote a normal body temperature. If body temperature is elevated, a minimum amount of bedding is used. The room may be cooled to 18.3°C (65°F). However, if the patient is an older adult and does not have an elevated temperature, a warmer environment is needed.

Because of damage to the temperature-regulating centre in the brain or severe intracranial infection, patients who are unconscious often develop very high temperatures. Such temperature elevations must be controlled, because the increased metabolic demands of the brain can exceed cerebral circulation and oxygen delivery, potentially resulting in cerebral deterioration (Hickey, 2014). Studies suggest that hyperthermia may contribute to poor outcome after brain injury but not through a decreased brain oxygen level (Madden & DeVon, 2015). Persistent hyperthermia with no identified clinical source of infection indicates brainstem damage and a poor prognosis.

> **NURSING ALERT**
>
> **The body temperature of a patient who is unconscious is never taken by mouth. Rectal or tympanic (if not contraindicated) temperature measurement is preferred to the less accurate axillary temperature.**

Strategies for reducing fever include:

- Removing all bedding over the patient (with the possible exception of a light sheet)
- Administering acetaminophen PRN as prescribed

- Giving cool sponge baths and allowing an electric fan to blow over the patient to increase surface cooling
- Using a hypothermia blanket
- Frequent temperature monitoring to assess the patient's response to the therapy and to prevent an excessive decrease in temperature and shivering.

Bladder Management of the Neuroscience Patient

The patient with an altered LOC is often incontinent or has urinary retention. The bladder is palpated or scanned at intervals to determine whether urinary retention is present, because a full bladder may be an overlooked cause of overflow incontinence. A portable bladder ultrasound instrument is a useful tool in bladder management and retraining programs.

If the patient is not voiding, a program of intermittent catheterization should be devised in order to reduce the patient's risk of urinary tract infection. A catheter may be inserted during the acute phase of illness to monitor urinary output. Because catheters are a major cause of urinary tract infection, the patient is observed for fever and cloudy urine. The area around the urethral orifice is inspected for drainage and cleansed routinely. The urinary catheter is usually removed if the patient has a stable cardiovascular system and if no diuresis, sepsis, or voiding dysfunction existed before the onset of coma. Although many patients who are unconscious urinate spontaneously after catheter removal, the bladder should be palpated or scanned with a portable ultrasound device periodically for urinary retention and to prevent autonomic dysreflexia.

An external catheter (condom catheter) for the male patient and absorbent pads for the female patient can be used for patients who are unconscious and can urinate spontaneously, although involuntarily. As soon as consciousness is regained, a bladder training program is initiated (Hickey, 2014). The patient who is incontinent is monitored frequently for skin irritation and skin breakdown. Appropriate skin care is implemented to prevent these complications.

Promoting Bowel Function

The abdomen is assessed by listening for bowel sounds and measuring the girth of the abdomen with a tape measure. There is a risk of diarrhea from infection, and administration of antibiotics, and hyperosmolar fluids in a patient's enteral feedings. Frequent loose stools may also occur with fecal impaction. Commercial fecal collection bags and rectal tubes are available for patients with fecal incontinence.

Immobility and lack of dietary fibre can cause constipation. The nurse monitors the number and consistency of bowel movements and performs a rectal examination for signs of fecal impaction. Stool softeners may be prescribed and can be administered orally or via internal feeding tubes. To facilitate bowel emptying, a glycerin suppository may be indicated. The patient may require an enema every other day to empty the lower colon.

Restoring Health Maintenance

Once increased ICP is not a problem, the nurse assists the patient and family to restore the health of the patient who is unconscious. This involves using auditory, visual, olfactory, gustatory, tactile, and kinesthetic activities to stimulate the patient emerging from coma (Megha, Harpreet, & Nayeem, 2013). Efforts are made to restore the sense of daily rhythm by maintaining usual day and night patterns for activity and sleep. The nurse touches and talks to the patient and encourages family members and friends to do so. Communication is extremely important and includes touching the patient and spending enough time with the patient to become sensitive to their needs. It is also important to avoid making any negative comments about the patient's status or prognosis in the patient's presence.

The nurse orients the patient to time and place at least once every 8 hours. Sounds from the patient's usual environment may be introduced using a tape recorder. Family members can read to the patient from a favourite book and may suggest radio and television programs that the patient previously enjoyed as a means of enriching the environment and providing familiar input.

When arousing from coma, many patients experience a period of agitation, indicating that they are becoming more aware of their surroundings but still cannot react or communicate in an appropriate fashion. Although this is disturbing for many family members, it is actually a positive clinical sign. At this time, it is necessary to minimize stimulation by limiting background noises, having only one person speak to the patient at a time, giving the patient a longer period of time to respond, and allowing for frequent rest or quiet times. After the patient has regained consciousness, videotaped family or social events may assist the patient in recognizing family and friends and allow him or her to experience missed events.

Programs of sensory stimulation for patients with brain injury have been developed in an effort to improve outcomes. Although these are controversial programs with inconsistent results, some research supports the concept of providing structured stimulation (Megha et al., 2013).

Meeting the Family's Needs

The family of the patient with altered LOC may be thrown into a sudden state of crisis and go through the process of severe anxiety, denial, anger, remorse, grief, and reconciliation. Depending on the disorder that caused the altered LOC and the extent of the patient's recovery, the family may be unprepared for the changes in the cognitive and physical status of their loved one. If the patient has significant residual deficits, the family may require considerable time, assistance, and support to come to terms with these changes. To help family members mobilize resources and coping skills, the nurse reinforces and clarifies information about the patient's condition, permits the family to be involved in care, and listens to and encourages ventilation of feelings and concerns while supporting decision-making about management and placement after hospitalization. Families may benefit from participation in support groups offered through the hospital, rehabilitation facility, or community organizations.

In some circumstances, the family may need to face the death of their loved one. A GCS of 3, no facial movement or grimacing in response to noxious stimuli with pupils that are either constricted or dilated, and are in a fixed position are clinical signs of increasing pressure on the brain stem leading to **brain death** (Arbour, 2013). The patient with a catastrophic neurologic disorder is often pronounced brain dead before the heart stops beating. The term brain death describes irreversible loss of all functions of the entire brain, including the brain stem (Arbour, 2013). The term may be misleading to the family because, although brain function has ceased, the patient appears to be alive, with the heart rate and blood pressure sustained by vasoactive medications and breathing continued by mechanical ventilation. When discussing a patient who is brain dead with family members, it is important to provide accurate, timely, understandable, and consistent information (Arbour, 2013). End-of-life care is discussed in Chapter 15.

Monitoring and Managing Potential Complications

Pneumonia, aspiration, and respiratory failure are potential complications in any patient who has a depressed LOC and who cannot protect the airway or turn, cough, and take deep breaths. The longer the period of unconsciousness, the greater the risk is of pulmonary complications.

Vital signs and respiratory function are monitored closely to detect any signs of respiratory failure or distress. Total blood count and arterial blood gas measurements are assessed to determine whether there are adequate red blood cells to carry oxygen and whether ventilation is effective. Chest physiotherapy and suctioning are initiated to prevent respiratory complications such as pneumonia. Oral care interventions are performed for patients receiving mechanical ventilation to decrease the incidence of pneumonia (Robertson & Carter, 2013). If pneumonia develops, cultures are obtained to identify the organism so that appropriate antibiotics can be administered.

The patient with altered LOC is monitored closely for evidence of impaired skin integrity, and strategies to prevent skin breakdown and pressure injuries are continued through all phases of care, including hospitalization, rehabilitation, and home care. Factors that contribute to impaired skin integrity (e.g., incontinence, inadequate dietary intake, pressure on bony prominences, edema) are addressed. Assessment and management of pressure injuries are discussed in Chapter 13.

The patient should also be monitored for signs and symptoms of VTE, which may manifest as a deep vein thrombosis (DVT) or pulmonary embolism (PE). Prophylaxis with subcutaneous heparin or low–molecular-weight heparin (dalteparin [Fragmin], danaparoid [Orgaran]) as well as antiembolism stockings or pneumatic compression devices are prescribed according to the patient's risk factors for thrombosis and bleeding (Foreman, Schmalz, & Griessenauer, 2014). The nurse observes for signs and symptoms of DVT or PE.

Patients with a prolonged decrease in LOC are at risk for developing contractures. During acute care, the patient is turned every 2 hours and passive range of motion performed at least twice a day. Splints, provided by occupational therapy, are applied to the hands and feet in a rotating manner to maintain functional joint alignment. Hand splints have been reported to be safe and beneficial for patients in decreasing spasticity and improving hand opening (Thibault, Deltombe, Wannez, et al., 2015). See Chapter 13 for further information about management of contractures.

Evaluation

Expected patient outcomes may include the following:

1. Maintains clear airway and demonstrates appropriate breath sounds
2. Experiences no injuries
3. Attains or maintains adequate fluid balance
   a. Has no clinical signs or symptoms of dehydration
   b. Demonstrates expected range of serum electrolytes
   c. Has no clinical signs or symptoms of overhydration
4. Achieves healthy oral mucous membranes
5. Maintains skin integrity
6. Has no corneal irritation
7. Attains or maintains thermoregulation
8. Has no urinary retention
9. Has no diarrhea or fecal impaction
10. Receives appropriate sensory stimulation
11. Has family members who cope with crisis
    a. Verbalize fears and concerns
    b. Participate in patient's care and provide sensory stimulation by talking and touching
12. Is free of complications
    a. Has arterial blood gas values and O_2 saturation levels within expected range
    b. Displays no signs or symptoms of pneumonia
    c. Exhibits intact skin over pressure areas
    d. Does not develop VTE such as DVT or PE

INCREASED INTRACRANIAL PRESSURE

The rigid cranial vault contains brain tissue (1,400 g), blood (75 mL), and CSF (75 mL). The volume and pressure of these three components are usually in a state of equilibrium and produce the ICP. ICP is usually measured in the lateral ventricles, with the usual pressure being 0 to 10 mm Hg, and 15 mm Hg being the upper limit of normal (Hickey, 2014).

The **Monro–Kellie hypothesis** states that, because of the limited space for expansion within the skull, an increase in any one of the components causes a change in the volume of the others. Because brain tissue has limited space to expand, compensation typically is accomplished by displacing or shifting CSF, increasing the absorption or diminishing the production of CSF, or decreasing cerebral blood volume. Without such changes, ICP begins to rise. Under usual circumstances, minor changes in blood volume and CSF volume occur constantly as a result of alterations in intrathoracic pressure (coughing, sneezing, straining), posture, blood pressure, and systemic oxygen and carbon dioxide levels (Hickey, 2014; Raboel, Bartek, Andresen, et al., 2012).

Pathophysiology

Increased ICP affects many patients with acute neurologic conditions because pathologic conditions alter the relationship between intracranial volume and ICP. Although elevated ICP is most commonly associated with head injury, it also may be seen as a secondary effect in other conditions, such as brain tumours, subarachnoid hemorrhage, subdural or epidural hematomas, and toxic and viral encephalopathies. Increased ICP from any cause decreases cerebral perfusion, stimulates further swelling (edema), and may shift brain tissue, or result in **herniation**, a dire and frequently fatal event.

Decreased Cerebral Blood Flow

Increased ICP may significantly reduce cerebral blood flow due to compressed cerebral vasculature, resulting in ischemia which eventually leads to cell death. In the early stages of cerebral ischemia, the vasomotor centres are stimulated and the systemic pressure rises to maintain cerebral blood flow. In later stages, this is often accompanied by a slow bounding pulse and respiratory irregularities. These changes in vital signs are important clinically because they suggest increased ICP.

The concentration of carbon dioxide in the blood and in the brain tissue also has a role in the regulation of cerebral blood flow. An increase in the arterial partial pressure of carbon dioxide ($PaCO_2$) causes cerebral vasodilation, leading to increased cerebral blood flow and increased ICP. A decrease in $PaCO_2$ has a vasoconstrictive effect, reducing blood flow to the brain (Olson, Lewis, Bader, et al., 2013; Stewart-Amidei & Klein, 2013). Decreased venous outflow may also increase cerebral blood volume, thus raising ICP.

Cerebral Edema

Cerebral edema or swelling is defined as an abnormal accumulation of water or fluid in the intracellular space, extracellular space, or both, associated with an increase in the volume of brain tissue. Edema can occur in the grey, white, or interstitial matter. As brain tissue swells within the rigid skull, several mechanisms attempt to compensate for the increasing ICP. These compensatory mechanisms include autoregulation as well as decreased production and flow of CSF. **Autoregulation** refers to the brain's ability to alter the cerebral vascular resistance to blood flow through changes in the diameter of its blood vessels, to maintain a constant cerebral blood flow despite fluctuations in mean arterial blood pressure. This mechanism is often impaired in patients who are experiencing a pathologic and sustained increase in ICP.

Cerebral Response to Increased Intracranial Pressure

As ICP rises, compensatory mechanisms in the brain work to maintain blood flow and prevent tissue damage. The brain can maintain a steady perfusion pressure if the arterial systolic blood pressure is 50 to 150 mm Hg and the ICP is less than 40 mm Hg. Changes in ICP are closely linked with cerebral perfusion pressure (CPP). The CPP is calculated by subtracting the ICP from the mean arterial pressure (MAP). For example, if the MAP is 100 mm Hg and the ICP is 15 mm Hg, then the CPP is 85 mm Hg. The usual CPP is 70 to 100 mm Hg (Hickey, 2014). As ICP rises and the autoregulatory mechanism of the brain is overwhelmed, the CPP can increase to greater than 100 mm Hg or decrease to less than 50 mm Hg. Patients with a sustained CPP of less than 50 mm Hg experience irreversible neurologic damage. Therefore, the CPP must be maintained at 70 to 80 mm Hg to ensure adequate blood flow to the brain. If ICP is equal to MAP, cerebral circulation ceases.

A clinical phenomenon known as the **Cushing's reflex** is seen when cerebral blood flow decreases significantly. With this decrease in blood flow, the vasomotor centre triggers an increase in arterial pressure in an effort to perfuse the brain tissue, despite the increased ICP. A sympathetically mediated response causes an increase in the systolic blood pressure with a widening of the pulse pressure and cardiac slowing (bradycardia). This response is seen clinically as an increase in systolic blood pressure (as high as 270 mm Hg), widening of the pulse pressure, and reflex slowing of the heart rate. It is a late sign requiring immediate intervention; however, cerebral perfusion may be recoverable if the Cushing's response is treated rapidly.

At a certain point, the brain's ability to autoregulate becomes ineffective and decompensation (ischemia and infarction) begins. When this occurs, the patient exhibits significant changes in LOC and vital signs. The bradycardia, hypertension, and irregular respiratory patterns associated with this deterioration are known as **Cushing's triad**, a grave clinical sign. At this point, herniation of the brain stem and occlusion of the cerebral blood flow occur if therapeutic intervention is not initiated. Herniation refers to the shifting of brain tissue from an area of high pressure to an area of lower pressure (Fig. 63-2). The herniated tissue exerts pressure on the brain area into which it has shifted, which interferes with the blood supply in that area. Cessation of cerebral blood flow results in cerebral ischemia, infarction, and brain death (Hickey, 2014).

Clinical Manifestations

If ICP increases to the point at which the brain's ability to adjust has reached its limits, neural function is impaired; this may be manifested at first by clinical changes in LOC and later by abnormal respiratory and vasomotor responses.

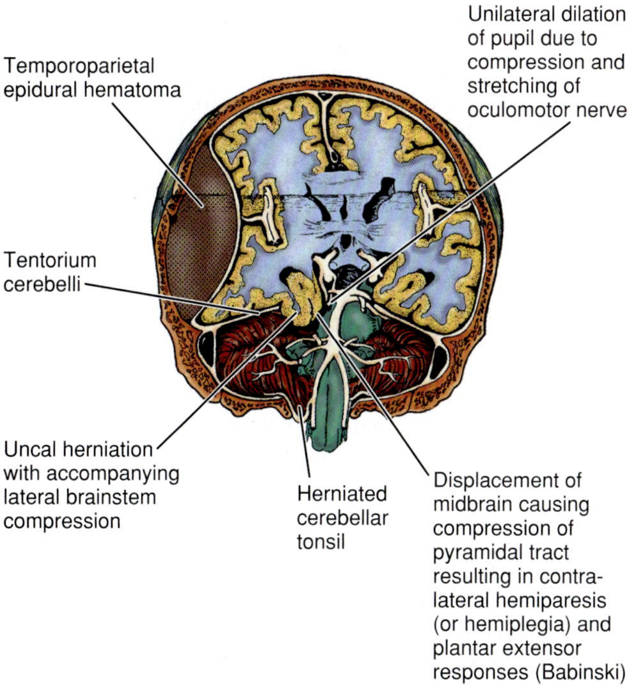

FIGURE 63-2. Cross-section of the brain showing herniation of part of the temporal lobe through the tentorium as a result of a temporoparietal epidural hematoma. (Reprinted with permission from Hickey, J. V. (2014). *The clinical practice of neurological and neurosurgical nursing* (7th ed.). Philadelphia, PA: Lippincott Williams & Wilkins.)

NURSING ALERT

The earliest sign of increasing ICP is a change in LOC. Slowing of speech and delay in response to verbal suggestions are other early indicators.

Any sudden change in the patient's condition, such as anxiety, irritability, restlessness (without apparent cause), confusion, or increasing drowsiness, has neurologic significance. These signs may result from decreased cerebral perfusion as a result of compression of the brain due to hemorrhage or edema, an expanding intracranial lesion (hematoma or tumour), or a combination of both.

As ICP continues to increase, the patient becomes stuporous, reacting only to loud or painful stimuli. At this stage, serious impairment of brain circulation is probably taking place, and immediate intervention is required. As neurologic function deteriorates further, the patient becomes **minimally conscious** and exhibits abnormal motor responses in the form of posturing—**decortication** (abnormal flexion of the upper extremities and extension of the lower extremities), or **decerebration** (extreme extension of the upper and lower extremities), or flaccidity (see Fig. 63-1). If the coma is profound, with the pupils dilated and fixed and respirations impaired or absent, death is usually inevitable (Arbour, 2013; Hickey, 2014).

Assessment and Diagnostic Findings

The diagnostic studies used to determine the underlying cause of increased ICP are discussed in detail in Chapter 65. The most common diagnostic tests are CT scanning and MRI. The patient may also undergo cerebral angiography, PET, or SPECT. Transcranial Doppler studies provide information about cerebral blood flow. The patient with increased ICP may also undergo electrophysiologic monitoring to observe cerebral blood flow indirectly. Evoked potential monitoring measures the electrical potentials produced by nerve tissue in response to external stimulation (auditory, visual, or sensory). Lumbar puncture is avoided in patients with increased ICP, because the sudden release of pressure in the lumbar area can cause the brain to herniate (Hickey, 2014).

Complications

Complications of increased ICP include brain stem herniation, diabetes insipidus (DI), cerebral salt-wasting syndrome (CSW), and syndrome of inappropriate antidiuretic hormone (SIADH).

DI is the result of **decreased** secretion of antidiuretic hormone (ADH) due to compression or injury to the pituitary gland. The patient has excessive urine output, decreased urine osmolality, and serum hyperosmolarity (Diepenbrock, 2012). Therapy consists of replacing fluids, correcting electrolyte abnormalities, and in severe cases medical management with vasopressin (desmopressin [DDAVP]) therapy. DI is discussed in Chapters 17 and 43.

SIADH is the result of increased secretion of ADH. The patient becomes volume overloaded, urine output diminishes, and serum sodium concentration becomes dilute. Treatment of SIADH includes fluid restriction (less than 800 mL/day with no free water), which is usually sufficient to correct the hyponatremia. In severe cases, careful administration of a 3% hypertonic saline solution may be therapeutic (Aylwin, Burst, Peri, et al., 2015). The change in serum sodium concentration should not exceed a correction rate of approximately 1.3 mEq/L/hr. Further discussion of SIADH is presented in Chapters 17 and 43.

Another less common cause of hyponatremia in people with intracranial conditions is CSW. There is a primary loss of extracellular water because of a sodium transport abnormality and subsequent loss of sodium and water through the renal system. This condition is treated with fluid and sodium replacement (Morton & Fontaine, 2013). It is important to distinguish this condition from SIADH as the treatments differ (Hickey, 2014). Refer to Table 63-2 for differentiation between CSW, SIADH, and DI.

Medical Management

Increased ICP is a true emergency and must be treated promptly. Invasive monitoring of ICP (20 mm Hg or greater) is an important component in identifying increased ICP. Immediate management to relieve increased ICP requires immediate indication of the offending cause. The three most common ones being cerebral edema, increased ventricle volume (CSF or blood), and increased cerebral blood flow. The goal of treatment then focuses on decreasing cerebral edema, lowering the volume of CSF, or decreasing cerebral blood volume while maintaining cerebral perfusion. These goals are accomplished by administering sedation and osmotic diuretics, restricting fluids,

TABLE 63-2 Comparison of Diabetes Insipidus, SIADH, Cerebral Salt Wasting

	DI	SIADH	CSW
Serum sodium	Hypernatremia	Hyponatremia	Hyponatremia
Vascular volume	Decreased	WNL or increased	Decreased
Extracellular fluid	Decreased	Increased	Decreased
Urine sodium	<20 mmol/d	>40 mmol/d	>40 mmol/d
Urine osmolality	Increased	Increased	Increased

SIADH, syndrome of inappropriate secretion of antidiuretic hormone; CSW, cerebral salt wasting; DI, diabetes insipidus; WNL, within expected limits.

draining CSF—via external ventricular drains, controlling fever, maintaining systemic blood pressure and oxygenation, and reducing cellular metabolic demands. Judicious use of hyperventilation is recommended only if the ICP is not responding to other measures (AANN, 2012). Management of increased ICP is discussed in Chapter 65.

Monitoring Intracranial Pressure and Cerebral Oxygenation

The purposes of ICP monitoring is to identify increased intracranial pressure early in its course (before cerebral damage occurs), to quantify the degree of ICP elevation, to initiate appropriate treatment, to provide access to CSF for sampling and drainage, and to evaluate the effectiveness of treatment. ICP can be monitored in many ways: intraventricular catheter (ventriculostomy), a subarachnoid bolt, an epidural or subdural catheter, or a fibre optic transducer-tipped catheter placed in the subdural space or in the ventricle (Fig. 63-3).

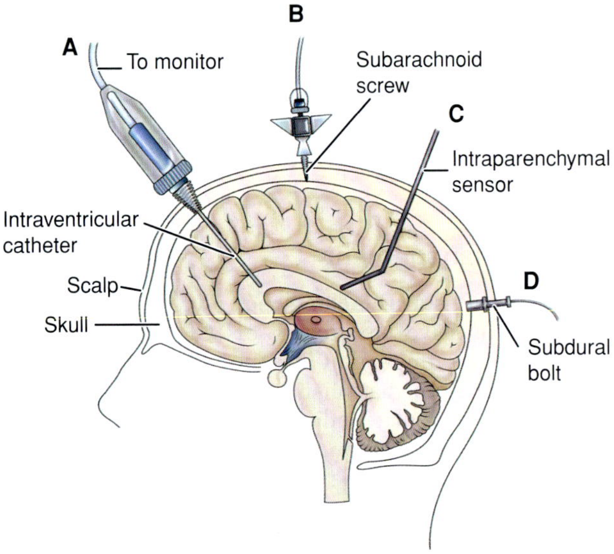

FIGURE 63-3. Intracranial pressure monitoring. A device may be placed in (**A**) the ventricle, (**B**) the subarachnoid space, (**C**) the intraparenchymal space, or (**D**) the subdural space.

When a **ventriculostomy** or ventricular catheter monitoring device is used for monitoring ICP, a fine-bore catheter is inserted into a lateral ventricle, preferably in the nondominant hemisphere of the brain (Hickey, 2014). The catheter is connected by a fluid-filled system to a transducer, which records the pressure in the form of an electrical impulse. In addition to obtaining continuous ICP recordings, the ventricular catheter allows CSF to drain, particularly during acute increases in pressure. The ventriculostomy can also be used to drain blood from the ventricles. Also, continuous drainage of CSF under pressure control is an effective method of treating intracranial hypertension. Another advantage of a ventricular catheter is access for the intraventricular administration of medications and the occasional instillation of air or a contrast agent for ventriculography. Complications associated with its use include ventricular infection, meningitis, ventricular collapse, occlusion of the catheter by brain tissue or blood, and problems with the monitoring system (Stewart-Amidei & Klein, 2013).

The **subarachnoid screw or bolt** is a hollow cylindrical device that is inserted through the skull and dura mater so that the tip protrudes into the cranial subarachnoid space (Hickey, 2014). It has the advantage of not requiring a ventricular puncture. The subarachnoid screw is attached to a pressure transducer, and the output is recorded on an oscilloscope. The hollow screw technique also has the advantage of avoiding complications from brain shift and small ventricle size. Complications include infection and blockage of the screw by clot or brain tissue, which leads to a loss of pressure tracing and a decrease in accuracy at high ICP readings.

A fibre optic monitor, or transducer-tipped catheter, is a newer alternative to other intraventricular, subarachnoid, and subdural systems (Stewart-Amidei & Klein, 2013). The miniature transducer reflects pressure changes, which are converted to electrical signals in an amplifier and displayed on a digital monitor. The catheter can be inserted into the ventricle, subarachnoid space, subdural space, or brain parenchyma or under a bone flap. If inserted into the ventricle, it can also be used in conjunction with a CSF drainage device.

Interpreting Intracranial Pressure Waveforms

Waves of high pressure and troughs of relatively normal pressure indicate changes in ICP. Waveforms are captured and recorded on an oscilloscope. These waves have been classified as A waves (plateau waves), B waves, and C waves (Fig. 63-4). The plateau waves (A waves) are transient, paroxysmal, recurring elevations of ICP that may last 5 to 20 minutes and range in amplitude from 40 to 100 mm Hg (Dias, Maia, Cerejo, et al., 2014). Plateau waves have clinical significance and indicate changes in vascular volume within the intracranial compartment that are beginning to compromise cerebral perfusion. The A waves may increase in amplitude and frequency, reflecting cerebral ischemia and brain damage that can occur before overt signs and symptoms of raised ICP are seen clinically. B waves are shorter (30 seconds to 2 minutes) and have smaller amplitude (up to 50 mm Hg). They have less clinical significance, but if seen in a series in a patient with depressed consciousness, they may precede the appearance of A waves. B waves may be seen in patients with

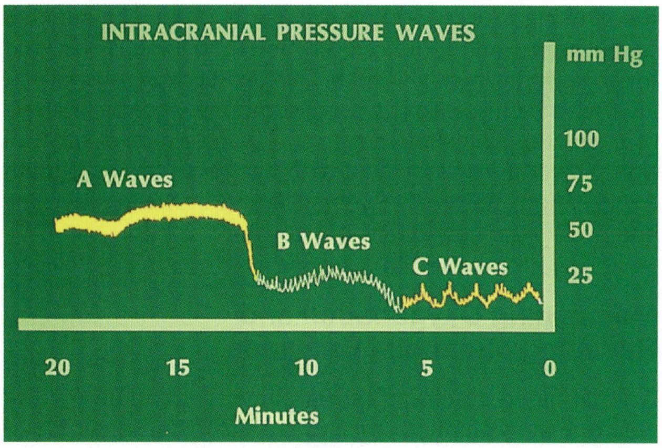

FIGURE 63-4. Intracranial pressure waves. Composite diagram of A (plateau) waves, which indicate cerebral ischemia; B waves, which indicate intracranial hypertension and variations in the respiratory cycle; and C waves, which relate to variations in systemic arterial pressure and respirations.

intracranial hypertension and decreased intracranial compliance. C waves are small, rhythmic oscillations with frequencies of 4 to 8 per minute and appear to be related to rhythmic variations of the systemic arterial blood pressure and respirations (Hickey, 2014).

Other Neurologic Monitoring Systems

Another trend in neurologic monitoring is **microdialysis** of the patient with a brain injury (de Lima Oliveira, Kairalla, Fonoff, et al., 2014). Cortical probes are placed near the injured area and are used to measure levels of glutamate, lactate, pyruvate, and glucose, substances that reflect the metabolic function of the brain. Some researchers theorize that direct measurements of glucose and energy by-products in the brain will lead to better management of these patients. Although cerebral microdialysis has reduced the mortality of patients who are brain injured, more study is needed to link it to improved outcomes (de Lima Oliveira et al., 2014).

An additional trend is monitoring of cerebral oxygenation through monitoring of the oxygen saturation in the jugular venous bulb ($SjvO_2$) or via a catheter in the brain. Cerebral oxygenation is thought to be important because changes in cerebral perfusion may reflect an increase in ICP. Readings taken from a catheter residing in the jugular outflow tract allow for a comparison of arterial and venous oxygen saturation, and the balance of cerebral oxygen supply and demand is demonstrated. Venous jugular desaturations can reflect early cerebral ischemia, alerting the clinician before an increase in ICP occurs. Minimizing cerebral desaturations can potentially improve outcomes (Sandsmark et al., 2012). This type of monitoring is now widely available and has been successfully used to identify secondary brain insults. A limiting factor is that this saturation reflects overall perfusion of the brain rather than that of a specific injured area (Oddo, Bosel, & Participants in the International Multidisciplinary Consensus Conference on Multimodality Monitoring, 2014).

Another method of measuring cerebral oxygenation and temperature is by inserting a fibre optic catheter into the brain matter (Oddo et al., 2014). The most common system is Licox (Fig. 63-5). The system includes a monitor with a screen for the display of oxygen and temperature values and cables that connect to the monitoring probes in the brain (Hickey, 2014).

Decreasing Cerebral Edema

Osmotic diuretics such as mannitol and hypertonic saline (3%) may be given to dehydrate the brain tissue and reduce cerebral edema (Ong, Keyrouz, & Diringer, 2015). They act by drawing water across intact membranes, thereby reducing the volume of the brain and extracellular fluid. An indwelling urinary catheter is usually inserted to monitor urinary output and to manage the resulting diuresis. If the patient is receiving osmotic diuretics, serum osmolality and electrolytes should be determined to assess hydration status. If a brain tumour is the cause of the increased ICP, corticosteroids (e.g., dexamethasone) help reduce the edema surrounding the tumour.

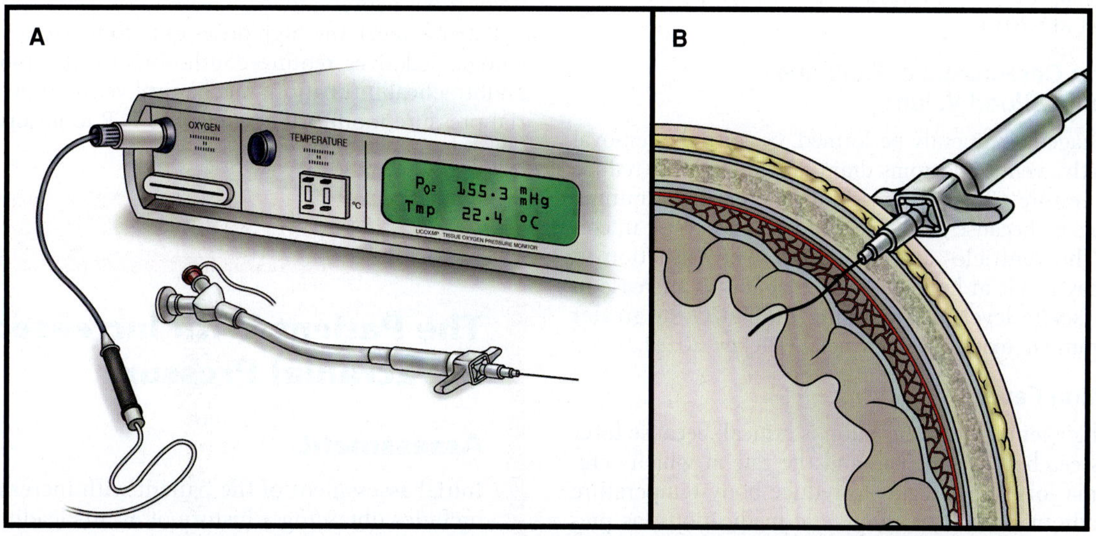

FIGURE 63-5. Licox catheter system. **A.** The brain tissue oxygen catheter and monitor. **B.** Placement of the catheter in brain white matter. (Redrawn with permission of Integra NeuroSciences, Plainsboro, NJ.)

Another method for decreasing cerebral edema is fluid restriction (Hickey, 2014). Limiting overall fluid intake leads to dehydration and hemoconcentration, which draws fluid across the osmotic gradient and decreases cerebral edema. Conversely, overhydration of the patient with increased ICP is avoided, because it increases cerebral edema.

Researchers have long hypothesized that lowering body temperature would decrease cerebral edema by reducing the oxygen and metabolic requirements of the brain, thus protecting the brain from continued ischemia. If body metabolism can be reduced by lowering the body temperature, the collateral circulation in the brain may be able to provide an adequate blood supply to the brain. The effect of hypothermia on ICP requires more study; thus far, induced hypothermia has not consistently been shown to be beneficial for patients with brain injury. Inducing and maintaining hypothermia is a major clinical treatment and requires knowledge and skilled nursing observation and management. The type and length of rewarming techniques after hypothermia may also be factors in the outcome of patients with neurologic injuries (Andrews, Sinclair, Rodriguez, et al., 2015; Madden & DeVon, 2015).

Maintaining Cerebral Perfusion

Cardiac output may be manipulated to provide adequate perfusion to the brain. Improvements in cardiac output are made using fluid volume and inotropic agents such as dobutamine (Dobutrex) and norepinephrine (Levophed). The effectiveness of the cardiac output is reflected in the CPP, which is maintained at greater than 70 mm Hg (Oddo et al., 2014). A lower CPP indicates that the cardiac output is insufficient to maintain adequate cerebral perfusion. $SjvO_2$ and Licox, described earlier, assist in monitoring cerebral perfusion.

Decompressive hemicraniectomy may also be considered as a surgical strategy to assist in the management of refractory intracranial hypertension. The removal of a part of the skull allows the brain to expand without the pressure constraints exerted by the cranial vault. Complications of this procedure include infection and increased potential for injury to the unprotected underlying brain structures. Once the patient is no longer at risk for increased ICP, the bone flap may be surgically replaced (Alali, Naimark, Wilson, et al., 2014).

Reducing Cerebrospinal Fluid and Intracranial Blood Volume

CSF drainage is frequently performed, because the removal of CSF with a ventriculostomy drain can dramatically reduce ICP and restore CPP. Caution should be used in draining CSF, however, because excessive drainage may result in collapse of the ventricles and herniation. The reduction in $PaCO_2$ may result in hypoxia, ischemia, and an increase in cerebral lactate levels. Maintaining the $PaCO_2$ at greater than 30 mm Hg may prove beneficial (Hickey, 2014).

Controlling Fever

Preventing a temperature elevation is critical, because fever increases cerebral metabolism and the rate at which cerebral edema forms. Strategies to reduce body temperature include administration of antipyretic medications, as prescribed, and the use of a hypothermia blanket. Additional strategies for reducing fever were discussed previously in the Nursing Process section on altered LOC. The patient's temperature is monitored closely, and the patient is observed for shivering, which should be avoided because it is associated with increased oxygen consumption, increased levels of circulating catecholamines, and increased vasoconstriction. Shivering is associated with decreased levels of brain oxygenation; however, the association between shivering and neurologic outcome is unknown.

Maintaining Oxygenation and Reducing Metabolic Demands

Arterial blood gases and pulse oximetry are monitored to ensure that systemic oxygenation remains optimal. Metabolic demands may be reduced through the administration of high doses of barbiturates if the patient is unresponsive to conventional treatment. The mechanism by which barbiturates decrease ICP and protect the brain is uncertain, but the resultant comatose state is thought to reduce the metabolic requirements of the brain, thus providing cerebral protection (Alali et al., 2014).

Another method of reducing cellular metabolic demand and improving oxygenation is the administration of medications causing sedation. The patient who receives these agents cannot move; this decreases the metabolic demands and results in a decrease in cerebral oxygen demand. The patient cannot respond to or report pain either. The most common agents used for sedation are pentobarbital (Nembutal), thiopental (Pentothal), propofol (Diprivan), and dexmedetomidine (Precedex) (Majdan, Mauritz, Wilbacher, et al., 2013; Wang, Ji, Fen, et al., 2013).

If sedative agents are used, the ability to perform serial neurologic assessments is lost. Therefore, other monitoring tools are needed to assess the patient's status and response to therapy. Important parameters that must be assessed include ICP, blood pressure, heart rate, respiratory rate, and the patient's response to ventilator therapy (e.g., "fighting or bucking the ventilator"). The level of pharmacologic paralysis is adjusted based on serum levels of the medications given and the assessed parameters. Potential complications of these medications include hypotension caused by decreased sympathetic tone and myocardial depression.

Patients receiving high doses of barbiturates or pharmacologic sedatives require continuous cardiac monitoring, endotracheal intubation, mechanical ventilation, and arterial pressure monitoring, as well as ICP monitoring.

Nursing Process

The Patient With Increased Intracranial Pressure

PRACTICE & LEARN

Assessment

Initial assessment of the patient with increased ICP includes obtaining a history of events leading to the present illness and the pertinent past medical history. Due to the patient's altered LOC it is usually necessary to obtain this information from family or friends. The neurologic examination should be as complete as the patient's condition allows. It includes an evaluation of mental status, LOC, cranial nerve function, cerebellar function (balance and coordination), reflexes, and motor and sensory functions. Because the patient is critically ill, ongoing assessment is more focused, including pupil checks, assessment of selected cranial nerves, frequent measurements of vital signs and ICP, and use of the Glasgow Coma Scale. Assessment of the patient with altered LOC is summarized in Table 63-1.

Nursing Priorities

Based on the assessment data, the major nursing priorities for patients with increased ICP include the following:

- Airway clearance
- Ineffective breathing
- Ineffective cerebral tissue perfusion
- Risk for hemodynamic imbalance
- Maintenance of body temperature
- Fluid volume abnormalities
- Risk for infection

Other relevant nursing diagnoses are included in the section on altered LOC.

Collaborative Problems/ Potential Complications

Based on the assessment data, potential complications include:

- Brain stem herniation
- DI
- Infection
- SIADH
- CSW

Planning and Goals

The goals for the patient include maintenance of a patent airway, normalization of respiration, adequate cerebral tissue perfusion through reduction in ICP, restoration of fluid balance, absence of infection, and absence of complications.

Nursing Interventions

Maintaining a Patent Airway

Airway patency is assessed regularly. Secretions that are obstructing the airway must be suctioned with care, and coughing is discouraged as transient elevations of ICP occur with coughing and suctioning (Hickey, 2014). Hypoxia caused by poor oxygenation leads to cerebral ischemia and subsequent edema. Coughing is discouraged because it increases ICP. The lung fields are auscultated at least every 8 hours to determine the presence of adventitious sounds or any areas of congestion. Elevating the head of the bed may aid in lung expansion and in clearing secretions and improve venous drainage of the brain.

Achieving an Adequate Breathing Pattern

The patient must be monitored constantly for respiratory irregularities. Increased pressure on the frontal lobes or deep midline structures may result in Cheyne–Stokes respirations, whereas pressure in the midbrain can cause hyperventilation. If the lower portion of the brain stem (the pons and medulla) is involved, respirations become irregular and eventually cease.

Hyperventilation therapy is a controversial therapy in traumatic brain injury used in some centres to reduce ICP by causing cerebral vasoconstriction and a decrease in cerebral blood volume. The nurse collaborates with the respiratory therapist in monitoring the $PaCO_2$, which is usually maintained at less than 30 mm Hg. Patients undergoing hyperventilation therapy also benefit from multimodality monitoring to determine the overall effect of this therapy on brain perfusion (de Lima Oliveira et al., 2014).

A neurologic observation record (Fig. 63-6) is maintained, and all observations are made in relation to the patient's baseline condition. Repeated assessments of the patient are made (sometimes minute by minute) so that improvement or deterioration may be noted immediately. If the patient's condition deteriorates, preparations are made for surgical intervention.

Optimizing Cerebral Tissue Perfusion

In addition to ongoing nursing assessment, strategies are initiated to reduce factors contributing to the elevation of ICP (Table 63-3).

Proper positioning helps reduce ICP. The patient's head is kept in a neutral (midline) position, maintained with the use of a cervical collar if necessary, to promote venous drainage. Elevation of the head is maintained at 30 to 45 degrees unless contraindicated. Extreme rotation of the neck and flexion of the neck are avoided, because compression or distortion of the jugular veins increases ICP. Extreme hip flexion is also avoided, because this position causes an increase in intra-abdominal and intrathoracic pressures, which can produce an increase in ICP. Relatively minor changes in position can significantly affect ICP. If monitoring reveals that turning the patient raises ICP, rotating beds, turning sheets, and holding the patient's head during turning may minimize the stimuli that increase ICP. Research suggests that patient response to position change is highly variable and requires close hemodynamic monitoring and individualized care (Mitchell, Kirkness, & Blissitt, 2015).

The Valsalva manoeuvre, which can be produced by straining at defecation, moving in bed, or sneezing contribute to spikes in ICP and are avoided. Stool softeners may be prescribed if the patient is alert and able to eat; a diet high in fibre may be indicated. Abdominal distention, which increases intra-abdominal and intrathoracic pressure and ICP, are noted. Enemas and cathartics are avoided if possible.

(text continued on page 2004)

NURSING NEUROLOGIC CRITICAL CARE FLOWSHEET

ADDRESSOGRAPH

	Date												
	Time												
	Initials												
Level of orientation (✓)	Person												
	Place												
	Date and time												
	No orientation												
Awakens to (✓)	Voice												
	Touch												
	Noxious stimuli												
	Painful stimuli												
	No response												
Best verbal response (✓)	Clear and appropriate												
	Clear and inappropriate												
	Difficulty speaking*												
	Perseveration												
	Aphasic expressive (nonfluent)												
	Aphasic receptive (fluent)												
	Sounds no speech												
	No verbal response												
	ETT/TRACH												
Best motor response (✓)	Moves all extremities purposefully												
	Withdraws and lifts to painful stimuli												
	Moves to painful stimuli												
	Decorticates (spinal reflex)												
	Decerebrates (spinal reflex)												
	No motor response												
Best motor strength upper extremities (✓)	No drifts (R/L)	R/L	R/L	R/L	R/L	R/L	R/L	R/L	R/L	R/L	R/L	R/L	R/L
	Drift (R/L)	R/L	R/L	R/L	R/L	R/L	R/L	R/L	R/L	R/L	R/L	R/L	R/L
	Can only lift forearm (R/L)	R/L	R/L	R/L	R/L	R/L	R/L	R/L	R/L	R/L	R/L	R/L	R/L
	Trace movement of hand or arm (R/L)	R/L	R/L	R/L	R/L	R/L	R/L	R/L	R/L	R/L	R/L	R/L	R/L
	Trace movement of fingers only (R/L)	R/L	R/L	R/L	R/L	R/L	R/L	R/L	R/L	R/L	R/L	R/L	R/L
	No motor response (R/L)	R/L	R/L	R/L	R/L	R/L	R/L	R/L	R/L	R/L	R/L	R/L	R/L
Best strength lower extremities (✓)	Raises leg off bed (R/L)	R/L	R/L	R/L	R/L	R/L	R/L	R/L	R/L	R/L	R/L	R/L	R/L
	Drags heel on bed and lifts knee (R/L)	R/L	R/L	R/L	R/L	R/L	R/L	R/L	R/L	R/L	R/L	R/L	R/L
	Trace movement of foot or leg (R/L)	R/L	R/L	R/L	R/L	R/L	R/L	R/L	R/L	R/L	R/L	R/L	R/L
	Trace movement of toes only (R/L)	R/L	R/L	R/L	R/L	R/L	R/L	R/L	R/L	R/L	R/L	R/L	R/L
	No response (R/L)	R/L	R/L	R/L	R/L	R/L	R/L	R/L	R/L	R/L	R/L	R/L	R/L
Seizure activity (✓)	No seizure activity												
	With loss of consciousness*												
	Without loss of consciousness*												
Ataxia (✓)	Gross ataxia												
	Fine motor ataxia												
	Does not apply												
ICP monitoring	Ventriculostomy mL												
	ICP mm Hg												
	Not applicable												

*= FURTHER DOCUMENTATION IS REQUIRED TO VALIDATE ASSESSMENT

FIGURE 63-6. A neurologic assessment flow chart.

PUPIL GAUGE (mm)

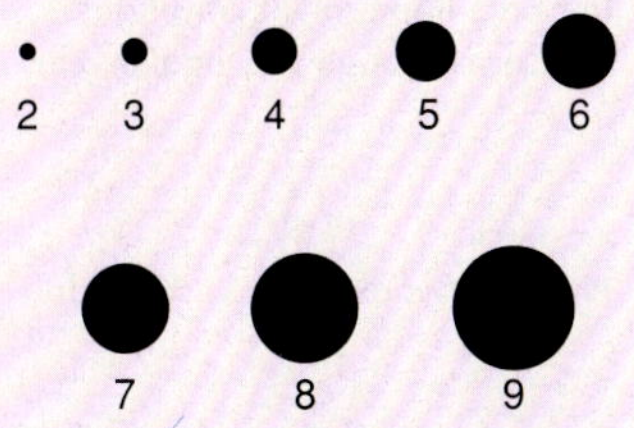

B=Brisk, S=Sluggish, F=Fixed

ADDRESSOGRAPH

	Date												
	Time												
	Initials												
Incision +/–	Dry and intact												
	Drainage												
Pupils: refer to above gauge (✓) (+)=Present (–)=Absent	Size (R/L)	R / L	R / L	R / L	R / L	R / L	R / L	R / L	R / L	R / L	R / L	R / L	R / L
	Regular (R/L)	R / L	R / L	R / L	R / L	R / L	R / L	R / L	R / L	R / L	R / L	R / L	R / L
	Irregular* (R/L)	R / L	R / L	R / L	R / L	R / L	R / L	R / L	R / L	R / L	R / L	R / L	R / L
	Reaction (R/L) (B) - (S) - (F)	R / L	R / L	R / L	R / L	R / L	R / L	R / L	R / L	R / L	R / L	R / L	R / L
	Ptosis (R/L) (+) (–)	R / L	R / L	R / L	R / L	R / L	R / L	R / L	R / L	R / L	R / L	R / L	R / L
	Gaze preference (R/L) (+)* (–)	R / L	R / L	R / L	R / L	R / L	R / L	R / L	R / L	R / L	R / L	R / L	R / L
Meningeal signs (+)=Present (–)=Absent	Headache												
	Nuchal rigidity												
	Photophobia												
Visual fields (+)=Present (–)=Absent* NA=Not applicable	Right upper outer												
	Right lower outer												
	Left upper outer												
	Left lower outer												
Nystagmus (+)=Present (–)=Absent	Lateral (R/L)	R / L	R / L	R / L	R / L	R / L	R / L	R / L	R / L	R / L	R / L	R / L	R / L
	Vertical (R/L)	R / L	R / L	R / L	R / L	R / L	R / L	R / L	R / L	R / L	R / L	R / L	R / L
Cranial nerves (+)=Present (–)=Absent	III, IV, VI, Extraocular movements												
	VII – Peripheral facial droop (R/L)	R / L	R / L	R / L	R / L	R / L	R / L	R / L	R / L	R / L	R / L	R / L	R / L
	XII – Tongue deviation (R/L)	R / L	R / L	R / L	R / L	R / L	R / L	R / L	R / L	R / L	R / L	R / L	R / L
	IX – Gag reflex												
	V, VII – Corneal reflex (R/L)	R / L	R / L	R / L	R / L	R / L	R / L	R / L	R / L	R / L	R / L	R / L	R / L
	X, IX – Cough reflex												
	Doll's eyes if appropriate												
Follows commands	Two step verbal command												
	One step verbal command												
	Unable to follow command												

*= **FURTHER DOCUMENTATION IS REQUIRED TO VALIDATE ASSESSMENT**

Initials	Signature	Title	Initials	Signature	Title

FIGURE 63-6. (*Continued*)

TABLE 63-3 Increased Intracranial Pressure and Interventions

Factor	Physiology	Interventions	Rationale
Cerebral edema	Can be caused by contusion, tumour, or abscess; water intoxication (hypo-osmolality); alteration in the blood–brain barrier (protein leaks into the tissue, causing water to follow)	Administer osmotic diuretics as prescribed (monitor serum osmolality). Maintain head of bed elevation at 30 degrees Maintain alignment of the head	Promotes venous return Prevents impairment of venous return through the jugular veins
Hypoxia	A decrease in PaO_2 to <60 mm Hg causes cerebral vasodilation	Maintain PaO_2 >60 mm Hg Maintain oxygen therapy Monitor arterial blood gas values Suction when needed Maintain a patent airway	Prevents hypoxia and vasodilation
Hypercapnia (elevated $PaCO_2$)	Causes vasodilation	Maintain $PaCO_2$ (normally 35–45 mm Hg) by establishing ventilation	Normalizing $PaCO_2$ minimizes vasodilation and thus reduces the cerebral blood volume
Impaired venous return	Increases the cerebral blood volume	Maintain head alignment Elevate head of bed 30 degrees	Hyperextension, rotation, or hyperflexion of the neck causes decreased venous return
Increase in intrathoracic or abdominal pressure	An increase in these pressures due to coughing, PEEP, or Valsalva manoeuvre causes a decrease in venous return	Monitor arterial blood gas values, and keep PEEP as low as possible Provide humidified oxygen Administer stool softeners as prescribed	To keep secretions loose and easy to suction or expectorate Soft bowel movements will prevent straining or Valsalva manoeuvre

PaO_2, partial pressure of arterial oxygen; $PaCO_2$, partial pressure of arterial carbon dioxide; PEEP, positive end-expiratory pressure.

Adapted from American Association of Neuroscience Nurses. (2012). *Care of the patient undergoing intracranial pressure monitoring/external ventricular drainage or lumbar drainage: AANN Clinical Practice Guideline Series*. Glenview, IL: Author; Hickey, J. V. (2014). *The clinical practice of neurological and neurosurgical nursing* (7th ed.). Philadelphia, PA: Lippincott Williams & Wilkins.

Mechanical ventilation presents unique problems for the patient with increased ICP. Before suctioning, the patient should be preoxygenated and briefly hyperventilated using 100% oxygen on the ventilator. Suctioning should not last longer than 15 seconds. High levels of positive end-expiratory pressure (PEEP) must be utilized cautiously, because they may decrease venous return to the heart and decrease venous drainage from the brain through increased intrathoracic pressure (Nemer, Caldeira, Santos, et al., 2015).

Activities that increase ICP, as indicated by changes in waveforms, should be avoided if possible. Spacing of nursing interventions may prevent transient increases in ICP. During nursing interventions, the ICP should not increase above 25 mm Hg, and it should return to baseline levels within 5 minutes. Patients with increased ICP should not demonstrate a significant increase in pressure or change in the ICP waveform. Patients with the potential for a significant increase in ICP may need sedation before initiation of nursing activities (Bader, Littlejohns, & Olson, 2016).

Emotional stress and frequent arousal from sleep are avoided. A calm atmosphere is maintained. Environmental stimuli (e.g., noise, conversation) should be minimal.

Maintaining Negative Fluid Balance

The administration of osmotic and loop diuretics is part of the treatment protocol to reduce ICP. Corticosteroids may be used to reduce cerebral edema (except when it results from trauma), and fluids may be restricted. All of these treatment modalities promote dehydration.

Skin turgor, mucous membranes, urine output, and serum and urine osmolality are monitored to assess fluid status. If IV fluids are prescribed, the nurse ensures that they are given at a slow to moderate rate with an IV infusion pump, to prevent too-rapid administration and avoid overhydration. For the patient receiving mannitol, the nurse observes for the possible development of heart failure and pulmonary edema. The intent of treatment is to promote a shift of fluid from the intracellular to the intravascular compartment and to control cerebral edema. However, this shift of fluid volume to the intravascular compartment may overwhelm the ability of the myocardium to increase workload sufficient to meet these demands, which may cause failure and pulmonary edema.

For patients undergoing dehydrating procedures, vital signs, including blood pressure, must be monitored to assess fluid volume status. An indwelling urinary catheter is inserted to permit assessment of renal function and fluid status. During the acute phase, urine output is monitored hourly. An output greater than 200 mL per hour for two consecutive hours may indicate the onset of diabetes insipidus (Hickey, 2014). These patients need careful oral hygiene, because mouth dryness occurs with dehydration. Frequently rinsing the mouth with nondrying solutions, lubricating the lips, and removing encrustations relieve dryness and promote comfort.

Preventing Infection

The risk of infection is greatest when ICP is monitored with an intraventricular catheter and increases with the duration of the monitoring. Most health care facilities have written protocols for managing these systems and maintaining their sterility; strict adherence to the protocols is essential.

Aseptic technique must be used when managing the system and changing the ventricular drainage bag. The drainage system is also checked for loose connections, because they can cause leakage and contamination of the CSF as well as inaccurate readings of ICP. The nurse observes the character of the CSF drainage and reports increasing cloudiness or blood. The patient is monitored for signs and symptoms of meningitis: fever, chills, nuchal (neck) rigidity, and increasing or persistent headache. (See Chapter 66 for a discussion of meningitis.)

Monitoring and Managing Potential Complications

The primary complication of increased ICP is brain herniation resulting in death (see Fig. 63-2). Nursing management focuses on detecting early signs of increasing ICP, because medical interventions are usually ineffective once later signs develop. Frequent neurologic assessments and documentation and analysis of trends will reveal the subtle changes that may indicate increasing ICP.

DETECTING INDICATIONS OF INCREASING INTRACRANIAL PRESSURE. The nurse assesses for and immediately reports any signs or symptoms of increasing ICP (Chart 63-1). The focus is on detecting early signs of increasing ICP.

MONITORING INTRACRANIAL PRESSURE. Because clinical assessment is not always a reliable guide in recognizing increased ICP, especially in patients who are comatose, monitoring of ICP and cerebral oxygenation is an essential part of management. ICP is monitored closely for continuous elevation or significant increase over baseline. The trend of ICP measurements over time is an important indication of the patient's underlying status. Vital signs are assessed when an increase in ICP is noted (Bader et al., 2016).

Careful attention to aseptic technique is needed when handling any part of the monitoring system. The insertion site is inspected for signs of infection. Temperature, pulse, and respirations are closely monitored for systemic signs of infection. All connections and stopcocks are checked for leaks, because even small leaks can distort pressure readings and lead to infection (AANN, 2012).

When ICP is monitored with a fluid system, the transducer is calibrated at a particular reference point, usually 2.5 cm (1 in) above the ear with the patient in the supine position; this point corresponds to the level of the foramen of Monro (Fig. 63-7). CSF pressure readings depend on the patient's position.

CHART 63-1

Detecting Increasing Intracranial Pressure (ICP)

Early Signs and Symptoms of Increasing ICP

- *Disorientation, restlessness, increased respiratory effort, purposeless movements, and mental confusion.* These are early clinical indications of increasing ICP because the brain cells responsible for cognition are extremely sensitive to decreased oxygenation.
- *Pupillary changes and impaired extraocular movements.* These occur as the increasing pressure displaces the brain against the oculomotor and optic nerves (cranial nerves II, III, IV, and VI), which arise from the midbrain and brainstem (see Chapter 66).
- *Weakness in one extremity or on one side of the body.* This occurs as increasing ICP compresses the pyramidal tracts.
- *Headache that is constant, increasing in intensity, and aggravated by movement or straining.* This occurs as increasing ICP causes pressure and stretching of venous and arterial vessels in the base of the brain.

Later Signs and Symptoms of Increasing ICP

- The level of consciousness continues to deteriorate until the patient is comatose (Glasgow Coma Scale score ≤8).
- The pulse rate and respiratory rate decrease or become erratic, and the blood pressure and temperature increase. The pulse pressure (the difference between the systolic and diastolic pressures) widens. The pulse fluctuates rapidly, varying from bradycardia to tachycardia.
- Altered respiratory patterns develop, including Cheyne–Stokes breathing (rhythmic waxing and waning of rate and depth of respirations alternating with brief periods of apnea) and ataxic breathing (irregular breathing with a random sequence of deep and shallow breaths).
- Projectile vomiting may occur with increased pressure on the reflex centre in the medulla.
- Hemiplegia or decorticate or decerebrate posturing may develop as pressure on the brainstem increases; bilateral flaccidity occurs before death.
- Loss of brainstem reflexes, including pupillary, corneal, gag, and swallowing reflexes, is an ominous sign of approaching death.

Adapted from Hickey, J. V. (2014). *The clinical practice of neurological and neurosurgical nursing* (7th ed.). Philadelphia, PA: Lippincott Williams & Wilkins.

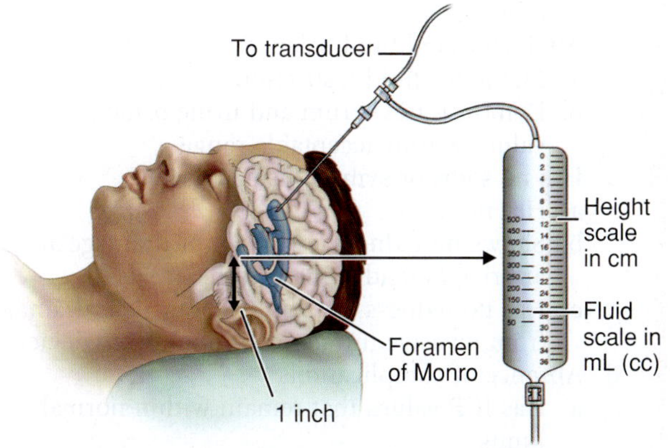

FIGURE 63-7. Location of the foramen of Monro for calibration of intracranial pressure monitoring system.

For subsequent pressure readings, the head should be in the same position relative to the transducer. Fibre optic catheters are calibrated before insertion and do not require further referencing; they do not require the head of the bed to be at a specific position to obtain an accurate reading.

When technology is associated with patient management, the nurse must be certain that the technologic equipment is functioning properly. The most important concern must be the patient to whom equipment is attached. The patient and family must be informed about the technology and the goals of its use. The patient's response is monitored, and appropriate comfort measures are implemented to ensure that the patient's stress is minimized.

ICP measurement is only one parameter; repeated neurologic checks and clinical examinations remain important measures. Astute observation, comparison of findings with previous observations, and interventions can assist in preventing life-threatening ICP elevations.

MONITORING FOR SECONDARY COMPLICATIONS. The nurse also assesses for complications of increased ICP, including DI, CSW, and SIADH (see Chapters 17 and 43). Urine output should be monitored closely. DI requires fluid and electrolyte replacement, and if severe may require further medical management with the administration of vasopressin, to replace and slow the urine output. Serum electrolyte levels are monitored closely for imbalances. SIADH requires fluid restriction and monitoring of serum electrolyte levels. CSW requires replacement of lost fluid and sodium.

Evaluation

Expected patient outcomes may include the following:

1. Maintains patent airway
2. Attains optimal breathing pattern
   a. Breathes in a regular pattern
   b. Attains or maintains arterial blood gas values within acceptable range
3. Demonstrates optimal cerebral tissue perfusion
   a. Increasingly oriented to time, place, and person
   b. Follows verbal commands; answers questions correctly
4. Attains desired fluid balance
   a. Maintains fluid restriction
   b. Demonstrates serum and urine osmolality values within acceptable range
5. Has no signs or symptoms of infection
   a. Has no fever
   b. Shows no redness, swelling, or drainage at arterial, IV, and urinary catheter sites
   c. Has no redness, swelling, or purulent drainage from invasive intracranial monitoring device
6. Absence of complications
   a. Has ICP values that remain within normal limits
   b. Demonstrates urine output and serum electrolyte levels within acceptable limits

INTRACRANIAL SURGERY

A **craniotomy** involves opening the skull surgically to gain access to intracranial structures. This procedure is performed to remove a tumour, relieve elevated ICP, evacuate a blood clot, or control hemorrhage. The surgeon cuts the skull to create a bony flap, which can be repositioned after surgery and held in place by periosteal or wire sutures. One of two approaches through the skull is used: (1) above the tentorium (supratentorial craniotomy) into the supratentorial compartment, or (2) below the tentorium into the infratentorial (posterior fossa) compartment. A third approach, the **transsphenoidal** approach (through the mouth and nasal sinuses) is often used to gain access to the pituitary gland (Bader et al., 2016). Table 63-4 compares these three different surgical approaches.

Alternatively, intracranial structures may be approached through burr holes (Fig. 63-8), which are circular openings made in the skull by either a hand drill or an automatic craniotome (which has a self-controlled system to stop the drill when the bone is penetrated). Burr holes may be used to determine the presence of cerebral swelling and injury and the size and position of the ventricles. They are also a means of evacuating an intracranial hematoma or abscess and for making a bone flap in the skull that allows access to the ventricles for decompression, ventriculography, or shunting procedures. Other cranial procedures include **craniectomy** (excision of a portion of the skull) and cranioplasty (repair of a cranial defect using a plastic or metal plate).

Supratentorial and Infratentorial Approaches

Preoperative Management

Medical Management

Preoperative diagnostic procedures may include a CT scan to demonstrate the lesion and show the degree of

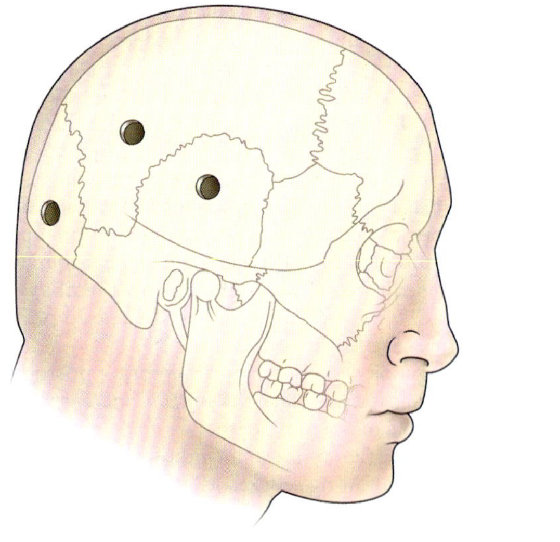

FIGURE 63-8. Burr holes may be used in neurosurgical procedures to make a bone flap in the skull, to aspirate a brain abscess, or to evacuate a hematoma.

TABLE 63-4 Comparison of Cranial Surgical Approaches

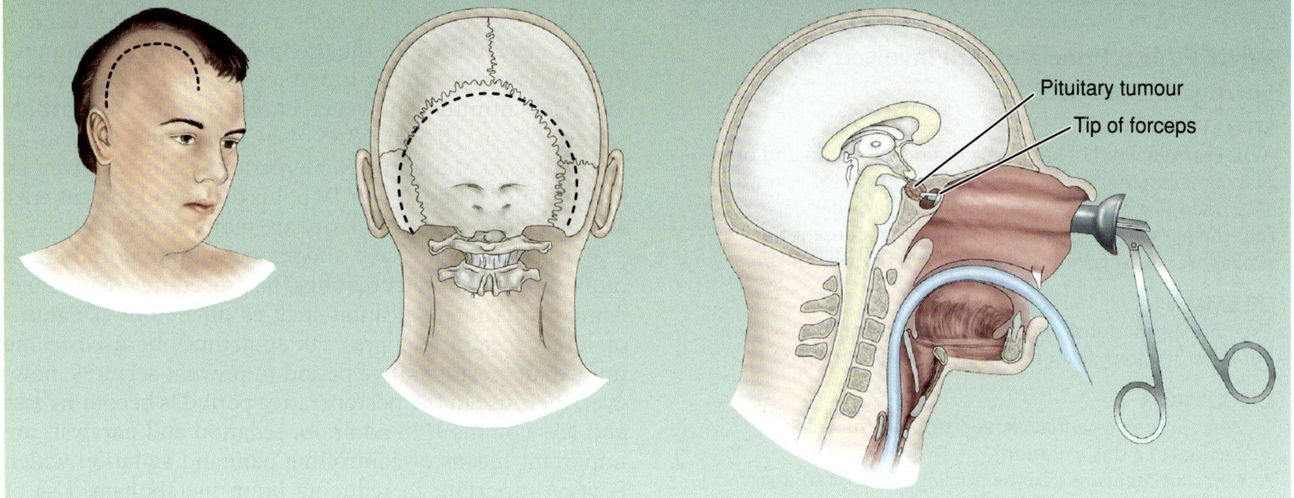

	Supratentorial	Infratentorial	Transsphenoidal
Site of Surgery	Above the tentorium	Below the tentorium, brain stem	Sella turcica and pituitary region
Incision Location	Incision is made above the area to be operated on; usually located behind the hairline	Incision is made at the nape of the neck, around the occipital lobe	Incision is made beneath the upper lip to gain access into the nasal cavity
Selected Nursing *Interventions*	Maintain head of bed elevated 30–45 degrees, with neck in neutral alignment Position patient on either side or back. (Avoid positioning patient on operative side if a large tumour has been removed)	Maintain neck in straight alignment Avoid flexion of the neck to prevent possible tearing of the suture line Position the patient on either side. (Check surgeon's preference for positioning of patient)	Maintain nasal packing in place and reinforce as needed Instruct patient to avoid blowing the nose Provide frequent oral care Keep head of bed elevated to promote venous drainage and drainage from the surgical site

surrounding brain edema, the ventricular size, and the displacement. An MRI scan provides information similar to that of a CT scan with improved tissue contrast, resolution, and anatomic definition. Cerebral angiography may be used to study a tumour's blood supply or obtain information about vascular lesions. Transcranial Doppler flow studies are used to evaluate the blood flow within intracranial blood vessels.

Most patients are prescribed an anticonvulsant medication such as phenytoin (Dilantin) or a phenytoin metabolite (Cerebyx) before surgery to reduce the risk of postoperative **seizures** (paroxysmal transient disturbances of the brain resulting from transient and abnormal electric discharge in the neurons of the cerebral cortex) (Diepenbrock, 2012; Hickey, 2014). Before surgery, corticosteroids such as dexamethasone (Decadron) may be administered to reduce cerebral edema if the patient has a space occupying lesion such as a brain tumour. A hyperosmotic agent (Mannitol) can also be given to decrease brain tension prior to opening the skull. Antibiotics may be administered if there is a chance of cerebral contamination; however, research does not support their use. Benzodiazepines such as diazepam (Valium) or lorazepam (Ativan) may be prescribed prior to surgery to allay anxiety.

Nursing Management

The preoperative assessment serves as a baseline against which postoperative status and recovery are compared. This assessment includes evaluating the LOC and responsiveness to stimuli and identifying any neurologic deficits, such as paralysis, visual dysfunction, alterations in personality or speech, and bladder and bowel disorders. Distal and proximal motor strength in both upper and lower extremities is recorded using the 5-point scale. Testing of motor function is discussed in Chapter 62.

The patient's and their family's understanding of and reactions to the anticipated surgical procedure and its possible sequelae are assessed, as is the availability of support systems for the patient and family. Adequate preparation for surgery, with attention to the patient's physical and emotional status, can reduce the risk of anxiety, fear, and postoperative complications. The patient is assessed for neurologic deficits and their potential impact after surgery.

Preparation of the patient and family includes providing information about what to expect during and after surgery. Hair is removed with the use of clippers and the surgical site prepared immediately before surgery (usually in the operating room), to decrease the chance of infection. An indwelling urinary catheter is inserted in the operating

CHART 63-2

Ethics and Related Issues

What Ethical Principles Are Involved With Surrogate Consent?

SITUATION

A 35-year-old woman has had a brain injury, is in and out of a comatose state, and needs a craniotomy for removal of an epidural hematoma. The health care provider determines that the patient is unable to give informed consent for the procedure, so consent is obtained from the next of kin.

DILEMMA

The principle of autonomy for the patient conflicts with the principle of paternalism for the health care providers.

DISCUSSION

1. What are the essential elements of informed consent pertinent to this situation?
2. What mechanisms can the nursing staff use to assist them in resolving any dilemma they have regarding the patient's right to autonomy?

room to drain the bladder during the administration of diuretics and to permit urinary output to be monitored. The patient may have central and arterial lines placed for fluid administration and monitoring of pressures after surgery.

An altered cognitive state may make the patient unaware of the impending surgery (Chart 63-2). Even so, encouragement and attention to the patient's needs are necessary. Whatever the state of awareness of the patient, the family needs reassurance and support, because they usually recognize the seriousness of brain surgery.

Postoperative Management

Postoperatively, an arterial line and a central venous pressure line may be in place to monitor and manage blood pressure and central venous pressure. The patient may be intubated and ventilated via a ventilator or may receive supplemental oxygen therapy via another respirator adjunct. Ongoing postoperative management is aimed at detecting and reducing cerebral edema, relieving pain and preventing seizures, monitoring ICP and neurologic status.

Postoperatively for motor deficits or weakness or paralysis of the arms or legs, trochanter rolls are applied to the extremities, and the feet are positioned against a footboard or the ankles are supported in a neutral position with orthotic boots. A patient who can ambulate is encouraged to do so. If the patient is aphasic, writing materials or picture and word cards showing the bedpan, glass of water, blanket, and other frequently used items may help improve communication.

The large head dressing applied after surgery may impair hearing temporarily. Vision may be limited if the eyes are swollen shut. If a tracheostomy or endotracheal tube is in place, the patient will be unable to speak until the tube is removed, so an alternative method of communication must be established.

Reducing Cerebral Edema, Preventing Seizures, and Relieving Pain

Medications to reduce cerebral edema in the postoperative patient are essentially the same as those which are used to reduce elevated ICP in the preoperative patient. Mannitol 20% IV is given rapidly to reduce cerebral edema within 10 to 20 minutes; however, more recently hypertonic saline (3% or 10% or 23.4% NaCl) is being used as an alternative to Mannitol. The hypertonic saline is given by continuous IV infusion or IV bolus doses and the patients' serum sodium and osmolarity are monitored closely.

For patients who have undergone supratentorial craniotomy, the risk of seizures after the procedure are possible. Anticonvulsant medication such as phenytoin (Dilantin) or levetiracetam (Keppra) can sometimes be used in the immediate postoperative period to prevent seizures; however, their use in the postoperative period is becoming less and less common. In addition, sedation and paralysis are important means of controlling pain and agitation which is very important in reducing brain metabolism. Use of medication such as morphine, propofol, and lorazepam are used for analgesia and sedation, while muscular paralytics such as vecuronium can be used with patients who require ventilatory support postoperatively to reduce the stress of mechanical ventilation.

Monitoring Intracranial Pressure

A patient undergoing intracranial surgery may have an ICP or cerebral oxygenation monitor inserted during surgery. Strict adherence to written protocols for managing these systems is essential, as discussed earlier, for preventing infection and managing ICP. The system is removed after the ICP or cerebral oxygenation is normal and stable. The neurosurgeon must be notified immediately if the system is not functioning.

Nursing Process

The Patient Who Has Undergone Intracranial Surgery

Assessment

After surgery, the frequency of postoperative monitoring is based on the patient's clinical status. Assessing respiratory function is essential, because even a small degree of hypoxia can increase cerebral ischemia. The respiratory rate and pattern are monitored, and arterial blood gas values are assessed frequently. Fluctuations in vital signs are carefully monitored and documented, because they may indicate increased ICP. The patient's temperature is measured to assess for hyperthermia. Neurologic checks are made frequently to assess the patient's condition in order to detect increased ICP, cerebral edema, or bleeding. A slight change in LOC or response to stimuli may be the first sign of increasing ICP.

The surgical dressing is inspected for evidence of bleeding and CSF drainage. The incision is monitored for redness, tenderness, bulging, separation, or foul odour. Sodium retention may occur in the immediate postoperative period. Serum and urine electrolytes, BUN, blood glucose, blood counts, arterial blood gases, weight, and clinical status are monitored. Intake and output are measured in view of losses associated with fever, respiration, and CSF drainage. The nurse must be alert to the development of complications; all assessments are carried out with these issues in mind. Seizures are a potential complication, and any seizure activity is carefully recorded and reported. Restlessness may occur as the patient becomes more responsive, or restlessness may be caused by pain, confusion, hypoxia, or other stimuli.

Nursing Priorities

Based on the assessment data, the patient's major nursing priorities after intracranial surgery may include the following:

- Risk for poor cerebral tissue perfusion
- Body temperature maintenance
- Airway and gas exchange
- Disturbed sensory perception
- Body image disturbance

Other nursing diagnoses may include impaired communication (aphasia) related to insult to brain tissue, and high risk for impaired skin integrity related to immobility, pressure, and incontinence; impaired physical mobility related to a neurologic deficit secondary to the neurosurgical procedure or to the underlying disorder may also occur.

Collaborative Problems/ Potential Complications

Potential complications include the following:

- Increased ICP
- Cerebral edema
- Bleeding
  - Postoperative hematoma
  - Hypovolemic shock
  - Deep vein thrombosis (DVT)
  - Gastric ulcer hemorrhage
- Fluid and electrolyte disturbances
  - SIADH
  - CSW
  - DI
- Hyperglycemia
- Infection
  - Pneumocephalus
  - Hydrocephalus
  - CSF leakage
- Seizures

Planning and Goals

The major goals for the postoperative patient include neurologic homeostasis to improve cerebral tissue perfusion, adequate thermoregulation, adequate ventilation and gas exchange, ability to cope with sensory deprivation, adaptation to changes in body image, and absence of complications.

Nursing Interventions

Maintaining Cerebral Tissue Perfusion

Attention to the patient's respiratory status is essential, because even slight decreases in the oxygen level (hypoxia) or slight increases in the carbon dioxide level (hypercarbia) can affect cerebral perfusion, the clinical course, and the patient's outcome. The endotracheal tube is left in place until the patient shows signs of awakening and has adequate spontaneous ventilation, as evaluated clinically and by arterial blood gas analysis. Secondary brain damage can result from impaired cerebral oxygenation.

Some degree of cerebral edema occurs after brain surgery; it tends to peak 24 to 72 hours after surgery. The control of cerebral edema was discussed earlier. Nursing strategies used to control factors that may raise ICP were presented in the previous Nursing Process section discussing increased ICP. Intraventricular drainage, if present, is carefully monitored, using strict asepsis when any part of the system is handled.

Vital signs and neurologic status (LOC and responsiveness, pupillary and motor responses) are assessed every 15 to 60 minutes depending on the physician's postoperative orders and the patient's condition. If the patient has an alteration in any assessment findings, more frequent assessments may be required. After surgery, the patient is placed on his or her back or side (on the unoperated side if a large lesion was removed) with one pillow under the head. The head of the bed may be elevated 30 degrees, depending on the level of the ICP and the neurosurgeon's preference. The patient may be turned on either side, keeping the neck in a neutral position. When the patient is being turned, the body is turned as a unit to prevent placing strain on the incision and possibly tearing the sutures. The head of the bed may be elevated slowly as tolerated by the patient.

The patient's position is changed every 2 hours, and skin care is given frequently. During position changes, care is taken to prevent disruption of the ICP monitoring system, if one is in place A turning sheet placed under the patient's head to midthigh makes it easier to move and turn the patient safely.

Regulating Temperature

Moderate temperature elevation can be expected after intracranial surgery because of the reaction to blood at the operative site or in the subarachnoid space. Injury to the hypothalamic centres that regulate body temperature can occur during surgery. Fever is treated vigorously to combat the effect of an elevated temperature on brain metabolism and function.

Nursing interventions include monitoring the patient's temperature and using the following measures to reduce body temperature: removing blankets, placing ice packs, and administering prescribed antipyretics to reduce fever (Rockett, Thompson, & Blissitt, 2015).

Conversely, hypothermia may be seen after lengthy neurosurgical procedures. Therefore, frequent measurements of rectal temperatures are necessary. Rewarming should occur slowly to prevent shivering, which increases cellular oxygen demands.

Improving Pulmonary Function/Gas Exchange

The patient undergoing neurosurgery is at risk for impaired gas exchange and pulmonary infections due to immobility, immunosuppression, decreased LOC, and fluid restriction. Immobility compromises the respiratory system by causing pooling and stasis of secretions in dependent areas and the development of atelectasis. The patient whose fluid intake is restricted may be more vulnerable to atelectasis as a result of inability to expectorate thickened secretions. Pneumonia can develop due to aspiration and restricted mobility.

Repositioning the patient every 2 hours helps to mobilize pulmonary secretions and prevent stasis. After the patient regains consciousness, additional measures to expand collapsed alveoli can be instituted, such as yawning, sighing, deep breathing, incentive spirometry, and coughing (unless contraindicated). If necessary, the oropharynx and trachea are suctioned to remove secretions that cannot be raised by coughing; however, coughing and suctioning cause sharp, but transient increases in ICP. Therefore, suctioning should be used cautiously. Increasing the humidity in the oxygen delivery system may help to loosen secretions. The nurse and the respiratory therapist work together to monitor the effects of chest physical therapy.

Managing Sensory Deprivation

Periorbital edema is a common consequence of intracranial surgery, because fluid drains into the dependent periorbital areas when the patient has been positioned in a prone position during surgery. A hematoma may form under the scalp and spread down to the orbit, producing an area of ecchymosis (black eye).

Before surgery, the patient and family are informed that one or both eyes may be edematous temporarily after surgery. After surgery, elevating the head of the bed (if not contraindicated) and applying ice packs over the eyes will help reduce the edema. If periorbital edema increases significantly, the surgeon is notified, because this may indicate that a postoperative clot is developing or that there is increasing ICP and poor venous drainage. Health care personnel should announce their presence when entering the room to avoid startling the patient whose vision is impaired due to periorbital edema or neurologic deficits.

Additional factors that can affect sensation include a bulky head dressing, the presence of an endotracheal tube, and effects of increased ICP. The timing of the first postoperative dressing change is usually ordered by the attending surgical team. In the absence of bleeding or a CSF leak, every effort is made to minimize the size of the head dressing. If the patient requires an endotracheal tube for mechanical ventilation, every effort is made to extubate the patient as soon as clinical signs indicate it is possible.

Enhancing Self-Image

The patient is encouraged to verbalize feelings and frustrations about any change in appearance. Nursing support is based on the patient's reactions and feelings. Factual information may need to be provided if the patient has misconceptions about puffiness about the face, periorbital bruising, and hair loss. Attention to grooming, and the use of the patient's own clothing are encouraged. Social interaction with close friends, family, and hospital personnel may increase the patient's sense of self-worth.

The family and social support system can be of assistance while the patient recovers from surgery.

Monitoring and Managing Potential Complications

The nurse must be vigilant for complications that may develop within hours of surgery and require close collaboration with the neurosurgeon. These include increased ICP, bleeding and hypovolemic shock, altered fluid and electrolyte balance (e.g., water intoxication and DI), infection, and seizures.

MONITORING FOR INCREASED INTRACRANIAL PRESSURE AND BLEEDING. Increased ICP and bleeding are life-threatening to the patient who has undergone intracranial surgery. The following points must be kept in mind when caring for any patient who has undergone such surgery:

- An increase in systolic blood pressure and decrease in pulse with respiratory failure may indicate increased ICP.
- An accumulation of blood under the bone flap (epidural, subdural, or intracerebral hematoma) may pose a threat to life. A clot must be suspected in any patient who does not awaken as expected or whose condition deteriorates. An intracranial hematoma is suspected if the patient has any new postoperative neurologic deficits (especially a dilated pupil on the operative side). In these circumstances an urgent CT scan of the brain is obtained and the patient is returned to the operating room immediately for evacuation of the clot if indicated.
- Cerebral edema, infarction, metabolic disturbances, and hydrocephalus are conditions that may mimic the clinical manifestations of a clot.

The patient is monitored closely for indicators of complications, and early signs and trends in clinical status are reported to the surgeon. Treatments are initiated promptly, and the nurse assists in evaluating the patient's response to treatment. The nurse also provides support to the patient and family.

If signs and symptoms of increased ICP occur, efforts to decrease the ICP are initiated: alignment of the head in a neutral position without flexion to promote venous drainage, elevation of the head of the bed to 30 degrees (when prescribed), decreasing stimulation, administration of mannitol or hypertonic saline (osmotic diuretics), and possible administration of pharmacologic paralyzing agents.

MANAGING FLUID AND ELECTROLYTE DISTURBANCES. Fluid and electrolyte imbalances may occur because of the patient's underlying condition and its management or as complications of surgery. These disturbances can contribute to the development of cerebral edema.

The postoperative fluid regimen depends on the type of neurosurgical procedure and is determined on an individual basis. The volume and composition of fluids are adjusted based on daily serum electrolyte values, along with fluid intake and output. Fluids may have to be restricted in patients with cerebral edema.

Oral fluids are usually resumed after the first 24 hours. The presence of gag and swallowing reflexes must be checked before initiation of oral fluids. Some patients with posterior fossa tumours have impaired swallowing, so fluids may need to be administered by alternative routes. The patient is observed for signs and symptoms of nausea and vomiting as the diet is progressed (Hickey, 2014).

Patients undergoing surgery for brain tumours often receive large doses of corticosteroids and therefore tend to develop hyperglycemia. Serum glucose levels are measured every 4 to 6 hours. These patients are also prone to stress ulcers, so histamine-2 receptor antagonists (H_2 blockers) are prescribed to suppress the secretion of gastric acid. Patients are also monitored for bleeding and assessed for GI discomfort.

If the surgical site is near to (or causes edema to) the pituitary gland and hypothalamus, the patient may develop symptoms of DI, which is characterized by excessive urinary output, elevated serum osmolality, decreased urine osmolality, hypernatremia, and a low urine specific gravity. The urine specific gravity is measured hourly, and fluid intake and output are monitored. Fluid replacement must compensate for urine output, and serum potassium levels must be monitored.

SIADH, which results in water retention with hyponatremia and serum hypo-osmolality, occurs in a wide variety of CNS disorders (e.g., brain tumour, head trauma) causing fluid disturbances. Nursing management includes careful intake and output measurements, specific gravity determinations of urine, and monitoring of serum and urine electrolyte levels while following directives for fluid restriction. SIADH is usually self-limited.

PREVENTING INFECTION. The patient undergoing neurosurgery is at risk for infection related to the neurosurgical procedure (brain exposure, bone exposure, wound hematomas) and the presence of IV and arterial lines for fluid administration and monitoring. Risk for infection is increased in patients who undergo lengthy intracranial operations and in those who have external ventricular drains in place.

The dressing is often stained with blood in the immediate postoperative period. Because blood is an excellent culture medium for bacteria, the dressing is reinforced with sterile pads so that contamination and infection are avoided. A heavily stained or displaced dressing should be reported immediately. A drain is sometimes placed in the craniotomy incision to facilitate drainage.

After suboccipital surgical procedures, CSF may leak through the incision. This complication is dangerous because of the possibility of meningitis. After a craniotomy, the patient is instructed to avoid coughing, sneezing, or nose blowing, which can cause CSF leakage by creating pressure on the operative site. Any sudden discharge of fluid from a cranial incision is reported at once, because a large leak requires surgical repair. Attention should be paid to the patient who complains of a salty taste or "postnasal drip," because this can be caused by CSF trickling down the throat.

Aseptic technique is used when handling dressings, drainage systems, IVs, and arterial lines. The patient is monitored carefully for signs and symptoms of infection, and cultures are obtained if infection is suspected. Appropriate antibiotics are administered as prescribed. Other causes of infection in the patient undergoing intracranial surgery, such as pneumonia and urinary tract infections, are similar to those in other postoperative patients.

MONITORING FOR SEIZURE ACTIVITY. Seizures may occur as complications after any intracranial neurosurgical procedure. Preventing seizures is essential to avoid further cerebral edema. Administering the prescribed anticonvulsant medication before and after surgery may prevent the development of seizures in subsequent months and years. **Status epilepticus** (prolonged seizures without recovery of consciousness in the intervals between seizures) may occur after craniotomy and also may be related to the development of complications (hematoma, ischemia). The management of status epilepticus is described later in this chapter.

MONITORING AND MANAGING OTHER COMPLICATIONS. Other complications may occur during the first 2 weeks or later and may compromise the patient's recovery. The most important of these are VTE (DVT, PE), pulmonary and urinary tract infections, and pressure ulcers. Most of these complications may be avoided with frequent changes of position, adequate suctioning of secretions, thrombosis prophylaxis, early removal of indwelling urinary catheter, early ambulation, and skin care.

Promoting Home, Community-Based, and Transitional Care

EDUCATING PATIENTS ABOUT SELF-CARE. The recovery of a neurosurgical patient at home depends on the extent of the surgical procedure and its success. The patient's strengths as well as limitations are assessed and explained to the family, along with the family's part in promoting recovery. Because administration of postoperative medications (steroids, pain medications, and anticonvulsants) is a priority, the patient and family are taught to use a check-off system,

CHART 63-3

HOME CARE CHECKLIST • Discharge After Intracranial Surgery

At the completion of education, the patient and/or caregiver will be able to:

- Name the procedure that was performed, any complications that occurred, and identify any permanent changes in anatomic structure or function as well as changes in ADLs, IADLs, roles, relationships, and spirituality.
- Identify interventions and strategies (e.g., durable medical equipment, adaptive equipment) used in recovery period.
- Describe ongoing postoperative therapeutic regimen, including diet and activities to perform (e.g., walking and breathing exercises) and to limit or avoid (e.g., lifting weights, driving a car, contact sports).
- State the name, dose, side effects, frequency, and schedule for all medications.
- State how to obtain medical supplies and carry out dressing changes, wound care, and other prescribed regimens.
- Identify durable medical equipment needs, proper usage, and maintenance necessary for safe utilization.
- Describe signs and symptoms of complications.
- State time and date of follow-up appointments.
- Relate how to reach primary provider with questions or complications.
- Identify community resources for peer and caregiver/family support:
  - Identify sources of support (e.g., friends, relatives, faith community).
  - Identify phone numbers, meeting locations/times of community resources for patients and their caregivers/families.
- Identify the need for health promotion (e.g., weight reduction, smoking cessation, stress management), disease prevention, and screening activities.

ADL, activities of daily living; IADL, independent activities of daily living.

pill boxes, calendars, and alarms to ensure that the medications are taken as prescribed.

The patient and family are taught what to expect after surgery (Chart 63-3). Dietary restrictions usually are not required unless another health problem necessitates a special diet. Although showering or tub bathing is permitted, the scalp should be kept dry until all the sutures have been removed. Avoiding the wearing of scarfs or caps until the craniotomy site has fully healed and sutures/staples have been removed. In rare cases if the skull bone has been removed, the neurosurgeon may prescribe a protective helmet. After a craniotomy, the patient may require rehabilitation, depending on the postoperative level of function. The patient may require physical therapy for residual weakness and mobility issues. An occupational therapist is consulted to assist with self-care issues. If the patient is aphasic, speech therapy may be necessary.

CONTINUING AND TRANSITIONAL CARE. Barring complications, patients are discharged from the hospital as soon as possible. Patients with severe motor deficits require extensive physical and occupational therapy and rehabilitation. Those with postoperative cognitive and speech impairments require psychological evaluation, speech therapy, and rehabilitation. The nurse collaborates with the physician and other health care professionals during hospitalization and home care to achieve as complete a rehabilitation as possible and to assist the patient and family to return to or as close to their previous level of functioning.

If tumour, injury, or disease makes the prognosis poor, care is directed toward making the patient as comfortable as possible and decreasing their burden of care. Other possible consequences include weakness or paralysis, blindness, and seizures. The home care nurse, hospice nurse, and social worker collaborate with the family to plan for additional home health care or hospice services or placement of the patient in an extended-care facility (see also the section on cerebral metastases in Chapter 67). The patient and family are encouraged to discuss end-of-life preferences for care; the patient's end-of-life preferences must be respected (see Chapter 15). The nurse involved in home and continuing care of patients after cranial surgery also needs to remind patients and family members of the need for health promotion and recommended health screening.

Evaluation

Expected patient outcomes may include the following:

1. Achieves optimal cerebral tissue perfusion
   a. Opens eyes on request; uses recognizable words, progressing to usual speech
   b. Obeys commands with appropriate motor responses

2. Maintains appropriate body temperature
   a. Registers normal body temperature
3. Has expected gas exchange
   a. Has arterial blood gas values within expected ranges
   b. Breathes easily; lung sounds are clear without adventitious sounds
   c. Takes deep breaths and changes position as directed
4. Copes with sensory deprivation
5. Demonstrates improving self-concept
   a. Pays attention to grooming
   b. Visits and interacts with others
6. Exhibits absence of complications
   a. Exhibits ICP within expected range
   b. Has minimal bleeding at surgical site; surgical incision is healing without evidence of infection
   c. Shows fluid balance and electrolyte levels within desired ranges
   d. Exhibits no evidence of seizures

Lesions of the Anterior Skull Base/Transsphenoidal Approach

Tumours within the sella turcica and small adenomas of the pituitary can be removed through a transsphenoidal approach (see Table 63-4). Although an otorhinolaryngologist may make the initial opening, the neurosurgeon completes the opening into the sphenoidal sinus and exposes the floor of the sella. Microsurgical techniques provide improved illumination, magnification, and visualization so that nearby vital structures can be avoided.

The transsphenoidal approach offers direct access to the sella turcica with minimal risk of trauma and hemorrhage (Bader et al., 2016). It avoids many of the risks of craniotomy, and the postoperative discomfort is similar to that of other transnasal surgical procedures. It may also be used for pituitary ablation (destruction) in patients with metastatic breast or prostatic cancer.

Complications

Manipulation of the posterior pituitary gland during surgery may produce transient normal imbalances such as DI, SIADH of several days' duration (Hickey, 2014). Other complications include CSF leakage, visual disturbances, postoperative meningitis, pneumocephalus (air in the intracranial cavity; see Chapter 43).

Preoperative Management

Medical Management

The preoperative workup of a lesion in the anterior skull base may include evaluations by an endocrinologist, ear nose and throat surgeons, and ophthalmologists. Complete endocrine, ophthalmological, and head and neck exams are all undertaken.

Nursing Management

Deep breathing is taught before surgery. The patient is instructed that after the surgery he or she will need to avoid vigorous coughing, blowing the nose, sucking through a straw, or sneezing, because these actions may place increased pressure at the surgical site and cause a CSF leak (Hickey, 2014).

Postoperative Management

Medical Management

Because the procedure disrupts the oral and nasal mucous membranes, management focuses on preventing infection and promoting healing. Medications include antimicrobial agents (which are continued until the nasal packing inserted at the time of surgery is removed), corticosteroids, analgesic agents for discomfort, and agents for the control of DI if necessary (Hickey, 2014).

Nursing Management

Vital signs are measured to monitor hemodynamic, cardiac, and ventilatory status. Because of the anatomic proximity of the pituitary gland to the optic chiasm, visual acuity and visual fields are assessed at regular intervals. One method is to ask the patient to count the number of fingers held up by the nurse. Evidence of decreasing visual acuity suggests an expanding hematoma.

The head of the bed is raised to decrease pressure on the sella turcica and to promote normal drainage. The patient is cautioned against blowing the nose or engaging in any activity that raises ICP, such as bending over or straining during urination or defecation.

Intake and output are measured as a guide to fluid and electrolyte replacement and to assess for DI. The urine specific gravity is measured after each voiding. Daily weight is monitored. Fluids are usually given after nausea ceases, and the patient then progresses to a regular diet.

The nasal packing inserted during surgery is checked frequently for blood or CSF drainage. The major discomfort is related to the nasal packing and to mouth dryness and thirst caused by mouth breathing. Oral care is provided every 4 hours or more frequently. Usually, the teeth are not brushed until the incision above the teeth has healed. Warm saline mouth rinses and the use of a cool mist vaporizer are helpful. Petrolatum is soothing when applied to the lips. A room humidifier assists in keeping the mucous membranes moist. The packing is removed in 3 to 4 days, and only then can the area around the nares be cleaned with the prescribed solution to remove crusted blood and moisten the mucous membranes (Hickey, 2014).

Home care considerations include advising the patient to use a room humidifier to keep the mucous membranes moist and to soothe irritation. The head of the bed is elevated at 30 degrees for at least 2 weeks after surgery. The patient is cautioned against blowing the nose or sneezing for at least 1 month (Hickey, 2014).

SEIZURE DISORDERS

Seizures are episodes of abnormal motor, sensory, autonomic, or psychic activity (or a combination of these) that result from sudden excessive discharge from cerebral

CHART 63-4

Classification of Seizures: 2016 Basic Scheme

Focal

- Motor
- Nonmotor
- Awareness
  - Aware
  - Impaired awareness
  - Unknown awareness

Generalized

- Motor
- Absence

Unknown

- Motor
- Nonmotor
- Awareness
  - Aware
  - Impaired awareness
  - Unknown awareness
- Unclassified

Adapted from Fisher, R., Cross, H., French, J., et al. (2016). Operational classification of seizure types by the International League Against Epilepsy (ILAE). Retrieved on September 29, 2016, from www.ilae.org/visitors/centre/documents/ClassificationSeizureILAE-2016.pdf

neurons (Hickey, 2014). A localized area or all of the brain may be involved. The International League Against Epilepsy (ILAE) has defined epilepsy as at least two unprovoked seizures occurring more than 24 hours apart (Fisher, Acevedo, Arzimanoglou, et al., 2014). The ILAE differentiates between three main seizure types: focal, generalized, and unknown seizures (Chart 63-4). Generalized seizures occur in and rapidly engage bilaterally distributed networks. Focal seizures are thought to originate within one hemisphere in the brain. The unknown type includes epileptic spasms. Unclassified seizures are so termed because of incomplete data but are not considered a classification (Fisher et al., 2014). Seizures may also be characterized as "provoked," or related to acute, reversible conditions such as structural, metabolic, immune, infectious, or unknown etiologies (Scheffer, French, Hirsch, et al., 2016).

Pathophysiology

The underlying cause is an electrical disturbance (dysrhythmia) in the nerve cells in one section of the brain; these cells emit abnormal, recurring, uncontrolled electrical discharges. The characteristic seizure is a manifestation of this excessive neuronal discharge. Associated loss of consciousness, excess movement or loss of muscle tone or movement, and disturbances of behaviour, mood, sensation, and perception may also occur.

The specific causes of seizures are varied and can be categorized as idiopathic (genetic, developmental defects) and acquired. Causes of acquired seizures include:

- Cerebrovascular disease
- Hypoxemia of any cause, including vascular insufficiency
- Fever (childhood)
- Head injury
- Hypertension
- CNS infections
- Metabolic and toxic conditions (e.g., renal failure, hyponatremia, hypocalcemia, hypoglycemia, pesticide exposure)
- Brain tumour
- Drug and alcohol withdrawal
- Allergies

Clinical Manifestations

Depending on the location of the discharging neurons, seizures may range from a simple staring episode (generalized absence seizure) to prolonged convulsive movements with loss of consciousness.

The initial pattern of the seizures indicates the region of the brain in which the seizure originates (see Chart 63-4). Only a finger or hand may shake, or the mouth may jerk uncontrollably. The person may talk unintelligibly; may be dizzy; and may experience unusual or unpleasant sights, sounds, odours, or tastes, but without loss of consciousness (Hickey, 2014).

Generalized seizures often involve both hemispheres of the brain, causing both sides of the body to react. Intense rigidity of the entire body may occur, followed by alternating muscle relaxation and contraction (generalized tonic–clonic contraction). The simultaneous contractions of the diaphragm and chest muscles may produce a characteristic epileptic cry. The tongue is often chewed, and the patient is incontinent of urine and feces. After 1 or 2 minutes, the convulsive movements begin to subside; the patient relaxes and lies in deep coma, breathing noisily. The respirations at this point are chiefly abdominal. In the postictal state (after the seizure), the patient is often confused and hard to arouse and may sleep for hours. Many patients report headache, sore muscles, fatigue, and depression (AANN, 2016a). Other generalized seizures may be absence types of seizures (Fisher, Cross, French, et al., 2016).

Focal seizures are subdivided into events characterized by both motor and nonmotor symptoms. There may be an impairment of consciousness or awareness or other dyscognitive features, localization, and progression of symptoms (Fisher et al., 2016).

Assessment and Diagnostic Findings

The diagnostic assessment is aimed at determining the type of seizures, their frequency and severity, and the factors that precipitate them. A developmental history is taken, including events of pregnancy and childbirth, to seek evidence of pre-existing injury. The patient is also questioned about illnesses or head injuries that may have affected the brain. In addition to physical and neurologic evaluations, diagnostic examinations include biochemical, hematologic, and serologic studies. MRI is used to detect structural lesions such as focal abnormalities, cerebrovascular abnormalities, and cerebral degenerative changes (AANN, 2016a).

The EEG furnishes diagnostic evidence for a substantial proportion of patients with epilepsy and assists in classifying the type of seizure. Abnormalities in the EEG usually continue between seizures or, if not apparent, may be elicited by hyperventilation or during sleep (AANN, 2016a). Microelectrodes (depth electrodes) can be inserted deep in the brain to probe the action of single brain cells. Some people with clinical seizures have normal EEGs, whereas others who have never had seizures have abnormal EEGs. Telemetry and computerized equipment are used to monitor electrical brain activity while the patient pursues their normal activities and to store the readings on computer tapes for analysis. Video recording of seizures taken simultaneously with EEG telemetry is useful in determining the type of seizure as well as its duration and magnitude (Updyke & Duryea, 2013).

SPECT is an additional tool that is sometimes used in the diagnostic workup. It is useful for identifying the epileptogenic zone so that the area in the brain giving rise to seizures can be removed surgically (AANN, 2016a).

Nursing Management

During a Seizure

A major responsibility of the nurse is to observe and record the sequence of signs. The nature of the seizure usually indicates the type of treatment required (AANN, 2016a). Before and during a seizure, the patient is assessed and the following items are documented:

- Circumstances before the seizure (visual, auditory, or olfactory stimuli; tactile stimuli; emotional or psychological disturbances; sleep; hyperventilation)
- Occurrence of an aura (a premonitory or warning sensation, which can be visual, auditory, or olfactory)
- First thing the patient does in the seizure—where the movements or the stiffness begins, conjugate gaze position, and the position of the head at the beginning of the seizure. This information gives clues to the location of the seizure origin in the brain. (In recording, it is important to state whether the beginning of the seizure was observed.)
- Type of movements in the part of the body involved
- Areas of the body involved (turn back bedding to expose patient)
- Size of both pupils and whether the eyes are open
- Whether the eyes or head are turned to one side
- Presence or absence of automatisms (involuntary motor activity, such as lip smacking or repeated swallowing)
- Incontinence of urine or stool
- Duration of each phase of the seizure
- Unconsciousness, if present, and its duration
- Any obvious paralysis or weakness of arms or legs after the seizure
- Inability to speak after the seizure
- Movements at the end of the seizure
- Whether or not the patient sleeps afterward
- Cognitive status (confused or not confused) after the seizure

In addition to providing data about the seizure, nursing care is directed at preventing injury and supporting the patient, not only physically but also psychologically. Consequences such as anxiety, embarrassment, fatigue, and depression can be devastating to the patient.

After a Seizure

After a patient has a seizure, the nurse's role is to document the events leading to and occurring during and after the seizure and to prevent complications (e.g., aspiration, injury). The patient is at risk for hypoxia, vomiting, and pulmonary aspiration. To prevent complications, the patient is placed in the side-lying position to facilitate drainage of oral secretions, and suctioning is performed, if needed, to maintain a patent airway and prevent aspiration (Chart 63-5). Seizure precautions are maintained, including having available functioning suction equipment with a suction catheter and oral airway. The bed is placed in a low position with side rails up and padded, if necessary, to prevent injury to the patient. The patient may be drowsy and may wish to sleep after the seizure; he or she may not remember events leading up to the seizure and for a short time thereafter.

The Epilepsies

Epilepsy is a group of syndromes characterized by unprovoked, recurring seizures (AANN, 2016a). Epileptic syndromes are classified by specific patterns of clinical features, including age at onset, family history, and seizure type. The epilepsies include electroclinical syndromes (a complex of clinical features, signs, and symptoms) and other epilepsies (Institute of Medicine [IOM], 2012). Epilepsy can be primary (idiopathic) or secondary (when the cause is known and the epilepsy is a symptom of another underlying condition, such as a brain tumour).

Epilepsy affects an estimated 3% of people during their lifetime, and most forms of epilepsy occur in children and older adults (England, Liverman, Schultz, et al., 2012). The improved treatment for cerebrovascular disorders, head injuries, brain tumours, meningitis, and encephalitis has increased the number of patients at risk for seizures after recovery from these conditions. In addition, advances in EEG have aided in the diagnosis of epilepsy. The general public has been educated about epilepsy, which has reduced the stigma associated with it; as a result, more people are willing to acknowledge that they have epilepsy.

Although some evidence suggests that susceptibility to some types of epilepsy may be inherited, the cause of seizures in many people is idiopathic (unknown). Epilepsy can follow birth trauma, asphyxia neonatorum, head injuries, some infectious diseases (bacterial, viral, parasitic), toxicity (carbon monoxide and lead poisoning), circulatory problems, fever, metabolic and nutritional disorders, or drug or alcohol intoxication. It is also associated with brain tumours, abscesses, and congenital malformations.

Pathophysiology

Messages from the body are carried by the neurons (nerve cells) of the brain by means of discharges of electrochemical energy that sweep along them. These impulses occur in bursts whenever a nerve cell has a task to perform. Sometimes, these cells or groups of cells continue firing after a task is finished. During the period of unwanted discharges, parts of the body controlled by the errant cells may perform erratically. Resultant

CHART 63-5

Care of the Patient During and After a Seizure

Nursing Care During a Seizure

- Provide privacy, and protect the patient from curious onlookers. (The patient who has an aura may have time to seek a safe, private place.)
- Ease the patient to the floor, if possible.
- Protect the head with a pad to prevent injury (from striking a hard surface).
- Loosen constrictive clothing and remove eyeglasses.
- Push aside any furniture that may injure the patient during the seizure.
- If the patient is in bed, remove pillows and raise side rails.
- *Do not attempt to pry open jaws that are clenched in a spasm or attempt to insert anything in the mouth during a seizure.* Broken teeth and injury to the lips and tongue may result from such an action.
- Do not attempt to restrain the patient during the seizure, because muscular contractions are strong and restraint can produce injury.
- If possible, place the patient on one side with head flexed forward, which allows the tongue to fall forward and facilitates drainage of saliva and mucus. If suction is available, use it if necessary to clear secretions.

Nursing Care After the Seizure

- Keep the patient on one side to prevent aspiration. Make sure the airway is patent.
- On awakening, reorient the patient to the environment.
- If the patient is confused or wandering, guide the patient gently to a bed or chair.
- If the patient becomes agitated after a seizure (postictal), stay a distance away, but close enough to prevent injury until the patient is fully aware.

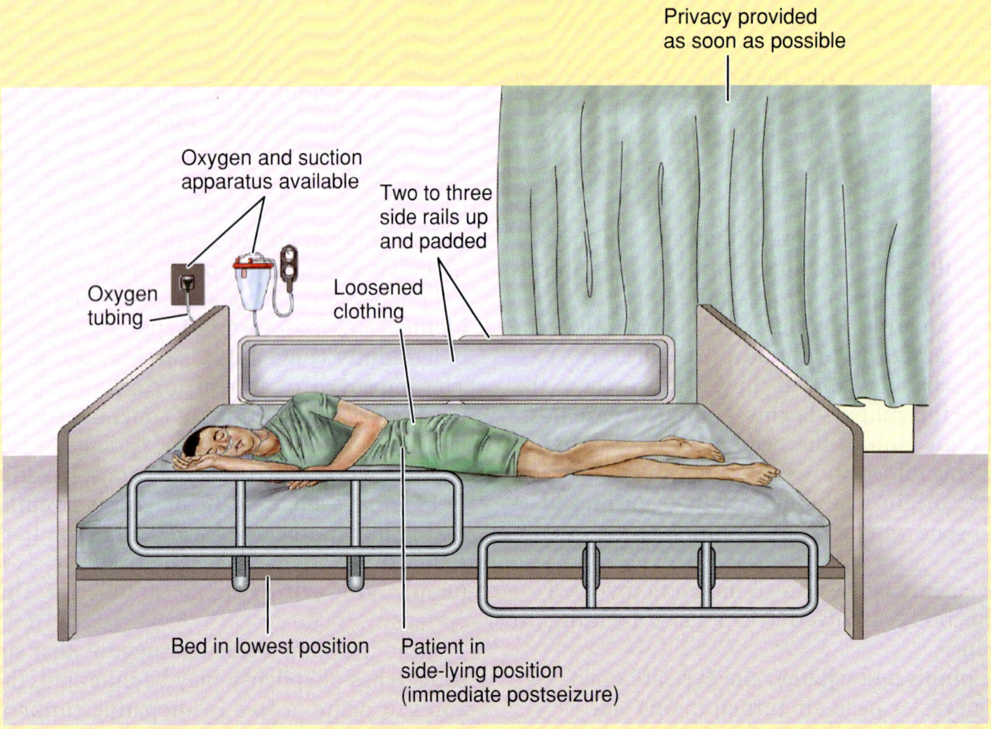

Adapted from American Association of Neuroscience Nurses (AANN). (2016a). *Care of adults and children with seizures and epilepsy: AANN clinical practice guideline series.* Chicago, IL: Author.

dysfunction ranges from mild to incapacitating and often causes loss of consciousness (Hickey, 2014). If these uncontrolled, abnormal discharges occur repeatedly, a person is said to have an epileptic syndrome. Epilepsy is not associated with intellectual level. People who have epilepsy without other brain or nervous system disabilities fall within the same intelligence ranges as the overall population. Epilepsy is not synonymous with mental retardation or illness. However, many people who have developmental disabilities because of serious neurologic damage also have epilepsy.

Clinical Manifestations

Depending on the location of the discharging neurons, seizures may range from a simple staring episode (absence seizure) to prolonged convulsive movements with loss of consciousness.

The initial pattern of the seizures indicates the region of the brain in which the seizure originates. In simple partial seizures, only a finger or hand may shake, or the mouth may jerk uncontrollably. The person may talk unintelligibly; may be dizzy; and may experience unusual or unpleasant sights, sounds, odours, or tastes, but without loss of consciousness (Hickey, 2014).

In complex partial seizures, the person either remains motionless or moves automatically but inappropriately for time and place, or he or she may experience excessive emotions of fear, anger, elation, or irritability. Whatever the manifestations, the person does not remember the episode when it is over.

Generalized seizures (previously referred to as grand mal seizures) involve both hemispheres of the brain, causing both sides of the body to react (Hickey, 2014). Intense rigidity of the entire body may occur, followed by alternating muscle relaxation and contraction (generalized tonic–clonic contraction). The simultaneous contractions of the diaphragm and chest muscles may produce a characteristic epileptic cry. The tongue is often chewed, and the patient may be incontinent of urine or stool. After seconds or minutes, the convulsive movements begin to subside; the patient relaxes and may become minimally conscious, breathing noisily. The respirations at this point are chiefly abdominal. In the postictal state (after the seizure), the patient is often confused and hard to arouse and may sleep for hours. Many patients report headache, sore muscles, fatigue, and depression after a seizure.

Assessment and Diagnostic Findings

The diagnostic assessment is aimed at determining the type of seizures, their frequency and severity, and the factors that precipitate them. A developmental history is taken, including events of pregnancy and childbirth, to seek evidence of pre-existing injury. The patient is also questioned about illnesses or head injuries that may have affected the brain. In addition to physical and neurologic evaluations, diagnostic examinations include biochemical, hematologic, and serologic studies. MRI is used to detect structural lesions such as focal abnormalities, cerebrovascular abnormalities, and cerebral degenerative changes (Gulanick & Myers, 2013).

The electroencephalograph (EEG) furnishes diagnostic evidence for a substantial proportion of patients with epilepsy and assists in classifying the type of seizure. Abnormalities in the EEG usually continue between seizures or, if not apparent, may be elicited by hyperventilation or during sleep (Urden et al., 2013). Microelectrodes (depth electrodes or subdural grids) can be inserted deep in the brain or along the outside of the brain in order to locate in which area of the brain the seizures are coming from. Some people with clinical seizures have normal EEGs, whereas others who have never had seizures have abnormal EEGs. Telemetry and computerized equipment are used to monitor electrical brain activity while the patient pursues his or her usual activities and to store the readings on computer tapes for analysis. Video recording of seizures taken simultaneously with EEG telemetry is useful in determining the type of seizure as well as its duration and magnitude. SPECT is an additional tool of nuclear medicine that is sometimes used in the diagnostic workup. It is useful for calculating regional and global cerebral blood flow, by measuring cerebral metabolic use of oxygen and glucose. This helps to identify the epileptogenic zone so that the area in the brain giving rise to seizures can be removed surgically or appropriate treatment can be determined (Urden et al., 2013).

Epilepsy in Women

Women who have epilepsy face particular needs associated with the syndrome. They often note an increase in seizure frequency during menses; this has been linked to the increase in sex hormones that alter the excitability of neurons in the cerebral cortex (Dworetzky, Townsend, Pennell, et al., 2012). The effectiveness of contraceptives is decreased by anticonvulsant medications. Therefore, patients are encouraged to discuss family planning with their neurologist or primary health care provider and to obtain preconception counselling if they are considering childbearing (Rauchenzauner, Ehrensberger, Prieschl, et al., 2013).

Women of childbearing age who have epilepsy require special care and guidance before, during, and after pregnancy. Many women note a change in the pattern of seizure activity during pregnancy. The risk of congenital fetal anomaly is two to three times higher in women with epilepsy. Maternal seizures, anticonvulsant medications, and genetic predisposition all contribute to possible congenital malformations in infants. Women who take certain anticonvulsant medications for epilepsy are at risk and need careful monitoring, including blood studies to detect the level of anticonvulsant medications taken throughout pregnancy (Ko, 2014). High-risk mothers (teenagers, women with histories of difficult deliveries, women who use illicit drugs [e.g., crack, cocaine], and women with diabetes or hypertension) should be identified and monitored closely during pregnancy, because damage to the fetus during pregnancy and delivery can increase the risk of epilepsy. All of these issues need further study (Thomas & Devi, 2012).

Gerontologic Considerations

Older adults have a high incidence of new-onset epilepsy (Chart 63-6) (Hickey, 2014; Miller, Buelow, & Bakas, 2014). Cerebrovascular disease is the leading cause of seizures in the older adult. The increased incidence is also associated with head injury, dementia, infection, alcoholism, and aging. Treatment depends on the underlying cause. Because many older adults have chronic health problems, they may be taking other medications that can interact with medications prescribed for seizure control. In addition, the absorption, distribution, metabolism, and excretion of medications are altered in the older adult as a result of age-related changes in renal and liver functions. Therefore, older adult patients must be monitored closely for adverse and toxic effects of anticonvulsant medications and for osteoporosis. The cost of anticonvulsant medications can lead to poor adherence to the prescribed regimen in older adult patients on fixed incomes.

Prevention

Society-wide efforts are the key to prevention of epilepsy. Head injury is one of the main causes of epilepsy that can be prevented. Through highway safety programs and occupational safety precautions, lives can be saved and

NURSING RESEARCH PROFILE

Chart 63-6. Experiences With a New Diagnosis of Epilepsy in Older Adults

Miller, W., Buelow, J., & Bakas, T. (2014). Older adults and new onset epilepsy: Experiences with diagnosis. *Journal of Neuroscience Nursing*, *46*(1), 2–10.

Purpose

Older adults in the United States have a high rate of new-onset epilepsy; however, most research focuses on children and young adults. Older adults may exhibit a different clinical presentation, display age-related cognitive and metabolic changes, and have comorbidities that increase the likelihood of polypharmacy, creating unique challenges. This research was undertaken to identify the experience and characteristics of the older adult with new-onset epilepsy.

Design

A qualitative descriptive approach was undertaken to describe the experiences of 20 community dwelling older adults with new-onset epilepsy living in both urban and rural settings. Eligible participants were diagnosed at or after the age of 60 years, diagnosed within the previous 3 months, took at least one anticonvulsant medication, and spoke and read English. Semistructured interviews were conducted by one researcher and analyzed and coded using conventional content analysis that identified clusters and themes.

Findings

The mean age of the participants was 70 years; 12 were women and 8 were men. Length of time until diagnosis was the most prominent theme during the interviews and split into two main themes: delayed diagnosis and nondelayed diagnosis. Participants with delayed diagnosis (epilepsy not diagnosed within 3 months of symptoms) attributed the delay to their primary providers not recognizing atypical symptoms or attributing symptoms to another neurologic process, or to their own delay in seeking care. The nondelayed participants reported typical seizure characteristics and rapid referral to a neurologic provider. The seizure events were obvious and interfered with daily life. Participants living in rural areas and women more often experienced delays in diagnosis.

Nursing Implications

Nurses need to be aware that older adults are the group at highest risk for developing new-onset epilepsy, and what might be identified as symptoms of aging may in fact be seizure-related events. Nurses can educate older adults regarding their risk of developing epilepsy and should describe both typical and atypical seizure presentations. Patients should be encouraged to seek specialized care for symptoms such as unexplained changes in mental status, Syncope, and dizziness.

epilepsy due to head injury prevented; these programs are discussed in Chapter 65.

Medical Management

The management of epilepsy is individualized to meet the needs of each patient and not just to manage and prevent seizures. Management differs from patient to patient, because some forms of epilepsy arise from brain dysfunction and others result from altered brain chemistry.

Pharmacologic Therapy

Many medications are available to control and prevent seizures, although the exact mechanisms of action are unknown. The objective is to achieve seizure control with minimal side effects. Medication therapy controls rather than cures seizures. Medications are selected on the basis of the type of seizure being treated, the effectiveness and safety of the medications, side effect profile and cost. If properly prescribed and taken, medications control seizures in 70% to 80% of patients with seizures. However, 20% of patients with generalized seizures and 30% of those with partial seizures do not demonstrate improvement with any prescribed medication or may be unable to tolerate the side effects of medications (Torbic, Forni, Anger, et al., 2013). These patients are diagnosed with refractory epilepsy and surgical options are then explored. Table 63-5 lists the medications in current use.

Treatment usually starts with a single medication. The starting dose and the rate at which the dosage is increased depend on the medication's effect and the occurrence of side effects. If possible the medication levels in the blood are monitored. Changing to another medication may be necessary if seizure control is not achieved, side effects are intolerable, or if toxicity makes it impossible to increase the dosage. These medications may need to be adjusted because of concurrent illness, weight changes, or increases in stress. Side effects of anticonvulsant medications may be divided into three groups: (1) idiosyncratic or allergic disorders, which manifest primarily as skin reactions; (2) acute toxicity, which may occur when the medication is initially prescribed; and (3) chronic toxicity, which occurs late in the course of therapy.

The manifestations of drug toxicity are variable, and any organ system may be involved. Gingival hyperplasia (swollen and tender gums) can be associated with long-term use of phenytoin (Dilantin), for example (Torbic et al., 2013). Periodic physical and dental examinations and laboratory tests are performed for patients receiving medications that are known to have hematopoietic, genitourinary, or hepatic effects.

Surgical Management

Surgery is indicated for patients whose epilepsy results from intracranial tumours, abscesses, cysts, or vascular or structural anomalies. Some patients have intractable seizure disorders that do not respond to medication. A focal atrophic process may occur secondary to trauma, inflammation, stroke, or anoxia. If the seizures originate in a reasonably well-circumscribed area of the brain that can be excised without producing significant neurologic deficits, the removal of the area generating the seizures may

TABLE 63-5 Major Anticonvulsant Medications

Medication	Dose-Related Side Effects	Toxic Effects
carbamazepine (Tegretol)	Dizziness, drowsiness, unsteadiness, nausea and vomiting, diplopia, mild leukopenia	Severe skin rash, blood dyscrasias, hepatitis
clonazepam (Rivotril)	Drowsiness, behaviour changes, headache, hirsutism, alopecia, palpitations	Hepatotoxicity, thrombocytopenia, bone marrow failure, ataxia
ethosuximide (Zarontin)	Nausea and vomiting, headache, gastric distress	Skin rash, blood dyscrasias, hepatitis, systemic lupus erythematosus
gabapentin (Neurontin)	Dizziness, drowsiness, somnolence, fatigue, ataxia, weight gain, nausea	Leukopenia, hepatotoxicity
lamotrigine (Lamictal)	Drowsiness, tremor, nausea, ataxia, dizziness, headache, weight gain	Severe rash (Stevens–Johnson syndrome)
levetiracetam (Keppra)	Somnolence, dizziness, fatigue	Unknown
oxcarbazepine (Trileptal)	Dizziness, somnolence, double vision, fatigue, nausea, vomiting, loss of coordination, abnormal vision, abdominal pain, tremor, abnormal gait	Hepatotoxicity
phenobarbital (Luminal)	Sedation, irritability, diplopia, ataxia	Skin rash, anemia
phenytoin (Dilantin)	Visual problems, hirsutism, gingival hyperplasia, dysrhythmias, dysarthria, nystagmus	Severe skin reaction, peripheral neuropathy, ataxia, drowsiness, blood dyscrasias
primidone (Mysoline)	Lethargy, irritability, diplopia, ataxia, impotence	Skin rash
topiramate (Topamax)	Fatigue, somnolence, confusion, ataxia, anorexia, depression, weight loss	Nephrolithiasis
valproate (Depakote, Depakene)	Nausea and vomiting, weight gain, hair loss, tremor, menstrual irregularities	Hepatotoxicity, skin rash, blood dyscrasias, nephritis
zonisamide (Zonegran, Excegran)	Somnolence, dizziness, anorexia, headache, nausea, agitation, rash	Leukopenia, hepatotoxicity

Adapted from Karch, A. (2015). *2015 Lippincott's nursing drug guide*. Philadelphia, PA: Lippincott Williams & Wilkins.

produce long-term control and improvement (Morton & Fontaine, 2013).

This type of neurosurgery has been aided by several advances, including microsurgical techniques, EEGs with depth electrodes, improved illumination and hemostasis, and the introduction of neuroleptanalgesic agents (droperidol and fentanyl). These techniques, combined with use of local anesthetic agents, enable the neurosurgeon to perform surgery on an alert and cooperative patient. Using special testing devices, electrocortical mapping, and the patient's responses to stimulation, the boundaries of the epileptogenic focus (i.e., abnormal area of the brain) are determined. Any abnormal epileptogenic focus is then excised (Morton & Fontaine, 2013). Resection surgery significantly reduces the incidence of seizures in patients with refractory epilepsy.

When seizures are refractory to medication in adolescents and adults with focal seizures, a vagal nerve stimulator (VNS) may be implanted under the clavicle. The device is connected to the vagus nerve in the cervical area, where it delivers electrical signals to the brain to control and reduce seizure activity. An external programming system is used by the physician to change stimulator settings (Wheless, 2013). Patients can activate the stimulator with a magnet at the time of a seizure or aura. Some patients report that use of the VNS diminishes the severity or duration of the seizure. Complications such as infection, cardiac dysrhythmias, hoarseness, cough, and laryngeal spasm can occur with the use of this device (AANN, 2016a; Wheless, 2013).

Another surgical option for patients with refractory seizure activity is the responsive neurostimulation system (RNS) (U.S. Food and Drug Administration, 2014). This is a surgically implanted device with electrodes that sense and record brain electrical activity. Electrodes deliver an electrical stimulation to the location of seizure origination within the brain. The RNS works by interrupting brainwave activity before a clinical seizure can occur (AANN, 2016a).

More research is needed to determine the effects of the various surgical approaches on complication rates, quality of life, anxiety, and depression, all of which are issues for patients with epilepsy.

Nursing Process

The Patient With Epilepsy

Assessment

The nurse elicits information about the patient's seizure history. The patient is asked about the factors or events that may precipitate the seizures. Alcohol intake is documented. The nurse determines whether the patient has an aura before an epileptic seizure, which may indicate the origin of the seizure (e.g., seeing a flashing light may indicate that the seizure originated in the occipital lobe) (Urden et al., 2013). Observation and assessment during and after a seizure assist in identifying the type of seizure and its management.

The effects of epilepsy on the patient's lifestyle are assessed. What limitations are imposed by the seizure disorder? Does the patient participate in any recreational activities? Have any social contacts? Is the patient working, and is it a positive or stressful experience? What coping mechanisms are used?

Nursing Priorities

Based on the assessment data, the patient's major nursing priorities may include the following:

- Risk for injury
- Fear
- Ineffective coping
- Deficient knowledge

Collaborative Problems/ Potential Complications

The major potential complications for patients with epilepsy are status epilepticus and medication side effects (toxicity).

Planning and Goals

The major goals for the patient may include prevention of injury, control of seizures, achievement of a satisfactory psychosocial adjustment, acquisition of knowledge and understanding about the condition, and absence of complications.

Nursing Interventions

Preventing Injury

Injury prevention for the patient with seizures is a priority. Patients for whom seizure precautions are instituted should have pads applied to the side rails while in bed. Steps to prevent or minimize injury are presented in Chart 63-5.

Reducing Fear of Seizures

Fear that a seizure may occur unexpectedly can be reduced by the patient's adherence to the prescribed treatment regimen. Cooperation of the patient and family and their trust in the prescribed regimen are essential for control of seizures. The nurse emphasizes that the prescribed anticonvulsant medication must be taken on a continuing basis and that drug dependence or addiction does not occur. Periodic monitoring is necessary to ensure the adequacy of the treatment regimen, to prevent side effects, and to monitor for drug resistance (Hickey, 2014).

In an effort to control seizures, factors that may precipitate them are identified, such as emotional disturbances, new environmental stressors, onset of menstruation in female patients, or fever (AANN, 2016a). The patient is encouraged to follow a regular and moderate routine in lifestyle, diet (avoiding excessive stimulants), exercise, and rest (sleep deprivation may lower the seizure threshold). Moderate activity is therapeutic, but excessive exercise should be avoided. An additional dietary intervention, referred to as the ketogenic diet, may be helpful for control of seizures in some patients. This high-protein, low-carbohydrate, high-fat diet is most effective in children whose seizures have not been controlled with two anticonvulsant medications, but it is sometimes used for adults who have had poor seizure control (Nei, Ngo, Sirven, et al., 2014).

Photic stimulation (e.g., bright flickering lights, television viewing) may precipitate seizures; wearing dark glasses or covering one eye may be preventive. Tension states (anxiety, frustration) induce seizures in some patients. Classes in stress management may be of value. Because seizures are known to occur with alcohol intake, alcoholic beverages should be avoided.

Improving Coping Mechanisms

The social, psychological, and behavioural problems that frequently accompany epilepsy can be more of a disability than the actual seizures. Epilepsy may be accompanied by feelings of stigmatization, alienation, depression, and uncertainty. The patient must cope with the constant fear of a seizure and the psychological consequences (Sung, Muller, Ditchman, et al., 2013). Children with epilepsy may be ostracized and excluded from school and peer activities. These problems are compounded during adolescence and add to the challenges of dating, not being able to drive, and feeling different from other people. Adults face these problems in addition to the burden of finding employment, concerns about relationships and childbearing, insurance problems, and legal barriers. Alcohol abuse may complicate matters. Family reactions may vary from outright rejection of the person with epilepsy to overprotection.

Counselling assists the patient and family to understand the condition and the limitations it imposes. Social and recreational opportunities are necessary for good mental health. Nurses can improve the quality of life for patients with epilepsy by teaching them and their families about symptoms and their management (Sung et al., 2013).

Providing Patient and Family Education

Perhaps the most valuable facets of care contributed by the nurse to the person with epilepsy are education and efforts to modify the attitudes of the patient and family toward the disorder. The person who experiences seizures may consider every seizure a potential source of humiliation and shame. This may result in anxiety, depression, hostility, and secrecy on the part of the patient and family. Ongoing education and encouragement should be given to patients to enable them to overcome these reactions. The patient with epilepsy should carry an emergency medical identification card or wear a medical information bracelet. The patient and family need to be educated about medications as well as care during a seizure.

Monitoring and Managing Potential Complications

Status epilepticus, the major complication, is described later in this chapter. Another complication is the toxicity of medications. The patient and family are instructed about side effects and are given specific guidelines to assess and report signs and symptoms that indicate medication overdose. Anticonvulsant medications require careful monitoring for therapeutic levels. However, not all anticonvulsant medication serum levels can be monitored. The patient should plan to have serum drug levels assessed at regular intervals. Many known drug interactions occur with anticonvulsant medications. A complete pharmacologic profile should be reviewed with the patient to avoid interactions that either potentiate or inhibit the effectiveness of the medications.

NURSING ALERT

Patients with epilepsy are at risk for status epilepticus from having their medication regimen interrupted.

Promoting Home, Community-Based, and Transitional Care

EDUCATING PATIENTS ABOUT SELF-CARE. Thorough oral hygiene after each meal, gum massage, daily flossing, and regular dental care are essential to prevent or control gingival hyperplasia in patients receiving phenytoin. The patient is also educated to inform all health care providers of the medication being taken, because of the possibility of drug interactions. An individualized comprehensive education plan is needed to assist the patient and family to adjust to this chronic disorder. Written patient education materials must be appropriate for the patient's reading level and must be provided in alternative formats if warranted. See Chart 63-7 for health promotion strategies for the patient with epilepsy.

CONTINUING AND TRANSITIONAL CARE. For many people with epilepsy, overcoming employment problems is a challenge. Vocational rehabilitation agencies can provide information about job training. According to the Canadian Human Rights Act, it is illegal for an employer (within federal jurisdiction) to discriminate on the basis of physical or mental disability, but barriers to employment still exist. Epilepsy Canada (2014), a national organization, works to advocate and lobby for people with disabilities.

Patients who have uncontrollable seizures accompanied by psychological and social difficulties should be referred as early as possible to a comprehensive epilepsy centre where continuous audio–video and EEG monitoring, specialized treatment, and rehabilitation services are available (AANN, 2016a). Patients and their families need to be reminded of the importance of participating in health promotion activities and recommended health screenings to promote a healthy lifestyle. Genetic and preconception counselling is advised.

CHART 63-7

Health Promotion: Strategies for the Patient With Epilepsy

- Take anticonvulsant medications daily as prescribed to keep the drug level constant to prevent seizures. Never discontinue medications, even if there is no seizure activity.
- Keep a medication and seizure record (in electronic or paper format), noting when medications are taken and any seizure activity.
- Notify the primary provider if unable to take medications due to illness.
- Have anticonvulsant medication serum levels checked regularly. When testing is prescribed, report to the laboratory for blood sampling before taking morning medication.
- Avoid activities that require alertness and coordination (driving, operating machinery) until after the effects of the medication have been evaluated.
- Report signs of toxicity so that dosage can be adjusted. Common signs include drowsiness, lethargy, dizziness, difficulty walking, hyperactivity, confusion, inappropriate sleep, and visual disturbances.
- Avoid over-the-counter medications unless approved by the primary provider.
- Carry a medical alert bracelet or identification card specifying the name of the anticonvulsant medication and primary provider.
- Avoid seizure triggers, such as alcoholic beverages, electrical shocks, stress, caffeine, constipation, fever, hyperventilation, and hypoglycemia.
- Take showers rather than tub baths to avoid drowning if seizure occurs; never swim alone.
- Exercise in moderation in a temperature-controlled environment to avoid excessive heat.
- Develop regular sleep patterns to minimize fatigue and insomnia.
- Be aware of and use the Epilepsy Foundation of America (EFA) special services, including help in obtaining medications, vocational rehabilitation, and coping with epilepsy.

Evaluation

Expected patient outcomes may include the following:

1. Sustains no injury during seizure activity
   a. Complies with treatment regimen and identifies the hazards of stopping the medication
   b. Can identify appropriate care during seizure; caregivers can also do so
2. Indicates a decrease in fear
3. Displays effective individual coping
4. Exhibits knowledge and understanding of epilepsy
   a. Identifies the side effects of medications
   b. Avoids factors or situations that may precipitate seizures (e.g., flickering lights, hyperventilation, alcohol)
   c. Follows a healthy lifestyle by getting adequate sleep and eating meals at regular times to avoid hypoglycemia
5. Absence of complications

Status Epilepticus

Status epilepticus (acute prolonged seizure activity) is a series of generalized seizures that occur without full recovery of consciousness between attacks (Trinka, Cock, Hesdorffer, et al., 2015). The term has been broadened to include continuous clinical or electrical seizures (on EEG) lasting at least 30 minutes, even without impairment of consciousness. It is considered a medical emergency. Status epilepticus produces cumulative effects. Vigorous muscular contractions impose a heavy metabolic demand and can interfere with respirations. Some respiratory arrest at the height of each seizure produces venous congestion and hypoxia of the brain. Repeated episodes of cerebral anoxia and edema may lead to irreversible and fatal brain damage. Factors that precipitate status epilepticus include interruption of anticonvulsant medication, fever, concurrent infection, or other illness.

Medical Management

The goals of treatment are to stop the seizures as quickly as possible, to ensure adequate cerebral oxygenation, and to maintain the patient in a seizure-free state. An airway and adequate oxygenation are established. If the patient remains unconscious and unresponsive, an endotracheal tube is inserted. IV diazepam (Valium), lorazepam (Ativan), or fosphenytoin is given slowly in an attempt to halt seizures immediately. Other medications (phenytoin, phenobarbital) are given later to maintain a seizure-free state.

An IV line is established, and blood samples are obtained to monitor serum electrolytes, glucose, and phenytoin levels. EEG monitoring may be useful in determining the nature of the seizure activity. Vital signs and neurologic signs are monitored on a continuing basis. An IV infusion of dextrose is given if the seizure is caused by hypoglycemia. If initial treatment is unsuccessful, general anesthesia with a short-acting barbiturate may be used. The serum concentration of the anticonvulsant medication is measured, because a low level suggests that the patient was not taking the medication or that the dosage was too low. Cardiac involvement or respiratory depression may be life-threatening. The potential for postictal cerebral edema also exists.

Nursing Management

The nurse initiates ongoing assessment and monitoring of respiratory and cardiac function because of the risk for delayed depression of respiration and blood pressure secondary to administration of anticonvulsant medications and sedatives to halt the seizures. Nursing assessment also includes monitoring and documenting the seizure activity and the patient's responsiveness.

The patient is turned to a side-lying position, if possible, to assist in draining pharyngeal secretions. Suction equipment must be available because of the risk of aspiration. The IV line is closely monitored, because it may become dislodged or occluded during seizures.

A person who has received long-term anticonvulsant therapy has a significant risk for fractures resulting from bone disease (osteoporosis, osteomalacia, and hyperparathyroidism), a side effect of therapy. Therefore, during seizures, the patient is protected from injury with the use of seizure precautions and is monitored closely. The patient having seizures can inadvertently injure nearby people, so nurses should protect themselves. Additional nursing interventions for the person having seizures are presented in Chart 63-5.

HEADACHE

Headache, or cephalalgia, is one of the most common of all human physical complaints. Headache is a symptom rather than a disease entity; it may indicate organic disease (neurologic or other disease), a stress response, vasodilation (migraine), skeletal muscle tension (tension headache), or a combination of factors. A **primary headache** is one for which no organic cause can be identified. This type of headache includes migraine, tension-type, and cluster headaches (Hickey, 2014). Cranial arteritis is another common cause of headache. A classification of headaches was issued first by the Headache Classification Committee of the International Headache Society in 1988. The International Headache Society revised the headache classification in (2013); an abbreviated list is shown in Chart 63-8.

Migraine is a complex of symptoms characterized by periodic and recurrent attacks of severe headache lasting from hours to days in adults. The cause of migraine has not been clearly demonstrated, but it is primarily a vascular disturbance that has a strong familial tendency. The typical time of onset is at puberty, and the incidence is higher in women than men (D'Arcy, 2014).

There are many subtypes of **migraine headache**, including migraine with and without aura. Most patients have

CHART 63-8

International Headache Society Classification of Headache

- Migraine
- Tension-type headache
- Trigeminal autonomic cephalalgias
- Other primary disorders
- Headache attributed to trauma or injury to the head and/or neck
- Headache attributed to cranial or cervical vascular disorder
- Headache attributed to nonvascular intracranial disorder
- Headache attributed to a substance or its withdrawal
- Headache attributed to infection
- Headache attributed to disorder of homeostasis
- Headache or facial pain attributed to disorder of cranium, neck, eyes, ears, nose, sinuses, teeth, mouth, or other facial or cranial structures
- Headache attributed to psychiatric disorder
- Painful cranial neuropathies and other facial pains
- Other headache disorders

Adapted from Headache Classification Committee of the International Headache Society. (2013). The international classification of headache disorders, 3rd edition (beta version). *Cephalalgia*, *33*(9), 629–808.

migraine without an aura. *Tension-type headaches* tend to be chronic and less severe and are probably the most common type of headache. *Trigeminal autonomic cephalalgias* include cluster headaches and paroxysmal hemicrania. Cluster headaches are relatively uncommon and seen more frequently in men than in women (Grossman & Porth, 2014). Types of headaches not subsumed under these categories fall into the *other primary headache* group and include headaches triggered by cough, exertion, and sexual activity.

Cranial arteritis is a cause of headache in the older population, reaching its greatest incidence in those older than 70 years of age. Inflammation of the cranial arteries is characterized by a severe headache localized in the region of the temporal arteries. The inflammation may be generalized (in which case cranial arteritis is part of a vascular disease) or focal (in which case only the cranial arteries are involved).

A **secondary headache** is a symptom associated with other causes, such as a brain tumour, an aneurysm, or lumbar puncture (Destrebecq, Terzoni, & Sala, 2014). Although most headaches do not indicate serious disease, persistent headaches require further investigation. Serious disorders related to headache include brain tumours, subarachnoid hemorrhage, stroke, severe hypertension, meningitis, and head injuries.

Pathophysiology

The cerebral signs and symptoms of migraine result from a hyperexcitable brain that is susceptible to a phenomenon known as cortical spreading depression, a wave of depolarization over the cerebral cortex, cerebellum, and hippocampus. This depolarization activates inflammatory neuropeptides and other neurotransmitters (including serotonin), resulting in the stimulation of meningeal nociceptors. Vascular changes, inflammation, and a continuation of pain signal stimulation occur (Charles, 2015). The initial phase of this process is known as the premonitory phase and may include light, sound, and smell sensitivity. If treatment is initiated at this point, the migraine may be fully terminated. As the attack progresses, central sensitization occurs, and the migraine becomes much harder to treat.

Attacks can be triggered by hormonal changes associated with menstrual cycles, bright lights, stress, depression, sleep deprivation, fatigue, or odours. Certain foods containing tyramine (especially aged cheese), monosodium glutamate, and chocolate may be food triggers (Grossman & Porth, 2014). The use of oral contraceptives may be associated with increased frequency and severity of attacks in some women.

Emotional or physical stress may cause contraction of the muscles in the neck and scalp, resulting in tension headache. The pathophysiology of cluster headache is not fully understood. One theory is that it is caused by dilation of orbital and nearby extracranial arteries. Cranial arteritis is thought to represent an immune vasculitis in which immune complexes are deposited within the walls of affected blood vessels, producing vascular injury and inflammation. A biopsy may be performed on the involved artery to make the diagnosis.

Clinical Manifestations

Migraine

The migraine with aura can be divided into four phases: prodrome, aura, the headache, and recovery (headache termination and postdrome).

Prodrome Phase

The prodrome phase is experienced by 60% of patients, with symptoms that occur hours to days before a migraine headache. Symptoms may include depression, irritability, feeling cold, food cravings, anorexia, change in activity level, increased urination, diarrhea, or constipation. Patients usually experience the same prodrome with each migraine headache.

Aura Phase

An aura may be a variable feature for patients who experience migraines (Charles & Hansen, 2015). An aura is characterized by focal neurologic symptoms. Visual disturbances (i.e., light flashes and bright spots) are most common and may be hemianopic (affecting only half of the visual field). Other symptoms that may follow include numbness and tingling of the lips, face, or hands; mild confusion; slight weakness of an extremity; drowsiness; and dizziness.

This period of aura was thought to correspond to the phenomenon of cortical spreading depression that is associated with reduced metabolic demand in abnormally functioning neurons. This can be associated with decreased blood flow; however, cerebral blood flow studies performed during migraine headaches demonstrate that although changes in blood vessels occur during phases of migraine, cerebral blood flow is not the main abnormality. In fact, some studies suggest that the aura and headache phases may occur simultaneously (Charles, 2013).

Headache Phase

As vasodilation and a decline in serotonin levels occur, a throbbing headache (unilateral in 60% of patients) intensifies over several hours. This headache is severe and incapacitating and is often associated with photophobia, nausea, and vomiting. Its duration varies, ranging from 4 to 72 hours (Hickey, 2014).

Recovery Phase

In the recovery phase (termination and postdrome), the pain gradually subsides. Muscle contraction in the neck and scalp is common, with associated muscle ache and localized tenderness, exhaustion, and mood changes. Any physical exertion exacerbates the headache pain. During this postheadache phase, patients may sleep for extended periods.

Other Headache Types

The tension-type headache is characterized by a steady, constant feeling of pressure that usually begins in the forehead, temple, or back of the neck. It is often bandlike or may be described as "a weight on top of my head."

Cluster headaches are unilateral and come in clusters of one to eight daily, with excruciating pain localized to the eye and orbit and radiating to the facial and temporal regions. The pain is accompanied by watering of the eye and nasal congestion. Each attack lasts 15 minutes to

3 hours and may have a crescendo–decrescendo pattern (Hickey, 2014). The headache is often described as penetrating.

Cranial arteritis often begins with general manifestations, such as fatigue, malaise, weight loss, and fever. Clinical manifestations associated with inflammation (heat, redness, swelling, tenderness, or pain over the involved artery) usually are present. Sometimes a tender, swollen, or nodular temporal artery is visible. Visual problems are caused by ischemia of the involved structures.

Assessment and Diagnostic Findings

The diagnostic evaluation includes a detailed history, a physical assessment of the head and neck, and a complete neurologic examination. Headaches may manifest differently in the same person over the course of a lifetime, and the same type of headache may manifest differently from patient to patient. The health history focuses on assessing the headache itself, with emphasis on the factors that precipitate or provoke it. The patient is asked to describe the headache in his or her own words. A headache diary is a very useful tool in the identification, diagnosis, treatment, and overall management of headaches.

Because headache is often the presenting symptom of various physiologic and psychological disturbances, a general health history is an essential component of the patient database. Headache may be a symptom of endocrine, hematologic, gastrointestinal, infectious, renal, cardiovascular, or psychiatric disease. Therefore, questions addressed in the health history should cover major medical and surgical illness as well as a body systems review.

The medication history can provide insight into the patient's overall health status and indicate medications that may be provoking headaches. Antihypertensive agents, diuretic medications, anti-inflammatory agents, and monoamine oxidase (MAO) inhibitors are a few of the categories of medications that can provoke headaches (Becker, Findlay, Moga, et al., 2015). Emotional factors can play a role in precipitating headaches. Stress is thought to be a major initiating factor in migraine headaches; therefore, sleep patterns, level of stress, recreational interests, appetite, diet, emotional or psychiatric problems, and family stressors are relevant. There is a strong familial tendency for headache disorders, and a positive family history may help in making a diagnosis (Latimer, 2013).

A direct relationship may exist between exposure to toxic substances and headache. Careful questioning may uncover chemicals to which a worker has been exposed. The Workplace Hazardous Materials Information System (WHMIS) is a national system established in 1988 that provides employees information on hazardous material used in the workplace. Employees have access to material safety data sheets (commonly referred to as MSDS) for all substances with which they come in contact in the workplace. The occupational history also includes assessment of the workplace as a possible source of stress and for a possible ergonomic basis of muscle strain and headache.

A complete description of the headache itself is crucial. The nurse reviews the age at onset of headache; the headache's frequency, location, and duration; the type of pain; factors that relieve and precipitate the event; and associated symptoms. The data obtained should include the patient's own words about the headache in response to the following questions:

- What is the location? Is it unilateral or bilateral? Does it radiate?
- What is the quality—dull, aching, steady, boring, burning, intermittent, continuous, paroxysmal?
- How many headaches occur during a given period of time?
- What are the precipitating factors, if any—environmental (e.g., sunlight, weather change), foods, exertion, other?
- What makes the headache worse (e.g., coughing, straining)?
- What time (day or night) does it occur?
- How long does a typical headache last?
- Are there any associated symptoms, such as facial pain, lacrimation (excessive tearing), or scotomas (blind spots in the field of vision)?
- What usually relieves the headache (aspirin, nonsteroidal anti-inflammatory drugs, ergot preparation, food, heat, rest, neck massage)?
- Does nausea, vomiting, weakness, or numbness in the extremities accompany the headache?
- Does the headache interfere with daily activities?
- Do you have any allergies?
- Do you have insomnia, poor appetite, loss of energy?
- Is there a family history of headache?
- What is the relationship of the headache to your lifestyle or physical or emotional stress?
- What medications are you taking?

Diagnostic testing often is not helpful in the investigation of headache, because often there are few objective findings. In patients who demonstrate abnormalities on the neurologic examination, CT, cerebral angiography, or MRI may be used to detect underlying causes, such as tumour or aneurysm. Electromyography (EMG) may reveal a sustained contraction of the neck, scalp, or facial muscles. Laboratory tests may include complete blood count, erythrocyte sedimentation rate, electrolytes, glucose, creatinine, and thyroid hormone levels.

Prevention

Prevention begins by having the patient avoid specific triggers that are known to initiate the headache syndrome. Preventive medical management of migraine involves the daily use of one or more agents that are thought to block the physiologic events leading to an attack. Treatment regimens vary greatly, as do patient responses; therefore, close monitoring is indicated.

Alcohol, nitrites, vasodilators, and histamines may precipitate cluster headaches. Elimination of these factors helps prevent the headaches.

Medical Management

Therapy for migraine headache is divided into abortive (symptomatic) and preventive approaches. The abortive approach, best used in those patients who have less frequent attacks, is aimed at relieving or limiting a headache at the onset or while it is in progress. The preventive approach is used in patients who experience more frequent attacks at

CHART 63-9

Patient Education: Migraine Headaches

The nurse instructs the patient to:

- Be aware of the definition of migraine headaches along with the characteristics and manifestations.
- Recognize triggers of migraine headaches and how to avoid such triggers as:
  - Foods that contain tyramine, such as chocolate, cheese, coffee, dairy products
  - Dietary habits that result in long periods between meals
  - Menstruation and ovulation (caused by hormone fluctuation)
  - Alcohol (causes vasodilation of blood vessels)
  - Fatigue and fluctuations in sleep patterns
- Develop and use a paper or electronic headache diary.
- Implement stress management and lifestyle changes to minimize the frequency of headaches.
- Ensure correct pharmacologic management: acute therapy and prophylaxis to include medication regimen and side effects.
- Use comfort measures during headache attacks, such as resting in a quiet and dark environment, applying cold compresses to the painful area, and elevating the head.
- Seek out resources for education and support, such as the National Headache Foundation.

regular or predictable intervals and may have a medical condition that precludes the use of abortive therapies (Becker et al., 2015). Medical management of migraine during pregnancy and lactation includes nonpharmacologic strategies in addition to safe medication practices (Wells, Turner, Lee, et al., 2016). Nonpharmacologic treatments include mainly avoidance of triggers (Chart 63-9) (Grossman & Porth, 2014).

The triptans, which are serotonin receptor agonists, are the most specific antimigraine agents available. These agents cause vasoconstriction, reduce inflammation, and may reduce pain transmission. The five triptans in routine clinical use include sumatriptan (Imitrex), naratriptan (Amerge), rizatriptan (Maxalt), zolmitriptan (Zomig), and almotriptan (Axert) (D'Arcy, 2014). Numerous serotonin receptor agonists are under study. Many of the triptan medications are available in a variety of formulations, such as nasal sprays, inhalers, conventional tablet, disintegrating tablet, suppositories, or injections. The nasal sprays are useful for patients experiencing nausea and vomiting (Dahlöf & Van Den Brink, 2012).

The triptans are considered first-line treatment of the management of moderate to severe migraine pain. Best results are achieved with early use of triptans; oral dosing takes effect within 20 to 60 minutes of taking the drug and if needed may be repeated in 2 to 4 hours. Triptans are contraindicated in patients with ischemic heart disease. Careful administration and dosing instructions to patients are important to prevent adverse reactions such as increased blood pressure, drowsiness, muscle pain, sweating, and anxiety. Interactions are possible if the medication is taken in conjunction with St. John's wort (Karch, 2015).

Ergotamine preparations (taken orally, sublingually, subcutaneously, intramuscularly, by rectum, or by inhalation) may be effective in aborting the headache if taken early in the migraine process. They are low in cost. Ergotamine tartrate acts on smooth muscle, causing prolonged constriction of the cranial blood vessels. Each patient's dosage is based on individual needs. Side effects include aching muscles, paresthesias (numbness and tingling), nausea, and vomiting. Pretreatment with antiemetic agents may be required. None of the triptan medications should be taken concurrently with medications containing ergotamine because of the potential for a prolonged vasoactive reaction (Karch, 2015).

Many widely used medications for the prevention of migraine are available. An analysis of research in the last decade reported the most effective medications for migraine treatment include anticonvulsant agents (divalproex sodium [Depakote], valproate [Depacon], topiramate [Topamax]), beta-blockers (metoprolol [Lopressor], propranolol [Inderal], timolol [Blocadren]), and triptans (frovatriptan [Frova]). Other medications prescribed for migraine prevention include antidepressant agents (amitriptyline [Elavil], venlafaxine [Effexor]) and additional beta-blockers (atenolol [Tenormin], nadolol [Corgard]) and triptans (naratriptan [Amerge], zolmitriptan [Zomig]) (D'Arcy, 2014).

The medical management of an acute attack of cluster headaches may include 100% oxygen by facemask for 15 minutes, subcutaneous sumatriptan, or intranasal zolmitriptan (Becker et al., 2015).

The medical management of cranial arteritis consists of early administration of a corticosteroid to prevent the possibility of loss of vision due to vascular occlusion or rupture of the involved artery. The patient is instructed not to stop the medication abruptly, because this can lead to relapse. Analgesic agents are prescribed for comfort.

Nursing Management

When migraine or the other types of headaches have been diagnosed, the goal of nursing management is to enhance pain relief. It is reasonable to try nonpharmacologic interventions first, but the use of medications should not be delayed. The goal is to treat the acute event of the headache and to prevent recurrent episodes. Prevention involves patient education regarding precipitating factors, possible lifestyle or habit changes that may be helpful, and pharmacologic measures.

Relieving Pain

Individualized treatment depends on the type of headache and differs for migraine, cluster headaches, cranial arteritis, and tension headache. Nursing care is directed toward treatment of the acute episode. A migraine or a cluster headache in the early phase requires abortive medication therapy instituted as soon as possible. Some headaches can be prevented if the appropriate medications are taken before the onset of pain. Nursing care during an attack includes comfort measures such as a quiet, dark environment; elevation of the head of the bed to 30 degrees; and symptomatic treatment (i.e., administration of antiemetic medication) (Hickey, 2014).

Symptomatic pain relief for tension headache may be obtained by application of local heat or massage. Additional strategies may include administration of analgesic agents, antidepressant medications, steroids, anti nauseates (Metoclopramide), and muscle relaxants.

Promoting Home, Community-Based, and Transitional Care

Educating Patients About Self-Care

Headaches, especially migraines, are more likely to occur when the patient is ill, overly tired, or stressed. Nonpharmacologic therapies are important and include patient education about the type of headache, its mechanism (if known), and appropriate changes in lifestyle to avoid triggers. Regular sleep, meals, exercise, relaxation, and avoidance of dietary triggers may be helpful in avoiding headaches (Hickey, 2014).

The patient with tension headaches needs teaching and reassurance that the headache is not the result of a brain tumour; this is a common unspoken fear. Stress reduction techniques, such as biofeedback, exercise programs, and meditation, are examples of nonpharmacologic therapies that may prove helpful. The patient and family need to be reminded of the importance of following the prescribed treatment regimen for headache and keeping follow-up appointments. In addition, the patient is reminded of the importance of participating in health promotion activities and recommended health screenings to promote a healthy lifestyle.

Continuing and Transitional Care

The Canadian Headache Society is a scientific society of health care professionals (see Resources) provides resources and information regarding latest research and care of headache.

Critical Thinking Exercises

1 A patient is admitted to your unit for a transsphenoidal cranial procedure. Identify the nursing interventions indicated before, during, and after the procedure. What patient and caregiver education is indicated in preparation for discharge? How will your nursing interventions and patient education change if a supratentorial surgical approach is used?

2 As a member of your unit's practice council, you are working on updating interventions to manage increased intracranial pressure. Using your knowledge of evidence-based practice guidelines, list the most important interventions for nurses to implement. Compare and contrast the options supported by the guidelines.

3 Identify the priorities, approach, and techniques you would use to provide care to a 25-year-old female patient with migraine headaches. How will your priorities, approach, and techniques differ if the patient is male, if the patient has tension-type or cluster headaches?

REFERENCES AND SELECTED READINGS

Books

American Association of Neuroscience Nurses (AANN). (2012). *Nursing management of adults with severe traumatic brain injury. AANN clinical practice guidelines series*. Glenview, IL: Author.

American Association of Neuroscience Nurses (AANN). (2016a). *Care of adults and children with seizures and epilepsy: AANN clinical practice guideline series*. Chicago, IL: Author.

American Association of Neuroscience Nurses (AANN). (2016b). *Care of the adult patient with a brain tumor: AANN clinical practice guideline series*. Chicago, IL: Author.

Bader, M., Littlejohns, L. R., & Olson, D. (2016). *AANN core curriculum for neuroscience nursing* (6th ed.). Chicago, IL: American Association of Neuroscience Nurses.

Bhatia, A., & Gupta, A. (2013). Neuromonitoring in the Intensive Care unit. In M. Pinsky, L. Brochard, G. Hedenstiema, et al. (Eds.). *Applied physiology in intensive care medicine* (pp. 145–151). New York: Springer.

Dudek, S. G. (2013). *Nutrition essentials for nursing practice* (7th ed.). Philadelphia, PA: Wolters Kluwer Health/Lippincott Williams & Wilkins.

Grossman, S. C., & Porth, C. M. (2014). *Pathophysiology: Concepts of altered health states* (9th ed.). Philadelphia, PA: Lippincott Williams & Wilkins.

Gulanick, M., & Myers, J. (2013). *Nursing care plans; nursing diagnosis and intervention*. St Louis, MO. Elsevier/Mosby.

Hickey, J. V. (2014). *The clinical practice of neurological and neurosurgical nursing* (7th ed.). Philadelphia, PA: Lippincott Williams & Wilkins.

Karch, A. (2015). *2015 Lippincott's nursing drug guide*. Philadelphia, PA: Lippincott Williams & Wilkins.

Wheless, J. (2013). Vagus nerve stimulation therapy. In E. Wyllie, G. D. Cascino, B. E. Gidal, et al. (Eds.). *Wyllie's treatment of epilepsy: Principles and practice* (5th ed.). Philadelphia, PA: Lippincott Williams & Wilkins.

Journals and Electronic Documents

Alali, A., Naimark, D., Wilson, J., et al. (2014). Economic evaluation of decompressive hemicraniectomy versus barbiturate coma for refractory intracranial hypertension following traumatic brain injury. *Critical Care Medicine*, *42*(10), 2235–2243.

Andrews, P., Sinclair, L., Rodriguez, A., et al. (2015). Hypothermia for intracranial hypertension after traumatic brain injury. *The New England Journal of Medicine*, *373*(25), 2403–2412.

Aylwin, S., Burst, V., Peri, A., et al. (2015). "Do's and dont's" in the management of hyponatremia. *Current Medical Research and Opinion*, *31*(9), 1755–1761.

Bauman, M., & McCourt, T. R. (2014). Assessing and managing patients with chronic subdural hematoma. *American Nurse Today*, *9*(9), 38–41.

Becker, W., Findlay, T., Moga, C., et al. (2015). Guideline for primary care management of headache in adults. *Canadian Family Physician*, *61*(8), 670–679.

Bruno, M., Laureys, S., & Demerttzi, A. (2013). Coma and disorders of consciousness. *Handbook of Clinical Neurology*, *118*(2013), 205–213.

Charles, A. (2013). The evolution of migraine attack—A review of recent evidence. *Headache*, *53*(2), 413–419.

Charles, A. (2015). Sounding out migraine-related interactions between the brainstem and the cortex. *Cephalalgia*, *35*(11), 941–943.

Charles, A., & Hansen, J. (2015). Migraine aura: New ideas about cause, classification, and clinical significance. *Current Opinion in Neurology*, *28*(3), 255–260.

Dahlöf, C., & Van Den Brink, A. (2012). Dihydroergotamine, ergotamine, methysergide and sumatriptan—Basic science in relation to migraine treatment. *Headache*, *52*(4), 707–714.

D'Arcy, Y. (2014). Preventing migraine headaches in adults. *Nursing*, *44*(1), 58–61.

de Lima Oliveira, M., Kairalla, A., Fonoff, E., et al. (2014). Cerebral microdialysis in traumatic brain injury and subarachnoid hemorrhage: State of the art. *Neurocritical Care*, *21*(1), 152–162.

Destrebecq, A., Terzoni, S., & Sala, E. (2014). Post-lumbar puncture headache: A review of issues for nursing practice. *Journal of Neuroscience Nursing*, *46*(3), 180–186.

Dias, C., Maia, I., Cerejo, A., et al. (2014). Pressures, flow, and brain oxygenation during plateau waves of intracranial pressure. *Neurocritical Care*, *21*(1), 124–132.

Dworetzky, B. A., Townsend, M. K., Pennell, P. B., et al. (2012). Female reproductive factors and risk of seizure or epilepsy: Data from the nurses' health study II. *Epilepsia*, *53*(1), e1–e4.

England, M., Liverman, C., Schultz, A., et al. (2012). Epilepsy across the spectrum: Promoting health and understanding. A summary of the Institute of Medicine report. *Epilepsy and Behavior*, *25*(2), 266–276.

Fisher, R., Acevedo, C., Arzimanoglou, A., et al. (2014). A practical clinical definition of epilepsy. *Epilepsia*, *55*(4), 475–482.

Fisher, R., Cross, H., French, J., et al. (2016). *Operational classification of seizure types by the International League Against Epilepsy (ILAE)*. Retrieved on September 29, 2016, from www.ilae.org/visitors/centre/documents/ClassificationSeizureILAE-2016.pdf

Foreman, P., Schmalz, P., & Griessenauer, C. (2014). Chemoprophylaxis for venous thromboembolism in traumatic brain injury: A review and evidence based protocol. *Clinical Neurology and Neurosurgery*, *123*, 109–116.

Headache Classification Committee of the International Headache Society. (2013). The international classification of headache disorders, 3rd edition (beta version). *Cephalalgia*, *33*(9), 629–808.

Institute of Medicine (IOM). (2012). *Epilepsy across the spectrum: Promoting health and understanding*. Retrieved January 5, 2017, from www.nationalacademies.org/hmd/Reports/2012/Epilepsy-Across-the-Spectrum.aspx

Johansson, R. M., Malmvall, B. E., Andersson-Gare, B., et al. (2012). Guidelines for preventing urinary retention and bladder damage during hospital care. *Journal of Clinical Nursing*, *22*(3–4), 347–355.

Kiyoshi-Teo, H., & Blegen, M. (2015). Influence of institutional guidelines on oral hygiene practices in intensive care units. *American Journal of Critical Care*, *24*(4), 309–318.

Lagana, A., Triolo, O., D'Amico, V., et al. (2016). Management of women with epilepsy: From preconception to post-partum. *Archives of Gynecology and Obstetrics*, *293*(3), 493–503.

Latimer, K. M. (2013). Chronic headache: stop the pain before it starts Familiarity with the risks associated with medication overuse and the importance of headache prophylaxis is key to easing your patient's pain. *Journal of Family Practice*, *62*(3), 126–134.

Lee, T. M., Savage, J., McKee, H., et al. (2013). How do you know when your patient is "waking up": coma recovery assessment in a complex continuing care setting. *Canadian Journal of Neuroscience Nursing*, *35*(2), 27–33.

Madden, L., & DeVon, H. (2015). A systematic review of the effects of body temperature on outcome after adult traumatic brain injury. *Journal of Neuroscience Nursing*, *47*(4), 190–203.

Majdan, M., Mauritz, W., Wilbacher, I., et al. (2013). Barbiturates use and its effects in patients with severe traumatic brain injury in five European countries. *Journal of Neurotrauma*, *30*(1), 23–29.

Megha, M., Harpreet, S., & Nayeem, Z. (2013). Effect of frequency of multimodal coma stimulation on the consciousness levels of traumatic brain injury comatose patients. *Brain Injury*, *27*(5), 570–577.

Miller, W., Buelow, J., & Bakas, T. (2014). Older adults and new onset epilepsy: Experiences with diagnosis. *Journal of Neuroscience Nursing*, *46*(1), 2–10.

Mitchell, P., Kirkness, C., & Blissitt, P. (2015). Chapter 5 cerebral perfusion pressure and intracranial pressure in traumatic brain injury. *Annual Review of Nursing Research*, *33*, 111–117.

Munro, N., & Ruggiero, M. (2014). Ventilator-associated pneumonia bundle. *AACN Advanced Critical Care*, *25*(2), 163–175.

Nei, M., Ngo, L., Sirven, J., et al. (2014). Ketogenic diet in adolescents and adults with epilepsy. *Seizure*, *23*(6), 439–442.

Nemer, S., Caldeira, J., Santos, R., et al. (2015). Effects of positive end-expiratory pressure on brain tissue oxygen pressure of severe traumatic brain injury patients with acute respiratory distress syndrome—A pilot study. *Journal of Critical Care*, *30*(6), 1263–1266.

Oddo, M., Bosel, J., & Participants in the International Multidisciplinary Consensus Conference on Multimodality Monitoring. (2014). Monitoring of brain and systemic oxygenation in neurocritical care patients. *Neurocritical Care*, *21*(Suppl 2), S103–S120.

Olson, D. M., Lewis, L. S., Bader, M. K., et al. (2013). Significant practice pattern variations associated with intracranial pressure monitoring. *Journal of Neuroscience Nursing*, *45*(4), 186–193.

Ong, C., Keyrouz, S., & Diringer, M. (2015). The role of osmotic therapy in hemispheric stroke. *Neurocritical Care*, *23*(2), 285–291.

Rauchenzauner, M., Ehrensberger, M., & Prieschl, M. (2013). Generalized tonic–clonic seizures and antiepileptic drugs during pregnancy—a matter of importance for the baby? *Journal of neurology*, *260*(2), 484–488.

Rockett, H., Thompson, H., & Blissitt, P. (2015). Fever management: Practices of neuroscience nurses: What has changed? *Journal of Neuroscience Nursing*, *47*(2), 66–75.

Sandsmark, D., Kumar, M., Park, S., et al. (2012). Multimodal monitoring in subarachnoid hemorrhage. *Stroke*, *43*(5), 1440–1445.

Scheffer, I. E., French, J., Hirsch, E., et al. (2016). Classification of the epilepsies: New concepts for discussion and debate—Special report of the ILAE classification task force of the commission for classification and terminology. *Epilepsia Open*, *1*(1–2), 37–44.

Thibault, A., Deltombe, T., Wannez, S., et al. (2015). Impact of soft splints on upper limb spasticity in chronic patients with disorders of consciousness: A randomized, single-blind, controlled trial. *Brain Injury*, *29*(7–8), 830–836.

Thomas, S. V., Syam, U., & Devi, J. S. (2012). Predictors of seizures during pregnancy in women with epilepsy. *Epilepsia*, *53*(5), e85–e88.

Torbic, H., Forni, A. A., Anger, K. E., et al. (2013). Use of antiepileptics for seizure prophylaxis after traumatic brain injury. *American Journal of Health-System Pharmacy*, *70*(9), 759–766.

Trinka, E., Cock, H., Hesdorffer, D., et al. (2015). A definition and classification of status epilepticus—Report of the ILAE Task Force on Classification of Status Epilepticus. *Epilepsia*, *56*(10), 1515–1523.

Updyke, M., & Duryea, B. (2013). To provoke or not to provoke: Ethical considerations in the epilepsy monitoring unit. *Journal of Neuroscience Nursing*, *45*(3), 133–138.

Van Der Naalt, J. (2015). Resting functional imaging tools (MRS, SPECT, PET, and PCT). *Handbook of Clinical Neurology*, *127*(2015), 295–308.

Wang, X., Dong, Y., Han, X., et al. (2013). Nutritional support for patients sustaining traumatic brain injury: A systematic review and meta-analysis of prospective studies. *PLoS ONE*, *8*(3), 1–14.

Wang, X., Ji, J., Fen, L., et al. (2013). Effects of dexmetetomidine on cerebral blood flow in critically ill patients with or without traumatic brain injury: A prospective controlled trial. *Brain Injury*, *27*(13–14), 1617–1622.

Wells, R., Turner, D., Lee, M., et al. (2016). Managing migraine during pregnancy and lactation. *Neurology and Neuroscience Reports*, *16*(4), 40.

Wijdicks, E. (2013). Brain death. *Handbook of Clinical Neurology*, *118*(2013), 191–203.

Resources

Brain Injury Association of Canada: http://biac-aclc.ca/en/
Brain Tumour Foundation of Canada: http://www.braintumour.ca
Canadian Association of Neuroscience Nurses: http://www.cann.ca
Canadian Epilepsy Alliance: http://www.canadianepilepsyalliance.org/
Canadian Headache Society: https://headachesociety.ca/about-us/
Canadian Human Rights Act: https://laws-lois.justice.gc.ca/eng/acts/h-6/page-1.html#h-3
Canadian League against Epilepsy: http://www.clae.org/
Canadian Neurological Sciences Federation: http://www.cnsfederation.org/
Council of Canadians with Disabilities: http://www.ccdonline.ca
Epilepsy Canada: http://www.epilepsy.ca
Epilepsy Foundation: http://www.epilepsyfoundation.org
Help for Headaches: http://www.headache-help.org
International Bureau for Epilepsy: http://www.ibe-epilepsy.org
International Headache Society: http://www.i-h-s.org/
International League against Epilepsy: http://www.ilae.org/
National Headache Foundation: http://www.headaches.org
Neuro-Patient Resource Centre: http://infoneuro.mcgill.ca
Spina Bifida and Hydrocephalus Association of Canada: http://www.sbhac.ca
Think First Foundation of Canada: http://www.thinkfirst.ca

64 Management of Patients With Cerebrovascular Disorders

Adapted by Ron Prince

Learning Objectives

On completion of this chapter, the learner will be able to:

1. Describe the incidence and social impact of cerebrovascular disorders.
2. Identify the risk factors for cerebrovascular disorders and related measures for prevention.
3. Compare the various types of cerebrovascular disorders: their causes, clinical manifestations, and medical management.
4. Apply the principles of nursing management to the care of a patient in the acute stage of an ischemic stroke.
5. Use the nursing process as a framework for care of a patient recovering from an ischemic stroke.
6. Use the nursing process as a framework for care of a patient with a hemorrhagic stroke.
7. Identify essential elements for family teaching and preparation for home care of the patient who has had a stroke.

Cerebrovascular disorders is an umbrella term that refers to a functional abnormality of the central nervous system (CNS) that occurs when the usual blood supply to the brain is disrupted. **Stroke** is caused by a blockage of blood vessels or by rupture of a blood vessel and bleeding into brain tissue.

Stroke is the third leading cause of death in Canada (Statistics Canada, 2017). It ranks third among women and fourth among men (Statistics Canada, 2013). The number of Canadian patients aged 20 and older who sustained a stroke rose gradually over the decade between 2003 to 2004 and 2012 to 2013 with the addition of over 215,000 survivors (Government of Canada, 2017). According to Canadian Heart and Stroke Foundation (2014), an estimated 50,000 strokes in Canada occur every year, and 315,000 Canadians are living with stroke and suffer from its disabilities.

The Canadian Heart and Stroke Foundation (2014) estimates that there is a death related to stroke or heart disease every 10 minutes. The Public Health Agency of Canada reports that stroke costs the Canadian economy $3.6 billion a year. The nature of these costs are associated with physician/medical services, the cost of hospitalization, and lost income and work productivity. A study conducted by Grant, Goldsmith and Anton (2014), revealed that the average length of stay for Canadians poststroke is 35 days in inpatient rehabilitative units. The costs associated with length of stay compound the annual expenditure.

Strokes, defined as an interruption of brain function due to vascular origin, are classed as ischemic in 80% of cases and hemorrhagic in the remaining 20% of cases (Catangui, 2013).

Although there are some similarities between the two broad types of stroke, differences exist in etiology, pathophysiology, medical management, surgical management, and nursing care. Table 64-1 compares ischemic and hemorrhagic strokes.

Ischemic Stroke

INTERACTIVE TUTORIALS

An ischemic stroke, cerebrovascular accident (CVA) is a sudden loss of function resulting from disruption of the blood supply to a part of the brain. With the approval of thrombolytic therapy for the treatment of acute ischemic stroke in 1996 came a revolution in the care of patients after a stroke. Early treatment with thrombolytic therapy

TABLE 64-1 Comparison of Major Types of Stroke

Types of Stroke	Causes	Main Presenting Symptoms	Functional Recovery
Ischemic	• Large artery thrombosis • Small penetrating artery thrombosis • Cardiogenic embolic • Cryptogenic (no known cause) • Other	Numbness or weakness of the face, arm, or leg, especially on one side of the body	Usually plateaus at 6 months
Hemorrhagic	• Intracerebral hemorrhage • Subarachnoid hemorrhage • Cerebral aneurysm • Arteriovenous malformation	• "Exploding headache" • Decreased level of consciousness	Slower, usually plateaus at about 18 months

Adapted from Hickey, J. V. (2014). *The clinical practice of neurological & neurosurgical nursing* (7th ed.). Philadelphia, PA: Lippincott Williams & Wilkins.

for ischemic stroke results in fewer stroke symptoms and less loss of function. Approved thrombolytic therapy initially had a treatment window of only 3 hours after the onset of a stroke. The time has now been extended to 4.5 hours. Rapid intervention in 4.5 hours or less is key to successful reperfusion of the ischemic penumbra region (Manning, Campbell, Oxley, et al., 2014; Rosso & Samson, 2014). Urgency is needed on the part of the public and health care practitioners for rapid transport of the patient to a hospital for assessment and administration of the medication.

Ischemic strokes are subdivided into five different types based on the cause: large artery thrombotic strokes (20%), small penetrating artery thrombotic strokes (25%), cardiogenic embolic strokes (20%), **cryptogenic strokes** (30%), and other (5%) (see Table 64-1). Thrombotic (large vessel) strokes are caused by sites of plaque formation along the vessel wall which leads to occlusion and resultant ischemia of the area being fed by the vessel (Hickey, 2014).

Small penetrating artery thrombotic strokes affect one or more vessels and are the most common type of ischemic stroke. Small artery thrombotic strokes are also called lacunar strokes because of the cavity that is created once the infarcted brain tissue disintegrates (Hickey, 2014). Recent knowledge has identified six underlying causes for the formation of **lacunar type strokes**: embolism, high blood pressure, blood dyscrasias, vasospasm, small brain vessel bleeds, and the occlusion of small vessels (Hickey, 2014).

Cardiogenic embolic strokes are associated with cardiac dysrhythmias, usually **atrial fibrillation**. Embolic strokes can also be associated with valvular heart disease and thrombi in the left ventricle. Emboli originate from the heart and circulate to the cerebral vasculature, most commonly the left middle cerebral artery (MCA), resulting in a stroke. Embolic strokes may be prevented by the use of anticoagulation therapy in patients with atrial fibrillation.

The last two classifications of ischemic strokes are cryptogenic strokes, which have no known cause, and strokes from other causes, such as illicit drug use, coagulopathies, migraine, birth control pills, and spontaneous dissection of the carotid or vertebral arteries.

Pathophysiology

In an ischemic stroke, there is disruption of the cerebral blood flow due to obstruction of a blood vessel. This disruption in blood flow initiates a complex series of cellular metabolic events referred to as the ischemic cascade (Fig. 64-1).

The ischemic cascade begins when cerebral blood flow decreases to less than 25 mL per 100 g of blood per minute. At this point, neurons are no longer able to maintain

Glossary

agnosia: failure to recognize familiar objects perceived by the senses
aneurysm: a weakening or bulge in an arterial wall
aphasia: inability to express oneself or to understand language
apraxia: inability to perform previously learned purposeful motor acts on a voluntary basis
atrial fibrillation: rapid irregular electrical activity in the atria of the heart, leading to irregular apical pulse rate
cryptogenic stroke: a stroke of unknown origin
dysarthria: defects of articulation due to neurologic causes
expressive aphasia: inability to express oneself; often associated with damage to the temporal lobe area
hemianopsia: blindness of half of the field of vision in one or both eyes
hemiplegia/hemiparesis: weakness/paralysis of one side of the body, or part of it, due to an injury in the **motor area of the brain:** infarction a zone of tissue deprived of blood supply
Korsakoff's syndrome: disorder characterized by psychosis, disorientation, delirium, insomnia, and hallucinations usually seen in alcoholics
lacunar type stroke: lack of blood flow through a small artery in the brain which results in decreased blood flow. A group of lacuna strokes can lead to dementia.
penumbra region: area of low cerebral blood flow, area surrounding a stroke
receptive aphasia: inability to understand what someone else is saying; often associated with damage to the temporal lobe area

Physiology/Pathophysiology

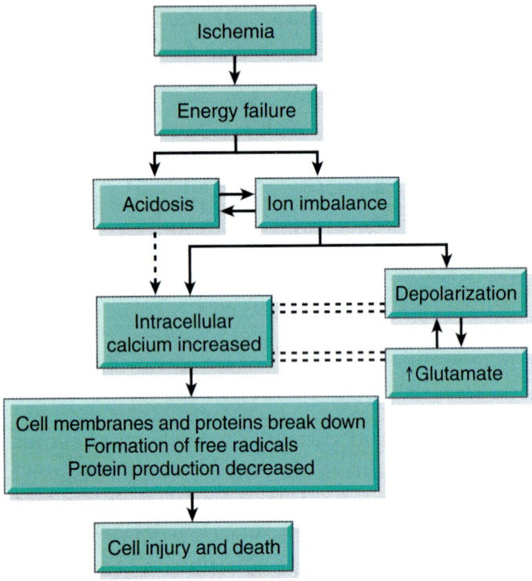

FIGURE 64-1. Processes contributing to ischemic brain cell injury.

aerobic respiration. The mitochondria must then switch to anaerobic respiration, which generates large amounts of lactic acid, causing a change in the pH. This switch to the less efficient anaerobic respiration also renders the neuron incapable of producing sufficient quantities of adenosine triphosphate (ATP) to fuel the depolarization processes. The membrane pumps that maintain electrolyte balances begin to fail, and the cells cease to function.

Early in the cascade, an area of low cerebral blood flow, referred to as the penumbra region, exists around the area of infarction. The **penumbra region** is ischemic brain tissue that may be salvaged with timely intervention. The ischemic cascade threatens cells in the penumbra because membrane depolarization of the cell wall leads to an increase in intracellular calcium and the release of glutamate. The influx of calcium and the release of glutamate, if continued, activate a number of damaging pathways that result in the destruction of the cell membrane, the release of more calcium and glutamate, vasoconstriction, and the generation of free radicals. These processes enlarge the area of infarction into the penumbra, extending the stroke. A person experiencing a stroke typically loses 1.9 million neurons each minute that a stroke is not treated, and the ischemic brain ages 3.6 years each hour without treatment (Saver, 2006). Rapid intervention, 4.5 hours or less, is key to successful reperfusion of the ischemic penumbra region (Rosso & Samson, 2014; Manning et al., 2014).

Each step in the ischemic cascade represents an opportunity for intervention to limit the extent of secondary brain damage caused by a stroke. The penumbra area may be revitalized by administration of tissue plasminogen activator (t-PA). Medications that protect the brain from secondary injury are called neuroprotectants. Neuroprotection involves pharmacotherapeutics and physical treatment strategies to improve the cellular environment following ischemic events. By improving environmental conditions, programmed apoptosis is inhibited. This allows for better health outcomes for stroke survivors (Mandel, Fonoff, Bor-Seng-Shu, et al., 2012). Ongoing research is investigating the role selective brain cooling can play in preventing stroke damage (Heart and Stroke Foundation, 2013).

Clinical Manifestations

An ischemic stroke can cause a wide variety of neurologic deficits, depending on the location of the lesion (which vessels are obstructed), the size of the area of inadequate perfusion, and the amount of collateral (secondary or accessory) blood flow (see Chapter 62 for discussion of anatomy and brain blood supply). The patient may present with any of the following signs or symptoms:

- Numbness or weakness of the face, arm, or leg, especially on one side of the body
- Confusion or change in mental status
- Trouble speaking or understanding speech
- Visual disturbances
- Difficulty walking, dizziness, or loss of balance or coordination
- Sudden severe headache

Motor, sensory, cranial nerve, cognitive, and other functions may be disrupted. Table 64-2 reviews the neurologic deficits frequently seen in patients with strokes. Table 64-3 compares the symptoms and behaviours seen in right hemispheric stroke with those seen in left hemispheric stroke.

Motor Loss

A stroke is an upper motor neuron lesion and results in loss of voluntary control over motor movements. Because the upper motor neurons decussate (cross), a disturbance of voluntary motor control on one side of the body may reflect damage to the upper motor neurons on the opposite side of the brain. The most common motor dysfunction is **hemiplegia** (paralysis of one side of the body) caused by a lesion of the opposite side of the brain. **Hemiparesis**, or weakness of one side of the body, is another sign. The concept of upper and lower motor neuron lesions is described in more detail in Chapter 62.

In the early stage of stroke, the initial clinical features may be flaccid paralysis and loss of or decrease in the deep tendon reflexes. When these deep reflexes reappear (usually by 48 hours), increased tone is observed along with spasticity (abnormal increase in muscle tone) of the extremities on the affected side.

Communication Disorders Poststroke

Other brain functions affected by stroke are language and communication. In fact, stroke is the most common cause of **aphasia**. The following are dysfunctions of language and communication:

- **Dysarthria** (difficulty in speaking), caused by paralysis of the muscles responsible for producing speech
- Dysphasia (impaired speech) or aphasia (loss of speech), which can be **expressive aphasia**, **receptive aphasia**, or global (mixed) aphasia
- **Apraxia** (inability to perform a previously learned action), as may be seen when a patient makes verbal substitutions for desired syllables or words

TABLE 64-2 Neurologic Deficits of Stroke: Manifestations and Nursing Implications

Neurologic Deficit	Manifestation	Nursing Implications/Patient Teaching Applications
Visual Field Deficits		
Homonymous hemianopsia (loss of half of the visual field)	• Unaware of persons or objects on side of visual loss • Neglect of one side of the body • Difficulty judging distances	Place objects within intact field of vision Approach the patient from side of intact field of vision Instruct/remind the patient to turn head in the direction of visual loss to compensate for loss of visual field Encourage the use of eyeglasses if available When teaching the patient, do so within patient's intact visual field
Loss of peripheral vision	• Difficulty seeing at night • Unaware of objects or the borders of objects	Place objects in centre of patient's intact visual field Encourage the use of a cane or other object to identify objects in the periphery of the visual field Driving ability will need to be evaluated
Diplopia	• Double vision	Explain to the patient the location of an object when placing it near the patient Consistently place patient care items in the same location
Motor Deficits		
Hemiparesis	• Weakness of the face, arm, and leg on the same side (due to a lesion in the opposite hemisphere)	Place objects within the patient's reach on the nonaffected side Instruct the patient to exercise and increase the strength on the unaffected side
Hemiplegia	• Paralysis of the face, arm, and leg on the same side (due to a lesion in the opposite hemisphere)	Encourage the patient to provide range-of-motion exercises to the affected side Provide immobilization as needed to the affected side Maintain body alignment in functional position Exercise unaffected limb to increase mobility, strength, and use
Ataxia	• Staggering, unsteady gait • Unable to keep feet together; needs a broad base to stand	Support patient during the initial ambulation phase Provide supportive device for ambulation (walker, cane) Instruct the patient not to walk without assistance or supportive device
Dysarthria	• Difficulty in forming words	Provide the patient with alternative methods of communicating Allow the patient sufficient time to respond to verbal communication Support patient and family to alleviate frustration related to difficulty in communicating
Dysphagia	• Difficulty in swallowing	Test the patient's pharyngeal reflexes before offering food or fluids Assist the patient with meals Place food on the unaffected side of the mouth Allow ample time to eat
Sensory Deficits		
Paresthesia (occurs on the side opposite the lesion)	• Numbness and tingling of extremity • Difficulty with proprioception	Instruct patient that sensation may be altered Provide range of motion to affected areas and apply corrective devices as needed
Verbal Deficits		
Expressive aphasia	• Unable to form words that are understandable; may be able to speak in single-word responses	Encourage patient to repeat sounds of the alphabet Explore the patient's ability to write as an alternative means of communication
Receptive aphasia	• Unable to comprehend the spoken word; can speak but may not make sense	Speak slowly and clearly to assist the patient in forming the sounds Explore the patient's ability to read as an alternative means of communication
Global (mixed) aphasia	• Combination of both receptive and expressive aphasia	Speak clearly and in simple sentences; use gestures or pictures when able Establish alternative means of communication
Cognitive Deficits	• Short- and long-term memory loss • Decreased attention span • Impaired ability to concentrate • Poor abstract reasoning • Altered judgment	Reorient patient to time, place, and situation frequently Use verbal and auditory cues to orient patient Provide familiar objects (family photographs, favorite objects) Use noncomplicated language Match visual tasks with a verbal cue; holding a toothbrush, simulate brushing of teeth while saying, "I would like you to brush your teeth now" Minimize distracting noises and views when teaching the patient Repeat and reinforce instructions frequently

continued >

TABLE 64-2 Neurologic Deficits of Stroke: Manifestations and Nursing Implications (Continued)

Neurologic Deficit	Manifestation	Nursing Implications/Patient Teaching Applications
Emotional Deficits	• Loss of self-control • Emotional lability • Decreased tolerance to stressful situations • Depression • Withdrawal • Fear, hostility, and anger • Feelings of isolation	Support patient during uncontrollable outbursts Discuss with the patient and family that the outbursts are due to the disease process Encourage patient to participate in group activity Provide stimulation for the patient Control stressful situations, if possible Provide a safe environment Encourage patient to express feelings and frustrations related to disease process

Adapted from Hickey, J. V. (2014). *The clinical practice of neurological & neurosurgical nursing* (7th ed.). Philadelphia, PA: Lippincott Williams & Wilkins.

Perceptual Disturbances

Perception is the ability to interpret sensation. Strokes can result in visual-perceptual dysfunctions, disturbances in visual-spatial relations, and sensory loss.

Visual-perceptual dysfunctions are caused by disturbances of the primary sensory pathways between the eye and visual cortex. Homonymous **hemianopsia** (loss of half of the visual field) may occur from stroke and may be temporary or permanent. The affected side of vision corresponds to the paralyzed side of the body. Disturbances in visual-spatial relations (perceiving the relationship of two or more objects in spatial areas) are frequently seen in patients with right hemispheric damage. Strokes affecting perception are typically localized to the occipital and parietal lobes of the brain.

Sensory Loss

The sensory losses from stroke may take the form of slight impairment of touch, or it may be more severe, with loss of proprioception (ability to perceive the position and motion of body parts) as well as difficulty in interpreting visual, tactile, and auditory stimuli. **Agnosias** are deficits in the ability to recognize previously familiar objects perceived by one or more of the senses.

Cognitive Impairment and Psychological Effects

If damage has occurred to the frontal lobe, learning capacity, memory, or other higher cortical intellectual functions may be impaired. Such dysfunction may be reflected in a limited attention span, difficulties in comprehension, forgetfulness, and a lack of motivation. These changes can cause the patient to become easily frustrated during rehabilitation. Depression is common and may be exaggerated by the patient's natural response to this catastrophic event. Emotional lability, hostility, frustration, resentment, lack of cooperation, and other psychological problems may occur.

TABLE 64-3 Comparison of Left and Right Hemispheric Strokes

Left Hemispheric Stroke	Right Hemispheric Stroke
Paralysis or weakness on right side of body	Paralysis or weakness on left side of body
Right visual field deficit	Left visual field deficit
Aphasia (expressive, receptive, or global)	Spatial-perceptual deficits
Increased distractibility	
Altered intellectual ability	Impulsive behaviour and poor judgment
Slow, cautious behaviour	Lack of awareness of deficits

Adapted from Hickey, J. V. (2014). *The clinical practice of neurological and neurosurgical nursing* (7th ed.). Philadelphia, PA: Wolters Kluwer Health/Lippincott Williams & Wilkins.

Assessment and Diagnostic Findings

Any patient with neurologic deficits needs a careful history and a complete physical and neurologic examination. Initial assessment focuses on airway patency, which may be compromised by loss of gag or cough reflexes and altered respiratory pattern; cardiovascular status (including blood pressure, cardiac rhythm and rate, carotid bruit); and gross neurologic deficits.

Patients may present to the acute care facility with temporary neurologic symptoms. A transient ischemic attack (TIA) is a neurologic deficit typically lasting less than 1 hour. A TIA is manifested by a sudden loss of motor, sensory, or visual function. The symptoms result from temporary ischemia (impairment of blood flow) to a specific region of the brain but when brain imaging is performed there is no evidence of ischemia. A TIA may serve as a warning of impending stroke. Quick response and timely intervention by skilled health care professionals can significantly reduce the potential of a stroke event and the negative sequelae that follow (Sander, 2013). All patients presenting to an emergency department with suspected stroke or TIA must have an immediate clinical evaluation and investigations to establish the diagnosis, rule out stroke and TIA, or determine eligibility for thrombolytic therapy, and develop a plan for further management (Casaubon & Suddes, 2013). Lack of evaluation and treatment of a patient who has experienced previous TIAs may result in a stroke and irreversible deficits. Quick response and timely intervention by skilled health care providers can significantly reduce the potential of a stroke event and the negative sequelae to follow (Sander, 2013).

The initial diagnostic test for a stroke is usually a noncontrast computed tomography (CT) scan performed emergently to determine if the event is ischemic or hemorrhagic (the category of stroke determines treatment). Further diagnostic workup for ischemic stroke involves attempting to identify the source of the thrombi or emboli (Anderson,

2016). A 12-lead electrocardiogram (ECG) and a carotid ultrasound are standard tests. Other studies may include CT angiography or magnetic resonance imaging and angiography (MRI and MRA) of the brain and neck vessels; transcranial Doppler flow studies; transthoracic or transesophageal echocardiography; xenon-enhanced CT scan; and single photon emission CT (SPECT) scan (Jauch, Saver, Adams, et al., 2013; Miller & Summers, 2014). CT scanning continues to be the most reliable and effective means of delineating between hemorrhagic and ischemic strokes because it is fast and readily available in most tertiary care centres. It is an integral component in stroke management (Catangui, 2013). It is vital to obtain brain imaging as soon as possible, as initial treatment decisions are made based on the initial imaging.

The emergence of Telestroke Networks in Canada has been instrumental in overcoming geographical barriers in the management of acute stroke care. Telestroke Networks are enhancing the model of care in rural and remote hospitals. Through this approach to care, patients receive an early diagnosis and early intervention which leads to much better health outcomes (Switzer, Demaerschalk, Xie, et al., 2012).

Prevention

Primary prevention of ischemic stroke remains the best approach. Preventive strategies including a healthy lifestyle reduces the risk of an initial stroke, and the risk of a subsequent stroke for patients with prior strokes. Hypertension is the single most important modifiable risk factor for stroke (Coutts & Kelloway, 2012). Leading a healthy lifestyle, which includes no smoking, maintaining a healthy weight, following a healthy diet (including low sodium [Appel, 2014] and modest alcohol consumption), and daily exercise, can reduce the risk of having a stroke by about one half (Coutts & Kelloway, 2012). Referral to a Stroke Prevention Clinic after an initial hospital visit for a TIA is associated with significantly lower mortality and with increased use of evidence-based therapies for secondary stroke prevention. Prevention includes diet/nutrition, fitness, monitoring of blood pressure, adherence to appropriate medication regimens, smoking cessation, and healthy sleep hygiene practices. Prevention also includes access to medical care in the form of diagnostics, interventions, and education (Heart and Stroke Foundation, 2013).

The risk of coronary heart disease and stroke has decreased in women on the Dietary Approaches to Stop Hypertension (DASH) diet. The DASH-style diet highlights the following consumption guidelines: increase the number of fruit and vegetable servings, reduce salt intake, and lower saturated fat intake. In addition to dietary modifications, physical exercise is a vital component in stroke prevention (Appel, 2014; Kokubo, 2012; Lahr, van der Zee, Luijckx, et al., 2013).

Stroke risk screenings are an ideal opportunity to lower stroke risk by identifying people or groups of people who are at high risk for stroke and by educating patients and the community about recognition and prevention of stroke. Recent research indicates that a dose of aspirin 100 mg every other day has the potential to reduce the risk of ischemic events, especially TIAs (Rist, Buring, Kase, et al., 2013).

Advanced age, gender, and race are well-known nonmodifiable risk factors for stroke (Heart and Stroke Foundation, 2014). High-risk groups include people older than 55 years of age, as the incidence of stroke more than doubles in each successive decade. Men have a higher rate of stroke than women. Additional research reveals that there should be a more focused look at stroke and its challenges when considering cultural differences. It is imperative that stroke risk factors, age of onset of stroke events, the degree of deficits at the onset of a stroke, and access to comprehensive stroke care centres be closely reviewed to provide for better clinical outcomes. For example, Hispanics have a higher incidence of metabolic syndrome and diabetes mellitus, and thus they are at greater risk for experiencing a stroke event (Qian, Fonarow, Smith, et al., 2013). First Nations, Inuit, and Métis, and people of African (Chart 64-1) and South Asian descent are more likely to have high blood pressure and diabetes and therefore are at greater risk of stroke than the general Canadian population (Heart and Stroke Foundation, 2014). The incidence of stroke in African Canadians is almost twice as high as in Caucasians. African Canadians also suffer more extensive physical impairments and are twice as likely to die from stroke than are Caucasians (Chart 64-1).

Modifiable risk factors for ischemic stroke include hypertension, atrial fibrillation, hyperlipidemia, obesity, smoking, and diabetes (Chart 64-2). For people who are at high risk, interventions that alter modifiable factors, such as treating hypertension and hyperglycemia and stopping smoking, significantly reduces stroke risk. Other treatable conditions that increase risk of stroke are carotid stenosis and valvular heart disease (e.g., endocarditis, prosthetic heart valves). Periodontal disease has also been linked to stroke risk. The association between periodontal disease and stroke may result from the host inflammatory response and the chronic bacterial infection, but the exact mechanism is not fully understood. Periodontal disease is a treatable and preventable condition.

Several methods of preventing recurrent stroke have been identified for patients who have experienced TIAs or ischemic stroke. New research involves investigating the effectiveness of carotid artery stenting (CAS) over the alternative method of endarterectomy (Coutts & Kelloway, 2012). In patients with atrial fibrillation, which increases the risk of emboli, administration of warfarin (Coumadin), or newer anticoagulants, inhibit clot formation, and may prevent both thrombotic and embolic strokes.

Medical Management

Patients who have experienced a TIA or stroke should have medical management for secondary prevention. Those with atrial fibrillation (or cardioembolic strokes) are treated with dose-adjusted warfarin (Coumadin) with a target international normalized ratio (INR) of 2 to 3. Other newer anticoagulants that may be prescribed as alternative drugs include dabigatran (Pradaxa), apixaban (Eliquis), edoxaban (Savaysa), or rivaroxaban (Xarelto), unless they are contraindicated. These newer drugs are also known as new or novel oral anticoagulants (NOACs) (Bentz, 2015). If anticoagulants are contraindicated, aspirin alone is the best option, although the addition of

NURSING RESEARCH PROFILE

Chart 64-1. Awareness of Stroke Risk in Young African Americans

Aycock, D. M., & Clark, P. C. (2016). Incongruence between perceived long-term risk and actual risk of stroke in rural African Americans. *Journal of Neuroscience Nursing*, *48*(1), 35–41.

Purpose

African Americans aged 20 to 44 years are twice as likely to have a stroke as Caucasians of the same age. African Americans aged 35 to 64 years also have a higher risk (three to four times) of dying from a stroke than Caucasians. When a stroke occurs in a younger adult, they live longer with disabilities with greater health care costs and loss of productivity. Because up to 80% of strokes can be prevented with recognition and elimination of risk factors, primary prevention is critically important. The purpose of this study was to examine the accuracy of perceived stroke risk of African Americans aged 19 to 54 years.

Design

This study used a descriptive-correlational design. Participants consisted of a nonrandom sample that was recruited from a mobile health clinic (traveling to four rural counties over 4 months). Participants self-identified as African American, were between 19 and 54 years of age, were current residents of a rural county, and could not have a physical impairment that could keep them from exercising. Sixty-six participants were enrolled in the study. Participants were asked to select the risk that represented their risk of having a stroke in the next 10 to 20 years (no risk, little risk, moderate risk, or high risk). This was compared to an individual actual risk assessment that was based on accepted risk factors for stroke. The form that was used included health, social and family histories, and biophysiologic health measures (blood pressure and glucose). A scoring system was used as a guide to obtain a risk factor score. Scores could range between 0 and 8 (zero would be no risk factors). The measures were compared and participants were placed into risk accuracy categories: accurate, underestimate, or overestimate.

Findings

The mean age of participants was 43.3 years. Most of the participants were female (71%). Comparisons of the scores showed that 44% underestimated their risk, 47% were accurate, and 9% overestimated their risk. Sixty-seven percent of participants with a family history of stroke and 69% with a history of hypertension did not identify these as risk factors. Eighty percent of those who smoked cigarettes, 93% of those with diabetes, and 88% of those who were either overweight or who had obesity did not identify these as risk factors. This sample had a high burden of risk factors for stroke. Of the 39 participants who had three or more risk factors, only 19 (49%) thought that they were moderate to high risk of stroke.

Nursing Implications

This study suggests that more public education about primary prevention and awareness of modifiable stroke risk factors is needed. Nurses are in an optimal position to provide this education. Nurses in all settings (hospital, community, rehabilitation, outpatient clinics, and industry) should be involved in prevention and wellness activities for the public. This study focused on a young to middle-aged African American sample. Awareness campaigns can be focused and individualized for a younger population, and this study indicates that this type of campaign is needed. More studies are needed to test educational materials and tools that can be of benefit to this young to middle-aged population.

CHART 64-2

Modifiable Risk Factors: Ischemic Stroke

- Asymptomatic carotid stenosis
- Atrial fibrillation
- Diabetes (associated with accelerated atherogenesis)
- Dyslipidemia
- Excessive alcohol consumption
- Hypercoagulable states
- Hypertension (controlling hypertension, the major risk factor, is the key to preventing stroke)
- Migraine
- Obesity
- Sedentary lifestyle
- Sleep apnea
- Smoking

Adapted from Meschia, J. F., Bushnell, C., Boden-Albala, B., et al. (2014). Guidelines for the primary prevention of stroke: A statement for healthcare professionals from the American Heart Association/American Stroke Association. *Stroke*, *45*(12), 3754–3832.

clopidogrel (Plavix) to aspirin is also a reasonable therapy (Kernan, Ovbiagele, Black, et al., 2014).

Platelet-inhibiting medications, including aspirin, extended-release dipyridamole plus aspirin (Aggrenox), and clopidogrel decrease the incidence of cerebral infarction in patients who have experienced TIAs and stroke from suspected embolic or thrombotic causes. The specific medication that is used is based on the patient's health history.

Research suggests that medications known as statins reduce coronary events and ischemic strokes. The most current stroke prevention guideline now includes the recommendation of a statin even if the low-density lipoprotein (LDL) cholesterol is below 100 mg/dL and there is no evidence of atherosclerotic cardiovascular disease (coronary artery disease/myocardial infarction, hypertensive heart disease and peripheral arterial disease) (Kernan et al., 2014). The Canadian Cardiovascular Society (2016) has included indications for statin medications, such as simvastatin (Zocor), to include secondary stroke prevention.

After the acute stroke period, antihypertensive medications are also used, if indicated, for secondary stroke prevention. Preferred drugs include angiotensin-converting enzyme (ACE) inhibitors and diuretics, or a combination of both (Kernan et al., 2014).

Medical management of acute ischemic stroke needs to include consideration for endovascular treatment (Powers, Derdeyn, Biller, et al., 2015). Health Canada has approved several devices that open the blocked artery and restore blood flow to the brain. These devices are used by specialists in the endovascular suite.

Endovascular Techniques

Ongoing research is focusing on several aspects of the medical management of acute ischemic stroke. Recanalization devices are receiving significant attention as a means of restoring blood flow following an ischemic stroke. The sooner the blood flow is restored, the better the health outcome will be for the patient who has had a stroke. Devices that aid in the retrieval and removal of a thrombus (thrombectomy) are collectively referred to clot retrieval devices. However, these devices also have a short window of efficacy; ideally, they need to be utilized within 6 hours of stroke onset. After 6 hours the brain tissue has already experienced irreversible damage. This damaged brain tissue has now become prone to a hemorrhagic stroke. This phenomenon is called hemorrhagic transformation. When hemorrhagic transformation occurs patients have even poorer outcomes. Research investigating the efficacy of the Solitaire Flow Restoration Device, Penumbra System, Merci, and TREVO devices compare the rate of recanalization and improved outcomes following the procedure. Recanalization refers to clearing the vessel passageway thereby restoring blood flow. In two studies the Solitaire Flow Restoration Device had the best rate of recanalization over the other thrombectomy devices (Hann, Chalouhi, Starke, et al., 2013; Almekhlafi, Menon, Freiheit, et al., 2013; Hussain, Zaidat, & Fitzsimmons, 2012). Transcranial ultrasound is proven to be useful in detecting further emboli that may be present postrecanalization. Transcranial ultrasound can be performed at the bedside (Demchuk & Bal, 2012).

Thrombolytic Therapy

Thrombolytic agents are used to treat ischemic stroke by dissolving the blood clot that is blocking blood flow to the brain (Catangui, 2013). Recombinant t-PA is a genetically engineered form of t-PA, a thrombolytic substance made naturally by the body. It works by binding to fibrin and converting plasminogen to plasmin, which stimulates fibrinolysis of the atherosclerotic lesion. Rapid diagnosis of stroke and initiation of thrombolytic therapy (within 3.0 to 4.5 hours) in patients with ischemic stroke leads to a decrease in the size of the stroke and an overall improvement in functional outcome after 3 months. The combination of fibrinolytics with antithrombotics works as a means of improving recanalization times (Bautista, 2012; Demchuk & Bal, 2012). Other research studies are currently reviewing the pharmacokinetics and pharmacodynamics associated with the direct factor Xa inhibitor, Apixaban. This anticoagulant agent shows promise as a means of reducing the risk of stroke associated with atrial fibrillation (Keating, 2013).

Canada's dispersed population presents numerous challenges, especially to the implementation of best practices for stoke care. To realize the full potential of thrombolytic therapy, community education directed at recognizing the symptoms of stroke and obtaining appropriate emergency care is necessary to ensure rapid transport to a hospital and initiation of therapy within the 3.0- to 4.5-hour period. Delays make the patient ineligible for thrombolytic therapy, because revascularization of necrotic tissue (which develops after 3 to 4.5 hours) increases the risk of cerebral edema and hemorrhage.

The Heart and Stroke Foundation of Canada (2018) has adopted a campaign to help educate Canadians on the symptoms of stroke. The organization has adopted the acronym FAST: Face—is it drooping; Arms—can you raise both; Speech—is it slurred or jumbled; Time—call 911 right away. This simple acronym can help the public to identify the signs and symptoms of stroke as quickly as possible, to maximize treatment options and improve health outcomes.

Enhancing Prompt Diagnosis

After being notified by emergency medical service personnel, the emergency department contacts the appropriate staff (neurologist, neuroradiologist, radiology department, nursing staff, ECG, and laboratory technicians) and informs them of the patient's imminent arrival at the hospital. Many acute care centres in Canada have an acute stroke triage team. This specialized team is on call 24 hours a day, 7 days a week and is specially trained to recognize and treat strokes as quickly as possible. A multidisciplinary approach to stroke management is vital in achieving positive rehabilitative outcome goals. Nurses, physiotherapists, occupational therapists, and speech therapists are instrumental in maximizing independence in stroke survivors (Shah, Tartaro, Chew, et al., 2013; Eissa, Krass, & Bajorek, 2012).

Initial management requires the definitive diagnosis of an ischemic stroke by brain imaging (CT scan) and a careful history to determine whether the patient meets the criteria for t-PA therapy (Chart 64-3). Some of the absolute contraindications for thrombolytic therapy include symptom onset greater than 4.5 hours before admission, a patient who is anticoagulated (with an INR above 1.7), or a patient who has recently had any type of intracranial pathology (e.g., previous stroke, head injury, trauma). Once it is determined that the patient is a candidate for t-PA therapy, no anticoagulants are administered for the next 24 hours.

Before receiving t-PA, the patient is assessed using the National Institutes of Health Stroke Scale (NIHSS), a standardized assessment tool that helps evaluate stroke severity (Table 64-4). NIHSS scores range from 0 (no stroke) to 42 (severe stroke) (Catangui, 2013). Certification in the administration of the scale is recommended and is available for nurses and other health care professionals. The NIH Stroke Scale continues to be the most reliable indicator in identifying functional outcome in poststroke survivors (Siegler, Boehme, Kumar, et al., 2013; Saposnik, Guzik, Reeves, et al., 2012; Specogna, Patten, Turin, et al., 2013).

Dosage and Administration

The patient is weighed to determine the dose of t-PA. The dosage for t-PA is 0.9 mg/kg, with a maximum dose of 90 mg. Ten percent of the calculated dose is administered

CHART 64-3

Eligibility Criteria for Tissue Plasminogen Activator Administration

- Age ≥18 years
- Clinical diagnosis of ischemic stroke
- Time of onset of stroke known and is less than 3 hours before treatment
- Systolic blood pressure ≤185 mm Hg; diastolic ≤110 mm Hg
- No minor stroke or rapidly resolving stroke
- No seizure at onset of stroke
- Prothrombin time ≤15 seconds or international normalized ratio ≤1.7 (if taking an anticoagulant, the same guidance is used)
- Not received heparin during the past 48 hours with elevated partial thromboplastin time
- Platelet count ≥100,000/mm^3
- Glucose >50 mg/dL
- No prior intracranial hemorrhage, neoplasm, arteriovenous malformation, or aneurysm
- No major surgical procedures or serious trauma within 14 days
- No stroke, serious head injury, or intracranial surgery within 3 months
- No gastrointestinal or urinary bleeding within 21 days
- No pregnancy

Some of these are relative contraindications (the provider administering the medication needs to weigh the risks and benefits of the therapy). There are more stringent criteria if t-PA is considered for those patients in the 3.0- to 4.5-hour time window.

Adapted from Jauch, E. C., Saver, J. L., Adams, H. P., et al. (2013). Guidelines for the early management of patients with ischemic stroke: A guideline from the American Heart Association/American Stroke Association. *Stroke, 44*(1), 870–947.

as an intravenous (IV) bolus over 1 minute. The remaining dose (90%) is administered via an infusion pump over 1 hour.

The patient is admitted to the intensive care unit or an acute stroke unit, where continuous cardiac monitoring and frequent neurologic assessments are conducted. Vital signs are obtained frequently, with particular attention to blood pressure (with the goal of lowering the risk of intracranial hemorrhage). An example of a standard protocol would be to obtain vital signs every 15 minutes for the first 2 hours, every 30 minutes for the next 6 hours, then every hour until 24 hours after treatment. Research suggests that the burden associated with hypertension and the increased risk associated with stroke warrants an aggressive approach to blood pressure control. Clinical trials reveal that control of systolic hypertension significantly reduces stroke mortality (Lackland, 2013; Weiss, Beloosesky, Kenett, et al., 2013). (See Chapter 33 on Hypertension.) Airway management is instituted based on the patient's clinical condition and arterial blood gas values.

Side Effects

Bleeding is the most common side effect of t-PA administration, and the patient is closely monitored for any signs or symptoms of bleeding (IV insertion sites, angiography sites, urinary catheter site, endotracheal tube, nasogastric tube, urine, stool, emesis, other secretions). A 24-hour delay in placement of nasogastric tubes, urinary catheters, and intra-arterial pressure catheters is recommended. Intracranial bleeding is a major complication that occurred in approximately 6.4% of patients in the initial t-PA study (NINDS, 1995). A number of factors are associated with the occurrence of symptomatic intracranial bleeding: age greater than 70 years, baseline NIHSS score greater than 20, serum glucose concentration 16.6 mmol/L or higher, and edema or mass effect observed on the patient's initial CT scan.

Therapy for Patients With Ischemic Stroke Not Receiving t-PA

Not all patients are candidates for t-PA therapy. In some centres, other treatments may include anticoagulant administration (IV heparin or low–molecular-weight heparin). Because of the risks associated with anticoagulation, their general use is no longer recommended for patients with acute ischemic stroke (Jauch et al., 2013). New research is looking at the use of dabigatran etexilate (a direct thrombin inhibitor). The pharmacologic safety associated with the administration of dabigatran shows great promise and more research is underway (Clemens, Ryn, Sennewald, et al., 2012).

Careful maintenance of cerebral hemodynamics to maintain cerebral perfusion is extremely important after a stroke. Increased intracranial pressure (ICP) from brain edema, and associated complications, may occur after a large ischemic stroke. Interventions during this period include measures to reduce ICP, such as administering an osmotic diuretic (e.g., mannitol), maintaining the partial pressure of carbon dioxide ($PaCO_2$) within the range of 30 to 35 mm Hg, and positioning to avoid hypoxia. Other treatment measures include the following:

- Elevation of the head of the bed to promote venous drainage and to lower increased ICP
- Possible hemicraniectomy for severe cerebral edema from a very large stroke
- Intubation with an endotracheal tube to establish a patent airway, if necessary
- Continuous hemodynamic monitoring (the goals for blood pressure remain controversial for a patient who has not received thrombolytic therapy; antihypertensive treatment may be withheld unless the systolic blood pressure exceeds 220 mm Hg or the diastolic blood pressure exceeds 120 mm Hg)
- Neurologic assessment to determine if the stroke is evolving and if other acute complications are developing; such complications may include seizures, bleeding from anticoagulation, or medication-induced bradycardia, which can result in hypotension and subsequent decreases in cardiac output and cerebral perfusion pressure

Managing Potential Complications

Adequate cerebral blood flow is essential for cerebral oxygenation. If cerebral blood flow is inadequate, the amount of oxygen supplied to the brain will decrease, and tissue ischemia will result. Adequate oxygenation begins with pulmonary care, maintenance of a patent airway, and administration of supplemental oxygen as needed. The importance of adequate gas exchange in these patients

TABLE 64-4 Summary of National Institutes of Health Stroke Scale (NIHSS)

Category	Description	Score
1a. Level of consciousness (LOC)	Alert	0
	Arousable by minor stimulation	1
	Obtunded, strong stimulation to attend	2
	Unresponsive, or reflexic responses only	3
1b. LOC questions (month, age)	Answers both correctly	0
	Answers one correctly	1
	Both incorrect	2
1c. LOC commands (open, close eyes; make fist, let go)	Obeys both correctly	0
	Obeys one correctly	1
	Both incorrect	2
2. Best gaze (eyes open—patient follows examiner's finger or face)	Normal	0
	Partial gaze palsy	1
	Forced deviation	2
3. Visual (introduce visual stimulus/threat to patient's visual field quadrants)	No visual loss	0
	Partial hemianopsia	1
	Complete hemianopsia	2
	Bilateral hemianopsia	3
4. Facial palsy (show teeth, raise eyebrows and squeeze eyes shut)	Normal	0
	Minor	1
	Partial	2
	Complete	3
5a. Motor; arm—left (elevate extremity to 90 degrees and score drift/movement)	No drift	0
	Drift but maintains in air	1
	Unable to maintain in air	2
	No effort against gravity	3
	No movement	4
	Amputation, joint fusion (explain)	N/A
5b. Motor; arm—right (elevate extremity to 90 degrees and score drift/movement)	No drift	0
	Drift but maintains in air	1
	Unable to maintain in air	2
	No effort against gravity	3
	No movement	4
	Amputation, joint fusion (explain)	N/A
6a. Motor; leg—left (elevate extremity to 30 degrees and score drift/movement)	No drift	0
	Drift but maintains in air	1
	Unable to maintain in air	2
	No effort against gravity	3
	No movement	4
	Amputation, joint fusion (explain)	N/A
6b. Motor; leg—right (elevate extremity to 30 degrees and score drift/movement)	No drift	0
	Drift but maintains in air	1
	Unable to maintain in air	2
	No effort against gravity	3
	No movement	4
	Amputation, joint fusion (explain)	N/A
7. Limb ataxia (finger-to-nose and heel-to-shin testing)	Absent	0
	Present in one limb	1
	Present in two limbs	2
8. Sensory (pinprick to face, arm, trunk, and leg—compare side to side)	Normal	0
	Mild to moderate loss	1
	Severe to total loss	2
9. Best language (name items, describe a picture and read sentences)	No aphasia	0
	Mild to moderate aphasia	1
	Severe aphasia	2
	Mute	3
10. Dysarthria (evaluate speech clarity by having patient repeat words)	Normal	0
	Mild to moderate dysarthria	1
	Severe dysarthria, mostly unintelligible or worse	2
	Intubated or other physical barrier	N/A
11. Extinction and inattention (use information from prior testing to score)	No abnormality	0
	Visual, tactile, auditory, or other extinction to bilateral simultaneous stimulation	1
	Profound hemiattention or extinction to more than one modality	2
Total score		—

Adapted from the version available at the National Institute of Neurological Disorders and Stroke, National Institutes of Health, Bethesda, MD 20892. Retrieved from www.ninds.nih.gov/sites/default/files/NIH_Stroke_Scale_Booklet.pdf. It is recommended that the full scale with all instructions be used.

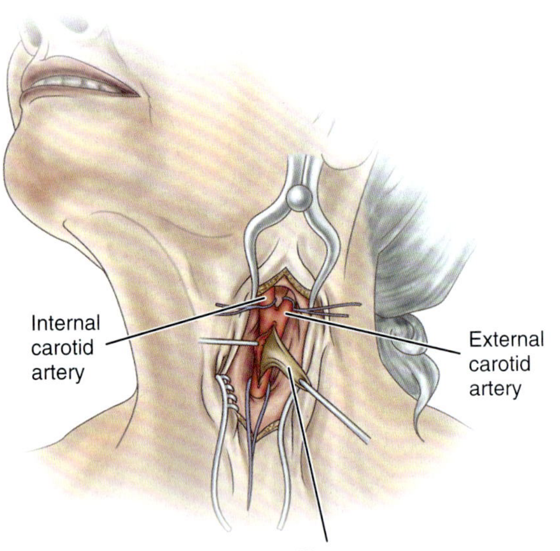

FIGURE 64-2. Plaque, a potential source of emboli in transient ischemic attack and stroke, is surgically removed from the carotid artery.

cannot be overemphasized as many patients are at risk for aspiration pneumonia. Other potential complications after a stroke include urinary tract infections, cardiac dysrhythmias, and complications of immobility.

Surgical Prevention of Ischemic Stroke

The gold standard surgical procedure for selected patients with TIAs and mild stroke is carotid endarterectomy (CEA), which is currently the most frequently performed noncardiac vascular procedure. A CEA is the removal of an atherosclerotic plaque from the carotid artery to prevent stroke in patients with occlusive disease of the extracranial cerebral arteries (Fig. 64-2). This surgery is indicated for patients with symptoms of TIA or mild stroke found to be caused by severe (70% to 99%) carotid artery stenosis or moderate (50% to 69%) stenosis with other significant risk factors (Gensicke, Zumbrunn, Jongen, et al., 2013).

CAS, with or without angioplasty, is a less invasive procedure that is used for treatment of carotid stenosis. This procedure has less discomfort for the patient and a shorter recovery time than CEA. Age can be considered when deciding which procedure will be best for the patient. For older patients (older than 70 years), CEA demonstrated improved outcomes in research studies; for those who were younger, outcomes between CAS and CEA were similar when comparing procedure complications (Kernan et al., 2014).

Nursing Management

The primary complications of CEA are stroke, postoperative hemorrhage/hematoma, cranial nerve injuries, infection, and carotid artery disruption. It is important to maintain adequate blood pressure levels in the immediate postoperative period. Hypotension is avoided to prevent cerebral ischemia and thrombosis. Uncontrolled hypertension may precipitate cerebral hemorrhage, edema, hemorrhage at the surgical incision, or disruption of the arterial reconstruction. Medications are used to reduce the blood pressure to previous levels. Close cardiac monitoring is necessary, because these patients have a high incidence of coronary artery disease.

After CEA, a neurologic flow sheet is used to monitor and document assessment parameters for all body systems, with particular attention to neurologic status. The surgeon is notified immediately if a neurologic deficit develops. Formation of a thrombus at the site of the endarterectomy is suspected if there is a sudden increase in neurologic deficits, such as weakness on one side of the body. The patient should be prepared for repeat endarterectomy.

Difficulty in swallowing, hoarseness, or other signs of cranial nerve dysfunction must be assessed. The nurse focuses on assessment of the following cranial nerves: facial (VII), vagus (X), spinal accessory (XI), and hypoglossal (XII). Some edema in the neck after surgery is expected; however, extensive edema and hematoma formation can obstruct the airway. Postoperatively nurses are required to measure neck circumference frequently in order to track small changes in the surgical site. Any increases greater than 3 cm should be reported to the attending service. Emergency airway supplies, including those needed for a tracheostomy, must be available at the bedside. Table 64-5 provides more information about potential complications of carotid surgery.

Nursing Process

The Patient Recovering From an Ischemic Stroke

PRACTICE & LEARN

The acute phase of an ischemic stroke may last from 24 to 72 hours, but ongoing monitoring of all body systems is essential as long as the patient requires care. The patient who has had a stroke is at risk for multiple complications, including deconditioning and other musculoskeletal problems, swallowing difficulties, bowel and bladder dysfunction, inability to perform self-care, and skin breakdown. After the stroke is complete, management focuses on the prompt initiation of rehabilitation for any deficits.

Assessment

During the acute phase, a neurologic flow sheet is maintained to provide data about the following important measures of the patient's clinical status:

- Change in level of consciousness or responsiveness as evidenced by movement, resistance to changes of position, and response to stimulation; orientation to time, place, and person
- Presence or absence of voluntary or involuntary movements of the extremities; muscle tone; body posture; and position of the head
- Stiffness or flaccidity of the neck
- Eye opening, comparative size and shape of pupils, and pupillary reactions to light, accommodation, and ocular position. At risk for dry eyes due to lack of spontaneous blink reflex

TABLE 64-5 Selected Complications of Carotid Endarterectomy and Nursing Interventions

Complication	Characteristics	Nursing Interventions
Incision hematoma	Occurs in 5.5% of patients. Large or rapidly expanding hematomas require emergency treatment. If the airway is obstructed by the hematoma, the incision may be opened at the bedside	Monitor neck discomfort and wound expansion. Report swelling, subjective feelings of pressure in the neck, difficulty breathing
Hypertension	Poorly controlled hypertension increases the risk of postoperative complications, including hematoma and hyperperfusion syndrome. There is an increased incidence of neurologic impairment and death due to intracerebral hemorrhage. May be related to surgically induced abnormalities of carotid baroreceptor sensitivity	Keep in mind that risk is highest in the first 48 hours after surgery. Check blood pressure frequently, and report deviations from baseline. Administer medications, as prescribed, to reduce hypertension. Observe for and report new onset of neurologic deficits
Postoperative hypotension	Occurs in approximately 5% of patients. Treated with fluids and low-dose phenylephrine infusion. Usually resolves in 24–48 hours. Patients with hypotension should have serial electrocardiograms to rule out myocardial infarction	Monitor blood pressure, and observe for signs and symptoms of hypotension
Hyperperfusion syndrome	Occurs when cerebral vessel autoregulation fails. Arteries accustomed to diminished blood flow may be permanently dilated; increased blood flow after endarterectomy coupled with insufficient vasoconstriction leads to capillary bed damage, edema, and hemorrhage	Observe for severe unilateral headache improved by sitting upright or standing
Intracerebral hemorrhage	Occurs infrequently but is often fatal (60%) or results in serious neurologic impairment. Can occur secondary to hyperperfusion syndrome. Increased risk with advanced age, hypertension, presence of high-grade stenosis, poor collateral flow, and slow flow in the region of the middle cerebral artery	Monitor neurologic status, and report any changes in mental status or neurologic functioning immediately

- Colour of the face and extremities; temperature and moisture of the skin
- Quality and rates of pulse and respiration; arterial blood gas values as indicated, body temperature, and arterial pressure
- Ability to speak
- Volume of fluids ingested or administered; volume of urine excreted each 24 hours
- Presence of bleeding
- Maintenance of blood pressure within the desired parameters

After the acute phase, the nurse assesses mental status (memory, attention span, perception, orientation, affect, speech/language), sensation/perception (the patient may have decreased awareness of pain and temperature), motor control (upper and lower extremity movement), swallowing ability, nutritional and hydration status, skin integrity, activity tolerance, and bowel and bladder function. Ongoing nursing assessment continues to focus on any impairment of function in the patient's daily activities, because the quality of life after stroke is closely related to the patient's functional status.

Nursing Priorities

Based on the assessment data, the major nursing priorities for a patient with a stroke may include the following:

- Impaired physical mobility
- Unilateral neglect
- Acute pain (painful shoulder)
- Self-care deficits (bathing, hygiene, toileting, dressing, grooming, and feeding)
- Disturbed sensory perception (kinesthetic, tactile, or visual)
- Impaired swallowing
- Impaired nutritional status
- Impaired urinary elimination
- Impaired bowel function—incontinence or constipation
- Disturbed thought processes
- Impaired verbal communication
- Impaired skin integrity
- Interrupted family processes
- Sexual dysfunction

Collaborative Problems/ Potential Complications

Potential complications include:

- Decreased cerebral blood flow due to increased ICP
- Inadequate oxygen delivery to the brain
- Pneumonia

Planning and Goals

Although rehabilitation begins on the day the patient has the stroke, the process is intensified during convalescence and requires a coordinated team effort. It is helpful for the team to know what the patient was like before the stroke, that is, the patient's baseline: his or her illnesses, abilities, mental and emotional state, behavioural characteristics, activities of daily living (ADLs), family dynamics, and socioeconomic status. The goal of rehabilitation is to reduce the level of dependency on others and to enable the stroke survivor to achieve a richer and more meaningful rehabilitative process. It is of utmost importance that the quality of life be restored (Shah et al., 2013).

The major goals for the patient and family may include improved mobility, avoidance of pain or discomfort, achievement of self-care, relief of sensory and perceptual deprivation, prevention of aspiration, continence of bowel and bladder, improved thought processes, achieving a form of communication, maintaining skin integrity, restored family functioning, maintained or satisfactory sexual function, and absence of complications.

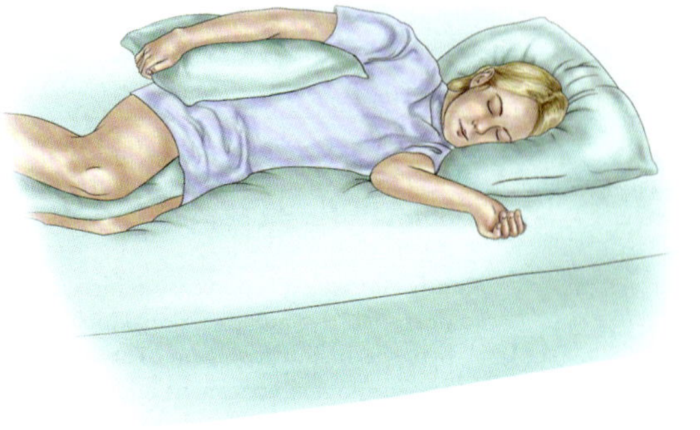

FIGURE 64-3. Correct positioning to prevent shoulder adduction.

Nursing Interventions

Nursing care plays a significant role in the patient's recovery. Often, many body systems are impaired as a result of the stroke, and conscientious care and timely interventions can prevent debilitating complications. During and after the acute phase, nursing interventions focus on the whole person and their family. In addition to providing physical care, the nurse encourages and fosters recovery by listening to the patient and asking questions to elicit the meaning of their stroke experience.

Improving Mobility and Preventing Joint Deformities

A patient with hemiplegia has unilateral paralysis (paralysis on one side). When control of the voluntary muscles is lost, the strong flexor muscles exert control over the extensors. The arm tends to adduct (adductor muscles are stronger than abductors) and to rotate internally. The elbow and the wrist tend to flex, the affected leg tends to rotate externally at the hip joint and flex at the knee, and the foot at the ankle joint supinates and tends toward plantar flexion.

Correct positioning is important to prevent contractures; measures are used to relieve pressure, assist in maintaining good body alignment, and prevent compressive neuropathies, especially of the ulnar and peroneal nerves. Because flexor muscles are stronger than extensor muscles, a splint applied at night to the affected extremity may prevent flexion and maintain correct positioning during sleep. (See Chapter 13 for additional information.)

PREVENTING SHOULDER ADDUCTION. To prevent adduction of the affected shoulder while the patient is in bed, a pillow is placed in the axilla when there is limited external rotation; this keeps the arm away from the chest. A pillow is placed under the arm, and the arm is placed in a neutral (slightly flexed) position, with distal joints positioned higher than the more proximal joints (i.e., the elbow is positioned higher than the shoulder and the wrist higher than the elbow). This helps to prevent edema and the resultant joint fibrosis that will limit range of motion if the patient regains control of the arm (Fig. 64-3).

POSITIONING THE HAND AND FINGERS. The fingers are positioned so that they are slightly flexed. The hand is placed in slight supination (palm faces upward), which is its most functional position. If the upper extremity is flaccid, a splint can be used to support the wrist and hand in a functional position. If the upper extremity is spastic, a hand roll is not used, because it stimulates the grasp reflex. In this instance a dorsal wrist splint is useful in allowing the palm to be free of pressure. Every effort is made to prevent hand edema and contractures.

Spasticity, particularly in the hand, can be a disabling complication after stroke. Botulinum toxin type A injected intramuscularly into wrist and finger muscles has been shown to be effective in reducing this spasticity (although the effect is temporary, typically lasting 2 to 4 months) (Teasell, Foley, Pereira, et al., 2012). Other treatments for spasticity may include stretching, splinting, and oral medications such as baclofen (Lioresal), diazepam (Valium), dantrolene (Dantrium), and tizanidine (Zanaflex).

CHANGING POSITIONS. The patient's position must be changed every 2 hours. To place a patient in a lateral (side-lying) position, a pillow is placed between the legs before the patient is turned. To promote venous return and prevent edema, the upper thigh should not be acutely flexed. The patient may be turned from side to side, but if sensation is impaired, the amount of time spent on the affected side should be limited.

If possible, the patient is placed in a prone position for 15 to 30 minutes several times a day. A small pillow or a support is placed under the pelvis, extending from the level of the umbilicus to the upper third of the thigh (Fig. 64-4). This position helps promote hyperextension of the hip joints, which is essential for usual gait and helps prevent knee and hip flexion contractures. The prone position also helps drain bronchial secretions and prevents contractural deformities of the shoulders and knees. During positioning, it is important to reduce pressure and change position frequently to prevent pressure ulcers.

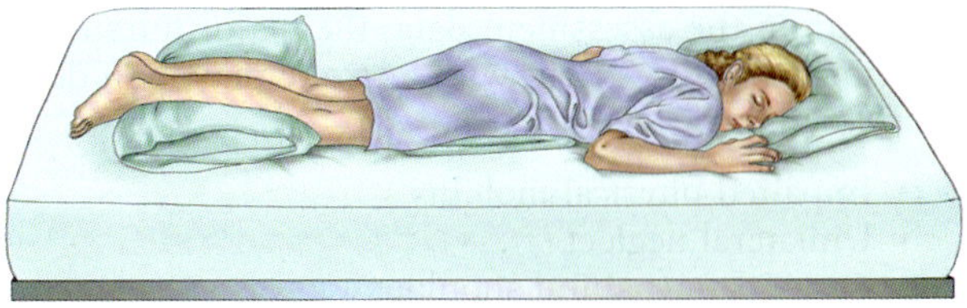

FIGURE 64-4. Prone position with pillow support helps prevent hip flexion.

ESTABLISHING AN EXERCISE PROGRAM. The affected extremities are exercised passively and put through a full range of motion four or five times a day to maintain joint mobility, regain motor control, prevent contractures in the paralyzed extremity, prevent further deterioration of the neuromuscular system, and enhance circulation. Exercise is helpful in preventing venous stasis, which may predispose the patient to venous thromboembolism (VTE). VTE includes deep vein thrombosis (DVT) and pulmonary embolus (PE).

Repetition of an activity forms new pathways in the CNS and therefore encourages new patterns of motion. At first, the extremities are usually flaccid. If tightness occurs in any area, the range-of-motion exercises should be performed more frequently (see Chapter 13).

The patient is observed for signs and symptoms that may indicate PE or excessive cardiac workload during exercise; these include shortness of breath, chest pain, cyanosis, and increasing pulse rate with exercise. Frequent short periods of exercise always are preferable to longer periods at infrequent intervals. Regularity in exercise is most important. Improvement in muscle strength and maintenance of range of motion can be achieved only through daily exercise.

The patient is encouraged and reminded to exercise the unaffected side at intervals throughout the day. It is helpful to develop a written schedule to remind the patient and family of the exercise activities. The nurse supervises and supports the patient during these activities. The patient can be taught to put the unaffected leg under the affected one to assist in moving it when turning and exercising. Flexibility, strengthening, coordination, endurance, and balancing exercises prepare the patient for ambulation. Quadriceps muscle setting and gluteal setting exercises are started early to improve the muscle strength needed for walking; these are performed at least five times daily for 10 minutes at a time.

PREPARING FOR AMBULATION. As soon as possible, the patient is assisted out of bed and an active rehabilitation program is started. The patient is first taught to maintain balance while sitting and then to learn to balance while standing. If the patient has difficulty in achieving standing balance, a tilt table, which slowly brings the patient to an upright position, can be used. Tilt tables are especially helpful for patients who have been on bed rest for prolonged periods and have orthostatic blood pressure changes.

If the patient needs a wheelchair, the folding type with hand brakes is the most practical because it allows the patient to manipulate the chair. The chair should be low enough to allow the patient to propel it with the uninvolved foot and narrow enough to permit it to be used in the home. Before the patient is transferred from the wheelchair, the brakes must be applied and locked on both sides of the chair. A customized wheelchair that has been measured and fit by an occupational therapist is optimal for patients who will require assistance to ambulate.

The patient is usually ready to walk as soon as standing balance is achieved. Parallel bars are useful in these first efforts. A chair or wheelchair is readily available in case the patient suddenly becomes fatigued or feels dizzy.

The training periods for ambulation should be short and frequent to allow the patient to gain strength and confidence. At first, a two-wheeled walker is used to provide stability and support. After a patient has demonstrated safe ambulation with a walker, a cane can be used to provide support and assist with balance. In general, a three- or four-pronged cane provides a stable support in the early phases of rehabilitation.

Preventing Shoulder Pain

A case-control study revealed that out of 107 participants, 49% reported shoulder pain on admission to a treatment facility, upon discharge and at the 1-month follow-up appointment. The pain was reported as more severe with spasticity. This study highlighted the importance for proper care and management of the affected limb. In addition to the care recommendations, the study gave credence to the importance of a multidisciplinary approach with the sharing of knowledge and expertise among all members of the care team. The benefits of a collaborative approach to care is to improve the quality of life of stroke survivors while enabling their recovery (Smith, 2012; Burr, Shephard, & Zehr, 2012).

Shoulder function is essential in achieving balance and performing transfers and self-care activities. Three situations can occur: painful shoulder, subluxation of the shoulder, and shoulder–hand syndrome. A flaccid shoulder joint may be overstretched by the use of excessive force in turning the patient or from overstrenuous arm and shoulder movement. To prevent shoulder pain, the nurse should never lift the patient by the flaccid shoulder, or pull on the affected arm or shoulder. Overhead pulleys should also be avoided. If the arm is paralyzed, subluxation (incomplete dislocation) at the shoulder can occur as a result of overstretching of the joint capsule and musculature by the force of gravity when the patient sits or stands. This results in severe pain. Shoulder–hand syndrome (painful shoulder and generalized swelling of the hand) can cause a frozen shoulder and ultimately atrophy of subcutaneous tissues. When a shoulder becomes stiff, it is usually painful.

Many shoulder issues can be prevented by proper patient movement and positioning. Muscle activation in the shoulder and arm is a priority focus of rehabilitation. Targeted motor training exercises are an essential part of rehabilitative protocols (Roh, Rymer, Perreault, et al., 2012). The flaccid arm is positioned on a table or with pillows while the patient is seated. Some clinicians advocate the use of a properly worn sling when the patient first becomes ambulatory, to prevent the paralyzed upper extremity from dangling without support. Range-of-motion exercises are important in preventing painful shoulder. Overstrenuous arm movements are avoided. The patient is instructed to interlace the fingers, place the palms together, and push the clasped hands slowly forward to bring the scapulae forward; he or she then raises both hands above the head. This is repeated throughout the day. The patient is instructed to flex the affected wrist at intervals and move all the joints of the affected fingers. The patient is encouraged to touch, stroke, rub, and look at both hands. Pushing the heel of the hand firmly down on a surface is useful. Elevation of the arm and hand is also important in preventing dependent edema of the hand. Patients with continuing pain after attempted movement and positioning may require the addition of analgesia to their treatment program. In addition to limb mobilization, other treatment modalities must be considered, such as pain analgesia, positioning of the limb at rest and during the day, high-intensity transcutaneous electrical nerve stimulation, and shoulder strapping (Smith, 2012). Other treatments to reduce shoulder pain may include massage, and aromatherapy combined with acupressure (Mehta, Teasell, & Foley, 2013).

Medications are helpful in the management of poststroke pain. Amitriptyline hydrochloride (Elavil) has been used, but it can cause cognitive problems, has a sedating effect, and is not effective in all patients. Antiepileptic drugs used for poststroke seizures are still under investigation by the research community. New-generation antiepileptic drugs are gaining more attention and more research efforts. The pharmacokinetic and pharmacodynamic properties associated with gabapentin, lamotrigine, topiramate, oxcarbazepine, and levetiracetam show great promise in the management of poststroke seizure activity. This is due to the fact that these medications have not shown to interfere or interact with anticoagulants or antiplatelet agents that are onboard (Gilad, 2012).

Enhancing Self-Care

As soon as the patient can sit up, personal hygiene activities are encouraged. The patient is helped to set realistic goals; if feasible, a new task is added daily. The first step is to carry out all self-care activities on the unaffected side. Such activities as combing the hair, brushing the teeth, shaving with an electric razor, bathing, and eating can be carried out with one hand and should be encouraged. Although the patient may feel awkward at first, these motor skills can be learned by repetition, and the unaffected side will become stronger with use. The nurse makes sure that the patient does not neglect the affected side. Assistive devices will help make up for some of the patient's deficits (Chart 64-4). A small towel is easier to control while drying after bathing, and boxed paper tissues are easier to use than a roll of toilet tissue.

Return of functional ability is important to the patient recovering after a stroke. An early baseline assessment of functional ability with an instrument such as the Functional Independence Measure (FIM) is important in team planning and goal setting for the patient. The FIM is an 18-item ordinal scale used to measure the functional ability within rehabilitative populations. Functional skills that are assessed include activities of daily living: dressing one's upper and lower body, toileting, bathing, grooming, transferring, walking, and negotiating stairs (Ward, Pivko, Brooks, et al., 2011). Perceptual problems may make it difficult for the patient to dress without assistance because of an inability to match the clothing to the body parts. To assist the patient, the nurse can take steps to keep the environment organized and uncluttered, because the patient with a perceptual problem is easily distracted. The clothing is placed on the affected side in the order in which the garments are to be put on. Using a large mirror while dressing promotes the patient's awareness of what he or she is putting on the affected side. The patient has to make many compensatory movements when dressing; these can produce fatigue and painful twisting of the intercostal muscles. Support and encouragement are provided to prevent the patient from becoming overly fatigued and discouraged. Even with intensive training, not all patients can achieve independence in dressing. The Stroke Rehabilitation Assessment of Movement (STREAM), a 30-item scale, is another tool that can be used to examine voluntary movement and basic mobility in poststroke survivors (Ward et al., 2011). The Stroke Impact Scale-16 is a questionnaire used to help the practitioner gain a better understanding about the patient's perception of his or her own recovery (Ward et al., 2011).

CHART 64-4

Assistive Devices to Enhance Self-Care After Stroke

Eating Devices
- Nonskid mats to stabilize plates
- Plate guards to prevent food from being pushed off plate
- Wide-grip utensils to accommodate a weak grasp

Bathing and Grooming Devices
- Long-handled bath sponge
- Grab bars, nonskid mats, handheld shower heads
- Electric razors with head at 90 degrees to handle
- Shower and tub seats, stationary or on wheels

Toileting Aids
- Raised toilet seat
- Grab bars next to toilet

Dressing Aids
- Velcro closures
- Elastic shoelaces
- Long-handled shoe horn

Mobility Aids
- Canes, walkers, wheelchairs
- Transfer devices such as transfer boards and belts

Adjusting to Physical Changes

Patients with a decreased field of vision are always approached on the side where visual perception is intact. All visual stimuli (e.g., clock, calendar, television) should be placed on this side. The patient can be taught to turn the head in the direction of the defective visual field to compensate for this loss. The nurse should make eye contact with the patient and draw his or her attention to the affected side by encouraging the patient to move the head. The nurse may also want to stand at a position that encourages the patient to move or turn to visualize who is in the room. Increasing the natural or artificial lighting in the room and providing eyeglasses if needed are important aids to increasing vision.

The patient with homonymous hemianopsia (loss of half of the visual field) turns away from the affected side of the body and tends to neglect that side and the space on that side; this is called amorphosynthesis. In such instances, the patient cannot see food on half of the tray, and only half of the room is visible. It is important for the nurse to constantly remind the patient of the other side of the body, to maintain alignment of the extremities, and, if possible, to place the extremities where the patient can see them.

Assisting With Nutrition

Stroke can result in swallowing issues (dysphagia) due to impaired function of the mouth, tongue, palate, larynx, pharynx, or upper esophagus. Patients must be observed for paroxysms of coughing, food dribbling out of or pooling in one side of the mouth, food retained for long periods in the mouth, or nasal regurgitation when swallowing liquids. Swallowing difficulties place the patient at risk for aspiration, pneumonia, dehydration, and malnutrition.

A speech therapist will evaluate the patient's swallowing ability. If swallowing function is partially impaired, it may return over time, or the patient may be taught alternative swallowing techniques, advised to take smaller boluses of food, and taught about types of foods that are easier to swallow. The patient may be started on a thick liquid or puréed diet, because these foods are easier to swallow than thin liquids. Having the patient sit upright, preferably out of bed in a chair, and instructing him or her to tuck the chin toward the chest as he or she swallows will help prevent aspiration. The diet may be advanced as the patient becomes more proficient at swallowing. If the patient cannot resume oral intake, a gastrointestinal feeding tube is placed for ongoing tube feedings and medication administration.

Enteral tubes can be either nasogastric (placed in the stomach) or nasoenteral (placed in the duodenum) to reduce the risk of aspiration. Nursing responsibilities in feeding include elevating the head of the bed at least 30 degrees to prevent aspiration, checking the position of the tube before feeding, ensuring that the cuff of the tracheostomy tube (if in place) is inflated, and giving the tube feeding slowly. The feeding tube is aspirated periodically to ensure that the feedings are passing through the gastrointestinal tract. Retained or residual feedings increase the risk of aspiration. Patients with retained feedings may benefit from the placement of a gastrostomy tube or a percutaneous endoscopic gastrostomy tube (PEG tube). In a patient with a nasogastric tube, the feeding tube should be placed in the duodenum to reduce the risk of aspiration. For long-term feedings, a gastrostomy tube is preferred. Management of patients with tube feedings is discussed in Chapter 36.

Attaining Bladder and Bowel Control

After a stroke, the patient may have transient urinary incontinence due to confusion, inability to communicate needs, and inability to use the washroom, urinal or bedpan because of impaired motor and postural control. Occasionally after a stroke, the bladder becomes atonic, with impaired sensation in response to bladder filling. Sometimes control of the external urinary sphincter is lost or diminished. During this period, intermittent catheterization with sterile technique is carried out. After muscle tone increases and deep tendon reflexes return, bladder tone increases and spasticity of the bladder may develop. The voiding pattern is analyzed, and the washroom, commode chair, urinal, or bedpan is offered on this pattern or schedule. If possible, male patients should be encouraged to stand because the upright position may help them void.

Patients may have problems with bowel control, particularly constipation. Unless contraindicated, a high-fibre diet and adequate fluid intake (2 to 3 L/day) should be provided and a regular time (usually after breakfast) should be established for toileting. Bowel incontinence is often observed in patients who have had a stroke, especially those requiring feeding tubes. Strict and frequent incontinence pads changes are required to maintain skin integrity. Pharmacologic management may be necessary for extreme cases; rectal tubes are often required as well. See Chapter 13 for additional information about bladder and bowel control.

Improving Thought Processes

After a stroke, the patient may have challenges with cognitive, behavioural, and emotional deficits related to brain damage. However, in many instances, a considerable degree of function can be recovered, because not all areas of the brain are equally damaged; some remain more intact and functional than others.

After assessment that delineates the patient's deficits, the neuropsychologist, in collaboration with the primary care physician, psychiatrist, nurse, and other professionals, structures a training program using cognitive-perceptual retraining, visual imagery, reality orientation, and cueing procedures to compensate for losses.

The role of the nurse is supportive. The nurse reviews the results of neuropsychological testing, observes the patient's performance and progress, gives positive feedback, and, most importantly, conveys an attitude of confidence and hope. Interventions capitalize on the patient's strengths and remaining abilities while attempting to improve performance of affected functions. Other interventions are similar to those for improving cognitive functioning after a head injury (see Chapter 65).

Improving Communication

Aphasia, which impairs the patient's ability to express himself or herself and to understand what is being said, may become apparent in various ways. The cortical area that is responsible for integrating the myriad pathways required for the comprehension and formulation of language is called Broca's area. It is located in the temporal lobe of the brain and is fed by one of the middle cerebral arteries. This area is responsible for control of the combinations of muscular movements needed to speak each word. Broca's area is so close to the left motor area that a disturbance in the motor area often affects the speech area. This is why so many patients who are paralyzed on the right side (due to damage or injury to the left side of the brain) cannot speak, whereas those paralyzed on the left side are less likely to have speech disturbances.

The speech therapist assesses the communication needs of the patient with a stroke, describes the precise deficit, and suggests the best overall method of communication. Most language intervention strategies can be tailored for the individual patient. The patient is expected to take an active part in establishing goals.

A person with aphasia may become depressed. The inability to talk on the telephone, answer a question, or participate in conversation often causes anger, frustration, fear of the future, and hopelessness. Nursing interventions include strategies to make the atmosphere conducive to communication. This includes being sensitive to the patient's reactions and needs and responding to them in an appropriate manner. The nurse provides strong emotional support and understanding to allay anxiety and frustration.

A common pitfall is for the nurse or other health care team member to complete the thoughts or sentences of the patient. This is to be avoided, because it causes the patient to become more frustrated at not being allowed to speak and may deter efforts to practice putting thoughts together and completing sentences. A consistent schedule, routines, and repetition help the patient to function despite significant deficits. A written copy of the daily schedule, a folder of personal information (birth date, address, names of relatives), checklists, and an audiotaped list help improve the patient's memory and concentration. The patient may also benefit from a communication board, which has pictures of common needs and phrases. The board may be translated into any language.

When talking with the patient, it is important for the nurse to gain the patient's attention, speak slowly, and keep the language of instruction consistent. One instruction is given at a time, and time is allowed for the patient to process what has been said. The use of gestures may enhance comprehension. Speaking is thinking out loud, and the emphasis is on thinking. Listening and sorting out incoming messages requires mental effort; the patient must struggle against mental inertia and needs time to organize a response.

In working with the patient with aphasia, the nurse must remember to talk to the patient during care activities. This provides social contact for the patient. Chart 64-5 describes points to keep in mind when communicating with the patient with aphasia. The use of simple yes and no questions should also be used in order to prevent patients from feeling frustrated by their inability to communicate effectively.

CHART 64-5

Communicating With the Patient With Aphasia

- Face the patient and establish eye contact
- Speak in a normal manner and tone
- Use short phrases, and pause between phrases to allow the patient time to understand what is being said
- Limit conversation to practical and concrete matters
- Use gestures, pictures, objects, and writing
- As the patient uses and handles an object, say what the object is. It helps to match the words with the object or action
- Be consistent in using the same words and gestures each time you give instructions or ask a question
- Keep extraneous noises and sounds to a minimum. Too much background noise can distract the patient or make it difficult to sort out the message being spoken

Maintaining Skin Integrity

The patient who has had a stroke may be at risk for skin and tissue breakdown because of altered sensation and inability to respond to pressure and discomfort by turning and moving. Preventing skin and tissue breakdown requires frequent assessment of the skin, with emphasis on bony areas and dependent parts of the body. During the acute phase, a specialty bed (e.g., low–air-loss bed) may be used until the patient can move independently or assist in moving.

A regular turning schedule (e.g., every 2 hours) is adhered to even if pressure-relieving devices are used to prevent tissue and skin breakdown. When the patient is positioned or turned, care must be used to minimize shear and friction forces, which cause damage to tissues and predispose the skin to breakdown. Nurses must pay special attention to body mechanics when turning or moving patients who are immobile to avoid injuring themselves.

The patient's skin must be kept clean and dry; gentle massage of healthy (nonreddened) skin and adequate nutrition are other factors that help to maintain skin and tissue integrity (see Chapter 12).

Improving Family Coping

Family members play an important role in the patient's recovery. Family members are encouraged to participate in counselling and to use support systems that will help with the emotional and physical stress of caring for the patient. Involving others in the patient's care and teaching stress management techniques and methods for maintaining personal health also facilitate family coping.

The family may have difficulty accepting the patient's disability and may be unrealistic in their expectations. They are given information about the expected outcomes and are counselled to avoid doing activities for patients that they can do themselves. Families are assured that their love, support and interest are part of the patient's therapy.

The family is informed that the rehabilitation of the patient with hemiplegia requires many months and that progress may be slow. The gains made by the patient in the hospital or rehabilitation unit must be maintained. All caregivers should approach the patient with a supportive and optimistic attitude, focusing on the patient's remaining abilities. The rehabilitation team, the medical and nursing team, the patient, and the family are all involved in developing attainable goals for the patient at home.

Most relatives of patients with stroke handle the physical changes better than the emotional aspects of care. The family is prepared to expect occasional episodes of emotional lability. The patient may laugh or cry easily and may be irritable and demanding or depressed and confused. The nurse can explain to the family that the patient's laughter does not necessarily connote happiness, nor does crying reflect sadness, and that emotional lability usually improves with time.

Helping the Patient Cope With Sexual Dysfunction

Sexual functioning can be profoundly altered by stroke. Although research in this area of stroke management is limited, it appears that patients who have had a stroke consider sexual function important, and many have sexual dysfunction. Impaired sexual activity in poststroke survivors not only includes sexual dysfunction but also impaired sexual satisfaction. Although there are assessment tools to evaluate the level of independence associated with activities of daily living; those to evaluate the presence and/or degree of depression and anxiety, methods to adequately assess sexual function poststroke are not available (Bugincourt, Hamy, Canaple, et al., 2014). Poststroke survivors can be faced with a number of barriers to sexual activity. These barriers may include physical limitations; discomfort and/or pain which may limit sexual positions; and decreased libido/arousal depending on the location of the stroke within the brain (Rosenbaum, Vadas, & Kalichman, 2014).

Nurses in the rehabilitation setting play a crucial role in beginning a dialogue between the patient and his or her partner about sexuality after a stroke. In-depth assessments to determine sexual history before and after the stroke are followed by appropriate interventions. Interventions related to impaired sexual activity should not be solely focused on the physical barriers, rather on exploring other alternatives that promote/enhance intimacy, pleasure, and ultimately self-confidence (Rosenbaum et al., 2014). An all-encompassing approach includes dialogue about impaired sexual activity by all members of the rehabilitative team—nurses, occupational therapists, physiotherapists, and speech pathologists (Rosenbaum et al., 2014).

Promoting Home, Community-Based, and Transitional Care

EDUCATING PATIENTS ABOUT SELF-CARE. Patient and family education is a fundamental component of rehabilitation. The nurse provides teaching about stroke, its causes and prevention, and the rehabilitation process. In both acute care and rehabilitation facilities, the focus is on teaching the patient to resume as much self-care as possible. This may entail using assistive devices or modifying the home environment to help the patient live with a disability. Decreasing burden of care for family members is also a very important goal of the rehabilitation process. Caregiver burden plays a significant role in how patients and families recover from a stroke.

An occupational therapist may be helpful in assessing the home environment and recommending modifications to help the patient become more independent. For example, a shower is more convenient than a tub for the patient with hemiplegia because most patients do not gain sufficient strength to get up and down from a tub. Sitting on a stool of medium height with rubber suction tips allows the patient to wash with greater ease. A long-handled bath brush with a soap container is helpful to the patient who has only one functional hand. If a shower is not available, a stool may be placed in the tub and a portable shower hose attached to the faucet. Handrails may be attached alongside the bathtub and the toilet. Other assistive devices include special utensils for eating, grooming, dressing, and writing (see Chart 64-4).

A program of physical therapy can be beneficial, whether it takes place in the home or in an outpatient program. Constraint-induced movement therapy has been used in stroke rehabilitation and involves constraint of the less affected upper limb with a mitt, and intensely training the more affected limb. Robotic-assisted therapy uses sensorimotor training of the upper limb. This method allows patients to train without the presence of a therapist. Recent research has focused on techniques using robotics, virtual reality and video game applications, transcranial magnetic stimulation, and ambulation with body weight support and treadmill training (Brainin & Zorowitz, 2013).

CONTINUING AND TRANSITIONAL CARE. The recovery and rehabilitation process after stroke may be prolonged and requires patience and perseverance on the part of both the patient and the family. Depending on the specific neurologic deficits resulting from the stroke, the patient at home may require the services of a number of health care professionals. The nurse often coordinates the care of the patient at home and considers the many educational needs of caregivers and patients. The family (often the spouse) requires education as well as assistance in planning and providing care.

The family is advised that the patient may tire easily, may become irritable and upset by small events, and may be less interested in events than expected. Emotional concerns associated with stroke are often related to speech dysfunction and the frustrations of being unable to communicate. A speech therapist allows the family to be involved and gives the family practical instructions to help the patient between therapy sessions.

Depression is a common and serious problem in the patient who has had a stroke. The incidence of depression in patients who have had a stroke ranges from 25% to 79%. Risk factors include social isolation, gender (more prevalent in women), a history of depression, and cognitive or physical impairment (Miller, Murray, Richards, et al., 2010). Because the length of hospital stays has shortened, depression may not be identified in the acute setting. Nurses in all care settings should identify patients who may be at risk for depression or who show depressive symptoms (Miller et al., 2010). In the home or in the rehabilitation setting, nurses may be involved in coordinating care and referring patients and family to appropriate resources. The family can help by continuing to support the patient and by giving positive reinforcement for the progress that is being made. Antidepressant therapy may be prescribed, and may help with recovery from stroke (Flaster, Sharma, & Rao, 2013).

Community-based stroke support groups may allow the patient and family to learn from others with similar problems and to share their experiences. Support groups take the form of in-person meetings as well as Internet-based support programs. The patient is encouraged to continue hobbies and recreational and leisure interests and to maintain contact with friends to prevent social isolation. All nurses coming in contact with the patient should encourage the patient to keep active, adhere to the exercise program, and remain as self-sufficient as possible.

The nurse should recognize the potential effects of caregiving on the family. Not all families have the adaptive coping skills and adequate psychological functioning necessary for the long-term care of another person. The patient's spouse may be older, with their own health concerns; in some instances, the patient may have been the provider of care to the spouse. A spouse may have to take on new roles and responsibilities in the relationship and around the home. He or she may also feel a sense of loss (of freedom and leisure time as well as of the marital relationship). Caregivers may also experience social isolation and financial burdens. Depression is common in caregivers of patients who have survived a stroke, with rates as high as 30% to 52% (Miller et al., 2010). Nurses should assess caregivers for signs of depression.

Caregivers may require reminders to attend to their own health concerns and well-being. Even healthy caregivers may find it difficult to maintain a schedule that includes being available around the clock. The nurse encourages the family to arrange for respite care services (planned short-term care to relieve the family from having to provide continuous 24-hour care), which may be available from an adult day care centre. Some hospitals also offer weekend respite care that can provide caregivers with needed time for themselves. The nurse involved in home and continuing care also needs to remind the patient and family of the need for respite care as well as continuing health promotion and screening practices.

A spouse may have to take on new roles and responsibilities in the relationship and around the home. He or she may also feel a sense of loss (of freedom and leisure time as well as of the marital relationship).

Evaluation

Expected patient outcomes may include the following:

1. Achieves improved mobility
   a. Avoids deformities (contractures and footdrop)
   b. Participates in prescribed exercise program
   c. Achieves sitting balance
   d. Uses unaffected side to compensate for loss of function of hemiplegic side
2. Reports absence of shoulder pain
   a. Demonstrates shoulder mobility; exercises shoulder
   b. Elevates arm and hand at intervals
3. Achieves self-care; performs hygiene care; uses adaptive equipment
4. Demonstrates techniques to compensate for altered sensory reception, such as turning the head to see people or objects
5. Demonstrates safe swallowing
6. Meets their daily nutritional needs
7. Achieves regular bowel and bladder elimination
8. Participates in cognitive improvement program
9. Demonstrates improved communication
10. Maintains intact skin without breakdown
    a. Demonstrates appropriate skin turgor
    b. Participates in turning and positioning activities
11. Family members demonstrate a positive attitude and coping mechanisms
    a. Encourage patient in exercise program
    b. Take an active part in rehabilitation process
    c. Contact respite care programs or arrange for other family members to assume some responsibilities for care
12. Develops alternative approaches to sexual expression

Hemorrhagic Stroke

Hemorrhagic strokes account for 15% to 20% of cerebrovascular disorders and are primarily caused by intracranial or subarachnoid hemorrhage. Hemorrhagic strokes are caused by bleeding into the brain tissue, the ventricles, or the subarachnoid space. Primary intracerebral hemorrhage from a spontaneous rupture of small vessels accounts for approximately 80% of hemorrhagic strokes and is caused chiefly by uncontrolled hypertension. Subarachnoid hemorrhage is caused by a tear in a cerebral artery. Bleeding from this site enters into the subarachnoid space. In 50% of the cases, bleeding is the result of a burst **aneurysm**.

Another common cause of intracerebral hemorrhage in older people is cerebral amyloid angiopathy, which involves damage caused by the deposit of beta-amyloid protein in the small- and medium-sized blood vessels of the brain. Secondary intracerebral hemorrhage is associated with arteriovenous malformations (AVMs), intracranial aneurysms, intracranial neoplasms, or certain medications (e.g., anticoagulants, amphetamines). Twenty percent of all strokes worldwide are of the intracerebral hemorrhage type. Of this group, there is a 32% to 50% mortality rate within 30-days poststroke (Martini, Flaherty, Brown, et al., 2012). Patients who survive the acute phase of care usually have more severe deficits and a longer recovery phase compared to those with ischemic stroke.

Pathophysiology

The pathophysiology of hemorrhagic stroke depends on the cause and type of cerebrovascular disorder. Symptoms are produced when a primary hemorrhage, aneurysm, or AVM presses on nearby cranial nerves or brain tissue or, more dramatically, when an aneurysm or AVM ruptures, causing subarachnoid hemorrhage (hemorrhage into the cranial subarachnoid space). Usual brain metabolism is disrupted by the brain's exposure to blood; by an increase in ICP resulting from the sudden entry of blood into the subarachnoid space, which compresses and injures brain tissue; or by secondary ischemia of the brain resulting from the reduced perfusion pressure and vasospasm that frequently accompany subarachnoid hemorrhage.

Intracerebral Hemorrhage

An intracerebral hemorrhage, or bleeding into the brain tissue, is most common in patients with hypertension and cerebral atherosclerosis, because degenerative changes from these diseases cause rupture of the blood vessel. An intracerebral hemorrhage may also result from certain types of vascular malformations, brain tumours, and the use of medications (e.g., oral anticoagulants, amphetamines, and illicit drug use).

There seems to be a correlation between hematoma location and the rate of mortality associated with an intracerebral hemorrhage. More research is needed; however, this sheds new light on the importance of diagnostic imaging to determine the extent and location of the bleed. Increased mortality is seen with hemorrhage isolated to regions such as the parietal lobe, basal ganglia, posterior insula, and posterolateral thalamus (Lee, King, Stradling, et al., 2014).

Intracranial (Cerebral) Aneurysm

An intracranial (cerebral) aneurysm is a dilation of the walls of a cerebral artery that develops as a result of weakness in the arterial wall. The cause of aneurysms is unknown, although research is ongoing. An aneurysm may be due to atherosclerosis, which results in a defect in the vessel wall with subsequent weakness of the wall; a congenital defect of the vessel wall; hypertensive vascular disease; head trauma; or advancing age or infection (mycotic aneurysms).

Any artery within the brain can be the site of a cerebral aneurysm, but these lesions usually occur at the bifurcations of the large arteries at the circle of Willis (Fig. 64-5). The cerebral arteries most commonly affected by an aneurysm are the internal carotid artery (ICA), anterior cerebral artery (ACA), anterior communicating artery (ACoA), posterior communicating artery (PCoA), posterior cerebral artery (PCA), and MCA. Multiple cerebral aneurysms are not uncommon.

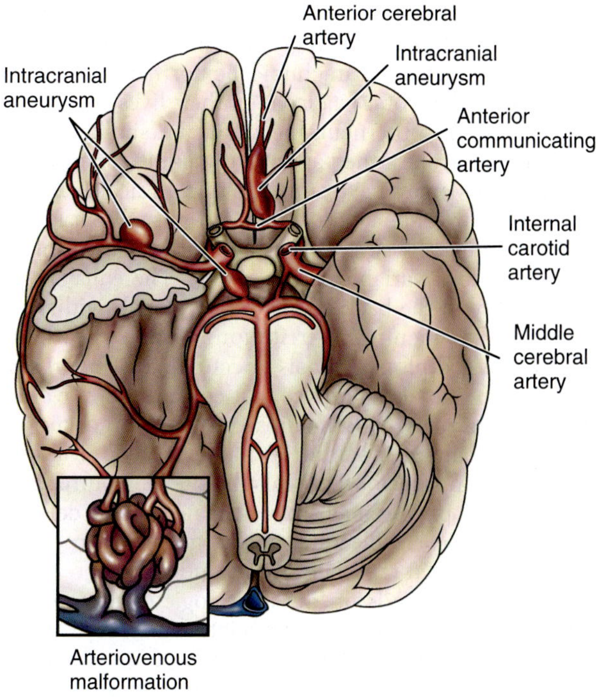

FIGURE 64-5. Common sites of intracranial aneurysms and an arteriovenous malformation.

Arteriovenous Malformations

Most AVMs are caused by an abnormality in embryonal development that leads to a tangle of arteries and veins in the brain that lacks a capillary bed (see Fig. 64-5). The absence of a capillary bed leads to dilation of the arteries and veins and eventual rupture. AVM is a common cause of hemorrhagic stroke in young people.

Subarachnoid Hemorrhage

A subarachnoid hemorrhage (hemorrhage into the subarachnoid space) may occur as a result of an AVM, intracranial aneurysm, trauma, dural arteriovenous fistulas, cavernomas, or hypertension. The most common causes are a leaking aneurysm in the area of the circle of Willis or a congenital AVM of the brain.

Clinical Manifestations

The patient with a hemorrhagic stroke can present with a wide variety of neurologic deficits, similar to the patient with ischemic stroke. The conscious patient most commonly reports a severe headache. A comprehensive assessment reveals the extent of the neurologic deficits. Many of the same motor, sensory, cranial nerve, cognitive, and other functions that are disrupted after ischemic stroke are also altered after a hemorrhagic stroke. Table 64-2 reviews the neurologic deficits frequently seen in patients with strokes. Table 64-3 compares the symptoms seen in right hemispheric stroke with those seen in left hemispheric stroke. Symptoms associated with subarachnoid hemorrhage include an atypical headache of sudden onset;

vomiting; neck stiffness; photophobia; hypertension; and cardiac arrhythmias. The most common complaint from a person who has a subarachnoid hemorrhage is that they are having "the worst headache of their lives."

In addition to the neurologic deficits (similar to those of ischemic stroke), the patient with an intracranial aneurysm or AVM may have some unique clinical manifestations. Rupture of an aneurysm or AVM usually produces a sudden, unusually severe headache and often loss of consciousness for a variable period of time. There may be pain and rigidity of the back of the neck (nuchal rigidity) and spine due to meningeal irritation. Visual disturbances (visual loss, diplopia, ptosis) occur if the aneurysm is adjacent to one of the nerves that control eye movement. Tinnitus, dizziness, and hemiparesis may also occur.

At times, an aneurysm or AVM leaks blood, leading to the formation of a clot that seals the site of rupture. In this instance, the patient may show little neurologic deficit. In other cases, severe bleeding occurs, resulting in cerebral damage, followed rapidly by coma and death.

Prognosis depends on the neurologic condition of the patient, the patient's age, associated diseases, and the extent and location of the hemorrhage or intracranial aneurysm. Subarachnoid hemorrhage from an aneurysm is a catastrophic event with significant morbidity and mortality. Chart 64-6 presents ethical issues related to the patient with a severe hemorrhagic stroke.

Assessment and Diagnostic Findings

Any patient with suspected stroke should undergo a CT scan or MRI to determine the type of stroke, the size and location of the hematoma, and the presence or absence of ventricular blood and hydrocephalus (Catangui, 2013). Cerebral angiography confirms the diagnosis of an intracranial aneurysm, AVM, or other vascular malformation. These tests show the location and size of the lesion and provide information about the affected arteries, veins, adjoining vessels, and vascular branches. Lumbar puncture is sometimes performed if there is no evidence of increased ICP, the CT scan results are negative, and subarachnoid hemorrhage must be confirmed. Once the CSF is obtained, it is examined for xanthochromia—blood. Lumbar puncture in the presence of increased ICP could result in brain stem herniation or rebleeding. When diagnosing a hemorrhagic stroke in a patient younger than 40 years of age, some clinicians obtain a toxicology screen for illicit drug use.

CHART 64-6

Ethics and Related Issues

What Are the Ethical Issues Related to DNR Orders After Severe Stroke?

SITUATION

An 85-year-old patient is admitted with a large intracerebral hemorrhage, severe neurologic deficits, and a past medical history of coronary artery bypass graft surgery, hypertension, atrial fibrillation, and gout. The patient does not have an advanced directive. The attending physician suggests a do-not-resuscitate (DNR) order to the family.

DILEMMA

The principle of autonomy for the patient (including death with dignity) conflicts with the principle of beneficence for the health care providers.

DISCUSSION

1. What arguments would you pose in favour of the DNR order?
2. What arguments would you pose against the DNR order?
3. Does the family have the right to refuse?
4. Is a DNR order an example of "patient abandonment" by health care workers, or an attempt to limit treatment and avoid CPR in a patient with an anticipated poor outcome?

Prevention

Primary prevention of hemorrhagic stroke is the best approach and includes managing hypertension and ameliorating other significant risk factors.

Blood pressure management of a daytime value of less than 139/80 mm Hg and a nighttime value of greater than 115/65 mm Hg along with healthy lifestyle choices significantly reduces the risk associated with intracerebral hemorrhage (Aronow, 2013; Canadian Hypertension Education Program [CHEP] recommendations for blood pressure management, 2014). Additional risk factors are increased age, male gender, and excessive alcohol intake. Stroke risk screenings provide an ideal opportunity to lower hemorrhagic stroke risk by identifying high-risk individuals or groups and educating patients and the community about recognition and prevention.

Complications

Potential complications of hemorrhagic stroke include rebleeding or hematoma expansion; cerebral vasospasm resulting in cerebral ischemia; hydrocephalus which results when free blood obstructs the reabsorption of cerebrospinal fluid (CSF) by the arachnoid villi; and seizures.

Cerebral Hypoxia and Decreased Blood Flow

Immediate complications of a hemorrhagic stroke include cerebral hypoxia, decreased cerebral blood flow, and extension of the area of injury. Providing adequate oxygenation of blood to the brain minimizes cerebral hypoxia. Brain function depends on delivery of oxygen to the tissues. Administering supplemental oxygen and maintaining the hemoglobin and hematocrit at acceptable levels will assist in maintaining tissue oxygenation.

Cerebral blood flow is dependent on the blood pressure, cardiac output, and integrity of cerebral blood vessels. Adequate hydration (IV fluids) must be ensured to reduce blood viscosity and improve cerebral blood flow. Extremes of hypertension or hypotension need to be avoided to prevent changes in cerebral blood flow and the potential for extending the area of injury.

A seizure can also compromise cerebral blood flow, resulting in further injury to the brain. Observing for seizure activity and initiating appropriate treatment are important components of care after a hemorrhagic stroke.

Vasospasm

The development of cerebral vasospasm (narrowing of the lumen of the involved cranial blood vessel) is a serious complication of subarachnoid hemorrhage and is a leading cause of morbidity and mortality in those who survive the initial subarachnoid hemorrhage. Of those with cerebral vasospasm, 15% to 20% die (Wuchner, Bakas, Adams, et al., 2012). The mechanism responsible for vasospasm is not clear, but it is associated with increasing amounts of blood in the subarachnoid cisterns and cerebral fissures, as visualized by CT scan. Monitoring for vasospasm may be performed through the use of bedside transcranial Doppler ultrasonography or follow-up cerebral angiography (Connolly, Rabinstein, Carhuapoma, et al., 2012).

Vasospasm most frequently occurs 7 to 10 days after initial hemorrhage (Connolly et al., 2012), when the clot undergoes lysis (dissolution), and the chance of rebleeding is increased. It leads to increased vascular resistance, which impedes cerebral blood flow and causes brain ischemia (delayed cerebral ischemia) and infarction. The signs and symptoms reflect the areas of the brain involved. Vasospasm is often heralded by a worsening headache, a decrease in level of consciousness (confusion, lethargy, and disorientation), or a new focal neurologic deficit (aphasia, hemiparesis).

Management of vasospasm remains difficult and controversial. It is believed that early surgery to clip the aneurysm prevents rebleeding and that removal of blood from the basal cisterns around the major cerebral arteries may prevent vasospasm.

Medication may be effective in the treatment and prevention of vasospasm. Based on the theory that vasospasm is caused by an increased influx of calcium into the cell, medication therapy may be used either to block or antagonize this action, or to prevent or reverse the action of vasospasm if already present. Nimodipine is the most studied calcium channel blocker for prevention of vasospasm in subarachnoid hemorrhage. An oral solution of nimodipine (Nymalize) was approved by the FDA in 2013; prior to this approval, the medication was only available in a liquid filled gel capsule (Nimotop). Current guidelines recommend that nimodipine be prescribed for all patients with subarachnoid hemorrhage (Connolly et al., 2012). This is currently the only drug approved by the FDA for the prevention and treatment of vasospasm in subarachnoid hemorrhage.

Another therapy for vasospasm and the resulting delayed cerebral ischemia, referred to as triple-H therapy, is aimed at minimizing the deleterious effects of the associated cerebral ischemia and includes: (1) fluid volume expanders (hypervolemia); (2) induced arterial hypertension; and (3) hemodilution. However, current research and guidelines now endorse euvolemia to prevent delayed cerebral ischemia and induced arterial hypertension for treatment of delayed cerebral ischemia (Connolly et al., 2012).

Increased Intracranial Pressure

An increase in ICP can occur after either an ischemic or a hemorrhagic stroke but almost always follows a subarachnoid hemorrhage, usually because of disturbed circulation of CSF caused by blood in the basal cisterns. Neurologic assessments are performed frequently, and if there is evidence of deterioration from increased ICP (due to cerebral edema, herniation, hydrocephalus, or vasospasm), CSF drainage may be instituted by ventricular catheter drainage. Mannitol may be administered to reduce ICP. When mannitol or hypertonic saline (3% or 5%) is used as a long-term measure to control ICP, dehydration and disturbances in electrolyte balance (hyponatremia or hypernatremia; hypokalemia or hyperkalemia) may occur.

Mannitol/hypertonic saline pulls water out of the brain tissue by osmosis and reduces total body water through diuresis. The patient is monitored for signs of dehydration and for rebound elevation of ICP. Hypertonic saline infusions significantly decrease water content in cerebral tissue by inducing a hypernatremic state. However, a recent study demonstrates that there is a rebound hypernatremic effect seen following the use of hyperosmolar therapies. This study reflects the importance of continued blood analysis of sodium levels throughout the hypertonic saline infusion (Ryu, Walcott, Kahle, et al., 2013).

Hypertension

Hypertension is the most common cause of intracerebral hemorrhage, and its treatment is critical. Specific goals for blood pressure management, which are individualized for each patient, remain controversial. New guidelines from the Canadian Hypertension Education Program (CHEP) (2014) recommend maintaining blood pressure at or below at 130/80 mm Hg. Elevated blood pressure during the initial phase of an acute intracerebral hemorrhage has a poorer health outcome for the stroke survivor (Rodriguez-Luna, Piñeiro, Rubiera, et al., 2013; Bautista, 2012).

Systolic blood pressure may be lowered to prevent rebleeding and hematoma enlargement. If blood pressure is elevated, antihypertensive therapy (labetalol [Trandate], nicardipine [Cardene], nitroprusside [Nitropress], hydralazine [Apresoline]) may be prescribed. During the administration of antihypertensives, arterial hemodynamic monitoring is important to detect and avoid a precipitous drop in blood pressure, which can produce brain ischemia. Stool softeners are used to prevent straining, which can elevate the blood pressure.

Medical Management

The goals of medical treatment for hemorrhagic stroke are to allow the brain to recover from the initial insult (bleeding), to prevent or minimize the risk of rebleeding, and to prevent or treat complications. Management may consist of bed rest with sedation to prevent agitation and stress, management of vasospasm, and surgical or medical treatment to prevent rebleeding. If the bleeding is caused by anticoagulation with warfarin (Coumadin), the INR may be corrected with fresh-frozen plasma and vitamin K. Because seizures can occur after intracerebral hemorrhage, anticonvulsant agents are often administered prophylactically for a brief period of time. Analgesic agents may be prescribed for head and neck pain. The patient is fitted with sequential compression devices or antiembolism stockings to prevent deep vein thrombosis (DVT). Fever should be treated. Hyperglycemia in the initial phase of a stroke is seen in nearly 48% of stroke patients. The concern associated with hyperglycemia during this phase is the inducement of a physiologic stress or inflammatory response. A study investigating the health outcomes of poststroke survivors who developed hyperglycemia in the early stages of their stroke revealed that nondiabetic persons experienced more negative health outcomes than their diabetic counterparts. This study concludes that efforts should be made to include hyperglycemia monitoring in the stroke protocol guidelines (Mitchell, Coates, Ryan, et al., 2012; Bautista, 2012).

After discharge most patients will require antihypertensive medications to decrease their risk of another intracerebral hemorrhage. Statins are also often prescribed.

Surgical Management

Surgical options for a ruptured aneurysm include surgical clipping or endovascular coil embolization (coiling). In a recent study of 2,143 patients with a definitive subarachnoid hemorrhage, half of the patients underwent coiling while the remaining half had the surgical clipping procedure done. Better success rates were evidenced in the clinical group who underwent the coiling procedure; however this group also exhibited increased rates of postprocedure rebleeding within the first year. This study highlights the existing controversy and the need for further research and randomized studies (Shivashankar, Miller, Jindal, et al., 2013; Bautista, 2012).

Surgical evacuation is most frequently accomplished via a craniotomy (see Chapter 65).

The patient with an intracranial aneurysm is prepared for surgical intervention as soon as his or her condition is considered stable. Surgical treatment of the patient with an unruptured aneurysm is an option. The goal of surgery is to prevent bleeding in an unruptured aneurysm or further bleeding in an already ruptured aneurysm. This objective is accomplished by isolating the aneurysm from its circulation or by strengthening the arterial wall. An aneurysm may be excluded from the cerebral circulation by means of a ligature or a clip across its neck. If this is not anatomically possible, the aneurysm can be reinforced by wrapping it with some substance to provide support and induce scarring.

Less invasive endovascular treatments are now being used for aneurysms. These procedures are performed by neurosurgeons or interventional neuroradiologists in neurointerventional radiology facilities. Two procedures include endovascular treatment (occlusion of the parent artery) and aneurysm coiling (obstruction of the aneurysm site with a coil). Although these techniques are associated with lower risks than intracranial surgery in general, secondary stroke and rupture of the aneurysm are still potential complications.

Postoperative complications include psychological symptoms (disorientation, amnesia, **Korsakoff's syndrome**, personality changes), intraoperative embolization, postoperative internal artery occlusion, fluid and electrolyte disturbances (from dysfunction of the neurohypophyseal system), and gastrointestinal bleeding.

Nursing Process

The Patient With a Hemorrhagic Stroke

Assessment

A complete neurologic assessment is performed initially and includes evaluation for the following:

- Altered level of consciousness
- Sluggish pupillary reaction
- Motor and sensory dysfunction
- Cranial nerve deficits (extraocular eye movements, facial droop, presence of ptosis, etc.)
- Speech difficulties and visual disturbance
- Headache and nuchal rigidity or other neurologic deficits

All patients should be monitored in the intensive care unit or a dedicated neurocritical care unit after an intracerebral or subarachnoid hemorrhage. Neurologic assessment findings are documented and reported as indicated. The frequency of these assessments varies depending on the patient's condition. Any changes in the patient's condition require reassessment and thorough documentation; changes should be reported immediately.

Alteration in level of consciousness often is the earliest sign of deterioration in a patient with a hemorrhagic stroke. Because nurses have the most frequent contact with patients, they are in the best position to detect subtle changes. Brief periods of confusion and mild drowsiness and slight slurring of speech may be early signs that the level of consciousness is deteriorating.

Nursing Priorities

Based on the assessment data, the patient's major nursing priorities may include the following:

- Ineffective tissue perfusion (cerebral)
- Disturbed sensory perception (aneurysm precautions)
- Anxiety

Collaborative Problems/ Potential Complications

Based on the assessment data, potential complications that may develop include the following:

- Vasospasm
- Seizures
- Hydrocephalus
- Rebleeding
- Electrolyte disorders

Planning and Goals

The goals for the patient may include improved cerebral tissue perfusion, relief of sensory and perceptual deprivation, relief of anxiety, and the absence of complications.

Nursing Interventions

Optimizing Cerebral Tissue Perfusion

The patient is closely monitored for neurologic deterioration resulting from recurrent bleeding, increasing ICP, or vasospasm. A neurologic flow record is maintained. The blood pressure, pulse, level of consciousness (an indicator of cerebral perfusion), pupillary responses, and motor function are checked hourly. Respiratory status is monitored, because a reduction in oxygen in areas of the brain with impaired autoregulation increases the chances of a cerebral infarction. Any changes are reported immediately.

IMPLEMENTING ANEURYSM PRECAUTIONS. Cerebral aneurysm precautions are implemented for the patient with a diagnosis of aneurysm to provide a nonstimulating environment, prevent increases in ICP, and prevent further bleeding. The patient is placed in a quiet, nonstressful environment, because activity, pain, and anxiety elevate the blood pressure, which increases the risk for bleeding. Visitors, except for family, are restricted.

The head of the bed is elevated 15 to 30 degrees to promote venous drainage and decrease ICP. Some neurosurgeons or intensivists, however, prefer that the patient remain flat to increase cerebral perfusion.

Any activity that suddenly increases the blood pressure or obstructs venous return is avoided. This includes the Valsalva manoeuvre, straining, forceful sneezing, pushing oneself up in bed, acute flexion or rotation of the head and neck (which compromises the jugular veins), and cigarette smoking. Any activity requiring exertion is contraindicated. The patient is instructed to exhale through the mouth during voiding or defecation to decrease strain. No enemas are permitted, but stool softeners and mild laxatives are prescribed. Both prevent constipation, which would cause an increase in ICP, as would enemas. Dim lighting is helpful, because photophobia (visual intolerance of light) is common. Coffee and tea, unless decaffeinated, are usually eliminated.

Antiembolism stockings or sequential compression devices may be prescribed to decrease the incidence of DVT resulting from immobility. The legs are observed for signs and symptoms of DVT (tenderness, redness, swelling, warmth, and edema), and abnormal findings are reported.

External stimuli are kept to a minimum. Visitors are restricted in an effort to keep the patient as quiet as possible. This precaution must be individualized based on the patient's condition and response to visitors. A sign indicating this restriction is placed on the door of the room, and the restrictions should be discussed with both patient and family. The purpose of aneurysm precautions are thoroughly explained to both the patient (if possible) and family.

Relieving Sensory Deprivation and Anxiety

Sensory stimulation is kept to a minimum for patients on aneurysm precautions. For patients who are awake, alert, and oriented, an explanation of the restrictions helps reduce the patient's sense of isolation.

Keeping the patient well informed of the plan of care provides reassurance and helps minimize anxiety. Appropriate reassurance also helps relieve the patient's fears and anxiety. The family also requires information and support.

Monitoring and Managing Potential Complications

VASOSPASM. The patient is assessed for signs of possible vasospasm: intensified headaches, a decrease in level of responsiveness (confusion, disorientation, lethargy), or evidence of aphasia or partial paralysis. These signs may develop several days after surgery or on the initiation of treatment and must be reported immediately. If vasospasm is diagnosed, calcium channel blockers or fluid volume expanders may be prescribed. If the vasospasm is severe the patient may undergo further endovascular procedures to ensure the cerebral vasculature stays patent.

SEIZURES. Seizure precautions are maintained for every patient who may be at risk for seizure activity. Should a seizure occur, maintaining the airway and preventing injury are the primary goals. Medication therapy is initiated at this time, if not already prescribed. The medication of choice for many years has been phenytoin (Dilantin). Recent studies demonstrate that phenytoin is perhaps not the best choice for seizure prophylaxis in patients with subarachnoid hemorrhage (intracerebral hemorrhage). Fever and diminishing scores on the NIHSS at 2 weeks poststroke are commonly seen in patients who are on phenytoin. Newer antiepileptic agents such as levetiracetam and lacosamide demonstrate reduced adverse effects and better health outcomes. More study is indicated in the area of seizure management (Rowe, Goodwin, Brophy, et al., 2013; Bautista, 2012).

HYDROCEPHALUS. Blood in the subarachnoid space or ventricles impedes the circulation of CSF, resulting in hydrocephalus. A CT scan that indicates dilated ventricles confirms the diagnosis. Hydrocephalus can occur within minutes after subarachnoid hemorrhage or several days (subacute) or up to several weeks (delayed) later. Symptoms vary according to the time of onset and may be nonspecific. Acute hydrocephalus is characterized by sudden onset of stupor or coma and is managed with a ventriculostomy drain to decrease ICP. Symptoms of subacute and delayed hydrocephalus include gradual onset of drowsiness, behavioural changes, and ataxic gait. A ventriculoperitoneal shunt is surgically placed to treat chronic hydrocephalus. Changes in patient responsiveness are reported immediately.

REBLEEDING. The rate of recurrent hemorrhage is approximately 2% after a primary intracerebral hemorrhage. Hypertension is the most serious risk factor, suggesting the importance of appropriate antihypertensive treatment. Rebleeding can also occur after the insertion of an external ventricular drain. If CSF is removed quickly the pressure within the brain changes and rebleeding may occur.

Aneurysm rebleeding occurs most frequently during the first 24 hours and up to 2 weeks after the initial hemorrhage and is considered a major complication. Symptoms of rebleeding include sudden severe headache, nausea, vomiting, decreased level of consciousness, and neurologic deficit. Rebleeding is confirmed by CT scan. Blood pressure is carefully maintained with medications. The most effective preventive treatment is to secure the aneurysm if the patient is a candidate for surgery or endovascular treatment. Rebleeding is rare as early intervention either surgically or via an endovascular procedure has become the standard of care.

ELECTROLYTE DISORDERS. The most common electrolyte imbalance in patients with subarachnoid hemorrhage is hyponatremia (Bautista, 2012). Hyponatremia occurs in upward of 50% of patients having suffered an aneurysmal subarachnoid hemorrhage (Bautista, 2012).

Laboratory data must be checked frequently, and hyponatremia (defined as a serum sodium concentration of less than 135 mmol/L) must be identified as early as possible. The patient's primary health care professional needs to be notified of a low serum sodium level that has persisted for 24 hours or longer. The patient is then evaluated for syndrome of inappropriate antidiuretic hormone (SIADH) or cerebral salt-wasting syndrome (CSW). (SIADH is described in Chapter 17.) CSW occurs when the kidneys are unable to conserve sodium and volume depletion results. The treatment most often is the use of hypertonic 3% saline.

Promoting Home, Community-Based, and Transitional Care

EDUCATING PATIENTS ABOUT SELF-CARE. The patient and family are provided with information

CHART 64-7

HOME CARE CHECKLIST • The Patient Recovering From a Stroke

At the completion of education, the patient and/or caregiver will be able to:

- State the impact of the stroke on physiologic functioning, ADLs, IADLs, roles, relationships, and spirituality
- State names, dose, side effects, frequency and schedule for all medications
- State how to contact all members of the treatment team (e.g., health care providers, home care professionals, rehabilitation team, and durable medical equipment and supply vendor)
- State changes in lifestyle (e.g., diet, ADLs, IADLs, activity) necessary for recovery and health maintenance as applicable
- Demonstrate environmental modifications and adaptive techniques for accomplishing activities of daily living
- Demonstrate home exercises, the use of splints or orthotics, proper positioning, and frequent repositioning
- Identify safety measures to prevent falls
- Identify holistic interventions for pain management (e.g., positioning, distraction)
- Describe procedures for maintaining skin integrity
- Demonstrate indwelling catheter care, if applicable. Describe a bowel and bladder elimination program as appropriate
- Verbalize dietary adjustments (e.g., thickened liquids, pureed diet, small frequent meals) during recovery
- Demonstrate swallowing techniques or care of enteral feeding tube
- Identify psychosocial consequences of stroke (e.g., depression, emotional lability, frustration, fatigue) and appropriate interventions
- Discuss measures to prevent subsequent strokes
- Identify potential complications and discuss measures to prevent them (blood clots, aspiration, pneumonia, urinary tract infection, fecal impaction, skin breakdown, contracture)
- Relate how to reach primary provider with questions or complications
- State time and date of follow-up medical appointments, therapy, and testing
- Identify resources and other sources of support (e.g., friends, relatives, faith community, stroke support groups, caregiver support)
- Identify the need for health promotion, disease prevention, and screening activities
- Identify appropriate recreational or diversional activities

ADL, activities of daily living; IADL, independent activities of daily living.

that will enable them to cooperate with the care and restrictions required during the acute phase of hemorrhagic stroke and to prepare them to return home. Patient and family teaching includes information about the causes of hemorrhagic stroke and its possible consequences. In addition, the patient and family are informed about the medical treatments that are implemented, including surgical intervention if warranted, and the importance of interventions taken to prevent and detect complications (i.e., aneurysm precautions, close monitoring of the patient). Depending on the presence and severity of neurologic impairment and other complications resulting from the stroke, the patient may be transferred to a rehabilitation unit or centre for additional patient and family teaching about strategies to regain self-care ability. Teaching addresses the use of assistive devices or modification of the home environment to help the patient live with the disability. Modifications of the home may be required to provide a safe environment.

CONTINUING AND TRANSITIONAL CARE. The acute and rehabilitation phase of care focuses on obvious needs, issues, and deficits for the patient with a hemorrhagic stroke. The patient and family are reminded of the importance of following recommendations to prevent further hemorrhagic stroke and keeping follow-up appointments with health care providers for monitoring of risk factors. Referral for home care may be warranted to assess the home environment and the ability of the patient and to ensure that the patient and family are able to manage at home. Home visits provide opportunities to monitor the physical and psychological status of the patient and the ability of the family to cope with any alterations in the patient's status. In addition, the home care nurse reminds the patient and family of the importance of continuing health promotion and screening practices. Chart 64-7 lists teaching points for the patient recovering from a stroke.

Evaluation

Expected patient outcomes may include the following:

1. Demonstrates intact neurologic status and appropriate vital signs and respiratory patterns
   a. Is alert and oriented to time, place, and person
   b. Demonstrates usual speech patterns and intact cognitive processes
   c. Demonstrates equal strength, movement, and sensation of all four extremities
   d. Exhibits expected deep tendon reflexes and pupillary responses
2. Demonstrates appropriate sensory perceptions
   a. States rationale for aneurysm precautions
   b. Exhibits clear thought processes
3. Exhibits reduced anxiety level
   a. Is less restless
   b. Exhibits absence of physiologic indicators of anxiety (e.g., has appropriate vital signs including respiratory rate; absence of excessive, fast speech)
4. Is free of complications
   a. Exhibits absence of vasospasm
   b. Exhibits expected vital signs and neuromuscular activity without seizures
   c. Verbalizes understanding of seizure precautions
   d. Exhibits appropriate mental status and expected motor and sensory status
   e. Reports no visual changes

Critical Thinking Exercises

1 A 72-year-old male is in the ED being evaluated for a suspected stroke. Identify the priorities, approach, and techniques you would use to provide care for him. What are specific time goals for obtaining a head CT scan? If he is eligible for t-PA, how will your priorities change? If his stroke is a hemorrhagic stroke, how will your approach, techniques, and priorities change?

2 You are caring for a patient after a large ischemic stroke. The patient has hemiplegia and is beginning to experience shoulder pain on the side affected by the stroke. Identify the priority nursing interventions that can be implemented to prevent shoulder pain. What education can you provide to the patient for interventions that can be done at home once discharged?

3 A 69-year-old woman has experienced a brainstem stroke. She has just arrived to the nursing unit from the ED and you are her nurse. She has not had a swallow assessment yet. What is the time goal for obtaining an evaluation of her swallowing function? Evaluate the strength of the evidence to support nurses performing dysphagia screening.

REFERENCES AND SELECTED READINGS

Books

Bader, M., Littlejohns, L. R., & Olson, D. (2016). *AANN core curriculum for neuroscience nursing* (6th ed.). Chicago, IL: American Association of Neuroscience Nurses.

Canadian Hypertension Education Program. (2014). *The 2014 Canadian hypertension education program recommendations*. Markham, ON: Author. Retrieved from https://www.hypertension.ca/images/CHEP_2014/2014_CHEPRecsFullVersion_EN_HCP1000.pdf

Hickey, J. V. (2013). *The clinical practice of neurological & neurosurgical nursing* (7th ed.). Philadelphia, PA: Wolters Kluwer Health/Lippincott Williams & Wilkins.

Hickey, J. V. (2014). *The clinical practice of neurological & neurosurgical nursing* (7th ed.). Philadelphia, PA: Lippincott Williams & Wilkins.

Karch, A. (2014). *2015 Lippincott's nursing drug guide*. Philadelphia, PA: Lippincott Williams & Wilkins.

Journals and Electronic Documents

Almekhlafi, M., Menon, B., Freiheit, E., et al. (2013). A meta-analysis of observational intra-arterial stroke therapy studies using the Merci Device, Penumbra System, and Retrievable Stents. *American Journal of Neuroradiology*, *34*, 140–145.

Anderson, J. (2016). Acute ischemic stroke: The golden hour. *Nursing Critical Care*, *11*(3), 28–36.

Appel, L. (2014). Reducing sodium intake to prevent stroke. *Stroke*, *45*, 909–911.

Aronow, W. (2013). Hypertension-related stroke prevention in the elderly. *Current Hypertension Reports*, *15*, 582–589.

Aycock, D. M., & Clark, P. C. (2016). Incongruence between perceived long-term risk and actual risk of stroke in rural African Americans. *Journal of Neuroscience Nursing, 48*(1), 35–41.

Bautista, C. (2012). Unresolved issues in the management of aneurysmal subarachnoid hemorrhage. *AACN Advanced Critical Care, 23*(2), 175–185.

Bentz, B. (2015). Nonvitamin K antagonist oral anticoagulants in everyday practice: Stroke prevention in atrial fibrillation and treatment of venous thromboembolism. *Journal of the American Association of Nurse Practitioners, 27*(12), 721–731.

Brainin, M., & Zorowitz, R. (2013). Advances in stroke: Recovery and rehabilitation. *Stroke, 44*(2), 311–313.

Bugincourt, J., Hamy, O., Canaple, S., et al. (2014). Impaired sexual activity in young ischaemic stroke patients: An observational study. *European Journal of Neurology, 21*, 140–146.

Burr, J., Shephard, R., & Zehr, E. (2012). Physical activity after stroke and spinal cord injury. *Canadian Family Physician, 58*, 1236–1239.

Casaubon, L. K., Suddes, M. (2013). Hyperacute stroke care. In Lindsay M.P., Gubitz G., Bayley M., et al. (Eds.) on behalf of the Canadian Stroke Best Practices and Standards Advisory Committee. *Canadian Best Practice Recommendations for Stroke Care.* Ottawa: Canadian Stroke Network and Heart and Stroke Foundation of Canada. Retrieved from http://www.strokebestpractices.ca/wp-content/uploads/2010/10/Ch3_SBP2013_Hyper-Acute-_23MAY13_EN_-FINAL5.pdf

Catangui, E. (2013). Knowledge and understanding of CT imaging in stroke: A case study approach. *British Journal of Neuroscience Nursing, 9*(5), 240–246.

Clemens, A., Ryn, J., Sennewald, R., et al. (2012). Switching from enoxaparin to dabigatran etexilate: Pharmacokinetics, pharmacodynamics, and safety profile. *European Journal of Clinical Pharmacology, 68*, 607–616.

Conference Board of Canada. (2014). Health, health care and wellness. Retrieved from http://www.conferenceboard.ca/topics/health/default.aspx

Connolly, E., Rabinstein, A., Carhuapoma, J., et al. (2012). Guidelines for the management of aneurysmal subarachnoid hemorrhage: A guideline for healthcare professionals from the American Heart Association/American Stroke Association. *Stroke, 43*(6), 1711–1737.

Coutts, S. B., & Kelloway, L. (2012). Chapter 2: Prevention of stroke. *Canadian Best Practice Recommendations for Stroke Care*. pp. 1–69.

Creasy, K. R., Lutz, B. J., Young, M. E., et al. (2015). Clinical implications of family-centered care in stroke rehabilitation. *Rehabilitation Nursing, 40*(6), 349–359.

Czernuszenko, A., & Czlonkowska, A. (2009). Risk factors for falls in stroke patients during inpatient rehabilitation. *Clinical Rehabilitation, 23*, 176–188.

Dawes, M. (2013). Why is controlling blood pressure after stroke so difficult? *Canadian Medical Association Journal, 185*(1), 11–12.

Demchuk, A., & Bal, S. (2012). Thrombolytic therapy for acute ischaemic stroke: What can we do to improve outcomes? *Current Opinion in Neurology, 72*(14), 1833–1845.

Denno, M., Gillard, P., Graham, G., et al. (2013). Anxiety and depression associated with caregiver burden in caregivers of stroke survivors with spasticity. *Archives of Physical Medicine and Rehabilitation, 94*, 1731–1736.

Eissa, A., Krass, I., & Bajorek, B. (2012). Barriers to the utilization of thrombolysis for acute ischemic stroke. *Clinical Pharmacology and Therapeutics, 37*, 399–409.

El-Kafy, E., Elshemy, S., & Alghamdi, M. (2014). Effect of constraint-induced therapy on upper limb functions: A randomized control trial. *Scandinavian Journal of Occupational Therapy, 21*, 11–23.

Ennen, K. A. (2013). Taking a second look at stroke in women. *American Nurse Today, 8*(5), 12–15.

Flaster, M., Meresh, E., Rao, M., et al. (2013). Central poststroke pain: Current diagnosis and treatment. *Topics in Stroke Rehabilitation, 20*(2), 116–123.

Flaster, M., Sharma, A., & Rao, M. (2013). Poststroke depression: A review emphasizing the role of prophylactic treatment and synergy with treatment for motor recovery. *Topics in Stroke Rehabilitation, 20*(2), 139–150.

García-Rodríguez, L., Gaist, D., Morton, J., et al. (2013). Antithrombotic drugs and risk of hemorrhagic stroke in the general population. *American Academy of Neurology, 81*, 566–574.

Gensicke, H., Zumbrunn, T., Jongen, L., et al. (2013). Characteristics of ischemic brain lesions after stenting or endarterectomy for symptomatic carotid artery stenosis: Results from the international carotid stenting study-magnetic resonance imaging substudy. *Stroke, 44*, 80–86.

Gilad, R. (2012). Management of seizures following a stroke: What are the options? *Drugs and Aging, 29*(7), 533–538.

Government of Canada (2017). Stroke in Canada Highlights From The Canadian Chronic Disease Surveillance System. Retrieved from https://www.canada.ca/content/dam/phac-aspc/documents/services/publications/diseases-conditions/stroke-vasculaires/stroke-vasculaires-canada-eng.pdf

Grant, C., Goldsmith, C., & Anton, H. (2014). Inpatient stroke rehabilitation lengths of stay in Canada derived from the national rehabilitation reporting system, 2008 and 2009. *Archives of Physical Medicine and Rehabilitation, 95*, 74–78.

Gupta, N., Pandia, M., & Dash, H. (2013). Research studies that have influenced practice of neuroanesthesiology in recent years: A literature review. *Indian Journal of Anaesthesia, 57*(2), 117–126.

Hann, S., Chalouhi, N., Starke, R., et al. (2013). Comparison of neurologic and radiographic outcomes for Solitaire versus Merci/Penumbra systems for acute stroke intervention. *BioMed Research International*, 1–9.

Heart and Stroke Foundation. (2013). Stroke prevention. Retrieved from http://www.heartandstroke.com/site/c.ikIQLcMWJtE/b.3483939/k.16FB/Stroke__Stroke_prevention_and_risk_factors.htm

Heart and Stroke Foundation. (2014). Stroke prevention. Retrieved from http://www.heartandstroke.com/site/c.ikIQLcMWJtE/b.3483939/k.16FB/Stroke__Stroke_prevention_and_risk_factors.htm

Heart and Stroke Foundation. (2014). 2014 stroke report. Together against a rising tide: Advancing stroke systems of care. Retrieved from https://www.heartandstroke.ca/-/media/pdf-files/canada/stroke-report/hsf-stroke-report-2014.ashx?la=en&hash=4FD2B18A0EEDA2A193EFDBBDB983F23B1FBD570D

Heart and Stroke Foundation of Canada (2018). https://www.strokebest-practices.ca/-/media/1-stroke-best-practices/resources/patient-resources/signs-of-stroke-and-heart-attack-bookmark-en.ashx

Hemphill, J. C., Greenberg, S. M., Anderson, C. S., et al. (2015). Guidelines for the management of spontaneous intracerebral hemorrhage: A guideline for healthcare professionals from the American Heart Association/American Stroke Association. *Stroke, 46*(7), 2032–2060.

Hussain, S., Zaidat, O., & Fitzsimmons, B. (2012). The penumbra system for mechanical thrombectomy in endovascular acute ischemic stroke therapy. *American Academy of Neurology, 79*(Supp 1), 135–140.

Jauch, E. C., Saver, J. L., Adams, H. P., et al. (2013). Guidelines for the early management of patients with ischemic stroke: A guideline from the American Heart Association/American stroke Association. *Stroke, 44*(1), 870–947.

Kaatz, S., Kouides, P. A., Garcia, D. A., et al. (2012). Guidance on the emergent reversal of oral thrombin and factor Xa inhibitors. *American Journal of Hematology, 87*(Suppl. 1), S141–S145.

Keating, G. (2013). Apixaban: A review of its use for reducing the risk of stroke and system embolism in patients with nonvalvular atrial fibrillation. *Drugs, 73*, 825–843.

Kernan, W. N., Ovbiagele, B., Black, H. R., et al. (2014). Guidelines for the prevention of stroke in patients with stroke and transient ischemic attack: A guideline for healthcare professionals from the American Heart Association/American Stroke Association. *Stroke, 45*(7), 2160–2236.

Kokubo, Y. (2012). Traditional risk factor management for stroke: A never-ending challenge for health behaviors of diet and physical activity. *Current Opinion in Neurology, 25*(1), 11–17.

Kouwenhoven, S., Kirkevold, M., Engedal, K., et al. (2011). 'Living a life in shades of grey': Experiencing depressive symptoms in the acute phase after stroke. *Journal of Advanced Nursing, 68*(8), 1726–1737.

Lackland, D. (2013). Hypertension: Joint national committee on detection, evaluation, and treatment of high blood pressure guidelines. *Current Opinion in Neurology, 26*(1), 8–12.

Lahr, M., van der Zee, D., Luijckx, G., et al. (2013). A simulation-based approach for improving utilization of thrombolysis in acute brain infarction. *Medical Care, 51*(12), 1101–1105.

Lee, J., King, C., Stradling, D., et al. (2014). Influence of hematoma location on acute mortality after intracerebral hemorrhage. *Journal of Neuroimaging, 24*, 131–136.

Lord, A., Fernandez, L., Schmidt, J., et al. (2012). Effect of rebleeding on the course and incidence of vasospasm after subarachnoid hemorrhage. *Neurology, 78*, 31–37.

Malhotra, K., Conners, J., Lee, V., et al. (2014). Relative changes in transcranial Doppler velocities are inferior to absolute thresholds in prediction of symptomatic vasospasm after subarachnoid hemorrhage. *Journal of Stroke and Cerebrovascular Diseases, 23*(1), 31–36.

Mandel, M., Fonoff, E., Bor-Seng-Shu, E., et al. (2012). Neurogenic neuroprotection: Clinical perspectives. *Functional Neurology, 27*(4), 207–216.

Manning, N., Campbell, B., Oxley, T., et al. (2014). Acute ischemic stroke: Time, penumbra, and reperfusion. *Stroke, 45*, 640–644.

Martini, S., Flaherty, M., Brown, W., et al. (2012). Risk factors for intracerebral hemorrhage differ according to hemorrhage location. *Neurology, 79*, 2275–2282.

Mehta, S., Teasell, R., & Foley, N. (2013). Painful hemiplegic Shoulder. In R. Teasell (Ed.). *Evidence based review of stroke rehabilitation*. http://www.ebrsr.com/sites/default/files/Chapter11_HemiplegicShoulder_FINAL__16ed.pdf

Meschia, J. F., Bushnell, C., Boden-Albala, B., et al. (2014). Guidelines for the primary prevention of stroke: A statement for healthcare professionals from the American Heart Association/American Stroke Association. *Stroke, 45*(12), 3754–3832.

Middleton, S., Grimley, R., & Alexandrov, A. W. (2015). Triage, treatment, and transfer: Evidence-based clinical practice recommendations and models of nursing care for the first 72 hours of admission to hospital for acute stroke. *Stroke, 46*(2), e18–e25.

Miller, E. L., Murray, L., Richards, L., Zorowitz, R. D., Bakas, T., Clark, P., & Billinger, S. A. (2010). Comprehensive overview of nursing and interdisciplinary rehabilitation care of the stroke patient: A scientific statement from the American Heart Association. *Stroke, 41*(10), 2402–2448.

Miller, E. T., & Summers, D. (2014). Update on transient ischemic attack nursing care. *Stroke, 45*(5), e71–e73.

Mitchell, E., Coates, V., Ryan, A., et al. (2012). Hyperglycaemia monitoring and management in stroke care: Policy versus practice. *Diabetic Medicine, 29*, 1108–1114.

Mozaffarian, D., Benjamin, E. J., Go, A. S., et al. (2016). AHA statistical update: Heart disease and stroke statistics—2016 update: A report from the American Heart Association. *Circulation, 133*(4), e38–e360.

NINDS, T. (1995). The National Institute of Neurological Disorders and Stroke rt-PA Stroke Study Group. Tissue plasminogen activator for acute ischemic stroke. *N Engl J Med, 333*(24), 1581–1587.

Powers, W. J., Derdeyn, C. P., Biller, J., Coffey, C. S., Hoh, B. L., Jauch, E. C.,...& Meschia, J. F. (2015). 2015 American Heart Association/American Stroke Association focused update of the 2013 guidelines for the early management of patients with acute ischemic stroke regarding endovascular treatment: A guideline for healthcare professionals from the American Heart Association/American Stroke Association. *Stroke, 46*(10), 3020–3035.

Puhr, M. I., & Thompson, H. J. (2015). The use of transitional care models in patients with stroke. *Journal of Neuroscience Nursing, 47*(4), 223–234.

Qian, F., Fonarow, G., Smith, E., et al. (2013). Racial and ethnic differences in outcomes in older patients with acute ischemic stroke. *Circulation: Cardiovascular Quality and Outcomes, 6*, 284–292.

Rist, P., Buring, J., Kase, C., et al. (2013). Effect of low-dose aspirin on functional outcome from cerebral vascular events in women. *Stroke, 44*, 432–436.

Rodriguez-Luna, D., Piñeiro, S., Rubiera, M., et al. (2013). Impact of blood pressure changes and course on hematoma growth in acute intracerebral hemorrhage. *European Journal of Neurology, 20*, 1277–1283.

Roh, J., Rymer, W., Perreault, E., et al. (2012). Alterations in upper limb muscle synergy structure in chronic stroke survivors. *Journal of Neurophysiology, 109*, 768–781.

Rosenbaum, T., Vadas, D., & Kalichman, L. (2014). Sexual function in post-stroke patients: Considerations for rehabilitation. *The Journal of Sexual Medicine, 11*, 15–21.

Rosso, C., & Samson, Y. (2014). The ischemic penumbra: The location rather than the volume of recovery determines outcome. *Current Opinion in Neurology, 27*(1), 35–41.

Rowe, A., Goodwin, H., Brophy, G., et al. (2013). Seizure prophylaxis in neurocritical care: A review of evidence-based support. *Pharmacotherapy*, 1–13.

Ryu, J., Walcott, B., Kahle, K., et al. (2013). Induced and sustained hypernatremia for the prevention and treatment of cerebral edema following brain injury. *Neurocritical Care Journal, 19*, 222–231.

Sander, R. (2013). Prevention and treatment of acute ischemic stroke. *Nursing Older People, 25*(8), 34–38.

Saposnik, G., Guzik, A., Reeves, M., et al. (2012). Stroke prognostication using age and NIH stroke scale. *American Academy of Neurology, 80*, 21–28.

Saver, J. L. (2006). Time is brain quantified. *Stroke, 37*(1), 263–266.

Scheitz, J., Seiffge, D., Tütüncü, S., et al. (2014). Dose-related effects of statins on symptomatic intracerebral hemorrhage and outcome after thrombolysis for ischemic stroke. *Stroke, 45*, 509–514.

Shackley, P., Shaw, L., Price, C., et al. (2012). Cost-effectiveness of treating upper limb spasticity due to stroke with botulinum toxin type A: Results from the botulinum toxin for the upper limb after stroke (BoTULS) trial. *Toxins, 4*, 1415–1426.

Shah, S., Tartaro, C., Chew, F., et al. (2013). Skilled nursing facility functional rehabilitation outcome: Analyses of stroke admissions. *International Journal of Therapy and Rehabilitation, 20*(7), 352–360.

Shivashankar, R., Miller, R., Jindal, G., et al. (2013). Treatment of cerebral aneurysms—surgical clipping or endovascular coiling: The guiding principles. *Seminars in Neurology, 33*(05), 476–487.

Siegler, J., Boehme, A., Kumar, A., et al. (2013). What change in the National Institute of Health Stroke Scale should define neurologic deterioration in acute ischemic stroke? *Journal of Stroke and Cerebravascular Diseases, 22*(5), 675–682.

Smith, M. (2012). Management of hemiplegic shoulder pain following stroke. *Nursing Standard, 26*(44), 35–44.

Specogna, A., Patten, S., Turin, T., et al. (2013). The reliability and sensitivity of the National Institute of Health Stroke Scale for spontaneous intracerebral hemorrhage in an uncontrolled setting. *PLOS ONE, 8*(12), 1–4.

Statistics Canada. (2013). Leading causes of death in Canada. Retrieved from http://www.statcan.gc.ca/pub/84-215-x/2012001/hl-fs-eng.htm

Statistics Canada. (2017). Table 102–0561—Leading causes of death, total population, by age group and sex, Canada. CANSIM (death database) [Internet]. Ottawa (Ontario): Statistics Canada; 2017 Mar 8 [cited 2017 June 6]. Available at: http://www5.statcan.gc.ca/cansim/a05?lang=eng&id=1020561

Switzer, J., Demaerschalk, B., Xie, J., et al. (2012). Cost-effectiveness of hub-and-spoke telestroke networks for the management of acute ischemic stroke from the hospitals' perspectives. *Circulation: Cardiovascular Quality and Outcome, 6*, 18–26.

Teasell, R., Foley, N., Pereira, S., Sequeira, K., & Miller, T. (2012). Evidence to practice: Botulinum toxin in the treatment of spasticity post stroke. *Topics in stroke rehabilitation, 19*(2), 115–121.

The Canadian Cardiovascular Society (2016). 2016 Canadian Cardiovascular Society Guidelines for the Management of Dyslipidemia for the Prevention of Cardiovascular Disease in the Adult. https://www.onlinecjc.ca/article/S0828-282X(16)30732-2/pdf

Thompson, B. G., Brown, R. J., Amin-Hanjani, S., et al. (2015). Guidelines for the management of patients with unruptured intracranial aneurysms: A guideline for healthcare professionals from the American Heart Association/American Stroke Association. *Stroke, 46*(8), 2368–2400.

Treat-Jacobson, D. J., Rich, K., DeVeaux, T., et al. (2013). Society for vascular nursing clinical practice guideline (CPG) for carotid artery stenting. *Journal of Vascular Nursing, 31*(1), 32–55.

Turner, J. (2012). Environmental factors of hospitalisation which contribute to post-stroke depression during rehabilitation for over 65 year olds. *Journal of the Australasian Rehabilitation Nurses Association, 15* (1), 11–15.

Ward, I., Pivko, S., Brooks, G., et al. (2011). Validity of the stroke rehabilitation assessment of movement scale in acute rehabilitation: A comparison with the Functional Independence Measure and Stroke Impact Scale-16. *American Academy of Physical Medicine and Rehabilitation, 3*(11), 1013–1021.

Weiss, A., Beloosesky, Y., Kenett, R., et al. (2013). Systolic blood pressure during acute stroke is associated with functional status and long-term mortality in the elderly. *Stroke, 44*, 2434–2440.

Wijdicks, E. M., Sheth, K. N., Carter, B. S., et al. (2014). Recommendations for the management of cerebral and cerebellar infarction with swelling: A statement for healthcare professionals from the American Heart Association/American Stroke Association. *Stroke, 45*(4), 1222–1238.

Wuchner, S., Bakas, T., Adams, G., et al. (2012). Nursing interventions and assessments for aneurysmal subarachnoid hemorrhage patients: A mixed methods study involving practicing nurses. *Journal of Neuroscience Nursing, 44*(4), 177–185.

Zanichkowsky, R., Nascimento, J. A., McCune, M., et al. (2016). Where does the time go? The effect of protocols for stroke last known well documentation on intravenous recombinant tissue plasminogen activator delivery in the northeast. *Journal of Neuroscience Nursing, 48*(2), 71–74.

Zheng, L., & Alexander, S. A. (2015). Current evidence in the management of poststroke hemiplegic shoulder pain: A review. *Journal of Neuroscience Nursing, 47*(1), 10–19.

Resources

American Association of Neuroscience Nurses: http://www.aann.org

American Stroke Association, a Division of the American Heart Association: http://www.strokeassociation.org

Canadian Association of Neuroscience Nurses: http://www.cann.ca/

Canadian Council of Cardiovascular Nurses: http://www.cccn.ca

Canadian Hypertension Education Program (CHEP) Recommendations: @http://www.hypertension.ca

Canadian Stroke Network: http://www.Canadian stroke network.ca

Heart and Stroke Foundation of Canada: http://www.heartandstroke.ca

National Institute of Neurological Disorders and Stroke: http://www.ninds.nih.gov

National Stroke Association: http://www.stroke.org

65 Management of Patients With Neurologic Trauma

Adapted by Ron Prince

Learning Objectives

On completion of this chapter, the learner will be able to:

1. Describe the mechanisms of injury, clinical signs and symptoms, diagnostic testing, and treatment options for patients with traumatic brain and spinal cord injuries.
2. Describe the nursing management of patients with brain injury.
3. Use the nursing process as a framework for care of patients with traumatic brain injury.
4. Identify the population at risk for spinal cord injury.
5. Describe the clinical features and management of the patient with neurogenic shock.
6. Discuss the pathophysiology of autonomic dysreflexia and describe the appropriate nursing interventions.
7. Use the nursing process as a framework for care of patients with spinal cord injury.

Trauma involving the central nervous system can be life-threatening. Even if it is not life-threatening, brain and **spinal cord injury** (SCI) may result in major physical and psychological dysfunction and can alter the patient's life completely. Neurologic trauma affects the patient, the family, the health care system, and society as a whole because of its major sequelae and the costs of acute rehabilitation and long-term care of patients with trauma to the brain and spinal cord.

Head Injuries

Head injury is a broad classification that includes injury to the scalp, skull, or brain. Head injury is a broad classification that encompasses any damage to the head as a result of trauma. A head injury does not necessarily mean a brain injury is present. **Traumatic brain injury** (TBI) or craniocerebral trauma describes an injury that is the result of an external force and is of sufficient magnitude to interfere with daily life and prompts the seeking of treatment.

Catastrophic head injuries account for one half of all trauma deaths and one half of trauma cases resulting in major disability. Head injuries in Canada are a significant portion of the burden of neurologic conditions. A head injury may lead to conditions ranging from scalp lacerations or mild **concussion** to coma and death; the most serious form is known as a TBI. The most common causes of TBIs for people under 75 years of age are motor vehicle crashes (50%), while violence, sports, and other causes make up the remainder. People at highest risk for TBI are those in the 15- to 19-year age group. Males are twice as likely as females to sustain a TBI. The best approach to head injury is prevention (Chart 65-1).

Pathophysiology

Research suggests that not all brain damage occurs at the moment of impact. Damage to the brain from traumatic injury takes two forms: **primary injury** and **secondary injury**. Primary injury is defined as the consequence of direct contact to the head/brain during the instant of initial injury, causing extracranial focal injuries (e.g., **contusions**, lacerations, external hematomas, skull fractures), as well as possible focal brain injuries from sudden movement of the brain within the cranial vault (e.g., subdural hematomas [SDHs], concussion, diffuse axonal injury [DAI]). The greatest opportunity for decreasing TBI is the implementation of prevention strategies (see Chart 65-1).

CHART 65-1

Health Promotion: Preventing Head and Spinal Cord Injuries

- Advise drivers to obey traffic laws, and to avoid speeding or driving when under the influence of drugs or alcohol.
- Advise all drivers and passengers to wear seat belts and shoulder harnesses. Children younger than 12 years of age should be restrained in an age/size-appropriate system in the back seat.
- Caution passengers against riding in the back of pickup trucks.
- Advise motorcyclists, scooter riders, bicyclists, skateboarders, and roller skaters to wear helmets.
- Promote educational programs that are directed toward violence and suicide prevention in the community.
- Provide water safety instruction.
- Teach patients steps that can be taken to prevent falls, particularly in older adults.
- Advise athletes to use protective devices. Recommend that coaches be educated in proper coaching techniques.
- Advise owners of firearms to keep them locked in a secure area where children cannot access them.

Secondary injury evolves over the ensuing hours and days after the initial injury and results from inadequate delivery of nutrients and oxygen to the cells. Identification, prevention, and treatment of secondary injury are the main foci of early management of severe TBI. Contributors to this process include intracranial pathologic processes such as intracranial hemorrhage, cerebral edema, intracranial hypertension, hyperemia, seizures, and vasospasm (Bader, Littlejohns, & Olson, 2016; Hickey, 2014). Systemic effects from hypotension, hyperthermia, hypoxia, hypercarbia, infection, electrolyte imbalances, and anemia can also be factors which add to the complex biochemical, metabolic, and inflammatory changes that further compromise an injured brain (Bader et al., 2016; Hickey, 2014).

The Monro–Kellie hypothesis, also known as the Monro–Kellie doctrine, explains the dynamic equilibrium of cranial contents. The cranial vault contains three main components: brain, blood, and cerebrospinal fluid (CSF). According to the Monro–Kellie hypothesis, the cranial vault is a closed system, and if one of the three components increases in volume, at least one of the other two must decrease in volume or the pressure will increase. Any bleeding or swelling within the skull increases the volume of contents within the skull and therefore causes increased intracranial pressure (ICP). If the pressure increases enough, it can cause displacement of the brain through or against the rigid structures of the skull. This causes restriction of blood flow to the brain, decreasing oxygen delivery and waste removal. Cells within the brain become anoxic and cannot metabolize properly, producing ischemia, infarction, irreversible brain damage, and eventually brain death (see Fig. 65-1).

Scalp Injury

Isolated scalp trauma is generally classified as a minor injury. Because its many blood vessels constrict poorly, the scalp bleeds profusely when injured. Trauma may result in an abrasion (brush wound), contusion, laceration, or hematoma beneath the layers of tissue of the scalp (subgaleal hematoma). A large avulsion (tearing away) of the scalp may be potentially life-threatening and is a true emergency due to excessive blood loss. Diagnosis of a

Glossary

autonomic dysreflexia: a life-threatening emergency in spinal cord injury patients that causes a hypertensive emergency; also called autonomic hyperreflexia

complete spinal cord lesion: a condition that involves total loss of sensation and voluntary muscle control below the level of the lesion

concussion: a temporary loss of neurologic function with no apparent structural damage to the brain

contusion: bruising of the brain

halo vest: external traction device that encircles the head like a halo and stabilizes the cervical spine

head injury: an injury to the scalp, skull, and/or brain

incomplete spinal cord lesion: a condition in which there is preservation of the sensory or motor fibres, or both, below the lesion

neurogenic bladder: bladder dysfunction that results from a disorder or dysfunction of the nervous system; may result in either urinary retention or incontinence

paraplegia: paralysis of the lower extremities with dysfunction of the bowel and bladder from a lesion in the thoracic, lumbar, or sacral region of the spinal cord

primary injury: initial damage to the brain that results from the traumatic event

secondary injury: an insult to the brain subsequent to the original traumatic event

spinal cord injury (SCI): an injury to the spinal cord, vertebral column, supporting soft tissue, or intervertebral disks caused by trauma

tetraplegia: varying degrees of paralysis of both arms and legs, with dysfunction of bowel and bladder from a lesion of the cervical segments of the spinal cord; formerly called *quadriplegia*

transection: severing of the spinal cord itself; transection can be complete (all the way through the cord) or incomplete (partially through)

traumatic brain injury: an injury to the skull or brain that is severe enough to interfere with normal functioning

traumatic brain injury, closed (blunt): occurs when the head accelerates and then rapidly decelerates or collides with another object and brain tissue is damaged, but there is no opening through the skull and dura

traumatic brain injury, open (penetrating): occurs when an object penetrates the skull, enters the brain, and damages the soft brain tissue in its path (penetrating injury), or when blunt trauma to the head is so severe that it opens the scalp, skull, and dura to expose the brain

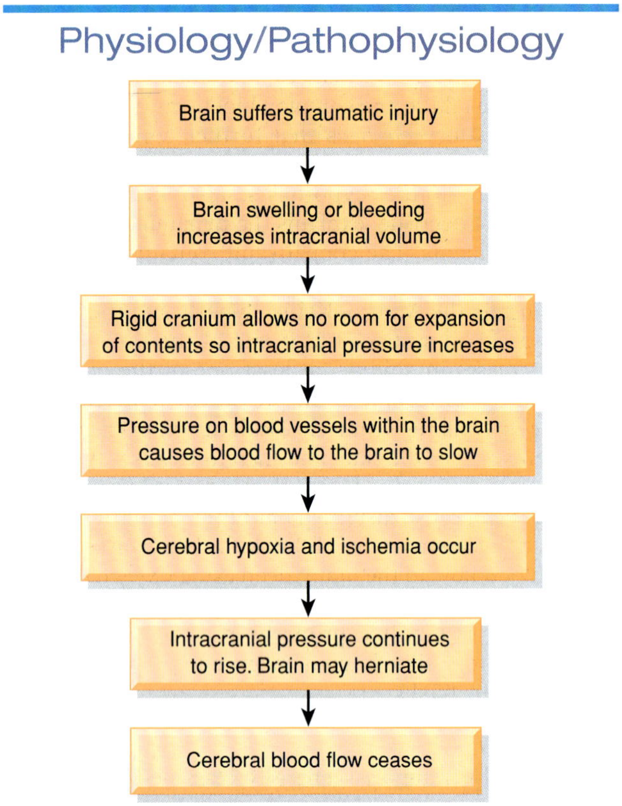

FIGURE 65-1. Pathophysiology of traumatic brain injury.

scalp injury is based on physical examination, inspection, and palpation. Scalp wounds are potential portals of entry for organisms that cause intracranial infections. Therefore, the area is irrigated before the laceration is sutured, to remove foreign material and to reduce the risk for infection. Subgaleal hematomas (hematomas below the outer covering of the skull) usually reabsorb and do not require any specific treatment.

Skull Fractures

A skull fracture is a break in the continuity of the skull caused by forceful trauma. It may occur with or without damage to the brain. Skull fractures are classified by type and location. Types include linear, comminuted, and depressed skull fractures, whereas location fractures include frontal, temporal, and basal skull fractures. A simple (linear) fracture is a break in the continuity of the bone. A comminuted skull fracture refers to a splintered or multiple fracture line. Depressed skull fractures occur when the bones of the skull are forcefully displaced downward, and can vary from a slight depression to bones of the skull being splintered and embedded within brain tissue. A fracture of the base of the skull is referred to as a basal skull fracture (Hickey, 2014) (see Fig. 65-2). A fracture may be open, indicating a scalp laceration or tear in the dura (e.g., from a bullet or an ice pick), or closed, in which case the dura is intact.

Clinical Manifestations

Symptoms, apart from those of the local injury, depend on the severity and the anatomic location of the underlying brain injury. Persistent, localized pain usually suggests that a fracture is present. Fractures of the cranial vault may or may not produce swelling in the region of the fracture; therefore, an x-ray or computed tomography (CT) scan is needed for diagnosis.

Fractures of the base of the skull tend to traverse the paranasal sinus of the frontal bone or the middle ear located in the temporal bone (see Fig. 65-2). Therefore, they frequently produce hemorrhage or fluid leakage (CSF) from the nose, pharynx, or ears, and blood may appear under the conjunctiva. An area of ecchymosis (bruising) may be seen over the mastoid (Battle's sign) and/or the eye orbits (raccoon eyes). Basilar skull fractures are suspected when CSF escapes from the ears (CSF otorrhea) and the nose (CSF rhinorrhea). A CSF leak is a serious problem, because meningeal infection can occur if organisms gain access to the cranial contents via the nose, ear, or sinus through a tear in the dura.

Assessment and Diagnostic Findings

A CT scan can be used to diagnose a skull fracture. The ease with which a diagnosis of skull fracture is made depends on the site of the fracture. If a fracture is found on CT scan, there is always the question of associated brain injury, and a magnetic resonance imaging (MRI) scan provides better resolution and clearer pictures of the injured area (Hickey, 2014).

Gerontologic Considerations

Older patients with head injuries differ from those who are younger in terms of etiology of injury, higher mortality rates, longer lengths of hospital stay, and poorer

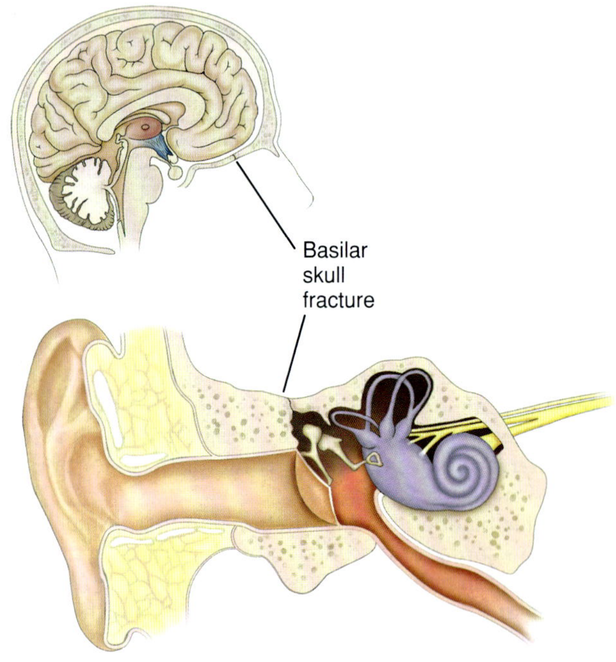

FIGURE 65-2. Basilar fractures allow cerebrospinal fluid to leak from the nose and ears. (Adapted from Hickey, J. V. (2014). *The clinical practice of neurological and neurosurgical nursing* (7th ed.). Philadelphia, PA: Wolters Kluwer Health/Lippincott Williams & Wilkins.)

functional outcomes. Neurologic assessment can be challenging, as the older adult patient with a TBI can have hearing and/or visual deficits or pre-existing dementia or cognitive issues, making establishment of a neurologic baseline difficult. The most common causes of injury in older adult patients are falls and motor vehicle crashes (Stocchetti & Maas, 2014). Approximately 61% of all TBIs among adults aged 65 years and older result from falls (CDC, 2016a). Physiologic changes related to aging may place the older adult at increased risk for injury, alter the type and severity of injury that occurs, or lead to complications. Two major factors place older adults at increased risk for hematomas. First, brain weight decreases, the dura becomes more adherent to the skull, and reaction times slow with increasing age (Eliopoulos, 2018). Second, many older adults take aspirin and anticoagulant agents as part of routine management of chronic conditions.

Medical Management

Nondepressed skull fractures generally do not require surgical treatment; however, close observation of the patient is essential. Nursing personnel may observe the patient in the hospital, but if no underlying brain injury is present, the patient may be allowed to return home. If the patient is discharged home, specific instructions must be given to the family (see later discussion of concussion).

Depressed skull fractures usually require surgery with elevation of the skull and debridement, usually within 24 hours of injury. Skull fractures can be a combination of open, compound, closed, or simple. Associated injuries include concurrent scalp laceration, dural tears, and brain injury directly below the fracture from compression of the tissue below the bony injury and from lacerations produced by the bony fragments (Hickey, 2014).

Brain Injury

The most important consideration in any **head injury** is whether the brain is injured. Even seemingly minor injury can cause significant brain damage secondary to obstructed blood flow and decreased tissue perfusion. The brain cannot store oxygen or glucose to any significant degree. Because the cerebral cells need an uninterrupted blood supply to obtain these nutrients, irreversible brain damage and cell death occur if the blood supply is interrupted for even a few minutes. Clinical manifestations of brain injury (injury to the brain that is severe enough to interfere with usual functioning) are listed in Chart 65-2. A TBI **closed (blunt)** occurs when the head accelerates and then rapidly decelerates or collides with another object (e.g., a wall, the dashboard of a car) and brain tissue is damaged but there is no opening through the skull and dura. A TBI **open (penetrating)** occurs when an object penetrates the skull, enters the brain, and damages the soft brain tissue in its path (penetrating injury), or when blunt trauma to the head is so severe that it opens the scalp, skull, and dura to expose the brain.

Types of Brain Injury

Injuries to the brain can be focal or diffuse. Focal injuries include contusions and several types of hematomas. Concussions and diffuse axonal injuries are the major diffuse injuries (Hickey, 2014).

CHART 65-2

Assessment: Assessing Traumatic Brain Injury

Be alert for the following signs and symptoms:

- Altered level of consciousness
- Confusion
- Pupillary abnormalities (changes in shape, size, and response to light)
- Altered or absent gag reflex
- Absent corneal reflex
- Sudden onset of neurologic deficits
- Changes in vital signs (altered respiratory pattern, widened pulse pressure, bradycardia, tachycardia, hypothermia, or hyperthermia)
- Vision and hearing impairment
- Sensory dysfunction
- Headache
- Seizures

Contusion

In cerebral contusion, the brain is bruised and damaged in a specific area because of severe acceleration–deceleration force or blunt trauma. The impact of the brain against the skull leads to a contusion. Clinical manifestations of a contusion are dependent on size, location, and the extent of surrounding cerebral edema. Although a contusion may occur in any area of the brain, most are usually located in the anterior portions of the frontal and temporal lobes, around the sylvian fissure, and at the orbital areas; less commonly, contusions are located at the parietal and occipital areas.

Contusions can be characterized by loss of consciousness associated with stupor and confusion. The effects of injury, particularly hemorrhage and edema, peak after about 18 to 36 hours. These effects, which can cause secondary effects resulting in increased ICP and possible herniation syndromes, are most pronounced in temporal lobe contusions. Patients are most often managed medically with interventions directed toward prevention of additional insults. Deep contusions are more often associated with hemorrhage and destruction of the reticular activating fibres, altering arousal (Hickey, 2014).

Intracranial Hemorrhage

Hematomas are collections of blood in the brain that may be epidural (above the dura), subdural (below the dura), or intracerebral (within the brain) (see Fig. 65-3). Major symptoms are frequently delayed until the hematoma is large enough to cause distortion of the brain and increased ICP. The signs and symptoms of cerebral ischemia resulting from compression by a hematoma are variable and depend on the speed with which vital areas are affected and the area that is injured. A rapidly developing hematoma, even if small, may be fatal, whereas a larger but slowly developing one may allow compensation for increases in ICP.

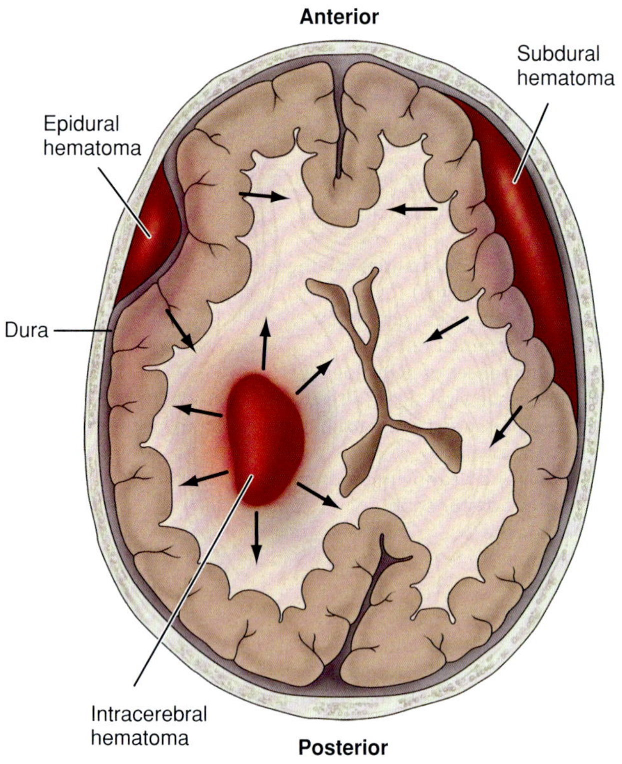

FIGURE 65-3. Location of epidural, subdural, and intracerebral hematomas.

Epidural Hematoma

After a head injury, blood may collect in the epidural (extradural) space between the skull and the dura mater. This can result from a skull fracture that causes a rupture or laceration of the middle meningeal artery, the artery that runs between the dura and the skull inferior to a thin portion of temporal bone. Hemorrhage from this artery causes rapid pressure on the brain. Epidural hematomas (EDHs) account for approximately 2.7% to 4% of traumatic head injuries (Hickey, 2014).

Symptoms are caused by the expanding hematoma. EDHs are often characterized by a brief loss of consciousness, followed by a lucid interval in which the patient is awake and conversant. During this lucid interval, compensation for the expanding hematoma takes place by rapid absorption of CSF and decreased intravascular volume, both of which help to maintain the ICP within normal limits. When these mechanisms can no longer compensate, even a small increase in the volume of the blood clot produces a marked elevation in ICP. The patient then becomes increasingly restless, agitated, and confused as the condition progresses to coma. Then, often suddenly, signs of herniation appear (usually deterioration of consciousness and signs of focal neurologic deficits, such as dilation and fixation of a pupil or paralysis of an extremity), and the patient's condition deteriorates rapidly. The most common type of herniation syndrome associated with an EDH is uncal herniation causing pressure on the midbrain (Hickey, 2014).

An EDH is considered an extreme emergency; marked neurologic deficit or even respiratory arrest can occur within minutes. Treatment consists of making openings through the skull (burr holes) to decrease ICP emergently, remove the clot, and control the bleeding. A craniotomy may be required to remove the clot and control the bleeding. A drain is usually inserted after creation of burr holes or a craniotomy to prevent reaccumulation of blood.

Subdural Hematoma

An SDH is a collection of blood between the dura and the brain, a space normally occupied by a thin cushion of fluid. The most common cause is trauma, but it can also occur as a result of coagulopathies or rupture of an aneurysm. An SDH is more frequently venous in origin and is caused by the rupture of small vessels that bridge the subdural space (Bauman & McCourt, 2014). SDHs may be acute or chronic depending on the size of the involved vessel and the amount of bleeding on CT scan.

ACUTE SDH. Approximately 50% of brain injuries and 60% of deaths in patients with brain injuries result from acute SDHs and are associated with major head injury involving contusion or laceration. Clinical symptoms develop rapidly (Bauman & McCourt, 2014). Signs and symptoms include changes in the level of consciousness (LOC), pupillary signs, and hemiparesis. There may be minor or even no symptoms with small collections of blood. Coma, increasing blood pressure, decreasing heart rate, and slowing respiratory rate are all signs of a rapidly expanding mass requiring immediate intervention.

If the patient can be transported rapidly to the hospital, an immediate craniotomy is performed to open the dura, allowing the subdural clot to be evacuated. Successful outcome also depends on the control of ICP and careful monitoring of respiratory function. The mortality rate for patients with acute SDH is high because of associated brain damage (Bauman & McCourt, 2014).

CHRONIC SDH. A chronic SDH can develop from seemingly minor head injuries and is seen most frequently in older adults who are prone to this type of head injury due to brain atrophy, which is a consequence of the aging process (Bauman & McCourt, 2014). Seemingly minor head trauma may produce enough impact to shift the brain contents abnormally. The time between injury and onset of symptoms can be lengthy (e.g., 3 weeks to months), so the actual injury may be forgotten.

A chronic SDH can resemble other conditions—for example, it may be mistaken for a stroke. The bleeding is less profuse, but compression of the intracranial contents still occurs. The blood within the brain changes in character in 2 to 4 days, becoming thicker and darker. In a few weeks, the clot breaks down and has the colour and consistency of motor oil. Eventually, calcification or ossification of the clot takes place. The brain adapts to this foreign body invasion, and the clinical signs and symptoms fluctuate. Symptoms include severe headache, which tends to come and go; alternating focal neurologic signs; personality changes; mental deterioration; and focal seizures (Bauman & McCourt, 2014).

The treatment for a chronic SDH consists of surgical evaluation for evacuation of the clot. Consideration must be made for reversal of coagulopathies and iatrogenic anticoagulation (Bauman & McCourt, 2014). The operative procedure may be carried out through multiple burr holes, or a craniotomy may be performed for a sizeable subdural mass that cannot be suctioned or drained through burr holes.

Intracerebral Hemorrhage and Hematoma

Intracerebral hemorrhage is bleeding into the parenchyma of the brain. It is commonly seen in head injuries when force is exerted to the head over a small area (e.g., missile injuries, bullet wounds, stab injuries). These hemorrhages within the brain may also result from the following:

- Systemic hypertension, which causes degeneration and rupture of a vessel
- Rupture of an aneurysm
- Vascular anomalies
- Intracranial tumours
- Bleeding disorders such as leukemia, hemophilia, aplastic anemia, and thrombocytopenia
- Complications of anticoagulant therapy

Nontraumatic causes of intracerebral hemorrhage are discussed in Chapter 64.

The onset may be insidious, beginning with the development of neurologic deficits, followed by headache. Management includes supportive care; control of ICP; and careful administration of fluids, electrolytes, and antihypertensive medications. Surgical intervention by craniotomy or craniectomy permits removal of the blood clot and control of hemorrhage, but may not be possible because of the inaccessible location of the bleeding or the lack of a clearly circumscribed area of blood that can be removed.

Concussion

A concussion is a temporary loss of neurologic function with no apparent structural damage to the brain. Of the 1.7 million TBIs that occur in the United States each year, it is estimated that approximately 80% of them are concussions, also referred to as "mild TBI" (CDC, 2016b; Hyatt, 2014). The mechanism of injury is usually blunt trauma from an acceleration–deceleration force, a direct blow, or a blast injury. If brain tissue in the frontal lobe is affected, the patient may exhibit bizarre irrational behaviour, whereas involvement of the temporal lobe can produce temporary amnesia or disorientation.

The duration of mental status abnormalities is an indicator of the grade of the concussion. The patient is discharged from the hospital or ED once he or she returns to baseline after a concussion. Monitoring includes observing the patient for a decrease in LOC, worsening headache, dizziness, seizures, abnormal pupil response, vomiting, irritability, slurred speech, and numbness or weakness in the arms or legs. The occurrence of these symptoms is a red flag indicating the need for further intervention. Recovery may appear complete, but long-term sequelae are possible and repeat injuries common.

Repeated concussive incidents can lead to a syndrome known as chronic traumatic encephalopathy. This syndrome has been recognized in those participating in contact sports such as football and boxing. The presentation is similar to Alzheimer's disease, characterized by personality changes, memory impairment, and speech and gait disturbances. Imaging findings show gross cerebral, particularly temporal lobe, atrophy (Bailes, Petraglia, Omalu, et al., 2013; Hickey, 2014).

Diffuse Axonal Injury

DAI results from widespread shearing and rotational forces that produce damage throughout the brain—to axons in the cerebral hemispheres, corpus callosum, and brainstem. The injured area may be diffuse with no identifiable focal lesion. DAI is associated with prolonged traumatic coma; it is more serious and is associated with a poorer prognosis than a focal lesion. The patient with DAI in severe head trauma experiences no lucid interval, immediate coma, decorticate and decerebrate posturing (see Chapter 66, Fig. 66-1), and global cerebral edema. Diagnosis is made by clinical signs in conjunction with a CT or MRI scan (Bodanapally, Sours, Zhuo, et al., 2015). Recovery depends on the severity of the axonal injury.

Medical Management

Assessment and diagnosis of the extent of injury are accomplished by the initial physical and neurologic examinations. CT and MRI scans are the main neuroimaging diagnostic tools and are useful in evaluating the brain structure (Bodanapally et al., 2015). Positron emission tomography (PET) is available in some trauma centres for assessing brain function.

Any patient with a head injury is presumed to have a cervical spine injury until proven otherwise. The patient is transported from the scene of the injury on a board with the head and neck maintained in alignment with the axis of the body. A cervical collar should be applied and maintained until cervical spine x-rays have been obtained and the absence of cervical SCI documented.

All therapy is directed toward preserving brain homeostasis and preventing secondary brain injury, which is injury to the brain that occurs after the original traumatic event (Bader et al., 2016). Common causes of secondary injury are cerebral edema, hypotension, and respiratory depression that may lead to hypoxemia and electrolyte imbalance. Treatments to prevent secondary injury include stabilization of cardiovascular and respiratory function to maintain adequate cerebral perfusion, control of hemorrhage and hypovolemia, and maintenance of optimal blood gas values.

Treatment of Increased Intracranial Pressure

As the damaged brain swells with edema or as blood collects within the brain, an increase in ICP occurs; this requires aggressive treatment (see Chapter 66 for a discussion of the relationship between ICP and cerebral perfusion pressure [CPP]). If the ICP remains elevated, it can decrease the CPP. Initial management is based on preventing secondary injury and maintaining adequate cerebral oxygenation.

Surgery is required for evacuation of blood clots, debridement and elevation of depressed fractures of the skull, and suture of severe scalp lacerations. ICP is monitored closely; if increased, it is managed by maintaining adequate oxygenation, elevating the head of the bed, and maintaining normal blood volume (Stocchetti & Maas, 2014). Devices to monitor ICP or drain CSF can be inserted during surgery or at the bedside using aseptic technique. The patient is cared for in the intensive care unit (ICU), where expert nursing care and medical treatment are readily available.

Supportive Measures

Treatment also includes ventilatory support, seizure prevention, fluid and electrolyte maintenance, nutritional support, and management of pain and anxiety. Patients who are comatose are intubated and mechanically ventilated to ensure adequate oxygenation and protect the airway.

Because seizures can occur after head injury and can cause secondary brain damage from hypoxia, anticonvulsant agents may be given. If the patient is very agitated, benzodiazepines are the most commonly used sedative agents and do not affect cerebral blood flow or ICP. Lorazepam (Ativan) and midazolam (Versed) are frequently used but have active metabolites that may cause prolonged sedation, making it difficult to conduct a neurologic assessment. Propofol (Diprivan), a sedative–hypnotic agent that is supplied in an intralipid emulsion for intravenous (IV) use, is the sedative of choice. It is an ultra–short-acting, rapid-onset drug with elimination half-life of less than an hour. It has a major advantage of being titratable to its desired clinical effect but still provides the opportunity for an accurate neurologic assessment (Hickey, 2014). A nasogastric tube may be inserted, because reduced gastric motility and reverse peristalsis are associated with head injury, making regurgitation and aspiration common in the first few hours.

Brain Death

When a patient has sustained a severe head injury incompatible with life, the patient is a potential organ donor. The nurse may assist in the clinical examination for determination of brain death and in the process of organ procurement. The three cardinal signs of brain death on clinical examination are coma, the absence of brainstem reflexes, and apnea. Adjunctive tests, such as cerebral blood flow studies, electroencephalogram (EEG), transcranial Doppler, and brainstem auditory–evoked potential, are often used to confirm brain death (Hickey, 2014). The health care team provides information to the family and assists them with the decision-making process about end-of-life care.

Nursing Process

The Patient With a Traumatic Brain Injury

Assessment

Depending on the patient's neurologic status, the nurse may elicit information from the patient, from the family, or from witnesses or emergency rescue personnel. Although all usual baseline data may not be collected initially, the immediate health history should include the following questions:

- When did the injury occur?
- What caused the injury? A high-velocity missile? An object striking the head? A fall?
- What was the direction and force of the blow?

A history of unconsciousness or amnesia after a head injury indicates a significant degree of brain damage, and changes that occur minutes to hours after the initial injury can reflect recovery or indicate the development of secondary brain damage. The nurse should determine if there was a loss of consciousness, the duration of the unconscious period, and if the patient could be aroused.

In addition to asking questions that establish the nature of the injury and the patient's condition immediately after the injury, the nurse examines the patient thoroughly. This assessment includes determining the patient's LOC using the Glasgow Coma Scale (GCS) and assessing the patient's response to tactile stimuli (if unconscious), pupillary response to light, corneal and gag reflexes, and motor function. The GCS is based on the three criteria of eye opening, verbal responses, and motor responses to verbal commands or painful stimuli. It is particularly useful for monitoring changes during the acute phase, the first few days after a head injury. It does not take the place of an in-depth neurologic assessment.

Detailed assessments are made initially and at frequent intervals throughout the acute phase of care (Hickey, 2014). Monitoring of ICP is crucial to decision making for patients with neurologic injuries, yet research findings indicate that practices for the measurement of ICP vary widely (Olson, Rogers, & Stutzman, 2015) (see Chart 65-3). Baseline and ongoing assessments are critical in nursing assessment of the patient with brain injury, whose condition can worsen dramatically and irrevocably if subtle signs are overlooked (Arciniegas, Zasler, Vanderploeg, et al., 2013; Booker, 2015). More information on assessment is provided in the following sections and in Figure 65-4 and Table 65-1.

Nursing Priorities

Based on the assessment data, the patient's major nursing priorities may include the following:

- Airway clearance
- Ineffective cerebral tissue perfusion
- Deficient fluid volume
- Nutrition
- Injury prevention
- Body temperature balance
- Prevention of pressure injuries
- Disturbed thought processes
- Disturbed sleep pattern
- Interrupted family processes
- Deficient knowledge

The nursing priorities for the unconscious patient and the patient with increased ICP also apply (see Chapter 63).

Collaborative Problems/Potential Complications

Based on all the assessment data, the major complications include the following:

- Decreased cerebral perfusion
- Cerebral edema and herniation

NURSING RESEARCH PROFILE

Chart 65-3. Validating the Electronic Medical Record for Measuring Increased Intracranial Pressure

Olson, D. M., Rogers, M. S., & Stutzman, S. (2015). Electronic medical record validation: Exploring the reliability of intracranial pressure data abstracted from the electronic medical record-pilot. *Journal of Nursing Measurement*, *23*(3), 532–540.

Purpose

The most reliable and valid methods of measuring and documenting intracranial pressure (ICP) monitoring for patients with neurologic injuries are not known. The purpose of this pilot study was to compare different methods of ICP monitoring.

Design

This was a nonrandomized, unblinded, observational study that compared three different technologies. The technologies for recording ICP included pen and paper (P&P), electronic medical record (EMR), and video data with continuous data acquisition (CDA).

Findings

Data were obtained from 11 patients who had ICP monitoring and 26 nurses who provided care to these patients. Patients' mean age was 50.7 years, six (54.4%) were female, and eight (72.7%) were White (two Black, and one not declared). Patient diagnoses included subarachnoid hemorrhage (six), intracranial hemorrhage (two), neoplasm (two), and one patient with cerebral edema following ischemic stroke. Nurses were primarily baccalaureate prepared (*n* 22, 84.6%) with a mean of 8.3 (*SD* 9.8) years of nursing experience and 7.5 (*SD* 1.7) years of experience in critical care. ICP values did not significantly differ between EMR and P&P records, despite an average of 16 minutes' difference in reporting times. ICP values did vary significantly when comparing CDA data to EMR or paper.

Nursing Implications

This pilot study called into question the validity of ICP values as they are currently recorded. Nurses caring for patients with neurologic injuries need to know that significant practice variation exists and there are no best practice standards for recording ICP. With EMRs becoming pervasive, more nursing research is essential in this area.

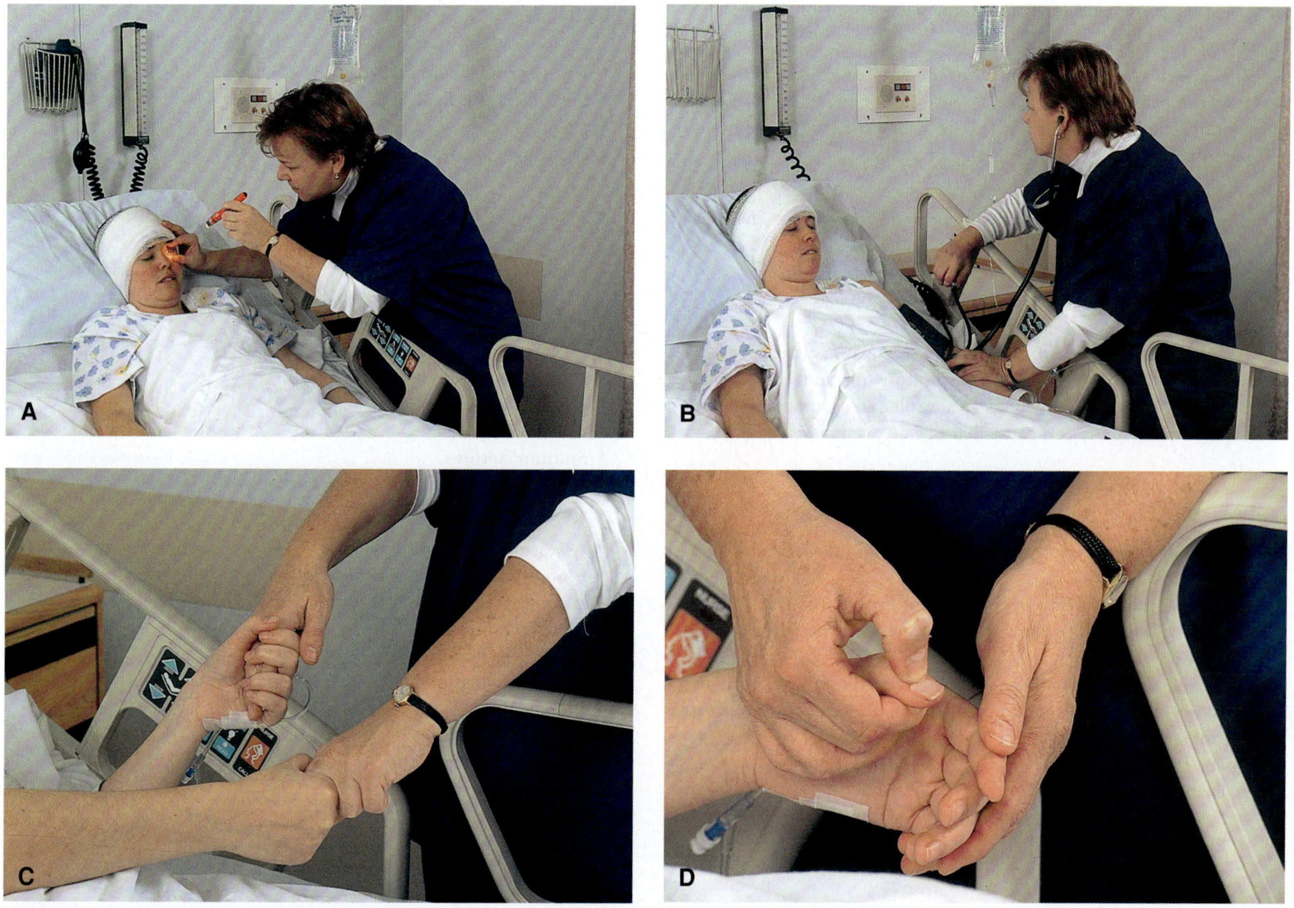

FIGURE 65-4. Assessment parameters for the patient with a head injury include eye opening and responsiveness (**A**), vital signs (**B**), and motor response reflected in hand strength or response to painful stimulus (**C**, **D**). (Photos by B. Proud.)

TABLE 65-1 Multisystem Assessment Measures for the Patient With Traumatic Brain Injury

System-Specific Considerations	Assessment Data
Neurologic System	
• Severe TBI results in unconsciousness and alters many neurologic functions. • All body functions must be supported. • Increased ICP and herniation syndromes are life threatening. • Measures are instituted to control elevated ICP.	• Assessment of neurologic status • Assessment for signs and symptoms of ICP elevation • Calculation of cerebral perfusion pressure if ICP monitor is in place • Monitoring of anticonvulsant medication blood levels
Integumentary System (Skin and Mucous Membranes)	
• Immobility secondary to TBI and unconsciousness contributes to the development of pressure areas and skin breakdown. • Intubation causes irritation of the mucous membrane and deterioration of oral health.	• Assessment of skin integrity and character of the skin • Assessment of oral mucous membrane and oral health
Musculoskeletal System	
• Immobility contributes to musculoskeletal changes. • Decerebrate or decorticate posturing makes proper positioning difficult.	• Assessment of range of motion of joints and development of deformities or spasticity
Gastrointestinal System	
• Injury to the GI tract can result in paralytic ileus. • Constipation can result from bed rest, NPO status, fluid restriction, and opioids given for pain control. • Bowel incontinence is related to the patient's unconscious state or altered mental state.	• Assessment of abdomen for bowel sounds and distention • Monitoring for decreased hemoglobin
Genitourinary System	
• Fluid restriction or the use of diuretic agents can alter the amount of urinary output. • Urinary incontinence is related to the patient's unconscious state.	• Intake and output record
Metabolic (Nutritional) System	
• The patient receives all fluids IV for the first few days until the GI tract is functioning. • A nutritional consultation is initiated within the first 24–48 hours; parenteral or enteral nutrition may be started.	• Assessment of fluid and electrolyte balance • Recording of weight, if possible • Hematocrit • Electrolyte studies
Respiratory System	

• Complete or partial airway obstruction will compromise the oxygen supply to the brain.
• An altered respiratory pattern can result in cerebral hypoxia.
• A short period of apnea at the moment of impact can result in spotty atelectasis.
• Systemic disturbances from head injury can cause hypoxemia.
• Brain injury can alter brainstem respiratory function.
• Shunting of blood to the lungs as a result of a sympathetic discharge at the time of injury can cause neurogenic pulmonary edema.
	• Assessment of respiratory function:
	  • Auscultate chest for breath sounds
	  • Note the respiratory pattern, if possible (not possible if a ventilator is being used)
	  • Note the respiratory rate
	  • Note whether the cough reflex is intact
	• Arterial blood gas levels
	• Complete blood count
	• Chest x-ray studies
	• Sputum cultures
	• Oxygen saturation using pulse oximetry

Cardiovascular System	

• The patient may develop cardiac dysrhythmias, tachycardia, or bradycardia.
• The patient may develop hypotension or hypertension.
• Because of immobility and unconsciousness, the patient is at high risk for DVT and PE.
• Fluid and electrolyte imbalance can be related to several problems, including alterations in antidiuretic hormone secretion, the stress response, or fluid restriction.
• Specific conditions may occur:
  • Diabetes insipidus
  • Syndrome of inappropriate secretion of antidiuretic hormone
  • Electrolyte imbalance
  • Hyperglycemic hyperosmolar syndrome
	• Assessment of vital signs
	• Monitoring for cardiac dysrhythmias
	• Assessment for venous thromboembolism including PE and DVT
	• Electrocardiogram
	• Electrolyte studies
	• Blood coagulation studies
	• Blood glucose level
	• Blood acetone level
	• Blood osmolality
	• Urine specific gravity

TABLE 65-1 Multisystem Assessment Measures for the Patient With Traumatic Brain Injury (Continued)

System-Specific Considerations	Assessment Data
Psychological/Emotional Response	
• The patient with TBI is unconscious. • The family needs emotional support to deal with the crisis.	• Alternative methods of assessment for pain are indicated in the patient who is unconscious • Collection of information about the family and the role within the family of the person with head injury • Assessment of the family to determine how functional it was before the injury occurred

TBI, traumatic brain injury; ICP, intracranial pressure; GI, gastrointestinal; NPO, nothing by mouth; IV, intravenous; DVT, deep vein thrombosis; PE, pulmonary embolism.

Adapted from Booker, K. (2015). *Critical care nursing: Monitoring and treatment for advanced nursing practice*. Oxford: Wiley Blackwell.

- Impaired oxygenation and ventilation
- Impaired fluid, electrolyte, and nutritional balance
- Risk of posttraumatic seizures

Planning and Goals

The goals for the patient may include maintenance of a patent airway, adequate CPP, fluid and electrolyte balance, adequate nutritional status, prevention of secondary injury, maintenance of normal body temperature, maintenance of skin integrity, improvement of cognitive function, prevention of sleep deprivation, effective family coping, increased knowledge about the rehabilitation process, and absence of complications.

Nursing Interventions

The nursing interventions for the patient with a TBI are extensive and diverse. They include making nursing assessments, setting priorities for nursing interventions, anticipating needs and complications, and initiating rehabilitation.

Maintaining the Airway

One of the most important nursing goals in the management of head injury is to establish and maintain an adequate airway. The brain is extremely sensitive to hypoxia, and a neurologic deficit can worsen if the patient is hypoxic. Therapy is directed toward maintaining optimal oxygenation to preserve cerebral function. An obstructed airway causes carbon dioxide retention and hypoventilation, which can produce cerebral vessel dilation and increased ICP (McNett & Olson, 2013; Mitchell, Kirkness, & Blissitt, 2015).

Interventions to ensure an adequate exchange of air are the following:

- Maintaining the patient who is unconscious in a position that facilitates drainage of oral secretions, with the head of the bed elevated about 30 degrees to decrease intracranial venous pressure
- Establishing effective suctioning procedures (pulmonary secretions produce coughing and straining, which increase ICP)
- Guarding against aspiration and respiratory insufficiency
- Closely monitoring arterial blood gas values to assess the adequacy of ventilation. The goal is to keep blood gas values within normal limits to ensure adequate cerebral blood flow
- Monitoring the patient who is receiving mechanical ventilation for pulmonary complications such as acute respiratory distress syndrome and pneumonia (Hickey, 2014)

The patient who is intubated is at high risk for ventilator-associated pneumonia, and providing good oral hygiene can help prevent this complication (Larrow & Klich-Heartt, 2016).

Monitoring Neurologic Function

Patients with severe TBI are admitted to the ICU for close assessment and monitoring (cardiac monitoring, pulse oximetry, invasive arterial blood pressure monitoring, end-tidal CO_2, and temperature monitoring). Parameters are assessed initially and as frequently as the patient's condition requires. As soon as the initial assessment is made, the use of a neurologic observational flow record is started and maintained.

The importance of ongoing assessment and monitoring of the patient with brain injury cannot be overstated.

LEVEL OF CONSCIOUSNESS. The GCS is used to assess LOC at regular intervals, because changes in the LOC precede all other changes in vital and neurologic signs. The patient's best responses to predetermined stimuli are recorded. Each response is scored (the greater the number, the better the functioning), and the sum of these scores gives an indication of the severity of coma and a prediction of possible outcome. The lowest score is 3 (least responsive); the highest is 15 (most responsive). A GCS score between 3 and 8 is generally accepted as indicating a severe head injury (Bader et al., 2016). The GCS is considered the most sensitive indicator of a lapse in neurologic functioning in patients with TBI and is often the earliest sign of acute change in ICP.

VITAL SIGNS. Although a change in LOC is the most sensitive neurologic indication of deterioration of the patient's condition, vital signs also are monitored at frequent intervals to assess the intracranial status. Table 65-1 depicts the general assessment parameters for the patient with a head injury.

Signs of increasing ICP include slowing of the heart rate (bradycardia), increasing systolic blood pressure, and widening pulse pressure (Cushing reflex). As brain compression increases, respirations become rapid, the blood pressure may decrease, and the pulse slows further. This is an ominous development, as is a rapid fluctuation of vital signs (Hickey, 2014). The temperature is maintained at less than 38°C (100.4°F) (Perez-Barcena, Llompart-Pou, & O'Phelan, 2014). Tachycardia and arterial hypotension may indicate that bleeding is occurring elsewhere in the body. In a patient with a head injury, a rapid increase in body temperature is regarded as unfavourable because hyperthermia increases the metabolic demands of the brain and may indicate brainstem damage—a poor prognostic sign.

MOTOR FUNCTION. Motor function is assessed frequently by observing spontaneous movements, asking the patient to raise and lower the extremities, and comparing the strength and equality of the upper and lower extremities at periodic intervals. To assess upper extremity strength, the nurse instructs the patient to squeeze the examiner's fingers tightly. The nurse assesses lower extremity motor strength by placing the hands on the soles of the patient's feet and asking the patient to push down against the examiner's hands. Examination of the motor system is discussed in more detail in Chapter 62. The presence or absence of spontaneous movement of each extremity is also noted, and speech and eye signs are assessed.

If the patient does not demonstrate spontaneous movement, responses to painful stimuli are assessed (Hickey, 2014). Motor response to pain is assessed by applying a central stimulus, such as pinching the pectoralis major muscle, to determine the patient's best response. Peripheral stimulation may provide inaccurate assessment data because it may result in a reflex movement rather than a voluntary motor response. Abnormal responses (lack of motor response; extension responses) are associated with a poorer prognosis.

OTHER NEUROLOGIC SIGNS. In addition to the patient's spontaneous eye opening, which is evaluated with the GCS, the size and equality of the pupils and their reaction to light are assessed (Booker, 2015). A unilaterally dilated and poorly responding pupil may indicate a developing hematoma, with subsequent pressure on the third cranial nerve due to shifting of the brain. If both pupils become fixed and dilated, this indicates acute injury and intrinsic damage to the upper brainstem and is a poor prognostic sign (Bader et al., 2016).

The patient with a head injury may develop deficits such as anosmia (lack of sense of smell), eye movement abnormalities, aphasia, memory deficits, and posttraumatic seizures or epilepsy. Patients may be left with residual psychological deficits (impulsiveness; emotional lability; or uninhibited, aggressive behaviours) and, as a consequence of the impairment, may lack insight into their emotional responses.

Monitoring Fluid and Electrolyte Balance

Brain damage can produce metabolic and hormonal dysfunctions. The monitoring of serum electrolyte levels is important, especially in patients receiving osmotic diuretics, those with syndrome of inappropriate antidiuretic hormone (SIADH) secretion, and those with posttraumatic diabetes insipidus.

Serial studies of blood and urine electrolytes and osmolality are carried out because head injuries may be accompanied by disorders of sodium regulation. Hyponatremia is common after head injury due to shifts in extracellular fluid, electrolytes, and volume. Hyperglycemia, for example, can cause an increase in extracellular fluid that lowers sodium. Hypernatremia may also occur as a result of sodium retention that may last several days, followed by sodium diuresis. Increasing lethargy, confusion, and seizures may be the result of electrolyte imbalance.

Endocrine function is evaluated by monitoring serum electrolytes, blood glucose values, and intake and output. Urine is tested regularly for acetone. A record of daily weights is maintained, especially if the patient has hypothalamic involvement and is at risk for the development of diabetes insipidus.

Promoting Adequate Nutrition

Head injury results in metabolic changes that increase calorie consumption and nitrogen excretion. Protein demand increases. Early initiation of nutritional therapy has been shown to improve outcomes in patients with head injury. Patients with brain injury are assumed to be catabolic, and nutritional support consultation should be considered as soon as the patient is admitted. Parenteral nutrition via a central line or enteral feedings given via a nasogastric or nasojejunal feeding tube should be considered, though enteral is the preferred route (Hickey, 2014). If CSF rhinorrhea occurs or if there is any suspicion of disruption to the skull base, an oral feeding tube should be inserted instead of a nasal tube.

Laboratory values should be monitored closely in patients receiving parenteral nutrition. Elevating the head of the bed can help prevent distention, regurgitation, and aspiration. A continuous-drip infusion or pump may be used to regulate the feeding. Enteral or parenteral feedings are usually continued until the swallowing reflex returns and the patient can meet caloric requirements orally. See Chapter 36 for the principles and technique of enteral feedings.

Preventing Injury

Often, as the patient emerges from coma, a period of lethargy and stupor is followed by a period of agitation. Each phase is variable and depends on the person, the location of the injury, the depth and duration of coma, and the patient's age. Restlessness may be caused by hypoxia, fever, pain, or a full bladder. It may indicate injury to the brain but may also be a sign that the patient is regaining consciousness. (Some restlessness may be beneficial because the lungs and extremities are exercised.) Agitation may also be the

CHART 65-4

Ethical Dilemma: When Is It Appropriate to Use Restraints?

Case Scenario

You work as a staff nurse on a rehabilitation unit. A 23-year-old man is admitted to the unit with a brain injury, which occurred as a result of a motorcycle crash. His severe brain injuries caused cerebral hypoxia and ischemia to occur. He has periods of severe agitation, has fallen out of bed twice, and an enclosed bed has been prescribed for his safety.

Discussion

Nurses must weigh carefully the risks of limiting autonomy and increasing the risks of injury by using restraints against the risks of injury if not using restraints, which have been documented as resulting in physical harm and death.

Analysis

- Describe the ethical principles that are in conflict in this case (see Chapter 3, Chart 3-3). Which principle should have pre-eminence when a treatment plan is devised for this patient?
- What are your professional obligations in this case? What steps might you take to ensure that the patient's autonomy is preserved?

result of discomfort from catheters, IV lines, restraints, and repeated neurologic checks. Alternatives to restraints must be used whenever possible.

Strategies to prevent injury include the following:

- Assessing the patient to ensure that oxygenation is adequate and the bladder is not distended. Dressings and casts are checked for constriction
- Using padded side rails or wrapping the patient's hands in mitts to protect the patient from self-injury and dislodging of tubes. Restraints are used judiciously, because straining against them can increase ICP or cause other injury. Enclosed or floor-level specialty beds may be indicated (see Chart 65-4)
- Avoiding opioids as a means of controlling restlessness, because they depress respiration, constrict the pupils, and alter responsiveness
- Reducing environmental stimuli by keeping the room quiet, limiting visitors, speaking calmly, and providing frequent orientation information (e.g., explaining where the patient is and what is being done)
- Providing adequate lighting to prevent visual hallucinations
- Minimizing disruption of the patient's sleep–wake cycles
- Lubricating the patient's skin with oil or emollient lotion to prevent irritation due to rubbing against the sheet
- Using an external sheath catheter for a male patient if incontinence occurs. Because prolonged use of an indwelling catheter inevitably produces infection, the patient may be placed on an intermittent catheterization schedule

Maintaining Body Temperature

Fever in the patient with a TBI can be the result of damage to the hypothalamus, cerebral irritation from hemorrhage, or infection. The nurse monitors the patient's temperature every 2 to 4 hours. If the temperature increases, efforts are made to identify the cause and to control it using acetaminophen and cooling devices to maintain normothermia (Madden & DeVon, 2015; Wilson & DellaPenna, 2015). Cooling devices should be used with caution so as not to induce shivering, which increases ICP. If infection is suspected, potential sites of infection are cultured and antibiotic agents are prescribed and given. Research about intentional hypothermia for patients with TBI suggests there is no clear evidence to guide therapy (Madden & DeVon, 2015; Wilson & DellaPenna, 2015).

Maintaining Skin Integrity

Patients with TBI often require assistance in turning and positioning because of immobility or unconsciousness. Prolonged pressure on the tissues decreases circulation and leads to tissue necrosis. Potential areas of breakdown need to be identified early to avoid the development of pressure ulcers. Specific nursing measures include the following:

- Assessing all body surfaces and documenting skin integrity every 8 hours
- Turning and repositioning the patient every 2 hours (Larrow & Klich-Heartt, 2016)
- Providing skin care every 4 hours
- Assisting the patient to get out of bed to a chair three times a day

Improving Coping

Although many patients with head injury survive because of resuscitative and supportive technology, they frequently have ineffective coping due to cognitive sequelae. Cognitive impairment includes memory deficits; decreased ability to focus and sustain attention to a task (distractibility); impulsivity; egocentricity; and slowness in thinking, perceiving, communicating, reading, and writing. Psychiatric, emotional, and relationship problems develop in many patients after head injury. Resulting psychosocial, behavioural, emotional, and cognitive impairments are devastating to the family as well as to the patient (Tam, McKay, Sloan, et al., 2015).

These problems require collaboration among many disciplines. A neuropsychologist (specialist in evaluating and treating cognitive problems) plans a program and initiates therapy or counselling to help the patient reach maximal potential. Cognitive rehabilitation activities help the patient devise new problem-solving strategies. The retraining is carried out over an extended period and may include the use of sensory stimulation and reinforcement, behaviour modification, reality orientation, computer training programs, and video games. Assistance from many disciplines is necessary during this phase of recovery. Even if intellectual ability does not improve, social and behavioural abilities may improve.

The patient recovering from a TBI may experience fluctuations in the level of cognitive function, with orientation, attention, and memory frequently affected. Many types of sensory stimulation programs have been tried, and research on these programs is ongoing (Hickey, 2014). When pushed to a level greater than the impaired cortical functioning allows, the patient may show symptoms of fatigue, anger, and stress (headache, dizziness). The Rancho Los Amigos Scale: Levels of Cognitive Functioning is frequently used to assess cognitive function and evaluate ongoing recovery from head injury. Progress through the levels of cognitive function can vary widely for individual patients (Hagen, Malkmus, & Durham, 1972).

Preventing Sleep Pattern Disturbance

Patients who require frequent monitoring of neurologic status may experience sleep deprivation as they are awakened hourly for assessment of LOC. To allow the patient longer times of uninterrupted sleep and rest, the nurse can group nursing care activities so that the patient is disturbed less frequently. Environmental noise is decreased, and the room lights are dimmed. Measures to increase comfort may promote sleep and rest (Giusti, Tuteri, & Giontella, 2016).

Supporting Family Coping

Having a loved one sustain a TBI produces a great deal of stress in the family. This stress can result from the patient's physical and emotional deficits, the unpredictable outcome, and altered family relationships. Families report difficulties in coping with changes in the patient's temperament, behaviour, and personality (Tam et al., 2015). Such changes are associated with disruption in family cohesion, loss of leisure pursuits, and loss of work capacity, as well as social isolation of the caretaker. The family may experience marital disruption, anger, grief, guilt, and denial in recurring cycles.

To promote effective coping, the nurse can ask the family how the patient is different now, what has been lost, and what is most difficult about coping with this situation. Helpful interventions include providing family members with accurate and honest information and encouraging them to continue to set well-defined short-term goals. Family counselling helps address the family members' acute feelings of loss and helplessness and gives them guidance for the management of inappropriate behaviours. Support groups help the family members share problems, develop insight, gain information, network, and gain assistance in maintaining realistic expectations, hope, and a good quality of life (Tam et al., 2015).

The Brain Injury Association of America (see the Resources section) serves as a clearinghouse for information and resources for patients with head injuries and their families, including specific information on coma, rehabilitation, behavioural consequences of head injury, and family issues. This organization can provide names of facilities and professionals who work with patients with head injuries and can assist families in organizing local support groups.

Many patients with severe head injury die of their injuries, and many of those who survive experience long-term disabilities that prevent them from resuming their previous roles and functions. During the most acute phase of injury, family members need factual information and support from the health care team.

Many patients with severe head injuries that result in brain death are young and otherwise healthy and are therefore considered for organ donation. Family members of patients with such injuries need support during this extremely stressful time and assistance in making decisions to end life support and permit donation of organs. They need to know that the patient who is brain dead and whose respiratory and cardiovascular systems are maintained through life support is not going to survive and that the severe head injury, not the removal of the patient's organs or the removal of life support, is the cause of the patient's death. Bereavement counsellors and members of the organ procurement team are often very helpful to family members in making decisions about organ donation and in helping them cope with stress.

Monitoring and Managing Potential Complications

DECREASED CEREBRAL PERFUSION PRESSURE. Maintenance of adequate CPP is important to prevent serious complications of head injury due to decreased cerebral perfusion. Adequate CPP is greater than 50 mm Hg. If CPP falls below a patient's threshold, a vasodilating cascade occurs, causing the volume of blood to increase inside the brain, which causes ICP to increase. Measures to maintain adequate CPP are essential because a decrease in CPP can impair cerebral perfusion and cause brain hypoxia and ischemia, leading to permanent brain damage. Once the threshold CPP is reached, vasoconstriction of the cerebral blood vessels occurs, causing ICP to decrease. Therapy (e.g., elevation of the head of the bed, increased IV fluids, CSF drainage) is directed toward decreasing cerebral edema and increasing venous outflow from the brain. Systemic hypotension, which causes vasoconstriction and a significant decrease in CPP, is treated with increased IV fluids or vasopressors (Griesdale, Ortenwall, Norena, et al., 2015; Perez-Barcena et al., 2014).

CEREBRAL EDEMA AND HERNIATION. The patient with a head injury is at risk for additional complications such as increased ICP and brainstem herniation. Cerebral edema is the most common cause of increased ICP in the patient with a head injury, with the swelling peaking approximately 48 to 72 hours

CHART 65-5

Controlling ICP in Patients With Severe Brain Injury

- Elevate the head of the bed as prescribed.
- Maintain the patient's head and neck in neutral alignment (no twisting or flexing the neck).
- Initiate measures to prevent the Valsalva manoeuvre (e.g., stool softeners).
- Maintain body temperature within normal limits.
- Administer oxygen (O_2) to maintain partial pressure of arterial oxygen (PaO_2) >90 mm Hg.
- Maintain fluid balance with normal saline solution.
- Avoid noxious stimuli (e.g., excessive suctioning, painful procedures).
- Administer sedation to reduce agitation.
- Maintain cerebral perfusion pressure of 50–70 mm Hg.

Adapted from Bader, M. K., Littlejohns, L. R., & Olson, D. (2016). *AANN core curriculum for neuroscience nursing* (6th ed.). Chicago, IL: American Association of Neuroscience Nurses.

after injury. Bleeding also may increase the volume of contents within the rigid, closed compartment of the skull, causing increased ICP and herniation of the brainstem and resulting in irreversible brain anoxia and brain death (Hickey, 2014; Perez-Barcena et al., 2014). Measures to control ICP are listed in Chart 65-5 and discussed in Chapter 66.

IMPAIRED OXYGENATION AND VENTILATION. Impaired oxygen and ventilation may require mechanical ventilatory support. The patient must be monitored for a patent airway, altered breathing patterns, and hypoxemia and pneumonia. Interventions may include endotracheal intubation, mechanical ventilation, and positive end-expiratory pressure. See Chapters 21 and 66 for a detailed discussion of these topics.

IMPAIRED FLUID, ELECTROLYTE, AND NUTRITIONAL BALANCE. Fluid, electrolyte, and nutritional imbalances are common in the patient with a head injury. Common imbalances include hyponatremia, which is often associated with SIADH (see Chapters 17 and 52), hypokalemia, and hyperglycemia. Modifications in fluid intake with tube feedings or IV fluids, including hypertonic saline, may be necessary to treat these imbalances (Hickey, 2014). Insulin administration may be prescribed to treat hyperglycemia; blood glucose levels are maintained between 80 and 160 mg/dL (Perez-Barcena et al., 2014).

Undernutrition is also a common problem in response to the increased metabolic needs associated with severe head injury. Decisions about early feeding should be individualized; options include IV hyperalimentation or placement of a feeding tube (jejunal or gastric). Caloric expenditure can increase up to 120% to 140% with TBI, requiring close monitoring of nutritional status, with a higher concentration of protein if tolerated (Horn, Kinikini, Moore, et al., 2015).

POSTTRAUMATIC SEIZURES. Patients with head injury are at an increased risk for posttraumatic seizures. Posttraumatic seizures are classified as immediate (within 24 hours after injury), early (within 1 to 7 days after injury), or late (more than 7 days after injury) (Hickey, 2014). Seizure prophylaxis is the practice of administering anticonvulsant medications to patients with head injury to prevent seizures. It is important to prevent posttraumatic seizures, especially in the immediate and early phases of recovery, because seizures may increase ICP and decrease oxygenation (Zaman, Dubiel, Driver, et al., 2017). However, many anticonvulsant medications impair cognitive performance and can prolong the duration of rehabilitation. Therefore, the overall benefits of these medications must be weighed against their side effects. Research evidence supports the use of prophylactic anticonvulsant agents to prevent immediate and early seizures after head injury, but not for prevention of late seizures (Hickey, 2014; Zaman et al., 2017). See Chapter 66 for the nursing management of seizures.

Promoting Home, Community-Based, and Transitional Care

EDUCATING PATIENT ABOUT SELF-CARE. Teaching early in the course of head injury often focuses on reinforcing information given to the family about the patient's condition and prognosis. As the patient's status and expected outcome change over time, family teaching may focus on interpretation and explanation of changes in the patient's physical and psychological responses.

If the patient's physical status allows discharge to home, the patient and family are instructed about limitations that can be expected and complications that may occur. The nurse explains to the patient and family, verbally and in writing, how to monitor for complications that merit contacting the neurosurgeon. Depending on the patient's prognosis and physical and cognitive status, the patient may be included in teaching about self-care management strategies.

If the patient is at risk for late posttraumatic seizures, anticonvulsant medications may be prescribed at discharge. The patient and family require instruction about the side effects of these medications and the importance of continuing to take them as prescribed.

CONTINUING AND TRANSITIONAL CARE. The rehabilitation phase of care for the patient with a TBI begins at hospital admission. Admission to the rehabilitation unit is a milestone in a patient's recovery and requires intense work by the patient to complete the daily schedule of therapies. The goals of rehabilitation are to maximize the patient's ability to return to his or her highest level of functioning and to his or her home and the community, address concerns before discharge for a smooth transition to home or rehabilitation, and promote independence with adaptation to deficits (Hickey, 2014). The patient is encouraged to continue the rehabilitation program after discharge, because improvement in status may continue 3 or more years after injury.

CHART 65-6

HOME CARE CHECKLIST • The Patient With a TBI

At the completion of education, the patient and/or caregiver will be able to:

- State the impact of TBI and treatment on physiologic functioning, ADLs, IADLs, roles, relationships, and spirituality.
- State the purpose, dose, route, schedule, side effects, and precautions for prescribed medications.
- State how to contact all members of the treatment team (e.g., health care providers, home care professionals, rehabilitation team, and durable medical equipment and supply vendor).
- State changes in lifestyle (e.g., ADLs, IADLs, activity) necessary for recovery and health maintenance, as applicable.
  - Demonstrate safe techniques to assist patient with self-care, hygiene, and ambulation.
  - Demonstrate safe techniques for eating, feeding patient, or assisting patient with eating.
  - Identify need for close monitoring of behaviour due to changes in cognitive functioning.
  - Describe strategies for reinforcing positive behaviours.
  - Describe household modifications needed to ensure a safe environment for the patient.
- Explain the need for monitoring for changes in neurologic status and for complications.
- Identify changes in neurologic status and signs and symptoms of complications (e.g., pneumonia, urinary tract infection, meningitis) that should be reported to the neurosurgeon or nurse.
- Relate how to reach primary provider with questions or complications.
- State importance of continuing follow-up by health care team.
- State time and date of follow-up medical appointments, therapy, and testing.
- Identify sources of support (e.g., friends, relatives, faith community, brain injury support groups, caregiver support).
- Identify the need for health promotion, disease prevention, and screening activities.

TBI, traumatic brain injury; ADL, activities of daily living; IADL, independent activities of daily living.

Changes in the patient with a TBI and the effects of long-term rehabilitation on the family and their coping abilities need ongoing assessment. Continued teaching and support of the patient and family are essential as their needs and the patient's status change. Teaching points to address with the family of the patient who is about to return home are described in Chart 65-6.

Depending on status, the patient is encouraged to return to usual activities gradually. Referral to support groups and to the Brain Injury Canada may be warranted (see the Resources section).

During the acute and rehabilitation phases of care, the focus of education is on obvious needs, issues, deficits, and complications. Complications after TBI include infections (e.g., pneumonia, urinary tract infection [UTI], sepsis, wound infection, osteomyelitis, meningitis, ventriculitis, brain abscess) and heterotopic ossification (painful bone overgrowth in weight-bearing joints).

The nurse needs to remind the patient and family of the need for continuing health promotion and screening practices after the initial phase of care. Patients who have not been involved in these practices in the past are educated about their importance and are referred to appropriate health care providers.

Evaluation

Expected patient outcomes may include the following:

1. Attains or maintains effective airway clearance, ventilation, and brain oxygenation
   a. Achieves expected blood gas values and has appropriate breath sounds on auscultation
   b. Mobilizes and clears secretions
2. Achieves satisfactory fluid and electrolyte balance
   a. Demonstrates serum electrolytes within expected range
   b. Has no clinical signs of dehydration or overhydration
3. Attains adequate nutritional status
   a. Is free of gastric distention and vomiting
   b. Maintains weight
4. Avoids injury
   a. Shows lessening agitation and restlessness
   b. Is oriented to time, place, and person
   c. Of self and caregivers
5. Maintains appropriate body temperature
   a. Absence of fever
   b. Absence of hypothermia
6. Demonstrates intact skin integrity
   a. Exhibits no redness or breaks in skin integrity
   b. Exhibits no pressure ulcers

7. Shows improvement in cognitive function and improved memory
8. Demonstrates usual sleep–wake cycle
9. Demonstrates absence of complications
   a. Exhibits expected vital signs and body temperature, and increasing orientation to time, place, and person
   b. Demonstrates usual or reduced ICP
10. Experiences no posttraumatic seizures
    a. Takes anticonvulsant medications as prescribed
    b. Identifies side effects/adverse effects of anticonvulsant medications
11. Family demonstrates adaptive family processes
    a. Joins support group
    b. Shares feelings with appropriate health care personnel
    c. Makes end-of-life decisions, if needed
12. Participates in rehabilitation process as indicated for patient and family members
    a. Takes active role in identifying rehabilitation goals and participating in recommended patient care activities
    b. Prepares for discharge

Spinal Cord Injury

SCI is a major health disorder. Approximately 86,000 Canadians live with SCI. Approximately 1,000 new injuries occur each year (Noonan, Chan, Santos, et al., 2017). SCI is primarily an injury of young adult males and an overwhelming majority of those injured are between 16 and 30 years of age (Urden et al., 2013).

Motor vehicle crashes account for 31.5% of reported cases of SCI, falls (25.3%), and with violence primarily from gunshot wounds, recreational sporting activities, and other events accounting for the remaining injuries (Chen, Tang, Vogel, et al., 2013). Paraplegia (paralysis of the lower body) and **tetraplegia** (formerly quadriplegia—paralysis of all four extremities) can occur, with incomplete tetraplegia the largest category, followed by complete paraplegia, complete tetraplegia, and paraplegia.

The predominant risk factors for SCI include young age, male gender, and alcohol and drug use. The frequency with which these risk factors are associated with SCI serves to emphasize the importance of primary prevention. The same interventions suggested earlier in this chapter for head injury prevention serve to decrease the incidence of SCI as well (see Chart 65-1).

Most (80%) people who live with SCIs are men. Life expectancy continues to increase for people with SCI because of improved health care but remains slightly lower than for those without SCI. The major causes of death are pneumonia, pulmonary emboli (PE), and septicemia (Hickey, 2014).

Pathophysiology

Damage in SCI ranges from transient concussion (from which the patient fully recovers) to contusion, laceration, and compression of the spinal cord tissue (either alone or in combination), to complete **transection** (severing) of the spinal cord (which renders the patient paralyzed below the level of the injury). The vertebrae most frequently involved are the 5th, 6th, and 7th cervical vertebrae (C5–C7), the 12th thoracic vertebra (T12), and the 1st lumbar vertebra (L1). These vertebrae are most susceptible because there is a greater range of mobility in the vertebral column in these areas (Hickey, 2014).

SCIs can be separated into two categories: primary injuries and secondary injuries. Primary injuries are the result of the initial insult or trauma and are usually permanent. Secondary injuries resulting from SCI include edema and hemorrhage (Bader et al., 2016; Mohit, 2016). The secondary injury is a major concern for critical care nurses. Early treatment is essential to prevent partial damage from becoming total and permanent.

Clinical Manifestations

Manifestations of SCI depend on the type and level of injury (Chart 65-7). The type of injury refers to the extent of injury to the spinal cord itself. **Incomplete spinal cord lesions** (the sensory or motor fibres, or both, are preserved below the lesion) are classified according to the area of spinal cord damage: central, lateral, anterior, or peripheral. The American Spinal Injury Association (ASIA) provides classification of SCI according to the degree of sensory and motor function present after injury. "Neurologic level" refers to the lowest level at which sensory and motor functions are appropriate. Below the neurologic level, there is total sensory and motor paralysis, loss of bladder and bowel control (usually with urinary retention and bladder distention), loss of sweating and vasomotor tone, and marked reduction of blood pressure from loss of peripheral vascular resistance. A **complete spinal cord lesion** (total loss of sensation and voluntary muscle control below the lesion) can result in **paraplegia** or **tetraplegia**.

If conscious, the patient may report acute pain in the back or neck, which may radiate along the involved nerve. However, absence of pain does not rule out spinal injury, and a careful assessment of the spine is conducted if there has been a significant force and mechanism of injury (i.e., concomitant head injury). Often the patient speaks of fear that the neck or back is broken.

Respiratory dysfunction is related to the level of injury. The muscles contributing to respiration are the diaphragm (C4), intercostals (T1–T6), and abdominals (T6–T12). Injuries at C4 or above (causing paralysis of the diaphragm) often will require ventilator support, since acute respiratory failure is a leading cause of death (Hickey, 2014). Injuries of T12 and above will have impact on respiratory function. Functional abilities by level of injury are described in Table 65-2.

Assessment and Diagnostic Findings

A detailed neurologic examination is performed. Diagnostic x-rays (lateral cervical spine x-rays) and CT scanning are usually performed initially. An MRI scan may be ordered as a further workup if a ligamentous injury is suspected, because significant spinal cord damage may exist even in the absence of bony injury (Hickey, 2014). If an MRI scan is contraindicated, a myelogram may be used to

CHART 65-7

Effects of Spinal Cord Injuries

Central Cord Syndrome

- Characteristics: Motor deficits (in the upper extremities compared to the lower extremities; sensory loss varies but is more pronounced in the upper extremities); bowel/bladder dysfunction is variable, or function may be completely preserved.
- Cause: Injury or edema of the central cord, usually of the cervical area. May be caused by hyperextension injuries. Seen frequently in patients with cervical spine stenosis.

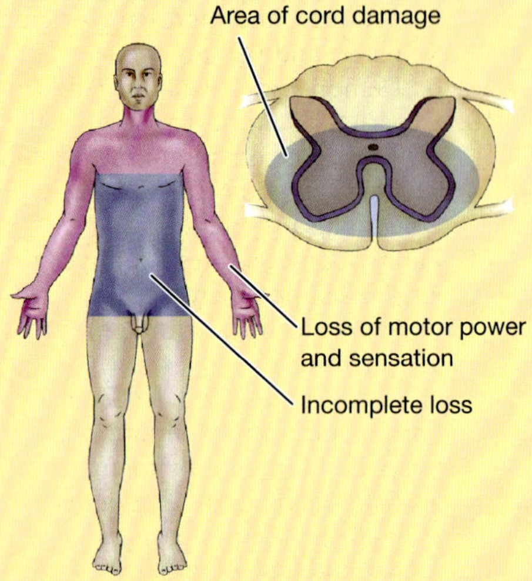

Central Cord Syndrome

Anterior Cord Syndrome

- Characteristics: Loss of pain, temperature, and motor function is noted below the level of the lesion; light touch, position, and vibration sensation remain intact.
- Cause: The syndrome may be caused by acute disk herniation or hyperflexion injuries associated with fracture-dislocation of vertebra. It also may occur as a result of injury to the anterior spinal artery, which supplies the anterior two thirds of the spinal cord.

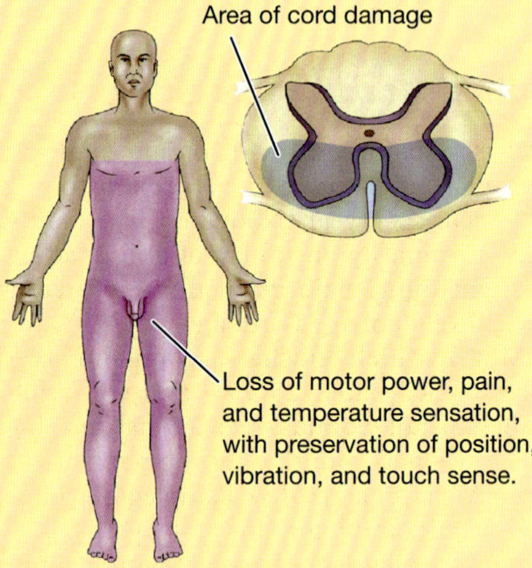

Anterior Cord Syndrome

Brown-Séquard Syndrome (Lateral Cord Syndrome)

- Characteristics: Ipsilateral paralysis or paresis is noted, together with ipsilateral loss of touch, pressure, and vibration and contralateral loss of pain and temperature.
- Cause: The lesion is caused by a transverse hemisection of the cord (half of the cord is transected from north to south), usually as a result of a knife or missile injury, fracture-dislocation of a unilateral articular process, or possibly an acute ruptured disk.

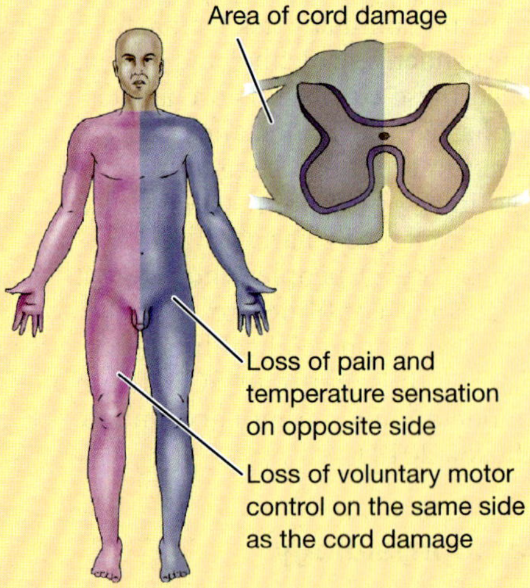

Brown-Séquard Syndrome

Adapted from Hickey, J. (2014). *The clinical practice of neurological & neurosurgical nursing* (7th ed.). Philadelphia, PA: Lippincott Williams & Wilkins.

TABLE 65-2 Functional Abilities by Level of Cord Injury

Injury Level	Segmental Sensorimotor Function	Dressing, Eating	Elimination	Mobility[a]
C1	Little or no sensation or control of head and neck; no diaphragm control; requires continuous ventilation	Dependent	Dependent	Limited. Voice or sip-n-puff controlled electric wheelchair
C2–C3	Head and neck sensation; some neck control; independent of mechanical ventilation for short periods	Dependent	Dependent	Same as for C1
C4	Good head and neck sensation and motor control; some shoulder elevation; diaphragm movement	Dependent, may be able to eat with adaptive sling	Dependent	Limited to voice, mouth, head, chin, or shoulder-controlled electric wheelchair
C5	Full head and neck control; shoulder strength; elbow flexion	Independent with assistance	Maximal assistance	Electric or modified manual wheelchair, needs transfer assistance
C6	Fully innervated shoulder; wrist extension or dorsiflexion	Independent or with minimal assistance	Independent or with minimal assistance	Independent in transfers and wheelchair
C7–C8	Full elbow extension; wrist plantar flexion; some finger control	Independent	Independent	Independent; manual wheelchair
T1–T5	Full hand and finger control; use of intercostal and thoracic muscles	Independent	Independent	Independent; manual wheelchair
T6–T10	Abdominal muscle control, partial to good balance with trunk muscles	Independent	Independent	Independent; manual wheelchair
T11–L5	Hip flexors, hip abductors (L1–L3); knee extension (L2–L4); knee flexion and ankle dorsiflexion (L4–L5)	Independent	Independent	Short distance to full ambulation with assistance
S1–S5	Full leg, foot, and ankle control; innervation of perineal muscles for bowel, bladder, and sexual function (S2–S4)	Independent	Normal to impaired bowel and bladder function	Ambulate independently with or without assistance

[a]Assistance refers to adaptive equipment, setup, or physical assistance.

Adapted from Hickey, J. V. (2014). *The clinical practice of neurological & neurosurgical nursing* (7th ed.). Philadelphia, PA: Lippincott Williams & Wilkins.

visualize the spinal axis. An assessment is made for other injuries, because spinal trauma often is accompanied by concomitant injuries, commonly to the head and chest. Continuous electrocardiographic monitoring may be indicated if an SCI is suspected, because bradycardia (slow heart rate) and asystole (cardiac standstill) can be seen in patients with acute spinal cord injuries.

Emergency Management

The immediate management at the scene of the injury is critical, because improper handling of the patient can cause further damage and loss of neurologic function. Any patient who is involved in a motor vehicle crash, a diving or contact sports injury, a fall, or any direct trauma to the head and neck must be considered to have SCI until such an injury is ruled out. Initial care must include a rapid assessment, immobilization, extrication, and stabilization or control of life-threatening injuries, and transportation to the most appropriate medical facility. Immediate transportation to a trauma centre with the capacity to manage major neurologic trauma is then necessary (Hickey, 2014).

At the scene of the injury, the patient must be immobilized on a spinal (back) board, with the head and neck maintained in a neutral position, to prevent an incomplete injury from becoming complete. One member of the team must assume control of the patient's head to prevent flexion, rotation, or extension; this is done by placing the hands on both sides of the patient's shoulders with the patient's head stabilized between the forearms; this position will limit movement and maintain alignment while a spinal board or cervical immobilizing device is applied. If possible, at least four people should slide the patient carefully onto a board for transfer to the hospital. Any twisting movement may irreversibly damage the spinal cord by causing a bony fragment of the vertebra to cut into, crush, or sever the cord completely.

The standard of care is that the patient is referred to a regional spinal injury or trauma centre because of the experienced multidisciplinary personnel and support services required to counteract the destructive changes that occur in the first 24 hours after injury. During treatment in the emergency and x-ray departments, the patient is kept on the transfer board. The patient must always be maintained in an extended position. No part of the body should be twisted or turned, and the patient is not allowed to sit up. Once the extent of the injury has been determined, the patient may be placed on a rotating specialty bed (Fig. 65-5) or in a cervical collar (Fig. 65-6). Later, if SCI and bone

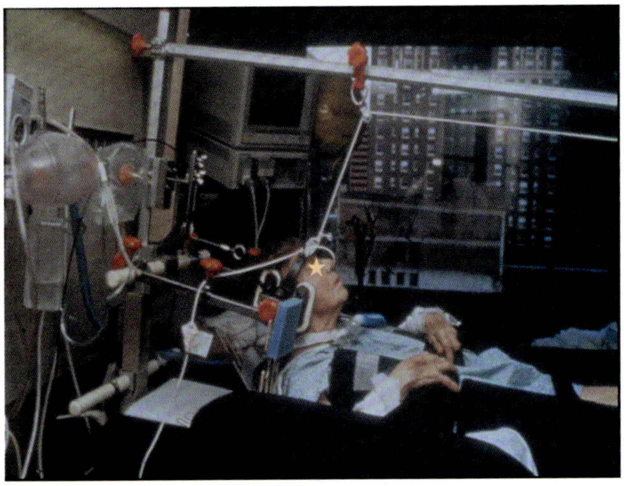

FIGURE 65-5. Patient in skeletal traction in a rotating specialty bed. (Adapted from Schwartz, E. D., Adam, E., & Flander, S. (2007). *Spinal trauma: Imaging, diagnosis, and management*. Philadelphia, PA: Lippincott Williams & Wilkins.)

instability have been ruled out, the patient may be moved to a conventional bed or the collar may be removed without harm. If a specialty bed is needed but not available, the patient should be placed in a cervical collar and on a firm mattress.

Medical Management (Acute Phase)

The goals of management are to prevent secondary injury, to observe for symptoms of progressive neurologic deficits, and to prevent complications. The patient is resuscitated as necessary, and oxygenation and cardiovascular stability are maintained. SCI is a devastating event; new treatment methods and medications are continually being investigated for the acute and chronic phases of care (Perez-Barcena et al., 2014; Stocchetti & Maas, 2014).

Pharmacologic Therapy

Administration of high-dose IV corticosteroids or methylprednisolone sodium succinate in the first 24 or 48 hours is controversial. Despite the ongoing controversy surrounding the practice, the use of IV high-dose methylprednisolone is accepted as standard therapy for SCI in many countries and remains an established clinical practice in most trauma centres in the United States (Hickey, 2014). However, in Canada, the use of steroids in the acute phase of an SCI is no longer the standard of care.

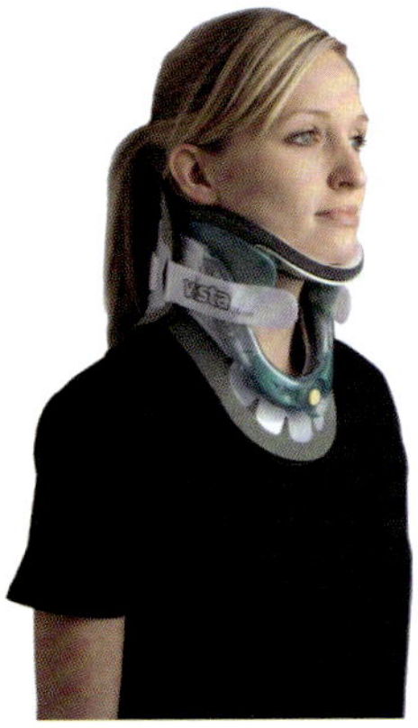

FIGURE 65-6. Cervical collar. (Used with permission from Aspen Medical Products.)

Respiratory Therapy

Oxygen is given to maintain a high partial pressure of arterial oxygen (PaO_2), because hypoxemia can create or worsen a neurologic deficit of the spinal cord. If endotracheal intubation is necessary, extreme care is taken to avoid flexing or extending the patient's neck, which can result in extension of a cervical injury.

In high cervical spine injuries, spinal cord innervation to the phrenic nerve, which stimulates the diaphragm, is lost. Diaphragmatic pacing (electrical stimulation of the phrenic nerve) attempts to stimulate the diaphragm to help the patient breathe. Intramuscular diaphragmatic pacing is currently in the clinical trial phase for the patient with a high cervical injury. This is implanted via laparoscopic surgery, usually after the acute phase.

Skeletal Fracture Reduction and Traction

Management of SCI requires immobilization and reduction of dislocations (restoration of preinjury position) and stabilization of the vertebral column. This can be accomplished by surgical and/or nonsurgical interventions; both aim to prevent new or worsening neurologic damage.

Cervical fractures can be reduced, and the cervical spine aligned with some form of skeletal traction, such as with skeletal tongs or with the use of the halo device (Bader et al., 2016). Traction is applied to the skeletal traction device by weights (ensuring the weights are unencumbered); the amount depends on the size of the patient and the degree of fracture displacement (see Fig. 65-5). The traction force is exerted along the longitudinal axis of the vertebral bodies, with the patient's neck in a neutral position. The traction is then gradually increased by adding more weights. As the amount of traction is increased, the spaces between the intervertebral discs widen and the vertebrae are given a chance to slip back into position. Reduction usually occurs after correct alignment has been restored. Once reduction is achieved, as verified by cervical spine x-rays and neurologic examination, the weights are gradually removed until the amount of weight needed to maintain the alignment is identified. Traction is sometimes supplemented with manual manipulation of the neck by a surgeon, to help achieve realignment of the vertebral bodies.

A halo device may be used initially with traction or may be applied after removal of the tongs. It consists of a titanium or stainless steel halo ring that is fixed to the skull by four pins, which are inserted into the outer table of the skull. The ring is attached to a removable **halo vest**, a device that suspends the weight of the unit circumferentially around the chest. A frame connects the ring to the chest. Halo devices provide immobilization of the cervical spine while allowing early ambulation (see Fig. 65-7) for patients with adequate function.

Thoracic and lumbar injuries are usually treated with surgical intervention, followed by immobilization with a fitted brace. Traction is often not indicated either before or after surgery, due to the relative stability of the spine in these regions.

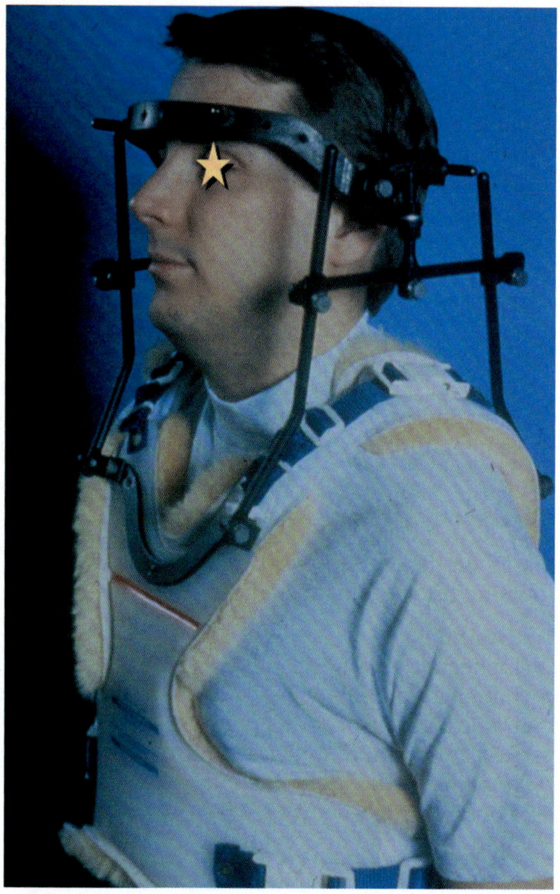

FIGURE 65-7. Halo and vest for cervical and thoracic injuries. (Adapted from Schwartz, E. D., Adam, E., & Flander, S. (2007). *Spinal trauma: Imaging, diagnosis, and management*. Philadelphia, PA: Lippincott Williams & Wilkins.)

NURSING ALERT

The patient's vital organ functions and body defenses must be supported and maintained until spinal and neurogenic shock abates and the neurologic system has recovered from the traumatic insult; this can take up to 4 months.

Surgical Management

Surgery is indicated in any of the following situations:

- Compression of the cord is evident.
- The injury results in a fragmented or unstable vertebral body.
- The injury involves a wound that penetrates the cord.
- Bony fragments are in the spinal canal.
- The patient's neurologic status is deteriorating.

Early surgical stabilization may improve the clinical outcome of patients compared to surgery performed later during the clinical course. The goals of surgical treatment are to preserve neurologic function by removing pressure from the spinal cord and to provide stability.

Management of Acute Complications of Spinal Cord Injury

Spinal and Neurogenic Shock

The spinal shock associated with SCI reflects a sudden depression of reflex activity in the spinal cord (areflexia) below the level of injury. The muscles innervated by the part of the spinal cord segment below the level of the lesion are without sensation, paralyzed, and flaccid, and the reflexes are absent. Blood pressure may be decreased and the patient may be bradycardic. Studies suggest that hypotension and shock can further damage the spinal cord and that the mean arterial pressure (MAP) should be maintained at 85 mm Hg or higher during the hyperacute phase (Jia, Kowalski, Sciubba, et al., 2013). The reflexes that initiate bladder and bowel function are affected. Bowel distention and paralytic ileus can be caused by depression of the reflexes and are treated with intestinal decompression by insertion of a nasogastric tube. A paralytic ileus most often occurs within the first 2 to 3 days after SCI and resolves within 3 to 7 days (Bader et al., 2016).

Neurogenic shock develops as a result of the loss of autonomic nervous system function below the level of the lesion. The vital organs are affected, causing decreases in blood pressure, heart rate, and cardiac output, as well as venous pooling in the extremities and peripheral vasodilation (Bader et al., 2016). In addition, the patient does not perspire in the paralyzed portions of the body, because sympathetic activity is blocked; therefore, close observation is required for early detection of an abrupt onset of fever. See Chapter 18 for further discussion of neurogenic shock.

With injuries to the cervical and upper thoracic spinal cord, innervation to the major accessory muscles of respiration is lost and respiratory problems develop. These include decreased vital capacity, retention of secretions, increased partial pressure of arterial carbon dioxide ($PaCO_2$) levels and decreased oxygen levels, respiratory failure, and pulmonary edema.

Venous Thromboembolism

The risk of venous thromboembolism (VTE) is a potential complication of immobility and occurs in patients with SCI at the same rate as those having had other types of traumatic injuries (Bader et al., 2016). Patients who develop VTE are at high risk for both deep vein thrombosis (DVT) and PE due to immobility, flaccidity, and decreased vasomotor tone (Jia et al., 2013).

Manifestations of PE include pleuritic chest pain, anxiety, shortness of breath, and abnormal blood gas values (increased $PaCO_2$ and decreased PaO_2). A fatal PE has been reported in up to 2% of patients with SCI within the first 3 months postinjury (Hickey, 2014).

Low-dose anticoagulation therapy usually is initiated to prevent DVT and PE, along with the use of antiembolism stockings or sequential pneumatic compression devices (SCDs). In some cases, permanent indwelling filters (see Chapter 23) may be placed prophylactically in the vena cava to prevent emboli (dislodged clots) from migrating to the lungs and causing PE. Prevention continues into the rehabilitation and chronic phases of SCI care (Abrams & Wakasa, 2014; Jia et al., 2013).

NURSING ALERT

The calves or thighs of a patient who is immobile should never be massaged because of the danger of dislodging an undetected thromboembolus.

Other Complications

In addition to respiratory complications (respiratory failure, pneumonia) and **autonomic dysreflexia** (characterized by pounding headache, profuse sweating, nasal congestion, piloerection ["goose bumps"], bradycardia, and hypertension), other complications that may occur include pressure ulcers and infection (urinary, respiratory, and local infection at the skeletal traction pin sites) (Morton & Fontaine, 2013).

Nursing Process

The Patient With Acute Spinal Cord Injury

Assessment

The patient's breathing pattern and the strength of the cough are assessed, and the lungs are auscultated, because paralysis of abdominal and respiratory muscles diminishes coughing and makes clearing of bronchial and pharyngeal secretions difficult. Reduced excursion of the chest also results.

The patient is monitored closely for any changes in motor or sensory function and for symptoms of progressive neurologic damage. In the early stages of SCI, determining whether the cord has been severed may not be possible, because signs and symptoms of cord edema are indistinguishable from those of cord transection. Edema of the spinal cord may occur with any severe cord injury and may further compromise spinal cord function.

Motor and sensory functions are assessed through careful neurologic examination. These findings are recorded on a flow sheet so that changes in the baseline neurologic status can be monitored closely and accurately. The ASIA classification is commonly used to describe level of function for patients with SCI. Chart 65-7 gives examples of the effects of altered spinal cord function. At the minimum:

- Motor ability is tested by asking the patient to spread the fingers, squeeze the examiner's hand, and move the toes or turn the feet.
- Sensation is evaluated by gently pinching the skin or touching it lightly with an object such as a tongue blade, starting at shoulder level and working down both sides of the extremities. The patient should have both eyes closed so that the examination reveals true findings, not what the patient hopes to feel. The patient is asked where the sensation is felt.
- Any changes in neurologic function are reported immediately.

The patient is also assessed for spinal shock, a complete loss of all reflex, motor, sensory, and autonomic activity below the level of the lesion that causes bladder paralysis and distention. The lower abdomen is palpated for signs of urinary retention and overdistention of the bladder. A bladder scanner is often used and strict intake and output is recorded. Further assessment is made for gastric dilation and paralytic ileus caused by an atonic bowel, a result of autonomic disruption.

Temperature is monitored, because the patient may have periods of hyperthermia as a result of alteration in temperature control due to autonomic disruption.

Nursing Priorities

Based on the assessment data, the patient's major nursing priorities may include the following:

- Breathing
- Ineffective airway clearance
- Impaired mobility
- Disturbed sensory perception
- Risk for pressure injuries
- Impaired urinary elimination
- Constipation
- Acute pain and discomfort

Collaborative Problems/ Potential Complications

Based on the assessment data, potential complications that may develop include:

- VTE
- Orthostatic hypotension
- Autonomic dysreflexia

Planning and Goals

The goals for the patient may include improved breathing pattern and airway clearance, improved mobility, improved sensory and perceptual awareness, maintenance of skin integrity, relief of urinary retention, improved bowel function, promotion of comfort, and absence of complications.

Nursing Interventions

Promoting Adequate Breathing and Airway Clearance

Possible impending respiratory failure is detected by observing the patient, measuring vital capacity, monitoring oxygen saturation through pulse oximetry, and monitoring arterial blood gases. Early and vigorous attention to clearing bronchial and pharyngeal secretions can prevent retention of secretions and atelectasis. Suctioning may be indicated, but it should be used with caution to avoid stimulating the vagus nerve and producing bradycardia and cardiac arrest.

If the patient cannot cough effectively because of decreased inspiratory volume and inability to generate sufficient expiratory pressure, chest physiotherapy and assisted coughing may be indicated. Specific breathing exercises are supervised by the nurse to increase the strength and endurance of the inspiratory muscles, particularly the diaphragm. Assisted coughing promotes clearing of secretions from the upper respiratory tract and is similar to the use of abdominal thrusts to clear an airway. Assisted coughing can be more effective than traditional suctioning because traditional suctioning clears the right mainstem bronchus, whereas sites for atelectasis and pneumonia are most commonly in the left lower lung lobe (Jia et al., 2013). Proper humidification and hydration are important to prevent secretions from becoming thick and difficult to remove even with coughing. The patient is assessed for signs of respiratory infection (e.g., cough, fever, dyspnea). Ascending edema of the spinal cord in the acute phase may cause respiratory difficulty that requires immediate intervention. Therefore, the patient's respiratory status must be monitored closely.

Improving Mobility

Proper body alignment is maintained at all times. If not on a specialized rotating bed, the patient should not be turned until the primary provider has indicated that it is safe to do so. Once safe for movement, the patient is repositioned frequently and is assisted out of bed as soon as the spinal column is stabilized. The feet are prone to footdrop; therefore, various types of splints are used to prevent footdrop. When used, the splints are removed and reapplied every 2 hours. Trochanter rolls, applied from the crest of the ilium to the midthigh of both legs, help prevent external rotation of the hip joints. Patients with lesions above the midthoracic level have loss of sympathetic control of peripheral vasoconstrictor activity, leading to hypotension. These patients may tolerate changes in position poorly and require monitoring of blood pressure when positions are changed.

Contractures can develop rapidly with immobility and muscle paralysis. A joint that is immobilized too long becomes fixed as a result of contractures of the tendon and joint capsule. Atrophy of the extremities results from disuse. Contractures and other complications may be prevented by range-of-motion exercises that help preserve joint motion and stimulate circulation. Passive range-of-motion exercises should be implemented as soon as possible after injury. Toes, metatarsals, ankles, knees, and hips should be put through a full range of motion at least four, or ideally five, times daily.

For most patients who have a cervical fracture without neurologic deficit, reduction in traction followed by rigid immobilization for 6 to 8 weeks restores skeletal integrity. These patients are allowed to move gradually to an erect position. A neck brace or moulded collar is applied when the patient is mobilized after traction is removed (see Fig. 65-6).

Preventing Injury due to Sensory and Perceptual Alterations

The nurse assists the patient to compensate for sensory and perceptual alterations that occur with SCI. The intact senses above the level of the injury are stimulated through touch, aromas, flavourful food and beverages, conversation, and music. Additional strategies include the following:

- Providing glasses to enable the patient to see from the supine position
- Encouraging the use of hearing aids, if indicated, to enable the patient to hear conversations and environmental sounds
- Providing emotional support to the patient and family
- Educating the patient and family about strategies to compensate for, or cope with, sensory deficits

Maintaining Skin Integrity

Pressure ulcers are a significant complication of SCI. The most common sites are over the sacrum (39.0%), heels (13.0%), ischial tuberosity (8.0%), and the occiput (back of head) (6.1%) (Jia et al., 2013). Pressure ulcers may begin within hours of an acute SCI where pressure is continuous and where the peripheral circulation is inadequate as a result of spinal shock and a recumbent position. It is important to move the patient from the backboard as soon as possible and inspect the skin. In addition, patients who wear cervical collars for prolonged periods may develop breakdown from the pressure of the collar under the chin, on the shoulders, and at the occiput. Pressure ulcers can add substantially to the personal and economic costs of living with SCI. The prevalence of this complication ranges from 17% for people 2 months after injury to 33% for those living with SCI.

The most effective approach to addressing this costly complication of SCI is prevention. The patient's position is changed at least every 2 hours (Bader et al., 2016). Turning not only assists in the prevention of pressure ulcers but also prevents pooling of blood and edema in the dependent areas. Careful inspection of the skin is made each time the patient is turned. The skin over the pressure points is assessed for redness or breaks; the perineum is checked for soilage, and the catheter is observed for adequate drainage. The patient's general body alignment and comfort are assessed. Special attention should be given to pressure areas in contact with the transfer board.

In addition, the patient's skin should be kept clean by washing with a mild soap, rinsing well, and blotting dry. Pressure-sensitive areas should be kept well lubricated and soft with oil or emollient lotion. The patient is educated about the danger of pressure ulcers and is encouraged to take control and make decisions about appropriate skin care. See Chapter 13 for other aspects of the prevention of pressure ulcers.

Maintaining Urinary Elimination

Immediately after SCI, the urinary bladder becomes atonic and cannot contract by reflex activity. Urinary retention is the immediate result. During the initial acute phase, a Foley catheter is inserted; however, prompt discontinuation is advised due to high risk of catheter-associated UTI. Once discontinued, the patient has no sensation of bladder distention and overstretching of the bladder and detrusor muscle may occur, delaying the return of bladder function.

Intermittent catheterization is carried out to avoid overdistention of the bladder and high risk for UTI due to retention of urine. At an early stage, family members are shown how to carry out intermittent catheterization and are encouraged to participate in this facet of care, because they will be involved in long-term follow-up and must be able to recognize complications so that treatment can be instituted.

The patient is educated to record fluid intake, voiding pattern, amounts of residual urine after voiding, characteristics of urine, and any unusual sensations that may occur. The management of a **neurogenic bladder** (bladder dysfunction that results from a disorder or dysfunction of the nervous system) is discussed in detail in Chapter 13.

Improving Bowel Function

Immediately after SCI, a paralytic ileus usually develops as a result of neurogenic paralysis of the bowel; therefore, a nasogastric tube is often required to relieve distention and to prevent vomiting and aspiration (Rodriguez, 2016).

Bowel activity usually returns within the first week. With the intake of nutrition, it is important to establish a bowel program. A bowel program can help to control bowel movements by establishing a pattern of planned evacuation (see Chapter 13). The nurse administers prescribed combinations of stool softeners, stimulant laxatives, bulking laxatives, and rectal laxatives along with rectal stimulation, to counteract the effects of immobility and analgesic agents (Rodriguez, 2016).

Providing Comfort Measures: The Patient in Traction With Tongs or a Halo Vest

A patient who has had pins, tongs, or calipers placed for cervical stabilization may have a headache or discomfort for several days after the pins are inserted. Patients initially may be bothered by the rather startling appearance of these devices, but usually they readily adapt to it because the device provides comfort for the unstable neck (see Fig. 65-7). The patient may complain of being caged in and of noise created by any object coming in contact with the frame of a halo device, but they can be reassured that adaptation will occur.

The areas around the four pin sites of a halo device are cleaned at least daily and observed for redness, drainage, and pain. The pins are observed for loosening, which may contribute to infection. If one of the pins becomes detached, the head is stabilized in a neutral position by one person, while another notifies the primary provider. A torque screwdriver should be readily available in case the screws on the frame need tightening.

The skin under the halo vest is inspected for excessive perspiration, redness, and skin blistering, especially on the bony prominences. The vest is opened at the sides to allow the torso to be washed. The liner of the vest should not become wet, because dampness causes skin excoriation. Powder is not used inside the vest, because it may contribute to the development of pressure ulcers. The liner should be changed periodically to promote hygiene and good skin care. If the patient is to be discharged with the vest, detailed instructions must be given to the family, with time allowed for them to demonstrate the necessary skills of halo vest care (see Chart 65-8).

Monitoring and Managing Potential Complications

Patients are at high risk for VTE after SCI. The patient must be assessed for symptoms of VTE including DVT and PE. Chest pain, shortness of breath, and changes in arterial blood gas values must be reported promptly to the primary provider. The circumferences of the thighs and calves are measured and recorded daily; further diagnostic studies are performed if a significant increase is noted. Patients remain at high risk for thrombophlebitis for several months after the initial injury. Patients with paraplegia or tetraplegia are at increased risk for the rest of their lives. Immobilization and the associated venous stasis, as well as varying degrees of autonomic disruption, contribute to the high risk and susceptibility for DVT.

Anticoagulation should be initiated within 72 hours of injury and continued for at least 3 months (Jia et al., 2013). The use of low–molecular-weight heparin or low-dose unfractionated heparin may be followed by long-term oral anticoagulation (i.e., warfarin [Coumadin]). Additional measures such as range-of-motion exercises, antiembolism stockings, and adequate hydration are important preventive measures. SCDs may also be used to reduce venous pooling and promote venous return. It is also important to avoid external pressure on the lower extremities that may result from flexion of the knees while the patient is in bed.

ORTHOSTATIC HYPOTENSION. For the first 2 weeks after SCI, the blood pressure tends to be unstable and can be quite low. It gradually returns to preinjury levels, but periodic episodes of severe orthostatic hypotension frequently interfere with efforts to mobilize the patient. Interruption in the reflex arcs that normally produce vasoconstriction in the upright position, coupled with vasodilation and pooling in abdominal and lower extremity vessels, can result in hypotension. Orthostatic hypotension is a particularly common problem for patients with lesions above T7. In some patients with tetraplegia, even slight elevations of the head can result in blood pressure dysregulation.

CHART 65-8

HOME CARE CHECKLIST • The Patient With a Halo Vest

At the completion of education, the patient and/or caregiver will be able to:

- Name the procedure that was performed and identify any permanent changes in anatomic structure or function as well as changes in ADLs, IADLs, roles, relationships, and spirituality.
  - Describe the rationale for the use of the halo vest.
- State how to contact all members of the treatment team (e.g., health care providers, home care professionals, rehabilitation team, durable medical equipment and supply vendor).
- State changes in lifestyle (e.g., diet, ADLs, IADLs, activity) necessary for recovery and health maintenance, as applicable.
  - Demonstrate safe techniques to assist the patient with self-care, hygiene, and ambulation.
  - Demonstrate assessment of frame, traction, tongs, and pins.
  - Demonstrate pin care using correct technique.
  - Demonstrate care of skin, including assessment (e.g., reddened or irritated areas, breakdown).
  - Identify signs and symptoms of infection.
  - Explain the reasons for and the method for changing the vest liner.
  - Identify holistic measures of pain management.
- Identify signs and symptoms of complications (e.g., venous thromboembolism, respiratory impairment, urinary tract infection).
- Describe emergency measures if respiratory or other complications develop while the patient is in the halo vest or if the frame becomes dislodged.
- Relate how to reach primary provider with questions or complications.
- State time and date of follow-up medical appointments, therapy, and testing.
- Identify sources of support (e.g., friends, relatives, faith community, spinal cord injury support groups, caregiver support).
- Identify the need for health promotion, disease prevention, and screening activities.

ADLs, activities of daily living; IADLs, independent activities of daily living.

A number of techniques can be used to reduce the frequency of hypotensive episodes. Close monitoring of vital signs before and during position changes is essential. Optimization of fluid status and vasopressor medication can be used to treat the profound vasodilation. Antiembolism stockings should be applied to improve venous return from the lower extremities. Abdominal binders may also be used to encourage venous return and provide diaphragmatic support when the patient is upright (Bader et al., 2016; Mills, Fung, Travios, et al., 2015). Activity should be planned in advance, and adequate time should be allowed for a slow progression of position changes from recumbent to sitting and upright. Tilt tables frequently are helpful in assisting patients to make this transition.

Recognizing Autonomic Dysreflexia

Autonomic dysreflexia, also known as autonomic hyperreflexia, is an acute life-threatening emergency that occurs as a result of exaggerated autonomic responses to stimuli that are harmless in people without SCI. It occurs only after spinal shock has resolved. This syndrome is characterized by a severe, pounding headache with paroxysmal hypertension, profuse diaphoresis above the spinal level of the lesion (most often of the forehead), nausea, nasal congestion, and bradycardia. It occurs among patients with cord lesions above T6 (the sympathetic visceral outflow level) after spinal shock has subsided (Bader et al., 2016). The sudden increase in blood pressure may cause retinal hemorrhage, hemorrhagic stroke, myocardial infarction, or seizures (Hickey, 2014). A number of stimuli may trigger this reflex: distended bladder (the most common cause); distention or contraction of the visceral organs, especially the bowel (from constipation, impaction); or stimulation of the skin (tactile, pain, thermal stimuli, pressure ulcer). Because this is an emergency situation, the objectives are to remove the triggering stimulus and to avoid the possibility of serious complications (Wan & Krassioukov, 2014).

The following measures are carried out:

- The patient is placed immediately in a sitting position to lower blood pressure.
- Rapid assessment is performed to identify and alleviate the cause.
- The bladder is emptied immediately via a urinary catheter. If an indwelling catheter is not patent, it is irrigated or replaced with another catheter.

- The rectum is examined for a fecal mass. If one is present, a topical anesthetic agent is inserted 10 to 15 minutes before the mass is removed, because visceral distention or contraction can cause autonomic dysreflexia.
- The skin is examined for any areas of pressure, irritation, or broken skin.
- Any other stimulus that could be the triggering event, such as an object next to the skin or a draft of cold air, must be removed.
- If these measures do not relieve the hypertension and excruciating headache, antihypertensive medications may be prescribed and given slowly by the IV route.
- The medical record is labeled with a clearly visible note about the risk of autonomic dysreflexia.
- The patient is instructed about prevention and management measures.
- Any patient with a lesion above the T6 segment is informed that such an episode is possible and may occur even many years after the initial injury (Bader et al., 2016).

Promoting Home, Community-Based, and Transitional Care

EDUCATING PATIENTS ABOUT SELF-CARE. In most cases, patients with SCI (i.e., patients with tetraplegia or paraplegia) need long-term rehabilitation. The process begins during hospitalization, as acute symptoms begin to subside or come under better control and the overall deficits and long-term effects of the injury become clear. The goals begin to shift from merely surviving the injury to learning strategies necessary to cope with the alterations that the injury imposes on activities of daily living (ADLs). The emphasis shifts from ensuring that the patient is stable and free of complications to specific assessment and planning designed to meet the patient's rehabilitation needs. Patient teaching may initially focus on the injury and its effects on mobility, dressing, and bowel, bladder, and sexual function. As the patient and family acknowledge the consequences of the injury and the resulting disability, the focus of teaching broadens to address issues necessary for carrying out the tasks of daily living and taking charge of their lives (Griffiths & Kennedy, 2012). Teaching begins in the acute phase and continues throughout rehabilitation and throughout the patient's life as changes occur, the patient ages, and problems arise.

Caring for the patient with SCI at home may at first seem a daunting task to the family. They will require dedicated nursing support to gradually assume full care of the patient. Although maintaining function and preventing complications will remain important, goals regarding self-care and preparation for discharge will assist in a smooth transition to rehabilitation and eventually to the community.

CONTINUING AND TRANSITIONAL CARE. The goal of the rehabilitation process is independence. The nurse becomes a support to both the patient and the family, assisting them to assume responsibility for increasing aspects of patient care and management. Care for the patient with SCI involves members of all the health care disciplines, which may include nursing, medicine, rehabilitation, respiratory therapy, physical and occupational therapy, case management, and social services. The nurse often serves as coordinator of the management team and as a liaison with rehabilitation centres and home care agencies. The patient and family often require assistance in dealing with the psychological impact of the injury and its consequences; referral to a psychiatric clinical nurse specialist or other mental health care professional often is helpful.

The nurse should reassure female patients with SCI that pregnancy is not contraindicated and fertility is relatively unaffected, but that women who are pregnant with acute or chronic SCI pose unique management challenges. The usual physiologic changes of pregnancy may predispose women with SCI to many potentially life-threatening complications, including autonomic dysreflexia, pyelonephritis, respiratory insufficiency, thrombophlebitis, PE, and unattended delivery. Preconception assessment and counselling are strongly recommended to ensure that the woman is in optimal health and to increase the likelihood of an uneventful pregnancy and healthy outcomes (Pebdani, Johnson, & Amtmann, 2014).

As more patients survive acute SCI, they face the changes associated with aging with a disability. Therefore, teaching in the home and community focuses on health promotion and addresses the need to minimize risk factors (e.g., smoking, alcohol and drug abuse, obesity). Routine health screening and preventive services are needed for the older adult with SCI. Home care nurses and others who have contact with patients with SCI are in a position to teach patients about healthy lifestyles, remind them of the need for health screenings, and make referrals as appropriate. Assisting patients to identify accessible health care professionals, clinical facilities, and imaging centres may increase the likelihood that they will participate in health screening.

Evaluation

Expected patient outcomes may include the following:

1. Demonstrates improvement in gas exchange and clearance of secretions, as evidenced by usual breath sounds on auscultation
   a. Breathes easily without shortness of breath
   b. Performs hourly deep-breathing exercises, coughs effectively, and clears pulmonary secretions
   c. Is free of respiratory infection (i.e., has appropriate temperature, respiratory rate, and pulse; normal breath sounds; absence of purulent sputum)
2. Moves within limits of the dysfunction and demonstrates completion of exercises within functional limitations
3. Demonstrates adaptation to sensory and perceptual alterations
   a. Uses assistive devices (e.g., prism glasses, hearing aids, computers) as indicated

   b. Describes sensory and perceptual alterations as a consequence of injury
4. Demonstrates optimal skin integrity
   a. Exhibits usual skin turgor; skin is free of reddened areas or breaks
   b. Participates in skin care and monitoring procedures within functional limitations
5. Regains urinary bladder function
   a. Exhibits no signs of UTI (i.e., has appropriate temperature; voids clear, dilute urine)
   b. Has adequate fluid intake
   c. Participates in bladder training program within functional limitations
6. Regains bowel function
   a. Reports regular pattern of bowel movement
   b. Consumes adequate dietary fibre and oral fluids
   c. Participates in bowel training program within functional limitations
7. Reports absence of pain and discomfort
8. Is free of complications
   a. Demonstrates no signs of thrombophlebitis, DVT, or PE
   b. Maintains blood pressure within expected limits
   c. Reports no lightheadedness with position changes
   d. Exhibits no manifestations of autonomic dysreflexia (i.e., absence of headache, diaphoresis, nasal congestion, bradycardia, or diaphoresis)

Medical Management of Long-Term Complications of Spinal Cord Injury

The patient faces a lifetime of disability, requiring ongoing follow-up and care. The expertise of a number of health professionals, including physicians (specifically a physiatrist), rehabilitation nurses, occupational therapists, physical therapists, psychologists, social workers, rehabilitation engineers, and vocational counsellors, is necessary at different times as the need arises.

The patient with an SCI has a shorter life expectancy compared to those who have not had an SCI (Abrams & Wakasa, 2014). As patients with SCI age, they have many of the same medical problems as others. In addition, they face the threat of complications associated with their disability (Hickey, 2014). Usually, patients are encouraged to follow up at an outpatient spinal cord clinic when complications and other issues arise. Lifetime care includes assessment of the urinary tract at prescribed intervals, because there is the likelihood of continuing alteration in detrusor and sphincter function, and the patient is prone to UTI (Abrams & Wakasa, 2014).

Long-term problems and complications of SCI include disuse syndrome, autonomic dysreflexia (discussed earlier), bladder and kidney infections, spasticity, and depression (Abrams & Wakasa, 2014). Pressure ulcers with potential complications of sepsis, osteomyelitis, and fistulas occur in about 10% of patients. Spasticity may be particularly disabling. Heterotopic ossification (overgrowth of bone) in the hips, knees, shoulders, and elbows occurs in many patients after SCI. Spasticity and heterotopic ossification of these complications are painful and can produce a loss of range of motion (Abrams & Wakasa, 2014). Management includes observing for and addressing any alteration in physiologic status and psychological outlook, as well as the prevention and treatment of long-term complications. The nursing role involves emphasizing the need for vigilance in self-assessment and care.

Nursing Process

The Patient With Tetraplegia or Paraplegia

Assessment

Assessment focuses on the patient's general condition, complications, and how the patient is managing at that particular point in time. A head-to-toe assessment and review of systems should be part of the database, with emphasis on the areas that are prone to problems in this population. A thorough inspection of all areas of the skin for redness or breakdown is critical. The nurse reviews the established bowel and bladder program with the patient, because the program must continue uninterrupted. Patients with tetraplegia or paraplegia have varying degrees of loss of motor power, deep and superficial sensation, vasomotor control, bladder and bowel control, and sexual function. They are faced with potential complications related to immobility, skin breakdown and pressure ulcers, recurring UTIs, and contractures. Knowledge about these particular issues can further guide the assessment in any setting. Nurses in all settings, including home care, must be aware of these potential complications in the lifetime management of these patients.

An understanding of the emotional and psychological responses to tetraplegia or paraplegia is achieved by observing the responses and behaviours of the patient and family and by listening to their concerns (Chuang, Yang, & Kuo, 2015). Documenting these assessments and reviewing the plan with the entire team on a regular basis provide insight into how both the patient and the family are coping with the changes in lifestyle and body functioning. Additional information frequently can be gathered from the social worker or psychiatric/mental health worker.

It takes time for the patient and family to comprehend the magnitude of the disability. They may go through stages of grief, including shock, disbelief, denial, anger, depression, and acceptance. During the acute phase of the injury, denial can be a protective mechanism to shield the patient from the acute reality of what has happened. As the patient realizes the permanent nature of paraplegia or tetraplegia, the grieving process may be prolonged and all-encompassing because of the recognition that long-held plans and expectations are interrupted or permanently altered. A period of depression often follows as the patient experiences a loss of self-esteem in areas of self-identity, sexual functioning, and social and emotional roles. Exploration and assessment of these issues can assist in developing a meaningful plan of care.

Nursing Priorities

Based on the assessment data, the major nursing priorities for the patient with tetraplegia or paraplegia may include the following:

- Impaired mobility
- Risk for disuse syndrome
- Risk for pressure injuries
- Impaired urinary elimination
- Constipation
- Sexual dysfunction
- Ineffective coping
- Deficient knowledge

Collaborative Issues/ Potential Complications

Based on all the assessment data, potential complications of tetraplegia or paraplegia that may develop include:

- Spasticity
- Infection and sepsis

Planning and Goals

The goals for the patient may include attainment of some form of mobility; maintenance of healthy, intact skin; achievement of bladder management without infection; achievement of bowel control; achievement of sexual expression; strengthening of coping mechanisms; and absence of complications.

Nursing Interventions

The patient requires extensive rehabilitation, which is less difficult if appropriate nursing management has been carried out during the acute phase of the injury or illness. Nursing care is one of the key factors determining the success of the rehabilitation program. The main objective is for the patient to live as independently as possible in the home and community.

Increasing Mobility

EXERCISE PROGRAMS. The unaffected parts of the body are built up to optimal strength to promote maximal self-care. The muscles of the hands, arms, shoulders, chest, spine, abdomen, and neck must be strengthened in the patient with paraplegia, because he or she must bear full weight on these muscles to ambulate. The triceps and the latissimus dorsi are important muscles used in crutch walking. The muscles of the abdomen and the back also are necessary for balance and for maintaining the upright position.

To strengthen these muscles, the patient can do push-ups when in a prone position and sit-ups when in a sitting position. Extending the arms while holding weights (traction weights can be used) also develops muscle strength. Squeezing rubber balls or crumbling newspaper promotes hand strength.

With encouragement from all members of the rehabilitation team, the patient with paraplegia can develop the increased exercise tolerance needed for gait training and ambulation activities. The importance of maintaining cardiovascular fitness is stressed to the patient. Alternative exercises to increase the heart rate to target levels are designed within the patient's abilities.

MOBILIZATION. After the spine is stable enough to allow the patient to assume an upright posture, mobilization activities are initiated. A brace or vest may be used, depending on the level of the lesion. A patient whose paralysis is a result of complete transection of the cord can begin weight bearing early, because no further damage can be incurred. The sooner muscles are used, the less chance there is of disuse atrophy. The earlier the patient is brought to a standing position, the less opportunity there is for osteoporotic changes to take place in the long bones. Weight bearing also reduces the possibility of renal calculi and enhances many other metabolic processes.

Braces and crutches enable some patients with paraplegia to ambulate for short distances. Ambulation using crutches requires a high expenditure of energy. Motorized wheelchairs and specially equipped vans can provide greater independence and mobility for patients with high-level SCI or other lesions. Every effort should be made to encourage the patient to be as mobile and active as possible.

Long-term risks include altered body composition, a decrease in lean body mass, decreased bone mineral density, and increased BMI. Patients are at high risk for obesity due to high fat intake combined with decreased physical activity (Lieberman, Goff, Hammond, et al., 2014). This puts patients at higher risk of developing comorbid conditions such as diabetes and cardiovascular disease. Patients benefit from nutrition counselling to prevent these secondary complications. For those who are overweight or who have obesity, weight-loss programs must be designed to accommodate the dietary and physical activity barriers that are unique to this population (Lieberman et al., 2014).

Preventing Disuse Syndrome

Patients are at high risk for development of contractures as a result of disuse syndrome due to the musculoskeletal system changes (atrophy) brought about by the loss of motor and sensory functions below the level of injury. Range-of-motion exercises must be provided at least four times a day, and care is taken to stretch the Achilles tendon with exercises. The patient is repositioned frequently and is maintained in proper body alignment whether in bed or in a wheelchair.

Contractures can complicate day-to-day care, increasing the difficulty of positioning and decreasing mobility. Medical management for contractures will include serial casting or splinting. The use of Botox is also becoming more and more frequent in this patient population. A number of surgical procedures have been tried with varying degrees of success. These techniques are used if more conservative approaches fail, but the best treatment is prevention. Severing of tendons or the implantation of baclofen pumps are also common surgical approaches utilized.

Promoting Skin Integrity

Because these patients spend a great portion of their lives in wheelchairs, pressure ulcers are an ever-present threat. Contributing factors are permanent sensory loss over pressure areas; immobility, which makes relief of pressure difficult; trauma from bumps (against the wheelchair, toilet, furniture, and so forth) that cause unnoticed abrasions and wounds; loss of protective function of the skin from excoriation and maceration due to excessive perspiration and possible incontinence; and poor general health (anemia, edema, malnutrition), leading to poor tissue perfusion. The prevention and management of pressure ulcers are discussed in detail in Chapter 13.

The person with tetraplegia or paraplegia must take responsibility for monitoring (or directing monitoring) of his or her skin status. This involves relieving pressure and not remaining in any position for longer than 2 hours, in addition to ensuring that the skin receives meticulous attention and cleansing. The patient is taught that ulcers develop over bony prominences that are exposed to unrelieved pressure in the lying and sitting positions. The most vulnerable areas are identified. The patient with paraplegia is instructed to use mirrors, if possible, to inspect these areas morning and night, observing for redness, slight edema, or any abrasions. While in bed, the patient should turn at 2-hour intervals and then inspect the skin again for redness that does not fade on pressure. The bottom sheet should be checked for wetness and for creases. The patient with tetraplegia or paraplegia who cannot perform these activities is encouraged to direct others to check these areas and prevent ulcers from developing.

The patient is taught to relieve pressure while in the wheelchair by performing frequent pressure relief manoeuvres, leaning from side to side to relieve ischial pressure, and tilting forward while leaning on a table. The caregiver for the patient with tetraplegia will need to perform these activities if the patient cannot do so independently. A wheelchair cushion is prescribed to meet individual needs, which may change in time with changes in posture, weight, and skin tolerance. A referral can be made to a rehabilitation engineer, who can measure pressure levels while the patient is sitting and then tailor the cushion and other necessary aids and assistive devices to the patient's needs.

The diet for the patient with tetraplegia or paraplegia should be high in protein, vitamins, and calories to ensure minimal wasting of muscle and the maintenance of healthy skin, and high in fluids to maintain well-functioning kidneys. Excessive weight gain and obesity should be avoided, because they further limit mobility.

Improving Bladder Management

The effect of the spinal cord lesion on the bladder depends on the level of injury, the degree of cord damage, and the length of time after injury. A patient with tetraplegia or paraplegia usually has either a reflex or a nonreflex bladder (see Chapter 12). Both bladder types increase the risk of UTI.

The nurse emphasizes the importance of maintaining an adequate flow of urine by encouraging a fluid intake of about 2.5 L daily. The patient should empty the bladder frequently so that there is minimal residual urine and should pay attention to personal hygiene, because infection of the bladder and kidneys almost always occurs by the ascending route. The perineum must be kept clean and dry, and attention must be given to the perianal skin after defecation. Underwear should be cotton (which is more absorbent) and should be changed at least once a day.

If an external catheter (condom catheter) is used, the sheath is removed nightly; the penis is cleansed to remove urine and is dried carefully, because warm urine on the periurethral skin promotes the growth of bacteria. Attention also is given to the collection bag. The nurse emphasizes the importance of monitoring for signs of UTI: cloudy, foul-smelling urine or hematuria (blood in the urine); fever; or chills.

The female patient who cannot achieve reflex bladder control or self-catheterization may need to wear pads or waterproof undergarments. Surgical intervention may be indicated in some patients to create a urinary diversion.

Establishing Bowel Control

The objective of a bowel training program is to establish bowel evacuation through reflex conditioning, a technique described in Chapter 12. If the SCI occurs above the sacral segments or nerve roots and there is reflex activity, the anal sphincter may be massaged (digital stimulation) to stimulate defecation. If the cord lesion involves the sacral segment or nerve roots, anal massage is not performed, because the anus may be relaxed and lack tone. Massage is also contraindicated if there is spasticity of the anal sphincter. The anal sphincter is massaged by inserting a gloved finger (which has been adequately lubricated) 2.5 to 3.7 cm into the rectum and moving it in a circular motion or from side to side. It soon becomes apparent which area triggers the defecation response. This procedure should be performed at regular time intervals (usually every 48 hours), after a meal, and at a time that will be convenient for the patient at home. The patient also is taught the symptoms of impaction (frequent loose stools; constipation) and is cautioned to watch for hemorrhoids. A diet with sufficient fluids and fibre is essential to developing a successful bowel training program, avoiding constipation, and decreasing the risk of autonomic dysreflexia.

Counselling on Sexual Expression

Many patients with tetraplegia and paraplegia can have some form of meaningful sexual relationship, although modifications are necessary. The patient and partner benefit from counselling about the range of sexual expression possible, special techniques and positions, exploration of body sensations offering sensual feelings, and urinary and bowel hygiene as related to sexual activity (Morton & Fontaine, 2013). For men with erectile failure, penile prostheses enable them to have and sustain an erection, and impotence drugs may be helpful. Sildenafil (Viagra), vardenafil (Levitra), and tadalafil (Cialis), for example, are oral smooth muscle relaxants that cause blood to flow into the penis, resulting in an erection (see Chapter 50).

Sexual education and counselling services are included in the rehabilitation services at spinal centres. Small group meetings in which patients can share their feelings, receive information, and discuss sexual concerns and practical aspects are helpful in producing effective attitudes and adjustments.

Enhancing Coping Mechanisms

The impact of the disability and loss becomes marked when the patient returns home. Each time something new enters the patient's life (e.g., a new relationship, going to work), the patient is reminded anew of his or her limitations. Grief reactions and depression are common.

To work through this depression, the patient must have some hope for relief in the future. The nurse can encourage the patient to feel confident in his or her ability to achieve self-care and relative independence. The role of the nurse ranges from caretaker during the acute phase to teacher, counsellor, and facilitator as the patient gains mobility and independence.

The patient's disability affects not only the patient but also the entire family. In many cases, family therapy is helpful in working through issues as they arise. Adjustment to the disability leads to the development of realistic goals for the future, making the best of the abilities that are left intact and reinvesting in other activities and relationships. Rejection of the disability causes self-destructive neglect and noncompliance with the therapeutic program, which leads to more frustration and depression. Crises for which interventions may be sought include social, psychological, marital, sexual, and psychiatric problems. The family usually requires counselling, social services, and other support systems to help them cope with the changes in their lifestyle and socioeconomic status.

A major goal of nursing management is to help the patient overcome his or her sense of futility and to encourage the patient in the emotional adjustment that must be made before he or she is willing to venture into the outside world. However, an excessively sympathetic attitude on the part of the nurse may cause the patient to develop an overdependence that defeats the purpose of the entire rehabilitation program. The patient is taught and assisted when necessary, but the nurse should avoid performing activities that the patient can do independently with a little effort. This approach to care more than repays itself in the satisfaction of seeing a patient who is demoralized and helpless become independent and find meaning in a newly emerging lifestyle.

Monitoring and Managing Potential Complications

SPASTICITY. Muscle spasticity can be a problematic complication of tetraplegia and paraplegia. Flexor or extensor spasms occur below the level of the spinal cord lesion and can interfere with the rehabilitation process, ADLs, and quality of life (Abrams & Wakasa, 2014). Spasticity results from an imbalance between the facilitatory and inhibitory effects on neurons that exist normally. The area of the cord distal to the site of injury or lesion becomes disconnected from the higher inhibitory centres located in the brain, so facilitatory impulses, which originate from muscles, skin, and ligaments, predominate.

Spasticity is defined as a condition of increased muscle tone in a muscle that is weak. Initial resistance to stretching is quickly followed by sudden relaxation. The stimulus that precipitates spasm can be obvious, such as movement or a position change, or subtle, such as a slight jarring of the wheelchair. Most patients with tetraplegia or paraplegia have some degree of spasticity. Because it increases muscle tone, some degree of spasticity can be beneficial in patients who are weak (Abrams & Wakasa, 2014). With SCI, the onset of spasticity usually occurs from a few weeks to 6 months after the injury. The same muscles that are flaccid during the period of spinal shock develop spasticity during recovery. The intensity of spasticity tends to peak approximately 2 years after the injury, after which the spasms tend to regress.

Management of spasticity is based on the severity of symptoms and the degree of incapacitation. The antispasmodic medication baclofen (Lioresal) is one of the most commonly used agents because it is available in an oral and an intrathecal form. Other medications such as diazepam (Valium) and dantrolene (Dantrium) are also effective in controlling spasm (Morton & Fontaine, 2013). All of the antispasmodic medications cause drowsiness, weakness, and vertigo in some patients. Passive range-of-motion exercises and frequent turning and repositioning are helpful, because stiffness tends to increase spasticity. These activities also are essential in the prevention of contractures, pressure ulcers, and bowel and bladder dysfunction. Baclofen pumps which are implanted surgically have proven to be quite beneficial in this patient population.

INFECTION AND SEPSIS. Patients with tetraplegia and paraplegia are at increased risk for infection and sepsis from a variety of sources: urinary tract, respiratory tract, and pressure ulcers. Sepsis remains a major cause of complications and death in these patients. Prevention of infection and sepsis is essential through maintenance of skin integrity, complete emptying of the bladder at regular intervals, and prevention of urinary and fecal incontinence. The risk for respiratory infection can be decreased by avoiding contact with people who have symptoms of respiratory infection, performing coughing and deep-breathing exercises to prevent pooling of respiratory secretions, receiving yearly influenza vaccines, and giving up smoking. A high-protein diet is important in maintaining an adequate immune system, as is avoiding factors that may reduce immune system function, such as excessive stress, drug abuse, and excessive alcohol intake.

If infection occurs, the patient requires thorough assessment and prompt treatment. Antibiotic therapy and adequate hydration, in addition to local measures (depending on the site of infection), are initiated immediately.

UTIs are minimized or prevented by aseptic technique in catheter management, adequate hydration, bladder training program, and prevention of overdistention of the bladder and urinary stasis.

Skin breakdown and infection are prevented by maintenance of a turning schedule; frequent back care; regular assessment of all skin areas; regular cleaning and lubrication of the skin; passive range-of-motion exercise to prevent contractures; pressure relief over broken skin areas, bony prominences, and heels; and wrinkle-free bedsheets.

Pulmonary infections are managed and prevented by frequent coughing, turning, and deep-breathing exercises and chest physiotherapy; aggressive respiratory care and suctioning of the airway if a tracheostomy is present; assisted coughing as needed; and adequate hydration.

Infections of any kind can be life-threatening. Aggressive nursing interventions are key to prevention, detection, and early management.

Promoting Home, Community-Based, and Transitional Care

EDUCATING PATIENTS ABOUT SELF-CARE. Patients with tetraplegia or paraplegia are at risk for complications for the rest of their lives. Therefore, a major aspect of nursing care is teaching the patient and family about these complications and about strategies to minimize risks. UTIs, contractures, infected pressure ulcers, and sepsis may necessitate hospitalization. Other late complications that may occur include lower extremity edema, joint contractures, respiratory dysfunction, and pain. To avoid these and other complications, the patient and a family member are taught skin care, catheter care, range-of-motion exercises, breathing exercises, and other care techniques. Teaching is initiated as soon as possible and extends into the rehabilitation or long-term care facility and home. In all aspects of care, it is important for the nurse and patient to set mutual goals and discuss the tasks the patient is capable of doing independently and which tasks the patient needs assistance to complete. (See Chapter 12 for a more detailed discussion of rehabilitation.)

CONTINUING AND TRANSITIONAL CARE. Referral for home care is often appropriate for assessment of the home setting, patient teaching, and evaluation of the patient's physical and emotional status. During visits by the home care nurse, teaching about strategies to prevent or minimize potential complications is reinforced. The home environment is assessed for adequacy for care and for safety. Environmental modifications are made, and specialized equipment is obtained, ideally before the patient goes home.

The home care nurse also assesses the patient's and the family's adherence to recommendations and their use of coping strategies. The use of inappropriate coping strategies (e.g., drug and alcohol use) is assessed, and referrals to counselling are made for the patient and family. Appropriate and effective coping strategies are reinforced. The nurse reviews previous teaching and determines the need for further physical or psychological assistance. The patient's self-esteem and body image may be very poor at this time. Because people with high levels of social support often report feelings of well-being despite major physical disability, it is beneficial for the nurse to assess and promote further development of the support system and effective coping strategies for each patient.

The patient requires continuing, lifelong follow-up by the physician, physical therapist, and other rehabilitation team members, because the neurologic deficit is usually permanent and new deficits, complications, and secondary conditions can develop. These require prompt attention before they take their toll in additional physical impairment, time, morale, and financial costs. It is also useful for the patient to meet with vocational counsellors as he or she may have to change occupation and may require assistance with additional educational or vocational training.

The nurse is in a good position to remind patients and family members of the need for continuing health promotion and screening practices. Referral to accessible health care providers and imaging centres is important in health promotion and health screening. Chapter 10 has more information on chronic illness and disability.

Evaluation

Expected patient outcomes may include the following:

1. Attains some form of mobility
2. Contractures do not develop
3. Maintains healthy, intact skin
4. Achieves bladder control, absence of UTI
5. Achieves bowel control
6. Reports sexual satisfaction
7. Shows improved adaptation to environment and others
8. Exhibits reduction in spasticity
    a. Reports understanding of the precipitating factors
    b. Uses measures to reduce spasticity
9. Describes long-term management required
10. Exhibits absence of complications

Critical Thinking Exercises

1 An 18-year-old man is brought to the ED by his family, who report that he was "dinged" in a football game 1 week ago. The patient does not recall the event. His family states that he is sleeping more than usual and seems forgetful. What is the evidence base for conducting a comprehensive and focused evaluation for a patient with a sports concussion injury? What evidence-based recommendations may guide return to sports for this patient? Identify the criteria used to evaluate the strength of the evidence for these practices.

2 A 90-year-old patient on anticoagulant therapy is admitted to your unit with a chronic SDH. Identify the priorities, approach, and techniques you would use to provide care for this patient in the preoperative phase of care. How will your priorities, approach, and techniques differ in the postoperative phase of care?

3 A 68-year-old woman was involved in a motor vehicle crash 2 days ago and sustained a T6 fracture with SCI. As a result, she has paraplegia and is in a neurologic intensive care unit. Identify the priorities, approach, and techniques you would use to provide care for this patient during the acute phase of care. Identify how your priorities, approach, and techniques will differ once the patient reaches the rehabilitation phase of care.

REFERENCES AND SELECTED READINGS

Books

Arciniegas, D. B., Zasler, N. D., Vanderploeg, R. D., et al. (Eds.). (2013). *Management of adults with traumatic brain injury*. Arlington, VA: American Psychiatric Association.

Bader, M. K., Littlejohns, L. R., & Olson, D. (2016). *AANN core curriculum for neuroscience nursing* (6th ed.). Chicago, IL: American Association of Neuroscience Nurses.

Booker, K. (2015). *Critical care nursing: Monitoring and treatment for advanced nursing practice*. Oxford: Wiley Blackwell.

Comerford, K. C. (2015). *Nursing 2015 drug handbook*. Philadelphia, PA: Wolters Kluwer.

Diepenbrock, N. (2012). *Quick reference to critical care*. Philadelphia, PA: Wolters Kluwer Health/Lippincott Williams & Wilkins.

Eliopoulos, C. (2018). *Gerontological nursing* (9th ed.). Philadelphia, PA: Wolters Kluwer.

Hagen, C., Malkmus, D., & Durham, P. (1972). *The Rancho levels of cognitive functioning scale*. Downey, CA: Communication Disorders Service, Rancho Los Amigos Hospital. Revised 11/15/74 by: Danese Malkmus and Kathryn Stenderup.

Hickey, J. V. (2014). *The clinical practice of neurological & neurosurgical nursing* (7th ed.). Philadelphia, PA: Lippincott Williams & Wilkins.

Urden, L. D., Stacy, K. M., & Lough, M. E. (2013). Critical Care Nursing, Diagnosis and Management, 7: Critical Care Nursing. Elsevier Health Sciences.

West, T. A., Bergman, A., Biggins, M. S., et al. (2011). *Care of the patient with mild traumatic brain injury: AANN and ARN clinical practice guidelines series*. Glenview, IL: American Association of Neuroscience Nurses.

Journals and Electronic Documents

Head Injury

Abrams, G. M., & Wakasa, M. (2014). Chronic complications of spinal cord injury and disease. UpToDate. Retrieved on 2/24/17 at www.uptodate.com/contents/chronic-complications-of-spinal-cord-injury-and-disease

American Spinal Injury Association (ASIA). (2016). International standards for neurological classification of spinal cord injury. Retrieved on 2/23/17 at www.asia-spinalinjury.org/wp-content/uploads/2016/02/International_Stds_Diagram_Worksheet.pdf

Arbour, R. B. (2013). Brain death: Assessment, controversy, and confounding factors. *American Journal of Critical Care Nurses, 33*(6), 27–48.

Asselin, G., Penning, J. H., Ramanujam, S., et al. (2012). Therapeutic horse back riding of a spinal cord injured veteran: A case study. *Rehabilitation Nursing, 37*(6), 270–276.

Bailes, J. E., Petraglia, A. L., Omalu, B. I., et al. (2013). Role of subconcussion in repetitive mild traumatic brain injury. *Journal of Neurosurgery, 119*(5), 1235–1245.

Bauman, M., & McCourt, T. R. (2014). Assessing and managing patients with chronic subdural hematoma. *American Nurse Today, 9*(9), 38–41.

Beauchamp, M. R., Scarlett, L. J., Ruissen, G. R., et al. (2016). Peer mentoring of adults with spinal cord injury: A transformational leadership perspective. *Disability & Rehabilitation, 38*(19), 1884–1892.

Bodanapally, U. K., Sours, C., Zhuo, J., et al. (2015). Imaging of traumatic brain injury. *Radiologic Clinics of North America, 53*(4), 695–715.

Centers for Disease Control and Prevention (CDC). (2016a). *Injury prevention & control: Traumatic brain injury & concussion*. Retrieved on 2/9/2017 at www.cdc.gov/traumaticbraininjury/get_the_facts.html

Centers for Disease Control and Prevention (CDC). (2016b). *CDC study finds that adoption of the Brain Trauma Foundation guidelines could result in a substantial reduction in traumatic brain-injury-related deaths*. Retrieved on 2/9/2017 at www.cdc.gov/traumaticbraininjury/brain_trauma_guidelines.html

Chen, Y., Tang, Y., Vogel, L., et al. (2013). Causes of spinal cord injury. *Topics in Spinal Cord Injury Rehabilitation, 19*(1), 1–8.

Chuang, C., Yang, Y., & Kuo, L. T. (2015). Finding a way to cope: A qualitative study of the experience of persons with spinal cord injury. *Journal of Neuroscience Nursing, 47*(6), 313–319.

Giusti, G. D., Tuteri, D., & Giontella, M. (2016). Nursing interactions with intensive care unit patients affected by sleep deprivation: An observational study. *Dimensions of Critical Care Nursing, 35*(3), 154–159.

Griesdale, D. E., Örtenwall, V., Norena, M., et al. (2015). Adherence to guidelines for management of cerebral perfusion pressure and outcome in patients who have severe traumatic brain injury. *Journal of Critical Care, 30*(1), 111–115.

Griffiths, H. C., & Kennedy, P. (2012). Continuing with life as normal: Positive psychological outcomes following spinal cord injury. *Topics in Spinal Cord Injury Rehabilitation, 18*(3), 241–252.

Hemphill, J. C., & Phan, N. (2016). Traumatic brain injury: Epidemiology, classification and pathophysiology. UpToDate. Retrieved on 2/18/2017 at www.uptodate.com/contents/traumatic-brain-injury-epidemiology-classification-and-pathophysiology

Hollander, J. E., & Camacho, M. (2014). Assessment and management of scalp lacerations. UpToDate. Retrieved on 2/17/2017 at www.uptodate.com/contents/assessment-and-management-of-scalp-lacerations

Horn, S. D., Kinikini, M., Moore, L. W., et al. (2015). Enteral nutrition for patients with traumatic brain injury in the rehabilitation setting: Associations with patient preinjury and injury characteristics and outcomes. *Archives of Physical Medicine and Rehabilitation, 96*(8), S245–S255.

Hyatt, K. S. (2014). Mild traumatic brain injury. *American Journal of Nursing, 114*(11), 36–42.

Jia, X., Kowalski, R. G., Sciubba, D. M., et al. (2013). Critical care of the traumatic spinal cord injury. *Journal of Intensive Care Medicine, 28*(1), 12–23.

Larrow, V., & Klich-Heartt, E. I. (2016). Prevention of ventilator-associated pneumonia in the intensive care unit: Beyond the basics. *Journal of Neuroscience Nursing, 48*(3), 160–165.

Lieberman, J., Goff, D., Hammond, F., et al. (2014). Dietary intake and adherence to the 2010 guidelines for Americans among individuals with chronic spinal cord injury: A pilot study. *Journal of Spinal Cord Medicine, 37*(6), 751–757.

Madden, L. K., & DeVon, H. A. (2015). A systematic review of the effects of body temperature on outcome after adult traumatic brain injury. *Journal of Neuroscience Nursing, 47*(4), 190–203.

McNett, M. M., & Olson, D. M. (2013). Evidence to guide nursing interventions for critically ill neurologically impaired patients with ICP monitoring. *Journal of Neuroscience Nursing, 45*(3), 120–123.

Mills, P. B., Fung, C. K., Travios, A., et al. (2015). Nonpharmacologic management of orthostatic hypotension: A systematic review. *Archives of Physical Medicine and Rehabilitation, 96*(2), 366–375.

Mitchell, P. H., Kirkness, C., & Blissitt, P. A. (2015). Cerebral perfusion pressure and intracranial pressure in traumatic brain injury. *Annual Review of Nursing Research, 33*(1), 111–183.

Mohit, A. A. (2016). Cellular events and pathophysiology of SCI. *Spine (Phila Pa 1976)*, *41*(Suppl 7), S28.
Morton, P., & Fontaine, D. (2013). Critical care nursing: A holistic approach. *Critical Care Nurse*, *33*(1), 75.
National Spinal Cord Injury Statistical Center (NSCISC). (2016). Spinal Cord Injury (SCI) facts and figures at a glance. Retrieved on 2/23/2017 at www.nscisc.uab.edu/Public/Facts%202016.pdf
Noonan, V. K., Chan, E., Santos, A., et al. (2017). Traumatic spinal cord injury care in Canada: a survey of canadian centers. *Journal of Neurotrauma*, *34*(20), 2848–2855.
Olson, D. M., Rogers, M. S., & Stutzman, S. E. (2015). Electronic medical record validation: Exploring the reliability of intracranial pressure data abstracted from the electronic medical record-pilot. *Journal of Nursing Measurement*, *23*(3), 532–540.
Pebdani, R. N., Johnson, K. L., & Amtmann, D. (2014). Personal experiences of pregnancy and fertility in individuals with spinal cord injury. *Sexuality and Disability*, *32*(1), 65–74.
Perez-Barcena, J., Llompart-Pou, J. A., & O'Phelan, K. H. (2014). Intracranial pressure monitoring and management of intracranial hypertension. *Critical Care Clinics*, *30*(4), 735–750.
Rodriguez, G. M. (2016). Bowel function after spinal cord injury. *Archives of Physical Medicine and Rehabilitation*, *97*(2), 339–340.
Saunders, L. L., Clarke, A., Tate, D. G., et al. (2015). Lifetime prevalence of chronic health conditions among persons with spinal cord injury. *Archives of Physical Medicine and Rehabilitation*, *96*(4), 673–679.
Stocchetti, N., & Maas, A. I. (2014). Traumatic intracranial hypertension. *New England Journal of Medicine*, *370*(22), 2121–2130.
Tam, S., McKay, A., Sloan, S., et al. (2015). The experience of challenging behaviours following a severe TBI: A family perspective. *Brain Injury*, *29*(7–8), 813–821.
Teasdale, G., & Jennett, B. (1974). Assessment of coma and impaired consciousness. A practical scale. *Lancet*, *2*(7872), 81–84.
Wan, D., & Krassioukov, A. V. (2014). Life-threatening outcomes associated with autonomic dysreflexia: A clinical review. *The Journal of Spinal Cord Medicine*, *37*(1), 2–10.
Wilson, M., & DellaPenna, A. (2015). Targeted temperature modulation in the neuroscience patient. *Critical Care Nursing Clinics of North America*, *28*(1), 125–136.
Zaman, A., Dubiel, R., Driver, S., et al. (2017). Seizure prophylaxis guidelines following traumatic brain injury: An evaluation of compliance. *Journal of Head Trauma Rehabilitation*, *32*(2), E13–E17.

Spinal Cord Injury

Resources

American Association of Neuroscience Nurses (AANN): http://www.aann.org
American Association of Spinal Cord Injury Nurses (AASCIN): http://www.geronurseonline.org/MainMenuCategory/PartnerOrganizations/AASCIN.html
American Spinal Injury Association (ASIA): http://www.asia-spinalinjury.org
Brain Injury Canada: https://www.braininjurycanada.ca
Canadian and American Spinal Research Organization: http://www.csro.com
Canadian Association of Neuroscience Nurses: http://www.cann.ca
Canadian Paraplegic Association: http://www.spinalcordinjurycanada.ca
World Federation of Neuroscience Nurses: http://www.wfnn.nu

66 Management of Patients With Neurologic Infections, Autoimmune Disorders, and Neuropathies

Adapted by Ron Prince

Learning Objectives

On completion of this chapter, the learner will be able to:

1. Differentiate among the infectious disorders of the nervous system according to causes, manifestations, medical care, and nursing management.
2. Describe the pathophysiology, clinical manifestations, and medical and nursing management of multiple sclerosis, myasthenia gravis, and Guillain–Barré syndrome.
3. Use the nursing process as a framework for care of patients with multiple sclerosis and Guillain–Barré syndrome.
4. Describe disorders of the cranial nerves, their manifestations, and indicated nursing interventions.
5. Develop a plan of nursing care for the patient with a cranial nerve disorder.

The diverse group of neurologic disorders that make up infectious and autoimmune disorders and cranial and peripheral neuropathies presents unique challenges for nursing care. Infectious processes of the nervous system may cause death or permanent dysfunction. Cranial and peripheral nerve disorders may affect the patient's comfort, functional independence, and self-esteem. Autoimmune disorders usually have a slow, progressive course which requires the nurse to manage symptoms and to facilitate the patient and family's understanding of the disease process. Nurses caring for patients with these disorders must have a clear understanding of the pathologic processes, clinical outcomes, and other issues patients and their families may confront, such as adaptation to the effects of the disease, potential changes in family dynamics, and, possibly, end-of-life issues.

INFECTIOUS NEUROLOGIC DISORDERS

The infectious disorders of the nervous system include meningitis, brain abscesses, various types of encephalitis, and Creutzfeldt–Jakob and variant Creutzfeldt–Jakob disease (CJD and vCJD). The clinical manifestations, assessment, and diagnostic findings as well as the medical and nursing management are related to the specific infectious process.

Meningitis

Meningitis is an inflammation of the pia mater, the arachnoid, and the cerebrospinal fluid (CSF)–filled subarachnoid space (Bader, Littlejohns, & Olson, 2016). Meningitis is classified as aseptic or septic. In aseptic meningitis, bacteria are not the cause of the inflammation; the cause is viral or secondary to lymphoma, leukemia, neurosurgical procedures, or brain abscess. Septic meningitis, also known as bacterial meningitis, refers to meningitis caused by bacteria, most commonly *Neisseria meningitidis*, although *Haemophilus influenzae* and *Streptococcus pneumoniae* are also causative agents.

Factors that increase the risk for developing bacterial meningitis include tobacco use and viral upper respiratory infection because they increase the amount of droplet production. Otitis media and mastoiditis increase the risk of bacterial meningitis because the bacteria can cross the blood brain barrier, epithelium membrane and enter the subarachnoid space. Persons with immune system deficiencies are also at greater risk for developing bacterial meningitis. Outbreaks of *N. meningitidis* infection are most likely to occur in dense community groups, such as college campuses and

CHART 66-1

Meningitis in Specific Populations

Meningitis can occur as a complication of other diseases and is an opportunistic infection seen with greater frequency in patients who are immunocompromised.

Meningitis in Patients With Acquired Immune Deficiency Syndrome (AIDS)

- Cryptococcal meningitis is the most common fungal infection of the central nervous system in patients with AIDS. Patients may experience headache, nausea, vomiting, seizures, confusion, and lethargy. Treatment consists of IV administration of amphotericin B followed by fluconazole. Maintenance therapy with fluconazole may be necessary to prevent relapse.
- Some patients who are immunosuppressed develop few if any symptoms because of blunted inflammatory responses; others develop atypical features.
- Onset of fever, headache, nausea, and malaise most often occur over a few weeks. Only 25% of patients present with stiff neck and photophobia.

Meningitis in Patients With Lyme Disease

- Lyme disease is a multisystem inflammatory process caused by the tick-transmitted spirochete *Borrelia burgdorferi*.
- Neurologic abnormalities are seen in later stages (stages 2 or 3). Stage 2 occurs with the start of a characteristic rash or 1 to 6 months after the rash has disappeared.
- Neurologic abnormalities include aseptic meningitis, chronic lymphocytic meningitis, and encephalitis.
- Cranial nerve inflammation, including Bell's palsy and other peripheral neuropathies, is common.
- Stage 3 (the chronic form of the disease) begins years after the initial tick infection and is characterized by arthritis, skin lesions, and neurologic abnormalities.
- Most patients with stage 2 and 3 Lyme disease are treated with IV antibiotics, usually ceftriaxone or penicillin G.
- Meningeal and systemic symptoms begin to improve within days, although other symptoms, such as headache, may persist for weeks.

Adapted from Theroux, N., Phipps, M., Zimmerman, L., et al. (2013). Neurological complications associated with HIV and AIDS: Clinical implications for nursing. *Journal of Neuroscience Nursing, 45*(1), 5–13.

military installations. Although infections occur year round, the peak incidence is in the winter and early spring.

Pathophysiology

Meningeal infections generally originate in one of two ways: through the bloodstream as a consequence of other infections or by direct spread, such as might occur after a traumatic injury to the facial bones or secondary to invasive procedures such as operations to the head, neck, or spine.

N. meningitidis concentrates in the nasopharynx and is transmitted by secretion or aerosol contamination. Bacterial or meningococcal meningitis also occurs as an opportunistic infection in patients with acquired immunodeficiency syndrome (AIDS) and as a complication of Lyme disease (Chart 66-1).

Once the causative organism enters the bloodstream, it crosses the blood–brain barrier and proliferates in the CSF. The host immune response stimulates the release of cell wall fragments and lipopolysaccharides, facilitating inflammation of the subarachnoid and pia mater. Because the cranial vault contains little room for expansion, the inflammation may cause increased intracranial pressure (ICP). CSF circulates through the subarachnoid space, where inflammatory cellular materials from the affected meningeal tissue enter and accumulate.

The prognosis for bacterial meningitis depends on the causative organism, the severity of the infection and illness, and the timeliness of treatment. Acute fulminant presentation may include adrenal damage, circulatory collapse, and widespread hemorrhages (Waterhouse–Friderichsen syndrome). This syndrome is the result of endothelial damage and vascular necrosis caused by the bacteria. Complications include visual impairment, deafness, seizures, paralysis, hydrocephalus, and septic shock.

Clinical Manifestations

Headache, fever, and neck stiffness are frequently the initial symptoms. Fever tends to remain high throughout the

Glossary

ataxia: impaired coordination of movement during voluntary movement

diplopia: double vision, or the awareness of two images of the same object occurring in one or both eyes

dysphagia: difficulty swallowing

dysphonia: voice impairment or altered voice production

hemiparesis: weakness of one side of the body, or part of it, due to an injury in the motor area of the brain

hemiplegia: paralysis of one side of the body, or part of it, due to an injury in the motor area of the brain

neuropathy: general term indicating a disorder of the nervous system

paresthesia: numbness, tingling, or a "pins and needles" sensation

prion: a pathogen smaller than a virus that is resistant to standard sterilization procedures

ptosis: drooping of the eyelids

spasticity: muscular hypertonicity with increased resistance to stretch often associated with weakness, increased deep tendon reflexes, and diminished superficial reflexes

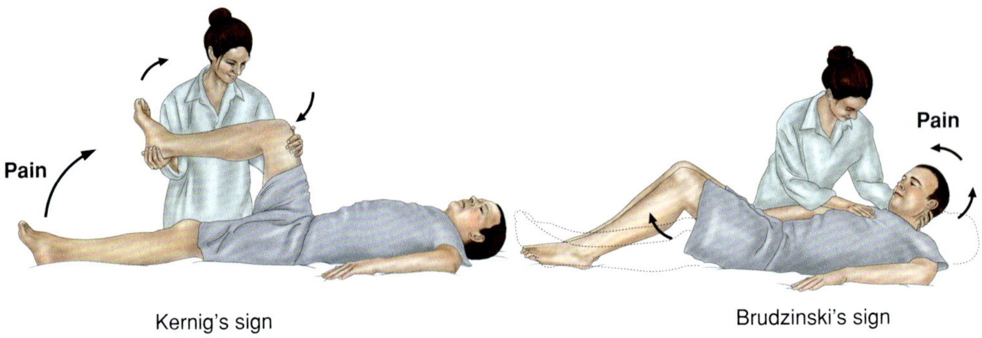

FIGURE 66-1. Testing for meningeal irritation. **A.** Kernig's sign. **B.** Brudzinski's sign.

course of the illness. The headache is usually either steady or throbbing and very severe as a result of meningeal irritation (Stephen, Skillen, & Day, 2012). Meningeal irritation results in a number of other well-recognized signs common to all types of meningitis:

- *Neck mobility:* A stiff and painful neck (nuchal rigidity) can be an early sign and any attempts at flexion of the head are difficult because of spasms in the muscles of the neck. Normally the neck is supple, and the patient can easily bend the head and neck forward.
- *Positive Kernig's sign:* When the patient is lying with the thigh flexed on the abdomen, the leg cannot be completely extended (Fig. 66-1).
- *Positive Brudzinski's sign:* When the patient's neck is flexed (after ruling out cervical trauma or injury), flexion of the knees and hips is produced; when the lower extremity of one side is passively flexed, a similar movement is seen in the opposite extremity (see Fig. 66-1). Brudzinski's sign is a more sensitive indicator of meningeal irritation than Kernig's sign.
- *Photophobia* (extreme sensitivity to light): This finding is common, although the cause is unclear.
- A rash can be a striking feature of *N. meningitidis* infection, occurring in about half of patients with this type of meningitis. Skin lesions develop, ranging from a petechial rash with purpuric lesions to large areas of ecchymosis.

Disorientation, confusion, and memory impairment are common early in the course of the illness. The changes depend on the severity of the infection as well as the individual response to the physiologic processes. Behavioural manifestations are also common. As the illness progresses, lethargy, unresponsiveness, and coma may develop.

Seizures can occur and are the result of areas of irritability in the brain. ICP increases secondary to diffuse brain swelling or hydrocephalus (Bader et al., 2016). The initial signs of increased ICP include increasing confusion, decreased level of consciousness (LOC), and focal motor deficits. If ICP is not controlled, the uncus of the temporal lobe may herniate through the tentorium, causing pressure on the brain stem. Brain stem herniation is a life-threatening event that causes cranial nerve dysfunction and depresses the centres of vital functions, such as the medulla. See Chapter 63 for discussion of the patient with a change in LOC or increased ICP.

An acute fulminant infection occurs in about 10% of patients with meningococcal meningitis, producing signs of overwhelming septicemia: an abrupt onset of high fever, extensive purpuric lesions (over the face and extremities), shock, and signs of disseminated intravascular coagulation (DIC). Death may occur within a few hours after onset of the infection.

Assessment and Diagnostic Findings

If the clinical presentation suggests meningitis, diagnostic testing is conducted to identify the causative organism. A computed tomography (CT) scan or magnetic resonance imaging (MRI) scan is used to detect a shift in brain contents (which may lead to herniation) prior to a lumbar puncture. Once signs of herniation have been ruled out via imaging, then a lumbar puncture can be performed to obtain CSF samples. Bacterial culture and Gram staining of CSF and blood are key diagnostic tests (Bader et al., 2016). An overview of CSF values and alterations in bacterial, viral, and fungal meningitis is presented in Table 66-1. CSF studies demonstrate low glucose, high protein levels, and

TABLE 66-1 Cerebrospinal Fluid Values Diagnostic for Meningitis

Parameter	Normal CSF	Bacterial Meningitis	Viral Meningitis	Fungal Meningitis
Opening pressure (mm H_2O)	100–180	200–500	≤250	>200
Leukocyte count (white blood cell/mm^3)	0–5	Increased 100–5,000	Increased 50–1,000	Increased >20
Neutrophils (%)	0	≥80	<40	
Protein (mg/dL)	18–45	Elevated 100–500	Elevated <200	Elevated >45
Glucose (mg/dL)	45–80; 0.6 times blood glucose level	<40; <0.4 times blood glucose level	>45	<40

CSF, cerebrospinal fluid.

Adapted from Bader, M., Littlejohns, L. R., & Olson, D. (2016). *AANN core curriculum for neuroscience nursing* (6th ed.). Chicago, IL: American Association of Neuroscience Nurses.

high white blood cell count. Gram staining allows for rapid identification of the causative bacteria and initiation of appropriate antibiotic therapy.

Prevention

There are five serogroups of invasive meningococcal disease (IMD): A, B, C, Y, and W135, with serogroup C being the most common cause of meningococcal outbreaks in Canada (National Advisory Committee on Communicable Diseases, 2013). Since 1985, the incidence of IMD in Canada is 2 per 100,000 people per year, or about 298 cases each year, occurring mainly during the winter months. Incidence is highest in children younger than 1 year of age, then declines, and then there is a smaller peak in the 15- to 19-year age group. While there have been no outbreaks of meningitis in college/university residences in Canada, increased numbers of cases have been noted in the United States and the United Kingdom. Routine immunization is recommended for military recruits: meningococcal C conjugate for those staying in Canada and quadrivalent polysaccharide meningococcal vaccine for those posted outside of Canada. For infants, two doses of meningococcal C conjugate vaccine are given 2 to 3 months apart, beginning at 3 months of age. Routine immunization for health care workers is not recommended. Household contacts of people with meningococcal meningitis should be treated with antimicrobial chemoprophylaxis using rifampin (Rifadin), ciprofloxacin hydrochloride (Cipro), or ceftriaxone sodium (Rocephin). Therapy should be started as soon as possible after contact; a delay in the initiation of therapy will limit the effectiveness of the prophylaxis. Vaccination should also be considered as an adjunct to antibiotic chemoprophylaxis for anyone living with a person who develops meningococcal infection. Vaccination for children and at-risk adults should be encouraged to avoid meningitis caused by *H. influenzae* and *S. pneumoniae*.

Medical Management

Successful outcomes depend on the early administration of an antibiotic that crosses the blood–brain barrier into the subarachnoid space in sufficient concentration to halt the multiplication of bacteria. Initial choices of antibiotics are broad-spectrum coverage with a third-generation cephalosporin, vancomycin, and a Penicillin antibiotic such as ampicillin, with adjustment of antibiotic regimen as required by CSF culture results (Bader et al., 2016). The resulting rapid death of the pathogen caused by the antibiotics may potentially produce inflammation which is treated with adjunctive corticosteroid therapy administered with the initial dose of antibiotics (Bader et al., 2016).

Dehydration and shock are treated with fluid volume expanders. Seizures, which may occur early in the course of the disease, are controlled with phenytoin (Dilantin). Increased ICP is treated as necessary (see Chapter 63).

Nursing Management

The patient with meningitis is critically ill; therefore, many of the nursing interventions are collaborative with the physician, respiratory therapist, and other members of the health care team. The patient's prognosis may depend on sound nursing judgment and supportive care.

Neurologic status and vital signs are continually assessed. Pulse oximetry +/– arterial blood gas values are used to quickly identify the need for respiratory support if increasing ICP compromises the brain stem. Insertion of a cuffed endotracheal tube (or tracheotomy) and mechanical ventilation may be necessary to maintain adequate tissue oxygenation.

Blood pressure (usually monitored using an arterial line) is assessed for shock, which precedes cardiac or respiratory failure. Rapid IV fluid replacement may be prescribed, but care is taken to prevent fluid overload. Fever also increases the workload of the heart and cerebral metabolism. ICP will increase in response to increased cerebral metabolic demands. Therefore, measures are taken to reduce body temperature as quickly as possible.

Other important components of nursing care include the following measures:

- Protecting the patient from injury secondary to seizure activity or altered LOC
- Monitoring daily body weight; serum electrolytes; and urine volume, specific gravity, and osmolality, especially if syndrome of inappropriate antidiuretic hormone (SIADH) is suspected
- Preventing complications associated with immobility, such as pressure ulcers and pneumonia
- Instituting droplet precautions until 24 hours after initiation of antibiotic therapy (oral and nasal discharge is considered infectious)
- Adequate pain management

Any sudden, critical illness can be devastating to the family. Because the patient's condition is often critical and the prognosis guarded, the family needs to be informed about the patient's condition and permitted to see the patient at intervals, even though the priority is to address the patient's need for immediate and intensive treatment. An important aspect of the nurse's role is to support the family and assist them in identifying others who can be supportive to them during the crisis.

Promoting Home, Community-Based, and Transitional Care

After the patient has achieved physiologic homeostasis and has demonstrated achievement of major health care goals, rehabilitation continues either in a rehabilitation facility, skilled nursing facility or at home. Continued support and evaluation by the nurse are essential.

Because patients may have been critically ill and focused on the most obvious needs and issues, the nurse reminds the patient and family about the importance of continuing health-promotion and screening practices, such as regular physical examinations and appropriate diagnostic screening tests.

Brain Abscess

Brain abscesses are rare in immunocompetent people; they are more frequently diagnosed in people who are immunosuppressed as a result of an underlying disease or use of immunosuppressive medications; for example, patients with HIV infection or hematologic malignancies.

Pathophysiology

A brain abscess is a collection of infectious material within the tissue of the brain. Bacteria are the most common causative organisms. An abscess may occur by direct contact with brain tissue from intracranial trauma or surgery, penetrating head injury, tongue piercing, or by the spread of infection from the lungs, gums, tongue, or heart, or from a wound or intra-abdominal infection (Bader et al., 2016). To prevent brain abscess, otitis media, mastoiditis, rhinosinusitis, dental infections, and systemic infections should be treated promptly.

Clinical Manifestations

The clinical manifestations of a brain abscess result from alterations in intracranial dynamics (edema, brain shift), infection, or the location of the abscess (Chart 66-2).

Headache, usually worse in the morning, is the most prevalent symptom. Fever and vomiting is also common. Focal deficits such as weakness and decreasing vision may occur, depending on the area of brain that is involved. As the abscess expands, symptoms of increased ICP such as decreasing LOC and seizures can occur.

Assessment and Diagnostic Findings

Neuroimaging studies such as magnetic resonance imaging (MRI) or computed tomography (CT) scanning identify the size and location of the abscess. The MRI or CT scans reveal a ring around a hypodense area (Slazinski, 2013). Aspiration of the abscess, guided by CT or MRI, is the best method to culture and identify the infectious organism. Blood cultures are obtained if the abscess is believed to arise from a distant source. Chest x-ray is performed to rule out predisposing lung infections and an electroencephalogram (EEG) may help localize the lesion (Hickey, 2014). As cerebral abscesses rarely originate within the brain, it is key to find the original source of the infection so that both the cerebral abscess and the original source can be treated promptly and accurately. Blood cultures are obtained if the abscess is believed to arise from a distant source.

CHART 66-2

Assessing for Brain Abscesses

Be alert for the following signs and symptoms:

Frontal Lobe

Hemiparesis
Aphasia (expressive)
Seizures
Frontal headache

Temporal Lobe

Localized headache
Changes in vision
Facial weakness
Receptive aphasia (inability to understand language)

Cerebellar Abscess

Occipital headache
Ataxia (inability to coordinate movements)
Nystagmus (rhythmic, involuntary movements of the eye)
Decreased LOC

Medical Management

Treatment is aimed at controlling increased ICP, draining the abscess, and providing antimicrobial therapy directed at the abscess and the primary source of infection. Large IV doses of antibiotics are administered to penetrate the blood–brain barrier and reach the abscess. The choice of the specific antibiotic medication is based on culture and sensitivity testing and directed at the causative organism. A stereotactic CT-guided aspiration may be used to drain the abscess and identify the causative organism. Corticosteroids may be prescribed to help reduce the inflammatory cerebral edema if the patient shows evidence of an increasing neurologic deficit. Anticonvulsant medications (phenytoin, phenobarbital, levetiracetam) may be prescribed to prevent or treat seizures.

Nursing Management

Nursing care focuses on continuing to assess the neurologic status, administering medications, assessing the response to treatment, and providing supportive care.

Ongoing neurologic assessment alerts the nurse to changes in ICP, which may indicate a need for more aggressive intervention. The nurse also assesses and documents the responses to medications. Blood laboratory test results, specifically blood glucose and serum potassium levels, need to be closely monitored when corticosteroids are prescribed. Sodium levels also need to be carefully monitored, as hyponatremia is commonly seen in this patients population. Administration of insulin or electrolyte replacement may be required to return these values to normal or acceptable levels.

Patient safety is another key nursing responsibility. Injury may result from decreased LOC or falls related to motor weakness or seizures.

The patient with a brain abscess is very ill, and neurologic deficits, such as **hemiparesis**, seizures, visual deficits, and cranial nerve palsies, may remain after treatment. Seizures are common sequelae. The nurse must assess the family's ability to express distress at the patient's condition, cope with the patient's illness and deficits, and obtain support.

Herpes Simplex Virus Encephalitis

Encephalitis is an acute inflammatory process of the brain tissue. Herpes simplex virus (HSV) encephalitis is the most common form of acute nonepidemic viral encephalitis in the world. There are two herpes simplex viruses: HSV-1 and HSV-2. HSV-1 typically affects children and adults. HSV-2 is commonly the cause of genital herpes.

Pathophysiology

The pathology of encephalitis involves local necrotizing hemorrhage that becomes more generalized, followed by edema. There is also progressive deterioration of nerve cell bodies (Grossman & Porth, 2014).

Clinical Manifestations

The initial symptoms of HSV-1 encephalitis include fever, headache, and confusion. Focal neurologic symptoms reflect the areas of cerebral inflammation and necrosis and include fever, headache, behavioural changes, focal seizures, dysphasia, hemiparesis, and altered LOC (Grossman & Porth, 2014).

Assessment and Diagnostic Findings

Neuroimaging studies such as CT and MRI, as well EEG and CSF studies, are used to diagnose HSV encephalitis. MRI is the neuroimaging study of choice for detection of early changes caused by HSV-1; the study shows edema in the temporal lobe. The EEG reveals diffuse slowing or focal changes in the temporal lobe. Lumbar puncture often reveals a high opening pressure and low glucose and high protein levels in CSF samples. Viral cultures are almost always negative. The polymerase chain reaction (PCR) is the standard test for early diagnosis of HSV-1 encephalitis. PCR identifies the DNA bands of HSV-1 in the CSF. The validity of PCR is very high between the 3rd and 10th days after symptom onset.

Medical Management

Acyclovir (Zovirax), an antiviral agent, is the medication of choice in the treatment of HSV (Grossman & Porth, 2014). However, new antiviral agents are becoming more common and are used depending on the patient's symptoms, severity of the disease, and response to treatment. Early administration of antiviral agents is usually well tolerated by the patient and improves the prognosis associated with HSV-1 encephalitis. The mode of action is inhibition of viral DNA replication. To prevent relapse, treatment should continue for up to 3 weeks. Slow IV administration over 1 hour prevents crystallization of the medication in the urine. The usual dose of acyclovir is decreased if the patient has a history of renal insufficiency. Studies are in progress to determine the effectiveness of an oral agent, valacyclovir hydrochloride (Valtrex), in the treatment of HSV-1 encephalitis.

Nursing Management

Assessment of neurologic function is key to monitoring the progression of disease. Comfort measures to reduce headache include dimming the lights, limiting noise and visitors, grouping nursing interventions, and administering analgesic agents. Opioid analgesic medications may mask neurologic symptoms; therefore, they are used cautiously. Seizures and altered LOC require care directed at injury prevention and safety. Nursing care addressing patient and family anxieties is ongoing throughout the illness. Monitoring of blood chemistry test results and urinary output alert the nurse to the presence of renal complications related to antiviral therapy.

Arthropod-Borne Virus Encephalitis

Arthropod vectors transmit several types of viruses that cause encephalitis. The primary vector in North America is the mosquito. In cases of West Nile virus, humans are the secondary host; birds are the primary host. Arbovirus infection (transmitted by arthropod vectors) occurs in specific geographic areas during the summer and fall. In the United States, West Nile and St. Louis are the most common types of arboviral encephalitis; both are members of the Japanese encephalitis serogroup. West Nile virus, which may cause encephalitis, was first detected in North America in 1999 and is now present in Canada, the United States, and Mexico.

Pathophysiology

Viral replication occurs at the site of the mosquito bite. The host immune response attempts to control viral replication. If the immune response is inadequate, viremia will ensue. The virus gains access to the central nervous system (CNS) via the cerebral capillaries, resulting in encephalitis. It spreads from neuron to neuron, predominantly affecting the cortical grey matter, the brain stem, and the thalamus. Meningeal exudates compound the clinical presentation by irritating the meninges and increasing ICP.

Clinical Manifestations

All arboviral encephalitis begins with early flulike symptoms, but specific neurologic manifestations depend on the viral type (Bader et al., 2016). A unique clinical feature of St. Louis encephalitis is SIADH with hyponatremia. Signs and symptoms specific to West Nile encephalitis include a maculopapular or morbilliform rash on the neck, trunk, and arms; enlarged lymph nodes and legs; and flaccid paralysis (Grossman & Porth, 2014). Both West Nile and St. Louis encephalitis can result in parkinsonianlike movements, reflecting inflammation of the basal ganglia. Seizures, a poor prognostic indicator, are present in both types of encephalitis but are more common in the St. Louis type (Bader et al., 2016).

Assessment and Diagnostic Findings

After a brief febrile prodrome, neurologic symptoms reflect the area of the brain that is involved. Neuroimaging and CSF evaluation are useful in the diagnosis of arboviral encephalitis. The MRI scan demonstrates inflammation of the basal ganglia in cases of St. Louis encephalitis and inflammation in the periventricular area in cases of West Nile encephalitis. Immunoglobulin M antibodies to West Nile virus are observed in serum and CSF. Serum cultures are not useful, because the viremia is brief. PCR evaluation of CSF may demonstrate viral ribonucleic acid (RNA).

Medical Management

No specific medication for arboviral encephalitis exists. Medical management focuses on symptom management, which includes controlling seizures and increased ICP. Interferon may be useful in treating St. Louis encephalitis. Neuropsychiatric complications, such as emotional outbursts and other behaviour changes, occur frequently.

Nursing Management

If the patient is very ill, hospitalization may be required. The nurse carefully assesses neurologic status and identifies improvement or deterioration in the patient's condition. Injury prevention is key in light of the potential for falls or seizures. Arboviral encephalitis may result in death or lifelong residual health issues such as neurologic deficits and seizures. The family will need support and teaching to cope with these outcomes.

Public education addressing the prevention of arboviral encephalitis is a key nursing role. Clothing that provides coverage and insect repellents containing 25% to 30% diethyltoluamide (DEET) should be used on exposed clothing and skin in high-risk areas to decrease mosquito and tick bites. Screens should be in good repair in the home, and standing water should be removed.

Fungal Encephalitis

Fungal infections of the CNS occur rarely in healthy people. The presentation of fungal encephalitis is related to geographic area or to an immune system that is compromised due to disease or immunosuppressive medication. Causes of fungal infections include *Cryptococcus neoformans*, *Blastomyces dermatitidis*, *Histoplasma capsulatum*, *Aspergillus fumigatus*, *Candida*, and *Coccidioides immitis* (Bader et al., 2016). *C. immitis* is found mainly in California, Arizona, New Mexico, and Texas. *B. dermatitidis* exists in the Southeastern United States and in the Ohio, St. Lawrence, and Mississippi River basins. It is a risk for coal miners, construction workers, and farmers. *C. neoformans* is associated with exposure to bird droppings and may be seen in bird handlers.

Pathophysiology

The fungal spores enter the body via inhalation. They initially infect the lungs, causing vague respiratory symptoms. The fungi then enter the bloodstream, causing a fungemia. If the fungemia overwhelms the person's immune system, the fungus may spread to the CNS. The fungal invasion may cause meningitis, encephalitis, or brain abscess.

Clinical Manifestations

The common symptoms of fungal encephalitis include fever, malaise, headache, meningeal signs, and change in LOC or cranial nerve dysfunction. Symptoms of increased ICP related to hydrocephalus often occur. *C. neoformans* and *C. immitis* are associated with specific skin lesions. *H. capsulatum* is associated with seizures, and *A. fumigatus* may cause ischemic or hemorrhagic strokes.

Assessment and Diagnostic Findings

A history of immunosuppression associated with AIDS or use of immunosuppressive medications may indicate fungal disease of the brain. Occupational and travel history may point to a fungal cause of CNS infection. Infections caused by *H. capsulatum* and *C. immitis* will demonstrate fungal antibodies in serologic tests. The CSF usually demonstrates elevated white cell and protein levels; glucose levels are decreased. *C. neoformans* is easily identified in CSF fungal cultures. *Candida* may be cultured from the blood or CSF. To identify *B. dermatitidis*, cisternal or ventricular cultures of CSF may need to be obtained. *A. fumigatus* is difficult to isolate in CSF and is diagnosed by lung biopsy. Neuroimaging is used to identify CNS changes related to fungal infection. MRI is the study of choice; it demonstrates areas of hemorrhage, abscess, or enhanced meninges indicating inflammation.

Medical Management

Medical management is directed at the causative fungus and the neurologic consequences of the infection. Seizures are controlled by standard anticonvulsant medications. Increased ICP is controlled by repeated lumbar punctures or shunting of CSF.

Antifungal agents are administered for a specific period to cure the infection in patients with competent immune systems. Patients with compromised immune systems receive antifungal therapy until the infection is controlled, after which they receive a maintenance dose of the medication for an indefinite period. Although the dose and duration of treatment depend on the causative fungi, amphotericin B is the standard antifungal agent used in treatment (Karch, 2014). Dosing depends on the causative organism, and it is usually administered by IV. The most common adverse reactions are fever, chills, nausea and vomiting, and hypokalemia (Karch, 2014). Renal insufficiency is a serious reaction to amphotericin B that can occur. Fluconazole (Diflucan) or flucytosine (Ancobon) may be administered orally in conjunction with amphotericin B as maintenance therapy. Potential side effects of fluconazole include nausea, vomiting, and a transient increase in liver enzymes. The most common adverse reaction to flucytosine is bone marrow suppression. Therefore, patients receiving flucytosine should have leukocyte and platelet counts monitored regularly.

Nursing Management

ICP will increase if hydrocephalus develops and the inflammatory response progresses. Nursing assessment aimed at early identification of increased ICP is necessary to ensure early control and management. (See Chapter 63 for management of the patient with increased ICP.) Administering nonopioid analgesic agents, limiting environmental stimuli, and positioning may optimize patient comfort. Administering diphenhydramine (Benadryl) and acetaminophen (Tylenol) approximately 30 minutes before giving amphotericin B may prevent flulike side effects. If renal insufficiency develops, the dose may need to be reduced. Increasing levels of serum creatinine and blood urea nitrogen (BUN) may alert the nurse to the development of renal insufficiency and the need to address the patient's renal status.

Providing support assists the patient and family to cope with the illness. Workup of the patient for immunodeficiency diseases such as AIDS may put additional stress on the family. The nurse may need to mobilize community support systems for the patient and family, because the recovery may be long.

Creutzfeldt–Jakob and Variant Creutzfeldt–Jakob Disease

CJD and vCJD belong to a group of degenerative, infectious neurologic disorders called transmissible spongiform encephalopathies (TSEs). CJD is very rare and has no identifiable cause. vCJD is the human variation of bovine spongiform encephalopathy (BSE); it results from the ingestion by humans of prions in infected beef. TSEs are caused by prions, proteinaceous particles that are smaller than a virus and are resistant to standard methods of sterilization. Although CJD and vCJD have distinct clinical features, one characteristic they share is a lack of CNS inflammation. In both diseases, the symptoms are progressive, there is no definitive treatment, and the outcome is fatal.

Approximately 1 to 2 persons per 1 million are affected worldwide. To date there have been about 676 definite or probable death from CJD in Canada (Public Health Agency of Canada, 2014).

Pathophysiology

The **prion** is a unique pathogen because it lacks nucleic acid, which enables the organism to withstand conventional means of sterilization. How the prion replicates in the absence of nucleic acid is unknown. In both CJD and vCJD, the prion crosses the blood–brain barrier and is deposited in brain tissue and causes degeneration of brain tissue. Cell death occurs, and spongy vacuoles are produced in the brain (spongiform changes). The spongiform vacuoles are surrounded by amyloid plaque (NINDS, 2016).

Ninety percent of the cases of CJD appear sporadically (Vacca, 2016). Although it is not transmittable by typical human contact, 5% of cases of sporadic CJD result from contaminated neurosurgical instruments, cadaver-derived growth factor, or corneal transplants. Ten percent of cases appear to be familial (Vacca, 2016).

In the mid-1980s, BSE was identified in dairy cattle herds in the United Kingdom. One-third of the cattle were infected, and 200,000 animals died of the disease. Researchers believed that BSE could not be transmitted to humans; however, in 1996, the first case of vCJD was described. The mode of transmission was linked to the ingestion of beef contaminated with neurologic tissue. As well, all of the people who develop vCJD have a specific, shared genotype (Vacca, 2016). Following an outbreak of BSE in Alberta in 2003, Canada now prohibits feeding cattle food containing ground-up animal materials, including neurologic tissue.

Clinical Manifestations

CJD and vCJD have several clinically distinct features. Psychiatric symptoms occur early in vCJD, whereas they are a late symptom in CJD. The presenting symptoms of vCJD include affective symptoms (i.e., behavioural changes), sensory disturbance, and limb pain. Muscle spasms and rigidity, dysarthria, incoordination, cognitive impairment, and sleep disturbances follow. Patients with sporadic CJD present with mental deterioration, **ataxia**, and visual disturbance. Memory loss, involuntary movement, paralysis, and mutism occur as the disease progresses. After clinical presentation, people with vCJD survive an average of 14 months; those with CJD survive for about 6 months (Bader et al., 2016).

Assessment and Diagnostic Findings

Historically, brain biopsy was used to diagnose CJD. The three diagnostic tests currently used in suspicious clinical presentations to support the diagnosis of CJD are immunologic assessment, EEG, and MRI scanning. Immunologic assessment of CSF detects a protein kinase inhibitor called 14-3-3. The presence of this inhibitor indicates neuronal cell death, which is not specific to CJD but does support the diagnosis. The EEG reveals a characteristic pattern over the duration of the disease. After initial slowing, the EEG shows periodic activity. Later in the course of the disease, the EEG shows burst-suppressions characterized by periodic spikes alternating with slow periods. The MRI scan demonstrates symmetric or unilateral hyperintense signals arising from the basal ganglia (Bader et al., 2016).

Patients with vCJD do not demonstrate EEG or CSF changes, and the MRI scan shows bilateral hyperintensity of the posterior thalamus. The prion associated with vCJD has been shown to accumulate in the tonsils and other lymphoreticular tissues; therefore, tonsillar biopsy may be used in the diagnosis of vCJD (Bader et al., 2016).

Medical Management

After the onset of specific neurologic symptoms, progression of disease occurs quickly. There is no effective treatment for CJD or vCJD (Public Health Agency of Canada, 2012). The care of the patient is supportive and palliative. Goals of care include prevention of injury related to immobility and dementia, promotion of patient comfort, and provision of support and education for the family.

Nursing Management

The nursing care of patients is primarily supportive and palliative. Psychological and emotional support of patients and families throughout the course of the illness is needed. Care includes providing for a dignified death and supporting the family through the processes of grief and loss. Early integration of a palliative care team and hospice services are appropriate either at home or at an inpatient facility. (See Chapter 15 for an in-depth discussion of end-of-life issues.)

Prevention of disease transmission is an important part of nursing care. Although patient isolation is not necessary, use of standard precautions is important. Institutional protocols are followed for blood and body fluid exposure and decontamination of equipment. In the operating room, it is recommended that disposable instruments be used and then incinerated, because conventional methods of sterilization do not destroy the prion. The World Health Organization has guidelines that outline the stringent sterilization methods that must be used to destroy prions on surfaces.

AUTOIMMUNE PROCESSES

Autoimmune nervous system disorders include multiple sclerosis (MS), myasthenia gravis, and Guillain–Barré syndrome.

Multiple Sclerosis

MS is an immune-mediated, progressive demyelinating disease of the CNS. Demyelination refers to the destruction of myelin, the fatty and protein material that surrounds certain nerve fibres in the brain and spinal cord; it results in impaired transmission of nerve impulses (Fig. 66-2). MS may occur at any age but typically manifests in young adults between the ages of 20 and 40 years; it affects women more frequently than men (Bader et al., 2016).

The precise cause of MS remains unknown (Ward-Abel, Vernon, & Warner, 2014). Autoimmune activity results in demyelination, but the sensitized antigen has not been identified. Multiple factors play a role in the initiation of the immune process. Geographic prevalence is highest in countries that are in Northern latitudes. It is believed that some environmental exposure at a young age may play a role in the development of MS later in life.

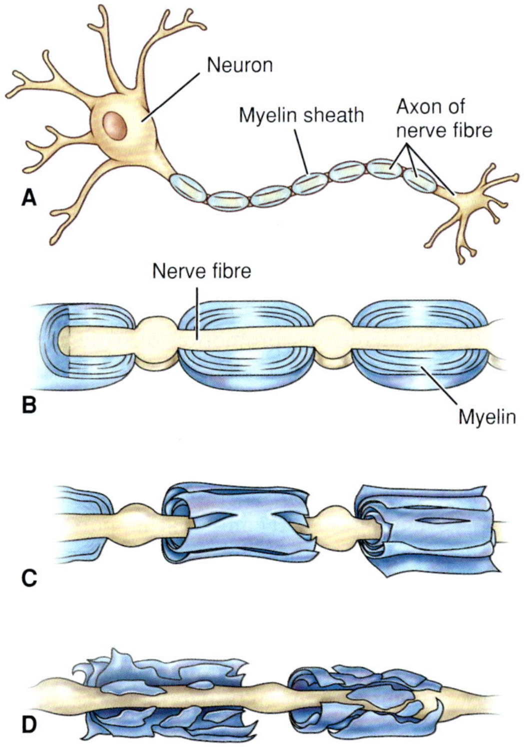

FIGURE 66-2. The process of demyelination. A and B depict a normal nerve cell and axon with myelin. C and D show the slow disintegration of myelin, resulting in a disruption in axon function.

Genetic predisposition is indicated by the presence of a specific cluster (haplotype) of human leukocyte antigens (HLAs) on the cell wall. Its presence may increase susceptibility to factors, such as viruses, that trigger the autoimmune response activated in MS. A specific virus capable of initiating the autoimmune response has not been identified. It is believed that DNA on the virus mimics the amino acid sequence of myelin, resulting in an immune system cross-reaction in the presence of a defective immune system. Environmental risks include smoking, lack of vitamin D exposure, and exposure to the Epstein–Barr virus (Bader et al., 2016).

Pathophysiology

Sensitized T and B lymphocytes cross the blood–brain barrier; their function is to check the CNS for antigens and then leave. In MS, sensitized T cells remain in the CNS and promote the infiltration of other agents that damage the immune system. The immune system attack leads to inflammation that destroys myelin (which normally insulates the axon and speeds the conduction of impulses along the axon) and the oligodendroglial cells that produce myelin in the CNS.

Demyelination interrupts the flow of nerve impulses and results in a variety of manifestations, depending on the nerves affected. Plaques appear on demyelinated axons, further interrupting the transmission of impulses. Demyelinated axons are scattered irregularly throughout the CNS. The areas most frequently affected are the optic nerves, chiasm, optic tracts; the cerebrum; the brain stem and cerebellum; and the spinal cord. The axons themselves begin to degenerate, resulting in permanent and irreversible damage (Wu & Alvarez, 2016).

Clinical Manifestations

The course of MS may assume many different patterns (Lublin & Reingold, 1996). In some patients, the disease follows a benign course, and symptoms are so mild that the patient does not seek health care or treatment. There are four types of MS: relapsing remitting (RR), primary progressive, secondary progressive, and progressive relapsing. Between 80% and 85% of MS cases begin with an RR course with complete recovery between clearly defined symptomatic exacerbations. With each relapse, recovery is usually complete; however, residual deficits may occur and accumulate over time, contributing to functional decline. About 50% of those with the RR course of MS progress to a secondary progressive course, in which disease progression occurs with or without relapses. Around 10% of patients have a primary progressive course, in which disabling symptoms steadily increase, with rare plateaus and temporary improvement. Primary progressive MS may result in quadriparesis, cognitive dysfunction, visual loss, and brain stem syndromes. The least common presentation (about 5% of cases) is the progressive relapsing course. It is characterized by relapses with continuous disabling progression between exacerbations (Hickey, 2014).

The signs and symptoms of MS are varied and multiple, reflecting the location of the lesion (plaque) or combination of lesions. The primary symptoms most commonly reported are fatigue, depression, weakness, numbness, difficulty in coordination, loss of balance, and pain. Visual disturbances due to lesions in the optic nerves or their connections may include blurring of vision, **diplopia** (double vision), patchy blindness (scotoma), and total blindness.

Fatigue is one of the most common problems affecting most people with MS and is often the most disabling symptom (Morrison & Stuifbergen, 2016; Riley & Vargus, 2015). Heat, depression, anemia, deconditioning, and medication may contribute to fatigue. Avoiding hot temperatures, effective treatment of depression and anemia, and occupational and physical therapies may help control fatigue. Additional strategies include a balance of rest and activities, good nutrition, and a healthy lifestyle including avoidance of alcohol and cigarette smoking (Lemon & Clark, 2014).

Pain is another common symptom of MS that can contribute to social isolation. Lesions on the sensory pathways cause pain. Additional sensory manifestations include **paresthesias**, dysesthesias, and proprioception loss. Many people with MS need daily analgesic medications. In some cases, pain is managed with opioids, anticonvulsant medications, or antidepressants. Rarely, surgery may be needed to interrupt pain pathways.

Among perimenopausal women, those with MS are more likely to have pain related to osteoporosis. In addition to estrogen loss, immobility and corticosteroid therapy play a role in the development of osteoporosis among women with MS. Bone mineral density testing is recommended for this high-risk group. Diagnosis and treatment of osteoporosis are discussed in Chapter 71.

Spasticity (muscle hypertonicity) of the extremities and loss of the abdominal reflexes result from disease involvement of the main motor pathways (pyramidal tracts) of the spinal cord. Disruption of the sensory axons may produce sensory dysfunction (paresthesias, pain). Cognitive and psychosocial problems may reflect frontal or parietal lobe involvement. Some degree of cognitive change (e.g., memory loss, decreased concentration) occurs in about half of patients, but severe cognitive changes with dementia (progressive organic mental disorder) are rare.

Involvement of the cerebellum or basal ganglia can produce ataxia (impaired coordination of movements) and tremor. Loss of the control connections between the cortex and the basal ganglia may occur and cause emotional lability and euphoria. Bladder, bowel, and sexual dysfunctions are common.

Secondary complications of MS include urinary tract infections, constipation, pressure ulcers, contracture deformities, dependent pedal edema, pneumonia, reactive depression, and osteoporosis. Emotional, social, marital, economic, and vocational problems may also occur.

Exacerbations and remissions are characteristic of MS. During exacerbations, new symptoms appear and existing ones worsen; during remissions, symptoms decrease or disappear. Relapses may be associated with emotional and physical stress.

Assessment and Diagnostic Findings

The diagnosis of MS is based on the presence of multiple plaques in the CNS observed with MRI. Electrophoresis of CSF identifies the presence of oligoclonal banding (several bands of immunoglobulin G bonded together, indicating an immune system abnormality). Electromylographs can help define the extent of the disease process and monitor changes. Underlying bladder dysfunction is diagnosed by urodynamic studies. Neuropsychological testing may be indicated to assess cognitive impairment. A sexual history helps identify changes in sexual function.

Gerontologic Considerations

The life expectancy for patients with MS is not dramatically different from that of patients without MS. Patients with MS who are older adults have specific physical and psychosocial challenges. They may have chronic health problems, for which they may be taking additional medications that could interact with medications prescribed for MS. The absorption, distribution, metabolism, and excretion of medications are altered in the older adults as a result of age-related changes in renal and liver functions. Therefore, older adult patients must be monitored closely for adverse and toxic effects of MS medications and for osteoporosis (particularly with frequent corticosteroid use that may be needed to treat exacerbations). The cost of medications may lead to poor adherence to the prescribed regimen in older adult patients on fixed incomes.

Older patients with MS are particularly concerned about increasing disability, family burden, marital concern, and the possible future need for nursing home care. Immobility resulting in fewer social opportunities contributes to loneliness and depression. Along with functional loss, spasticity, pain and bladder dysfunction, impaired sleep, and an increased need for assistance with self-care contribute to the physical challenges experienced by the older patient with MS.

Medical Management

No cure exists for MS. An individual treatment program is indicated to relieve the patient's symptoms and provide continuing support, particularly for patients with cognitive changes, who may need more structure and support. The goals of treatment are to delay the progression of the disease, manage chronic symptoms, and treat acute exacerbations. Many patients with MS have a stable disease course and require only intermittent treatment, whereas others experience steady progression of their disease. Symptoms requiring intervention include spasticity, fatigue, bladder dysfunction, and ataxia. Management strategies target the various motor and sensory symptoms and effects of immobility that can occur.

Pharmacologic Therapy

Interferon medications are the mainstay of medical treatment for MS. Interferon beta-1a (Rebif) and interferon beta-1b (Betaseron) are administered subcutaneously.

Researchers have investigated the clinical effectiveness of beta-1b compared with beta-1a. Another preparation of interferon beta-1a, Avonex, is administered intramuscularly once a week. Side effects of all interferon beta medications include flulike symptoms that can be managed with acetaminophen and ibuprofen and resolve after a few months. Additional side effects include potential liver damage, fetal abnormalities, and depression. For optimal control of disability, disease-modifying medications should be started early in the course of the disease (Hickey, 2014).

Glatiramer acetate (Copaxone) reduces the rate of relapse in the RR course of MS. It decreases the number of plaques noted on MRI and increases the time between relapses. Copaxone is administered subcutaneously daily. It acts by increasing the antigen-specific suppressor T cells. Side effects are minimal and manageable (Hickey, 2014). Copaxone is an option for those with an RR course; however, it may take 6 months for evidence of an immune response to appear.

Steroids are the main treatment modality for the treatment of acute relapses in RR MS. IV methylprednisolone shortens the duration of relapse. It exerts anti-inflammatory effects by acting on T cells and cytokines. One gram is administered IV daily for 3 days, followed by an oral taper of prednisone. Side effects include mood swings, weight gain, and electrolyte imbalances (Karch, 2014).

The medication mitoxantrone (Novantrone) is administered via IV infusion every 3 months. Novantrone can reduce the frequency of clinical relapses in patients with secondary-progressive or worsening relapsing-remitting MS. Patients must be very closely monitored for side effects, especially cardiac toxicity (Karch, 2014).

Medications are also prescribed for management of specific symptoms. Baclofen (Lioresal), a gamma-aminobutyric acid (GABA) agonist, is the medication of choice for treating spasticity. It can be administered orally or by intrathecal injection for severe spasticity (Karch, 2014). Benzodiazepines (Valium), tizanidine (Zanaflex), and dantrolene (Dantrium) may also be used to treat spasticity. Patients with disabling spasms and contractures may require nerve blocks or surgical intervention. When patients have severe MS and spasticity affects their quality of life, Baclofen (Lioresal) pumps are inserted to provide a continuous dose of medication and decrease spasticity. Fatigue that interferes with activities of daily living (ADLs) may be treated with amantadine (Symmetrel), pemoline (Cylert), or fluoxetine (Prozac). Ataxia is a chronic problem most resistant to treatment. Medications used to treat ataxia include beta-adrenergic blockers (Inderal), anticonvulsant agents (Neurontin), and benzodiazepines (Klonopin).

Bladder and bowel problems are often among the most difficult ones for patients, and a variety of medications (anticholinergic agents, alpha-adrenergic blockers, antispasmodic agents) may be prescribed. Nonpharmacologic strategies also assist in establishing effective bowel and bladder elimination (see later discussion).

Urinary tract infection is often superimposed on the underlying neurologic dysfunction. Ascorbic acid (vitamin C) may be prescribed to acidify the urine, making bacterial growth less likely. Antibiotics are prescribed when appropriate.

Nursing Process

The Patient With Multiple Sclerosis

Assessment

Nursing assessment addresses neurologic deficits, secondary complications, and the impact of the disease on the patient and family. The patient's mobility and balance are observed to determine whether there is risk of falling. Assessment of function is carried out both when the patient is well rested and when fatigued. The patient is assessed for weakness, spasticity, visual impairment, incontinence, and disorders of swallowing and speech. Additional areas of assessment include how MS has affected the patient's lifestyle, how the patient is coping, and what the patient would like to improve.

Nursing Priorities

Based on the assessment data, the patient's major nursing priorities may include the following:

- Decreased physical mobility due to weakness, muscle paresis, spasticity
- Sensory and visual impairment
- Urgency, frequency, incontinence, and constipation due to nervous system dysfunction
- Altered speech and aspiration
- Loss of memory, dementia, euphoria due to cerebral dysfunction
- Lack of coping
- Inability to perform home maintenance management due to physical, psychological, and social limits imposed by MS
- Sexual dysfunction

Planning and Goals

The major goals for the patient may include promotion of physical mobility, avoidance of injury, achievement of bladder and bowel continence, promotion of speech and swallowing mechanisms, improvement of cognitive function, development of coping strengths, improved home maintenance management, and adaptation to sexual dysfunction.

Nursing Interventions

An individualized program of physical therapy, rehabilitation, and education is combined with emotional support. An educational plan of care is developed to enable the person with MS to deal with the physiologic, social, and psychological problems that accompany chronic disease. Research shows that depression, pain, fatigue, and walking difficulty all decrease physical activity. Assisting patients with management of these symptoms may help increase

NURSING RESEARCH PROFILE

Chart 66-3. Predictors of Fatigue in Patients With MS

Morrison, J. D., & Stuifbergen, A. K. (2016). Predictors of fatigue impact in persons with long-standing multiple sclerosis. *Journal of Neuroscience Nursing, 48*(3), 143–150.

Purpose

Fatigue is very common among those with MS and has a negative impact on many aspects of their lives. The underlying mechanisms are poorly understood and treatment is a challenge. The purpose of this study was to explain the physical, cognitive, and psychosocial dimensions of fatigue among those with long-standing MS.

Design

More than 300 people with long-standing MS (for 17 years or more) were surveyed to measure fatigue impact, MS-related functional limitations, depressive symptoms, barriers to health promotion, personal resources, and health-promoting behaviours. The relationships among fatigue impact, age, MS duration, MS-related functional limitations, depressive symptoms, barriers to health promotion, personal resources, and health-promoting behaviours were also explored.

Findings

Age and MS duration were not significantly related to fatigue impact. Moderate to strong positive, linear relationships were reported among fatigue impact measures and MS functional limitations (range: $r = 0.41–0.58$, $p < 0.01$), depressive symptoms (range: $r = 0.58–0.63$, $p < 0.01$), and barriers (range: $r = 0.55–0.63$, $p < 0.01$). Moderate inverse linear relationships were reported among fatigue impact measures and personal resources (range: $r = -0.40–0.50$, $p < 0.01$) and health-promoting behaviours (range: $r = -0.34–0.44$, $p < 0.01$). MS functional limitation was reported as the strongest predictor of physical and psychosocial fatigue impact, while depressive symptoms was the strongest predictor of total and cognitive fatigue impact.

Nursing Implications

Nurses working with patients with MS should know that functional limitations and depressive symptoms were strong predictors of fatigue impact in this study. This illustrates the importance of nurses assessing and monitoring depressive symptoms, functional status, and dimensions of fatigue at each encounter with patients, whether in the in-patient or out-patient setting.

the level of physical activity and overall sense of well-being (Chart 66-3).

Promoting Physical Mobility

Relaxation and coordination exercises promote muscle efficiency. Progressive resistive exercises are used to strengthen weak muscles, because diminishing muscle strength is often significant in MS. Utilization of a specialized team of physical, occupational, and recreational therapists who specialize in treating MS patients is beneficial in improving patients'/families' quality of life.

EXERCISES. Walking improves the gait, particularly the problem of loss of position sense of the legs and feet (proprioception). If certain muscle groups are irreversibly affected, other muscles can be trained to compensate. Instruction in the use of assistive devices may be needed to ensure their safe and correct use.

MINIMIZING SPASTICITY AND CONTRACTURES. Muscle spasticity is common and, in its later stages, is characterized by severe adductor spasm of the hips with flexor spasm of the hips and knees. Without relief, fibrous contractures of these joints occur. Warm packs may be beneficial, but hot baths should be avoided because of risk of burn injury secondary to sensory loss and increasing symptoms that may occur with elevation of the body temperature.

Daily exercises for muscle stretching are prescribed to minimize joint contractures. Special attention is given to the hamstrings, gastrocnemius muscles, hip adductors, biceps, and wrist and finger flexors. Muscle spasticity is common and interferes with normal function. A stretch–hold–relax routine is helpful for relaxing and treating muscle spasticity. Swimming and stationary bicycling are useful, and progressive weight bearing can relieve spasticity in the legs. The patient should not be hurried in any of these activities, because this often increases spasticity.

ACTIVITY AND REST. The patient is encouraged to work and exercise to a point just short of fatigue. Very strenuous physical exercise is not advisable, because it raises the body temperature and may aggravate symptoms. The patient is advised to take frequent short rest periods, preferably lying down. Extreme fatigue may contribute to the exacerbation of symptoms.

Similar to the population at large, many patients with MS are overweight or have obesity. Contributing factors include the use of corticosteroids for exacerbations of symptoms and mobility impairments as a result of the disease. Interventions to promote healthy eating and weight reduction need to take into account that fatigue and mobility impairments are barriers to engagement in nutritional behaviours for people with MS. Nurses also need to be certain to include family members in interventions and nutrition education, because they are often the gatekeepers for food preparation and selection. Additional strategies include avoidance of alcohol and cigarette smoking (Bader et al., 2016).

MINIMIZING EFFECTS OF IMMOBILITY. Because of the decrease in physical activity that often occurs with MS, complications associated with immobility, including pressure ulcers, expiratory muscle weakness, and accumulation of bronchial secretions, need to be considered and steps taken to prevent them.

Measures to prevent such complications include assessing and maintaining skin integrity and having the patient perform coughing and deep-breathing exercises.

Preventing Injury

If motor dysfunction causes problems of incoordination and clumsiness, or if ataxia is apparent, the patient is at risk for falling. To overcome this disability, the patient is taught to walk with feet apart to widen the base of support and to increase walking stability. If loss of position sense occurs, the patient is taught to watch the feet while walking. Gait training may require assistive devices (walker, cane, braces, crutches, parallel bars) and instruction about their use by a physical therapist. If the gait remains inefficient, a wheelchair or motorized scooter may be the solution. The occupational therapist is a valuable resource person in suggesting and securing aids to promote independence. If incoordination is a problem and tremor of the upper extremities occurs when voluntary movement is attempted (intention tremor), weighted bracelets or wrist cuffs are helpful. The patient is trained in transfer and activities of daily living (ADLs).

Because sensory loss may occur in addition to motor loss, pressure ulcers are a continuing threat to skin integrity. The need to use a wheelchair continuously increases the risk. See Chapter 13 for a discussion of the prevention and treatment of pressure ulcers.

Enhancing Bladder and Bowel Control

Generally, bladder symptoms fall into the following categories: (1) inability to store urine (hyperreflexic, uninhibited); (2) inability to empty the bladder (hyporeflexic, hypotonic); and (3) a mixture of both types. The patient with urinary frequency, urgency, or incontinence requires special support. The sensation of the need to void must be heeded immediately, so the bedpan or urinal should be readily available. A bladder protocol is set up (every 1.5 to 2 hours initially, with gradual lengthening of the interval). The patient is instructed to drink a measured amount of fluid every 2 hours and then attempt to void 30 minutes after drinking. Use of a timer or wristwatch with an alarm may be helpful for the patient who does not have enough sensation to signal the need to empty the bladder. The nurse encourages the patient to take the prescribed medications to treat bladder spasticity, because this allows greater independence. Intermittent self-catheterization (see Chapter 13) has been successful in maintaining bladder control in patients with MS. If a female patient has permanent urinary incontinence, urinary diversion procedures may be considered. The male patient may wear a condom catheter for urine collection.

Bowel problems include constipation, fecal impaction, and incontinence. Adequate fluids, dietary fibre, and a bowel-training program are frequently effective in solving these problems. See Chapter 13 for a discussion of promoting bowel continence.

Enhancing Communication and Managing Swallowing Difficulties

When the cranial nerves that control the mechanisms of speech and swallowing are affected, dysarthrias (defects of articulation) marked by slurring, low volume of speech, and difficulties in phonation may occur. **Dysphagia** (difficulty swallowing) may also occur. A speech therapist evaluates speech and swallowing and instructs the patient, family, and health team members about strategies to compensate for speech and swallowing problems.

NURSING ALERT

Impaired swallowing increases the patient's risk of aspiration. To reduce that risk, the nurse implements strategies such as having suction apparatus available, ensuring careful feeding, confirming correct food and liquid consistency, and positioning properly for eating.

Improving Sensory and Cognitive Function

Measures may be taken if visual defects or changes in cognitive status occur.

VISION. The cranial nerves affecting vision may be affected by MS. An eye patch or a covered eyeglass lens may be used to block the visual impulses of one eye if the patient has diplopia (double vision). Prism glasses may be helpful for patients who are confined to bed and have difficulty reading in the supine position. People who are unable to read regular-print materials may obtain large-print or audio books from local libraries and from the Canadian National Institute for the Blind (CNIB). The CNIB also has books available in Braille.

COGNITION AND EMOTIONAL RESPONSES. Cognitive impairment and emotional lability occur early in MS in some patients and may impose numerous stresses on the patient and family. Some patients with MS are forgetful and easily distracted and may exhibit emotional lability.

Patients adapt to illness in a variety of ways, including denial, depression, withdrawal, and hostility. Emotional support assists patients and their families to adapt to the changes and uncertainties associated with MS and to cope with the disruption in their lives. The patient is assisted to set meaningful and realistic goals, to remain as active as possible, and to maintain interests and activities. Hobbies may help the patient's morale and provide satisfying interests if the disease progresses to the stage in which formerly enjoyed activities can no longer be pursued. The family should be made aware of the nature and degree of cognitive impairment. The occupational therapist can be helpful in formulating a structured daily routine.

STRENGTHENING COPING MECHANISMS. The diagnosis of MS is always distressing to the patient and family. They need to know that no two patients with MS have identical symptoms or courses of illness. Although some patients do experience significant disability early, others have a near-normal lifespan with minimal disability. Some families, however, face overwhelming frustrations and problems. MS affects people who are often in a productive stage of life and concerned about career and family responsibilities. Family conflict, disintegration, separation, and divorce are not uncommon. Often, very young family members assume the responsibility of caring for a parent with MS. Nursing interventions in this area include alleviating stress and making appropriate referrals for counselling and support to minimize the adverse effects of dealing with chronic illness.

The nurse, mindful of these complex problems, initiates home care and coordinates a network of services, including social services, speech therapy, physical therapy, and homemaker services. To strengthen the patient's coping skills, as much information as possible is provided. Patients need an updated list of available assistive devices, services, and resources.

Coping through problem solving involves helping the patient define the problem and develop alternatives for its management. Careful planning and maintaining flexibility and a hopeful attitude are useful for psychological and physical adaptation.

Improving Self-Care Abilities

MS can affect every facet of daily living. Certain abilities are often impossible to regain after they are lost. Physical function may vary from day to day. Modifications that allow independence in self-care should be implemented (e.g., assistive eating devices, raised toilet seat, bathing aids, telephone modifications, long-handled comb, tongs, modified clothing). Physical and emotional stresses should be avoided as much as possible, because these may worsen symptoms and impair performance. Exposure to heat increases fatigue and muscle weakness, so air conditioning is recommended in at least one room. Exposure to extreme cold may increase spasticity.

Promoting Sexual Functioning

Patients with MS and their partners face problems that interfere with sexual activity, both as a direct consequence of nerve damage and also from psychological reactions to the disease. Easy fatigability, conflicts arising from dependency and depression, emotional lability, and loss of self-esteem compound the problem. Erectile and ejaculatory disorders in men and orgasmic dysfunction and adductor spasms of the thigh muscles in women can make sexual intercourse difficult or impossible. Bladder and bowel incontinence and urinary tract infections add to the difficulties.

An experienced sexual counsellor can help bring into focus the patient's or partner's sexual resources and suggest relevant information and supportive therapy. Sharing and communicating feelings, planning for sexual activity (to minimize the effects of fatigue), and exploring alternative methods of sexual expression may open up a wide range of sexual enjoyment and experiences.

Promoting Home, Community-Based, and Transitional Care

EDUCATING PATIENTS ABOUT SELF-CARE. As the disease progresses, the patient and family need to learn new strategies to maintain optimal independence. Teaching of new self-care techniques may be initiated in the hospital or clinic setting and reinforced in the home. Self-care education may address the use of assistive devices, self-catheterization, and administration of medications that affect the course of the disease or treat complications. Although the disease-modifying medications (the "ABC and R medications") may slow the progression of disease and disability in many persons with MS, they are not effective in all patients. Patients who receive these medications will require teaching and support, while those unable to take them or for whom the medications have not been effective need continued support and assistance in coping with this reality. Exercises that enable the patient to continue some form of activity or that maintain or improve swallowing, speech, or respiratory function may be taught to the patient and family (Chart 66-4).

CONTINUING AND TRANSITIONAL CARE. After discharge, the home care nurse often provides teaching and reinforcement of new interventions in the patient's home. Nurses in the home setting assess for changes in the patient's physical and emotional status, provide physical care to the patient if required, coordinate outpatient services and resources, and encourage health promotion, appropriate health screenings, and adaptation. If changes in the disease or its course are noted, the home care nurse encourages the patient to contact the primary care provider, because treatment of an acute exacerbation or new problem may be indicated. Continuing health care and follow-up are recommended.

The patient with MS is encouraged to contact the local chapter of the Multiple Sclerosis Society of Canada for services, publications, and contact with others who have MS (see Resources). Local chapters also provide direct services to patients. Through group participation, the patient has an opportunity to meet others with similar problems, share experiences, and learn self-help methods in a social environment.

Evaluation

Expected patient outcomes may include the following:

1. Improves physical mobility
    a. Participates in gait-training and rehabilitation program
    b. Establishes a balanced program of rest and exercise
    c. Uses assistive devices correctly and safely
2. Is free of injury
    a. Uses visual cues to compensate for decreased sense of touch or position
    b. Asks for assistance when necessary

CHART 66-4

HOME CARE CHECKLIST • The Patient With MS

At the completion of education, the patient and/or caregiver will be able to:

- State the impact of MS and treatment on physiologic functioning, ADLs, IADLs, roles, relationships, and spirituality.
- State the purpose, dose, route, schedule, side effects, and precautions for prescribed medications.
    - Demonstrate correct techniques of administering injectable medications, if prescribed.
- State how to contact all members of the treatment team (e.g., health care providers, home care professionals, and durable medical equipment and supply vendor).
- State changes in lifestyle (e.g., exercise, activity) necessary to maintain health.
    - Demonstrate environmental modifications and adaptive techniques for accomplishing activities of daily living.
    - Identify strategies to manage symptoms (pain, cognitive responses, dysphagia, tremors, visual disturbances).
    - State how to prevent complications (e.g., pressure ulcers, pneumonia, depression).
    - Identify coping strategies.
    - Identify ways to minimize fatigue.
    - Explain how to prevent injury.
    - Identify optimal nutritional intake; consider weight reduction as indicated if patient is overweight or has obesity.
    - State ways to promote sexual function.
    - Discuss ways to manage bowel and bladder function.
    - Name benefits of exercise and physical activity.
    - Identify ways to minimize immobility and spasticity.
- Relate how to reach primary provider with questions or complications.
- State time and date of follow-up medical appointments, therapy, and testing.
- Identify sources of support (e.g., friends, relatives, faith community, National MS Society and MS support groups, caregiver support).
- Identify the need for health-promotion, disease prevention, and screening activities.

3. Attains or maintains control of bladder and bowel patterns
    a. Monitors self for urine retention and employs intermittent self-catheterization technique, if indicated
    b. Identifies the signs and symptoms of urinary tract infection
    c. Maintains adequate fluid and fibre intake
4. Participates in strategies to improve speech and swallowing
    a. Practices exercises recommended by speech therapist
    b. Maintains adequate nutritional intake without aspiration
5. Compensates for altered thought processes
    a. Uses lists and other aids to compensate for memory losses
    b. Discusses problems with trusted advisor or friend
    c. Substitutes new activities for those that are no longer possible
6. Demonstrates effective coping strategies
    a. Maintains sense of control
    b. Modifies lifestyle to fit goals and limitations
    c. Verbalizes desire to pursue goals and developmental tasks of adulthood
7. Adheres to plan for home maintenance management
    a. Uses appropriate techniques to maintain independence
    b. Engages in health-promotion activities and health screenings as appropriate
8. Adapts to changes in sexual function
    a. Is able to discuss problem with partner and appropriate health professional
    b. Identifies alternative means of sexual expression

Myasthenia Gravis

Myasthenia gravis, an autoimmune disorder affecting the myoneural junction within the CNS, is characterized by varying degrees of weakness of the voluntary muscles. Women are affected more frequently than men, and they tend to develop the disease at an earlier age (20 to 30 years of age, vs. 60 to 70 years for men) (Bader et al., 2016).

Pathophysiology

Normally, a chemical impulse precipitates the release of acetylcholine from vesicles on the nerve terminal at the myoneural junction. The acetylcholine attaches to receptor sites on the motor endplate and stimulates muscle contraction. Continuous binding of acetylcholine to the receptor site is required for muscular contraction to be sustained.

In myasthenia gravis, antibodies directed at the acetylcholine receptor sites impair transmission of impulses across the myoneural junction. Therefore, fewer receptors

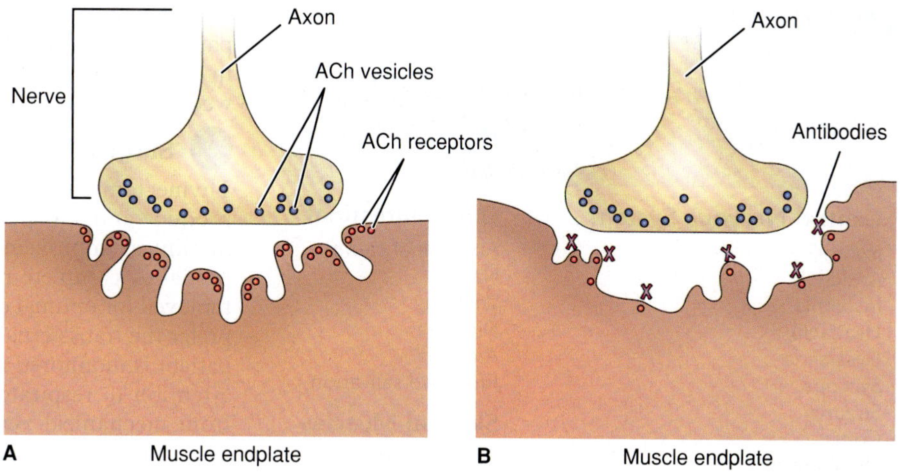

FIGURE 66-3. Myasthenia gravis. **A.** Normal acetylcholine (Ach) receptor site. **B.** ACh receptor site in myasthenia gravis.

are available for stimulation, resulting in voluntary muscle weakness that escalates with continued activity (Fig. 66-3). These antibodies are found in 80% to 90% of people with myasthenia gravis (Hickey, 2014). Eighty percent of people with myasthenia gravis have either thymic hyperplasia or a thymic tumour, and the thymus gland is believed to be the site of antibody production. In patients who are antibody negative, researchers believe that the offending antibody is directed at a portion of the receptor site rather than the whole complex (American Association of Neuroscience Nurses [AANN], 2013).

Clinical Manifestations

The initial manifestation of myasthenia gravis in two thirds of patients involves the ocular muscles. Diplopia (double vision) and **ptosis** (drooping of the eyelids) are common (Bader et al., 2016). Many patients also experience weakness of the muscles of the face and throat (bulbar symptoms) and generalized weakness. Weakness of the facial muscles results in a bland facial expression. Laryngeal involvement produces **dysphonia** (voice impairment) and increases the risk of choking and aspiration. Generalized weakness affects all the extremities and the intercostal muscles, resulting in decreasing vital capacity and respiratory failure (Mcilvoy, 2014). Myasthenia gravis is purely a motor disorder with no effect on sensation or coordination.

Assessment and Diagnostic Findings

An acetylcholinesterase inhibitor test (stim test) is used to diagnose myasthenia gravis. The acetylcholinesterase inhibitor stops the breakdown of acetylcholine, thereby increasing availability at the neuromuscular junction. Edrophonium chloride (Tensilon), a fast-acting acetylcholinesterase inhibitor, is administered IV to diagnose myasthenia gravis. Thirty seconds after injection, facial muscle weakness and ptosis should resolve for about 5 minutes (Hickey, 2014). Immediate improvement in muscle strength after administration of this agent represents a positive test and usually confirms the diagnosis. Atropine should be available to control the side effects of edrophonium, which include bradycardia, sweating, and cramping (Karch, 2014).

The acetylcholine receptor antibody titres are elevated as indicated previously. Repetitive muscle stimulation demonstrates a decrease in successive action potentials. The thymus gland, a site of acetylcholine receptor antibody production, may be enlarged in myasthenia gravis, and may be identified by MRI scan. A single-fibre electromyography (EMG) detects a delay or failure of neuromuscular transmission and is about 99% sensitive in confirming the diagnosis of myasthenia gravis (Hickey, 2014).

Medical Management

Management of myasthenia gravis is directed at improving function and reducing and removing circulating antibodies. Therapeutic modalities include administration of anticholinesterase medications and immunosuppressive therapy, plasmapheresis, and thymectomy. There is no cure for myasthenia gravis; treatments do not stop the production of the acetylcholine receptor antibodies.

Pharmacologic Therapy

Pyridostigmine bromide (Mestinon), an anticholinesterase medication, is the first line of therapy. It provides symptomatic relief by inhibiting the breakdown of acetylcholine and increasing the relative concentration of available acetylcholine at the neuromuscular junction. The dosage is gradually increased to a daily maximum and is administered in divided doses (usually four times a day). Adverse effects of anticholinesterase medications include fasciculations, abdominal pain, diarrhea, and increased oropharyngeal secretions (Mcilvoy, 2014). Pyridostigmine tends to have fewer side effects than other anticholinesterase medications (Chart 66-5).

If pyridostigmine bromide does not improve muscle strength and control fatigue, the next agents used are the immunomodulating drugs. The goal of immunosuppressive therapy is to reduce production of the antibody. Corticosteroids suppress the patient's immune response, decreasing the amount of antibody production, and this correlates with clinical improvement. An initial dose of prednisone is given daily; as symptoms improve, the medication is tapered and a maintenance dose may be given indefinitely (Bader et al., 2016). As the corticosteroid medications take effect the dosage of anticholinesterase medication can usually be

CHART 66-5

Pharmacology: Potential Adverse Effects of Anticholinesterase Medications

Central Nervous System
Irritability
Anxiety
Insomnia
Headache
Dysarthria
Syncope
Seizures
Coma
Diaphoresis

Respiratory
Bronchial relaxation
Increased bronchial secretions

Cardiovascular
Tachycardia
Hypotension

Gastrointestinal
Abdominal cramps
Nausea
Vomiting
Diarrhea
Anorexia
Increased salivation

Skeletal Muscles
Fasciculations
Spasms
Weakness

Genitourinary
Frequency
Urgency

Integumentary
Rash
Flushing

lowered. Cytotoxic medications are used to treat myasthenia gravis if there is inadequate response to steroids. Azathioprine (Imuran) inhibits T lymphocytes and reduces acetylcholine receptor antibody levels. Therapeutic effects may not be evident for 3 to 12 months. Leukopenia and hepatotoxicity are serious adverse effects, so monthly evaluation of liver enzymes and white blood cell count is necessary.

Intravenous immune globulin (IVIG) is also used to treat exacerbations, and, in selected patients, it is used on a long-term adjunctive basis. IVIG treatment is easy to administer and involves the administration of pooled human gamma-globulin, and improvement occurs in a few days (Hickey, 2014).

A number of medications are contraindicated for patients with myasthenia gravis because they exacerbate the symptoms. The physician and the patient should weigh risks and benefits before any new medications are prescribed, including antibiotics, cardiovascular medications, anticonvulsant and psychotropic medications, morphine, quinine and related agents, beta-blockers, and nonprescription medications. Procaine (Novocain) should be avoided, and the patient's dentist is informed of the diagnosis of myasthenia gravis.

Therapeutic Plasma Exchange

A technique called TPE, formerly referred to as plasmapheresis, is used to treat exacerbations. The patient's plasma and plasma components are removed through a centrally placed large-bore double-lumen catheter. The blood cells and antibody-containing plasma are separated, after which the cells and a plasma substitute are reinfused. Plasma exchange produces a temporary reduction in the level of circulating antibodies. The typical course of plasmapheresis consists of daily or alternate-day treatment, and the number of treatments is determined by the patient's response. Plasma exchange improves symptoms in 75% of patients; however, improvement lasts only a few weeks after treatment is completed (Stephen et al., 2012).

Surgical Management

Thymectomy (surgical removal of the thymus gland) can produce antigen-specific immunosuppression and result in clinical improvement. The procedure results in either partial or complete remission. The entire gland must be removed for optimal clinical outcomes; therefore, surgeons prefer the transsternal surgical approach. After surgery, the patient is monitored in an intensive care unit, with special attention to respiratory function. The patient is weaned from mechanical ventilation after thorough respiratory assessment. After the thymus gland is removed, it may take up to 3 years for the patient to benefit from the procedure, because of the long life of circulating T cells (Hickey, 2014).

Complications

A myasthenic crisis is an exacerbation of the disease process characterized by severe generalized muscle weakness and respiratory and bulbar weakness that may result in respiratory failure. Crisis may result from disease exacerbation or a specific precipitating event. The most common precipitator is respiratory infection; others include medication change, surgery, pregnancy, and medications that exacerbate myasthenia. A cholinergic crisis caused by overmedication with cholinesterase inhibitors is rare; atropine sulphate should be on hand to treat bradycardia or respiratory distress (Karch, 2014).

Neuromuscular respiratory failure is the critical complication in myasthenic and cholinergic crises. Respiratory muscle and bulbar weakness combine to cause respiratory compromise. Weak respiratory muscles do not support inhalation. An inadequate cough and an impaired gag reflex, caused by bulbar weakness, result in poor airway clearance. A downward trend of two respiratory function tests, the negative inspiratory force and vital capacity, is the first clinical sign of respiratory compromise. Respiratory therapists are actively involved in the care of myasthenia patients. These members of the care team perform frequent vital capacity tests in order to track the patient's clinical course and response to therapy. A decreasing trend in a patient's vital capacities will trigger closer monitoring of the patient's condition.

Endotracheal intubation and mechanical ventilation may be needed (see Chapter 25). Noninvasive positive-pressure ventilation uses an external device that provides respiratory support without endotracheal intubation. Cholinesterase inhibitors are stopped when respiratory failure occurs and gradually restarted after the patient demonstrates improvement with a course of plasmapheresis or IVIG. Nutritional support may be needed if the patient is intubated for a long period.

Nursing Management

Because myasthenia gravis is a chronic disease and most patients are seen on an outpatient basis, much of the nursing care focuses on patient and family teaching. Educational topics for outpatient self-care include medication management, energy conservation, strategies to help with ocular manifestations, and prevention and management of complications.

Medication management is a crucial component of ongoing care. Understanding the actions of the medications and taking them on schedule is emphasized, as are the consequences of delaying medication and the signs and symptoms of myasthenic and cholinergic crises. The patient can determine the best times for daily dosing by keeping a diary to determine fluctuation of symptoms and to learn when the medication is wearing off. The medication schedule can then be manipulated to maximize strength throughout the day.

NURSING ALERT

Maintenance of stable blood levels of anticholinesterase medications is imperative to stabilize muscle strength. Therefore, the anticholinesterase medications must be administered on time. Any delay in administration of medications may exacerbate muscle weakness and make it impossible for the patient to take medications orally.

Regular administration of IVIG or subcutaneous immunoglobulin (SCIG) may be prescribed. The patient and family are educated about managing immunoglobulin therapy (Chart 66-6).

The patient is also taught strategies to conserve energy. To do this, the nurse helps the patient identify the optimal times for rest throughout the day. If the patient lives in a two-storey home, the nurse can suggest that frequently used items (e.g., hygiene products, cleaning products, snacks) be kept on each floor to minimize travel between floors. The patient is encouraged to apply for a handicapped license plate to minimize walking from parking spaces, and to schedule activities to coincide with peak energy and strength levels.

To minimize the risk of aspiration, mealtimes should coincide with the peak effects of anticholinesterase medication. In addition, rest before meals is encouraged to reduce muscle fatigue. The patient is advised to sit upright during meals, with the neck slightly flexed to facilitate swallowing. Soft foods in gravy or sauces can be swallowed more easily; if choking occurs frequently, the nurse can suggest puréed food with a puddinglike consistency. Suction should be available at home, with the patient and family instructed in its use. Supplemental feedings may be necessary in some patients to ensure adequate nutrition.

Impaired vision results from ptosis of one or both eyelids, decreased eye movement, or double vision. To prevent corneal damage when the eyelids do not close completely, the patient is instructed to tape the eyes closed for short intervals and to regularly instill artificial tears. Patients who wear eyeglasses can have "crutches" attached to help lift the eyelids. Patching of one eye can help with double vision.

The patient is reminded of the importance of maintaining health-promotion practices and of following health care screening recommendations. Factors that exacerbate symptoms and potentially cause crisis should be noted and avoided: emotional stress, infections (particularly respiratory infections), vigorous physical activity, some medications, and high environmental temperature. The Myasthenia Gravis Foundation of Canada provides support groups, services, and educational materials for patients, families, and health care providers (see Resources).

Myasthenic Crisis

Respiratory distress and varying degrees of dysphagia (difficulty swallowing), dysarthria (difficulty speaking), eyelid ptosis, diplopia, and prominent muscle weakness are symptoms of myasthenic crisis. The patient is placed in an intensive care unit for constant monitoring because of associated intense and sudden fluctuations in clinical condition.

Providing ventilatory assistance takes precedence in the immediate management of the patient with myasthenic crisis. Ongoing assessment for respiratory failure is essential. The nurse assesses the respiratory rate, depth, and breath sounds and monitors pulmonary function parameters (vital capacity and negative inspiratory force) to detect pulmonary problems before respiratory dysfunction progresses. Blood is drawn for arterial blood gas analysis. Endotracheal intubation and mechanical ventilation may be needed (see Chapter 26).

If the abdominal, intercostal, and pharyngeal muscles are severely weak, the patient cannot cough, take deep breaths, or clear secretions. Chest physical therapy, including postural drainage to mobilize secretions and suctioning to remove secretions, may have to be performed frequently. (Postural drainage should not be performed for 30 minutes after feeding.)

Assessment strategies and supportive measures include the following:

- Arterial blood gases, serum electrolytes, input and output, and daily weight are monitored.
- If the patient cannot swallow, nasogastric tube feedings may be prescribed.
- Sedatives and tranquilizers are avoided, because they aggravate hypoxia and hypercapnia and can cause respiratory and cardiac depression.

Guillain–Barré Syndrome

Guillain–Barré syndrome is an autoimmune attack on the peripheral nerve myelin. The result is acute, rapid segmental demyelination of peripheral nerves and some cranial nerves, producing ascending weakness with dyskinesia (inability to execute voluntary movements), hyporeflexia, and paresthesias (numbness). An antecedent event (most often a viral infection) precipitates clinical presentation (Winer, 2014). *Campylobacter jejuni*, cytomegalovirus, Epstein–Barr virus, *Mycoplasma pneumoniae, H. influenzae*, and HIV are the most common infectious agents that are associated with the development of Guillain–Barré syndrome. Results of studies on recovery rates differ, but most indicate that 60% to 75% of patients recover completely. Residual deficits of varying degree occur in 20% to 25% of patients. Residual deficits are most likely in patients with rapid disease

CHART 66-6

GUIDELINES for Managing Immunoglobulin Therapy

Immunoglobulin therapy is an important treatment for a variety of disease states that are characterized by deficient production of antibodies. Immunoglobulin can be administered for replacement therapy as an IV infusion or subcutaneous (SQ) injection. It can safely be administered in outpatient as well as inpatient settings.

Equipment (as Needed)

- Single-use tourniquet
- Single-use scissors or clippers for hair removal
- IVIG solution, tubing, connector, catheter, or syringe
- Chlorhexidine gluconate, povidone-iodine, or alcohol swabs
- Nonlatex gloves
- Transparent dressing, bandage, or sterile gauze
- Padded, appropriate-length arm board
- Tape
- Topical analgesics
- Preservative-free 0.9% NaCl flush solution
- Padded, appropriate-length arm board or finger splint
- Electronic infusion pump

Implementation

NURSING ACTIONS	RATIONALE
1. Verify prescription for IVIG therapy and identify patient.	1. Serious errors can be avoided by careful checking. Immunoglobulin is supplied in a 5% solution or a lyophilized powder with a reconstituting diluent prepared from Cohn fraction II obtained from pools of 1,000–20,000 donors. Currently, a number of different IV preparations are approved for use and have been shown to be effective and safe by the U.S. Food and Drug Administration. Immunoglobulin can also be administered via SQ injection.
2. Check for allergies (i.e., latex, iodine).	2. Checking for allergies reduces risk of allergic reaction.
3. Explain procedure to patient.	3. Knowledge increases patient comfort and cooperation.
4. Perform hand hygiene, and put on disposable nonlatex gloves.	4. Asepsis is essential to prevent infection. The use of nonlatex gloves prevents exposure of nurse to patient's blood and of patient and nurse to latex.
5. Obtain Ht. and Wt. of patient before treatment.	5. Obtaining Ht. and Wt. helps verify accurate dosing.
6. Assess baseline vital signs before, during, and after treatment.	6. An elevated temperature at the beginning of treatment may be an indication to delay the therapy to avoid misinterpreting this as an adverse reaction.
7. Premedicate with acetaminophen (Tylenol) and diphenhydramine (Benadryl) as prescribed 30 minutes before the start of infusion therapy. Corticosteroids may be prescribed as well.	7. Premedicating may help avert adverse reactions. Corticosteroids may be used to prevent possible severe reactions in patients who are perceived to be at risk.
8. Verify the route and dose of IVIG therapy.	8. IVIG can be administered via the IV or SQ routes. The optimal dose is determined by the patient's response. In most instances, an IV dose of 200–800 mg/kg of body weight is administered every 3–4 weeks to ensure adequate serum levels of immunoglobulin G (IgG).
9. Insert IV cannula or catheter according to Guidelines for Starting a Peripheral Intravenous Infusion, as needed.	9. Patient may need IV access, may have a port or long-term catheter for an IV infusion.
10. Administer the IV infusion at a slow rate, not to exceed 3 mL/min, usually at 100–200 mL/h.	10. Administer according to manufacturer's instructions. Beginning at a slow rate helps minimize adverse reactions.
11. Continually assess the patient for adverse reactions.	11. Be aware of complaints of a tickle or lump in the throat as the precursor to laryngospasm that precedes bronchoconstriction. Caution should be exercised when changing IVIG products, because they are not biologically equivalent. Understand that long-term tolerance of an older IVIG product does not necessarily imply tolerance to a newer product, even if it is technically superior.
12. Stop IV infusion at the first sign of reaction.	12. Initiate the institutional protocol to be followed in an emergent situation. Patients who have an IgA deficiency have IgE antibodies to IgA, which requires administration of plasma or immunoglobulin replacement from IgA-deficient patients. Because all IV immunoglobulin preparations contain some IgA, they may cause an anaphylactic reaction in patients with IgE anti-IgA antibodies.
13. Administer SQ immunoglobulin as orders.	13. The pharmacokinetics of IgG differ when smaller doses are given more frequently, as is commonly done with SQ regimens.

Ht., height; Wt., weight.

Adapted from Cherin, P., Marie, I., Michallet, M., et al. (2016). Management of adverse events in the treatment of patients with immunoglobulin therapy: A review of evidence. *Autoimmunity Reviews*, *15*, 71–81.

progression, those who require mechanical ventilation, and those 60 years of age or older.

There are several types of GBS. With the most well-known type, the patient experiences weakness in the lower extremities, which progresses upward and has the potential for respiratory failure. The second type is purely motor with no altered sensation. A third type, called descending GBS, is much more difficult to diagnose; it mostly affects the head and neck muscles. The rarest type, the Miller–Fisher variant, presents with ataxia, areflexia, and ophthalmoplegia (McNair, 2013).

Pathophysiology

Myelin is a complex substance that covers nerves, providing insulation and speeding the conduction of impulses from the cell body to the dendrites. The cell that produces myelin in the peripheral nervous system is the Schwann cell. In Guillain–Barré syndrome, the Schwann cell is spared, allowing for remyelination in the recovery phase of the disease.

Guillain–Barré syndrome is the result of a cell-mediated and humoral immune attack on peripheral nerve myelin proteins that causes inflammatory demyelination. The best-accepted theory of cause is molecular mimicry, in which an infectious organism contains an amino acid that mimics the peripheral nerve myelin protein. The immune system cannot distinguish between the two proteins and attacks and destroys peripheral nerve myelin. The exact location of the immune attack within the peripheral nervous system is the ganglioside GM1b. With the autoimmune attack, there is an influx of macrophages and other immune-mediated agents that attack myelin and cause inflammation and destruction, interruption of nerve conduction, and axonal loss (Hickey, 2014).

Clinical Manifestations

Guillain–Barré syndrome typically begins with muscle weakness and diminished reflexes of the lower extremities. Hyporeflexia and weakness may progress to tetraplegia. Demyelination of the nerves that innervate the diaphragm and intercostal muscles results in neuromuscular respiratory failure. Sensory symptoms include paresthesia of the hands and feet and pain related to the demyelination of sensory fibres.

The antecedent event usually occurs 2 weeks before symptoms begin. Weakness usually begins in the legs and progresses upward. Maximum weakness, the plateau, varies in length but usually includes neuromuscular respiratory failure and bulbar weakness. The duration of the symptoms is variable; complete functional recovery may take up to 2 years. Any residual symptoms are permanent and reflect axonal damage from demyelination.

Cranial nerve demyelination can result in a variety of clinical manifestations. Optic nerve demyelination may result in blindness. Bulbar muscle weakness related to demyelination of the glossopharyngeal and vagus nerves results in the inability to swallow or clear secretions. Vagus nerve demyelination results in autonomic dysfunction, manifested by instability of the cardiovascular system. The presentation is variable and may include tachycardia, bradycardia, hypertension, or orthostatic hypotension. The symptoms of autonomic dysfunction occur and resolve rapidly. Guillain–Barré syndrome does not affect cognitive function or LOC.

Although the classic clinical features include areflexia and ascending weakness, variation in presentation occurs. There may be a sensory presentation, with progressive sensory symptoms; an atypical axonal destruction; or the Miller–Fisher variant, which includes paralysis of the ocular muscles, ataxia, and areflexia (McNair, 2013).

Assessment and Diagnostic Findings

The patient presents with symmetric weakness, diminished reflexes, and upward progression of motor weakness. A history of a viral illness in the previous few weeks suggests the diagnosis. Changes in vital capacity and negative inspiratory force are assessed to identify impending neuromuscular respiratory failure. Serum laboratory tests are not useful in the diagnosis. However, elevated protein levels are detected in CSF evaluation, without an increase in other cells. Evoked potential studies demonstrate a progressive loss of nerve conduction velocity.

Medical Management

Because of the possibility of rapid progression and neuromuscular respiratory failure, Guillain–Barré syndrome is a medical emergency, requiring management in an intensive care unit. After baseline values are identified, assessment of changes in muscle strength and respiratory function alert the clinician to the physical and respiratory needs of the patient. Respiratory therapy or mechanical ventilation may be necessary to support pulmonary function and adequate oxygenation. Mechanical ventilation may be required for an extended period. The patient is weaned from mechanical ventilation after the respiratory muscles can again support spontaneous respiration and maintain adequate tissue oxygenation.

Other interventions are aimed at preventing the complications of immobility. These may include the use of anticoagulant agents and antiembolism stockings or sequential compression boots to prevent thrombosis and pulmonary emboli.

Plasmapheresis and IVIG are used to directly affect the peripheral nerve myelin antibody level. Both therapies decrease circulating antibody levels and reduce the amount of time the patient is immobilized and dependent on mechanical ventilation. Studies indicate that IVIG and plasmapheresis are equally effective in treating Guillain–Barré syndrome; however, IVIG is the therapy of choice because it is associated with fewer side effects. The cardiovascular risks posed by autonomic dysfunction require continuous electrocardiographic (ECG) monitoring. Tachycardia and hypertension are treated with short-acting medications such as alpha-adrenergic blocking agents. The use of short-acting agents is important, because autonomic dysfunction is very labile. Hypotension is managed by increasing the amount of IV fluid administered.

Nursing Process

The Patient With Guillain–Barré Syndrome

Assessment

Ongoing assessment for disease progression is critical. The patient is monitored for life-threatening complications (respiratory failure, cardiac dysrhythmias, deep vein thrombosis [DVT]) so that appropriate interventions can be initiated. Because of the threat to the patient in this sudden, potentially life-threatening disease, the nurse must assess the patient's and family's ability to cope and their use of coping strategies.

Nursing Priorities

Based on the assessment data, the patient's major nursing priorities may include the following:

- Ineffective breathing pattern and decreased gas exchange
- Decreased physical mobility likely due to paralysis
- Nutrition less than body requirements likely due to inability to swallow
- Aspiration risk likely due to cranial nerve impairment
- Change in verbal communication likely due to cranial nerve dysfunction
- Fear and anxiety likely due to loss of control and paralysis

Collaborative Problems/ Potential Complications

Based on the assessment data, potential complications that may develop include the following:

- Respiratory failure
- Autonomic dysfunction

Planning and Goals

The major goals for the patient may include improved respiratory function, increased mobility, improved nutritional status, effective communication, decreased fear and anxiety, and absence of complications.

Nursing Interventions

Maintaining Respiratory Function

Respiratory function can be maximized with incentive spirometry and chest physiotherapy. Monitoring for changes in vital capacity and negative inspiratory force are key to early intervention for neuromuscular respiratory failure. Mechanical ventilation is required if the vital capacity falls, making spontaneous breathing impossible and tissue oxygenation inadequate.

The potential need for mechanical ventilation should be discussed with the patient and family on admission to provide time for psychological preparation and decision making. Intubation and mechanical ventilation result in less anxiety if they are initiated on a nonemergency basis to a well-informed patient. The patient may require mechanical ventilation for a long period. Nursing management of the patient requiring mechanical ventilation is discussed in Chapter 26.

Bulbar weakness that impairs the ability to swallow and clear secretions is another factor in the development of respiratory failure in the patient with Guillain–Barré syndrome. Suctioning may be needed to maintain a clear airway.

The nurse assesses the blood pressure and heart rate frequently to identify autonomic dysfunction, so that interventions can be initiated quickly if needed. Medications are administered or a temporary pacemaker is placed for clinically significant bradycardia.

Enhancing Physical Mobility

Nursing interventions to enhance physical mobility and prevent the complications of immobility are key to the function and survival of patients. The paralyzed extremities are supported in functional positions, and passive range-of-motion exercises are performed at least twice daily. DVT and pulmonary embolism are threats to the paralyzed patient. Nursing interventions are aimed at preventing DVT. Range-of-motion exercises, position changes, anticoagulation, the use of antiembolism stockings or sequential compression boots, and adequate hydration will decrease the risk of DVT.

Padding may be placed over bony prominences, such as the elbows and heels, to reduce the risk of pressure ulcers. The need for consistent position changes every 2 hours cannot be overemphasized. The nurse evaluates laboratory test results that may indicate malnutrition or dehydration, both of which increase the risk of pressure ulcers. The nurse collaborates with the physician and dietitian to develop a plan to meet the patient's nutritional and hydration needs.

Providing Adequate Nutrition

Paralytic ileus may result from insufficient parasympathetic activity. In this event, the nurse administers IV fluids and parenteral nutrition as a supplement and monitors for the return of bowel sounds. If the patient cannot swallow due to bulbar paralysis (immobility of muscles), a gastrostomy tube may be placed to administer nutrients. The nurse carefully assesses the return of the gag reflex and bowel sounds before resuming oral nutrition.

Improving Communication

Because of paralysis, the patient cannot talk, laugh, or cry and therefore has no method for communicating needs or expressing emotion. Establishing some form of communication with picture cards or an eye blink system provides a means of communication.

Collaboration with the speech therapist may be helpful in developing a communication mechanism that is most effective for a specific patient.

Decreasing Fear and Anxiety

The patient and family are faced with a sudden, potentially life-threatening disease, and anxiety and fear are constant themes for them. The impact of disease on the family depends on the patient's role within the family. Referral to a support group may provide information and support to the patient and family.

The family may feel helpless in caring for the patient. Mechanical ventilation and monitoring devices may frighten and intimidate them. Family members often want to participate in physical care; with instruction and support by the nurse, they should be allowed and encouraged to do so.

In addition to fear, the patient may experience isolation, loneliness, and lack of control. Nursing interventions that increase the patient's sense of control include providing information about the condition, emphasizing a positive appraisal of coping resources, and teaching relaxation exercises and distraction techniques. The positive attitude and atmosphere of the multidisciplinary team are important to promote a sense of well-being.

Diversional activities are encouraged to decrease loneliness and isolation. Encouraging visitors, engaging visitors or volunteers to read to the patient, listening to music or audio-books, and watching television are ways to alleviate the patient's sense of isolation.

Monitoring and Managing Potential Complications

Thorough assessment of respiratory function at regular and frequent intervals is essential, because respiratory insufficiency and subsequent failure due to weakness or paralysis of the intercostal muscles and diaphragm may develop quickly. Respiratory failure is the major cause of mortality. In addition to the respiratory rate and the quality of respirations, vital capacity is monitored frequently and at regular intervals, so that respiratory insufficiency can be anticipated. Decreasing vital capacity with associated muscle weakness indicates impending respiratory failure. Signs and symptoms include breathlessness while speaking, shallow and irregular breathing, use of accessory muscles, tachycardia, weak cough, and changes in respiratory pattern.

Other complications include cardiac dysrhythmias, which necessitate ECG monitoring; transient hypertension; orthostatic hypotension; DVT; pulmonary embolism; urinary retention; and other threats to any immobilized and paralyzed patient. These require monitoring and attention to prevent them and prompt treatment if indicated.

Promoting Home, Community-Based, and Transitional Care

EDUCATING PATIENTS ABOUT SELF-CARE. Patients with Guillain–Barré syndrome and their families are usually frightened by the sudden onset of life-threatening symptoms and their severity. Therefore, teaching the patient and family about the disorder and its generally favourable prognosis is important (Chart 66-7).

During the acute phase of the illness, the patient and family are instructed about strategies they can implement to minimize the effects of immobility and other complications. As function begins to return, family members and other home care providers are instructed about care of the patient and their role in the rehabilitation process. Preparation for discharge is an interdisciplinary effort requiring family or caregiver education by all team members, including the nurse, physician, occupational and physical therapists, speech therapist, and respiratory therapist.

CONTINUING AND TRANSITIONAL CARE. Most patients with Guillain–Barré syndrome experience complete recovery. Patients who have experienced total or prolonged paralysis require intensive rehabilitation; the extent depends on the severity of the damage and the patient's needs. Approaches include a comprehensive inpatient program if deficits are significant, an outpatient program if the patient can travel by car, or a home program of physical and occupational therapy. The recovery phase may be long and requires patience as well as involvement on the part of the patient and family.

During acute care, the focus is on immediate issues and deficits. The nurse needs to remind or instruct patients and family members of the need for continuing health-promotion and screening practices after this initial phase of care.

Evaluation

Expected patient outcomes may include the following:

1. Maintains effective respirations and airway clearance
   a. Has normal breath sounds on auscultation
   b. Demonstrates gradual improvement in respiratory function
2. Shows increasing mobility
   a. Regains use of extremities
   b. Participates in rehabilitation program
   c. Demonstrates no contractures and minimal muscle atrophy
3. Receives adequate nutrition and hydration
   a. Consumes diet adequate to meet nutritional needs
   b. Swallows without aspiration
4. Demonstrates recovery of speech
   a. Communicates needs through alternative strategies
   b. Practices exercises recommended by the speech therapist
5. Shows lessening fear and anxiety
6. Has absence of complications
   a. Breathes spontaneously
   b. Has vital capacity within normal range
   c. Exhibits normal arterial blood gases and pulse oximetry

CHART 66-7

HOME CARE CHECKLIST • The Patient With GBS

At the completion of education, the patient and/or caregiver will be able to:

- State the impact of GBS and treatment on physiologic functioning, ADLs, IADLs, roles, relationships, and spirituality.
- State the purpose, dose, route, schedule, side effects, and precautions for prescribed medications.
- State how to contact all members of the treatment team (e.g., health care providers, home care professionals, and durable medical equipment and supply vendor).
- State what types of environmental and safety changes or supports are needed for optimum functioning in the home.
  - State changes in lifestyle (e.g., nutrition, skin care, exercise, activity) necessary during recovery period and to maintain health as indicated.
  - Demonstrate environmental modifications and adaptive techniques for accomplishing ADLs (e.g., bathing, hygiene, grooming, dressing) and safely managing self-care.
  - Manage respiratory needs—tracheostomy care, suctioning.
  - Verbalize dietary adjustments and optimum nutrition during recovery.
  - Demonstrate proper body mechanics regarding lifting and transfers.
  - Practice gait training and strength endurance.
  - Perform range-of-motion exercises.
  - Discuss bowel and bladder management.
  - Operate and explain function of medical equipment and mobility aids—walkers, wheelchairs, bedside commodes, tub transfer benches, adaptive devices.
  - Describe coping mechanisms and diversional activities appropriately.
- Relate how to reach primary provider with questions or complications.
- State time and date of follow-up medical appointments, therapy, and testing.
- Identify sources of support (e.g., friends, relatives, faith community, GBS Foundation International, support groups, caregiver support).
- Identify the need for health-promotion, disease prevention, and screening activities.

CRANIAL NERVE DISORDERS

Because the brain stem and cranial nerves involve vital motor, sensory, and autonomic functions of the body, these nerves may be affected by conditions arising primarily within these structures or in secondary extension from adjacent disease processes. The cranial nerves are examined separately and in sequence (see Chapter 61). Some cranial nerve deficits can be detected by observing the patient's face, eye movements, speech, and swallowing. EMG is used to investigate motor and sensory dysfunction. An MRI scan is used to obtain images of the cranial nerves and brain stem. An overview of disorders that may affect each of the cranial nerves, including clinical manifestations and nursing interventions, is presented in Table 66-2. The following discussion centres on the most common disorders of the cranial nerves: trigeminal neuralgia, a condition affecting the fifth cranial nerve; and Bell's palsy, caused by involvement of the seventh cranial nerve.

Trigeminal Neuralgia (Tic Douloureux)

Trigeminal neuralgia is a condition of the fifth cranial nerve that is characterized by paroxysms of pain in the area innervated by any of the three branches of the fifth cranial nerve—V1, V2, V3, but most commonly the second and third branches of the trigeminal nerve (Fig. 66-4) (Grossman & Porth, 2014). The pain ends as abruptly as it starts and is described as a unilateral shooting and stabbing sensation. The unilateral nature of the pain is an important feature. Associated involuntary contraction of the facial muscles can cause sudden closing of the eye or twitching of the mouth, hence the former name *tic douloureux* (painful twitch). Although the cause of trigeminal neuralgia is not always clear structural abnormalities along the course of the nerve are often found. As the brain ages, a loop of a cerebral artery or vein may compress the nerve root entry point, which can be identified on MRI scan (Grossman & Porth, 2014).

Trigeminal neuralgia is most likely to occur after age 40 and is more common in women and in people with MS compared to the general population (Bader et al., 2016). Pain-free intervals may be measured in terms of minutes, hours, days, or longer. With advancing years, the painful episodes tend to become more frequent and agonizing. The patient lives in constant fear of attacks. And the disease itself can have a very significant effect on a patient's quality of life.

Attacks can occur with any stimulation of the terminals of the affected nerve branches, such as washing the face, shaving, brushing the teeth, eating, and drinking. A draft of cold air or direct pressure against the nerve trunk may

TABLE 66-2 Disorders of Cranial Nerves

Disorder	Clinical Manifestations	Nursing Interventions
Olfactory Nerve—I		
Head trauma Intracranial tumour Intracranial surgery	Unilateral or bilateral anosmia (temporary or persistent) Diminished taste for food	Assess sense of smell. Assess for cerebrospinal fluid rhinorrhea if patient has sustained head trauma.
Optic Nerve—II		
Optic neuritis Increased intracranial pressure Pituitary tumour	Lesions of optic tract producing homonymous hemianopsia	Assess visual acuity. Restructure environment to prevent injuries. Teach patient to accommodate for visual loss.
Oculomotor Nerve—III		Assess extraocular movement and for nonreactive pupil
Trochlear Nerve—IV		Assess extraocular movement and for nonreactive pupil.
Abducens Nerve—VI		
Vascular Brain stem ischemia Hemorrhage and infarction Neoplasm Trauma Infection	Dilation of pupil with loss of light reflex on one side Impairment of ocular movement Diplopia Gaze palsies Ptosis of eyelid	Assess extraocular movement and for nonreactive pupil.
Trigeminal Nerve—V		
Trigeminal neuralgia Head trauma Cerebellopontine lesion Sinus tract tumour and metastatic disease Compression of trigeminal root by tumour	Pain in face Diminished or loss of corneal reflex Chewing dysfunction	Assess for pain and triggering mechanisms for pain. Assess for difficulty in chewing. Discuss trigger zones and pain precipitants with patient. Protect cornea from abrasion. Ensure good oral hygiene. Educate patient about medication regimen.
Facial Nerve—VII		
Bell's palsy Facial nerve tumour Intracranial lesion Herpes zoster	Facial dysfunction; weakness and paralysis Hemifacial spasm Diminished or absent taste Pain	Recognize facial paralysis as emergency; refer for treatment as soon as possible. Teach protective care for eyes. Select easily chewed foods; patient should eat and drink from unaffected side of mouth. Emphasize importance of oral hygiene. Provide emotional support for changed appearance of face.
Vestibulocochlear Nerve—VIII		
Tumours and acoustic neuroma Vascular compression of nerve Ménière's syndrome	Tinnitus Vertigo Hearing difficulties	Assess pattern of vertigo. Provide for safety measures to prevent falls. Ensure that patient can maintain balance before ambulating. Caution patient to change positions slowly. Assist with ambulation. Encourage use of assistive devices.
Glossopharyngeal Nerve—IX		
Glossopharyngeal neuralgia from neurovascular compression of cranial nerves IX and X Trauma Inflammatory conditions Tumour Vertebral artery aneurysms	Pain at base of tongue Difficulty in swallowing Loss of gag reflex Palatal, pharyngeal, and laryngeal paralysis	Assess for paroxysmal pain in throat, decreased or absent swallowing, and gag and cough reflexes. Monitor for dysphagia, aspiration, and nasal dysarthric speech. Position patient upright for eating or tube feeding.
Vagus Nerve—X		
Spastic palsy of larynx; bulbar paralysis; high vagal paralysis Guillain-Barré syndrome Vagal body tumours Nerve paralysis from malignancy, surgical trauma such as carotid endarterectomy	Voice changes (temporary or permanent hoarseness) Vocal paralysis Dysphagia	Assess for airway obstruction/provide airway management. Prevent aspiration. Support patient having voice reconstruction procedures.

TABLE 66-2 Disorders of Cranial Nerves (Continued)

Disorder	Clinical Manifestations	Nursing Interventions
Spinal Accessory Nerve—XI		
Spinal cord disorder Amyotrophic lateral sclerosis Trauma Guillain-Barré syndrome	Drooping of affected shoulder with limited shoulder movement Weakness or paralysis of head rotation, flexion, extension; shoulder elevation	Support patient undergoing diagnostic tests.
Hypoglossal Nerve—XII		
Medullary lesions Amyotrophic lateral sclerosis Polio and motor system disease, which may destroy hypoglossal nuclei Multiple sclerosis Trauma	Abnormal movements of tongue Weakness or paralysis of tongue muscles Difficulty in talking, chewing, and swallowing	Observe swallowing ability. Observe speech pattern. Be aware of swallowing or vocal difficulties. Prepare for alternate feeding methods (tube feeding) to maintain nutrition.

Adapted from Bader, M., Littlejohns, L. R., & Olson, D. (2016). *AANN core curriculum for neuroscience nursing* (6th ed.). Chicago, IL: American Association of Neuroscience Nurses; Hickey, J. V. (2014). *The clinical practice of neurological & neurosurgical nursing* (7th ed.). Philadelphia, PA: Lippincott Williams & Wilkins.

also cause pain. Certain areas are called trigger points because the slightest touch immediately starts an attack or episode. To avoid stimulating these areas, patients with trigeminal neuralgia try not to touch or wash their faces, shave, chew, or do anything else that might cause an attack. These behaviours are a key factor in coming up with the diagnosis.

Medical Management

Pharmacologic Therapy

Anticonvulsant medications, such as carbamazepine (Tegretol), are often helpful in relieving pain in most patients with trigeminal neuralgia. They work by reducing the transmission of impulses at certain nerve terminals. Carbamazepine is taken with meals. Serum levels must be monitored to avoid toxicity in patients who require high doses to control the pain. Side effects include nausea, dizziness, drowsiness, and aplastic anemia. The patient is monitored for bone marrow depression during long-term therapy. Gabapentin

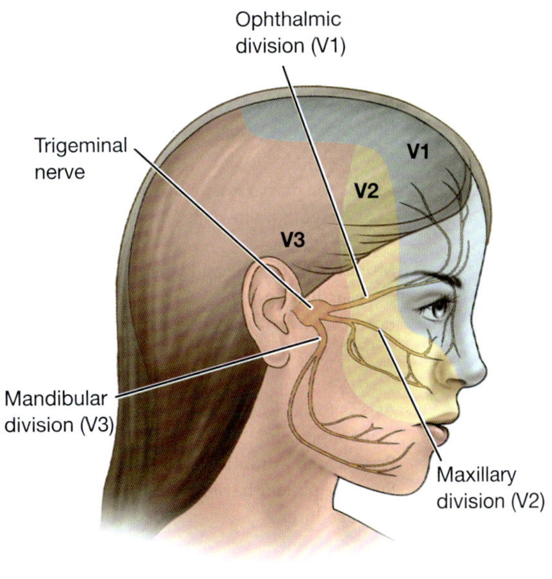

FIGURE 66-4. Distribution of trigeminal nerve branches.

(Neurontin) and baclofen (Lioresal) are also used for pain control. If pain control is still not achieved, phenytoin (Dilantin) may be used as adjunctive therapy.

Surgical Management

If pharmacologic management fails to relieve pain, a number of surgical options are available. Although these procedures may relieve facial pain for a few years, recurrence and complication rates are high (Hickey, 2014). The choice of procedure depends on the patient's preference, health status, and location of the surgical lesion.

Microvascular Decompression of the Trigeminal Nerve

An intracranial approach is used to relieve the contact between the cerebral vessel and the trigeminal nerve root entry. With the aid of an operating microscope, the artery loop is lifted from the nerve to relieve the pressure, and a small prosthetic device such as Teflon is inserted between the artery and the nerve to prevent recurrence of impingement on the nerve. The postoperative management is the same as for other intracranial surgeries (see Chapter 63).

Radiofrequency Thermal Coagulation

Percutaneous radiofrequency produces a thermal lesion on the trigeminal nerve. Although immediate pain relief is experienced, dysesthesia of the face and loss of the corneal reflex may occur. Use of stereotactic MRI for identification of the trigeminal nerve followed by gamma knife radiosurgery is being used at some medical centres.

Percutaneous Balloon Microcompression

Percutaneous balloon microcompression disrupts large myelinated fibres in all three branches of the trigeminal nerve. After its placement, the balloon is filled with a contrast material for fluoroscopic identification. The balloon compresses the nerve root for 1 minute and provides microvascular decompression.

Nursing Management

Preventing Pain

Preoperative management of a patient with trigeminal neuralgia occurs mostly on an outpatient basis and includes recognizing factors that may aggravate excruciating facial pain, such as food that is too hot or too cold or jarring of the patient's bed or chair. Even washing the face, combing the hair, or brushing the teeth may produce acute pain. The nurse can assist the patient in preventing or reducing this pain by providing instructions about preventive strategies. Providing cotton pads and room temperature water for washing the face, instructing the patient to rinse with mouthwash after eating if tooth brushing causes pain, and performing personal hygiene during pain-free intervals are all effective strategies. The patient is instructed to take food and fluids at room temperature, to chew on the unaffected side, and to ingest soft foods. The nurse recognizes that anxiety, depression, and insomnia often accompany chronic painful conditions and uses appropriate interventions and referrals. See Chapter 16 for management of patients with chronic pain.

Providing Postoperative Care

Postoperative neurologic assessments are conducted to evaluate the patient for facial motor and sensory deficits in each of the three branches of the trigeminal nerve. If the surgery results in sensory deficits to the affected side of the face, the patient is instructed not to rub the eye because the pain of a resulting injury will not be detected. The eye is assessed for irritation or redness. Artificial tears may be prescribed to prevent dryness in the affected eye. The patient is cautioned not to chew on the affected side until numbness has diminished. The patient is observed carefully for any difficulty in eating or swallowing foods of different consistencies.

Bell's Palsy

Bell's palsy (facial paralysis) is caused by unilateral inflammation of the seventh cranial nerve, which results in weakness or paralysis of the facial muscles on the affected side (Fig. 66-5). Although the cause is unknown, theories about causes include vascular ischemia, viral disease (herpes simplex, herpes zoster), autoimmune disease, or a combination of all of these factors. Most adults with Bell's palsy are younger than 45 years of age (Greco, Gallo, Fusconi, et al., 2012).

Bell's palsy may be a type of pressure paralysis. The inflamed, edematous nerve becomes compressed to the point of damage, or its blood supply is occluded, producing ischemic necrosis of the nerve. The face is distorted from paralysis of the facial muscles; increased lacrimation (tearing); and painful sensations in the face, behind the ear, and in the eye. The patient may experience speech difficulties and may be unable to eat on the affected side because of weakness or paralysis of the facial muscles. Most patients recover completely, and Bell's palsy rarely recurs (Greco et al., 2012).

Medical Management

The objectives of treatment are to maintain the muscle tone of the face and to prevent or minimize denervation. The patient should be reassured that no stroke has occurred and that spontaneous recovery occurs within 3 to 5 weeks in most patients.

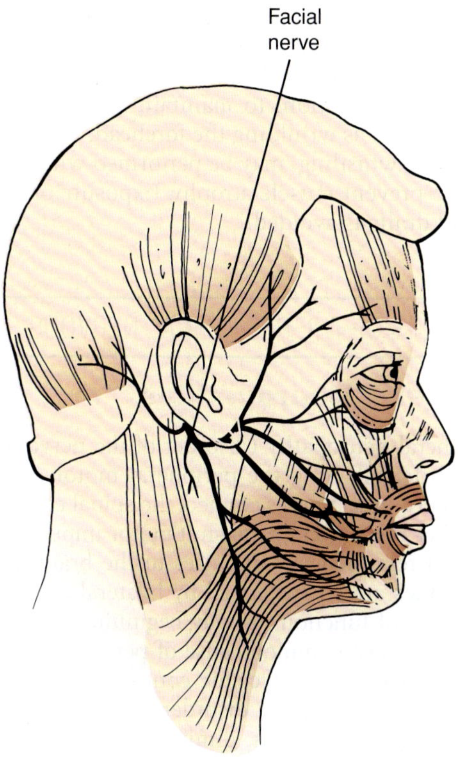

FIGURE 66-5. Distribution of the facial nerve.

Corticosteroid therapy (prednisone) may be prescribed to reduce inflammation and edema; this reduces vascular compression and permits restoration of blood circulation to the nerve. Early administration of corticosteroid therapy appears to diminish the severity of the disease, relieve the pain, and prevent or minimize denervation (Gagyor, Madhok, Daly, et al., 2016). Facial pain is controlled with analgesic agents. Heat may be applied to the involved side of the face to promote comfort and blood flow through the muscles. Electrical stimulation may be applied to the face to prevent muscle atrophy. Although most patients recover with conservative treatment, surgical exploration of the facial nerve may be indicated if a tumour is suspected, for surgical decompression of the facial nerve, or for surgical treatment of a paralyzed face.

Nursing Management

While the paralysis lasts, nursing care involves protection of the eye from injury. Frequently, the eye does not close completely and the blink reflex is diminished, so the eye is vulnerable to injury from dust and foreign particles. Corneal irritation and ulceration may occur. Distortion of the lower lid alters the proper drainage of tears. To prevent injury, the eye should be covered with a protective shield at night. The eye patch may abrade the cornea, however, because there is some difficulty in keeping the partially paralyzed eyelids closed. Moisturizing eye drops during the day and eye ointment at bedtime may help prevent injury (Hickey, 2014). The patient can be taught to close the paralyzed eyelid manually before going to sleep. Wraparound sunglasses or goggles may be worn during the day to decrease normal evaporation from the eye.

After the sensitivity of the nerve to touch decreases and the patient can tolerate touching the face, the nurse can suggest massaging the face several times daily, using a gentle upward motion, to maintain muscle tone. Facial exercises, such as wrinkling the forehead, blowing out the cheeks, and whistling, may be performed with the aid of a mirror to prevent muscle atrophy. Exposure of the face to cold and drafts is avoided.

DISORDERS OF THE PERIPHERAL NERVOUS SYSTEM

Peripheral Neuropathies

A peripheral **neuropathy** (disorder of the nervous system) is a disorder affecting the peripheral motor and sensory nerves. Peripheral nerves connect the spinal cord and brain to all other organs. They transmit motor impulses from the brain and relay sensory impulses to the brain. Peripheral neuropathies are characterized by bilateral and symmetric disturbance of function, usually beginning in the feet and hands. The most common cause of peripheral neuropathy is diabetes with poor glycemic control. The major symptoms of peripheral nerve disorders are loss of sensation, muscle atrophy, weakness, diminished reflexes, pain, and paresthesia (numbness, tingling) of the extremities.

Peripheral nerve disorders are diagnosed by history, physical examination, and electrodiagnostic studies such as EEG. The diagnosis of peripheral neuropathy in the geriatric population is challenging because many symptoms, such as decreased reflexes, can be associated with the normal aging process (Eliopoulos, 2018).

No specific treatment exists for peripheral neuropathy. Elimination or control of the cause may slow progression. Patients with peripheral neuropathy are at risk for falls, thermal injuries, and skin breakdown. The plan of care includes inspection of the lower extremities for skin breakdown. Assistive devices such as a walker or cane may decrease the risk of falls. Bath water temperature is checked to avoid thermal injury. Footwear should be accurately sized. Driving may be limited or eliminated, thereby disrupting the patient's sense of independence.

Mononeuropathy

Mononeuropathy is limited to a single peripheral nerve and its branches. It arises when the trunk of the nerve is compressed or entrapped (as in carpal tunnel syndrome), traumatized (as when bruised by a blow), overstretched (as in joint dislocation), punctured by a needle used to inject a drug or damaged by the drugs thus injected, or inflamed because an adjacent infectious process extends to the nerve trunk. Mononeuropathy is frequently seen in patients with diabetes.

Pain is seldom a major symptom of mononeuropathy when the condition is due to trauma, but in patients with complicating inflammatory conditions such as arthritis, pain is prominent. Pain is increased with all body movements that tend to stretch, strain, or cause pressure on the injured nerve and sudden jarring of the body (e.g., from coughing or sneezing). The skin in the areas supplied by nerves that are injured or diseased may become reddened and glossy, the subcutaneous tissue may become edematous, and the nails and hair in this area are altered. Chemical injuries to a nerve trunk, such as those caused by drugs injected into or near it, are often permanent.

The objective of treatment of mononeuropathy is to remove the cause, if possible (e.g., freeing the compressed nerve). Local corticosteroid injections may reduce inflammation and the pressure on the nerve. Aspirin or codeine may be used to relieve pain.

Nursing care involves protection of the affected limb or area from injury, as well as appropriate patient teaching about mononeuropathy and its treatment.

Critical Thinking Exercises

1 A 19-year-old patient is admitted with suspected meningitis. Describe the pathophysiology of meningitis. What are the signs of meningeal irritation the nurse should watch for and how are they tested? What is the priority nursing diagnosis in the patient with meningitis? What history and physical findings are common in the patient with meningitis?

2 Identify the priorities, approach, and techniques you would use to provide care to the patients in your assignment on an intermediate neuroscience unit. Two of the patients have a diagnosis of myasthenia gravis, one is intubated and on a ventilator, one patient has a diagnosis of GBS and the other has meningitis. What tasks can you delegate and to whom?

3 A 35-year-old woman is newly diagnosed with Bell's palsy. Identify her treatment options. Describe the evidence base for the options that you have identified and the criteria used to evaluate the strength of the evidence for her various treatment options.

REFERENCES AND SELECTED READINGS

Books

American Association of Neuroscience Nurses (AANN). (2013). *Care of the patient with myasthenia gravis: AANN patient guideline series*. Glenview, IL: Author.

Bader, M., Littlejohns, L. R., & Olson, D. (2016). *AANN core curriculum for neuroscience nursing* (6th ed.). Chicago, IL: American Association of Neuroscience Nurses.

Comerford, K. C. (2015). *Nursing 2015 drug handbook*. Philadelphia, PA: Wolters Kluwer.

Eliopoulos, C. (2018). *Gerontological nursing* (9th ed.). Philadelphia, PA: Lippincott Williams & Wilkins.

Grossman, S. C., & Porth, C. M. (2014). *Pathophysiology: Concepts of altered health states* (9th ed.) Philadelphia, PA: Lippincott Williams & Wilkins.

Hickey, J. V. (2014). *The clinical practice of neurological & neurosurgical nursing* (7th ed.). Philadelphia, PA: Lippincott Williams & Wilkins.

Lemon, C. A., & Clarke, R. (2014). Nursing management: Chronic neurological problems. In S. L. Lewis, S. R. Derksen, M. M. Heitkemper, et al. (Eds.). *Medical surgical nursing in Canada* (3rd Can. ed.). Toronto, ON: Elsevier Canada.

Public Health Agency of Canada. (2012). Creutzfeldt-Jacob disease. Ottawa, ON: Author. Retrieved from http://www.phac-aspc.gc.ca/hcai-iamss/cjd-mcj/cjd-eng.php

Public Health Agency of Canada. (2014). Creutzfeldt-Jacob disease, CJD Surveillance System. Ottawa: Author, Retrieved from http://www.phac-aspc.gc.ca/hcai-iamss/cjd-mcj/cjdss-ssmcj/stats-eng.php

Stephen, T. C., Skillen, D. L., Day, R. A., et al. (2012). *Canadian Jensen's nursing health assessment: A best practice approach* (1st ed.). Philadelphia, PA: Wolters Kluwer Health/Lippincott Williams & Wilkins.

Weber, J., & Kelley, J. (2014). *Health assessment in nursing* (5th ed.). Philadelphia, PA: Lippincott Williams & Wilkins.

Journals and Electronic Documents

Cherin, P., Marie, I., Michallet, M., et al. (2016). Management of adverse events in the treatment of patients with immunoglobulin therapy: A review of evidence. *Autoimmunity Reviews*, *15*(1), 71–81.

Digre, K., & Brennan, K. (2012). Shedding light on photophobia. *Journal of Neuroophthalmology*, *32*(1), 68–81.

Filipi, M., Beavin, J., Brillante, R., et al. (2014). Nurses' perspective on approaches to limit flu-like symptoms during interferon therapy for multiple sclerosis. *International Journal of MS Care*, *16*(1), 55–60.

Gagyor, I., Madhok, V., Daly, F., et al. (2016). Corticosteroids for Bell's palsy (idiopathic facial paralysis). *Cochrane Database of Systematic Reviews*, *7*, CN-01208827.

Gagyor, I., Madhok, V., Daly, F., et al. (2016). Corticosteroids for Bell's palsy (idiopathic facial paralysis). *Cochrane Database of Systematic Reviews*, *7*, CN-01208827.

Lublin, F. D., & Reingold, S. C. (1996). Defining the clinical course of multiple sclerosis: Results of an international survey. National Multiple Sclerosis Society (USA) Advisory Committee on Clinical Trials of New Agents in Multiple Sclerosis. *Neurology*, *46*(4), 907–911.

Mcilvoy, L. (2014). Respiratory failure from a myasthenic crisis. *American Nurse Today*, *9*(9), 28.

McNair, N. (2013). Treatment of Guillain-Barré syndrome. *The Art and Science of Infusion Nursing*, *36*(6), 397–400.

Morrison, J. D., & Stuifbergen, A. K. (2016). Predictors of fatigue impact in persons with long-standing multiple sclerosis. *Journal of Neuroscience Nursing*, *48*(3), 143–150.

National Advisory Committee on Communicable Diseases. (2013). Update on the use of quadrivalent conjugate meningococcal vaccines. *Canada Communicable Disease Report CCDR 39*, ACS-1, 1–40. Public Health Agency of Canada. Retrieved from http://www.phac-aspc.gc.ca/publicat/ccdr-rmtc/13vol39/acs-dcc-1/index-eng.php

National Institute of Allergies and Infectious Diseases (NIAID). (2008). NIAID research on West Nile Virus. Retrieved from http://www.niaid.nih.gov/topics/westnile/Pages/default.aspx

National Institute of Neurological Disorders and Stroke (NINDS). (2016). Creutzfeldt-Jakob Disease Fact Sheet. Retrieved on October 3, 2016, from www.ninds.nih.gov/disorders/cjd/detail_cjd.htm.N

Newland, P., Jensen, M. P., Budhathoki, C., et al. (2015). Secondary health conditions in individuals with multiple sclerosis: A cross-sectional web-based survey analysis. *Journal of Neuroscience Nursing*, *47*(3), 124–130.

Riley, C., & Vargus, W. (2015). Multiple sclerosis in the elderly: Considerations in the geriatric population for diagnosis and management. *Current Geriatrics Reports*, *4*(2), 131–141.

Slazinski, T. (2013). Brain abscess. *Critical Care Nursing Clinics of North America*, *25*(3), 381–388.

Theroux, N., Phipps, M., Zimmerman, L., et al. (2013). Neurological complications associated with HIV and AIDS: Clinical implications for nursing. *Journal of Neuroscience Nursing*, *45*(1), 5–13.

Vacca, V. (2016). CJD: Understanding Creutzfeldt-Jakob disease. *Nursing*, *46*(3), 36–42; quiz 42–43.

Ward-Abel, N., Vernon, K., & Warner, R. (2014). An exciting era of treatments for relapsing-remitting multiple sclerosis. *British Journal of Neuroscience Nursing*, *10*(1), 21–28.

Winer, J. B. (2014). An update in Guillain-Barré syndrome. *Autoimmune Diseases*, *2014*, 793024.

Wu, G., & Alvarez, E. (2016). The immune-pathophysiology of MS. Retrieved on October 3, 2016, from www.ncbi.nlm.nih.gov

Resources

Guillain-Barré Syndrome Foundation International: http://gbs-cidp.org/
Multiple Sclerosis Society of Canada: http://mssociety.ca/en/
Myasthenia Gravis Foundation of America: http://www.myasthenia.org
The Neuropathy Association, Inc.: http://www.neuropathy.org

67 Management of Patients With Oncologic or Degenerative Disorders

Adapted by Ron Prince

Learning Objectives

On completion of this chapter, the learner will be able to:

1. Identify the pathophysiologic processes responsible for oncologic disorders.
2. Describe brain and spinal cord tumours: their classification, clinical manifestations, diagnosis, and medical and nursing management.
3. Use the nursing process as a framework for care of patients with cerebral metastases or inoperable brain tumours.
4. Identify the pathophysiologic processes responsible for various degenerative neurologic disorders.
5. Use the nursing process as a framework for care of patients with Parkinson's disease.
6. Identify resources for patients and families with oncologic and degenerative neurologic disorders.
7. Use the nursing process as a framework for care of patients following a cervical discectomy.

The occurrence of oncologic or degenerative disease processes in the neurologic system produces a unique set of nursing challenges. Oncologic disorders include brain and spinal cord tumours. Degenerative neurologic disorders include Parkinson's disease, Huntington's disease, Alzheimer's disease, amyotrophic lateral sclerosis (ALS), muscular dystrophies, and degenerative disc disease. Postpolio syndrome is thought to be degenerative in nature and is included in this chapter.

ONCOLOGIC DISORDERS OF THE BRAIN AND SPINAL CORD

Oncologic disorders of the brain and spinal cord include several types of neoplasms, each with its own biology, prognosis, and treatment options. Because of the unique anatomy and physiology of the central nervous system (CNS), this collection of neoplasms is challenging to diagnose and treat.

Primary Brain Tumours

A brain tumour is a localized intracranial lesion that occupies space within the skull. A tumour usually grows as a spherical mass, but it also can grow diffusely and infiltrate tissue. The effects of neoplasms are caused by the compression and infiltration of tissue as well as by cerebral edema. A variety of physiologic changes result, causing any or all of the following pathophysiologic events:

- Increased intracranial pressure (ICP)
- Cerebral edema
- Seizure activity
- Focal neurologic deficits
- Hydrocephalus
- Altered pituitary function

Primary brain tumours originate from cells and structures within the brain. Secondary, or metastatic, brain tumours develop from structures outside the brain and occur in 10% to 20% of patients with cancer (American Brain Tumor Association [ABTA], 2014). Primary brain tumours rarely metastasize outside the CNS. Metastatic lesions to the brain can occur from the lung, breast, lower gastrointestinal tract, pancreas, kidney, and skin (melanomas).

The cause of primary brain tumours is unknown. The only known risk factor is exposure to ionizing radiation. Both glial and meningeal neoplasms have been linked to irradiation of the cranium. The risk is 1% to 3% with a latency period of 10 to 20 years after exposure (American Association of Neuroscience Nurses [AANN], 2014a). Environmental risk factors, such as cell phone use, have been investigated, but results suggest that they are not associated with primary brain tumours. A history of any allergy has also been investigated and preliminary results suggest a decreased incidence of glioma, meningioma, and acoustic neuroma (Turner, Krewski, Armstrong, et al., 2013).

The incidence of brain tumours appears to have increased in the past few decades. Epidemiologic data, however, suggest that this is due more to aggressive and accurate diagnosis rather than to an actual rise in incidence. In Canada, it is estimated that 1,650 men and 1,200 women will develop brain cancer in 2013 (Canadian Cancer Society's Advisory Committee on Cancer Statistics, 2013). Secondary tumours or metastases to the brain from a systemic primary cancer are even more common than new cases of primary malignant brain and other nervous system tumours. The highest incidence of brain tumours in adults occurs in the fifth, sixth, and seventh decades. In adults, most brain tumours originate from glial cells (cells that make up the structure and support system of the brain and spinal cord) and are supratentorial (located above the cerebellum). Neoplastic lesions in the brain ultimately cause death by impairing vital functions, such as respiration, or by increasing ICP.

Types of Primary Brain Tumours

Brain tumours may be classified into several groups: those arising from the coverings of the brain the dura (e.g., meningiomas), those developing in or on the cranial nerves (e.g., acoustic neuroma, schwannomas), those originating within brain tissue (e.g., glioma), and metastatic lesions originating elsewhere in the body. Tumours of the pituitary and pineal glands and of cerebral blood vessels are also types of brain tumours. Relevant clinical considerations include the location and the histologic character of the tumour. Tumours may be benign or malignant. A benign tumour, such as a meningioma or a colloid cyst, can occur in a vital area and can grow large enough to have serious effects (Hickey, 2014). See Chart 67-1 for the classification of brain tumours.

CHART 67-1

Classification of Brain Tumours in Adults

I. Intracerebral tumours
  A. Gliomas—Infiltrate any portion of the brain; most common type of brain tumour
    1. Astrocytomas (grades I and II)
    2. Glioblastoma multiforme (astrocytoma grades III and IV)
    3. Oligodendrocytoma (low and high grades)
    4. Ependymoma (grades I to IV)
    5. Medulloblastoma
II. Tumours arising from supporting structures
  A. Meningiomas
  B. Neuromas (acoustic neuroma, schwannoma)
  C. Pituitary adenomas
III. Developmental tumours
  A. Angiomas
  B. Dermoid, epidermoid, teroma, craniopharyngioma
IV. Metastatic lesions

Gliomas

Glial tumours, the most common type of intracerebral brain neoplasm, account for approximately half of brain tumours, and are divided into many categories (Lawler & Chiocca, 2013). Astrocytomas, which are the most common type of glioma, are graded on a scale from I to IV to indicate the degree of malignancy (American Brain Tumor Association [ABTA], 2014). For the first time, the World Health Organization (WHO) has introduced changes in the classification of CNS tumours; they are now including molecular parameters in addition to histology to classify many tumour entities, thus formulating a concept for how CNS tumour diagnoses, management and treatment should be structured in the molecular era (Louis, Perry, Reinfenberger, et al., 2016).

The grading scale looks at the following factors: cell mitosis, necrosis, cellular atypia, neovascularization, infiltration, and molecular genetics. Usually, these tumours

Glossary

bradykinesia: abnormally slow voluntary movements and speech
chorea: rapid, jerky, involuntary, purposeless movements of the extremities or facial muscles, including facial grimacing
dementia: broad term for a syndrome characterized by a general decline in higher brain functioning, such as reasoning, with a pattern of eventual decline in ability to perform even basic activities of daily living, such as toileting and eating
dyskinesia: impaired ability to execute voluntary movements
dysphonia: voice impairment or altered voice production
neurodegenerative: a disease, process, or condition leading to deterioration of cells or function of the nervous system
papilledema: edema of the optic nerve usually due to increased intracranial pressure (ICP)
paresthesia: numbness, tingling, or a "pins and needles" sensation
sciatica: pain and tenderness that radiates along the sciatic nerve that runs through the thigh and leg
spondylosis: degenerative changes occurring in a disc and adjacent vertebral bodies; can occur in the cervical or lumbar vertebrae

spread by infiltrating into the surrounding neural connective tissue and therefore cannot be totally removed without causing considerable damage to vital structures.

Oligodendroglial tumours represent 20% of gliomas and are categorized as low grade or high grade (anaplastic) (American Brain Tumour Association [ABTA], 2012a). The histologic distinction between astrocytomas and oligodendrogliomas is difficult to make, but important, because oligodendrogliomas are more sensitive than astrocytomas to chemotherapy (Lawler & Chiocca, 2013).

Meningiomas

Meningiomas, which represent 15% to 20% of all primary brain tumours, are common benign encapsulated tumours of arachnoid cells on the meninges (Ostrom et al., 2015). They are slow growing and occur most often in middle-aged adults (more often in women). Meningiomas most often occur in areas proximal to the venous sinuses. Manifestations depend on the area involved and are the result of compression rather than invasion of brain tissue. Standard treatment is surgery with complete removal or partial dissection. Although meningiomas are often thought to be benign tumours, they can be atypical and often have a high morbidity secondary to their location within the brain.

Acoustic Neuromas

An acoustic neuroma is a tumour of the eighth cranial nerve, the cranial nerve most responsible for hearing and balance. It usually arises just within the internal auditory meatus, where it frequently expands before filling the cerebellopontine recess. An acoustic neuroma may grow slowly and attain considerable size before it is correctly diagnosed. The patient usually experiences loss of hearing, tinnitus, and episodes of vertigo and staggering gait. As the tumour becomes larger, painful sensations of the face may occur on the same side, as a result of the tumour's compression of the fifth cranial nerve (American Brain Tumor Association [ABTA], 2014). Many acoustic neuromas are benign and can be managed conservatively. Many that continue to grow can be surgically removed and have a good prognosis (see Chapter 61). Some acoustic neuromas may be suitable for stereotactic radiotherapy rather than open craniotomy. Stereotactic radiotherapy is discussed later in this chapter.

Pituitary Adenomas

Pituitary tumours represent about 9% to 12% of all brain tumours, making them the third most common primary brain tumour (ABTA, 2012b). They cause symptoms as a result of pressure on adjacent structures (the pituitary gland or stalk) or hormonal changes (hyperfunction or hypofunction of the pituitary). The pituitary gland, also called the *hypophysis*, is a relatively small gland located in the sella turcica. It is attached to the hypothalamus by a short stalk (hypophyseal stalk) and is divided into two lobes: the anterior (adenohypophysis) and the posterior (neurohypophysis).

Pressure Effects of Pituitary Adenomas

Pressure from a pituitary adenoma may be exerted on the optic nerves, optic chiasm, or optic tracts or on the hypothalamus or the third ventricle if the tumour invades the cavernous sinuses or expands into the sphenoid bone. These pressure effects produce headache, visual dysfunction, hypothalamic disorders (disorders of sleep, appetite, temperature, and emotions), increased ICP, and enlargement and erosion of the sella turcica.

Hormonal Effects of Pituitary Adenomas

Functioning pituitary tumours can produce one or more hormones normally produced by the anterior pituitary. There are prolactin-secreting pituitary adenomas (prolactinomas), growth hormone–secreting pituitary adenomas that produce acromegaly in adults, and adrenocorticotropic hormone (ACTH)–producing pituitary adenomas that result in Cushing's disease (Melmed, 2016). Adenomas that secrete thyroid-stimulating hormone or follicle-stimulating hormone and luteinizing hormone occur infrequently, whereas adenomas that produce both growth hormone and prolactin are relatively common.

The female patient whose pituitary gland is secreting excessive quantities of prolactin presents with amenorrhea or galactorrhea (excessive or spontaneous flow of milk). Male patients with prolactinomas may present with impotence and hypogonadism. Acromegaly, caused by excess growth hormone, produces enlargement of the hands and feet, distortion of the facial features, and pressure on peripheral nerves (entrapment syndromes). The clinical features of Cushing's disease, a condition associated with prolonged overproduction of cortisol, occur with excessive production of ACTH. Manifestations include a form of obesity with redistribution of fat to the facial, supraclavicular, and abdominal areas; hypertension; purple striae and ecchymoses; osteoporosis; elevated blood glucose levels; and emotional disorders. Endocrine disorders resulting from these tumours are discussed in Chapter 43.

Gerontologic Considerations

The most frequent tumour types in the elderly are glioblastoma multiforme, anaplastic astrocytoma, and cerebral metastases from other sites (Perkins & Liu, 2016). The incidence of primary brain tumours and the likelihood of malignancy increases with age. Intracranial tumours can produce personality changes, confusion, speech dysfunction, or disturbances of gait. In elderly patients, early signs and symptoms of intracranial tumours can be easily overlooked or incorrectly attributed to cognitive and neurologic changes associated with normal aging. Neurologic signs and symptoms in the elderly must be carefully evaluated, because 10% of brain metastases occur in patients with no history of prior cancer. Researchers are investigating patterns of care and clinical outcomes of elderly patients with primary brain tumours (Gallego Perez-Larraya & Delattre, 2014).

Clinical Manifestations

Brain tumours can produce both focal or generalized neurologic signs and symptoms. Generalized symptoms reflect increased ICP, and the most common focal or specific signs and symptoms result from tumours that interfere with functions in specific brain regions. Figure 67-1 indicates common tumour sites in the brain.

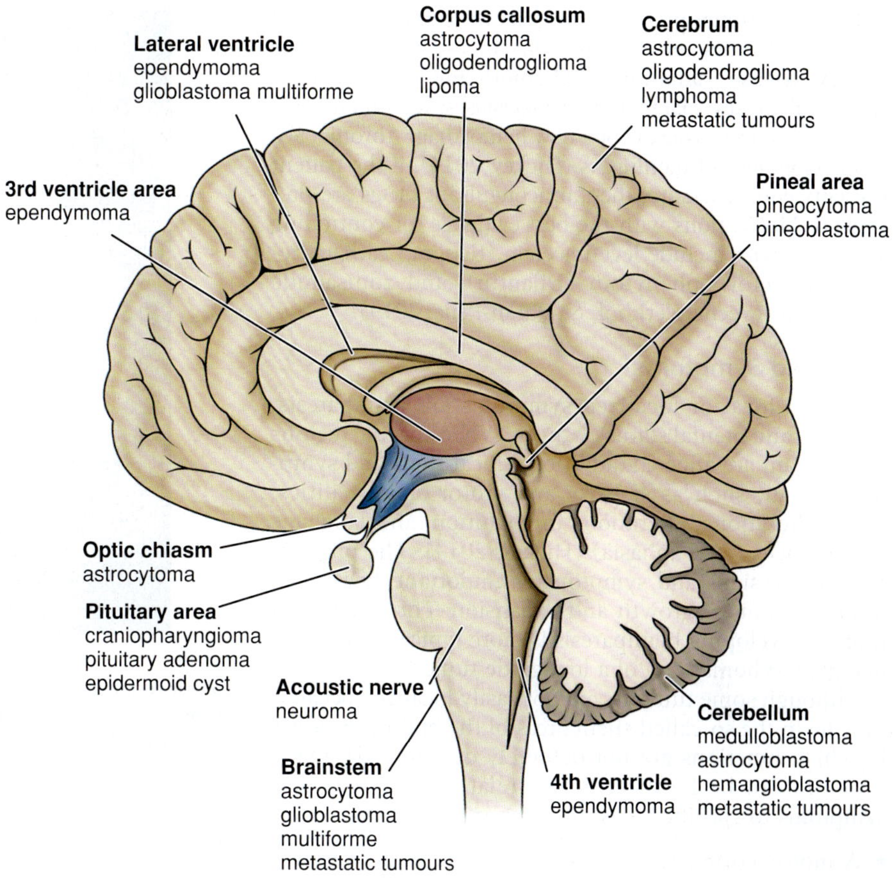

FIGURE 67-1. Common brain tumour sites.

Increased Intracranial Pressure

As discussed in Chapter 62, the skull is a rigid compartment containing essential noncompressible contents: brain matter, intravascular blood, and cerebrospinal fluid (CSF). According to the modified Monro–Kellie hypothesis, if any one of these skull components increases in volume, ICP increases unless one of the other components decreases in volume. Consequently, any change in volume occupied by the brain (as occurs with disorders such as brain tumour or cerebral edema) produces signs and symptoms of increased ICP.

Symptoms of increased ICP result from a gradual compression of the brain by the enlarging tumour. The effect is a disruption of the equilibrium that exists between the brain, the CSF, and the cerebral blood. As the tumour grows, compensatory adjustments may occur through compression of intracranial veins, reduction of CSF volume (by increased absorption or decreased production), a modest decrease in cerebral blood flow, or reduction of intracellular and extracellular brain tissue mass. When these compensatory mechanisms fail, the patient develops signs and symptoms of increased ICP, most often including headache, nausea with or without vomiting, and **papilledema** (edema of the optic disc) (Hickey, 2014). Personality changes and a variety of focal deficits, including motor, sensory, and cranial nerve dysfunction, are common.

Headache

Headache, although not always present, is most common in the early morning and is made worse by coughing, straining, or sudden movement. It is thought to be caused by the tumour's invading, compressing, or distorting the pain-sensitive structures or by edema that accompanies the tumour. Headaches are usually described as deep or expanding or as dull but unrelenting. Frontal tumours usually produce a bilateral frontal headache; pituitary gland tumours produce pain radiating between the two temples (bitemporal); in cerebellar tumours, the headache may be located in the suboccipital region at the back of the head.

Vomiting

Vomiting, seldom related to food intake, is usually the result of irritation of the vagal centres in the medulla which is often caused by obstructive hydrocephalus. A common presentation for patients with brain tumours is forceful vomiting, also described as projectile vomiting.

Visual Disturbances

Papilledema is present in 70% to 75% of patients and is associated with visual disturbances such as decreased visual acuity, diplopia (double vision), and visual field deficits (Rigi, Almarzbuqi, Morgan, et al., 2015).

Seizures

Seizures are common, occurring in 60% of patients with brain tumours either initially or throughout their disease process (AANN, 2014a). Seizures may be focal or generalized. Tumours of the frontal, parietal, and temporal lobes carry the greatest risk of seizures; seizures are unusual with brain stem or cerebellar tumours. See Chapter 66 for discussion about seizures and related management.

If not the initial presentation, seizures can be a result of metabolic factors (electrolyte imbalances, liver failure or kidney disease, radiation or chemotherapy side effects), structural causes (parenchymal metastases, leptomeningeal disease, dural metastases) or a new hemorrhage, thrombosis, or development of meningitis (Hickey, 2014). If the patient presents with a seizure, then anticonvulsant drugs are prescribed. Medications with the best evidence for controlling seizure activity include levetiracetam (Keppra), carbamazepine (Tegretol), phenytoin (Dilantin), and zonisamide (Zonegran) (Vecht, Kerkhof, & Duran-Pena, 2014).

Localized Symptoms

Common focal or localized symptoms are hemiparesis, seizures, and mental status changes. When specific regions of the brain are affected, additional local signs and symptoms occur, such as sensory and motor abnormalities, visual alterations, alterations in cognition, and language disturbances (e.g., aphasia) (Hickey, 2014). The progression of the signs and symptoms is important, because it indicates tumour growth and expansion. For example, a rapidly developing hemiparesis is more typical of a highly malignant glioma than of a low-grade tumour.

Although some tumours are not easily localized because they lie in the so-called silent areas of the brain (i.e., areas in which functions are not definitely determined), many tumours can be localized by correlating the signs and symptoms to specific areas in the brain, as follows:

- A motor cortex tumour produces seizure like movements localized on one side of the body, called jacksonian seizures.
- An occipital lobe tumour produces visual manifestations: Contralateral homonymous hemianopsia (visual loss in half of the visual field on the opposite side of the tumour) and visual hallucinations.
- A cerebellar tumour causes dizziness, an ataxic or staggering gait with a tendency to fall toward the side of the lesion, marked muscle incoordination, and nystagmus (involuntary rhythmic eye movements), usually in the horizontal direction.
- A frontal lobe tumour frequently produces personality disorders, changes in emotional state and behaviour, and an apathetic mental attitude. The patient often becomes extremely untidy and careless and may use obscene language.
- A cerebellopontine angle tumour usually originates in the sheath of the acoustic nerve and gives rise to a characteristic sequence of symptoms. Tinnitus and vertigo appear first, soon followed by progressive nerve deafness (eighth cranial nerve dysfunction). Numbness and tingling of the face and tongue occur (due to involvement of the fifth cranial nerve). Later, weakness or paralysis of the face develops (seventh cranial nerve involvement). Finally, because the enlarging tumour presses on the cerebellum, abnormalities in motor function may be present. Nausea and vomiting are also common findings in patients with these kinds of tumours.

Assessment and Diagnostic Findings

The history of the illness and the manner and time frame in which the symptoms evolved are key components in the diagnosis of brain tumours. A neurologic examination indicates the areas of the CNS that are involved. To assist in the precise localization of the lesion, a battery of tests is performed. Computed tomography (CT) scans, enhanced by a contrast agent, can give specific information concerning the number, size, and density of the lesions and the extent of secondary cerebral edema. CT scans can provide information about the ventricular system and whether the lesions are causing obstructive hydrocephalus. A magnetic resonance imaging (MRI) scan is the most helpful diagnostic tool for detecting brain tumours, particularly smaller lesions, and tumours in the brain stem and pituitary regions, where bone is thick (Fig. 67-2). MRI is also useful in monitoring response to treatment.

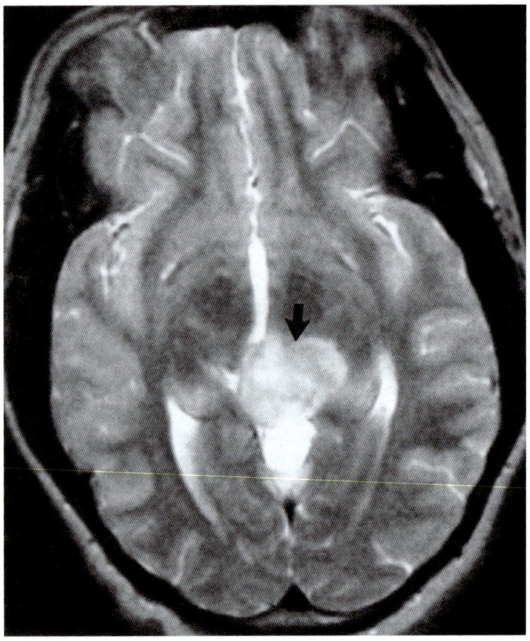

FIGURE 67-2. Magnetic resonance image of the brain shows an exophytic tectal glioma (*arrow*) in this patient with neurofibromatosis type 1. (From Brant, W. E., & Helms, C. A. [2006]. *Fundamentals of diagnostic radiology* [3rd ed.]. Philadelphia, PA: Lippincott Williams & Wilkins.)

Computer-assisted stereotactic (three-dimensional) biopsy is used to diagnose deep-seated brain tumours and to provide a basis for treatment and prognosis. Stereotactic approaches involve the use of a three-dimensional frame that allows very precise localization of the tumour; a stereotactic frame and multiple imaging studies (x-rays, CT scans, or MRIs) are used to localize the tumour and verify its position (see Fig. 67-3). Brain-mapping technology helps determine the proximity of diseased areas of the brain to structures essential for normal brain function.

Positron emission tomography (PET) is used to supplement MRI or CT scanning in centres where it is increasingly available. Newer PET scans are being used concurrently with CT scans (hybrid scans) to produce a fused image of the PET and CT scan. On PET scans, low-grade tumours are associated with hypometabolism and high-grade tumours show hypermetabolism. This information can be useful in making treatment decisions (ABTA, 2012). Cerebral angiography allows for the visualization of cerebral blood vessels and measurement of blood flow into the brain and tumours (ABTA, 2012).

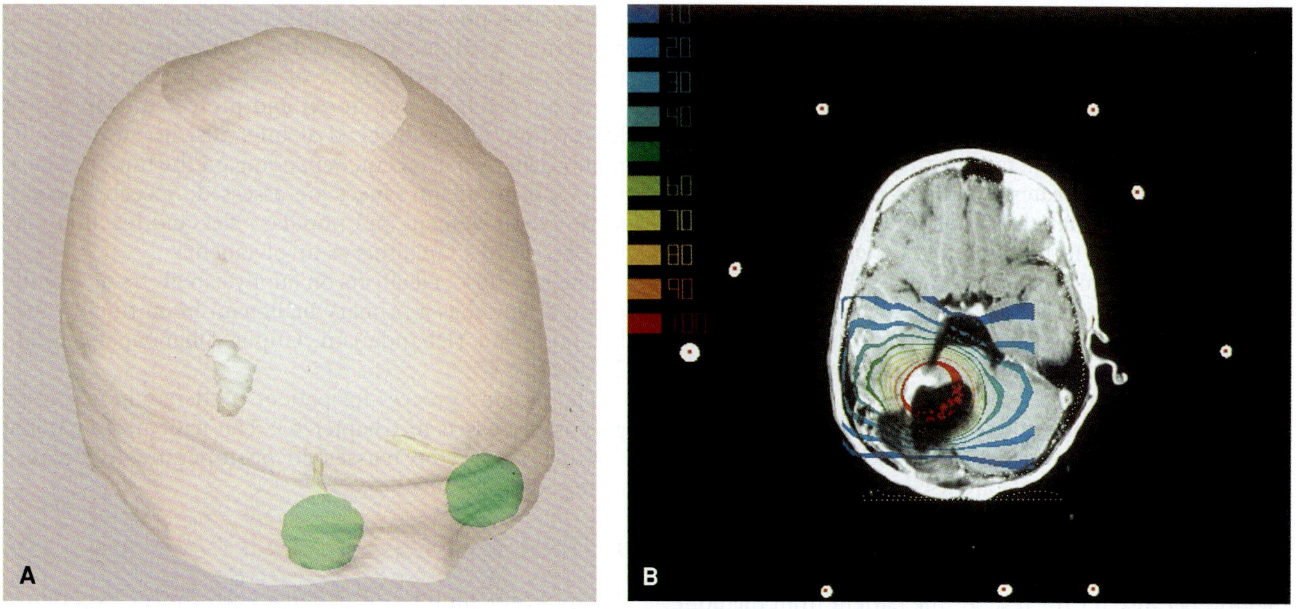

FIGURE 67-3. **A.** Using stereotactic or "brain-mapping" guided approach, a three-dimensional computer image fuses the computed tomography image and magnetic resonance image to pinpoint the exact location of the brain tumour. This low-grade astrocytoma is localized adjacent to the brain stem, is nonoperable, and is treated with radiation. Note the optic chiasm and optic nerves. **B.** Computerized image of the prescribed radiation dose.

An electroencephalogram (EEG) can detect an abnormal brain wave in regions occupied by tumour; it is used to evaluate temporal lobe seizures and to assist in ruling out other disorders. Cytologic studies of the CSF may be performed to detect malignant cells, because CNS tumours can shed cells into the CSF.

Medical Management

A variety of medical management approaches, including surgery, chemotherapy, and external-beam radiation therapy, are used alone or in combination (AANN, 2014a).

Secreting tumours may be treated with medications that suppress hormones. Nonfunctioning tumours may have no effect on pituitary function or may suppress hormone production and release. Hormone replacement may be necessary for these patients to restore normal endocrine function.

Surgical Management

The objective of surgical management is to remove as much tumour as possible without increasing the neurologic deficit (paralysis, blindness), or to relieve symptoms by partial removal (decompression). Surgery also provides tissue to establish a definitive diagnosis. A variety of surgical approaches may be used; the specific approach depends on the type of tumour, its location, and its accessibility. Conventional surgical approaches require a craniotomy (incision into the skull). See Chapter 63 for a discussion of care of the patient who has undergone a craniotomy. This approach is used in patients with meningiomas, acoustic neuromas, cystic astrocytomas of the cerebellum, colloid cysts of the third ventricle, congenital tumours such as dermoid cyst, and some of the granulomas. With improved imaging techniques and the availability of the operating microscope and microsurgical instrumentation, even large tumours can be removed through a relatively small craniotomy. For patients with malignant glioma, complete removal of the tumour and cure are not possible, but the rationale for resection includes relief of ICP, removal of any necrotic tissue, and reduction in the bulk of the tumour, which theoretically leaves behind fewer cells to become resistant to radiation or chemotherapy. Most pituitary adenomas are treated by transsphenoidal microsurgical removal (see Chapter 63), and the remainder of tumours that cannot be removed completely are treated by radiation (Hickey, 2014).

Radiation Therapy

Radiation therapy—the cornerstone of treatment for many brain tumours—decreases the incidence of recurrence of incompletely resected tumours (AANN, 2014a). Gamma radiation is delivered via an external beam to the tumour in multiple fractions. Brachytherapy (the surgical implantation of radiation sources to deliver high doses at a short distance) is an option for some types of tumours depending on their location. It is usually used as an adjunct to conventional radiation therapy or as a rescue measure for recurrent disease. Radioisotopes such as iodine 131 (^{131}I) are used to minimize effects on surrounding brain tissue.

Stereotactic procedures may be performed using a linear accelerator or gamma knife to perform radiosurgery (Hickey, 2014). These procedures allow treatment of deep, inaccessible tumours, often in a single session. Precise localization of the tumour is accomplished by the stereotactic approach and by minute measurements and precise positioning of the patient. Multiple narrow beams then deliver a very high dose of radiation. An advantage of this method is that no surgical incision is needed. Disadvantages include the lag time between treatment and the desired result as well as the potential for developing radiation necrosis (AANN, 2014a).

Chemotherapy

Chemotherapy may be used in conjunction with radiation therapy, or as the sole therapy, with the goal of increasing survival time. The greatest challenge in chemotherapy of brain tumours is that the blood–brain barrier prevents drugs from getting to the tumour in effective doses without causing systemic toxicity (AANN, 2014a).

Malignant glioma is usually treated with 6 weeks of oral temozolomide (Temodar) during radiation therapy, followed by 6 to 12 months of oral temozolomide. Low-grade gliomas may be treated with 6 months of oral temozolomide alone. Temozolomide is the first oral chemotherapy that crosses the blood–brain barrier (Hickey, 2014). Several other chemotherapy agents are used alone or in combination depending on the type of tumour (see Chapter 68).

Autologous bone marrow transplantation is used in some patients who will receive chemotherapy or radiation therapy, because it can "rescue" the patient from the bone marrow toxicity associated with high doses of chemotherapy and radiation. A fraction of the patient's bone marrow is aspirated, usually from the iliac crest, and stored. The patient receives large doses of chemotherapy or radiation therapy to destroy large numbers of malignant cells. The marrow is then reinfused intravenously after treatment is completed. See Chapter 54 for discussion of bone marrow transplant.

Pharmacologic Therapy

Corticosteroids are useful in relieving headache and alterations in level of consciousness. Corticosteroids such as dexamethasone (Decadron) are thought to reduce inflammation and edema around tumours (AANN, 2014a). Other medications used include osmotic diuretics (e.g., mannitol [Osmitrol] and hypertonic saline) to decrease the fluid content of the brain, which leads to a decrease in ICP. Anticonvulsant medications are used to treat and control seizures (Vecht et al., 2014). Venous thromboembolic events, such as deep vein thrombosis and pulmonary embolism, occur in about 15% of patients and are associated with significant morbidity. Patients receiving anticoagulant agents must be closely monitored because of the risk of CNS hemorrhage (Farge, 2013).

Nursing Management

The patient with a brain tumour may be at increased risk for aspiration as a result of cranial nerve dysfunction. Preoperatively, the gag reflex and ability to swallow are evaluated. In patients with diminished gag response, care includes teaching the patient to direct food and fluids toward the unaffected side, having the patient sit upright to eat, offering a semisoft diet, and having suction readily available. The effects of increased ICP caused by the tumour mass are reviewed in Chapter 63. The nurse performs neurologic checks, monitors vital signs, maintains a neurologic flow chart, spaces nursing interventions to prevent rapid increase in ICP, and reorients the patient when necessary to person, time, and place. Patients with changes in cognition caused by their lesion require frequent reorientation and the use of orienting devices (e.g., personal possessions, photographs, lists, clock), supervision of and assistance with self-care, and ongoing monitoring and intervention for prevention of injury. Patients with seizures are carefully monitored and protected from injury. Motor function is checked at intervals, because specific motor deficits may occur, depending on the tumour's location. Sensory disturbances are assessed. Speech is evaluated. Eye movement and pupillary size and reaction may be affected by cranial nerve involvement.

The psychosocial effects on family caregivers of a family member who has a primary malignant brain tumour may be significant (Dhandapani, Gupta, Dhandapani, et al., 2015).

The nursing process for patients undergoing neurosurgery is discussed in Chapter 63. The patient's functional abilities should be reassessed postoperatively, because changes can occur.

Cerebral Metastases

A significant number of patients with cancer experience neurologic deficits caused by metastasis to the brain. Although metastatic lesions to the brain are the most common intracerebral tumour, their exact incidence is unknown (Ostrom et al., 2015). This high rate of occurrence is clinically important as more patients with all forms of cancer live longer because of improved therapies to treat their original cancer source. Neurologic signs and symptoms include headache, gait disturbances, visual impairment, personality changes, altered mentation (memory loss and confusion), focal weakness, paralysis, aphasia, and seizures. These signs and symptoms can be devastating to both patient and family. Metastases to the CSF and meninges, known as leptomeningeal metastases, can produce symptoms of headache and isolated cranial nerve deficits.

Medical Management

The treatment of metastatic nervous system cancer is palliative and involves eliminating or reducing serious symptoms. Even when palliation is the goal, distressing signs and symptoms can be relieved, thereby improving the quality of life for both patient and family. Patients with intracerebral metastases who are not treated have a steady downhill course with a limited survival time. The therapeutic options include whole brain radiation therapy (the foundation of treatment) for multiple metastases or stereotactic radiosurgery for up to three sites of metastases. Surgery may be considered for a single symptomatic metastasis. Systemic chemotherapy directed at the primary cancer may be ineffective in crossing the blood–brain barrier, but chemotherapy that crosses this barrier may be added. Intrathecal chemotherapy, with direct injection of chemotherapy agents into the CSF of the brain or spinal canal, may be useful in persons with leptomeningeal metastases (Lukas, Buerki, & Mrugula, 2016). Some combination of these treatments is usually the optimal method.

Pain can be a significant problem and is managed by means of a stepped progression in the doses and type of analgesic agents needed for relief. If the patient has severe pain, morphine can be infused into the epidural or subarachnoid space through a spinal needle and a catheter placed as near as possible to the spinal segment where the pain is projected. Small doses of morphine are given at prescribed intervals.

Nursing Process

The Patient With Nervous System Metastases or Primary Brain Tumour

Assessment

The nursing assessment includes a baseline neurologic examination and focuses on how the patient is functioning, moving, and walking; adapting to weakness or paralysis and to loss of vision and speech; and dealing with seizures. Assessment addresses symptoms that cause distress to the patient and affect the quality of life, including pain, respiratory problems, bowel and bladder disorders, sleep disturbances, and impairment of skin integrity, fluid balance, and temperature regulation (Hickey, 2014). Tumour invasion, compression, or obstruction may cause these disorders.

Nutritional status is assessed, because cachexia (weak and emaciated condition) is common in patients with metastases. The nurse explores changes associated with poor nutritional status (anorexia, pain, weight loss, altered metabolism, muscle weakness, malabsorption, and diarrhea) and asks the patient about altered taste sensations that may be secondary to dysphagia, weakness, and depression and about distortions and impaired sense of smell (anosmia).

The nurse takes a dietary history to assess food intake, intolerance, and preferences. Calculation of body mass index can confirm the loss of subcutaneous fat and lean body mass (see Chapter 5). Biochemical measurements are reviewed to assess the degree of malnutrition, impaired cellular immunity, and electrolyte balance. A dietitian assists in determining the caloric needs of the patient.

The nurse works with other members of the health care team to assess the impact of the illness on the family in terms of home care, altered relationships, financial problems, time pressures, and family problems. This information is important in helping family members cope with the diagnosis and the changes associated with it.

Nursing Priorities

Based on the assessment data, the patient's major nursing priorities may include the following:

- Self-care deficit (feeding, bathing, and toileting) and decreased cognitive abilities
- Nutrition, less than body requirements
- Anxiety and fear of dying
- Anticipatory grief and increased need for family support due to the burdens imposed by the care of the person with a terminal illness

Other nursing priorities of the patient with cerebral metastases may include acute pain related to tumour compression; impaired gas exchange related to dyspnea; constipation related to decreased fluid and dietary intake and medications; impaired urinary elimination related to reduced fluid intake, vomiting, and side effects of medications; sleep pattern disturbances related to discomfort and fear of dying; impairment of skin integrity related to cachexia, poor tissue perfusion, and decreased mobility; deficient fluid volume related to fever, vomiting, and low fluid intake; and ineffective thermoregulation related to hypothalamic involvement, fever, and chills. See Chapter 16 for assessment and nursing interventions for the patient with cancer.

Planning and Goals

The goals for the patient may include compensating for self-care deficits, improving nutrition, reducing anxiety, enhancing family coping skills, and absence of complications.

Interventions

Compensating for Self-Care Deficits

The patient may have difficulty participating in goal setting as the tumour metastasizes and affects cognitive function. The nurse should encourage the family to keep the patient as independent as possible for as long as possible. Increasing assistance with self-care activities is required. Because the patient with cerebral metastasis and the family live with uncertainty, they are encouraged to plan for each day and to make the most of each day. The tasks and challenges are to assist the patient to find useful coping mechanisms, adaptations, and compensations for solving problems that arise. This helps patients maintain some sense of control. An individualized exercise program helps maintain strength, endurance, and range of motion. Eventually, referral for home or hospice care may be necessary (see Chapter 18).

Improving Nutrition

Patients with nausea, vomiting, diarrhea, breathlessness, and pain are rarely interested in eating. These symptoms are managed or controlled through assessment, planning, and care. The nurse teaches the family how to position the patient for comfort during meals. Meals are planned for times when the patient is rested and in less distress from pain or the effects of treatment.

The patient needs to be clean, comfortable, and free of pain for meals, in an environment that is as attractive as possible. Oral hygiene before meals helps to improve appetite. Offensive sights, sounds, and odours are eliminated. Creative strategies may be required to make food more palatable, provide enough fluids, and increase opportunities for socialization during meals. The family may be asked to keep a daily weight chart and to record the quantity of food eaten to determine the daily calorie count. Dietary supplements, if acceptable to the patient, can be provided to meet increased caloric needs. If the patient is not interested in most usual foods, those foods preferred by the patient should be offered. When the patient shows marked deterioration as a result of tumour growth and effects, some other form of nutritional support (e.g., tube feeding, parenteral nutrition) may be indicated if consistent with the patient's end-of-life preferences (AANN, 2014a). Nursing interventions include assessing the patency of the central and IV lines or feeding tube, monitoring the insertion site for infection, checking the infusion rate, monitoring intake and output, and changing the IV tubing and dressing. Family members are instructed in these techniques if they will be providing care at home. Parenteral nutrition can be provided at home if indicated.

The patient's quality of life may guide the selection, initiation, maintenance, and discontinuation of nutritional support. The nurse and family should not place too much emphasis on eating or on discussions about food, because the patient may not desire aggressive nutritional intervention. The subsequent course of action must be congruent with the wishes and choices of the patient and family.

Relieving Anxiety

Patients with cerebral metastases may be restless, with changing moods that may include intense depression, euphoria, paranoia, and severe anxiety. The response of patients to terminal illness reflects their pattern of reaction to other crisis situations. Serious illness imposes additional strains that often bring other unresolved problems to light. The patient's own coping strategies can help deal with anxious and depressed feelings. Health care providers need to be sensitive to the patient's concerns and fears.

Patients need the opportunity to exercise some control over their situation. A sense of mastery can be gained as they learn to understand the disease and its treatment and how to deal with their feelings. The presence of family, friends, a spiritual advisor, and health professionals may be supportive. Support groups such as the Brain Tumour Support Group may provide a feeling of support and strength.

Spending time with patients allows them time to talk and to communicate their fears and concerns. Open communication and acknowledgement of fears are often therapeutic. Touch is also a form of communication. These patients need reassurance that continuing care will be provided and that they will not be abandoned. The situation becomes more endurable when others share in the experience of dying. If a patient's emotional reactions are very intense or prolonged, additional help from a spiritual advisor, social worker, or mental health professional may be indicated.

Enhancing Family Processes

Nursing should ensure that palliative care services are introduced early in the patient's course of treatment. Early introduction to palliative care services have proven to improve both quality and quantity of life. The family needs to be reassured that their loved one is receiving optimal care and that attention will be paid to the patient's changing symptoms and concerns. When the patient can no longer carry out self-care, the family and additional support systems (social worker, home health aide, home care nurse, hospice nurse) may be needed. End-of-life care is provided with respect, and reassurance is provided by communicating the plan of care to the family (Dhandapani et al., 2015).

Promoting Home, Community-Based, and Transitional Care

EDUCATING PATIENTS ABOUT SELF-CARE. The patient and family often have major responsibility for care at home. Therefore, teaching includes pain management strategies, prevention of complications related to treatment strategies, and methods to ensure adequate fluid and food intake (Chart 67-2). Teaching needs of the patient and family regarding care priorities are likely to change as the disease progresses. The nurse should assess the changing needs of the patient and the family and inform them about resources and services early, to assist them in dealing with changes in the patient's condition.

CONTINUING AND TRANSITIONAL CARE. Home care nursing and hospice services are valuable resources that should be made available to the patient and the family early in the course of a terminal illness. Anticipating needs before they occur can assist in smooth initiation of services. Home care needs and interventions focus on four major areas: palliation of symptoms and pain control, assistance in self-care, control of treatment complications, and administration of specific forms of treatment, such as parenteral nutrition. The home care nurse assesses pain management, respiratory status, complications of the disorder and its treatment, and the patient's cognitive and emotional status. Additionally, the nurse assesses the family's ability to perform necessary care and notifies the physician about changing needs or complications if indicated (Warnoch & Tod, 2013).

The patient and family who elect to care for the patient at home as the disease progresses benefit from the care and support provided through hospice and palliative care services (Ownsworth, Goadby, & Chambers, 2015). Steps to initiate hospice care, including discussion of hospice care as an option, should not be postponed until death is imminent. Exploration of hospice care as an option should be initiated at a time when hospice services can provide support and care to the patient and family consistent with their end-of-life decisions and can assist in allowing death with dignity. End-of-life care is further described in Chapter 15.

CHART 67-2

HOME CARE CHECKLIST • The Patient With Nervous System Metastases

At the completion of education, the patient and/or caregiver will be able to:

- State effects of the tumour according to its type and location in the brain or spinal cord.
- State the impact of the tumour and treatment on physiologic functioning, ADLs, IADLs, roles, relationships, and spirituality.
  - Describe goals and side effects of treatment and suggested management approaches.
- State the name, dose, side effects, frequency, and schedule for all medications.
  - When indicated, use nonpharmacologic pain management techniques in addition to prescribed pharmacologic methods.
- State how to contact all members of the treatment team (e.g., health care providers, home care professionals, and durable medical equipment and supply vendor).
- State changes in lifestyle (e.g., nutritional needs, ADL assistance) necessary to maintain health.
- Identify coping strategies, such as:
  - Taking control, setting daily goals, and staying positive.
  - Rehabilitation to improve self-care.
  - Relaxation techniques.
  - Family support.
  - Support groups.
  - American Brain Tumor Association.
  - Faith community/religious practices and rituals.
- Identify community resources, including palliative care, home health service, hospice, as appropriate.
- List complications of medications/therapeutic regimen necessitating a call to the nurse or primary provider.
- List complications of medications/therapeutic regimen necessitating a visit to the emergency department.
- Relate how to reach primary provider with questions or complications.
- State time and date of follow-up medical appointments, therapy, and testing.

Evaluation

Expected patient outcomes may include the following:

1. Engages in self-care activities as long as possible
   a. Uses assistive devices or accepts assistance as needed
   b. Schedules periodic rest periods to permit maximal participation in self-care
2. Maintains as optimal a nutritional status as possible
   a. Eats and accepts food within limits of condition and preferences
   b. Accepts alternative methods of providing nutrition if indicated
3. Reports being less anxious
   a. Is less restless and is sleeping better
   b. Verbalizes concerns and fears about death
   c. Participates in activities of personal importance as long as feasible
4. Family members seek help as needed
   a. Demonstrate ability to bathe, feed, and care for the patient and participate in pain management and prevention of complications
   b. Express feelings and concerns to appropriate health professionals
   c. Discuss and seek hospice care as an option

Spinal Cord Tumours

Tumours within the spinal canal are classified according to their anatomic relation to the spinal cord (Bader, Littlejohns, Olson, et al., 2016). They include intramedullary lesions (within the spinal cord), extramedullary-intradural lesions (within or under the spinal dura), and extramedullary-extradural lesions (outside the dural membrane). Primary tumours are usually intramedullary, consisting of astrocytoma or ependymoma; meningiomas can occur as extramedullary-intradural lesions. Secondary tumours are far more common and are usually extramedullary-extradural lesions. Tumours that occur within the spinal canal or exert pressure on it cause symptoms ranging from localized or shooting pains, weakness and loss of reflexes below the tumour level to progressive loss of motor function and paralysis. Usually, sharp pain occurs in the area innervated by the spinal roots that arise from the cord in the region of the tumour. In addition, increasing sensory deficits develop below the level of the lesion. Loss of bowel and bladder function is common.

Assessment and Diagnostic Findings

Neurologic examination and diagnostic studies are used to make the diagnosis. Neurologic examination includes assessment of pain, loss of reflexes, loss of sensation or motor function, and the presence of weakness and paralysis. Additional assessment findings usually include pain duration for longer than 1 month and an elevated erythrocyte sedimentation rate. Helpful diagnostic studies include x-rays, radionuclide bone scans, CT scans, MRI scans, and biopsy.

The MRI scan is the most commonly used and the most sensitive diagnostic tool (Hickey, 2014) and it is particularly helpful in detecting epidural spinal cord compression and metastases.

Medical Management

Treatment of specific intraspinal tumours depends on the type and location of the tumour and the presenting symptoms and physical status of the patient. Surgical intervention is the primary treatment for most spinal cord tumours (Mechtler & Nandigam, 2013). Other treatment modalities include partial removal of the tumour, decompression of the spinal cord, chemotherapy, and radiation therapy, particularly for intramedullary tumours and metastatic lesions.

Extramedullary-extradural spinal cord compression occurs in 5% to 7% of patients who die of cancer and is considered a neurologic emergency. For the patient with spinal cord compression resulting from metastatic cancer (most commonly from breast, prostate, or lung), high-dose dexamethasone (Decadron) combined with radiation therapy is effective in relieving pain of the patient with spinal cord compression). Palliative care may be an option for the medical management of some patients. Chemotherapy specific to the tumour type may be considered (Perkins & Liu, 2016). Palliative care may be an option for the medical management of some patients.

Surgical Management

Tumour removal is desirable but not always possible. The goal is to remove as much tumour as possible while sparing uninvolved portions of the spinal cord. Microsurgical techniques have improved the prognosis for patients with intramedullary tumours. Prognosis is related to the degree of neurologic impairment at the time of surgery, the speed with which symptoms occurred, and the origin of the tumour. Patients with extensive neurologic deficits before surgery usually do not make significant functional recovery even after successful tumour removal (Mechtler & Nandigam, 2013).

Nursing Management

Providing Preoperative Care

The objectives of preoperative care include recognition of neurologic changes through ongoing assessments, pain control, and management of altered activities of daily living (ADLs) resulting from sensory and motor deficits and bowel and bladder dysfunction. The nurse assesses for weakness, muscle wasting, spasticity, sensory changes, bowel and bladder dysfunction, and potential respiratory problems, especially if a cervical tumour is present. The patient is also evaluated for coagulation deficiencies. A history of aspirin intake is obtained and reported, because the use of aspirin may impede hemostasis postoperatively. Breathing exercises are taught and demonstrated preoperatively. Postoperative pain management strategies are discussed with the patient before surgery.

Assessing the Patient After Surgery

The patient is monitored for deterioration in neurologic status. A sudden onset of neurologic deficit is an ominous sign and may be due to vertebral collapse associated with spinal cord infarction. Frequent neurologic checks are carried out, with emphasis on movement, strength, and sensation of the upper and lower extremities. Assessment of sensory function involves pinching the skin of the arms, legs, and trunk to determine if there is loss of feeling and, if so, at what level. Vital signs are monitored at regular intervals.

Managing Pain

The prescribed pain medication should be administered in adequate amounts and at appropriate intervals to relieve pain and prevent its recurrence. Pain is the hallmark of spinal metastasis. Patients with sensory root involvement or vertebral collapse may suffer excruciating pain, which requires effective pain management (Hickey, 2014).

If the tumour has caused the patient's spine to become unstable, the bed is usually kept flat initially. The nurse turns the patient as a unit, keeping shoulders and hips aligned and the back straight. The side-lying position is usually the most comfortable, because this position imposes the least pressure on the surgical site. Placement of a pillow between the knees of the patient in a side-lying position helps to prevent extreme knee flexion.

Monitoring and Managing Potential Complications

If the tumour was in the cervical area, respiratory compromise due to postoperative edema may occur. The nurse monitors the patient for asymmetric chest movement, abdominal breathing, and abnormal breath sounds. For a high cervical lesion, the endotracheal tube remains in place until adequate respiratory function is ensured. The patient is encouraged to perform deep-breathing and coughing exercises.

The area over the bladder is palpated or a bladder scan is performed to assess for urinary retention. The nurse also monitors for incontinence, because urinary dysfunction usually implies significant decompensation of spinal cord function. An intake and output record is maintained. Additionally, the abdomen is auscultated for bowel sounds.

Staining of the dressing may indicate leakage of CSF from the surgical site, which may lead to serious infection or to an inflammatory reaction in the surrounding tissues that can cause severe pain in the postoperative period.

Promoting Home, Community-Based, and Transitional Care

Educating Patients About Self-Care

In preparation for discharge, the patient is assessed for the ability to function independently in the home and for the availability of resources such as family members to assist in caregiving. Patients with residual sensory involvement are cautioned about the dangers of extremes in temperature. They should be alerted to the dangers of heating devices (e.g., hot water bottles, heating pads, space heaters). The patient is taught to check skin integrity daily. Patients with impaired motor function related to motor weakness or paralysis may require training in ADLs and safe use of assistive devices, such as a cane, walker, or wheelchair.

The patient and family members are instructed about pain management strategies, bowel and bladder management, and assessment for signs and symptoms that should be reported promptly.

Continuing and Transitional Care

Referral for inpatient or outpatient rehabilitation may be warranted to improve self-care abilities. A home care referral may be indicated and provides the home care nurse with the opportunity to assess the patient's physical and psychological status and the patient's and family's ability to adhere to recommended management strategies. During the home visit, the nurse determines whether changes in neurologic function have occurred. The patient's respiratory status and nutritional status are assessed. The adequacy of pain management is assessed, and modifications are made to ensure adequate pain relief. The need for hospice services or placement in an extended-care facility is discussed with the patient and family if warranted, and the patient is asked about preferences for end-of-life care. Additionally, social workers may be consulted to assist the patient and family members in identifying support groups and agencies that can provide help in coping with the disease process.

Physiology/Pathophysiology

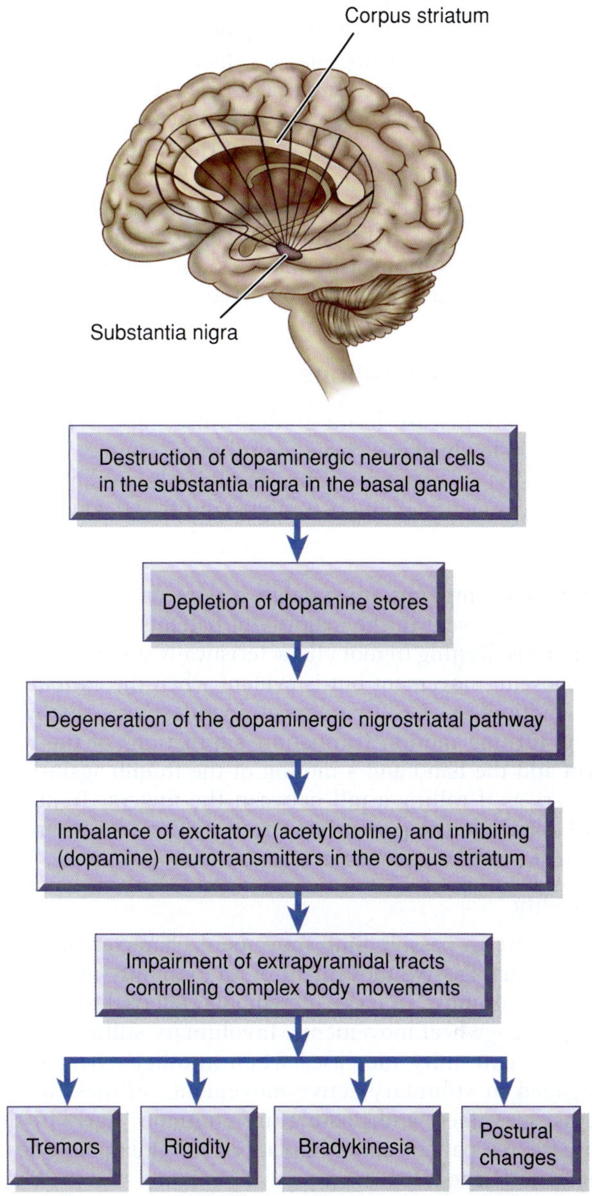

FIGURE 67-4. Pathophysiology of Parkinson's disease. The nuclei in the substantia nigra project fibres to the corpus striatum. The nerve fibres carry dopamine to the corpus striatum. The loss of dopamine nerve cells from the brain's substantia nigra is thought to be responsible for the symptoms of parkinsonism.

DEGENERATIVE DISORDERS

Disorders of the central and peripheral nervous system that are **neurodegenerative** (leading to deterioration of normal cells or function of the nervous system) are characterized by the slow onset of signs and symptoms. Patients are managed at home for as long as possible and are admitted to the acute care setting for exacerbations, treatments, and surgical interventions as needed.

Parkinson's Disease

Parkinson's disease is a slowly progressing neurologic movement disorder that eventually leads to disability. It is the second most common neurodegenerative disease, and an estimated 5,500 new cases are reported each year in Canada (Parkinson Society British Columbia, 2014). The disease affects men more often than women. Symptoms usually first appear in the fifth decade of life; however, cases have been diagnosed as early as 30 years of age.

The degenerative or idiopathic form of Parkinson's disease is the most common; there is also a secondary form with a known or suspected cause. Although the cause of most cases is unknown, research suggests a multifactorial combination of age, environment, and heredity (Moore et al., 2017).

Pathophysiology

Parkinson's disease is associated with decreased levels of dopamine within the CNS resulting from destruction of pigmented neuronal cells in the substantia nigra in the basal ganglia region of the brain (Fig. 67-4). Fibres or neuronal pathways project from the substantia nigra to the corpus striatum, where neurotransmitters are key to the control of complex body movements. Through the neurotransmitters acetylcholine (excitatory) and dopamine (inhibitory), striatal neurons relay messages to the higher motor centres that control and refine motor movements. The loss of dopamine stores in this area of the brain results in more excitatory neurotransmitters than inhibitory neurotransmitters, leading to an imbalance that affects voluntary movement.

Clinical symptoms do not appear until 60% of the pigmented neurons are lost and the striatal dopamine level is decreased by 80%. Cellular degeneration impairs the extrapyramidal tracts that control semiautomatic functions and coordinated movements; motor cells of the motor cortex and the pyramidal tracts are not affected. Current theories suggest a combined and complicated interweaving of both environmental and genetic factors that affect numerous fundamental cellular processes. Fifteen percent of early PD cases are associated with multiple genetic mutations (Gopalakrishna & Alexander, 2015). Ongoing research includes recognition of biomarkers and development of individualized treatment options (Kalia & Lang, 2015).

Clinical Manifestations

Parkinson's disease has a gradual onset, and symptoms progress slowly over a chronic, prolonged course. The cardinal signs are tremor, rigidity, **bradykinesia** (abnormally slow movements), and postural instability (Hickey, 2014).

Tremor

Although symptoms are variable, a slow, unilateral resting tremor is present in the majority of patients at the time of diagnosis. Resting tremor characteristically disappears with purposeful movement but is evident when the extremities are motionless. The tremor may manifest as a rhythmic, slow turning motion (pronation–supination) of the forearm and the hand and a motion of the thumb against the fingers as if rolling a pill between the fingers. Tremor is present while the patient is at rest; it increases when the patient is walking, concentrating, or feeling anxious.

Rigidity

Resistance to passive limb movement characterizes muscle rigidity. Passive movement of an extremity may cause the limb to move in jerky increments, referred to as lead-pipe or cogwheel movements. Involuntary stiffness of the passive extremity increases when another extremity is engaged in voluntary active movement. Stiffness of the arms, legs, face, and posture are common. Early in the disease, the patient may complain of shoulder pain due to rigidity (Hickey, 2014).

Bradykinesia

One of the most common features of Parkinson's disease is bradykinesia, which refers to the overall slowing of active movement (Gopalakrishna & Alexander, 2015). Patients may also take longer to complete activities and have difficulty initiating movement, such as rising from a sitting position or turning in bed.

Postural Instability

The patient commonly develops postural and gait problems. A loss of postural reflexes occurs, and the patient stands with the head bent forward and walks with a propulsive gait. The posture is caused by the forward flexion of the neck, hips, knees, and elbows. The patient may walk faster and faster, trying to move the feet forward under the body's centres of gravity (shuffling gait). Difficulty in pivoting causes loss of balance (either forward or backward). Gait impairment and postural instability place the patient at increased risk for falls (Kalia & Lang, 2015).

Other Manifestations

The effect of Parkinson's disease on the basal ganglia often produces autonomic symptoms that include excessive and uncontrolled sweating, paroxysmal flushing, orthostatic hypotension, gastric and urinary retention, constipation, and sexual dysfunction. Psychiatric changes include personality changes, depression, **dementia** (progressive mental deterioration), delirium, hallucinations, and anxiety (Kalia & Lang, 2015). Depression is common; whether it is a reaction to the disorder or is related to a biochemical abnormality is uncertain (Moore et al., 2017). Mental changes may appear in the form of cognitive, perceptual, and memory deficits, although intellect is not usually affected. Dementia affects up to 75% of patients over the course of the disease. Auditory and visual hallucinations have been reported in up to 40% of people with Parkinson's disease and may be associated with depression, dementia, lack of sleep, or adverse effects of medications (Kalia & Lang, 2015). Additionally, sleep disturbances are common.

Hypokinesia (abnormally diminished movement) is also common and may appear after the tremor. The freezing phenomenon refers to a transient inability to perform active movement and is thought to be an extreme form of bradykinesia. Additionally, the patient tends to shuffle and exhibits a decreased arm swing. As dexterity declines, micrographia (small handwriting) develops. The face becomes increasingly masklike and expressionless, and the frequency of blinking decreases. **Dysphonia** (soft, slurred, low-pitched, and less audible speech) may occur as a result of weakness and incoordination of the muscles responsible for speech. In many cases, the patient develops dysphagia, begins to drool, and is at risk for choking and aspiration.

Complications associated with Parkinson's disease are common and are typically related to disorders of movement. As the disease progresses, patients are at risk for respiratory and urinary tract infection, skin breakdown, and injury from falls. The adverse effects of medications used to treat the symptoms are associated with numerous complications such as **dyskinesia** or orthostatic hypotension (Karch, 2014).

Assessment and Diagnostic Findings

Although laboratory tests and imaging studies are not helpful to the clinician in diagnosing Parkinson's disease, ongoing research with PET and single photon emission computed tomography (SPECT) scanning has been helpful in understanding the disease and advancing treatment. Currently, the disease is diagnosed clinically from the patient's history and the presence of two of the four cardinal manifestations: tremor, rigidity, bradykinesia, and postural changes.

Early diagnosis can be difficult because patients rarely are able to pinpoint when the symptoms started. Often, a family member notices a change such as stooped posture, a stiff arm, a slight limp, tremor, or slow, small handwriting. The medical history, presenting symptoms, neurologic examination, and response to pharmacologic management are carefully evaluated when making the diagnosis (Hickey, 2014). With advances in neuroimaging techniques investigators are seeking to identify early warning symptoms or a prodromal phase of Parkinson's disease. For example,

Parkinson's disease not only affects the substantia nigra, but extends to regions such as the anterior olfactory site well before cardinal symptoms appear. Extensions to other regions are associated with a loss of smell, decreased contrast sensitivity to colours, and altered sleep cycles called REM behaviour disorder.

Medical Management

Treatment is directed at controlling symptoms and maintaining functional independence, because no medical or surgical approaches in current use prevent disease progression. Care is individualized for each patient based on presenting symptoms and social, occupational, and emotional needs. Pharmacologic management is the mainstay of treatment, although advances in research have led to increased surgical options. Patients are usually cared for at home and are admitted to the hospital only for complications or to initiate new treatments.

Pharmacologic Therapy

Antiparkinsonian medications act by (1) increasing striatal dopaminergic activity; (2) reducing the excessive influence of excitatory cholinergic neurons on the extrapyramidal tract, thereby restoring a balance between dopaminergic and cholinergic activities; or (3) acting on neurotransmitter pathways other than the dopaminergic pathway.

Levodopa (Larodopa) is the most effective agent and the mainstay of treatment. Levodopa is converted to dopamine in the basal ganglia, producing symptom relief. Levodopa is available in three forms: immediate-release, orally disintegrating, and sustained-release tablets (Kalia & Lang, 2015). The beneficial effects of levodopa are most pronounced in the first few years of treatment. Benefits begin to wane and adverse effects become more severe over time. Confusion, hallucinations, depression, and sleep alterations are associated with prolonged use.

Within 5 to 10 years, most patients develop a response to the medication characterized by dyskinesia (abnormal involuntary movements), including facial grimacing, rhythmic jerking movements of the hands, head bobbing, chewing and smacking movements, and involuntary movements of the trunk and extremities. The patient may experience an on–off syndrome in which sudden periods of near immobility ("off effect") are followed by a sudden return of effectiveness of the medication ("on effect"). Various adjunctive therapies are used to minimize dyskinesias (Hickey, 2014). Another potential complication of long-term dopaminergic medication use is neuroleptic malignant syndrome, which is characterized by severe rigidity, stupor, hyperthermia, and elevated creatine kinase levels (Musselman & Saely, 2013). Additional medications used to treat Parkinson's disease are described in Table 67-1.

Surgical Management

The limitations of levodopa therapy, improvements in stereotactic surgery, and new approaches in transplantation

TABLE 67-1 Selected Medications Used to Treat Parkinson's Disease

Medications	Indications and Therapeutic Effects	Common Side Effects
Anticholinergic Agents		
trihexyphenidyl hydrochloride (Apo-Trihex)	Control of tremor in patients with early-onset disease	Blurred vision, flushing, rash, constipation, urinary retention, and acute confusional states
benztropine mesylate (Cogentin)	Counteract the action of acetylcholine	Contraindicated in patients with narrow-angle glaucoma
Antiviral Agent		
amantadine hydrochloride (Symmetrel)	Reduce rigidity, tremor, bradykinesia, and postural changes in early Parkinson's disease (PD)	Psychiatric disturbances (mood changes, confusion, depression, hallucinations), lower extremity edema, nausea, epigastric distress, urinary retention, headache, and visual impairment
Dopamine Agonists		
bromocriptine mesylate (Parlodel)	Early PD as well as secondary drug therapy after carbidopa or levodopa loses effectiveness	Nausea, vomiting, diarrhea, lightheadedness, hypotension, impotence, and psychiatric effects
pergolide (Permax)		
Nonergot Derivatives		
ropinirole hydrochloride (Requip)	Early stages of PD	May cause drowsiness or dizziness
pramipexole (Mirapex)		
Monoamine Oxidase-Inhibitors		
selegiline (Emsam)	Inhibit dopamine breakdown	Agitation, dizziness, nausea, headache, rhinitis, back pain, stomatitis, postural hypotension, insomnia
rasagiline (Azilect)		
Catechol-O-Methyltransferase Inhibitors		
entacapone (Comtan)	Increase the duration of action of carbidopa or levodopa	Abdominal pain, back pain, constipation, nausea, diarrhea, blood in urine
tolcapone (Tasmar)	Reduce motor fluctuations in patients with advanced PD	

Adapted from Moore, D. J., Smith, B. M., & Cho, M. H. (2017). Managing meditations for hospital patients with Parkinson disease. *American Nurse Today*, *12*(1), 9–12.

have renewed interest in the surgical treatment of Parkinson's disease. In patients with disabling tremor, rigidity, or severe levodopa-induced dyskinesia, surgery may be considered. Although surgery provides symptom relief in selected patients, it has not been shown to alter the course of the disease or to produce permanent improvement.

Stereotactic Procedures

Thalamotomy and pallidotomy are effective in relieving many of the symptoms of Parkinson's disease (Hickey, 2014). Patients eligible for these procedures are those who have had an inadequate response to medical therapy; they must meet strict criteria to be eligible. Candidates eligible for these procedures are patients with idiopathic Parkinson's disease who are taking maximum doses of antiparkinsonian medications. Patients with dementia and atypical Parkinson's disease are usually not considered for stereotactic procedures. Parkinson's disease rating scales and specific neurologic tests are used to identify eligible patients.

The intent of thalamotomy and pallidotomy is to interrupt the nerve pathways and thereby alleviate tremor or rigidity. During thalamotomy, a stereotactic electrical stimulator damages part of the ventrolateral portion of the thalamus in an attempt to reduce tremor; the most common complications are ataxia and hemiparesis. Pallidotomy involves destruction of part of the ventral aspect of the medial globus pallidus through electrical stimulation in patients with advanced disease (Hickey, 2014). The procedure is effective in reducing rigidity, bradykinesia, and dyskinesia, thus improving motor function and ADLs in the immediate postoperative course. Potential complications include hemiparesis and stroke, as well as cognitive, speech, swallowing, and visual changes.

A CT scan, x-ray, or MRI scan is used to localize the appropriate surgical site in the brain. Then the patient's head is positioned in a stereotactic frame (Fig. 67-5). After the surgeon makes an incision in the skin and a burr hole is made into the skull, an electrode is passed through to the target area into the thalamus or globus pallidus. The desired response of the patient to the electrical stimulation (i.e., a decrease in rigidity) is the basis for the selection of the area of the brain to be altered.

Pacemakerlike brain implants are used to relieve tremors (AANN, 2014b). The stimulation can be bilateral or unilateral; bilateral stimulation of the subthalamic nucleus is thought to be of greater benefit to patients than results achieved with thalamotomy, pallidotomy, or fetal nigral transplantation. In deep brain stimulation, an electrode is placed in the thalamus and connected to a pulse generator that is implanted in a subcutaneous subclavicular or abdominal pouch (Kalia & Lang, 2015). The battery-powered pulse generator sends high-frequency electrical impulses through a wire placed under the skin to a lead anchored to the skull (Fig. 67-6). The electrode blocks nerve pathways in the brain that cause tremors. These devices are not without complications that can result from both the surgical procedure needed for implantation and the device itself (e.g., lead leakage and accidental deactivation by electromagnetic fields from electrical items such as an electrical toothbrush) (Tousi & Wilson, 2013).

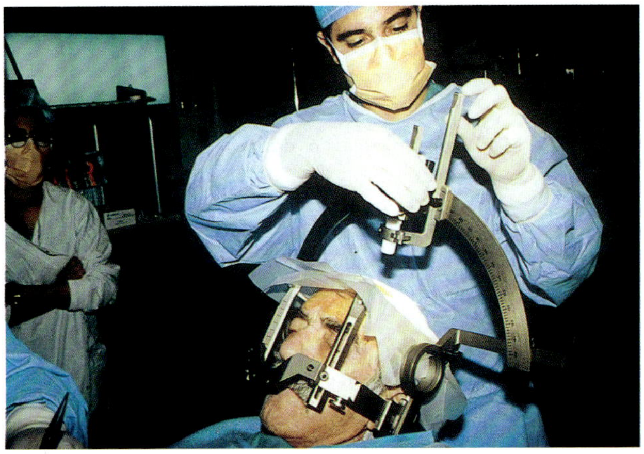

FIGURE 67-5. A stereotactic frame is applied to a patient's head in preparation for pallidotomy. The frame immobilizes the head.

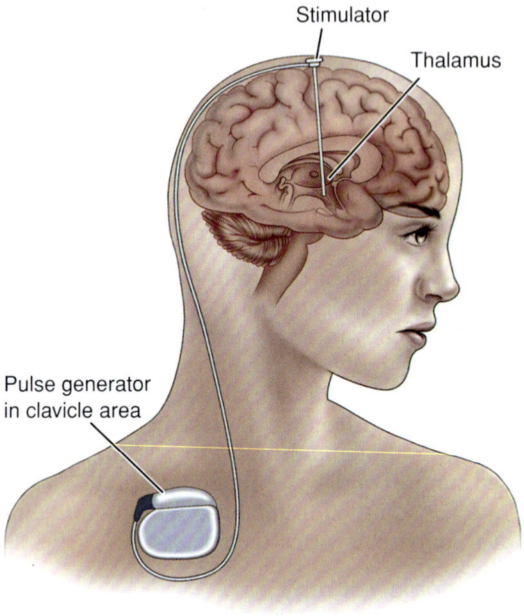

FIGURE 67-6. Deep brain stimulation is provided by a pulse generator surgically implanted in a pouch beneath the clavicle. The generator sends high-frequency electrical impulses to the thalamus, thereby blocking the nerve pathways associated with tremors in Parkinson's disease.

Neural Transplantation

Ongoing research is exploring transplantation of porcine neuronal cells, human fetal cells, and stem cells (Kim, Lee, & Kim, 2013). Legal, ethical, and political concerns surrounding the use of fetal brain cells and stem cells have limited the implementation of these procedures.

Nursing Process

The Patient With Parkinson's Disease

Assessment

Assessment focuses on how the disease has affected the patient's ADLs and functional abilities. The patient is observed for degree of disability and functional changes that occur throughout the day, such as responses to medication. Almost every patient with a movement disorder has some functional alteration and may have some type of behavioural dysfunction. The following questions may be useful to assess alterations:

- Do you have leg or arm stiffness?
- Have you experienced any irregular jerking of your arms or legs?
- Have you ever been "frozen" or rooted to the spot and unable to move?
- Does your mouth water excessively? Have you (or others) noticed yourself grimacing or making faces or chewing movements?
- What specific activities do you have difficulty doing?

During this assessment, the nurse observes the patient for quality of speech, loss of facial expression, swallowing deficits (drooling, poor head control, coughing), tremors, slowness of movement, weakness, forward posture, rigidity, evidence of mental slowness, and confusion. Parkinson's disease symptoms, as well as side effects of medications, put these patients at high risk for falls; therefore, a fall risk assessment should be conducted.

Nursing Priorities

Based on the assessment data, the patient's major nursing priorities may include the following:

- Altered physical mobility likely due to muscle rigidity and motor weakness
- Inability to self-care such as feeding, dressing, hygiene, and toileting
- Constipation likely due to medication and reduced activity
- Decreased nutrition, less than body requirements likely due to tremor, slowness in eating, difficulty in chewing and swallowing
- Altered verbal communication likely due to decreased speech volume, slowness of speech, inability to move facial muscles
- Lack of coping likely due to depression

Other nursing priorities may include sleep pattern disturbances, deficient knowledge, risk for injury, risk for activity intolerance, disturbed thought processes, and compromised family coping.

Planning and Goals

The goals for the patient may include improving functional mobility, maintaining independence in ADLs, achieving adequate bowel elimination, attaining and maintaining acceptable nutritional status, achieving effective communication, and developing positive coping mechanisms.

Nursing Interventions

Improving Mobility

A progressive program of daily exercise will increase muscle strength, improve coordination and dexterity, reduce muscular rigidity, and prevent contractures that occur when muscles are not used. Walking, riding a stationary bicycle, swimming, and gardening are all exercises that help maintain joint mobility. Stretching (stretch–hold–relax) and range-of-motion exercises promote joint flexibility. Postural exercises are important to counter the tendency of the head and neck to be drawn forward and down. A physical therapist may be helpful in developing an individualized exercise program and can provide instruction to the patient and caregiver on exercising safely. Faithful adherence to an exercise and walking program helps delay the progress of the disease. Warm baths and massage, in addition to passive and active exercises, help relax muscles and relieve painful muscle spasms that accompany rigidity.

Balance may be adversely affected because of the rigidity of the arms (arm swinging is necessary in normal walking). Special walking techniques must be learned to offset the shuffling gait and the tendency to lean forward. The patient is taught to concentrate on walking erect, to watch the horizon, and to use a wide-based gait (i.e., walking with the feet separated). A conscious effort must be made to swing the arms, raise the feet while walking, and use a heel–toe placement of the feet with long strides. The patient is advised to practice walking to marching music or to the sound of a ticking metronome, because this provides sensory reinforcement. Performing breathing exercises while walking helps move the rib cage and aerate parts of the lungs. Frequent rest periods aid in preventing frustration and fatigue.

Enhancing Self-Care Activities

Encouraging, teaching, and supporting the patient during ADLs promote self-care. See Chapter 12 for rehabilitation techniques.

Environmental modifications are necessary to compensate for functional disabilities. Patients may have severe mobility problems that make normal activities impossible. Adaptive or assistive devices may be useful. A hospital bed at home with bedside rails, an overbed frame with a trapeze, or a rope tied to the foot of the bed can provide assistance in pulling up without help. An occupational therapist can evaluate the patient's needs in the home, make recommendations regarding adaptive devices, and teach the patient and caregiver how to improvise.

Improving Bowel Elimination

The patient may have severe problems with constipation. Among the factors causing constipation are weakness of the muscles used in defecation, lack of exercise, inadequate fluid intake, and decreased autonomic nervous system activity. The medications used for the treatment of the disease also inhibit normal intestinal secretions. A regular bowel routine may be established by encouraging the patient to follow a regular time pattern, consciously increase fluid intake, and eat foods with moderate fibre content. Laxatives should be avoided. Psyllium (Metamucil), for example, decreases constipation but carries the risk of bowel obstruction (Karch, 2014). A raised toilet seat is useful, because the patient has difficulty in moving from a standing to a sitting position.

Improving Nutrition

Patients may have difficulty maintaining their weight. Eating becomes a very slow process, requiring concentration due to a dry mouth from medications and difficulty chewing and swallowing. These patients are at risk for aspiration because of impaired swallowing and the accumulation of saliva. They may be unaware that they are aspirating; subsequently, bronchopneumonia may develop.

Monitoring weight on a weekly basis indicates whether caloric intake is adequate. Supplemental feedings increase caloric intake. As the disease progresses, a nasogastric tube or percutaneous endoscopic gastroscopy may be necessary to maintain adequate nutrition. A dietitian can be consulted regarding nutritional needs.

Enhancing Swallowing

Swallowing difficulties and choking are common in Parkinson's disease (Hickey, 2014). These can lead to problems with poor head control, tongue tremor, hesitancy in initiating swallowing, difficulty in shaping food into a bolus, and disturbances in pharyngeal motility. To offset these problems, the patient should sit in an upright position during mealtime. A semisolid diet with thick liquids is easier to swallow than solids; thin liquids should be avoided. Thinking through the swallowing sequence is helpful. The patient is taught to place the food on the tongue, close the lips and teeth, lift the tongue up and then back, and swallow. The patient is encouraged to chew first on one side of the mouth and then on the other. To control the buildup of saliva, the patient is reminded to hold the head upright and make a conscious effort to swallow. Massaging the facial and neck muscles before meals may be beneficial.

Encouraging the Use of Assistive Devices

An electric warming tray keeps food hot and allows the patient to rest during the prolonged time that it may take to eat. Special utensils also assist at mealtime. A plate that is stabilized, a nonspill cup, and eating utensils with built-up handles are useful self-help devices. The occupational therapist can assist in identifying appropriate adaptive devices.

Improving Communication

Speech disorders are present in most patients with Parkinson's disease. The low-pitched, monotonous, soft speech of patients requires that they make a conscious effort to speak slowly, with deliberate attention to what they are saying. The patient is reminded to face the listener, exaggerate the pronunciation of words, speak in short sentences, and take a few deep breaths before speaking. A speech therapist may be helpful in designing speech improvement exercises and assisting the family and health care personnel to develop and use a method of communication that meets the patient's needs. A small electronic amplifier is helpful if the patient has difficulty being heard.

Supporting Coping Abilities

Support can be given by encouraging the patient and pointing out that activities will be maintained through active participation. A combination of physiotherapy, psychotherapy, medication therapy, and support group participation may help reduce the depression that often occurs. Patients with Parkinson's disease can become withdrawn. It is best if patients are active participants in their therapeutic program, including social and recreational events. A planned program of activity throughout the day prevents too much daytime sleeping as well as disinterest and apathy.

Patients often feel embarrassed, apathetic, inadequate, bored, and lonely. In part, these feelings may result from physical slowness and the great effort that even small tasks require. The patient is assisted and encouraged to set achievable goals (e.g., improvement of mobility). Every effort should be made to encourage patients to carry out the tasks involved in meeting their own daily needs and to remain independent. Doing things for the patient merely to save time undermines the basic goal of improving coping abilities and promoting a positive self-concept.

Promoting Home, Community-Based, and Transitional Care

EDUCATING PATIENTS ABOUT SELF-CARE. Patient and family education is important in the management of Parkinson's disease. Teaching needs depend on the severity of symptoms and the stage of the disease. Care must be taken not to overwhelm the patient and family with too much information early in the disease process. The patient's and family's need for information is ongoing as adaptations become necessary. The education plan should include a clear explanation of the disease and the goal of assisting the patient to remain functionally independent as long as possible. Every effort is made to explain the nature of the disease and its management to offset disabling anxieties and fears. The patient and family must be taught about the effects and side effects of medications and about the importance of reporting side effects to the physician (Chart 67-3). Nurses in the home help patients and their families enhance self-management and quality of life (Shin & Habermann, 2016a).

CONTINUING AND TRANSITIONAL CARE. In the early stages, the patient can be managed well at home. Family members often serve as caregivers, with home care or community services available to assist in meeting health care needs as the disease progresses. The family caregiver may be under considerable stress from living with and caring for a person with a significant disability. Providing information about treatment and care prevents many unnecessary problems. The

CHART 67-3

Health Promotion: Strategies for the Patient With PD

To promote optimal health, the nurse works closely with the patient and family to ensure that they understand:

- How PD and its treatment impact physiologic functioning, ADLs, IADLs, roles, relationships, and spirituality
- The importance of adhering to the prescribed medication regimen; including knowing the purpose, dose, route, schedule, side effects, and precautions for all medications
- How and when to contact all members of the treatment team (e.g., health care providers, home care professionals, and durable medical equipment and supply vendors)
- Specific types of environmental and safety changes or support that will allow optimum functioning in the home
- The risk of falls/injury and how to implement fall prevention and adaptive measures in the home

In addition, the nurse advises the patient and family about lifestyle changes that are necessary to maintain health and promote self-care and independence. These include:

- Ensuring nutritional needs, including adhering to dietary restrictions, managing dysphagia, and preventing aspiration
- Promoting speech and communication skills: speech exercises, communication techniques, breathing exercises
- Managing constipation: fluid intake, bowel routine
- Managing urinary problems: functional incontinence, retention (indwelling urinary catheter care, suprapubic catheter care)
- Avoiding the effects of immobility and promoting the advantages of preventive care: skin breakdown (frequent turning, pressure release, skin care), pneumonia (deep breathing, movement), contractures (range-of-motion exercises)
- Promoting the benefits of a daily exercise program
- Ensuring safe walking and balancing
- Using appropriate coping mechanisms and diversional activities

PD, Parkinson's disease; ADL, activities of daily living; IADL, independent activities of daily living.

caregiver is included in the plan and may be advised to learn stress reduction techniques, to include others in the caregiving process, to obtain periodic relief from responsibilities, and to have a yearly health assessment. Allowing family members to express feelings of frustration, anger, and guilt is often helpful to them (see Chart 67-4).

The patient should be evaluated in the home for adaptation and safety needs and compliance with the plan of care. In the advanced stages, patients usually enter long-term care facilities if family support is absent. Periodically, admission to an acute care facility may be necessary for changes in medical management or treatment of complications. Nurses provide support, education, and monitoring of patients over the course of the illness.

The nurse involved in home and continuing care needs to remind the patient and family members of the importance of addressing health-promotion needs such as screening for hypertension and stroke risk

NURSING RESEARCH PROFILE

Chart 67-4. When a Partner Has Parkinson's Disease

Martin, S. C. (2015). Psychosocial challenges experienced by partners of people with Parkinson disease. *Journal of Neuroscience Nursing*, *47*(4), 211–222.

Purpose

Persons with PD may experience devastating effects that impact those individuals who are close to them as well as the person experiencing the disease. The purpose of this study was to investigate the psychosocial experience of partners of people with PD.

Design

This qualitative descriptive study used in-depth interviews to investigate the psychosocial experience of partners of people with PD. A semistructured interview guide was used with 23 participants (15 women, 8 men) who identified that they were in a committed, romantic relationship with a person with PD.

Findings

Data analysis revealed a multitude of challenges for partners of people with PD. Some challenges included having the person with PD withdraw from communication, being unable to "rescue" the person from their disease (PD), and being the recipient of the person with PD's frustration. Additional challenges included becoming impatient with the person with PD, shouldering increased responsibilities, being confronted with the prospect of losing the person with PD, losing valued activities, being unable to predict the person with PD's daily well-being, and experiencing uncertainty about future caregiving and disease progression.

Nursing Implications

Partners of persons with PD face significant psychosocial challenges related to both caregiving and noncaregiving issues. Nurses should be prepared to provide reassurance to partners of persons with PD that their feelings are normal, as well as offer direction on how to enlist the support of family and friends and access additional support services.

assessments in this predominantly elderly population. Patients are taught about the importance of these activities and are referred to appropriate health care providers. Informational booklets and a newsletter for patient education are published by the Parkinson's Society of Canada and the National Parkinson's Foundation (see Resources).

Evaluation

Expected patient outcomes may include the following:

1. Strives toward improved mobility
   a. Participates in exercise program daily
   b. Walks with wide base of support; exaggerates arm swinging when walking
   c. Takes medications as prescribed
2. Progresses toward self-care
   a. Allows time for self-care activities
   b. Uses self-help devices
3. Maintains bowel function
   a. Consumes adequate fluid
   b. Increases dietary intake of fibre
   c. Reports regular pattern of bowel function
4. Attains improved nutritional status
   a. Swallows without aspiration
   b. Takes time while eating
5. Achieves a method of communication
   a. Communicates needs
   b. Practices speech exercises
6. Copes with effects of Parkinson's disease
   a. Sets realistic goals
   b. Demonstrates persistence in meaningful activities
   c. Verbalizes feelings to appropriate person

Huntington's Disease

Huntington's disease is a chronic, progressive, hereditary disease of the nervous system that results in progressive involuntary choreiform movement and dementia. The disease affects approximately 1 in 10,000 men or women of all races at midlife. Every person has the gene that causes Huntington's disease; however, only those who inherit the expansion of the gene will develop the disease and pass it onto their children. Because it is transmitted by an autosomal dominant gene, each child of a parent with Huntington's disease has a 50% risk of inheriting the disorder (Bader et al., 2016).

A genetic mutation in Huntington's disease, the presence of a repeat in the Huntington gene (*HTT*), has been identified. Genetic testing can identify people who will develop this disease but cannot predict timing of disease onset. Although the gene was mapped in 1983, patients may choose not to be tested because of concerns about employment and health care discrimination. People of childbearing age with a family history of Huntington's disease often seek information about their risk of disease transmission. Genetic counselling is crucial, and patients and their families may require long-term psychological counselling and emotional, financial, and legal support (see Chapter 11).

Pathophysiology

The basic pathology involves premature death of cells in the striatum (caudate and putamen) of the basal ganglia, the region deep within the brain that is involved in the control of movement. Cells also are lost in the cortex, the region of the brain associated with thinking, memory, perception, and judgment, and in the cerebellum, the area that coordinates voluntary muscle activity. Cell loss is associated with a mutant variety of the protein called huntingtin. Huntingtin normally concentrates in neurons and is involved in vital cellular processes. The mutant huntingtin protein disrupts neuronal cellular functioning in areas such as the mitochondria, transport of axon critical factors, calcium signalling, and transcription of various genes (Bordelon, 2013; Ha & Fung, 2012). One possible theory is that glutamine, a building block for protein, abnormally collects in the cell nucleus, causing cell death (Ferrer, 2016).

Clinical Manifestations

The most prominent clinical features of the disease are **chorea** (abnormal involuntary movements), intellectual decline, and, often, emotional disturbance (Bader et al., 2016). As the disease progresses, a constant writhing, twisting, uncontrollable movement may involve the entire body. These motions are devoid of purpose or rhythm, although patients may try to turn them into purposeful movement. All of the body musculature is involved. Facial movements produce tics and grimaces. Speech becomes slurred, hesitant, often explosive, and eventually unintelligible. Chewing and swallowing are difficult, and there is a constant danger of choking and aspiration. Choreiform movements persist during sleep but are diminished (Wilson, Pollock, & Aubeeluck, 2014).

As with speech, the gait becomes disorganized to the point that ambulation eventually is impossible. Although independent ambulation should be encouraged for as long as possible, a wheelchair usually becomes necessary. Eventually, the patient is confined to bed when the chorea interferes with walking, sitting, and all other activities. Bladder and bowel control is lost. Cognitive function is usually affected, with dementia usually occurring. Initially, the patient is aware that the disease is responsible for the myriad dysfunctions that are occurring. The mental and emotional changes that occur may be more devastating to the patient and family than the abnormal movements. Personality changes may result in nervous, irritable, or impatient behaviours. In the early stages, patients are particularly subject to uncontrollable fits of anger; profound, often suicidal depression; apathy; anxiety; psychosis; or euphoria. Judgment and memory are impaired, and dementia eventually ensues. Hallucinations, delusions, and paranoid thinking may precede the appearance of disjointed movements. Emotional and cognitive symptoms often become less acute as the disease progresses (Bader et al., 2016).

Onset usually occurs between 35 and 45 years of age, although about 10% of patients are children. The disease progresses slowly. Despite a ravenous appetite, patients usually become emaciated and exhausted. Patients succumb in

10 to 20 years to heart failure, pneumonia, or infection, or as a result of a fall or choking.

Assessment and Diagnostic Findings

The diagnosis is made based on the clinical presentation of characteristic symptoms, a positive family history, the known presence of a genetic marker, and exclusion of other causes. The use of a genetic test has been available since 1993 and genetic counselling is recommended prior to and following the genetic test (Andersson, Juth, Petersen, et al., 2012; Bader et al., 2016). CT or MRI scans show symmetrical striatal atrophy before motor symptoms appear (Ross et al., 2014).

Medical Management

No treatment halts or reverses the underlying process; therefore, the focus is on optimizing quality of life with available medication and supportive treatment. Patients experience the most benefit when they have integrated expertise of a Huntington's disease multidisciplinary team (Smith, D'Cruz, Gray, et al., 2015). The only medication that is approved by the Food and Drug Administration to treat the symptom of chorea is tetrabenazine (Xenazine) (Kumar, Singh, Kumar, et al., 2015).

Benzodiazepines and neuroleptic drugs have also been reported to control chorea. Motor signs must be assessed and evaluated on an ongoing basis so that optimal therapeutic drug levels can be reached. Akathisia (motor restlessness) in the patient who is overmedicated is dangerous because it may be mistaken for the restless fidgeting of the illness and consequently may be overlooked. In certain types of the disease, hypokinetic motor impairment resembles PD. In patients who present with rigidity, some temporary benefit may be obtained from antiparkinsonian medications, such as levodopa.

Selective serotonin reuptake inhibitors and tricyclic antidepressants have been recommended for control of psychiatric symptoms. The threat of suicide is present particularly early in the course of the disease. Psychotic symptoms usually respond to antipsychotic medications. Psychotherapy aimed at allaying anxiety and reducing stress may be beneficial. Nurses must look beyond the disease to focus on the patient's needs and capabilities (Chart 67-5).

Patients who have emotional disturbances, particularly depression, may be helped by antidepressant medications. Several new treatments, such as stem cell transplantation and gene therapy are under investigation (Bordelon, 2013).

Promoting Home, Community-Based, and Transitional Care

Educating Patients About Self-Care

The needs of the patient and family for education depend on the nature and severity of the physical, cognitive, and psychological changes experienced by the patient. The patient and family members are taught about the medications prescribed and about signs indicating a need for change in medication or dosage. The teaching plan addresses strategies to manage symptoms such as chorea, swallowing problems, limitations in ambulation, and loss of bowel and bladder function. Consultation with a speech therapist may be indicated to assist in identifying alternative communication strategies if speech is affected.

Continuing and Transitional Care

A program combining medical, nursing, psychological, social, occupational, speech, and physical rehabilitation services and palliative care is needed to help the patient and family cope with this severely disabling illness. Huntington's disease exacts enormous emotional, physical, social, and financial tolls on every member of the patient's family. The family needs supportive care as they adjust to the impact of the illness. Regular follow-up visits help allay the fear of abandonment.

Home care assistance, day care centres, respite care, and eventually skilled long-term care can assist the patient and family in coping with the constant strain of the illness. Although the relentless progression of the disease cannot be halted, families can benefit from the supportive care of knowledgeable health care workers who endeavour to provide excellence in care during all phases of the disease (Harding, Stewart, & Knight, 2012).

Voluntary organizations can be major aids to families and have been largely responsible for bringing the illness to national attention. The Huntington's Society of Canada helps patients and families by providing information, referrals, family and public education, and support for research.

Amyotrophic Lateral Sclerosis

ALS is a disease where there is a loss of motor neurons (nerve cells controlling muscles) in the anterior horns of the spinal cord and the motor nuclei of the lower brain stem. It is often referred to as Lou Gehrig's disease after the famous baseball player who suffered from the disease. As motor neuron cells die, the muscle fibres that they supply undergo atrophic changes. Neuronal degeneration may occur in both the upper and lower motor neuron systems (see Chapter 63). ALS is theorized to be a complex genetic disorder that interacts with environmental factors. Among the 90% of cases that are classified as sporadic ALS, genetic mutation is thought to play a causative role (Harms & Baloh, 2013).

Approximately 2,500 to 3,000 Canadians live with ALS (ALS Society of Canada, 2014). ALS affects more men than women, with onset occurring usually in the fifth or sixth decade of life. Several risk factors have been identified, such as cigarette smoking and aluminum exposure, but the exact cause is still unknown (Antao & Horton, 2012; Bellomo & Cichminski, 2015; de Jong, Huisman, Sutedja, et al., 2012; Fitzgerald, O'Reilly, Fondell, et al., 2013). Whatever the cause, once ALS is initiated, numerous cellular events such as, oxidative stress, overexcitation of nerve cells by the neurotransmitter glutamate, mitochondrial dysfunction, and growth factor deficiency, occur. Eventually the affected motor neuron cells die.

The majority of cases of ALS arise sporadically, but 5% to 10% of cases are familial ALS resulting from an autosomal dominant trait carried by one parent. Familial ALS occurs 10 years earlier than the ALS average, and those afflicted tend to have a shorter life span (Bellomo & Cichminski, 2015). About 30% of patients with ALS live for 5 years after

CHART 67-5

Care of the Patient With Huntington's Disease

Nursing Priorities: Injury from falls and skin breakdown (pressure ulcers, abrasions), resulting from constant movement

Nursing Interventions

Pad the sides and head of the bed; ensure that the patient can see over the sides of bed.
Use padded heel and elbow protectors.
Keep the skin meticulously clean.
Apply emollient cleansing agent and skin lotion as needed.
Use soft sheets and bedding.
Have patient wear football padding or other forms of padding.
Encourage ambulation with assistance to maintain muscle tone.
Secure the patient (only if necessary) in bed or chair with padded protective devices, making sure that they are loosened frequently.

Nursing Priorities: Lack of nutrition, less than body requirements, likely due to inadequate intake and dehydration resulting from swallowing or chewing disorders and danger of choking or aspirating food

Nursing Interventions

Administer phenothiazines as prescribed before meals (appears to calm some patients).
Talk to the patient before mealtime to promote relaxation; use mealtime for social interaction. Provide undivided attention and help the patient enjoy the mealtime experience.
Use a warming tray to keep food warm.
Learn the position that is best for *this* patient. Keep patient as close to upright as possible while feeding. Stabilize patient's head gently with one hand while feeding.
Show the food and explain what the foods are (e.g., whether hot or cold).
Encircle the patient with one arm and get as close as possible to provide stability and support while feeding. Use pillows and wedges for additional support.
Do not interpret stiffness, turning away, or sudden turning of the head as rejection; these are uncontrollable choreiform movements.
For feeding, use a long-handled spoon (iced-tea spoon). Place spoon on middle of tongue and exert slight pressure.
Place bite-sized food between patient's teeth. Serve stews, casseroles, and thick liquids.
Disregard messiness and treat the person with dignity.
Wait for the patient to chew and swallow before introducing another spoonful. Make sure that bite-sized food is small.
Give between-meal feedings. Constant movement expends more calories. Patients often have voracious appetites, particularly for sweets.
Use blenderized meals if patient cannot chew; do not repeatedly give the same strained baby foods; gradually introduce increased textures and consistencies to the diet.
For swallowing difficulties:
  Apply gentle deep pressure around the patient's mouth.
  Rub fingers in circles on the patient's cheeks and then down each side of the patient's throat.
Develop skill in Heimlich manoeuvre (to be used in the event of choking).

Nursing Priorities: Anxiety and impaired communication

Nursing Interventions

Read to the patient.
Employ biofeedback and relaxation therapy to reduce stress.
Consult with speech therapist to help maintain and prolong communication abilities.
Try to devise a communication system, perhaps using cards with words or pictures of familiar objects, before verbal communication becomes too difficult. Patients can indicate correct card by hitting it with hand, grunting, or blinking the eyes.
Learn how this particular patient expresses needs and wants—particularly nonverbal messages (widening of eyes, responses).
Patients can understand even if unable to speak. Do not isolate patients by ceasing to communicate with them.

Nursing Priorities: Disturbed thought processes and impaired social interaction

Nursing Interventions

Reorient the patient after awakening.
Have clock, calendar, and wall posters in view to assist in orientation.
Use every opportunity for one-to-one contact.
Use music for relaxation.
Have the patient wear a medical identification bracelet.
Keep the patient in the social mainstream.
Recruit and train volunteers for social interaction. Role-model appropriate and creative interactions.
Do not abandon a patient because the disease is eventually terminal. Patients are *living* until the end.

diagnosis, with 10% to 20% surviving for up to 10 years and 5% surviving greater than 20 years postdiagnosis.

Clinical Manifestations

Clinical manifestations depend on the location of the affected motor neurons, because specific neurons activate specific muscle fibres. The chief symptoms are fatigue, progressive muscle weakness, cramps, fasciculations (twitching), and incoordination. Loss of motor neurons in the anterior horns of the spinal cord results in progressive weakness and atrophy of the muscles of the arms, trunk, or legs. Spasticity usually is present, and the deep tendon stretch reflexes become brisk and overactive. Usually, the function of the anal and bladder sphincters remains intact, because the spinal nerves that control muscles of the rectum and urinary bladder are not affected.

In about 25% of patients, weakness starts in the muscles supplied by the cranial nerves, and difficulty in talking, swallowing, and ultimately breathing occurs. When the patient ingests liquids, soft palate and upper esophageal weakness causes the liquid to be regurgitated through the nose. Weakness of the posterior tongue and palate impairs the ability to laugh, cough, or even blow the nose. If bulbar muscles are impaired, speaking and swallowing are progressively difficult, and aspiration becomes a risk. The voice assumes a nasal sound, and articulation becomes so disrupted that speech is unintelligible. Some emotional liability may be present. It was traditionally believed that ALS spared cognitive function, but it is now recognized that some patients experience cognitive impairment.

The prognosis generally is based on the area of CNS involvement and the speed with which the disease progresses. Eventually, respiratory function is compromised. Death usually occurs as a result of infection, respiratory failure, or aspiration.

Assessment and Diagnostic Findings

ALS is diagnosed on the basis of the signs and symptoms, because no clinical or laboratory tests are specific for this disease. Electromyography and muscle biopsy studies of the affected muscles indicate reduction in the number of functioning motor units. An MRI scan may show high signal intensity in the corticospinal tracts; this differentiates ALS from a multifocal motor neuropathy. Neuropsychological testing can assist in assessment and diagnosis (Hickey, 2014).

Management

No specific therapy exists for ALS. The main focus of medical and nursing management is on interventions to maintain or improve function, well-being, and quality of life. The average survival time is 3 to 5 years with death due, most commonly, to respiratory insufficiency (Majmuder, Wu, & Paganoni, 2014).

The medication riluzole (Rilutek), which is a glutamate antagonist, and Nuedexta, which is used to treat emotional lability, are both approved by the Food and Drug Administration for treatment of ALS (ALS Society of Canada, 2014). The action of riluzole is not clear, but its use has prolonged survival by 3 to 6 months (Hickey, 2014). Symptomatic treatment and rehabilitative measures are used to support the patient and improve the quality of life. Baclofen (Lioresal), dantrolene sodium (Dantrium), or diazepam (Valium) may be useful for patients troubled by spasticity, which causes pain and interferes with self-care. Research continues to test new drugs, such as tirasemtiv (ALS Society of Canada, 2014) and novel therapies such as stem cell transplants in an effort to treat ALS (Prabhakar, Marwaha, Lal, et al., 2012). Most patients with ALS are managed at home and in the community, with hospitalization for acute problems. The most common reasons for hospitalization are dehydration and malnutrition, pneumonia, and respiratory failure; recognizing these problems at an early stage in the illness allows for the development of preventive strategies. End-of-life issues include pain, dyspnea, and delirium (Hickey, 2014). Mechanical ventilation (using negative-pressure ventilators) is an option if alveolar hypoventilation develops. Noninvasive positive-pressure ventilation is also an option. The use of noninvasive positive-pressure ventilation is particularly helpful at night and postpones the decision about whether to undergo a tracheotomy for long-term mechanical ventilation.

A patient experiencing aspiration and swallowing may require enteral feeding. A percutaneous endoscopic gastrostomy tube is inserted before the forced vital capacity drops below 50% of the predicted value. The tube can be safely placed in patients who are using noninvasive positive-pressure ventilation for ventilatory support (Hickey, 2014).

Decisions about life support measures are made by the patient and family and should be based on a thorough understanding of the disease, the prognosis, and the implications of initiating such therapy. Patients are encouraged to complete an advance directive or "living will" to preserve their autonomy in decision making. See Chapter 15 for additional discussion of end-of-life care.

The ALS Society of Canada provides information and support to patients and their families. In partnership with other organizations and agencies, the ALS Society also supports research activities.

Muscular Dystrophies

Muscular dystrophies are a group of genetic, incurable muscle disorders characterized by progressive weakening and wasting of the skeletal or voluntary muscles (Shieh, 2013). They have been classified according to their clinical presentation and affected muscle regions. For example, Duchenne muscular dystrophy, the most common type, which occurs in 1 of every 4,700 male births (Bader et al., 2016), delays motor development, enlarges calf muscles, weakens proximal muscles, and causes cardiomyopathy (Allen, Thrush, Hoffman, et al., 2012). Another type, limb girdle muscular dystrophy, which refers to a large group of genetics subtypes, causes proximal muscle weakness while sparing facial and distal muscles. Recent genetic advances have increased the identification of specific genetic syndromes for limb girdle muscular dystrophy. Similarly, knowledge of cellular dysfunctioning has expanded (Shieh, 2013). Concomitantly, there has been development of novel therapies such as viral gene therapy, stem cell transplants, and new pharmaceuticals that seek to interrupt the altered cellular pathways (Leung & Wagner, 2013). The therapeutic safety and efficacy of novel therapies are being researched through clinical trials (Kang, Morrison, Iannaccone, et al., 2015).

The pathologic features of all muscular dystrophies include degeneration and loss of muscle fibres, variation in muscle fibre size, phagocytosis and regeneration, and replacement of muscle tissue by connective tissue. The common characteristics of these diseases include varying degrees of muscle wasting and weakness and abnormal elevation in serum levels of muscle enzymes. Differences among these diseases centre on the genetic pattern of inheritance, the muscles involved, the age at onset, and the rate of disease progression. The unique needs of these patients, who in the past did not live to adulthood, must be addressed as they live longer as a result of better supportive care.

Medical Management

Treatment of the muscular dystrophies at this time focuses on supportive care and prevention of complications in the absence of a cure or specific pharmacologic interventions (Kang, Morrison, Iannaccone, et al., 2015). The goal of supportive management is to keep the patient active and functioning as normally as possible and to minimize functional deterioration. An individualized therapeutic exercise program is prescribed to prevent muscle tightness, contractures, and disuse atrophy. Night splints and stretching exercises are used to delay contractures of the joints, especially the ankles, knees, and hips. Braces may compensate for muscle weakness.

Spinal deformity is a severe problem. Weakness of trunk muscles and spinal collapse occur almost routinely in patients with severe neuromuscular disease. To help prevent spinal deformity, the patient is fitted with an orthotic jacket or brace to improve sitting stability and reduce trunk deformity. This measure also supports cardiovascular status. In time, spinal fusion is performed to maintain spinal stability. Other procedures may be carried out to correct deformities or help alleviate pain.

Compromised pulmonary function may result either from progression of the disease or from deformity of the thorax secondary to severe scoliosis. Upper respiratory infections and fractures from falls must be vigorously treated in a way that minimizes immobilization because joint contractures become worse when the patient's activities are more restricted than usual.

Other difficulties may be manifested in relation to the underlying disease. Weakness of the facial muscles makes it difficult to attend to dental hygiene and to speak clearly. Gastrointestinal tract problems may include gastric dilation, rectal prolapse, and fecal impaction. Finally, cardiomyopathy appears to be a common complication in all forms of muscular dystrophy (Kang, Morrison, Iannaccone, et al., 2015).

Genetic counselling is advised for parents and siblings of the patient because of the genetic nature of this disease. The Muscular Dystrophy Association works to combat neuromuscular disease through research, programs of patient services and clinical care, and professional and public education (see Resources).

Nursing Management

The goals of the patient and the nurse are to maintain function at optimal levels and to enhance the quality of life. Therefore, the patient's physical requirements, which are considerable, are addressed without losing sight of emotional and developmental needs. The patient and family are actively involved in decision making, including end-of-life decisions.

During hospitalization for treatment of complications, the knowledge and expertise of the patient and family members responsible for caregiving in the home are assessed. Because the patient and family caregivers often have developed caregiving strategies that work effectively for them, these strategies need to be acknowledged and accepted, and provisions must be made to ensure that they are maintained during hospitalization.

Families of adolescents and young adults with muscular dystrophy need assistance to shift the focus of care from pediatric to adult care and to understand the usual disease course. Nursing goals include assisting the adolescent to make the transition to adult values and expectations while providing age-appropriate ongoing care. The nurse may need to help build the confidence of an older adolescent or adult patient by encouraging him or her to pursue job training to become economically independent. Other nursing interventions might include guidance in accessing adult health care and finding appropriate programs in sex education.

Promoting Home, Community-Based, and Transitional Care

Educating Patients About Self-Care

The management goals are addressed in special rehabilitation programs or in the patient's home and community. Therefore, the patient and family require information and instruction about the disorder, its anticipated course, and care and management strategies that will optimize the patient's growth and development and physical and psychological status. Members of a variety of health-related disciplines are involved in patient and family teaching; recommendations are communicated to all members of the health care team so that they may work toward common goals.

Continuing and Transitional Care

Both the neuromuscular disease and the associated deformities may progress in adolescence and adulthood. Self-help and assistive devices can aid in maintaining maximum independence. These devices, recommended by physical and occupational therapists, often become necessary as more muscle groups are affected.

The family is taught to monitor the patient for respiratory problems, because respiratory infection and cardiac failure are the most common causes of death (Dalton & Sampson, 2015). As respiratory difficulties develop, patients and their families need information regarding respiratory support. Options currently exist that can provide ventilatory support (e.g., negative-pressure devices, positive-pressure ventilators) while allowing mobility. Patients can remain relatively independent in a wheelchair, for example, while being maintained on a ventilator at home for many years.

The patient is encouraged to continue with range-of-motion exercises to prevent contractures, which are particularly disabling. Practical adaptations must be made, however, to cope with the effects of chronic neuromuscular disability. The patient at various stages of the disease may require a manual or an electric wheelchair, gait aids, upper and lower extremity and spinal orthoses, seating systems, bathroom equipment, lifts, ramps, and additional assistive devices, all of which require a team approach. The home care nurse assesses how the patient and family are managing, makes referrals, and coordinates the activities of the physical therapist, occupational therapist, and social services.

The patient is greatly concerned about issues surrounding the threat of increasing disability and dependence on others, accompanied by a significant deterioration in health-related quality of life. The patient is faced with a progressive loss of function, leading eventually to death. Feelings of helplessness and powerlessness are common. Each functional loss is accompanied by grief and mourning. The patient and family are assessed for depression, anger, or denial. The patient and family are assisted and encouraged to address decisions about end-of-life options before their need arises.

A psychiatric nurse counsellor or other mental health professional may assist the patient to cope and adapt to the disease. By understanding and addressing the physical and psychological needs of the patient and family, the nurse provides a hopeful, supportive, and nurturing environment

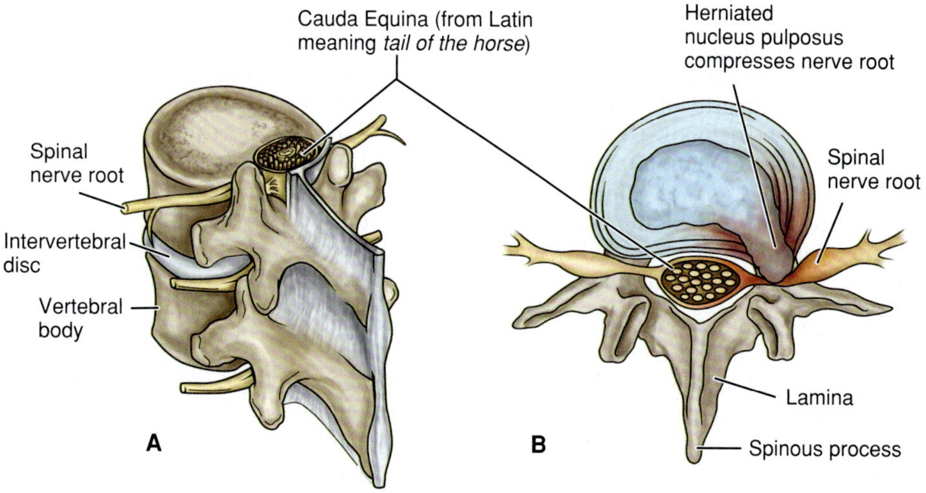

FIGURE 67-7. **A.** Normal lumbar spine vertebrae, intervertebral discs, and spinal nerve root. **B.** Ruptured vertebral disc.

(LaDonna et al., 2016). One study reported that adult patients' illness perceptions are directly connected to their quality of life in muscular dystrophy, and these perceptions influence their overall mood (Graham, Weinman, Sadjadi, et al., 2014).

Degenerative Disc Disease

In Canada, low back pain is a significant public health disorder. It is estimated that 80% of Canadians will develop back pain during their lifetime (Back Pain Canada, 2014). This results in significant economic and social costs. Acute low back pain lasts less than 3 months; chronic or degenerative disc disease has a duration of 3 months or longer. Most back problems are related to disc disease.

Pathophysiology

The intervertebral disc is a cartilaginous plate that forms a cushion between the vertebral bodies (Fig. 67-7A). This tough, fibrous material is incorporated in a capsule. A ball-like cushion in the centre of the disc is called the nucleus pulposus. In herniation of the intervertebral disc (ruptured disc), the nucleus of the disc protrudes into the annulus (the fibrous ring around the disc), with subsequent nerve compression. Protrusion or rupture of the nucleus pulposus usually is preceded by degenerative changes that occur with aging. Loss of protein polysaccharides in the disc decreases the water content of the nucleus pulposus. The development of radiating cracks in the annulus weakens resistance to nucleus herniation. After trauma (falls and repeated minor stresses such as lifting incorrectly), the cartilage may be injured.

For most patients, the immediate symptoms of trauma are short lived, and those resulting from injury to the disc do not appear for months or years. Then, with degeneration in the disc, the capsule pushes back into the spinal canal, or it may rupture and allow the nucleus pulposus to be pushed back against the dural sac or against a spinal nerve as it emerges from the spinal column (see Fig. 67-7B). This sequence produces pain due to radiculopathy (pressure in the area of distribution of the involved nerve endings). Continued pressure may produce degenerative changes in the involved nerve, such as changes in sensation and deep tendon reflexes.

Clinical Manifestations

A herniated disc with accompanying pain may occur in any portion of the spine: cervical, thoracic (rare), or lumbar. The clinical manifestations depend on the location, the rate of development (acute or chronic), and the effect on the surrounding structures.

Assessment and Diagnostic Findings

A thorough health history and physical examination are important to rule out potentially serious conditions that may manifest as low back pain, including fracture, tumour, infection, or cauda equina syndrome (Hickey, 2014).

The MRI scan has become the diagnostic tool of choice for localizing even small disc protrusions, particularly for lumbar spine disease. If the clinical symptoms are not consistent with the pathology seen on MRI, CT scanning, and myelography are performed. A neurologic examination is carried out to determine whether reflex, sensory, or motor impairment from root compression is present and to provide a baseline for future assessment. Electromyography may be used to localize the specific spinal nerve roots involved.

Medical Management

Herniations of the cervical and the lumbar discs occur most commonly and are usually managed conservatively with bed rest and medication (Hickey, 2014). Surgery is sometimes necessary.

Surgical Management

Surgical excision of a herniated disc is performed if there is evidence of a progressing neurologic deficit (muscle weakness and atrophy, loss of sensory and motor function, loss of sphincter control) and continuing pain or **sciatica** (leg pain resulting from sciatic nerve involvement) that are unresponsive to conservative management. The goal of surgical treatment is to reduce the pressure on the nerve root to relieve pain and reverse neurologic deficits (Hickey, 2014). Microsurgical techniques make it possible to remove only the amount of tissue that is necessary, which preserves the integrity of normal tissue better and imposes less trauma on the body. During these procedures, spinal cord function can be monitored electrophysiologically.

To achieve the goal of pain relief, several surgical techniques are used, depending on the type and location of disc herniation, surgical morbidity, and results of previous surgery. Some of the surgical techniques available include:

- Microdiscectomy: removal of herniated or extruded fragments of intervertebral disc material
- Laminectomy: removal of the bone between the spinal process and facet–pedicle junction to expose the neural elements in the spinal canal (Hickey, 2014); this allows the surgeon to inspect the spinal canal, identify and remove pathologic tissue, and relieve compression of the cord and roots
- Hemilaminectomy: removal of part of the lamina and part of the posterior arch of the vertebra
- Partial laminectomy or laminotomy: creation of a hole in the lamina of a vertebra
- Discectomy with fusion: fusion of the vertebral spinous process with a bone graft (from iliac crest or bone bank); the object of spinal fusion is to bridge over the defective disc to stabilize the spine and reduce the rate of recurrence
- Foraminotomy: opening up of the intervertebral foramen to increase the space for exit of a spinal nerve, resulting in reduced pain, compression, and edema

Herniation of a Cervical Intervertebral Disc

The cervical spine is subjected to stresses that result from disc degeneration (due to aging, occupational stresses) and **spondylosis** (degenerative changes occurring in a disc and adjacent vertebral bodies). Cervical disc degeneration may lead to lesions that can cause damage to the spinal cord and its roots (Bader et al., 2016).

Clinical Manifestations

A cervical disc herniation usually occurs at the C5–C6 or C6–C7 interspaces. Pain and stiffness may occur in the neck, the top of the shoulders, and the region of the scapulae. Sometimes patients interpret these signs as symptoms of heart trouble or bursitis. Pain may also occur in the upper extremities and head, accompanied by **paresthesia** (tingling or a "pins and needles" sensation) and numbness of the upper extremities. Cervical MRI usually confirms the diagnosis. Occasionally, the disc herniates centrally onto the spinal cord, causing Lhermitte's syndrome, an electriclike shock sensation in the extremities or spine with neck flexion or straining, and bilateral arm and leg weakness (myelopathy).

Medical Management

The goals of treatment are to rest and immobilize the cervical spine to give the soft tissues time to heal and to reduce inflammation in the supporting tissues and the affected nerve roots in the cervical spine. Bed rest (usually 1 to 2 days) is important because it eliminates the stress of gravity and relieves the cervical spine of the need to support the head. It also reduces inflammation and edema in soft tissues around the disc, relieving pressure on the nerve roots. Proper positioning on a firm mattress may bring dramatic relief from pain.

The cervical spine may be rested and immobilized by a cervical collar, cervical traction, or a brace. A collar allows maximal opening of the intervertebral foramina and holds the head in a neutral or slightly flexed position. The patient may have to wear the collar 24 hours a day during the acute phase. The skin under the collar is inspected for irritation. After the patient is free of pain, cervical isometric exercises are started to strengthen the neck muscles.

Pharmacologic Therapy

Analgesic agents (nonsteroidal anti-inflammatory agents [NSAIDs], propoxyphene [Darvon], oxycodone [Tylox], or hydrocodone [Vicodin]) are prescribed during the acute phase to relieve pain, and sedatives may be administered to control the anxiety that is often associated with cervical disc disease. Muscle relaxants (cyclobenzaprine [Flexeril], methocarbamol [Robaxin], metaxalone [Skelaxin]) and benzodiazepines (Valium) are administered to interrupt muscle spasm and to promote comfort. NSAIDs (aspirin, ibuprofen [Motrin, Advil], naproxen [Naprosyn, Anaprox], Toradol) or corticosteroids are prescribed to treat the inflammation that usually occurs in the affected nerve roots and supporting tissues. Occasionally, a corticosteroid is injected into the epidural space for relief of radicular (spinal nerve root) pain. NSAIDs are administered with food and antacids to prevent gastrointestinal irritation (Karch, 2014). Hot, moist compresses (for 10 to 20 minutes) applied to the back of the neck several times daily increase blood flow to the muscles and help relax the patient and reduce muscle spasm.

Surgical Management

Surgical excision of the herniated disc may be necessary if there is a significant neurologic deficit, progression of the deficit, evidence of cord compression, or pain that either worsens or fails to improve. A cervical discectomy, with or without fusion, may be performed to alleviate symptoms (Gebremariam, Koes, Peul, et al., 2012). An anterior surgical approach may be used through a transverse incision to remove disc material that has herniated into the spinal canal and foramina, or a posterior approach may be used at the appropriate level of the cervical spine. Potential complications with the anterior approach include carotid or vertebral artery injury, recurrent laryngeal nerve dysfunction, esophageal perforation, and airway obstruction. Complications of the posterior approach include damage to the nerve root or the spinal cord due to retraction or contusion of either of these structures, resulting in weakness of muscles supplied by the nerve root or cord.

Microsurgery, such as endoscopic microdiscectomy, may be performed in selected patients through a small incision, using magnification techniques. This usually results in less tissue trauma and pain, and patients consequently have a shorter hospital stay compared with those who have conventional surgery.

Nursing Process

The Patient Undergoing a Cervical Discectomy

Assessment

The patient is asked about past injuries to the neck (whiplash), because unresolved trauma can cause persistent discomfort, pain and tenderness, and symptoms of arthritis in the injured joint of the cervical spine. Assessment includes determining the onset, location, and radiation of pain and assessing for paresthesias, limited movement, and diminished function of the neck, shoulders, and upper extremities. It is important to determine whether the symptoms are bilateral; with large herniations, bilateral symptoms may be caused by cord compression. The area around the cervical spine is palpated to assess muscle tone and tenderness. Range of motion in the neck and shoulders is evaluated.

The patient is asked about any health issues that may influence the postoperative course and quality of life. It is also important to assess mood and stress levels. The nurse determines the patient's need for information about the surgical procedure and reinforces what the physician has explained. Strategies for pain management are discussed with the patient (Hickey, 2014).

Nursing Priorities

Based on the assessment data, the patient's major nursing diagnoses may include the following:

- Acute pain likely due to surgical procedure
- Altered physical mobility
- Difficulty in Swallowing
- Lack of knowledge

Other nursing priorities may include preoperative anxiety, postoperative constipation, urinary retention related to the surgical procedure, self-care deficits related to use of a neck orthosis, and sleep pattern disturbance related to disruption in lifestyle.

Collaborative Problems/ Potential Complications

Based on all the assessment data, the potential complications may include the following:

- Hematoma at the surgical site, resulting in cord compression and neurologic deficit
- Recurrent or persistent pain after surgery

Planning and Goals

The goals for the patient may include relief of pain, improved mobility, increased knowledge and self-care ability, and prevention of complications.

Nursing Interventions

Relieving Pain

If the patient has had anterior cervical discectomy and fusion with bone removed from the iliac crest, considerable pain may be experienced at the donor site. Interventions consist of monitoring the donor site for hematoma formation, administering the prescribed postoperative analgesic agent, positioning for comfort, and reassuring the patient that the pain can be relieved. If the patient experiences a sudden increase in pain, extrusion of the graft may have occurred, requiring reoperation. A sudden increase in pain should be promptly reported to the surgeon.

The patient may experience a sore throat, hoarseness, and dysphagia due to temporary edema. These symptoms are relieved by throat lozenges, voice rest, and humidification. A puréed diet may be given if the patient has dysphagia.

Patients with degenerative disc disease are often prescribed numerous opioids and nonopioid medications.

Improving Mobility

Postoperatively, a cervical collar (neck orthosis) may be ordered which contributes to limited neck motion and altered mobility. The patient is instructed to turn the body instead of the neck when looking from side to side. The neck should be kept in a neutral (midline) position. The patient is assisted during position changes, to make sure that head, shoulders, and thorax are kept aligned. When assisting the patient to a sitting position, the nurse supports the patient's neck and shoulders. To increase stability, the patient should wear shoes when ambulating.

Monitoring and Managing Potential Complications

The patient is evaluated for bleeding and hematoma formation by assessing for excessive pressure in the neck or severe pain in the incision area. The dressing is inspected for serosanguineous drainage which suggests a dural leak. If this occurs, meningitis is a threat. A complaint of headache requires careful evaluation. Neurologic checks are made for swallowing deficits and upper and lower extremity weakness, because cord compression may produce rapid or delayed onset of paralysis. The patient who has had an anterior cervical discectomy is also assessed for a sudden return of radicular (spinal nerve root) pain, which may indicate instability of the spine.

Throughout the postoperative course, the patient is monitored frequently to detect any signs of respiratory difficulty, because retractors used during surgery may injure the recurrent laryngeal nerve, resulting in hoarseness and the inability to cough effectively and clear pulmonary secretions. In addition, the blood pressure and pulse are monitored to evaluate cardiovascular status.

Bleeding at the surgical site and subsequent hematoma formation may occur. Severe localized pain not relieved by analgesic agents should be reported to the surgeon. A change in neurologic status (motor or sensory function) should be reported promptly, because it suggests hematoma formation that may necessitate surgery to prevent irreversible motor and sensory deficits.

Promoting Home, Community-Based, and Transitional Care

EDUCATING PATIENTS ABOUT SELF-CARE. The patient's hospital stay is likely to be short; therefore, the patient and family should understand the care that is important for a smooth recovery. A cervical collar is usually worn for 6 weeks or longer depending on the patient's bone quality, or surgical procedure performed. The patient is instructed in use and care of the cervical collar. The patient is instructed to alternate tasks that involve minimal body movement (e.g., reading) with tasks that require greater body movement.

The patient is instructed about strategies for pain management and about signs and symptoms that may indicate complications that should be reported to the physician. The nurse assesses the patient's understanding of these management strategies, limitations, and recommendations. Additionally, the nurse assists the patient in identifying strategies to cope with ADLs (e.g., self-care, childcare) and minimize risks to the surgical site (Chart 67-6). A discharge teaching plan is developed collaboratively by members of the health care team to decrease the risk of recurrent disc herniation. Topics include those previously discussed as well as proper body mechanics, maintenance of optimal weight, proper exercise techniques, and modifications in activity.

CONTINUING AND TRANSITIONAL CARE. The patient is instructed to see the physician at prescribed intervals so that the physician can document the disappearance of old symptoms and assess the range of motion of the neck. Recurrent or persistent pain may occur despite removal of the offending disc or disc fragments. Patients who undergo discectomy usually have consented to surgery after prolonged pain; they have often undergone repeated courses of ineffective conservative management and previous surgeries to relieve the pain. Therefore, the recurrence or persistence of symptoms postoperatively, including pain and sensory deficits, is often discouraging for the patient and family. The patient who experiences recurrence of symptoms requires emotional support and understanding. Additionally, the patient is assisted in modifying activities and in considering options for subsequent treatment. The nurse reminds the patient and family members of the need to participate in health-promotion and health screening practices.

Evaluation

Expected patient outcomes may include the following:

1. Reports decreasing frequency and severity of pain
2. Demonstrates improved mobility
   a. Demonstrates progressive participation in self-care activities
   b. Identifies prescribed activity limitations and restrictions
   c. Demonstrates proper body mechanics
3. Is knowledgeable about postoperative course, medications, and home care management
   a. Lists the signs and symptoms to be reported postoperatively
   b. Identifies dose, action, and potential side effects of medications
   c. Identifies appropriate home care management activities and any restrictions
4. Has absence of complications
   a. Reports no increase in incision pain or sensory symptoms
   b. Demonstrates normal findings on neurologic assessment

Herniation of a Lumbar Disc

Approximately 90% to 95% of lumbar disc herniations occur at the L5–S1 region (Hickey, 2014). A herniated lumbar disc produces low back pain accompanied by varying degrees of sensory and motor impairment.

Clinical Manifestations

The patient complains of low back pain with muscle spasms, followed by radiation of the pain into one hip and down into the leg (sciatica). Pain is aggravated by actions that increase intraspinal fluid pressure, such as bending, lifting, or straining (as in sneezing or coughing), and usually is relieved by bed rest. Usually there is some type of postural deformity, because pain causes an alteration of the normal spinal mechanics. If the patient lies on the back and attempts to raise a leg in a straight position, pain radiates into the leg; this manoeuvre, called the straight leg-raising test, stretches the sciatic nerve. Additional signs include muscle weakness, alterations in tendon reflexes, and sensory loss.

Assessment and Diagnostic Findings

The diagnosis of lumbar disc disease is based on the history and physical findings and the use of imaging techniques such as MRI, CT, and myelography.

Medical Management

The objectives of treatment are to relieve pain, slow disease progression, and increase the patient's functional ability (AANN, 2014c). Bed rest, previously a standard in treatment of back pain, is no longer recommended. The American College of Physicians recommends patients remain active.

Because muscle spasm is prominent during the acute phase, muscle relaxants are used. Evidence supports the use of NSAIDs, which may be administered to counter the inflammation that usually occurs in the supporting

CHART 67-6

HOME CARE CHECKLIST • The Patient With Cervical Discectomy and Cervical Collar

At the completion of education, the patient and/or caregiver will be able to:

- Name the procedure that was performed and identify any permanent changes in anatomic structure or function as well as changes in ADLs, IADLs, roles, relationships, and spirituality.
- Identify interventions and strategies (e.g., durable medical equipment, adaptive equipment) used in adapting to any permanent changes in structure or function to promote safety and optimum functioning.
  - Use adequate mattress and chair support.
- State the name, dose, side effects, frequency, and schedule for all medications.
  - Describe nonpharmacologic interventions for pain relief used in conjunction to prescribed pain relief preparations.
- State how to obtain medical supplies and carry out dressing changes, wound care, and other prescribed regimens.
- State how to contact all members of the treatment team (e.g., health care providers, home care professionals, and durable medical equipment and supply vendor).
- Describe ongoing postoperative therapeutic regimen, including diet and activities to perform (e.g., exercises) and to limit or avoid (e.g., lifting, stair climbing, driving a car) during rehabilitation.
- Describe care for the surgical incision site.
- Keep staples or sutures clean and dry and cover with dry dressing.
- Demonstrate proper body mechanics and prescribed exercise techniques.
  - Describe how to modify activity for optimum functioning.
  - Avoid sitting or standing for more than 30 minutes.
  - Avoid twisting, flexing, extending, or rotating the neck.
  - Avoid sleeping in a prone position or the use of pillows to minimize neck flexion in bed; keep head in a neutral position.
  - Wear low-heeled shoes.
  - Place a wrinkle-free silk scarf under the collar to increase comfort.
  - **For men:** Shave without twisting or moving the neck. This may be done with help while lying flat or sitting. Remove only the front part of the collar for shaving.
- Practice stress reduction and relaxation techniques.
- Care of the cervical collar:
  - Wear the collar at all times until directed otherwise by the primary provider.
  - Wash the neck under the collar twice a day with mild soap.
  - Keep the neck still while the collar is open.
  - With the assistance of a helper, wash the neck in steps.
  - Lie flat and supine.
  - Open the Velcro tabs on each side of the collar and remove its front portion.
  - Gently wash and dry the neck.
  - Replace the front part of the collar and refasten the tabs.
  - Turn to one side with a thin pillow under the head.
  - Open one tab.
  - Gently wash and dry the back of the neck. Refasten the tab.
  - Turn to the other side and wash and dry this side. Refasten the tab.
- Notify primary provider if any signs or symptoms of infection occur, such as fever, redness or irritation, drainage, increased pain.
- Relate how to reach primary provider with questions or complications.
- State time and date of follow-up medical appointments, therapy, and testing.
- Identify sources of support (e.g., friends, relatives, faith community, support groups, caregiver support).
- Identify the need for health-promotion, disease prevention, and screening activities.

ADL, activities of daily living; IADL, independent activities of daily living.

tissues and the affected nerve roots. Contrarily, recent evidence suggests the use of systemic corticosteroids is ineffective for pain relief (Hickey, 2014). Short-term epidural injections of steroids have some beneficial effect. Moist heat and massage help relax muscles. Strategies for increasing the patient's functional ability include weight reduction, physical therapy, and biofeedback. Exercises, prescribed by physical therapists, can help strengthen back muscles and decrease pain (Hickey, 2014). Chapter 16 describes nursing interventions for the patient with pain.

Surgical Management

In the lumbar region, surgical treatment includes lumbar disc excision through a posterolateral laminotomy and the newer techniques of microdiscectomy and percutaneous discectomy. In microdiscectomy, an operating microscope is used to visualize the offending disc and compressed nerve roots; it permits a small incision (2.5 cm [1 in]) and minimal blood loss and takes about 30 minutes of operating time. Generally, the hospital stay is short, and the patient makes a rapid recovery. Several minimally invasive techniques in spinal surgery have led to improved patient outcomes and lower hospital costs, and research on these techniques is ongoing. Research suggests that intraoperative wound infiltration with bupivacaine hydrochloride solution decreases pain and the need for opioids postoperatively (Hickey, 2014).

Complications of Disc Surgery

A patient undergoing a disc procedure at one level of the vertebral column may have a degenerative process at other levels. A herniation relapse may occur at the same level or elsewhere, so the patient may become a candidate for another disc procedure. Arachnoiditis (inflammation of the arachnoid membrane) may occur after surgery (and after myelography); it involves an insidious onset of diffuse, frequently burning pain in the lower back, radiating into the buttocks. Disc excision can leave adhesions and scarring around the spinal nerves and dura, which then produce inflammatory changes that create chronic neuritis and neurofibrosis. Disc surgery may relieve pressure on the spinal nerves, but it does not reverse the effects of neural injury and scarring and the pain that results. Failed disc syndrome (recurrence of sciatica after lumbar discectomy) remains a cause of disability (Hickey, 2014).

Nursing Management

Providing Preoperative Care

Most patients fear surgery on any part of the spine and therefore need explanations about the surgery and reassurance that it will not weaken the back. When data are being collected for the health history, any reports of pain, paresthesia, or muscle spasm are recorded to provide a baseline for comparison after surgery. Health issues that may influence the postoperative course and quality of life (e.g., fatigue, mood, stress, patient expectations) are important to assess (Hickey, 2014). Preoperative assessment also includes an evaluation of movement of the extremities as well as bladder and bowel function. To facilitate the postoperative turning procedure, the patient is taught to turn as a unit (called logrolling) as part of the preoperative preparation (see Fig. 67-8). Before surgery, the patient is also encouraged to take deep breaths, cough, and perform muscle-setting exercises to maintain muscle tone.

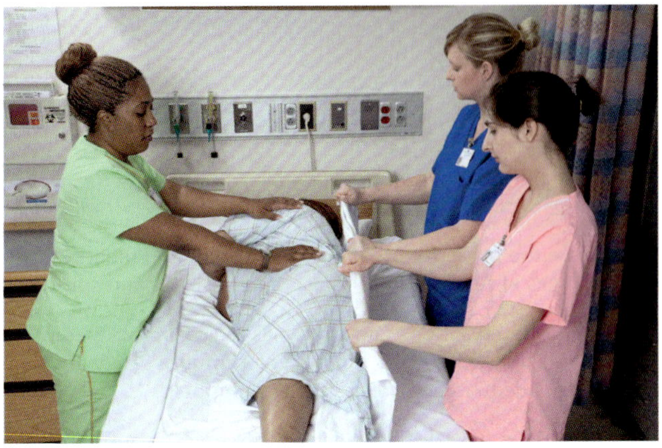

FIGURE 67-8. Before the patient undergoes laminectomy surgery, the logrolling technique that will be used for turning the patient should be demonstrated. The patient's arms will be crossed and the spine aligned. To avoid twisting the spine, the head, shoulders, knees, and hips are turned at the same time so that the patient rolls over like a log. When in a side-lying position, the patient's back, buttocks, and legs are supported with pillows.

Assessing the Patient After Surgery

After lumbar disc excision, vital signs are checked frequently and the wound is inspected for hemorrhage, because vascular injury is a complication of disc surgery. Because postoperative neurologic deficits may occur from nerve root injury, the sensation and motor strength of the lower extremities are evaluated at specified intervals, along with the colour and temperature of the legs and sensation of the toes. It is important to assess for urinary retention, another sign of neurologic deterioration.

In discectomy with fusion, the patient has an additional surgical incision if bone fragments were taken from the iliac crest or fibula to serve as wedges in the spine. The recovery period is longer than for those patients who underwent discectomy without spinal fusion, because bony union must take place.

Positioning the Patient

To position the patient, a pillow is placed under the head, and the knee rest is elevated slightly to relax the back muscles. When the patient is lying on one side, however, extreme knee flexion must be avoided. The patient is encouraged to move from side to side to relieve pressure and is reassured that no injury will result from moving. When the patient is ready to turn, the bed is placed in a flat position and a pillow is placed between the patient's legs. The patient turns as a unit (logrolls) without twisting the back.

To get out of bed, the patient lies on one side while pushing up to a sitting position. At the same time, the nurse or family member eases the patient's legs over the side of the bed. Coming to a sitting or standing posture is accomplished in one long, smooth motion. Most patients walk to the bathroom on the same day as the surgery. Sitting is discouraged except for defecation.

Promoting Home, Community-Based, and Transitional Care

Educating Patients About Self-Care

The patient is advised to increase activity gradually, as tolerated, because it takes up to 6 weeks for the ligaments to heal. Excessive activity may result in spasm of the paraspinal muscles.

Activities that produce flexion strain on the spine (e.g., driving a car) should be avoided until healing has taken place. Heat may be applied to the back to relax muscle spasms. Scheduled rest periods are important, and the patient is advised to avoid heavy work for 2 to 3 months after surgery. Exercises are prescribed to strengthen the abdominal and erector spinal muscles. A back brace or corset may be necessary if back pain persists.

Continuing and Transitional Care

Referral for inpatient or outpatient rehabilitation may be warranted to improve self-care abilities after medical or surgical treatment for herniation of a lumbar disc. A home care referral may be indicated and provides the home care nurse with the opportunity to assess the patient's physical and psychological status, as well as his or her ability to adhere to recommended management strategies. During the home visit, the nurse determines whether changes in neurologic function have occurred. The adequacy of pain management is assessed, and modifications are made to ensure adequate pain relief.

Postpolio Syndrome

People who survived the polio epidemic of the 1950s, many of whom are now elderly, are developing new symptoms of weakness, fatigue, and musculoskeletal pain. Researchers estimate that between 25% and 40% (Groce, Banks, & Stein, 2014) of the 1,000,000 polio survivors are experiencing the phenomenon known as postpolio syndrome. Women and greater severity of acute paralytic poliomyelitis are associated with an increased risk of developing postpolio syndrome (Bertolasi, Acler, dall'Ora, et al., 2012).

Pathophysiology

The exact cause of postpolio syndrome is not known, but researchers have proposed three main hypotheses. These include, overstress/overuse-induced degeneration of remaining neurons, the persistence of the polio virus, and neuroinflammation or immune-related damage (Bertolasi et al., 2012).

Assessment and Diagnostic Findings

No specific diagnostic test exists for postpolio syndrome. Clinical diagnosis is made on the basis of the history and physical examination and exclusion of other medical conditions that could be causing the new symptoms. Patients report a history of paralytic poliomyelitis followed by partial or complete recovery of function, with a plateau of function and then the recurrence of symptoms. Signs and symptoms may occur decades after the original onset of poliomyelitis (Woodward, 2014).

Management

No specific medical or surgical treatment is available for this syndrome, and therefore nurses play a pivotal role in the team approach to assisting patients and families in dealing with the symptoms of progressive loss of muscle strength and significant fatigue. Other health care professionals who may assist in patient care include physical, occupational, speech, and respiratory therapists. Nursing interventions are aimed at maintaining the patient's strength as well as physical, psychological, and social well-being (Woodward, 2014).

The patient needs to plan and coordinate activities to conserve energy and reduce fatigue. Rest periods should be planned and assistive devices used to reduce weakness and fatigue. Lifestyle changes and pacing are also used to cope with fatigue.

Pain in muscles and joints may be a problem. Nonpharmacologic techniques such as the application of heat and cold are most appropriate, because older patients may not tolerate or may have strong reactions to medications.

Maintaining a balance between adequate nutritional intake and avoiding excess calories that can lead to obesity in this sedentary group of patients is a challenge. Pulmonary hygiene and adequate fluid intake can help with airway management. Several interventions can improve sleep, including limiting caffeine intake before bedtime and assessing for nocturia. If nocturia is an issue, the patient needs to be evaluated for obstructive sleep apnea. Supportive ventilation may be appropriate, with continuous positive airway pressure if sleep apnea is a problem.

Bone density testing in patients with unilateral low limb involvement postpolio syndrome has revealed low bone mass and osteoporosis of the hips (Oncu, Atamaz, Durmas, et al., 2013). Therefore, the importance of identifying risks, preventing falls, and treating osteoporosis must be discussed with patients and families. Families also need to be made aware of the possibility of changes in individual and family relationships due to the many symptoms of postpolio syndrome (Woodward, 2014). The nurse also needs to remind patients and family members of the need for health-promotion activities and health screening.

Critical Thinking Exercises

1 A 34-year-old woman, working, married, with three children has been newly diagnosed with a spinal cord tumour. Assess and prioritize the patient's physiologic and psychosocial needs. What nursing interventions and actions would you suggest to assist in managing the treatment of and coping with a spinal cord tumour? How would this be different if the patient lives alone?

2 A 65-year-old man is newly diagnosed with ALS. Identify the evidence-based practices for the management of ALS. Describe the evidence base for the practices that you have identified and the criteria used to evaluate the strength of that evidence. Identify the health-promotion activities you would recommend to this patient and the rationale for your recommendations.

3 A 72-year-old woman is admitted for low back pain that radiates down her leg. What are your priorities for providing care for this patient? Give your rationale. What further diagnostic testing is needed? How will your priorities change if the patient is scheduled for back surgery?

REFERENCES AND SELECTED READINGS

Books

American Association of Neuroscience Nurses (AANN). (2014a). *Care of the adult patient with a brain tumor: AANN clinical practice guideline series*. Chicago, IL: Author.

American Association of Neuroscience Nurses (AANN). (2014b). *Care of movement disorder patient with deep brain stimulation: AANN clinical practice guideline series*. Chicago, IL: Author.

American Association of Neuroscience Nurses (AANN). (2014c). *Thoracolumbar spine surgery: A guide to preoperative and postoperative care: AANN clinical practice guideline series*. Chicago, IL: Author.

American Brain Tumor Association (ABTA). (2014). From https://www.abta.org/wp-content/uploads/2018/03/glioblastoma-brochure.pdf

Back Pain Canada. (2014). *Health professional*. Toronto: Author. Retrieved from http://www.backcarecanada.ca/site.php?sec_id=439&msid=3

Bader, M., Littlejohns, L. R., & Olson, D. (2016). *AANN core curriculum for neuroscience nursing* (6th ed.). Chicago, IL: American Association of Neuroscience Nurses.

Dalton, J., & Sampson, J. B. (2015). Chapter 18. Overview of adult muscular dystrophies. In: *Genetic counseling for adult neurodegenerative disease*. New York: Springer Science and Business.

Hickey, J. V. (2014). *The clinical practice of neurological & neurosurgical nursing* (7th ed.). Philadelphia, PA: Lippincott Williams & Wilkins.

Karch, A. M. (2014). *Lippincott's nursing drug guide* (12th ed.). Philadelphia, PA: Lippincott Williams & Wilkins.

Kennedy-Malone, L., Martin-Plank, L., & Duffy, E. (2018). *Advanced practice nursing in the care of older adults*. FA Davis.

Lawler, S., & Chiocca, E. (2013). Brain tumours and gliomas. In S. Geoffrey, Ginsburg, F. Huntington, et al. (Eds.), *Genomic and personalized medicine* (2nd ed., pp. 749–769). San Diego, CA: Elsevier.

Journals and Electronic Documents

Alzheimer Society of Canada. (2012). A new way of looking at the impact of dementia in Canada. Retrieved March 8, 2014, from http://www.alzheimer.ca/~/media/Files/national/Media-releases/asc_factsheet_new_data_09272012_en.ashx

Bellomo, T., & Cichminski, L. (2015). Amyotrophic lateral sclerosis: What nurses need to know. *Nursing*, *45*(10), 47–51.

Dhandapani, M., Gupta, S., Dhandapani, S., et al. (2015). Study of factors determining caregiver burden among primary caregivers of patients with intracranial tumors. *Surgical Neurology International*, *6*, 160.

Gallego Perez-Larraya, J., & Delattre, J. Y. (2014). Management of the elderly patient with gliomas. *Oncologist*, *19*(12), 1258–1267.

Gopalakrishna, A., & Alexander, S. A. (2015). Understanding Parkinson disease: A complex and multifaceted illness. *Journal of Neuroscience Nursing*, *47*(6), 320–326.

Graham, C. D., Weinman, J., Sadjadi, R., et al. (2014). A multicentre postal survey investigating the contribution of illness perceptions, coping and optimism to quality of life and mood in adults with muscle disease. *Clinical Rehabilitation*, *28*(5), 508–519.

Groce, N. E., Banks, L. M., & Stein, M. A. (2014). Surviving polio in a post-polio world. *Social Science and Medicine*, *107*, 171–178.

Kalia, L. V., & Lang, A. E. (2015). Parkinson's disease. *Lancet*, *386*(9996), 896–912.

Kang, P. B., Morrison, L., Iannaccone, S. T., et al. (2015). Evidence-based guideline summary: Evaluation, diagnosis, and management of congenital muscular dystrophy: Report of the Guideline Development Subcommittee of the American Academy of Neurology and the Practice Issues Review Panel of the American Association of Neuromuscular & Electrodiagnostic Medicine. *Neurology*, *84*(13), 1369–1378.

Kim, S. U., Lee, H., & Kim, Y. B. (2013). Neural stem cell-based treatment for neurodegenerative diseases. *Neuropathology*, *33*(5), 491–501.

Lin, N. U., Lee, E. Q., Aoyama, H., et al. (2015). Response assessment criteria for brain metastases: proposal from the RANO group. *The Lancet Oncology*, *16*(6), e270–e278.

Louis, D., Perry, A., Reinfenberger, G., et al. (2016). The 2016 World Health Organization Classification of Tumors of the Central Nervous System: A summary. *Acta Neuropathology*, *131*(6), 803–820.

Lukas, R. V., Buerki, R., & Mrugula, M. M. (2016). Management of leptomeningeal disease from solid tumors. *Oncology*, *30*(8), 724–730.

Majmuder, S., Wu, J., & Paganoni, S. (2014). Rehabilitation in amyotrophic lateral sclerosis: Why it matters. *Muscle Nerve*, *50*, 4–13.

Melmed, S. (2016). Pituitary medicines from discovery to patient focused outcomes. *Journal of Clinical Endocrinology and Metabolism*, *101*(3), 769–779.

Moore, D. J., Smith, B. M., & Cho, M. H. (2017). Managing meditations for hospital patients with Parkinson disease. *American Nurse Today*, *12*(1), 9–12.

Ostrom, Q. T., Gittleman, H., Fulop, J., et al. (2015). CBTRUS statistical report: Primary brain and central nervous system tumors diagnosed in the United States in 2008–2012. *Neuro-Oncology*. 2015;(17 Suppl 4): iv1–iv62.

Ownsworth, T., Goadby, E., & Chambers, S. K. (2015). Support after brain tumor means different things: Family caregivers' experiences of support and relationship changes. *Frontiers in Oncology*, *5*(33), 1–13.

Perkins, A., & Liu, G. (2016). Primary brain tumors in adults: Diagnosis and treatment. *American Family Physician*, *93*(3), 211–217.

Rigi, M., Almarzbuqi, S. J., Morgan, M. L., et al. (2015). Papilledema: Epidemiology, etiology, and clinical management. *Eye and Brain*, (7), 45–57.

Shank, C. D., Lepard, J. R., Walters, B. C., & Hadley, M. N. (2018). Towards evidence-based guidelines in neurological surgery. *Neurosurgery*. From https://doi.org/10.1093/neuros/nyy414

Smith, E. E. (2017). Clinical presentations and epidemiology of vascular dementia. *Clinical Science*, *131*(11), 1059–1068.

Woodward, S. (2014). Shining the spotlight on post-polio syndrome. *British Journal of Neuroscience Nursing*, *10*(1), 5.

World Health Organization & Alzheimer's Disease International. (2012). Dementia: A public health priority. Geneva: Publications of the World Health Organization. Retrieved March 7, 2014, from http://www.who.int/mental_health/publications/dementia_report_2012/en/

Amyotrophic Lateral Sclerosis

ALS Society of Canada. (2014). ALS Quick Facts. Retrieved March 8, 2014, from http://www.als.ca/sites/default/files/files/Fact%20Sheets/2011Research_Facts%20Sheet_Apr%2017.pdf

Antao, V. C., & Horton, D. K. (2012). The national amyotrophic lateral sclerosis registry. *Journal of Environmental Health*, *75*(1), 28–30.

de Jong, S. W., Huisman, M., Sutedja, N., et al. (2012). Smoking, alcohol consumption, and the risk of amyotrophic lateral sclerosis: A population-based study. *American Journal of Epidemiology*, *176*(3), 233–239.

Fitzgerald, K., O'Reilly, E., Fondell, E., et al. (2013). Intakes of vitamin C and careteniods and risk of amyotrophic lateral sclerosis: Pooled results from 5 cohort studies. *Annuals of Neurology*, *73*(2), 236–245.

Harms, M., & Baloh, R. (2013). Clinical neurogenetics. *Neurologic Clinics*, *31*(4), 929–950.

Prabhakar, S., Marwaha, N., Lal, V., et al. (2012). Autologous bone-marrow-derived stem cells in amyotrophic lateral sclerosis: A pilot study. *Neurology India*, *60*(5), 465–469.

Degenerative Disc Disease

Debono, B., Bousquet, P., Sabatier, P., et al. (2016). Postoperative monitoring with a mobile application after ambulatory lumbar discectomy: An effective tool for spine surgeons. *European Spine Journal*, *25*(11), 3536–3542.

Díaz-Arribas, M. J., Fernández-Serrano, M., Royuela, A., et al. (2017). Minimal clinically important difference in quality of life for patients with low back pain. *Spine*, *42*(24), 1908–1916.

Faught, R. W., Church, E. W., Halpern, C. H., et al. (2016). Long-term quality of life after posterior cervical foraminotomy for radiculopathy. *Clinical Neurology and Neurosurgery*, *142*, 22–25.

Gebremariam, L., Koes, B. W., Peul, W. C., et al. (2012). Evaluation of treatment effectiveness for the herniated cervical review. *Spine (Phila Pa 1976)*, *37*(2), E109–E118.

Li, X., Han, Y., Di, Z., et al. (2016). Percutaneous endoscopic lumbar discectomy for lumbar disc herniation. *Journal of Clinical Neuroscience*, *33*, 19–27.

Schroeder, G. D., Boody, B. S., Kepler, C. K., et al. (2018). Comparing health-related quality of life outcomes in patients undergoing either primary or revision anterior cervical discectomy and fusion. *Spine, 43*(13), E752–E757.

Wilson, C. A., Roffey, D. M., Chow, D., et al. (2016). A systematic review of preoperative predictors for postoperative clinical outcomes following lumbar discectomy. *The Spine Journal, 16*(11), 1413–1422.

Huntington's Disease

Allen, H. D., Thrush, P. T., Hoffman, T. M., et al. (2012). Cardiac management in neuromuscular diseases. *Physical Medicine and Rehabilitation Clinics of North America, 23*(4), 855–868.

American Brain Tumour Association (ABTA). (2012a). About brain tumours: A primer for patients and caregivers: 2012. Retrieved February 28, 2014, from http://www.abta.org/secure/about-brain-tumours-a-primer.pdf

American Brain Tumour Association (ABTA). (2012b). Pituitary tumour: 2012. Retrieved February 27, 2014, from http://www.abta.org/secure/pituitary-tumours-brochure.pdf

Andersson, P., Juth, N., Petersen, A., et al. (2012). Ethical aspects of undergoing a predictive genetic testing for Huntington's disease. *Nursing Ethics, 20*(2), 189–199.

Armstrong, T. S., Shade, M. Y., Breton, G., et al. (2017). Sleep-wake disturbance in patients with brain tumors. *Neuro-Oncology, 19*(3), 323–335.

Bertolasi, L., Acler, M., dall'Ora, E., et al. (2012). Risk factors for post-polio syndrome among an Italian population: A case-control study. *Neurological Sciences, 33*, 1271–1275.

Bjornestad, A., Tysnes, O. B., Larsen, J. P., et al. (2016). Loss of independence in early Parkinson disease: A 5-year population-based incident cohort study. *Neurology*, 10–1212.

Bordelon, Y. (2013). Clinical neurogenetics. *Neurologic Clinics, 31*(4), 1085–1094.

Canadian Cancer Society's Advisory Committee on Cancer Statistics. (2013). *Canadian Cancer Statistics 2013*. Toronto, ON: Canadian Cancer Society.

Comelli, I., Lippi, G., Campana, V., et al. (2017). Clinical presentation and epidemiology of brain tumors firstly diagnosed in adults in the Emergency Department: A 10-year, single center retrospective study. *Annals of Translational Medicine, 5*(13), 269.

Domingos, J., Sarkozy, A., Scoto, M., et al. (2017). Dystrophinopathies and limb-girdle muscular dystrophies. *Neuropediatrics, 48*(04), 262–272.

Farge, D. (2013). International clinical practice guidelines for the treatment and prophylaxis of venous thromboembolism in patients with cancer. *Journal of Thrombosis and Haemostasis, 11*(1), 56–70.

Ferrer, I. (2016). Mini-symposium: Huntington's disease. *Brain Pathology, 26*(6), 724–725.

Goncalves, P. H., Peterson, S. L., Vigneau, F. D., et al. (2016). Risk of brain metastases in patients with nonmetastatic lung cancer: Analysis of the Metropolitan Detroit Surveillance, Epidemiology, and End Results (SEER) data. *Cancer, 122*(12), 1921–1927.

Ha, A., & Fung, V. (2012). Huntington's disease. *Current Opinion in Neurology, 25*(4), 491–498.

Harding, V., Stewart, I., & Knight, C. (2012). Health-care workers' perceptions of contributors to quality of life for people with Huntington's disease. *British Journal of Neuroscience Nursing, 8*(4), 191–197.

Hickey, P., & Stacy, M. (2016). Deep brain stimulation: A paradigm shifting approach to treat Parkinson's disease. *Frontiers in Neuroscience, 10*, 173.

Hohenberger, C., Schmidt, C., Höhne, J., et al. (2018). Effect of surgical decompression of spinal metastases in acute treatment—Predictors of neurological outcome. *Journal of Clinical Neuroscience, 52*, 74–79.

Johnson, M. O., Frank, S., Mendlik, M., et al. (2018). Utilization of hospice services in a population of patients with Huntington's disease. *Journal of Pain and Symptom Management, 55*(2), 440–443.

Kumar, A., Singh, S. K., Kumar, V., et al. (2015). Huntington's disease: An update of therapeutic strategies. *Gene, 556*(2), 91–97.

LaDonna, K. A., Koopman, W. J., Ray, S. L., et al. (2016). Hard to swallow: A phenomenological exploration of the experience of caring for individuals with myotonic dystrophy and dysphagia. *Journal of Neuroscience Nursing, 48*(1), 42–51

Leung, D. G., & Wagner, K. R. (2013). Therapeutic advances in muscular dystrophy. *Annals of Neurology, 74*, 404–411.

Lozano, C. S., Tam, J., & Lozano, A. M. (2018). The changing landscape of surgery for Parkinson's disease. *Movement Disorders, 33*(1), 36–47.

Lyman, G. H., Bohlke, K., Khorana, A. A., et al. (2015). Venous thromboembolism prophylaxis and treatment in patients with cancer: American Society of Clinical Oncology clinical practice guideline update 2014. *Journal of Clinical Oncology, 33*(6), 654–656.

Martin, S. C. (2015). Psychosocial challenges experienced by partners of people with Parkinson disease. *Journal of Neuroscience Nursing, 47*(4), 211–222.

Mechtler, L. L., & Nandigam, K. (2013). Spinal cord tumours. *Neurologic Clinics, 31*(1), 241–268.

Mestre, T. A., & Shannon, K. (2017). Huntington disease care: From the past to the present, to the future. *Parkinsonism & Related Disorders, 44*, 114–118.

Molitch, M. E. (2017). Diagnosis and treatment of pituitary adenomas: A review. *JAMA, 317*(5), 516–524.

Moskowitz, C. B., & Rao, A. K. (2017). Making a measurable difference in advanced Huntington disease care. In *Handbook of clinical neurology* (Vol. 144, pp. 183–196). Elsevier.

Musselman, M., & Saely S. (2013). Diagnosis and treatment of drug-induced hyperthermia. *American Journal of Health-System Pharmacy, 70*(1), 34–42.

Oncu, J., Atamaz, F., Durmas, B., et al. (2013). Psychometric properties of fatigue severity and fatigue impact scales in postpolio patients. *International Journal of Rehabilitation Research, 36*(4), 339–345.

Park, J. K., Vernick, D. M., Ramakrishna, N., & Wen, P. Y. (2016). *Vestibular schwannoma (acoustic neuroma)*. UpToDate, Waltham, MA.

Parkinson Society British Columbia. (2014). Parkinson's disease Fact Sheet. Retrieved March 2, 2014, from http://www.parkinson.bc.ca/Parkinsons-Disease-Fact-Sheet

Pasarikovski, C. R., Alotaibi, N. M., Al-Mufti, F., et al. (2017). Hypertonic saline for increased intracranial pressure after aneurysmal subarachnoid hemorrhage: A systematic review. *World Neurosurgery, 105*, 1–6.

Patel, T., Yu, J., & Piepmeier, J. (2012). Role of neurosurgery and radiation therapy in the management of brain tumours. *Hematology/Oncology Clinics of North America, 26*(4), 757–777.

Picillo, M., & Fasano, A. (2016). Recent advances in essential tremor: surgical treatment. *Parkinsonism & Related Disorders, 22*, S171–S175.

Postuma, R. B., Berg, D., Stern, M., et al. (2015). MDS clinical diagnostic criteria for Parkinson's disease. *Movement Disorders, 30*(12), 1591–1601.

Quelhas, R. (2013). Psychiatric care in Parkinson's disease. *Journal of Psychiatric Practice, 19*(2), 119–141.

Richards, J., & Ballard, N. (2008). Colloid cyst: A case study. *Journal of Neuroscience Nursing, 40*(2), 103–105.

Ross, C. A., Aylward, E. H., Wild, E. J., et al. (2014). Huntington's disease: National history, biomarkers and prospects for therapeutics. *Nature Reviews Neurology, 10*, 204–216.

Safarpour, D., Thibault, D. P., DeSanto, C. L., et al. (2015). Nursing home and end-of-life care in Parkinson disease. *Neurology, 85*(5), 413–419.

Schwarz, S., Thon, N., Nikolajek, K., et al. (2012). Iodine-125 brachytherapy for brain tumours—A review. *Radiation Oncology, 7*, 1–30.

Shieh, P. B. (2013). Muscular dystrophies and other genetic myopathies. *Neurologic clinics, 31*(4), 1009–1029.

Shin, J. Y., & Habermann, B. (2016a). Medication adherence in people with Parkinson disease. *Journal of Neuroscience Nursing, 48*(4), 185–204.

Shin, J. Y., & Habermann, B. (2016b). Nursing research in Parkinson's disease from 2006–2015: A systematic review. *Clinical Nursing Research*, (2016), 1–15.

Smith, S., D'Cruz, G., Gray, R., et al. (2015). A concept map of what helps people with HD live with their condition. *Journal of Huntington's Disease,4*(3), 261–270.

Srivanitchapoom, P., & Hallett, M. (2016). Camptocormia in Parkinson's disease: Definition, epidemiology, pathogenesis and treatment modalities. *Journal of Neurology, Neurosurgery, Psychiatry, 87*(1), 75–85.

Thompson, R., & Straub, V. (2016). Limb-girdle muscular dystrophies—International collaborations for translational research. *Nature Reviews Neurology, 12*(5), 294–309.

Tousi, B., & Wilson, K. (2013). Falls related to accidental deactivation of deep brain stimulators in patients with Parkinson's disease living in long term care facilities. *Journal of the American Medical Directors Association, 14*, 58–59.

Turner, M. C., Krewski, D., Armstrong, B. K., et al. (2013). Allergy and brain tumors in the INTERPHONE study: Pooled results from Australia, Canada, France, Israel, and New Zealand. *Cancer Causes and*

Control: An International Journal of Studies of Cancer in Human Populations, *24*(5), 949–960.
Varghese, M., Nymoen, H. G., Saxhaug, C., et al. (2016). Symptomatic spinal metastasis from intracranial glioblastoma multiforme—Two illustrative cases and a review of the literature. *Acta Oncologica*, *55*(9–10), 1236–1238.
Vecht, C. J., Kerkhof, M., & Duran-Pena, A. (2014). Seizure prognosis in brain tumors: New insights and evidence-based management. *The Oncologist*, *19*(7), 751–759.
Vermeulen, S., Prueter, J., Meier, R., Loiselle, C., & Landis, D. (2018). Clinical outcomes of acoustic neuromas patients treated with single fraction Vs multi-fraction radiosurgery. *Journal of Oncology Research and Therapy*: JONT-169. DOI, 10.
Warnoch, C., & Tod, A. (2013). A descriptive exploration of the experiences of patients with significant functional impairment following a recent diagnosis of metastatic spinal cord compression. *Journal of Advanced Nursing*, *70*(3), 564–574.
Wefel, J. S., Parsons, M. W., Gondi, V., et al. (2018). Neurocognitive aspects of brain metastasis. *Handbook of Clinical Neurology*, *149*, 155–165.
Wilson, E., Pollock, K., & Aubeeluck, A. (2014). Providing care services to people affected by Huntington's disease an overview of the challenges. *British Journal of Neuroscience Nursing*, *10*(3), 139–143.
Wilson, M. H. (2016). Monro-Kellie 2.0: The dynamic vascular and venous pathophysiological components of intracranial pressure. *Journal of Cerebral Blood Flow & Metabolism*, *36*(8), 1338–1350.
Winder, J. Y., Achterberg, W. P., & Roos, R. A. (2018). Marriage as protector for nursing home admission in Huntington's disease. *Journal of Huntington's Disease*, *7*(3), 263–269.

Resources

ALS Society of Canada/Société canadienne de la SLA: http://www.als.ca.
Brain Tumour Foundation of Canada: http://www.braintumour.ca.
British Columbia Cancer Agency: http://www.bccancer.bc.ca.
Canadian Cancer Society: http://www.cancer.ca.
Canadian Chiropractic Association: http://www.ccachiro.org.
Huntington Society of Canada/Société Huntington du Canada: http://www.huntingtonsociety.ca.
Michael J. Fox Foundation for Parkinson's Research: http://www.michaeljfox.org/index.cfm.
Muscular Dystrophy Canada: http://www.muscle.ca.
Parkinson Society Canada/Société Parkinson Canada: http://www.parkinson.ca.
Polio Canada: http://www.marchofdimes.ca/EN/programs/PolioCanada/Pages/default.aspx.

68 Oncology: Nursing Management in Cancer Care

Adapted by Alice S.W. Khin

Learning Objectives

On completion of this chapter, the learner will be able to:

1. Compare the structure and function of the normal cell and the cancer cell.
2. Differentiate between benign and malignant tumours.
3. Identify agents and factors that have been found to be carcinogenic.
4. Describe the significance of health education and preventive care in decreasing the incidence of cancer.
5. Differentiate among the purposes of surgical procedures used in cancer treatment, diagnosis, prophylaxis, palliation, and reconstruction.
6. Describe the roles of surgery, radiation therapy, chemotherapy, targeted therapy, hematopoietic stem cell transplantation, and other therapies in treating cancer.
7. Describe the special nursing needs of patients receiving chemotherapy.
8. Describe nursing care related to common nursing diagnoses associated with cancer: impaired skin integrity, alopecia, nutritional problems, and altered body image.
9. Identify potential complications for the patient with cancer and discuss associated nursing care.
10. Describe the concept of hospice in providing care for patients with advanced cancer.
11. Identify assessment parameters and nursing management of patients with oncologic emergencies.

Cancer is not a single disease with a single cause; rather, it is a group of distinct diseases with different causes, manifestations, treatments, and prognoses. Cancer nursing practice covers all age groups and nursing specialties and is carried out in a variety of health care settings, including the home, community, acute care institutions, outpatient centres, rehabilitation, and long-term care facilities. The scope, responsibilities, and goals of cancer nursing, also called **oncology** nursing, are as diverse and complex as those of any nursing specialty. Because many people associate cancer with pain and death, nurses need to identify their own reactions to cancer and set realistic goals to meet the challenges inherent in caring for patients with cancer.

The scope, responsibilities, and goals of cancer nursing, also called oncology nursing, are as diverse and complex as those of any nursing specialty. Nursing management of the patient with oncologic disorders includes care of patients throughout the cancer trajectory from prevention through end-of-life care (see Fig. 68-1).

Precision medicine is now possible because of the recent development of biologic databases (e.g., human genome sequencing), technologic advances that can identify unique characteristics of individual persons (e.g., genomics, cellular assay tests), and computer-driven systems that can mine and analyze datasets. This is an exciting time for oncology as the immediate goal of the precision medicine initiative is to focus on preventing and curing cancers (Collins & Varmus, 2015).

Epidemiology of Cancer

Although cancer affects people of all ages, cancer is more likely to occur in people older than 65 years of age. Overall, the incidence of cancer is higher in men than in women and higher in industrialized sectors and nations.

The Canadian Cancer Society estimates nearly 1 in 2 Canadians is expected to be diagnosed with cancer at some point during their lifetime. In 2017 alone, about 206,200 new cases of cancer were diagnosed in Canada. Although an increasing number of Canadians are surviving at least 5 years past their cancer diagnosis, cancer continues to be the leading cause of death in Canada. About 1 in 4 Canadians is expected to die from cancer (Canadian Cancer Society's Steering Committee, 2018). In 2017, an estimated:

- 103,100 Canadian men were diagnosed with cancer and 42,600 men died from cancer.
- 103,200 Canadian women were diagnosed with cancer and 38,200 women died from cancer.
- On average, 565 Canadians were diagnosed with cancer every day.
- On average, 221 Canadians died from cancer every day.

Glossary

alopecia: hair loss

anaplasia: cells that lack normal cellular characteristics and differ in shape and organization with respect to their cells of origin; usually, anaplastic cells are malignant

angiogenesis: growth of new blood vessels that allow cancer cells to grow

apoptosis: programmed cell death

benign: not cancerous; benign tumours may grow but are unable to spread to other areas

biologic response modifier (BRM) therapy: use of agents or treatment methods that can alter the immunologic relationship between the tumour and the host to provide a therapeutic benefit

biopsy: a diagnostic procedure to remove a small sample of tissue to be examined microscopically to detect malignant cells

brachytherapy: delivery of radiation therapy through internal implants

cancer: a disease process whereby cells proliferate abnormally, ignoring growth-regulating signals in the environment surrounding the cells

carcinogenesis: process of transforming normal cells into malignant cells

chemotherapy: use of medications to kill tumour cells by interfering with cellular functions and reproduction

control: containment of the growth of cancer cells

cure: prolonged survival and disappearance of all evidence of disease so that the patient has the same life expectancy as anyone else in his or her age group

cytokines: substances produced by cells of the immune system to enhance production and functioning of components of the immune system

dysplasia: bizarre cell growth resulting in cells that differ in size, shape, or arrangement from other cells of the same type of tissue

extravasation: leakage of medication from the veins into the subcutaneous tissues

grading: identification of the type of tissue from which the tumour originated and the degree to which the tumour cells retain the functional and structural characteristics of the tissue of origin

graft-versus-host disease (GVHD): an immune response initiated by T lymphocytes of donor tissue against the recipient's tissues (skin, gastrointestinal tract, liver); an undesirable response

graft-versus-tumour effect: the donor cell response against the malignancy; a desirable response

hyperplasia: increase in the number of cells of a tissue; most often associated with periods of rapid body growth

malignant: having cells or processes that are characteristic of cancer

metaplasia: conversion of one type of mature cell into another type of cell

metastasis: spread of cancer cells from the primary tumour to distant sites

myelosuppression: suppression of the blood cell–producing function of the bone marrow

nadir: lowest point of white blood cell depression after therapy that has toxic effects on the bone marrow

neoplasia: uncontrolled cell growth that follows no physiologic demand

neutropenia: abnormally low absolute neutrophil count

oncology: field or study of cancer

palliation: relief of symptoms and promotion of comfort and quality of life

precision medicine: using advances in research, technology, and policies to develop individualized plans of care to prevent and treat disease

radiation therapy: use of ionizing radiation to interrupt the growth of malignant cells

staging: process of determining the extent of disease, including tumour size and spread or metastasis to distant sites

stomatitis: inflammation of the oral tissues, often associated with some chemotherapeutic agents and radiation therapy to the head and neck region

targeted therapies: cancer treatments that seek to minimize the negative effects on healthy tissues by disrupting specific cancer cell functions, such as malignant transformation, communication pathways, processes for growth and metastasis, and genetic coding

thrombocytopenia: decrease in the number of circulating platelets; associated with the potential for bleeding

tumour-specific antigen (TSA): protein on the membrane of cancer cells that distinguishes the malignant cell from a benign cell of the same tissue type

vesicant: substance that can cause tissue necrosis and damage, particularly when extravasated

xerostomia: dry oral cavity resulting from decreased function of salivary glands

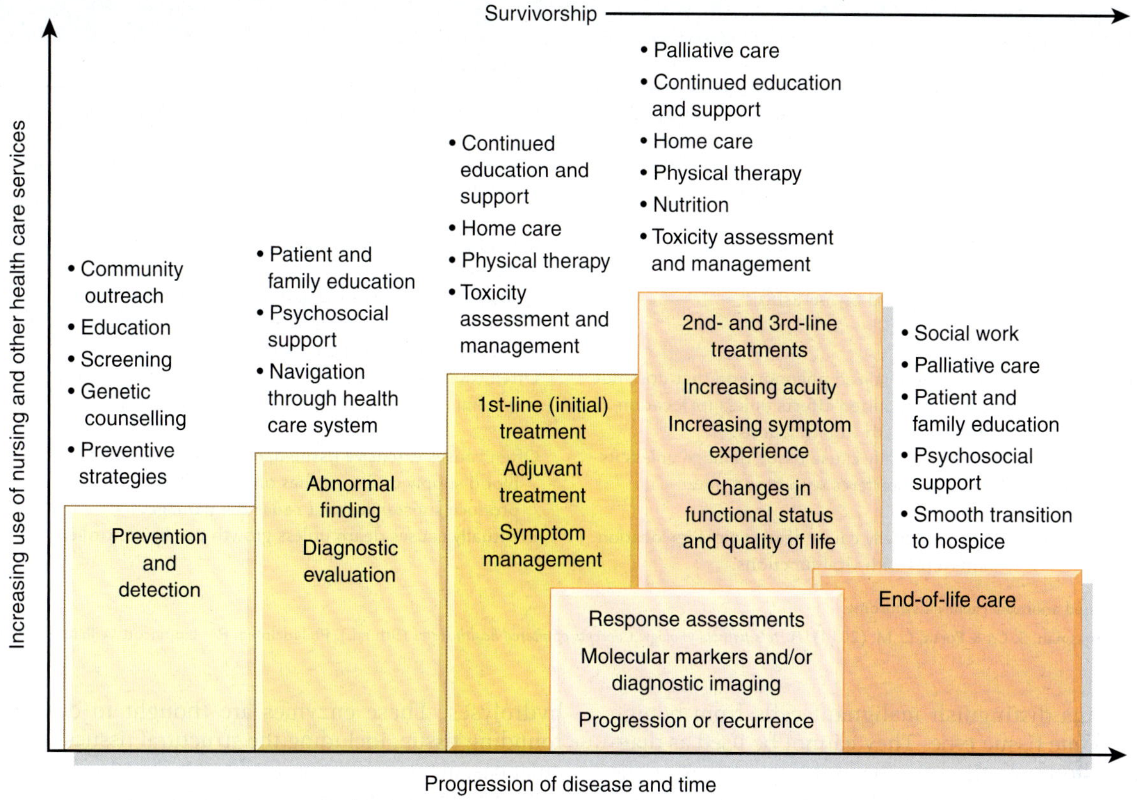

FIGURE 68-1. Cancer care trajectory. The cancer care trajectory reflects the phases and care required during the continuum of the cancer experience from prevention and early detection through end-of-life care. Specialized nursing care is provided throughout the entire trajectory.

Lung, breast, colorectal, and prostate cancers are the most common types of cancer in Canada (excluding nonmelanoma skin cancer) (Canadian Cancer Society, 2019).

Pathophysiology of the Malignant Process

Cancer is a disease process that begins when a cell is transformed by genetic mutations of the cellular deoxyribonucleic acid (DNA). Genetic mutations may be inherited and/or acquired, leading to abnormal cell behaviour (Grossman & Porth, 2014). The initial genetically altered cell forms a clone and begins to proliferate abnormally, evading normal intracellular and extracellular growth-regulating processes or signals as well as the immune system defence mechanisms of the body. Genetic mutations may lead to abnormalities in cell signalling transduction processes (signals from outside and within cells that turn cell activities either on or off) that can in turn lead to cancer development. Ultimately, cells acquire a variety of capabilities that allow them to invade surrounding tissues and/or gain access to lymph and blood vessels, which carry the cells to other areas of the body resulting in metastasis or spread of the cancer (Acharyya, Matrisian, Welch, et al., 2015).

Proliferative Patterns

During the life span, various body tissues normally undergo periods of rapid or proliferative growth that must be distinguished from **malignant** growth activity. Several patterns of abnormal cell growth exist: **hyperplasia, metaplasia, dysplasia, anaplasia**, and **neoplasia**. Cancerous cells are described as malignant neoplasms. They demonstrate uncontrolled cell growth that follows no physiologic demand (neoplasia). **Benign** (noncancerous) and malignant growths (cancerous) are classified and named by tissue of origin (e.g., benign tumours of the meninges are called meningioma and malignant tumours of the meninges are called meningeal sarcoma).

Characteristics of Malignant Cells

Benign and malignant cells differ in many cellular growth characteristics, including the method and rate of growth, ability to metastasize or spread, general effects, destruction of tissue, and ability to cause death. These differences are summarized in Table 68-1. The degree of anaplasia (cells that lack normal cellular characteristics and differ in shape and organization with respect to their cells of origin) ultimately determines the malignant potential.

Despite their individual differences, all cancer cells share some common cellular characteristics related to the cell membrane, special proteins, the nuclei, chromosomal abnormalities, and the rate of mitosis and growth. The cell membranes are altered in cancer cells, which affect fluid movement in and out of the cell. The cell membrane of malignant cells also contains proteins called **tumour-specific antigens (TSAs)**, such as (e.g., carcinoembryonic antigen [CEA] and prostate-specific antigen [PSA]), which develop over time as the cells become less differentiated.

TABLE 68-1 Characteristics of Benign and Malignant Tumours

Characteristics	Benign	Malignant
Cell	Well-differentiated cells resemble normal cells of the tissue from which the tumour originated.	Cells are undifferentiated and may bear little resemblance to the normal cells of the tissue from which they arose.
Mode of growth	Tumour grows by expansion and does not infiltrate the surrounding tissues; usually encapsulated.	Grows at the periphery and overcomes contact inhibition to invade and infiltrate surrounding tissues.
Rate of growth	Rate of growth is usually slow.	Rate of growth is variable and depends on level of differentiation; the more anaplastic the tumour, the faster its growth.
Metastasis	Does not spread by metastasis.	Gains access to the blood and lymphatic channels and metastasizes to other areas of the body or grows across body cavities such as the peritoneum.
General effects	Is usually a localized phenomenon that does not cause generalized effects unless its location interferes with vital functions.	Often causes generalized effects, such as anemia, weakness, systemic inflammation, weight loss, and CACS.
Tissue destruction	Does not usually cause tissue damage unless its location interferes with blood flow.	Often causes extensive tissue damage as the tumour outgrows its blood supply or encroaches on blood flow to the area; may also produce substances that cause cell damage.
Ability to cause death	Does not usually cause death unless its location interferes with vital functions.	Eventually causes death unless growth can be controlled.

CACS, cancer-related anorexia–cachexia syndrome.

Adapted from Grossman, S. C., & Porth, C. M. (2014). *Porth's pathophysiology: Concepts of altered health states* (9th ed.). Philadelphia, PA: Lippincott Williams & Wilkins.

These proteins distinguish malignant cells from benign cells of the same tissue type. They cannot be used as diagnostic tools; however, they may be useful in measuring the extent and tracking the course of disease in a person during diagnosis, treatment, or relapse. Malignant cellular membranes also contain less fibronectin, a cellular cement. They are therefore less cohesive and do not adhere to adjacent cells readily.

Typically, nuclei of cancer cells are large and irregularly shaped (pleomorphism). Nucleoli, structures within the nucleus that house ribonucleic acid (RNA), are larger and more numerous in malignant cells, perhaps because of increased RNA synthesis. Chromosomal abnormalities (translocations, deletions, additions) and fragility of chromosomes are commonly found when cancer cells are analyzed.

Mitosis (cell division) occurs more frequently in malignant cells than in normal cells. As the cells grow and divide, more glucose and oxygen are needed. If glucose and oxygen are unavailable, malignant cells use anaerobic metabolic channels to produce energy, which makes the cells less dependent on the availability of a constant oxygen supply.

Invasion and Metastasis

Malignant disease processes have the ability to allow the spread or transfer of cancerous cells from one organ or body part to another by invasion and **metastasis**.

Invasion, which refers to the growth of the primary tumour into the surrounding host tissues, occurs in several ways. Mechanical pressure exerted by rapidly proliferating neoplasms may force fingerlike projections of tumour cells into surrounding tissue and interstitial spaces. Malignant cells are less adherent and may break off from the primary tumour and invade adjacent structures. Malignant cells are thought to possess or produce specific destructive enzymes (proteinases), such as collagenases (specific to collagen), plasminogen activators (specific to plasma), and lysosomal hydrolyses. These enzymes are thought to destroy surrounding tissue, including the structural tissues of the vascular basement membrane, facilitating invasion of malignant cells. The mechanical pressure of a rapidly growing tumour may enhance this process.

Metastasis is the dissemination or spread of malignant cells from the primary tumour to distant sites by direct spread of tumour cells to body cavities or through lymphatic and blood circulation. Tumours growing in or penetrating body cavities may shed cells or emboli that travel within the body cavity and seed the surfaces of other organs. This can occur in ovarian cancer when malignant cells enter the peritoneal cavity and seed the peritoneal surfaces of such abdominal organs, such as the liver or pancreas. Patterns of metastasis can be partially explained by circulatory patterns and by specific affinity for certain malignant cells to bind to molecules in specific body tissue.

Lymphatic and Hematogenous Spread

Lymph and blood are key mechanisms by which cancer cells spread. Lymphatic spread (the transport of tumour cells through the lymphatic circulation) is the most common mechanism of metastasis. Tumour emboli enter the lymph channels by way of the interstitial fluid, which communicates with lymphatic fluid. Malignant cells also may penetrate lymphatic vessels by invasion. After entering the lymphatic circulation, malignant cells either lodge in the lymph nodes or pass between the lymphatic and venous circulations. Tumours arising in areas of the body with rapid and extensive lymphatic circulation are at high risk for metastasis through lymphatic channels. Breast tumours frequently metastasize in this manner through axillary, clavicular, and thoracic lymph channels.

Hematogenous spread is the dissemination of malignant cells via the bloodstream and is directly related to the vascularity of the tumour. Few malignant cells can survive the turbulence of arterial circulation, insufficient oxygenation, or destruction by the body's immune system. In addition, the structure of most arteries and arterioles is far too secure to permit malignant invasion. Those malignant cells that do survive are able to attach to endothelium and attract fibrin, platelets, and clotting factors to seal themselves from immune system surveillance. The endothelium retracts, allowing the malignant cells to enter the basement membrane and secrete lysosomal enzymes. These enzymes destroy surrounding body tissues, allowing implantation.

Angiogenesis

Angiogenesis is the growth of new capillaries from the host tissue by the release of growth factors and enzymes such as vascular endothelial growth factor (VEGF). These proteins rapidly stimulate formation of new blood vessels, which helps malignant cells obtain the necessary nutrients and oxygen. It is also through this vascular network that tumour emboli can enter the systemic circulation and travel to distant sites. Large tumour emboli that become trapped in the microcirculation of distant sites may further metastasize to other sites. Therapies that target VEGF or its receptors are being used to treat many cancers effectively (see Targeted Therapies).

Carcinogenesis

Molecular Process

Malignant transformation, or **carcinogenesis**, is thought to be at least a three-step cellular process, involving initiation, promotion, and progression. During *initiation*, initiators (carcinogens), such as chemicals, physical factors, and biologic agents, escape normal enzymatic mechanisms and alter the genetic structure of the cellular DNA. Normally, these alterations are reversed by DNA repair mechanisms or the changes initiate programmed cellular death. Occasionally, cells escape these protective mechanisms, and permanent cellular mutations occur. These mutations usually are not significant to cells until the second step of carcinogenesis.

During *promotion*, repeated exposure to promoting agents (cocarcinogens) causes the expression of abnormal or mutant genetics information even after long latency periods. Latency periods for the promotion of cellular mutations vary with the type of agent and the dosage of the promoter as well as the innate characteristics of the target cell.

Cellular oncogenes are responsible for the vital cellular functions of growth and differentiation. Cellular proto-oncogenes act as an "on switch" for cellular growth. Proto-oncogenes are influenced by multiple growth factors that stimulate cell proliferation, such as epidermal growth factor (EGF) and transforming growth factor alpha. Another proto-oncogene that plays an important role in cancer development is the *k-ras (KRAS2)* oncogene located on chromosome 12.

Just as proto-oncogenes "turn on" cellular growth, cancer suppressor genes "turn off," or regulate, unneeded cellular proliferation. When suppressor genes mutate or lose their regulatory capabilities, malignant cells are allowed to reproduce uncontrollably. The *p53 (TP53)* gene is a tumour suppressor gene that is frequently implicated in many human cancers. This gene determines whether cells will live or die after their DNA is damaged. **Apoptosis** is the innate cellular process of programmed cell death. Alterations in *TP53* may decrease apoptotic signals, thus giving rise to a survival advantage for mutant cell populations. Mutant *TP53* is associated with a poor prognosis and may be associated with determining response to treatment. Once this genetic expression occurs in cells, the cells begin to produce mutant cell populations that are different from their original cellular ancestors.

During *progression*, the altered cells exhibit increasingly malignant behaviour. These cells acquire the ability to stimulate angiogenesis (growth of new blood vessels that allow cancer cells to grow), to invade adjacent tissues, and to metastasize. Cellular oncogenes are responsible for vital cell functions, including proliferation and differentiation. Cellular proto-oncogenes, such as those for the epidermal growth factor receptor (EGFR), transcription factors such as *c-Myc*, or cell-signalling proteins such as *Kirsten ras* (*KRAS*), act as "on switches" for cellular growth. Amplification of proto-oncogenes or overexpression of growth factors, such as EGF, can lead to uncontrolled cell proliferation. Mutations that increase the activity of oncogenes also deregulate cell proliferation. Genetic alterations in the gene for *KRAS* have been associated with pancreatic, lung, and colorectal cancers (Lovly, Horn, & Pao, 2015).

Just as proto-oncogenes "turn on" cellular growth, cancer suppressor genes "turn off," or regulate, unneeded cellular proliferation. When suppressor genes are mutated, resulting in loss of function or expression, the cells begin to produce mutant cell populations that are different from their original cellular ancestors. See Chart 68-1 for further discussion of genetics concepts and cancer.

Etiology

Categories of agents or factors implicated in carcinogenesis include viruses and bacteria, physical agents, chemical agents, genetic or familial factors, dietary factors, and hormonal agents. Additional research is needed for a better understanding of the relationships between etiologic factors and cancer.

Viruses and Bacteria

Viruses are difficult to evaluate as a cause of human cancers because they are difficult to isolate. However, infectious causes are considered or suspected when specific cancers appear in clusters. Viruses are thought to incorporate themselves in the genetic structure of cells, thus altering future generations of that cell population, perhaps leading to cancer. It is estimated that about 11% of all cancers worldwide are linked to viral infections (Schiller & Lowy, 2014). For example, the Epstein–Barr virus is highly suspect as a cause in Burkitt lymphoma, nasopharyngeal cancers, and some types of non-Hodgkin and Hodgkin lymphomas. Herpes simplex virus type 2, cytomegalovirus, and human papillomavirus (HPV) types 16, 18, 31, and 33 are associated with dysplasia and cancer of the cervix. The hepatitis B virus is implicated in cancer of the liver; the human T-cell lymphotropic virus may be a cause of some lymphocytic leukemias and lymphomas; and the human immunodeficiency virus (HIV) is associated with Kaposi sarcoma.

Bacteria have been evaluated as a cause of cancer over the years but with little evidence to support the link of bacteria to cancer. Chronic inflammatory reactions to bacteria and

GENETICS IN NURSING PRACTICE

Chart 68-1. Genetics Concepts and Oncologic Disorders

Cancer is a genetic disease. Every phase of carcinogenesis is affected by multiple gene mutations. Some of these mutations are inherited (present in germ-line cells) and present a greater risk for a person to develop oncologic disorders; however, most (90%) are somatic mutations that are acquired mutations in specific cells. Examples of cancers influenced by genetics include:

Autosomal dominant:

- Breast and ovarian cancer
- Colorectal cancer
- Familial adenomatous polyposis
- Cowden syndrome
- Li-Fraumeni syndrome
- Lynch Syndrome (Hereditary nonpolyposis colon cancer)
- Multiple endocrine neoplasia types 1 and 2
- Neurofibromatosis types 1 and 2
- Prostate cancer
- Retinoblastoma
- von Hippel-Lindau syndrome
- Wilms tumour

Autosomal recessive:

- Ataxia telangiectasia
- Endometrial cancer
- Gastrointestinal stromal tumour
- Familial melanoma syndrome
- Xeroderma pigmentosum

Nursing Assessments

Refer to Chapter 11.

FAMILY HISTORY ASSESSMENT SPECIFIC TO ONCOLOGIC DISORDERS

- Obtain information about both maternal and paternal sides of family for three generations.
- Obtain cancer history for at least three generations.
- Look for clustering of cancers that occur at young ages, multiple primary cancers in one individual, cancer in paired organs, and two or more close relatives with the same type of cancer suggestive of hereditary cancer syndromes.

PATIENT ASSESSMENT

- Assess for the following:
  - Physical findings that may predispose the patient to cancer, such as multiple colon polyps or the presence of more than one tumour. If a tumour was previously diagnosed, inquire about the age of the patient when the first tumour was noted.
  - Skin findings, such as atypical moles, that may be related to familial melanoma syndrome.
  - Multiple café-au-lait spots, axillary freckling, and two or more neurofibromas associated with neurofibromatosis type 1.
  - Facial trichilemmomas, mucosal papillomatosis, multinodular thyroid goiter or thyroid adenomas, macrocephaly, fibrocystic breasts, and other fibromas or lipomas related to Cowden syndrome.
- Assess for lifestyle risks (e.g., smoking, obesity, alcohol use).
- Determine potential occupational or environmental hazards that may generate exposure to inhaled chemicals, gases, or other irritants (e.g., toxic metals, asbestos, radon).

Management Issues Specific to Oncologic Disorders

- Assess patient's understanding of genetic factors related to their cancer.
- Offer appropriate genetics information and resources.
- Refer for cancer risk assessment when a hereditary cancer syndrome is suspected so that patient and family can discuss inheritance risk with other family members and availability of genetic testing.
- Provide support to patients and families with known genetic test results for hereditary cancer syndromes. Refer to support groups as appropriate.
- Participate in the management and coordination of risk reduction measures for those with known gene mutations.

Genetics Resources Specific to Oncologic Disorders

American Cancer Society: www.cancer.org
National Cancer Institute: www.cancer.gov
See also Chapter 11 for additional components of genetic counselling.

the production of carcinogenic metabolites are possible mechanisms under investigation. In the early 1990s, the International Agency for Research on Cancer (IARC) identified *Helicobacter pylori* (*H. pylori*) as the first bacterium to be termed a definite cause of cancer in humans. *H. pylori* has been associated with an increased incidence of gastric malignancy related to chronic superficial gastritis, with resultant atrophic and metaplastic changes to the gastric mucosa (Feller, Altini, & Lemmer, 2013).

Physical Agents

Physical factors associated with carcinogenesis include exposure to sunlight or radiation, chronic irritation or inflammation, and tobacco use.

Excessive exposure to the ultraviolet rays of the sun, especially in fair-skinned, blue- or green-eyed people, increases the risk of skin cancers. Factors such as clothing styles (sleeveless shirts or shorts); use of sunscreens; occupation; recreational habits; and environmental variables, including humidity, altitude, and latitude, all play a role in the amount of exposure to ultraviolet light.

Exposure to ionizing radiation can occur with repeated diagnostic x-ray procedures or with radiation therapy used to treat disease. Fortunately, improved x-ray equipment minimizes the risk of extensive radiation exposure. Radiation therapy used in disease treatment and exposure to radioactive materials at nuclear weapon manufacturing sites or nuclear power plants are associated with a higher incidence of leukemias, multiple myeloma, and cancers of the lung, bone, breast, thyroid, and other tissues. Background radiation from the natural decay processes that produce radon has also been associated with lung cancer.

Homes with high levels of trapped radon should be ventilated to allow the gas to disperse into the atmosphere.

Chemical Agents

About 75% of all cancers are thought to be related to the environment. Most hazardous chemicals produce their toxic effects by altering DNA structure in body sites distant from chemical exposure. The liver, lungs, and kidneys are the organ systems most often affected, presumably because of their roles in detoxifying chemicals.

Tobacco smoke, thought to be the single most lethal chemical carcinogen, accounts for at least 30% of cancer deaths. Smoking is strongly associated with cancers of the lung, head and neck, esophagus, stomach, pancreas, cervix, kidney, and bladder and with acute myeloblastic leukemia. More than 60 individual carcinogenic chemicals have been identified in tobacco and tobacco smoke. Tobacco may also act synergistically with other substances, such as alcohol, asbestos, uranium, and viruses, to promote cancer development. Chewing tobacco is associated with cancers of the oral cavity, which primarily occur in men younger than 40 years of age. Considerable research has also substantiated the effect of secondhand cigarette smoke as an environmental risk factor for both smokers and nonsmokers (Raja & Sultana, 2013).

Many chemical substances found in the workplace have proved to be carcinogens or cocarcinogens. Most hazardous chemicals produce their toxic effects by altering DNA structure in body sites distant from chemical exposure. The liver, lungs, and kidneys are the organ systems most often affected, presumably because of their roles in detoxifying chemicals.

Genetics and Familial Factors

Almost every cancer type has been shown to run in families. This may be due to genetics, shared environments, cultural or lifestyle factors, or chance alone. Genetic factors play a role in cancer cell development. Abnormal chromosomal patterns and cancer have been associated with extra chromosomes, too few chromosomes, or translocated chromosomes. Specific cancers with underlying genetic abnormalities include Burkitt lymphoma, chronic myelogenous leukemia, meningiomas, acute leukemias, retinoblastomas, Wilms tumour, and skin cancers, including malignant melanoma. In addition, there are syndromes that represent a cluster of cancers that are identified by a specific genetic alteration that is inherited across generations of a family. In these families, the associated genetic mutation is found in all cells and represents an inherited susceptibility to cancer for all family members who carry the mutation.

Approximately 5% of cancers in adults display a pattern of cancers suggestive of a familial predisposition. The hallmarks of families with a hereditary cancer syndrome include cancer in two or more first- or second-degree relatives, early onset of cancer in family members younger than 50 years of age, the same type of cancer in several family members, individual family members with more than one type of cancer, and a rare cancer in one or more family members. There is also evidence of an autosomal dominant inheritance pattern of cancers affecting several generations of the family.

Since the early 1990s, there have been considerable advances in the recognition of inherited cancer susceptibility syndromes and in the ability to isolate and identify the inherited genetic mutation responsible for the cancer patterns. Discoveries of mutations in genes related to critical cell control functions, such as tumour suppression, DNA repair mechanisms, and oncogenes, have enabled the appropriate identification of families at risk for these syndromes. Examples of these syndromes include hereditary breast and ovarian cancer syndrome (*BRCA1* and *BRCA2*) and multiple endocrine neoplasia syndrome (*MEN1* and *MEN2*) (Chart 68-1). Other cancers associated with familial inheritance syndromes include nephroblastomas, pheochromocytomas, and colorectal, stomach, thyroid, renal, prostate, and lung cancers (National Cancer Institute [NCI], 2016).

Dietary Factors

Dietary factors are also linked to environmental cancers. Dietary substances can be proactive (protective), carcinogenic, or cocarcinogenic. The risk of cancer increases with long-term ingestion of carcinogens or cocarcinogens or chronic absence of protective substances in the diet.

Dietary substances that appear to increase the risk of cancer include fats, alcohol, salt-cured or smoked meats, nitrate-containing and nitrite-containing foods, and red and processed meats. Alcohol increases the risk of cancers of the mouth, pharynx, larynx, esophagus, liver, colorectum, and breast. Greater consumption of vegetables and fruits is associated with a decreased risk of cancer in general (Boeing, Bechthold, Bub, et al., 2012). A high-caloric dietary intake is also associated with an increased cancer risk. Obesity is associated with endometrial cancer, postmenopausal breast cancers, and colon, esophagus, and kidney cancers. There is evidence that obesity also increases the risk for cancers of the esophagus, breast, endometrium, colon and rectum, kidney, pancreas, thyroid, and gallbladder (Lu, Clague, & Bernstein, 2015; Thomson, McCullough, Wertheim, et al., 2014).

Hormonal Agents

Tumour growth may be promoted by disturbances in hormonal balance, either by the body's own (endogenous) hormone production or by administration of exogenous hormones. Cancers of the breast, prostate, and uterus are thought to depend on endogenous hormonal levels for growth. Diethylstilbestrol (DES) has long been recognized as a cause of vaginal carcinomas. Oral contraceptives and prolonged estrogen therapy are associated with an increased incidence of hepatocellular, endometrial, and breast cancers, but they decrease the risk of ovarian cancer. The combination of estrogen and progesterone appears safer than estrogen alone in decreasing the risk of endometrial cancers; however, studies support discontinuing hormonal therapy containing both estrogen and progestin because of the increased risk of breast cancer, coronary heart disease, stroke, and blood clots (Chlebowski, Anderson, Pettinger, et al., 2013).

Hormonal changes related to the female reproductive cycle are also associated with cancer incidence. Early onset of menses under age 12 and delayed onset of menopause after age 55, nulliparity (never giving birth), and delayed childbirth after age 30 are all associated with an increased risk of breast cancer. Increased numbers of pregnancies are associated with a decreased incidence of breast, endometrial, and ovarian cancers.

Women who take estrogen after menopause appear to have an increased risk of ovarian cancer. Combination estrogen and progesterone therapy is linked to a higher risk of breast cancer. The longer the combined therapy is used, the higher the risk. However, within 3 years of stopping the hormones, the risk returns to that of a woman who never used this therapy. Women who have taken hormonal therapy appear to have a lower risk of getting colorectal cancer, but when cancers are found, it may be more advanced (more likely to have spread to lymph nodes or distant sites) than the cancers found in women not taking hormones (American Cancer Society [ACS], 2014).

Role of the Immune System

In humans, transformed cells arise on a regular basis, but are recognized by surveillance cells of the immune system that destroy them before cell growth becomes uncontrolled (immune surveillance). When the immune system fails to identify and stop the growth of transformed cells, a tumour can develop and progress.

Patients who are immunocompromised have an increased incidence of cancer. Transplant recipients who receive immunosuppressive therapy to prevent rejection of the transplanted organ have an increased incidence of cancer (Grossman & Porth, 2014). Patients with acquired immune deficiency syndrome (AIDS) have an increased incidence of Kaposi sarcoma and other cancers. Patients who were previously treated for one cancer are at increased risk for secondary cancers (Grossman & Porth, 2014).

Normal Immune Responses

Through the process of immune surveillance, an intact immune system usually has the ability to recognize and combat cancer cells through multiple, interacting cells and actions of the innate, humoral, and cellular components of the immune system. Tumour-associated antigens (TAAs; also called *tumour cell antigens*) are found on the membranes of many cancer cells. TAAs are processed by antigen-presenting cells (APCs) (e.g., macrophages and dentritic cells [very specialized cells of the immune system] that present antigens to both T and B lymphocytes) and are presented to T lymphocytes that recognize the antigen-bearing cells as foreign. Multiple TAAs have been identified—some are found in many types of cancer, some exist in the normal tissues of origin as well as the cancer cells, some exist in both normal and cancer cells but are overexpressed (exist in higher concentrations) in cancer cells, and others are very specific to certain cancer types (Kasper, Fauci, Hauser, et al., 2015).

In response to recognizing TAAs as foreign, T-cell lymphocytes release several cytokines that elicit various immune system actions, including (1) proliferation of cytotoxic (cell-killing) T lymphocytes capable of direct destruction of cancer cells, (2) induction of cancer cell apoptosis, and (3) recruitment of additional immune system cells (B-cell lymphocytes that produce antibodies, natural killer [NK] cells, and macrophages) that contribute to the destruction and degradation of cancer cells.

NK cells are a major component of the body's defence against cancer. NK cells are a subpopulation of lymphocytes that act by directly destroying cancer cells or by producing lymphokines and enzymes that assist in cell destruction.

Immune System Failure

Several theories postulate how malignant cells survive and proliferate, evading the elaborate immune system defence mechanisms (Grossman & Porth, 2014). If the body fails to recognize the TAAs on cancer cells or the function of the APCs is impaired, the immune response is not stimulated. Some cancer cells have been found to have altered cell membranes that interfere with APC binding and presentation to T lymphocytes. Tumours can also express molecules that induce T-lymphocyte anergy or tolerance such as PD-1 ligand. These molecules bind to PD-1 proteins on T lymphocytes and either block the killing of the tumour or induce cell death in the lymphocyte. In addition, cancer cells have been found to release cytokines that inhibit APCs as well as other cells of the immune system. When tumours do not possess TAAs that label them as foreign, the immune response is not alerted. This allows the tumour to grow too large to be managed by normal immune mechanisms.

The immunogenicity (immunologic appearance) of cancer cells can be altered through genetic mutations, allowing the cells to evade immune cell recognition. Conversely, mutations are the source for some TAAs. Tumour antigens may combine with the antibodies produced by the immune system and hide or disguise themselves from normal immune defence mechanisms. The tumour antigen–antibody complexes that evade recognition lead to a false message to decrease further production of antibodies as well as other immune system components.

Overexpression (abnormally high concentrations) of host suppressor T lymphocytes induced through the release of cytokines by malignant cells is thought to downregulate the immune response, thus permitting uncontrolled cell growth (Kasper et al., 2015). Suppressor T lymphocytes normally assist in regulating lymphocyte production and diminishing immune responses (i.e., antibody production) when they are no longer required. Low levels of antibodies and high levels of suppressor cells have been found in patients with multiple myeloma, which is a cancer associated with hypogammaglobulinemia (low amounts of serum antibodies). Conversely, there is evidence that proliferation of helper T lymphocytes, which promote the immune response, is impaired by cytokines produced by cancer cells (Kasper et al., 2015). Without helper T lymphocytes, the immune system response is limited and the cancer cells continue to proliferate. Understanding the role of the immune system and identification of the ways in which cancer evades the body's natural defences provide the foundation for therapeutic approaches that seek to support and enhance the immune system's role in combating cancer (see Chapters 51, 52, and 68).

Detection and Prevention of Cancer

Nurses and physicians have traditionally been involved with tertiary prevention, the care, and rehabilitation of patients after cancer diagnosis and treatment. However, the Canadian Cancer Society, the NCI, clinicians, and researchers also place emphasis on primary and secondary prevention of cancer. Nurses must be aware of factors such as race, cultural influences, access to care, patient–physician and patient–nurse relationships, level of education, income, and age that influence the knowledge, attitudes, and beliefs individuals have about cancer. These factors also may affect the health-promoting behaviours that people practice.

Primary Prevention

Primary prevention is concerned with reducing the risks of disease through health promotion strategies. The majority of risk factors that place humans at risk for cancer are modifiable (Yarbro, Wujcik, & Holmes Gobel, 2013). By acquiring the knowledge and skills necessary to educate the community about cancer risk, nurses in all settings play a key role in cancer prevention. One way to reduce the risk of cancer is to help patients avoid known carcinogens. Another strategy involves encouraging patients to make dietary and lifestyle changes (smoking cessation, decreased caloric intake, increased physical activity) that studies show influence the risk for cancer. Nurses use their teaching and counselling skills to provide patient education and support public education campaigns through organizations, such as the Canadian Cancer Society, that guide patients and families in taking steps to reduce cancer risks through health promotion behaviours.

An example of primary prevention is the use of immunization to reduce the risk of cancer through prevention of infections associated with cancer. The HPV vaccine is recommended to prevent cervical and head and neck cancers (Chen, Hsu, Yang, et al., 2014). The vaccine to prevent HBV infection is recommended by the Centers for Disease Control and Prevention (CDC) (2015) and Health Canada to reduce the risk of hepatitis and subsequent development of liver cancer.

Secondary Prevention

Secondary prevention programs promote screening and early detection activities such as breast and testicular self-examination and Papanicolaou (Pap) tests. Many organizations conduct cancer screening events that focus on cancers with the highest incidence rates or those that have improved survival rates if diagnosed early, such as breast or prostate cancer. These events offer education and examinations such as mammograms, digital rectal examinations, and PSA blood tests for minimal or no cost. These programs often target people who lack access to health care insurance or who cannot afford to participate on their own.

The evolving understanding of the role of genetics in cancer cell development has contributed to prevention and screening efforts. Many centres across the country are offering innovative cancer risk evaluation programs that provide in-depth screening and follow-up screening for people who are found to be at high risk for cancer. Nurses in all settings can develop programs that identify risks for patients and families and that incorporate teaching and counselling into all educational efforts, particularly for patients and families with a high incidence of cancer. Nurses and physicians can encourage individuals to comply with detection efforts as suggested by the Canadian Cancer Society (Table 68-2).

Unfolding Patient Stories: Doris Bowman • Part 2

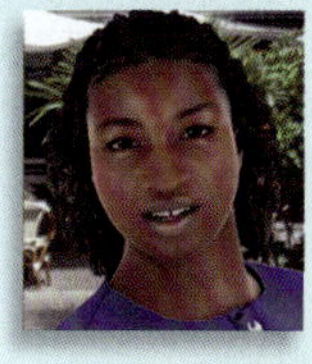

Recall from Chapter 48 Doris Bowman, a 39-year-old diagnosed with uterine fibroids, dysmenorrhea, and menorrhagia; she is now scheduled for a total abdominal hysterectomy with bilateral salpingo-oophorectomy. She has a family history of uterine and ovarian cancer. She asks the nurse what she can do to further reduce her risk for cancer and is also concerned for her family members. What patient and family education should the nurse present on risk reduction strategies, health promotion, and cancer screening?

Care for Doris and other patients in a realistic virtual environment: *vSim for Nursing* (**thepoint.lww.com/vSimMedicalSurgical**). Practice documenting these patients' care in DocuCare (**thepoint.lww.com/DocuCareEHR**).

Tertiary Prevention

Tertiary prevention efforts focus on monitoring for and preventing recurrence of the primary cancer as well as screening for the development of second malignancies in cancer survivors. Survivors are assessed for the development of second malignancies such as lymphoma and leukemia, which have been associated with certain **chemotherapy** agents and the use of radiation therapy. Survivors may also develop second malignancies not related to treatment but genetic mutations related to inherited cancer syndromes, environmental exposures, and lifestyle factors.

Diagnosis of Cancer

A cancer diagnosis is based on an assessment of physiologic and functional changes and results of the diagnostic evaluation. Patients with suspected cancer undergo extensive testing to (1) determine the presence and extent of tumour, (2) identify possible spread (metastasis) of disease or invasion of other body tissues, (3) evaluate the function of involved and uninvolved body systems and organs, and (4) obtain tissue and cells for analysis, including evaluation of tumour stage and grade. The diagnostic evaluation includes a review of systems, physical examination, imaging studies, laboratory tests of blood, urine and other body fluids, and surgical and pathology reports. Knowledge of suspicious symptoms and of the behaviour of particular types of cancer assists in determining relevant diagnostic tests (Table 68-3).

Patients undergoing extensive testing may be fearful of the procedures and anxious about the possible test results. Nurses help relieve the patient's fear and anxiety by explaining the tests to be performed, the sensations likely to be experienced, and the patient's role in the test procedures. The nurse encourages the patient and family to voice their fears about the test results, supports the patient and family throughout the test period, and reinforces and clarifies information conveyed by the physician. The nurse also encourages the patient and family to communicate and share their concerns and to discuss their questions and concerns with one another.

TABLE 68-2 Canadian Cancer Society Recommendations for Early Detection of Cancer in Asymptomatic, Average-Risk People[a]

Site	Gender	Age	Evaluation	Frequency
Colon/rectum	Male (M)/ female (F)	50 years and older	Fecal occult blood test	Every 2 years; high-risk individuals should discuss an individual plan of surveillance with their physician
Prostate	M	50 years and older and asymptomatic for prostate cancer or over 40 years of age and high risk	Discuss potential benefits of prostate-specific antigen (PSA) testing and digital rectal examination (DRE) with physician	
Skin	M/F	All ages	Watch skin for changes in birthmarks or moles; any new skin growths; sores that do not heal; or patches of skin that bleed, ooze, swell, itch, or become red and bumpy	
Testicles	M	15 years and older	Testicular self-examination (TSE)	Regularly
Breast	F	40–49 years	Clinical breast examination (CBE)	Every 2 years
			Breast self-examination (BSE)	Regularly
			Discuss risks and benefits of mammography with physician	
		50–74 years	CBE	Every 2 years
			BSE	Regularly
			Mammography	Every 2 years
		75 years and older	Discuss with physician; regarding frequency of testing for breast cancer	
Cervix	F	Women who are sexually active at 21 Women who are no longer sexually active should continue to have this test.	Pap test	1–3 years, depending on provincial/territorial guidelines

[a]See the Canadian Cancer Society's Web site (http://www.cancer.ca) for more detailed recommendations for each cancer type.

Tumour Staging and Grading

A complete diagnostic evaluation includes identifying the stage and grade of the tumour. This is accomplished prior to treatment to provide baseline data for evaluating outcomes of therapy and to maintain a systematic and consistent approach to ongoing diagnosis and treatment. Treatment options and prognosis are based on **staging** and **grading**.

Staging determines the size of the tumour and the existence of local invasion and distant metastasis. Several systems exist for classifying the anatomic extent of disease. The tumour, nodes, and metastasis (TNM) system is frequently used (Acharyya et al., 2015) (Chart 68-2). A variety of other staging systems are also used to describe the extent of cancers, such as central nervous system (CNS) cancers, hematologic cancers, and malignant melanoma, which are not well described by the TNM system. Staging systems also provide a convenient shorthand notation that condenses lengthy descriptions into manageable terms for comparisons of treatments and prognoses.

Grading refers to the classification of the tumour cells. Grading systems seek to define the type of tissue from which the tumour originated and the degree to which the tumour cells retain the functional and histologic characteristics of the tissue of origin (differentiation). Samples of cells used to establish the grade of a tumour may be obtained from tissue scrapings, body fluids, secretions, or washings, **biopsy**, or surgical excision. This information helps the health care team predict the behaviour and prognosis of various tumours. The tumour is assigned a numeric value ranging from I to IV. Grade I tumours, also known as well-differentiated tumours, closely resemble the tissue of origin in structure and function. Tumours that do not clearly resemble the tissue of origin in structure or function are described as poorly differentiated or undifferentiated and are assigned grade IV. These tumours tend to be more aggressive and less responsive to treatment than well-differentiated tumours.

Anatomic Stage Group

Once the diagnosis, clinical stage, and histologic grade have been determined, the anatomic stage group, designated by I through IV (representing increasing severity of disease), is assigned to facilitate communication, treatment decisions, and estimation of prognosis. The anatomic stage group is also useful for comparing clinical outcomes.

Management of Cancer

Treatment options offered to cancer patients should be based on realistic and achievable goals for each specific

TABLE 68-3 Selected Diagnostic Tests Used to Detect Cancer

Test	Description	Examples of Diagnostic Uses
Tumour marker identification	Analysis of substances found in tumour tissue, blood, or other body fluids that are indicative of cancer cells or specific characteristics of cancer cells. These substances may also be found in some normal body tissues	Breast, colon, lung, ovarian, testicular, prostate cancers
Genetic tumour markers (Also called prognostic indicators)	Analysis for the presence of mutations (alterations) in genes found in tumours or body tissues. Assists in diagnosis, selection of treatment, prediction of response to therapy, and risk of progression or recurrence	Breast, lung, kidney, ovarian, brain cancers; leukemia; and lymphoma. Many uses of genetic profiling are considered investigational
Mammography	Use of x-ray images of the breast	Breast cancer
Magnetic resonance imaging (MRI)	Use of magnetic fields and radiofrequency signals to create sectioned images of various body structures	Neurologic, pelvic, abdominal, thoracic, breast cancers
Computed tomography (CT) scan	Use of narrow-beam x-ray to scan successive layers of tissue for a cross-sectional view	Neurologic, pelvic, skeletal, abdominal, thoracic cancers
Fluoroscopy	Use of x-rays that identify contrasts in body tissue densities; may involve the use of contrast agents	Skeletal, lung, gastrointestinal cancers
Ultrasonography (ultrasound)	High-frequency sound waves echoing off body tissues are converted electronically into images; used to assess tissues deep within the body	Abdominal and pelvic cancers
Endoscopy	Direct visualization of a body cavity or passageway by insertion of an endoscope into a body cavity or opening; allows tissue biopsy, fluid aspiration, and excision of small tumours. Used for diagnostic and therapeutic purposes	Bronchial, gastrointestinal cancers
Nuclear medicine imaging	Uses IV injection or ingestion of radioisotope substances, followed by imaging of tissues that have concentrated the radioisotopes	Bone, liver, kidney, spleen, brain, thyroid cancers
Positron emission tomography (PET)	Through the use of a tracer, provides black-and-white or colour-coded images of the biologic activity of a particular area, rather than its structure. Used in detection of cancer or its response to treatment	Lung, colon, liver, pancreatic, head and neck cancers; Hodgkin and non-Hodgkin lymphoma and melanoma
PET fusion	Use of a PET scanner and a CT scanner in one machine to provide an image combining anatomic detail, spatial resolution, and functional metabolic abnormalities	See PET
Radioimmunoconjugates	Monoclonal antibodies are labeled with a radioisotope and injected IV into the patient; the antibodies that aggregate at the tumour site are visualized with scanners	Colorectal, breast, ovarian, head and neck cancers; lymphoma and melanoma
Vascular imaging	Use of contrast agents that are injected into veins or arteries and monitored by fluoroscopy, CT, or MRI imaging in order to assess tumour vasculature. Used to assess tumour vascularity prior to surgical procedures. Use in assessing the efficacy of antiangiogenesis (preventing new blood vessel formation) drugs is largely investigational	Liver and brain cancers

CHART 68-2

TNM Classification System

T The extent of the primary tumour
N The absence or presence and extent of regional lymph node metastasis
M The absence or presence of distant metastasis
The use of numerical subsets of the TNM components indicates the progressive extent of the malignant disease.

Primary Tumour (T)

Tx Primary tumour cannot be assessed
T0 No evidence of primary tumour
Tis Carcinoma in situ
T1, T2, T3, T4 Increasing size and/or local extent of the primary tumour

Regional Lymph Nodes (N)

Nx Regional lymph nodes cannot be assessed
N0 No regional lymph node metastasis
N1, N2, N3 Increasing involvement of regional lymph nodes

Distant Metastasis (M)

Mx Distant metastasis cannot be assessed
M0 No distant metastasis
M1 Distant metastasis

Adapted from American Cancer Society (ACS). (2015). Cancer facts and figures 2015. Retrieved February 22, 2016, from www.cancer.org/acs/groups/content/@editorial/documents/document/acspc-044552.pdf

type of cancer. The range of possible treatment goals may include complete eradication of malignant disease (**cure**), prolonged survival and containment of cancer cell growth (**control**), or relief of symptoms associated with the disease (**palliation**).

The health care team, the patient, and the patient's family must have a clear understanding of the treatment options and goals. Open communication and support are vital as the patient and family periodically reassess treatment plans and goals when complications of therapy develop or disease progresses.

Multiple modalities are commonly used in cancer treatment. A variety of approaches, including surgery, radiation therapy, chemotherapy, and biologic response modifier (BRM) therapies, may be used at various times throughout treatment. Understanding the principles of each and how they interrelate is important in understanding the rationale and goals of treatment.

Surgery

Surgical removal of the entire cancer remains the ideal and most frequently used treatment method. The specific surgical approach, however, may vary for several reasons. Diagnostic surgery is the definitive method of identifying the cellular characteristics that influence all treatment decisions. Surgery may be the primary method of treatment, or it may be prophylactic, palliative, or reconstructive.

Diagnostic Surgery

Diagnostic surgery, such as a biopsy, is usually performed to obtain a tissue sample for analysis of cells suspected to be malignant. In most instances, the biopsy is taken from the actual tumour, but in some situations, it is necessary to biopsy lymph nodes near the suspicious tumour. Knowing whether adjacent lymph nodes contain tumour cells helps physicians plan for systemic therapies instead of or in addition to surgery or radiation, to combat tumour cells that have gone beyond the primary tumour site. The use of injectable dyes and nuclear medicine imaging can help the surgeon identify the sentinel lymph node to which the primary tumour and surrounding tissue drains. Sentinel lymph node biopsy (SLNB), also known as sentinel lymph node mapping, is a minimally invasive surgical approach that in some instances has replaced more invasive lymph node dissections (lymphadenectomy) and their associated complications such as lymphedema and delayed healing. SLNB has been widely adopted for regional lymph node staging in selected cases of melanoma and breast cancer (Canadian Cancer Society, 2014).

Biopsy Types

The three most common biopsy methods are the excisional, incisional, and needle methods. The choice of biopsy is determined by the size and location of the tumour, the type of treatment anticipated if the cancer diagnosis is confirmed, and the need for surgery and general anesthesia. The biopsy method that allows for the least invasive approach while permitting the most representative tissue sample is chosen. Occasionally, diagnostic imaging techniques are used to assist in locating the suspicious lesion and to facilitate accurate tissue sampling. The patient and family are given the opportunity and time to discuss the options before definitive plans are made. The nurse serves as the patient's advocate and liaison between the patient and physician to facilitate this process.

Excisional biopsy is most frequently used for easily accessible tumours of the skin, breast, and upper or lower gastrointestinal and upper respiratory tracts. In many cases, the surgeon can remove the entire tumour as well as the surrounding marginal tissues. The removal of normal tissue beyond the tumour area decreases the possibility that residual microscopic disease cells may lead to a recurrence of the tumour. This approach not only provides the pathologist, who stages and grades the cells, with the entire tissue specimen but also decreases the chance of seeding the tumour (disseminating cancer cells throughout surrounding tissues).

Incisional biopsy is performed if the tumour mass is too large to be removed. In this case, a wedge of tissue from the tumour is removed for analysis. The cells of the tissue wedge must be representative of the tumour mass so that the pathologist can provide an accurate diagnosis. If the specimen does not contain representative tissue and cells, negative biopsy results do not guarantee the absence of cancer.

Excisional and incisional approaches are often performed through endoscopy. However, surgical incision may be required to determine the anatomic extent or stage of the tumour. For example, a diagnostic or staging laparotomy (the surgical opening of the abdomen to assess malignant abdominal disease) may be necessary to assess malignancies such as gastric cancer.

Needle biopsies are performed to sample suspicious masses that are easily accessible, such as some growths in the breasts, thyroid, lung, liver, and kidney. Needle biopsies are most often performed on an outpatient basis. They are fast, relatively inexpensive, easy to perform, and usually require only local anesthesia. In general, the patient experiences slight and temporary physical discomfort. In addition, the surrounding tissues are disturbed only minimally, thus decreasing the likelihood of seeding cancer cells. Needle aspiration biopsy involves aspirating tissue fragments through a needle guided into an area suspected of bearing disease. Occasionally, x-ray, computed tomography (CT) scanning, ultrasonography, or magnetic resonance imaging (MRI) is used to help locate the suspicious area and guide the placement of the needle. In some instances, the aspiration biopsy does not yield enough tissue to permit accurate diagnosis. A needle core biopsy uses a specially designed needle to obtain a small core of tissue. Most often, this specimen is sufficient to permit accurate diagnosis.

Surgery as Primary Treatment

When surgery is the primary approach in treating cancer, the goal is to remove the entire tumour or as much as is feasible (a procedure sometimes called *debulking*) and any involved surrounding tissue, including regional lymph nodes.

Two common surgical approaches used for treating primary tumours are local and wide excisions. When the mass is small, local excision is often performed on an outpatient basis. It includes removal of the mass and a small margin of normal tissue that is easily accessible. Wide or radical excisions (en bloc dissections) include removal of the primary tumour, lymph nodes, adjacent involved structures, and surrounding tissues that may be at high risk for tumour spread (this surgical method can result in disfigurement and altered functioning, necessitating rehabilitation or reconstructive procedures). However, wide excisions are considered if the tumour can be removed completely and the chances of cure or control are good.

Minimally invasive surgical techniques are increasingly replacing traditional surgery associated with large incisions for a variety of cancers. The advantages of minimally invasive approaches include minimization of surgical trauma, decreased blood loss, decreased incidence of wound infection and other complications associated with surgery, decreased surgical time and requirement for anesthesia, decreased postoperative pain and limited mobility, and shorter periods of recovery (Nguyen, Summers, & Finkelstein, 2015).

Video-assisted endoscopic surgery, an example of a minimally invasive procedure, uses an endoscope with intense lighting and an attached multichip mini-camera is inserted into the body through a small incision. The surgical instruments are inserted into the surgical field through one or two additional small incisions, each about 3 cm in length. The camera transmits the image of the involved area to a monitor so the surgeon can manipulate the instruments to perform the necessary procedure. Such surgery is used for many thoracic and abdominal procedures. The use of robotics during laparoscopic procedures permits the removal of tumours with more precision and dexterity than could be accomplished by laparoscopic surgery alone (Niklas, Saar, Berg, et al., 2016). Laparoscopic robotic–assisted surgery has been used for prostate and gynecologic cancers. Transoral robotic–assisted surgery is being used for certain types of oral and laryngeal cancers (Chung, Rosenthal, Magnuson, et al., 2015).

Salvage surgery is an additional treatment option that uses an extensive surgical approach to treat the local recurrence of a cancer after the use of a less extensive primary approach. A mastectomy to treat recurrent breast cancer after primary lumpectomy and radiation is an example of salvage surgery.

Surgery may completely excise limited areas of metastatic disease (referred to as oligometastatic disease) as well. An example would be colon cancer with one to three small areas of liver metastasis and no evidence of cancer elsewhere. In the past, patients with recurrent or metastatic disease were treated with palliation only as their disease was considered incurable. However, evidence suggests possible cure or prolonged disease-free survival for patients with controlled or completely removed primary cancer and completely removed, limited, metastatic disease (Corbin, Hellman, & Weichselbaum, 2013; Di Lascio & Pagani, 2014).

In addition to surgery that uses surgical blades or scalpels to excise the mass and surrounding tissues, several other types of surgical techniques are available. Table 68-4 identifies these techniques and provides examples of their use in the patient with cancer. A multidisciplinary approach to patient care is essential for the patient undergoing cancer-related surgery. The effects of surgery on the patient's body image, self-esteem, and functional abilities are addressed. If necessary, a plan for postoperative rehabilitation is made before the surgery is performed.

The growth and dissemination of cancer cells may have produced distant micrometastases by the time the patient seeks treatment. Therefore, attempting to remove wide margins of tissue in the hope of "getting all the cancer" may not be feasible. This reality substantiates the need for a coordinated multidisciplinary approach to cancer therapy.

Once the surgery has been completed, one or more additional (or adjuvant) modalities may be chosen to increase the likelihood of eradicating the remaining microscopic cancer cells that are undetectable by available diagnostic procedures. However, some cancers that are treated surgically in the very early stages (e.g., skin and testicular cancers) are considered to be curable without additional therapy.

Prophylactic Surgery

Prophylactic or risk reduction surgery involves removing nonvital tissues or organs that are at increased risk of

TABLE 68-4 Selected Techniques Used for Localized Destruction of Tumour Tissue

Type of Procedure	Description	Examples of Use
Chemosurgery	Use of chemicals or chemotherapy applied directly to tissue to cause destruction	Intraperitoneal chemotherapy for ovarian cancer involving the abdomen and peritoneum
Cryoablation	Use of liquid nitrogen or a very cold probe to freeze tissue and cause cell destruction	Cervical, prostate, and rectal cancers
Electrosurgery	Use of an electric current to destroy tumour cells	Basal and squamous cell skin cancers
Laser surgery	Use of light and energy aimed at an exact tissue location and depth to vaporize cancer cells (also referred to as photocoagulation or photoablation)	Dyspnea associated with endobronchial obstructions
Photodynamic therapy	IV administration of a light-sensitizing agent (hematoporphyrin derivative [HPD]) that is taken up by cancer cells, followed by exposure to laser light within 24 to 48 hours; causes cancer cell death	Palliative treatment of dysphagia associated with esophageal and dyspnea associated with endobronchial obstructions
Radiofrequency ablation (RFA)	Uses localized application of thermal energy that destroys cancer cells through heat: temperatures exceed 50°C (122°F)	Nonresectable liver tumours, pain control with bone metastasis

developing cancer. The following factors are considered when discussing possible prophylactic surgery:

- Family history and genetic predisposition
- Presence or absence of signs and symptoms
- Potential risks and benefits
- Ability to detect cancer at an early stage
- Alternative options for managing increased risk
- The patient's acceptance of the postoperative outcome

Colectomy, mastectomy, and oophorectomy are examples of prophylactic surgeries. Identification of genetic markers indicative of inherited cancer syndromes or a predisposition to develop some types of cancer plays a role in decisions concerning prophylactic surgeries. However, what is adequate justification for prophylactic surgery remains controversial. For example, several factors are considered when deciding to proceed with a prophylactic mastectomy, including a strong family history of breast cancer; positive *BRCA1* or *BRCA2* findings; an abnormal physical finding on breast examination, such as progressive nodularity and cystic disease; a proven history of breast cancer in the opposite breast; abnormal mammography findings; abnormal biopsy results; and individual factors that may influence the patient's decision-making process (Mahon, 2014). Prophylactic surgery is discussed with patients and families along with other approaches for managing increased risk of cancer development. Preoperative education and counselling, as well as long-term follow-up, are provided.

Palliative Surgery

When cure is not possible, the goals of treatment are to make the patient as comfortable as possible and to promote quality of life as defined by the patient and his or her family. Palliative surgery is performed in an attempt to relieve complications of cancer, such as ulceration, obstruction, hemorrhage, pain, and malignant effusion (Table 68-5). Honest and informative communication with the patient and family about the goal of surgery is essential to avoid false hope and disappointment.

TABLE 68-5 Types of Palliative Surgery and Interventions

Procedure	Indications
Abdominal shunt placement	Ascites
Biliary stent placement	Biliary obstruction
Bone stabilization	Displaced bone fracture related to metastatic disease
Colostomy or ileostomy	Bowel obstruction
Cordotomy	Pain
Epidural catheter placement (for administering epidural analgesics)	Pain
Excision of solitary metastatic lesion	Metastatic lung, liver, or brain lesion
Gastrostomy, jejunostomy tube placement	Upper gastrointestinal tract obstruction
Hormone manipulation (removal of ovaries, testes, adrenals, pituitary)	Tumours that depend on hormones for growth
Nerve block	Pain
Percutaneous enteral gastrostomy (PEG) tube placement	Enteral nutrition
Pericardial drainage tube placement	Pericardial effusion
Peritoneal drainage tube placement	Ascites
Pleural drainage tube placement	Pleural effusion
Ureteral stent placement	Ureteral obstruction
Venous access device placement (for administering parenteral analgesics)	Pain

Reconstructive Surgery

Reconstructive surgery may follow curative or radical surgery in an attempt to improve function or obtain a more desirable cosmetic effect. It may be performed in one operation or in stages. The surgeon who will perform the surgery discusses possible reconstructive surgical options with the patient before the primary surgery is performed. Reconstructive surgery may be indicated for breast, head and neck, and skin cancers.

The nurse recognizes the patient's needs and the impact that altered functioning and body image may have on quality of life. The nurse provides the patient and family with opportunities to discuss these issues. The individual needs of the patient undergoing reconstructive surgery must be accurately assessed and addressed.

Nursing Management

Patients undergoing surgery for cancer require general perioperative nursing care, as described in Unit 4 of this text, as well as specific care related to age, organ impairment, nutritional deficits, disorders of coagulation, and altered immunity that may increase the risk of postoperative complications. Combining other treatment methods, such as radiation and chemotherapy, with surgery also contributes to postoperative complications, such as infection, impaired wound healing, altered pulmonary or renal function, and the development of deep vein thrombosis. In these situations, the nurse completes a thorough preoperative assessment for factors that may affect the patient undergoing the surgical procedure.

Patients who are undergoing surgery for the diagnosis or treatment of cancer are often anxious about the surgical procedure, possible findings, postoperative limitations, changes in normal body functions, and prognosis. The patient and family require time and assistance to deal with the possible changes and outcomes resulting from the surgery.

The nurse provides education and emotional support by assessing the needs of the patient and family and by discussing their fears and coping mechanisms. The nurse encourages the patient and family to take an active role in decision making when possible. If the patient or family asks about the results of diagnostic testing and surgical procedures, the nurse's response is guided by the information the physician has previously conveyed to the patient and family. The patient and family may ask the nurse to explain and clarify information that the physician initially provided but that they did not grasp because they were anxious and overwhelmed at the time. It is important that the nurse communicates frequently with the physician and other members of the health care team to be certain that the information provided is consistent.

Postoperatively, the nurse assesses the patient's responses to the surgery and monitors the patient for possible complications, such as infection, bleeding, thrombophlebitis, wound dehiscence, fluid and electrolyte imbalance, and organ dysfunction. The nurse also provides for the patient's comfort. Postoperative teaching addresses wound care, activity, nutrition, and medication information.

Plans for discharge, follow-up, home care, and treatment are initiated as early as possible to ensure continuity of care from hospital to home or from a cancer referral centre to the patient's local hospital and health care provider. Patients and families are encouraged to use community resources such as the Canadian Cancer Society for support and information.

Radiation Therapy

More than half of patients with cancer receive a form of **radiation therapy** at some point during treatment. Radiation may be used to cure cancer, as in thyroid carcinomas, localized cancers of the head and neck, and cancers of the uterine cervix. Radiation therapy may also be used to control malignant disease when a tumour cannot be removed surgically or when local nodal metastasis is present, or it can be used neoadjuvantly (prior to local definitive treatment) with or without chemotherapy to reduce the size of a tumour to enable surgical resection. Radiation therapy may be used prophylactically to prevent the spread of a primary cancer to a distant area (e.g., irradiating the brain to prevent leukemic infiltration or metastatic lung cancer). Palliative radiation therapy is used to relieve the symptoms of metastatic disease, especially when the cancer has spread to the brain, bone, or soft tissue, or to treat oncologic emergencies, such as superior vena cava syndrome, bronchial airway obstruction, or spinal cord compression.

Two types of ionizing radiation—electromagnetic radiation (x-rays and gamma rays) and particulate radiation (electrons, beta particles, protons, neutrons, and alpha particles)—can lead to tissue disruption. The most harmful tissue disruption is the direct alteration of the DNA molecule within the cells of the tissue. Ionizing radiation breaks the strands of the DNA helix, leading to cell death. It can also lead to the formation of free radicals and irreversibly damage DNA. If the DNA is incapable of repair, the cell may die immediately, or it may initiate cellular suicide, a genetically programmed cell death (apoptosis) (Datta, Kundu, Ghosh, et al., 2014; Montezano, Dulak-Lis, Tsiropoulou, et al., 2015).

Replicating cells are most vulnerable to the disruptive effects of radiation (during DNA synthesis and mitosis, i.e., early S, G_2, and M phases of the cell cycle; see Fig. 68-2). Therefore, those body tissues that undergo frequent cell division are most sensitive to radiation therapy. These tissues include bone marrow, lymphatic tissue, epithelium of the gastrointestinal tract, hair follicles, and gonads. Slower-growing tissues and tissues at rest (e.g., muscle, cartilage, nervous system, and connective tissues) are relatively radioresistant (less sensitive to the effects of radiation). However, it is important to remember that radiation therapy is localized treatment, and only the tissues that are within the treatment field are affected.

A radiosensitive tumour is one that can be destroyed by a dose of radiation that still allows for cell regeneration in the normal tissue. Tumours that are well oxygenated also appear to be more sensitive to radiation. In theory, therefore, radiation therapy may be enhanced if more oxygen

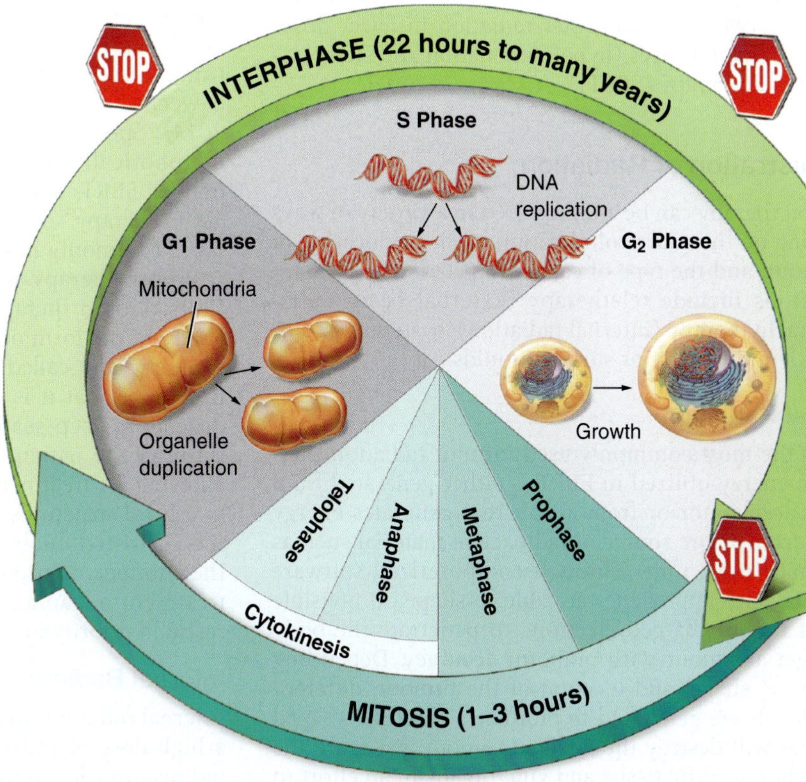

FIGURE 68-2. Cell cycle. The cell cycle's four steps are illustrated beginning with G_1 and proceeding to M. The first growth phase (G_1), DNA synthesis phase (S), second growth phase (G_2), and mitosis (M) are illustrated. (Reprinted with permission from Grossman, S. C., & Porth, C. M. (2014). *Porth's pathophysiology: Concepts of altered health states* [9th ed.]. Philadelphia, PA: Lippincott Williams & Wilkins.)

can be delivered to tumours. In addition, if the radiation is delivered when most tumour cells are cycling through the cell cycle, the number of cancer cells destroyed (cell kill) is maximal. Radiation sensitivity is also enhanced in tumours that are smaller in size and that contain cells that are rapidly dividing (highly proliferative) and poorly differentiated (no longer resembling the tissue of origin) (Ryan, Iwamoto, Haas, et al., 2012; Yarbro et al., 2013).

Certain chemicals, including chemotherapy agents, act as radiosensitizers and sensitize hypoxic (oxygen-poor) tumours to the effects of radiation therapy. Combinations of chemotherapy and radiation therapy are typically used to take advantage of the radiosensitizing effects of chemotherapy and achieve an improved survival benefit while minimizing side effects of such therapy.

Radiation Dosage

The radiation dosage depends on the sensitivity of the target tissues to radiation, the size of the tumour, tissue tolerance of the surrounding normal tissues, and critical structures adjacent to the tumour target. The lethal tumour dose is defined as that dose that will eradicate 95% of the tumour yet preserve normal tissue. In external beam radiation therapy (EBRT), the total radiation dose is delivered over several weeks in daily doses called fractions. This allows healthy tissue to repair and to achieve greater cell kill by exposing more cells to the radiation as they begin active cell division. Repeated radiation treatments over time (fractionated doses) also allow for the periphery of the tumour to be reoxygenated repeatedly, because tumours shrink from the outside inward. This increases the radiosensitivity of the tumour, thereby increasing tumour cell death (Morgan, Ten Haken, & Lawrence, 2015; Ryan et al., 2012; Yarbro et al., 2013). Newer approaches take advantage of increased radiation beam conformality (better tumour targeting) to administer radiation in fewer doses with larger fraction sizes (hypofractionation and stereotactic body radiotherapy [SBRT]).

Administration of Radiation

Radiation therapy can be administered in a variety of ways depending on the source of radiation used, the location of the tumour, and the type of cancer targeted. The primary applications include teletherapy (external beam radiation), brachytherapy (internal radiation), systemic (radioisotopes), and contact or surface moulds.

External Radiation

EBRT is the most commonly used form of radiation therapy. The energy utilized in EBRT is either generated from a linear accelerator or from a unit that generates energy directly from a core source of radioactive material such as a Gamma Knife® unit. Through computerized software programs, both approaches are able to shape an invisible beam of highly charged electrons to penetrate the body and target a tumour with pinpoint accuracy. Depending on the size, shape, and location of the tumour, different energy levels are generated to produce a carefully shaped beam that will destroy the targeted tumour, yet spare the surrounding healthy tissue and vital organs in an effort to reduce the treatment toxicities for the patient. With advances in computer technology, these beams can be shaped to a two- or three-dimensional shape to conform to the exact shape of the tumour as measured by imaging studies such as positron emission tomography (PET), CT, or MRI scans. Recent treatment enhancements in EBRT include the ability to direct different energy levels at different angles directed at the tumour, called intensity-modulated radiation therapy (IMRT), which enables higher doses to be delivered to the tumour while sparing the important healthy structures surrounding the tumour. IMRT can be administered as standard daily fractions or as "hyperfractionated" twice-daily fractions, which shortens the duration of the patient's treatment schedule. Image-guided radiation therapy (IGRT) uses continuous monitoring of the tumour with ultrasound or CT scans during the treatment to allow for automatic adjustment of the target as the tumour changes shape or position, again in an effort to spare the healthy surrounding tissue and reduce side effects (Christodoulou, Bayman, McCloskey, et al., 2014). The most recent treatment enhancements now include respiratory gating, where the treatment delivery is actually synchronized with the patient's respiratory cycle, enabling the beam to be adjusted as the tumour moves (Christodoulou et al., 2014).

Gamma rays generated from the spontaneous decay of naturally occurring solid source of radioactivity, such as cobalt-60, as one of the oldest forms of EBRT. With the advent of modern linear accelerators, the use of solid radioactive elements are confined primarily to the Gamma Knife® stereotactic radiosurgery unit, which is used as a one-time, high-dose delivery of EBRT for treatment of benign and malignant intracranial lesions.

SBRT is another form of EBRT using higher doses of radiation to penetrate very deeply into the body to control deep-seated tumours that cannot be treated by other approaches such as surgery. SBRT is delivered with considerably higher treatment fraction doses over a short span of time, usually 1 to 5 treatment days, in contrast to 6 to 8 weeks for conventional EBRT (Christodoulou et al., 2014). Specialized linear accelerators with the capability of robotically moving around the patient are used to deliver SBRT, such as the CyberKnife®, Trilogy™, and TomoTherapy® delivery systems, which are being utilized more commonly in community hospital settings.

Proton therapy is another very different approach to EBRT. Proton therapy utilizes high-linear energy transfer (LET) in the form of charged protons generated by a large magnetic unit called a cyclotron. The advantage of proton therapy is that it is capable of delivering its high-energy dose to a deep-seated tumour, with no energy exiting through the patient's healthy tissue behind the tumour, allowing for treatment of deep tumours in close proximity to critical structures such as the heart or major blood vessels (Christodoulou et al., 2014). With recent expansion in the number of proton therapy centres, investigation of treatment advantages utilizing proton therapy will be a research priority in the future (Christodoulou et al., 2014).

Internal Radiation

Internal radiation implantation, or brachytherapy, delivers a high dose of radiation to a localized area. The specific radioisotope for implantation is selected on the basis of its half-life, which is the time it takes for half of its radioactivity to decay. Internal radiation can be implanted by means of needles, seeds, beads, or catheters into body cavities (vagina, abdomen, pleura) or interstitial compartments (breast, prostate). Patients may have many fears or concerns about internal radiation and the nurse must be prepared to explain the various approaches and safety precautions that will be used to protect both the patient and the staff.

Brachytherapy

Brachytherapy is the placement of radioactive sources within or immediately next to the cancer site in order to provide a highly targeted, intense dose of radiation beyond a dose that is usually provided by EBRT. In addition, this form of radiation delivery helps to spare exposure to normal surrounding tissue. The radiation source can be implanted by means of needles or rods, seeds, beads, ribbons, or catheters placed into body cavities (vagina, abdomen, pleura), lumens within organs, or interstitial tissue compartments (breast, prostate). Multiple imaging techniques such as ultrasound, CT, or MRI are used to guide placement of radiation sources. Patients may have many fears or concerns about internal radiation, and the nurse explains the various approaches and safety precautions that will be used to protect the patient, family, and health care staff.

Brachytherapy may be delivered as a temporary or a permanent implant. Temporary applications may be delivered as high-dose radiation (HDR) for short periods of time or low-dose radiation (LDR) for a more extended period of time. The primary advantage of HDR sources of brachytherapy is that treatment time is shorter, there is reduced exposure to personnel, and the procedure can typically be performed as an outpatient procedure over several days. HDR brachytherapy can be used for intraluminal, interstitial, intracavitary, and surface lesions.

Intraluminal brachytherapy involves the insertion of catheters or hollow tubes into the lumens of organs so that the radioisotope can be delivered as close to the tumour bed as possible. Obstructive lesions in the bronchus, esophagus, or bile duct can be treated with this approach. Contact or surface application is used for treatment of tumours of the eye such as retinoblastoma in children or ocular melanoma in adults.

Interstitial HDR implants, used in treating such malignancies as prostate, pancreatic, or breast cancer, may be temporary or permanent, depending on the site and radioisotope used. Based on the dose to be delivered (LDR or HDR), the implants may consist of seeds, needles, wires, strands, or small catheters positioned to provide a local radiation source. Prostate HDR therapy is one form of interstitial brachytherapy, in which radioactive strands or wires are placed, while the patient is under anesthesia, into hollow catheters that have been inserted in the perineum close to the prostate gland (Halperin, Wazer, Perez, et al., 2013).

Intracavitary radioisotopes are frequently used to treat gynecologic cancers. In these malignancies, the radioisotopes are inserted into specially positioned applicators after their placement is verified by x-ray. Treatment can be achieved with either HDR or LDR brachytherapy sources depending on the extent of disease. LDR therapy requires hospitalization as the patient is treated over several days. Nursing care of the hospitalized LDR patient is essential to maximize effective safe delivery of the therapy and prevention of complications. The patient is maintained on bed rest in a specially prepared private room typically for 72 hours and logrolled to prevent displacement of the intracavitary delivery device. An indwelling urinary catheter is inserted to ensure that the bladder remains empty. Low-residue diets and antidiarrheal agents are provided to prevent bowel movements during therapy, which would displace the radioisotopes. Visitors and personnel must limit their time and proximity to the patient due to the risk of radiation exposure. HDR intracavitary brachytherapy is typically delivered as an outpatient procedure in the radiation therapy department over several days. HDR intraoperative radiotherapy (IORT) has been used as a treatment approach for advanced gynecologic cancer that has spread to the para-aortic area or pelvic wall (Lukens, Gamez, Hu, et al., 2014).

Systemic brachytherapy involves the IV or oral administration of a therapeutic radioactive isotope targeted to a specific tumour. Radioactive iodine (I^{131}) is a widely used form of systemic brachytherapy and is the primary treatment for thyroid cancer. Others include strontium 89 for bone metastases, samarium 153 metastatic bone lesions, and phosphorus 32 for malignant ascites associated with ovarian cancer. Radioisotopes are now also being used as radioimmunotherapy for the treatment of refractory non-Hodgkin lymphoma (NHL). Radioimmunotherapy involves the administration of a radionuclide chemically conjugated (bound) to a monoclonal antibody (MoAb) (discussed later in this chapter) that specifically targets NHL Tumour cells, delivering the radionuclide directly to the tumour and sparing the surrounding healthy tissue.

Toxicity

Toxicity of radiation therapy is localized to the region being irradiated. Toxicity may be increased if concomitant chemotherapy is administered. Acute local reactions occur when normal cells in the treatment area are also destroyed and cellular death exceeds cellular regeneration. Body tissues most affected are those that normally proliferate rapidly, such as the skin; the epithelial lining of the gastrointestinal tract, including the oral cavity; and the bone marrow. Altered skin integrity is a common effect and can include **alopecia** (hair loss). Skin reactions are identified and graded by severity along a continuum ranging from erythema and dry desquamation (flaking of skin), to moist desquamation (dermis exposed, skin oozing serous fluid), and potentially, ulceration. Re-epithelialization occurs after treatments have been completed.

Alterations in oral mucosa secondary to radiation therapy include **stomatitis** (inflammation of the oral tissues), **xerostomia** (dryness of the mouth), change and loss of taste, and decreased salivation. The entire gastrointestinal mucosa may be involved, and esophageal irritation with chest pain and dysphagia may result. Anorexia, nausea, vomiting, and diarrhea may occur if the stomach or colon is in the irradiated field. Symptoms subside and gastrointestinal re-epithelialization occurs after treatments have been completed.

Bone marrow cells proliferate rapidly, and if sites containing bone marrow (e.g., the iliac crest, sternum) are included in the radiation field, anemia, leukopenia (decreased white blood cells [WBCs]), and **thrombocytopenia** (a decrease in platelets) may result. The patient is then at increased risk for infection and bleeding until blood cell counts return to normal. Chronic anemia may occur (Ryan et al., 2012; Yarbro et al., 2013).

Research to develop cytoprotective agents that can protect normal tissue from radiation damage continues. The most commonly used cytoprotectant is amifostine, which is utilized in head and neck cancer patients to reduce acute and chronic xerostomia while preserving antitumour efficacy (Ryan et al., 2012; Yarbro et al., 2013).

Certain systemic side effects are also commonly experienced by patients receiving radiation therapy. These side effects include fatigue, malaise, and anorexia and may be secondary to substances released when tumour cells break down. The effects are temporary and most often subside with the cessation of treatment.

Late effects (months to years after treatment) of radiation therapy may also occur in various body tissues. These effects are chronic, usually produce fibrotic changes secondary to a decreased vascular supply, and are irreversible. Severe late effects may affect the lungs, heart, CNS, and bladder. Toxicities may intensify when radiation is combined with other treatment modalities.

Nursing Management

Nurses anticipate, prevent, and work collaboratively with other providers to manage symptoms associated with radiation therapy in order to promote healing, patient comfort, and quality of life. Symptoms that are not appropriately managed may lead to poor outcomes as a result of interruptions, decreased doses, or early cessation of treatment (Fogh & Yom, 2014). Ideally, nurses consider factors that may be predictive of radiation toxicities or radiosensitivity of tissues. In particular, diminished body mass index (BMI) and elevated radiation doses have been associated with greater toxicity and symptoms (O'Gorman, Sasiadek, Denieffe, et al., 2015). The area of the body being irradiated partially guides the focus of nursing assessments.

In patients receiving EBRT, the nurse assesses the patient's skin regularly throughout the course of treatment. In addition, nutritional status and general feelings of well-being are assessed throughout the course of treatment. Evidence-based protocols for nursing management of the toxicities associated with radiation therapy are used. If systemic symptoms, such as weakness and fatigue, occur, the nurse explains that these symptoms are a result of the treatment and do not represent deterioration or progression of the disease.

Assessment and management of these problems are discussed in more detail in Chart 68-3.

Protecting Caregivers

When the patient has a radioactive implant in place, the nurse and other health care providers need to protect themselves as well as the patient from the effects of radiation. Patients receiving internal radiation emit radiation while the implant is in place; therefore, contact with the health care team is guided by principles of time, distance, and shielding to minimize exposure of personnel to radiation. Specific instructions are usually provided by the radiation safety officer and specify the maximum time that can be spent safely in the patient's room, the shielding equipment to be used, and special precautions and actions to be taken if the implant is dislodged. Safety precautions used in caring for a patient receiving brachytherapy include assigning the patient to a private room, posting appropriate notices about radiation safety precautions, having staff members wear dosimeter badges, making sure that pregnant staff members are not assigned to the patient's care, prohibiting visits by children or pregnant visitors, limiting visits from others, and seeing that visitors maintain a safe distance from the radiation source.

Patients with seed implants typically are able to return home; radiation exposure to others is minimal. Information about any precautions, if needed, is provided to the patient and family members to ensure safety. Depending on the dose and energy emitted by a systemic radionuclide, patients may or may not require special precautions or hospitalization (Ryan et al., 2012). The nurse should explain the rationale for these precautions to keep the patient from feeling unduly isolated.

Chemotherapy

In chemotherapy, antineoplastic agents are used in an attempt to destroy tumour cells by interfering with cellular functions, including replication. Chemotherapy is used primarily to treat systemic disease rather than localized lesions that are amenable to surgery or radiation. Chemotherapy may be combined with surgery, radiation therapy, or both to reduce tumour size preoperatively (neoadjuvant), to destroy any remaining tumour cells postoperatively (adjuvant), or to treat some forms of leukemia or lymphoma (primary). The goals of chemotherapy (cure, control, palliation) must be realistic because they will determine the medications that are used and the aggressiveness of the treatment plan.

Cell Kill and the Cell Cycle

Each time a tumour is exposed to a chemotherapy agent, a percentage of the tumour cells (20% to 99%, depending on dosage) is destroyed. Repeated doses of chemotherapy are necessary over a prolonged period to achieve regression of the tumour. Eradication of 100% of the tumour is almost impossible. Instead, the goal of treatment is eradication of enough of the tumour so that the remaining tumour cells can be destroyed by the body's immune system.

Actively proliferating cells within a tumour are the most sensitive to chemotherapeutic agents (the ratio of dividing cells to resting cells is referred to as the growth fraction). Nondividing cells capable of future proliferation are the least sensitive to antineoplastic medications and consequently are potentially dangerous. However, the nondividing cells must be destroyed to eradicate a cancer. Repeated cycles of chemotherapy or sequencing of multiple chemotherapeutic agents are used to kill more tumour cells by destroying these nondividing cells as they begin active cell division.

Reproduction of both healthy and malignant cells follows the cell cycle pattern (see Fig. 68-2). The cell cycle

(text continued on page 2177)

Plan of Nursing Care

Chart 68-3. The Patient With Cancer

Nursing Priority: Risk for infection
Goal: Prevention of infection

NURSING INTERVENTIONS	RATIONALE
1. Assess patient for evidence of infection: a. Check vital signs every 4 hours. b. Monitor white blood cell (WBC) count and differential each day. c. Inspect all sites that may serve as entry ports for pathogens (intravenous sites, wounds, skin folds, bony prominences, perineum, and oral cavity).	1. Signs and symptoms of infection may be diminished in the immunocompromised host. Prompt recognition of infection and subsequent initiation of therapy will reduce morbidity and mortality associated with infection.
2. Report fever (≥38.3°C or ≥38°C for longer than 1 hour), chills, diaphoresis, swelling, heat, pain, erythema, exudate on any body surfaces. Also report change in respiratory or mental status, urinary frequency or burning, malaise, myalgias, arthralgias, rash, or diarrhea.	2. Early detection of infection facilitates early intervention.
3. Obtain cultures and sensitivities as indicated before initiation of antimicrobial treatment (wound exudate, sputum, urine, stool, blood).	3. Tests identify the organism and indicate the most appropriate antimicrobial therapy. Use of inappropriate antibiotics enhances proliferation of additional flora and encourages growth of antibiotic-resistant organisms.
4. Initiate measures to minimize infection.	4. Exposure to infection is reduced.
a. Discuss with patient and family (1) Placing patient in private room if absolute WBC count <1,000/mm³. (2) Importance of patient avoiding contact with people who have known or recent infection or recent vaccination.	a. Preventing contact with pathogens helps prevent infection.
b. Instruct all personnel in careful hand hygiene before and after entering room.	b. Hands are a significant source of contamination.
c. Avoid rectal or vaginal procedures (rectal temperatures, examinations, suppositories; vaginal tampons).	c. Incidence of rectal and perianal abscesses and subsequent systemic infection is high. Manipulation may cause disruption of membrane integrity and enhance progression of infection.
d. Use stool softeners to prevent constipation and straining.	d. Minimizes trauma to tissues.
e. Assist patient in practice of meticulous personal hygiene.	e. Prevents skin irritation.
f. Instruct patient to use electric razor.	f. Minimizes skin trauma.
g. Encourage patient to ambulate in room unless contraindicated.	g. Minimizes chance of skin breakdown and stasis of pulmonary secretions.
h. Avoid fresh fruits, raw meat, fish, and vegetables if absolute WBC count <1,000/mm³; remove fresh flowers and potted plants.	h. Fresh fruits and vegetables harbour bacteria not removed by ordinary washing. Flowers and potted plants are sources of organisms.
i. Each day: change water pitcher, denture cleaning fluids, and respiratory equipment containing water.	i. Stagnant water is a source of infection.

EXPECTED OUTCOMES

- Demonstrates normal temperature and vital signs.
- Exhibits absence of signs of inflammation: local edema, erythema, pain, and warmth.
- Exhibits normal breath sounds on auscultation.
- Takes deep breaths and coughs every 2 hours to prevent respiratory dysfunction and infection.
- Exhibits absence of pathologic bacteria on cultures.
- Avoids contact with others with infections.
- Avoids crowds.
- All personnel carry out hand hygiene after each voiding and bowel movement.
- Excoriation and trauma of skin are avoided.
- Trauma to mucous membranes is avoided (avoidance of rectal thermometers, suppositories, vaginal tampons, perianal trauma).
- Uses recommended procedures and techniques if participating in management of invasive lines or catheters.
- Uses electric razor.
- Is free of skin breakdown and stasis of secretions.
- Adheres to dietary and environmental restrictions.
- Exhibits no signs of septicemia or septic shock.
- Exhibits normal vital signs, cardiac output, and arterial pressures when monitored.
- Demonstrates ability to administer colony-stimulating factor.

continued >

Plan of Nursing Care

Chart 68-3. The Patient With Cancer, *Continued*

NURSING INTERVENTIONS	RATIONALE	EXPECTED OUTCOMES
5. Assess intravenous sites every day for evidence of infection:	5. Nosocomial staphylococcal septicemia is closely associated with intravenous catheters.	
a. Change peripheral short-term intravenous sites every other day.	a. Incidence of infection is increased when catheter is in place >72 hours.	
b. Cleanse skin with povidone-iodine before arterial puncture or venipuncture.	b. Povidone-iodine is effective against many gram-positive and gram-negative pathogens.	
c. Change central venous catheter dressings every 48 hours.	c. Allows observation of site and removes source of contamination.	
d. Change all solutions and infusion sets every 72–96 hours.	d. Once introduced into the system, microorganisms are capable of growing in infusion sets despite replacement of container and high flow rates.	
e. Follow Infusion Nursing Society guidelines for care of peripheral and central venous access devices.	e. Infusion nursing society collaborates with other nursing subspecialties in determining guidelines for intravenous access care.	
6. Avoid intramuscular injections.	6. Reduces risk for skin abscesses.	
7. Avoid insertion of urinary catheters; if catheters are necessary, use strict aseptic technique.	7. Rates of infection greatly increase after urinary catheterization.	
8. Teach patient or family member to administer granulocyte (or granulocyte-macrophage) colony-stimulating factor when prescribed.	8. Granulocyte colony-stimulating factor decreases the duration of neutropenia and the potential for infection.	
9. Advise patient to avoid exposure to animal excreta; discuss dental procedures with physician; avoid vaginal douche; and avoid vaginal or rectal manipulation during sexual contact during period of neutropenia	9. Minimizes exposure to potential sources of infection and disruption of skin integrity.	
Nursing Priority: Impaired skin integrity **Goal:** To maintain skin integrity		
1. In erythematous areas:	1. Care to the affected areas must focus on preventing further skin irritation, drying, and damage.	• Avoids use of soaps, powders, and other cosmetics on site of radiation therapy. • States rationale for special care of skin. • Exhibits minimal change in skin. • Avoids trauma to affected skin region (avoids shaving, constricting and irritating clothing, extremes of temperature, and use of adhesive tape). • Reports change in skin promptly. • Demonstrates proper care of blistered or open areas. • Exhibits absence of infection of blistered and opened areas. • Wound is free from development of eschar.
a. Avoid the use of soaps, cosmetics, perfumes, powders, lotions and ointments, deodorants.	a. These substances may cause pain and additional skin irritation and damage.	
b. Use only lukewarm water to bathe the area.	b. Avoiding water of extreme temperatures minimizes additional skin damage, irritation, and pain.	
c. Avoid rubbing or scratching the area.	c. Rubbing and or scratching will lead to additional skin irritation, damage, and increased risk of infection.	
d. Avoid shaving the area with a straight-edged razor.	d. Use of razors may lead to additional irritation and disruption of skin integrity and increased risk of infection.	
e. Avoid applying hot-water bottles, heating pads, ice, and adhesive tape to the area.	e. Avoiding extreme temperatures minimizes additional skin damage, irritation, burns, and pain.	
f. Avoid exposing the area to sunlight or cold weather.	f. Sun exposure or extreme cold weather may lead to additional skin damage and pain.	

Plan of Nursing Care

Chart 68-3. The Patient With Cancer, *Continued*

NURSING INTERVENTIONS	RATIONALE	EXPECTED OUTCOMES
g. Avoid tight clothing in the area. Use cotton clothing.	g. Allows air circulation to affected area.	
h. Apply vitamin A and D ointment to the area.	h. Aids healing.	
2. If wet desquamation occurs:	2. Open weeping areas are susceptible to bacterial infection. Care must be taken to prevent introduction of pathogens.	
a. Do not disrupt any blisters that have formed.	a. Disruption of skin blisters disrupts skin integrity and may lead to increased risk of infection.	
b. Avoid frequent washing of the area.	b. Frequent washing may lead to increased irritation and skin damage, with increased risk for infection.	
c. Report any blistering.	c. Blistering of skin represents progression of skin damage.	
d. Use *prescribed* creams or ointments.	d. Decreases irritation and inflammation of the area.	
e. If area weeps, apply a nonadhesive absorbent dressing.	e. Enhances drying.	
f. If the area is without drainage, use moisture and vapour-permeable dressings such as hydrocolloids and hydrogels on noninfected areas.	f. Promotes healing.	
g. Consult with enterostomal therapist (ET) and physician if eschar forms.	g. Eschar must be removed to promote healing and prevent infection. ET nurses have expertise in the care of wounds.	

Nursing Priority: Mouth care
Goal: Maintenance of intact oral mucous membranes

NURSING INTERVENTIONS	RATIONALE	EXPECTED OUTCOMES
1. Assess oral cavity daily.	1. Provides baseline for later evaluation.	• States rationale for frequent oral assessment and hygiene.
2. Instruct patient to report oral burning, pain, areas of redness, open lesions on the lips, pain associated with swallowing, or decreased tolerance to temperature extremes of food.	2. Identification of initial stages of stomatitis will facilitate prompt interventions, including modification of treatment as prescribed by physician.	• Identifies signs and symptoms of stomatitis to report to nurse or physician. • Participates in recommended oral hygiene regimen.
3. Encourage and assist in oral hygiene.	3. Patients who are having discomfort or pain, or other symptoms related to the disease and treatment may require encouragement and assistance in performing oral hygiene.	• Avoids mouthwashes with alcohol. • Brushes teeth and mouth with soft toothbrush. • Uses lubricant to keep lips soft and nonirritated.
Preventive		• Avoids hard-to-chew, spicy, and hot foods.
a. Advise patient to avoid irritants such as commercial mouthwashes, alcoholic beverages, and tobacco.	a. Alcohol content of mouthwashes will dry oral tissues and potentiate breakdown.	• Exhibits clean, intact oral mucosa. • Exhibits no ulcerations or infections of oral cavity.
b. Brush with soft toothbrush; use nonabrasive toothpaste after meals and bedtime; floss every 24 hours unless painful or platelet count falls below 40,000 cu/mm. **Mild stomatitis** (generalized erythema, limited ulcerations, small white patches: *Candida*)	b. Limits trauma and removes debris.	• Exhibits no evidence of bleeding. • Reports absent or decreased oral pain. • Reports no difficulty swallowing. • Exhibits healing (re-epithelialization) of oral mucosa within 5–7 days (mild stomatitis). • Exhibits healing of oral tissues within 10–14 days (severe stomatitis).
c. Use normal saline mouth rinses every 2 hours while awake; every 6 hours at night.	c. Assists in removing debris, thick secretions, and bacteria.	• Exhibits no bleeding or oral ulceration. • Consumes adequate fluid and food.
d. Use soft toothbrush or toothette.	d. Minimizes trauma.	• Exhibits absence of dehydration and weight loss.

continued >

Plan of Nursing Care

Chart 68-3. The Patient With Cancer, *Continued*

NURSING INTERVENTIONS	RATIONALE	EXPECTED OUTCOMES
e. Remove dentures except for meals; be certain dentures fit well.	e. Minimizes friction and discomfort.	
f. Apply water-soluble lip lubricant.	f. Promotes comfort.	
g. Avoid foods that are spicy or hard to chew and those with extremes of temperature.	g. Prevents local trauma.	
Severe stomatitis (confluent ulcerations with bleeding and white patches covering more than 25% of oral mucosa)		
h. Obtain tissue samples for culture and sensitivity tests of areas of infection.	h. Assists in identifying need for antimicrobial therapy.	
i. Assess ability to chew and swallow; assess gag reflex.	i. Patient may be in danger of aspiration.	
j. Use oral rinses (may combine in solution saline, anti-*Candida* agent, such as Mycostatin, and topical anesthetic agent as described below) as prescribed or place patient on side and irrigate mouth; have suction available.	j. Facilitates cleansing, provides for safety and comfort.	
k. Remove dentures.	k. Prevents trauma from ill-fitting dentures.	
l. Use toothette or gauze soaked with solution for cleansing.	l. Limits trauma, promotes comfort.	
m. Use water-soluble lip lubricant.	m. Promotes comfort.	
n. Provide liquid or pureed diet.	n. Ensures intake of easily digestible foods.	
o. Monitor for dehydration.	o. Decreased oral intake and ulcerations potentiate fluid deficits.	
4. Minimize discomfort.		
a. Consult physician for use of topical anesthetic, such as dyclonine and diphenhydramine, or viscous lidocaine.	a. Alleviates pain and increases sense of well-being; promotes participation in oral hygiene and nutritional intake.	
b. Administer systemic analgesics as prescribed.	b. Adequate management of pain related to severe stomatitis can facilitate improved quality of life, participation in other aspects of activities of daily living, oral intake, and verbal communication.	
c. Perform mouth care as described.	c. Promotes removal of debris, healing, and comfort.	
Nursing Priority: Skin integrity **Goal:** Maintenance of skin integrity		
Prevention		
1. Instruct patients to avoid sunlight through use of protective clothing, use of sunscreen with SPF of 30 with physical blockers (zinc oxide, titanium dioxide), or avoidance of direct sun exposure.	1. Many agents are associated with photosensitivity; sunburn would intensify inflammation associated with rash and potentiate loss of skin integrity.	• Sun exposure will be limited; no development of sunburn. • Absence of dehydration. • Participates in skin care regimen as instructed. • Absence of dryness, flaking.
2. Maintain adequate oral hydration.	2. Prevents skin dryness related to dehydration.	• Rash severity does not interfere with level of comfort and adherence to targeted therapy as prescribed; absence of local or systemic infection.
3. Avoid long hot showers or baths, harsh soaps and laundry detergents, perfumes, and nonhypoallergenic cosmetics.	3. Prevents skin irritation, dryness, flaking, and inflammation.	

Plan of Nursing Care

Chart 68-3. The Patient With Cancer, *Continued*

NURSING INTERVENTIONS	RATIONALE	EXPECTED OUTCOMES
4. Apply emollients; apply hydrocortisone 1% cream with moisturizer at least twice daily; administer doxycycline 100 mg twice per day or minocycline, as prescribed.	4. Minimizes dryness, flaking, and disruption of skin integrity.	• Rash severity does not interfere with level of comfort and adherence to targeted therapy as prescribed; absence of local or systemic infection. • Local infection is controlled; absence of bacteremia and sepsis.
Treatment		
1. Apply topical treatment as prescribed: clindamycin 1%, fluocinonide 0.05% cream twice a day, or alclometasone 0.05% cream twice a day.	1. Recommended by Multinational Association of Supportive Care in Cancer (MASCC) as treatment to minimize skin disruption and prevent infection.	
2. For severe papulopustular rash: Administer systemic treatment as prescribed: doxycycline 100 mg twice per day; minocycline 100 mg daily; or isotretinion at low doses of 20–30 mg/day.	2. Recommended by Multinational Association of Supportive Care in Cancer (MASCC) as treatment to minimize skin disruption and prevent infection.	
Assess for development of infection: obtain cultures of pustules and administer appropriate antibiotics as prescribed by the physician.	Prompt recognition and treatment of infection are necessary to prevent bacteremia, sepsis, and further patient compromise.	

Nursing Priority: Alopecia
Goal: Maintenance of tissue integrity; coping with hair loss

NURSING INTERVENTIONS	RATIONALE	EXPECTED OUTCOMES
1. Discuss potential hair loss and regrowth with patient and family; advise that hair loss may occur on body parts other than the head.	1. Provides information so patient and family can begin to prepare cognitively and emotionally for loss.	• Identifies alopecia as potential side effect of treatment. • Identifies positive and negative feelings and threats to self-image. • Verbalizes meaning that hair and possible hair loss have for him or her. • States rationale for modifications in hair care and treatment. • Uses mild shampoo and conditioner and shampoos hair only when necessary. • Avoids hair dryer, curlers, sprays, and other stresses on hair and scalp. • Wears hat or scarf over hair when exposed to sun. • Takes steps to deal with possible hair loss before it occurs; purchases wig or hairpiece. • Maintains hygiene and grooming. • Interacts and socializes with others. • States that hair loss and necessity of wig are temporary.
2. Explore potential impact of hair loss on self-image, interpersonal relationships, and sexuality.	2. Facilitates coping.	
3. Prevent or minimize hair loss through the following:	3. Retains hair as long as possible.	
a. Use scalp hypothermia and scalp tourniquets, if appropriate.	a. Decreases hair follicle uptake of chemotherapy (not used for patients with leukemia or lymphoma because tumour cells may be present in blood vessels or scalp tissue).	
b. Cut long hair before treatment.	b. Minimizes hair loss due to the weight and manipulation of hair.	
c. Use mild shampoo and conditioner, gently pat dry, and avoid excessive shampooing.		
d. Avoid electric curlers, curling irons, dryers, clips, barrettes, hair sprays, hair dyes, and permanent waves.		
e. Avoid excessive combing or brushing; use wide-toothed comb.		
4. Prevent trauma to scalp.	4. Preserves tissue integrity.	
a. Lubricate scalp with vitamin A and D ointment to decrease itching.	a. Assists in maintaining skin integrity.	
b. Have patient use sunscreen or wear hat when in the sun.	b. Prevents ultraviolet light exposure.	
5. Suggest ways to assist in coping with hair loss:	5. Minimizes change in appearance.	
a. Purchase wig or hairpiece before hair loss.	a. Wig that closely resembles hair colour and style is more easily selected if hair loss has not begun.	

continued >

Plan of Nursing Care

Chart 68-3. The Patient With Cancer, *Continued*

NURSING INTERVENTIONS	RATIONALE	EXPECTED OUTCOMES
b. If hair loss has occurred, take photograph to wig shop to assist in selection.	b. Facilitates adjustment.	
c. Begin to wear wig before hair loss.	c. Enables patient to be prepared for loss and facilitates adjustment.	
d. Contact the Canadian Cancer Society for donated wigs, or a store that specializes in this product.	d. Provides options to patient.	
e. Wear hat, scarf, or turban.	e. Conceals loss.	
6. Encourage patient to wear own clothes and retain social contacts.	6. Assists in maintaining personal identity.	
7. Explain that hair growth usually begins again once therapy is completed.	7. Reassures patient that hair loss is usually temporary.	
Nursing Priority: Imbalanced nutrition **Goal:** Patient experiences less nausea and vomiting associated with chemotherapy; weight loss is minimized		
1. Assess the patient's previous experiences and expectations of nausea and vomiting, including causes and interventions used.	1. Identifies patient concerns, misinformation, potential strategies for intervention. Also gives patient sense of empowerment and control.	• Identifies previous triggers of nausea and vomiting. • Exhibits decreased apprehension and anxiety. • Identifies previously used successful interventions for nausea and vomiting. • Reports decrease in nausea. • Reports decrease in incidence of vomiting. • Consumes adequate fluid and food when nausea subsides. • Demonstrates use of distraction, relaxation, and imagery when indicated. • Exhibits normal skin turgor and moist mucous membranes. • Reports no additional weight loss.
2. Adjust diet before and after drug administration according to patient preference and tolerance.	2. Each patient responds differently to food after chemotherapy. A diet containing foods that relieve the patient's nausea or vomiting is most helpful.	
3. Prevent unpleasant sights, odours, and sounds in the environment.	3. Unpleasant sensations can stimulate the nausea and vomiting centre.	
4. Use distraction, music therapy, biofeedback, self-hypnosis, relaxation techniques, and guided imagery before, during, and after chemotherapy.	4. Decreases anxiety, which can contribute to nausea and vomiting. Psychological conditioning may also be decreased.	
5. Administer prescribed antiemetics, sedatives, and corticosteroids before chemotherapy and afterward as needed.	5. Administration of antiemetic regimen before onset of nausea and vomiting limits the adverse experience and facilitates control. Combination drug therapy reduces nausea and vomiting through various triggering mechanisms.	
6. Ensure adequate fluid hydration before, during, and after drug administration; assess intake and output.	6. Adequate fluid volume dilutes drug levels, decreasing stimulation of vomiting receptors.	
7. Encourage frequent oral hygiene.	7. Reduces unpleasant taste sensations.	
8. Provide pain relief measures, if necessary.	8. Increased comfort increases physical tolerance of symptoms.	
9. Consult with dietitian as needed.	9. Interdisciplinary collaboration is essential in addressing complex patient needs.	
10. Assess and address other contributing factors to nausea and vomiting, such as other symptoms, constipation, gastrointestinal irritation, electrolyte imbalance, radiation therapy, medications, and central nervous system metastasis.	10. Multiple factors may contribute to nausea and vomiting.	

Plan of Nursing Care

Chart 68-3. The Patient With Cancer, *Continued*

Nursing Priority: Imbalanced nutrition

Goal: Maintenance of nutritional status and of weight within 10% of pretreatment weight

NURSING INTERVENTIONS	RATIONALE
1. Teach patient to avoid unpleasant sights, odours, sounds in the environment during mealtime.	1. Anorexia can be stimulated or increased with noxious stimuli.
2. Suggest foods that are preferred and well tolerated by the patient, preferably high-calorie and high-protein foods. Respect ethnic and cultural food preferences.	2. Foods preferred, well tolerated, and high in calories and protein maintain nutritional status during periods of increased metabolic demand.
3. Encourage adequate fluid intake, but limit fluids at mealtime.	3. Fluids are necessary to eliminate wastes and prevent dehydration. Increased fluids with meals can lead to early satiety.
4. Suggest smaller, more frequent meals.	4. Smaller, more frequent meals are better tolerated because early satiety does not occur.
5. Promote relaxed, quiet environment during mealtime with increased social interaction as desired.	5. A quiet environment promotes relaxation. Social interaction at mealtime increases appetite.
6. If patient desires, serve wine at mealtime with foods.	6. Wine often may stimulate appetite and add calories.
7. Consider cold foods, if desired.	7. Cold, high-protein foods are often more tolerable and less odorous than hot foods.
8. Encourage nutritional supplements and high-protein foods between meals.	8. Supplements and snacks add protein and calories to meet nutritional requirements.
9. Encourage frequent oral hygiene.	9. Oral hygiene stimulates appetite and increases saliva production.
10. Provide pain relief measures.	10. Pain impairs appetite.
11. Provide control of nausea and vomiting.	11. Nausea and vomiting increase anorexia.
12. Increase activity level as tolerated.	12. Increased activity promotes appetite.
13. Decrease anxiety by encouraging verbalization of fears, concerns; use of relaxation techniques; imagery at mealtime.	13. Relief of anxiety may increase appetite.
14. Position patient properly at mealtime.	14. Proper body position and alignment are necessary to aid chewing and swallowing.
15. For collaborative management, provide enteral tube feedings of commercial liquid diets, elemental diets, or blenderized foods as prescribed.	15. Tube feedings may be necessary in the severely debilitated patient who has a functioning gastrointestinal system.
16. Provide parenteral nutrition with lipid supplements as prescribed.	16. Parenteral nutrition with supplemental fats supplies needed calories and proteins to meet nutritional demands, especially in the nonfunctional gastrointestinal system.
17. Administer appetite stimulants as prescribed by physician.	17. Although the mechanism is unclear, medications such as megestrol acetate (Megace) have been noted to improve appetite in patients with cancer and human immunodeficiency virus (HIV) infection.

EXPECTED OUTCOMES

- Patient and family identify minimal nutritional requirements.
- Exhibits weight loss no greater than 10% of pretreatment weight.
- Reports decreasing anorexia and increased interest in eating.
- Demonstrates normal skin turgor.
- Identifies rationale for dietary modifications. Patient and family verbalize strategies to address and minimize nutritional deficits.
- Participates in calorie counts and diet histories.
- Uses appropriate relaxation and imagery before meals.
- Exhibits laboratory and clinical findings indicative of adequate nutritional intake: normal serum protein and transferrin levels; normal serum iron levels; normal hemoglobin, hematocrit, and lymphocyte levels; normal urinary creatinine levels.
- Consumes diet high in required nutrients.
- Carries out oral hygiene before meals.
- Reports that pain does not interfere with meals.
- Reports decreasing episodes of nausea and vomiting.
- Participates in increasing levels of activity.
- States rationale for use of tube feedings or parenteral nutrition.
- Participates in management of tube feedings or parenteral nutrition, if prescribed.

continued >

Plan of Nursing Care — Chart 68-3. The Patient With Cancer, *Continued*

NURSING INTERVENTIONS	RATIONALE	EXPECTED OUTCOMES
18. Encourage family and friends not to nag or cajole patient about eating.	18. Pressuring patient to eat may cause conflict and unnecessary stress.	
19. Assess and address other contributing factors to nausea, vomiting, and anorexia such as other symptoms, constipation, GI irritation, electrolyte imbalance, radiation therapy, medications, and central nervous system metastasis.	19. Multiple factors contribute to anorexia and nausea.	

Nursing Priority: Fatigue
Goal: Increased activity tolerance and decreased fatigue level

NURSING INTERVENTIONS	RATIONALE	EXPECTED OUTCOMES
1. Encourage rest periods during the day, especially before and after physical exertion.	1. During rest, energy is conserved and levels are replenished. Several shorter rest periods may be more beneficial than one longer rest period.	• Reports decreasing levels of fatigue. • Increases participation in activities gradually. • Rests when fatigued. • Reports restful sleep. • Requests assistance with activities appropriately. • Reports adequate energy to participate in activities important to him or her (e.g., visiting with family, hobbies). • Consumes diet with recommended protein and caloric intake. • Uses relaxation exercises and imagery to decrease anxiety and promote rest. • Participates in planned exercise program gradually. • Reports no breathlessness during activities. • Exhibits acceptable hemoglobin and hematocrit levels. • Exhibits normal fluid and electrolyte balance. • Reports decreased discomfort. • Exhibits improved mobility.
2. At minimum, promote patient's normal sleep habits.	2. Sleep helps to restore energy levels. Prolonged napping during day may interfere with sleep habits.	
3. Rearrange daily schedule and organize activities to conserve energy expenditure.	3. Reorganization of activities can reduce energy losses and stressors.	
4. Encourage patient to ask for others' assistance with necessary chores, such as housework, child care, shopping, cooking.	4. Conserves energy.	
5. Encourage reduced job workload, if necessary and possible, by reducing number of hours worked per week.	5. Reducing workload decreases physical and psychological stress and increases periods of rest and relaxation.	
6. Encourage adequate protein and calorie intake.	6. Protein and calorie depletion decreases activity tolerance.	
7. Encourage use of relaxation techniques, mental imagery.	7. Promotion of relaxation and psychological rest decreases physical fatigue.	
8. Encourage participation in planned exercise programs.	8. Proper exercise programs increase endurance and stamina and lower fatigue.	
9. For collaborative management, administer blood products as prescribed.	9. Lowered hemoglobin and hematocrit predispose patient to fatigue due to decreased oxygen availability.	
10. Assess for fluid and electrolyte disturbances.	10. May contribute to altered nerve transmission and muscle function.	
11. Assess for sources of discomfort.	11. Coping with discomfort requires energy expenditure.	
12. Provide strategies to facilitate mobility.	12. Impaired mobility requires increased energy expenditure.	

Nursing Priority: Chronic pain
Goal: Relief of pain and discomfort

NURSING INTERVENTIONS	RATIONALE	EXPECTED OUTCOMES
1. Use pain scale to assess pain and discomfort characteristics: location, quality, frequency, duration, etc.	1. Provides baseline for assessing changes in pain level and evaluation of interventions.	• Reports decreased level of pain and discomfort on pain scale. • Reports less disruption from pain and discomfort. • Explains how fatigue, fear, anger, etc., contribute to severity of pain and discomfort.
2. Assure patient that you know that pain is real and will assist him or her in reducing it.	2. Fear that pain will not be considered real increases anxiety and reduces pain tolerance.	

Plan of Nursing Care — Chart 68-3. The Patient With Cancer, *Continued*

NURSING INTERVENTIONS	RATIONALE	EXPECTED OUTCOMES
3. Assess other factors contributing to patient's pain: fear, fatigue, anger, etc.	3. Provides data about factors that decrease patient's ability to tolerate pain and increase pain level.	• Accepts analgesia as prescribed. • Exhibits decreased physical and behavioural signs of pain and discomfort in acute pain (no grimacing, crying, moaning; displays interest in surroundings and activities around him or her). • Takes an active role in administration of analgesia. • Identifies additional effective pain relief strategies. • Uses alternative pain relief strategies appropriately. • Reports effective use of new pain relief strategies and decrease in pain intensity. • Reports that decreased level of pain permits participation in other activities and events.
4. Administer analgesics to promote optimum pain relief within limits of physician's prescription.	4. Analgesics tend to be more effective when administered early in pain cycle.	
5. Assess patient's behavioural responses to pain and pain experience.	5. Provides additional information about patient's pain.	
6. Collaborate with patient, physician, and other health care team members when changes in pain management are necessary.	6. New methods of administering analgesia must be acceptable to patient, physician, and health care team to be effective; patient's participation decreases the sense of powerlessness.	
7. Encourage strategies of pain relief that patient has used successfully in previous pain experience.	7. Encourages success of pain relief strategies accepted by patient and family.	
8. Teach patient new strategies to relieve pain and discomfort: distraction, imagery, relaxation, cutaneous stimulation, etc.	8. Increases number of options and strategies available to patient.	

Nursing Priority: Anticipatory grieving
Goal: Appropriate progression through grieving process

NURSING INTERVENTIONS	RATIONALE	EXPECTED OUTCOMES
1. Encourage verbalization of fears, concerns, and questions regarding disease, treatment, and future implications.	1. An increased and accurate knowledge base decreases anxiety and dispels misconceptions.	• The patient and family progress through the phases of grief as evidenced by increased verbalization and expression of grief. • The patient and family identify resources available to aid coping strategies during grieving. • The patient and family use resources and supports appropriately. • The patient and family discuss the future openly with each other. • The patient and family discuss concerns and feelings openly with each other. • The patient and family use nonverbal expressions of concern for each other.
2. Explore previous successful coping strategies.	2. Provides frame of reference and examples of coping.	
3. Encourage active participation of patient or family in care and treatment decisions.	3. Active participation maintains patient independence and control.	
4. Visit family frequently to establish and maintain relationships and physical closeness.	4. Frequent contacts promote trust and security and reduce feelings of fear and isolation.	
5. Encourage ventilation of negative feelings, including projected anger and hostility, within acceptable limits.	5. This allows for emotional expression without loss of self-esteem.	
6. Allow for periods of crying and expression of sadness.	6. These feelings are necessary for separation and detachment to occur.	
7. Involve spiritual advisor as desired by the patient and family.	7. This facilitates the grief process and spiritual care.	
8. Advise professional counselling as indicated for patient or family to alleviate pathologic grieving.	8. This facilitates the grief process.	
9. Allow for progression through the grieving process at the individual pace of the patient and family.	9. Grief work is variable. Not every person uses every phase of the grief process, and the time spent in dealing with each phase varies with every person. To complete grief work, this variability must be allowed.	

Nursing Priority: Disturbed body image
Goal: Improved body image and self-esteem

NURSING INTERVENTIONS	RATIONALE	EXPECTED OUTCOMES
1. Assess patient's feelings about body image and level of self-esteem.	1. Provides baseline assessment for evaluating changes and assessing effectiveness of interventions.	• Identifies concerns of importance. • Takes active role in activities. • Maintains previous role in decision making.

continued >

Plan of Nursing Care

Chart 68-3. The Patient With Cancer, *Continued*

NURSING INTERVENTIONS	RATIONALE	EXPECTED OUTCOMES
2. Identify potential threats to patient's self-esteem (e.g., altered appearance, decreased sexual function, hair loss, decreased energy, role changes). Validate concerns with patient.	2. Anticipates changes and permits patient to identify importance of these areas to him or her.	• Verbalizes feelings and reactions to losses or threatened losses. • Participates in self-care activities. • Permits others to assist in care when he or she is unable to be independent. • Exhibits interest in appearance and uses aids (cosmetics, scarves, etc.) appropriately. • Participates with others in conversations and social events and activities. • Verbalizes concern about sexual partner and/or significant others. • Explores alternative ways of expressing concern and affection.
3. Encourage continued participation in activities and decision making.	3. Encourages and permits continued control of events and self.	
4. Encourage patient to verbalize concerns.	4. Identifying concerns is an important step in coping with them.	
5. Individualize care for the patient.	5. Prevents or reduces depersonalization and emphasizes patient's self-worth.	
6. Assist patient in self-care when fatigue, lethargy, nausea, vomiting, and other symptoms prevent independence.	6. Physical well-being improves self-esteem.	
7. Assist patient in selecting and using cosmetics, scarves, hairpieces, and clothing that increase his or her sense of attractiveness.	7. Promotes positive body image.	
8. Encourage patient and partner to share concerns about altered sexuality and sexual function and to explore alternatives to their usual sexual expression.	8. Provides opportunity for expressing concern, affection, and acceptance.	
9. Refer to collaborating specialists as needed.	9. Interdisciplinary collaboration essential in meeting patient needs.	
Collaborative Problem: Potential complication: risk for bleeding problems **Goal:** Prevention of bleeding		
1. Assess for potential for bleeding: monitor platelet count.	1. Mild risk: 50,000–100,000/mm^3 (0.05–0.1 × 10^{12}/L) Moderate risk: 20,000–50,000/mm^3 (0.02–0.05 × 10^{12}/L) Severe risk: less than 20,000/mm^3 (0.02 × 10^{12}/L)	• Signs and symptoms of bleeding are identified. • Exhibits no blood in feces, urine, or emesis. • Exhibits no bleeding of gums or of injection or venipuncture sites. • Exhibits no ecchymosis (bruising). • Patient and family identify ways to prevent bleeding. • Uses recommended measures to reduce risk of bleeding (uses soft toothbrush, shaves with electric razor only). • Exhibits normal vital signs. • Reports that environmental hazards have been reduced or removed. • Consumes adequate fluid. • Reports absence of constipation. • Avoids substances interfering with clotting. • Absence of tissue destruction. • Exhibits normal mental status and absence of signs of intracranial bleeding. • Avoids medications that interfere with clotting (e.g., aspirin). • Absence of epistaxis and cerebral bleeding.
2. Assess for bleeding:	2. Early detection promotes early intervention.	
a. Petechiae or ecchymosis	a. Indicates injury to microcirculation and larger vessels.	
b. Decrease in hemoglobin or hematocrit	b–e. Indicates blood loss.	
c. Prolonged bleeding from invasive procedures, venipunctures, minor cuts or scratches		
d. Frank or occult blood in any body excretion, emesis, sputum		
e. Bleeding from any body orifice		
f. Altered mental status	f. Indicates neurologic involvement.	
3. Instruct patient and family about ways to minimize bleeding:	3. Patient can participate in self-protection.	
a. Use soft toothbrush or toothette for mouth care.	a. Prevents trauma to oral tissues.	
b. Avoid commercial mouthwashes.	b. Contain high alcohol content that will dry oral tissues.	
c. Use electric razor for shaving.	c. Prevents trauma to skin.	
d. Use emery board for nail care.	d. Reduces risk of trauma to nail beds.	
e. Avoid foods that are difficult to chew.	e. Prevents oral tissue trauma.	

Plan of Nursing Care

Chart 68-3. The Patient With Cancer, *Continued*

NURSING INTERVENTIONS	RATIONALE	EXPECTED OUTCOMES
4. Initiate measures to minimize bleeding.	4. Preserves circulating blood volume.	
a. Draw all blood for lab work with one daily venipuncture.	a. Minimizes trauma and blood loss.	
b. Avoid taking temperature rectally or administering suppositories and enemas.	b. Prevents trauma to rectal mucosa.	
c. Avoid intramuscular injections; use smallest needle possible.	c. Prevents intramuscular bleeding.	
d. Apply direct pressure to injection and venipuncture sites for at least five minors.	d. Minimizes blood loss.	
e. Lubricate lips with petrolatum.	e. Prevents skin from drying.	
f. Avoid bladder catheterizations; use smallest catheter if catheterization is necessary.	f. Prevents trauma to urethra.	
g. Maintain fluid intake of at least 3 L/24 hours unless contraindicated.	g. Hydration helps to prevent skin drying.	
h. Use stool softeners or increase bulk in diet.	h. Prevents constipation and straining that may injure rectal tissue.	
i. Avoid medications that will interfere with clotting (e.g., aspirin).	i. Minimizes risk of bleeding.	
j. Recommend use of water-based lubricant before sexual intercourse.	j. Prevents friction and tissue trauma.	
5. When platelet count is less than 20,000/mm^3, institute the following:	5. Platelet count of less than 20,000/mm^3 (0.02×10^{12}/L) is associated with increased risk of spontaneous bleeding.	
a. Bed rest with padded side rails.	a. Reduces risk of injury.	
b. Avoidance of strenuous activity.	b. Increases intracranial pressure and risk of cerebral hemorrhage.	
c. Platelet transfusions as prescribed; administer prescribed diphenhydramine hydrochloride or hydrocortisone sodium succinate to prevent reaction to platelet transfusion.	c. Allergic reactions to blood products are associated with antigen–antibody reaction that causes platelet destruction.	
d. Supervise activity when out of bed.	d. Reduces risk of falls.	
e. Caution against forceful nose blowing.	e. Prevents trauma to nasal mucosa and increased intracranial pressure.	

Adapted from Eaton, L. H., Mitchell, D. H., & Doorenbos, A. Z. (2015). Evidence-based practice beliefs and behaviors of nurses providing cancer pain management: A mixed-methods approach. *Oncology Nursing Forum, 42*(2), 165–173; Eilers, J., Harris, D., Henry, K., et al (2014). Evidence-based interventions for cancer treatment-related mucositis: Putting evidence into practice. *Clinical Journal of Oncology Nursing, 18*(6), 80–96; Fogh, S., & Yom, S. S. (2014). Symptom management during the radiation oncology treatment course: A practical guide for the oncology clinician. *Seminars in Oncology, 41*(6), 764–775; Heston, A. H., Schwartz, A. L., Justice-Gardiner, H., et al. (2015). Addressing physical activity needs of survivors by developing a community-based exercise program: LIVESTRONG® at the YMCA. *Clinical Journal of Oncology Nursing, 19*(2), 213–217; and Mazanec, P., & Prince-Paul, M. (2014). Integrating palliative care into active cancer treatment. *Seminars in Oncology Nursing, 30*(4), 203–211.

time is the time required for one tissue cell to divide and reproduce two identical daughter cells. The cell cycle of any cell has four distinct phases, each with a vital underlying function:

1. G_1 phase—RNA and protein synthesis occur
2. S phase—DNA synthesis occurs
3. G_2 phase—premitotic phase; DNA synthesis is complete, mitotic spindle forms
4. Mitosis—cell division occurs

The G_0 phase, the resting or dormant phase of cells, can occur after mitosis and during the G_1 phase. Within the G_0 phase are those dangerous cells that are not actively dividing but have the potential for replicating. The administration of certain chemotherapeutic agents (as well as some other forms of therapy) is coordinated with the cell cycle.

Classification of Chemotherapeutic Agents

Chemotherapeutic agents may be classified by their relationship to the cell cycle. Certain chemotherapeutic agents that are specific to certain phases of the cell cycle are termed *cell cycle–specific* agents. These agents destroy cells that are actively reproducing by means of the cell cycle; most affect cells in the S phase by interfering with DNA and RNA synthesis. Other agents, such as the vinca or plant alkaloids, are specific to the M phase, where they halt mitotic spindle formation. Chemotherapeutic agents that act independently of the cell cycle phases are termed *cell cycle–nonspecific* agents. These agents usually have a prolonged effect on cells, leading to cellular damage or death. Many treatment plans combine cell cycle–specific and cell cycle–nonspecific agents to increase the number of vulnerable tumour cells killed during a treatment period (Polovich, Olsen, & Lefebvre, 2014; Yarbro et al., 2013).

Chemotherapeutic agents are also classified by chemical group, each with a different mechanism of action. These include the alkylating agents, nitrosoureas, antimetabolites, antitumour antibiotics, plant alkaloids, hormonal agents, and miscellaneous agents. The classification, mechanism of action, common drugs, cell cycle specificity, and common side effects of selected antineoplastic agents are listed in Table 68-6.

Chemotherapeutic agents from every category may be used to enhance tumour cell kill during therapy by creating multiple cellular lesions. Combined chemotherapy relies on agents of differing toxicities and with synergistic actions. Use of combination therapy also prevents the development of drug-resistant mechanisms.

Adjunct Chemotherapeutic Agents

In certain regimens, additional medications are given with chemotherapy agents to enhance activity or protect normal cells from injury. For example, leucovorin (Wellcovorin) is often given with fluorouracil (5-FU) to treat colorectal cancer. Leucovorin, a compound similar to folic acid, helps fluorouracil bind with an enzyme inside of cancer cells and enhances the ability of fluorouracil to remain in the intracellular environment. Leucovorin also rescues normal cells from the toxic effects of high doses of methotrexate (Trexall). When given at certain doses for the treatment of some forms of leukemia or lymphoma, methotrexate causes a folic acid deficiency in cells, resulting in cell death. Significant toxicity, including severe bone marrow suppression, mucositis, diarrhea and liver, and lung and kidney damage, can occur. Leucovorin helps to prevent or lessen these toxicities.

Administration of Chemotherapeutic Agents

Chemotherapeutic agents may be administered in the hospital, outpatient centre, or home setting by topical, oral, intravenous, intramuscular, subcutaneous, arterial, intracavitary, and intrathecal routes. The route of administration depends on the type of agent; the required dose; and the type, location, and extent of tumour being treated. Guidelines for the safe administration of chemotherapy have been developed by the Canadian Association of Nurses in Oncology (Polovich et al., 2014). Patient education is essential to maximize safety if chemotherapy is administered in the home (Chart 68-4).

Dosage

Dosage of antineoplastic agents is based primarily on the patient's total-body surface area, previous response to chemotherapy or radiation therapy, and function of major organ systems. Dosages are determined to maximize cell kill while minimizing impact on healthy tissues and subsequent toxicities. The therapeutic effect may be compromised if inadequate dosing is required due to toxicities. Modification of dosage is often required if critical laboratory values or the patient's symptoms indicate unacceptable or dangerous toxicities. Various laboratory tests are performed prior to, during, and after chemotherapy to determine optimal treatment options, evaluate the patient's response, and monitor toxicity. Laboratory and physical assessments of the hematologic, hepatic, renal, cardiovascular, and pulmonary systems are critical in evaluating the response to chemotherapy (Yarbro et al., 2013). Chemotherapy treatment regimens include standard dosage therapy, dose-dense regimens, and myeloablative regimens with bone marrow or peripheral stem cell transplant. For certain chemotherapeutic agents, there is a maximum lifetime dose limit that must be adhered to because of the danger of long-term irreversible organ complications (e.g., because of the risk of cardiomyopathy, doxorubicin has a cumulative lifetime dose limit of 550 mg/m^2).

Extravasation

Antineoplastic chemotherapeutic agents are additionally classified by their potential to damage soft tissue if they inadvertently leak from a vein (**extravasation**). The consequences of extravasation range from mild discomfort to severe tissue destruction, depending on whether the agent is classified as a nonvesicant, irritant, or vesicant. Irritant agents induce inflammatory reactions but usually cause no permanent tissue damage (Schulmeister, 2014).

Vesicants are those agents that, if deposited into the subcutaneous tissue (extravasation), cause tissue necrosis and damage to underlying tendons, nerves, and blood vessels. Although the complete mechanism of tissue destruction is unclear, it is known that the pH of many antineoplastic agents is responsible for the severe inflammatory reaction as well as the ability of these agents to bind to tissue DNA. Sloughing and ulceration of the tissue progresses to tissue necrosis and may be so severe that skin grafting may be necessary. The full extent of tissue damage may take several weeks to become apparent. Medications classified as vesicants include many of the commonly used agents: cisplatin, dactinomycin, daunorubicin, doxorubicin, epirubicin, melphalan, mitomycin, paclitaxel, vinblastine, vincristine, and vinorelbine (Polovich et al., 2014).

Chemotherapy is given only by those who have the knowledge and established competencies for vesicant and extravasation management (Schulmeister, 2014). Prevention and management of extravasation are essential. Vesicant chemotherapy should never be given in peripheral veins involving the hand or wrist. Peripheral

TABLE 68-6 Select Antineoplastic Agents

Drug Class and Examples	Mechanism of Action	Cell Cycle Specificity	Common Side Effects
Alkylating Agents			
Busulfan (Busulfex, Myleran), carboplatin (Paraplatin), chlorambucil (Leukeran), cisplatin (Platinol-AQ), cyclophosphamide (Cytoxan), dacarbazine (DTIC-Dome), altretamine (Hexalen), ifosfamide (Ifex), melphalan (Alkeran), nitrogen mustard (Mustargen), oxaliplatin (Eloxatin), thiotepa (Thioplex)	Bond with DNA, RNA, and protein molecules leading to impaired DNA replication, RNA transcription, and cell functioning; all resulting in cell death	Cell cycle—nonspecific	Bone marrow suppression, nausea, vomiting, cystitis (cyclophosphamide, ifosfamide), stomatitis, alopecia, gonadal suppression, renal toxicity (cisplatin), and development of secondary malignancies
Nitrosoureas			
Carmustine (BCNU [BiCNU, Gliadel]), lomustine or CCNU (CeeNU), semustine (methyl-CCNU [MeCCNU]), streptozocin (Zanosar)	Similar to alkylating agents; cross the blood–brain barrier	Cell cycle—nonspecific	Delayed and cumulative myelosuppression, especially thrombocytopenia; nausea, vomiting, pulmonary, hepatic and renal damage
Topoisomerase I Inhibitors			
Irinotecan (Camptosar) Topotecan (Hycamtin) ***Topoisomerase II Inhibitors*** Etoposide (Etopophos, VePesid) Teniposide (Vumon, VM-26)	Induce breaks in the DNA strand by binding to enzyme topoisomerase, preventing cells from dividing	Cell cycle—specific (S phase)	Bone marrow suppression, diarrhea, nausea, vomiting, flulike symptoms (topotecan), rash (etoposide), hepatotoxicity (teniposide)
Antimetabolites			
5-Azacitidine (Vidaza), capecitabine (Xeloda), cytarabine (DepoCyt, Tarabine), edatrexate, fludarabine (Fludara), 5-fluorouracil (5-FU), gemcitabine (Gemzar), hydroxyurea (Droxia, Hydrea), cladribine (Leustatin), 6-mercaptopurine (Purinethol), methotrexate (Trexall, Rheumatrex), pentostatin (Nipent), 6-thioguanine (Tabloid)	Interferes with the biosynthesis of metabolites or nucleic acids necessary for RNA and DNA synthesis; inhibits DNA replication and repair	Cell cycle—specific (S phase)	Nausea, vomiting, diarrhea, bone marrow suppression, stomatitis, renal toxicity (methotrexate), hepatotoxicity (6-thioguanine), hand–foot syndrome (capecitabine)
Antitumour Antibiotics			
Bleomycin (BLM, Blenoxane), dactinomycin (Cosmegen), daunorubicin (DaunoXome), doxorubicin (Adriamycin), epirubicin, idarubicin (Idamycin), mitomycin (Mutamycin), mitoxantrone (Novantrone), plicamycin (Mithracin)	Interfere with DNA synthesis by binding DNA; prevent RNA synthesis	Cell cycle—nonspecific	Bone marrow suppression, nausea, vomiting, alopecia, anorexia, cardiac toxicity (daunorubicin, doxorubicin), red urine (doxorubicin, idarubicin, epirubicin), pulmonary fibrosis (bleomycin)
Mitotic Spindle Inhibitors			
Plant alkaloids: vinblastine (Velban), vincristine (VCR [Oncovin]), vinorelbine (Navelbine)	Arrest metaphase by inhibiting mitotic tubular formation (spindle); inhibit DNA and protein synthesis	Cell cycle—specific (M phase)	Bone marrow suppression (mild with VCR), peripheral neuropathies, nausea and vomiting
Taxanes: paclitaxel (Taxol), docetaxel (Taxotere)	Arrest metaphase by inhibiting tubulin depolymerization	Cell cycle—specific (M phase)	Hypersensitivity reactions, bone marrow suppression, alopecia, peripheral neuropathies, **mucositis**
Epothilones: ixabepilone (Ixempra)	Alters microtubules and inhibits mitosis	Cell cycle—specific (M phase)	Peripheral neuropathies, bone marrow suppression, hypersensitivity reactions, hepatic impairment
Hormonal Agents			
Androgens and antiandrogens, estrogens and antiestrogens, progestins and antiprogestins, aromatase inhibitors, luteinizing hormone–releasing hormone analogues, steroids	Bind to hormone receptor sites that alter cellular growth; block binding of estrogens to receptor sites (antiestrogens); inhibit RNA synthesis; suppress cytochrome P450 system	Cell cycle—nonspecific	Hypercalcemia, jaundice, increased appetite, masculinization, feminization, sodium and fluid retention, nausea, vomiting, hot flashes, vaginal estrogen dryness

continued >

TABLE 68-6 Select Antineoplastic Agents (Continued)

Drug Class and Examples	Mechanism of Action	Cell Cycle Specificity	Common Side Effects
Miscellaneous Agents			
Asparaginase (Elspar), procarbazine (Matulane)	Inhibits protein, DNA, and RNA synthesis	Varies	Anorexia, nausea, vomiting, bone marrow suppression, hepatotoxicity, hypersensitivity reaction, pancreatitis
Arsenic trioxide (Trisenox)	Causes fragmentation of DNA resulting in cell death; in acute promyelocytic leukemia, it corrects protein changes and changes malignant cells into normal white blood cells.		Nausea, vomiting, electrolyte imbalances, fever, headache, cough, dyspnea, electrocardiogram abnormalities

DNA, deoxyribonucleic acid; RNA, ribonucleic acid.

Adapted from Comerford, K. C. (2015). *Nursing 2015 drug handbook*. Philadelphia, PA: Wolters Kluwer; Neuss, M. N., Polovich, M., McNiff, K., et al. (2013). 2013 Updated American Society of Clinical Oncology/Oncology Nursing Society chemotherapy administration safety standards including standards for the safe administration and management of oral chemotherapy. *Oncology Nursing Forum*, *40*(3), 225–233.

CHART 68-4

HOME CARE CHECKLIST • The Patient Receiving Care for an Oncologic Disorder

At the completion of education, the patient and/or caregiver will be able to:

- State the impact of cancer treatment on physiologic functioning, ADLs, IADLs, roles, relationships, and spirituality.
- State changes in lifestyle (e.g., diet, activity) necessary to maintain health.
- State the name, dose, side effects, frequency, and schedule for all medications.
- Demonstrate how to administer the chemotherapy agent in the home:
  - Describe safe storage and handling of oral chemotherapy/targeted agents in the home.
  - Demonstrate safe disposal of needles, syringes, IV supplies, or unused chemotherapy medications.
  - List possible side effects of chemotherapeutic agents and suggested management approaches.
- List possible side effects of radiation therapy and suggested management approaches.
- List complications of medications/therapeutic regimen necessitating a call to the nurse or primary provider.
- List complications of medications/therapeutic regimen necessitating a visit to the emergency department.
- Locate list of names and telephone numbers of resource personnel involved in care (e.g., home care nurse, infusion services, IV vendor, equipment company, radiation therapy department).
- Explain treatment plan and importance of upcoming visits to the primary provider.
- State how to obtain medical supplies after discharge.
- Identify durable medical equipment needs, proper usage, and maintenance necessary for safe utilization.
- Demonstrate usage of adaptive equipment for ADLs.
- Identify community resources for peer and caregiver/family support:
  - Identify sources of support (e.g., friends, relatives, faith community).
  - Identify phone numbers of support groups for people with cancer and their caregivers/families.
  - State meeting locations and times.
- Identify the need for health promotion, disease prevention, and screening activities.

ADL, activities of daily living; IADL, independent activities of daily living.

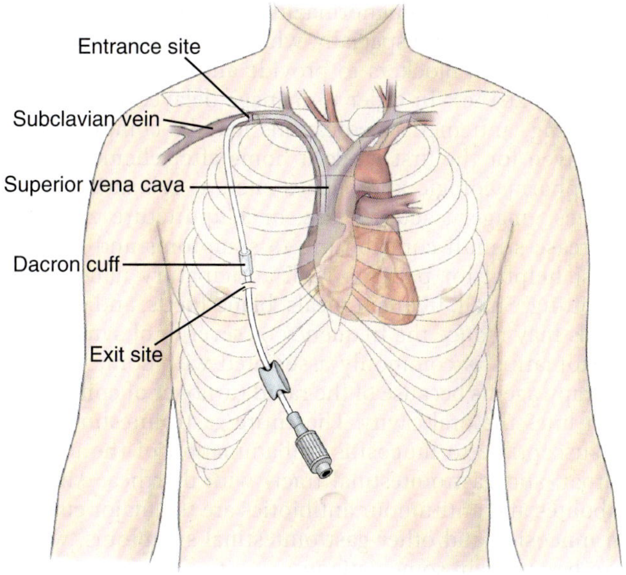

FIGURE 68-3. Right atrial catheter. The right atrial catheter is inserted into the subclavian vein and advanced until its tip lies in the superior vena cava just above the right atrium. The proximal end is then tunnelled from the entry site through the subcutaneous tissue of the chest wall and brought out through an exit site on the chest. The Dacron cuff anchors the catheter in place and serves as a barrier to infection.

administration is permitted for short-duration infusions only, and placement of the venipuncture site should be on the forearm area using a soft, plastic catheter. For any frequent or prolonged administration of antineoplastic vesicants, right atrial silastic catheters, implanted venous access devices, or peripherally inserted central catheters (PICCs) should be inserted to promote safety during medication administration and reduce problems with access to the circulatory system (Figs. 68-3 and 68-4).

Hypersensitivity Reactions

Most of the available chemotherapeutic agents have the potential to cause hypersensitivity reactions; however, the overall incidence of hypersensitivity reactions to these agents is only about 5%. Understanding and managing hypersensitivity reactions is critical when caring for patients receiving chemotherapy because these reactions are potentially life threatening. Prevention is the first line of defence, and nurses need to have a clear understanding of which agents have the potential for precipitating hypersensitivity reactions, determining the patient's responses to certain agents via skin testing, and providing appropriate premedication before administering agents with a high potential for causing hypersensitivity reactions. Education of patients should emphasize the importance of adhering to prescribed self-administered premedication before presenting to the infusion centre and recognizing and reporting the signs and symptoms to the nurse once their infusion has started. Early intervention can prevent progression of a reaction to systemic anaphylaxis. Most reactions coincide with chemotherapy agent administration, but some reactions can be delayed or occur after several uneventful courses of therapy. Although patients may react to the first infusion of a chemotherapy agent, repeated exposure increases the likelihood of a reaction along with other predisposing risk factors such as pre-existing allergic reactions

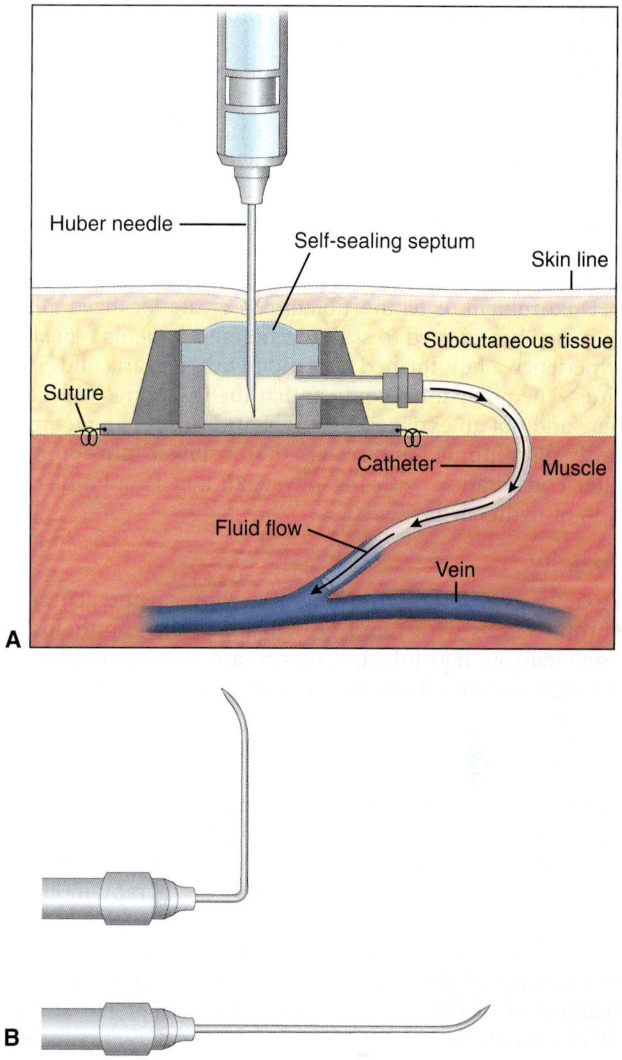

FIGURE 68-4. Implanted vascular access device. **A.** A schematic diagram of an implanted vascular access device used for administration of medications, fluids, blood products, and nutrition. The self-sealing septum permits repeated puncture by Huber needles without damage or leakage. **B.** Two Huber needles used to enter the implanted vascular port. The 90-degree needle is used for top-entry ports for continuous infusions.

to food, blood products, and other medications. Emergency medication and resuscitation equipment should be easily accessible.

The usual chemotherapy hypersensitivity reaction is categorized as a type 1 immediate, immunoglobulin E–mediated reaction. Type 1 hypersensitivity reactions may present as a local reaction and then rapidly progress to systemic anaphylaxis, or the initial presentation may be an acute life-threatening anaphylaxis. Symptoms include generalized itching with localized or generalized urticaria; flushing of the face, hands, or feet; chest tightness; agitation; nausea and vomiting; dyspnea and bronchospasm; difficulty speaking; feeling of impending doom; and hypotension (Wilkes & Barton-Burke, 2014). The medication should be discontinued immediately and emergency procedures initiated. Many institutions have developed specific protocols for responding to hypersensitivity reactions including standing orders for administration of emergency medications (Castells, 2015). Chapter 53 presents further discussion of allergic reaction.

For some chemotherapeutic agents, especially if they are essential in the treatment plan, desensitization procedures may be possible, and the patient is retreated with the agent at reduced dosages or slower infusion rates. Premedication regimens including corticosteroids, histamine-1 and histamine-2 antagonists, and antipyretics are routinely preadministered for certain chemotherapy agents to prevent or minimize potential reactions.

Doxorubicin or daunorubicin can create localized allergic reactions referred to as flare reactions. Patients typically experience a hot, flushed sensation with urticaria and pruritus. The nurse must confirm that the reaction is indeed a flare and not an extravasation. The infusion can be temporarily discontinued and restarted at a slower infusion rate after consultation with the physician and IV administration of hydrocortisone.

Toxicity

Toxicity associated with chemotherapy can be acute or chronic. Cells with rapid growth rates (e.g., epithelium, bone marrow, hair follicles, sperm) are very susceptible to damage, and the effects may manifest in virtually any body system.

Gastrointestinal System

The most common side effects of chemotherapy are nausea and vomiting, which may persist for 24 to 48 hours; delayed nausea and vomiting may occur up to 1 week after administration. The experience of chemotherapy-induced nausea and vomiting (CINV) may affect quality of life, psychological status, nutrition, fluid and electrolyte status, functional ability, compliance with treatment, and utilization of health care resources (Gonella & Di Giulio, 2015). Comorbidities, the underlying malignancy, other treatment approaches, and medications, as well as symptoms (i.e., pain), may contribute to CINV. Acute CINV is experienced in the first 24 hours after chemotherapy with a maximal intensity after 5 to 6 hours; delayed CINV occurs 24 hours posttreatment and may last as many as 7 days with a maximal intensity 48 to 72 hours after drug administration (Gonella & Di Giulio, 2015). Anticipatory nausea and vomiting, occurring prior to administration of chemotherapy, may be a conditioned response triggered by a stimulus such as the smell of the infusion setting, the sight of the nurse, or the outpatient centre waiting room.

Several mechanisms are responsible for the occurrence of nausea and vomiting, including activation of multiple receptors found in the vomiting centre of the medulla, the chemoreceptor trigger zone, the gastrointestinal tract, the pharynx, and the cerebral cortex. Activation of neurotransmitter receptors in these areas is thought to induce CINV. Stimulation may originate through peripheral, autonomic, vestibular, or cognitive pathways. The primary neuroreceptors known to be implicated in CINV are 5-hydroxytryptamine (5-HT or serotonin) and dopamine receptors (National Comprehensive Cancer Network [NCCN], 2015e).

The approach for managing CINV is based on the knowledge of the probability of emesis of the chemotherapy agents used. Algorithms are used to prevent and treat CINV based on national guidelines that consider this classification of chemotherapy agents (NCCN, 2015e).

Corticosteroids, phenothiazines, sedatives, and histamines are helpful, especially when used in combination with serotonin blockers to provide antiemetic protection (NCCN, 2015e). In order to manage delayed nausea and vomiting, antiemetic medications may be combined and are given for the first week at home after chemotherapy. Nonpharmacologic approaches such as relaxation techniques, imagery, acupressure, or acupuncture can help decrease stimuli contributing to symptoms and may be most helpful for patients with anticipatory nausea and vomiting. Small, frequent meals, bland foods, and comfort foods may reduce the frequency or severity of symptoms.

Stomatitis is commonly associated with some chemotherapy agents because of the rapid turnover of epithelium that lines the oral cavity. The entire gastrointestinal tract is susceptible to mucositis (inflammation of the mouth, throat, and gastrointestinal tract) with diarrhea. Antimetabolites and antitumour antibiotics are the major culprits in mucositis and other gastrointestinal symptoms, which can be severe in some patients.

Hematopoietic System

Many chemotherapy agents cause some degree of **myelosuppression** (depression of bone marrow function), resulting in decreased WBCs (leukopenia), granulocytes (neutropenia), red blood cells (RBCs) (anemia), and platelets (thrombocytopenia) and increased risk of infection and bleeding. Depression of these cells is the usual reason for limiting the dose of the chemotherapy. Myelosuppression is predictable; for most agents, patients usually reach the point at which blood counts are lowest 7 to 14 days after chemotherapy has been given. During these 2 weeks, nurses anticipate associated toxicities, especially a fever associated with neutrophil count less than 1,500 cells/mm^3. Frequent monitoring of blood cell counts is essential, and patients are educated about strategies to protect against infection, injury, and blood loss, particularly while counts are low (Manea, 2014).

Other agents—colony-stimulating factors (granulocyte colony-stimulating factor [G-CSF] and granulocyte-macrophage colony-stimulating factor [GM-CSF])—can be given after chemotherapy to stimulate the bone marrow to produce WBCs, especially neutrophils, at an accelerated rate, thus decreasing the duration of neutropenia. G-CSF and GM-CSF decrease the episodes of infection and the need for antibiotics and allow for more timely treatment cycles of chemotherapy with less need to reduce the dosage. Erythropoietin (EPO) stimulates RBC production, thus decreasing the symptoms of treatment-induced chronic anemia and reducing the need for blood transfusions. Interleukin 11 (IL-11) (oprelvekin [Neumega]) stimulates the production of megakaryocytes (precursors to platelets) and can be used to prevent and treat severe thrombocytopenia but has had limited use because of toxicities, such as HSR; capillary leak syndrome; pulmonary edema; atrial dysrhythmias; and nausea, vomiting, and diarrhea (Kuter, 2015).

Renal System

Some chemotherapy agents damage the kidneys because they impair water secretion, leading to syndrome of inappropriate secretion of antidiuretic hormone (SIADH), decrease renal perfusion, precipitate end products after cell lysis, and cause interstitial nephritis (Comerford,

2015). Cisplatin (Platinol), methotrexate, and mitomycin (Mutamycin) are particularly toxic to the kidneys. Rapid tumour cell lysis after chemotherapy results in increased urinary excretion of uric acid, which can cause renal damage. In addition, intracellular contents are released into the circulation, resulting in hyperkalemia, hyperphosphatemia, and hypocalcemia and obstructive nephropathy. (See later discussion of tumour lysis syndrome.)

Monitoring laboratory values of blood urea nitrogen (BUN), serum creatinine, creatinine clearance, and serum electrolytes is essential (Comerford, 2015). Adequate hydration, diuresis, alkalinization of the urine to prevent formation of uric acid crystals, and administration of allopurinol (Zyloprim) may be used to prevent renal toxicity. Amifostine has demonstrated an ability to minimize renal toxicities associated with cisplatin, cyclophosphamide (Cytoxan), and ifosfamide (Ifex) therapies.

Hemorrhagic cystitis is a bladder toxicity that can result from cyclophosphamide and ifosfamide therapies. Hematuria can range from microscopic to frank bleeding with symptoms ranging from transient irritation during urination, dysuria, and suprapubic pain to life-threatening hemorrhage. Protection of the bladder focuses on aggressive IV hydration, frequent voiding, and diuresis. Mesna (Mesnex) is a cytoprotectant agent that binds with the toxic metabolites of cyclophosphamide or ifosfamide in the kidneys to prevent hemorrhagic cystitis.

Cardiopulmonary System

Several agents are associated with cardiac toxicity. Anthracyclines (e.g., daunorubicin, doxorubicin) are known to cause irreversible cumulative cardiac toxicities, especially when total dosage reaches 300 mg/m^2 and 550 mg/m^2, respectively (Comerford, 2015). If these agents are given in the presence of thoracic radiation therapy or other agents with cardiotoxicity potential, the cumulative dose limit is lower. Patients at increased risk for the development of cardiopulmonary toxicities include those older than 70 years, those with a history of pre-existing cardiac disease, hypertension, tobacco use, renal or hepatic dysfunction, and longer survival time. Dexrazoxane (Zinecard) has been used on a limited basis as a cardioprotectant when doxorubicin is needed in individuals who have already received a cumulative dose limit and continuation of therapy is deemed beneficial. Patients with known cardiac disease (e.g., heart failure) are treated with lower doses or agents not known to be associated with cardiac toxicity. Cardiac ejection fraction (volume of blood ejected from the heart with each beat) and other signs of heart failure must be monitored closely.

Bleomycin (Blenoxane), carmustine (BCNU), busulfan (Busulfex, Myleran), mitomycin, and paclitaxel/docetaxel, among other agents, have toxic effects on lung function, such as alveolar damage, bronchospasm, pneumonitis, and pulmonary fibrosis. Therefore, patients are monitored closely for changes in pulmonary function, including pulmonary function test results. Patients with known lung disease are treated with alternative agents not known to cause pulmonary toxicity. When pulmonary toxicity occurs, the agent is stopped and patients are treated with steroids and other supportive therapies (Schulmeister, 2014).

Capillary leak syndrome with resultant pulmonary edema is an effect of cytarabine (DepoCyt, Tarabine, Ara-C), mitomycin C, cyclophosphamide, and carmustine. Subtle onset of dyspnea and cough may progress rapidly to acute respiratory distress and subsequent respiratory failure. Patients who are at significant risk for capillary leak syndrome are monitored closely.

Reproductive System

Testicular and ovarian functions can be affected by chemotherapeutic agents, resulting in possible sterility. Women may develop problems with ovulation or early menopause, whereas men may develop temporary or permanent azoospermia (absence of spermatozoa). Because treatment may damage reproductive cells, banking of sperm is often recommended for men before treatment is initiated (Frankel Kelvin, 2015). Options available for women prior to initiation of chemotherapy include freezing (cryopreservation) of oocytes, embryos, or ovarian tissue (Frankel Kelvin, 2015). Patients and their partners are informed about potential changes in reproductive function resulting from chemotherapy. In addition, many chemotherapy agents are known or thought to be teratogenic. Therefore, patients are advised to use reliable methods of birth control while receiving chemotherapy and not to assume that sterility has resulted.

Neurologic System

Chemotherapy-induced neurotoxicity, a potentially dose-limiting toxicity, can affect the CNS, peripheral nervous system, and/or the cranial nerves. Neurotoxicity characterized by metabolic encephalopathy can occur with ifosfamide, high-dose methotrexate, and cytarabine. With repeated doses, the taxanes and plant alkaloids, especially vincristine, can cause cumulative peripheral nervous system damage with sensory alterations in the feet and hands. These sensations can be described as tingling, pricking, or numbness of the extremities; burning or freezing pain; sharp, stabbing, or electric shock–like pain; and extreme sensitivity to touch. If unreported by patients or undetected, progressive motor axon damage can lead to loss of deep tendon reflexes, with muscle weakness, loss of balance and coordination, and paralytic ileus.

Severe peripheral neuropathies may lead to diminished quality of life and functional abilities and result in dose reductions, a change in chemotherapy regimen, or early cessation of treatment (Tofthagen, Visovsky, & Hopgood, 2013). Although often reversible, these side effects may take many months to resolve or persist indefinitely. Along with the usual paresthesias of the hands and feet, oxaliplatin has a unique and frightening neurotoxicity presentation that is often precipitated by exposure to cold and is characterized by pharyngolaryngeal dysesthesia consisting of lip paresthesia, discomfort or tightness in the back of the throat, inability to breathe, and jaw pain.

NURSING ALERT

Patients receiving oxaliplatin must be instructed to avoid drinking cold fluids or going outside with hands and feet exposed to cold temperatures to avoid exacerbation of these symptoms. Cisplatin may cause peripheral neuropathies and hearing loss due to damage to the acoustic nerve.

Cognitive Impairment

Many patients with cancer experience difficulty with remembering dates, multitasking, managing numbers and finances, organization, face or object recognition, inability to follow directions, feeling easily distracted, and motor and behavioural changes. Although not completely understood, these are viewed as symptoms of cognitive impairment, defined as a decline in the information-handling processes of attention and concentration, executive function, information processing speed, language, visual–spatial skill, psychomotor ability, learning, and memory (Von Ah, 2015). Commonly referred to by patients as "chemo brain," cognitive impairment has been associated with both cancer and cancer treatments, including surgery, radiation, chemotherapy, and targeted agents (Bender & Thelen, 2013). The symptoms may be subtle or profound with potential negative effects on functional abilities, employment, independence, quality of life, and psychosocial status. Comorbidities, age, medications, pain, impaired nutrition, anemia, fatigue, fluid and electrolyte disturbances, organ dysfunction, infection, and hormonal imbalances are factors that may contribute to the experience of cognitive impairment and make it difficult to fully understand. Underlying mechanisms of cognitive impairment in patients with cancer being explored include neurotoxic effects, oxidative stress, hormonal changes, immune dysregulation, cytokine release, clotting, genetic predisposition, and accelerated aging processes (Merriman, Von Ah, Miaskowski, et al., 2013; Von Ah, 2015).

Fatigue

Cancer-related fatigue has been defined as an unusual, persistent, and subjective sense of tiredness that is not proportional to recent activity and interferes with usual functioning (NCCN, 2015f). Fatigue is a distressing side effect for most patients that greatly affects quality of life during treatment and for months after treatment. The health care team works together to identify effective pharmacologic and nonpharmacologic approaches for fatigue management.

Nursing Management

Nurses play an important role in assessing and managing many of the problems experienced by patients receiving chemotherapy. Chemotherapy agents affect both normal and malignant cells; therefore, their effects are often widespread, affecting many body systems.

Laboratory and physical assessments of metabolic indices and the dermatologic, hematologic, hepatic, renal, cardiovascular, neurologic, and pulmonary systems are critical in evaluating the body's response to chemotherapy. These assessments are performed prior to, during, and after a course of chemotherapy to determine optimal treatment options, evaluate the patient's response, and monitor toxicity. Patients are monitored for long-term effects of chemotherapy after active treatment has been completed during the period of survivorship (see Chart 68-5).

Assessing Fluid and Electrolyte Status

Anorexia, nausea, vomiting, altered taste, mucositis, and diarrhea put patients at risk for nutritional and fluid and electrolyte disturbances. Therefore, it is important for the nurse to assess the patient's nutritional and fluid and electrolyte status frequently and to use creative ways to encourage an adequate fluid and dietary intake.

Assessing Cognitive Status

Nurses should assess patients routinely for indications of cognitive impairment. Prior to the initiation of treatment, patients and families should be informed about the possibility of cognitive impairment. Nursing assessment plays an important role in determining the need for referral for neurocognitive evaluation and intervention (Jansen, 2013).

Modifying Risks for Infection and Bleeding

Suppression of the bone marrow and immune system is expected and frequently serves as a guide in determining appropriate chemotherapy dosage but increases the risk of anemia, infection, and bleeding disorders. Nursing assessment and care address factors that would further increase the patient's risk. The nurse's role in decreasing the risk of infection and bleeding is discussed further in the Nursing Care of Patients With Cancer section (see Chart 68-3).

Administering Chemotherapy

Nurses must be aware of chemotherapy and other agents most associated with HSRs, strategies for prevention, signs and symptoms characteristic of HSRs, and the appropriate early and time-sensitive interventions for preventing progression to anaphylaxis. Nurses provide patient and family

CHART 68-5

Potential Long-Term Complications of Cancer Chemotherapy

- Abnormalities in senses of taste, smell, and touch
- Abnormal balance, tremors, or weakness
- Avascular necrosis
- Cardiovascular toxicity (coronary artery disease, myocardial infarction, congestive heart failure, valvular heart disease, peripheral arterial disease)
- Decreased libido
- Dental caries
- Dry mouth
- Dysphagia
- Dyspnea on exertion
- Growth retardation in children
- Herpes infections (zoster and varicella)
- Hypothyroidism
- Immune dysfunction
- Infertility
- Osteoporosis
- Pericarditis (acute or chronic)
- Pneumococcal sepsis
- Pneumonitis (acute or chronic)
- Secondary cancers:
  - Acute myeloid leukemia
  - Myelodysplastic syndromes
  - Non-Hodgkin lymphoma
  - Solid tumours (especially bone and soft tissue, lung, breast)
  - Thyroid cancer
  - Thymic hyperplasia

education that emphasizes two key points: the importance of adhering to prescribed self-administered premedication before presenting to the infusion centre, and recognizing and reporting the signs and symptoms to the nurse once the infusion has started. Patients and families are also educated about signs and symptoms that may occur at home following discharge from the infusion area that may warrant medication administration or immediate transport to the emergency department for further assessment and treatment.

The local effects of the chemotherapeutic agent are also of concern. The patient is observed closely during administration of the agent because of the risk and consequences of extravasation. Prevention of extravasation is essential and relies on vigilant nursing care (Neuss, Polovich, McNiff, et al., 2013). Selection of peripheral veins, skilled venipuncture, and careful administration of medications are essential. Peripheral administration is limited to short-duration (less than 1 hour; IV push or bolus) infusions using only a soft, plastic catheter placed in the forearm area. Continuous infusion of vesicants that take longer than 1 hour or are given frequently is given only via a central line, such as a right atrial silastic catheter, implanted venous access device, or PICC. These long-term venous access devices promote safety during medication administration and reduce problems with repeated access to the circulatory system (see Figs. 68-3 and 68-4). Indwelling or subcutaneous venous access devices require consistent nursing care. Complications include infection and thrombosis (Cotogni, Barbero, Garrino, et al., 2015).

Indications of extravasation during administration of vesicant agents include the following:

- Absence of blood return from the IV catheter
- Resistance to flow of IV fluid
- Burning or pain, swelling, or redness at the site

NURSING ALERT

If extravasation is suspected, the medication administration is stopped immediately.

An extravasation kit should be readily available with emergency equipment and antidote medications, as well as a quick reference for how to properly manage an extravasation of the specific vesicant agent used (although evidence-based data regarding effective antidotes are limited) (Gonzalez, 2013). Nurses should refer to their organization's policy and procedures for reporting, managing, and documenting extravasation. Safety standards require the availability of defined extravasation management procedures, including antidote order sets and accessibility of antidotes in all settings where vesicant chemotherapy is given (Neuss et al., 2013). Recommendations and guidelines for managing vesicant extravasation, which vary with each agent, have been issued by individual medication manufacturers, pharmacies, and the Oncology Nursing Society (ONS) (Neuss et al., 2013; Schulmeister, 2014).

Difficulties or problems with administration of chemotherapeutic agents are brought to the attention of the primary provider promptly so that corrective measures can be taken to minimize local tissue damage.

The nurse evaluates the patient receiving neurotoxic chemotherapy, communicates findings with the medical oncologist, provides education to patients and families, and makes appropriate referrals for complete neurologic evaluation and occupational or rehabilitative therapies (Coyle, Griffie, & Czaplewski, 2014).

Preventing Nausea and Vomiting

Nurses are integral to the prevention and management of CINV. They collaborate with other members of the oncology care team to identify factors contributing to the experience of CINV and select effective antiemetic regimens that maximize currently available therapies. Nurses provide education for patients and families regarding antiemetic regimens and care for delayed CINV that may continue at home after the chemotherapy infusion has completed (NCCN, 2015e).

Managing Cognitive Changes

Although several approaches have been explored, no evidence-based guidelines for the prevention, treatment, or management of cognitive impairment have been established. Examples of nonpharmacologic approaches that nurses recommend to patients include exercise, natural restorative environmental intervention (walking in nature or gardening), and cognitive training programs (Merriman et al., 2013; Von Ah, 2015). Nurses should assist patients to address factors such as fluid and electrolyte imbalances, nutrition deficits, fatigue, pain, and infection to minimize their contribution to cognitive impairment.

Managing Fatigue

Fatigue is a common side effect of chemotherapy. Nurses assist patients to explore the role that the underlying disease processes, combined treatments, other symptoms, and psychosocial distress play in the patient's experience of fatigue. In addition, nurses work with the patient and other team members to identify effective approaches for fatigue management (NCCN, 2015f).

Protecting Caregivers

Nurses involved in handling chemotherapeutic agents may be exposed to low doses of the agents by direct contact, inhalation, or ingestion. Urinalyses of personnel repeatedly exposed to cytotoxic agents have demonstrated mutagenic activity. Although long-term studies of nurses who handle chemotherapeutic agents have not been conducted, it is known that chemotherapeutic agents are associated with secondary formation of cancers and chromosome abnormalities. In addition, nausea, vomiting, dizziness, alopecia, and nasal mucosal ulcerations have occurred in health care personnel who have handled chemotherapeutic agents. Various organizations have developed specific precautions for health care providers involved in the preparation and administration of chemotherapy (Chart 68-6) (Polovich et al., 2014; Wilkes & Barton-Burke, 2014). Nurses must be familiar with their institutional policies regarding personal protective equipment, handling and disposal of chemotherapeutic agents and supplies, and management of accidental spills

CHART 68-6

Safety in Handling Chemotherapy for Health Care Providers

- When preparing (compounding, reconstituting) chemotherapy for administration, use the following safety equipment to prevent exposure through inhalation, direct contact, and ingestion:
  - Class II or III biologic safety cabinet (BSC)
  - Closed system transfer devices
  - Puncture and leak-proof containers, IV bags
  - Needleless systems (i.e., IV tubing and syringes)
- If BSC is not available when preparing chemotherapy for administration, use the following safety equipment to minimize exposure:
  - Surgical N-95 respirator to provide respiratory and splash protection
  - Eye and face protection (both face shield and goggles) working at or above eye level or cleaning a spill
- When preparing or administering chemotherapy or handling linens and other materials contaminated with chemotherapy or blood and body fluids of patients receiving chemotherapy, wear the following for personal protection:
  - Double layer of powder-free gloves specifically designated for chemotherapy handling (the inner glove is worn under the gown cuff and the outer glove is worn over the cuff)
  - Long sleeve, disposable gowns (without seams or closures that can allow drugs to pass through) made of polyethylene-coated polypropylene or other laminate materials
- Linens contaminated with chemotherapy or blood and body fluids of patients receiving chemotherapy should be placed in the following:
  - Closed-system, puncture- and leak-proof containers labeled "hazardous: chemotherapy-contaminated linens"
  - Above referenced container maintained in the infusion centre soiled utility room for outpatient settings
  - Above referenced container maintained in the patient room and/or soiled utility room for inpatient settings
- Chemotherapy preparation equipment (i.e., syringes, tubing, empty vials, etc.), gowns, and gloves should be disposed of in:
  - Closed-system, puncture- and leak-proof containers labeled "hazardous: chemotherapy-contaminated waste"
- Wash hands with soap and water after removing gloves used to prepare or administer chemotherapy or clean contaminated linens and other materials
- "Spill kits" with the appropriate gowns, gloves, disposable absorbent materials for cleansing large areas, and hazard sign should be kept in all areas where chemotherapy is prepared and given
- Implement a quality improvement program addressing safe chemotherapy handling that includes the following:
  - Standard operating policies and procedures for:
    - Chemotherapy handling, preparation, and disposal
    - Handling and disposal of chemotherapy spills
    - Handling and disposal of blood and body fluids and contaminated materials of patients receiving chemotherapy
  - Conduct competency-based education, training, and performance evaluations regarding chemotherapy safety procedures at orientation and at subsequent regular intervals
  - Medical monitoring program to identify indicators of exposure
  - Root cause analysis for all chemotherapy spills and exposure incidents

Adapted from National Institute for Occupational Safety and Health. (2010). *Personal protective equipment for health care workers who work with hazardous drugs.* Retrieved from www.cdc.gov/niosh/docs/wp-solutions/2009-106/pdfs/2009-106.pdf; http://search.ccinfoweb.ccohs.ca/ccohs/jsp/search/ccohs.jsp?QueryText=personal±protective±equipment±for±health±care±workers&MaxDocs=500&ResultStart=1&SortSpec=Score±desc&hTab=0&wb-srch-sub=

or exposures. Emergency spill kits are readily available in any treatment area where chemotherapy is prepared or administered. Precautions must also be taken when handling any bodily fluids or excreta from the patient, as many agents are excreted unaltered in urine and feces. Nurses have a responsibility to educate patients, caregivers, assistive personnel, and housekeepers concerning these precautions.

Hematopoietic Stem Cell Transplantation

Hematopoietic stem cell transplantation (HSCT) has been used to treat several malignant and nonmalignant diseases for many years. The use of HSCT for solid tumours is limited to clinical trials (Maziarz & Schubach-Slater, 2015). However, the use of HSCT in the treatment of certain adult hematologic malignancies (i.e., malignant myeloma, acute leukemia, and NHL) is considered standard of care.

The process of obtaining hematopoietic stem cells (HSCs) has evolved over the years. Historically, HSCs were obtained in the operating room by harvesting large amounts of bone marrow tissue from a donor under general anesthesia. However, peripheral blood stem cell collection using the process of apheresis has gained widespread use. The cells collected are specially processed and ultimately reinfused into the patient. This method of collecting HSCs is a safe and a more cost-effective means of collection than the process of harvesting of marrow (Maziarz & Schubach-Slater, 2015). Stem cells can also be collected from umbilical cord blood harvested from the placenta of newborns at birth.

Types of Hematopoietic Stem Cell Transplantation

Types of HSCT are based on the source of donor cells and the treatment (conditioning) regimen used to prepare the patient for stem cell infusion and eradicate malignant cells. These include:

- *Allogeneic HSCT* (AlloHSCT): From a donor other than the patient (may be a related donor such as a family member or a matched unrelated donor from the National Bone Marrow Registry or Cord Blood Registry)
- *Autologous:* From the patient
- *Syngeneic:* From an identical twin
- *Myeloablative:* Consists of giving patients high-dose chemotherapy and, occasionally, total-body irradiation
- *Nonmyeloablative:* Also called *mini-transplants;* does not completely destroy bone marrow cells

AlloHSCTs are used primarily for diseases of the bone marrow and are dependent on the availability of a human leukocyte antigen–matched donor, which greatly limits the number of possible transplants. An advantage of AlloHSCT is that the transplanted cells should not be immunologically tolerant of a patient's malignancy and should cause a lethal **graft-versus-tumour effect** in which the donor cells recognize the malignant cells and act to eliminate them.

AlloHSCT may involve either myeloablative (high-dose) or nonmyeloablative (mini-transplant) chemotherapy. In ablative AlloHSCT, the recipient receives high doses of chemotherapy and possibly total-body irradiation to completely eradicate (ablate) the bone marrow and any malignant cells and help prevent rejection of the donor stem cells. The collected HSCs that are infused IV into the recipients travel to sites in the body where they produce bone marrow and establish themselves through the process of engraftment. Once engraftment is complete (2 to 4 weeks, sometimes longer), the new bone marrow becomes functional and begins producing RBCs, WBCs, and platelets. In nonablative AlloHSCT, the chemotherapy doses are lower and are aimed at destroying malignant cells (without completely eradicating the bone marrow), thus suppressing the recipient's immune system to allow engraftment of donor stem cells. The lower doses of chemotherapy, associated with less organ toxicity and infection, can be used for older patients or those with underlying organ dysfunction for whom high-dose chemotherapy would be prohibitive. After engraftment, it is hoped that the donor cells will create a graft-versus-tumour effect. Before engraftment, patients are at high risk for infection, sepsis, and bleeding. Side effects of the high-dose chemotherapy and total-body irradiation can be acute and chronic. Acute side effects include alopecia, hemorrhagic cystitis, nausea, vomiting, diarrhea, encephalopathy, pulmonary edema, acute kidney injury, fluid and electrolyte imbalances, and severe mucositis (Maziarz & Schubach-Slater, 2015). Chronic side effects include sterility; pulmonary, cardiac, renal, neurologic, and hepatic dysfunction; osteoporosis; avascular bone necrosis; diabetes; and secondary malignancy (Maziarz & Schubach-Slater, 2015).

During the first 30 days after the conditioning regimen, AlloHSCT patients are at risk for developing hepatic sinusoidal obstructive syndrome (HSOS) (previously referred to as veno-occlusive disease) related to chemotherapy-induced inflammation of the sinusoidal epithelium. Inflammation causes embolization of RBCs, resulting in destruction, fibrosis, and occlusion of the sinusoids (Maziarz & Schubach-Slater, 2015). Signs and symptoms of HSOS may include weight gain, hepatomegaly, increased bilirubin, and ascites. Although various approaches have been used to treat HSOS, evidence-based strategies have not emerged. The use of peripheral stem cells, specific chemotherapy dosing, and nonmyeloablative regimens has been associated with a decreased incidence (Maziarz & Schubach-Slater, 2015).

Graft-versus-host disease (GVHD), a major cause of morbidity and mortality in 30% to 50% of the allogeneic transplant population, occurs when the donor lymphocytes initiate an immune response against the recipient's tissues (skin, gastrointestinal tract, liver) during the beginning of engraftment (Maziarz & Schubach-Slater, 2015). The donor cells view the recipient's tissues as foreign or immunologically different from what they recognize as "self" in the donor. To prevent GVHD, patients receive immunosuppressant drugs, such as cyclosporine (Sandimmune), methotrexate, tacrolimus (Prograf), or mycophenolate mofetil (MMF).

GVHD may be acute, occurring within the first 100 days, or chronic, occurring after 100 days (Barbarotta, 2015). Clinical manifestations of acute GVHD include diffuse rash progressing to blistering and desquamation similar to second-degree burns; mucosal inflammation of the eyes and the entire gastrointestinal tract with subsequent diarrhea that may exceed 2 L/day; and biliary stasis with abdominal pain, hepatomegaly, and elevated liver enzymes progressing to obstructive jaundice. The first 100 days or so after AlloHSCT is crucial for patients; the immune system and blood-making capacity (hematopoiesis) must recover sufficiently to prevent infection and hemorrhage. Most acute side effects, such as nausea, vomiting, and mucositis, resolve during this period of time. However, there are some complications that may occur, such as encephalopathy, hemolytic uremia syndrome, hemolytic anemia, and thrombotic thrombocytopenic purpura (Maziarz & Schubach-Slater, 2015).

Autologous HSCT (AuHSCT) is considered for patients with disease of the bone marrow who do not have a suitable donor for AlloHSCT or for patients who have healthy bone marrow but require bone marrow–ablative doses of chemotherapy to cure an aggressive malignancy. The most common malignancies treated with AuHSCT include lymphoma and multiple myeloma. However, the use of AuHSCT has gained increasing acceptance in treating neuroblastoma, Ewing sarcoma, and germ cell tumours (Maziarz & Schubach-Slater, 2015). Stem cells are collected from the patient and preserved for reinfusion; if necessary, they are treated to kill any malignant cells within the marrow, called *purging*. The patient is then treated with ablative chemotherapy and, possibly, total-body irradiation to eradicate any remaining tumour. Stem cells are then reinfused. Until engraftment occurs in the bone marrow sites of the body, there is a high risk of infection, sepsis, and bleeding. Acute and chronic toxicities from chemotherapy and radiation therapy may be severe. The risk of HSOS is also present after autologous transplantation. No immunosuppressant medications are necessary after AuHSCT, because the patient does not receive foreign tissue. A disadvantage of AuHSCT is the risk that tumour cells may remain in the bone marrow despite high-dose chemotherapy (conditioning regimens).

Syngeneic transplants result in less incidence of GVHD and graft rejection; however, there is also less graft-versus-tumour effect to fight the malignancy. Syngeneic transplant is associated with transmission of genetic defects (Maziarz & Schubach-Slater, 2015). For this reason, even when an identical twin is available for marrow donation, another matched sibling or even an unrelated donor may be the most suitable donor to combat an aggressive malignancy.

Nursing Management

Nursing care of patients undergoing HSCT is complex and demands a high level of skill. Transplantation nursing can be extremely rewarding yet extremely stressful. The success of BMT is greatly influenced by nursing care throughout the transplantation process.

Implementing Pretransplantation Care

All patients must undergo extensive pretransplantation evaluations to assess the current clinical status of the disease. Nutritional assessments, extensive physical examinations, organ function tests, and psychological evaluations are conducted. Blood work includes assessing past antigen exposure (e.g., hepatitis virus, cytomegalovirus, herpes simplex virus, HIV). The patient's social support systems and financial resources are also evaluated. Informed consent and patient teaching about the procedure and pretransplantation and posttransplantation care are vital.

Providing Care During Treatment

Skilled nursing care is required during the treatment phase of HSCT when high-dose chemotherapy (conditioning regimen) is administered. The acute toxicities of nausea, diarrhea, mucositis, and hemorrhagic cystitis require close monitoring and constant attention by the nurse.

Nursing management during bone marrow infusion or stem cell reinfusions consists of monitoring the patient's vital signs and blood oxygen saturation; assessing for adverse effects, such as fever, chills, shortness of breath, chest pain, cutaneous reactions, nausea, vomiting, hypotension or hypertension, tachycardia, anxiety, and taste changes; and providing ongoing support and patient teaching. During stem cell reinfusion, patients may experience adverse reactions to the cryoprotectant dimethyl sulfoxide (DMSO) used to preserve the harvested stem cells. These reactions may include nausea, vomiting, chills, dyspnea, cardiac dysrhythmias, and hypotension progressing to cardiac or respiratory arrest (Maziarz & Schubach-Slater, 2015).

NURSING ALERT

Until engraftment of the new marrow occurs, the patient is at high risk for death from sepsis and bleeding and death.

A cluster of symptoms referred to as engraftment syndrome may occur during the neutrophil recovery phase in both allogeneic and autologous transplants. Clinical features of this syndrome vary widely but may include noninfectious fever associated with skin rash, weight gain, diarrhea, and pulmonary infiltrates, with improvement noted after the initiation of corticosteroid therapy rather than antibiotic therapy (Maziarz & Schubach-Slater, 2015). Until engraftment is well established, the patient requires support with blood products and hematopoietic growth factors.

Potential infections may be bacterial, viral, fungal, or protozoan in origin. During the first 30 days following transplant, the patient is most at risk for developing reactivations of viral infections, including herpes simplex, EBV, cytomegalovirus, and varicella zoster. Mucosal denudement poses a risk for *Candida* (yeast) infection locally and systemically. Pulmonary toxicities offer the opportunity for fungal infections such as *Aspergillus*. Renal complications arise from the nephrotoxic chemotherapy agents used in the conditioning regimen or those used to treat infection (amphotericin B, aminoglycosides). A neutropenic diet is usually prescribed for patients to decrease the risk of exposure to foodborne infections from bacteria, yeast, molds, viruses, and parasites (Lassiter & Schneider, 2015). Whether a neutropenic diet decreases rates of infection is currently in question; see the nursing research profile in Chart 68-7.

NURSING RESEARCH PROFILE

Chart 68-7. Do Neutropenic Diets Prevent Infection?

Lassiter, M., & Schneider, S. M. (2015). A pilot study comparing the neutropenic diet to a non-neutropenic diet in the allogeneic hematopoietic stem cell transplantation population. *Oncology Nursing Forum, 19*(3), 273–278.

Purpose

Despite years of implementation on oncology units, there is little evidence to support the use of a neutropenic diet. The purpose of this pilot study was to determine whether a neutropenic diet compared to a diet without restrictions made a difference in the incidence of infections and nutritional status of patients receiving myeloablative allogeneic hematopoietic stem cell transplantation (HSCT).

Design

This was a prospective randomized pilot study. A variety of laboratory measurements were collected for indications of infection (blood cultures) and to assess nutritional status. Laboratory measurements were compared between the control (neutropenic diet) and experimental (regular diet) arms using the two-sided Wilcoxon rank sum test. Chi square was used to compare the percentage of patients with positive blood cultures in the two groups.

Findings

No significant differences between the control group ($n = 21$) and experimental group ($n = 25$) were found for demographic variables or patients who required total parenteral nutrition. Across all time points, no significant differences were found in any of the laboratory values with the exception of the total protein level. The median in the total protein level across all time points was 20% in the control arm and 16% in the experimental group, a significant difference ($p = 0.023$). Analysis of positive blood cultures failed to demonstrate any significant difference between the experimental and control groups.

Nursing Implications

Nurses should know that this pilot study provides beginning evidence that the neutropenic diet does not contribute to differences in infection rates or nutrition when compared to unrestricted diets in patients undergoing HSCT. Nurses need to conduct additional research with larger samples and multi-institutional involvement before the safety of changing this long-standing practice can be established.

Tumour lysis syndrome and acute tubular necrosis are also risks after HSCT. Nursing assessment for signs of these complications is essential for early identification and treatment. GVHD requires skilful nursing assessment to detect early effects on the skin, liver, and gastrointestinal tract. HSOS resulting from the conditioning regimens used can result in fluid retention, jaundice, abdominal pain, ascites, tender and enlarged liver, and encephalopathy. Pulmonary complications, such as pulmonary edema, interstitial pneumonia, and other pneumonias, often complicate recovery.

Providing Care After Treatment

Caring for Recipients

Ongoing nursing assessment in follow-up visits is essential to detect late effects of therapy after HSCT, which can occur 100 days or more after the procedure. Late effects include infections (e.g., varicella zoster infection), restrictive pulmonary abnormalities, and recurrent pneumonias. Chronic GVHD involves the skin, liver, intestine, esophagus, eyes, lungs, joints, and vaginal mucosa. Cataracts may also develop after total-body irradiation.

Psychosocial assessments by nursing staff must be ongoing. In addition to the stressors affecting patients at each phase of the transplantation experience, stem cell donors and family members also have psychosocial needs that must be addressed.

Caring for Donors

Like HSCT recipients, donors also require nursing care. They commonly experience mood alterations, decreased self-esteem, and guilt from feelings of failure if the transplantation fails. Family members must be educated and supported to reduce anxiety and promote coping during this difficult time. In addition, they must also be assisted to maintain realistic expectations of themselves as well as of the patient. As HSCT becomes more prevalent, many ethical issues become apparent, including those related to informed consent, allocation of resources, and quality of life.

Hyperthermia

Hyperthermia (thermal therapy), the generation of temperatures greater than physiologic fever range (greater than 41.5°C), has been used for many years to destroy cancerous tumours. Malignant cells may be more sensitive than normal cells to the harmful effects of high temperatures for several reasons. Malignant cells lack the mechanisms necessary to repair damage caused by elevated temperatures. Most tumour cells lack an adequate blood supply to provide needed oxygen during periods of increased cellular demand, such as during hyperthermia. Cancerous tumours lack blood vessels of adequate size for dissipation of heat. In addition, the body's immune system may be indirectly stimulated when hyperthermia is used.

Hyperthermia is most effective when combined with radiation therapy, chemotherapy, or biologic therapy. Hyperthermia and radiation therapy are thought to work well together because hypoxic tumour cells and cells in the S phase of the cell cycle are more sensitive to heat than radiation; the addition of heat damages tumour cells so that they cannot repair themselves after radiation therapy. Hyperthermia is thought to alter cellular membrane permeability when used with chemotherapy, allowing for an increased uptake of the chemotherapeutic agent. Hyperthermia may enhance the function of immune system cells, such as macrophages and T cells.

Heat can be produced by using radio waves, ultrasound, microwaves, magnetic waves, hot-water baths, or even hot-wax immersions. Hyperthermia may be local or regional, or it may include the whole body. Local or regional hyperthermia may be delivered to a cancerous extremity (for malignant melanoma) by regional perfusion, in which the affected extremity is isolated by a tourniquet and an extracorporeal circulator heats the blood flowing through the affected part. Hyperthermia probes may also be inserted around a tumour in a local area and attached to a heat source during treatment. Chemotherapeutic agents, such as melphalan, may also be heated and instilled into the region's circulating blood. Local or regional hyperthermia may also include infusion of heated solutions into cancerous body organs. Whole-body hyperthermia to treat disseminated disease may be achieved by extracorporeal circulation, immersion of the patient in heated water or paraffin, or enclosure in a heated suit (Ryan et al., 2012).

Side effects of hyperthermia treatments include skin burns and tissue damage, fatigue, hypotension, peripheral neuropathies, thrombophlebitis, nausea, vomiting, diarrhea, and electrolyte imbalances. Resistance to hyperthermia may develop during the treatment because cells adapt to repeated thermal insult. Research into the effectiveness of hyperthermia is ongoing.

Nursing Management

Although hyperthermia has been used for many years, many patients and their families are unfamiliar with this cancer treatment. Consequently, they need explanations about the procedure, its goals, and its effects. The nurse assesses the patient for adverse effects and acts to reduce the occurrence and severity of adverse effects. Local skin care at the site of the implanted probes is necessary.

Targeted Therapies

Recent scientific advances have led to an improved understanding of cancer development. Traditional therapies such as chemotherapy and radiation affect all actively proliferating cells. As a result, both healthy cells and malignant cells are subject to harmful systemic effects of treatment. **Targeted therapies** seek to minimize the negative effects on healthy tissues by disrupting specific cancer cell functions such as malignant transformation, cell communication pathways (called signal transduction), processes for growth and metastasis, and genetic coding. Actions of targeted therapies include stimulation or augmentation of immune responses through the use of BRMs, targeting of cancer cell growth factors, promotion of apoptosis, and genetic manipulation through gene therapy (Polovich et al., 2014). Most of the currently available targeted therapies are categorized as either MoAbs or small molecule tyrosine kinase inhibitors.

Biologic Response Modifiers

Biologic response modifier (BRM) therapy involves the use of naturally occurring or recombinant (reproduced through genetic engineering) agents or treatment methods that can alter the immunologic relationship between the tumour and the cancer patient (host) to provide a therapeutic benefit. Although the mechanisms of action vary with each type of BRM, the goal is to destroy or stop the malignant growth. The basis of BRM treatment lies in the restoration, modification, stimulation, or augmentation of the body's natural immune defences against cancer (Yarbro et al., 2013).

Nonspecific Biologic Response Modifiers

Some of the early investigations of the stimulation of the immune system involved nonspecific agents such as bacillus Calmette–Guérin (BCG) and *Corynebacterium parvum*. When injected into the patient, these agents serve as antigens that stimulate an immune response. The hope is that the stimulated immune system will then eradicate malignant cells. Extensive animal and human investigations with BCG have shown promising results, especially in treating localized malignant melanoma. In addition, BCG bladder instillation (intravesicular) is a standard form of treatment for localized bladder cancer (Blix, 2014). However, use of nonspecific agents in advanced cancer remains limited, and research is ongoing to identify other uses and other agents.

Monoclonal Antibodies

MoAbs, another type of BRM, are targeted antibodies for specific malignant cells (Fig. 68-5). This type of specificity allows MoAbs to destroy the cancer cells and spare normal cells. The specificity of MoAbs is dependent on identifying key antigen proteins on the surface of tumours that are not present on normal tissues. Blocking these targets leads to apoptosis by disrupting communication between cells. There are several categories of these TAAs: CEA, a prominent tumour marker identified in colon cancer; growth factors such as EGFs and VEGFs; and oncogenes such as *C-erb* or *Bcr-Abl* (Polovich et al., 2014). MoAbs bind with specific tumour cell antigens and block the ability of the tumour cell to reproduce, or deliver cytotoxic agents directly to the tumour cell causing cell death.

MoAbs are being used as aids in diagnostic evaluation of both primary and metastatic tumours through radiologic techniques. For example, MoAbs are used to assist in diagnosing ovarian and colorectal cancers. Their use in detecting breast, gastric, and prostate cancers and lymphoma is

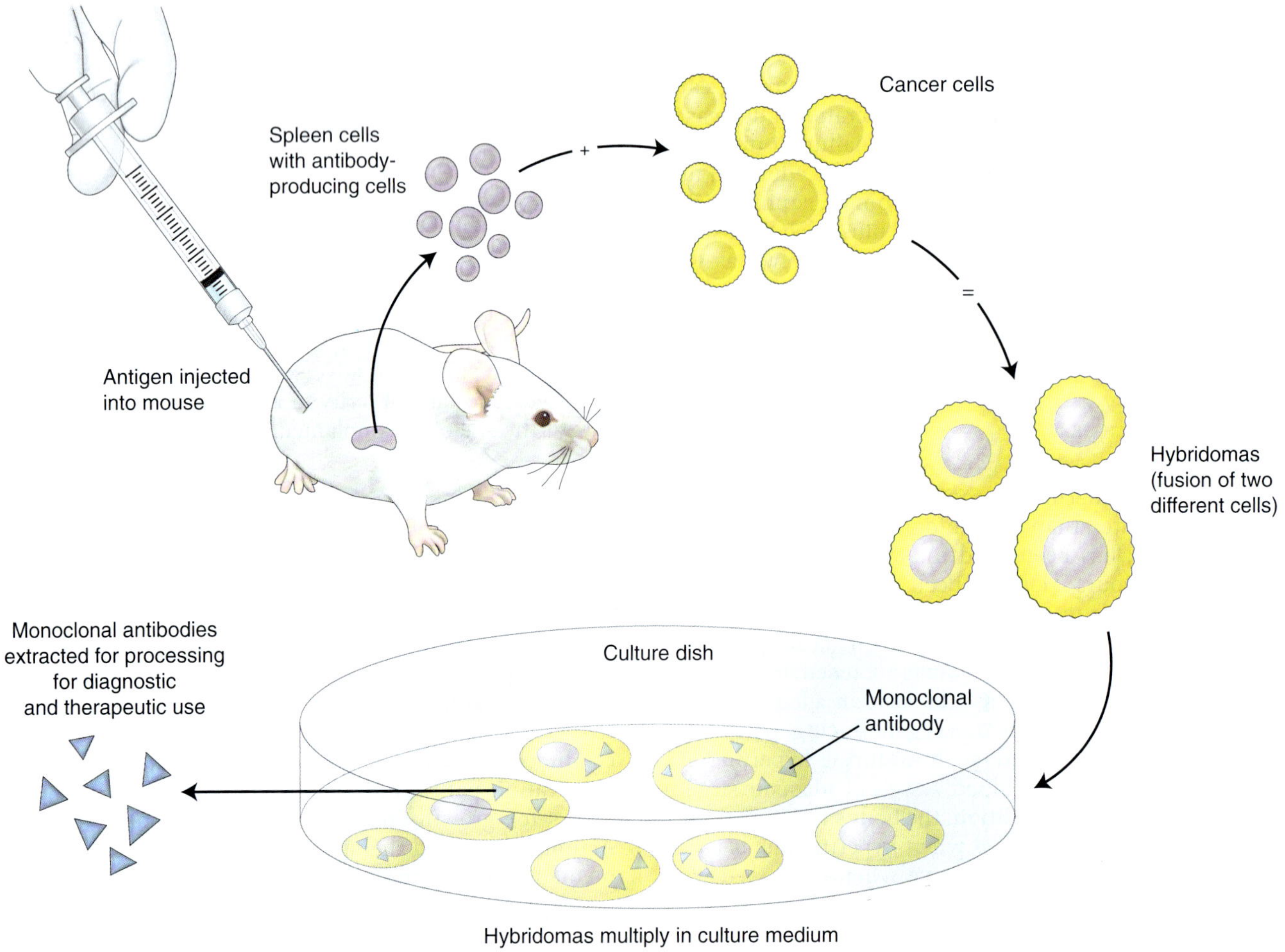

FIGURE 68-5. Antibody-producing spleen cells are fused with cancer cells. This process produces cells called hybridomas. These cells, which can grow indefinitely in a culture medium, produce antibodies that are harvested, purified, and prepared for diagnostic or treatment purposes.

under investigation. MoAbs are also used in purging residual tumour cells from the bone marrow or peripheral blood of patients who are undergoing BMT or peripheral stem cell rescue after high-dose cytotoxic therapy.

Several MoAbs have been approved for treatment of cancer using a variety of extracellular (outside the cell membrane) and intracellular (inside the cell membrane) targets. Some of the MoAbs are used alone, whereas others are used in combination with agents that facilitate their antitumour actions. For example, gemtuzumab ozogamicin is used for the treatment of a specific type of acute myeloid leukemia (Wilkes & Barton-Burke, 2014); ibritumomab tiuxetan and tositumomab are used for the treatment of specific types of NHL. Some MoAbs target specific genetic mutations expressed by certain tumours, as in chronic myelogenous leukemia with the Philadelphia chromosome abnormality (*Bcr-Abl*). Imatinib mesylate was developed to specifically bind with the *Bcr-Abl* abnormality, thus inhibiting cell proliferation.

EPIDERMAL GROWTH FACTOR RECEPTORS AND TYROSINE KINASE PATHWAYS. Normal cell growth is regulated by well-defined communication pathways between the environment surrounding the cell and the internal cell environment, the nucleus, and the intracellular cytoplasm. The cell membrane contains important protein receptors that respond to signals transmitted from the external environment and transmit that signal to the internal cell environment using enzymatic pathways called signal transduction pathways. Advances in understanding the genetic nature of cancers have resulted in these protein receptors and the cellular communication pathways to be used as targets for new cancer treatment agents. New drugs are being developed that will target these specific receptors and pathways and prevent the continued growth of the cancer cells. The family of EGFRs has been proven to be a critical communication pathway. EGFRs are widely expressed by many normal cell types and in certain cancers. Tumours can be overexpressed or underexpressed (Polovich et al., 2014). Overexpression of EGFR is associated with advanced tumour stage, more aggressive tumours, a predictor of resistance to standard chemotherapy, and a poor patient prognosis. Recent scientific advances have enabled the development of numerous new targeted therapy drugs that bind to a specific protein receptor or block a specific signal transduction pathway expressed by a tumour but not by a normal cell, enabling a very targeted, specific cell kill. MoAbs bind to the extracellular protein receptors and are larger molecules that are administered by IV. Tyrosine kinase inhibitors are smaller molecules that target the intracellular signalling pathways and are given orally. The efficacy of these new targeted agents depends on consistent and reliable delivery, and because they involve the patient's natural immune system, they can precipitate very significant adverse events specific to each agent. It is important for nurses to be familiar with the administration issues related to patient education about self-administered oral agents and patient safety related to adverse events (Yarbro et al., 2013).

VASCULAR ENDOTHELIAL GROWTH FACTORS. Angiogenesis requires growth factors, cytokines, enzymes, and proteins, all generated by the tumour to stimulate the formation of new capillaries to deliver oxygen and other nutrients to the hypoxic tumour. The major pathway for angiogenesis is activation of the VEGF family of proteins (Polovich et al., 2014). VEGF is essential for the growth and proliferation of malignant cells and when activated, stimulates growth of new blood vessels. These new blood vessels differ greatly from normal vessels with less well-organized structure, increased permeability allowing migration of tumour cells, and increased interstitial pressure preventing chemotherapy from reaching the tumour. VEGF is overexpressed in many solid tumours and colorectal cancers and is associated with advanced tumour stage and poor prognosis (Polovich et al., 2014).

Bevacizumab is a MoAb directed toward VEGF. It is currently the only U.S. Food and Drug Administration (FDA)-approved angiogenesis inhibitor and is used for the treatment of colorectal cancer. Research is ongoing to evaluate its effectiveness with other solid tumours. Side effects of bevacizumab include delays in wound healing, hemorrhage, hypertension, thromboembolism, and proteinuria. Newer agents such as sorafenib and sunitinib have shown multitargeted activity against VEGF cell receptors and tyrosine kinase pathways and have been approved for metastatic renal cell carcinoma.

Cytokines

Cytokines, substances produced by cells of the immune system to enhance the production and functioning of components of the immune system, are also the focus of cancer treatment research. Cytokines are grouped into families, such as interferons (IFNs), ILs, colony-stimulating factors, and tumour necrosis factors. Colony-stimulating factors have been described earlier in this chapter for their supportive role in myelosuppressive treatment modalities. Refer to Chapter 51 for a more detailed discussion of the immune system.

Interferons

IFNs are cytokines with both antiviral and antitumour properties. Multiple antitumour effects of IFNs include antiangiogenesis, direct destruction of tumour cells, inhibition of growth factors, and disruption of the cell cycle. IFN-α is used in treatment of hairy-cell leukemia, Kaposi sarcoma, chronic myelogenous leukemia, high-grade NHL, renal cell cancer, cutaneous T-cell lymphoma, and melanoma. IFN is administered by subcutaneous, intramuscular, intravenous, and intracavitary routes. Efforts are under way to establish the effectiveness of IFN in combination with other treatment regimens for treatment of various malignancies.

Interleukins

ILs are cytokines produced by subsets of T-cell lymphocytes, NK cells, and dendritic cells (cells that present antigens to the immune system). Similar to IFNs, ILs have immunomodulatory effects on other components of the immune response. IL-2 has been approved by the U.S. FDA as a treatment option for renal cell cancer and metastatic melanoma in adults. However, because toxicities may be severe and life threatening, the role of ILs as cancer treatment has been limited (Weber, 2014).

Retinoids

Retinoids are vitamin A derivatives (retinol, all-*trans*-retinoic acid [ATRA], and 13-*cis*-retinoic acid) that play a role in growth, reproduction, apoptosis, epithelial cell differentiation, and immune function. Retinoids are believed to have a role in cancer prevention as well as treatment. Specific receptors in the cell nucleus are retinoid dependent, thus when retinoids bind with these receptors, cell differentiation and replication are affected.

ATRA is used in treating acute promyelocytic leukemia, a rare form of leukemia, and cutaneous T-cell lymphoma. Synthetic retinoid agents such as 4-HRP have been shown to play a role in cellular apoptosis and are being evaluated for prevention of second breast cancers. Retinoids are being tested for treatment of various epithelial cancers, leukemias, melanoma, and neuroblastoma, and for prevention of breast, lung, prostate, and brain cancers (Wilkes & Barton-Burke, 2014).

Cancer Vaccines

Cancer vaccines are used to mobilize the body's immune response to recognize and attack cancer cells. Cancer vaccines contain either portions of cancer cells alone or portions of cells in combination with other substances (adjuvants) that can augment or boost immune responses. *Autologous* vaccines are made from the patient's own cancer cells, which are obtained during diagnostic biopsy or surgery. The cancer cells are killed and prepared for injection back into the patient. *Allogeneic* vaccines are made from cancer cells that are obtained from other people who have a specific type of cancer. These cancer cells are grown in a laboratory and eventually killed and prepared for injection.

Prophylactic vaccines are given to prevent disease. Quadrivalent HPV recombinant vaccine (Gardasil) protects against types of HPV associated with common genital warts and development of cervical cancer. HPV9 (Gardasil-9), recommended for both males and females, protects against nine HPV types associated with cervical, anal, vaginal, and vulvar cancers. HPV9 also protects against genital warts. All of the HPV vaccines are given as a series of three doses over 6 months. Although the role of HPV vaccines in prevention of oropharyngeal cancers related to HPV 16 has not been fully established, there are preliminary data to suggest effectiveness (Herrero, Quint, Hildesheim, et al., 2015).

Therapeutic vaccines are given to kill existing cancer cells and to provide long-lasting immunity against further cancer development. Challenges to the therapeutic activity of cancer vaccines include the size of the tumour burden, the mechanisms that allow tumour cells to avoid recognition as "nonself" by the immune system, and immune tolerance as the result of previous exposure to the tumour antigens.

Gene Therapy

Gene therapy includes approaches that correct genetic defects, manipulate genes to induce tumour cell destruction, or assist the body's immune defences in the hope of preventing or combating disease. One of the challenges confronting cancer gene therapy is the multiple somatic mutations involved in the development of cancer, making it difficult to identify the most effective gene therapy approach.

Considerable advances have been made in the identification of effective tumour cell targets and evaluation of the most appropriate vectors. Vectors serve as a vehicle or carrier to transport a gene into the target cell. With improved understanding of cell surface proteins and signalling pathways, many clinical trials are underway.

At this time, there are no FDA-approved gene therapies for cancer. Three approaches have been used in the development of gene therapies, with adenoviruses showing the most promise in each:

- *Tumour-directed therapy* is the introduction of a therapeutic gene (suicide gene) into tumour cells in an attempt to destroy them. This approach is challenging because it is difficult to identify the gene that would cause optimal tumour destruction, and patients with widespread disease would require multiple injections to treat every site of disease.
- *Active immunotherapy* is the administration of genes that will invoke the antitumour responses of the immune system.
- *Adoptive immunotherapy* is the administration of genetically altered lymphocytes that are programmed to cause tumour destruction.

Nursing Management

Patients receiving targeted therapies have many of the same needs as patients undergoing other cancer treatments. However, manipulation and stimulation of the immune system create unique challenges. Consequently, the nurse must assess the need for education, support, and additional resources for both the patient and the family and assist in planning and evaluating patient care. Patient education is important, as many of the toxicities associated with targeted therapies are not only a source of physical discomfort, but they also impact the quality of life, and potentially impact patient adherence to oral drug regimens (Vioral, Leslie, Best, et al., 2014; Yagasaki & Komatsu, 2013).

Monitoring Therapeutic and Adverse Effects

The nurse must become familiar with each agent given and its potential effects. Adverse effects such as fever, myalgia, nausea, and vomiting, as seen with IFN therapy, may not be life-threatening. Other adverse effects (e.g., capillary leak syndrome, pulmonary edema, hypotension) that may become life-threatening can occur with BRM approaches such as high-dose IL-2 therapy. MoAbs are associated with both common and unique adverse effects. Although mild to moderate infusion reactions are more commonly associated with chimeric MoAbs, severe HSRs have been seen with MoAb infusions. Nurses must be aware of the adverse effects of BRMs and recognize the signs and symptoms of serious reactions to emergently institute appropriate interventions and supportive care. Nurses monitor patients for the impact of adverse effects on performance status and quality of life so that appropriate measures can be implemented to improve patient outcomes.

Promoting Home, Community-Based, and Transitional Care

The nurse educates patients about self-care and assists in providing for continuing care. Some targeted therapies can be given subcutaneously by the patient or family members at home. As needed, the home care nurse educates the patient and family how to administer these agents and monitors the use of appropriate technique as well as safe disposal of sharps and contaminated materials. The nurse also provides instructions about side effects and helps the patient and family identify strategies to manage many of the common side effects of BRM therapy, such as fatigue, anorexia, and flulike symptoms.

The use of oral medications to treat cancer has risen greatly in the past several years, especially with advances in targeted therapies, many of which are given by mouth. It has been estimated that almost half of the new antineoplastic drugs are oral agents (IMS, 2014). Of over 700 drugs in development, 80% are based on targeted approaches and about 35% are oral agents. The rising use of oral therapies shifts the responsibility for delivery of treatment to patients and families in the home setting. Treatment approaches with newer mechanisms of action and associated toxicities, as well as the transition of responsibility to patients and families, increase the need for nurses to identify factors affecting adherence and develop strategies to address adherence barriers (see Table 68-7).

The nurse collaborates with physicians, social workers, third-party payers, and pharmaceutical companies to help the patient obtain reimbursement or support for the cost of oral targeted therapies and other required medications. The nurse also reminds the patient about the importance of keeping follow-up appointments with the physician and assesses the patient's need for symptom management related to the underlying diseases and/or adverse effects of treatment. Home care nurses maintain communication with the physician regarding patient adherence and tolerance of treatment so that changes in care can be implemented in a timely fashion.

Complementary, Alternative, and Integrative Health Therapies

For many patients and their clinicians, a challenge in managing their cancer treatments is in finding the balance between achieving a reasonable quality of life while undergoing potentially toxic and life-saving modalities. Many patients seek a more holistic or nontraditional approach, turning to complementary and alternative therapies while continuing to utilize conventional medicine.

The National Center for Complementary and Alternative Medicine (NCCAM) at the National Institutes of Health defines Complementary and Alternative Medicine (CAM) as diverse medical and health care systems, practices, and products that are not presently considered to be part of conventional medicine. Complementary medicine denotes therapies in conjunction with conventional medicine, whereas alternative medicine denotes therapies used instead of conventional medicine. More recently, the term Integrative Medicine has been used, which denotes a combination of conventional medicine and CAM that have a strong scientific base for use and safety. The use of complementary strategies is influenced by age, race, ethnicity, and geography (Clarke, Black, Stussman, et al., 2015). However, patients do not routinely communicate complementary practices to their health care providers because they usually are not asked about their use; they withhold the information, fearing that their physicians would not approve, or they feel that the use of these approaches will not affect the conventional treatment they are receiving.

Although many complementary modalities can be a source of comfort and emotional support for patients, assessment of complementary therapy use is important for patient safety. Patients often perceive vitamins and

TABLE 68-7 Strategies for Promoting Adherence to Oral Antineoplastic Agents

Assess for factors that may interfere with adherence to oral antineoplastic agents; develop plan of care that addresses specific assessment findings.

Barriers to Adherence	Strategies for Promoting Adherence
Sociodemographic Factors • Limited financial resources • Competing priorities for financial resources • Joblessness • Limited or no insurance • Racial or ethnic disparities • Lower level of education • Poor health literacy • Illiteracy • Non-English speaking • Lack of transportation • Lack of or limited social support • Rural residence	• Refer to financial counselling through health care facility, local nonprofit health/oncology support/advocacy, or other nonprofit community advocacy organizations. • Refer to social worker for referrals as described above and/or for disability applications through employer or Social Security Administration, Medicaid, or Medicare applications. • Explore patient assistance programs for costs of health care, copays, medications, household costs, transportation services (costs or availability), and home care available through nonprofit organizations, oncology support/advocacy or other nonprofit community advocacy organizations, religious institutions, philanthropic organizations, pharmaceutical industry-sponsored programs, health care institution-specific programs; assist with financial documentation and application procedures as needed. • Explore assistance programs for other priorities competing for financial resources (i.e., for utility costs, gas, child care, food). • Assist patient to identify family, friends, or other available supports to assist with activities of daily living, household responsibilities, errands, shopping, meals, transportation or other responsibilities; assist with delegation of needs and schedules of availability if needed. • Assess preferred method of learning (i.e., verbal, visual, written materials); tailor instructional materials to patient needs, including language. • Include family, significant other, and friends in education whenever feasible. • Use return demonstration of behaviours and devices used to support adherence. • Provide contact information that spans 24 hours for questions or problems. • Contact patient by phone or other means (e-mail) to assess for concerns in between follow-up visits to physician.

continued >

TABLE 68-7 Strategies for Promoting Adherence to Oral Antineoplastic Agents (Continued)

Barriers to Adherence	Strategies for Promoting Adherence
	• Encourage patient to use adherence reminders, such as pill boxes, medication calendars, checklists, medication diaries, alarms on cell phone or other devices/timers; explore availability of programmed telephone reminder services, text messages from family member, friend, or other caregiver; review diary at each visit. • Instruct patient to bring pill bottles to each follow-up visit; perform pill counts to monitor adherence. • Send postcard reminder to patient weekly (or less often) or 1 week prior to due date for medication refill. • Refer to home care for continued education, and follow up on adherence. • Identify local pharmacies that supply oral cancer therapies. Instruct patients to contact nurse if the pharmacy cannot fill the prescription within 24 hours. • Remind patients to anticipate need for adequate supply of medications prior to travel or vacation.
Age • Older adults; especially those >75 years	• Ensure that printed education materials and instructions are printed in black using at least 14-point sans-serif font such as Arial or Calibri. • Use illustrated education materials. • Review and revise adherence strategies if patient status declines or changes. • Explore availability of alarmed medication box.
Beliefs • Oral medications less effective or important than IV treatments • Fatalism about disease outcomes	• Provide education regarding oral versus IV medications. • Discuss goals of care and ongoing assessment of response to treatment.
Comorbidities • Pre-existing chronic disease • Vision or hearing impairments	• Communicate with primary care and other providers involved in care of patient regarding current cancer disease status and treatment; collaborate with other providers for ongoing management of nononcology issues or exacerbation of issues that may impact cancer treatment adherence. • Collaborate with appropriate resources to assist with special needs and assistive devices for vision or hearing impairments.
Polypharmacy • Multiple medications for comorbidities and/or cancer treatment and symptom management	• Review all medications prescribed by oncology physicians and other providers involved in care of patient for pre-existing chronic disease. • Assess patient use of over-the-counter medications and other agents. • Consult with pharmacist to identify medications and other agents that may be contraindicated or that may interfere with antineoplastic regimen. • Collaborate with all providers prescribing medications in order to simplify and/or reduce number of required medications if possible. • Provide patient, family, or other caregiver education regarding specific instructions when multiple medications are required. • Provide written checklist for patient to utilize daily to check off each medication when taken. • Do not give patients prescriptions that allow for refills; prescriptions should be for a finite period of time that concludes with next scheduled visit.
Psychiatric, Psychological, or Cognitive Concerns • Psychiatric disease • Depression • Cognitive impairments • Anxiety	• Avoid initial education regarding oral medications at the same time of first physician visit; have patient and other learners return for another appointment to see nurse for education, and follow up with subsequent visit if deemed to be at high risk for adherence challenges. • Discuss with physician the necessity for referral to psychiatrist to evaluate need for psychotropic medications. • Refer patient for professional mental health counselling as needed. • Identify additional supports for care and education as discussed earlier.
Disease Factors • Symptoms such as pain, nausea, fatigue, skin rashes, etc. • Impaired mobility	• Proactively assess and manage symptoms related to underlying disease and/or treatments. • Provide patient, family, or other caregivers education about expected side effects and management strategies. • Instruct patient to premedicate with antiemetic as prescribed 30 minutes prior to taking oral antineoplastic agent if needed for nausea and/or vomiting. • Identify additional supports for care as discussed earlier. • Assess need for referral to home physical and/or occupational therapy to address impaired mobility and need for assistive devices.
Communication Issues • Patient–Clinician • Clinician–Clinician	• Establish rapport and allow patients, families, and other caregivers time and opportunity to ask questions. • Do not assume adherence to oral antineoplastic agents; assess potential barriers consistently throughout course of treatment at each follow-up visit. • Communicate with primary provider regarding current cancer disease status, treatment and information regarding antineoplastic agents, such as drug–drug interactions, expected toxicities, and toxicities requiring prompt intervention.

Adapted from Vioral, A., Leslie, M., Best, R., et al. (2014). Patient adherence with oral oncolytic therapies. *Seminars in Oncology Nursing, 30*(3), 190–199.

dietary supplements as harmless, natural products that have no side effects or potential toxicities. Deep tissue massage and other manipulative therapies are contraindicated in patients with open wounds, radiation dermatitis, thrombocytopenia, VTE, and coagulation disorders, and in those taking anticoagulants. See Chapter 8 for more information on complementary, alternative, and integrative health therapies.

Mind–body and biofield therapies have a holistic focus on channelling positive energy, promoting relaxation, and reducing stress and have been reported as being beneficial to patients as measured by wound healing and reduction in pain, edema, and anxiety (Perlman, Lontok, Huhmann, et al., 2013). There is, however, risk associated with some of the CAM modalities. Because of the possibility of herb–vitamin–drug interactions, there is concern about the use of biologics and dietary supplements, which are neither regulated by the FDA nor subjected to rigorous scientific evaluation. Patients often perceive vitamins and dietary supplements as harmless, natural products that have no side effects or potential toxicities. One example of herbal–drug interaction is the effect of St. John's wort on the efficacy of irinotecan, cyclophosphamide, tamoxifen, cyclosporine, and warfarin. Each nursing assessment should include an open discussion with patients about their use of CAM. This requires that nurses develop the appropriate familiarity and knowledge related to CAM in order to direct patients to safe, reliable, and credible sources for information.

Unproven and Unconventional Therapies

Despite increasing 5-year survival rates with the use of traditional methods of treatment, a significant number of patients use or seriously consider using some form of unconventional treatment. Hopelessness, desperation, unmet needs, lack of factual information, and family or social pressures are major factors that motivate patients to seek unconventional methods of treatment and allow them to fall prey to deceptive practices and quackery.

Unconventional treatments are those without scientific evidence of the ability to cure or control cancer. In addition to being ineffective, some unconventional treatments may also be harmful to the patient and may cost thousands of dollars.

In the age of the Internet, patients have unlimited access to frequently unreliable claims of "miracle cures" that range from plant remedies to metabolic therapy using special diets, supplements, or "detoxification" regimens involving unconventional enemas and colonic cleansing procedures. The ACS maintains a list of potentially dangerous and harmful unproven therapies on its Web site.

Nursing Care of Patients With Cancer

INTERACTIVE TUTORIALS

The outlook for patients with cancer has greatly improved because of scientific and technologic advances. However, as a result of the underlying disease or various treatment modalities, patients with cancer may experience a variety of secondary problems such as infection, reduced WBC counts, bleeding, skin problems, nutritional problems, pain, fatigue, and psychological stress. Chart 68-3 provides a nursing care plan for patients with cancer.

Maintaining Tissue Integrity

Some of the most frequently encountered disturbances of tissue integrity, in addition to stomatitis, include skin and tissue reactions to radiation therapy, alopecia, and metastatic skin lesions.

Stomatitis

Mucositis is a common side effect of radiation and some types of chemotherapy that may lead to inflammation and ulceration of any portion of the gastrointestinal tract from the oral cavity throughout the alimentary canal. One form of mucositis, stomatitis, is an inflammatory response of the oral tissues that is characterized by mild redness (erythema) and edema or, if severe, by painful ulcerations, bleeding, and secondary infection. Stomatitis commonly develops 5 to 14 days after patients receive certain chemotherapeutic agents, such as doxorubicin and 5-fluorouracil, and BRMs, such as IL-2 and IFN. As many as 40% of patients receiving chemotherapy experience some degree of stomatitis during treatment. Patients receiving high-dose chemotherapy are at increased risk. Stomatitis may also occur after radiation treatments to the head and neck. Oropharyngeal mucositis may be worse in patients with head and neck cancers who receive combined modality therapy of both radiation and chemotherapy.

The destruction of cells in the oral cavity initiates the inflammatory process, leading to further tissue damage and ulceration of oral tissues. Normal flora invades the ulcerations and causes additional damage. Poor oral hygiene, existing dental disease, use of other medications that dry mucous membranes, advanced age, smoking, previous cancer treatment, diminished renal function, and impaired nutritional status further contribute to the severity of stomatitis. Radiation-induced xerostomia associated with decreased function of the salivary glands may contribute to stomatitis in patients who have received radiation to the head and neck.

Myelosuppression predisposes the patient to oral bleeding and infection. Severe oral pain can significantly affect swallowing, nutritional intake, speech, and a willingness to maintain oral hygiene. As a result of the ability to give higher doses of chemotherapy due to improvements in managing neutropenia with growth factors, stomatitis is a common reason for treatment delays and dose reductions (Yarbro et al., 2013). Advanced stomatitis may cause or prolong hospitalizations, significantly reduce the patient's quality of life, and ultimately lead to poor patient outcomes.

It is important for nurses to assess the oropharyngeal cavity of patients prior to, throughout the course of, and after treatment. It is important that the same tool or method of assessment is used by all clinicians involved in the patient's care. Nursing assessment begins with understanding the patient's usual practices for oral hygiene and identification of individuals at risk for stomatitis. The patient is also assessed for dehydration, infection, pain, and nutritional impairment resulting from stomatitis.

Ongoing studies are addressing the inflammation and release of chemical substances that lead to stomatitis. At this time, most clinicians agree that good oral hygiene, including brushing, flossing, and rinsing, is necessary to minimize the risk of oral complications associated with cancer therapies.

Palifermin, a synthetic form of human keratinocyte growth factor, is an IV medication for treatment of oral mucositis in patients with hematologic cancer who are undergoing radiation conditioning regime prior to HSC support. Palifermin promotes epithelial cell repair and more rapid replacement of cells in the mouth and gastrointestinal tract (Wilkes & Barton-Burke, 2014). It is not yet been approved for use in patients with other types of cancer. Careful timing of administration and monitoring are essential for maximum effectiveness and to detect adverse effects.

Radiation-Associated Impairment of Skin Integrity

Although advances in radiation therapy have resulted in decreased incidence and severity of skin impairments, patients may still develop skin reactions that lead to pain, irritation, pruritus, burning, and diminished quality of life. Nursing care for patients with skin reactions includes maintaining skin integrity, cleansing the skin, promoting comfort, reducing pain, preventing additional trauma, and preventing and managing infection. Although a variety of methods and products are used in clinical practice for patients with radiation-induced skin reactions, there is limited evidence to support their value. Patients with skin and tissue reactions to radiation therapy require careful skin care to prevent further skin irritation, drying, and damage, as discussed in the nursing care plan (see Chart 68-3), under Impaired skin integrity.

Alopecia

The temporary or permanent thinning or complete loss of hair is a potential adverse effect of whole-brain radiation therapy, various chemotherapies, and targeted agents. Alopecia usually begins 2 to 3 weeks after the initiation of chemotherapy and radiation therapy; regrowth most often begins within 8 weeks after the last treatment. Some patients who undergo radiation to the head may sustain permanent hair loss. The onset of gradually progressing alopecia and body hair loss associated with targeted therapies generally occurs 1 to 3 months after the start of treatment and may be patchy appearing as temporal or frontal hair loss. This type of hair loss is usually reversible after the end of therapy and in some cases beginning sooner. Several targeted agents are associated with changes in hair growth rate, curliness, texture, and pigmentation. Although health care providers may view hair loss as a minor issue, for many patients it is a major assault on body image, challenging to self-esteem, and resulting in psychosocial distress and depression. Despite the significant psychosocial impact of alopecia, few studies have addressed methods to prevent or minimize the impact of alopecia. The use of cryotherapy to the head during the administration of chemotherapy has been explored but is not consistently used because of concern about later development of scalp metastasis. When cryotherapy is offered, its use is avoided in patients with hematologic malignancies. Nurses provide information about hair loss and support the patient and family in coping with changes in body image. Patients are assisted to identify proactive choices that may empower them to improve responses to cancer and perceived lack of control as discussed in the nursing care plan (see Chart 68-3).

Malignant Skin Lesions

Skin lesions may occur with local extension or metastasis of the tumour into the epithelium and its surrounding lymph and blood vessels. Either locally invasive or metastatic cancer to the skin may result in erythema, discoloured nodules, or progression to wounds involving edema, exudates, and tissue necrosis. The most extensive lesions may ulcerate with an overgrowth of microorganisms that results in a very distressing malodour. These lesions are a source of considerable pain, discomfort, and embarrassment.

Ulcerating skin lesions usually indicate widely disseminated disease that is unlikely to be eradicated. Managing these lesions becomes a nursing priority. Nurses carefully assess malignant skin lesions for the size, appearance, condition of the surrounding tissue, odour, bleeding, drainage, and associated pain or other symptoms including evidence of infection. The potential for serious complications such as hemorrhage, vessel compression/obstruction, or airway obstruction should be noted so that the caregiver can be instructed in palliative measures to maintain patient comfort. Since this type of lesion is associated with advanced disease, the nurse assesses the wound for progression over time.

Nursing care also includes cleansing the skin, reducing superficial bacteria, controlling bleeding, reducing odour, protecting the skin from further trauma, and relieving pain. The patient and family require emotional support, assistance, and guidance to care for these skin lesions and to address comfort measures at home. Referral for home care is indicated.

Promoting Nutrition

Nutritional Impairment

Most patients with cancer experience some weight loss during their illness. Anorexia, malabsorption, and cachexia are common examples of nutritional problems. Impaired nutritional status may contribute to both physical and psychosocial consequences (Chart 68-8). Nutritional concerns include decreased protein and caloric intake, metabolic or mechanical effects of the cancer, systemic disease, side effects of the treatment, or the patient's emotional status.

CHART 68-8

Potential Consequences of Impaired Nutrition in Patients With Cancer

- Decreased survival
- Immune incompetence
- Anemia
- Increased incidence of infection
- Delayed tissue and wound healing
- Fatigue
- Diminished functional ability
- Decreased capacity to continue antineoplastic therapy
- Increased hospital admissions
- Increased length of hospital stay
- Impaired psychosocial functioning

Anorexia

Among the many causes of anorexia in patients with cancer are alterations in taste, manifested by increased salty, sour, and metallic taste sensations, and altered responses to sweet and bitter flavours. Taste alterations may result from mineral deficiencies, increases in circulating amino acids and cellular metabolites, or the administration of chemotherapeutic agents. Taste changes contribute to decreased appetite and nutritional intake and protein–calorie malnutrition. Patients undergoing radiation therapy to the head and neck may experience "mouth blindness," which is a severe impairment of taste.

Anorexia may occur because people feel full after eating only a small amount of food. This sense of fullness occurs secondary to a decrease in digestive enzymes, abnormalities in the metabolism of glucose and triglycerides, and prolonged stimulation of gastric volume receptors, which convey the feeling of being full. Psychological distress throughout illness may also have a negative impact on appetite. Patients may develop an aversion to food because of the nausea associated with treatment.

Malabsorption

Many patients with cancer are unable to absorb nutrients from the gastrointestinal system as a result of tumour activity and cancer treatment. Tumours may impair enzyme production or produce fistulas. Some tumours secrete hormones and enzymes, such as gastrin, that lead to increased gastrointestinal irritation, peptic ulcer disease, and decreased fat digestion. Tumours may interfere with protein digestion.

Chemotherapy and radiation may irritate and damage mucosal cells of the bowel, inhibiting absorption. Radiation therapy has been associated with sclerosis of the blood vessels in the bowel and fibrotic changes in the gastrointestinal tissue. Surgical intervention may change peristaltic patterns, alter gastrointestinal secretions, and reduce the absorptive surfaces of the gastrointestinal mucosa, all leading to malabsorption.

Cancer-Related Anorexia–Cachexia Syndrome

Cancer-related anorexia–cachexia syndrome (CACS) is a complex biologic process that results from a combination of increased energy expenditure and decreased intake (Alt-Epping & Nauck, 2015; Bozzetti, 2013). This syndrome can occur in both the curative and palliative stages of treatment and care. Combined immunologic, neuroendocrine, and metabolic processes give rise to anorexia, unintentional weight loss, and increased metabolic demand with impaired metabolism of glucose and lipids. As this syndrome continues, altered metabolic processes and tumour responses lead to cytokine release, causing generalized systemic inflammation. The patient experiences continued weight loss and malnutrition characterized by loss of adipose tissue, visceral protein, and skeletal muscle mass. Patients with CACS complain of loss of appetite, early satiety, and fatigue. As many as 80% of all patients with cancer experience some degree of cachexia (Alt-Epping & Nauck, 2015; Bozzetti, 2013). Protein losses are associated with the development of anemia, peripheral edema, and progressive debilitation. The signs and symptoms of cancer cachexia and progressive debilitation appear to result in decreased quality of life, psychological distress, and anxiety for both patient and family as they respond to actual and perceived impending losses, fear, lack of control, and helplessness.

Nursing care is integral to an interdisciplinary approach that addresses the multiple factors contributing to impaired nutritional status in patients with cancer (see Chart 68-3).

General Nutritional Considerations

Assessment of the patient's nutritional status is conducted at diagnosis and throughout the course of treatment and the disease process. The patient's weight and caloric intake are monitored closely. Diet history, episodes of anorexia, changes in appetite, situations and foods that aggravate or relieve anorexia, and medication history are assessed. Difficulty in chewing or swallowing and the presence of nausea, vomiting, or diarrhea are noted.

Clinical and laboratory data useful in assessing nutritional status include anthropometric measurements (triceps skin fold and middle-upper arm circumference), serum protein levels (albumin and transferrin), serum electrolytes, lymphocyte count, skin response to intradermal injection of antigens, hemoglobin levels, hematocrit, urinary creatinine levels, and serum iron levels. Whenever possible, every effort is made to maintain adequate nutrition through the oral route. Prokinetic agents such as metoclopramide are used in some settings to increase gastric emptying in patients with early satiety and delayed gastric emptying.

If adequate nutrition cannot be maintained by oral intake, nutritional support via the enteral route may be necessary. Patients with head and neck cancers who receive radiation therapy or combination therapies are at particularly high risk for impaired oral intake and inadequate fluid and nutritional status. Increasingly, patients at risk for significantly impaired nutrition have prophylactic percutaneous endoscopic gastrostomy (PEG) tubes inserted prior to initiation of antineoplastic treatment and the onset of weight loss and other consequences of limited oral intake (Bozzetti, 2013). When needed, the patient and family are taught to administer enteral nutrition in the home.

If malabsorption is a problem, enzyme and vitamin replacement may be instituted. Additional strategies include changing the feeding schedule, using simple diets, and relieving diarrhea. If malabsorption is severe, parenteral nutrition may be necessary (Fig. 68-6).

However, patients receiving parenteral nutrition are at increased risk for complications, including catheter-related and systemic infections. The use of parenteral nutrition in patients with advanced or end-stage cancer is rare and controversial (Bozzetti, 2013). Parenteral nutrition can be given in several ways: by a long-term venous access device such as a right atrial catheter (see Fig. 68-3), implanted venous port (see Fig. 68-4), or PICC (see Fig. 68-6). The nurse educates the patient and family to care for the venous access device and to administer parenteral nutrition. Home care nurses provide education and assist with or supervise parenteral nutrition administration in the home.

Interventions to reduce cachexia usually do not prolong survival or improve nutritional status significantly. Before invasive nutritional strategies are instituted, the nurse

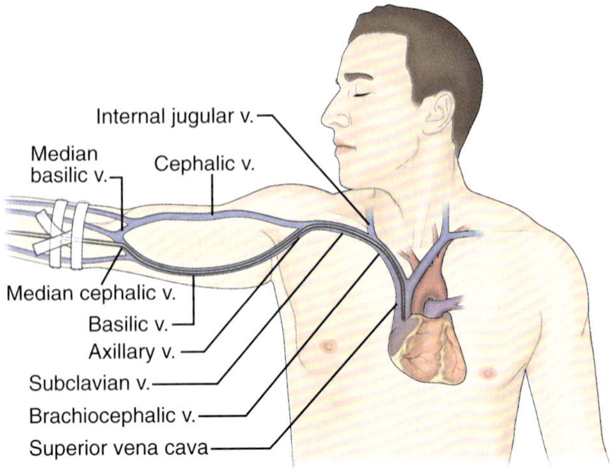

FIGURE 68-6. A peripherally inserted central catheter (PICC) is advanced through the cephalic or basilic vein to the axillary, subclavian, or brachiocephalic vein or the superior vena cava.

should assess the patient carefully and discuss options with the patient and family. Creative dietary therapies, enteral (tube) feedings, or parenteral nutrition may be necessary to ensure adequate nutrition. Care is also directed toward preventing trauma, infection, and other complications that increase metabolic demands.

Relieving Pain

More than half of patients with cancer experience pain throughout the cancer trajectory. Moderate to severe pain is reported by approximately 30% to 70% of patients with cancer during treatment and by as many as 80% of those with advanced disease (Eaton, Mitchell, & Doorenbos, 2015). Although cancer pain may be acute, it is more frequently characterized as chronic. (For more information on cancer-related pain, see Chapter 16.) As in other situations involving pain, the experience of cancer pain is influenced by physical, psychosocial, cultural, and spiritual factors.

Pain is also associated with various cancer treatments. Acute pain is linked with trauma from surgery. Occasionally, chronic pain syndromes, such as postsurgical neuropathies (pain related to nerve tissue injury), occur. Some chemotherapeutic agents cause tissue necrosis, peripheral neuropathies, and stomatitis—all potential sources of pain—whereas radiation therapy can cause pain secondary to skin or organ inflammation. Cancer patients may have other sources of pain, such as arthritis or migraine headaches, that are unrelated to the underlying cancer or its treatment (see Table 68-8).

The nurse assesses the patient for the source and site of pain as well as those factors that increase the patient's perception of pain, such as fear and apprehension, fatigue, anger, and social isolation. Pain assessment scales (see Chapter 16) are useful for assessing the patient's pain and for evaluating the effectiveness of any interventions. Other symptoms that contribute to the pain experience, such as nausea and fatigue, are assessed as well.

Although it is often controllable, advanced cancer pain is commonly irreversible and not quickly resolved. For many patients, pain is often seen as a signal that the tumour is growing and that death is approaching. As patients anticipate the pain and their anxiety increases, pain perception heightens, producing fear and further pain. Chronic cancer pain, then, can lead to a cycle progressing from pain to anxiety to fear and back to pain. Inadequate pain management is most often the result of misconceptions and insufficient knowledge about pain assessment and pharmacologic interventions on the part of patients, families, and health care providers (Eaton et al., 2015). Chapter 16 provides information concerning factors contributing to the pain experience, pain perception, and tolerance as well as pharmacologic and nonpharmacologic nursing interventions addressing pain. The nursing care plan (see Chart 68-3) also provides strategies for nursing assessment and management.

The World Health Organization advocates a three-step approach to treat cancer pain (Fig. 68-7). Analgesics are administered based on the patient's level of pain.

No reasonable pharmacologic and nonpharmacologic approaches, even those that may be invasive, should be overlooked because of a poor or terminal prognosis. The nurse helps the patient and family take an active role in managing pain. The nurse provides education and support to correct fears and misconceptions about opioid use. Inadequate pain control leads to a diminished quality of life characterized by suffering, anxiety, fear, immobility, isolation, and depression. Improving the patient's quality of life through palliative care is as important as preventing a painful death.

Decreasing Fatigue

Fatigue is one of the most frequent and distressing symptoms experienced by patients receiving cancer therapy. Patients report that fatigue persists and interferes with activities of daily living for months to years after the

TABLE 68-8 Examples of Sources of Cancer Pain

Source	Descriptions	Underlying Cancer
Bone metastasis	Throbbing, aching	Breast, prostate, myeloma
Ischemia	Sharp, throbbing	Kaposi sarcoma
Lymphatic or venous obstruction	Dull, aching, tightness	Lymphoma, breast, Kaposi sarcoma
Nerve compression, infiltration	Burning, sharp, tingling	Breast, prostate, lymphoma
Organ obstruction	Dull, crampy, gnawing	Colon, gastric
Organ infiltration	Distention, crampy	Liver, pancreatic
Skin inflammation, ulceration, infection, necrosis	Burning, sharp	Breast, head and neck, Kaposi sarcoma

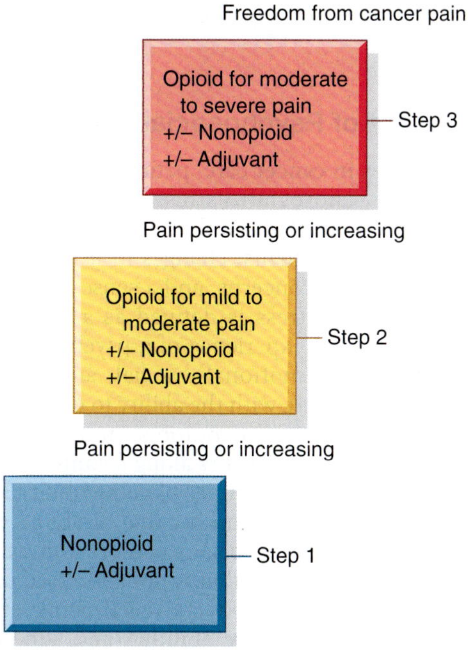

FIGURE 68-7. Various opioid (narcotic) and nonopioid medications may be combined with other medications to control pain. (Adapted from the World Health Organization's three-step ladder approach to relieving cancer pain.)

CHART 68-9

Sources of Fatigue in Patients With Cancer

- Pain, pruritus
- Imbalanced nutrition related to nausea, vomiting, cancer-related anorexia–cachexia syndrome
- Electrolyte imbalance related to vomiting, diarrhea
- Ineffective protection related to neutropenia, thrombocytopenia, anemia
- Impaired tissue integrity related to stomatitis, mucositis
- Impaired physical mobility related to neurologic impairments, surgery, bone metastasis, pain, and analgesic use
- Uncertainty and deficient knowledge related to disease process, treatment
- Anxiety related to fear, diagnosis, role changes, uncertainty of future
- Ineffective breathing patterns related to cough, shortness of breath, and dyspnea
- Disturbed sleep pattern related to cancer therapies, anxiety, and pain

Adapted from Bryant, A. L., Walton, A. L., & Phillips, B. (2015). Cancer-related fatigue: Scientific progress has been made in 40 years. *Clinical Journal of Oncology Nursing, 19*(2), 137–139; National Comprehensive Cancer Network. (2015f). *NCCN guidelines for supportive care: Cancer-related fatigue.* Retrieved March 24, 2016, from www.nccn.org/professionals/physician_gls/f_guidelines.asp#fatigue

completion of treatment (Pachman, Price, & Carey, 2014). Fatigue rarely exists in isolation; patients typically experience other symptoms concurrently, such as pain, dyspnea, anemia, sleep disturbances, or depression.

In assessing fatigue, the nurse distinguishes between *acute fatigue,* which occurs after an energy-demanding experience, and *cancer-related fatigue,* which is defined as "a distressing persistent, subjective sense of physical, emotional, and/or cognitive tiredness or exhaustion related to cancer or cancer treatment that is not proportional to recent activity and interferes with usual functioning" (NCCN, 2015f). Acute fatigue serves a protective function, whereas cancer-related fatigue does not. The exact mechanisms of fatigue are not well understood and are multifactorial in nature.

Despite the commonly occurring experience of fatigue in patients with cancer, a reliable assessment tool has not been identified. The experience of fatigue is highly subjective, with patient descriptors varying greatly (NCCN, 2015f). The nurse assesses physiologic and psychological factors that can contribute to fatigue (see Chart 68-9).

Exercise and physical activity are effective approaches to the management of cancer-related fatigue (Pachman et al., 2014). Psychoeducational approaches, cognitive–behavioural therapy to address sleep, progressive muscle relaxation, yoga, and mindfulness meditation may be effective measures to facilitate fatigue management (Mitchell, Hoffman, Clark, et al., 2014). Nurses assist patients with strategies to minimize fatigue or help the patient cope with fatigue as described in the nursing care plan (see Chart 15-7, Fatigue). Occasionally, pharmacologic interventions are utilized, including antidepressants for patients with depression, anxiolytics for those with anxiety, hypnotics for patients with sleep disturbances, and psychostimulants for some patients with advanced cancer or fatigue that does not respond to other interventions (NCCN, 2015f).

Improving Body Image and Self-Esteem

The nurse identifies potential threats to the patient's body image and assesses the patient's ability to cope with the many bodily changes that may be experienced throughout the course of disease and treatment. Entry into the health care system is often accompanied by depersonalization. Threats to self-concept occur as the patient faces the realization of illness, disfigurement, possible disability, and death. To accommodate treatments or because of the disease, many patients with cancer are forced to alter their lifestyles. Priorities and values change when body image is threatened. Disfiguring surgery, hair loss, cachexia, skin changes, altered communication patterns, and sexual dysfunction can threaten the patient's self-esteem and body image.

A creative and positive approach is essential when caring for patients with altered body image. Nursing strategies for addressing issues related to body image and self-esteem are included in the nursing care plan (see Chart 68-3). The nurse serves as a listener and counsellor to both the patient and the family. Possible influences of the patient's culture and age are considered when discussing concerns and potential interventions.

Addressing Sexuality

The physiologic processes associated with cancer; potential short- and long-term effects of cancer treatments; and psychosocial, emotional, and spiritual responses to the entire experience may lead patients to confront a variety of sexuality-based issues. Patients at the greatest risk of sexual dysfunction are those with tumours that involve the sexual or pelvic organs and those whose treatment affects the hormonal systems mediating sexual function (Goldfarb, Mulhall, Nelson, et al., 2013). Although sexuality is an important component of overall health, many nurses and other health professionals are hesitant to include sexuality in their discussions with patients (Kelvin, Steed, & Jarrett, 2014). Workshops have been developed to help nurses overcome barriers to discussing sexuality (Smith, 2015). In offering a holistic approach to the care of patients with cancer, nurses should initiate discussions about sexuality and assess sexual health.

Infertility, a common consequence of cancer and cancer treatments, can be of concern to patients and their partners. The potential for impaired fertility is discussed and options are reviewed for fertility preservation (Frankel Kelvin, 2015). Fertility plans are discussed and determined prior to the initiation of any therapy that may compromise reproductive abilities.

Referrals are made as needed for specialized evaluation and interventions that are beyond the scope of nursing intervention.

Assisting in the Grieving Process

A cancer diagnosis need not indicate a fatal outcome. Many forms of cancer are curable, and others may be controlled for long periods of time similar to the course of other chronic diseases. Despite the tremendous advances in cancer, many patients and their families still view cancer as a fatal disease that is inevitably accompanied by pain, suffering, debilitation, and emaciation. Grieving is a normal response to these fears and to actual or potential losses: loss of health, normal sensations, body image, social interaction, intimacy, independence, and usual social roles. Patients, families, and friends may grieve for the loss of quality time to spend with others, the loss of future and unfulfilled plans, and the loss of control over the patient's body and emotional reactions. Nurses continue to assess the patient and family for positive or maladaptive coping behaviours, interpersonal communication, and evidence of the need for additional psychosocial support or interventions such as referral for professional counselling.

If the patient enters the terminal phase of disease, the nurse may assess that the patient and family members are at different stages of grief. In such cases, the nurse assists the patient and family to acknowledge and cope with their reactions and feelings. The nurse also empowers the patient and family to explore preferences for issues related to end-of-life care, such as withdrawal of active disease treatment, desire for the use of life-support measures, and symptom management approaches. Oncology nurses respectfully support the patient's spiritual or religious views and facilitate contact with their preferred clergy member, if desired. In addition, nurses consider the patient's cultural beliefs and practices when addressing issues related to grief. After the death of a patient with cancer, home care and/or hospice nurses follow up with surviving family members for bereavement counselling to facilitate expression and coping with feelings of loss and grief. (See Chapter 15 for further discussion of end-of-life issues.)

Management of Psychosocial Distress

Despite advances in cancer care, patients experience varying levels of psychosocial distress related to actual or potential losses, fear of the unknown, symptoms due to cancer or cancer treatments, changes in usual family and social roles, financial concerns, and a sense of loss of control. Psychosocial distress is defined as a multifactorial unpleasant emotional experience of a psychological (cognitive, behavioural, emotional), social, and/or spiritual nature that may interfere with the ability to cope effectively with cancer, its physical symptoms, and its treatment (NCCN, 2015g). Distress occurs along a continuum, ranging from common normal feelings of vulnerability, sadness, and fears to problems that can become disabling, such as depression, anxiety, panic, social isolation, and existential and spiritual crises. Distress that is not addressed can have a significant impact on the overall well-being, interpersonal relationships, cognitive abilities, and adherence to treatment regimens, leading to poor outcomes.

Nurses need to screen patients for psychosocial distress during the course of the cancer experience. Patients are supported in managing various sources and levels of distress. Referral to mental health providers may be helpful to address specific concerns (Schilli, 2014).

Monitoring and Managing Potential Complications

Infection

For patients in all stages of cancer, the nurse assesses factors associated with the development of infection. Although infection-associated morbidity and mortality have greatly decreased, prevention and prompt treatment of infection are essential in patients with cancer. Often, more than one predisposing factor is present in patients with cancer. The nurse monitors laboratory studies to detect early changes in WBC counts. Common sites of infection, such as the pharynx, skin, perianal area, urinary, and respiratory tracts, are assessed on a regular basis. However, the typical signs of infection (swelling, redness, drainage, and pain) may not occur in myelosuppressed patients because of decreased circulating WBCs and a diminished local inflammatory response. Fever may be the only sign of infection (NCCN, 2015h). The nurse monitors the patient for sepsis, particularly if invasive catheters or long-term IV catheters are in place.

WBC function is often impaired in patients with cancer. Among the five types of WBCs (neutrophils [granulocytes], lymphocytes, monocytes, basophils, and eosinophils), neutrophils serve as the body's primary initial defence against invading organisms. Comprising 60% to 70% of the body's WBCs, neutrophils act by engulfing and destroying infective organisms through phagocytosis. Both the total WBC count and the concentration of neutrophils are important in determining the patient's ability to fight infection. A decrease in circulating WBCs is referred to as leukopenia. Granulocytopenia is a decrease in neutrophils.

A differential WBC count identifies the relative numbers of WBCs and permits tabulation of polymorphonuclear neutrophils (PMNs) or segmented neutrophils (mature neutrophils, reported as "polys," PMNs, or "segs") and immature forms of neutrophils (reported as bands, metamyelocytes, and "stabs"). The absolute neutrophil count (ANC) is calculated by the following formula:

$$\text{ANC} = \frac{(\text{Total WBC}) \times [\%\ \text{segmented neutrophils} + \text{bands}]}{100}$$

Neutropenia, an abnormally low ANC, is associated with an increased risk of infection. The risk of infection rises as the ANC decreases. As the ANC declines below 1,500 cells/mm^3, the risk of infection rises. An ANC less than 500 cells/mm^3 reflects a severe risk of infection (NCCN, 2015h; Segal, Walsh, Gea-Banacloche, et al., 2015). The **nadir** is the lowest ANC following chemotherapy, targeted therapy, or radiation therapy that suppresses bone marrow function. Severe neutropenia may necessitate delays in administration of myelosuppressive therapies or treatment dose adjustments, although the use of the hematopoietic growth factors (i.e., colony-stimulating factors; see previous discussion) has reduced the severity and duration of treatment-associated neutropenia as well as infection-related morbidity and early death (Smith, Bohlke, Lyman, et al., 2015). The administration of these growth factors assists in maintaining treatment schedules, drug dosages, treatment effectiveness, and quality of life.

Febrile patients who are neutropenic are assessed for factors that increase the risk of infection and for sources of infection through cultures of blood, sputum, urine, stool, IV and urinary or other catheters, and wounds, if appropriate (see Table 68-9). In addition, a chest x-ray is usually obtained to assess for pulmonary infection.

Defence against infection is compromised in many different ways. The integrity of the skin and mucous membranes is challenged by multiple invasive diagnostic procedures, by the adverse effects of all cancer treatment modalities, and by the detrimental effects of immobility. Impaired nutrition as a result of CACS, nausea, vomiting, diarrhea, and the underlying disease alters the body's ability to combat invading organisms. Medications such as antibiotics disturb the balance of normal flora, allowing the overgrowth of normal flora and pathogenic organisms. Other medications can also alter the immune response (see Chapters 51 and 52). Cancer itself may lead to defects in cellular and humoral immunity. Advanced cancer may cause obstruction of hollow viscera (e.g., intestines), blood, and lymphatic vessels, creating a favourable environment for proliferation of pathogenic organisms. In some patients, tumour cells infiltrate bone marrow and prevent normal production of WBCs.

Nurses are in a key position to assist in preventing and identifying symptoms of infection, as discussed in the nursing care plan (see Chart 68-3). Clinical practice guidelines developed by the ONS, the Infusion Nurses Society (INS), the NCCN, and the American Society of Clinical Oncology (ASCO) are used to guide prevention and management of infection. Interventions to prevent infection and alternative patient education formats for infection-related instruction are high nursing research priorities.

Gram-positive bacteria (*Streptococcus, enterococci*, and *Staphylococcus* species) and gram-negative organisms (*Escherichia coli, Klebsiella pneumoniae, Enterobacter*, and *Pseudomonas aeruginosa*) are the most frequently isolated causes of infection. Fungal organisms, such as *Candida albicans*, also contribute to the incidence of serious infection. Viral infections in immunocompromised patients are caused most often by herpes simplex, respiratory syncytial, parainfluenza, and influenza A and B viruses.

Fever is reported promptly as it is an important sign of infection in patients when associated with neutropenia. Patients with neutropenic fever (see Table 68-9) are assessed for infection and reported promptly (NCCN, 2015h). Antibiotics may be prescribed after cultures of wound drainage, exudates, sputum, urine, stool, or blood are obtained. Careful consideration is given to the underlying malignancy, prior antineoplastic treatment, ANC, comorbidities, and other patient-related factors prior to the identification of the most appropriate antibiotic therapy. Evidence-based guidelines are available for prevention and treatment of cancer-related infections (NCCN, 2015h). Patients with neutropenia are treated with broad-spectrum antibiotics before the infecting organism is identified because of the increased risk of mortality associated with untreated infection. Broad-spectrum antibiotic therapy targets the most likely major pathogenic organisms. It is important for these medications to be given and taken promptly as scheduled, to achieve adequate blood levels. Once the offending organism is identified, more specific antimicrobial therapy is prescribed as appropriate. Nurses provide education for patients and families regarding prevention of infection, signs and symptoms to report, and the importance of adherence to prescribed antimicrobial therapy.

Septic Shock

The nurse assesses the patient frequently for infection and inflammation throughout the course of the disease and treatment. Septicemia and septic shock are life-threatening complications that must be prevented or detected and treated promptly. Although all patients with cancer are at risk, patients who are neutropenic or who have hematologic malignancies are at the greatest risk. Patients with signs and symptoms of impending sepsis and septic shock require immediate hospitalization and aggressive treatment.

Signs and symptoms of septic shock (see Chapter 18) include altered mental status, either subnormal or elevated temperature, cool and clammy skin, decreased urine output, hypotension, tachycardia, other dysrhythmias, electrolyte imbalances, tachypnea, and abnormal arterial blood gas values. Patients and family members are educated about signs of septicemia, methods for preventing infection, and actions to take if signs and symptoms of infection or septicemia occur.

Although septic shock is most often associated with overwhelming gram-negative bacterial infections, there is an increasing incidence of gram-positive infections related to the use of long-term venous access devices. Patients with prolonged neutropenia or hematologic malignancies are also more susceptible to fungal and viral sources of sepsis as well. In a patient with impending shock, the nurse monitors temperature and hemodynamic and respiratory status on a regular and frequent basis. Neurologic

TABLE 68-9 Assessment of Neutropenic Fever in Patients With Cancer

Fever Criteria	Neutropenia Criteria
• Any one-time temperature of 38.3°C (101°F) or • Any temperature of ≥38°C (100.4°F) or ≥1 hour	• <500 neutrophils/mcL or • <1,000 neutrophils/mcL and predicted to decline to ≤500 neutrophils/mcL over the next 48 hours

Assessment Targets for Neutropenic Fever Evaluation

Infection Risk Factors	Physical Assessment	Diagnostic Procedures	Microbiologic Cultures
• Chronic comorbid illnesses • Underlying hematologic malignancies • Immunosuppression related to factors other than neutropenia (i.e., immunosuppressive therapy following allogeneic HSCT or hypogammaglobulinemia [decreased gammaglobulin production]) • Solid tumours causing obstructions of the bronchial tree, ureters, colon, or biliary ducts • Advanced or refractory underlying malignancy • Prolonged duration of neutropenia • Age ≥65 years • Limited mobility and/or debilitation • Medications (e.g., corticosteroids such as prednisone) • Antibiotic therapy or prophylaxis • Recent surgery for diagnosis or treatment • Chemotherapy or targeted therapy received within the last 7–10 days • Prior treatment with multiple types of chemotherapy regimens • Recent radiation therapy; especially to areas associated with bone marrow reserves • Prior documented infections • Impaired skin integrity • Invasive drainage or urinary catheters • Peripheral or central venous access devices • Exposures (travel, others with infection, blood administration, pets) • Diarrhea • Poor nutritional status • Recent lumbar puncture or indwelling Ommaya reservoir™ (long-term intraventricular catheter for administration of chemotherapy into CSF and ventricles)	• Skin, pressure points, wounds • Surgical or biopsy incision sites • IV access or reservoir sites • Drainage catheter sites • Tracheostomy site • Lungs and sinuses • Perivaginal and perirectal areas • Alimentary canal, abdomen • Neurologic assessment • Vital signs	• Diagnostic imaging as appropriate to identify abscesses, fistulas, pneumonia, obstruction, etc. • Complete blood count/differential • Serum chemistries, liver function tests • Renal function tests • Pulse oximetry or arterial blood gases • Lumbar puncture for CSF analysis	• Blood (peripheral and central venous access if applicable) • Urine (especially with indwelling catheter) • Skin wounds, lesions, incision sites, catheter exit sites • Catheter tips when feasible • Drainage from catheters • Stool, diarrhea • Sputum • CSF

CSF, cerebrospinal fluid.

Adapted from National Comprehensive Cancer Network. (2015h). *Clinical practice guidelines: Prevention and treatment of cancer related infections (v2.2015)*. Retrieved from www.nccn.org/professionals/physician_gls/pdf/infections.pdf; Segal, B. H., Walsh, T. J., Gea-Banacloche, J. C., et al. (2015). Infections in the cancer patient. In V. T. DeVita, T. S. Lawrence, & S. A. Rosenberg (Eds.). *Cancer: Principles & practice of oncology*. Philadelphia, PA: Lippincott Williams & Wilkins.

assessments are carried out to detect changes in orientation and responsiveness. Fluid and electrolyte status is monitored by measuring fluid intake and output and serum electrolytes. Arterial blood gas values and pulse oximetry are monitored to determine tissue oxygenation. Nurses administer IV fluids, blood products, vasopressor and inotropic agents as prescribed to maintain blood pressure and tissue perfusion, as well as broad-spectrum antibiotics, which may be prescribed initially to combat the underlying infection (see Chapter 18). Supplemental oxygen and sometimes mechanical ventilation are necessary. Systemic steroids and drotrecogin alfa have been used in some centres for patients who have severe and prolonged septic shock or those that are at risk for development of clotting disturbances.

Bleeding and Thrombocytopenia

Platelets are essential for normal blood clotting and coagulation (hemostasis). Thrombocytopenia, a decrease in the circulating platelet count, is the most common cause of bleeding in patients with cancer and is usually defined as a platelet count less than $100,000/mm^3$ $(0.1 \times 10^{12}/L)$.

The risk of bleeding increases when the platelet count decreases below 50,000/mm^3 (0.05×10^{12}/L). At platelet counts lower than 10,000/mm^3 (0.02×10^{12}/L), the risk for spontaneous bleeding is increased (Barbarotta, 2015).

Thrombocytopenia often results from bone marrow depression after certain types of chemotherapy and radiation therapy and with tumour infiltration of the bone marrow. In some cases, platelet destruction is associated with an enlarged spleen (hypersplenism) and abnormal antibody function, which occur with leukemia and lymphoma. Bacterial and viral infections may lead to early platelet destruction or impaired bone marrow production of platelets and subsequent thrombocytopenia. Some medications (i.e., heparin, vancomycin) may cause bone marrow toxicity, leading to decreases in circulating platelets. Less commonly, posttransfusion complications may lead to antibody destruction of platelets, causing profound thrombocytopenia. Lastly, coagulopathies associated with infection or malignancies, such as gastric and pancreatic cancers, may result in thrombocytopenia (Kuter, 2015). The nursing care plan addresses nursing assessment parameters and interventions for patients at risk for bleeding (see Chart 68-3).

NURSING ALERT

Although laboratory test results confirm the diagnosis of thrombocytopenia, the patient who is developing thrombocytopenia may display early signs and symptoms. Thus, nurses need to observe keenly for petechiae and ecchymoses, which are early indicators of decreasing platelet levels. Early detection promotes early intervention.

Additional medications may be prescribed to address bleeding or thrombocytopenia based on the underlying etiology. (Refer to Chapter 54 for further discussion of assessment and treatment of thrombocytopenia and coagulopathies.)

Venous thromboembolism (VTE), a common problem for patients with cancer, includes deep venous thrombosis (DVT), pulmonary embolism (PE), superficial venous thrombosis (SVT), and thrombosis in other abdominal or thoracic venous tributaries such as the mesenteric veins or the superior vena cava. The incidence of VTE has been linked to an increased likelihood of death in patients with cancer (NCCN, 2015i). Factors associated with risk for VTEs in cancer patients include pre-existing underlying or cancer-related coagulopathies, medications including chemotherapy, hospitalizations, surgical procedures, increased age, debilitation, immobility, infection, and peripheral and central venous catheters (NCCN, 2015i). Patients with cancer are monitored for associated risk factors and are assessed on an ongoing basis for VTE. Nurses provide patient and family education regarding symptoms of VTE to report to the provider. Recommendations for prophylaxis are based on national guidelines and patient risk factors. Nursing assessment findings associated with VTE are reported promptly so that VTE evaluation and treatment can be initiated expeditiously.

Promoting Home, Community-Based, and Transitional Care

Educating Patients About Self-Care

Most commonly, patients with cancer are diagnosed and treated in the outpatient setting. Nurses in outpatient settings often have the responsibility for patient education and helping coordinate care in the home (see Chart 68-4). The shift of care from acute care facilities to the home or outpatient settings as well as the increasing use of oral antineoplastic agents places significant responsibility for care on the patient and family. In order to maintain optimal patient outcomes and quality of life, patients and families require support and information that will prepare them to engage in self-care. Education initially focuses on the most immediate care needs likely to be encountered at home.

Approaches to preparing patients for self-care responsibilities are chosen with consideration of the patient's preferred learning strategies, level of education, and health literacy. Knobf (2013) suggests that patient education is best achieved through a nurse–patient relationship that involves an exchange of information to support patient needs that can vary across time points of the cancer continuum. Easily understood, concrete, objective information that assists patients to understand what to expect and includes sensory and temporal components is important. Symptoms, side effects of treatment, and changes in the patient's status that should be reported are discussed and reinforced with printed materials that can be referred to in the home. Nurses help to empower patients by sharing strategies to manage side effects or other symptoms. Additional learning needs are based on the priorities conveyed by the patient and family as well as on the complexity of care required.

Technologic advances allow home administration of IV chemotherapy, blood products, and antibiotics; enteral or parenteral nutrition; and parenteral analgesics. Patients and families are taught to care for vascular access devices, infusion pumps, various types of drainage catheters, and on occasion, complex wounds. The importance of patient safety and infection control is included in patient and family education. Although nurses are often available to provide some assistance with cancer care in the home, patients and families need information that will enable them to have a sense of comfort, decrease distress, improve coping, foster self-management, promote adherence, and enhance quality of life (Knobf, 2013).

Continuing and Transitional Care

Referral for home or transitional care is often indicated for patients with cancer. The responsibilities of the nurse include assessing the home environment and suggesting modifications in the home or in care to help address the patient's physical and safety needs. Home care nurses also assess the psychosocial impact of cancer on the patient and family so that appropriate interventions can be identified and/or referrals for support services are instituted.

Ongoing nursing visits and/or phone contact from the home or transitional care nurse assist in prevention, early identification, prompt reporting, and management of patient problems. Timely modifications in therapy to manage symptoms and adverse effects of treatment may decrease patient suffering and decrease emergency department visits or hospital admissions. Continued contact facilitates evaluation of the patient's progress, responses to treatment, and assessment of the ongoing needs of the patient and family. It is necessary to assess the patient's and family's understanding of the treatment plan and management strategies and to reinforce previous education. The nurse facilitates coordination of patient care by maintaining close communication with all involved health care providers. The nurse may make referrals and coordinate available community resources (e.g., local office of the ACS, home aides, church groups, faith community nurses, support groups) to assist patients and caregivers.

Gerontologic Considerations

More than 70% of all new cancers occur in people older than 60 years of age (Canadian Cancer Society's Advisory Committee on Cancer Statistics, 2013). The rising numbers of individuals over age 65 with cancer have led to the emergence of geriatric oncology, a multidimensional and multidisciplinary approach to treating growing numbers of older adults with cancer.

Nurses working with the older adult population must understand the normal physiologic changes that occur with aging and that these changes may ultimately influence older patients' responses to cancer treatment (Table 68-10). In addition, many older adult patients have comorbidities and multiple medications that may contribute to drug interactions and toxicities in older adult patients.

The understanding of the effects and tolerance of chemotherapy, targeted therapies, and radiation in the older adult is limited, as older adults have been underrepresented in oncology clinical trials. Potential chemotherapy–related toxicities, such as renal impairment, myelosuppression, fatigue, and cardiomyopathy, may increase as a result of declining organ function and diminished physiologic reserves. The recovery of normal tissues after radiation therapy may be delayed, and older adult patients may experience more severe adverse effects, such as mucositis, nausea and vomiting, and myelosuppression. Because of impaired healing and declining pulmonary and cardiovascular functioning, older patients are slower to recover from surgery. Older patients are also at increased risk for complications, such as atelectasis, pneumonia, and wound infections.

Access to quality cancer care for the older adult patients may be limited by discriminatory or fatalistic attitudes of health care providers, caregivers, and patients themselves. Issues such as the gradual loss of supportive resources, declining health or loss of a spouse, and unavailability of relatives or friends may result in limited access to care and unmet needs for assistance with activities of daily living. In addition, the economic impact of health care may be difficult for those living on fixed incomes.

It is not uncommon for older adult patients to delay reporting symptoms, attributing them to "old age." Many do not want to report illness for fear of losing their independence or financial security. Sensory losses (e.g., hearing and visual losses) and memory deficits are considered when planning patient education, because they may affect the patient's ability to process and retain information. In such cases, the nurse acts as a patient advocate, encouraging independence and identifying resources for support when indicated. Nurses must be aware of the special needs of the aging population and work collaboratively with other disciplines to address identified needs.

Providing Care to the Patient With Advanced Cancer

Providing Care in Oncologic Emergencies

Table 68-11 discusses selected nursing and medical care of oncologic emergencies.

As a result of advances in all aspects of cancer care, it is more common that individuals are living with cancer that has advanced beyond the original site of development to regional or distant sites. Patients with advanced cancer are

TABLE 68-10 Age-Related Changes and Their Effects on Patients With Cancer

Age-Related Changes	Implications
Impaired immune system	Use special precautions to avoid infection; monitor for atypical signs and symptoms of infection.
Altered drug absorption, distribution, metabolism, and elimination	Mandates careful calculation of chemotherapy and frequent assessment for drug response and side effects; dose adjustments may be necessary.
Increased prevalence of other chronic diseases	Monitor for effect of cancer or its treatment on patient's other chronic diseases; monitor patient's tolerance for cancer treatment; monitor for interactions with medications used to treat chronic diseases.
Diminished renal, respiratory, and cardiac reserves	Be proactive in prevention of decreased renal function, atelectasis, pneumonia, and cardiovascular compromise; monitor for side effects of cancer treatment.
Decreased skin and tissue integrity; reduction in body mass; delayed healing	Prevent pressure ulcers secondary to immobility; monitor skin and mucous membranes for changes related to radiation or chemotherapy; monitor nutritional status.
Decreased musculoskeletal strength	Prevent falls; assess support for performing activities of daily living in home setting; encourage safe use of assistive mobility devices.
Decreased neurosensory functioning: loss of vision, hearing, and distal extremity tactile senses	Provide teaching and instructions modified for patient's hearing and vision changes; provide instruction concerning safety and skin care for distal extremities; assess home for safety.
Altered social and economic resources	Assess for financial concerns, living conditions, and resources for support.
Potential changes in cognitive and emotional capacities	Provide teaching and support modified for patient's level of functioning and safety.

TABLE 68-11 Oncologic Emergencies: Manifestations and Management

Emergency	Clinical Manifestations and Diagnostic Findings	Management
Superior Vena Cava Syndrome (SVCS) Compression or invasion of the superior vena cava by tumour; enlarged lymph nodes; intraluminal thrombus that obstructs venous circulation; or drainage of the head, neck, arms, and thorax. Most often associated with lung cancer, SVCS is also associated with lymphoma, thymoma, and testicular cancers and mediastinal metastases from breast cancer. If untreated, SVCS may lead to cerebral anoxia (because not enough oxygen reaches the brain), laryngeal edema, bronchial obstruction, and death.	***Clinical*** Gradually or suddenly impaired venous drainage giving rise to: Progressive shortness of breath (dyspnea), cough, hoarseness, chest pain, and facial swelling Edema of the neck, arms, hands, and thorax and reported sensation of skin tightness, difficulty swallowing, and stridor Possibly engorged and distended jugular, temporal, and arm veins Dilated thoracic vessels causing prominent venous patterns on the chest wall Increased intracranial pressure, associated visual disturbances, headache, and altered mental status	***Medical*** Radiation therapy to shrink tumour or enlarged lymph nodes and relieve symptoms Chemotherapy for sensitive cancers (e.g., lymphoma, small cell lung cancer) or when the mediastinum has been irradiated to maximum tolerance Anticoagulant or thrombolytic therapy for central venous catheter–related intraluminal thrombosis Percutaneously placed intravascular stents may be a priority consideration rather than surgery, unless symptoms are rapidly progressing. Supportive measures such as oxygen therapy, corticosteroids, and diuretics (in cases of fluid overload)
	Diagnostic Diagnosis is confirmed by: Clinical findings Chest x-ray Thoracic computed tomography (CT) scan Thoracic magnetic resonance imaging (MRI) Venogram if intraluminal thrombosis is suspected	***Nursing*** Identify patients at risk for SVCS. Provide patient education regarding signs and symptoms to report. Monitor and report clinical manifestations of SVCS. Monitor cardiopulmonary and neurologic status. Avoid upper extremity venipuncture and blood pressure measurement; instruct patient to avoid tight or restrictive clothing and jewellery on fingers, wrist, and neck. Facilitate breathing and drainage from upper portion of body by instructing patient to maintain some elevation of head and upper body with semi-Fowler position; avoid completely supine or prone positions (this helps to promote comfort and reduce anxiety associated with dependent and progressive edema). Promote energy conservation to minimize shortness of breath. Monitor the patient's fluid volume status; administer fluids cautiously to minimize edema. Assess for thoracic radiation–related problems such as mucositis with resultant dysphagia (difficulty swallowing) and esophagitis. Monitor for chemotherapy-related problems, such as myelosuppression. Provide postoperative care as appropriate.
Spinal Cord Compression Most commonly caused by compression of the cord and its nerve roots by a metastatic paravertebral tumour that extends into the epidural space; vertebral bone metastasis leading to bone collapse and displacement impinging on the spinal cord or nerve roots; and less commonly, primary malignancy of the cord. May potentially lead to significant and permanent neurologic impairment associated with multiple physical, psychosocial consequences. Most often associated with cancers that metastasize to the bone such as breast, lung, and prostate cancers and lymphoma. Also seen in nasopharyngeal cancer and multiple myeloma.	***Clinical*** Local inflammation, edema, venous stasis, and impaired blood supply to nerve tissues Local or radicular back or neck pain along the dermatomal areas innervated by the affected nerve root (e.g., thoracic radicular pain extends in a band around the chest or abdomen) Pain exacerbated by movement, supine recumbent position, coughing, sneezing, or the Valsalva maneuver Neurologic dysfunction and related motor and sensory deficits (numbness, tingling, feelings of coldness in the affected area, inability to detect vibration, loss of positional sense) Motor loss ranging from subtle weakness to flaccid paralysis	***Medical*** Radiation therapy to reduce tumour size and halt progression; corticosteroid therapy to decrease inflammation and swelling at the compression site Surgery to debulk tumour and stabilize the spine if symptoms progress despite radiation therapy or if vertebral fracture or bone fragments lead to additional nerve damage; surgery is also an option when the tumour is not radiosensitive or is located in an area that was previously irradiated Minimally invasive surgical procedures, referred to as vertebral augmentation, may be used for patients with vertebral fractures to attain stability of the bone, prevent nerve compression, and decrease pain. Procedures include: Vertebroplasty: involves percutaneous injection of polymethyl methacrylate (PMMA), a bone cement filler, into the vertebral body

continued >

TABLE 68-11 Oncologic Emergencies: Manifestations and Management (Continued)

Emergency	Clinical Manifestations and Diagnostic Findings	Management
About 70% of compressions occur at the thoracic level, 20% in the lumbosacral level, and 10% in the cervical and sacral regions. The prognosis depends on the severity and rapidity of onset.	Bladder and/or bowel dysfunction depending on level of compression (above S2, overflow incontinence; from S3 to S5, flaccid sphincter tone and bowel incontinence) ***Diagnostic*** Percussion tenderness at the level of compression Abnormal reflexes Sensory and motor abnormalities MRI is a preferred diagnostic tool; may also utilize x-rays, bone scans, and CT scan	Kyphoplasty: a balloon is inserted into the damaged vertebral body and then inflated to create a cavity within the bone that can be filled with bone cement. The balloon helps to compress the fracture fragments together as the cavity is created Radiofrequency vertebral augmentation: similar to kyphoplasty; instead of the balloon, a small navigational cannula is inserted into the vertebra to create small pathways for cement. The cement is heated with radiofrequency to create an ultra-high viscosity that is thought to promote bone stability Chemotherapy as adjuvant to other local therapies for patients with chemosensitive cancers such as lymphoma or small cell lung cancer *Note:* Despite treatment, patients with poor neurologic function before treatment are less likely to regain complete motor and sensory function; patients who develop complete paralysis usually do not regain all neurologic function ***Nursing*** Perform ongoing assessment of neurologic function to identify existing and progressing dysfunction Control pain with pharmacologic and nonpharmacologic measures Prevent complications of immobility resulting from pain and decreased function (e.g., skin breakdown, urinary stasis, thrombophlebitis, decreased clearance of pulmonary secretions) Maintain muscle tone by assisting with range-of-motion exercises in collaboration with physical and occupational therapists; patients with unstable vertebral fractures do not initiate physical therapy until spine stabilization procedures have been completed Institute intermittent urinary catheterization and bowel training programs for patients with bladder or bowel dysfunction Provide encouragement and support to patient and family coping with pain and altered functioning, lifestyle, roles, and independence Institute appropriate referrals for home care and physical and occupational therapy
Hypercalcemia Hypercalcemia is a potentially life-threatening metabolic abnormality resulting when the calcium released from the bones is more than the kidneys can excrete or the bones can reabsorb. It may result from production of cytokines, hormonal substances, and growth factors by cancer cells, or by the body in response to substances produced by cancer cells, which lead to bone breakdown and calcium release. Most commonly seen in breast, lung, and renal cancers; myeloma; and some types of leukemia.	***Clinical*** Fatigue, weakness, confusion, decreased level of responsiveness, hyporeflexia, nausea, vomiting, constipation, ileus, polyuria (excessive urination), polydipsia (excessive thirst), dehydration, and dysrhythmias ***Diagnostic*** Total serum calcium level >10.5 mg/dL (2.74 mmol/L) Ionized serum calcium >1.29 mmol/L	***Medical*** Identify patients at risk for hypercalcemia and assess for signs and symptoms of hypercalcemia Educate patient and family; prevention and early detection can prevent fatality Educate at-risk patients to recognize and report signs and symptoms of hypercalcemia Provide patient and family education regarding: Need to consume 2–4 L of fluid daily unless contraindicated by existing renal or cardiac disease Use of dietary and pharmacologic interventions such as stool softeners and laxatives for constipation Maintenance of nutritional intake without restricting normal calcium intake Antiemetic therapy for nausea and vomiting Promotion of mobility and emphasis on importance in preventing demineralization and breakdown of bones Safety precautions for patients with impaired mental and mobility status

TABLE 68-11 Oncologic Emergencies: Manifestations and Management (Continued)

Emergency	Clinical Manifestations and Diagnostic Findings	Management
Tumour Lysis Syndrome (TLS) Potentially fatal complication that occurs spontaneously or more commonly following radiation, biotherapy, or chemotherapy-induced cell destruction of large or rapidly growing cancers such as leukemia, lymphoma, and small cell lung cancer. The release of tumour intracellular contents (nuclei acids, electrolytes, and debris) leads to rapidly induced electrolyte imbalances—hyperkalemia, hyperphosphatemia (leading to hypocalcemia), and hyperuricemia—that can have life-threatening end-organ effects on the myocardium, kidneys, and central nervous system	***Clinical*** Clinical manifestations depend on the extent of metabolic abnormalities. Clinical TLS is diagnosed when ≥1 of 3 conditions arise either 3 days prior to or 7 days after cytotoxic cancer therapy: acute kidney injury (defined as a rise in creatinine to ≥1.5 times the upper limit of normal that is not attributable to medications), dysrhythmias (including sudden cardiac death), and seizures *Neurologic:* Fatigue, weakness, memory loss, altered mental status, muscle cramps, tetany, paresthesias (numbness and tingling), seizures *Cardiac:* Elevated blood pressure, shortened QT complexes, widened QRS waves, altered T waves, dysrhythmias, cardiac arrest GI: Anorexia, nausea, vomiting, abdominal cramps, diarrhea, increased bowel sounds Renal: Flank pain, oliguria, anuria, kidney injury, acidic urine pH Other: Gout, malaise, pruritus ***Diagnostic*** Electrolyte imbalances identified by serum electrolyte measurement and urinalysis (see Chapter 13); electrocardiogram to detect cardiac dysrhythmias	***Medical*** To prevent kidney injury and restore electrolyte balance, aggressive fluid hydration is initiated 24–48 hours before and after the initiation of cytotoxic therapy to increase urine volume and eliminate uric acid and electrolytes; urine is alkalinized by adding sodium bicarbonate to IV fluid to maintain a urine pH of 7–7.5; this prevents kidney injury secondary to uric acid precipitation in the kidneys. Diuresis with a loop diuretic or osmotic diuretic if urine output is not sufficient Allopurinol (Zyloprim) therapy to inhibit the conversion of nucleic acids to uric acid; rasburicase (Elitek) may be used to convert already formed uric acid to allantoin, which is highly water soluble and eliminated in urine. Administration of a cation-exchange resin, such as sodium polystyrene sulfonate (Kayexalate), to treat hyperkalemia by binding and eliminating potassium through the bowel Administration of IV sodium bicarbonate, hypertonic dextrose, and regular insulin temporarily shifts potassium into cells and lowers serum potassium levels if a rapid decrease in potassium is necessary. Administration of phosphate-binding gels, such as aluminum hydroxide, to treat hyperphosphatemia by promoting phosphate excretion in the feces Hemodialysis when patients are unresponsive to the standard approaches for managing uric acid and electrolyte abnormalities. Identify at-risk patients. Institute essential preventive measures (e.g., fluid hydration, medications) as prescribed. Assess patient for signs and symptoms of electrolyte imbalances. Assess urine pH to confirm alkalization. Monitor serum electrolyte and uric acid levels for evidence of fluid volume overload secondary to aggressive hydration. Instruct patients to monitor for and report symptoms indicating electrolyte disturbances.

MRI, magnetic resonance imaging; CT, computed tomography.

Adapted from Baehring, Y. (2015). Oncologic emergencies: Spinal cord compression. In V. T. DeVita, T. S. Lawrence, & S. A. Rosenberg (Eds.). *Cancer: Principles & practice of oncology*. Philadelphia, PA: Lippincott Williams & Wilkins; Wallace, A., Robinson, C., Myer, J., et al. (2015). The metastatic spine disease multidisciplinary working group algorithms. *The Oncologist, 20*(9), 1–11; Wang, L., Jian, Y., Yang, G., et al. (2015). Management of tumor lysis syndrome in patients with multiple myeloma during bortezomib treatment. *Clinical Journal of Oncology Nursing, 19*(1), E4–E7; and Yahalom, J. (2015). Oncologic emergencies: Superior vena cava syndrome. In V. T. DeVita, T. S. Lawrence, & S. A. Rosenberg (Eds.). *Cancer: Principles & practice of oncology*. Philadelphia, PA: Lippincott Williams & Wilkins.

likely to experience many of the problems described previously, although more often and to a greater degree. Symptoms of pain, anorexia, weight loss, CACS, fatigue, and impaired functional status and mobility make patients more susceptible to depressive symptoms, skin breakdown, fluid and electrolyte imbalances, and infection.

Treatment for the patient with advanced cancer is likely to be palliative rather than curative, with an emphasis on prevention and appropriate management of pain. The use of long-acting analgesic agents at set intervals, rather than on an "as-needed" basis, is recommended in addressing pain management. Working with the patient and family, as well as with other health care providers, to manage pain is essential to increase the patient's comfort and offer some sense of control. Other medications (e.g., sedatives, tranquilizers, muscle relaxants, antiemetics) are added to assist in palliating additional symptoms and promoting quality of life.

If the patient is a candidate for radiation therapy or surgical interventions to relieve pain or other symptoms, the potential benefits and risks of these procedures (e.g., percutaneous nerve block, cordotomy) are explained to the patient and family. Measures are taken to prevent complications that result from altered sensation, immobility, and changes in bowel and bladder function.

Weakness, altered mobility, fatigue, and inactivity typically increase with advanced cancer as a result of the disease, treatment, inadequate nutritional intake, or dyspnea. The nurse works with the patient and family to identify realistic goals and promote comfort. Measures include use of energy conservation methods to accomplish tasks and activities that the patient values most.

Efforts are made to provide the patient with as much control and independence as desired but with assurance that support and assistance are available when needed. In addition, health care teams work with the patient and family to ascertain and comply with the patient's wishes about treatment methods and care as the terminal phases of illness and death approach.

Hospice

For many years, society was unable to cope appropriately with patients in the most advanced stages of cancer, and patients died in acute care settings rather than at home or in facilities better designed to meet their needs. The needs of patients with terminal illnesses are best met by a comprehensive multidisciplinary specialty program that focuses on quality of life, palliation of symptoms, and provision of psychosocial and spiritual support for patients and families when cure and control of the disease are no longer possible. The concept of hospice best addresses these needs. Most important, the focus of care includes the family, as well as the patient. Hospice care can be provided in several settings: free-standing, hospital-based, and community- or home-based settings.

Because of the high costs associated with maintaining freestanding hospices, care is often delivered through coordination of services provided by hospitals, home care programs, and the community. Patients should be referred to palliative care and hospice services in a timely fashion so that complex patient needs can be addressed. Although physicians, social workers, clergy, dietitians, pharmacists, physical therapists, and volunteers are involved in patient care, nurses often coordinate hospice services.

Hospice programs strive to facilitate clear communication among patients, family members, and health care providers. Most patients and families are informed of the prognosis and are encouraged to participate in decisions regarding pursuing or terminating cancer treatment. Through collaboration with other support disciplines, the nurse helps the patient and family cope with changes in role identity, family structure, grief, and loss. Hospice nurses are actively involved in bereavement counselling. See Chapter 15 for a detailed discussion of end-of-life care.

Cancer Survivorship

Over 850,000 Canadians are alive today who have been previously diagnosed with cancer (Canadian Cancer Society's Advisory Committee on Cancer Statistics, 2013). Largely as a result of increased screening programs for breast, cervical, and prostate cancers and advances in treatment, the numbers of cancer survivors have tripled over the past 37 years. Cancer survivorship refers to a distinct phase of cancer care that follows primary treatment for cancer and lasts until cancer recurrence or end of life. Although individuals vary and there are many types of cancers and treatments, the acute, long-term, and late effects of cancer and its treatment may have multiple physical and psychosocial consequences.

Survivorship care is often based on expert opinion and experience rather than on evidence-based practices. Knowledge regarding survivorship concerns continues to evolve. The Institute of Medicine has identified four components of survivorship care, the period that follows primary treatment for cancer and lasts until end of life. In addition to a summary of prior diagnosis and treatment, survivorship care includes monitoring and treatment for late effects related to disease and prior treatments, physical and vocational rehabilitation, psychosocial support and counselling as necessary, and surveillance and screening for new and recurrent cancer (Hewitt, Greenfield, & Stovall, 2006) (see Table 68-12). Advocacy organizations across the country have recommended that a survivorship care plan be provided to all patients with cancer and their primary provider at the completion of treatment. The survivorship care plan includes a summary of cancer diagnosis and treatment and recommendations for follow-up and care, including approaches to treat symptoms, rehabilitative needs, monitoring for late effects, and surveillance and screening for new and recurrent cancer. Referrals for specific services such as lymphedema therapy, chronic pain management, and genetic counselling are also provided. Nurses assist in the development of the survivorship care plan and provide education and care for cancer survivors. Nurses, other health care providers, public health professionals, and patient advocates design and conduct research to identify needs of cancer survivors and evidence-based approaches to care.

TABLE 68-12 Components of Survivorship Care

Component	Examples of Care
Prevention and detection of new and recurrent cancer	• Mammography (Canadian Cancer Society guidelines) • Papanicolaou (Pap) smears (Canadian Cancer Society guidelines) • Smoking cessation programs • Nutrition counselling
Surveillance for cancer spread, recurrence or second cancers	• Colonoscopy post-colon cancer • Mammography post-breast cancer • Liver function tests post-colon cancer • Prostate specific antigen post-prostate cancer
Intervention for consequences of cancer and its treatments	• Lymphedema therapy • Pain management • Enterostomal therapy • Fertility care
Coordination between specialists and primary care providers to meet health needs	• Care for comorbidities (e.g., diabetes) • Influenza vaccination • Bone densitometry

From Canadian Cancer Society. (2019). *Life after cancer treatment.* Retrieved May 23, 2019, from https://www.cancer.ca/en/cancer-information/cancer-journey/life-after-cancer/?region=on; Hewitt, M., Greenfield, S., & Stovall, E. (Eds.). (2006). *From cancer patient to cancer survivor.* Washington, DC: Institute of Medicine and National Research Council, The National Academies Press. Components of survivorship care provided by the Institute of Medicine report on cancer survivorship.

Critical Thinking Exercises

1 A 63-year-old man previously treated for stage III prostate cancer with HDR brachytherapy and androgen deprivation therapy returns to the cancer centre for a follow-up visit. While you are assessing his vital signs, he tells you that he has been having back pain for the last 3 weeks that he attributes to sleeping on an old mattress. What are the priorities to include in your nursing assessment of this patient? Identify the diagnostic procedures that you anticipate will be required to further evaluate this patient's back pain. What are your priorities for care of this patient?

2 An 80-year-old woman, who lives alone, was just recently diagnosed with stage IV colon cancer. She is being discharged from the hospital following a palliative colon resection. What will be the focus of educating this patient for self-care? Describe at least three age-related implications that will be important to consider. What type of referrals might be appropriate for this woman?

3 You are caring for a 32-year-old woman who is a breast cancer survivor. The patient takes tamoxifen 20 mg orally once daily and this will continue for the next 5 years. Are there any preventive measures that should be considered to address survivorship needs? What is the evidence for these interventions and education that you identified? How strong is that evidence, and what criteria did you use to assess the strength of that evidence?

REFERENCES AND SELECTED READINGS

Books

Acharyya, S., Matrisian, L., Welch, D. R., et al. (2015). Invasion and metastasis. In J. Mendelsohn, P. M. Howley, M. A. Israel, et al. (Eds.). *The molecular basis of cancer*. Philadelphia, PA: Elsevier-Saunders.

Alt-Epping, B., & Nauck, F. (Eds.). (2015). *Palliative care in oncology*. Berlin: Springer.

Baehring, Y. (2015). Oncologic emergencies: Spinal cord compression. In V. T. DeVita, T. S. Lawrence, & S. A. Rosenberg (Eds.). *Cancer: Principles & practice of oncology*. Philadelphia, PA: Lippincott Williams & Wilkins.

Barbarotta, L. M. (2015). Oncologic emergencies in critical care. In Booker, K. J. *Critical care nursing: Monitoring and treatment for advanced nursing practice*. Oxford, UK: Wiley Blackwell.

Comerford, K. C. (2015). *Nursing 2015 drug handbook*. Philadelphia, PA: Wolters Kluwer.

DeNavas-Walt, C., Proctor, B. D., & Smith, J. C. (2013). *Income, poverty, and health insurance coverage in the United States: 2012*. Washington, DC: U.S. Government Printing Office, Report # P60–245.

Grossman, S. C., & Porth, C. M. (2014). *Porth's pathophysiology: Concepts of altered health states* (9th ed.). Philadelphia, PA: Lippincott Williams & Wilkins.

Halperin, E. C., Wazer, D. E., Perez, C. A., et al. (Eds.). (2013). *Perez and Brady's principles and practice of radiation oncology* (6th ed.). Philadelphia, PA: Lippincott Williams & Wilkins.

Hannon, R. A., & Porth, C. M. (2017). *Porth's pathophysiology: Concepts of altered health states* (2nd ed.). Philadelphia, PA: Lippincott Williams & Wilkins.

Hewitt, M., Greenfield, S., & Stovall, E. (Eds.). (2006). *From cancer patient to cancer survivor*. Washington, DC: Institute of Medicine and National Research Council, The National Academies Press.

Kaplan, M. (2012a). Hypercalcemia of malignancy. In M. Kaplan (Ed.). *Understanding and managing oncologic emergencies: A resource for nurses* (2nd ed.). Pittsburgh, PA: Oncology Nursing Society.

Kaplan, M. (2012b). Spinal cord compression. In M. Kaplan (Ed.). *Understanding and managing oncologic emergencies: A resource for nurses* (2nd ed.). Pittsburgh, PA: Oncology Nursing Society.

Kasper, D. L., Fauci, A. S., Hauser, S. L., et al. (Eds.). (2015). *Harrison's principles of internal medicine* (19th ed.). New York: McGraw-Hill Education.

Lu, Y., Clague, J., & Bernstein, L. (2015). Cancer etiology: Obesity and physical activity. In V. T. DeVita, T. S. Lawrence, & S. A. Rosenberg (Eds.). *Cancer: Principles & practice of oncology*. Philadelphia, PA: Lippincott Williams & Wilkins.

Maziarz, R. T., & Schubach-Slater, S. (Eds.). (2015). *Blood and marrow transplant handbook: Comprehensive guide for patient care*. New York: Springer.

Morgan, M. A., Ten Haken, R. K., & Lawrence, T. S. (2015). Essentials of radiation therapy. In V. T. DeVita, T. S. Lawrence, & S. A. Rosenberg (Eds.). *Cancer: Principles & practice of oncology*. Philadelphia, PA: Lippincott Williams & Wilkins.

Nguyen, D. M., Summers, R. M., & Finkelstein, S. E. (2015). Cancer diagnosis: Respiratory tract. In V. T. DeVita, T. S. Lawrence, & S. A. Rosenberg (Eds.). *Cancer: Principles & practice of oncology*. Philadelphia, PA: Lippincott Williams & Wilkins.

Polovich, M., Olsen, M., & Lefebvre, K. (2014). *Chemotherapy and biotherapy guidelines and recommendations for practice* (4th ed.). Pittsburgh, PA: Oncology Nursing Society.

Ryan, R., Iwamoto, M., Haas, M. L., et al. (2012). *Manual for radiation oncology nursing practice and education* (4th ed.). Pittsburgh, PA: Oncology Nursing Society.

Schulmeister, L. (2014). Safe management of chemotherapy: Infusion-related complications. In M. Polovich, M. Olsen, & M. LeFebvre (Eds.). *Chemotherapy and biotherapy guideline and recommendations for practice* (4th ed.). Pittsburgh, PA: Oncology Nursing Society.

Segal, B. H., Walsh, T. J., Gea-Banacloche, J. C., et al. (2015). Infections in the cancer patient. In V. T. DeVita, T. S. Lawrence, & S. A. Rosenberg (Eds.). *Cancer: Principles & practice of oncology*. Philadelphia, PA: Lippincott Williams & Wilkins.

Story, K. T. (2012). Cardiac tamponade. In M. Kaplan (Ed.). *Understanding and managing oncologic emergencies: A resource for nurses* (2nd ed.). Pittsburgh, PA: Oncology Nursing Society.

Wilkes, G. M., & Barton-Burke, M. (2014). *2014 oncology nursing drug handbook*. Sudbury, MA: Jones & Bartlett.

Yahalom, J. (2015). Oncologic emergencies: Superior vena cava syndrome. In V. T. DeVita, T. S. Lawrence, & S. A. Rosenberg (Eds.). *Cancer: Principles & practice of oncology*. Philadelphia, PA: Lippincott Williams & Wilkins.

Yarbro, C., Wujcik, D., & Holmes Gobel, B. (Eds). (2013). *Cancer symptom management* (4th ed.). Sudbury, MA: Jones & Bartlett.

Journals and Electronic Documents

Alesi, E. R., & del Fabbro, E. (2014). Opportunities for targeting the fatigue-anorexia-cachexia symptom cluster. *The Cancer Journal, 20*(5), 325–329.

American Cancer Society (ACS). (2014). *Cancer treatment and survivorship: Facts and figures 2014–2015*. Retrieved March 22, 2016, from www.cancer.org/acs/groups/content/@research/documents/document/acspc-042801.pdf

Beck, M. (2015). Radiation safety in the management of patients undergoing radioactive iodine ablation therapy. *Clinical Journal of Oncology Nursing, 19*(1), 44–46.

Bender, C. M., & Thelen, B. D. (2013). Cancer and cognitive changes: The complexity of the problem. *Seminars in Oncology Nursing, 29*(4), 232–237.

Benito, L., Binefa, G., Lluch, T., et al. (2014). Defining the role of the nurse in population-based cancer screening programs: A literature review. *Oncology Nursing Forum, 18*(2), 77–83.

Bessede, E., Dubus, P., Megraud, F., et al. (2014). Helicobacter pylori infection and stem cells at the origin of gastric cancer. *Oncogene, 34*(20), 2547–2555.

Blix, A. (2014). Personalized medicine, genomics, and pharmacogenomics: A primer for nurses. *Clinical Journal of Oncology Nursing, 18*(4), 437–441.

Boeing, H., Bechthold, A., Bub, A., et al. (2012). Critical review: Vegetables and fruit in the prevention of chronic diseases. *European Journal of Nutrition, 51*(6), 637–663.

Bozzetti, F. (2013). Nutritional support of the oncology patient. *Critical Reviews in Oncology & Hematology, 87*(2), 172–200.

Braskett, M., & Cohen, M. (2014). *Diagnosis and management of chemotherapy induced hypersensitivity reactions*. American College of Physicians Hospitalist, Retrieved March 11, 2016, from www.acphospitalist.org/archives/2014/06/expert_analysis.htm

Brittain, K., & Murphy, V. P. (2015). Sociocultural and health correlates related to colorectal cancer screening adherence among urban African Americans. *Cancer Nursing, 38*(2), 118–124.

Bryant, A. L., Walton, A. L., & Phillips, B. (2015). Cancer-related fatigue: Scientific progress has been made in 40 years. *Clinical Journal of Oncology Nursing, 19*(2), 137–139.

Canadian Cancer Society's Advisory Committee on Cancer Statistics. (2013). Canadian Cancer Statistics 2013. Toronto, Canada: Canadian Cancer Society. Retrieved from http://www.cancer.ca/~/media/cancer.ca/CW/cancer%20information/cancer%20101/Canadian%20cancer%20statistics/canadian-cancer-statistics-2013-EN.pdf

Canadian Cancer Society. (2014). Melanoma: Deadliest type of skin cancer is on the rise. Toronto, Canada: Canadian Cancer Society. Retrieved from https://www.cancer.ca/en/about-us/for-media/media-releases/national/2014/2014-canadian-cancer-statistics/?region=on

Canadian Cancer Society. (2019). Cancer statistics at a glance.Toronto, Canada: Canadian Cancer Society. Retrieved from https://www.cancer.ca/en/cancer-information/cancer-101/cancer-statistics-at-a-glance/?region=on

Canadian Cancer Society's Steering Committee. (2018). Canadian cancer statistics: A 2018 special report on cancer incidence by stage. Toronto, Canada, Canadian Cancer Society. Retrieved from:http://www.cancer.ca/~/media/cancer.ca/CW/cancer%20information/cancer%20101/Canadian%20cancer%20statistics/Canadian-Cancer-Statistics-2018-EN.pdf?la=en

Caruana, I., Diaconu, I., & Dottia, G. (2014). From monoclonal antibodies to chimeric antigen receptors for the treatment of human malignancies. *Seminars in Oncology, 41*(5), 661–666.

Castells, M. C. (2015). Anaphylaxis to chemotherapy and monoclonal antibodies in anaphylaxis. *Immunology and Allergy Clinics of North America, 35*(2), 335–348.

Centers for Disease Control and Prevention (CDC). (2015). *Hepatitis B FAQs for health professionals.* Retrieved March 7, 2016, from www.cdc.gov/hepatitis/hbv/hbvfaq.htm#D4

Chen, C. J., Hsu, W. L., Yang, H. I., et al. (2014). Epidemiology of virus infection and human cancer. *Recent Results in Cancer Research, 193*, 11–32.

Chlebowski, R. T., Anderson, G., Manson, J. E., et al. (2010). Estrogen alone in postmenopausal women and breast cancer detection by means of mammography and breast biopsy. *Journal of Clinical Oncology, 28*(16), 2690–2697.

Christodoulou, M., Bayman, N., McCloskey, P., et al. (2014). New radiotherapy approaches in locally advanced non-small cell lung cancer. *European Journal of Cancer, 50*(3), 525–534.

Chung, T. K., Rosenthal, E. L., Magnuson, J. S., et al. (2015). Transoral robotic surgery for oropharyngeal and tongue cancer in the United States. *Laryngoscope, 125*(1), 140–145.

Citrin, D. E., & Mitchell, J. B. (2014). Altering the response to radiation: Sensitizers and protectors. *Seminars in Oncology, 41*(6), 848–859.

Clarke, T. C., Black, L. I., Stussman, B. J., et al. (2015). Trends in the use of complementary health approaches among adults: United States, 2002–2012. *National Health Statistics Reports, 79*, 1–16.

Collins, F. S., & Varmus, H. (2015). A new initiative on precision medicine. *New England Journal of Medicine, 372*(9), 793–795.

Corbin, K. S., Hellman, S., & Weichselbaum, R. R. (2013). Extracranial oligometastases: A subset of metastases curable with stereotactic radiotherapy. *Journal of Clinical Oncology, 31*(11), 1384–1390.

Cotogni, P., Barbero, C., Garrino, C., et al. (2015). Peripherally inserted central catheters in non-hospitalized cancer patients: 5-year results of a prospective study. *Supportive Care in Cancer, 23*(2), 403–409.

Coyle, C. E., Griffie, J., & Czaplewski, L. M. (2014). Eliminating extravasation events: A multidisciplinary approach. *Journal of Infusion Nursing, 37*(3), 157–164.

Damsky-Dell, D., Held-Warmkessel, J., Jakubek, P., et al. (2014). Care of the open abdomen after cytoreductive surgery and hyperthermic intraperitoneal chemotherapy for peritoneal surface malignancies. *Oncology Nursing Forum, 41*(4), 438–441.

Datta, S., Kundu, S., Ghosh, P., et al. (2014). Correlation of oxidant status with oxidative tissue damage in patients with rheumatoid arthritis. *Clinical Rheumatology, 33*(11), 1557–1564.

Di Lascio, S., & Pagani, O. (2014). Oligometastatic breast cancer: A shift from palliative to potentially curative treatment? *Breast Care, 9*(1), 7–14.

Eaton, L. H., Mitchell, D. H., & Doorenbos, A. Z. (2015). Evidence-based practice beliefs and behaviors of nurses providing cancer pain management: A mixed-methods approach. *Oncology Nursing Forum, 42*(2), 165–173.

Eilers, J., Harris, D., Henry, K., et al. (2014). Evidence-based interventions for cancer treatment-related mucositis: Putting evidence into practice. *Clinical Journal of Oncology Nursing, 18*(6), 80–96.

Eilers, J., & Million, R. (2007). Prevention and management of oral mucositis in patients with cancer. *Seminars in Oncology Nursing, 23*(3), 201–212.

Feller, L., Altini, M., & Lemmer, J. (2013). Inflammation in the context of oral cancer. *Oral Oncology, 49*(9), 887–892.

Flynn, K. E., Reese, J. B., Jeffery, D. D., et al. (2012). Patient experiences with communication about sex during and after treatment for cancer. *Psycho-Oncology, 21*(6), 594–601.

Fogh, S., & Yom, S. S. (2014). Symptom management during the radiation oncology treatment course: A practical guide for the oncology clinician. *Seminars in Oncology, 41*(6), 764–775.

Frankel Kelvin, J. (2015). Sperm banking: Fertility preservation for male patients with cancer. *Clinical Journal of Oncology Nursing, 19*(1), 108–110.

Fritz, A., Percy, C., Jack, A., et al. (2013). *International classification of diseases for oncology (ICD-O)—3rd edition, 1st revision.* Retrieved February 25, 2016, from apps.who.int/iris/bitstream/10665/96612/1/9789241548496_eng.pdf?ua=1

Gibson, R. J., Keefe, D. M., Lalla, R. V., et al. (2013). Systematic review of agents for the management of gastrointestinal mucositis in cancer patients. *Supportive Care in Cancer, 21*(1), 313–326.

Given, B. (2015). Prevention, identification, and management of late effects through risk reduction. *Seminars in Oncology Nursing, 31*(1), 31–41.

Goldfarb, S., Mulhall, J., Nelson, C., et al. (2013). Sexual and reproductive health in cancer survivors. *Seminars in Oncology, 40*(6), 726–744.

Gonella, S., & Di Giulio, P. (2015). Delayed chemotherapy-induced nausea and vomiting in the hematology population: A review of the literature. *Clinical Journal of Oncology Nursing, 19*(4), 438–443.

Gonzalez, T. (2013). Chemotherapy extravasations: Prevention, identification, management and documentation. *Clinical Journal of Oncology Nursing, 17*(1), 61–66.

Herrero, R., Quint, W., Hildesheim, S., et al. (2015). Reduced prevalence of oral human papillomavirus (HPV) 4 years after bivalent HPV vaccination in a randomized clinical trial in Costa Rica. *PLoS One, 8*(7), 1–9.

Heston, A. H., Schwartz, A. L., Justice-Gardiner, H., et al. (2015). Addressing physical activity needs of survivors by developing a community-based exercise program: LIVESTRONG® at the YMCA. *Clinical Journal of Oncology Nursing, 19*(2), 213–217.

IMS Institute. (2014). Innovation in cancer care and implications for health systems: Global oncology trend report. Retrieved from www.imshealth.com/vgn-ext-templating/v/index.jsp?vgnextoid=f8d4df7a5e8b5410VgnVCM10000076192ca2RCRD

Jansen, C. E. (2013). Cognitive changes associated with cancer and cancer therapy: Patient assessment and education. *Seminars in Oncology Nursing, 29*(4), 270–279.

Kannan, R., Madden, K., & Andrews, S. (2014). Primer on immuno-oncology and immune response. *Clinical Journal of Oncology Nursing, 18*(3), 311–317, 326.

Kelvin, J. F., Steed, R., & Jarrett, J. (2014). Discussing safe sexual practices during cancer treatment. *Clinical Journal of Oncology Nursing, 18*(4), 449–453.

Knobf, M. (2013). Being prepared: Essential to self-care and quality of life for the person with cancer. *Clinical Journal of Oncology Nursing, 17*(3), 255–261.

Kohler, B. A., Sherman, R. L., Howlader, N., et al. (2015). Annual report to the nation on the status of cancer, 1975–2011. *Journal of the National Cancer Institute, 107*(6), 1–25.

Kuter, D. J. (2015). Managing thrombocytopenia associated with cancer chemotherapy. *Oncology, 29*(4), 282–294.

Lassiter, M., & Schneider, S. M. (2015). A pilot study comparing the neutropenic diet to a non-neutropenic diet in the allogeneic hematopoietic stem cell transplantation population. *Oncology Nursing Forum, 19*(3), 273–278.

Leduc-Souville, B., Bertrand, E., & Schlatter, J. (2013). Risk management of excreta in a cancer unit. *Clinical Journal of Oncology Nursing, 17*(3), 248–252.

Lovly, C. M., Horn, L., & Pao, W. (2015). *KRAS in non-small cell lung cancer (NSCLC).* My Cancer Genome. Retrieved February 25, 2016, from www.mycancergenome.org/content/disease/lung-cancer/kras

Lukens, N. J., Gamez, M., Hu, K., et al. (2014). Modern brachytherapy. *Seminars in Oncology, 41*(6), 831–847.

Mack, F., Ritchie, M., & Sapra, P. (2014). The next generation of antibody drug conjugates. *Seminars in Oncology, 41*(5), 637–652.

Mahon, S. M. (2014). Providing care for previvors: Implications for oncology nurses. *Clinical Journal of Oncology Nursing, 18*(1), 21–24.

Manea, P. (2014). Optimizing the management of patients with myelofibrosis. *Clinical Journal of Oncology Nursing, 18*(3), 330–337.

Mazanec, P., & Prince-Paul, M. (2014). Integrating palliative care into active cancer treatment. *Seminars in Oncology Nursing, 30*(4), 203–211.
Merriman, J. D., Von Ah, D., Miaskowski, C., et al. (2013). Proposed mechanisms for cancer and treatment-related cognitive changes. *Seminars in Oncology Nursing, 29*(4), 260–269.
Miceli, T., Lilleby, T., Noonan, K., et al. (2013). Autologous hematopoietic stem cell transplantation for patients with multiple myeloma: An overview for nurses in community practice. *Clinical Journal of Oncology Nursing, 17*(6), 13–24.
Mitchell, S. A., Hoffman, A. J., Clark, J. C., et al. (2014). Putting evidence into practice: An update of evidence-based interventions for cancer-related fatigue during and following treatment. *Clinical Journal of Oncology Nursing, 18*(6), S38–S58.
Montezano, A. C., Dulak-Lis, M., Tsiropoulou, S., et al. (2015). Oxidative stress and human hypertension: Vascular mechanisms, biomarkers, and novel therapies. *Journal of Canadian Cardiology, 31*(5), 631–641.
National Cancer Institute (NCI). (2012a). *Hormone therapy for breast cancer*. Retrieved from http://www.cancer.gov/cancertopics/factsheet/therapy-breast
National Cancer Institute (NCI). (2012b). *Obesity and cancer risk*. Retrieved from http://www.cancer.org/cancertopics/factsheet/Risk/obesity
National Cancer Institute (NCI). (2016). *Cancer genetics overview for health professionals*. Retrieved March 2, 2016, from www.cancer.gov/cancertopics/pdq/genetics/overview/healthprofessional
National Comprehensive Cancer Network (NCCN). (2015a). Clinical practice guidelines in oncology: Genetic/familial high risk assessment: Breast and ovarian. Retrieved from www.nccn.org/professionals/physician_gls/pdf/genetics_screening.pdf
National Comprehensive Cancer Network (NCCN). (2015b). Clinical practice guidelines in oncology: Genetic/familial high risk assessment: Colorectal. Retrieved from www.nccn.org/professionals/physician_gls/pdf/genetics_colon.pdf
National Comprehensive Cancer Network (NCCN). (2015c). Clinical practice guidelines: Breast. Retrieved from www.nccn.org/professionals/physician_gls/PDF/infections.pdf
National Comprehensive Cancer Network (NCCN). (2015d). NCCN clinical practice guidelines in oncology: Prostate cancer. Retrieved from www.nccn.org/professionals/physician_gls/pdf/prostate.pdf
National Comprehensive Cancer Network (NCCN). (2015e). NCCN clinical practice guidelines in oncology: Antiemesis. Retrieved from www.nccn.org/professionals/physician_gls/pdf/antiemesis.pdf
National Comprehensive Cancer Network (NCCN). (2015f). NCCN guidelines for supportive care: Cancer related fatigue. Retrieved from www.nccn.org/professionals/physician_gls/f_guidelines.asp#fatigue
National Comprehensive Cancer Network (NCCN). (2015g). NCCN clinical practice guidelines in oncology: Distress [v.2.2015]. Retrieved from http://www.nccn.org/professionals/physician_gls/pdf/distress.pdf
National Comprehensive Cancer Network (NCCN). (2015h). NCCN clinical practice guidelines in oncology: Prevention and treatment of cancer-related infection [v.2.2015]. Retrieved from http://www.nccn.org/professionals/physician_gls/pdf/infections.pdf
National Comprehensive Cancer Network (NCCN). (2015i). NCCN clinical practice guidelines in oncology: Cancer-associated thromboembolic disease [v.1.2015]. Retrieved from http://www.nccn.org/professionals/physician_gls/pdf/vte.pdf
National Institutes of Health, National Center for Complementary and Integrative Health (NCCIH). (2015). *Complementary, alternative, or integrative health: What's in a name?* Retrieved October 10, 2015, from nccih.nih.gov/health/integrative-health
Navari, R. M. (2013). Management of chemotherapy-induced nausea and vomiting. *Drugs, 73*(3), 249–262.
Neuss, M. N., Polovich, M., McNiff, K., et al. (2013). 2013 Updated American Society of Clinical Oncology/Oncology Nursing Society chemotherapy administration safety standards including standards for the safe administration and management of oral chemotherapy. *Oncology Nursing Forum, 40*(3), 225–233.
Niklas, C., Saar, M., Berg, B., et al. (2016). da Vinci and open radical prostatectomy: Comparison of clinical outcomes and analysis of insurance costs. *Urologia International, 96*(3), 287–294.
Oeffinger, K. C. (2013). Introduction: The science of survivorship: Moving from risk to risk reduction. *Seminars in Oncology, 40*(6), 662–665.
O'Gorman, C., Sasiadek, W., Denieffe, S., et al. (2015). Predicting radiotherapy-related clinical toxicities in cancer: A literature review. *Clinical Journal of Oncology Nursing, 18*(3), 37–44.
Pachman, D., Price, K. A., & Carey, E. C. (2014). Nonpharmacologic approach to fatigue in patients with cancer. *The Cancer Journal, 20*(5), 313–318.
Perlman, A., Lontok, O., Huhmann, M., et al. (2013). Prevalence and correlates of postdiagnosis initiation of complementary and alternative medicine among patients at a comprehensive cancer center. *Journal of Oncology Practice, 9*(1), 34–41.
Raja, D., & Sultana, B. (2013). Health risk of environmental tobacco smoke. *Internet Journal of Allied Health Sciences & Practice, 11*(2), 6.
Schiller, J. T., & Lowy, D. R. (2014). Virus infection and human cancer: An overview. *Recent Results in Cancer Research, 193*, 1–10.
Schilli, S. M. (2014). Screening for distress in patients with cancer. *Clinical Journal of Oncology Nursing, 18*(6), E103–E106.
Shackelford, J. A., Weyhenmeyer, D. P., & Mabus, L. K. (2015). Fostering early breast cancer detection: Faith community nurses reaching at-risk populations. *Oncology Nursing Forum, 18*(6), 113–118.
Siegel, R. L., Miller, K. D., & Jemal, A. (2015). Cancer statistics, 2015. *Cancer Journal for Clinicians, 65*(1), 5–29.
Smith, A. (2015). A workshop for educating nurses to address sexual health in patients with breast cancer. *Clinical Journal of Oncology Nursing, 19*(3), 248–250.
Smith, T. J., Bohlke, K., Lyman, G. H., et al. (2015). Recommendations for the use of WBC growth factors: American Society of Clinical Oncology clinical practice guideline update. *Journal of Clinical Oncology, 33*(28), 3199–3212.
Suzuki, H., Asakawa, A., Amitani, H., et al. (2013). Cancer cachexia-pathophysiology and management. *Journal of Gastroenterology, 48*(5), 574–594.
Tayyem, A. Q. (2014). Cryotherapy effect on oral mucositis severity among recipients of bone marrow transplantation: A literature review. *Clinical Journal of Oncology Nursing, 18*(4), E84–E87.
Thomson, C. A., McCullough, M. L., Wertheim, B., et al. (2014). Nutrition and physical activity cancer prevention guidelines, cancer risk, and mortality in the Women's Health Initiative. *Cancer Prevention Research, 7*(1), 42–53.
Tipian, C. (2014). Brushing up on mouth care for cancer patients with mucositis. *American Nurse Today, 9*(11), 38–40.
Tofthagen, C., Visovsky, C. M., & Hopgood, R. (2013). Chemotherapy-induced peripheral neuropathy: An algorithm to guide nursing management. *Clinical Journal of Oncology Nursing, 17*(2), 138–144.
Vadhan-Raj, S., Goldberg, J. D., Perales, M. A., et al. (2013). Clinical applications of palifermin: Amelioration of oral mucositis and other potential indications. *Journal of Cell & Molecular Medicine, 17*(11), 1371–1384.
Violral, A., Leslie, M., Best, R., et al. (2014). Patient adherence with oral oncolytic therapies. *Seminars in Oncology Nursing, 30*(3), 190–199.
Von Ah, D. (2015). Cognitive changes associated with cancer and cancer treatment: State of the science. *Clinical Journal of Oncology Nursing, 19*(1), 47–56.
Weber, J. S. (2014). Immuno-oncology comes of age. *Seminars in Oncology, 41*(5), S1–S2.
Yagasaki, K., & Komatsu, H. (2013). The need for a nursing presence in oral chemotherapy. *Clinical Journal of Oncology Nursing, 17*(5), 512–516.

Resources

Alberta Health Services, Alberta Cancer Board: http://www.cancerboard.ab.ca
BC Cancer: http://www.bccancer.bc.ca
Canadian Breast Cancer Network: http://www.cbcn.ca
Canadian Cancer Society: http://www.cancer.ca
Canadian Prostate Cancer Network: http://www.cpcn.org
CancerCare Manitoba: http://www.cancercare.mb.ca
Cancer Care Ontario: http://www.cancercare.on.ca
Cancer Care Nova Scotia: http://www.cancercare.ns.ca
Cancer Information Network: http://www.cancernetwork.com
Colorectal Cancer Association of Canada: http://www.colorectal-cancer.ca
Fondation québécoise du cancer: http://www.fqc.qc.ca
Horizon Health Network, New Brunswick: http://www.rhab-rrsb.ca
Hospice and Palliative Care Nurses Association (HPNA): http://www.hpna.org
National Cancer Institute, Cancer Topics: http://cancernet.nci.nih.gov/cancertopics
National Center for Complementary and Alternative Medicine (NCCAM): http://www.nccam.nih.gov
National Comprehensive Cancer Network: http://www.nccn.org
Newfoundland Cancer Treatment and Research Foundation: http://www.easternhealth.ca/nctrf
Oncology Nursing Society (ONS): http://www.ons.org

UNIT 15

Musculoskeletal Function

Case Study

DEVELOPING A TEAM APPROACH TO CARE IN THE HOME SETTING

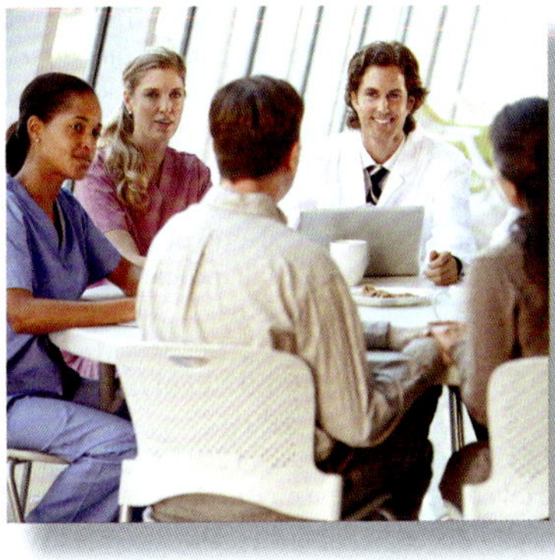

The nurse is participating in an interdisciplinary team meeting discussing patients in an inpatient acute rehabilitation unit. The team consists of a physician, nurse, pharmacist, social worker, occupational therapist, physical therapist, and registered dietician. The team is discussing the interdisciplinary management plan for a patient recently admitted for transitional care from the hospital, where he had an above-the-knee amputation of the right leg as a result of poorly controlled diabetes. The team has concerns for the patient because he lives alone and is unable to care for himself to achieve an optimal recovery. In addition, his last hemoglobin A1c was 9.8%, indicating that his diabetes is still not well controlled. The team must develop strategies necessary to help the patient recover from his recent surgery and develop a plan of care for controlling his diabetes before he can transition to home care.

QSEN Competency Focus: Teamwork and Collaboration

The complexities inherent in today's health care system challenge nurses to demonstrate integration of specific interdisciplinary core competencies that are aimed at ensuring the delivery of safe and quality patient care (Institute of Medicine, 2003). The Quality and Safety Education for Nurses project (QSEN, 2017; Cronenwett, Sherwood, Barnsteiner, et al., 2007) provides a framework for the knowledge, skills, and attitudes (KSAs) required for nurses to demonstrate competency in these key areas, which include ***patient-centred care***, ***interdisciplinary teamwork and collaboration***, ***evidence-based practice***, ***quality improvement***, ***safety***, and ***informatics.***

Teamwork and Collaboration Definition: Function effectively within nursing and interprofessional teams, fostering open communication, mutual respect, and shared decision making to achieve quality patient care.

SELECTED PRE-LICENSURE KSAs	APPLICATION AND REFLECTION
Knowledge	
Recognize contributions of other individuals and groups in helping patient/family achieve health goals.	Collaborative problems require nursing interventions as well as those of other health care providers on the team. What are nursing interventions for managing diabetes? What contributions might the pharmacist and dietician have in regard to managing diabetes?
Skills	
Integrate the contributions of others who play a role in helping patient/family achieve goals.	Think of an example of a collaborative problem for this patient with both medical and nursing interventions. How does the nurse integrate the contributions of other team members into the nursing plan of care? What are some common goals that the team may share for this patient?
Attitudes	
Value the perspectives and expertise of all health team members. Value teamwork and the relationship upon which it is based.	Reflect on your experience with teamwork. What is the value of each team member's different area of expertise for this patient? How might perspectives differ between interdisciplinary team members? Considering these differences in perspectives, how might each individual member of this team foster a relationship for teamwork?

Cronenwett, L., Sherwood, G., Barnsteiner, J., et al. (2007). Quality and safety education for nurses. *Nursing Outlook, 55*(3), 122–131; Institute of Medicine. (2003). *Health professions education: A bridge to quality*. Washington, DC: National Academies Press; and QSEN Institute. (2017). *QSEN competencies: Definitions and pre-licensure KSAs*. Retrieved June 12, 2019, from www.qsen.org/competencies/pre-licensure-ksas

69 Assessment of Musculoskeletal Function

Adapted by Jennifer Densmore

Learning Objectives

On completion of this chapter, the learner will be able to:

1. Describe the anatomy and physiology of the musculoskeletal system.
2. Relate the significance of the health history to the assessment of musculoskeletal health.
3. Describe the physical examination of the musculoskeletal system.
4. Discuss the significance of assessment for the nursing diagnosis of musculoskeletal dysfunction.
5. Demonstrate knowledge of the diagnostic tests used for assessment of musculoskeletal function.

The musculoskeletal system comprises the bones, **joints**, muscles, **tendons**, **ligaments**, menisci, and **bursae** of the body. Their functions are highly integrated. Disease and/or injury of one component adversely affect the others. For instance, an infection in a joint (septic arthritis) causes degeneration of the articular surfaces of the bones within the joint and local muscle **atrophy**.

Diseases and injuries involving the musculoskeletal system are commonly implicated in disability and death. Across the Canadian life span, these are broadly grouped into five categories: genetic, traumatic, infectious, neoplastic, and rheumatologic. Musculoskeletal disorders can significantly affect overall productivity, independence, and quality of life. Nurses in all practice areas encounter patients with disturbances in the musculoskeletal system. Among those are the many types of arthritis. In Canada, more than 4.6 million individuals aged 15 years or older report having arthritis. Two out of three are women, and for them arthritis is the leading cause of disability; in men, it is the third cause (The Arthritis Society, 2014). To complicate disability, arthritis has a significant impact on mental health. Another condition, osteoporosis, is associated with risk for fractures among Canadians who are 40 years of age or more. A common complication of osteoporosis is the fracture of a hip, pelvis, spine, upper arm, or wrist. Many Canadians are at risk, especially because they are not being screened for the condition, do not report regular physical activity, and/or are not taking calcium or vitamin D supplements (PHAC, 2010b). In 2005 to 2006, 132,000 hospitalizations in Canada were associated with arthritis (PHAC, 2010a).

Anatomic and Physiologic Overview

The musculoskeletal system protects vital organs, including the brain, heart, lungs, and spinal cord; provides a sturdy framework to support body structures; and makes mobility possible. Muscles and tendons hold the bones together; **tendons** attach muscles to bones. They also move to produce heat that helps maintain body temperature. Joints permit body movement that facilitates the return of deoxygenated blood to the right side of the heart by massaging the venous vasculature. The musculoskeletal system serves as a reservoir for immature blood cells and essential minerals, including calcium, phosphorus, magnesium, and fluoride. Over 98% of total body calcium is present in bone (Martini, Timmons, & Tallitsch, 2012).

Structure and Function of the Skeletal System

The human body has 206 bones divided into four categories: long bones (e.g., femur), short bones (e.g., metacarpals), flat bones (e.g., sternum), and irregular bones (e.g., vertebrae). The function and forces exerted on a specific bone determine its construction and shape. Bones are constructed of **cancellous** (trabecular) or **cortical** (compact) bone tissue. Long bones are shaped like rods or shafts with rounded ends (Fig. 69-1). The shaft (**diaphysis**) is primarily **cortical bone**. The ends of the long bones (**epiphyses**) are primarily **cancellous bone**. The epiphyseal plate, which separates the epiphyses from the diaphysis, is calcified in adults and is the centre for longitudinal growth in children.

The ends of long bones are covered at the joints by articular **cartilage** (dense, tough, avascular tissue). Long bones are designed for weight bearing and movement.

Short bones consist of cancellous bone covered by a layer of compact bone. Flat bones (cancellous bone layered between compact bone) are important sites of hematopoiesis and protect several vital organs (e.g., the heart). Irregular bones have unique shapes related to their function, but generally their structure is similar to that of flat bones.

Bone is composed of cells, protein matrix, and mineral deposits. Three basic types of cells exist: **osteoblasts**, **osteocytes**, and **osteoclasts**. Osteoblasts secrete bone matrix for bone formation. Matrix consists of collagen and ground substances (glycoproteins and proteoglycans) that provide a framework for deposit of inorganic mineral salts (primarily calcium and phosphorus). Osteocytes (mature bone cells) support bone maintenance and lie in lacunae (bone matrix units). Osteoclasts, located in shallow Howship's lacunae (small pits in bones), are multinuclear cells active in bone **resorption**. The microscopic and fundamental functional unit of mature cortical bone is the **osteon** (haversian system). The centre of the osteon, the haversian canal, contains a capillary. Around the capillary are circles of mineralized bone matrix called **lamellae**. Within the lamellae are osteocyte-containing lacunae. Tiny canaliculi (canals) communicate with adjacent blood vessels in the haversian system to nourish the lacunae. Layers of lacunae in cancellous bone form an irregular lattice network (**trabeculae**) that is filled with red bone marrow. Capillaries nourish the osteocytes located in the lacunae (Porth, 2017). A dense, fibrous membrane known as the **periosteum** covers the bone, but not the articular ends. This membranous structure nourishes bone and facilitates its growth. The periosteum contains nerves, blood vessels, and lymphatics, and makes possible the attachment of tendons and ligaments (Porth, 2017). The **endosteum** is a thin, vascular membrane that lines

Glossary

atonic: without tone; denervated muscle that atrophies
atrophy: wasting; decrease in the size of a muscle
bursa: fluid-filled sac found in connective tissue, commonly but not always in the area of joints
callus: osseous material at a fracture site; replaced by bone during healing
cancellous bone: latticelike bone structure; network of osseous material
cartilage: dense, tough, avascular connective tissue in joints, at ends of bone
clonus: rapid, rhythmic muscular contractions associated with a significant hyperactive deep tendon reflex
contracture: fibrosis of connective tissue found in fascia, joint, muscle, or skin; a shortening
cortical bone: dense rigid layer of a bone; also called compact bone
crepitus: grating or crackling sounds or sensations; may occur when bone fragments move against each other, cartilage erodes and joint surfaces grind on each other, inflamed tendons move, or air is trapped in subcutaneous tissues
diaphysis: shaft (middle section) of a long bone
effusion: excess fluid in joint or other body structure
endosteum: a thin, vascular membrane covering the marrow cavity of long bones and the network of osseous tissue (trabeculae) in cancellous bone
epiphysis: end of a long bone
fascia (epimysium): a fibrous membrane that covers, supports, and separates muscles; superficially, connects skin to muscle
fasciculation: involuntary twitching of muscle fibres
flaccid: limp; without muscle tone
hypertrophy: enlargement; increase in size or bulk of muscle
isometric contraction: increased muscle tension, muscle length unchanged, no joint motion
isotonic contraction: muscle tension unchanged, muscle length shortened, joint motion
joint: articulation between two bones; type of joint determines amount of movement
joint capsule: fibrous connective tissue that encloses joints
kyphosis: exaggeration of the convex curvature of the thoracic spine
lamella: a thin layer, membrane, plate, or scale; may be bone, cellular, or tissue
ligament: band of fibrous connective tissue connecting bones, cartilages, or organs
lordosis: exaggeration of the concave curvature of the lumbar spine
ossification: formation of bone matrix
osteoblast: bone-forming cell of mesodermal origin
osteoclast: bone resorption cell; absorbs calcium salts
osteocyte: mesodermal bone-forming cell; maintains bone as living structure
osteogenesis: bone formation
osteon: microscopic functional unit of compact bone
paresthesia: unpleasant numb, tingling, stinging, burning, or prickly sensation
periosteum: dense fibrous membrane covering bone, but not articular surfaces; serves as attachment for tendons and ligaments
remodelling: process that ensures bone maintenance through simultaneous bone resorption and formation
resorption: removal/destruction of tissue, such as bone
scoliosis: lateral curvature of the spine; congenital, functional, idiopathic, or disease related
spastic: increased muscle tone
synovium: membrane in joint that secretes lubricating fluid
tendon: band of fibrous connective tissue connecting muscle to bone
tone (tonus): residual tension in relaxed muscle
trabeculae: latticelike bone structure; network of osseous tissue in cancellous bone

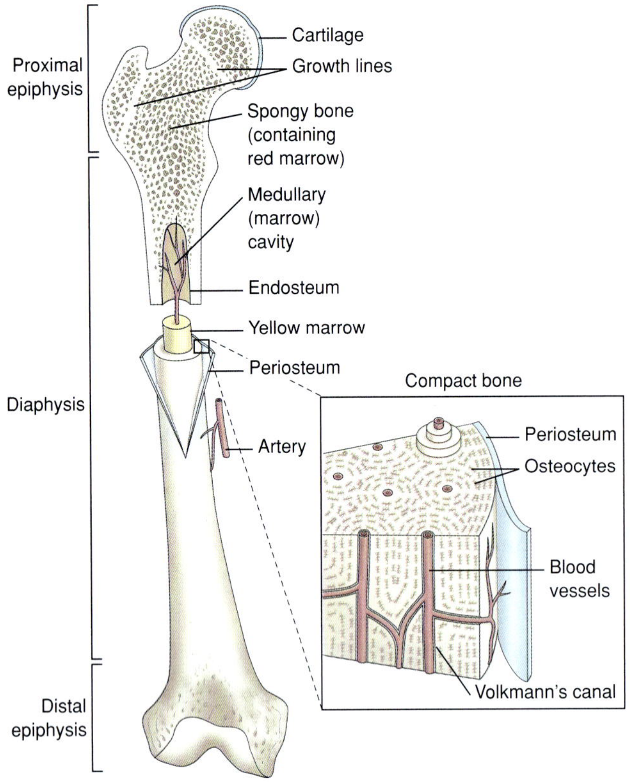

FIGURE 69-1. Structure of a long bone; composition of compact bone.

the marrow cavity of long bones and the trabeculae in cancellous bone. Located near the endosteum in Howship's lacunae are osteoclasts that dissolve bone matrix to maintain the marrow cavity (Porth, 2017).

Vascular bone marrow is located in flat bones and the medullary (shaft) cavity of long bones. In adults, red bone marrow, found mainly in the sternum, ilium, vertebrae, and ribs, produce red blood cells, white blood cells, and platelets in a process called hematopoiesis. Adult long bones are filled with fatty yellow marrow (Porth, 2017).

Bone tissue is highly vascular. Cancellous bone receives a rich blood supply from epiphyseal vessels. Periosteal vessels carry blood to compact bone through minute Volkmann's canals. In addition, nutrient arteries penetrate the periosteum and enter the medullary cavity through foramina (small openings). Arteries supply blood to the marrow and bone. Veins may accompany arteries or exit separately (Porth, 2017).

Bone Formation

Osteogenesis (bone formation) begins long before birth. Bone matrix is formed during **ossification** and hard mineral crystals composed of calcium and phosphorus (e.g., hydroxyapatite) are bound to the collagen fibres. The minerals give bone its characteristic strength and the proteinaceous collagen gives bone its resilience (Porth, 2017).

Bone Maintenance

Bone is a dynamic tissue in a constant state of turnover. During childhood, bones grow and form by a process called modelling. During an individual's early 20s, **remodelling** is the primary process. Remodelling maintains bone structure and function through simultaneous resorption and osteogenesis (Porth, 2017). Each year, almost 20% of the adult skeleton is replaced (Martini et al., 2012). Every 10 years, the adult skeleton is totally replaced (Coates, 2013). At the same time, bone turnover *rates* are affected by many diseases and conditions. Bone turnover markers assist in the management of osteoporosis and fracture prediction (Dreyer & Vieira, 2010; Naylor & Eastell, 2012).

In healthy individuals, several factors influence the balance between bone resorption and formation: physical activity; dietary intake of certain nutrients, especially calcium; and various hormones, including calcitriol (i.e., activated vitamin D), parathyroid hormone (PTH), calcitonin, thyroid hormone, cortisol, growth hormone, estrogen, and testosterone (Porth, 2017).

Physical activity, particularly weight-bearing activity, stimulates bone formation and remodelling. Bones subjected to frequent weight bearing tend to be thick and strong. Conversely, bones become osteopenic and weak in individuals who are unable to engage in regular weight-bearing activities, are on prolonged bed rest, or have some physical disabilities. They have increased bone resorption from calcium loss and their weakened bones may fracture easily.

NURSING ALERT

Weight-bearing activity or exercise should not be confused with weight-resistance exercise. Weight-bearing activity, which supports bone maintenance, is any activity done while a person is on their feet that works a person's bones and muscles against gravity (e.g., walking, tennis). Weight-resistance exercise, on the other hand, uses weights or resistance to strengthen muscles.

Dietary habits are important for bone health. The body requires calcium from dairy products (e.g., milk, yogurt, cheese, custards) and nondairy alternatives (e.g., soy, almonds, calcium-enriched orange juice, canned salmon, or sardines) to build bone mass. Vitamin D is essential to ensure strong bones, in part by promoting the absorption of the mineral calcium. It also protects against fractures by improving muscle function which helps to maintain balance and prevent falls. Canadians do not produce enough vitamin D from sun exposure due to Canada's northern geographical location, the use of sunscreen, and the decreasing ability to synthesize vitamin D with age. Osteoporosis Canada recommends that all Canadian adults use vitamin D supplements daily year-round (Osteoporosis Canada, 2014d). Several hormones are vital for ensuring that calcium is properly absorbed and available for bone mineralization and matrix formation. Calcitriol increases the amount of calcium in the blood by promoting absorption of calcium from the gastrointestinal tract. It also facilitates mineralization of osteoid tissue. A vitamin D deficiency results in a bone mineralization deficit, deformity, and fracture (Osteoporosis Canada, 2014a; Porth, 2017).

Calcitonin and PTH are the major hormonal regulators of calcium homeostasis. Secreted by the thyroid gland in response to elevated blood calcium levels, calcitonin inhibits bone resorption and increases calcium deposit in bone (Porth, 2017). Partly by promoting movement of calcium from the bone, PTH regulates the concentration of calcium in the blood. Responding to low blood calcium levels, increased levels of PTH prompt the mobilization of calcium, demineralization of bone, and formation of bone cysts.

Both thyroid hormones and cortisol have multiple systemic effects with specific effects on bones. Excessive thyroid hormone production in adults (e.g., Graves' disease) can increase bone resorption and decrease bone formation. Increased levels of cortisol have the same effects. Individuals receiving long-term synthetic cortisol or corticosteroids (e.g., prednisone) are at increased risk for steroid-induced osteopenia and fractures.

Growth hormone has direct and indirect effects on skeletal growth and remodelling. It stimulates the liver and to a lesser degree the bones to produce insulin-like growth factor-1 (IGF-I) that accelerates bone modelling in children and adolescents. Growth hormone also directly stimulates skeletal growth in children and adolescents. Likely, the low levels of both growth hormone and IGF-I that occur with aging are partly responsible for decreased bone formation and resultant osteopenia (Porth, 2017).

Estrogen and testosterone have important effects on bone remodelling (Porth, 2017). Estrogen stimulates osteoblasts and inhibits osteoclasts, enhancing bone formation and inhibiting resorption. Testosterone has both direct and indirect effects on bone growth and formation. Directly, it causes skeletal growth in adolescence and has continued effects on skeletal muscle growth throughout the life span. Increased muscle mass creates greater weight-bearing stress on bones, resulting in increased bone formation. Indirectly, testosterone converts to estrogen in adipose tissue, providing an additional source of bone-preserving estrogen for aging men.

During bone remodelling, osteoblasts produce a receptor activator of nuclear factor–kappa beta ligand that binds to the receptor activator of nuclear factor–kappa beta present on the cell membranes of osteoclast precursors. This causes them to differentiate and mature into osteoclasts, which trigger bone resorption. Conversely, osteoblasts may produce osteoprotegerin (OPG) that blocks the action of RANKL, stopping the process of bone resorption. As a result of the inflammatory process, T cells may become activated and also produce RANKL, overriding the effects of OPG and causing continued bone resorption during times of stress and injury. This can lead to loss of bone matrix and fractures (Porth, 2014). The bone blood supply also affects bone formation. With diminished blood supply or hyperemia (congestion), osteogenesis and bone density decrease. Bone necrosis occurs when the bone is deprived of blood.

Bone Healing

Most fractures heal with a combination of intramembranous and endochondral ossification processes. When a bone is fractured, it regenerates itself without scarring, but a thickened area on the bone surface could indicate a healed fracture (Porth, 2014).

Fracture healing occurs in the bone marrow, bone cortex, periosteum, and adjacent soft tissue. In the marrow, endothelial cells rapidly differentiate into osteoblasts. In the bone cortex, new osteons are formed. In the periosteum, a hard **callus** (fibrous tissue) forms during intramembranous ossification peripheral to the fracture and cartilage forms during endochondral ossification close to the fracture site. In adjacent soft tissue, a bridging callus forms that provides stability to the fractured bones.

The process of fracture healing may be structured over three phases:

Phase I: Reactive phase: When the fracture occurs, the body responds by bleeding into the injured tissue and forming of a hematoma at the fracture site. The release of cytokines initiates the fracture healing processes by causing proliferation of fibroblasts and angiogenesis to ensue (i.e., the growth of new blood vessels). Dense granulation tissue begins to form within the clot.

Phase II: Reparative phase: Granulation tissue is initially replaced with procallus (a callus precursor). Fibroblasts invade the procallus and produce a denser type of callus composed mostly of fibrocartilage. Approximately 3 to 4 weeks postinjury, denser bony calluses replace the fibrocartilaginous callus. Lamellar bone then forms as the bony callus calcifies months postinjury.

Phase III: Remodelling phase: Finally, remodelling creates new bone in its former structural arrangement and may take months to years. It is contingent on the extent of bone modification required, the function of the bone, and the functional stresses on the bone.

Serial x-rays are used to monitor the progress of bone healing. The rate of fracture healing depends on the type of bone fractured, the adequacy of blood supply, the surface contact of the fragments, age and the general health of the injured individual, and immobility of the fracture site. Adequate immobilization is essential until x-rays confirm bone formation with ossification. Immobilization may occur with an external fibreglass cast or an orthopedic surgeon may use hardware (e.g., pins, plates, screws, nails) to perform an open reduction and internal fixation.

When fractures are treated with open rigid compression plate fixation techniques, the bony fragments can be placed in direct contact. Primary bone healing occurs during cortical bone (haversian) remodelling. Little or no cartilaginous callus develops. Immature bone develops from the endosteum. An intensive regeneration of new osteons occurs in the fracture line by a process similar to that of regular bone maintenance. Fracture strength is obtained when the new osteons have become established.

Structure and Function of the Articular System

The junction of two or more bones is called a joint (articulation). One method of classifying joints is according to the type of cartilage in the joint: synarthrotic, amphiarthrotic, and diarthrotic (Martini et al., 2012). Synarthrotic joints are immovable and fibrous (e.g., the skull sutures). Amphiarthrotic joints (e.g., the vertebral joints, costal cartilages, symphysis pubis) allow limited motion; their bones are

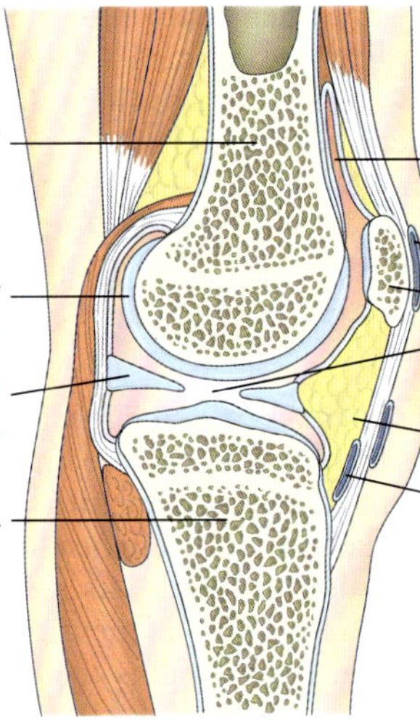

FIGURE 69-2. Hinge joint of the knee.

joined by fibrous cartilage. Diarthrotic joints are freely movable, synovial, and the most common (Fig. 69-2).

Diarthrotic joints include:

- *Ball-and-socket* joints (e.g., the hip, the shoulder) that permit full freedom of movement (flexion, extension, abduction, adduction, internal rotation, external rotation).
- *Hinge* joints that permit flexion and extension in one plane (e.g., the elbow, the knee, interphalangeal joints).
- *Saddle* joints that allow movement in two planes at right angles to each other (flexion, extension, abduction, adduction, circumduction). The joint at the base of the thumb is a saddle, biaxial joint.
- *Pivot* joints in the neck that permit rotation of the atlas on the axis.
- *Gliding* joints that permit limited movement in all directions (e.g., the joints of the carpal bones in the wrist, intervertebral joints) (Martini et al., 2012).

Smooth hyaline cartilage covers the ends of articulating bones of diarthrotic (movable) joints. A tough, fibrous sheath called the **joint capsule** surrounds articulating bones. The **synovium**, a membrane that lines the capsule, secretes lubricating and shock-absorbing synovial fluid into the joint capsule and prevents direct contact of bone surfaces. In some synovial joints (e.g., the knee), fibrocartilage discs (e.g., medial meniscus, lateral meniscus) are located between the articular cartilage surfaces and provide shock absorption (Porth, 2017).

Ligaments (fibrous connective tissue bands) bind articulating bones together. Ligaments and muscle tendons, which pass over the joint, provide joint stability. In some joints, interosseous ligaments (e.g., the cruciate ligaments of the knee) are found within the capsule and add anterior and posterior stability to the joint.

A bursa is a sac filled with synovial fluid that cushions the movement of tendons, ligaments, and bones at a point of friction. For example, bursae are found in the joints of the elbow, shoulder, hip, and knee.

A **meniscus** is a crescent-shaped (semilunar) fibrocartilage found in joints (e.g., the knee, acromioclavicular joint, radiocarpal joint). It partly divides a joint cavity and is a shock absorber. In the knee, it disperses friction between the tibia and femur (Martini et al., 2012).

Structure and Function of the Skeletal Muscle System

Muscles are attached by tendons to bones, connective tissue, other muscles, soft tissue, or skin. The muscles of the body are composed of parallel groups of muscle cells (fasciculi) encased in fibrous tissue called **fascia (epimysium)**. The more fasciculi contained in a muscle, the more precise its movements. Muscles vary in shape and size according to the activities for which they are responsible. Contractions of skeletal (striated) muscles facilitate body movement, posture, and heat production.

Skeletal Muscle Contraction

Each muscle cell (muscle fibre) contains myofibrils which are composed of a series of sarcomeres, the actual contractile units of skeletal muscle. Sarcomeres contain thick (myosin) and thin (actin) filaments.

Muscle cells contract in response to electrical impulses delivered by an effector nerve cell at the motor end plate. When stimulated, the muscle cell depolarizes and generates an action potential—similar to that described for nerve cells. Action potentials propagate along the muscle cell membrane, leading to the release of calcium ions that are stored in specialized organelles called sarcoplasmic reticula. A local increase in calcium ion concentration causes the myosin and actin filaments to slide across one another. Shortly after the muscle cell membrane depolarizes, it recovers its resting membrane voltage. Calcium is rapidly removed from the sarcomeres by active reaccumulation in the sarcoplasmic reticulum. When the calcium concentration in the sarcomere decreases, the myosin and actin filaments cease to interact, and the sarcomere returns to its original resting length (relaxation). Actin and myosin do not interact in the absence of calcium (Grossman & Porth, 2014).

Energy consumption occurs during muscle contraction and relaxation. The primary source of energy for muscle cells is adenosine triphosphate (ATP), which is generated through cellular oxidative metabolism. At low levels of activity (i.e., sedentary activity), the skeletal muscle synthesizes ATP from the oxidation of glucose to water and carbon dioxide. During strenuous activity, when sufficient oxygen may not be available, glucose is metabolized primarily to lactic acid, an inefficient process compared to that of oxidative pathways. Stored muscle glycogen is used to supply glucose during periods of activity. Muscle fatigue has various proposed explanations and is distinct from delayed-onset muscle soreness (Martini et al., 2012). One cause of muscle fatigue is thought to be depletion of glycogen and accumulation of lactic acid, resulting in failure of the cycle of muscle contraction and relaxation. During muscle contraction, the excess energy released from ATP is dissipated in the form of heat. During **isometric contraction**, almost all the energy released is in the form of heat; during **isotonic contraction**, some energy is expended in mechanical work. In certain situations (e.g., shivering), the primary stimulus for muscle contraction is the need to generate heat.

The contraction of muscle fibres results in either isotonic or isometric contractions. In isometric contractions, the length of the muscles remains constant but the force generated by the muscles increases; an example of this is pushing against an immovable wall. Isotonic contractions are characterized by shortening of the muscle with no increase in tension within the muscle; an example of this is flexing the forearm. In daily activities, many muscle movements are a combination of isometric and isotonic contractions. For example, during walking, isotonic contraction results in shortening of the leg, and isometric contraction causes the stiff leg to push against the floor. The speed of muscle contraction is variable. Myoglobulin is a hemoglobin-like protein pigment present in striated muscle cells and transports oxygen. Muscles containing large quantities of myoglobulin (red muscles) have been observed to contract slowly and powerfully (e.g., respiratory and postural muscles). Muscles containing little myoglobulin (white muscles) contract quickly (e.g., extraocular eye muscles). Most muscles contain both red and white muscle fibres (Grossman & Porth, 2014).

Muscle Tone

Relaxed muscles demonstrate a state of readiness to respond to contraction stimuli known as residual tension. This state of readiness (muscle **tone [tonus]**) is produced by maintaining some muscle fibres in a contracted state. Muscle spindles, which are sense organs in the muscles, monitor muscle tone. Muscle tone is minimized during sleep and increased when an individual is anxious. A **flaccid** muscle is limp and without tone; a **spastic** muscle has greater-than-expected tone. In conditions characterized by lower motor neuron destruction (e.g., polio), denervated muscle becomes **atonic** (soft and flabby) and atrophies (Grossman & Porth, 2014).

Muscle Actions

Muscles accomplish movement by contraction. Using coordinated muscle groups, the body performs a wide variety of movements.

The prime mover is the muscle (agonist) that causes a particular motion. The muscles assisting the prime mover are known as synergists; those causing movement opposite to that of the prime mover are antagonists (Martini et al., 2012). An antagonist must relax to allow the prime mover to contract, producing motion. For example, when contraction of the biceps causes flexion of the elbow joint, the biceps are the prime movers, and the triceps are the antagonists. A person with muscle paralysis (a loss of movement, possibly from nerve damage) may be able to retrain functioning muscles within the synergistic group to produce the needed movement. Muscles of the synergistic group then become the prime movers (Fig. 69-3).

Exercise, Disuse, and Repair

Muscles need to be exercised to maintain function and strength. When muscle repeatedly reaches maximum or close to maximum tension over a long time (e.g., in regular exercise with weights), the cross-sectional area of the muscle enlarges. This **hypertrophy** results from an increase in the size, but not the number, of individual muscle fibres. Hypertrophy persists only if exercise continues. The opposite phenomenon occurs with disuse of muscle over a long period of time. Age and disuse cause loss of muscular function and fibrotic tissue replaces contractile muscle tissue. Decrease in muscle size is called atrophy. Bed rest and immobility cause loss of muscle mass and strength. When a treatment modality (e.g., casting, traction, or bed rest) results in immobility, the patient can counteract the effects by performing isometric exercise of the muscles of the immobilized part. Quadriceps contraction exercises (tightening the muscles of the anterior thigh) and gluteal setting exercises (tightening of the muscles of the buttocks) help maintain the larger muscle groups important in ambulation. Active and weight-resistance exercises of uninjured parts of the body maintain muscle strength. Injured muscles need rest and immobilization for tissue repair. Healed muscle then requires progressive exercise to resume its strength and function.

Gerontologic Considerations

Multiple changes in the musculoskeletal system occur with aging (Table 69-1).

Height diminishes due to osteoporosis (excessive bone loss), **kyphosis**, thinned intervertebral discs, compressed vertebral bodies, and flexion of the knees and hips. Numerous metabolic changes, including menopausal withdrawal of estrogen, and decreased activity contribute to osteoporosis (Fertleman, Levy, & Meredith, 2018). Women lose more bone mass than men. Bones change shape and have reduced strength. Fractures are common. Collagen structures absorb less energy. Increased inactivity, diminished neuron stimulation, and nutritional deficiencies contribute to reduced muscle strength. Earlier musculoskeletal challenges for which the patient has compensated may become new conditions because of age-related changes. For example, individuals who had polio and have functioned by using synergistic muscle groups may experience increasing incapacity because of a reduced compensatory ability. Fortunately, many effects of aging can be slowed by pursuing positive lifestyle behaviours. Regular exercise improves the quality of life and makes the bones stronger (Martini et al., 2012).

Assessment

Assessment of the patient with musculoskeletal alterations includes evaluation of the effects on the patient and his or her activities of daily living. The nurse assists patients with musculoskeletal concerns to maintain their general health and manage their treatment programs. This includes encouraging optimal nutrition and addressing risks related to immobility. After completing a health history and physical examination, the nurse creates an individualized plan of nursing care to help the patient optimize health.

Health History

Obtain an overall impression of the patient's health status. After collecting identifying data, conduct a symptom/sign analysis of the patient's presenting concern(s). Inquire about the location/radiation, nature (quality) of the symptom, the severity, and its timing (onset, frequency, duration). Ask about the factors that aggravate or alleviate the symptom, and any associated symptoms. Finally, determine if environmental factors are influencing the symptom, the significance to the patient of having the symptom,

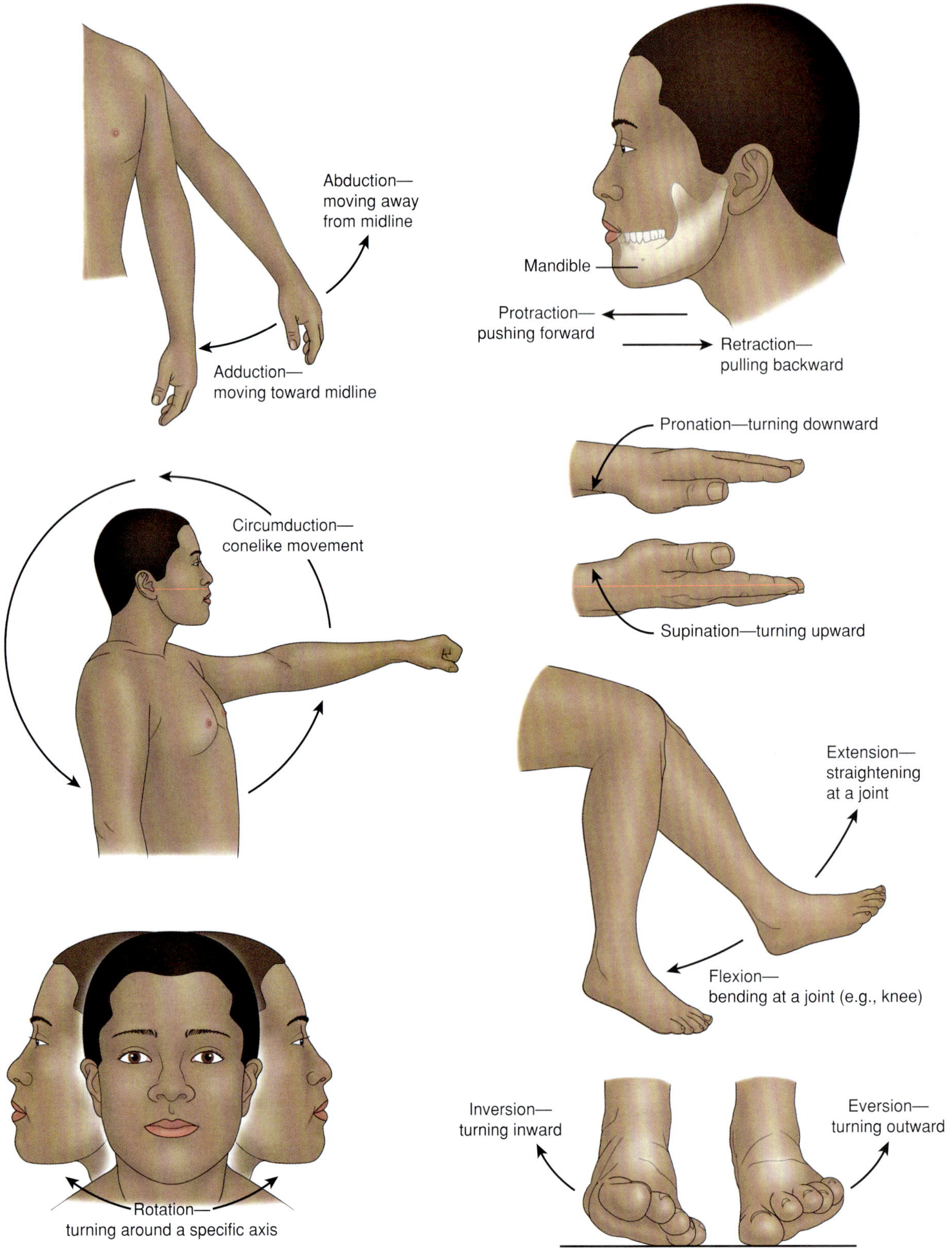

FIGURE 69-3. Body movements produced by muscle contraction.

and what the patient believes is causing the symptom (Stephen, 2012).

List the patient's medications (name, dosage, frequency, purpose, and response) and document any allergies. Inquire about concurrent health conditions (e.g., diabetes, heart disease, chronic obstructive pulmonary disease [COPD], rheumatoid arthritis, infection, disability), past surgeries, and history of genetic or familial disorders (Stephen, 2012) (Chart 69-1).

Explore the patient's expectations related to health, and his or her lifestyle behaviours such as tobacco use, exercise patterns, alcohol consumption, and street and over-the-counter medications. Review dietary habits, including calcium intake and use of a vitamin D supplement

TABLE 69-1 Age-Related Changes of the Musculoskeletal System

Musculoskeletal System	Structural Changes	Functional Changes	History and Physical Findings
Bones	Gradual, progressive loss of bone mass after 30 years of age Vertebrae collapse	Bones fragile and prone to fracture: vertebrae, hip, wrist	Loss of height Posture changes Kyphosis Loss of flexibility Flexion of hips and knees Back pain Osteoporosis Fracture
Muscles	Increase in collagen and resultant fibrosis Muscles diminish in size (atrophy); wasting Tendons less elastic	Loss of strength and flexibility Weakness Fatigue Stumbling Falls	Loss of strength Diminished agility Decreased endurance Prolonged response time (diminished reaction time) Diminished tone Broad base of support History of falls
Joints	Cartilage—progressive deterioration Thinning of intervertebral discs	Stiffness, reduced flexibility, and pain interfere with activities of daily living	Diminished range of motion Stiffness Loss of height
Ligaments	Lax ligaments (less strength; weakness)	Postural joint alteration Weakness	Joint pain on motion; resolves with rest Crepitus Joint swelling/enlargement Osteoarthritis (degenerative joint disease)

(Stephen, 2012). Consider the patient's learning ability, current occupation, and economic status in the preliminary plan of care. Update initial interview data as interactions with the patient continue. Subjective data (detailed information obtained from the patient) always guide the physical examination.

Common Symptoms

Nurses usually perform a focused musculoskeletal assessment if patients report symptoms such as muscle or joint pain, stiffness, joint swelling, weakness, altered sensations, or difficulty with mobility. In the event of a potential dislocation, fracture, or rupture, the nurse conducts an emergency (very focused) assessment. In contrast, when acquiring baseline data, the nurse performs a comprehensive assessment (Stephen, 2012).

Pain

Pain is considered to be the fifth vital sign (Skillen, 2012) (see Chapter 16 for a thorough discussion of pain). Most patients with diseases, traumatic conditions, or disorders of the muscles, bones, and joints experience pain. Characteristically, they describe bone pain as a dull, deep ache, "boring" in nature; they report muscular pain as a soreness, aching, or cramping. Fracture pain is sharp, piercing, and relieved by immobilization; a bone infection, muscle spasm, or pressure on a sensory nerve may also produce sharp pain. Pain may be related to systemic disease. Although pain is subjective, the nurse also may observe signs of pain (e.g., restlessness, legs flexed tightly against buttocks, distressed facial features, irritability) (Urden, Stacy, & Lough, 2017). It is vital that the nurse observe for signs of pain in individuals who are developmentally challenged, verbally stoic, suffering a form of dementia, or unable to communicate in English (and translation is not available). Related signs that the nurse assesses for include alignment of the body; indications of pressure from traction, bed lines, a cast, or other appliances; and signs of tension on the skin at a pin site. Rest, elevation, hot/cold packs, and analgesia relieve most mechanical musculoskeletal pain. Pain that increases with activity may indicate joint sprain, muscle strain, or compartment syndrome. Steadily increasing pain points to an infectious process (osteomyelitis), a malignant tumour, or neurovascular complication. Radiating pain occurs when pressure is exerted on a nerve root. Pain is exhausting and if prolonged, it can make the patient increasingly preoccupied and dependent. See Chapter 16. Questions that the nurse asks during a symptom analysis of pain include:

- Is the body in proper alignment?
- Are the joints symmetrical or are bony deformities present?
- Is there any inflammation or arthritis, swelling, warmth, tenderness, or redness?
- Is there pressure from traction, bed linens, a cast, or other appliances?
- Is there tension on the skin at a pin site?

The patient's pain and discomfort must be managed successfully. Not only is pain exhausting, but also, if prolonged, it can force the patient to become increasingly withdrawn and dependent on others as the musculoskeletal disorder continues.

Stiffness

The symptom of stiffness may be a challenge to assess, as patients report the symptom differently. It can be tightness

GENETICS IN NURSING PRACTICE

Chart 69-1. Musculoskeletal Disorders

When assessing a patient with musculoskeletal concerns, nurses assess for the possibility of a genetic component to the patient's condition(s).

Musculoskeletal Impairments Influenced by Genetic Factors

Autosomal Dominant:
- Achondroplasia
- Nail–patella syndrome
- Osteogenesis imperfecta
- Polydactyly
- van der Woude's syndrome

Autosomal Recessive:
- Tay-Sachs disease

Forms of Muscular Dystrophy:
- Becker's muscular dystrophy
- Congenital muscular dystrophy
- Distal muscular dystrophy
- Duchenne muscular dystrophy (X-linked)
- Emery–Dreifuss muscular dystrophy (X-linked)
- Facioscapulohumeral muscular dystrophy (autosomal dominant)
- Limb–girdle muscular dystrophy (autosomal dominant and autosomal recessive forms)

Other genetic disorders that impact the musculoskeletal system:
- Amyotrophic lateral sclerosis (neurologic disorder)
- Ehlers–Danlos syndrome (connective tissue disorder)
- Marfan's syndrome (connective tissue disorder)
- Spina bifida (neurologic disorder)
- Stickler's syndrome (connective tissue disorder)

Nursing Assessments

FAMILY HISTORY
- Assess for other similarly affected family members.
- Assess for the presence of other related genetic conditions (e.g., hematologic, cardiac, integumentary conditions).
- Determine the age at onset (e.g., fractures present at birth as in osteogenesis imperfecta, hip dislocation present at birth in developmental dysplasia of the hip, or early-onset osteoporosis).

PATIENT ASSESSMENT
- Assess stature for general screening purposes (unusually short stature may be related to achondroplasia; unusually tall stature may be related to Marfan's syndrome).
- Assess for disease-specific skeletal findings (e.g., pectus excavatum, **scoliosis**, long fingers [Marfan's syndrome], osteoarthritis of the hip, waddling gait [DDH]).
- Assess for disease-specific skin findings (e.g., velvety texture with unusual scarring and/or thin fragile skin [Ehlers–Danlos syndrome]).
- Assess for other common disease-specific findings (e.g., vision impairment [Stickler's syndrome, Marfan's syndrome], blue/grey sclerae, opalescent dentin, hearing impairment [osteogenesis imperfecta]).

Management Issues Specific to Genetics
- Inquire whether DNA gene mutation or other genetic testing has been performed on affected family members.
- If indicated, refer patient for further genetic counselling and evaluation so that family members can discuss gene inheritance, risk to other family members, and the availability of genetic testing and gene-based interventions.
- Offer appropriate genetic information and resources.
- Assess patient's understanding of genetic information.
- Provide support and information to families with newly diagnosed genetic-related musculoskeletal disorders.
- Participate in management and coordination of care of patients with genetic conditions and people predisposed to develop or pass on a genetic condition.

Genetics Resources

Canadian Association of Genetic Counsellors (CAGC), http://cagc-accg.ca—Listing of genetic centres across Canada

Canadian Directory of Genetic Support Groups, https://www.lhsc.on.ca/canadian-directory-of-genetic-support-groups/introduction-to-the-directory—Resource guide for families and professionals

Canadian Genetic Diseases Network, http://www.cihr-irsc.gc.ca/e/51277.html—Its stated mission is to be the primary catalyst in advancing Canada's scientific and commercial competitiveness in genetic research and the application of genetic discoveries to the prevention, diagnosis, and treatment of human disease

Canadian Organization for Rare Disorders (CORD), http://www.cord.ca—Information on over 6,000 rare disorders and links individuals/families together with the same rare disorder

Genetics Society of Canada (GSC), http://life.biology.mcmaster.ca/GSC/news.html—Promotion of research and communication of the results and implications of genetics to the public

Genetic Alliance, http://www.geneticalliance.org—Directory of support groups for patients and families with genetic conditions

Gene Clinics, https://www.ncbi.nlm.nih.gov/pubmed/11968082—Listing of common genetic disorders with up-to-date clinical summaries, genetic counselling, and testing information

National Organization for Rare Disorders, http://www.rarediseases.org—Directory of support groups and information for patients and families with rare genetic disorders

OMIM: Online Mendelian Inheritance in Man, https://www.ncbi.nlm.nih.gov/omim—Complete listing of inherited genetic conditions

and discomfort with movement after a period of inactivity—a common description. In contrast, it has been described as "my legs are poisoned" and still refers to the same discomfort. If the stiffness lasts less than 30 minutes after arising in the morning, it is often associated with osteoarthritis, which can be monoarticular, aggravated by activity, and relieved by rest. If stiffness persists more than an hour and occurs regularly for at least 6 weeks, it is associated with rheumatoid arthritis, especially if polyarticular and symmetric in nature. Stiffness may also be one of the symptoms of fibromyalgia or another condition, polymyalgia rheumatica, that presents in older adults, usually over 60 years of age (Partington, Helliwell, Muller, et al., 2018). Careful and sensitive questioning during the health history interview is required. A comprehensive symptom analysis is essential.

Joint Swelling

Nonarticular swelling may be associated with constrictive clothing, lymphedema, trauma, or cardiac conditions. When the swelling is in a joint, it restricts the motion of the joint. If ligaments are torn (e.g., collateral or cruciate ligaments of the knee), the swelling subsides slowly and responds to elevation and cold applications. If swelling is associated with redness and pain, it may be related to a gout syndrome that results from elevated serum uric acid levels and is aggravated by purine-rich foods (e.g., liver, sardines) and alcohol. A serious infection, osteomyelitis, may display evidence of redness, swelling, and loss of movement. It requires blood and bone cultures to determine the causative organism; it may be difficult to treat (Grossman & Porth, 2014).

Weakness

Weakness in proximal muscles is often a myopathy; weakness in distal muscle groups is more likely related to neuropathy. See Chapter 63 for a discussion of neurologic disorders. Chronic use of corticosteroids tends to cause myopathies and muscle weakness. A reversible condition, hypothyroidism, can cause muscle weakness. Conversely, a progressive disease, amyotrophic lateral sclerosis (ALS), is irreversible. If muscle weakness fluctuates, it may be related to myasthenia gravis, a gradually progressive disorder with fatigue. A mild paralysis may be observed in multiple sclerosis. Weakness can lead to gait disturbances, the risk of falls, and difficulty with some aspects of self-care.

Altered Sensations

Sensory disturbances are frequently associated with musculoskeletal conditions. The patient may describe **paresthesias** (burning, tingling, numbness). These sensations may be caused by pressure on nerves or by circulatory impairment. Soft tissue swelling or direct trauma to these structures can impair their function (e.g., compartment syndrome). In addition to the questions of a symptom/sign analysis (Stephen, 2012), always assess the neurovascular status of the involved musculoskeletal area (see Chapter 63). Ask the patient to compare the sensation in the unaffected extremity and inquire about tight or constricting clothing or footwear. Determine if elevation of the affected part affects the symptom. Inspect the affected area and the area distal to it for colour (e.g., pallor, cyanosis, duskiness), and swelling. Palpate for peripheral pulses and pitting edema and compare sides. Assess capillary refill by pressing on the nail until it blanches, releasing it quickly, and observing for return of colour within 3 seconds.

Past Health, Social, and Family History

When assessing the musculoskeletal system, the nurse should gather pertinent data to include in the patient's health history, such as occupation (e.g., does the patient's work require physical activity or heavy lifting?), exercise patterns, alcohol consumption, tobacco use, and dietary intake (e.g., calcium and vitamin D). Concurrent health conditions (e.g., diabetes, heart disease, COPD, infection, pre-existing disability) and related problems (e.g., familial or genetic abnormalities [see Chart 69-1]) need to be considered when developing and implementing the plan of care. Any previous history of trauma or injury to the musculoskeletal system or a history of falls should be included as well (Weber & Kelley, 2014).

The Fracture Risk Assessment Tool

The Fracture Risk Assessment Tool (FRAX®) was developed in 2008 by a task force convened by the World Health Organization (WHO). It is a tool that predicts a patient's 10-year risk of fracturing a hip or other major bone, which includes the spine, forearm, or shoulder (National Osteoporosis Foundation [NOF], 2014). The tool may be accessed online, where it automatically calculates a patient's odds of fracture. Data entered are validated risks for fracture, and include:

- age (risk increases with increasing age)
- gender (risk is higher in females)
- body mass index (risk is higher with lower body mass indices)
- history of a previous fracture
- parental history of hip fracture
- current cigarette smoker
- current use of a corticosteroid (e.g., prednisone)
- history of rheumatoid arthritis
- alcohol intake of three or more drinks per day
- history of secondary causes/risks for osteoporosis, which include any of the following:
  - type I diabetes
  - osteogenesis imperfecta
  - untreated long-standing hyperthyroidism
  - hypogonadism or premature menopause
  - chronic malnutrition or malabsorption syndrome
  - chronic liver disease

An additional validated risk factor that may be entered into the FRAX® is the patient's bone mineral density (BMD), based on bone densitometry results, if those results are hip based (see later discussion). However, while entering BMD results in the FRAX® provides a more accurate fracture risk calculation, it is not necessary (American College of Rheumatology, 2016). Thus, the FRAX® provides a good estimate of fracture risk in patients who may not have submitted to BMD testing. Patients who should be assessed for hip or major bone fracture risk include men and postmenopausal women over the age of 50, patients with known low BMD, and patients with known secondary causes/risks for osteoporosis.

Physical Assessment

Examination of the musculoskeletal system ranges from a basic assessment of functional capabilities to sophisticated physical examination manoeuvres that facilitate diagnosis of specific bone, muscle, and joint disorders. The extent of assessment depends on the patient's physical concerns, health history, and physical clues that warrant further exploration. Nursing assessment is primarily a functional evaluation, focusing on the patient's ability to perform activities of daily living, manage treatment regimens, and progress to recovery, but it also considers potential risks, and observations to share with the interprofessional team.

Use inspection and palpation to evaluate the patient's posture, gait, balance, bone integrity, range of motion (joint function), and muscle strength and size. In addition, assess the integument (skin, hair, nails) and neurovascular status as they are important parts of a complete musculoskeletal assessment (Stephen, Skillen, & Day, 2013–2014). Understand and be able to perform correct assessment techniques on patients with musculoskeletal trauma. When specific symptoms or physical findings of musculoskeletal dysfunction are apparent, carefully document the examination findings and share the information with the physician or nurse practitioner who may decide that a more extensive examination and a diagnostic workup are necessary.

Posture

The vertebral column (spine) supports the trunk and back, transfers upper body weight to the pelvis and legs, and cushions the effects of movements such as walking or running (Grossman & Porth, 2014). It has concave curvatures in its cervical and lumbar sections, and convex curvatures in the thoracic and sacrococcygeal sections. Common deformities of the spine include kyphosis, an increased convex curvature of the thoracic spine; **lordosis** (swayback), an exaggerated concave curvature of the lumbar spine; and scoliosis, a lateral curvature of the spine (Fig. 69-4).

Kyphosis is common in older patients with osteoporosis and in some patients with neuromuscular diseases. Lordosis is frequently seen during pregnancy as a woman adjusts her posture in response to changes in her centre of gravity. Scoliosis may be congenital, functional, idiopathic (without an identifiable cause), or the result of damage to the paraspinal muscles, as in polio.

During inspection of the spine, expose the entire back, buttocks, and legs. Inspect the spinal curvatures and trunk symmetry from posterior and lateral views. Standing behind the patient, note any differences in the height of the shoulders, scapulae, iliac crests, posterior superior iliac spines, or gluteal folds (Stephen et al., 2013–2014). Shoulder and hip symmetry, as well as alignment of the vertebral column, are usually inspected with the patient erect, and flexed forward. Scoliosis is evidenced by a lateral curvature of the spine, shoulders that are not level, an asymmetric waistline, and one prominent scapula, accentuated by bending forward. Due to older adults' experience of a loss in height from reduced water content in discs between vertebrae and osteoporosis-related vertebral compression fractures, measure the adults' height annually during health screenings (Osteoporosis Canada, 2014b).

Gait

Inspect gait by having the patient walk away for a short distance. Observe for a smooth, rhythmic gait. Unsteadiness or irregular movements (frequently noted in older patients) are not expected. Limping is most frequently caused by painful weight bearing. In such instances, the patient can usually pinpoint the area of discomfort, thus guiding further examination. If one extremity is shorter than another, a limp may be created as the patient's pelvis drops downward on the affected side with each step. Limited joint motion may affect gait and a knee may be implicated. Evaluate the knee (joints, bones, ligaments, tendons, and cartilage), and consider tests of the anterior and posterior cruciate ligaments, medial and lateral collateral ligaments, and medial and lateral menisci. A variety

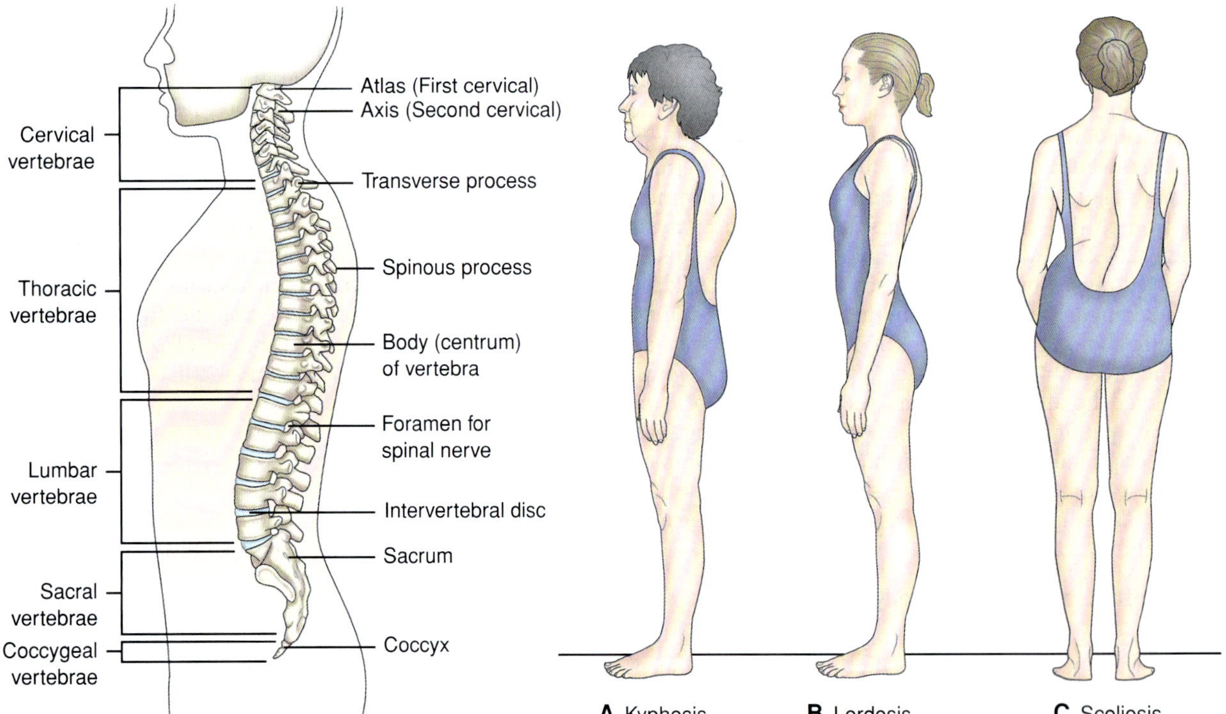

FIGURE 69-4. A normal spine and three abnormalities. **A.** Kyphosis: an increased convexity of the spine's thoracic curvature. **B.** Lordosis: exaggeration of the lumbar spine concave curvature. **C.** Scoliosis: a lateral curvature of the spine.

of neurologic conditions affect gait, such as stroke (spastic hemiparesis gait), lower motor neuron disease (steppage gait), and Parkinson's disease (shuffling gait).

Bone Integrity

The bony skeleton is assessed for deformities and alignment. Symmetric parts of the body, such as extremities, are compared. Abnormal bony growths due to bone tumours may be observed. Shortened extremities, amputations, and body parts that are not in anatomic alignment are noted. Fracture findings may include abnormal angulation of long bones, motion at points other than joints, and **crepitus** (a grating or crackling sound or sensation) at the point of abnormal motion. Movement of fracture fragments must be minimized to avoid additional injury. The nurse should include the following observations (Weber & Kelley, 2014):

- If the affected part is an extremity, how does its overall appearance compare to the unaffected extremity?
- Can the patient move the affected part? If an extremity is involved, does each toe or finger have normal sensation and motion (flexion and extension), and is the skin warm or cool?
- What is the colour of the part distal to the affected area? Is it pale? Dusky? Mottled? Cyanotic?
- Does rapid capillary refill occur? (The nurse can gently squeeze a nail until it blanches, then release the pressure. The amount of time for the colour under the nail to return to normal is noted. Colour normally returns within 3 seconds. The return of colour is evidence of capillary refill.)
- Is a pulse distal to the affected area palpable? If the affected area is an extremity, how does the pulse compare to the pulse of the unaffected extremity?
- Is edema present?
- Is any constrictive device or clothing causing nerve or vascular compression?
- Does elevating the affected part or modifying its position affect the symptoms?

Integument

Before focusing further on the musculoskeletal system, inspect the skin, hair, and nails of the upper and lower extremities. Compare sides and inspect for colour and edema. Palpate for warmer or cooler temperatures, comparing distal to proximal sites as well as sides. It is important to detect increased or decreased tissue perfusion. Cuts, bruises, skin colour, hair loss, decreased circulation, inflammation, and swelling can influence nursing assessment and management of musculoskeletal conditions.

Joint Function

Inspect the articular system by noting range of motion, deformity, stability, and nodular formation. Range of motion is evaluated both actively (the joint is moved by the patient using the muscles surrounding the joint) and passively (the relaxed joint is moved by the nurse). Be familiar with the expected range of motion of major joints (see Chapter 56). Precise measurement of range of motion can be made using a goniometer (a protractor designed for evaluating the degree of joint motion). Limited range of motion may be the result of skeletal deformity, joint pathology, or **contracture** (shortening) of the surrounding muscles, tendons, and joint capsule. In older patients, limited range of motion associated with osteoarthritis may reduce their ability to perform activities of daily living.

If joint motion is compromised or the joint is painful, palpate the joint for **effusion** (excessive fluid within the capsule), swelling, and increased temperature that may reflect active inflammation. An effusion is suspected if the joint is swollen and bony landmarks are obscured. The most common site for joint effusion is the knee. Use the balloon sign and ballottement of the patella (Fig. 69-5) to identify large amounts of fluid in the joint spaces beneath the patella.

Consult with a physician or nurse practitioner if inflammation or fluid is suspected in a joint.

Joint deformity may be caused by contracture, dislocation (complete separation of joint surfaces), subluxation (partial separation of articular surfaces), or disruption of structures surrounding the joint. Weakness or disruption of joint-supporting structures may result in a weak joint that requires an external supporting appliance (e.g., brace).

Palpation of the joint during passive motion provides information about the integrity of the joint. Usually, the joint moves smoothly. A snap or crack may indicate that a ligament is slipping over a bony prominence. Slightly roughened surfaces, as in arthritic conditions, result in crepitus (grating, crackling sounds or sensation) as the irregular joint surfaces move across one another.

Inspect and palpate the tissues surrounding the joints for nodule formation. Rheumatoid arthritis, gout, and osteoarthritis may produce characteristic nodules. The subcutaneous nodules of rheumatoid arthritis are soft; they occur within and along tendons that provide extensor function to the joints. The nodules related to gout are hard, lying within and immediately adjacent to the joint capsule itself. They may rupture, exuding white uric acid crystals onto the skin surface. Osteoarthritic nodules are also hard, but they represent bony overgrowth that has resulted from destruction of the cartilaginous surface of bone within the joint capsule. While actively forming, they may be painful to palpation. Heberden's nodes are palpated medially and laterally at the distal interphalangeal joints of the hand; Bouchard's nodes are located at the proximal interphalangeal joints. Both are common in older adults (Grossman & Porth, 2014).

Often, the size of the joint is exaggerated by atrophy of the muscles proximal and distal to that joint. This is seen in rheumatoid arthritis of the knees, in which the quadriceps muscle may atrophy dramatically. In rheumatoid arthritis, joint involvement assumes a symmetric pattern (Fig. 69-6) (see Chapter 56 for further information about rheumatoid arthritis).

Muscle Strength and Size

Inspect the size (bulk) of individual muscles, the patient's ability and method for changing position, and coordination of the upper and lower extremities. Compare bilaterally. Various conditions may cause weakness to a group of muscles, such as polyneuropathy, electrolyte disturbances (particularly potassium and calcium), myasthenia gravis, poliomyelitis, and muscular dystrophy. Palpate for muscle tone (residual tension) by moving the relaxed extremity through passive range of motion. After assessing muscle

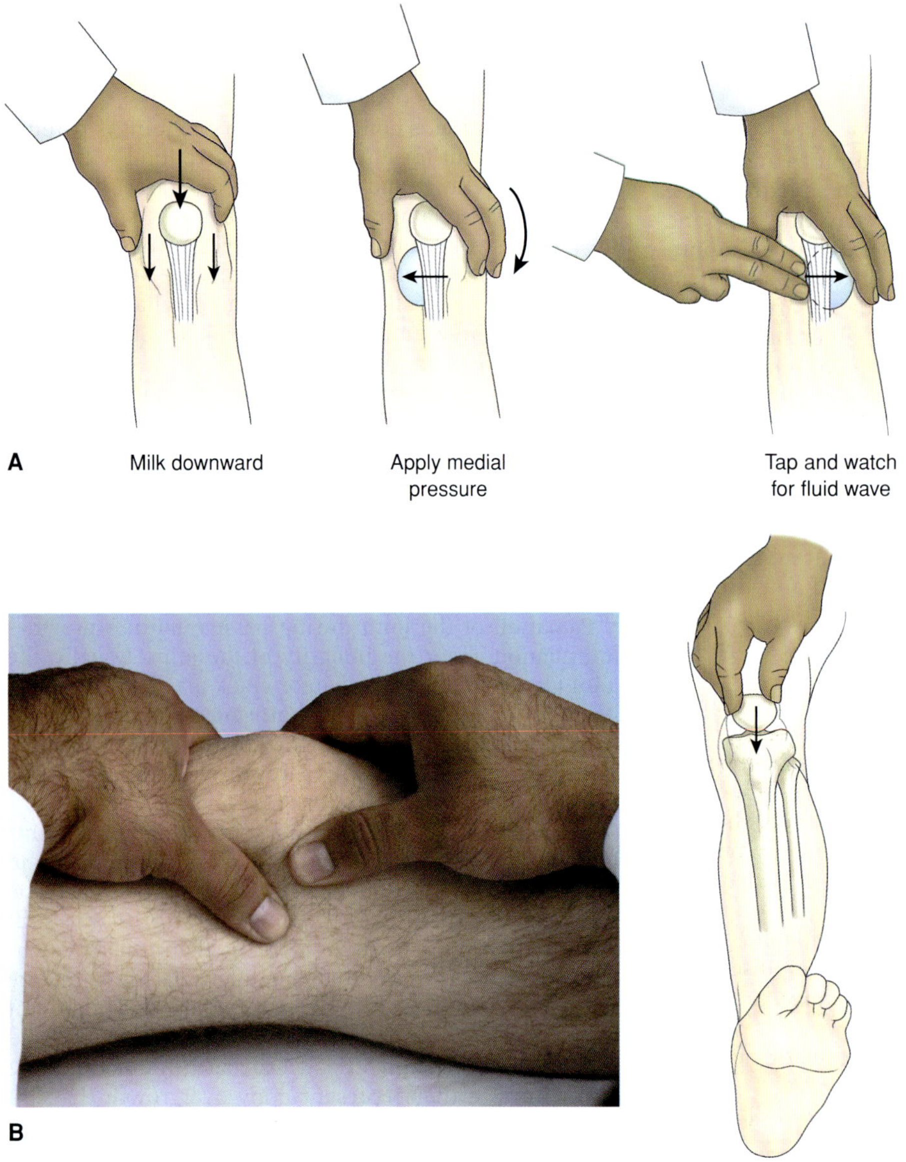

FIGURE 69-5. Tests for detecting fluid in the knee. **A.** Technique for balloon sign. The medial and lateral aspects of the extended knee are milked firmly in a downward motion, which displaces any fluid downward. The examiner feels for any fluid entering the space directly inferior to the patella. When larger amounts of fluid are present, the subpatellar region feels as if it is "ballooning," and the balloon sign test is positive. **B.** Technique for ballottement sign. The medial and lateral aspects of the extended knee are milked firmly in a downward motion. The examiner pushes the patella toward the femur and observes for fluid return to the region superior to the patella. When larger amounts of fluid are present, the patella elevates, there is visible return of fluid to the region directly superior to the patella, and the ballottement test is positive. (Photograph used with permission from Bickley, L. S. [2017]. *Bates' guide to physical examination and history taking* [12th ed.]. Philadelphia, PA: Lippincott Williams & Wilkins.)

tone, evaluate muscle strength by having the patient perform certain manoeuvres with and without your resistance. For example, when testing the biceps, ask the patient to extend the arm fully and then to flex it against your resistance. A simple handshake may provide an indication of grasp strength. Grade muscle strength using a 0 to 5 point scale (0 = no detectable contraction, 5 = complete range of motion against gravity and full resistance) (Bickley, 2017).

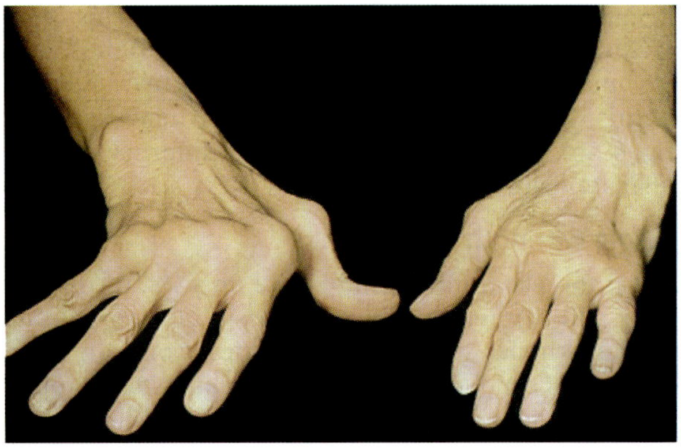

FIGURE 69-6. Rheumatoid arthritis joint deformity with ulnar deviation of fingers and "swan-neck" deformity of fingers (i.e., hyperextension of proximal interphalangeal joints with flexion of distal interphalangeal joints).

Be alert to muscle **clonus** (rhythmic contractions of a muscle) in the ankle or wrist associated with sudden, forceful, sustained dorsiflexion of the foot or extension of the wrist. Observe for **fasciculation** (involuntary twitching of muscle fibre groups).

Measure the girth of an extremity to monitor increased size due to exercise, edema, bleeding into the muscle, or decreased size because of atrophy. Measure the unaffected extremity as the reference standard for the affected extremity. Take measurements at the same (corresponding) location on each extremity, and with the extremity in the same position, with the muscle at rest. Document the distance from a specific anatomic landmark (e.g., 10 cm below the inferior border of the patella for measurement of the calf muscle) in the patient's health record so that subsequent measurements can be made at the same point. For ease of serial assessment, mark the skin at the point

CHART 69-2

Indicators of Peripheral Neurovascular Dysfunction

Circulation

Colour: Pale, cyanotic, or mottled
Temperature: Cool
Capillary refill: More than 3 seconds

Motion

Weakness
Paralysis

Sensation

Paresthesia
Unrelenting pain
Pain on passive stretch
Absence of feeling

of measurement. Consider variations in size greater than 1 cm to be significant.

Neurovascular Status

Assessment of neurovascular status (Chart 69-2) is frequently referred to as assessment of circulation, motion, and sensation (CMS).

Perform frequent neurovascular assessments of patients with musculoskeletal disorders (especially those with fractures) because of the risk for tissue and nerve damage. Chart 69-3 describes tests of peripheral nerve function.

Be especially alert to compartment syndrome, a complication described in detail later in this unit. This serious neurovascular condition is caused by pressure within a muscle compartment that increases to such an extent that microcirculation diminishes, leading to nerve and muscle anoxia, and necrosis. Function can be permanently lost if the anoxic situation continues for longer than 6 hours (Grossman & Porth, 2014).

CHART 69-3

Assessment: Assessing for Peripheral Nerve Function

Assessment of peripheral nerve function has two key elements: evaluation of sensation and evaluation of motion. Perform one or all of the following during a musculoskeletal assessment. Use a splintered tongue blade for the prick.

Nerve	Test of Sensation	Test of Movement
Peroneal nerve	Prick the skin midway between the great and second toes. 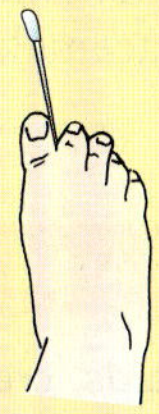	Ask the patient to dorsiflex the foot and extend the toes. 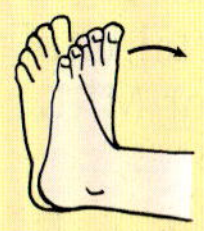
Tibial nerve	Prick the medial and lateral surface of the sole. 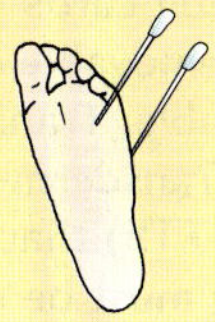	Ask the patient to plantar flex toes and foot. 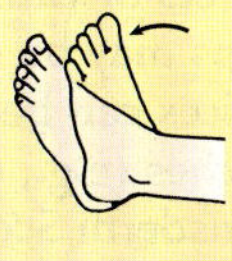
Radial nerve	Prick the skin midway between the thumb and the second finger. 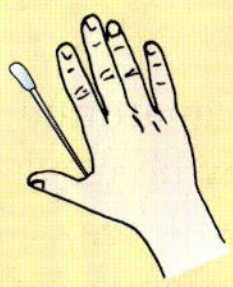	Ask the patient to stretch out the thumb, then the wrist, and then the fingers at the metacarpal joints. 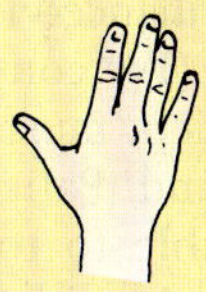
Ulnar nerve	Prick the distal fat pad of the little finger. 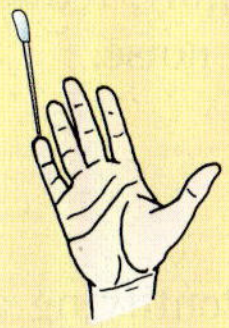	Ask the patient to abduct all fingers. 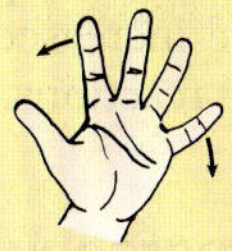
Median nerve	Prick the top or distal surface of the index finger. 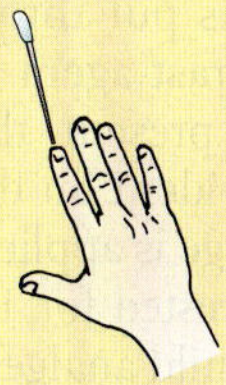	Ask the patient to touch the thumb to the little finger. Also observe whether the patient can flex the wrist. 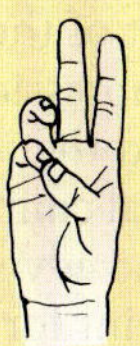

Diagnostic Evaluation

X-Ray Studies

X-ray studies are important for evaluating patients with musculoskeletal disorders. Bone x-rays determine bone density, texture, erosion, and changes in bone relationships. X-ray study of the cortex of the bone reveals any widening, narrowing, or signs of irregularity. Joint x-rays reveal fluid, irregularity, spur formation, narrowing, and changes in the joint structure. Multiple x-rays, with multiple views (e.g., anterior–posterior, lateral, oblique), are needed for full assessment of the structure being examined. Serial x-rays may be indicated to determine the status of the healing process. After being positioned for the study, the patient must remain still while the x-rays are obtained.

Computed Tomography

A computed tomography (CT) scan, which may be performed with or without the use of contrast agents, shows in detail a specific plane of involved bone and can reveal tumours of soft tissue or injuries to ligaments or tendons. It is used to identify the location and extent of fractures in areas that are difficult to evaluate (e.g., acetabulum). The patient must remain still during the procedure.

Magnetic Resonance Imaging

Magnetic resonance imaging (MRI) is a noninvasive imaging technique that uses magnetic fields, radio waves, and computers to demonstrate alterations (i.e., tumours or narrowing of tissue pathways through bone) of soft tissues such as muscle, tendon, cartilage, nerve, and fat. Because an electromagnet is used, patients with any metal implants, clips, or pacemakers are not candidates for MRI.

NURSING ALERT

Jewellery, hair clips, hearing aids, credit cards with magnetic strips, and other metal-containing objects must be removed before the MRI is performed because they can become dangerous projectile objects or cause burns. Credit cards with magnetic strips may be erased; nonremovable cochlear devices can become inoperable. Transdermal patches (e.g., NicoDerm, Transderm-Nitro, Transderm Scop, Catapres-TTS) that have a thin layer of aluminized backing must be removed because they also can cause burns. Notify the physician or nurse practitioner before the patches are removed.

To enhance visualization of anatomic structures, intravenous (IV) contrast agent may be used. During the MRI, the patient must lie still and will hear a rhythmic knocking sound. Patients who experience claustrophobia may be unable to tolerate the confinement of closed MRI equipment without sedation. Open MRI systems are available, but they use lower-intensity magnetic fields, which produce lower-quality images. Advantages of open MRI include increased patient comfort, reduction of claustrophobic reactions, and reduced noise.

Arthrography

Arthrography is useful for identifying acute or chronic tears of the joint capsule or supporting ligaments of the knee, shoulder, ankle, hip, or wrist. A radiopaque contrast agent or air is injected into the joint cavity to visualize irregular surfaces. The joint is put through its range of motion to distribute the contrast agent while a series of x-rays is obtained. If a tear is present, the contrast agent leaks out of the joint and is evident on the x-ray image.

A compression elastic bandage is applied after an arthrogram and the joint is usually rested for 12 hours. Provide additional comfort measures (mild analgesia, ice) as appropriate and advise the patient to expect clicking or crackling in the joint for a day or two after the procedure, until the contrast agent or air is absorbed.

Bone Densitometry

Bone densitometry is used to estimate BMD. This can be performed using x-rays or ultrasound. The most common modalities include dual-energy x-ray absorptiometry (DXA or DEXA), quantitative computed tomography (QCT), and quantitative ultrasound (QUS). Measures of the hip and spine using DXA BMD are very accurate for estimating the extent of osteoporosis and monitoring a patient's response to treatment for osteoporosis. Peripheral DXA (pDXA) is an alternative test that measures BMD of the forearm, finger, or heel, but its ability to project hip or spine fracture risk is less accurate than DXA. While the BMD of the heel can be used to diagnose and monitor osteoporosis, predicting hip fracture risk related to osteoporosis is best achieved through DXA of the hip and is the most commonly prescribed diagnostic test for determining BMD (Insight Medical Imaging, 2014). Men and women 65 years and over need to have the BMD test which is accurate, painless, and safe (Osteoporosis Canada, 2014c) (see Chapter 71 for a further discussion of osteoporosis risks).

Nursing Interventions

Before the patient undergoes any of the imaging studies described previously (i.e., x-rays, CT scans, MRIs, arthrography, bone densitometry), the nurse prepares the patient. For these studies, the patient must lie still. During an MRI study, the patient may hear a knocking sound. In addition, the nurse assesses for conditions that may require special consideration during the study or that may be contraindications to the study (e.g., pregnancy; claustrophobia; inability to tolerate required positioning due to age, debility, or disability; metal implants). If contrast agents will be used for the CT scan, MRI, or arthrography, the patient is assessed for possible allergies (Van Leeuwen & Bladh, 2016).

The patient having an arthrogram may feel some discomfort or tingling during the procedure. After the arthrogram, a compression elastic bandage may be applied if prescribed, and the joint is usually rested for 12 hours. Strenuous activity should be avoided until approved by the primary provider. The nurse provides additional comfort measures (e.g., mild analgesia, ice) as appropriate and explains to the patient that it is normal to experience clicking or crackling in the joint for 24 to 48 hours after the procedure until the contrast agent or air is absorbed.

Bone Scan

A bone scan is performed to detect metastatic and primary bone tumours, osteomyelitis, some fractures (e.g., not visible with traditional x-rays), and aseptic necrosis. Two to three hours after a bone-seeking radioisotope is injected intravenously, the scan is performed. Distribution and concentration of the isotope (radionuclide) in the bone are measured. The degree of nuclide uptake is related to the metabolism of the bone. An increased uptake is observed in primary skeletal disease (osteosarcoma), metastatic bone disease, inflammatory skeletal disease (osteomyelitis), and fractures that do not heal as expected.

Nursing Interventions

Inquire about possible allergies to the radioisotope before the patient undergoes a bone scan. Assess for any condition that would contraindicate performing the procedure (e.g., pregnancy). Before the scan, ask the patient to empty the bladder, because a full bladder interferes with accurate scanning of the pelvic bones. Afterward, encourage the patient to drink plenty of fluids to help distribute and eliminate the isotope.

Arthroscopy

Arthroscopy is a procedure that allows direct visualization of a joint to diagnose joint disorders. Treatment of tears, defects, and disease processes may be performed through the arthroscope. The procedure occurs in the operating room under sterile conditions; a local anesthetic agent is injected into the joint or general anesthesia is used. A large-bore needle is inserted, and the joint is distended with saline. The arthroscope is introduced to visualize joint structures, synovium, and articular surfaces. After the procedure, the puncture wound is closed with sterile adhesive strips or sutures and covered with a sterile dressing. Complications are rare, but may include infection, hemarthrosis, neurovascular compromise, thrombophlebitis, stiffness, effusion, adhesions, and delayed wound healing.

Nursing Interventions

At the end of the arthroscopic procedure, the joint is wrapped with a compression dressing to control swelling. Apply ice if prescribed to control edema and enhance comfort. Frequently, the joint is kept extended and elevated to reduce swelling. Monitor and document the neurovascular status. Administer analgesic agents as needed. Teach the patient about activities and exercises that may be performed. Inform the patient and family regarding the symptoms (e.g., swelling, numbness, cool skin) of complications and the importance of notifying the physician or nurse practitioner if experiencing any of these symptoms.

Arthrocentesis

Arthrocentesis (joint aspiration) is carried out to obtain synovial fluid for purposes of examination or relief of pain due to effusion. Examination of synovial fluid is helpful in the diagnosis of septic arthritis and other inflammatory arthropathies and reveals the presence of hemarthrosis (bleeding into the joint cavity), which suggests trauma or a bleeding disorder. Usually, synovial fluid is clear, pale, straw coloured, and scant in volume. Using aseptic technique, the physician inserts a needle into the joint and aspirates fluid. Anti-inflammatory medications may be injected into the joint. A sterile dressing is applied after aspiration to reduce the risk of infection.

Nursing Interventions

After the arthroscopic procedure, the joint is wrapped with a compression dressing to control swelling. In addition, ice may be applied to control edema and enhance comfort. Frequently, the joint is kept extended and elevated to reduce swelling. The nurse monitors and documents the neurovascular status (see Chart 69-2). Analgesic agents are given as needed. The patient is instructed to avoid strenuous activity of the joint, and exercises must be approved by the primary provider. The patient and family are instructed to monitor for signs and symptoms of complications (e.g., fever, excessive bleeding, swelling, numbness, cool skin) and the importance of notifying the primary provider should any of these occur (Van Leeuwen & Bladh, 2016).

Electromyography

Electromyography (EMG) provides information about the electrical potential of the muscles and the nerves innervating them. The test is performed to evaluate muscle weakness, pain, and disability. The purpose of the procedure is to determine any alteration of function and differentiate muscle and nerve disorders. Needle electrodes are inserted into selected muscles, and responses to electrical stimuli are recorded on an oscilloscope. Warm compresses may relieve residual discomfort after the study.

Nursing Interventions

Before the patient undergoes an EMG, the nurse inquires if the patient is taking any anticoagulant medications and assesses for any active skin infection. An EMG is usually contraindicated in patients receiving anticoagulant therapy (e.g., warfarin) because the needle electrodes may cause bleeding within the muscle. EMG also may be contraindicated in patients with extensive skin infections due to the risk of spreading infection from the skin to the muscle. The nurse instructs the patient to avoid using any lotions or creams on the day of the test (Van Leeuwen & Bladh, 2016). If the nurse finds that the patient is taking an anticoagulant or has a skin infection, the primary provider is notified.

Biopsy

To aid with diagnosis, a biopsy may be performed to determine the structure and composition of bone marrow, bone, muscle, or synovium. Teach the patient about the procedure and assure the patient that analgesic agents will be provided. Monitor the biopsy site for edema, bleeding, pain, and infection. Apply ice as prescribed to control bleeding and edema and administer prescribed analgesic agents for comfort.

Nursing Interventions

The nurse educates the patient about the procedure and assures the patient that analgesic agents will be provided. The nurse monitors the biopsy site for edema, bleeding, pain, hematoma formation, and infection. Ice is applied as prescribed to control bleeding and edema. In addition, antibiotics and analgesic agents are given as prescribed. The patient is instructed to report signs of redness, bleeding, or pain at the biopsy site as well as fever or chills to the primary provider (Van Leeuwen & Bladh, 2016).

Laboratory Studies

Examination of the patient's blood and urine can provide information about a primary musculoskeletal problem (e.g., Paget's disease of the bone), a developing complication (e.g., infection), the baseline for instituting therapy (e.g., anticoagulant therapy), or the response to therapy. Before surgery, coagulation studies are performed to detect bleeding tendencies because bone is vascular tissue.

Serum calcium levels are altered in patients with osteomalacia, parathyroid dysfunction, Paget's disease, metastatic bone tumours, or prolonged immobilization. Serum phosphorus levels are inversely related to calcium levels and are diminished in osteomalacia associated with malabsorption syndrome. Acid phosphatase is elevated in Paget's disease and metastatic cancer. Alkaline phosphatase (ALP) is elevated during early fracture healing and in diseases with increased osteoblastic activity (e.g., metastatic bone tumours) (HealthLink BC, 2012a). Bone metabolism may be evaluated using thyroid studies and determination of calcitonin, PTH, and vitamin D levels. Serum enzyme levels of creatine kinase and aspartate aminotransferase become elevated with muscle damage. Serum osteocalcin (bone GLA protein) indicates the rate of bone turnover. Urine calcium levels increase with bone destruction (e.g., parathyroid dysfunction, metastatic bone tumours, multiple myeloma) (HealthLink BC, 2012b). Specific urine and serum biochemical markers can be used to provide information about bone formation. These include urinary *N*-telopeptide of type 1 collagen (N-Tx) and deoxypyridinoline (Dpd), both of which reflect increased osteoclast activity and increased bone resorption. Conversely, elevated serum levels of bone-specific ALP, osteocalcin, and intact *N*-terminal propeptide of type 1 collagen (P1NP) reflect increased activity of osteoblasts and enhanced bone-remodelling activity (Coates, 2013).

Critical Thinking Exercises

1 You are a nurse working in a primary care office. You assess a 79-year-old man who complains of back pain for the past "month or so." The patient reports that the pain has been increasing and is no longer relieved with ibuprofen (Motrin). Vital signs are within normal limits. The patient weighs 118 lb, and you note that he is 2 in shorter than he was 5 years ago. What additional assessment information would you want to obtain from this patient? What appropriate diagnostic tests would you anticipate for this patient? What is your priority nursing diagnosis and plan of care for this patient? What musculoskeletal disorder is this patient at risk for?

2 You are a nurse working in the Emergency Department (ED) and caring for a 75-year-old woman who arrived via ambulance after falling at home. She tells you she slipped on a rug and hurt her wrist trying to brace herself from the fall. You notice an obvious deformity of her right wrist. Her current weight is 90 lb; she admits to smoking a half a pack of cigarettes a day for the past 45 years, and drinks one alcoholic drink a day. She has a medical history of COPD and hypertension. X-ray confirms a fractured right distal radius. What other health concerns should be evaluated for this patient? What is the evidence base that supports strategies for educating and planning care for this patient? In particular, what strategies can be implemented in order to educate this patient about fall prevention and maximize her musculoskeletal health? What is the strength of the evidence of the effectiveness of these strategies?

3 You are a nurse working at an assisted living facility. You are developing an educational program regarding bone health and aging. What are the current evidence-based recommendations to maintain bone health? What is the level of evidence that supports each of the recommendations and strategies for reducing musculoskeletal risk for the aging adult?

REFERENCES AND SELECTED READINGS

Books

Bickley, L. S. (2017). *Bates' guide to physical examination and history taking* (12th ed.). Philadelphia, PA: Lippincott Williams & Wilkins.
Grossman, S. C., & Porth, C. M. (2014). *Porth's pathophysiology: Concepts of altered health states* (9th ed.). Philadelphia, PA: Lippincott Williams & Wilkins.
Hannon, R. A. (2017). *Porth pathophysiology: Concepts of altered health states*. Wolters Kluwer.
Martini, F. H., Timmons, M. J., & Tallitsch, R. B. (2012). *Human anatomy* (7th ed.). Toronto, ON: Pearson Benjamin Cummings.
National Osteoporosis Foundation (NOF). (2014). *Clinician's guide to prevention and treatment of osteoporosis*. Washington, DC: Author.
Skillen, D. L. (2012). General survey and vital signs assessment. In T. C. Stephen, D. L. Skillen, R. A. Day, et al. (Eds.). *Canadian Jensen nursing health assessment: A best practice approach* (1st ed., pp. 91–124). Philadelphia, PA: Wolters Kluwer Health/Lippincott Williams & Wilkins.
Stephen, T. C. (2012). The health history. In T. C. Stephen, D. L. Skillen, R. A. Day, et al. (Eds.). *Canadian Jensen nursing health assessment: A best practice approach* (1st ed., pp. 37–51). Philadelphia, PA: Wolters Kluwer Health/Lippincott Williams & Wilkins.
Stephen, T. C., Skillen, D. L., & Day, R. A. (2013–2014). *A syllabus for adult health assessment*. Edmonton, AB: University of Alberta, Faculty of Nursing.
Swartz, M. (2014). *Textbook of physical diagnosis: History and examination* (7th ed.). Philadelphia, PA: Saunders.
Urden, L. D., Stacy, K. M., & Lough, M. E. (2017). *Critical care nursing: Diagnosis and management*. Maryland Heights, MO: Elsevier Health Sciences.
Van Leeuwen, A., & Bladh, M. (2016). *Textbook of laboratory and diagnostic testing: Practical application of nursing process at the bedside*. Philadelphia, PA: F. A. Davis.
Weber, J., & Kelley, J. (2014). *Health assessment in nursing* (5th ed.). Philadelphia, PA: Lippincott Williams & Wilkins.

Journals and Electronic Documents

American College of Rheumatology. (2016). *Fracture Risk Assessment Tool (FRAX)*. Retrieved May 5, 2016, from www.rheumatology.org/I-Am-A/Rheumatologist/Research/Clinician-Researchers/Fracture-Risk-Assessment-Tool-FRAX
Coates, P. (2013). *Bone turnover markers*. Retrieved from http://www.racgp.org.au/alp/2013/may/bone-turnover-markers
Dreyer, P., & Vieira, J. G. (2010). *Bone turnover assessment: A good surrogate marker?* Retrieved from http://www.ncbi.nlm.nih.gov/pubmed/20485896
Fertleman, M., Levy, S., & Meredith, G. (2018). Metabolic bone diseases. *ABC of Orthopaedics and Trauma*, 173.
González-Gay, M. A., Matteson, E. L., & Castañeda, S. (2017). Polymyalgia rheumatica. *The Lancet*, *390*(10103), 1700–1712.
HealthLink BC. (2012a). *Alkaline phosphatase: Test overview*. Retrieved from http://www.healthlinkbc.ca/kb/content/medicaltest/hw1717.html
HealthLink BC. (2012b). *Calcium (Ca) in urine*. Retrieved from http://www.healthlinkbc.ca/kb/content/medicaltest/hw27965.html
Insight Medical Imaging. (2014). *Densitometry*. Retrieved from http://www.insightimaging.ca/scr-densitometry.htm
Naylor, K., & Eastell, R. (2012). *Bone turnover markers: Use in osteoporosis*. Retrieved from http://www.Ncbi.nlm.nih.gov/pubmed/22664836
O'Donnell, S., Lagacé, C., McRae, L., et al. (2011). *Report summary—Life with arthritis in Canada: A personal and public health challenge*. Retrieved from http://www.phac-aspc.gc.ca/publicat/cdic-mcbc/31-3/ar-08-eng.php
Osteoporosis Canada. (2014a). *Calcium: An important nutrient that builds stronger bones*. Retrieved from http://www.osteoporosis.ca/osteoporosis-and-you/nutirtion/calcium-requirements

- Pulselessness (This is a very late sign, as there has to be a significant increase in pressure to overcome arterial pressure)
- Polar or Poikilothermia (i.e., cold; is sometimes added as the sixth "P")

Of these clinical manifestations, the first two are the most reliable. By the time a limb is pulseless, severe and often permanent damage has occurred.

In many institutions, it is common practice for the patient to have a posterior slab (i.e., the posterior component of a cast) held in position with a Tensor-type bandage. In this way, pressure is reduced on the limb, and pressure can be relieved even more by removing the bandage while maintaining the alignment of the limb in the posterior slab. In the setting of a full cast, pressure is relieved by bivalving the cast (cut in half longitudinally, see Chart 70-2) while maintaining alignment, and the extremity must be elevated.

If the compartment syndrome is due to increased pressure within the fascial compartment, an orthopedic surgeon will perform a **fasciotomy**, which is a surgical procedure in which the fascia is incised to relieve the pressure. The wound is then left open to allow the fluid to drain from the compartment. Closure of the wound may involve the use of a Vac dressing and skin grafting; the wound usually takes months to completely heal. It is therefore important to closely monitor the patient's response to conservative and surgical management of compartment syndrome. The nurse records neurovascular responses and promptly reports changes to the orthopedic surgeon.

PRESSURE ULCERS. Pressure of the cast on soft tissues may cause tissue anoxia and pressure ulcers. Lower extremity sites most susceptible to pressure are the heel, malleoli, dorsum of the foot, head of the fibula, and anterior surface of the patella. The main pressure sites on the upper extremity are located at the medial epicondyle of the humerus and the ulnar styloid (see Fig. 70-1).

Usually, the patient with a pressure ulcer reports pain and tightness in the area. The drainage may stain the cast and emit an odour. Even if discomfort does not occur with tissue breakdown and necrosis, there may still be extensive loss of tissue. The nurse must monitor the patient with a cast for pressure ulcer development and report findings to the most responsible health care provider.

To inspect the pressure area, the orthopedic surgeon may bivalve the cast or cut an opening (window) in the cast. The portion of the cast is replaced and held in place by an elastic compression dressing or tape. This prevents the underlying tissue from swelling through the window and creating pressure areas around its margins.

DISUSE SYNDROME. The patient needs to learn to contract the muscles of the limb in the cast (i.e., isometric muscle contraction). This helps to reduce muscle atrophy and maintain muscle strength. The nurse teaches patients with a leg cast to "push the knee into the bed" while lying on their backs and for those patients with an arm cast instruct them to "make a fist." Muscle-setting exercises (e.g., quadriceps-setting and gluteal-setting exercises) are important in maintaining muscles essential for walking (Chart 70-3). Isometric exercises should be performed hourly while the patient is awake.

CHART 70-2

GUIDELINES for Univalving or Bivalving a Cast

Equipment

- Cast knife or cutter
- Bandage scissors
- Cast spreader
- Elastic compression bandage

Implementation

NURSING ACTIONS	RATIONALE
1. With a cast cutter, make a longitudinal cut to divide the cast in half.	1. The cast cutter provides the quickest and safest means to cut the cast and relieve pressure.
2. Cut the underpadding with scissors.	2. The padding between the cast and the scissors must also be cut to relieve pressure; using bandage scissors ensures that the skin underlying the padding is not abraded or cut inadvertently.
3. Spread the cast apart with cast spreaders.	3. Spreading the cut ends of the cast apart relieves pressure and permits inspection of the underlying skin without interrupting the reduction and alignment of the bone.
4. Secure the anterior and posterior parts of the cast together with an elastic compression bandage.	4. This maintains immobilization.
5. Elevate the extremity (but no higher than heart level).	5. This diminishes edema formation and promotes circulation.

Adapted from Caple, C., & Woten, M. (2016). Cast care: Performing. In D. Pravikoff (Ed.). *Nursing practice and skill*. Glendale, CA: CINAHL Information Systems; Smith, N. (2016). Caring for an adult with a body cast. In: D. Pravikoff (Ed.). *Nursing practice and skill*. Glendale, CA: CINAHL Information Systems.

CHART 70-3

Muscle-Setting Exercises

Isometric contractions of the muscle maintain muscle mass and strength and prevent atrophy.

Quadriceps-Setting Exercise

- Position the patient supine with leg extended.
- Instruct the patient to push knee back onto the mattress by contracting the anterior thigh muscles.
- Encourage the patient to hold the position for 10 seconds, relax for 10 seconds, and repeat 10 times per hour.
- Let the patient relax.
- Have the patient repeat the exercise 10 times each hour when awake.

Gluteal-Setting Exercise

- Position the patient supine with legs extended, if possible.
- Instruct the patient to contract the muscles of the buttocks.
- Encourage the patient to hold the contraction for 10 seconds, relax for 10 seconds, and repeat 10 times per hour.
- Let the patient relax.
- Have the patient repeat the exercise 10 times each hour when awake.

Promoting Home, Community-Based, and Transitional Care

EDUCATING THE PATIENT ABOUT SELF-CARE. The nurse encourages the patient to participate actively in personal care and to use assistive devices safely. The nurse must assist the patient to identify areas of concern and develop strategies to achieve independence in activities of daily living (ADLs) (Chart 70-4). The patient's participation in planning and accomplishing ADLs are an important aspect of independence and maintaining control.

When the cast is dry, the nurse instructs the patient as follows:

- Move as normally as possible, avoiding excessive use of the injured extremity and walking on wet, slippery floors or sidewalks.
- Perform prescribed exercises regularly, as scheduled.
- Elevate the casted extremity to heart level frequently to prevent swelling.
- Do not scratch the skin under the cast. This may cause a break in the skin and result in the formation of an ulcer. Cool air from a hair dryer may alleviate an itch.
- Cushion rough edges of the cast with tape.
- Keep the cast dry, but do not cover it with plastic or rubber, as this causes condensation, which dampens the cast and skin. Moisture softens a plaster cast. (A wet fibreglass cast must be dried thoroughly with a hair dryer on a cool setting to avoid skin problems.)
- Report any of the following to the orthopedic surgeon: persistent pain, swelling that does not respond to elevation, changes in sensation, decreased ability to move exposed fingers or toes, and changes in skin colour and temperature.

CHART 70-4

HOME CARE CHECKLIST • The Patient With a Cast

At the completion of education, the patient and/or caregiver will be able to:

- Promote cast drying specifically: do not cover, leave exposed to circulating air; handle damp plaster cast with palms of hands and do not rest the cast on hard surfaces or sharp edges that can dent a soft cast.
- Manage swelling and pain: elevate casted limb to heart level, apply ice bag intermittently, take analgesics as prescribed, and do isometric exercises.
- Report pain that is not relieved by elevating the casted limb or by analgesics as this is an indicator of impaired tissue perfusion leading to compartment syndrome.
- Demonstrate ability to transfer.
- Use mobility aids safely.
- Avoid excessive use of injured extremity and adhere to weight-bearing limitations.
- Manage minor skin irritations from cast: pad rough edges of cast with tape and blow cool air from hair dryer to relieve itching.
- Demonstrate exercises to promote circulation and minimize disuse syndrome.
- State indicators of complications and report promptly to orthopedic surgeon: uncontrolled swelling and pain; cool, pale extremities; paresthesia; paralysis; purulent drainage staining cast; and signs of systemic infection
- Describe care of extremity following cast removal:
- Skin care; gradual resumption of normal activities

CHART 70-5

GUIDELINES for Removing a Cast

When removing a cast, the orthopedic surgeon or nurse practitioner proceeds as follows:

PROCEDURE	RATIONALE
1. Inform patient about the procedure.	1. Facilitates cooperation and reduces fear about the procedure
2. Reassure patient that the electric saw or cast cutter will not cut skin. (Explain that blade oscillates to cut cast and vibrations will be felt.)	2. Reduces anxiety
3. Wear eye protection (patient and operator of the cast cutter).	3. Protects eyes from cast particles
4. Bivalve cast using a series of alternating pressures and linear movements of blade along the line to be cut.	4. Cuts cast in halves; avoids burning sensation from prolonged contact of oscillating blade with padding
5. Cut padding with scissors.	5. Releases all of the casting materials
6. Support body part as it is removed from the cast.	6. Reduces stresses on body part that has been immobilized
7. Gently wash and dry area that has been immobilized.[a] Apply emollient lotion.	7. Removes dead skin that has accumulated during immobilization; keeps skin supple
8. Teach patient to avoid rubbing and scratching skin.	8. Protects skin integrity
9. Collaborates with physical therapist to teach patient to resume gradual use of limb within the guidelines prescribed.	9. Protects weakened part from excessive stress; progressive exercises reduce stiffness and restore muscle strength and function
10. Teach patient to control swelling by elevating the extremity or using elastic bandage if prescribed.	10. Facilitates circulation (i.e., venous return) and controls fluid pooling

[a]If a new cast is to be applied, follow guidelines for application of a cast and associated nursing care.

- Note odours around the cast, stained areas, warm spots, and pressure areas. Report them to the most responsible health care provider.

The nurse prepares the patient for cast removal or cast changes by explaining what to expect (Chart 70-5). The cast is cut with a vibrating blade rather than a rotating blade. The patient can feel the vibration and pressure. The blade does not injure the patient's skin. The cotton padding is cut with scissors.

The casted limb is weak from disuse, the joint will be stiff, and the muscles may appear atrophied. The skin will be dry and scaly from accumulated dead skin and is vulnerable to injury from scratching. The skin needs to be washed gently and lubricated with an emollient lotion.

The patient is taught to resume activities gradually within the prescribed therapeutic regimen. The limb that has been casted cannot withstand normal stresses because the muscles are weak from disuse. In addition, it is important for the patient to continue to elevate the affected extremely after the cast is removed.

Evaluation

Expected patient outcomes may include the following:

1. Understands therapeutic regimen
   a. Elevates affected extremity
   b. Exercises according to instructions
   c. Keeps cast dry
   d. Reports any problems that develop
   e. Keeps cast clinic appointments
2. Reports less pain
   a. Elevates extremity that is in cast
   b. Repositions self
   c. Uses occasional oral analgesic
3. Demonstrates increased mobility
   a. Uses assistive devices safely
   b. Exercises to increase strength
   c. Changes position frequently
   d. Performs range-of-motion exercises of joints not in cast
4. Exhibits healing of abrasions and lacerations
   a. No signs of local or systemic infection (e.g., fever, local discomfort, purulent drainage, cast staining, or odour from cast)
   b. Intact skin when cast is removed
5. Maintains adequate neurovascular function of affected extremity
   a. Normal skin colour and temperature
   b. Minimal swelling
   c. Satisfactory capillary refill on testing
   d. Active movement of fingers or toes if they are not casted
   e. Normal sensations in casted body part
   f. Adequate pain management
6. Exhibits absence of complications
   a. Normal neurovascular status of casted extremity
   b. No pressure ulcers
   c. Minimal muscle wasting
7. Participates in regular activities of living (ADLs)
   a. Performs ADLs independently or with minimal assistance
   b. Adheres to prescribed exercise regimen

Specific Cast Management Considerations

Arm Casts

The nurse, in consultation with an occupational therapist, suggests devices designed to aid in one-handed activities. The patient may experience fatigue due to modified activities and the weight of the cast. Frequent rest periods are necessary.

Nursing Interventions

To control swelling, the nurse elevates the immobilized arm. When the patient is lying down, the arm is elevated so that each joint is positioned higher than the preceding proximal joint (e.g., elbow higher than the shoulder, hand higher than the elbow).

A **sling** may be used when the patient ambulates. To prevent pressure on the cervical spinal nerves, the sling should distribute the supported weight over a large area and not on the back of the neck. The nurse encourages the patient to remove the arm from the sling and elevate the arm frequently.

Circulatory disturbances in the hand may become apparent with signs of cyanosis, swelling, and an inability to move the fingers. A serious complication of impaired circulation in the arm is Volkmann's ischemic contracture, which is a form of compartment syndrome. Contracture of the fingers and wrist occurs as the result of obstructed arterial blood flow to the forearm and hand. The patient is unable to extend the fingers, describes abnormal sensation (e.g., unrelenting pain, pain on passive stretch), and exhibits signs of diminished circulation to the hand. Permanent damage develops within a few hours if action is not taken.

This serious complication can be identified early with nursing surveillance and proper care. The nurse makes frequent neurovascular checks (see Chapters 62 and 69). As previously mentioned, compartment syndrome may be managed by bivalving the cast to release external compression. A fasciotomy may be necessary to improve vascular status.

Leg Casts

The application of a leg cast imposes a degree of immobility on the patient. The cast may be a short leg cast, extending to below the knee, or a long leg cast, extending to the groin. The fresh cast must be handled in a manner that will not cause denting.

> **NURSING ALERT**
>
> **Injury to the peroneal nerve as a result of pressure is a cause of footdrop (the inability to maintain the foot in a normally flexed position). Consequently, the patient drags the foot when ambulating.**

The nurse and physical therapist instruct the patient how to transfer and ambulate safely with assistive devices (e.g., crutches, walker) (see Chapter 13). The gait to be used depends on whether the patient is permitted to bear weight. If weight bearing is allowed, the cast, splint, or brace is reinforced to withstand the body weight. A cast boot or shoe, which is worn over the casted foot, provides a broad, nonskid walking surface.

Nursing Interventions

The nurse supports the patient's leg on pillows to heart level to control swelling and applies ice packs over the fracture site as prescribed. The patient should elevate the casted leg when seated. The patient should also assume a recumbent position several times a day with the casted leg elevated to promote venous return and manage swelling.

The nurse assesses neurovascular status of the limb as previously described. Nerve function is assessed by observing the patient's ability to move the toes and by asking about sensation in the foot. Neuropathic symptoms may be caused at the head of the fibula by pressure on the peroneal nerve.

When the cast is hard and dry, the nurse teaches the patient how to transfer and ambulate safely with assistive devices (e.g., crutches, walker). If weight bearing is allowed, the cast is reinforced to withstand body weight. A cast boot provides a broad, nonskid walking surface.

Body or Spica Casts

Body casts and spica casts of the hip or shoulder are rarely used. The emphasis now is on **open reduction and internal fixation** (ORIF) techniques and early mobilization.

> **NURSING ALERT**
>
> **The nurse monitors the patient in a large body cast for potential physiologic cast syndrome, noting bowel sounds every 4 to 8 hours, and reports abdominal discomfort and distention, nausea, and vomiting to the primary provider.**

Caring for a patient with a body or spica cast at home can be very stressful for the caregiver(s); therefore, it is essential that nurses provide appropriate support and discharge education. To minimize complications after the cast is applied, the nurse should give the patient a comprehensive discharge package that supplements home care instructions with visual training instructions, as well as provide telephone counselling after discharge (Demir, Erden, Bulut, et al., 2015). Specifically, the nurse educates the family about how to care for the patient, which includes providing hygienic, cast and skin care, ensuring proper positioning, preventing complications, and recognizing symptoms that should be reported to the primary provider.

Managing the Patient With Splints and Braces

Contoured **splints** of plaster or pliable thermoplastic materials may be used for conditions that do not require rigid immobilization. The splint needs to immobilize and support the body part in a functional position. The splint must be well padded to prevent pressure, skin abrasion, and skin breakdown. The splint is overwrapped with an elastic bandage applied in a spiral fashion and with pressure uniformly distributed so that the circulation is not restricted. The nurse frequently assesses the neurovascular status and skin integrity of the splinted extremity as previously documented.

For long-term use, custom-fitted plastic **braces** (orthoses) are used to provide support, control movement, and prevent additional injury. An orthotist adjusts the brace for fit, positioning, and motion.

The nurse teaches the patient how to apply the brace and to protect the skin from irritation and breakdown. The nurse also assesses neurovascular integrity and the patient's general comfort.

Managing the Patient With an External Fixator

External fixators are used to manage open fractures with soft tissue damage. They provide stable support for severe comminuted (crushed or splintered) fractures while permitting active treatment of damaged soft tissues (Fig. 70-3). The fracture is reduced, aligned, and immobilized by a series of pins inserted in the bone. Pin position is maintained through attachment to a frame. The fixator facilitates patient comfort, early mobility, and movement of uninvolved joints.

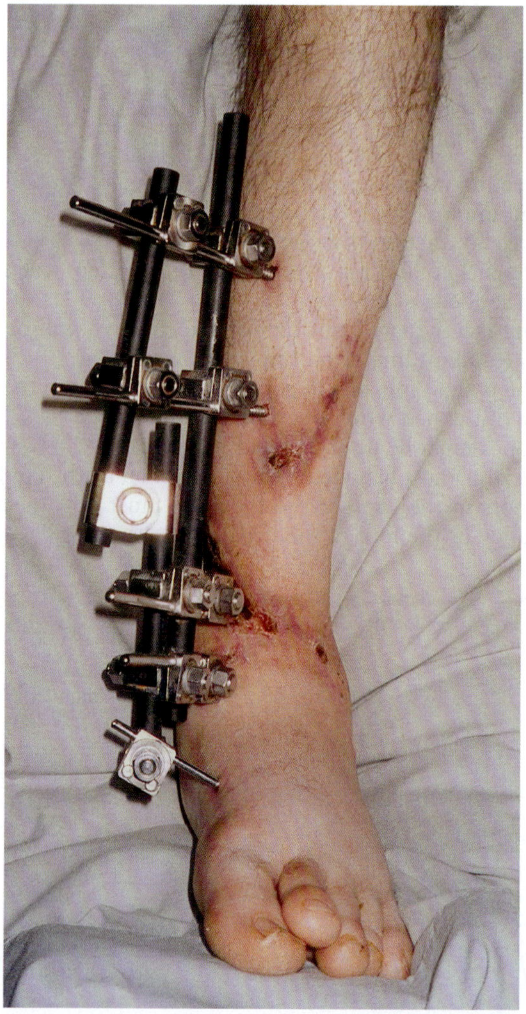

FIGURE 70-3. External fixation device. Pins are inserted into bone. The fracture is reduced and aligned and then stabilized by attaching the pins to a rigid portable frame. The device facilitates treatment of soft tissue damaged in complex fractures.

> **NURSING ALERT**
>
> **It is the orthopedic surgeon's responsibility to adjust the external fixator device.**

Nursing Interventions

The external fixator appears clumsy and unwieldly, therefore it is important to prepare the patient psychologically for the application of the device. Reassurance that early mobility is anticipated promotes acceptance of the device.

As with other limb injuries the extremity is elevated to reduce swelling. Sharp points on the fixator are covered to prevent device-induced injuries. The nurse monitors the neurovascular status of the extremity every 2 to 4 hours and assesses each pin site for redness, drainage, tenderness, pain, and loosening of the pin. Serous drainage from the pin sites is to be expected. The nurse must be alert for potential problems caused by pressure from the device on the skin, nerves, or blood vessels and for the development of compartment syndrome. The nurse carries out pin care as prescribed to prevent pin-track infection. This typically includes cleaning each pin site separately three times a day with cotton-tipped applicators soaked in a cleansing solution.

It is important to note that there is no clear evidence with respect to what cleansing agent should be used or indeed whether the pin sites should be cleaned at all (Kazmers, Fragomen, & Rozbruch, 2016). If signs of infection are present or if the pins or clamps seem loose, the nurse notifies the orthopedic surgeon.

The nurse encourages isometric and active exercises within the limits of tissue damage. When limb swelling subsides, the nurse encourages the patient's mobility within the prescribed weight-bearing limits. The fixator is removed after the soft tissue heals. The fracture may require additional stabilization by a cast while healing.

The Ilizarov external fixator is a special device used to correct angulation and rotational defects, to treat nonunion (failure of bone fragments to heal), and to lengthen limbs. Tension wires are attached to fixator rings, which are joined by telescoping rods. Bone formation is stimulated by prescribed daily adjustment of the telescoping rods. It is important to teach the patient how to adjust the telescoping rods and how to perform skin care. Generally, the nurse can encourage weight bearing. After the desired correction has been achieved, no additional adjustments are made, and the fixator is left in place until the bone heals.

Promoting Home, Community-Based, and Transitional Care

Educating Patients About Self-Care

The nurse teaches the patient to perform pin-site care according to the prescribed protocol and to report any signs of pin-site infection including redness,

CHART 70-6

HOME CARE CHECKLIST • The Patient With an External Fixator

At the completion of education, the patient and/or caregiver will be able to:

- Demonstrate pin site care.
- State signs of pin site infection: redness, tenderness, increased or purulent pin-site drainage and report promptly.
- Describe approaches to controlling swelling and pain: elevate limb to heart level, take analgesics as prescribed.
- Report pain uncontrolled by elevation and analgesics: may be an indicator of impaired tissue perfusion, compartment syndrome, or pin tract infection.
- Demonstrate ability to transfer.
- Use mobility aids safely.
- Avoid excessive use of injured extremity; adhere to weight-bearing limitations.
- State indicators of complications and report promptly to orthopedic surgeon: uncontrolled swelling and pain; cool, pale fingers or toes; paresthesia; paralysis; purulent drainage; signs of systemic infection; loose fixator pins or clamps.
- Describe care of extremity after fixator removal: gradual resumption of normal activities to protect limb from undue stresses.

tenderness, increased or purulent pin-site drainage, or fever. The nurse instructs the patient and family to monitor neurovascular status and report any changes. The nurse teaches the patient or family member to check the integrity of the fixator frame daily and to report loose pins or clamps. A physical therapist may teach the patient to transfer, use ambulatory aids, and adjust to weight-bearing limits and altered gait patterns (Chart 70-6).

Managing the Patient in Traction

Traction uses a pulling force to promote and maintain alignment to an injured part of the body. The goals of traction include decreasing muscle spasms and pain, realignment of bone fractures, and correcting or preventing deformities. The type of traction, amount of weight, and whether traction can be removed for nursing care must be determined to obtain its therapeutic effects.

At times, traction needs to be applied in more than one direction to achieve the desired line of pull. When this is done, one of the lines of pull counteracts the other. These lines of pull are known as the vectors of force. The actual resultant pulling force is somewhere between the two lines of pull (see Fig. 70-4). The effects of traction are evaluated with x-ray studies, and adjustments are made if necessary.

Traction is used primarily as a short-term intervention until other modalities, such as external or internal fixation, are possible. These modalities reduce the risk of disuse syndrome and minimize hospital lengths of stay, often allowing the patient to be cared for in the home setting.

Principles of Effective Traction

Whenever traction is applied, countertraction must be used to achieve effective results. Countertraction is the force acting in the opposite direction. Usually, the patient's body weight and bed position adjustments supply the needed countertraction.

When caring for the patient in traction, the nurse should follow these additional principles:

- Traction must be continuous to be effective in reducing and immobilizing fractures.
- Skeletal traction is *never* interrupted.
- Weights are not removed unless intermittent traction is prescribed.
- Any factor that might reduce the effective pull or alter its resultant line of pull must be eliminated.
- The patient must be in good body alignment in the centre of the bed when traction is applied.
- Ropes must be unobstructed.
- Weights must hang freely and not rest on the bed or floor.
- Knots in the rope or the footplate must not touch the pulley or the foot of the bed.

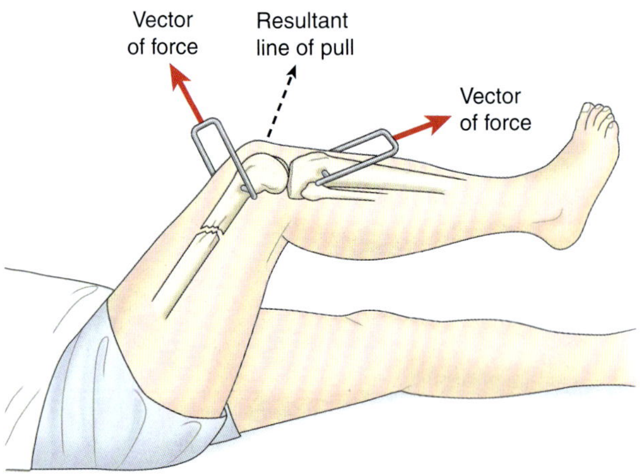

FIGURE 70-4. Traction may be applied in different directions to achieve the desired therapeutic line of pull. Adjustments in applied forces may be prescribed over the course of treatment.

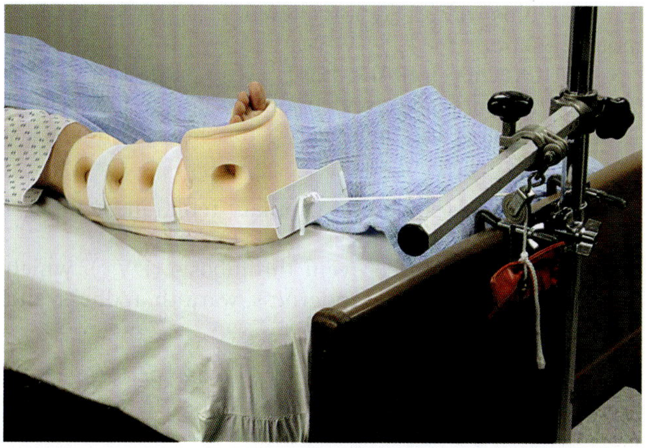

FIGURE 70-5. Buck's extension traction. Lower extremity in unilateral Buck's extension traction is aligned in a foam boot and traction applied by the free-hanging weight. The Heelift Traction Boot is shown here. (Photo courtesy of DM Systems, Inc.)

Types of Traction

The use of traction has decreased significantly due to advances in the surgical reduction of fractures, shortened lengths of hospital stay, and research that queries the effectiveness of its use (Newton-Triggs, Pugh, Rogers, et al., 2014). However, a basic working knowledge of the use of traction is necessary, because some orthopedic surgeons still prescribe traction for their patients (Hajbaghery & Moradi, 2013).

There are several types of traction. *Straight* or *running traction* applies the pulling force in a straight line with the body part resting on the bed. The countertraction is provided by the patient's body and movement can alter the traction provided. Buck's extension traction (discussed later; see Fig. 70-5) is an example of straight traction. *Balanced suspension traction* (see Fig. 70-6) supports the affected extremity off the bed and allows for some patient movement without disruption of the line of pull. With this traction, the countertraction is produced by devices such as slings or splints.

Traction may be applied to the skin (*skin traction*) or directly to the bony skeleton (*skeletal traction*). The mode of application is determined by the purpose of the traction. Traction can be applied with the hands (*manual traction*). This is temporary traction that may be used when applying a cast, giving skin care under a Buck's extension foam boot, or adjusting the traction apparatus.

Skin Traction

Skin traction is used less frequently than in years past; the AAOS (2014) recently reported that there was no reduction in pain or complications associated with its use compared with other standard interventions. Nonetheless, skin traction may be prescribed for short-term use to stabilize a fractured leg, control muscle spasms, and immobilize an area before surgery. The pulling force is applied by weights that are attached to the client with Velcro, tape, straps, boots, or cuffs. The amount of weight applied must not exceed the tolerance of the skin. No more than 2 to 3.5 kg (4.5 to 8 lb) of traction can be used on an extremity. Pelvic traction is usually limited to 4.5 to 9 kg (10 to 20 lb), depending on the weight of the patient.

Types of skin traction used for adults include Buck's extension traction (applied to the lower leg) (described next), the chin halter strap (occasionally used to treat chronic neck pain), and the pelvic belt (sometimes used to treat lower back pain).

Buck's Extension Traction

Buck's extension traction (unilateral or bilateral) is skin traction to the lower leg. The pull is exerted in one plane when partial or temporary immobilization is desired (see Fig. 70-5). It is used as a temporary measure to overcome muscle spasms and promote immobilization of hip fractures in adult patients waiting for more definitive treatment such as surgery. However, current data show no direct benefit to using this traction with patients with hip fractures (AAOS, 2014).

Before the traction is applied, the nurse inspects the skin for abrasions and circulatory disturbances. The skin and circulation must be in healthy condition to tolerate the traction. The extremity should be clean and dry before the foam boot or traction tape is applied.

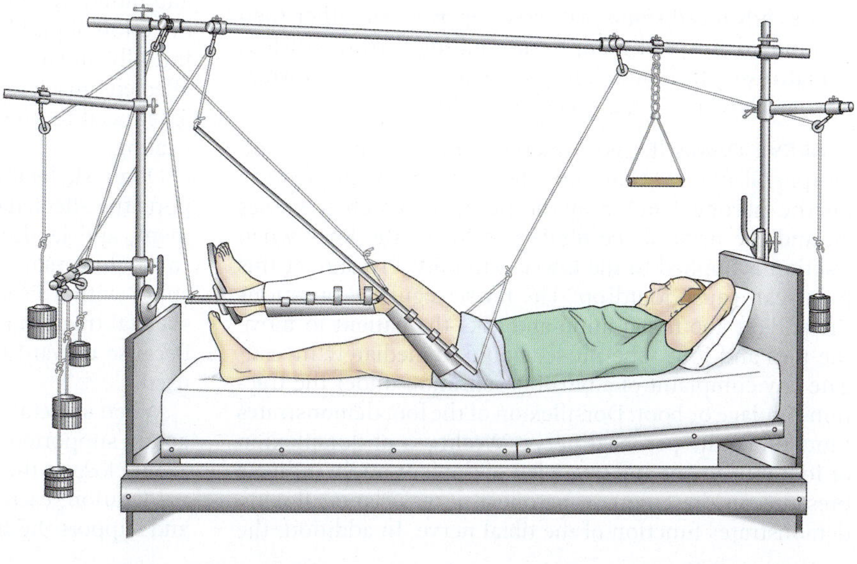

FIGURE 70-6. Balanced suspension skeletal traction with Thomas leg splint. The patient can move vertically as long as the resultant line of pull is maintained. Note the use of overhead trapeze.

To apply Buck's traction, the extremity is elevated and supported under the patient's heel and knee while the foam boot is placed under the leg, with the patient's heel in the heel of the boot. Next, the Velcro straps are secured around the leg. Traction tape that is overwrapped with an elastic bandage in a spiral fashion may be used instead of the boot. Excessive pressure is avoided over the malleolus and proximal fibula during application to prevent pressure ulcers and nerve damage. The rope is then affixed to the spreader or footplate over a pulley fastened to the end of the bed and attaches the prescribed weight—usually 5 to 8 lb—to the rope. The weight should hang freely, not touching the bed or the floor as this compromises the efficiency of the traction system (Newton-Triggs et al., 2014).

Nursing Interventions

Ensuring Effective Skin Traction

To ensure effective skin traction, it is important to avoid wrinkling and slipping of the traction bandage and to maintain countertraction. Proper positioning must be maintained to keep the leg in a neutral position. To prevent bony fragments from moving against one another, the patient should not turn from side to side; however, the patient may shift position slightly with assistance.

Monitoring and Managing Potential Complications

SKIN BREAKDOWN. During the initial assessment, the nurse identifies sensitive, fragile skin (common in older adults). The nurse also inspects the skin area that is in contact with tape, foam, or shearing forces, at least every 8 hours, for signs of irritation or inflammation. The nurse performs the following procedures to monitor and prevent skin breakdown:

Removes the foam boots to inspect the skin, the ankle, and the Achilles tendon three times a day. A second person is needed to support the extremity during the inspection and skin care.

- Palpates the area of the traction tapes daily to detect underlying tenderness.
- Provides frequent repositioning to alleviate pressure and discomfort, because the patient who must remain in a supine position is at increased risk for development of a pressure ulcer.
- Uses advanced static mattresses or overlays rather than standard hospital foam or alternating–air/low–air-loss mattresses to reduce the risk of pressure ulcer formation (Qaseem, Mir, Starkey, et al., 2015).

NERVE DAMAGE. Skin traction can place pressure on peripheral nerves. Care must be taken to avoid pressure on the peroneal nerve at the point at which it passes around the neck of the fibula just below the knee when traction is applied to the lower extremity. Pressure at this point can cause footdrop. The nurse regularly questions the patient about sensation and asks the patient to move the toes and foot. The nurse should immediately investigate any complaint of a burning sensation under the traction bandage or boot. Dorsiflexion of the foot demonstrates function of the peroneal nerve. Weakness of dorsiflexion or foot movement and inversion of the foot might indicate pressure on the common peroneal nerve. Plantar flexion demonstrates function of the tibial nerve. In addition, the nurse should promptly report altered sensation or impaired motor function.

CIRCULATORY IMPAIRMENT. After skin traction is applied, the nurse assesses circulation of the foot within 15 to 30 minutes and then every 1 to 2 hours. Circulatory assessment consists of:

- Peripheral pulses, colour, capillary refill, and temperature of the fingers or toes.
- Manifestations of deep vein thrombosis (DVT), which include unilateral calf tenderness, warmth, redness, and swelling.

The nurse also encourages the patient to perform active foot exercises every hour when awake.

Skeletal Traction

Skeletal traction is often used when continuous traction is desired to immobilize, position, and align a fracture of the femur, tibia, and cervical spine. It is used when traction is to be maintained for a significant amount of time, when skin traction is not possible, and when greater weight (11 to 18 kg [25 to 40 lb]) is needed to achieve the therapeutic effect. Skeletal traction involves passing a metal pin or wire (e.g., Steinmann pin, Kirschner wire) through the bone (e.g., proximal tibia or distal femur) under local anesthesia, avoiding nerves, blood vessels, muscles, tendons, and joints. Traction is then applied using ropes and weights attached to the end of the pin. Alternatively, skeletal traction may involve the application of tongs to the head that are fixed to the skull to immobilize cervical fractures (see Chapter 65).

The surgeon applies skeletal traction using surgical asepsis. The insertion site is prepared with a surgical scrub agent such as chlorhexidine solution. A local anesthetic agent is given at the insertion site and periosteum. The surgeon makes a small skin incision and drills the sterile pin or wire through the bone. The patient feels pressure during this procedure and possibly some pain when the periosteum is penetrated.

After insertion, the pin or wire is attached to the traction bow or caliper. The ends of the pin or wire are covered with caps to prevent injury to the patient or caregivers. The weights are attached to the pin or wire bow by a rope and pulley system that exerts the appropriate amount and direction of pull for effective traction. The weights applied initially must overcome the shortening spasms of the affected muscles. As the muscles relax, the traction weight is reduced to prevent fracture dislocation and to promote healing.

Often, skeletal traction is balanced traction, which supports the affected extremity, allows for some patient movement, and facilitates patient independence and nursing care while maintaining effective traction. The Thomas splint with a Pearson attachment is frequently used with skeletal traction for fractures of the femur (see Fig. 70-6). Because upward traction is required, an overbed frame is used.

When skeletal traction is discontinued, the extremity is gently supported while the weights are removed. The pin is cut close to the skin and removed by the surgeon. Internal fixation, casts, or splints are then used to immobilize and support the healing bone.

Nursing Interventions

Maintaining Effective Skeletal Traction

When skeletal traction is used, the nurse checks the traction apparatus to see that the ropes are in the wheel grooves of the pulleys, the ropes are not frayed, the weights hang freely, and the knots in the rope are tied securely. The nurse also evaluates the patient's position, because slipping down in bed results in ineffective traction (Zhang, 2015).

> **NURSING ALERT**
>
> **The nurse must never remove weights from skeletal traction unless a life-threatening situation occurs. Removal of the weights defeats their purpose and may result in injury to the patient.**

Maintaining Positioning

The nurse must maintain alignment of the patient's body in traction as prescribed to promote an effective line of pull (Zhang, 2015). The nurse positions the patient's foot to avoid footdrop (plantar flexion), inward rotation (inversion), and outward rotation (eversion). The patient's foot may be supported in a neutral position by orthopedic devices (e.g., foot supports).

If the patient reports severe pain from muscle spasm, the weights may be too heavy or the patient may need realignment. Pain must be reported to the primary provider if body alignment fails to reduce discomfort. Opioid and nonopioid analgesics may be used to control pain. Muscle relaxants may be prescribed to relieve muscles spasms as needed.

Preventing Skin Breakdown

The patient's elbows frequently become sore, and nerve injury may occur if the patient repositions by pushing on the elbows. In addition, patients frequently push on the heel of the unaffected leg when they raise themselves. This digging of the heel into the mattress may injure the tissues. It is important to instruct patients not to use their heels or elbows to push themselves up in bed (Levin & Morris, 2013). To encourage movement without using the elbows or heel, a **trapeze** can be suspended overhead within easy reach of the patient (see Fig. 70-6). The trapeze helps the patient move about in bed and move on and off the bedpan. Transparent film, hydrocolloid dressings, or skin sealants may also be applied to bony prominences (such as elbows) or critical areas to decrease the force of shearing and friction (Clark, Black, Alves, et al., 2014).

Specific pressure points are assessed for irritation and inflammation at least every 8 hours. Patients at high risk for skin breakdown (e.g., older adults, malnourished patients) may need to be assessed more frequently (Call, Pedersen, Bill, et al., 2015). Areas that are particularly vulnerable to pressure caused by a traction apparatus applied to the lower extremity include the ischial tuberosity, popliteal space, Achilles tendon, and heel. If the patient is not permitted to turn on one side or the other, the nurse must make a special effort to provide back care and to keep the bed dry and free of crumbs and wrinkles. The patient can assist by holding the overhead trapeze and raising the hips off the bed. If the patient cannot do this, the nurse can push down on the mattress with one hand to relieve pressure on the back and bony prominences and to provide for some shifting of weight. Advanced static mattresses or overlays should be used rather than foam or alternating–air/low–air-loss mattresses to reduce the risk of pressure ulcer formation (Qaseem et al., 2015). The patient's heel should be placed on a pillow or heel suspension device to keep the heel from the bed's surface (Baath, Engstrom, Gunningberg, et al., 2016).

For change of bed linens, the patient raises the torso while caregivers on both sides of the bed roll down and replace the upper mattress sheet. Then, as the patient raises the buttocks off the mattress, the sheets are slid under the buttocks. Finally, the lower section of the bed linens is replaced while the patient rests on the back. Sheets and blankets are placed over the patient in such a way that the traction is not disrupted.

Monitoring Neurovascular Status

The nurse evaluates the body part to be placed in traction and compares its neurovascular status (e.g., colour, temperature, capillary refill, edema, pulses, ability to move, and sensations) to the unaffected extremity every hour for the first 24 hours after traction is applied and every 4 hours thereafter. The nurse instructs the patient to report any changes in sensation or movement immediately so that they can be promptly evaluated. Venous thromboembolus (VTE) formation is a significant risk for the immobilized patient. The nurse encourages the patient to do active flexion–extension ankle exercises and isometric contraction of the calf muscles (calf-pumping exercises) 10 times an hour while awake to decrease venous stasis. In addition, antiembolism stockings, compression devices, and anticoagulant therapy may be prescribed to help prevent thrombus formation.

> **NURSING ALERT**
>
> **The nurse must immediately investigate every report of discomfort expressed by the patient in traction. Prompt recognition of a developing neurovascular problem is essential so that corrective measures can be instituted quickly.**

PROVIDING PIN-SITE CARE. The wound at the pin insertion site requires attention, and it is important to follow the facility's specific policy pertaining to skeletal pin care. The goal is to avoid infection and development of osteomyelitis (see Chapter 71). For the first 48 hours after insertion, the site is covered with a sterile absorbent nonstick dressing and a rolled gauze or Ace-type bandage. After this time, a loose cover dressing or no dressing is recommended (a bandage is necessary if the patient is exposed to airborne dust). Evidence-based recommendations (Smith & Dahlen, 2013) for pin-site care include the following:

- Pins located in areas with soft tissue are at greatest risk for infection.
- After the first 48 to 72 hours following skeletal pin placement, pin-site care should be performed daily or weekly.

- Chlorhexidine 2 mg/mL solution is the most effective cleansing solution. If chlorhexidine is contraindicated (due to known sensitivity or skin reaction), saline solution should be used for cleansing.
- Strict handwashing before and after skeletal pin-site care should always take place.

The nurse must inspect the pin sites every 8 hours for reaction (i.e., normal changes that occur at the pin site after insertion) and infection. Signs of reaction may include redness, warmth, and serosanguineous drainage at the site, which tend to subside after 72 hours. Signs of infection may mirror those of reaction but also include the presence of purulent drainage, pin loosening, tenting of skin at pin site, odour, and fever. Prophylactic broad-spectrum IV antibiotics may be given for 24 to 48 hours postinsertion to prevent infection; however, the evidence is confounding and there is no general consensus on the advisability of this practice (Smith & Dahlen, 2013). Minor infections may be readily treated with antibiotics, and infections that result in systemic manifestations may additionally warrant pin removal until the infection resolves.

NURSING ALERT

The nurse must inspect the pin site at least every 8 hours for signs of inflammation and evidence of infection.

Due to a lack of evidence-based research findings, controversy exists about skeletal pin care, showering, and the use of massage to release skin adherence to pins. Some evidence suggests that crusting at the pin site should be retained as long as the pin site remains uninfected as the retained crusts provide a natural barrier from bacterial contamination (Britten, Ghoz, Duffield, et al., 2013). The patient and family should be taught to perform any prescribed pin-site care prior to discharge from the hospital and should be provided with written follow-up instructions that include the signs and symptoms of infection.

PROMOTING EXERCISE. Patient exercises, within the therapeutic limits of the traction, assist in maintaining muscle strength and tone, and in promoting circulation. Active exercises include pulling up on the trapeze, flexing and extending the feet, and range-of-motion and weight-resistance exercises for noninvolved joints. Isometric exercises of the immobilized extremity (quadriceps and gluteal setting exercises) are important for maintaining strength in major ambulatory muscles (see Chart 70-3). Without exercise, the patient will lose muscle mass and strength, and rehabilitation will be greatly prolonged.

Nursing Management

Assessing Anxiety

The nurse must consider the psychological and physiologic impact of the musculoskeletal problem, traction device, and immobility. Traction restricts mobility and independence. The equipment can look threatening, and its application can be frightening. Confusion, disorientation, and behavioural problems may develop in patients who are confined in a limited space for an extended time. Therefore, the nurse must assess and monitor the patient's anxiety level and psychological responses to traction.

Assisting With Self-Care

Initially, the patient may require assistance with self-care activities. The nurse helps the patient eat, bathe, dress, and toilet. Convenient arrangement of items such as the telephone, tissues, water, and assistive devices (e.g., reachers, overbed trapeze) may facilitate self-care. With resumption of self-care activities, the patient feels less dependent and less frustrated and experiences improved self-esteem. Because some assistance is required throughout the period of immobility, the nurse and the patient can creatively develop routines that maximize the patient's independence.

Monitoring and Managing Potential Complications

Immobility-related complications may include pressure ulcers (see Chapter 13), atelectasis, pneumonia, constipation, loss of appetite, urinary stasis, urinary tract infections, and VTE formation. Early identification of pre-existing or developing conditions facilitates prompt interventions to resolve them.

Atelectasis and Pneumonia

The nurse auscultates the patient's lungs every 4 to 8 hours to assess respiratory status and educates the patient about performing deep breathing and coughing exercises to aid in fully expanding the lungs and clearing pulmonary secretions. If the patient history and baseline assessment indicate that the patient is at risk for development of respiratory complications, specific therapies (e.g., the use of an incentive spirometer) may be indicated. If a respiratory complication develops, prompt institution of prescribed therapy is needed.

Constipation and Anorexia

Reduced gastrointestinal motility results in constipation and anorexia. A diet high in fibre and fluids may help stimulate gastric motility. If constipation develops, therapeutic measures may include stool softeners, laxatives, suppositories, and enemas. To improve the patient's appetite, the patient's food preferences are included, as appropriate, within the prescribed therapeutic diet.

Urinary Stasis and Infection

Incomplete emptying of the bladder related to positioning in bed can result in urinary stasis and infection. In addition, the patient may find the use of a bedpan uncomfortable and may limit fluids to minimize the frequency of urination. The nurse monitors the fluid intake and the character of the urine. Adequate hydration is important; therefore, the nurse instructs the patient to consume adequate amounts of fluid and to void every 3 to 4 hours. If the patient exhibits signs or symptoms of urinary tract infection (e.g., burning or pain on urination, hematuria), the nurse notifies the primary provider.

Venous Thromboembolism

Venous stasis that predisposes the patient to VTE occurs with immobility. The nurse educates the patient about how to perform ankle and foot exercises within the limits of the traction therapy every 1 to 2 hours when awake to prevent DVT. Involving family members in performing these exercises can increase adherence and promote the family's involvement with the patient's care (Miller & Walsh, 2015). The patient is encouraged to drink fluids to prevent dehydration and associated hemoconcentration, which contribute to stasis. The nurse monitors the patient for signs of DVT, including unilateral calf tenderness, warmth, redness, and swelling (increased calf circumference). The nurse promptly reports findings to the primary provider for evaluation and therapy.

During traction therapy, the nurse encourages the patient to exercise muscles and joints that are not in traction to prevent deterioration, deconditioning, and venous stasis. The physical therapist can design bed exercises that minimize loss of muscle strength. During the patient's exercise, the nurse ensures that traction forces are maintained and that the patient is properly positioned to prevent complications resulting from poor alignment.

Managing the Patient Undergoing Orthopedic Surgery

Patients with musculoskeletal conditions such as fractures, joint disease, necrotic or infected tissue, and tumours require orthopaedic surgery. Surgical procedures include ORIF, arthroscopy, arthroplasty, fasciotomy, amputation, and bone grafting. The goals include improving function by restoring motion and stability and relieving pain and disability. Chart 70-7 presents descriptions of orthopedic surgeries.

CHART 70-7

Orthopedic Surgeries

Open reduction: correction and alignment of the fracture after surgical dissection and exposure of the fracture
Internal fixation: stabilization of the reduced fracture by the use of metal screws, plates, nails, and pins
Arthroscopy: repair of joint conditions using an arthroscope. A minimally invasive procedure that allows the surgeon to operate within a joint.
Hemiarthroplasty: replacement of one of the articular surfaces (e.g., in a hip hemiarthroplasty, the femoral head and neck are replaced with a femoral prosthesis—the acetabulum is not replaced)
Joint arthroplasty: surgical insertion of metal and synthetic prostheses
Total joint arthroplasty: surgical insertion of metal and synthetic prostheses to replace both articular surfaces within a joint
Meniscectomy: complete or partial excision of meniscal fibrocartilage in the knee
Amputation: removal of a body part
Bone graft: placement of bone tissue from autologous or homologous grafts to promote healing, to stabilize, or replace diseased bone
Tendon transfer: movement of tendon insertion to improve function
Fasciotomy: incision and diversion of the muscle fascia to relieve muscle constriction, as in compartment syndrome, or to reduce fascia contracture

Joint surgery is one of the most frequently performed orthopedic surgeries. Joint disease or deformity may necessitate surgical intervention to relieve pain, improve stability, and improve function. Surgical procedures include excision of damaged and diseased tissue, repair of damaged structures (e.g., ruptured tendon), removal of loose bodies (débridement), **arthroplasty** (joint replacement), and **arthrodesis** (fusion of a joint).

The procedure is based on the patient's underlying orthopedic condition, general physical health, impact of joint disability on daily activities, and age. Timing of these procedures is important to ensure maximum function. Surgery should be performed before surrounding muscles become contracted and atrophied and serious structural abnormalities occur. The orthopedic surgeon carefully evaluates the patient so that the most appropriate procedure is performed. In the operating room a pneumatic tourniquet may be applied after exsanguination of the limb with bandages to produce a "bloodless field."

Joint Replacement

Patients with severe joint pain and disability may undergo joint replacement. Conditions contributing to joint degeneration include osteoarthritis, rheumatoid arthritis, trauma, and congenital deformity. Some fractures (e.g., femoral neck fracture) may cause disruption of the blood supply and subsequent **avascular necrosis** (death of tissue due to insufficient blood supply); management with joint replacement may be elected over ORIF. Joints frequently replaced include the hip, knee (see Fig. 70-7), and finger joints. More complex joints (shoulder, elbow, wrist, ankle) are replaced less frequently.

Joint arthroplasty refers to the surgical removal of an unhealthy joint and replacement of joint surfaces with metal or synthetic materials. Total joint arthroplasty, also known as total joint replacement, involves the replacement of all components of an articulating joint. Most joint replacements consist of metal (e.g., stainless steel, cobalt-chromium, titanium) and high-density polyethylene components. In order to achieve fixation of components, the material can be cemented, cementless, or a hybrid of both of these materials. Cemented fixation uses a fast-curing bone cement (polymethylmethacrylate [PMMA]) to hold implants in place. Cementless fixation relies on new bone growing into the surface of the implant by using a press-fit, porous-coated prosthesis. There is also a hybrid fixation technique for TKA where the femoral component is inserted without cement, and the tibial and patellar components are inserted with cement. Use of each of these materials and techniques have different benefits and risks. Current research evidence supports the use of either component fixation methods (cemented or cementless) because postoperative functional outcomes, rates of complications, and rates of reoperations are similar (AAOS, 2015b; Karachalios & Antoniou, 2015). Identifying patient-specific factors that may inform the decision to utilize a particular fixation technique is important. Considerations include gender, age, diagnosis, weight, and activity level as well as the presence of healthy bone with adequate blood supply (Khan, Osman, Green, et al., 2016). Issues of cost and cost-effectiveness should also be considered (Mullaji & Shetty, 2015).

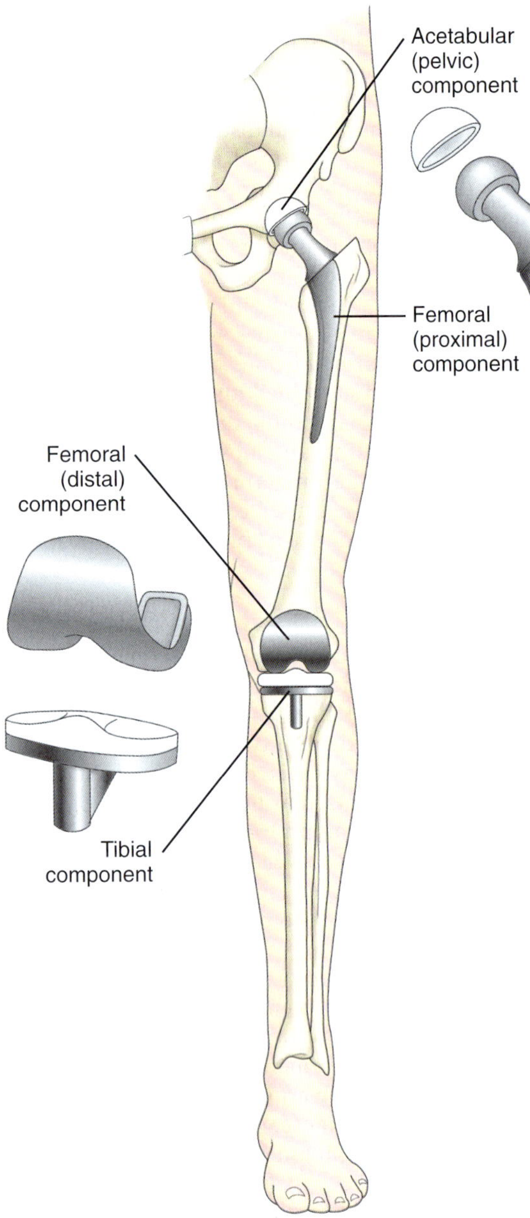

FIGURE 70-7. Examples of hip and knee replacement.

With joint replacement, patients may expect pain relief, return of joint motion, and improved functional status and quality of life. The scope of these improvements depends in part on patients' preoperative soft tissue condition and general muscle strength. Serious complications seldom occur, and recent innovations in total joint replacement surgery have made this a safer and more routinely performed surgery (AAOS, 2015b). In fact, minimally invasive surgical techniques, biomaterials, postoperative rehabilitation protocols, and multimodal analgesia strategies have led to earlier hospital discharge and quicker recovery (Lee, 2016). The American Joint Replacement Registry (AJRR) monitors the performance of devices and evaluates the cost-effectiveness of procedures. The data generated from the AJRR can provide orthopedic researchers and practitioners with the information necessary to improve the quality of health care among patients in need of knee and hip replacement procedures (Dy, Bumpass, Makhni, et al., 2016; Smith & Smith, 2012).

Nursing Interventions

Assessment of the patient and preoperative management are aimed at having the patient in optimal health at the time of surgery (see Chapter 19). If a patient is at risk for postoperative bleeding or is anemic, epoetin alfa (Epogen, Procrit) or iron supplements (e.g., ferrous sulphate) may be prescribed preoperatively to increase hemoglobin (Loftus, Spratling, Stone, et al., 2016).

Preventing Infection

Recent infections prior to the planned surgery may result in postponement of surgery. Preoperative skin preparation prior to surgery is done to reduce the risk of infection. As with any surgery, there is strict adherence to aseptic technique. Laminar air-flow (LAF) systems are often used in orthopedic ORs. However, there is debate in the literature whether LAF ventilation provides any significant benefit with respect to reduction in intraoperative infections (McHugh, Hill, & Humphreys, 2015). Prophylactic antibiotics are administered perioperatively as a single preoperative or short perioperative course (Dhammi, Haq, & Kumar, 2015).

Osteomyelitis is a difficult condition to treat. Chronic infection of the prosthesis usually requires removal of the implant and joint revision.

Managing Pain

Assessment of the patient's pain preoperatively and any cultural and personal preferences are important components related to the control of pain following joint surgery. Assessing the patient's level of understanding of the surgery and explaining what to expect in the postoperative period (e.g., incentive spirometry, pain control methods, activity limits) can improve outcomes. In particular, research findings suggest that patients who attend structured preoperative education classes report feeling better prepared for surgery and better able to control their pain after surgery (Louw, Diener, Butler, et al., 2013) (see Chart 70-8) (see Chapter 16).

Promoting Ambulation

Patients with total hip or total knee replacement begin ambulation with a walker or crutches within a day after surgery. The nurse and the physical therapist assist the patient in achieving independent ambulation. Specific weight-bearing limits on the prosthesis are determined by the orthopedic surgeon and are based on the patient's condition, the procedure, and the fixation method. Usually, patients with cemented prostheses can proceed to weight bearing as tolerated. If the patient has a press-fit, cementless, ingrowth prosthesis, weight bearing immediately after surgery may be limited to minimize micromotion of the prosthesis in the bone. As the patient is able to tolerate more activity, the nurse encourages transferring to a chair several times a day for short periods and walking for progressively greater distances.

Total Hip Arthroplasty (Replacement)

Total hip arthroplasty involves the surgical replacement of a damaged hip with a prosthesis that has a plastic acetabular component in the socket and a metal femoral

NURSING RESEARCH PROFILE

Chart 70-8. Guided Imagery for Pain Relief after Total Knee Replacement

Draucker, C., Jacobson, A. F., Umberger, W. A., et al. (2015). Acceptability of a guided imagery intervention for persons undergoing a total knee replacement. *Orthopaedic Nursing, 34*(6), 356–364.

Purpose

Complementary health modalities with mind–body approaches can be valid and effective adjuncts used by the patient with orthopedic conditions. Guided imagery (GI), the generation of positive sensory and affective images to promote healing outcomes, has been shown to be an effective intervention for the reduction of pain and anxiety in patients having orthopedic surgery. Despite its popularity, little is known about the acceptability of the intervention. The purpose of this study was to describe the perceptions of patients undergoing total knee replacement (TKR) surgery regarding the acceptability of a customized GI intervention to promote TKR outcomes.

Design

This study was part of a larger mixed methods study involving a randomized controlled trial (RCT) to evaluate a GI intervention for patients undergoing TKR. Eighty-two participants were randomly assigned to receive a GI ($n = 42$) or placebo (audiobook) ($n = 40$) intervention. Eligible participants were recruited from an orthopedic practice that performs a large volume of total joint replacements using a standardized approach. Participants who met the inclusion criteria (first-time TKR; no history of autoimmune disease or steroid use; no current use of GI; body mass index <40; no sensory or cognitive impairment) were randomly assigned to the treatment (GI) or control (audiobook) intervention. For this study, only narrative and interview data were analyzed to assess the acceptability of the intervention from only the individuals that experienced the GI intervention.

Findings

Overall, most participants were generally satisfied and felt actively engaged with the GI intervention. Participants specifically liked the content of the GI messages and appreciated hearing that their pain before and after surgery was temporary. The majority of participants in the study described that the GI intervention improved relaxation, enhanced pain management, and improved outlook and mood during the pre-, intra-, and postoperative time periods. Many participants reported being engaged with the intervention and enjoyed it; very few individuals were nonadherent or dropped out of the study. A smaller subgroup of participants did not find the intervention to be acceptable and described their reasons for dissatisfaction and disengagement. One aspect of the intervention that the participants did not find satisfactory was that the CDs were too repetitious. These comments provide helpful information for refining the intervention in the future.

Nursing Implications

The results of this study suggest that the utilization of a GI intervention is an acceptable approach to promote positive outcomes for patients undergoing TKR. The qualitative findings enhanced the understanding of the participants' experience. The findings of this study may be useful as nurses can play a pivotal role in helping patients understand complementary therapies that can help them recover from orthopedic surgery. A tailored GI intervention to meet individual patient needs and preferences warrants further research.

component that has a shaft, neck, and head (see Fig. 70-7). Patients tend to be 60 years of age or older, have unremitting pain or irreversibly damaged hip joints. With the advent of improved prosthetic materials and operative techniques, the life of the prosthesis has been extended, and today younger patients with severely damaged and painful hip joints are undergoing total hip replacement.

Nursing Interventions

The nurse must be aware of potential complications associated with total hip arthroplasty (see Chart 70-9). Complications that may occur include loosening of the prosthesis, dislocation of the prosthesis, abnormal wound drainage, thromboembolism, infection, immobility, and heel ulcers.

Gerontologic Considerations

The older adult patient who has had THA merits special postoperative care considerations. Early THA surgery for hip fractures (within 24 to 36 hours) is recommended for most patients once a medical assessment has been made and the patient's condition has been stabilized appropriately. If there are no contraindications (e.g., history of a bleeding disorder), these patients should receive LMWH for DVT prophylaxis; mechanical devices should be used for patients in whom anticoagulants and antiplatelet agents are contraindicated. Providing an appropriate postoperative analgesic regimen for older adults can be challenging in the presence of impaired cognition, medical comorbidities, and possible drug interactions. Consulting with a pain management specialist to specifically tailor the analgesic type and dose may be helpful (see Chapter 16).

All older adult patients' post-THA should be placed on a higher-specification, foam pressure-relieving mattress rather than a standard hospital mattress (Qaseem et al., 2015). A major goal following surgery in this patient population is early mobilization, in an effort to prevent the complications associated with prolonged immobility and to return the patient to functional activity (Mohanty, Rosenthal, Russell, et al., 2016). Early assisted mobilization and ambulation on the day of surgery can decrease hospital length of stay, complications, and hospital costs and can prepare patients to care for themselves at home with a higher level of independent functioning (Yager & Stichler, 2015). Patients who are assigned to restricted hip precautions have slower rehabilitation and return to usual ADLs (Barnsley, Barnsley, & Page, 2015).

Preventing Dislocation of the Hip Prosthesis

The patient's leg must be maintained in **abduction** to prevent dislocation of the prosthesis. The use of an abduction

(text continued on page 2253)

Plan of Nursing Care

Chart 70-9. The Patient With a Total Hip Arthroplasty

NURSING INTERVENTIONS	RATIONALE	EXPECTED OUTCOMES
Nursing Priority: Postoperative pain management **Goal:** Relief of pain		
1. Assess for pain using standard pain intensity scale.	1. Pain is expected after surgery due to tissue trauma. Muscle spasms occur after total hip replacements. Immobility causes discomfort at pressure points.	• Patient describes discomfort • Expresses confidence in efforts to control pain • States pain is reduced; pain intensity scores are decreasing • Appears comfortable and relaxed • Uses physical, psychological, and pharmacologic measures to reduce pain and discomfort
2. Ask patient to describe discomfort.	2. Pain characteristics may help to determine the cause of discomfort. Pain may be due to complications (hematoma, infection, dislocation). Pain is an individual experience.	
3. Acknowledge pain; inform patient of available analgesics or muscle relaxants.	3. The nurse can reduce patient stress by communicating concern and availability of pain management resources.	
4. Use pain-modifying techniques.	4.	
a. Use analgesics.	a. Parenteral opioids for first 24 to 48 hours and progress to oral analgesics.	
b. Change position within prescribed limits.	b. Use pillows to provide support and relief of pressure on bony prominences assists in minimizing pain.	
c. Modify environment.	c. Interactions with others, distractions, and sensory overload or deprivation may affect the pain experience.	
d. Notify surgeon about persistent pain.	d. Surgical intervention may be necessary if the pain is due to hematoma or excessive edema.	
5. Evaluate and record discomfort and effectiveness of pain-modifying techniques.	5. Effectiveness of action is based on experience; data provide a baseline about pain experiences, management, and pain relief.	
Nursing Priority: Mobility impaired due to activity restrictions after hip replacement **Goal:** Adequate pain management to do ADLs		
1. Maintain proper positioning of hip joint (abduction, neutral rotation, limited flexion).	1. Prevents dislocation of hip prosthesis.	• Prescribed position maintained • No heel pressure • Patient assists in position changes • Shows increased independence in transfers • Exercises hourly • Participates in progressive ambulation program • Actively participates in exercise regimen • Uses ambulatory aids correctly and safely
2. Relieve heel pressure.	2. Prevents pressure ulcer on heel.	
3. Instruct and assist in position changes and transfers.	3. Encourages active participation and prevents dislocation.	
4. Instruct and supervise isometric quadriceps- and gluteal-setting exercises.	4. Strengthens muscles for walking.	
5. Together with physical therapist, instruct and supervise progressive safe ambulation within limitations of weight-bearing prescription.	5. Amount of weight-bearing depends on patient's condition and prosthesis; ambulatory aids are used to assist the patient with non–weight-bearing and partial weight-bearing ambulation.	
6. Offer encouragement, and support exercise regimen.	6. Reconditioning exercises can be uncomfortable and fatiguing; encouragement helps patient comply with the exercise program.	
7. Instruct and supervise safe use of ambulatory aids.	7. Prevents injury from unsafe use.	

Plan of Nursing Care

Chart 70-9. The Patient With a Total Hip Arthroplasty, *Continued*

NURSING INTERVENTIONS	RATIONALE	EXPECTED OUTCOMES
Collaborative Problems: Hemorrhage; neurovascular compromise; dislocation of prosthesis; deep vein thrombosis; infection related to surgery **Goal:** Prevent complications		
Hemorrhage		
1. Monitor vital signs, observe for shock.	1. Changes in pulse, blood pressure, and respirations may indicate the development of shock. Blood loss and stress of surgery may contribute to the development of shock.	• Vital signs stabilize within normal limits • Amount of drainage decreases • No bright red bloody drainage • Hematology values are within normal limits
2. Note character and amount of drainage.	2. Within 48 hours, bloody drainage collected in a portable suction device should decrease to 25 to 30 mL per 8 hours. Excessive drainage (more than 250 mL in first 8 hours after surgery) and bright red drainage may indicate active bleeding.	
3. Notify surgeon if patient develops shock or excessive bleeding, and prepare for administration of fluids, blood component therapy, and medications.	3. Corrective measures need to be instituted.	
4. Monitor hemoglobin and hematocrit values.	4. Anemia due to blood loss may develop. Blood replacement or iron supplementation may be needed.	
Neurovascular Compromise		
1. Assess affected extremity for colour, sensation, and temperature and movement.	1. Pale, cool skin with decreased tissue perfusion. Sensation and movement indicates neurovascular compromise.	• Colour normal • Extremity warm • Palpable pedal pulses • Normal sensation and movement • Dorsiflex ankle and extend toes indicate peroneal nerve function. Plantar flex ankle and flex toes indicate tibial nerve function. • Normal capillary refill • Moderate edema and swelling; tissue not palpably tense • Pain controllable • Normal sensations • No paresthesia • Normal motor abilities • No paresis or paralysis • Pulses strong and equal
2. Assess toes for capillary refill response.	2. After compression of the nail, rapid return of pink colour indicates good capillary perfusion.	
3. Assess extremity for edema and swelling. Report patient complaints of leg tightness.	3. The trauma of surgery will cause edema. Swelling and hematoma can compromise circulation and function.	
4. Elevate extremity (keep leg lower than hip when in chair).	4. Minimizes dependent edema.	
5. Assess for deep, throbbing, unrelenting pain.	5. Surgical pain can be controlled; pain due to neurovascular compromise is not relieved by treatment.	
6. Assess for pain on passive flexion of foot.	6. With nerve ischemia, there will be pain on passive stretch.	
7. Notify surgeon if neurovascular status is altered.	7. Function of extremity needs to be preserved.	
Dislocation of Prosthesis		
1. Position patient as prescribed.	1. Femoral component maintained in acetabular component	• Prosthesis not dislocated
2. Use abductor splint or pillows to maintain position and support extremity.	2. Keep the hip in abduction and in a neutral rotation to prevent dislocation.	
3. Support leg and place pillows between legs when patient is turning and side-lying; turn to unaffected side.	3–5. Prevent dislocation.	
4. Avoid acute flexion of hip (head of bed at 60 degrees or less).		
5. Avoid crossing legs.		

continued >

Plan of Nursing Care

Chart 70-9. The Patient With a Total Hip Arthroplasty, *Continued*

NURSING INTERVENTIONS	RATIONALE	EXPECTED OUTCOMES
6. Observe for severe hip pain. Assess for shortened extremity, internally or externally rotated leg, inability to move extremity.	6. Findings may indicate dislocation of the prosthesis.	
7. Notify surgeon of possible dislocation.	7. Joint dislocations compromise neurovascular status and future function of the extremity.	
Deep Vein Thrombosis		
1. Administer prescribed anticoagulant therapy.	1. Reduces risk of venous clotting	• Wears elastic stockings; uses compression device • No skin breakdown • Pulses equal and strong • Skin temperature normal • Changes position with assistance • Participates in exercise regimen • Well hydrated • No chest pain; lungs clear to auscultation;
2. Use elastic compression stocking or sequential compression device as prescribed.	2. This aids in venous blood return and prevents stasis.	
3. Remove stocking for 20 minutes twice a day, and provide skin care.	3. Skin care is necessary to avoid breakdown. Extended removal of stockings defeats the purpose of stockings.	
4. Assess skin temperature of legs.	4. Local inflammation will increase local skin temperature.	
5. Avoid pressure on leg veins from equipment (e.g., abductor splint straps, sequential compression stockings) or pillows.	5. Compression of blood vessels diminishes blood flow.	
6. Change position and increase activity as prescribed.	6. Activity promotes circulation and diminishes venous stasis.	
7. Supervise ankle exercises hourly.	7. Muscle exercise promotes circulation.	
8. Monitor body temperature.	8. Body temperature increases with inflammation.	
9. Encourage fluids.	9. Dehydration increases blood viscosity	
Infection Related to Surgery		
1. Monitor vital signs.	1. Temperature, pulse, and respirations increase in response to infection. Magnitude of response may be decreased in older adult.	• Vital signs normal • Well-approximated incision without drainage or excessive inflammatory response • Minimal discomfort; no hematoma • Patient tolerates antibiotics
2. Use aseptic technique for dressing changes and emptying of portable drainage.	2. Reduces risk of introducing organisms.	
3. Assess wound appearance and character of drainage.	3. Red, swollen, draining incision with indurated skin is indicative of infection.	
4. Assess pain.	4. Pain may be due to wound hematoma—a possible locus of infection—that needs to be surgically evacuated.	
5. Administer prophylactic antibiotics as prescribed, and observe for side effects.	5. Reduced risk of infected prosthesis.	
Nursing Priority: Risk for ineffective health maintenance related to surgery **Goal:** Cares for self at home		
1. Assess home environment for discharge planning.	1. Physical barriers such as stairs, may limit ambulation and self-care at home.	• Home is accessible for patient at time of discharge. • Patient appears relaxed and develops strategies to deal with identified problems. • Personal assistance is available. • Patient demonstrates ability to provide necessary assistance within therapeutic prescription.
2. Encourage patient to express concerns about care at home; explore possible solutions.	2. Patient may have special problems that need to be identified and resolved.	
3. Assess availability of physical assistance for health care activities.	3. Patient may require assistance in routine health care due to limited mobility and hip range of motion.	

Plan of Nursing Care

Chart 70-9. The Patient With a Total Hip Arthroplasty, *Continued*

NURSING INTERVENTIONS	RATIONALE	EXPECTED OUTCOMES
4. Provide caregiver home health care information.	4. Understanding of rehabilitative regimen contributes to patient adherence.	• Patient practices home care program. • Patient keeps follow up health care appointments.
5. Instruct patient on posthospital care: a. Activity limitations (hip precautions, weight-bearing limits) b. Exercise instructions c. Safe use of ambulatory aids d. Wound care e. Measures to promote healing f. Medications, if any g. Potential problems h. Continuing health care supervision and management	5. Lack of knowledge and poor preparation for care at home contribute to patient anxiety, insecurity, and nonadherence to the therapeutic regimen.	

wedge pillow (Fig. 70-8), or pillows between the legs keeps both hips in abduction. It is important to keep the operative hip in abduction when repositioning the patient in bed. Depending on the surgeon's preference, some patients are not permitted to be turned onto the affected side, whereas others may be turned to either side.

The patient's hip is never flexed more than 90 degrees, therefore the head of the bed is never elevated more than 60 degrees. Limited flexion is maintained during transfers and when sitting. When the patient is initially assisted out of bed the abduction wedge pillow or pillows are kept between the legs. The patient should maintain the affected hip in extension and pivot on the unaffected leg with assistance of the nurse. The nurse protects the affected hip from **adduction**, flexion, and internal or external rotation.

High-seat (orthopedic) chairs, semi-reclining wheelchairs, and raised toilet seats are used to minimize hip joint flexion. When sitting, the patient's hips should be higher than the knees and the affected leg should not be elevated; the patient may flex the knees.

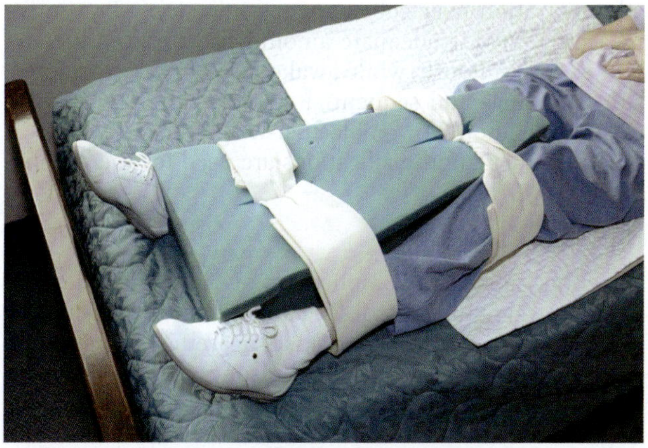

FIGURE 70-8. An abduction pillow may be used after a total hip replacement to prevent dislocation of the prosthesis.

At no time should patients cross their legs and they must avoid acute flexion of the hip. The patient should not bend at the waist to put on shoes and socks. Occupational therapists can provide the patient with devices to assist with dressing below the waist. Hip precautions are needed for 3 to 4 months after surgery (Chart 70-10).

Dislocation may occur with positioning that exceeds the limits of the prosthesis. The nurse must recognize dislocation of the prosthesis. Signs of dislocation include:

- Increased pain in the affected hip or groin
- Shortening of the leg with abnormal external or internal rotation
- Acute pain on moving the affected leg
- A "popping" sensation in the hip

If a prosthesis becomes dislocated, the nurse (or the patient, if at home) immediately notifies the most responsible health care provider, because the hip must be reduced and stabilized promptly so that the leg does not sustain circulatory and nerve damage. After closed reduction, the hip may be stabilized with traction or a brace to minimize the risk of recurrent dislocation. As the muscles and joint capsule heal, the chance of dislocation diminishes. Undue stress to the new hip joint should be avoided for the first 3 to 6 months (e.g., sitting in a low chair and bending forward).

Monitoring Wound Drainage

Fluid and blood accumulating at the surgical site are usually drained with a portable suction device (e.g., hemovac drain). This prevents accumulation of fluid, which could contribute to discomfort and provide a site for infection. Drainage of 200 to 500 mL in the first 24 hours is expected; by 48 hours postoperatively, the total drainage in 8 hours usually decreases to 30 mL or less, and the suction device is then removed. The nurse should notify the most responsible provider of any drainage volumes greater than anticipated.

Preventing Venous Thromboembolism

The term venous thromboembolism (VTE) refers to two separate but interrelated conditions: **deep vein**

CHART 70-10

Patient Education: Avoiding Hip Dislocation After Replacement Surgery

Until the hip prosthesis stabilizes after hip replacement surgery, the patient needs to learn about proper positioning so that the prosthesis remains in place. Dislocation of the hip is a serious complication of surgery that causes pain and loss of function and necessitates reduction under anesthesia to correct the dislocation. Desirable positions include abduction, neutral rotation, and flexion of less than 90 degrees. When the patient is seated, the knees should be lower than the hip.

Methods for avoiding dislocation include:

- Keep the knees apart at all times.
- Put a pillow between the legs when sleeping.
- Never cross the legs when seated.
- Avoid bending forward when seated in a chair.
- Use a high-seated chair and a raised toilet seat.
- Do not flex the hip to put on clothing such as pants, stockings, socks, or shoes.

Positions to avoid after total hip replacement are illustrated below.

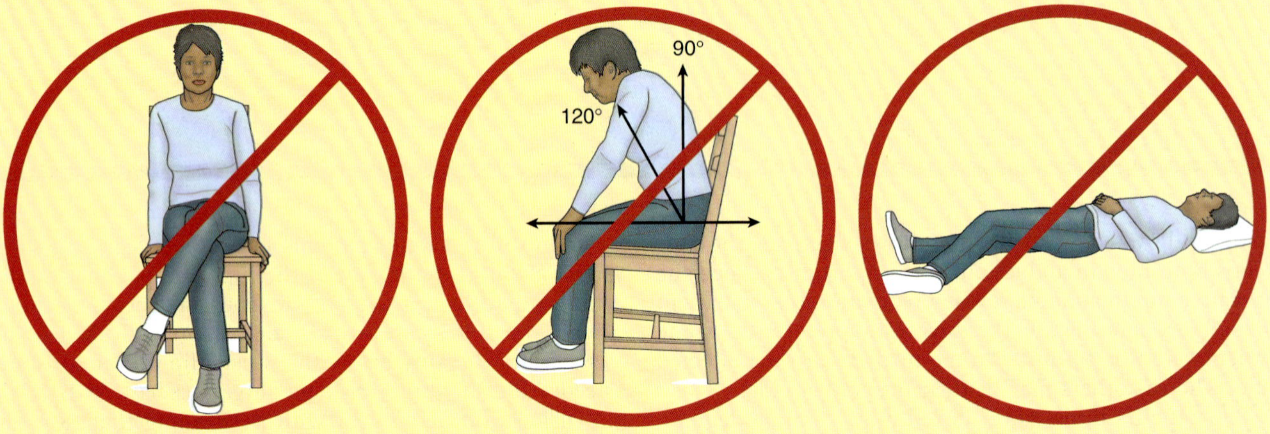

Affected leg should not cross the centre of the body

Hip should not bend more than 90 degrees

Affected leg should not turn inward

thrombosis (DVT) and **pulmonary embolism (PE)**. As the name implies a DVT occurs when a blood clot forms in the deep (and large) veins of the leg. A pulmonary embolism occurs when a portion of the clot breaks off and travels in the venous circulation, through the heart lodging in a pulmonary artery. According to the Canadian Venous Thromboembolism Clinical Trials and Outcomes Research (CanVECTOR), the development of a PE is the most serious type of VTE and represents the third leading cause of mortality in patients in hospital (CanVECTOR) hence the importance of prevention in orthopedic surgery patients.

There have been advances in surgical techniques and postoperative management; however, VTE is still a major risk for orthopedic patients having lower limb arthroplasty surgery. In the absence of prophylactic therapy, the incidence of DVT is 40% to 60% and 5% to 10% for PE after THA (Thrombosis Canada, 2018).

With the advent of routine prophylactic anticoagulant therapy the incidence of fatal PE has declined, however VTE that is symptomatic is still reported up to 3 months after surgery. It is interesting to note that most cases of symptomatic VTE occur *after* discharge from hospital (Thrombosis Canada, 2018).

It is therefore important to routinely assess the patient for development of VTE. Signs of DVT include calf pain/tenderness, swelling, warm and erythematous skin. Patients experiencing a PE may have a sudden onset of shortness of breath, pleuritic type chest pain, cough, hemoptysis, disorientation, and confusion. It is also important to emphasize to the patient the importance of adhering to the anticoagulant therapy for the prescribed period of time after discharge. Most patients need to continue with anticoagulant therapy for 30 to 35 days. The patient's perceptions must be taken into account in order to improve VTE prophylaxis therapy (Yaping, Jing, & Yuzhao, 2018).

Low–molecular-weight heparins such as enoxaparin are used for VTE prophylaxis; however, direct oral anticoagulant therapy is now being used (e.g., Rivaroxaban) more frequently as adherence increased with once-daily oral administration over subcutaneous injections. Preventive measures include adequate amounts of fluids, ankle and foot exercises hourly while awake, use of elastic compression stockings and sequential compression devices, and early ambulation. Low–molecular-weight heparin or direct oral anticoagulation medications are used for the prophylaxis of DVT.

Preventing Infection

Infection—a serious complication of THA—may necessitate removal of the prosthesis. Patients who are older, have obesity, poorly nourished, smoke cigarettes, or use corticosteroid medications (e.g., prednisone) and patients who have diabetes, rheumatoid arthritis, concurrent infections (e.g., urinary tract infection, dental abscess), carry MRSA, or have hematomas are at high risk for infection (Smith & Dahlen, 2013).

Over time, 1 in 5 patients with THA will undergo revision of the prosthesis, most commonly because of aseptic loosening, infection, instability, or a mechanical complication. Because these joint infections are difficult to treat, strategies for preventing infections should be implemented at various steps of the process of care. Strict hand hygiene and utilization of appropriate infection control practices can prevent transmission of infectious organisms. Proper preoperative patient skin cleansing reduces risk of bacteria entering sites caused by invasive devices or procedures. Appropriate antibiotic administration and discontinuation, as well as thorough patient education regarding subsequent antibiotic use is important. The presence of drains provides a means by which bacteria may enter the body and attach to prosthetic equipment (Smith & Dahlen, 2013; Tsang, 2015). Using a standard recording document to note and describe wound drainage may improve physician and nurse communication and promote decreased infection rates (Tsang, Cheng, Ho, et al., 2016). Moreover, caution should be exercised during the drain removal process to prevent the drain from breaking. After the drain is removed, the nurse should clean the drain tube site with an antiseptic solution and apply a small gauze dressing if there is any oozing at the site (Kneedler, Moss, Pfister, et al., 2015).

Acute infections may occur within 3 months after surgery and are associated with progressive superficial infections or hematomas. Delayed surgical infections may appear 4 to 24 months after surgery and may cause return of discomfort in the hip. Previously, prophylactic antibiotics were prescribed if the patient needed any future surgical or invasive procedures, such as tooth extraction or cystoscopic examination. However, the routine use of antibiotic prophylaxis prior to dental procedures for patients with total joint prostheses remains controversial and is not recommended (Sollecito, Abt, Lockhart, et al., 2015). Antibiotic prophylaxis can still be prescribed for some patients considered at higher risk of infection (e.g., patients who are immunosuppressed) (Jevsevar, Cummins, Azar, et al., 2015).

Infections occurring more than 2 years after surgery are attributed to the spread of infection through the bloodstream from another site in the body. If an infection occurs, antibiotics are prescribed. Severe infections may require surgical débridement or removal of the prosthesis.

Promoting Home, Community-Based, and Transitional Care

EDUCATING THE PATIENT ABOUT SELF-CARE. Before the patient leaves the acute care setting, the nurse provides thorough education to promote continuity of the therapeutic regimen and active participation in the rehabilitation process (see Chart 70-11). The patient may be discharged to their home, a rehabilitation unit, a transitional care unit, or a long-term care facility. The nurse advises the patient of the importance of a daily exercise program in maintaining the functional motion of the hip joint and strengthening the abductor muscles of the hip, and reminds the patient that it will take time to strengthen and retrain the muscles.

CHART 70-11

Patient Education: Providing Home Care After Hip Replacement

Considerations

- Pain management
- Wound care
- Mobility
- Self-care (activities of daily living)
- Potential problems

Nursing Interventions

Discuss with patient methods to reduce pain:

- Periodic rest
- Distraction and relaxation techniques
- Medication therapy (e.g., nonsteroidal anti-inflammatory drugs, opioid analgesics): actions of medications, administration, schedule, side effects

Instruct patient in the following:

- Keeping incision clean and dry
- Cleansing incision daily with soap and water and changing the dressing
- Recognizing signs of wound infection (e.g., pain, swelling, drainage, fever)

Explain that sutures or staples will be removed 10 to 14 days after surgery.

Educate patient about the following:

- Safe use of assistive devices
- Weight-bearing limitations
- How to change positions frequently
- Limitations on hip flexion and adduction (e.g., avoid acute flexion and crossing legs)
- How to stand without flexing hip acutely
- Avoidance of low-seated chairs
- Sleeping with pillow between legs to prevent adduction
- Gradual increase in activities and participation in prescribed exercise regimen
- Use of important medications for anticoagulant therapy
- Assess home environment for physical barriers.

Instruct patient to use elevated toilet seat and to use reachers to aid in dressing.

Encourage patient to accept assistance with activities of daily living during early convalescence until mobility and strength improve.

Arrange services and accommodations to address the patient's disability or illness.

Assess patient for development of potential problems, and instruct patient to report signs of potential problems:

- Dislocation of prosthesis: severe pain, shortening of leg, inability to move leg, popping sensation in hip, abnormal rotation
- Deep vein thrombosis (e.g., unilateral calf pain, swelling, redness)
- Wound infection: swelling, purulent drainage, pain, fever, erythematous skin and induration.
- Pulmonary embolism: sudden shortness of breath, tachypnea, pleuritic chest pain, disorientation and confusion.

Discuss with patient the need to continue regular health care (routine physical examinations) and screenings.

The patient will need physical therapy to regain mobility. Assistive devices (crutches, walker, or cane) may be used for a time. After sufficient muscle tone has developed to permit a normal gait without discomfort, these devices are not necessary. In general, by 3 months, the patient can resume routine ADLs. Stair climbing typically may resume within 3 to 6 weeks following surgery (AAOS, 2015b). Some discomfort with activity and at night is common for several weeks. Frequent walks, swimming, and the use of a high rocking chair are excellent for hip exercises.

Restrictions must be kept in mind when resuming sexual activity. Patients should be questioned about sexual concerns and counselled on physical and functional aspects of sexual activity. Sexual intercourse can be resumed based upon the surgeon's recommendation (typically 3 to 6 months postoperatively) and should be carried out with the patient in the supine position (flat on the back) to avoid excessive adduction and flexion of the new hip (Meiri, Rosenbaum, & Kalichman, 2014). Attention to positioning and comfort may enhance the intimacy of the experience.

At no time during the first 4 months should the patient cross the legs or flex the hip more than 90 degrees. Assistive devices should be used for dressing, such as long-handled shoehorns or dressing sticks for putting on shoes and socks. The patient should avoid low chairs and sitting for longer than 45 minutes at a time. These precautions minimize hip flexion and the risks of prosthetic dislocation, hip stiffness, and flexion contracture. Driving requires sufficient range of motion and muscle strength; most patients are given permission to drive 4 to 6 weeks postoperatively. Travelling long distances should be avoided unless frequent position changes are possible. Other activities to avoid include tub baths, jogging, lifting heavy loads, and excessive bending and twisting (e.g., lifting, shovelling snow, forceful turning). The primary provider may give the patient a card indicating that he or she has had a joint replacement; this card may be used to alert security personnel who use screening devices at airports or malls.

CONTINUING AND TRANSITIONAL CARE. A nurse may assess the patient's home for potential problems and monitor wound healing. The nurse, physical therapist, or occupational therapist assesses the home environment for physical barriers that may impede the patient's rehabilitation. In addition, the nurse or therapist may need to assist the patient in acquiring devices such as reachers and long-handled shoehorns or tongs to help with dressing or a toilet seat extender to elevate the toilet seat. After successful surgery and rehabilitation, the patient can expect a hip joint that is free or almost free of pain, has good motion, is stable, and permits normal or near-normal ambulation and function.

Total Knee Replacement

Total knee arthroplasty surgery is performed on patients with functional disabilities related to conditions such as osteoarthritis and rheumatoid arthritis. Similar to the hip prosthesis, there are metal and plastic components.

Nursing Interventions

Postoperatively, the knee is dressed with a compression bandage. Ice or cold packs may be applied to reduce postoperative swelling and bleeding. The nurse assesses the neurovascular status (movement, sensation, colour, pulse, capillary refill) of the surgical extremity and compares it with the contralateral extremity every 2 to 4 hours. It is important to encourage active flexion of the foot every hour when the patient is awake. Postoperative efforts are directed at preventing complications (VTE, peroneal nerve palsy, infection, bleeding, limited range of motion).

A wound suction drain may be present to remove fluid accumulating in the joint. If a drain is used, it is usually left in place for only 24 to 48 hours to reduce the risk of infection (Tsang, 2015). Antibiotics are given prophylactically and continued for 24 hours postoperatively (Smith & Dahlen, 2013). If extensive bleeding is anticipated, an autotransfusion drainage system may be used during the immediate postoperative period. All blood must be transfused within 6 hours of collection (Tsang, 2015). The colour, type, and amount of drainage are documented, and any excessive drainage or change in characteristics of the drainage is promptly reported to the primary provider.

A **continuous passive motion (CPM) device** may be prescribed to promote range of motion, circulation, and healing, and to prevent scar tissue from forming in the knee, which could decrease mobility and increase postoperative pain. The patient's leg is usually placed in this device immediately after surgery. The degree of flexion and extension of the joint and the cycle rate (the number of revolutions per minute) are prescribed by the surgeon, but it is often the responsibility of the nurse to maintain the device and monitor the patient's response to the therapy.

Recent research findings suggest that CPM has no influence on functional recovery, drainage, pain, or decreasing adverse outcomes in patients post-TKA; in fact, it necessitates that the patient spend more time in bed (Tabor, 2013). Additional considerations include the time it takes for staff to repeatedly place the patient in and out of the machine. Additionally, care and maintenance of the machine can be costly, time consuming, and burdensome.

The physical therapist supervises exercises for strength and range of motion and educates the patient about how to use assistive devices based on weight-bearing restrictions. To avoid flexion contractures, patients are instructed to limit positions of flexion. A knee gatch position (i.e., raising the hospital bed so that the knee is flexed) and pillows placed behind the knee are both avoided. If satisfactory flexion is not achieved, gentle manipulation of the knee joint under general anesthesia may be necessary about 2 weeks after surgery.

Patients who are postoperative for TKA should mobilize and ambulate by the first postoperative day (Yager & Stichler, 2015). The patient's weight-bearing status is determined by the primary provider. The knee is usually protected with a knee immobilizer and is elevated when the patient sits in a chair. The typical requirements for discharge to home may include evidence of wound stability (e.g., no erythema, discharge, or redness), appropriate anticoagulation status by laboratory results (i.e., international normalized ratio [INR] between 1.5 and 2), progress toward physical therapy goals (e.g., appropriate use of walker), and satisfactory pain control with oral medications (Newton-Triggs et al., 2014).

Acute rehabilitation usually takes about 1 to 2 weeks; length of time and discharge destination (e.g., home, acute rehabilitation unit) depend on the age and tolerance of the patient. If discharge is to home, the patient may continue to use the CPM device if prescribed and may undergo physical therapy on an outpatient basis. Total recovery takes 6 weeks or longer, especially for those older than 75 years. Late complications that may occur include polyethylene-induced breakdown infection (osteolysis), periprosthetic joint infections, and aseptic loosening of prosthetic components (Osmon, Berbari, Berendt, et al., 2013).

More than 95% of patients who have TKA will still have a functioning prosthesis 15 to 20 years after surgery (Lee, 2016). TKA is a viable option for improving both disease-specific and generic health-related quality of life, especially pain and function, leading to positive patient satisfaction (Shan, Shan, Suzuki, et al., 2015). Patients usually can achieve a pain-free, functional joint and participate more fully in life activities than before the surgery.

Nursing Process

Preoperative Care of the Patient Undergoing Orthopedic Surgery

Assessment

Assessment of the patient is focused on hydration status, current medication history, pain, and risk for infection. Immobilization and bed rest contribute to the development of DVT, urinary stasis and risk for bladder infections. Adequate hydration decreases blood viscosity and venous stasis and ensures adequate urine flow. Hydration status is assessed by examining the patient's skin and mucous membranes, vital signs, urinary output, and appropriate laboratory values.

Pain assessment is as important as assessing the patient's temperature, pulse, respirations, and blood pressure. Assessment of pain is referred to as the "fifth vital sign." Location, quality, and intensity of pain are three important parameters to assess. The nurse asks the patient to identify the exact location of pain; this may provide essential diagnostic clues. For instance, a patient with compartment syndrome might identify the location of pain as distal to the fracture or surgical repair site. (Compartment syndrome was discussed earlier in this chapter, and in Chapter 70.) Quality of pain is determined by asking for a description of the pain (e.g., "burning," "throbbing," or "stabbing"). Intensity of pain might be described as mild to excruciating and is rated using a variety of intensity pain scales, such as the numeric pain scale or FACES pain scale. (See Chapter 16 for a discussion of pain intensity scales.)

The medication history provides information for perioperative management. The patient with chronic illness such as rheumatoid arthritis or chronic pulmonary disease may have received corticosteroid medications. The patient's use of other medications, such as anticoagulants, cardiovascular agents, or insulin, needs to be documented and discussed with the surgeon and anesthesiologist to ensure adequate management.

The nurse asks the patient specifically about the occurrence of colds, dental problems, urinary tract infections, and other infections 2 weeks prior to surgery. Pre-existing infections must be resolved before elective orthopedic surgery is performed. Other areas of preoperative assessment are similar to those for any patient undergoing surgery.

Nursing Priorities

Based on nursing assessment data, the patient's major preoperative nursing priorities related to orthopedic status may include the following:

- Acute pain
- Risk for peripheral neurovascular dysfunction
- Impaired physical mobility
- Disturbed body image

Planning and Goals

The major goals for the patient before orthopedic surgery may include relief of pain, adequate neurovascular function, health promotion, improved mobility, and positive self-esteem.

Nursing Interventions

Relieving Pain

Specific strategies for managing perioperative pain are tailored to the patient's needs. Pain is decreased with immobilization of a fractured bone or an injured, inflamed joint. Elevation of an edematous extremity promotes venous return and reduces associated discomfort. Ice relieves swelling and directly reduces discomfort by diminishing nerve stimulation.

Analgesics are frequently prescribed to manage the acute pain of musculoskeletal injury and associated muscle spasm. Alternative methods of pain management (e.g., distraction, focusing, guided imagery, quiet environment, back rubs) may be used to decrease pain perception.

Maintaining Adequate Neurovascular Function

Trauma, edema, or immobilization devices may interrupt tissue perfusion. The nurse must frequently assess neurovascular status (i.e., colour, temperature, capillary refill, pulses, edema, pain, sensation, motion) of the extremity and document the findings. If circulation is compromised, the nurse institutes measures to restore adequate circulation. These include promptly notifying the most responsible health care provider, elevating the extremity, and releasing constricting wraps or casts as prescribed.

Promoting Health

The nurse assists the patient in activities that promote health during the perioperative period. The nurse assesses nutritional status and hydration. The preoperative fasting regimen is usually tolerated well. If the patient has diabetes, is older adults and frail, or is the victim of multiple trauma, special fluid and nutritional provisions may be necessary.

The nurse monitors fluid intake, urinary output, urinalysis findings, and complaints of burning on urination. Coughing, deep breathing, and the use of an incentive spirometer are used to improve respiratory function during the perioperative period. Ongoing smoking cessation should be promoted and smoking cessation resources and medications should be offered to the patient.

The nurse provides skin care, paying special attention to pressure points. It is important to institute the use of pressure-reducing surfaces (i.e., special mattresses) for patients at high risk for skin breakdown who may be immobilized longer than normal. With elective surgeries, the patient may be instructed to use a germicidal soap for several days before hospitalization.

The nurse discusses with the patient and the family the need for assistance with ADLs and the therapeutic regimen during convalescence so that adequate support is available when the patient is discharged. Modification of the home environment may be necessary to accommodate the altered mobility of the patient after surgery. Referral to the social worker, transition coordinator, and the case manager may be needed to ensure a smooth transition to home care.

Improving Mobility

Preoperatively, the patient's mobility may be impaired by pain, swelling, and immobilizing devices (e.g., splints and casts). The nurse should elevate and adequately support edematous extremities with pillows. It is important to manage pain by promptly administering medication before moving the injured limb. The patient should perform active range-of-motion exercises of uninvolved joints, and, unless contraindicated, the nurse teaches gluteal-setting and quadriceps-setting isometric exercises to maintain the muscles needed for ambulation (see Chart 70-3). The patient exercises to strengthen upper extremities in preparation for using assistive devices postoperatively. If the patient has an opportunity to practice using assistive devices (e.g., crutches, walker, wheelchair) before surgery, this may improve patient safety and promote independent mobility in the postoperative period.

Helping the Patient Maintain Self-Esteem

The degree of assistance required in maintaining self-esteem is dependent on events preceding hospitalization and the surgery and rehabilitation planned. Orthopedic patients may need assistance in accepting changes in body image, diminished self-esteem, or inability to perform their roles and responsibilities. The nurse encourages patients to express concerns and anxieties and helps them to develop coping strategies in relation to alterations in physical capacity that may impact their self-esteem.

Evaluation

Expected patient outcomes may include the following:

1. Reports adequate pain management
   a. Uses multiple approaches to manage pain
   b. States that medication is effective in managing pain
   c. Progressively mobilizes with less discomfort
2. Exhibits adequate neurovascular function
   a. Exhibits normal skin colour, sensation and movement, temperature, and capillary refill
   b. Demonstrates reduced swelling
3. Promotes healthy recovery
   a. Eats balanced diet appropriate to meet nutritional needs
   b. Maintains adequate hydration
   c. Abstains from smoking
   d. Continues to practice deep breathing and coughing and uses incentive spirometry
   e. Engages in progressive mobilization and strengthening exercises
   f. Plans for appropriate postoperative home support
4. Maximizes appropriate mobility
   a. Requests assistance as required
   b. Elevates edematous extremity routinely
   c. Uses appropriate immobilizing and assistive devices

Nursing Process

Postoperative Care of the Patient Undergoing Orthopedic Surgery

Assessment

In the postoperative period the nurse assesses the patient in relation to pain management, neurovascular status, mobility, health promotion, and self-esteem. Skeletal trauma and surgery performed on bones, muscles, and joints produces significant pain, especially during the first 48 hours postoperatively.

Tissue perfusion must be monitored closely, because edema and bleeding into the tissues can compromise circulation and result in compartment syndrome. There are three factors (known as Virchow's triad) that contribute to deep vein thrombosis: venous stasis from immobility, endothelial injury from the surgery, and hypercoagulability from immobility and inflammation (Patel & Chun, 2017).

General anesthesia, regional anesthesia, analgesia, and immobility can result in altered functioning of the respiratory, gastrointestinal, and urinary systems. The nurse assesses the patient's understanding of the mobility restrictions, discusses the plan of care with the patient, and encourages active participation. Frequent assessment of vital signs, level of consciousness, neurovascular status, wound drainage, breath sounds, bowel sounds, fluid balance, and pain provides the nurse with data that may suggest the possible development of complications. The nurse reports abnormal findings to the orthopedic surgeon promptly.

In major orthopedic surgery, there is a risk of hypovolemic shock due to blood loss. Muscle dissection frequently produces wounds in which hemostasis is poor. Wounds that were not evident under tourniquet control in the operating room may bleed during the postoperative period. The nurse must be alert for a sudden decrease in blood pressure combined with a rapid thready pulse as these are two common observations in blood loss leading to hypovolemic shock.

Changes in the patient's pulse rate, respiratory rate, or colour may indicate pulmonary or cardiovascular complications. Atelectasis and pneumonia may occur and may be related to pre-existing pulmonary disease, deep anesthesia, decreased activity, analgesics, and reduced respiratory reserve due to advanced age or an underlying musculoskeletal disorder (e.g., restrictive lung expansion secondary to kyphosis, rheumatoid arthritis, or osteoporosis).

Voiding in unnatural positions may contribute to urinary retention. In addition, older adults men usually have some degree of prostate enlargement and may already have difficulty voiding. Therefore, it is important to monitor urinary output.

Temperature elevations and decreased oxygen saturation within the first 48 hours are frequently related to atelectasis or other respiratory problems. Temperature elevations during the next few days are associated with urinary tract infections. Superficial wound infections take 4 to 6 days to develop. Fever from phlebitis usually occurs during the end of the first week through the second week.

Venous thromboembolism (see discussions of pulmonary embolism in Chapter 24 and DVT in Chapter 32) is one of the most common and dangerous of all complications occurring in the postoperative orthopedic patient (Bateman, Dow, Brzezinski, et al., 2017). In addition to Virchow's triad, advanced age, lower extremity orthopedic surgery, and immobilization are significant risk factors. The nurse assesses the patient daily for calf swelling, tenderness, warmth, and redness. The nurse promptly reports abnormal findings to the orthopedic surgeon.

In addition, fat embolus syndrome (FES) (see Chapter 72) may occur with orthopedic surgery. The nurse must be alert to changes in respiration, behaviour, and level of consciousness that suggest the development of fat emboli.

Nursing Priorities

Based on assessment data, the patient's major nursing priorities may include the following:

- Acute pain
- Peripheral neurovascular dysfunction
- Risk for ineffective therapeutic regimen management
- Impaired physical mobility
- Situational low self-esteem

Collaborative Problems/ Potential Complications

Based on assessment data, potential complications may include the following:

- Hypovolemic/hemorrhagic shock
- Atelectasis; pneumonia
- Urinary retention/urinary tract infection
- Wound infection
- Venous thromboembolism

Planning and Goals

The major goals for the patient after orthopedic surgery include relief of pain, adequate neurovascular function, health promotion, improved mobility, positive self-esteem, and absence of complications.

Nursing Interventions

Relieving Pain

Edema, hematomas, and muscle spasms contribute to the pain experienced in the postoperative period. Some patients report that the pain is less than that experienced preoperatively, and only moderate amounts of analgesics are needed. The nurse closely monitors the patient's pain level and response to therapeutic measures and makes every effort to manage the pain.

There are multiple pharmacologic approaches to pain management. It has been found that local infiltration analgesia can be effective in managing the patient's pain in the immediate postoperative period (Li, Qu, Pan, et al., 2018). Patient-controlled analgesia (PCA) and epidural analgesia may be prescribed to manage the pain. If intramuscular and oral analgesics are prescribed on an as-needed basis (PRN), it is preferable for the nurse to provide the medication at regular intervals. The nurse rotates intramuscular injection sites, avoiding the operative hip and thigh. The nurse may administer medications on a preventive basis within the prescribed intervals if the onset of pain can be predicted (e.g., 30 minutes before planned activity such as transfer or exercise).

In addition to pharmacologic approaches to controlling pain, elevation of the operative extremity and application of ice, if prescribed, help to control edema and pain. Portable suction of the wound decreases fluid accumulation and hematoma formation. The nurse may find that repositioning, relaxation, distraction, and guided imagery help in reducing the patient's pain.

The nurse should report increasing and unmanageable pain to the orthopedic surgeon for evaluation. After 2 to 3 days, most patients require only occasional oral analgesia for residual muscle soreness and spasm.

Maintaining Adequate Neurovascular Function

The nurse monitors the neurovascular status of the involved body part and notifies the orthopedic surgeon promptly of any indications of diminished tissue perfusion. The patient is reminded to perform muscle-setting, ankle, and calf-pumping exercises hourly while awake to enhance circulation.

Maintaining Health

It is important to encourage the patient to participate in the postoperative treatment regimen. A well-balanced diet with adequate protein and vitamins is needed for wound healing. The patient progresses to a regular diet as soon as possible. The nurse assesses the patient's skin integrity on a regular basis for pressure ulcers. Patients at risk for pressure ulcers include those who spend an extended time in bed, older adults, patients who are malnourished, and those unable to move without assistance. Turning, washing, and drying the skin and minimizing pressure over bony prominences are necessary to maintain skin integrity.

Improving Physical Mobility

It is not uncommon for patients to be reluctant to move after orthopedic surgery. They often increase their mobility once they have been reassured that movement within therapeutic limits is beneficial, that the nurse will provide assistance, and that every effort will be made to manage their postoperative pain.

Metal pins, screws, rods, and plates used for internal fixation are designed to maintain the position of the bone until ossification occurs. They are not designed to support the body's weight, and they can bend, loosen, or break if stressed. The estimated strength of the bone, the stability of the fracture, reduction and fixation, and the amount of bone healing are important considerations in determining weight-bearing limits. The incision may appear healed, but the underlying bone requires much more time to repair and regain normal strength. Some orthopedic procedures require weight-bearing restrictions. The orthopedic surgeon will prescribe the weight-bearing limits and the use of protective devices (orthoses), if necessary, after surgery.

The physical therapist tailors the exercise program to the patient's needs. The goal is the patient's return to the highest level of function in the shortest time possible. Rehabilitation involves progressive increases in the patient's activities and exercises. Assistive devices such as crutches walkers are used to assist postoperative mobility. The nurse makes sure that the patient uses these devices safely (see discussions of crutch walking and use of a walker in Chapter 13).

Maintaining Self-Esteem

The nurse and the patient set realistic goals in the postoperative period. Increased self-care activities within the limits of the therapeutic regimen and resumption of roles facilitate recognition of abilities and promote self-esteem, personal identity, and role performance. Acceptance of altered body image is facilitated by support provided by the nurse and the patient's support system.

Monitoring and Managing Potential Complications

HYPOVOLEMIC SHOCK. Excessive loss of blood during or after surgery can result in shock. The nurse monitors the patient for signs and symptoms of hypovolemic shock: increased pulse rate, decreased blood pressure, urine output less than 30 mL/hour, restlessness, change in mentation, thirst, and decreased hemoglobin and hematocrit. The nurse reports these findings to the orthopedic surgeon and assists in appropriate management. (Refer to Chapter 18 for a discussion of managing shock.)

ATELECTASIS AND PNEUMONIA. The nurse auscultates the patient's lungs and encourages deep-breathing and coughing exercises. Full expansion of the lungs prevents the accumulation of pulmonary secretions and the development of atelectasis and pneumonia. Incentive spirometry is encouraged. Signs of respiratory abnormalities such as increased respiratory rate, productive cough, diminished or adventitious breath sounds and fever should be reported to the surgeon.

URINARY RETENTION. The nurse monitors the patient's urinary output after surgery. The nurse encourages the patient to void every 3 to 4 hours to prevent urinary retention and bladder distention. It is important to provide privacy during toileting. The patient may need assistance to void in an unusual position. If the patient is unable to stand to void or sit on a toilet seat, fracture bedpans are a little more comfortable than conventional bedpans. Voiding in the side-lying position is helpful to the male patients. Some male patients have difficulty voiding in bed, in which case they will need assistance and support to stand. Intermittent catheterizations may be required until the patient is able to void independently. Indwelling urinary catheters are to be used only when absolutely necessary and should be removed as soon as possible.

INFECTION. Infection is a risk after any surgery; however, it is of particular concern for the patient who has undergone arthroplasty, as periprosthetic joint infections (PJI) are a major cause of prosthetic joint revision surgery (Ratto, Arrigoni, Rosso, et al., 2016). The incidence of PJI is 0.3% to 1.7% of all THAs and 0.8% to 1.9% of all TKAs (Kamath, Ong, Lau, et al., 2015).

At times, infected bone and prosthesis are surgically removed. It may be several months before joint revision surgery can be performed. Major preoperative risk factors for infection include morbid obesity (BMI >40 kg/m^2), poor glycemic control (HbA1c >7%), smoking (≥1 pack/day), inflammatory joint disease (e.g., rheumatoid arthritis), and chronic renal disease. Patients undergoing elective arthroplasty are routinely assessed at preoperative assessment clinic by general internal medicine specialists to mitigate the effects of the risk factors prior to surgery.

Intravenous antibiotics are given preoperatively and, on occasion, in the postoperative period. It is therefore important to use aseptic technique for dressing changes and emptying wound drain

containers. The nurse monitors the patient's vital signs, incision, and drainage.

In addition, the nurse assesses the patient for signs of other infections involving the urinary tract, lungs, the GI tract, and blood (septicemia). Osteomyelitis is an inflammation of the bone and bone marrow that is usually due to infection. A common infectious organism is *Staphylococcus aureus*. Osteomyelitis usually does not present until several months and sometimes several years after arthroplasty surgery (Tande & Patel, 2014).

VENOUS THROMBOEMBOLISM. Prophylactic anticoagulant therapy is the mainstay of reducing the risk of venous thromboembolism. It is important for patients to do ankle and calf-pumping exercises, and make use of elastic compression stockings, and sequential compression devices. Adequate hydration and early mobilization are also important. The nurse monitors the patient for signs of DVT and promptly reports findings to the orthopedic surgeon for management.

Promoting Home, Community-Based, and Transitional Care

EDUCATING THE PATIENT ABOUT SELF-CARE. The average length of stay in hospital after elective arthroplasty surgery is 3 to 5 days (El Bitar, Illingworth, Scaife, et al., 2015; Burn, Edwards, Murray, et al., 2018). Convalescence and rehabilitation take place at home or in a nonacute care setting. The nurse teaches the patient and the family to recognize postoperative complications such as wound infection or dislocation of the prosthesis. The patient must understand the prescribed medication regimen. The patient gradually resumes physical activities and adheres to weight-bearing limitations. The patient must be able to perform transfers and to use mobility aids safely. If the patient has a cast or other immobilizing device, family members should be instructed on safely assisting the patient. Specific exercises are taught and practiced before discharge. The nurse discusses recovery and health promotion, emphasizing a healthy lifestyle and diet.

CONTINUING AND TRANSITIONAL CARE. Every effort is made to have special equipment and home modifications completed before the patient is discharged home. The nurse, physical therapist, and social worker assist the patient and family in identifying their needs in preparation for care of the patient at home.

Home health nursing and physical therapy may be part of discharge planning. A follow-up appointment is arranged for 6 weeks after discharge for the patient to be seen by the orthopedic surgeon. See Chart 70-11 for home health education for the patient.

Evaluation

Expected patient outcomes may include the following:

1. Reports decreased level of pain
   a. Uses multiple approaches to manage pain
   b. Uses oral analgesia to manage pain
   c. Elevates extremity to control edema and discomfort
   d. Moves with greater comfort
2. Exhibits adequate neurovascular function
   a. Exhibits normal colour and temperature of skin with normal capillary refill (<2 seconds)
   b. Demonstrates intact sensory and motor function
   c. Demonstrates reduced swelling of affected limb
3. Promotes health
   a. Eats diet appropriate for nutritional needs and maintains hydration
   b. Abstains from smoking
   c. Practices deep breathing and coughing exercises
   d. Repositions self to relieve pressure on skin
   e. Engages in strengthening exercises
4. Maximizes mobility within therapeutic limits
   a. Requests assistance when moving
   b. Elevates edematous extremity
   c. Uses immobilizing devices
   d. Complies with weight-bearing limitations
5. Expresses positive self-esteem
   a. Discusses temporary or permanent changes in body image
   b. Discusses role performance
   c. Views self as capable of assuming responsibilities
   d. Actively participates in planning care and in therapeutic regimen
6. Experiences no postoperative complications
   a. Maintains normal vital signs
   b. Has breath sounds equal to the bases. No adventitia
   c. Demonstrates wound healing with no signs of infection
   d. Does not experience urinary retention
   e. Voids clear urine
   f. Exhibits no signs of venous thromboembolism

Critical Thinking Exercises

1 An 84-year-old woman has had an internal fixation for her fractured hip. On her second postoperative day, she complains that her elastic stockings feel tight and hot and asks you to remove them. How would you respond to this request? What is the rationale for your action? Role-play your explanation to her regarding the purpose of the stockings.

2 A 68-year-old man has had a repair of a fracture of his right tibia. During the evening of his second postoperative day, he complains of increasing pain and paresthesias of his toes. Opioid analgesics have only moderately relieved his pain. The night-shift nurse documents her findings and asks you, as the oncoming day-shift nurse, to report these findings to the orthopedic surgeon when he makes his rounds. You assess the patient after report and find that he now describes his right lower leg as "very painful." The skin on his leg is shiny, capillary refill is more than 3 seconds, and his right toes feel much cooler than the left toes. The pain is unremitting despite regular analgesia.
What condition are you most concerned about?

3 An 80-year-old woman with multiple trauma has had an ORIF of her right hip. On the second postoperative day, a physical therapy assistant helps the patient get out of bed. She has been sitting out of bed for approximately an hour and a half when she requests to be placed back in bed. What is the best way to accomplish this transfer from chair to bed? What specific precautions might you follow?

REFERENCES AND SELECTED READINGS

Books

Alisangco, J., Asplund, C., & Benjamin, H. (2016). Splinting and casting. In R. B. Birrer, F. G. O'Connor, & S. F. Kane (Eds.). *Musculoskeletal and sports medicine for the primary care practitioner* (4th ed.). Boca Raton, Florida: CRC Press.

Barker, D. M., & Murray, P. A. (2013). Orthopaedic pain. In L. Schoenly (Ed.). *Core curriculum for orthopaedic nursing* (7th ed.). Chicago, IL: National Association of Orthopaedic Nurses.

Clarke, S., & Santy-Tomlinson, J. (2014). *Orthopaedic and trauma nursing: An evidence-based approach to musculoskeletal care*. Chichester, UK: John Wiley & Sons, Ltd.

Herdman, T. H., & Kamitsuru, S. (2014). *NANDA International nursing diagnoses: Definitions and classification, 2015–17*. Oxford, UK: Wiley-Blackwell.

Hovius, S. E., & Nijhuis, T. H. (2015) Compartment syndrome in the extremities. In R. D. Farhadieh, N. W. Bulstrode, & S. Cugno (Eds.). *Plastic and reconstructive surgery: Approaches and techniques*. Chichester, UK: John Wiley & Sons, Ltd.

Karachalios, T., & Antoniou, I. (2015). Long term outcome of total knee arthroplasty. The effect of implant fixation (cementless). In T. Karachalios (Ed.). *Total knee arthroplasty*. London: Springer.

Magee, D. (2014). *Orthopedic physical assessment* (6th ed.). Philadelphia, PA: Elsevier.

Newton-Triggs, L., Pugh, H., Rogers, J., et al. (2014). Key musculoskeletal interventions. In S. Clarke., & J. Santy-Tomlinson (Eds.). *Orthopedics and nursing trauma, an evidence-based approach to musculoskeletal care*. Oxford, UK: Wiley-Blackwell.

Scott, R. (2015). *Total knee arthroplasty* (2nd ed.). Philadelphia, PA: Elsevier.

Journals and Documents

Ali, P., Santy-Tomlinson, J., & Watson, R. (2014). Assessment and diagnosis of acute limb compartment syndrome: A literature review. *International Journal of Orthopaedic and Trauma Nursing, 18*(4), 180–190.

American Academy of Orthopaedic Surgeons (AAOS). (2014). *Management of hip fractures in the elderly evidence-based clinical practice guideline*. Retrieved February 24, 2016, from www.aaos.org/research/guidelines/HipFxGuideline.pdf

American Academy of Orthopaedic Surgeons (AAOS). (2015a). *OrthoInfo. Care of casts and splints*. Retrieved February 24, 2016, from orthoinfo.aaos.org/topic.cfm?topic=A00095

American Academy of Orthopaedic Surgeons (AAOS). (2015b). *Surgical management of osteoarthritis of the knee evidence-based clinical practice guideline*. Retrieved February 24, 2016, from www.aaos.org/uploadedFiles/PreProduction/Quality/Guidelines_and_Reviews/SMOAK%20CPG__12.4.15.pdf

Baath, C., Engstrom, M., Gunningberg, L., et al. (2016). Prevention of heel pressure ulcers among older patients—from ambulance care to hospital discharge: A multi-centre randomized controlled trial. *Applied Nursing Research, 30*, 170–175.

Barnsley, L., Barnsley, L., & Page, R. (2015). Are hip precautions necessary post total hip arthroplasty? A systematic review. *Geriatric Orthopaedic Surgery & Rehabilitation, 6*(3), 230–235.

Bateman, D. K., Dow, R. W., Brzezinski, A., et al. (2017). Correlation of the Caprini score and venous thromboembolism incidence following primary total joint arthroplasty-results of a single-institution protocol. *Journal of Arthroplasty, 32*(12), 3735–3741.

Bosco, J. A., Bookman, J., Slover, J., et al. (2015). Principles of antibiotic prophylaxis in total joint arthroplasty: Current concepts. *Journal of the American Academy of Orthopaedic Surgeons, 23*(8), e27–e35.

Britten, S., Ghoz, A., Duffield, B., et al. (2013). Ilizarov fixator pin site care: The role of crusts in the prevention of infection. *Injury, 44*(10), 1275–1278.

Brown, A., Boshers, B., Chapman, L. F., et al. (2015). Do elderly patients use patient-controlled analgesia medication delivery systems correctly?. *Orthopaedic Nursing, 34*(4), 203–208.

Brubacher, J. W., Karg, J., Weinstock, P., et al. (2016). A novel cast removal training simulation to improve patient safety. *Journal of Surgical Education, 73*(1), 7–11.

Budhiparama, N. C., Abdel, M. P., Ifran, N. N., et al. (2014). Venous thromboembolism (VTE) prophylaxis for hip and knee arthroplasty: Changing trends. *Current Review of Musculoskeletal Medicine, 7*(2), 108–116.

Burn, E., Edwards, C. J., Murray, D. W., et al. (2018). Trends and determinants of length of stay and hospital reimbursement following knee and hip replacement: Evidence from linked primary care and NHS hospital records from 1997 to 2014. *BMJ Open, 8*, e019146.

Call, E., Pedersen, J., Bill, B., et al. (2015). Enhancing pressure ulcer prevention using wound dressings: What are the modes of action? *International Wound Journal, 12*(4), 408–413.

Clark, M., Black, J., Alves, P., et al. (2014). Systematic review of the use of prophylactic dressings in the prevention of pressure ulcers. *International Wound Journal, 11*(5), 460–471.

Demir, S. G., Erden, S., Bulut, H., et al. (2015). The problems experienced by parents providing postoperative home care following their child's surgery for developmental dysplasia of the hip. *Orthopaedic Nursing, 34*(5), 280–286.

Dennis, D. A, Kittleson, A. J., Yang, C. C., et al. (2016). Does tourniquet use in TKA affect recovery of lower extremity strength and function? A randomized trial. *Clinical Orthopaedics and Related Research, 474*(1), 69–77.

Dhammi, I. K., Haq, R. U., & Kumar, S. (2015). Prophylactic antibiotics in orthopedic surgery: Controversial issues in its use. *Indian journal of orthopaedics, 49*(4), 373.

Donaldson, J., Haddad, B., & Khan, W. S. (2014). The pathophysiology, diagnosis and current management of acute compartment syndrome. *Open Orthopaedic Journal, 8*, 185–193.

Draucker, C. B., Jacobson, A. F., Umberger, W. A., et al. (2015). Acceptability of a guided imagery intervention for persons undergoing a total knee replacement. *Orthopaedic Nursing, 34*(6), 356–364.

Dy, C. J., Bumpass, D. B., Makhni, E. C., et al. (2016). The evolving role of clinical registries: Existing practices and opportunities for orthopaedic surgeons. *The Journal of Bone & Joint Surgery, 98*(2), e7.

El Bitar, Y. F., Illingworth, K. D., Scaife, S. L., et al. (2015). Hospital length of stay following primary total knee arthroplasty: Data from the nationwide inpatient sample database. *Journal of Arthroplasty, 30*(10), 1710–1715.

Garner, M. R., Taylor, S. A. Gausden, E., et al. (2014). Compartment syndrome: Diagnosis, management, and unique concerns in the twenty-first century. *HSSJ: The Musculoskeletal Journal of Hospital for Special Surgery, 10*(2), 143–152.

Gebhart, T. (2015). Superior mesenteric artery syndrome. *Gastroenterology Nursing, 38*(3), 189–193.

Hajbaghery, M. A., & Moradi, T. (2013). Quality of care for patients with traction in Shahid Beheshti Hospital in 2012. *Archives of Trauma Research, 2*(2), 85–90.

Hanna-Bull, D. (2015). Preventing heel pressure ulcers: Sustained quality improvement initiative in a Canadian acute care facility. *Journal of Wound, Ostomy and Continence Nursing, 43*(2), 129–132.

Hazel, D., Bern, J., Bono, J., et al. (2015). Effect of preoperative autologous blood donation coupled with fluid resuscitation on transfusion requirements following orthopedic surgery. *Journal of Hematology, 4*(2), 157–163.

Hickey, B. A., Morgan, A., Pugh, N., et al. (2014). The effect of lower limb cast immobilization on calf muscle pump function: A simple strategy of exercises can maintain flow. *Foot & Ankle International, 35*(5), 429–433.

Horn, P. L., & Badowski, E. (2015). To improve nurses' knowledge base and increase their comfort level when caring for patients in a spica cast. *Orthopaedic Nursing, 34*(6), 334–337.

Jennison, T., McNally, M., & Pandit. H. (2014). Prevention of infection in external fixator pin sites. *Acta Biomaterialia, 10*(2), 595–603.

Jevsevar, D. S., Cummins, D. S., Azar, F. M., et al. (2015). One size does not fit all: Involve orthopaedic implant patients in deciding whether to use prophylactic antibiotics with dental procedures. *Journal of the American Academy of Orthopaedic Surgeons, 23*(3), 141–142.

Kamath, A. F., Ong, K. L., Lau, E., et al. (2015). Quantifying the burden of revision total joint arthroplasty for periprosthetic infection. *Journal of Arthroplasty*, *30*(9), 1492–1497.

Kazmers, N. H., Fragomen, A. T., & Rozbruch, S. R. (2016). Prevention of pin site infection in external fixation: A review of the literature. *Strategies in Trauma and Limb Reconstruction*, *11*(2), 75–85.

Khan, M., Osman, K., Green, G., et al. (2016). The epidemiology of failure in total knee arthroplasty avoiding your next revision. *Bone & Joint Journal*, *98*(1), 105–112.

Kneedler, J. A., Moss, R., Pfister, J. I., et al. (2015). Wound drainage systems in perioperative nursing. Retrieved May 9, 2015, from www.pfiedler.com/ce/1200/files/assets/common/downloads/Wound%20Drain%20Systems%20in%20Perioperative%20Nursing.pdf

Korean Knee Society. (2012). Guidelines for the management of postoperative pain after total knee arthroplasty. *Knee Surgery and Related Research*, *24*(4), 201–207.

Ktistakisa, J., Gueradob, E., & Giannoudis, P. V. (2015). Pin-site care: Can we reduce the incidence of infections? *Injury*, *46*(3), S35–S39.

Lee, G. C. (2016). What's new in adult reconstructive knee surgery. *Journal of Bone & Joint Surgery American*, *98*(2), 156–165.

Lethaby, A., Temple, J., & Santy-Tomlinson, J. (2013). Pin site care for preventing infections associated with external bone fixators and pins. *Cochrane Database of Systematic Reviews*, (12):CD004551. doi: 10.1002/14651858.CD004551.pub3.

Levin, B., & Morris, N. (2013). *Practice points: Pressure ulcer. National Association of Orthopaedic Nurses*. Retrieved May 24, 2016, from www.orthonurse.org/p/do/sd/sid=1140&type=0

Li, C., Qu, J., Pan, S, et al. (2018). Local infiltration anesthesia versus epidural analgesia for postoperative pain control in total knee arthroplasty: A systematic review and meta-analysis. *Journal of Orthopaedic Surgery and Research*, *13*(1), 112.

Lieberman, J. R., & Pensak, M. J. (2013). Prevention of venous thromboembolic disease after total hip and knee arthroplasty. *Journal of Bone & Joint Surgery American*, *95*(19), 1801–1811.

Liu, D., Dan, M., & Adivi, N. (2015). Blood conservation strategies in total hip and knee arthroplasty. *Reconstructive Review*, *4*(4), 39–45.

Loftus, T. J., Spratling, L., Stone, B. A., et al. (2016). A patient blood management program in prosthetic joint arthroplasty decreases blood use and improves outcomes. *The Journal of Arthroplasty*, *31*(1), 11–14.

Louw, A., Diener, I., Butler, D. S., et al. (2013). Preoperative education addressing postoperative pain in total joint arthroplasty: Review of content and educational delivery methods. *Physiotherapy Theory and Practice*, *29*(3), 175–194.

McHugh, S. M., Hill, A. D., & Humphreys, H. (2015). Laminar airflow and the prevention of surgical site infection. More harm than good? *Surgeon*, *13*(1), 52–58.

Meiri, R., Rosenbaum, T. Y., & Kalichman, L. (2014). Sexual function before and after total hip replacement: Narrative review. *Sexual Medicine*, *2*(4), 159–167.

Miller, A., & Walsh, C. (2015). *Clinical practice guideline thromboembolic disease prevention. National Association of Orthopaedic Nurses*. Retrieved May 24, 2016, from www.orthonurse.org/p/do/vi/sid=2254

Mohanty, S., Rosenthal, R. A., Russell, M. M., et al. (2016). Optimal perioperative management of the geriatric patient: A best practices guideline from the American College of Surgeons NSQIP and the American Geriatrics Society. *Journal of the American College of Surgeons*, *222*(5), 930–947.

Mullaji, A., & Shetty, G. (2015). Cemented total knee arthroplasty remains the "gold standard." *Seminars in Arthroplasty*, *26*(2), 62–64.

National Association of Orthopedic Nurses (NAON). (2014). *NAON position statement: Preventing infection in the inpatient orthopaedic patient*. Retrieved May 24, 2016, from www.orthonurse.org/p/do/sd/sid=1601&type=0

Oron, A., Lindner, D., Bergman, A., et al. (2013). Molding significantly affects the mechanical properties of plaster of Paris in orthopaedic use. *Current Orthopaedic Practice*, *24*(6), 647–650.

Orthopaedic patient education resources. http://coa-aco.org/for-patients/patient-education-resources

Osmon, D. R., Berbari, E. F., Berendt, A. R., et al. (2013). Diagnosis and management of prosthetic joint infection: Clinical practice guidelines by the Infectious Diseases Society of America. *Clinical Infectious Diseases*, *56*(1), e1–e25.

Park, J. H., Rasouli, M. R., Mortazavi, S. M., et al. (2013). Predictors of perioperative blood loss in total joint arthroplasty. *The Journal of Bone & Joint Surgery American*, *95*(19), 1777–1783.

Patel, K., & Chun, B. E. (2017). What is the Virchow Triad? *Medscape*. https://www.medscape.com/answers/1911303-22988/what-is-the-virchow-triad

Pechar, J., & Lyons, M. M. (2016). Acute compartment syndrome of the lower leg: A review. *The Journal for Nurse Practitioners*, *12*(4), 265–270.

Qaseem, A., Mir, T. P., Starkey, M., et al. (2015). Risk assessment and prevention of pressure ulcers: A clinical practice guideline from the American College of Physicians. *Annals of Internal Medicine*, *162*, 359–369.

Rasouli, M. R., Maltenfort, M. G., Erkocak, O. F., et al. (2016). Blood management after total joint arthroplasty in the United States: 19 year trend analysis. *Transfusion*, *56*(5), 1112–1120.

Ratto, N., Arrigoni, C., Rosso, F., et al. (2016). Total knee arthroplasty and infection: How surgeons can reduce the risks. *EFORT Open Review*, *1*, 339–344.

Ruda, S. (2013). NAON practice points: Fat embolism syndrome. Retrieved May 24, 2016, from www.orthonurse.org/p/do/sd/sid=875&type=0

Shan, L., Shan, B., Suzuki, A., et al. (2015). Intermediate and long-term quality of life after total knee replacement. *Journal of Bone & Joint Surgery American*, *97*(2), 156–168.

Smith, M., & Smith, T. (2012). The American joint replacement registry. *Orthopaedic Nursing*, *31*(5), 296–299.

Smith, M. A., & Dahlen, N. R. (2013). Clinical practice guideline surgical site infection prevention. *Orthopaedic Nursing*, *32*(5), 242–248.

Sollecito, T. P., Abt, E., Lockhart, P. B., et al. (2015). The use of prophylactic antibiotics prior to dental procedures in patients with prosthetic joints: Evidence-based clinical practice guideline for dental practitioners—a report of the American Dental Association Council on Scientific Affairs. *The Journal of the American Dental Association*, *146*(1), 11–16.

Suggs, S., & Holt, K. (2015). The use of tranexamic acid in joint replacement surgery. *Orthopaedic Nursing*, *34*(2), 89–92.

Tabor, D. (2013). An empirical study using range of motion and pain score as determinants for continuous passive motion: Outcomes following total knee replacement surgery in an adult population. *Orthopaedic Nursing*, *32*(5), 261–265.

Tande, A. J., & Patel, R. (2014). Prosthetic joint infection. *Clinical microbiology reviews*, *27*(2), 302–345.

Thomas, K., Barrett, B., Tupper, R., et al. (2014). Pain management after total knee arthroplasty: A case–control study of continuous nerve block therapy. *Orthopaedic Nursing*, *33*(5), 268–276.

Thrombosis Canada. (2018). http://thrombosiscanada.ca/guides/pdfs/ThromboprophylaxisOrthopedic_Surgery.pdf

Tsang, L. F. (2015). Developing an evidence-based nursing protocol on wound drain management for total joint arthroplasty. *International Journal of Orthopaedic and Trauma Nursing*, *19*(2), 61–73.

Tsang, L. F., Cheng, H. C., Ho, H. S., et al. (2016). Translating evidence-based protocol of wound drain management for total joint arthroplasty into practice: A quasi-experimental study. *International Journal of Orthopaedic and Trauma Nursing*, *21*, 49–61.

Turney, J., Noble, D., & Kim, S. C. (2013). Orthopaedic nurses' knowledge and interrater reliability of neurovascular assessments with 2-point discrimination test. *Orthopaedic Nursing*, *32*(3), 167–172.

Unver, B., Karatosun, V., & Tuncali, B. (2013). Effects of tourniquet pressure on rehabilitation outcomes in patients undergoing total knee arthroplasty. *Orthopaedic Nursing*, *32*(4), 217–222.

van der Weegen, W., Kornuijt, A., & Das, D. (2016). Do lifestyle restrictions and precautions prevent dislocation after total hip arthroplasty? A systematic review and meta-analysis of the literature. *Clinical Rehabilitation*, *30*(4), 329–339.

Vanderbeck, K. (2013). NAON practice points: Acute pain management. Retrieved May 24, 2016, from www.orthonurse.org/p/do/sd/sid=1542&type=0

Wilson, R. A., Watt-Watson, J., Hodnett, E., et al. (2016). A randomized controlled trial of an individualized preoperative education intervention for symptom management after total knee arthroplasty. *Orthopaedic Nursing*, *35*(1), 20–29.

Wittig-Wells, D., Higgins, M., Davis, E., et al. (2015). Impact of a focused approach for discharge teaching regarding the use of aspirin as anticoagulant after joint replacement surgery. *Orthopaedic Nursing*, *34*(4), 211–220.

Wu, C. T., Chen, I. L., Wang, J. W., et al. (2016). Surgical site infection following total knee arthroplasty: Risk factors in patients with timely administration of systemic prophylactic antibiotics. *The Journal of Arthroplasty*, *31*(7), 1568–1573.

Yager, M., & Stichler, J. (2015). The effect of early ambulation on patient outcomes for total joint replacement. *Orthopaedic Nursing*, *34*(4), 197–200.

Yaping, X., Jing, Z., & Yuzhao, C. (2018). Prevention of venous thromboembolism in patients undergoing major orthopedic surgery in China: A qualitative study of patients' perceptions. *Journal of Orthopaedic Surgery and Research*, *13*(98), 1–5.

Zhang, Y. (2015). The perioperative nursing of treating the elderly patients of femoral intertrochanteric fracture with PFNA. *Journal of Nursing*, *4*(1), 1–4.

Zhou, X., Tao, L., Li, J., et al. (2013). Do we really need tranexamic acid in total hip arthroplasty? A meta-analysis of nineteen randomized controlled trials. *Archives of Orthopaedic and Trauma Surgery*, *133*(7), 1017–1027.

Resources

A patient's guide to total joint replacement and complete care. Cleveland Clinic: https://my.clevelandclinic.org/ccf/media/Files/Ortho/patient-education/total-joint-replacement-patient-guide.pdf?la=en

Canadian Institutes of Health Research, Institute of Musculoskeletal Health and Arthritis: http://www.cihr-irsc.gc.ca/e/13217.html

Canadian Orthopaedic Association: http://www.coa-aco.org/

Canadian Orthopaedic Foundation: http://www.canorth.org/

Canadian Orthopaedic Nurses Association: http://www.cona-nurse.org/

Cast care: Do's and don'ts. Mayo Clinic: https://www.mayoclinic.org/healthy-lifestyle/childrens-health/in-depth/cast-care/art-20047159

National Association of Orthopaedic Nurses (NAON): http://www.orthonurse.org/

National Institute of Arthritis and Musculoskeletal and Skin Diseases: http://www.niams.nih.gov/

Thrombo prophylaxis: Orthopedic Surgery (2018): https://thrombosiscanada.ca/clinicalguides/# http://thrombosiscanada.ca/wp-content/uploads/2018/03/Thromboprophylaxis-Orthopedic-2018Feb21-Final.pdf

Venous thromboembolism: https://www.canvector.ca/venous-thrombo-embolism

71 Management of Patients With Musculoskeletal Disorders

Adapted by James A. Rankin and Karen Lynn Then

Learning Objectives

On completion of this chapter, the learner will be able to:

1. Use the nursing process as a framework for care of the patient with musculoskeletal disorders.
2. Describe rehabilitation and health education needs of the patient with low back pain; pharmacologic therapy for Paget's disease; and causes and medical management of osteomalacia.
3. Describe conditions of the upper extremities and nursing care of the patient undergoing surgery of the hand or wrist.
4. Use the nursing process as a framework for care of the patient undergoing foot surgery.
5. Explain the pathophysiology, pathogenesis, prevention, and management of osteoporosis.
6. Identify the causes and related medical management of osteomalacia.
7. Describe the medication therapy program for the patient with Paget's disease.
8. Use the nursing process as a framework for care of the patient with osteomyelitis.
9. Use the nursing process as a framework for care of the patient with a bone tumour.

Musculoskeletal disorders constitute major health problems and causes of disability. The onset of these disorders usually occurs during an adult's most productive years of life. Musculoskeletal diseases are second only to cardiovascular diseases in terms of cost to the Canadian health care system. Examples of direct health care costs are remuneration of health professionals, supplies, and service-related equipment costs. Indirect costs are those associated with loss of work, worker replacement, and decreased productivity due to disease. In addition, the limitations imposed on individuals are severe, and the economic cost, in terms of loss of productivity, medical expenses, and other costs that are not compensated, is in the billions of dollars.

Acute Low Back Pain

The International Association for the Study of Pain (IASP) has defined chronic pain as lasting for a long period that persists beyond the usual time of healing and has no identifiable cause (IASP, 1986; Treede, 2018). For the purpose of the International Classification of Diseases (ICD) coding system, this was pragmatically defined as pain that persists or recurs for more than 12 weeks. In contrast, acute low back pain is defined as pain lasting 1 to 4 weeks. Pain that lasts longer than 6 weeks raises a "red flag" as 80% to 90% of all episodes of low back pain resolve within 6 weeks.

The number of medical visits resulting from low back pain is second only to the number of visits for upper respiratory illnesses. In the primary care setting, the cause of low back pain cannot be attributed to a specific disease or spinal abnormality in more than 85% of patients. Typically, patients have significant improvement after the first month of presentation. Most low back pain is caused by one of many musculoskeletal problems, including acute lumbosacral strain, unstable lumbosacral ligaments, weak muscles, osteoarthritis, spinal stenosis, intervertebral disc degeneration, inflammatory spondyloarthropathies, and unequal leg length.

Older patients may experience back pain associated with osteoporotic vertebral fractures or bone metastases. Other causes include pregnancy, kidney disorders, pelvic conditions, retroperitoneal tumours, abdominal aneurysms, and psychosomatic problems.

In addition, obesity, stress, and occasionally depression may contribute to low back pain. Mechanical back pain is usually aggravated by activity, whereas pain due to inflammatory conditions is worse at night. Individuals with chronic low back pain are at risk of developing a dependence on alcohol or analgesics in an attempt to cope and self-treat the pain. In patients who have had low back pain for more than 6 weeks, the nurse should be aware of the possibility of serious spine pathology. Indicators of serious pathology are known as low back pain "red flags." In the setting of pain for more than 6 weeks, red flags according to Williams, Henschke, Maher, et al. (2013) include:

- Pain in patients younger than 18 years or older than 50 years (e.g., ankylosing spondylitis, spinal stenosis from degenerative disc disease)
- Pain continuing to radiate below the knee (e.g., spinal cord compression)
- History of trauma or malignancy
- Constitutional symptoms—fever, chills, night sweats, weight loss (e.g., infection, malignancy)
- Unrelenting pain (e.g., malignancy)
- Pain at night or that is unrelenting (e.g., inflammatory spondyloarthropathy, malignancy)
- Severe or rapidly progressive neurologic deficit (e.g., cauda equina syndrome)
- Urinary and/or fecal incontinence (e.g., severe cord compression)

Pathophysiology

The spinal column can be thought of as an elastic rod constructed of rigid units (vertebrae) and flexible units (intervertebral discs) held together by complex facet joints, multiple ligaments, and paravertebral muscles. The unique construction allows for flexibility while providing maximum protection for the spinal cord. The muscles of the torso stabilize the spine. The abdominal and thoracic muscles are recruited in lifting activities. Obesity, poor posture, structural degeneration, and overstretching of the spinal support tissue result in back pain (Grossman & Porth, 2014).

There are 24 intervertebral discs in the human spine that separate and cushion the spinal vertebrae. The discs are tough fibrocartilage that consists of a matrix of chondrocytes and collagen fibres. The outer part of the disc, known as the annulus fibrosis (fibrous ring), is made of concentric sheets of collagen. The inner core of the disc, known as the nucleus pulposus, comprises a mucoprotein gel of water and loosely arranged collagen.

As we age, the gel gradually dessicates leading to degenerative disc disease and the shock-absorbing capability of the discs decreases. The outer layer of annulus fibrosus also deteriorates with age, weakens, and may tear. In individuals who lift and twist their lumbar spine, part of the nucleus pulposus may bulge out beyond the annulus fibrosus and compress a spinal nerve root (radiculopathy). This is known as a herniated disc, colloquially termed a "slipped disc." However, it is important to appreciate that although the disc can be compressed, torn, and stretched, it cannot "slip" out from between two vertebrae as it is firmly and tightly attached to the bony structures (Grossman & Porth, 2014). The lumbar discs at L4–L5 and L5–S1 are subject to the greatest mechanical stress and the greatest degenerative changes. Management of intervertebral disc disease is discussed in Chapter 65.

Clinical Manifestations

The patient complains of either acute back pain (0 to 4 weeks) or chronic back pain (lasting more than 3 months without improvement) and fatigue. The patient may report pain radiating from the spine along the distribution of a nerve. **Radiculopathy** occurs where there is significant pressure on one or more nerve roots as they exit the spine. **Myelopathy** refers to any neurologic symptoms due to disease or injury to the spinal cord. It is important to note that, on occasion, myelopathy may be accompanied by radiculopathy.

A common presentation of radiculopathy is pressure on the sciatic nerve root at L5 causing pain in the lumbar spine radiating to the foot, also known as **sciatica**. The patient's gait, spinal mobility, reflexes, leg length, leg motor strength, and sensory perception may be altered. Physical examination may disclose paravertebral muscle spasm (greatly increased muscle tone of the back postural muscles) with a loss of the normal lumbar curve (lordosis) and possible spinal deformity.

Assessment and Diagnostic Findings

One of the most comprehensive overviews for the assessment and management of acute low back pain is the *Clinic on Low-Back Pain in Interdisciplinary Practice* (CLIP) guidelines (Rossignol et al., 2007).

Glossary

bursitis: inflammation of a fluid-filled sac in a joint
contracture: abnormal shortening of muscle or fibrosis of joint structures
involucrum: new bone growth around a sequestrum
myelopathy: any neurologic condition affecting the spinal cord; in inflammatory conditions, it is known as myelitis
radiculopathy: compression, inflammation, or injury to a spinal nerve root
sciatica: sciatic nerve pain; pain travels down back of thigh into foot
sequestrum: dead bone in abscess cavity
tenosynovitis: inflammation of a tendon and its sheath; occurs most commonly in hands and feet

CHART 71-1

Diagnostic Procedures for Low Back Pain

X-ray of the spine: may demonstrate a fracture, dislocation, infection, osteoarthritis, or scoliosis
Bone scan and blood studies: may disclose infections, tumours, and bone marrow abnormalities
Computed tomography (CT scan): useful in identifying underlying problems, such as obscure soft tissue lesions adjacent to the vertebral column and problems of vertebral discs
Magnetic resonance imaging (MRI): visualization of location of spinal pathology
Electromyogram (EMG) and nerve conduction studies: used to evaluate spinal nerve root disorders (radiculopathies)

The initial evaluation of acute low back pain includes a focused history and physical examination, including general observation of the patient, back examination, and neurologic testing (reflexes, sensory impairment, straight-leg raising, muscle strength, and muscle atrophy). The findings may suggest nonspecific back symptoms, sciatica, spinal fracture, cancer, infection, inflammation, or rapidly progressing neurologic deficit.

Diagnostic procedures described in Chart 71-1 are indicated for the patient with potentially serious or prolonged low back pain. The nurse prepares the patient for these studies, provides the necessary support during the testing period, and monitors the patient for any adverse responses to the procedures.

Medical Management

Most back pain is self-limited and resolves within 4 to 6 weeks with analgesics, rest, and avoidance of strain. Based on initial assessment findings indicating nonspecific back symptoms, the patient is reassured that the pain is not due to a serious condition and x-rays or other imaging modalities are not necessary (American Board of Internal Medicine [ABIM], 2015). Management focuses on relief of discomfort, activity modification, and patient education. The presence of other medical problems complicates the picture and has higher cost, less favourable outcomes, and more long-term disability (Schaafsma, Anema, & van der Beek, 2015).

Nonprescription analgesics such as nonsteroidal anti-inflammatory drugs (NSAIDs) and short-term prescription muscle relaxants (e.g., cyclobenzaprine [Flexeril]) are effective in relieving acute low back pain, but no one medication is considered superior to another (Michigan Quality Improvement Consortium [MQIC], 2016a). Tricyclic antidepressants (e.g., amitriptyline [Elavil]) and the dual-action serotonin–norepinephrine reuptake inhibitors (e.g., duloxetine [Cymbalta]) (National Institute of Neurological Disorders [NINDS], 2014) or atypical anticonvulsant medications (e.g., gabapentin [Neurontin], which is prescribed for pain from radiculopathy) are used effectively in chronic low back pain. Opioid medications are indicated only short term for acute moderate to severe cases of low back pain, except in older adults, those with kidney disease, or those who must avoid chronic NSAID exposure because of its adverse gastric effects. Systemic corticosteroids and acetaminophen (Tylenol) are not effective in alleviating low back pain (Morgan, Dhruva, Wright, et al., 2015).

Effective nonpharmacologic interventions include thermal applications (hot or cold) and spinal manipulation (e.g., chiropractic therapy). Lumbar support belts are not recommended to treat acute low back pain but may be marginally effective devices for preventing low back pain in occupational health settings (MQIC, 2016a). Orthopedic shoe inserts are not recommended for prevention, but may help correct an underlying issue contributing to the problem (e.g., unequal leg length). Cognitive–behavioural therapy (e.g., biofeedback), exercise regimens, spinal manipulation, physical therapy, acupuncture, massage, and yoga are all effective nonpharmacologic interventions for treating chronic low back pain (Schaafsma et al., 2015).

Most patients need to alter their activity patterns to avoid aggravating the pain. They should avoid twisting, bending, lifting, and reaching—all of which stress the back. The patient is taught to change position frequently. Sitting should be limited to 20 to 50 minutes based on level of comfort. Absolute bed rest is no longer recommended; typical activities of daily living (ADLs) should be resumed as soon as possible. A quick return to normal activities and a program of low-stress aerobic exercise are recommended (MQIC, 2016a). Conditioning exercises for both back and trunk muscles are begun after about 2 weeks to help prevent recurrence of pain.

Nursing Process

The Patient With Acute Low Back Pain

Assessment

Observation of the patient's posture, position changes, and gait should be done. Often, the patient's movements are guarded, with the back kept as still as possible. The patient often selects a chair of standard seat height with arms for support. The patient may sit and stand in an unusual position, leaning away from the most painful side, and may ask for assistance when undressing for the physical examination.

It is important to obtain an accurate description of the location, severity, duration, characteristic (e.g., dull, sharp, burning), and radiation together with any associated weakness in the legs. It is also important to determine if the pain is worse with activity, after activity, or at night when resting. Descriptions of how the pain occurred—with a specific action (e.g., opening a garage door) or with an activity in which weak muscles were overused (e.g., weekend gardening)—and how the patient has dealt with the pain often suggest areas for intervention and patient teaching.

CHART 71-2

Health Promotion: Strategies for Preventing Acute Low Back Pain

Prevention

- Weight reduction as needed: Modify diet to achieve ideal body weight
- Avoid high heels
- Walk daily and gradually increase the distance and pace of walking
- Avoid jumping and jarring activities
- Stretch to enhance flexibility. Do strengthening exercises

Body Mechanics

- Practice good posture
- Avoid twisting, lifting above waist level, and reaching up for any length of time
- Push objects rather than pull them
- Keep load close to your body when lifting
- Lift with the large leg muscles, not the back muscles
- Squat while keeping the back straight when it is necessary to pick something up off the floor
- Bend your knees and tighten abdominal muscles when lifting
- Avoid overreaching or a forward flexion position
- Use a wide base of support

Work Modifications

- Adjust height of chair using a footstool to position knees higher than hips
- Adjust height of work area to avoid stress on back
- Avoid bending, twisting, and lifting heavy objects
- Avoid prolonged standing and repetitive tasks
- Avoid work involving continuous vibrations
- Use lumbar support in straight back chair with armrests
- When standing for any length of time, rest one foot on a small stool or box to relieve lumbar lordosis

The patient is assessed using the OPQRST approach to pain assessment:

O nset—Sudden, gradual
P rovocation/Palliation—What makes the pain better or worse?
Q uality—How would you describe the pain (stabbing, throbbing, dull ache)?
R adiation/Region—Does the pain radiate (chest to jaw and left arm)? Is it localized to one area?
S everity—Rate the pain on a scale of 1 to 10; 10 is the worst pain ever. Does the pain vary in intensity?
T iming—Is the pain constant or intermittent? How long does it last? Is it worse in the morning or during the night? What were you doing when it happened? Does it happen after a meal?

If back pain is a recurrent problem, information about previous successful pain management methods helps in planning current management. The nurse also asks how the back pain affects the patient's lifestyle. Assess work and recreational activities in relation to health education, as stress and anxiety can induce muscle spasms and pain. It is important to determine the effect of any limitations in movement on activities of daily living (ADLs).

In addition, the nurse assesses the effect of acute pain on the emotional well-being of the patient, work situations, and family relationships. Referral to an acute pain service nurse clinician for assessment and management of stressors contributing to the low back pain and related depression may be appropriate.

On physical examination, the nurse assesses the spine (cervical concavity, thoracic convexity, and lumbar concavity), any leg length discrepancy, iliac crest, and shoulder symmetry. The nurse palpates the paraspinal muscles and notes spasm and tenderness. The paraspinal muscles relax and spasm decreases with the patient in a prone position. The nurse assesses range of motion of the spine (flexion, extension, lateral flexion, and rotation). The nurse also evaluates nerve involvement by assessing deep tendon reflexes, sensations (e.g., paresthesia), and muscle strength. With the patient supine, the nurse passively flexes the patient's hip with the knee extended (commonly known as a straight-leg raise). If this manoeuvre provokes pain, then this might suggest nerve root involvement.

Nursing Priorities

Major nursing priorities include the following:

- Acute low back pain
- Impaired physical mobility
- The need for patient education related to proper body mechanics
- Low self-esteem
- Poor nutritional status
- Obesity

Planning and Goals

The major goals for the patient are pain management, improved physical mobility, the proper use of body mechanics, physical therapy for spinal and abdominal muscle strengthening, improved self-esteem, and weight reduction (Chart 71-2).

Nursing Interventions

Managing Pain

The nurse assesses the patient's response to medications such as acetaminophen, oral and topical NSAIDs, opioid analgesics, and adjuvant medications (e.g., nortriptyline). As the acute pain subsides, medications are reduced as prescribed. The nurse encourages the patient to reduce stress on the paravertical muscles and to change position frequently. Patients are taught to manage pain through behavioural therapies that reduce muscular and psychological tension. Diaphragmatic breathing and relaxation help to reduce muscle tension contributing to low back pain. Diverting the patient's attention from the pain to another activity (e.g., reading, conversation, watching television) may be helpful in some instances. Guided imagery, in which the relaxed patient learns to focus on a pleasant event, may be used along with other pain relief strategies (Chart 71-2).

Self-applied intermittent heat or cold may reduce the pain. The nurse evaluates and notes the patient's response to various pain management modalities.

Improving Physical Mobility

The nurse assesses the patient's movement and posture. As the pain subsides, self-care activities are resumed with minimal strain on the injured area. Position changes should be made slowly and carried out with assistance. Twisting and jarring motions are avoided. The nurse encourages the patient to alternate lying, sitting, and walking activities frequently and advises the patient to avoid sitting, standing, or walking for long periods. Sitting in a chair with armrests to support body weight with a soft support at the small of the back provides comfort.

With severe pain, the patient limits activity for 1 to 2 days. Extended periods of inactivity are not effective and result in deconditioning. The patient rests in bed on a firm mattress (a bed board may be used). Lumbar flexion is increased by elevating the head and thorax 30 degrees using pillows or a foam wedge and slightly flexing the knees supported on a pillow. Alternatively, the patient assumes a lateral position with knees and hips flexed (curled position) with a pillow between the knees and legs and a pillow supporting the head (Fig. 71-1). A prone position is avoided because it accentuates lordosis. The nurse instructs the patient to get out of bed by rolling to one side and placing the legs down while pushing the torso up, keeping the spine straight.

Low-stress aerobic exercises, such as short walks or swimming, are gradually introduced. After 2 weeks, conditioning exercises for the abdominal and trunk muscles are started. The physical therapist designs an exercise program for the patient to reduce lordosis, increase flexibility, and reduce strain on the spine. The program involves hyperextension exercises to strengthen the paravertebral muscles, flexion exercises to increase spinal range of motion, and isometric flexion exercises to strengthen trunk muscles. Each exercise period begins with relaxation. Exercise begins twice a day and increases as the patient recovers. Activities should not cause excessive lumbar strain, twisting, or discomfort; for example, activities such as horseback riding and weight lifting are avoided.

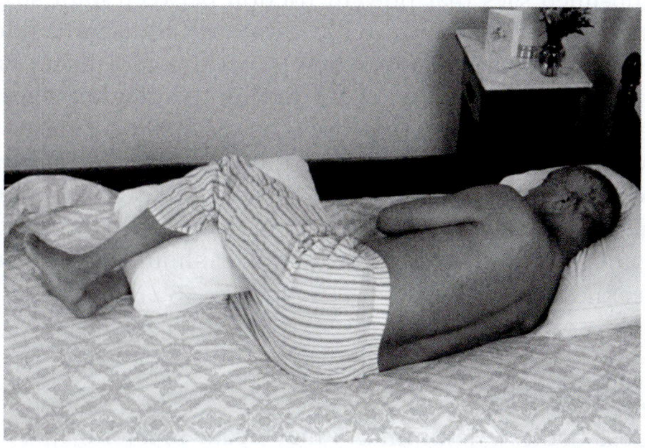

FIGURE 71-1. Positioning to promote lumbar flexion. (© B. Proud.)

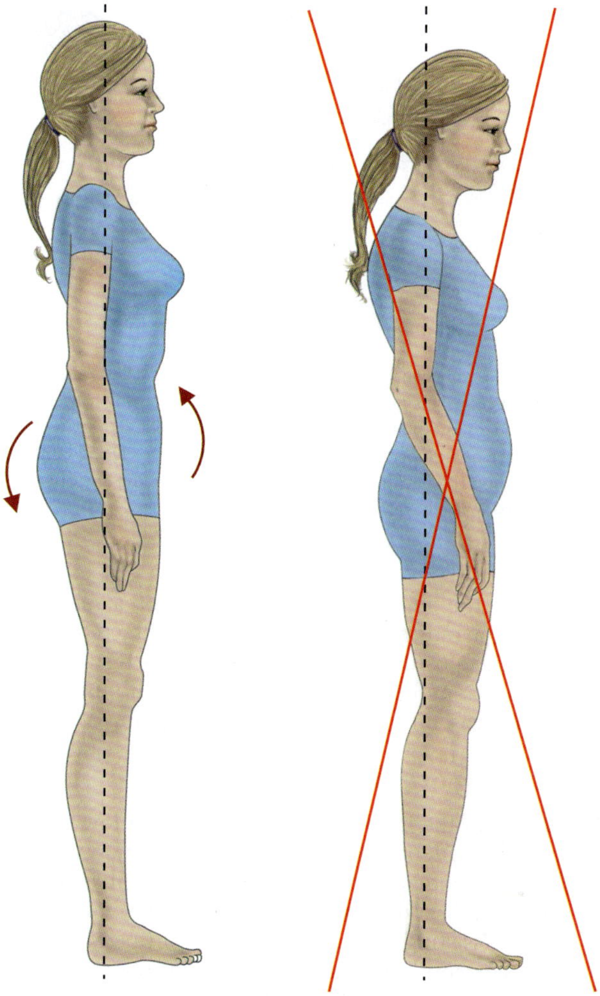

FIGURE 71-2. Proper and improper standing postures. (**Left**) Abdominal muscles contracted, giving a feeling of upward pull, and gluteal muscles contracted, giving a downward pull. (**Right**) Slouch position, showing abdominal muscles relaxed and body out of proper alignment.

Using Proper Body Mechanics

Proper body mechanics and posture are essential to avoid recurrence of back pain. The patient must be taught how to stand, sit, lie, and lift properly (Figs. 71-2 and 71-3). The patient should shift weight frequently and rest one foot on a low stool, which decreases lumbar lordosis. The proper posture and alignment can be verified by looking in a mirror. Locking the knees when standing and bending forward for long periods should be avoided.

When the patient is sitting, the knees and hips should be flexed, and the knees should be level with the hips to minimize lordosis; the feet should be flat on the floor. The patient should sleep on the side with knees and hips flexed or supine with knees supported in a flexed position. Sleeping prone should be avoided.

The patient should use the strong quadriceps muscles rather that the weaker paravertebral muscles of the spine for lifting. With feet placed shoulder width apart to provide a wide base of support, the patient bends the knees, tightens the abdominal muscles,

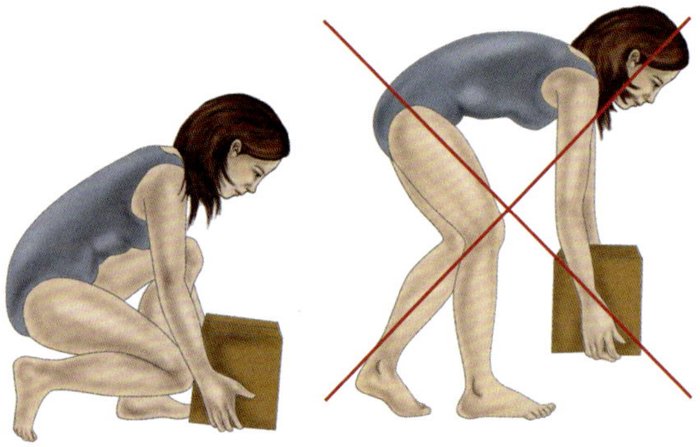

FIGURE 71-3. Proper and improper lifting techniques. (**Left**) Correct position for lifting. This person is using the long and strong muscles of the arms and legs and holding the object so that the line of gravity falls within the base of support. (**Right**) Incorrect position for lifting because pull is exerted on the back muscles, and leaning causes the line of gravity to fall outside the base.

and lifts the object close to the body with a smooth motion, avoiding twisting and jerking. Practicing protective postures, and body mechanics results in natural strengthening of the paravertebral muscles and decreased recurrence of low back pain.

Improving Self-Esteem

Because of the immobility associated with low back pain, the patient may depend on others to do various tasks. Dependency may continue beyond physiologic needs and become a way to fulfill psychosocial needs. Assisting the patient and support people to recognize continued dependency helps the patient identify and cope with the underlying reason for the dependency.

Role-related responsibilities may have been modified with the onset of low back pain. As recovery from acute low back pain and mobility progresses, the patient should cautiously resume their former ADLs.

The patient may need help in coping with specific stressors and in learning how to control stressful situations. When people successfully deal with stress, they develop confidence in their abilities to manage other stressful situations. Psychotherapy or counselling may be needed to assist the person in resuming a full, productive life. Back clinics use multidisciplinary approaches to help the patient with pain and with resumption of role-related responsibilities.

Modifying Nutrition for Weight Reduction

Obesity contributes to back strain by stressing the relatively weak back muscles. Exercises are less effective and more difficult to perform when the patient is overweight. Weight reduction through diet modification may prevent recurrence of back pain. Weight reduction is based on a sound nutritional plan that includes a change in eating habits to maintain a desirable weight. Monitoring weight reduction, noting achievement, and providing encouragement and positive reinforcement facilitate adherence. Frequently, back problems resolve as normal weight is achieved.

Evaluation

Expected patient outcomes may include the following:

1. Experiences pain relief
   a. Rests and changes positions comfortably
   b. Obtains adequate pain management through the use of physical modalities, psychological techniques, and medications
   c. Avoids drug dependency
2. Demonstrates resumption of physical mobility
   a. Resumes activities
   b. Avoids positions that cause pain and muscle spasm
   c. Plans recumbent rest periods throughout the day
3. Demonstrates back-conserving body mechanics
   a. Improves posture
   b. Positions self to minimize stress on back
   c. Demonstrates use of good body mechanics
   d. Participates in exercise program
4. Resumes role-related responsibilities
   a. Uses coping techniques to deal with stressful situations
   b. Demonstrates decreased dependence on others for self-care
   c. Resumes role responsibilities as low back pain resolves
   d. Resumes a full, productive lifestyle
5. Achieves weight loss
   a. Sets realistic goals
   b. Participates in development of weight reduction plan
   c. Adheres to weight reduction regimen

Common Problems of the Upper Extremity

The structures in the upper extremity are frequently the sites of painful syndromes. The structures most often affected are the shoulder, wrist, and hand.

Bursitis and Tenosynovitis

Bursitis and **tenosynovitis** are painful inflammatory conditions that commonly occur in the shoulder. Bursae are fluid-filled sacs that prevent friction between joint structures during joint activity. Similarly, muscle tendon sheaths become inflamed with repetitive movement and strain. The synovial tissue lining the tendon sheath becomes inflamed, giving rise to tenosynovitis. Conservative treatment includes rest of the extremity, intermittent ice to the joint, NSAIDs, and cortisone injections around the sheath but not into the tendon itself. Arthroscopic synovectomy may be considered if shoulder pain and weakness persist.

Loose Bodies

Loose bodies ("joint mice") may occur in a joint space as a result of articular cartilage wear and bone erosion. These fragments can interfere with joint movement ("locking the joint"). Loose bodies are removed by arthroscopic surgery if they cause pain or mobility issues.

Shoulder Impingement Syndrome

Shoulder impingement syndrome is a chronic pain condition involving entrapment and inflammation of one or more of the tendons of the rotator cuff muscle as they traverse the subacromial space or from inflammation of the shoulder bursae. It is caused by repetitive use with combined abduction, forward flexion, and internal rotation of the shoulder or injury to the shoulder. It may occur in anyone but more commonly in individuals involved in prolonged physical work at or above shoulder level (e.g., construction workers, house painters, swimmers, baseball players or injury/trauma to the rotator cuff).

The shoulder consists of two joints, the humerus and glenoid cavity of the scapula form the glenohumeral joint, and the clavicle and acromion process of the scapula form the acromioclavicular joint. The ball and socket arrangement of the glenohumeral joint is very shallow and prone to dislocation. The rotator cuff is a collection of muscles and tendons that are responsible for maintaining the humeral head in the glenoid cavity and for the complete range of movement of the shoulder. The muscles and tendons of the rotator cuff are the supraspinatus, infraspinatus, teres minor, and subscapularis (also known as the SITS muscle). The rotator cuff muscles are attached to the head of the humerus by their tendons.

The tendons have the same names as the rotator cuff muscles, that is, supraspinatus tendon, infraspinatus tendon, teres minor tendon, and subscapularis tendon. In addition, while not part of the rotator cuff arrangement, the biceps muscle allows for forward flexion and the long head of the biceps tendon is attached to the labrum of the glenoid.

Impingement occurs when one or more of the rotator cuff tendons in the subacromial space are intermittently rubbed against the acromion process of the scapula during movement of the shoulder. The impingement results in tendinitis (e.g., supraspinatus tendinitis) or bursitis (e.g., subacromial bursitis). Conservative treatment includes rest, NSAIDs, joint injections, and physical therapy (Chart 71-3). Arthroscopic debridement is used for persistent pain. Gentle joint motion is begun after surgery. (Refer to Chapter 72 for a discussion of rotator cuff injury.)

Carpal Tunnel Syndrome

Carpal tunnel syndrome (CTS) is a neuropathy of the median nerve due to compression at the wrist. The vast majority of CTS cases are idiopathic. The median nerve courses through the carpal tunnel in the wrist, which is surrounded by bone on three sides and a transverse carpal ligament on the fourth. Compression of the median nerve may occur from a thickening of the flexor tendon sheath, skeletal encroachment, edema, or a soft tissue mass and is associated with arthritis, hypothyroidism, and pregnancy. The patient experiences pain, numbness, and paresthesia along the median nerve distribution (thumb and first two fingers). Later in the condition, there may be evidence of muscle atrophy in particular of the thenar eminence.

CHART 71-3

Patient Education: Measures to Promote Shoulder Healing of Impingement Syndrome

The nurse instructs the patient to:

- Rest the joint in a position that minimizes stress on the joint structures to prevent further damage and the development of adhesions.
- Support the affected arm on pillows while sleeping, to keep from turning onto the shoulder.
- Gradually resume motion and use of the joint. Assistance with dressing and other activities of daily living (ADLs) may be needed.
- Avoid working and lifting above shoulder level or pushing an object against a "locked" shoulder.
- Perform the prescribed daily range-of-motion and strengthening exercises.

Tinel's sign may be used to help identify CTS (Fig. 71-4); however, the hand elevation test (HET) has been found to be more sensitive (88%) and specific (98%) (Amirfeyz, Gozzard, & Leslie, 2005). The HET is a provocative test that simply involves elevating the arm of the hand that is affected for 1 to 2 minutes, to determine if the symptoms of CTS can be replicated.

Pain at night is common, and patients frequently report resting the affected limb above the head. Treatment of CTS is based on the underlying cause. Splints prevent hyperextension and prolonged flexion of the wrist, avoidance of repetitive flexion of the wrist (e.g., the use of ergonomic changes at work to reduce wrist strain), NSAIDs, and carpal canal cortisone injections may relieve the symptoms. Specific yoga postures, relaxation, and acupuncture may provide nontraditional alternatives to relieve carpal tunnel symptoms. Traditional or endoscopic laser surgical release of the transverse carpal ligament may be necessary. The patient wears a hand splint after surgery and limits hand

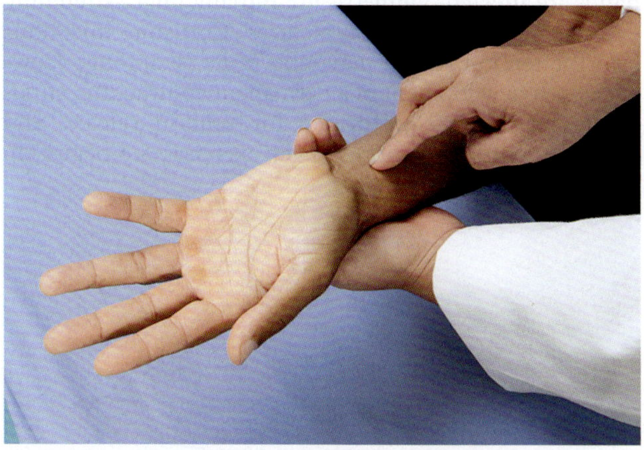

FIGURE 71-4. Tinel's sign may be elicited in patients with carpal tunnel syndrome by percussing lightly over the median nerve, located on the inner aspect of the wrist. If the patient reports tingling, numbness, and pain, the test for Tinel's sign is considered positive. (From Weber, J. W., & Kelley, J. [2014]. *Health assessment in nursing* [5th ed.]. Philadelphia, PA: Lippincott Williams & Wilkins. Photo by B. Proud.)

use during healing. The patient may need assistance with personal care and ADLs. Full recovery of motor and sensory functions after nerve release surgery may take several weeks or months.

Ganglion

A ganglion is a collection of gelatinous material associated with tendons and joints believed to be due to an outpouching of the synovial membrane. It is a round, firm, cystic swelling, usually found on the dorsum of the wrist along the extensor carpi radialis brevis tendon. A ganglion can be as small as a pea or larger than 5 cm in diameter. The *cyst* contains a viscous, sticky, clear, colourless, gelatinous material that mainly consists of hyaluronic acid, globulins, and protein. It most frequently occurs in women between 20 and 40 years. Ganglion cysts are usually painless; however, they can be painful if they impinge on a nerve. Treatment includes watchful waiting, aspiration, corticosteroid injection, or surgical excision. After treatment, a compression dressing and immobilization splint are used. Unfortunately, treatment by aspiration and steroid injection is not always effective, leading to recurrence of the ganglion.

Dupuytren's Contracture

Dupuytren's contracture results from insidious and progressive fibrosis of the palmar fascia, which causes flexion of the fourth and fifth fingers and frequently the middle finger. This renders the fingers more or less useless (Fig. 71-5). It is caused by an inherited autosomal dominant trait and occurs most frequently in men who are older than 50 years and who are of Scandinavian or Celtic origin. It is also associated with arthritis, diabetes, gout, and alcoholism. It starts as a nodule of the palmar fascia. The nodule may not change, or it may progress so that the fibrous thickening extends to involve the skin in the distal palm and produces a **contracture** of the fingers. The patient may experience dull aching discomfort, morning numbness, cramping, and stiffness in the affected fingers. This condition starts in one hand, but eventually both hands are affected symmetrically. Initially, finger-stretching exercises may prevent contractures. Cortisone injections into the tendon sheath may relieve the symptoms. However, with development of a permanent contracture, surgical fasciotomy is performed for tendon release and improvement in function. Finger exercises are begun on postoperative day 1 or 2.

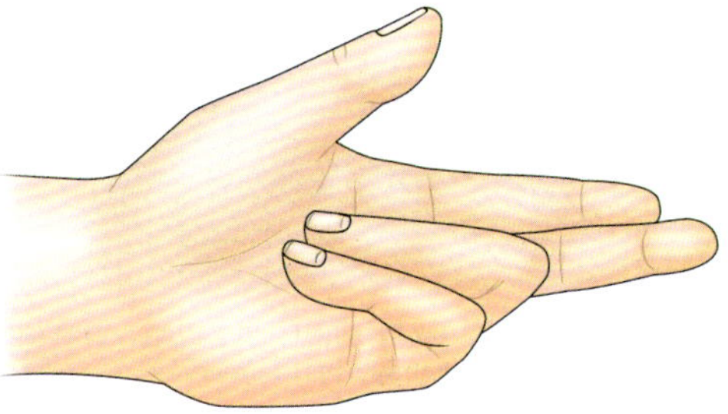

FIGURE 71-5. Dupuytren's contracture, a flexion deformity caused by an inherited trait, is a slowly progressive contracture of the palmar fascia, which severely impairs the function of the fourth, fifth, and sometimes the middle fingers.

Nursing Process

The Patient Undergoing Surgery of the Hand or Wrist

Assessment

Surgery of the hand or wrist, unless related to major trauma, is generally an outpatient procedure. Before surgery, the nurse assesses the patient's level of discomfort and limitations in function caused by the ganglion, CTS, Dupuytren's contracture, or other condition of the hand.

Nursing Priorities

The nursing priorities for the patient undergoing surgery of the hand may include the following:

- Peripheral neurovascular dysfunction
- Acute pain
- Self-care deficit
- Risk for infection

Planning and Goals

The goals of patient care include pain management, improved self-care, and absence of infection.

Nursing Interventions

Promoting Neurovascular Function

Neurovascular assessment of the exposed fingers every hour for the first 24 hours is essential for monitoring function of the nerves and perfusion of the hand. The nurse assesses colour, warmth, sensation, and movement. The nurse also compares the affected hand with the unaffected hand and the postoperative status with the documented preoperative status. The patient is asked to describe the sensations in the hands and demonstrate motor function. Dressings are to be supportive and nonconstrictive. Pain that is not well managed by appropriate analgesic use suggests that there may be compromised neurovascular functioning.

Managing Pain

Pain may be caused by edema, hematoma formation, or restrictive bandages. Swelling is managed by elevating the hand to heart level with pillows. An elevating sling may be attached to an IV pole. When the patient is ambulatory, the arm is elevated in a conventional sling with the hand at heart level.

Ice packs may be applied intermittently to the surgical area during the first 24 to 48 hours. Unless contraindicated, active extension and flexion of the fingers to promote circulation is encouraged, even though movement is limited by the bulky dressing.

Generally, the pain can be controlled by oral analgesics. The nurse evaluates the patient's response to analgesics and to other pain management measures.

Improving Self-Care

During the first few days after surgery, the patient will need assistance with ADLs as independent self-care is impaired. The patient may need assistance with feeding, dressing, and personal hygiene. Within a few days, the patient develops skills in one-handed ADLs and is usually able to function with minimal assistance and the use of assistive devices. The nurse encourages use of the involved hand, unless contraindicated, within the limits of discomfort. As rehabilitation progresses, the patient resumes the use of the injured hand. Physical or occupational therapy–directed exercises may be prescribed.

Preventing Infection

As with all surgery, there is a risk of infection. The nurse teaches the patient to monitor temperature and signs and symptoms that suggest an infection. It also is important to instruct the patient to keep the dressing clean and dry and to report any drainage, foul odour, or increased pain and swelling. Patient education includes aseptic wound care as well as education related to prescribed antibiotics.

Promoting Home, Community-Based, and Transitional Care

EDUCATING PATIENTS ABOUT SELF-CARE. After the patient has undergone hand surgery, the nurse teaches the patient how to monitor neurovascular status and the signs of complications that need to be reported to the surgeon (e.g., paresthesia, paralysis, uncontrolled pain, coolness of fingers, extreme swelling, excessive bleeding, purulent drainage, fever). The nurse reviews prescribed medications with the patient. In addition, the nurse teaches the patient to elevate the hand above the elbow and to apply ice to control swelling. Unless contraindicated, the nurse encourages extension and flexion exercises of the fingers to promote circulation. For bathing, the nurse instructs the patient to keep the dressing dry by covering it with a plastic bag secured by water proof tape. Generally, the wound is not redressed until the patient's follow-up visit with the surgeon (Chart 71-4).

CHART 71-4

HOME CARE CHECKLIST • **Hand or Foot Surgery**

At the completion of education, the patient and/or caregiver will be able to:

- Name the procedure that was performed and identify any permanent changes in anatomic structure or function as well as changes in ADLs, IADLs, roles, relationships, and spirituality.
- Identify modification of home environment, interventions, and strategies (e.g., durable medical equipment, adaptive equipment) used in safely adapting to changes in structure or function and promote effective recovery and rehabilitation.
- Describe ongoing postoperative therapeutic regimen, including diet and activities to perform (e.g., immobilization) and to limit or avoid (e.g., lifting weights, driving a car, contact sports).
- Describe methods to prevent wound infection (e.g., keeping dressing clean and dry during ADLs).
- Demonstrate how to assess neurovascular status.
- Demonstrate control of edema by elevating extremity and applying ice intermittently if prescribed.
- Observe prescribed weight-bearing, activity, and exercise limits.
- Demonstrate safe use of assistive devices, if appropriate.
- Consume a healthy diet to promote healing.
- State the name, dose, side effects, frequency, and schedule for all prescribed therapeutic and prophylactic medications (e.g., antibiotics and analgesic agents).
- State indicators of wound infections (e.g., redness, swelling, tenderness, purulent drainage, fever, signs of systemic infection) to report promptly to primary provider.
- State indicators of other potential complications to report promptly to primary provider (e.g., uncontrolled swelling and pain; cool, pale fingers or toes; paresthesia; paralysis; purulent drainage; signs of deep vein thrombosis or pulmonary embolism).
- Relate how to reach primary provider with questions or complications.
- Verbalize the need to keep appointment with surgeon for initial dressing change.
- State time and date of follow-up appointments and testing.
- Identify the need for health promotion (e.g., weight reduction, smoking cessation, stress management), disease prevention, and screening activities.

Evaluation

Expected patient outcomes may include the following:

1. Maintains peripheral tissue perfusion
   a. Demonstrates normal skin temperature, capillary refill, sensation, and movement
2. Achieves pain relief
   a. Reports decreased pain level
   b. Controls edema by elevating hand
   c. Experiences decreased discomfort with movement
3. Demonstrates self-care
   a. Secures assistance with ADLs during first few days postoperatively
   b. Adapts to using one hand for ADLs
   c. Uses injured hand within its functional capability
4. Demonstrates absence of wound infection
   a. Adheres to treatment protocol and prevention strategies
   b. Reports temperature and pulse within normal limits
   c. Experiences no wound inflammation or purulent discharge

Common Foot Problems

Repetitive strain leading to inflammation of the bones and soft tissue, osteoarthritis, and injury are the most common causes of foot problems. In addition, systemic diseases such as diabetes, peripheral arterial disease, and dermatologic conditions may also lead to a variety of foot conditions. Patients with peripheral arterial disease and arteriosclerosis complain of burning and itching feet, resulting in scratching and skin breakdown. Dermatology problems commonly affect the feet in the form of fungal infections and plantar warts. Foot deformities may occur with rheumatoid arthritis and osteoarthritis.

Pain from foot strain is treated with rest, elevation, physiotherapy, supportive strappings, and orthotic devices. The patient must inspect the foot and skin under pads and orthotic devices for pressure and skin breakdown daily. Active foot exercises promote the circulation and help to strengthen the feet. Walking in properly fitting shoes is an excellent exercise.

Plantar Fasciitis

Plantar fasciitis, an inflammation of the foot-supporting fascia, presents as an acute onset of heel pain experienced with the first steps in the morning and after periods of sitting. The pain is localized to the anteromedial aspect of the heel and diminishes with gentle stretching of the Achilles tendon. Management includes stretching exercises and wearing shoes with support and cushioning to relieve pain. Orthotic devices (e.g., heel cups, arch supports), insoles, and splints of different types worn during sleep to keep the foot and ankle dorsiflexed are helpful. Walking in bare feet is to be avoided whenever possible. Oral and topical NSAIDs, and occasionally cortisone injections, may be helpful. Unresolved plantar fasciitis may progress to fascial tears at the heel and eventual development of heel spurs.

Corn

A corn is an overgrowth of epidermis known as hyperkeratosis that is produced by internal pressure. The underlying bone is prominent because of congenital or acquired abnormalities or external pressure due to ill-fitting shoes. The fifth toe is most frequently affected.

Corns are treated by soaking and scraping off the horny layer by a podiatrist, by application of a protective shield or pad, or by surgical modification of the underlying offending osseous structure. Soft corns are located between the toes and are kept soft by moisture. Treatment consists of drying the affected spaces and separating the affected toes with lamb's wool or gauze. A wider shoe may be helpful.

Callus

A callus is a discretely thickened area of the skin that has been exposed to persistent pressure or friction. Faulty foot mechanics usually precede the formation of a callus. Treatment consists of eliminating the underlying causes and having the callus treated by a podiatrist. A keratolytic ointment may be applied and a thin plastic cup is worn over the heel if the callus is on this area. Felt padding with adhesive backing is also used to prevent and relieve pressure. Orthotic devices decrease the pressure from bony protuberances, or the protuberance may be excised.

Ingrown Toenail

An ingrown toenail (onychocryptosis) is a condition in which the free edge of a nail plate penetrates the surrounding skin; a localized infection may develop. This painful condition is caused by external pressure (tight shoes), internal pressure (deformed toes, growth under the nail), trauma, or infection. An ingrown toenail can be prevented by clipping nails straight across and filing the corners consistent with the contour of the toe. Active treatment consists of washing the foot twice a day, followed by the application of a local antibiotic ointment, and relieving the pain by decreasing the pressure of the nail plate on the surrounding soft tissue. Warm, wet soaks help to drain an infection. In the presence of severe infection, the toenail may need to be excised by a podiatrist.

Hammer Toe

Hammer toe is a flexion deformity of the interphalangeal joint (Fig. 71-6). Tight socks or shoes may push an overlying toe into the line of the other toes. The toes are pulled upward, forcing the metatarsal joints (ball of the foot) downward. Corns develop on top of the toes, and tender calluses develop under the metatarsal area. The treatment consists of conservative measures: wearing open-toed sandals or shoes that conform to the shape of the foot and protecting the protruding joints with pads. Surgical correction (osteotomy) may be necessary to correct an established deformity.

Hallux Valgus

Hallux valgus, commonly called a *bunion*, is a deformity in which the great toe deviates laterally (see Fig. 71-6). It is associated with a marked prominence of the medial aspect

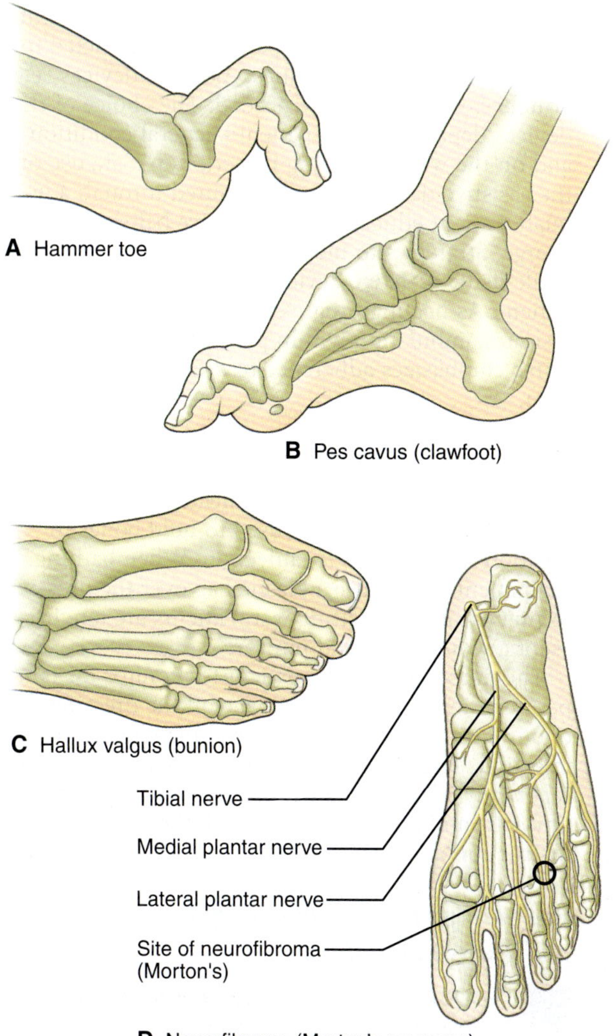

FIGURE 71-6. Common foot deformities. **A.** Hammer toe. **B.** Pes cavus (clawfoot). **C.** Bunion (hallux valgus). **D.** Neurofibroma (Morton's neuroma).

of the first metatarsophalangeal joint. There is osseous enlargement (exostosis) of the medial side of the first metatarsal head, over which a bursa may form (secondary to pressure and inflammation). Acute bursitis symptoms include a reddened area, edema, and tenderness.

Factors contributing to bunion formation include heredity, ill-fitting shoes, and gradual lengthening and widening of the foot associated with aging. Osteoarthritis is frequently associated with hallux valgus. Treatment depends on the patient's age, the degree of deformity, and the severity of symptoms. If a bunion deformity is uncomplicated, wearing a shoe that conforms to the shape of the foot or that is moulded to the foot to prevent pressure on the protruding portions may be all the treatment that is needed. Surgical removal of the bunion (exostosis) and osteotomies to realign the toe may be required to improve function and appearance. Complications related to bunionectomy include limited range of motion, paresthesias, tendon injury, and recurrence of deformity.

Postoperatively, the patient may have intense throbbing pain at the operative site, requiring liberal doses of analgesic medication. The foot is elevated to the level of the heart to decrease edema and pain. The neurovascular status of the toes is assessed. Toe flexion and extension exercises are initiated to facilitate walking. Shoes that fit the shape and size of the foot are recommended.

Pes Cavus

Pes cavus (clawfoot) refers to a foot with an abnormally high arch and a fixed equinus deformity of the forefoot (see Fig. 71-6). The shortening of the foot and increased pressure produce calluses on the metatarsal area and on the plantar aspect of the foot. Causes of pes cavus include Charcot–Marie–Tooth disease, a peripheral neuromuscular disease associated with a familial degenerative disorder, diabetes mellitus, and tertiary syphilis. Exercises are prescribed to manipulate the forefoot into dorsiflexion and relax the toes. Bracing to protect the foot may be used. Arthrodesis (fusion) is performed to reshape and stabilize the foot.

Morton's Neuroma

Morton's neuroma (plantar digital neuroma, neurofibroma) is a swelling of the third (lateral) branch of the median plantar nerve (see Fig. 71-6). The third digital nerve, which is located in the third intermetatarsal (web) space, is most commonly involved. Microscopically, digital artery changes cause an ischemia of the nerve.

The result is a throbbing, burning pain in the foot that is usually relieved when the patient rests. Conservative treatment consists of inserting innersoles and metatarsal pads designed to spread the metatarsal heads and balance the foot posture. Local injections of hydrocortisone and a local anesthetic may provide relief. If these fail, surgical excision of the neuroma is necessary. Pain relief and loss of sensation are immediate and permanent.

Flatfoot

Flatfoot (pes planus) is a common disorder in which the longitudinal arch of the foot is diminished. It may be caused by congenital abnormalities or associated with bone or ligament injury, muscle and posture imbalances, excessive weight, muscle fatigue, poorly fitting shoes, or arthritis. Symptoms include a burning sensation, fatigue, clumsy gait, edema, and pain.

Exercises to strengthen the muscles and to improve posture and walking habits are helpful. A number of foot orthoses are available to give the foot additional support. Orthopedic surgeons and podiatrists treat severe flatfoot problems.

Nursing Process

The Patient Undergoing Foot Surgery

Assessment

Surgery of the foot may be necessary because of various conditions, including neuromas and foot deformities (bunion, hammer toe, clawfoot). Generally, foot surgery is performed on an outpatient basis. Before surgery, the nurse assesses the patient's ambulatory ability and balance and the neurovascular status of the foot. Additionally, the nurse considers the availability of assistance at home and the structural characteristics of the home in planning for care during the first few days after surgery. The nurse uses these data, in addition to knowledge of the usual medical management of the condition, to formulate an appropriate nursing care plan.

Nursing Priorities

Priorities for the patient undergoing foot surgery may include the following:

- Decreased peripheral tissue perfusion
- Acute pain
- Impaired physical mobility
- Infection

Planning and Goals

The goals for the patient may include adequate tissue perfusion, relief of pain, improved mobility, and absence of infection.

Nursing Interventions

Promoting Tissue Perfusion

Neurovascular assessment of the exposed toes every 1 to 2 hours for the first 24 hours is essential to monitor the function of the nerves and the perfusion of the tissues. If the patient is discharged within several hours after the surgery, the nurse teaches the patient and family how to assess for swelling and neurovascular status (colour, sensation, warmth, and movement). Compromised neurovascular function can increase the patient's pain. (Refer to Chart 69-3 in Chapter 69.)

Managing Pain

Pain experienced by patients who undergo foot surgery is related to inflammation and edema. Formation of a hematoma may contribute to the discomfort. To manage the swelling, the foot is elevated on several pillows when the patient is sitting or lying. Ice packs applied to the surgical area intermittently during the first 24 to 48 hours help manage swelling and provide some pain relief. As activity increases, dependent positioning of the foot is uncomfortable; elevating the foot relieves the discomfort. Oral analgesics may be used to manage the pain. The nurse instructs the patient and family about the appropriate use of these medications.

Improving Mobility

After surgery, the patient will have a bulky dressing on the foot, protected by a light cast or a special protective boot. Limits for weight bearing on the foot will be prescribed by the surgeon. Some patients are allowed to walk on the heel and progress to weight bearing as tolerated; other patients are restricted to non–weight-bearing activities. Assistive devices (e.g., crutches, walker) may be needed. The choice of the devices depends on the patient's general condition and on the weight-bearing prescription. Safe use of the assistive devices must be ensured through adequate patient education and practice before discharge. Strategies to move around the house safely while using assistive devices are discussed with the patient. As healing progresses, the patient gradually resumes ambulation within prescribed limits. The nurse emphasizes adherence to the therapeutic regimen.

Preventing Infection

Any surgery carries a risk for infection. In addition, percutaneous pins may be used to hold bones in position and are sites for infection. When bathing, the patient can secure a plastic bag over the dressing to prevent it from getting wet. Patients are taught aseptic wound care and pin care.

The nurse teaches the patient to monitor for temperature and infection. Drainage on the dressing, foul odour, or increased pain and swelling could indicate infection. The nurse instructs the patient to promptly report any of these findings to the physician. If prophylactic antibiotics are prescribed, the nurse provides instruction about their correct use.

Promoting Home, Community-Based, and Transitional Care

EDUCATING PATIENTS ABOUT SELF-CARE. The nurse plans patient teaching for home care, focusing on neurovascular status, pain management, mobility, and wound care (see Chart 71-4).

Evaluation

Expected patient outcomes may include the following:

1. Maintains peripheral tissue perfusion
   a. Demonstrates normal skin temperature, capillary refill, normal sensations, and motor function
2. Obtains pain relief
   a. Elevates foot to control edema
   b. Applies ice to foot
   c. Uses oral analgesics
   d. Reports decreased pain and increased comfort
3. Demonstrates increased mobility
   a. Uses assistive devices safely
   b. Resumes weight bearing gradually as prescribed
   c. Exhibits gradual increase in mobility
4. Develops no infection
   a. Reports temperature and pulse within normal limits
   b. Reports no purulent drainage or signs of wound inflammation
   c. Maintains clean and dry dressing
   d. Takes prophylactic antibiotics as prescribed

Metabolic Bone Disorders

Osteoporosis

Osteoporosis is a disease that threatens more than 2 million Canadians (Osteoporosis Canada, 2019). One in four women and at least one in eight men in Canada have osteoporosis (Osteoporosis Canada, 2019). Characteristics of osteoporosis include a reduction of bone density and a change in bone structure, both of which increase susceptibility to fracture. The normal homeostatic bone turnover is altered: The rate of bone resorption is greater than the rate of bone formation, resulting in a reduced total bone mass. Suboptimal bone mass development in children and teens contributes to the development of osteoporosis.

Patients are susceptive to fragility fractures as bone becomes progressively porous and brittle. Osteoporosis frequently results in compression fractures (Fig. 71-7) of the thoracic and lumbar spine, fractures of the neck and intertrochanteric region of the femur, and Colles' fractures of the wrist. Osteoporosis is responsible for more than 80% of fractures in people over 60 years of age (Wright, Hooker, Nielson, et al., 2018). The risk that a 50-year-old white woman will experience a hip, vertebra, or wrist fracture during her lifetime is 40% (Wright, Looker, Saag, et al., 2018).

Men and black Canadians have a lower rate of osteoporosis. Multiple compression fractures of the vertebrae result in skeletal deformity. Osteoporosis is a costly disorder in terms of human suffering, long-term disability, reduced mobility, decreased independence, and death. It is very costly in terms of Canadian health care dollars. With the increasing age of the population, by 2025, there will be four times more hip fractures in Canada.

The gradual collapse of a vertebra may be asymptomatic; it is observed as progressive kyphosis. With the development of kyphosis, also known as "dowager's hump," there is an associated loss of height (Fig. 71-8). Postmenopausal women lose height from vertebral collapse. The postural changes result in relaxation of the abdominal muscles and a protruding abdomen. The deformity may also produce pulmonary insufficiency.

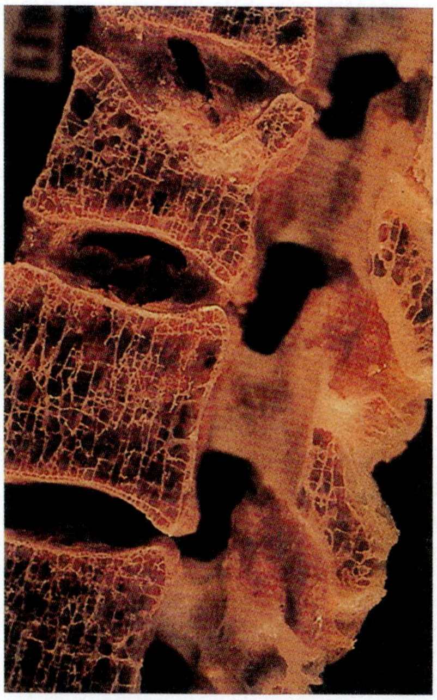

FIGURE 71-7. Progressive osteoporotic bone loss and compression fractures. (From Rubin, E., Gorstein, F., Schwarting, R., et al. [2004]. *Pathology* [4th ed.]. Philadelphia, PA: Lippincott Williams & Wilkins.)

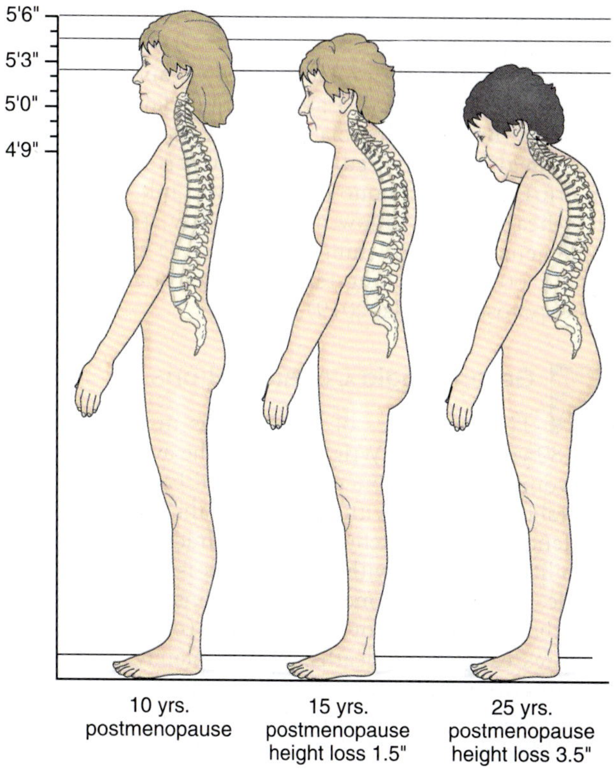

FIGURE 71-8. Typical loss of height associated with osteoporosis and aging.

Prevention

It is thought that 60% to 80% of a person's peak bone mass is genetically determined. Up to 90% of peak adult bone mass is achieved by age 20; this can be affected by factors such as diet, physical activity, and medications. Primary osteoporosis occurs in women after menopause (usually between 45 and 55 years) and later in life in men, but it is not merely a consequence of aging.

Failure to develop optimal peak bone mass during childhood, adolescence, and young adulthood contributes to the development of osteoporosis without resultant bone loss. Early identification of at-risk teenagers and young adults is important. A prevention program includes increased calcium, vitamin D, and protein; participation in regular weight-bearing impact exercise such as walking but not long-distance running. Lifestyle modification (e.g., reduced use of caffeine, salt, cigarettes, carbonated soft drinks, alcohol) is needed to decrease the risk for osteoporosis, fractures, and associated disability (Cosman, de Beur, LeBoff, et al., 2014; Dhaliwal, Mikhail, Usera, et al., 2018). Secondary osteoporosis is the result of medications or other conditions and diseases that affect bone metabolism and is more common in men. Specific disease states (e.g., celiac disease, hypogonadism) and medications (e.g., corticosteroids, anticonvulsant medications) that place patients at risk need to be identified and therapies instituted to reverse the development of osteoporosis.

Examples of health promotion/disease and injury prevention initiatives across Canada include falls prevention programs (British Columbia, Manitoba, and Nova Scotia), bone health public education (Alberta, Manitoba, Ontario), a health phone line (Health Link Alberta) for identification and follow-up of fragility fractures, and implementation of calcium and vitamin D supplementation in 60% of all long-term care facilities (Ontario) (Osteoporosis Canada, 2019).

Gerontologic Considerations

The prevalence of osteoporosis in women older than 80 years is 50% (Wright, 2014). The average 75-year-old woman has lost 25% of her cortical bone and 40% of her trabecular bone. With the aging of the population, the incidence of hip, vertebra and wrist fractures, pain, and disability associated with osteoporosis is increasing. The female lifetime risk (one in six) is considerably greater than the lifetime risk for breast cancer (one in nine); hip fractures cause more deaths. Approximately, 30,000 hip fractures occur in Canada each year, and 70% are osteoporosis related (Bone and Joint Canada [BJC], 2014). The mortality rate less than 1 year after hip fracture is 27% (Cenzer, Tang, Boscardin, et al., 2016), with men more likely to die than women. For patients with hip fracture, 50% will never regain their prefracture level of functioning and will require assistance with daily activities. Another 20% will need placement in long-term care facilities.

Older adults absorb dietary calcium less efficiently and excrete it more readily through their kidneys; therefore, postmenopausal women and the older adults actually need to consume liberal amounts of calcium. As much as 1,500 mg daily of elemental calcium for postmenopausal women is required. Most residents of long-term care facilities have a low bone mineral density (BMD) and are at risk for fracture. Hip protectors had been found to reduce the incidence of hip fracture in older adults; however, adherence in wearing these hip protectors is low. Evidence suggests that they are not effective in preventing fractures.

Pathophysiology

Normal bone remodelling in the adult results in gradually increased bone mass until the early 30s. Gender, race, genetics, aging, low body weight, body mass index (BMI), nutrition, lifestyle choices (e.g., smoking, caffeine, alcohol consumption), and physical activity influence peak bone mass and the development of osteoporosis.

Loss of bone mass is a universal phenomenon associated with aging. Age-related loss begins soon after the peak bone mass is achieved (i.e., in the third decade of life) (Cosman et al., 2014). Calcitonin, which inhibits bone resorption and promotes bone formation, is decreased. Estrogen, which inhibits bone breakdown, decreases with aging. On the other hand, parathyroid hormone (PTH) increases with aging, increasing bone turnover, and resorption. The consequence of these changes is net loss of bone mass over time.

The loss of estrogens at menopause or with oophorectomy causes an accelerated bone resorption that continues during the postmenopausal years. More than half of all women over 50 years of age show evidence of osteopenia (Cosman et al., 2014).

Secondary osteoporosis is associated with many disease states, nutritional deficiencies, and medications. Coexisting medical conditions (e.g., malabsorption syndromes, lactose intolerance, alcohol abuse, renal failure, liver failure, Cushing's syndrome, hyperthyroidism, hyperparathyroidism) contribute to bone loss and the development of osteoporosis (Cosman et al., 2014). Medications (e.g., corticosteroids, anticonvulsant medications, heparin, tetracycline, aluminum-containing antacids, thyroid supplements) affect the body's use and metabolism of calcium. The degree of osteoporosis is related to the duration of medication therapy. When the therapy is discontinued or the metabolic problem is corrected, the progression of osteoporosis is halted, but restoration of lost bone mass usually does not occur.

Risk Factors

Small-framed women are at greatest risk for osteoporosis. Men have a greater peak bone mass and do not experience a sudden midlife estrogen reduction. As a result, osteoporosis occurs about one decade later, but one in four men still sustain an osteopenic fracture (Cosman et al., 2014; Fasolino & Whitright, 2015). It is believed that both testosterone and estrogen are important in achieving and maintaining bone mass in men, although the risk profile for men is not as well established as it is for women (see Chart 71-5). Risk for osteoporosis rises with increasing age for both genders (Fasolino & Whitright, 2015; Wong & McGirt, 2013) (see Chart 71-6).

Nutritional factors contribute to the development of osteoporosis. A diet that includes adequate calories and nutrients needed to maintain bone, calcium, and vitamin D must be consumed. Patients who have had bariatric surgery are at increased risk for osteoporosis as the duodenum is bypassed, which is the primary site for absorption of calcium. Patients who have gastrointestinal diseases that cause malabsorption (e.g., celiac disease, alcoholism) may benefit from additional magnesium supplements (González-Reimers, Quintero-Platt, Rodríguez-Rodríguez, et al., 2015).

Bone formation is enhanced by the stress of weight and muscle activity. When immobilized by casts, general inactivity, paralysis, or other disability, the bone is resorbed faster than it is formed, and osteoporosis results (Grossman & Porth, 2014). Immobility contributes to the development of osteoporosis. Resistance and impact exercises are most beneficial in developing and maintaining bone mass (Fasolino & Whitright, 2015).

Testing for osteoporosis is recommended for persons over 50 years with at least one major risk factor or two or more minor risk factors and for all women and men over 65 years of age (Osteoporosis Canada, 2019).

Assessment and Diagnostic Findings

Osteoporosis may be undetectable on routine x-rays until there has been significant demineralization, resulting in radiolucency of the bones (Cosman et al., 2014). When the vertebrae collapse, causing compression fractures, the

NURSING RESEARCH PROFILE

Chart 71-5. Osteoporosis Risks in Men

Fasolino, T., & Whitright, T. (2015). A pilot study to identify modifiable and non-modifiable variables associated with osteopenia and osteoporosis in men. *Orthopaedic Nursing, 34*(5), 289–293.

Purpose

Modifiable and nonmodifiable risk factors for women with osteoporosis have been identified. However, one in four men over the age of 60 will have an osteoporotic fracture in their lifetime; scant evidence focuses on their risks, hampering the development of male-specific osteoporosis screening and prevention programs. The purpose of this study was to identify risk factors that lead to osteoporosis in men.

Design

This was an exploratory pilot study conducted among patients affiliated with an internal medicine practice. Self-report surveys were completed by male participants between the ages of 65 and 75 years who had not previously been diagnosed with osteopenia or osteoporosis, were not taking bisphosphonate medications, and did not have a history of hyperthyroidism or parathyroid disease. Self-report measures on the survey included use of tobacco, alcohol consumption, exercise history, fracture history in adulthood, and family history of osteoporosis. Body mass indices (BMIs) were calculated based on participants' height and weight. Bone mineral density (BMD) studies using DEXA imaging were completed on each participant.

Findings

Ninety-two of 101 participants (99% Caucasian; mean age 70.7 years) completed all portions of the study. Thirty-nine (38.6%) participants had normal BMDs, 43 (42.6%) participants had osteopenia, and 19 (18.8%) participants had previously undiagnosed osteoporosis. Among potential modifiable risk factors analyzed, only a lower BMI was significantly associated with lower BMD ($p = 0.02$). Tobacco use, alcohol consumption, and self-reported exercise levels were not statistically related to BMD results. None of the potential non-modifiable risk factors, including age, history of fracture, and family history, correlated with BMD.

Nursing Implications

Over half of the men in this study had low BMDs, with 18.8% found to have osteoporosis that had not been previously diagnosed. These findings suggest that current recommendations set by the U.S. Preventive Services Task Force to not screen men for osteopenia and osteoporosis before the age of 70 should be reconsidered. However, results from this study do not clearly illuminate which osteoporosis risk factors are of significance to men. This research must be replicated with a larger sample and include men from more diverse ethnic backgrounds that better mirror the diversity among American men.

CHART 71-6

Risk Factors for Osteoporosis

Major Risk Factors

- Increased age (65 years or older)
- Sex (female)
- Low body weight
- Decreased bone mineral density
- History of a parent who had a hip fracture
- Fracture with minimum trauma (fragility fracture) after age 40 years
- Estrogen deficiency or early menopause (before age 45 years); testosterone deficiency in men
- Primary hyperparathyroidism
- Osteopenia or vertebral compression fracture visible on x-ray
- Tendency to fall
- Contributing, coexisting medical conditions (e.g., celiac disease, Crohn's disease), which reduce absorption of nutrients
- Corticosteroid therapy of 7.5 mg a day for 3 months or more

Minor Risk Factors

- Rheumatoid arthritis
- Hyperthyroidism
- Caffeine (more than 1,000 mL of coffee per day)
- Poor nutrition with low calcium and vitamin D
- Smoking
- Alcohol (more than 2 drinks per day)
- Prolonged use of medications (anticonvulsants or heparin)
- Medications that increase risk of falling (e.g., sedatives)

Risk-Lowering Strategies

- Increased dietary calcium, vitamin D, and protein intake
- Follow Canada's Food Guide
- Smoking cessation
- Reduced salt intake
- Alcohol and caffeine consumption in moderation
- Regular weight-bearing impact exercise regimen
- Regular exercise (e.g., walking)
- Review:
  Osteoporosis Canada's Web site https://osteoporosis.ca/about-the-disease/what-is-osteoporosis/secondary-osteoporosis/how-to-minimize-the-harmful-effects
  Osteoporosis Canada's fact sheet *Exercise for Healthy Bones*

Adapted from Osteoporosis Canada. (2009c). Retrieved January 2019, from https://osteoporosis.ca

thoracic vertebrae become wedge shaped and the lumbar vertebrae become biconcave. Osteoporosis is diagnosed by dual-energy x-ray absorptiometry (DEXA), which provides information about BMD at the spine and hip. The DEXA scan data are analyzed and reported as T-scores (the number of standard deviations above or below the average BMD value for a 30-year-old healthy Caucasian woman). T-scores that are gender specific for men are not yet available.

Baseline DEXA testing is recommended for all women older than 65 years, for women who are postmenopausal older than 50 years with osteoporosis risk factors, and for all people who have had a fracture thought to occur as a consequence of osteoporosis (Cosman et al., 2014). BMD studies are also useful in assessing response to therapy and are recommended 3 months post any osteoporotic fracture. There is no evidence to support basic screening of men or for the optimal time interval to repeat studies following a normal baseline report.

Fracture risk can be estimated using the World Health Organization (WHO) Fracture Risk Assessment Tool (FRAX). Treatment is now reserved for those with a 10-year risk of more than 3% for hip fracture or 20% risk for other major fractures. The risk scores are based on BMD, personal and family history of fractures, BMI, gender, age, and secondary factors such as medication use, smoking, and history of rheumatoid disease (Cosman et al., 2014).

Laboratory studies (e.g., serum calcium, serum phosphate, serum alkaline phosphatase [ALP], urine calcium excretion, urinary hydroxyproline excretion, hematocrit, erythrocyte sedimentation rate [ESR]), and x-ray studies are used to exclude other possible disorders (e.g., multiple myeloma, osteomalacia, hyperparathyroidism, malignancy) that contribute to bone loss. In men, low testosterone levels may be part of the cause (Cosman et al., 2014).

Medical Management

A diet rich in calcium and vitamin D throughout life, with an increased calcium intake during adolescence and the middle years, protects against skeletal demineralization. Such a diet includes three glasses of skimmed vitamin D–enriched milk or other foods high in calcium (e.g., cheese and other dairy products, steamed broccoli, canned salmon with bones) daily. A cup of milk or calcium-fortified orange juice contains about 300 mg of calcium.

The recommended adequate intake level of calcium for men 50 to 70 years is 1,000 mg daily, and for women aged 51 and older and men aged 71 and older is 1,200 mg daily (Cosman et al., 2014). Some researchers are challenging these levels as too low for patients with low baseline values, while others express concern of administering higher dosages, noting that they are associated with adverse events (e.g., renal calculi) (Hansen, Johnson, Chambers, et al., 2015; Veugelers & Ekwaru, 2014). The recommended vitamin D intake for adults up to 70 years of age is 600 IU daily, and 800 IU daily for those over the age of 70 (Cosman et al., 2014).

Regular weight-bearing exercise promotes bone formation. Recommendations include 20 to 30 minutes of aerobic, bone-stressing exercise daily (e.g., not swimming). Weight training stimulates an increase in BMD. In addition, exercise improves balance, reducing the incidence of falls and fractures (Cosman et al., 2014). Women who are postmenopausal and men aged 50 and older should be advised to avoid excessive intake of alcohol. Those who use tobacco products should be advised to quit (Cosman, de Beur, LeBoff, et al., 2015).

Pharmacologic Therapy

To ensure adequate calcium intake, a calcium supplement (e.g., Caltrate, Citracal) with vitamin D may be prescribed and taken with meals or with a beverage high in vitamin C to promote absorption. The recommended daily dose should be split and not taken as a single dose. Common side effects of calcium supplements are abdominal distention and constipation. Calcium from foods is better absorbed, but calcium supplements may be necessary for patients who are lactose intolerant. Meta-analysis findings demonstrate that vitamin D taken alone is not effective in primary prevention of fractures. However, vitamin D plus calcium does reduce the risk of fractures (Avenell, Mak, & O'Connell, 2014). Calcium and vitamin D may be taken to prevent osteoporosis, or may be taken as supplements to drugs prescribed to prevent or treat osteoporosis. These types of drugs include bisphosphonates, estrogen agonist/antagonists, and receptor activator of nuclear factor kappa-B ligand (RANKL) inhibitors (see Table 71-1).

In Canada, three bisphosphonates are approved for the treatment of osteoporosis: alendronate (Fosamax, Fosavance), risedronate (Actonel), and etidronate (Didronel). Absorption of bisphosphonates by the oral route is poor, even when taken on an empty stomach. These drugs are considered first-line prevention therapies for low BMD in postmenopausal women and the prevention of glucocorticoid-induced osteoporosis in men and women. They also are first-line treatment therapies for postmenopausal women with osteoporosis and vertebral fractures, for glucocorticoid-induced osteoporosis in both sexes, and for men with low bone mass or osteoporosis.

Alendronate produces increased bone mass by inhibiting osteoclast function and decreased bone loss. Weekly dosing of alendronate is available and has been shown to be as effective as daily dosing. Adequate calcium and vitamin D intake is needed for maximum effect, but these supplements should not be taken at the same time of day as bisphosphonates. Side effects of alendronate include gastrointestinal symptoms (e.g., dyspepsia, nausea, flatulence, diarrhea, constipation), and some patients may develop esophageal ulcers, gastric ulcers, or osteonecrosis of the jaw related to bisphosphonate use. Patients must take these medications with a full glass of water, on an empty stomach in the morning, and must sit upright for 30 to 60 minutes after administration. Risedronate can also be taken daily or weekly and is well tolerated. Side effects may include headache and diarrhea. Taken daily, risedronate reduces the incidence of hip and vertebral fractures in women with postmenopausal osteoporosis. Risedronate and alendronate are effective in reducing the number of hip and vertebral fractures. Etidronate is generally well tolerated; diarrhea is the main side effect. The drug is taken in an intermittent pattern daily for 2 weeks every 3 months. Etidronate has produced significant increases in BMD of the lumbar spine with a decrease in vertebral fractures but has not decreased the risk of hip fractures.

TABLE 71-1 Selected Osteoporosis Medications

Medication	Therapeutic Effects and Indications	Key Nursing Considerations
Bisphosphonates	Inhibit osteoclasts, causing decreased bone loss and increased bone mass	Adequate calcium and vitamin D intake is needed to assure maximum effect; however, these supplements should not be taken at the same time as the bisphosphonates Side effects include gastrointestinal symptoms, including dyspepsia, nausea, flatulence, diarrhea, and constipation Adverse effects may include esophageal or gastric ulcers, osteonecrosis of the jaw, and atypical femur fractures; these effects may be mitigated by instituting a 1–2-year drug-free holiday in patients with mild osteoporosis after 4–5 years of treatment, and in patients with higher fracture risk after 10 years of treatment
Alendronate (Fosamax) Risedronate (Actonel)	• Prevention and treatment of osteoporosis in women who are postmenopausal • Treatment of osteoporosis in men, and in women and men taking corticosteroids	Administer PO, either daily or weekly Advise patient to take in the morning on empty stomach with 250 mL of water while sitting upright and to remain upright for at least 30 minutes Effects of alendronate may be diminished in older adult patients who take proton pump inhibitors
Ibandronate (Boniva)	• Treatment of osteoporosis in women who are postmenopausal • IV dosing may be a good option for patients either intolerant of PO bisphosphonates or nonadherent to prescribed therapy	May be given PO monthly or IV every 3 months
Zoledronic acid (Reclast)	• Prevention and treatment of osteoporosis in women who are postmenopausal • Treatment of osteoporosis in men and in both men and women taking corticosteroids for at least 12 months	Administer IV once yearly for osteoporosis treatment or once every 2 years for osteoporosis prevention This is the most potent bisphosphonate and is associated with acute kidney injury; therefore, it is contraindicated in patients with creatinine clearances less than 35 mL/min or in patients with chronic kidney disease
Estrogen Agonist/ Antagonist (formerly called selective estrogen receptor modulator [SERM]) Raloxifene (Evista)	Promotes estrogenic effects on bone, preserving BMD, with concomitant antiestrogenic effects on the uterus and breasts • Prevention and treatment of osteoporosis in women who are postmenopausal, particularly those with breast cancer • May also reduce the risk of breast cancer in patients at risk	Administer PO once daily. May be given in tandem with calcium and vitamin D Side effects include hot flashes and leg cramps Adverse effects include VTE formation
RANKL Inhibitor Denosumab (Prolia)	Monoclonal antibody that increases BMD and reduces the porosity of cortical bone by inhibiting the effects of TNF on osteoclasts, inhibiting their activity • Treatment of osteoporosis in men and women who are postmenopausal at high risk of fracture; also indicated for women with osteoporosis and breast cancer receiving aromatase inhibitors and for men with osteoporosis and prostate cancer receiving gonadotropin-reducing hormones	Given once every 6 months SQ Side effects include skin rashes Adverse effects include hypocalcemia, cellulitis, osteonecrosis of the jaw, and atypical femur fracture Note: when treatment with denosumab is stopped, loss of BMD can be rapid; other drugs should be started to mitigate this response

BMD, bone mineral density; PO, orally; IV, intravenously; SQ, subcutaneous; TNF, tissue necrosis factor; VTE, venous thromboembolism.

Adapted from Cosman, F., de Beur, S. J., LeBoff, M. S., et al. (2014). Clinician's guide to prevention and treatment of osteoporosis. *Osteoporosis International*, *25*(10), 2359–2381.

Calcitonin (Salmon synthetic) (Miacalcin) primarily suppresses bone loss through direct action on osteoclasts and reduced bone turnover. Calcitonin is administered daily, primarily by nasal spray and less often by subcutaneous or intramuscular injection. Side effects include nasal irritation, flushing, gastrointestinal disturbances, and urinary frequency. Nasal calcitonin is used to reduce the pain of acute vertebral fractures for postmenopausal women with severe osteoporosis. Calcitonin is effective in the prevention of vertebral fractures but not other types of fractures. BMD of the hip and spine is maintained or slightly improved. Calcitonin can be used for patients on glucocorticoid drugs or who have glucocorticoid-induced osteoporosis to maintain or increase BMD of the hip.

In clinical trials, small daily subcutaneous injections of PTH or PTH bioactive fragments (1–34; 1–38), have been found to stimulate bone formation. In July 2004, the

Therapeutic Products Directorate of Health Canada approved PTH (with teriparatide as the active ingredient), under the name Forteo, as a bone formation agent for the treatment of osteoporosis. It stimulates osteoblasts to build bone matrix and facilitates overall calcium absorption. Route of administration is by subcutaneous injection daily for 18 months, and the use of this drug has improved BMD in men.

In addition, antilipid medications, such as statins (HMG-CoA reductase inhibitors), reduce the incidence of fractures in patients who take these medications to control their hyperlipidemia. The statins promote bone growth, thereby preventing the development of osteoporosis.

Provincial/territorial drug plans have three categories of coverage: Open Access (drugs are covered by the plan); Restricted Access (drugs are covered but a specific authorization request by the prescriber or pharmacist has to be submitted); and Not Accessible (drugs not covered by the plan).

Fracture Management

Fractures of the hip are managed surgically by joint replacement or by closed or open reduction and internal fixation (e.g., hip pinning). Surgery, early ambulation, intensive physical therapy, and adequate nutrition result in decreased morbidity and improved outcomes. In addition, since 80% of fractures are due to osteoporosis, it is essential that patients are evaluated for osteoporosis and treated (Cosman et al., 2014). Currently, fewer than 38% are evaluated and receive adequate treatment. One strategy is to give patients who are suffering a fracture a card with information about their fracture to take to their health care provider and to notify health care providers that one of their patients has had a fracture.

Osteoporotic compression fractures of the vertebrae are managed conservatively. Additional vertebral fractures and progressive kyphosis are common. Pharmacologic and dietary treatments are aimed at increasing vertebral bone density. A new procedure, percutaneous vertebroplasty/kyphoplasty (injection of polymethylmethacrylate bone cement into the fractured vertebra), is reported to provide rapid acute pain relief and improved quality of life. The long-term effect of this procedure is unknown. Patients who have not responded to first-line approaches to the treatment of vertebral compression fracture can be considered for the procedure. It is contraindicated in the presence of infection, old fractures, and certain coagulopathies.

Nursing Process

The Patient With a Spontaneous Vertebral Fracture Related to Osteoporosis

Assessment

Health promotion, identification of people at risk for osteoporosis, and recognition of problems associated with osteoporosis form the basis for nursing assessment. The health history includes the occurrence of osteopenia and osteoporosis and focuses on family history of both conditions and any fractures in parents and grandparents; previous fractures including fragility fractures; dietary consumption of calcium, vitamin D, and protein; exercise patterns; onset of menopause; and the use of corticosteroids as well as alcohol, smoking, and salt and caffeine intake. Four main risk factors for fractures related to osteoporosis are low BMD, prior fragility fractures, increasing age, and family history of osteoporosis. Questions are asked about previous falls and risk factors for falling such as reduced muscle strength (seen as problems getting up from a chair unassisted), impaired balance, low body mass, and decreased visual acuity. Symptoms such as back pain, constipation, or altered body image, are explored.

Physical examination may disclose a fracture, kyphosis of the thoracic spine, or shortened stature. A loss of more than 2 cm in height over 1 year or a total loss of more than 4 cm suggests possible vertebral fractures and the need for x-ray confirmation. Factors that have been identified in predicting increased risk of hip fracture in postmenopausal women include increasing age, fair to poor self-reported health, relatively greater height, relatively lighter weight, any fracture after age 54 years, white or Asian ancestry, sedentary lifestyle, current smoker, parental hip fracture, current corticosteroid use, and treatment for diabetes.

Nursing Priorities

Major nursing priorities for the patient who experiences a spontaneous vertebral fracture related to osteoporosis may include the following:

- Decreased awareness of osteoporosis and treatment
- Acute pain
- Constipation
- Additional fractures related to osteoporosis

Planning and Goals

The major goals for the patient include knowledge about osteoporosis and the treatment regimen, relief of pain, improved bowel elimination, prevention of falls, and absence of additional fractures.

Nursing Interventions

Promoting Understanding of Osteoporosis and the Treatment Regimen

Patient teaching focuses on factors influencing the development of osteoporosis, interventions to arrest or slow the process, and measures to relieve symptoms. Adequate dietary or supplemental calcium and vitamin D, regular weight-bearing impact exercise, and modification of lifestyle, if necessary (e.g., cessation of smoking, reduced use of caffeine [less than 4 cups per day], salt, alcohol), help to maintain bone mass. Diet, exercise, and physical activity are the primary keys to developing high-density bones that are resistant to osteoporosis. It is emphasized that all people continue to need sufficient calcium, vitamin D, sunshine, and weight-bearing impact exercise to slow the progression of osteoporosis.

Patient teaching related to medication therapy is important. Because gastrointestinal symptoms and abdominal distention are frequent side effects of calcium supplements, the nurse instructs the patient to take the calcium supplements with meals. Also, it is important to teach the patient to drink adequate fluids to reduce the risk of renal calculi. If HRT is prescribed, the nurse teaches the patient about the importance of adherence and periodic screening for breast and endometrial cancer. Alendronate must be taken on an empty stomach with water and then the patient must not consume foods or liquids or assume a reclining position for 30 to 60 minutes. Nasal calcitonin is administered daily, alternating the nares. An adequate daily intake of dietary calcium and vitamin D is needed along with these prescribed medications.

Managing Pain

Managing back pain resulting from compression fracture involves resting in bed in a supine or side-lying position several times a day. Knee flexion increases comfort by relaxing back muscles. Nasal calcitonin is the treatment of choice to relieve the pain of vertebral fractures. Intermittent local heat and back rubs promote muscle relaxation. The nurse instructs the patient to move the trunk as a unit and to avoid bending and twisting. Patients are taught to pick up an object from the floor by holding onto something for support and positioning one leg behind them while bending over ("golfer method" of picking up golf balls). This manoeuvre keeps the back straight. The nurse encourages good posture and teaches body mechanics. When the patient is assisted out of bed, a lumbosacral corset may be worn for temporary support and immobilization, although such a device is frequently uncomfortable and is poorly tolerated by many older patients. The patient gradually resumes activities as pain diminishes. Vertebroplasty may be considered for some patients.

Improving Bowel Elimination

Constipation is a problem related to immobility and medications. Early institution of a high-fibre diet, increased fluids, and the use of prescribed stool softeners help to prevent or minimize constipation. If the vertebral collapse involves the T10–L2 vertebrae, the patient may develop a paralytic ileus. The nurse therefore monitors the patient's intake, bowel sounds, and bowel activity.

Preventing Injury

Physical activity is essential to strengthen muscles, improve balance, prevent disuse atrophy, and retard progressive bone demineralization. Isometric exercises can strengthen trunk muscles. The nurse encourages walking, good body mechanics, and good posture. Daily weight-bearing activity, preferably outdoors in the sunshine to enhance the body's ability to produce vitamin D, is encouraged. Sudden bending, jarring, twisting, and strenuous lifting are avoided.

Gerontologic Considerations

Older adults fall because a hip has fractured (fragility fracture) or as a result of environmental hazards, neuromuscular disorders, diminished senses, syncope, and responses to medications. The patient and family need to be included in planning for care and preventive management regimens. For example, the home environment should be assessed for safety and elimination of potential hazards (e.g., scatter rugs, cluttered rooms and stairwells, toys on the floor, pets underfoot). A safe environment can then be created (e.g., well-lit staircases with secure handrails, grab bars in the bathroom, properly fitting footwear).

Evaluation

Expected patient outcomes may include the following:

1. Acquires knowledge about osteoporosis and treatment regimen
   a. States relationship of calcium and vitamin D intake and of exercise to bone mass
   b. Consumes adequate dietary calcium, vitamin D, and protein for age group
   c. Increases level of weight-bearing impact exercise
   d. Takes prescribed medication therapy
   e. Adheres to prescribed screening and monitoring procedures
2. Achieves pain management
   a. Experiences decreased pain at rest
   b. Experiences minimal discomfort during ADLs
   c. Demonstrates decreased tenderness at fracture site
3. Demonstrates usual bowel elimination
   a. Has active bowel sounds and reports regular bowel movements
4. Experiences no new fractures
   a. Maintains good posture and uses appropriate body mechanics
   b. Consumes a diet high in calcium, vitamin D, and protein
   c. Engages in weight-bearing impact exercises (walks daily)
   d. Rests by lying down several times a day
   e. Maintains a safe home environment
   f. Accepts assistance and supervision as needed

Osteomalacia

Osteomalacia is a metabolic disease affecting bone formation due to inadequate mineralization. As a result of faulty mineralization, there is softening and weakening of bone, causing pain, tenderness, bowing of the bones, and pathologic fractures. Osteomalacia in children is known as rickets. The term "osteomalacia" is used to refer to the disease in adults. On physical examination, skeletal deformities (spinal kyphosis and bowed legs) give patients an unusual appearance and a waddling or limping gait. These patients may be uncomfortable with their appearance. As a result of calcium deficiency, muscle weakness, and unsteadiness, there is an increased risk for falls and fractures.

Pathophysiology

The most common cause of osteomalacia is vitamin D (cholecalciferol) deficiency. Vitamin D is derived from exposure to sunlight and from a healthy diet. Vitamin D promotes calcium absorption from the gastrointestinal tract and facilitates mineralization of bone by calcium and phosphate. Osteomalacia due to poor dietary intake of vitamin D and calcium may be associated with low socioeconomic status/poverty, food faddism, or general lack of knowledge about nutrition. It occurs most frequently in areas where vitamin D is not added to food, where dietary deficiencies exist, and where there is less exposure to sunlight. Babies that are exclusively breastfed are at risk for rickets, as mother's milk does not have sufficient amounts of vitamin D; therefore, the babies require vitamin D supplementation.

Osteomalacia may result from poor calcium absorption (e.g., malabsorption syndrome) or from excessive loss of calcium from the body. Vitamin D (as well as vitamins A, E, and K) is fat soluble. Patients with gastrointestinal disorders such as celiac disease, chronic biliary tract obstruction, inflammatory bowel disease, and chronic pancreatitis are at risk for osteomalacia, as vitamin D is poorly absorbed. In addition, liver and kidney diseases can produce a lack of vitamin D, as these organs convert vitamin D to the active form (calcitriol).

Renal tubular acidosis and chronic renal failure are associated with osteomalacia. The body uses available calcium to combat the acidosis, and PTH stimulates the release of skeletal calcium in an attempt to reestablish a physiologic pH. During this continual drain of skeletal calcium, bony fibrosis occurs and bony cysts form. Chronic glomerulonephritis, obstructive uropathies, and heavy metal poisoning result in a reduced serum phosphate level and demineralization of bone.

Hyperparathyroidism leads to skeletal decalcification and thus to osteomalacia by increasing phosphate excretion in the urine. Prolonged use of anticonvulsant medication (e.g., phenytoin, phenobarbital) poses a risk for osteomalacia, as does insufficient vitamin D (dietary, sunlight).

Gerontologic Considerations

A nutritious diet with adequate amounts of vitamin D and calcium is particularly important in older adults. Prevention, identification, and management of osteomalacia in older people is thought to reduce the risk of fractures. The occurrence of osteomalacia and osteoporosis increases the risk of fractures. In community-dwelling individuals, taking a vitamin D supplement (with or without calcium) has been shown to reduce skeletal complications by only 15% (Bolland, Grey, Gamble, et al., 2014).

Assessment and Diagnostic Findings

On x-ray studies, generalized demineralization of bone is evident. Studies of the vertebrae may show a compression fracture with indistinct vertebral end plates. Laboratory studies show low serum calcium and phosphorus levels and a moderately elevated ALP. Urine excretion of calcium and creatinine is low. Bone biopsy demonstrates an increased amount of osteoid, a demineralized, cartilaginous bone matrix that is sometimes referred to as prebone.

Medical Management

Physical, psychological, and pharmaceutical measures are used to reduce the patient's discomfort and pain. If the underlying cause of osteomalacia is corrected, the disorder may resolve. If kidney disease prevents activation of absorbed vitamin D, then supplementation requires the activated form (calcitriol). If osteomalacia is caused by malabsorption, increased doses of vitamin D, along with supplemental calcium, are usually prescribed. Exposure to sunlight may be recommended; ultraviolet radiation transforms a cholesterol substance (7-dehydrocholesterol) present in the skin into vitamin D (Singer, Bone, Hosking, et al., 2014).

Osteomalacia due to dietary deficiencies is similarly treated by a diet rich in protein, calcium, and vitamin D. The patient is instructed about dietary sources of calcium (almonds, canned salmon, fortified milk, soy, and orange juice) and vitamin D (fortified milk, cereals, eggs, salmon, and vitamin D3 supplements). Osteoporosis Canada recommends 1,000 mg of calcium a day for adults between 19 and 50 years of age (including breastfeeding and pregnant women) and 1,200 mg a day for those over 50. For the same age groups, 400 to 1,000 IU and 800 to 2,000 IU of vitamin D is recommended, respectively (see Chart 71-7). The American Academy of Pediatrics recommends 400 IU of vitamin D daily for infants, children, and adolescents. Extremely high doses of vitamin D are toxic and can enhance the risk of hypercalcemia.

Physical, psychological, and pharmaceutical measures are used to reduce the patient's discomfort and pain. When assisting the patient to change positions, the nurse handles the patient gently, and pillows are used to support the body. As the patient responds to therapy, the skeletal discomfort decreases.

Appropriate treatment of the underlying nutritional deficiency will resolve the skeletal problems associated with osteomalacia. Long-term monitoring of the patient is appropriate to ensure stabilization or reversal of osteomalacia. Some orthopedic deformities may need to be treated with braces or surgery (e.g., osteotomy may be performed to correct long bone deformity).

Paget's Disease

Pathophysiology

The etiology of Paget's disease (osteitis deformans) is unknown. It is a disorder of localized rapid bone turnover, most commonly affecting the skull, femur, tibia, pelvis, and vertebrae. There is a primary proliferation of osteoclasts causing bone resorption. This is followed by a compensatory increase in osteoblastic activity that replaces the bone. As bone turnover continues, a classic mosaic (disorganized) pattern of bone develops. The diseased bone in Paget's disease is highly vascularized and structurally weak, leading to pathologic fractures. Structural bowing of the legs causes malalignment of the hip, knee, and

CHART 71-7

HOME CARE CHECKLIST • Osteoporosis and Osteomalacia

At the completion of education, the patient and/or caregiver will be able to:

Infants, Children, and Adolescents

- List risk factors for osteoporosis.
- Identify calcium- and vitamin D–rich foods.
- Consume diet with adequate calcium: 1,000 mg/day between 19 and 50 years of age, including breastfeeding and pregnant women and vitamin D (800–1,000 IU/day).
- The American Academy of Pediatrics recommends 400 IU of vitamin D daily for infants, children, and adolescents.
- Engage in weight-bearing exercise daily.
- Modify lifestyle choices—avoid smoking, alcohol, caffeine, carbonated beverages, and salt.

Menopausal and Postmenopausal Women

- List risk factors for osteoporosis.
- Identify calcium- and vitamin D–rich foods.
- Consume diet with adequate calcium (1,200–1,500 mg/day) and vitamin D (800–2,000 IU/day).
- Knowledge of calcium supplements.
- Engage in weight-bearing impact exercise at least three times weekly.
- Engage in exercise that improves balance and strength to reduce the incidence of falls.
- Demonstrate good body mechanics.
- Modify lifestyle choices—avoid smoking, and use of alcohol, caffeine, salt, and carbonated beverages.
- Participate in screening for osteoporosis (age 50 years with risk factors or 65 years of age).
- Discuss pharmacologic agents to maintain and enhance bone mass.
- Review concurrent medical conditions and medications with health care provider to identify factors that contribute to bone mass loss.
- Assess home environment for hazards contributing to falls.

Men

- List risk factors associated with osteoporosis in men, including medications (e.g., corticosteroids, anticonvulsant medications, aluminum-containing antacids), chronic diseases (e.g., kidney, lung, gastrointestinal), and undiagnosed low testosterone levels.
- Modify lifestyle choices to avoid smoking and excessive intake of alcohol, caffeine, salt, and carbonated beverages.
- Engage in weight-bearing impact exercise daily, such as walking, and exercise to improve balance and strength to limit falls.
- Consume diet with adequate calcium (1,200–1,500 mg/day) and vitamin D (800–2,000 IU/day).
- Participate in screening for osteoporosis.
- Talk with health care provider about use of medications (e.g., alendronate) to enhance bone mass or to correct testosterone deficiency.
- Assess home for hazards contributing to falls.

ankle joints, which contributes to the development of arthritis and back and joint pain.

Paget's disease occurs in about 2% to 3% of the population older than 50 years. The incidence is slightly greater in men than in women and increases with aging. A family history has been noted, with siblings developing the disease.

Clinical Manifestations

Paget's disease is insidious to the extent that many patients are not aware that they have the condition. Some patients do not experience symptoms but have skeletal deformity. A few patients have symptomatic deformity and pain. The condition is most frequently identified on x-ray during a routine physical examination or in the course of an assessment for another medical issue. Sclerotic changes, skeletal deformities (e.g., bowing of the femur and tibia, enlargement of the skull, deformity of the pelvic bones), and cortical thickening of the long bones occur.

In most patients, skeletal deformity involves the skull or long bones. The skull may thicken, and the patient may report that a hat no longer fits. In some cases of Paget's disease, the cranium, but not the face, is enlarged. This gives the face a small, triangular appearance. Most patients with skull involvement have impaired hearing from cranial nerve compression and dysfunction. Other cranial nerves may also be compressed.

The femurs and tibiae tend to bow, producing a waddling gait. The spine is flexed and is rigid; the chin rests on the chest. The thorax is compressed and immobile on respiration. The trunk is flexed on the legs to maintain balance; the arms are bent outward and forward and appear long in relation to the shortened trunk, giving the patient an apelike posture.

Pain, tenderness, and warmth over the bones may be noted. The pain is mild to moderate, deep, and aching; it increases with weight bearing if the lower extremities are involved. Pain and discomfort may precede skeletal deformities of Paget's disease by years and are often wrongly attributed by the patient to old age or arthritis.

The temperature of the skin overlying the affected bone increases because of increased bone vascularity. Patients with large, highly vascular lesions may develop high-output cardiac failure because of the increased vascular bed and metabolic demands.

Assessment and Diagnostic Findings

Elevated serum alkaline phosphatase concentration and urinary hydroxyproline excretion reflect increased osteoblastic activity. Higher values suggest more active disease. Patients with Paget's disease have normal blood calcium levels. X-rays confirm the diagnosis of Paget's disease. Local areas of demineralization and bone overgrowth produce characteristic mosaic patterns and irregularities. Bone scans demonstrate the extent of the disease. Bone biopsy may aid in the differential diagnosis.

Medical Management

Pain is managed by the administration of NSAIDs. Gait problems from bowing of the legs are managed with walking aids, shoe lifts, and physical therapy. Weight is controlled to reduce stress on weakened bones and malaligned joints. Asymptomatic patients may be managed with diets adequate in calcium and vitamin D and periodic monitoring.

Fractures, arthritis, and hearing loss are complications of Paget's disease. Fractures are managed according to location. Healing occurs if fracture reduction, immobilization, and stability are adequate. Severe degenerative arthritis may require total joint replacement. Loss of hearing is managed with hearing aids and communication techniques used with the hearing-impaired person (e.g., lip reading, body language).

Pharmacologic Therapy

Patients with moderate to severe disease may benefit from specific antiosteoclastic therapy. Several medications reduce bone turnover, reverse the course of the disease, relieve pain, and improve mobility.

Calcitonin, a polypeptide hormone, retards bone resorption by decreasing the number and availability of osteoclasts. Calcitonin therapy facilitates remodelling of abnormal bone into normal lamellar bone, relieves bone pain, and helps to alleviate neurologic and biochemical signs and symptoms. Calcitonin is administered subcutaneously or by nasal inhalation. Side effects include flushing of the face and nausea. The effect of calcitonin therapy is evident in 3 to 6 months.

Bisphosphonates, such as risedronate (Actonel) and alendronate (Fosamax), produce rapid reduction in bone turnover and relief of pain. They reduce serum alkaline phosphatase and urinary hydroxyproline levels. Bisphosphonates should be taken on an empty stomach to increase absorption. Patients also require elemental calcium (1,500 mg a day) and 1,000 IU of vitamin D daily during therapy.

Gerontologic Considerations

Careful assessment of the patient's pain and discomfort is necessary. Patient teaching helps the patient understand the treatment regimen, the need for a diet with adequate calcium and vitamin D, and how to compensate for altered musculoskeletal functioning. The home environment is assessed for safety to prevent falls and to reduce the risk for fracture. Strategies for coping with a chronic health problem and its effect on quality of life need to be developed.

Musculoskeletal Infections

Osteomyelitis

Osteomyelitis is an infection of the bone that results in inflammation, necrosis, and formation of new bone. Osteomyelitis is classified as:

- Hematogenous osteomyelitis (i.e., due to bloodborne spread of infection)
- Contiguous-focus osteomyelitis, from contamination from bone surgery, open fracture, or traumatic injury (e.g., gunshot wound)
- Osteomyelitis with vascular insufficiency, seen most commonly among patients with diabetes and peripheral vascular disease, most commonly affecting the feet (Grossman & Porth, 2014)

Patients who are at high risk for osteomyelitis include older adults and those who are poorly nourished or have obesity. Other patients at risk include those with impaired immune systems, those with chronic illnesses (e.g., diabetes, rheumatoid arthritis), those receiving long-term corticosteroid therapy or immunosuppressive agents, and those who use IV drugs (Lalani, 2016).

Postoperative surgical wound infections typically occur within 30 days after surgery. They are classified as incisional (superficial, located above the deep fascia layer) or deep (involving tissue beneath the deep fascia). If an implant has been used, deep postoperative infections may occur within a year. Osteomyelitis may become chronic and may affect the patient's quality of life.

Pathophysiology

More than 50% of bone infections are caused by *Staphylococcus aureus* and increasingly of the variety that is methicillin resistant (i.e., methicillin-resistant *Staphylococcus aureus* [MRSA]) (Kaplan, 2014). Surgical site ink markers have been linked to infections by cross-contamination between preoperative patients who use their markers; therefore, these items are now considered one patient or one-time use items (Driessche, 2012). Other pathogens include the gram-positive organisms *streptococci* and *enterococci*, followed by gram-negative bacteria, including *pseudomonas* (Kaplan, 2014).

The initial response to infection is inflammation, increased vascularity, and edema. After 2 or 3 days, thrombosis of the local blood vessels occurs, resulting in ischemia with bone necrosis. The infection extends into the medullary cavity and under the periosteum and may spread into adjacent soft tissues and joints. Unless the infective process is treated promptly, a bone abscess forms. The resulting abscess cavity contains **sequestrum** (i.e., dead bone tissue), which does not easily liquefy and drain. Therefore, the cavity cannot collapse and heal, as it does in soft tissue abscesses. New bone growth, the **involucrum**, forms and surrounds the sequestrum. Although healing appears to take place, a chronically infected sequestrum remains and produces recurring abscesses throughout the patient's life. This is referred to as chronic osteomyelitis.

Clinical Manifestations

In bloodborne infection, onset is sudden and is associated with the clinical manifestations of septicemia (e.g., chills, fever, night sweats, tachycardia, and general malaise). The infection extends through the cortex of the bone into the periosteum and the soft tissues. The infected area becomes painful, swollen, and extremely tender. The patient may describe a constant, pulsating pain that intensifies with movement as a result of the pressure caused by a collection of pus. In osteomyelitis due to spread of adjacent infection or from direct contamination, there may be no generalized symptoms of septicemia. The area is swollen, warm, painful, and tender to touch.

The patient with chronic osteomyelitis presents with a continuously draining sinus or experiences recurrent periods of pain, inflammation, swelling, and drainage. The low-grade infection thrives in scar tissue because it has a reduced blood supply.

Assessment and Diagnostic Findings

In acute osteomyelitis, early x-ray findings demonstrate soft tissue swelling. In about 2 weeks, areas of irregular decalcification, bone necrosis, periosteal elevation, and new bone formation are evident. Radioisotope bone scans, particularly with isotope-labelled white blood cell (WBC) scan, and magnetic resonance imaging (MRI) facilitate early definitive diagnosis. Blood tests reveal an elevated WBC and C-reactive protein. Wound and blood cultures are taken to identify the offending microorganism and guide appropriate antibiotic therapy.

With chronic osteomyelitis, large, irregular cavities, raised periosteum, sequestra, or dense bone formations are seen on x-ray. Bone scans may be performed to identify areas of infection. The sedimentation rate and the WBC count are usually normal. Anemia, associated with chronic infection, may be evident. The abscess is cultured to determine the infective organism and appropriate antibiotic therapy.

Prevention

Elective orthopedic surgery is postponed if the patient has a current infection (e.g., urinary tract infection, sore throat) or a recent history of infection. During orthopedic surgery, careful attention is paid to the surgical environment and to techniques to decrease direct bone contamination. Prophylactic antibiotics, administered to achieve adequate tissue levels at the time of surgery and for 24 hours after surgery, are helpful. Urinary catheters and drains are removed as soon as possible to decrease the incidence of hematogenous spread of infection.

Treatment of focal infections diminishes hematogenous spread. Aseptic postoperative wound care reduces the incidence of superficial infections and osteomyelitis. Prompt management of soft tissue infections reduces extension of infection to the bone. When patients who have had joint replacement surgery undergo dental procedures or other invasive procedures (e.g., cystoscopy), prophylactic antibiotics are frequently recommended.

Medical Management

The initial goal of therapy is to control and halt the infectious process. Antibiotic therapy depends on the results of blood and wound cultures. Frequently, the infection is caused by more than one pathogen. General supportive measures (e.g., hydration, a diet high in vitamins and protein, correction of anemia) should be instituted. The area affected with osteomyelitis is immobilized to decrease discomfort and to prevent pathologic fracture of the weakened bone. Warm wet soaks for 20 minutes several times a day may be prescribed to increase circulation.

Pharmacologic Therapy

Bone infections are more difficult to eradicate than soft tissue infections because bone is mostly avascular and less accessible to the body's natural immune response. Because there is decreased penetration by medications, antibiotic therapy is longer term than with other infections; typically, it continues for 3 to 6 weeks. After the infection appears to be controlled, the antibiotic may be given orally. However, there is little evidence to support optimal length of therapy (Conterno & Turchi, 2013).

Obtaining culture and sensitivity is the ideal scenario for antibiotic therapy. However, IV empiric therapy can be initiated. For example, with methicillin-sensitive *Staphylococcus aureus* (MSSA), a cephalosporin such as ceftriaxone may be used. The aim is to control the infection before the blood supply to the area diminishes as a result of thrombosis. Around-the-clock dosing is necessary to achieve a sustained therapeutic serum concentration of the antibiotic. An antibiotic to which the causative organism is sensitive is prescribed after results of the culture and sensitivity studies are known. IV antibiotic therapy continues for 3 to 6 weeks. After the infection appears to be controlled, the antibiotic may be administered orally for up to 3 months; however, it is not clear that subsequent oral therapy improves the outcome. To enhance absorption of the orally administered medication, antibiotics should not be administered with food.

Surgical Management

If the patient does not respond to antibiotic therapy, the infected bone is surgically exposed, the purulent and necrotic material is removed, and the area is irrigated with sterile saline solution. Antibiotic-impregnated beads may be placed in the wound for direct application of antibiotics for 2 to 4 weeks and IV antibiotic therapy is continued.

In chronic osteomyelitis, antibiotics are adjunctive therapy to surgical debridement. A sequestrectomy (removal of enough involucrum to enable the surgeon to remove the sequestrum) is performed. In many cases, sufficient bone is removed to convert a deep cavity into a shallow saucer (saucerization). All dead, infected bone and cartilage must be removed before permanent healing can occur. A closed-suction irrigation system may be used to remove debris. Wound irrigation using sterile physiologic saline solution may be performed for 7 to 8 days.

The wound is either closed tightly to obliterate the dead space or packed and closed later by granulation or possibly by grafting. The debrided cavity may be packed with cancellous bone graft to stimulate healing. With a large defect, the cavity may be filled with a vascularized bone transfer or muscle flap (in which a muscle is moved from an adjacent area with blood supply intact). These microsurgery techniques enhance the blood supply. The improved blood supply facilitates bone healing and eradication of the infection. The surgical procedures may be staged over time to ensure healing. Surgical debridement weakens the bone; internal fixation or external supportive devices may be needed to stabilize or support the bone to prevent pathologic fracture.

Nursing Process

The Patient With Osteomyelitis

Assessment

The patient with osteomyelitis reports an acute onset of signs and symptoms (e.g., localized pain, swelling, erythema, fever) or recurrent drainage of an infected sinus with associated pain, swelling, and low-grade fever. The nurse assesses the patient for risk factors (e.g., older age, diabetes, long-term corticosteroid therapy) and for a history of previous injury, infection, or orthopedic surgery. The patient avoids pressure on the area and guards movement. In acute hematogenous osteomyelitis, the patient exhibits generalized weakness due to the systemic reaction to the infection.

Physical examination reveals an inflamed, markedly swollen, warm area that is tender. Purulent drainage may be noted. The patient has an elevated temperature. With chronic osteomyelitis, the temperature elevation may be minimal, occurring in the afternoon or evening.

Nursing Priorities

Nursing priorities for the patient with osteomyelitis may include:

- Acute pain
- Impaired physical mobility
- Increased risk for extension of infection and bone abscess formation
- Lack of knowledge

Planning and Goals

The patient's goals include pain management, improved physical mobility within therapeutic limitations, control and eradication of infection, and increased knowledge of the treatment regimen.

Nursing Interventions

Managing Pain

The affected part may be immobilized with a splint to decrease pain and muscle spasm. The nurse monitors the neurovascular status of the affected extremity. The wounds are frequently very painful, and the extremity must be handled with great care and gentleness. Elevation reduces swelling and associated discomfort. Pain is controlled with prescribed analgesics and other pain-reducing techniques.

Improving Physical Mobility

Treatment regimens restrict activity. The bone is weakened by the infectious process and must be protected by immobilization devices and avoidance of stress on the bone. The patient must understand the rationale for the activity restrictions. The joints above and below the affected part should be gently placed through their range of motion. The nurse encourages full participation in ADLs within the physical limitations to promote general well-being.

Controlling the Infectious Process

The nurse monitors the patient's response to antibiotic therapy and observes the IV access site for evidence of phlebitis, infection, or infiltration. With long-term, intensive antibiotic therapy, the nurse monitors the patient for signs of superinfection (e.g., oral or vaginal candidiasis, loose or foul-smelling stools).

In those patients requiring surgery, the nurse promotes adequate circulation by wound suction to prevent fluid accumulation, elevating the affected area to facilitate venous drainage and avoidance of pressure on grafted area. The patient will continue to require immobilization of the limb and to adhere to weight-bearing restrictions. The nurse changes dressings using aseptic technique to promote healing and to prevent cross-contamination.

The nurse continues to monitor the general health and nutrition of the patient. A diet high in protein and vitamin C provides a positive nitrogen balance and promotes healing. The nurse encourages adequate hydration as well.

Promoting Home, Community-Based, and Transitional Care

EDUCATING PATIENTS ABOUT SELF-CARE. The patient and family must learn and recognize the importance of strictly adhering to the therapeutic regimen of antibiotics and preventing falls or other injuries that could result in bone fracture. The patient needs to know how to maintain and manage the IV access and IV administration equipment in the home. Major centres in Canada have outpatient home parenteral therapy programs (HPTPs) that patients attend intermittently. Infectious disease specialists and RNs at HPTP clinics provide supervision, advice, and management for the patient's parenteral therapy. Medication education includes the medication name, dosage, frequency, administration rate, safe storage, handling, adverse reactions, and laboratory testing. In addition, aseptic dressing and warm compress techniques are taught.

The nurse carefully monitors the patient for the development of additional painful areas or sudden increases in body temperature. The nurse instructs the patient and family to observe and report elevated temperature, drainage, odour, increased inflammation, adverse reactions, and signs of superinfection.

CONTINUING AND TRANSITIONAL CARE. Management of osteomyelitis, including wound care and IV antibiotic therapy, is usually performed at home with supervision at an HPTP clinic. The patient must be medically stable, physically able, and motivated to adhere strictly to the therapeutic regimen of antibiotic therapy. The home care environment needs to be conducive to promotion of health and to the requirements of the therapeutic regimen.

If the patient is unable to attend the HPTP clinic, a home care nurse may be needed to assist with IV administration of the antibiotics. The nurse monitors the patient for response to the treatment, signs and symptoms of superinfections, and adverse drug reactions. The nurse stresses the importance of follow-up health care appointments (Chart 71-8).

Evaluation

Expected patient outcomes may include the following:

1. Experiences pain management
   a. Reports decreased pain and discomfort
   b. Experiences no tenderness at the site of infection
2. Increases physical mobility
   a. Participates in self-care activities
   b. Maintains full function of unimpaired extremities
   c. Demonstrates safe use of immobilizing and assistive devices
   d. Modifies environment to promote safety and to avoid falls
3. Shows absence of infection
   a. Takes antibiotics as prescribed
   b. Reports normal temperature, no swelling, and no wound drainage
   c. Laboratory results indicate WBC and CRP are in normal range
   d. Wound cultures are negative
4. Adheres to therapeutic plan
   a. Takes medications as prescribed
   b. Protects affected limb
   c. Demonstrates proper wound care
   d. Reports signs and symptoms of complications promptly
   e. Eats a diet high in protein and vitamin C
   f. Keeps follow-up health appointments
   g. Reports increased strength
   h. Reports no elevation of temperature or recurrence of pain, swelling, or other symptoms at site

Septic (Infectious) Arthritis

The successful invasion and proliferation of microbial organisms in joints cause a septic arthritis. The most common type of microbes causing septic arthritis are bacteria; however, joints may also be infected by viruses, mycobacteria, fungi, and parasites. Joints can become infected through spread of infection from other parts of the body (hematogenous spread) or directly through trauma or surgical instrumentation. Previous trauma to joints, joint replacement, coexisting arthritis, and diminished host resistance contribute to the development of an infected joint. The bacterium *S. aureus* causes most adult joint infections, followed by streptococci and gram-negative organisms. The older adult, patients who use IV drugs, and patients who are seriously immunocompromised may be infected by *Escherichia coli*. Prompt recognition and treatment of an infected joint are important as an accumulation of pus results in chondrolysis (destruction of hyaline cartilage) and destruction of the joint.

Clinical Manifestations

The patient with acute septic arthritis usually presents with a hot, painful, swollen joint with decreased range of motion. Systemic chills, fever, and leukocytosis are present. Risk factors include advanced age, diabetes mellitus, rheumatoid arthritis, and pre-existing joint disease or joint replacement.

Gerontologic Considerations

Older patients and patients taking corticosteroids or immunosuppressive medications may not exhibit

CHART 71-8

HOME CARE CHECKLIST • The Patient With Osteomyelitis

At the completion of education, the patient and/or caregiver will be able to:

- State the impact of osteomyelitis on physiologic functioning, ADLs, IADLs, roles, relationships, and spirituality.
- Identify modification of home environment, interventions, and strategies (e.g., durable medical equipment, adaptive equipment) used in safely adapting to changes in structure or function and promote effective recovery and rehabilitation.
- State how to obtain medical supplies and carry out dressing changes, wound care, and other prescribed regimens.
- Describe ongoing postoperative therapeutic regimen, including diet and activities to perform (e.g., exercises) and to limit or avoid (e.g., lifting weights, driving a car, contact sports).
    - Consume a healthy diet to promote wound and bone healing.
    - Observe prescribed weight-bearing and activity limits.
    - Demonstrate proper wound care.
    - Demonstrate safe use of ambulatory aids and assistive devices.
- State the name, dose, side effects, frequency, and schedule for all medications.
    - Demonstrate accurate and safe administration of medications.
- When indicated, identify the benefits and expected outcomes of intravenous antibiotic therapy and IV access management.
    - Demonstrate how to prepare, infuse, maintain, and clean IV access and equipment.
    - Identify adverse effects of antibiotic therapy and actions to take for adverse effects.
    - Describe to whom, how, and when to report adverse effects.
- Relieve pain with pharmacologic and nonpharmacologic interventions.
- State indicators of wound infections (e.g., redness, swelling, tenderness, purulent drainage, fever) and systemic infection (e.g., fever, chills, rapid pulse, general malaise) to report promptly to primary provider.
- Relate how to reach primary provider with questions or complications.
- State time and date of follow-up appointments and testing.
- Identify the need for health promotion (e.g., weight reduction, smoking cessation, stress management), disease prevention, and screening activities.

typical clinical manifestations of infection. Therefore, they require ongoing assessment to detect infection as early as possible in the infectious process.

Assessment and Diagnostic Findings

An assessment for the source and cause of infection is performed. Diagnostic studies include aspiration, examination, and culture of the synovial fluid. Computed tomography (CT) and MRI may show damage to the joint lining. Radioisotope scanning may be useful in localizing the infectious process.

Medical Management

Prompt treatment is essential and may save a joint prosthesis for patients who already have one. Broad-spectrum IV antibiotics are started promptly and then changed to organism-specific antibiotics after culture results are available. The IV antibiotics are continued until symptoms resolve.

In addition to prescribing antibiotics, the primary provider may aspirate the joint with a needle, to remove excessive joint fluid, exudate, and debris. This promotes comfort and decreases joint destruction caused by the action of proteolytic enzymes in the purulent fluid. Occasionally, arthrotomy is performed to drain the joint and remove dead tissue.

The inflamed joint is supported and immobilized in a functional position by a splint that increases the patient's comfort. Analgesics, such as codeine, may be prescribed to manage pain. The patient's nutrition and fluid status are monitored. Progressive range-of-motion exercises are ordered after the infection subsides.

If septic joints are treated promptly, recovery of normal function is expected. The patient is assessed periodically for recurrence. If the articular cartilage was damaged during the inflammatory reaction, joint fibrosis and diminished function may result.

Nursing Management

The nurse educates the patient and family about the septic arthritis physiologic process and explains the importance of supporting the affected joint, adhering to the prescribed antibiotic regimen, inspecting the skin under any splints that may be prescribed, and observing weight-bearing and activity restrictions. The patient is also educated that recurrence of infection in the near and far future is possible, and is educated about signs and symptoms to observe and report to the primary provider. The same interventions used for the patient with osteomyelitis are planned for the patient with septic arthritis. See previous discussion.

Bone Tumours

Neoplasms of the musculoskeletal system are of various types, including osteogenic, chondrogenic, fibrogenic, muscle (rhabdomyogenic), and marrow (reticulum) cell tumours as well as nerve, vascular, and fatty cell tumours. They may be primary tumours or metastatic tumours from primary cancers elsewhere in the body (e.g., breast, lung, prostate, kidney). Metastatic bone tumours are more common than primary bone tumours.

Benign Bone Tumours

Benign tumours of the bone and soft tissue are more common than malignant primary bone tumours. Benign bone tumours generally are slow growing and well circumscribed, present few symptoms, and are not a cause of death.

Benign primary neoplasms of the musculoskeletal system include osteochondroma, enchondroma, bone cyst (e.g., aneurysmal bone cyst), osteoid osteoma, rhabdomyoma, and fibroma. Some benign tumours, such as giant cell tumours, have the potential to become malignant.

Osteochondroma is the most common benign bone tumour. It usually occurs as a large projection of bone at the end of long bones (at the knee or shoulder). It develops during growth and then becomes a static bony mass. In fewer than 1% of patients, the cartilage cap of the osteochondroma may undergo malignant transformation after trauma, and a chondrosarcoma or osteosarcoma may develop.

Enchondroma is a common tumour of the hyaline cartilage that develops in the hand, femur, tibia, or humerus. Usually, the only symptom is a mild ache. Pathologic fractures may occur.

Bone cysts are expanding lesions within the bone. Aneurysmal (widening) bone cysts are seen in young adults, who present with a painful, palpable mass of the long bones, vertebrae, or flat bone. Unicameral (single cavity) bone cysts occur in children and cause mild discomfort and possible pathologic fractures of the upper humerus and femur, which may heal spontaneously.

A painful tumour that occurs in children and young adults is the osteoid osteoma. The neoplastic tissue is surrounded by reactive bone formation that assists in its identification by x-ray.

Giant cell tumours (osteoclastomas) are benign for long periods but may invade local tissue and cause destruction. They occur in young adults and are soft and hemorrhagic. Eventually, giant cell tumours may undergo malignant transformation and metastasize.

Malignant Bone Tumours

Primary malignant musculoskeletal tumours are relatively rare and arise from connective and supportive tissue cells (sarcomas) or bone marrow elements (multiple myeloma; see Chapter 68). Malignant primary musculoskeletal tumours include osteosarcoma, chondrosarcoma, Ewing's sarcoma, and fibrosarcoma. Soft tissue sarcomas include liposarcoma, fibrosarcoma of soft tissue, and rhabdomyosarcoma. Bone tumour metastasizing to the lungs is common.

Osteogenic sarcoma (osteosarcoma) is the most common and most often fatal primary malignant bone tumour. Prognosis depends on whether the tumour has metastasized to the lungs at the time the patient seeks health care. Osteogenic sarcoma appears most frequently in males between the ages of 10 and 25 years (in bones that grow rapidly), in older people with Paget's disease, and as a result of radiation exposure. Clinical manifestations include pain, swelling, limited motion, and weight loss—which is considered an ominous finding. The bony mass may be palpable, tender, and fixed, with an increase in skin temperature over the mass and venous distention. The primary lesion may involve any bone, but the most common sites are the distal femur, the proximal tibia, and the proximal humerus.

Malignant tumours of the hyaline cartilage are called *chondrosarcomas*. These tumours are the second most common primary malignant bone tumour. They are large, bulky, slow-growing tumours that affect adults. The usual tumour sites include the pelvis, femur, humerus, spine, scapula, and tibia. Metastases to the lungs occur in fewer than half of patients. When these tumours are well differentiated, large bloc excision or amputation of the affected extremity results in increased survival rates; however, these tumours may recur.

Metastatic Bone Disease

Metastatic bone disease (secondary bone tumour) is more common than any primary bone tumour. Tumours arising from tissues elsewhere in the body may invade the bone and produce localized bone destruction (lytic lesions) or bone overgrowth (blastic lesions). The most common primary sites of tumours that metastasize to bone are the kidney, prostate, lung, breast, ovary, and thyroid. Metastatic tumours most frequently attack the skull, spine, pelvis, femur, and humerus and involve more than one bone (polyostotic).

Pathophysiology

A tumour in the bone causes the normal bone tissue to react by osteolytic response (bone destruction) or osteoblastic response (bone formation). Primary tumours cause bone destruction, which weakens the bone, resulting in bone fractures. Adjacent normal bone responds to the tumour by altering its normal pattern of remodelling. The surface of the bone changes, and the contours enlarge in the tumour area.

Malignant bone tumours invade and destroy adjacent bone tissue. Benign bone tumours, in contrast, have a symmetric, controlled growth pattern and place pressure on adjacent bone tissue. Malignant invading bone tumours weaken the structure of the bone until it can no longer withstand the stress of ordinary use; pathologic fracture commonly results.

Clinical Manifestations

Patients with metastatic bone tumour may have a wide range of associated clinical manifestations. They may be symptom-free or have pain (mild and occasional to constant and severe); varying degrees of disability; and, at times, obvious bone growth. Weight loss, malaise, and fever may be present. The tumour may be diagnosed only after pathologic fracture has occurred.

With spinal metastasis, spinal cord compression may occur. It can progress rapidly or slowly. Neurologic deficits (e.g., progressive pain, weakness, gait abnormality, paresthesia, paraplegia, urinary retention, loss of bowel or bladder control) must be identified early and treated with decompressive laminectomy to prevent permanent spinal cord injury.

Assessment and Diagnostic Findings

The differential diagnosis is based on the history, physical examination, and diagnostic studies, including CT, bone scans, myelography, arteriography, MRI, biopsy, and biochemical assays of the blood and urine. Serum alkaline phosphatase levels are frequently elevated with osteogenic sarcoma. With metastatic carcinoma of the prostate, serum acid phosphatase levels are elevated. Hypercalcemia is present with breast, lung, or kidney cancer bone metastases. Symptoms of hypercalcemia include muscle weakness, fatigue, anorexia, nausea, vomiting, polyuria, cardiac dysrhythmias, seizures, and coma. Hypercalcemia must be identified and treated promptly. Surgical biopsy is performed for histologic identification. Extreme care is taken during biopsy to prevent seeding and resultant recurrence after excision of the tumour.

Chest x-rays are performed to determine the presence of lung metastases. Surgical staging of musculoskeletal tumours is based on tumour grade and site (intracompartmental or extracompartmental) as well as on metastasis. Staging is used for planning treatment.

During the diagnostic period, the nurse explains the diagnostic tests and provides psychological and emotional support to the patient and family. The nurse assesses coping behaviours and encourages the use of support systems.

Medical Management

Primary Bone Tumours

Treatment of bone tumours includes surgical excision (ranging from local excision to amputation and disarticulation), radiation therapy, and chemotherapy (preoperative, intraoperative [neoadjuvant], postoperative, and adjunctive for possible micrometastases). Major gains are being made in the use of wide bloc excision with restorative grafting technique (Muscolo, Ayerza, Aponte-Tinao, et al., 2005). Survival and quality of life are important considerations in procedures that attempt to save the involved extremity.

Limb-sparing (salvage) procedures are used to remove the tumour and adjacent tissue. A customized prosthesis, total joint arthroplasty, or bone tissue from the patient (autograft) or from a cadaver donor (allograft) replaces the resected tissue. Soft tissue and blood vessels may need grafting because of the extent of the excision. Complications include infection, loosening or dislocation of the prosthesis, allograft nonunion, fracture, devitalization of the skin and soft tissues, joint fibrosis, and recurrence of the tumour. Function and rehabilitation after limb salvage depend on positive encouragement and reducing the risk for complications.

Surgical removal of the tumour may require amputation of the affected extremity, with the amputation extending well above the tumour to achieve local control of the primary lesion (refer to Nursing Process: The Patient Undergoing an Amputation in Chapter 72).

Because of the danger of metastases with malignant bone tumours, combined chemotherapy is started before and continued after surgery in an effort to eradicate micrometastatic lesions. The goal of combined chemotherapy is greater therapeutic effect at a lower toxicity rate with reduced resistance to the medications. There is an improved long-term survival rate when a localized osteosarcoma is removed and chemotherapy is initiated. Soft tissue sarcomas are treated with radiation, limb-sparing excision, and adjuvant chemotherapy (see Chapter 68).

Secondary Bone Tumours

The treatment of metastatic bone cancer is palliative. The therapeutic goal is to relieve the patient's pain and discomfort while promoting quality of life.

Surgical interventions may be needed. If metastatic disease weakens the bone, structural support and stabilization are needed to prevent pathologic fracture. At times, large bones with metastatic lesions are strengthened by prophylactic internal fixation. Internal fixation of pathologic fractures, arthroplasty, or methyl methacrylate (bone cement) reconstruction minimizes associated disability and pain. Patients with metastatic disease are at higher risk for pulmonary congestion, hypoxemia, deep vein thrombosis, and hemorrhage than are other patients after orthopedic surgery.

Hypercalcemia resulting from breakdown of bone requires to be recognized promptly. Treatment includes hydration with IV administration of normal saline solution, diuresis, mobilization, and medications such as bisphosphonates, pamidronate, and calcitonin. Because inactivity leads to loss of bone mass and increased calcium in the blood, the nurse assists the patient to increase activity and ambulation.

Hematopoiesis is frequently disrupted by tumour invasion of the bone marrow or by treatment (chemotherapy or radiation). Blood product transfusions restore hematologic factors. Pain can result from multiple factors, including the osseous metastasis, surgery, chemotherapy or radiation side effects, and arthritis. Pain must be assessed accurately and managed with adequate and appropriate opioid, nonopioid, and nonpharmaceutical interventions. External beam radiation to involved metastasis sites may be used. Patients with multiple bony metastases may achieve pain management with systemically administered "bone-seeking" isotopes (e.g., strontium 89). Refer to Chapter 16 for more information about pain management.

Additional therapies are used to treat the original cancer. Radiation and hormonal therapy may be effective in promoting healing of osteolytic lesions. Chemotherapy is used to control the primary disease (see Chapter 68).

Nursing Process

The Patient With a Bone Tumour

Assessment

The nurse asks the patient about the onset and course of symptoms. During the assessment, the nurse notes the patient's understanding of the disease process, how the patient and the family have been coping, and how the patient has managed the pain. On physical examination, the nurse gently palpates the mass and notes the size and associated soft tissue swelling, pain, and tenderness. Assessment of the neurovascular status and range of motion of the extremity provides baseline data for future comparisons. The nurse evaluates the patient's mobility and ability to perform ADLs.

Nursing Priorities

The major nursing priorities for the patient with a bone tumour may include the following:

- Lack of knowledge
- Pain
- Increased risk for injury
- Ineffective coping
- Increased risk for situational low self-esteem

Collaborative Problems/ Potential Complications

Potential complications may include the following:

- Delayed wound healing
- Nutritional deficiency
- Infection
- Hypercalcemia

Planning and Goals

The major goals for the patient include knowledge of the disease process and treatment regimen, control of pain, absence of pathologic fractures, effective patterns of coping, improved self-esteem, and absence of complications.

Nursing Interventions

The nursing care of a patient who has undergone excision of a bone tumour is similar in many respects to that of other patients who have had skeletal surgery. Vital signs are monitored; blood loss is assessed; and observations are made to assess for the development of complications such as deep vein thrombosis, pulmonary emboli, infection, contracture, and disuse atrophy. The affected part is elevated to control swelling, and the neurovascular status of the extremity is assessed.

Promoting Understanding of the Disease Process and Treatment Regimen

Patient and family teaching about the disease process and diagnostic and management regimens is essential. Explanation of diagnostic tests, treatments (e.g., wound care), and expected results (e.g., decreased range of motion, numbness, change of body contours) helps the patient deal with the procedures and changes. Cooperation and adherence to the therapeutic regimen are enhanced through understanding. The nurse can most effectively reinforce and clarify information provided by the physician by being present during these discussions.

Managing Pain

Accurate pain assessment is the foundation for pain management. Pharmacologic and nonpharmacologic techniques are used to manage pain and increase the patient's comfort level. The nurse works with the patient in designing the most effective pain management regimen, thereby increasing the patient's control over the pain. The nurse prepares the patient and gives support during painful procedures. Prescribed IV or epidural analgesics are used during the early postoperative period. Later, oral or transdermal opioid or nonopioid analgesics are usually adequate to relieve pain. In addition, external radiation or systemic radioisotopes may be used to control pain (refer to Chapter 16 for further discussion of pain management).

Preventing Pathologic Fracture

Bone tumours weaken the bone to a point at which normal activities or even position changes can result in fracture. During nursing care, the affected extremities must be supported and handled gently. External supports (e.g., splints) may be used for additional protection. At times, the patient may elect to have surgery (e.g., open reduction and internal fixation, joint replacement) in an attempt to prevent pathologic fracture. Prescribed weight-bearing restrictions must be followed. The nurse teaches the patient how to use assistive devices safely and how to strengthen unaffected extremities.

Promoting Coping Skills

The nurse encourages the patient and family to verbalize their fears, concerns, and feelings. They need to be supported as they deal with the impact of the malignant bone tumour. Feelings of shock, despair, and grief are expected. Referral to a psychiatric nurse liaison, psychologist, counsellor, or spiritual advisor may be indicated for specific psychological help and emotional support.

Promoting Self-Esteem

Independence versus dependence is an issue for the patient who has a malignancy. Lifestyle is dramatically changed, at least temporarily. It is important to support the family in working through the adjustments that must be made. The nurse assists the patient in dealing with changes in body image due to surgery and possible amputation. It is helpful to provide realistic reassurance about the future and resumption of role-related activities and to encourage self-care and socialization. The patient participates in planning daily activities. The nurse encourages the patient to be as independent as possible. Involvement of the patient and family throughout treatment encourages confidence, restoration of self-concept, and a sense of being in control of one's life.

Monitoring and Managing Potential Complications

DELAYED WOUND HEALING. Wound healing may be delayed because of tissue trauma from surgery, previous radiation therapy, inadequate nutrition, or infection. The nurse minimizes pressure on the wound site to promote circulation to the tissues. An aseptic, nontraumatic wound dressing promotes healing. Monitoring and reporting of laboratory findings facilitate initiation of interventions to promote homeostasis and wound healing.

Repositioning the patient at frequent intervals reduces the incidence of skin breakdown due to pressure. Special therapeutic beds may be needed to prevent skin breakdown and to promote wound healing after extensive surgical reconstruction and skin grafting.

INADEQUATE NUTRITION. Because loss of appetite, nausea, and vomiting are frequent side effects of chemotherapy and radiation therapy, it is necessary to provide adequate nutrition for healing and health promotion. Antiemetics and relaxation techniques reduce the gastrointestinal reaction. Stomatitis is controlled with anesthetic or antifungal mouthwash (see Chapter 68). Adequate hydration is essential. Nutritional supplements or total parenteral nutrition may be prescribed to achieve adequate nutrition.

OSTEOMYELITIS AND WOUND INFECTIONS. Prophylactic antibiotics and strict aseptic dressing techniques are used to diminish the occurrence of osteomyelitis and wound infections. During healing, other infections (e.g., upper respiratory infections) need to be prevented so that hematogenous spread does not result in osteomyelitis. If the patient is receiving chemotherapy, it is important to monitor the WBC count and to instruct the patient to avoid contact with people who have colds or other infections.

HYPERCALCEMIA. Hypercalcemia is a dangerous complication of bone cancer. The symptoms must be recognized and treatment initiated promptly. Symptoms include muscular weakness, incoordination, anorexia, nausea and vomiting, constipation, electrocardiographic changes (e.g., shortened QT interval and ST segment, bradycardia, heart blocks), and altered mental states (e.g., confusion, lethargy, psychotic behaviour). Refer to Chapter 17 for a full discussion of hypercalcemia and its management.

Promoting Home, Community-Based, and Transitional Care

EDUCATING PATIENTS ABOUT SELF-CARE. Preparation for and coordination of continuing health care are begun early as a multidisciplinary effort. Patient teaching addresses medication, dressing, treatment regimens, and the importance of physical and occupational therapy programs. The nurse teaches weight-bearing limitations and special handling to prevent pathologic fractures. It is important that the patient and family know the signs and symptoms of possible complications as well as resources available for continuing care (Chart 71-9).

CONTINUING AND TRANSITIONAL CARE. Frequently, arrangements are made for home, community-based, or transitional care supervision and follow-up. The nurse assesses the patient's and family's abilities to meet the patient's needs and determines whether the services of other agencies are needed. The nurse advises the patient to have readily available the telephone numbers of people to contact in case concerns arise.

The nurse emphasizes the need for long-term health supervision to ensure cure or to detect tumour recurrence or metastasis. If the patient has metastatic disease, end-of-life issues may need to be explored. Referral for hospice care is made if appropriate.

Evaluation

Expected patient outcomes may include the following:

1. Describes disease process and treatment regimen
   a. Describes pathologic condition
   b. States goals of therapeutic regimen
   c. Seeks clarification of information
2. Achieves adequate pain management
   a. Uses multiple pain management techniques, including prescribed medications
   b. Experiences no pain or decreased pain at rest, during ADLs, or at surgical sites
3. Decreases risk of pathologic fracture
   a. Avoids stress to weakened bones
   b. Uses assistive devices safely and appropriately
   c. Strengthens uninvolved extremities with exercise
4. Demonstrates effective coping patterns
   a. Verbalizes feelings
   b. Identifies strengths and abilities
   c. Requests assistance as needed
5. Demonstrates positive self-concept
   a. Identifies home and family responsibilities that can be accomplished
   b. Exhibits confidence in own abilities
   c. Demonstrates acceptance of altered body image
   d. Demonstrates independence in ADLs
6. Decreases risk of complications
   a. Demonstrates wound healing and maintenance of skin integrity
   b. Experiences no skin breakdown
   c. Maintains or increases body weight
   d. Experiences no infections
   e. Does not experience hypercalcemia
   f. Manages side effects of therapies

CHART 71-9

HOME CARE CHECKLIST • The Patient With a Bone Tumour

At the completion of education, the patient and/or caregiver will be able to:

- State the impact of the bone tumour growth process and treatment on physiologic functioning, ADLs, IADLs, roles, relationships, and spirituality.
- Identify modification of home environment, interventions, and strategies (e.g., durable medical equipment, wound care/dressings, adaptive equipment, ADL assistance) used in safely adapting to changes in structure or function and promote effective recovery and rehabilitation.
- Describe ongoing therapeutic regimen, including diet and activities to perform (e.g., exercises) and to limit or avoid (e.g., lifting weights, driving a car, contact sports).
  - Consume a healthy diet to promote healing and health.
  - State weight-bearing and activity restrictions.
  - Support affected musculoskeletal area; position to decrease risk of skin breakdown.
  - Demonstrate safe use of ambulatory aids and assistive devices.
  - Engage in exercise that improves balance to reduce risk of falls.
- State the name, dose, side effects, frequency, and schedule for all prescribed therapeutic and prophylactic medications (e.g., antibiotics, analgesic agents).
- Control pain with pharmacologic and nonpharmacologic interventions.
- State indicators of complications to report promptly to primary provider such as:
  - Wound infection/delayed wound healing (e.g., redness, swelling, tenderness, purulent drainage, fever).
  - Osteomyelitis (e.g., localized pain, edema, erythema, fever).
  - Hypercalcemia (e.g., muscular weakness, anorexia, decreased coordination, nausea, vomiting, constipation).
- Relate how to reach primary provider with questions or complications.
- State time and date of follow-up appointments, therapy, and testing.
- Identify community resources for peer and caregiver/family support:
  - Identify sources of support (e.g., friends, relatives, faith community).
  - Identify phone numbers, meeting locations, and times of support groups (e.g., cancer support groups, caregiver support groups).
- Identify the need for health promotion, disease prevention, and screening activities.

ADLs, activities of daily living; IADLs, independent activities of daily living.

g. Reports symptoms of medication toxicity or complications

7. Participates in continuing health care at home
   a. Complies with prescribed regimen (i.e., takes prescribed medications, continues physical and occupational therapy programs)
   b. Acknowledges need for long-term health supervision
   c. Keeps follow-up health care appointments
   d. Reports occurrence of symptoms or complications

Critical Thinking Exercises

1 A 30-year-old nurse seeks treatment for acute low back pain in the hospital occupational health clinic after a lifting injury sustained from transferring a patient with obesity the previous evening. He tells you that his fellow nurses always ask him to help with heavy lifts. He wants to know if a lumbar brace will help to diminish his back pain. He also wonders if he should wear one all the time while at work. What is the strength of the evidence that supports or does not support the use of a lumbar brace for this patient, in either alleviating his pain or in preventing further lumbar strain?

2 A college student presents to the student health centre after she jammed the first digit of her right foot on her dormitory room door. Describe the priority assessment process that you would follow when you examine her right foot. What is the expected care for a possible broken toe?

3 At the medical clinic where you work as a nurse, a 65-year-old man who is overweight presents with persistent low-grade pain along his lumbar spine. He believes it is related to moving around some boxes about a month ago. He has a history of heavy cigarette smoking, alcohol consumption, and a personal history of prostatic cancer. What are the risk factors for problems other than muscle strain that must be considered, based on his medical history?

REFERENCES AND SELECTED READINGS

Books

Czerniak, B. (2016). *Dorfman and Czerniak's bone tumors* (2nd ed.). Philadelphia, PA: WB Saunders.

Davis, A., James, S., & Saifuddin, A. (2015). Bone tumours (2): Malignant bone tumours. In A. Grainger & P. O'Connor (Eds.). *Grainger and Allison's diagnostic radiology: The musculosketetal system*. New York: Elsevier.

Grossman, S., & Porth, C. (2014). *Porth's pathophysiology: Concepts of altered health states* (9th ed.). Philadelphia, PA: Lippincott Williams & Wilkins.

Rubin, E., Gorstein, F., Schwarting, R., et al. (2004). *Pathology* (4th ed.). Philadelphia, PA: Lippincott Williams & Wilkins.

Weber, J. W., & Kelley, J. (2014). *Health assessment in nursing* (5th ed.). Philadelphia, PA: Lippincott Williams & Wilkins.

Journals and Electronic Documents

American Board of Internal Medicine (ABIM). (2015). Choosing wisely campaign. Retrieved February 13, 2016, from choosingwisely.org

American College of Foot and Ankle Surgeons (ACFAS). (2009). Clinical practice guideline for the diagnosis and treatment of forefoot disorders. *Journal of Food and Ankle Surgery*, *48*(2), 230–272.

American College of Foot and Ankle Surgeons (ACFAS). (2010). Diagnosis and treatment of heel pain. *Journal of Foot and Ankle Surgeons*, *49*(3 Suppl.), S1–S19.

American College of Occupational and Environmental Medicine. (2011). Carpal tunnel syndrome. Retrieved February 13, 2016, from www.guideline.gov/content.aspx?id=34436&search=carpal+tunnel+syndrome

Amirfeyz, R., Gozzard, C., & Leslie, I. J. (2005). Hand elevation test for assessment of carpal tunnel syndrome. *Journal of hand surgery, 30*(4), 361–364.

Avenell, A., Mak, J. C., & O'Connell, D. (2014). Vitamin D and vitamin D analogues for preventing fractures in postmenopausal women and older men. *Cochrane Database of Systematic Reviews*, *4*, CD000227.

Ball, T., Butler, M., & Parsons, S. (2013). Pes-cavus—not just a clinical sign. Diagnosis, aetiology and management. *Advances in Clinical Neuroscience and Rehabilitation—Rehabilitation articles*, *12*(6), 16–19.

Banwell, H., Mackintosh, S., & Thewlis, D. (2014). Foot orthoses for adults with flexible pes planus: A systematic review. *Journal of Foot & Ankle Research*, *7*(1), 23.

Bolland, M. J., Grey, A., Gamble, G. D., et al. (2014). The effect of vitamin D supplementation on skeletal, vascular, or cancer outcomes: A trial sequential meta-analysis. *The Lancet Diabetes & Endocrinology*, *2*(4), 307–320.

Bries, A., Kerr, B., & George, L. (2015). Osteomyelitis: An overview of imaging modalities. *Critical Care Nursing Quarterly*, *38*(2), 154–164.

Buchman, A. S., Shah, R. C., Leurgans, S. E., et al. (2010). Musculoskeletal pain and incident disability in community-dwelling older adults. *Arthritis Care and Research*, *62*(9), 1287–1293.

Canadian Agency for Drugs and Technologies in Health. (2014). *Mattresses for chronic back or neck pain: A review of the clinical effectiveness and guidelines. Summary of evidence*. Retrieved November 29, 2016, from www.ncbi.nlm.nih.gov/books/NBK263383

Cenzer, I. S., Tang, V., Boscardin, W. J., et al. (2016). One-Year mortality after hip fracture: Development and validation of a prognostic index. *Journal of the American Geriatrics Society*, *64*(9), 1863–1868.

Cicci, J., Buie, L., Bates, J., et al. (2014). Denosumab for the management of hyperglycemia of malignancy in patients with multiple myeloma and renal dysfunction. *Clinical Lymphoma, Myeloma & Leukemia*, *14*(6), e207–e211.

Coleman, R., Body, J. J., Aapro, M., et al. (2014). Bone health in cancer patients: ESMO clinical practice guidelines. *Annals of Oncology*, *25*(Suppl. 3), 124–137.

Conterno, L. O., & Turchi, M. D. (2013). Antibiotics for treating chronic osteomyelitis in adults. *Cochrane Database of Systematic Reviews*, *9*, CD004439.

Cosman, F., de Beur, S. J., LeBoff, M. S., et al. (2014). Clinician's guide to prevention and treatment of osteoporosis. *Osteoporosis International*, *25*(10), 2359–2381.

Cosman, F., de Beur, S. J., LeBoff, M. S., et al. (2015). Erratum to: Clinician's guide to prevention and treatment of osteoporosis. *Osteoporosis International*, *26*(7), 2045–2047.

de Heer, E., Gerrits, M., Beekman, A., et al. (2014). The association of depression and anxiety with pain: A study from NESDA. *PLoS One*, *9*(10), e106907.

Dhaliwal, R., Mikhail, M., Usera, G., et al. (2018). The relationship of physical performance and osteoporosis prevention with vitamin D in older African Americans (PODA). *Contemporary Clinical Trials*, *65*, 39–45.

Dong, W., Goost, H., Lin, X. B., et al. (2015). Treatments for shoulder impingement syndrome: A PRISMA systematic review and network meta-analysis. *Medicine (Baltimore)*, *94*(10), e510.

Driessche, A. M. (2012). Surgical site markers: Potential source of infection. *Orthopaedic Nursing*, *31*(6), 344–347.

Fasolino, T., & Whitright, T. (2015). A pilot study to identify modifiable and nonmodifiable variables associated with osteopenia and osteoporosis in men. *Orthopaedic Nursing*, *34*(5), 289–293.

Goldenberg, D. L., & Sexton, D. J. (2016). Septic arthritis in adults. *UpToDate*. Retrieved December 11, 2016, from www.uptodate.com/contents/septic-arthritis-in-adults

González-Reimers, E., Quintero-Platt, G., Rodríguez-Rodríguez, E., et al. (2015). Bone changes in alcoholic liver disease. *World Journal of Hepatology*, *7*(9), 1258–1264.

Hansen, K. E., Johnson, R. E., Chambers, K. R., et al. (2015). Treatment of vitamin D insufficiency in postmenopausal women: A randomized clinical trial. *JAMA Internal Medicine*, *175*(10), 1612–1621.

Henschke, N., Maher, C. G., Osteolo, R. W., et al. (2013). Red flags to screen for malignancy in patients with low-back pain. *Cochrane Database of Systematic Reviews*, 2, CD008686.

Huppins, L. (2011). Evidence-based medicine (EBM) and orthotic therapy. *Podiatry Management*, *4*(100), 97–102.

International Association for the Study of Pain. (1986). Classification of chronic pain. Descriptions of chronic pain syndromes and definitions of pain terms. *Pain. Supplement*, *3*, s1–s226.

Johnson, R. E., Haas, K., Lindow, K., et al. (2014). Plantar fasciitis: What is the diagnosis and treatment? *Orthopaedic Nursing*, *33*(4), 198–204.

Kaplan, S. L. (2014). Recent lessons for the management of bone and joint infections. *Journal of Infection*, *68*(Suppl. 1), S51–S56.

Lalani, T. (2016). Overview of osteomyelitis in adults. *UpToDate*. Retrieved April 4, 2016, from www.uptodate.com/contents/overview-of-osteomyelitis-in-adults

Lee, W. J., Lee, S. M., Won, C. H, et al. (2014). Efficacy of intralesional bleomycin for the treatment of plantar hard corns. *International Journal of Dermatology*, *53*(12), e572–e577.

Malhotra, R., Chan, C., & Nather, A. (2014). Osteomyelitis in the diabetic foot. *Medical Clinics of North America*, *97*(5), 947–956.

Michigan Quality Improvement Consortium (MQIC). (2016a). *Management of acute low back pain in adults*. Retrieved November 29, 2016, from www.mqic.org/pdf/mqic_2016_lbp_guideline_update_alert.pdf

Michigan Quality Improvement Consortium (MQIC). (2016b). *Management and prevention of osteoporosis*. Retrieved November 29, 2016, from www.guideline.gov/summaries/summary/47804/management-and-prevention-of-osteoporosis?q=Michigan+Quality+Improvement+Consortium

Morgan, D. J., Dhruva, S. S., Wright, S. M., et al. (2015). Update on medical practices that should be questioned in 2015. *JAMA Internal Medicine*, *175*(12), 1960–1964.

Muscolo, D. L., Ayerza, M. A., Aponte-Tinao, L. A., et al. (2005). Use of distal femoral osteoarticular allografts in limb salvage surgery. *JBJS*, *87*(11), 2449–2455.

National Institute of Neurological Disorders (NINDS). (2014). *Low back pain fact sheet*. Retrieved February 13, 2016, from www.ninds.nih.gov/disorders/backpain/detail_backpain.htm

NPS Medicinewise. (2015). *Osteoporosis: Not just a woman's disease*. Retrieved April 4, 2016, from www.nps.org.au/publications/health-professional/health-news-evidence/2015/osteoporosis

Osteoporosis Canada. (2019). https://osteoporosis.ca/about-the-disease/

Rodriguez, J. A. (2014). Corticosteroid versus platelet-rich plasma injection in epicondylitis. *Orthopaedic Nursing*, *33*(5), 257–265.

Rossignol, S., Schwab, M., Schwartz, M., et al. (2007). Spinal cord injury: time to move?. *Journal of Neuroscience*, *27*(44), 11782–11792.

Schaafsma, F. G., Anema, J. R., & van der Beek, A. J. (2015). Back pain: Prevention and management in the workplace. *Best Practice & Research Clinical Rheumatology*, *29*(3), 483–494.

Sharff, K. A., Richards, E. P., & Townes, J. M. (2013). Clinical management of septic arthritis. *Current Rheumatology Reports*, *15*(6), 332.

Shemory, S. T., Pfefferle, K. J., & Gradisar, I. M. (2015). Modifiable risk factors in patients with low back pain. Paper presented at the 2015 Annual Meeting of the American Academy of Orthopaedic Surgeons (AAOS), Las Vegas, NV.

Shirzad, K., Kiesau, C. D., DeOrio, J. K., et al. (2011). Lesser toe deformities. *Journal of the American Academy of Orthopaedic Surgeons*, *19*(8), 505–514.

Singer, F., Bone, H., Hosking, D., et al. (2014). Paget's disease of the bone: An endocrine society clinical practice guideline. *The Journal of Clinical Endocrinology & Metabolism, 99*(12), 4408–4422.

Smeltzer, S. C., & Qi, B. B. (2014). Practical implications for nurses caring for patients being treated for osteoporosis. *Nursing: Research and Reviews, 4*(4), 19–33.

Smith, M. A., & Dahlen, N. R. (2013). Clinical practice guideline: Surgical site infection prevention. *Orthopaedic Nursing, 32*(5), 249–250.

Song, D., Meng, B., Gan, M., et al. (2015). The incidence of secondary vertebral fracture of vertebral augmentation techniques versus conservative treatment for painful osteoporotic vertebral fractures: A systematic review and meta-analysis. *Acta Radiologica, 56*(8), 970–979.

Sood, A., Paik, A., & Lee, E. (2013). *Dupuytren's contracture. Eplasty, 13, ic1*. Retrieved November 29, 2016, from www.ncbi.nlm.nih.gov/pmc/articles/PMC3552604

Treede R. D. (2018). The International Association for the Study of Pain definition of pain: As valid in 2018 as in 1979, but in need of regularly updated footnotes. *Pain Reports, 3*(2), e643.

United States Preventive Services Task Force (USPSTF). (2013). Menopausal hormone therapy for the primary prevention of chronic conditions. *Annals of Internal Medicine, 158*(1), 47–54.

van Vugt, T. A., Geurts, J., & Arts, J. J. (2016). Clinical application of antimicrobial bone graft substitute in osteomyelitis treatment: A systematic review of different bone graft substitutes available in clinical treatment of osteomyelitis. *BioMed Research International*, doi:10.1155/2016/6984656.

Veugelers, P., & Ekwaru, J. (2014). A statistical error in the estimation of the recommended dietary allowance for vitamin D. *Nutrients, 6*(10), 4472–4475.

Vitamin D Council. (2016). *How do I get the vitamin D my body needs?* Retrieved December 11, 2016, from www.vitamindcouncil.org/about-vitamin-d/how-do-i-get-the-vitamin-d-my-body-needs

Williams, C., Henschke, N., Maher, C., et al. (2013). Red flags to screen for vertebral fracture in patients presenting with low-back pain. *Cochrane Database of Systematic Reviews, 1*, CD008643.

Wong, C. C., & McGirt, M. J. (2013). Vertebral compression fractures: A review of current management and multimodal therapy. *Journal of Multidisciplinary Healthcare, 6*, 205–214.

Wright, N. C., Hooker, E. R., Nielson, C. M., et al. Osteoporotic Fractures in Men (MrOS) Study Research Group. (2018). The epidemiology of wrist fractures in older men: The Osteoporotic Fractures in Men (MrOS) study. *Osteoporosis International, 29*(4), 859–870.

Wright, N. C., Looker, A. C., Saag, K. G., et al. (2014). The recent prevalence of osteoporosis and low bone mass in the United States based on bone mineral density at the femoral neck or lumbar spine. *Journal of Bone and Mineral Research: The Official Journal of the American Society for Bone and Mineral Research, 29*(11), 2520–2526.

Resources

Arthritis Society: http://www.arthritis.ca

Canadian Cancer Society: http://www.cancer.ca

Canadian Institutes of Health Research: http://www.cihr-irsc.gc.ca/e/13217.html

Canadian Orthopaedic Association: http://www.coa-aco.org

Canadian Orthopaedic Foundation: http://www.canorth.org

Canadian Rheumatology Association: http://www.rheum.ca

National Institute of Arthritis and Musculoskeletal and Skin Diseases, Office of Communications and Public Liaison: http://www.niams.nih.gov

Osteoporosis Canada: http://www.osteoporosis.ca

Paget Foundation: http://www.paget.org

Spondylitis Association of America: https://www.spondylitis.org/About-Spondylitis/Inflammatory-vs-Mechanical-Back-Pain

The Impact of Arthritis in Canada: Today and Over the Next 30 Years. Arthritis Alliance of Canada: www.arthritisalliance.ca

Therapeutic Products Directorate, Health Canada; Drug Product Database: http://www.hc-sc.gc.ca/dhp-mps/prodpharma/databasdon/index-eng.php

72 Management of Patients With Musculoskeletal Trauma

Adapted by James A. Rankin and Karen Lynn Then

Learning Objectives

On completion of this chapter, the learner will be able to:

1. Differentiate among contusions, strains, sprains, and dislocations.
2. Describe selected sports injuries and their nursing management.
3. Describe the clinical manifestations of a fracture and the emergency management of the patient with a fracture.
4. Describe the principles of fracture reduction, fracture immobilization, and management of open fractures.
5. Use the nursing process as a framework for care of the older adult patient with a fracture and amputation.
6. Describe the prevention and management of immediate and delayed complications of fractures.
7. Describe the rehabilitative needs of patients with fractures of the clavicle, upper and lower extremities, pelvis, hips, ribs, and thoracolumbar spine.
8. Describe the rehabilitative and health education needs of the patient who has had an amputation.

Injury to the musculoskeletal (MSK) system results in injury or dysfunction to adjacent structures and of structures. In severe fractures there is muscle spasm, and laceration to blood vessels, nerves as well as other adjacent soft tissues.

Treatment of MSK injury involves providing support to the injured part until healing is complete. Conservative treatment includes the use of bandages, adhesive strapping, splints, or casts. In severe trauma, orthopedic surgeons perform open reduction and internal fixation (ORIF) of the bone using hardware such as pins, plates, and screws. At times, traction is used to correct deformity or shortening.

Emphasis is on early mobilization of the patient in order to prevent complications of extended bed rest such as pneumonia, pressure ulcers, joint contractures, constipation, and urinary tract infections. In addition to the appropriate nursing care, physical and occupational therapists contribute to the patients timely recovery.

Contusions, Strains, and Sprains

A *contusion* is a soft tissue injury caused by blunt force to the skin; small blood vessels rupture and bleed into the soft tissue, resulting in a bruise known as an ecchymosis. A hematoma develops when the bleeding is sufficient to cause a solid swelling of blood in the tissues. Localized symptoms of pain, swelling, and discolouration are managed with intermittent application of cold. Most contusions resolve in 1 to 2 weeks.

A joint **strain** occurs with overuse or overstretching, of muscles or tendons resulting in microscopic, incomplete tears causing muscle spasm. The patient experiences sudden pain, with localized tenderness on moving the joint. The hamstring and lower lumbar region are common sites for strains.

A **sprain** involves overstretching or tearing of ligaments surrounding a joint caused by a wrenching or twisting motion. Ligaments are strong bands of fibrous tissue that connect bones in a joint providing stability while permitting mobility. Torn ligaments make the joint much less stable; bleeding and inflammation cause swelling, pain, and loss of joint function. The degree of disability and pain increases during the first 2 to 3 hours after the injury because of the associated swelling and bleeding. Diagnostic imaging is taken to assess for an avulsion fracture as the stretching of the ligament is severe enough to pull (avulse) part of the bone.

Nursing Management

Treatment of contusions, strains, and sprains consists of resting and elevating the affected part, applying cold, and, on occasion, using a compression bandage. (The acronym PRICE—*P*rotection, *R*est, *I*ce, *C*ompression, *E*levation—is helpful for remembering treatment interventions.) Protection from further injury is accomplished through support of the affected area (e.g., sling) and/or splinting. Rest prevents additional injury and promotes healing. Ice applied intermittently for 20 to 30 minutes during the first 24 to 48 hours after injury produces vasoconstriction, which decreases bleeding, edema, and discomfort. Care must be taken to avoid skin and tissue damage from excessive cold application. An elastic compression bandage may be used to reduce swelling and provides support for the injured tissues. However, the bandage must not be applied too tightly as this may impact the normal inflammatory response; the nurse should assess the patient's extremities for colour, temperature, sensation, and movement. Elevation helps to reduce the swelling. In a severe sprain with torn muscles and ligaments, a surgical repair or casting of the limb may be necessary to immobilize the limb. As with the use of elastic bandages, the neurovascular status of the injured extremity is monitored frequently.

After 24 to 48 hours the acute inflammatory stage gradually resolves and heat may be applied for 15 to 30 minutes, four times/day to relieve muscle spasm and to promote vasodilation, and facilitate healing. Depending on the severity of injury, progressive passive and active exercises may begin in 2 to 5 days. Severe sprains may require 1 to 3 weeks of immobilization before protected exercises are initiated. Excessive exercise early in the course of treatment delays recovery. Ligaments and tendons do not have a very good blood supply, therefore strains and sprains take weeks or months to heal.

Joint Dislocations

A **dislocation** of a joint is a condition in which the articular surfaces of the bones forming the joint are no longer in anatomic contact. The bones are literally "out of joint." A **subluxation** is a partial dislocation of the articulating surfaces. Traumatic dislocations are orthopedic emergencies because the associated joint structures, blood supply, and nerves are distorted and severely stressed. If the dislocation is not treated promptly, *necrosis* (tissue death due to anoxia and diminished blood supply) and nerve palsy may occur.

Dislocations may be congenital (most often the hip is effected), spontaneous, or pathologic, caused by disease of the articular or periarticular structures, or traumatic, resulting from injury in which the joint is disrupted by force.

Signs and symptoms of a traumatic dislocation are pain, change in contour of the joint, change in the length of the extremity, loss of normal range of motion (ROM), and change in the axis of the dislocated bones. X-rays confirm the diagnosis and demonstrate any associated fracture.

Medical Management

The affected joint needs to be immobilized while the patient is transported to the hospital. The dislocation is promptly reduced by bringing the displaced bones and tissues into normal alignment to preserve joint function. Analgesia, muscle relaxants, and anesthesia are used to facilitate closed reduction. The joint is immobilized by bandages, splints, casts, or traction and is maintained in a stable position. Neurovascular status is monitored. After reduction gentle, progressive, active and passive movement is begun to preserve ROM and restore strength.

Nursing Management

Nursing care is directed at providing comfort, evaluating the patient's neurovascular status, and protecting the joint during healing. The nurse teaches the patient how to manage the immobilizing devices and how to protect the joint from reinjury.

Sports-Related Musculoskeletal Injuries

Unfortunately, some recreational athletes push themselves beyond the level of their physical conditioning and incur

Glossary

allograft: tissue harvested from a donor for use in another person
amputation: removal of a body part, usually a limb or part of a limb
arthroscope: surgical instrument used to examine internal joint structures
autograft: tissue harvested from one area of the body and used for transplantation to another area of the body
débridement: surgical removal of contaminated and devitalized tissues and foreign material
dislocation: separation of joint surfaces
fracture: break in the continuity of a bone
fracture reduction: restoration of fracture fragments into anatomic alignment and rotation
malunion: healing of a fractured bone in a malaligned position
meniscus: crescent-shaped fibrocartilage found in certain joints, such as the knee joint
nonunion: failure of fragments of a fractured bone to heal together
phantom limb pain: pain perceived as being in the amputated limb
PRICE: acronym for Protection, Rest, Ice, Compression, Elevation
rotator cuff: shoulder muscles (supraspinatus, subscapularis, infraspinatus, and teres minor) and their tendons
sprain: overstretching or tearing injury to ligaments
strain: torn muscles or tendons
subluxation: partial separation of joint surfaces
tendinitis: inflammation of a tendon

injuries. Injuries to the MSK system may be acute (e.g., sprains, strains, dislocations, fractures), or they may be gradual, resulting from repetitive overuse (e.g., chondromalacia patella, tendinitis, stress fractures). Professional athletes are also susceptible to injury, even though their training is supervised closely to minimize the occurrence of injury.

- Contusions result from direct falls or blows. The initial dull pain becomes greater, with swelling and stiffness occurring within 24 to 48 hours.
- Sprains commonly occur in fingers, ankles, and knees. If the ligament damage is major, the joint becomes unstable, and surgical repair may be required. In addition, an avulsion fracture may occur.
- Strains cause a sharp, stabbing pain caused by bleeding and immediate protective muscle contraction. Tennis players often suffer calf muscle strains; soccer players often experience hamstring strains; and swimmers, weight lifters, and tennis players often suffer shoulder strains.
- **Tendinitis** (inflammation of a tendon) is caused by overuse and is seen in tennis players (epicondylar tendinitis, or "tennis elbow"), in runners and gymnasts (Achilles tendinitis), and in basketball players (infrapatellar tendinitis).
- Meniscal injuries of the knee occur when the foot is planted firmly in the ground and there is excessive rotation of the knee (skiers and soccer players are prone to this type of injury).
- Dislocations are seen with sports that involve throwing or lifting.
- Fractures. Skaters, bikers and older women are prone to have a fracture of the distal radius, known as a Colles' fracture. Colloquially this is known as a FOOSH (Fall On Out-Stretched Hands) injury. Ballet dancers and track-and-field athletes may experience metatarsal fractures. Stress fractures occur with repeated bone trauma from activities such as jogging, gymnastics, basketball, and aerobics. The tibiae, fibulae, and metatarsals are most vulnerable.

Management

Patients who have experienced a sports-related injury are often highly motivated to return to their previous level of activity. Compliance with restriction of activities and gradual resumption of activities may be a significant problem for these patients. They need to be taught how to avoid further injury or cause a new injury. With recurrence of symptoms, they need to diminish their level and intensity of activity to a comfortable level and to treat the symptoms with PRICE. The time required to recover from a sports-related injury take a few days to several months.

Prevention

Sports-related injuries can be prevented by the use of proper equipment (e.g., running shoes, wrist guards) and by effectively training and conditioning the body. Specific training needs to be tailored to the person and the sport. Warm-up routines generally include walking or slow jogging for about 5 minutes, followed by slow, gradual stretching. The athlete holds the stretch for 10 seconds before relaxing and repeating the stretch. Preparing the body for sports activities increases the person's flexibility and decreases the incidence of strains and sprains.

After exercise, the body needs to cool off to prevent cardiovascular problems such as hypotension, syncope, and dysrhythmias. The athlete needs to be taught to "tune in" to body symptoms that indicate stress and to modify activities to minimize injury and promote healing.

Injuries to the Tendons, Ligaments, and Menisci

Rotator Cuff Tears

A **rotator cuff** tear is a rip in a tendon that connects one of the rotator muscles to the humeral head. The rotator cuff stabilizes the humeral head and is composed of four muscles and their tendons that include the supraspinatus, infraspinatus, teres minor, and subscapularis muscles (National Association of Orthopedic Nurses [NAON], 2013). Rotator cuff tears may result from acute or chronic stresses on the joint and from intrinsic (e.g., age-related factors) or extrinsic (e.g., overuse, fracture, etc.) factors. Physical examination should include bilateral evaluation of the joint. The patient complains of aching pain that is typically insidious in nature (unless related to an acute injury) and worsens with use. The patient will complain of tenderness to palpation and difficulty sleeping on affected side, and will exhibit decreased ROM and decreased strength. X-rays and MRIs aid in confirming diagnosis and extent of injury, but the most accurate diagnostic modality is arthroscopic (NAON, 2013).

Medical Management

Initial conservative management includes use of nonsteroidal anti-inflammatory drugs (NSAIDs); rest with modification of activities; injection of a corticosteroid into the shoulder joint; and progressive stretching, ROM, and strengthening exercises. Some rotator cuff tears require arthroscopic **débridement** (removal of devitalized tissue) or arthroscopic or open acromioplasty with tendon repair. Postoperatively, the shoulder is immobilized for several weeks. Physical therapy with shoulder exercises is begun as ordered, and the patient is instructed to perform the exercises at home. Full recovery is expected in 6 to 12 months.

Epicondylitis (Tennis Elbow)

Epicondylitis is a chronic, painful condition that is caused by excessive, repetitive extension, flexion, pronation, and supination activities of the forearm. Excessive, repetitious activities result in inflammation (tendinitis) and minor tears in the tendons at the origin of the muscles on the medial or lateral epicondyles. Activities contributing to the development of epicondylitis include tennis, racket sports, pitching, gymnastics, and repetitive use of tools such as a screwdriver. Typically the pain radiates down the extensor (dorsal) surface of the forearm. The patient may have decreased grip strength. Most often, relief is obtained by rest and avoidance of the aggravating activity.

Medical Management

Application of ice after the activity and administration of oral and topical NSAIDs are useful for pain management. In some instances, the arm is immobilized in a moulded splint or cast. A local injection of a corticosteroid is reserved for patients with severe pain who do not respond to NSAIDs and immobilization. After pain subsides, rehabilitation exercises include gentle and gradually increased stretching of the tendons. A tennis elbow counterforce strap to limit extension of the elbow may be prescribed when activity is resumed. Occasionally, surgery may be needed to release strictures or to débride the joint.

Lateral and Medial Collateral Ligament Injury

Lateral collateral ligament (LCL) connects the distal end of the femur to the proximal end of the fibula. The medial collateral ligament (MCL) connects the distal end of the femur to the proximal end of the tibia. The knee ligaments provide stability to the knee (Fig. 72-1) by preventing overstretching of the knee outward (LCL) and inward (MCL). Injury to the ligaments occurs when the foot is firmly planted and there is a direct blow to the knee—either medially, causing stretching and tearing injury to the LCL, or laterally, causing stretching and tearing injury to the MCL. The patient immediately experiences severe pain, joint instability, and requires assistance to walk. Football players are at risk for LCL and MCL injuries.

Medical Management

Early management includes PRICE. The joint is evaluated for fracture. Hemarthrosis (bleeding into the joint) may develop, contributing to the pain; should this occur, the joint fluid may be aspirated to relieve pressure.

Treatment depends on the severity of the injury. Conservative management includes PRICE, weight bearing as tolerated (WBAT), and the use of a hinged brace for support. Crutches may be indicated to assist ambulation until weight bearing can be tolerated. Exercises to strengthen the supportive muscles to the knee without straining the ligaments are beneficial. Severe MCL injuries are initially treated with non–weight-bearing status with progression to WBAT in a hinged brace for a lengthy time frame; the healing process may take 8 to 12 weeks. Severe LCL injuries usually require surgical intervention, followed by bracing and physical therapy (Agranoff, 2015). A progressive rehabilitation program helps restore the function and strength of the knee. Rehabilitation occurs over many months, and the patient may need to wear a derotational brace while engaging in sports to prevent reinjury.

Nursing Management

The nurse provides patient teaching about the proper use of ambulatory devices, the healing process, and activity limitation to promote healing. The nurse teaches the surgical patient about pain management, medications (analgesics, antibiotics), brace use, wound care, possible complications (e.g., altered neurovascular status, infection, skin breakdown), and self-care.

Cruciate Ligament Injury

The anterior cruciate ligament (ACL) and the posterior cruciate ligament (PCL) of the knee stabilize forward and backward motion of the femur and tibia (see Fig. 72-1). The ligaments form a cross or 'X' in the centre of the knee. Injury occurs when the foot is firmly planted, the knee is hyperextended, and there is severe torsion (twisting) stress on the joint. ACL and MCL injuries also occur with the knee flexed and being struck on the dashboard of a car in a vehicle collision. The patient reports a pop or tearing sensation with this twisting injury. The patient experiences severe pain, joint instability, and pain with ambulation.

Emergency management includes PRICE. The bones are radiographically assessed for fractures. Joint effusion and hemarthrosis require joint aspiration and wrapping with a compression elastic dressing.

Treatment depends on the severity of the injury and the effect of the injury on daily activities. Conservative treatment involves application of a brace, physical therapy, and avoiding undue stress on the knee. Surgical ACL reconstruction includes tendon repair with grafting and is performed as ambulatory arthroscopic surgery. After surgery, the patient is taught to manage pain with oral opioid analgesics, NSAIDs, and cryotherapy (a cooling pad incorporated in a dressing). The patient is taught about monitoring neurovascular status of the leg, wound care, and signs of complications that need to be reported promptly to the surgeon. Exercises (ankle pumps, quadriceps sets, and hamstring sets) are encouraged during the early postoperative period. The nurse reinforces instruction about

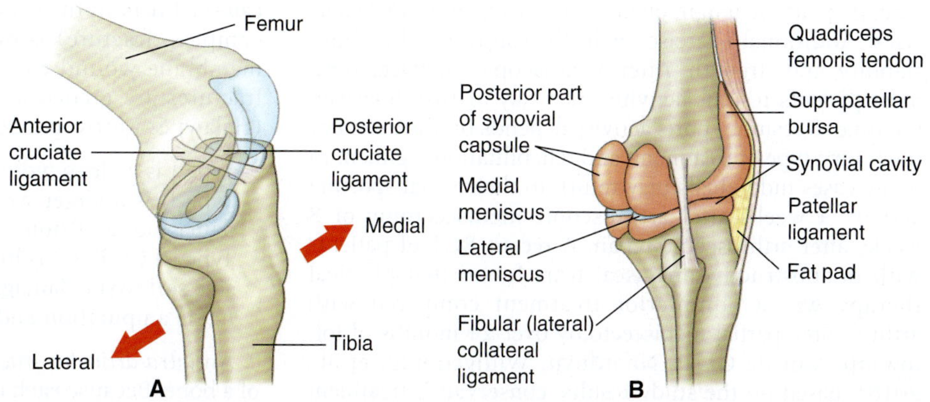

FIGURE 72-1. Knee ligaments. **A.** Anterolateral view. **B.** Posterolateral view.

weight-bearing limitation, exercise restrictions, and the use of a knee brace or immobilizer. The patient must protect the graft by complying with exercise restrictions. The physical therapist supervises progressive ROM and weight bearing (as the patient is permitted). Rehabilitation after surgery typically takes 6 to 12 months.

Meniscal Injuries

In the knee, there are two crescent-shaped (semilunar) cartilages, called *menisci*, attached to the edge of the shallow articulating surface of the head of the tibia (see Fig. 72-1). Each **meniscus** moves slightly backward and forward to accommodate the condyles of the femur when the leg is flexed or extended. Normally, there is some torsional movement permitted in the knee joint. In sports or accidents, twisting of the knee or repetitive squatting may result in either tearing or detachment of the cartilage from the tibial plateau.

These injuries leave loose cartilage in the knee joint that may slip between the femur and the tibia, preventing full extension of the leg. If this happens during walking or running, patients often describe their leg as "giving way" under them. Patients may hear or feel a click in the knee when they walk, especially when they extend the leg that is bearing weight, as in going upstairs. When the cartilage is attached to the front and back of the knee but torn loose laterally (bucket-handle tear), it may slide between the bones to lie between the condyles and prevent full flexion or extension. As a result, the knee "locks." The torn cartilage is an irritant in the joint, causing inflammation, chronic synovitis, and effusion. Meniscal injuries produce pain, disability, and anxiety as the patient never knows when the knee will malfunction.

Medical Management

Conservative treatment includes immobilization of the knee, the use of crutches, anti-inflammatory agents, analgesics, modification of activities, and physical therapy. If symptoms persist, the damaged cartilage is surgically removed (meniscectomy) through a procedure in which the orthopedic surgeon uses an **arthroscope** to visualize and repair the damage. After surgery, a pressure dressing is applied, and a knee-immobilizing splint may be required. The most common complication is an effusion into the knee joint, which produces pain. The physician may need to aspirate the joint to remove fluid and relieve the pressure. Patients are taught quadriceps-setting and ROM exercises. Additional exercises help to restore full function, stability, and strength. After arthroscopic meniscectomy, most patients resume activities in a day or two; however, the time to resume sports activity depends on the extent of the injury, type of treatment, and rehabilitation regimen. In many cases individuals may return to their usual sporting activity 4 weeks after arthroscopic meniscectomy or 8 weeks after arthroscopic repair. A recent RCT of patients with nonobstructive meniscal tears found that physical therapy was a noninferior treatment compared with arthroscopic partial meniscectomy over 24 months of follow-up (van de Graaf, Noorduyn, Willigenburg, et al., 2018). Based on the study results, conservative treatment with physiotherapy is an alternative to arthroscopic surgery for patients with nonobstructive meniscal tears.

Rupture of the Achilles Tendon

Traumatic rupture of the Achilles tendon, generally within the tendon sheath, occurs during activities when there is a sudden contraction of the calf muscle with the foot fixed firmly to the floor or ground. The patient experiences sharp pain and is unable to plantar flex the foot. There is debate among MSK health professionals concerning conservative or surgical treatment for this type of injury. In a meta-analysis of randomized controlled trials, the authors concluded that consideration should be given to conservative treatment in centres that can provide functional rehabilitation. The rates of rerupture of the tendon were similar between conservative and surgical treatment (Soroceanu, Sidhwa, Aarabi, et al., 2012).

After surgery, a cast or brace is used to immobilize the joint. Conservative management involves a plantar-flexed cast or "Achilles boot" for 6 to 8 weeks. After immobilization, a heel lift is worn and progressive physical therapy is instituted to promote strengthening and ankle ROM.

Fractures

A **fracture** is a complete or incomplete disruption in the continuity of bone structure and is defined according to its type and extent. Fractures occur when the bone is subjected to stress greater than it can absorb (Porth, 2015). Fractures may be caused by direct blows, crushing forces, sudden twisting motions, and extreme muscle contractions. When the bone is broken, adjacent structures are also affected, which may result in soft tissue edema, hemorrhage into the muscles and joints, joint dislocations, ruptured tendons, severed nerves, and damaged blood vessels. Body organs may be injured by the force that caused the fracture or by fracture fragments.

Types of Fractures

Fracture types are classified by location (e.g., proximal, midshaft, distal) and type (Porth, 2015). Fractures are also described according to the degree of break (e.g., a *greenstick fracture* refers to a partial break) or the character of any fractured bone fragments (e.g., a *comminuted fracture* has more than two fragments). Select specific types of fractures are displayed in Figure 72-2.

A *closed fracture* (simple fracture) is one that does not cause a break in the skin. An *open fracture* (compound, or complex, fracture) is one in which the skin or mucous membrane wound extends to the fractured bone. Open fractures are graded according to the following criteria (Halawi & Morwood, 2015):

- Type I is a clean wound less than 1 cm long.
- Type II is a larger wound without extensive soft tissue damage or avulsions.
- Type III (A, B, C) is highly contaminated and has extensive soft tissue damage. It may be accompanied by traumatic amputation and is the most severe.

An *intra-articular fracture* extends into the joint surface of a bone. Because each end of a long bone is cartilaginous,

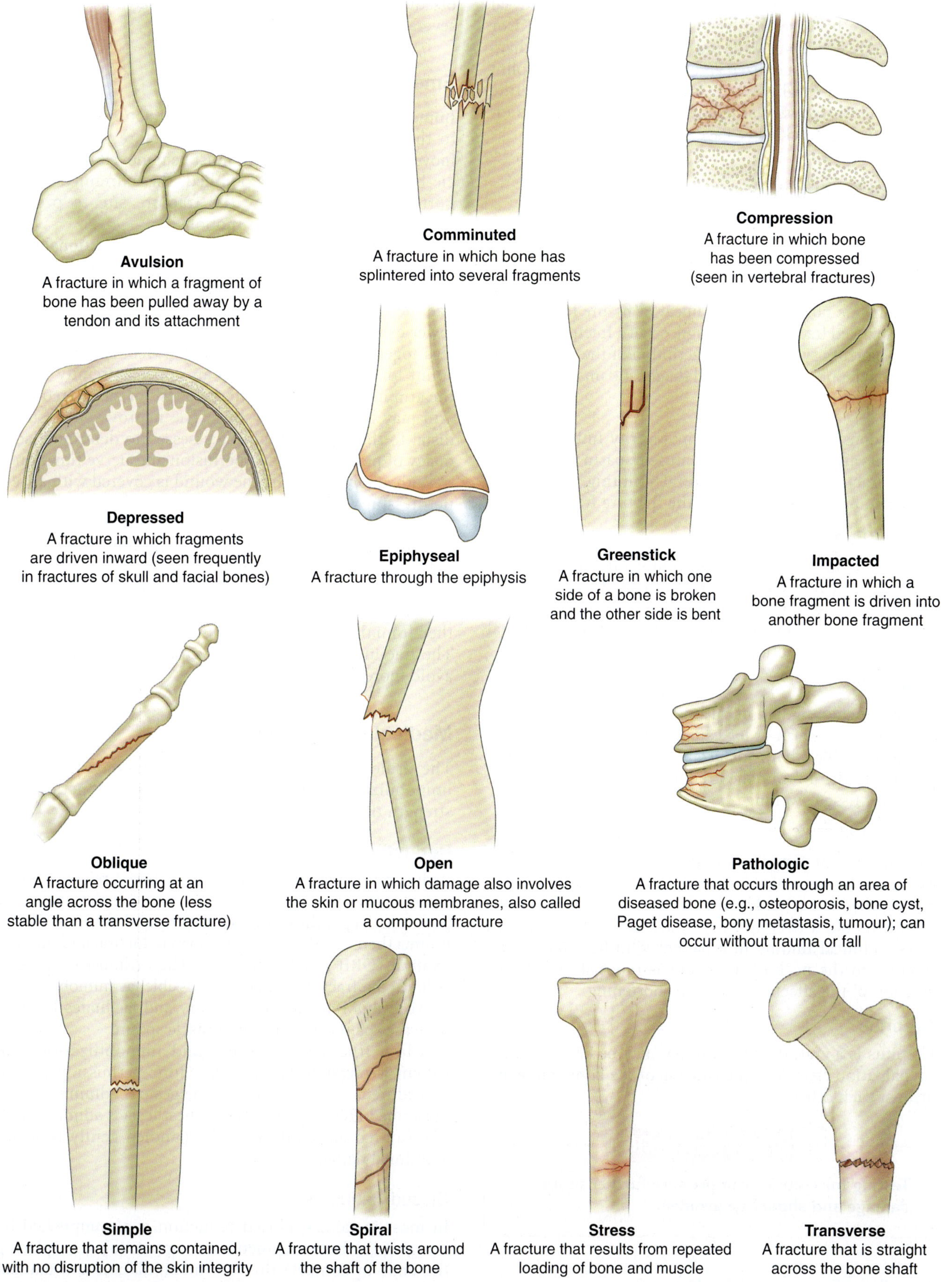

FIGURE 72-2. Specific types of fractures.

if the fracture is nondisplaced, x-rays will not always reveal the fracture because cartilage is nonradiopaque. MRI or arthroscopy will identify the fracture and confirm the diagnosis. The joint is stabilized and immobilized with a splint or cast, and no weight bearing is allowed until the fracture has healed. Intra-articular fractures often lead to posttraumatic arthritis (Buckley & Page, 2016).

Clinical Manifestations

The clinical manifestations of a fracture are pain, loss of function, deformity, shortening of the extremity, crepitus, and local swelling and discolouration. Not all of these clinical manifestations are present in every fracture. For example, many are not present with linear or fissure fractures or with impacted fractures. The diagnosis of a fracture is based on the patient's symptoms, a description of the mechanism of injury, the physical signs, and diagnostic imaging.

Pain

Pain is constant and increases in severity until the bone fragments are immobilized. The muscle spasm that accompanies fracture is a type of natural splinting designed to minimize further movement of the fracture fragments.

Loss of Function

After a fracture, the extremity cannot function properly because normal function of the muscles depends on the integrity of the bones to which they are attached. Pain contributes to the loss of function. In addition, abnormal movement (false motion) may be present.

Deformity

Displacement, angulation, or rotation of the fragments in a fracture of the arm or leg causes a deformity (either visible or palpable) that is detectable when the limb is compared with the uninjured extremity. Deformity also results from soft tissue swelling.

Shortening

In fractures of long bones, there is shortening of the extremity because of the contraction of the muscles that are attached above and below the site of the fracture. The fragments often overlap by as much as 2.5 to 5.0 cm. A classic clinical finding in a patient who has sustained a fracture to the neck of the femur is internal or external rotation of the affected limb with shortening.

Crepitus

Crepitus is a grating sensation that may be heard and felt on palpation caused by the rubbing of the bone fragments against each other.

> **NURSING ALERT**
>
> **Testing for crepitus can produce further tissue damage and should be avoided.**

Localized Edema and Ecchymosis

Localized edema and discolouration of the skin (ecchymosis) occur after a fracture as a result of trauma and bleeding into the tissues. These signs may not develop for several hours after the injury.

Emergency Management

Immediately after injury, whenever a fracture is suspected, to the limb must be immobilized before the patient is moved. If an injured patient must be removed from a vehicle before splints can be applied, the extremity is supported above and below the fracture site to prevent rotation as well as angular motion.

Movement of fracture fragments causes additional pain, soft tissue damage, and bleeding. Temporary, well-padded splints, firmly bandaged over clothing, serve to immobilize the fracture. Immobilization of the long bones of the lower extremities may be accomplished by bandaging the legs together, with the unaffected extremity serving as a splint for the injured one. In an upper extremity injury, the arm may be bandaged to the chest, or an injured forearm may be placed in a sling. The neurovascular status distal to the injury should be assessed to determine adequacy of peripheral tissue perfusion and nerve function.

With an *open fracture*, the wound is covered with a sterile dressing to prevent contamination of deeper tissues. No attempt is made to reduce the fracture, even if one of the bone fragments is protruding through the wound. Splints are applied for immobilization.

In the emergency department, clothes are gently removed, first from the uninjured side of the body and then from the injured side by cutting patient's clothing off. The fractured extremity is moved as little as possible to avoid more damage.

Medical Management

The principles of fracture treatment include reduction, immobilization, and regaining of normal function and strength through rehabilitation.

Reduction

Reduction of a fracture ("setting" the bone) refers to restoration of the fracture fragments to anatomic alignment and position. Depending on the nature and severity of the trauma there is either closed or open reduction and internal fixation (ORIF) of the fracture. The orthopedic surgeon reduces the fracture as soon as possible, as immobilization restricts ROM at the site of injury and facilitates healing, decreases pain, swelling, and muscle spasm.

Before **fracture reduction** and immobilization, the patient is prepared for the procedure; permission for the procedure is obtained, and an analgesic is administered as prescribed. Regional or general anesthesia is administered. The injured extremity must be handled gently to avoid additional damage.

Closed Reduction

In most instances, closed reduction is accomplished by bringing the bone fragments into apposition (i.e., placing the ends in contact) through manipulation and manual traction. The extremity is held in the desired position while the orthopedic surgeon applies a cast, splint, or other device. Reduction under anesthesia with percutaneous pinning may be used. The immobilizing device maintains the reduction and stabilizes the extremity for bone healing. X-rays are obtained to verify that the bone fragments are correctly aligned.

Skin or skeletal traction is a much less common intervention to effect fracture reduction and immobilization. It may be used in children and is used in fractures to the cervical spine (halo traction). Traction is used to provide some comfort until the patient is physiologically stable and able to withstand an ORIF. The use of traction and the nursing management of a patient in traction are described in Chapter 70.

Open Reduction

Some fractures require ORIF where the fracture fragments are surgically reduced and fixed in place. Internal fixation hardware (metal pins, wires, screws, plates, nails, or rods) are used to hold the bone fragments in position until bone healing occurs. The hardware may be screwed to the bone or inserted through the bony fragments or directly into the medullary cavity (Fig. 72-3). Internal fixation devices ensure firm approximation and fixation of the bony fragments and facilitate early mobilization of the patient.

Immobilization

After the fracture has been reduced, the bone fragments must be immobilized until union occurs. Immobilization may be accomplished by external or internal fixation.

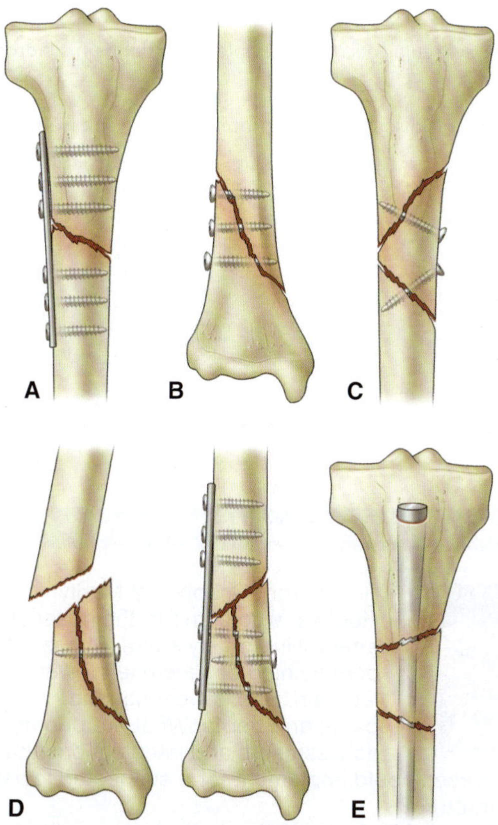

FIGURE 72-3. Techniques of internal fixation. **A.** Plate and six screws for a transverse or short oblique fracture. **B.** Screws for a long oblique or spiral fracture. **C.** Screws for a long butterfly fragment. **D.** Plate and six screws for a short butterfly fragment. **E.** Medullary nail for a segmental fracture.

Methods of external fixation include bandages, casts, splints, continuous traction, and external fixators. Metal implants used for internal fixation serve as internal splints to immobilize the fracture. It is important to emphasize that *immobilization of the limb* is a fundamental principle in fracture healing; however, the goal is *early mobilization of the patient* in order to prevent complications of bed rest.

Maintaining and Restoring Function

Reduction and immobilization are maintained as prescribed to promote bone and soft tissue healing. Swelling is controlled by elevating the injured extremity and applying ice. Neurovascular status is monitored, and the orthopedic surgeon is notified immediately if signs of neurovascular compromise are identified. Restlessness, anxiety, and discomfort are controlled with a variety of approaches, such as reassurance, position changes, and pain management strategies, including the use of analgesics. Isometric and muscle-setting exercises are encouraged to minimize disuse atrophy and to promote circulation. Participation in activities of daily living (ADLs) is encouraged to promote independent functioning and self-esteem. Gradual resumption of activities is promoted within the therapeutic prescription. With internal fixation, the surgeon determines the amount of movement and weight bearing the extremity can withstand and orders the level of activity.

Nursing Management

Patients With Closed Fractures

The nurse encourages patients with closed (simple) fractures to return to their usual activities as rapidly as possible. The nurse teaches patients how to control swelling and pain associated with the fracture and with soft tissue trauma and encourages them to be active within the limits of the fracture immobilization (Chart 72-1). It is important to teach exercises to maintain the health of unaffected muscles and to increase the strength of muscles needed for transferring and for using assistive devices (e.g., crutches, walker, special utensils). The nurse and physical therapist teach patients how to use assistive devices safely. Plans are made to help patients modify their home environment as needed and to secure personal assistance if necessary. Patient teaching includes self-care, medication information, monitoring for potential complications, and the need for continuing health care supervision. Fracture healing and restoration of full strength and mobility may take several months.

Patients With Open Fractures

In severe open fractures in which the patient has been in contact with road surfaces or soil there is risk of osteomyelitis, tetanus infection, and gas gangrene from anaerobic bacteria such as *Clostridium perfringens*. The objectives of management are to prevent infection of the wound, soft tissue, and bone and to promote healing. The nurse administers tetanus prophylaxis, as indicated. Serial irrigation and débridement are used to remove anaerobic organisms. Intravenous antibiotics are prescribed to prevent or treat infection.

Prompt, thorough wound irrigation and débridement in the operating room are necessary. The wound is cultured and devitalized bone fragments are removed. The fracture is carefully reduced and stabilized by internal or external

CHART 72-1

HOME CARE CHECKLIST • The Patient With a Closed Fracture

At the completion of education, the patient and/or caregiver will be able to:

- Name the procedure that was performed and identify any changes in anatomic structure or function as well as changes in ADLs, IADLs, roles, relationships, and spirituality.
- Identify modification of home environment, interventions, and strategies (e.g., durable medical equipment, adaptive equipment) used in safely promoting effective recovery and rehabilitation.
- Describe ongoing therapeutic regimen, including diet and activities to perform (e.g., exercises) and to limit or avoid (e.g., lifting weights, driving a car, contact sports).
  - Describe approaches to control swelling (e.g., elevate extremity to heart level).
  - Consume a healthy diet to promote bone healing.
  - Observe prescribed weight bearing and activity limits.
  - Participate in prescribed exercise regimen to maintain the health of unaffected muscles and those muscles now needed for safe transfer, mobility, etc.
  - If indicated, demonstrate safe use of mobility aid, assistive device, immobilizing device, and transfer technique.
- State the name, dose, side effects, frequency, and schedule for all prescribed therapeutic and prophylactic medications (e.g., antibiotics, analgesic agents).
- Control pain with pharmacologic and nonpharmacologic interventions.
- Report pain uncontrolled by elevation and analgesics (may be an indicator of impaired tissue perfusion or compartment syndrome).
- State indicators of complications to report promptly to primary provider (e.g., uncontrolled swelling and pain; cool, pale fingers or toes; paresthesia; paralysis; signs of local and systemic infection; signs of venous thromboembolism; problems with immobilization device).
- State possible complications of fractures (i.e., delayed union; nonunion; avascular necrosis; complex regional pain syndrome, formerly called *reflex sympathetic dystrophy syndrome;* heterotopic ossification).
- Describe gradual resumption of normal activities when medically cleared, and discuss how to protect fracture site from undue stresses.
- Relate how to reach primary provider with questions or complications.
- State time and date of follow-up appointments, therapy, and testing.
- Identify the need for health promotion, disease prevention, and screening activities.

ADL, activities of daily living; IADL, independent activities of daily living.

fixation (see Chapter 70). Damage to blood vessels, soft tissues, muscles, nerves, and tendons is treated.

With open fractures, primary wound closure may be delayed. Heavily contaminated wounds are left unsutured and dressed with sterile gauze to permit swelling and wound drainage. Wound irrigation and débridement may be repeated, removing infected and devitalized tissue and increasing vascularity in the region. After it has been determined that infection is not present, the wound is closed, and dead space is eliminated by grafting of autogenous skin or a flap.

The nurse elevates the extremity to reduce edema. It is important to assess neurovascular status frequently. The nurse monitors the patient's vital signs at regular intervals and assesses the patient for signs of infection. In 4 to 8 weeks, bone grafting may be necessary to bridge bone defects and to stimulate bone healing.

Unfolding Patient Stories: Marilyn Hughes • Part 2

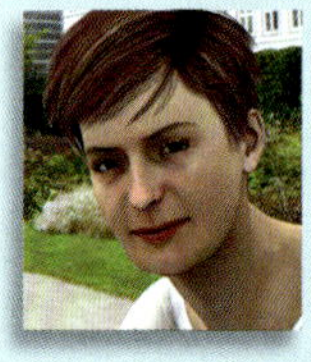

Recall from Chapter 62 Marilyn Hughes, who came to the hospital after falling on icy stairs. She is complaining of severe left lower leg pain. She is wearing long pants and boots. What are priority assessments and interventions that the nurse should implement for a suspected lower leg fracture?

Care for Marilyn and other patients in a realistic virtual environment: ***vSim** for Nursing* (**thepoint.lww.com/vSimMedicalSurgical**). Practice documenting these patients' care in DocuCare (**thepoint.lww.com/DocuCareEHR**).

CHART 72-2

Factors That Affect Fracture Healing

Factors That Enhance Fracture Healing

- Immobilization of fracture fragments
- Maximum bone fragment contact
- Sufficient blood supply
- Proper nutrition
- Exercise: weight bearing for long bones
- Hormones: growth hormone, thyroid, calcitonin, vitamin D, anabolic steroids
- Electric potential across fracture

Factors That Inhibit Fracture Healing

- Age >40 years
- Avascular necrosis
- Bone loss
- Cigarette smoking
- Comorbidities (e.g., diabetes, rheumatoid arthritis)
- Corticosteroids, nonsteroidal anti-inflammatory drugs
- Extensive local trauma
- Inadequate immobilization
- Infection
- Local malignancy
- Malalignment of the fracture fragments

Adapted from Buckley, R., & Page, J. L. (2016). General principles of fracture care. Medscape. Retrieved February 15, 2016, from emedicine.medscape.com/article/1270717-overview#showall; Porth, C. M. (2015). *Essentials of pathophysiology: Concepts of altered health states* (4th ed.). Philadelphia, PA: Lippincott Williams & Wilkins.

Fracture Healing and Complications

Weeks to months are required for most fractures to heal. Many factors influence the time frame of the healing process (see Chart 72-2). With a comminuted fracture, fragments must be properly aligned to attain the best healing possible. It is essential for the fractured bone to have blood supply to the area to facilitate the healing process. In general, fractures of flat bones (pelvis, sternum, and scapula) heal rapidly. A complex, comminuted fracture may heal slowly. Fractures at the ends of long bones, where the bone is more vascular and cancellous, heal more quickly than do fractures in areas where the bone is dense and less vascular (midshaft). Fractures typically heal more quickly in younger patients (Porth, 2015).

If fracture healing is disrupted, bone union may be delayed or stopped completely. Factors that can impair fracture healing include inadequate fracture immobilization, inadequate blood supply to the fracture site or adjacent tissue, extensive space between bone fragments, interposition of soft tissue between bone ends, infection, and metabolic problems.

Early complications from fractures include shock, fat embolism, compartment syndrome, deep vein thrombosis (DVT), pulmonary embolism (PE), disseminated intravascular coagulopathy (DIC), and infection. Later complications include delayed union, nonunion, necrosis of bone, reaction to internal fixation devices, complex regional pain syndrome (CRPS) (formerly called *reflex sympathetic dystrophy* [RSD]), and heterotrophic ossification.

Early Complications

Shock

Hypovolemic or traumatic shock resulting from hemorrhage (both visible and nonvisible blood loss) and from loss of extracellular fluid into damaged tissues may occur in fractures of the extremities, thorax, pelvis, or spine. Bone is very vascular, and large quantities of blood may be lost (e.g., 2 to 3 L) as a result of trauma, especially in fractures of the femur and pelvis. Treatment of shock consists of restoring blood volume and circulation, pain management, providing adequate splinting, and protecting the patient from further injury and other complications. (Refer to Chapter 18 for a discussion of shock.)

Fat Embolism Syndrome

Fat embolism syndrome (FES) describes the clinical manifestations that occur when fat emboli enter circulation following orthopedic trauma, especially long bone (e.g., femur) fractures. At the time of fracture, fat globules may diffuse from the marrow into the vascular compartment. The fat globules (i.e., emboli) may occlude the small blood vessels that supply the lungs, brain, kidneys, and other organs. The onset of symptoms is rapid, typically within 12 to 72 hours of injury (Kosova, Bergmark, & Piazza, 2015; Porth, 2015). FES occurs more frequently in males between the ages of 10 and 40 years after a traumatic injury. Although only a small percentage of patients who survive multitrauma have a diagnosis of FES by the time of hospital discharge (0.17% to 1.29%), fat emboli have been found in as many as 82% of trauma patient autopsies (Kosova et al., 2015).

CLINICAL MANIFESTATIONS. The classic triad of clinical manifestations of FES include hypoxemia, neurologic compromise, and a petechial rash (Porth, 2015). The typical first manifestations are pulmonary and include hypoxia, tachypnea, and dyspnea accompanied by tachycardia, substernal chest pain, low-grade fever, crackles, and additional manifestations of respiratory failure. Chest x-ray may show evidence of acute respiratory distress syndrome (ARDS) or it may be normal. Petechial rash may develop 2 to 3 days after the onset of symptoms. This rash is secondary to dysfunction in the microcirculation and/or thrombocytopenia and is typically located in nondependent regions (e.g., chest, mucous membranes) of the body. There may be varying degrees of neurologic deficits that can include restlessness, agitation, seizures, focal deficits, and encephalopathy (Kosova et al., 2015; Porth, 2015). Diagnosis relies on clinical examination (Kosova et al., 2015).

NURSING ALERT

Subtle personality changes, restlessness, irritability, or confusion in a patient who has sustained a fracture are indications for immediate arterial blood gas testing.

In systemic embolization, the patient appears pale, there are petechiae, (possibly due to a transient thrombocytopenia), in the buccal membranes, conjunctival sacs, the hard palate, and over the chest and anterior axillary folds. The patient develops a temperature of more than 39.5°C. Free fat may be found in the urine with emboli in the kidneys and acute renal failure develops.

PREVENTION AND MANAGEMENT. Immediate immobilization of fractures, including early surgical fixation, minimal fracture manipulation, and adequate support for fractured bones during turning and positioning, and maintenance of fluid and electrolyte balance are measures that may reduce the incidence of fat emboli. There is no specific treatment for FES; the treatment is supportive. Vasopressors, mechanical ventilation, and sometimes corticosteroids are used as supportive therapy (Kosova et al., 2015; Porth, 2015).

The objectives of management are to support the respiratory system, to prevent respiratory and metabolic acidemia, and to correct homeostatic disturbances. Cardiorespiratory failure is the most common cause of death. Respiratory support is provided with oxygen given in high concentrations. Controlled-volume ventilation with positive end-expiratory pressure may be used to prevent or treat pulmonary edema. Corticosteroids may be administered to treat the inflammatory lung reaction and to control cerebral edema. Vasoactive medications to support cardiovascular function are administered to prevent hypotension, shock, and interstitial pulmonary edema. Accurate fluid intake and output records facilitate adequate fluid replacement therapy. Morphine may be prescribed for pain and anxiety for the patient who is on a ventilator. In addition, the nurse provides reassurance to allay apprehension. The patient's response to therapy is closely monitored.

Fat emboli are a major cause of death for patients with fractures, therefore the nurse must recognize early indications of FES and report them promptly to the orthopedic surgeon. Respiratory support must be instituted early.

Acute Compartment Syndrome

An anatomic compartment is an area of the body encased by bone or fascia (e.g., the fibrous membrane that covers and separates muscles) that contains muscles, nerves, and blood vessels. The human body has 46 anatomic compartments, and 36 of these are located in the extremities (see Fig. 72-4). Compartment syndrome is characterized by the elevation of pressure within an anatomic compartment that is above normal perfusion pressure. Compartment syndrome arises from an increase in compartment volume (e.g., from edema or bleeding), a decrease in compartment size (e.g., from a restrictive cast), or aspects of both. When the pressure within an affected compartment rises above normal, perfusion to the tissues is impaired, causing cell death, which may lead to tissue necrosis and permanent dysfunction (Porth, 2015). Compartment syndrome occurs more frequently in young adults, and although it may take up to 48 hours for symptoms to present, it typically develops quickly, within 6 to 8 hours after the initial injury or after fracture repair (NAON, 2013).

ASSESSMENT AND DIAGNOSTIC FINDINGS. Frequent assessment of neurovascular function after fracture is essential. Sensory deficits include unrelenting pain despite narcotic analgesia being administered, paresthesia, and hypoesthesia. Severe, unrelenting pain is the most important sign in ACS. *Paresthesia* (tingling "pins and needle" sensation) and numbness along the involved nerve are early signs of nerve involvement. ROM is evaluated by asking the patient to move fingers or toes distal to the problem. Motor weakness is a late sign of nerve ischemia. No movement (*paralysis*) is indicative of nerve damage.

Peripheral circulation is evaluated by assessing colour, temperature, capillary refill time, swelling, and pulses. Swelling in the compartment contributes to reduction in tissue perfusion. Cyanotic (blue-tinged) nail beds suggest venous congestion. Pale, dusky cold fingers or extremities and prolonged capillary refill time indicate significantly decreased arterial perfusion. Swelling makes palpation of the peripheral pulses difficult and Doppler ultrasonography may be used to identify a pulse. It is extremely important to note that a decreased or absent pulse is a very late sign of a compromised blood supply to the limb. Passive stretching of the muscle causes severe, acute pain. With continued nerve ischemia and edema, the patient experiences sensations of hypoesthesia (diminished sensitivity to stimulation) progressing to loss of sensation. The muscles are swollen and hard to palpation. The pressure can be measured by inserting a tissue pressure–measuring device into the muscle compartment. (Normal pressure is 8 mm Hg or less.) Nerve and muscle tissues deteriorate as compartment pressure increases. Prolonged pressure of more than 30 mm Hg can result in compromised microcirculation. Nerve tissue is more sensitive than muscle to elevated tissue pressures.

MEDICAL MANAGEMENT. Prompt management of acute compartment syndrome is essential. The orthopedic surgeon must be notified immediately if ACS is suspected. Delay results in permanent nerve and muscle damage, necrosis, rhabdomyolysis, acute tubular necrosis, loss of limb and death.

Acute compartment syndrome is managed by elevation of the extremity to the heart level and release of restrictive devices (dressings or cast). If conservative measures do not restore tissue perfusion and relieve pain within 1 hour, a fasciotomy (surgical decompression with incision of the fibrous membrane that covers and separates muscles) must be done to relieve the pressure caused by the constrictive muscle fascia. After fasciotomy, the wound is left open to permit the muscle tissues to expand and excess tissue fluid to drain; it is covered with moist, sterile saline dressings. The limb is splinted in a functional position and elevated. Passive ROM exercises are performed every 4 to 6 hours. In 3 to 5 days, when the swelling has resolved and tissue perfusion has been restored, the wound is débrided and closed with skin grafts.

NURSING MANAGEMENT. The nurse should frequently assess pain and neurovascular status of the affected limb and report any negative changes that may suggest compartment syndrome immediately to the primary provider. The limb should be maintained in a functional position at the level of the heart to promote optimal blood flow.

NURSING ALERT

Compartment syndrome is managed by maintaining the extremity at the heart level (*not above heart level*), and opening and bivalving the cast or opening the splint, if one or the other is present.

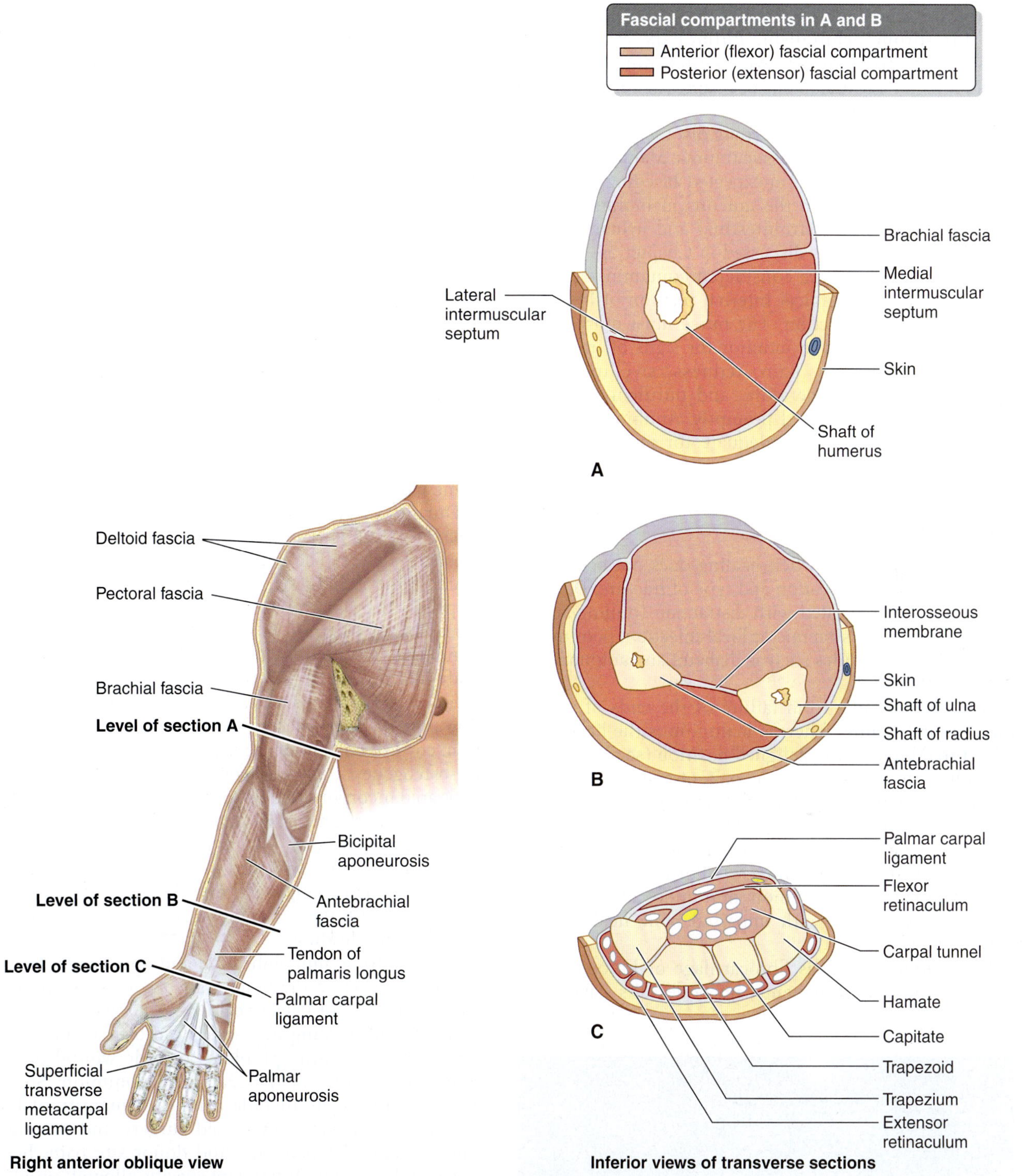

FIGURE 72-4. Cross-sections of anatomic compartments. Compartments of the right forearm. (From Moore, K. L., Agur, A. M. R., & Dalley, A. F. II. (2015). *Essential clinical anatomy* (5th ed.). Philadelphia, PA: Lippincott Williams & Wilkins.)

Pain management is essential and is accomplished with opioid analgesia, as prescribed. Careful assessment of intake and output and urinalysis could alert the nurse to the development of rhabdomyolysis (see Chapter 45).

Education is necessary for those patients discharged to home-based or community settings with fractures and casts and should include recognition of the unique characteristics of acute compartment syndrome (increasing, refractory pain and neurovascular manifestations) and instructions when to contact the primary provider for emergent follow-up.

Other Early Complications

Venous thromboembolism, which includes DVT and PE, is associated with Virchow's triad of hypercoagulability, venous stasis and endothelial injury all of which can occur in orthopedic patients due to the nature of their injury and having decreased mobility. Patients with fractures of the lower extremities and pelvis are at high risk for thromboembolism. Pulmonary emboli may cause death several days to weeks after injury. (Refer to Chapter 24 for discussion of PE, Chapter 32 for discussion of thromboembolism.)

DIC includes a group of bleeding disorders with diverse causes, including massive tissue trauma. Manifestations of DIC include ecchymoses; unexpected bleeding after surgery; and bleeding from the mucous membranes, venipuncture sites, and gastrointestinal and urinary tracts. The treatment of DIC is discussed in Chapter 54.

All open fractures are considered contaminated until proven otherwise. Surgical internal fixation of fractures carries a risk for infection. The nurse must monitor for and teach the patient to monitor for signs of infection, including tenderness, pain, redness, swelling, local warmth, elevated temperature, and purulent drainage. Infections must be treated promptly. Antibiotic therapy must be appropriate and adequate for prevention and treatment of infection.

Delayed Complications

Delayed Union and Nonunion

Delayed union occurs when healing does not occur at a normal rate for the location and type of fracture. Delayed union may be associated with distraction (pulling apart) of bone fragments, systemic or local infection, poor nutrition, and comorbidities such as diabetes and autoimmune diseases.

Nonunion results from failure of the ends of a fractured bone to unite, whereas malunion is the healing of a fractured bone in a malaligned position (see Fig. 72-5). In both of these instances, the patient complains of persistent discomfort and abnormal movement at the fracture site. Nonunion occurs most commonly in tibial fractures, whereas malunion occurs most commonly in fractures of the hand (or fingers) (Porth, 2015). Factors contributing to delayed union, nonunion, and malunion are those associated with impaired bone healing (see Chart 72-2).

In nonunion, there is fibrocartilage or fibrous tissue between the bone fragments; no bone salts have been deposited. A false joint (pseudarthrosis) develops at the site of the fracture. Nonunion most commonly occurs with fractures of the middle third of the humerus and the lower third of the tibia; nonunion most commonly occurs in the neck of the femur in older adults.

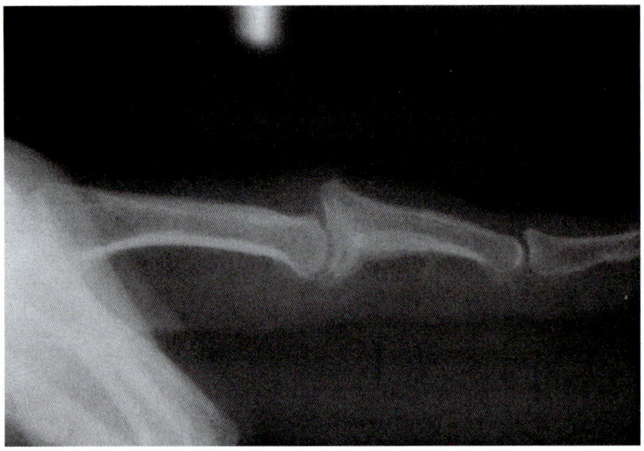

FIGURE 72-5. Eight-month-old ring finger malunion in a 19-year-old female patient. (From Strickland, J. W., & Graham, T. J. (2005). *Master techniques in orthopaedic surgery: The hand* (2nd ed.). Philadelphia, PA: Lippincott Williams & Wilkins.)

MEDICAL MANAGEMENT. The surgeon treats nonunion with internal fixation, bone grafting, electrical bone stimulation, or a combination of these therapies. Internal fixation stabilizes the bone fragments and ensures bone contact.

Bone grafts provide for osteogenesis, osteoconduction, and osteoinduction. *Osteogenesis* (bone formation) occurs after transplantation of bone containing osteoblasts. *Osteoconduction* is provision by the graft of the structural matrix for ingrowth of blood vessels and osteoblasts. *Osteoinduction* is the stimulation of host stem cells to differentiate into osteoblasts by several growth factors, including bone morphogenetic proteins. Bone transplants undergo creeping substitution, which is a reconstructive process in which the bone transplant is gradually replaced by new bone.

During surgery, the bone fragments are trimmed, infected tissue is removed, and a bone graft is placed in the bony defect. The bone graft may be an **autograft**, in which bone is harvested from the patient from one site (typically the iliac crest) and grafted at the fracture site, or it may be an **allograft**, in which bone is harvested from a donor that is grafted to the patient's fracture site. The bone graft fills the bone gap, provides a lattice structure for invasion by bone cells, and actively promotes bone growth. The type of bone selected for grafting depends on function: cortical bone for structural strength, cancellous bone for osteogenesis, and corticocancellous bone for strength and rapid incorporation. Bone grafts may be chips, wedges, blocks, bone segments, or demineralized bone matrix. At times, autograft bone, allograft bone, and demineralized cortical matrix are combined to optimize graft incorporation and bone healing. Free vascularized bone autografts are grafted with their own blood supply, allowing for primary fracture healing.

After grafting, immobilization and non–weight bearing are required while the bone graft becomes incorporated and the fracture or defect heals. Depending on the type of bone grafted, healing may take from 6 to 12 months or longer. Bone grafting problems include wound or graft infection, fracture of the graft, and nonunion. Specific autograft problems include a limited quantity of bone available for harvest; increased surgery and anesthesia time; increased blood loss; and donor site pain, hematoma, and infection. Infrequent specific allograft problems include partial acceptance (lack of host and donor histocompatibility, which retards graft incorporation), graft rejection (rapid and complete resorption of the graft), and transmission of disease (rare).

Osteogenesis in nonunion may be stimulated by electrical impulses; the effectiveness is similar to that of bone grafting. The use of electrical impulses is not effective with large bone gaps or synovial pseudarthrosis. The electrical stimulation modifies the tissue environment, making it electronegative, which enhances mineral deposition and bone formation.

In some situations, pins that act as cathodes are inserted percutaneously, directly into the fracture site, and

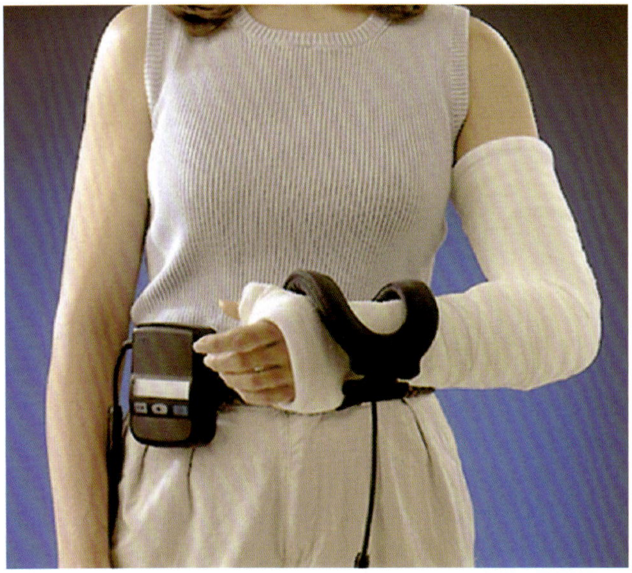

FIGURE 72-6. Bone-healing stimulator applied to the arm. (Reprinted with permission from EBI Medical Systems, Parsippany, New Jersey.)

electrical impulses are directed to the fracture continuously. Direct current methods cannot be used when infection is present.

Another method for stimulating osteogenesis is noninvasive inductive coupling. Pulsing electromagnetic fields are delivered to the fracture for approximately 10 hours each day by an electromagnetic coil over the nonunion site (Fig. 72-6). During the electrical stimulation treatment period, which takes 3 to 6 months or longer, rigid fracture fixation with adequate support is needed.

NURSING MANAGEMENT. The patient with a nonunion has experienced an extended time in fracture treatment and frequently becomes frustrated with prolonged therapy. The nurse provides emotional support and encouragement to the patient and encourages compliance with the treatment regimen. The orthopedic surgeon evaluates the progression of bone healing with periodic x-rays.

Nursing care for the patient with a bone graft include pain management, monitoring the patient for signs of infection at the donor and recipient sites, and patient education. The nurse needs to reinforce information concerning the objectives of the bone graft, immobilization, non–weight bearing, wound care, signs of infection, and follow-up care with the orthopedic surgeon.

Nursing care for the patient with electrical bone stimulation focuses on patient education that addresses immobilization, weight-bearing restrictions, and correct daily use of the stimulator as prescribed.

Avascular Necrosis of Bone (AVN; Osteonecrosis)

AVN occurs when the bone loses its blood supply and dies. It may occur after a fracture with disruption of the blood supply to the distal area. It is also seen with prolonged high-dose corticosteroid therapy, radiation therapy, sickle cell disease, rheumatoid arthritis, and other diseases. The patient develops pain with movement that progresses to pain at rest. Diagnostics include history and physical examination with x-rays, CT scans, and bone scans. Medical management of AVN includes administration of NSAIDs, exercises, and limiting weight bearing of the affected region; however, total joint replacement is the definitive treatment when located in the hip or knee (Porth, 2015).

Reaction to Internal Fixation Devices (Delayed)

Internal fixation devices may be removed after bony union has taken place. In most patients, however, the device is not removed unless there are symptoms affecting the patient's ADLs. Pain and decreased function are the prime indications that a problem has developed. Problems may include mechanical failure (inadequate insertion and stabilization); material failure (faulty or damaged device); corrosion of the device, causing local inflammation; allergic response to the metallic alloy used; and osteoporotic remodelling adjacent to the fixation device (in which stress needed for bone strength is transferred to the device, causing a disuse osteoporosis). If the device is removed, the bone needs to be protected from refracture related to osteoporosis, altered bone structure, and trauma. Bone remodelling reestablishes the bone's structural strength.

Complex Regional Pain Syndrome

CRPS (formerly known as reflex sympathetic dystrophy) is an infrequent but severely painful condition involving the sympathetic nervous system that typically affects women and involves an upper extremity. CRPS type 1 occurs after an injury or illness that did not directly involve any nerves of the affected limb. CRPS type 2 has similar symptoms; however, there is a distinct history of injury to the nerves of the affected limb. Clinical manifestations of CRPS include severe burning pain, local edema, hyperesthesia, stiffness, discolouration, fluctuating vasomotor skin changes (i.e., warm, red, dry and cold, sweaty, cyanotic), and trophic changes (i.e., glossy, shiny skin; increased hair and nail growth). This syndrome is frequently chronic, with extension of symptoms to adjacent areas of the body. Disuse muscle atrophy and bone deossification (osteoporosis) occur with persistence of CRPS. The ADLs of patients are severely affected due to the severe, intractable, chronic pain they experience.

NURSING MANAGEMENT. Prevention includes elevation of the extremity after injury or surgery and selection of an immobilization device (e.g., external fixator) that allows for the greatest ROM and functional use of the rest of the extremity. The primary focus is early effective pain management with analgesics, anesthetic nerve blocks, and the intravenous bisphosphonate pamidronate. NSAIDs, corticosteroids, muscle relaxants, and antidepressants are also used. With adequate pain management, the patient can participate in ROM exercises and functional use of the affected area. The nurse helps the patient cope with CRPS manifestations and explores different ways to manage the pain (see Chapter 16).

NURSING ALERT

The nurse avoids using the involved extremity for blood pressure measurements and venipunctures.

Heterotrophic Ossification

Heterotrophic ossification (myositis ossificans) is the abnormal formation of bone, near bones or in muscle, in response to soft tissue trauma after blunt trauma, fracture, or total joint replacement. The muscle is painful, and normal muscular contraction and movement are limited. Early mobilization has been recommended. Indomethacin (Indocin) may be used prophylactically if deep muscle contusion has occurred. Usually, the bone lesion resorbs over time, but the abnormal bone eventually may need to be excised if symptoms persist.

Concept Mastery Alert

For further review of fractures, visit thePoint for an Interactive Tutorial.

Fractures of Specific Sites

Injuries to the skeletal structure may vary from a simple linear fracture to a severe crush injury. The type and location of the fracture and the extent of damage to surrounding structures determine the therapeutic management. Maximum functional recovery is the goal of management.

Clavicle

Fracture of the clavicle (collarbone) is a common injury that results from a direct blow to the shoulder or a fall. Head or cervical spine injuries are associated with these fractures. The clavicle serves as a rigid support structure to hold the shoulder upward, outward, and backward from the thorax. The patient tends to assume a protective position when the clavicle is fractured by slumping the shoulders and immobilizing the arm to prevent shoulder movements. The treatment goal is to align the shoulder in its normal position by means of closed reduction and immobilization.

More than 80% of these fractures occur in the middle third of the clavicle. A clavicular strap, also called a *figure-of-eight bandage* (Fig. 72-7), is used to pull the shoulders back, reducing and immobilizing the fracture. When a clavicular strap is used, the axillae are well padded to prevent a compression injury to the brachial plexus and the axillary artery. The nurse monitors the circulation and nerve function of both arms. A sling may be used to support the arm and to decrease pain. The patient may be permitted to use the arm for light activities within the range of comfort.

Fracture of the distal third of the clavicle, without displacement and ligament disruption, is treated with a sling and restricted motion of the arm. When a fracture in the distal third is accompanied by a disruption of the coracoclavicular ligament, there is displacement, which is treated by ORIF.

Complications of clavicular fractures include trauma to the nerves of the brachial plexus, injury to the subclavian vein or artery from a bony fragment, and **malunion** (poorly aligned healing of the fractured bone). Malunion may be a cosmetic problem (e.g., when low-neckline clothing is worn).

The nurse cautions the patient not to elevate the arm above shoulder level until the ends of the bone have united (about 6 weeks) but encourages the patient to exercise the elbow, wrist, and fingers as soon as possible. When prescribed, shoulder exercises (Fig. 72-8) are performed to obtain full shoulder motion. Vigorous activity is limited for 3 months.

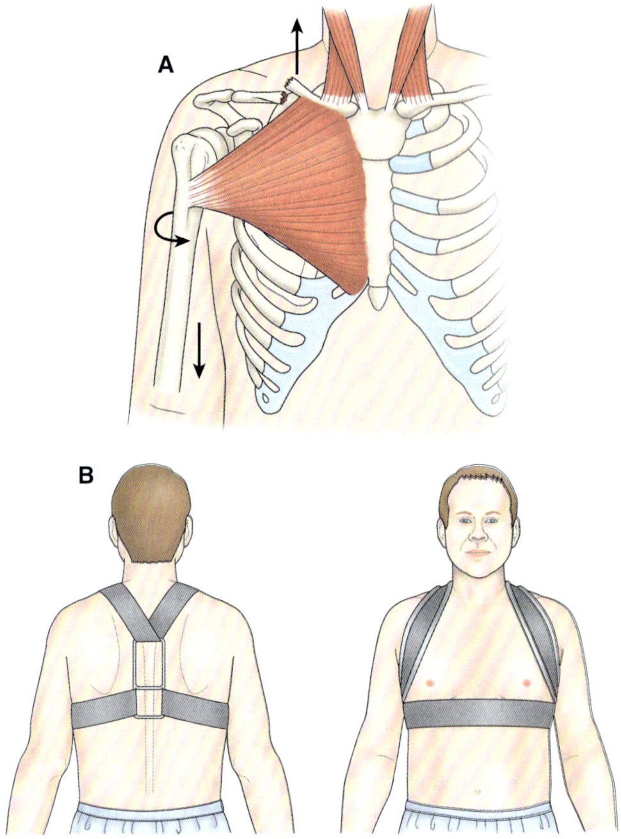

FIGURE 72-7. Fracture of the clavicle. **A.** Anteroposterior view shows typical displacement in midclavicular fracture. **B.** Immobilization is accomplished with a clavicular strap.

Humeral Neck

Fractures of the proximal humerus may occur through either the anatomic or the surgical neck of the humerus. The anatomic neck is located just below the humeral head. The surgical neck is the region below the tubercles. Impacted fractures of the surgical neck of the humerus are seen most frequently in older women after a fall on an outstretched arm; by definition impacted fractures are nondisplaced. Active middle-aged patients who are injured in a fall may suffer severely displaced humeral neck fractures with associated rotator cuff damage.

The patient presents with the affected arm hanging limp at the side and supported by the uninjured hand. Neurovascular assessment of the extremity is essential to evaluate fully the extent of injury and the possible involvement of the neurovascular bundle (nerves and blood vessels) of the arm.

Many impacted fractures of the surgical neck of the humerus are not displaced and do not require reduction. The arm is supported and immobilized by a sling and swathe that secure the supported arm to the trunk (Fig. 72-9). A soft pad is placed in the axilla to absorb moisture and avoid skin breakdown. Limitation of motion and stiffness

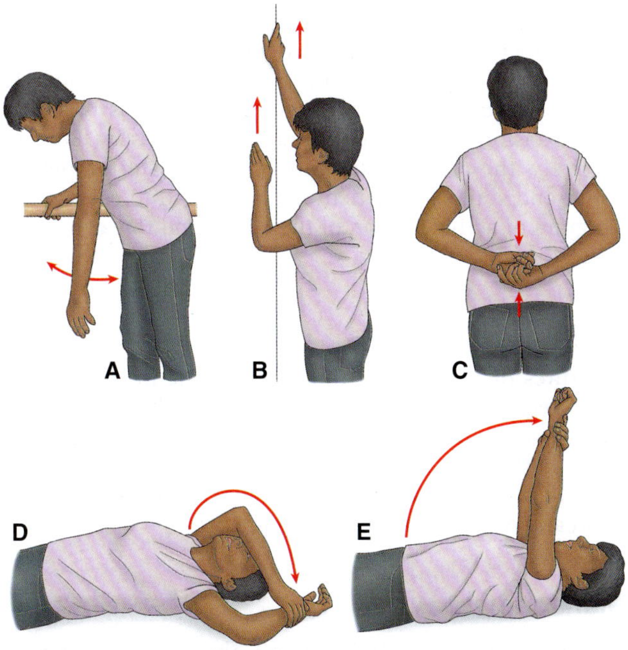

FIGURE 72-8. Exercises that promote shoulder range of motion include pendulum exercise (**A**) and wall climbing (**B**). The unaffected arm is used to assist with internal rotation (**C**), external rotation (**D**), and elevation (**E**). In **C**, **D**, and **E**, the unaffected arm is used for power.

of the shoulder occur with disuse. Therefore, pendulum exercises are begun as soon as tolerated by the patient. In pendulum or circumduction exercises, the nurse or physical therapist instructs the patient to lean forward and allow the affected arm to abduct and rotate. Early motion of the joint does not displace the fragments if motion is carried out within the limits imposed by pain.

These fractures require 6 to 10 weeks to heal, and the patient should avoid vigorous activity (e.g., tennis) for an additional 4 weeks. Residual stiffness, aching, and some limitation of ROM may persist for 6 months or longer.

When a humeral neck fracture is displaced, treatment consists of closed reduction, ORIF, or replacement of the humeral head with a prosthesis. In this type of fracture, exercises are started only after a prescribed period of immobilization.

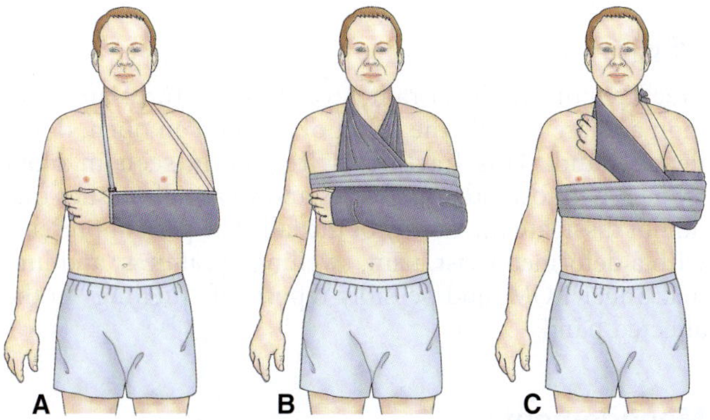

FIGURE 72-9. Immobilizers for proximal humeral fractures. **A.** Commercial sling with immobilizing strap permits easy removal for hygiene and is comfortable on the neck. **B.** Conventional sling and swathe. **C.** Stockinette–Velpeau and swathe are used when there is an unstable surgical neck component. This position relaxes the pectoralis major.

Humeral Shaft

Fractures of the shaft of the humerus are most frequently caused by direct trauma that results in a transverse, oblique, or comminuted fracture or by an indirect torsion force that results in a spiral fracture. The nerves and brachial blood vessels may be injured with these fractures. Wrist drop is indicative of radial nerve injury. Initial neurovascular assessment is essential to identify nerve or blood vessel injury, which requires immediate attention.

Initially, well-padded splints, overwrapped with an elastic bandage, are used to immobilize the upper arm and to support the arm in 90 degrees of flexion at the elbow. A sling or collar and cuff support the forearm. The weight of the hanging arm and splints reduce the fracture. External fixators are used to treat open fractures of the humeral shaft (see Chapter 70). ORIF of a fracture of the humerus is necessary with nerve palsy, blood vessel damage, comminuted fracture, or pathologic fracture.

Functional bracing is another form of treatment used for these fractures. A contoured thermoplastic sleeve is secured in place with interlocking fabric (Velcro) closures around the upper arm, immobilizing the reduced fracture. As swelling decreases, the sleeve is tightened, and uniform pressure and stability are applied to the fracture. The forearm is supported with a collar and cuff sling (Fig. 72-10). Functional bracing allows active use of muscles, shoulder and elbow motion, and good approximation of fracture fragments. Pendulum shoulder exercises are performed as prescribed to provide active movement of the shoulder, thereby preventing adhesions of the shoulder joint capsule. Isometric exercises may be prescribed to prevent muscle atrophy. The callus that develops is substantial, and the sleeve can be discontinued in about 8 weeks. Complications seen with humeral shaft fractures include delayed union and nonunion.

Elbow

Fractures of the distal humerus result from motor vehicle crashes, falls on the elbow (in the extended or flexed

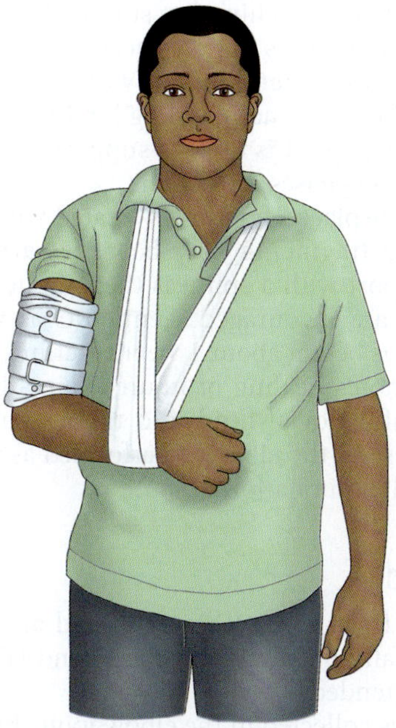

FIGURE 72-10. Functional humeral brace with collar and cuff sling.

CHART 72-3

Volkmann's Ischemic Contracture

- Observe the distal extremity for swelling, skin colour, nail bed capillary refill, and temperature. Compare affected and unaffected hands.
- Assess radial pulse.
- Assess for paresthesia (tingling and burning sensations) in the hand, which may indicate nerve injury or impending ischemia.
- Evaluate the patient's ability to move the fingers.
- Explore the intensity and character of the pain.
- Directly measure tissue pressure as prescribed.
- Report indications of diminished nerve function or diminished circulatory perfusion promptly before irreparable damage occurs; fasciotomy may become necessary.

position), or a direct blow. These fractures may result in injury to the median, radial, or ulnar nerves.

The patient is evaluated for paresthesia and signs of compromised circulation in the forearm and hand. The most serious complication of a supracondylar fracture of the humerus is Volkmann's ischemic contracture (a compartment syndrome), which results from antecubital swelling or damage to the brachial artery (Chart 72-3). The nurse needs to monitor the patient regularly for compromised neurovascular status and signs of compartment syndrome.

Other potential complications are damage to the joint articular surfaces and hemarthrosis (blood in the joint). If hemarthrosis is present, the physician may aspirate the joint to remove the blood, thereby relieving the pressure and pain.

Management

The goal of therapy is prompt reduction and stabilization of the distal humerus fracture, followed by controlled active motion after swelling has subsided and healing has begun. If the fracture is not displaced, the arm is immobilized in a cast or posterior splint with the elbow at 45 to 90 degrees of flexion and in a sling for 4 to 6 weeks. Then, a thermoplastic splint is used to support the fracture, and rehabilitation exercises are begun.

Usually, a displaced fracture is treated with ORIF. Excision of bone fragments may be necessary. Additional external support with a splint is then applied. Active finger exercises are encouraged. Gentle ROM exercise of the injured joint is begun about 1 week after internal fixation. Motion promotes healing of injured joints by producing movement of synovial fluid into the articular cartilage. Active exercise of the elbow is performed as prescribed to prevent residual limitation of motion.

Radial Head

Radial head fractures are common and are usually produced by a fall on the outstretched hand (FOOSH) with the elbow extended.

If blood has collected in the elbow joint (hemarthrosis), it is aspirated to relieve pain and to allow early active elbow and forearm ROM. Immobilization for these undisplaced fractures is accomplished with a splint. The patient is instructed not to lift with the arm for approximately 4 weeks. If the fracture is displaced, surgery is required, with excision of the radial head when necessary. Postoperatively, the arm is immobilized in a posterior plaster splint and sling. The patient is encouraged to carry out a program of active motion of the elbow and forearm when prescribed.

Radial and Ulnar Shafts

Fractures of the shaft of the bones of the forearm occur most frequently in children. The radius or the ulna may be fractured at any level. Frequently, displacement occurs when both bones are broken. The forearm's unique functions of pronation and supination must be preserved with good anatomic position and alignment.

Management

If the fragments are not displaced, the fracture is treated by closed reduction with a long arm cast applied from the upper arm to the proximal palmar crease. A loop may be incorporated in the cast near the elbow and a sling pulled through it to prevent the cast from sagging against the forearm.

The circulation, motion, and sensation of the hand are assessed after the cast is applied. The arm is elevated to control edema. Frequent finger flexion and extension are encouraged to reduce edema. Active motion of the involved shoulder is essential. The reduction and alignment are monitored closely by x-rays to ensure adequate immobilization. The fracture is immobilized for about 12 weeks; during the last 6 weeks, the arm may be in a functional forearm brace that allows exercise of the wrist and elbow. Lifting and twisting are avoided.

Displaced fractures are managed by ORIF, using a compression plate with screws, intramedullary nails, or rods. The arm is usually immobilized in a plaster splint or cast. Open fractures may be managed with external fixation devices. The arm is elevated to control swelling. Neurovascular status is monitored. Elbow, wrist, and hand exercises are begun as permitted by the immobilization device.

Wrist

Fractures of the distal radius (Colles' fracture) are common and are usually the result of a fall on an open, dorsiflexed hand. This fracture is frequently seen in older women with osteoporotic bones and weak soft tissues that do not dissipate the energy of the fall. The patient presents with a deformed wrist, pain, swelling, weakness, and limited finger ROM, and possibly reports of "tingling" in the affected hand.

Management

Treatment usually consists of closed reduction and immobilization with a short arm cast. For fractures with extensive comminution or impaction, ORIF, arthroscopic percutaneous pinning, or external fixation is used to achieve and maintain reduction and to allow for early functional rehabilitation. The wrist and forearm are elevated for 48 hours after reduction to control swelling.

Active motion of the fingers and shoulder should begin promptly. The patient is taught to do the following exercises to reduce swelling and prevent stiffness:

- Hold the hand at the level of the heart.
- Move the fingers from full extension to flexion. Hold and release. (Repeat at least 10 times every hour when awake.)
- Use the hand in functional activities.
- Actively exercise the shoulder and elbow, including complete ROM exercises of both joints.

The fingers may swell due to diminished venous and lymphatic return. The nurse assesses the sensory function of the median nerve by pricking the distal aspect of the index finger. The motor function is assessed by the patient's ability to touch the thumb to the little finger. Diminished circulation and nerve function must be treated promptly by release of constricting bandages.

Hand

Trauma to the hand often requires extensive reconstructive surgery. The objective of treatment is always to regain maximum function of the hand.

Management

For an undisplaced fracture of the phalanx (finger bone), the finger is splinted for 3 to 4 weeks to relieve pain and to protect the finger from further trauma. Displaced fractures and open fractures may require ORIF, using wires or pins.

The neurovascular status of the injured hand is evaluated. Swelling is controlled by elevation of the hand. Functional use of the uninvolved portion of the hand is encouraged.

Pelvis

The sacrum, ilium, pubis, and ischium bones form the pelvic bone, which is a fused, stable, bony ring in adults (Fig. 72-11). Falls, motor vehicle crashes, and crush injuries can cause pelvic fractures. Pelvic fractures are serious as at least two thirds of affected patients have significant and multiple injuries. Management of severe, life-threatening pelvic fractures is coordinated with the trauma team. Hemorrhage and thoracic, intra-abdominal, and cranial injuries have priority over treatment of fractures. There is a high mortality rate associated with pelvic fractures, related to hemorrhage, pulmonary complications, fat emboli, intravascular coagulation, thromboembolic complications, and infection.

Pelvic fracture symptoms include ecchymosis; tenderness over the symphysis pubis, anterior iliac spines, iliac crest, sacrum, or coccyx; local swelling; numbness or tingling of pubis, genitals, and proximal thighs; and inability to bear weight without discomfort. Computed tomography of the pelvis helps to determine the extent of injury by demonstrating sacroiliac joint disruption, soft tissue trauma, pelvic hematoma, and fractures. Neurovascular assessment of the lower extremities is completed to detect injury to pelvic blood vessels and nerves.

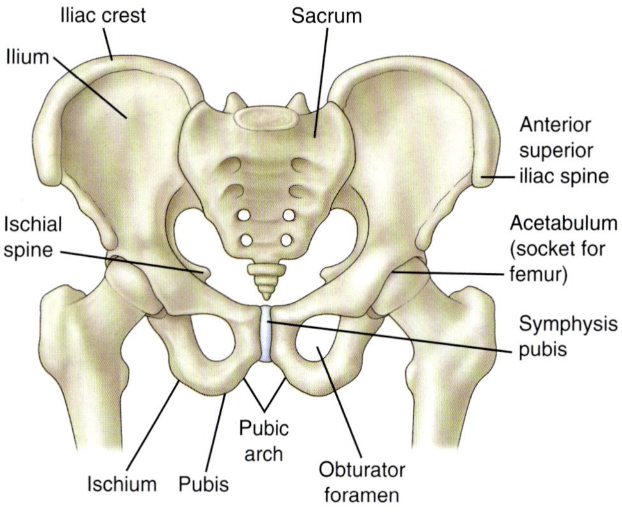

FIGURE 72-11. Pelvic bones.

Hemorrhage and shock are two of the most serious consequences that may occur. Bleeding arises from the cancellous surfaces of the fracture fragments, from laceration of veins and arteries by bone fragments, and possibly from a torn iliac artery. The peripheral pulses of both lower extremities are palpated; absence of pulses may indicate a torn iliac artery or one of its branches. Peritoneal lavage may be performed to detect intra-abdominal hemorrhage. The patient is handled gently to minimize further bleeding and shock.

The nurse assesses for injuries to the bladder, rectum, intestines, other abdominal organs, and pelvic vessels and nerves. To assess for urinary tract injury, the patient's urine is examined for blood. A voiding cystourethrogram and an intravenous urogram may be performed. Laceration of the urethra is suspected in males with anterior fracture of the pelvis and blood at the urethral meatus. (Females rarely experience a lacerated urethra.) A catheter should not be inserted until the status of the urethra is known. Abdominal pain and signs of peritonitis suggest injury to the intestines or abdominal bleeding. Paralytic ileus may accompany pelvic fractures.

Numerous classification systems have been used to describe pelvic fractures in relation to anatomy, stability, and mechanism of injury. Some fractures of the pelvis do not disrupt the pelvic ring; others disrupt the ring, which may be rotationally or vertically unstable. The severity of pelvic fractures varies. Long-term complications of pelvic fractures include malunion, nonunion, residual gait disturbances, and back pain from ligament injury.

Stable Pelvic Fractures

Stable fractures of the pelvis (Fig. 72-12) include fracture of a single pubic or ischial ramus, fracture of ipsilateral pubic and ischial rami, fracture of the pelvic wing of ilium (i.e., Duverney's fracture), and fracture of the sacrum or coccyx. Also, if injury results in only a slight widening of the pubic symphysis or the anterior sacroiliac joint and the pelvic ligaments are intact, the disrupted pubic symphysis is likely to heal spontaneously with conservative management. Most fractures of the pelvis heal rapidly because the pelvic bones are mostly cancellous bone, which has a rich blood supply.

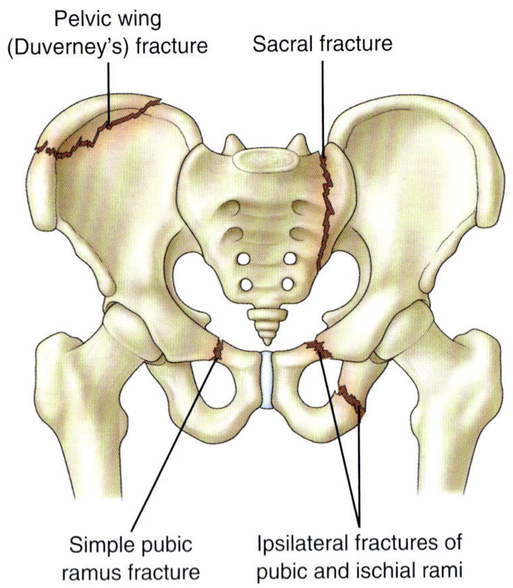

FIGURE 72-12. Stable pelvic fractures.

Stable pelvic fractures are treated with a few days of bed rest and symptom management until the pain and discomfort are controlled. The patient on bed rest is at risk for complications from immobility, including constipation, venous stasis, and pulmonary complications. Fluids, dietary fibre, ankle and leg exercises, elastic compression stockings to aid venous return, logrolling, coughing and deep breathing, and skin care reduce the risk for complications and increase the patient's comfort. The patient with a fractured sacrum is at risk for paralytic ileus, and bowel sounds should be monitored.

The patient with fracture of the coccyx experiences pain on sitting and with defecation. Sitz baths may be prescribed to relieve pain, and stool softeners may be given to prevent the need to strain on defecation. As pain resolves, activity is gradually resumed with the use of ambulatory aids (e.g., crutches, walker) for protected weight bearing. Early mobilization reduces problems related to immobility.

Unstable Pelvic Fractures

Unstable fractures of the pelvis (Fig. 72-13) may result in rotational instability (the open book type, in which a separation occurs at the symphysis pubis with some sacral ligament disruption), vertical instability (the vertical shear type, with superior–inferior displacement), or a combination of both. Lateral or anteroposterior compression of the pelvis produces rotationally unstable pelvic fractures. Vertically unstable pelvic fractures occur when force is exerted on the pelvis vertically, as when the person falls from a height onto extended legs or is struck from above by a falling object. Vertical shear pelvic fractures involve the anterior and posterior pelvic ring with vertical displacement, usually through the sacroiliac joint. There is generally complete disruption of the posterior sacroiliac, sacrospinous, and sacrotuberous ligaments. Vertical displacement of the hemipelvis is usually evident.

Treatment of unstable pelvic fractures generally involves external fixation or ORIF. This promotes hemostasis, hemodynamic stability, comfort, and early mobilization.

Acetabulum

Fractures of the acetabulum are seen in motor vehicle crashes in which the femur is jammed into the dashboard. Treatment depends on the pattern of fracture. Stable, nondisplaced fractures and fractures that involve minimal articular weight bearing may be managed with traction and protective (toe touch) weight bearing. Displaced and unstable acetabular fractures are treated with open reduction, joint débridement, and internal fixation or arthroplasty. Internal fixation permits early non–weight-bearing ambulation and ROM exercise. Complications seen with acetabular fractures include nerve palsy, heterotopic ossification, and posttraumatic arthritis.

Hip

There is a high incidence of hip fracture among older people, who have brittle bones from osteoporosis (particularly women) and who tend to fall frequently. Weak quadriceps muscles, general frailty due to age, and conditions that produce decreased cerebral arterial perfusion (transient ischemic attacks, anemia, emboli, cardiovascular disease, effects of medications) contribute to the incidence of falls. The patient who has sustained a hip fracture frequently has a comorbidity (e.g., cardiovascular, pulmonary, renal, endocrine). Often, a fractured hip is a catastrophic event that will have a negative impact on the patient's lifestyle (i.e., loss of ability to live independently) and quality of life.

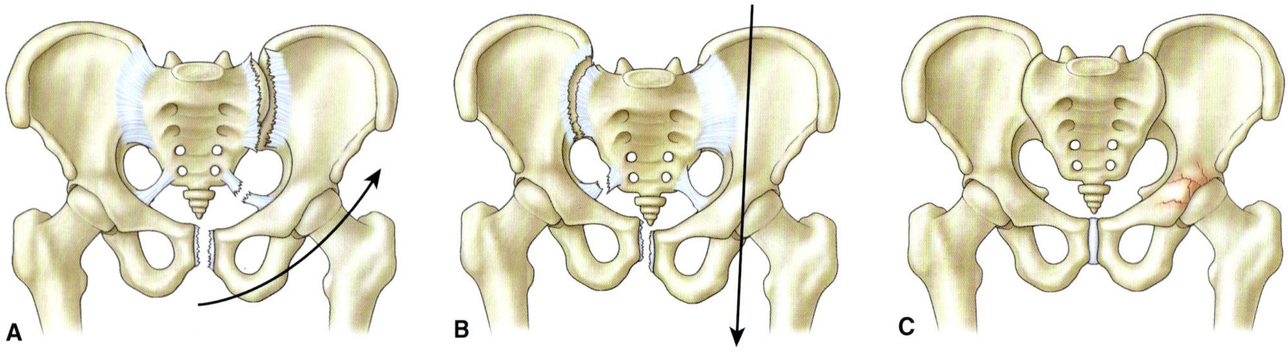

FIGURE 72-13. Unstable pelvic fracture. A. Rotationally unstable fracture: The symphysis pubis is separated and the anterior sacroiliac, sacrotuberous, and sacrospinous ligaments are disrupted. B. Vertically unstable fracture: The hemipelvis is displaced anteriorly and posteriorly through the symphysis pubis, and the sacroiliac joint ligaments are disrupted. C. Undisplaced fracture of the acetabulum.

It is important to listen carefully to the patient's description of the fall. For example, an 85-year-old woman reported that she was standing in her bathroom at home cutting her fingernails when all of a sudden she fell to her knees and was unable to get up. Fortunately, she had an alert system in place and pushed the button on her wrist bracelet and assistance arrived. She arrived at the hospital reporting severe pain in her right thigh. X-rays revealed a longitudinal fracture of the femur. On her fourth postoperative day, as analgesics were reduced, she reported severe pain in her left hip area to her nurses. X-rays revealed a hip fracture. In this case, it was determined that her hip had fractured and was the reason for her initial fall. Patients may provide a history of falling and fracturing their hips; it is important for health care professionals to be alert to the possibility that an osteoporotic hip fracture may cause the fall in the first instance. This case also highlights the need for nurses to complete a thorough symmetrical assessment in patients for other fractures.

There are three major types of hip fracture. *Extracapsular fractures* are fractures of the trochanteric region (between the base of the neck and the lesser trochanter of the femur) and of the subtrochanteric region. *Intracapsular fractures* are fractures of the neck of the femur. Fractures of the neck of the femur may damage the vascular system that supplies blood to the head and the neck of the femur, and the bone may become ischemic. For this reason, AVN is common in patients with femoral neck fractures (see Fig. 72-14). *Periprosthetic fractures* are fractures to the regions surrounding prosthetics joints (NAON, 2013).

Extracapsular intertrochanteric fractures have an excellent blood supply and heal readily. However, extensive soft tissue damage may have occurred at the time of injury. It is not uncommon for the fracture to be comminuted and unstable. There is a fairly high mortality rate after intertrochanteric hip fractures, as the patients are usually older (70 to 85 years of age), have other medical comorbidities, and are poor surgical candidates.

Clinical Manifestations

With fractures of the femoral neck, the leg is shortened, adducted, and externally or internally rotated. The patient complains of pain in the hip and groin or in the medial side of the knee. With most fractures of the femoral neck, the patient is unable to move the leg without a significant increase in pain. The patient is most comfortable with the leg slightly flexed in external rotation. Impacted intracapsular femoral neck fractures cause moderate discomfort (even with movement), may allow the patient to bear weight, and may not demonstrate obvious shortening or rotational changes. With extracapsular femoral fractures of the trochanteric or subtrochanteric regions, the extremity is significantly shortened, externally rotated to a greater degree than intracapsular fractures, exhibits muscle spasm that resists positioning of the extremity in a neutral position, and has an associated large hematoma or area of ecchymosis. The diagnosis of fractured hip is confirmed with x-ray.

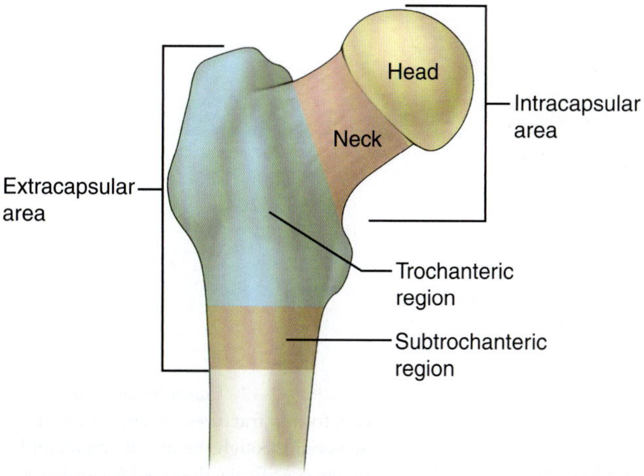

FIGURE 72-14. Regions of the proximal femur.

Gerontologic Considerations

Older adults (particularly women) who have low bone density from osteoporosis and who tend to fall frequently have a high incidence of hip fracture. Stress and immobility related to the trauma predispose the older adult to atelectasis, pneumonia, sepsis, VTE, pressure ulcers, and reduced ability to cope with other health problems. Many older adults hospitalized with hip fractures exhibit delirium as a result of stress of the trauma, pain, unfamiliar surroundings, sleep deprivation, and medications. In addition, delirium that develops in some older adult patients may be caused by mild cerebral ischemia or mild hypoxemia. Other factors associated with delirium include responses to malnutrition, dehydration, infectious processes, mood disturbances, and blood loss (Holly, Rittenmeyer, & Weeks, 2014). The same factors that may cause delirium may superimpose delirium on dementia in the older adult with a fractured hip, further complicating recovery.

To prevent complications, the nurse must assess the older patient for chronic conditions that require close monitoring. Examination of the legs may reveal edema due to heart failure or absence of peripheral pulses from peripheral vascular disease. Similarly, chronic respiratory problems may be present and may contribute to the possible development of atelectasis or pneumonia. Coughing and deep-breathing exercises are encouraged. Frequently, older adults take cardiac, antihypertensive, or respiratory medications that need to be continued. The patient's responses to these medications should be monitored.

Dehydration and poor nutrition may be present. At times, older adults who live alone cannot call for help at the time of injury. A day or two may pass before assistance is provided, and as a result, dehydration occurs. Nutritional status may have been poor prior to admission, so the nurse should monitor for complications of dehydration and poor nutrition (e.g., pressure ulcers). Nutritional supplements are effective in improving outcomes in older adults and should be incorporated into the plan of care (American Academy of Orthopaedic Surgeons [AAOS], 2014b).

Muscle weakness may have initially contributed to the fall and fracture. Bed rest and immobility cause an additional loss of muscle strength unless the nurse encourages the patient to move all joints except the involved hip and knee. Patients are encouraged to use their arms and the overhead trapeze to reposition themselves. This strengthens the arms and shoulders, which facilitates walking with assistive devices.

Medical Management

The goal of surgical treatment of hip fractures is to obtain a satisfactory fixation so that the patient can be mobilized quickly and avoid secondary postoperative complications. Surgical treatment consists of (a) open or closed reduction of the fracture and internal fixation, (b) replacement of the femoral head with a prosthesis (hemiarthroplasty), or (c) closed reduction with percutaneous stabilization for an intracapsular fracture. Surgical intervention is carried out as soon as possible after injury. The preoperative objective is to ensure that the patient is in as favourable a condition as possible for the surgery. Displaced femoral neck fractures may be treated as emergencies, with reduction and internal fixation performed within 12 to 24 hours after fracture. This minimizes the effects of diminished blood supply and reduces the risk for avascular necrosis.

After general or spinal anesthesia, the hip fracture is reduced under x-ray visualization using an image intensifier. A stable fracture is usually fixed with nails, a nail-and-plate combination, multiple pins, or compression screw devices (Fig. 72-15). The orthopedic surgeon determines the specific fixation device based on the fracture site or sites. Adequate reduction is important for fracture healing (the better the reduction, the better the healing).

Hemiarthroplasty (replacement of the head of the femur with a prosthesis) is usually reserved for fractures that cannot be satisfactorily reduced or securely nailed or to avoid complications of nonunion and avascular necrosis of the head of the femur. Total hip replacement (see Chapter 70) may be used in selected patients with acetabular defects.

Nursing Management

The immediate postoperative care for a patient with a hip fracture is similar to that for other patients undergoing major surgery (refer to Chapter 19 as well as the Nursing Process section on Preoperative Care of the Patient Undergoing Orthopedic Surgery in Chapter 70). Attention is given to pain management, prevention of secondary medical problems, and early mobilization of the patient so that independent functioning can be restored.

During the first 24 to 48 hours, relief of pain and prevention of complications are priorities. The nurse encourages deep-breathing, coughing, and foot flexion exercises every 1 to 2 hours. Thigh-high elastic compression stockings and pneumatic compression devices are used to prevent venous stasis. The nurse administers prescribed intravenous prophylactic antibiotics and monitors the patient's hydration, nutritional status, and urine output. A pillow is placed between the legs to maintain abduction and alignment and to provide needed support when turning the patient.

Repositioning the Patient

The nurse may turn the patient onto the affected or unaffected extremity as prescribed by the physician. The standard method involves placing a pillow between the patient's legs to keep the affected leg in an abducted position. The patient is then turned onto the side while proper alignment and supported abduction are maintained.

Promoting Strengthening Exercises

The patient is encouraged to exercise as much as possible by means of an overbed trapeze. This device helps to strengthen the arms and shoulders in preparation for protected ambulation (e.g., toe touch, partial weight bearing). On the first postoperative day, the patient transfers to a chair with assistance and begins assisted ambulation. The amount of weight bearing that can be permitted depends on the stability of the fracture reduction. The physician prescribes the degree of weight bearing and the rate at which the patient can progress to full weight bearing. Physical therapists work with the patient on transfers, ambulation, and the safe use of a walker and crutches.

The patient who has experienced a fractured hip can anticipate discharge to home or to an extended care facility with the use of an ambulatory aid. Some modifications

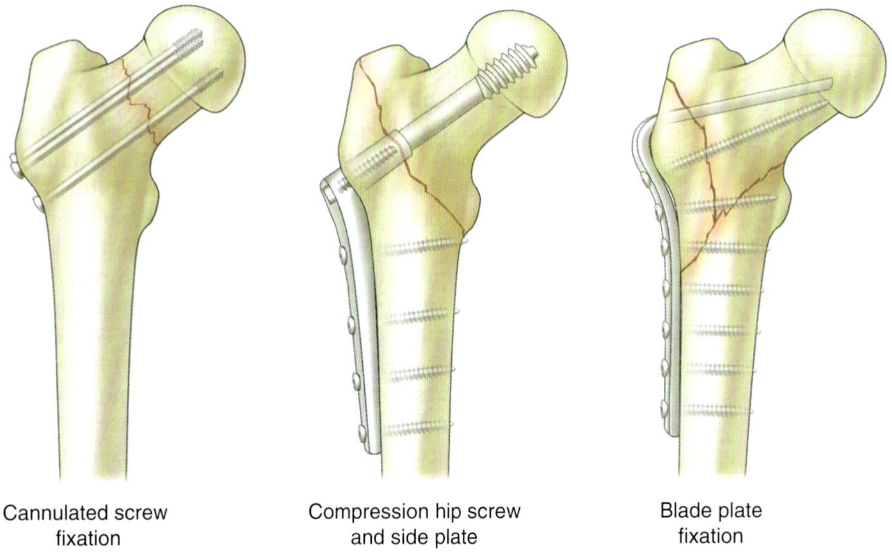

FIGURE 72-15. Examples of internal fixation for hip fractures. Internal fixation is achieved through the use of screws and plates specifically designed for stability and fixation.

in the home may be needed to permit safe use of walkers and crutches and for the patient's continuing care.

Monitoring and Managing Potential Complications

Older adults with hip fractures are particularly prone to complications that may require more vigorous treatment than the fracture. In some instances, shock proves fatal. Achievement of homeostasis after injury and after surgery is accomplished through careful monitoring and collaborative management, including adjustment of therapeutic interventions as indicated.

Neurovascular complications may occur from direct injury to nerves and blood vessels or from increased tissue pressure. With hip fracture, bleeding into the tissues is expected. Excessive swelling may be observed. Therefore, the nurse must monitor the neurovascular status of the affected leg.

To prevent VTE, the nurse encourages intake of fluids and ankle and foot exercises. Antiembolism stockings, pneumatic compression devices, and prophylactic anticoagulant therapy are indicated and should be prescribed. During hospitalization, the patient or the patient's caregiver should be educated regarding the signs, symptoms, and risks of VTE, and how to administer anticoagulant prophylaxis as prescribed (see Chart 72-4). Intermittent assessment of the patient's legs for signs of DVT, which may include unilateral calf tenderness, warmth, redness, and swelling, is indicated.

Pulmonary complications (e.g., atelectasis, pneumonia) are a threat to older patients undergoing hip surgery. Coughing and deep-breathing exercises, intermittent changes of position, and the use of an incentive spirometer may help prevent respiratory complications. Pain must be treated with analgesic agents, typically opioids; otherwise, the patient may not be able to cough, deep breathe, or engage in prescribed activities. The nurse assesses breath sounds to detect adventitious or diminished sounds.

A break in the integrity of the skin breakdown is seen in older patients with hip fracture. Blisters caused by tape are related to the tension of soft tissue edema under the nonelastic tape. An elastic hip spica wrap dressing or elastic tape applied in a vertical fashion may reduce the incidence of tape blisters. Patients with hip fractures need to be assisted in changing their position while in bed every 2 to 4 hours as they are at risk for pressure ulcers. Proper skin care, especially on the heels, back, sacrum, and shoulders, helps to relieve pressure. High-density foam, static air, or another type of special mattress may provide protection by distributing pressure more evenly.

Issues of bladder continence may occur. In general, the routine use of an indwelling catheter is avoided because of the high risk for urinary tract infection. If a catheter is inserted at the time of surgery, it usually is removed on the morning of the first postoperative day. Urinary retention is common after surgery; the nurse must assess the patient's voiding patterns. To ensure proper urinary tract function, the nurse encourages liberal fluid intake within the cardiovascular tolerance of the patient.

Delayed complications of hip fractures include infection, nonunion, avascular necrosis of the femoral head (particularly with femoral neck fractures), and issues with the fixation device (e.g., protrusion of the fixation device through the acetabulum, loosening of hardware). Infection is suspected if the patient complains of persistent, moderate discomfort in the hip and has a mildly elevated sedimentation rate. The nursing management of the older patient with a hip fracture is summarized in the Plan of Nursing Care (Chart 72-5).

(text continued on page 2325)

NURSING RESEARCH PROFILE

Chart 72-4. Venous Thromboembolism Knowledge of Older Adults After Hip Fracture

Lee, J., Donaldson, J., Drake, D., et al. (2014). Venous thromboembolism knowledge among older post-hip fracture patients and their caregivers. *Geriatric Nursing, 35*(5), 374–380.

Purpose

Venous thromboembolism (VTE) is a serious complication following hip fracture injury in older adults. As VTE risk extends beyond the acute hospital phase, prevention of VTE should also be assured postdischarge. The purpose of this study was to assess older adults' knowledge of VTE prophylaxis after hip fracture and their satisfaction with VTE prophylaxis education provided during their hospitalization.

Design

The researchers used a survey to complete this descriptive cross-sectional study with adults older than 65 years of age following a hip fracture with surgical intervention. Patients ($n = 30$) or their caregivers ($n = 30$) consented to serve as participants and answered questions regarding VTE prophylaxis prior to discharge from the hospital.

Findings

Both patients and caregivers expressed the desire for more education on VTE prophylaxis, particularly information on medications used for VTE prevention and possible side effects and drug–drug interactions of these medications. The participants were also found to have insufficient knowledge of VTE risk factors, symptoms, and prevention measures.

Nursing Implications

Patients post hip fracture surgery or their caregivers may need to administer anticoagulant prophylaxis for several weeks postdischarge. Nurses administer medications to older adult patients post hip fracture surgery, and are in a prime position to educate patients about the indications, side effects, and risks involved with anticoagulant prophylaxis. These researchers assert that nurses should not only verbally instruct patients about anticoagulant prophylaxis, but also involve family members in education sessions and supplement verbal instruction with dissemination of written materials for future reference.

Plan of Nursing Care — Chart 72-5. Care of the Older Patient With a Fractured Hip

NURSING INTERVENTIONS	RATIONALE	EXPECTED OUTCOMES
Nursing Priority: Acute pain **Goal:** Pain management		
1. Assess type and location of patient's pain.	1. Pain is expected after fracture; soft tissue damage and muscle spasm contribute to discomfort; pain is subjective and is evaluated through description of characteristics and location, which are important for determining cause of discomfort and for proposing interventions. Continuing pain may indicate development of neurovascular problems.	• Patient describes discomfort • Expresses confidence in efforts to control pain • Expresses little discomfort with position changes • Expresses comfort when leg is positioned and immobilized • Minimizes movement of extremity before reduction and fixation • Uses physical, psychological, and pharmacologic measures to reduce discomfort • Describes a decrease in pain in 24 to 48 hours after surgery • Requests pain medications, and uses pain relief measures early in pain cycle • States that positioning provides comfort • Appears comfortable and relaxed • Moves with increasing comfort as healing progresses
2. Acknowledge the patient's pain; inform patient of available analgesics; record patient's baseline discomfort.	2. Reduces stress experienced by the patient by communicating concern and availability of help in dealing with pain. Documentation provides baseline data.	
3. Handle the affected extremity gently, supporting it with hands or pillow.	3. Movement of bone fragments is painful; muscle spasms occur with movement; adequate support diminishes soft tissue tension.	
4. Apply Buck's traction as ordered. Use trochanter roll.	4. This immobilizes fracture to decrease pain, muscle spasm, and external rotation of hip.	
5. Use pain-modifying strategies.	5. Pain perception can be diminished by distraction and refocusing of attention.	
a. Modify the environment.	a. Interaction with others, distraction, and environmental stimuli may modify pain experiences.	
b. Administer prescribed analgesics as needed.	b. Analgesics reduce the pain; muscle relaxants may be prescribed to decrease discomfort associated with muscle spasm.	
c. Encourage patient to use pain relief measures before pain is "unbearable."	c. Mild pain is easier to control than severe pain.	
d. Evaluate patient's response to medications and other pain reduction techniques.	d. Assessment of effectiveness of measures provides basis for future management interventions; early identification of adverse reactions is necessary for corrective measures and care plan modifications.	
e. Consult with surgeon if relief of pain is not obtained.	e. Change in treatment plan may be necessary.	
6. Position for comfort and function.	6. Alignment of body facilitates comfort; positioning for function diminishes stress on musculoskeletal system.	
7. Assist with frequent changes in position.	7. Change of position relieves pressure and associated discomfort.	
Nursing Priority: Decreased physical mobility **Goal:** Independent mobilization with functional, stable hip		
1. Maintain neutral positioning of hip. 2. Use trochanter roll. 3. Place pillow between legs when turning.	1. Prevents stress on fixation 2. Minimizes external rotation 3. Supports leg; prevents adduction	• Patient engages in therapeutic positioning • Uses pillow between legs when turning

Plan of Nursing Care

Chart 72-5. Care of the Older Patient With a Fractured Hip, *Continued*

NURSING INTERVENTIONS	RATIONALE	EXPECTED OUTCOMES
4. Instruct and assist in position changes and transfers.	4. Encourages patient's active participation while preventing stress on hip fixation.	• Assists in position changes; shows increased independence in transfers • Exercises every 2 hours while awake • Uses trapeze • Participates in progressive ambulation program • Actively participates in exercise regimen • Uses ambulatory aids correctly and safely
5. Instruct in and supervise isometric, quadriceps-setting, and gluteal-setting exercises.	5. Strengthens muscles needed for walking.	
6. Encourage use of trapeze.	6. Strengthens shoulder and arm muscles necessary for use of ambulatory aids.	
7. In consultation with physical therapist, instruct in and supervise progressive safe ambulation within limitations of weight-bearing prescription.	7. Amount of weight bearing depends on the patient's condition, fracture stability, and fixation device; ambulatory aids are used to assist the patient with non–weight-bearing and partial–weight-bearing ambulation.	
8. Offer encouragement, and support exercise regimen.	8. Reconditioning exercises can be uncomfortable and fatiguing; encouragement helps patient comply with the program.	
9. Instruct in and supervise safe use of ambulatory aids.	9. Prevents injury from unsafe use.	

Nursing Priority: Risk for impaired skin integrity
Goal: Wound healing

NURSING INTERVENTIONS	RATIONALE	EXPECTED OUTCOMES
1. Monitor vital signs.	1. Temperature, pulse, and respiration increase in response to infection. (Magnitude of response may be minimal in older patients.)	• Patient's vital signs are within normal range • Well-approximated incision without drainage or excessive inflammatory response • Relates minimal discomfort; demonstrates no hematoma • Tolerates antibiotics; with no evidence of osteomyelitis.
2. Perform aseptic dressing changes.	2. This avoids introducing infectious organisms.	
3. Assess wound appearance and character of drainage.	3. Red, swollen, draining incision is indicative of infection.	
4. Assess report of pain.	4. Pain may be due to wound hematoma, a possible locus of infection, which needs to be surgically evacuated.	
5. Administer prophylactic antibiotic, if prescribed, and observe for side effects.	5. Antibiotics reduce the risk for infection.	

Nursing Priority: Risk for urinary continence and elimination issues
Goal: Normal urinary elimination patterns

NURSING INTERVENTIONS	RATIONALE	EXPECTED OUTCOMES
1. Monitor intake and output.	1. Adequate fluid intake ensures hydration; adequate urinary output minimizes urinary stasis.	• Intake and output are adequate; patient exhibits normal voiding patterns • Demonstrates no evidence of urinary tract infection
2. Avoid/minimize use of indwelling catheter.	2. Source of bladder infection.	
3. Perform intermittent catheterization for urinary retention.	3. Empties bladder; reduces urinary tract infections	

Nursing Priority: Difficulty coping with injury
Goal: Stress modification by using effective coping mechanisms

NURSING INTERVENTIONS	RATIONALE	EXPECTED OUTCOMES
1. Encourage patient to express concerns and to discuss the possible impact of fractured hip.	1. Verbalization helps patient deal with problems and feelings. Clarification of thoughts and feelings promotes problem solving.	• Patient describes feelings concerning fractured hip and implications for lifestyle

continued >

Plan of Nursing Care — Chart 72-5. Care of the Older Patient With a Fractured Hip, *Continued*

NURSING INTERVENTIONS	RATIONALE	EXPECTED OUTCOMES
2. Support use of coping mechanisms. Involve significant others and support services as needed.	2. Coping mechanisms modify disabling effects of stress; sharing concerns lessens the burden and facilitates necessary modification.	• Uses available resources and coping mechanisms; develops health promotion strategies • Uses community resources as needed • Participates in development of health care plan
3. Contact social services, if needed.	3. Anxiety may be related to financial or social problems; facilitates management of problems associated with continuing care.	
4. Explain anticipated treatment regimen and routines to facilitate positive attitude in relation to rehabilitation.	4. Understanding of plan of care helps to diminish fears of the unknown.	
5. Encourage patient to participate in planning.	5. Participating in care provides for some control of self and environment.	
Nursing Priority: Risk for disorientation **Goal:** Remains oriented and participates in decision making		
1. Assess orientation status.	1. Evaluate presenting orientation of patient; confusion may result from stress of fracture, unfamiliar surroundings, coexisting systemic disease, cerebral ischemia, or other factors. Baseline data are important for determining change.	• Patient establishes effective communication • Demonstrates orientation to time, place, and person • Participates in self-care activities • Remains mentally alert • Avoids episodes of confusion
2. Interview family regarding patient's orientation and cognitive abilities before injury.	2. Provides data for evaluation of current findings.	
3. Assess patient for auditory and visual deficits.	3. Diminished vision and auditory acuity frequently occur with aging; glasses and hearing aid may increase patient's ability to interact with environment.	
a. Assist patient with use of sensory aids (e.g., glasses, hearing aid)	a. Aids must be in good working order and available for use.	
b. Control environmental distractors	b. Facilitates communication.	
4. Orient to and stabilize environment a. Use orientation activities and aids (e.g., clock, calendar, pictures, introduction of self). b. Minimize number of staff working with patient.	4. Reorientation is important because: a. Short-term memory may be faulty in older adults; frequent reorientation helps. b. Consistency of caregivers promotes trust.	
5. Give simple explanations of procedures and plan of care.	5. Promotes understanding and active participation.	
6. Encourage participation in hygiene and nutritional activities.	6. Participation in routine activities promotes orientation and increases awareness of self.	
7. Provide for safety. a. Keep side rails up when patient is in bed. b. Keep light on at night. c. Have call bell available. d. Provide prompt response to requests for assistance.	7. Side rails decrease chance for additional injury from falls; mechanism for securing assistance is available to patient; independent activities based on faulty judgment may result in injury.	
8. Assess mental responses to medications, especially sedatives and analgesics.	8. Older people tend to be more sensitive to medications; abnormal responses (e.g., hallucinations, depression) may occur.	

Plan of Nursing Care

Chart 72-5. Care of the Older Patient With a Fractured Hip, *Continued*

Collaborative Problems: Hemorrhage; pulmonary complications; peripheral neurovascular dysfunction; deep vein thrombosis; pressure ulcers related to surgery and immobility
Goal: Decrease risk of complications

NURSING INTERVENTIONS	RATIONALE	EXPECTED OUTCOMES
Hemorrhage		
1. Monitor vital signs, observing for shock.	1. Changes in pulse, blood pressure, and respirations may indicate development of shock; blood loss and stress may contribute to development of shock.	• Vital signs stabilized within normal limits • Experiences no excessive or bright red drainage • Hemoglobin and hematocrit values within normal limits
2. Consider preinjury blood pressure values and management of coexisting hypertension, if present.	2. Necessary for interpretation of current blood pressure determinations	
3. Note character and amount of drainage.	3. Excessive drainage and bright red drainage may indicate active bleeding.	
4. Notify surgeon if patient develops shock or excessive bleeding.	4. Corrective measures need to be instituted.	
5. Note hemoglobin and hematocrit values, and report decreases in values.	5. Anemia due to blood loss may develop; bleeding into tissues after hip fracture may be extensive; blood replacement may be needed.	
Pulmonary Complications		
1. Assess respiratory status: respiratory rate, depth, and duration; breath sounds; sputum. Monitor temperature.	1. Anesthesia and bed rest diminish respiratory effort and cause pooling of respiratory secretions. Adventitious breath sounds, pain on respiration, shortness of breath, blood-tinged sputum, cough, and so forth indicate pulmonary problems.	• Patient has clear breath sounds • Breath sounds present in all fields • Exhibits no shortness of breath, chest pain, or elevated temperature • PaO_2 on room air within normal limits • Performs respiratory exercises; uses incentive spirometer as instructed • Changes position frequently • Consumes adequate fluids
2. Report adventitious and diminished breath sounds and elevated temperature.	2. Elevated temperature in the early postoperative period may be due to a respiratory problem.	
3. Supervise deep-breathing and coughing exercises. Encourage use of incentive spirometer if prescribed.	3. Promote optimal ventilation. Coexisting respiratory conditions diminish lung expansion.	
4. Administer oxygen as prescribed.	4. Reduced ventilatory efforts may diminish PaO_2 when patient is on room air.	
5. Turn and reposition patient at least every 2 hours. Mobilize patient (assist patient out of bed) as soon as possible.	5. Promotes optimal ventilation; diminishes pooling of respiratory secretions.	
6. Ensure adequate hydration.	6. Liquefies respiratory secretions; facilitates expectoration.	
Peripheral Neurovascular Dysfunction		
1. Assess affected extremity for colour and temperature.	1. The skin becomes pale and feels cool with decreased tissue perfusion. Venous congestion may cause cyanosis.	• Patient has normal colour, and the extremity is warm. • Demonstrates normal capillary refill response • Exhibits moderate swelling; tissue not palpably tense • States pain is controllable • Reports no pain with passive dorsiflexion • Reports normal sensations and no paresthesia
2. Assess toes for capillary refill response.	2. After compression of the nail, rapid return of pink colour indicates good capillary perfusion.	
3. Assess affected extremity for edema and swelling.	3. The trauma of surgery will cause swelling; excessive swelling and hematoma formation can compromise circulation and function; edema may be due to coexisting cardiovascular disease.	

continued >

Plan of Nursing Care

Chart 72-5. Care of the Older Patient With a Fractured Hip, *Continued*

NURSING INTERVENTIONS	RATIONALE	EXPECTED OUTCOMES
4. Elevate affected extremity.	4. This minimizes dependent edema.	• Demonstrates normal motor abilities and no paresis or paralysis • Has strong and equal pulses
5. Assess for deep, throbbing, unrelenting pain.	5. Surgical pain can be controlled; pain due to neurovascular compromise is refractory to treatment with analgesics.	
6. Assess for pain on passive flexion of foot.	6. With nerve ischemia, there will be pain on passive stretch.	
7. Assess for sensations and numbness.	7. Diminished pain and paresthesia may indicate nerve damage. Sensation in web between great and second toe—peroneal nerve; sensation on sole of foot—tibial nerve.	
8. Assess ability to move foot and toes.	8. Dorsiflexion of ankle and extension of toes indicate function of peroneal nerve. Plantar flexion of ankle and flexion of toes indicate functioning of tibial nerve.	
9. Assess pedal pulses in both feet.	9. This indicates circulatory status of extremities.	
10. Notify surgeon if diminished neurovascular status occurs.	10. Function of extremity needs to be preserved.	
Deep Vein Thrombosis or VTE		
1. Apply thigh-high elastic compression stockings and/or sequential compression device as prescribed.	1. Compression aids venous blood return and prevents stasis.	• Wears thigh-high elastic compression stockings • Uses sequential compression device • Experiences no skin breakdown • Experiences no more warmth than usual in skin areas • Exhibits no increase in calf circumference • Changes position with assistance and supervision • Participates in exercise regimen • Experiences no chest pain; has lungs clear to auscultation; presents no evidence of pulmonary emboli • Exhibits no signs of dehydration; has normal hematocrit • Maintains normal body temperature
2. Remove stockings for 20 minutes twice a day, and provide skin care.	2. Skin care is necessary to avoid skin breakdown. Extended removal of stocking or device defeats purpose.	
3. Assess popliteal, dorsalis pedis, and posterior tibial pulses.	3. Pulses indicate arterial perfusion of extremity. With coexisting arteriosclerotic vascular disease, pulses may be diminished or absent.	
4. Assess skin temperature of legs.	4. Local inflammation increases local skin temperature.	
5. Measure calf circumference twice daily.	5. Increased calf circumference indicates edema or altered perfusion.	
6. Avoid pressure on popliteal blood vessels from appliances or pillows.	6. Compression of blood vessels diminishes blood flow.	
7. Change patient's position and increase activity as prescribed.	7. Activity promotes circulation and diminishes venous stasis.	
8. Supervise ankle exercises hourly while patient is awake.	8. Muscle exercise promotes circulation.	
9. Ensure adequate hydration.	9. Older people may become dehydrated because of low fluid intake, resulting in hemoconcentration.	
10. Monitor body temperature.	10. Body temperature increases with inflammation (magnitude of response minimal in older adults).	
Pressure Ulcers Related to Surgery and Immobility		
1. Monitor condition of skin at pressure points (e.g., heels, sacrum, shoulders); inspect heels at least twice a day.	1. Older patients are subject to skin breakdown at points of pressure because of diminished subcutaneous tissue.	• Patient exhibits no signs of skin breakdown • Skin remains intact • Repositions self frequently • Uses protective devices
2. Reposition patient at least every 2 hours. Avoid skin shearing.	2. This avoids prolonged pressure and trauma to the skin.	
3. Administer skin care, especially to pressure points.	3. Immobility causes pressure at bony prominences; position changes relieve pressure.	

Plan of Nursing Care

Chart 72-5. Care of the Older Patient With a Fractured Hip, *Continued*

NURSING INTERVENTIONS	RATIONALE	EXPECTED OUTCOMES
4. Use special care mattress and other protective devices (e.g., heel protectors); support heel off the mattress.	4. Devices minimize pressure on skin at bony prominences.	
5. Institute care according to protocol at first indication of potential skin breakdown.	5. Early interventions prevent tissue destruction and prolonged rehabilitation.	

Nursing Priority: Reduction in independent ADLs related to fractured hip and impaired mobility
Goal: Maintains independent ADLs/promotion behaviours

NURSING INTERVENTIONS	RATIONALE	EXPECTED OUTCOMES
1. Assess home environment for discharge planning.	1. Physical barriers (especially stairs, bathrooms) may limit patient's ability to ambulate and care for self at home.	• Home is accessible for patient at time of discharge. • Patient appears relaxed and develops strategies to deal with identified problems. • Has personal assistance available • Demonstrates ability to use necessary assistance within therapeutic prescription • Complies with home care program; keeps follow-up health care appointments
2. Encourage patient to express concerns about care at home; explore with patient possible solutions to problems.	2. Patient may have special problems that need to be identified and dealt with.	
3. Assess availability of physical assistance for health care activities.	3. Because of limitation of mobility, patient requires some assistance in routine health care.	
4. Teach caregiver the home health care regimen.	4. Understanding of rehabilitative regimen is necessary for compliance.	
5. Instruct patient in posthospital care: a. Activity limitations b. Reinforce exercise instructions c. Safe use of ambulatory aids d. Wound care e. Measures to promote healing (nutrition, wound care) f. Medications, if any g. Potential problems h. Continuing health care supervision	5. Lack of knowledge and poor preparation for care at home contribute to patient anxiety, insecurity, and nonadherence to therapeutic regimen.	

Health Promotion

Osteoporosis screening of patients who have experienced hip fracture is important for prevention of future fractures. With dual-energy x-ray absorptiometry (DEXA) scan screening, the 10-year risk for additional fracture is quantified. Specific patient education regarding dietary requirements, lifestyle changes, and exercise to promote bone health is needed. Specific therapeutic interventions are initiated to decrease additional bone loss and build bone mineral density. Studies have shown that health care providers caring for patients with hip fractures fail to diagnose or treat these patients for osteoporosis despite the high probability that hip fractures are secondary to osteoporosis. Fall prevention is important and is facilitated through exercises to improve muscle tone and balance and through the elimination of environmental hazards. In addition, the use of hip protectors that absorb or shunt impact forces may help to prevent an additional hip fracture in the event a patient falls.

Femoral Shaft

Considerable force is required to break the shaft of the femur in adults. Most femoral fractures are seen in young adults who have been involved in a motor vehicle crash or who have fallen from a high place. Frequently, these patients have associated multiple traumas.

The patient presents with an enlarged, deformed, painful thigh and cannot move the hip or the knee. The fracture may be transverse, oblique, spiral, or comminuted. Frequently, the patient develops shock because the loss of 2 to 3 L of blood into the tissues. An increase in diameter of the thigh may indicate continued bleeding. Refer to Figure 72-16A for the types of femoral fractures.

Assessment and Diagnostic Findings

Assessment includes checking the neurovascular status of the extremity, especially circulatory perfusion of the lower leg and foot (popliteal, posterior tibial, and pedal pulses and toe capillary refill time). A Doppler ultrasound monitoring device may be needed to assess blood flow. Dislocation of the hip and knee may accompany these fractures. Knee effusion suggests ligament damage and possible instability of the knee joint.

Medical Management

Continued neurovascular monitoring is needed. The fracture is immobilized so that additional soft tissue damage

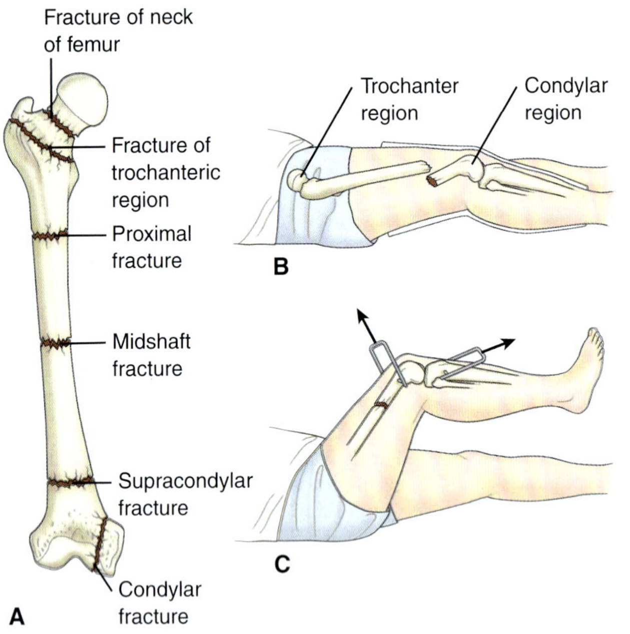

FIGURE 72-16. **A.** Types of femoral fractures. One method of correction for a fracture of the femur in the distal third is two-wire skeletal traction. **B.** Example of deformity on admission to hospital. **C.** Adequate reduction is achieved when additional wire is inserted in the lower femoral fragment, and vertical lift is secured.

does not occur. Generally, splinting is used to immobilize fracture fragments until the patient is physiologically stable and ready for ORIF procedures.

ORIF is performed as soon as possible after injury. Intramedullary locking nail devices are used for midshaft (diaphyseal) fractures. Depending on the supracondylar fracture pattern, intramedullary nailing or screw plate fixation may be used. Internal fixation permits early mobilization. A thigh cuff orthosis may be used for external support. To preserve muscle strength, the patient is instructed to exercise the lower leg, foot, toes, and hip on a regular basis. Active muscle movement enhances healing by increasing blood supply and electrical potentials at the fracture site. Prescribed weight-bearing limits are based on the fracture pattern. Physical therapy includes ROM and strengthening exercises, safe use of ambulatory aids, and gait training. Functional ambulation stimulates fracture healing. Healing for a fractured shaft of femur depends on the type of fracture and severity of the injury and may take 3 to 12 months.

Compression plates and intramedullary nails may need to be removed after 12 to 18 months due to reaction or loosening. After plates are removed, a thigh cuff orthosis is used for several months to provide support while bone remodelling occurs.

An external fixator may be used if the patient has an open fracture with extensive soft tissue trauma, bone loss, and infection, or has hip and tibial fractures.

A common complication after fracture of the femoral shaft is restriction of knee ROM. Active and passive knee exercises begin as soon as possible, depending on the management approach and the stability of the fracture and knee ligaments. Other complications include malunion, delayed union or nonunion, pudendal nerve palsy, and infection.

Tibia and Fibula

The most common fracture below the knee involves the tibia and fibula that results from a direct blow, a fall with the foot in a flexed position, or a violent twisting motion. Fractures of the tibia and fibula often occur in association with each other. The patient presents with pain, deformity, obvious hematoma, and considerable edema. Frequently, these fractures are open and involve severe soft tissue damage because there is little subcutaneous tissue in the area.

Assessment and Diagnostic Findings

Peroneal nerve damage is assessed. If nerve function is impaired, the patient is unable to dorsiflex the great toe and has diminished sensation in the first web space. Tibial artery damage is assessed by evaluating pulses, skin temperature, and colour and by testing the capillary refill response. Hemarthrosis or ligament damage may occur with fracture near the joint.

The patient is monitored for acute compartment syndrome. Symptoms include severe, intractable pain that is unrelieved by medications and increases with plantar flexion, tense and tender muscle lateral to tibial crest, and paresthesia.

Medical Management

Most closed tibial fractures are treated with closed reduction and initial immobilization in a long leg walking cast or a patellar tendon–bearing cast. Reduction must be relatively accurate in relation to angulation and rotation. As with other lower extremity fractures, the leg should be elevated to manage edema. Partial weight bearing is usually prescribed after 7 to 10 days. Activity decreases edema and increases circulation. The cast is changed to a short leg cast or brace in 3 to 4 weeks, which allows for knee motion. Fracture healing takes 6 to 10 weeks. At times, it is difficult to maintain reduction, and percutaneous pins may be placed in the bone and held in position by an external fixator.

Comminuted fractures are treated with ORIF using intramedullary nails or plates and screws, or external fixation. External support may be used with internal fixation. Hip, foot, and knee exercises are encouraged within the limits of the immobilizing device. Partial weight bearing is begun when prescribed and is progressed as the fracture heals in 4 to 8 weeks.

Open fractures are treated with external fixation. Distal fractures with extensive soft tissue damage heal slowly and may require bone grafting.

Continued neurovascular evaluation is needed. The development of compartment syndrome requires prompt recognition and resolution to prevent permanent functional deficit. Other complications include delayed union, infection, impaired wound edge healing due to limited soft tissue, and loosening of the internal fixation hardware.

Rib

Uncomplicated fractures of the lower ribs occur frequently in adults of all ages, typically from either motor vehicle crashes or falls, and usually result in no impairment of function. They are typically diagnosed based on clinical presentation and confirmed with x-rays or ultrasound scans (Melendez, 2015). Because these fractures cause pain with respiratory effort, the patient tends to decrease respiratory excursions and refrains from coughing. As a result, tracheobronchial secretions are not mobilized, aeration of the lung is diminished, and a predisposition to atelectasis and pneumonia results. To help the patient cough and take deep breaths and use an incentive spirometer, the nurse may splint the chest with their hands, or may educate the patient on using a pillow to temporarily splint the affected site. NSAIDs may be prescribed to provide analgesic relief. Occasionally, an anesthesia care provider administers intercostal nerve blocks or epidural analgesia to relieve pain and to improve respiratory function (Melendez, 2015).

Chest strapping to immobilize the rib fracture is *not* used, because decreased chest expansion may result in pneumonia and atelectasis. The pain associated with rib fracture diminishes significantly in 3 or 4 days, and the fracture heals within 6 weeks. In addition to pneumonia and atelectasis, complications include a flail chest, pneumothorax, and hemothorax. The management of patients with these conditions is discussed in Chapter 24.

Gerontologic Considerations

Older adults sustaining rib fractures are at an increased risk for complications. Even in the presence of isolated rib trauma, hospital admission is recommended for the older adult with multiple rib fractures or for the older adult who cannot effectively cough and mobilize sputum (Melendez, 2015). Careful monitoring of respiratory status and encouraging the patient to mobilize early, and, for the bedfast patient, encouraging turning, coughing, and deep breathing and use of an incentive spirometer, can prevent respiratory complications (see Chapter 26).

Thoracolumbar Spine

Fractures of the thoracolumbar spine may involve (a) the vertebral body, (b) the laminae and articulating processes, and (c) the spinous processes or transverse processes. The T12–L2 area of the spine is most vulnerable to fracture. Fractures generally result from indirect trauma caused by excessive loading, sudden muscle contraction, or excessive motion beyond physiologic limits. Osteoporosis contributes to vertebral body collapse resulting in a compression fracture.

Stable spinal fractures are caused by flexion, extension, lateral bending, or vertical loading. The anterior structural column (vertebral bodies and disks) or the posterior structural column (neural arch, articular processes, ligaments) have been disrupted. Unstable fractures occur with fracture dislocations and exhibit disruption of both anterior and posterior structural columns. The potential for neural damage exists.

The patient with a spinal fracture presents with acute tenderness, swelling, paravertebral muscle spasm, and change in the normal curves or in the gap between spinous processes. Pain is increased with moving, coughing, or weight bearing. Immobilization is essential until initial assessments have determined whether there is any spinal cord injury and whether the fracture is stable or unstable. Few spinal fractures are associated with neurologic deficits. If spinal cord injury with neurologic deficit does occur, it requires immediate surgery (laminectomy with spinal fusion) to decompress the spinal cord.

Medical Management

Stable spinal fractures are treated conservatively with limited bed rest. The head of the bed is elevated less than 30 degrees until the acute pain subsides (several days). Analgesics are prescribed for pain relief. The patient is monitored for a transient *paralytic ileus* caused by associated retroperitoneal hemorrhage. Sitting is avoided until the pain subsides. A spinal brace or plastic thoracolumbar orthosis may be applied for support during progressive ambulation and resumption of activities.

The patient with an unstable fracture is treated with bed rest and on occasion with the use of a special turning device (e.g., Stryker frame) to maintain spinal alignment. Neurologic status is monitored closely during the preoperative and postoperative periods. Within 24 hours after fracture, open reduction, decompression, and fixation with spinal fusion and instrument stabilization are usually accomplished. Postoperatively, the patient may be cared for on the turning device or in a bed with a firm mattress. Progressive ambulation is begun a few days after surgery, with the patient using a body brace orthosis. Patient teaching emphasizes good posture; good body mechanics; and, after healing is sufficient, back-strengthening exercises. (Spinal cord injury is discussed in Chapter 65.)

Amputation

Amputation of a lower extremity is necessary due to progressive peripheral arterial disease (often a sequelae of diabetes mellitus), fulminating gas gangrene, trauma (crushing injuries, burns, frostbite, electrical burns), congenital deformities, chronic osteomyelitis, or malignant tumour. Of all the causes, peripheral arterial disease accounts for most amputations of lower extremities.

Amputation is done to relieve symptoms, improve function, and save or improve the patient's quality of life. If the health care team communicates a positive attitude, the patient adjusts to the amputation more readily and actively participates in the rehabilitative plan, learning how to modify activities and how to use assistive devices for ADLs and mobility.

Levels of Amputation

Amputation is performed at the most distal point that will heal successfully. The site of amputation is determined by two factors: adequacy of circulation and functional usefulness (i.e., meets the requirements for the use of a prosthesis).

The circulatory status of the extremity is evaluated through physical examination and specific studies. Muscle and skin perfusion is important for healing. Doppler flowmetry, segmental blood pressure determinations, and transcutaneous PaO_2 are valuable diagnostic aids. CT

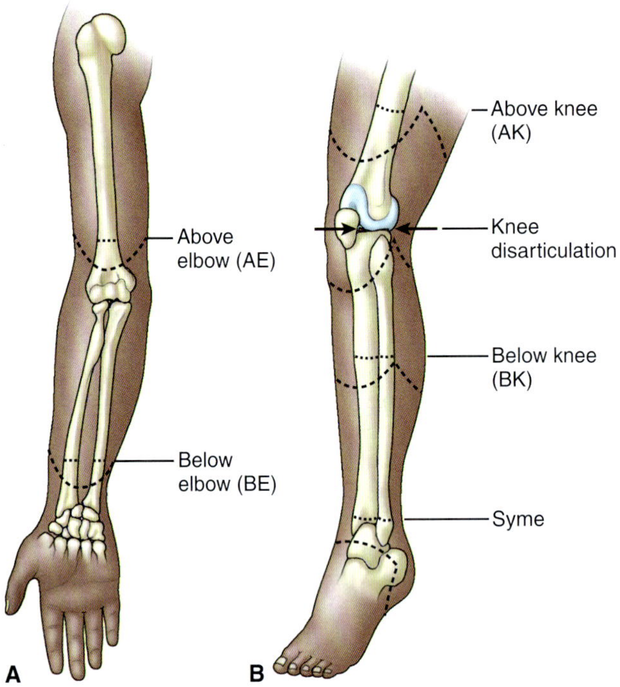

FIGURE 72-17. Levels of amputation are determined by circulatory adequacy, type of prosthesis, function of the part, and muscle balance. **A.** Levels of amputation of upper extremity. **B.** Levels of amputation of lower extremity.

angiography is performed if revascularization is considered an option.

The objective of surgery is to conserve as much extremity length as possible. Preservation of knee and elbow joints is desired. Figure 72-17 shows the levels at which an extremity may be amputated. Almost any level of amputation can be fitted with a prosthesis.

The amputation of toes and portions of the foot causes minor changes in gait and balance. A Syme amputation (modified ankle disarticulation amputation) is performed most frequently for extensive foot trauma and produces a painless, durable extremity that can withstand full weight bearing.

Below-knee amputations are preferred to above-knee amputations because of the importance of the knee joint and the energy requirements for walking. Knee disarticulations are most successful with young, active patients who are able to develop precise control of the prosthesis. When above-knee amputations are performed, all possible length is preserved, muscles are stabilized and shaped, and hip contractures are prevented for maximum ambulatory potential. Most people who have a hip disarticulation amputation must rely on a wheelchair for mobility.

Upper extremity amputations are performed to preserve the maximum functional length. The prosthesis is fitted early for maximum function.

A *staged amputation* may be used when there is gangrene and infection. Initially, a guillotine amputation is performed to remove the necrotic and infected tissue. The wound is débrided and allowed to drain. Sepsis is treated with systemic antibiotics. In a few days, after the infection has been controlled and the patient's condition has stabilized, a definitive amputation with skin closure is performed.

Complications

Complications that may occur with amputation include *hemorrhage, infection, skin breakdown, phantom limb pain,* and *joint contracture.* Because major blood vessels have been severed, there is an increased risk hemorrhage. Infection is a risk with all surgical procedures. The risk for infection increases with contaminated wounds after traumatic amputation. Skin irritation caused by the prosthesis may result in skin breakdown. **Phantom limb pain** is caused by the severing of peripheral nerves. Joint contracture is caused by positioning and a protective flexion withdrawal pattern associated with pain and muscle imbalance.

Medical Management

The objective of treatment is to achieve healing of the amputation wound, the result is a nontender residual limb (stump) with healthy skin for prosthetic attachment. Healing is enhanced by gentle handling of the residual limb, control of residual limb edema through rigid or soft compression dressings, and the use of aseptic technique in wound care to avoid infection.

A *closed rigid cast dressing* is frequently used to provide uniform compression, to support soft tissues, to control pain, and to prevent joint contractures. Immediately after surgery, a sterilized residual limb sock is applied to the residual limb. Felt pads are placed over pressure-sensitive areas. The residual limb is wrapped with elastic plaster of Paris bandages while firm, even pressure is maintained. Care is taken not to constrict circulation.

For the patient with a lower extremity amputation, the plaster cast may be equipped to attach a temporary prosthetic extension (pylon) and an artificial foot. This rigid dressing technique is used as a means of creating a socket for immediate postoperative prosthetic fitting. The length of the prosthesis is tailored to the patient. Early minimal weight bearing on the residual limb with a rigid cast dressing and a pylon attached produces little discomfort. The cast is changed in about 10 to 14 days. Elevated body temperature, severe pain, or a loose-fitting cast may necessitate earlier replacement.

A *removable rigid dressing* may be placed over a soft dressing to control edema, to prevent joint flexion contracture, and to protect the residual limb from unintentional trauma during transfer activities. This rigid dressing is removed several days after surgery for wound inspection and is then replaced to control edema. The dressing facilitates residual limb shaping.

A *soft dressing* with or without compression may be used if there is significant wound drainage and frequent inspection of the residual limb (stump) is needed. An immobilizing splint may be incorporated in the dressing. Stump (wound) hematomas are controlled with wound drainage devices to minimize infection.

Rehabilitation

The multidisciplinary rehabilitation team (patient, nurse, physician, social worker, physical therapist, occupational therapist, psychologist, prosthetist, vocational rehabilitation worker) helps the patient achieve the highest possible

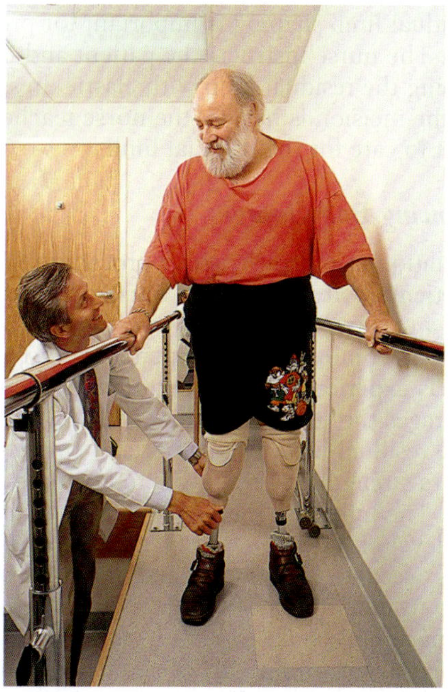

FIGURE 72-18. Many patients who have had amputations receive prostheses soon after surgery and begin learning how to use them with the help and support of the rehabilitation team, which includes nurses, physicians, physical therapists, and others.

level of function and participation in life activities (see Fig. 72-18). Prosthetic clinics and support groups for people with amputations facilitate this rehabilitation process (Geertzen, van der Linde, Rosenbrand, et al., 2015).

Patients who undergo amputation need support as they grieve the loss and change in body image. Their reactions can include anger, bitterness, and hostility. Psychological issues (e.g., denial, anxiety, avoidance) may be influenced by the type of support the patient receives from the rehabilitation team, the effectiveness of pain management, and by how quickly ADLs and the use of the prosthesis are learned. Knowing the full options and capabilities available with the various prosthetic devices can give the patient a sense of control over the resulting disability (Geertzen et al., 2015).

Patients who require amputation because of severe trauma can be young and healthy. These patients heal rapidly and are physically able to participate in a vigorous rehabilitation program. Because the amputation is the result of an injury, the patient needs psychological support in accepting the sudden change in body image and in dealing with the stresses of hospitalization, long-term rehabilitation, and modification of lifestyle.

Nursing Process

The Patient Undergoing an Amputation

Assessment

Before surgery, the nurse must evaluate the neurovascular and functional status of the limb through history and physical assessment. If the patient has experienced a traumatic amputation, the nurse assesses the function and condition of the residual limb. The nurse also assesses the circulatory status and function of the unaffected limb. If infection or gangrene develops, the patient may have associated enlarged lymph nodes, fever, and purulent drainage. A culture and sensitivity test is obtained to determine the appropriate antibiotic therapy.

The nurse evaluates the patient's nutritional status and develops a plan for nutritional care in consultation with a dietitian or metabolic or nutrition support team, if indicated. A diet with adequate protein and vitamins is essential to promote wound healing.

Any concurrent health problems (e.g., dehydration, anemia, cardiac insufficiency, chronic respiratory problems, diabetes) need to be identified and treated so that the patient is in the best possible condition to withstand the surgical procedure. The use of corticosteroids, anticoagulants, vasoconstrictors, or vasodilators may influence management and prolong or delay wound healing.

The nurse assesses the patient's psychological status. Evaluation of the patient's emotional reaction to amputation is important. Grief responses to permanent alterations in body image, function, and mobility are likely. Professional counselling can help the patient cope in the aftermath of amputation surgery.

Nursing Priorities

Based on assessment data, the patient's major nursing priorities may include the following:

- Acute pain
- Risk for disturbed sensory perception
- Impaired skin integrity
- Issues with body image related to amputation
- Ineffective coping
- Risk for anticipatory and/or dysfunctional grieving
- Self-care issues: feeding, and personal hygiene related to loss of extremity
- Independent mobility issues

Collaborative Problems/ Potential Complications

Based on assessment data, potential complications that may develop include the following:

- Postoperative hemorrhage
- Infection
- Skin breakdown

Planning and Goals

The major goals of the patient may include pain management, decreased altered sensory perceptions, wound healing, acceptance of altered body image, resolution of the grieving process, independence in self-care, restoration of physical mobility, and absence of complications.

Nursing Interventions

Managing Pain

Surgical pain can be effectively managed with opioid analgesics, nonpharmaceutical interventions, or evacuation of the hematoma or accumulated fluid. Pain may be incisional or may be caused by inflammation, infection, pressure on a bony prominence, or hematoma. Muscle spasms may add to the patient's discomfort. Changing the patient's position or placing a light sandbag on the residual limb to counteract the muscle spasm may improve the patient's level of comfort. Evaluation of the patient's pain and responses to interventions is an important part of the nurse's role in pain management. The pain may be an expression of grief and alteration of body image.

Minimizing Altered Sensory Perceptions

Amputees may experience phantom limb pain soon after surgery or 2 to 3 months after amputation. It occurs more frequently in above-knee amputations. The patient describes pain or unusual sensations, such as numbness, tingling, or muscle cramps as well as a feeling that the extremity is present, crushed, cramped, or twisted in an abnormal position. When a patient describes phantom pains or sensations, the nurse acknowledges these feelings and helps the patient modify these perceptions.

Phantom sensations may diminish over time; however, some patients experience phantom pain for the rest of their lives. The pathogenesis of the phantom limb phenomenon is unknown. Keeping the patient active helps decrease the occurrence of phantom limb pain. Early intensive rehabilitation and stump desensitization with kneading massage brings some relief. Distraction techniques and activity are helpful. Transcutaneous electrical nerve stimulation (TENS), ultrasound, or local anesthetics may provide relief for some patients. In addition, beta blockers may relieve dull, burning discomfort; anticonvulsant medications control stabbing and cramping pain; and tricyclic antidepressants are used to improve mood and coping ability.

Promoting Wound Healing

The residual limb must be handled gently. Whenever the dressing is changed, aseptic technique is required to prevent wound infection and possible osteomyelitis.

> **NURSING ALERT**
>
> **If the cast or elastic dressing inadvertently comes off, the nurse must immediately wrap the residual limb with an elastic compression bandage. If this is not done, excessive edema will develop in a short time, resulting in a delay in rehabilitation. The nurse notifies the surgeon if a cast dressing comes off so that another cast can be applied.**

Residual limb shaping is important for prosthesis fitting. The nurse instructs the patient and family in wrapping the residual limb with elastic dressings. After the incision is healed, the nurse teaches the patient to care for the residual limb.

Enhancing Body Image

Amputation is a reconstructive procedure that alters the patient's body image. The nurse who has established a trusting relationship with the patient is better able to communicate acceptance of the patient who has experienced an amputation. The nurse encourages the patient to look at, feel, and then care for the residual limb. It is important to identify the patient's strength and resources to facilitate rehabilitation. The nurse assists the patient to regain the previous level of independent functioning. The patient who is accepted as a whole person is more readily able to resume responsibility for self-care; self-concept improves, and body-image changes are accepted. Even with highly motivated patients, this process may take months.

Helping the Patient Resolve Grieving

The loss of an extremity (or part of one) may come as a shock even if the patient was prepared preoperatively. The patient's behaviour (e.g., crying, withdrawal apathy, anger) and expressed feelings (e.g., depression, fear, helplessness) will reveal how the patient is coping with the loss and working through the grieving process. The nurse acknowledges the loss by listening and providing support.

The nurse creates an accepting and supportive atmosphere in which the patient and family are encouraged to express and share their feelings and work through the grief process. The support from family and friends promotes the patient's acceptance of the loss. The nurse helps the patient deal with immediate needs and become oriented to realistic rehabilitation goals and future independent functioning. Mental health and support group referrals may be appropriate.

Promoting Independent Self-Care

Amputation of an extremity affects the patient's ability to provide adequate self-care. The patient is encouraged to be an active participant in self-care. The patient needs time to accomplish these tasks and must not be rushed. Practicing an activity with consistent, supportive supervision in a relaxed environment enables the patient to learn self-care skills. The patient and the nurse need to maintain positive attitudes and to minimize fatigue and frustration during the learning process.

Independence with dressing and personal hygiene depends on balance, transfer abilities, and physiological tolerance of the activities. The nurse works with the physical therapist and occupational therapist to teach and supervise the patient in these self-care activities.

The patient with an upper extremity amputation will have issues with feeding and personal hygiene.

Assistance is provided only as needed; the nurse encourages the patient to learn to perform these tasks independently. The nurse, therapists, and prosthetist work with the patient to achieve maximum independence.

Helping the Patient Achieve Physical Mobility

Positioning assists in preventing the development of hip or knee joint contracture in the patient with a lower extremity amputation. Abduction, external rotation, and flexion of the lower extremity are avoided. Depending on the surgeon's preference, the residual limb may be placed in an extended position or elevated for a brief period after surgery. The foot of the bed is raised to elevate the residual limb.

NURSING ALERT

The residual limb should not be placed on a pillow, as a flexion contracture of the hip may result.

The nurse encourages the patient to turn from side to side and to assume a prone position, if possible, to stretch the flexor muscles and to prevent flexion contracture of the hip. The nurse discourages sitting for prolonged periods, to prevent flexion contracture. The legs should remain close together to prevent an abduction deformity.

Postoperative ROM exercises are started early, because contracture deformities develop rapidly. ROM exercises include hip and knee exercises for below-knee amputations and hip exercises for above-knee amputations. It is important that the patient understands the importance of exercising the residual limb.

The upper extremities, trunk, and abdominal muscles are exercised and strengthened. The extensor muscles in the arm and the depressor muscles in the shoulder play an important part in crutch walking. The patient uses an overhead trapeze to change position and strengthen the biceps. The patient may flex and extend the arms while holding weights. Doing push-ups while seated strengthens the triceps muscles. Exercises, such as hyperextension of the residual limb, conducted under the supervision of the physical therapist or occupational therapist, also aid in strengthening muscles as well as increasing circulation, reducing edema, and preventing atrophy.

A patient with an upper extremity amputation uses both shoulders to operate the prosthesis; therefore, the muscles of both shoulders are exercised. A patient with an above-the-elbow amputation or shoulder disarticulation is likely to develop a postural abnormality caused by loss of the weight of the amputated extremity; postural exercises are helpful.

Strength and endurance are assessed, and activities are increased gradually to prevent fatigue. As the patient progresses to independent use of the wheelchair, the use of ambulatory aids, or ambulation with a prosthesis, the nurse emphasizes safety considerations. Environmental barriers (e.g., steps, inclines, doors, wet surfaces) are identified, and methods of managing them are practiced. It is important to anticipate, identify, and manage problems associated with the use of the mobility aids (e.g., pressure on the axillae from crutches, skin irritation of the hands from wheelchair use, residual limb irritation from a prosthesis).

Amputation of the leg changes the centre of gravity; therefore, the patient may need to practice position changes (e.g., standing from sitting, standing on one foot). The patient is taught transfer techniques early and is reminded to maintain good posture when getting out of bed. A well-fitting shoe with a nonskid sole should be worn. During position changes, the patient should be guarded and stabilized with a transfer belt at the waist to prevent falling.

As soon as possible, the patient with a lower extremity amputation is assisted to stand between parallel bars to allow extension of the temporary prosthesis to the floor with minimal weight bearing. How soon after surgery the patient is allowed to touch down the artificial foot depends on the patient's physical status and wound healing. As endurance increases and balance is achieved, ambulation is started with the use of parallel bars or crutches. The patient learns to use a normal gait, with the residual limb moving back and forth while the patient is walking with the crutches. To prevent a permanent flexion deformity from occurring, the residual limb should *not* be held up in a flexed position.

The patient with an upper extremity amputation is taught how to carry out the ADLs with one arm. The patient is started on one-handed self-care activities as soon as possible. The use of a temporary prosthesis is encouraged. The patient who learns to use the prosthesis soon after the amputation is less dependent on one-handed self-care activities.

A patient with an upper extremity amputation may wear a cotton T-shirt to prevent contact between the skin and shoulder harness and to promote absorption of perspiration. The prosthetist advises about cleaning the washable portions of the harness. Periodically, the prosthesis is inspected for potential problems.

The residual limb must be conditioned and shaped into a conical form to permit accurate fit, maximum comfort, and function of the prosthetic device. Elastic bandages, an elastic residual limb shrinker, or an air splint is used to condition and shape the residual limb. The nurse teaches the patient or a member of the family the correct method of bandaging.

Bandaging supports the soft tissue and minimizes the formation of edema while the residual limb is in a dependent position. The bandage is applied in such a manner that the remaining muscles required to operate the prosthesis are as firm as possible, whereas those muscles that are no longer useful atrophy. An improperly applied elastic bandage contributes to circulatory problems and a poorly shaped residual limb.

Effective preprosthetic care is important to ensure proper fitting of the prosthesis. The major problems that can delay prosthetic fitting during this period are (a) flexion deformities, (b) nonshrinkage of the residual limb, and (c) abduction deformities of the hip.

The physician usually prescribes activities to condition or "toughen" the residual limb in preparation for a prosthesis. The patient begins by pushing the residual limb into a soft pillow, then into a firmer pillow, and finally against a hard surface. The patient is taught to massage the residual limb to mobilize the surgical incision site, decrease tenderness, and improve vascularity. Massage is usually started once healing has occurred and is first done by the physical therapist. Skin inspection and preventive care are taught.

The prosthesis socket is custom moulded to the residual limb by the prosthetist. Prostheses are designed for specific activity levels and patient abilities. Types of prostheses include hydraulic, pneumatic, biofeedback-controlled, myoelectrically controlled, and synchronized prostheses.

Adjustments of the prosthetic socket are made by the prosthetist to accommodate the residual limb changes that occur during the first 6 months to 1 year after surgery. A light plaster cast, an elastic bandage, or a shrinking sock is used to limit edema during periods when the patient is not wearing the permanent prosthesis.

Some patients are not candidates for a prosthesis and are thus patients with amputations who are *nonambulatory*. If use of a prosthesis is not possible, the patient is instructed in the use of a wheelchair to achieve independence. A special wheelchair designed for patients who have had amputations is recommended. Because of the decreased weight in the front, a regular wheelchair may tip backward when the patient sits in it. In wheelchairs designed for patients who have had amputations, the rear axle is set back about 5 cm to compensate for the change in weight distribution.

Monitoring and Managing Potential Complications

After any surgery, efforts are made to reestablish homeostasis and to prevent problems related to surgery, anesthesia, and immobility. The nurse assesses body systems (e.g., respiratory, gastrointestinal, genitourinary) for problems associated with immobility (e.g., pneumonia, anorexia, constipation, urinary stasis) and institutes corrective management. Avoiding problems associated with immobility and restoring physical activity are necessary for maintenance of health.

> **NURSING ALERT**
>
> **Immediate postoperative bleeding may develop slowly or may take the form of a massive hemorrhage resulting from a loosened suture. A large tourniquet should be in plain sight at the patient's bedside so that if severe bleeding occurs, it can be applied to the residual limb to control the hemorrhage. The nurse immediately notifies the surgeon in the event of excessive bleeding.**

Massive *hemorrhage* due to a loosened suture is a serious problem. The nurse monitors the patient for any signs or symptoms of bleeding. It is also important to monitor the patient's vital signs and to observe the suction drainage.

Infection is a complication of amputation. Patients who have undergone traumatic amputation most likely have a contaminated wound. The nurse administers antibiotics as prescribed. It is important to monitor the incision, dressing, and drainage for indications of infection (e.g., change in colour, odour, or consistency of drainage; increasing discomfort). The nurse also monitors for systemic indicators of infection (e.g., elevated temperature) and promptly reports indications of infection to the surgeon.

Skin breakdown may result from immobilization or from pressure from various sources. The prosthesis may cause pressure areas to develop. The nurse and the patient assess for breaks in the skin. Careful skin hygiene is essential to prevent skin irritation, infection, and breakdown. The healed residual limb is washed and dried (gently) at least twice daily. The skin is inspected for pressure areas, dermatitis, and blisters. If they are present, they must be treated before further skin breakdown occurs. Usually, a residual limb sock is worn to absorb perspiration and to prevent direct contact between the skin and the prosthetic socket. The sock is changed daily and must fit smoothly to prevent irritation caused by wrinkles. The socket of the prosthesis is washed with a mild detergent, rinsed, and dried thoroughly with a clean cloth. The nurse advises the patient that the socket must be thoroughly dry before the prosthesis is applied.

Promoting Home, Community-Based, and Transitional Care

EDUCATING PATIENTS ABOUT SELF-CARE. Before discharge to the home or to a rehabilitation facility, the nurse encourages the patient and family to become active participants in care. They participate, as appropriate, in skin care and residual limb care and in the management of the prosthesis. The patient receives ongoing instructions and practice sessions in learning how to transfer and how to use mobility aids and other assistive devices safely. The nurse explains the signs and symptoms of complications that must be reported to the physician (Chart 72-6).

CONTINUING AND TRANSITIONAL CARE. After the patient has achieved physiologic homeostasis and has demonstrated achievement of major health care goals, rehabilitation continues either in a rehabilitation facility or at home. Continued support and supervision by the home care nurse are essential.

Before the patient's discharge to the home, the nurse should assess the home environment. Modifications are made to ensure the patient's continuing care, safety, and mobility. An overnight or weekend experience at home may be tried to identify problems that were not identified on the assessment visit. Physical therapy and occupational therapy may

CHART 72-6

HOME CARE CHECKLIST • The Patient With an Amputation

At the completion of education, the patient and/or caregiver will be able to:

- Name the procedure that was performed and identify any permanent changes in anatomic structure or function as well as changes in ADLs, IADLs, roles, relationships, and spirituality.
- Identify modification of home environment, interventions, and strategies (e.g., durable medical equipment, adaptive equipment, ADL assistance), used in safely adapting to changes in structure or function and promote effective recovery and rehabilitation.
  - Identify professionals and community agencies to help with transition to home.
- Describe ongoing postoperative therapeutic regimen, including diet and activities to perform (e.g., exercises) and to limit or avoid (e.g., lifting weights, driving a car, contact sports).
  - Describe care of residual limb and conditioning for prosthesis.
  - Consume a healthy diet to promote wound healing.
  - Participate in rehabilitation program to regain functional independence, promote circulation, maintain the health of unaffected muscles and those muscles now needed for safe transfer, mobility, etc.
  - If indicated, demonstrate safe use of mobility aid, assistive device, and transfer technique.
  - Observe prescribed weight bearing and activity limits.
- State the name, dose, side effects, frequency, and schedule for all prescribed therapeutic and prophylactic medications (e.g., antibiotics, anticoagulants, analgesic agents).
- State how to obtain medical supplies and carry out dressing changes, wound care, and other prescribed regimens.
- Describe approaches to controlling pain (e.g., take analgesics as prescribed; use nonpharmacologic interventions).
- State indicators of complications to report promptly to primary provider (e.g., uncontrolled pain; signs of local or systemic infection; residual limb skin breakdown).
- Relate how to reach primary provider with questions or complications.
- State time and date of follow-up appointments, therapy, and testing.
- Identify community resources for peer and caregiver/family support:
  - Identify sources of support (e.g., friends, relatives, faith community).
  - Identify phone numbers, meeting locations and times of support groups (e.g., amputee support groups, caregiver support groups).
- Identify the need for health promotion, disease prevention, and screening activities.

Resources

ADLs, activities of daily living; IADLs, independent activities of daily living.

continue in the home or on an outpatient basis. Transportation to continuing health care appointments must be arranged. The social service department of the hospital or the community agency managing continued health care may be of great assistance in securing personal assistance and transportation services.

During follow-up health visits, the nurse evaluates the patient's physical and psychosocial adjustment. Periodic preventive health assessments are necessary. Frequently, an elderly spouse is unable to provide the assistance required, and additional help at home is needed. Modifications in the plan of care are made on the basis of such findings. Often, the patient and family find involvement in a support group for patients who have had amputations to be of value; here, they are able to share problems, solutions, and resources. Talking with those who have successfully dealt with a similar problem may help the patient develop a satisfactory solution.

Patients, family members, and health care providers tend to focus on the most obvious needs and issues; however, the nurse reminds the patient and family about the importance of continuing health promotion and screening practices, such as regular physical examinations and diagnostic screening tests. Those patients who have not been involved in these practices in the past are instructed in their importance and are referred to appropriate health care providers.

Evaluation

Expected patient outcomes may include the following:

1. Experiences decreased/manageable pain
   a. Appears relaxed, uses measures to increase comfort and verbalizes comfort

b. Participates in self-care and rehabilitative activities
2. Experiences reduction in phantom limb pain
   a. Reports decreased phantom sensations
   b. Uses distraction techniques
   c. Performs stump desensitization massage
3. Achieves wound healing
   a. Controls residual limb edema
   b. Achieves nontender, nonadherent scar
   c. Demonstrates residual limb care
4. Demonstrates improved body image and effective coping
   a. Acknowledges change in body image
   b. Participates in self-care activities
   c. Demonstrates increasing independence
   d. Projects self as a whole person
   e. Resumes role-related responsibilities
   f. Reestablishes social contacts
   g. Demonstrates confidence in abilities
5. Exhibits resolution of grieving
   a. Expresses grief
   b. Works through feelings with family and friends
   c. Focuses on future functioning
   d. Participates in support group
6. Moves toward independent self-care
   a. Asks for assistance when needed
   b. Uses aids and assistive devices to facilitate self-care
   c. Verbalizes satisfaction with abilities to perform ADLs
7. Achieves maximum independent mobility
   a. Avoids positions contributing to contracture development
   b. Demonstrates full active ROM
   c. Maintains balance when sitting and transferring
   d. Increases strength and endurance
   e. Demonstrates safe transferring technique
   f. Achieves functional use of prosthesis
   g. Overcomes environmental barriers to mobility
   h. Uses community services and resources as needed
8. Reduces risk of complications of hemorrhage, infection, and skin breakdown
   a. Does not experience excessive bleeding
   b. Maintains normal blood values
   c. Is free of local or systemic signs of infection
   d. Repositions self frequently
   e. Is free of pressure-related problems
   f. Reports any skin discomfort and irritations promptly

Critical Thinking Exercises

1 You are a medical-surgical nurse working on a busy orthopedic unit caring for a 78-year-old female patient admitted one evening with a femoral neck fracture after a fall. The patient lives alone in her own home but remains very active within her community doing volunteer work. She is scheduled for surgery tomorrow. The patient tells you that she feels, "This is the beginning of the end for me." Identify this patient's unique nursing, medical, physical therapy, occupational therapy, social, and emotional needs. Devise a nursing plan of care that addresses these needs. What is the strength of the evidence that supports your plan of care for this patient?

2 A female college student athlete injures her knee during a soccer game the first week of the season. The trainer tells the student that she probably has an ACL injury and potentially also a meniscus injury. The student presents to the Student Health Center, where you work as a clinic nurse, unsure of the treatment plan for her injury. She expresses concern about how this injury will affect her chances at playing soccer for the remainder of the season. Describe the collaboration necessary to provide a comprehensive treatment plan for this patient. How will you, as the clinic nurse, support the student in this plan?

3 After a motorcycle crash, a 28-year-old male sustained a tibial fracture, which was surgically repaired yesterday afternoon. He was admitted to the inpatient orthopedic unit postoperatively, where you work as a staff nurse. During morning shift report, the night nurse reports to you, the oncoming day shift nurse, that the patient has been complaining of continuing pain all night that has not been alleviated despite administration of prescription opioid pain medication. The night shift nurse reports to you that she feels that the patient may have a high tolerance for pain medication due to his history of drug abuse. Describe your immediate assessments and interventions as you prioritize care for this patient.

REFERENCES AND SELECTED READINGS

Books

Emergency Nurses Association (ENA). (2013). *Sheehy's manual of emergency care*. St. Louis, MO: Mosby.
Moore, K. L., Agur, A. M. R., & Dalley, A. F. II (2015). *Essential clinical anatomy* (5th ed.). Philadelphia, PA: Lippincott Williams & Wilkins.
National Association of Orthopedic Nurses (NAON). (2013). *Core curriculum for orthopaedic nursing* (7th ed.). Boston, MA: Pearson.
Porth, C. M. (2015). *Essentials of pathophysiology: Concepts of altered health states* (4th ed.). Philadelphia, PA: Lippincott Williams & Wilkins.
Strickland, J. W., & Graham, T. J. (2005). *Master techniques in orthopaedic surgery: The hand* (2nd ed.). Philadelphia, PA: Lippincott Williams & Wilkins.

Journals and Electronic Documents

Agranoff, A. B. (2015). Medial collateral and lateral collateral ligament injury treatment and management. *Medscape*. Retrieved February 15, 2016, from emedicine.medscape.com/article/307959-treatment#d9
American Academy of Orthopaedic Surgeons (AAOS). (2014a). *Muscle contusion (bruise)*. Retrieved February 15, 2016, from orthoinfo.aaos.org/topic.cfm?topic=a00341
American Academy of Orthopaedic Surgeons (AAOS). (2014b). *Management of hip fractures in the elderly: Evidenced based clinical practice guidelines*. Retrieved February 15, 2016, from www.aaos.org/Research/guidelines/HipFxGuideline.pdf
Amputee Coalition. (2015). *Limb loss statistics*. Retrieved February 15, 2016, from www.amputee-coalition.org/resources/limb-loss-statistics/
Baker, B., Lubowitz, J. H., & Wolf, B. T. (2015). Meniscus injuries treatment and management. *Medscape*. Retrieved February 15, 2016, from emedicine.medscape.com/article/90661-treatment#d11
Buckley, R., & Page, J. L. (2016). General principles of fracture care. *Medscape*. Retrieved on February 14, 2016, from emedicine.medscape.com/article/1270717-overview#showall

Cooper, M. T. (2015). Acute Achilles tendon ruptures: Does surgery offer superior results (and other confusing issues)? *Clinical Sports Medicine, 34*(4), 595–606.

Dingemanse, R., Randsdorp, M., Koes, B., et al. (2014). Evidence for the effectiveness of electrophysical modalities for treatment of medial and lateral epicondylitis: A systematic review. *The British Journal of Sports Medicine, 48*(12), 957–965.

Duckworth, A. D., McQueen, M. M., & Ring, D. (2013). Fractures of the radial head. *The Bone & Joint Journal, 95-B*(2), 151–159.

Geertzen, J., van der Linde, H., Rosenbrand, K., et al. (2015). Dutch evidence-based guidelines for amputation and prosthetics of the lower extremity: Rehabilitation process and prosthetics. Part 2. *Prosthetics and Orthotics International, 39*(5) 361–371.

Haentjens, P., Magaziner, J., Colón-Emeric, C. S., et al. (2010). Meta-analysis: Excess mortality after hip fracture among older women and men. *Annals of Internal Medicine, 152*(6), 380–390.

Halawi, M., & Morwood, M. (2015). Acute management of open fractures: An evidence-based review. *Orthopedics, 38*(11), e1025–e1033.

Highsmith, M. J., Kahle, J. T., Miro, R. M., et al. (2016). Prosthetic interventions for people with transtibial amputation: Systematic review and meta-analysis of high-quality literature and systematic reviews. *Journal of Rehabilitation Research and Development, 53*(2), 157–184.

Holly, C., Rittenmeyer, L., & Weeks, S. (2014). Evidenced-based clinical audit criteria for the prevention and management of delirium in the postoperative patient with hip fracture. *Orthopaedic Nursing, 33*(1), 27–34.

Kare, J. A. (2015). Volkmann contracture. *Medscape*. Retrieved February 15, 2016, from emedicine.medscape.com/article/1270462-overview

Kent, M., Hsia, H., Van de Ven, T., et al. (2017). Perioperative pain management strategies for amputation: A topical review. *Pain Medicine, 18*(13), 504–519.

Kleinhenz, B. P. (2014). Clavicle fractures. *Medscape*. Retrieved February 15, 2016, from emedicine.medscape.com/article/92429-overview#a7

Kodde, I., Kaas, L., Flipsen, M., et al. (2015). Current concepts in the management of radial head fractures. *World Journal of Orthopedics, 6*(11), 954–960.

Kosova, E., Bergmark, B., & Piazza, G. (2015). Fat embolism syndrome. *Circulation, 131*(3), 317–320.

Lee, J., Donaldson, J., Drake, D., et al. (2014). Venous thromboembolism knowledge among older post-hip fracture patients and their caregivers. *Geriatric Nursing, 35*(5), 374–380.

Melendez, S. L. (2015). Rib fracture treatment and management. *Medscape*. Retrieved February 15, 2016, from emedicine.medscape.com/article/825981-overview

Morris, C., Potter, B., Athanasian, E., et al. (2015). Extremity amputations: Principles, techniques, and recent advancements. *Instructional Course Lectures, 64*, 105–117.

Paschos, N., Mitsionis, G., Vasiliadis, H., et al. (2013). Comparison of early mobilization protocols in radial head fractures. *Journal of Orthopaedic Trauma, 27*(3), 134–139.

Paulson, S., Comfort, C. P., Lee, B. C., et al. (2014). Prolonging life: Legal, ethical, and social dilemmas. *Annals of the New York Academy of Sciences, 1330*, 19–39.

Pirowska, A., Wloch, T., Nowobilski, R., et al. (2014). Phantom phenomena and body scheme after amputation: A literature review. *Neurologia I Neurochirurgia Polska, 48*(1), 52–59.

Russell, G. V., & Jarrett, C. A. (2016). Pelvic fractures. *Medscape*. Retrieved February 15, 2016, from emedicine.medscape.com/article/1247913-overview#a10

Saccomano, S., & Ferrara, L. (2015). Fall prevention in older adults. *Nurse Practitioner, 40*(6), 40–47.

Schaller, T. M. (2016). Open fractures. *Medscape*. Retrieved February 15, 2016, from emedicine.medscape.com/article/1269242-overview

Sobolev, B., Guy, P., Sheehan, K. J., et al; for the Canadian Collaborative Study of Hip Fractures (2018). Mortality effects of timing alternatives for hip fracture surgery. *Canadian Medical Association Journal, 190*(31), E923–E932.

Soroceanu, A., Sidhwa, F., Aarabi, S., et al. (2012). Surgical versus nonsurgical treatment of acute Achilles tendon rupture: A meta-analysis of randomized trials. *Journal of Bone & Joint Surgery American Volume, 94*(23), 2136–2143.

Speed, J. (2015). Heterotopic ossification. *Medscape*. Retrieved on February 15, 2016, from emedicine.medscape.com/article/327648-overview#showall

Street, P., Thompson, J., & Bailey, M. (2015). Management of urinary catheters following hip fracture. *Australasian Journal on Ageing, 34*(4), 241–246.

Thacker, M. M., Tejwani, N., & Thakkar, C. (2014). Acetabulum fractures. *Medscape*. Retrieved February 15, 2016, from emedicine.medscape.com/article/1246057-overview

van de Graaf, V. A., Noorduyn, J. C. A., Willigenburg, N. W., et al; ESCAPE Research Group. (2018). Effect of early surgery vs physical therapy on knee function among patients with nonobstructive meniscal tears: The ESCAPE randomized clinical trial. *Journal of the American Medical Association, 320*(13), 1328–1337.

Vinas, F. (2015). Lumbar spine fracture and dislocations. *Medscape*. Retrieved February 15, 2016, from emedicine.medscape.com/article/1264191-overview

Vincent, H., Horodyski, M., Vincent, K., et al. (2015). Psychological distress after orthopedic trauma: Prevalence in patients and implications for rehabilitation. *Physical Medicine and Rehabilitation, 7*(9), 978–989.

von Keudell, A. G., Weaver, M. J., Appleton, P. T., et al. (2015). Diagnosis and treatment of acute extremity compartment syndrome. *The Lancet, 386*(1000), 1299–1310.

Walczak, B., Johnson, C., & Howe, B. M. (2015). Myositis ossificans. *Journal of the American Academy of Orthopaedic Surgeons, 23*(10), 612–622.

Resources

Amputee and Disability Resource Directory for Canadian Amputees: http://www.amputee.ca

Canadian Orthopaedic Association: http://www.coa-aco.org

Canadian Orthopaedic Foundation: http://www.canorth.org

Easter Seal Society of Canada, c/o The Easter Seals/March of Dimes National Council: http://www.easterseals.ca

National Institute of Arthritis and Musculoskeletal and Skin Diseases: http://www.niams.nih.gov/

Reflex Sympathetic Dystrophy Syndrome Association of America (RSDSA): http://www.rsds.org

War Amps: http://www.waramps.ca

UNIT 16

Other Acute Problems

Case Study

ENSURING EQUITABLE PATIENT ASSIGNMENTS IN AN EMERGENCY DEPARTMENT

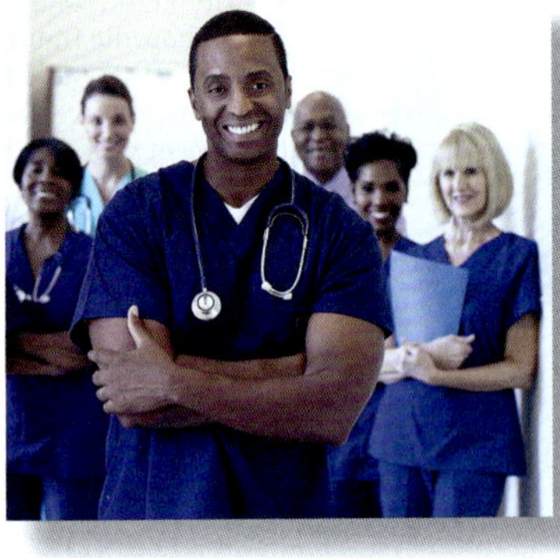

A new charge nurse has just started a 12-hour night shift in a community emergency department (ED). The first order of business is to make patient assignments for the 32-bed unit. Staffing for this shift includes 3 RNs (1 new and 2 seasoned), 1 LPN, and 1 unlicensed/unregulated assistant. What would be a fair assignment and what can be delegated to each of these staff members? How can the nurse foster open communication, mutual respect, and shared decision making with the team to achieve quality patient care?

QSEN Competency Focus: Teamwork and Collaboration

The complexities inherent in today's health care system challenge nurses to demonstrate integration of specific interdisciplinary core competencies that are aimed at ensuring the delivery of safe and quality patient care (Institute of Medicine, 2003). The Quality and Safety Education for Nurses project (QSEN, 2017; Cronenwett, Sherwood, Barnsteiner, et al., 2007) provides a framework for the knowledge, skills, and attitudes (KSAs) required for nurses to demonstrate competency in these key areas, which include ***patient-centred care***, ***interdisciplinary teamwork and collaboration***, ***evidence-based practice***, ***quality improvement***, ***safety***, and ***informatics.***

Teamwork and Collaboration Definition: Function effectively within nursing and interprofessional teams, fostering open communication, mutual respect, and shared decision making to achieve quality patient care.

SELECTED PRE-LICENSURE KSAs	APPLICATION AND REFLECTION
Knowledge	
Describe own strengths, limitations, and values in functioning as a member of the team.	Describe the charge nurse's priorities in making a fair assignment for this night shift. How would these intersect with those of other members of the team? Describe roles of each of the team members and how these roles interplay with each other.
Skills	
Function competently within own scope of practice as a member of the healthcare team.	As a novice charge nurse in the ED setting, whom would you rely on to help you develop your skill set? Identify your professional development growth goals so that you would be an effective member of the emergency health care team.
Attitudes	
Contribute to resolution of conflict and disagreement.	Reflect upon your preferred communication style and approach to conflict. How might you react if a seasoned nurse challenges the assignment? What skills might you wish to develop to be most effective in this setting with seasoned nurses and other members of the team?

Cronenwett, L., Sherwood, G., Barnsteiner, J., et al. (2007). Quality and safety education for nurses. *Nursing Outlook, 55*(3), 122–131; Institute of Medicine. (2003). *Health professions education: A bridge to quality*. Washington, DC: National Academies Press; and QSEN Institute. (2017). *QSEN competencies: Definitions and pre-licensure KSAs*. Retrieved June 12, 2019, from www.qsen.org/competencies/pre-licensure-ksas

73 Emergency Nursing

Adapted by Holly A. Feist

Learning Objectives

On completion of this chapter, the learner will be able to:

1. Describe emergency care as a collaborative, holistic approach that includes the patient, the family, and significant others.
2. Discuss priority emergency measures instituted for the patient with an emergency condition.
3. Identify the priorities of care for the patient with multiple system injuries.
4. Compare and contrast the emergency management of patients with heat stroke, frostbite, and hypothermia.
5. Specify the similarities and differences of the emergency management of patients with swallowed or inhaled poisons, skin contamination, and food poisoning.
6. Explain the emergency management of patients with drug overdose, those with acute alcohol intoxication, those who have been sexually assaulted, and those who have been victims of human trafficking.
7. Differentiate between the emergency care of patients who are overactive, those who are violent, those who are depressed, and those who are suicidal.

The term *emergency management* traditionally refers to care given to patients with urgent and critical needs. However, because many people lack access to health care, the emergency department (ED) is increasingly used for nonurgent problems. Therefore, the philosophy of emergency management has broadened to include the concept that an emergency is whatever the patient or the family considers it to be.

Large numbers of people seek emergency care for serious life-threatening conditions, such as cardiac dysrhythmias, acute coronary syndrome (ACS), acute heart failure, pulmonary edema, and stroke. Priorities for managing these cardiac and other conditions are discussed in Chapters 28, 29, 31, and 63. Emergency management of trauma and conditions not found elsewhere in this book are discussed in this chapter. It is assumed that care and treatment are provided under the direction of a physician or emergency nurse practitioner. Facts about ED visits in Canada are presented in Chart 73-1.

Scope and Practice of Emergency Nursing

Emergency nursing is a speciality that encompasses all demographics and physiologic processes from birth to death and everywhere in between (National Emergency Nurses Association [NENA], 2018). It includes assessment, intervention, and management of perceived, actual, or potential health problems of a physical, psychological, or social nature that occur suddenly and require urgent intervention and management (NENA, 2018).

The emergency nurse has specialized education, training, experience, and expertise in assessing and identifying patients' health care problems in emergent and urgent situations. In addition, the emergency nurse establishes priorities, monitors and continuously assesses acutely ill and injured patients, supports and attends to families, supervises allied health personnel, and teaches patients and families within a time-limited, high-pressured care environment (NENA, 2018). Nursing interventions are accomplished interdependently, in consultation with or under the direction of a physician or nurse practitioner. The roles of nursing and medicine are complementary in an emergency situation. Appropriate nursing and medical interventions are anticipated based on assessment data. The emergency health care staff members work as a team in performing the highly technical, hands-on skills required to care for patients in emergency situations.

CHART 73-1

Facts About Emergency Department Visits in Canada

- In 2017–2018, there were 11.4 million visits to emergency departments (EDs) in Canada.
- Average ED waiting time before being seen by a health care provider was 3.2 hours.
- Average length of stay in the ED was 2.5 hours.
- One in 10 ED visits resulted in hospital admission.
- CTAS response rates were met for only 10% of ED visits.
- Nine of 10 patients spent less than 7.9 hours in the ED.
- The top 3 reasons for coming to the Emergency Department include abdominal and pelvic pain, pain in the throat or chest, and acute respiratory infections

Sources: CIHI (2019). Emergency department (ED) visits: Volumes and median length of stay by triage level, visit disposition and main problem. Retrieved from https://apps.cihi.ca/mstrapp/asp/Main.aspx?evt=2048001&hiddensections=header%2Cpath%2CdockTop%2CdockLeft%2Cfooter&documentID=5C3D461F11E8D6F520190080EFE53D3B&Server=apmstrextprd_i.cihi.ca&Project=Quick±Stats&; CIHI (2018). NACRS Emergency department visits and length of stay, 2017–2018. Retrieved from https://www.cihi.ca/en/access-data-reports/results?f%5B0%5D=field_primary_theme%3A2050

The nursing process provides a logical framework for problem solving in this environment. Patients in the ED have a wide variety of actual or potential problems, and their condition may change rapidly. Therefore, nursing assessment must be frequent, and nursing diagnoses change with the patient's condition. Although a patient may have several diagnoses at a given time, the focus is on the most life-threatening ones; often, both independent and interdependent nursing interventions are required.

Challenges in Emergency Nursing

Wait Times (Crowding)

The Canadian Institute for Health Information (CIHI, 2019) reported wait times for patients to be seen by emergency health care professionals was around 3.25 hours, and the average stay in the ED was around 2.5 hours (see Chart 73-1). In general, patients are staying longer in the ED when compared to previous years (CIHI, 2019). Most patients are seen in a teaching or large community hospital. The majority of patients seen will be between the ages of 20 and 64 years old; 9.2% of patients are classed as "frequent users," or which includes patients have been to an ED four or more times in the past year (CIHI, 2019). Ninety percent of emergency patients will go home, while the remaining 10% will be admitted to the hospital (CIHI, 2019).

A systematic review on the effects of emergency room crowding revealed that not only are more patients leaving without being seen, but staff also have difficulty meeting recommended guidelines for treatment delivery such as antibiotics and analgesics (Morley, Unwin, Peterson, et al., 2018). This systematic review also found that emergency room crowding also resulted in increased exposed to a medical error, increased likelihood of death, and increased wait time for medical procedures such as cardiac catheterization (Morley et al., 2018). Staff in overcrowded emergency rooms are more likely to have increased stress and be exposed to violence when compared to inpatient staff (Morley et al., 2018).

Vital Signs

A core nursing activity in the ED is assessing vital signs (Lambe, Currey, & Considine, 2016). This includes heart rate (and rhythm where appropriate), blood pressure, temperature, and peripheral oxygen saturation. The

Glossary

antivenin: antitoxin manufactured from venom of poisonous snakes to assist the patient's immune system response to an envenomation

Canadian Triage and Acuity Scale (CTAS): The sorting or prioritizing of patients within the emergency department. This scale is used in Canadian ERs and many other centres internationally to categorize patients in relation to their illness and when they should be seen by an emergency physician.

carboxyhemoglobin: hemoglobin that is bound to carbon monoxide and therefore is unable to bind with oxygen, resulting in hypoxemia

corrosive poison: alkaline or acidic agent; causes tissue destruction after contact

cricothyroidotomy: surgical opening of the cricothyroid membrane to obtain an airway that is maintained with a tracheostomy or endotracheal tube

emergent: triage category signifying potentially life-threatening injuries or illnesses requiring immediate treatment

envenomation: injection of a poisonous material by sting, spine, bite, or other means

fasciotomy: surgical incision of the extremity to the level of the fascia to relieve pressure and restore neurovascular function to the extremity

Hare traction: portable in-line traction applied to the lower extremity to manage femur or hip fractures or dislocations

minor: triage category signifying non–life-threatening injuries or illnesses that can be routinely managed in a clinic or physician's office or that require no medical care

nonurgent: triage category signifying episodic or minor injury or illness in which treatment may be delayed several hours or longer without increased morbidity

rapid sequence intubation (RSI): medical procedure involving a prompt induction of medications in order to facilitate insertion of a breathing tube in to the trachea

resuscitation: triage category signifying life-threatening injuries or illnesses requiring immediate intervention

triage: process of assessing patients to determine management priorities. In Canada the CTAS system is usually used.

urgent: triage category signifying serious illness or injury that is not immediately life-threatening

Canadian Association of Emergency Physicians (CAEP) has recommended how often patients should have their vital signs taken prior to when a physician examines the patient. This frequency is based on Canadian Triage and Acuity Scale (CTAS), or how sick the patient is presumed to be when first seen at triage. The CTAS recommends continuous vital signs measurement for patients with CTAS 1, every 15 minutes for patients with CTAS 2, and every 30 minutes for patients with CTAS 3. If a patient is categorized as CTAS 4, vital signs are taken every hour. Vital signs are measured every 2 hours for patients in the CTAS 5 category (CTAS, 2013).

Once the patient is seen by the emergency physician, standards for frequency of vital signs will differ depending on the hospital.

Issues in Emergency Nursing Care

Emergency nursing is demanding because of the diversity of conditions and situations that present unique challenges. These challenges include legal issues, occupational health and safety risks for ED staff, and the challenge of providing holistic care in the context of a fast-paced, technology-driven environment in which serious illness and death are encountered on a daily basis. Another dimension of emergency nursing is nursing in disasters. With the increasing use of weaponry, the emergency nurse must recognize and treat patients exposed to biologic and other weapons and anticipate nursing care in the event of a mass casualty incident. Refer to Chapter 74 for a full discussion of nursing care in disasters, mass casualties, and epidemics/pandemics, including caring for victims of terrorism.

Documentation of Consent and Privacy

Consent to examine and treat the patient is part of the ED record. The patient must consent to invasive procedures (e.g., angiography, lumbar puncture) unless he or she is unconscious or in critical condition and unable to make decisions. If the patient is unconscious and brought to the ED without family or friends, this fact must be documented. Monitoring of the patient's condition, as well as all instituted treatments and the times at which they were performed, must be documented. After treatment, a notation is made on the record about the patient's condition, response to the treatment, and condition at discharge or transfer and about instructions given to the patient and family for follow-up care.

Patients of high profile are often provided with an alias, and access to the medical record, both paper and electronic, is limited to protect the privacy of the patient. A patient may also request extra privacy by limiting access to his or her room and by choosing not to receive phone calls, mail, flowers, other gifts, or certain visitors. These practices relate to the federally mandated privacy policy stipulated in the Personal Health Information Protection Act (PHIPA, 2018).

Limiting Exposure to Health Risks

Because of the increasing numbers of people infected with communicable diseases such as human immunodeficiency virus (HIV), tuberculosis (TB), hepatitis B, and severe respiratory infections (SRIs), health care providers are at an increased risk for exposure to communicable diseases through blood or other body fluids. This risk is further compounded in the ED because of the common use of invasive treatments in patients who may have a wide range of conditions and who frequently cannot provide a comprehensive medical history. Furthermore, many EDs do not have multiple enclosed spaces that limit exposure of communicable diseases to others. All emergency health care professionals must adhere strictly to standard precautions to mitigate exposure.

Recent communicable disease outbreaks in Canada have been linked to increased international travel (Bhatia, Sarwal, Robinson, et al., 2015) and increased vaccine hesitancy (Dubé, Bettinger, Fisher, et al., 2016). For instance, a 2014 measles outbreak in British Columbia resulted in approximately 2,600 reported cases of measles, 182 hospitalizations, and 1 death from measles complications in a community that is known to have low vaccination rates (Naus, Puddicombe, Murti, et al., 2015).

Early identification and adherence to transmission-based precautions for patients who are potentially infectious are crucial. Nurses in the ED are usually fitted with personal high-efficiency particulate air (HEPA) filter masks to use when treating patients with airborne diseases. In some jurisdictions, occupational health regulations govern the fitting and use of such equipment.

The potential for exposure to highly contagious organisms, hazardous chemicals or gases, and radiation related to acts of terrorism or natural or manmade disasters presents additional risks to ED staff (see Chapter 74 for information about decontamination procedures).

Violence in the Emergency Department

Not only do ED staff members encounter patients who may be violent because of the effects of substance abuse, injury, or other emergencies, but they may also encounter other violent situations. Frequently, patients and families waiting for assistance are emotionally volatile. Often, waiting rooms are the sites where feelings of dissatisfaction, fear, and anger are channelled violently. Some EDs assign security officers to the area and have installed silent alarm systems or metal detectors to identify weapons in order to protect patients, families, and staff. Most urban EDs are locked units, as safety is the first priority.

Patients or family members may come to the ED armed. To avoid angry confrontations, members of gangs and feuding families need to be separated in the ED, in the waiting room, and later in the inpatient nursing unit. Nurses and other personnel must be prepared to deal with these circumstances. If situations escalate and security is questionable the ED should be placed in lockdown, denying entrance and departure of nonpatients. Patients from prison and those who are under guard need to be handcuffed to the bed and appropriately assessed to ensure the safety of hospital staff and other patients. The following precautions are taken:

- The hand or ankle restraint (handcuff) is never released.
- Always have a guard is present in the room.
- The patient is placed face down on the stretcher to avoid injury from head-butting, spitting, or biting.

- Use of restraints on patients who are violent are used according to the institutional policy.
- Medication is administered as necessary to control violent behaviour until definitive treatment can be obtained.

In the case of gunfire in the ED, self-protection is a priority. There is no advantage to protecting others if medical caregivers are injured. Security officers and police must gain control of the situation first, and then care is provided to the injured.

Providing Comprehensive Care

Patients and families experiencing sudden injury or illness are often overwhelmed by anxiety because they have not had time to adapt to the crisis. They experience real and terrifying fear of death, mutilation, immobilization, and other assaults on their personal identity and body integrity. When confronted with trauma, severe disfigurement, severe illness, or sudden death, the family experiences several stages of crisis. The stages begin with anxiety and progress through denial, remorse and guilt, anger, grief, and reconciliation. The initial goal for the patient and family is anxiety reduction, a prerequisite to effective and appropriate coping. During this stressful time, safety is of prime importance. Close observation and preplanning are essential and security personnel are stationed nearby in the event that a patient or family member responds to stress with physical violence.

Assessment of the patient and family's psychological function includes evaluating emotional expression, degree of anxiety, and cognitive functioning.

Possible nursing diagnoses include:

- General anxiety or death anxiety related to uncertain potential outcomes of the illness or trauma
- Defensive coping related to acute situational crisis

Possible nursing diagnoses for the family include:

- Grieving
- Interrupted family processes
- Compromised or disabled family coping related to acute situational crises

Patient-Focused Interventions

Clinicians caring for the patient act confidently and competently to relieve anxiety and promote a sense of security. Reacting and responding to the patient in a warm manner promotes a sense of security. Explanations should be given on a level that the patient can understand, because an informed patient is better able to cope positively with stress. Human contact and supportive words reduce the panic of the severely injured or ill person and aid in dispelling fear of the unknown.

The unconscious patient should be treated as if conscious; that is, the patient should be touched, called by name, and given an explanation of every procedure that is performed. As the patient regains consciousness, the nurse orients the patient by stating his or her name, the date, and the location. This basic information should be provided repeatedly, as needed, in a reassuring way.

Family-Focused Interventions

The family is kept informed about where the patient is, how he or she is doing, and the care that is being given.

CHART 73-2

Helping Family Members Cope With Sudden Death

The nurse takes the following actions:

- Take the family to a private place.
- Talk to the family together, so that they can grieve together.
- Reassure the family that everything possible was done; inform them of the treatment rendered.
- Avoid using euphemisms such as "passed on." Show the family that you care by touching, offering coffee, water, and the services of a chaplain.
- Encourage family members to support each other and to express emotions freely (grief, loss, anger, helplessness, tears, disbelief).
- Avoid giving sedation to family members; this may mask or delay the grieving process, which is necessary to achieve emotional equilibrium and to prevent prolonged depression.
- Encourage the family to view the body if they wish; this action helps to integrate the loss. Cover disfigured and injured areas before the family sees the body. Go with the family to see the body. Show acceptance by touching the body to give the family "permission" to touch.
- Spend time with the family, listening to them and identifying any needs that they may have for which the nursing staff can be helpful.
- Allow family members to talk about the deceased and what he or she meant to them; this permits ventilation of feelings of loss. Encourage the family to talk about events preceding admission to the ED. Do not challenge initial feelings of anger or denial.
- Avoid volunteering unnecessary information (e.g., the patient was drinking).

Allowing family members to stay with the patient, when possible, also helps alleviate their anxieties. In many facilities, family presence during resuscitation is permitted to assist the family to cope through this difficult time. Many family members respond very well to this approach, and it provides some answers to the question "Was everything done?" (Chan, 2018). Family presence during resuscitation and all aspects of care is a common practice in EDs across Canada (Chan, 2018). Additional interventions are based on the assessment of the stage of crisis that the family is experiencing. Measures to help family members cope with sudden death are presented in Chart 73-2.

Anxiety and Denial

During these crises, family members are encouraged to recognize and talk about their feelings of anxiety. Asking questions is encouraged. Honest answers given at the level of the family's understanding must be provided. Although denial is an ego-defence mechanism that protects one from recognizing painful and disturbing aspects of reality, prolonged denial is not encouraged or supported. The family must be prepared for the reality of what has happened and what may come.

Remorse and Guilt

Expressions of remorse and guilt are common, with family members accusing themselves (or each other) of negligence or minor omissions. Family members are urged to verbalize their feelings to help them cope appropriately.

Anger

Expressions of anger, common in crisis situations, are a way of handling anxiety and fear. Anger is frequently directed by the family at the patient, but it is also often expressed toward the physician, the nurse, or admitting personnel. The therapeutic approach is to allow the anger to be expressed and to assist the family members to identify their feelings of frustration.

Grief

Grief is a complex emotional response to anticipated or actual loss. The key nursing intervention is to help family members work through their grief and to support their coping mechanisms, letting them know that it is usual and acceptable for them to cry, feel pain, and express loss. The hospital chaplain and social services staff serve as invaluable members of the team when assisting families to work through their grief. It is critical for the nurse to understand that all reactions to a crisis are individual and normal.

Caring for Emergency Personnel

Concerted efforts have been made to focus on the needs of the ED staff, especially after serious and stressful events (Kenney Powell & Hentzen Daniels, 2018). Events can range from a local trauma case involving children; to treating someone known to the emergency worker, such as a colleague or family member; to a more complex natural disaster or multicasualty situation. It is important to remember that all staff members may not necessarily respond in the same way; an event that is stressful for one person may not be as stressful for another. In addition, because stress is a daily occurrence in the ED, the staff may not recognize the personal effect of any one event. The availability of nonjudgmental counselling is essential to promoting a healthy staff. After serious events, critical incident stress debriefing is necessary to critique individual and group performance. In addition, personal and group stress debriefing is also essential.

EMERGENCY NURSING AND THE CONTINUUM OF CARE

A key principle underlying emergency care is that the patient is rapidly assessed, treated, and referred to the appropriate setting for ongoing care. This makes the ED a temporary point on the continuum of care. Most patients who receive emergency care are discharged directly from the ED to their homes, and emergency nurses plan and facilitate the patient's safe discharge and follow-up care in the home and the community.

Discharge Planning

Before discharge, verbal and written instructions for continuing care are given to the patient and the family or significant others. Many EDs have preprinted standard instruction sheets for the more common conditions, which can then be individualized for each patient. Discharge instructions should be available in a variety of languages. A language interpreter is used as necessary to provide both written and verbal instructions.

Instructions should include information about prescribed medications, treatments, diet, activity, and when to contact a health care professional or schedule follow-up appointments. It is imperative that instructions are written legibly, use simple language, and are clear in their teaching. When providing discharge instructions, the nurse also considers any special needs the patient may have related to hearing or visual impairments. Where possible, alternate formats of instruction (e.g., large print, Braille, audiotape) should be available to meet the needs of patients with hearing or visual impairments.

Community and Transitional Services

Before discharge, some patients require the services of a social worker to help them meet continuing health care needs. Home care resources may be contacted before discharge to arrange services. This is particularly important for patients who are older or have a disability and who need assistance. Identifying continuing health care needs and making arrangements for meeting these needs can prevent return visits to the ED or readmission to the hospital.

For patients who are returning to long-term care facilities and for those who already rely on community agencies for continuing health care, communication about the patient's condition and any changes in health care needs that have occurred are provided to the appropriate facilities or agencies. This communication is essential to promote continuity of care and to ensure ongoing care to meet the patient's changing health care needs.

Gerontologic Considerations

The ED is a common point of entry into the health care system for patients 65 years and older. In fact, patients in this age group account for more than 45% of the admissions to the hospital from the ED. Of the 11 million ED visits in Canada in 2017/2018, 1.1 million people were admitted, and 50% were over the age of 65 (see Chart 73-1). Older patients typically arrive with one or more presenting conditions and chronic illness diagnoses. Nonspecific symptoms, such as weakness and fatigue, episodes of falling, incontinence, and change in mental status, may be manifestations of acute, potentially life-threatening illness in the older person. Emergencies in this age group may be more difficult to manage because older patients may have an atypical presentation, an altered response to treatment, a greater risk of developing complications, or a combination of these factors.

The older patient may perceive the emergency as a crisis signaling the end of an independent lifestyle or even resulting in death. The nurse gives attention to the patient's feelings of anxiety and fear.

The older patient may have limited sources of social and financial support during these times of crises. The nurse assesses the psychosocial resources of the patient (and of the caregiver, if necessary) and anticipates discharge needs. Referrals for support services (e.g., to the social service department, or a gerontologic nurse specialist) may be necessary.

Obesity Considerations

The growing rate of obesity in Canada has implications for treating patients with obesity within the ED, in terms of stocking appropriately sized equipment, gowns, and stretchers; ensuring that equipment (e.g., computed tomography [CT] scanners) is able to handle a greater weight capacity; and recognizing specific disorders and complications that may occur in these patients. For instance, research suggests that increased mortality is associated with the degree of obesity (ENA, 2013). Other considerations in ED management of patients with obesity include an understanding that it is generally more challenging to insert IV lines and airways. Ventilation also can be a challenge from the increased weight of the chest wall and the increased incidence of hypoventilation and sleep apnea among patients with obesity. Special consideration must be taken with lipophilic medications, as they take longer to clear from the larger volume of adipose tissue. Weight-based medications must be calculated carefully using ideal body mass. X-rays may be difficult to visualize because of poor penetration.

Complications that patients with obesity are more prone to experience during hospitalization include respiratory failure, acute kidney injury, pneumonia, deep vein thrombosis, and pressure ulcers. Patients with severe obesity who have femur fractures have a significantly higher risk of death, as well as a higher risk of acute respiratory distress syndrome (ARDS) and sepsis than patients of normal weight (Weinlein, Deaderick, & Murphy, 2015). Although many of these complications do not occur until later in the hospital stay, some preventive measures (e.g., encouraging turning, coughing, and deep-breathing exercises to prevent atelectasis) may be initiated in the ED. Functional recovery time is extended in patients with obesity, resulting in longer lengths of stay and increased hospital costs. Initiating prevention measures in the ED, such as early backboard removal and providing early preventive respiratory care, are targeted to improve recovery time (Childs, Nahm, Dolenc, et al., 2015; Dhungel, Liao, Raut, et al., 2015). Arranging transfers of patients with obesity must also take into consideration the availability of appropriately sized equipment.

PRINCIPLES OF EMERGENCY CARE

By definition, emergency care is care that must be rendered without delay. In an ED, several patients with diverse health problems—some life-threatening, some not—may present to the ED simultaneously. One of the first principles of emergency care is triage.

Triage

The word **triage** comes from the French word *trier*, meaning "to sort." In the daily routine of the ED, triage is used to sort patients into groups based on the severity of their health concerns and the immediacy with which these concerns must be treated.

A basic and widely used triage system that has been in use for many years has three categories: emergent, urgent, and nonurgent (Beveridge et al., 2018). Emergent patients have the highest priority—their conditions are life-threatening and they must be seen immediately. Urgent patients have serious health problems but not immediately life-threatening ones; they must be seen within 1 hour. Nonurgent patients have episodic illnesses that can be addressed within 24 hours without increased morbidity (Beveridge et al., 2018). A fourth category that is increasingly used is "fast-track." These patients require simple first aid or basic primary care and may be treated in the ED or safely referred to a clinic or physician's office.

In Canadian EDs, a more refined and comprehensive triage system is used. The **Canadian Triage and Acuity Scale (CTAS)** is a five-level triage score developed in the emergency care setting to prioritize patient care requirements and examine patient care processes, workload, and resource requirements relative to the case mix and community needs (Beveridge et al., 2018). The CTAS allows ED nurses and physicians to triage patients according to the type and severity of their presenting signs and symptoms, ensure that the sickest patients are seen first when ED capacity has been exceeded due to visit rates or reduced access to other services, and to ensure that a patient's need for care is reassessed while in the ED.

The five-level triage scores are Level I Resuscitation; Level II **Emergent**; Level III **Urgent**; Level IV Less Urgent; Level V **Non-Urgent**. Triage is defined by the Canadian Association of Emergency Physicians and the National Emergency Nurses Affiliation as an operational process applied in the ED where an experienced RN uses critical thinking skills and a standardized set of guidelines to assess and prioritize patients and decide how long they can safely wait for treatment. Due to the increasing demand on ED services, triage must now face the question of "How long can they safely wait?" whereas in the past, the triage nurses faced the decision of where to locate the patient. The triage nurse will base his or her decision on acute level by the following steps: Critical look on arrival, chief concern, first-order modifiers such as vital signs, pain score, and mechanism of injury, and potentially second-order modifiers such as hypertension and blood glucose levels (Beveridge et al., 2018). Various documentation templates are available to capture the relevant data collected at the triage station. There is an increasing ability to utilize electronic triage systems during the arrival phase of patient care in the ED. This five-level triage system is also used in the United States, Australia, and the United Kingdom.

In the five-level system, patients in the emergent category identified in the previously used three-level system have been divided into two distinct groupings, resuscitation and emergent. Patients in the **resuscitation** category need treatment immediately to prevent death. Patients in the emergent category may deteriorate rapidly and develop a major life-threatening situation or require time-sensitive treatment. Patients in the urgent category have non–life-threatening conditions but require two or more resources (defined below) to provide their care. If these patients' vital signs deviate significantly from their baseline, they may require "up-triaging" to the emergent category. Patients in the nonurgent category have non–life-threatening conditions and likely need only one resource to provide for their needs. Patients in the **minor** category have no life-threatening conditions and likely require no resources to provide their evaluation and management.

Triage is an advanced skill. Emergency nurses spend many hours learning to classify different illnesses and injuries to ensure that patients most in need of care do not needlessly wait. Protocols may be followed to initiate laboratory or x-ray studies while the patient is in the triage area. Collaborative protocols are developed and used by the triage nurse based on his or her level of experience. Nurses in the triage area collect additional crucial baseline data: full vital signs including pain assessment, history of the current event and past medical history, neurologic assessment findings, weight, allergies (especially to latex and medications), domestic violence screening, and necessary diagnostic data. Some facilities collect these data in a computerized system, which helps guide the nurse through assessment and documentation. The following questions reflect the minimum information that should be obtained from the patient or from the person who accompanied the patient to the ED and then are documented.

- What were the circumstances, precipitating events, location, and time of the injury or illness?
- When did the symptoms appear?
- Was the patient unconscious after the injury or onset of illness?
- How did the patient get to the ED?
- What was the health status of the patient before the injury or illness?
- Is there a history of medical illness or previous surgeries? A history of admissions to the hospital?
- Is the patient currently taking any medications, especially hormones, insulin, digitalis, or anticoagulants? Is the patient using any complementary or alternative therapies such as herbology, naturopathy, reiki, massage, or acupuncture?
- Does the patient have any allergies, especially to latex, medications, eggs, or nuts?
- Does the patient smoke or use recreational drugs? How frequently? What type? When was the last time they were used?
- Does the patient have any fears? Does the patient feel that he or she is in danger or in an unsafe situation?
- When was the last meal eaten? (This is important if general anesthesia is to be given or if the patient is unconscious.)
- When was the last menstrual period?
- Is the patient under a physician's care? What are the name and contact information for the physician?
- What was the date of the patient's most recent tetanus immunization?

In addition to the collection of initial vital signs and medical history, triage consists of providing basic first aid, which may include application of ice, bleeding control, and basic wound care, as well as initiating protocol-based orders (e.g., x-rays, administering antipyretics or mild analgesics, obtaining an electrocardiogram [ECG] or urinalysis, removing sutures). The triage nurse also is responsible for and monitors the waiting area, maintains a safe environment, reassesses waiting patients, and is the initial liaison to the families of patients.

Routine ED triage protocols differ significantly from the triage protocols used in disasters and mass casualty incidents (field triage). Routine triage directs all available resources to the patients who are most critically ill, regardless of potential outcome. In field triage (or hospital triage during a disaster), scarce resources must be used to benefit the most people possible. This distinction affects triage decisions (see Chapter 74).

Assess and Intervene

For the patient assigned to a resuscitation, emergent, or urgent triage category, stabilization, provision of critical treatments, and prompt transfer to the appropriate setting (intensive care unit, operating room, general care unit) are the priorities of emergency care. Although treatment is initiated in the ED, ongoing definitive treatment of the underlying problem is provided in other settings, and the sooner the patient is stabilized and moved to that area, the better the outcome.

A systematic approach to effectively establishing and treating health priorities is the primary survey/secondary survey approach. The primary survey focuses on stabilizing life-threatening conditions. The ED staff work collaboratively and follow the ABCD (***a***irway, ***b***reathing, ***c***irculation, ***d***isability) method:

- Establish a patent airway.
- Provide adequate ventilation, employing resuscitation measures when necessary. (Trauma patients must have the cervical spine protected and chest injuries assessed first, immediately after the airway is established.)
- Evaluate and restore cardiac output by controlling hemorrhage, preventing and treating shock, and maintaining or restoring effective circulation. This includes the prevention and management of hypothermia. In addition, peripheral pulses are examined, and any immediate closed reductions of fractures or dislocations are performed if an extremity is pulseless.
- Determine neurologic disability by assessing neurologic function using the Glasgow Coma Scale and a motor and sensory evaluation of the spine (see Chapter 62).

After these priorities have been addressed, the ED team proceeds with the secondary survey. This includes the following:

- A complete health history and head-to-toe assessment (includes a reassessment of airway and breathing parameters)
- Diagnostic and laboratory testing
- Insertion or application of monitoring devices such as ECG electrodes, arterial lines, or urinary catheters
- Splinting of suspected fractures
- Cleansing, closure, and dressing of wounds
- Performance of other necessary interventions based on the patient's condition

Once the patient has been assessed, stabilized, and tested, appropriate medical and nursing diagnoses are formulated, initial important treatment is started, and plans for the proper disposition of the patient are made. Many emergent and urgent conditions and priority emergency

interventions are discussed in detail in the remaining sections of this chapter.

In addition to the management of the illness or injury, the ED nurse must also focus on providing comfort and emotional support to the patient and family. Included in this is pain management. Effective pain management must be instituted early and should include rapid-acting agents that result in minimal sedation so that the patient can continue to interact with the staff for continued assessment. Moderate sedation can help facilitate short procedures in the ED; the patient will not remember the procedure later. The patient is closely monitored during the procedure and then rapidly awakens when it is complete (see Chapter 21).

AIRWAY OBSTRUCTION

Acute upper airway obstruction is a life-threatening medical emergency.

Pathophysiology

The airway may be partially or completely occluded. Partial obstruction of the airway can lead to progressive hypoxia, hypercarbia, and respiratory and cardiac arrest. If the airway is completely obstructed, permanent brain injury or death will occur within 3 to 5 minutes secondary to hypoxia. Air movement is absent in the presence of complete airway obstruction. Oxygen saturation of the blood decreases rapidly because obstruction of the airway prevents entry of air into the lungs. Oxygen deficit occurs in the brain, resulting in unconsciousness, with death following rapidly.

Upper airway obstruction has a number of causes, including aspiration of foreign bodies, anaphylaxis, viral or bacterial infection, trauma, and inhalation or chemical burns. For older patients, especially those in extended-care facilities, sedatives and hypnotic medications, diseases affecting motor coordination (e.g., Parkinson's disease), and mental dysfunction (e.g., dementia, mental retardation) are risk factors for asphyxiation by food. In adults, aspiration of a bolus of meat is the most common cause of airway obstruction. Peritonsillar abscesses, epiglottitis, and other acute infectious processes of the posterior pharynx can also result in airway obstruction (Solheim, 2018).

Clinical Manifestations

Typically, a person with a foreign body airway obstruction cannot speak, breathe, or cough. The patient may clutch the neck between the thumb and fingers (i.e., universal distress signal). Other common signs and symptoms include choking, apprehensive appearance, refusing to lie flat, inspiratory and expiratory stridor, laboured breathing, use of accessory muscles (suprasternal and intercostal retraction), flaring nostrils, increasing anxiety, restlessness, and confusion. Cyanosis and loss of consciousness develop as hypoxia worsens. Cyanosis and loss of consciousness are late signs. Action must be taken before these manifestations develop, if possible, or immediately if the patient has already exhibited these signs.

Assessment and Diagnostic Findings

Assessment of the patient who has a foreign object occluding the airway may involve simply asking the person whether he or she is choking and requires help. If the person is unconscious, inspection of the oropharynx may reveal the offending object. X-rays, laryngoscopy, or bronchoscopy also may be performed.

Management

If the patient can breathe and cough spontaneously, a partial obstruction should be suspected. The victim is encouraged to cough forcefully and to persist with spontaneous coughing and breathing efforts as long as good air exchange exists. There may be some wheezing between coughs. If the patient demonstrates a weak, ineffective cough, high-pitched noise while inhaling, increased respiratory difficulty, or cyanosis, the patient should be managed as if there were complete airway obstruction.

After the obstruction is removed, rescue breathing is initiated if respirations are not spontaneous. If the patient also has no pulse, cardiac compressions are instituted. These measures provide oxygen to the brain, heart, and other vital organs until definitive medical treatment can restore and support usual heart and ventilatory activity.

Establishing an Airway

Establishing an airway may be as simple as repositioning the patient's head to prevent the tongue from obstructing the pharynx. Alternatively, other manoeuvres, such as abdominal thrusts, the head-tilt–chin-lift manoeuvre, the jaw-thrust manoeuvre, or insertion of specialized equipment, may be needed to open the airway, remove a foreign body, or maintain the airway. In all manoeuvres, the cervical spine must be protected from injury. After these manoeuvres are performed, the patient is assessed for breathing by watching for chest movement and listening and feeling for air movement. In such a case, nursing diagnoses would include ineffective airway clearance related to obstruction of the airway by the tongue, an object, or fluids (blood, saliva) and ineffective breathing pattern related to airway obstruction or injury.

Abdominal Thrusts

The terms *subdiaphragmatic abdominal thrusts, abdominal thrusts*, and *Heimlich manoeuvre* are used interchangeably. This manoeuvre causes elevation of the diaphragm, forcing air from the lungs to create an artificial cough that can move and expel an obstructing foreign body from the airway.

Head-Tilt–Chin-Lift Manoeuvre

The patient is placed supine on a firm, flat surface. If the patient is lying face down, the body is turned as a unit so that the head, shoulders, and torso move simultaneously with no twisting (i.e., logroll). Next, the airway is opened using either the head-tilt–chin-lift manoeuvre or the jaw-thrust manoeuvre. In the head-tilt–chin-lift manoeuvre, one hand is placed on the victim's forehead, and firm backward pressure is applied with the palm to tilt the head back. The fingers of the other hand are placed under the bony part of the lower jaw near the chin and lifted up. The chin and the teeth are brought forward almost to occlusion to support the jaw.

NURSING ALERT

The head-tilt–chin-lift manoeuvre, which helps tilt the head back, should be used only if it is determined that the patient's cervical spine is not injured.

Jaw-Thrust Manoeuvre

After one hand is placed on each side of the patient's jaw, the angles of the patient's lower jaw are grasped and lifted, displacing the mandible forward. This is a safe approach to opening the airway of a patient with suspected spinal cord injury because it can be accomplished without extending the neck.

Oropharyngeal Airway Insertion

An oropharyngeal airway is a semicircular tube or tubelike plastic device that is inserted over the back of the tongue into the lower posterior pharynx in a patient who is breathing spontaneously but who is unconscious (Chart 73-3). This type of airway prevents the tongue from falling back against the posterior pharynx and obstructing the airway. It also allows health care providers to suction secretions.

NURSING ALERT

In the case of potential facial trauma or basal skull fracture, the nasopharyngeal airway should not be used because it could enter the brain cavity instead of the pharynx.

Endotracheal Intubation

The purpose of endotracheal intubation is to establish and maintain the airway in patients with respiratory insufficiency or hypoxia. Endotracheal intubation is indicated to establish an airway in the following situations:

- for a patient who cannot be adequately ventilated with an oropharyngeal airway
- to bypass an upper airway obstruction
- to prevent aspiration
- to permit connection of the patient to a resuscitation bag or mechanical ventilator
- to facilitate the removal of tracheobronchial secretions (Fig. 73-1).

Because the procedure requires skill, endotracheal intubation is performed only by those who have had extensive training. These may include physicians, nurse anesthetists, respiratory therapists, flight nurses, and nurse practitioners. However, the emergency nurse is commonly called on to assist with intubation.

Rapid sequence intubation (RSI) may be indicated in any of the above situations. RSI is a medical procedure

CHART 73-3

Inserting an Oropharyngeal Airway

1. Measure the oral airway alongside the head. The airway should reach from lip to ear.
2. Extend the patient's head by placing one hand under the bony chin (*only if the cervical spine is uninjured*). With the other hand, tilt the head backward by applying pressure to the forehead while simultaneously lifting the chin forward.
3. Open the patient's mouth.
4. **(A)** Insert the oropharyngeal airway with the tip facing up toward the roof of the mouth until it passes the uvula.
   (B) Rotate the tip 180 degrees so that the tip is pointed down toward the pharynx. This displaces the tongue anteriorly, and the patient then breathes through and around the airway.
5. The distal end of the oropharyngeal airway is in the hypopharynx, and the flange is approximately at the patient's lips. Make sure that the tongue has not been pushed into the airway.

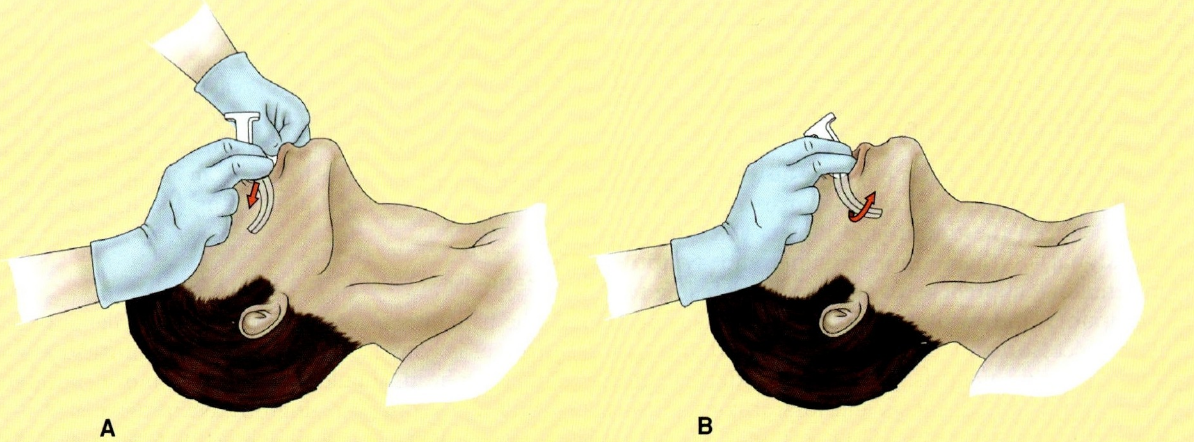

Adapted from Walsh, K., & Woten, M. (2016). Oropharyngeal airway: Inserting in adults. In D. Pravikoff (Ed.). *Nursing practice and skill*. Glendale, CA: CINAHL Information Systems.

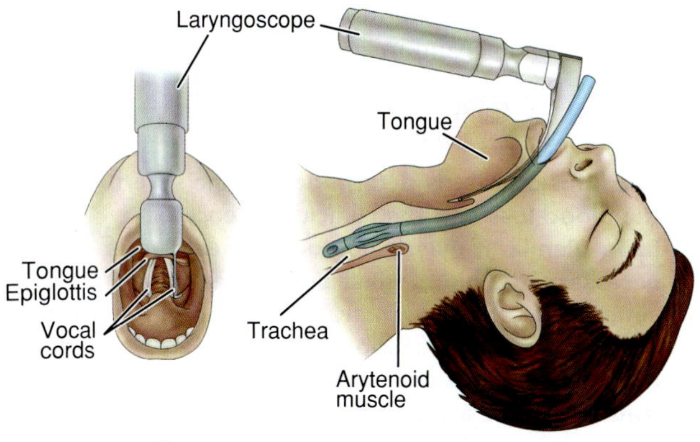

FIGURE 73-1. Endotracheal intubation in a patient without a cervical spine injury. A. The primary glottic landmarks for tracheal intubation as visualized with proper placement of the laryngoscope. B. Positioning the endotracheal tube.

involving a prompt induction of medications to support the subsequent intubation of the trachea. Medications used to facilitate RSI include a sedative, an analgesic, and a neuromuscular blockade agent; these are usually administered by the practitioner performing the intubation.

Intubation With a King (Combitube) or Laryngeal Mask Airway

If the patient is not hospitalized and cannot be intubated in the field, emergency medical personnel may insert a King, which rapidly provides pharyngeal ventilation. When the tube is inserted into the trachea, it functions like an endotracheal tube (Fig. 73-2).

The two balloons that surround the tube are inflated after the tube is inserted. One balloon is large (100 mL) and occludes the oropharynx. This permits ventilation by forcing air through the larynx. The smaller balloon is inflated with 15 mL of air and is supposed to anchor the device in the esophagus at a site distal to the glottis; however, it can occlude the trachea if it is inadvertently placed there. Breath sounds are auscultated after balloon inflation to make sure that the oropharyngeal balloon (or cuff) does not obstruct the glottis. The patient can be ventilated through either one of the two ports (e.g., tracheal or esophageal) of the tube, depending on whether the tube is placed in the trachea or esophagus.

If it is difficult to establish an airway, a laryngeal mask airway (LMA) may be inserted as an interim airway device. The design of the LMA provides a "mask" in the subglottic airway with a cuff inflated within the esophagus. It allows easy insertion for rapid airway control until a more definitive airway can be placed. Some LMAs also permit removal of secretions from the esophagus (see Chapter 20).

Cricothyroidotomy (Cricothyroid Membrane Puncture)

Cricothyroidotomy is the opening of the cricothyroid membrane to establish an airway. This procedure is used in emergency situations in which endotracheal intubation is either not possible or contraindicated, as in airway obstruction from extensive maxillofacial trauma, cervical spine injuries, laryngospasm, laryngeal edema (after an allergic reaction or extubation), hemorrhage into neck

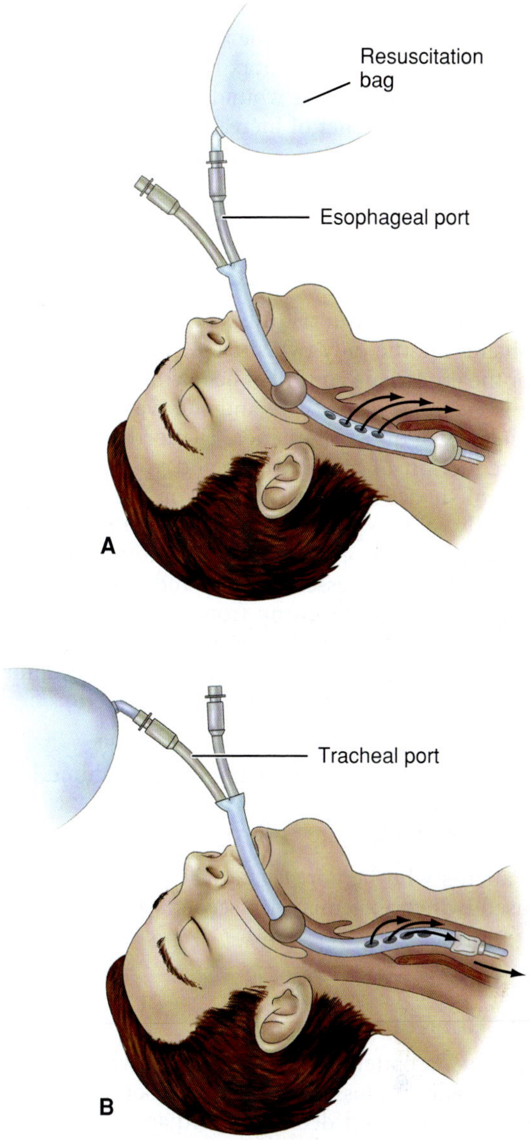

FIGURE 73-2. A. Combitube in esophageal position. B. Combitube tracheal position.

tissue, or obstruction of the larynx. After these manoeuvres are performed, the patient is assessed for breathing by watching for chest movement and listening and feeling for air movement.

In such a case, nursing priorities would include monitoring airway clearance and breathing patterns as these may be altered as a result of an obstruction of the tongue, object, or fluids (blood, saliva). After a cricothyroidotomy and the patient is stable a tracheostomy is performed.

Maintaining Ventilation

After the airway is determined to be unobstructed, the nurse must ensure that ventilation is adequate by checking for equal bilateral breath sounds. Satisfactory management of ventilations may prevent hypoxia and hypercapnia. The nurse must quickly assess for absent or diminished breath sounds, open chest wounds, and difficulty delivering artificial breaths for the patient. The nurse should monitor pulse oximetry, capnography, and arterial blood gases if the patient requires airway or ventilatory assistance. A tension pneumothorax can mimic hypovolemia, so ventilatory assessment precedes assessment for hemorrhage. A pneumothorax (both simple and tension) or sucking (open) chest wound is managed with a chest tube; immediate relief of increasing positive intrathoracic pressure and maintenance of adequate ventilation should occur immediately.

HEMORRHAGE

Assessment and intervention of airway and breathing problems are the only two situations that take precedence over the immediate control of hemorrhage. Stopping bleeding is essential to the care and survival of patients in an emergency or disaster situation. Hemorrhage that results in the reduction of circulating blood volume is a primary cause of shock. Minor bleeding, which is usually venous, generally stops spontaneously unless the patient has a bleeding disorder or has been taking anticoagulants.

The patient is assessed for signs and symptoms of shock: cool, moist skin (resulting from poor peripheral perfusion), decreasing blood pressure, increasing heart rate, delayed capillary refill, and decreasing urine volume.

The goals of emergency management are to:

- control the bleeding,
- maintain adequate circulating blood volume for tissue oxygenation,
- prevent shock.

Patients who hemorrhage are at risk for cardiac arrest caused by hypovolemia with secondary anoxia.

Management

Fluid Replacement

Whenever a patient is hemorrhaging—whether externally or internally—a loss of circulating blood results in a fluid volume deficit and decreased cardiac output. Therefore, fluid replacement is imperative to maintain circulation. Typically, two large-gauge IV catheters are inserted to provide a means for fluid and blood replacement, and blood samples are obtained for analysis, typing, and cross-matching. Replacement fluids are administered as prescribed, depending on clinical estimates of the type and volume of fluid lost. Replacement fluids may include isotonic electrolyte solutions (e.g., lactated Ringer's, normal saline), colloids (e.g., volume expanders), and blood component therapy.

Packed red blood cells are infused when there is massive blood loss, which may also necessitate transfusion of other blood components, including platelets and clotting factors. In emergencies, O-negative blood is used for women of childbearing age, and O-positive or O-negative blood is used for men and for postmenopausal women. In an emergent situation, there is no time to type and cross-match or type and screen blood. O-negative blood provides safe administration of blood immediately without sensitizing an Rh-negative woman to Rh-positive blood. Sensitization can result in difficulties during pregnancy later.

Additional platelets and clotting factors are given when large amounts of blood are needed, because replacement blood is deficient in clotting factors.

See Chapter 54 for full discussion of blood component therapy indications and treatment.

> **NURSING ALERT**
>
> **The infusion rate is determined by the severity of the blood loss and the clinical evidence of hypovolemia. If massive blood replacement is necessary, the blood must be warmed in a commercial blood warmer, because administration of large amounts of blood that has been refrigerated has a core cooling effect that may lead to cardiac arrest and coagulopathy.**

Control of External Hemorrhage

If a patient is hemorrhaging externally (e.g., from a wound), a rapid physical assessment is performed as the patient's clothing is cut away in an attempt to identify the area of hemorrhage. Direct, firm pressure is applied over the bleeding area or the involved artery at a site that is proximal to the wound (Fig. 73-3). Most bleeding can be stopped or at least controlled by application of direct pressure. Otherwise, unchecked arterial bleeding results in death. A firm pressure dressing is applied, and the injured part is elevated to stop venous and capillary bleeding if possible. If the injured area is an extremity, the extremity is immobilized to control blood loss.

A tourniquet is applied to an extremity only as a *last resort* when the external hemorrhage cannot be controlled in any other way and immediate surgery is not feasible. Care must be taken when applying a tourniquet because of the risk of loss of the extremity. The tourniquet is applied just proximal to the wound and tied tightly enough to control arterial blood flow. If there is no arterial bleeding, the tourniquet is removed and a pressure dressing is applied. If the patient has suffered a traumatic amputation with uncontrollable hemorrhage, the tourniquet remains in place until the patient is in the operating room.

Control of Internal Bleeding

If the patient shows no external signs of bleeding but exhibits tachycardia, falling blood pressure, thirst, apprehension, cool and moist skin, or delayed capillary refill, internal hemorrhage is suspected. Typically, packed red blood cells are administered at a rapid rate, and the patient is prepared for more definitive treatment (e.g., surgery, pharmacologic therapy). In addition, arterial blood gas specimens are obtained to evaluate pulmonary function and tissue perfusion and to establish baseline hemodynamic parameters, which are then used as an index for determining the amount of fluid replacement the patient can tolerate and the response to therapy. The patient is maintained in the supine position and monitored closely until hemodynamic or circulatory parameters improve, or until he or she is transported to the operating room or intensive care unit.

HYPOVOLEMIC SHOCK

Shock is a condition in which there is loss of effective circulating blood volume. Inadequate organ and tissue perfusion

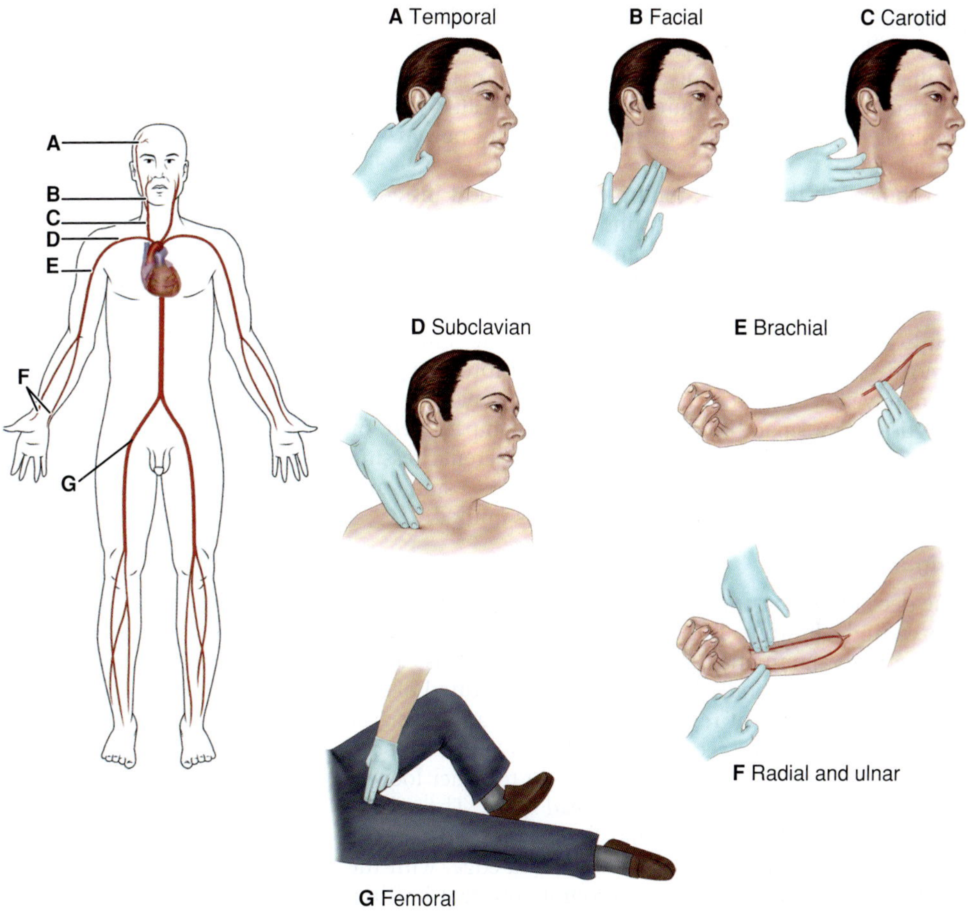

FIGURE 73-3. Pressure points for control of hemorrhage.

follows, ultimately resulting in cellular metabolic derangements. In any emergency situation, the onset of shock should be anticipated by assessing all injured people immediately. The underlying cause of shock (hypovolemic, cardiogenic, neurogenic, anaphylactic or septic) must quickly be determined in order to initiate treatment. Of these, hypovolemia is the most common cause (see Chapter 18 for further discussion of management of hypovolemic shock).

WOUNDS

Wounds involving injury to soft tissues can vary from minor tears to severe crushing injuries. The types of wounds that may occur are defined in Chart 73-4. The primary goal of treatment is to restore the physical integrity and function of the injured tissue while minimizing scarring and preventing infection. Proper documentation of the characteristics of the wound, using precise descriptions, accurate measurements, and correct terminology, is essential. Such information may be needed in the future for forensic evidence. If consent is obtained, photographs are helpful because they provide an accurate, visible depiction of the wound. Patients involved in domestic violence or trauma may need the photographs later to visually describe the extent of injury.

Determining *when* and *how* the wound occurred is important because a treatment delay increases infection risk. Using aseptic technique, the clinician inspects the wound to determine the extent of damage to underlying structures or the presence of a foreign body. Sensory, motor, and vascular functions are evaluated for changes that might indicate complications.

Management

Wound Cleansing

Hair around the wound may be clipped (only as directed) if it is anticipated that the hair will interfere with wound closure. Typically, the area around the wound is cleansed with normal saline solution. Antibacterial agents, such as

CHART 73-4

Definition of Terms: Wounds

Laceration: skin tear with irregular edges and vein bridging
Avulsion: tearing away of tissue from supporting structures
Abrasion: denuded skin
Ecchymosis/contusion: blood trapped under the surface of the skin
Hematoma: tumourlike mass of blood trapped under the skin
Stab: incision of the skin with well-defined edges, usually caused by a sharp instrument; a stab wound is typically deeper than long
Cut: incision of the skin with well-defined edges, usually longer than deep
Patterned: wound representing the outline of the object (e.g., steering wheel) causing the wound

povidone-iodine (Betadine) or hydrogen peroxide, should not be allowed to get deep into the wound without thorough rinsing. These agents are used only for the initial cleansing because they injure exposed and healthy tissue, resulting in further tissue damage and delay new tissue granulation.

If indicated, the area is infiltrated with a local intradermal anesthetic through the wound margins or by regional block. Patients with soft tissue injuries usually have localized pain at the site of injury. The nurse then assists with cleaning and débriding the wound. The wound is irrigated gently and copiously with sterile isotonic saline solution to remove surface dirt. Devitalized tissue and foreign matter are removed because they impede healing and may promote infection. Any small bleeding vessels are clamped, tied, or cauterized. After wound treatment, a nonadherent dressing is applied to protect the wound and to serve as a splint and as a reminder to the patient that the area is injured.

Primary Closure

The decision to suture a wound depends on the nature of the wound, the time since the injury was sustained, the degree of contamination, and the vascularity of tissues. If primary closure is indicated, the wound is sutured or stapled, with the patient receiving either local anesthesia or moderate sedation (see Chapter 20). Wound closure begins when subcutaneous fat is brought together loosely with a few sutures to close off the dead space. The subcuticular layer is then closed, and finally the epidermis is closed. Sutures are placed near the wound edge, with the skin edges levelled carefully to promote optimal healing. Instead of sutures, sterile strips of reinforced microporous tape or a bonding agent (skin glue) may be used to close clean, superficial wounds.

Delayed Primary Closure

Delayed primary closure may be indicated if tissue has been lost or there is a high potential for infection. A thin layer of gauze (to ensure drainage and prevent pooling of exudate), covered by an occlusive dressing, may be used. The wound is splinted in a functional position to prevent motion and decrease the possibility of contracture.

If there are no signs of suppuration (formation of purulent drainage), the wound may be sutured (with the patient receiving a local anesthetic). Use of antibiotics to prevent infection depends on factors such as how the injury occurred, the age of the wound, and the risk of contamination. The site is immobilized and elevated to limit accumulation of fluid in the interstitial spaces of the wound.

Tetanus prophylaxis is administered as prescribed, based on the condition of the wound and the patient's immunization status.

The patient is instructed about signs and symptoms of infection and is instructed to contact the health care professional or clinic if there is sudden or persistent pain, fever or chills, bleeding, rapid swelling, foul odour, drainage, or redness surrounding the wound.

TRAUMA

Trauma an unintentional or intentional wound or injury inflicted on the body from a mechanism against which the body cannot protect itself. In Canada, trauma is the leading cause of death of individuals under 45 years of age. In 2016/2017, 2 million individuals were treated in Canadian ED hospitals for some form of traumatic injury (CIHI, 2018). The majority of patients seen for a trauma type injury were between the ages of 18 and 64 and were struck by or against an object or person (CIHI, 2018). Of the 2 million people seen in Canada's emergency rooms for a trauma, 26,519 of them will be seen because of a sport-related injury (CIHI, 2018). Only 5% of all trauma patients will be admitted to the hospital (CIHI, 2018).

Collection of Forensic Evidence

In assessing and managing any patient with an emergency condition, but especially the patient experiencing trauma, meticulous documentation is essential. Included in documentation are descriptions of all wounds, mechanism of injury, time of events, and collection of evidence. In trauma care, the nurse must be exceedingly careful with all potential evidence, handling and documenting it properly.

The basics of care management for patients with traumatic injury include an understanding that trauma in any patient (living or dead) has potential legal or forensic implications if criminal activity is suspected. Hence, proper management from both a medical and forensic perspective is essential.

When clothing is removed from the patient who has experienced trauma, the nurse is very careful not to cut through or disrupt any tears, holes, blood stains, or dirt present on the clothing if criminal activity is suspected. Each piece of clothing should be placed in an individual paper bag. If the clothing is wet, it should be hung to dry. Clothing is not given to families. Valuables should be inventoried and either placed in the hospital safe or it should be clearly documented to which family member they were given. If a police officer is present to collect clothing or any other items from the patient, each item is labelled. The transfer of custody to the officer, the officer's name, the date, and the time are documented.

If suicide or homicide is suspected in a deceased trauma patient, the medical examiner examines the body on site or has the body moved to the coroner's office for autopsy. All tubes and lines must remain in place. The patient's hands must be covered with paper bags to protect evidence on the hands or under the fingernails. In the surviving patient, tissue specimens may be swabbed from the hands and nails as potential evidence. Photographs of wounds or clothing are essential and should include a reference ruler in one photo and one without the ruler.

Documentation also includes any statements made by the patient in the patient's own words and surrounded by quotation marks. A chain of evidence is essential. If the patient's case is reviewed in a court of law in the future, clear documentation assists the judicial process and helps to identify the activities that occurred in the ED.

Injury Prevention

Any discussion of trauma management must address injury prevention. A component of the emergency nurse's daily role is to provide injury prevention information to every

patient with whom there is contact, including patients admitted for reasons other than injury. The only way to reduce the incidence of trauma is through prevention.

There are three components of injury prevention: education, legislation, and automatic protection. Providing educational information and materials to help prevent violence and to maintain safety at home and in vehicles is important. Involvement in local injury prevention organizations, nursing organizations, and health fairs promotes wellness and safety. In practice, nursing and other health care professionals should avoid using the word "accident," because trauma events are *preventable* and should be viewed as such rather than as "fate" or "happenstance." Responsibility and accountability must be assigned to traumatic incidents, particularly because of the high rate of trauma recidivism (repeated trauma). People who are at risk for trauma and trauma recidivism should be identified and provided with education and counselling directed toward altering risky behaviours and preventing further trauma (Kenney Powell & Hentzen Daniels, 2018).

The second component of injury prevention is legislation. Nurses are actively involved in safety legislation at the local, provincial/territorial, and federal levels. Such legislation is meant to provide universal safety measures, not to infringe on rights.

The third component is automatic protection. Airbags and automotive design are included in this category. These mechanisms provide for safety without requiring personal intervention.

Multiple Trauma

Multiple trauma is caused by a single catastrophic event that causes life-threatening injuries to at least two distinct organs or organ systems. Patients with single-system trauma still receive full assessment, because even single-system injuries can be life-threatening or more severe than they initially appear. Mortality in patients with multiple trauma is related to the severity of the injuries and the number of systems and organs involved. Immediately after injury, the body is hypermetabolic, hypercoagulable, and severely stressed.

Care of the patient with multiple injuries requires a team approach, with one person responsible for coordinating the treatment. The nursing staff assumes responsibility for assessing and monitoring the patient, ensuring airway and IV access, administering prescribed medications, collecting laboratory specimens, and documenting activities and the patient's subsequent responses.

Assessment and Diagnostic Findings

Evidence of trauma may be sparse or absent. Patients with multiple trauma are assumed to have a spinal cord injury until it is proven otherwise. The injury regarded as the least significant in appearance may be the most lethal. For example, the pelvic fracture not identified until an x-ray is obtained may cause rapid and massive hemorrhage into the pelvic cavity, but an obvious amputation of the arm may have already stopped bleeding from the body's normal response of vasoconstriction, despite being obvious and a devastating injury; meanwhile, the patient may be dying from an internal, not so visible, injury.

CHART 73-5

Priority Management in Patients With Multiple Injuries

1. Establish airway and ventilation

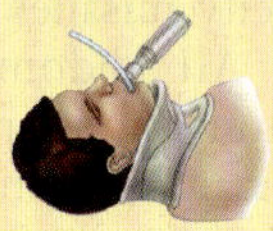

2. Control hemorrhage

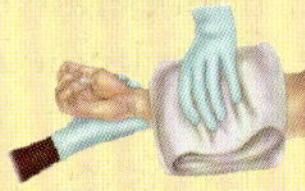

3. Prevent and treat hypovolemic shock

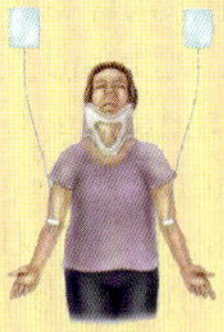

4. Assess for head and neck injuries

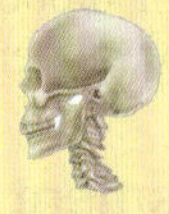

5. Evaluate for other injuries - reassess head and neck, chest, assess abdomen, back, and extremities

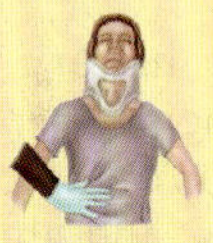

6. Splint fractures

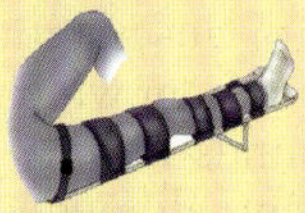

7. Perform a more thorough and ongoing examination and assessment

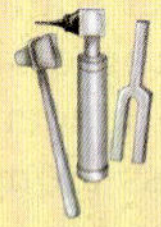

Adapted from American College of Surgeons. (2013). *Advanced trauma life support* (9th ed.). Chicago, IL: Author.

Management

The goals of treatment are to determine the extent of injuries and to establish priorities of treatment. Any injury interfering with a vital physiologic function (e.g., airway, breathing, circulation) is an immediate threat to life and has the highest priority for immediate treatment. Essential life-saving procedures are performed simultaneously by the emergency team. As soon as the patient is resuscitated, clothes are removed or cut off and a rapid physical assessment is performed. Transfer from field management to the ED must be orderly and controlled, with attention given to the verbal report from emergency medical services. Treatment in a trauma centre is appropriate for patients experiencing major trauma. Treatment priorities are presented in Chart 73-5.

Intra-Abdominal Injuries

Intra-abdominal injuries are categorized as penetrating or blunt trauma. *Penetrating* abdominal injuries (i.e., gunshot wounds, stab wounds) are serious and usually require surgery. Penetrating abdominal trauma results in a high incidence of injury to hollow organs, particularly the small bowel. The liver is the most frequently injured solid organ. In gunshot wounds, the most important prognostic factor is the velocity at which the missile enters the body. High-velocity missiles (bullets) produce extensive tissue damage. All abdominal gunshot wounds that cross the peritoneum or are associated with peritoneal signs require surgical exploration. Conversely stab wounds may be managed nonoperatively due to low velocity and less penetration of the implement (i.e., weapon).

Blunt trauma to the abdomen may result from motor vehicle crashes, falls, blows, or explosions. Blunt trauma is commonly associated with extra-abdominal injuries to the chest, head, or extremities. Patients with blunt trauma are a challenge because injuries may be difficult to detect. The incidence of delayed and trauma-related complications is greater than for penetrating injuries. This is especially true of blunt injuries involving the liver, kidneys, spleen, or blood vessels, which can lead to massive blood loss into the peritoneal cavity.

Assessment and Diagnostic Findings

As the history of the traumatic event is obtained, the abdomen is inspected as a part of the secondary survey for obvious signs of injury, including penetrating injuries, bruises, and abrasions. Abdominal assessment continues with auscultation of bowel sounds to provide baseline data from which changes can be noted. Absence of bowel sounds may be an early sign of intraperitoneal involvement, although stress can also decrease or halt peristalsis and bowel sounds. Further abdominal assessment may reveal progressive abdominal distention, involuntary guarding, tenderness, pain, muscular rigidity, or rebound tenderness along with changes in bowel sounds, all of which are signs of peritoneal irritation. Hypotension and signs and symptoms of shock may also be noted. Additionally, the chest and other body systems are assessed for injuries that frequently accompany intra-abdominal injuries.

Laboratory studies that aid in assessment include the following:

- Urinalysis to detect hematuria (indicative of a urinary tract injury)
- Serial hemoglobin and hematocrit levels to evaluate trends reflecting the presence or absence of bleeding
- White blood cell (WBC) count to detect elevation (generally associated with trauma)
- Serum amylase analysis to detect increasing levels, which suggest pancreatic injury or perforation of the gastrointestinal tract

Internal Bleeding

Hemorrhage frequently accompanies abdominal injury, especially if the liver or spleen has been traumatized. Therefore, the patient is assessed continuously for signs and symptoms of external and internal bleeding. The front of the body, flanks, and back are inspected for bluish discolouration, asymmetry, abrasion, and contusion. Abdominal CT scans permit detailed evaluation of abdominal contents and retroperitoneal examination. Bedside thoracic and abdominal ultrasounds can rapidly assess hemodynamically unstable patients to detect intraperitoneal bleeding (Montoya, Stawicki, Evans, et al., 2016). This is referred to as the focused assessment sonography for trauma (FAST) examination (Montoya et al., 2016).

NURSING ALERT

The location of pain can indicate certain types of intra-abdominal injuries. Pain in the left shoulder is common in a patient with bleeding from a ruptured spleen, whereas pain in the right shoulder can result from laceration of the liver.

Intraperitoneal Injury

The abdomen is assessed for tenderness, rebound tenderness, guarding, rigidity, spasm, increasing distention, and pain. Referred pain is a significant finding because it suggests intraperitoneal injury. To determine if there is intraperitoneal injury and bleeding, the patient is usually prepared for diagnostic procedures, such as abdominal ultrasonography, or abdominal CT scanning.

In patients with stab wounds, sinography may be performed to detect peritoneal penetration; a purse-string suture is placed around the wound and a small catheter is introduced through the wound. A contrast agent is then introduced through the catheter, and x-rays are taken to identify any peritoneal penetration.

Genitourinary Injury

A focused genitourinary examination, which typically includes a rectal and/or vaginal examination, is performed to determine any injury to the pelvis, bladder, urethra, vagina, or intestinal wall. In the male patient, a high-riding prostate gland (abnormal position) discovered during a rectal examination indicates a potential urethral injury. A digital vaginal examination is performed on female patients to determine if there is an open pelvic fracture that has torn the vagina.

NURSING ALERT

To decompress the bladder and monitor urine output in a patient with a genitourinary injury, an indwelling catheter is inserted after a rectal examination has been completed, not before the examination. In addition, urethral catheter insertion when a possible urethral injury is present is contraindicated; a urology consultation and further evaluation of the urethra are required.

Management

As indicated by the patient's condition, resuscitation procedures (restoration of airway, breathing, and circulation) are initiated. A patent airway is maintained, and attempts to stabilize the respiratory, circulatory, and nervous systems are made. Bleeding is controlled by application of direct pressure to any external bleeding wounds and by occlusion of any chest wounds. Circulating blood volume is maintained with intravenous fluid replacement, including blood component therapy. The patient is monitored for signs and symptoms of shock after an initial response to transfusion therapy, because these are often the first signs of internal hemorrhage.

With blunt trauma, the patient is kept on a stretcher to immobilize the spine. A backboard may be used for transporting the patient to the x-ray department, to the operating room, or to the intensive care unit. Cervical spine immobilization is maintained until cervical x-rays have been obtained and cervical spine injury has been ruled out. Likewise, once the patient has arrived at the definitive destination, the backboard is removed, and logrolling can be used to protect the spine until x-rays are obtained and confirm there is no evidence of injuries.

Knowing the mechanism of injury (e.g., penetrating force from a gunshot or knife, blunt force from a blow) is essential to determining the type of management needed. All wounds are located, counted, and documented. If abdominal viscera protrude, the area is covered with sterile, moist saline dressings to keep the viscera from drying.

Typically, oral fluids are withheld in anticipation of surgery, and the stomach contents are aspirated with a nasogastric tube to reduce the risk of aspiration and to decompress the stomach in preparation for diagnostic procedures.

Trauma predisposes the patient to infection by disruption of mechanical barriers, exposure to exogenous bacteria from the environment at the time of injury, aspiration of vomitus, and diagnostic and therapeutic procedures (hospital-acquired infection). Tetanus prophylaxis and broad-spectrum antibiotics are administered as prescribed.

Throughout the stay in the ED, the patient's condition is continuously monitored for changes. If there is continuing evidence of shock, blood loss, free air under the diaphragm, evisceration, hematuria, severe head injury, or suspected or known abdominal injury, the patient is rapidly transported to surgery. In most cases, blunt liver and spleen injuries are managed nonsurgically.

Crush Injuries

Crush injuries occur when a person is caught between opposing forces (e.g., run over by a moving vehicle, crushed between two cars, crushed under a collapsed building).

Assessment and Diagnostic Findings

The patient is observed for the following:

- Hypovolemic shock resulting from extravasation of blood and plasma into injured tissues after compression has been released
- Paralysis of a body part
- Erythema and blistering of skin
- Damaged body part (usually an extremity) appearing swollen, tense, and hard
- Renal dysfunction (prolonged hypotension causes kidney damage and acute renal insufficiency; myoglobinuria secondary to muscle damage can cause acute tubular necrosis and acute renal failure)

Management

In conjunction with maintaining the airway, breathing, and circulation, the patient is observed for acute renal insufficiency. Injury to the back can cause kidney damage. Severe muscular damage may cause rhabdomyolysis, which signifies a release of myoglobin from ischemic skeletal muscle, resulting in acute tubular necrosis. In addition, major soft tissue injuries are splinted promptly to control bleeding and pain. Serum lactate is monitored and normalizing levels indicate successful resuscitation. While monitoring serum lactate has been the gold standard of successful resuscitation for many years, new evidence suggests that monitoring peripheral perfusion status may be another method to gauge resuscitation (Hernández, Ospina-Tascón, Petri Damiani, et al., 2019). At this time additional research on this is needed on this monitoring parameter (Hernández et al., 2019).

If an extremity is injured, it is elevated to relieve swelling and pressure. If the patient reports extreme pain in an extremity, the nurse immediately assesses for compartment syndrome using the 6 Ps: **Pain**—severe, **Pallor**, of skin (pale or mottled look), **Pulselessness**, **Poikilothermic** (or **Polar)** sensation (cold to the touch), **Paresthesia** (burning, numb, or tingling), and **Paralysis** (lack of purposeful movement) (Kiser-Larson, 2017). See also Chapter 70. If compartment syndrome develops, the physician may perform a **fasciotomy** (i.e., surgical incision to the level of the fascia) to restore neurovascular function (see Chapters 70 and 71). Medications for pain and anxiety are then administered as prescribed, and the patient is quickly transported to the operating suite for wound débridement and fracture repair. A hyperbaric oxygen chamber (if available) may be used to hyperoxygenate crushed tissue, if indicated.

Fractures

Immediate appropriate management of a fracture may determine the patient's eventual outcome and may mean the difference between recovery and disability. When the patient is being examined for fracture, the body part is handled gently and as little as possible. Clothing is cut off to visualize the affected body part. Assessment is conducted for pain over or near a bone, swelling (from blood, lymph, and exudate infiltrating the tissue), and circulatory disturbance. The patient is assessed for ecchymosis, tenderness, and crepitation (see Chapter 72). The nurse must remember that the patient may have multiple fractures accompanied by head, chest, spine, or abdominal injuries.

Management

Immediate attention is given to the patient's general condition. Assessment of airway, breathing, and circulation (which includes pulses in the extremities) is conducted. The patient is also evaluated for neurologic or abdominal injuries before the extremity is treated, unless a pulseless extremity is detected.

If a pulseless extremity is identified, repositioning of the extremity to proper alignment is required. If the pulseless extremity involves a fractured hip or femur, **Hare** traction (a portable in-line traction device) may be applied to assist with alignment. If repositioning is ineffective in restoring the pulse, a rapid total-body assessment must be completed, followed by transfer of the patient to the operating room for arteriography and possible arterial repair.

After the initial evaluation has been completed, all injuries identified are evaluated and treated. The fractured body part is inspected. Using a systematic head-to-toe approach, the nurse inspects the entire body, observing for lacerations, swelling, and deformities, including angulation (bending), shortening, rotation, and asymmetry. All peripheral pulses, especially those distal to the fractured extremity, are palpated. The extremity is also assessed for coolness, blanching, and decreased sensation and motor function, which are indicative of injury to the extremity's neurovascular supply.

A splint is applied before the patient is moved. Splinting immobilizes the joint at a site distal and proximal to the fracture, relieves pain, restores or improves circulation, prevents further tissue injury, and prevents a closed fracture from becoming an open one. To splint an extremity, one hand is placed distal to the fracture and some traction is applied while the other hand is placed beneath the fracture for support. The splints should extend beyond the joints adjacent to the fracture. Upper extremities must be splinted in a functional position. If the fracture is open, a moist, sterile dressing is applied.

After splinting, the vascular status of the extremity is checked by assessing colour, temperature, pulse, and blanching of the nail bed. In addition, the patient is assessed for neurovascular compromise if pain or pressure is reported. (See Chapter 72 for a complete description of fracture management.)

ENVIRONMENTAL EMERGENCIES

Heat Stroke

Heat stroke is an acute medical emergency caused by failure of the heat-regulating mechanisms of the body. The most common cause of heat stroke is prolonged exposure to an environmental temperature of greater than 39.2°C. It usually occurs during extended heat waves, especially when they are accompanied by high humidity.

People at risk for heat stroke are those not acclimatized to heat, those who are older or very young, those unable to care for themselves, those with chronic and debilitating diseases, and those taking certain medications (e.g., major tranquilizers, anticholinergics, diuretics, beta blockers). Exertional heat stroke occurs in healthy individuals during sports or work activities (e.g., exercising in extreme heat and humidity). Another form of heat stroke is heat exhaustion in which the patient's temperature may be normal to 40°C (104°F). The patient demonstrates weakness, hypotension, increased heart rate, and increased thirst. Hyperthermia results because of inadequate heat loss. This type of heat stroke can also cause death. Strategies used to prevent heat stroke are reviewed in Chart 73-6.

Gerontologic Considerations

Most heat-related deaths occur in older people because their circulatory systems are unable to compensate for stress imposed by heat. Older people have a decreased ability to perspire as well as a decreased ability to vasodilate and vasoconstrict. They have less subcutaneous tissue, a decreased thirst mechanism, and a diminished ability to concentrate urine to compensate for heat. Many older people do not drink adequate amounts of fluid, partly because of fear of incontinence, and thus have a greater risk of heat stroke.

CHART 73-6

Health Promotion: Preventing Heat-Induced Illnesses

The nurse provides the following advice for the patient treated for heat-induced illness:

- Avoid immediate re-exposure to high temperatures; hypersensitivity to high temperatures may remain for a considerable time.
- Maintain adequate fluid intake, wear loose clothing, and reduce activity in hot weather.
- Monitor fluid losses and weight loss during workout activities or exercise and replace fluids and electrolytes.
- Use a gradual approach to physical conditioning, allowing sufficient time for return to baseline temperature.
- Plan outdoor activities to avoid the hottest part of the day (between 10 AM and 2 PM).

For older patients living in urban settings with high environmental temperatures:

- The nurse directs these patients to places where air conditioning is available (e.g., shopping mall, library, church) and advises them that fans alone are not adequate to prevent heat-induced illness.

Assessment and Diagnostic Findings

Heat stroke causes thermal injury at the cellular level, resulting in coagulopathies and widespread damage to the heart, liver, and kidneys. Recent patient history reveals exposure to elevated ambient temperature or excessive exercise during extreme heat. When assessing the patient, the nurse notes the following symptoms: profound central nervous system (CNS) dysfunction (manifested by confusion, delirium, bizarre behaviour, coma); elevated body temperature (40.6°C or higher); hot, dry skin; and usually anhidrosis (absence of sweating), tachypnea, hypotension, and tachycardia.

Management

The primary goal is to reduce the high body temperature as quickly as possible, because mortality is directly related to the duration of hyperthermia. Simultaneous treatment focuses on stabilizing oxygenation using the ABCs (*a*irway, *b*reathing, and *c*irculation) of basic life support. This includes establishing IV access for fluid administration.

After the patient's clothing is removed, the core (internal) temperature is reduced to 39°C as rapidly as possible, preferably within 1 hour (Flarity, 2018). One or more of the following methods may be used as prescribed:

- Cool sheets and towels or continuous sponging with cool water

- Ice applied to the neck, groin, chest, and axillae while spraying with tepid water
- Cooling blankets

Additional methods that may be used with caution (Flarity, 2018):

- Ice water immersion
- Gastric lavage
- Rectal lavage
- Cardiopulmonary bypass
- Hemodialysis

During cooling procedures, an electric fan is positioned so that it blows on the patient to augment heat dissipation by convection and evaporation. The patient's temperature is constantly monitored with a thermistor placed in the rectum, bladder, or esophagus to evaluate core temperature. Caution is used to avoid hypothermia and to prevent hyperthermia, which may recur spontaneously within 3 to 4 hours. The cooling process should stop at 39°C in order to avoid iatrogenic hypothermia (Flarity, 2018).

Throughout treatment, the patient's status is monitored carefully, including vital signs, ECG findings (for possible myocardial ischemia, myocardial infarction, and dysrhythmias), central venous pressure (CVP), and level of responsiveness, all of which may change with rapid alterations in body temperature. A seizure may be followed by recurrence of hyperthermia. To meet tissue needs exaggerated by the hypermetabolic condition, 100% oxygen is administered. Endotracheal intubation and mechanical ventilation to support failing cardiopulmonary systems may be required.

IV infusion therapy of normal saline or lactated Ringer's solution is initiated as directed to replace fluid losses and maintain adequate circulation. Fluids are administered carefully because of the dangers of myocardial injury from high body temperature and poor renal function. Cooling redistributes fluid volume from the periphery to the core.

Urine output is also measured frequently, because acute tubular necrosis may occur as a complication of heat stroke from rhabdomyolysis (myoglobin in the urine). Blood specimens are obtained for serial testing to detect bleeding disorders, such as disseminated intravascular coagulation (DIC), and for serial enzyme studies to estimate thermal hypoxic injury to the liver, heart, and muscle tissue. Permanent liver, cardiac, and CNS damage may occur.

Additional supportive care may include dialysis for renal failure, anticonvulsant medications to control seizures, potassium for hypokalemia, and sodium bicarbonate to correct metabolic acidosis. Benzodiazepines (e.g., diazepam [Valium]) or chlorpromazine (Thorazine) may be prescribed to suppress seizure activity. Patient education regarding the prevention of heat stroke (see Chart 73-6) is also important to prevent a recurrence.

Frostbite

Frostbite is trauma from exposure to freezing temperatures and freezing of the intracellular fluid and fluids in the intercellular spaces. It results in cellular and vascular damage. Frostbite can result in venous stasis and thrombosis. Body parts most frequently affected by frostbite include the feet, hands, nose, and ears. Frostbite ranges from first degree (redness and erythema) to fourth degree (full-depth tissue destruction).

Assessment and Diagnostic Findings

A frozen extremity may be hard, cold, and insensitive to touch and may appear white or mottled blue-white. The extent of injury from exposure to cold is not always initially known. The patient history should include environmental temperature, duration of exposure, humidity, and the presence of wet conditions.

Management

The goal of management is to restore usual body temperature. Constrictive clothing and jewellery that could impair circulation are removed. Wet clothing is removed as rapidly as possible. If the lower extremities are involved, the patient should not be allowed to ambulate.

Controlled yet rapid rewarming is instituted. Frozen extremities are usually placed in a 37° to 40°C circulating bath for 30- to 40-minute spans. This treatment is repeated until circulation is effectively restored. Early rewarming appears to decrease the amount of ultimate tissue loss. During rewarming, an analgesic for pain is administered as prescribed, because the rewarming process may be very painful. To avoid further mechanical injury, the body part is not handled. Massage is contraindicated.

Once rewarmed, the part is protected from further injury and is elevated to help control swelling. Sterile gauze or cotton is placed between affected fingers or toes to prevent maceration, and a bulky dressing is placed on the extremity. A foot cradle may be used to prevent contact with bedclothes if the feet are involved. Hemorrhagic blebs, which may develop 1 hour to a few days after rewarming, are left intact and not ruptured. Nonhemorrhagic blisters are débrided to decrease the inflammatory mediators found in the blister fluid.

A physical assessment is conducted with rewarming to observe for concomitant injury, such as soft tissue injury, dehydration, alcohol coma, or fat embolism. Problems such as hyperkalemia (e.g., from release of potassium in the damaged cells) and hypovolemia, which occur frequently in people with frostbite, are corrected. Risk of infection is also great; therefore, strict aseptic technique is used during dressing changes, and tetanus prophylaxis is administered as indicated. Nonsteroidal anti-inflammatory medication is prescribed for its anti-inflammatory effects and to control pain.

Additional measures that may be carried out when appropriate include the following:

- Whirlpool bath for the affected body parts to aid circulation and débridement of necrotic tissue to help prevent infection
- Escharotomy (incision through the eschar) to prevent further tissue damage, to allow for normal circulation, and to permit joint motion
- Fasciotomy to treat compartment syndrome

After rewarming, hourly active motion of any affected digits is encouraged to promote maximal restoration of function and to prevent contractures. Discharge instructions also include encouraging the patient to avoid tobacco, alcohol, and caffeine because of their vasoconstrictive effects, which further reduce the already deficient blood supply to injured tissues.

Hypothermia

Hypothermia is a condition in which the core (internal) temperature is 35°C or less as a result of exposure to cold or an inability to maintain body temperature in the absence of low ambient temperatures. Urban hypothermia (extreme exposure to cold in an urban setting) is associated with a high mortality rate; older people, infants, people with concurrent illnesses, and people who are homeless are particularly susceptible. Alcohol ingestion increases susceptibility because it causes systemic vasodilation. Some medications (e.g., phenothiazines) or medical conditions (e.g., hypothyroidism, spinal cord injury) decrease the ability to shiver, hampering the body's innate ability to generate body heat. Trauma victims are also at risk for hypothermia resulting from treatment with cold fluids, unwarmed oxygen, and exposure during examination. The patient may also have frostbite, but hypothermia takes precedence in treatment.

Assessment and Diagnostic Findings

Hypothermia leads to physiologic changes in all organ systems. There is progressive deterioration, with apathy, poor judgment, ataxia, dysarthria, drowsiness, pulmonary edema, acid–base abnormalities, coagulopathy, and eventual coma. Shivering may be suppressed at a temperature of less than 32.2°C, because the body's self-warming mechanisms become ineffective. The heartbeat and blood pressure may be so weak that peripheral pulses become undetectable. Cardiac dysrhythmias may also occur. Other physiologic abnormalities include hypoxemia and acidosis.

Management

Management consists of continuous monitoring of all vital signs (including cardiac monitoring), and temperature, along with rewarming, removal of wet clothing, insulation, and supportive care.

Monitoring

The ABCs of basic life support are a priority. The patient's vital signs, CVP, urine output, arterial blood gas levels, blood chemistry determinations (blood urea nitrogen, creatinine, glucose, electrolytes), and chest x-rays are evaluated frequently. Body temperature is monitored with an esophageal, bladder, or rectal thermistor. Continuous ECG monitoring is performed, because cold-induced myocardial irritability leads to conduction disturbances, especially ventricular fibrillation. An arterial line is inserted and maintained to record blood pressure and to facilitate blood sampling.

Rewarming

Rewarming methods include active internal (core) rewarming and passive or active external (spontaneous) rewarming.

Active internal (core) rewarming methods are used for moderate to severe hypothermia (less than 28° to 32.2°C) and include cardiopulmonary bypass, warm fluid administration, warm humidified oxygen by ventilator, and warmed peritoneal lavage. Monitoring for ventricular fibrillation as the patient's temperature increases from 31° to 32°C is essential.

Passive or active external rewarming is used for mild hypothermia (32.2° to 35°C). Passive active rewarming uses over-the-bed heaters to the extremities and increases blood flow to the acidotic, anaerobic extremities. The cold blood from peripheral tissues has high lactic acid levels. As this blood returns to the core, it causes a significant drop in the core temperature (i.e., core temperature afterdrop) and can potentially cause cardiac dysrhythmias and electrolyte disturbances. Active external rewarming uses forced air warm blankets. Care must be taken to prevent extremity burn from these devices, because the patient may not have effective sensation to feel the burn.

Supportive Care

Supportive care during rewarming includes the following as directed:

- External cardiac compression (typically performed only as directed in patients with temperatures higher than 31°C).
- Defibrillation of ventricular fibrillation. A patient whose temperature is less than 32°C experiences spontaneous ventricular fibrillation if moved or touched. Defibrillation is ineffective in patients with temperatures lower than 31°C; therefore, the patient must be rewarmed first.
- Mechanical ventilation with positive end-expiratory pressure (PEEP) and heated humidified oxygen to maintain tissue oxygenation.
- Administration of warmed IV fluids to correct hypotension and to maintain urine output and core rewarming, as described previously.
- Administration of sodium bicarbonate to correct metabolic acidosis if necessary.
- Administration of antiarrhythmic medications.
- Insertion of an indwelling urinary catheter to monitor urinary output and renal function.

Nonfatal Drowning

Nonfatal drowning is defined as survival for at least 24 hours after submersion that caused a respiratory arrest. The most common consequence is hypoxemia. Drowning is the second most common cause of unintentional death in children younger than 14 years (Drowning Prevention Research Centre Canada, 2016). In 2015 there were 313 drownings in Canada (Drowning Prevention Research Centre Canada, 2016). Unintentional water-related fatalities have shown a decline since 1998 (Drowning Prevention Research Centre Canada, 2016).

Factors associated with drowning and nonfatal drowning include alcohol ingestion, inability to swim, diving injuries, hypothermia, and exhaustion. The majority of drowning events occur in lakes, rivers, oceans, and bathtubs (Drowning Prevention Research Centre Canada, 2016). Young adults aged 20 to 35 and seniors (over 65 years of age) are the population with the highest number of reported deaths related to drowning and over 80% of the reported cases in Canada occurred among men (Drowning Prevention Research Centre Canada, 2016). With regard to ethnicity, newcomers to Canada and Aboriginal peoples are at higher risk of drowning (Drowning Prevention Research Centre Canada, 2016).

Efforts to save the patient should not be abandoned prematurely. Successful resuscitation with full neurologic recovery has occurred in patients who have experienced nonfatal drowning after prolonged submersion in cold water. This is possible because of a decrease in metabolic demands and/or the diving reflex. The nonfatal drowning process involves the onset of hypoxia, hypercapnia, bradycardia, and dysrhythmias. If there is a violent struggle associated with the near-drowning episode, exercise-induced acidosis and tachypnea can result in aspiration. Hypoxia and acidosis cause eventual apnea and loss of consciousness. When the victim loses consciousness and makes a final effort to breathe, the terminal gasp occurs. Water then moves passively into the airways prior to death.

After resuscitation, hypoxia and acidosis are the primary complications experienced by a person who has experienced nonfatal drowning; immediate intervention in the ED is essential. Resultant pathophysiologic changes and pulmonary injury depend on the type of fluid (fresh or salt water) and the volume aspirated. Fresh water aspiration results in a loss of surfactant and, therefore, an inability to expand the lungs. Salt water aspiration leads to pulmonary edema from the osmotic effects of the salt within the lungs. If a person survives submersion, ARDS, resulting in hypoxia, hypercarbia, and respiratory or metabolic acidosis, can occur.

Management

Therapeutic goals include maintaining cerebral perfusion and adequate oxygenation to prevent further damage to vital organs. Immediate cardiopulmonary resuscitation is the factor with the greatest influence on survival. The most important priority in resuscitation is to manage the hypoxia, acidosis, and hypothermia. Prevention and management of hypoxia are accomplished by ensuring an adequate airway and respiration, thus improving ventilation (which helps correct respiratory acidosis) and oxygenation. Arterial blood gases are monitored to evaluate oxygen, carbon dioxide, bicarbonate levels, and pH. These parameters determine the type of ventilatory support needed. Use of endotracheal intubation with PEEP improves oxygenation, prevents aspiration, and corrects intrapulmonary shunting and ventilation–perfusion abnormalities (caused by aspiration of water). If the patient is breathing spontaneously, supplemental oxygen may be administered by mask. However, an endotracheal tube is necessary if the patient does not breathe spontaneously.

Because of submersion, the patient is usually hypothermic. A rectal probe is used to determine the degree of hypothermia. Prescribed rewarming procedures (e.g., extracorporeal warming, warmed peritoneal dialysis, inhalation of warm aerosolized oxygen, torso warming) are started during resuscitation. The choice of warming method is determined by the severity and duration of hypothermia and available resources. Intravascular volume expansion and inotropic agents are used to treat hypotension and impaired tissue perfusion. ECG monitoring is initiated, because dysrhythmias frequently occur. An indwelling urinary catheter is inserted to measure urine output. Hypothermia and accompanying metabolic acidosis may compromise renal function. Nasogastric intubation is used to decompress the stomach and to prevent the patient from aspirating gastric contents.

Even if the patient appears healthy, close monitoring continues with serial vital signs, serial arterial blood gas values, ECG monitoring, intracranial pressure assessments, serum electrolyte levels, intake and output, and serial chest x-rays. After a nonfatal drowning, the patient is at risk for complications such as hypoxic or ischemic cerebral injury, ARDS, pulmonary damage secondary to aspiration, and life-threatening cardiac arrest.

Decompression Sickness

Decompression sickness, also called “the bends,” occurs in patients who have engaged in diving (lake, as well as ocean, diving), high-altitude flying, or flying in commercial aircraft within 24 hours after diving. Although decompression sickness occurs in relatively few divers compared with the number of divers worldwide, its effects can be hazardous. Being aware of decompression sickness and assessing the patient properly ensures proper management and results in the least morbidity possible.

Decompression sickness results from formation of nitrogen bubbles that occur with rapid changes in atmospheric pressure. They may occur in joint or muscle spaces, resulting in musculoskeletal pain, numbness, or hypesthesia. More significantly, nitrogen bubbles can become air emboli in the bloodstream and thereby produce stroke, paralysis, or death. Taking a rapid history about the events preceding the symptoms is essential. Recompression is necessary as soon as possible and may necessitate a low-altitude flight to the nearest hyperbaric chamber.

Assessment and Diagnostic Findings

To identify decompression sickness, a detailed history is obtained from the patient or diving partner. Evidence of rapid ascent, loss of air in the tank, buddy breathing, recent alcohol intake or lack of sleep, or a flight within 24 hours after diving suggests possible decompression sickness. Some patients describe a perfect dive yet still have the signs and symptoms of decompression sickness, and they must receive treatment for the condition.

Signs and symptoms include joint or extremity pain, numbness, hypesthesia, and loss of range of motion. Neurologic symptoms mimicking those of a stroke or spinal cord injury can indicate an air embolus. Cardiopulmonary arrest can also occur in severe cases and is usually fatal. Any neurologic symptoms should be rapidly assessed. All patients with decompression sickness need rapid transfer to a hyperbaric chamber.

Management

A patent airway and adequate ventilation are established, as described previously, and 100% oxygen is administered throughout treatment and transport. A chest x-ray is obtained to identify aspiration, and at least one IV line is started with lactated Ringer’s or normal saline solution.

The cardiopulmonary and neurologic systems are supported as needed. If an air embolus is suspected, the head of the bed should be lowered. The patient's wet clothing is removed, and the patient is kept warm. Transfer to the closest hyperbaric chamber for treatment is initiated. If air transport is necessary, low-altitude flight (below 1,000 ft) is required. However, the patient who is awake and alert without central neurologic deficits may be able to travel by ground ambulance or by automobile, depending on the severity of symptoms. Throughout treatment, the patient is continually assessed, and changes are documented. If aspiration is suspected, antibiotics and other treatment may be prescribed. Canadian hyperbaric facilities and diving medicine centres are located in Victoria, Vancouver, Burnaby, Edmonton, Calgary, Moose Jaw, Winnipeg, Toronto, Hamilton, Ottawa, Tobermory, Les Escoumins, Montral, Lévis, Rimouski, Pincourt, St. John's, and Halifax (Canadian Undersea and Hyperbaric Medical Association [CUHMA], 2019).

Anaphylactic Reaction

An anaphylactic reaction is an acute systemic hypersensitivity reaction that occurs within seconds or minutes after exposure to certain foreign substances, such as medications (e.g., penicillin, iodinated contrast material), and other agents, such as latex, insect stings (e.g., bee, wasp, yellow jacket, hornet), or foods (e.g., eggs, peanuts). Repeated administration of parenteral or oral therapeutic agents (e.g., repeated exposures to penicillin) may also precipitate an anaphylactic reaction when initially only a mild allergic response occurred. Anaphylaxis prevention strategies are provided in Chart 73-7.

An anaphylactic reaction is the result of an antigen–antibody interaction in a sensitized person who, as a consequence of previous exposure, has developed a special type of antibody (immunoglobulin) that is specific for that particular allergen. Immunoglobulin E (IgE) is responsible for most of the immediate types of human allergic responses. A second exposure to the same antigen results in a more severe and more rapid response (see Chapter 53).

An anaphylactic reaction produces a wide range of clinical manifestations, especially respiratory symptoms (difficulty breathing and stridor secondary to laryngeal edema), fainting, itching, swelling of mucous membranes, and a sudden decrease in blood pressure secondary to massive vasodilation that may progress to shock (Chart 73-8). (See Chapters 18 and 53 for additional discussion and management of anaphylactic reactions.)

CHART 73-7

Nursing Interventions for Preventing Anaphylactic Reactions

- Be aware of the danger of anaphylactic reactions and the early signs of anaphylaxis.
- Ask the patient about previous allergies to medications, foods, stings, latex, pollen, peanuts, nuts from trees, eggs, and so on.
- Before giving a foreign serum or other type of antigenic agent, ask the patient or caregiver whether the agent was received at some earlier time.
- Avoid giving medications to patients with hay fever, asthma, or other allergic disorders unless necessary.
- Avoid giving parenteral medications unless absolutely necessary, because anaphylactic reactions are more likely to occur when the agent is given parenterally.
- Perform a skin test before administration of certain materials known to produce anaphylactic reactions (e.g., horse serum). Remember that negative skin test results do not always indicate safety and that skin testing can precipitate anaphylaxis in highly sensitive patients. Have epinephrine, intravenous infusions, and intubation and tracheostomy equipment available as precautionary measures.
- If the patient is an outpatient, keep him or her in the office, hospital, or clinic for at least 30 minutes after injection of any agent. Caution the patient to return if symptoms develop.
- Caution patients who are highly sensitive (e.g., to insect bites and stings) to carry kits equipped to treat insect stings (epinephrine). Instruct the patient, family, and significant others in the use of the emergency supplies.
- Encourage patients with allergies to wear medical identification tags or bracelets.

Latex Allergy

Emergency nurses frequently deal with latex allergies. The number of products that contain latex is staggering. Nurses must be aware of latex allergy (health care providers have died from anaphylaxis related to latex allergy) and the potential for patients to react to latex.

There is an increased awareness among manufacturers of the need for products that are latexfree. Latexfree gloves are provided for nurses who have latex allergy or who have signs of allergy, such as itching, redness, or rash associated with use of a latex product. Severe anaphylaxis can occur even on first exposure; therefore, recognition of the signs and symptoms of anaphylaxis is essential. Treatment must be rapid, and the latex product must be removed promptly. Refer to Chapters 20 and 53 for more information about latex allergy.

Insect Stings

A person may have an extreme sensitivity to the venoms of insects in the order Hymenoptera (bees, hornets, yellow jackets, fire ants, and wasps). Venom allergy is thought to be an IgE-mediated reaction, and it constitutes an acute emergency. Although stings in any area of the body can trigger anaphylaxis, stings of the head and neck or multiple stings are especially serious.

Clinical manifestations range from generalized urticaria, itching, malaise, and anxiety due to laryngeal edema to severe bronchospasm, shock, and death. Generally, the shorter the time between the sting and the onset of severe symptoms, the worse the prognosis.

Management includes stinger removal if the sting is from a bee because the venom is associated with sacs around the barb of the stinger itself. The stinger is removed with one quick scrape of a fingernail over the site. Wound care with soap and water is sufficient for stings. Scratching is avoided because it results in a histamine response. Ice application reduces swelling and also decreases venom absorption. An oral antihistamine and analgesic will decrease the itching and pain.

CHART 73-8

Assessment: Anaphylaxis

Be alert for the following signs and symptoms:

Respiratory Signs

- Nasal congestion
- Itching
- Sneezing and coughing
- Possible respiratory distress that progresses rapidly (caused by bronchospasm or edema of the larynx)
- Chest tightness
- Other respiratory difficulties, such as wheezing, dyspnea, and cyanosis

Skin Manifestations

- Flushing with a sense of warmth and diffuse erythema
- Generalized itching over the entire body (indicates developing general systemic reaction)
- Urticaria (hives)
- Massive facial angioedema possible with accompanying upper respiratory edema

Cardiovascular Manifestations

- Tachycardia or bradycardia
- Peripheral vascular collapse as indicated by
  - Pallor
  - Imperceptible pulse
  - Decreasing blood pressure
  - Circulatory failure, leading to coma and death

Gastrointestinal Problems

- Nausea
- Vomiting
- Colicky abdominal pains
- Diarrhea

In the case of an anaphylactic or severe allergic response, epinephrine is administered to the patient as discussed previously in Chapter 53. Desensitization therapy should be given to people who have had systemic or significant local reactions. Patient and family education is an important measure in preventing exposure to stinging insects (Chart 73-9).

Animal and Human Bites

Bites are a common reason for visits to the ED. Dog bites constitute 90% of these bites and are responsible for the majority of deaths from bites by a nonvenomous animal. Cat bites have a high risk of infection because of the presence of *Pasteurella* in their saliva. All animal bites must be reported to public health authorities, which must provide follow-up screening of the offending animal for rabies. If the animal cannot be located and rabies vaccination verified, rabies prophylaxis for the person who has been bitten must be instituted.

Human bites are frequently associated with rapes, sexual assaults, or other forms of battery. The human mouth contains more bacteria than that of most other animals, so a high risk of bite-related infection exists. Depending on the circumstances surrounding the event, the victim may delay seeking treatment. The ED nurse should inspect any bitten tissue for pus, erythema, or necrosis. A health care provider should take photographs, which can be used as evidence in criminal and legal proceedings. Cleansing with soap and water is then necessary, followed by the administration of antibiotics and tetanus toxoid as prescribed.

CHART 73-9

Patient Education: Limiting Exposure to Stinging Insects

To Minimize Your Chances of Being Stung:

- Avoid places where stinging insects congregate, such as camp and picnic sites, and insect feeding areas, such as flower beds, ripe fruit orchards, garbage, and fields of clover.
- Wear covering on the feet, and avoid going barefoot outdoors, because yellow jackets nest and pollinate on the ground.
- Avoid perfumes, scented soaps, and bright colours, which attract bees.
- Keep car windows closed.
- Spray garbage cans with quick-acting insecticide.
- Secure a professional exterminator to dispose of wasp and hornet nests or beehives in the home area.
- Remain motionless if an insect is buzzing around. Motion, especially running, increases the likelihood of being stung.
- If allergic, carry a self-treatment kit containing injectable (Epi-Pen) and inhalant forms of epinephrine, an oral antihistamine, and written instructions. Carry it with you at all times.

If You are Stung, Do the Following:

1. Inject self immediately with epinephrine if allergy is known or allergic response occurs.
2. Remove the stinger with one quick scrape of the fingernail. *Do not* squeeze the venom sac because this may cause injection of additional venom.
3. Clean the area with soapy water, and apply ice.
4. Report to the nearest health care facility for further examination if allergic response or allergy is suspected.

Snakebites

1. Venomous (poisonous) snakes caused more than 2,000 of the 6,000 snakebites in the United States annually (Tintinalli, Stapczyski, Ma, et al., 2016). In Canada, an estimated 300 people are bitten each year, with none dying from the bite. Across the globe, more than 400,000 snakebites occur each year with a 5% mortality rate (Smith, Sammons, Carr, et al. 2014). Children between 1 and 9 years of age are the most likely victims (Maclean, 2016). The greatest number of bites occurs during the daylight hours and early evening of the summer months. The most frequent poisonous snakebite in the United States occurs from Crotalidae, otherwise called pit vipers, such as water moccasins, copperheads, and rattlesnakes. The most common site is the upper extremity (ENA, 2013). Of pit viper bites, 75% to 80% result in **envenomation** (injection of a poisonous material by sting, spine, bite, or other means); the rest result in what are called *dry bites* (Tintinalli et al., 2016). Venomous snakebites are medical

emergencies. In Canada of the 26 native species of snakes, only four are venomous.
2. The northern pacific rattlesnake—also known as the western rattlesnake, in British Columbia.
3. The massasauga in the Georgian Bay area of Ontario.
4. The prairie rattlesnake in southern Saskatchewan and Alberta.

The desert nightsnake, a rare species, found only in the southern Okanagan valley of British Columbia. Though considered venomous, it is only potent enough to kill small prey (Orkin Canada, 2018).

Nineteen different species of venomous snakes are found in various regions within the United States. Nurses should be familiar with the types of snakes common to the geographic region in which they practice. However, the exotic pet industry sells atypical snakes as "pets." Because of this, venomous snakes such as cobras and asps may be found outside of their native region (Maclean, 2016).

Clinical Manifestations

Snake venom consists primarily of proteins and has a broad range of physiologic effects. It may affect multiple organ systems, especially the neurologic, cardiovascular, and respiratory systems.

Classic clinical signs of envenomation are edema, ecchymosis, and hemorrhagic bullae, leading to necrosis at the site of envenomation. Symptoms include lymph node tenderness, nausea, vomiting, numbness, and a metallic taste in the mouth. Without decisive treatment, these clinical manifestations may progress to include fasciculations, hypotension, paresthesias, seizures, and coma (Smith et al., 2014).

Management

Initial first aid at the site of the snakebite includes having the person lie down, removing constrictive items such as rings, providing warmth, cleansing the wound, covering the wound with a light sterile dressing, and immobilizing the injured body part below the level of the heart. Airway, breathing, and circulation are the priorities of care. Ice, incision and suction, or a tourniquet is *not* applied. Tetanus and analgesia should be given as necessary. Initial evaluation in the ED is performed quickly and includes information about the following:

- Whether the snake was venomous or nonvenomous; discourage bringing the snake for identification—even a dead snake's venom is poisonous. Do *not* handle any snake brought to the ED. If the snake is transported to the ED, caution should be taken because the snake is frequently in a stunned, not dead, state. The bite reflex can remain intact for up to 90 minutes after the death of the snake (Auerbach, 2017).
- Where and when the bite occurred and the circumstances of the bite.
- Sequence of events, signs, and symptoms (fang punctures, pain, edema, and erythema of the bite and nearby tissues).
- Severity of poisonous effects. Call the local poison control phone number to gain access to information about an exotic snakebite presentation and management, as necessary. The poison control centre may also be able to assist with retrieving antivenin for these particular species (Smith et al., 2014).
- Vital signs.
- Circumference of the bitten extremity or area at several points. The circumference of the extremity that was bitten is compared with the circumference of the opposite extremity.
- Laboratory data (complete blood count, urinalysis, and coagulation studies).

The course and prognosis of snakebite injuries depend on the kind and amount of venom injected; where on the body the bite occurred; and the general health, age, and size of the patient. There is no one specific protocol for treatment of snakebites. In general, ice, tourniquets, heparin, and corticosteroids are not used during the acute stage. Corticosteroids are contraindicated in the first 6 to 8 hours after the bite because they may depress antibody production and hinder the action of **antivenin** (antitoxin manufactured from the snake venom and used to treat snakebites).

Parenteral fluids may be used to treat hypotension. If vasopressors are used to treat hypotension, their use should be short term. Surgical exploration of the bite is rarely indicated. Typically, the patient is observed closely for at least 6 hours. The patient is *never* left unattended.

Administration of Antivenin (Antitoxin)

Although envenomation does not always occur, it should always be suspected with snakebites. An assessment of progressive signs and symptoms is essential before considering administration of antivenin, which is most effective if given within 4 hours and no greater than 12 hours after the snakebite. The decision to administer antivenin depends on worsening tissue injury and evidence of systemic and coagulopathic symptoms. Rattlesnakes are more likely to cause coagulation abnormalities as well as more systemic effects. Coagulation abnormalities are not restricted to severe envenomation (Auerbach, 2017).

The most readily available antivenin in the United States and Canada is Crotalidae polyvalent immune Fab antivenom (FabAV or CroFab) (Auerbach, 2017). The dose depends on the type of snake and the estimated severity of the bite. Indications for antivenin depend on the progression of symptoms, including coagulopathy and systemic reaction.

Crotalidae polyvalent immune Fab antivenom does not require pretesting (i.e., skin sensitivity screening for an allergic reaction), albeit monitoring for a hypersensitivity reaction is still necessary. Outside of the United States, however, other antivenin formulas that may be commercially available may still result in severe serum sickness. If the dose exceeds 10 vials, serum sickness will most likely occur. Serum sickness is a type of hypersensitivity response that results in fever, arthralgias, pruritus, lymphadenopathy, and proteinuria and can progress to neuropathies (Auerbach, 2017). However, FabAV must be given cautiously to patients receiving anticoagulation therapy. Administration of FabAV may result in a recurring coagulopathy. The dosage and administration of FabAV are different from previously manufactured types of antivenin and should be reviewed carefully before the medication is given.

Before administering antivenin and every 15 minutes thereafter, the circumference of the affected part is measured. Premedication with diphenhydramine (Benadryl) or cimetidine (Tagamet) may be indicated, because these antihistamines may decrease the allergic response to antivenin. Antivenin is given as an IV infusion whenever possible, although intramuscular administration can be used.

Depending on the severity of the snakebite, the antivenin is diluted in 500 to 1,000 mL of normal saline solution. The infusion is started slowly, and the rate is increased after 10 minutes if there is no reaction. The total dose should be infused during the first 4 to 6 hours after the bite. The initial dose is repeated until symptoms decrease, after which time the circumference of the affected part should be measured every 30 to 60 minutes for the next 48 hours to detect symptoms of compartment syndrome (swelling, loss of pulse, increased pain, and paresthesias).

There is no limit to the number of antivenin vials that can be given. The decision to continue to administer vials is based upon patient symptoms. Consultation with a snakebite expert is essential at this point; this consultant may be identified and found through contacting the Poison Control Centre (see Resources section) or a local zoo reptile centre. The most common cause of allergic reaction to the antivenin is too-rapid infusion. Reactions may consist of a feeling of fullness in the face, urticaria, pruritus, malaise, and apprehension. These symptoms may be followed by tachycardia, shortness of breath, hypotension, and shock. In this situation, the infusion should be stopped immediately and IV diphenhydramine given. Vasopressors are used for patients in shock, and resuscitation equipment must be on standby while antivenin is infusing. It is important to note that serum sickness (hypersensitivity) can occur within the first few weeks after discharge. The patient and the patient's family members should be educated about the clinical manifestations of serum sickness (i.e., fever; rash starting on the chest and spreading to the back; arthralgia; GI disturbances [e.g., nausea, vomiting, diarrhea, abdominal pain], and headache) and return to the ED if they occur (Auerbach, 2017; Tintinalli et al., 2016).

Spider Bites

There are two venomous spiders found in the United States and Canada that may interact with humans: the brown recluse and the black widow. Both are usually found in dark places such as closets, woodpiles, and attics, as well as in shoes (ENA, 2013).

Brown recluse spider bites are painless. Systemic effects such as fever and chills, nausea and vomiting, malaise, and joint pain develop within 24 to 72 hours. The site of the bite may appear reddish to purple in colour within 2 to 8 hours after the bite. Necrosis occurs in the next 2 to 4 days in approximately 10% of cases. The centre of the bite may become necrotic, and surgical débridement may be necessary. Wound care consists of cleansing with soap and water, and hyperbaric oxygen treatments may be helpful. Most wounds heal within 2 to 3 months (ENA, 2013; Tintinalli et al., 2016).

Black widow spider bites feel like pinpricks. Systemic effects usually occur within 30 minutes—much more rapidly than with brown recluse spider bites. Signs and symptoms include abdominal rigidity, nausea and vomiting, hypertension, tachycardia, and paresthesias. Severe pain also develops within 60 minutes and increases over 1 to 2 days. Treatment involves application of ice to the site to decrease swelling and discomfort, along with elevation and assessment of tetanus immunization status. Analgesic agents and benzodiazepines may relieve muscle spasms. Cardiopulmonary monitoring is essential. Antivenin is effective for severe black widow spider bites. This antivenin is horse serum based; therefore, testing for sensitivity must be performed prior to administration (Auerbach, 2017; ENA, 2013).

Tick Bites

Tick bites are common in many areas of Canada, and they usually occur in grassy or wooded areas. It is important to learn the place where the bite occurred as well as the location of the bite on the body. The patient may demonstrate weakness; joint pain; skin rash, especially on the palms and soles of feet; headache; and fever. Ticks can carry diseases such as Rocky Mountain spotted fever, tularemia, and Lyme disease. The tick bite itself is not usually the problem; rather, it is the pathogen transmitted by the tick that can cause serious disease. The tick should be removed with tweezers using a straight upward pull (see Fig. 73-4), and the patient should be informed of the signs and symptoms of diseases carried by ticks, especially if the patient lives in an area endemic for tick-related diseases (e.g., Lyme disease).

Lyme disease has three stages. Stage I presents with a "bull's eye" rash (i.e., erythema migrans) that typically can be found in the axilla, groin, or thigh area and that appears within 4 weeks after the tick bite, with a peak manifestation time of 7 days after the bite. Classically, this rash is at least 5 cm in diameter with bright red borders. It is accompanied by flulike signs and symptoms that may include chills, fever, myalgia, fatigue, and headache. Without treatment, the rash subsides within 3 to 4 weeks. However, the rash and flulike manifestations can be significantly reduced within days if prompt treatment with antibiotics is initiated. If antibiotics are not administered, stage II Lyme disease may present within 4 to 10 weeks following the tick bite and may manifest with joint pain, memory loss, poor motor coordination, and meningitis. Stage III can begin anywhere from weeks to more than a year after the bite and has serious long-term chronic sequelae, including arthritis, neuropathy, myalgia, and myocarditis.

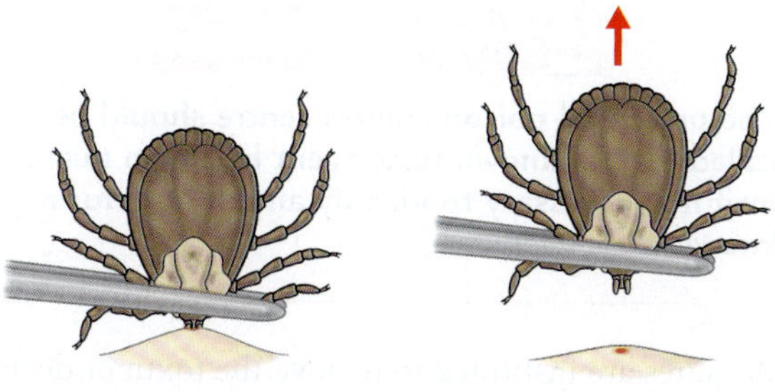

FIGURE 73-4. Removal of tick with tweezers using a straight upward pull.

POISONING

A poison is any substance that, when ingested, inhaled, absorbed, applied to the skin, or produced within the body in relatively small amounts, injures the body by its chemical action. Poisoning from inhalation and ingestion of toxic materials, both intentional and unintentional, constitutes a major health hazard and an emergency situation. Emergency treatment is initiated with the following goals:

- To remove or inactivate the poison before it is absorbed
- To provide supportive care in maintaining vital organ function
- To administer a specific antidote to neutralize a specific poison
- To implement treatment that hastens the elimination of the absorbed poison

Ingested (Swallowed) Poisons

Swallowed poisons may be corrosive. **Corrosive poisons** include alkaline and acid agents that can cause tissue destruction after coming in contact with mucous membranes. Alkaline products include lye, drain cleaners, toilet bowl cleaners, bleach, nonphosphate detergents, oven cleaners, and button batteries (batteries used to power watches, calculators, or cameras). Acid products include toilet bowl cleaners, pool cleaners, metal cleaners, rust removers, and battery acid.

Control of the airway, ventilation, and oxygenation are essential. In the absence of cerebral or renal damage, the patient's prognosis depends largely on successful management of respiration and circulation. Measures are instituted to stabilize cardiovascular and other body functions. ECG, vital signs, and neurologic status are monitored closely for changes. Shock may result from the cardiodepressant action of the substance ingested, from venous pooling in the lower extremities, or from reduced circulating blood volume resulting from increased capillary permeability. An indwelling urinary catheter is inserted to monitor renal function. Blood specimens are obtained to determine the concentration of a drug or poison.

Efforts are made to determine what substance was ingested; the amount; the time since ingestion; signs and symptoms, such as pain or burning sensations, any evidence of redness or burn in the mouth or throat, pain on swallowing or an inability to swallow, vomiting, or drooling; age and weight of the patient; and pertinent health history.

NURSING ALERT

The provincial poison control centre should be called if an unknown toxic agent has been taken or if it is necessary to identify an antidote for a known toxic agent.

Measures are instituted to remove the toxin or decrease its absorption. The patient who has ingested a corrosive poison, which can be a strong acid or alkaline substance, is given water or milk to drink for dilution. However, dilution is not attempted if the patient has acute airway edema or obstruction or if there is clinical evidence of esophageal, gastric, or intestinal burn or perforation. The following gastric emptying procedures may be used as prescribed:

- Syrup of ipecac to induce vomiting in the alert patient (*never* use with corrosive poisons)
- Gastric lavage for the obtunded patient (Chart 73-10); gastric aspirate is saved and sent to the laboratory for testing (toxicology screens)
- Activated charcoal administration if the poison is one that is absorbed by charcoal Cathartic, when appropriate

NURSING ALERT

Vomiting is NEVER induced after ingestion of caustic substances (acid or alkaline) or petroleum distillates.

If there is a specific chemical or physiologic antagonist (antidote), it is administered as early as possible to reverse or diminish the effects of the toxin. If this measure is ineffective, procedures may be initiated to remove the ingested substance. These procedures include administration of multiple doses of charcoal, diuresis (for substances excreted by the kidneys), dialysis, or hemoperfusion. Hemoperfusion involves detoxification of the blood by processing it through an extracorporeal circuit and an adsorbent cartridge containing charcoal or resin, after which the cleansed blood is returned to the patient.

Throughout detoxification, the patient's vital signs, CVP, and fluid and electrolyte balance are monitored closely. Hypotension and cardiac dysrhythmias are possible. Seizures are also possible because of CNS stimulation from the poison or from oxygen deprivation. If the patient reports pain, analgesics are administered cautiously. Severe pain causes vasomotor collapse and reflex inhibition of usual physiologic functions.

After the patient's condition has stabilized and discharge is imminent, written material is given to the patient indicating the signs and symptoms of potential issues related to the poison ingested and signs or symptoms requiring evaluation by a physician. If poisoning was determined to be a suicide or self-harm attempt, a psychiatric consultation should be requested before the patient is discharged. In cases of inadvertent poison ingestion, poison prevention and home poison-proofing instructions is provided to the patient and family.

Carbon Monoxide Poisoning

Carbon monoxide poisoning may occur as a result of industrial or household incidents or attempted suicide. It is implicated in more deaths than any other toxin except alcohol. Carbon monoxide exerts its toxic effect by binding to circulating hemoglobin and thereby reducing the oxygen-carrying capacity of the blood. Hemoglobin absorbs carbon monoxide 200 times more readily than it absorbs oxygen. Carbon monoxide–bound hemoglobin, called **carboxyhemoglobin**, does not transport oxygen.

CHART 73-10

GUIDELINES for Assisting With Gastric Lavage

Gastric lavage is the aspiration of stomach contents and washing out of the stomach by means of a large-bore gastric tube. Gastric lavage is contraindicated after acid or alkali ingestion, in the presence of seizures, or after ingestion of hydrocarbons or petroleum distillates. It is particularly dangerous after ingestion of strong corrosive agents.

Purposes

- For urgent removal of ingested substance to decrease systemic absorption
- To empty the stomach before endoscopic procedures
- To diagnose gastric hemorrhage and to arrest hemorrhage

Equipment

- Large-bore Levin tubes or large-bore Ewald tube
- Large irrigating syringe with adapter
- Large plastic funnel with adapter to fit tube
- Water-soluble lubricant
- Tap water or appropriate antidote (milk, saline solution, sodium bicarbonate solution, fruit juice, activated charcoal)
- Container for aspirate; suction apparatus
- Nasotracheal or endotracheal tubes with inflatable cuffs
- Containers for specimens

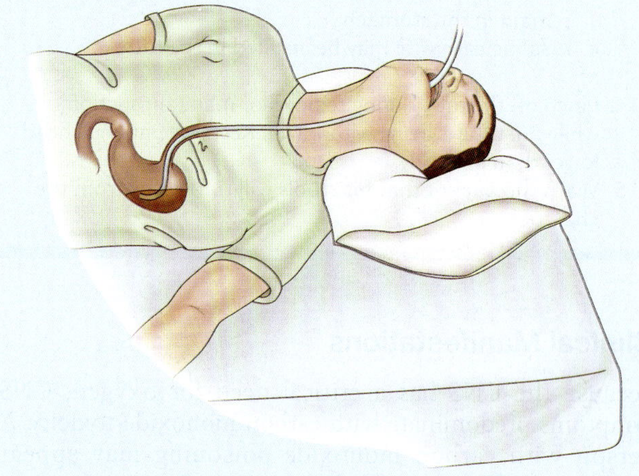

During gastric lavage, the patient is positioned on the left side, which allows the gastric contents to pool and decreases the passage of fluid into the duodenum.

ACTION	RATIONALE
1. Remove dentures and inspect the oral cavity for loose teeth.	1. This will prevent aspiration of teeth.
2. Measure the distance between the tip of the nose and the xiphoid process. Mark the tube with indelible pencil or tape.	2. This distance is a rule-of-thumb measurement of the distance the tube must be passed to reach the stomach. This avoids curling and kinking of excess tubing in the stomach.
3. Lubricate the tube with water-soluble lubricant.	3. Lubrication eases insertion of the tube.
4. If comatose, the patient is intubated with a cuffed nasotracheal or endotracheal tube before placement of the nasogastric tube.	4. A cuffed nasotracheal or endotracheal tube decreases the risk of aspiration of gastric contents.
5. Place the patient in a left lateral position with the head lowered about 15 degrees.	5. This position decreases passage of gastric contents into the duodenum during lavage.
6. Pass the tube orally while keeping the patient's head in a neutral position. Pass the tube to the adhesive marking. Encourage patient to swallow to assist with passage of the tube. Then lower the head of the stretcher or bed. Have standby suction available.	6. The depth of insertion of the tube varies according to the size of the patient. If the tube enters the trachea instead of the esophagus, the patient will experience coughing, dyspnea, stridor, and cyanosis. Positive confirmation of tube placement is accomplished by x-ray.
7. Aspirate the stomach contents with the syringe attached to the tube before instilling water or an antidote. Save the specimen for analysis. Ensure correct placement before installation.	7. Aspiration is carried out to determine that the tube is in the stomach and to remove the stomach contents. Positive confirmation of tube placement is accomplished by x-ray.
8. Remove the syringe. Attach the funnel to the end of the tube, or use a 50-mL syringe to instill solution in the gastric tube. The volume of fluid placed in the stomach should be small.	8. Overfilling of the stomach may cause regurgitation and aspiration or force the stomach contents through the pylorus.
9. Elevate the funnel above the patient's head and pour 150 to 200 mL of solution into the funnel.	9. Gravity allows the solution to flow into the tube.
10. Lower the funnel and siphon the gastric contents into the container or connect to suction.	10. The fluid should flow in freely and drain by gravity.
11. Save samples of the first two washings.	11. Keep the first washing sample isolated from other washings for toxicologic analysis.
12. Repeat the lavage procedure until the returns are relatively clear and no particulate matter is seen.	12. This usually requires a total volume of at least 2 L; some clinicians advocate the use of 5 to 20 L.

continued >

GUIDELINES for Assisting With Gastric Lavage (Continued)

ACTION	RATIONALE
13. At the completion of lavage:	13.
a. The stomach may be left empty.	a. The stomach is kept empty if no further medications are required.
b. An adsorbent (powder form of activated charcoal mixed with water to form a liquid the consistency of thick soup) may be instilled in the tube and allowed to remain in the stomach.	b. Activated charcoal reduces absorption by adsorbing (attaching to its surface) a wide range of substances; it renders the poison inaccessible to the circulation, thereby reducing its toxicity.
c. A saline cathartic may be instilled in the tube.	c. A cathartic may be given to hasten the elimination of remaining ingested material.
14. Pinch off the tube during removal or maintain suction while the tube is being withdrawn. Keep the patient's head lower than the body.	14. Pinching off the tube prevents aspiration and the initiation of the gag reflex. Keeping the patient's head lower than the body also helps to prevent initiation of the gag reflex.
15. Warn the patient that his stools will turn black from the charcoal.	15. Patient teaching is important to reduce anxiety.

Clinical Manifestations

Because the CNS has a critical need for oxygen, CNS symptoms predominate with carbon monoxide toxicity. A person with carbon monoxide poisoning may appear intoxicated (from cerebral hypoxia). Other signs and symptoms include headache, muscular weakness, palpitation, dizziness, and confusion, which can progress rapidly to coma. Skin colour, which can range from pink or cherry red to cyanotic and pale, is **NOT** a reliable sign. Pulse oximetry is also **NOT** valid, because the hemoglobin is well saturated. It is not saturated with oxygen, but the pulse oximeter indicates only if the hemoglobin is saturated; in this case, it is saturated with carbon monoxide rather than with oxygen.

Management

Carbon monoxide poisoning requires immediate treatment. Goals of management are to reverse cerebral and myocardial hypoxia and to hasten elimination of carbon monoxide. Whenever a patient inhales a poison, the following general measures apply:

- Carry the patient to fresh air immediately; open all doors and windows.
- Loosen all tight clothing.
- Initiate cardiopulmonary resuscitation if required; administer 100% oxygen.
- Prevent chilling; wrap the patient in blankets.
- Keep the patient as quiet as possible.
- Do not give alcohol in any form or permit the patient to smoke.

In addition, for the patient with carbon monoxide poisoning, carboxyhemoglobin levels are analyzed on arrival in the ED and before treatment with oxygen if possible. Oxygen at 100% is administered at atmospheric or preferably hyperbaric pressures to reverse hypoxia and accelerate the elimination of carbon monoxide. Oxygen is administered until the carboxyhemoglobin level is less than 5%. The patient is monitored continuously. Psychoses, spastic paralysis, ataxia, visual disturbances, and deterioration of mental status and behaviour may persist after resuscitation and may be symptoms of permanent brain damage.

When unintentional carbon monoxide poisoning occurs, the health department should be contacted so that the dwelling or building in question can be inspected. A psychiatric consultation is warranted if poisoning was determined to be a suicide attempt.

Skin Contamination Poisoning (Chemical Burns)

Skin contamination injuries from exposure to chemicals are challenging because of the large number of possible offending agents with diverse actions and metabolic effects. The severity of a chemical burn is determined by the mechanism of action, the penetrating strength and concentration, and the amount and duration of exposure of the skin to the chemical.

The skin should be drenched immediately with running water from a shower, hose, or faucet, except in the case of lye and white phosphorus, which should be brushed off the skin, dry.

> **NURSING ALERT**
>
> **Water should not be applied to burns from lye or white phosphorus because of the potential for an explosion or for deepening of the burn. All evidence of these chemicals should be brushed off the patient before any flushing occurs.**

The skin should be flushed with a constant stream of water as the patient's clothing is removed. The skin of health care personnel assisting the patient should be appropriately protected if the burn is extensive or if the agent is significantly toxic or is still present. Prolonged lavage with generous amounts of tepid water is important.

Attempts to determine the identity and characteristics of the chemical agent are necessary in order to specify future treatment. The standard burn treatment appropriate for the size and location of the wound (antimicrobial treatment, débridement, tetanus prophylaxis, antidote administration as prescribed) is instituted (see Chapter 59). The patient may require plastic surgery for further wound management. The patient is instructed to have the affected area reexamined at 24 and 72 hours and in 7 days because of the risk of underestimating the extent and depth of these types of injuries. Some urban centres will have outpatient burn clinics that will manage the patient post burn.

Food Poisoning

Food poisoning is a sudden illness that occurs after ingestion of contaminated food or drink. Botulism is a serious form of food poisoning that requires continual surveillance. Assessment questions for patients with food poisoning are discussed in Chart 73-11.

The key to treatment is determining the source and type of food poisoning. If possible, the suspected food should be brought to the medical facility and a history obtained from the patient or family.

Food, gastric contents, vomitus, serum, and feces are collected for examination. The patient's respirations, blood pressure, level of consciousness, CVP (if indicated), and muscular activity are monitored closely. Measures are instituted to support the respiratory system. Death from respiratory paralysis can occur with botulism, fish poisoning, and some other food poisonings.

Because large volumes of electrolytes and water are lost by vomiting and diarrhea, fluid and electrolyte status must be assessed. Severe vomiting produces alkalosis, and severe diarrhea produces acidosis. Hypovolemic shock may also occur from severe fluid and electrolyte losses. The patient is assessed for signs and symptoms of fluid and electrolyte imbalances, including lethargy, rapid pulse rate, fever, oliguria, anuria, hypotension, and delirium. Weight and serum electrolyte levels are obtained for future comparisons.

CHART 73-11

Assessment: Food Poisoning

Use the following questions to elicit information about the circumstances surrounding the possibility of food poisoning:

- How soon after eating did the symptoms occur? (Immediate onset suggests chemical, plant, or animal poisoning.)
- What was eaten in the previous meal? Did the food have an unusual odour or taste? (Most foods causing bacterial poisoning *do not* have unusual odour or taste.)
- Did anyone else become ill from eating the same food?
- Did vomiting occur? What was the appearance of the vomitus?
- Did diarrhea occur? (Diarrhea is usually absent with botulism and with shellfish or other fish poisoning.)
- Are any neurologic symptoms present? (These occur in botulism and in chemical, plant, and animal poisoning.)
- Does the patient have a fever? (Fever is characteristic in salmonella, ingestion of fava beans, and some fish poisoning.)

Measures to control nausea are also important to prevent vomiting, which could exacerbate fluid and electrolyte imbalances. An antiemetic medication is administered parenterally as prescribed if the patient cannot tolerate fluids or medications by mouth. For mild nausea, the patient is encouraged to take sips of weak tea, carbonated drinks, or tap water. After nausea and vomiting subside, clear liquids are usually prescribed for 12 to 24 hours, and the diet is gradually progressed to a low-residue, bland diet.

SUBSTANCE ABUSE

Substance abuse is the misuse of specific substances, such as drugs or alcohol, to alter mood or behaviour. Drug abuse is the use of drugs for other than legitimate medical purposes. People who abuse drugs often take a variety of drugs simultaneously (such as alcohol, barbiturates, opioids, and tranquilizers), and the combination may have additive and addictive effects. "Rave" parties are large-scale parties attended by hundreds of people, often teenagers, involved in drug use. At these events, one of the most commonly used drugs is 3,4-methylenedioxymethamphetamine (MDMA), or Ecstasy, a methamphetamine-based drug that users believe produces a "harmless high." ED nurses should be aware of "rave" parties in their geographic area so they can prepare for a potential influx of patients who abuse this drug. Others may combine Ecstasy with sildenafil (Viagra); this drug combination is nicknamed "sextasy." People who abuse IV/injection drugs are at increased risk for HIV infection, acquired immunodeficiency syndrome (AIDS), hepatitis B and C, and tetanus.

Clinical manifestations vary with the substance used, but the underlying principles of management are essentially the same. Table 73-1 identifies commonly abused drugs, listing their clinical manifestations and therapeutic management. Treatment goals for a patient with a drug overdose are to support the respiratory and cardiovascular functions, to enhance clearance of the agent, and to provide for safety of the patient and staff.

Opioid abuse and related deaths have become a crisis in Canada recently. Between January 2016 and June 2018, more than 9,000 opioid related deaths were reported (Government of Canada, 2018). In 2017, an average of 17 people per day in Canada were hospitalized due to an opioid overdose, and smaller communities saw a 2.5 times higher rate of hospitalizations for opioid overdoses than Canada's largest cities (Government of Canada, 2018). Canadians aged 20 to 29 are the highest group to suffer from an opioid related overdose; 71% of them will be male (Government of Canada, 2018). In general, western provinces (British Columbia, Alberta and Saskatchewan) and Ontario have higher rates of opioid-related deaths when compared to the rest of the country (Government of Canada, 2018).

Acute Alcohol Intoxication

Alcohol is a psychotropic drug that affects mood, judgment, behaviour, concentration, and consciousness. There is a high prevalence of alcoholism among ED patients.

(text continued on page 2370)

TABLE 73-1 Emergency Management of Patients With Drug Overdose

Drug	Clinical Manifestations	Therapeutic Management
Cocaine *Routes may include:* • Intranasally ("snorting")—inhaled into nostrils through straws • By smoking ("freebasing")—cocaine hydrochloride dissolved in ether to yield a pure cocaine alkaloid base ("crack," "rocks"); smoking in a small pipe delivers large quantities of cocaine to lungs. • IV • Polysubstance (cocaine and heroin)	Cocaine is a CNS stimulant that can cause: • Increased heart rate and blood pressure • Hyperpyrexia • Seizures • Sluggish, dilated pupillary response • Muscle rigidity • Increased energy, agitation, aggression • Ventricular dysrhythmias • Intense euphoria, then anxiety, sadness, insomnia, and sexual indifference • Cocaine hallucinations with delusions • Psychosis with extreme paranoia and ideas of persecution • Hypervigilance Chronic psychotic symptoms may persist. Overall psychotic symptoms are short-lived compared to methamphetamines	1. Maintain airway and provide respiratory support. 2. Control seizures. 3. Monitor cardiovascular effects; have antiarrhythmic drugs and defibrillator available. 4. Treat for hyperthermia. 5. If cocaine was ingested, evacuate stomach contents and use activated charcoal to treat. Whole bowel irrigation may be necessary to treat body packers ("mules"). 6. Refer for psychiatric evaluation and treatment in an inpatient unit that eliminates access to the drug. Include drug rehabilitation counselling.
Opioids Heroin Opium or paregoric Morphine, codeine, semisynthetic derivatives: oxycodone (OxyContin), methadone, meperidine (Demerol), tramadol (Ultram), fentanyl (Sublimaze)	Acute intoxication (overdose) can result in: • Pinpoint pupils (may be dilated with severe hypoxia) • Decreased blood pressure • Marked respiratory depression/arrest • Pulmonary edema • Stupor → coma • Seizures Fresh needle marks along course of any superficial vein Skin abscesses (from "popping")	1. Support respiratory and cardiovascular functions. 2. Establish IV lines; obtain blood for chemical and toxicologic analysis. Patient may be given bolus of glucose to eliminate possibility of hypoglycemia. 3. Administer narcotic antagonist (naloxone hydrochloride IV, IM [Narcan]) as prescribed to reverse severe respiratory depression and coma. 4. Continue to monitor level of responsiveness and respirations, pulse, and blood pressure. Duration of action of naloxone hydrochloride is shorter than that of heroin; repeated dosages may be necessary. 5. Send urine for analysis; opioids can be detected in urine. 6. Obtain an ECG. 7. Do not leave patient unattended; he or she may lapse back into coma rapidly. Clinical status may change from minute to minute. Hemodialysis may be indicated for severe drug intoxication. Activated charcoal may be considered if opioids were taken orally and if the patient is alert. 8. Monitor for pulmonary edema, which is frequently seen in patients who abuse/overdose on narcotics. 9. Refer patient for psychiatric and drug rehabilitation evaluation before discharge.
Barbiturates Pentobarbital (Nembutal), secobarbital (Seconal), amobarbital (Amytal), gamma-hydroxybutyrate (GHB, "liquid Ecstasy")	*Acute intoxication (may mimic alcohol intoxication):* • Respiratory depression • Flushed face • Decreased pulse rate; decreased blood pressure • Increasing nystagmus (to vertical and horizontal gaze) • Sluggish pupils • Lack of convergence of eyes • Depressed deep tendon reflexes • Decreasing mental alertness • Difficulty in speaking • Poor motor coordination and flaccid muscles • Coma, death *GHB:* • Sexual disinhibition • Amnesia, myoclonus, agitation • Overdoses when mixed with alcohol	1. Maintain airway and provide respiratory support. 2. Endotracheal intubation or tracheostomy is considered if there is any doubt about the adequacy of airway exchange. a. Check airway frequently. b. Perform suctioning as necessary. 3. Support cardiovascular and respiratory functions; most deaths result from respiratory depression or shock. 4. Start infusion through large-gauge needle or IV catheter to support blood pressure; coma and dehydration result in hypotension and respond to infusion of IV fluids with elevation of blood pressure. 5. Evacuate stomach contents or lavage if within 1 hour of ingestion to prevent absorption; repeated doses of activated charcoal may be given. 6. Assist with hemodialysis for patient with severe overdose. 7. Maintain neurologic and vital sign flow sheet. 8. Patient awakening from overdose may demonstrate combative behaviour. 9. Refer for psychiatric and drug rehabilitation consultation to evaluate suicide potential and drug abuse.

TABLE 73-1 Emergency Management of Patients With Drug Overdose (Continued)

Drug	Clinical Manifestations	Therapeutic Management
Inhalants		
Amyl nitrate Freon Propane Trichloroethylene Gasoline Perchloroethylene Toluene (metallic paint spray) HeliumCanned air Hand sanitizer *Routes may include:* • Sniffing/snorting—direct inhalation of fumes • "Bagging"—sniff from a bag • "Huffing"—sniff from a rag/cloth • "Dusting"—direct spray into the nostrils	Effects mimic those of alcohol, with dizziness and imbalance: • Euphoria, headache, disinhibition, altered level of consciousness to coma • Renal, hepatic, and cardiac toxicity • Aplastic anemia • Fetal growth retardation • Respiratory depression, arrest from CNS depression • Vasodilation • Nosebleeding • Vertical and horizontal nystagmus • Lack of convergence of eyes • Sluggish pupils • Temperature fluctuations • Circumoral red spots/rash • Air embolus	1. Provide airway support, ventilation, and oxygen. 2. Treat cardiac dysrhythmias and hypotension. 3. Provide advanced cardiac life support as needed. 4. Monitor for profound hypotension when amyl nitrate is combined with MDMA and sildenafil or with anesthetic agents. 5. Monitor for hypertension when volatile solvents used.
Amphetamine-Type Drugs (pep pills, "uppers," "speed," "crystal meth")		
amphetamine (Benzedrine) dextroamphetamine (Dexedrine) methamphetamine (Desoxyn, "speed") 3,4-methylenedioxymethamphetamine (MDMA) ("Ecstasy," "Adam")[a] 3,4-methylenedioxy-*N*-ethylamphetamine (MDEA) ("Eve") 3,4-methylenedioxyamphetamine (MDA); methylphenidate (Ritalin) "ice," "rocks," "crystal meth" 3,4-methylenedioxypyrovalerone (MDPV) or 4-methylmethcathinone (mephedrone); "Bath salts" (synthetic stimulant)	• Nausea, vomiting, anorexia • Palpitations, tachycardia • Increased blood pressure • Tachypnea, anxiety • Nervousness • Diaphoresis, mydriasis • Repetitive or stereotyped behaviour • Irritability, insomnia, agitation • Visual misperceptions, auditory hallucinations • Fearfulness, anxiety, depression, hostility, paranoia • Hyperactivity, rapid speech, euphoria, hyperalertness • Decreased inhibition • Seizures, coma, hyperthermia • Cardiovascular collapse • Rhabdomyolysis • MDMA is both a hallucinogenic and stimulant. • MDPV and mephedrone effects last >24 hours.	1. Provide airway support, ventilation, cardiac monitoring; insert IV line. 2. Use GI evacuation in cases of oral overdose; activated charcoal, gastric lavage if within 1 hour of ingestion. 3. Keep in calm, cool, quiet environment; elevated temperature potentiates amphetamine toxicity. Maintain normothermia, cooling the patient as necessary. 4. Administer small doses of diazepam (Valium) (IV) or haloperidol (Haldol) as prescribed for CNS and muscular hyperactivity. 5. Administer appropriate pharmacologic therapy as prescribed for severe hypertension and ventricular dysrhythmias. 6. Treat seizures with benzodiazepines (e.g., diazepam) as prescribed. 7. Treat sympathetic stimulation with beta-blocker agents as prescribed. 8. Try to communicate with patient if delusions or hallucinations are present. 9. Place in a protective environment (preferably psychiatric security room with video monitoring) to observe for suicide attempt. 10. Refer for psychiatric and drug rehabilitation evaluation.
Hallucinogens or Psychedelic-Type Drugs		

Lysergic acid diethylamide (LSD)
Phencyclidine HCl (PCP, "angel dust")
Mescaline, psilocybin
Cannabinoids (marijuana)
Ketamine ("special K")
Synthetic cannabinoids ("spice," "incense," "K2")
Butane honey oil (BHo)—"dabs," "shatter"
	• Nystagmus
	• Pupil dilation
	• *Psychedelics*
	  • Sluggish pupillary response
	  • Increased pulse and temperature
	  • Muscle rigidity
	• Mild hypertension
	• Marked confusion bordering on panic
	• Incoherence, hyperactivity
	• Withdrawn
	• Combative behaviour; delirium, mania, self-injury (lasts 6–12 hours)
	• Hallucinations, body image distortion
	• Hypertension, hyperthermia, acute kidney injury
	• Flashback—recurrence of LSD-like state without having taken the drug; may occur weeks or months after drug was taken
		1. Evaluate and maintain patient's circulation, airway, and breathing.
		2. Determine by urine or serum drug screen whether the patient has ingested hallucinogenic drug or has a toxic psychosis.
		3. Try to communicate with and reassure the patient.
		a. "Talking down" involves understanding the process through which the patient is proceeding and helping the patient overcome fears while establishing contact with reality.
		b. Remind the patient that fear is common with this problem.
		c. Reassure the patient that he is not losing his mind but is experiencing the effect of drugs and that this will wear off.
		d. Instruct the patient to keep the eyes open; this reduces the intensity of reaction.
		e. Reduce sensory stimuli by minimizing noise, lights, movement, tactile stimulation.

continued >

TABLE 73-1 Emergency Management of Patients With Drug Overdose (Continued)

Drug	Clinical Manifestations	Therapeutic Management
	• Ketamine—"out-of-body" experience; increased aggressiveness • Synthetic cannabinoids—euphoria, increased sensory experience, relaxation • Manufacturing can result in burns	4. Sedate the patient as prescribed if hyperactivity cannot be controlled; diazepam or a barbiturate may be prescribed. 5. Search for evidence of trauma; patients who use hallucinogens have a tendency to "act out" their hallucinations. 6. Manage seizures with benzodiazepines (e.g., diazepam) as necessary. 7. Observe patient closely; patient's behaviour may become hazardous. Have safety officers stationed near the patient's room. 8. Monitor for hypertensive crisis if patient has prolonged psychosis due to drug ingestion. 9. Place patient in a protected environment under proper medical supervision to prevent self-inflicted bodily harm. **Management for Phencyclidine Abuse** 1. Place patient in a calm, supportive environment to minimize stimuli; protect from self-injury. 2. Avoid talking down. 3. Do not leave patient unobserved. Treat symptoms as they occur. a. Drug effects are unpredictable and prolonged. b. Symptoms are likely to exacerbate; patient becomes out of control. 4. Refer all patients in this category for psychiatric and drug evaluation/rehabilitation.
Drugs Producing Sedation, Intoxication, or Psychological and Physical Dependence (nonbarbiturate sedatives)		
diazepam (Valium) chlordiazepoxide (Librium) oxazepam (Serax) lorazepam (Ativan) midazolam (Versed) flunitrazepam (Rohypnol, "roofies," "date rape drug")[a]	Seizures, coma, circulatory collapse, death *Acute intoxication:* • Respiratory depression • Decreasing mental alertness • Confusion • Slurred speech, decreased blood pressure • Ataxia • Pulmonary edema • Coma, death **Flunitrazepam:** • Disinhibition with antegrade amnesia • Weakness and unsteadiness with impaired judgment • Powerlessness	1. Endotracheal tube is inserted as a precaution; use assisted ventilation to stabilize and correct respiratory depression. Observe for sudden apnea and laryngeal spasm. 2. Assess for hypotension. a. Insert indwelling urinary catheter for patient who is comatose; decreased urinary volume is an index of reduced renal flow associated with reduced intravascular volume or vascular collapse. b. Start volume expansion with saline or dextrose as prescribed. 3. Evacuate stomach contents; lavage (if within 1 hour of ingestion); activated charcoal. 4. Start ECG monitoring. Observe for dysrhythmias. 5. Administer flumazenil (Romazicon), a benzodiazepine antagonist (reversal agent). 6. Refer patient for psychiatric evaluation (potential suicide intent).
Salicylate Poisoning		
Aspirin (present in compound analgesic tablets) • Toxic levels (150–200 mg/kg body weight) • Chronic toxicity (occurs in older adults due to decreased kidney function) • Long-term intoxication (>100 mg/kg/day for more than 2 days)	• Restlessness • Tinnitus, deafness • Blurring of vision • Hyperpnea • Hyperpyrexia • Sweating • Epigastric pain, vomiting • Dehydration • Respiratory alkalosis and metabolic acidosis • Disorientation, coma • Cardiovascular collapse • Coagulopathy	1. Treat respiratory depression. 2. Induce gastric emptying by lavage (if within 1 hour after ingestion). 3. Give activated charcoal to adsorb aspirin. 4. Support patient with IV infusions as prescribed to establish hydration and correct electrolyte imbalances, including administration of sodium bicarbonate. 5. Enhance elimination of salicylates as directed by forced diuresis, alkalinization of urine, peritoneal dialysis, or hemodialysis, according to severity of intoxication. 6. Monitor serum salicylate level for efficacy of treatment. 7. Administer specific prescribed pharmacologic agent for bleeding and other problems. 8. Recognize that concretions formed in the gut may result in prolonged exposure as they are digested. 9. Refer patient for psychiatric evaluation (potential suicide intent). 10. Monitor thromboelastography for platelet function.

TABLE 73-1 Emergency Management of Patients With Drug Overdose (Continued)

Drug	Clinical Manifestations	Therapeutic Management
Acetaminophen (present in prescription and nonprescription analgesics, antipyretics, and cold remedies)	Lethargy to encephalopathy and death GI upset, diaphoresis Right upper quadrant pain Abnormal liver function tests, prolonged prothrombin time, increased bilirubin, disseminated intravascular coagulation Hepatomegaly leading to liver failure Metabolic acidosis Hypoglycemia Stage I—within 24 hours; GI irritation, possible metabolic acidosis and coma if severe ingestion Stage II—24–48 hours; monitor liver and coagulation studies. Stage III—after 48 hours; hepatic encephalopathy/jaundice, vomiting, right upper quadrant pain, coagulopathy, hypoglycemia, acute kidney injury	1. Maintain airway. 2. Obtain acetaminophen level. Levels ≥140 mg/kg are toxic. 3. Laboratory studies—liver function tests, prothrombin time/partial thromboplastin time, complete blood count, blood urea nitrogen, creatinine. 4. Lavage (if within 1 hour after ingestion); activated charcoal. 5. Prepare for possible hemodialysis, which clears acetaminophen but does not halt liver damage. 6. Administer N-acetylcysteine (Mucomyst) as soon as possible. N-acetylcysteine replenishes essential liver enzymes and requires a total of 18 doses every 4 hours. Charcoal absorbs N-acetylcysteine; do not administer together. Repeat N-acetylcysteine dose if patient vomits. 7. Refer patient for psychiatric evaluation (potential suicide intent).
Tricyclic Antidepressants		
amitriptyline (Elavil) doxepin (Sinequan) nortriptyline (Aventyl) imipramine (Tofranil)	Dysrhythmia: ventricular fibrillation/tachycardia, sinus tachycardia Hypotension Pulmonary edema, hypoxemia, acidosis Confusion, agitation, coma Visual hallucinations Clonus, tremors, hyperactive reflexes, nystagmus, myoclonic jerking Seizures Blurred vision, flushing, hyperthermia	1. Provide airway support, ventilation, cardiac monitoring; insert IV line with normal saline solution. 2. If within 1–2 hours after overdose, insert a nasogastric tube and instill activated charcoal every 4 hours × 3. 3. Administer a sodium bicarbonate drip to decrease dysrhythmias; the alkaline environment increases the protein binding of the metabolite. Synchronized cardioversion may be indicated with some dysrhythmias refractory to sodium bicarbonate. Torsades de pointes should be treated with IV magnesium sulphate. 4. Administer vasopressors. 5. Manage seizure activity with benzodiazepines (e.g., diazepam) as necessary. 6. Refer patient for psychiatric evaluation for potential suicide intent and evaluation of medication regimen for effectiveness.
Selective Serotonin Reuptake Inhibitors and Other Antidepressants		
trazodone (Desyrel) fluoxetine (Prozac) paroxetine (Paxil) sertraline (Zoloft) venlafaxine (Effexor) escitalopram (Lexapro) bupropion (Wellbutrin)	Decreased level of consciousness, confusion Respiratory depression Increased heart rate Serotonin syndrome may occur if the SSRI was taken in conjunction with dextromethorphan or meperidine Agitation, seizures Hyperthermia, diaphoresis Hypertension, headache, shivering, "goose flesh," cardiac dysrhythmias, loss of consciousness	1. Administer activated charcoal with possibly whole bowel irrigation if a sustained-release medication was taken. 2. Use seizure precautions and administer benzodiazepines (e.g., diazepam) as prescribed.
Anabolic Steroids "roids," "juice," methandrostenolone, stanozolol, nandrolone Synthetic testosterone	Increase in LDL, decrease in HDL Alter carbohydrate metabolism Hyponatremia, hypokalemia Hypocalcemia/osteoporosis Mood swings/violent behaviours Invincibility, depression, potential for suicide attempts Memory loss, cognitive disabilities Immunosuppression Used to bulk up muscles, so skeletal muscle hypertrophy is a common manifestation.	1. Provide supportive therapy appropriate to patient's emotional manifestations. 2. Protect the patient from self-harm/harming others. 3. Encourage the patient to stop use; refer patient for psychiatric evaluation.

CNS, central nervous system; →, precedes; IV, intravenous; IM, intramuscular; ECG, electrocardiogram; GI, gastrointestinal; SSRI, selective serotonin reuptake inhibitor; LDL, low-density lipoprotein; HDL, high-density lipoprotein.

[a]Polydrug use at "rave clubs" frequently involves MDMA, alcohol, amphetamines, LSD, and sometimes dextromethorphan. Terms such as "Ecstasy" may refer to flunitrazepam (Rohypnol), GHB, ephedrine, and/or caffeine, in addition to MDMA.

Adapted from Emergency Nurses Association. (2013). *Sheehy's manual of emergency care* (7th ed.). St. Louis, MO: Mosby; National Institute on Drug Abuse. (2015a). Drug facts. Retrieved February 20, 2017, from www.drugabuse.gov/publications/drugfacts/; and Tintinalli, J. E., Stapczyski, J. S., Ma, O. J, et al. (2016). *Tintinalli's emergency medicine manual* (8th ed.). New York: McGraw-Hill Medical.

Because patients who abuse alcohol return frequently to the ED, they present a challenge to those who care for them. Their management requires nurses to have patience and thoughtfulness. Long-term treatment is achieved with decision-making skills, commitment, and intensive treatment programs on the patient's part (Moraleda Barreno et al., 2019).

The economic burden of alcohol-related harm accounts for approximately $14.6 billion per year in Canada (Canadian Centre on Substance Use and Addiction [CCDUS], 2019). After tobacco, alcohol is the substance that causes the most harm to Canadians (CCDUS, 2019). Aboriginal communities, youth, seniors, and pregnant woman are specifically at risk for alcohol-related harm (CCDUS, 2019).

Alcohol, or ethanol, is a multisystem toxin and CNS depressant that causes drowsiness, impaired coordination, slurring of speech, sudden mood changes, aggression, belligerence, grandiosity, and uninhibited behaviour. In excess, it can also cause stupor, coma, and death. Increasingly, underage minors and college students arrive at the ED with alcohol poisoning from binge drinking. All too frequently, the result is death.

In the ED, the patient is assessed for head injury, hypoglycemia (which mimics intoxication), and other health problems. Possible nursing diagnoses include ineffective breathing pattern related to CNS depression and risk for violence (self-directed or other-directed) related to severe intoxication from alcohol.

Treatment involves detoxification of the acute poisoning, recovery, and rehabilitation. Commonly, the patient uses mechanisms of denial and defensiveness. The nurse should approach the patient in a nonjudgmental manner, using a firm, consistent, accepting, and reasonable attitude. Speaking in a calm and slow manner is helpful because alcohol interferes with thought processes. If the patient appears intoxicated, hypoxia, hypovolemia, and neurologic impairment must be ruled out before it is assumed that the patient is intoxicated. Typically, a blood specimen is obtained for analysis of the blood alcohol level.

If drowsy, the patient should be allowed to sleep off the state of alcoholic intoxication. During this time, maintenance of a patent airway and observation for symptoms of CNS depression are essential. The patient should be undressed and kept warm with blankets. On the other hand, if the patient is noisy or belligerent, sedation may be necessary. If sedation is used, the patient should be monitored carefully for hypotension and decreased level of consciousness.

In addition, the patient is examined for alcohol withdrawal delirium and also for injuries and organic disease (such as head injury, seizures, pulmonary infections, hypoglycemia, and nutritional deficiencies) that may be masked by alcoholic intoxication. People with alcoholism suffer more injuries than the general population. Also, acute alcohol intoxication is the cause of trauma for many nonalcoholic patients. Pulmonary infections are also more common in patients with alcoholism, resulting from respiratory depression, an impaired defence system, and a tendency toward aspiration of gastric contents. The patient may show little increase in temperature or WBC count. The patient may be hospitalized or admitted to a detoxification centre in an effort to examine problems underlying the substance abuse.

Alcohol Withdrawal Syndrome/ Delirium Tremens

Alcohol withdrawal syndrome is an acute toxic state that occurs as a result of sudden cessation of alcohol intake after a bout of heavy drinking or, more typically, after prolonged intake of alcohol. Severity of symptoms depends on how much alcohol was ingested and for how long.

Patients who are heavy alcohol consumers are more likely to access health care (Wood, Albarquoni, Tkachuk, et al., 2018). Delirium tremens (DTs), the most severe type of alcohol withdrawal, may not be present in patients for up to 6 days after they present to the ED as many medications given in the ED or OR (e.g., analgesics, anaesthetics, beta blockers) may mask signs and symptoms of DTs (Efre, 2018).

Patients with alcohol withdrawal syndrome show signs of anxiety, uncontrollable fear, tremor, irritability, agitation, insomnia, and incontinence. They are talkative and preoccupied and experience visual, tactile, olfactory, and auditory hallucinations that often are terrifying. Autonomic overactivity occurs and is evidenced by tachycardia, dilated pupils, and profuse perspiration. Usually, all vital signs are elevated in the alcoholic toxic state. Delirium tremens is a life-threatening condition and carries a high mortality rate.

The goals of management are to give adequate sedation and support to allow the patient to rest and recover without danger of injury or peripheral vascular collapse. A physical examination is performed to identify pre-existing or contributing illnesses or injuries (e.g., head injury, pneumonia). A drug history is obtained to elicit information that may facilitate adjustment of any sedative requirements. Baseline blood pressure is determined, because the patient's subsequent treatment may depend on blood pressure changes.

Usually, the patient is sedated as directed with a sufficient dosage of benzodiazepines to establish and maintain sedation, which reduces agitation, prevents exhaustion, prevents seizures, and promotes sleep. The patient should be calm, able to respond, and able to maintain an airway safely on his or her own. A variety of medications and combinations of medications are used (e.g., diazepam [Valium], chlordiazepoxide [Librium], lorazepam [Ativan], and clonidine [Catapres]). Haloperidol (Haldol) or droperidol (Inapsine) may be administered for severe acute alcohol withdrawal syndrome. Dosages are adjusted according to the patient's symptoms (agitation, anxiety) and blood pressure response.

The patient is placed in a calm, nonstressful environment (usually a private room) and observed closely. The room remains lighted to minimize the potential for illusions (visual misrepresentations) and hallucinations. Homicidal or suicidal responses may result from hallucinations. Closet and bathroom doors are closed to eliminate shadows. Someone is designated to stay with the patient as much as possible. The presence of another person has a reassuring and calming effect, which helps the patient maintain contact with reality. Any visual misrepresentations (illusions) are explained in attempts to orient the patient to reality.

NURSING ALERT

Restraints are used as prescribed, if necessary, if the client is aggressive or violent, but only when other alternatives have been unsuccessful. The least restrictive device that will prevent the patient from injuring self or others is used. Caution is taken to ensure that restraints are applied properly and that they are not impairing circulation to any part of the body or interfering with respirations. Restraints should be used in tandem with verbal intervention to calm the patient and promote compliance. Restraints must be released according to protocol. Physical observation (e.g., skin integrity, circulatory status, respiratory status) is ongoing, and the patient's response is documented.

Fluid losses may result from gastrointestinal losses (vomiting), profuse perspiration, and hyperventilation. In addition, the patient may be dehydrated as a result of alcohol's effect of decreasing antidiuretic hormone. The oral or IV route is used to restore fluid and electrolyte balance.

Temperature, pulse, respiration, and blood pressure are recorded frequently (every 30 minutes in severe forms of delirium) to monitor for peripheral circulatory collapse or hyperthermia (the two most serious complications). Phenytoin (Dilantin) or other anticonvulsant medications may be prescribed to prevent repeated withdrawal seizures.

Frequently seen complications include infections (e.g., pneumonia), trauma, hepatic failure, hypoglycemia, and cardiovascular problems. Hypoglycemia may accompany alcohol withdrawal, because alcohol depletes liver glycogen stores and impairs gluconeogenesis; many patients with alcoholism also are malnourished. Parenteral dextrose may be prescribed if the liver glycogen level is depleted. Orange juice, electrolyte supplement drinks, or other sources of carbohydrates are given to stabilize the blood glucose level and counteract tremulousness. Supplemental vitamin therapy and a high-protein diet are provided as prescribed to counteract nutritional deficits. The patient should be referred to an alcoholic treatment centre for follow-up care and rehabilitation.

VIOLENCE, ABUSE, AND NEGLECT

Family Violence, Abuse, and Neglect

EDs are often the first place where victims of family violence, abuse, or neglect go to seek help.

In Canada, there has been a decline in the rate of family violence against youth and intimate partners since 2009 (Statistics Canada, 2018). Statistically, rates of physical assault among youth girls and boys is similar; however, the rate of sexual abuse is significantly higher in girls (Statistics Canada, 2018). People aged 25 to 34 are most vulnerable to intimate partner violence (Statistics Canada, 2018). It is estimated that up to one third of all patients in the ED have experienced intimate partner violence (IPV) at some point in their lives. In Canada, certain women groups are more at risk for family violence. This includes young women, Aboriginal women, women with disabilities, women with poor mental health, women who are gay or bisexual and women who live in more remote areas (Conroy, 2018). Research studies suggest that as many as 44% of all women murdered by a partner had visited an ED within the 2 years prior to death. According to self-reported data from the 2014 General Social Survey on Victimization, only 5% (1 in 20) of incidents of sexual assault were reported to police (Conroy, 2018). ED nurses need to be vigilant in their assessments of both women and men who present with injuries that may be consistent with IPV. In addition, ED nurses must be aware that men and women with disabilities are at higher risk of domestic violence and abuse than nondisabled people and should include questions to that effect in their evaluations.

In a 2015 Canadian survey, 7% to 9% of seniors 65 or older reported mistreatment of some form (McDonald, 2018). Thirty-three percent of seniors encounter family violence from their own children (Statistics Canada, 2018). There are reasons to believe that family violence against older adults is underestimated, as elders may be more hesitant than younger adults to report incidents affecting them. Data reveal that older women are more likely than older men to be abused by family members. Elder abuse takes many forms, including physical and psychological abuse, neglect, violation of personal rights, and financial abuse (see Chapter 14).

Clinical Manifestations

When people who have been abused seek treatment, they may present with physical injuries or with health concerns such as anxiety, insomnia, or gastrointestinal symptoms that are related to stress. The possibility of abuse should be investigated whenever a person presents with multiple injuries that are in various stages of healing, when injuries are unexplained, and when the explanation does not fit the physical picture (Chart 73-12). The possibility of neglect should be investigated whenever a dependent person shows evidence of inattention to hygiene, to nutrition, or to known medical needs (e.g., unfilled medication prescriptions, missed appointments with health care providers). In the ED, the most common physical injuries seen are unexplained bruises, lacerations, abrasions, head injuries, or fractures. The most common clinical manifestations of neglect are malnutrition and dehydration.

Assessment and Diagnostic Findings

Nurses in EDs are in an ideal position to provide early detection and interventions for victims of IPV. This requires an acute awareness of the signs of possible abuse, maltreatment, and neglect. Nurses must be skilled in interviewing techniques that are likely to elicit accurate information. A careful history is crucial in the screening process. Asking questions in private—away from others—may be helpful in eliciting information about abuse, maltreatment, and neglect (Chart 73-13).

Whenever evidence leads one to suspect abuse or neglect, an evaluation with careful documentation of descriptions of events and drawings or photographs of

CHART 73-12

Assessment: Assessing for Abuse, Maltreatment, and Neglect

The following questions may be helpful when assessing a patient for abuse, maltreatment, and neglect:

- I noticed that you have a number of bruises. Can you tell me how they happened? Has anyone hurt you?
- You seem frightened. Has anyone ever hurt you?
- Sometimes patients tell me that they have been hurt by someone at home or at work. Could this be happening to you?
- Are you afraid of anyone at home or work, or of anyone with whom you come in contact?
- Has anyone failed to help you to take care of yourself when you needed help?
- Has anyone prevented you from seeing friends or other people whom you wish to see?
- Have you signed any papers that you did not understand or did not wish to sign?
- Has anyone forced you to sign papers against your will?
- Has anyone forced you to engage in sexual activities within the past year?
- Has anyone prevented you from using an assistive device (e.g., wheelchair, walker) within the past year?
- Has anyone you depend on refused to help you take your medicine, bathe, groom, or eat within the past year?

injuries is important, because the medical record may be used as part of a legal proceeding. Assessment of the patient's general appearance and interactions with significant others, an examination of the entire surface area of the body, and a mental status examination are crucial.

Management

Whenever abuse, maltreatment, or neglect is suspected, the health care provider's primary concern is the safety and welfare of the patient. Treatment focuses on the consequences of the abuse, violence, or neglect and on prevention of further injury. Protocols of most EDs require that a multidisciplinary approach be used. Nurses, physicians, social workers, and community agencies work collaboratively to develop and implement a plan for meeting the patient's needs.

If the patient is in immediate danger, he or she should be separated from the abusing or neglecting person whenever possible. Referral to a shelter may be the most appropriate action, but many shelters are inaccessible to people with mobility limitations.

When abuse or neglect is the result of stress experienced by a caregiver who is no longer able to cope with the burden of caring for an older person or a person with chronic disease or a disability, respite services may be necessary. Support groups may be helpful to these caregivers. When mental illness of the abuser or neglecter is responsible for the situation, alternative living arrangements may be required.

Nurses are mindful that competent adults are free to accept or refuse the help that is offered to them. Some patients insist on remaining in the home environment where the abuse or neglect is occurring. The wishes of patients who are competent and not cognitively impaired should be respected. However, all possible alternatives, available resources, and safety plans are explored with the patient.

Mandatory reporting laws are in place in all provinces in Canada for health care workers to report *suspected* child or

NURSING RESEARCH PROFILE

Chart 73-13. Barriers to Nurses Screening for Intimate Partner Violence

DeBoer, M. I., Kothari, R., Kothari, M. A., et al. (2013). What are barriers to nurses screening for intimate partner violence? *Journal of Trauma Nursing*, *20*(3), 155–160.

Purpose

Intimate partner violence (IPV) is a common comorbidity among women who present to emergency departments (EDs) for treatment. It is estimated that between 15% and 30% of all women who present to EDs have experienced IPV within the past year, though few seek care for treatment of IPV-related injuries. Nurses are in a prime position to screen patients for IPV. The purpose of this study was to identify barriers to nurses screening patients for IPV.

Design

This was a descriptive cross-sectional study. Registered nurses (RNs) who worked in a 450-bed level 1 trauma centre and who were employed in positions that provided direct patient care were invited to anonymously complete a survey. The survey consisted of 7 demographic and 22 attitude- and knowledge-based Likert scale items. A total of 156 RNs completed the survey, after Institutional Review Board approval was obtained.

Findings

The mean age of participants ($N = 156$) was 43.2 years, with 16.8 mean years of nursing experience. The majority of participants (82.6%) reported taking care of 2 or fewer patients who had been subject to IPV within the past year. The majority (81%) affirmed their feeling that they had sufficient time to screen patients for IPV. However, nearly half (44%) disagreed that they were adequately trained to recognize signs and symptoms of IPV. The majority (95%) affirmed their belief that it is the RN's responsibility to recognize IPV. Results of knowledge-based survey items that confirmed the participants' ability to recognize IPV risks were mixed.

Nursing Implications

Most RNs who participated in this study expressed the belief that recognizing and screening patients for IPV was a key nursing role and felt that they had sufficient time to do so. However, the majority perceived that they cared for few patients with IPV within the past year, although IPV is a prevalent problem. Moreover, many felt that they lacked adequate training to screen for IPV. Many also did not correctly identify knowledge of IPV risks. Providing RNs with education that can enhance their ability to screen patients for IPV may result in earlier detection of patients who have been subjected to IPV.

elder abuse to an official agency, usually Adult (or Child) Protective Services. All that is required for reporting is the suspicion of abuse; the health care worker is not required to prove abuse or neglect. Likewise, health care workers who report suspected abuse are immune from civil or criminal liability if the report is made in good faith. Subsequent home visits resulting from the report of suspected abuse are a part of gathering information about the patient in the home environment. In addition, there are resource hotlines for use by health care workers and by patients who seek answers to questions about abuse and neglect.

Sexual Assault

The definition of *rape* is forced sexual acts, especially if these acts involve vaginal or anal penetration. Perpetrators and victims may be either male or female. Society is focused on the rights and care of people who have been sexually assaulted, and law enforcement agencies are increasingly sensitive and aggressive in managing these crimes. Rape crisis centres offer support and education and help people who have been sexually assaulted through the subsequent police investigation and courtroom experience.

The manner in which the patient is received and treated in the ED is important to his or her future psychological well-being. Crisis intervention begins when the patient enters the health care facility. The patient should be seen immediately. Most hospitals have a written protocol that addresses the patient's physical and emotional needs as well as collection of forensic evidence.

In Canada there is a growing opportunity for emergency nurses to become prepared as a sexual assault nurse examiner (SANE). Preparing for this role requires specific training in forensic evidence collection, history taking, documentation, and ways to approach the patient and family. Specialized training also includes learning proper photographic methods and the use of colposcopy. Colposcopy facilitates assessment by magnifying tissues and looking for evidence of microtrauma. Evidence is collected through photography, videography, and analysis of specimens. Another tool useful to the SANE is the light-staining microscope, which enables the examiner to identify motile and nonmotile sperm and infectious organisms. This tool saves time and also enhances assessment. The SANE complements the ED staff and they can spend more time with both the patient and police officers investigating the incident (Hugo Nielson, 2018).

Assessment and Diagnostic Findings

The patient's reaction to rape has been termed *rape trauma syndrome* and is seen as an acute stress reaction to a life-threatening situation. The nurse performing the assessment is aware that the patient may go through several phases of psychological reactions, often described as two stages: acute and long-term (King County Sexual Assault Resource Center, n.d.).

- An acute disorganization phase, which may manifest as an expressed state in which shock, disbelief, fear, guilt, humiliation, anger, and other such emotions are encountered or as a controlled state in which feelings are masked or hidden and the victim appears composed.
- A phase of denial and unwillingness to talk about the incident, followed by a phase of heightened anxiety, fear, flashbacks, sleep disturbances, hyperalertness, and psychosomatic reactions that is consistent with post-traumatic stress disorder (PTSD) (see Chapter 10 for further discussion of PTSD).
- A long-term phase of reorganization, in which the incident is put into perspective; some victims never fully recover and go on to develop chronic stress disorders and phobias.

Management

The goals of management are to provide support, to reduce the patient's emotional trauma, and to gather available evidence for possible legal proceedings. All of the interventions are aimed at encouraging the patient to gain a sense of control over his or her life.

Throughout the patient's stay in the ED, the patient's privacy and sensitivity must be respected. The patient may exhibit a wide range of emotional reactions, such as hysteria, stoicism, or feelings of being overwhelmed. Support and caring are crucial. The patient should be reassured that anxiety is natural and asked whether a support person may be called. Appropriate support is available from professional and community resources. The Rape Victim Companion Program, if available in the community, can be contacted, and the services of a volunteer can be requested. The patient should never be left alone.

Physical Examination

A written, witnessed informed consent must be obtained from the patient (or parent or guardian if the patient is a minor) for examination, for taking of photographs, and for release of findings to police. A history is obtained only if the patient has not already talked to a police officer, social worker, or crisis intervention worker. The patient should not be asked to repeat the history. Any history of the event that is obtained should be recorded in the patient's own words. The patient is asked whether he or she has bathed, douched, brushed his or her teeth, changed clothes, urinated, or defecated since the attack, because these actions may alter interpretation of subsequent findings. The time of admission, time of examination, date and time of the alleged rape, and the patient's emotional state and general appearance (including any evidence of trauma, such as discolouration, bruises, lacerations, secretions, or torn and bloody clothing) are documented.

For the physical examination, the patient is helped to undress and is draped properly. Each item of clothing is placed in a separate paper bag. Plastic bags are not used because they retain moisture; moisture may promote mould and mildew formation, which can destroy evidence. The bags are labelled and given to appropriate law enforcement authorities.

The patient is examined (from head to toe) for injuries, especially injuries to the head, neck, breasts, thighs, back, and buttocks. Body diagrams and photographs aid in documenting the evidence of trauma. The physical examination focuses on the following:

- External evidence of trauma (bruises, contusions, lacerations, stab wounds)

- Dried semen stains (appearing as crusted, flaking areas) on the patient's body or clothes
- Broken fingernails and body tissue and foreign materials under nails (if found, samples are taken)
- Oral examination, including a specimen of saliva and cultures of gum and tooth areas

Pelvic and rectal examinations are also performed. The perineum and other areas are examined with a Wood lamp or other filtered ultraviolet light. Areas that appear fluorescent may indicate semen stains. The colour and consistency of any discharge present is noted. A water-moistened rather than a lubricated vaginal speculum is used for the examination. Lubricant contains chemicals that may interfere with later forensic testing of specimens and acid phosphatase determinations. The rectum is examined for signs of trauma, blood, and semen. During the examination, the patient is advised of the nature and necessity of each procedure and given the rationale for each question asked.

Specimen Collection

During the physical examination, numerous laboratory specimens may be collected, including the following:

- Vaginal aspirate, examined for presence or absence of motile and nonmotile sperm
- Secretions (obtained with a sterile swab) from the vaginal pool for acid phosphatase, blood group antigen of semen, and precipitin test against human sperm and blood
- Separate smears from the oral, vaginal, and anal areas
- Culture of body orifices for gonorrhea
- Blood serum for syphilis and HIV testing and DNA analysis; a sample of serum for syphilis may be frozen and saved for future testing
- Pregnancy test if there is a possibility that the patient may be pregnant
- Any foreign material (leaves, grass, dirt), which is placed in a clean envelope
- Pubic hair samples obtained by combing or trimming. Several pubic hairs with follicles are placed in separate containers and identified as the patient's hair

To preserve the chain of evidence, each specimen is labelled with the name of the patient, the date and time of collection, the body area from which the specimen was obtained, and the names of personnel collecting specimens. Then the specimens are given to a designated person (e.g., forensic laboratory technician), and an itemized receipt is obtained.

Treating Potential Consequences of Rape

After the initial physical examination is completed and specimens have been obtained, any associated injuries are treated as indicated. The patient is given the option of prophylaxis against sexually transmitted infection (STI). A single oral dose of Cefixime may be prescribed as prophylaxis for gonorrhea. In addition, a single oral dose of azithromycin (if poor adherence is expected) or a 7 day course of Doxycycline may be prescribed as prophylaxis for syphilis and chlamydia (Government of Canada, 2014). Treatment for Hepatitis B and C and HIV may also be included in some cases.

Antipregnancy measures may be considered if the patient is of childbearing age (Government of Canada, 2014). A postcoital contraceptive medication, such as an oral contraceptive medication that contains levonorgestrel and ethinyl estradiol (Alesse, Seasonique), may be prescribed after a pregnancy test. To promote effectiveness, the contraceptive medication should be administered within 12 to 24 hours and no later than 72 hours after intercourse. The 21-day package rather than the 28-day package is prescribed so that the patient does not take the inert tablets by mistake. An antiemetic may be administered as prescribed to decrease discomfort from side effects. Fresh clothing and supplies for hygienic cleaning are usually offered to the patient once the collection of evidence has been completed.

Follow-Up Care

The patient is informed of counselling services to prevent long-term psychological effects. Counselling services are made available to both the patient and the family. A referral is made to the Rape Victim Companion Program, if available. Appointments for follow-up surveillance for pregnancy and for STD and HIV testing also are made.

The patient is encouraged to return to his or her previous level of functioning as soon as possible. When leaving the health care facility, the patient should be accompanied by a family member or friend.

Human Trafficking

The most rapidly growing area of criminal activity in the world is human trafficking, or modern day slavery (ENA, 2015b). Human trafficking is defined as the use of force, fraud, or coercion for the purpose of subjection to involuntary servitude (Solheim, 2016). Human trafficking may involve forced sex or labour or both. Data show approximately 20 million people are trafficked in this form of slavery, with at least 17,000 of these in the United States. These people have limited access to health care and the ED may be the only access point to identify their situation (ENA, 2015b). The statistics as of April 2012 found at https://www.publicsafety.gc.ca/cnt/rsrcs/pblctns/ntnl-ctn-pln-cmbt provide some context for the extent of human trafficking in Canada.

A victim of trafficking may present to the ED with injury, accompanied by a significantly older boyfriend or travel partner. The victim may have a history of being a chronic runaway, or of homelessness, and of self-mutilation. Common behaviours exhibited by these patients may include cowering or deferring to the person accompanying them, who may appear controlling, and appearing frightened or agitated. The patient may have a special mark/tattoo present, poor dentition, and multiple injuries in various stages of healing. Common physical complaints include injuries, poor healing or poorly healed old injuries, abdominal pain, dizziness, headaches, rashes or sores. Patients may demonstrate addiction, panic attacks, impulse control, hostility, and suicidal ideation.

The ED nurse may be well positioned to offer an opportunity for the patient to speak, alone without an accompanying companion, who could be a perpetrator of abuse. Targeted, appropriate questions may include asking patients if they are in control of their own money; whether or not they are able to come and go as they please; and who is the person or persons accompanying them (Solheim, 2016).

PSYCHIATRIC EMERGENCIES

A psychiatric emergency is an urgent, serious disturbance of behaviour, affect, or thought that makes the patient unable to cope with life situations and interpersonal relationships. A patient presenting with a psychiatric emergency may display overactive or violent, underactive or depressed, or suicidal behaviours.

The most important concern of the ED personnel is determining whether the patient is at risk for injuring self or others. The aim is to try to maintain the patient's self-esteem (and life, if necessary) while providing care. Determining whether the patient is currently under psychiatric care is important so that contact can be made with the therapist or physician who works with the patient.

Patients Who Are Overactive

Patients who display disturbed, uncooperative, and paranoid behaviour and those who feel anxious and panicky may be prone to assaultive and destructive impulses and abnormal social behaviour. Intense nervousness, depression, and crying are evident in some patients. Disturbed and noisy behaviour may be exacerbated or compounded by alcohol or drug intoxication.

A reliable source for obtaining an accurate history is needed to identify events leading to the crisis. Past mental illness, hospitalizations, injuries, serious illnesses, use of alcohol or drugs, crises in interpersonal relationships, or intrapsychic conflicts are explored. Because abnormal thoughts and behaviour may be manifestations of an underlying physical disorder, such as hypoglycemia, drug or alcohol toxicity, a stroke, a seizure disorder, or head injury, a physical assessment is also performed.

The immediate goal is to gain control of the situation. If the patient is potentially violent, security or local police should be nearby. Restraints are used as a *last* resort and only as prescribed. Approaching the patient with a calm, confident, and firm manner is therapeutic and has a calming effect. Helpful interventions include the following:

- Introduce yourself by name.
- Tell the patient, "I am here to help you."
- Repeat the patient's name from time to time.
- Speak in one-thought sentences and be consistent.
- Give the patient space and time to slow down.
- Show interest in, listen to, and encourage the patient to talk about personal thoughts and feelings.
- Offer appropriate and honest explanations.

A psychotropic agent (e.g., one that exerts an effect on the mind) may be prescribed for emergency management of functional psychosis. However, a patient with a personality disorder should not be treated with psychotropic medications, and psychotropic medications should not be used if the patient's behaviour results from the use of hallucinogens (e.g., lysergic acid diethylamide [LSD]).

Agents such as chlorpromazine and haloperidol act specifically against psychotic symptoms of thought fragmentation and perceptual and behavioural aberrations. The initial dose depends on the patient's body weight and the severity of the symptoms. After administration of the initial dose, the patient is observed closely to determine the degree of change in psychotic behaviour. Subsequent doses depend on the patient's response. Typically, after stabilization, the patient is transferred to an inpatient psychiatric unit or psychiatric outpatient treatment is arranged.

Violent Behaviour

Violent and aggressive behaviour, often episodic, is a means of expressing feelings of anger, fear, or hopelessness about a situation. Usually, the patient has a history of outbursts of rage, temper tantrums, or impulsive behaviour. People with a tendency for violence frequently lose control when intoxicated with alcohol or drugs. Family members are the most frequent victims of their aggression. Patients with a propensity for violence include those intoxicated by drugs or alcohol; those going through drug or alcohol withdrawal; and those diagnosed with acute paranoid schizophrenic state, acute organic brain syndrome, acute psychosis, paranoid character, borderline personality, or antisocial personality disorders.

The goal of treatment is to bring the violence under control. A specially designated room with at least two exits should be used for the interview. The door of the room should be kept open, and the nurse remains in clear view of the staff, *staying between the patient and the door*. However, the patient's exit to the door must not be blocked, because the patient may feel trapped and threatened. No objects that could be used as weapons should be in sight, in the room, or carried in with health care personnel. If the interviewer feels anxious or uneasy about the patient's response, security staff, a family member, or another health care worker should be asked to remain in the hall nearby in the event that additional help is needed. The patient should never be left alone, because this may be interpreted as rejection or provide an opportunity for self-harm.

To bring the violence under control, it is crucial to use a calm, noncritical approach while remaining in control of the situation. Sudden movements are avoided. If the patient is carrying a weapon, the emergency health care provider should ask that it be surrendered. If the patient is unwilling to surrender the weapon, the security staff is called. If necessary, the security staff may seek further assistance from the local police department.

The patient's violent behaviour is a crisis situation for the patient and the ED. Crisis intervention, achieved by talking and listening to the patient, is best accomplished by expressing an interest in the patient's well-being while attempting to tune in to the patient and remain firm. The patient's agitated state is acknowledged by statements such as, "I want to work with you to relieve your distress."

The patient is allowed the opportunity to express anger verbally. If the patient is delusional, challenging the patient is avoided. Trying to hear what the patient is saying, conveying an expectation of appropriate behaviour, and making the patient aware that help is available are key. The patient is informed that violent behaviour may be frightening to others and that violence is not acceptable.

Help that is available in crisis situations (from a clinic or mental health facility) should be described and offered. Often, the offer of protection by hospitalization is welcomed by the patient, who fears losing control or harming self or others. If the patient does not calm down, security personnel or police intervention may be necessary.

If these measures fail to alleviate the patient's tension, medication may be prescribed (rapid sedation with haloperidol, diazepam, or chlorpromazine) to reduce tension, anxiety, and hyperactivity. Soft restraints must be prescribed by a physician only if other measures to calm the patient have failed. After combativeness, agitation, and fear have decreased, the patient is referred for further mental health treatment.

Posttraumatic Stress Disorder

Posttraumatic stress disorder (PTSD) is the development of characteristic symptoms after a psychologically stressful event that is considered outside the range of usual human experience (e.g., rape, combat, motor vehicle crash, natural catastrophe, terrorist attack). Symptoms of this disorder include intrusive thoughts and dreams, phobic avoidance reaction (avoidance of activities that arouse recollection of the traumatic event), heightened vigilance, exaggerated startle reaction, generalized anxiety, and societal withdrawal. PTSD may be acute (beginning within 1 month of stressful event), chronic (ongoing signs and symptoms), or delayed (beginning several years after the stressful event) (Mayo Clinic, 2019) and recent research shows that it is more prevalent in women (Takahashi, McCance, & Clayton, 2019). PTSD often presents as multiple readmissions to the ED for minor or recurring concerns without evidence of injury. Refer to Chapter 10 for further discussion of assessment, diagnostic findings, and management of patients with PTSD.

Patients Who Are Underactive or Depressed

In the ED, depression may be seen as the primary condition bringing the patient to the health care facility or it may be masked by anxiety and somatic complaints. The person who is depressed has a mood disturbance. Clinical manifestations may include sadness, apathy, feelings of worthlessness, self-blame, suicidal thoughts, desire to escape, avoidance of simple problems, anorexia and weight loss, decreased interest in sex, sleeplessness, and ceaseless activity or reduction in activity. The agitated depressed individual may exhibit motor restlessness and severe anxiety.

Any patient who is depressed may be at risk of suicide. Attempts are made to find out whether the patient has thought about or attempted suicide. Questions such as, "Have you ever thought about taking your own life?" may be helpful. Generally, the patient is relieved to have an opportunity to discuss personal feelings. If the patient is seriously depressed, relatives are notified. The patient should never be left alone, because suicide is usually committed in solitude, and has occurred in Canadian EDs. See Chapter 10 for further discussion of assessment, diagnostic findings, and management of patients with depression.

Patients Who Are Suicidal

Attempted suicide is an act that stems from depression (e.g., loss of a loved one, loss of body integrity or status, poor self-image) and can be viewed as a cry for help and intervention. Males are at greater risk than females. Others at risk are older people; young adults; people who are enduring unusual loss or stress; those who are unemployed, divorced, widowed, or living alone; those showing signs of significant depression (e.g., weight loss, sleep disturbances, somatic concerns, suicidal preoccupation); and those with a history of a previous suicide attempt, suicide in the family, or psychiatric illness.

Being aware of people at risk and assessing for specific factors that predispose a person to suicide are key management strategies. Specific signs and symptoms of potential suicide include the following:

- Communication of *suicidal intent*, such as preoccupation with death or talking of someone else's suicide (e.g., "I'm tired of living. I've put my affairs in order. I'm better off dead. I'm a burden to my family.")
- History of a previous suicide attempt (the risk is much greater in these cases)
- Family history of suicide
- Loss of a parent at an early age
- Specific plan for suicide
- A means to carry out the plan

Emergency management focuses on treating the consequences of the suicide attempt (e.g., gunshot wound, drug overdose) and preventing further self-injury. A patient who has made a suicidal attempt may do so again. Crisis intervention is used to determine suicidal potential, to discover areas of depression and conflict, to find out about the patient's support system, and to determine whether hospitalization or psychiatric referral is necessary. Depending on the patient's potential for suicide, the patient may be admitted to the intensive care unit, referred for follow-up care, or admitted to the psychiatric unit.

Unfolding Patient Stories: Carl Shapiro • Part 2

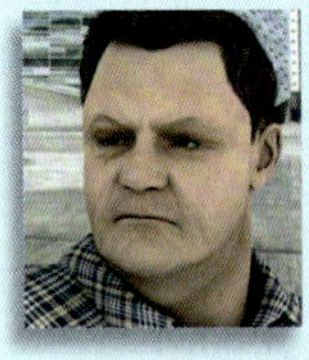

Recall from Chapter 29 Carl Shapiro, who was diagnosed with hypertension and hyperlipidemia during a routine visit to his primary provider. He arrives in the ED with a blood pressure of 210/110. The nurse discovers that he stopped his antihypertensive medication due to erectile dysfunction. How does the nurse maintain patient privacy in the ED during discussion of personal issues? What topics should be included in an individualized discharge plan to address his concerns, educational needs, and continuity of care when the nurse receives orders for an ACE inhibitor, captopril (Capoten), and discharge home?

Care for Carl and other patients in a realistic virtual environment: ***vSim** for Nursing* (**thepoint.lww.com/vSimMedicalSurgical**). Practice documenting these patients' care in DocuCare (**thepoint.lww.com/DocuCareEHR**).

Critical Thinking Exercises

1 After falling down the stairs, a 25-year-old woman arrives at the ED by car accompanied by an older male. Various parts of her body have bruises, some of which appear to be in various stages of healing. When asked to step to the waiting room, the male refuses; security is required to remove him from the room so that the patient examination can occur privately. The patient is particularly quiet and does not actively participate in her history or questions regarding her injuries. As the nurse interviewing and assessing this patient, what do you suspect? You also note that the patient jumps at a knock on the door and pulls away from touch. She states her occupation is a waitress. How do you evaluate the patient situation? What is expected of the nurse in terms of reporting the patient situation? What strategies should be used to provide sensitive care for this patient?

2 A 28-year-old male with a gunshot wound arrives to the hospital lobby after being dropped off by an unknown driver who has abandoned him. He is actively bleeding from multiple wounds in his chest and abdomen and is having difficulty breathing and speaking. The security guard in the lobby calls the ED and a "trauma alert lobby" is announced. The patient is brought rapidly to the ED for assessment and disposition. What are the first measures of the primary survey that you will use to assess and stabilize the patient? Will you expect to administer blood products? What do you anticipate in terms of the ED disposition for this patient? What security measures need to be in place to maintain patient, staff, and visitor safety?

3 Two males in their thirties are transported by EMS to the ED after a house-fire. The EMS agency states suspicious evidence was found in the kitchen, which seemed to be the source of the fire. The patients are hesitant to discuss the events prior to the fire. Both suffered multiple full-thickness burns to their upper extremities, face, neck, and chest. EMS personnel expressed concern about contaminants at the scene, which may be on the patients' clothing. What decision must be made regarding decontamination versus immediate burn care? What is the possible source of the contaminants? As with all patients who have experienced trauma, what is the strength of the evidence that dictates first priorities? In addition to the contaminants, to what other chemical were the patients exposed that may result in inadequate ventilation?

4 It is midsummer and you work in an urban ED. The community includes a large low income and older adult population, and many local residents are concerned about the degree of crime in the area. An 80-year-old woman is brought to the ED unresponsive, skin very dry, pale, with low blood pressure, and with slight tachycardia. Her history includes that she takes a beta blocker and a diuretic for hypertension. Her family states that she lives alone without air conditioning. She rarely opens windows or uses a fan in a window due to fear of a break-in. What do you suspect is the primary problem for this patient? What would you expect her core temperature to be? What will be the immediate treatment for this disorder from which she is suffering? What do you expect her ED disposition to be?

REFERENCES AND SELECTED READINGS

Books

American College of Surgeons. (2013). *Advanced trauma life support* (9th ed.). Chicago, IL: Author.

Auerbach, P. S. (2017). *Wilderness medicine* (7th ed.). St. Louis, MO: Elsevier Mosby.

Black, M. C., Basile, K. C., Breiding, M. J., et al. (2011). *The National Intimate Partner and Sexual Violence Survey (NISVS): 2010 Summary Report*. Atlanta, GA: National Center for Injury Prevention and Control, Centers for Disease Control and Prevention.

Chan, G. K. (2018). Chapter 5: Palliative and end-of-life care. In V. Sweet (Ed.). *Emergency nursing core curriculum* (7 ed., pp. 52–68). St. Louis, MO: Elsevier.

Efre, A. (2018). Chapter 42: Chemical dependency. In V. Good, P. Kirkwood (Eds.). *Advanced critical care nursing* (2nd ed., pp. 800–822). St. Louis, MO: Elsevier.

Emergency Nurses Association. (2013). *Sheehy's manual of emergency care* (7th ed.). St. Louis, MO: Mosby.

Flarity, K. (2018). Chapter 15: Environmental emergencies. In V. Sweet (Ed.). *Emergency nursing core curriculum* (7 ed., pp. 219–244). St. Louis, MO: Elsevier.

Gilboy, N., Tanabe, P., Travers, D., et al. (2012). *Emergency severity index (ESI): A triage tool for emergency department care, version 4. Implementation handbook. Publication No. 12–0014*. Rockville, MD: Agency for Healthcare Research and Quality, Publication.

Hugo Nielson, M. (2018). Chapter 3: Abuse and neglect. In V. Sweet (Ed.). *Emergency nursing core curriculum* (7 ed., pp. 36–46). St. Louis, MO: Elsevier.

Kenney Powell, K., & Hentzen Daniels, J. (2018). Chapter 42: Professional, patient and community. In V. Sweet (Ed.). *Emergency nursing core curriculum* (7 ed., pp. 647–656). St. Louis, MO: Elsevier.

Solheim, J. (2016). *Emergency nursing: The profession/the pathway/the practice*. Indianapolis: Sigma Theta Tau International Honor Society of Nursing.

Solheim, J. (2018). Chapter 13: Dental, ear, nose and throat emergencies. In V. Sweet (Ed.). *Emergency nursing core curriculum* (7 ed., pp. 183–205). St. Louis, MO: Elsevier.

Takahashi, L., McCance, K., & Clayton, M. (2019). Chapter 11: Stress and disease. In S. Huether, K. McCance (Eds.). *Pathophysiology* (8 ed., pp. 323–345). St. Louis, MO: Elsevier.

Tintinalli, J. E., Stapczyski, J. S., Ma, O. J., et al. (2016). *Tintinalli's emergency medicine manual* (8th ed.). New York: McGraw-Hill Medical.

Walsh, K., & Woten, M. (2016). Oropharyngeal airway: Inserting in adults. In D. Pravikoff (Ed.). *Nursing practice and skill*. Glendale, CA: CINAHL Information Systems.

Journals and Electronic Documents

Amerson, R., Whittington, R., & Duggan, L. (2014). Intimate partner violence affecting Latina women and their children. *Journal of Emergency Nursing*, *40*(6), 531–536.

Avander, K., Heikki, A., Bjersa, K., et al. (2016). Trauma nurses' experience of workplace violence and threats: Short- and long-term consequences in a Swedish setting. *Journal of Trauma Nursing*, *23*(2), 51–57.

Baumann, M. H., Patilla, J. S., Lehner, K. R., et al. (2013). Powerful cocaine-like actions of 3,4-methylenedioxypyrovalerone (MDPV), a principal constituent of psychoactive 'bath salts' products. *Neuropsychopharmacology*, *38*(4), 552–562.

Beveridge, R., Clarke, B., Janes, L., et al. (2018). CTAS: Implementation guidelines. Retrieved from https://caep.ca/resources/ctas/implementation-guidelines/#level1

Bhatia, N., Sarwal, S., Robinson, H., et al. (2015). Federal public health strategies to minimize the importation of communicable diseases into Canada. *Canadian Communicable Disease Report*, *41*(Suppl 6), 3–8.

Cadogan, M. P., Phillips, L. R., & Ziminski, C. E. (2016). A perfect storm: Care transitions for vulnerable older adults discharged home from the emergency department without a hospital admission. *The Gerontologist*, *56*(2), 326–334.

Canadian Centre on Substance Use and Addition. (2019). Alcohol. Retrieved from http://www.ccdus.ca/Eng/topics/alcohol/Pages/default.aspx

Canadian Institute for Health Information (CIHI). (2019). Injury and trauma emergency department hospitalization statistics, 2016–2017. Retrieved from https://www.cihi.ca/en/access-data-reports/results?query=injury+and+trauma&Search+Submit=

Canadian Institute for Health Information (CIHI). (2018). NACRS Emergency department visits and length of stay by province/territory, 2017–2018. Retrieved from https://www.cihi.ca/en/access-data-reports/results?f%5B0%5D=field_primary_theme%3A2050

Canadian Undersea and Hyperbaric Medical Association (CUHMA). (2019). Hyperbaric map of Canada. Retrieved from https://cuhma.ca/facilities/facilities

Centers for Disease Control and Prevention (CDC). (2013). Emergency department visits by persons aged 65 and over: United States, 2009–2010. NCHS Data Brief 130. Retrieved February 16, 2017, from www.cdc.gov/nchs/data/databriefs/db130.htm

Centers for Disease Control and Prevention (CDC). (2014). Unintentional drowning deaths in the United States, 2009–2010. NCHS Data Brief 149. Retrieved February 16, 2017, from www.cdc.gov/nchs/data/databriefs/db149.pdf

Childs, B. R., Nahm, N. J., Dolenc, A. J., et al. (2015). Obesity is associated with more complications and longer hospital stays after orthopaedic trauma. *Journal of Orthopaedic Trauma, 29*(11), 504–509.

Conroy, S. (2018). Police-reported violence against girls and young women in Canada, 2017. Retrieved from https://www150.statcan.gc.ca/n1/pub/85-002-x/2018001/article/54981-eng.htm

Day, S., Fox, J., Majercik, S., et al. (2015). Implementing a domestic violence screening program. *Journal of Trauma Nursing, 22*(3), 176–181.

DeBoer, M. I., Kothari, R., Kothari, M. A., et al. (2013). What are barriers to nurses screening for intimate partner violence? *Journal of Trauma Nursing, 20*(3), 155–160.

Dhungel, V., Liao, J., Raut, H., et al. (2015). Obesity delays functional recovery in trauma patients. *Journal of Surgical Residency, 193*(1), 415–420.

Drowning Prevention Research Centre Canada. (2016). Canadian drowning report—2016 Edition. Retrieved from http://www.lifesavingsociety.com/media/241812/canadiandrowningreport_english_web.pdf

Dubé, E., Bettinger, J. A., Fisher, W. A., et al. (2016). Vaccine acceptance, hesitancy and refusal in Canada: Challenges and potential approaches. *Canada Communicable Disease Report, 42*(12), 246–251.

Edwards, C., Stephens-Stidham, S., Contreras, M. A., et al. (2016). Building the conversation for hospital-based injury prevention program capacity. *Journal of Emergency Nursing, 42*(2), 174–176.

Emergency Nurses Association (ENA). (2015a). Emergency nursing interface with mobile integrated health (MIH) and community paramedicine (CP) programs position statement. Retrieved January 14, 2017, from www.ena.org/SiteCollectionDocuments/Position%20Statements/MIHAndCP.pdf

Emergency Nurses Association (ENA). (2015b). Human trafficking patient awareness in the emergency setting: Position statement. Retrieved January 15, 2017, from www.ena.org/SiteCollectionDocuments/Position%20Statements/HumanTrafficking.pdf

Foresman-Capuzzi, J. (2014). CSI & U: Collection and preservation of evidence in the emergency department. *Journal of Emergency Nursing, 40*(3), 229–236.

Government of Canada. (2014). Section 6-6: Canadian guidelines on sexually transmitted infections—specific populations—sexual assault in post-pubertal adolescents and adults. Retrieved from https://www.canada.ca/en/public-health/services/infectious-diseases/sexual-health-sexually-transmitted-infections/canadian-guidelines/sexually-transmitted-infections/canadian-guidelines-sexually-transmitted-infections-43.html

Government of Canada. (2018). Opioids related harms in Canada. Retrieved from https://www.canada.ca/content/dam/hc-sc/documents/services/publications/healthy-living/infographic-opioid-related-harms-december-2018/infographic-opioid-related-harms-december-2018.pdf

Hernández, G., Ospina-Tascón, G., Petri Damiani, L., et al. (2019). Effect of a resuscitation strategy targeting peripheral perfusion status vs serum lactate levels on 28-day mortality among patients with septic shock: The ANDROMEDA-SHOCK randomized clinical trial. *Journal of the American Medical Association, 321*(7), 654–664.

Hess, J. J., Saha, S., & Luber, G. (2014). Summertime acute heat illness in U.S. emergency departments from 2006 through 2010: Analysis of a nationally representative sample. *Environmental Health Perspectives, 122*(11), 1209–1215.

Inaba, K., Siboni, S., Resnick, S., et al. (2015). Tourniquet use for civilian extremity trauma. *Journal of Trauma, 79*(2), 232–237.

Jabre, P., Belpomme, V., Azoulay, E., et al. (2013). Family presence during cardiopulmonary resuscitation. *The New England Journal of Medicine, 368*(11), 1008–1018.

Kane, I., Mitchell, A. M., Aiello, J., et al. (2016). Screening, brief intervention, and referral to treatment education for emergency nurses in 5 hospitals: Implementation steps and hurdles. *Journal of Emergency Nursing, 42*(1), 53–60.

King County Sexual Assault Resource Center. (n.d.). Rape trauma syndrome. Retrieved from https://www.kcsarc.org/sites/default/files/Resources%20-%20Rape%20Trauma%20Syndrome.pdf

Kisser-Larson, N. (2017). The experience of intense pain: Nursing management and interventions. *Journal of Christian Nursing, 34*(2), 88–96.

Lachs, M., & Pillemer, K. (2015). Elder abuse. *New England Journal of Medicine, 373*(20), 1947–1956.

Lambe, K., Currey, J., & Considine, J. (2016). Emergency nurses' decisions regarding frequency and nature of vital sign assessment. *Journal of Clinical Nursing, 26*, 1949–1959. doi: 10.1111jocn.13597

Leske, J. S., McAndrew, N. S., & Brasel, K. J. (2013). Experiences of families when present during resuscitation in the emergency department after trauma. *Journal of Trauma Nursing, 20*(1), 77–85.

Maclean. (2016). Snakebites on the rise in Canada due to global warming, study says. *Canteach Letter*. Retrieved from https://www.cantechletter.com/2016/03/snakebite-rise-canada/

Mayo Clinic. (2019). Post-traumatic stress disorder. Retrieved from https://www.mayoclinic.org/diseases-conditions/post-traumatic-stress-disorder/symptoms-causes/syc-20355967

McDonald, L. (2018). The mistreatment of older Canadians: Findings from the 2015 national prevalence study. *Journal of Elder Abuse & Neglect, 30*(3), 176–208.

Molina, G. (2017). Butane hash. Los Angeles Times. Retrieved February 20, 2017, from www.latimes.com/local/la-me-butane-hash-pictures-20140201-photogallery.html

Montoya, J., Stawicki, S., Evans, D., et al. (2016). From FAST to E-FAST: An overview of the evolution of ultrasound-based traumatic injury assessment. *European Journal of Trauma and Emergency Surgery, 42*(2), 119–126.

Moore, K. (2015). Hot topics: Chemical burns in the emergency department. *Journal of Emergency Nursing, 41*(4), 364–365.

Moraleda Barreno, E., Domínguez-Salas, S., Díaz-Batanero, C., et al. (2019). Specific aspects of cognitive impulsivity are longitudinally associated with lower treatment retention and greater relapse in therapeutic community treatment. *Journal of Substance Abuse Treatment, 96*, 33–38. doi: https://doi.org/10.1016/j.jsat.2018.10.004

Morley, C., Unwin, M., Peterson, G., et al. (2018). Emergency department crowding: A systemic review of causes, consequences and solutions. *PLoS One, 13*(8).

Musccal, E., & DeGuzman, M. M. (2016). Rhabdomyolysis. *Medscape*. Retrieved May 5, 2017, from www.emedicine.medscape.com/article/1007814-overview

National Center on Elder Abuse. (2016). What we do: Research—Statistics/data. Retrieved February 20, 2017, from ncea.acl.gov/whatwedo/research/statistics.html

National Emergency Nurses Association. (2018). *Emergency nursing: Scope and standards of Canadian practice* (6th ed.). Retrieved from http://nena.ca/w/wp-content/uploads/2018/11/Standards-of-ED-Nursing-Practice-2018.pdf

National Institute on Drug Abuse. (2015a). Drug facts. Retrieved February 20, 2017, from www.drugabuse.gov/publications/drugfacts

National Institute on Drug Abuse. (2015b). Drug facts: What are synthetic cannabinoids? Retrieved February 20, 2017, from www.drugabuse.gov/publications/drugfacts/synthetic-cannabinoids

Naus, M., Puddicombe, D., Murti, M., et al. (2015). Outbreak of measles in an unvaccinated population, British Columbia, 2014. *Canada Communicable Disease Report, 41*(7), 169–174.

Oode, Y., Yanagawa, Y., Omori, K., et al. (2015). Analysis of patients with decompression illness transported via physician-staffed emergency helicopters. *Journal of Emergency Trauma Shock, 8*(1), 26–29.

Orkin Canada. (2018). The top venomous snakes in Canada. Retrieved from https://www.orkincanada.ca/blog/venomous-snakes-in-canada/

Personal Health Information Protection Act (PHIPA). (2018). Retrieved from www.ontario.ca/laws/statue/04p03/v27

Rui, P., Kang, K., & Albert, M. (2013). National Hospital Ambulatory Medical Care Survey: 2013 emergency department summary tables. Retrieved February 22, 2017, from www.cdc.gov/nchs/data/ahcd/nhamcs_emergency/2013_ed_web_tables.pdf

Slain, T., Rickard-Aasen, S., Pringle, J. L., et al. (2014). Incorporating screening, brief intervention, and referral to treatment into emergency nursing workflow using an existing computerized physician order entry/clinical decision support system. *Journal of Emergency Nursing, 40*(6), 568–574.

Smith, S., Sammons, S. S., Carr, J., et al. (2014). Bedside management considerations in the treatment of pit viper envenomation. *Journal of Emergency Nursing, 40*(6), 537–545.

Speroni, K. G., Fitch, T., Dawson, E., et al. (2014). Incidence and cost of nurse workplace violence perpetrated by hospital patients or patient visitors. *Journal of Emergency Nursing*, *40*(3), 218–228.

Statistics Canada. (2018). Police-reported family violence in Canada, 2017. Retrieved from https://www150.statcan.gc.ca/n1/pub/11-627-m/11-627-m2018054-eng.htm

The Canadian Triage and Acuity Scale. (2013). Combined Adult/pediatric Educational Program. Retrieved from http://ctas-phctas.ca/wp-content/uploads/2018/05/participant_manual_v2.5b_november_2013_0.pdf.

The Pest Blog (2019). Five most dangerous pests in Canada. Retrieved from http://www.pestblog.ca/most-dangerous-pests-in-canada/

Weinlein, J. C., Deaderick, S., & Murphy, R. F. (2015). Morbid obesity increases the risk for systemic complications in patients with femoral shaft fractures. *Journal of Orthopaedic Trauma*, *29*(3), e91–e95.

Wood, E., Albarquoni, L., Tkachuk, S., et al. (2018). Will this hospitalized patient develop severe alcohol withdrawal syndrome? The rational clinical examination systematic review. *Journal of the American Medical Association*, *320*(8), 825–833.

World Health Organization (WHO). (2016). Drowning: Fact sheet. Retrieved February 16, 2017, from www.who.int/mediacentre/factsheets/fs347/en/

Zafren, K. (2013). Frostbite: Prevention and initial management. *High Altitude Medical Biology*, *14*(1), 9–12.

Resources

Air & Surface Transport Nurses Association: https://www.astna.org/
American College of Surgeons, Committee on Trauma: http://www.facs.org
Canadian Association of Critical Care Nurses: https://www.caccn.ca/
Canadian Association of Emergency Physicians: http://www.caep.ca/
Canadian Centre for Abuse Awareness (CCAA): http://www.ccfaa.com
Canadian Centre on Substance Abuse: http://www.ccsa.ca
Canadian Centre on Substance Use and Addiction: http://www.ccdus.ca
Canadian Institute for Health Information: www.cihi.ca
Canadian Nurses Association: http://www.cna-nurses.ca
Canadian Poison Control Centres: http://www.safekid.org/pcc.htm
Centers for Disease Control and Prevention: http://www.cdc.gov
Emergency Nurses Association: http://www.ena.org
Heart and Stroke Foundation of Canada: http://www.heartandstroke.com
National Emergency Nurses Affiliation: http://www.nena.ca
National Safety Council: http://www.nsc.org
National Trauma Registry: http//secure.cihi.ca/ntr
Public Health Agency of Canada: http://www.phac-aspc.gc.ca.
Registered Nurses Association of Ontario Practice Guidelines: http://rnao.ca/bpg/guidelines
Society of Trauma Nurses: http://traumanursesoc.org
Statistics Canada: http://www.statcan.gc.ca/start-debut-eng.html
Trauma Association of Canada: http//tac.medical.org

74 Terrorism, Mass Casualty, and Disaster Nursing

Adapted by Lance Hoddinott

Learning Objectives

On completion of this chapter, the learner will be able to:

1. Identify the necessary components of an emergency operations plan.
2. Discuss how triage in a disaster differs from triage in an emergency.
3. Develop a plan of care for a patient experiencing short- or long-term psychological effects after a disaster.
4. Describe chemical, biologic, radiologic, nuclear, and explosives (CBRNE) events.
5. Describe isolation precautions necessary for biologic agents.
6. Evaluate the different levels of personal protection and decontamination procedures that may be necessary during an event involving mass casualties or weapons of mass destruction (WMD).
7. Identify physical injuries that may occur after blast events.
8. Identify the differences among the various chemical agents used in terrorist events, their effects, and the decontamination and treatment procedures that are necessary.
9. Determine the injuries associated with varying levels of radiation or chemical exposure and the associated decontamination processes.

Canadian health care providers need to be prepared to deal with mass casualties that can tax the resources of health care organizations and their communities. **Disasters** arise as a result of either natural or human-made circumstances. Natural disasters can include phenomena such as floods, tornadoes, forest fires, blizzards, ice storms, earthquakes, hurricanes, and tsunamis. While human-made disasters can include events such as radiation leaks or other toxic substance spillages in industrial accidents, dangerous infectious diseases, **terrorism**, and biologic warfare, as well as more common events such as airplane crashes, train crashes, and motor vehicle accidents.

The possibility and reality of mass casualties associated with disasters, terrorism, and biologic warfare are not new to human history, nor is the concept of using **weapons of mass destruction (WMDs)**. The use of WMDs dates as far back as the 6th century BCE for biologic weapons and the year 423 BCE for chemical weapons (U.S. Army Medical Research Institute of Chemical Defense, 2000). However, geopolitical forces and interests, religious differences, the "shrinking globe," and the availability of destructive technology have brought the possibility of more terrorist events close to home. Examples include the bombing of subway trains and a double-decker bus in London (July 7, 2005); bombing of commuter trains in Spain (March 11, 2004); the nightclub bombing in Bali (October 12, 2002); the total destruction of the World Trade Center towers (New York) and damage to the Pentagon (Washington, DC) (September 11, 2001), and the release of anthrax in the United States in 2001. It is no longer a question of *whether* it will happen again but *when* it will happen again. In Canada in 2013, an alleged al-Qaeda terrorist conspiracy was narrowly averted, in the form of disruption, potential destruction, and derailment of trains operated by Canada's national passenger railway service (Blackwell, 2013).

Following the September 11, 2001 attacks, the U.S. government created the Department of Homeland Security to coordinate federal and state efforts to combat terrorist activity. Similarly, in 2003 the Canadian government created Public Safety Canada. This agency helps Canadians and their communities protect themselves from emergencies and disasters related to all kinds of hazards through

national leadership in the development and implementation of policies, plans, and a range of programs (Public Safety Canada, 2013a). In Canada, emergency preparedness and management is directed at addressing all forms of disasters, be they natural or human induced. The Canadian emergency management framework has four functions: prevention and mitigation, preparedness, response, and recovery, all of which act together as a part of a continuum framework. *Prevention and mitigation* relates to eliminating or reducing risk, *preparedness* relates to being ready to respond to disasters, *response* relates to being able to act during disasters and manage consequences, and *recovery* relates to restoring conditions after a disaster (Public Safety Canada, 2016). Canadians expect that all levels of government (federal, provincial/territorial, and municipal) will protect them from health crises. The Canadian health care organizations must be prepared for any and all types of emergencies. The focus of this chapter is on emergency preparedness and the process of responding to disasters, both natural and human-made, mass casualties, **epidemics/pandemics**, and terrorism.

Emergency Preparedness

Federal, Provincial/Territorial, and Local Responses to Emergencies

Many resources are available at the federal, provincial/territorial, and local levels to assist with the management of emergencies, **mass casualty incidents (MCIs)**, and disasters. An MCI is defined as disasters and major incidents characterized by quantity, severity, and diversity of patients that can rapidly overwhelm the ability of local medical resources to deliver comprehensive and definitive medical care (Edgerly, 2016).

Disasters are often assigned levels, which indicate the anticipated level of response (Chart 74-1). A list of the local resources with specific instructions about how and when to contact them should be readily available and frequently reviewed for needed updates as a part of routine and ongoing preparation activities.

Emergency response is initially managed at the local level, for example, hospitals, EMS, fire departments, police, and municipalities. If additional assistance is required, it is requested from the provinces or territories. If the emergency escalates beyond their capabilities, the

CHART 74-1

Disaster Levels

Disasters are often classified by the resultant anticipated necessary response:

Level I: Local emergency response personnel and organizations can contain and effectively manage the disaster and its aftermath.

Level II: Regional efforts and aid from surrounding communities are sufficient to manage the effects of the disaster.

Level III: Local and regional assets are overwhelmed; statewide or federal assistance is required.

Glossary

CBRNE event: an event that involves a potential, perceived, or actual act with chemical, biologic, radiologic, nuclear, or explosive materials that are, or are suspected to be, used in a deliberate or intentional way to cause harm.

decontamination: process of removing, or rendering harmless, contaminants that have accumulated on personnel, patients, equipment, and contaminated clinical areas.

disaster: a social phenomenon that results when a hazard intersects with a vulnerable community in a way that exceeds or overwhelms the community's ability to cope and may cause serious harm to the safety, health, welfare, property or environment of people; may be triggered by a naturally occurring phenomenon which has its origins within the geophysical or biologic environment or by human action or error, whether malicious or unintentional, including technologic failures, accidents, and terrorist acts (Public Safety Canada, 2016).

disaster nursing: adaptation of professional nursing skills in regards to disaster and the disaster management continuum, which includes all associated prevention and mitigation, preparedness, response, and recovery activities

epidemic: outbreak of a disease or illness that spreads rapidly throughout a segment of a human population, affecting a significantly large number of individuals at the same time

mass casualty incident (MCI): situation in which the number of casualties exceeds the number of available resources

pandemic: outbreak of a disease over a wide geographic area or worldwide and affecting an exceptionally high proportion of the population

personal protective equipment (PPE): the clothing or equipment that a health worker handling any hazardous products, or working in a hazardous environment wears to reduce or prevent exposure to the product or environment.

safety data sheet (SDS): provides information to employees and health care providers regarding a given specific chemical agent that includes Product Identification, Hazard Identification, Composition/Information on Ingredients, First-aid measures, Fire-fighting measures, Accidental release measures, Handling and storage, Exposure controls/Personal protection, Physical and chemical properties; also known as the Worker's Right to Know

terrorism: unlawful use of violence or threats of violence against individuals in order to coerce or intimidate

weapons of mass destruction (WMD): weapons used to cause widespread death and destruction provinces or territories seek assistance from the National Emergency Response System (NERS) which was approved by the Federal, Provincial, and Territorial (FPT) Ministers in January 2011. During any chemical, biologic, radiologic, nuclear, and explosives (CBRNE) disaster, the coordination and provisioning of resources can move quickly from the local to the national level as required (Public Safety Canada, 2013b). There is a network of Federal and Regional Offices across Canada that serves as a link to emergency management counterparts.

Federal Agencies and Other National Organizations

Health Canada, Public Health Canada, Public Safety Canada, and National Defence and the Canadian Forces are some of the key federal agencies involved in emergency preparedness. Chart 74-2 provides a list of selected agencies. In addition to the agencies listed in Chart 74-2, federal departments also directly oversee aspects that do not fall under specific agencies. For example, Health Canada is responsible for the Canada–United States Joint International Coordination of Nuclear Emergency Preparedness and Response. This plan, ratified in 1996, would ensure collaboration between the two countries in case of a nuclear incident. This cooperation would be particularly important considering the nature of radiologic events.

Under the Public Health Agency of Canada (PHAC), the Centre for Emergency Preparedness and Response (CEPR) coordinates public health security issues. It is organized in a number of specialized offices (PHAC, 2012a). One of these offices, the Office of Emergency Response Services, has the responsibility to support emergency health and social services in the provinces/territories in the event of a national health emergency or disaster (PHAC, 2013). Its web site includes a number of publications that are useful in planning for emergency situations. Disaster Assistance Response Team (DART), a well-known team of the Canadian Forces, can be deployed to provide humanitarian relief and care, including producing large quantities of safe water. The DART is equipped to conduct emergency relief operations for up to approximately 40 days to bridge the gap until national and international aid agencies arrive to provide long-term help. For example, within 24 hours of the 2010 Haiti earthquake, the first reconnaissance elements of the DART landed in Port-au-Prince as part of Canada's whole-of government response to the catastrophic earthquake (National Defence and the Canadian Armed Forces, 2013).

A number of nongovernmental, not-for-profit agencies that have a national scope are also involved in emergency preparedness; the Canadian Risk and Hazards (Knowledge and Practice) Network (CRHNet), and the Canadian Red Cross are examples of these. The Canadian Risk and Hazards Network provides an environment for hazards research, education and emergency management practitioner communities to effectively share knowledge and innovate approaches that reduce vulnerability (Canadian Risk and Hazards Network, 2018). The Canadian Red Cross is another organization that devotes energy to helping Canadians prepare for disasters and provides relief to those affected by disasters both nationally and internationally.

CHART 74-2

Federal Departments and Selected Agencies

Health Canada
Public Health Agency of Canada
Infectious Disease and Emergency Preparedness Branch
Centre for Infectious Disease Prevention and Control
Centre for Emergency Preparedness and Response
Office of Emergency Preparedness
National Emergency Stockpile System
Office of Emergency Response Services
National Office of Health Emergency Response Teams
Office of Laboratory Security
Office of Public Health Security
Counter-Terrorism Coordination and Health Information Networks
Office of Management and Administrative Services
Public Safety Canada
Emergency Management
Emergency Preparedness
Joint Emergency Preparedness Program
National Defence and the Canadian Forces
Office of Critical Infrastructure Protection and Emergency Preparedness
Canadian Forces Disaster Assistance Response Team

Provincial/Territorial and Local Agencies

There are several provincial and local agencies that are devoted to emergency preparedness. Provincial and territorial emergency management organizations (EMOs) are an excellent source of information about how to prepare for emergencies in your particular region. EMOs' activities include planning and research, training, response operations, and the administration and delivery of disaster financial assistance programs. EMOs are most familiar with the natural hazards and other risks of your region. Students should be well informed about the role of the EMO in the province or territory that they are working in. For a complete list of all provincial/territorial EMOs see http://www.getprepared.gc.ca/cnt/rsrcs/mrgnc-mgmt-rgnztns-eng.aspx. The Alberta Emergency Management Agency (AEMA) provides an example of a provincial agency devoted to emergency preparedness. Its role is to "lead the coordination, collaboration and cooperation of all organizations involved in the prevention, preparedness, and response to disasters and emergencies" in Alberta (AEMA, 2017). Like other provincial agencies, it includes generic disaster plans that are similar from province to province and programs/plans that are specific to its geography and industrial activities. For example, during the June 2013 Calgary flood the organization immediately initiated its emergency preparedness plan to help deal with the disaster. Like other jurisdictions, Alberta has learned from previous disasters; for example, the creation of an Emergency Public Warning System followed the 1987 Edmonton Tornado—one of the most important natural disasters to have occurred in Canada. Through the media, this system is designed to warn Albertans about severe weather, flood, wildfire, hazardous material release, terrorist threat, and other threats to human life or safety. Most recently, a technologic upgrade has been made to the alert system that includes an advanced text-to-speech service that improves the clarity and pronunciation of audio alerts (AEMA, 2013).

Within communities, existing social service agencies are responsible for emergency social services planning. Agencies such as municipal and provincial departments of social services, public health, mental health, family and children's services, service clubs, church groups, and business and professional associations are involved. Other resources may include local Canadian Red Cross chapters, poison control centres, and other types of volunteer organizations.

The Incident Command System

The Incident Command System (ICS) Canada is a standardized on-site command and control system used to manage emergency incidents and planned events. ICS enhances incident management response through improved interoperability. The ICS System is a management tool for organizing personnel, facilities, equipment, and communication for any emergency situation. It consists of a structure with well-defined roles and responsibilities that other agencies recognize. The three primary goals of the ICS are to provide for the orderly and predictable division of labour; provide for the overall safety at the incident or event; and, ensure that the work at the incident or event is performed efficiently and effectively (Incident Command System Canada [ICSC], 2012). Under this structure, one individual is designated as Incident Commander (IC) or, if the disaster covers more than one jurisdiction, a Unified Commander (UC) system may be used (ICSC, 2012). In a cross-jurisdictional emergency situation, individuals designated by their jurisdictional or organizational authorities must jointly determine objectives, strategies, plans, resource allocations, and priorities and work together to execute integrated incident operations and maximize the use of assigned resources (ICSC, 2012). Although the ICS is primarily a field structure and process, aspects of it are used at the level of an individual hospital or health care organization's emergency response plan as well.

Health Care Emergency Preparedness Plans

Health care organizations are required by Accreditation Canada to create and test a plan for emergency preparedness (Accreditation Canada, 2013). Additionally, the need for such plans may also be required as a result of governmental regulation. Generally, health care organizations develop and test emergency preparedness plans through the oversight of a senior administrator and/or emergency preparedness officer or committee.

Before the basic emergency management plan (EMP) can be developed, the planning committee of the organization first evaluates the community to anticipate the types of natural and man-made disasters that might occur. Effective emergency management planning includes the integration of mandate-specific all-hazards risk assessment (AHRA) as the planning premise (Public Safety Canada, 2013c). The AHRA will assist the committee to identify, analyze, and prioritize the full range of potential threats. The process takes into account vulnerabilities associated with specific threats, identifies potential consequences should a threat be realized, and considers means to mitigate the risks. This information can be gathered by questioning local law enforcement and fire departments and assessing the amount of air or train traffic; automobile traffic; transportation of dangerous goods by truck or train; and flood, earthquake, tornado, blizzard, or hurricane activity. Consideration is given to special situations such as proximity to chemical plants, oil refineries, nuclear facilities, or military bases that may enhance the community's potential for man-made disasters. Federal, judicial, or financial buildings, schools, and any places where large groups of individuals gather can be considered high-risk areas.

Based on the AHRA, the planning committee must identify what supplies are necessary. If the situation requires additional resources beyond the local level, provincial/territorial agencies are contacted, and, if necessary, the CEPR of the PHAC can be contacted. The CEPR immediately sends out two field hospitals along with extra cots and bedding for shelters. These supplies along with medical supplies and medications are part of Canada's National Emergency Stockpile System (NESS). If needed, the CEPR can send a field medical response team that can provide medical services, counselling, and mental health services (PHAC, 2012b).

Another scenario that might be anticipated is the dispersal of a pulmonary intoxicant or choking agent, which requires that the planners find out the numbers and types of **personal protective equipment (PPE)** required and available to protect health care providers as well as how many ventilators would be available for patients within the organization and in the community. The committee might also outline how staff within an organization would triage and assign priority to patients when the number of ventilators is limited. Information should be available about local resources for stocking and restocking any of the basic and special supplies, how those supplies are requested, and the time required to receive those supplies. Multiple factors influence a facility's ability to respond effectively to a sudden influx of injured patients, and the committee must anticipate various scenarios to improve its preparedness.

The Public Health Agency of Canada maintains a NESS that provides health and social service supplies quickly to provinces and territories when their own resources are not enough during an emergency within a 24-hour response time frame (PHAC, 2012b). NESS is responsible to assess and refurbish stockpile units, and distribute medical and pharmaceutical supplies when requested by provinces and territories in emergency situations and supports the response to a variety of emergencies with health impacts, including influenza pandemics, terrorism events, and natural disasters (PHAC, 2012b).

Components of the Emergency Operations Plan

The principles of emergency management must be a part of the Emergency Operations Plan (EOP) that is designed and includes a comprehensive plan for tackling all potential and actual hazards. Emergency management adopts an all-hazards approach in every jurisdiction in Canada by addressing vulnerabilities exposed by both natural and human-induced hazards and disasters. The all-hazards approach increases efficiency by recognizing and integrating common emergency management elements across all hazard types, and then supplementing these common elements with hazard-specific subcomponents to fill gaps only as required. The EOP should be integrated with local, provincial/territorial, and federal government plans. The primary goal is protection of the community. Predetermined organization is essential to minimize confusion, ensure that all key operations are directed, and promote a well-coordinated response. Canadian EOPs are based upon the four basic principles of emergency management: prevention and mitigation, preparedness, response, and recovery. Essential components of the EOP include the following:

- *An activation response/trigger:* The EOP activation response of a health care facility defines where, how, and when the response is initiated.
- *An internal/external communication plan:* Communication is critical for all parties involved, including communication to and from the prehospital area. A sharing and coordination of information is extremely important during the response phase of a disaster.
- *A plan for coordinated patient care:* A response is planned for coordinated patient care into and out of the facility, including transfers to other facilities. The site of the disaster can determine where the greater number of patients may self-refer (e.g., in the Edmonton Tornado in 1987, the wounded from a badly damaged trailer park began arriving at a hospital for individuals with mental illnesses [the nearest facility] before the institution even knew there was a disaster).
- *Security plans:* A coordinated security plan involving facility and community agencies is key to the control of an otherwise chaotic situation.
- *Identification of external resources:* External resources are identified, including local, provincial/territorial, and federal resources and information about how to activate these resources.
- *A plan for people management and traffic flow:* "People management" includes strategies to manage the patients, the public, the media, and the personnel. Specific areas are assigned, and a designated individual is delegated to manage each of these groups
- *A data management strategy:* A data management plan for every aspect of the disaster will save time at every step. If a computerized system is used for charting, tracking, and staffing, a backup system is necessary.
- *Deactivation response:* Deactivation of the response is as important as activation; resources should not be overused. The individual who decides when the facility is able to go from the disaster response back to daily activities is clearly identified.
- *A post incident response:* Post incident response must include a critique and a debriefing for all parties involved, immediately and again at a later date. Often, facilities see increased volumes of patients up to 3 months after an incident.
- *A plan for practice drills:* Practice drills that include community participation allow for troubleshooting any issues before a real-life incident occurs.
- *Anticipated resources:* Food and water must be available for staff, families, and others who may be at the health care facility for an extended period.
- *MCI planning:* MCI planning includes such issues as planning for mass fatalities and morgue readiness.
- *An education plan for all of the above:* A strong educational plan for all personnel regarding each step of the plan allows for improved readiness and additional input for fine-tuning of the EOP.

The EOP should also include a structure that defines roles for all employees in each emergency situation. The most common structure is the ICS described earlier but applied at the level of the health care organization itself rather than at the site of the disaster. For example, an administrator, possibly the nurse executive, will act as the IC and coordinate all aspects of the implementation of the plan. Other personnel will be designated to perform key roles, such as resource manager or patient disposition coordinator. Such a predetermined organization is essential to minimize confusion, ensure that all key operations are directed, and promote a well-coordinated response.

Initiating the Emergency Management Plan

Notification of a disaster situation to a health care organization varies with each situation. Generally, the notification to the organization comes from outside sources unless the initial incident occurred on site. The disaster activation plan should clearly state how the EMP is to be initiated. If communication is functioning, field incident command will give notice of the approximate number of arriving patients, although the number of self-referring patients will not be known.

Identifying Patients and Documenting Patient Information

Patient tracking is a critical component of casualty management. Disaster tags, which are numbered and include triage priority, name, address, age, location and description of injuries, and treatments or medications given, are used to communicate patient information. The tag should be securely placed on the patient and remain with the patient at all times. The tag number and the patient's name, if known, are recorded in a disaster log. The log is used by the command centre to track patients, assign beds, and provide families with information. An important additional consideration for patient tracking is in regards to those unable to speak for themselves because of injury or perhaps a language barrier. These unidentified/unknown patients will also need a means of tracking. As a result, a system of identification for such patients must also be planned and created in advance and must also be able to function in conjunction with the regular patient tracking system.

Triage

Triage is the sorting of patients to determine the priority of their health care needs and the proper site for treatment. Under normal operational circumstances, health care workers assign a high priority and allocate the most resources to those who are the most critically ill. For example, a young adult who has a chest injury and is in full cardiac arrest would receive advanced cardiopulmonary resuscitation, including medications, chest tubes, intravenous (IV) fluids, blood, and possibly emergency surgery in an effort to restore life. The Canadian Emergency Department Triage and Acuity Scale (CTAS) is a tool used in emergency departments to triage (rank) patients based on the seriousness of presenting signs and symptoms to be sure that the sickest patients are seen first and that patients are reassessed during their time in an emergency department. See Chapter 73 for a detailed description of the CTAS. However, in a disaster, when health care providers are faced with a large number of casualties, the fundamental principle guiding resource allocation is to do the greatest good for the greatest number of individuals. Decisions are based on the likelihood of survival and consumption of available resources. Therefore, this same patient, and others with conditions associated with a high mortality rate, would be assigned a low triage priority in a disaster situation, even if the individual is conscious. Although this may sound uncaring, from an ethical standpoint the expenditure of limited resources on individuals with a low chance of survival, and denial of those resources to others with serious but treatable conditions, cannot be justified.

Triage categories separate patients according to severity of injury and use a colour-coded tagging system so that the triage category is immediately obvious. There are several triage systems in use across the country, and every nurse should be aware of the system used by his or her organization and community.

There is not one consistent triage system in use in Canada during mass casualty emergencies; however, many agencies are using the Simple Triage and Rapid Treatment (START) and JumpSTART methods of triage. START is a five-step triage method: it begins with the triage officer asking all individuals who can walk to go to a certain area. They are all initially tagged as green, ambulatory. Secondly, assess respirations: if present, go to step 3; if absent, open airway and breathe. If respirations resume, tag Red; if no respirations, tag Black. Step 3 is an assessment of the respiratory rate: if 30 rpm or less, proceed to Step 4; if greater than 30 rpm, tag Red. Step 4, assesses capillary refill. If less than or equal to 2 seconds, go to Step 5; if greater than 2 seconds, tag as Red. The final step assesses mental status: if able to follow commands, tag as Yellow; if not able to obey commands, tag as Red. Unless deceased, victims tagged in the BLACK category should be reassessed once critical interventions have been completed for RED and YELLOW patients. The JumpSTART method is similar but has made adjustments for its use on children 1 to 8 years of age. Table 74-1 includes the Triage Colour Codes used by Emergency Medical Services during mass casualty emergencies and aligns with the START Triage method.

Staff should control all entrances to the acute care organization so that incoming patients are directed to the triage area first. The triage area may be outside the entry or just at the door of the ED. This facilitates the triage of all patients, including those arriving by medical transport and those who walk into the ED. Some patients who have already been seen in the field may be reclassified in the triage area, based on their current presentation. This practice also ensures that if there is a CBRNE/HAZMAT component to the incident, all patients can be decontaminated prior to entering the facility, thereby reducing the risk of cross-contamination to health care staff, equipment, and facilities.

Managing Internal Problems

Each facility must determine its supply lists based on its own needs assessment. The Red Cross has developed a basic survival/shelter resource kit. The EOP committee should determine the top 10 critical medications used during normal day-to-day operations and then anticipate

TABLE 74-1 Triage Categories During a Mass Casualty Incident

Triage Category	Priority	Colour	Typical Conditions
Immediate: Injuries are life threatening but survivable with minimal intervention. Individuals in this group can progress rapidly to expectant if treatment is delayed.	1	Red	Sucking chest wound, airway obstruction secondary to mechanical cause, shock, hemothorax, tension pneumothorax, asphyxia, unstable chest and abdominal wounds, incomplete amputations, open fractures of long bones, and 2nd/3rd-degree burns of 15–40% total body surface area
Delayed: Injuries are significant and require medical care but can wait hours without threat to life or limb. Individuals in this group receive treatment only after immediate casualties are treated.	2	Yellow	Stable abdominal wounds without evidence of significant hemorrhage; soft tissue injuries; maxillofacial wounds without airway compromise; vascular injuries with adequate collateral circulation; genitourinary tract disruption; fractures requiring open reduction, débridement, and external fixation; most eye and central nervous system injuries
Minimal: Injuries are minor, and treatment can be delayed hours to days. Individuals in this group should be moved away from the main triage area.	3	Green	Upper extremity fractures, minor burns, sprains, small lacerations without significant bleeding, behavioural disorders or psychological disturbances
Expectant: Injuries are extensive, and chances of survival are unlikely even with definitive care. Persons in this group should be separated from other casualties, but not abandoned. Comfort measures should be provided when possible.	4	Black	Patients who are unresponsive with penetrating head wounds, high spinal cord injuries, wounds involving multiple anatomic sites and organs, 2nd/3rd-degree burns in excess of 60% of body surface area, seizures or vomiting within 24 hours after radiation exposure, profound shock with multiple injuries, agonal respirations; no pulse, no blood pressure, pupils fixed and dilated

Adapted from American College of Surgeons. (2010). *Disaster management and emergency preparedness course*. Chicago, IL: Author.

which other medications may be required in a disaster or an MCI. For example, the health care facility might plan to have available a stockpile of antidotes (e.g., cyanide kits), antibiotics used in treating biologic agents, or immunizations (e.g., flu vaccines). Information should be available about stocking or restocking any of the basic and special supplies, how those supplies are requested, and the time required to receive those supplies.

Communicating With the Media and Family

Communication is a key component of disaster management. Communication within the vast team of disaster responders is paramount; however, effective, informative communication with the media and worried family members is also crucial.

Managing Media Requests for Information

Although the media have an obligation to report the news and can play a significant positive role in communication, the number of reporters and newscasters and their support teams can be overwhelming, possibly compromising operations and patient confidentiality. A clearly defined process for managing media requests that includes a designated spokesperson, the public information officer, a site for the dissemination of information (away from patient care areas), and a regular schedule for providing updates should be part of the disaster plan.

The EOP helps prevent the release of contradictory or inaccurate information. Initial statements should focus on current efforts and what is being done to better understand the scope and impact of the situation. Information about casualties should not be released. Security staff should not allow media personnel access to patient care areas.

Caring for Families

Friends and family members converging on the scene must be cared for by the organization. The public information officer's role is to provide direction for the families and provide them with information as it becomes available. They may be feeling intense anxiety, shock, or grief and should be provided with information and updates about their loved ones as soon as possible and regularly thereafter. They should not be in the triage or treatment areas but in a designated area staffed by available social workers, counsellors, therapists, or clergy. Access to this area should be controlled to prevent families from being disturbed. Chart 74-3 discusses cultural variables to consider when coping with disaster-related injuries and death.

> CHART 74-3
>
> **Cultural Considerations**
>
> Any disaster or mass casualty incident can be expected to involve members of diverse religious, ethnic, and cultural groups or may be targeted at and predominately affect a specific religious or ethnic group. Health care providers likewise include members of all religious, ethnic, and cultural backgrounds and should bear in mind that victims may have:
>
> - Language difficulties that increase fears and frustrations
> - Specific religious practices related to medical treatment, hygiene, or diet
> - Specific places/times for prayer
> - Rituals about handling the dead
> - Timing of funeral services
>
> Some religious communities have plans for emergencies and disasters, and local hospitals should integrate these plans to the extent possible into their emergency operations plans.

The Nurses Role in Responding to a Disaster

The role of the nurse during a disaster varies. In rural or remote settings where there are few providers, the nurse may be asked to perform outside his or her area of expertise and may take on responsibilities normally held by physicians or advanced practice nurses. For example, a critical care nurse may intubate a patient or even insert chest tubes. Wound débridement or suturing may be performed by registered nurses. A nurse may serve as the triage officer.

During disasters in Canada, registered nurses have a duty to provide care (Canadian Nurses Association [CNA], 2019). In addition, many provincial nursing associations provide direction for providing nursing care during a disaster. Canadian competencies for entry-level Registered nurses in Canada are required to have knowledge of nursing in disaster situations (College of Nurses of Ontario [CNO], 2014).

Although the exact role of a nurse in disaster management depends on the specific needs of the facility at the time, it should be clear which nurse or physician is in charge of a given patient care area and which procedures each individual nurse may or may not perform. Assistance can be obtained through the incident command centre, and nonmedical personnel can provide services where possible. For example, family members can provide nonskilled interventions for their loved ones. Nurses should remember that nursing care in a disaster focuses on essential care from a perspective of what is best for all patients.

New settings and atypical roles for nurses arise during a disaster; for example, the nurse may provide shelter care in a temporary housing area or bereavement support and assistance with identification of deceased loved ones. Individuals may require crisis intervention, or the nurse may participate in counselling other staff members and in Critical Incident Stress Management (CISM). Special care may be warranted for vulnerable populations during a disaster (Chart 74-4).

Considering Ethical Conflicts

Disasters can present a disparity between the resources of the health care agency and the needs of the victims. This generates ethical dilemmas for nurses and other health care providers. Issues include conflicts related to the following:

- Rationing care
- Futile therapy
- Consent
- Duty
- Confidentiality
- Resuscitation
- Assisted suicide

CHART 74-4

Caring for Vulnerable Individuals During a Disaster

When a disaster occurs, the multiple agencies involved attempt to provide food, water, and shelter to all those affected. There are some populations that are considered as vulnerable during mass casualty incidents. The terms "at-risk individuals," "vulnerable populations," and "special-needs populations" are often used interchangeably. These groups often include people who are older or young, have limited or no English proficiency, experience geographic or cultural isolation, or suffer from addiction. During mass casualty incidents it is important to consider the needs of vulnerable populations, including, but not limited to, individuals with mental illness, disabilities, the older people, pregnant women, and children. They all have specific needs that require attention. It is recommended that individuals with disabilities have a personal support network to check on them after a disaster and to provide needed assistance. They should also have a back-up system and an evacuation plan. Agencies need to be aware that service animals are also affected during a disaster and may be brought to shelters with their companions.

It is important to do advance planning and preparation for vulnerable groups and include local agencies into emergency management plans that can be utilized to assist those that may be at a disadvantage. On its web site, the Canadian Red Cross has a document that provides recommendations that can be implemented while integrating emergency management and high-risk populations. This can be retrieved from http://www.redcross.ca/cmslib/general/dm_high_risk_populations.pdf

Nurses may find it difficult to not provide care to the dying or to withhold information to maintain patient confidentiality. Clinical scenarios that are unimaginable in normal circumstances may confront the nurse in extreme instances. Other ethical dilemmas may arise out of health care providers' instincts for self-protection and protection of their families. For example, what should a pregnant nurse do when incoming disaster victims have been exposed to radiation yet too few nurses are available? Chart 74-5 presents an ethical dilemma related to mass casualty response.

Nurses can prepare for the ethical distress and/or dilemmas they will face during disasters by establishing a framework for evaluating ethical questions before they arise and by identifying and exploring possible responses to difficult clinical situations. They can refer to the *Code of Ethics for Registered Nurses* (CNA, 2017). They can consider how the fundamental ethical principles of utilitarianism, beneficence, and justice will influence their decisions and care in disaster response (see Chapter 3).

Managing Behavioural Issues

While many individuals pull together and function well during a disaster, both individuals and communities may also still suffer immediate and sometimes long-term psychological trauma. Common responses to disaster include the following:

- Depression
- Anxiety
- Somatization (fatigue, general malaise, headaches, gastrointestinal disturbances, skin rashes)
- Posttraumatic stress disorder (PTSD)

CHART 74-5

Ethical Dilemma: Who Receives Care First During a Mass Casualty?

Case Scenario

You work as a staff nurse in the emergency department (ED) of a 75-bed community hospital. The unit is notified that an armed man entered the local social security office building and began shooting people in the lobby. There were numerous casualties, including the perpetrator, who was shot by a police officer. Within minutes of the notification, several patients are transported into the trauma bay area with gunshot wounds and other traumatic injuries. A young man appears to be hallucinating and attempts to assault a staff nurse. The perpetrator of the violent assault is transported into the trauma bay on a gurney, with an apparent gunshot wound to the head. An older woman grabs your arm and yells, "You have to take care of my husband first! He has a bad heart and may not be able to survive!" Another patient points at the perpetrator and yells, "He is the one who is responsible for this! How can you treat him?! He doesn't deserve to live!"

Discussion

One of the most difficult and morally distressing situations that nurses working in the ED may face is how to triage and treat patients when medical resources are scarce. Participating in disaster drills may prepare nurses working in the ED in how to respond if an emergency operations plan needs to be executed for a true mass casualty situation. These drills are intended to assist nurses in the ED to triage and prioritize care in a way that is unbiased. The key principle of triage in these situations is to do the greatest good for the greatest number of people. Medical resources must be distributed to patients in a fair and equitable manner.

Analysis

- Describe the ethical principles that are in conflict in this case (see Chapter 3, Chart 3-3). Which principle should have preeminence as you respond to the patient who feels the perpetrator does not have a right to receive medical care?
- Reflect upon your own desire to do good (i.e., practice beneficence) and how this desire to help an older couple may affect your triage decision. How would you respond to the wife? Should the age of her husband and his past medical history influence the triage process?
- How would you most appropriately triage the patient who has no visible physical injuries but is apparently experiencing a mental health crisis?

Resources

See Chapter 3, Chart 3-2 for ethics resources.

Abbasi, J. (2016). Expanding the health care response to mass violence. *JAMA, 316*(10), 1031–1033.

- Substance abuse
- Interpersonal conflicts
- Impaired performance

Factors that influence an individual's response to disaster include the degree and nature of the exposure to the disaster, loss of friends and loved ones, existing coping strategies, available resources and support, and the personal meaning attached to the event. Other factors, such as loss of home and valued possessions, extended exposure to danger, and exposure to toxic contamination, also influence response and increase the risk of adjustment problems. Those exposed to the dead and injured, those endangered by the event, the older people, children, emergency first responders, and health care personnel caring for victims are considered to be at higher risk for emotional sequelae.

Nurses can assist disaster victims through active listening and providing emotional support, giving information, and referring patients to therapists or social workers. Health care workers need to be aware that they should either provide information for or refer individuals to mental health care services because experience has shown that few disaster victims seek these services, and early intervention minimizes psychological consequences. Nurses can also discourage victims from subjecting themselves to repeated exposure to the event through media replays and news articles, and encourage them to return to normal activities and social roles when appropriate.

Critical Incident Stress Management

CISM is an approach to preventing and treating the emotional trauma that can affect emergency responders as a consequence of their jobs and that can also occur to anyone involved in a disaster or MCI. CISM is handled by its own teams, which are available to the OEM. All branches of emergency services have CISM teams, as do the military, health care organizations, and many industries (e.g., airline industry).

Components of a management plan include education before an incident occurs about critical incident stress and coping strategies; field support (ensuring that staff get adequate rest, food, and fluids, and rotating workloads) during an incident; and defusings, debriefings, demobilization, and follow-up care after the incident.

Defusing is a process by which the individual receives education about recognition of stress reactions and management strategies for handling stress. Debriefing is a more complicated intervention; it involves a 2- to 3-hour process during which participants are asked about their emotional reactions to the incident, what symptoms they may be experiencing (e.g., flashbacks, difficulty sleeping, intrusive thoughts), and other psychological ramifications. In follow-up, members of the CISM team contact the participants of a debriefing and schedule a follow-up meeting if necessary. Individuals with ongoing stress reactions are referred to mental health specialists.

Emergency Debriefing

Just as planning for a disaster or an MCI is critical, debriefing after the event is equally important. Debriefing provides the opportunity to examine what went well and what went wrong. For example, in the days and weeks following Hurricane Katrina and Hurricane Rita in the United States (in 2005), television and print sources provided details of the lack of preparedness to respond to a major disaster. Offers to provide aid came from around the world, including from developing countries.

In one Alberta natural disaster, a tornado hit a campground at Pine Lake Alberta at 17:00 hours on a sunny summer weekend in 2000. Winds of 300 km/hr tossed cars, trailers, trees, and individuals into the air and some into the lake. Survivors immediately began searching and rescuing others; other survivors left the scene. The first responders were the Royal Canadian Mounted Police (RCMP) and EMS personnel. Other EMS units, the Shock Trauma Air Rescue Society (STARS) helicopter system, and the Red Deer Regional Hospital (RDH) were all notified. STARS immediately initiated their disaster plan, sent two helicopters, and updated the RDH and large hospitals in Edmonton and Calgary.

Some patients were treated at nearby local hospitals. Less urgent "green" category patients (Table 74-1) were evaluated and treated by EMS personnel at a local community centre. Others with more serious injuries were sent to RDH. Once additional physicians arrived from Edmonton, a staging centre (like a mini emergency room) was established in an empty hangar at the Red Deer airport. There, patients received blood transfusions, reduction of fractures, intubations, and placement of chest tubes. RDH activated its emergency plan and expected a large number of category "blue" or "red" patients. One hospital in Calgary and two in Edmonton implemented full disaster plans. By the end of the first night, over 130 individuals were injured and 9 were dead. Three more victims died of their injuries in intensive care units. Most injuries were from blunt trauma to the head, torso, and extremities. Critical incident stress debriefing was offered to rescue workers and personnel. Sookram et al. (2001) have analyzed the emergency response to the Tornado at Pine Lake and conclude the following:

What Went Wrong

- The disaster response grew out of control with too many ambulances lined up trying to get into the campground, leaving surrounding communities without service.
- All phone communication failed between the disaster site and receiving hospitals. Although communication was sent via STARS, hospitals waited for other confirmation before acting. A mobile communication vehicle was needed.
- Regional receiving hospitals overreacted and fully activated their disaster plans rather than a staged response.

What Went Right

- Survivors helped each other.
- The first STARS physician to arrive at the site became the "triage master."
- Physicians functioned well at the site and at the staging centre to complement EMS personnel.
- Patients were classified according to colour coding (Table 74-1) and received treatment from appropriate personnel.
- Following changes due to regionalization, the RDH had recently revised its disaster plan.

Preparedness and Response

Recognition and Awareness

Preparedness for terrorism and other disasters includes awareness of the potential for covert use of WMD, self-protection, and early detection, containment, or **decontamination** of substances and agents that may affect others by secondary exposure. The strength of many toxins, today's mobile society, and long incubation periods for some organisms and substances can result in an epidemic that can quickly and silently spread across the entire country. For example, there must be awareness that the healthy individual with a rapid onset of flulike symptoms can have an ominous illness such as SARS (2002–2003) and as occurred with the anthrax exposures in 2001.

Nurses should have a heightened awareness of trends that may suggest the beginning of an epidemic/pandemic or a deliberate dispersal of toxic or infectious agents, including the following:

- An unusual increase in the number of individuals seeking care for fever, respiratory, or gastrointestinal symptoms.
- Clusters of patients who present with the same unusual illness from a single location. For example, clusters can be from a specific geographic location, such as a city, or from a single sporting or entertainment event.
- A large number of rapidly fatal cases, especially when death occurs within 72 hours after hospital admission.
- Any increase in disease incidence in a normally healthy population. These cases should be reported to the local or provincial/territorial medical officer of health.

If any of these trends are noted, an extensive patient history is taken in an attempt to identify the possible agent involved. This history includes an occupational, work, and environmental assessment, in addition to the regular admission history. An exposure history contains, at a minimum, information about current and past exposures to possible hazards and an assessment of the patient's typical day and any deviations in routines. The work history includes, at a minimum, a description of all previous jobs, including short-term, seasonal, and part-time employment and any military service. The environmental history includes assessment of present and previous home locations, water supply, and any hobbies, to name a few factors. The admission history should include such information as recent travel and contact with others who have been ill or have recently died of a fatal illness. This is just a brief review of the extensive history that may need to be obtained to identify an exposure agent and should become a universal part of admission processes at all health care organizations (Agency for Toxic Substances and Disease Registry, 2016).

Suspicions or findings are reported to the appropriate resources in the facility and to proper authorities in the community. Resources can include the Infection Control Department, the local or provincial/territorial medical officer of health, **safety data sheets (SDS)**, the PHAC, the local poison control centre, and many Internet sites. Reporting furnishes data elements to those agencies responsible for epidemiology and response. Reporting also allows for sharing of information among facilities and jurisdictions and can help determine the source of infections or exposure and prevent further exposures and even deaths.

Personal Protective Equipment

Another component of preparedness and response involves the protection of the health care provider by additional **personal protective equipment (PPE)**. Chemical or biologic agents and radiation are silent killers and are generally colourless and odourless. The purpose of PPE is to shield health care workers from the chemical, physical, biologic, and radiologic hazards that may exist when caring for contaminated patients. The U.S. Environmental Protection Agency (EPA) has divided protective clothing and respiratory protection into the following four categories, levels A through D:

- Level A protection is worn when the highest level of respiratory, skin, eye, and mucous membrane protection is required. This includes a self-contained breathing apparatus (SCBA) and a fully encapsulating, vapour-tight, chemical-resistant suit with chemical-resistant gloves and boots.
- Level B protection requires the highest level of respiratory protection but a lesser level of skin and eye protection than with level A situations. This level of protection includes the SCBA and a chemical-resistant suit, but the suit is not vapour tight.
- Level C protection requires the air-purified respirator, which uses filters or sorbent materials to remove harmful substances from the air. A chemical-resistant coverall with splash hood, chemical-resistant gloves, and boots are included in level C protection.
- Level D protection is the typical work uniform.

Levels C and D PPE are the levels most often used in hospital facilities.

Protective equipment must be donned before contact with a contaminated patient. The acute care facility's standard precaution PPE (level D) generally is not adequate for protection from a chemically, biologically, or radiologically contaminated patient. Level C PPE is adequate for the average patient exposure. The health care provider must use equipment that is capable of providing protection against the agent involved. This may mean using a splash suit along with a full-face positive-pressure or negative-pressure respirator (a filter-type gas mask) or even an SCBA for medical personnel in the field. Most emergency response plans in Canada have adopted the U.S. Occupational Health and Safety Administration PPE levels.

No single PPE is capable of protecting against all hazards. Under no circumstances should responders wear any PPE without proper training, practice, and fit testing of respirator masks as necessary (Valdez, 2015). For example, since SARS (2002–2003), nursing students in most programs in Canada must be fit-tested for masks before beginning any acute care clinical placement.

Decontamination

Decontamination, the process of removing accumulated contaminants, is critical to the health and safety of health care providers by preventing secondary contamination.

The decontamination plan should establish procedures and educate employees about decontamination procedures, identify the equipment needed and methods to be used, and establish methods for disposal of contaminated materials (Veenema, 2013).

Canadian researchers are piloting a new HazMat decontamination protocol to help civilians during a disaster (Quan, 2014). The protocol is for first responders to help civilians in the critical moments after a mass-casualty chemical, biologic, or radiologic incident. The protocol is applicable in many disaster scenarios, for example, chemical leaks from truck spills or train derailments, mishandling of pesticides in agricultural settings and terrorist attacks.

Although many principles and theories surround decontamination of a patient, authorities agree that, to be effective, decontamination must include a minimum of two steps. The first step is removal of the patient's clothing and jewellery and then rinsing the patient with water. Depending on the type of exposure, this step alone can remove a large amount of the contamination and decrease secondary contamination. The second step consists of a thorough soap-and-water wash and rinse. When patients arrive at the organization after being assessed and treated by a prehospital provider, it should not be assumed that they have been thoroughly decontaminated. The hospital must be prepared to perform additional decontamination prior to entry into the facility. The hospital personnel may also treat "walking wounded" or "worried well" who did not receive any decontamination at the scene.

NURSING ALERT

When patients arrive at the facility after being assessed and treated by a prehospital provider, it should not be assumed that they have been thoroughly decontaminated.

Natural Disasters

Natural disasters may result in mass casualties. Natural disasters can occur anywhere at any time and include events such as tornadoes, hurricanes, floods, avalanches, tidal waves (e.g., tsunamis), earthquakes, and volcanic eruptions. In the event of a natural disaster, loss of communications, potable water, and electricity is usually the greatest obstacle to a well-coordinated emergency response, and preparatory planning is essential. Communications systems such as wireless technology (e.g., cellular phones, computers, other communication devices) and hardwired technology (traditional telephone, fax machines, etc.) may or may not be functional. Recent information has indicated that the use of social media may, in fact, save lives in a disaster. With 27 million cell phone users in Canada, the use of social media in disaster situations is of great importance (Canadian Wireless Telecommunications Association, 2013). Using Twitter, tweets about an East Coast USA earthquake actually outran the quake itself, meaning people were informed *before* the quake even hit. Although it was only, on average, a 30-second warning, that was likely time for people to move to safer locations within their home or workplace.

The majority of the immediate casualties are trauma related. These mass casualties tax the trauma system to its limits to provide triage, transport of patients (in poor weather and road conditions), and management within the trauma centres. The majority of patients usually begin arriving within an hour of the event. However, the "walking wounded" may not seek care for 5 days to 2 weeks after the event or may seek care for injuries received during clean-up activities. Casualties arrive at hospitals in three waves. The first wave consists of minimally (generally) injured individuals who arrive of their own accord. The second wave consists of severely injured patients. The third wave consists of injured patients who arrive after they are discovered by rescuers. For example, in the event of earthquakes, buildings collapse and cause the majority of fatalities from injuries that primarily involve the head and chest (Veenema, 2013). The majority of the patients usually begin arriving within an hour of the event; the "walking wounded" may not seek care for 5 days to 2 weeks after the event or may seek care for injuries inflicted during the clean-up activities.

Excessive exposure to the natural elements and the need for food and water (by both patients and emergency responders) are critical issues. Without cover (e.g., buildings may be unsafe or destroyed) or potable water (e.g., water may be either contaminated or unavailable), injuries from exposure to heat, cold, or contaminated food or water can occur. Safety equipment that protects rescue workers from injury, exposure, and potentially dangerous animals (e.g., snakes, alligators, spiders) must be readily available. Rescue workers may also injure themselves in the process of extrication or cleanup (e.g., chain saws, building collapse). Hypothermia can occur rapidly in workers who are exposed to water at temperatures of 23.9°C or less. As is true during all disasters, mental health workers and shelters are needed throughout the community. Veterinary assistance is also essential because pets are frequently abandoned and injured. In addition, emergency response workers must be prepared to treat the most common ailments experienced after exposure to a specific natural disaster. For instance, pulmonary problems peak with earthquakes and volcanic eruptions because of the increased particulate matter in the air. Most volcano-related deaths are from suffocation. After floods or water disasters, waterborne transmission of agents such as *Escherichia coli*, *Salmonella*, *Shigella*, typhoid, leptospirosis, malaria, and tularemia are common and cause widespread disease. In addition, other waterborne hazards can include human exposure to poisonous snakes and alligators in the flood waters. The Lac-Mégantic derailment in July 2013 was the fourth deadliest train crash in Canadian history, killing 47 people, destroying 40 buildings, and spilling millions of litres of crude oil in the town and nearby lake and rivers (Beaudin, 2014).

In some instances, early warning systems have assisted in decreasing the number of deaths from tornadoes and hurricanes. However, even with the advent of early warning systems, some individuals are unable or unwilling to leave prior to the occurrence of the natural disaster. When buildings collapse, rapid response to identify and remove trapped victims is the only means of improving survivability. There is a direct relationship between time trapped and survival; fewer than 50% of individuals survive if they are trapped more than 2 to 6 hours. Water-damaged buildings are not safe and require extensive examination before experts can ensure safe occupancy. Larger-scale issues that can cause significant later morbidity and mortality include the absence of water purification, waste removal, removal of human and animal remains, and vector control. Removal or disposal of biologic, chemical, and nuclear agents must also be considered.

Weapons of Terror

Although biologic, chemical, and radiologic events are not everyday events, they can occur at any organization, and every nurse needs to know the basics of caring for affected patients. An explosion may spread the dangerous material. Therefore, treatment of blast injuries must be anticipated and planned.

Blast Injury

Examples of recent highly publicized bombings that have caused significant injuries or loss of lives include those in a disco in Tel Aviv in 2001, in the London subway system in 2005, and on the Mumbai (India) commuter trains in 2006. Terrorist bombings occur frequently throughout the Middle East today, particularly in Iraq and Afghanistan. Several types of bombs are typically used, resulting in various injuries.

Types of Explosive Devices

Commonly used bombs include pipe bombs, Molotov cocktails, fertilizer bombs, and "dirty" bombs (so-called because they spread radiation). The most commonly utilized bomb is the pipe bomb, which consists of relatively low-velocity explosives and may also contain nails or other implements that cause more damage when the explosive ignites. Another type of commonly used explosive device is the Molotov cocktail, which uses a common flammable liquid such as gasoline in a glass bottle and a source of ignition, such as a rag. This forms a simple yet effective incendiary device. Other common explosive devices include fertilizer bombs, which were used in the Oklahoma City bombing in 1995, and dirty bombs, which include a radioactive source that spreads radiation after the initial blast. Common hazards following a bombing include secondary devices (set to explode at a predetermined time, typically after the arrival of rescue personnel), building collapse, contamination from biologic, chemical, or radiologic weapons, and the presence of terrorists among the patients and bystanders. The entire scene of the bombing is a crime scene and is treated as such. Triage of patients involved in a bombing is the same as for all disasters, with a heightened awareness that serious internal injuries from the blast wave may not be evident.

Physical Injuries

The actual blast that occurs during the initial seconds of the bombing causes a pressure wave or primary blast wave. Injuries can result from the impact of the explosion, the primary blast wave, or shrapnel within the bomb. The majority of injuries are caused by the primary blast wave. A blast wave has four effects. These include spalling, which refers to the pressure wave; implosion, which refers to rupture of organs from entrapped gases; shearing, which refers to the blast response of different body tissues dependent on their density; and irreversible work, which refers to the presence of forces that exceed the tensile strength of an organ or tissue.

Different phases of the blast may result in common injuries that include blast lung, tympanic membrane (TM) rupture, and head and abdominal injuries (Table 74-2). Although approximately 50% to 70% of deaths result from head injuries, the majority of head injuries are not life threatening. Bombings that occur in enclosed spaces amplify the blast wave, resulting in more pressure wave injuries. Distance from the blast, whether the blast space was enclosed, composition of the explosive, whether a building collapsed, and the efficiency of medical resources available after the blast all affect patient outcomes after a blast injury.

TABLE 74-2 Phases of Blasts and Associated Common Injuries

Phase of Blast Injury	Common Injuries
Primary: Results from pressure wave	Pulmonary barotraumas, including pulmonary contusions Head injuries, including concussion, other severe brain injuries Tympanic membrane rupture, middle ear injury Abdominal hollow organ perforation, hemorrhage
Secondary: Results from debris from the scene or shrapnel from the bomb	Penetrating trunk, skin, and soft tissue injuries Fractures, traumatic amputations
Tertiary: Results from pressure wave that causes the victim to be thrown	Head injuries Fractures, including skull
Quaternary: Results from pre-existing conditions exacerbated by the force of the blast or by postblast injury complications	Severe injuries with complex injury patterns—burns, crush injuries, head injuries Common pre-existing conditions that become exacerbated—COPD, asthma, cardiac conditions, diabetes, and hypertension

COPD, chronic obstructive pulmonary disease.
Adapted from Pennardt, A., & Lavonas, E. J. (2016). Blast injuries. *Medscape*. Retrieved April 2, 2017, from emedicine.medscape.com/article/822587-overview

Blast Lung

Blast lung results from the blast wave as it passes through air-filled lungs. The result is hemorrhage and tearing of the lung, ventilation–perfusion mismatch, and possible air emboli. Typical signs and symptoms include dyspnea, hypoxia, tachypnea or apnea (depending on severity), cough, chest pain, and hemodynamic instability. Management involves providing respiratory support that includes administration of supplemental oxygen, but may also require intubation and mechanical ventilation. If a hemothorax or pneumothorax is present, a chest tube must be inserted to re-expand the lung. In the event of an air embolus, the patient should be immediately placed in the prone left lateral position to prevent migration of the embolus and will require emergent treatment in a hyperbaric chamber. Complications following blast lung can include respiratory failure as well as acute respiratory distress syndrome (ARDS) (see Chapter 24 for further discussion).

Tympanic Membrane Rupture

The TM is the most frequent injury after subjection to a pressure wave because it is the body's most sensitive organ to pressure. There is an increased incidence of TM rupture when a blast occurs in close proximity to the patient and when it occurs in an enclosed space. Signs and symptoms include hearing loss, tinnitus, pain, dizziness, and otorrhea. The majority of TM ruptures heal spontaneously. A chest radiograph is recommended in the presence of TM rupture since this may indicate exposure to significant overpressure. In a large series of victims of terrorist bombings, mostly involving closed spaces, 22% of patients with eardrum perforation had other significant injuries (Pennardt & Lavonas, 2014). Other ear injuries may include ossicular disruption and impaction of foreign bodies.

Abdominal and Head Injuries

Blast abdomen may be evidenced by abdominal hemorrhage and internal organ injury. The typical signs and symptoms of internal abdominal injury can include pain, guarding, rebound tenderness, rectal bleeding, nausea, and vomiting (see Chapter 73 for further discussion of abdominal trauma) (CDC, 2012).

Head injuries are typically minor but those that are severe result in the majority of postblast deaths. These injuries can occur without a direct blow to the head and may result from the blast itself, building collapse, or flying debris. Concussions commonly occur postblast and the usual follow-up evaluation and treatment for postconcussive syndrome is indicated (see Chapter 65 for further discussion of head injuries). Approximately 30% of head injuries involve vascular structures (e.g., arteriovenous fistula, pseudoaneurysm, or dissection) (Veenema, 2013).

Special Populations

Special populations may have different blast-associated risks. For instance, the older people are particularly susceptible to bone fractures because they tend to have decreased bone density. They also tend to have more preexisting morbid conditions that may be exacerbated by the explosion. Pregnant patients' abdomens are particularly susceptible to placental shear forces that may result in abruptio placentae. Individuals with mobility disabilities may have difficulty extricating themselves from the site of the blast (CDC, 2012).

Biologic Weapons

Biologic weapons are weapons that spread disease among the general population or the military.

Effects of Biologic Weapons

Biologic warfare is a covert method of severely affecting the target. Biologic weapons are easily obtained and easily disseminated and can result in significant mortality and morbidity. The potential use of biologic agents calls for continuous increased surveillance by health care organizations and ministries of health and an increased index of suspicion by clinicians. Many biologic weapons result in signs and symptoms similar to those of common disease processes. Appropriate management of a biologic threat includes rapid recognition of the potential agent; use of proper PPE; decontamination, isolation or quarantine of infected patients when appropriate; and the administration of appropriate vaccinations, antidotes, or medications to individuals at risk.

Biologic agents are delivered in either a liquid or dry state, applied to foods or water, or vaporized for inhalation or direct contact. Vaporization may be accomplished through spray or explosives loaded with the agent. With increased travel, an agent could be released in one city and affect individuals in other cities thousands of miles away. The vector can be an insect, animal, or individual, or there may be direct contact with the agent itself.

The following is a discussion of two of the agents most likely to be used or weaponized. Table 74-3 describes other easily weaponized biologic agents.

Types of Biologic Agents

Anthrax

Anthrax is recognized as the most likely weaponized biologic agent available and has been recognized as a highly debilitating agent for centuries. *Bacillus anthracis* is a naturally occurring gram-positive, encapsulated rod that lives in the soil in the spore state throughout the world. The bacterium sporulates (i.e., is liberated) when exposed to air and is infective only in the spore form. Contact with infected animal products (raw meat) or inhalation of the spores results in infection. Cattle and other herbivores are vaccinated against anthrax to prevent transmission through contaminated meat.

The number of spores needed to cause inhalational anthrax varies, as evidenced by anthrax cases in the United States in 2001, indicating that fewer spores of weapon-grade anthrax may be required to cause inhalational anthrax (Cunha, 2014). As an aerosol, anthrax is odourless and invisible and can travel a great distance before disseminating; hence, the site of release and the site of infection can be kilometres apart.

CLINICAL MANIFESTATIONS. Anthrax is caused by replicating bacteria that release toxin, resulting in hemorrhage, edema, and necrosis. The incubation period is 1 to 6 days. There are three primary methods of infection: skin contact, inhalation, and gastrointestinal ingestion. Skin lesions (the most common infection) cause edema with pruritus and macule or papule formation, resulting in ulceration with 1- to 3-mm vesicles. A painless eschar develops, which falls off in 1 to 2 weeks (Auerbach, 2017).

Ingestion of anthrax results in fever, nausea and vomiting, abdominal pain, bloody diarrhea, and occasionally ascites. If severe diarrhea develops, decreased intravascular volume becomes the primary treatment concern. The bacterium affects the terminal ileum and cecum. Sepsis can occur.

The inhalation form of anthrax results in the most severe clinical manifestations. Its symptoms mimic those

TABLE 74-3 Selected Examples of Biologic Agents That Can Be Used as Weapons

Agent/Organism	Contagion	Decontamination and Protective Equipment	Signs and Symptoms	Treatment (Mortality Rate)
Tularemia—*Francisella tularensis:* Gram-negative coccobacillus, one of the most infectious bacteria known.	Direct contact with infected animals or aerosolized as a bioterror weapon; bites Not contagious through human-to-human contact Found in Oklahoma, Missouri, Arkansas	Standard barrier precautions. Clothing and linens should be laundered under the usual hospital protocol.	*Initial:* Abrupt onset of fever, fatigue, chills, headache, lower backache, malaise, rigour, coryza, dry cough, and sore throat without adenopathy. Nausea and vomiting or diarrhea possible. *As disease progresses:* Sweating, fever, progressive weakness, anorexia, and weight loss demonstrate continued illness. *Mortality secondary to:* Pneumonitis (if inhalation is the source) with copious watery or purulent sputum, hemoptysis, respiratory insufficiency, sepsis, and shock.	Streptomycin or gentamicin/aminoglycoside for 10–14 days. Inhalation tularemia must be treated within 48 hours of onset. In mass casualty situations, doxycycline or ciprofloxacin is recommended. For persons exposed to tularemia, tetracycline or doxycycline is recommended for 14 days. (Mortality rate = 2%)
Botulism—*Clostridium botulinum:* Botulinum blocks acetylcholine-containing vesicles from fusing with the terminal membranes of the motor neuron end-plate, resulting in a flaccid paralysis.	Direct contact Not contagious through human-to-human contact	Any skin exposure to the botulism toxin can be treated with soap and water or a 0.1% hypochlorite solution. Standard precautions are used when treating patients with botulism.	*Gastrointestinal botulism:* Abdominal cramps, nausea, vomiting, and diarrhea *Inhalation botulism:* Fever; symmetric descending flaccid paralysis with multiple cranial nerve palsies. *Classic signs and symptoms include* diplopia, dysphagia, dry mouth, lack of fever, and alert mental status. *Other possible symptoms include* ptosis of the eyelids, blurred vision, enlarged sluggish pupils, dysarthria, and dysphonia. *Mortality secondary to:* Airway obstruction and inadequate tidal volume	Supportive ventilatory therapy is necessary if respiratory infection occurs. Aminoglycosides and clindamycin are contraindicated because they exacerbate neuromuscular blockage. Equine antitoxin is used to minimize subsequent nerve damage. There is a 2% rate of anaphylaxis to the antitoxin; therefore, diphenhydramine (Benadryl) and epinephrine must be immediately available for use. Supportive care—mechanical ventilation, nutrition, fluids, prevention of complications (Mortality rate = 5%).
Plague—*Yersinia pestis:* nonsporulating gram-negative coccobacillus. The bacterium causes destruction and necrosis of the lymph nodes.	Contagious *Bubonic plague:* Transmitted through flea bites with no person-to-person transmission *Pneumonic plague:* Transmitted through respiratory droplet contact	Isolation barrier precautions with full face respirators; the patient should wear a mask. Rooms should receive a terminal cleaning. Clothing and linens with body fluids on them should be cleaned with the usual disinfectant. Routine precautions should be used in the case of death.	*Bubonic plague:* Sudden fever and chills, weakness, a swollen and tender lymph node (bubo) in the groin, axilla, or cervical area. The resultant bacteremia progresses to septicemia from the endotoxin and, finally, shock and death. *Primary septicemic plague:* Disseminated intravascular coagulation, necrosis of small vessels, purpura, and gangrene of the digits and nose (black death). *Pneumonic plague:* Severe bronchospasm, chest pain, dyspnea, cough, and hemoptysis. There is a 100% mortality associated with pneumonic plague if not treated within the first 24 hours.	Streptomycin or gentamicin for 10–14 days. Start within 12–24 hours. Tetracycline or doxycycline is an acceptable alternative if an aminoglycoside cannot be given. People with close contact exposure (<2 m) require prophylaxis with doxycycline for 7 days. (Mortality rate = 50%)

Adapted from Dire, D. J. (2016). CBRNE—Biological warfare agents. *Medscape.* Retrieved November 26, 2016, from emedicine.medscape.com/article/829613-overview; Emergency Nurses Association. (2013). *Sheehy's manual of emergency care* (7th ed.). St. Louis, MO: Elsevier Mosby; Emergency Nurses Association. (2014). *Trauma nursing core course* (7th ed.). Chicago, IL: Author; and Veenema, T. G. (2013). *Disaster nursing and emergency preparedness* (3rd ed.). New York: Springer.

of the flu, and usually treatment is sought only when the second stage of severe respiratory distress occurs. At this point, even antibiotic therapy will not halt the progress of the disease. Inhaled anthrax can incubate for up to 60 days, making it difficult to identify its source. Initial signs and symptoms include cough, headache, fever, vomiting, chills, weakness, mild chest discomfort, dyspnea, and syncope, without rhinorrhea or nasal congestion. Most patients have a brief recovery period followed by the second stage within 1 to 3 days, characterized by fever, severe respiratory distress, stridor, hypoxia, cyanosis, diaphoresis, hypotension, and shock. These patients require optimization of oxygenation, correction of electrolyte imbalances, and ventilatory and hemodynamic support. The majority of these patients may have hemorrhagic mediastinitis on a chest x-ray (a hallmark sign). The disease can also progress to include meningitis with subarachnoid hemorrhage. Death results approximately 24 to 36 hours after the onset of severe respiratory distress. The mortality rate approaches 100% (Auerbach, 2017).

TREATMENT. Presently, anthrax is penicillin sensitive; however, strains of penicillin-resistant anthrax are thought to exist. Recommended treatment includes penicillin (Penicillin V), erythromycin (E-mycin, Erythrocin), gentamicin (Garamycin), or doxycycline (Vibramycin). If antibiotic treatment begins within 24 hours after exposure, death can be prevented. In a mass casualty situation, treatment with ciprofloxacin (Cipro) or doxycycline is recommended. Treatment is continued for 60 days. For patients who have been directly exposed to anthrax but have no signs and symptoms of disease, ciprofloxacin or doxycycline is used for prophylaxis for 60 days (Auerbach, 2017).

Standard precautions are the only ones indicated to protect the caregiver exposed to a patient infected with anthrax. The patient is not contagious, and the disease cannot spread from individual to individual. Equipment should be cleaned using standard hospital disinfectant. After death, cremation is recommended because the spores can survive for decades and represent a threat to morticians and forensic medicine personnel.

There is a vaccine for anthrax however, it is not yet widely used because it requires multiple time-interval–sensitive boosters and has up to a 48% systemic reaction rate. The anthrax vaccine is given in a series of six shots over 18 months and each year a booster dose is given. Only people at high risk of exposure should be given the anthrax vaccine. This may include certain laboratory workers, people who work with imported animals where preventive standards are lacking (such as veterinarians who travel to work in other countries), and certain military personnel (Healthwise, 2012).

Smallpox

Smallpox (variola) is classified as a DNA virus. It has an incubation period of approximately 10 to 14 days (PHAC, 2014). It is extremely contagious and is spread by direct contact, by contact with clothing or linens, or by droplets from individual to individual only after the fever has decreased and the rash phase has begun. There is an associated 30% case fatality rate (i.e., the likelihood of fatality per case diagnosed). Aerosolization of the virus would result in widespread dissemination.

The World Health Organization declared smallpox eradicated in 1977 and stopped worldwide vaccination in 1980. In Canada, the last children were vaccinated in the 1970s. Therefore, a large portion of the current population has no immunity to the virus. A smallpox vaccination plan introduced in 2003 proposed that a designated number of ED staff receive the first vaccinations to ensure that ED staff would be immunized in the event of a smallpox outbreak. The government estimated that 0.1% of those individuals receiving the vaccine would have serious side effects. Of these, approximately 4% would have life-threatening complications, and 0.1% would die. Canada supports the recommendation to not routinely immunize the general Canadian population against smallpox, thus, as a result, smallpox vaccination is highly restricted (PHAC, 2014). The Canadian Smallpox Contingency Plan (PHAC, 2014) provides recommendations for actions to be taken if smallpox occurs in Canada or elsewhere in the world.

CLINICAL MANIFESTATIONS. Signs and symptoms of smallpox infection include high fever, malaise, headache, backache, and prostration. After 1 to 2 days, a maculopapular rash appears, evolving at the same rate, beginning on the face, mouth, pharynx, and forearms. Only then does the rash progress to the trunk and also become vesicular to pustular (Veenema, 2013). There is a large amount of the virus in the saliva and pustules. Smallpox is contagious only after the appearance of the rash. There are two forms of smallpox, variola major and variola minor. Variola major is more common, results in a higher fever and more extensive rash, and has a 30% case fatality rate. Hemorrhagic smallpox, a subtype of variola major, includes all of the above signs and symptoms plus a dusky erythema and petechiae leading to frank hemorrhage of the skin and mucous membranes, and it results in death by day 5 or 6 (Veenema, 2013).

TREATMENT. Treatment includes supportive care with antibiotics for any additional infection. The patient must be isolated with the use of transmission precautions. Laundry and biologic wastes should be autoclaved before being washed with hot water and bleach. Standard decontamination of the room is effective. All individuals who have household or face-to-face contact with the patient after the fever begins should be vaccinated within 4 days to prevent infection and death. A patient with a temperature of 38°C or higher within 17 days after exposure must be placed in isolation. Cremation is preferred for all deaths because the virus can survive in scabs for up to 13 years (Veenema, 2013).

Severe Acute Respiratory Syndrome

Not all mass casualty biologic events are terrorist based. The SARS outbreak in 2003 is a prime example of a non–terrorist-based mass casualty biologic event. The disease started as "atypical" pneumonia in China in February and spread to 29 countries throughout the world by July. Air travel and worldwide trade have increased the possibility that any contagious disease may spread rapidly.

SARS is caused by a virus, officially named SARS-CoV. Its incubation period is 2 to 10 days. Individuals at risk include health care workers who have had unprotected exposure to SARS-CoV. See Chapter 24 for further discussion of SARS.

TABLE 74-4 Common Chemical Agents

Agent	Action	Signs and Symptoms	Decontamination and Treatment
Nerve Agents			
Sarin Soman	Inhibition of cholinesterase	Increased secretions (salivation, lacrimation, emesis, urination), gastrointestinal motility, diarrhea, bronchospasm	Soap and water Supportive care Benzodiazepines Pralidoxime Atropine
Blood Agent			
Cyanide	Inhibition of aerobic metabolism	Inhalation—tachypnea, tachycardia, coma, seizures; bright red skin; can progress to respiratory arrest, respiratory failure, cardiac arrest, death	Soap and water Sodium nitrite Sodium thiocyanate Amyl nitrate Hydroxocobalamin
Vesicant Agents			
Lewisite Sulphur mustard Nitrogen mustard Phosgene	Blistering agents	Superficial to partial-thickness burn with vesicles that coalesce; conjunctivitis, nasal irritation	Soap and water Blot; do not rub dry
Pulmonary Agents			
Phosgene Chlorine	Separation of alveoli from capillary bed	Pulmonary edema, bronchospasm, chest tightness, burning sensation, blurry vision; Phosgene can result in pain then blisters followed by partial- to full-thickness burn	Copious flushing Move to fresh air—away from gases Airway management Ventilatory support Bronchoscopy

Adapted from Ciottone, G. R., & Arnold, J. L. (2015). CBRNE—Chemical warfare agents. *Medscape.* Retrieved November 26, 2015, from emedicine.medscape.com/article/829454-overview; Emergency Nurses Association. (2013). *Sheehy's manual of emergency care* (7th ed.). St Louis, MO: Elsevier Mosby; Emergency Nurses Association. (2014). *Trauma nursing core course* (7th ed.). Chicago, IL: Author; and Veenema, T. G. (2013). *Disaster nursing and emergency preparedness* (3rd ed.). New York: Springer.

Chemical Weapons

Agents that may be used in **chemical warfare** are overt agents in that the effects are more apparent and occur more quickly than those caused by biologic weapons. Refer to Table 74-4 for an overview of common chemical agents.

Characteristics of Chemicals

Volatility

Volatility is the tendency for a chemical to become a vapour. The most common volatile agents are phosgene and cyanide. Most chemicals are heavier than air, except for hydrogen cyanide. Therefore, in the presence of most chemicals, individuals should stand up to avoid heavy exposure (because the chemical will sink toward the floor or ground).

Persistence

Persistence means that the chemical is less likely to vaporize and disperse. More volatile chemicals do not evaporate very quickly. Most industrial chemicals (e.g., cyanide) are not very persistent. Weaponized agents (chemicals developed as weapons by the military or terrorists [e.g., mustard gas]) are more likely than industrial chemicals to penetrate skin and mucous membranes and also cause secondary exposure.

Toxicity

Toxicity is the potential of an agent to cause injury to the body. The median lethal dose (LD_{50}) is the amount of the chemical that will cause death in 50% of those who are exposed. The median effective dose (ED_{50}) is the amount of the chemical that will cause signs and symptoms in 50% of those who are exposed. The concentration time (CT) is the concentration released multiplied by the time exposed (mg/min). For example, if 1,000 mg of a chemical is released and the time an individual is exposed to this amount of chemical is 10 minutes, then the CT would be 10,000 mg/min.

Latency

Latency is the time from absorption to the appearance of signs and symptoms. Sulphur mustards and pulmonary agents have the longest latency, whereas other vesicants, nerve agents, and cyanide produce signs and symptoms within seconds.

Limiting Exposure

Evacuation is essential, as is the removal of the individual's clothing and decontamination as close to the scene as possible and before transport of the exposed individual. Soap and water are effective means of decontamination in most cases. Staff involved in decontamination efforts must wear PPE and contain and dispose of the runoff after decontamination procedures.

Types of Chemicals

Vesicants

Vesicants are chemicals that cause blistering and result in burning, conjunctivitis, bronchitis, pneumonia, hematopoietic suppression, and death. Examples of vesicants include lewisite, phosgene, nitrogen mustard, and sulphur mustard. In World War I and in the Iran–Iraq conflict of

1980 to 1988, vesicants were used to disable opponents. Vesicants were the primary incapacitating agents, resulting in minimal (less than 5%) death but large numbers of injuries (Veenema, 2013). Liquid sulphur mustard was the most frequently used vesicant in these conflicts. The skin damage is irreversible but is seldom fatal (2% to 3% mortality).

CLINICAL MANIFESTATIONS. The initial presentation after exposure to a vesicant is similar to that of a large superficial to partial-thickness burn in the warm and moist areas of the body (i.e., perineum, axillae, antecubital spaces). There is stinging and erythema for approximately 24 hours, followed by pruritus, painful burning, and small vesicle formation after 2 to 18 hours. These vesicles can coalesce into large, fluid-filled bullae. Lewisite and phosgene result in immediate pain after exposure. Tissue damage occurs within minutes.

If the eye is exposed, there is pain, photophobia, lacrimation, and decreased vision. This progresses to conjunctivitis, blepharospasm, corneal ulcer, and corneal edema.

Respiratory effects are more serious and often are the cause of mortality with vesicant exposure. Purulent fibrinous pseudomembrane discharge may cause obstruction of the airways. Gastrointestinal exposure may cause nausea and vomiting, leukopenia, and upper gastrointestinal bleeding.

TREATMENT. Appropriate decontamination includes soap and water. Scrubbing and the use of hypochlorite solutions should be avoided because they increase penetration. Once the substance has penetrated, it cannot be removed. Eye exposure requires copious irrigation. For respiratory exposure, intubation and bronchoscopy to remove necrotic tissue are essential. With lewisite exposure, dimercaprol (BAL in oil) is administered intravenously for systemic toxicity and topically for skin lesions. All individuals with sulphur mustard exposures should be monitored for 24 hours for delayed (latent) effects.

Nerve Agents

The most toxic agents in existence are the nerve agents such as sarin, soman, tabun, VX, and organophosphates (pesticides). They are inexpensive, effective in small quantities, and easily dispersed. In the liquid form, nerve agents evaporate into a colourless, odourless vapour. Organophosphates are similar in nature to the nerve agents used in warfare and are readily available. Nerve agents can be inhaled or absorbed percutaneously or subcutaneously. These agents bond with acetylcholinesterase, so that acetylcholine is not inactivated; the adverse result is continuous stimulation (hyperstimulation) of the nerve endings. Carbamates, which are insecticides originally extracted from the Calabar bean, are derivatives of carbamic acid; they are nerve agents that specifically inhibit acetylcholinesterase for several hours and then spontaneously become unbound from the acetylcholinesterase. However, organophosphates require the formation of new enzyme (acetylcholinesterase) before nervous system function can be restored.

A very small drop of a nerve agent is enough to result in sweating and twitching at the site of exposure. A larger amount results in more systemic symptoms. Effects can begin anywhere from 30 minutes up to 18 hours after exposure. The more common organophosphates and carbamates (e.g., sevin, malathion) that are used in agriculture result in less severe symptoms than do those used in warfare. In an ordinary situation (e.g., nonwarfare, nonterrorist attack situation), a patient could arrive at the ED having been unintentionally or intentionally exposed to organophosphates in a suicidal attempt.

CLINICAL MANIFESTATIONS. Signs and symptoms of nerve gas exposure are those of cholinergic crisis and include bilateral miosis, visual disturbances, increased gastrointestinal motility, nausea and vomiting, diarrhea, substernal spasm, indigestion, bradycardia and atrioventricular block, bronchoconstriction, laryngeal spasm, weakness, fasciculations, and incontinence. The patient must be examined in a dark area to truly identify miosis. Neurologic responses include insomnia, forgetfulness, impaired judgment, depression, and irritability. A lethal dose results in loss of consciousness, seizures, copious secretions, fasciculations, flaccid muscles, and apnea.

TREATMENT. Decontamination with copious amounts of soap and water or saline solution for 8 to 20 minutes is essential. The water is blotted off, not wiped off, the skin. Fresh 0.5% hypochlorite solution (bleach) can also be used. The airway is maintained, and suctioning is frequently required. One must be aware that plastic airway equipment will absorb sarin gas, resulting in continued exposure to the agent.

IV atropine 2 to 4 mg is administered, followed by 2 mg every 3 to 8 minutes for up to 24 hours of treatment. Alternatively, IV atropine 1 to 2 mg/hr may be administered until clear signs of anticholinergic activity have returned (decreased secretions, tachycardia, and decreased gastrointestinal motility). Another medication that may serve as an antidote is pralidoxime (2-PAM), which allows cholinesterase to become active against acetylcholine. Pralidoxime 1 to 2 g in 100 to 150 mL of normal saline solution is administered over 15 to 30 minutes. Pralidoxime has no effect on secretions and may have any of the following side effects: hypertension, tachycardia, weakness, dizziness, blurred vision, and diplopia. Diazepam (Valium) or other benzodiazepines are used to control seizures, to decrease fasciculations, and to alleviate apprehension and agitation. Military personnel believed to be at risk for chemical attack are provided with Mark I automatic injectors, which contain 2-mg atropine and 600-mg pralidoxime chloride. Diazepam may be administered by a partner.

Blood Agents

Blood agents such as hydrogen cyanide and cyanogen chloride have a direct effect on cellular metabolism, resulting in asphyxiation through alterations in hemoglobin. Cyanide is an agent that has profound systemic effects. It is commonly used in the mining of gold and silver and in the plastics and dye industries. In 1984, the Union Carbide pesticide plant in Bhopal, India, inadvertently released large amounts of cyanide in an industrial disaster and hundreds of deaths occurred.

A cyanide release is often associated with the odour of bitter almonds. In house fires, cyanide is released during the combustion of plastics, rugs, silk, furniture, and other construction materials. There is a significant correlation between blood cyanide and carbon monoxide levels in patients who survive fires, and in many cases, the cause of death is cyanide poisoning.

CLINICAL MANIFESTATIONS. Cyanide can be ingested, inhaled, or absorbed through the skin and mucous membranes. Cyanide is protein bound and inhibits aerobic metabolism, leading to respiratory muscle failure, respiratory arrest, cardiac arrest, and death. Its inhalation results in flushing, tachypnea, tachycardia, nonspecific neurologic symptoms, stupor, coma, and seizure preceding respiratory arrest.

TREATMENT. Rapid administration of amyl nitrate, sodium nitrite, and sodium thiosulphate is essential to the successful management of cyanide exposure. First, the patient is intubated and placed on a ventilator. Next, amyl nitrate pearls are crushed and placed in the ventilator reservoir to induce methemoglobinemia. Cyanide has a 20% to 25% higher affinity for methemoglobin than it does for hemoglobin; it binds methemoglobin to form either cyanomethemoglobin or sulphmethemoglobin. The cyanomethemoglobin is then detoxified in the liver by the enzyme rhodanese. Next, sodium nitrite is administered intravenously to induce the rapid formation of methemoglobin. IV sodium thiosulphate is then administered; it has a higher affinity for cyanide than methemoglobin does and stimulates the conversion of cyanide to sodium thiocyanate, which can be excreted by the kidneys. Although they may be lifesaving, these emergency medications do have side effects: sodium nitrite can result in severe hypotension, and thiocyanate can cause vomiting, psychosis, arthralgia, and myalgia.

The production of methemoglobin is contraindicated in patients with smoke inhalation, because they already have decreased oxygen-carrying capacity secondary to the carboxyhemoglobin produced by smoke inhalation. In facilities where a hyperbaric chamber is available, it may be used to provide oxygenation while the previously discussed therapies are initiated. An alternative suggested treatment for cyanide poisoning is hydroxocobalamin (vitamin B_{12a}). Hydroxocobalamin binds cyanide to form cyanocobalamin (vitamin B_{12}). It must be administered intravenously in large doses. Administration of vitamin B_{12a} can result in a transient pink discolouration of mucous membranes, skin, and urine. In high doses, tachycardia and hypertension can occur, but they usually resolve within 48 hours.

Pulmonary Agents

Pulmonary agents such as phosgene and chlorine destroy the pulmonary membrane that separates the alveolus from the capillary bed, disrupting alveolar–capillary oxygen transport mechanisms. Capillary leakage results in fluid-filled alveoli. Phosgene and chlorine both vaporize, rapidly causing this pulmonary injury. Phosgene has the odour of fresh-mown hay.

Signs and symptoms include pulmonary edema with shortness of breath, especially during exertion. An initial hacking cough is followed by frothy sputum production. Phosgene poisoning results in severe pulmonary distress, and death may occur between 6 and 24 hours after exposure. There are no specific treatments for this type of poisoning other than supportive measures. A particulate air-filter mask is the only protection required to protect health care personnel. Phosgene does not injure the eyes.

Nuclear Radiation Exposure

The threat of **nuclear warfare** or radiation exposure is very real with the availability of nuclear material and easily concealed simple devices, such as the so-called dirty bomb, for dispersal. A dirty bomb is a conventional explosive (e.g., dynamite) that is packaged with radioactive material that scatters when the bomb is detonated. It disperses radioactive material and may be called a radiologic weapon, but is not a nuclear weapon, which uses a complex nuclear fission reaction that is thousands of times more devastating than the dirty bomb.

Sources of radioactive material include not only nuclear weapons but also reactors and simple radioactive samples, such as weapons-grade plutonium or uranium, freshly spent nuclear fuel, or medical supplies (e.g., radium, certain cesium isotopes) used in cancer treatments and radiology. Exposure of a large number of individuals can be accomplished by placing a radioactive sample in a public place. Thousands may be exposed this way; some may be immediately affected, and others may require health monitoring for many years to assess long-term effects. The effectiveness of these weapons was demonstrated in the devastating results of the bombings of Hiroshima and Nagasaki in World War II.

Nuclear reactor incidents have occurred in the Fukushima Daiichi (2011), the Chernobyl (1986), and the Three Mile Island (1979) nuclear facilities. Three hundred thousand people were evacuated and approximately 18,500 deaths occurred from the earthquake and tsunami that caused the Fukushima Daiichi nuclear meltdown (NPAJ, 2014). In comparison, in Chernobyl there were 31 official deaths on the day of the Chernobyl incident, which involved a core meltdown and explosion, releasing radiation throughout the community. The long-term effects of this incident, including increased incidence of thyroid cancers and leukemia, continue to be evaluated. Reactors, however, follow very strict security measures and protocols for prevention of core meltdown. These measures decrease the possibility of a radiation incident from a reactor.

Any terrorist-sponsored or unintentional radiation release can be sizable and may require the entire hospital and prehospital staff to be prepared, recognize signs and symptoms of exposure, and rapidly treat victims without contamination of personnel, visitors, patients, or the facility itself.

Types of Radiation

Atoms consist of protons, neutrons, and electrons. The protons and neutrons are in balance in the nucleus. The protons repel each other because they are all positively charged. The number of protons is specific for each element in the periodic table. There is a specific ratio of protons and neutrons for each different atom, and the result is element stability. When an element is radioactive, there is an imbalance in the nucleus, resulting from an excess of neutrons.

To achieve stability, a radioactive nuclide can eject particles until the most stable number (an even number) of protons and neutrons exists. A proton can become a neutron by ejecting a positron; conversely, a neutron can become a proton by ejecting a negative electron. An alpha particle is released when two protons and two electrons are ejected.

Alpha particles cannot penetrate the skin. A thin layer of paper or clothing is all that is necessary to protect the skin from alpha radiation. However, this low-level radiation can enter the body through inhalation, ingestion, or injection (open wound). Only localized damage occurs.

Beta particles have the ability to moderately penetrate the skin to the layer in which skin cells are being produced. This high-energy radiation can cause skin damage if the skin is exposed for a prolonged period and can cause injury if beta particles penetrate the skin.

Gamma radiation is a short-wavelength electromagnetic energy that is emitted when there is excess core nucleus energy. Gamma particles are penetrating. Therefore, it is difficult to shield against gamma radiation. X-rays are an example of gamma radiation. Gamma radiation often accompanies both alpha- and beta-particle emission.

Measurement and Detection

Radiation is measured in several different units. The *rad* is the basic unit of measurement. A rad is equivalent to 0.01 J of energy per kilogram of tissue. To determine the damaging effect of the rad, a conversion to the *rem* (roentgen equivalents human) is necessary. The rem reflects the type of radiation absorbed and the potential for damage. For example, 200,000 mrem results in mild radiation sickness (1 rem = 1,000 mrem) (ACS, 2010). Typical natural yearly exposure for an individual is 360 mrem. Another important concept is *half-life*. The half-life of a radioactive product is the time it takes to lose half of its radioactivity.

The only way to detect radiation is through a device that determines the exposure per minute. There are various devices for this purpose. The Geiger counter (or Geiger–Mueller survey meter) can measure background radiation quickly through detection of gamma radiation and some beta radiation. With high-level radiation, the Geiger counter may underestimate exposure. Other devices include the ionization chamber survey meter, alpha monitors, and dose rate meters. Personal dosimeters are simple tools that identify radiation exposure and are worn by radiology personnel.

Exposure

Exposure is affected by time, distance, and shielding. The longer the individual is within the radiation area, the higher the exposure. Also, the larger the amount of radioactive material in the area, the greater the exposure. The farther away the individual is from the radiation source, the lower the exposure. Shielding from the radiation source also decreases exposure. One should never touch radioactive materials directly.

Three types of radiation-induced injury can occur: external irradiation, contamination with radioactive materials, and incorporation of radioactive material into body cells, tissues, or organs:

- *External irradiation* exposure occurs when all or part of the body is exposed to radiation that penetrates or passes completely through the body. In this type of exposure, the individual is not radioactive and does not require special isolation or decontamination measures. Irradiation does not necessarily constitute a medical emergency.
- *Contamination* occurs when the body is exposed to radioactive gases, liquids, or solids either externally or internally. If internal, the contaminant can be deposited within the body. Contamination requires immediate medical management to prevent incorporation.
- *Incorporation* is the actual uptake of radioactive material into the cells, tissues, and susceptible organs. The organs involved are usually the kidneys, bones, liver, and thyroid.

Sequelae of contamination and incorporation can occur days to years later. The thyroid gland can be largely protected from radiation exposure by administration of stable iodine (potassium iodide, or KI) before or promptly after the intake of radioactive iodine.

Priorities in the treatment of any type of radiation exposure are always treatment of life-threatening injuries and illnesses first, followed by measures to limit exposure, contamination control, and finally decontamination.

Decontamination

Hospital and community disaster plans should be in effect when managing a radiation disaster. Access restriction is essential to prevent contamination of other areas of the hospital. Triage outside the hospital is the most effective means of preventing contamination of the facility itself. Floors are covered to prevent tracking of contaminants throughout the treatment areas. Strict isolation precautions should be in effect. All air ducts and vents must be sealed to prevent spread. Waste is controlled through double-bagging and the use of plastic-lined containers outside of the facility.

Staff are required to wear protective clothing, such as water-resistant gowns, two pairs of gloves, masks, caps, goggles, and booties. Dosimetry devices should be worn by all staff members participating in patient care. The radiation safety officer in the hospital should be notified immediately to assist with surveys (using a radiation survey meter) of the incoming patients and to provide dosimeters to all staff personnel involved in direct care of exposed patients. There is minimal risk to staff if the patients are properly surveyed and decontaminated. The majority of patients can be safely decontaminated with soap and water.

Each patient arriving at the hospital should first be surveyed with the radiation survey meter for external contamination and then directed toward the decontamination area as needed. Decontamination occurs outside of the emergency department with a shower, collection pool, tarp, and collection containers for patient belongings, as well as soap, towels, and disposable paper gowns for patients. Water runoff needs to be contained. Patients who are uninjured can perform self-decontamination with handheld showers. After the patient has showered, a resurvey is conducted to determine whether the radioactive contaminants have been removed. Additional washings should occur until the patient is free of contamination. It is important to ensure that during showers previously clean areas are not contaminated with runoff from the washed contaminated areas (e.g., hair should be washed in a position that protects the body from contamination). Wounds are irrigated and then covered with a water-resistant dressing prior to total body decontamination.

Internal contamination or incorporation requires decontamination through catharsis, gastric lavage with chelating agents (agents that bind with radioactive substances and are then excreted), or both. Samples of urine, feces, and vomitus are surveyed to determine internal contamination levels. Biologic samples are taken through nasal and throat swabs, and a complete blood count with differential is obtained.

Acute Radiation Syndrome

Acute radiation syndrome (ARS) can occur after exposure to radiation. It is the dose, rather than the source, that determines whether ARS develops. Factors that determine whether the patient's response to exposure will result in ARS include a high dose (minimum 100 rad) and rate of radiation with total body exposure and penetrating-type radiation. Age, medical history, and genetics also affect the outcome after exposure. The course is predictable. Table 74-5 identifies the phases of ARS.

Each body system is affected differently in ARS. Systems with cells that rapidly reproduce are most commonly affected. The effects on the hematopoietic system include decreased numbers of lymphocytes, granulocytes, thrombocytes, and reticulocytes. It is the first system affected and serves as an indicator of the severity of radiation exposure (Veenema, 2013). A predictor of outcome is the absolute lymphocyte count at 48 hours after exposure. A significant exposure would be indicated by blood lymphocyte counts of 300 to 1,200/mm^3. Barrier precautions should be implemented to protect the patient from infection. Neutrophils decrease within 1 week, platelets decrease within 2 weeks, and red blood cells decrease within 3 weeks. Hemorrhagic complications, fever, and sepsis are common.

The gastrointestinal system, with its rapidly reproducing cells, is also readily affected by radiation. Doses of radiation required to produce symptoms are approximately 600 rad or higher. The gastrointestinal symptoms usually occur at the same time as the changes in the hematopoietic system. Nausea and vomiting occur within 2 hours after exposure. Sepsis, fluid and electrolyte imbalance, and opportunistic infections can occur as complications. An ominous sign is the presence of high fever and bloody diarrhea; these typically appear on day 10 after exposure.

The central nervous system is affected when the dose exceeds 1,000 rad (ENA, 2014). The symptoms occur when damage to the blood vessels of the brain results in fluid leakage. Signs and symptoms include cerebral edema, nausea, vomiting, headache, and increased intracranial pressure (ICP). Increased ICP heralds a poor outcome and imminent death. Central nervous system injury with this amount of exposure is irreversible and occurs before hematopoietic or gastrointestinal system symptoms appear. Cardiovascular collapse is usually seen in conjunction with these injuries.

Skin effects can also indicate the dose of radiation exposure. With exposure of 600 to 1,000 rad, erythema occurs; it can disappear within hours, and then reappear. The exposed patient must be evaluated hourly for the presence of erythema. With exposures greater than 1,000 rad, desquamation (radiation dermatitis) of the skin occurs. Necrosis becomes evident within a few days to months at doses greater than 5,000 rad.

Secondary injury can occur when the radiation exposure occurs during a traumatic event such as a blast or burn. Trauma in addition to radiation exposure increases patient mortality. Attention must first be directed toward the primary assessment for trauma. Airway, breathing, circulation, and fracture reduction require immediate attention. All definitive treatments must occur within the first 48 hours. Thereafter, all surgical procedures should be delayed for 2 to 3 months because of the potential for delayed wound healing and the possible development of opportunistic infections several weeks after exposure.

Survival

There are three categories of predicted survival after radiation exposure: probable, possible, and improbable. Triage of victims at the scene, after decontamination, is conducted using the routine system for disaster triage. Presenting signs and symptoms determine the potential for survival and therefore the category of predicted survival during triage.

Probable survivors have either no initial symptoms or only minimal symptoms (e.g., nausea and vomiting), or

TABLE 74-5 Phases of Effects of Radiation Exposure

Phase	Time of Occurrence	Signs and Symptoms
Prodromal phase (presenting symptoms)	48–72 hours after exposure	Nausea, vomiting, loss of appetite, diarrhea, fatigue High-dose radiation—fever, respiratory distress, and increased excitability
Latent phase (a symptom-free period)	After resolution of prodromal phase; can last up to 3 weeks With high-dose radiation, latent period is shorter	Decreasing lymphocytes, leukocytes, thrombocytes, red blood cells
Manifest Illness phase	After latent period phase	Infection, fluid and electrolyte imbalance, bleeding, diarrhea, shock, and altered level of consciousness
Recovery phase	After manifest illness phase	Can take weeks to months for full recovery
OR		
Death	After manifest illness phase	Increased intracranial pressure is a sign of impending death

Adapted from Centers for Disease Control and Prevention (CDC). (2015). *Acute radiation syndrome: A fact sheet for clinicians*. Retrieved November 26, 2016, from www.emergency.cdc.gov/radiation/arsphysicianfactsheet.asp

these symptoms resolve within a few hours. These patients should have a complete blood count drawn and may be discharged with instructions to return if any symptoms recur.

Possible survivors present with nausea and vomiting that persist for 24 to 48 hours. They experience a latent period, during which leukopenia, thrombocytopenia, and lymphocytopenia occur. Barrier precautions and protective isolation are implemented if the patient's lymphocyte count is less than 1,200/mm^3. Supportive treatment includes administration of blood products, prevention of infection, and provision of enhanced nutrition.

Improbable survivors have received more than 800 rad of total body penetrating irradiation. Individuals in this group demonstrate an acute onset of vomiting, bloody diarrhea, and shock. Any neurologic symptoms will suggest a lethal dose of radiation (ENA, 2014). These patients still require decontamination to prevent further contamination of the area and of others. Personal protection is essential, because it is virtually impossible to fully decontaminate these patients; all of their internal organs have been irradiated. The survival time is variable; however, death usually occurs swiftly due to shock. If there are no neurologic symptoms, patients may be alert and oriented, similar to a patient with extensive burns. In a mass casualty situation, these patients would be triaged into the black category, where they will receive comfort measures and emotional support. If it is not a mass casualty situation, aggressive fluid and electrolyte therapies are essential.

Critical Thinking Exercises

1. You work in an occupational health clinic that provides support to a chemical plant that manufactures chlorine. A patient walks to the clinic after being told to report for an examination by his supervisor since he temporarily removed his PPE while at work. Although he walked to the clinic, he tells you that now his eyes are burning and he is experiencing blurry vision. What evidence-based assessments and interventions would you now implement and why?
2. You are a home health nurse. Several patients who comprise your caseload are dependent upon electronic medical equipment, including one patient who requires home mechanical ventilation and three who require home intravenous therapy. You live in a coastal area and a category 4 hurricane is threatening to hit your community within the next 48 hours. Describe the precautions you would take to ensure that these patients are not deprived of the use of their electronic medical equipment in case of a loss of power.
3. You are working in the emergency department (ED) of a community hospital. One evening, a radio call from EMS sends an alert that there is a possible multiple shooting at a restaurant a block away from the hospital. What are your priorities and first actions? What might be done to ensure safety of the ED staff and patients? How would you prepare for the arrival of patients who may have been injured from this event?

REFERENCES AND SELECTED READINGS

Books

Auerbach, P. S. (2017). *Wilderness medicine* (6th ed.). Philadelphia, PA: Mosby Elsevier.

Emergency Nurses Association (ENA). (2013). *Sheehy's manual of emergency care* (7th ed.). St. Louis, MO: Elsevier Mosby.

Emergency Nurses Association (ENA). (2014). *Trauma nursing core course* (7th ed). Chicago: Emergency Nurses Association.

Tintinalli, J. E., Stapczyski, J. S., Ma, O. J., et al. (2016). *Tintinalli's emergency medicine manual* (8th ed.). New York: McGraw-Hill Medical.

Veenema, T. G. (2013). *Disaster nursing and emergency preparedness* (3rd ed.). New York: Springer.

Journals and Electronic Documents

Accreditation Canada. (2013). *Required Organization Practices Handbook 2014*. Ottawa, ON: Author. Retrieved from http://www.accreditation.ca/sites/default/files/rop-handbook-2014-en.pdf

Alberta Emergency Management Agency (AEMA). (2012). *About Us: AEMA*. Edmonton, AB: Author. Retrieved from http://www.aema.alberta.ca/about_us_main.cfm

Alberta Emergency Management Agency (AEMA). (2013). *New voice technology for Alberta Emergency Alert*. Edmonton, AB: Author. Retrieved from http://alberta.ca/release.cfm?xID=338186A747386-94AB-749E-E369F5D17A09EBDC

American College of Surgeons (ACS). (2010). *Disaster management and emergency preparedness course*. Chicago, IL: Author.

Beaudin, M. (2014). Lac-Mégantic disaster: Where things stand today. *The Gazette*. 23 January, 2014. Retrieved from http://www.montrealgazette.com/news/M%C3%A9gantic+disaster+Where+things+stand+today/9418300/story.html

Bharosa, N., Lee, J., & Janssen, M. (2010). Challenges and obstacles in sharing and coordinating information during multi-agency disaster response: Propositions from field exercises. *Information Systems Frontiers*, *12*(1), 49–65.

Blackwell, T. (2013). Two men arrested over 'al-Qaeda inspired' plan to attack a Via Rail train in Toronto area: RCMP. *National Post*. 22 April, 2013.

Canadian Nurses Association. (2019). Emergency and pandemic preparedness. Retrieved from https://www.cna-aiic.ca/en/nursing-practice/evidence-based-practice/emergency-and-pandemic-preparedness Canadian

Canadian Wireless Telecommunications Association. (2013). *Facts and figures*. Retrieved from http://cwta.ca/facts-figures/

Centers for Disease Control and Prevention (CDC). (2012). *Blast injuries: Fact sheets for professionals*. Retrieved from stacks.cdc.gov/view/cdc/21571/Print

College of Nurses of Ontario (CNO). (2014). *Competencies for entry-level Registered nurse practice*. Ottawa, ON: Author. Retrieved from http://ww2.cno.org/Global/docs/reg/41037_EntryToPracitic_final.pdf

Cunha B. (2014). Anthrax clinical presentation. *Medscape*. 27 January, 2014. Retrieved from http://emedicine.medscape.com/article/212127-clinical

Edgerly D. (2016). The basics of mass casualty triage. *Journal of Emergency Medical Services*. Retrieved from https://www.jems.com/articles/print/volume-41/issue-5/departments-columns/back-to-basics/the-basics-of-mass-casualty-triage.html

Genes, N. (2011). *Medscape: How Twitter has reshaped emergency responses*. Retrieved from http://www.medscape.com/viewarticle/749183_2

Government of Canada. (2017). *An emergency management framework for Canada* (3rd ed.). Retrieved from https://www.publicsafety.gc.ca/cnt/rsrcs/pblctns/2017-mrgnc-mngmnt-frmwrk/index-en.aspx

Healthwise. (2012). Anthrax vaccine. Retrieved from https://myhealth.alberta.ca/health/pages/conditions.aspx?hwid = zb1243&

Hogarth, W. D., & Neil, G. F. (2001). Tornado at Pine Lake, Alberta—July 14, 2000. Anatomy of a disaster: One hospital's experience and recommendations. *Canadian Journal of Emergency Medicine*, *3*(1), 38–40.

Incident Command System Canada (ICSC). (2012). *Incident Command System*. Retrieved from http://www.icscanada.ca/images/upload//ICS%20OPS%20Description2012.pdf

National Defence and the Canadian Armed Forces. (2013). *The Disaster Assistance Response Team (DART)*. Ottawa, ON: Author. Retrieved from http://www.forces.gc.ca/en/operations-abroad-recurring/dart.page

National Police Agency of Japan (NPAJ). (2014). *Damage situation and police countermeasures*. Tokyo, Japan: Author. Retrieved from https://www.npa.go.jp/english/index.htm

Pennardt, A., & Lavonas, E. (2014). Blast injuries clinical presentation. *Medscape. 19* February, 2014. Retrieved from http://emedicine.medscape.com/article/822587-clinical#a0217

Public Health Agency of Canada. (2012a). *Emergency Preparedness and Response*. Ottawa, ON: Author. Retrieved from http://www.phac-aspc.gc.ca/ep-mu/index-eng.php

Public Health Agency of Canada. (2012b). *National Emergency Stockpile System*. Ottawa, ON: Author. Retrieved from http://www.phac-aspc.gc.ca/ep-mu/ness-eng.php

Public Health Agency of Canada. (2013). *Emergency response services*. Ottawa, ON: Author. Retrieved from http://www.phac-aspc.gc.ca/emergency-urgence/index-eng.php

Public Health Agency of Canada. (2014). *Canadian Immunization Guide*. Ottawa, ON: Author. Retrieved from http://www.phac-aspc.gc.ca/publicat/cig-gci/p04-spox-vari-eng.php

Public Safety Canada. (2011). *An emergency management framework for Canada* (2nd ed.). Ottawa, ON: Author. Retrieved from http://www.publicsafety.gc.ca/cnt/rsrcs/pblctns/mrgnc-mngmnt-frmwrk/mrgnc-mngmnt-frmwrk-eng.pdf

Public Safety Canada. (2013a). *Emergency management*. Retrieved from http://www.publicsafety.gc.ca/cnt/mrgnc-mngmnt/index-eng.aspx

Public Safety Canada. (2013b). *Responding to emergency events*. Retrieved from http://www.publicsafety.gc.ca/cnt/mrgnc-mngmnt/rspndng-mrgnc-vnts/index-eng.aspx

Public Safety Canada. (2013c). *All-hazards risk assessment*. Retrieved from http://www.publicsafety.gc.ca/cnt/mrgnc-mngmnt/mrgnc-prprdnss/ll-hzrds-rsk-ssssmnt-eng.aspx

Public Safety Canada. (2016). *An emergency management framework for Canada*. (2nd ed.). Ministers Responsible for Emergency Management. Retrieved from https://www.publicsafety.gc.ca/cnt/rsrcs/pblctns/mrgnc-mngmnt-frmwrk/index-en.aspx

Quan, D. (2014). HazMat specialists set to roll out decontamination protocol to help civilians in a disaster. *Postmedia News*. January 12, 2014. Retrieved from http://www.canada.com/HazMat±specialists±roll±decontamination±protocol±help±civilians±disaster/9377840/story.html

Risk and Hazards Network. (2013). *Welcome to CRHNet.ca*. Toronto, ON: Author. Retrieved from http://host.jibc.ca/crhnet/index.htm

Sookram, S., Borkent, H., Powell, G., Hogarth, W. D., & Shepherd, L. (2001). Tornado at Pine Lake, Alberta—July 14, 2000: Assessment of the emergency medicine response to a disaster. *Canadian journal of emergency medicine, 3*(1), 34–37.

U.S. Army Medical Research Institute of Chemical Defense. (2000). Retrieved from https://ccc.apgea.army.mil/products/info/obtainmaterials.htm

Valdez, A. M. (2015). Are you covered? Safe practices for the use of personal protective equipment. *Journal of Emergency Nursing, 41*(2), 154–157.

Resources

Alberta Emergency Management Agency (AEMA): https://www.alberta.ca/alberta-emergency-management-agency.aspx?utm_source=redirector

Agency for Toxic Substances and Disease Registry: https://www.atsdr.cdc.gov/

Canadian Association of Emergency Physicians: http://www.caep.ca

Canadian Centre for Emergency Preparedness: http://www.ccep.ca

Canadian Red Cross: http://www.redcross.ca

Canadian Risk and Hazards Network (CRHNet): https://www.crhnet.ca/symposiums/crhnet-conference-2018

Centre for Emergency Preparedness and Response: http://www.phac-aspc.gc.ca/cepr-cmiu

Centers for Disease Control and Prevention (CDC), Emergency Preparedness and Response: www.emergency.cdc.gov

Health Canada: http://www.hc-sc.gc.ca

National Emergency Nurses Affiliation: http://www.nena.ca

National Microbiology Laboratory: http://www.nml.ca

Public Health Agency of Canada: http://www.phac-aspc.gc.ca/index-eng.php

Public Safety Canada: http://publicsafety.gc.ca

U.S. Centers for Disease Control and Prevention, 1600 Clifton Road NE, Atlanta, GA 30333, (404) 639-3311: http://www.cdc.gov

World Health Organization: http://www.who.int/

Index

Note: Page number followed by c, f, and indicates text from chart, figure and table respectively.

A

AAI. *See* Ankle-arm index (AAI)
ABCDEs of moles, 1824c
ABCD method, in ED, 2344
Abciximab (ReoPro), 742
Abdomen
  assessment, 672
  auscultation, 905
  four-quadrant method, 905, 905f
  inspection, 905–906
  percussion, 905
Abdominal aortic aneurysms, 856, 857f
  assessment and diagnostic findings, 857
  clinical manifestations, 857
  medical management, 857
    endovascular and surgical management, 857
    pharmacologic therapy, 857
  nursing management, 857–858
  pathophysiology, 857
  rupture, 858
Abdominal binder, 432, 1428, 2079
Abdominal breathing, 291
Abdominal cavity, 1114
Abdominal compartment syndrome (ACS), 350, 356
Abdominal discomfort, gastritis, 978
Abdominal distention, 672, 2001
Abdominal guarding, 1120
Abdominal obesity, 1141, 1144
Abdominal pain, 903f
  abdominal aortic aneurysm, 858
  acute pancreatitis, 1120
  chronic pancreatitis, 1126
  hepatic dysfunction, 1055
Abdominal thrusts, 491c, 2345
Abdominal ultrasonography, 907–908
  nursing interventions, 908
Abdominal x-rays, 911
  gallbladder disease, 1111
Abduction, 2233
Ablation, 692, 705
  of hepatocellular carcinoma, 1097
Abnormal heart sound, 653, 669–670
Abnormal uterine bleeding, 1396
Aboriginal Canadians, 8, 91–92
Abortion, 1402–1404
  elective, 1404c
  habitual, 1403
  induced, 1403–1404
  spontaneous, 1402–1403
ABPM. *See* Ambulatory blood pressure monitoring (ABPM)
Abrasion, 2349c
Abscess, 998, 1009, 1015, 1017, 1412
  after intestinal surgery, 1041t
  anorectal, 1045
  appendicitis, 1009
  blind dental, 923
  chronic dentoalveolar, 923
  Crohn's disease, 1016
  crypt, 1017
  diverticulitis, 1013
  formation, 1010, 1011
  liver, 1102–1103
  pelvic, 1011t
  periapical, 919, 922–923
  secondary, 1010
  ulcerative colitis, 1017
Absolute neutrophil count (ANC), 1599, 1632
  calculation of, 2201
Absorption, 899
Absorption atelectasis, 603
Abstinence, 1397
Abuse, 2371–2373
  alcohol, 224–225
  elder, 233
  substance (*See* Substance abuse)
Acalculous cholecystitis, 1108
Acarbose (Glucobay), 1157
Accelerated idioventricular rhythm (AIVR), 710
Accessory muscles, use of, 454
Access to Assistive Technology in Canada: A Jurisdictional Scan of Programs, 179
Access to Information Act, 1892
Accountability, 73, 75
Accreditation Canada, 176, 386, 396
Accreditation of Rehabilitation Facilities (CARF), 176
Acculturation, 93
Accuzyme, 1784
Acebutolol
  antiarrhythmic medication, 699t
  hypertension, 885t
ACE inhibitors. *See* Angiotensin-converting enzyme (ACE) inhibitors
Acesulfame-K (Ace-K), 1147
Acetabulum, fractures of, 2316
Acetaminophen (Tylenol), 858, 2094
  hematologic disorders, 1607
  hepatic dysfunction, 1054
  herpes labialis, 474c
  kidney cancer, 1291
  pain management, 285, 477
  rheumatic diseases, 1743
  toxicity, 2369t
Acetazolamide, 1062
  for sleep apnea, 488
  urinary stone formation, 1351
Acetic acid, 1856
Acetylcholine, gastrointestinal regulatory substances, 901t
Acetylcholinesterase inhibitor test (stim test), 2103
N-Acetylcysteine, 842
Achalasia, 899, 914, 919, 934
  assessment and diagnostic findings, 934
  clinical manifestations, 934
  esophagomyotomy, 935
  management, 934–935
  treatment of, 935f
Achieving Health for All, 46
Achilles boot, 2302
Achilles reflex, 1976–1978
Achilles tendinitis, 2300
Achilles tendon, rupture of, 2302
Achlorhydria, 977, 978
Acid–base balance, 1122
  regulation of, 1267
Acid–base disturbances, 329
  and compensation, 333t
  homeostatic mechanisms and, 329
  metabolic acidosis, 329–330
  metabolic alkalosis, 330–331
  mixed acid–base disorders, 332–333
  respiratory acidosis, 331–332
  respiratory alkalosis, 332
Acidosis, 316
  end-stage kidney disease, 1297
  metabolic, 329–330, 330t
  respiratory, 331–332
Acinetobacter baumannii, 1854
Acne
  nutritional management, 1793
  quality of life among women with, 1790c
  surgery, 1795
Acne-Specific QOL Questionnaire (Acne-QOL), 1790c
Acne vulgaris, 1790c, 1792–1795
  assessment and diagnostic findings, 1793
  clinical manifestations, 1792–1793
  educating patients about self-care, 1795
  medical management
    nutrition and hygiene therapy, 1793
    prevention of scarring, 1795
  nursing management, 1794–1795
  pathophysiology, 1792
  pharmacologic treatments
    benzoyl peroxide preparations, 1793–1794
    estrogen therapy, 1794
    first-line medications, 1793t
    oral antibiotics, 1794
    oral retinoids, 1794
    salicylic acid preparations, 1794
    topical antibiotic therapy, 1794
  surgical treatment, 1794
Acoustic gel, 840
Acoustic neuroma, 2118. *See also* Primary brain tumours
Acoustic trauma, 1935
Acquired/adaptive immunity, 1519
  active, 1519
  passive, 1519
Acquired coagulation disorders, 1668–1689
  acquired thrombophilias, 1675–1678
  activated protein C resistance, 1674–1675
  antithrombin deficiency, 1674
  blood disorders, therapies for, 1678–1680
  bone marrow transplantation, 1689
  disseminated intravascular coagulation, 1668–1671, 1672c–1673c
  hematopoietic stem cell transplantation, 1689
  hyperhomocysteinemia, 1671, 1674
  liver disease, 1668
  procuring blood and blood products, 1680–1683
  protein C deficiency, 1674
  protein S deficiency, 1674
  thrombotic disorders, 1671
  transfusion, 1683–1689
  vitamin K deficiency, 1668

Acquired cold urticaria (ACU), 1592
Acquired disabilities, 166
Acquired drug resistance, 525
Acquired immunodeficiency syndrome (AIDS), 905, 927, 1001, 1422–1423, 1537
  assessment and diagnostic findings, 1544–1545
  from blood transfusion, 1681c
  care of patient with, 1556c–1561c
  clinical manifestations, 1550–1553
  complementary, alternative and integrative modalities, 1554–1555
  Cryptococcus neoformans, 1552
  cytomegalovirus retinitis, 1554
  depression, 1553
  description, 1537–1538
  emotional and ethical concerns, 1568–1569
  epidemiology, 1538
  gerontologic considerations, 1539
  Kaposi's Sarcoma, 1551
  Legionella infection, 1727
  lymphomas, 1551
  medical management, 1553–1554
  nursing process, 1556, 1561–1568
  nutrition therapy, 1554
  pathophysiology, 1541–1543
  pneumocystis pneumonia, 1553
  prevention, 1539–1540, 1540c
  reducing risk of transmission, 1540–1541
  stages, 1543–1544
  standard precautions, 1541c
  supportive care, 1555–1556
  transmission, 1538
  treatment, 1545–1550
Acquired thrombophilias, 1675–1678
  etiology, 1675
  medical management, 1675–1678
  nursing management, 1678
Acrocyanosis, 861
ACS. *See* Acute coronary syndrome (ACS); American Cancer Society (ACS)
ACT. *See* Activated clotting time (ACT)
Actinic cheilitis, lip abnormalities, 920t
Actinic keratoses, 1819
Activated clotting time (ACT), 864
Activated partial thromboplastin time (aPTT), 741, 864, 1606
Activated protein C (APC) resistance, 1674–1675
Active dressings, 1783
Active immunotherapy, 2192
Activities of daily living (ADLs), 157, 167, 178, 179c, 218, 853, 1085, 2039, 2080
  self-care deficits in, 178–180
    assessment, 178
    expected outcomes, 180
    nursing diagnosis, 178
    nursing interventions, 179–180
    planning and goals, 178
Activity
  and exercise, 663
  pacing, 573
Activity tolerance, 575
  cardiomyopathy, 793
  heart failure, 818–819
Acute abdomen, 1008
  appendicitis, 1009–1010
  diverticular disease, 1010–1013
  nursing process, 1013–1014
  peritonitis, 1014–1015
Acute arterial embolism, symptoms of, 859
Acute bacterial rhinosinusitis (ABRS), 475
Acute chest syndrome, 1621–1622
Acute cholecystitis, 1110, 1111, 1115
Acute coronary syndrome (ACS), 653, 658, 744
  assessment and diagnostic findings, 745, 745c
    cardiac biomarkers, 746–747, 747t
    echocardiogram, 746
    electrocardiogram, 745–746, 746f
    patient history, 745
  cardiac rehabilitation programs, 749–750
  clinical manifestations, 745
  continuing and transitional care, 754
  emergent PCI, 749
  ethical considerations, 739c
  inpatient management, 748
  medical management, 747–750
  Non–ST-segment elevation MI (NSTEMI), 744
  nursing process, 750–754
  in older adults, 738–739, 739c
  pathophysiology, 744–745
  pharmacologic therapy, 747–748, 748c
    ACE inhibitors, 748
    analgesics, 748
    thrombolytics (fibrinolytics), 748, 748c
  plan of nursing care, 751–753
  promoting health after, 755c
  self-care, 754
  ST-segment elevation myocardial infarction (STEMI), 744
  symptom presentation in, 739
  unstable angina, 744
Acute fatigue, defined, 2199
Acute heart failure, 824–826
Acute hemolytic reaction, 1685–1686
Acute hypertension, 1922
Acute idiopathic pancreatitis, 1119
Acute intermittent peritoneal dialysis, 1314
Acute kidney failure, 1283
Acute kidney injury (AKI), 1282, 1292–1297
  assessment and diagnostic findings, 1293–1294
  categories of, 1292–1293
  causes of, 1293c
  characteristics of, 1294t
  classifications, 1292
  clinical manifestations, 1293
  contrast-induced, 842
  gerontologic considerations, 1295
  hospital-acquired, 1295
  intrarenal, 1292
  medical management, 1295
  nursing management, 1296–1297
  nutritional therapy, 1296
  pathophysiology, 1292
  pharmacologic therapy, 1295–1296
  phases, 1293
    diuresis period, 1293
    initiation period, 1293
    oliguria period, 1293
    recovery period, 1293
  postrenal, 1293
  prerenal, 1292
  prevention, 1294–1295, 1294c
  RIFLE classification for, 1292t
  in shock, 347
Acute low back pain, 2265–2270
  assessment and diagnostic findings, 2266–2267
  clinical manifestations, 2266
  definition, 2265
  diagnostic procedures for, 2267c
  medical management, 2267
  nursing process for, 2267–2270
    assessment, 2267–2268
    nursing interventions, 2268–2270
    nursing priorities, 2268
    planning and goals, 2268
  pathophysiology, 2266
  prevention strategies, 2268c
Acute lung injury (ALI), 505
  in shock, 347
Acute lymphocytic leukemia (ALL), 1640
  clinical manifestations, 1640
  medical management, 1640
  nursing management, 1640
Acute myeloid leukemia (AML), 1636–1638
  assessment and diagnostic findings, 1637
  clinical manifestations, 1636, 1636f
  complications, 1637
  medical management, 1637–1638
  nursing management, 1638
Acute nephritic syndrome, 1283, 1286–1287
  assessment and diagnostic findings, 1286–1287
  clinical manifestations, 1286
  complications, 1287
  medical management, 1287
  nursing management, 1287
  pathophysiology, 1286, 1286f
Acute otitis externa, 1937
  clinical features, 1939t
Acute otitis media, 1939
  clinical features, 1939t
Acute pancreatitis
  abdominal pain, 1120
  antacids, 1120
  assessment, 1120
  cardiac dysfunction, 1122
  clinical manifestations, 1120
  continuing care, 1123
  diagnosis, 1120
  gerontologic considerations, 1119
  hemorrhagic shock, 1122
  home, community-based, and transitional care, 1122–1123
  hypovolemic shock, 1122
  medical management, 1120–1121
  multiple organ failure, 1122
  nursing management, 1121–1123
  nutrition, 1120
  pathophysiology, 1119
  self-care, 1122–1123
  shock, 1122
  transitional care, 1123
Acute pharyngitis. *See also* Pharyngitis
  assessment/diagnostic findings, 480
  clinical manifestations, 480
  medical management
    nutritional therapy, 480
    pharmacologic therapy, 480
  nursing management, 480–481
  pathophysiology, 479–480
Acute promyelocytic leukemia (APL), 1637
Acute pyelonephritis, 1339
  assessment and diagnostic findings, 1339
  clinical manifestations, 1339
  medical management, 1339
  pharmacologic therapy, 1339
Acute renal failure (ARF), 1922
Acute respiratory distress syndrome (ARDS), 534–537
  assessment/diagnostic findings, 535
  clinical manifestations, 535
  defined, 505
  medical management, 535–536
  nursing management, 536

pathophysiology, 535, 535f
risk factors, 535c
in shock, 347
Acute respiratory failure (ARF), 533–534. *See also* Pleural conditions
clinical manifestations, 534
decreased respiratory drive
dysfunction of chest wall, 534
dysfunction of lung parenchyma, 534
medical management, 534
nursing management, 534
pathophysiology, 534
Acute rhinosinusitis. *See also* Rhinosinusitis
assessment/diagnostic findings, 475–476
clinical manifestations, 475
complications, 476
medical management, 476, 476t
nursing management, 476–477
pathophysiology, 475
Acute tracheobronchitis. *See also* Respiratory infections
clinical manifestations, 508
medical management, 508
nursing management, 508
pathophysiology, 508
Acute tubular necrosis (ATN), 1283, 1292
Acute vascular occlusion, 859
Acute viral rhinosinusitis (AVRS), 475
Acyclovir (Zovirax), 1797, 1799, 1894
herpes labialis, 474c
herpes simplex virus 2, 1418
proctitis, 1044
AD. *See* Alzheimer's disease (AD)
Adaptation, 101, 103
Selye's theory of, 105
stress and, 103
Adaptive devices, 178, 179
Addiction, 286
Addison disease, 1001, 1773t. *See* Adrenocortical insufficiency
Addisonian crisis, monitoring and managing, 1249
Additional precautions (AP), 1698, 1703
Adduction, 2233
A-delta nociceptor fibres, 271
Adenocarcinoma, tumour cells, 943
Adenoiditis
assessment/diagnostic findings, 481–482
clinical manifestations, 481
medical management, 482
nursing management, 482
Adenoids, 439
Adenomyosis, 1431
Adenosine triphosphate (ATP), 342, 2030, 2218
Adequate compression therapy, 869
ADH. *See* Antidiuretic hormone (ADH)
Adherence to therapeutic regimen, 38–40
Adiposopathy, 1192
Adjunct chemotherapeutic agents, 2178
Adjunctive modalities/management, dysrhythmias
cardioversion and defibrillation, 715–717
electrophysiology studies, 717–718
implantable cardioverter defibrillator, 723–725, 726c
pacemaker therapy, 718–723, 722t
Adjuvant chemotherapy, 1446, 1468
Adjuvant hormonal therapy, 1446, 1470, 1471t
ADLs. *See* Activities of daily living (ADLs)
Adnexa, 1373, 1375
Adnexal palpation, 1390
Adolescents, nutritional assessment in, 65
Adoptive immunotherapy, 2192
Adrenal cortex, 1245
Adrenal glands
anatomic and physiologic overview, 1244, 1245f
adrenal cortex, 1245
adrenal medulla, 1245
disorders of
adrenocortical insufficiency, 1248–1250
Cushing syndrome, 1250–1252
pheochromocytoma, 1246–1248
primary aldosteronism, 1255
homeostasis, role in, 301
Adrenaline rush, 107
Adrenal insufficiency, preoperative assessment, 380–381
Adrenal medulla, 1245
Adrenal sex hormones, 1245–1246
Adrenergic, 1966
Adrenergic agents, in allergic rhinitis, 1583
Adrenergic antagonists, in hypertension, 892
Adrenocortical insufficiency, 1248–1250
assessment and diagnostic findings, 1249
clinical manifestations, 1248–1249
home care checklist, 1250
medical management, 1249
nursing management, 1249
Adrenocorticotropic hormone (ACTH), 105, 301
Adult-onset conditions, testing and screening for, 140, 141t–143t, 143
nursing role in, 144
Adult polycystic disease. *See* Autosomal dominant polycystic kidney disease (ADPKD)
Adult voiding dysfunction, 1340, 1340t. *See also* Urinary tract infection (UTI)
Advance care planning, 240
Advanced cardiovascular life support, 831
Advance directives, 28, 234–235, 240
Advanced nursing practice, 11
Adventitia, arterial wall, 835
Adventitious sounds, 457, 458t
Aerobic metabolism, 342
Aerosol delivery devices, 571t
Aerosol masks, 606
Afferent impulses, 1969
Aflatoxin, and hepatocellular carcinoma, 1095
AFP. *See* Alpha-fetoprotein (AFP)
Afterload, 653, 740
Ageism, 24, 220
Age-related macular degeneration, 219, 1908–1910, 1910f
Agglutination, 1517, 1522
Aging, 210. *See also* Older adults
in blood vessels walls and blood flow, 839
cellular replacement, 1770
changes associated with, 42–43
cognitive aspects of, 221–222, 222c
demographics of, 210–211
diabetes and management, effect on, 1149c
with disability, 234
gastrointestinal tract, 903t
health care costs of, 234
hepatobiliary system, 1054c
pharmacologic aspects of, 222–224
physical aspects of, 212–219
psychosocial aspects of, 219–221
related changes in eye, 1889t
skin changes, 1769–1770, 1769f, 1770c
theories of, 212
Aging population, and health care delivery, 8
Agitation, 989
Agnogenic myeloid metaplasia. *See* Primary myelofibrosis
Agnosia, 1975–1976
Agranulocytes, 1603–1604
lymphocytes, 1603
monocytes, 1603
AIDS. *See* Acquired immunodeficiency syndrome (AIDS)
AIDS-related pain, 269c
Air embolism
complications of, 336
IV therapy and, 336
parenteral nutrition, 969, 970t
Air plethysmography, 872
Air pressure variances, 442
Air trapping, 564
Airway clearance, 527, 574–575
Airway management. *See also* Respiratory care modalities
emergency management of, 612, 613c
endotracheal intubation, 612–614
mechanical ventilation, 619–622
neck dissection, 930
nursing process, 622–632
tracheostomy, 614–619
Airway obstruction, 2345–2348
assessment and diagnostic findings, 2345
clinical manifestations, 2345
management, 2345
abdominal thrusts, 2345
cricothyroidotomy, 2347
endotracheal intubation, 2346–2347, 2347f
establishing airway, 2345–2347
head-tilt–chin-lift manoeuvre, 2345–2346
jaw-thrust manoeuvre, 2346
King (Combitube)/laryngeal mask airway, 2347, 2347f
maintaining ventilation, 2344–2346
oropharyngeal airway insertion, 2346, 2346c
pathophysiology, 2345
Airway pressure release ventilation (APRV), 602, 620
Airway resistance, 442, 442c
AKI. *See* Acute kidney injury (AKI)
Alanine aminotransferase (ALT), 1056, 1060
Al-Anon, 1095
Alaryngeal communication, 471, 495
Albinism, 1773t
Albumin, 351, 1056, 1179
administration, 1063
levels, measurement of, 67
Albumin to creatinine ratio (ACR), 1179
Albuterol, 588t, 591t
Alcohol, 112
ingestion, 981
intoxication, 2365, 2370
Alcohol-based hand rub (ABHR), 1698, 1702
Alcohol consumption
chronic pancreatitis, 1123
hypertension, 883t
irritable bowel syndrome, 1005
jaundice, 1060
older people, 224–225
oral cancer, 925
and risk of cancer, 2155
type 2 diabetes, 1146–1147
Alcoholic cirrhosis, 1084
Alcoholics Anonymous, 1095
Alcoholism, and hypomagnesemia, 323
Alcohol screening questionnaires, 59
Alcohol septal ablation, cardiomyopathy, 789

Alcohol withdrawal syndrome, 378, 2370–2371
in postoperative phase, 378
Aldosterone, 107, 301, 313
antagonists, 813
deficiency of, 310
Aldosterone receptor blockers, hypertension, 884t
Aleve, in premenstrual syndrome, 1395
Alfentanil (Alfenta), 401t
Alfuzosin (Uroxatral), in benign prostatic hyperplasia, 1491
Algorithm, 10
Aliskiren (Tekturna), hypertension, 887t
Alkaline pH, 900
Alkaline phosphatase, 1056, 1095
Alkalosis, 313
metabolic, 330–331
potassium distribution and, 314
respiratory, 332
Alkylating agents, 551, 2179t
ALL. *See* Acute lymphocytic leukemia (ALL)
Alleles, 133
Allen's test, 926
Allergen, 1571, 1572
Allergic contact dermatitis, 1787
Allergic disorders, 1579
allergic rhinitis, 1581–1587
anaphylaxis, 1580–1581
angioneurotic edema, 1591–1592
assessment, 1575
form, 1577c–1578c
physiologic overview, 1571–1575
atopic dermatitis, 1590–1591
B cells, 1572
cold urticaria, 1592
contact dermatitis, 1589–1590
dermatitis medicamentosa, 1591
diagnostic evaluation
complete blood count with differential, 1575
eosinophil count, 1576
provocative testing, 1579
serum-specific IgE test, 1579
skin tests, 1576–1578
total serum IgE levels, 1576
food allergy, 1592–1593
hereditary angioedema, 1592
home care checklist, 1589c
latex allergy, 1593–1596
T cells, 1572
urticaria (hives), 1591–1592
Allergic rhinitis, 1581–1587
assessment and diagnostic findings, 1583
clinical manifestations, 1582
medical management, 1583–1587
nursing process, 1587–1589
pathophysiology, 1582
Allergy, 1571, 1572. *See also* Allergic disorders
preoperative assessment, 381, 381f
Alliance for Equality of Blind Canadians, 1892
Alloantibodies, 1628
AlloDerm, 1786
Allodynia, 273
Allogeneic HSCT (AlloHSCT), 2186, 2187
Allogeneic vaccines, 2192
Allografts, 778, 786, 1859, 2310
Allopurinol (Zyloprim), 1637
gout, 1758
polycythemia, 1631
All-trans retinoic acid (ATRA), 1637, 2191, 2192
Alma-Ata Declaration of 1978, 7
Almotriptan (Axert), 2025
Alopecia, 1768, 1778, 2150, 2165, 2196
Alpha-adrenergic receptors, 351–352
Alpha1-antitrypsin augmentation therapy, for COPD, 570
Alpha-1 antitrypsin deficiency, 142t, 564
Alpha$_1$-blockers, hypertension, 885t
Alpha-fetoprotein (AFP), 1096
Alpha FIM, 178
Alpha-glucosidase inhibitors, 1137, 1157
Alpha-interferon, hepatitis B, 1080
Alpha-Keri oil, 1789
Alpha thalassemia, 1627
Alprostadil, in erectile dysfunction, 1485
ALS. *See* Amyotrophic lateral sclerosis (ALS)
ALT. *See* Alanine aminotransferase (ALT)
Alteplase (Activase), 748
Altered level of consciousness (LOC), 1987
assessment and diagnostic findings, 1989
care for patient with
assessment, 1990, 1991t
goals of care, 1992
nursing priorities, 1990–1992
patient outcomes, 1995
potential complications, 1992
clinical manifestations, 1989
complications, 1989
medical management, 1989–1990
nursing interventions, 1992–1995
airway maintenance, 1992
bladder management, 1994
body temperature maintenance, 1993–1994
fluid balance maintenance, 1992–1993
managing nutritional needs, 1992–1993
meeting family's needs, 1994–1995
monitoring and managing potential complications, 1995
oral care, 1993
preserving corneal integrity, 1993
promoting bowel function, 1994
protection of patient, 1992
restoring health maintenance, 1994
skin and joint integrity maintenance, 1993
pathophysiology, 1989
Aluminum-based antacids, constipation, 998
Aluminum hydroxide
antacids, 978
gastroesophageal reflux disease, 939t
Aluminum hydroxide gel, antacid, 993
Aluminum–magnesium liquid antacids, 927
Alveoli, 441–442
Alvimopan (Entereg), for opioid-induced constipation, 288
Alzheimer's disease (AD), 121, 227–230
assessment and diagnostic findings, 228
clinical manifestations, 228
familial AD, 227
medical management, 228
nursing management, 228–230
balanced activity and rest, 230
communication, 229
home, community-based, and transitional care, 230
independence in self-care activities, 229
promoting adequate nutrition, 229–230
promoting physical safety, 229
reducing anxiety and agitation, 229
socialization and intimacy needs, 229–230
supporting cognitive function, 229
pathophysiology, 227–228, 227f
risk factor for, 227
sporadic AD, 227
Alzheimer Society of Canada, 230
Amantadine (Symmetrel), 2097, 2098
Ambulation
impaired physical mobility, 187–188
ischemic stroke, 2041
orthopedic surgery, 2248
parenteral nutrition, 971
Ambulatory blood pressure monitoring (ABPM), 882
Ambulatory electrocardiography, 676
Ambulatory health care, 18–19
Ambulatory surgery, 376
preoperative education, 386
Ambulatory surgical centres, 418
Amenorrhea, 1373, 1395–1396
primary, 1395
secondary, 1396
American Academy of Allergy, Asthma, & Immunology (AAAAI), 1579
American Cancer Society (ACS), 926, 1129, 1482
American College of Obstetricians and Gynecologists (ACOG), 1417
American Joint Committee on Cancer (AJCC) Stage Groupings, 1036c
American Joint Replacement Registry (AJRR), 2248
American Society for Parenteral and Enteral Nutrition (ASPEN), 957
American Society of Anesthesiologists (ASA) Physical Status Classification System, 396
Amikacin, in acute kidney injury, 1294
Amiloride (Midamor)
heart failure, 820t
hypertension, 884t
Aminoglycoside, 1336
acute kidney injury, 1294
antibiotic agents, 1950c
5-aminolevulinic acid (ALA-PDT), 1822
Aminopeptidase, 901t
Aminosalicylates, in inflammatory bowel disease, 1018
Amiodarone
antiarrhythmic medication, 699t
atrial fibrillation prevention, 704
Amitriptyline (Elavil), 2025
rheumatoid arthritis, 1745
for sleep, 1736
urinary incontinence, 1342
AML. *See* Acute myeloid leukemia (AML)
Amlodipine (Norvasc), 741
heart failure, 813
hypertension, 887t
Ammonia, 300
Ammonia conversion, role of liver, 1053
Ammonium chloride, 1062
Amnion, 1859
Amoxicillin (Amoxil), 983
chronic *H. pylori* gastritis, 995
peptic ulcer disease and gastritis, 979t
Amoxicillin-clavulanate, 1339
Amphetamine-type drugs, 2367t
Amphiarthrotic joints, 2217–2218
Amphotericin B, in acute kidney injury, 1294
Ampicillin, 1336
Amputation, 2327
above-knee, 2328
below-knee, 2328
complication, 2328
levels of, 2327–2328, 2328f
of lower extremity, 2327
medical management, 2328

closed rigid cast dressing, 2328
removable rigid dressing, 2328
soft dressing, 2328
nursing interventions
continuing and transitional care, 2332–2333
enhancing body image, 2330
helping patient resolve grief, 2330
home care checklist, 2333c
monitoring and managing complications, 2332
pain management, 2330
phantom pains or sensations, 2330
physical mobility, help in, 2331–2332
promoting independent self-care, 2330–2331
self-care, 2332
wound healing, promoting, 2330
nursing process, 2329–2334
assessment, 2329
expected patient outcomes, 2333–2334
interventions, 2330–2333
nursing priorities, 2329
planning and goals, 2329
potential complications, 2329
rehabilitation, 2328–2329, 2329f
staged, 2328
upper extremity, 2328
Amsler grid, 1886–1887
Amylase, 899, 900, 901t, 1107
Amyotrophic lateral sclerosis (ALS), 2112t, 2135–2137. *See also* Degenerative disorders
assessment/diagnostic findings, 2137
clinical manifestations, 2136–2137
Anabolic steroids, abuse of, 2368t
Anaerobic metabolism, 342, 349
Anagrelide (Agrylin), for polycythemia, 1630
Anal canal, examination, 906
Anal fissures, 999, 1045
Anal fistula, 1045
Analgesia
patient-controlled, 423
in percutaneous needle biopsy, 468
Analgesics
esophageal disorder, 942c
gastritis, 978
neck surgery, 933c
parotitis, 924
periapical abscess, 923
pericarditis, 799, 800
peripheral arterial insufficiency, 849
peritonitis, 1015
relieving pain, 993
Anal lesions, types of, 1045f
Anal sphincter, 915
Anal veins, 999
Analysis, 22
Anaphylactic (type I) hypersensitivity, 1574
Anaphylactic reaction, 2358, 2358c
assessment, 2359c
clinical manifestations, 2358
nursing interventions for prevention of, 2358
Anaphylactic shock, 359, 365–366
medical management, 365
nursing management, 365–366
Anaphylaxis, 1572, 1580–1581
causes of, 1580c
clinical manifestations, 1580
intraoperative, 406
medical management, 1581
nursing management, 1581
pathophysiology, 1580
prevention, 1580–1581
Anaplasia, 2150
Anaprox, in premenstrual syndrome, 1395
Anasarca, 309
Anastomosis, 835, 1037f, 1099
Anastrozole (Arimidex), in breast cancer, 1458, 1471
Androgens, 1373, 1375
Android obesity, 1196, 1196f
Anemia, 194, 1599, 1602, 1607–1611
aplastic, 1616–1617
assessment and diagnostic findings, 1610–1611
of chronic disease, 1615–1616
cirrhosis and, 1085
classification of, 1607–1610, 1609t
clinical manifestations, 1610
complications, 1611
end-stage kidney disease, 1298
gerontologic considerations, 1611
and heart failure, 807
hemolytic, 1610c, 1620–1621
hypoproliferative, 1613–1615
iron deficiency, 1613–1615
medical management, 1611
megaloblastic, 1617–1618
nursing process, 1611–1613
pernicious, 1617
pruritus in, 1790
in renal disease, 1615
skin colour change in, 1773t
Anemic hypoxia, 603c
Anergy, 67, 1599
Anesthesia, 398–399
advances in, 373
general anesthesia, 399–403
inhalation anesthetic agent, 399, 400f, 400t
intravenous administration, 399–400, 401t–403t, 403
stages, 399
intrapleural, 423
local anesthesia, 405
monitored anesthesia care, 405
regional anesthesia, 403–405
report to nurse, by provider, 413
Anesthesia awareness, 399, 405–406
Anesthesiologist, 392, 396
Anesthetist, 396
Aneurysmal subarachnoid hemorrhage, 2052
Aneurysms, 835, 842, 855, 2046. *See also* Abdominal aortic aneurysms
coiling, 2050
medical management, 858
nursing management, 858
rebleeding, 2051
Angina pectoris, 731, 738
assessment and diagnostic findings, 739–740
clinical manifestations, 738
gerontologic considerations, 738–739, 739c
home care checklist, 744c
intractable/refractory angina, 738c
medical management, 740–742
nursing process, 742–743
assessment, 742, 742c
continuing and transitional care, 743
interventions, 742–743
nursing priorities, 742
planning and goals, 742
potential complications, 742
self-care program, 743
oxygen therapy, 742
pathophysiology, 738
pharmacologic therapy
aspirin, 741
beta-adrenergic blocking agents, 740–741
calcium channel blockers, 741
clopidogrel, 741
glycoprotein IIb/IIIa agents, 742
heparin, 741–742
nitroglycerin, 740, 740c
physical exertion and, 738
severity of, 738
silent ischemia, 738c
stable angina, 738c
unstable angina, 738, 738c
variant angina, 738c
Angiogenesis, 1599, 2150, 2153, 2191. *See also* Cancer
Angiography, 1887
pancreatic tumour, 1128
Angiomas, 1777, 1777t, 1819
Angioneurotic edema, 1572, 1591–1592
Angioplasty, 835
Angiotensin-converting enzyme (ACE), 301
Angiotensin-converting enzyme (ACE) inhibitors, 448, 704, 811, 838, 893, 1100, 1285
acute kidney injury, 1296
aortic regurgitation, 781
heart failure, 811–812, 811t
hypertension, 886t
mitral regurgitation, 780
nephropathy, 1180
Angiotensin I, 807, 812, 837
Angiotensin II, 301, 812, 838
Angiotensin receptor blockers (ARBs), 1101
heart failure, 812
mitral regurgitation, 780
Angular cheilosis, 1599, 1611
Anhidrosis, 1181
Animal and human bites, 2359
Anion gap, 328, 329
Ankle-arm index (AAI), 835, 840
Ankle-brachial index (ABI), 185, 835, 840, 841c
Ankle exercises, 182
Ankle systolic pressure, 841
Ankylosing spondylitis (AS), 1756
Ankylosis, 1732
Annuloplasty, 778, 784, 784f
Anorectal abscess, 1045
Anorectal disorders, 1044
anal fissure, 1045
anal fistula, 1045
anorectal abscess, 1045
cyst, 1046–1047
hemorrhoids, 1045–1046
nursing management, 1047
pilonidal sinus, 1046–1047
proctitis, 1044–1045
Anorectal manometry, 914, 999
Anorectal reflex, 202
Anorexia, 902, 994, 1002, 2197, 2246
chronic constipation, 1011
colorectal cancer, 1043
gastritis, 978
hepatic dysfunction, 1055
peritonitis, 1014
Anoscopy, proctoscopy, and sigmoidoscopy, 913–914
Anoxia, 1059
ANP. *See* Atrial natriuretic peptide (ANP)

Antacids
acid neutralizing agents, 939t
acute pancreatitis, 1120
aluminum–magnesium liquid, 927
esophagus, 940, 941, 944
GERD, pharmacologic management of, 938, 939t
Anterior cerebral artery (ACA), 2047
Anterior cingulate cortex (ACC), 272
Anterior communicating artery (ACoA), 2047
Anterior cord syndrome, 2072c
Anterior cruciate ligament (ACL), 2301
Anterior pituitary gland
abnormalities of, 1218–1219
hormones of, 1218
Anthracyclines, for cardiac toxicity, 2183
Antiallergy medications, 1894
Antiarrhythmic medications, 692, 699t, 723
cardiogenic shock, 358
diarrhea, 1001
Antibiotics, 869, 874, 875, 924
acne vulgaris, 1794, 1795
anal fistula, 1045
appendicitis, 1010
burn wound, 1854
constipation, 998
diarrhea, 1001
diverticular disease, 1012
doxycycline, 1794
exfoliative dermatitis, 1813
folliculitis, 1796
impetigo, 1795–1796
infective endocarditis, 795, 796, 797
minocycline, 1794
neutropenic fever, 2201
ostomy, 1023
peptic ulcer disease and gastritis, 979t
peritonitis, 1015
pilonidal sinus, 1046
proctitis, 1044
rhytidectomy (face-lift), 1830
sepsis, 1871
Stevens–Johnson syndrome, 1816
tetracycline, 1794
tetraplegia or paraplegia, 2085
toxic epidermal necrolysis, 1816
Antibody, 1517, 1519, 1571, 1572
Anticentromere antibody (ACA), 1751
Anticholinergics
asthma, 592
constipation, 998
Anti-citrullinated peptide antibody (ACPA), 1743
Anticoagulants
contraindications, 864c
heart failure, 815
medications, 867c
patient education, 867c
pulmonary embolism, 544
Anticonvulsants, 289
end-stage kidney disease, 1299
Antidepressants, 224, 289
abuse, 2368t
irritable bowel syndrome, 1005
Antidiarrheal therapy, in HIV infection, 1554
Antidiuretic hormone (ADH), 107, 301, 343, 1266
functions of, 301, 302f
secretion, 1063
and thirst mechanism, 301
Antiembolism (AE) stockings, 185
myocarditis, 798
Antiemetics, 1039
Antigen, 1516, 1517, 1571, 1572
Antigenic determinant, 1516, 1517
Antihistamine, 1572, 1574
allergic rhinitis, 1583, 1584t
Antihyperglycemic agents, oral/ injectable, 1156
alpha-glucosidase inhibitors, 1157
biguanides, 1158
dipeptidyl peptidase-IV inhibitors, 1157
general considerations for, 1158
meglitinides, 1157
sites of action of, 1158f
sulfonylureas, 1156
thiazolidinediones, 1157
Antihypertensives
constipation, 998
diarrhea, 1001
end-stage kidney disease, 1299
medications, 883
therapy, 887
Anti-IL-12, 1018
Anti-inflammatory medications, 1110
Antimetabolites, 2179t
Antimicrobial-resistant organisms (ARO), 1706
Antineoplastic agents, 1950, 2179t–2180t
Antiobesity medications, 1199, 1200t
Antioxidants, for oxygen toxicity, 602
Antiphospholipid syndrome, 1675
Antireflux valve, 948, 949
Antiretroviral therapy (ART), 1537
adherence to, 1548c–1549c
Antiseborrheic shampoos, 1792
Antispas, 1345
Antispasmodics, 1005, 1012
Antithrombin deficiency, 1674
Antithrombotic drugs, for atrial fibrillation, 703
Antithymocyte globulin (ATG), 1098, 1101, 1616
Antithyroid medications, hyperthyroidism, 1233
Antitissue transglutaminase (tTG), 1007
Antitumour antibiotics, 2182
Antivenin, 2360–2361
Antrectomy, 977, 984
Anuria, 804, 818, 1283, 1292
Anus, 899
endoscopic examination, 913
Anxiety
assessment of, 122c
cardiomyopathy, 793, 794
gastric cancer, 990
gastritis, 978
heart failure, 819–821
illness and, 121–122, 122c
management of, 122c
mitral valve prolapse, 778, 779
nursing implications, 121–122
patient during surgery, 408
patient undergoing bariatric surgery, 1206
patient with newly diagnosed diabetes, 1171
peptic ulcer disease, 981
preoperative, 383
pulmonary edema, 824
Anxiety, relieving, 416, 546, 634
nursing process for, 2124
AOBP. *See* Automated office blood pressure (AOBP)
Aortic aneurysm
aortic valve replacement, repair of, 856f
endograft repair, 857f
repair of, 856f
Aortic area, 668
Aortic balloon valvuloplasty, 783
Aortic regurgitation, 781
Aortic stenosis
assessment and diagnostic findings, 782
clinical manifestations, 782
medical management, 782
pathophysiology, 781–782
Aortic valve, 777, 778, 781
autografts, 786
replacement, repair of, 856f
Aortoiliac disease, 855
medical management, 855
nursing management, 855
Apheresis, 1678
types of, 1679t
Aphonia, 471, 483
Aphthous stomatitis, mouth abnormalities, 920t
Apical impulse, 653
Apixaban (Eliquis), 2033
acquired thrombophilias, 1676
atrial fibrillation, 864, 875
Aplastic anemia, 1616–1617
assessment and diagnostic findings, 1616
clinical manifestations, 1616
medical management, 1616
nursing management, 1616–1617
pathophysiology, 1616
Aplastic crisis, 1621. *See also* Sickle cell crisis
Apligraf, 870, 1786
Apnea, 439, 471
Apocrine sweat glands, 1768
Apoptosis, 1517, 1519, 2150, 2153
Appendectomy, 1010, 1011t
Appendicitis, 998, 1009–1010
assessment and diagnostic findings, 1009
clinical manifestations, 1009
complications, 1009
McBurney's point, 1009f
medical management, 1010
nursing management, 1010
pathophysiology, 1009
peritonitis, 1015
Appetite, 904
Applied ethics, 25
Appraisal of stressful event, 104
and development of emotion, 104
primary appraisal, 104
reappraisal, 104
secondary appraisal, 104
Appropriate use criteria (AUC), 723
Apraxia, 2030
Aprepitant (Emend), in breast cancer, 1469
aPTT. *See* Activated partial thromboplastin time (aPTT)
Aqueous solutions, for eyes, 1893
Arachnoid villi, 1962
Arboviral encephalitis, 2094
ARBs. *See* Angiotensin receptor blockers (ARBs)
ARDS. *See* Acute respiratory distress syndrome (ARDS)
ARF. *See* Acute respiratory failure (ARF)
Argatroban
heparin-induced thrombocytopenia, 865
pulmonary embolism, 544
Arginine vasopressin (AVP), 309
Argon laser
for cutaneous lesions, 1831
photocoagulation, 1178
Arm
casts, 2240
exercises, 643c

Aromatase inhibitor, 1446, 1470
endometriosis, 1431
Aromatherapy, for postoperative nausea/vomiting, 417c
Arrhythmogenic right ventricular cardiomyopathy (ARVC), 787, 788
Arsenic trioxide, 2180t
Arterial aneurysms, etiologic classification of, 855c
Arterial blood gas, 333, 333t, 460–461
evaluation of, steps in, 334c
metabolic acidosis, 330
metabolic alkalosis, 330–331
respiratory acidosis, 331
respiratory alkalosis, 332
Arterial disorders, 843
aneurysms, 855–858
aortoiliac disease, 855
arterial embolism and arterial thrombosis, 859–860
arteriosclerosis and atherosclerosis, 843–850
dissecting aorta, 858–859
peripheral arterial occlusive disease, 850–853
Raynaud's phenomenon, 860–861
thromboangiitis obliterans, 854–855
upper extremity arterial occlusive disease, 853–854
Arterial embolism, 859
assessment and diagnostic findings, 859–860
clinical manifestations, 859
medical management, 860
endovascular management, 860
pharmacologic therapy, 860
surgical management, 860
nursing management, 860
pathophysiology, 859
Arterial insufficiency, ulcers, 838t
Arterial occlusions, 858
upper (*See* Upper extremity arterial occlusive disease)
Arterial pulses
palpation of, 667
pulse amplitude, 667
pulse contour, 667
pulse rate, 667
pulse rhythm, 667
Arterial thrombosis
assessment and diagnostic findings, 859–860
clinical manifestations, 859
medical management, 860
endovascular management, 860
pharmacologic therapy, 860
surgical management, 860
nursing management, 860
pathophysiology, 859
Arteries, 834–836, 1962–1963
atherosclerotic obstruction, 851f
Arteriolar narrowing, 881
Arteriolar vasoconstriction, 838
Arterioles, 834–836
Arteriosclerosis, 835, 843, 1819
clinical manifestations, 846
medical management, 846
improving peripheral arterial circulation, 846–848
maintaining tissue integrity, 849
radiologic interventions, 846
relieving pain, 849
surgical management, 846
pathophysiology, 843–844
prevention, 845–846
risk factors, 844–845
Arteriovenous fistula (AVF), 1283, 1306, 1307f
Arteriovenous graft, 1283, 1306–1307, 1307f
Arteriovenous malformations (AVMs), 2047
Artery, location of, 841f
Arthritis, 1731, 1732, 1759–1760
in older adults, 375
Arthritis pain, 269c
Arthrocentesis, 2229
Arthrodesis, 2233, 2247
Arthrography, 2228
Arthroplasty, 1732, 1755, 2233, 2247
Arthropod-borne virus encephalitis
assessment and diagnostic findings, 2093
clinical manifestations, 2093
medical management, 2094
nursing management, 2094
pathophysiology, 2093
Arthroscope, 2302
Arthroscopy, 2229
Articular cartilage, 2215
Artificial fingernails, 397
Artificial insemination, 1405–1406
Artificial larynx, 495
Artificial sphincters, 1344
Artificial tears, 1894
Artificial urinary sphincter, 1344
Arytenoid cartilages, 440
Asbestosis. *See also* Pneumoconiosis
clinical manifestations, 548
defined, 505
medical management, 548
pathophysiology, 548
Ascites, 304, 309, 989, 1052, 1061–1065
assessment and diagnostic findings, 1061
cirrhosis and, 1084
clinical manifestations, 1061
dietary control of, 1062
gastric cancer, 989
hepatic disorders, 1061–1065
home care checklist, 1066
medical management, 1061–1065
bed rest, 1062
nutritional therapy, 1062
paracentesis, 1062–1063
pharmacologic therapy, 1062
transjugular intrahepatic portosystemic shunt, 1063, 1065f
treatment method, 1065
nursing management, 1065
home and community-based care, 1065
pancreatic cancer, 1128
pathophysiology, 1061
right ventricular failure, 810
Ascorbic acid (vitamin C), 197, 2098
Asepsis, 1297
Aseptic technique, 927
Asparaginase, 2180t
acute lymphocytic leukemia, 1640
Aspartame (NutraSweet, Equal), 1147
Aspartate aminotransferase (AST), 1056, 1060, 1095
Aspergillus fumigatus, 2094
Aspiration, 505, 948, 958. *See also* Respiratory infections
pathophysiology, 521
pneumonia, 511
enteral therapy, 956t
patients at risk, 952
prevention, 521–522
absent reflexes, compensating for, 521, 521c
delayed stomach emptying, 522
feeding tube placement, 522
prolonged intubation, effects of, 522
risk factors, 520c
risk of, 941
Aspirin, 741, 1950, 1950c, 2034, 2059
acquired thrombophilias, 1678
coronary artery disease, 662, 663
enteric-coated, 1786
gastritis, 976
heart failure, 832
intoxication, 2368t
for pain management, 285
pericarditis, 799
peripheral arterial occlusive disease, 852
premenstrual syndrome, 1395
before surgery, 382
urinary stone formation, 1351
Assessment, 22, 1076. *See also* Physical assessment
abdomen, 672
acute pancreatitis, 1120
acute pharyngitis, 480
acute rhinosinusitis, 475–476
adenoiditis, 481–482
amyotrophic lateral sclerosis, 2137
aortic regurgitation, 781
aortic stenosis, 782
appendicitis, 1009
ARDS, 535
ascites, 1061
asthma, 585
atelectasis, 506
blunt trauma, 554
bronchiectasis, 577, 583
cancer of larynx, 492, 493c
cardiac tamponade, 829
cardiogenic shock, 826–827
cardiomyopathy, 788–789, 792
care of patient in cast, 2234
celiac disease, 1007–1008
cervical discectomy, 2141
chronic heart failure, 810
chronic inflammatory bowel disease, 1020
chronic rhinosinusitis, 477–478
colorectal cancer, 1034, 1038
constipation, 999
COPD, 567–569, 568c
cystic fibrosis, 597
degenerative disc disease, 2139
diabetes mellitus, 1170–1172
diarrhea, 1002
diverticular disease, 1011
dysrhythmias, 713
empyema, 532
esophageal varices, 1066–1067
esophagus, 940
fecal incontinence, 1003
food poisoning, 2365c
of functional capacity, 177–178
gallbladder disease, 1115–1116
gastric cancer, 990
gastrostomy and jejunostomy, 961
GI function, 429
health history in (*See* Health history)
heart failure, 809c, 810, 817–818
hepatic cirrhosis, 1085
hepatic disorders
health history, 1054–1055
physical assessment, 1055–1056
hepatic encephalopathy, 1072
hepatitis A virus, 1076
hepatitis B virus, 1078–1079
herniation of lumbar disc, 2142, 2144
in home and community, 70, 70c
hospitalized patient after surgery, 421

Assessment (*continued*)
infective endocarditis, 795–796
irritable bowel syndrome, 1005
laryngeal obstruction, 491
liver metastases, 1095–1096
lung abscess, 529
lung cancer, 550–551
mitral regurgitation, 780
mitral stenosis, 780
mitral valve prolapse, 779
myocarditis, 797
neck dissection, 929
nose fracture, 490
in nursing process, 28, 29–30, 30c
nutritional (*See* Nutritional assessment)
obstructive sleep apnea, 487
pancreatic cancer, 1128–1129
parenteral nutrition, 969
Parkinson's disease, 2130–2131
of patient, in PACU, 413
of patient undergoing laryngectomy, 495–496
peptic ulcer disease, 984–986
pericarditis, 799, 800
peritonitis, 1014–1015
peritonsillar abscess, 483
physical (*See* Physical examination)
pleural effusion, 531
pleurisy, 530
pneumonia, 512–513, 517–518
postpolio syndrome, 2145
primary brain tumours, 2120–2121, 2123
pulmonary contusion, 557
pulmonary edema, 533, 824
pulmonary embolism, 545
pulmonary hypertension, 538–539
pulmonary tuberculosis, 524–525, 525–526
recurrent acute rhinosinusitis, 477–478
sarcoidosis, 546
spinal cord tumours, 2125–2126
status asthmaticus, 595
sternal/rib fractures, 555
tonsillitis, 481–482
tube feeding, 955
ulcerative colitis, 1017–1018
upper airway infections, 484
Assist–control ventilation (A/C), 602, 620
Assisted-living facilities, 221
Assisted reproductive technologies, 1406
Assisted suicide, 242
Assistive device, 179
for PD patients, 2132
AST. *See* Aspartate aminotransferase (AST)
Astereognosis, 1975–1976
Asterixis, in hepatic encephalopathy, 1052, 1055
Asthma. *See also* Chronic pulmonary disease
about, 583–584
assessment/diagnostic findings, 585
clinical manifestations, 584–585
complications, 585, 587
defined, 564
medical management, 586f, 587–594
bronchodilator medications for COPD, 587t
of exacerbations, 592–593, 592f
long-term medications, 588t–590t
peak flow meters, 593, 593f, 594c
quick-relief medications, 591t, 592
nursing management, 593–594
pathophysiology, 584, 584f
prevention, 585
Astigmatism, 1888
Astrocytes, 1963
Asynchronous pacemaker, 720
Ataxia, 2031t, 2098
Atelectasis, 504–507, 2246, 2260. *See also* Chest and lower respiratory tract disorders
assessment/diagnostic findings, 506
clinical manifestations, 506
defined, 505
management, 507–508, 507c
pathophysiology, 505–506, 506f
prevention, 507, 507c
Atenolol, 740, 2025
antiarrhythmic medication, 699t
hypertension, 885t
Aterior lamellar keratoplasty (ALK), 1905
Atheromas, 730
Atherosclerosis, 729, 835, 843–850. *See also* Coronary atherosclerosis
clinical manifestations, 846
development of, 730
diabetes-related, 1175–1176
home and community-based care, 850
medical management, 846
improving peripheral arterial circulation, 846–848
maintaining tissue integrity, 849
promoting vasodilation and preventing vascular compression, 848–849
radiologic interventions, 846
relieving pain, 849
surgical management, 846
pathophysiology, 843–844
prevention, 845–846
risk factors, 844–845
thoracic aortic aneurysm, 855
Atherosclerotic lesions, 844
Atopic dermatitis, 1572, 1579, 1590–1591
medical management, 1591
nursing management, 1591
Atopy, 1572
Atorvastatin (Lipitor), 735t, 736
Atracurium besylate (Tracrium), 401t
Atrial dysrhythmias. *See also* Dysrhythmias
atrial fibrillation, 701–706, 702c, 702t, 703c
atrial flutter, 701
premature atrial complex, 700–701
Atrial fibrillation, 701–706, 2029
assessment/diagnostic findings, 703
cardiac complications, 944
cardiac rhythm therapies
catheter ablation therapy, 704–705
convergent procedure, 705
maze and mini-maze procedures, 705
classification system, 702c
medical management
electrical cardioversion for, 704
pharmacologic therapy, 703–704, 703c
risk factors, 702c
Wolff–Parkinson–White (WPW) syndrome, 706
Atrial flutter, 701
Atrial gallop, 809
Atrial natriuretic peptide (ANP), 302–303
fluid balance, role in, 303, 304f
Atrial septal defect, 783
Atrioventricular blocks, and infective endocarditis, 795
Atrioventricular nodal reentry tachycardia (AVNRT), 704, 706–707
Atrioventricular (AV) node, 653
Atrioventricular (AV) valves, 654–655, 654f
Atrophic pharyngitis, 481
Atrophy, 110, 110t
of muscles, 1968
Atropine, 912
cardiopulmonary resuscitation, 832t
Atropine sulphate, 2104
urinary retention, 1345
Atypical hyperplasia, 1446, 1456
Audiometry, 1933
AUDIT (Alcohol Use Disorders Identification Test), 59
Auditory brain stem implants (ABIs), 1953
Auditory brain stem response, 1933–1934
Augmentation mammoplasty, 1476
Auscultation, 905
in physical assessment, 65
Australasian Society of Clinical Immunology and Allergy (ASCIA), 1578
Authorized agent–controlled analgesia, 294
Autoantibodies, 1628
Autografts, 778, 786, 1857, 1860–1861, 2310
Autoimmune hemolytic anemias, 1628
Autoimmune nervous system disorders
Guillain–Barré syndrome, 2105–2109, 2110c
multiple sclerosis, 2096–2102
myasthenia gravis, 2102–2105
Autologous HSCT (AuHSCT), 2186, 2187
Autologous vaccines, 2192
Autolytic debridement, 1784
Automated office blood pressure (AOBP), 877, 882
Automaticity, 692
Autonomic hyperreflexia (dysreflexia), 200
Autonomic nervous system, 902, 1965
anatomy, 1967f
effects of, 1966t
functions of, 1965
hypothalamus, 1965
inhibitory–excitatory role, 1965
neurons, 1965
parasympathetic division, 1965
sympathetic and parasympathetic portions, 900
sympathetic division, 1965
Autonomic neuropathy, 1181
hypoglycemic unawareness, 1181
management, 1182
manifestations of, 1181
sexual dysfunction, 1181
sudomotor neuropathy, 1181
Autonomy, 25, 25c, 241
Autoregulation, 343
Autosomal dominant inheritance, 135–136, 135f
complete penetrance, 136
incomplete penetrance, 136
variable expression, 136
Autosomal dominant polycystic kidney disease (ADPKD), 1289
Autosomal recessive inheritance, 136–137, 137f
Autosomal recessive PKD. *See* Autosomal dominant polycystic kidney disease (ADPKD)
Autosomes, 133
Avascular necrosis, 1640, 2233, 2247
Avascular necrosis of bone (AVN), 2311
Avian influenza pandemic, 1710
Avitaminosis, 111
AVNRT. *See* Atrioventricular nodal reentry tachycardia (AVNRT)
Avoidance therapy, for allergic rhinitis, 1583

Avonex, 2098
AVP receptor antagonists, for hyponatremia, 311
Avulsion, 2349c
Awareness, Motivation, Skills, and Opportunity (AMSO) Model, 46
Axial flow VADs, 792
Axillary freckling, 1820
Axillary lymph node dissection (ALND), 1459
Axons, 1958
of lower motor neurons, 1968
of primary neuron, 1969
of secondary neuron, 1969
of spinal cord, 1969
Aygestin, 1431
Azacitidine, in myelodysplastic syndrome, 1619
Azathioprine, 1098, 1101, 1814
anal fistula, 1045
immune hemolytic anemia, 1629
immunomodulators, 1018
rheumatoid arthritis, 1745
Azilsartan (Edarbi), hypertension, 886t
Azithromycin (Zithromax)
chlamydia, 1420
Ebola virus disease, 1727
mycobacterium avium complex, 1553
sexual assault, 1384
Azotemia, 1283, 1286
enteral therapy, 956t

B

Babinski reflex, 1978
Babinski response, 1968
Babinski sign, 1978f
Bacille Calmette–Guerin (BCG), 1357
Bacillus Calmette–Guérin (BCG), 2190
Bacitracin, 1855
Back pain. *See* Acute low back pain
Baclofen (Lioresal), 2098, 2112
Bacteremia, 1698, 1707–1708, 1721
bacterial endocarditis, 795
Bacteria
in carcinogenesis, 2153–2154
Helicobacter pylori, 907
into large intestine, 902
person-to-person transmission, 981
into small intestine, 899
Bacterial peritonitis, cirrhosis and, 1084
Bacterial vaginosis, 1414
clinical manifestations, 1414
medical management, 1414
Bacteriuria, 1332, 1334
Bactrim, 1336
thalassemia, 1628
Bad cholesterol, 732
Balance control and coordination, 1975
Ball-and-socket joints, 2218
Balloon tamponade, esophageal varices, 1068
Balloon valvuloplasty, 783–784, 783f, 786
Balneotherapy, 1786, 1786t
Band cell, 1599, 1603
Banking sperm, 1510
Bariatric surgery
insurance coverage for, 1203
patient selection criteria for, 1204, 1204c
patient undergoing
assessment of, 1204
body image changes, 1207
bowel habits maintenance, 1207–1208
collaborative problems, 1206
evaluation, 1209
fluid volume balance of, 1206
home, community-based, and transitional care, 1209
infection prevention, 1206–1207
nursing interventions, 1206
nursing priorities for, 1204, 1206
nutritional status of, 1207
planning and goals, 1206
potential complications, 1206, 1208
reducing anxiety of, 1206
relieving pain of, 1206
procedures, 1203, 1205f
Barium enema, 1002, 1005
Barium sulphate suspension, 909
Barium swallow, 934, 936, 937, 938, 944
Baroreceptors, 301, 343, 653
Barotrauma and pneumothorax, 626
Barrel chest, 452
Barrett's esophagus (BE), 907, 934, 939
assessment and diagnostic findings, 940
clinical manifestations, 940
management, 940
Barthel Index, 178
Bartholin glands, 1374
Bartholin's cyst, 1412, 1427
Basal cell carcinoma (BCC), 1821f
clinical manifestations, 1820–1821
in immunocompromised population, 1826
medical management
nonsurgical alternative therapies, 1822
surgical, 1821–1822
nursing management, 1822
prognosis for, 1821
Basal ganglia, 1961
disorders affecting, 1969
functions, 1969
Base bicarbonate deficit. *See* Metabolic acidosis
Base bicarbonate excess. *See* Metabolic alkalosis
Basilar skull fractures, 2058
Basiliximab (Simulect), 1098, 1101
Basophils, 1518
Bath oils, 1789
Bath water, reflex vasodilation, 848
Battle's sign, 2058
BCC. *See* Basal cell carcinoma (BCC)
B cells, 1516, 1517, 1572
BCG Matrix, 1860
BE. *See* Barrett's esophagus (BE)
Beau's lines, 1777
Beclomethasone Propionate (QVAR), 588t
Beconase, in allergic rhinitis, 1585
Bed rest
ascites, 1062
constipation, 1000
hepatitis B, 1080
myocarditis, 798
Beers Criteria for Potentially Inappropriate Medication Use in the Elderly, 222
Belladonna, in urinary retention, 1345
Bell's palsy, 2111t, 2113–2114
medical management, 2113
nursing management, 2113–2114
Benazepril (Lotensin)
heart failure, 811t
hypertension, 886t
Bendamustine (Treanda), in chronic lymphocytic leukemia, 1642
Bendroflumethiazide (Naturetin), 820t
Bends. *See* Decompression sickness
Beneficence, 25, 25c
Benign disorders, of female reproductive system
adenomyosis, 1431
chronic pelvic pain, 1431
endometrial hyperplasia, 1431
endometriosis, 1430–1431
ovarian cysts, 1428–1429
uterus, benign tumours of, 1429–1430
vulvar cysts, 1427–1428
vulvar dystrophy, 1428
vulvitis, 1427
vulvodynia, 1427
Benign nephrosclerosis, 1285
Benign primary neoplasms of musculoskeletal system, 2291
Benign proliferative breast disease, 1446, 1456
Benign prostatic hyperplasia (BPH), 216, 1480, 1481, 1483
assessment and diagnostic findings, 1490–1491
clinical manifestations, 1490
medical management, 1491–1494
Benign tumours
characteristics of, 2152t
of esophagus, 940
Benson relaxation response, 116, 116c
Bentonite, 1787
Benzalkonium chloride, 1893
Benzodiazepines, 2007, 2098
Benzoyl erythromycin, 1794
Benzoyl peroxide, 1793–1794
Benzoyl sulphur, 1794
Benzthiazide (exna), 820t
Bereavement, 240, 257
Bernard, Claude, 102
Beta-adrenergic receptors, 351–352
Beta-2 agonists, in hyperkalemia, 317
Beta-blockers, 812, 1862
in angina, 740–741
blood pressure, 892
heart failure, 812
heart rate control, 704
hypertension, 885t
mitral regurgitation, 780
myocardial infarction, 747c
Betadine, for cleaning urinary catheters, 1350
Beta-glucan, 1860
Beta thalassemia, 1627
Betaxolol (Kerlone), hypertension, 885t
Bethanechol (Urecholine)
gastroesophageal reflux disease, 939t
neurogenic bladder, 1346
neuromuscular disorders, 939
Bevacizumab, 2191
Bicarbonate–carbonic acid buffer system, 329
Biceps reflex, 1976
Biguanides, 1157
Bile, 901t
Bile acid
sequestrant, 735t, 736, 998
synthesis, 1109
Bile duct
blockage of, 1111
injury, 1115
stone, 1115
Bile formation, role of liver, 1053–1054
Bile leak, 1114, 1115
Bile peritonitis, 1112, 1114
Bile reflux, 1208
gastritis, 993
Bile stasis, 1109
Bilevel positive airway pressure (BiPAP) therapy, 487, 602, 620
Biliary anastomoses, 1099
Biliary cholesterol saturation, 1109
Biliary colic, 1110

Biliary disorders
gallbladder, 1106–1107
anatomy and function, 1106–1108, 1107f
cholecystitis, 1108–1109
cholelithiasis, 1109–1115
pancreas, 1107f
cancer, 1128–1129
chronic, 1123–1127
cysts, 1127–1128
endocrine, 1107–1108
enzymes, 1107
exocrine, 1107
hyperinsulinism, 1131
necrosis, 1122
pancreatic islet tumours, 1131
tumours of pancreas head, 1126–1131
ulcerogenic tumours, 1131
Biliary drainage
gallbladder disease, 1116–1117
procedure, 1130
Biliary system, 1107f
Biliary tract, diagnosis of, 1110t
Bilingualism, 91
Bilirubin
concentration, 1054
excretion, 1054
Billroth II procedure, 989
Billroth I (gastroduodenostomy), peptic ulcer disease, 985t
Bilobectomy, 551c
Bimanual palpation, 1388
Bioartificial liver (BAL), 1083
Biobrane, 1859, 1859f
Biochemical assessment, 66–67
Biochemical mediators, 342, 343
Bioengineered skin, 1786
Biofeedback, 201, 1000, 1003
Biologic response modifier (BRM) therapy, 2150, 2160, 2190
Biologic therapies, 1018
Biologic valves, 786
Biologic variations, 95–96
Biologic wound dressings, 1859
Biopsy, 926
core needle, 1453
defined, 2150
excisional, 1453
forceps, 912, 1044
incisional, 1453
liver, 1057–1058
lung, 466, 468
lymph node, 468
magnetic resonance imaging-guided core, 1453
pleural, 466
stereotactic core, 1453
tissue, 1011
types of, 2160
ultrasound-guided core, 1453
Bisacodyl (Dulcolax), 288
laxative medications, 1001t
Bismuth subsalicylate (Pepto-Bismol), 979t
Bisoprolol (Zebeta), hypertension, 885t
Bites
animal, 2359
human, 2359
snakebites, 2359–2361
spider, 2361
tick, 2361, 2361f
Black keratosis, 1819
Black widow spider bites, 2361
Bladder
cancer, 1356–1358
assessment and diagnostic findings, 1357
clinical manifestations, 1357
medical management, 1357–1358
risk factors, 1356c
distention, 672
flaccid, 1346
spastic, 1346
training, 201
trauma, 1355
Bladder emptying, 1268
Bladder scanner, 201
Bladder ultrasonography, 1277
Blast cell, 1599, 1603
Blastomyces dermatitidis, 2094
Bleeding
anticoagulant therapy, 865
cirrhosis, 1094
diverticulitis, 1011, 1013
duodenal tumours, 995
esophageal varices, 1065, 1067f, 1071t
hepatic cirrhosis, 1094
hepatic disorders, 1074
liver transplantation, 1100
monitoring and managing complications, 865
thrombocytopenia and, 2202–2203
ulcerative colitis, 1016t
vitamin K deficiency, 1110
Bleeding disorders, 1657–1668
clinical manifestations, 1657–1658
essential thrombocythemia, 1658–1660
hemophilia, 1663–1666
immune thrombocytopenic purpura, 1661–1663
medical management, 1658
nursing management, 1658
platelet defects, 1663
secondary thrombocytosis, 1660
thrombocytopenia, 1660–1661
von Willebrand's disease, 1666–1668
Blenderized formulas, 954
Bleomycin
cardiac toxicity, 2183
Hodgkin lymphoma, 1649
Blindness, 1888–1889
assessment and diagnostic testing, 1889
contrast-sensitivity testing measures, 1889
glare testing, 1889
history taking, 1889
common causes of, 1888–1889
definition, 1888
gerontologic considerations, 1889
medical management, 1889–1890
vision restoration, 1890
nursing management, 1890–1892
coping strategy, 1890–1891
home, community-based, and transitional care, 1892
spatial orientation and mobility, 1891–1892
strategies for interacting with people, 1891c
Blistering diseases
assessment, 1814
bullous pemphigoid, 1814
dermatitis herpetiformis, 1814
nursing interventions
anxiety reduction, 1815
enhancing skin integrity and relieving discomfort, 1815
monitoring and managing complications, 1815
oral health restoration, 1814–1815
patient outcomes, 1815
nursing priorities, 1814
pemphigus vulgaris, 1813–1814
planning and goals, 1814
Stevens–Johnson syndrome, 1816
toxic epidermal necrolysis, 1816
ulcerations, 1819
Blood
chemistry, for CVD, 672–674, 673t–674t
pressure
postural, 666–667
pulse pressure, 666
Blood–brain barrier, 1083, 1963, 2091
Blood cells, 1600–1604, 1600t. *See also* Hematologic disorders
red, 1600–1603
white, 1603–1604
Blood clots, in IV line, 338
Blood component therapy, 1679
Blood disorders, therapies for, 1678–1680
Blood donation, 1680–1681
complications of, 1682
Blood flow
cardiogenic shock, 826
left ventricular failure, 808
mitral regurgitation, 779
nicotine, 845
thromboembolus obstructing, 838
vascular disorders, 837
Blood glucose monitors, 1148
Blood–ocular barriers, 1892
Blood pressure (BP)
ASH and ISH standards, 889
autoregulation of, 1267
cuffs, 841c
diets, 883
follow-up, recommendations, 892t
measuring, 890c
medications, 891c
physical examination, 881
regulation, 343–344
treatment for, 891c
World Health Organization, 883t
Blood processing, 1682–1683
Bloodstream infections, 336
Blood transfusions
diseases transmission by, 1681c
in hypovolemic shock, 355, 356
Blood urea nitrogen (BUN), 299, 300, 881, 1286, 1624
Bloody stools, liver disease, 1055
Blue pigtail, 949
Blunt trauma, 555. *See also* Chest trauma
assessment/diagnostic findings, 554
flail chest
medical management, 555–556
pathophysiology, 555
kidney, 1328
contusion, 1328
major laceration, 1328
minor laceration, 1328
vascular injury, 1328
medical management, 554–555
pathophysiology, 554
pulmonary contusion
assessment/diagnostic findings, 557
clinical manifestations, 556
medical management, 557
pathophysiology, 556
sternal/rib fractures
assessment/diagnostic findings, 555
clinical manifestations, 555
medical management, 555

Body fluids, 296–297. *See also* Fluid and electrolytes
electrolytes in, 297–298
fluid compartments, 297
extracellular fluid (ECF), 297
intracellular fluid (ICF), 297
third-space fluid shift, 297
Body image
in cancer, 2199
enhancing, 963
patient undergoing bariatric surgery, 1207
Body mass index (BMI), 66, 1191–1192
classification for overweight and obesity, 1196t
measurement of, 66
radiation doses and, 2166
table, 1195f
Body mechanics and posture, 2269–2270
Body movements, in physical assessment, 63
Body or spica casts, 2240
Body temperature, in older people, 232
Body temperature maintenance, hyperthyroidism, 1236
Body weight
and hypertension, 883t
medications affecting, 1197c
Boerhaave's syndrome, 919, 937
Bolus, 948
feedings, 954
gastrostomy feeding, by gravity, 964f
Bone-anchored hearing aid (BAHA), 1953
Bone cement, 2247
Bone cysts, 2291
Bone densitometry, 2228
Bone grafts, 924, 2310
Bone-healing stimulator, 2311f
Bone marrow, 1516, 1518f, 1600. *See also* Hematologic disorders
Bone marrow transplant (BMT), 1616, 1689
Bone mineral density (BMD), 143, 2223
Bone(s), 2214
cancellous, 2214–2215
cells, 2215
cortical, 2214
flat, 2215
formation, 2216
haversian system, 2215
healing, 2217
health, diet and, 2216
long, 2214, 2215f
maintenance, 2216–2217
pain, 2221
remodelling, 2216, 2217
short, 2215
tissue, 2216
Bone scan, 2228–2229
Bone tumours, 2291–2295
assessment and diagnostic findings, 2292
benign, 2291
clinical manifestations, 2292
home care checklist for, 2295c
malignant, 2291
medical management, 2292
metastatic bone disease, 2291
nursing process for, 2293–2294
pathophysiology, 2291
Borborygmus, 998, 1002
Bortezomib (Velcade), for multiple myeloma, 1654, 1655
Bosentan (Tracleer), for scleroderma, 1752
Boston keratoprosthesis, 1905
Botulinum toxin, 934
urinary incontinence, 1342
Bougienage, 938
Bowel cleansing, 913
Bowel continence, promotion of, 202–203
Bowel elimination
in PD, 2131
tube feeding, 958
Bowel habits
change, 904
maintenance, 1207–1208
Bowel incontinence, 200
Bowel obstruction, 1209
Bowel preparation, preoperative, 387
Bowel training programs, 202, 1003
Bowel tumours, 998
Bowen disease, 1480
Bowman's space, 1287
BP. *See* Blood pressure (BP)
Braces, 2233, 2234
patient with, 2240–2241
Brachial plexus block, 405
Brachioradialis reflex, 1976
Brachytherapy, 1412, 1434, 1446, 1468, 2150, 2165
Bracketing, 23
Braden scale, 195
Bradykinesia, 2117, 2128
Bradykinin, 838, 1572, 1574
Braille, 1892
Brain
blood–brain barrier, 1963, 2091
cerebellum, 1961
cerebral circulation, 1962–1963
cerebrospinal fluid, 1962
cerebrum, 1960–1961
external surface of, 196of
spinal cord, 1963–1964
spinal tracts, 1963–1964
vertebral column, 1964
stem, 1961
structures for protecting, 1961–1962
Brain abscesses, 2091–2092
assessment and diagnostic findings, 2092, 2092c
clinical manifestations, 2092
medical management, 2092
nursing management, 2092
pathophysiology, 2092
Brain death, 1996
Brain Injury Association of America, 2068
Brain natriuretic peptide (BNP), 303, 674
Brain stem auditory evoked responses (BAERs), 1984
Brain stem herniation, 2090
Brain stem ischemia, 2111t
Branch retinal vein occlusion, 1908
Bravelle, 1405c
BRCA1, 1446
BRCA2, 1446
Breakthrough pain, 280
Breast
assessment
anatomic and physiologic overview, 1445–1446, 1447f
health history, 1446
physical assessment, 1447–1449, 1449f
benign conditions of
benign proliferative breast disease, 1456
breast pain, 1455
cysts, 1455
fibroadenomas, 1455–1456
biopsies, types, 1453t
conditions affecting nipple
fissure, 1454
nipple discharge, 1454
diagnostic evaluation, 1449f
magnetic resonance imaging, 1452
mammography, 1450–1452
procedures for tissue analysis, 1452–1454
self examination, 1449–1450
ultrasonography, 1452
infections
lactational abscess, 1455
mastitis, 1454
inspection of, 1448c
male, 1476–1477
malignant conditions of, 1456–1461, 1467–1476
nursing process, 1461–1467
reconstruction, 1473f
self-examination, 1451c
surgery, reconstructive, 1476
Breast and ovarian cancer syndrome, 2155
Breast cancer, 142t
assessment and diagnostic findings, 1459
clinical manifestations, 1459
gerontologic considerations, 1475
hormone therapy, 1496, 1500
management
genetic testing, 1474
pregnancy, 1474–1475
quality of life and survivorship, 1475
nurse navigators, 1463c
nursing management, 1469–1470
pathologic factors associated with, 1459c
patient undergoing surgery for
assessment, 1461
evaluation, 1467
exercise after, 1466c
home care checklist, 1470c
planning and goals, 1461
postoperative nursing interventions, 1462–1467
preoperative nursing interventions, 1461–1462
prevention strategies in high-risk patient
chemoprevention, 1458
long-term surveillance, 1457–1458
prophylactic mastectomy, 1458
prognosis, 1459
protective factors, 1457
reconstructive breast surgery, 1476
recurrent and metastatic, treatment of, 1472
risk factors, 1457, 1458t
staging, 1459
surgical management
breast conservation treatment, 1460
modified radical mastectomy, 1459–1460
prosthetics, 1474
radiation therapy, 1467–1468
reconstructive procedures after mastectomy, 1472–1474
sentinel lymph node biopsy, 1460–1461
systemic treatments, 1468–1472
total mastectomy, 1460
types of
ductal carcinoma in situ, 1456
invasive cancer, 1456–1457
Breast-conservation treatment, 1446, 1460
Breast self-examination (BSE), 1386, 1446
Breathing
exercises, 573, 608c
patterns, 575
and respiratory rates, 452, 453t, 454
problems, in lung cancer, 552

Breathing (*continued*)
retraining, 612 (*See also* Chest physiotherapy (CPT))
nursing management, 612
Breath sounds, 457, 457t
left ventricular failure, 809
Brentuximab vedotin (Adcetris), Hodgkin's lymphoma, 1649
Bridging technique, 196
Brightness Acuity Tester, 1889
Brilinta (Ticagrelor), 741
Bristol Stool Chart, 202
Bristol Stool Form Scale, 1005
British North America Act of 1867, 4, 6
Broca's area, 1960
Bromocriptine (Parlodel), 1405c
Bronchi and bronchioles, 440–441
Bronchiectasis, 564. *See also* Chronic pulmonary disease
assessment/diagnostic findings, 577, 583
clinical manifestations, 577
medical management, 583
nursing management, 583
pathophysiology, 577
Bronchiole constriction, 812
Bronchodilator, 569–570, 571t
medications, for COPD, 587t
Bronchogenic carcinoma. *See* Lung cancer
Bronchophony, 439, 457
Bronchoplastic or sleeve resection, 633
Bronchoscopy, 439, 464–465, 464f
nursing interventions, 465
procedure, 464–465
Brown recluse spider bites, 2361
Brown-Séquard syndrome (Lateral cord syndrome), 2072c
Brudzinski's sign, 2090, 2090f
Bruit, 835, 836
Brushing, mechanical cleansing, 922
Bubble mask, 398
Bucket-handle tear, 2302
Buck's extension traction, 2243–2244
Budd-Chiari syndrome, 1070, 1083
Budesonide, 588t, 589t, 1018
allergic rhinitis, 1585
Buerger's disease, 854–855
assessment and diagnostic findings, 854
clinical manifestations, 854
medical management, 854
nursing management, 854–855
Buffer systems, 329
Bulbar paralysis, 2111t
Bullectomy, 572
Bullous impetigo, 1795
Bullous pemphigoid, 1814
Bull's eye rash, 2361
Bumetanide (Burinex, Bumex)
heart failure, 820t
hypertension, 884t
Bupivacaine (Marcaine, Sensoricaine), 404t
Buprenorphine, for pain management, 282, 287
Bupropion (Wellbutrin), 224
Bupropion SR, 569
Buried bumper syndrome, 963
Burn care
acute or intermediate phase of
dressing changes, 1856
fluid and electrolyte changes, 1854t
infection prevention, 1854
medical management, 1849–1854
modulation of hypermetabolism, 1862
nonpharmacologic measures, 1862
nursing interventions, 1864–1871
nursing priorities, 1863
nutrition management, 1862
pain management, 1861–1862
patient assessment, 1863
patient outcomes, 1871–1872
planning and goals, 1864
plan of nursing care, 1865c–1869c
potential complications, 1864
topical antibacterial therapy, 1855–1856
wound cleansing, 1854–1855
wound débridement, 1857
wound dressing, 1856–1861
emergent/resuscitative phase of, 1843–1844
case scenario, 1846c
fluid and electrolyte changes in, 1847t
fluid replacement therapy, 1845–1848
gerontologic considerations, 1848–1849
medical management, 1844–1848
nursing management, 1849
plan of nursing care, 1850c–1853c
transfer to burn centre, 1845, 1847c
gerontologic considerations, 1857–1861
outpatient, 1876
rehabilitation phase
nursing interventions, 1874–1875
nursing priorities, 1873
patient assessment, 1873
patient outcomes, 1875–1876
planning and goals, 1873–1874
potential complications, 1873
prevention of hypertrophic scarring, 1872
Burns
characteristics according to depth, 1838t
classification
deep partial-thickness burn, 1837–1838
depth of tissue destruction, 1837–1838
factors determining depth, 1838
full-thickness burn, 1838
superficial burn injury, 1837
superficial partial-thickness burn, 1837
disorders of wound healing, 1862–1863
electrical, 1839–1840
incidence, 1835–1836
local and systemic responses to, 1840
cardiovascular response, 1840
edema, 1840
fluids, electrolytes, and blood volume, effects on, 1840–1841
pulmonary response, 1841–1842
systemic responses, 1842–1843
management of, 1842–1843
method to estimate inujry
Lund and Browder method, 1838–1839
Palmer method, 1839–1840
rule of nines, 1838, 1839f
outlook for survival and recovery, 1837
gerontologic considerations, 1837
pathophysiology of, 1837
pathophysiologic changes with severe burn, 1838t
prevention of, 1836–1837, 1836c
rehabilitation programs, 177
zones of injury, 1839f
Burr holes, 2006, 2006f
Bursa, 2218
Bursitis and tenosynovitis, 2270
Busulfan
cardiac toxicity, 2183
chronic myeloid leukemia, 1639
Butrans, 287
Bypass grafts, peripheral arterial occlusive disease, 852

C

CA. *See* Cancer antigen (CA)
CABG. *See* Coronary artery bypass graft (CABG)
Cachexia, heart failure and, 810
CACS. *See* Cancer-related anorexia-cachexia syndrome (CACS)
Cadaver allografts, 1859
CAD risk equivalents, 732
Café-au-lait spots, 1773t
Caffeine, 1121
CAGE (Cutting down, Annoyance by criticism, Guilty feelings, and Eye-openers), 59
CAGE Questions Adapted to Include Drugs (CAGEAID), 59
Calamine lotion, 1787
Calcipotriene (Dovonex), 1808
Calcitonin, 318, 321, 2216–2217
Calcitriol, 2216
Calcium, 318
deficit (hypocalcemia), 318–320, 318t
excess (hypercalcemia), 318t, 320–322
normal total serum level, 318
Calcium acetate, for end-stage kidney disease, 1299
Calcium alginates, 870, 1045, 1786
Calcium and phosphorus binders, 1299
Calcium and phosphorus imbalance, in end-stage kidney disease, 1298
Calcium carbonate
end-stage kidney disease, 1299
gastroesophageal reflux disease, 939t
Calcium channel blockers, 813, 935
in angina, 741
aortic regurgitation, 781
hypertension, 886t
peripheral arterial occlusive disease, 860
Calcium chloride, 320
Calcium gluconate, 317, 320
Calcium stones, 1351
Calcium supplements, 320
Calculi, 925
Calculous cholecystitis, 1108
Calf pain, 839
Calicivirus, 1719
Callus, 2217, 2274
Caloric intake, in diabetic meal plan, 1144
Campylobacter infections, 1718
Canada
Aboriginal communities in, 8
cross-cultural health encounters in, 14
health care services in, 6, 13
history of nursing in, 4
nursing care delivery models in, 6
Canada Food and Drug Act, 1402
Canada Health Act, 6, 13, 221, 926, 931, 1043, 1357, 1431
Canada Post Corporation Act, 1892
Canadian Anesthesiologists' Society (CAS), 386
Canadian Association Disability Service Providers in Post Secondary Education, 1892
Canadian Association of Emergency Physicians (CAEP), 2340
Canadian Breast Cancer Network (CBCN), 1475
Canadian Cancer Society, 2150
Canadian Cardiovascular Society (CCS), 732
Canadian Centre for Occupational Health and Safety (CCOHS), 1783
Canadian Charter of Human Rights and Freedoms, 1892
Canadian College of Medical Geneticists, 146

Canadian Council on Health Services Accreditation, 9
Canadian Digestive Health Foundation, 997
Canadian Gerontological Nursing Association, 212
Canadian HIV Vaccine Initiative (CHVI), 1541
Canadian Hospice Palliative Care Nurses Group (CHPC-NG), 243
Canadian Human Rights Act, 1892
Canadian Hypertension Education Program, 888
The Canadian Institute for Health Information (CIHI), 2339
Canadian Interprofessional Health Collaborative (CIHC), 11
Canadian Liver Foundation, 1058
Canadian Mammogram Quality Guidelines, 1450
Canadian Multiculturalism Act, 91
Canadian Nurses Association (CNA), 83, 239
  Code of Ethics for Registered Nurses, 5, 165
Canadian Nurses Protective Society, on delegation, 73
Canadian Patient Safety Institute (CPSI), 1345
Canadian Standards Association, 396
Canadian Task Force for Preventative Health Care (CTFPHC), 1447
Canadian Triage and Acuity Scale (CTAS), 2340, 2343
  Level II Emergent, 2343
  Level III Less Urgent, 2343
  Level III Urgent, 2343
  Level I Resuscitation, 2343
  Non-Urgent, 2343
Canadian Urological Association (CUA), 1355
Canadian Venous Thromboembolism Clinical Trials and Outcomes Research (CanVECTOR), 2254
Canaliculi, 1053
Cancer
  bladder, 1356–1358
  breast, 1456–1461, 1467–1476
  carcinogenesis
    chemical agents, 2155
    dietary factors, 2155
    genetics/familial factors, 2155
    hormonal agents, 2155–2156
    molecular process, 2153–2156, 2154c
    physical agents, 2154–2155
    viruses/bacteria, 2153–2154
  caregivers, protection of, 2185–2195, 2186c
    complementary, alternative, and integrative health therapies, 2193, 2195
    hematopoietic stem cell transplantation, 2186–2189
    hyperthermia, 2189
    targeted therapies, 2189–2193, 2193t–2194t
  cell kill and cell cycle, 2166, 2178–2185
    adjunct chemotherapeutic agents, 2178
    chemotherapy agents, administration of, 2178–2184
    chemotherapy agents, classification of, 2178, 2179t–2180t
    nursing management, 2184–2185
  cervix, 1432–1434
  chemotherapy, 2166
  defined, 2150, 2151
  diagnosis of, 2157, 2159t
  epidemiology of, 2150–2151
  esophagus (*See* Esophagus cancer)
  fallopian tubes, 1438
  immune system, role of
    failure, 2156
    normal immune responses, 2156
  and immunotherapy, 1525
  invasion and metastasis
    angiogenesis, 2153
    lymphatic/hematogenous spread, 2152–2153
  kidney, 1290–1291
  of larynx, 491–502
    assessment/diagnostic findings, 492, 493c
    medical management, 492–495
    nursing process for, 495–502
    risk factors for, 492c
  of lungs (*See* Lung cancer)
  malignant cells, characteristics of, 2151–2152, 2152t
  management of, 2158
  nursing care of cancer patients
    bleeding, thrombocytopenia and, 2202–2203
    body image and self-esteem, 2199
    fatigue, 2198–2199, 2199c
    gerontologic considerations, 2204, 2204t
    grieving process, 220
    hospice, 2208
    infection management, 2200–2201, 2202t
    nutrition promotion, 2196–2198, 2196c
    oncologic emergencies, 2204–2208, 2205t–2207t
    patient education, 2203–2204
    psychosocial distress, 2200
    relieving pain, 2198, 2198t
    septic shock, 2201–2202
    sexuality, 2199–2200
    tissue integrity, 2195–2196
  oncology nursing, defined, 2149
  oral (*See* Oral cancer)
  ovary, 1438–1440
  pathophysiology of malignant process, 2151–2153
  pharynx (*See* Pharynx cancer)
  precision medicine, 2149
  prevention of, 2156–2156
    primary, 2157
    secondary, 2157, 2158t
    tertiary, 2157
  proliferative patterns, 2151
  radiation therapy, 2163–2166
    administration of radiation, 2164–2165
    nursing management, 2166
    protecting caregivers, 2166
    radiation dosage, 2164
    toxicity of, 2165–2166
  surgery, 2160–2163
    diagnostic, 2160
    nursing management, 2162–2163
    palliative, 2162, 2162t
    as primary treatment, 2160–2161, 2161t
    prophylactic, 2161–2162
    reconstructive, 2162
  survivorship care, 2208, 2208t
  tumour staging and grading, 2158
    anatomic stage group, 2158
    TNM classification system, 2159c
  uterus, 1434–1435
  vaccines
    allogeneic, 2192
    autologous, 2192
    prophylactic, 2192
    therapeutic, 2192
  vagina, 1437–1438
  vulva, 1435–1437
Cancer antigen (CA), 906
Cancer Control: Knowledge into Action for Effective Programmes—Palliative Care, 243
Cancer rehabilitation, 177
Cancer-related anorexia-cachexia syndrome (CACS), 2197
Cancer-related fatigue, defined, 2199
Cancer-related pain, 269
Candesartan (Atacand), hypertension, 886t
Candida albicans, 1413
Candida (yeast) infections, 1779
Candida species, 1818, 2094
Candidiasis, 1412, 1413–1414, 1534, 1551
  clinical manifestations, 1413
  medical management, 1414
  mouth abnormalities, 920t
Cane, walking with, 192
Canine companion programs, 206
Canker sore, mouth abnormalities, 920t
Cannabinoids, 272, 289
CAP. *See* Community-acquired pneumonia (CAP)
Capacitance vessels, 836
CAPD. *See* Continuous ambulatory peritoneal dialysis (CAPD)
Capecitabine, 1035
Capillaries, anatomic of, 836
Capillary endothelial cells, 1963
Capillary leak syndrome, 2183
Capsaicin (Capsaicin cream), 1181, 1789
Capsule colonoscopy, 913
Capsule endoscopy, 914
Captopril (Capoten)
  heart failure, 811t
  hypertension, 886t
Capture, 719
Caput medusae, 1085
Capzasin, 1789
Carbamazepine (Tegretol), 2112
  interaction with anesthetics, 382t
Carbohydrate antigen (CA 19-9), 989
Carbohydrates
  broken into, 902
  counting, 1145
  in diabetic diet, 1145
  metabolism, endocrine control of, 1108
Carbon dioxide laser, 1831
Carbon dioxide narcosis, 331
Carbon dioxide transport, 446
Carbonic acid deficit. *See* Respiratory alkalosis
Carbonic acid excess. *See* Respiratory acidosis
Carbonic anhydrase inhibitors, in metabolic alkalosis, 331
Carbon monoxide poisoning, 2362, 2364
Carboplatin (Paraplatin), in ovarian cancer, 1439
Carboxymethylcellulose (MCM), 1004, 1894
Carbuncles, 1796–1797
Carcinoembryonic antigen (CEA), 906, 989, 1034, 1096
Carcinogenesis. *See also* Cancer
  chemical agents, 2155
  defined, 2150
  dietary factors, 2155
  genetics and familial factors, 2155
  hormonal agents, 2155–2156
  molecular process, 2153–2156, 2154c
  physical agents, 2154–2155
  viruses and bacteria, 2153–2154
Carcinogens, 471
  associated with laryngeal cancer, 492
Cardiac action potential, 656

Cardiac arrest
clinical manifestations, 830
emergency assessment and management, 830–832
advanced cardiovascular life support, 831
defibrillation, 831
follow-up monitoring, 831–832
maintaining airway and breathing, 830–831
Cardiac biomarker analysis, 672
Cardiac biomarkers, 746–747, 747t
Cardiac catheterization, 653, 682–684
heart failure, 810
left heart, 683
nursing interventions, 683–684
right heart, 683
self-management after, 685c
Cardiac conduction system, 653, 655, 655f
Cardiac dysfunction, acute pancreatitis, 1122
Cardiac dysrhythmias, heart failure, 807
Cardiac electrophysiology
cardiac action potential, 656
overview, 655–656, 655f
refractory period, 656
Cardiac event recorders, 677
Cardiac failure, 554
Cardiac hemodynamics, 803–805
cardiac cycle, 657
cardiac output, 657–658
invasive assessment of, 804–805
noninvasive assessment of, 804
Cardiac implantable electronic devices, 677
Cardiac output (CO), 343, 999
alterations in, 625
cardiomyopathy, 792
defined, 653
heart rate on cardiac output, effect of, 657
stroke volume on cardiac output, effect of, 657–658
Cardiac rehabilitation, 177, 749–750
Cardiac resynchronization therapy (CRT), 721
Cardiac rhythm therapies. *See also* Atrial fibrillation
catheter ablation therapy, 704–705
convergent procedure, 705
maze and mini-maze procedures, 705
Cardiac sphincter, 934
Cardiac stress test, 653
exercise stress testing, 679
pharmacologic stress testing, 679–680
Cardiac tamponade, 560, 829c. *See also* Chest trauma
assessment and diagnostic findings, 829
clinical manifestations, 829
medical management, 829–830
pathophysiology, 828–829
pericarditis, 800
Cardiac transplantation, heart failure and, 811, 816
Cardiogenic embolic strokes, 2029
Cardiogenic shock, 341, 356–359
assessment and diagnostic findings, 826–827
clinical manifestations, 356, 826
coronary, 356
medical management, 356–358, 827–828
circulatory assist devices, 827
correction of underlying causes, 357
fluid therapy, 357
hemodynamic monitoring, 357
laboratory marker monitoring, 357
mechanical assistive devices, 358
oxygenation, 357
pain control, 357
pharmacologic therapy, 357–358
noncoronary, 356
nursing management, 358–359, 828
family presence during procedures, 359, 360c
fluids and medications administration, 358–359
intra-aortic balloon counterpulsation, 359
monitoring hemodynamic status, 358
prevention of shock, 358
safety and comfort enhancement, 359
pathophysiology, 356, 356f, 826, 826f
Cardiomegaly, 1288
Cardiomyopathy, 778, 787–794
arrhythmogenic right ventricular, 788
assessment, 788–789
clinical manifestations, 788
diagnostic findings, 788–789
dilated, 787–788
and heart failure, 807
hypertrophic, 788
medical management, 789
nursing process, 792–794
pathophysiology, 787–788
restrictive, 788
surgical management, 789–792
heart transplantation, 789–791
left ventricular outflow tract surgery, 789
mechanical assist devices, 791–792
total artificial hearts, 791
unclassified, 788
Cardiopulmonary bypass (CPB), 358, 758–759, 759f
Cardiopulmonary resuscitation (CPR), 709, 830–832, 832t
chest compressions, 830–832, 831f
chin-lift and bag-and-mask technique, 831f
follow-up monitoring and care in, 831–832
maintaining airway and breathing in, 830–832, 831f, 832t
medications used in, 832t
Cardiopulmonary system, chemotherapy and, 2183
Cardiovascular age, 888
Cardiovascular agents, in end-stage kidney disease, 1299
Cardiovascular death, 852
Cardiovascular disease, 142t, 662c, 729
and end-stage kidney disease, 1297
metabolic syndrome and, 732
Cardiovascular function
anatomy of heart
coronary arteries, 655
heart chambers, 652–654
heart valves, 654–655
cardiovascular disorders, 662c
diagnostic evaluation
cardiac catheterization, 682–684
cardiac stress testing, 679–680
chest x-ray and fluoroscopy, 675
CT, 681
echocardiography, 682
electrocardiography, 675–679
electrophysiologic testing, 684
hemodynamic monitoring, 685–689
laboratory tests, 672–675, 673t–674t
MRA, 681–682
radionuclide imaging, 680–681
function of heart
cardiac electrophysiology, 655–657
cardiac hemodynamics, 657–658
gender considerations, 658
gerontologic considerations, 658, 659t, 672
health history, 658–659
past health, family, and social history, 662–664
physical assessment, 664–672
abdomen, 672
arterial pulses, 667
blood pressure, 666–667, 667c
general appearance, 665
heart auscultation, 669–671
heart inspection and palpation, 668–669
jugular venous pulsations, 668
lungs, 671–672
of skin and extremities, 665–666, 665t
signs and symptoms
chest pain, 660, 660t–661t
types of, 659
Cardiovascular overload, fluid replacement and, 351
Cardiovascular risk
assessment of, 888–893
helping patients, 888–889
hypertension, 881
nursing process, 889–893
Cardiovascular stability
dysrhythmias, 416
hemorrhage, 415–416, 415t
hypertension, 416
hypotension and shock, 415
Cardiovascular system, age-related changes in, 213, 214t, 215
Cardioversion/defibrillation
defibrillation, 717
electrical cardioversion, 716–717
overview, 715–716, 715f, 716f
Cardizem. *See* Diltiazem
Caregiver role, 10
Caregivers, protection of, 2185–2195, 2186c. *See also* Cancer
complementary, alternative, and integrative health therapies, 2193, 2195
hematopoietic stem cell transplantation, 2186–2189
hyperthermia, 2189
targeted therapies, 2189–2193, 2193t–2194t
Care mapping, 10
Care of patient in cast. *See also* Musculoskeletal care modalities
casting materials
non-plaster, 2232–2233
plaster, 2233
nursing process for, 2234, 2235c, 2237c, 2238c
splints and braces, 2233–2234
Carfilzomib (Kyprolis), for multiple myeloma, 1654, 1655
Carmustine, for cardiac toxicity, 2183
Carotenemia, 1773t
Carotid endarterectomy (CEA), 2038, 2111t
complications of, 2039t
Carpal tunnel syndrome (CTS), 2271–2272
Carriers, 136
Carrier testing, 139
Carvedilol (Coreg)
heart failure, 812
hypertension, 885t
Case management, 10
Case manager, 10
Cast
defined, 2233
management (*See also* Musculoskeletal care modalities)
arm casts, 2240
body or spica casts, 2240
leg casts, 2240
removal, 2239c

Casting materials
non-plaster, 2232–2233
plaster, 2233
Cataracts
assessment and diagnostic findings, 1901
clinical manifestations, 1900
common types of, 1900
medical management, 1901–1903
nursing management, 1903
postoperative care, 1903
preoperative care, 1903
promoting home, community-based, and transitional care, 1903
pathophysiology, 1900
risk factors for formation, 1901c
surgical management, 1901–1903
lens replacement, 1902–1903
patient safety, 1922
phacoemulsification, 1901–1902
Cataract surgery, 1922
Catastrophic head injuries, 2056
Catastrophic reaction, 229
Catch-up vaccination, 1079
Catecholamines, 105
Catheter ablation therapy, 704–705
Catheter-associated urinary tract infection (CAUTI), 1337
risk factors for, 1338c
Catheterization
indwelling catheters, 1347
nursing management, 1347–1350
assessing the patient, 1347–1348
gerontologic considerations, 1348, 1348f
intermittent self-catheterization, 1349–1350
minimizing trauma, 1348
preventing infection, 1348, 1349c
retraining the bladder, 1348–1349
purpose of, 1346
suprapubic catheters, 1347, 1347f
urinary tract infections, 1346–1347
Catheters
Arrow, and Hohn, 968
central, 969
displacement, parenteral nutrition, 970t
feeding tubes, 955
Hickman and Groshong, 969
indwelling, 1347
percutaneous (nontunnelled) central, 967
peripherally inserted central, 969
polyurethane, 947
suprapubic, 1345, 1347, 1347f
triple-lumen, 1347
triple-lumen central, 968
Cation exchange resins, 317
Cauda equina, 1963
CBC. *See* Complete blood count (CBC)
CCK-PZ. *See* Cholecystokinin-pancreozymin (CCK-PZ)
CCPD. *See* Continuous cyclic peritoneal dialysis (CCPD)
CCRCs. *See* Continuing care retirement communities (CCRCs)
CEA. *See* Carcinoembryonic antigen (CEA); Carotid endarterectomy (CEA)
Cefixime
proctitis, 1044
sexual assault, 1384
Ceftriaxone (Rocephin), 1339, 2091
pelvic inflammatory disease, 1421
proctitis, 1044
Celiac disease, 1007t
assessment and diagnostic findings, 1007–1008
clinical manifestations, 1007
malabsorption, disorders of, 1006–1008
medical management, 1008
nursing management, 1008
pathophysiology, 1006–1007
Celiac nerve block, endoscopic ultrasound (EUS)-guided placement, 1127
Cell cycle–specific agents, 2178
Cell division, 134
Cell function, normal, 342
Cell kill and cell cycle, 2166, 2178–2185. *See also* Cancer
adjunct chemotherapeutic agents, 2178
chemotherapeutic agents
administration of, 2178–2184
classification of, 2178, 2179t–2180t
nursing management, 2184–2185
Cell regeneration, 1059
Cells of nervous system, 1958
Cellular changes, in shock, 342–343, 343f
Cellular fibrinolytic system, 1605
Cellular immune response, 1517, 1519, 1522
Cellular immunity, 1604
Cellular injury, 111–114
chemical agents, 112
disordered immune responses, 112
genetic disorders, 112
hypoxia, 111
infectious agents, 112
nutritional imbalance, 111
physical agents, 111
electrical shock, 112
mechanical trauma, 112
radiation, 112
temperature extremes, 111–112
response to injury, 113–114 (*See also* Inflammation)
Cellular oncogenes, 2153
Cellular proto-oncogenes, 2153
Cellulitis, 874–875
clinical manifestations, 874
medical management, 875
nursing management, 875
pathophysiology, 874
Cemented fixation, 2247
Centers for Disease Control and Prevention (CDC), 397, 1538
Central alpha$_2$-agonists, hypertension, 884t
Central Cord Syndrome, 2072c
Central cyanosis, 505
Central line–associated bloodstream infection (CLABSI), 351
evidence-based interventions for prevention of, 352c
Central nervous system (CNS), 900, 1960–1964, 1987
brain
blood–brain barrier, 1963
cerebellum, 1961
cerebral circulation, 1962–1963
cerebrospinal fluid (CSF), 1962
cerebrum, 1960–1961
spinal cord, 1963–1964
stem, 1961
structures for protecting, 1961–1962
depression, during ERCP, 1111
function, effect of hypoglycemia on, 1164
Central parenteral nutrition (CPN) solutions, 967
Central retinal artery occlusion, 1908
Central retinal vein occlusions (CRVOs), 1908
Central venous access device (CVAD), 948, 967
Central venous pressure (CVP), 351
monitoring of, 686
Centre for Infectious Disease Prevention and Control (CIDPC), 1538
Cephalalgia. *See* Headaches
Cephalexin (Keflex), 1830
Cephalosporins, 1336, 1339, 1796
Ceramide, 1806
CeraVe, 1806
Cerebellar tumour, 2120
Cerebellopontine angle tumour, 2120
Cerebellopontine lesion, 2111t
Cerebral angiography, 1982
Cerebral circulation, 1962–1963
arteries, 1962–1963, 1963f
veins, 1963
Cerebral dominance, 1961
Cerebral edema, 1996
patient with newly diagnosed diabetes, 1172
Cerebral hemispheres, 1960
Cerebral hypoxia, cardiogenic shock, 824, 826
Cerebral metastases, 2122–2123. *See also* Oncologic disorders of brain and spinal cord
Cerebral oxygenation, 1998–1999
Cerebral salt wasting, 1998t, 2006
Cerebral salt-wasting syndrome (CSW), 2052
Cerebrospinal fluid (CSF), 1962
basilar skull fractures and, 2058, 2058f
examination of, 1984
in fungal encephalitis, 2094
leak, 2058
rhinorrhea, 2058
Cerebrovascular accident (CVA), 1625
Cerebrovascular disorders
definition, 2028
diabetes and, 1175
Cerebrum, 1960–1961
Certified registered nurse anesthetist (CRNA), 392
Cerumen impaction, 1937
Ceruminous glands, 1768
Cervical cancer, 1431
assessment and diagnostic findings, 1432–1433
clinical manifestations, 1432
medical management, 1433–1434
Pap smear test, 1390
risk factors, 1432c
surgical procedures for, 1433c
Cervical cap, 1400
Cervical palpation, 1388–1389
Cervicitis, 1419–1420
Cervix, 1373, 1374
cancer of, 1432–1434
inspecting, 1388
speculum examination of, 1387f
Cetaphil, 1806
Cetirizine/pseudoephedrine (Zyrtec-D), 1583
CF. *See* Cystic fibrosis (CF)
Chancre, lip abnormalities, 920t
Chandelier sign, 1373, 1389
Charcot joints, 1180
Charleston pouch, 1332, 1363
Checklists, preoperative, 388, 388f
Cheilitis, 1794
Chelation therapy, 1623
Chemical agents, in carcinogenesis, 2155
Chemical burns, 938, 2364–2365
Chemical débridement, 1857

Chemical face peeling
  complications, 1829
  management, 1829–1830
Chemo brain, 2184
Chemolysis, 1352
Chemoreceptors, 343
Chemotherapeutic agents, 1035
  classification of, 2178, 2179t–2180t
  dosage, 2178
  extravasation, 2178, 2181
  home care checklist, 2180c
  hypersensitivity reactions, 2181–2182
  toxicity
    cardiopulmonary system, 2183
    cognitive impairment, 2184
    fatigue, 2184
    gastrointestinal system, 2182
    hematopoietic system, 2182
    neurologic system, 2183
    renal system, 2182–2183
    reproductive system, 2183
Chemotherapy, 925, 995, 1129, 2150
  breast cancer, 1468–1470, 1468t
  cancer management, 2166
  diarrhea, 1001
  liver tumours, 1096
  lung cancer, 551–552
  primary brain tumours, 2122
  prostate cancer, 1500–1501
Chemotherapy-induced nausea and vomiting (CINV), 2182, 2185
Cherry angioma, 1777t
Chest
  pain, 448–449, 659, 660, 660t–661t (*See also* Cardiovascular function)
    mitral valve prolapse, 778–779
    with pneumonia, 449
    in shock, 347
  percussion, 602
Chest and lower respiratory tract disorders
  atelectasis, 504–508, 507c
  chest trauma
    blunt trauma, 554–557
    cardiac tamponade, 560
    penetrating trauma (stab/gunshot wounds), 557
    pneumothorax, 557–560
    subcutaneous emphysema, 560
  chest tumours
    lung cancer, 548–553, 551c, 553c
    tumours of mediastinum, 553–554
  occupational lung diseases, 547–548
    asbestosis, 548
    coal worker's pneumoconiosis, 548
  pleural conditions
    acute respiratory distress syndrome, 534–537, 535c, 537c
    acute respiratory failure, 533–534
    empyema, 532–533
    pleural effusion, 531–532
    pleurisy, 530–531
    pulmonary edema, 533
    pulmonary embolism, 541–546, 541c, 543c
    pulmonary heart disease, 540–541
    pulmonary hypertension, 537–540, 538c
    sarcoidosis, 546–547
  respiratory infections
    acute tracheobronchitis, 508
    aspiration, 520–522, 520c, 521c
    lung abscess, 529–530
    pneumonia, 508–520, 509c, 510t, 513t, 514–516t, 520c, 521c
    pulmonary tuberculosis, 522–525, 523c
Chest compressions, in cardiopulmonary resuscitation, 830, 831f
Chest configuration. *See also* Thoracic inspection
  barrel chest, 452
  funnel chest, 452
  kyphoscoliosis, 452
  pigeon chest, 452
Chest drainage system. *See also* Thoracic surgery
  comparison, 635t
  defined, 602
  dry suction systems with one-way valve, 639
  dry suction water seal systems, 639
  features of, 638–639
  guidelines for management, 636c–637c
  postoperative complication management, 638c
  water seal system, 639
Chest percussion and vibration, 610–612
  nursing management
    continuing and transitional care, 611–612
    educating patient about self-care, 611
Chest physiotherapy (CPT), 944
  about, 608
  breathing retraining, 612
  Chest percussion and vibration, 610–612
  defined, 602
  postural drainage, 609–610
    nursing management, 610, 610c
Chest trauma
  blunt trauma, 554–557
  cardiac tamponade, 560
  penetrating trauma (stab/gunshot wounds), 557
  pneumothorax, 557–560
  subcutaneous emphysema, 560
Chest tumours
  lung cancer, 548–553, 551c, 553c
  tumours of mediastinum, 553–554
Chest wall resection, 551c
Chest x-rays, 462, 2092
  and fluoroscopy, 675
  pericardial effusion, 829
  pulmonary edema, 824
  thoracic aortic aneurysm, 856
Chewing tobacco, 845c
Cheyne–Stokes respirations, 2001
CHF. *See* Congestive heart failure (CHF)
Childhood sexual abuse, 1384
Child–Pugh classification, 1099
Chlamydia, 1420
  medical management, 1420
  nursing management, 1420
Chlamydia trachomatis, 1044, 1723
  assessment and diagnostic findings, 1723
  clinical manifestations, 1723
  complications, 1723
  medical management, 1723
  nursing management, 1723–1724
Chlorambucil (Leukeran), in chronic lymphocytic leukemia, 1642
Chloramphenicol (Chloromycetin), in thalassemia, 1628
Chlorhexidine gluconate, 763
Chlorhexidine-impregnated disc, 968
Chloride, 327
  and bicarbonate, 327
  deficit (hypochloremia), 327–328, 327t
  excess (hyperchloremia), 327t, 328
Chloroquine (Aralen), in thalassemia, 1628
Chlorothiazide (Diuril)
  heart failure, 820t
  hypertension, 884t
  thalassemia, 1628
Chlorpromazine hydrochloride, interaction with anesthetics, 382t
Chlorpromazine (Thorazine), nipple discharge, 1454
Chlorthalidone (Hygroton)
  heart failure, 820t
  hypertension, 884t
Chlortrimazole, 1856
Cholecystectomy, 1107, 1112
  open, 1115
  percutaneous, 1115
  small-incision, 1115
  surgical, 1115
Cholecystitis, 1107, 1108
Cholecystography
  gallstones, 1111
  liver dysfunction and jaundice, 1111
Cholecystojejunostomy, 1107, 1130
Cholecystokinin, gastrointestinal regulatory substances, 901t
Cholecystokinin-pancreozymin (CCK-PZ), 1106, 1107
Cholecystostomy, 1107, 1115
Choledochostomy, 1107, 1115
Cholelithiasis, 1107, 1108
Cholescintigraphy, cholelithiasis, 1111
Cholesteatoma, 1940
Cholesterol
  coronary atherosclerosis and, 732–736, 734f
  gallstones, 1109, 1109f
  granuloma, 1943
  levels, 674
Cholesterol-lowering drugs, 704
Cholesterol-saturated bile predisposes, 1109
Cholestyramine (Questran), 735t, 736, 993
Cholinesterase inhibitors (CEIs), 228, 1000
Chordae tendineae, 777, 778, 780, 784
Chordoplasty, 778, 784
Chorea, 2117, 2134
Chromosomal differences, 138
  and genetic conditions, 138
Chromosomes, 133, 133f
Chronic arterial disease, 868
Chronic bronchitis, 565
  defined, 564
The Chronic Care Model, 165
Chronic conditions, 155. *See also* Chronic illness
  challenges of living with, 161
  characteristics of, 158–160
  definition of, 156–157
  home and community-based care, 165–166
  management of, 157, 164
  multiple, 161
  nursing care of people with, 162–165
    direct care, 162–163
    holistic approach to care, 163
    nursing process, 163–165
    supportive care, 163
  phenomenon of chronicity, 155–156
  prevalence and causes of, 157–158
  and quality of life, 156
  reactions to, 156
Chronic dentoalveolar abscess, 923
Chronic dermatosis, 1788
Chronic diarrhea, 1002
Chronic diseases, 155. *See also* Chronic conditions
  as global issue, 157

interventions for prevention of, 158, 159c
myths and truths about, 158t
patient education for, 158, 165
risk factors for, 157
Chronic gastric ulcers, 981
Chronic glomerulonephritis, 1287
assessment and diagnostic findings, 1288
clinical manifestations, 1287–1288
medical management, 1288
nursing management, 1288
pathophysiology, 1287
Chronic heart failure, 805–824
assessment and diagnostic findings, 810
clinical manifestations, 808–810
etiology, 806–807
medical management, 811–816
nursing management, 816–824
pathophysiology, 807–808
Chronic hyperlipidemia, vascular endothelial cell injury, 844
Chronic hypertension, 1922
Chronic idiopathic jaundice, 1061
Chronic illness, 155
acute phase, 162c
adjustment to, factors affecting, 156
characteristics of, 158–160
collaborative process, 159
development of other chronic conditions, 159
ethical issues, 160
family life, 159
health care costs, 159–160
home life, 159
living with uncertainty, 160
loss in income, 160
phases of illness, 159
psychological and social issues, 158–159
self-management, 159
therapeutic regimens, 159
comeback phase, 162c
continuing care, 165–166
crisis phase, 162c
downward phase, 162c
dying phase, 162c
health education for people with, 38
holistic approach to care, 162
implications for nursing, 162
nursing care for special populations with, 166
phases of, 161, 162c
pretrajectory phase, 162c
stable phase, 162c
teaching self-care, 165
trajectory phase, 162c
identification of, 163
understanding, 161
Paterson's Shifting Perspectives Model, 161
Trajectory Model of Chronic Illness, 161, 162c
unstable phase, 162c
Chronic inflammatory bowel disease
assessment, 1020
collaborative problems, 1020
evaluation, 1023
nursing interventions, 1020–1023
nursing priorities, 1020
planning and goals, 1020
ulcerative colitis, 1018
nutritional therapy, 1018
pharmacologic therapy, 1018–1019
surgical management, 1019–1020
Chronic kidney disease (CKD), 1282–1285, 1297–1300
assessment and diagnostic findings, 1297–1298
acidosis, 1297
anemia, 1298
calcium and phosphorus imbalance, 1298
sodium and water retention, 1297
clinical manifestations, 1297
complications, 1298–1299
gerontologic considerations, 1300
hypertension, 878
medical management, 1285, 1299–1300
dialysis, 1300
nutritional therapy, 1299
pharmacologic therapy, 1299
nursing management, 1300
continuing and transitional care, 1300
promoting home, community-based, and transitional care, 1300
pathophysiology, 1284, 1297
stages, 1285, 1285c
Chronic laxative, 998
Chronic liver disease, hepatic disorders, 1058
Chronic lymphocytic leukemia (CLL), 1641–1642
clinical manifestations, 1641, 1641f
medical management, 1641–1642
pathophysiology, 1641
Chronic myeloid leukemia (CML), 1638–1640
clinical manifestations, 1638
medical management, 1638–1639
nursing management, 1639–1640
oral therapy for, 1639t
risk factors, 1639t
Chronic obstructive pulmonary disease (COPD), 440, 443t, 448, 849, 1620
assessment and diagnostic findings, 567–569, 568c
bronchodilator medications for, 587t
chronic bronchitis, 565
clinical manifestations, 567
complications, 569
defined, 564
emphysema, 565–566
grades of, 568t
medical management, 569–573, 571t
nursing management, 573–577, 576c, 577c, 578c–582c
overview, 563–564
pathophysiology, 564, 565f
risk factors for, 566, 566c
Chronic otitis media
clinical manifestations, 1940
medical management, 1940–1941
Chronic pain, 2265. *See also* Pain
Chronic pancreatitis
nonsurgical management, 1126–1127
surgical management, 1127
Chronic pelvic pain, 1431
Chronic pharyngitis. *See also* Pharyngitis
clinical manifestations, 481
medical management, 481
nursing management, 481
Chronic pulmonary disease
asthma, 583–594
bronchiectasis, 577–583
chronic obstructive pulmonary disease, 563–577
cystic fibrosis, 596–598
status asthmaticus, 595–596
Chronic pyelonephritis, 1339–1340
assessment and diagnostic findings, 1339
clinical manifestations, 1339
complications, 1340
medical management, 1340
nursing management, 1340
Chronic rhinosinusitis (CRS). *See also* Rhinosinusitis
assessment/diagnostic findings, 477–478
clinical manifestations, 477
complications, 478
medical management, 478–479
nursing management, 479
occurrence, 477
pathophysiology, 477
Chronic sialadenitis, 925
Chronic thromboembolic pulmonary hypertension (CTEPH), 538c
Chronic venous insufficiency, 867–868
clinical manifestations, 867
complications, 867–868
medical and nursing management, 868
Chronotropy, 692, 693
Chvostek's sign, 319, 319f
Chyle fistula, neck dissection, 933
Chylomicrons, 733
Chyme, 899, 900
Ciclesonide (Alvesco), 588t
Cidofovir (Vistide), 1921
Cigarette smoking, 125, 845, 845c, 878
and CAD, 736
irritable bowel syndrome, 1005
pancreatic cancer, 1128
risk factors for cancer, 925
Cigar, risk factors for cancer, 925
Cilia, 439
Cilostazol (Pletal), in peripheral arterial occlusive disease, 852
Cimetidine (Tagamet), 331, 907
gastric acid, 1120
in peptic ulcer disease, 1574
peptic ulcer disease and gastritis, 979t
Ciprofloxacin, 1339, 2091
proctitis, 1045
sexual assault, 1384
CircAid, 866, 869
Circle of Willis, 1963, 2047
Circulating nurse, 392, 394–395
Circulatory hypoxia, 603c
Circulatory impairment, skin traction, 2244
Circulatory overload, signs of, 312
Circumcision, 1480, 1481, 1511
Cirrhosis. *See* Hepatic cirrhosis
Cisatracurium besylate (Nimbex), 401t
Cisplatin, 989
bladder cancer, 1357
13-*cis*-retinoic acid, 2191
CJD. *See* Creutzfeldt-Jakob disease (CJD)
CKD. *See* Chronic kidney disease (CKD)
Clarithromycin (Biaxin), 983
chronic *H. pylori* gastritis, 995
mycobacterium avium complex, 1553
peptic ulcer disease and gastritis, 979t
Classic aging pattern of intelligence, 222
Classic KS, 1826
Clavicle, fracture of, 2312, 2312f, 2313f
Clavicular strap, 2312, 2312f
Clergyman's sore throat, 481
Clevidipine (Cleviprex)
hypertension, 887t
hypertensive emergencies, 893
Client. *See* Patient
Clindamycin (Cleocin), 483
bacterial vaginosis, 1414
Clinical breast exam (CBE), 1384

Clinical guidelines, 10
Clinical manifestations, 481
  abscess, 922
  achalasia, 934
  acne vulgaris, 1792–1793
  acquired immune deficiency syndrome, 1550–1553
  acute coronary syndrome, 745
  acute low back pain, 2266
  acute lymphocytic leukemia, 1640
  acute myeloid leukemia, 1636, 1636f
  acute otitis media, 1939
  acute pancreatitis, 1120
  acute pharyngitis, 480
  acute respiratory failure, 534
  acute rhinosinusitis, 475
  acute tracheobronchitis, 508
  adenoiditis, 481
  adrenocortical insufficiency, 1248–1249
  altered level of consciousness (LOC), 1989
  amyotrophic lateral sclerosis, 2136–2137
  anemia, 1610
  angina pectoris, 738
  aplastic anemia, 1616
  appendicitis, 1009
  ARDS, 535
  asbestosis, 548
  ascites, 1061
  atelectasis, 506
  Barrett's esophagus, 940
  basal cell carcinoma, 1820–1821
  bleeding disorders, 1657–1658
  bone tumours, 2292
  brain abscesses, 2092
  bronchiectasis, 577
  cancer of larynx, 492
  cardiac arrest, 830
  cardiac tamponade, 829
  cardiogenic shock, 356, 826
  cataracts, 1900
  celiac disease, 1007
  Chlamydia trachomatis, 1723
  chronic heart failure, 808–810
  chronic lymphocytic leukemia, 1641, 1641f
  chronic myeloid leukemia, 1638
  chronic otitis media, 1940
  chronic pharyngitis, 481
  chronic rhinosinusitis, 477
  coal worker's pneumoconiosis, 548
  colorectal cancer, 1034
  conjunctivitis, 1915
  constipation, 999
  contact dermatitis, 1589–1590
  COPD, 567
  coronary atherosclerosis, 731–732
  Creutzfeldt–Jakob disease, 2095
  Cushing syndrome, 1250–1251, 1251c
  cystic fibrosis, 596–597
  degenerative disc disease, 2139
  diabetes insipidus, 1221
  diabetes mellitus, 1142
  diabetic ketoacidosis, 1166
  diabetic retinopathy, 1178
  diarrhea, 1002
  disseminated intravascular coagulation, 1668–1669
  diverticular disease, 1011
  diverticulum, 937
  dry eye syndrome, 1914
  Ebola virus disease, 1726
  empyema, 532
  epilepsy, 2016–2017
  esophageal spasm, 935
  esophageal varices, 1066
  esophagus cancer, 943
  essential thrombocythemia, 1659
  external otitis (otitis externa), 1937
  fecal incontinence, 1003
  food allergy, 1593
  fungal encephalitis, 2094
  gastric cancer, 989
  gastritis, 978
  gastroesophageal reflux disease, 938
  generalized exfoliative dermatitis, 1812
  giant cell arteritis, 1753
  glaucoma, 1897, 1897t
  gout, 1758
  Guillain–Barré syndrome, 2107
  headaches, 2023–2024
  hearing loss, 1934–1936
  hemophilia, 1665
  hemorrhagic stroke, 2047–2048
  hepatic cirrhosis, 1084–1085
  hepatic encephalopathy, 1072
  hepatitis A virus, 1076
  hepatitis B virus, 1078
  hereditary angioedema, 1592
  hereditary hemochromatosis, 1629
  herniation of cervical intervertebral disc, 2140
  herniation of lumbar disc, 2142
  herpes simplex virus (HSV) encephalitis, 2093
  herpes zoster, 1797–1798
  hiatal hernia, 936
  hidradenitis suppurativa, 1791
  hip fracture, 2317
  Hodgkin lymphoma, 1648–1649, 1649f
  human immune deficiency virus, 1550–1553
  Huntington's disease, 2134–2135
  hypercalcemia, 321
  hyperglycemic hyperosmolar nonketotic syndrome, 1163
  hyperkalemia, 316
  hypermagnesemia, 324
  hypernatremia, 312
  hyperparathyroidism, 1241
  hyperphosphatemia, 326
  hyperthyroidism, 1231
  hypervolemia, 305t, 307
  hypocalcemia, 319, 319f
  hypokalemia, 314
  hypomagnesemia, 323
  hyponatremia, 310–311, 310f
  hypophosphatemia, 325
  hypothyroidism, 1226
  hypovolemia, 304, 305t
  immune hemolytic anemia, 1628
  immune thrombocytopenic purpura, 1661–1662
  impetigo, 1795
  increased intracranial pressure, 1996–1997
  iron deficiency anemia, 1614
  irritable bowel syndrome, 1004
  irritant contact dermatitis, 1806
  ischemic stroke, 2030–2032
  jaw disorders, 923
  labyrinthitis, 1946
  laryngeal obstruction, 490–491
  laryngitis, 483–484
  latex allergy, 1595–1596, 1595t
  liver metastases, 1095
  lower urinary tract infection, 1334
  lung abscess, 529
  lung cancer, 550
  malignant melanoma, 1823
  megaloblastic anemias, 1617
  Ménière's disease, 1945
  metabolic acidosis, 329–330
  metabolic alkalosis, 330
  motion sickness, 1944
  multiple myeloma, 1653–1654
  multiple sclerosis, 2096–2097
  myelodysplastic syndrome, 1619
  nasal fracture, 490
  Neisseria gonorrhoeae, 1723
  nephropathy, 1179
  neutropenia, 1632
  non-Hodgkin lymphomas, 1651
  obstructive sleep apnea, 486–487, 487c
  oral cavity cancer, 926
  oral cavity disorders, 922
  osteoarthritis, 1755
  osteomyelitis, 2287
  otosclerosis, 1943
  Paget's disease, 2286
  pancreatic cancer, 1128
  pancreatic tumours, 1129
  Parkinson's disease, 2128
  pediculosis capitis, 1800
  pemphigus vulgaris, 1813
  peptic ulcer disease, 982
  perforation, 937
  peritonitis, 1014
  peritonsillar abscess, 483
  pertussis, 1728
  pharynx cancer, 926
  pheochromocytoma, 1246
  pituitary tumours, 1220
  platelet defects, 1663
  pleural effusion, 531
  pleurisy, 530
  pneumonia, 512
  pneumothorax, 558
  polycythemia, 1630
  polymyalgia rheumatica, 1753
  polymyositis, 1752
  primary aldosteronism, 1255
  primary brain tumours, 2118–2120
    increased intracranial pressure, 2119–2120
    localized symptoms, 2120
  psoriasis, 1807
  pulmonary contusion, 556
  pulmonary edema, 533, 824
  pulmonary embolism, 542
  pulmonary heart disease, 540
  pulmonary hypertension, 538
  pulmonary tuberculosis, 524
  respiratory acidosis, 331
  respiratory alkalosis, 332
  retinal detachment, 1907
  rheumatic diseases, 1733
  rheumatoid arthritis, 1743–1744
  rhinitis, 472–473
  sarcoidosis, 546
  scabies, 1801–1802
  scleroderma, 1751
  seborrheic dermatoses, 1791–1792
  seizure disorders
    focal seizures, 2014
    generalized absence seizure, 2014
    generalized seizures, 2014
  septic (infectious) arthritis, 2289
  serous otitis media, 1940
  sickle cell disease, 1621–1622
  Sjögren's syndrome, 1750
  spinal cord injury, 2071
  squamous cell carcinomas, 1820–1821
  status asthmaticus, 595

Stevens–Johnson syndrome, 1816
systemic lupus erythematosus, 1748–1749
thalassemia, 1628
thrombocytopenia, 1660
toxic epidermal necrolysis, 1816
traumatic brain injury, 2059
tumours of mediastinum, 553
ulcerative colitis, 1017
variant Creutzfeldt–Jakob disease, 2095
viral rhinitis, 474, 474c
von Willebrand's disease, 1667
Clinical nurse specialist (CNS), 11
Clinical pathways, 9–10
Clinical photographs, 1780
Clinic managers, 18
CLL. *See* Chronic lymphocytic leukemia (CLL)
Clomid, 1405c
Clomiphene citrate (Clomid), 1429
infertility, 1405, 1406
ovulation, 1405c
Clomipramine (Anafranil), for premature ejaculation, 1488
Clonal stem cell disorders, 1633–1634
Clonidine (Catapres), 569
Clonidine (Catapres-TTS), 910
hypertension, 884t
Clonus, 1978
Clopidogrel, 741, 2034
peripheral arterial occlusive disease, 852
Closed commissurotomy, 783
Clostridium difficile, 906, 958, 1001
Clostridium perfringens, 2305
Clothing
constrictive, 849
peripheral vascular disease, 848
Clotrimazole (Gyne-Lotrimin), for candidiasis, 1414
Clotted catheter line, parenteral nutrition, 970t
Cloxacillin, 1796
Clubbing of fingers, 450–451, 451f
Cluster headaches, 2023–2024
medical management, 2025
CML. *See* Chronic myeloid leukemia (CML)
CNS. *See* Central nervous system (CNS)
Coagulation studies, 672–674, 673t–674t
Coal worker's pneumoconiosis. *See also* Pneumoconiosis
clinical manifestations, 548
medical management, 548
nursing management, 548
pathophysiology, 548
Cobblestone, 1016
Cobicistat, 1547
Cocaine, 2366t
Coccidioides immitis, 2094
Cochlear implants, 1953–1954, 1953f, 1980
selection of patients, 1953
Cochlear Ménière's disease, 1945
Codeine, 281t, 287
Code of Ethics for Registered Nurses, 26, 27
Cognitive appraisal, 104
Cognitive behaviour therapy (CBT), for pain relief, 290
Cognitive coping strategies, 384
Cognitive impairment, after chemotherapy, 2184
Cognitive–motivational–relational theory, 104
Coitus interruptus, 1401
Cola and cranberry juice, 951
Colchicine
cirrhosis, 1085
gout, 1758
pericarditis, 799
Colds/cold sores, 474c, 1798
Cold sore/fever blister, lip abnormalities, 920t
Cold urticaria, 1592
clinical manifestations, 1592
medical management, 1592
Colectomy, 2162
Colicky pains and kidney cancer, 1290
Colistimethate, in acute kidney injury, 1294
Collaborative problems, 28, 30c, 31–32
cardiomyopathy, 792
chronic inflammatory bowel disease, 1020
colorectal cancer, 1039
diverticular disease, 1013
gallbladder disease, 1116
gastrostomy and jejunostomy, 962
heart failure, 818
hypertension, 889
leg ulcer, 870
and nursing diagnoses, differences between, 32, 32f
parenteral nutrition, 969
patient with newly diagnosed diabetes, 1171
peptic ulcer disease, 986
pericarditis, 800
tube feeding, 956
Collagen-vascular diseases, 780
College of Family Physicians of Canada, 49
College of Nurses of Ontario, on delegation, 73
Colles' fracture, 2300, 2314–2315
Colloids, in shock, 350–351, 354
Colon cancers, 912
in older people, 1035
Colonic function, disorders of, 902
Colonic J-pouch, 1036
Colonic transit studies, 911, 999
Colonization, 1698
Colonoscopy, 913, 1018
Colony-forming units (CFU), 1335
Colony-stimulating factors, 1524–1525
Colorectal cancer, 1033–1038, 1035
assessment and diagnostic findings, 1034
clinical manifestations, 1034
collaborative problems, 1039
complications, 1035
diagnosis of, 906
evaluation, 1043–1044
medical management
adjuvant therapy, 1035–1036
surgical management, 1036–1037
nursing interventions
body image, 1041
colostomy appliance, 1040–1041
emotional support, 1039–1040
home and community-based care, 1043
postoperative care, 1040
preparing the patient for surgery, 1039
sexuality issues, 1043
nursing priorities, 1038
nursing process, 1038–1044
pathophysiology, 1034
planning and goals, 1039
prevention, 1035
risk factors, 1034c
staging of, 1036c
Colorectal neoplasms
colon, polyps of, 1044
colorectal cancer, 1033–1038
rectum, polyps of, 1044
Colostomy, 998, 1027, 1037
appliances, 1041
irrigation, 1027, 1041, 1042c–1043c
Colour changes of skin, 1772
light and dark skin, 1773t
Colour flow techniques, 841
Colour fundus photography, 1887
Colour vision testing, 1886
Colpexin Sphere, 1425
Colposcopy and cervical biopsy, 1391
CoLyte, 913
Coma, 1060
Combitube, 2347, 2347f
Comedones, 1794
Commercial heel protector, 196
Commissurotomy, 778, 783–784
closed, 783–784
open, 784
Common cold. *See* Viral rhinitis
Communicable disease outbreaks, in Canada, 2340
Communication
cross-cultural, 93, 94c
multiple organ dysfunction syndrome, 366–367
in Parkinson's disease, 2132
with patients and families within palliative hospice, 244–245
Community-acquired pneumonia (CAP), 509–510, 510t
Community-associated methicillin-resistant *Staphylococcus aureus* (CA-MRSA), 1698, 1707
Community-based care
diabetes as secondary diagnosis, 1188
diabetes mellitus, 1163–1164
diabetic retinopathy, 1178–1179
hypoglycemia, 1165
neck dissection, 933
patient undergoing bariatric surgery, 1209
patient with newly diagnosed diabetes, 1172
Community-based nursing, 13–14
ambulatory settings, 18–19
community health nurse, functions of, 14–15
and community health nursing, 14
community resources and referrals, 16
home care, 15–16
discharge planning for, 16
nursing in home setting, 15–16
safety precautions in, 17c
homeless people, care of, 19–20
home visit, 16–18
agency's policies and, 16
assessment in, 17
bag with supplies and equipment, 16
documentation considerations for, 17
ending the visit, 18
initial home visit, 17
medication management in, 17
need for future visits, assessment of, 17–18, 18c
patient's referral form, 16
personal safety precautions, 17, 17c
occupational health programs, 19
preventive care in, 14
primary prevention, 14
secondary prevention, 14
tertiary prevention, 14
school health programs, 19
Community resources, 16
Community wellness, education for, 37. *See also* Health education
Comorbidity, 222
Compartment syndrome, 2227, 2236, 2308–2309, 2309f
Compensation, acid–base disorders and, 332–333, 333t

Compensatory mechanisms, 101
Compensatory stage, of shock, 344
clinical manifestations, 344–345, 344t
medical treatment, 345
nursing management, 345–346
anxiety reduction, 346
safety promotion, 346
tissue perfusion assessment, 345–346
Complement, 1517, 1521
Complementary and alternative medicine (CAM), 96
for cancer treatment, 2193, 2195
defined by National Institutes of Health, 2193
mind and body practices, 96
natural products, 96
Complete blood count (CBC), 904
Complex regional pain syndrome (CRPS), 269c, 2307, 2311
Compliance, 439
in lungs, 442
Compression of trigeminal root by tumour, 2111t
Computed tomography (CT), 462–463, 681, 908, 989, 1980, 2058
brain abscess, 2092
colonography, 912
gallbladder, 1115
hepatic disorders, 1058
meningitis, 2090
pancreatic tumour, 1128
for pelvic examination, 1393
pericarditis, 799
scanning, ulcerative colitis, 1018
Computed tomography angiography (CTA), 842
thoracic aortic aneurysm, 856
Computer-aided detection (CAD), 1452
Computer-assisted stereotactic biopsy, 2120
Concentrated (fluorinated) corticosteroids, 1788
Concomitant lactose intolerance, tube feeding, 958
Concussion, 2056, 2061
Condom
female, 1400, 1401f, 1539
male, 1401, 1539
use, 1540c
Condom catheters, 202
Conduction abnormalities, 710–713. *See also* Dysrhythmias
first-degree AV block, 711
medical management of, 713
second-degree AV block
type I, 711–712
type II, 712
third-degree AV block, 712–713
Conductive keratoplasty, 1906
Condylomata, 1412, 1416, 1819
Cone biopsy, 1391
Confidentiality, 25, 25c
and ethical issues in nursing, 26
Confidentiality of genomic information, 146
Confusion, 989
Confusion Assessment Method for the ICU (CAM-ICU), 349, 772
Congestive heart failure (CHF), 804, 805, 849
Conjunctival sac, 1892
Conjunctivitis
assessment and diagnostic findings, 1915
clinical manifestations, 1915
medical management
allergic conjunctivitis, 1916
bacterial conjunctivitis, 1916
patient education, 1917c
toxic conjunctivitis, 1916
viral conjunctivitis, 1916
types
allergic conjunctivitis, 1916
bacterial conjunctivitis, 1915
toxic conjunctivitis, 1916
viral conjunctivitis, 1915–1916
Connective tissue disorders, 998
Consequentialism, 24
Conservative therapy, 935
Consolidation, 505
Consolidation therapy, 1637
Constipation, 429, 898, 997–1000, 998, 2246
assessment and diagnostic findings, 999
clinical manifestations, 999
complications, 999
enteral therapy, 956t
irregularity of defecation, 997
medical management, 1000
in older adults, 217
opioid-induced, 288
pathophysiology, 998–999
patient education, 1000c
prevention of, 203
Constitutional Act of 1982, 6
Constrictive pericarditis, 798, 799
Constructional apraxia, 1052, 1072
Consultation, with dietitian, 924
Contact dermatitis, 1589–1590, 1788
assessment and diagnostic findings, 1590
clinical manifestations, 1589–1590
lip abnormalities, 920t
types, testing, and treatment of, 1590t
Contact lenses, 1893
Continent ileal urinary reservoir, 1363
Continent urinary diversion (Kock or Charleston pouch), 1332, 1358, 1363–1364
continent ileal urinary reservoir, 1363
ureterosigmoidostomy, 1363–1364
Continuing care, 2138–2139
acute coronary syndrome, 754
acute pancreatitis, 1123
adrenocortical insufficiency, 1250
angina pectoris, 743
ascites, 1065
for bone tumours, 2294
cardiomyopathy, 793–794
cervical discectomy, 2142
chronic illness, 165–166
cirrhosis, 1095
coronary artery bypass graft, 774
corticosteroid therapy, 1258
Cushing syndrome, 1253–1254
diabetes mellitus, 1163–1164
as secondary diagnosis, 1188
diabetic retinopathy, 1179
gallbladder disease, 1117
gastric cancer, 991
gastric surgery, 994
gastritis, 980
heart failure, 823
hepatic encephalopathy, 1074
hepatitis B virus, 1080–1081
Huntington's disease, 2135
hyperthyroidism, 1236
inflammatory bowel disease, 1022
IV therapy, 338
liver transplantation, 1102
liver tumour, 1098
orthopedic surgery, 2261
osteomyelitis, 2289
ostomy, 1031
pancreatic tumours, 1129, 1131
Parkinson's disease, 2132–2133, 2133c
patient undergoing bariatric surgery, 1209
patient with newly diagnosed diabetes, 1172
peptic ulcer disease, 987, 988
pheochromocytoma, 1248
shock, 367
total hip arthroplasty, 2256
tube feeding, 959
Continuing care retirement communities (CCRCs), 220–221
Continuous ambulatory peritoneal dialysis (CAPD), 1283, 1314–1315, 1315c
complications, 1315
procedure, 1315
Continuous central venous oximetry monitoring, in shock, 346
Continuous cyclic peritoneal dialysis (CCPD), 1283, 1314, 1315–1316
home, community-based, and transitional care, 1316, 1317c
nursing management, 1316
Continuous ECG monitoring. *See also* Electrocardiography (ECG)
ambulatory electrocardiography, 676
cardiac event recorders, 677
cardiac implantable electronic devices, 677
continuous monitors, 676–677
continuous real-time monitors, 677
hardwire cardiac monitoring, 675
lead systems, 676
telemetry, 675–676
Continuous glucose monitoring system (CGMS), 1150
Continuous kidney replacement therapy (CRRT), 1282, 1283, 1311, 1311f
Continuous mandatory ventilation (CMV), 602
Continuous monitors, 676–677
Continuous palliative sedation therapy, 254
Continuous passive motion (CPM), 182, 2233, 2256
Continuous positive airway pressure (CPAP), 376, 487, 602, 603
Continuous quality improvement (CQI), 9
Continuous real-time monitors, 677
Continuous subcutaneous insulin infusion, 1137, 1155–1156
Continuous venovenous hemodiafiltration (CVVHDF), 1311
Continuous venovenous hemodialysis (CVVHD), 1311
Continuous venovenous hemofiltration (CVVH), 1311
Continuous wave (CW) Doppler ultrasound device, 840
Contraception, 1396–1397
contraindications, 1397
Contraceptives
injectable, 1399–1400
transdermal, 1399
vaginal, 1399
Contractility, 653
Contracture, 2225
Contractures, 180, 1857, 1863
prevention of, 181
Contrast agents, 909
patient care during urologic testing with, 1278c
Contrast-enhanced digital mammography (CEDM), 1452
Contrast-induced nephropathy (CIN), 1295

Control, 2160
Controlled ventilation, 602
Contusions, 2056, 2059, 2298–2299, 2349c
Conus medullaris, 1963
Convergent procedure, 705
Conversion tables, for TD systems, 282
Cooley's anemia, 1627
Coombs test, 1628
Cooper's ligaments, 1445
Coordination of movement, 1968–1969
COPD. *See* Chronic obstructive pulmonary disease (COPD)
Coping, 104–105, 108, 125
  enhancement, 115–116
  hyperthyroidism, measures, 1235
  measures, 574
  neck dissection, 930
  in Parkinson's disease, 2132
  and stress tolerance
    in cardiac disease, 664
  tube feeding, 959
Cordectomy, 493
Core needle biopsy, 1453
Corn, 2274
Corneal disorders
  corneal dystrophies, 1903
  fuchs endothelial dystrophy, 1904
  keratoconus, 1904
Corneal dystrophies, 1903
Corneal reflex, 1978
Corneal surgeries
  anterior lamellar keratoplasty (ALK), 1905
  Boston keratoprosthesis, 1905
  deep anterior lamellar keratoplasty (DALK), 1905
  Descemet's stripping endothelial keratoplasty (DSEK), 1905
  keratoprosthesis, 1905
  nursing management, 1905–1906
  penetrating keratoplasty (PKP), 1905
  phototherapeutic keratectomy (PKT), 1904–1905
  posterior lamellar keratoplasty (PLK), 1905
  tissue for corneal transplantation, donor characteristics, 1905c
Cornstarch base, 1787
Coronary arteries, 655, 731, 731f
Coronary artery bypass graft (CABG), 733, 757
  alternative CABG techniques, 759, 759f
  blockage in coronary arteries, 758
  cardiac output, decrease in, 771–772
  cardiopulmonary bypass, 758–759, 759f
  cerebral circulation after, 771
  common used conduits in, 758, 758f
  complications of, 759–761, 760t–761t
  fluid and electrolyte imbalance after, 771, 772
  for high-risk patients, 758
  impaired gas exchange after, 771, 772
  indications for, 757–758
  intraoperative nursing management, 763
  nursing interventions
    monitoring and managing complications, 763
    patient education, 763
    reducing fear and anxiety, 762–763
  plan of nursing care, 765–760c
  postoperative nursing management, 764, 764f, 770
    assessment, 770–771
    fluid and electrolyte balance, 772
    home, community-based, and transitional care, 774
    maintaining adequate tissue perfusion, 773
    maintaining cardiac output, 771–772
    maintaining normal body temperature, 773–774
    managing complications, 771
    minimizing confusion, 772–773
    monitoring for complications, 771
    promoting adequate gas exchange, 772
    relieving pain, 773
  preoperative management, 761–763
    aspirin and beta-blockers, 761–762
    assessment, 762
    health history, 762
    physical examination, 762
  psychosocial assessment, 762
  traditional, 758–759, 758f, 759f
  vein commonly used for, 758, 758f
Coronary artery disease (CAD), 729, 881, 1068. *See also specific diseases*
  diabetes, 1175
Coronary atherosclerosis, 729–730. *See also* Angina pectoris
  clinical manifestations, 731–732
  gender and, 737
  pathophysiology, 730–731, 731f, 732f
  prevention, 732–737
    controlling cholesterol abnormalities, 732–736
    diabetes control, 737
    dietary measures, 733–734, 735t
    hypertension management, 736–737
    medications, 735–736, 735t
    physical activity, 734–735
    tobacco use, cessation of, 736
  psychosocial factors and behaviour patterns, 737
  risk factors, 732, 733c
    modifiable, 732, 733c
    nonmodifiable, 733c
Cor pulmonale, 505. *See also* Pulmonary heart disease
Corpus callosum, 1961, 1961f
Corpus luteum, 1373, 1375
Corrosive poisons, 2362
Cortical cataract, 1900
Corticospinal tracts, 1967–1968
Corticosteroid insufficiency, in critically ill patients, 353
Corticosteroids, 1018, 1082, 1098, 1101, 1787–1788
  allergic rhinitis, 1585
  anti-inflammatory and antiallergy actions, 1255
  applications, 1255
  asthma, 587, 588t
  Bell's palsy, 2113
  blistering diseases, 1813–1814
  bullous pemphigoid, 1814
  commonly used, 1256t
  COPD, 570
  dosage, 1256
  glaucoma, 1894
  head and pubic lice, 1801
  herpes zoster, 1798
  methylprednisolone, 1830
  mononeuropathy, 2114
  nursing management, 1257–1258
  pericarditis, 799
  pruritus, 1789
  psoriasis, 1808–1809
  rhytidectomy (face-lift), 1830
  sickle cell crisis, 1624
  side effects, 1256, 1257t
  status asthmaticus, 596
  tapering, 1257
  TEN and SJS, 1816
  therapeutic uses, 1256
Cortisol, 106, 301
Corynebacterium parvum, 2190
Costovertebral angle, 1273f
Cotton-wool spots, 881
Cough, 448, 672
  left ventricular failure, 809
  pulmonary complications, signs/symptoms of, 952
  pulmonary edema, 824, 825
  thoracic aortic aneurysm, 856
Cough etiquette, 1702
Coughing exercises, preoperative instructions, 384, 385c
Coughing technique, 610c
Covermark, 1819
Cowden's syndrome, 143t
Cowper's gland, 1479
CPB. *See* Cardiopulmonary bypass (CPB)
CPN solutions. *See* Central parenteral nutrition (CPN) solutions
CPR. *See* Cardiopulmonary resuscitation (CPR)
CPT. *See* Chest physiotherapy (CPT)
Cracking, arterial lumen, 846
Crackles, 439, 672, 817
Cramping pains, dumping syndrome, 993
Cranial arteritis, 2022, 2023, 2024
  medical management, 2025
Cranial mononeuropathies, in diabetes, 1180
Cranial nerve disorders
  abducens nerve, 2111t
  Bell's palsy, 2113–2114
  facial nerve, 2111t
  glossopharyngeal nerve, 2111t
  hypoglossal nerve, 2112t
  oculomotor nerve, 2111t
  olfactory nerve, 2111t
  optic nerve, 2111t
  spinal accessory nerve, 2112t
  trigeminal nerve, 2111t
  trigeminal neuralgia (tic douloureux), 2110–2113
  trochlear nerve, 2111t
  vagus nerve, 2111t
  vestibulocochlear nerve, 2111t
Cranial nerves, 1961, 1964, 1964t
  assessment of, 1973c–1974c
Craniocerebral trauma, 2056
Craniotomy, 2006
C-reactive protein (CRP), 674, 845, 922, 1005
Creams, 1787
Creatine kinase (CK), 746
  isoenzymes, 747
Creatinine, 300, 1099
  clearance, 1285
  serum creatinine levels, 300
Creatinine/height index, 67
Crepitus, 2304
CREST syndrome, 1751
Creutzfeldt–Jakob disease (CJD)
  assessment and diagnostic findings, 2095
  clinical manifestations, 2095
  medical management, 2095
  nursing management, 2095–2096
  pathophysiology, 2095
Cricoid cartilage, 440
Cricothyroid membrane puncture, 2347
Cricothyroidotomy, 2347
Crinone, 1405c

Critical-Care Pain Observation Tool (CPOT), 279
Critical illness–related corticosteroid insufficiency, 353
Critically ill patient
respiratory function in, assessment of
inspiratory force, 460
minute ventilation, 459, 460c
tidal volume, 459
vital capacity, 459–460
Critical thinkers, 22–23
Critical thinking, 21
in action, 24c
action plan, development of, 22, 23
and clinical decision making, 21, 22
cognitive/mental activities in, 22
definitions of, 21
exercises, 23
intellectual integrity in, 22
metacognition in, 21, 22
in nursing practice, 22–23
skills, 22, 23
development of, 21, 23
use of, 21, 22
Crohn's disease, 1017, 1018, 1019, 1027, 1045
inflammatory bowel disease, 1016–1017
vs. ulcerative colitis, 1016
Cromolyn sodium (NasalCrom), 587, 589t, 1585
Cross-cultural communication, 93, 94c
Crotalidae polyvalent immune Fab antivenom, 2360
Crotamiton (Eurax), 1802
Crowe, Cathy, 20
CRP. *See* C-reactive protein (CRP)
CRPS. *See* Complex regional pain syndrome (CRPS)
Cruciate ligament injury, 2301–2302
Crutch gaits, 190, 191c
Crutch walking, 180, 188, 190, 191c
CRVO. *See* Central retinal vein occlusions (CRVOs)
Cryoablation, 705
Cryopreserved saphenous veins, 852
Cryosurgery, 1794, 1822
of prostate, 1480, 1496
Cryosurgical hemorrhoidectomy, 1046
Cryotherapy, 1412, 1417, 2196
and laser therapy, 1391
Crypt abscesses, 1017
Cryptococcal meningitis, 1553–1554
Cryptococcus neoformans, 1552
Cryptogenic strokes, 2029
Cryptorchidism, 1480, 1506
Cryptosporidium, 1719
Crystallized intelligence, 222
Crystalloids
3:1 rule, 354
in shock, 350–351, 354
CSF. *See* Cerebrospinal fluid (CSF)
CSW. *See* Cerebral salt-wasting syndrome (CSW)
CT. *See* Computed tomography (CT)
CTA. *See* Computed tomography angiography (CTA)
CTAS. *See* Canadian Triage and Acuity Scale (CTAS)
C-type natriuretic peptide (CNP), 303
Cultural blindness, 93
Cultural competence, 92, 93
Cultural diversity, 91
influence of, on health care delivery, 8
Cultural/ethnic patterns, 59
Cultural humility, 91
Cultural imposition, 93
Culturally competent nursing care, 91
Culturally safe nursing care, 91
Cultural nursing assessment, 97, 99c
Cultural taboos, 93
Cultural values and beliefs
preoperative assessment, 383
preoperative teaching, 386
Culture, 90. *See also* Transcultural nursing
definition of, 8, 90
and dietary history, 68
diversity within, 91
ethnic, 90–91
food and, 95, 96c
and health care, 92, 93
influence on readiness to learn, 40
nursing assessment of, 97, 99c
role of, in community-based practice, 14
subcultures, 91, 92
Culture care accommodation, 93
Culture Care Diversity and Universality, 92–93
Culture care restructuring, 93
Cultured epithelial autograft (CEA), 1860
Cure, 2160
Curling's ulcers, 982
Curreiri formula, 1862
Cushing's reflex, 1996
Cushing's triad, 1996
Cushing syndrome, 1218, 1250–1252, 1768, 1788
assessment and diagnostic findings, 1251–1252
clinical manifestations, 1250–1251, 1251c
home care checklist, 1254c
medical management, 1252
nursing process, 1252–1254
ulcers, 982
Cutaneous manifestations of systemic diseases, 1767t
Cutaneous neurofibromas, 1820
Cutaneous ureterostomy, 1363
Cutaneous urinary diversions, 1358–1363, 1359f, 1360f
cutaneous ureterostomy, 1363
ileal conduit, 1358–1363
nursing care, 1361c
patient education, 1362
Cuticle, 1768
Cutting. *See* Female genital mutilation (FGM)
Cut wound, 2349c
CVAD. *See* Central venous access device (CVAD)
CW. *See* Continuous wave (CW)
CyA. *See* Cyclosporine A (CyA)
Cyanoacrylate embolization, 872
Cyanosis, 451, 795, 809, 839, 1772
bluish hue of, 1772
colour changes in, 1773t
detection of, 1772
CyberKnife, 2164
Cyclamate, 1147
Cyclic feeding, 948, 954
Cyclic guanosine monophosphate (cGMP), 1484
Cyclic infusions, 955
Cyclobenzaprine (Amrix), fibromyalgia, 1759
Cyclo-oxygenase 2 (COX-2), 1745
Cyclophosphamide, 1814, 2183
breast cancer, 1469
chronic lymphocytic leukemia, 1642
immune hemolytic anemia, 1629
rheumatoid arthritis, 1745
Cycloplegics, 1893–1894, 1893t
Cyclosporine
acute kidney injury, 1294
anal fistula, 1045
heart transplantation, 789
immunomodulators, 1018
liver transplantation, 1098
Cyclosporine A (CyA), 1809
Cyproterone acetate (Androcur), in prostate cancer, 1500
Cystectomy, 1332, 1350
Cystic fibrosis (CF). *See also* Chronic pulmonary disease
assessment/diagnostic findings, 597
clinical manifestations, 596–597
medical management, 597–598
nursing management, 598
pathophysiology, 596
Cystine stones, 1351
Cystitis, 1331, 1332
Cystocele, 1373, 1387, 1412, 1424
Cystography, 1279
Cystolitholapaxy, 1352
Cystoscopic examination, 1279, 1279f
Cysts, 1455, 1455t
anorectal disorders, 1046–1047
of skin, 1819
Cytarabine (Cytosar), 2183
acute myeloid leukemia, 1637
Cytochrome P450 enzyme system, 144, 145, 1100
variations, clinical effects of, 145t
Cytogenetics, 138
Cytokines, 1517, 1518, 1599, 1603. *See also* Targeted therapies, in cancer
and biologic activity, 1523t
defined, 2150
interferons, 2191
interleukins, 2191
retinoids, 2191–2192
Cytomegalovirus, 1418
retinitis, 1554, 1921
Cytotoxic agents, 1788
Cytotoxic (type II) hypersensitivity, 1574
Cytotoxic T cells, 1517

D

Dabigatran (Pradaxa), 864, 865, 2033
acquired thrombophilias, 1676
Dacarbazine (DTIC), in Hodgkin lymphoma, 1649
Daclizumab (Zenapax), 1098, 1101
DAI. *See* Diffuse axonal injury (DAI)
Daily fluid intake, 978
Dakin's solution, 1856
DALK. *See* Deep anterior lamellar keratoplasty (DALK)
Dalteparin, 741
venous thromboembolism, 864
Danazol (Danocrine)
endometriosis, 1430–1431
immune hemolytic anemia, 1629
Dandruff, 1792
Dapoxetine (Priligy), premature ejaculation, 1488
Dapsone, 1814
thalassemia, 1628
Daratumumab (Darzalex), multiple myeloma, 1655
Darbepoetin alfa (Aranesp)
breast cancer, 1470
myelodysplastic syndrome, 1619
Dasabuvir (Viekira Pak), 1081

Dasatinib (Sprycel), in chronic myeloid leukemia, 1638
Daunorubicin, 2182
  acute myeloid leukemia, 1637
Dawn phenomenon, 1155
DBE. *See* Double-balloon enteroscopy (DBE)
DBP. *See* Diastolic blood pressure (DBP)
DCM. *See* Dilated cardiomyopathy (DCM)
D-dimer, 1599
  pulmonary embolism, 828
Death
  clinicians' attitudes toward, 241
  coping With, 260
  patient and family attitudes toward, 241
  signs of approaching, 254–255, 256c
  time of, 257
On Death and Dying, 241
Débridement, 2300
  leg ulcers, 869
Debulking, 2160
Decitabine (Dacogen), in myelodysplastic syndrome, 1619
Decompression (intestinal), 948
Decompression sickness, 2357–2358
  assessment and diagnostic findings, 2357
  management, 2357–2358
Decompressive hemicraniectomy, 2000
Decongestants, 476
Deep abrasive therapy, 1794
Deep anterior lamellar keratoplasty (DALK), 1905
Deep breathing
  before coughing, 384
  preoperative instructions, 384, 385c
Deep inferior epigastric perforator flap (DIEP), 1474
Deep peptic ulcer, 981f
Deep-seated bacterial rhinosinusitis, 476
Deep tendon reflexes, 1976–1978, 1977t–1978t
Deep vein thrombosis (DVT), 430–431, 843, 1323, 2041, 2203, 2254
  complications of, 863c
  endovascular management, 864
  providing comfort, 865–866
  risk factors, 862c
  treatment for, 863
  unfractionated heparin, 863
DEET. *See* Diethyltoluamide (DEET)
Defecatory disorders, 999
Defecography, 915, 999
Deferasirox (Exjade), in myelodysplastic syndrome, 1620
Deferoxamine (Desferal), in myelodysplastic syndrome, 1620
Defibrillation, 717
  chest and heart rhythm, 831
  defined, 692
Degenerative disc disease. *See also* Degenerative disorders
  assessment/diagnostic findings, 2139
  clinical manifestations, 2139
  medical management, 2139–2140
  pathophysiology, 2139
  surgical management, 2139–2140
Degenerative disorders. *See also* Oncologic disorders of brain and spinal cord
  amyotrophic lateral sclerosis, 2135–2137
    assessment/diagnostic findings, 2137
    clinical manifestations, 2136–2137
  degenerative disc disease
    assessment/diagnostic findings, 2139
    clinical manifestations, 2139
    medical management, 2139–2140
    pathophysiology, 2139
  herniation of cervical intervertebral disc
    clinical manifestations, 2140
    medical management, 2140
    nursing process for cervical discectomy, 2141–2142, 2143c
  herniation of lumbar disc
    assessment/diagnostic findings, 2142
    clinical manifestations, 2142
    medical management, 2142, 2144
    nursing management, 2144–2145
  Huntington's disease
    assessment/diagnostic findings, 2135
    care of patient with, 2136c
    clinical manifestations, 2134–2135
    medical management, 2135
    pathophysiology, 2134
  muscular dystrophies
    medical management, 2137–2138
    nursing management, 2138–2139
  Parkinson's disease
    assessment/diagnostic findings, 2128–2129
    clinical manifestations, 2128
    medical management, 2129–2130, 2129t
    nursing process for, 2130–2134
    pathophysiology, 2127–2128
  postpolio syndrome
    assessment/diagnostic findings, 2145
    management, 2145
    pathophysiology, 2145
Degenerative joint disease, 923
Dehiscence, 413
Dehydration
  and acidosis, 1032
  enteral therapy, 956t
Delayed gastric emptying, and diabetes, 1181
Delayed hemolytic reaction, 1687–1688
Delayed-type hypersensitivity (DTH), 1574
Delayed union, 2310
Delayed wound healing, 2294
Delegatee, 73
Delegation, 73
  benefits of, 75
    for delegatee, 75
    for organization, 75
    for regulated nurses, 75
  definitions of, 73
  delegation decision tree for assessment of, 77f
  delegator's self-reflection, 76c
  effective, 75
    strategies for, 77c
  factors hindering, 77
    inadequate staffing, 77
    overdelegating, 77–78
    resistance to delegation, 78
    underdelegating, 77
  five rights of
    right circumstance, 76
    right direction and communication, 76–77
    right person, 76
    right supervision and evaluation, 77
    right task, 76
  guiding principles of, 75
    evaluating delegation, 75
    promoting collaboration and teamwork, 76
    remembering accountability, 75
    setting priorities, 75
  of nursing care, 73–75
  skills, 77
    strategies for learning skills for, 78
    success or failure of, 74
    and work assignment, 75
Delegator, 73, 76c
Delirium, 224, 225, 519, 626
  assessment tools, 349
  in cardiac surgery patients, 772
  dementia and, differences between, 226t
  postoperative, 432, 433c
  in shock, 347, 349
Delirium tremens, 2370–2371
Delta agent, 1081
Delta agonists, 272
Demand oxygen delivery system (DODS), 606
Dementia, 224, 225, 2117, 2128
Demyelination, 2096f
Dendrites, 1958
Denial, 241
Denial of care, 27
Denuded skin, 1782
Deodorants, 1791
Deodorizers, 610
Deontologic theory, 24
Deoxyribonucleic acid (DNA), 133, 133f, 1525
Depolarization, 653, 692
Depo-Provera, 1399–1400
Depressed skull fractures, 2059
Depression, 1004
  constipation, 1000
  heart failure, 821
  illness and, 122–123, 123c
  manifestations of, 122
  nursing implications, 123
  in older adults, 224
  psychoeducational programs, 123
  risk factors for, 123c
Dermablend, 1819
Dermabrasion, 1794, 1795, 1830
Dermagraft, 1786
Dermatitis herpetiformis, 1007, 1814
Dermatitis medicamentosa, 1591
Dermatofibroma, 1820
Dermatophyte infections, 1779
Dermatosis, 1776
Dermis, 1766
  blood and lymph vessels, 1766
  papillary layer, 1766
  reticular layer, 1766
Dermis–epidermis junction, 1768
DES. *See* Diffuse esophageal spasm (DES)
Desaturate, 564
Descemet's stripping endothelial keratoplasty (DSEK), 1905
Descending GBS, 2107
Desensitization therapy, 2359
Desflurane (Suprane), 400t
Desipramine (Norpramin), 1554
Desloratadine/pseudoephedrine (Claritin-D), 1583
Desmopressin acetate (DDAVP), 313, 355
  diabetes insipidus, 1221
Desquamation (shedding of epidermis), 928
Developmental disabilities, 166
Dexamethasone, 1999, 2007
  breast cancer, 1469
  interaction with anesthetics, 382t
Dexlansoprazole (Dexilant), for gastroesophageal reflux disease, 939t
Dexmedetomidine, 631
Dexrazoxane, for cardiac toxicity, 2183
Dextrose 5% in water (D_5W), 313, 334
Diabetes Canada guidelines, 882

Diabetes Control and Complications Trial (DCCT), 1143
Diabetes insipidus, 313, 1220, 1998t
  assessment and diagnostic findings, 1221
  clinical manifestations, 1221
  medical management, 1221
Diabetes mellitus, 111, 1003, 1137
  assessment and diagnostic findings, 1142–1143, 1143c
  care in, special issues in, 1183–1187
    hospitalized diabetic patients, 1183–1187
  classification, 1138, 1139t
    gestational diabetes, 1138
    type 1 diabetes, 1138
    type 2 diabetes, 1138
  clinical manifestations, 1142
  complications, 1164
    diabetic ketoacidosis, 1165–1169
    hyperglycemic hyperosmolar nonketotic syndrome, 1169–1170
    hypoglycemia, 1164
    long-term, 1175–1183
  consequences, 1138
  diagnosis of, 1140c
  diarrhea, 1001
  economic cost, 1138
  education, 1159–1163
  exercise, 1147–1148
    benefits, 1147
    guidelines for, 1148c
    precautions, 1148
    recommendations, 1147–1148
  foot and leg problems, 1182–1183
  gerontologic considerations, 1143
  and heart disease, 737
  heart failure, 806
  incidence, 1136, 1138
  macrovascular complications, 1175–1176
  management, 1143–1148
  microvascular complications and diabetic retinopathy, 1176–1180
  monitoring, 1148–1150
  nephropathy, 1179–1180
  neuropathies, 1180–1182
  nursing management, 1158–1164
    diabetic education plan, development of, 1159–1160, 1159c
    education, 1159–1163
    home and community-based care, 1163–1164
    implementing plan, 1160–1161
    in-depth and continuing education, 1160
    survival skill, teaching of, 1161
    transitional care, 1163–1164
  nursing process
    diabetes as secondary diagnosis, 1187–1189
    newly diagnosed diabetes mellitus, 1170–1175
  nutrition, 1144–1147
    caloric distribution, 1145–1146
    Diabetic Canada's guidelines and recommendations, 1144
    food classification systems, 1146
    goals of nutritional management, 1144
    meal planning and education, 1144–1146
  ocular complications of, 1177t
  overview, 1138–1140
  peripheral arterial disease, 845
  pharmacologic therapy, 1150–1158
    complications of insulin therapy, 1152, 1155
    insulin delivery methods, 1155–1156
    insulin regimens, 1151–1152, 1153t–1154t
    insulin therapy and insulin preparations, 1150–1156
    oral antihyperglycemic agents, 1156
  physiology and pathophysiology, 1140
  primary goals of treatment, 1138
  pruritus in, 1790
  risk factors, 1138c
  screening for, 1143
  skin disorders in, 1779
  type 2, 142t
Diabetic Canada, 1144–1146
Diabetic dermopathy (shin spots), 1779
Diabetic ketoacidosis (DKA), 1137, 1141, 1165
  assessment and diagnostic findings, 1166–1167
  clinical features, 1165
  clinical manifestations, 1166
  and hyperglycemic hyperosmolar nonketotic syndrome, 1169t
  medical management, 1167–1168
    rehydration, 1167–1168
    restoring electrolytes, 1168
    reversing acidosis, 1168
  nursing management, 1169
  pathophysiology, 1165
  prevention, 1166
Diabetic macrovascular complications, 1175
  cerebrovascular disease, 1175
  coronary artery disease, 1175
  peripheral vascular disease, 1175
  prevention and treatment, 1175–1176
Diabetic neuropathy, 1180
  autonomic neuropathy, 1181–1182
  peripheral neuropathy, 1181
Diabetic retinopathy, 1176–1180, 1177f, 1177t, 1921
  assessment and diagnostic findings, 1178
  clinical manifestations, 1178
  medical management, 1178
  non-proliferative retinopathy, 1177
  nursing management, 1178–1179
  preproliferative retinopathy, 1177
  proliferative retinopathy, 1177
Diagnosis
  acute pancreatitis, 1120
  appendicitis, 1009
  ascites, 1061
  cardiac tamponade, 829
  cardiogenic shock, 826–827
  celiac disease, 1007–1008
  chronic heart failure, 810
  colorectal cancer, 1034
  constipation, 999
  diarrhea, 1002
  diverticular disease, 1011
  esophageal varices, 1066–1067
  fecal incontinence, 1003
  gastric cancer, 989
  hepatic cirrhosis, 1085
  hepatic encephalopathy, 1072
  hepatitis A virus, 1076
  hepatitis B virus, 1078–1079
  irritable bowel syndrome, 1005
  liver metastases, 1095–1096
  pancreatic cancer, 1128
  pancreatic tumours, 1129
  peptic ulcer disease, 982
  peritonitis, 1014–1015
  pulmonary edema, 824
  ulcerative colitis, 1017–1018
Diagnosis-related groups (DRGs), 10
Diagnostic surgery, for cancer, 2160
Dialysate, 1283, 1305
Dialysis, 1300, 1305–1319
  acute, 1300
  end-stage kidney disease, 1300
  hemodialysis, 1305–1311
  nursing management of hospitalized patient on, 1316–1319
    administering medications, 1319
    cardiac and respiratory complications, 1318
    catheter site, 1318–1319
    electrolyte levels and diet, 1318
    managing discomfort and pain, 1318
    monitoring blood pressure, 1318
    preventing infection, 1318
    protecting vascular access, 1316–1318
    providing psychological support, 1319
    taking precautions during intravenous therapy, 1318
    uremia, monitoring symptoms of, 1318
  for patient with diabetes, 1180
  peritoneal, 1311–1316
  quality of life in patients receiving, 1309c
Dialyzer, 1283, 1295, 1305, 1306f
Diamox, for sleep apnea, 488
Diaphoresis, dumping syndrome, 993
Diaphragm, 1400
Diaphragmatic breathing, 385c, 608c, 612
Diaphragmatic excursion, 456
Diarrhea, 898, 902, 904, 909, 982, 1000–1003
  acute, 1000
  assessment and diagnostic findings, 1002
  chronic, 1000
  clinical manifestations, 1002
  colorectal cancer, 1043
  complications, 1002
  dumping syndrome, 993
  enteral therapy, 956t
  exudative, 1002
  inflammatory bowel disease, 1000
  malabsorptive, 1001
  medical management, 1002
  nursing management, 1002–1003
  pathophysiology, 1001–1002
  perianal skin care, 1003
  secretory, 1001
Diarrheal diseases
  Calicivirus, 1719
  Campylobacter infections, 1718
  causes, 1712, 1718
  Cryptosporidium, 1719
  Escherichia coli, 1719
  Giardia, 1719
  Salmonella infection, 1718–1719
  Shigella infection, 1719
  transmission, 1712
  Vibrio cholerae, 1719–1720
Diarthrotic joints, 2218, 2218f
Diastole, 653, 692
Diastolic blood pressure (DBP), 882
  hypertension urgency, 882
Diastolic dysfunction, 805, 813, 815
Diastolic heart failure, 804, 805
Diazepam (Valium), 402t, 2007
  cervical cancer, 1391
  interaction with anesthetics, 382t
DIC. *See* Disseminated intravascular coagulation (DIC)
Dicloxacillin, 1796
Dicyclomine hydrochloride, 1345

Diet
celiac disease, 1008
chronic inflammatory bowel disease, 1022
constipation, 1000
diarrhea, 1002
diverticulitis, 1012, 1013
gluten-free, 1008
hospitalized diabetic patients, 1185–1186
irritable bowel syndrome, 1004
patient with newly diagnosed diabetes, 1171
Dietary Approaches to Stop Hypertension (DASH) diet, 883, 883t, 2033
Dietary data, 68
Dietary factors, in carcinogenesis, 2155
Dietary guidelines, for bariatric surgery patients, 1207c
Dietary interview, 68
Dietary self-management, gastric surgery, 994
Dietary sodium, 821c
hypertension, 883t
Diet compatibility, 984
Diethylstilbestrol (DES), 1437, 2155
Diethyltoluamide (DEET), 2094
Differentiation, 1599, 1600
Diffuse axonal injury (DAI), 2056, 2061
Diffuse connective tissue diseases, 1743–1754
giant cell arteritis, 1753–1754
polymyalgia rheumatica, 1753–1754
polymyositis, 1752–1753
rheumatoid arthritis, 1743–1747
scleroderma, 1751–1752
Sjögren's syndrome, 1750–1751
systemic lupus erythematosus, 1748–1750
Diffuse esophageal spasm (DES), 935
Diffusion, 298, 298f, 299, 1283, 1305
pulmonary, 443
Diffusion-weighted imaging (DWI), 1980
Digest fat (triglyceride), 901t
Digestion, 899, 900
Digestive disorders, 908c
Digestive system, organs of, 899f
Digital dislodgement, 999
Digitalis, 813
heart failure, 813, 814c
toxicity, 798
Digital mammography, 1452
Digital rectal examination (DRE), 1482, 1482f
Digital vaginal examination, 2352
Digoxin (Lanoxin), 813, 814c
acute kidney injury, 1296
end-stage kidney disease, 1299
Dihydrotestosterone (DHT), 1491
Dilated cardiomyopathy (DCM), 787–788
Dilation and curettage, 1391
Diltiazem, 741
antiarrhythmic medication, 699t
heart failure, 813
hypertension, 886t
Dimenhydrinate (Dramamine), 1944
for postoperative nausea/vomiting, 416t
Dimethicone (Cetaphil), 1806
Dimethyl sulfoxide (DMSO), 2188
Dipeptidase, 901t
Dipeptidyl peptidase-IV inhibitors (gliptins), 1157
Diphenhydramine (Benadryl), 1318, 1789, 2094
Diphenoxylate (Lomotil), in diarrhea, 1002
Diplopia, 2031t
Direct ophthalmoscopy, 1884–1886
of retina, 1908
Direct renin inhibitors, hypertension, 887t
Direct thrombin inhibitors, in venous thromboembolism, 864
Disability, 155
acquired, 166
age-associated, 166
aging with, 234
characteristics of, 166–167
chronic health conditions and, 155, 156
coping with, 168, 169c
definitions of, 166
developmental, 166
versus disabling disorders, 167–168
and fatigue, 170
health promotion education classes for people with, 168
models of, 167, 167c
biopsychosocial model, 167c
functional model, 167c
medical model, 167c
rehabilitation model, 167c
social model, 167c
nurse, role of, 168
nursing care of patients with, 170
health promotion and prevention, 170–171
during hospitalization, 170
older adults and, 160c, 169c
patient education, 169c
patient responses to, 168
people-first language, use of, 168
secondary health conditions, 167
and sexuality issues, 168–170
Disability Rating Scale (DRS), 178
Discharge from PACU
continuing and transitional care, 419
direct discharge, 418–419
preparation, 419
readiness for, 417–418
Discharge planning
bowel surgery for colorectal cancer, 1043
emergency department, 2342
for home care, 16
Disease Activity Score-28 (DAS28), 1744
Dislocations, 2299
Dissecting aorta, 858
assessment and diagnostic findings, 859
clinical manifestations, 859
medical management, 859
nursing management, 859
pathophysiology, 858–859
Dissection, 835
Disseminated intravascular coagulation (DIC), 865, 1668–1671, 2090
assessment and diagnostic findings, 1669–1670
clinical manifestations, 1668–1669
medical management, 1670–1671
nursing care plan, 1672c–1673c
nursing management, 1671
pathophysiology, 1668
in shock, 348
Dissolution therapy, 1107, 1111
Distal interphalangeal (DIP), 1755
Distal occlusive disease, 850
Distal radius, fractures of, 2314–2315
Distraction, 384
Distributive shock, 341, 359–364
anaphylactic shock, 359, 365–366
neurogenic shock, 359, 364–365
pathophysiology, 359, 359f
risk factors for, 361c
septic shock, 359, 360–364
Disuse syndrome, 2237
Diuretics, 812–813, 924
cardiogenic shock, 827
constipation, 998
heart failure, 806t, 812–813, 820t
hypertension, 884t
for hypervolemia, 308
lymphedema, 874
pulmonary edema, 825
side effects of, 813
therapy, 1062
Divalproex sodium (Depakote), 2025
Diverticular disease, 1010–1013
assessment and diagnostic findings, 1011
clinical manifestations, 1011
collaborative problems, 1013
complications, 1011–1012
evaluation, 1014
medical management
dietary and pharmacologic management, 1012
surgical management, 1012–1013
nursing interventions
elimination patterns, 1013
home and community-based care, 1013
relieving pain, 1013
nursing priorities, 1013
pathophysiology, 1011
planning and goals, 1013
saclike herniation, 1010
Diverticulitis, 998, 1011, 1027
acute, complication of, 1012t
Hartmann's procedure, 1012f
Diverticulosis, 998, 1010
Diverticulum, 936–937, 998, 1010
assessment and diagnostic findings, 937
clinical manifestations, 937
management, 937
Dizziness, 659, 892, 999, 1971
dumping syndrome, 993
hypertension, 881
jaw pain, 923
in older adults, 231
DNA mismatch repair genes (MMR), 1035
Dobutamine, 2000
cardiogenic shock, 357
end-stage kidney disease, 1299
heart failure, 813
pulmonary edema, 825
shock, 353t
Dobutrex. *See* Dobutamine
Docetaxel (Taxotere), in breast cancer, 1469
Documentation, in ED, 2340
Docusate (Colace), laxative medications, 1001t
DOE. *See* Dyspnea on exertion (DOE)
Dofetilide
antiarrhythmic medication, 699t
atrial fibrillation prevention, 704
Domperidone (Motilium), for neuromuscular disorders, 939
Donepezil hydrochloride (Aricept), for Alzheimer's disease, 227
Do Not Resuscitate (DNR), 240
Door-to-balloon time, 749
Dopamine
in cardiogenic shock, 358
in shock, 353t
Doppler echocardiography
aortic regurgitation, 781
aortic stenosis, 780
hypertrophic cardiomyopathy, 788
infective endocarditis, 796
mitral regurgitation, 780
mitral stenosis, 780

Doppler transducer, 840
Dorsal recumbent position, for surgery, 408, 409f
Dosage of antineoplastic agent, 2178
Dose-dense chemotherapy, 1446
Double-balloon enteroscopy (DBE), 914
Double effect, 25, 25c
Double gloving, 398
Double/triple-lumen tubes, 951
Douche, 1412
Down's syndrome, 134, 138
Doxazosin (Cardura)
  benign prostatic hyperplasia, 1491
  hypertension, 885t
Doxepin (Sinequan), in urinary retention, 1345
Doxorubicin, 989, 2182
  bladder cancer, 1357
  breast cancer, 1469
  chemotherapeutic agents, 552
  Hodgkin lymphoma, 1649
  ovarian cancer, 1439
Doxycycline (Vibramycin), 1794
  chlamydia, 1420
  pelvic inflammatory disease, 1421
  proctitis, 1044
  sexual assault, 1384
Dressings, 1784–1786, 1785t
  active, 1783
  autografts, 1860–1861
  axillary, 1788
  biologic, 1859
  biosynthetic and synthetic, 1859–1860
  in burn care, 1856–1861
  calcium alginates, 1786
  change, 427–428, 428c
  to cover topical corticosteroid, 1788
  dermal substitutes, 1860
  foam, 1786
  hydrocolloids, 1785
  Hydrofiber™ Technology, 1785–1786
  hydrogels, 1785
  interactive, 1783
  moisture-retentive, 1784–1786
  occlusive, 1784, 1856
  plastic wrap, 1788
  quick guide to function and action of, 1785t
  telfa pads, 1788
  temporary and permanent burn wound coverings, 1858t
  for topical medications, 1788
  vinyl gloves, 1788
  wet, 1784
Dressler syndrome, 798
Dromotropy, 692, 693
Dronabinol (Marinol), in AIDS-related anorexia, 1554
Drug-induced hepatitis, 1082
Drug-induced liver disease, 1082
Drug metabolism, role of liver, 1054
Dry eye syndrome
  assessment and diagnostic findings, 1914
  clinical manifestations, 1914
  medical management, 1914–1915
Dry mouth, older adults, 922c
Dry powder inhaler, 570
Dry suction systems with one-way valve, 635t, 639
Dry suction water seal systems, 635t, 639
D-type natriuretic peptide (DNP), 303
Dual-chamber pacing (DDD), 720
Dual-energy x-ray absorptiometry (DEXA), 2325
Dubin–Johnson syndrome, 1061
Ductal carcinoma in situ (DCIS), 1446, 1456–1457
  medical management, 1456
Duloxetine (Cymbalta)
  fibromyalgia, 1759
  for pain relief, 289
Dumping syndrome, 948, 954, 977, 993, 1192, 1208
  preventing symptoms, 958c
  tube feeding, 958
Duodenal tumours, 994
  assessment and diagnostic findings, 995
  clinical manifestations, 994–995
  management, 995
Duodenal ulcers
  comparison of, 981t
  heart failure, 915
Duodenum, 948, 949, 977
DuoDERM, 1783, 1860
Duplex ultrasonography, 835, 841–842
  colour flow duplex image, 842f
Dupuytren's contracture, 2272, 2272f
Durable power of attorney, 28
Dura mater, 1961–1962
Duration of sound, 1933
Dutasteride (Avodart), in benign prostatic hyperplasia, 1491
DVT. *See* Deep vein thrombosis (DVT)
DWI. *See* Diffusion-weighted imaging (DWI)
Dying and death, 125. *See also* Death
Dying for a Home: Homeless Activists Speak Out, 20
Dyna-Care, 866
Dysarthria, 2030, 2031t
Dysautonomia, 779
Dysentery, 1001
Dysesthesias, 2097
Dysfunctional cervix, 1403
Dysfunctional uterine bleeding (DUB), 1396
Dyskinesia, 2117, 2128
Dyslipidemia, hypertension, 878
Dysmenorrhea, 1373, 1380, 1395
  assessment and diagnostic findings, 1395
  management, 1395
  primary, 1395
  secondary, 1395
Dyspareunia, 1373, 1380, 1396
Dyspepsia (indigestion), 899, 902, 989
  abdominal discomfort, 903
Dysphagia, 471, 902, 919, 923, 934, 935, 937, 943, 1192, 1208, 2031t
  benign tumours, 940
  chemical burns, 938
  diverticulum, 937
  esophageal perforation, 937
  esophageal spasm, 935
  esophagus cancer, 942
  esophagus disorders, 934
  foreign bodies, 938
  gastric surgery, 993
  hiatal hernia, 936
  in older adults, 217
  temporomandibular disorders, 923
  thoracic aortic aneurysm, 856
Dysphasia, 2030
Dysphonia, 2103, 2117, 2128
Dysplasia, 110, 110t, 1412, 1417, 2150
  gastroesophageal reflux disease, 919
Dyspnea, 439, 447–448
  thoracic aortic aneurysm, 842
Dyspnea on exertion (DOE), 804, 809
Dysrhythmias, 1002
  adjunctive modalities/management
    cardioversion and defibrillation, 715–717
    electrophysiology studies, 717–718
    implantable cardioverter defibrillator, 723–725, 726c
    pacemaker therapy, 718–723, 722t
  cardiogenic shock, 825
  conduction abnormalities, 710–713
  defined, 691, 692
  ECG rhythm strip, 696, 697c
  electrocardiogram, 694–696
  and heart failure, 809
  on heart rate and contractility, 693–694
  hypertension and, 416
  normal electrical conduction, 692
  normal sinus rhythm, 696–697
  nursing process for, 713–715
  types of
    atrial, 700–706, 702c, 703c
    junctional, 706–707
    sinus node, 697–700, 699t
    ventricular, 707–710
Dysuria, 1332

E

Ear, 1926f
  assessment of hearing and balance, 1928–1929
    common symptoms/signs, 1929–1931
    evaluation of gross auditory acuity, 1932–1933
    health history, 1928–1929
    otoscopic examination, 1931, 1931f
    vestibular dysfunction testing, 1933
  aural rehabilitation, 1951–1954
  conditions
    external ear, 1937–1938
    inner ear, 1943–1951
    middle ear, 1938–1943
  diagnostic evaluation of hearing and balance
    audiometry, 1933
    auditory brain stem response, 1933–1934
    electronystagmography, 1934
    middle ear endoscopy, 1934
    platform posturography, 1934
    sinusoidal harmonic acceleration, 1934
    tympanogram, 1933
  external
    auricle, 1925
    external auditory canal, 1927
  functions of
    assessment of hearing and balance, 1928–1929
    balance and equilibrium, 1928
    hearing, 1928
  inner, 1927–1928
    membranous labyrinth, 1928
    organ of Corti, 1928
  middle
    ossicles, 1927
    tympanic membrane (eardrum), 1927
  physical examination, 1931
Earaches, jaw pain, 923
Early goal-directed therapy (EGDT), 364
Early-onset familial Alzheimer's disease (EOFAD), 141t
Eating well with Canada's Food Guide, 68
Ebixa, for Alzheimer's disease, 227
Ebola virus disease, 1726–1727
  clinical manifestation, 1726
  medical management, 1726
  nursing management, 1726–1727
  pathophysiology, 1726
Ecchymosis, 1777, 1777t, 2298, 2349c

Ecchymosis (bruising), 1120
ECG. *See* Electrocardiography (ECG)
Echocardiography. *See also* Cardiovascular function
  heart failure, 810
  traditional, 682
  transesophageal, 682
Echo off, 840
e-Cigarettes, 845, 845c
Ecstasy, 2365
Ectopic pregnancy, 1407–1409
  assessment and diagnostic findings, 1407–1408
  causes, 1407
  clinical manifestations, 1407
  medical management, 1408
    pharmacologic therapy, 1408
    surgical management, 1408
  nursing process, 1408–1409
  sites, 1407f
Eczema herpeticum, 1798, 1799
ED. *See* Erectile dysfunction (ED)
Edema, 1286, 2233
  cirrhosis and, 1085
  generalized, 309
  hepatic disorders, 1074
  hepatic dysfunction, 1055
  hypervolemia and, 308–309
  insufficient vascular blood flow, 837
  of limbs, 185
  localized, 309
  right ventricular failure, 810
  treatment, 309
Edoxaban (Savaysa), 2033
  acquired thrombophilias, 1676
Edrophonium chloride (Tensilon), 2103
Effluent, 1283, 1314
EGD. *See* Esophagogastroduodenoscopy (EGD)
Egophony, 439, 457
EHR. *See* Electronic health record (EHR)
Ejaculation, disorders of, 1487–1488
Ejection fraction, 653
Elastic compression stockings, 185
Elastin fibres, 839
Elder abuse, 233
Elective abortions, 1404c
Elective replacement indicator (ERI), 692, 719
Electrical alternans, 800
Electrical burns, 1839–1840
  ABCs of emergency care, 1839
  acute renal failure in, 1839–1840
  administration of intravenous (IV) fluids and, 1839–1840
Electrical cardioversion
  for atrial fibrillation, 704
  tachydysrhythmia treatment, 716–717
Electrical conduction, normal, 692
Electrical-mechanical dissociation (EMD), 830
Electrical relaxation, 692
Electrical stimulation, 291
Electric/electromagnetic VADs, 791
Electrocardiography (ECG), 1113
  components of
    waveforms/compexes/intervals, 695–696
  continuous ECG monitoring
    ambulatory electrocardiography, 676
    cardiac event recorders, 677
    cardiac implantable electronic devices, 677
    continuous monitors, 676–677
    continuous real-time monitors, 677
    hardwire cardiac monitoring, 675
    lead systems, 676
    telemetry, 675–676
  heart failure, 810
  mitral stenosis, 780
  nursing interventions for, 677–679
  obtaining, 694–695, 694f
  pericarditis, 799
  peripheral arterial occlusive disease, 860
  rhythm strip
    heart rate determination, 696
    heart rhythm determination, 696
Electrode application, for cardiac rhythm analysis, 676c
Electroencephalography, 1983, 2092
Electrogastrography, 915
Electrohydraulic lithotripsy, 1352
Electrolarynx, 931
Electrolyte imbalances, 309
  calcium, 318
    hypercalcemia, 318t, 320–322
    hypocalcemia, 318–320, 318t
  chloride, 327
    hyperchloremia, 327t, 328
    hypochloremia, 327–328, 327t
  magnesium, 322
    hypermagnesemia, 322t, 324
    hypomagnesemia, 322–324, 322t
  phosphorus, 324
    hyperphosphatemia, 325t, 326–327
    hypophosphatemia, 324–326, 325t
  potassium, 313
    hyperkalemia, 314t, 315–318
    hypokalemia, 313–315, 314t
  sodium, 309
    hypernatremia, 310t, 312–313
    hyponatremia, 309–312, 310t
Electrolytes (CoLyte, GoLYTELY), 954
  diabetic ketoacidosis, 1168
  excretion, regulation of, 1266–1267
  heart failure, assessment in, 824
  laxative medications, 1001t
  patient with newly diagnosed diabetes, 1171
Electromagnetic interference (EMI), 722
Electromagnetic radiation, 2163
Electromyography (EMG), 1983
  irritable bowel syndrome, 1005
Electronic cigarettes, 549
Electronic health record (EHR), 30, 53
Electronic pulse generator, 718
Electronystagmography, 1934
Electrophysiology study (EPS), 683, 717–718. *See also* Adjunctive modalities/management
Electrosurgery, 1821–1822
Elephantiasis, 873
  medical management
    pharmacologic therapy, 874
    surgical management, 874
  nursing management, 874
Elimination, 899
  in cardiac disease, 663
  of stool, 902
  of undigested unabsorbed foodstuffs, 900
Elimination patterns, altered
  assessment, 200
  expected outcomes, 203
  gerontological considerations, 200
  nursing diagnoses, 200–201
  nursing interventions, 201
    bowel continence, promotion of, 202–203
    constipation, prevention of, 203
    urinary continence, promotion of, 201–202
  nursing process for, 200–203
Eltrombopag (Promacta), in myelodysplastic syndrome, 1619
Embolectomy catheter, 860
EMD. *See* Electrical-mechanical dissociation (EMD)
Emergency care
  definition of, 2343
  principles of, 2343
    assess and intervene, 2344
    triage, 2343–2344
Emergency contraception, 1402
  methods of, 1402
  nursing management, 1402
  pills, 1402
Emergency management, 2338. *See also* Emergency nursing
  cardiac arrest, 830–832
Emergency nursing, 2338. *See also* Emergency care
  airway obstruction, 2345–2348
  anaphylactic reaction, 2358, 2358c
  animal and human bites, 2359
  challenges in
    vital signs, 2339–2340
    wait times, 2339
  and continuum of care, 2342
    community and transitional services, 2342
    discharge planning, 2342
    gerontologic considerations, 2342–2343
    obesity considerations, 2343
  decompression sickness, 2357–2358
  family-focused interventions, 2341, 2341c
    anger, 2342
    anxiety and denial, 2341
    caring for emergency personnel, 2342
    grief, 2342
    remorse and guilt, 2341–2342
  family violence, abuse, and neglect, 2371–2373
  frostbite, 2355–2356
  heat stroke, 2354–2355
  hemorrhage, 2348
  human trafficking, 2374–2375
  hypothermia, 2356
  hypovolemic shock, 2348–2349
  insect stings, 2358–2359
  issues in, 2340
    documentation of consent and privacy, 2340
    limiting exposure to health risks, 2340
    violence in ED, 2340–2341
  latex allergy, 2358
  nonfatal drowning, 2356–2357
  patient-focused interventions, 2341
  poisoning, 2362
    carbon monoxide poisoning, 2362, 2364
    chemical burns, 2364–2365
    food poisoning, 2365, 2365c
    swallowed poisons, 2362
  providing comprehensive care, 2341
  psychiatric emergencies, 2375
    depressed/underactive patient, 2376
    overactive patient, 2375
    posttraumatic stress disorder, 2376
    suicidal patient, 2376
    violent behaviour, 2375–2376
  scope and practice of, 2338–2339
  sexual assault, 2373–2374
  snakebites, 2359–2361
  spider bites, 2361
  substance abuse, 2365
    acute alcohol intoxication, 2365, 2370

Emergency nursing (*continued*)
alcohol withdrawal syndrome, 2370–2371
drug overdose, 2366–2369
tick bites, 2361, 2361f
trauma, 2350
crush injuries, 2353
documentation, 2350
fractures, 2353–2354
injury prevention, 2350–2351
intra-abdominal injuries, 2351–2353
multiple trauma, 2351
visits to emergency departments (EDs) in Canada, 2339c
wounds, 2349–2350
Emergency preparedness
debriefing, 2388
disaster levels, 2381c
emergency management plan, initiating, 2384–2386
identifying patients/documenting patient information, 2386
managing internal problems, 2385–2386
triage, 2384–2385
emergency operations plan, 2383–2384
federal agencies/national organizations, 2382
federal, provinical/territorial, and local responses, 2382–2383
Incident Command System, 2383
media/family, communicating, 2386
caring for families, 2386
critical incident stress management, 2388
media requests for information, 2386
nurse's role in disaster response plans, 2386–2388
natural disasters, 2390–2391
provincial/territorial/local agencies, 2381–2382
terrorism, preparing
decontamination, 2389–2390
personal protective equipment, 2389
recognition/awareness, 2389
weapons of terror, 2391
biologic weapons, 2392–2394
blast injury, 2391–2392
chemical weapons, 2395–2397
nuclear radiation exposure, 2397–2400
Emerging infectious diseases, 1698
Ebola virus disease, 1726–1727
Legionnaires' disease, 1727
pertussis, 1727–1728
West Nile virus, 1726
Zika virus, 1725–1726
EMG. *See* Electromyography (EMG)
Emotional support, 117
Emphysema, 564, 565–566
Empyema, 505
assessment/diagnostic findings, 532
clinical manifestations, 532
medical management, 532
nursing management, 532–533
pathophysiology, 532
Emtricitabine (Truvada), HIV infection, 1539
Enalapril (Vasotec)
heart failure, 811t
hypertension, 886t
Enalaprilat (Vasotec IV)
heart failure, 811t
hypertension, 886t
hypertensive emergencies, 893
Enamel hypoplasia, 1794
Encephalitis
arboviral, 2094
arthropod-borne virus, 2093–2094
fungal, 2094–2095
herpes simplex virus (HSV), 2092–2093
St. Louis, 2093
West Nile, 2093
Enchondroma, 2291
Endarterectomy, in peripheral arterial occlusive disease, 852
Endemic (iodine-deficient) goitre, 1237–1238
Endemic (African) KS, 1826
Endocervicitis, 1412, 1419–1420
Endocrine disorders, 998, 1107, 1217c
assessment
health history, 1217
physical examination, 1217
diagnostic evaluation
blood tests, 1217
genetic screening, 1218
imaging studies, 1218
stimulation tests, 1218
suppression tests, 1218
urine tests, 1217, 1218
metabolic and, 1217c
Endocrine system
anatomic and physiologic overview, 1213
hormones
action and source of, 1216t
classification and action of, 1215–1217
function and regulation of, 1215
hormone-secreting glands of, 1215f
importance of, 1213
End-of-life care, 238
assisted suicide, 242
clinician attitudes toward death, 241
coping with death and dying:, 260
culturally competent care, 245–246, 246c
euthanasia, 241–242
general considerations in, 243
communication, 243–245
psychosocial issues, 243
goal setting in, 246–247, 247c, 247f
hope, enabling and supporting, 248
hospice palliative care, 238–242
palliative sedation, principles of, 254
patient and family attitudes toward death, 241
perceptions of helpful interventions during, 255c
principles and components, 242–243
signs of approaching death, 254–255, 256c
spiritual care, 247–248
support to dying patients and families, 254–260
after-death care, 257
anticipatory grief and mourning, 257–258
complicated grief and mourning, 259
grief and mourning after death, 258–259, 260t
imminently dying, 255–257
physiologic changes close to death, 254–255
respiratory changes at end of life, 255
symptoms management, 248–249
anorexia, dehydration, and cachexia, 251–253, 252t
delirium, 253
depression, 253–254
dyspnea, 250, 250c
fatigue, 251
pain, 249–250
End-of-life issues, and ethical dilemmas, 27
Endolymph, 1928
Endolymphatic sac decompression, 1946
Endometrial ablation, 1373, 1392
Endometrial biopsy, 1391
Endometrial hyperplasia, 1431
Endometriosis, 1373, 1389, 1412, 1430–1431
assessment and diagnostic findings, 1430
clinical manifestations, 1430
medical management, 1430–1431
nursing management, 1431
pathophysiology, 1430
Endometrium, 1373, 1375
Endomyocardial biopsy, 789
Endophthalmitis, 1898
Endorphins, 272
Endoscopic/injection sclerotherapy, 1068
esophageal varices, 1068f
Endoscopic procedures
bronchoscopy, 464–465, 464f
thoracentesis, 466
thoracoscopy, 465–466, 465f
Endoscopic retrograde cholangiopancreatography (ERCP), 908, 1107, 1111, 1111f
fluoroscopy and multiple x-rays, 1111
nursing implications, 1111
pancreatic tumour, 1128
percutaneous transhepatic cholangiography, 1112
Endoscopic therapies, esophageal varices, 1068–1069
Endoscopic ultrasonography (EUS), 907, 943, 989
Endoscopic variceal ligation (EVL), 1052, 1069
Endoscopy, 934, 937, 938, 940, 1002
Endosteum, 2215
Endotracheal intubation, 602, 612–614, 614c, 1068, 2346–2347, 2347f. *See also* Airway management
Endovascular techniques, 2035
End-stage kidney disease (ESKD), 1283, 1284, 1297–1300
assessment and diagnostic findings, 1297–1298, 1298c
acidosis, 1297
anemia, 1298
calcium and phosphorus imbalance, 1298
sodium and water retention, 1297
clinical manifestations, 1297
complications, 1298–1299
gerontologic considerations, 1300
medical management, 1299–1300
dialysis, 1300
nutritional therapy, 1299
pharmacologic therapy, 1299
nursing management, 1300
continuing and transitional care, 1300
promoting home, community-based, and transitional care, 1300
pathophysiology, 1297
patient with, 1301c–1304c
Enduring power of attorney, 235
Enema administration, 999
Energy metabolism, 342
ENFit, 952
Enflurane (Ethrane), 400t
Enkephalins, 272
Enoxaparin, 741
venous thromboembolism, 864
Entamoeba histolytica, 1018, 1102
Entecavir (ETV), 1080
Enteral feeding. *See also* Enteral therapy
hospitalized diabetic patients, 1185–1186
in sepsis, 363
in shock, 348, 353
Enteral pumps, 954

Enteral therapy
complications of, 956t
conditions, 953t
Enteric-coated aspirin, 1786
Enteric feeding tube, 948t
Enterocele, 1412
Enteroclysis, 977, 995
GI tract, 909
Enucleation, 1919–1920
Envenomation, 2359
Environmental emergencies
anaphylactic reaction, 2358, 2358c
animal and human bites, 2359
decompression sickness, 2357–2358
frostbite, 2355–2356
heat stroke, 2354–2355
hypothermia, 2356
insect stings, 2358–2359
latex allergy, 2358
nonfatal drowning, 2356–2357
snakebites, 2359–2361
spider bites, 2361
tick bites, 2361, 2361f
Environmental exposure, and lung cancer, 549–550
Enzymatic debriding agents, 1784
Enzyme immunoassay (EIA), 1534, 1538
Enzyme-linked immunosorbent assay (ELISA), 1534, 1538
Enzymes secretions, 901t
Enzyme tests, liver cell damage, 1085
Eosinophil, 1518, 1572, 1574
count, 1576
Ephedrine sulphate
nasal congestion, 481
urinary retention, 1345
Epicel, 1786
Epicondylitis, 2300–2301
Epicutaneous immunotherapy (EPIT), 1586
allergic rhinitis, 1586–1587
Epidermal cysts, 1819
Epidermal growth factor receptors, 2191
Epidermis, 1764–1765, 1765–1766, 1768
characteristics of, 1766
of dark-skinned people, 1766
dead cells in, 1765
fibrous protein of, 1765
in irritant contact dermatitis, 1802
Langerhans cells of, 1766
layers, 1765
melanocytes, 1766
merkel cells of, 1766
Epidermopoiesis, 1808
Epididymitis, 1480
medical management, 1506
nursing management, 1506–1507
Epidural analgesia, for normal respiratory function, 634
Epidural anesthesia, 403, 404f
Epidural catheter bolus, 384
Epidural catheters, for pain control, 294
Epidural hematoma, 2060
Epidural infusions, 423
Epigastric area, 668
Epigastric distress, 1110
Epigenetics, 130
Epiglottis, 440
Epilepsy
assessment and diagnostic findings, 2017
clinical manifestations, 2016–2017
collaborative problems/potential complications, 2020
definition, 2015
diagnosis of, 2015
gerontologic considerations, 2017
incidence, 2015
in women, 2017
medical management, 2018–2019
nursing interventions
continuing and transitional care, 2021
improving coping mechanism, 2020
monitoring and managing potential complications, 2021
patient outcomes, 2021
planning and goals, 2020
promoting home, community-based, and transitional care, 2021
providing patient and family education, 2020
reducing fear of seizures, 2020
nursing priorities, 2020
pathophysiology, 2015–2016
patient assessment, 2019–2020
pharmacologic therapy, 2018
prevention of, 2017–2018
strategies for patients with, 2021c
surgical management, 2018–2019
susceptibility to, 2015
Epinephrine, 106
cardiopulmonary resuscitation, 832t
peripheral vascular resistance, 837
self-administration of, 1582c
in shock, 353t
EpiPen, 1581
Epiphrenic diverticula, 937
Epirubicin (Ellence), in breast cancer, 1469
Epispadias, 1510
Epistaxis. *See also* Obstruction and trauma
defined, 471
medical management, 488
nursing management, 488–489
risk factors for, 488c
Epitope, 1516, 1517
Eplerenone (Inspra), hypertension, 884t
Epoetin alfa
breast cancer, 1470
myelodysplastic syndrome, 1619
Epoprostenol (Flolan), in scleroderma, 1752
Eprex, in end-stage kidney disease, 1299
Eprosartan (Teveten), hypertension, 886t
Epstein–Barr virus, 1060, 1418
Eptifibatide (Integrilin), 742
Equilibrium radionuclide angiocardiography (ERNA), 681
Erb's point, 668
ERCP. *See* Endoscopic retrograde cholangiopancreatography (ERCP)
Erectile dysfunction (ED), 1480, 1483–1487, 1484c
assessment and diagnostic findings, 1484
medical management, 1484–1487
medications classes, 1484c
nursing management, 1487
treatment, 1486t–1487t
Ergotamine preparations, 2025
Erosion, mucous membrane, 981
Erosive gastritis, endoscopic view, 997f
Erythema, 1572, 1573, 1772
Erythema nodosum, 1017
Erythroblasts, 1602
Erythrocytes (red blood cells), 1599, 1600–1603
sedimentation rate, 1599
Erythrocyte sedimentation rate (ESR), 1011
Erythroderma, 1812
Erythroid cells, 1599, 1615
Erythromelalgia, 1760
Erythromycin, 1796
proctitis, 1045
Erythroplakia, mouth abnormalities, 921t
Erythropoiesis, 1599, 1602–1603
Erythropoietin, 1599, 1602, 2182
end-stage kidney disease, 1299
sickle cell crisis, 1624
Escharotomy, 2355
Escherichia coli, 1014, 1094, 1108, 1719, 1818
ESKD. *See* End-stage kidney disease (ESKD)
Esmolol, as antiarrhythmic medication, 699t
ESO2 camera, 911
Esomeprazole (Nexium)
gastric acid, 939
gastroesophageal reflux disease, 939t
peptic ulcer disease and gastritis, 979t
Esophageal adenocarcinoma (EAC), 939
Esophageal banding, 1069, 1069f
Esophageal cancer, risk factors, 942
Esophageal disorder, home care checklist, 942
Esophageal manometry, 914, 934, 935
Esophageal motility studies, 914
Esophageal mucosa, 943
Esophageal perforation, 937
Esophageal peristalsis, 909
Esophageal problems, 918
Esophageal reconstruction, with free jejunal transfer, 943f
Esophageal reflux, of gastric acid, 915
Esophageal spasm
assessment and diagnostic findings, 935
clinical manifestations, 935
management, 935–936
Esophageal speech, 495
Esophageal ulcers, 981
Esophageal varices
assessment and diagnostic findings
endoscopy, 1066–1067
laboratory tests, 1067
portal hypertension measurements, 1067
bleeding esophageal varices, 1067f, 1071t
clinical manifestations, 1066
endoscopic/injection sclerotherapy, 1068f
esophageal banding, 1069f
hepatic disorders, 1065–1071
medical management
balloon tamponade, 1068
endoscopic therapies, 1068–1069
esophageal banding therapy, 1069
pharmacologic therapy, 1067–1068
transjugular intrahepatic portosystemic shunting (TIPS), 1069
nursing management, 1070–1071
pathophysiology, 1065–1066
portal systemic shunts, 1070f
surgical management, 1069–1070
bypass procedures, 1070
devascularization and transection, 1070
treatment modality, 1071t
Esophagectomy, 943
Esophagogastrectomy, 989
Esophagogastroduodenoscopy (EGD), 911, 919, 936, 989
Esophagojejunostomy, 989
Esophagoscopy, 937
Esophagus cancer, 942–945
assessment and diagnostic findings, 943
clinical manifestations, 943
medical management, 943–944
nursing management, 944–945
pathophysiology, 942–943

Esophagus disorders, 899, 903t
  achalasia
    assessment and diagnostic findings, 934
    clinical manifestations, 934
    management, 934–935
  benign tumours, 940
  chemical burns, 938
  diverticulum, 936–937
    assessment and diagnostic findings, 937
    clinical manifestations, 937
    management, 937
  emergency conditions, 940
  esophageal spasm
    assessment and diagnostic findings, 935
    clinical manifestations, 935
    management, 935–936
  foreign bodies, 938
  gastroesophageal reflux disease
    assessment and diagnostic findings, 938–939, 940
    clinical manifestations, 938, 940
    management, 939, 940
  hiatal hernia, 936
    assessment and diagnostic findings, 936
    clinical manifestations, 936
    management, 936
  nonemergency symptoms, 940
  perforation, 937
    assessment and diagnostic findings, 937
    clinical manifestations, 937
    management, 937–938
  risk factors for cancer, 925
ESR. *See* Erythrocyte sedimentation rate (ESR)
Essential hypertension, 878
Essentials of Genetics and Genomic Nursing, 131
Essential thrombocythemia (ET), 1658–1660
  assessment and diagnostic findings, 1659
  clinical manifestations, 1659
  complications, 1659
  medical management, 1659–1660
  nursing management, 1660
Estrogen, 1373, 1375, 1794
  after menopause, and ovarian cancer risk, 2156
  and progesterone therapy, combination, 2156
ET. *See* Essential thrombocythemia (ET)
Ethacrynic acid (Edecrin)
  acute kidney injury, 1295
  heart failure, 820t
  hypertension, 884t
Ethambutol
  antituberculosis medication, 526t
  mycobacterium avium complex, 1553
  TB and HIV infection, 1551
Ethical analysis, steps of, 28, 29c
  assessment, 29c
  evaluation, 29c
  implementation, 29c
  planning, 29c
Ethical decision making, 28
  guidelines for, 29c
Ethical dilemm, 24
Ethical principles, 25, 25c
Ethics
  approaches to
    applied ethics, 25
    meta-ethics, 24
    relational ethics, 25
  charts, 28
  in health care, 23–24
  and morality, 24
  moral situations and, 25–26
  preventive, 27–28
    advance directives, 28
    ethics committees, 28
  principles of, 25, 25c
  problems related to, 26
    confidentiality, 26
    end-of-life issues, 27
    palliative care, 27
    refusing care, 27
    restraints, use of, 27
    trust, 27
    truth-telling, 27
  theories
    deontologic/formalist theory, 24
    teleologic theory/consequentialism, 24
Ethnic culture, 90–91. *See also* Culture
Ethoglucid, bladder cancer, 1357
Etiology, chronic heart failure, 806–807
Etomidate (Amidate), 402t
Etoposide, 989
  chemotherapeutic agents, 552
Etretinate, 1809
European Pressure Ulcer Advisory Panel (EPUAP), 195
EUS. *See* Endoscopic ultrasonography (EUS)
Euthanasia, 241–242
Everolimus (Afinitor), 1098
Evidence-based practice (EBP), 9, 11
Evisceration, 413, 1919
EVL. *See* Endoscopic variceal ligation (EVL)
Evoked potential studies, 1983–1984
Exacerbation
  of asthma, 592–593, 592f
  of COPD, 570–572
Excimer lasers, 1809
Excisional biopsy, 1453, 2160
Exemestane (Aromasin), in breast cancer, 1458, 1471
Exenteration, 1920
Exercise-associated hyponatremia, 310
Exercise of extremities, preoperative instructions, 384, 385c
Exercise promotion, 2246
Exercises
  after head and neck surgery, 932f
  body positioning, 866
  diabetes mellitus, 1147–1148
  to strengthen abdominal muscles, 1000
  type 2 diabetes, 1142
Exercise stress testing, 679
Exocrine, 1107
Expanded polytetrafluoroethylene (ePTFE), 852
Expectoration, 461
Explanation, 22
Exploratory laparoscopy, in esophageal cancer, 943
Expressive aphasia, 2030, 2031t
External beam radiation therapy (EBRT), 2164
External catheters, 202
External ear. *See also* Ear
  auricle, 1925
  conditions
    cerumen impaction, 1937
    gaping earring puncture, 1938
    malignant external otitis, 1938
  external auditory canal, 1927
  physical examination, 1931
  specialized apocrine glands, 1768
External fixator
  defined, 2233
  patient with, 2241–2242, 2242c
External genitalia, 1374, 1374f. *See also* Female reproductive system
External hemorrhoids, 1046
External otitis (otitis externa)
  clinical features, 1939t
  clinical manifestations, 1937
  medical management, 1937
  nursing management, 1938
  prevention of, 1938c
External radiation, 2164
External rotation deformity of hip, prevention of, 182
Extra-articular disorders, 1760
Extracellular fluid (ECF) compartment, 297
  interstitial space, 297
  intravascular space, 297
  transcellular space, 297
Extracorporeal liver assist devices (ELAD), 1083
Extracorporeal membrane oxygenation (ECMO), 791
Extracorporeal shock wave lithotripsy (ESWL), 1352
Extraovarian primary peritoneal carcinoma (EOPPC), 1438
Extravasation, 337, 2150, 2178, 2181
Extremities
  arterial insufficiency, 850
  blood flow, 839
  circulatory insufficiency of, 838
Exudates, 881
Exudative retinal detachments, 1907
Eye
  anatomic and physiologic overview, 1882f
    aqueous-filled anterior chamber, 1882
    aqueous humour (transparent nutrient-containing fluid, 1882
    choroid, 1883
    ciliary body, 1883
    conjunctiva, 1882
    cornea, 1883
    dilator muscles, 1883
    epithelium, 1883
    iris, 1883
    macula, 1883
    nerve fibres, 1883
    optic disc, 1883
    optic nerve, 1883
    retina, 1883
    retinal pigment epithelium, 1883
    retinal vessels, 1883
    sclera, 1882–1883
    sensory retina, 1883
    uveal tract, 1883
  assessment, 1884c
    external eye examination, 1884
    ocular history, 1883
    visual acuity, 1883–1884
  diagnostic evaluation
    Amsler grid, 1886–1887
    angiography, 1887
    colour fundus photography, 1887
    colour vision testing, 1886
    direct ophthalmoscopy, 1884–1886
    indirect ophthalmoscopy, 1886
    laser scanning polarimetry, 1887
    optical coherence tomography, 1887
    perimetry testing, 1887–1888
    slit-lamp examination, 1886
    tonometry, 1886
    ultrasonography, 1887

Eye and vision disorders, 1885c
cataracts, 1900–1903
corneal disorders, 1903–1906
glaucoma, 1896–1900
impaired vision, 1888–1892
infectious and inflammatory conditions, 1913–1918
ocular consequences of systemic disease, 1921–1922
orbital and ocular tumours, 1918–1919
retinal disorders, 1906–1913
Eye prostheses, 1920, 1920f
Ezetimibe, 735t, 736

F

Faces, Legs, Activity, Cry, and Consolability (FLACC) scale, 279
Faces pain scale-revised (FPS-R), 278
Face tents, 606
Facial edema, 1085
Facial lipoatrophy, 1548f
Facial molluscum contagiosum, 1779
Facial nerve neuroma, 1943
Facial nerve tumour, 2111t
Facial paralysis. *See* Bell's palsy
Facial reconstructive surgery, 1830
Factor V Leiden thrombophilia, 142t
Factor Xa, in venous thromboembolism, 864
Faintness, dumping syndrome, 993
Fallopian tubes, cancer of, 1438
Falls, in older adults, 231–232
Famciclovir (Famvir), 1797, 1799
herpes simplex virus 2, 1418
Familial amyotrophic lateral sclerosis, 141t
Familial atypical cold urticaria (FACU), 1592
Family education, for patient with chronic conditions, 165
Family-focused interventions, in ED, 2341, 2341c
anger, 2342
anxiety and denial, 2341
caring for emergency personnel, 2342
coping with sudden death, 2341c
grief, 2342
remorse and guilt, 2341–2342
Family history, 56, 56f, 57c
Family, support to, in shock, 349
Famotidine (Pepcid), 907
antacids, 939
peptic ulcer disease and gastritis, 979t
Fasciotomy, 2233, 2353
FAST acronym, 2035
Fasting plasma glucose (FPG), 1137, 1143
Fat, 732–733, 1766
in diabetic diet, 1146
metabolism and development of heart disease, 733
necrosis, 1456
Fat embolism syndrome (FES), 2307–2308
Fatigue
in cancer
decreasing, 2198–2199
sources of, 2199c
cancer-related, 2184
chronic constipation, 1011
colorectal cancer, 1043
diabetes mellitus, 1143
hepatic dysfunction, 1055
left ventricular failure, 811
management, after chemotherapy, 2185
mitral valve prolapse, 778
people with disabilities and, 170
reduction, 552
Fat intake, in nutritional assessment, 68
Fat metabolism, role of liver, 1053
Fat redistribution syndrome (lipodystrophy), 1548
Fatty liver disease, 1060
lifestyle behaviours, 1054
Fatty streaks, atherosclerotic lesions, 844
Febrile nonhemolytic reaction, 1685
Febuxostat (Uloric), in gout, 1758
Fecal elimination, abnormalities of
constipation, 997–1000
diarrhea, 1000–1003
fecal incontinence, 1003–1004
irritable bowel syndrome, 1004–1005
Fecal immunochemical test (FIT), 1034
Fecal impaction, 999
Fecal incontinence, 200, 998, 1003–1004
assessment and diagnostic findings, 1003
clinical manifestations, 1003
medical management, 1003
nursing management, 1003–1004
pathophysiology, 1003
Fecal leukocytes, 906
Fecal matter, 1019
Fecal occult blood testing (FOBT), 907
Feces, 902
Feedback, 41
Feeding tube placement, 522
Felodipine (Plendil), 741
heart failure, 813
hypertension, 887t
Female condom, 1400, 1401f
Female genital mutilation (FGM), 1380, 1382
Female physiologic processes, management of
abnormal uterine bleeding, 1396
abortion, 1402–1404
amenorrhea, 1395–1396
coitus interruptus, 1401
contraception, 1396–1397
dysmenorrhea, 1395
dyspareunia, 1396
ectopic pregnancy, 1407–1409
emergency contraception, 1402
fertility awareness, 1401–1402
infertility, 1404–1406
mechanical barriers, 1400–1401
menopause, 1377–1380
menorrhagia, 1396
menstrual disorders, 1394–1396
menstruation, 1393–1394
metrorrhagia, 1396
nurses role, 1372–1373
periconception health care, 1406–1407
perimenopause, 1376–1377
postmenopausal bleeding, 1396
premenstrual syndrome, 1394–1395
Female reproductive disorders
bacterial vaginosis, 1414
benign disorders
adenomyosis, 1431
chronic pelvic pain, 1431
endometrial hyperplasia, 1431
endometriosis, 1430–1431
ovarian cysts, 1428–1429
uterus, benign tumours of, 1429–1430
vulvar cysts, 1427–1428
vulvar dystrophy, 1428
vulvitis, 1427
vulvodynia, 1427
candidiasis, 1413–1414
cervicitis, 1419–1420
endocervicitis, 1419–1420
herpes simplex virus 2, 1417–1418
HIV and AIDS, 1422–1423
human papillomavirus, 1416–1417
malignant conditions, 1431–1432
cervix, cancer of, 1432–1434
fallopian tubes, cancer of, 1438
hysterectomy, 1440
ovary, cancer of, 1438–1440
radiation therapy, 1442–1443
uterus, cancer of, 1434–1435
vagina, cancer of, 1437–1438
vulva, cancer of, 1435–1437
pelvic inflammatory disease, 1420–1422
structural disorders
pelvic organ prolapse, 1424–1425
uterine prolapse, 1425–1427
vagina, fistulas of, 1423–1424
trichomoniasis, 1414–1415
vulvovaginal infections, 1411–1412
Female reproductive process, 1382c
Female reproductive system
age related changes in, 1377t
anatomy, 1373–1375
external genitalia, 1374, 1374f
internal reproductive structures, 1374–1375
diagnostic evaluation
colposcopy and cervical biopsy, 1391
computed tomography, 1393
cone biopsy and loop electrosurgical excision procedure, 1391
cryotherapy and laser therapy, 1391
dilation and curettage, 1391
endometrial (aspiration) biopsy, 1391
endoscopic examinations, 1391–1392
hysterosalpingography/uterotubography, 1393
magnetic resonance imaging, 1393
Pap smear, 1390
ultrasonography, 1393
function, 1375–1376
Femoral shaft, fracture of, 2325–2326, 2326f
Fenofibrate (TriCor), 735t
Fentanyl, 281–282, 286, 401t, 1120, 1861
TD patch, 286
Fertility awareness, 1401–1402
Fetor hepaticus, 1052, 1072
Fever, 1010, 1012
blisters, 1798
in burn injury, 1854
hepatic dysfunction, 1055
infective endocarditis, 794–797
neutropenic, 2201, 2202t
Fexofenadine (Allegra), 1789
Fibre bundles, 1963
Fibre, in diabetic diet, 1146
Fibreoptic bronchoscopy, 464, 551
Fibreoptic endoscopy, 951, 978
Fibric acid, 735t, 736
Fibrin, 1599, 1604
Fibrinogen, 1598, 1599
Fibrinolysis, 1599, 1600
Fibrinolytic action, 1786
Fibrinolytic therapy, 737
Fibroadenomas, 1455–1456
Fibrocystic breast changes, 1446, 1455
Fibroid, 1429–1430
clinical manifestations, 1429, 1429f
medical management, 1429–1430
tumour, 1412
Fibromyalgia, 269c, 1004, 1758, 1759
assessment and diagnostic findings, 1759
medical management, 1759
nursing management, 1759
pathophysiology, 1759

Fibroscopy, 899
upper GI tract, 911
Fibrous plaques, atherosclerotic lesions, 844
FICA Spiritual History Tool, 83, 85
FICE. *See* Flexible imaging spectral colour enhancement (FICE)
Fidelity, 25, 25c
Fight-or-flight reaction, 106, 107, 344
Figure-of- eight bandage, 2312, 2312f
Filgrastim (Neupogen)
acute myeloid leukemia, 1637
breast cancer, 1469
Filtration, 299
FIM. *See* Functional Independence Measure (FIM)
Finasteride (Proscar), for benign prostatic hyperplasia, 1491
Fine-needle aspiration (FNA), 505, 1225, 1446, 1452
Fingerprints, 1766
First-degree atrioventricular block, 711
First heart sound, 653, 669
First-intention healing, 413
First-line antituberculosis medications, 526t
Fish oil capsules, 735t
Fissures, 998
Fistulas, 909, 998, 1011, 1017, 1412, 1423
Crohn's disease, 1017
ulcerative colitis, 1016t, 1017
Fistulectomy, 1045
FIT. *See* Fecal immunochemical test (FIT)
Fitz-Hugh–Curtis syndrome, 1420
Flaccid bladder, 1346
Flaccidity, 1969, 1974
Flaccid paralysis, 1968
Flail chest
medical management, 555–556
pathophysiology, 555
Flaps, 1829
Flatfoot, 2275
Flatline. *See* Ventricular asystole
Flecainide
antiarrhythmic medication, 699t
for atrial fibrillation prevention, 704
Fleet's enema, 914
Flexible fibreoptic colonoscope, 912, 912f
Flexible imaging spectral colour enhancement (FICE), 911
Flexi-Seal Fecal Management System, 1004, 1004f
Flucloxacillin, 1796
Fluconazole (Diflucan), 2094
candidiasis, 1414
cryptococcal meningitis, 1553
Flucytosine (Ancobon), 2094
Fludarabine (Fludara), for chronic lymphocytic leukemia, 1642
Fluid
and electrolyte status, after chemotherapy, 2184
intake in pneumonia, 519
Fluid and electrolytes, 296
body fluids, amount and composition of, 296–297
electrolytes in body fluids, 297–298
gerontologic considerations, 303–304
homeostatic mechanisms, 301
adrenal glands, 301
antidiuretic hormone and thirst, 301
baroreceptors, 301
heart and blood vessel, 301
kidneys, 301
lungs, 301
osmoreceptors, 302
parathyroid glands, 301
pituitary gland, 301
release of atrial natriuretic peptide, 302–303
renin–angiotensin–aldosterone system, 301
laboratory tests, 299–300
management
blistering diseases, 1815
emergent/resuscitative phase of burn injury, 1851c
exfoliative dermatitis, 1812
intracranial surgery, 2011
role of skin, 1768
Stevens–Johnson syndrome, 1816–1817
toxic epidermal necrolysis, 1816–1817
traumatic brain injury, 2061–2062, 2066
regulation of body fluid compartments
diffusion, 299
filtration, 299
osmosis and osmolality, 298–299, 298f
sodium–potassium pump, 299
routes of gains and losses, 299, 299t
GI tract, 299
kidneys, 299
lungs, 299
skin, 299
Fluid attenuation inversion recovery (FLAIR), 1980
Fluid balance
adrenocortical insufficiency, 1249
parenteral nutrition, 971
promoting, 978
Fluid challenge test, 305
Fluid intake and output (I&O), 299, 299f
monitoring in critically ill patients, 303c
Fluid intake, parotitis, 924
Fluid loss, organs of, 299
Fluid overload, 335–336
heart failure, 805
parenteral nutrition, 970t
patient with newly diagnosed diabetes, 1171
Fluid replacement therapy
in burn patients, 1845–1848
additional gauges of fluid requirements, 1846
goal of optimal fluid resuscitation, 1846–1847
guidelines and formulas for fluid replacement, 1848c
projected fluid requirements, 1847–1848
in sepsis, 362
in shock, 350, 355t
complications of, 351
crystalloid and colloid solutions, 350–351
Fluid retention, 1094
Fluid therapy, parenteral, 333
intravenous solutions, types of, 333
hypertonic fluids, 335
hypotonic fluids, 335
isotonic fluids, 333–335
local complications, 336
clotting and obstruction, 338
hematoma, 338
infiltration and extravasation, 336–337, 337c
phlebitis, 337, 338c
thrombophlebitis, 337–338
medications by IV route, 335
nursing management, 335–338
purpose of, 333
systemic complications, 335
air embolism, 336
circulatory overload, 335–336
febrile reaction, 335
infection, 336
Fluid volume, 1094–1095
balance, patient undergoing bariatric surgery, 1206
cirrhosis, 1094–1095
heart failure, 819
Fluid volume deficit (FVD)
hypovolemia, 304–307
intravascular, 297
NG intubation and, 952
Fluid volume disturbances
hypervolemia, 307–309
hypovolemia, 304–307
Fluid volume excess (FVE). *See* Hypervolemia
Flunisolide, 588t
allergic rhinitis, 1585
Fluorescein angiography, 1178, 1908
Fluorescent in situ hybridization (FISH), 138, 1641
Fluorescent treponemal antibody absorption test (FTA-ABS), 1723
Fluoridated water, 922
Fluoride varnish, 922
Fluoroscopic examination, 909
Fluoroscopy, 463
chest x-ray and, 675
Fluorouracil, 1898
bladder cancer, 1357
breast cancer, 1469
5-Fluorouracil (5-FU), 989, 1129
Fluoxetine (Prozac), 1789, 2097, 2098
antidepressant therapy, 1554
fibromyalgia, 1759
in premenstrual syndrome, 1395
Flutamide (Euflex), 1496
Fluticasone, 588t
Fluticasone furoate, 589t
Fluticasone/salmeterol (Advair), 589t
Flutter valve, 602, 611
Foam dressings, 1786
leg ulcer, 869
FOBT. *See* Fecal occult blood testing (FOBT)
Focal photocoagulation, 1178
Focal seizures, 2014
Focused assessment sonography for trauma (FAST) examination, 2352
Folate deficiency, 1074, 1618
Folfirinox, 1129
Folic acid deficiency, 1617
Folk healers, 97
and ethical dilemma, 98c
Follicle-stimulating hormone (FSH), 1373, 1375
Follicular Lymphoma International Prognostic Index (FLIPI), 1651
Folliculitis
medical management, 1796–1797
nursing management, 1797
promoting home, community-based, and transitional care, 1797
Follistim, 1405c
Fondaparinux (Arixtra), 864
Food allergy, 1592–1593
assessment and diagnostic findings, 1593
clinical manifestations, 1593
medical management, 1593, 1593c
nursing management, 1593
Food and Drug Administration (FDA), 1008
Food poisoning, 1001, 2365, 2365c
Food record, 68

Foods labels, 1147
FOOSH (Fall On Out-Stretched Hands) injury, 2300
Foot and leg problems, in diabetes, 1182–1183, 1182f
Foot care, in diabetes, 1182–1183
Foot cramps, 854
Footdrop, 182
  prevention of, 182
Foot problems, common, 2274–2276
  callus, 2274
  corn, 2274
  flatfoot (pes planus), 2275
  hammer toe, 2274, 2275f
  ingrown toenail, 2274
  Morton's Neuroma, 2275
  nursing process, 2275–2276
  pes cavus, 2275
  plantar fasciitis, 2274
Forced expiratory techniques (FET), 634
Forced vital capacity (FVC), 460
Forearm claudication, 853
Foreign bodies, in esophagus, 938
Formalist theory, 24
Formoterol, 588t, 589t
Fornix, 1373, 1374
Fortamet, 1405c
Foscarnet (Foscavir), 1921
Fosinopril (Monopril)
  in heart failure, 811t
  hypertension, 886t
Fossae, 1961
Fourth heart sound, 670
Fowler position, 1010
Fractional Er:YAG laser resurfacing, 1831
Fraction of inspired oxygen, 602
Fracture, 2233, 2302, 2312, 2353
  acetabulum, 2316
  assessment, 2353
  clavicle, 2312, 2312f, 2313f
  clinical manifestations, 2304
    crepitus, 2304
    deformity, 2304
    localized edema and ecchymosis, 2304
    loss of function, 2304
    pain, 2304
    shortening, 2304
  closed, 2302
  complications, 2307
    acute compartment syndrome, 2308–2309, 2309f
    avascular necrosis of bone, 2311
    complex regional pain syndrome, 2311
    delayed union and nonunion, 2310–2311
    fat embolism, 2307–2308
    heterotrophic ossification, 2312
    internal fixation devices, reaction to, 2311
    shock, 2307
    venous thromboembolism, 2309–2310
  elbow, 2313–2314
  emergency management, 2304
  femoral shaft, 2325–2326
  greenstick, 2302
  hand, 2315
  healing, 2217, 2307, 2307c
  hip, 2316–2319, 2320–2325c, 2325
  humeral neck, 2312–2313, 2313f
  humeral shaft, 2313, 2313f
  intra-articular, 2302, 2304
  management of, 2353–2354
    osteoporosis, 2282
  medical management, 2304
    closed reduction, 2304–2305
    immobilization, 2305
    internal fixation technique, 2305, 2305f
    maintaining and restoring function, 2305
    open reduction, 2305
    reduction, 2304
  nursing management
    home care checklist, 2305, 2306c
    patients with closed fractures, 2305, 2306c
    patients with open fractures, 2305–2306
  open, 2302
  pain, 2221
  pelvic fracture, 2315–2316, 2316f
  radial and ulnar shafts, 2314
  radial head, 2314
  rib, 2326–2327
  thoracolumbar spine, 2327
  tibia and fibula, 2326
  types, 2302, 2303f
  wrist, 2314–2315
Fracture Risk Assessment Tool (FRAX), 2223
Fragrance-free deodorants, 1791
Frail older adults, 231
Fraser Health Authority, 249
Fraser Institute Canada, 96
Free flap, 1829
Fremitus, 439
Frequency, 1332, 1334
Frey's syndrome, 919, 925
Friction rub, 670, 905
Frontal lobe, 1960, 1967
  tumour, 2120
Frontotemporal dementia with parkinsonism-17, 141t
Frostbite, 1819, 2355–2356
  assessment and diagnostic findings, 2355
  management, 2355–2356
  venous stasis and thrombosis, 2355
Frovatriptan (Frova), 2025
5-FU. *See* 5-Fluorouracil (5-FU)
Fuchs endothelial dystrophy, 1904
Full-length sterile drapes, 968
Fulminant hepatic failure, 1052
  drug-induced liver disease, 1082–1083
  hepatitis B, 1078
  liver transplantation, 1099, 1102
Functional bracing, 2313
Functional constipation, 999
Functional incontinence, 1332, 1341. *See also* Urinary incontinence
Functional Independence Measure (FIM), 178
Functional residual capacity (FRC), 443
Fundus, 1373, 1374
Fungal encephalitis
  assessment and diagnostic findings, 2094
  clinical manifestations, 2094
  medical management, 2094
  nursing management, 2094–2095
Fungal (mycotic) skin infections, 1800
Fungemia, 1698, 1707–1708
Funnel chest (pectus excavatum), 452
Furantoin, 1336
Furosemide (Lasix), 311, 321, 1323
  acute kidney injury, 1295
  hypertension, 884t
  pulmonary edema, 825
Furuncles, 1796–1797
Fusiform aneurysm, 855
FVD. *See* Fluid volume deficit (FVD)

G

Gabapentin (Neurontin), 2112
  fibromyalgia, 1759
Gadolinium-based contrast agents, 463
Gait, in physical assessment, 63
Galantamine hydrobromide (Razadyne), for Alzheimer's disease, 227
Gallbladder, 1106–1107
  cholecystitis, 1108–1109
  cholelithiasis, 1109
    assessment and diagnostic findings, 1110–1112
    clinical manifestations, 1110
    medical management, 1112–1115
    pathophysiology, 1109
    risk factors, 1109c
  with gallstones, 1108
  laparoscopic cholecystectomy, 1113–1114
  monitoring and managing complications, 1117
  nursing process, 1115–1118
  preoperative measures, 1113
  removal of, 915
  surgical treatment of, 1113
Gallium scan, 464
Gallstones, 1108, 1110, 1119
  dissolving, 1112–1113
  nonsurgical techniques, 1112–1113, 1113f
  obstructs, 1110
Gamete intrafallopian transfer (GIFT), 1406
Gamma-aminobutyric acid (GABA), 272
  neurotransmission, 1072
Gamma-glutamyl transferase (GGT), 1056, 1060, 1095
Gamma Knife unit, 2164
Gamma rays, 2164
Ganciclovir, 1894, 1921
Ganglion, 2272
Gangrene, 844f
  of gallbladder, 1108
  of toe, 854, 868f
Gaping earring puncture, 1938
Gas/bloating/cramping, enteral therapy, 956t
Gas exchange, 438
  oxyhemoglobin dissociation curve, 445–446, 446c
  partial pressure of gases, 444, 445c, 445f
  pressure on oxygen transport, effects of, 445
Gastrectomy, dietary intervention, 991c
Gastric acid stimulation test, 915
Gastric aspiration, 950, 951
Gastric cancer, 988–992
  assessment and diagnostic findings, 989
  clinical manifestations, 989
  home care checklist, 992c
  medical management, 989
  nursing interventions, 990–992
    home and community-based care, 991–992
    optimal nutrition, 990
    psychosocial support, 991
    reducing anxiety, 990
    relieving pain, 990
  nursing priorities, 990
  nursing process, 990–992
  pathophysiology, 989
  planning and goals, 990
Gastric emptying procedures, 2362
Gastric hyperacidity, 981
Gastric intubation, pulmonary complications, 952
Gastric juice yields, 915
Gastric lavage, 2362, 2363–2364c

Gastric mucosa, 978
Gastric outlet obstruction (GOO), 977, 984, 987, 1209
  peptic ulcer disease, 987
Gastric perforation, 989
Gastric resection, with gastrojejunostomy, 1007t
Gastric residual volumes (GRVs), 956
Gastric retention, 993
Gastric secretion, 900
Gastric secretory studies, 982
Gastric stoma, 960
Gastric sump tubes, 949
Gastric surgery
  home care checklist, 995c
  nursing management, 993
    adequate nutrition, 993–994
    dietary self-management, 994
    home and community-based care, 994
    increasing knowledge, 993
    monitoring and managing complications, 994
    reducing anxiety, 993
    relieving pain, 993
    resuming enteral intake, 993
  peptic ulcers, 992
Gastric triangle, 982
Gastric tubes, 948t
  gastric sump, 949
  Levin tube, 949
Gastric ulcers
  comparison of, 981t
  duodenal, comparison of, 981t
Gastrin
  gastrointestinal regulatory substances, 901t
  secreting, 981
Gastritis, 976, 977
  acute, 976, 978
  assessment and diagnostic findings, 978
  chronic, 976, 978
  clinical manifestations, 978
  home care checklist, 980c
  medical management, 978
  nursing management
    home and community-based care, 980–981
    promoting fluid balance, 978
    promoting optimal nutrition, 978
    reducing anxiety, 978
    relieving pain, 978–980
  pathophysiology, 976–977
  pharmacotherapy, 979t–980t
Gastroduodenal, 914
Gastroesophageal reflux disease (GERD), 914, 919, 934, 936, 938, 981, 1004
  assessment and diagnostic findings, 938–939, 940
  clinical manifestations, 938, 940
  management, 939, 940
  pharmacologic management, 939t
Gastroesophageal sphincter, 934
Gastrografin, 909
Gastrohepatic omentum, 987
Gastrointestinal disorders, 908c
Gastrointestinal intubation
  enteral therapy
    complications of, 956t
    conditions, 953t
  enteric tubes, 949
  gastric tubes, 948–949, 948t
    for decompression, drainage, aspiration, and lavage, 948–949
    gastric sump (Salem) tube, 949
    Levin tube, 949
  gastrostomy and jejunostomy, 960–961
  nasoenteric tube feeding, 955f
  nursing management, 949
    confirming placement, 950–951
    inserting the tube, 949–950
    maintaining tube function, 951–952
    oral and nasal hygiene, 952
    patient monitoring, 951–952
    preparing the patient, 949
    securing the tube, 951
    tube removing, 952
  nursing research profile
    enteral feedings, 953c
  parenteral nutrition
    administration methods, 967–969
    clinical indications, 966
    discontinuing parenteral nutrition, 969
    formulas, 966
    initiating therapy, 967
    nitrogen balance, 966
  tube feedings with nasogastric/nasoenteric devices, 952–960
    administration methods, 954–955
    formulas, 954
    osmosis and osmolality, 953–954
  variety of tubes, 947
Gastrointestinal regulatory substances, 901
Gastrointestinal system
  age-related changes in, 214t, 216–217
  effects of chemotherapy on, 2182
Gastrointestinal (GI) tract, 976
  abdominal pain, 903f
  abnormalities of, 898
  age-related changes, 903t
  anatomy of, 898–900
    blood supply of large intestine, 900f
  assessment of, 902–906
  bleeding, 914
  denture care, 904c
  diagnostic evaluation, 906–915
    abdominal ultrasonography, 907–908
    breath test, 907
    computed tomography, 909–910
    DNA testing, 908
    gastric acid stimulation test, 915
    gastric analysis, 915
    gastrointestinal motility studies, 911
    imaging studies, 908–911
    laparoscopy (peritoneoscopy), 915
    lower gastrointestinal tract study, 909
    magnetic resonance imaging, 910
    manometry and electrophysiologic studies, 914–915
    nursing interventions, 909
    nursing practice, 908c
    pH monitoring, 915
    positron emission tomography, 910
    scintigraphy (radionuclide testing), 910–911
    serum laboratory studies, 906
    stool tests, 906–907
    upper gastrointestinal tract study, 909
  digestive system, function of
    chewing and swallowing, 900
    colonic function, 902
    gastric function, 900
    organs, 899f
    small intestine function, 900–902
    waste products, 902
  effluent, 1019
  endoscopic procedures, 911
    anoscopy, proctoscopy, and sigmoidoscopy, 913–914
    endoscopy through ostomy, 914
    fibreoptic colonoscopy, 912–913
    small bowel enteroscopy, 914
    upper gastrointestinal fibroscopy/esophagogastroduodenoscopy, 911–912
  health history assessment, 902
    bowel habits changes, 904
    dyspepsia, 903
    intestinal gas, 903
    nausea and vomiting, 903–904
    pain, 903
    past health, family, and social, 904
    stool characteristics, 904
  hemorrhage, 993
  integrity, 943
  motility, 902
  physical assessment
    abdominal inspection, 905–906
    auscultation, 905–906
    gums, 905
    lips, 904
    oral cavity inspection and palpation, 904
    palpation, 905–906
    percussion, 905–906
    rectal inspection, 906
    tongue, 905
  physiologic overview, 898–902
  primary functions, 900
  treatment modalities, 947
Gastrointestinal varices, cirrhosis and, 1085
Gastroscopy, 911, 911f, 912
Gastrostomy, 948, 960
  assessment, 961
  collaborative problems, 962
  gastrointestinal intubation, 960–961
  nursing priorities, 961–962
  nursing process, 961–965
  planning and goals, 962
Gate control theory, of pain, 273–274, 274f, 290
Gatorade, 1029
GBS. *See* Guillain–Barré syndrome (GBS)
G-button, 948, 961
GBV-C. *See* Hepatitis GB virus-C (GBV-C)
GCA. *See* Giant cell arteritis (GCA)
GCS. *See* Glasgow Coma Scale (GCS)
Geenius HIV-1/2 Confirmatory Assay, 1544
Gelfoam, 1046
Gemcitabine, 552, 1129
Gemfibrozil (Lopid), 735t, 736
Gender chromosome, 133
Gene mutations, 134–135, 134f, 135f
  acquired, 135, 135f
  carriers of, 136
  germline/hereditary, 134, 134f
  spontaneous, 134–135
General adaptation syndrome (GAS), 105
Generalized absence seizure, 2014
Generalized exfoliative dermatitis
  assessment and diagnostic findings, 1812
  clinical manifestations, 1812
  medical management, 1812–1813
Generalized seizures, 2014
Genes, 132
  and chromosomes, 133, 133f
  role in human variation, 132–135
Gene therapy, 2192. *See also* Cancer
Genetic counselling, 150
  across life span, 151c
  communicating information to patients, 151–152
  components of, 150c
  follow-up, 152

informed consent for, 151
precounselling information, 151
preparing patients for genetics evaluation, 151
providing support during, 152
Genetic engineering, 1517, 1525
Genetic makeup, 130
Genetics, 130–131
adult-onset conditions, 140, 141t–143t, 143
advances in, 9
ancestry, cultural, social, and piritual concerns, 146–147
applications in nursing practice, 147–148
family history assessment, 148–149
follow-up after genetic evaluation, 152
genetic counselling and evaluation services, 150–152, 150c, 151c
health assessment, 148
physical assessment, 149
psychosocial assessment, 149–150, 150c
digestive and gastrointestinal disorder, 908c
ethical concerns relating to, 146
hypertension, 879
integration with genomics, 132–138
nursing competencies for, 132c
and older adult, 213c
technologies in practice, 138–144
Genetic screening, 139–140, 140t
Genetics family history, 148–149, 148c
Genetics-related nursing care, 23
Genetics services, 150
Genetic testing, 138–139, 139c
genotypic methods, 139
phenotypic approach, 139
Genetic tests, 139, 140t
Genetic variations, 135
Genital herpes, 1797, 1798
medical management, 1799
nursing process, 1418–1419
Genitourinary injury, 2352
Genitourinary system, age-related changes in, 214t, 216
Genitourinary trauma, 1355–1356
medical management, 1356
nursing management, 1356
surgical management, 1356
Genogram, 56, 56f
Genome, 130
Genomic profiles, 130
Genomics, 130–131. *See also* Genetics
applications in nursing practice, 147–148
family history assessment, 148–149
follow-up after genetic evaluation, 152
genetic counselling and evaluation services, 150–152, 150c, 151c
health assessment, 148
physical assessment, 149
psychosocial assessment, 149–150, 150c
framework for nursing practice, 131–132
future perspective, 152
integration with genetics, 132–138
nursing competencies for, 132c
personalized treatments, 144–146
technologies in practice, 138–144
Genotype, 133
Gentamicin, 1339
acute kidney injury, 1294
Gentamicin sulphate, 1856
GERD. *See* Gastroesophageal reflux disease (GERD)
Geriatric Depression Scale (GDS), 224
Geriatric syndromes, 231
Germinal tumours, 1507
Gerontologic considerations, 517, 1148
abdominal aortic aneurysm, 857
acute kidney injury, 1295
acute pancreatitis, 1119
anemia, 1611
anemia of chronic disease, 1616
angina pectoris, 738–739, 739c
blindness and visual impairment, 1889
blood pressure, 892
breast cancer, 1475
burns, 1837, 1848–1849, 1857, 1876
cancer, 2204, 2204t
cardiovascular function, 658, 659t, 672
catheterization, 1348, 1348f
changes in blood vessels walls and blood flow, 839
cholelithiasis, 1115
chronic kidney disease, 1300
colorectal cancer, 1035, 1037–1038
complications, 1009–1010
constipation, 999–1000
diabetes mellitus, 1143
diarrhea, 1002
diastolic blood pressure, 882
diverticular disease, 1012
emergency nursing, 2342–2343
end-stage kidney disease, 1300
epilepsy, 2017
fluid and electrolytes, 303–304
gastric cancer, 989–990
GI disorders, 902
hearing difficulties, 1935–1936
heart failure, 816
heat stroke, 2354
hemophilia, 1666
hepatitis B virus, 1078
hip fracture, 2317–2318
hospitalized diabetic patients, 1186–1187
human immune deficiency virus, 1539
hypertension, 880–881
hypoglycemia, 1164
hypovolemia, 304–305
immune system, 1525–1526
impaired skin integrity, 195
indwelling catheters, 1348–1350
kidney disorder, 1283–1284
liver functions, 1054
lower urinary tract infection, 1334–1335, 1335c
lung cancer, 552–553
male reproductive function, 1482–1483
multiple myeloma, 1655–1656
multiple sclerosis, 2097
nervous system, 1978–1979
obesity, 1201
osteomalacia, 2284
osteoporosis, 2278
PACU, 416
pancreas, 1108
perioperative period, 375
peripheral arterial disease, 839, 849
primary brain tumours, 2118
pruritus, 1789
pulmonary tuberculosis, 525
rheumatic diseases, 1739, 1742–1743
rib fracture, 2327
scabies, 1802
septic (infectious) arthritis, 2289–2290
skin, 1769–1770, 1769f, 1770c
total hip arthroplasty, 2249
traumatic brain injury, 2058–2059
urinary incontinence, 1341–1342
Gerontologic/geriatric nursing, 212
Gerontology, 212
Gerota's fascia, 1290
Gestational diabetes, 1139t, 1142
gFOBT. *See* Guaiac-based fecal occult blood test (gFOBT)
GGT. *See* Gamma-glutamyl transferase (GGT)
Giant cell arteritis (GCA), 1753–1754
assessment and diagnostic findings, 1753
clinical manifestations, 1753
medical management, 1753
nursing management, 1753–1754
pathophysiology, 1753
Giant cell tumours, 2291
Giardia, 1719
GI bleeding, in shock, 347
GI ischemia, in shock, 347–348
Gilbert's syndrome, 1060
Gingivitis, gum abnormalities, 921t
Glands of skin
apocrine sweat glands, 1768
eccrine sweat glands, 1768
sebaceous glands, 1768
sweat glands, 1768
Glasgow Coma Scale (GCS), 363, 2062
Glatiramer acetate (Copaxone), 2098
Glaucoma
assessment and diagnostic findings, 1897–1898
clinical manifestations, 1897, 1897t
incidence, 1896
medical management, 1898–1899
nursing management, 1899–1900
continuing and transitional care, 1899–1900
patient education, 1900c
promoting home, community-based, and transitional care, 1899
pathophysiology, 1896
pharmacologic therapy, 1898, 1899t
physiology, 1896
risk factors for, 1896c
stages, 1896c
surgical management, 1898–1899
drainage implants or shunts, 1899
filtering procedures for chronic glaucoma, 1898
laser iridotomy, 1898
laser trabeculoplasty, 1898
trabeculectomy, 1898
treatment, 1897t
types, 1897, 1897t
Gliding joints, 2218
Gliomas, 2117–2118. *See also* Primary brain tumours
Glisson's capsule, 1084
Global (mixed) aphasia, 2030, 2031t
Global Oral Health Programme, 922
Globulins, 1056
Glomerular filtration, 1265–1266
Glomerular filtration rate (GFR), 1284
end-stage kidney disease, 1297–1298
Glomerulonephritis, 1283, 1284, 1286, 1287
Glomus jugulare, 1943
Glomus tumour, 1943
Glomus tympanicum, 1943
Glossectomy, 926
Glossopharyngeal neuralgia, 2111t
Glottis, 440
Glucagon, 1108, 1140, 1165
foreign bodies in esophagus, 938
Glucagon-like peptide (GLP), 1157–1158
Glucocorticoids, 106, 1245
Gluconeogenesis, 106, 342

Glucophage, 1405c
Glucose, 342
Glucose metabolism
abnormalities of, 1075
role of liver in, 1053
Glucose-6-phosphate dehydrogenase deficiency, 1627–1628, 1814
Glucose tolerance test, 1123
Glucosuria, 1141
Gluteal setting exercises, 2219, 2238c
Gluten, 1008c
celiac disease, 1006
free foods, 1008
Gluten-free diet, 1814
Glyburide (Micronase), in thalassemia, 1628
Glycated hemoglobin (A1c), 1137, 1143
Glycemic control
insulin therapy, 1121
in shock, 348
Glycemic index, 1145
Glycerin suppository, laxative medications, 1001t
Glycogenolysis, 1053, 1141
Glycoprotein (GP) IIb/IIIa agents, 742
Glycosaminoglycan (GAG), 1332
Glycosylated hemoglobin, 1150
Goals of Care Designations (GCD) Order, 240
Goals of Care (GOC) Orders, 240
Go-LYTELY, 913
Gonadotropin-releasing hormone (GnRH), 1375
Gonal-F, 1405c
Gonorrhea, 1420
medical management, 1420
nursing management, 1420
Good cholesterol, 732
Goodpasture's syndrome, 1574
Gore-Tex, 856
Goserelin (Zoladex), 1496
Gout, 1757–1759
clinical manifestations, 1758
medical management, 1758, 1758t
nursing management, 1759
pathophysiology, 1757–1758
Graafian follicle, 1373, 1375
Grading of tumour, 2158
Graduated compression stockings, for deep vein thrombosis, 866
Grafting of burn wound, 1857–1861
autografts, 1860–1861
biologic dressings, 1859
biosynthetic and synthetic dressings, 1859–1860
dermal substitutes, 1860
types
allogeneic or homograft, 1827
heterograft, 1827
split-thickness and full-thickness graft, 1828f
xenograft, 1827
Graft-*versus*-host disease (GVHD), 1638, 2150, 2187
Graft-*versus*-tumour effect, 2150
Gram-positive bacteria, 2201
Granisetron (Kytril), for breast cancer, 1469
Granulex, 1784
Granulocyte, 1599, 1603
Granulocyte colony-stimulating factor (G-CSF), 2182
Granulocyte-macrophage colony-stimulating factor (GM-CSF), 2182
Granulocytopenia, 2200
Granulomatous uveitis, 1917
Grapefruit, 815
Graves disease, 1231
Grief, 257. *See also* End-of-life care
after death, 258–259
anticipatory, 257–258
complicated, 259
factors influencing grieving, 124
illness and, 123–124
Kübler-Ross's five stages of, 257, 258t
nursing implications, 124
nursing interventions for, 260t
physical response to, 124
Grieving process, in cancer, 220
Gross auditory acuity
Rinne test, 1932–1933
vestibular dysfunction testing, 1933
Weber test, 1932, 1933f
whisper test, 1932
Group A beta-hemolytic streptococcus (GABHS), 479, 1286
Group A streptococcus (GAS), 479
Group teaching, 41
G tube, 960–961
Guaiac-based fecal occult blood test (gFOBT), 1034
Guanfacine (Tenex), hypertension, 885t
Guided imagery, 116
Guide dogs, 1892
hearing, 1954
Guillain–Barré syndrome (GBS), 1725, 2105–2109, 2110c, 2111t, 2112t
assessment and diagnostic findings, 2107
autonomic dysfunction in, 2107
clinical manifestations, 2107
collaborative problems/potential complications, 2108
demyelination of nerves, 2107
home care checklist, 2110c
immunoglobulin therapy, 2106c
medical management, 2107
nursing interventions
continuing and transitional care, 2109
decreasing anxiety and fear, 2109
diversional activities, 2109
enhancing physical mobility, 2108
improving communication, 2108–2109
monitoring and managing potential complications, 2109
nutrition management, 2108
patient outcomes, 2109
promoting home, community-based, and transitional care, 2109
respiratory function maintenance, 2108
nursing priorities, 2108
planning and goals, 2108
pathophysiology, 2107
patient assessment, 2108
plasmapheresis and IVIG in, 2107
types, 2107
Guillotine amputation, 2328
Gum Arabic (GA), 1004
Gums, inspection of, 905
Gunshot wounds, 557
abdominal, 2352
Gynecomastia, 1446, 1449, 1476–1477

H

Habilitation, 174. *See also* Rehabilitation
Habit training, 201
Habitual abortion, 1403
Hair
alopecia, 1768
anagen phase (growth), 1766
colour, 1766, 1777–1778
loss of, 1766–1768
of different parts of body, 1766
estimated daily loss of, 1766
of eyes, 1766
follicles, 1766
growth, 1770
hypothyroidism and changes in, 1768
inflammation and damages to, 1766
loss, 1778, 1778f
quantity and distribution, 1766–1767
shaft, 1766
of skin, 1766
Hair assessment
body hair distribution, 1778
colour and texture, 1777–1778
hair loss, 1778
pattern hair distribution, 1779
Hair loss. *See* Alopecia
Hairy leukoplakia, 920t
Hallucinogens, 2367t
Haloperidol (Haldol), 772
Halothane (Fluothane), 400t
Halo traction, 2305
Hammer toe, 2274, 2275f
Hand–foot syndrome, 1035
Hand hygiene methods, 1702c
Hand or foot surgery, home care checklist of, 2273c
HAP. *See* Hospital-acquired pneumonia (HAP)
Hapten, 1572
Haptoglobin, 1599
Hardwire cardiac monitoring, 675
Hare traction, 2353–2354
Hartmann's procedure, 1013
HAV. *See* Hepatitis A virus (HAV)
Havrix and Vaqta (HAV vaccines), 1076
HBO. *See* Hyperbaric oxygenation (HBO)
HBPM. *See* Home blood pressure monitoring (HBPM)
HBsAg, 1079
HBV. *See* Hepatitis B virus (HBV)
HCAP. *See* Health care-associated pneumonia (HCAP)
HCC. *See* Hepatocellular carcinoma (HCC)
HCl. *See* Hydrochloric acid (HCl)
HCM. *See* Hypertrophic cardiomyopathy (HCM)
HCV. *See* Hepatitis C virus (HCV)
HDL. *See* High-density lipoprotein (HDL)
HDR. *See* High-dose radiation (HDR)
HDV. *See* Hepatitis D virus (HDV)
Headaches, 2119. *See also* Increased intracranial pressure (ICP)
assessment and diagnostic findings, 2024
cause of, 2022
classification, 2022c
cluster headaches, 2023–2024
cranial arteris, 2023
cranial arteritis, 2024
migraine, 2022
primary headache, 2022
secondary headache, 2023
tension-type headache, 2023
trigeminal autonomic cephalalgias, 2023
clinical manifestations, 2023–2024
definition, 2022
disorders related to, 2023
gastritis, 978
jaw pain, 923
medical management, 2024–2025
nursing management
continuing and transitional care, 2026

pain management, 2025–2026
promoting home, community-based, and transitional care, 2026
pathophysiology, 2023
prevention of, 2024
spinal anesthesia and, 404
Head and neck
cancers, 925, 929
lymphatic drainage, 929f
rehabilitation exercises, 932f
Head injuries
assessment and diagnostic findings, 2058
catastrophic, 2056
classification, 2056
gerontologic considerations, 2058–2059
medical management, 2059
pathophysiology, 2056–2058
primary injury, 2056
scalp injury, 2057–2058
secondary injury, 2056–2057
skull fracture, 2058
prevention of, 2057c
Head-tilt–chin-lift manoeuvre, 2345–2346
Head trauma, 2111t
Health, 6–7
determinants of, 46
optimal, 46
WHO definition of, 6–7
Health assessment, genetics and genomics in, 148
Health Belief Model, 46
Health care
ambulatory, 18–19
changes in, 5–6, 13
patient/client in, 5
Health care–associated infection (HAI), 1698
Health care-associated pneumonia (HCAP), 510
Health care costs of aging, 234
Health care delivery, influences on, 7
changing patterns of disease, 8–9
population demographics, 7–8
aging population, 8
cultural diversity, 8
quality health care, demand for, 9
quality improvement and evidence-based practice, 9
case management, 10
clinical pathways and care mapping, 9–10
continuous quality improvement, 9
evidence-based practice, 9
technology and genetics, advances in, 9
Health disparities, 92
in minorities, 92
Health education, 37
educational environments, 38
in nursing care, 37
for people with chronic illness, 38
purpose of, 37
adherence to therapeutic regimen, 38–40
informed decision making and self-care, 38
Health fairs, 49
Health field, 157
Health history, 29–30, 52, 54
components of, 54–55
biographical data, 55
chief complaint, 55
family history, 56, 56f, 57c
past health history, 55
present health concern/illness, 55
review of systems, 56
considerations in obtaining of
communication, 53, 53f
ethical use of data, 53
nurse, role of, 52–53
use of technology, 53–54
gastrointestinal system assessment, 902
heart failure, 817
immune system, 1525–1531
age-related changes, 1527t
allergy, 1528
disorders and diseases, 1528–1529
gender, 1525
gerontologic considerations, 1525–1526
immunization, 1527
infection, 1527–1528
medications and blood transfusions, 1530–1531
nutrition, 1526–1527
informant in, 54
from older adult, 54c
other formats, 62
patient profile in, 56, 58c
cultural environment, 58–59
current medications, 56
disability, 59, 60c
education and occupation, 56–57
family relationships and support system, 59
lifestyle, 59
past life events related to health, 56
physical environment, 57
risk for abuse, 61
self-concept, 61
sexuality, 61
spiritual environment, 57–58
stress and coping responses, 61–62
in respiratory diseases
chest pain, 448–449
cough, 448
dyspnea, 447–448
hemoptysis, 449
risk factors, 449c
signs and symptoms, 447–449
sputum production, 448
wheezing, 449
therapeutic communication techniques, 31t
Health–illness continuum, 6–7
Health information technology (HIT), 9
Health literacy, 39
Health promotion, 7, 42, 45
components of, 46–47
nutritional awareness, 47
physical fitness, 47
self-responsibility, 47
stress reduction and management, 47
definition of, 7, 45
genetics in, 46c
health and wellness, 45
hepatitis, 1077c
Lalonde report, 7
models, 45–46
nursing implications of, 49–50
for older people, 49
for PD patient, 2133t
of people with disabilities, 170–171
purpose of, 45
screening for adults, 48, 48t
strategies, 47–49
adolescents, 48–49
young and middle-aged adults, 49
Health-protecting behaviour, 45–46
Hearing aids, 1951–1953, 1952t
concerns, 1952c
options and features of, 1951c
tips for care, 1952c
Hearing and balance
assessment of, 1928–1929
common symptoms/signs, 1929–1931
evaluation of gross auditory acuity, 1932–1933
health history, 1928–1929
otoscopic examination, 1931, 1931f
vestibular dysfunction testing, 1933
diagnostic evaluation of
audiometry, 1933
auditory brain stem response, 1933–1934
electronystagmography, 1934
middle ear endoscopy, 1934
platform posturography, 1934
sinusoidal harmonic acceleration, 1934
tympanogram, 1933
Hearing guide dogs, 1954
Hearing loss. *See also* Ear
causes of, 1930
clinical manifestations, 1934–1936
common symptoms/signs, 1929–1931
definition, 1933
environmental factors responsible for, 1935
gerontologic considerations, 1935–1936
guidelines for communicating with hearing impaired people, 1936c
interferon medications and, 1950c
medical management, 1936
in Ménière's disease, 1945
nursing management, 1936
prevention of, 1935
risk factors, 1935c
severity of, 1933t
signs and symptoms of, 1935c
WHO estimate, 1935
Hearing problems, jaw pain, 923
Heart
age, 888
auscultation
abnormal heart sounds, 669–670
auscultation procedure, 670–671
heart sounds, interpretation of, 671
murmurs, 670, 671c
normal heart sounds, 669
chambers, 652–654
infectious diseases of, 794
infective endocarditis, 794–797
myocarditis, 797–798
pericarditis, 798–799
rheumatic endocarditis, 794
inspection and palpation, 668–669
sounds
abnormal, 669–670
interpretation of, 671
normal, 669
valves
atrioventricular, 654–655, 654f
semilunar, 655
Heart and Stroke Foundation of Canada, 2035
Heartburn (pyrosis), 934
Heart disease, in older adults, 213
Heart failure (HF)
assessment and diagnostic findings, 810
chronic, 805–824
assessment and diagnostic findings, 810
clinical manifestations, 808–810
etiology, 806–807
medical management, 811–816
nursing management, 816–824
pathophysiology, 807–808

Heart failure (*continued*)
classification, 806, 806t
clinical manifestations, 808–810, 808f, 815c
diastolic, 804, 805
dietary sodium, 821c
diuretic medications, 820t
diuretic therapy, 813c
gerontologic considerations, 816
home care checklist, 822c
hypertension, 878
infective endocarditis, 796, 797
management, 810–816
lifestyle recommendations, 811
nutritional therapy, 815
other procedures and surgical approaches, 816
pharmacologic therapy, 811–815
supplemental oxygen, 815–816
nursing management, 816–817
nursing process, 817–818, 817–824
pathophysiology, 807–808, 808f
risk factors, 805, 806, 881
systolic, 804, 805, 814c
toxicity, 814c
vicious cycle of HF, 808
Heart murmurs, infective endocarditis, 795
Heart rate
on cardiac output, effect of, 657
and contractility, dysrhythmias on, 693–694
determination from ECG, 696
in shock, 347
Heart rhythm determination from ECG, 696
Heart transplantation, 789–791, 790f
complications, 789
indications for, 789
orthotopic method of, 790f
risk of rejection, 790
Heat stroke, 2354–2355
assessment and diagnostic findings, 2354
gerontologic considerations, 2354
management, 2354–2355
prevention, 2354c
Heberden's nodes, 2225
Heimlich manoeuvre, 2345
Helicobacter pylori, 907, 938, 977, 981
antigen, 982
infection, 978, 983t
Helper T cells, 1517, 1522
Hematemesis, 904, 977, 978
hepatic dysfunction, 1055
Hematochezia, hepatic dysfunction, 1055
Hematocrit, 1120, 1599, 1606
Hematogenous spread, cancer, 2152–2153. *See also* Cancer
Hematologic disorders
acquired coagulation disorders, 1668–1689
acute lymphocytic leukemia, 1640
acute myeloid leukemia, 1636–1638
anatomic and physiologic overview, 1598–1605
anemia, 1607–1611
aplastic, 1616–1617
of chronic disease, 1615–1616
classification of, 1607–1610, 1609t
hemolytic, 1620–1621
hypoproliferative, 1613–1615
megaloblastic, 1617–1618
in renal disease, 1615
assessment, 1605
bleeding disorders, 1657–1668
blood cells, 1600–1604, 1600t, 1602f
bone marrow, 1600, 1609f
aspiration and biopsy, 1606–1607
chronic lymphocytic leukemia, 1641–1642
chronic myeloid leukemia, 1638–1640
clonal stem cell disorders, 1633–1634
diagnostic evaluation, 1605–1607
health history and physical assessment in, 1608t
hereditary hemochromatosis, 1629–1630
home care checklist, 1634c
immune hemolytic anemia, 1628–1629
leukemia, 1634–1636
leukopenia, 1632–1633
lymphoma, 1648–1652
lymphopenia, 1633
multiple myeloma, 1652–1657
myelodysplastic syndrome, 1618–1620
nursing practice, 1606c
pathophysiology, 1601f
polycythemia, 1630–1632
primary myelofibrosis, 1646–1648
risk factors, 1633c
sickle cell disease, 1621–1624
nursing process, 1624–1627
thalassemia, 1627–1628
Hematology, 672–674, 673t–674t
Hematoma, 431, 1464, 2298, 2349c
IV therapy and, 338
Hematopoiesis, 1599, 1600
Hematopoietic stem cells (HSC), 2186
Hematopoietic stem cell transplantation (HSCT), 1534, 1616, 1623, 1679, 1689
nursing management, 2187–2189, 2188c
types of, 2186–2187
use of, 2186
Hematuria, 1276, 1286
Hemiparesis, 2031t
Hemiplegia, 881, 1968
Hemiplegia-associated shoulder pain, 269c
Hemoccult II, 907
Hemochromatosis, 1629
Hemodialysis, 1283, 1295, 1305–1311
complications, 1307–1308
continuous kidney replacement therapies, 1311, 1311f
continuous venovenous hemodialysis, 1311
continuous venovenous hemofiltration, 1311
dialyzers, 1305, 1306f
home, 1309–1310
home care checklist, 1310c
nursing management
home, community-based, and transitional care, 1309–1310
nutritional and fluid therapy, 1308
pharmacologic therapy, 1308
psychosocial needs, 1308–1309, 1309c
for patient with diabetes, 1180
vascular access
arteriovenous fistula, 1306, 1307f
arteriovenous graft, 1306–1307, 1307f
devices, 1305–1306, 1307f
Hemodynamic monitoring, 685–689. *See also* Cardiovascular function
central venous pressure monitoring, 686
defined, 653
intra-arterial blood pressure monitoring, 687
minimally invasive cardiac output monitoring devices, 687–689
pulmonary artery pressure monitoring, 686–687
Hemodynamic resistance, 837
Hemoglobin, 1599, 1600
Hemolysis, 1599, 1610
Hemolytic anemias, 1610c, 1620–1624
acquired forms, 1621
causes, 1610c
inherited forms, 1620–1621
sickle cell disease, 1621–1624, 1621f
Hemolytic jaundice, 1060
Hemophilia, 1663–1666
clinical manifestations, 1665
gerontologic considerations, 1666
medical management, 1665–1666
nursing management, 1666
Hemophilic arthropathy, 1665f
Hemoporphyrin assays, 907
Hemoptysis, 439, 449, 505, 671
HemoQuant, 907
Hemorrhage, 858, 881, 932, 1208, 1968
abdominal injury and, 2352
assessing and monitoring anticoagulant therapy, 865
and blood transfusions, 416
causes of, 416
cirrhosis, 1094
complicates gastric surgery, 994
defined, 415
emergency management, 2348
external hemorrhage, control of, 2348
fluid replacement, 2348
hepatic cirrhosis, 1094
internal bleeding, control of, 2348
neck dissection, 932
peptic ulcer disease, 986–987
pressure points for control of, 2349f
types of, 415t
Hemorrhagic chemosis, 1913
Hemorrhagic cystitis, 2183
Hemorrhagic shock, acute pancreatitis, 1122
Hemorrhagic stroke
arteriovenous malformations, 2047
assessment and diagnostic findings, 2048
cause of, 2046
clinical manifestations, 2047–2048
collaborative problems/potential complications, 2050
electrolyte imbalance in, 2052
ethics and related issues, 2048c
hydrocephalus in, 2051
incidence, 2046
intracerebral hemorrhage, 2047
intracranial (cerebral) aneurysm, 2047
medical management, 2049–2050
statins, 2050
nursing interventions, 2050–2053
continuing and transitional care, 2053
home care checklist, 2052c
implementing aneurysm precautions, 2051
monitoring and managing potential complications, 2051–2052
optimizing cerebral tissue perfusion, 2050–2051
patient outcomes, 2053
promoting home, community-based, and transitional care, 2052–2053
relieving sensory deprivation and anxiety, 2051
seizure precautions, 2051
vasospasm prevention, 2051
nursing planning and goals, 2050
nursing priorities, 2050
pathophysiology, 2047
patient assessment, 2050
potential complications, 2048–2049
cerebral hypoxia and decreased blood flow, 2048

cerebral vasospasm, 2048–2049
deleterious effects, 2049
hypertension, 2049
increased intracranial pressure, 2049
prevention of, 2048
rate of recurrent hemorrhage, 2051
rebleeding in, 2051–2052
subarachnoid hemorrhage, 2046, 2047
surgical management, 2050
Hemorrhagic transformation, 2035
Hemorrhoids, 998, 999, 1045, 1790
anorectal disorders, 1045–1046
Nd:YAG laser, 1046
Hemosiderin, 1599, 1629
Hemostasis, 1599, 1600, 1605
primary, 1605
secondary, 1605
Hemothorax, 505
Heparin, 741–742, 865
for pulmonary embolism, 544
therapy, 860
Heparin-induced thrombocytopenia (HIT), 741, 864, 1676
Hepatic artery port, liver metastases, 1097, 1098
Hepatic cirrhosis, 1052
assessment and diagnostic findings, 1084c, 1085
bleeding and hemorrhage, 1094
clinical manifestations, 1084
edema, 1085
gastrointestinal varices, 1085
infection and peritonitis, 1084–1085
mental deterioration, 1085
portal obstruction and ascites, 1084
vitamin deficiency and anemia, 1085
fluid volume excess, 1094–1095
hepatic encephalopathy, 1094
medical management, 1085
nursing management, 1085–1095
home and community-based care, 1095
nutritional status, 1094
rest, 1093–1094
risk of injury, 1094
skin care, 1094
pathophysiology, 1083–1084
Hepatic disorders
ascites, 1061–1065
assessment
health history, 1054–1055
physical assessment, 1055–1056
chronic liver disease, 1058
diagnostic evaluation
computed tomography, 1058
liver biopsy, 1057–1058
liver function tests, 1056–1057
magnetic resonance imaging, 1058
ultrasonography, 1058
edema and bleeding, 1074
esophageal varices, 1065–1071
hemolytic jaundice, 1060
hepatic encephalopathy and coma, 1071–1074
hepatocellular jaundice, 1060
hereditary hyperbilirubinemia, 1060–1061
jaundice, 1060
liver biopsy, 1058c–1059c
metabolic abnormalities, 1075
nursing practice, 1055
obstructive jaundice, 1060
portal hypertension, 1061
pruritus and skin changes, 1075
vitamin deficiency, 1074–1075
Hepatic encephalopathy, 1052, 1060, 1094
assessment and diagnostic findings, 1072
cirrhosis, 1094
clinical manifestations, 1072
and coma, 1071–1074
management principles, 1073
medical management, 1072–1073
nursing management, 1073–1074
home and community-based care, 1074
pathophysiology, 1071–1072
^{99m}Tc-hepatic iminodiacetic acid (HIDA), 1111
Hepatic sinusoidal obstructive syndrome (HSOS), 2187
Hepatic venous pressure gradient (HVPG), 1067
Hepatitis A virus (HAV), 1076–1078
assessment and diagnostic findings, 1076
clinical manifestations, 1076
medical management, 1077–1078
nursing management, 1078
prevention, 1076–1077
Hepatitis B immune globulin (HBIG), 1384
Hepatitis B virus (HBV), 1078–1081
assessment and diagnostic findings, 1078–1079
clinical manifestations, 1078
immunization, 1079–1080
medical management, 1080
nursing management, 1080–1081
home and community-based care, 1080
passive immunity, 1080
risk factors, 1078c
transmission of, 1079
Hepatitis C virus (HCV), 1081
Hepatitis, dietary management of, 1077c
Hepatitis D virus (HDV), 1081
Hepatitis E virus (HEV), 1081
Hepatitis GB virus-C (GBV-C), 1082
Hepatitis G virus, 1082
Hepatobiliary system, age-related changes, 1054c
Hepatocellular carcinoma (HCC), 1078
Hepatocellular jaundice, 1060
Hepatojugular reflux, 672
Hepatomegaly
gastric cancer, 989
right ventricular failure, 810
Hepatotoxins, 1054, 1082
Herbal products, use of, before surgery, 382–383
Hereditary angioedema (HAE), 490, 1592
clinical manifestations, 1592
medical management, 1592
Hereditary colon cancer, 1034
Hereditary hemochromatosis, 141t, 1629–1630
assessment and diagnostic findings, 1629
clinical manifestations, 1629
medical management, 1629–1630
nursing management, 1630
Hereditary hyperbilirubinemia, 1060–1061
HER-2/neu, 1446, 1453
Hernia, 919
Herniation of cervical intervertebral disc. *See also* Degenerative disorders
clinical manifestations, 2140
medical management
pharmacologic therapy, 2140
surgical management, 2140
nursing process for cervical discectomy, 2141–2142, 2143c
Herniation of lumbar disc
assessment/diagnostic findings, 2142
clinical manifestations, 2142
medical management, 2142, 2144
nursing management, 2144–2145
surgical management
complications of disc surgery, 2144
Herpes simplex
assessment and diagnostic findings, 1798–1799
complications, 1799
medical management, 1799
types, 1798
Herpes simplex virus, 471, 474, 474c, 1044
Herpes simplex virus 2 (HSV-2), 1417–1418
clinical manifestations, 1418
medical management, 1418
pathophysiology, 1417–1418
Herpes simplex virus (HSV) encephalitis, 2092–2093
assessment and diagnostic findings, 2093
clinical manifestations, 2093
medical management, 2093
nursing management, 2093
pathophysiology, 2093
Herpes simplex virus-1, lip abnormalities, 920t
Herpes zoster, 1797, 1797f, 2111t
clinical manifestations, 1797–1798
medical management, 1798
nursing management, 1798
Herpes zoster ophthalmicus (HZO), 1798
Herpetic gingivostomatitis, gum abnormalities, 921t
Heterografts, 786
Heterotopic ossification, 2233, 2312
HEV. *See* Hepatitis E virus (HEV)
HF. *See* Heart failure (HF)
HGD. *See* High-grade dysplasia (HGD)
Hiatal hernia, 936
assessment and diagnostic findings, 936
clinical manifestations, 936
management, 936
Hiccupping, gastritis, 978
Hidradenitis suppurativa (HS), 1791
High blood pressure, hypertension, 878
High-density lipoprotein (HDL), 732, 878, 882
High-dose chemotherapy, 2187
High-dose radiation (HDR), 2165
High-efficiency particulate air (HEPA) filter, 397, 1583, 2340
High-flow oxygen delivery systems, 604
High-frequency chest wall oscillation (HFCWO), 610
High-frequency oscillatory support ventilators, 619–620
High-grade dysplasia (HGD), 940
High-grade squamous intraepithelial lesions (HGSIL), 1433
Highly active antiretroviral drug therapies (HAART), 1537
High-sensitivity assay for C-reactive protein (hs-CRP), 674
High vagal paralysis, 2111t
Hinchey classification, 1011
Hinge joints, 2218
Hip dislocation after replacement surgery, 2254c
Hip fracture, 2316–2319, 2320–2325c, 2325
care of older patient, nursing care plan, 2320–2325c
clinical manifestations, 2317
extracapsular fractures, 2317
gerontologic considerations, 2317–2318
intracapsular fractures, 2317
nursing management, 2318–2319
health promotion, 2325

Hip fracture (*continued*)
monitoring and managing complications, 2319
prevention of VTE, 2319, 2319c
promoting strengthening exercises, 2318–2319
repositioning the patient, 2318
periprosthetic fractures, 2317
surgical treatment, 2318, 2318f
Hip spica cast, 2232
Hirschsprung's disease, 998
Hirsutism, 1766
Histamine, 113, 838, 915, 1572, 1573–1574
gastrointestinal regulatory substances, 901t
Histamine-2 (H_2) antagonists, 1120
receptor, 939t, 983
Histiocytes, 1599, 1604
Histoplasma capsulatum, 2094
Histotoxic hypoxia, 603c
HIT with thrombosis (HITT), 865
thrombocytopenia, 865
HLA. *See* Human leukocyte antigen (HLA)
HMG-CoA reductase inhibitors, 735t, 736, 845
Hodgkin lymphoma, 1648–1650
assessment and diagnostic findings, 1649
clinical manifestations, 1648–1649, 1649f
medical management, 1649–1650
nursing management, 1650
pathophysiology, 1648
Hohn catheters, 968
Holding space, 83
Hollow screw technique, 1998
Holter monitors. *See* Continuous monitors
Holy writings, 85
Homans' sign, 863
Home blood pressure monitoring (HBPM), 882
Home care, 15–16
discharge planning for, 16
home visit, 16–18
agency's policies and, 16
assessment in, 17
bag with supplies and equipment, 16
documentation considerations for, 17
ending the visit, 18
initial home visit, 17
medication management in, 17
need for future visits, assessment of, 17–18, 18c
patient's referral form, 16
personal safety precautions, 17, 17c
nursing in home setting, 15–16
safety precautions in, 17c
Home care checklist
adrenocortical insufficiency, 1250
angina pectoris, 744c
ascites, 1066
asthma management, 594c
bone tumours, 2295c
cervical discectomy/cervical collar, 2143c
Cushing syndrome, 1254c
discharge after surgery, 419c
esophageal disorder, 942
gastric cancer, 992c
gastric surgery, 995c
gastritis, 980c
hand or foot surgery, 2273c
heart failure, 822c
hyperparathyroidism, 1243
hyperthyroidism, 1237c
hypoparathyroidism, 1244
hypothyroidism, 1230c
inflammatory bowel disease, 1022c
neck surgery, 933c
nervous system metastases, 2125c
oncologic disorder, 2180c
oral cavity disorders, 928c
osteoporosis and osteomalacia, 2285c
ostomy care, 1031c
oxygen therapy, 607c
parenteral nutrition, 973c
patients with closed fractures, 2305, 2306c
patient with amputation, 2333c
patient with cast, 2238c
patient with ICD, 726
patient with laryngectomy, 501c
patient with newly diagnosed diabetes, 1174c
peptic ulcer disease, 988c
recurrent pulmonary embolism prevention, 543c
rehabilitation, 204–205c
thoracotomy, 645c
ventilator care, 628c
Home care nurses, 234
Home, community-based, and transitional care
acute pancreatitis, 1122–1123
adrenocortical insufficiency, 1249
ascites, 1065
for bone tumours, 2294
cardiomyopathy, 793–794
cirrhosis, 1095
colorectal cancer, 1043
common problems of upper extremity, 2273
corticosteroid therapy, 1257–1258
Cushing syndrome, 1253–1254
diabetes as secondary diagnosis, 1188
diabetes mellitus, 1163–1164
diabetic retinopathy, 1178–1179
diverticular disease, 1013
gallbladder disease, 1117
gastric cancer, 991–992
gastric surgery, 994
gastritis, 980–981
heart failure, 821–823
hepatic encephalopathy, 1074
hepatitis B virus, 1080
hypertension, 891–892
hyperthyroidism, 1236
hypoglycemia, 1165
jaw disorders, 924
liver transplantation, 1102
in liver tumour, 1097–1098
oral cavity disorders, 928–929
osteomyelitis, 2289
pancreatic cancer, 1129
patient undergoing bariatric surgery, 1209
patient with newly diagnosed diabetes, 1172
pericarditis, 800
pheochromocytoma, 1248
thyroid cancer, 1240
tube feeding, 959
Home environment, assessment of, 70, 70c
Home health care agencies, 15
Home hemodialysis, 1309–1310
Homeless people
health conditions of, 19
nursing care for, 19–20
Homeostasis, 102–103, 296
Homeostatic mechanisms, 301, 329
adrenal glands, 301
antidiuretic hormone and thirst, 301
baroreceptors, 301
heart and blood vessel, 301
kidneys, 301
lungs, 301
osmoreceptors, 302
parathyroid glands, 301
pituitary gland, 301
release of atrial natriuretic peptide, 302–303
renin–angiotensin–aldosterone system, 301
Home ventilator care, criteria for, 627c
Home visits, 16–18
Homocysteine, 675
Homografts, 786
Homonymous hemianopsia, 2031t
HOPE Questions for Spiritual Assessment, 83, 85
Hormonal agents
antineoplastic, 2179t
in carcinogenesis, 2155–2156
Hormonal contraception
benefits and risks, 1397–1398, 1398c, 1399c
contraindications, 1398–1399
implants, 1400
injectable contraceptives, 1399–1400
intrauterine device, 1400
oral hormonal contraception, 1399
transdermal contraceptives, 1399
vaginal contraceptives, 1399
Hormone replacement therapy (HRT), 1379, 1446
Hormones
action and source of, 1216t
classification and action of, 1215–1217
function and regulation of, 1215
Hormone therapy (HT), 737, 1446, 1496, 1500
breast cancer, 1470–1471
in menopause, 1379
prostate cancer, 1496, 1500
Hospice, 2208
Hospice nursing, 15
Hospice palliative care, 238
focus of, 242
historical context, 238–239
legal and ethical contexts, 240
principles and components, 242–243
sociocultural context, 240–241
technologic context, 239–240
Hospice Palliative Care Nursing Standards of Practice, 239
Hospice services, 234
Hospital-acquired infections, 678
Hospital-acquired infective endocarditis, 795
Hospital-acquired pneumonia (HAP), 510–511
Hospital Insurance and Diagnostic Act of 1957, 6
Hospitalized postoperative patient, care of, 419–421
after surgery, 420–421
nursing process for, 421–434, 430t, 431t
receiving patient in clinical unit, 420
Host, 1698
Hot/cold theory of health and illness, 97
Hôtel-Dieu de Québec, 4
HPV-16, 926
HSCT. *See* Hematopoietic stem cell transplantation (HSCT)
Human B-lymphotropic virus, 1418
Human Genome Project, 112, 130, 132
Human immune deficiency virus (HIV), 1422–1423, 1537, 1542c
assessment and diagnostic findings, 1544–1545
care, aboriginal women's view, 1555c
clinical manifestations, 1550–1553
complementary, alternative and integrative modalities, 1554–1555
emotional and ethical concerns, 1568–1569

encephalopathy, 1534, 1552, 1552c
epidemiology, 1538
ethics and related issues, 1568c
gerontologic considerations, 1539
infection, 927, 937, 1080
acute, 1543
stages, 1543t
life with, 1423c
medical management, 1553–1554
nursing process, 1556, 1561–1568
assessment, 1561–1562
complications, 1562
evaluation, 1568
improving knowledge of, 1565–1568
nursing interventions, 1562–1565
nursing priorities, 1562
planning and goals, 1562
pathophysiology, 1541–1543
prevention, 1539–1540
reducing the risk of transmission, 1540–1541
risk factors, 1539c
stages, 1543–1544
standard precautions, 1541c
supportive care, 1555–1556
test, 1538, 1544–1545, 1545c
transmission, 1538
treatment, 1545–1550
Human immune deficiency virus type 1 (HIV-1), 1538
structure of, 1542f
Human insulins, 1152
Human leukocyte antigen (HLA), 1006, 1141, 1733
Human papillomavirus (HPV), 1390, 1416–1417
medical management, 1417
pathophysiology, 1416–1417
prevention, 1417
Human trafficking, 2374–2375
Humeral neck, fractures of, 2312–2313, 2313f
Humeral shaft, fractures of, 2313, 2313f
Humoral immune response, 1517, 1519
Humoral immunity, 1604
Huntington's disease, 141t, 143, 1969. *See also* Degenerative disorders
assessment/diagnostic findings, 2135
care of patient with, 2136c
clinical manifestations, 2134–2135
medical management, 2135
pathophysiology, 2134
HVPG. *See* Hepatic venous pressure gradient (HVPG)
Hydralazine (Apresoline), 813, 2049
in heart failure, 813
hypertension, 886t
Hydration therapy
ethical dilemma, 962c
hyperparathyroidism, 1242
tube feeding, 959
Hydrocele, 1480, 1509
Hydrochloric acid (HCl), 899, 900, 901t
Hydrochlorothiazide (HydroDIURIL), 820t
hypertension, 884t
thalassemia, 1628
Hydrochlorothiazide (Microxide), interaction with anesthetics, 382t
Hydrocodone (Vicodin), 281t
Hydrocolloids, 1785
Hydrocortisone (Solu-Cortef), 1018
Hydrofiber™ Technology dressings, 1785–1786
Hydrofibre, 1045
Hydroflumethiazide (Diucardin, Saluron), 820t
Hydrogels, 1785
Hydrogen breath test, 907
Hydrogen peroxide, 2350
Hydromer, 949
Hydromorphone (Dilaudid), 287, 1120
Hydrophilic colloids, 1005
Hydrophilic (water-absorbing) surface, 1786
Hydrophobic (water-resistant) surface, 1786
Hydrostatic force, 837
Hydrostatic pressure, 298, 299
Hydrotherapy, 1854
Hydroxychloroquine (Plaquenil), in rheumatoid arthritis, 1744
Hydroxypropyl methylcellulose, 1894
Hydroxyurea, 1623, 1809
Hydroxyzine (Atarax), 1789, 1813
for postoperative nausea/vomiting, 416t
Hygiene, of hospitalized diabetic patients, 1186
Hygroscopic agents, 1787
Hymen, 1373
Hyperaldosteronism, 314
hypertension, 878
Hyperbaric oxygen therapy, 199, 606, 870
Hyperbilirubinemia, 1060
Hypercalcemia, 318t, 320–322, 1350, 2206t, 2294
assessment and diagnostic findings, 321
clinical manifestations, 321
medical management, 321–322
nursing management, 322
pathophysiology, 320–321
Hypercalcemic crisis, 321, 1242
Hyperchloremia, 327t, 328
assessment and diagnostic findings, 328
clinical manifestations, 328
medical management, 328
nursing management, 328
pathophysiology, 328
Hyperchloremic acidosis, 329. *See also* Metabolic acidosis
Hyperchlorhydria, 978
Hypercholesterolemia, 133
Hypercontractile esophagus, 935
Hyperdynamic cardiomyoplasty, 789
Hyperemia, 1773t
Hyperglycemia, 380, 2049, 2066
enteral therapy, 956t
in hospitalized diabetic patients, 1184
parenteral nutrition, 970t
patient with newly diagnosed diabetes, 1172
in shock, 342
Hyperglycemic hyperosmolar nonketotic syndrome (HHNS), 1169, 1169t
assessment and diagnostic findings, 1169–1170
clinical manifestations, 1169
insulin resistance in, 1169, 1169t
medical management, 1170
nursing management, 1170
Hyperglycemic hyperosmolar syndrome (HHS), 1137
Hyperhomocysteinemia, 845, 1671, 1674
Hyperinsulinism, 1131
Hyperkalemia, 314t, 315–318, 1288, 1294
assessment and diagnostic findings, 316
clinical manifestations, 316
medical management, 316–317
metabolic acidosis and, 330
nursing management, 317–318
pathophysiology, 316
Hyperlipidemia, 142t
and heart failure, 806, 815
Hypermagnesemia, 322t, 324
assessment and diagnostic findings, 324
clinical manifestations, 324
medical management, 324
nursing management, 324
pathophysiology, 324
Hypermetabolism, 1862
Hypernatremia, 310t, 312–313, 343
assessment and diagnostic findings, 313
clinical manifestations, 312
medical management, 313
nursing management, 313
pathophysiology, 312
Hyperopia, 1888
Hyperparathyroidism, 1350
assessment and diagnostic findings, 1241
causes of, 1241
clinical manifestations, 1241
complications, 1242
home care checklist, 1243
medical management, 1241–1242
nursing management, 1242
Hyperphosphatemia, 325t, 326–327
assessment and diagnostic findings, 326
clinical manifestations, 326
medical management, 326
nursing management, 326–327
pathophysiology, 326
Hyperpigmentation, 1772–1773, 1795
Hyperplasia, 110, 110t, 2150
Hyperpnea, 301
Hyperresonance, 65
Hypersensitivity, 1571, 1572
chemical mediators of, 1573t
Hypersensitivity reactions, by chemotherapeutic agents, 2181–2182
Hypertension, 845, 877, 889, 999, 1100, 1922
assessment and diagnostic findings, 882–888
and cardiovascular disease, 736–737
cardiovascular risk, assessment of, 888–893
clinical manifestations, 881
collaborative problems/potential complications, 889
complications of, 881–882
defined, 653, 736
diagnosis of, 882
diets, 883
and dysrhythmias, 416
follow-up, 888
and health behaviours, 879c
heart failure, 805, 806
lifestyle modifications, 883t
liver transplantation, 1100–1101
masked, 881
measuring blood pressure, 890c
medical management
global vascular protection therapy, 887
pharmacologic therapy, 883–887
medication therapy, 884t
monitoring and managing complications, 892
nursing interventions, 889–890
nursing priorities, 889
nursing research profile, 879c
pathophysiology, 879–881
primary, 879–880
secondary, 880
patient outcomes, 892–893
peripheral arterial disease, 845
planning and goals, 889
primary, 878
promoting adherence to therapeutic regimen, 890
risk factors, 878c

Hypertension (*continued*)
self-care, 891–892
therapeutic program, 890
transitional care, 892
white coat, 881
Hypertension Canada, 887
Hypertension-related eye changes, 1922
Hypertension urgency, diastolic blood pressure, 882
Hypertensive crises, 893
Hypertensive emergency, 878, 893
Hypertensive encephalopathy, 1287
Hypertensive peristalsis, 935
Hypertensive urgency, 878, 893
Hyperthermia (thermal therapy), 2189
Hyperthermia, in sepsis, 364
Hyperthyroidism, 1223
assessment and diagnostic findings, 1231
clinical manifestations, 1231
definition, 1231
gerontologic considerations, 1234–1235
home care checklist, 1237c
medical management, 1231–1234
adjunctive therapy, 1233–1234
antithyroid medications, 1233, 1233t
pharmacotherapy, 1232
radioactive iodine therapy, 1232–1233
surgical management, 1234
nursing process, 1235–1236
pruritus in, 1790
Hypertonic crystalloid solution, 350–351
Hypertonic fluids, 333, 335
Hypertrichosis, 1788
Hypertrophic cardiomyopathy (HCM), 788
Hypertrophic pharyngitis, 481
Hypertrophy, 110, 110t, 878
Hyperuricemia, 813, 817
Hyperventilation therapy, 2001
Hypervolemia, 307–309
assessment and diagnostic findings, 307
and azotemia, 308
clinical manifestations, 305t, 307
medical management, 308
dialysis, 308
nutritional therapy, 308
pharmacologic therapy, 308
nursing management, 308–309
detecting hypervolemia, 309
edema assessment, 308–309
patient education, 309
preventing hypervolemia, 309
pathophysiology, 307
Hyphae, 1412
Hyphema, 1913
Hypnosis, for pain relief, 291
Hypoalbuminemia, 1017, 1288, 1318
in blistering diseases, 1813
Hypocalcemia, 318–320, 318t
assessment and diagnostic findings, 319–320, 320c
clinical manifestations, 319
Chvostek's sign, 319, 319f
osteoporosis, 319
seizures, 319
tetany, 319
Trousseau's sign, 319, 319f
kidney injury and, 319
medical management, 320
emergency pharmacologic therapy, 320
nutritional therapy, 320
nursing management, 320
pathophysiology, 319
transient, 319
Hypochloremia, 327–328, 327t
assessment and diagnostic findings, 328
clinical manifestations, 327–328
medical management, 328
nursing management, 328
pathophysiology, 327
Hypochlorhydria, 978
Hypochromia, 1599, 1627
Hypoglycemia, 380, 1137, 1144, 1164
assessment and diagnostic findings, 1164
clinical manifestations, 1164
CNS function, impairment of, 1164
gerontologic considerations, 1164
in hospitalized diabetic patients, 1184
management
home and community-based care, 1164
immediate treatment, 1164
initiating emergency measures, 1165
patient education, 1165
patient with newly diagnosed diabetes, 1172
sulfonylurea and, 1156
Hypoglycemic effect, 1108
Hypoglycemic unawareness, in autonomic neuropathy, 1181
Hypokalemia, 313–315, 314t, 1002
assessment and diagnostic findings, 314–315
clinical manifestations, 314
medical management, 315
and metabolic alkalosis, 330
nursing management, 315
pathophysiology, 314
patient with newly diagnosed diabetes, 1172
Hypokinesia, 2128
Hypomagnesemia
assessment and diagnostic findings, 323
clinical manifestations, 323
medical management, 323
nursing management, 323–324
pathophysiology, 322–323
Hyponatremia, 309–312, 310t, 2066
acute, 309
assessment and diagnostic findings, 311
chronic, 309–310
clinical manifestations, 310–311, 310f
exercise-associated, 310
medical management, 311
pharmacologic therapy, 311
sodium replacement, 311
water restriction, 311
nursing management, 311–312
detection and control, 312
fluid needs, 312
neurologic signs, 312
pathophysiology, 310
and SIADH, 310
Hypoparathyroidism
home care checklist, 1244
nursing management, 1244
Hypopharyngeal sphincter, 934
Hypophosphatemia, 324–326, 325t
assessment and diagnostic findings, 325
clinical manifestations, 325
in malnourished patients, 325
medical management, 326
nursing management, 326
pathophysiology, 325
Hypophysectomy, pituitary tumours, 1220
Hypophysis. *See* Pituitary gland
Hypopigmentation, 1772, 1795
Hypoproliferative anemia, 1613–1615
anemia of chronic disease, 1615–1616
anemias in renal disease, 1615
aplastic anemia, 1616–1617
iron deficiency anemia, 1613–1615
megaloblastic anemias, 1617
Hypospadias, 1510
Hypotension
defined, 653
during ERCP, 1111
and shock, 415
Hypothalamic–pituitary–thyroid axis, 1222f
Hypothalamus, 1961, 1965
in stress response, 105, 106f
Hypothermia, 406, 2356
active external rewarming, 2356
active internal rewarming, 2356
assessment and diagnostic findings, 2356
in exfoliative dermatitis, 1813
prevention of, 1817
supportive care, 2356
urban, 2356
vital signs monitoring, 2356
Hypothyroidism, 998, 1223
causes of, 1225–1226, 1225c
clinical manifestations, 1226
gerontologic considerations, 1230–1231
home care checklist, 1230c
medical management
cardiac dysfunction prevention, 1227
medication interactions prevention, 1227
pharmacologic therapy, 1226
nursing care plan, 1229c, 1230c
nursing management
continuing care and transitional care, 1227
self-care, patient education about, 1227
Hypotonic fluids, 333, 335
Hypoventilation, risk factors for, 460
Hypovolemia, 304–307, 554, 1015, 1021, 1030, 1039
assessment and diagnostic findings, 304
clinical manifestations, 304, 305t
gerontologic considerations, 304–305
medical management, 305
fluid challenge test, 305
water and electrolyte solutions, 306t
nursing management, 307
assessment for FVD, 307
mental function, 307
prevention and correction, 307
skin and tongue turgor, 307
urine concentration, 307
vital signs, 307
pathophysiology, 304
Hypovolemic shock, 341, 353–356, 415, 1721, 2260, 2348–2349
acute pancreatitis and, 1122
medical management, 354–355
fluid and blood replacement, 354–355, 355t
fluid redistribution, 355
patient positioning, 355, 355f
pharmacologic therapy, 355
treatment of underlying cause, 354
nursing management, 355–356
blood transfusions, 356
fluids and medications administration, 356
oxygen administration, 356
pathophysiology, 354, 354f
Hypoxemia, 439, 447, 554, 601
defined, 602
Hypoxemic hypoxia, 603c
Hypoxia, 109, 111, 439, 602, 1120
general anesthesia and, 406
types of, 603

Hysterectomy, 1412, 1440
  nursing process, 1440–1442
Hysterosalpingography (HSG), 1393
  for pelvic examination, 1393
Hysteroscopy, 1373, 1392

I

IABP. *See* Intra-aortic balloon pump (IABP)
IADLs. *See* Instrumental activities of daily living (IADLs)
Iatrogenic incontinence, 1332, 1341. *See also* Urinary incontinence
IBD. *See* Inflammatory bowel disease (IBD)
Ibritumomab tiuxetan (Zevalin), for non-Hodgkin's lymphomas, 1651
Ibrutinib (Imbruvica), for chronic lymphocytic leukemia, 1642
IBS. *See* Irritable bowel syndrome (IBS)
Ibuprofen, 858
  breast pain, 1455
  chronic lower back pain, 996
  pain management, 285
  pericarditis, 799
  premenstrual syndrome, 1395
  rheumatoid arthritis, 1745
Ibutilide, antiarrhythmic medication, 699t
ICD. *See* Implantable cardioverter defibrillator (ICD)
ICDSC. *See* Intensive Care Delirium Screening Checklist
Ice therapy, for pain relief, 290
Idarubicin (Idamycin), for acute myeloid leukemia, 1637
Idarucizumab (Praxbind), 865
Idelalisib (Zydelig), for chronic lymphocytic leukemia, 1642
Idionodal rhythm, 706
Idiopathic inflammatory myopathies, 1752
Idioventricular rhythm, 709–710
IFN. *See* Interferons (IFN)
Ifosfamide. *See* Alkylating agents
IgA. *See* Immunoglobulin A (IgA)
IL. *See* Interleukins (IL)
Ileal conduit, 1332, 1358–1363
  complications, 1358–1359
  nursing management, 1359–1363
Ileal dysfunction, 1007t
Ileocecal valve, 898, 902
Ileostomy, 998, 1019, 1030c
  continent, 1019, 1027, 1030c
  Crohn's disease, 1016t
  proctocolectomy, 1019
  total colectomy, 1019
  ulcerative colitis, 1016t
Illness
  causes of, 96
    biomedical/scientific view, 96
    magico-religious view, 97
    naturalistic/holistic perspective, 96–97
  course of, 121
  extenuating circumstances
    dying and death, 125
    healthy and unhealthy coping strategies, 125
    posttraumatic stress disorder, 124–125
    substance abuse, 125–126
  family considerations in, 126–127
  and incapacitation, 121
  onset of, 120
  outcome, 121
  psychosocial typology of, 120–121
  responses to, 120, 121
    anxiety, 121–122, 122c
    depression, 122–123, 123c
    loss and grief, 123–124
    suicide, 123, 123c
  and stigma, 121
  stress and maladaptation in models of, 108
Image-guided radiation therapy (IGRT), 2164
Imagery, 384
Imatinib mesylate (Gleevec), for chronic myeloid leukemia, 1638
Imipramine (Tofranil)
  antidepressant therapy, 1554
  urinary retention, 1345
Imiquimod (Aldara), for human papillomavirus, 1417
Immigration and tuberculosis, 1728–1729
Immune, 1698
Immune complex (type III) hypersensitivity, 1574
Immune dysfunction, assessing for, 1526c
Immune functions of skin, 1769
Immune globulin, 1076
Immune hemolytic anemia, 1628–1629
  assessment and diagnostic findings, 1628
  clinical manifestations, 1628
  medical management, 1628–1629
  nursing management, 1629
Immune reconstitution inflammatory syndrome (IRIS), 1534, 1550
Immune response, 1517, 1518
Immune system, 112, 1517
  anatomy
    bone marrow, 1516
    lymphoid tissues, 1517
  assessment of
    health history, 1525–1531
  diagnostic evaluation, 1531
  disorder, 1517t
  function, 1517–1518
    acquired immunity, 1519
    cellular immune response, 1522–1523
    complement system, 1523–1524
    humoral immune response, 1521–1522
    immunomodulators, 1524–1525
    natural immunity, 1518–1519
    response to invasion, 1519–1521, 1520f, 1521f
  medications and effects on, 1530t
  role of, in cancer, 2156
    normal immune responses and, 2156
Immune thrombocytopenic purpura (ITP), 1661–1663
  assessment and diagnostic findings, 1662
  clinical manifestations, 1661–1662
  medical management, 1662
  nursing management, 1663
  pathophysiology, 1661
Immunity, 1516, 1517
  acquired, 1518
  natural, 1518
Immunization, hepatitis B virus, 1079–1080
Immunocompromised host, pneumonia in, 511
Immunofluorescence testing, 1780
Immunogenicity, 2156
Immunoglobulin, 1521, 1572
  characteristics, 1522c
  therapy, managing, 1536c
Immunoglobulin A (IgA), 1007, 1333
Immunoglobulin G (IgG), 1285
Immunoglobulinopathy, 1007t
Immunologic disorders, 1529c
Immunologic status, 1531c
Immunology, advances in, 1525
Immunomodulators, 1524–1525, 1654
  asthma, 591
  inflammatory bowel disease, 1018
Immunopathology, 1516, 1517
Immunoregulation, 1517, 1519
Immunosenescence, 1517, 1525
Immunosuppressant drugs, 2187
Immunosuppression-associated KS, 1826
Immunotherapy
  allergic rhinitis, 1585–1587
  indications and contraindications, 1586c
  liver tumours, 1096
Impaired cerebellar function, 1969
Impaired fasting glucose (IFG), 1137, 1138
Impaired glucose tolerance (IGT), 1137, 1138, 1139t
Impaired liver function, nursing care, 1086c–1093c
Impaired physical mobility. *See* Physical mobility, impaired
Impaired skin integrity, 193–200. *See also* skin integrity, impaired
Impaired vision, hypertension, 878
Impairment, 166, 174
Impetigo, 1286
  clinical manifestations, 1795
  medical management, 1795–1796
  nursing management, 1796
Implantable cardioverter defibrillator (ICD), 692, 709. *See also* Adjunctive modalities/management
  cardiomyopathy, 789
  effective coping, 725, 726c
  home care checklist, 726c
  home, community-based/transitional care, 725
  infection prevention, 725
  nursing management with, 724–725
  overview, 723–724, 723f
Implanted hearing devices, 1953
Implanted ports, 967, 969
  vascular access, 969
Implants, 1400
Impotence and priapism, 1626
Impruv, 1806
Inadequate water intake, tube feeding, 958
Incapacitation, 121
Incentive spirometry, 384, 602
  indications, 607
  nursing management, 607, 608c
  patient education about, 608c
Incisional biopsy, 1453, 2160
Incontinence pads, 202
Increased intracranial pressure (ICP), 1987, 1995–1996, 2057, 2111t. *See also* Primary brain tumours
  assessment and diagnostic findings, 1997
  cerebral response to, 1996
  clinical manifestations, 1996–1997
  collaborative problems/potential complications, 2001
  complications, 1997
  detecting
    early signs and symptoms, 2005c
    later signs and symptoms, 2005c
  effect of hypothermia, 2000
  electronic medical record for measuring, 2063c
  headache, 2119
  management during intracranial surgery, 2010–2011
  medical management, 1997–2000
    controlling fever, 2000
    decreasing cerebral edema, 1999–2000

Increased intracranial pressure (*continued*)
maintaining cerebral perfusion, 2000
maintaining oxygenation and reducing metabolic demands, 2000
monitoring intracranial pressure and cerebral oxygenation, 1998–1999
reducing cerebrospinal fluid and intracranial blood volume, 2000
monitoring, 1998
cerebral oxygenation, 1998–1999
epidural monitor in, 1998
fibre optic, 1998
interpreting intracranial pressure waveforms, 1998–1999
intracranial pressure, 1998–1999, 1998f, 2005–2006
LICOX catheter system, 1999f
microdialysis, 1999
neurologic, 1999
oxygen saturation in jugular venous bulb, 1999
secondary complications, 2006
subarachnoid screw or bolt for, 1998
of venous jugular esaturations, 1999
ventriculostomy for, 1998
Monro–Kellie hypothesis, 1996
nursing interventions
achieving adequate breathing pattern, 2001
airway maintenance, 2001
for cerebral edema, 2004t
cerebral tissue perfusion, optimization of, 2001–2004
for hypercapnia, 2004t
hyperventilation therapy, 2001
for hypoxia, 2001, 2004t
for impaired venous return, 2004t
for increase in intrathoracic or abdominal pressure, 2004t
infection prevention, 2005
monitoring and managing potential complications, 2005–2006
negative fluid balance maintenance, 2004
neurologic assessment flow chart, 2002f–2003f
patient outcomes, 2006
planning and goals, 2001
nursing priorities, 2001
pathophysiology, 1996
cerebral edema, 1996
decreased cerebral blood flow, 1996
patient assessment, 2000–2001
seizures, 2119–2120
SIADH and, 1997
visual disturbances, 2119
vomiting, 2119
Incubation period, 1697, 1698
Indapamide (Lozol), hypertension, 884t
Indiana Pouch, 1363
Indigestion, 903
Indirect ophthalmoscopy, 1886
Indolent neoplasms, 1633
Indomethacin (Indocin), for gout, 1758
Induced abortion, 1403–1404
medical management, 1403
nursing management, 1404
Induration, 505
Indwelling catheters, 1347
gerontologic considerations
intermittent self-catheterization, 1349–1350
minimizing trauma, 1348
preventing infection, 1348
retraining the bladder, 1348–1349
nursing management, 1347–1348
suprapubic catheters, 1347
Infections, 1698, 2111t
bacterial skin
folliculitis, 1796–1797
impetigo, 1795–1796
Candida (yeast), 1779
dermatophyte, 1779
of eye structures, 1913–1918, 1914t
fungal (mycotic) skin, 1799
IV therapy and, 336
liver transplantation, 1101
microorganisms for catheter-related, 971
parasitic skin infestation
pediculosis corporis, 1801
pediculosis pubis, 1801
pediculus humanus capitis, 1799–1801
scabies, 1801–1802
prevention, 967c, 1206–1207
primary skin, 1795
pulmonary, 2085
secondary candidal (yeast), 1792
secondary skin, 1782–1783, 1795
skin, 1779
stages of, 923
tinea (ringworm), 1798, 1799t
UTIs, 2085
viral skin
herpes simplex, 1798–1799
herpes zoster, 1797–1798
Infectious dermatoses
bacterial skin infections, 1795–1797
fungal (mycotic) skin infections, 1799
parasitic skin infestation, 1799–1802
viral skin infections, 1797–1799
Infectious disease, 1698, 1705–1706
care of patient with, 1713c–1718c
causative organisms, routes of transmission, 1699t–1700t
chain of infection, 1697–1700
Chlamydia trachomatis, 1723
assessment and diagnostic findings, 1723
clinical manifestations, 1723
complications, 1723
medical management, 1723
nursing management, 1723–1724
colonization, 1705
diarrheal diseases
Calicivirus, 1719
Campylobacter infections, 1718
causes, 1712, 1718
Cryptosporidium, 1719
Escherichia coli, 1719
Giardia, 1719
Salmonella infection, 1718–1719
Shigella infection, 1719
transmission, 1712
vibrio cholerae, 1719–1720
emerging infectious diseases
Ebola virus disease, 1726–1727
Legionnaires' disease, 1727
pertussis, 1727–1728
West Nile virus, 1726
Zika virus, 1725–1726
hand hygiene methods, 1702c
health care–associated infection potential
antimicrobial-resistant organisms, 1706–1707
bloodstream infections, 1707–1708
home care checklist, 1705c
minimize the risk of infection
additional precautions, 1703
administrative measures, 1701
engineering measures, 1700–1701
home-based care, 1703–1705
routine practices, 1701–1703
Neisseria gonorrhoeae, 1723
assessment and diagnostic findings, 1723
clinical manifestations, 1723
complications, 1723
medical management, 1723
nursing management, 1723–1724
nursing process, 1720–1721
preventing infection
avian influenza pandemic, 1710
immunization programs, 1709–1710
influenza pandemic, 1710
prevention and control, 1697
sexually transmitted infection, 1721–1722
HIV, 1722
nursing process, 1724–1725
syphilis
assessment and diagnostic findings, 1722–1723
medical management, 1723
nursing management, 1723
stages, 1722
travel and immigration
AIDS, 1728
immigration and tuberculosis, 1728–1729
immigration and vector-borne diseases, 1729
Infectious neurologic disorders
arthropod-borne virus encephalitis, 2093–2094
brain abscesses, 2091–2092
Creutzfeldt–Jakob disease, 2095–2096
fungal encephalitis, 2094–2095
herpes simplex virus (HSV) encephalitis, 2092–2093
meningitis, 2088–2091
variant Creutzfeldt–Jakob disease, 2095–2096
Infective endocarditis, 780, 787, 794–797
assessment and diagnostic findings, 795–796
clinical manifestations, 795
medical management, 796
nursing management, 797
pathophysiology, 795
prevention, 796
risk factors for, 795c
surgical management, 796–797
Inference, 22
Infertility, 1404–1406, 2200
diagnostic findings
male factors, 1405
ovarian and ovulation factors, 1404
tubal and uterine factors, 1404–1405
medical management
artificial insemination, 1405–1406
assisted reproductive technologies, 1406
pharmacologic therapy, 1405, 1405c
nursing management, 1406
primary, 1404
secondary, 1404
Infertility Awareness Association of Canada (IAAC), 1406
Infiltrating ductal carcinoma, 1457. *See also* Breast cancer
Infiltrating lobular carcinoma, 1457. *See also* Breast cancer
Infiltration, 336
assessing for, 337c

monitoring of insertion site for, 336
treatment, 337
Inflammation, 113–114
acute, 113–114
and atherosclerosis, 730
chemical mediators of, 113
chronic, 114
of cranial arteries, 2023
of eye structures, 1913–1918, 1914t
subacute, 114
systemic response to, 113
Inflammatory bowel disease (IBD), 998, 1000, 1015
Crohn's disease, 1016–1017, 1016t
diarrhea, 1000
gallbladder, 1108
home care checklist, 1022c
nursing process, 1020–1023
ulcerative colitis, 1017–1020
Inflammatory carcinoma, 1457. *See also* Tubular ductal carcinoma
Inflammatory disease, 909
Inflammatory response, 113, 113f
Infliximab, anal fistula, 1045
Influenza vaccine, 232, 570, 1710
Informed consent, 24, 376–377
emancipated minor and, 377
signed consent form, 377
valid, 377c
voluntary consent, 376
in writing, 376
Infrapatellar tendinitis, 2300
Infratentorial approach, to intracranial surgery, 2006–2013
ethics and related issues, 2008c
home care checklist after, 2012c
nursing interventions
aseptic technique, 2011
cerebral edema, management of, 2010
cerebral tissue perfusion maintenance, 2009
continuing and transitional care, 2012
enhancing self-image, 2010
fluid and electrolyte disturbances, management of, 2011
improving pulmonary function/gas exchange, 2010
infection prevention, 2011
intracranial hematoma, management of, 2010
monitoring and managing potential complications, 2010–2011
monitoring for increased intracranial pressure and bleeding, 2010–2011
monitoring for seizure activity, 2011
pressure ulcers, management of, 2011
promoting home, community-based, and transitional care, 2011–2012
sensory deprivation management, 2010
SIADH, management of, 2011
status epilepticus, management of, 2011
temperature regulation, 2009–2010
patient assessment, 2008–2009
patient outcomes, 2012–2013
postoperative management
anticonvulsant medication for, 2008
cerebral edema, reduction of, 2008
collaborative problems/potential complications, 2009
medical management, 2013
monitoring intracranial pressure, 2008
nursing priorities, 2009
pain management, 2008
planning and goals, 2009
seizure prevention, 2008
ventilatory support, 2008
preoperative management
medical management, 2006–2007
nursing management, 2007–2008
risk of postoperative seizures, 2007
Infundibulum of hypothalamus, 1961
Infusion Nurses Society (INS), 2201
Ingestion, 899
of food, 900
Ingrown toenail, 2274
Inhalants abuse, 2367t
Inhaled anesthetic agents, 399
delivery methods, 399, 400f
gases, 399, 400t
volatile liquid agents, 399, 400t
Inheritance patterns, 135
autosomal dominant inheritance, 135–136, 135f
dominant and recessive, 135
multifactorial genetic conditions, 137–138, 137f, 138f
nontraditional inheritance, 138
patterns of Mendelian inheritance, 136t
Inhibited, defined, 692
Injectable contraceptives, 1399–1400
Injury prevention, 2350–2351
automatic protection, 2351
education for, 2351
legislation for, 2351
surgical patient, 409–410
Innate immune functions of skin, 1769
Inner ear, 1927–1928. *See also* Ear
conditions
Ménière's disease, 1944–1946
motion sickness, 1944
membranous labyrinth, 1928
organ of Corti, 1928
perfusion, 1946
Inotropic medications, cardiogenic shock, 827
Inotropy, 692, 693
INR. *See* International normalized ratio (INR)
Insect stings, 2358–2359, 2359c
Insensible perspiration, 1768
Inspection, in physical assessment, 64
Inspiratory force, 460
Inspiratory muscle training, 573
Institute for Safe Medication Practices (ISMP), 952
Institutional ethics committees, 28
Instrumental activities of daily living (IADLs), 167, 178, 218
Insufflation, 1392
Insulin, 1137, 1150
complications of therapy
insulin resistance, 1152
lipodystrophy, 1152
local allergic reaction, 1152
morning hyperglycemia, 1155, 1155t
systemic allergic reactions, 1152
delivery methods
insulin pens, 1155
transplantation of pancreatic cells, 1156
delivery methods, alternate
insulin pumps, 1155–1156
insulin syringe, 1155f
jet injectors, 1155
diabetic ketoacidosis, 1165–1166
to lower blood glucose, 1107–1108
misconceptions related to treatment, 1171
regimens, 1151–1152, 1153t–1154t, 1156
conventional, 1152
intensive, 1152
resistance, 1138, 1152
self administration of, education of, 1161–1163
inserting needle, 1163
preparing injection, 1162
selecting and rotating injection site, 1162–1163, 1162f
selecting syringes, 1161–1162
skin preparation, 1163
storing insulin, 1161
withdrawing insulin, 1162
self administration of, teaching of
selecting and rotating injection site, 1162f
syringe, 1155f
therapy and preparations, 1150–1156
time course of action, 1150–1151
types of insulin, 1151t
waning, 1152
Insulin aspart (NovoRapid), 1151
Insulin detemir (Levemir), 1151
Insulin glargine (Lantus), 1151
Insulin (Humalog), interaction with anesthetics, 382t
Insulin-like growth factor-1 (IGF-I), 2217
Insulin lispro (Humalog), 1151
Insulinoma, 1131
Intake and output (I&O), 952
Integra, 1860
Integrase strand transfer inhibitors (INSTI), 1545
Integument. *See also* Skin
anatomic and physiologic overview, 1764–1770
assessment of, 1770–1779
colour changes, 1772, 1772f, 1773t
cyanosis, 1772
erythema, 1772
health history, 1770
inspection and palpation, 1772
patients with dark skin, 1773
physical examination, 1772–1779
rashes, 1772
conditions influenced by genetic factors, 1771c
Integumentary system, age-related changes in, 214t, 216
Intellectual integrity, 22
Intelligence test, 222
Intensity, 1933
Intensity-modulated radiation therapy (IMRT), 2164
Intensive Care Delirium Screening Checklist (ICDSC), 349
Interactive dressings, 1783
Interdisciplinary team, in rehabilitation practice, 175–176, 176c
Interferon alfa-2b (Intron-A), in polycythemia, 1631
Interferon beta-1a (Rebif), 2097
Interferon beta-1b (Betaseron), 2097
Interferons (IFN), 1517, 1524, 2191
Interleukin-5 (IL-5), 1524
Interleukin 2 (IL-2), in kidney cancer, 1291
Interleukins (IL), 2191
Intermittent claudication, 835, 839
Intermittent mandatory ventilation (IMV), 602, 620
Intermittent pneumatic compression devices, 866
Intermittent self-catheterization, 201–202
Internal capsule, 1967
Internal carotid artery (ICA), 2047
Internal radiation implantation, 2164–2165

International Association for the Study of Pain, 266
International Council of Nurses (ICN), 4, 26
International Federation of Gynecology and Obstetrics (FIGO), 1433
International normalized ratio (INR), 704, 864, 1099, 1606
International Prognostic Index (IPI), 1651
Internet learning, 41
Interpretation, 22
Interpreter, use of, 93
Interprofessional collaboration, 243
Interprofessional collaborative practice, 11
Interstitial cystitis, 1332, 1350
Interstitial HDR, 2165
Interstitial nephritis, 1283, 1295, 1331, 1332
Interventions
 cardiomyopathy, 793–794
 colorectal cancer
  body image, 1041
  colostomy appliance, 1040–1041
  emotional support, 1039–1040
  home and community-based care, 1043
  postoperative care, 1040
  preparing the patient for surgery, 1039
  sexuality issues, 1043
 diabetes as secondary diagnosis, 1188–1189
 esophagus, 940
 gallbladder disease, 1116–1118
 gastric cancer, 990–992
 heart failure, 818–819, 818–823
 liver transplantation, 1101–1102
 neck dissection, 930–934
 patient with newly diagnosed diabetes, 1171–1172
 peptic ulcer disease, 986
 pericarditis, 800
Intestinal gas, gastrointestinal tract, 903
Intestinal obstruction, 1031–1033
 causes of, 1032f
 functional, 1031
 large bowel
  assessment and diagnostic findings, 1033
  clinical manifestations, 1033
  medical management, 1033
  nursing management, 1033
  pathophysiology, 1033
 mechanical, 1031, 1032t
 small bowel
  assessment and diagnostic findings, 1032
  clinical manifestations, 1032
  medical management, 1032–1033
  nursing management, 1033
  pathophysiology, 1031–1032
Intestinal peristalsis, 902
Intestinal surgery, complications and nursing interventions, 1041t
Intimal hyperplasia, 852
Intima, of arterial wall, 730
Intimate partner violence (IPV), 1382–1384, 2371–2373, 2372c
Intra-aortic balloon counterpulsation, in cardiogenic shock, 358
Intra-aortic balloon pump (IABP), 827, 827f
Intra-arterial blood pressure monitoring, 687
Intracavitary radioisotopes, 2165
Intracerebral hemorrhage, 2047
Intracranial aneurysms, 2047
 surgical intervention, 2050
Intracranial hemorrhage, 2059–2061
Intracranial neoplasms, 2047
Intracranial surgery, 2111t
 approaches
  comparison of, 2007t
  infratentorial, 2006–2013
  supratentorial, 2006–2013
  transsphenoidal, 2006, 2013
 burr holes in, 2006, 2006f
 craniotomy, 2006
 ethics and related issues, 2008c
 home care checklist after, 2012c
 medical management
  supratentorial and infratentorial approaches, 2006–2007
  transsphenoidal approach, 2013
 monitoring
  for increased intracranial pressure and bleeding, 2010–2011
  of potential complications, 2010–2011
  for seizure activity, 2011
 nursing interventions
  aseptic technique, 2011
  cerebral edema, management of, 2010
  cerebral tissue perfusion maintenance, 2009
  continuing and transitional care, 2012
  enhancing self-image, 2010
  fluid and electrolyte disturbances, management of, 2011
  improving pulmonary function/gas exchange, 2010
  increased intracranial pressure and bleeding, monitoring for, 2010–2011
  infection prevention, 2011
  intracranial hematoma, management of, 2010
  potential complications, monitoring and managing, 2010–2011
  pressure ulcers, management of, 2011
  promoting home, community-based, and transitional care, 2011–2012
  seizure activity, monitoring for, 2011
  sensory deprivation management, 2010
  SIADH, management of, 2011
  status epilepticus, management of, 2011
  temperature regulation, 2009–2010
 nursing management
  supratentorial and infratentorial approaches, 2007–2008
  transsphenoidal approach, 2013
 patient assessment, 2008–2009
 patient outcomes, 2012–2013
 postoperative management
  anticonvulsant medication for, 2008
  cerebral edema, reduction of, 2008
  collaborative problems/potential complications, 2009
  medical management, 2013
  monitoring intracranial pressure, 2008
  nursing priorities, 2009
  pain management, 2008
  planning and goals, 2009
  seizure prevention, 2008
  transsphenoidal approach, 2013
  ventilatory support, 2008
 preoperative management
  medical management, 2006–2007, 2013
  nursing management, 2007–2008, 2013
  transsphenoidal approach, 2013
Intracranial tumour, 2111t
Intracytoplasmic sperm injection (ICSI), 1406
Intraductal papilloma, 1456
Intragastric balloon therapy, 1201
Intralesional therapy, 1788
Intralipids, 948
Intraluminal brachytherapy, 2165
Intramural diverticulosis, 937
Intranasal corticosteroids, 476, 476t
Intraoperative nursing management, 392
 anesthesia and sedation, 398–399
  general anesthesia, 399–403
  local anesthesia, 405
  moderate sedation, 405
  monitored anesthesia care, 405
  regional anesthesia, 403–405
 complications and, 405–407
  anaphylaxis, 406
  hypothermia, 406
  hypoxia and other respiratory complications, 406
  intraoperative awareness, 405–406
  malignant hyperthermia, 406–407
  nausea and vomiting, 406
 nursing process, 407–410
 surgical environment, 396–397
  blood and body fluids, exposure to, 398
  health hazards associated with, 398
  laser risks, 398
  robot-assisted technology, 398
  surgical asepsis, 397–398
 surgical team, 392
  anesthesiologist, 392, 396
  anesthetist, 396
  circulating nurse, 392, 394–395
  patient, 392–394
  registered nurse first assistant, 396
  scrub role, 392, 395
  surgeon, 395–396
Intraoperative radiation therapy (IORT), 1129, 1442, 2165
Intraoral orthotics, 924
Intraotologic catheters, 1946
Intrapleural anesthesia, 423
Intrarenal azotemia, 1295
Intrauterine device (IUD), 1400
Intravenous (IV)
 fluid therapy, 1003
 infusion, 813–815, 842
  pulmonary edema, 825
 inotropes, 813
Intravenous anesthetic agents, 399–400, 401t–403t, 403
Intravenous fat emulsion (IVFE), 948
Intravenous urography, 1278–1279
Intrinsic factor, 899, 900
Introitus, 1373, 1374
Invasion, 2152
Invasive cancer, 1456
 infiltrating ductal carcinoma, 1457
 infiltrating lobular carcinoma, 1457
 medullary carcinoma, 1457
Invasive meningococcal disease (IMD), 2091
Involuntary motor activity, 1968
Iodine-deficient goitre, 1237–1238
Ionizing radiation, exposure to, 2154
IORT. *See* Intraoperative radiation therapy (IORT)
Ipratropium (Atrovent), 591t
IPV. *See* Intimate partner violence (IPV)
Irbesartan (Avapro), hypertension, 886t
Irinotecan (Camptosar), 552, 1129
Iron deficiency anemia, 1613–1615
 assessment and diagnostic findings, 1614
 cause of, 1613
 clinical manifestations, 1614
 medical management, 1614, 1614c
 nursing management, 1614–1615, 1615c
Iron preparations, constipation, 998
Iron storage, role of liver, 1053

Iron stores and metabolism, 1602–1603
Irritable bowel syndrome (IBS), 998, 1004–1005, 1005f
assessment and diagnostic findings, 1005
clinical manifestations, 1004
medical management, 1005
nursing management, 1005
pathophysiology, 1004
Quality of Life, 1006c
spastic contractions, 1005f
Irritant contact dermatitis, 1802
clinical manifestations, 1806
medical management, 1806
plan of nursing care, 1803c–1806c
strategies for avoiding, 1806c
Ischemia, 111, 731, 835
Ischemic bowel, 855, 858
Ischemic cardiomyopathy, 787, 789
Ischemic cascade, 2029–2030
Ischemic heart disease, heart failure, 815
Ischemic necrosis, 843
Ischemic stroke
assessment and diagnostic findings, 2032–2033
cardiogenic embolic strokes, 2029
clinical manifestations, 2030–2032
cognitive impairment and psychological effects, 2032
communication disorders poststroke, 2030
motor loss, 2030
perceptual disturbances, 2032
sensory losses, 2032
definition, 2028
high-risk groups, 2033
African Canadians, 2033
Asians, 2033
Hispanics, 2033
ischemic brain cell injury, 2030f
large artery thrombotic strokes, 2029
medical management, 2033–2038
angiotensin-converting enzyme (ACE) inhibitors and diuretics, 2034–2035
anticoagulants, 2033
antihypertensive medications, 2034–2035
carotid endarterectomy (CEA), 2038
CAS with or without angioplasty, 2038
dosage and administration, 2035–2036
endovascular techniques, 2035
enhancing prompt diagnosis, 2035
maintenance of cerebral hemodynamics, 2036
management of potential complications, 2036–2038
new or novel oral anticoagulants (NOACs), 2033
platelet-inhibiting medications, 2034
side effects, 2036
statins, 2034
surgical prevention of ischemic stroke, 2038
therapy for patients with ischemic stroke not receiving t-PA, 2036
thrombolytic therapy, 2035
modifiable risk factors, 2033, 2034c
nursing interventions
adjusting to physical changes, 2042–2043
assisting with nutrition, 2043
attaining bladder and bowel control, 2043
changing patient's position, 2040
communication, improving, 2044
continuing and transitional care, 2045–2046
enhancing self-care, 2042, 2042c
establishing an exercise program, 2041
family coping, improving, 2044–2045
improving mobility, 2040
joint deformity prevention, 2040
patient outcomes, 2046
positioning hand and fingers, 2040
preparing for ambulation, 2041
promoting home, community-based, and transitional care, 2045–2046
sexual dysfunction coping, helping with, 2045
shoulder adduction prevention, 2040
shoulder pain prevention, 2041–2042
skin integrity maintenance, 2044
thought processes, improving, 2043
nursing management, 2038–2046
collaborative problems/potential complications, 2039
nursing priorities, 2039
patient assessment, 2038–2039
planning and goals, 2039–2040
pathophysiology, 2029–2030, 2030f
prevention of, 2033
referral to Stroke Prevention Clinic, 2033
small penetrating artery thrombotic strokes, 2029
thrombolytic therapy, 2029
treatment for, 2028–2029
Islet cell transplants, 1137, 1156
Isoflurane (Forane), 400t
Isolated systolic hypertension, 878
Isometric contractions, 2218
Isoniazid
antituberculosis medication, 526t
TB and HIV infection, 1551
Isosorbide dinitrate, in heart failure, 813
Isosorbide (Isordil), for erectile dysfunction, 1485
Isotonic contraction, 2218
Isotonic fluids, 333–335
D_5W, 334
lactated Ringer's solution, 335
normal saline solution, 334–335
Isotretinoin (Accutane), 1794–1795
Isradipine (Dynacirc CR), hypertension, 887t
Itching (pruritus), 1772
ITP. *See* Immune thrombocytopenic purpura (ITP)
IV. *See* Intravenous (IV)
Ivabradine (Corlanor), 812
IV cidofovir (Vistide), 1554
IV conivaptan hydrochloride (Vaprisol), 311
IV diazepam (Valium), in end-stage kidney disease, 1299
IV fat emulsions (IVFEs), 966
IVFE. *See* Intravenous fat emulsion (IVFE)
IVFEs. *See* IV fat emulsions (IVFEs)
IV foscarnet (Foscavir), 1554
IV ganciclovir (Cytovene), 1554
Ixazomib (Ninlaro), for multiple myeloma, 1655

J

Jackhammer esophagus, 935
Jackson–Pratt tubes, 1102, 1358
Janeway lesions, 795
Jaundice, 1052, 1060, 1766, 1772
alcohol intake, 1060
chronic idiopathic, 1061
colour changes in, 1773t
gallbladder disease, 1110
hemolytic, 1060
hepatic dysfunction, 1055
hepatocellular, 1060
obstructive, 1060
serum bilirubin levels, 1060, 1061
in shock, 347
Jawbone, 923
Jaw disorders, 923
surgical management, 924
home and community-based care, 924
nursing management, 924
temporomandibular disorders, 923
assessment and diagnostic findings, 923
clinical manifestations, 923
medical management, 923–924
Jaw-thrust manoeuvre, 2346
J-cloths, 1791
Jejunostomy
assessment, 961
collaborative problems, 962
gastrointestinal intubation, 960–961
nursing priorities, 961–962
nursing process, 961–965
planning and goals, 962
Jejunostomy tube (J tube), 961
Jejunum, 948
Jet injectors, 1155
Joint active system (JAS) splints, 182
Joint pain, hepatic dysfunction, 1055
Joint(s), 2214, 2217
amphiarthrotic, 2217–2218
arthroplasty, 2247
capsule, 2218
deformity, 2225
diarthrotic, 2218, 2218f
dislocations, 2299
effusion, 2225
function, assessment of, 2225
infection in, 2214
replacement, 2247–2248 (*See also* Orthopedic surgery)
surgery, 2247
swelling, 2223
synarthrotic, 2217
Joint space, 1754
J tube, 963
Jugular venous distention (JVD), 804, 818
Jugular venous pulsations, 668
Junctional dysrhythmias
AVNRT, 706–707
junctional or idionodal rhythm, 706
nonparoxysmal junctional tachycardia, 706
premature junctional complex, 706
Junctional rhythm, 706
Justice, 25, 25c
JVD. *See* Jugular venous distention (JVD)

K

Kaposi's sarcoma (KS), 1534, 1551, 1551f, 1826
mouth abnormalities, 921t
Kayexalate, 317, 1295–1296
acute kidney injury, 1295–1296
retention enema, 1296
Kegel exercises, 201, 1342, 1425c
Keloids, 1820
Keratin, 1765, 1768
Keratinocytes, 1764, 1768
Keratoconjunctivitis, 1750, 1816
Keratoconus, 1904
Keratoprosthesis, 1905
Kernig's sign, 2090
Ketamine, 289, 402t
Ketoconazole, hepatic dysfunction, 1054

Ketone, 1137
testing for, 1150
Ketone bodies, 1141
fatty acids, 1053
Kidney and urinary disorders. *See* Renal and urologic disorders
Kidney artery embolization, 1291
kidney biopsy, 1280
Kidney cancer, 1290–1291
clinical manifestations, 1290c
medical management, 1290–1291
nursing management, 1291
risk factors, 1290c
Kidney disorders, 1291–1292
acute kidney injury, 1292–1297
chronic kidney disease, 1284–1285
end-stage kidney disease, 1297–1300
fluid and electrolyte imbalances
clinical manifestation, 1282–1284, 1284t
nephrosclerosis, 1285
polycystic kidney disease, 1289–1290
primary glomerular diseases, 1285–1289
Kidney donation, 1324c
Kidney replacement therapies
dialysis, 1300, 1305–1319
Kidneys, 1262–1264
blood supply to, 1263
functions of, 1263c
functions of, in fluid balance, 301
nephrons, 1263–1264, 1264f
regulation of BP by, 343
Kidney stones
nursing process, 1354–1355
preventing, 1352c
treating methods, 1353f
Kidneys, ureters, and bladder (KUB), 1351, 1393
Kidney surgery
care of patient undergoing, 1321c–1323c
management of patients, 1319–1323
nursing management, 1320, 1323
perioperative concerns, 1319, 1319f
postoperative management, 1319–1320
preoperative considerations, 1319
transplantation, 1324–1328, 1324f
postoperative management, 1325–1328, 1327t
preoperative management, 1325
rejection and infection, 1325c
Kidney transplantation, in patient with diabetes, 1180
Kidney trauma, 1328–1329, 1328f
blunt, 1328
medical management, 1329
nursing management, 1329
Kinins, 113
Kirsten ras (KRAS), 2153
Klebsiella pneumoniae, 970
Klebsiella species, 1818
Knee ligaments, 2301, 2301f
Knitted Dacron, 855
Kock pouch, 998, 1019, 1027, 1030c, 1332, 1363
Korsakoff's syndrome, 2050
KS. *See* Kaposi's sarcoma (KS)
Kupffer cells, 1052, 1054, 1078
Kyphoscoliosis, 452
Kyphosis, 2219, 2224, 2224f

L

LABA. *See* Long-acting beta2-agonists (LABA)
Labetalol, 2049
antiarrhythmic medication, 699t
hypertension, 885t, 893
Labia majora, 1374
Labia minora, 1374
Laboratory tests. *See also* Cardiovascular function
blood chemistry, 672–674, 673t–674t
brain natriuretic peptide, 674
cardiac biomarker analysis, 672
coagulation studies, 672–674, 673t–674t
c-reactive protein, 674
heart failure, 810
hematology, 672–674, 673t–674t
homocysteine, 675
lipid profile
cholesterol levels, 674
triglycerides, 674
Labyrinthitis, 1946
Lacerations, 2056, 2349c
Lactase, 901t
Lactated Ringer's solution, 328, 335
Lactational abscess, 1455
Lactic acid, 342
Lactic acidosis, biguanide therapy and, 1157
Lactic dehydrogenase, 1056
Lactobacillus acidophilus, 1411
Lactose intolerance, 1000, 1007t, 1008c
Lactulose (Cephulac), 1073
Lacunar type strokes, 2029
Lalonde report, 7
Langerhans cells, 1766, 1769
Langerhans islets, 1107
Lansoprazole (Prevacid), 983
gastric acid, 939
gastroesophageal reflux disease, 939t
peptic ulcer disease and gastritis, 979t
Laparoscopic cholecystectomy, 1112, 1113, 1114f, 1117
Laparoscopic robotic–assisted surgery, 2161
Laparoscopy, 915, 1033, 1058, 1391–1392, 1392f
exploratory, 943
in GI disease diagnosis, 915
pancreatic tumour, 1128
Large artery thrombotic strokes, 2029
Large bowel obstruction
assessment and diagnostic findings, 1033
clinical manifestations, 1033
medical management, 1033
nursing management, 1033
pathophysiology, 1033
Large intestine, 899
Laryngeal mask airway (LMA), 2347
Laryngeal nerve, damage to, 63
Laryngeal obstruction. *See also* Obstruction and trauma
assessment/diagnostic findings, 491
causes of, 491t
clinical manifestations, 490–491
medical management, 491, 491c
Laryngeal preservation, 926
Laryngectomy
defined, 471
partial, 494
total, 494, 494f
undergoing, nursing process for, 495–502, 496c, 501c
Laryngitis. *See also* Upper airway infections
clinical manifestations, 483–484
defined, 471
medical management, 484
nursing management, 484
Larynx
anatomy, 440
cancer of, 491
assessment/diagnostic findings, 492, 493c
clinical manifestations, 492
medical management, 492–495
nursing process for, 495–502
risk factors for, 492c
risk factors for cancer, 925
Laser-Assisted In Situ Keratomileusis (LASIK), 1906
Laser-compatible scopes, 911
Laser hyperthermia, liver tumours, 1096
Laser panretinal photocoagulation, 1908
Laser safety, practices for, 398
Laser scanning polarimetry, 1887
Laserskin, 1786
Laser surgery, 494
Laser treatment of cutaneous lesions, 1831–1832
LASIK. *See* Laser-Assisted In Situ Keratomileusis (LASIK)
Lassitude, gastritis, 978
Latency, 1698
Latent reservoir, 1534, 1544
Late-onset familial Alzheimer's disease, 141t
Lateral collateral ligament (LCL) injury, 2301
Lateral horn, 1963
Latex allergy, 1593–1596, 1594t, 2358
assessment and diagnostic findings, 1596
clinical manifestations, 1595–1596, 1595t
medical management, 1596
nursing management, 1596
surgical patient with, 408
Latex allergy screening questionnaire, 381, 381f
Lavage, 948
Laxatives
diarrhea, 1000
urinary stone formation, 1351
LDL. *See* Low-density lipoprotein (LDL)
LDLT. *See* Living donor liver transplantation (LDLT)
LDR. *See* Low-dose radiation (LDR)
Lead poisoning, 998
Leads, 718
Lead systems, 676
Leaflet plication, 784
Leaflet repair, 778, 784, 784f
Learning. *See also* Teaching
definition of, 40
environment, 41
motivation for, 39, 40
readiness to learn (*See* Learning readiness)
teaching and, 40
Learning contract, 39
Learning readiness, 40–41
culture, influence of, 40
emotional readiness, 40–41
experiential readiness, 41
personal values and, 40
physical readiness, 40
teachable moment, 40
Lectures, 41
Ledipasvir-sofosbuvir (Harvoni), 1081
Leflunomide (Arava), for rheumatoid arthritis, 1744
Left heart catheterization, 683
Left internal mammary artery (IMA), 758
Left shift, or shift to the left, 1599, 1603
Left-sided heart failure, 804, 808–809
Left ventricular failure, 838
Left ventricular outflow tract surgery, 789
Legal blindness, 1888
Leg and foot ulcers, 1779
Leg bags, 202

Leg casts, 2240
Leg crossing, 853
Leg exercises, 385c, 863, 866
Legionnaires' disease, 1727
Leg ulcers, 1626
  assessment and diagnostic findings, 869
  clinical manifestations
    arterial ulcers, 868
    venous ulcers, 868–869
  complications, 870
  evaluation, 871
  medical management, 869
    compression therapy, 869
    débridement, 869
    hyperbaric oxygenation (HBO), 870
    negative pressure wound therapy, 870
    pharmacologic therapy, 869
    stimulated healing, 870
    topical therapy, 869
    wound dressing, 869–870
  nursing history and assessment, 870
  nursing interventions, 871
  nursing process, 870–871
  pathophysiology, 868
  planning and goals, 870
Leininger, Madeleine, 90
Lenalidomide
  multiple myeloma, 1654
  myelodysplastic syndrome, 1619
Lentigo maligna melanomas, 1823
Lepirudin, 865
  for pulmonary embolism, 544
Lesbian, gay, bisexual, transgender and queer (LGBTQ), 1384
  health care, 1385c
  HIV prevention in, 1540
  isolation in, 1386c
Letrozole (Femara), for breast cancer, 1471
Leucovorin, 1129, 2178
Leukemia, 1599, 1634–1636
  cutis, 1636, 1636f
Leukocyte, 1599, 1600, 1603–1604
  agranulocytes, 1603
  esterase test, 1335
  function of, 1604
  granulocytes, 1603
Leukocyte tagging, ulcerative colitis, 1018
Leukocytosis, 113, 1010, 1012, 1095
Leukopenia, 927, 1599, 1605, 1632–1633
  neutropenia
    clinical manifestation, 1632
    medical management, 1632–1633
    nursing management, 1633
Leukoplakia, 920t, 1391
Leukotriene modifiers, 1585t
  allergic rhinitis, 1585
Leukotrienes, 1572, 1574
  for asthma, 591
Leuprolide, 1496
  fibroids, 1430
  ovulation, 1405c
Levator ani, 1374
Levetiracetam (Keppra), 2008
Levin tube, 949
Levothyroxine sodium (Synthroid), interaction with anesthetics, 382t
Lice infestation, 1799
Licensed practical nurse, 4
Lichenification (leathery thickening), 1787
Lichen planus, mouth abnormalities, 920t
LICOX catheter system, 1999f
Lidocaine, 404t, 1789
  antiarrhythmic medication, 699t
  for herpes labialis, 474c
  oral cavity conditions, 927
  for pain at chest tube insertion site, 643
Lifestyle changes, 853, 854, 863, 871
  blood pressure, 891c
  heart failure, 811
Lifestyle modification, for obesity, 1196–1199
  healthy diets, 1198–1199
  physical activity, 1198
  plan for caloric deficit, 1197
  sleep habits, 1199
Lifestyle patterns, assessment of, 59
Li–Fraumeni syndrome, 143t
Lifting techniques, 2270f
Ligaments, 2214, 2218, 2298
Lindane (Kwell), 1802
Liniments, 1787
Lipase, 899, 900, 1107
Lipid-lowering medications, 735–736, 735t
Lipid profile
  cholesterol levels, 674
  triglycerides, 674
Lipids, 966
Lipoatrophy, 1152
Lipodystrophy, 1152
Lipolysis, 1166
Lipoproteins, 733, 734f
Lips, inspection of, 904
Lipsticks, 1008
Liquid diet, of hospitalized diabetic patients, 1185
Lisinopril (Prinivil, Zestril)
  heart failure, 811t
  hypertension, 886t
Lithium toxicity, 312
Lithotomy position, for surgery, 408, 409f
Lithotripsy, 919, 925, 1107, 1111
Liver, 1107f
  anatomy, 1051–1053
  and biliary system, 1052f
  enlargement, 1056
  functions of
    ammonia conversion, 1053
    bile formation, 1053–1054
    bilirubin excretion, 1054
    drug metabolism, 1054
    fat metabolism, 1053
    glucose metabolism, 1053
    iron storage, 1053
    protein metabolism, 1053
    vitamin, 1053
  glucagon, 1108
  lobe removal, 1097
  technique for palpating, 1056f
Liver abscess, 1102
  assessment and diagnostic findings, 1103
  clinical manifestations, 1103
  medical management, 1103
  nursing management, 1103
  pathophysiology, 1103
Liver assessment, 1054
  health history, 1054–1055
  physical assessment, 1055–1056
Liver biopsy, 1057–1058
  hepatic disorders, 1057–1058, 1058c–1059c
Liver cancer, 1095
  liver metastases
    assessment and diagnostic findings, 1095–1096
    clinical manifestations, 1095
    medical management, 1096
    nursing management, 1097–1098
    surgical management, 1096–1097
  primary liver tumours, 1095
Liver diseases, 1060, 1668
  child–pugh classification, 1084t
Liver enlargement, cirrhosis and, 1084
Liver function tests, 1113
  clinical functions, 1057t
  hepatic disorders, 1056–1057
Liver metastases
  assessment and diagnostic findings, 1095–1096
  clinical manifestations, 1095
  medical management, 1096
  nursing management, 1097–1098
  surgical management, 1096–1097
Liver transplantation
  anastomosis to donor liver bile duct, 1100f
  complication, 1100–1101
  ethical dilemma, 1099c
  immunosuppression, 1098
  liver cancer, 1097
  nursing management, 1101–1102
  orthotopic liver transplantation, 1098
  severe GI bleeding, 1099
  surgical procedure, 1099–1100
Living donor liver transplantation (LDLT), 1100
  liver transplantation, complications of, 1101
LMWH. *See* Low-molecular-weight heparin (LMWH)
Lobectomy, 551c, 633
  in liver tumour, 1097
Lobes, 440
Lobular carcinoma in situ (LCIS), 1446, 1456
Local ablation, in liver tumour, 1097
Local adaptation syndrome, 105
Local anesthesia, 394, 404t, 405
  advantages of, 405
  contraindications to, 405
  epinephrine, 405
Local anesthetics
  long-acting, 289
  for pain relief, 289
Local conduction blocks, 405
Local hyperthermia, 2189
Long-acting beta2-agonists (LABA), 570, 588t, 591
Long-acting muscarinic antagonists (LAMA), 570
Long arm cast, 2232
Long leg cast, 2232
Long-term care facilities, 221
Loop diuretics, 812, 820t
  for hypervolemia, 308
Loop electrocautery excision procedure (LEEP), 1391, 1412, 1433
Loose bodies, 2270–2271
Loperamide, 907, 1002
Lorazepam (Ativan), 1862, 2007, 2008, 2062
  breast cancer, 1469
  before cardiac surgery, 763
Lordosis, 2224, 2224f
Losartan (Cozaar), hypertension, 886t
Lotions, 1787
Low back pain, 2265. *See also* Acute low back pain
  abdominal aortic aneurysm, 858
Low-density lipoprotein (LDL), 732, 878, 882
Low-dose radiation (LDR), 2165
Lower gastrointestinal tract study, 909
Lower motor neurons, 1968
Lower respiratory structures and breathing
  physical findings, 457, 458t
  positioning, 452
  thoracic auscultation, 456–457

Lower respiratory structures and breathing (*continued*)
adventitious sounds, 457, 458t
breath sounds, 457, 457t
voice sounds, 457
thoracic inspection
accessory muscles, use of, 454
breathing patterns/respiratory rates, 452, 453t, 454
chest configuration, 452
thoracic palpation
respiratory excursion, 454–455
tactile fremitus, 455
thoracic percussion, 455–456, 456t
diaphragmatic excursion, 456
Lower respiratory tract. *See also* Respiratory system
lungs, 440–442
Lower urinary tract infections. *See also* Urinary tract infection (UTI)
assessment and diagnostic findings, 1335–1336
clinical manifestation, 1334
gerontologic considerations, 1334–1335, 1335c
medical management, 1336
nursing process, 1336–1338
pathophysiology, 1332–1334
Lower urinary tract symptoms (LUTS), 1490
Low-flow oxygen delivery systems, 604
Low-molecular-weight heparin (LMWH), 741, 863
protamine sulphate, 865
in venous thromboembolism, 864
Low-profile gastrostomy device (LPGD), 948, 960, 961
Low-profile jejunostomy devices (LPJDs), 961
Low sodium diets, 308
LPGD. *See* Low-profile gastrostomy device (LPGD)
LPJDs. *See* Low-profile jejunostomy devices (LPJDs)
Lubath oil, 1789
Lubiprostone (Amitiza), 1000
laxative medications, 1001t
Lumbar puncture, 1984–1985
Luminal disorders, 1006
Lung abscess
assessment/diagnostic findings, 529
clinical manifestations, 529
medical management, 529–530
nursing management, 530
pathophysiology, 529
patient education about self-care, 530
pharmacologic therapy, 529–530
prevention, 529
Lung cancer, 548–553. *See also* Chest tumours
assessment/diagnostic findings, 550–551
classification and staging, 549
clinical manifestations, 550
gerontologic considerations, 552–553
medical management, 551–552, 551c
nursing management, 552, 553c
pathophysiology, 549
risk factors
dietary factors, 550
electronic cigarettes, 549
environmental/occupational exposure, 549–550
genetics, 550
second-hand (passive) smoke, 549
tobacco smoke, 549
treatment-related complications, 552
Lung(s)
alveoli, 441–442
assessment of, 671–672
biopsy
nursing interventions, 468
procedure, 466, 468
bronchi and bronchioles, 440–441
homeostasis, role in, 301
lobes, 440
mediastinum, 440
pleura, 440
resection, types of, 551c
scans, 463–464
transplantation, 573
volumes and capacities, 442–443, 443t
Lung sounds, fluid replacement and, 351
Lung volume, reduction surgery, 572
Lupron, 1405c
Luteal phase, 1373, 1376
Luteinizing hormone (LH), 1373, 1375
Luteinizing hormone–releasing hormone (LHRH), 1496
Lyme disease, 2361
Lymphadenectomy, 2160
Lymphangiography, 843
Lymphatic disorders
lymphangitis and lymphadenitis, 873
lymphedema and elephantiasis, 873–874
Lymphatic obstruction, 1006
Lymphatic spread, cancer, 2152–2153. *See also* Cancer
Lymphatic vessels
anatomic of, 836
obstruction of, 838
transport lymph, 834
Lymphedema, 873, 1446, 1460, 1463–1464
medical management
pharmacologic therapy, 874
surgical management, 874
nursing management, 874
Lymph node biopsy
nursing interventions, 468
procedure, 468
Lymphocyte, 1599, 1600, 1603. *See also* Agranulocytes
in immune response, 1524t
Lymphoid, 1599, 1600
tissues, 1517
Lymphokines, 1517, 1522
Lymphoma, 1554, 1648–1652
Hodgkin, 1648–1650
Non-Hodgkin, 1650–1652
Lymphopenia, 1633
Lymphoscintigraphy, 843
Lynch syndrome, 142t
Lysis, 1599, 1637

M

Macrodantin, 1336
thalassemia, 1628
Macrophage, 1599
Macular degeneration, 219
Macular edema, 1177, 1178
Macular translocation, 1910
Mafenide acetate, 1855, 1855t
Magnesium, 322
antacids, diarrhea, 1001
cardiopulmonary resuscitation, 832t
deficit (hypomagnesemia), 322–324, 322t
excess (hypermagnesemia), 322t, 324
Magnesium-based antacids, 324
Magnesium hydroxide (milk of magnesia), 1001t
Magnesium sulphate, for status asthmaticus, 596
Magnetic resonance angiography (MRA), 681–682, 842, 1980
Magnetic resonance–guided focused ultrasound surgery (MRgFUS), 1429–1430
Magnetic resonance imaging (MRI), 908, 1123, 1980–1981
brain abscess, 2092
breast, 1452
fluoroscopic studies, 463
hepatic disorders, 1058
kidney cancer, 1290
meningitis, 2090
nursing interventions, 463, 464
for pelvic examination, 1393
pelvic floor, 999
pericarditis, 799
pulmonary angiography, 463
radioisotope diagnostic procedures, 463–464
of spine, 2071–2073
ulcerative colitis, 1018
Magnetic resonance imaging–guided core biopsy, 1453
Magnetic resonance spectroscopy, 1980
MAID. *See* Medical assistance in dying (MAID)
Major histocompatibility complex (MHC), 1006
Malabsorption, 998, 2197
cause, 1006
celiac disease, 1006
chronic pancreatitis, 1123
Crohn's disease, 1017
diarrhea, 1001, 1002
disorders of, 1005–1008
celiac disease, 1006–1008
of vitamin B_{12}, 978, 980
Maladaptation, diseases of, 108
Maladaptive responses, 107–108
Malaise, hepatic dysfunction, 1055
Male breast
cancer, 1477
diseases of, 1476–1477
physical assessment of, 1449
Male condom, 1401
Male hypogonadism, 1483
Male pattern baldness, 1778f
Male reproductive function
age-related change in, 1482t
anatomic and physiologic overview, 1479–1481
assessment, 1479–1483
diagnostic evaluation
prostate fluid or tissue analysis, 1483
prostate-specific antigen test, 1483
ultrasonography, 1483
disorders, 1488c
ejaculation concerns, 1487–1488
erectile dysfunction, 1483–1487
genitourinary tract infections, 1488–1489
penis, 1510–1511
prostate conditions, 1489–1496, 1500–1501
testes and adjacent structures, 1506–1510
genitourinary tract, 1488–1489
gerontologic considerations, 1482–1483
health history and clinical manifestations, 1481–1482
physical assessment
digital rectal examination, 1482
gerontologic considerations, 1482–1483
testicular examination, 1482
prostate-specific antigen test, 1483
prostatic disorders, 1489–1496, 1500–1501

Male sexual function, tests of, 1483
Malignant, 2150
Malignant cells, characteristics of, 2151–2152, 2152t
Malignant essential hypertension, 1922
Malignant external otitis, 1938
Malignant hyperthermia (MH), 405, 406
  clinical manifestations, 407
  medical management, 407
  nursing management, 407
  pathophysiology, 407
Malignant melanoma
  assessment and diagnostic findings, 1823–1824
  care of patient with, 1824–1826
    patient outcomes, 1826
  clinical manifestations, 1823
  medical management, 1824
  nursing interventions
    monitoring and managing potential complications, 1825
    promoting home, community-based, and transitional care, 1825
    reducing anxiety and depression, 1825
    relieving pain and discomfort, 1825
  risk factors, 1822–1823, 1823c
  staging of tumour, 1823
Malignant nephrosclerosis, 1285
Malignant skin lesions, 2196
Malignant transformation, 2153
Malignant tumours, 1095
  characteristics of, 2152t
Malnutrition, 69, 375, 1102
  oral cavity conditions, 927
  preoperative assessment, 378
  sialadenitis, 924
  tube feeding, 958
Malocclusion, 923
Maltase, 901t
Malunion, clavicular fractures, 2312
Mammography, 1450–1452, 1450f
  contrast, 1452
  digital, 1452
  three-dimensional (3D), 1452
Mammoplasty, 1446, 1476
Mandibular advancement devices (MAD), 487
Mandibular fractures, 924
Mandibular structural abnormalities, 924
Mannitol, 2007, 2008
Mannitol (Osmitrol), for acute kidney injury, 1295
Manometry, 914
  constipation, 999
  esophageal, 934, 935, 936
Mantoux test
  for tuberculosis, 524, 524f
Masking cosmetics, 1819
Masks, in surgical department, 397
Maslow's hierarchy of needs, 5, 6f, 32
Massage, for pain relief, 290
Mass spectrometer, 396
MAST (Michigan Alcohol Screening Test), 59
Mastalgia, 1446, 1455
Mast cell, 1572
  stabilizers, 1585
Mastectomy, 1446, 1456, 2161, 2162
Mastication (chewing), 922
Mastitis, 1446, 1454
Mastoidectomy/mastoid surgery
  nursing interventions, 1941–1942
    altered sensory perception, prevention of, 1942
    home, community-based, and transitional care, 1942
    improving hearing and communication, 1942
    infection prevention, 1941–1942
    injury prevention, 1942
    reducing anxiety, 1941
    releieving pain, 1941
    wound healing, promoting, 1942
  nursing priorities, 1941
  patient assessment, 1941
  patient outcomes, 1942–1943
  planning and goals, 1941
  self care after, 1942c
Mastopexy, 1476
Maxillomandibular fixation, 924
Maze and mini-maze procedures, 705
MDCT. *See* Multidetector-computed tomography (MDCT)
MDS. *See* Myelodysplastic syndrome (MDS)
Meal planning, for patients with diabetes, 1144–1146
Mean arterial pressure (MAP), 343, 1996
Mean corpuscular volume (MCV), 1610
Measles, mumps, and rubella (MMR) vaccines, 1709–1710
Mechanical assistive devices, in cardiogenic shock, 358
Mechanical barriers
  cervical cap, 1400
  diaphragm, 1400
  female condom, 1400
  male condom, 1401
  spermicides, 1400–1401
Mechanical débridement, 1857
Mechanical stimulation, 202
Mechanical valves, 786
Mechanical ventilation
  adjusting, 622, 622c
  classification of ventilators, 619–620
  indications, 619, 619c
  monitoring, 622
  nursing process for patient in
    assessment, 622–623
    collaborative problems, 623, 623t, 624c
    evaluation, 628–632
    nursing interventions, 623–628, 626c, 627c, 628c
    nursing priorities, 623
    planning and goals, 623
  thoracic surgery and, 635
  ventilator mode, 620–622, 621f
Mechanical ventilator, 602
  defined, 619
Meclizine hydrochloride (Antivert), 1944
Medial collateral ligament (MCL) injury, 2301
Mediastinoscopy, 468
Mediastinum, 440
Medical assistance in dying (MAID), 85, 242
Medical Care Act of 1968, 6
Medical management, 482
  abdominal aortic aneurysm, 857
  abscess, 922
  acne vulgaris
    nutrition and hygiene therapy, 1793
    prevention of scarring, 1795
  acquired immune deficiency syndrome, 1553–1554
  acquired thrombophilias, 1675–1678
  acute coronary syndrome, 747–750
  acute low back pain, 2267
  acute lymphocytic leukemia, 1640
  acute myeloid leukemia, 1637–1638
  acute or intermediate phase of burn care, 1849–1854
  acute otitis media, 1939
  acute pancreatitis, 1120–1121
  of acute pharyngitis
    nutritional therapy, 480
    pharmacologic therapy, 480
  of acute respiratory failure, 534
  of acute rhinosinusitis, 476, 476t
  of acute tracheobronchitis, 508
  of adenoiditis, 482
  adrenocortical insufficiency, 1249
  allergic rhinitis, 1583–1587
  altered level of consciousness (LOC), 1989–1990
  Alzheimer's disease, 228
  amputation, 2328
  anaphylactic shock, 365
  anaphylaxis, 1581
  anemia, 1611
  aneurysms, 858
  angina pectoris, 740–742
  aortic regurgitation, 781
  aortic stenosis, 781
  aortoiliac disease, 855
  aplastic anemia, 1616
  appendicitis, 1010
  of ARDS, 535–536
  arterial embolism, 860
  of asbestosis, 548
  ascites, 1061–1065
  of asthma, 586f, 587–594
    bronchodilator medications for COPD, 587t
    of exacerbations, 592–593, 592f
    long-term medications, 588t–590t
    peak flow meters, 593, 593f, 594c
    quick-relief medications, 591t, 592
  atopic dermatitis, 1591
  of atrial fibrillation, 703–704, 703c
  of atrial flutter, 701
  of AVNRT, 707
  bacterial vaginosis, 1414
  basal cell carcinoma (BCC)
    nonsurgical alternative therapies, 1822
    surgical, 1821–1822
  Bell's palsy, 2113
  benign prostatic hyperplasia, 1491–1494
  bladder cancer, 1357–1358
  bleeding disorders, 1658
  blindness, 1889–1890
    vision restoration, 1890
  of blunt trauma, 554–555
  bone tumours, 2292
  brain abscesses, 2092
  of bronchiectasis, 583
  Buerger's disease, 854
  bullous pemphigoid, 1814
  of cancer of larynx, 492–495
  candidiasis, 1414
  cardiac tamponade, 829–830
  cardiogenic shock, 356–358, 827–828
    circulatory assist devices, 827
  cataracts, 1901–1903
  celiac disease, 1008
  cellulitis, 875
  cerebral metastases, 2122–2123
  cervical cancer, 1433–1434
  chlamydia, 1420
  Chlamydia trachomatis, 1723
  chronic heart failure, 811–816
  chronic lymphocytic leukemia, 1641–1642
  chronic myeloid leukemia, 1638–1639

Medical management (*continued*)
chronic otitis media, 1940–1941
of chronic pharyngitis, 481
of chronic rhinosinusitis, 478–479
cluster headaches, 2025
of coal worker's pneumoconiosis, 548
colorectal cancer
adjuvant therapy, 1035–1036
surgical management, 1036–1037
of conduction abnormalities, 713
conjunctivitis
allergic conjunctivitis, 1916
bacterial conjunctivitis, 1916
patient education, 1917c
toxic conjunctivitis, 1916
viral conjunctivitis, 1916
constipation, 1000
of COPD
alpha1-antitrypsin augmentation therapy, 570
bronchodilators, 569–570, 571t
bullectomy, 572
corticosteroids, 570
exacerbation of COPD, 570–572
lung transplantation, 573
lung volume reduction surgery, 572
oxygen therapy, 572
pharmacologic therapy, 569–570, 571t
pulmonary rehabilitation, 573
risk reduction, 569
surgical management, 572–573
vaccines, 570
cranial arteritis, 2025
Creutzfeldt–Jakob disease (CJD), 2095
cushing syndrome, 1252
of cystic fibrosis, 597–598
cytomegalovirus retinitis, 1921
degenerative disc disease, 2139–2140
dermatitis herpetiformis, 1814
diabetes insipidus, 1221
diabetic ketoacidosis, 1167–1168
rehydration, 1167–1168
restoring electrolytes, 1168
reversing acidosis, 1168
diabetic retinopathy, 1178
diarrhea, 1002
dissecting aorta, 859
disseminated intravascular coagulation, 1670–1671
diverticular disease
dietary and pharmacologic management, 1012
surgical management, 1012–1013
dry eye syndrome, 1914–1915
ductal carcinoma in situ, 1456
Ebola virus disease, 1726
ectopic pregnancy, 1408
emergent/resuscitative phase of burn care, 1844–1848
of empyema, 532
endometriosis, 1430–1431
epilepsy, 2018–2019
of epistaxis, 488
erectile dysfunction, 1484–1487
esophageal varices, 1068–1069
esophagus cancer, 943–944
essential thrombocythemia, 1659–1660
external otitis (otitis externa), 1937
fecal incontinence, 1003
fibroids, 1429–1430
fibromyalgia, 1759
folliculitis, 1796–1797
food allergy, 1593, 1593c
fracture, 2304–2305
fungal encephalitis, 2094
gastric cancer, 989
gastritis, 978
generalized exfoliative dermatitis, 1812–1813
genital herpes, 1799
giant cell arteritis, 1753
glaucoma, 1898–1899
gonorrhea, 1420
gout, 1758, 1758t
Guillain–Barré syndrome, 2107
headaches, 2024–2025
head injuries, 2059
hearing loss, 1936
hemophilia, 1665–1666
hemorrhagic stroke, 2049–2050
statins, 2050
hepatic cirrhosis, 1085
hepatic encephalopathy, 1072–1073
hepatitis A virus, 1077–1078
hepatitis B virus, 1080
hereditary angioedema, 1592
hereditary hemochromatosis, 1629–1630
herniation of cervical intervertebral disc
pharmacologic therapy, 2140
surgical management, 2140
of herniation of lumbar disc, 2142, 2144
herpes simplex, 1799
herpes simplex virus 2, 1418
herpes simplex virus (HSV) encephalitis, 2093
herpes zoster, 1798
hidradenitis suppurativa (HS), 1791
Hodgkin lymphoma, 1649–1650
human immune deficiency virus, 1553–1554
human papillomavirus, 1417
of Huntington's disease
continuing/transitional care, 2135
patient education about self-care, 2135
hypercalcemia, 321–322
hyperglycemic hyperosmolar nonketotic syndrome, 1170
hyperkalemia, 316–317
hypermagnesemia, 324
hypernatremia, 313
hyperparathyroidism, 1241–1242
hyperphosphatemia, 326
hyperthyroidism, 1231–1234
adjunctive therapy, 1233–1234
antithyroid medications, 1233, 1233t
pharmacotherapy, 1232
radioactive iodine therapy, 1232–1233
surgical management, 1234
hypervolemia, 308
hypocalcemia, 320
hypokalemia, 315
hypomagnesemia, 323
hyponatremia, 311
hypoparathyroidism, 1243–1244
hypophosphatemia, 326
hypothyroidism
cardiac dysfunction prevention, 1227
medication interactions prevention, 1227
pharmacologic therapy, 1226
hypovolemia, 305
hypovolemic shock, 354–355
of idioventricular rhythm, 710
immune hemolytic anemia, 1628–1629
immune thrombocytopenic purpura, 1662
impetigo, 1795–1796
increased intracranial pressure (ICP), 1997–2000
induced abortion, 1403
infective endocarditis, 796
infertility, 1405–1406
intracranial surgery
postoperative management, 2013
preoperative management, 2006–2007, 2013
supratentorial and infratentorial approaches, 2006–2007
transsphenoidal approach, 2013
iron deficiency anemia, 1614
irritable bowel syndrome, 1005
irritant contact dermatitis, 1806
ischemic stroke, 2033–2038
ACE inhibitors and diuretics, 2034–2035
anticoagulants, 2033
antihypertensive medications, 2034–2035
carotid endarterectomy, 2038
CAS with or without angioplasty, 2038
dosage and administration, 2035–2036
endovascular techniques, 2035
enhancing prompt diagnosis, 2035
maintenance of cerebral hemodynamics, 2036
management of potential complications, 2036–2038
new or novel oral anticoagulants, 2033
platelet-inhibiting medications, 2034
side effects, 2036
statins, 2034
surgical prevention of ischemic stroke, 2038
therapy for patients with ischemic stroke not receiving t-PA, 2036
thrombolytic therapy, 2035
jaw disorders, 923–924
of junctional rhythm, 706
labyrinthitis, 1946
of laryngeal obstruction, 491, 491c
of laryngitis, 484
lateral and medial collateral ligament injury, 2301
latex allergy, 1596
leg ulcers, 869
liver metastases, 1096
lower urinary tract infections, 1336
of lung abscess, 529–530
of lung cancer
chemotherapy, 551–552
palliative therapy, 552
radiation therapy, 551
surgical management, 551, 551c
malignant melanoma, 1824
megaloblastic anemias, 1618
Ménière's disease, 1945–1946
meniscal injuries, 2302
menopause, 1378–1379
metabolic acidosis, 330
metabolic alkalosis, 331
mitral regurgitation, 796
mitral stenosis, 780
mitral valve prolapse, 779
motion sickness, 1944
multiple myeloma, 1654–1655
multiple organ dysfunction syndrome, 366
multiple sclerosis (MS), 2097–2098
myasthenia gravis, 2103–2104
myelodysplastic syndrome, 1619–1620
myocarditis, 797–798
of nasal fracture, 490
of nasal obstruction, 489
Neisseria gonorrhoeae, 1723
nephrolithiasis, 1351–1352
nephropathy, 1180

neurogenic bladder, 1346
neurogenic shock, 364
neutropenia, 1632–1633
non-Hodgkin lymphomas, 1651
obesity, 1196–1201
lifestyle modification, 1196–1199
nonsurgical interventions, 1201
pharmacologic therapy, 1199, 1200t
obstructive sleep apnea
pharmacologic therapy, 488
surgical management, 487–488
oral cavity cancer, 926
oral cavity disorders, 922
orbital cellulitis, 1918
orbital implants and conformers, 1920
orbital trauma
foreign bodies and corneal abrasions, 1912–1913
ocular burns, 1913
penetrating injuries and contusions, 1913
splash injuries, 1912
orchitis, 1506
osteoarthritis, 1755
osteomalacia, 2284
osteomyelitis, 2287–2288
osteoporosis, 2280–2282, 2281t
otosclerosis, 1943
ototoxicity, 1951
ovarian cancer, 1439
ovarian cysts, 1429
Paget's disease, 2286
pancreatic cancer, 1129
pancreatic tumours, 1129–1130
of Parkinson's disease
pharmacologic therapy, 2129, 2129t
surgical management, 2129–2130
pediculosis capitis, 1800
pelvic inflammatory disease, 1421
pemphigus vulgaris, 1813–1814
of penetrating trauma, 557
penile cancer, 1511
peptic ulcer disease, 982–984
pericarditis, 799
peritonitis, 1015
of peritonsillar abscess, 483
pertussis, 1728
pharynx cancer, 926
pheochromocytoma, 1247
pituitary tumours, 1220
platelet defects, 1663
of pleural effusion, 531–532
of pleurisy, 530
of pneumonia, 513–517, 514t–516t
of pneumothorax, 558–560
polycythemia, 1630–1631
polymyalgia rheumatica, 1753
polymyositis, 1752
of premature atrial complex, 701
premenstrual syndrome, 1394–1395
primary aldosteronism, 1255
of primary brain tumours
chemotherapy, 2122
pharmacologic therapy, 2122
radiation therapy, 2121–2122
surgical management, 2121
primary immune deficiency diseases, 1534–1535, 1536c
primary myelofibrosis, 1647
prostate cancer, 1496, 1500
prostatitis, 1490
pruritus (itching), 1789–1790
psoriasis, 1807–1808
of pulmonary edema, 533
of pulmonary heart disease, 540
of pulmonary hypertension, 539
of pulmonary tuberculosis, 525, 526t
of PVC, 708
refractive errors, 1889–1890
respiratory acidosis, 332
respiratory alkalosis, 332
rheumatic diseases, 1733–1736, 1739
rheumatoid arthritis, 1744–1745
of rhinitis, 473
of sarcoidosis, 547
scabies, 1802
scleroderma, 1752
seborrheic dermatoses, 1792
sepsis, 362–363
septic (infectious) arthritis, 2290
serous otitis media, 1940
sickle cell disease, 1623–1624
of sinus bradycardia, 697–698
of sinus tachycardia, 698–700, 699t
Sjögren's syndrome, 1751
skin disorders, 1786–1788
balneotherapy, 1786, 1786t
creams, 1787
gels, 1787
lotions, 1787
ointments, 1787
pastes, 1787
powders, 1787
spray and aerosols, 1787
topical corticosteroids, 1787–1788, 1788t
spinal cord injury (SCI), acute phase
pharmacologic therapy, 2074
respiratory therapy, 2074
skeletal fracture reduction and traction, 2074
surgical management, 2075
spinal cord injury (SCI), long-term complications, 2081
spinal cord tumours, 2126
spondyloarthropathies, 1756–1757
spontaneous abortion, 1403
squamous cell carcinomas (SCC)
nonsurgical alternative therapies, 1822
surgical, 1821–1822
of status asthmaticus, 595–596
status epilepticus, 2022
Stevens–Johnson syndrome (SJS), 1816
supratentorial approach, to intracranial surgery, 2006–2007, 2013
syphilis, 1723
systemic lupus erythematosus, 1749–1750
testicular cancer, 1508–1509
thalassemia, 1628
thrombocytopenia, 1661
thyroid cancer, 1239
toxic epidermal necrolysis (TEN), 1816
traumatic brain injury (TBI)
brain death, 2062
fluid and electrolyte maintenance, 2061–2062
increased intracranial pressure, 2061
management of pain and anxiety, 2062
nutritional support, 2062
seizure prevention, 2061–2062
ventilatory support, 2061–2062
trichomoniasis, 1414
trigeminal neuralgia (tic douloureux), 2112
of tumours of mediastinum, 554
tympanic membrane perforation, 1938–1939
urethral trauma, 1356
urolithiasis, 1351–1352
uterine cancer, 1435
uveitis, 1917
vagina, fistulas of, 1424
vaginal cancer, 1437–1438
variant Creutzfeldt–Jakob disease (CJD), 2095
vasospasm, 2049
of ventricular asystole, 710
of ventricular fibrillation, 709
of ventricular tachycardia, 708–709
of viral rhinitis, 474–475
vision impairment, 1889–1890
vision restoration, 1890
von Willebrand's disease, 1668
vulvar cancer, 1435–1436
vulvar dystrophy, 1428
vulvitis, 1427
vulvodynia, 1427
Medicare, 13
Medicated shampoos, 1792
Medication therapy, tube feeding, 958
Medicinal marijuana, use of, 177
Meditation, 384
Mediterranean diet, 733
Medroxyprogesterone acetate, for sleep apnea, 488
Medulla, 1967
Medullary carcinoma, 1457. *See also* Breast cancer
Medullary lesions, 2112t
Mefenamic acid (Ponstel), premenstrual syndrome, 1395
Megacolon, 999
Megaloblastic anemias, 1617
assessment and diagnostic findings, 1618
clinical manifestations, 1617
medical management, 1618
nursing management, 1618
pathophysiology, 1617
Megestrol acetate (Megace), for AIDS-related anorexia, 1554
Meglitinides, 1156
Meiosis, 134
Melanin, 1766, 1773
Melanocytes, 1766
Melanocyte-stimulating hormone, 1766
Melena, 904, 977, 982
hepatic dysfunction, 1055
Melphalan (Alkeran), for leukemia, 1636
Membranous labyrinth, 1928
Memory cells, 1517, 1521
Menarche, 1373, 1393
Mendelian conditions, 135
Ménière's disease, 1931, 1944–1946
assessment and diagnostic findings, 1945
clinical manifestations, 1945
dietary guidelines for patients with, 1945c
medical management, 1945–1946
pharmacologic therapy, 1945–1946
surgical management
endolymphatic sac decompression, 1946
intraotologic catheters, 1946
middle and inner ear perfusion, 1946
vestibular nerve sectioning, 1946
Ménière's syndrome, 2111t
Meningeal irritation, 2090
Meningeal sarcoma, 2151
Meninges, 1961
Meningioma, 2151
Meningiomas, 2118. *See also* Primary brain tumours
Meningitis, 2088
assessment and diagnostic findings, 2090–2091

Meningitis (*continued*)
cerebrospinal fluid values diagnostic for, 2090t
clinical manifestations, 2089–2090
increased ICP in, 2090
medical management, 2091
nursing management, 2091
promoting home, community-based, and transitional care, 2091
pathophysiology, 2089
prevention, 2091
seizures in, 2090
in specific populations, 2089c
vaccination for, 2091
Meniscal injuries, 2300, 2302
Meniscus, 2218
Menometrorrhagia, 1396
Menopausal period, 1376
Menopause, 1373, 1377–1380, 1378c
clinical manifestations, 1378, 1378c
medical management, 1378–1379
nursing management, 1379–1380
postmenopausal bleeding, 1377–1378
psychological considerations, 1378
Menorrhagia, 1396
Menotropins, 1405c
Menstruation, 1373, 1376, 1376f, 1393–1394
cultural considerations, 1394
disorders, 1375–1376, 1394–1396
abnormal uterine bleeding, 1396
amenorrhea, 1395–1396
dysmenorrhea, 1395
hormonal changes during, 1377t
premenstrual syndrome, 1394–1395
psychosocial considerations, 1393–1394
Mental deterioration, cirrhosis and, 1085
Men who have sex with men (MSM), 1489, 1538
Meperidine (Demerol), 281t, 287, 290
diverticulitis, 1013
Mercaptans, 1072
Mercaptopurine (6-MP), 1018
Merci device, 2035
Merkel cells, 1766
Mesna (Mesnex), 2183
Mesocaval shunt, 1070
Metabolic acidosis, 329–330
anion gap in, 330t
assessment and diagnostic findings, 330
chronic, 330
clinical manifestations, 329–330
high anion gap acidosis, 329
medical management, 330
normal anion gap acidosis, 329
pathophysiology, 329
Metabolic alkalosis, 330–331, 1032
assessment and diagnostic findings, 330–331
chronic, 330
clinical manifestations, 330
medical management, 331
pathophysiology, 330
Metabolic bone disorders, 2277–2286
osteomalacia, 2283–2284
assessment and diagnostic findings, 2284
gerontologic considerations, 2284
medical management, 2284
pathophysiology, 2284
osteoporosis, 2277–2283
assessment and diagnostic findings, 2278, 2280
gerontologic considerations, 2278
loss of height associated with, 2277f
medical management, 2280–2282, 2281t
nursing process for, 2282–2283
pathophysiology, 2278
prevention, 2277–2278
risk factors, 2278, 2279c
risks in men, 2279c
Paget's disease, 2284–2286
Metabolic disorders, 1059, 1217c
hepatic disorders, 1075
Metabolic syndrome, 730, 732, 1141
heart failure, 806
Metacognition, 22
Meta-ethics, 24
Metal-containing electrodes, 678
Metaplasia, 110–111, 110t, 2150
Metastasis, 2150, 2152
Metastatic bone disease, 2291
Metastatic skin tumours, 1826
Metformin, 1157
thalassemia, 1628
type 2 diabetes, 1142
Methadone, 287
for pain management, 287
Methicillin-resistant *Staphylococcus aureus* (MRSA), 924, 1698, 1706–1707, 1854
Methicillin-susceptible *Staphylococcus aureus*, 1854
Methohexital sodium (Brevital), 403t
Methotrexate, 1809
bladder cancer, 1357
breast cancer, 1469
immunomodulators, 1018
rheumatoid arthritis, 1744, 1745
Methyclothiazide (Enduron)
heart failure, 820t
hypertension, 884t
Methylcellulose (Citrucel), 1001t
N-methyl-D-aspartate (NMDA), 271
Methyldopa (Aldomet), hypertension, 885t
3,4-methylenedioxymethamphetamine (MDMA), 2365
Methylnaltrexone (Relistor), for opioid-induced constipation, 288
Methylphenidate (Ritalin), antidepressant therapy, 1554
Methylprednisolone (Medrol), 588t, 591t
Methyl tertiary butyl ether (MTBE), 1113
Metoclopramide (Reglan), 939, 951
breast cancer, 1469
gastric motility, 944
neuromuscular disorders, 939
postoperative nausea/vomiting, 416t
Metoclopramide hydrochloride (Reglan), 993
Metocurine (Metubine), 402t
Metolazone (Zaroxolyn, Mykrox)
heart failure, 812, 820t
hypertension, 884t
Metoprolol, 740, 2025
antiarrhythmic medication, 699t
heart failure, 812
hypertension, 885t
Metoprolol extended release (Toprol-XL), hypertension, 885t
Metrodin, 1405c
Metronidazole (Flagyl), 983, 1018
bacterial vaginosis, 1414
pelvic inflammatory disease, 1421
peptic ulcer disease and gastritis, 979t
proctitis, 1044
sexual assault, 1384
Metrorrhagia, 1396
MHC. *See* Major histocompatibility complex (MHC)
MI. *See* Myocardial infarction (MI)
Michigan Alcohol Screening Test (MAST), 126
Miconazole, 1856
candidiasis, 1414
Microbiome, 1192
Microbiota, 1192
Microcytosis, 1599, 1627
Microhemagglutination test (MHA-TP), 1723
Microvascular decompression of trigeminal nerve, 2112
Micturition, 1332, 1340
Micturition (voiding), 1268
Midazolam (Versed), 402t, 912, 1862, 2062
cervical cancer, 1391
Midbrain, 1961
Middle ear. *See also* Ear
conditions
masses, 1943
otosclerosis, 1943
tympanic membrane perforation, 1938–1939
endoscopy, 1934
implantation (MEI), 1953
ossicles, 1927
perfusion, 1946
tympanic membrane (eardrum), 1927
Middle ear effusion. *See* Serous otitis media
Middle fossa, 1961
Midesophageal diverticula, 937
Mifepristone (Mifeprex)
fibroids, 1430
induced abortion, 1403
Migraine, 2022
aura phase, 2023
cause of, 2022
headache phase, 2023
patient education, 2025c
prodrome phase, 2023
recovery phase, 2023
with and without aura, 2022–2023
Migraine headaches, 1004
Milk thistle (*Silybum marianum*), 1085
Miller–Fisher variant GBS, 2107
Milnacipran (Savella), for fibromyalgia, 1759
Milrinone, 814
cardiogenic shock, 358, 827
pulmonary edema, 825
in shock, 353t
Mind–body and biofield therapies, 2195
Mindfulness, 384
Mineralocorticoids, 1245
hypertension, 878
Mineral oil, laxative medications, 1001t
Mini-cholecystectomy, 1115
Minimally invasive cardiac output monitoring devices, 687–689
Minimally invasive surgery, 373
Minimally invasive surgical techniques, 2161
Mini-Mental State Examination (MMSE), 222, 224
Mini-nebulizer therapy. *See* Small-volume nebulizer therapy
Mini-transplants, 2186, 2187
Minocycline, 1794
Minorities, 92
Minoxidil (Loniten), hypertension, 886t
Minute ventilation, 459, 460c
Mirtazapine (Remeron), 224
Misoprostol (Cytotec)
peptic ulcer disease and gastritis, 980t
spontaneous abortion, 1403
Mithramycin, 321
Mitomycin, 1898–1899
bladder cancer, 1357
for cardiac toxicity, 2183

Mitomycin-C, 989, 2183
Mitosis (cell division), 134, 2152
Mitotic spindle inhibitors, 2179t
Mitoxantrone (Novantrone), 2098
acute myeloid leukemia, 1637
Mitral (apical) area, 668
Mitral balloon valvuloplasty, 783–784
Mitral click, 779
Mitral regurgitation, 779–780
assessment and diagnostic findings, 780
clinical manifestations, 780
medical management, 780
pathophysiology, 780
Mitral stenosis, 780–781
assessment and diagnostic findings, 780
clinical manifestations, 780
medical management, 781
pathophysiology, 780
Mitral valve, 777, 778, 784f
Mitral valve prolapse, 778–779
assessment and diagnostic findings, 779
clinical manifestations, 778–779
medical management, 779
nursing management, 779
pathophysiology, 778, 779f
Mivacurium (Mivacron), 401t
Mixed acid–base disorders, 332–333
Mixed incontinence, 1332, 1344
Mixed urinary incontinence, 1341. *See also* Urinary incontinence
MoAb. *See* Monoclonal antibodies (MoAb)
Mobility improvement
after orthopedic surgery, 2258
in cervical discectomy, 2141
for PD patient, 2131
Mobility, in older adults, 231
Model of end-stage liver disease (MELD), 1099
A Model to Guide Hospice and Palliative Care: Based on the National Principles and Norms of Practice, 239
Moderate sedation, 405
Modified Early Warning System (MEWS), 364
Modified radical mastectomy, 1446, 1459–1460
MODS. *See* Multiple organ dysfunction syndrome
Moexipril (Univasc)
in heart failure, 811t
hypertension, 886t
Mohs' micrographic surgery, 1821
Moisture-retentive dressings, 1784–1786
Moldable stomal skin barrier, 1038f
Molecular process, in carcinogenesis, 2153–2156, 2154c
Moles, 1819–1820
Mometasone furoate (Asmanex), 588t
Moniliasis/thrush, mouth abnormalities, 920t
Monitored anesthesia care (MAC), 405
Monoclonal antibodies (MoAb), 736, 1524, 1525, 2165, 2190–2191. *See also* Targeted therapies, in cancer
epidermal growth factor receptors, 2191
tyrosine kinase pathways, 2191
vascular endothelial growth factors, 2191
Monocyte, 1599, 1603. *See also* Agranulocytes
Mononeuropathy, 2114
Monooctanoin, 1112
Monosomy, 134
Monotherapy, 878, 892
Monro–Kellie hypothesis, 1996, 2057
Montelukast (Singulair), 590t
Moral dilemmas, 25
Moral distress, 26
Morality, 24. *See also* Ethics
Moral problems, 25, 26
Moral uncertainty, 25
Morning hyperglycemia, 1155, 1155t
Morphine, 286, 1120, 2008
in cardiogenic shock, 357
for chest discomfort, 544
diverticulitis, acute, 1012
for pain management, 281t, 282, 286
pulmonary edema, 825
Morphine sulphate (MS Contin), 401t, 1861
acute MI, 748
interaction with anesthetics, 382t
Mortality rate
hepatitis A, 1076
hepatitis B, 1078
surgical resection of esophagus, 942, 943
vague clinical symptoms, 1103
Morton's Neuroma, 2275
Motion sickness, 1944
Motivational interviewing, 41
Motor ability, evaluation of, 1973–1974
Motor cortex tumour, 2120
Motor fibres, 1961
Motor pathways of nervous system, 1967–1969
Mourning, 240, 257–259, 260t. *See also* Grief
Mouth care, oral cavity disorders, 927
Mouth, physical assessment, 451
Moxifloxacin (Avelox), in Ebola virus disease, 1727
MRA. *See* Magnetic resonance angiography (MRA)
MRI. *See* Magnetic resonance imaging (MRI)
MS. *See* Multiple sclerosis (MS)
MS Contin or oxycodone (OxyContin), 1861
MTBE. *See* Methyl tertiary butyl ether (MTBE)
MTX. *See* Methotrexate (MTX)
Mucinous carcinoma, 1457
Mucomyst, 910
Mucosal disorders, 1006
Mucosal proctectomy, 1020
Mucous membranes, 1002
Multiculturalism, 91
Multidetector computed tomographic angiography (MDCTA), 544
Multidetector-computed tomography (MDCT), 842
Multidisciplinary action plans (MAPs), 10
Multidrug resistance, 525, 527
Multifactorial genetic conditions, 137–138, 137f, 138f
Multimodal analgesia, 280–284
Multiple chronic conditions (MCC), 161
Multiple endocrine neoplasia, 142t, 2155
Multiple-gated acquisition (MUGA) scanning, 681
Multiple myeloma, 1652–1657
assessment and diagnostic findings, 1654
clinical manifestations, 1653–1654
gerontologic considerations, 1655–1656
medical management, 1654–1655
nursing management, 1656–1657
pathophysiology, 1652–1653
Multiple organ dysfunction syndrome (MODS), 345c, 366–367
clinical manifestations, 366
medical management, 366
nursing management, 366
effective communication, 366–367
pathophysiology, 366
Multiple organ failure, acute pancreatitis, 1122
Multiple sclerosis (MS), 120, 998, 2112t
assessment and diagnostic findings, 2097
cause of, 2096
clinical manifestations, 2096–2097
gerontologic considerations, 2097
life expectancy for patients with, 2097
medical management, 2097–2098
nursing interventions, 2098
bladder and bowel control, enhancing, 2100
cognition and emotional responses, 2100
communication and managing swallowing difficulties, enhancing, 2100
improving self-care abilities, 2101
improving sensory and cognitive function, 2100–2101
injury prevention, 2100
minimizing spasticity and contractures, 2099
patient outcomes, 2101
promoting home, community-based, and transitional care, 2101
promoting physical mobility, 2099–2100
promoting sexual functioning, 2101
strengthening coping mechanisms, 2100–2101
nursing priorities, 2098
planning and goals, 2098
pathophysiology, 2096
patient assessment, 2098
pharmacologic therapy, 2097–2098
predictors of fatigue in patients with, 2099c
primary progressive, 2096
progressive relapsing, 2096
relapsing remitting (RR), 2096
secondary progressive, 2096
signs and symptoms of, 2097
Multistrip dipstick testing, 1335
Mumps (epidemic parotitis), 924
Mupirocin, 1796
Mural thrombi, 797, 798
Murmurs, 670, 671c. *See also* Heart
defined, 653
Muscle metabolites, 838
Muscle relaxants, 403
constipation, 998
Muscles, 2218
actions, 2219
antagonists, 2219
atonic, 2219
atrophy, 851, 2214, 2219
clonus, 2226
fascia (epimysium), 2218
fasciculation, 2226
fatigue, 2218
flaccid, 2219
hypertrophy, 2219
skeletal muscle contraction, 2218–2219, 2220f
spastic, 2219
strength and size, 2225–2227
synergists, 2219
tone, 2219
Muscle-setting exercises, 2238c
Muscle strength, 1974–1975
balance control and coordination, 1975
grading, 1974c
Muscle weakness, 1002
Muscular dystrophies. *See also* Degenerative disorders
medical management, 2137–2138
nursing management
continuing/transitional care, 2138–2139
patient education about self-care, 2138

Musculoskeletal assessment, 2219
Fracture Risk Assessment Tool, 2223
health history, 2219–2223
past health, social, and family history, 2223
physical assessment, 2223–2224
bone integrity, 2225
gait, 2224–2225
integument, 2225
joint function, 2225
muscle strength and size, 2225–2227
neurovascular status, 2227, 2227c
posture, 2224
symptoms, 2221
altered sensations, 2223
joint swelling, 2223
pain, 2221
stiffness, 2221–2223
weakness, 2223
Musculoskeletal care modalities
cast management
arm casts, 2240
body or spica casts, 2240
leg casts, 2240
in cast, patient care
casting materials, 2232–2233
nursing process for, 2234, 2235c, 2237c, 2238c
splints and braces, 2233–2234
external fixator, patient with, 2241–2242, 2242c
orthopedic surgery
descriptions, 2247c
joint replacement, 2247–2248
nursing interventions, 2248, 2249c
nursing process for, 2257–2261
total hip arthroplasty, 2249–2256, 2250c–2253c, 2255c
total knee replacement, 2256–2257
splints and braces, patient with, 2240–2241
traction
nursing management, 2246–2247
principles of effective traction, 2242
skeletal traction, 2244–2246
skin traction, 2243–2244
Musculoskeletal disorders
acute low back pain, 2265–2270
assessment and diagnostic findings, 2266–2267
clinical manifestations, 2266
definition, 2265
diagnostic procedures for, 2267c
medical management, 2267
nursing process for, 2267–2270
pathophysiology, 2266
prevention strategies, 2268c
bone tumours, 2291–2295
assessment and diagnostic findings, 2292
benign, 2291
clinical manifestations, 2292
malignant, 2291
medical management, 2292
metastatic bone disease, 2291
nursing process for, 2293–2294
pathophysiology, 2291
common foot problems, 2274–2276
callus, 2274
corn, 2274
flatfoot (pes planus), 2275
hammer toe, 2274, 2275f
ingrown toenail, 2274
Morton's Neuroma, 2275
nursing process, 2275–2276
pes cavus, 2275
plantar fasciitis, 2274
common problems of upper extremity, 2270–2274
bursitis and tenosynovitis, 2270
carpal tunnel syndrome (CTS), 2271–2272
Dupuytren's contracture, 2272, 2272f
ganglion, 2272
loose bodies, 2270–2271
nursing process for, 2272–2274
shoulder impingement syndrome, 2271
diagnostic evaluation
arthrocentesis, 2229
arthrography, 2228
arthroscopy, 2229
biopsy, 2229
bone densitometry, 2228
bone scan, 2228–2229
CT scan, 2227–2228
electromyography, 2229
laboratory studies, 2229–2230
magnetic resonance imaging, 2228
x-ray studies, 2227
genetics and, 2222c
metabolic bone disorders, 2277–2283
osteomalacia, 2283–2284
osteoporosis, 2277–2283
Paget's disease, 2284–2286
musculoskeletal infections, 2286–2291
osteomyelitis, 2286–2289
septic (infectious) arthritis, 2289–2291
onset of, 2265
Musculoskeletal system, 2214
age-related changes in, 214t, 218, 2219, 2221t
articular system, structure and function of, 2217–2218, 2218f
function of, 2214
skeletal muscle system, structure and function of, 2218–2219
exercise, disuse, and repair, 2219
muscle actions, 2219
muscle tone, 2219
skeletal muscle contraction, 2218–2219
skeletal system, structure and function of, 2214–2217
bone formation, 2216
bone healing, 2217
bone maintenance, 2216–2217
Music therapy, 384
for pain relief, 291
Mutant *TP53*, 2153
Mutations, 132, 134–135, 134f, 135f
Myasthenia gravis, 1813
assessment and diagnostic findings, 2103
clinical manifestations, 2103
complications, 2104
endotracheal intubation and mechanical ventilation, 2104
medical management, 2103–2104
nursing management, 2104–2105
pathophysiology, 2102–2103
pharmacologic therapy, 2103–2104
anticholinesterase medications, 2104c
Myasthenic crisis, 2105
Mycobacterium avium complex (MAC), 1534, 1550, 1553
Mycophenolate mofetil (CellCept), 1098, 1101
Mycotic aneurysms, 855
Mydriasis, 1893
Mydriatics, 1893–1894, 1893t, 1905
Myectomy, 789
Myeloablative HSCT, 2186
Myelodysplastic syndrome (MDS), 1611, 1618–1620
assessment and diagnostic findings, 1619
clinical manifestations, 1619
medical management, 1619–1620
nursing management, 1620
primary, 1619
secondary, 1619
Myelography, 1982
Myeloid, 1599, 1600
Myelopoiesis, 1599, 1603
Myeloproliferative neoplasms, 1648t
Myelosuppression, 2150, 2182, 2195
Myocardial contractility, 740
Myocardial infarction (MI), 653, 731, 744, 844f, 852. *See also* Acute coronary syndrome (ACS)
biomarkers of, 746–747, 747t
diabetes, 1175
hypertension, 878
promoting health after, 755c
in shock, 347
treatment guidelines for, 747c
Myocardial perfusion imaging. *See also* Radionuclide imaging
nursing interventions, 680–681
positron emission tomography (PET), 680
procedure, 680
single photon emission computed tomography (SPECT), 680
Myocarditis, 797
assessment and diagnostic findings, 797
clinical manifestations, 797
medical management, 797–798
nursing management, 798
pathophysiology, 797
prevention, 797
Myocardium, 655
defined, 653
Myofascial pain, 923
Myoglobin, 747
Myomectomy, 1412, 1429
Myositis ossificans, 2312
Myotomy-myectomy, 789
Myotonic muscular dystrophy type 1, 141t
Myringotomy, 1939
Myxedema coma, 1226

N

Nabothian cysts, 1388
Nadir, 2150, 2201
Nadolol, 2025
antiarrhythmic medication, 699t
hypertension, 885t
Nail
assessment of, 1777–1778
colour changes, 1772
clubbing of, 1777
disorders, 1778f
growth, 1768
role in sensory functions, 1768
Naloxone hydrochloride (Narcan), in pulmonary edema, 826
Nanoparticle albumin-bound paclitaxel (nab-paclitaxel), 1129
Naproxen
pain management, 285
premenstrual syndrome, 1395
rheumatoid arthritis, 1745
Naratriptan (Amerge), 2025
Nasal cannula, 604
Nasal hygiene, 952

Nasal obstruction. *See also* Obstruction and trauma
- medical management, 489
- nursing management, 489

Nasal oxygen, 544
Nasal saline sprays, 476
Nasoduodenal tubes, 948, 949, 953
Nasoenteric intubation, 952
Nasogastric (NG)
- drainage, 993, 994
- intubation, 978, 993
- secretions, 1122
- suction, 855, 1023, 1112
- tube, 937, 947, 948, 951f, 1130
  - measuring length of, 950f

Nasogastric/nasoenteric devices
- tube feeding, 952–960, 955f
  - administration methods, 954–955
  - formulas, 954
  - osmosis and osmolality, 953–954

Nasojejunal feeding, 953
Nasojejunal tube, 948
Nasopharyngeal cancer, 1940
Nasopharyngeal irritation, enteral therapy, 956t
Nasopharynx, 950
Nasotracheal suction, guidelines for, 641c
NASPE-BPEG code, for pacemaker generator function, 719, 720c, 724
Natalizumab (Tysabri), for Crohn's disease, 1018
National Asthma Education and Prevention Program (NAEPP), 1585
National Cancer Institute (NCI), 925
National Center for Complementary and Alternative Medicine (NCCAM), 2193
National Comprehensive Cancer Network (NCCN), 1456, 1483
National Educational Association of Disabled Students, 1892
National High Blood Pressure Education Program, 891
National Institute of Allergy and Infectious Disease (NIAID), 1418, 1533, 1585
National Institute of Dental and Craniofacial Research (NIDCR), 923
National Kidney Foundation (NKF), 1285
Natriuretic peptide hormones, 302–303
Natural débridement, 1857
Natural health products (NHPs), preoperative assessment, 382–383
Natural immunity, 1518
- immune regulation, 1519
- inflammatory response, 1518–1519
- physical and chemical barriers, 1519
- white blood cell action, 1518

Natural killer (NK) cells, 1517, 1518, 1523, 2156
Nausea and vomiting
- enteral therapy, 956t
- gastritis, 978
- gastrointestinal (GI) tract, 903
- during intraoperative period, 406
- opioid-induced, 288
- in PACU, controlling, 416–417, 416t, 417c
- peritonitis, 1014
- prevention, after chemotherapy, 2185
- thoracic aortic aneurysm, 842

Nd:YAG laser, hemorrhoids, 1046
Nebivolol
- antiarrhythmic medication, 699t
- hypertension, 885t

Neck dissection
- assessment, 929–930
- collaborative problems, 930
- evaluation of, 934
- nursing interventions, 930–934
- nursing priorities, 930
- nursing process, 929–934
- planning and goals, 930
- postoperative care, 930

Neck surgery, home care checklist, 933c
Necrotizing gingivitis, gum abnormalities, 921t
Nedocromil, 587, 589t
Needle biopsies, 2160
Nefazodone (Serzone), 224
Negative emotions, 104
Negative feedback, 109–110
Negative inotropic effect, 741
Negative pressure (vacuum) devices
- erectile dysfunction, 1485, 1487

Neglect, 233, 2371–2373
- assessment, 2372c

Neighbourhood health centres, 18
Neisseria gonorrhoeae, 1044, 1723
- assessment and diagnostic findings, 1723
- clinical manifestations, 1723
- complications, 1723
- medical management, 1723
- nursing management, 1723–1724

Neoplasia, 2150
Neovascularization of iris, 1908
Nephrectomy, 1290–1291
Nephrolithiasis, 1350
- assessment and diagnostic findings, 1351
- clinical manifestations, 1351
- defined, 1350
- medical management, 1351–1352
- pathophysiology, 1350–1351

Nephron-sparing surgery, 1291
Nephropathy, 1137, 1144
- assessment and diagnostic findings, 1179–1180
- clinical manifestations, 1179
- diabetes and, 1179
- medical management, 1180

Nephrosclerosis, 1283, 1285
- assessment and diagnostic findings, 1285
- benign, 1285
- malignant, 1285
- medical management, 1285
- pathophysiology, 1285

Nephrotic syndrome, 1283, 1288–1289
- assessment and diagnostic findings, 1289
- clinical manifestations, 1289
- complications, 1289
- medical management, 1289
- nursing management, 1289
- pathophysiology, 1289, 1289f

Nephrotoxic, 1283
- agents, 1293

Nerve cell bodies, 1958
Nerve conduction studies, 1983
Nerve injury, neck dissection, 933
Nerve paralysis from malignancy, 2111t
Nervous system
- age-related changes in, 214t, 218–219
- assessment, 1969
  - health history, 1970–1971
  - physical examination, 1971–1979
- cells of, 1958
- diagnostic evaluation
  - cerebral angiography, 1982
  - computed tomography (CT) scanning, 1980
  - electroencephalography, 1983
  - electromyography, 1983
  - evoked potential studies, 1983–1984
  - examination of cerebrospinal fluid, 1984
  - lumbar puncture, 1984–1985
  - magnetic resonance imaging (MRI), 1980–1981
  - myelography, 1982
  - nerve conduction studies, 1983
  - noninvasive carotid flow studies, 1982
  - positron emission tomography (PET), 1981
  - single photon emission computed tomography (SPEC), 1981
  - transcranial Doppler, 1982–1983

Nesiritide (Natrecor), for pulmonary edema, 825
Neural transplantation, for Parkinson's disease, 2130
Neurodegenerative, 2117, 2127
Neurofibromatosis, 1820
Neurogenic bladder, 1332
- assessment and diagnostic findings, 1346
- cause, 1346
- complications, 1346
- defined, 1346
- description, 1346
- flaccid bladder, 1346
- medical management, 1346
- pathophysiology, 1346
- spastic bladder, 1346

Neurogenic shock, 359, 364–365
- medical management, 364
- nursing management, 364–365

Neuroglial cells, 1958
Neurologic disorders
- genetic factors, 1970c
- health history, 1970–1971
- neurologic examination, 1971–1979
  - consciousness and cognition, 1972
  - cranial nerves, 1973
  - emotional status, 1972
  - gerontologic considerations, 1978–1979
  - impact on patient's lifestyle and relationships, 1972
  - intellectual function, 1972
  - language ability, 1972
  - level of consciousness, 1972
  - mental status, 1972, 1979
  - motor alterations, 1979
  - motor system, 1973–1975
  - nursing implications, 1979
  - reflexes, 1976–1978
  - sensory alterations, 1979
  - sensory system, 1975–1976
  - structural and physiologic changes, 1979
  - temperature regulation and pain perception, 1979
  - thought content, 1972
- symptoms and signs of, 1971
  - dizziness, 1971
  - muscle weakness, 1971
  - pain, 1971
  - seizures, 1971
  - sensory alterations, 1971
  - vertigo, 1971

Neurologic function
- anatomy and physiology overview
  - cells of nervous system, 1958
  - central nervous system, 1960–1964
  - motor pathways of nervous system, 1967–1969
  - neurotransmitters (chemical messengers), 1958–1960, 1960t

Neurologic function (*continued*)
peripheral nervous system, 1964–1967
sensory pathways of nervous system, 1969
diagnostic evaluation
cerebral angiography, 1982
CT scan, 1980
electroencephalography, 1983
electromyography, 1983
evoked potential studies, 1983–1984
examination of cerebrospinal fluid, 1984
lumbar puncture, 1984–1985
magnetic resonance imaging, 1980–1981
myelography, 1982
nerve conduction studies, 1983
noninvasive carotid flow studies, 1982
positron emission tomography (PET), 1981
single photon emission computed tomography (SPEC), 1981
transcranial Doppler, 1982–1983
nervous system assessment, 1969
health history, 1970–1971
physical examination, 1971–1979
Neurologic system, chemotherapy-induced neurotoxicity, 2183
Neurologic trauma, 2056
Neuromodulation, 291
Neuromuscular blockade (NMB), 1083
Neuron, 1959f
Neuropathic pain, 269, 273
central mechanism of, 273
peripheral mechanism of, 273
Neuropathic pain syndromes, 269c
Neuropathy, 1137, 1144
Neuroprotectants, 2030
Neuroscience nursing, 1988
Neurotransmitters (chemical messengers), 1958–1960, 1960t
functions, 1958–1959
imbalance of, 1959
major, 1960t
Neurovascular disorders, 1760
Neurovascular status
defined, 2233
monitoring, 2245
Neutral protamine Hagedorn (NPH) insulin, 1151
Neutropenia, 1599, 1616, 2150, 2201
causes, 1632c
clinical manifestation, 1632
medical management, 1632–1633
nursing management, 1633
precautions, 1635c
Neutropenic fever, 2201, 2202t
Neutrophil, 1518, 1599, 1600
Newborn screening, 140t
New or novel oral anticoagulants (NOACs), 2033
A New Perspective on the Health of Canadians, 157
New York Heart Association (NYHA), 806
NHL. *See* Non-Hodgkin lymphomas (NHL)
Nicardipine (Cardene), 2049
hypertension, 887t, 893
NicoDerm, 910
Nicotine
patch, 736
for peripheral arterial insufficiency, 845
replacement, 569
stomatitis, mouth abnormalities, 920t
Nifedipine
heart failure, 813
hypertension, 887t
Nightingale, Florence, 4
Nikolsky's sign, 1813
Nimodipine, 2049
Nimotop, 2049
Nipple–areola reconstruction, 1474
NIPPV. *See* Noninvasive positive-pressure ventilation (NIPPV)
Nissen fundoplication, in gastroesophageal reflux disease, 939
Nitrate reduction test, 1335
Nitrofurantoin, 1336
thalassemia, 1628
Nitrofurazone (Furacin), 1856
Nitroglycerin
for angina pectoris, 740, 740c, 743
in cardiogenic shock, 357
intermittent IV infusion of, 740
in shock, 353t
sublingual, 740, 740c
Nitroglycerine (Transderm-Nitro), 910
hypertension, 886t
hypertensive emergencies, 893
pulmonary edema, 825
Nitroprusside, 2049
hypertension, 886t
shock, 353t
Nitrosoureas, as antineoplastic agent, 2179t
Nitrous oxide, as gas anesthetic agent, 300, 400t
Nizatidine (Axid)
antacids, 939
peptic ulcer disease and gastritis, 979t
NMB. *See* Neuromuscular blockade (NMB)
Nociception, 270f, 271
Nociceptive pain, 269, 270f, 271–273
modulation, 272
perception, 272–273
transduction, 271
transmission, 271
Nociceptive pain syndromes, 269c
Nociceptors, 271
Nocturia, 663, 1332, 1334, 1480, 1481
left ventricular failure, 809
Nocturnal penile tumescence test, 1484
Nodular goitre, 1238
Nodular melanoma, 1823
Noise, exposure limit of, 1935
Noise-induced hearing loss (NIHL), 1935
Nolvadex, breast disease, 1456
Nonalcoholic fatty liver disease (NAFLD), 1056
Nonalcoholic steatohepatitis (NASH), 1056
Non-AOBP, 882
Nonbullous impetigo, 1795
Noncommunicable diseases, 155
Non–contrast-enhanced study, 910
Noncytotoxic wound-cleansing agent, 869
Nondihydropyridine calcium channel blocker, 704
Nondisjunction, 134
Nonfatal drowning, 2356–2357
complications, 2357
defined, 2356
factors associated with, 2356
management, 2357
Nongerminal tumours, 1507
Non-GI functional disorders, 1004
Non-HDL cholesterol, 882
Non-Hodgkin lymphomas (NHL), 1650–1652, 1650f, 2165
assessment and diagnostic findings, 1651
clinical manifestations, 1651
medical management, 1651
nursing management, 1651–1652
Noninfectious inflammatory dermatoses
generalized exfoliative dermatitis, 1812–1813
irritant contact dermatitis, 1802–1806
psoriasis, 1806–1810
Noninvasive carotid flow studies, 1982
Noninvasive positive-pressure ventilation (NIPPV), 620
Noninvasive respiratory therapies. *See also* Respiratory care modalities
chest physiotherapy, 608–612
incentive spirometry, 607–608
oxygen therapy, 601–607
small-volume nebulizer therapy, 608
Nonmaleficence, 25, 25c
Nonmyeloablative HSCT, 2186
Nonneoplastic polyps, 1044
Nonnucleoside reverse transcriptase inhibitors (NNRTI), 1545
Nonopioid pre-emptive analgesic agents, for breathing problems, 634
Nonparoxysmal junctional tachycardia, 706
Nonpharmacologic measures, 423
Non-plaster cast, 2232–2233
Nonrebreathing masks, 605
Nonspecific biologic response modifiers, 2190
Nonsteroidal anti-inflammatory drugs (NSAIDs), 924, 1011, 1295, 1394
acute low back pain, 2267
glaucoma, 1894
hidradenitis suppurativa (HS), 1791
kidney stone pain, 1351
pain management, 285
pericarditis, 799
Non–ST-segment elevation MI (NSTEMI), 744, 746. *See also* Acute coronary syndrome (ACS); Myocardial infarction (MI)
Nonsurgical septal reduction therapy, for cardiomyopathy, 789
Non treponemal tests (NTT), 1722
Nonunion, 2310–2311, 2310f
Nonviral hepatitis, 1082
drug-induced liver disease, 1082
toxic hepatitis, 1082
Norcuron. *See* Vecuronium
Norepinephrine, 106, 2000
gastrointestinal regulatory substances, 901t
shock, 353t
No-rinse cleanser, 198
Normal electrical conduction, 692
Normal flora, 1698, 1705
Normal heart sounds, 653, 669
Normal sinus rhythm, 696–697
Normochromic anemia, 1599, 1615
Normocytic anemia, 1599, 1615
North American Nursing Diagnosis Association (NANDA) International, 31, 36, 62
Norton scale, 195
Nortriptyline, 569
Norwalk virus, 1001
Nose
anatomy, 438–439
fracture of, 489–490 (*See also* Obstruction and trauma)
assessment/diagnostic findings, 490
clinical manifestations, 490
medical management, 490
nursing management, 490
physical assessment, 451
Nosebleed. *See* Epistaxis
Nosocomial, 505

Nothing by mouth (NPO)
in hospitalized diabetic patients, 1185
from midnight, 909, 910, 912
status, 993
Novarel, 1405c
NPO. *See* Nothing by mouth (NPO)
NSAIDs. *See* Nonsteroidal anti-inflammatory drugs (NSAIDs)
N-Terface, 1860
Nuchal rigidity, 471, 477
Nuclear cataract, 1900
Nuclear scans, 1278
Nucleated RBC, 1599, 1602
Nucleic acid amplification test (NAAT), 1544, 1545, 1723
Nuclei for cranial nerves, 1961
Nucleoli, 2152
Nucleotide reverse transcriptase inhibitors (NRTI), 1545
Nuedexta, 231
Null lymphocytes, 1517, 1523
Nu-Lytely, 913
Numeric rating scale, 277–278
Nurse
in ambulatory care settings, 18–19
in community settings, 13–15
culturally competent, 14
as patient advocate, 410
roles of, 10
caregiver role, 10
leadership role, 10
research role, 10–11
school, 19
spirituality of, 85
Nurse practitioners (NP), 4, 11
Nurse-to-nurse report, in PACU, 413c
Nursing, 4, 26
community-based (*See* Community-based nursing)
defined, 4
ethical problems in, 26
confidentiality, 26
end-of-life issues, 27
refusing care, 27
restraints, use of, 27
trust, 27
truth-telling, 27
ethics (*See* Ethics)
history of, in Canada, 4
home care, 15–16
Nursing care of cancer patients
bleeding, thrombocytopenia and, 2202–2203
body image and self-esteem, 2199
fatigue, 2198–2199, 2199c
gerontologic considerations, 2204, 2204t
grieving process, 220
hospice, 2208
infection management, 2200–2201, 2202t
nutrition promotion, 2196–2198, 2196c
oncologic emergencies, 2204–2208, 2205t–2207t
patient education, 2203–2204
psychosocial distress, 2200
relieving pain, 2198, 2198t
septic shock, 2201–2202
sexuality, 2199–2200
tissue integrity, 2195–2196
Nursing diagnoses, 28, 30c, 31
cardiomyopathy, 792
choosing, 31
and collaborative problems, differences between, 32, 32f
heart failure, 817–818
neck dissection, 930
patient with newly diagnosed diabetes, 1170–1172
pericarditis, 800
Nursing interventions
acute low back pain, 2268–2270
bone tumours, 2293
bowel function, 429
bronchoscopy, 465
cardiac output promotion, 423–424
cardiomyopathy, 793–794
chest x-ray, 462
chronic inflammatory bowel disease, 1020–1023
colorectal cancer
body image, 1041
colostomy appliance, 1040–1041
emotional support, 1039–1040
home and community-based care, 1043
postoperative care, 1040
preparing the patient for surgery, 1039
sexuality issues, 1043
common problems of upper extremity, 2272–2273
computed tomography (CT), 463
Cushing syndrome, 1252–1253
deep vein thrombosis, 430–431
diabetes as secondary diagnosis, 1188–1189
diverticular disease
elimination patterns, 1013
home and community-based care, 1013
relieving pain, 1013
emotional support to patient/family, 430
in encouraging activity, 424–425
esophagus, 940
gastric cancer, 990–992
gastrostomy and jejunostomy, 962–964
gerontologic considerations, 432
GI function management, 428
heart failure, 818–823
hematoma, 431
home/community-based/transitional care, 433
hypertension, 889–890
hyperthyroidism, 1235
for inpatient cardiac monitoring, 677–679, 678c
managing voiding, 429–430
MRI, 463, 464
neck dissection, 930–934
normal body temperature maintenance, 428
in nutrition, 428–429
orthopedic surgery
ambulation promotion, 2248
infection prevention, 2248
pain management, 2248, 2249c
osteomyelitis, 2288–2289
osteoporosis, 2282–2283
parenteral nutrition, 969–972
for patient during surgery, 408–410
patient undergoing bariatric surgery, 1206
patient with newly diagnosed diabetes, 1171–1172
pericarditis, 800
postoperative, immediate, 420c
in relieving pain, 422–423
epidural infusions, 423
intrapleural anesthesia, 423
opioid analgesics, 423
patient-controlled analgesia, 423
renal and urologic disorders, 1280
respiratory complications prevention, 422
safe environment maintenance, 430
skeletal traction
effective, 2245
exercise promotion, 2246
neurovascular status monitoring, 2245
pin-site care, 2245–2246
positioning maintenance, 2245
skin breakdown, preventing, 2245
skin traction
circulatory impairment, 224
effectiveness, 2244
nerve damage, 2244
skin breakdown, 2244
for stress management, 114–117
thoracoscopy, 465–466
total hip arthroplasty
continuing/transitional care, 2256
dislocation of hip prosthesis, preventing, 2249, 2253
gerontologic considerations, 2249
infection prevention, 2254–2255
patient education about self-care, 2255–2256
potential complications, 2250c–2253c
VTE prevention, 2253–2254
wound drainage, 2253
tube feeding, 956–959
wound
care, 425–428, 425c, 426t, 428c
dehiscence/evisceration, 432
infection, 431
Nursing Interventions Classification (NIC), 33, 36
Nursing leadership, 10
Nursing management, 949, 1047
abscess, 922
acne vulgaris, 1794–1795
acquired thrombophilias, 1678
acute lymphocytic leukemia, 1640
acute myeloid leukemia, 1638
acute pancreatitis, 1121–1123
acute respiratory failure, 534
acute rhinosinusitis, 476–477
acute tracheobronchitis, 508
adenoiditis, 482
adrenocortical insufficiency, 1249
after surgery, in PACU, 420–421
Alzheimer's disease, 228–230
anaphylactic shock, 365–366
anaphylaxis, 1581
anorectal disorders, 1047
aplastic anemia, 1616–1617
appendicitis, 1010
ARDS
general measures, 536
ventilator considerations, 536–537, 537c
ascites, 1065
assessments, 413
asthma
continuing and transitional care, 594
patient education about self-care, 593–594
atopic dermatitis, 1591
atrial fibrillation, 705
basal cell carcinoma (BCC), 1822
Bell's palsy, 2113–2114
bleeding disorders, 1658
blindness, 1890–1892
coping strategy, 1890–1891
promoting home, community-based, and transitional care, 1892
promoting spatial orientation and mobility, 1891–1892
brain abscesses, 2092

Nursing management (*continued*)
breast cancer, 1469–1470
breathing retraining, 612
bronchiectasis, 583
cardiogenic shock, 358–359, 828
cardiovascular stability, 415–416
cataracts, 1903
postoperative care, 1903
preoperative care, 1903
promoting home, community-based, and transitional care, 1903
catheterization, 1347–1350
celiac disease, 1008
chemotherapy
administering of, 2184–2185
cognitive change management, 2185
cognitive status assessment, 2184
fatigue management, 2185
fluid and electrolyte status, 2184
long-term complications of, 2184c
nausea and vomiting prevention, 2185
risks for infection/bleeding, 2184
chest percussion and vibration, 610–612
Chlamydia trachomatis, 1723–1724
chronic heart failure, 816–824
chronic myeloid leukemia, 1639–1640
chronic pharyngitis, 481
chronic rhinosinusitis, 479
coal worker's pneumoconiosis, 548
confirming placement, 950–951
considerations in cosmetic procedures, 1827t
COPD
activity pacing, 573
activity tolerance, 575
airway clearance, 574–575
breathing exercises, 573
breathing patterns, 575
continuing/transitional care, 576–577, 578c–581c
coping measures, 574
inspiratory muscle training, 573
nutritional therapy, 574
oxygen therapy, 574
palliative care, 574
patient assessment, 574
patient education, 573
patient education about self-care, 575–576, 576c, 577c
physical conditioning, 574
of potential complications, 575
self-care activities, 573–574
corneal surgeries, 1905–1906
corticosteroid therapy, 1257–1258
Creutzfeldt–Jakob disease (CJD), 2095–2096
cystic fibrosis, 598
dermabrasion, 1830
diabetes insipidus, 1221
diabetes mellitus, 1158–1164
diabetic ketoacidosis, 1169
diabetic retinopathy, 1178–1179
diarrhea, 1002–1003
disseminated intravascular coagulation, 1671
Ebola virus disease, 1726–1727
emergency contraception, 1402
emergent/resuscitative phase of burn care, 1849
empyema, 532–533
endometriosis, 1431
epistaxis, 488–489
erectile dysfunction, 1487
esophageal varices, 1070–1071
esophagus cancer, 944–945
essential thrombocythemia, 1660
external otitis (otitis externa), 1938
fecal incontinence, 1003–1004
fibromyalgia, 1759
folliculitis, 1797
food allergy, 1593
fracture, 2305–2306
fungal encephalitis, 2094–2095
gastritis, 978–981
gastrointestinal intubation, 949
giant cell arteritis, 1753–1754
glaucoma, 1899–1900
continuing and transitional care, 1899–1900
patient education, 1900c
promoting home, community-based, and transitional care, 1899
gout, 1759
headaches
continuing and transitional care, 2026
pain management, 2025–2026
promoting home, community-based, and transitional care, 2026
hearing loss, 1936
hemophilia, 1666
hepatic cirrhosis, 1085–1095
hepatic encephalopathy, 1073–1074
hepatitis A virus, 1078
hepatitis B virus, 1080–1081
hereditary hemochromatosis, 1630
herniation of lumbar disc
assessing patient after surgery, 2144
continuing/transitional care, 2145
educating patients about self-care, 2145
positioning patient, 2144
providing preoperative care, 2144–2145
herpes simplex virus (HSV) encephalitis, 2093
herpes zoster, 1798
hip fracture, 2318–2319
Hodgkin lymphoma, 1650
HSCT
care during treatment, 2188–2189
caring for donors, 2189
caring for recipients, 2189
neutropenic diets for infection prevention, 2188c
pretransplantation care implementation, 2188
hypercalcemia, 322
hyperglycemic hyperosmolar nonketotic syndrome, 1170
hyperkalemia, 317–318
hypermagnesemia, 324
hypernatremia, 313
hyperphosphatemia, 326–327
hyperthermia, 2189
hypervolemia, 308–309
hypocalcemia, 320
hypokalemia, 315
hypomagnesemia, 323–324
hyponatremia, 311–312
hypoparathyroidism, 1244
hypophosphatemia, 326
hypovolemia, 307
hypovolemic shock, 355–356
immune hemolytic anemia, 1629
immune thrombocytopenic purpura, 1663
impetigo, 1796
induced abortion, 1404
infective endocarditis, 797
infertility, 1406
infratentorial approach, to intracranial surgery, 2007–2008
inserting the tube, 949–950
intracranial surgery, 2007–2008, 2013
supratentorial and infratentorial approaches, 2007–2008
transsphenoidal approach, 2013
iron deficiency anemia, 1614–1615, 1615c
irritable bowel syndrome, 1005
ischemic stroke, 2038–2046
jaw disorders, 924
laryngitis, 484
lateral and medial collateral ligament injury, 2301
latex allergy, 1596
liver metastases, 1097–1098
lung abscess, 530
lung cancer
breathing problems, relieving, 552
fatigue reduction, 552
psychological support, providing, 552
symptom management, 552
maintaining tube function, 951–952
megaloblastic anemias, 1618
menopause, 1379–1380
mitral valve prolapse, 779
monitoring the patient, 951–952
multiple myeloma, 1656–1657
multiple organ dysfunction syndrome, 366–367
myasthenia gravis, 2104–2105
myelodysplastic syndrome, 1620
myocarditis, 798
nasal fracture, 490
nasal obstruction, 489
Neisseria gonorrhoeae, 1723–1724
neurogenic shock, 364–365
neutropenia, 1633
non-Hodgkin lymphomas, 1651–1652
obesity, 1201–1203
obstructive sleep apnea, 488
ocular medication administration, 1894–1896
oral and nasal hygiene, 952
oral cancer, 926
oral cavity, 927–929, 928–929
orbital implants and conformers, 1920–1921
patient education, 1920
promoting home, community-based, and transitional care, 1920–1921
osteoarthritis, 1755–1756
ostomy, 1023–1031
ovarian cancer, 1439–1440
oxygen therapy, 606–607
in PACU, 413–418, 415t, 416t
gerontologic considerations, 417
nausea and vomiting, controlling, 416–417, 416t, 417c
pain and anxiety, relieving, 416
readiness for discharge from PACU, 417–418
pancreatic cancer, 1129
pancreatic tumours, 1130–1131
parenteral fluid therapy, 335–338
patent airway maintenance, 414–415
pediculosis capitis, 1800–1801
pediculosis corporis and pubis, 1801
pelvic inflammatory disease, 1421–1422
perianal itching, 1791
pericarditis, 799
perimenopause, 1376–1377
perineal itching, 1791
peritonitis, 1015

peritonsillar abscess, 483
pertussis, 1728
pharynx cancer, 926
platelet defects, 1663
pleural effusion, 532
pleurisy, 531
polycythemia, 1631–1632
polymyalgia rheumatica, 1753–1754
polymyositis, 1752–1753
postoperative, for thoracic surgery, 639–648
airway clearance, 640–642, 641c
continuing/transitional care, 644, 645c–648c
fluid volume/nutrition, 644
gas exchange/breathing, 640
mobility/shoulder exercises, 643
pain/discomfort, relieving, 642–643
patient education about self-care, 644, 645c
potential complications monitoring, 644
respiratory/cardiovascular status, 640
postural drainage, 610, 610c
premenstrual syndrome, 1395
preoperative, thoracic surgery and, 632–634
preparing the patient, 949
primary aldosteronism, 1255
primary brain tumours, 2122
primary immune deficiency diseases, 1537
primary myelofibrosis, 1647–1648
prostatitis, 1490
pruritus (itching), 1790, 1791
psoriasis, 1809–1810
pulmonary edema, 533, 825–826
pulmonary embolism
anxiety, relieving, 546
continuing/transitional care, 546
monitoring for complications, 546
oxygen therapy management, 546
pain management, 545–546
patient education about self-care, 546
postoperative nursing care, 546
potential assessment, 545
risk minimization, 545
thrombolytic therapy monitoring, 545
thrombus formation prevention, 545
pulmonary heart disease, 540–541
pulmonary hypertension, 539–540
radiation therapy, 2166, 2167c–2177c
refractive errors, 1890–1892
refractive surgeries, 1906
removing the tube, 952
retinal detachment, 1908
rheumatoid arthritis, 1745–1747
rhinitis, 473
rhytidectomy (face-lift), 1830–1831
scabies, 1802
scleroderma, 1752
seborrheic dermatoses, 1792
securing the tube, 951
seizure disorders
after seizure, 2015
during seizure, 2015
sepsis, 363–364
septic (infectious) arthritis, 2290–2291
Sjögren's syndrome, 1751
skin conditions, 1788–1789
skin disorders, 1788–1789
skin grafting, 1828–1829
small-volume nebulizer therapy, 608
spinal cord tumours, 2126–2127
spondyloarthropathies, 1757
spontaneous abortion, 1403
squamous cell carcinomas (SCC), 1822
status asthmaticus, 596
status epilepticus, 2022
supratentorial approach, to intracranial surgery, 2007–2008
surgery in cancer, 2162–2163
syndrome of inappropriate antidiuretic hormone, 1222
syphilis, 1723
systemic lupus erythematosus, 1750
targeted therapies, in cancer
home, community-based/transitional care, 2192–2195
oral antineoplastic agents, 2193t–2194t
therapeutic and adverse effects, 2192
unproven/unconventional therapies, 2195
testicular cancer, 1509
thalassemia, 1628
thrombocytopenia, 1661
thyroid cancer
home, community-based, and transitional care, 1240
postoperative care, 1239–1240
potential complications, 1240
preoperative care, 1239
tonsillitis
educating patients about self-care, 482
postoperative care, providing, 482
tracheostomy, 615–617
traction
anxiety assessment, 2246
atelectasis/pneumonia, 2246
constipation/anorexia, 2246
self-care, assisting with, 2246
urinary stasis/infection, 2246
venous thromboembolism, 2248–2249
trigeminal neuralgia (tic douloureux), 2112–2113
urethral trauma, 1356
urinary retention, 1345–1346
valvuloplasty and replacement, 799–800
variant Creutzfeldt–Jakob disease (CJD), 2095–2096
vasectomy, 1510
viral rhinitis, 475
vision impairment, 1890–1892
coping strategy, 1890–1891
promoting home, community-based, and transitional care, 1892
promoting spatial orientation and mobility, 1891–1892
vulvar cancer, 1436–1437
vulvar dystrophy, 1428
Nursing Outcomes Classification (NOC), 32, 36
Nursing priorities
for acute low back pain, 2268
for bone tumours, 2293
chronic inflammatory bowel disease, 1020
colorectal cancer, 1038
for common problems of upper extremity, 2272
Cushing syndrome, 1252
diverticular disease, 1013
gallbladder disease, 1116
gastrostomy and jejunostomy, 961–962
heart failure, 818
hyperthyroidism, 1235
osteomyelitis, 2288
osteoporosis, 2282
parenteral nutrition, 969
patient undergoing bariatric surgery, 1204, 1206
tube feeding, 955
Nursing process, 21, 28–29, 29f
acute abdomen, 1013–1014
acute coronary syndrome, 750–754
for acute low back pain, 2267–2270
assessment, 2267–2268
nursing interventions, 2268–2270
nursing priorities, 2268
planning and goals, 2268
altered elimination patterns, 200–203
amputation, 2329–2334
angina pectoris, 742–743
assessment in, 28, 29, 30c
health history, 29–30, 31t
other important and relevant information, 30
physical assessment, 30
recording data, 30
for bone tumours, 2293–2294
cardiomyopathy, 792–794
assessment, 792
diagnosis, 792
evaluation, 794
nursing interventions, 793–794
planning and goals, 792
for cervical discectomy
assessment, 2141
collaborative problems, 2141
evaluation, 2142
nursing interventions, 2141–2142
nursing priorities, 2141
planning and goals, 2141
colorectal cancer, 1038–1044
for common foot problems, 2275–2276
for common problems of upper extremity, 2272–2274
infection prevention, 2273
neurovascular assessment, 2272
nursing interventions, 2272–2273
nursing priorities, 2272
pain management, 2272
patient evaluation, 2274
planning and goals, 2272
self-care, 2273
critical thinking and ethical principles in, use of, 29
Cushing syndrome, 1252–1254
diabetes as secondary diagnosis, 1187–1189
assessment, 1187
diagnosis, 1187
nursing interventions, 1188–1189
planning and goals, 1187–1188
diabetes mellitus
diabetes as secondary diagnosis, 1187–1189
newly diagnosed diabetes mellitus, 1170–1175
diagnosis in, 28, 31
collaborative problems, 28, 30c, 31–32
nursing diagnoses, 28, 30c, 31
documentation of outcomes and revision of plan, 34, 36
for dysrhythmias
assessment, 713
collaborative problems, 713
nursing interventions, 713–715, 714c
nursing priorities, 713
planning and goals, 713
evaluation in, 28, 30c, 33–34
gallbladder disease, 1115–1118
gastric cancer, 990–992
heart failure, 817–818, 817–824
assessment, 817–818
diagnosis, 817–818

Nursing process (*continued*)
evaluation, 823–824
nursing interventions, 818–823
planning and goals, 818
for hospitalized patient after surgery
assessment, 421
bowel function, 429
cardiac output, 423–424
emotional support to patient/family, 430
encouraging activity, 424–425
gastrointestinal function/nutrition, 428–429
normal body temperature, maintaining, 428
nursing priorities, 421
pain, relieving, 422–423
planning and goals, 421–422
potential complications, 430–433, 430t, 431t
respiratory complications, 422
safe environment maintenance, 430
voiding, management, 429–430
wound care, 425–428, 425c, 426t, 428c
hyperthyroidism, 1235–1236
impaired physical mobility, 180–193
impaired skin integrity, 193–200
implementation phase in, 28, 30c, 33
nursing interventions, execution of, 33
inflammatory bowel disease, 1020–1023
leg ulcers, 870–871
neck dissection, 929–934
newly diagnosed diabetes mellitus, 1170–1175
assessment, 1170–1172
diagnosis, 1170–1171
evaluation, 1172–1175
nursing interventions, 1171–1172
planning and goals, 1171
for osteoporosis, 2282–2283
parenteral nutrition, 969–972
for Parkinson's disease
assessment, 2130–2131
evaluation, 2134
nursing interventions, 2131–2133, 2133c
nursing priorities, 2131
planning and goals, 2131
patient during surgery, 407
assessment, 407
evaluation, 410
nursing interventions, 408–410
nursing priorities, 407–408
planning and goals, 408
potential complications, 408
in patient education, 43–45, 43c
for patient in cast
assessment, 2234
cast removal, 2239c
collaborative problems, 2234
compartment syndrome, 2236
disuse syndrome, 2237
evaluation, 2239
home care checklist, 2238c
muscle-setting exercises, 2238c
nursing interventions, 2234–2239
nursing priorities, 2234
planning and goals, 2234
pressure ulcers, 2237
univalving or bivalving cast, 2237c
patient undergoing bariatric surgery
assessment of, 1204
body image changes, 1207
bowel habits maintenance, 1207–1208
collaborative problems, 1206
evaluation, 1209
fluid volume balance of, 1206
home, community- based, and transitional care, 1209
infection prevention, 1206–1207
nursing interventions, 1206
nursing priorities for, 1204, 1206
nutritional status of, 1207
planning and goals, 1206
potential complications, 1206, 1208
reducing anxiety of, 1206
relieving pain of, 1206
for patient undergoing laryngectomy
assessment, 495–496
collaborative problems, 496
evaluation, 501–502
nursing interventions, 497–501
nursing priorities, 496
planning and goals, 497
peptic ulcer disease, 984–988
pericarditis, 799
assessment, 799
diagnosis, 800
evaluation, 800
nursing interventions, 800
planning in, 28, 30c, 32
establishing expected outcomes, 32–33
establishing goals, 33
nursing actions, determination of, 33
setting priorities, 32
plan of nursing care, example of, 34–35c
for pneumonia
assessment, 517–518
collaborative problems, 518
evaluation, 520
nursing interventions, 518–520
nursing priorities, 518
planning and goals, 518
for primary brain tumours
assessment, 2123
continuing/transitional care, 2124
evaluation, 2124
family processes, enhancing, 2124
home care checklist, 2125c
nursing priorities, 2123
nutrition, 2123–2124
patient education about self-care, 2124
planning and goals, 2123–
relieving anxiety, 2124
self-care deficits, compensating for, 2123
for pulmonary tuberculosis
assessment, 525–526
collaborative problems, 526
evaluation, 528–529
nursing interventions, 527
nursing priorities, 526
planning and goals, 526–527
potential complications management, 527–528
self-care deficits in ADLs, 178–180
sickle cell disease, 1624–1627
steps of, 28, 30c
surgical procedures, 984t–985t
taxonomy of nursing practice, 36
for upper airway infections
assessment, 484
collaborative problems, 484
nursing interventions, 484–485
planning and goals, 484
potential complications, 484
priorities, 484
Nursing research, 10–11
Nursing research profile
chronic heart failure patient, 815c
diabetes education, 1159c
with gastrectomy, 991c
living with total artificial heart, 790c
low-sodium diet, in heart failure, 815c
pressure ulcers among critically ill patients with extreme obesity, 1203c
Nutcracker esophagus (NE), 935
Nutrition, 41, 574
acute gallbladder, 1112
acute pancreatitis, 1120
for acute pharyngitis, 480
in ARDS, 536
ascites, 1062
in cancer
anorexia, 2197
cancer-related anorexia–cachexia syndrome, 2197
general considerations, 2197–2198
malabsorption, 2197
nutritional impairment, 2196–2197, 2196c
for cardiac disease, 663
chronic inflammatory bowel disease, 1018
colorectal cancer, 1039
coma, 1074
Crohn's disease, 1017
diabetes as secondary diagnosis, 1188
diabetes mellitus, 1144–1147
ethical dilemma, 962c
gastric cancer, 990
gastric surgery
bile reflux, 993
dumping syndrome, 993–994
dysphagia and gastric retention, 993
vitamin and mineral deficiencies, 994
hepatic cirrhosis, 1085, 1094
hepatic encephalopathy, 1074
for hospitalized patient after surgery, 428–429
hyperparathyroidism, 1242
hyperthyroidism, 1235
maintaining, 931
oral cavity and pharynx, 926, 928
Parkinson's disease, 2132
parotitis, 924
patient undergoing bariatric surgery, 1207
peripheral vascular disease, 849
pneumonia, 519
primary brain tumours, 2123–2124
pulmonary tuberculosis, 527
respiratory weaning and, 631–632
sialadenitis, 924
thoracic surgery, postoperative, 644
Nutritional assessment, 65
in adolescents, 65
components of, 66
biochemical assessment, 66–67
body mass index, 66
clinical examination, 67, 67t
dietary data, 68
waist circumference measurement, 66, 66f
in older adults, 65–66
Nutritional awareness, 47
Nutritional balance, tube feeding, 956–957
Nutritional deficiency, 65
Nutritional imbalance, 111
Nutritional status
analysis of, 69–70
assessment of, 65 (*See also* Nutritional assessment)
factors influencing, 69

in physical assessment, 63
physical indicators of, 67t
preoperative assessment, 378
pressure injuries and, 194, 197
unhealthy/poor nutrition, 65, 69, 69t
Nutritional supplements, 924
Nutritional therapy
acne vulgaris, 1795
acute kidney injury, 1296
HIV infection and ART, 1554
hypervolemia, 308
hypocalcemia, 320
in hypocalcemia, 320
nephrolithiasis, 1351–1352
osteomalacia, 2284
rheumatoid arthritis, 1745
in sepsis, 363
in shock, 353
traumatic brain injury, 2066
urolithiasis, 1351–1352
Nutrition support, assessment of, 972c
NuvaRing, 1399
Nystagmus, 1944
Nystatin (Mycostatin), 1027
candidiasis, 1414

O

Obesity, 63, 65
among children and adolescents, 1192
assessment and diagnostic findings, 1195–1196
considerations in ED, 2343
definition of, 65
diseases and disorders associated, 1194, 1194c, 1194f
gerontologic considerations, 1201
health risks of, 1192–1193
patient education on, 1193c
medical management, 1196–1201
lifestyle modification, 1196–1199
nonsurgical interventions, 1201
pharmacologic therapy, 1199, 1200t
nursing management, 1201–1203
pathophysiology, 1194–1195
accumulation of body fat, 1194
metabolic imbalance, 1194
"thrifty gene" hypothesis, 1194
and perioperative considerations, 375–376
pressure ulcers among critically ill patients with extreme, nursing research profile of, 1203c
prevalence, 1191–1192, 1192f
surgical management, 1203–1204
type 2 diabetes, 1144
Obinutuzumab (Gazyra), 1642
Obstruction, 998
Obstruction and trauma. *See also* Upper respiratory tract disorders
cancer of larynx, 491–495, 492c, 493c
epistaxis (nosebleed), 488–489, 488c
laryngeal obstruction, 490–491, 491c, 491t
nasal fracture, 489–490
nasal obstruction, 489
obstructive sleep apnea, 486–488, 486c
Obstructive jaundice, 1060
Obstructive sleep apnea (OSA), 376, 439. *See also* Obstruction and trauma
assessment/diagnostic findings, 487
clinical manifestations, 486–487, 487c
medical management
pharmacologic therapy, 488
surgical management, 487–488
nursing management, 488
pathophysiology, 486
Occipital lobe, 1961
tumour, 2120
Occlusive dressings, 1856
Occupational exposure, and lung cancer, 549–550
Occupational health nurses, 19
Occupational lung diseases. *See* Pneumoconiosis
Octreotide (Sandostatin), 983, 1068
in bleeding from esophageal varices, 1067
Ocular irrigants and lubricants, 1894
Ocular medication administration, 1892–1896
antiallergy medications, 1894
anti-infective medications, 1894
corticosteroids, 1894
medications for glaucoma, 1894
mydriatics and cycloplegics, 1893–1894, 1893t
nonsteroidal anti-inflammatory drugs (NSAIDs), 1894
nursing management, 1894–1896
ocular irrigants and lubricants, 1894
patient education, 1895c
topical anesthetic agents, 1893
Ocular trauma, 1912
assessment and diagnostic findings, 1912
Odynophagia, 483, 919, 934, 935
Ofatumumab (Arzerra), for chronic lymphocytic leukemia, 1642
Official Languages Act of 1969, 91
Off-pump coronary artery bypass (OPCAB), 759, 759f
Oil droplets, 1002
Oil-in-water creams, 1787
Ointments, 1787
Older adults
age-related changes, in body systems, 212–213, 214–215t
cardiovascular system, 213, 215
gastrointestinal system, 216–217
genitourinary system, 216
integumentary system, 216
musculoskeletal system, 218
nervous system, 218–219
reproductive system, 216
respiratory system, 215–216
sensory system, 219
altered drug responses in, 223, 223c
altered pain and febrile responses in, 233
altered systemic response of, 233
cardiovascular reflexes, 892
cognitive function, changes in, 222
intelligence, 222
learning and memory, 222
considerations in perioperative period, 375
dehydration in, 304
and disability, 160c
dizziness in, 231
emotional component of illness in, 233
ethical and legal issues affecting, 234–235
exercise program for, 218, 218c
falls and falling, 231–232
fluid and electrolyte disturbances in, 303–304
frail, 231
genetics and, 213c
geriatric syndromes, 231
health assessment in, 54c
health care needs of, 8
health promotion programs for, 49, 49f
health status of, 211–212
heart failure, 805, 816, 823
home care services for, 15, 234
hospice services, 234
impaired mobility in, 231
liver decreases, 1054
living arrangements, 220–221
with adult children, 220, 221f
assisted-living facilities, 221
continuing care retirement communities, 220–221
long-term care facilities, 221
mental health issues in, 224
alcohol and drug abuse, 224–225
delirium, 225, 225f
dementia, 225–230
depression, 224
neglect and abuse of, 233–234
nonadherence to therapeutic regimens by, 39–40
nursing care of, 212
nutritional assessment in, 65–66
nutritional health of, 217
preoperative assessment and education for, 386c
with pseudobulbar affect, 231
renal function in, 303
role of family, 221
sexual health of, assessment of, 61
shock in, 345c
skin breakdown in, risk of, 195
sleep in, 217–218
stress and coping in, 220
surgical patient, 393–394
susceptibility to infection, 232–233
teaching strategies for, 42–43
upper respiratory tract disorders in, 471c
urinary incontinence in, 232
Oligometastatic disease, 2161
Oliguria, 804, 809, 818, 1286
Olmesartan (Benicar), hypertension, 886t
OLT. *See* Orthotopic liver transplantation (OLT)
Omalizumab, for asthma, 590t, 591–592
Omega-3 polyunsaturated fatty acids, 815
Omentum, 977
Omeprazole (Prilosec), 907, 983
chronic *H. pylori* gastritis, 995
gastric acid, 939
gastroesophageal reflux disease, 939t
peptic ulcer disease and gastritis, 979t
rheumatic diseases, 1743
Oncologic disorders of brain and spinal cord. *See also* Degenerative disorders
cerebral metastases
medical management, 2122–2123
primary brain tumours, 2116–2122
assessment/diagnostic findings, 2120–2121
clinical manifestations, 2118–2120
gerontologic considerations, 2118
medical management, 2121–2122
nursing management, 2122
nursing process for, 2123–2125
types of, 2117–2118
spinal cord tumours
assessment/diagnostic findings, 2125–2126
medical management, 2126
nursing management, 2126–2127
surgical management, 2126
Oncologic emergencies, 2204–2208, 2205t–2207t
Oncology, 2150
Oncology nursing, defined, 2149
Oncotic pressure, 299

Ondansetron (Zofran)
breast cancer, 1469
for postoperative nausea/vomiting, 416t
On-demand pacing, 720, 720f
Onychocryptosis. *See* Ingrown toenail
Oocytes, 134
Oophorectomy, 1412, 1431, 2162
OPCAB. *See* Off-pump coronary artery bypass (OPCAB)
Open commissurotomies, 784
Opening snaps, 653, 669, 670
Open Invite Mnemonic, 83
Open lung biopsy, 505
Open reduction and internal fixation (ORIF), 2233, 2240, 2298, 2304
Operating Room Nurses Association of Canada (ORNAC), 373, 396
Ophthalmic herpes zoster, 1798
Ophthalmic ointments, 1893
Ophthalmology. *See also* Eye
issues in, 1922
patient safety practices, 1922
Opioid abuse, 2365, 2366t. *See also* Substance abuse
Opioid analgesics, 423
Opioids, 281t, 285–289
addiction, physical dependence, and tolerance, 286
adverse effects of, 287–288
constipation, 288
nausea and vomiting, 288
pruritus, 288
respiratory depression, 287–288
sedation, 288
analgesics, diverticulitis, 1013
buprenorphine, 287
Canadian Opioid Guidelines 2017, 285
constipation, 998
equianalgesia, 285–286
factors influencing use of, 288–289
fentanyl, 286
hydromorphone, 287
methadone, 287
morphine, 286
morphine equivalents daily (MED), 285
opioid formulations, 286
opioids to avoid, 287
oxycodone, 287
titration of opioid dose, 285
tramadol, 287
Opioid suppositories, urinary retention, 1345
Opportunistic infection, 1534, 1537
Op-Site, 951
Opsonization, 1517, 1522
Optical coherence tomography, 1887
Optic chiasm, 1961
Optic neuritis, 2111t
Optimal health, 46
Oral acetyl cysteine, 910
Oral anticoagulants
drug interactions, 865
in venous thromboembolism, 864
Oral antineoplastic agents, 2193t–2194t
Oral cancer, 925
assessment and diagnostic findings, 926
clinical manifestations, 926
head and neck, anatomy of, 919f
human papillomavirus prevention, 926
medical management, 926
mouth, structures of, 919f
nursing management, 926
pathophysiology, 925–926
Oral candidiasis, 1779
Oral care, 931
Oral cavity disorders, 903t
dental plaque and caries, 918–922
dental health and disease, 922
prevention, 922
nursing management
ensuring adequate food and fluid intake, 927
home and community-based care, 928–929
home care checklist, 928c
minimizing pain and discomfort, 927
preventing infection, 927–928
promoting mouth care, 927
self-care, educating patients, 928
self-image, 927
transitional care, 928–929
periapical abscess, 922–923
clinical manifestations, 922
medical management, 922
nursing management, 922
risk factors for cancer, 925
Oral cholecystography, 1111
Oral contraceptives, 862, 863
Oral diphenoxylate atropine (Lomotil), 1027
Oral disorder, home care checklist, 928c
Oral hairy leukoplakia, 1779
mouth abnormalities, 920t
Oral hormonal contraception, 1399
Oral hygiene
infective endocarditis, 796
parotitis, 924
Oral lesions, 927
Oral morning medications, 909
Oral rehydration solutions, 307
Oral suction, 945
Orbital and ocular tumours
benign tumours
conjunctiva, 1918
eyelid, 1918
orbit, 1918
malignant tumours
conjunctiva, 1919
eyelid, 1918–1919
ocular melanoma, 1919
orbit, 1918
rhabdomyosarcoma, 1918
Orbital cellulitis, 1917–1918
Orbital implants and conformers, 1920
medical management, 1920
nursing management, 1920–1921
patient education, 1920
promoting home, community-based, and transitional care, 1920–1921
Orbital surgeries, 1919
Orbital trauma, 1910–1911
assessment and diagnostic findings, 1912
foreign bodies, 1912
fractures, 1911–1912
medical management
foreign bodies and corneal abrasions, 1912–1913
ocular burns, 1913
penetrating injuries and contusions, 1913
splash injuries, 1912
soft tissue injury and hemorrhage, 1911
Orchiectomy, 1480
Orchitis, 1480, 1506
medical management, 1506
Organ of Corti, 1928
Organs of homeostasis or adjustment, 109
Orientation, 228
ORNAC. *See* Operating Room Nurses Association of Canada (ORNAC)
Orogastric tubes, 947
Orolabial herpes, 1797
Oropharyngeal airway insertion, 2346, 2346c
Oropharyngeal catheter, 604
Oropharynx, 440
Ortho Evra, 1399
Orthopedic rehabilitation programs, 177
Orthopedic surgery. *See also* Musculoskeletal care modalities
descriptions, 2247c
joint replacement, 2247–2248
nursing interventions, 2248, 2249c
nursing process for, 2257–2261
total hip arthroplasty, 2249–2256, 2250c–2253c, 2255c
total knee replacement, 2256–2257
Orthopnea, 439, 505
Orthoses and prostheses, assisting with, 192
Orthostasis, 999
Orthostatic (postural) hypotension, 184
Orthotopic neobladder, 1364
Orthotopic transplantation
heart, 778, 790, 790f
liver, 1052
Osler nodes, 795
Osmolality, 298, 299–300, 948, 953, 1266
factors affecting, 300t
serum, 300
urine, 300
Osmolarity, 300, 1266
Osmoles, 299
Osmoreceptors, 302
Osmosis, 298–299, 298f, 948, 953, 1283, 1305
Osmotic diuresis, 299, 1141
Osmotic pressure, 299
Ossicles, 1927
Ossiculoplasty, 1941
Osteitis deformans. *See* Paget's disease
Osteoarthritic nodules, 2225
Osteoarthritis (OA), 1731, 1732, 1754–1756
assessment and diagnostic findings, 1755
clinical manifestations, 1755
medical management, 1755
nursing management, 1755–1756
pathophysiology, 1754, 1754f
Osteoblasts, 2215
Osteochondroma, 2291
Osteoclasts, 2215
Osteoconduction, 2310
Osteocytes, 2215
Osteogenesis, 2216, 2310
in nonunion, 2310
Osteogenic sarcoma (osteosarcoma), 2291
Osteoinduction, 2310
Osteomalacia, 2283–2284
assessment and diagnostic findings, 2284
gerontologic considerations, 2284
home care checklist, 2285c
medical management, 2284
pathophysiology, 2284
Osteomyelitis, 2233, 2248, 2286–2289, 2294
assessment and diagnostic findings, 2287
classification, 2286
clinical manifestations, 2287
medical management
pharmacologic therapy, 2287–2288
surgical management, 2288
nursing process, 2288–2289
pathophysiology, 2287
prevention, 2287
Osteonecrosis, 2311

Osteopenia, 1008
Osteophyte, 1732, 1754
Osteoporosis, 2277–2283
assessment and diagnostic findings, 2278, 2280
gerontologic considerations, 2278
home care checklist, 2285c
hypocalcemia and, 319
loss of height associated with, 2277f
medical management, 2280–2282, 2281t
nursing process for, 2282–2283
pathophysiology, 2278
prevention, 2277–2278
risk factors, 2278, 2279c
risks in men, 2279c
Osteoprotegerin (OPG), 2217
Osteotomy, 2233
Ostomy, 1023–1031
home care checklist, 1031c
intestinal obstruction, 1031–1033
irrigating, colostomy, 1027–1031
nursing management, 1023–1031
postoperative care, 1023–1027
preoperative care, 1023
surgery, 1024c–1026c
Ostomy appliance, guidelines for changing, 1028c–1029c
Otosclerosis, 1943
Otoscopic examination, 1931, 1931f
Ototoxicity, 1950–1951
assessment and diagnostic findings, 1950–1951
medical management, 1951
selected ototoxic substances, 1950c
Ottawa Charter for Health Promotion, 7, 45, 157
Ovarian cancer, 1438–1440
assessment and diagnostic findings, 1438
clinical manifestations, 1438
epidemiology, 1438
medical management, 1439
nursing management, 1439–1440
pathophysiology, 1438
stages of, 1439c
Ovarian cysts, 1428–1429
medical management, 1429
Ovarian hyper stimulation syndrome (OHSS), 1405
Ovary, 1373, 1375
cancer of, 1438–1440
Overflow incontinence, 1332, 1344
Oversedation, during ERCP, 1111
Over-the-counter (OTC) medications, preoperative assessment, 382
Ovidrel, 1405c
Ovulation, 1373, 1375
detection methods, 1402
Oxaliplatin (Eloxatin), 1129
Oxidant drugs, glucose-6-phosphate dehydrogenase deficiency, 1628
Oxybutynin chloride (Ditropan), urinary retention, 1345
Oxycel gauze, 1046
Oxycodone, 287, 849, 1861
for pain management, 281t, 287
Oxycodone controlled release (OxyNeo), 287
Oxycodone plus acetaminophen (Tylenol), 849
Oxygen
administration methods, 604–606, 604t
cardiopulmonary resuscitation, 831
delivery systems, 604
as gas anesthetic agent, 400t
heart failure, 815–816
left ventricular failure, 809
masks, 605
pulmonary edema, 825
saturation, 439
therapy, 572, 574, 1015, 1093
complications, 603–604
continuing and transitional care, 607
educating patients about self-care, 606–607
gerontologic considerations, 606
hypoxia, types of, 603
indications, 601–603
management, 546
toxicity, and absorption atelectasis, 603
transport
effects of pressure on, 445
respiratory system and, 442
Oxygenation, intracranial pressure and cerebral, 1998–2000
Oxyhemoglobin, 1599, 1601
Oxyhemoglobin dissociation curve, 445–446, 446c

P

Pacemaker
cardiomyopathy, 789
electrodes, 718
malfunction, 722t
spike, 719
syndrome, 720, 721
therapy (*See also* Adjunctive modalities/ management)
complications of, 721–722, 722t
design/types, 718–719
pacemaker generator functions, 719–721
pacemaker surveillance, 722–723
Packed red blood cells (PRBC), 1611
Paclitaxel, 756
breast cancer, 1469
for cardiac toxicity, 2183
ovarian cancer, 1439
PACU. *See* Postanesthesia care unit (PACU)
PAD. *See* Peripheral arterial disease (PAD)
Paget's disease, 1446, 1457, 2284–2286. *See also* Tubular ductal carcinoma
assessment and diagnostic findings, 2286
clinical manifestations, 2286
gerontologic considerations, 2286
medical management, 2286
pathophysiology, 2284, 2286
Pain, 266, 1971
acute, 267
adjuvant analgesic agents for, 284–285
local anesthetics, 289
assessment, 276f, 277
patient interview, 277–279
in physical examination, 63
breakthrough, 280
in cancer, 269
relieving, 2198
sources of, 2198t
cholecystitis, 1110
cholelithiasis, 1110
chronic, 268–273
on defecation, 1009
definition of, 266
duodenal tumours, 995
effects of, 274
at end of life, 268c
ethics and related issues, 277c
evaluation of management strategies, 291
gallbladder disease, 1116
gate control theory, 273–274, 274f
gerontologic considerations, 289–290
GI disease, 903
intensity scales, 272f, 277–278
laparoscopic cholecystectomy, 1118c
management, 279
after total knee replacement, 2248, 2249c
bone tumours, 2293
burn injury, 1861–1862
common problems of upper extremity, 2272
malignant melanoma, 1825
osteoporosis, 2283
patient undergoing bariatric surgery, 1206
pericarditis, 800
peripheral arterial insufficiency, 847c
peripheral neuropathy, 1181
preoperative education, 384
relieving, gastric cancer, 990
Stevens–Johnson syndrome, 1817–1818
toxic epidermal necrolysis, 1817–1818
trigeminal neuralgia (tic douloureux), 2112–2113
multimodal analgesia, 280–284
intraspinal and epidural routes, 283–284, 283f
oral administration, 280
parenteral administration, 280
patient-controlled analgesia, 284
rectal route, 280
timing of administration, 280
transdermal route, 280–281
transmucosal/intranasal route, 283
neuropathic, 269, 273
nociceptive, 269, 270f, 271–273
non-opioid analgesic agents, 285
acetaminophen, 285
NSAIDs, 285
nonopioid pharmacotherapy
anticonvulsants, 289
antidepressants, 289
cannabinoids, 289
ketamine, 289
nonpharmacologic methods for
cognitive behaviour therapy, 290
exercise, 290
hypnosis, 291
massage, 290
music therapy, 291
physical therapy, 290
relaxation techniques, 291
thermal therapies, 290
transcutaneous electrical nerve stimulation, 290
novel medical interventions for
interventional pain injections, 291
stimulation procedures, 291
nurse's role in management of, 274–275
opioid analgesic agents, 281t, 285–289
addiction, physical dependence, and tolerance, 286
adverse effects of, 287–288
buprenorphine, 287
equianalgesia, 285–286
factors influencing use of, 288–289
fentanyl, 286
hydromorphone, 287
methadone, 287
morphine, 286
opioid formulations, 286
opioids to avoid, 287
oxycodone, 287
titration of opioid dose, 285
tramadol, 287

Pain (*continued*)
plan of nursing care, 292c
procedural, 267
reassessing, 279
referred, 277
relief measures, 423
in cervical discectomy, 2141
in PACU, 416
syndromes, 269c
and temperature sensations, evaluation of, 1975
Pain Assessment *IN* Advanced Dementia (PAINAD), 279
Palifermin, 2196
Palliation, 2150, 2160
Palliative approach, 240
Palliative care, 242–243, 574
Palliative sedation, 254
Palliative surgery, for cancer, 2162, 2162t. *See also* Cancer
Palliative therapy, 1045
for lung cancer, 552
Pallor, 1772, 1773t
Palmar–plantar erythrodysesthesia (PPE), 1035
Palonosetron (Aloxi), in breast cancer, 1469
Palpation
of arterial pulses, 667
of bladder, 1273f
in physical assessment, 64, 64f
Palpitations, 659
dumping syndrome, 993
Pamidronate (Aredia), in multiple myeloma, 1655
Pancreatic cancer
clinical manifestations, 1128
malignant cells, 1128
medical management, 1129
nursing management, 1129
home and community-based care, 1129
Pancreatic cells, transplantation of, 1156
Pancreatic cysts, 1127–1128
Pancreatic disease, diagnosis of, 1110t
Pancreatic enzymes, secretion of, 1107
Pancreatic insufficiency, 1007t
Pancreatic islet tumours
nursing management, 1131
surgical management, 1131
Pancreatic lipase, 901t
Pancreatic necrosis, 1122
Pancreaticoduodenectomy, 1130, 1130f
Pancreaticojejunostomy, 1127
Pancreatic secretions, 900
Pancreatic tumours
assessment and diagnostic findings, 1129
clinical manifestations, 1129
medical management, 1129–1130
nursing management, 1130–1131
Pancreatitis, 1107, 1118
acute (*See* Acute pancreatitis)
chronic (*See* Chronic pancreatitis)
severity criteria, 1119c
Pancuronium (Pavulon), 402t
Pancytopenia, 1599, 1616
Panhypopituitarism, 1219
Pannus, 1732
Panobinostat (Farydak), multiple myeloma, 1655
Pan Pacific Pressure Injury Advisory Panel (PPPIAP), 195
Panretinal photocoagulation, 1178
Pantoprazole (Protonix)
gastric acid, 939
gastroesophageal reflux disease, 939t
histamine-2 (H_2) antagonists, 1120
peptic ulcer disease and gastritis, 979t
Papaverine, for erectile dysfunction, 1485
Papillary layer of dermis, 1766
Papilledema, 1887, 2117, 2119
Pap smear, 1388, 1388f
optimal, 1389c
Paracentesis
ascites, 1062–1063
guidelines for assisting with, 1063c–1064c
Paranasal sinuses, anatomy, 439, 440f
Paraplegia, 1968
collaborative issues/potential complications, 2082
nursing interventions
bladder management, 2083
enhancing coping mechanisms, 2084
establishing bowel control, 2083
exercise programs, 2082
increasing mobility, 2082
infection and sepsis, prevention of, 2084–2085
for mobilization, 2082
monitoring and managing potential complications, 2084–2085
patient outcomes, 2085
preventing disuse syndrome, 2082–2083
promoting home, community-based, and transitional care, 2085
sexual education and counselling services, 2083–2084
skin integrity, promoting, 2083
spasticity management, 2084
nursing priorities, 2082
planning and goals, 2082
patient assessment, 2081–2082
thoracic aneurysms repair and, 856
Parasitic skin infestation
lice infestation
pediculosis capitis, 1799–1801
pediculosis corporis, 1801
pediculosis pubis, 1801
scabies, 1801–1802
Parasympathetic nerve stimulation, 900
Parasympathetic nervous system, 1967
Parathormone (parathyroid hormone), 1240. *See also* Hyperparathyroidism; Hypoparathyroidism
Parathyroid glands
anatomic and physiologic overview, 1240, 1241f
homeostasis, role in, 301
hyperparathyroidism
assessment and diagnostic findings, 1241
causes of, 1241
clinical manifestations, 1241
complications, 1242
home care checklist, 1243
medical management, 1241–1242
nursing management, 1242
hypoparathyroidism
assessment and diagnostic findings, 1243
causes, 1242
clinical manifestations, 1243
home care checklist, 1244
medical management, 1243–1244
nursing management, 1244
pathophysiology, 1240–1241
Parathyroid hormone (PTH), 301, 318, 320
Paravertebral anesthesia, 405
Parenteral calcium salts, 320
Parenteral iron formulations, 1614c
Parenteral nutrition (PN), 928, 933, 937, 941, 947, 948, 972
administration methods, 967–969
clinical indications, 966
collaborative problems, 969
complications of, 970t
discontinuing parenteral nutrition, 969
educating patients, 972c
formulas, 966
home care checklist, 973c
hospitalized diabetic patients, 1186
initiating therapy, 967
nitrogen balance, 966
nursing interventions, 969–972
nursing priorities, 969
older adult patient, 973c
pain and diarrhea, 1018
planning and goals, 969
Paresthesia, 1181, 2031t, 2097, 2117, 2140, 2308
Paresthesias, 2223
Parietal lobe, 1960–1961
Parkinson's disease (PD), 939, 998, 1959, 1969. *See also* Degenerative disorders
assessment/diagnostic findings, 2128–2129
clinical manifestations
bradykinesia, 2128
dysphonia, 2128
hypokinesia, 2128
postural instability, 2128
psychiatric changes, 2128
rigidity, 2128
tremor, 2128
medical management, 2129–2130, 2129t
nursing process for, 2130–2134
pathophysiology, 2127–2128
Parotid gland, inflammation of, 924
Parotitis, 919
Paroxetine (Paxil), 224
fibromyalgia, 1759
rheumatoid arthritis, 1745
Paroxysmal atrial tachycardia (PAT), 707
Paroxysmal dysrhythmia, 692
Paroxysmal nocturnal dyspnea (PND), 804, 809
Paroxysmal supraventricular tachycardia (PSVT), 707
Partial laryngectomy, 494
Partial pressure of carbon dioxide ($PaCO_2$), 1996
Partial pressure of oxygen, 445
Partial-rebreathing masks, 605
Particulate radiation, 2163
Passive immunity, hepatitis B virus, 1080
Passive smoke, 549
Pastes, 1787
Past health history, 55
PAT. *See* Preadmission testing (PAT)
Patch testing, 1780
Patellar reflex, 1976
Patent airway maintenance, 414–415
Paternalism, 25, 25c
Pathogen associated molecular patterns (PAMP), 1520
Pathologic reflexes, 1978
Pathologic sounds, 65
Pathophysiologic processes, 101–102
Pathophysiology
abdominal aortic aneurysm, 857
acquired immune deficiency syndrome, 1541–1543
acute coronary syndrome, 744–745
acute low back pain, 2266

acute pancreatitis, 1119
acute pharyngitis, 479–480
acute respiratory failure, 534
acute rhinosinusitis, 475
acute tracheobronchitis, 508
allergic rhinitis, 1582
Alzheimer's disease, 227–228, 227f
anaphylaxis, 1580
aortic regurgitation, 781
aortic stenosis, 780
aplastic anemia, 1616
appendicitis, 1009
ARDS, 535, 535f
arterial embolism, 859
arterial thrombosis, 859
arteriosclerosis, 843–844
asbestosis, 548
ascites, 1061
aspiration, 521
asthma, 584, 584f
atelectasis, 505–506, 506f
atherosclerosis, 843–844
blunt trauma, 554
bone tumours, 2291
bronchiectasis, 577
cardiac tamponade, 828–829
cardiogenic shock, 356, 356f, 826
celiac disease, 1006–1007
cellulitis, 874
chronic heart failure, 807–808
chronic lymphocytic leukemia, 1641
chronic rhinosinusitis, 477
coal worker's pneumoconiosis, 548
colorectal cancer, 1034
constipation, 998–999
COPD, 564, 565f
coronary atherosclerosis, 730–731, 731f
cystic fibrosis, 596
diabetes mellitus, 1140
diabetic ketoacidosis, 1165
diabetic ketoacidosis (DKA), 1165
diarrhea, 1001–1002
dissecting aorta, 858–859
disseminated intravascular coagulation, 1668
distributive shock, 359, 359f
diverticular disease, 1011
Ebola virus disease, 1726
endometriosis, 1430
esophageal varices, 1065–1066
esophagus cancer, 942–943
fecal incontinence, 1003
fibromyalgia, 1759
gastric cancer, 989
gastritis, 976–977
giant cell arteritis, 1753
gout, 1757–1758
heart failure, 807–808, 808f
hematologic disorders, 1601f
hepatic cirrhosis, 1083–1084
hepatic encephalopathy, 1071–1072
Hodgkin lymphoma, 1648
human immune deficiency virus, 1541–1543
Huntington's disease, 2134
hypercalcemia, 320–321
hyperkalemia, 316
hypermagnesemia, 324
hypernatremia, 312
hyperphosphatemia, 326
hypertension, 879–881
hypervolemia, 307
hypocalcemia, 319
hypokalemia, 314
hypomagnesemia, 322–323
hyponatremia, 310
hypophosphatemia, 325
hypovolemia, 304
hypovolemic shock, 354, 354f
immune thrombocytopenic purpura, 1661
infective endocarditis, 795
irritable bowel syndrome, 1004
leg ulcers, 868
lower urinary tract infections
  bacterial invasion, 1332–1333
  reflux, 1333
  routes of infection, 1334
  uropathogenic bacteria, 1334
lung abscess, 529
lung cancer, 549
of malignant process, 2151–2153
megaloblastic anemias, 1617
metabolic acidosis, 329
metabolic alkalosis, 330
mitral regurgitation, 780
mitral stenosis, 780
mitral valve prolapse, 778, 779f
multiple myeloma, 1652–1653
multiple organ dysfunction syndrome, 366
myocarditis, 797
nephrolithiasis, 1350–1351
neurogenic bladder, 1346
obesity, 1194–1195
obstructive sleep apnea, 486
oral cavity cancer, 925–926
osteoarthritis, 1754, 1754f
osteomalacia, 2284
osteomyelitis, 2287
osteoporosis, 2278
ovarian cancer, 1438
Paget's disease, 2284, 2286
parathyroid glands, 1240–1241
Parkinson's disease, 2127–2128
pelvic inflammatory disease, 1421, 1421f
peptic ulcer disease, 982
pericarditis, 798
peritonitis, 1014
pertussis, 1728
pharynx cancer, 925–926
pituitary function, abnormalities of, 1218
pleural effusion, 531
pleurisy, 530
pneumonia, 511–512
polymyalgia rheumatica, 1753
polymyositis, 1752
postpolio syndrome, 2145
primary immune deficiency diseases, 1533
pulmonary contusion, 556
pulmonary edema, 533, 824
pulmonary embolism, 541–542
pulmonary heart disease, 540
pulmonary hypertension, 538
pulmonary tuberculosis, 522–524
recurrent acute rhinosinusitis, 477
respiratory acidosis, 331
respiratory alkalosis, 332
rheumatoid arthritis, 1743
rhinitis, 471–472, 472c, 472t
sarcoidosis, 546
scleroderma, 1751
sepsis, 361–362
shock, 342–344
Sjögren's syndrome, 1750
status asthmaticus, 595
systemic lupus erythematosus, 1748
ulcerative colitis, 1017
urinary retention, 1345
urolithiasis, 1350–1351
uterine cancer, 1434–1435
varicose veins (varicosities), 872
venous thromboembolism, 862
Patient, 5
  basic needs of, 5
  cultural diversity, 394
  fears and risks, 392–393, 394c
  identification, 395
  nursing care, 394
  older adult, 393–394
  surgical, 392–394
Patient-centred care, 23
Patient-controlled analgesia (PCA), 284, 384, 423, 1624, 1861
  normal respiratory function, 634
Patient-controlled epidural analgesia (PCEA), 384
Patient-controlled perineurial anesthesia (PCPA), 384
Patient-directed music (PDM), effects of, 275c
Patient education
  about activities of daily living, 179, 179c
  before and after urodynamic testing, 1274c
  breathing exercises, 608c
  chronic conditions, 165
  coronary artery bypass graft, 763
  coughing technique, 610c
  diabetes mellitus, 1159–1163
  dietary guidelines for bariatric surgery patients, 1207c
  edema, 309
  foot care tips, 1173c
  health risks of obesity, 1193c
  hepatic encephalopathy, 1074
  hypoglycemia, 1165
  incentive spirometry, 608c
  IV therapy, 338
  liver transplantation, 1102
  preoperative, 383–386
    ambulatory surgical patient, 386
    cognitive coping strategies, 384
    deep breathing, coughing, and incentive spirometry, 384, 385c
    mobility and active body movement, 384, 385c
    pain management, 384
    preparation procedures and, 383
  self-injection of insulin, 1163
  weight loss, 1198c
Patient Evaluation Conference System (PECS), 178
Patient-focused interventions, in emergency department, 2341
Patient Health Questionnaire (PHQ), 664
Patient Health Questionnaire-4 (PHQ-4), 1790c
Patient positioning
  in bed, 181, 181c
    side-lying (lateral) position, 181c
    supine (dorsal) position, 181c
  external rotation deformity of hip, prevention of, 182
  footdrop, prevention of, 182
  to prevent musculoskeletal complications, 181–182
Patient profile, 56–62, 58c. *See also* Health history
Patient safety, in preoperative area, 389
Patient Safety Institute of Canada, 27
Patient seclusions, 27
Patterned wound, 2349c
PCA. *See* Patient-controlled analgesia (PCA)

PCIs. *See* Percutaneous coronary interventions (PCIs)
PD. *See* Parkinson's disease (PD); Peritoneal dialysis (PD)
PDT, 1822
PE. *See* Pulmonary embolism (PE)
Peak flow meters, 593, 593f, 594c
Pectus carinatum, 452
Pectus excavatum, 452
Pediatric rehabilitation programs, 177
Pediculosis capitis, 1799–1801
  clinical manifestations, 1800
  medical management, 1800
  nursing management, 1800–1801
Pediculosis pubis, 1801
Pedigree, 135
PEG. *See* Percutaneous endoscopic gastrostomy (PEG); Polyethylene glycol (PEG)
Pegfilgrastim (Neulasta), breast cancer, 1469
Pegloticase (Krystexxa), gout, 1758
Pelvic examination, 1386c
Pelvic exenteration, 1412, 1434
Pelvic floor dysfunction, 998
Pelvic floor exercises, 201
Pelvic floor muscle exercises, 1342
Pelvic inflammatory disease (PID), 1412, 1420–1422, 1553
  clinical manifestations, 1421
  complications, 1421
  home care checklist, 1422c
  medical management, 1421
  nursing management, 1421–1422
  pathophysiology, 1421, 1421f
Pelvic muscles, 999
Pelvic organ prolapse, 1424–1425
  clinical manifestations, 1424–1425
  Kegel exercise, 1425c
  medical management, 1425
Pelvic peritoneoscopy, 1391–1392
Pelvis, 2315
  fractures of, 2315–2316
  Pelvic bones, 2315, 2315f
  stable fractures of, 2315–2316, 2316f
  unstable fractures of, 2316, 2316f
Pemoline (Cylert), 2097, 2098
Pemphigus vulgaris, 1788, 1813–1814
  clinical manifestations, 1813
  complications, 1813
  medical management, 1813–1814
Penbutolol (Levatol), hypertension, 885t
Penetrating keratoplasty, 1905
Penetrating trauma (stab/gunshot wounds), 557
Penetration, peptic ulcer disease, 987
Penicillin, for pharyngitis, 480
Penicillin G, proctitis, 1044
Penile cancer, 1480, 1510–1511
  medical management, 1511
  prevention, 1511
Penile implants, 1485. *See also* Erectile dysfunction (ED)
Penis, 1480
  disorders affecting
    epispadias, 1510
    hypospadias, 1510
    phimosis, 1510
Penrose drain, 1363
Pentagastrin, 915
Pentobarbital, 2366t
Pentoxifylline (Trental), 1786
  peripheral arterial occlusive disease, 852
Penumbra region, 2030
Penumbra System, 2035
People-first language, 168
People with disabilities, health assessment of, 59, 60c
Peppermint oil, 1005
Pepsin, 899, 900, 901t
Peptic ulcer disease, 981–988, 983t
  assessment and diagnostic findings, 982
  clinical manifestations, 982
  collaborative problems, 986
  deep, 981f
  drug regimens, 983t
  evaluation, 988
  home care checklist, 988c
  medical management, 982–984
    dietary modification, 984
    follow-up care, 984
    pharmacologic therapy, 983
    smoking cessation, 983
    stress reduction and rest, 983
    surgical management, 984
  nursing interventions
    complications, 986–987
    home and community-based care, 987–988
    monitoring, 986–987
    nutritional status, 986
    reducing anxiety, 986
    relieving pain, 986
  nursing priorities, 986
  nursing process, 984–988
  pathophysiology, 982
  pharmacotherapy, 979t–980t
  planning and goals, 986
  surgical procedures, 984t–985t
Pepto-Bismol, 983
Percussion, in physical assessment, 64–65, 64f
Percutaneous balloon microcompression, 2112
Percutaneous balloon valvuloplasty, 783
Percutaneous biliary drainage, 1096
  liver tumours, 1096
Percutaneous (nontunnelled) central catheters, 967
Percutaneous coronary interventions (PCIs), 664, 733, 755
  complications, 756, 757t
  postprocedure care, 756–757
  procedures
    coronary artery stent, 756
    percutaneous transluminal coronary angioplasty, 755–756, 756f
Percutaneous endoscopic gastrostomy (PEG), 948, 960
  insertion of, 960
  tube, 960
Percutaneous liver biopsy, 1058c–1059c
Percutaneous mechanical thrombectomy devices, 860
Percutaneous needle biopsy, 468
Percutaneous nephrolithotomy, 1352
Percutaneous transhepatic cholangiography, 1111, 1128
Percutaneous transluminal angioplasty (PTA), 846
Percutaneous transluminal coronary angioplasty (PTCA), 740, 755–756, 756f, 757t
Perforation, 937
  assessment and diagnostic findings, 937
  clinical manifestations, 937
  management, 937–938
  peptic ulcer disease, 987
  peritonitis, 1015
Perfusion, pulmonary, 443
Perfusion-weighted imaging (PWI), 1980
Pergonal, 1405c
Perianal itching, 1790–1791
Periapical abscess, 919, 922–923
  analgesics, 923
  clinical manifestations, 922
  medical management, 922
  nursing management, 922
Pericardial effusion, 798, 799, 800
  assessment and diagnostic findings, 829
  clinical manifestations, 829
  medical management, 829–830
  pathophysiology, 828–829
Pericardial fluid, 799
Pericardial friction rub, 799
Pericardial window, 799
Pericardiectomy, 799
Pericardiocentesis, 799, 800
Pericardiotomy, 804, 830
Pericarditis, 798, 1318
  assessment and diagnostic findings, 799
  causes of, 798c
  clinical manifestations, 798–799
  medical management, 799
  nursing management, 799
  nursing process, 799–800
  pathophysiology, 798
Periconception health care, 1406–1407, 1407c
Perimenopause, 1373, 1376–1377
  nursing management, 1376–1377
Perimetry testing, 1887–1888
Perindopril (Aceon), hypertension, 886t
Perineal itching, 1790–1791
Perineum, 1374
Periodontal disease, 2033
Periodontitis, gum abnormalities, 921t
Perioperative nursing, 373
Perioperative period, 373, 373f
  special considerations during, 375
    ambulatory surgery, 376
    emergency surgeries, 376
    gerontologic considerations, 375
    obese patient, 375–376
    patients with disabilities, 376
Perioperative phase, 373
  nursing activities in, 374c
Periosteum, 2215
Peripheral arterial disease (PAD), 839
  diabetes, 845
  symptoms of, 839
  vascular problems, 847c–848c
Peripheral arterial occlusive disease
  assessment, 851
  clinical manifestations, 850–851
  diagnostic findings, 851
  medical management, 851
    endovascular management, 852
    home and community-based care, 853
    maintaining circulation, 853
    monitoring and managing complications, 853
    pharmacologic therapy, 852
    surgical management, 852–853
Peripheral immune response (PIR), 1527
  trajectories, 1528c
Peripherally inserted central catheters (PICCs), 948, 967, 969, 2181
Peripheral nerve function, assessment of, 2227
Peripheral nervous system, 1964–1967
  autonomic nervous system, 1965
  cranial nerves, 1964, 1964t
  disorders of, 2114
  spinal nerves, 1964–1965
  sympathetic nervous system, 1966

Peripheral neuropathy, 269c, 1181, 1288, 1297, 1534, 1552, 1657t, 2114
clinical manifestations, 1181
management, 1181
Peripheral parenteral nutrition (PPN), 967
Peripheral pulses, assessing, 840f
Peripheral resistance, 343
Peripheral vascular disease, 1175, 1819
foot and leg care, 850c
home care checklist, 850c
Periprosthetic joint infections (PJI), 2260
Peristalsis, 948, 949
Peristomal hernias, 1027
Peristomal skin irritation, 1029
Peritoneal dialysis (PD), 1283, 1295, 1311–1316, 1312f
approaches
acute intermittent peritoneal dialysis, 1314
continuous ambulatory peritoneal dialysis, 1314–1315
continuous cyclic peritoneal dialysis, 1315–1316
complications
acute, 1313–1314
long term, 1314
nursing management
home, community-based, and transitional care, 1316
psychosocial needs, 1316
for patient with diabetes, 1180
procedure
inserting the catheter, 1312–1313, 1313f
performing the exchange, 1313
preparing the equipment, 1312
preparing the patient, 1312
Peritoneum, 977, 981
Peritonitis, 998, 1008, 1011, 1014–1015, 1283, 1312, 1313–1314, 1366–1367
assessment and diagnostic findings, 1014–1015
bacterial, 1084
category, 1014
cirrhosis and, 1084
clinical manifestations, 1014
common gastrointestinal, 1014f
complications, 1015
medical management, 1015
nursing management, 1015
pathophysiology, 1014
Peritonsillar abscess, 482–483. *See also* Upper airway infections
assessment/diagnostic findings, 483
clinical manifestations, 483
medical management
surgical management, 483
nursing management, 483
Periumbilical pain, 1009
Periurethral bulking, 1342
Permanent colostomies, placement of, 1038f
Permanent pacemaker generators, 719
Permethrin (Elimite), 1802
Pernicious anemia, 915, 1617
Per-oral endoscopic myotomy (POEM), 935
Personal directive, 240
Personalized health care, legal aspects of, 146
Personalized medicine, 130, 131t
Pertussis, 1727–1728
assessment and diagnostic findings, 1728
clinical manifestations, 1728
medical management, 1728
nursing management, 1728
pathophysiology, 1728
Pes cavus, 2275
Pes planus. *See* Flatfoot
Pessaries, 1342
PET. *See* Positron emission tomography (PET)
Petechiae, 1599, 1658f, 1777, 1777t
Pet therapy, 206
Peyronie disease, 1480, 1511
Phacoemulsification, 1901–1902
Phagocytic cells, 1517, 1518
Phagocytic immune response, 1517, 1519
Phagocytosis, 113, 1599, 1603
Phakic intraocular lenses, 1906
Phantom limb pain, 273, 2328, 2330
Pharmacogenetics, 130
Pharmacogenomics, 144–146
Pharmacogenomic testing, 145
Pharmacokinetics, 144
Pharmacologic stress testing, 679–680
Pharmacologic therapy
abdominal aortic aneurysm, 857
acute pharyngitis, 480
allergic rhinitis, 1583–1585
arterial embolism, 860
arterial thrombosis, 860
ascites, 1062
benign prostatic hyperplasia, 1491
bladder cancer, 1357–1358
diabetes insipidus, 1221
diabetes mellitus, 1150–1158
ectopic pregnancy, 1408
elephantiasis, 874
endometriosis, 1430–1431
erectile dysfunction, 1484–1485
esophageal varices, 1067–1068
gastritis, 979t–980t
heart failure, 811–815
herniation of cervical intervertebral disc, 2140
hyperthyroidism, 1232
infertility, 1405, 1405c
leg ulcers, 869
lymphedema, 874
obstructive sleep apnea, 488
osteoarthritis, 1755
osteoporosis, 2280–2282
Paget's disease, 2286
Parkinson's disease, 2129, 2129t
peptic ulcer disease, 979t–980t
peripheral arterial occlusive disease, 852
primary aldosteronism, 1255
primary brain tumours, 2122
primary immune deficiency diseases, 1535
rheumatic diseases, 1736
sickle cell disease, 1623
Pharyngeal lipase, 901t
Pharyngitis. *See also* Upper airway infections
acute pharyngitis, 479–481
chronic pharyngitis, 481
defined, 471
Pharyngoesophageal pulsion diverticulum, 936
Pharynx
anatomy, 439
physical assessment, 451
Pharynx cancer, 903t, 952
assessment and diagnostic findings, 926
clinical manifestations, 926
human papillomavirus prevention, 926
medical management, 926
nursing management, 926
pathophysiology, 925–926
Phase I/II/III PACU, 413
Phenazopyridine, in thalassemia, 1628
Phenotype, 133
Phentolamine, in erectile dysfunction, 1485
Phenylephrine hydrochloride, for nasal congestion, 481
Phenylephrine (Neo-Synephrine), in shock, 353t
Phenytoin (Dilantin), 2007, 2008, 2112
end-stage kidney disease, 1299
Pheochromocytoma, 998, 1246–1248, 1922
assessment and diagnostic findings, 1246–1247
clinical manifestations, 1246
hypertension, 878
medical management
pharmacologic therapy, 1247
surgical management, 1247–1248
nursing management, 1248
Phimosis, 1480, 1510
Phlebitis, 337
assessing for, 338c
chemical, 337
mechanical, 337
treatment, 337
Phlebotomy, 1629, 1630
pH method, 948, 951
Phosphodiesterase type 5 (PDE-5) inhibitors, in erectile dysfunction, 1484–1485
Phosphorus, 324
deficit (hypophosphatemia), 324–326, 325t
excess (hyperphosphatemia), 325t, 326–327
Phosphorus supplements, 326
Phospho-Soda, 914
Photoaging, 1770
Photodynamic therapy (PDT), in bladder cancer, 1358
Photophobia, 1917, 2090
Photorefractive keratectomy (PRK), 1906
Phototherapy, 1809
Physical activity
hypertension, 883t
myocarditis, 798
Physical agents, in carcinogenesis, 2154–2155
Physical assessment. *See also* Physical examination
cardiovascular function, 664–672
abdomen, 672
arterial pulses, 667
blood pressure, 666–667, 667c
general appearance, 665
heart auscultation, 669–671
heart inspection and palpation, 668–669
jugular venous pulsations, 668
lungs, 671–672
of skin and extremities, 665–666, 665t
heart failure, 817–818
of mouth and pharynx, 451
of nose, 451
of pharynx, 451
of respiratory system
clubbing of fingers, 450–451, 451f
cyanosis, 451
lower respiratory structures/breathing, 452–457, 453c, 454t, 456t, 458t
upper respiratory structures, 451–452
of sinus, 451, 451f
of trachea, 451–452
of upper respiratory tract, 451–452, 451f
Physical dependence, 286
Physical examination, 30, 52, 62
blood pressure, 881
components of, 62–65
considerations in, 62
communication, 53, 53f
ethical use of data, 53

Physical examination (*continued*)
nurse, role of, 52–53
use of technology, 53–54
focused assessment, 63–64
auscultation, 65
in head to toe format, 64
inspection, 64
palpation, 64, 64f
percussion, 64–65, 64f
general inspection, 63
body movements, 63
gait, 63
nutritional status, 63
posture, 63
speech pattern, 63
vital signs and pain assessment, 63
purpose of, 30
tools of, 63
Physical fitness, and health, 47
Physical mobility, 2269
impaired (*See* Physical mobility, impaired)
Physical mobility, impaired
assessment, 180
evaluation, 193
nursing diagnoses, 180
nursing interventions
ambulating with assistive device, 188–192, 189–190t
assisting patient out of bed, 187c
assisting the patient with transfer, 185–187
cane, ambulating with, 190, 192
crutch walking, 188, 188f, 190
independent mobility, promotion of, 184–188
muscle strength and joint mobility, maintenance of, 182–184, 183–184c
orthoses and prostheses, assisting with, 192
patient transfer from bed to wheelchair, 186f
preparing for ambulation, 187–188
proper positioning, 181–182, 181c
therapeutic exercises, 184, 185t
walker, ambulating with, 190, 192
nursing process for, 180–193
planning and goals, 180
Physical restraint, 27
Physiologic dead space, 439
Physiologic sounds, 65
Physiotherapy, for pain relief, 290
Pia mater, 1962
Pics, 1611
PID. *See* Pelvic inflammatory disease (PID)
PIDD. *See* Primary immune deficiency diseases (PIDD)
Pigeon chest (pectus carinatum), 452
Pigmented nevi, 1819–1820
Pigskin-based dressing, 1859
Pike's Peak pattern, 1945
Pilar cysts, 1819
PillCam ESO, 913
Pilocarpine (Piloptic), in Sjögren's syndrome, 1751
Piloerector response, 1766
Pilonidal sinus
anorectal disorders, 1046–1047
on lower sacrum, 1046f
Pindolol (Visken), hypertension, 885t
Pin-site care, 2245–2246
Pioglitazone, 1157
Pipe smoking, and cancer, 925
Pit and fissure sealants, 922
Pitch, 1933
Pitting edema, 810, 810f
Pituitary adenomas. *See also* Primary brain tumours
hormonal effects of, 2118
pressure effects of, 2118
Pituitary function, abnormalities of, 1218
Pituitary gland, 1219f
anterior, 1218
definition, 1218
posterior, 1218
Pituitary portal blood system, 1218
Pituitary tumours, 2111t
assessment and diagnostic findings, 1220
clinical manifestations, 1220
medical management, 1220
types of, 1220
Pivot joints, 2218
PKD. *See* Polycystic kidney disease (PKD)
Placebos, use of, 27
Plantar fasciitis, 2274
Plantar reflex, 1978
Plaques, 730
Plasma, 1598, 1599
exchange, 1287
fibrinolytic system, 1605
and plasma proteins, 1604
Plasma pH, 329
Plasmapheresis, 1083, 1814
Plasminogen, 1599, 1605
Plaster cast, 2233
Platelet, 1599
Platelet-activating factor, 1574
Platelet defects, 1663
clinical manifestations, 1663
medical management, 1663
nursing management, 1663
Platelets (thrombocytes), 1604
transfusion of, 1685c
Platform posturography, 1934
Platinol. *See* Cisplatin
Platinum analogues, 551
Plavix. *See* Clopidogrel
Pleura, 440
Pleural biopsy, 466
Pleural conditions. *See also* Chest and lower respiratory tract disorders
acute respiratory distress syndrome, 534–537, 535c, 537c
acute respiratory failure, 533–534
empyema, 532–533
pleural effusion, 531–532
pleurisy, 530–531
pulmonary edema, 533
pulmonary embolism, 541–546, 541c, 543c
pulmonary heart disease, 540–541
pulmonary hypertension, 537–540, 538c
sarcoidosis, 546–547
Pleural effusion, 505, 517, 519. *See also* Pneumonia
assessment/diagnostic findings, 531
clinical manifestations, 531
medical management, 531–532
nursing management, 532
pathophysiology, 531
Pleural friction rub, 505
Pleural space, 505
Pleurisy
assessment/diagnostic findings, 530
clinical manifestations, 530
medical management, 530
nursing management, 531
pathophysiology, 530
PLISSIT model, 169
Plus acetylsalicylic acid (Aspirin), 849
Plus sofosbuvir (Sovaldi), 1081
PMS. *See* Premenstrual syndrome (PMS)
PN. *See* Parenteral nutrition (PN)
PND. *See* Paroxysmal nocturnal dyspnea (PND)
Penetrating keratoplasty (PKP), 1905
Pneumatic retinopexy, 1908
Pneumatic VADs, 791
Pneumococcal vaccination, 232, 570
Pneumoconiosis. *See also* Chest and lower respiratory tract disorders
asbestosis, 548
coal worker's pneumoconiosis, 548
overview, 547–548
Pneumocystis pneumonia (PCP), 1534, 1550, 1553
Pneumonectomy, 551c, 633
Pneumonia, 930, 2246, 2260. *See also* Respiratory infections
aspiration pneumonia, 511
assessment/diagnostic findings, 512–513
classification, 508–509, 509c
clinical manifestations, 512
community-acquired pneumonia, 509–510, 510t
complications
pleural effusion, 517
shock and respiratory failure, 517
health care–associated pneumonia (HCAP), 510
hospital-acquired pneumonia (HAP), 510–511
in immunocompromised host, 511
medical management, 513–517, 514t–516t
gerontologic considerations, 517
nursing process for, 517–520
pathophysiology, 511–512
prevention, 513
risk factors, 512, 513t
ventilator-associated pneumonia (VAP), 511
Pneumoperitoneum, 915
Pneumothorax, 557–560. *See also* Chest trauma
clinical manifestations, 558
defined, 505, 602
medical management, 558–560
parenteral nutrition, 970t
simple, 558
tension, 558
traumatic, 558
Podocon, for HPV infection, 1417
Podofilox, for HPV infection, 1417
Podofin, for HPV infection, 1417
POEM. *See* Per-oral endoscopic myotomy (POEM)
Poikilocytosis, 1599
Point of care (POC), 1544
Point-of-care risk assessment (PCRA), 1698, 1702
Point of maximal impulse (PMI), 653, 1624
Poisoning, 2362
carbon monoxide, 2362, 2364
chemical burns, 2364–2365
food poisoning, 2365, 2365c
swallowed poisons, 2362
Polio and motor system disease, 2112t
Polycystic kidney disease (PKD), 1284, 1289–1290
assessment and diagnostic findings, 1290
clinical manifestations, 1290
dominant, 142t

medical management, 1290
pathophysiology, 1289–1290
Polycystic ovary syndrome (PCOS), 1412, 1428
Polycythemia, 564, 1599, 1630–1632, 1773t
assessment and diagnostic findings, 1630
clinical manifestations, 1630
complications, 1630
medical management, 1630–1631
nursing management, 1631–1632
polycythemia vera, 1630
primary, 1630
secondary, 1632
vera, 1630
Polydipsia, diabetes mellitus, 1142
Polyethylene glycol (PEG)
electrolyte lavage solutions, 913
laxative medications, 1001t
Polymerase chain reaction, 1534
Polymorphonuclear neutrophils (PMN), 2201
Polymyalgia rheumatica (PMR), 1753–1754
assessment and diagnostic findings, 1753
clinical manifestations, 1753
medical management, 1753
nursing management, 1753–1754
pathophysiology, 1753
Polymyositis, 1752–1753
assessment and diagnostic findings, 1752
clinical manifestations, 1752
medical management, 1752
nursing management, 1752–1753
pathophysiology, 1752
Polymyxin B, in acute kidney injury, 1294
Polyp, 1373, 1388
Polyphagia, and diabetes mellitus, 1142
Polypharmacy, 222
Polyps of colon and rectum, 1044
Polysaccharide meningococcal vaccine, 2091
Polysporin, 1855
Polythiazide (Renese), 820t
Polyuria
diabetes mellitus, 1142
diabetic ketoacidosis, 1165
Pomalidomide, in multiple myeloma, 1654
Pons, 1961
Population screening, 143–144
Portacaval shunts, 1070
Porta hepatis, 1114
Portal hypertension, 1052, 1060
hepatic disorders, 1061
measurements, 1067
Portal hypotension, 1061
Portal of exit, 1698
Portal systemic shunts, in esophageal varices, 1070f
Portosystemic encephalopathy (PSE), 1071
Port-wine angiomas, 1819
Posaconazole (Noxafil), in acute myeloid leukemia, 1637
Positioning injury, perioperative, prevention of, 408–409, 409f
Positioning, patient
lower respiratory structure assessment, 452
pulmonary edema, 825
Positive end-expiratory pressure (PEEP), 602, 603
Positive feedback, 110
Positive pressure gradient (PPG) test, 185
Positive-pressure ventilators. *See also* Mechanical ventilation
high-frequency oscillatory support ventilators, 619–620
noninvasive positive-pressure ventilation, 620
pressure-cycled ventilator, 620
volume-cycled ventilators, 620
Positron emission tomography (PET), 463, 680, 908, 943, 1960, 1981, 2120
Postanesthesia care unit (PACU), 372
admitting patient to, 412–413
defined, 413
direct discharge, preparing for, 418–419
nursing management in, 413–418, 415t, 416t
phases of postanesthesia care, 412
Postanesthesia recovery room, 412
Postcoital intrauterine device insertion, 1402
Posterior cerebral artery (PCA), 2047
Posterior communicating artery (PCoA), 2047
Posterior cruciate ligament (PCL), 2301
Posterior fossa, 1961
Posterior pituitary gland
abnormalities of, 1219–1220
diabetes insipidus, 1220–1221
hormones of, 1218
Posterior subcapsular cataracts, 1900
Postexposure prophylaxis (PEP), 1384, 1534
Postganglionic nerve fibres, 1966
Postganglionic neuron, 1965
Postherpetic neuralgia, 269c
Postinfarction syndrome, 1291
Post–intensive care syndrome, 349
Post–lumbar puncture headache, 1984
Postmenopausal bleeding, 1396
Postoperative delirium, 432, 433c
Postoperative nausea and vomiting (PONV), 416–417, 416t, 417c
Postoperative nursing management
hospitalized postoperative patient, care of, 419–421
after surgery, 420–421
nursing process for, 421–434, 430t, 431t
receiving patient in clinical unit, 420
postanesthesia care unit
admitting patient to, 412–413
direct discharge, preparing for, 418–419
nursing management in, 413–418, 415t, 416t
phases of postanesthesia care, 412
Postpericardiotomy syndrome, 773, 774
Postpolio syndrome
assessment/diagnostic findings, 2145
management, 2145
pathophysiology, 2145
Postprocedural patient education, 909
Postpyloric enteric tubes, 957
Postthrombotic syndrome, 867–868
clinical manifestations, 867
complications, 867–868
medical and nursing management, 868
Posttraumatic growth, 82
Posttraumatic stress disorder (PTSD), 124–125, 2373, 2376
acute, 124
assessment of, 124c
chronic, 124
nursing implications, 124–125
and resilience in intensive care nurses, 125c
symptoms of, 124
Postural blood pressure changes, 666–667
Postural drainage, 602, 609–610. *See also* Chest physiotherapy (CPT)
nursing management, 610, 610c
Postural hypotension, 653, 666, 667c
Postural instability, 2128
Posture, in physical assessment, 63
Postvoid residual (PVR), 200, 201
Potassium, 313
deficit (hypokalemia), 313–315, 314t
diabetic ketoacidosis, 1168
excess (hyperkalemia), 314t, 315–318
intravenous, administration of, 315
Potassium-losing diuretics, 314
Potassium-sparing diuretics, 812, 813, 820t
hypertension, 884t
Potassium supplements, 315, 316
Phototherapeutic keratectomy (PKT), 1904–1905
Pouchitis, 1020
Povidone-iodine ointment (Betadine), 1796, 1855–1856, 2350
Powders, 1787
Powerlessness, heart failure, 821
PP interval, 692, 696
PPIs. *See* Proton pump inhibitors (PPIs)
PPN. *See* Peripheral parenteral nutrition (PPN)
PPPD. *See* Pylorus-preserving pancreaticojejunostomy (PPPD)
Practical nurses, 4
Prayer blankets, 84
Prazosin (Minipress), hypertension, 885t
Preadmission testing (PAT), 373, 383
Prealbumin, 67
Preanesthetic medication, 388
on call to OR, 388
Precedex, 631
Precision medicine, 2149, 2150
Precision Medicine Initiative, 130
Preconception screening, 140t
Prediabetes, 1138, 1139t
Prednisolone (Prelone), 588t, 591t
Prednisone, 588t, 591t, 1018
for nasal obstruction, 489
Preeclampsia, 1287
Pre-exposure prophylaxis (PrEP), 1534, 1539
Pregabalin (Lyrica), for fibromyalgia, 1759
Preganglionic neuron, 1965
Pregnancy and breast cancer, 1474–1475
Pregnancy-induced hypertension, 1922
Pregnyl, 1405c
Prehabilitation, 174
Preload, 653, 740
Premature atrial complex (PAC), 700–701
Premature ejaculation (PE), 1487–1488
Premature junctional complex, 706
Premature ventricular complex (PVC), 707–708
Premenstrual syndrome (PMS), 1394–1395
causes and treatment of, 1394c
clinical manifestations, 1394
medical management, 1394–1395
nursing management, 1395
Prenatal counselling and testing, 138
Prenatal screening, 139, 140t
Preoperative assessment, 377–378
cardiovascular status, 379
dentition, 378
drugs or alcohol use, 378
endocrine function, 380–381
genetic considerations, 377, 379c
health history, 377
hepatic and renal function, 379–380
immune function, 381–382, 381f
nutritional and fluid status, 378
nutrients for wound healing, 378, 380t
physical examination, 377
previous medication use, 382–383, 382t
psychosocial factors, 383
respiratory status, 378–379
risk factors for surgical complications, 378c
signs of abuse, 377–378
spiritual and cultural safety, 383

Preoperative education, 383–386
ambulatory surgical patient, 386
cognitive coping strategies, 384
deep breathing, coughing, and incentive spirometry, 384, 385c
mobility and active body movement, 384, 385c
pain management, 384
preparation procedures and, 383
Preoperative nursing interventions, 383
bowel preparation, 387
expected patient outcomes, 389, 389c
immediate, 387–388
attending to family needs, 389
patient transfer to presurgical area, 389
preanesthetic medication, 388
preoperative record, 388–389, 388f
injury prevention, 386
nutrition and fluids, 386–387
patient education, 383–386
ambulatory surgical patient, 386
cognitive coping strategies, 384
deep breathing, coughing, and incentive spirometry, 384, 385c
mobility and active body movement, 384, 385c
pain management, 384
patient safety, 386
psychosocial interventions
anxiety and fear reduction, 386
respecting cultural, spiritual, and religious beliefs, 386
skin preparation, 387
Preoperative record, 388–389, 388f
Presbycusis, 219
Presbyopia, 219, 1889
Pressure-cycled ventilator, 620
Pressure gradient stockings (PGS), 185
Pressure injuries, 193. *See also* Skin integrity, impaired
from friction and shear, 194, 194f, 197–198
healing, 198–199
risk factors for development of, 195, 195c
stage I, 198
stage II, 198
stage III, 198
stage IV, 198
Pressure-relieving devices, 196–197, 197f
Pressure support ventilation (PSV), 602, 620
Pressure ulcers, 1819, 2237
in critically ill patients with extreme obesity, 1203c
Pressurized metred-dose inhaler (pMDI), 569, 570
defined, 564
examples/use, 577f
patient education about, 577c
Presymptomatic testing, 143
Prevention
colorectal cancer, 1035
hepatitis A virus, 1076–1077
infective endocarditis, 796
myocarditis, 797
pulmonary edema, 825
Prevention and Treatment of Pressure Ulcers; Clinical Practice Guideline, 195
Preventive ethics, 27–28
advance directives, 28
institutional ethics committees, 28
Prevertebral ganglia, 1966
Priapism, 1480, 1511
PRICE (Protection, Rest, Ice, Compression, Elevation), 2299, 2301
Prilocaine, 1789
for pain at chest tube insertion site, 643
Primaquine, in thalassemia, 1628
Primary aldosteronism, 1255
Primary brain tumours
acoustic neuroma, 2118
assessment/diagnostic findings, 2120–2121
cause of, 2117
classification of, in adults, 2117c
clinical manifestations, 2118–2120
increased intracranial pressure, 2119–2120
localized symptoms, 2120
gerontologic considerations, 2118
gliomas, 2117–2118
incidence of, 2117
medical management
chemotherapy, 2122
pharmacologic therapy, 2122
radiation therapy, 2121–2122
surgical management, 2121
meningiomas, 2118
nursing management, 2122
nursing process for, 2123–2125
origin of, 2116
pituitary adenomas
hormonal effects of, 2118
pressure effects of, 2118
types of, 2117–2118, 2117c
Primary drug resistance, 525
Primary glomerular diseases, 1285–1289, 1286c
acute nephritic syndrome, 1286–1287
chronic glomerulonephritis, 1287–1288
nephrotic syndrome, 1288–1289
Primary health care (PHC), 7
Primary hypertension, 878
Primary immune deficiency diseases (PIDD), 1535t
assessment and diagnostic findings, 1533–1534
clinical manifestations, 1533
home care checklist, 1537c
medical management, 1534–1535, 1536c
nursing management, 1537
pathophysiology, 1533
prevention, 1534
Primary injury, 2056
Primary myelofibrosis, 1646–1648, 1647f
medical management, 1647
nursing management, 1647–1648
Primary prevention, 14
of cancer, 2157
intervention, 723
Primary skin infections, 1795
Primary survey, in ED, 2344
Primary thrombocythemia. *See* Essential thrombocythemia (ET)
PriMatrix, 870
PR interval, 692
Prinzmetal's angina, 738c
Proarrhythmic, 692
Probenecid (Benemid), in gout, 1758
Probiotics, use of, 1094
Problem-focused coping, 104
Procainamide, 699t
Procaine (Novocaine), 404t
Procarbazine, 2180t
Prochlorperazine (Compazine)
breast cancer, 1469
for postoperative nausea/vomiting, 416t
Proctitis, anorectal disorders, 1044–1045
Proctosigmoidoscopy, in Crohn's disease, 1017
Profore, 866
Progesterone, 1373, 1375
Progressive multifocal leukoencephalopathy (PML), 1534, 1552
Progressive muscle relaxation, 116
Progressive osteoporotic bone loss, 2277f
Prokinetic agents, 1000, 2197
Prolapse (of valve), 778
Proliferative phase, 1373, 1376
Promethazine (Phenergan), for postoperative nausea/vomiting, 416t
Prometrium, 1405c
Propafenone
antiarrhythmic medication, 699t
for atrial fibrillation prevention, 704
Proparacaine hydrochloride, 1893
Prophylactic antibiotics, 931
Prophylactic brain irradiation, 551
Prophylactic mastectomy, 1458. *See also* Breast cancer
Prophylactic surgery, for cancer, 2161–2162
Prophylactic therapy, for NSAID ulcers, 983t
Prophylactic vaccines, 2192
Propionibacterium acnes, 1792
Propofol, 402t, 1861, 2008, 2062
Proportional assist ventilation (PAV), 602, 621
Propoxyphene (Darvon), 281t
Propranolol, 2025
antiarrhythmic medication, 699t
hypertension, 885t
urinary retention, 1345
Propranolol long acting (Inderal LA), hypertension, 885t
Proprioception, 1961
evaluation of, 1975
Proprotein convertase subtilisin-kexin type 9 (PCSK9) agents, 736
Proptosis, 1911
Prostacyclin, 838
Prostaglandin inhibitors, in premenstrual syndrome, 1395
Prostaglandins, 113, 271, 838, 1267, 1572, 1574
Prostate cancer, 1480, 1494–1495
assessment and diagnostic findings, 1495
chemotherapy, 1500–1501
clinical manifestations, 1495
home care checklist, 1505c
hormonal therapy, 1496, 1500
impact of, 1504c
medical management, 1496, 1500
patient with, 1497c–1500c
sexual complications, 1495
treatment, 1495–1496, 1500–1501
Prostatectomy, patient undergoing, 1501–1504
Prostate fluid or tissue analysis, 1483
Prostate gland, 1480
Prostate HDR therapy, 2165
Prostate-specific antigen (PSA), 1480
test, 1483
Prostatism, 1480, 1490
Prostatitis, 1331, 1332, 1480
assessment and diagnostic findings, 1489–1490
clinical manifestations, 1489
medical management, 1490
nursing management, 1490
Prostatodynia, 1489
Prosthetics, 1474
Prostones, 1000
Protease inhibitors (PI), 1545
Protective boots, 871
Protein–calorie malnutrition, 325

Protein C deficiency, 1674
Protein metabolism, role of liver in, 1053
Protein S deficiency, 1674
Proteinuria, 1276, 1287
Prothrombin time (PT), 1606
Proton pump inhibitors (PPIs), 939, 939t, 977, 983, 1120
  gastric acid, 979t
Proton therapy, 2164
Proto-oncogenes, 2153
Protriptyline, 488
Proventil, 588t
Provincial poison control centre, 2362
Provirus, 1542
Proximal humeral fractures, 2312–2313, 2313f
Proximal interphalangeal (PIP), 1755
Prozac, in premenstrual syndrome, 1395
Pruritus (itching), 288
  general, 1789
    common oral medications for, 1789
    gerontologic considerations, 1789
    medical management, 1789–1790
    nursing management, 1790
    pathophysiology, 1789
    pharmacologic therapy, 1789–1790
    systemic disorders associated with generalized, 1789c
  hepatic disorders, 1075
  hepatic dysfunction, 1055
  perineal and perianal itching, 1790–1791
    nursing management, 1791
PSE. *See* Portosystemic encephalopathy (PSE)
Pseudobulbar affect, 231
Pseudoephedrine sulphate (Sudafed), 1342
Pseudofolliculitis barbae (shaving bumps), 1796
Pseudohyperkalemia, 316
Pseudomonas aeruginosa, 970, 1854, 1938
Pseudomonas species, 1818
Psoriasis, 1806–1807, 1807f
  assessment and diagnostic findings, 1807
  care of patient
    assessment, 1810
    nursing priorities, 1810
    planning and goals, 1810
  clinical manifestations, 1807
  complications, 1807
  medical management, 1807–1808
  nursing interventions
    home care checklist, 1812c
    increasing skin integrity, 1811
    monitoring and managing potential complications, 1811
    patient outcomes, 1811–1812
    promoting home, community-based, and transitional care, 1811
    promoting understanding, 1810–1811
    self-concept and body image, improving, 1811
  nursing management, 1809–1810
  pathophysiology, 1807
  pharmacologic therapy
    topical agents, 1808–1809
  treatment plan for, 1808t
Psoriatic arthritis, 1756
Psterior lamellar keratoplasty (PLK), 1905
Psychedelic-type drugs, 2367t
Psychiatric changes, 2128
Psychiatric emergencies, 2375
  overactive patient, 2375
  patient with suicidal potential, 2376
  posttraumatic stress disorder, 2376
  underactive/depressed patient, 2376
  violent behaviour, 2375–2376
Psychiatric rehabilitation, 177
Psychodermatosis, 1789
Psychogenic disorder, 904
Psychological distress, 383
Psychological support
  in lung cancer, 552
  in pulmonary edema, 825–826
Psychoneuroimmunology, 107
Psychosocial assessment, 383
Psychosocial distress
  defined, 2200
  management, 220
Psychosocial genetic health, assessment of, 149, 150c
Psychosocial support
  in acute kidney injury, 1297
  gastric cancer, 991
Psychosocial typology of illness, 120–121
Psyllium (Metamucil)
  diarrhea, 1003
  laxative medications, 1001t
PTA. *See* Percutaneous transluminal angioplasty (PTA)
PTCA. *See* Percutaneous transluminal coronary angioplasty (PTCA)
PTH. *See* Parathyroid hormone (PTH)
Ptosis, 2103
PTSD. *See* Posttraumatic stress disorder (PTSD)
Ptyalin (salivary amylase), 901t
Public Health Agency of Canada (PHAC), 7, 45, 1384, 1538, 1697
Public health nursing, 14
Pudendal, 1003
Pulmonary angiography, 463
Pulmonary arterial hypertension (PAH), 538c
Pulmonary artery catheter, 804, 814
Pulmonary artery pressure monitoring, 686–687
Pulmonary care activities, 993
Pulmonary circulation, oxygen-rich blood, 835f
Pulmonary complications, 1040
  signs and symptoms of, 952
Pulmonary congestion, 808, 809, 811, 815, 817, 819, 824, 826
Pulmonary contusion
  assessment/diagnostic findings, 557
  clinical manifestations, 556
  medical management, 557
  pathophysiology, 556
Pulmonary diffusion, 439, 443
Pulmonary edema, 347, 804, 824
  assessment and diagnostic findings, 824
  assessment/diagnostic findings, 533
  clinical manifestations, 533, 824
  defined, 505
  fluid replacement and, 351
  management, 825
  medical management, 533
  nursing management, 533, 825–826
  pathophysiology, 533, 824
  prevention, 825
Pulmonary embolism (PE), 505, 828, 828f, 861, 2041, 2203, 2254
  assessment/diagnostic findings, 542–544
  clinical manifestations, 542
  home care checklist, 543c
  medical management, 544–545
  nursing management, 545–546
  pathophysiology, 541–542
  risk factors, 541
Pulmonary function, 1297
Pulmonary function tests (PFT), 460, 461t
Pulmonary heart disease. *See also* Pleural conditions
  clinical manifestations, 540
  medical management, 540
  nursing management, 540–541
  pathophysiology, 540
Pulmonary hypertension (PH), 537–540, 1622
  assessment/diagnostic findings, 538–539
  causes of, 538c
  clinical classification of, 538c
  clinical manifestations, 538
  medical management, 539
  nursing management, 539–540
  pathophysiology, 538
Pulmonary infection, 626
Pulmonary perfusion, 439, 443
Pulmonary rehabilitation, 573
  programs, 177
Pulmonary tuberculosis. *See also* Respiratory infections
  assessment/diagnostic findings
    classification of tuberculosis, 525
    interpretation of results, 524
    QuantiFERON-TB Gold In-Tube (QFT-GIT) test/T-SPOT, 524–525
    tuberculin skin test, 524
  clinical manifestations, 524
  gerontologic considerations, 525
  medical management
    multidrug resistance, 525
    pharmacologic therapy, 525, 526t
    primary drug resistance, 525
    secondary/acquired drug resistance, 525
  nursing process for, 525–529
  pathophysiology, 522–524
  prevalence of, 522
  transmission and risk factors, 522, 523c
Pulmonary vascular resistance, 653
Pulmonic area, 668
Pulse amplitude, 667
Pulse contour, 667
Pulsed carbon dioxide laser, 1831
Pulsed erbium/yttrium-aluminum-garnet (Er:YAG) laser, 1831
Pulse-dye laser, 1831–1832
Pulseless electrical activity (PEA), 710
Pulse oximetry, 461
Pulse pressure, 345–346, 666
  aortic regurgitation, 781
  narrowing of, 345, 346
  normal, 346
  in shock, 345
Pulse rate, 667
Pulse rhythm, 667
PULSES profile, 178
Pulsion diverticulum, 936
Pulsus paradoxus, 792, 800, 1318
Pump failure, 838
Purging, 2187
Purified protein derivative (PPD), 1527
Pursed-lip breathing, 608c
Purulent, 505
Push-and-pull enteroscopy, 914
PUVA therapy, 1809–1810
PVC. *See* Premature ventricular complex (PVC)
P wave, 692, 695
PWI. *See* Perfusion-weighted imaging (PWI)
Pyelonephritis, 1283, 1293c, 1331, 1332, 1339, 1364
  acute, 1339
  chronic, 1339–1340
Pyloric obstruction, peptic ulcer disease, 987

Pyloroplasty, 977, 984
peptic ulcer disease, 985t
Pylorus, 977, 981
Pylorus-preserving pancreaticojejunostomy (PPPD), 1130
Pyogenic liver abscesses, 1102
Pyrazinamide
antituberculosis medication, 526t
TB and HIV infection, 1551
Pyridostigmine bromide (Mestinon), 2103
Pyridoxine (Aminoxin), in peripheral neuropathy, 1550
Pyrosis, 977, 982
gastroesophageal reflux disease, 919, 934, 938
Pyuria, 1332, 1335

Q

Qnasl, in allergic rhinitis, 1585
QOL. *See* Quality of Life (QOL)
QRS complex, 692, 695
QT interval, 692, 696
Quad canes, 192
Quadriceps contraction exercises, 2219
Quadriceps-setting exercise, 2238c
Quadrivalent HPV recombinant vaccine (Gardasil), 2192
Quality assurance (QA), 9
Quality of Life (QOL), 1000
QuantiFERON-TB Gold In-Tube (QFT-GIT) test, 524–525
Quick-relief medications, for asthma, 591t, 592
Quick SOFA (qSOFA) scale, 364
Quinapril (Accupril)
heart failure, 811t
hypertension, 886t
Quinethazone (Hydromox), 820t
Quinidine, 699t
Quinine, 1950, 1950c
Quinsy. *See* Peritonsillar abscess

R

Rabeprazole (AcipHex), 983
gastric acid, 939
gastroesophageal reflux disease, 939t
peptic ulcer disease and gastritis, 980t
Radial and ulnar shafts, fractures of, 2314
Radial head fractures, 2314
Radiation-associated impairment of skin integrity, 2196
Radiation-induced thyroid cancer, 1238
Radiation therapy, 995, 1035, 1043, 1442–1443, 1443f, 2150. *See also* Cancer
administration of radiation
brachytherapy, 2165
external radiation, 2164
internal radiation implantation, 2164–2165
bladder cancer, 1358
breast cancer, 1467–1468, 1468c
for cancer of larynx, 494–495
in cancer treatment, 2154
liver tumours, 1096
for lung cancer, 551
nursing management, 2166, 2167c–2177c
primary brain tumours, 2121–2122
protection for caregivers, 2166
radiation dosage, 2164
toxicity of, 2165–2166
Radical cystectomy, 1357
Radical neck dissection, 929, 929f
Radical prostatectomy, prostate cancer, 1495–1496
Radioactive iodine therapy, hyperthyroidism, 1232
Radioactive iodine uptake test, 1224–1225
Radioallergosorbent test (RAST), 1575
Radiofrequency nerve ablation, 291
Radiofrequency thermal coagulation, 2112
Radioimmunotherapy, 2165
Radioisotope diagnostic procedures (lung scans), 463–464
Radioisotopes, 653, 680
Radionuclide imaging. *See also* Cardiovascular function
cholelithiasis, 1111
myocardial perfusion imaging, 680–681
ventricular function and wall motion, test of, 681
Radionuclide testing, 910–911
Radioscan, 1225
Radiosensitive tumour, 2163
Radiosensitizers, 2164
Raloxifene (Evista), for breast cancer, 1458
Ramipril (Altace)
heart failure, 811t
hypertension, 886t
Range-of-motion exercises, 182
active, 182
passive, 182
performing, 183–184c
related terminology, 182c
Ranitidine (Zantac), 907
antacids, 939
gastric acid, 1120
peptic ulcer disease, 979t, 1574
Rape, 2373–2374
Rape crisis centres, 2373
Rape trauma syndrome, 1384, 2373
Rape Victim Companion Program, 2373, 2374
Rapid plasma reagin (RPR), 1722
Rapid sequence intubation (RSI), 2346–2347
Rapid strep tests, 461
Rapid streptococcal antigen test (RSAT), 481
Rasburicase (Elitek), 1637
Rash, 1772
N. meningitidis infection, 2090
Raynaud's disease, 849, 1819
Raynaud's phenomenon, 860, 1760
clinical manifestations, 861
medical management, 861
nursing management, 861
Raynaud's syndrome, 861
RCM. *See* Restrictive cardiomyopathy (RCM)
Reappraisal, 104
Rebound hypertension, 878
Rebound hypoglycemia, parenteral nutrition, 970t
Rebound tenderness, 1009, 1014, 1017
24-hour recall method, 68
Recanalization, 2035
Recent Life Changes Questionnaire, 104
Receptive aphasia, 2030, 2031t
Recombination, 134
Recombivax HB, 1079
Reconstructive surgery, for cancer, 2162
Reconstructive techniques, 929
Recovery room, 412
Rectal prolapse, 1003
Rectal sensory functioning tests, 914
Rectocele, 1373, 1387, 1412, 1424
Rectum carcinoma, abdominoperineal resection, 1037f
Recurrent acute rhinosinusitis. *See also* Rhinosinusitis
assessment/diagnostic findings, 477–478
clinical manifestations, 477
complications, 478
medical management, 478–479
nursing management, 479
pathophysiology, 477
Red blood cell (RBC), 1286, 1599, 1619
destruction, 1603
production, regulation of, 1267
transfusion of, 1684c
Red cell distribution width (RDW), 1610–1611
Reduction mammoplasty, 1476
Reed–Sternberg cell, 1648f
Re-epithelialization, 2165
Referred pain, 277
Reflex centres, 1961
Reflexes
Achilles reflex, 1976–1978
Babinski reflex, 1978
biceps reflex, 1976
brachioradialis reflex, 1976
clonus, 1978
corneal reflex, 1978
deep tendon reflexes, 1976–1978, 1977t–1978t
documenting, 1976c
involuntary movements, 1968
patellar reflex, 1976
plantar reflex, 1978
superficial reflexes, 1978
triceps reflex, 1976
Reflex incontinence, 1332
Reflux vomiting, 1032
Refraction ophthalmology, 1888
Refractive errors, 1888–1892
assessment and diagnostic testing, 1889
contrast-sensitivity testing measures, 1889
glare testing, 1889
history taking, 1889
blindness, 1888–1889
determining, 1888
gerontologic considerations, 1889
medical management, 1889–1890
nursing management, 1890–1892
vision impairment, 1888–1889
Refractive surgeries
conductive keratoplasty, 1906
nursing management, 1906
perioperative complications, 1906
phakic intraocular lenses, 1906
photorefractive keratectomy (PRK), 1906
Refractory period, defined, 656
Regeneration, 114
Regional anesthesia, 403–405, 404t
epidural anesthesia, 403, 404f
injection sites for, 404f
local conduction blocks, 405
spinal anesthesia, 403–405, 404f
Regional enteritis, 1016–1017
Regional hyperthermia, 2189
Regional pain block, 291
Registered nurse first assistant (RNFA), 396
Registered nurses (RNs), 4, 5
Registered practical nurse, 4
Registered psychiatric nurses, 4–5
REGRANEX Gel, 1786
Regulated Health Professions Act, 5
Regurgitation, 777, 778
Rehabilitation, 174
activities of daily living, self-care deficits in, 178–180
complementary and alternative therapies, 206

    continuing and transitional care, 203–206
    disability/impairment and, 174
    ethics and related issues, 175c
    follow-up care, 206–207
    functional capacity, assessment of, 177–178
    goal of, 174–175
    home care checklist, 204–205c
    nursing process
        altered elimination patterns, 200–203
        impaired physical mobility, 180–193
        impaired skin integrity, 193–200
        self-care deficits in ADLs, 178–180
    people with amputations, 2328–2329, 2329f
    self-care programs, 203
    specialty rehabilitation programs, 176–177
        burn rehabilitation programs, 177
        cancer rehabilitation, 177
        cardiac rehabilitation, 177
        orthopedic rehabilitation programs, 177
        pain management programs, 177
        pediatric rehabilitation programs, 177
        psychiatric rehabilitation, 177
        pulmonary rehabilitation programs, 177
        spinal cord injury rehabilitation programs, 177
        stroke recovery programs, 176–177
        for substance abuse, 177
        traumatic brain injury rehabilitation, 176–177
    team, 175–176, 176c
Rehabilitation services, 175
    access to, 175c
Reiter's syndrome, 1756
Rejection, liver transplantation, 1101
Relational ethics, 25, 93
Relationships, in cardiac disease, 664
Relaxation exercises, 206
Relaxation techniques, 116
    Benson relaxation response, 116, 116c
    guided imagery, 116
    for pain relief, 291
    progressive muscle relaxation, 116
Remifentanil (Ultiva), 401t
Renal and urinary systems
    anatomy of
        kidneys, 1262–1264
        ureters, 1264–1265
        urethra, 1265
        urinary bladder, 1265
    function of, 1262
        tubular reabsorption and tubular secretion, 1266–1269
        urine formation, 1265–1266
Renal and urologic disorders, 1272c
    assessment of
        changes in voiding, 1270, 1271t
        gastrointestinal symptoms, 1270
        genitourinary pain, 1270, 1270t
        health history, 1269–1270
        physical assessment, 1271–1273, 1273f
        unexplained anemia, 1270, 1271
    diagnostic evaluation
        bladder ultrasonography, 1277
        CT scanning, 1277
        cystography, 1279
        intravenous urography, 1278–1279
        kidney biopsy, 1280
        magnetic resonance imaging, 1277–1278
        MAG3 renogram, 1279
        nuclear scans, 1278
        osmolality, 1276
        renal and ureteral brush biopsy, 1280
        renal angiography, 1279
        renal function tests, 1277, 1277t
        retrograde pyelography, 1279
        specific gravity, 1276
        ultrasonography, 1277
        urinalysis and urine culture, 1274, 1276
        urologic endoscopic procedures, 1279–1280
        voiding cystourethrography, 1279
        x-ray study, 1277
    genetics in, 1272c
    nursing care plan for, 1275c
    risk factors for, 1269, 1269c
Renal angiography, 1279
Renal artery stenosis, hypertension, 878
Renal biopsy, 1280
Renal clearance, 1267
Renal disease, anemias in, 1615
Renal disorders, diabetes and, 1179–1180
Renal failure, 858
Renal function tests, 1277, 1277t
Renal system, chemotherapy agents on, 2182–2183
Renal tubular acidosis, 1350
Renin–angiotensin system, 1266f
Repaglinide (GlucoNorm), 1156
Repeated radiation treatments, 2164
Replacement, 114
Repolarization, 653, 692
Reproductive system
    age-related changes in, 214t, 216
    chemotherapeutic agents on, 2183
Repronex, 1405c
Required organizational practices (ROPs), 386
Reservoir, 1698
Residential schools, 91
Residual urine, 1332, 1344
Resonance, 65
Resource model of preventive health behaviour, 46
Respect for people, 25, 25c
Respiration, 439, 442
Respiratory acidosis, 331–332
    assessment and diagnostic findings, 331–332
    clinical manifestations, 331
    medical management, 332
    pathophysiology, 331
Respiratory alkalosis, 332
    assessment and diagnostic findings, 332
    clinical manifestations, 332
    medical management, 332
    pathophysiology, 332
Respiratory care modalities
    airway management
        emergency management of, 612, 613c
        endotracheal intubation, 612–614
        mechanical ventilation, 619–622
        nursing process, 622–632
        tracheostomy, 614–619
    noninvasive respiratory therapies
        chest physiotherapy, 608–612
        incentive spirometry, 607–608
        oxygen therapy, 601–607
        small-volume nebulizer therapy, 608
    in thoracic surgery
        postoperative management, 634–648
        preoperative management, 632–634, 633c, 634c
Respiratory centre, 1958
Respiratory depression
    by anesthetic agents, 406
    opioid-induced, 287–288
Respiratory disorders, 450c
Respiratory distress, 1120
Respiratory excursion, 454–455
Respiratory function assessment
    in acutely or critically ill patient, 457, 459–460, 460c
        inspiratory force, 460
        minute ventilation, 459, 460c
        tidal volume, 459
        vital capacity, 459–460
Respiratory hygiene, 1702
Respiratory infections. *See also* Chest and lower respiratory tract disorders
    acute tracheobronchitis, 508
    aspiration, 520–522, 520c, 521c
    lung abscess, 529–530
    pneumonia, 508–520, 509c, 510t, 513t, 514–516t, 520c, 521c
    pulmonary tuberculosis, 522–525, 523c
Respiratory status, gallbladder disease, 1116
Respiratory system
    age-related changes in, 214t, 215–216
    anatomy of
        lower respiratory tract, 440–442
        upper respiratory tract, 438–440
    diagnostic evaluation
        arterial blood gas (ABG) studies, 460–461
        biopsy, 466, 467–468
        chest x-ray, 462
        CT, 462–463
        cultures, 461
        endoscopic procedures, 464–466, 466c–467c
        MRI, 463
        pulmonary function tests, 460, 461t
        pulse oximetry, 461
        sputum studies, 461–462
    function of
        carbon dioxide transport, 446
        gas exchange, 444–446, 445c, 445f, 446c
        neurologic control of ventilation, 446
        oxygen transport, 442
        pulmonary diffusion and perfusion, 443
        respiration, 442
        ventilation, 442–443, 442c, 443t
        ventilation and perfusion balance/imbalance, 443–444, 444c
    gerontologic considerations, 446–447, 447t
    health history
        chest pain, 448–449
        cough, 448
        dyspnea, 447–448
        hemoptysis, 449
        signs and symptoms, 447–449
        sputum production, 448
        wheezing, 449
    past health, family, and social history, 449–450, 449c, 450c
    physical assessment of
        clubbing of fingers, 450–451, 451f
        cyanosis, 451
        lower respiratory structures and breathing, 452–457, 453c, 454t, 456t, 458t
        upper respiratory structures, 451–452
Respiratory weaning
    about, 630, 630c
    criteria for, 630
    defined, 602
    methods of, 630–631
    nutrition, 631–632
    from oxygen, 631
    patient preparation, 630
    tracheostomy tube removal, 631

Rest, 983
ascites, 1062
hepatic cirrhosis, 1093–1094
hepatitis B, 1080
pain, 835, 839
Restenosis, 756
Restless leg syndrome, 1297
Restorative proctocolectomy, 1019, 1020
Restraints, use of, 27
Restrictive cardiomyopathy (RCM), 788
Restrictive lung disease, 505
Reteplase (Retavase), 748
Rete (epidermal) ridges, 1766
Reticular activating system (RAS), 105
Reticular layer of dermis, 1766
Reticulocytes, 1599, 1601
Reticuloendothelial system (RES), 1598, 1599, 1604–1605
Reticulospinal tracts, 1964
Retinal detachment, 1906–1908, 1907f
assessment and diagnostic findings, 1907
clinical manifestations, 1907
exudative, 1907
nursing management, 1908
rhegmatogenous, 1907
surgical management
pneumatic retinopexy, 1908
scleral buckle, 1907
vitrectomy, 1907–1908
traction, 1907
Retinal vascular disorders, 1908
Retinoids, 1794, 2191–2192
Retinol-binding protein, 67
Retinopathy, 1137, 1144
Retirement homes act, 232
Retransplantation, 1101
Retroflexion, 1426
Retrograde pyelography, 1279
Retroperitoneal lymph node dissection (RPLND), 1508
Retroversion, 1426
Retrovirus, 1534, 1538
Reverse transcriptase, 1534, 1542
Reverse transcriptase–polymerase chain reaction (RT-PCR), 1545
Review of systems, 56
Rewarming
methods, 2356
supportive care during, 2356
Rhabdomyolysis, 325
Rhegmatogenous detachment, 1906, 1907
Rheumatic diseases, 1732
arthritis, 1759–1760
assessment and diagnostic findings, 1733, 1734c
laboratory studies, 1733
blood studies for, 1735t
clinical manifestations, 1733
diffuse connective tissue diseases, 1743–1754
exercise to promote mobility, 1739t
extra-articular disorders, 1760
fibromyalgia, 1759
gerontologic considerations, 1739, 1742–1743
hemolytic anemias, 1620–1624
home care checklist, 1747c
management goals and strategies, 1736t
medical management, 1733–1736, 1737t–1738t
exercise and activity, 1736
nonpharmacologic pain management, 1736
pharmacologic therapy, 1736
sleep, 1736, 1739
metabolic and endocrine diseases, 1757–1759
miscellaneous disorders, 1760
myelodysplastic syndrome, 1618–1620
neoplasms, 1760
neurovascular disorders, 1760
nursing care, 1740c–1742c
nursing management, 1739
older patients, 1742
osteoarthritis, 1754–1756
pathophysiology, 1732f
autoimmunity, 1733
degeneration, 1733
inflammation, 1732–1733
spondyloarthropathies, 1756–1757
unmet needs of patients with, 1746c
Rheumatic endocarditis, 794
Rheumatic fever, 794, 794c
Rheumatoid arthritis (RA), 1732, 1736, 1743–1747
assessment and diagnostic findings, 1744
clinical manifestations, 1743–1744
medical management, 1744–1745
nursing management, 1745–1747
pathophysiology, 1743
Rhinitis. *See also* Upper airway infections
clinical manifestations, 472–473
defined, 471
medical management
pharmacologic therapy, 473
nursing management
patient education for self-care, 473
overview, 470–471
pathophysiology, 471–472, 472c, 472t
Rhinitis medicamentosa, 471, 474
Rhinorrhea, 471, 472
Rhinosinusitis. *See also* Upper airway infections
acute
assessment/diagnostic findings, 475–476
clinical manifestations, 475
complications, 476
medical management, 476, 476t
nursing management, 476–477
pathophysiology, 475
chronic/recurrent acute
assessment/diagnostic findings, 477–478
clinical manifestations, 477
complications, 478
medical management, 478–479
nursing management, 479
pathophysiology, 477
defined, 471
Rhonchi, 439
Rhytidectomy (face-lift), 1830–1831
management, 1830–1831
prophylactic antibiotic for, 1830
psychological preparation, 1830
Ribavirin (Rebetol), 1081
Rib fracture, 2326–2327
Rifabutin, antituberculosis medication, 526t
Rifampin, 2091
antituberculosis medication, 526t
TB and HIV infection, 1551
Rifapentine, antituberculosis medication, 526t
RIFLE classification system, 1292, 1292t
Right heart catheterization, 683
Right kidney, technique for palpating, 1273f
Right lymphatic duct, 836
Right-sided heart failure, 804, 808, 809–810
Rigidity, 2128. *See also* Parkinson's disease
Ringer's lactate, 350
Ringworm, 1798
Rinne test, 1932–1933
comparison with Weber, 1932t
Risk reduction surgery. *See* Prophylactic surgery, for cancer
Ritonavir, 1547
Rituximab
chronic lymphocytic leukemia, 1642
immune hemolytic anemia, 1629
non-Hodgkin's lymphomas, 1651
Rivaroxaban (Xarelto), 864, 2033
acquired thrombophilias, 1676
Rivastigmine tartrate (Exelon), for Alzheimer's disease, 227
Rizatriptan (Maxalt), 2025
Robot-assisted technology, 8
Robotic-assisted laparoscopic radical prostatectomy (RALP), 1496
Rocuronium (Zemuron), 402t
Romiplastim (Nplate), for myelodysplastic syndrome, 1619
Rooke Vascular boot, 871
Rosiglitazone (Avandia), 1157
Rotator cuff tears, 2300
Roth spots, 795
Rotor's syndrome, 1061
Routine Practices (RP), 1698
Roux-en-Y gastric bypass (RYGB), 1204
RR interval, 692, 696
RSI. *See* Rapid sequence intubation (RSI)
Rubber-band ligation procedure, 1046
Rubor, 835, 839
Rubrospinal tracts, 1964
Runway Slider Sets, 196
Rupture of Achilles tendon, 2302

S

SABA. *See* Short-acting beta-adrenergic agonists (SABA)
Sabigatran (Pradaxa), 865
Saccharin, 1147
Saccharomyces boulardii, 1002
Saccular aneurysm, 855
Saclike herniation, diverticular disease, 1010
Sacral edema, 810
Sacred objects, 85
Sacred space, 83
Saddle joints, 2218
Salagen, 927
Salbutamol sulphate (Ventolin HFA)
acute kidney injury, 1296
kidney cancer, 1296
Salem Sump, 949
Salicylate poisoning, 2368t
Salicylic acid preparations, 1794
Saline cleansing enema, 914
Saline solution, 334–335
Salivary glands disorders
calculi, 924, 925
inflammation of, 924
neoplasms, 925
parotitis, 924
salivary calculus (sialolithiasis), 925
sialadenitis, 924–925
Salivary gland tumours, management of, 925
Salivary gland ultrasonography, 925
Salmeterol (Serevent Diskus), 588t
Salmonella infection, 1718–1719
Salpingitis, 1412
Salpingo-oophorectomy, 1412, 1431
Salvage surgery, 2161
Sanctity of life, 25, 25c

SANS. *See* Subacute necrotizing sialadenitis (SANS)
Sarafem
in premenstrual syndrome, 1395
Sarcoidosis. *See also* Pleural conditions
assessment/diagnostic findings, 546
clinical manifestations, 546
medical management, 547
pathophysiology, 546
Sarcomeres, 2218
Sargramostim (Leukine)
acute myeloid leukemia, 1637
myelodysplastic syndrome, 1619
Saturation of oxygen, 445
Savory dilators, 938
Saw palmetto, 1491
SBP. *See* Spontaneous bacterial peritonitis (SBP)
Scabies
assessment and diagnostic findings, 1802
clinical manifestations, 1801–1802
gerontologic considerations, 1802
medical management, 1802
nursing management, 1802
Scalded skin syndrome, 1816
Scalene lymph nodes, 468
Scalp injury, 2057–2058
Scanned carbon dioxide laser, 1831
Scarring, prevention of, 1795
SCC. *See* Squamous cell carcinoma (SCC); Squamous cell carcinomas (SCC)
SCD. *See* Sickle cell disease (SCD)
Schilling test, 1618
School health programs, 19
Sciatica, 2117, 2139
Scintigraphy, 910–911
radionuclide imaging, 908
Scintiscan, 1225
Scleral buckle, 1907
Scleroderma, 998, 1003, 1751–1752
assessment and diagnostic findings, 1751
clinical manifestations, 1751
medical management, 1752
nursing management, 1752
pathophysiology, 1751
Sclerotherapy, 873, 1046, 1052
varicose vein, 873
Scopolamine (Transderm Scop), 416t, 910
Scrub role, 395
Sebaceous cysts, 1819
Sebaceous glands, 1768
Seborrheic dermatoses, 1791–1792
clinical manifestations, 1791–1792
medical management, 1792
nursing management, 1792
secondary candidal (yeast) infection in, 1792
Seborrheic keratoses, 1819
Secondary drug resistance, 525
Secondary headache, 2023
Secondary hypertension, 878
Secondary injury, 2056–2057
Secondary prevention, 14
of cancer, 2157, 2158t
intervention, 723
Secondary skin infections, 1795
Secondary survey, in ED, 2344
Secondary testicular tumours, 1507
Second-degree atrioventricular block
type I, 711–712
type II, 712
Second-hand (passive) smoke, 549
Second heart sound, 653, 669
Second-intention healing, 413
Secretin, 1107
gastrointestinal regulatory substances, 901t
Secretory diarrhea, 1001
Secretory disorders
acne vulgaris, 1792–1795
hidradenitis suppurativa (HS), 1791
seborrheic dermatoses, 1791–1792
Secretory phase, 1373, 1376
Sedation vacation, 631
Sedative-hypnotic medications, in heart failure, 824
Segmentation contractions, 902
Segmentectomy, 551c, 633
Segmented bronchial drainage. *See* Postural drainage
Seizure disorders
assessment and diagnostic findings, 2014–2015
computerized equipment, 2015
EEG recordings, 2015
telemetry, 2015
video recording of seizures, 2015
classification of, 2014c
clinical manifestations
focal seizures, 2014
generalized absence seizure, 2014
generalized seizures, 2014
nursing management
after seizure, 2015
during seizure, 2015
pathophysiology, 2014
Seizures, 1971, 2119–2120. *See also* Increased intracranial pressure (ICP)
Selected antibiotics, constipation, 998
Selective estrogen receptor modulators (SERM), 1456
Selective serotonin reuptake inhibitors (SSRI), in premenstrual syndrome, 1395
Self-care, 2124
acne vulgaris, 1795
acute coronary syndrome, 754
acute pancreatitis, 1122–1123
acute rhinosinusitis, 476–477
adrenocortical insufficiency, 1249
angina pectoris, 743
ascites, 1065
burns, 1875
cancer, 2203–2204
cardiomyopathy, 793–794
cervical discectomy, 2142, 2143c
chest percussion and vibration, 611
cholecystectomy, 1118c
chronic illness, 165
chronic inflammatory bowel disease, 1021
chronic rhinosinusitis, 479
cirrhosis, 1095
colorectal cancer, 1043
for common problems of upper extremity, 2273
COPD, 573–574, 575–576, 576c, 577c
coronary artery bypass graft, 774
corticosteroid therapy, 1257–1258
Cushing syndrome, 1253
diabetes as secondary diagnosis, 1188
diabetes mellitus, 1161–1163
diabetic retinopathy, 1178–1179
dysrhythmias, 714
education programs, 7
epilepsy, 2021
epistaxis, 489
eye patch, 1903
gallbladder disease, 1117
gastric cancer, 991
gastric surgery, 994
glaucoma, 1899
Guillain–Barré syndrome, 2109
headaches, 2026
heart failure, 821–823
hemorrhagic stroke, 2952–2053
hepatic encephalopathy, 1074
hepatitis B virus, 1080
hospitalized diabetic patients, 1183
Huntington's disease, 2135
hyperthyroidism, 1236
hypoglycemia, 1165
intracranial surgery, 2011–2012
irritable bowel syndrome, 1006c
ischemic stroke, 2045–2046
IV therapy, 338
laparoscopic cholecystectomy, 1118, 1118c
leg ulcers, 871
liver transplantation, 1102
in liver tumour, 1097–1098
lumbar puncture, 1984
malignant melanoma, 1825
mastoid surgery, 1942
neck dissection, 933
oral cavity disorders, 928
orthopedic surgery, 2261
osteomyelitis, 2289
pancreatic cancer, 1129
pancreatic tumours, 1130–1131
paraplegia, 2085
in Parkinson's disease, 2132
patient education for, 38
patient undergoing bariatric surgery, 1209
patient with newly diagnosed diabetes, 1171, 1172
PD patients, 2131
peptic ulcer disease, 987
peripheral vascular disease, 850
pheochromocytoma, 1248
in pneumonia, 519
postoperative nursing, for thoracic surgery, 644, 645c
prosthetic eye, 1920–1921
psoriasis, 1811
pulmonary heart disease, 541
pulmonary tuberculosis, 528
rhinitis, 473
SCI, 2080
shock, 367
skin cancer, 1822
staphylococcal skin infections, 1797
Stevens-Johnson Syndrome, 1818
tetraplegia, 2085
tonsillitis, 482
total hip arthroplasty, 2255–2256
toxic epidermal necrolysis, 1818
tracheostomy, 617
tube feeding, 959
viral rhinitis, 475
Self-care abilities, fostering of, 179, 179c
Self-care deficits, compensating for, 2123
Self-catheterization, 202
Self-concept, 61
Self-esteem improvement
for acute low back pain, 2270
for bone tumours, 2293–2294
hyperthyroidism, 1235–1236
Self-esteem, in cancer, 2199
Self-help groups, 177
Self-monitoring of blood glucose (SMBG), 1137, 1148–1149
advantages, 1149
candidates for, 1149

Self-monitoring of blood glucose (*continued*)
disadvantages, 1149
frequency of, 1149
methods for, 1149
responding to results, 1149–1150
Self-perception/self-concept, in cardiac disease, 663–664
Self-recitation, optimistic, 384
Self-reflection, 22
Self-regulation, 22
Self-responsibility, for health promotion, 47
Self-transcendence, 81–82
Selye's theory of adaptation, 105
Semilunar valves, 655
Semiocclusive/occlusive wound dressings, 869
Semipermeable film dressings, 870
Sengstaken–Blakemore tube, 947
Senile (age-related) cataracts, 1900
Senna derivatives (Senokot), 288, 1001t
Sense of powerlessness, 793
Sensitivity, 692, 718
Sensitization, 273
Sensory deficits
from peripheral neuropathy or spinal cord injury, 1976
tactile discrimination, 1975
Sensory disabilities, 167
Sensory impulses, 1969
Sensory losses, 1969
Sensory pathways of nervous system, 1969
Sensory system
age-related changes in, 215t, 219
hearing, 219
sensory loss *versus* sensory deprivation, 219
taste and smell, 219
vision, 219
evaluation of, 1975–1976
functions of, 1969
Sentinel lymph node, 1446, 1460–1461
Sentinel lymph node biopsy (SLNB), 1460–1461, 2160
Sentinel lymph node dissection (SLND), 1464
Sentinel lymph node mapping, 2160
Sepsis, 350, 360–364, 1015, 1816, 1818
acute abdomen, 1008
community-acquired, 360
deaths from, 360
definition of, 360
health care–associated infections and, 360–361
medical management, 362–363
correction of underlying causes, 362
fluid replacement therapy, 362
nutritional therapy, 363
pharmacologic therapy, 362–363
Surviving Sepsis Campaign Bundles, 362, 363c
nursing management, 363–364
parenteral nutrition, 970t
pathophysiology, 361–362
peritonitis, 1015
Sepsis-3, 362, 363
Sepsis-Related Organ Failure Assessment Score. *See* Sequential Organ Failure Assessment (SOFA) score
Septal defects, 783
Septal tissue, 789
Septic arthritis, 2214
Septic (infectious) arthritis, 2289–2291
assessment and diagnostic findings, 2290
clinical manifestations, 2289
gerontologic considerations, 2289–2290
medical management, 2290
nursing management, 2290–2291
Septicemia, 1011, 1015
in cancer, 2201
Septic shock, 341, 359, 360–364, 1112
acute abdomen, 1008
in cancer, 2201–2202
Septorhinoplasty, 490
Septra, 1336
thalassemia, 1628
Sequential Organ Failure Assessment (SOFA) score, 363
Sequestration crisis, 1621. *See also* Sickle cell crisis
Seroma formation, 1464
Serophene, 1405c
Serosa, 977
Serotonin, 1572, 1574
Serotonin and norepinephrine reuptake inhibitors (SNRI), for pain relief, 289
Serous membrane lining, 1014
Serous otitis media, 1939–1940
clinical manifestations, 1940
medical management, 1940
Serratia species, 1818
Sertraline (Zoloft), 1789
fibromyalgia, 1759
rheumatoid arthritis, 1745
Serum, 1599, 1604
Serum albumin, 194
Serum aminotransferases, 1056
Serum bilirubin levels, 1060
Serum Free T_4, 1224
Serum osmolality, 300
Serum sickness, 2360
Serum thyroid-stimulating hormone (TSH), 1223–1224
Sevelamer hydrochloride (Renagel), for end-stage kidney disease, 1299
Severe chronic atrophic gastritis, 915
Sevoflurane (Ultane), 400t
Sex counsellor, 1043
Sextasy, 2365
Sexual assault, 1384, 2373–2374
assessment and diagnostic findings, 2373
follow-up care, 2374
management, 2373–2374
physical examination, 2373–2374
specimen collection, 2374
treating potential consequences, 2374
Sexual assault nurse examiner (SANE), 2373
Sexual assessment, 61
Sexual dysfunction, diabetes and, 1181
Sexual function, disabilities and, 168–170
Sexual health, 169
Sexual history, 61
Sexuality
in cancer, 2199–2200
and reproduction, in cardiac disease, 664
Sexually transmitted diseases (STDs), 1044
Sexually transmitted infection (STI), 1044, 1079, 1721–1722, 2374
condoms, 1722
HIV, 1722
nursing process, 1724–1725
routes of transmission, 1721t
Shigella infection, 1719
Shigellosis, 1001
Shingles, 1797
Shock, 341, 415, 1015, 2307. *See also* Multiple organ dysfunction syndrome (MODS)
acute pancreatitis, 1122
anaphylactic, 365–366
cardiogenic, 356–359
compensatory mechanisms in, 344, 344f
compensatory stage, 344
clinical manifestations, 344–345, 344t
medical treatment, 345
nursing management, 345–346
definition of, 341
distributive, 359–364
earlier indicator of, 345
and end-organ dysfunction, 342
fluid resuscitation in, 350, 355t
complications of, 351
crystalloid and colloid solutions, 350–351
hypovolemic, 353–356
irreversible stage, 349
medical management, 349
nursing management, 349–350
neurogenic, 364–365
nutritional support in, 353
in older patients, 345c
overview, 341–342
pathophysiology
blood pressure regulation, 343–344
cellular changes, 342–343, 343f
vascular responses, 343
physiologic responses to, 341–342
progressive stage, 346–347
cardiovascular effects, 347
gastrointestinal effects, 347–348
hematologic effects, 348
hepatic effects, 347
medical management, 348
neurologic effects, 347
nursing management, 348–349
pathophysiology, 347
renal effects, 347
respiratory effects, 347
rest and comfort promotion in, 349
and respiratory failure, 517 (*See also* Pneumonia)
in pneumonia, 519
septic, 341
stages of, 344, 344t
tissue hypoperfusion and, 341
vasoactive medications in, 351–353, 353t
Short-acting beta2-agonists (SABA), 570
for asthma, 592
Short arm cast, 2232
Short leg cast, 2232
Shortnes of breath on exertion (SOBE), 809
Shortness of breath, 659
Shoulder exercises, 643, 643c
Shoulder spica cast, 2232
SIADH. *See* Syndrome of inappropriate antidiuretic hormone (SIADH)
Sialadenitis, 919, 924
Sialography, 925
Sialolithiasis, 925
Sickle cell anemia, 134
Sickle cell crisis, 1621
Sickle cell disease (SCD), 1621–1624, 1621f
assessment and diagnostic findings, 1622–1623
attitudes toward patients with, 1626c
clinical manifestations, 1621–1622
complications in, 1622t
medical management, 1623–1624
nursing process, 1624–1627
prognosis, 1623
Sickle cell hemoglobin C (SC), 1621
Sickle cell hemoglobin D (SD), 1621
Sickle hemoglobin (HbS), 1621
Sick role identity, 157

Sick sinus syndrome, 721
Sigmoidoscopy, 1044
Signal transduction, 2189
Sildenafil (Viagra), 2084, 2365
  erectile dysfunction, 1485
  scleroderma, 1752
Silent killer, hypertension as, 878
Silver-impregnated alginate dressings, 1791
Silver-impregnated dressings, 1855t
Silver nitrate, 1855, 1855t
Silver sulfadiazine (Flamazine), 1855, 1855t
Simeprevir (Olysio), 1081
Simple cystectomy, 1357
Simple pneumothorax, 558
Sims/lateral position, for surgery, 409, 409f
Simvastatin (Zocor), 735t, 736, 2034
Single-chamber atrial pacing (AAI), 720
Single-lumen central catheter, 968
Single nucleotide polymorphisms (SNPs), 135, 145
Single photon emission computed tomography (SPECT), 680, 1981, 2015
Sinoatrial (SA) node, 653
Sinus
  physical assessment, 451, 451f
  rhythm, 692
Sinus arrhythmia, 700, 700f
Sinus bradycardia, 697–698
Sinus node dysrhythmias. *See also* Dysrhythmias
  sinus arrhythmia, 700, 700f
  sinus bradycardia, 697–698
  sinus tachycardia, 698–700, 699t
Sinusoidal harmonic acceleration, 1934
Sinus tachycardia, 698–700, 699t
Sinus tract tumour and metastatic disease, 2111t
Sirolimus (Rapamune), 756
Sirolimus/rapamycin (Rapamune), 1098, 1101
Sitagliptin (Januvia), 1157
Sitz baths, 1047
Six Ps, 859
Sjögren's syndrome, 1750–1751
  assessment and diagnostic findings, 1750–1751
  clinical manifestations, 1750
  medical management, 1751
  nursing management, 1751
  pathophysiology, 1750
SJS. *See* Stevens–Johnson syndrome (SJS)
Skeletal traction, 2244–2246
Skene's duct cysts, 1427
Skin
  anatomy, 1765f
    dermis, 1766
    epidermis, 1764–1765, 1765–1766
    glands, 1768
    hair, 1766–1768
    nails, 1768
    subcutaneous tissue (hypodermis), 1766
  assessment
    colour changes, 1772, 1772f, 1773t
    health history, 1770
    nail and hair, 1777–1779
    physical examination, 1772–1779
    skin lesions, 1774–1777, 1774t–1775t
    vascular changes, 1777
  benign changes in adults, 1770t
  breakdown prevention, 2245
  cancer, 1820–1824
    exposure to UV radiation and, 1820
    prevention of, 1822c
    risk factors, 1820c
  conditions
    nursing management, 1788–1789
    topical corticosteroids, 1787–1788, 1788t
    wound care for, 1783–1784
  dark skin assessment, 1773, 1773t
  dermis–epidermis junction, 1768
  diagnostic evaluation, 1779–1780
    clinical photographs, 1780
    immunofluorescence testing, 1780
    patch testing, 1780
    skin biopsy, 1780
    skin scrapings, 1780
    Tzanck smear, 1780
    Wood's light examination, 1780
  evaporation from, 1769
  and extremities, assessment of, 665–666, 665t
  functions of
    fluid balance, 1768
    immune response function, 1769
    protection, 1768
    sensation, 1768
    temperature regulation, 1768–1769
    vitamin production, 1769
  gerontologic considerations, 1769–1770, 1770c
  hair assessment
    body hair distribution, 1778
    colour and texture, 1777–1778
    hair loss, 1778
    pattern hair distribution, 1779
  lesions, assessment of, 1774–1777
    ABCDE method for screening, 1776–1777
    ABCDE method for screening moles, 1776–1777
    anatomic distribution of eruption, 1776
    atrophy, 1775t
    configurations, 1776f
    crust, 1775t
    cyst, 1774t
    erosion, 1775t
    fissure, 1775t
    keloid, 1775t
    lichenification, 1775t
    macule, patch, 1774t
    nodule, tumour, 1774t
    papule, plaque, 1774t
    primary and secondary, 1774t–1775t
    pustule, 1774t
    scales, 1775t
    scar, 1775t
    size of lesions, 1776
    surrounding skin, 1776
    texture, shape, and border, 1776
    ulcer, 1775t
    vesicle, bulla, 1774t
    wheal, 1774t
    wound bed, 1776
    wound edges and margins, 1776
    wound size, 1776
  lesions, malignant, 2196
  traction (*See also* Traction)
    Buck's extension traction, 2243–2244
    circulatory impairment, 2244
    nerve damage, 2244
    nursing interventions, 2244
    skin breakdown, 2244
  vascularity and hydration, 1777
Skin biopsy, 1780
Skin care, 1782–1789
  in acute kidney injury, 1297
  autolytic debridement, 1784
  choosing soaps, 1782
  diabetes as secondary diagnosis, 1188
  hepatic cirrhosis, 1094
  reversing inflammatory process, 1783
  secondary infection prevention, 1782–1783
  skin protection, 1782
  wound care, 1783–1784
  wound dressing, 1784–1786
Skin contamination poisoning, 2364–2365
Skin disorders, 1764
  anatomic distribution of, 1776f
  assessment of, 1770, 1770c
  cutaneous signs of manifestation of human immunodeficiency virus (HIV), 1779
  in diabetes, 1779
  infections, 1779
  medical management, 1786–1788
    balneotherapy, 1786, 1786t
    creams, 1787
    gels, 1787
    lotions, 1787
    ointments, 1787
    pastes, 1787
    powders, 1787
    spray and aerosols, 1787
    topical corticosteroids, 1787–1788, 1788t
  nursing management, 1788–1789
  skin lesion configurations, 1776f
Skin excoriation, 1027
Skin grafting
  application, 1827
  donor site and care, 1827, 1828f
  nursing management, 1828–1829
  survival of, 1828
  types
    allogeneic or homograft, 1827
    heterograft, 1827
    split-thickness and full-thickness graft, 1828f
    xenograft, 1827
Skin integrity, gallbladder disease, 1116–1117
Skin integrity, impaired
  assessment, 193
    altered nutritional status, 194
    decreased tissue perfusion, 194
    friction and shear, 194, 194f
    immobility, 193
    impaired sensory perception/cognition, 193–194
    moisture, 194
    of risk for pressure injury development, 195, 195c
  bariatric considerations, 195
  expected patient outcomes, 199–200
  gerontologic considerations, 195
  nursing diagnosis, 195
  nursing interventions
    frequent changes of position, 196
    improving mobility, 197
    minimizing irritating moisture, 198
    nutritional status, improving, 197
    positioning the patient, 196
    pressure injury healing, 198–199
    recurrence of pressure injuries, prevention of, 199
    reducing friction and shear, 197–198
    relieving pressure, 196
    sensory perception, improving, 197
    tissue perfusion, improving, 197
    using pressure-relieving devices, 196–197, 197f
  nursing process, 193–200
  planning and goals, 196

Skin integrity maintenance
blistering diseases, 1815
ischemic stroke, 2044
paraplegia, 2083
psoriasis, 1811
spinal cord injury (SCI), 2077
tetraplegia, 2083
traumatic brain injury (TBI), 2067
Skin irritation, 1040
Skin, of older person, 1003
Skin preparation, preoperative, 387
Skin scrapings, 1780
Skin tests, 1576–1579
clinical photographs, 1780
immunofluorescence testing, 1780
interpretation of, 1578–1579
patch testing, 1780
skin biopsy, 1780
skin scrapings, 1780
types of, 1578
Tzanck smear, 1780
Wood's light examination, 1780
Skull, 1961, 1962f
Skull fracture, 2058
depressed, 2059
SLE. *See* Systemic lupus erythematosus (SLE)
Sleep
in COPD, 576c
and rest
in cardiac disease, 663
and rheumatic diseases, 1736, 1739
Sleep apnea, hypertension, 878
Sleep apnea, in older adults, 218
Sleep–wake cycle, 1074, 1961
Sleeve resection, 551c
Sliding esophageal hernia, 936f
Sliding hiatal hernia, 936
Sling, 2233, 2240
Slit-lamp examination, 1886
Slow continuous ultrafiltration (SCUF), 1311
Slow-transit constipation, 999
Small bowel obstruction
assessment and diagnostic findings, 1032
clinical manifestations, 1032
medical management, 1032–1033
nursing management, 1033
pathophysiology, 1031–1032
Small intestine, 899
Small penetrating artery thrombotic strokes, 2029
Small-volume nebulizer therapy
indications, 608
nursing management, 608
Smart-e-Pants, 197
SMAST (Short Michigan Alcohol Screening Test), 59
Smoke evacuators, 398
Smoker's patch, mouth abnormalities, 920t
Smoking cessation, 569
gastritis, 978
peptic ulcer disease, 981, 987
Smoking cessation, preoperative, 378–379
Snakebites, 2359–2361
clinical signs, 2360
management, 2360–2361
venomous snakebites, 2359–2360
Snares, 1044
SOBE. *See* Shortnes of breath on exertion (SOBE)
Social support, 117
in intracranial surgery, 2010
for patients with tetraplegia or paraplegia, 2085
for patient with burns, 1845, 1872
in skin cancer, 1825
Social workers, 16
Societal participation, 166
Society of Critical Care Medicine (SCCM), 957
Society of Obstetricians and Gynaecologists of Canada (SOGC), 1390
Sodium, 309
deficit (hyponatremia), 309–312, 310t
diuresis, 2066
excess (hypernatremia), 310t, 312–313
hyponatremia, 309–312, 310t
imbalances, 309, 310t
and SIADH, 309
retention, 1945, 2009, 2066
Sodium and water retention, in end-stage kidney disease, 1297
Sodium bicarbonate, cardiopulmonary resuscitation, 832t
Sodium, dietary, 821c
Sodium nitroprusside (Nitropress), in hypertensive emergencies, 893
Sodium phosphate tablet, 913
Sodium polystyrene sulphonate (Kayexalate), for end-stage kidney disease, 1299
Sodium–potassium pump, 299
Sodium-restricted diet, 308
Sodium restriction, 1095
heart failure, 806t, 815, 815c
Sodium solutions, highly hypertonic, administration of, 311
Sodium, urine, 300
Solar plexus, 1966
Solitaire Flow Restoration Device, 2035
Soltamox, for breast disease, 1456
Somatosensory evoked responses (SERs), 1984
Somatostatin, 1108
in bleeding from esophageal varices, 1068
Somogyi effect, 1155
Sotalol, 699t
Spasm, 1119
of gallbladder, 1030
Spastic bladder, 1346
Spastic contractions, irritable bowel syndrome, 1005f
Spasticity, 1974, 2097
management, 2084
Spastic palsy of larynx, 2111t
Specialty certification, 387c
Specificity, 1571
Speech disorders, in Parkinson's disease, 2132
Speech pattern, in physical assessment, 63
Speech therapy, for cancer of larynx
artificial larynx, 495
esophageal speech, 495
tracheoesophageal puncture, 495, 495f
Sperm, 134
Spermatogenesis, 1479, 1480
Spermicides, 1400–1401
Sphincterotomy, 1111, 1114, 1121, 1127
Spider angioma, 1777t
Spider bites, 2361
Spinal anesthesia, 403–405, 404f
Spinal cord, 1963–1964
disorder, 2112t
spinal tracts, 1963–1964, 1963f
vertebral column, 1964
Spinal cord compression, 2205t
Spinal cord injury (SCI), 2056
assessment and diagnostic findings, 2071–2073
clinical manifestations, 2071
collaborative problems/potential complications, 2076
effects of, 2072c
emergency management, 2073
functional abilities by level, 2073t
management of acute complications
autonomic dysreflexia, 2076
respiratory complications, 2076
spinal and neurogenic shock, 2075
venous thromboembolism (VTE), 2075
medical management (acute phase)
pharmacologic therapy, 2074
respiratory therapy, 2074
skeletal fracture reduction and traction, 2074
surgical management, 2075
medical management (long-term complications), 2081
nursing interventions
autonomic dysreflexia, management of, 2079–2080
bowel function improvement, 2078
injury prevention, 2077
mobility improvement, 2077
monitoring and managing potential complications, 2078–2079
patient outcomes, 2080–2081
promoting adequate breathing and airway clearance, 2076–2077
promoting home, community-based, and transitional care, 2080
providing comfort measures, 2078
skin integrity maintenance, 2077
urinary elimination maintenance, 2078
nursing priorities, 2076
planning and goals, 2076
pathophysiology, 2071
patient assessment, 2076
risk factors for, 2071
Spinal Cord Injury Pressure Ulcer Scale (SCIPUS), 195
Spinal cord injury rehabilitation programs, 177
Spinal cord tumours. *See also* Oncologic disorders of brain and spinal cord
assessment/diagnostic findings, 2125–2126
medical management, 2126
nursing management, 2126–2127
surgical management, 2126
Spinal fractures, 2327
Spinal nerves, 1964–1965
Spinal reflex, 902
Spinocerebellar ataxia
type 1, 141t
type 2, 141t
type 3, 141t
type 6, 141t
Spinoreticular tract, 271
Spinothalamic tracts, 271, 1964
Spiral (helical) CT, 1128
Spiritual advisor, 82
Spiritual assessment, 58, 84
of terminally ill patients, 248
Spiritual beliefs
preoperative assessment, 383
preoperative teaching, 386
Spiritual distress, 82–83, 248
Spiritual environment, 57–58
Spirituality, 57, 80, 247–248
aging adults and, 81
definition of, 80–81
expressions of, 81
and health, relationship between, 81–82
modes of expression by patients, 82

less obvious expressions, 82–83
overt expressions, 82
of nurse, 85
and posttraumatic growth, 82
referral to spiritual care professional, 85–86
religion and, 80
ways to address spiritual needs of patients, 83
dignified care by staff, 84, 84c
formalized ways, 83
gerontologic considerations, 83
nonformalized ways, 83–85
respecting patients' beliefs, 83
Spiritual teddy bears, 84
Spirometer, 459, 460
Spirometry, 564
Spironolactone (Aldactone), 812, 813, 817, 820t
hypertension, 884t
Splenectomy, 1629, 1678
Splenomegaly, 1067
Splenoportography, 1067
Splinter hemorrhages, 795
Splints, 2233–2234
defined, 2233
patient with, 2240–2241
Spondyloarthropathies, 1756–1757
ankylosing spondylitis, 1756
medical management, 1756–1757
nursing management, 1757
psoriatic arthritis, 1756–1757
reactive arthritis, 1756
Spondylosis, 2117, 2140
Spontaneous abortion, 1402–1403
habitual abortion, 1403
medical management, 1403
nursing management, 1403
Spontaneous bacterial peritonitis (SBP), 1014, 1084
Sports-related musculoskeletal injuries, 2299–2300
contusions, 2300
dislocations, 2300
fractures, 2300
management, 2300
meniscal injuries of knee, 2300
prevention, 2300
sprains, 2300
strains, 2300
tendinitis, 2300
Sprain, 2298–2299
Spray and aerosol preparations, 1787
Sputum
production, 448
studies, 461–462
Squamous cell carcinoma (SCC), 942, 1821f
clinical manifestations, 1820–1821
in immunocompromised population, 1826
medical management
nonsurgical alternative therapies, 1822
surgical, 1821–1822
nursing management, 1822
promoting home, community-based, and transitional care, 1822
prognosis for, 1821
Stab wounds, 557, 2349c
abdominal, 2352
Stages of Change Model, 46, 46t
Staging, 2150
of tumour, 2158
Standing postures, 2269f
Stapedectomy, 1943, 1944f
Stapes surgery, 1943
Staphylococcal endocarditis infections of valves, 795
Staphylococcus aureus, 924, 970, 1795
Staphylococcus epidermidis, 970
Staphylococcus scabiei, 1802
Staphylokinase, 860
Stapled hemorrhoidopexy, 1046
Stasis dermatitis, 1779
Stasis syndromes, 1007t
State rehabilitation administration agencies, 205–206
Static support devices, 196
Statins, 845
endothelial function, 852
Status asthmaticus. *See also* Chronic pulmonary disease
assessment/diagnostic findings, 595
clinical manifestations, 595
medical management, 595–596
nursing management, 596
pathophysiology, 595
Status epilepticus
medical management, 2022
nursing management, 2022
STDs. *See* Sexually transmitted diseases (STDs)
Steady state, 102–103
control of, 109–110
Steapsin, 901t
Steatorrhea, 998, 1017, 1107, 1123
fatty stools, 994
gastric surgery, 982
Stem cell, 1516, 1517, 1525, 1599, 1600
Stem cell transplant (SCT), 1619
Stenosis, 777, 778, 780, 781, 783, 835, 839, 977
Stent, flexible, 846f
Step-Up Approach, 1122
Stereotactic core biopsy, 1446, 1453
Stereotactic procedures, for Parkinson's disease, 2130
Sterile endophthalmitis, 1903
Sterilization, 1397
tubal ligation, 1397
vasectomy, 1397
Sterilization methods, 1398t
Sternal/rib fractures
assessment/diagnostic findings, 555
clinical manifestations, 555
medical management, 555
Steroid-induced acne, 1788
Stethoscope, 669
Stevens–Johnson syndrome (SJS), 1816
assessment and diagnostic findings, 1816
care of patient
assessment, 1816–1817
nursing priorities, 1817
planning and goals, 1817
clinical manifestations, 1816
complications, 1816
medical management, 1816
nursing interventions
maintaining fluid balance, 1817
maintaining skin and mucous membrane integrity, 1817
monitoring and managing potential complications, 1818
patient outcomes, 1818–1819
preventing hypothermia, 1817
promoting home, community-based, and transitional care, 1818
reducing anxiety, 1818
relieving pain, 1817–1818
STI. *See* Sexually transmitted infection (STI)
St. John's wort, 222, 2025
St. Louis encephalitis, 2093
Stocking, 866
Stoma, 948
Stomach, 899
enzyme/secretion, 901t
ingestion of food, 900
peristaltic contractions, 900, 902
Stomach growling, 905
Stomach mucosa, inflammation of, 976
Stoma ischemia and necrosis, 1367
Stoma retraction and separation, 1367
Stoma skin barriers, 1038
Stomatitis, 919, 927, 2150, 2165, 2182, 2195–2196
mouth abnormalities, 921t
Stones
calcium, 1351
cystine, 1351
struvite, 1351
uric acid, 1351
Stools, 982
abnormal hardening of, 997
blood, 904
liver disease, 1055
characteristics of, abnormalities in, 904
colour, 904t
changes, 1110
DNA test, 907
foods and medications, 904t
softeners
diarrhea, 1000
and laxatives, 1000
watery, 1002
Strains, 2298–2299, 2300
Stratum corneum, 1765, 1768
Stratum germinativum, 1765
Stratum granulosum, 1765
Stratum lucidum, 1765
Stratum spinosum, 1765
Strawberry angiomas, 1819
Streptococcal pharyngitis, 479
Streptococcal skin diseases, 1795
Streptococcus pyogenes, 1522
Streptococcus viridans, 924
Stress, 103. *See also* Stressors
and adaptation, 103
at cellular level, 109, 109f
cellular adaptation, 110–111, 110t
cellular healing, 114
cellular injury, 111–114
control of steady state, 109–110
hospitalized diabetic patients, 1186
indicators of, 108–109, 108c
liver transplantation, 1101
maladaptive responses to, 107–108
management, 114–117, 115c
coping enhancement, 115–116
educational interventions, 116–117
enhancing social support, 117
promoting healthy lifestyle, 115, 115c
support and therapy groups, 117
teaching relaxation techniques, 116
nursing implications, 114
physiologic response to, 105, 106f
brain, role of, 105, 106f
hypothalamic–pituitary response, 106–107
immunologic response, 107
Selye's theory of adaptation, 105
sympathetic–adrenal–medullary response, 106, 107t

Stress (*continued*)
sympathetic nervous system response, 105–106
psychological responses to, 104
appraisal of stressful event, 104
coping with stressful event, 104–105
reduction, 983
role of, in health patterns, 117
as stimulus for disease, 103–104
Stress fractures, 2300
Stress incontinence, 1332, 1341. *See also* Urinary incontinence
Stressors
categories on, 103
cellular adaptation, 110–111, 110t
chronic, 103
daily hassles, 103
definition of, 103
identification of, 109
of old age, 220
physical, 103
physiologic, 103
psychosocial, 103
Stress reduction and management, for health promotion, 47
Stress ulcers, 982, 983
in acutely ill patients, 353
mucosal ulceration, 982
Stretch–hold–relax routine, 2099
Stridor, 439
String sign, in Crohn's disease, 1017
Stroke, 1622
awareness of stroke risk in young African Americans, 2034c
cognitive deficits of, 2031t
comparison of left and right hemispheric, 2032t
death related to, 2028
definition, 2028
emotional deficits of, 2032t
hemorrhagic
arteriovenous malformations, 2047
assessment and diagnostic findings, 2048
cause of, 2046
clinical manifestations, 2047–2048
collaborative problems/potential complications, 2050
ethics and related issues, 2048c
incidence, 2046
intracerebral hemorrhage, 2047
intracranial (cerebral) aneurysm, 2047
medical management, 2049–2050
nursing interventions, 2050–2053
nursing planning and goals, 2050
nursing priorities, 2050
pathophysiology, 2047
patient assessment, 2050
potential complications, 2048–2049
prevention of, 2048
subarachnoid hemorrhage, 2046, 2047
surgical management, 2050
incidence rate, 2028
ischemic
assessment and diagnostic findings, 2032–2033
cardiogenic embolic strokes, 2029
clinical manifestations, 2030–2032
definition, 2028
ischemic brain cell injury, 2030f
large artery thrombotic strokes, 2029
medical management, 2033–2038
nursing management, 2038–2046
pathophysiology, 2029–2030, 2030f
prevention of, 2033
small penetrating artery thrombotic strokes, 2029
thrombolytic therapy, 2029
treatment for, 2028–2029
methods of preventing recurrent, 2033
motor deficits of, 2031t
National Institutes of Health Stroke Scale (NIHSS), 2037t
neurologic deficits of, 2031t–2032t
risk of coronary heart disease and, 2033
risk screenings, 2033
sensory deficits of, 2031t
sexuality after, 2045
types of, 2029t
verbal deficits of, 2031t
visual field deficits of, 2031t
Stroke recovery programs, 176–177
Stroke Rehabilitation Assessment of Movement (STREAM), 2042
Strokes, 781, 783, 787, 797, 844f, 852, 881
hypertension, 878
Stroke volume, 653
on cardiac output, effect of, 657–658
Stromal tumours, 1507
Struvite stones, 1351
ST segment, 692, 695
ST-segment elevation myocardial infarction (STEMI), 744, 746. *See also* Acute coronary syndrome (ACS); Myocardial infarction (MI)
Stylet, 1491
Subacute necrotizing sialadenitis (SANS), 925
Subarachnoid hemorrhage, 2046–2047
Subarachnoid screw or bolt, 1998
Subchondral bone, 1732, 1754
Subclavian triple-lumen catheter, parenteral nutrition and adjunctive therapies, 968f
Subconjunctival injection, 1893
Subcultures, 91, 92
Subcutaneous emphysema, 560. *See also* Chest trauma
Subcutaneous immunoglobulin (SCIG), 1535
Subcutaneous immunotherapy (SIT), 1586
allergic rhinitis, 1586
Subcutaneous pain management system, 423f
Subcutaneous tissue (hypodermis), 1766
functions of, 1766
Subdiaphragmatic abdominal thrusts, 2345
Subdural hematomas, 2056, 2060
acute, 2060
chronic, 2060
Subgaleal hematomas, 2058
Sublingual immunotherapy (SLIT), 1586
allergic rhinitis, 1586
Subluxation, 2299
Substance abuse, 122, 125–126, 177, 2365
acute alcohol intoxication, 2365, 2370
alcohol withdrawal syndrome, 2370–2371
assessment for, 126c
drug overdose, 2366–2369
nursing implications, 126
in rehabilitation, 177
Substance dependence, 280
Substance P, 271
Succinylcholine, 401t
Sucralfate (Carafate), 907
peptic ulcer disease and gastritis, 980t
Sucralose (Splenda), 1147
Sucrase, 901t
Sudden cardiac death, 731
Sudden fall, 881
Sudomotor neuropathy, and diabetes, 1181
Sufentanil (Sufenta), 401t
Suicide, 123
risk factors for, 123, 123c
Sulfamethoxazole, 1336
Sulfasalazine (Azulfidine), 1018
rheumatoid arthritis, 1744
Sulfonamides, in thalassemia, 1628
Sulfonylureas, 1137, 1157–1158
Sumatriptan (Imitrex), 2025
Summation gallop, 653
Sun damage, 1820
Sundowning, 229
Sunlight, exposure to, 2154
Superficial inferior epigastric artery flap (SIEA), 1474
Superficial reflexes, 1978
Superficial thrombophlebitis, 1456
Superficial venous thrombosis (SVT), 2203
Superior vena cava syndrome (SVCS), 2205t
Super-normal vision, 1888
Supervision, 75
direct, 75
indirect, 75
Supplemental oxygen, in cardiogenic shock, 357
Supportive therapy, in sickle cell disease, 1624
Suppositories, 1047
Suppressor T cells, 1517, 1522, 2156
Suppurative lymphadenitis, 873
Suprapubic catheter, 1332, 1345, 1347, 1347f
Suprapubic prostatectomy, 1494
Suprapubic tapping, 201
Supratentorial approach, to intracranial surgery, 2006–2013
ethics and related issues, 2008c
home care checklist after, 2012c
nursing interventions
aseptic technique, 2011
cerebral edema, management of, 2010
cerebral tissue perfusion maintenance, 2009
continuing and transitional care, 2012
enhancing self-image, 2010
fluid and electrolyte disturbances, management of, 2011
improving pulmonary function/gas exchange, 2010
infection prevention, 2011
intracranial hematoma, management of, 2010
monitoring and managing potential complications, 2010–2011
monitoring for increased intracranial pressure and bleeding, 2010–2011
monitoring for seizure activity, 2011
pressure ulcers, management of, 2011
promoting home, community-based, and transitional care, 2011–2012
sensory deprivation management, 2010
SIADH, management of, 2011
status epilepticus, management of, 2011
temperature regulation, 2009–2010
patient assessment, 2008–2009
patient outcomes, 2012–2013
postoperative management
anticonvulsant medication for, 2008
cerebral edema, reduction of, 2008
collaborative problems/potential complications, 2009
medical management, 2013
monitoring intracranial pressure, 2008
nursing priorities, 2009

pain management, 2008
planning and goals, 2009
seizure prevention, 2008
ventilatory support, 2008
preoperative management
medical management, 2006–2007
nursing management, 2007–2008
risk of postoperative seizures, 2007
Supraventricular tachycardia (SVT), 692, 707
Surgeon, 395–396
Surgery
anesthesia, advances in, 373
in cancer, 2160–2163 (*See also* Cancer)
nursing management, 2162–2163
palliative surgery, 2162, 2162t
as primary treatment, 2160–2161, 2161t
prophylactic, 2161–2162
reconstructive surgery, 2162
classifications of, 373, 375, 375t
informed consent, 376–377, 377c
technology, advances in, 373
Surgical abdomen, 1008. *See* Acute abdomen
Surgical area
restricted zone, 396
semirestricted zone, 396
unrestricted zone, 396
Surgical asepsis, 396, 397
environmental controls, 397
OR ventilation, 397
sterilized equipment, 397
movement around sterile field, 398
principles of, 397–398
sterile drapes, use of, 397–398, 398f
Surgical attire, 396–397
Surgical biopsy, 1446, 1452, 1453
Surgical checklist, 409
Surgical débridement, 1857
Surgical drains, 427, 427f
Surgical environment, 396–397
blood and body fluids, exposure to, 398
health hazards associated with, 398
laser risks, 398
robot-assisted technology, 398
surgical asepsis, 397–398
Surgically placed central catheters, 969
Surgical management
abdominal aortic aneurysm, 857
arterial thrombosis, 860
atherosclerosis, 846
benign prostatic hyperplasia, 1491, 1491t–1492t, 1493
bladder cancer, 1357
breast cancer, 1459–1461, 1460t, 1467–1476
for cancer of larynx
ckordectomy, 493
laser surgery, 494
partial laryngectomy, 494
total laryngectomy, 494
vocal cord stripping, 493
chronic inflammatory bowel disease, 1019–1020
chronic rhinosinusitis (CRS), 478–479
colorectal cancer, 1036–1037
degenerative disc disease, 2139–2140
diverticular disease, 1012–1013
ectopic pregnancy, 1408
elephantiasis, 874
endometriosis, 1431
esophageal varices, 1069–1070
genitourinary trauma, 1356
herniation of cervical intervertebral disc, 2140
herniation of lumbar disc, 2144
infective endocarditis, 796–797
jaw disorders, 924
liver metastases, 1096–1097
of lung cancer, 551, 551c
lymphedema, 874
medical management, 860
obstructive sleep apnea, 487–488
osteoarthritis, 1755
Parkinson's disease, 2129–2130
neural transplantation, 2130
stereotactic procedures, 2130
peptic ulcer disease, 984
peripheral arterial occlusive disease, 852–853
peritonsillar abscess, 483
primary brain tumours, 2121
prostate cancer, 1495–1496
spinal cord tumours, 2126
spondyloarthropathies, 1757
urinary incontinence, 1342–1344, 1344f
Surgical safety checklist, 395, 395f
Surgical site, marking of, 395
Surgical team, 392
anesthesiologist, 392, 396
anesthetist, 396
circulating nurse, 392, 394–395
patient, 392–394
registered nurse first assistant, 396
scrub role, 392, 395
surgeon, 395–396
Survivorship care, in cancer, 2208, 2208t. *See also* Cancer
Susceptibility testing, 143
Susceptible, 1698
host, 1698
Suspensions, 1787
Sustained maximal inspiration. *See* Incentive spirometry
Swallowing, 900
Swallowing difficulties, in Parkinson's disease, 2132
Sweat glands, 1768
Sweating, 299, 859, 1769
thoracic aortic aneurysm, 842
Sweeteners, for patients with diabetes, 1147
nonnutritive sweeteners, 1147
nutritive, 1147
Swelling and cellulitis, 923
Sympathectomy, 861
Sympathetic–adrenal–medullary response, to stress, 106, 107t
Sympathetic nervous system regulating mechanisms of peripheral vascular blood flow, 837
Sympathetic neurons, 1966
Sympathetic syndromes, 1966
Symptom management, in lung cancer, 552
Synarel, 1405c
Synarthrotic joints, 2217
Synchronized intermittent mandatory ventilation (SIMV), 602, 620
Syncope, 999, 1944
Syndrome of inappropriate antidiuretic hormone (SIADH), 309, 1221–1222, 1998, 1998t, 2006, 2052, 2091, 2182
management after intracranial surgery, 2011
Syndrome X, 1141
Syngeneic HSCT, 2186
Syngeneic transplants, 2187
Synovium, 2218
Synthetic casts, 2232
Syphilis
assessment and diagnostic findings, 1722–1723
medical management, 1723
nursing management, 1723
stages, 1722
Syphilitic ulcers, 1819
Systemic arteriovenous oxygen difference, 836
Systemic brachytherapy, 2165
Systemic circulation, 834
Systemic lupus erythematosus (SLE), 998, 1731, 1748–1750
assessment and diagnostic findings, 1749
clinical manifestations, 1748–1749
medical management, 1749–1750
nursing management, 1750
pathophysiology, 1748
Systemic medications, 1788
Systemic vascular resistance, 653
Systems, constellation of, 102, 102f
Systole, 653, 692
Systolic Blood Pressure Intervention Trial (SPRINT), 888
Systolic click, 653, 670
Systolic crescendo-decrescendo murmur, 782
Systolic dysfunction, 805, 813
Systolic heart failure, 804, 805

T

TACE. *See* Transarterial chemoembolization (TACE)
Tachycardia, 809, 859
thoracic aortic aneurysm, 842
Tachypnea, 439, 447
Tacrolimus (Prograf), 1098
Tactile discrimination, 1975
Tactile fremitus, 64, 455
Tactile sensations, evaluation of, 1975
Tadalafil (Cialis), 2084
benign prostatic hyperplasia, 1491
erectile dysfunction, 1485
T'ai chi classes, 206
Tail of Spence, 1445
Talc, 1787
Tamoxifen
breast cancer, 1458
breast disease, 1456
cervical cancer, 1391
endometrial hyperplasia, 1431
Tampon, 1393
test, 1424
Tamsulosin (Flomax), for benign prostatic hyperplasia, 1491
Targeted therapies, 144, 2150
in cancer (*See also* Cancer)
about, 2189
biologic response modifiers, 2190
cancer vaccines, 2192
cytokines, 2191–2192
gene therapy, 2192
monoclonal antibodies, 2190–2191
nonspecific biologic response modifiers, 2190
nursing management, 2192–2193
Taxanes
breast cancer, 1469
chemotherapeutic agents, 551
Taxol. *See* Paclitaxel
Taxonomy of nursing practice, 36
Tazarotene (Tazorac), 1808–1809
TBI. *See* Traumatic brain injury (TBI)
TB, in older adults, 232
T-cell prolymphocytic leukemia, 1641

T cells, 1516, 1517, 1572
Teach-back technique, 41
Teaching, 37
  nursing process in patient education, 43–45, 43c
  older adults, 42–43
  people with disabilities, 42, 42t
  techniques and methods, 41
    demonstration and practice, 41
    electronic or Internet information, 41
    group teaching, 41
    lectures, 41
    motivational interviewing, 41
    reinforcement and follow-up, 41
    teaching aids, 41
Teaching aids, 41
Teaching–learning process, 40
  assessment in, 43–44
  evaluation in, 44–45
  implementation in, 44
  nursing diagnosis in, 44
  planning in, 44
Technology, advances in, 373
TED stockings, 866
TEE. *See* Transesophageal echocardiography (TEE)
Tegaderm, 1783, 1860
Tegaserod (Zelnorm), 1000
Telangiectasias (venous stars), 1777, 1777t, 1831
Telehealth, 15, 166
Telemetry, 653, 675–676
  transmitters, 679
Teleologic theory, 24
Telestroke Networks, 2033
Telfa pads, 1788
Telmisartan (Micardis), hypertension, 886t
Temperature regulation, 1768–1769
Temporal lobe, 1961
Temporomandibular disorders, 919, 923
  assessment and diagnostic findings, 923
  clinical manifestations, 923
  dysphagia, 923
  and jaw surgery, 923
  medical management, 923–924
Temporomandibular joint (TMJ), 923
TEN. *See* Toxic epidermal necrolysis (TEN)
Tendinitis, 2300
Tendons, 2214
Tenecteplase (TNKase), 748, 860
Tenesmus, 998, 1002
Tennis elbow, 2300–2301
Tenofovir (TDF), 1080
Tenofovir disoproxil fumarate, for human immune deficiency virus, 1539
Tenosynovitis, 2270
Tension pneumothorax, 558
  defined, 505
Tension-type headache, 2023
  symptomatic pain relief for, 2025–2026
Terazosin (Hytrin)
  benign prostatic hyperplasia, 1491
  hypertension, 885t
Terconazole (Terazol)
  candidiasis, 1414
Terminal ganglia, 1966
Terminal illness, 240
Tertiary prevention, 14
  of cancer, 2157
Testes, 1479, 1480
Testicular cancer, 1480
  assessment and diagnostic findings, 1507
  classification, 1507
  clinical manifestation, 1507
  medical management, 1508–1509
  nursing management, 1509
  risk factors, 1507
Testicular self-examination (TSE), 1482, 1508c
Testosterone, 1480
Tetany, 319, 326
Tetracaine (Pontocaine), 404t
Tetracaine hydrochloride, 1893
Tetracycline, 983, 1794
  peptic ulcer disease and gastritis, 979t
Tetrahydrocannabinol (THC), 1554
Tetraplegia, 1968
  collaborative issues/potential complications, 2082
  nursing interventions
    bladder management, 2083
    enhancing coping mechanisms, 2084
    establishing bowel control, 2083
    exercise programs, 2082
    increasing mobility, 2082
    infection and sepsis, prevention of, 2084–2085
    for mobilization, 2082
    monitoring and managing potential complications, 2084–2085
    patient outcomes, 2085
    preventing disuse syndrome, 2082–2083
    promoting home, community-based, and transitional care, 2085
    sexual education and counselling services, 2083–2084
    skin integrity, promoting, 2083
    spasticity management, 2084
  nursing priorities, 2082
    planning and goals, 2082
  patient assessment, 2081–2082
THA. *See* Total hip arthroplasty (THA)
Thalamus, 1961
Thalassemia, 1627–1628
  alpha, 1627
  assessment and diagnostic findings, 1628
  beta, 1627
  clinical manifestations, 1628
  glucose-6-phosphate dehydrogenase deficiency, 1627–1628
  major, 1627
  medical management, 1628
  nursing management, 1628
Thalidomide, for multiple myeloma, 1654
Theophylline, 589t
  for asthma, 591
Therapeutic baths, 1786, 1786t
Therapeutic bronchoscopy, 464
Therapeutic communication techniques, 31t
Therapeutic exercises, 182, 184, 185t
Therapeutic hypothermia, 357
Therapeutic lifestyle changes diet, 733, 735t
Therapeutic phlebotomy, 1679
Therapeutic regimen
  adherence to, 38–40
  nonadherence to, 39
Therapeutic vaccines, 2192
Thermal therapy. *See* Hyperthermia
Thiazide diuretics, 812, 820t
  for hypervolemia, 308
  thalassemia, 1628
Thiazolidinediones (TZDs), 1137, 1157
Thin-layer Rapid Use Epicutaneous (TRUE) test, 1590
Thiopental sodium (Pentothal), 403t
Thiotepa, for bladder cancer, 1357
Third-degree atrioventricular block, 712–713
Third heart sound, 670
Third-intention healing, 413
Third-space fluid shift, 297
Thirst, 1002
Thoracentesis, 466, 466c–467c, 505
Thoracic aortic aneurysm, 855
  assessment and diagnostic findings, 856
  clinical manifestations, 856
  medical management, 856
Thoracic auscultation, 456–457. *See also* Lower respiratory structures and breathing
  adventitious sounds, 457, 458t
  breath sounds, 457, 457t
  voice sounds, 457
Thoracic inspection
  accessory muscles, use of, 454
  breathing patterns/respiratory rates, 452, 453t, 454
  chest configuration, 452
Thoracic palpation. *See also* Lower respiratory structures and breathing
  respiratory excursion, 454–455
  tactile fremitus, 455
Thoracic percussion, 455–456, 456t. *See also* Lower respiratory structures and breathing
  diaphragmatic excursion, 456
Thoracic surgery
  postoperative management, 634–639
    chest drainage, 635–639, 635t, 636c–637c, 638c
    mechanical ventilation, 635
  postoperative nursing management, 639–648
  preoperative management
    assessment/diagnostic findings, 632
    nursing management, preoperative, 632–634
  and procedures, 633c
Thoracolumbar spine, fractures of, 2327
Thoracoscopy, 465–466, 465f
  nursing interventions, 465–466
  procedure, 465
Thoracotomy
  care after, 645c–648c
  defined, 602
Three-dimensional (3D) mammography, 1452
Thrills, 64
Throat cultures, 461
Throat lozenges, 952
Thrombin, 1599, 1605
Thromboangiitis obliterans, 854–855
  assessment and diagnostic findings, 854
  clinical manifestations, 854
  medical management, 854
  nursing management, 854–855
Thrombocyte, 1599, 1600
Thrombocytopenia, 1599, 1616, 1660–1661, 2150, 2202–2203
  assessment and diagnostic findings, 1660–1661
  causes and management, 1661t
  clinical manifestations, 1660
  heparin therapy, 865
  medical management, 1661
  nursing management, 1661
Thrombocytosis, 1599
Thromboembolus obstructing venous blood flow, 838
Thrombolytic therapy, 828, 860, 2029
  myocardial infarction, 748, 748c
  for pulmonary embolism, 545
  in venous thromboembolism, 864

Thrombolytic therapy monitoring, 545
Thrombophlebitis, IV infusion and, 337–338
Thrombopoietin, 1604
Thrombosis, risk factors for, 1674t
Thrombotic disorders, 1671
Thromboxane A_2, 838
Thrombus formation, 730–731
  prevention, 545
Thymectomy, 2104
Thyroglobulin (Tg), 1225
Thyroid antibodies, 1224
Thyroid cancer
  assessment and diagnostic findings, 1238–1239
  medical management, 1239
  nursing management
    home, community-based, and transitional care, 1240
    postoperative care, 1239–1240
    potential complications, 1240
    preoperative care, 1239
  prevalence, 1238
  radiation-induced, 1238
  types, 1238, 1238t
Thyroid cartilage, 440
Thyroid gland
  assessment
    diagnostic evaluation, 1223–1224
    physical examination, 1223
  calcitonin, 1223
  and surrounding structures, 1222f
  thyroid hormone
    composition, 1222
    function, 1223
    inadequate secretion, pathophysiology of, 1223
    regulation, 1222
    synthesis, 1222
Thyroid hormone replacement, diarrhea, 1000
Thyroid scan, 1225
Thyroid storm, 1232c
Thyroid tests, 1223–1225
  medications altering, 1225c
Thyroid tumours
  classification of, 1237
  endemic (iodine-deficient) goitre, 1237–1238
  nodular goitre, 1238
Thyrotoxic crisis. *See* Thyroid storm
Thyrotoxicosis, diarrhea, 1001
Thyrotropin-releasing hormone (TRH), 1222, 1222f
Thyroxin-binding protein, 67
TIA. *See* Transient ischemic attack (TIA)
Tiazac. *See* Diltiazem
Tibia and fibula, fracture of, 2326
Tick bites, 2361, 2361f
Tidal volume, 603
  of breath, 443, 459
  defined, 602
Timbre, 1933
Timolol (Blocadren), 2025
  antiarrhythmic medication, 699t
  hypertension, 885t
Tinea (ringworm) infections, 1798, 1800t
Tinnitus, 1930, 1945
TIPS. *See* Transjugular intrahepatic portosystemic shunt (TIPS)
Tirofiban (Aggrastat), 742
Tissue expander followed by a permanent implant, 1446, 1472–1473, 1473f
Tissue integrity
  alopecia, 2196
  malignant skin lesions, 2196
  radiation-associated impairment of, 2196
  stomatitis, 2195–2196
Tissue ischemia, 836
Tissue perfusion, left ventricular failure, 809
Tissue plasminogen activator (t-PA), 2030
Tissue turgor, 306
Tissue valves, 785, 786. *See also* Biologic valves
T Lymphocytes, 1522–1523
T lymphocytes, 1766
TMJ. *See* Temporomandibular joint (TMJ)
TNA. *See* Total nutrient admixture (TNA)
TNM system. *See* Tumour, nodes, and metastasis (TNM) system
Tobacco smoke, 549
  and risk of cancer, 2155
Tobacco use
  atherosclerotic lesions, 845
  Buerger's disease, 854
  cessation of, 736
  and oral cancer, 925
  peripheral arterial occlusive disease, 852
  risk factors, 857
Tobramycin, for acute kidney injury, 1294
Tolerance, 286
  to medication, 280
  to opioids, 286
TomoTherapy, 2164
Tongue, inspection of, 905
Tongue turgor, 306
Tonicity, 298–299
Tonometry, 1886
Tonsillectomy, 482
Tonsillitis
  assessment/diagnostic findings, 481–482
  clinical manifestations, 481
  defined, 471
  medical management, 482
  nursing management
    educating patients about self-care, 482
    providing postoperative care, 482
Tonsils, 439
Tonsil tip suction, 930
Tophi, 1732, 1757
Topical corticosteroids, 1787–1788, 1788t
Topiramate (Topamax), 2025
Topoisomerase I/II inhibitors, 2179t
Torsades de pointes, 709
Torsemide (Demadex)
  heart failure, 820t
  hypertension, 884t
Total artificial hearts, 777, 791–792
Total-body irradiation, 2187
Total colectomies, and ulcerative colitis, 1019
Total gastrectomy, 989, 994
Total hip arthroplasty (THA), 2248–2257
  nursing interventions, 2249–2256, 2250c–2253c
  total knee replacement, 2256–2257
Total iron-binding capacity (TIBC), 1611
Total knee replacement, 2256–2257
  continuous passive motion (CPM) device, 2256
  nursing interventions, 2256
Total laryngectomy, 494, 494f
Total mastectomy, 1460
Total nutrient admixture (TNA), 948, 966, 968
Total pain, 83
Total serum immunoglobulin E levels, 1576
Toxic anterior segment syndrome, 1903
Toxic endothelial cell destruction, 1903
Toxic epidermal necrolysis (TEN), 1816
  assessment and diagnostic findings, 1816
  care of patient
    assessment, 1816–1817
    nursing priorities, 1817
    planning and goals, 1817
  clinical manifestations, 1816
  complications, 1816
  medical management, 1816
  nursing interventions
    maintaining fluid balance, 1817
    maintaining skin and mucous membrane integrity, 1817
    monitoring and managing potential complications, 1818
    patient outcomes, 1818–1819
    preventing hypothermia, 1817
    promoting home, community-based, and transitional care, 1818
    reducing anxiety, 1818
    relieving pain, 1817–1818
Toxic hepatitis, 1082
Toxicity. *See also* Cancer
  chemotherapy-associated
    cardiopulmonary system, 2183
    cognitive impairment, 2184
    fatigue, 2184
    gastrointestinal system, 2182
    hematopoietic system, 2182
    neurologic system, 2183
    renal system, 2182–2183
    reproductive system, 2183
  of radiation therapy, 2165–2166
Toxic megacolon, in ulcerative colitis, 1018
Toxic shock syndrome, 1393
T-pieces, 606, 660f
TP interval, 692, 696
Trabeculae, 2215
Tracers, 680
Trachea
  anatomy, 440
  physical assessment, 451–452
Tracheal suction, guidelines for, 618c
Tracheoesophageal puncture, 495, 495f
Tracheostomy, 614–619. *See also* Airway management
  collars, 606, 606f
  complications, 615, 615c
  guidelines
    for tracheal suction, 618c
    for tracheostomy tube, 616c–617c
  nursing management
    continuing and transitional care, 617
    cuff management, 617
    patient education about self-care, 617
    suctioning tracheal tube, 615–617
  surgical procedure, 615
  tube, 602
    guidelines for, 616c–617c
    removal, in respiratory weaning, 631
Tracheostomy tube, 928
Tracheotomy, 491
  defined, 602
Traction. *See also* Musculoskeletal care modalities
  defined, 2233
  nursing management, 2246–2247
  principles of effective traction, 2242
  skeletal traction, 2244–2246
    nursing interventions, 2245–2246
  skin traction
    Buck's extension traction, 2243–2244
    circulatory impairment, 2244
    nerve damage, 2244
    nursing interventions, 2244
    skin breakdown, 2244
  types of, 2243

Traction retinal detachment, 1907
Traditional echocardiography, 682
Tramacet, 287
Tramadol, 287
  for pain management, 281t, 287
Trandolapril (Mavik)
  heart failure, 811t
  hypertension, 886t
Tranquilizers, 924
  constipation, 998
Transarterial chemoembolization (TACE), 1096
Transbronchial needle aspiration, 468
Transcatheter arterial embolization, 1096
  liver tumours, 1096
Transcervical intrauterine endoscopy, 1392
Transcranial Doppler, 1982–1983
Transcultural nursing, 90–99. *See also* Culture
  causes of illness, views on, 96–97
  cross-cultural communication, 93, 94c
  cultural concepts, 90–92
  culturally appropriate care, guidelines for, 98
  culturally competent and culturally safe care, 93
  culturally mediated characteristics, 94
    biologic variations, 95–96
    complementary therapies, 96
    diet, 95, 96c
    eye contact, 95
    observance of holidays, 95
    space and distance, 94
    time, 95
    touch, 95
  cultural nursing assessment, 97, 99c
  culture care accommodation, 93
  culture care restructuring, 93
  folk healers, 97, 98c
  future of, 98
  meaning of, 92
  overcoming language barriers, 94c
  underlying focus of, 92
Transcutaneous electrical nerve stimulation (TENS), 290, 1625, 1736
  devices, 910
  for pain relief, 290
Transdermal contraceptives, 1399
Transesophageal echocardiography (TEE), 682, 856
  mitral regurgitation, 780
  thoracic aortic aneurysm, 856
Trans fats, 68
Transferrin, 67, 1614
Transformational leadership, 76
Transfusion, 1683–1689
  complications, 1684–1688
  nursing management, 1688
  patient education, 1684
  pharmacologic alternatives, 1689
  pretransfusion assessment, 1683–1684
  setting, 1683
  therapy, 1623
Transfusion-associated circulatory overload (TACO), 356, 1686–1687
Transfusion dependence, 1619
Transfusion-related acute lung injury (TRALI), 356, 1687
Transfusion therapy
  blood and blood components in, 1680t
  sickle cell disease, 1623–1624
Transhiatal esophagectomy, 944f
Transient flora, 1698
Transient ischemic attack (TIA), 881, 1527
Transient/permanent paralysis, in hypertension, 881
Transitional care, 2138–2139
  acute coronary syndrome, 754
  acute pancreatitis, 1123
  adrenocortical insufficiency, 1249, 1250
  angina pectoris, 743
  ascites, 1065
  blood pressure, 892
  cervical discectomy, 2142
  chronic illness, 165–166
  cirrhosis, 1095
  coronary artery bypass graft, 774
  corticosteroid therapy, 1258
  Cushing syndrome, 1253–1254
  gallbladder disease, 1117
  gastric cancer, 991–992
  gastric surgery, 994
  gastritis, 980–981
  hepatic encephalopathy, 1074
  hepatitis B virus, 1080–1081
  Huntington's disease, 1235
  hyperthyroidism, 1236
  inflammatory bowel disease, 1022
  IV therapy, 338
  liver transplantation, 1102
  in liver tumour, 1097–1098
  orthopedic surgery, 2261
  ostomy, 1031
  pancreatic cancer, 1129
  pancreatic tumours, 1131
  in Parkinson's disease, 2132–2133, 2133c
  patient undergoing bariatric surgery, 1209
  peptic ulcer disease, 988
  pheochromocytoma, 1248
  shock, 367
  total hip arthroplasty, 2256
  tube feeding, 959
Transjugular intrahepatic portosystemic shunt (TIPS), 1063, 1065f
  ascites, 1063, 1065f
  esophageal varices, 1069
Transmissible spongiform encephalopathies (TSEs), 2095
Transmission, hepatitis B virus, 1079
Transnational nursing, 92
Transplantation
  heart, 789–791, 790f
    complications, 789
    indications for, 789
    orthotopic method, 790f
    risk of rejection, 790
  kidney, in patient with diabetes, 1180
  orthotopic
    heart, 778, 790
Transrectal ultrasound (TRUS), 1483
Transsacral (caudal) block, 405
Transsphenoidal approach, to intracranial surgery, 2006
Transtelephonic transmission, 722
Transtheoretical Model of Change, 46, 46t
Transtracheal oxygen catheter, 606
Transurethral incision of the prostate (TUIP), 1493–1494, 1493f
Transurethral microwave thermotherapy (TUMT), 1494
Transurethral needle ablation, 1494
Transurethral resection of the prostate (TURP), 1480, 1493, 1493f
Transverse rectus abdominis myocutaneous (TRAM) flap, 1446, 1473
Trapeze, 2233, 2245
Trastuzumab (Herceptin)
  breast cancer, 1471, 1472
Trauma, 2350
  bladder, 1355
  crush injuries, 2353
    assessment and diagnostic findings, 2353
    compartment syndrome, 2353
    management, 2353
    6 Ps, assessment by, 2353
  documentation, 2350
  fractures, 2353–2354
  genitourinary, 1355–1356
  injury prevention, 2350–2351
  intra-abdominal injuries, 2351–2353
    assessment and diagnostic findings, 2352
    blunt trauma, 2352
    genitourinary injury, 2352
    internal bleeding, 2352
    intraperitoneal injury, 2352
    location of pain, 2352
    management, 2352–2353
    penetrating, 2351–2352
  multiple, 2351
  multiple trauma, 2351
    assessment and diagnostic findings, 2351
    management, 2351
    treatment priorities, 2351c
  repeated, 2351
  ureteral, 1355
  urethral, 1355–1356
Traumatic brain injury (TBI), 2056
  clinical manifestations, 2059
  closed (blunt), 2059
  collaborative problems/potential complications, 2062–2065
  medical management
    brain death, 2062
    fluid and electrolyte maintenance, 2061–2062
    increased intracranial pressure, 2061
    management of pain and anxiety, 2062
    nutritional support, 2062
    seizure prevention, 2061–2062
    ventilatory support, 2061–2062
  multisystem assessment measures for, 2064t–2065t
  nursing interventions
    adequate CPP, maintenance of, 2068
    airway maintenance, 2065
    body temperature maintenance, 2067
    cerebral edema and herniation, management of, 2068–2069
    continuing and transitional care, 2069–2070
    controlling of ICP, 2069c
    fluid and electrolyte balance monitoring, 2066
    fluid, electrolyte, and nutritional balance, maintenance of, 2069
    home care checklist, 2070c
    impaired oxygen and ventilation, management of, 2069
    improving coping, 2067–2068
    injury prevention, 2066–2067
    monitoring and managing potential complications, 2068–2069
    neurologic function monitoring, 2065–2066
    patient outcomes, 2070–2071
    posttraumatic seizures, management of, 2069
    preventing sleep pattern disturbance, 2068
    promoting adequate nutrition, 2066

promoting home, community-based, and transitional care, 2069–2070
skin integrity maintenance, 2067
supporting family coping, 2068
nursing priorities, 2062
open (penetrating), 2059
pathophysiology, 2058f
patient assessment, 2062
rehabilitation, 176–177
types
concussion, 2061
contusion, 2059
diffuse axonal injury (DAI), 2061
epidural hematoma, 2060
intracerebral hemorrhage and hematoma, 2061
intracranial hemorrhage, 2059–2061
subdural hematoma, 2060
Traumatic dislocations, 2299
Traumatic pneumothorax, 558
Treatment modality, esophageal varices, 1071t
Tremor, 2128. *See also* Parkinson's disease
Trench mouth, gum abnormalities, 921t
Trendelenburg position, for surgery, 408, 409f
Treponema pallidum, 1044
Treponema pallidum and syphilis, 1722
T_3 resin uptake test, 1224
TREVO device, 2035
Triage, 2343–2344. *See also* Canadian Triage and Acuity Scale (CTAS)
data collection, 2344
definition of, 2343
field triage, 2344
five-level triage scores, 2343
protocols, 2344
Triamcinolone, 1798
allergic rhinitis, 1585
Triamcinolone acetonide, 588t
injections, 1809
Triamterene (Dyrenium), 820t, 1085
hypertension, 884t
Triceps reflex, 1976
Trichlormethiazide (Metahydrin, Naqua), 820t
Trichomonas vaginalis, 1414
Trichomoniasis, 1414–1415
clinical manifestations, 1414
medical management, 1414
Tricuspid area, 668
Tricuspid valve, 777, 778
Tricyclic antidepressants (TCA), 224
intoxication, 2368t
for pain relief, 289
Trigeminal autonomic cephalalgias, 2023
Trigeminal neuralgia (tic douloureux), 2110–2113, 2111t
medical management, 2112
nursing management, 2112–2113
pain management, 2112–2113
postoperative neurologic assessments, 2113
pharmacologic therapy, 2112
surgical management, 2112
Triggered, defined, 692
Triglycerides, 674, 733, 882
Trilogy, 2164
Trimethoprim, 1336
Trimethoprim–sulfamethoxazole (TMP–SMZ), 1490, 1553
thalassemia, 1628
Triple-H therapy, 2049
Triple-lumen catheters, 1347
Trisomy, 134
Trisomy 21, 138
Trochanter roll, 182
Tropical sprue, 1007t
Troponin, 746–747
Trousseau's sign, 319, 319f
Trust issues, 26
Truth and Reconciliation Commission, 8, 91
Truth-telling, in nurse–patient relationship, 27
Trypsin, 899, 900, 901t, 1107
T-SPOT, 524–525
tTG. *See* Antitissue transglutaminase (tTG)
T-tube, 1102
fistula, 1109
tract, 1113
Tubal embryo transfer (TET), 1406
Tube aspirate, pH of, 950, 951
Tube displacement, enteral therapy, 956t
Tube feeding, 952
administering medications, 957
advantages, 953
assessing patients, 958c
attachment device, 951
home care checklist, 965c
maintaining delivery systems, 957–958
medication for delivery, 957t
with nasogastric/nasoenteric devices, 952–960
administration methods, 954–955
formulas, 954
osmosis and osmolality, 953–954
nasojejunal, 953
nursing process, 955–960
planning and goals, 956
polyurethane or silicone rubber, 949
solutions, 955
types of medications, 957
Tube obstruction, enteral therapy, 956t
Tuberculin skin test (TST), 524, 1706
Tuberculosis, 1550–1551
Tuberculosis-associated–immune reconstitution inflammatory syndrome (TB-IRIS), 1550
Tuberculous ulcers, 1819
Tubergrip, 185
d-Tubocurarine, 402t
Tubular ductal carcinoma, 1457
inflammatory carcinoma, 1457
Paget's disease, 1457
Tubular reabsorption and tubular secretion, 1266–1269
Tumour-associated antigens (TAA), 2156
Tumour cell antigens. *See* Tumour-associated antigens (TAA)
Tumour-directed therapy, 2192
Tumour lysis syndrome (TLS), 316, 2189, 2207t
Tumour, nodes, and metastasis (TNM) system, 2158
classification system, 2159c
Tumours
and acoustic neuroma, 2111t
head of pancreas
assessment and diagnostic findings, 1129
clinical manifestations, 1129
medical management, 1129–1130
nursing management, 1130–1131
of mediastinum (*See also* Chest tumours)
assessment/diagnostic findings, 553
clinical manifestations, 553
medical management, 554
Tumours of skin
benign
actinic keratoses, 1819
angiomas, 1819
cysts, 1819
dermatofibroma, 1820
keloids, 1820
moles, 1819–1820
neurofibromatosis, 1820
seborrheic keratoses, 1819
warts, 1819
cosmetic procedures
chemical face peeling, 1829–1830
dermabrasion, 1830
Kaposi's sarcoma (KS), 1826
laser treatment of cutaneous lesions, 1831–1832
malignant
basal cell and squamous cell carcinomas, 1820–1822, 1826
malignant melanoma, 1822–1824
metastatic skin tumours, 1826
skin cancer, 1820–1824
plastic or reconstructive surgery, 1826–1827
facial, 1830
rhytidectomy (face-lift), 1830–1831
Tumour-specific antigen (TSA), 2150, 2151
Turbinate hypertrophy, 489
Turbulent blood flow, 837
Turgor, 306
Turner's syndrome, 134, 138
T wave, 692, 695
TWEAK (*T*olerance, *W*orry, *E*ye-opener, *A*mnesia, *K*ut down on drinking), 59
Tylenol, for pain relief, 477
Tympani, 905
Tympanic membrane (eardrum), 1927
Tympanic membrane perforation, 1938–1939
medical management, 1938–1939
surgical management, 1938–1939
Tympanogram, 1933
Tympanoplasty, 1940–1941
Tympanosclerosis, 1943
Tympanotomy, 1939
Tympany, 65
Type 1 diabetes, 1137, 1138, 1140
autoimmune response in, 1141
beta cell destruction, 1141
genetic predisposition, 1140–1141
hyperglycemia in, 1141
Type 2 diabetes, 1137, 1138, 1141–1142
insulin resistance in, 1141
prevention, 1142
Tyrosine kinase pathways, 2191
Tzanck smear, 1780

U

Ulcerative colitis, 1018
assessment and diagnostic findings, 1017–1018
chronic IBD, medical management of, 1018
nutritional therapy, 1018
pharmacologic therapy, 1018–1019
surgical management, 1019–1020
clinical manifestations, 1017
complications, 1018
inflammatory bowel disease, 1017–1020
nutritional therapy, 1018
pathophysiology, 1017
pharmacologic therapy, 1018–1019
surgical management, 1019–1020
Ulcerogenic tumours, 1131
Ulcers, 838t, 1819
from arterial emboli, 868f
healing, 983t
Ultrafiltration, 1283, 1305

Ultrasonography/Ultrasound, 1111, 1483, 1887
abdominal, 907
appendicitis, 1009
breast, 1452
gallbladder, 1115
hepatic disorders, 1058
and kidney failure, 1294
liver dysfunction and jaundice, 1111
pancreatic tumour, 1128
pelvic examination, 1393
peritonitis, 1015
salivary gland, 925
ulcerative colitis, 1018
Ultrasound-guided core biopsy, 1453
Umbilical veins, 852
Unclassified cardiomyopathies, 788
Undernutrition, in older adults, 217
Unfractionated heparin, 741
deep vein thrombosis, 863
in venous thromboembolism, 863–864
United Network for Organ Sharing (UNOS), 1101
United Ostomy Associations of Canada (UOAC), 1027
Unna boot, 866, 869
UNOS. *See* United Network for Organ Sharing (UNOS)
Unregulated health worker, 73–74
Upper airway infections
adenoiditis, 481–482
laryngitis, 483–484
nursing process for, 484–485
peritonsillar abscess, 482–483
pharyngitis, 479–481
rhinitis, 470–473, 472c, 472t
rhinosinusitis, 475–479, 476t
tonsillitis, 481–482
viral rhinitis, 473–475, 474c
Upper airway obstruction. *See* Airway obstruction
clearing, 613c
Upper extremity arterial occlusive disease
assessment and diagnostic findings, 853
clinical manifestations, 853
medical management, 853
nursing management, 853–854
Upper extremity, common problems of, 2270–2274
bursitis and tenosynovitis, 2270
carpal tunnel syndrome, 2271–2272
Dupuytren's contracture, 2272, 2272f
ganglion, 2272
loose bodies, 2270–2271
nursing process for, 2272–2274
infection prevention, 2273
neurovascular assessment, 2272
nursing interventions, 2272–2273
nursing priorities, 2272
pain management, 2272
patient evaluation, 2274
planning and goals, 2272
self-care, 2273
shoulder impingement syndrome, 2271
Upper GI fibroscopy, 911
Upper motor neurons, 1968
lesions, 1968
paralysis associated with, 1968
Upper respiratory tract. *See also* Respiratory system
larynx, 440
nose, 438–439
paranasal sinuses, 439, 440f
pharynx, tonsils, and adenoids, 439
physical assessment of
mouth and pharynx, 451
nose, 451
sinuses, 451, 451f
trachea, 451–452
trachea, 440
Upper respiratory tract disorders
nursing process
in laryngectomy, 495–502, 496c, 501c
for upper airway infections, 484–485
obstruction and trauma
cancer of larynx, 491–495, 492c, 493c
epistaxis (nosebleed), 488–489, 488c
laryngeal obstruction, 490–491, 491c, 491t
nasal fracture, 489–490
nasal obstruction, 489
obstructive sleep apnea, 486–488, 486c
in older adults, 471c
upper airway infections
adenoiditis, 481–482
laryngitis, 483–484
peritonsillar abscess, 482–483
pharyngitis, 479–481
rhinitis, 470–473, 472c, 472t
rhinosinusitis, 475–479, 476t
tonsillitis, 481–482
viral rhinitis, 473–475, 474c
Upper urinary tract infection
acute pyelonephritis, 1339
chronic pyelonephritis, 1339–1340
Urea breath tests, 907
Uremia, 1283, 1285, 1287, 1297, 1773t
Ureteral brush biopsy, 1280
Ureteral trauma, 1355
Ureterosigmoidostomy, 1332, 1363–1364
nursing management, 1364
Ureterovesical or vesicoureteral reflux, 1332
Ureterovesical/vesicoureteral reflux, 1333
Ureters, 1264–1265
Urethra, 1265
Urethral stricture, 1511
Urethral trauma, 1355–1356
Urethritis, 1331, 1332
Urethrovesical reflux, 1332, 1333, 1333f
Urge incontinence, 1332, 1341. *See also* Urinary incontinence
Uric acid stones, 1351
Urinary albumin excretion, 882
Urinary bladder, 1265
Urinary casts, 1283, 1288
Urinary continence, promotion of, 201–202
Urinary diversions
continent, 1363–1364
cutaneous urinary diversions, 1358–1363
nursing process, 1364–1368
orthotopic neobladder, 1364
Urinary incontinence, 200, 1269, 1332
assessment and diagnostic findings, 1342
description, 1341
gerontologic considerations, 1341–1342
interventions for, 1343c
medical management, 1342–1344
behavioural therapy, 1342
pharmacologic therapy, 1342
surgical management, 1342–1344, 1344f
nursing management, 1344, 1344c
in older adults, 232
risk factors, 1341c
transient incontinence, 1342c
types, 1341
Urinary output, in shock, 347
Urinary retention, 1344, 2260
after surgery, 429
assessment and diagnostic findings, 1345
autonomic neuropathy, 1181
chronic, 1344
complications, 1345
defined, 1344
nursing management, 1345–1346
pathophysiology, 1345
Urinary stasis/infection, 2246
Urinary systems. *See* Renal and urinary systems
Urinary tract cancers, bladder cancer, 1356–1358
Urinary tract infection (UTI), 1288, 1331–1332
acute bacterial sepsis, 1334
adult voiding dysfunction, 1340, 1340t
catheterization, 1334
causes, 1331
classifying, 1331–1332, 1333c
indwelling catheters and, 1347
lower
assessment and diagnostic findings, 1335–1336
clinical manifestation, 1334
gerontologic considerations, 1334–1335
medical management, 1336
pathophysiology, 1332–1334
older adults, 1334
preventing recurrent, 1338c
recurrent, 1338c
risk factors for, 1333c
uncomplicated, 1331, 1333c
upper
acute pyelonephritis, 1339
chronic pyelonephritis, 1339–1340
Urine colour, changes in, 1110, 1276c
Urine cultures, 1335
Urine dipstick test, 1150, 1179
Urine formation, 1265–1266
Urine ketone testing, 1150
Urine osmolality, 300
Urine output, aortoiliac disease and, 855
Urine sodium, 300, 310
Urine specific gravity, 300
Urine storage, 1268
Urine testing, for glucose, 1150
Urobilinogen, 1106
Urodynamic testing, patient education before and after, 1274c
Urofollitropin, 1405c
Urolithiasis, 1350
assessment and diagnostic findings, 1351
clinical manifestations, 1351
defined, 1350
medical management, 1351–1352
pathophysiology, 1350–1351
Urologic endoscopic procedures, 1279–1280
Urosepsis, 1332
Ursodeoxycholic acid (UDCA), and gallstones, 1112
Urticaria (hives), 1572, 1591–1592
Urticarial, 1578
U.S. National Pressure Ulcer Advisory Panel (NPUAP), 195
Uterine artery embolization (UAE), 1429
Uterine cancer
assessment and diagnostic findings, 1435
medical management, 1435
pathophysiology, 1434–1435
risk factors, 1435c
Uterine palpation, 1389–1390

Uterine prolapse, 1373, 1387, 1425–1427, 1426f
medical management, 1426
nursing management, 1426–1427
Uterotubography, for pelvic examination, 1393
Uterus, 1374–1375
benign tumours of, 1429–1430
cancer of, 1434–1435
UTI. *See* Urinary tract infection (UTI)
Utilitarianism, 24
Uveitis, 1917
Uvulopalatopharyngoplasty, 488
U wave, 692, 695

V

Vaccines
for cancer
allogeneic, 2192
autologous, 2192
prophylactic, 2192
therapeutic, 2192
catch-up, 1079
for COPD, 570
hepatitis A and B, 1078
VAC devices. *See* Vacuum-assisted closure (VAC) devices
Vacuum-assisted closure (VAC), 199, 870
Vagal blocking therapy, 1201
Vagal nerve fibres, 945
Vagina, 1374
cancer of, 1437–1438
fistulas of, 1423–1424, 1423f
assessment and diagnostic findings, 1423–1424
clinical manifestation, 1423
medical management, 1424
inspecting, 1388
speculum examination of, 1387f
Vaginal and rectal palpation, 1390
Vaginal cancer, 1437–1438
medical management, 1437–1438
Vaginal contraceptives, 1399
Vaginal infections, 1413t
Vaginitis, 1412, 1413t
Vagotomy
peptic ulcer disease, 984t
syndrome, 919
Vague epigastric, 1009
Valacyclovir, 1797, 1799
herpes labialis, 474c
herpes simplex virus 2, 1418
Valganciclovir (Valcyte)
cytomegalovirus retinitis, 1554
Valproate (Depacon), 2025
hepatic dysfunction, 1054
Valsalva manoeuvre, 968, 998, 999, 1940, 2001, 2051
constipation, 999
Valsartan (Diovan), hypertension, 886t
Valtrex, for herpes labialis, 474c
Valve leaflet resection, 784f
Valve prostheses, 785, 787
Valve replacement, 778, 780, 785–786
complications, 785
mechanical valves, 786
minimally invasive techniques, 785
procedure, 785, 785f
robot assisted, 785
tissue valves, 786
Valves, blood flow patterns, 867f
Valvular disorders, 777
aortic regurgitation, 781
aortic stenosis, 781
infectious diseases, 795
pericarditis, 798–799
rheumatic endocarditis, 794
mitral regurgitation, 777
mitral stenosis, 777
mitral valve prolapse, 777
nursing management, 782
repair and replacement procedures
nursing management, 786–787
valve replacement, 785–786
valvuloplasty, 782–784
septal defects, 783
Valvular heart disorders, 782
Valvuloplasty, 778, 782–783
annuloplasty, 784, 784f
cardiopulmonary bypass, 783
chordoplasty, 784
commissurotomy, 783, 783f
leaflet repair, 784, 784f
Vancomycin, for acute kidney injury, 1294
Vancomycin-resistant *Enterococcus* (VRE), 1698, 1707, 1854
Vancomycin-resistant *Staphylococcus aureus (VRSA)*, 1698
Vancyclovir (Valacyclovir), for chronic lymphocytic leukemia, 1642
Vardenafil (Levitra), 2084
erectile dysfunction, 1485
Varenicline, 569, 736
Variable expression, 136
Variant Creutzfeldt–Jakob disease (vCJD)
assessment and diagnostic findings, 2095
clinical manifestations, 2095
medical management, 2095
nursing management, 2095–2096
pathophysiology, 2095
Varicella-zoster viruses, 1797
Varicocele, 1480, 1509
Varicose veins (varicosities), 871
assessment and diagnostic findings, 872
clinical manifestations, 872
medical management
ligation and stripping, 872
sclerotherapy, 873
thermal ablation, 872–873
nursing management
home and community-based care, 873
promoting comfort, 873
pathophysiology, 872
prevention, 872
Vas Cath, 968
Vascular age, 888
Vascular bone marrow, 2216
Vascular compression of nerve, 2111t
Vascular dementia, 230
Vascular disorders
assessment of, 839
diagnostic evaluation, 839
air plethysmography, 843
angiography, 842
computed tomography angiography (CTA), 842
computed tomography scanning, 842
contrast phlebography (venography), 843
Doppler ultrasound flow studies, 840–841
duplex ultrasonography, 841–842
exercise testing, 841
lymphangiography, 843
lymphoscintigraphy, 843
magnetic resonance angiography (MRA), 842–843
health history, 839
physical assessment, 839
palpation of pulses, 839
skin inspection, 839
Vascular endothelial growth factor (VEGF), 2153, 2191
Vascular lesions, 1777t
Vascular system
anatomic of, 834
arteries and arterioles, 834–836
capillaries, 836
lymphatic vessels, 836
veins and venules, 836
assessment of, 834
function of
blood flow, 837
blood pressure, 837
capillary filtration and reabsorption, 837
circulatory needs of tissues, 836
hemodynamic resistance, 837
peripheral vascular regulating mechanisms, 837–838
gerontologic considerations, 839
pathophysiology of
alterations, in blood/lymphatic vessels, 838
extremities, circulatory insufficiency of, 838
pump failure, 838
Vasectomy, 1480, 1509–1510, 1509f
nursing management, 1510
Vasoactive medications, in shock, 351–353, 353t
Vasodilators, 854
hypertension, 886t
Vasomotor symptoms, 994
Vasopressin, 1068
in cardiogenic shock, 358
cardiopulmonary resuscitation, 832t
in shock, 353t
Vasopressors, in cardiogenic shock, 827
Vasospasm, 731, 849, 2048–2049
medical management, 2049
prevention, 2051
Vasospastic disorders, 849
Vasovasostomy, 1510
vCJD. *See* Variant Creutzfeldt–Jakob disease (vCJD)
Vecuronium, 402t, 2008
Vein graft, 852
Veins, 1963
anatomic of, 836
Vena cava filter, 864
Venereal disease research laboratory (VDRL), 1722
Venlafaxine (Effexor), 224, 2025
fibromyalgia, 1759
menopause, 1379
Venography, 843, 872
Venous blood flow, thromboembolus obstructing, 838
Venous disorders
chronic venous insufficiency/postthrombotic syndrome, 867–868
leg ulcer, 868–871
varicose veins (varicosities), 871–873
venous thromboembolism, 861–867
Venous hypertension, 869
Venous insufficiency, ulcers, 838t
Venous jugular desaturations, 1999
Venous stasis, 424, 773, 862, 862c, 867, 868, 872
Venous thromboembolism (VTE), 845, 1208, 2041, 2203, 2248–2249, 2261
assessment and diagnostic findings, 863

Venous thromboembolism (*continued*)
clinical manifestations, 862–863
deep veins, 863
superficial veins, 863
formation, 1010
medical management, 863–864
neurogenic shock and, 364–365
nursing management, 864–867
assessing and monitoring anticoagulant therapy, 865
monitoring and managing complications, 865
providing comfort, 865–866
pathophysiology, 862
prevention, 863, 2253–2254
Venous ulceration, chronic venous insufficiency, 867
Ventilation, 439. *See also* Respiratory system
air pressure variances, 442
airway resistance, 442, 442c
compliance, 442
lung volumes and capacities, 442–443, 443t
neurologic control of, 446
Ventilation-perfusion (V/Q) ratios, 443–444, 444c, 505, 545
Ventilator-associated pneumonia (VAP), 348, 511
Ventricular assist devices (VADs)
in cardiogenic shock, 358
Ventricular asystole, 710, 710f
Ventricular catheter monitoring device, 1998
Ventricular dysrhythmias
idioventricular rhythm, 709–710
premature ventricular complex, 707–708
ventricular asystole, 710, 710f
ventricular fibrillation, 709, 709f
ventricular tachycardia, 708
Ventricular escape rhythm. *See* Idioventricular rhythm
Ventricular fibrillation, 709, 709f
Ventricular function and wall motion, test of, 681
Ventricular gallop, 809
Ventricular hypertrophy, 806t, 807
Ventricular remodeling, 807, 811, 816
Ventricular tachycardia (VT), 692, 705
defined, 708
medical management, 708–709
Ventriculostomy, 1998
Venturi mask, 605
Venules, anatomic of, 836
Veracity, 25, 25c
Verapamil
antiarrhythmic medication, 699t
calcium channel blockers, 813
hypertension, 886t
Verbal communication, 926
Verbal descriptor scale (VDS), 278
Vertebral artery aneurysms, 2111t
Vertebral column, 1964
Vertigo, 1945, 1971
balance disturbance or true, 1943
benign paroxysmal positional vertigo (BPPV), 1946–1947
definition, 1944
labyrinthitis, 1946
plan of nursing care, 1947c–1949c
Vesicants, 2150, 2178
Vessel radius, and resistance in vascular system, 837
Vestibular cysts, 1427
Vestibular disorders, 904
Vestibular dysfunction testing, 1933
Vestibular gland, 1374
Vestibular Ménière's disease, 1945
Vestibular nerve sectioning, 1946
"V" formation, 905
Vibration
defined, 602
evaluation of, 1975
Vibrio cholerae, 1719–1720
Video-assisted endoscopic surgery, 2161
Video-assisted thoracoscopy (VATS), 465, 633
Vigilon, 1816
Vilanterol, 589t
Villi, 902
Vinblastine
bladder cancer, 1357
Hodgkin lymphoma, 1649
Vinca alkaloids, as chemotherapeutic agents, 552
Vinegar, 978
Vinorelbine, as chemotherapeutic agents, 552
Violence
in emergency department, 2340–2341
intimate partner, 2371–2373, 2372c
Viral hepatitis, 1075
hepatitis A virus (HAV), 1076–1078
hepatitis B virus (HBV), 1078–1081
hepatitis C virus (HCV), 1081
hepatitis D virus (HDV), 1081
hepatitis E virus (HEV), 1081
hepatitis GB virus-C (GBV-C), 1082
hepatitis G virus (HEV), 1082
Viral laryngitis, 483
Viral load test, 1534, 1545
Viral rhinitis. *See also* Upper airway infections
clinical manifestations, 474, 474c
medical management, 474–475
nursing management
patient education about self-care, 475
overview, 473–474
Viral set point, 1534, 1544
Virchow's triad, 862
Virtual colonoscopy, 908
Virulence, 1698
Viruses, in carcinogenesis, 2153–2154
Visceral afferent stimulation, 904
Visceral obesity, 1141
Visible neck depression, 929
Vision impairment, 1888–1889
activities affected by, 1889, 1890t
assessment and diagnostic testing, 1889
contrast-sensitivity testing measures, 1889
glare testing, 1889
history taking, 1889
common causes of, 1888–1889
definition, 1888
gerontologic considerations, 1889
medical management, 1889–1890
vision restoration, 1890
nursing management, 1890–1892
coping strategy, 1890–1891
promoting home, community-based, and transitional care, 1892
promoting spatial orientation and mobility, 1891–1892
strategies for interacting with people, 1891c
Vision/speech, hypertension, 881
Visual acuity, 1883–1884
Visual analogue scale (VAS), 277, 278
Visual disturbances, 2119. *See also* Increased intracranial pressure (ICP)
Vital capacity, 443, 459–460
Vital fatigue, 659
Vital signs
in emergency department, 2339–2340
in physical assessment, 63
Vitamin A acid (tretinoin), 1794
Vitamin B_{12}, 900
deficiency, 1617
and folic acid metabolism, 1603
malabsorption, 978, 980
Vitamin C, 849
Vitamin D
deficiency and associated deformities, 1769
in hypocalcemia, 320
production, 1769
recommended daily intake, 1769
synthesis, 1267
urinary stone formation, 1351
Vitamin deficiency
and anemia, 1085
cholelithiasis, 1110
cirrhosis and, 1085
gastritis, 978
hepatic disorders, 1074–1075
role of liver in, 1053
Vitamin K antagonist, 864
Vitamin K deficiency, 1085, 1668
Vitamins A, 1005
Vitamins B_{12}, 1005
Vitamins B_6 (pyridoxine), in premenstrual syndrome, 1395
Vitiligo, 1618, 1772, 1773t
Vitrectomy, 1178, 1907–1908
Vocal cord, 440
stripping, 493
Voice sounds, 457
Voiding cystourethrography, 1279
Volkmann's ischemic contracture, 2314, 2314c
Volume-cycled ventilators, 620
Voluntary motor system, 1968
Vomiting, 1032, 2119. *See also* Increased intracranial pressure (ICP)
colorectal cancer, 1043
during ERCP, 1111
gastritis, 978
gastrointestinal (GI) tract, 903
peritonitis, 1014
thoracic aortic aneurysm, 842
Von Recklinghausen's disease, 1820
von Willebrand's disease (vWD), 1666–1668
assessment and diagnostic findings, 1667
clinical manifestations, 1667
medical management, 1668
VTE. *See* Venous thromboembolism (VTE)
Vulvar cancer, 1435–1437
clinical manifestations, 1435
medical management, 1435–1436
nursing management, 1436–1437
Vulvar cysts, 1427–1428
medical management, 1428
Vulvar dystrophy, 1412, 1428
medical management, 1428
nursing management, 1428
Vulvectomy, 1412, 1428
Vulvitis, 1412, 1414, 1427
medical management, 1427
Vulvodynia, 1412, 1427
medical management, 1427
Vulvovaginal candidiasis, 1413
Vulvovaginal infections, 1411–1412
nursing process, 1415–1416
risk factors, 1412c

W

Waist circumference measurement, 66, 66f
Walker, ambulating with, 190, 192
Walking
  aortoiliac disease, 855
  arteriosclerosis, 846
  effect of muscle, 866
  exercise testing, 841
  peripheral arterial disease, 851
  peripheral vascular problem, 847c
  sclerotherapy, 873
Walking cast, 2232
Warfarin (Coumadin), 786, 2049
  acquired thrombophilias, 1676
  venous thromboembolism, 828, 864, 865, 867c
Warm compress, 327
Warm water mouth rinse, 923
Warts, 1819
Waste products
  of digestion, 902
  excretion of, 1267–1268
Wasting syndrome, 1534, 1551
Water, daily intake and output of, 299, 299f
Water excretion, regulation of, 1266
Water-hammer (Corrigan) pulse, 781
Water-in-oil emulsions, 1787
Water seal system, 635t, 639
Water-soluble contrast study, 909
Watery stools, 1002
Weakness
  chronic constipation, 1011
  constipation, 1000
  diabetes mellitus, 1142
  dumping syndrome, 993
  hepatic dysfunction, 1055
  hypertension, 881
  in proximal muscles, 2223
Weaning from ventilator. *See* Respiratory weaning
Weber test, 1932, 1932f
  comparison with Rinne, 1932t
Wedged pressure, 1067
Wedge resection, 551c, 633
WeeFIM instrument, 178
Weight-bearing activity, 2216
Weight bearing as tolerated (WBAT), 2301
Weight gain
  hepatic dysfunction, 1055
  medications associated with, 1197c
Weight loss
  acute low back pain, 2270
  chronic pancreatitis, 1123
  duodenal and gastric ulcers, 981t
  gastric cancer, 989
  hypertension, 883t
  patient education, 1198c
  peptic ulcer disease, 986
  type 2 diabetes, 1142
Weight-resistance exercise, 2216
Wellness, 7, 38, 45
Weapons of mass destruction (WMDs), 2380
West Nile encephalitis, 2093
West Nile fever, 1726
West Nile virus, 1726, 2093
Wet suction, 639
Wheat dextrin (Benefiber), laxative medications, 1001t
Wheelchair push-up, 196, 197f
Wheezes, 439, 672
Whiff test, 1414
Whipple's disease, 1007t, 1127, 1130, 1130f
Whirlpool bath, 2355
Whispered pectoriloquy, 439, 457
Whisper test, 1932
White blood cell (WBC), 1575, 1599, 2200, 2201
  action, 1518
White coat hypertension, 878
Whooping cough. *See* Pertussis
Wire needle localization, 1453
Wiring the jaw shut, 924
Wiskott–Aldrich syndrome, 1534
WOCN. *See* Wound-ostomy-continence nurse (WOCN)
Wolff-Parkinson-White (WPW) syndrome, 706
Women, health screening and counselling issues for, 1381c
Women with disabilities
  assessing, 1385c
  breast health of, 1475–1476
  health issues of, 1384
Wong-Baker FACES pain rating scale, 278
Wood's light examination, 1780, 1799
Workplace, health promotion programs at, 49
World Health Organization (WHO), 922, 1538
  definition of health by, 6
  on disability, 166
  obesity, definition of, 65
  on palliative care, 242
Wound, 2349–2350
  care for hospitalized postoperative patient
    dressing change, 427–428, 428c
    instructions for, 428c
    surgical drains, 427, 427f
    wound healing, factors affecting, 426, 426t
    wound-healing mechanisms, 425–426, 425c
  classification/surgical site infection risk, 431t
  cleansing, 2349–2350
  dehiscence and evisceration, 432
  delayed primary closure, 2350
  drainage, 2253
  dressings, 869
  healing
    factors affecting, 426, 426t
    mechanisms, 425–426, 425c
  infection, 962, 2294
  inspection, 2349
  primary closure, 2350
  related documentation, 2349
  sepsis, 431, 431t
  suction drain, 2256
  tetanus prophylaxis, 2350
  types of, 2349c
Wound care
  colon resection, 1040
  laparoscopic cholecystectomy, 1118c
Wound care for skin conditions
  burn care, 1854–1857
  disorders of wound healing, 1862–1863
  products, 1784c
  rules, 1783–1784
    categorization, 1783
    change practices, 1784
    evolution, 1784
    practice, 1784
    selection, 1783–1784
  wound coverage
    flaps, 1829
    skin grafts, 1827–1829
  wound dressing functions and categories, 1784–1786, 1785t
    autografts, 1860–1861
    biologic dressings, 1859
    biosynthetic and synthetic dressings, 1859–1860
    in burn care, 1856–1861
    dermal substitutes, 1860
    moisture-retentive dressings, 1784–1786
    occlusive dressings, 1784, 1856
    temporary and permanent burn wound coverings, 1858t
    wet dressings, 1784
Wound care specialist, 1332, 1347
Wound drainage tubes, 931
Wound healing
  disorders of, 1862–1863
    contractures, 1863
    failure of wound to heal, 1863
    keloids, 1863
    scars, 1863
  factors affecting, 426, 426t
  mechanisms, 425–426, 425c
  nutrients for, 378, 380t
Wound-ostomy-continence nurse (WOCN), 998, 1021, 1023, 1039, 1122, 1332, 1626

X

Xenografts, 778, 786, 1052, 1083, 1859
Xeroform, 1861
Xerostomia, 471, 495, 919, 927, 1750, 2150, 2165
X-linked inheritance, 137, 137f
X-rays
  appendicitis, 1009
  diverticular disease, 1011
  fecal incontinence, 1003
  irritable bowel syndrome, 1005, 1005f
  large bowel obstruction, 1033
  peritonitis, 1015
  small bowel obstruction, 1032
  ulcerative colitis, 1018
Xylocaine. *See* Lidocaine
Xylocaine, for herpes labialis, 474c

Y

Yankauer suction, 930
Yeast vaginitis, 1336
Yellow fever virus, 1060
Yin/yang theory, 97

Z

Zafirlukast (Accolate), 590t
Zeasorb (Stiefel), 1791
Zenker's diverticulum, 936
ZES. *See* Zollinger-Ellison syndrome (ZES)
Zika virus, 1725–1726
Zileuton (Zyflo), 590t
Zinc deficiency, tube feeding, 958
Zinc oxide, 1787
Zoledronic acid (Zometa), in multiple myeloma, 1655
Zollinger-Ellison syndrome (ZES), 915, 981, 1001, 1007t, 1107, 1131
Zolmitriptan (Zomig), 2025
Zovirax, for herpes labialis, 474c
Zymase, 1784

CCS0919